TABLE OF LOGARITHMS

Natural Numbers 10–54

N	0	1	2	3	4	5	6	7	8	9	P.P. 1	2	3	4	5	6	7	8	9
10	0000	0043	0086	0128	0170	0212	0253	0294	0334	0374	4	8	12	17	21	25	29	33	37
11	0414	0453	0492	0531	0569	0607	0645	0682	0719	0755	4	8	11	15	19	23	26	30	34
12	0792	0828	0864	0899	0934	0969	1004	1038	1072	1106	3	7	10	14	17	21	24	28	31
13	1139	1173	1206	1239	1271	1303	1335	1367	1399	1430	3	6	10	13	16	19	23	26	29
14	1461	1492	1523	1553	1584	1614	1644	1673	1703	1732	3	6	9	12	15	18	21	24	27
15	1761	1790	1818	1847	1875	1903	1931	1959	1987	2014	3	6	8	11	14	17	20	22	25
16	2041	2068	2095	2122	2148	2175	2201	2227	2253	2279	3	5	8	11	13	16	18	21	24
17	2304	2330	2355	2380	2405	2430	2455	2480	2504	2529	2	5	7	10	12	15	17	20	22
18	2553	2577	2601	2625	2648	2672	2695	2718	2742	2765	2	5	7	9	12	14	16	19	21
19	2788	2810	2833	2856	2878	2900	2923	2945	2967	2989	2	4	7	9	11	13	16	18	20
20	3010	3032	3054	3075	3096	3118	3139	3160	3181	3201	2	4	6	8	11	13	15	17	19
21	3222	3243	3263	3284	3304	3324	3345	3365	3385	3404	2	4	6	8	10	12	14	16	18
22	3424	3444	3464	3483	3502	3522	3541	3560	3579	3598	2	4	6	8	10	12	14	15	17
23	3617	3636	3655	3674	3692	3711	3729	3747	3766	3784	2	4	6	7	9	11	13	15	17
24	3802	3820	3838	3856	3874	3892	3909	3927	3945	3962	2	4	5	7	9	11	12	14	16
25	3979	3997	4014	4031	4048	4065	4082	4099	4116	4133	2	3	5	7	9	10	12	14	15
26	4150	4166	4183	4200	4216	4232	4249	4265	4281	4298	2	3	5	7	8	10	11	13	15
27	4314	4330	4346	4362	4378	4393	4409	4425	4440	4456	2	3	5	6	8	9	11	13	14
28	4472	4487	4502	4518	4533	4548	4564	4579	4594	4609	2	3	5	6	8	9	11	12	14
29	4624	4639	4654	4669	4683	4698	4713	4728	4742	4757	1	3	4	6	7	9	10	12	13
30	4771	4786	4800	4814	4829	4843	4857	4871	4886	4900	1	3	4	6	7	9	10	11	13
31	4914	4928	4942	4955	4969	4983	4997	5011	5024	5038	1	3	4	6	7	8	10	11	12
32	5051	5065	5079	5092	5105	5119	5132	5145	5159	5172	1	3	4	5	7	8	9	11	12
33	5185	5198	5211	5224	5237	5250	5263	5276	5289	5302	1	3	4	5	6	8	9	10	12
34	5315	5328	5340	5353	5366	5378	5391	5403	5416	5428	1	3	4	5	6	8	9	10	11
35	5441	5453	5465	5478	5490	5502	5514	5527	5539	5551	1	2	4	5	6	7	8	10	11
36	5563	5575	5587	5599	5611	5623	5635	5647	5658	5670	1	2	4	5	6	7	8	9	11
37	5682	5694	5705	5717	5729	5740	5752	5763	5775	5786	1	2	3	5	6	7	8	9	10
38	5798	5809	5821	5832	5843	5855	5866	5877	5888	5899	1	2	3	5	6	7	8	9	10
39	5911	5922	5933	5944	5955	5966	5977	5988	5999	6010	1	2	3	4	5	7	8	9	10
40	6021	6031	6042	6053	6064	6075	6085	6096	6107	6117	1	2	3	4	5	6	7	9	10
41	6128	6138	6149	6160	6170	6180	6191	6201	6212	6222	1	2	3	4	5	6	7	8	9
42	6232	6243	6253	6263	6274	6284	6294	6304	6314	6325	1	2	3	4	5	6	7	8	9
43	6335	6345	6355	6365	6375	6385	6395	6405	6415	6425	1	2	3	4	5	6	7	8	9
44	6435	6444	6454	6464	6474	6484	6493	6503	6513	6522	1	2	3	4	5	6	7	8	9
45	6532	6542	6551	6561	6571	6580	6590	6599	6609	6618	1	2	3	4	5	6	7	8	9
46	6628	6637	6646	6656	6665	6675	6684	6693	6702	6712	1	2	3	4	5	6	6	7	8
47	6721	6730	6739	6749	6758	6767	6776	6785	6794	6803	1	2	3	4	5	5	6	7	8
48	6812	6821	6830	6839	6848	6857	6866	6875	6884	6893	1	2	3	4	4	5	6	7	8
49	6902	6911	6920	6928	6937	6946	6955	6964	6972	6981	1	2	3	4	4	5	6	7	8
50	6990	6998	7007	7016	7024	7033	7042	7050	7059	7067	1	2	3	3	4	5	6	7	8
51	7076	7084	7093	7101	7110	7118	7126	7135	7143	7152	1	2	2	3	4	5	6	7	8
52	7160	7168	7177	7185	7193	7202	7210	7218	7226	7235	1	2	2	3	4	5	6	6	7
53	7243	7251	7259	7267	7275	7284	7292	7300	7308	7316	1	2	2	3	4	5	5	6	7
54	7324	7332	7340	7348	7356	7364	7372	7380	7388	7396	1	2	2	3	4	5	5	6	7

Natural Numbers 55–99

N	0	1	2	3	4	5	6	7	8	9	P.P. 1	2	3	4	5	6	7	8	9
55	7404	7412	7419	7427	7435	7443	7451	7459	7466	7474	1	2	2	3	4	5	5	6	7
56	7482	7490	7497	7505	7513	7520	7528	7536	7543	7551	1	2	2	3	4	5	5	6	7
57	7559	7566	7574	7582	7589	7597	7604	7612	7619	7627	1	2	2	3	4	5	5	6	7
58	7634	7642	7649	7657	7664	7672	7679	7686	7694	7701	1	1	2	3	4	4	5	6	7
59	7709	7716	7723	7731	7738	7745	7752	7760	7767	7774	1	1	2	3	4	4	5	6	7
60	7782	7789	7796	7803	7810	7818	7825	7832	7839	7846	1	1	2	3	4	4	5	6	7
61	7853	7860	7868	7875	7882	7889	7896	7903	7910	7917	1	1	2	3	4	4	5	6	6
62	7924	7931	7938	7945	7952	7959	7966	7973	7980	7987	1	1	2	3	4	4	5	6	6
63	7993	8000	8007	8014	8021	8028	8035	8041	8048	8055	1	1	2	3	3	4	5	6	6
64	8062	8069	8075	8082	8089	8096	8102	8109	8116	8122	1	1	2	3	3	4	5	5	6
65	8129	8136	8142	8149	8156	8162	8169	8176	8182	8189	1	1	2	3	3	4	5	5	6
66	8195	8202	8209	8215	8222	8228	8235	8241	8248	8254	1	1	2	3	3	4	5	5	6
67	8261	8267	8274	8280	8287	8293	8299	8306	8312	8319	1	1	2	2	3	4	5	5	6
68	8325	8331	8338	8344	8351	8357	8363	8370	8376	8382	1	1	2	2	3	4	4	5	6
69	8388	8395	8401	8407	8414	8420	8426	8432	8439	8445	1	1	2	2	3	4	4	5	6
70	8451	8457	8463	8470	8476	8482	8488	8494	8500	8506	1	1	2	2	3	4	4	5	5
71	8513	8519	8525	8531	8537	8543	8549	8555	8561	8567	1	1	2	2	3	4	4	5	5
72	8573	8579	8585	8591	8597	8603	8609	8615	8621	8627	1	1	2	2	3	4	4	5	5
73	8633	8639	8645	8651	8657	8663	8669	8675	8681	8686	1	1	2	2	3	4	4	5	5
74	8692	8698	8704	8710	8716	8722	8727	8733	8739	8745	1	1	2	2	3	4	4	5	5
75	8751	8756	8762	8768	8774	8779	8785	8791	8797	8802	1	1	2	2	3	3	4	5	5
76	8808	8814	8820	8825	8831	8837	8842	8848	8854	8859	1	1	2	2	3	3	4	5	5
77	8865	8871	8876	8882	8887	8893	8899	8904	8910	8915	1	1	2	2	3	3	4	4	5
78	8921	8927	8932	8938	8943	8949	8954	8960	8965	8971	1	1	2	2	3	3	4	4	5
79	8976	8982	8987	8993	8998	9004	9009	9015	9020	9026	1	1	2	2	3	3	4	4	5
80	9031	9036	9042	9047	9053	9058	9063	9069	9074	9079	1	1	2	2	3	3	4	4	5
81	9085	9090	9096	9101	9106	9112	9117	9122	9128	9133	1	1	2	2	3	3	4	4	5
82	9138	9143	9149	9154	9159	9165	9170	9175	9180	9186	1	1	2	2	3	3	4	4	5
83	9191	9196	9201	9206	9212	9217	9222	9227	9232	9238	1	1	2	2	3	3	4	4	5
84	9243	9248	9253	9258	9263	9269	9274	9279	9284	9289	1	1	2	2	3	3	4	4	5
85	9294	9299	9304	9309	9315	9320	9325	9330	9335	9340	1	1	2	2	3	3	4	4	5
86	9345	9350	9355	9360	9365	9370	9375	9380	9385	9390	1	1	2	2	3	3	4	4	5
87	9395	9400	9405	9410	9415	9420	9425	9430	9435	9440	0	1	1	2	3	3	4	4	5
88	9445	9450	9455	9460	9465	9469	9474	9479	9484	9489	0	1	1	2	2	3	4	4	5
89	9494	9499	9504	9509	9513	9518	9523	9528	9533	9538	0	1	1	2	2	3	3	4	4
90	9542	9547	9552	9557	9562	9566	9571	9576	9581	9586	0	1	1	2	2	3	3	4	4
91	9590	9595	9600	9605	9609	9614	9619	9624	9628	9633	0	1	1	2	2	3	3	4	4
92	9638	9643	9647	9652	9657	9661	9666	9671	9675	9680	0	1	1	2	2	3	3	4	4
93	9685	9689	9694	9699	9703	9708	9713	9717	9722	9727	0	1	1	2	2	3	3	4	4
94	9731	9736	9741	9745	9750	9754	9759	9763	9768	9773	0	1	1	2	2	3	3	4	4
95	9777	9782	9786	9791	9795	9800	9805	9809	9814	9818	0	1	1	2	2	3	3	4	4
96	9823	9827	9832	9836	9841	9845	9850	9854	9859	9863	0	1	1	2	2	3	3	4	4
97	9868	9872	9877	9881	9886	9890	9894	9899	9903	9908	0	1	1	2	2	3	3	4	4
98	9912	9917	9921	9926	9930	9934	9939	9943	9948	9952	0	1	1	2	2	3	3	4	4
99	9956	9961	9965	9969	9974	9978	9983	9987	9991	9996	0	1	1	2	2	3	3	3	4

Remington's

Pharmaceutical Sciences

RPS XIV

Remington's
PHARMACEUTICAL SCIENCES

A treatise on the theory and practice of pharmaceutical sciences, with essential information about pharmaceutical and medicinal agents; also a guide to the professional responsibilities and services of the pharmacist as a member of the health team . . . . A textbook and reference work for pharmacists, physicians, and other medical scientists

EDITORIAL BOARD MEMBERS

Arthur Osol, *Chairman* Richard A. Deno Alfonso R. Gennaro

Stewart C. Harvey Harold S. Hutchison Alfred N. Martin

Ewart A. Swinyard Linwood F. Tice Clarence T. Van Meter

SECTION EDITORS

Grafton D. Chase Richard A. Deno Alfonso R. Gennaro

Melvin R. Gibson Stewart C. Harvey Robert E. King Alfred N. Martin

Ewart A. Swinyard Clarence T. Van Meter Bernard Witlin

MANAGING EDITOR

John E. Hoover

With the cooperation of more than 300 editors, associate editors, and contributors

Over 1,000 Illustrations

FOURTEENTH EDITION

1970

Published in the 150th Anniversary Year
of the
Philadelphia College of Pharmacy and Science

MACK PUBLISHING COMPANY

Easton, Pennsylvania 18042

Remington Biographical Data

The following is a record of the editors and the dates of publication of successive editions of this book, prior to the Thirteenth Edition known as *Remington's Practice of Pharmacy* and subsequently as *Remington's Pharmaceutical Sciences*.

First Edition, 1886
Second Edition, 1889
Third Edition, 1897
Fourth Edition, 1905

Joseph P. Remington

Fifth Edition, 1907
Sixth Edition, 1917

Joseph P. Remington

Assisted by
E. Fullerton Cook

Seventh Edition, 1926

Editors
E. Fullerton Cook
Charles H. LaWall

with 37 Collaborators

Eighth Edition, 1936

Editors
E. Fullerton Cook
Charles H. LaWall

Associate Editors
Ivor Griffith
Adley B. Nichols
Arthur Osol

with 32 Collaborators

Ninth Edition, 1948

Editors
E. Fullerton Cook
Eric W. Martin

with 40 Associate Editors

Tenth Edition, 1951

Editors
E. Fullerton Cook
Eric W. Martin

with 49 Associate Editors

Eleventh Edition, 1956

Editors
Eric W. Martin
E. Fullerton Cook

Associate Editors
E. Emerson Leuallen
Arthur Osol
Linwood F. Tice
Clarence T. Van Meter

with the cooperation of more than 200 Assistant Editors and Contributors

Twelfth Edition, 1961

Editors
Eric W. Martin
E. Fullerton Cook
E. Emerson Leuallen
Arthur Osol
Linwood F. Tice
Clarence T. Van Meter

Assistant to the Editors
John E. Hoover

with the cooperation of more than 250 Assistant Editors and Contributors

Thirteenth Edition, 1965

Editor-in-Chief
Eric W. Martin

Editors
Grafton D. Chase
Herald R. Cox
Richard A. Deno
Alfonso R. Gennaro
Stewart C. Harvey
Robert E. King
E. Emerson Leuallen
Arthur Osol
Ewart A. Swinyard
Clarence T. Van Meter

Managing Editor
John E. Hoover

with the cooperation of more than 300 Editors, Assistant Editors and Contributors

Associate Editors

The following individuals either prepared original manuscript or revised one or more chapters for the FOURTEENTH EDITION OF REMINGTON'S PHARMACEUTICAL SCIENCES

Mary Celeste Alessandri, BA / Free-lance Writer. Co-author of Chapter 31, *Drug Nomenclature—United States Adopted Names.*

Kenneth E. Avis, DSc / Professor of Pharmaceutics, College of Pharmacy, The University of Tennessee. Author of Chapter 82, *Parenteral Preparations.*

Berton E. Ballard, PhD / Associate Professor of Pharmacy and Pharmaceutical Chemistry, University of California, San Francisco Medical Center. Co-author of Chapter 89, *Prolonged-Action Pharmaceuticals.*

Otto K. Behrens, PhD / Associate Director of Research, Eli Lilly and Co. Co-author of Chapter 8, *Research.*

Seymour M. Blaug, PhD / Professor of Pharmacy, College of Pharmacy, University of Iowa. Co-author of Chapter 85, *Medicated Applications.*

J. William Boehne, BS / Division of Nutrition, Food and Drug Administration. Co-author of Chapter 56, *Vitamins and Other Nutrients.*

John H. Brewer, PhD / Senior Microbiological Consultant, Becton, Dickinson & Co. Co-author of Chapter 81, *Sterilization.*

Harold H. Bryant, PhD / Director, Huntingdon Research Center, Inc. Author of Chapter 91, *Plastics.*

Arthur Cammarata, PhD / Associate Professor of Physical Medicinal Chemistry, School of Pharmacy, Temple University. Author of Chapter 17, *Quantum Chemistry,* and Chapter 18, *Thermodynamics.*

Joseph L. Ciminera, ScD / Manager, Statistical Services, Merck Sharp and Dohme Research Laboratories. Co-author of Chapter 11, *Statistics.*

Jack Cooper, PhG / Consultant, Pharmacy Research and Development, Sandoz, Ltd., Basle, Switzerland. Author of Chapter 5, *Pharmacists in Industry.*

Dwight L. Deardorff, PhD / Professor of Manufacturing Pharmacy, College of Pharmacy, University of Illinois. Author of Chapter 83, *Ophthalmic Solutions.*

Ara H. Der Marderosian, PhD / Associate Professor of Pharmacognosy, Philadelphia College of Pharmacy and Science. Author of Chapter 69, *Pesticides.*

Alan K. Done, MD / Director, Poison Information and Therapy Center, University of Utah Medical Center. Author of Chapter 100, *Poison Control.*

John C. Drach, PhD / Research Biochemist, Research Laboratories, Parke, Davis and Co. Author of Chapter 40, *Chromatography.*

Robert W. Elkas, PhD / Manager, Pharmaceutical Quality Control and Services, Lederle Laboratories. Co-author of Chapter 92, *Control.*

Alvin Felmeister, PhD / Associate Professor of Pharmacy, College of Pharmacy, Rutgers University. Author of Chapter 86, *Powders.*

James W. Gibb, PhD / Assistant Professor of Pharmacology, College of Pharmacy and College of Medicine, University of Utah. Author of Chapter 57, *Enzymes.*

Samuel W. Goldstein, PhD / Executive Secretary, Academy of Pharmaceutical Sciences, American Pharmaceutical Association. Author of Chapter 9, *Metrology.*

David E. Guttman, PhD / Associate Director, Analytical and Physical Chemistry, Smith Kline and French Laboratories. Co-author of Chapter 16, *Complexation.*

William I. Higuchi, PhD / Professor of Pharmacy, College of Pharmacy, University of Michigan. Co-author of Chapter 25, *Particle Phenomena.*

Richard A. Huebner, VMD / Director, Veterinary Service, Wyeth Laboratories. Author of Chapter 96, *Veterinary Services,* and Veterinary Editor of Part VI, *Pharmaceutical and Medicinal Agents.*

Daniel A. Hussar, PhD / Associate Professor of Pharmacy, Philadelphia College of Pharmacy and Science. Author of Chapter 94, *The Prescription.*

Joseph B. Jerome, PhD / Secretary, United States Adopted Names Council. Co-author of Chapter 31, *Drug Nomenclature—United States Adopted Names.*

Lloyd Kennon, PhD / Vice President—Director of Research and Development, Menley and James Laboratories. Author of Chapter 14, *Matter—Its States and Selected Properties.*

O. L. Kline, PhD / American Institute of Nutrition. Co-author of Chapter 56, *Vitamins and Other Nutrients.*

Adelbert M. Knevel, PhD / Professor of Medicinal Chemistry, School of Pharmacy and Pharmacal Sciences, Purdue University. Author of Chapter 27, *Separation.*

Harry B. Kostenbauder, PhD / Professor of Medicinal search, College of Pharmacy, University of Kentucky. Author of Chapter 21, *Reaction Kinetics.*

Allen M. Kratz, PharmD / Assistant Professor of Clinical Pharmacy, Philadelphia College of Pharmacy and Science. Pharmacy Co-editor of Part VI, *Pharmaceutical and Medicinal Agents.*

Austin H. Kutscher, DDS / Head, Section on Therapeutics and Clinical Pharmacology, School of Dental and Oral Surgery, Columbia University. Author of Chapter 95, *Dental Services.*

Clifton J. Latiolais, MSc / Director of Pharmacy, The Ohio State University Hospitals. Author of Chapter 93, *Hospital Pharmacy.*

Eric Jung-chi Lien, PhD / Assistant Professor of Pharmacy, School of Pharmacy, University of Southern California. Co-author of Chapter 15, *Atomic and Molecular Structure.*

Werner Lowenthal, PhD / Associate Professor of Pharmacy, School of Pharmacy, Medical College of Virginia, Health Science Division, Virginia Commonwealth University. Author of Chapter 10, *Calculation.*

Thomas J. Macek, PhD / Director of Revision, the United States Pharmacopeia. Author of Chapter 79, *Formulation.*

Gordon E. Mallett, PhD / Director of Fermentation Products Research, Eli Lilly and Co. Co-author of Chapter 8, *Research.*

John N. McDonnell, DSc / Consultant to the Pharmaceutical Industry. Author of Chapter 99, *Health Accessories.*

Robert H. Moser, MD / Col., US Army, Chief, Department of Medicine, Walter Reed General Hospital. Author of Chapter 72, *Adverse Effects and Interactions of Drugs.*

George Motoasca, BS / Manager, Product Development Department, S. B. Penick and Co. Co-author of Chapter 84, *Extraction and Extractives*.

Maven J. Myers, LLB, PhD / Associate Professor of Pharmacy Administration, Philadelphia College of Pharmacy and Science. Author of Chapter 3, *Ethics*.

Eino Nelson,* PhD / Late Professor of Pharmaceutics and Medicinal Chemistry, School of Pharmacy, State University of New York at Buffalo. Co-author of Chapter 89, *Prolonged-Action Pharmaceuticals*.

Jay Nematollahi, PhD / Assistant Professor of Pharmaceutical Chemistry, College of Pharmacy, The University of Texas. Author of Chapter 41, *Instrumental Methods of Analysis*.

Paul J. Niebergall, PhD / Associate Professor of Pharmacy, Philadelphia College of Pharmacy and Science. Author of Chapter 20, *Ionic Solutions and Electrolytic Equilibria*.

M. Pernarowski, PhD / Professor of Pharmaceutical Chemistry, Faculty of Pharmaceutical Sciences, The University of British Columbia. Author of Chapter 80, *Solutions, Emulsions, and Suspensions*.

G. Briggs Phillips, PhD / Director, Becton, Dickinson Research Center, Becton, Dickinson & Co. Co-author of Chapter 81, *Sterilization*.

George L. Phillips, MS / Director of Pharmacy Service, University of Michigan Hospital. Author of Chapter 77, *Allergenic Extracts*.

Henry D. Piersma, PhD / Director, Quality Control Section, Lederle Laboratories. Co-author of Chapter 92, *Control*.

Lila K. Randolph,* BS / Mathematical Statistician, Office of the Assistant Commissioner for Planning, US Food and Drug Administration. Co-author of Chapter 11, *Statistics*.

Louis A. Reber, PhD / Director of Graduate Studies, Philadelphia College of Pharmacy and Science. Author of Chapter 23, *Colloidal Dispersions*.

James W. Richards, MBA / Associate Professor of Pharmacy Administration, College of Pharmacy, University of Michigan. Author of Chapter 102, *Pharmaceutical Economics and Management*.

Edward G. Rippie, PhD / Professor of Pharmaceutics, College of Pharmacy, University of Minnesota. Author of Chapter 13, *Calculus*.

G. Victor Rossi, PhD / Professor of Pharmacology, Philadelphia College of Pharmacy and Science. Author of Chapter 38, *Biological Testing*.

Paul G. Sanders, MS / Manager, Applied Mathematics, Abbott Laboratories. Author of Chapter 12, *Computer Science*.

Louis C. Schroeter, PhD / Assistant Manager, Pharmacy Research, The Upjohn Co. Author of Chapter 88, *Coating of Tablets, Capsules, and Pills*.

* Deceased.

John J. Sciarra, PhD / Director, Graduate Division, and Professor of Pharmaceutical Chemistry, College of Pharmacy, St. John's University. Author of Chapter 90, *Aerosols*.

Eli Shefter, PhD / Associate Professor of Pharmaceutics, School of Pharmacy, State University of New York at Buffalo. Co-author of Chapter 15, *Atomic and Molecular Structure*.

Anthony P. Simonelli, PhD / Associate Professor of Pharmacy, College of Pharmacy, University of Michigan. Co-author of Chapter 25, *Particle Phenomena*.

Milton W. Skolaut, BS / Chief, Pharmacy Department, Clinical Center, National Institutes of Health. Author of Chapter 6, *Pharmacists in Government*.

Robert D. Smyth, MSc / Manager, Department of Biological Chemistry, William H. Rorer, Inc. Author of Chapter 39, *Clinical Analysis*.

Theodore D. Sokoloski, PhD / Associate Professor of Pharmacy, College of Pharmacy, The Ohio State University. Author of Chapter 19, *Solutions and Phase Equilibria*.

Glenn Sonnedecker, PhD / Director, American Institute of the History of Pharmacy. Author of Chapter 2, *Evolution of Pharmacy*.

Albert A. Stonehill, PhD / Manager, Product Research Department, Ethicon, Inc. Author of Chapter 97, *Surgical Supplies*, and Chapter 98, *Medical Emergencies*.

Douglas M. Surgenor, PhD / Provost, Faculty of Health Sciences, State University of New York at Buffalo. Author of Chapter 45, *Blood, Fluids, and Electrolytes*.

James Swarbrick, PhD / Professor, and Chairman, Division of Pharmaceutics, School of Pharmacy, University of Connecticut. Author of Chapter 24, *Coarse Dispersions*.

George C. Walker, PhD / Head, Department of Pharmacy, Faculty of Pharmacy, University of Toronto. Co-author of Chapter 84, *Extraction and Extractives*.

Sidney H. Willig, JD / Director of Drug Law Unit, Temple University. Author of Chapter 101, *Laws Governing Pharmacy*.

Charles O. Wilson, PhD / Dean, School of Pharmacy, Oregon State University. Author of Chapter 7, *Literature*.

Murray Zanger, PhD / Associate Professor of Chemistry, Philadelphia College of Pharmacy and Science. Co-author of Chapter 32, *Structure–Activity Relationship and Drug Design*.

George Zografi, PhD / Associate Professor, College of Pharmacy, University of Michigan. Author of Chapter 22, *Interfacial Phenomena*.

Louis C. Zopf, DSc / Dean, College of Pharmacy, University of Iowa. Co-author of Chapter 85, *Medicated Applications*.

Editorial Assistants

Frances F. Curran, MSc / Assistant in Pharmacology, Philadelphia College of Pharmacy and Science. Assisted Dr. Rossi, the author of Chapter 38, *Biological Testing*.

Peter Clemens Kronfeld, MD / Professor Emeritus' Department of Ophthalmology, University of Illinois. Assisted Dr. Deardorff, the author of Chapter 83, *Ophthalmic Solutions*.

Joseph F. McDonnell, Jr., MSc / Assistant Director of Technical Services, The Borden Co. Assisted Dr. McDonnell, the author of Chapter 99, *Health Accessories*, in the technical presentation on nutritional aspects of baby foods.

Contributors

The editors wish to express their deep appreciation to the following contributors who supplied suggestions, information, and illustrations, who read proof, and who assisted in many other ways during the preparation of the Fourteenth Edition of REMINGTON'S PHARMACEUTICAL SCIENCES. In addition to the individuals appearing below, the many pharmaceutical manufacturers which graciously supplied extensive information concerning specialties, methods of manufacture, and other data are listed in the *Appendix* under *Manufacturers Index* (page 2023).

W. K. Abbott, Wilmington, Del.
Margaretta E. Aeugle, Philadelphia, Pa.
Howard C. Ansel, Athens, Ga.
Robert B. Aron, Lodi, N. J.
Norman W. Atwater, Chicago, Ill.
Raphael O. Bachmann, Morgantown, W. Va.
Gilbert S. Banker, Lafayette, Ind.
Andrew J. Bartilucci, Jamaica, N. Y.
William E. Baum, Syracuse, N. Y.
James G. Beasley, Memphis, Tenn.
Henry W. Beck, Madison, Wis.
Karl Beck, North Chicago, Ill.
Charles H. Becker, Gainesville, Fla.
J. M. Beiler, Philadelphia, Pa.
Patrick F. Belcastro, Lafayette, Ind.
Ignatius J. Bellafiore, Jamaica, N. Y.
Leroy D. Beltz, Ada, Ohio
Leslie Z. Benet, Pullman, Wash.
Byrl E. Benton, Des Moines, Iowa
John V. Bergen, Washington, D. C.
Martin I. Blake, Chicago, Ill.
Charles W. Blissitt, St. Louis, Mo.
R. R. Blumenthal, Orange, N. J.
Rudolph H. Blythe, Gainesville, Fla.
David M. Bolton, West Point, Pa.
Mildred D. Bray, Lansdowne, Pa.
Harold Breslow, Garden City, N. Y.
Gary L. Brewer, Middletown, Ohio
Willis R. Brewer, Tucson, Ariz.
Richard C. Brogle, Morris Plains, N. J.
Virginia T. Brown, Middletown, Ohio
Charles A. Brownlee, Jr., Summit, N. J.
H. D. Bryan, Evansville, Ind.
Constance Bungart, Morton Grove, Ill.
Elmon L. Cataline, Albuquerque, N. M.
Elizabeth W. Chase, Philadelphia, Pa.
John H. Coleman, Rouses Point, N. Y.
Torrence J. Collier, Union, N. J.
Rosa Conlon, Orangeburg, N. Y.
E. M. Cook, North Branch, N. J.
Benjamin F. Cooper, Monroe, La.
Charles B. Cowling, Easton, Pa.
Barbara A. Craddock, Philadelphia, Pa.
Paul Creager, Detroit, Mich.
J. William Crosson, Chicago, Ill.
Mary Lou Dailey, Easton, Pa.
H. R. Dettelbach, Cincinnati, Ohio
J. L. Deuble, Philadelphia, Pa.
Walter L. Dickison, Weatherford, Okla.
Allan H. Doane, Morris Plains, N. J.
Durward F. Dodgen, Washington, D. C.
Evelyn B. Draper, Columbia, S. C.
William R. Ebert, Columbus, Ohio
Durward N. Entrekin, Athens, Ga.
Kenneth Ericson, Morristown, N. J.
Joseph C. Estes, Jr., Reidsville, N. C.
Darrell E. Favrhow, Fullerton, Calif.

Edward G. Feldmann, Washington, D. C.
C. W. Ferry, Tuckahoe, N. Y.
Mildred T. Fisher, Middletown, Ohio
Bryant W. Fitzgerald, Missoula, Mont.
Herbert L. Flack, Philadelphia, Pa.
Robyn A. Flye, Middletown, Ohio
Norman H. Francke, Atlanta, Ga.
William A. Fredell, Rochester, N. Y.
Bernard Friedland, Miami, Fla.
Salvatore A. Fusari, Detroit, Mich.
Robert J. Gerraughty, Kingston, R. I.
Ellen P. Gilligan, Philadelphia, Pa.
G. R. Goetchius, New York, N. Y.
Marvin Goldberg, Drexel Hill, Pa.
Allan M. Goodeve, Vancouver, B. C., Canada
C. L. Graham, Kalamazoo, Mich.
Philip A. Greth, Tuxedo, N. Y.
George B. Griffenhagen, Washington, D. C.
Mary C. Griffiths, Bethesda, Md.
Harry W. Grodon, New York, N. Y.
William Haas, West Allis, Wis.
S. Z. Haidri, New Brunswick, N. J.
Esther Jane W. Hall, Austin, Tex.
G. Vinton Hallock, Worcester, Mass.
Martin E. Hamner, Memphis, Tenn.
Robert A. Hardt, Chicago, Ill.
John W. Harmon, Newark, Del.
Loyd E. Harris, Norman, Okla.
R. V. Hauck, New York, N. Y.
Lois S. Hazel, Fort Washington, Pa.
Ruth Heil, St. Louis, Mo.
Arnold J. Henning, Boulder, Colo.
Jerome F. Hensiak, Omaha, Neb.
Donald O. Hensler, Middletown, Ohio
William T. Hensler, Hanover, N. J.
William F. Hewitt, Norwich, N. Y.
Eugene Hickman, Houston, Tex.
Bernard E. Hietbrink, Brookings, S. D.
W. W. Hilty, Indianapolis, Ind.
David L. Hiner, Salt Lake City, Utah
C. F. Hiskey, Garden City, N. Y.
F. A. Hochstein, Groton, Conn.
R. D. Holloman, Morton Grove, Ill.
Lola V. Hopkins, Laramie, Wyo.
Raymond E. Hopponen, Brookings, S. D.
Donald Hudson, Piscataway, N. J.
Karen E. Hudson, Middletown, Ohio
Mervyn J. Huston, Edmonton, Alta., Canada
Albert E. Hyers, West Orange, N. J.
R. D. Johnson, Palo Alto, Calif.
Hurd M. Jones, Jr., Tallahassee, Fla.
Wilbur R. Jones, Bristol, Tenn.
William R. Jones, Fort Washington, Pa.
Joseph L. Kanig, New York, N. Y.
Karl L. Kaufman, Indianapolis, Ind.
James D. Keiser, Bryan, Ohio
Louis D. King, Newark, N. J.

Thomas L. King, West Point, Pa.
Oscar Klioze, Richmond, Va.
Harold C. Krahnke, Milwaukee, Wis.
Robert S. Kreisler, New York, N. Y.
Ray R. Kriner, New Brunswick, N. J.
Ronald J. Landry, Northridge, Calif.
William J. Latham, Middletown, Ohio
James O. Lawrence, Kalamazoo, Mich.
Beverly A. Leamon, Easton, Pa.
J. B. Lesh, Kankakee, Ill.
Phillip J. Levine, Des Moines, Iowa
Richard L. Lewis, Middletown, Ohio
G. L. Lindsay, St. Louis, Mo.
Louis Malspeis, Columbus, Ohio
C. E. Manaresi, Toledo, Ohio
Dennie W. McClanahan, Middletown, Ohio
Edwin C. McCormick, Middletown, Ohio
W. B. McDowell, New York, N. Y.
Mary Jane McEntee, Philadelphia, Pa.
William S. McGregor, New York, N. Y.
F. J. McGroarty, New York, N. Y.
Edward C. McKeon, Yonkers, N. Y.
J. A. McNeilly, Philadelphia, Pa.
Robert W. Mendes, Boston, Mass.
Lloyd C. Miller, Bethesda, Md.
John J. Moir, Vancouver, B. C., Canada
B. Mollov, New York, N. Y.
Kenneth E. Moore, Richmond, Va.
Finlay A. Morrison, Vancouver, B. C., Canada
Robert W. Morrison, Columbia, S. C.
Howard E. Mossberg, Lawrence, Kan.
J. D. Mullins, Fort Worth, Tex.
R. A. Nash, Pearl River, N. Y.
Robert J. Nessel, Rahway, N. J.
J. Gerald O'Hern, Syracuse, N. Y.
Gary W. Omodt, Brookings, S. D.
Jack E. Orr, Seattle, Wash.
Albert M. Packman, Fort Washington, Pa.
John W. Palmer, Los Angeles, Calif.
Charles F. Peterson, Philadelphia, Pa.
Margareta Philip, Uppsala, Sweden
William F. Pillow, Jr., Indianapolis, Ind.
James M. Plaxco, Jr., Columbia, S. C.
I. Porush, Northridge, Calif.
L. H. Possley, Mount Prospect, Ill.
H. E. Post, Terre Haute, Ind.
Harold D. Powell, San Antonio, Tex.
William P. Purcell, Memphis, Tenn.
Ronald P. Quintana, Memphis, Tenn.
Charles W. Rahner, Jr., New York, N. Y.
B. K. Murahari Rao, Brookings, S. D.
B. E. Reidel, Vancouver, B. C., Canada
Wilhelm Reiss, New York, N. Y.
P. J. Rhodes, Lincoln, Neb.
Sidney Riegelman, San Francisco, Calif.
E. W. Roberson, Easton, Pa.
M. John Romer, Philadelphia, Pa.

John S. Ruggiero, Pittsburgh, Pa.
Janis O. Runikis, Vancouver, B. C., Canada
Sidney A. Sadin, Yonkers, N. Y.
Witold Saski, Lincoln, Neb.
John W. Schermerhorn, Boston, Mass.
R. Marilyn Schmidt, Union, N. J.
Richard H. Schneider, Chicago, Ill.
Richard L. Sedam, West Point, Pa.
Irwin S. Shupe, Rensselaer, N. Y.
H. I. Silverman, Orange, N. J.
Walter Singer, Albany, N. Y.
Gertrude H. Sink, Middletown, Ohio
Lloyd P. Sink, Middletown, Ohio
L. P. Sinotte, West Point, Pa.
G. E. H. Skrimshire, London, England
Evelyn M. Sloyer, Easton, Pa.
John H. Speer, Chicago, Ill.
A. B. Spradling, Kalamazoo, Mich.
Joseph B. Sprowls, Austin, Tex.
R. Srinivas, Brooklyn, N. Y.
Ludmila K. Stass, New Orleans, La.
A. W. Stewart, Fullerton, Calif.
Audrey H. Stein, Lynbrook, N. Y.
C. E. Sundberg, Cedar Rapids, Iowa
William B. Swafford, Memphis, Tenn.
Joseph V. Swintosky, Lexington, Ky.
Stephen A. Szumski, Pearl River, N. Y.
S. K. Talwar, Ghaziabad, India
Elmore H. Taylor, Memphis, Tenn.
Herman O. Thompson, Chapel Hill, N. C.
James M. Tio, Hines, Ill.
C. M. Todaro, Easton, Pa.
Robert G. Tucker, Morton Grove, Ill.
Beulah H. Tullar, Lansdowne, Pa.
E. E. Vannatta, Columbus, Ohio
H. Leslie Varley, Easton, Pa.
A. Verheecke, Ghent, Belgium
J. W. Wallace, Marcus Hook, Pa.
Alexander T. Warren, New Brunswick, N. J.
J. Ritner Weaver, Morris Plains, N. J.
Lawrence C. Weaver, Minneapolis, Minn.
G. F. Whattam, Baltimore, Md.
Keith W. Wheeler, Cincinnati, Ohio
Allen I. White, Pullman, Wash.
Hugh P. Wilder, Middletown, Ohio
Leon O. Wilken, Jr., Auburn, Ala.
William L. Williams, Upper Darby, Pa.
Lyle W. Willits, Kansas City, Mo.
Robert G. Wilson, Houston, Tex.
D. C. Wimer, North Chicago, Ill.
E. G. Wollish, Nutley, N. J.
E. L. Woroch, North Chicago, Ill.
N. C. Zacharias, Vancouver, B. C., Canada
Seymour Zelmanoff, Philadelphia, Pa.
Albert J. Zimmerman, North Chicago, Ill.
Henry B. Zimmerman, Cranbury, N. J.
Arthur G. Zupko, Brooklyn, N. Y.

Preface to the Fourteenth Edition

THE ACADEMIC DISCIPLINES comprising the pharmaceutical sciences as well as the practice of the specialized professions that constitute the broad field of pharmacy have undergone great change. The greatest changes, however, are in the making.

The need for greater understanding of the actions and reactions of drugs is imperative. The utility of a drug depends on the predominance of some biochemical reaction that produces in a particular patient a therapeutic effect. But other simultaneous reactions of the drug may be adverse, or its expected therapeutic reaction may be nullified or modified by a reaction with food, or a second drug given concomitantly may accentuate or diminish the actions of both drugs. Effective use of drugs requires full knowledge of such reactions, and its intelligent communication both to the patient, when necessary, and to his physician. The pharmacist is the health professional best qualified to provide this service.

Confirming this role for pharmacists, the Task Force on Prescription Drugs of the Department of Health, Education, and Welfare stated, in its *Final Report*, published in 1969:

> "... it is also becoming evident that appropriately trained pharmacists may become new and vital members of the total health team by serving as drug information specialists.
>
> "Some community pharmacists are already providing such services. They do not prescribe, but they discuss practical details of drug administration, possible side-effects, and other facets of drug use with each patient to whom a prescription drug is dispensed. They maintain patient or family records which contain data on drugs which have been dispensed to each patient, allergic responses, and adverse reactions. They call to the attention of the physician any prescriptions which may have been written for the same patient by other physicians, and they refer to him any prescriptions which may involve drug-interaction, synergism, or similar effects."

This edition of Remington anticipates both the new role for pharmacists, especially those who serve in community and hospital practice, and also the growing sophistication of all the pharmaceutical sciences. It reflects the over-all present progress of the profession of pharmacy, and at the same time prepares for future requirements of the profession.

The book has undergone extensive revision. More new material has been added than ever before, space for it having been provided by deleting or condensing the text on subjects of decreasing relevance.

This edition represents the effort of persons from academic institutions, hospitals, research laboratories, industrial establishments, and government agencies who have served as authors and contributors.

We are pleased to welcome as new editors Dr. Melvin R. Gibson, of Washington State University, for Part I, *Orientation;* Dr. Alfred N. Martin, of Temple University, for Part II, *Pharmaceutics* (formerly *Physical Pharmacy*); and Dr. Bernard Witlin, of the Philadelphia College of Pharmacy and Science, for Part VII, *Biological Products.*

The veteran editors are Dr. Clarence T. Van Meter, of the University of Pennsylvania, for Part III, *Pharmaceutical Chemistry*, plus the chemical formulas, nomenclature, and methods of synthesis throughout the book; Dr. Grafton D. Chase, of the Philadelphia

College of Pharmacy and Science, for Part IV, *Radioisotopes in Pharmacy and Medicine*, plus Chapter 26, *Rheology;* Dr. Alfonso R. Gennaro, of the Philadelphia College of Pharmacy and Science, for Part V, *Testing and Analysis*, also serving as co-editor of Part III and co-author of Chapter 32, *Structure-Activity Relationship and Drug Design;* Dr. Ewart A. Swinyard and Dr. Stewart C. Harvey, of the University of Utah, for Part VI, *Pharmaceutical and Medicinal Agents*, plus Chapter 42, *Drug Absorption, Action, and Disposition* (Dr. Harvey), and Chapter 73, *Introduction of New Drugs* (Dr. Swinyard); Dr. Robert E. King, of the Philadelphia College of Pharmacy and Science, for Part VIII, *Pharmaceutical Preparations and Their Manufacture*, plus Chapter 87, *Tablets, Capsules, and Pills;* and Dr. Richard A. Deno, of the University of Michigan, for Part IX, *General Practice.*

Thirteen new chapters have been introduced in this edition. Titles of the chapters added to Part II, *Pharmaceutics*, are *Computer Science, Calculus, Atomic and Molecular Structure, Solutions and Phase Equilibria, Interfacial Phenomena, Coarse Dispersions,* and *Particle Phenomena.* Much new material has been incorporated in other chapters in this part, notably those on *Complexation, Quantum Chemistry, Thermodynamics, Ionic Solutions and Electrolytic Equilibria,* and *Reaction Kinetics.*

The new chapters in Part III, *Pharmaceutical Chemistry*, are on *Drug Nomenclature—United States Adopted Names* and *Structure-Activity Relationship and Drug Design.* In Part V, *Testing and Analysis*, a new chapter on *Instrumental Methods of Analysis* has been added.

The new chapters in Part VI, *Pharmaceutical and Medicinal Agents*, are titled *Drug Absorption, Action, and Disposition; Adverse Effects and Interactions of Drugs;* and *Introduction of New Drugs.*

In Part IX, *General Practice*, Chapter 94, *The Prescription*, has been substantially enlarged by the inclusion of much new material on therapeutic incompatibility and of a table on drug interactions.

The contributions of the editors and authors and of the many other persons who participated in the preparation of the text and the publication of the Fourteenth Edition are gratefully acknowledged. Special thanks are due Managing Editor John E. Hoover, who ably planned, performed, and coordinated the editorial operations in producing this book.

The continuing cooperation of the Mack Publishing Company and especially of Harold S. Hutchison, executive vice-president of the Company, is hereby acknowledged, with deep gratitude. The Company's support of Remington in underwriting editorial and production costs in advance of publication is a very important contribution to the success of the work.

We deeply appreciate the meticulous care with which Mrs. Beulah H. Tullar, assisted ably by Mrs. Mildred D. Bray, prepared our comprehensive index.

The Philadelphia College of Pharmacy and Science extends to the heirs of Professor Joseph P. Remington its thanks for their assignment of the copyright of this book to the College, which has used the income from sales of the book to endow the Joseph Price Remington Memorial Chair of Pharmacy.

ARTHUR OSOL
Chairman of the Editorial Board

Preface to the First Edition

The rapid and substantial progress made in Pharmacy within the last decade has created a necessity for a work treating of the improved apparatus, the revised processes, and the recently introduced preparations of the age.

The vast advances made in theoretical and applied chemistry and physics have much to do with the development of pharmaceutical science, and these have been reflected in all the revised editions of the Pharmacopœias which have been recently published. When the author was elected in 1874 to the chair of Theory and Practice of Pharmacy in the Philadelphia College of Pharmacy, the outlines of study which had been so carefully prepared for the classes by his eminent predecessors, Professor William Procter, Jr., and Professor Edward Parrish, were found to be not strictly in accord, either in their arrangement of the subjects or in their method of treatment. Desiring to preserve the distinctive characteristics of each, an effort was at once made to frame a system which should embody their valuable features, embrace new subjects, and still retain that harmony of plan and proper sequence which are absolutely essential to the success of any system.

The strictly alphabetical classification of subjects which is now universally adopted by pharmacopœias and dispensatories, although admirable in works of reference, presents an effectual stumbling block to the acquisition of pharmaceutical knowledge through systematic study; the vast accumulation of facts collected under each head being arranged lexically, they necessarily have no connection with one another, and thus the saving of labor effected by considering similar groups together, and the value of the association of kindred subjects, are lost to the student. In the method of grouping the subjects which is herein adopted, the constant aim has been to arrange the latter in such a manner that the reader shall be gradually led from the consideration of elementary subjects to those which involve more advanced knowledge, whilst the groups themselves are so placed as to follow one another in a natural sequence.

The work is divided into six parts. Part I is devoted to detailed descriptions of apparatus and definitions and comments on general pharmaceutical processes.

The Official Preparations alone are considered in Part II. Due weight and prominence are thus given to the Pharmacopœia, the National authority, which is now so thoroughly recognized.

In order to suit the convenience of pharmacists who prefer to *weigh solids* and *measure liquids*, the official formulas are expressed, in addition to parts by weight, in *avoirdupois weight* and *apothecaries' measure*. These equivalents are printed in *bold type* near the margin, and arranged so as to fit them for quick and accurate reference.

Part III treats of Inorganic Chemical Substances. Precedence is of course given to official preparations in these. The descriptions, solubilities, and tests for identity and impurities of each substance are systematically tabulated under its proper title. It is confidently believed that by this method of arrangement the valuable descriptive features of the Pharmacopœia will be more prominently developed, ready reference facilitated, and close study of the details rendered easy. Each chemical operation is accompanied by equations, whilst the reaction is, in addition, explained in words.

The Carbon Compounds, or Organic Chemical Substances, are considered in Part IV. These are naturally grouped according to the physical and medical properties of their principal constituents, beginning with simple bodies like cellulin, gum, etc., and progressing to the most highly organized alkaloids, etc.

Part V is devoted to Extemporaneous Pharmacy. Care has been taken to treat of the practice which would be best adapted for the needs of the many pharmacists who conduct operations upon a moderate scale, rather than for those of the few who manage very large establishments. In this, as well as in other parts of the work, operations are illustrated which are conducted by manufacturing pharmacists.

Part VI contains a formulary of Pharmaceutical Preparations which have not been recognized by the Pharmacopœia. The recipes selected are chiefly those which have been heretofore rather difficult of access to most pharmacists, yet such as are likely to be in request. Many private formulas are embraced in the collection; and such of the preparations of the old Pharmacopœias as have not been included in the new edition, but are still in use, have been inserted.

In conclusion, the author ventures to express the hope that the work will prove an efficient help to the pharmaceutical student as well as to the pharmacist and the physician. Although the labor has been mainly performed amidst the harassing cares of active professional duties, and perfection is known to be unattainable, no pains have been spared to discover and correct errors and omissions in the text. The author's warmest acknowledgments are tendered to Mr. A. B. Taylor, Mr. Joseph McCreery, and Mr. George M. Smith for their valuable assistance in revising the proof sheets, and to the latter especially for his work on the index. The outline illustrations, by Mr. John Collins, were drawn either from the actual objects or from photographs taken by the author.

Philadelphia, October, 1885   J.P.R.

Table of Contents

GENERAL NOTICES OF
Remington's Pharmaceutical Sciences

A GUIDE TO THE USE OF RPS XIV

1. Guidance to the Reader: The attention of the reader is directed to Chapter 36 on *Official Requirements and Tests* (page 585), especially to the selected and abstracted material from the *General Notices of the USP and NF* (pages 585 and 587). This material provides interpretations and general statements which attach special significance to official monographs and standards, tests, assays, and other requirements contained in this text. Chapter 36 also assists the reader in correlating the contents of RPS XIV with related subject matter in the official compendia. The primary authorities for the drug standards found in this text are the *USP XVIII, NF XIII*, recent editions of *New Drugs*, the *Food, Drug, and Cosmetic Act* of 1939 and its Regulations, the *Federal* or *Harrison Narcotic Law* and its Regulations, the *Federal Insecticide, Fungicide, and Rodenticide Act* of 1947 and its Regulations, and the *Federal Public Health Service Act* of 1944 and its Regulations.

Correlations among various types of pharmaceutical information, eg, therapeutic activity and chemical composition, have been facilitated by arranging the contents of RPS XIV into well-defined areas (see page (xi)), and by classifying all official and important unofficial drugs both chemically and pharmacologically.

2. Use of Text: Permission to use in this volume certain portions of the text of the *United States Pharmacopeia, Eighteenth Revision*, the *National Formulary, Thirteenth Edition*, and recent editions of *New Drugs* has been granted by the appropriate authorities (page iv).

3. Patents and Trademarks: The inclusion in the USP, NF, or RPS of any drug in respect to which patent or trademark rights may exist shall not be deemed, and is not intended as, a grant of, or authority to exercise, any right or privilege protected by such patent or trademark. All such rights and privileges are vested in the patent or trademark owner, and no other person may exercise the same without express permission, authority, or license secured from such patent or trademark owner.

It is to be understood that compilation of these trademarks herein must not be interpreted as constituting or implying authority to dispense any product other than the one prescribed or ordered under the trademark specified in the prescription or order. Substitution of one trademarked product for another, even though both trademarks are listed herein as synonyms for the official preparation, is a breach of professional pharmacy ethics and is to be condemned.

When a drug is prescribed, or otherwise ordered, by an official or other nonproprietary name, followed by a trademark, the product supplied under the trademark of the manufacturer specified must be dispensed. When a drug is specified in a prescription, or is otherwise ordered by an official or other nonproprietary name without reference to a specific trademark, any product bearing the official name may be dispensed.

4. Compliance with Federal Statutes: The fact that a drug appears in the USP or NF does not exempt it from compliance with requirements of Acts of Congress or with regulations and rulings issued by agencies of the United States Government under authority of these Acts. Revisions of the federal requirements that affect the official standards will be made the subject of USP or NF Supplements as promptly as practicable.

5. Synonyms: Comprehensive lists of chemical, trade, and other names have been included under the official titles as an aid in identifying pharmaceutical products. Note the statements concerning patent rights and substitution in paragraph 3 above.

6. Metric System: The use of the metric system to express doses and quantities in formulas has received almost universal acceptance, and the use of the ancient and cumbersome apothecary system has been almost completely abandoned. Tables of exact equivalents (pages 86 and 87) and approximate equivalents (page 84 and inside the front cover) have been retained for ready reference in the occasional instances when conversion from one system to the other is desired.

7. Temperatures: For USP and NF drugs, unless otherwise specified, all temperatures are expressed in centigrade degrees; all measurements are made at 25° unless otherwise stated, except for alcohol (15.56°) or other special cases.

8. Other Requirements: Certain official requirements such as identification tests, the various tests for purity, and requirements for packaging and storage have been deleted from the individual monographs in Part VI. Chapter 36, *Official Requirements and Tests*, provides information relevant to these requirements; the appropriate official compendia should be consulted for the individual specific requirements.

Part
I

ORIENTATION

EDITOR

Melvin R. Gibson, PhD, *Professor of Pharmacognosy, College of Pharmacy, Washington State University, Pullman, Wash. 99163*

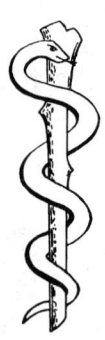

MEDICINE

Symbolized by the staff of Æsculapius, ancient god of healing. The serpent entwined about the staff denotes wisdom and the ability to heal, cure diseases, and prolong life.

Symbolized by the Bowl of Hygeia, the Goddess of Health in Greek Mythology. This bowl has rapidly gained international recognition as a symbol of pharmacy corresponding to the caduceus of the physician. Pharmacy is symbolized also by ℞, an abbreviation of "recipe," the Latin word for "take thou."

PHARMACY

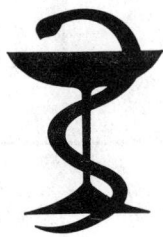

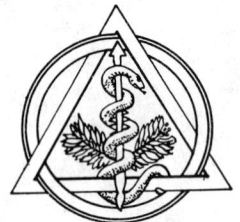

DENTISTRY

Symbolized by the serpent encircled about an ancient cautery. The leaves and berries in the background represents the two sets of teeth, while the triangle and circle are derived from the Greek letters—delta for "dens" and omicron for "odons," both words meaning tooth.

Symbolized by the lamp of Florence Nightingale. During the Crimean War, she introduced many hospital improvements, including new standards of comfort and cleanliness. The profession of nursing owes much to the pioneering work of "The Lady of the Lamp."

NURSING

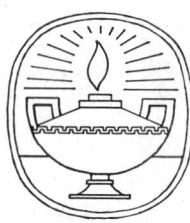

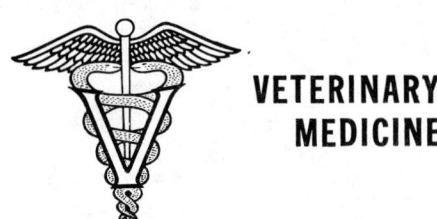

VETERINARY MEDICINE

Symbolized by a staff (caduceus) whose extended wings denote the Greek god Hermes. The intertwined serpents represent immortality, renovation of life, and vigor, as typified by the periodical changes of their skin.

ADAPTED, WITH PERMISSION, FROM ILLUSTRATIONS PREPARED BY PARKE, DAVIS & CO. AND THE AMERICAN VETERINARY MEDICAL ASSOCIATION

Scope

Pharmacy careers—pharmaceutical education—The American Foundation for Pharmaceutical Education—licensure—colleges of pharmacy

This chapter was prepared by

Melvin R. Gibson, PhD, *Professor of Pharmacognosy, College of Pharmacy, Washington State University, Pullman, Wash. 99163*

Pharmacy has been defined[1] as that profession which is concerned with the art and science of preparing from natural and synthetic sources suitable and convenient materials for distribution and use in the treatment and prevention of disease. It embraces a knowledge of the identification, selection, pharmacologic action, preservation, combination, analysis, and standardization of drugs and medicines. It also includes their proper and safe distribution and use, whether dispensed on the prescription of a licensed physician, dentist, or veterinarian, or, in those instances where it may legally be done, dispensed or sold directly to the consumer.

The word pharmacy is derived from the Greek word *pharmakon*, meaning medicine or drug. A pharmacist, then, is the person of drugs, or, the expert on drugs. He is the *only* expert on drugs. For expertise regarding drugs requires knowledge in depth in all the facets of pharmacy as outlined in the definition of the term pharmacy above.

The physician, dentist, and veterinarian may prescribe drugs and be primarily interested in the effect of those drugs on the patient, their therapeutic value, and toxicology. The nurse may administer the drug and be concerned with dosage forms, routes of administration, and toxic manifestations. But the pharmacist *is the only expert on drugs.* It is his legally granted responsibility to handle drugs. It is his professional responsibility to know *all about* those drugs. No educational program other than that in pharmacy provides the background to completely understand all there is to understand about drugs. The pharmacist, and the pharmacist alone, is in that unique position of embracing complete drug expertise.

Pharmacy Careers

Most persons when thinking of pharmacy tend to think first of the community pharmacist. And this generalization is numerically justified. There are approximately 121,500 registered pharmacists now in practice. About 85% are community pharmacists, 8% are hospital pharmacists, and the rest are in other areas of the profession.[2]

The *community pharmacist* in the US is a unique hybrid of businessman and professional. Born out of the necessity for back-up income, the business aspects of some pharmacies now all but inundates and obscures the primary unit of the pharmacy—the prescription laboratory. The supermarket and cut-rate pharmacies may be important factors in forcing a future dichotomy of pharmacy practice into stores selling merchandise, and professionally oriented pharmacies of the Pharmaceutical Center type. An extensive coverage of the current practice of pharmacy and its future may be found in Chapter 4, *Pharmacists in Practice.*

Hospital pharmacy, the practice of pharmacy in private and government-owned hospitals, is emerging as one of the most important areas of pharmacy practice. The number of pharmacists in the hospitals of the future will increase for three principal reasons:

1. There will be a great increase in population.
2. There will be a greater utilization of hospitals by those who need hospitalization and, hence, will receive better medical care. Hospitalization insurance, both private- and government-sponsored, will foster this trend. There is little question that more adequate care of the sick by government-sponsored programs will increase greatly in the years ahead requiring more of all medical facilities.
3. The pharmacist in the hospital will be given a greater role in all aspects of the use and monitoring of the use of drugs; this is related to the health manpower shortage brought about by the two conditions mentioned above. Current trends of progressive hospitals make the need for pharmacists per hospital much greater than ever before, because of their involvement in assuring better and safer[3] use of drugs.

A very active American Society of Hospital Pharmacists with special studies,[4] imagination, and zeal vigorously promotes this vital aspect of American pharmacy. A comprehensive study of hospital pharmacy may be found in Chapter 93, *Hospital Pharmacy.*

Wholesale pharmacy offers opportunities for a limited number of pharmacists. Like most wholesalers, the pharmacy wholesaler serves as the middle-man between manufacturer and retailer. Because of the special nature of the products handled and their legal restrictions, all wholesale drug firms employ registered pharmacists in supervisory capacities. These wholesale firms may specialize in a broad range of products sold in a pharmacy, both prescription and nonprescription drugs as well as merchandise items, or sometimes they deal in a limited line of quick-moving items.

Whatever their scope, the wholesale drug firms play a vital role in assuring the retail pharmacist of a quick and convenient source of supplies from a multiplicity of manufacturers. This makes possible better service by the pharmacist to his patients of those drugs which may be vital to the patient's welfare. It also lessens the retail pharmacists' financial burden of carrying large volumes of stock and the necessity of negotiations with hundreds of manufacturers. Recently, the larger wholesalers have assumed advisory roles to pharmacists in providing them with information and consultants on store redecorating and remodeling. The Pharmaceutical Center concept described in Chapter 4 is a project of one wholesaler, McKesson-Robbins and Co.

Industrial pharmacy offers opportunities to pharmacists of all educational levels. The greatest number of

3

pharmacists are involved in marketing and administration. The medical service representative, or detail man, who is in contact with physicians and pharmacists regarding his company's products may or may not be a pharmacist. But the most effective use is made of a pharmaceutically trained detail man because he is the only person educated as an expert on drugs. Some manufacturers employ pharmacists almost exclusively in this capacity; others do not.[5] The shortage of pharmacists is usually given as the reason why companies do not employ more pharmacists in detailing. This can be a rewarding career for persons with the right personality and inclinations.[6] It also is sometimes a steppingstone to supervisory positions in sales and to integration into the administrative and sales structure of a pharmaceutical firm.

Pharmacists with master's degrees in business or additional bachelor's degrees in law find ample opportunities in the pharmaceutical industry in the marketing, sales, and legal departments. Production and quality control supervisory positions in the industrial plant are often held by pharmacists with bachelor's degrees. Research and development personnel often have more advanced degrees, but not necessarily so. A more complete discussion of pharmacists in industry may be found in Chapter 5, *Pharmacists in Industry*.

Government service offers opportunities to pharmacists in various capacities. They may serve as noncommissioned officers and commissioned officers in the Army, Navy, and Air Force. Also, they may serve as commissioned officers in the United States Public Health Service, which furnishes pharmacists for the Coast Guard and Bureau of Prisons. Civil Service appointments are available for pharmacists in various capacities: in the Bureau of Narcotics and Dangerous Drugs of the Department of Justice, National Institutes of Health, Social Security Administration, Food and Drug Administration, Department of Labor, Department of Agriculture, and various other areas. See Chapter 6, *Pharmacists in Government*.

Pharmaceutical education offers an excellent opportunity for pharmacists with advanced degrees in any of the professional specialties. Expanding enrollments in colleges to meet the manpower needs of the future offer excellent opportunities for careers in college teaching. Higher salaries, more freedom for research and writing, independence of action, and cultural surroundings in pharmaceutical education make teaching each year more attractive than ever before. The shortage in all areas of pharmaceutical education is acute and will become more so in the foreseeable future. A survey conducted by the American Association of Colleges of Pharmacy indicated that there were 124 unfilled positions in pharmaceutical education at the beginning of the 1968–1969 school year. Persons interested in a future in pharmaceutical education should read *Graduate Study in Pharmaceutical Science*[7] and the issues of the *American Journal of Pharmaceutical Education*.[8]

For a limited number of pharmacists with writing and editing talent, *pharmaceutical journalism* offers rewarding experiences. National, regional, state, and industrial publications require a pharmaceutical background for their effective publishing, editing, and writing.

Organizational management also offers an opportunity for those pharmaceutically educated persons who wish to be officers of national and state associations and boards of pharmacy. With the increase in number of pharmacists, the increase in responsibilities of associations and boards will increase and be complicated by the greater involvement of the state and federal government in health care. The demand for such personnel will be limited, but persons with organizational interests and talents will be in great demand and will play important roles in the *future of pharmacy* in this country.

Pharmaceutical Education

The first school in the US to include pharmacy in the title of one of its professors was the Medical School of the College of Philadelphia in 1789. Pharmacy at this institution was taught by physicians for physicians. Prior to the founding of the Philadelphia College of Pharmacy in 1821 only a few attempts to provide instruction in pharmacy for pharmacists had been made.[9]

The education in medicine and law as in pharmacy evolved from entirely apprenticeship training to the current extensive collegiate education. At the beginning of the century minimal standards for colleges of pharmacy which were members of the AACP (known as the American Conference of Pharmaceutical Faculties prior to 1925) were unspecified until 1904 when grade school plus a 40-week course was the requirement. This was increased to grade school plus 50 weeks to be done in two years in 1907. In 1908 the one year of high school plus a two-year course was the requirement which was changed to two years of high school prerequisite in 1918. The entrance to pharmacy curricula prerequisite was raised to high school graduation in 1923. In 1925 the pharmacy curriculum was increased to three years and the PhG degree given, four years in 1932 with the BS (or BS in Pharmacy) degree, and five years in 1960 giving the BS in Pharmacy (or BPhar) degree.

Most colleges of pharmacy today offer the five-year program which is often so formulated that either the first year or the first two years may be taken at junior colleges or liberal arts colleges. Three years is the minimal requirement for registration in a college of pharmacy as prescribed by the AACP. The state of California requires four years of registration in a college of pharmacy for those applying for registration in that state. If all five years are not to be taken at an institution where pharmacy is taught, students are strongly advised to communicate with the college of pharmacy they are to enter to insure that their pre-pharmacy curriculum meets the prerequisite requirements for entrance into the formal pharmacy instruction years.

Two schools in California (University of California, University of Southern California) require a total of six years of education for the lowest degree offered (DPharm). Other colleges in the US offer six-year programs on an optional basis.

The undergraduate curriculum in pharmacy is intended to prepare men and women for the profession of pharmacy. The *Pharmaceutical Curriculum*[10] defines this:

Undergraduate education in pharmacy is intended to prepare men and women for the profession of pharmacy. Stated in another way, it trains students to think and act like pharmacists. These general objectives need to be comprehended in light of the activities which are required (1) to recognize, identify, select, procure, create, process, standardize, stabilize, fabricate, test, evaluate, and preserve all substances of whatever kind and combinations used in preventive, palliative, and curative medicine, and (2) to distribute them to other members of the health professions and to the public. No single individual today engages in all of these activities, but every pharmacist has to do with one or more of them. Out of these specific activities arise a number of others, such as (1) acting as the informed and readily accessible adviser to health-service personnel and the health-seeking public; (2) contributing to the continuing improvement in professional service and sharing his contributions freely with other professionals; (3) assisting in training the manpower for the profession of pharmacy; and (4) evaluating the numerous proposals for social and political improvement and actively supporting those which his informed judgment can approve.

The curriculum is divided into a number of areas to provide the future pharmacist with the background to achieve the goals quoted above.

General Education—One of the principal objectives of the extension of the curriculum to five years in 1960 was to provide the pharmacy student with more general education so that he could, as a practicing pharmacist, more easily take his place in society as a more well-rounded individual whose formal education was not so completely monolithic. As the pressures for more pharmacists in the future become more apparent, there well may be arguments presented to reverse the upward historical trend in the length of time required to educate a pharmacist. This probably would be done at the expense of general education. History has shown that more educational requirements have consistently attracted more students, not less. There are no ways to test the increased caliber of the students attracted by a longer, more well-rounded education, but those who have seen the progress of pharmaceutical education over the years have expressed subjective judgment that the general caliber of pharmacy students has increased along with increased educational requirements.

The pharmacist of the future will need in his ever-increasing responsibilities to evince ever-increasing intellectual powers to meet the demand of moral, political, and social problems. Only a broad general education can provide the background for that responsibility.

Prerequisite Courses—Any professional curriculum must be based upon a firm foundation of basic courses. To provide the background for the professional pharmacy courses, the basic courses can be classified into the physical sciences and mathematics, and the biological sciences. It is generally agreed that to be able to present many of the professional courses in pharmacy on a professional plane it is necessary to build upon a firm foundation of the principles of mathematics, chemistry, and physics. The application of these principles find their way into many of the professional pharmacy courses.

As the future pharmacist becomes less product-oriented and more patient-oriented his education will shift necessarily to a greater biological orientation. The basic biological courses dealing with the fundamental phenomena of biological systems will play an ever-increasing role in his background for professional education.

Students of pharmacy often fail to recognize the importance of prerequisite courses in the physical sciences, mathematics, and biological sciences in their search for "instant relevance." These courses are rightly taught most commonly by non-pharmacists. "Rightly" because the complexity of the pure sciences today can be taught best by specialists in those pure sciences. Once the fundamentals of these sciences are entrenched in the mind of the pharmacy student, he often fails to recognize from whence they came in his application of them in his professional courses.

Professional Courses—These vary in scope and content in the different schools and colleges of pharmacy. In recent years many institutions have made and are now making serious attempts to gear their curricula more closely to the demands of the future pharmacist. A study by the American Association of Colleges of Pharmacy Committee on Curriculum published in 1968 under the title *Studies of a Core Curriculum*[11] has as its purpose the stimulation of pharmacy faculties to re-evaluate their individual curricula in light of the future basic needs of the pharmacist in the practice of pharmacy.

Basic to all pharmacy professional curricula are offerings in *pharmacognosy*, the study of the biology, biochemistry, and commerce of natural drugs; *pharmacology*, the study of the action and use of drugs; *pharmaceutical chemistry*, the application of basic organic and inorganic chemistry to pharmaceuticals and the relation of these principles to drug use; *pharmacy* (*pharmaceutics*), the broad term which includes offerings in introductory pharmacy, calculations, preparations, techniques, dispensing pharmacy, physical pharmacy, biopharmaceutics (defined as the study of the influence of formulation on the therapeutic activity of a drug product[12]), and clinical pharmacy;* and *pharmacy administration* which deals with the principles and practices of business and law as they apply to pharmacy practice. Not yet generally accepted among the basic professional areas of pharmacy is the area of sociology of pharmacy. Undoubtedly the socioeconomic problems of pharmacy are part of its heritage and future. Just what part this area will play in pharmaceutical education is yet to be determined.

Opportunities for undergraduate students to specialize in certain professional areas beyond the core of courses is becoming increasingly prevalent in pharmaceutical education. Most prominent among the areas of specialization will be hospital pharmacy and research. Pharmacy faculties who have determined what core material is necessary for *all* pharmacists have supported various programs aimed at better preparing the student for specific special functions among the variety of career opportunities available to the pharmaceutically educated individual. A greater trend for this type of education specialization is foreseen in the future.

The American Foundation for Pharmaceutical Education—No discussion of pharmaceutical education, no matter how brief, would be complete without appropriate credit to the American Foundation for Pharmaceutical Education (AFPE). The AFPE was incorporated in 1942. Its objectives are set forth as follows:[14]

The principal objectives of the American Foundation for Pharmaceutical Education, in brief, are: (1) To encourage and assist in providing improved educational standards and facilities for the adequate training of competent personnel in the practice of pharmacy and all related fields; (2) to supply the pharmaceutical and allied manufacturing industries, hospitals, government agencies, college faculties and other professional fields with technically and scientifically trained personnel; (3) to help colleges develop strong undergraduate programs; (4) to support graduate work in properly qualified colleges;

---

* Clinical pharmacy because of its newness should be defined. Tyler[13] defined it as ". . . that division of pharmacy which deals with patient care with particular emphasis on drug therapy. In practice it is patient oriented and includes not only the dispensing of required medication but also advising the patient on the proper use of all medications, both prescribed and patient selected. It also utilizes the pharmacist as an information source for members of the medical and other health professions on all matters pertaining to drugs and their dosage forms."

and (5) to encourage scientific research as a necessary component of graduate work and as special projects.

The AFPE derives its income from individuals, former Fellows, and the voluntary contributions of the drug trade and allied manufacturing industries.

The accomplishments of the AFPE in the interest of pharmaceutical education are impressive and are summarized for the 1943–1968 period in Table I.[15]

The support of pharmaceutical education by the AFPE has become a vital necessity for progress of pharmaceutical education and, hence, the profession itself.

Licensure Requirements

The practice of pharmacy within each state is regulated by the laws of that state. This includes the regulation of licensure for pharmacy practice. To practice pharmacy in any state, a pharmacist must be a registered pharmacist (RPh) in that state. A "registered pharmacist" is also known as a "licensed pharmacist." Administration of pharmacy laws and the granting of registration to practice pharmacy are authorities vested in each state board of pharmacy. A graduate of any accredited college of pharmacy is eligible to take the examination for registration in any of the 50 states in the US providing he fulfills the requirements of citizenship and internship for the state. (See special California educational requirement below.) In recent years these examinations have been oriented more toward the application of theoretical material to actual practice rather than an examination of fact and theory alone.

A pharmacist registered in one of the 47 reciprocating states (California, Florida, and Hawaii are nonreciprocating states) may gain registration in any of the other reciprocating states by fulfilling the reciprocity requirements of the other states. Information about the reciprocity requirements of individual states may be obtained from the National Association of Boards of Pharmacy, 77 W. Washington St., Chicago, Ill. 60602.

Registration in the nonreciprocating states of California, Florida, and Hawaii is governed by each state's regulations which usually involves, in addition to fulfilling residence and internship requirements, the taking of each state's complete licensure examination. Reciprocating states sometimes waive all but that part of the licensing examination which deals with state law. California also requires a minimum of *four years* registration *in an accredited college of pharmacy*, whereas the requirement for all other states is a minimum of three years in an accredited college of pharmacy, allowing two years of the five-year program to be taken in junior colleges or liberal arts colleges. Colleges of pharmacy sometimes vary in their recommended programs allowing only one year to be taken in such junior or liberal arts colleges for the student to make normal progress toward graduation.

Additional information regarding pharmacy regulations may be found in Chapter 101, *Laws Governing Pharmacy*.

Accredited Colleges of Pharmacy

The following colleges hold membership in the American Association of Colleges of Pharmacy and were accredited by the American Council on Pharmaceutical Education as of July 1, 1969:

Alabama	Auburn University, School of Pharmacy, Auburn
	Samford University, School of Pharmacy, Birmingham
Arizona	University of Arizona, College of Pharmacy, Tucson
Arkansas	University of Arkansas, School of Pharmacy, Little Rock
California	University of California, School of Pharmacy, San Francisco
	University of Southern California, School of Pharmacy, Los Angeles
	University of the Pacific, School of Pharmacy, Stockton
Colorado	University of Colorado, School of Pharmacy, Boulder
Connecticut	University of Connecticut, School of Pharmacy, Storrs
District of Columbia	Howard University, College of Pharmacy, Washington
Florida	Florida Agricultural and Mechanical University, School of Pharmacy, Tallahassee
	University of Florida, College of Pharmacy, Gainesville
Georgia	Mercer University, Southern School of Pharmacy, Atlanta
	University of Georgia, School of Pharmacy, Athens
Idaho	Idaho State University, College of Pharmacy, Pocatello
Illinois	University of Illinois, College of Pharmacy, Chicago
Indiana	Butler University, College of Pharmacy, Indianapolis
	Purdue University, School of Pharmacy and Pharmacal Sciences, West Lafayette
Iowa	Drake University, College of Pharmacy, Des Moines
	University of Iowa, College of Pharmacy, Iowa City
Kansas	University of Kansas, School of Pharmacy, Lawrence
Kentucky	University of Kentucky, College of Pharmacy, Lexington
Louisiana	Northeast Louisiana State College, School of Pharmacy, Monroe
	Xavier University of Louisiana, College of Pharmacy, New Orleans
Maryland	University of Maryland, School of Pharmacy, Baltimore
Massachusetts	Massachusetts College of Pharmacy, Boston
	Northeastern University, College of Pharmacy, Boston
Michigan	Ferris State College, School of Pharmacy, Big Rapids
	University of Michigan, College of Pharmacy, Ann Arbor
	Wayne State University, College of Pharmacy, Detroit
Minnesota	University of Minnesota, College of Pharmacy, Minneapolis
Mississippi	University of Mississippi, School of Pharmacy, University
Missouri	St. Louis College of Pharmacy, St. Louis
	University of Missouri at Kansas City, School of Pharmacy, Kansas City

Table I—Summary Report of AFPE Grants in Support of Education—1943–1968

Graduate Fellowships (1946–1968) (736 fellowships)	$2,566,000
Undergraduate Scholarships (1943–1968) (3,367 scholarships)	739,000
Student Recruitment Programs (1944–1947; 1955–1968)	339,500
World War II Aid to Colleges (1944–1946)	97,000
American Journal of Pharmaceutical Education (1946–1968)	180,000
Pharmacy Teachers' Seminar (1949–1968)	154,500
American Council on Pharmaceutical Education (1945–1968)	566,500
The Pharmaceutical Survey (1946–1950)	178,400
Visiting Lecturers Program	15,500[a]
Educational Survey (AACP)	37,000
Grand Total	$4,879,900[a]

[a] Corrected figures supplied by AFPE.

Montana	University of Montana at Missoula, School of Pharmacy, Missoula		University of South Carolina, School of Pharmacy, Columbia
Nebraska	Creighton University, School of Pharmacy, Omaha	South Dakota	South Dakota State University, College of Pharmacy, Brookings
	University of Nebraska, College of Pharmacy, Lincoln	Tennessee	University of Tennessee, College of Pharmacy, Memphis
New Jersey	Rutgers—The State University, College of Pharmacy, Newark	Texas	Texas Southern University, School of Pharmacy, Houston
New Mexico	University of New Mexico, College of Pharmacy, Albuquerque		University of Houston, College of Pharmacy, Houston
New York	Columbia University, College of Pharmaceutical Sciences in the City of New York, New York		University of Texas, College of Pharmacy, Austin
	Fordham University, College of Pharmacy, Bronx	Utah	University of Utah, College of Pharmacy, Salt Lake City
	Long Island University, Brooklyn College of Pharmacy, Brooklyn	Virginia	Medical College of Virginia, School of Pharmacy, Richmond
	St. John's University, College of Pharmacy, Jamaica	Washington	University of Washington, College of Pharmacy, Seattle
	State University of New York at Buffalo, School of Pharmacy, Buffalo		Washington State University, College of Pharmacy, Pullman
	Union University, Albany College of Pharmacy, Albany	West Virginia	West Virginia University, School of Pharmacy, Morgantown
North Carolina	University of North Carolina, School of Pharmacy, Chapel Hill	Wisconsin	University of Wisconsin, School of Pharmacy, Madison
North Dakota	North Dakota State University, College of Pharmacy, Fargo	Wyoming	University of Wyoming, College of Pharmacy, Laramie
Ohio	Ohio Northern University, College of Pharmacy, Ada		

Ohio State University, College of Pharmacy, Columbus

University of Cincinnati, College of Pharmacy, Cincinnati

University of Toledo, College of Pharmacy, Toledo

Oklahoma — Southwestern State College, School of Pharmacy, Weatherford

University of Oklahoma, College of Pharmacy, Norman

Oregon — Oregon State University, School of Pharmacy, Corvallis

Pennsylvania — Duquesne University, School of Pharmacy, Pittsburgh

Philadelphia College of Pharmacy and Science, Philadelphia

Temple University, School of Pharmacy, Philadelphia

University of Pittsburgh, School of Pharmacy, Pittsburgh

Puerto Rico — University of Puerto Rico, College of Pharmacy, Rio Piedras

Rhode Island — University of Rhode Island, College of Pharmacy, Kingston

South Carolina — Medical College of South Carolina, School of Pharmacy, Charleston

References

1. Deno, R. A., et al, *The Profession of Pharmacy*, 2nd ed., Lippincott, Philadelphia, 1966, p. 1.
2. *Licensure Statistics and Census of Pharmacy*, Natl. Assoc. of Boards of Pharm., Chicago, Jan. 1, 1968.
3. Lader, L., *Look*, 76 (Nov. 26, 1968).
4. Francke, D. E., et al, *Mirror to Hospital Pharmacy*, Am. Soc. of Hosp. Pharmacists, Washington, D.C., 1964.
5. Gibson, M. R., *Am. J. Pharm. Educ.*, **23**, 461 (1959).
6. Peterson, A. F., *Pharmaceutical Selling, "Detailing" and Sales Training*, Heathcote-Woodbridge, Scarsdale, N.Y., 1959.
7. Brodie, D. C., ed., *Graduate Study in the Pharmaceutical Sciences*, Am. Assoc. of Coll. of Pharm., Silver Spring, Md., 1964.
8. Lyman, R. A., et al, eds., *Am. J. Pharm. Educ.*, (1937–present).
9. Sonnedecker, G., *Kremers' and Urdang's History of Pharmacy*, Lippincott, Philadelphia, 1963, p. 203.
10. Blauch, L. E., and Webster, G. L., *The Pharmaceutical Curriculum*, Am. Council on Educ., Washington, D.C., 1952, p. 47.
11. Gibson, M. R., ed., *Studies of a Core Curriculum*, Am. Assoc. of Coll. of Pharm., Silver Spring, Md., 1968.
12. Wagner, J. G., *Drug Intelligence*, **2**, 31 (1968).
13. Tyler, V. E., *Am. J. Pharm. Educ.*, **22**, 764 (1968).
14. *American Foundation for Pharmaceutical Education, Roster and Programs, 1968*, Washington, D.C., 1968, p. ix.
15. *American Foundation for Pharmaceutical Education, Roster and Programs, 1968*, Washington, D.C., 1968, p. 173.

2 | Evolution of Pharmacy

Antiquity—middle ages—modern Europe—American pharmacy—
organizations—education—legal controls—ethics—mixed trends—
bibliographic notes—a chronology for pharmacists

This chapter was prepared by

Glenn Sonnedecker, PhD, *Director, American Institute of the History of
Pharmacy, Madison, Wisc. 53706*

Pharmacy in some guise has been inseparable from mankind's history since it fulfils one of our most basic needs. As man made his way through remote times or places, he shielded himself against disease as best he could, often reaching out blindly toward the resources of nature, but sometimes using elaborate pharmaceutical theories, techniques, and implements. The person supplying this essential service may not be recognizable always as a pharmacist in our sense of the term; conversely, the pharmacist as such has been designated in a variety of ways throughout the ages. However named, it is mainly the community practitioner of pharmacy who stands within the focus of this short socio-historical essay.

Primitive Probings—How men fend off disease depends largely on how they define its cause. In the world still are millions who see the patient as a victim of evil forces or of a god's anger, who see disease as punishment for sin. So we can imagine, in the absence of much surviving evidence, how terrifying and supernatural seemed the afflictions of primitive men in the dawn of history. Afflictions that came in such mysterious ways and with such uncanny effects certainly called for supernatural as well as natural countermeasures.

Thus the healing practitioner, be he shaman or priest, had best know how to command the resources of the spirit world, and know what substances from the natural world convey or reinforce the countervailing powers. From such blind empirical groping, extending over many millennia, it came to be appreciated that some herbs were more powerful than others, whether with or without incantations. Yet, up to the present moment, there have been people who sought healing not from medication but from religion; indeed, most patients rely partly—and wholly when medical science fails—on their faith. Nevertheless, the changing relationship between empiricism (later, science) and religion is one significant strand in the history of therapeutics through antiquity and into the Middle Ages.

Antiquity

By the second millennium B.C. the civilizations of Babylonia and Egypt had produced the small clay tablets and the long scrolls (see Fig. 1) that survive as the oldest pharmaceutical records known. They show that these river-valley peoples knew, however crudely, many of the basic forms of drug administration employed today (eg, gargles, suppositories, inhalations, poultices, ointments) and knew hundreds of different substances used as drugs (eg, asafoetida, dates, garlic, castor beans, hellebore). In application, the theurgical and magical potentiation of the medications may never have been thrust aside entirely by practitioners in the ancient Near East, although the emphasis varied with the ebb and flow of civilization.

When no pressing need for specialization was felt, pharmacy and medicine have tended to coalesce, and a steadily progressive development of two cleanly separated fields scarcely can be traced before the late Middle Ages. However, from fragmentary pharmacomedical records so far deciphered, it appears that at one time, at least, a Babylonian class of preparers of remedies and cosmetics was quartered in a special street, and westward in Egypt, according to newer interpretation, the collectors, preparers, and conservators of drug resources became more specialized and separated than had been previously supposed.

Within another millennium the Greeks living around the Aegean Sea and on its islands, nourished by the intellectual produce of the fertile basins of the Nile and the Tigris and Euphrates, burst the old mold and created a distinctive intellectual life that today still commands admiration. Greek medicine was no exception.

Looking nature full in the face, without being blinded by either the divine or the customary, Greek intellectuals sought rational explanations of all within man's ken. In the medical field perhaps this was exemplified best by the followers of Hippocrates (born ca. 460 B.C. on Cos). Their best writings and practices showed the fundamentals of scientific method—observation and classification, rejection of unsupported theory and superstition, and a cautious generalization and induction that remained open to critical discussion and revision.

This produced less rather than more reliance on drug therapy among many practitioners, and in neither the drug armamentarium nor the cadre of pharmacomedical work were advances as startling as might be expected.

Hippocratic insistence on rational treatment of the individual did not require rejection of religion, but it did place the supernatural in a separate category of the patient's resources, and the practitioner himself typically relied on his natural resources whether for explanation, diagnosis, or treatment. This so limited the scope of claimed effectiveness that we are not surprised to find that ancient Greeks, rich and poor alike, streamed into the temples for aid when lay medicine failed, as it often did.

Beginning in the 7th century before Christ, the wise and kind Asklepios gradually superseded Apollo as the greatest of the healing gods. At the touch of his hand or staff or of the tongue of his sacred serpent, miraculous things happened to the afflicted. Medical practitioners were tolerant; indeed, in Asklepios they saw symbolic embodiment of an ideal perfection of their calling which reality could never be. The staff of Asklepios, entwined by a sacred serpent, gradually emerged as the official symbol of medicine around the world. On the right hand of Asklepios, helping to minister to the afflicted, stood Hygeia, one of his daughters, her arm entwined by a serpent and holding a bowl, now thought to have contained a healing potion. In modern times her bowl entwined by the serpent gradually emerged as the official symbol of pharmacy, through most of the Western world and, more recently, in the United States. How the virgin goddess and her divine, powerful father were envisioned may be seen in the classical statue depicted as Fig. 2.

Middle Ages

With the advent of Christianity the healing temples of Asklepios eventually fell into disuse. During the medieval millennium, however, religious medicine within Christian concepts gave the healing power of faith and divine intervention new scope. Moreover, the practice of pharmacy and medicine in the Western world largely passed from the hands of lay practitioners to clerics, under the impact of cultural barbarization and political fragmentation.

Monasteries became the centers of intellectual life, including pharmacomedical study as well as practice. Greco-Roman treatises were preserved, and fragments and epitomes, handwritten in Latin, were passed about as a basis for health services. Two widely used treatises on simple drugs were a condensate from Galen's medical writings, perhaps compiled by Gariopontus in the 11th century, and the herbal of a so-called Pseudo-Apuleius (an anonymous work from the 6th century or earlier, influenced by Dioscorides). The monks often cultivated medicinal plants outside the monastery, as well as collecting them from the countryside. Inside was an "armarium pigmentarium," a

room where the drugs were kept, to which a laboratory sometimes was added. Some monastic laboratories were renowned for expert distillation of aromatic and cordial waters.

As a guide to preparing compound drugs, two traditional types of Latin compilations, which evolved into modern counterparts, were the "Antidotaria" (similar to dispensatories) and "Receptaria" (more modest formularies). It was a practical literature for both medicine and pharmacy, copied by scribes who added, omitted, and revised to suit local needs.

During the second half of the European Middle Ages pharmacy gradually moved outside the monasteries, became better separated from medicine, and began to evolve independent standards and responsibilities in the more urbanized centers. This trend first becomes noticeable in Italy, Spain, and France, which provided transit points for drugs and for pharmacomedical knowledge flowing along Mediterranean trade routes from the burgeoning Arabic civilization.

Scholars working in Islamic lands after the 8th century assimilated old Greco-Roman wisdom more thoroughly than could be done in Europe; the best of them produced a pharmacomedical amalgam of their own that became authoritative treatises in Europe. Translation centers put many of these intellectual treasures of the Arabic world into Latin during the 11th and 12th centuries.

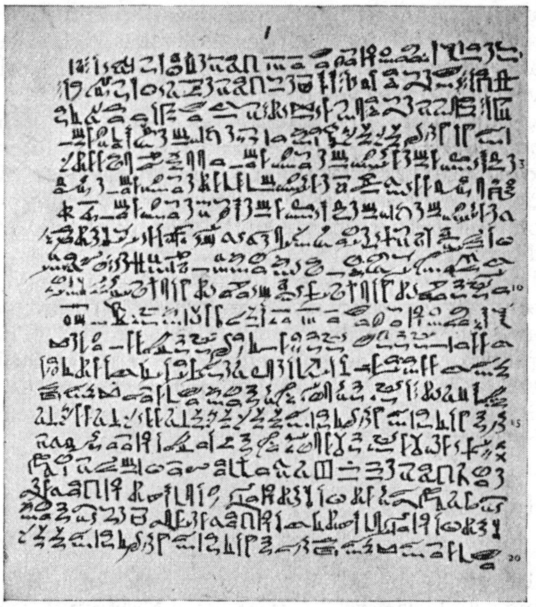

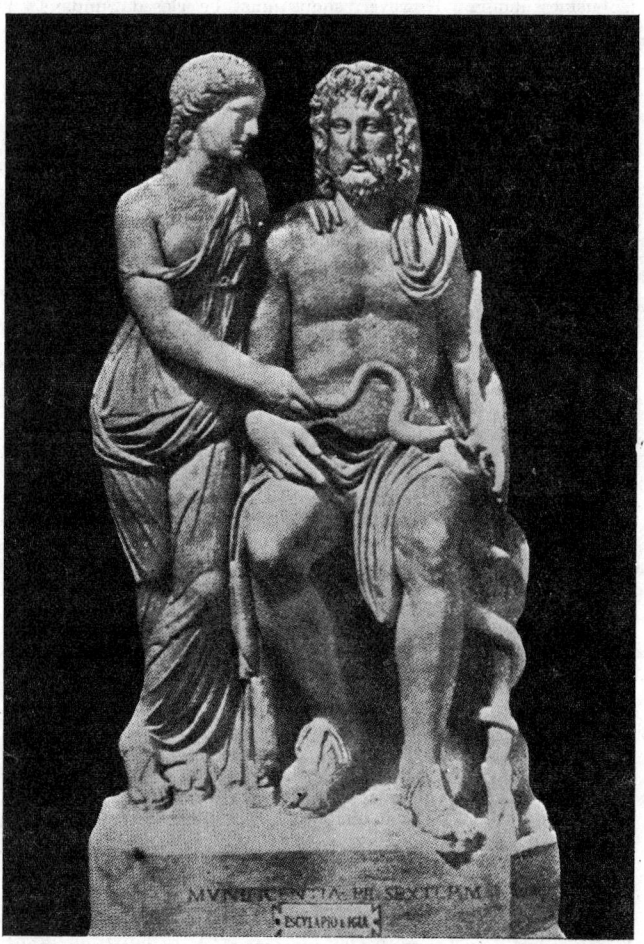

Fig. 1. Since the dawn of recorded history, the pharmaceutical efforts of man against disease are attested on scroll, stone, parchment, and paper. Illustrated is an excerpt from one of the most important pharmaceutical records of the ancient Near East, a papyrus more than 21 yards long, largely filled with information on drugs of the Egyptians. (Ebers Papyrus, about 1500 B.C.)

Fig. 2. Asklepios and his daughter Hygeia with a sacred serpent, are shown in this classical statue. Together they healed the afflicted of ancient Greece who sought their supernatural aid, and from them arose the international symbols of pharmacy and medicine still used today. (From Osler's *Evolution of Modern Medicine*.)

For pharmacy, the Arabic influence was important also because we can discern the rise of the qualified pharmacist (al-Saidalani) as a separate functionary, beginning around Baghdad not later than the first half of the 9th century. The richer Arabic materia medica and more refined and elegant polypharmacal modes of administering drugs (as compared with antiquity) intensified the need for a specialist in pharmaceutical work. This may be considered a pharmaceutical reflection of a general elaborative tendency of Arabic intellectualism.

Therapeutic effectiveness advanced only modestly, however, and the rationale of drug therapy, which was chiefly botanic, remained congealed in the Galenic mold of humoural pathology.

By the 12th century public pharmacies probably had begun to appear in the south of Italy and France and perhaps elsewhere. Some pharmacies apparently remained under church control since information about them appears in old monastic documents. Hospitals, however, were being secularized under municipal authority by the 13th century. While it is debated to what extent modern pharmacy—as part of a governmentally supervised system of health care—grew directly from monastic medicine, it is clear that the influence was pervasive.

By the 13th century the lay practice of pharmacy had developed sufficiently in the Kingdom of the Two Sicilies to justify legislation. These edicts became so influential elsewhere that they have been called the "magna charta" of pharmacy. This was part of serial health legislation (completed by 1240) that provided for the separation of pharmacy from medicine, for official supervision, and for obligating the pharmacist by oath to prepare drugs reliably, according to skilled art, in a uniform, suitable quality. Two further provisions placed a legal limitation on the number of pharmacies and on the prices of drugs.

Some of the responsibilities and some of the problems of a late-medieval pharmacist in Genoa are suggested by the code reproduced in the box on this page. A further glimpse of an acceptable pharmacist in 15th-century Italy can be seen in requirements stated by a contemporary physician, Saladin di Asculo, in his . . . *Compendium for Pharmacists.* He said that a pharmacist must know Latin to understand the pharmaceutical literature and the physicians' prescriptions. His main task is to prepare drugs (by such processes as rubbing, levigating, infusing, decocting, and distilling) and to compound and preserve them well. A pharmacist should be mature and modest, a pious and honest man, with compassion toward the poor. He must not be avaricious, and ask only reasonable fees. He must not be unskilled; he neither keeps deteriorated drugs in his shop, nor substitutes one drug for another against the patient's interest or the physician's expressed wish. If a young and inexperienced physician chooses unsuitable drugs on occasion, the pharmacist should "advise the physician to prescribe more placable and better ones . . . ." A pharmacist needs at hand at least six books, to practice his art properly, for which Saladin particularly recommended treatises on simple drugs by Avicenna and Serapion, on synonyms by Simon Januensis, on compound drugs by Pseudo-Mesuë and Nicolaus.

The late Middle Ages strengthened pharmacy functionally, legally, and as an independent calling often organized and disciplined within early guilds. This development was uneven, regionally, and periodically marred by friction (usually jurisdictional disputes) with medicine on one side or with spicers, grocers, or the like, on the other.*

The Pharmacists' Code of Genoa, As Revised 1407

from *Historiae Patriae Monumenta* . . . (Vol. 18, col. 674*ff*); adapted from a translation by Robert L. Reynolds, Professor of History, University of Wisconsin—see *Am. J. Pharm. Educ.*, 5: 330 (1941).

We fix and ordain that no outsider may take over, conduct or hold a pharmacy (or house or warehouse for a drug business) unless he has been licensed by the Master Pharmacists ["Speciarii"].

Nor shall any pharmacist break the rules of the profession under penalty.

No one save a licensed pharmacist may sell at retail syrups, elixirs, pills or other pharmacist's preparations. Except that merchants from overseas may sell small consignments of pharmaceutical materials.

Pharmacists are expected to keep their shops open during business hours. However, shops must be closed Sundays, Feasts of the Apostles and San Lorenzo's day. Save, however, that on such holy days they shall keep a [dispensing] window open at one table of only two palms size.

No quantity of arsenic or poisons may be sold, given away, allowed to be used or transferred except by a Master Pharmacist or his licensed employee who may be in charge. A pharmacist's son of over twenty years of age, trained in the profession, may suffice in such a case.

Since in the pharmacist's profession no personal advantages or prerogatives may be permitted, but only that whoever is best and produces the best products should be esteemed, and so that each may have incentive to improve and grow steadily from good to better: We fix and ordain that no pharmacist shall dare or presume to place or stamp, or cause to be placed or stamped, the label of another pharmacist on any bottle or pill-box. Rather, every pharmacist having or wishing to have a trade-mark which he might make, affix or stamp—or have made, affixed or impressed—on bottles and pill-boxes of preparations and other goods, may have such a trade-mark made or placed or impressed, but it must be different from every other pharmacist's mark.

No pharmacist may fill the bottle or pill-box bearing the label of any other pharmacist. If a purchaser comes with a bottle or box bearing another pharmacist's label, such label must be taken off or scratched over and the second pharmacist must affix his own label or trademark.

All materials from which remedies are compounded must be kept in the windows of the shop, in view of the public, continuously for eight days after the compound has been mixed.

No Turk or Tartar slave may be taught how to be a pharmacist. Other slaves may be taught the profession, but they may not be left in charge of shops even if they have been liberated, nor may they hold guild offices.

We fix and ordain—to prevent any pharmacist from having temptation or reason for sinning, and to keep them from raising prices higher than is becoming—that no pharmacist may keep shop in partnership or agreement with any physician. All pharmacists must swear an oath before the Masters of the Craft, each year, to observe completely and precisely the letter and spirit of this prohibition.

No one may peddle drugs, pills, or elixirs through the streets or from door to door, unless specially licensed. Sailors, mariners, and merchants coming from overseas may, however, seek purchasers for small consignments of pharmacist's wares.

No pharmacist or agent may receive, purchase, take, or accept as gift any merchandise from a city inspector or agent of such inspector or city warehouse supervisor.

Modern Europe

During the Renaissance, medicine moved more boldly outside the rather rigid framework of clerical and Arabic scholasticism. A year after Columbus reached America, there was born in a Swiss village a boy who

---

* Apparently some interchange of titles and of personnel among these groups occurred (at least in certain regions), until a clearer structuring of pharmacy and related occupations took place after the Middle Ages.

would become a medical iconoclast of far-reaching influence on the practice of pharmacy. Paracelsus, as he was later called, introduced the idea of the body as a chemical laboratory and railed against outmoded authorities. Through the Paracelsians, his followers, alchemical processes became more widely applied in pharmacy, chemicals were used more boldly for internal therapy, and extraction of medicinally active "quintessences" from nature's resources became a goal. Thus eventually the chemical role of the pharmacist overshadowed his more traditional art rooted in botanic science.

Through mastery of practical chemistry the best European pharmacists of the early modern period made discoveries important not only to drug therapy but also to the youthful science of chemistry (Fig. 3). The specialized development of sciences basic to pharmacy of the later 18th and 19th centuries would be needed, however, to mount the therapeutic revolution that meanwhile has replaced most of the centuries-old accretion of materia medica.

The scope and importance of guilds for pharmacy had varied markedly with the social circumstance of various cultural areas, but even in Italy and France they were being superseded by the 18th century. In their place rose modern professional societies, which also offered varying degrees of self-government. Frequently they either opened schools of pharmacy or encouraged established institutions of higher learning to do so. The traditional entrance to pharmacy through prolonged apprenticeship (often four to eight years as apprentice and clerk) gradually was modified by academic study. For example, pharmacy gained a better-defined place among scientific professions in Prussia when in 1725 obligatory examinations based on academic standards were instituted. During the later 18th century private institutes for formal education in pharmacy arose on German territory, leading to establishment of required pharmacy curricula in the regular universities, first in Bavaria (1808), then in other German states. In Italy by the early 19th century academic study and examination were required for pharmacy throughout the peninsula. About the same time, French legislation provided six higher schools of pharmacy for the country (1803), although there had been local and uneven development of academic courses there since the 16th century.

The maturing of West European pharmacy during the 17th century had given its best qualified practitioners a part in the early organized activities of science and its periodical literature. The pattern was set and ambitions nurtured for purely pharmaceutical organizations, and then specialized pharmaceutical periodicals, such as a German annual (f. 1780) and Trommsdorff's *Journal der Pharmacie* (f. 1794), and the French *Journal de la société des pharmaciens de Paris* (f. 1797).

Pharmaceutical manuals and reference works that began to come from the pens of pharmacists themselves by the 16th century also signalized a profession ascendant. The proliferation of formulas and the risk of varying composition in compound drugs of the same name stimulated a trend toward drug standardization. This was expressed in the adoption of the *Dispensatorium* of Valerius Cordus (1546) as official for the imperial city of Nuremberg, followed by other local pharmacopeias still in the 16th century. Still earlier (1499), the *Nuovo receptario* was published as a standard for the city-state of Florence, but its "officiality" rested on guild rather than government authority—a reminder

that the question of defining the term "pharmacopeia" affects pharmacopeial history.

Descendants of this literature would be used eclectically by American practitioners, especially the British pharmacopeias. The *Pharmacopoeia Londinensis* (1st ed., 1618), intended for the whole realm of England, was the first for so large a political unit. (Earlier pharmacopeias had been for Continental city-states or principalities.) Several British dispensatories, based on this and other pharmacopeias, made the dispensatory seem almost a British specialty. Duncan's *Edinburgh New Dispensatory* provided the basis for the first dispensatory published on American soil, the *American Dispensatory* (1806), compiled by John Redman Coxe, a Philadelphia physician.

Symptomatic of the *laissez-faire* development in Britain, which hindered orderly professional structuring, was the fact that the original apothecaries evolved into legally recognized medical practitioners (confirmed, 1703, by the Rose case). Although these general practitioners only slowly gave up drug dispensing (mostly in the present century), during the 19th century a modern profession of pharmacy was fashioned anew out of the "chymists" and "druggists." Education as well as organization was created through the present Pharmaceutical Society of Great Britain (founded 1841,

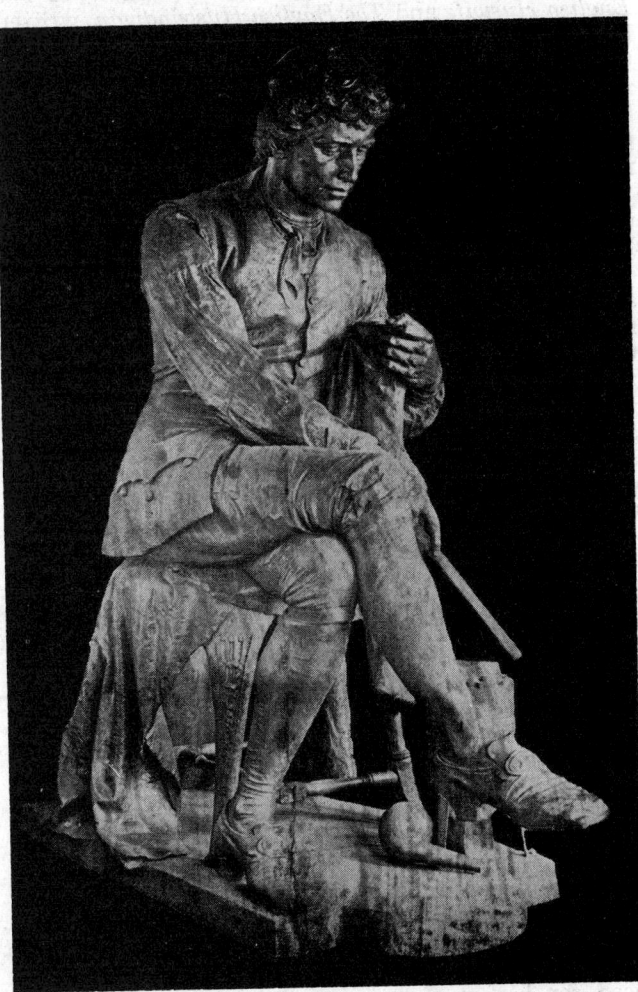

Fig. 3. This monument in Stockholm memorializes Carl Wilhelm Scheele, one of the most distinguished of the 18th-century pharmacist–chemists who made important contributions to science. Scheele discovered oxygen (a year before Priestley) and chlorine; he paved the way to the isolation of tungsten, manganese, and molybdenum; and through his method of isolating organic acids, opened a new era of organic chemistry. These and many other discoveries were made in the pharmacies where he worked.

after the old Society of Apothecaries of London, f. 1617, had become preoccupied with the medical ambitions of its members). The now-traditional designation of the British practitioner as a "chemist-and-druggist" (rather than apothecary or pharmacist) finds explanation in his unusual antecedents.

A dominant pharmaceutical influence from England, until long after the Revolution, helped shape the particular character of American pharmacy, fed by the availability of literature in the mother tongue, the immigration of ideas as well as men, and the heavy import of British drugs.

American Pharmacy*

In New England the settler often had to serve as his own physician and pharmacist. As the frontier moved amoeba-like west and south, a primitive battle against disheartening health conditions repeated itself again and again. In an emergency a man of more medical experience was sought, perhaps the clergyman or teacher. But the settler could meet many contingencies with some medical lore picked up from the Indians, a few store-bought remedies that were either imports or imitations of those popular in England, and a household herbal or medical book. Some brought over the volumes called *Countrey Contentments*, or *The English Huswife* and *The English Husbandman*, written by that prolific literary figure Gervase Markham. Others had *The English Physician* from the pen of that raucous medical pretender, Nicolas Culpeper. English herbals, such as those by John Parkinson and by John Gerarde, often guided the colonial cultivation and use of medicinal plants.

In the larger settlements men appeared who called themselves physician or apothecary—a title often self-bestowed, signifying only a bold medical pretension and courage. There were also isolated men, especially after the Revolution in the few maturing cities, who had qualified in Europe by professional experience and training. Both the qualified and the unqualified practitioners ordinarily practiced pharmacy as well as medicine. Their public pharmaceutical shops served as a base for medical practice, like the shops of the so-called apothecaries in 18th-century England. It was a pattern only slowly outgrown in New England as in the Olde.

The physician–pharmacist, whatever his knowledge or lack of it, multiplied his kind through a system of indentured apprenticeship imported from the mother country. The word "system" may be too strong, for a system already decadent in Europe had to be transplanted without the organized controls and standards that gave it measurable meaning within the old guilds.

By the early 19th century pharmacy began to show some independence from medicine. Here and there medical practice was disappearing from public drug shops into private offices. More pharmacists from abroad were venturing to America. Some Americans who had trained under a physician–pharmacist came to specialize increasingly in pharmaceutical service. A few of the drug merchants, importers, or operators of general stores grew more knowledgeable and ambitious as opportunity for pharmaceutical service grew. The need for higher competence and standards was felt

particularly among the so-called "druggists," men who imported drugs, developed small-scale manufacturing, operated a dispensing shop, and distributed drugs wholesale to physicians and to the general stores at country crossroads. These men began the long process of professionalization by helping to found the first associations and schools.

At first the independence of pharmacy and a feeling of interdependence among its practitioners were nurtured entirely through local associations. These "colleges," as they were called, sprang up in a few highly developed urban centers during the second quarter of the 19th century, setting a pattern for others later on. In the local associations, formerly isolated dispensers found mutual encouragement for improving their knowledge, technique, and ethical standards.

Pharmaceutical Organizations

As iron rails fanned out across the states and better communications tied towns more closely together, larger pharmaceutical organizations flourished and the pioneering local associations declined in importance. In 1852 the local associations were instrumental in founding the American Pharmaceutical Association (APhA). It in turn fostered pharmaceutical associations in the individual states. Most of the state associations in the present United States were born during the last 30 years of the 19th century. Today their combined membership far exceeds that of any single national organization. The activities of state associations embrace all aspects of dispensing pharmacy, although as a generality the main orientation had tended to be commercial.

The professional interests of pharmacists have always centered in the American Pharmaceutical Association. Its membership lies open to any pharmacy graduate who wishes to foster its aims. Kremers and Urdang succinctly characterized the role of the APhA in saying,

"It represented, defended and promoted, during the decades in which the calling gained its distinctive shape, all fields of pharmaceutical enterprise and interest, the scientific and educational as well as the commercial, the ethical, and the legal. It always has been the guardian, although not always the initiator, of all progressive movements concerning American pharmacy."

The initiative was increasingly divided after the end of the 19th century, as organized pharmacy splintered and developed more specialized organizations. Some of these offshoots remained affiliated or closely oriented to the mother society; others went separate, sometimes divergent ways. For example, the American Pharmaceutical Association could not focus sufficiently on economic interests to satisfy pharmacy owners, for whom a free economic system offered perplexing problems in the late 19th century. Therefore such problems have been dealt with since 1898 through the National Association of Retail Druggists (NARD), which limits its active membership to pharmacy owners. The NARD has demonstrated the compelling need for organized cooperation on questions of business and finance, just as the APhA has done in the professional and scientific sphere (see Fig. 4).

The fact that these two major national organizations have never contained more than a minority of the pharmacists in community practice illustrates a chronic organizational problem persisting since the 19th century. For the group-conscious segment of practicing pharmacists, this problem has been painfully intensified by periodic disharmony between the NARD and APhA, ranging from erratic coordination of effort

---

* The discussion of American pharmacy is adapted in part from an address at an Evening Meeting of the Pharmaceutical Society of Great Britain by Glenn Sonnedecker, "Structure and Stress of American Pharmacy," *Pharm. J.* **176**,171 (1956), which is utilized here with permission of the publisher.

to open clashes, especially after the 1940's. The roots of this organizational dilemma have never been carefully evaluated, but the record seems to imply an inadequate definition of the respective commercial and professional spheres of action and influence, ineffective diplomacy, and fundamental differences as to the goals of American pharmacy.

Less dissension, although only a tenuous coordination, has characterized the relations of 20-odd national societies, councils, and conferences that have come to serve the branches of dispensing pharmacy, manufacture, wholesale distribution, education, and legal control. With such a compartmented subdivision of power and functions, organized effort remained "uncoordinated, oft-times in conflict," concluded The Pharmaceutical Survey of 1946–1949. The two principal efforts toward the exchange and harmonizing of varied views are the House of Delegates of the APhA and the National Drug Trade Conference (of more selective representation and limited function).

Education

The associations of pharmacists have been instrumental in erecting an educational system, which must nourish every viable profession. Local pharmaceutical associations that sponsored the early pioneering instruction during the second quarter of the 19th century drew a certain stimulus from the burgeoning public interest in education generally, from the lead taken by medicine, and from a popular fascination with science at the time. The Philadelphia College of Pharmacy launched instruction in 1821, the same year it was founded as the first local association. It was 20 years before a similar beginning in England, for in the mother country the cord of professional continuity had been broken and pharmacy still steered an unsteady course in the cross currents of her particular historical circumstance.

In America by the end of the Civil War, five of the seven local associations were offering some academic instruction to those apprentices who had the desire, time, and money for formal schooling. Classes usually were held at night in rented rooms. There were no laboratories. Finances were uncertain. The pharmacists who controlled the new schools saw their purpose largely as a "rounding-off" and systematizing of the traditional apprenticeship. Students heard series of

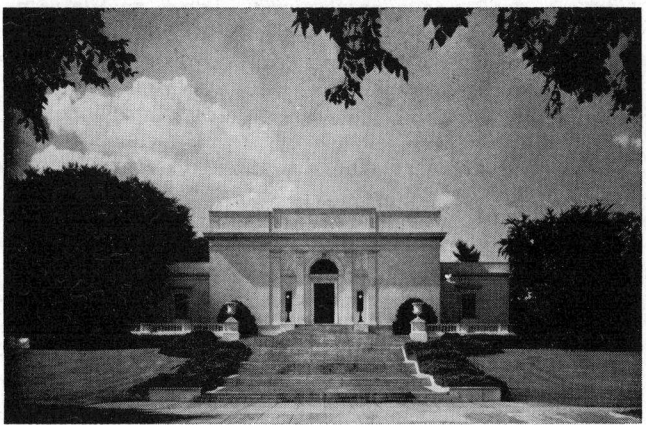

Fig. 4. The headquarters building of the American Pharmaceutical Association in Washington, D.C. (dedicated in 1934) symbolizes the professional development and aspirations of American pharmacy. The Association (founded in 1852) was the first national organization of pharmacy in the United States.

lectures in chemistry, in materia medica—and later on in pharmacy, as inadequacies of the apprenticeship were more frankly faced. The evolution of the instructional pattern closely paralleled that in England. Moreover, the most popular textbooks were of British origin. The lack of an American literature was a gap not quickly closed; and competent British texts were at hand in the mother tongue, no doubt preferred also, because French and German works tended to be more theoretical.

The early association schools in urban centers made their fundamental contribution by establishing an educational system, by raising the sights of pharmacy, by sending graduates into the more sparsely settled areas who might serve as foci around which professional endeavors could crystallize. However, perhaps not more than 1 in 20 of those entering pharmacy before the 1860's were able or willing to obtain a diploma.

After the war between the states came an upsurge in the founding of schools. At least 83 schools of various types opened their doors to pharmacy students during the 1800's, and about 60 of them survived the century. A student could choose among a wide array of standards, degrees, and curricula. Within this wild, mixed growth emerged an entirely new outlook for American pharmaceutical education, when it began to make connection with vigorous general institutions of higher learning.

The first significant break from the old pattern had come in 1868 when the state University of Michigan established a pharmacy course. It was infused with laboratory work. It demanded practically the full time of the student. It ignored the traditional apprenticeship requirement. The consequences were revolutionary as one state university after the other put pharmacy into its constellation of curricula.

This developing structure represented a promise rather than its fulfilment. For nowhere in the USA at the end of the 19th century, among all the states and schools was any *formal* professional education actually required for licensure. The first half of the present century brought sweeping changes. There was a consolidation and reintegration of pharmaceutical education, on the plane largely set by the schools of pharmacy in state universities. Cooperation and reasonable uniformity among the schools replaced the rugged individualism and wide disparity. The United States was growing up culturally, and nationally. The era of westward expansion had come to an end, and the more uniform social conditions emerging among the states, across this 3000-mile expanse, made it easier to cooperate in setting and maintaining standards.

When a new student walked through the door of a pharmacy school in 1900 he was expected to have at least an elementary school preparation—although standards of the different schools varied widely. Then in little more than two decades, recognized pharmacy schools erased a severe handicap to adequate instruction when they agreed upon high-school graduation as an entrance prerequisite. In 1900 the pharmacy student commonly took a two-year course of study, but he could find schools where he would graduate after studying only 40 weeks or so. The University of Wisconsin was already pioneering the four-year course, as an optional curriculum to the two-year course. After another three decades, all recognized schools agreed to make the four-year course a minimum standard (1932). The present five-year course was adopted as the minimum, after sharp controversy, for all students entering accredited schools after the spring of 1960. With encouragement from The Pharmaceutical Survey of 1946–1949, a six-year curriculum (leading to the professional degree of Doctor of Pharmacy) has been offered more recently by a few schools (first inaugurated in 1950 at the University of Southern California).

Research degrees presuppose a standard baccalaureate as preparation; hence it was at the University of Wisconsin where the first American pharmacists were given this foundation, that the first Doctor of Philosophy degree associated with a school of pharmacy was awarded in 1902.

A hesitant growth of graduate departments gained more momentum after the early 1930's. During the subsequent three decades the number of postgraduate students undertaking pharmaceutical research specialties multiplied about 15-fold, by 1963–1964 numbering 1339 in 54 schools.

Since 1932 an accrediting agency, the American Council on Pharmaceutical Education, has been active in maintaining standards of pharmaceutical education and fostering improvements. Because of modern demands on schools of pharmacy, at both the undergraduate and graduate level, the recent tendency has been toward strengthening the educational system rather than expanding it and toward consolidation of independent schools with general institutions of higher learning.

Legal Controls

While the development of pharmaceutical education represented a voluntary effort to help men take more effective advantage of the liberty and opportunity of young America, legal controls then seemed to smack of oppressive restriction, if not even of class distinction. But the British *laissez-faire* spirit, so congenial to American conditions, was gradually modified during the 19th century, without being lost.

In most states the original laws that effectively defined American pharmacy for the first time and delimited its practice were adopted in the period between 1870 and 1900. Earlier attempts here and there to regulate pharmacy by local and state laws typically were not enforced sufficiently to give much support for the development of professional standards.

After the Civil War the APhA promulgated a model state pharmacy act and fostered the founding of state pharmaceutical associations, which frequently played a key role in securing passage of a pharmacy law in the individual states. These laws were sufficiently disparate to make reciprocity of licenses difficult, if not impossible. The need to develop and coordinate a system expediting the transfer of pharmacists from one state to another therefore was one of the principal functions that gave life to the National Association of Boards of Pharmacy (f. 1904).

In modern form the state pharmacy acts mainly establish standards for pharmacists and pharmacies (and for other conditions of drug dispensing), typically leaving to additional legislation the setting of standards for drug products as such (including particularly the ramifications of adulteration and misbranding).

Early state regulation in this latter field proved to be gravely inadequate, thus increasing social pressures after the turn of the century for Federal legislation. The movement led by the physician–chemist Harvey W. Wiley, which culminated in the Federal Food and Drug Act of 1906, was strengthened by exposés of bad conditions in the food industry and, later, of uncontrolled quackery that infested much of the patent-medicine industry. The Federal law repeatedly has had strengthening revision and amendment (notably 1938, 1952, and 1962), supplemented by a separate statute governing biological products (since 1902; renovated 1944).

Because of the abuse of narcotics, and the frightening thraldom of addiction, the Federal (Harrison) Narcotic Act was passed in 1914, placing the United States in the vanguard of nations pledged to build an effective control mechanism, based on international agreement and cooperation. State laws analogous to both the national narcotic law and the food and drug law soon were adopted in most states, protecting against intrastate violators who are constitutionally beyond the reach of Federal agents.

This complex of laws, evolving in their modern form during the past century, have relied on pharmacists to fulfil important responsibilities, and in so doing help create a professionalized role for pharmacists in society. These legal controls are supplemented by the self-control represented by professional ethics.

The Ethics of Pharmacy

Characteristic of professions is a common concern with collective self-discipline of the group. As part of the *quid pro quo* for certain legal prerogatives granted to his profession by society, the practitioner has accepted responsibilities for an ethical standard of conduct going beyond conformity with law or technical skill. This has seemed particularly needful in health professions, such as pharmacy, where the services meet one of mankind's basic needs and where the patient often has no reliable means of judging the standard of service for himself.

In a profession this ethical obligation cannot be superseded by passage of laws; moreover, however wide the net may be woven for controlling a profession through force (law), an area of activities always remains for control through voluntary self-discipline (ethics). For the pharmacist that means essentially a willingness to help assure that a patient, at whatever time or place, may assume that a qualified practitioner invariably will use his professional knowledge in the best interests of the patient and of society—within a framework of interlaced technical, legal, and ethical standards of practice.

In pharmacy, as in other health professions, the ethical standards have been expressed through a professional oath and a professional code (although, historically, these forms sometimes hybridize). The oath ordinarily is brief and general, intended to obligate and inspire the pharmacist to abide by applicable laws, codified ethics, and the dictates of conscience and religious principles.

The Hippocratic Oath is a classical example in the health field. A modern version is still administered, internationally, to neophytes of the medical profession; and a pharmaceutical version has had some usage in the pharmaceutical profession. The oath gradually gaining wider use in American pharmacy has been developed by the American Association of Colleges of Pharmacy (reproduced on page 15). It is administered in various states either upon graduation from a school of pharmacy or upon conferral of the state license to practice.

The codes of ethics, compared with an oath, have been much more detailed and explicit. In well-elaborated form, a code provides an operational blueprint of the norms of professional conduct, a concrete recital of desirable and undesirable actions having recognized impact on the profession's character and functional reliability. If a codified ethos becomes too abstract or idealized—for the sake of brevity or of avoiding public acknowledgment of problem areas—the document becomes correspondingly handicapped as a practical instrument of self-government. An alternative (as employed by American medicine, for example) supplements a relatively concise and generalized code with a manual of currently valid interpretations and case histories concerning individual clauses or principles contained in the basic public-oriented document.

In American pharmacy, professional ethics were first codified (1848) by the first association, the Philadelphia College of Pharmacy. Four years later the American Pharmaceutical Association, still in the year of founding promulgated the document antecedent to the present Code of Ethics. At first too far ahead of its time for general application, the Code was given renewed life through major revisions in 1922, 1952, and 1969.

The APhA's Code has been considered the basic guide and document for American pharmacists, although pharmaceutical manufacturers, wholesalers, and other specialized groups have sufficiently specialized problems to make separate codes seem necessary. Even among practicing pharmacists themselves, there are sufficiently divergent interests and ideas so that some organizations have adopted their own version of the code of ethics—although ordinarily based on or harmonized with the principles codified by the APhA.

American pharmacy has not developed a widespread and effective program for encouraging compliance and adjudicating violations, in connection with its well-developed sense of professional ethics; but it seemed symptomatic of a new level of maturity when, in 1968, the APhA inaugurated a Judicial Board to take responsibility in this field. Moreover, several state pharmaceutical associations in recent years have developed a mechanism for doing so (eg, New York and Wisconsin), while other states have experimented with using the regulatory power of state boards to enforce ethical standards (eg, Louisiana and Connecticut).

Pharmacists differ on details of improving the expression of, or the extent of compliance with, a codified ethos. Yet they are united in recognizing, through the

centuries, that scientific competence becomes meaningful only when the practitioner's services are mediated by a sense of social responsibilities.

Mixed Trends

The legal and ethical controls, a more uniform education and competence among practitioners, organizational structuring, the solidification of traditions and group-consciousness concerned with norms of responsibility and performance—all these suggest a professional maturing of American pharmacy during the past century. Countervailing influences have been an almost complete loss of the practitioner's central function of preparing medication from the individual constituents and a commercializing development which tended to depreciate the average practitioner's valuation of the function for which he was educated and on which his claim as an independent professional largely depends.

Although large-scale industrialization of drug production occurred already in the 19th century, the withdrawal of prescription compounding as such occurred mainly between the 1920's and 1960's. Thus, while drugs became dramatically more effective during the present century, the practicing pharmacist lost much of his creative identification with the prescriptions he dispensed. At the same time the multiplicity and complexness of the new materia medica gave the

---

Oath and Prayer for Health Practitioners

Written in the spirit of the medieval physician-philosopher Moses Maimonides, but attributed to a German physician Marcus Hertz, in the late 18th century. Designed for medicine, the inspiring lines (below) are equally applicable and popular in pharmacy. (See F. Rosner, *Bull. Hist. Med.*, **41**, 440–454 (1967).)

Thy Eternal Providence has appointed me to watch over the life and health of Thy creatures. May the love for my art actuate me at all times; may neither avarice, nor miserliness, nor thirst for glory, or for a great reputation engage my mind for the enemies of Truth and Philanthropy could easily deceive me and make me forgetful of my lofty aim of doing good to Thy children.

May I never see in the patient anything but a fellow creature in pain.

Grant me strength, time, and opportunity always to correct what I have acquired, always to extend its domain; for knowledge is immense and the spirit of man can extend infinitely to enrich itself daily with new requirements. Today he can discover his errors of yesterday, and tomorrow he may obtain a new light on what he thinks himself sure of today.

O God, Thou hast appointed me to watch over the life and death of Thy creatures; here am I ready for my vocation.

And now I turn unto my calling:

O stand by me, my God, in this truly important task;
Grant me success! For—
Without Thy loving counsel and support,
Man can avail but naught.
Inspire me with true love for this my art
And for Thy creatures,
O, grant—
That neither greed for gain, nor thirst for fame, nor vain ambition,
May interfere with my activity.
For these I know are enemies of truth and love of men.
And might beguile one in profession,
From furthering the welfare of Thy creatures.
O strengthen me,
Grant energy unto both body and the soul
That I might e'er unhindered ready be
To mitigate the woes,
Sustain and help
The rich and poor, the good and bad, enemy and friend,
O let me e'er behold in the afflicted and the suffering,
Only the human being.

The American Pharmacist's Professional Oath*

I (your name) do solemnly swear:

That I will abide by the Code of Ethics of the American Pharmaceutical Association in my relations with the public, the other health professions, and fellow pharmacists,

That I will obey all the laws governing the practice of pharmacy, and that I will encourage the enforcement of these laws against all persons, pledging to assist the proper authorities in correcting any unlawful or unethical conduct among members of my profession,

That I will do my best to develop and maintain professional stature by keeping abreast of developments in my own and related professions, and

That I will hold the citizen's health and welfare paramount in all considerations relative to the practice of my profession.

---

* Developed and approved, 1963, by the American Association of Colleges of Pharmacy. For suggestions on use of the oath, see Bowers, R. A., *Am. J. Pharm. Educ.*, **28**, 269 (1964).

practitioner more potential as an expert advisor on pharmaceutical products to other health practitioners and, in a different sense, to lay patrons. Although by mid-century this role had become well defined as an objective, the transition into practice has developed slowly as a trend.

A corollary of this advisory function was the emergence of another goal: making the American pharmacy a center of health-education literature for the laity. Begun in an organized way through a collaborative project (1940) with the American Social Hygiene Association, such service has been fostered, meanwhile, by the APhA, as sporadic funds permit. The scope and effectiveness of "the community pharmacy as a community health education center" was given its most definitive test by the Association through a grant from the US Public Health Service (1963).

Two other trends that helped to blunt the impact of the withdrawal of the preparation of drugs from pharmacies, into remote manufacturing laboratories, were the rising number of prescriptions dispensed and some retrenching in the number of pharmacies. For example, prescriptions that nationally numbered close to 165,000,000 in 1931, had risen to at least 741,400,000 by 1963. Reflected in these estimates are such changes as less physician dispensing, greater economic prosperity, and more prescribing of drugs individually (ie, fewer complexly compounded medications). While the estimated number of prescriptions nationally was increasing about 4½ times, the network of pharmacies was decreasing numerically in relation to the population, from about 1 pharmacy to 2000 persons (1930) to about 1 to 3360 (1960). Such a noticeable increase in the average patronage potential seems large until compared with that in other highly developed Western countries. It is the unused capacity in the average American prescription department that has permitted pharmacy to fulfil the increased demand for pharmaceutical service without comparable increases in facilities. The trend toward larger establishments since World War II reflected more directly the influence of the concept of a supermarket or variety store, which could have a pharmacy as one of its units. A drift toward this type of "drugstore" design has not been resisted as strongly in America as it has among pharmacists in other highly developed countries, partly because of a tradition associating drug dispensing with a general store, a concept with roots in an earlier America, and associating the practitioner with extensive nonpharmaceutical work as an accepted norm.

An equally noteworthy countertrend (countertrends have not been uncommon in American pharmacy) runs in the direction of devoting a higher proportion of the pharmacy to health-related services. For example, in 1930 fewer than 1% of all pharmacies were estimated to be receiving half or more of their dollar volume from the prescription department. During the period up to the 1960's this percentage rose sharply, probably somewhere between 12 and 25% of all pharmacies (although there is a lack of agreement or verification of the exact figure).

These developments as a whole remind us that the community practice of pharmacy in America has retained its variegated nature even though evolving to a new level and character. A more complete description of modern pharmacy and its trends appears in Chapter 4, *Pharmacists in Practice.*

The concise compass of an introductory essay limits discussion largely to an interpretive overview of the evolution of the community practice of pharmacy.

Even within this scope, the individual pharmacists who most decisively shaped or altered the course of pharmacy's history have had to remain in the background. The lives of some of the leading American pharmacists have been briefly reported in biographical sketches in the 13th Edition of this book.

For accounts of the rise of smaller specialties within the profession, of the contributions from pharmacists to science and society, and of the development of the drug trade and industry, the reader may consult other, more specialized or more comprehensive, historical writings. The section *Bibliographic Notes*, beginning on this page, provides one key to finding many of these publications in libraries.

Here has been a glimpse of how pharmacy freed itself from superstition and quackery on one hand and, on the other, from domination by either religion or medicine. It has been noted how the pharmacist became less of a craftsman and more of a professional, although disadvantaged as well as advantaged by pressures from deep-going social, economic, and technologic change, particularly during the past century. A brilliant application of science to pharmaceutical endeavor has made the pharmacist's service qualitatively more effective and valuable to society, although the demand for his distinctively professional functions has been insufficient quantitatively to give the average practitioner a full-time occupation, especially in America.

The American pharmacist, like his counterpart in other countries, has earned increasing responsibilities within the legal structure regulating society. The extent to which pharmaceutical accomplishments have been given a place by historians in the record of man's endeavor permits practitioners and laymen alike to appreciate the persisting and essential quality of pharmacy.

Bibliographic Notes

History

Besides giving recognition to sources on which the historical essay is based, these references suggest further readings and reference materials. English-language publications are cited unless there is no approximate counterpart of a foreign-language publication. For those with deeper historical interests, bibliographies in some of the publications mentioned will open a wide range of more specialized and often more meaningful literature.

A few general guides to the historical literature are: Glenn Sonnedecker, J. H. Hoch, and Wolfgang Schneider, *Some Pharmaco-Historical Guidelines to the Literature*, American Institute of the History of Pharmacy, Madison, Wis., 1959 (also in *Am. J. Pharm. Educ.*, **23**, 143 (1959)); *Index-Catalogue of the Library of the Surgeon-General's Office*, US Army, Washington, D.C., 4 series, 1880–1936; E.-H. Guitard, *Manuel d'Histoire de la Littérature pharmaceutique*, Paris, 1942; *Bibliography of the History of Medicine*, National Library of Medicine, USPHS, Bethesda, Md., No. 1 (1965), *et seq.* (annual; includes pharmacy); *Current Work in the History of Medicine*, quarterly from The Wellcome Historical Medical Library, London, since 1954 (includes pharmacy internationally); "Bibliography of the History of Medicine of the United States and Canada," annually 1939–1966 in *Bulletin of the History of Medicine* (includes pharmacy section); E.-H. Guitard, *Index des Travaux d'Histoire de la Pharmacie de 1913 à 1963*, Societe d'Histoire de la Pharmacie, Paris, [1968]; "Pharmaziegeschichtliche Rundschau" (G. E. Dann, ed.), Vol. I, 1954–1957, *et seq.* (historical abstracts) as periodic supplement to the *Pharmazeutische Zeitung.* Glenn Sonnedecker and Alex Berman, *Some Bibliographic Aids for Historical Writers in Pharmacy*, American Institute of the History of Pharmacy, Madison, Wis., 1958; and David L. Cowen, *America's Pre-Pharmacopoeial Literature*, American Institute of the History of Pharmacy, Madison, Wis., 1961.

The book of most comprehensive scope in English is *Kremers and Urdang's History of Pharmacy*, revised by Glenn Sonnedecker, Lippincott, Philadelphia, 1963 (see "Glossary" as well as "Notes and References" for bibliographic material). Hermann Schelenz, *Geschichte der Pharmazie*, Berlin, 1904, republished by Oscar Rothacker, Berlin, 1961, a monumental reference work, is now outdated in many details, but richly documented to the earlier literature.

On antiquity: The most definitive paper of general scope on Egypt is by Frans Jonckheere, "Le 'Préparateur de Remèdes' dans l'Organisation de la Pharmacie égyptienne," Deutsche Akademie der Wissenschaften zu Berlin, Institut für Orientforschung, Veröffentlichung Nr. 29, Berlin, 1955 (Sonderdruck aus "Aegyptologische Studien..."). C. D. Leake, *The Old Egyptian Medical Papyri*, Lawrence, Kans., 1952, gives an overview of the documents; and for a first-hand impression of the papyrus most important pharmaceutically, see B. Ebbell, *The Papyrus Ebers*, Copenhagen, 1937. Henry Sigerist, *A History of Medicine, Vol. 1: Primitive and Archaic Medicine*, New York, 1955, is the best general survey. On Mesopotamia, an excellent book of breadth, relevant to pharmacy, is by Martin Levey, *Chemistry and Chemical Technology in Ancient Mesopotamia*, Amsterdam (Van Nostrand, distributor, Princeton), 1959; on Assyria, see monographs by Reginald C. Thompson. The best sociohistorical view of its scope in English is Henry E. Sigerist, *A History of Medicine, Vol. II: Early Greek, Hindu and Persian Medicine*, Oxford University Press, New York, 1961; more specifically on pharmacy are J. Berendes, *Die Pharmacie bei den alten Culturvölkern*, 2 vols., Halle a.S., 1891 and Alfred Schmidt, *Drogen und Drogenhandel im Altertum*, Leipzig, 1924. The Hippocratic treatises have been translated into English by W. H. S. Jones and E. T. Withington, *Hippocrates*, 4 vols., London, 1923–1931, while a compilation on Hippocratic drugs was published by Johann H. Dierbach, *Die Arzneimittel des Hippokrates...*, Heidelberg, 1824. For modern scholarship, from a different viewpoint, see Jerry Stannard, "Hippocratic Pharmacology," *Bull. Hist. Med.*, **35**, 497 (1961); see also his "Materia Medica and Philosophical Theory in Aretaeus," *Sudhoffs Arch. Gesch. Med. Naturw.*, **48**, 27 (1964). For a first-hand impression of the classical materia medica, see, eg, the three translations: Robert T. Gunther, ed., *The Greek Herbal of Dioscorides*, Oxford, 1934, republished Hafner Publ. Co., New York, 1959; Francis Adams, trans., *The Seven Books of Paulus Aegineta...*, 3 vols., Sydenham Society, London, 1844–1847; and W. G. Spencer, trans., *Celsus, De Medicina*, 3 vols., Loeb Classical Library, London and Cambridge, Mass., 1935–1938. On Greek temple medicine, see Ch. Kerenyi, *Le Medecin divin*, Basle, 1948, and E. J. Edelstein and L. Edelstein, *Asclepius, A. Collection and Interpretation of the Testimonies*, 2 vols., Baltimore, 1945.

On the Middle Ages: For a general survey of *medieval Islam* and its influence, see Lucien Leclerc, *Histoire de la Médecine Arabe*, 2 vols., Paris, 1876; also Donald Campbell, *Arabian Medicine and Its Influence on the Middle Ages*, 2 vols., London, 1926, and Cyril Elgood, *A Medical History of Persia and the Eastern Caliphate*, Cambridge, England, 1951. Much has been translated or written about Arabic materia medica and drug therapy, to which the principal key is a bibliographic volume by Sami K. Hamarneh, published in 1964 by the Internationale Gesellschaft für Geschichte der Pharmazie, Stuttgart, 1964. Of Hamarneh's other publications, an article of much general interest is "The Rise of Professional Pharmacy in Islam," *Medical History*, **6**, 59 (1962); and for a detailed view into 10th-century Spain (with a useful bibliography), see S. K. Hamarneh and G. Sonnedecker, *A Pharmaceutical View of Abulcasis al-Zahrawi in Moorish Spain*, E. J. Brill, Leiden, 1963. Important works by Max Meyerhof include several on materia medica, such as his monographs on al-Ghâfiqî, Publication No. 4, The Egyptian University Faculty of Medicine, Cairo, 1932, on al-Beruni in *Studien zur Geschichte des Naturwissenschaften und der Medizin*, Vol. 3, Berlin, 1943, pp. 159–208, and his four articles in *Ciba Symposia*, 6, Nos. 5 and 6 (1944). See likewise the writings of Martin Levey, such as *The Medical Formulary or Agrabadhin of al-Kindi*, University of Wisconsin Press, Madison, [ca. 1965]. For *medieval Europe*, a volume still not superseded (although outdated in details) is George F. Fort, *Medical Economy During the Middle Ages...*, New York, 1883; see also, David Riesman, *The Story of Medicine in the Middle Ages*, New York, 1935. A valuable guide and commentary is by Henry E. Sigerist, "The Latin Medical Literature of the Early Middle Ages," *J. Hist. Med.*, **13**, 127 (1958). Of more specifically pharmacomedical interest: The definitive work on the renowned pharmacomedical edicts in the Kingdom of the Two Sicilies is by Wolfgang-Hagen Hein and Kurt Sappert, *Die Medizinalordnung Friedrichs II. Eine pharmaziehistorische Studie*, Internationale Gesellschaft für Geschichte der Pharmazie, Eutin, 1957. In the periodical literature, note particularly the writings of Alfons Lutz (eg, "Der verschollene frühsalernitanische Antidotarius magnus...," Veröffentlichungen der Internationalen Gesellschaft für Geschichte der Pharmazie, n.s. V. 16, Stuttgart, 1960, pp. 97–133, with a rich bibliography), and of Rudolf Schmitz (eg, "...Apothekerstandes im Hoch- und Spät-Mittelalter," *ibid.*, V. 13, 1958, pp. 157–165) and "Ueber deutsche mittelalterliche Quellen zur Geschichte von Pharmazie und Medizin," *Deut. Apotheker-Ztg.*, **100**, 980 (1960). Writings of unusual value and clarity in English-language literature are by G. E. Trease, such as "The Spicers and Apothecaries of the Royal Household in the Reigns of Henry III, Edward I and Edward II," in *Nottingham Mediaeval Studies*, **3**, 19 (1959) and abridged in *Pharm. J.*, 4 April 1949, pp. 246–248. Sister Mary Francis Xavier [Welhoefer], *Statutes of the Guild of Physicians, Apothecaries and Merchants in Florence (1313–1316); a Brief Com-*

mentary, with an Introduction and Translation, unpublished PhD dissertation, University of Wisconsin, 1935, is uniquely useful, even though dated as to many details. On medieval European materia medica, see Henry E. Sigerist, "Materia Medica in the Middle Ages," *Bull. Hist. Med.*, **7**, 417 (1939) and his "Studien und Texte zur frühmittelalterlichen Rezeptliteratur," *Studien zur Geschichte der Medizin*, V. 13, Leipzig, 1923, pp. 187 *ff.*; probably the earliest pharmacist's textbook and manual has been translated into German by Leo Zimmermann, *Saladini de Asculo...Compendium aromatariorum*, Leipzig, 1919 (for Hebrew, see Suessmann Muntner, ed., Tel-Aviv, 1953).

On modern Europe: For a reliable and concise medical overview, see Erwin Ackerknecht, *A Short History of Medicine*, Ronald Press Co., New York, 1955; supplemented for detailed reference by Fielding H. Garrison, *An Introduction to the History of Medicine*, 4th ed, Philadelphia, 1929; republished 1960 (note the bibliographic essays of Appendix III). Some international survey volumes on pharmacy, with particular reference to the modern period, are listed by Sonnedecker and Berman, *Some Bibliographic Aids...* (cited above). A gap has been closed, meanwhile, by Leslie G. Matthews, *History of Pharmacy in Britain*, E. & S. Livingstone Ltd., Edinburgh and London, 1962, and Cecil Wall, H. C. Cameron, and E. A. Underwood, *A History of the Worshipful Society of Apothecaries of London, Vol. I: 1617–1815*, Oxford University Press, London, 1963. There is not yet a history both up to date and dealing comprehensively with European pharmacy; general bibliographic guides, such as those cited at the beginning of this essay, will yield books and monographs from particular topical and national viewpoints. On the question of early pharmacopeias, see two articles by Alfons Lutz, on the Florentine *Nuovo Receptario* in *Veröffentlichungen der Internationale Gesellschaft für Geschichte der Pharmazie*, V. 13, Stuttgart, 1958, pp. 113–128, and on the *Dispensatorium* of Valerius Cordus in *Festschrift zur 75. Geburtstag von Ernst Urban*, Stuttgart, 1949, pp. 107–125; see also, with caution, Jean Volckringer, *Evolution et Unification des Formulaires et des Pharmacopées*, Paris [1953]. D. A. Wittop Koning discusses the historically important question, "Was ist eine Pharmakopöe?" in *Veröff. der Interntl. Gesel. f. Gesch. d. Pharm.*, n.s. V. 22, Stuttgart, 1963, pp. 181–191.

On the United States: The standard volume in English, *Kremers and Urdang's History of Pharmacy*, revised by Glenn Sonnedecker, Lippincott, Philadelphia, 1963, devotes approximately two-thirds of the main text to the United States; and its bibliographies open up a wide range of other American literature. Noteworthy are the anniversary issues of *Druggists Circular*, **51** (Jan. 1907), and *Pharmaceutical Era*, **16**, No. 27 [Dec. 31] (1896). An article particularly drawn upon in the preceding chapter is my address, "Structure and Stress of American Pharmacy," *Pharm. J.*, 14 April 1956, pp. 3–8. A useful bibliography still in print is by George Griffenhagen, *Bibliography of Papers Published by the American Pharmaceutical Association that were presented before the Association's Section on Historical Pharmacy, 1904–1957*, American Institute of the History of Pharmacy, Madison, Wis., n.d. (includes subject and author indexes; emphasizes American history, but by no means restricted thereto). The "Pharmacy" section of the annual bibliography in the *Bulletin of the History of Medicine*, previously offered an important key to the literature, which was cumulated in *Bibliography of the History of Medicine of the United States and Canada*, Genevieve Miller, ed., Johns Hopkins, Baltimore, 1964; see also other "General Guides" listed (supra). Also noteworthy is the "Bookshelf" section of *Pharmacy in History* (a quarterly of the American Institute of the History of Pharmacy), and the sections on "History and Ethics," "Sociology and Economics," and "Literature," in *International Pharmaceutical Abstracts*.

Ethics

For useful cross-sections from history concerning ethics, see Charles LaWall, "Pharmaceutical Ethics," *J. APhA*, **10**, 895 and 961 (1921); George F. Archambault, "Ethical Standards...," *Bull. Am. Soc. Hosp. Pharm.*, **13**, 446 (1956); for a Catholic viewpoint, William L. Wolkovich, *Norms of Conduct for Pharmacists*, (17 Loring Street), Hudson, Mass., 1962; from a sociologist, Isador Thorner, "Pharmacy: The Functional Significance of an Institutional Pattern," *Am. J. Pharm. Educ.*, **6**, 305 (1942), or *Social Forces*, **20**, 321 (1942), and Urdang's commentary, *Am. J. Pharm. Educ.*, **6**, 319 and 617 (1942); Karl L. Kaufman, "Ethics for the Pharmacy Student," *Am. J. Pharm. Educ.*, **17**, 225 (1953); Theodore Greiner, "The Ethics of Drug Research on Human Subjects," *J. New Drugs*, **2**, 7 (1962); Allen I. White, "The Development of Professional Morality in Pharmacy Students," *Am. J. Pharm. Educ.*, **17**, 222 (1953); Frank Arnal, "International Code of Ethics for Pharmacists," in *Commission de l'Exercice de la Pharmacie d'Officine: Rapports, Federation Internationale Pharmaceutique*, Brussels, 1958, pp. 157–168.

On medical ethics see, for example, *Manual on Medical Ethics and Discipline* [American Medical Association, Chicago, 1966; restricted circulation], and supplements; Willard L. Sperry, *The Ethical Basis of Medical Practice*, New York, 1950; Joseph F. Fletcher, *Morals and Medicine*, Princeton University Press, Princeton, 1954 (Protestant–Catholic dialectic on perplexing issues); Ludwig Edelstein, *The Hippocratic Oath, Text, Translation, and Interpretation* (Suppl. to *Bull. Hist. Med.*), Baltimore, 1943; Chauncey D. Leake, *Percival's Medical Ethics*, Williams & Wilkins, Baltimore, 1927; see also special issue of *The Annals*, American Academy of Political and Social Science, **297** (Jan. 1955).

Some American Pharmaceutical Leaders

For biographical sketches of some American pharmaceutical leaders, the interested reader is referred to the 13th Edition of this text, page 20.

A Chronology for Pharmacists

Many dates involve uncertainties, approximations, and questions of meaning, which are not apparent in a concise table such as that below. Dates before the 18th century often are unverifiable or estimated.

B.C.
2000? **Earliest formulary** known in man's recorded history (Sumerian).
1500 **Ebers Papyrus,** Egyptian manuscript pertaining to pharmacy and therapy.
460 **Hippocrates,** famous Greek physician, was born.
350 **Diocles** wrote an important treatise on materia medica.
372 **Theophrastus** (372–285), the "father of botany," was born.
A.D.
50 **Dioscorides** wrote an important book on materia medica.
131 **Galen** (131–201), born, Roman physician who experimented with compounded drugs.
350 **Cosmas** and **Damian,** who became patron saints of pharmacy and medicine, persecuted.
585 Death of **Marcus Aurelius Cassiodorus** (490–585) who wrote a book on medieval science.
857 **Johann Mesue Senior,** Arabian physician (777–857) dies.
925 Death of **Rhazes,** the Persian physician (865–925).
1035 **Avicenna** (980–1035), famous physician and philosopher dies.
1178 **Mention of pharmacists in French records.**
1180 **Guild of Pepperers** in London.
1225 **Apothecary shop** established at Cologne.
1297 **Guild of Pharmacists** organized in Bruges.
1345 **Apothecary shop** established in London.
1348 **The Black Death**—Great Plague struck Europe.
1480 **Poison law** enacted by James I of Scotland.
1499 **Guild Pharmacopœia** published in Florence, Italy.
1529 **Paracelsus** (1493–1541) published his first treatise.
1546 **Nuremburg Pharmacopœia** (Dispensatory of Valerius Cordus), perhaps the first to be "official."
1548 **Charles V** issued decree regulating pharmacy. Jacques du Bois (Sylvius) first used title "Pharmacopœia" for a formulary.
1565 **Jean Nicot** (from whose name we have derived "nicotine") introduced **tobacco** plant in France.
1589 **Galileo** demonstrated the **law of falling bodies.**
1604 **Louis Hébert,** first pharmacist to settle in North America.
1617 **Society of Apothecaries** in London organized.
1618 **First London Pharmacopœia** published.
1620 **Pilgrims** settled at Plymouth, Mass.
1628 **Harvey** published his book on the **circulation of the blood.**
1646 **William Davis** operating apothecary shop that probably was one of the first in America (Boston).
1665 **Sir Isaac Newton** discovered the **law of gravitation.**
1680 **Leeuwenhoeck** discovered **yeast** plants.
1699 First edition of **Edinburgh Pharmacopœia** issued.
1703 English **apothecaries authorized to prescribe** as well as dispense.
1715 **Bartram's Botanical Gardens** established at Philadelphia. First tabulation of relationship between chemical substances issued by French pharmacist **E. Fr. Geoffroy.**
1731 **Philadelphia Hospital** founded.
1736 **First law related to pharmacy** in America enacted in Virginia.
1752 **Hospital pharmacy** in America established, at Pennsylvania Hospital in Philadelphia. **Jonathan Roberts** was first apothecary.
1762 **Antoine Baumé** publishes his *Élémens de Pharmacie* in France.
1765 **John Morgan** becomes influential advocate of **prescription writing** in United States.
1770 Three million people die of **smallpox** in the West Indies.
1772 **Nitrogen** discovered by **Rutherford.**
1773 **Scheele** isolates **oxygen** about 1773, **Priestley** by 1774.
1774 **Scheele** discovers **chlorine.**
1775 **First American Army hospital** established.
1776 **Declaration of Independence;** position of Apothecary-General created in army of the patriots.
1776 **Christopher Marshall,** famous American pharmacist, cares for wounded soldiers.
1777 **Collège de Pharmacie** established in Paris.

1783 **Pilâtre de Rozier,** a pharmacist, makes **first human flight** in a balloon.
1785 **Fowler** introduces **Fowler's Solution; Withering** publishes his treatise on **digitalis.**
1787 **Ergot** introduced in obstetrics by **Paullitzsky.**
1790 **First United States patent law** passed. Elisha Perkins took out first medical patent in 1796.
1793 **Plague** strikes Philadelphia.
1793 **Trommsdorff's** *Journal der Pharmazie* founded; first professional-scientific journal devoted to **pharmacy.**
1798 **Jenner** publishes his work on **vaccination.**
1805 **Sertürner** reports isolation of **morphine.**
1809 *Journal de Pharmacie et de Chimie* founded; first published as *Bulletin de Pharmacie.*
1811 **Iodine** discovered by **Courtois,** a French pharmacist.
1818 **Caventou** and **Pelletier** isolated **strychnine.**
1820 **Quinine** isolated by **Pelletier** and **Caventou.**
1820 **First edition of United States Pharmacopœia** published.
1821 **Philadelphia College of Pharmacy** founded by **Henry Troth** and associates.
1823 **Massachusetts College of Pharmacy** founded.
1825 First American pharmaceutical journal, *American Journal of Pharmacy*, published.
1826 **Bromine** discovered by pharmacist **Balard. Ethyl alcohol** synthesized by **Hennel.**
1828 **Wöhler** synthesizes **urea,** thus bridging gulf between organic and inorganic chemistry.
1829 **New York College of Pharmacy** founded.
1831 **Chloroform** prepared independently by **Liebig** and by **Soubeiran.**
1832 **Codeine** isolated by French pharmacist **Pierre Robiquet.**
1834 **Carbolic acid** and **aniline** prepared by German pharmacist **F. F. Runge.**
1841 **Maryland College of Pharmacy** founded.
1842 **Long** performed first operation under **anesthesia** using ether.
1843 **Oliver Wendell Holmes** points out that puerperal fever is contagious.
1848 **First American code of pharmaceutical ethics** prepared by Philadelphia College of Pharmacy.
1848 **First drug import law** enacted.
1852 **American Pharmaceutical Association** founded.
1852 **Darwin** publishes his *Origin of Species.*
1865 **First International Pharmaceutical Conference** in Brunswick, Germany.
1868 **University of Michigan** opens pharmacy course that will have far-reaching influence in modernizing American pharmaceutical education.
1883 **First National Retail Druggists Association** founded.
1888 **First National Formulary** issued by American Pharmaceutical Association.
1890 **Serum therapy** introduced by **von Behring** and **Kitasato.**
1893 **Aspirin** discovered by **A. Eichengrün** and **Felix Hoffman.**
1895 **Roentgen** discovered **X-rays.**
1898 **Radium** discovered by the **Curies.**
1898 **National Association of Retail Druggists** founded in USA.
1899 **Walter Reed** proved mosquitoes carried **yellow fever.**
1900 **American Association of Colleges of Pharmacy** founded.
1902 **First International Pharmacopœial Conference** held at Brussels; first American PhD supervised in pharmacy granted at University of Wisconsin.
1906 **Federal Food and Drug Act** passed.
1910 **Paul Ehrlich** and **S. Hata** introduce **arsphenamine** ("606") in widespread clinical trial.
1912 First Assembly of **International Pharmaceutical Federation** (The Hague).
1922 **Banting** and **Best** isolated **Insulin.**
1928 **Sir Alexander Fleming** discovers **Penicillin,** the first antibiotic.
1935 **Prontosil,** the first "sulfa" drug, introduced by **G. Domagk.**
1937 **American Journal of Pharmaceutical Education** founded; first periodical devoted to pharmaceutical education.
1938 **League of Nations Commission on International Pharmacopœial Standards** held conferences. Important revision of Federal Food and Drug Act (USA).

1942 **American Society of Hospital Pharmacists** founded.
1944 **Antibiotic activity of streptomycin** announced.
1945 **Atomic energy** released for use in warfare and medicine.
1947 **Medical Service Corps** created in US Army, with pharmacy represented by special group of commissioned officers.
1948 **First Pan American Congress of Pharmacy and Biochemistry.**

1949 **Cortisone and ACTH** introduced for rheumatic arthritis.
1951 **First International Pharmacopœia.**
1955 **Salk poliomyelitis vaccine** released for general use.
1959 **Synthetic modifications of natural penicillin** introduced; **American Society of Pharmacognosy** founded.
1962 Important amendments of the Federal Food and Drug Act.

3 | Ethics

Concept of professions—professional characteristics—the ethical code—
functional performance—relationship of trust—emerging conflicts—
encouraging adherence

This chapter was prepared by

Maven J. Myers, LLB, PhD, *Associate Professor of Pharmacy Administration,
Philadelphia College of Pharmacy and Science, Philadelphia, Pa.   19104*

The role of ethics in the advancement of pharmacy was succinctly stated by Elliott in *The General Report of the Pharmaceutical Survey (1946–1949)* when he observed:

> "After all has been said and done, it may be concluded that the outstanding factor determining the future of the profession of pharmacy is fundamentally moral in nature. The profession must contain a far greater proportion of members who are ever sharply jealous of the high reputation of the profession and who, by energetic cooperation, are determined ever to protect that reputation."[1]

Ethics and law are related in that both share the social purpose of encouraging "right" conduct. Law attempts to achieve its purpose through the sovereign power of government while ethics, in particular the ethics of a profession, attempts to achieve its purpose without the intervention of government.

Concept of Professions

Since pharmacy lays claim to being among the elite group known as the professions and since ethics are an inherent characteristic of professional behavior, an examination of the concept of professions provides the basis for a study of ethics in pharmacy.

Many occupations seek to be classified as professional. The designation implies that the practitioners of the occupation are performing an essential function in society. As Parsons has noted, "many of the most important features of our society are to a considerable extent dependent on the smooth functioning of the professions."[2]

Other reasons, derived from the first and perhaps more significant in contemporary society, also provide motivation to an occupational group seeking classification as a profession. Smith observed:

> "We trust our health to the physician, our fortune and sometimes our life and reputation to the lawyer and attorney. Such confidence could not safely be reposed in people of a very mean or low condition."[3]

Because of the importance of the professional functions and the inability of the receiver of these functions to assess the quality of service, a relationship of trust must exist between the professional and the patient. When the physician recommends surgery, the patient (having little ability to validate the professional's conclusion) must trust that the recommendation is made in the best interest of the patient and not merely to provide a monetary gain to the physician providing the service.

Smith recognized, and society in general appears to have agreed, that if the professional is to place the patient's interest above the professional's immediate pecuniary gain, the professional must enjoy an income sufficiently high so that the gain from exploiting an individual patient becomes an insignificant part of the professional's total income.   Thus, the average income of the professional usually is higher than that of the nonprofessional.

Yet, even in a highly materialistic society, monetary wealth is not the sole goal of the people.   How the wealth was earned frequently is as important as the amount of wealth.   Thus, a physician and a racketeer may have equal monetary wealth, yet society pays homage only to the physician.

Marshall points out that in the evolution of professions, those most likely to engage in the professions were aristocrats or men of leisure.[4]   Professions, thus, evolved as occupations connected with high status. The functional relationship of professions to society reinforces the status position of the professions, while the status itself acts as a motivating factor in an occupation's drive for recognition as a profession.

A third relevant motivating factor is man's desire for power.   Within the sphere of his professional activities, the professional exercises an authoritative power over his patient.   As explained by Greenwood:

> "(T)he professional dictates what is good or evil for the client, who has no choice but to accede to professional judgment.   Here the premise is that, because he lacks the requisite theoretical background, the client cannot diagnose his own needs or discriminate among the range of possibilities for meeting them."[5]

Thus, the functional relationship of the professions to social progress places them in an important position in the social framework.   The desire to serve a highly useful function in society is one of the main stimuli to professional behavior.   Flowing from the important positions the professions occupy in society are the income, status, and power possessed by professional practitioners.   The extent to which these goals are achieved is intimately related to the degree to which an occupation can validate its claim to being a profession.

Professional Characteristics

Based on Sonnedecker's criteria for professions[6] two groups of related professional characteristics appear. In applying these characteristics to an occupation it should be observed that the criteria are relative rather than absolute.   That is, an occupation is more or less professional than another occupation because it possesses these characteristics to a greater or lesser degree.

Specialized Knowledge and Social Utility—The first group of professional characteristics is the existence of a specialized body of knowledge, possession and utilization of which enable the practitioner to perform a highly useful social function. It will be observed that all occupations, except criminals, provide some positive benefit to society and are based on specialized knowledge. Thus, the functions performed by a garbage collector are important to the health of society and, through experience, garbage collectors likely have gained some knowledge which permits them to perform their functions more efficiently than the inexperienced layman.

Generally, the professions are more socially useful than other occupations; however, social utility alone does not make an occupation a profession. The social utility of an occupation must be based on the possession and utilization of a specialized body of knowledge.

An applied body of knowledge may be composed of knowledge of a manual skill or intellectual knowledge. It is the latter which is of primary significance as a criteria for professions. Thus, the pharmacist is not considered a professional because he can rapidly type a prescription label. Rather, the relevant professional function involved in this operation is the pharmacist's ability, based on his specialized knowledge of drugs, to properly interpret the prescriber's directions.

The exercise of proper judgment is a key element in this first group of professional characteristics. Traditionally, professional services are rendered to an individual rather than on a group basis. Using the specialized body of knowledge of the profession and the intellectual abilities of the professional practitioner, the practitioner makes a judgment as to the best course of treatment for the particular individual.

The first group of professional characteristics are related to ethics in that a major function of the ethics of a profession is to increase the social value of the profession by encouraging the development, acquisition, and proper utilization of the specialized knowledge of the profession.

Attitudes and Professional Behavior—The second group of characteristics of a profession is the possession by its practitioners of a set of attitudes which influences their professional behavior. The basic component of this set of attitudes is altruism, an unselfish concern for the welfare of others. Marshall summarized this thought in the following words:

"The professional man, it has been said, does not work in order to be paid: he is paid in order that he may work. Every decision he takes in the course of his career is based on his sense of what is right, not on his estimate of what is profitable."[4]

In the development of professions, one finds a strong historical base for altruism. Carr-Saunders and Wilson[7] point out that in Greece and Rome the functions of the lawyer were not performed by specially trained advocates, but by (presumably unpaid) friends of the litigants. The physician in the Roman Empire was not a free-lance practitioner, but a slave attached to a rich man's household. When training for the professions became formalized in the universities of the Middle Ages, not only were the universities controlled by the church but professional men were required to take religious orders. Thus, one would expect to find that the early professionals did not practice for personal financial gain.

The contemporary bases for altruism as a characteristic of professions already has been alluded to. The professions are concerned with matters that are vital to the health or well being of their patients. In

practicing a profession... specialized technical kno... patient or client does not p... patient's lack of knowledge, opportun... exploitation of the patient by the professi... cause of the vital nature of professional servi... consequences to the patient of such exploitation...e severe. Thus, the smooth functioning of the professions requires that the practitioner consider the needs of the patient as paramount, relegating the material needs of the practitioner to an inferior position.

Social Sanction—What might be thought of as a third group of professional characteristics, although they are actually the resultant effect of the two groups previously discussed, is social sanction. Ultimately, whether or not an occupation is a profession depends, to a large degree, on whether society views it as a profession. One measure of social sanction is the granting of exclusive rights of practice through the licensing power of the state. While such licensing attempts to protect the public from incompetent practitioners, frequently it also creates a relationship of trust between society and the professionals.

The extent of this trust also is a measure of the degree of social sanction; however, it is measured by a lack of the exercise of sovereign power. Given the legal monopoly inherent in professional licensing, the failure of society to impose further controls on the profession by implication sanctions the performance and self regulation of the profession.

Another measure of social sanction is the status, income, and power with which society rewards the professional. Thus, given either the altruistic goal of service to mankind or the egoistic goals of status, income, or power, a means of goal achievement is professionalization of the occupation. This professionalization is accomplished through adherence on the part of practitioners to ethical precepts which encourage qualitative increases in, for example, pharmacists' occupational role performance.

The Ethical Code

The foundation of all ethical behavior is the basic precept, "Do good and avoid evil." The ethics of pharmacy attempt to relate this basic precept to the practice of pharmacy. An initial problem, as pointed out by Barber, is "to specify how such rules are to be applied in the everyday, real-life, concrete situations that present us with ethical dilemmas."[8]

A first step in this specification is the codification of more particularized principles relating the basic ethic to pharmaceutical practice. Such a code "makes explicit what man already knows implicitly. It puts at his fingertips a concrete expression of principles already familiar to him . . . ."[9]

The first code of ethics for pharmacists in the United States was adopted in 1848 by the Philadelphia College of Pharmacy. Having felt that they had "erected a standard of scientific attainments, which there is a growing disposition of the part of candidates for the profession to reach," the code was adopted because of a desire "that in relation to professional conduct and probity, there should be a corresponding disposition to advance . . . ."[10]

When the American Pharmaceutical Association (APhA) was founded in 1852 it adopted a code of ethics[11] modeled after that of the Philadelphia College of Pharmacy. The code of the APhA, the national

... society of pharmacists, is generally recognized as establishing the guidelines of conduct for American pharmacists.

Initially, members of the Association were required to subscribe to the code, but in 1855 "the obligation to subscribe to the APhA code as a prerequisite of membership was dropped and the code itself disappeared from the literature for over half a century."[12] Relating the 1852 code to 20th-century pharmacy, Sletten observed:

"The old code obviously referred to a by-gone day. The colleges had taken over many of the educational functions of the apothecary and planned to take over most of the remainder. Uniformity of performance among pharmacists was to be engendered by a uniform educational program among the schools, examinations, and a common ethical code. The USP and NF had now become official standards. In addition, the growth of pharmaceutical manufacturers had greatly advanced product uniformity. No doubt the emphasis on fraud and quackery were thought to be inappropriate for the current situation. In addition, the old code had long been dormant in its written form. Rather than merely to give it renewed publicity, a new code reflecting more closely the current ideals of the APhA could be drawn up."[13]

The new code adopted by the Association in 1922[14] with modifications in 1952[15] was divided into three parts: the pharmacist in his relations to (1) the public, (2) other health practitioners, and (3) other pharmacists and the profession. Although the code was quite detailed, there was a need for an authoritative interpretation of its broad provisions as well as a mechanism to secure adherence to its principles. Thus, in 1966 there was established within the framework of APhA:

"A judicial board with full powers to discipline members and render advisory opinions and interpretative statements, reprimanding, suspending or expelling a member in any category for violation of the obligations of the constitution or bylaws, or for unprofessional conduct."[16]

In 1967 the APhA convened a Conference on Ethics. The sentiments expressed by the conferees likely reflect the thinking of the leadership of American pharmacy concerning the form and role of professional ethics in pharmacy's future. Excerpts from the summary of the conferees' discussions[17] follow:

"It was generally agreed that the Association and the profession require a code of ethics stated in broad principles with the APhA Judicial Board applying the principles to specific situations. Further, it was proposed that the new code of ethics encourage and guide the pharmacist in the performance of his professional duty rather than present him with nothing more than a compilation of 'thou shalt nots.' "
"The most important aim of the new code of ethics was considered to be the protection of the public—not the profession . . . .
"(T)he new code should be general rather than specific, positive rather than negative and should stress the integrity and professional judgment of the individual pharmacist.
"It was recommended that in the process of revising the code, an entirely new document be drafted rather than attempting to "patch up" the present code. Such an effort, it was pointed out, would allow greater emphasis in the new code on the expanding role of the pharmacist . . . ."

Relations to the Public

"In addition to 'drugs of good quality,' as presently specified in the code, it was recommended that a new code include 'efficacy' as a standard for drugs which the pharmacist may dispense ethically . . . .
"The present code of ethics states that the pharmacist seeks to merit the confidence of his patrons and zealously guards this confidence . . . . It was suggested that the new code require that the treatment received by the patient as well as the patient's ailments be kept in confidence. The prohibition on the release of information, however, was found in need of modification, particularly in light of the increase of third-party payments . . . .

"Although there was disagreement as to whether the pharmacist should recommend over-the-counter medication for routine disorders, participants generally agreed that the pharmacist should not diagnose but could aid the patron by offering guidance in the selection of medication . . . .
"The prohibition of participation by the pharmacist in any plan which eliminates the pharmacist–patient–prescriber relationship was considered to be of key importance—especially because of the risk of mail-order prescription schemes. Similarly, the personal relationship of the pharmacist to his patrons was considered important and should not be eliminated by the use of clerks . . . .
"There was general approval of the principle that the pharmacist seeks "only fair and honest remuneration for his services." Advertising by the pharmacist which stresses his professional fees or which implies a "professional superiority" was suggested for identification in the new code as unprofessional conduct . . . ."

Relations to Other Health Professions

"Many felt the new code should reflect the competence of the pharmacist and allow him to recommend remedies as indicated by his professional judgment. Also considered was the role of the pharmacist in the future and this prompted the suggestion that the new code allow for the continuing expansion of the contribution of the pharmacist. This expansion could perhaps go so far, it was noted, as to involve the pharmacist in the diagnosis–prescribing function with the physician . . . .
"The prohibition on discussion of therapeutic effect and composition of prescribed drugs with a patient also was critically attacked. It was recommended that the pharmacist be allowed to increase his opportunity to assist both practitioner and patient. In this regard, it was generally felt that the side effects of a drug, such as drowsiness, should be brought to the patient's attention although it would not be necessary to make the patient aware of the therapeutic effect of a prescribed drug. Consequently, modification of the inflexible prohibition on discussion was suggested to allow the pharmacist to use professional judgment in deciding whether to discuss medication with the patient . . . .
"Arrangements which could interfere with the patient's free choice of pharmacy or which could tend to an exploitation of the patient were opposed. Examples of arrangements discussed included divided fees, renting space from a physician on other than a flat rental basis, direct telephone lines, imprinted prescription blanks, and advertising of professional services . . . ."

Relations to Fellow Pharmacists

" 'The pharmacist's relation to the profession of pharmacy' was suggested as a more appropriate title for this section because it would include but subordinate the collegial relationship of one pharmacist to another . . . .
"The principle that the pharmacist will 'aid in driving the unworthy out of the calling' was approved. In addition, it was felt that the responsibility of the pharmacist to aid in this effort, beyond that of placing a charge, should be included in the new code.
"A statement encouraging the pharmacist to provide assistance to a fellow pharmacist was accepted for inclusion in the new code . . . .
"A suggested addition to this section in the new code would cover the obligations of the employer–employee relationship. For example, it was pointed out that the new code should provide that a pharmacist should not engage in any practice forbidden by the code of ethics as a condition of his employment. Another addition suggested for the new code would prohibit advertising which reflected adversely on a fellow pharmacist or which emphasized the price of professional services. And a question raised but not decided concerned the pharmacist's ownership of stock in a small repackaging firm."

In response to the sentiments expressed at the 1967 Conference on Ethics, the Judicial Board began to rewrite the profession's code on ethics. The code of ethics adopted by the Association in 1969 is shown on page 23.

Functional Performance

A principal factor contributing to the importance of professions is the functions they perform based on the possession and utilization of a specialized body of knowledge. On the one hand, the patients of the professional do not possess this body of knowledge; therefore, they must trust that the professional does. On the other hand, the ability of the professional to serve his patients as well as the income, status, and

Code of Ethics

American Pharmaceutical Association

Preamble

These principles of professional conduct for pharmacists are established to guide the pharmacist in his relationship with patients, fellow practitioners, other health professionals, and the public.

Section 1

A pharmacist should hold the health and safety of patients to be of first consideration; he should render to each patient the full measure of his ability as an essential health practitioner.

Section 2

A pharmacist should never condone the dispensing, promoting or distributing of drugs or medical devices, or assist therein, which are not of good quality, which do not meet standards required by law or which lack therapeutic value for the patient.

Section 3

A pharmacist should always strive to perfect and enlarge his professional knowledge. He should utilize and make available this knowledge as may be required in accordance with his best professional judgment.

Section 4

A pharmacist has the duty to observe the law, to uphold the dignity and honor of the profession, and to accept its ethical principles. He should not engage in any activity that will bring discredit to the profession and should expose, without fear or favor, illegal or unethical conduct in the profession.

Section 5

A pharmacist should seek at all times only fair and reasonable remuneration for his services. He should never agree to or participate in transactions with practitioners of other health professions or any other person under which fees are divided or which may cause financial or other exploitation in connection with the rendering of his professional services.

Section 6

A pharmacist should respect the confidential and personal nature of his professional records; except where the best interest of the patient requires or the law demands, he should not disclose such information to anyone without proper patient authorization.

Section 7

A pharmacist should not agree to practice under terms or conditions which tend to interfere with or impair the proper exercise of his professional judgment and skill, which tend to cause a deterioration of the quality of his service or which require him to consent to unethical conduct.

Section 8

A pharmacist should not solicit professional practice by means of advertising or by methods inconsistent with his opportunity to advance his professional reputation through service to patients and to society.

Section 9

A pharmacist should associate with organizations having for their objective the betterment of the profession of pharmacy; he should contribute of his time and funds to carry on the work of these organizations.

power of the professional are dependent on the ability to perform his professional functions.

Thus, a profession serves itself and society by giving high-quality performance in its professional role. A principal feature of ethics is to encourage a high level of role performance. Professional ethics are concerned not merely with the moral conduct of the practitioner in his professional relations but also with the function the profession performs and the quality of this performance.

The precept that, "A pharmacist should always strive to perfect and enlarge his professional knowledge," has, with minor changes, been part of pharmacy's code of ethics since its 1922 revision. The increased institutionalization of training for professions through colleges, formalized internship programs, and state licensing examinations does not decrease the significance of this ethic but does effect a change in its implementation.

The ethic that the pharmacist should perfect and enlarge his professional knowledge combined with his duty to support "organizations having for their objectives the betterment of the profession" imposes a duty on the pharmacist to encourage the proper functioning of the training institutions.

Of more direct import to the individual practitioner are the gaps which exist in the institutionalized structure. The structure has operated primarily as a means of assuring that when a student emerges from the structure (through college graduation or state licensure) he possesses the minimum technical knowledge which will permit him to perform the functions of the profession as they then exist.

However, the main tool of the professions (knowledge) is being constantly expanded and changed and, in some cases, the function of the profession itself is being modified. The technical training of 50 years ago, or even 5 years ago, does not assure that the previously trained professional has even the minimal technical competence to function effectively in his present or future professional role. In recent years the institutionalized training structure of pharmacy has become more aware of this gap and through voluntary or compulsory continuing education is making a strong effort to reduce the gap between prior training and current needs.

The possible institutionalization of continuing education does not, however, diminish the necessity of a commitment on the part of all practitioners to possess the body of knowledge on which the practice of the profession is based. While institutionalization may make the continuing education process more efficient, this merely makes it easier for the practitioner to maintain his proficiency and does not reduce the necessity for proficiency.

The position of pharmacy (and, thus of individual pharmacists) in our society depends on the service the profession renders to the members of society. Perfecting and enlarging his professional knowledge is an essential prerequisite to providing high-quality professional service. However, the mere possession of the requisite technical knowledge makes no contribution to the well being of society unless this knowledge is used for the benefit of the pharmacist's patients. Thus, the pharmacist is directed to "utilize and make available this knowledge as may be required in accordance with his best professional judgment."

While proper functioning of the professional in his role is important, of equal importance are the functions of the pharmacist as "an essential health practitioner." Thus, even though a practitioner performs his function with great technical competence, his role and the role of his occupation in society depend on the contributon of his function to the achievement of society's objectives.

That health is one of these objectives and that drugs are important in the attempt to attain this objective seem beyond dispute. Pharmacy's function has, over the period of its existence, undergone changes and the stated ethics of the profession have been modified to reflect these changes.

Thus, in 1852, when a main function of the pharmacist was compounding medicinal agents into dosage forms, the pharmacist was told that his first duty "after duly preparing himself for his profession" was "to procure good drugs and preparations ... ." In 1922, when the community pharmacist received many of his drugs already manufactured into dosage forms, the primary object of pharmacy was expanded and redefined as "the service it can render to the public in safeguarding the handling, sale, compounding, and dispensing of medicinal substances." The 1952 revision of the code expanded this to include the storage of drugs.

The proposed revision of the code still proscribes "the dispensing ... of drugs ... which are not of good quality" and offering for sale any drug or medical device that "lack therapeutic value."; however, the functional role of the pharmacist is now introduced with the broad statement that, "A pharmacist should hold the health and safety of patients to be of first consideration; he should render to each patient the full measure of his ability as an essential health practitioner."

While the proper performance of the physical act of dispensing drugs requires a high degree of skill and is an important function in society, the broad function expressed in the first section of the proposed revision of the code indicates a feeling that pharmacy's contribution to society can be more than that which is embodied in the physical act of dispensing drugs. The demands for health care are increasing much more rapidly than the supply of health-care practitioners and facilities. At the same time community pharmacists in their work situation are performing functions unrelated to health care resulting in the submaximal utilization of their professional knowledge at a time when other health-care resources are inadequate to optimally service the burgeoning demand. As Sister Emmanuel has expressed it:

"Undoubtedly, current health-care problems demand that new roles for the pharmacist be sought out in addition to his present one as dispenser of drugs. Cognizant of this, pharmaceutical educators are emphasizing the significance of flexibility as a quality in today's pharmacist. They also are fostering exploration of new roles where the pharmacist extends himself in a more personal manner to meet the needs of society and his colleagues—members of the health-care team."[18]

Thus, the professional ethics of pharmacy seek not only to encourage the adequate performance of the existing accepted role of the pharmacist but also to facilitate the expansion of this role to increase the functional contribution of pharmacy to society.

Relationship of Trust

In writing about the relation between professionalism and social structure, Marshall explained the necessity of the existence of a relationship of trust between the professional and patient:

"Ethical codes are based on the belief that between professional and client there is a relationship of trust, and between buyer and seller there is not ... .
"There are two reasons for this. One is that professional service is not standardized. It is unique and personal ... . It is hardly possible to be satisfied with a doctor or a lawyer unless one likes and respects him as a man ... . These essential qualities cannot be specified in a contract, they cannot be bought. They can only be given... .
"The second reason for the relationship of trust ... is the ignorance of the client. He often hardly knows what to ask for, let alone how it can be provided. He must surrender all initiative and put himself in his lawyer's hands or under his doctor's orders."[4]

These reasons justify the extension of the scope of professional ethics, beyond the technical performance of an occupational role, to the personal characteristics of the practitioner. Thus, we find that, "A pharmacist has the duty to observe the law ... . He should not engage in any activity that will bring discredit to the profession ... ."

Offenses directly related to the professional role, such as the illegal sale of narcotics by a pharmacist or falsification of claims for prepaid prescription insurance, clearly violate the ethic. The ethic, however, is not limited to such offenses but, presumably, includes all conduct which reflects adversely on the trustworthiness of a practitioner.

Ideal of Service—The necessity of a relationship of trust to the smooth functioning of the professions also imposes other restrictions on the professional practitioner. As the first section of the proposed code dictates, "A pharmacist should hold the health and safety of patients to be of first consideration." Thus, the ideal of service embodied in the professional ethic places the financial gain of the professional in a position secondary to the service he renders. As Kohn expressed it:

"(T)he professions in the finest sense do actually get their inspiration from a motive other than the money-getting motive ... . The earning of a livelihood is naturally the result of competent practice of a profession. But that is not its prime purpose in the best sense. The prime purpose is the perfection of a service ... ."[19]

This altruistic subordination of the practitioner's personal gain to the best interest of the patient is a dominant factor in distinguishing professions from other occupations. As has been observed, historically professions developed in an environment in which the practitioners had little interest in financial gain. In addition, since the professions usually deal with vital matters and because of the ignorance of the patient, it is likely that society demands that the professional be disinterested in personal gain as a continuing condition of the legal monopoly found in most professions. Finally, since altruism is a characteristic of professions and since the income of professionals usually is greater than that of nonprofessionals, the altruistic attitude may merely be a sacrificing of short-term gain in the interest of maintaining the existing professional structure with its above-average income level for professional practitioners.

This subordination of the practitioner's private interest does not mean that the professional must be oblivious to materialistic goals. A distinction should be made between a practitioner's total professional income and his income from a given patient transaction. With respect to the latter, the professional ethic requires that the needs and welfare of the patient are superior to the practitioner's immediate financial interest. Such an ethic is, however, difficult to adhere to unless the practitioner's total professional income is at a satisfactory level.

Indirect Remuneration—One of the main ethics derived from the required altruistic attitude is a prohibition on indirect remuneration of the practitioner. According to Carr-Saunders and Wilson:

"The fiduciary relationship between professional and client involves certain restrictions on the professional man's methods of charging. It requires that the practitioner shall be financially disinterested in the advice he gives, or, at least, that the possibility of conflict between duty and self-interest shall be reduced to a minimum."[20]

The 1848 code of the Philadelphia College of Pharmacy declared it unjust to medicine and injurious to the public for an apothecary to allow "any physician a percentage or commission on his prescriptions." Through various mutations, this prohibition has continued through the present code.

The obvious dangers of a prescriber standing to profit (whether through a direct commission, percentage rental in a prescriber owned building, or other mechanisms) from having the prescriptions he writes dispensed in a given pharmacy include the possible denial to the patient of freedom of choice of pharmacist and the ordering of unnecessary medication by the prescriber.

The bases of the prohibition against fee-splitting can also be interpreted as discouraging certain widely used practices, such as gifts to prescribers at Christmas or other occasions and even the granting of a professional discount to prescribers on their purchases in a pharmacy. There is a thin line which separates these practices from ethical gestures of friendship or professional respect and the unethical practice of attempting to influence the prescriber to steer his patients to a particular pharmacy.

Although the code specifically prohibits "arrangements with practitioners of other health professions" involving fee-splitting or other methods of patient exploitation, the indirect remuneration ethic is not limited to arrangements with other health professionals. The code also prohibits splitting of fees for professional services with persons in addition to health professionals, such as granting rebates to operators of nursing homes or extended-care facilities.

Conflict of Interest—By the very nature of the professional relationship and the trust that is required, conflict of interest situations which could lead to

patient exploitation are inevitable. A distinction should be made between those conflicts which are inherent in the professional relationship and those which are voluntarily created by the practitioner. The former require restraint by the professional to insure that there is no patient exploitation. The latter, since they are an unnecessary part of the professional relationship, should be avoided.

For example, if a pharmacist receives a prescription written generically for reserpine, he must exercise his professional judgment to determine which of the available reserpine products he will dispense. Depending on his method of charging for his professional services, the pharmacist might make more profit from dispensing one brand of reserpine than from another. Although this conflict could be avoided by the use of the professional fee, the choice among available reserpine products is a part of the professional service of the pharmacist and requires that he restrain his profit motive to dispense the product which best satisfies the patient's needs rather than the product which is most profitable.

An unnecessary part of the community pharmacist's professional relationship would be an ownership interest in a drug repackaging firm which distributes reserpine or other products which he could use to dispense generic prescriptions. The conflict of interest in this latter case differs from that in the former in that the ownership interest is a voluntarily acquired conflict which is not necessary to the proper performance of the professional.

To avoid these potential conflicts of interest a pharmacist likely should not have an influential ownership interest in a company which distributes products that he would use to dispense prescriptions written generically.

Also, great care should be observed in recommending nonprescription medication to patients to insure that the best product is dispensed. The use of high-margin private-label medication, which is sometimes of questionable quality, and participation in various promotional schemes, such as the use of "PM's" or push money, present ethical problems for the pharmacist. Whether such conduct is or is not ethical depends on the motivation of the pharmacist. From the pharmacist's point of view it is difficult, if not impossible, for him to objectively define his motive. In addition, the mere existence of unnecessary action which could result in patient exploitation can do much to destroy the public's trust in pharmacists, regardless of whether or not exploitation occurs. To avoid these problems, the pharmacist should refuse to participate in any unnecessary scheme whereby his professional judgment may become clouded by considerations of personal financial gain.

Commercial Practices—The relationship of trust that must exist between professional and patient also imposes restrictions on the methods used by the professional to attract patients. According to Carr-Saunders and Wilson:

"When the position of trust is regarded as extending to a profession as a whole, it is seen that certain common commercial practices are incompatible with the rendering of professional services; and from these practices the professional man is required to abstain. In particular professional men may only compete with one another in reputation for ability, which implies that advertisement, price-cutting, and other methods familiar to the business world are ruled out."[21]

If the patient is to have the required degree of trust in the professional whose services he utilizes, the primary motivating factor in determining patronage must be the quality of service, and not its price. In the commercial world, advertising has two basic purposes: to inform a consumer who has already decided to purchase of the availability of a product or service and to stimulate demand for the product or service. In the professional environment the use of advertising for the former purpose usually is allowed within reasonable limits while for the latter purpose advertising is almost universally discouraged.

The relationship of trust between professional and patient also requires that information about his patients which the practitioner obtains in the course of rendering his professional services be treated as confidential. To properly render his service, the professional frequently must know information which the patient might be unwilling to publicly disclose. The patient will give the professional this necessary information only if assured that its confidential nature will be respected.

Emerging Conflicts

The conflict between the personal interests of the professional and his duty to subordinate this interest to the best interest of his patient presents one of the major unresolved problems of the professions. In addition, changing patterns in pharmacy and health-care delivery present additional ethical conflicts.

The traditional unit of professional service has been the individual. Thus, professional services have not been mass produced, but each rendering of a service is specifically tailored to the individual needs of a specific patient. In general, the ethics of professions have evolved on the basis of primacy of the individual with the general welfare of society relegated to a secondary position. Marshall has summarized the situation as follows:

"The professional man cannot spread his services .... He is unable to go in for mass production and is forbidden to offer cheap lines for slender purses. Since he works for a limited market it is not surprising that he should choose one which is solvent and concentrate on the wealthy individual client. In other words he must find an employer, and the general public was not organized for his employment .... (T)his state of affairs led to a maldistribution of professional services in terms of social need, a maldistribution due to economic motives among professional men but not necessarily implying any disloyalty to the principle that service must not be sacrificed to profit .... Big-scale social activities only became possible when the initiative was taken by the state and the local authorities, by public corporations and rich charities. And by that time the professions had built up their tradition of individualism, which meant not so much the pursuit of individual self-interest as the service of individual clients in a relationship of individual trust. They were therefore disinclined to press for the establishment of corporate agencies for the distribution of professional services and reluctant to work for them when they appeared."[4]

The correction of this maldistribution likely can be effected only with structural changes in the health-care system and a resulting alteration of the professional–patient relationship. A system appears to be emerging in which frequently someone other than the recipient of the service provides the payment to the professional. The resulting third-party-payment programs likely will produce a system in which the third party exercises some control over the professional practice.

For example, traditionally the pharmacist has considered as confidential information about a patient which is contained in his prescription files and patient record cards. However, if a third party is to pay the prescription charges for a patient, the third party usually will require access to the information contained in these records.

Another problem related to the existing maldistribution is the supply of health personnel. Traditionally, health personnel have been trained in quantities sufficient only to meet the effective demand projections for their services in the near future with effective demand being defined as a want for the service and the ability to pay for the satisfaction of this want. Assuming the removal or drastic lowering of economic barriers to health care, the resulting demand for services likely will exceed the existing supply of personnel. As a result, pharmacists may be required to perform tasks different from those performed today and the ethical precepts of the profession may require modifications to achieve high-quality service in this different occupational role.

The increasing incidence of pharmacists not practicing in the community pharmacy environment gives some indication of the nature of the problem. Thus, the problems relating to professional ethics which are encountered by the institutional pharmacist, the industrial pharmacist, or the pharmacist functioning in an administrative capacity frequently are quite different from those encountered by the pharmacist in community practice.

Emerging systems of health care as well as other factors indicate the likelihood that an increased percentage of health practitioners will have an employee rather than an independent status. As with third-party payment, this can present situations in which the professional's duty to his patient is in conflict with his duty to his employer. Although this is not a new situation for pharmacy, the changing nature of the employer may present additional conflicts. Traditionally, the employed pharmacist has been an employee of another pharmacist in a community pharmacy. However, with increasing frequency the employer is a non-pharmacist—a corporate chain of pharmacies, an industrial corporation, a hospital, or a Government agency. Thus, the pharmacist–pharmacist employment relationship, with the attendant obligation of both employer and employee to adhere to pharmacy's ethics, is being replaced in many instances with a pharmacist–non-pharmacist employment relationship, in which only the pharmacist is obligated to adhere to the profession's ethical precepts.

Encouraging Adherence

One characteristic of ethics is that they are a mechanism of self regulation for a profession. As Sonnedecker expressed it:

"However far governmental regulation of pharmacy may reach, room remains for a set of moral expectations and injunctions in some form—for an institutionalized action pattern that makes it normal for the pharmacist to accept social responsibilities going beyond legal compulsion."[6]

Thus, in the primary sense ethics are not enforced by law, but they are adhered to because of an "institutionalized action pattern that makes it normal for the pharmacist to accept social responsibilities ...." The strengthening of this institutionalized action pattern leads to the advancement of the profession through its own self regulation. A failure of this system necessitates Government intervention in order to maintain pharmacy standards at a level required for the protection of the public health.

Reasons for Ethical Failures—As developed in previous sections, adherence to the ethics of pharmacy by a practitioner frequently is an example of enlightened self interest. Thus, by all practitioners maintaining high professional standards, the profession as a whole advances and each practitioner benefits. There appear to be two reasons why this enlightened self-interest does not always occur.

The first is lack of knowledge. There are two aspects to this reason for failure: ignorance on the part of practitioners of the existence or meaning of pharmacy's ethical precepts and concentration by practitioners on short-term goals. With respect to the first aspect, it is to be hoped that with a new code of ethics, a judicial board to supply interpretations of the code, and the attendant publicity the significance of this aspect will decrease. It is, nevertheless, important for all pharmacists and pharmacy organizations to do whatever they can to see that every pharmacist is aware of the ethical principles and their proper interpretation.

The second aspect can be reduced only by a reorientation of practitioner's thinking to concentrate on long-range, rather than short-range, goals. For example in the short run, it is to a pharmacist's advantage not to take the time to "perfect and enlarge" his professional knowledge. With the rapid increases in health knowledge that are occurring, however, the long-run result is that the pharmacist becomes so outdated that he is unable to perform his professional duties effectively and the state of knowledge in the profession has changed so drastically that, even if he tries, he is unable to learn the new technology.

The second reason why enlightened self interest does not always occur is, as one economist put it, "In the long-run we are all dead." Thus, a pharmacist might prostitute the heritage of the profession which has accumulated over the centuries by, for example, advertising low prescription prices to attract patronage. In doing so, the pharmacist takes a calculated risk that he will be able to continue profitably prostituting the profession and that the over-all effects of his actions will not be felt until succeeding generations take over the profession.

This type of ethical failure is much more difficult to correct and, likely, the optimum approach would be to prevent its occurrence rather than attempting to deal with it after it has occurred. To a considerable extent, this is a purpose of pharmacy education. As Bullough observed:

"It seems obvious that professional status for the individual is achieved only after long training . . . . One of the chief purposes of such training is to initiate the candidate into a set of professional attitudes and controls, to give him a professional conscience."[22]

The reference groups with which an individual identifies can have a profound effect on his actions.[23] If the group as a whole accepts the ethical standards, an individual who desires further association with the group (or fears disassociation from the group) will be likely to conform to the group standard. The effect of increasing the reference groups which accept the ethical standards of the profession likely is cumulative, since as more ethical groups emerge there is a smaller probability that a pharmacist will select a nonethical group as his reference group.

Sanctions—In spite of these actions, there still will remain a small proportion of pharmacists who do not adhere to the ethical precepts. Sanctions against members of this group by the professional association can range from censure to revocation of membership. The imposition of such sanctions must, of course, be in accordance with the member's right to due process.[24]

Potentially, the result of disciplinary action may be to increase, rather than decrease, the nonconformity of the offender. As Toby has noted:

"The status degradation inherent in punishment makes it more difficult to induce the offender to play a legitimate role instead of a nonconforming one. Whatever the offender's original motivations for nonconformity, punishment adds to them by neutralizing his fear of losing the respect of the community—he has already lost it."[25]

An additional limitation on sanctions by professional associations is the general limitation of their effect to members of the association. Thus, an association obviously cannot revoke the membership of a nonmember. In many cases, those most likely to commit offenses against the ethical code are not likely to have acquired membership in the professional association. A further deficiency is the failure of many members of the profession to expose unethical practice. In a study of discipline in the American Medical Association it was observed that:

"First and foremost, the Committee found apathy, substantial ignorance, and a lack of a sense of individual responsibility by physicians as a whole. The latter is demonstrated by the 'hear no evil, see no evil' attitude of many doctors and through the complaints which are received concerning physicians when the complaining physician later refuses to testify or give a deposition."[26]

In spite of the deficiencies of self regulation, there remains much that can be done within pharmacy to increase the service contribution of pharmacists through ethics. The situation was summarized by the late Dean LaWall when he described pharmacy as:

"(A) highly specialized calling, which may rise to the dignity of a true profession or sink to the level of the lowest commercialism, according to the ideals, the ability, and the training of the one who practices it."[27]

References

1. Elliott, E. C., dir., *The General Report of the Pharmaceutical Survey (1946–1949)*, American Council on Education, Washington, D.C., 1950, p. 4.
2. Parsons, T., *Social Forces*, **17**, 457 (1939).
3. Smith, A., *An Inquiry Into the Nature and Causes of the Wealth of Nations*, P. F. Collier & Son, New York, 1937, p. 107.
4. Marshall, T. H., *Can. J. Econ. Political Sci.*, **5**, 325 (1939).
5. Greenwood, E., in Nosow, S., and Form, W. H., eds., *Man, Work, and Society*, Basic Books, New York, 1962, p. 210.
6. Sonnedecker, G., *Am. J. Pharm.*, **133**, 243 (1961).
7. Carr-Saunders, A. M., and Wilson, P. A., in Nosow, S., and Form, W. H., eds., *Man, Work, and Society*, Basic Books, New York, 1962, pp. 199–200.
8. Barber, B., *J. APhA*, NS8, 137 (1968).
9. Giuliano, C., *J. APhA*, NS3, 73 (1963).
10. *Am. J. Pharm.*, **20**, 148 (1848).
11. *Am. J. Pharm.*, **25**, 16 (1853).
12. *J. APhA*, NS3, 65 (1963).
13. Sletten, C. A., *The Social Structure and Ideology of Organized Pharmacy*, unpublished PhD dissertation, Harvard University, 1959, pp. 329–330.
14. *J. APhA*, **11**, 728 (1922).
15. *J. APhA*, Pract Ed., **13**, 721 (1952).
16. *J. APhA*, NS6, 293 (1966).
17. *J. APhA*, NS8, 142 (1968).
18. Emmanuel, Sr., *J. APhA*, NS8, 284 (1968).
19. Kohn, R. D., *Ann. Am. Acad. Political Social Sci.*, **101**, 1 (May, 1922).
20. Carr-Saunders, A. M., and Wilson, P. A., *The Professions*, The Clarendon Press, Oxford, 1933, p. 426.
21. *Ibid*, p. 432.
22. Bullough, V. L., *The Development of Medicine as a Profession*, Hafner, New York, 1966, p. 2.
23. Krech, D. *et al*, *Individual in Society*, McGraw-Hill, New York, 1962, p. 197.
24. *Establishment and Maintenance of Membership Standards in Professional Societies of Pharmacists*, APhA, Washington, D.C., 1967.
25. Toby, J., *J. Criminal Law, Criminol. Police Sci.*, **55**, 332 (1964).
26. *Report of the Medical Disciplinary Committee to the Board of Trustees*, American Medical Association, Chicago, 1961, p. 52.
27. LaWall, C. H., *Four Thousand Years of Pharmacy*, Lippincott, Philadelphia, 1920, p. v.

4 | Pharmacists in Practice

The pharmacist and the pharmacy—the pharmacist and his principal roles—nursing homes and extended-care facilities—problems in pharmacy practice—the future of pharmacy and professional trends—the pharmacy and its products

This chapter was prepared by

Melvin R. Gibson, PhD, *Professor of Pharmacognosy, College of Pharmacy, Washington State University, Pullman, Wash. 99163*

The Pharmacist and the Pharmacy

The pharmacist and his function in the last quarter century have undergone dramatic changes in both personal orientation and professional activity. He is no longer a handmaiden of medicine filling secret prescriptions containing medication of often questionable value requiring manipulative arts and techniques. Today, he is a professional in his own right—a partner in the health team who handles drugs of great potency and value manufactured by a highly sophisticated industry. He handles these drugs in open consultation with physicians and patients with the confidence his advanced knowledge as an expert on drugs demands that he should.

In this last quarter century, also, there has been a marked increase in the type and quantity of convenience goods distributed by pharmacies, some of which have no relation to health. It is this commercialization of pharmacy which has created many of the problems now faced by the profession. Not the least part of this problem is the public image of pharmacy practice. The late distinguished pharmaceutical educator, Dr. Rufus A. Lyman (himself a physician and staunch Presbyterian) said, "There is commercialism in medicine and in the Presbyterian Church, as well as in pharmacy. The only difference is that commercialism in pharmacy is on display on every main street in the country."

Displayed as it is and exploited as it is, commercialization of pharmacy has created problems at all levels of pharmaceutical engagement. The glimmer of a reverse trend to strictly professional practice will be discussed later in this chapter.

The commercialization of retail pharmacy, whether motivated by a desire to be of greater service or by profits, has yet failed to completely besmirch the image of the pharmacist as a dedicated professional who holds the respect of the community at large and the business and professional persons of our towns and cities. The pharmacist is still the professional on main street most accessible to the public whose image remains as that of a reliable person with whom the public can talk in confidence on a variety of subjects who does not send a bill for this counsel. He is the person who is active in community affairs and often a community leader in worthwhile projects as well as giving generously of his time and efforts for the community good.

The separation of professional and business functions are today clouded in the public's mind. They are also clouded in the minds of many pharmacists. It is often easier to slip into commercialism than to

develop the professional aspects of pharmaceutical practice. White[1] put it this way:

Observations made throughout my thirty years in the profession suggest that motivation rather than education is the quality most lacking when pharmacists fail to achieve important new goals. The demands made day after day in a routine job allow the years to slip by without time taken for a self-analysis or a periodic evaluation of one's business. Soon both pharmacist and pharmacy have slipped into a decadence from which there is no easy escape.

Pharmacy is at a critical era in its history. At the center of interest is the pharmacist himself. He is well paid. (The average retail self-employed proprietor in 1967 had an income of $24,168.)[2] He is in a big profession which ranks fifth in size of all health professions.[3] He is well educated. A five-year curriculum is a minimum and some curricula require six years. The rest of this chapter will deal with the pharmacist, his practice, his problems, and his challenges; in short, where he is, what he is doing, and what he can do to affect his future in this critical period of the profession.

The Pharmacist and His Principal Roles

The Pharmacist, the Prescription, and the OTC Drugs—Hager[4] has said, "Adequate communications of information about drugs to persons who need such information by persons who are in a position and are qualified to supply that information is today a most important factor in the improvement of the health, strength, and vigor of the people of this country."

The people who know most about drugs are pharmacists. That is their province; that is their responsibility. Primary in this responsibility are prescription drugs. The physician must diagnose; he must prescribe. But the pharmacist handles that all-important commodity—the drug that alleviates or cures. His approach to the handling of this important commodity must not be taken lightly. In some instances he may be a consultant to the physician on drugs. But before he can really function as a partner with the physician in therapy, both his training and experience must be so directed. *Now his most important service* can be rendered to the person who wants and needs it most—the patient. Every new prescription should be discussed privately with the patient. Every prescription renewal which the pharmacist feels needs discussing with the patient should be discussed in private.[5]

The pharmacist is not in a position to discuss diagnoses and the ramification of diseases. However, he is capable of discussing the drug as a drug with the

28

patient. He does know how the drug is taken. He does know the side reactions of it which may be of concern to the patient. He does know its stability under various conditions. He does know its toxicity and dosage. He does understand its route of administration. He is an expert on drugs. The physician is not. The information which the pharmacist is able to supply can be of great assurance, interest, and need to the patient.

The second most important responsibility the pharmacist has to the patient is in the area of over-the-counter (OTC) drugs. The pharmacist's responsibility in this regard is well summarized by Penna[6] in his address to the Conference of Teachers of Pharmacy of the American Association of Colleges of Pharmacy:

> The necessity that practicing pharmacists take on a more professional attitude toward non-prescription medication is practically axiomatic. Likewise, the need which exists on behalf of the public for such professional pharmaceutical activity is self-evident. We see in the area of non-prescription medication, a new field of professional involvement, a new endeavor where the pharmacist can perform professional functions without first receiving instructions from a physician.
>
> In handling a case dealing with self-diagnosis and a non-prescription drug, the pharmacist has the total responsibility for all the professional decisions. He decides which products he carries in his pharmacy. He decides whether or not a patient has accurately self-diagnosed his condition. The pharmacist decides whether or not to recommend that the patient consult a physician or recommend a product, and finally, the pharmacist makes the decision as to which product to recommend in a given case.
>
> These decisions—all professional acts—are the reasons why pharmacists must take a more active and professional interest in non-prescription medication. These decisions are also the reasons why pharmacists in increasing numbers are becoming more involved in this specialty—they recognize the potential for professional service, the need and the professional satisfaction which are inherent in the specialty of non-prescription medication.
>
> Certainly non-prescription medication will play an ever-increasing role in the medical treatment of the future. Self-diagnosis and self-medication will continue to increase as the public becomes more knowledgeable about diseases and drugs. While this is intrinsically good and will have an immediate effect on reducing the physician work load, self-diagnosis and medication must be subject to professional guidance. The pharmacist who is available, accessible, knowledgeable and concerned is the logical choice for the individual on whom this responsibility should fall.

With greater pharmacist–patient orientation and patient–drug record-keeping the pharmacist becomes the only person who has *all* the information regarding the patient's drug consumption—prescription and nonprescription. He must use that information about drug consumption, coupled with his own singular drug expertise, to advise the patient, and if necessary, the patient's physician so that the patient benefits most and does not suffer from the multiple-drug therapy from prescription and nonprescription drugs.

The Pharmaceutical Center—Probably no event in the recent history of pharmacy has caught more dramatically the imagination of the professionally minded student than the Pharmaceutical Center concept. It was originally the 1960 realization of the dream of one man, Eugene V. White of Berryville, Va. Through the promotion of the American Pharmaceutical Association and McKesson & Robbins, the Pharmaceutical Center has become a thriving concept of the epitome of professional pharmacy practice. Its most eloquent evangelist is Mr. White himself.[7]

The professional store devoted almost exclusively to handling prescriptions is not new. It has its counterpart all over Europe. But the need for multipurpose retail establishments of all kinds in a rapidly developing and often sparsely settled US made the multipurpose pharmacy (business and professional)

the common trend in this country. The trend of overcommercialization often outweighed the professional development until the pharmacist found himself the educational product of professionalism and the in-practice victim of overcommercialization. This dichotomy of education and practice led to the disillusionment of many young pharmacists.

The disillusionment of Mr. White brought forth the Pharmaceutical Center. Figs. 5–7 illustrate interior and exterior views of such centers.

A departure from the usual strictly prescription store, the Pharmaceutical Center is an innovation not only in pharmacy interiors but also in the pharmacist–patient relationship. Placed in a relaxed and professional setting, and devoid of merchandise on display, the pharmacist has as his primary interest the patient and what he, the pharmacist, can do to serve the patient's best health interests. As Mr. White has emphasized in his many talks on the subject, a Pharmaceutical Center cannot be successful without the genuine interest of the pharmacist in the health needs of the patient. This pharmacist–patient relationship must be genuine, personal, and performed in the interest of the patient's welfare. There is no place for commercialism in such an establishment. The author of this chapter has even suggested[5] that all Pharmaceutical Centers have a consultation room so that each new prescription, and refills where indicated, should be discussed with the patient by the pharmacist.

The Pharmaceutical Center is the setting for the practice of pharmacy in its most professional context. Without the merchandise as a prop for financial security, it should not be entered into without thorough evaluation of prescription volume. But more important an evaluation is that of the sincerity of the pharmacist in his motives. The success of the Pharmaceutical Center is most determined by the dedication of the pharmacist to the best interests of the patients requiring his services.

What might be considered the creed of the Pharmaceutical Center has been expressed by an owner of such a center, Mr. Ralph S. Kuhn of Doylestown, Pa.:[7]

> Society creates a profession because of the need of the services rendered by said profession. Such a profession will only live so long as it renders the services required by the society that created it. Therefore, a profession is a trust and a privilege given by society to render a specialized service for members of society. If the profession refuses to recognize its responsibility or exploits its trust, then society will find other means for acquiring the necessary services. Pharmacists must be made to realize that they have not been fulfilling the very purpose for which they exist. They have been very cleverly diverted from doing the will of pharmacy to doing the will of the self-schooled, diabolical and articulate huckster and merchandiser. If pharmacy were fulfilling its obligation to society, we would not have to fight for ourselves because they would do it for us and do it better.

In small communities there will always be the need for a multipurpose pharmacy to serve the needs of the people and supply the pharmacist with diversified sources of income. These can be attractive, profitable establishments meeting the needs of these communities (Figs. 8 and 9).

In metropolitan areas the large diverse-product pharmacies will continue to be part of the pharmacy picture (Figs. 10–12). There is something undeniably attractive about wide selections of many lines of merchandise open for public view and selection. The super-market pharmacy will find its place in shopping centers and metropolitan centers. However, as the Pharmaceutical Center concept gains public acceptance and appreciation, it is predicted that the dichotomy of merchandising from strictly professional practice will become more evident. This is seen in the rapidly growing areas of the West Coast. The US eventually may see the pattern which exists in Europe—one class of pharmacy devoted to merchandise, another devoted to strictly professional practice.

Patient Orientation—The breakaway of the professional practice of pharmacy from the business image will neither be quick nor easy. However, it is believed by many that such a separation is critical for the survival of pharmacy as a professional entity. It is believed that the deciding factor in the emergence of a new professional image will depend upon the ability of the pharmacist to alter his image from that of simply a purveyor of drugs and merchandise to one of being a purveyor of advice and counsel both to the patient and to the public at large. The pharmacist's role as a consultant on drugs to the physician is often not well developed. The pharmacist has often viewed himself as subservient to the physician and his almighty prescription. In the future health-care picture the pharmacist will need to become a full-time partner to the physician. For he is the only expert on drugs today. This is expertise which is not being effectively utilized in the average pharmacy.

Where there is the greatest need for counsel and advice on drugs is to the patient. To emerge as a full-fledged professional the pharmacist must divest himself of the image and practice of product-orientation and become patient-oriented.

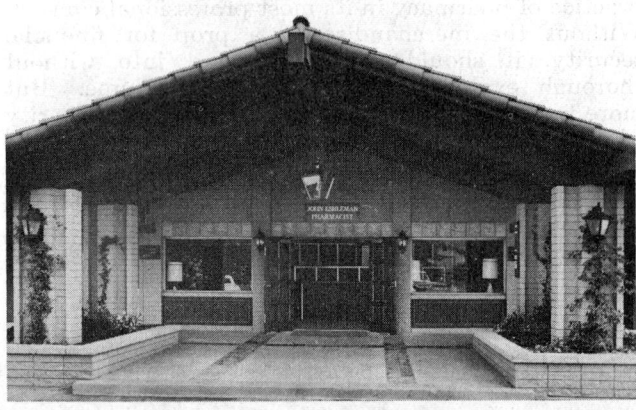

Fig. 5. Pharmaceutical Center, John J. Eshleman, owner, San Jose, Calif.

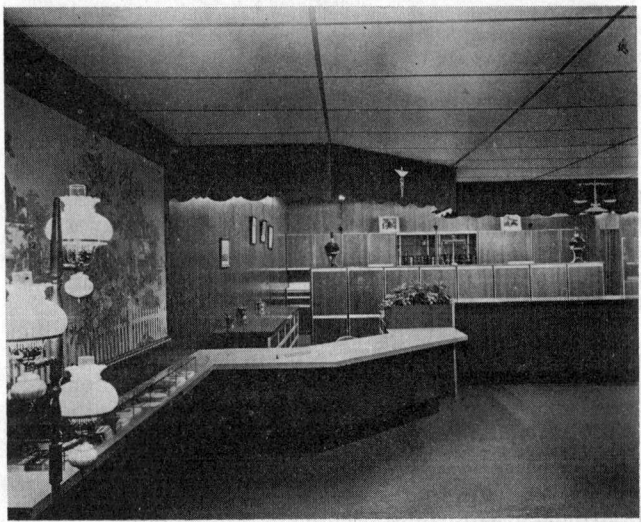

Fig. 6. Pharmaceutical Center (courtesy, McKesson & Robbins).

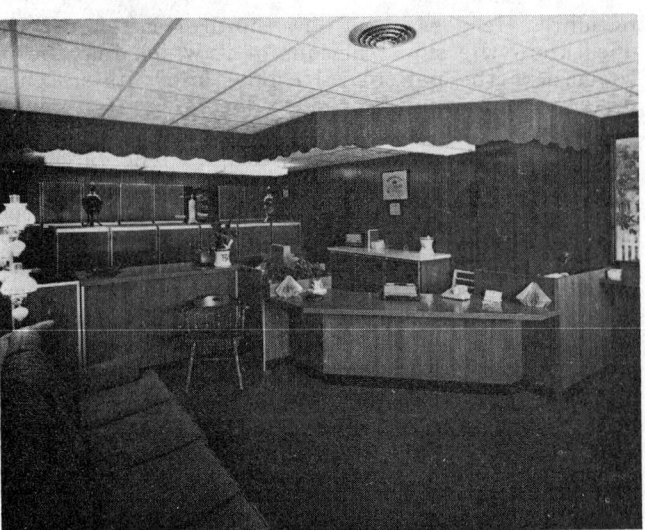

Fig. 7. Pharmaceutical Center (courtesy, McKesson & Robbins).

The pharmacist is in a unique position in the community. He is usually the best-educated and informed person on main street. He is the most "available" professional. No appointments are necessary to talk with him. He doesn't charge for his advice. This unique availability is appreciated and deserved by the public, but it is not always utilized to its fullest by the pharmacist as a means of service to the public.

The orientation of the pharmacist to the patient is often impersonal and businesslike. The patient is quick to sense this, and to form his impression of the pharmacist as a result. The "business" impression tags the pharmacist as a business man rather than a professional. One needs only to observe the functioning of a successful physician or attorney to know why they enjoy the prestige and confidence of people in general. In their functioning they have an intense *interest* in *you* and *your* problems—or they seem to. The *professional* pharmacist must also exhibit this interest and concern.

The physician sees his patient as a body of order and disorder. The attorney sees his client as an accumulation of personal and business assets and liabilities. The pharmacist should see his patient as a consumer of a multiplicity of drugs, the subject of numerous physician proddings and administrations. In this regard the pharmacist, like the physician and

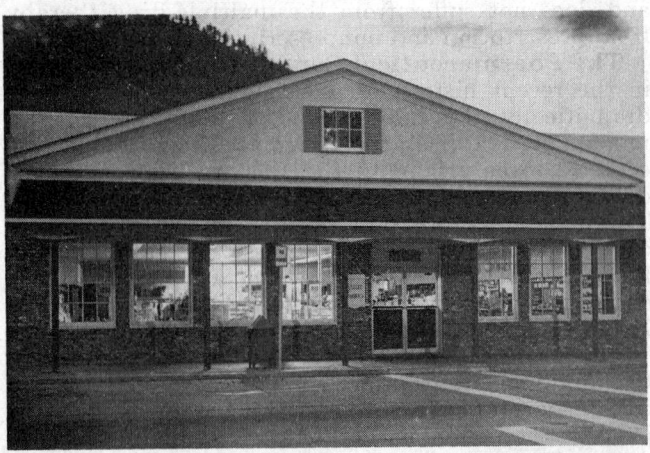

Fig. 8. Valley Pharmacy, Ron and Wayne Doane, owners, Cashmere, Wash. (population: 1,950).

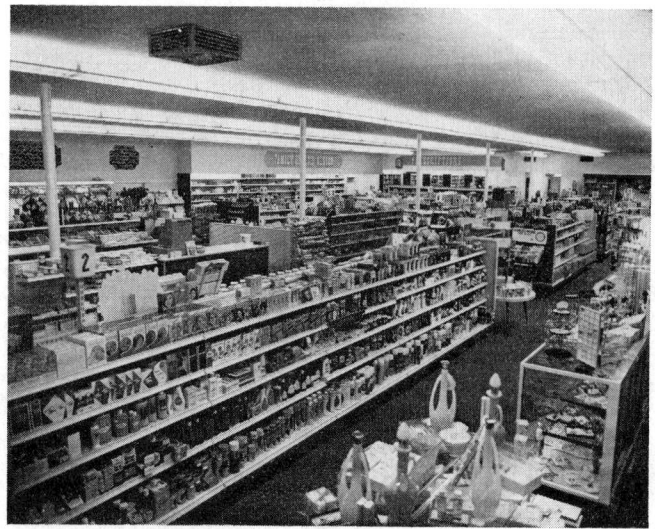

Fig. 9. Valley Pharmacy interior.

attorney, is unique. He sees one specialized aspect of a person's functioning. However, unlike the physician and attorney, he often does not put this information to use for the good of the patient or client.

The pharmacist *alone* knows what drugs a patient is taking—nonprescriptions, old prescriptions, new prescriptions, or multiple prescriptions from multiple physicians. In this age of specialization a patient may be seeing several physicians at one time. Physician's ethics, the reason for which seems somewhat obscure, seem to militate against mutual consultation on what each is doing for an individual patient. This often complicates the medication picture and may lead to serious drug interactions and untoward side effects. The *pharmacist knows this*. He must take steps in the patient's interest to use his drug knowledge to aid the physicians in their drug regimen for individual patients.

Another peculiarity of medical practice seems to be the lack of follow-up of patients. Unless a physician knows a patient very well he will usually make no effort to recontact a patient. The patient must always take the initiative to contact the physician. Often a patient may have a prescription refilled for years without the knowledge of the physician. The *pharmacist knows this*. Both the physician and patient should be informed of dangers which may result from such a practice. The pharmacist is in a unique position to recommend a revisit to a physician. Often that is all that is needed. There is a natural reluctance in all of us to go to a physician.

Not only can the pharmacist be of great value to the patient in suggesting revisits to a physician for medication purposes, but he also can be of great assistance to a person who needs a physician's care. Americans are an independent lot. They like "to do things themselves." Whether this be car repair, home repairs, building, or picture framing. The "do it yourself" industry is tremendous. The same applies to medication. A survey a few years ago indicated that about ⅓ of the people in the US got their health information from their neighbors!

Persons experiencing some physical problem often come first to the pharmacist. He is readily available and accessible. The individual may be only in need of advice or he may be in need of either minor or major medical attention. In any event the pharmacist can be of considerable value to the individual, and also of assistance to the physician. Minor complaints often can be helped with nonprescription items, thus saving the physician's time from unnecessary patient visitations.

Advice on *when* a patient should see a physician can be most valuable. Many patients wait too long, until their condition becomes so complex as to be dangerous to the patient and to require considerable time of the physician. In a conference at the Uni-

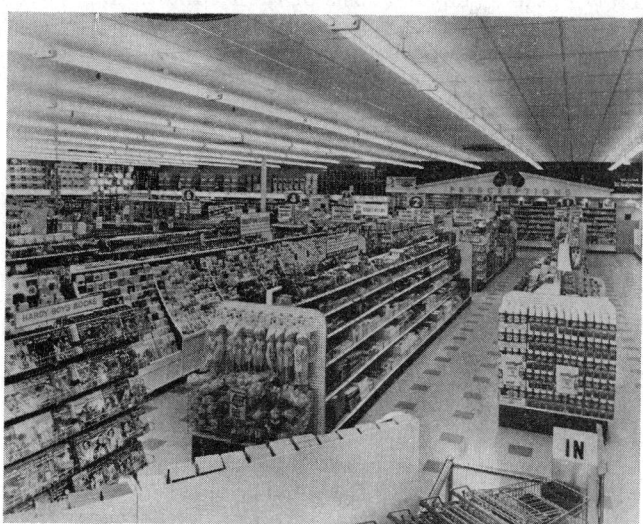

Fig. 11. Walgreen's Drugs, Tri-City Plaza, Gary, Ind.

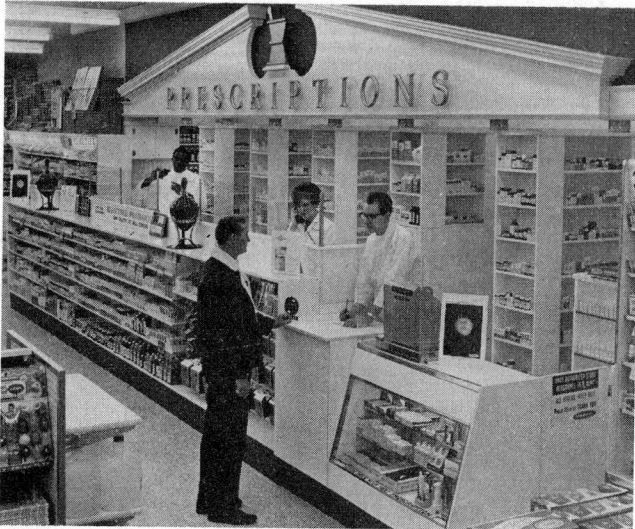

Fig. 12. Walgreen's Drugs, Pilsen Park Plaza Center, Chicago, Ill.

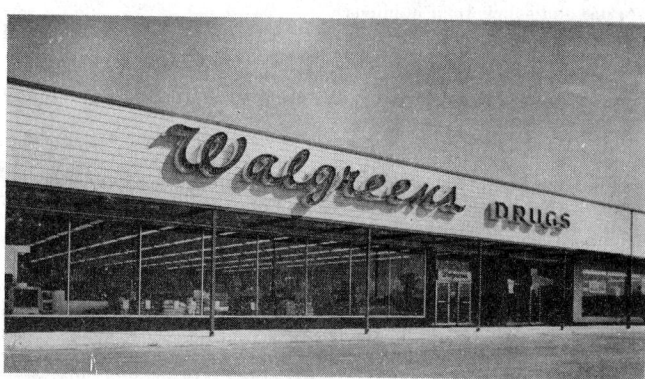

Fig. 10. Walgreen's Drugs, Mount Prospect, Ill.

versity of Michigan in 1967[8] it was recognized by physicians that the pharmacist can be of considerable assistance to the physician by intelligent screening of physical complaints of persons seeking the advice of the pharmacist. Often in the past the pharmacist has been reluctant to assume this responsibility. With his education properly oriented, the pharmacist can function efficiently in this regard.

The pharmacist is not a diagnostician, and his education will never be so oriented. Whereas, he cannot diagnose cancer, he can certainly inform others of the danger signs of cancer. The pharmacist's optimal functioning as a referral source will become even more critical as the physician shortage becomes more acute in the future.

The pharmacist can serve also as an important referral person to health facilities in a community as well as a referral agent to physicians. Few laymen know about and how to approach county, state, and federal health agencies. The effective utilization of these facilities can be enhanced greatly by a pharmacist who has the information regarding these facilities and recognizes in his patients the desirability of their use for persons in need of such agencies.

The *Survey of Sickness*[9] found that three out of four people who felt ill did not go to their physician. They made a self-diagnosis of their condition. There is evidence that such self-diagnosis can be disastrously wrong. Teeling-Smith pointed out that the pharmacist can be a most effective source of "health publicity." The APhA in an extensive survey[10] proved that pharmacists could be an effective source of information and literature regarding health.

As early as 1928 Surgeon General Cumming[11] recognized the important role pharmacists can play in educating the public in community health.

The usually strategic position and the familiar association of the drug store with medical matters in the popular mind place pharmacists in a position to render a material service to the community in connection with public health activities. It is the privilege, as well as the duty, of pharmacists to cooperate with public health agencies in the dissemination of reliable information concerning the public health and to assist the public health authorities especially as relates to communicable diseases and the protection of biological products.

It should be recognized that in any attempt at pharmacist–patient professional orientation there must be a genuine and personal interest by the pharmacist in the patient. Without such interest the association will be unsuccessful. In the words of the former Food and Drug Administration Commissioner Goddard,[12] the pharmacist must cooperate to see that the public is "well cared for—and *cared about.*"

Nursing Homes and Extended-Care Facilities

The US Public Health Service[13] defines a nursing home as "a facility or unit which is equipped for the accommodation of individuals not requiring hospital care but needing nursing care and related medical services."

The extended-care facilities are varied and essential as custodial institutions for those unable to care for themselves. They bridge the gap between nursing homes and self-care facilities.

The aged population in this country is about 20 million and increasing at the rate of about 1000 a day. Medicare and various forms of insurance provide hospitalization for large numbers of the aged population. This strain on hospital facilities finds partial respite with the growing nursing home and extended-care facilities. The future strain on hospital facilities will demand a tremendous increase in the number of hospitals but also a concomitant increase in nursing home and extended-care facilities.

Hospital pharmacy is the topic for another chapter, but nursing homes and extended-care facilities represent a relatively recent opportunity for the pharmacist to assure the intelligent utilization of drugs. This opportunity for the community pharmacist to be of service is discussed here in some detail. It is safe to say that in the near future every community will have one or more of these health facilities. It is the responsibility of the pharmacists in the community to make sure the persons in these facilities have efficient and supervised drug service. Thudium[14] has outlined the steps the pharmacist should take to institute properly supervised drug service in these health facilities:

Let me list some initial steps which can be taken in developing pharmacy service for your community hospital or extended care facility.

1. Determine how much time you are willing to devote to the institution or institutions on both a daily and weekly basis.

2. If possible, confer with or visit another pharmacist who is presently offering such services.

3. Write to national, state and local pharmaceutical associations to obtain information concerning pharmacy services in the smaller hospital or nursing home. Available from the American Pharmaceutical Association or the American Society of Hospital Pharmacists is the booklet, *Pharmaceutical Services in the Nursing Home*. Available from the American Society of Hospital Pharmacists are the following at a nominal cost:

a. *Minimum Standards for Pharmacies in Hospitals with a Guide to Application.*

b. *Statement on the Pharmacy and Therapeutics Committee.*

c. *Guidelines Relative to the Safe Use of Medications in Hospitals.*

d. *Regulations for Handling Narcotics.*

e. *Statement on Hospital Drug Distribution Systems.*

f. *Relationship between Smaller Hospitals and Part-time Pharmacists.*

These are a few of the publications you will find of help to you. You can get a complete list of publications and their cost by writing to the American Society of Hospital Pharmacists, 4630 Montgomery Avenue, Washington, D.C. 20014.

4. If possible, review pharmacy and hospital journals to find additional information concerning the need for pharmacy service in the small hospital and nursing home, and what services are being offered.

5. Develop your own concepts of what pharmacy service needs to be provided in your hospital and what services you would be able to provide.

6. Approach the hospital or nursing home administrator with a definite offer to organize a pharmacy service for him. Explain how you hope to improve the drug situation in his institution.

7. Make a personal survey of the hospital or nursing home, preferably with the administrator or the nursing supervisor; get a clear picture of its total operation.

8. Check all areas where medications are stored or used. Check all drug stock as to quantity and condition. An actual inventory may be advantageous in some cases. Determine disposition of outdated and obsolete products. Talk to nursing personnel to determine their opinions concerning the need for pharmacy service.

9. Contact physicians in the hospital whom you know from community practice, and present them with your ideas for pharmacy service and solicit their opinions.

10. Prepare a comprehensive plan for the pharmacy operation and present it to the administrator. Set up a working agreement which will recognize the pharmacist as the hospital agent for drug procurement and authorize him to control drug distribution in the hospital or nursing home.

11. If necessary, apply for a permit for the hospital pharmacy.

12. Sort out the drug stock and arrange it in a consistent and convenient manner. Consistency is particularly important if other people will have need to enter the pharmacy. If finances permit, build or install a small dispensing counter preferably with wall cabinets.

13. Arrange the stock at the nursing stations in uniform, properly labled containers. A list of the drugs stocked on the nursing station, if it applies, should be drawn up and posted.

14. Draw up a schedule of hours when pharmaceutical service will be provided, and outline a plan by which your retail pharmacy can be called for emergency items or information at other times.

15. Have a short meeting with the hospital or nursing home staff and explain the new arrangement. Your position and responsibilities should be formally announced.

Only the very large nursing homes and extended-care facilities will be able to employ a full-time pharmacist. The pharmacy service to these installations become a retail pharmacist's opportunity and responsibility.

The pharmacist's services to nursing homes and extended-care facilities have been outlined by William E. Dudley[15] of the Department of Health, Education, and Welfare:

Matters covered under the consulting role will be of interest to you—let me list some items the surveyor from the state health department will be making inquiry:

a. The automatic stop order policy on drug administration.

b. Control systems for (1) narcotics, (2) alcohol and spirituous liquors, and (3) barbiturate, amphetamine, and certain stimulant and depressant medications (medications controlled by the FDA Drug Abuse Act of 1965).

c. Controls on investigational drugs.

d. Handling of physicians' medication samples.

e. Policy on use of medication at patient's bedside. (Self-administration of medications by patients is *not* permitted except for emergency drugs on special orders of patient's physician or in a pre-discharge program under the supervision of licensed nurse.)

f. Emergency drug kits (contents and inspection procedure).

g. Period inspection of nursing station medication centers and type report required to insure—

(1) That external medications are kept apart from internal use drugs.

(2) That biological refrigerator has a thermometer, that temperature range of refrigerator is 35.5° to 50° Fahrenheit. (Ice cube section used for smallpox, yellow fever, measles, and polio vaccines, if stocked, and of types required below freezing storage.)

(3) That there are no out-dated medications (antibiotics, biologicals, etc.).

(4) That medication cabinets are kept locked.

(5) That metric-English weight and measure conversion charts are at each nursing station medication center.

(6) That working text references on drug uses, side effects, and contraindication, such as the American Hospital Formulary Service of the American Society of Hospital Pharmacists, are at nursing station medication centers.

h. Policy on medication labeling and changing containers (only by a pharmacist using light-resistant, tight containers).

i. Policy and procedure on removal of medications from pharmacy (or drug room) in the absence of the pharmacist (only by a nurse).

j. Policy and procedure on medications to be taken home by the patient (only on written authority of physician and only to use up supply already issued and properly labeled or sufficient to last until community pharmacy can be contacted).

k. Reporting adverse drug reactions to FDA or AMA.

l. Reporting medication errors.

m. Pharmacy or store room inventory control system including the dating of stocks on receipt.

n. Macroscopical (light-testing) examinations of parenterals (a good pharmacy practice).

o. Policy concerning additives to parenterals (by pharmacist only, if possible).

p. The creation and activities of the pharmacy and drug therapeutics committee including the keeping of written minutes of meetings (at least four meetings a year).

q. The establishment and maintenance of a formulary or drug list.

r. Fire control provisions, (1) alcohol vault, (2) types of fire extinguishers, (3) fire blankets, (4) fire sprinklers.

s. Qualifications of pharmacist (must be licensed in state, etc).

t. Policy on record-keeping (five years—federal statute).

u. Policy on poison control center communications and references. (How and whom to contact, etc.)

v. Audit of narcotics and other special drugs at nursing stations.

w. An "official" list of medical-drug abbreviations approved by the medical staff of the institution, such as, t.i.d., p.r.n., a.c., p.c., etc.

Besides these fundamental operating procedures the pharmacist can assist these health-care facilities in many other helpful ways. These have been outlined by Kabat and associates.[16,17] The nonresident community pharmacist can provide same-day prescription delivery service, immediate emergency delivery service, telephone consultation service for staff, 24-hour on-call service and pick-up of written orders and prescriptions. The pharmacist can establish personal contact with the physicians for needed

prescription renewal authorizations, provide in-person conferences with the nursing staff regarding drug problems, institute conferences with administration or medical staff to establish medication policies, provide drug reference source material for use in the facility, and prepare sterile irrigating solutions.

A truly ambitious pharmacist can make himself a most welcome asset to an extended-care facility by providing such services as extending credit to the facility and individual occupants, supplying equipment and sundries information, providing a shopping service for residents (candy and reading material are much appreciated). The personal acquaintance of the pharmacist with the residents can provide an excellent means of determining their needs for both materials and consultation.

Problems in Pharmacy Practice

Pharmacy, like any profession, has its problems. Those mentioned here are limited to those not mentioned elsewhere in this chapter but still having a direct bearing on the practice of pharmacy itself.

Continuing Education—Pharmacy has not really seriously faced up to the problem of continuing education. The rapid advances in medicine and in drug therapy dictate that the pharmacist keep abreast of developments in his science after his formal education is completed. To do otherwise is to deny his patients full benefits of modern science. As Bowers has said,[18] "Nothing less than the welfare of the profession and the health of the public is involved."

Colleges of pharmacy have offered token practical services and considerable lip service to this problem. Many have provided seminars or symposia once or twice a year. These have been mixed bags of heterogeneous subject matter. Enrollment usually has been small, with justification. They accomplished little. Extension courses have met with some success—either correspondence courses or courses brought to the vicinity of the pharmacists.

The colleges are not wholly to blame for this failure of continuing education—they have tried to do it on a shoestring, both as far as money and personnel. A major effort in this area needs to be made, possibly with national coordination and guidance. The program will require a great deal of money. Every new method of instruction should be evaluated as a possible means of promoting this program: closed-circuit TV, video tapes, telephone lectures, taped lectures, programed correspondence courses, coordinated lecture series, distributive newsletters, and literature search and review services.

Until such times as continuing education is truly a *continuing* education, the pharmacist will function at a level below what reasonably can be expected of him as a public servant acting in the best health interests of the public.

The preparation for a lifetime of continuing education must begin while the student is in college. He must be given the responsibility while a student to learn the tools and techniques of self-education. Cartter[19] has underlined this need in his statement, "The standard commencement ceremony, with its invitation to lifelong self-education, has too often been an initiation ceremony for which the initiates have no real preparation."

The Professional Fee and Third-Party Payment—In the rapidly developing US there developed in its early history a type of pharmacy practice which was unique—and necessary. Sparse population made prescription pharmacies economically unfeasible. Merchandise became the economic backstop for the pharmacist. The relationship of this merchandise to health and drugs was sometimes real, sometimes not. Often the needs of the community determined the inventory. After all, the commercial outlets in frontier America were few. The American pharmacist has been loathe to give up the economic backstop of "up-front" merchandise. Just as he has too often spent an inordinate amount of his time with up-front things, so his orientation toward prescription drugs has been commodity-oriented. Prescriptions have been priced on the cost of the commodity. It has been recognized only recently that he, unlike any other professional, has been selling "things" and giving away his most valuable property—his professional expertise of drugs. This expertise is in no way related to the price of the drug.

As the necessity in more populated areas for the merchandise-prescription dual-purpose store diminishes, this country has witnessed the advent of the supermarket drugstore, the cut-rate drugstore, and other mass merchandisers. The community pharmacist has lost ground in his attempts to successfully compete with these operations. He will probably continue to do so. His recourse is to a greater involvement in prescription practice and the professional promotion of expertise on drugs and de-emphasis of his product orientation. By emphasizing his professional function to the public and other members of the health team, he is on firm ground to charge a professional fee for prescriptions. This should be a common fee for all prescriptions regardless of cost to him. The products would be dispensed at cost plus a set professional fee determined on the basis of the cost of the operation of his pharmacy, including professional services rendered. The rationale of this practice is presented in an excellent article by Myers,[20] and in other articles by Myers.[21-24]

This country has seen only the beginning of health insurance plans which include prescriptions and the involvement of the state and federal government in this "third-party" payment trend for prescriptions and other health services. Vendor payments for prescribed drugs under Medicaid and welfare programs jumped from about $146 million in the year ending June 30, 1966, to $182 million for the 12-month period ending June 30, 1967.[25] Nearly 3.3 million people are enrolled in programs with prescription drug coverage.[26] Whether private or public, these plans will continue to insist on getting prescriptions priced at the lowest possible denomination. The pharmacist in the future more than ever will need to justify his profits on prescriptions. His most legitimate recourse is his professional fee for professional services he renders. He will be forced to become service-oriented rather than product-oriented. This well may be the most effective catalyst to his functioning more effectively in the area for which he is best trained—professional service.

Pharmacy Technicians—There is no question that health manpower will be a critically short commodity in the future. Whether pharmacists will be in that category is yet to be proved. Yet, there is a segment of the profession which believes we must have technicians trained to help the pharmacist. Just what he will do is as yet undefined. However, everyone seems disturbed that his functions will neither be adequately defined nor contained. Some educators

believe that colleges of pharmacy should train these technicians before community colleges pre-empt the privilege and pharmaceutical education has no control. Others believe that pharmaceutical education should have no part of the training. Some legalists believe that any technician produced should be licensed; others believe that to license would only give a foothold to prerogatives which would go beyond training.

As the controversy continues one can only suggest that someone define what a technician is supposed to do before one attempts to determine whether he should do it or be licensed to do it. This would also determine what formal training he should have (if any) and hence how it should be recognized (licensed?). However, the need for such a technician has not been shown and one wonders why the need for the discussion prevails.

This author can only advise that the community pharmacist's greatest need is to concentrate more on his professional functions and less on merchandising. In so doing he could make better use of his time and education. If he needs a technician he might consider training him to sell those items out front which don't need his expertise. He also might spend some time recruiting students for pharmaceutical education. The colleges are far from full of top-notch students!

The pharmaceutical profession might be advised to gain a lesson from nursing. It has three categories of registered nurses (associate, diploma, and baccalaureate)—all are RN's, and their problems have multiplied rather than diminished as a result of recognizing various levels of education. It will take generations to bring up the educational standards in nursing to where they should be.

Pharmaceutical education and pharmaceutical practice have been on the upward path for many years. The profession should be wary of vested interests who may wish to see pharmacy's future prostituted for selfish gain.

The Future of Pharmacy and Professional Trends

I think a keynote for the function of pharmacy might be best expressed in the words of Surgeon General Stewart:[27] "We have more to offer than we are delivering. We have more people to serve than we are serving."

Bernzweig of the USPHS has placed the responsibility for the future of pharmacy in more direct terms:[28]

Apparently, the major affliction facing pharmacists . . . is a disease of near epidemic proportions, which might be labeled *professional inertia*. Its chief symptom is a general attitude of indifference to what is going on . . . unfortunately, too many community pharmacists today . . . just don't seem to care. This laissez-faire attitude poses a real danger, for unless these individuals begin to enlarge their horizons and strive for greater professional identity not only their *skills* but their *services* will soon become obsolete!

The increase in this country's population at a rapid rate is a certainty. The shortage of personnel in many health professions is also a certainty. This shortage will be particularly critical in the medical profession. The health professions will need to find answers to the problem of treating those who are ill and advising those who are well. To do this the health professionals will need to start talking to each other more often and more productively. There will need to be a realignment of responsibilities and a coordination of those responsibilities. The maximum use will need to be made of the education and experience of all in the health professions. Pharmacists should not let this challenge go unheeded.

It has been mentioned before in this chapter that the pharmacist will need to change his orientation from product to patient. The physician seeks a patient as an organism of functioning and malfunctioning parts. The pharmacist should see the patient as a consumer of a multiplicity of drugs and respondent to those drugs. The pharmacist of the future must emerge as a consultant on drugs to the public. He must maintain current records of his patients which indicate the total regimen of drug consumption by the patient, both prescribed and non-prescribed drugs. The records must further indicate any untoward reactions of these patients to drugs and/or physical conditions which preclude the use of certain drugs.

The pharmacist of the future will need to take a more active role in health education of the public. He is the most accessible of all health professionals and is in the position of knowing most about the patient's general health problems, and even his economic status, which may have a direct bearing on his total health. His pharmacy can effectively serve as a distribution center for the free literature made available by a multiplicity of health agencies. The pharmacist can serve as an effective referral agent for patients in need of county, state, and federal health units.

In case of disaster the pharmacist should be prepared in supplies and technical orientation to be an effective source of assistance in emergencies and recognize his responsibilities to organized disaster programs.

The pharmacist of the future should take a more active role in poison control programs. He should be the most readily accessible source of emergency information and be able to use organized poison control centers for the most efficient benefit of those in need of such services.

The pharmacist should take full advantage of his potential to be of assistance to nursing homes and other extended-care facilities so that they have the appropriate pharmaceutical services.

These are some of the opportunities which await the community pharmacist in the immediate future. The opportunities for greater service open to hospital pharmacists are discussed in Chapter 93, *Hospital Pharmacy.*

The Pharmacy and Its Products

Personnel and Drug Statistics

The National Association of Boards of Pharmacy[29] estimates that there are 121,500 licensed pharmacy practioners in the US. Of these approximately 85% are in community pharmacy practice, 8% in hospital pharmacy practice, and the rest in education, manufacturing, or other pursuits.

In this chapter we have been concerned primarily with the community pharmacist. Community pharmacy viewed on a nationwide scale is big business. In 1968 pharmacists working in US drugstores filled 1,179,470,000 prescriptions.[30] This record high exceeded the 1967 sum by 7.6% and by more than 83 million prescriptions. The average retail price of a prescription rose 2.7% in 1968 over the 1967 figures ($3.41 in 1968 compared to $3.32 in 1967). This amounted to an increase in total prescription sales of more than $385,000,000 for a one-year total of

Table I—Number of Prescriptions Filled in US Pharmacies—1963–1968

	All Pharmacies			
	Total R̸ (000)	New R̸ (000)	Refills (000)	Refill ratio
1968....	1,179,470	527,880	651,590	55.3
1967....	1,096,280	490,910	605,370	55.2
1966....	1,025,870	466,080	559,790	54.6
1965....	964,780	426,850	537,930	55.8
1964....	875,760	403,620	472,140	53.9
1963....	823,200	388,180	435,020	52.8
% Change 1968				
vs 1967	Up 7.6%	Up 7.5%	Up 7.6%	
vs 1963	Up 43.3%	Up 36.0%	Up 49.8%	

	Average Pharmacy			
	Average R̸ expenditure	Total R̸	New R̸	Refills
1968....	3.41	22,960	10,280	12,680
1967....	3.32	21,170	9,480	11,690
1966....	3.26	19,660	8,930	10,730
1965....	3.20	18,240	8,070	10,170
1964....	3.12	16,510	7,610	8,900
1963....	3.09	15,370	7,250	8,120
% Change 1968				
vs 1967	Up 2.7%	Up 8.5%	Up 8.4%	Up 8.5%
vs 1963	Up 10.4%	Up 49.4%	Up 41.8%	Up 56.2%

$4,024,630,000. These statistics compared to the last six-year totals are in Table I.

These figures show that in just five years between 1963 and 1968 the average US pharmacy filled 49.4% more prescriptions (15,370 in 1963 and 22,960 in 1968) and increased prescription dollar sales by 65.1% ($47,460 in 1963 and $78,350 in 1968).

The total sales in pharmacies in 1968 exceeded $12 billion. The figure given is $12,065,000,000.[31] Sales broken down by types of stores for 1967 and 1968 are shown in Table II. The breakdown of sales for 1967 classified into general categories is shown in Table III.

Evolution and Trends

The American pharmacy has been a unique entity which has developed out of a necessity for multipurpose community needs in a rapidly growing frontier country. There are many who question the need for such multipurpose establishments in a rapidly urbanizing country. There are many who say, with some justification, that the professional training of a pharmacist is wasted on merchandising nondrug items. It is predicted that there will be fewer pharmacies in the future which combine merchandising and prescription service. This will be particularly obvious in areas of population concentration. The Pacific area of the US with its rapid growth of population is a microcosm of this trend. Table IV[33] illustrates population trends in the next decade. Table V[34] shows the location of pharmacies by types.

It has been estimated that there will be fewer pharmacies per capita in the future[35] and that the ratio of pharmacy owners to employed pharmacists will change with the number of employed pharmacists increasing in proportion to pharmacy owners. This is an expected trend with the larger number of prescription stores being opened.

It is predicted that there will be a gradual increase in the Pharmaceutical Center-type operation with the emphasis on patient orientation of the pharmacist.

Table II—Pharmacy Sales by Independents[a] and Chains[b] 1967–1968

	1968	1967	% Change 1968 vs 1967
Total Sales			
All pharmacies....	$12,065,000,000	$11,102,800,000	Up 8.7%
Independents...	8,051,000,000	7,522,150,000	Up 7.0%
Chains........	4,014,000,000	3,580,650,000	Up 12.1%
Chain %	33.3%	32.2%	...
Number of Stores			
All pharmacies....	51,369	51,657	Down 0.6%
Independents....	44,695	45,320	Down 1.4%
Chains........	6,674	6,337	Up 5.3%
Chain %.....	13.0%	12.3%	...
Sales per store			
All pharmacies....	$ 234,870	$ 214,930	Up 9.3%
Independents....	180,130	165,980	Up 8.5%
Chains........	601,440	565,040	Up 6.4%

[a] Units of 1, 2, and 3 store companies.
[b] Stores of companies operating 4 or more pharmacies.

Table III—Summary of 1967 Sales of Drugs

Departments	Spending in all outlets	Spending in pharmacies only	% of total store	% pharmacy to total spending
(Add 000 to all dollar figures)				
Drugs; other health aids:				
Prescriptions....................	$ 3,932,020	$ 3,639,460	32.78	93
Packaged medication.............	2,268,800	1,474,190	13.28	65
Prescription accessories...........	268,090	107,660	.97	40
First aid........................	205,860	116,040	1.05	56
Foot products....................	88,620	53,960	.48	61
Baby needs......................	306,750	160,760	1.45	52
Feminine needs..................	344,110	144,410	1.30	42
Veterinary......................	280,360	82,480	.74	29
Dieting aids....................	149,080	55,590	.50	37
Subtotal....................	$ 7,843,690	$ 5,834,550	52.55	..
Duplication..................	361,300	326,300	2.94	..
Subtotal for drugs, other health aids..........	$ 7,482,390	$ 5,508,250	49.61	74
Toiletries:				
Oral hygiene....................	$ 688,790	$ 203,800	1.84	30
Hair products...................	1,307,210	454,260	4.09	35
Shaving products................	745,880	243,800	2.20	33
Hand products..................	186,360	63,210	.57	34
Cosmetics......................	830,950	244,370	2.20	29
Other toiletries.................	1,777,790	233,060	2.10	13
Subtotal for toiletries..............	$ 5,536,980	$ 1,442,500	13.00	26
Total for drugs, other health aids, toiletries.....	$13,019,370	$ 6,950,750	62.61	53
Other products:				
Home sanitation.................	$ 241,010	$ 45,390	.41	19
Household supplies...............	522,400	45,870	.42	9
Stationery......................	1,634,460	266,100	2.40	16
Magazines and newspapers........	2,186,850	356,150	3.21	16
Photographic....................	2,196,210	704,190	6.34	32
Sundries.......................	3,899,010	381,290	3.43	10
Household glassware..............	309,700	11,960	.10	4
Subtotal for other products..................	$10,989,640	$ 1,810,950	16.31	16
Fountain and luncheonette......................	$ 2,792,080	$ 415,300	3.74	15
Packaged ice cream.............................	$ 955,890	$ 54,090	.49	6
Candy, tobacco:				
Confectionery....................	$ 3,087,070	$ 256,490	2.31	8
Tobacco and accessories.............	7,990,870	814,250	7.33	10
Subtotal for confectionery, tobacco, and accessories	$11,077,940	$ 1,070,740	9.64	10
Alcoholic beverages............................	$14,043,420	$ 168,320	1.51	1
Subtotal for pharmacy products and services individually listed above.....................	$52,878,340	$10,470,150	94.30	20
Unclassified..................................	nd	632,650	5.70	nd
Grand Total..............................	...	$11,102,800	100.00	..

Table IV—Important Population Trends in Future Decade 1970–1980[a]

	Total pop. increases	Increases in young homemakers 18–24 age group	Increase in people 65 and over
Total US	17%	20%	18%
New England	15%	20%	12%
Middle Atlantic	13	19	17
East Central	14	17	14
West Central	15	20	9
Southeast	19	16	28
Southwest	17	18	20
Pacific	28	29	29

[a] Bureau of Census figures.

This trend will see its greatest development when pharmaceutical education reorients its curricula to more patient-oriented education.

A very realistic review of pharmacy as it is and as it will need to become is presented in a recent publication of the US Dept. of Health, Education and Welfare.[36]

Table V—Locations of New Pharmacies

	100%	100%
In separate locations	45%	34%
In shopping centers	32%	36%
Prescription shops in all locations	13%	19%
In mass merchandisers	6%	7%
In super markets	4%	4%
	1966	1st 6 months 1967

References

1. White, A. I., *The Washington-Alaska Pharmacist*, **9** (9), 8 (1967).
2. *The Lilly Digest*, Eli Lilly & Co., Indianapolis, Ind., 1968, p. 62.
3. *33rd Annual Nielsen Review of Retail Drug Store Trends*, A. C. Nielsen Co., Chicago, 1967, p. 29.
4. Hager, G. P., *J. APhA*, **NS5**, 72 (1965).
5. Gibson, M. R., *J. APhA*, **NS6**, 632 (1966).
6. *The APhA Newsletter*, **7** (12), 1 (1968).
7. White, E. V., *J. APhA*, **NS5**, 532 (1965).
8. Deno, R. A., ed., *Proceedings, Pharmacy-Medicine-Nursing Conference on Health Education*, Univ. of Michigan, 1967.
9. Teeling-Smith, G., *J. APhA*, **NS6**, 22 (1966).
10. Griffenhagen, G. B., *The Pharmacy as a Health Education Center*, APhA, Washington D.C. 1964.
11. Cumming, H. S., *J. APhA*, **17**, 325 (1928).
12. Goddard, J. L., *J. APhA*, **NS6**, 358 (1966).
13. *Nursing Home Standards Guide*, US Dept. of Health, Education and Welfare, Washington, D.C., 1961, p. 1.
14. Thudium, V. F., *Pharmacy Services in Nursing Homes and Smaller Hospitals*, Proceedings of the Conference, Univ. of Michigan, 1966, p. 51.
15. Dudley, W. E., *Proceedings of District 8, AACP-NABP*, 1966, p. 34.
16. Herath, J. H., and Kabat, H. F., *J. APhA*, **NS5**, 315 (1965).
17. Bertin, R. J., and Kabat, H. F., *J. APhA*, **NS7**, 626 (1967).
18. Bowers, R. A., *Am. J. Pharm. Educ.*, **23**, 4 (1959).
19. Cartter, A. M., in Lee, C. B. T., ed., *Improving College Teaching*, Am. Council on Educ., Washington, D.C., 1967, p. 113.
20. Myers, M. J., *Am. J. Pharm.*, **140**, 101 (1968).
21. Myers, M. J., *J. APhA*, **NS8**, 628 (1968).
22. Myers, M. J., *J. APhA*, **NS8**, 632 (1968).
23. Myers, M. J., *J. APhA*, **NS8**, 636 (1968).
24. Myers, M. J., *J. APhA*, **NS8**, 639 (1968).
25. *Weekly Pharmacy Reports (The Green Sheet)*, **17** (47), 1 (1968).
26. *Digest of Drug Prescription Programs (Public Health Publ. 1489)*, US Govt. Printing Office, Washington, D.C., 1966, p. 2.
27. Stewart, W. H., *J. APhA*, **NS7**, 366 (1967).
28. Bernzweig, E. P., *Bull. Ontario Coll. Pharm.*, **XVII**(4), 61 (1968).
29. *Licensure Statistics and Census of Pharmacy*, Natl. Assoc. of Boards of Pharm., Chicago, Jan. 1, 1968.
30. Leibson, R. A., *Drug Topics*, **113**, 38 (Feb. 3, 1969).
31. Leibson, R. A., *Drug Topics*, **113**, 40 (Jan. 6, 1969).
32. Leibson, R. A., *Drug Topics*, **112**, 38 (Aug. 5, 1968).
33. *33rd Nielsen Review of Retail Drug Store Trends*, A. C. Nielsen Co., Chicago, Illinois, 1967, p. 22.
34. *33rd Nielsen Review of Retail Drug Store Trends*, A. C. Nielsen Co., Chicago, 1967, p. 24.
35. Deno, R. A., *et al*, *The Profession of Pharmacy*, 2nd ed., Lippincott, 1966, p. 238.
36. *The Drug Makers and the Drug Distributors*, US Dept. of Health, Education, and Welfare, US Govt. Printing Office, Washington, D.C., 1968.

5 | Pharmacists in Industry

Current therapeutics—profile of the industry—utilization of
pharmacists—research and development—pharmaceutical analysis and
control—pharmaceutical production—pharmaceutical sales—related
fields—education for industry—on-the-job training—salary—summary

This chapter was prepared by

Jack Cooper, PhG, *Consultant, Pharmacy Research and Development,
Sandoz, Ltd., Basle, Switzerland*

The historical role of the pharmacist in industry,
like that of the profession in general, is characterized
by a shifting blend of traditionalism and dynamism.
The earliest written records clearly demonstrate the
ingenuity and imagination with which our ancestors
utilized animal, vegetable, and mineral sources in providing a diversified armamentarium of therapeutic
agents. For thousands of years empiricism remained
the primary working tool of drug formulators whether
dressed in priestly or secular garments. Before the
practice of scientific pharmacy and rational therapy
could energetically move ahead, the experimental
philosophy of Claude Bernard,[1] as related to the accomplishments of organic chemistry, required general
acceptance. The scientific discoveries of the 19th
century provided the foundation upon which a progressive pharmaceutical industry could be built. Successful isolation of the active principles of botanical
drugs, the synthesis of coal-tar derivatives, and engineering advances in machinery were primary factors
in this development. Although the introduction of
arsphenamine in 1910 ushered in the chemotherapeutic
era, it was the discovery of the chemical effect of the
sulfonamides a quarter of a century later which destroyed the remaining influence of the therapeutic
nihilists and revolutionized the practice of medicine
and pharmacy.

As the experimental range and scientific precision
of pharmacologists, microbiologists, and biochemists
accelerated, the industrial pharmacist engaged in the
formulation of drug preparations found it necessary to
broaden the multidisciplinary foundation of his
training and to redirect his methodology from empirical compounding to experimentally developed compositions geared to therapeutic objectives. Rapid advances in analytical techniques and instrumentation
have had profound effects upon the training and practice of pharmacists serving in analytical and control
positions in the pharmaceutical industry.

The impact of social and economic change upon the
industry and industrial pharmacists has been, and will
continue to be, of the greatest importance. With alterations in the mode of medical practice, government
regulation, and health care payment schemes, the role
of industrial pharmacists in every aspect of professional activity cannot be expected to remain unaltered.
This chapter focuses upon pharmacists in industry
utilizing facts and attitudes obtained directly from
many educators and specialists, as well as from recently published documents.

Current Therapeutics

Although the key role played by drugs in the extension of life expectancy and in the alleviation of a host
of distressing symptoms accompanying minor or
chronic illness is generally recognized, it is only occasionally that one comes across physicians or even pharmacists who are conscious of the range and scope of
scientific collaboration involved in the development of
modern pharmaceuticals. The contributions of academic and industrial laboratories have been of the
greatest importance to drug research with each supporting and complementing the other. Even at the
level of quality the standards and accomplishments
are equivalent and when this fact is accepted collaboration between industry and universities operates
smoothly and efficiently, with public health the beneficiary of such interdependent association.

The organization and resources of industrial laboratories permit the planning and carrying out of specific
projects. The synthesis of large numbers of compounds, the highly organized mass biological screening
for pharmacological activity or toxicity, and the application of pharmacy research skills along diversified
dosage-form lines cannot be effectively pursued by
academic laboratories.

The productive, lifesaving, life-enhancing role of the
pharmaceutical industry during the past century is
spasmodically recognized and applauded, but unfortunately public opinion in this regard has recently
been distorted by the play of powerful economic, social, and political forces. The role of government in
controlling the content and quality of the available
therapeutic armamentarium has steadily increased,
and the total impact of the passage of the Kefauver–
Harris amendments to the Federal Food, Drug and
Cosmetic Act remains to be seen. The challenge imposed by stricter requirements relative to demonstrating the safety and efficacy of drugs has initiated
powerful efforts by industry scientists to evolve new
concepts and tools capable of attaining such objectives. Increasing recognition of biopharmaceutics as
a field of study representing the effort to link the
physical properties of a chemical substance and its pharmaceutical milieu—ie, the dosage form—with observed biological effects has enlarged the contributions
which the pharmacist can make to modern therapeutics. More than ever the patient remains the focus of
attention at all levels of pharmacist participation in
the development, production, and control of pharmaceutical preparations.

Profile of the Industry

The pharmaceutical industry is made up of approximately 1000 companies varying widely in plant size,
volume of business, and number of employees. Total
employment in the drug industry in 1966 was estimated to be almost 127,000. During the same year,

sales of prescription products reached $4.7 billion, with about 25% representing foreign sales by US-based companies. Although the sales of almost all therapeutic classes of pharmaceutical preparations have shown a steady increase over the past 5 years, the availability of new drugs for the treatment of cardiovascular, endocrine, neoplastic, and central nervous system diseases provided the greatest impetus for the growth of the prescription products' market.

In 1964, when the industry's investment in research and development was approximately $300 million, a National Science Foundation report[2] indicated that the drug industry was a leader among US industries in this area of investment. Two years later, research and development expenditures directed towards the discovery and introduction of new drugs in human and veterinary medicine passed the $400 million mark. This rapid increase in research and development costs did not result in a corresponding rise in new drug introductions. Probably as a direct consequence of requirements imposed by the New Drug Regulations of 1962 only 92 new drugs (single chemical entities) were permitted to reach the US market during the five year period from 1962–1966. During the preceding 5-year period 261 new drugs were introduced.

An increase of research and development expenditures to $476 million during 1967 demonstrated that the reaction of the industry to this decreased ratio of new drug introduction to expenditures has not been cost reduction but rather an effort to increase efficiency by improved administrative procedures. Strong pressure on drug prices by various governmental agencies has stimulated some pharmaceutical companies to enter into such diversified fields as medical instrumentation, hospital and laboratory supplies, and optics. In some of these businesses, as well as the older allied fields of proprietaries and cosmetics, the training of the pharmacist provides a sound basis for additional career opportunities.

Utilization of Pharmacists

The composition of the work force in the pharmaceutical industry is unusually diversified. Individuals trained in a variety of scientific disciplines and trades, professionals requiring licensure, and experts in business practices are essential elements in the companies developing, manufacturing, and distributing the bulk of prescription drugs.

Precise data concerning the number of pharmacists in active practice and their distribution in terms of career opportunities are not available. Multiple-state registration and practice in some types of pharmaceutical service without registration tend to confuse the statistical picture. More reliable and useful information will be available upon the completion of the "Survey of Pharmacy Manpower" by the National Association of Boards of Pharmacy.

Out of a national total of 122,421, a relatively recent compilation[3] lists 4496 registered pharmacists engaged in manufacturing or wholesale activities. Estimates based on other sources indicate that the actual number of graduate pharmacists in industry is probably twice that figure.

As a consequence of the large differences in company size, research involvement, product line, and type of distribution there exists considerable variability in the utilization of pharmacists within the industry. Although precise figures are not available at this time, a rough estimate would indicate that approximately

Table I—Pharmacy Graduates Classified by Type of Technical Work and Educational Level

	BS	MS	PhD	Totals
Research and development	96	42	45	183
Production	128	10	9	147
Quality control	65	3	1	69
Totals	289	55	55	399
% of total	72	14	14	

three-fourths of all graduate pharmacists employed in industry are engaged in nontechnical areas such as marketing or administration. The remainder are involved almost exclusively in research and development, production, and quality control. The proportion of pharmacists in each of these technical occupations is illustrated in Table I. These figures were obtained at the end of 1968 from seven pharmaceutical companies representing a mixture of two firms with an annual sales volume under $50 million; two firms with an annual sales volume of $50–100 million; and three firms with an annual sales volume exceeding $100 million.

Research and Development

In spite of some recent efforts to publicize the facts, the public in general and a large sector of practicing professionals remain unaware of the interdisciplinary nature of pharmaceutical research and tend to associate progress in therapeutics with the medical profession alone. This distortion of the true nature of the complex scientific and technological basis for modern drug development undoubtedly inhibits the entrance of qualified pharmacists into the ranks of research workers in the pharmaceutical industry.

The sequence of events leading towards the evolution of a new drug from synthesis to approval for marketing by the Food and Drug Administration is a long but necessary one. En route an observer will meet chemists, a variety of biologists, pharmacists, and, towards the end of the journey, physicians. Although group or team research has become respectable even in some academic institutions, it is the pharmaceutical industry which provides an outstanding example of a diversity of scientific skills united and directed towards the achievement of therapeutic goals.

A 1969 estimate of industry personnel engaged in research and development based upon extrapolation from 1965 data[4] shows that out of a total research and development staff comprising 19,000 individuals, approximately 10,500 are scientists and professionals; the remainder represent technicians and supporting personnel. About 10% of the scientific–professional group are classified as employed in pharmacy or pharmaceutical chemistry; 40% in the biological sciences; 30% as chemists; with the remainder divided among physicians, research administrators, engineers, and other types of specialists. Since some scientists in the chemical and biological groups are pharmacists, a total of 1200–1500 pharmacy-trained individuals employed in research and development would probably represent a more accurate estimate.

The composition of the research and development staff, and the proportional representation of the disciplines and professions which comprise it, depend on current interests and programs in pharmaceutical research, of which the following are the most important:

1. The synthesis of new compounds directed towards their utilization as drugs.

2. The isolation and purification of the active principles of plant and animal tissues and organs; the determination of their chemical composition and eventual synthesis.

3. Research on the cultivation of medicinal plants.

4. Research on the pharmacodynamics and toxicology of new drugs.

5. The biological, chemical, and physical standardization of drugs.

6. The preparation of drugs in dosage forms designed and tested to attain the therapeutic objective.

The preponderance of chemists, pharmacologists, biochemists, microbiologists, and other non-pharmacist specialists in an industry which represents an outgrowth of pharmacy is surprising but can be deduced from an investigation[5] of pharmacy education and organization since the turn of the century. However, as a result of the diverse training directed towards an understanding of therapeutic agents and their mode of use, the pharmacist is ideally suited for so-called "product development" in the pharmaceutical industry. Indeed, it is in this area of pharmacy research and development where the majority of technically oriented pharmacists can be found. As part of an effective pharmacy research group these scientists are busy with many basic and applied problems. Expressed in broad terms the following areas best illustrate their role:

1. Establishment of those physicochemical properties of drug substances and dosage forms which will influence their uniformity, stability, and physiological availability.

2. Development of the final formula and full-scale manufacturing process for all forms of administration of new drugs.

3. The improvement of existing formulas and processes in terms of quality or cost on the basis of scientific investigation.

4. The evaluation of new raw materials—ie, excipients, solvents, preservatives, etc. — with potential value in pharmaceutical formulation.

5. The preparation, packaging, and control of new drugs during the entire period of clinical investigation.

6. The scientific investigation of the stability and recommended storage conditions for all new products.

7. The scientific investigation of the merits and faults of new equipment preliminary to routine use in pharmaceutical production.

8. The investigation of the suitability of proposed packaging materials and containers.

The combination of an accelerated rate of technological progress and governmental intervention has made it crystal clear that empiric formulation and classic processing methods are no longer acceptable. Although group organization allows for variability in educational background and specific experience, the modern research pharmacist finds himself in a weak position unless his knowledge of a variety of disciplines remains adequate for his role. This does not mean that he need be an expert in these scientific areas, but it is difficult to see how he can manage without more than a nodding acquaintance with anatomy, physiology, pharmacology, biochemistry, bacteriology, analytical and physical chemistry, and, of course, advanced mathematics.

The combination of curiosity and perseverance supported by an analytical, logical mind provides the personality basis for successful performance in research and development. In addition, the ability to organize flexible but scientifically sound research protocols, to work easily and effectively with others, and to utilize communications skills efficiently represent attributes of great value in the complex research and development organizations within the pharmaceutical industry.

Education beyond the baccalaureate level is obviously advantageous in view of the multidisciplinary core of pharmacy research and development activi-

Table II—Pharmacy Graduates Classified by Educational Level
Research and Development (all phases)

	BS	MS	PhD	Totals
	2	0	1	3
	2	1	3	6
	6	2	7	15
	10	6	9	25
	13	13	8	34
	22	14	13	49
	41	6	4	51
Totals	96	42	45	183
% of Total	52	23	25	

ties. The present status of advanced degree programs as related to industrial pharmacy is discussed in a subsequent section of this chapter.

Although advancement to leadership positions is often related to the extent of educational training, opportunities in research and development exist for all levels of pharmacists.

A survey in 1968 of two small, two medium, and three large pharmaceutical companies demonstrates the relationship between educational level of pharmacists and the number employed in the research and development departments. The data are listed in Table II.

Pharmaceutical Analysis and Control

The important contributions made by pharmaceutical analysts in the development of new drug substances and dosage forms have received increasing recognition during the past decade. The enormous range of medicinal substances in terms of chemical structure and properties, the multiplicity of auxiliary agents which accompany them in dosage forms, and the variety, complexity, and sensitivity of modern analytical instruments require highly specialized skills. Organized as an Analytical Research and Development group, such specialists and supporting staff evolve a complete spectrum of physical and chemical properties of the drug substance, undertake degradation and kinetic studies for use in the stability-testing program, and develop the testing methods and specifications for the pharmaceutical dosage form. In addition, senior personnel in this group are involved in the preparation of pertinent sections of New Drug Applications, labeling specifications and liaison with the Food and Drug Administration, the *US Pharmacopeia*, and the *National Formulary*.

The Pharmaceutical Manufacturers Association has defined total control of quality as it applies to the drug industry as the organized effort within an entire establishment to design, produce, maintain, and assure the specified quality in each unit of product distributed. Although total control is a plantwide activity, a specialized group of scientific and technical personnel evaluates product quality and audits the control system. Since the exercise of independent judgment in the release of products for commercial distribution is a vital factor in such a control system, the head of Quality Control generally reports to a level of management other than Production.

A large portion of the activities of quality-control personnel involves laboratory procedures, ie, physical and chemical tests on raw materials, drug substances, dosage forms, and packaging components. The implementation of the Current Good Manufacturing

Practices section of the Food, Drug and Cosmetic Act in 1963 has broadened the inspection, record-keeping, and production-monitoring role of the Quality-Control group. Associated with, but not solely as a result of governmental regulations, an expansion of quality-control activities requiring biological tests has taken place within the past five years. Not only must there be provision for specific tests of potency or microbiological status of products, but bacteriological monitoring of water, equipment, operating environment, and personnel are now recognized as essential elements of total quality control. Such surveillance is no longer limited to sterile product manufacturing areas but literally covers the entire production operation.

In view of the broad scope of technical and administrative responsibilities in Analytical Research and Quality Control, differences of opinion exist among executives as to the role of pharmacists in these areas. For individuals with a BS degree a preference for chemists at the laboratory bench level is apparent. The reason generally presented is the absence of adequate training in analytical chemistry in most pharmacy schools. However, an equivalent preference for pharmacists is apparent in such activities as inspection, auditing of control records, complaint analyses, in-process control review, label control, and liaison work with government agencies. Pharmacists with advanced degrees and interests in analytical chemistry have achieved notable success in analytical-research or quality-control careers in the pharmaceutical industry.

Pharmaceutical Production

As considered in this section pharmaceutical production comprises a variety of activities, the most important being production planning and inventory control, warehousing, manufacturing, and packaging. Except in relatively small companies the pharmacist generally serves in a supervisory capacity with emphasis upon technical skills in actual manufacturing operations or administrative abilities as he assumes broader departmental responsibilities. Improvements in pharmaceutical education, advances in technology, and new federal requirements for quality of the man-

ufacturing operations have served to make the pharmacist an even more attractive candidate for positions in pharmaceutical production.

The potency of modern drug substances permits no laxity in the technical control of manufacturing operations; cross contamination must be prevented and unit-to-unit and batch-to-batch uniformity must be kept within extremely narrow limits. Manufacturing procedures must be meticulously followed and the reliability and reproducibility of a process can be assured only by clear understanding of the principles involved and the absence of deviation from prescribed controls. During the course of his education and training the pharmacist is imbued with a strong sense of responsibility concerning the handling of drugs and the absolute necessity for concentration and accuracy.

Most production executives agree that recent graduates from pharmacy schools are somewhat better qualified as a consequence of more thorough undergraduate training in the basic sciences. In a few institutions courses in manufacturing technology are available, generally as electives. Increasing use of automated equipment and in-process controls, the application of management techniques, and the necessity for comprehending and complying with regulations issued by Governmental agencies render the possession of advanced degrees highly desirable for those who seek to reach the higher levels of management.

Probably as a consequence of the specialized machinery used in packaging operations and the absence in pharmacy schools of educational programs in materials science, relatively few pharmacists are employed in the packaging sections of pharmaceutical production. Staffing at the supervisory level usually includes packaging specialists or industrial engineers.

In many companies the experimental program related to process improvement or development as well as well-planned studies of new machinery are carried out by pharmacists and/or engineers in the Development Division. Such groups also are frequently utilized for troubleshooting in the Production Department. In spite of differences in the assignment of authority and responsibility within different companies, collaboration and coordination between these technical groups is essential to smooth performance.

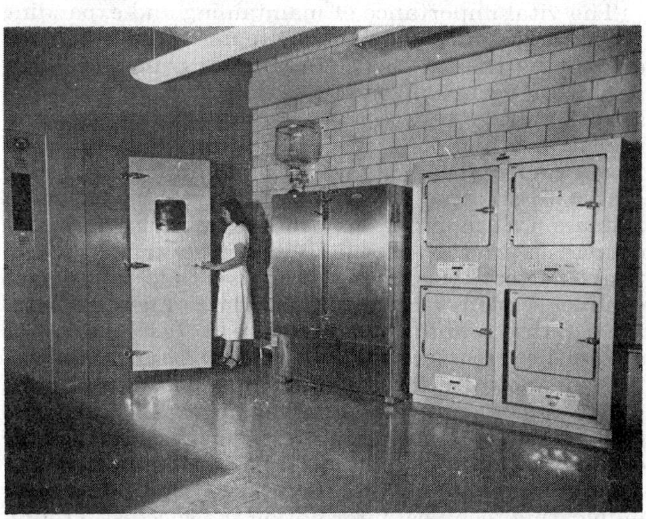

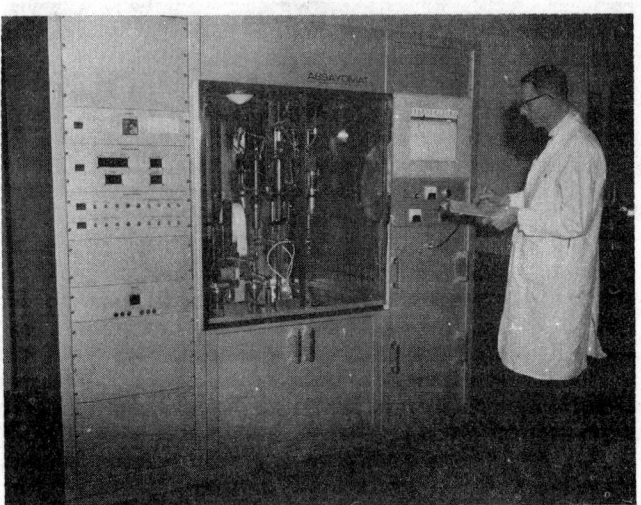

Fig. 13. Sample-storage area for stability testing program. The maintenance and periodic testing of drug substances and dosage forms under accelerated conditions of storage permits more rapid and precise evaluation of their stability under average or normal exposure to temperature, humidity, and light (courtesy, Ciba).

Fig. 14. The Assayomat. This unique, automated, analytical instrument is capable of handling the spectrophotometric assay of 160 individual capsules or tablets per day. Operated by a technician, it provides analytical data equivalent to the output of four chemists (courtesy, Ciba).

Pharmaceutical Sales

The appearance of salesmen, also known as detail men or professional service representatives, on the pharmaceutical scene can be traced back to the beginnings of the drug-manufacturing era about a century ago. Not only are these men important in the establishment of a favorable company image in the minds of physicians who prescribe drug preparations and pharmacists who dispense them, but, if properly trained, they are in a position to convey important and useful scientific information relative to specific products.

In spite of some criticism from within and outside the medical profession, the role of the professional service representative continues to be recognized as a necessary and useful adjunct to the existing pattern of drug marketing and distribution. The dissemination of information relative to drug usage in an environment where pharmaceutical and medical research are constantly expanding is so important that the accompanying sales effort produces little annoyance. In fact, many leaders in medicine feel that a representative is helpful when he brings new products to the attention of physicians or obtains from the scientific and technical staff of his company specific information concerning the properties, clinical experience, or adverse reactions of a particular drug. Through his contacts with other doctors, pharmacists, and hospitals, the representative acquires a broader view of why, how, and when his company's products are being used. When the circumstances are special, or in emergencies, the instincts and training of the representative respond to the need for service. The dialogue between a well-educated and well-trained representative and an inquiring physician cannot be replaced by an advertisement, a package insert (even with an officially approved text), or a brochure. Questioning, and being questioned, the qualified representative can sometimes stimulate either laboratory or clinical research.

As with physicians, many community and hospital pharmacists have found the professional service representative a valuable ally in the acquisition of knowledge about drug products and their place in therapeutics. In addition, the assistance of representatives in inventory control, the removal of outdated prepara-

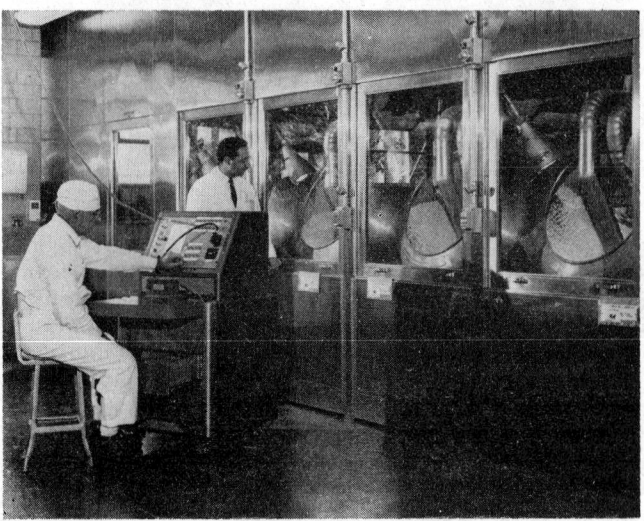

Fig. 16. Automated coating system. Automation of the tablet-coating process has improved the uniformity of coated tablets, reduced the process time, and eliminated operator variability. Punched tapes transmitting signals through a solid-state controller handle the sequential steps in the process (courtesy, Ciba).

tions, professional matters in the community, and in public-health affairs has been sought and obtained.

To function effectively the representative must be in a position to comprehend and communicate technical information of a multidisciplinary nature in the sensitive area of medical care. Consequently, applicants with educational backgrounds in pharmacy, chemistry, or biology represent the favored pool of potential representatives. In general, most marketing executives prefer pharmacists as candidates because so much of the pharmacy curriculum is directly related to the scientific aspects of therapeutics. However, competition for the available supply of pharmacists due to other career opportunities has increased the proportion of non-pharmacists entering pharmaceutical sales. Current estimates indicate that although the range of pharmacist employment in the professional service representative category is 5–90% in individual companies, the industry average may have dropped to 10–15%. However, the proportion of pharmacists attaining executive status in marketing or promotion from marketing to administration is much higher.

The vital importance of maintaining and expanding the technical knowledge of the representative is made evident by the extensive training programs currently organized and supported by manufacturers of prescription drugs. Elaborate training centers are maintained and equipped with the most modern audio-visual aids. Teaching is highly professional and geared to securing competence and reliability in the trainees. Such programs are ongoing with refresher courses on product knowledge and general pharmaceutical matters. Company scientists and physicians conduct sessions related to the release of new preparations. In the words of one executive, "such programs are a type of postgraduate education planned and totally financed by the employer that has, as a per employee price tag, an amount comparable to the tuition charges for four years at a prestigious Eastern college or university."

In addition to the capacity for acquiring and communicating technical information the successful representative demonstrates personally factors and interest patterns of a definite type. As with other sales-oriented individuals he is outgoing, gregarious, and

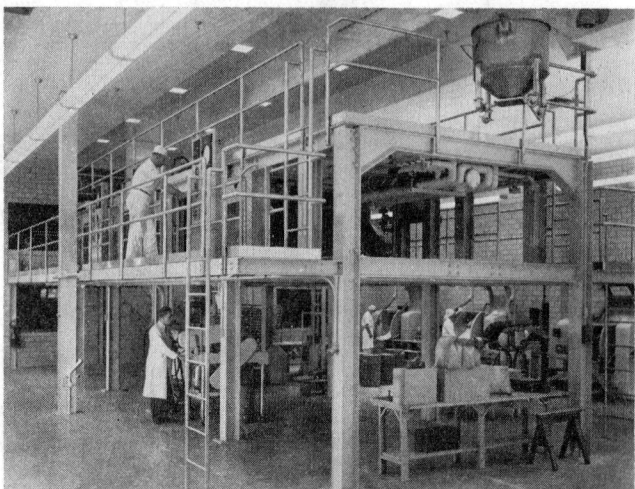

Fig. 15. Tablet manufacturing area (partial view). Powerful powder mixers and granulators are on the right, lower level. The three-level platform system in the center utilizes gravity loading (top level), rotary vacuum drying (middle level), and screening (bottom level). Rotational speed, drying temperature, and pressure levels are automatically controlled (courtesy, Ciba).

willing to become the center of attention. Careful planning, good judgment, and attention to detail must accompany ease of expression and satisfaction of the craving for personal achievement.

Although the five-year curriculum leading to the BS degree in Pharmacy has increased the number of non-technical electives available to students, relatively few courses are directed towards the specific needs of professional service representatives. Inclusion in the curriculum of electives directed towards the marketing aspects of the pharmaceutical industry rather than the commercial component of community pharmacy operations would be helpful in this regard.

Upon superficial analysis it appears as though starting salaries for representatives are often not competitive with those for pharmacists entering community pharmacy. However, other benefits such as incentive bonuses, stock purchase plans, insurance and pension plans, etc. frequently offset the salary differential. Also, because salaries for experienced representatives and sales managers are often higher than salaries for practicing pharmacists with as many years of experience, the long-range salary outlook may actually favor the professional service representative.

Aside from the financial rewards associated with the career of a representative, frequent expression has been given to gratification associated with acceptance of personal responsibility and discipline, craving for personal achievement, and the psychological effect of accomplishment through personal contact.

Pharmacy students seeking career guidance can turn to faculty advisers, experienced professional service representatives, or company interviewers. Special psychological tests useful in gauging sales potential are sometimes employed. A paper by Chavkin and Kanig[6] describes such tests with specific reference to requirements for success in pharmaceutical sales.

Related Fields

During the course of undergraduate training in pharmacy a number of students develop a keen interest in one of the basic science subjects in the curriculum. Upon graduation they elect to expand that interest by entering into a program leading to a graduate degree in such disciplines as pharmacology, pharmacognosy, microbiology, organic chemistry, or biochemistry. With an educational background of this type attractive career openings in schools of pharmacy or industry are readily available. The broader albeit less-concentrated training of the pharmacist is sought as a counterbalance to the narrow sectarianism often encountered in highly specialized fields. Alert pharmacists with sufficient initiative to maintain technical competence and capable of relating experimental data to practical therapeutics possess distinct advantages in competing with non-pharmacists in similar posts.

Although relatively few in numbers pharmacists with special interests, aptitudes, or personality traits find their pharmacy training extremely helpful in obtaining industrial positions which need such attributes. These individuals can be found in the ranks of medical correspondents, copywriters, scientific information specialists, purchasing agents, or in public, trade, or professional relations. In general, greater awareness of the existence of these peripheral career opportunities among pharmacy students would probably tend to increase the proportion of pharmacists to non-pharmacists employed in these specialized occupations.

Pharmacy Education for Industry

In spite of widespread agreement that excellent opportunities for rewarding careers exist in many facets of pharmaceutical industry operations, the majority of colleges of pharmacy fail to provide educational programs directed to interesting and preparing students for such careers. Analysis of 50 replies to letters addressed to the deans of all colleges of pharmacy (74) in 1968 clearly demonstrates this fact. Among the explanations most frequently offered, the following are the most interesting:

1. The college is geographically distant from the centers of pharmaceutical industry operations.
2. The primary role of colleges of pharmacy is the training of community pharmacists.
3. The numerical proportion of pharmacists in industry is too small to warrant special attention.
4. The financial investment of the pharmaceutical industry in colleges of pharmacy is too small.
5. The requirement of experience in community pharmacy as a condition of registration is a barrier to seeking industrial employment immediately following graduation.

It should be pointed out that in principle and by example quite a few colleges are unwilling to accept such explanations and that efforts are under way to correct deficiencies of this type in a profession which is fortunate enough to provide a variety of career opportunities. The location of a college should not be prejudicial to the training of students interested in industrial pharmacy. As long as pharmacy education is almost completely geared to the larger manpower needs of community pharmacy the industry will perforce seek its personnel elsewhere. Most colleges of pharmacy are tax supported and there is little evidence that private support from community or hospital pharmacists is significantly related to career opportunities in these fields. The requirement for "apprenticeship" training in community pharmacy as a condition for registration is considered by some as a dubious relic of outmoded pharmacy practice.

Regardless of the number of pharmacy students who might wish to accept career opportunities in industry, the shift from the manipulative compounding of prescriptions to the dispensing of manufactured dosage forms has introduced a new element into the practice of community and hospital pharmacy. Every pharmacy student should be more than superficially exposed to the methodology of modern drug development including dosage-form design, process research, packaging materials and properties, industrial organization and practices, principles of quality control, and legal requirements for pharmaceutical research and production. Except in relation to number of courses and depth of content, all pharmacy students would benefit from training in industrial pharmacy. It is difficult to see how a pharmacist can be considered, or consider himself, as an expert in drug quality in the absence of such educational experience. Even more difficult to accept in the presence of an educational deficiency of this nature would be the proposed role of "therapeutic consultant" to the physician.

As a consequence of a concentrated analysis of the educational needs of the pharmacist of the present and the future, a number of the colleges have adopted a core curriculum program. This system permits the adoption of certain options at an appropriate point during undergraduate training. The availability of an option in industrial pharmacy defined in its broadest sense would provide an attractive career potential as well as an opportunity for an exchange of teaching personnel and industry specialists in a cooperative program.

At the present time a number of colleges offer a required or, in most cases, an elective course in manufacturing pharmacy to undergraduate students. In a few cases the preparations manufactured in these laboratories are supplied to state institutions for dispensing to patients. Most undergraduate students are provided with the opportunity of participating in group visits to one or two large pharmaceutical companies as a means of exposing them to industrial pharmacy. Unfortunately such tours are too brief, too social, and far too often oriented towards the students' future roles as community pharmacists.

Far more progress has been made in graduate training in colleges of pharmacy. The range and depth of course work has been strengthened; the quality of research programs has been elevated by stricter requirements, better equipment, and a more progressive attitude towards technological changes. The radical revision of curricular and research projects which followed the elevation of physical pharmacy and biopharmaceutics to their proper roles in the teaching programs of schools of pharmacy has served to bring graduate students closer to the level of skills utilized by other scientists in industrial research and development. As a consequence the pharmacist possessing a graduate degree has become a more attractive candidate for employment in the pharmaceutical industry.

A professor of industrial pharmacy who has carefully analyzed the role of pharmacists in industry explains his teaching role as follows:

"The purpose of a graduate program is to help the student gain a new approach or outlook towards knowledge. It is the process by which he becomes a perpetual student. The basic structure of any graduate course must be theory whether the course involves physical, chemical or biological systems. However, I feel that graduate work in pharmaceutics must also contain sufficient experience in technology for the student to see how this theory is to be applied, as well as to facilitate the use of his hands in experimentation. In a graduate program he must also gain experience in expressing himself orally and in written form. These are our objectives and I feel that a student passing through this program successfully does have the potential of becoming a valuable man for the industry."

At least one university is offering an MS degree in Industrial Pharmacy, utilizing a cooperative educational plan under which graduate students supplement the lecture and laboratory courses on campus with practical experience gained while employed in pharmaceutical research or production laboratories in industry. A small number of pharmaceutical companies regularly employ selected pharmacy students as trainees during summer periods. Attitudes towards such cooperative programs were surveyed and discussed in a paper by Silverman and Cooper.[7]

The broad objectives and activities of the American Foundation for Pharmaceutical Education (AFPE) are financially supported mainly by the pharmaceutical industry in recognition of the importance of pharmacy as a profession and also in response to the contributions which well-trained pharmacists can make to the growth of the industry. Approximately one-third of the AFPE recipients of graduate fellowships are actively engaged in the pharmaceutical industry; more than half of the Directors of the Foundation are industry executives, and industry scientists participate in the Visiting Lecturers program of the American Association of Colleges of Pharmacy.

A number of colleges of pharmacy, recognizing their obligations to the continuing education of graduates and their faculty have developed extension programs of recognized value and importance to industrial pharmacy. Among the most prominent of these are the Land O'Lakes Conferences on Industrial Pharmaceutical Research and Pharmaceutical Analysis, the Arden House Educational Conferences for Industrial Pharmacists, and the Industrial Pharmacy Conferences of the University of Texas. Several colleges offer special courses and seminars in specific industrial areas of interest, such as sterile-products manufacturing, pharmacology, and good manufacturing practices. One college in a large urban center offers a Certificate Program in Applied Pharmaceutical Sciences with a choice of 24 evening courses, including such topics as Mathematics for the Researcher, Biological Cosmetic Science, Unit Operations, Modern Dosage-Form Analysis, Computer Techniques and Market Research.

Opportunities for continuing education are also provided by organizations such as the Industrial Pharmaceutical Technology Section of the Academy of Pharmaceutical Sciences which sponsors symposia and papers at two national and three regional meetings every year. Local groups in some parts of the country are providing informal round table sessions for educational purposes.

Additional opportunities for communication between industrial pharmacists and educators are provided by an exchange of lecturers, consultantships, research grants, and the provision of technical information in the form of books, reprints, and scientific films.

On-The-Job Training

The highly complex nature of pharmaceutical operations, the numerous disciplines and professions comprising the scientific and technical staff, the extensive requirements of the regulatory agencies, and the specialized nature of the marketing and distribution system make on-the-job training an essential component in the management of a pharmaceutical company. The customary student–preceptor, worker–supervisor relationship, while important, is hardly adequate and much more must be done to obtain a satisfactory level of safety and efficiency. In some companies these educational programs approach the pedagogic activities of a small university and many professional employees regard the plant and laboratory area as a miniature campus.

Lectures, seminars, round tables, films, and demonstrations take place regularly and are frequently participated in by small or large groups with subjects of the narrowest or broadest interest. Speakers are either highly qualified employee specialists or visiting experts from universities, government, or industry. Production workers receive training in good manufacturing practices, safety, and hygiene; junior chemists receive instruction in the most advanced types of instrumental analyses; research pharmacists learn about the use of computers in experimental design; and executives discuss management techniques with university professors.

Many companies, in response to the pressure of advancing technology in all areas of their operations, support the continuing formal education of employees. Tuition for relevant courses in colleges or universities is frequently reimbursed, and employees are encouraged to obtain advanced degrees or acquire superior vocational skills. Active membership in scientific or professional societies is encouraged and supported, and many industry employees have attained high office in such organizations.

The necessity for training professional sales representatives along scientific as well as marketing lines has resulted in the establishment of programs utilizing the most progressive teaching techniques. Such centers generally possess facilities and equipment capable of enriching the quality of communication between teachers and students.

On-the-job training, whether undertaken within or outside the plant, is recognized as an essential obligation in meeting the social and scientific requirements of pharmaceutical development, production, sales, and distribution.

Salaries

Variability in the availability of pharmacists in certain areas of the country, local differences in the cost of living, and current inflationary trends make it difficult to accurately present salary levels for industrial pharmacists. A survey (1968) of 18 leading pharmaceutical manufacturers shows average annual starting salaries for BS pharmacists without industrial experience to be $8500; for those with MS degrees, $11,000; and for PhD graduates, $13,000. The general tendency to broaden fringe benefits as part of industrial incentive planning and labor relations adds as much as 15–25% to the basic hiring salary.

From the point of view of increased opportunities for promotion, accompanied by financial rewards, possession of an advanced degree certainly makes the necessary investment in time and costs worthwhile. This additional educational effort is particularly important at the present time in view of the increasing scientific and technological complexity of drug development, production, and control. It should be noted, however, that many pharmacists not in possession of advanced degrees have through the exercise of native ability and energy achieved notable success in all phases of industrial operations.

Summary

In spite of an unparalleled assault upon the character and performance of the pharmaceutical industry, comprehensible in part as a reaction to the thalidomide tragedy, the growth of the industry has continued its upward trend. The difficulties of the past decade have undoubtedly left their mark but in general most executives and industry scientists remain confident of the future. Those changes already under way or contemplated will enhance rather than reduce the role of pharmacists in almost all areas of research, production, control, and marketing.

The proximity of industrial pharmacists to the actual development and production of therapeutic agents adds a stimulating and satisfying professional character to their daily work. For well-trained pharmacists entering any of the existing industrial career areas previously described, the opportunities for financial and psychological rewards are manifold.

Pharmacy students, teachers, and practitioners possess an equity in, and a responsibility for, the future health and potential contributions of the pharmaceutical industry. As eloquently expressed by Nobel Laureate Ernst B. Chain[8] of penicillin fame:

"... let us put an end to the prejudiced, irresponsible and tendentious denigration of the pharmaceutical industry and let us work quite intentionally and consciously towards creating an atmosphere which destroys distrust and promotes understanding between the industry, government and university circles and the general public, and which ensures opportunities for still closer and more intensified contacts between academic and industrial scientists. Let us be sure to deploy all our available resources, intellectual and material, in the most expedient manner so that we can give the scientists concerned with drug research, both in the universities and in industry, the most favorable conditions in which they can advance more speedily and with the least impediment towards their one great aim, to which they devote their lives and in which all of us have the highest stakes: to combat and conquer pain and an ever-increasing range of diseases through the discovery of new and more efficacious drugs."

For the industrial pharmacist the stake is equally high but the rewards of participation are also his to enjoy.

References

1. Bernard, C., *An Introduction to the Study of Experimental Medicine*, Henry Schuman, Inc., New York, 1949.
2. *Basic Research, Applied Research and Development in American Industry, 1965*, National Science Foundation, Washington, D.C., June, 1967.
3. *1967 Proceedings, NABP*, National Association of Boards of Pharmacy, Chicago, Ill.
4. *Resources for Medical Research*, Report No. 8, US Dept. of Health, Education and Welfare, Washington, D.C., March, 1966.
5. Cooper, J., *Am. J. Pharm.*, **132**, 158 (1960).
6. Chavkin, L. T., and Kanig, J. L., *Am. J. Pharm. Educ.*, **27**, 213 (1963).
7. Silverman, J. I., and Cooper, J., *J. APhA, NS5*, 214 (1965).
8. Chain, E. B., *J. Royal Soc. Arts*, **111**, 856 (1963).

6 | Pharmacists in Government

Career opportunities for pharmacists in government agencies

This chapter was prepared by

Milton W. Skolaut, BS, *Chief, Pharmacy Department, Clinical Center,*
National Institutes of Health, Bethesda, Md. 20014

The emphasis on health services for the population of the US has increased the importance of pharmacist participation in health programs. Many new doors have been opened for careers in the clinical practice of pharmacy in Federal hospitals, outpatient clinics, extended-care facilities, administrative, or health-related programs.

The pharmacists have a unique and broad-based education which will allow them to function effectively in a new and broader scope than ever before. Certain pharmacists, oriented to patients by their education rather than to products, can fulfil a rewarding career in a Federal hospital or related health program. All pharmacists have a wide range of opportunities for rewarding careers in health programs requiring the pharmacists basic knowledge.

Career Opportunities

Career opportunities in the Federal services are unlimited for the pharmacist with an excellent educational background and armed with a desire to serve. Increasing numbers of commissioned officers are required by the Army, Navy, Air Force, and Public Health Service. The Public Health Service also supplies the health services, including pharmacists, to the Coast Guard and the Bureau of Prisons.

Pharmacists' opportunities for Civil Service employment are available in the Veterans Administration; Health, Education and Welfare; Department of Commerce; Department of Labor; Department of Justice; and the staffs of Congressional Committees. The Department of Health, Education and Welfare offers Civil Service positions in the Food and Drug Administration of the Consumer Protection Environmental Health Service, National Institutes of Health, Social Security Administration, and the Office of Equal Opportunity. The Department of Justice utilizes pharmacists in the Bureau of Narcotics and Dangerous Drugs.

While it is not compulsory to have pharmacists in some of these positions, the fact that their talents are made available has contributed measurably to the efficiency and quality of the service rendered in a number of important governmental activities.

More and more it becomes evident to those who study the structure and function of government that there are certain positions of responsibility and trust where pharmaceutical training is of especial usefulness.

Often pharmacists who come into the military or civilian service as pharmacists find that the logical line of advancement takes them out of actual dispensing or compounding of drugs and medicines and leads them into administrative positions. This is, of course, comparable to what takes place in private practice and in the drug industry. The heads of large government agencies have found pharmacists invaluable in administrative positions because of their broad knowledge and experience in the professional and scientific phases of pharmaceutical practice. In government service, as well as in private industry, it is the ability of the individual to adapt himself to expanding services and new applications of his professional training and techniques which marks him for promotion and assignment to tasks of continually wider importance.

Recruitment—Broadly speaking, the positions in government service which require pharmaceutical training can be classified into *military* and *civilian* pursuits. In the military, the services of pharmacists are provided either by enlistment or commissioning of qualified persons and also, to a more limited extent, through civil service employment.

In the nonmilitary phases of government service pharmacists are recruited through the Civil Service Commission. The Public Health Service, which also provides service to the Coast Guard and the Bureau of Prisons, largely depends on its commissioned corps for the professional services of pharmacists, although it also calls on civil service for recruitment when necessary.

Armed Forces Requirements—While the Armed Forces are in a position to set up their medical services without reference to civilian pharmacy requirements, the modern tendency is to follow the standards of civilian pharmacy to the greatest extent possible, adapting them to the exigencies of military situations as indicated. Station hospitals and medical centers maintained by the Army, Navy, and Air Force make use of the same type of facilities and services found in civilian hospitals.

The pharmaceutical service in mobile units, such as those of the Navy and Air Force, and such as is required when armies are on the move, like every other phase of medical care, is adapted to the requirements of the armed forces which are being served.

Although the Medical Service Corps of the Army, Navy, and Air Force stem from the Medical Service Corps Act of 1947, each service is governed to a considerable extent by the provisions of the Officer Personnel Act of 1947. It is this latter Act which establishes rank structure and promotion procedure which are designed to place all officers on common ground within their services, but not necessarily on common ground with their contemporaries of sister services.

Qualifications—Anyone aspiring to make a professional career of service in the Armed Forces must bear in mind that professional knowledge by itself will not characterize him as a good officer. He must have other qualifications to fit him as a commissioned officer. These include ability to exhibit cooperation, judgment, leadership, promotion potential, and management effectiveness. The extent to which he possesses these is determined by selection boards within the respective services.

Once a pharmacist has been commissioned his advancement in any of the military services depends on his ability to progress continuously in his training as an officer. Each of the services maintains its own training schools and facilities, and while it is important for the pharmacist to keep abreast of progress in his own profession, if he is in the military service, he must also work constantly toward improving his military fitness because it is recognition of an officer's military fitness which leads to the most tangible rewards.

Selective Service System

Compulsory military service in peace time was unknown in our country until the threat of World War II required a change in the policy of preparedness to defend our way of life. The position of the United States in world affairs following World War II has necessitated a continuing policy of compulsory military service.

Selective Service—As a result of new responsibilities for leadership in world affairs which were thrust upon our government following World War II, it has been necessary to keep in force the Universal Military Training and Service Act, which provided the war manpower for both World War I and World War II. The Congress has continued to extend the Act each year, although not without controversy. Virtually all qualified and available young men between the ages of 18 and 26 must continue to look forward to giving a part of their lives to military service. However, the law recognizes the need for preparation for and practice of vital civilian activities, and provides for deferment for such endeavors.

Exemptions and Deferments—Considerable discussion in the Congress of the United States and among educators has been devoted to the question of whether universal military training should be made an accepted policy, or whether there should continue to be deferments from such training for those desiring to study for scientific and professional pursuits which are essential for the preservation of our democratic institutions as the fighting of battles.

Under the Universal Military Training and Service Act, deferments are continuing to be provided for those who are attending college, and are maintaining satisfactory progress.

The student must request his 2-S student deferment in writing, in order to be sure of being deferred. The college cannot do it. It is legally up to the student himself to provide his local board each year with proof that he is satisfactorily "pursuing a full-time course of instruction at a college, university or similar institution of learning."

As a general rule, pharmacy students have been deferred in order to permit them to complete their courses of study and further deferments are generally afforded those who must complete their apprentice or internship training in order to qualify for state board examinations.

No general rule may be applied to graduate students. Each case will be considered by the student's local draft board with which he is registered.

The law also provides for occupational deferments, and many practicing pharmacists are deferred to continue their civilian professional pursuits.

There is not sufficient pharmaceutical work in the Army to assure every drafted pharmacist the opportunity to practice pharmacy or a closely related vocation after completion of his basic military training.

He can, of course, enlist in the Navy or in the Air Force for specific pharmaceutical duty, but this requires a 3- or 4-year period of service, as compared with the 2-year period required under the draft. At present, the Army is the only branch of the military service which obtains men through Selective Service. Neither the Navy nor the Air Force at present draws upon Selective Service for personnel and many young men of draft age enlist in the Navy or the Air Force for specific pharmaceutical duty in order to meet their military service obligations.

College Students and Selective Service—Selective Service Law authorizes the deferment of college students whose "activity in study is found to be necessary to the maintenance of the national health, safety or interest." A student should interpret his deferment not as a right, but as a privilege granted in order that he might become a more useful citizen to himself and his nation.

Army

Revolutionary War—As far back as 1775 the Continental Congress established a hospital for the Army with an apothecary as one of the officers. In 1776 the Congress created the office of "druggist." He was to "receive and deliver all medicines, instruments, and shop furniture of the United States" and in 1777, when the Continental Congress reorganized the medical department, it divided the country into four districts and stated that there should be "one apothecary general for each district whose duty it shall be, to receive, prepare, and deliver medicines, and other articles of his department to the hospitals and Army, as shall be ordered by the director general."

During the Revolutionary War a central laboratory was established to manufacture the pharmaceutical products needed in the Army which were prepared and compounded mostly in the shop of the apothecary-general at Carlisle, Pa. This led to the publication of the first pharmacopœia in America, the *Lititz Pharmacopœia*, which was prepared for use in the military hospitals.

Civil War—During the Civil War the purchase and distribution of medicines was in the hands of medical officers. Pharmacists were employed in the volunteer regiments; however, their rank and pay were unsatisfactory. In peacetimes, no progress was made in providing for pharmaceutical service in the Army which came anywhere near the equivalent of such service in civilian life.

The American Pharmaceutical Association took cognizance of this situation in 1894 by appointing a "Committee on The Status of Pharmacists in the Service of the United States." The title of this committee was later changed to the "Committee on Status of Pharmacists in Government Service" and such a committee has been functioning continuously ever since with the aim of improving the rank of pharmacists called on to serve in the Armed Forces and to assure to the armed forces a quality of pharmaceutical service comparable to that given in civilian life.

Spanish–American War—The Committee on Status of Pharmacists in Government Service was active during the Spanish–American War in endeavoring to secure commissions for pharmacists in the National Guard of the various states. In 1900 it succeeded in having the State of New York pass an act which assigned a pharmacist to each regiment in the National

Guard with the rank of lieutenant, but this law was repealed in 1901.

World War I—It is quite understandable that in the absence of emergencies the interest of civilian pharmacists in serving in a military capacity has never been very great. Accordingly there was very little activity on the part of the Committee on Status of Pharmacists in Government Service until the advent of World War I. It had become a matter of routine for the Army to train personnel to dispense drugs and to provide for noncommissioned grades for such personnel. All of the pharmaceutical service in the Army was given under the direction of medical officers, and to this day the Medical Department of the Army has maintained that medical supply projects should come under the personal supervision of medical officers because of their understanding of the use of surgical instruments and medical supplies in addition to drugs.

World War I was probably the first occasion for the drafting of pharmacists in sufficiently large numbers to cause concerted action to improve their rank and assignment in the Armed Forces. Not only did this stimulate the APhA Committee on Status of Pharmacists in Government Service to become more active, but it also caused the formation of a separate organization known as the National Pharmaceutical Service Association, which urged the organization of a *Pharmacy Corps* in the Medical Department of the Army, and led Congressman Edmonds of Pennsylvania, in 1917, to introduce a bill in the House of Representatives to accomplish this.

The public hearing on this measure assembled one of the largest groups of pharmacists and pharmaceutical educators ever brought together to sponsor such legislation. The hearing focused attention on the fact that the basic education of pharmacists would have to be brought to a 4-year college level in order for the profession to receive consideration in the matter of commissioning its members directly from civilian life. The bill did not reach the stage of action by the House of Representatives. However, a number of pharmacists were commissioned in the *Sanitary Corps* of the Medical Department of the Army during World War I, and they were assigned to supervise pharmaceutical and medical supply procurement. An effort was also made to place pharmacists, who were obtained by the Army through the draft, in positions where their pharmaceutical background could be utilized.

In 1920 the Army organized a *Medical Administrative Corps* in which it commissioned men with various backgrounds in the ancillary medical professions and with experience in medical supply and administration, who could relieve medical officers of many nonmedical duties, thus freeing them for more strictly medical services.

World War II—When the United States became involved in the second world war, and the Selective Service draft again brought into the service a very large number of pharmacists, the pressure on the part of the profession for providing a separate *Pharmacy Corps* became more and more pronounced, and in 1942 Congressman Carl Durham of North Carolina, who had introduced a bill to establish a Pharmacy Corps in the Army, succeeded in having it passed. This bill provided specific assignments for a limited number of commissioned pharmacists, and for the transfer of all officers in the Medical Administrative Corps to the Pharmacy Corps. The Bill became a law on July 12, 1943, but the Corps was never properly organized or implemented during the war years because of strong opposition to it on the part of the Medical Department of the Army supported by the War Department.

Army Medical Service Corps

The unsatisfactory situation, with respect to organization and proper utilization of the Pharmacy Corps, which existed at the end of World War II, was finally resolved by the passage of new legislation in 1947. This legislation provided for a *Medical Service Corps* in both Army and Navy, and the consolidation within this Corps of the Pharmacy Corps, the Medical Administration Corps, and the Sanitary Corps. The Medical Service Corps organization provided for sections on Pharmacy, Supply, and Administration; Optometry; Sanitary Engineering; and Medical Allied Sciences. The Act creating the Corps is known as Public Law 337 of the 80th Congress, and became a law on August 4, 1947. The Air Force has also created a Medical Service Corps patterned along the same lines.

The first chief of the Medical Service Corps in the Army was a pharmacist.* He was succeeded after a 4-year tour of duty by a nonpharmacist who had come up through the ranks as a medical administrator, and he, in turn, was succeeded by a pharmacist whose term expired in 1959. It is the present policy of the Surgeon General of the Army to limit the tours of duty of Chiefs of the Corps to 4 years and to rotate this office to some extent among the 4 sections of the Corps. There is also a Pharmacy Consultant to the Surgeon General, who is a member of the Corps, with direct access to the Chief at all times for the purpose of maintaining proper liaison between the profession of pharmacy and the Surgeon General. In the 22 years in which this Corps has been functioning, a pattern has been established which will assure a more satisfactory future for commissioned pharmacists in the Army.

It is necessary for the profession of pharmacy to have a sufficient number of pharmacy officers in the Medical Service Corps at all times on a career basis, in order to establish a proper nucleus for expansion of the commissioned pharmacy service in times of war.

Organization of the Medical Service Corps—The Corps is divided into four major Sections: *Pharmacy, Supply, and Administration; Sanitary Engineering; Optometry;* and *Medical Allied Sciences.* The Corps consists of officers trained in 18 career fields, with many related occupational specialties. In addition to pharmacy these disciplines include hospital administration, biochemistry, optometry, nutrition, psychology, bacteriology, engineering, management, etc, all vitally necessary to the proper function of the Army Medical Service.

The initial strength of the Regular Corps was set at 1022. Based on the best experience tables then available, certain percentages of that strength were suballotted to these Sections by the Surgeon General. These percentages were: Pharmacy, Supply, and Administration: 60%; Optometry: 2%; Sanitary Engineering: 8%; and Medical Allied Sciences: 30%. These percentages were flexible, and therefore subject to change. The current approximate percentages are as follows: Pharmacy, Supply, and Administra-

---

*Current personnel are as follows—*Army:* Brigadier General William A. Hamrick, Chief, Medical Service Corps; Colonel Jack W. McNamara, Consultant in Pharmacy, Office of the Surgeon General. *Navy:* Captain E. L. Van Landingham, Chief, Medical Service Corps. *Air Force:* Colonel J. W. Polkinghorn, Chief, Medical Service Corps; Colonel A. Meyer, Chief, Biomedical Sciences Corps. *US Public Health Service:* Pharmacist Director Allen W. Brands, Pharmacy Liaison Representative. *Veterans Administration:* Mr. Robert A. Statler, Director of Pharmacy Service.

tion: 75%; Medical Allied Sciences: 16%; Sanitary Engineering: 3%; and Optometry: 6%.

The astonishing progress the Medical Service Corps has made is well illustrated by the fact that today there are approximately 5580 officers on active duty in the Corps. Almost every medical specialty except the professional practice of medicine, dentistry, nursing, diatetics, occupational and physical therapy, or veterinary medicine is being performed by the MSC officer. This fact is demonstrated in the increased size, responsibilities, and areas of utilization of the Corps. The prestige and caliber of the Corps, with its over 15 scientific specialties and over 50 administrative and tactical specialties, have grown progressively ever since its formation in 1947.

Pharmacy Officers—Pharmacists by their background, diversified professional training in the sciences, business, merchandising, and management, together with their close working relationships with the medical profession, make an ideal source of officer material for the army medical team headed by the physician whose mission is the preservation of the health of the Army.

At present there are approximately 276 pharmacist officers on active duty in the Army. Of this number approximately 137 are classified as pharmacy officers who are engaged either in pharmacy operations or in closely allied positions.

The number of pharmacy graduates subject to call to duty through Selective Service is greater than the Army requirement for commissioned officers in the field of pharmacy. However, pharmacy graduates who are drafted into the Army through Selective Service are classified as pharmacists and every attempt is made to assign them to pharmacy duties.

Currently, the Army is unable to meet its worldwide requirement for pharmacy personnel through the Selective Service system. This situation is not unique to the pharmacy graduate but also applies to thousands of college graduates, such as lawyers, engineers, biochemists, optometrists, hospital and business administrators, and economists and geologists, to name only a few.

Pharmacy officers have complete charge of supervision, training, and administration of enlisted and civilian personnel and, in general, concern themselves with the orderly management of pharmacies in Army treatment facilities. Pharmacy officers may expect to have a challenging and rewarding professional career in the US Army. The practice of pharmacy in the station hospitals is at a high professional level and the general area of supply and materiel management offers many opportunities.

Advanced training is available to regular Army officers leading to Master of Science and to Doctor of Philosophy degrees for certain specialty areas. The Army has developed a career planning program for use by the Medical Service Corps. The purpose and scope of the Army Career planning program is as follows:*

"1. Career planning for Army officers involves the entire field of personnel management and facilitates the realization of three primary objectives: First, it provides for the maximum development and utilization of an officer's inherent abilities, aptitudes, and interests, as well as for the best utilization of his acquired skills and accumulated knowledge. It recognizes that an officer makes significant use of his talents when his duty requirements are consistent with his capabilities and preferences. Second, career planning assists in building and maintaining a corps of highly motivated and competent

officers which results in a more efficient and proficient Army. Third, career planning assists in fulfilling the Army's obligation to the Nation by developing competent military leaders who are qualified to occupy positions of great responsibility in periods of peace and war.

2. Career planning requires the establishment of a program of duty assignments and formal schooling designed to meet the current needs of the Army and develop skills for future requirements. The success of the program depends upon the energetic support and cooperation given by each officer, and all the echelons of command.

3. To assure success, the policies and plans outlined herein must be administered so as to insure that—

    a. All officers are classified according to their qualifications, and such qualifications are made a matter of record.

    b. The professional capabilities of officers are developed to the highest level through intelligently planned and progressive rotation of assignments in order that the Army will always have a sufficient number of qualified officers to successfully accomplish its many assigned missions and functions.

    c. All officers have equal opportunity for selection for promotion, and significant assignments on the basis of demonstrated merit."

Enlisted Pharmacists—The utilization of pharmacists in an enlisted status should be mentioned also. Due to legislative and budgetary limitations, many skilled jobs must necessarily be filled by noncommissioned officers and enlisted personnel. Only positions of the greatest responsibility and requiring the highest type of leadership are necessarily filled by officers. The pharmacy colleges in the United States annually graduate about 4000 pharmacists. After screening out those with previous service, and those physically or otherwise disqualified, there remain 1000 to 1500 who are draft eligible. The Army has the job of classifying and assigning by numerical quotas of physically and mentally qualified men these inductees who have been placed in the Army to serve their country by Congressional direction. This classification and assignment job is to place them as nearly as possible where their special talents may be best utilized. The Army requirement for pharmacists does not compare with proportionate needs in civilian life. A distinct improvement of manpower utilization is that an Army regulation directs that all pharmacy inductees be assigned to Army medical service. This assures that no pharmacy graduate will go, for example, to Infantry, unless he is an Army medical man assigned to that type of unit. In September of 1961 it became necessary to reopen the Army Pharmacy Technicians School since the number of pharmacists being inducted under Selective Service was insufficient to meet the requirements for pharmacy technicians. This school is continuing with an annual output of approximately 150 trained pharmacy technicians. Many of these pharmacy technicians are being trained also as laboratory technicians, operating room technicians, medical record specialists, etc. All these positions go up to the highest noncommissioned officer rating, subject to vacancies being available. The enlisted staff also compounds and manufactures prescriptions under the supervision of the Pharmacy Officer. Commissioned officers who are graduates of recognized colleges of pharmacy, and duly licensed to practice pharmacy in the United States or its territories or possessions, are in charge of pharmacies in Army treatment facilities.

Navy

The US Navy organization for medical care is considerably different from that of the Army because of the nature of the basic service rendered by this branch of the Armed Forces. It does have some training stations and medical centers in various parts of the United States and its possessions, and here the general pattern

---

* Army Medical Service Corps, Career Planning Program, Department of the Army, Washington, D.C. 20315.

of excellent pharmaceutical service in hospitals is followed.

However, medical service on ships takes on a different form and only the larger units of the aircraft carrier class carry major equipment and personnel for complete medical service. The smaller units rely on emergency facilities, and the Navy, since its formal beginning in 1775, has relied on a *Hospital Corps,* which is trained specifically to care for the sick and injured.

In the early days of the Navy it was the practice to buy stocks of drugs from pharmacies and to have such prescriptions as were compounded made up by the surgeon's assistants, who were in many cases trained pharmacists.

In 1894 the APhA Committee on Status of Pharmacists in the Government Service reported that graduates of schools of pharmacy were assigned to the position of apothecary in the Navy following examination by a board of medical officers. In 1898, an Act of Congress was passed providing for the establishment of a Hospital Corps in the Navy consisting of pharmacists, hospital stewards, and hospital apprentices in the US Navy, and authorized the Secretary of the Navy to appoint 25 pharmacists with the rank, pay, and privileges of warrant officers. This Act was approved on June 17, 1898.

It was not until 1916 that any worthwhile progress was made in improving the status of pharmacists in the Navy. In that year the Naval Appropriation Act provided that pharmacists could, after 6 years of service as warrant officers, be commissioned as chief pharmacists "after passing satisfactorily such examinations as the Secretary of the Navy may prescribe."

During World War II pharmacists enlisting in the Navy were assigned to the Hospital Corps and were advanced in both noncommissioned and commissioned grades for duties involving first aid, minor surgery, general hospital work, prescription compounding, chemical analysis, and bacteriological work.

Navy Medical Service Corps

When the Medical Service Corps Act was passed in 1947, the Surgeon General of the Navy provided for a Pharmacy Section in the Medical Service Corps and a number of pharmacists have been commissioned for service in this Section. The *US Navy Medical Service Corps* numbers about 1688 officers, organized in 6 sections: Supply and Administration, Medical and Allied Sciences, Pharmacy, Optometry, Podiatry, and a Medical Specialist Section. The largest section is the Supply and Administration Section with 965 officers; the smallest is Podiatry, with 9 officers. There are 106 officers in the Pharmacy Section, 367 in the Medical Allied Science Section, 70 in the Optometrist Section, and 112 in the Medical Specialist Section. The total figure given above (1695) includes 59 commissioned warrant officers. There are many pharmacists who have transferred to the Allied Sciences Section and are assigned various duties in research and in atomic, chemical, and biological warfare activities.

Commissioned pharmacists have been used in the Navy as instructors for hospital corpsmen and as chiefs of pharmacy service in naval hospitals. Pharmacists who have entered upon graduate study and have special qualifications have also been commissioned in the Allied Science Section of the Medical Service Corps of the Navy.

This Corps also has a chief who could be selected from among the pharmacist officers of the Corps, although up to the present time no pharmacist has served in that capacity. See footnote on page 48.

Air Force

The United States Air Force Medical Service was activated on July 1, 1949. Although young in comparison with other federal medical services, the Air Force Medical Service has developed and matured rapidly. Pharmacists actively participated in the development of an excellent Air Force Medical Service.

In March 1965, the Medical Service Corps was reorganized into a Medical Service Corps and a Biomedical Sciences Corps. The pharmacist commissioned officers assigned to pharmacy duties were transferred to the Biomedical Sciences Corps. Pharmacy officers assigned to medical administration and medical supply duties remain in the Medical Service Corps.

The number of airmen in the Department of the Air Force, who are pharmacy graduates, is exceedingly small because the Air Force does not obtain any of its personnel through the Selective Service System. Personnel inducted into the Military Service through the Selective Service System have a 2-year period of obligated service. The Air Force, which obtains its airmen through the voluntary enlistment system, has a very firm policy which requires such personnel to agree to serve for a period of at least 4 years upon their initial entrance on active duty. In view of the firmness of this policy the average pharmacy graduate would prefer to complete 2 years of service in the Army as a draftee and return to his home pursuits. Many graduate pharmacists are utilized by the Air Force as Civil Service employees, but the preponderance of pharmacists in the Air Force are serving as commissioned officers in the Biomedical Sciences Corps.

Air Force Biomedical Sciences Corps

The objectives of the Biomedical Sciences Corps program was, and continues to be to provide a management structure for more adequate career planning, career development, and long-range programs for the most effective utilization of allied health professionals within the Air Force Medical Service.

Authorized specialties besides pharmacy in the Air Force Biomedical Sciences Corps are optometry, biomedical laboratory, bioenvironmental engineering, entomology, aviation physiology, clinical psychology, social worker, health physicist, dietitian, occupational therapy, physical therapy, biomedical scientist, and biomedical therapy.

Major progress has been achieved on the pharmacy element of the BSC program. In accordance with policies issued by the Department of Defense, necessary action has been taken to establish authorizations for pharmacists at major fixed medical facilities of the Air Force Medical Service. Commissioned officers on active duty serving in the line of the Air Force or in the MSC, and properly qualified airmen may apply for appointment or reappointment in the Biomedical Sciences Corps for duty as pharmacists. A total of 90 new authorizations for 1967 resulted from this special action.

There are 104 commissioned pharmacy officers in the Biomedical Sciences Corps assigned to pharmacy duties. Additional commissioned pharmacy officers function in the area of medical administration and medical supply. There are also men with a degree in pharmacy who have elected to become pilots or navigators serving with other components of the Air Force.

Graduate licensed pharmacists may be commissioned as Reserve officers in the Air Force Biomedical Sciences Corps, with concurrent active duty for a minimum period of 3 years which begins on the date they are ordered to active duty. Appointment in the Regular Air Force is highly competitive and is limited to Reserve officers on extended active duty. Applicants for a Reserve commission must be citizens of the United States, of good moral character, physically and professionally qualified, and at least 18 years of age. Individuals must have a license to practice pharmacy in one of the states or the District of Columbia and a baccalaureate degree in pharmacy from an accredited institution.

Commissioned pharmacists may be assigned duty primarily as pharmacy officers, but opportunities are available in other specialty fields of the Biomedical Sciences Corps and the Medical Service Corps. Pharmacists, by virtue of their educational background, attitude, and motivation, make excellent medical administrators, clinical laboratory officers, and medical supply officers. A few pharmacists are actively engaged in aerospace medical research. Each pharmacist is filling a position where his training and education help him to better accomplish his mission or one where he is fully utilizing his training in pharmacy. Many of the officers are in charge of pharmacies on an additional duty basis. Pharmacists are considered essential to the Air Force Biomedical Sciences Corps and are contributing to its success.

The Air Force provides selected Biomedical Sciences Corps officers with the opportunity for further education at some of the finest civilian and military schools in the country without the worry of heavy personal or financial burdens. A career in the Air Force Medical Service Corps also provides a life of rich professional experience, travel, and rewarding friendships, combined with personal dignity and security.

Department of Health, Education and Welfare

The United States Public Health Service of the Department of Health, Education and Welfare (HEW) is an outgrowth of the *Marine Hospital Service*, which was established in 1798 to provide hospital service and medical treatment for American merchant seamen. Pharmacists were employed in the Marine hospitals from the beginning under various titles including apothecaries, hospital stewards, pharmacists, and chemists. Those employed in the early days of the Marine Hospital Service under the title of apothecaries were engaged fully in pharmaceutical work except for such administrative duties as were part of the operation of the pharmacy.

In 1902 the name of the Marine Hospital Service was changed to the *Public Health and Marine Hospital Service* and the head of the service was designated as the Surgeon-General. Although an effort was made at that time by the APhA Committee on Status of Pharmacists in Government Service to provide commissioned rank for pharmacists in the service, this was not accomplished. However, the Surgeon-General created a position with the title of Pharmacist in the Service and there was general recognition of the pharmaceutical and administrative activities of pharmacists in the Public Health Service from that time on. As a result, a number of pharmacists entered the Public Health Service in a career capacity and when, in 1912, the name of the Public Health and Marine Hospital Service was changed to the Public Health Service,

pharmacists obtained professional recognition based on the education and training of the individual. This recognition has varied in accordance with the progress of pharmaceutical education as reflected in the minimum course requirements for the accredited undergraduate degree.

The Public Health Service has drawn its personnel from the Civil Service lists and by granting commissions. Legislation (The Parker Act) passed in 1930 for the purpose of coordinating the public health activities of the government authorized the appointment of pharmacists, as well as physicians, dentists, nurses, sanitary engineers, and other health professionals, as commissioned officers in the Public Health Service, by the President. These commissioned officers rank with the Army, Navy, and Air Force and are frequently assigned for duty with the Armed Forces in time of war or in national emergencies.

Experience over many years has shown the expediency and effectiveness of having a mobile corps of pharmacists. For the proper performance of their remarkably varied duties, they must have a broad understanding of the methods and functions of the Service, an understanding gained only by training and background of actual participation in field work. Thus, it is the practice to assign pharmacists, upon appointment, to the smaller stations, and later transfer them to more important posts.

The availability of the individual pharmacist for whatever duty might be assigned to him and the changes of duty and station have the collective effect of creating a permanent mobile corps of trained pharmacist officers who are essential to effective operation of Service activities.

As the Service expanded through the years, pharmacists have served at most of its field stations, including hospitals, quarantine stations, supply depots, research stations, and the like, both in the US and abroad.

The Department of Health, Education, and Welfare employs a considerable number of pharmacists in a variety of assignments, both as commissioned officers of the US Public Health Service and as Civil Service pharmacists. The National Institutes of Health employs pharmacists in the clinical research area, in the Division of Biologics Standards, in personnel assignments, in research assignments, and as grant administrators.

The Health Services and Mental Health Administration utilizes pharmacists in the clinical area of the National Institutes of Mental Health, Indian Health Service, and the Federal Health Programs Service. Pharmacists also fill responsible positions in the Community Health Service, Health Facilities Planning and Construction Service, and the Regional Medical Programs Service.

Many pharmacists are utilized effectively in the Food and Drug Administration of the Consumer Protection Environmental Health Service as new drug application reviewers, pharmacologists, computer programers, and in administration. The Social Security Administration has pharmacists filling responsible positions dealing with drug reimbursements and drug distribution problems.

The Public Health Service offers 1-year pharmacy residences at seven hospitals: Baltimore, Md.; Boston, Mass.; Gallup, N. Mex.; New Orleans, La.; San Francisco, Calif.; Seattle, Wash.; and Staten Island, N.Y. The Public Health Service pharmacy residencies begin on or about July 1 of each year. They afford graduate pharmacists opportunities to obtain the specialized training necessary to manage pharmacy departments and to become drug therapy consultants to the medical and dental staffs in today's modern hospitals.

Seniors in accredited schools of pharmacy may apply for these residencies provided they will have received a degree in pharmacy and met all other requirements prior to July 1. Each of the US Public Health Service hospitals offering pharmacy residency programs has a minimum of 200 general medical and surgical beds plus an outpatient department.

At US Public Health Service hospitals the pharmaceutical activities constitute a professional service within the clinical branch. The chief of the pharmacy department is responsible for the efficient administration of his service, and he is a voting member and secretary of the hospital's pharmacy and therapeutics committee.

The pharmacy residency program of the Public Health Service is coordinated jointly by the Chief, Pharmacy Branch, Federal Health Programs Service, and a senior pharmacist who serves as advisor for the training of pharmacy officers. Within the hospital, the chief of the pharmacy department directs the pharmacy residency program.

The residency consists of a postgraduate program of organized training and "at work" experiences in the varied activities of hospital pharmacy. Through a series of lectures and conferences the practice and theory of hospital pharmacy administration are covered in depth.

During the year a program of planned visits among the other departments of the hospital—such as internal medicine, surgery, pathology, radiology, nursing, and administration—are made. The resident participates in meetings of the pharmacy staff, the pharmacy and therapeutics committee, and journal conferences. He also attends many professional meetings of the hospital, both educational and administrative in nature, and has the opportunity to work with interns and residents from other services on joint studies.

Thus, the resident pharmacist gains firsthand knowledge of the professional and management activities that comprise not only hospital pharmacy but the total hospital function, with special reference to drug evaluation, selection, storage, and utilization; also to clinical drug studies, drug movement, and control.

The chiefs of pharmaceutical services in the USPHS hospitals serve on therapeutics committees, participate in staff discussions, and give instruction to interns and residents in other specialties on pharmaceutical aspects of medical care. They operate pharmacy service in general hospitals, outpatient clinics, and hospitals specializing in tuberculosis, leprosy, mental diseases, and narcotic addiction.

The function of the Pharmacy Branch of the Federal Health Programs Service is to promote the technical development of professional standards for pharmaceutical service; integrate the pharmacy service in the medical team; expand and develop bulk-compounding and prepackaging procedures; economize through more efficient procurement, storage, and use of pharmaceutical supplies; develop professional techniques and procedures; and establish teaching, training, and advisory services.

The Pharmacy Branch of the Indian Health Service provides pharmaceutical service in a system of 51 hospitals (ranging from 6 to 330 beds, each with a large outpatient department), 55 health centers, and several hundred field health stations.

Federal health services for American Indians date back to the early 1800's when Army physicians undertook to curb smallpox and other contagious diseases among Indian tribes living near military posts. The present-day program has grown out of treaties subsequently negotiated, which included various provisions for medical services. In 1849 the Bureau of Indian Affairs was transferred from the War Department to the Department of the Interior, and in 1955 the health program was transferred to the Public Health Service, US Department of Health, Education and Welfare.

Indians receive the full range of curative, preventive, and rehabilitative health services, including public health nursing, maternal and child health, dental, pharmacy, nutrition services, and health education.

In 1968 there were 398 pharmacists in the Department of Health, Education and Welfare. The greater number of these were assigned to positions within the Public Health Service. Of those pharmacists on active duty, 18 were in the Civil Service status and 380 held commissions in the Public Health Service Commissioned Corps. Grade distribution of the Civil Service pharmacists were as follows: GS-9:5; GS-10:4, GS-11:6; GS-12:1; GS-13:2. Rank distribution of the commissioned officers was as follows: Assistant Pharmacist (First Lieutenant): 44; Senior Assistant Pharmacist (Captain): 182; Pharmacist (Major): 81; Senior Pharmacist (Lt. Colonel): 37; and Pharmacist Director (Colonel): 36.

Veterans Administration

Rapid expansion of the Veterans Administration began immediately following World War II, with the tremendous increase in the veteran population. Today the Veterans Administration operates 166 hospitals and 200 outpatient clinics with over 700 pharmacists providing a professional pharmacy service to these activities.

VA Department of Medicine and Surgery

With the reorganization of the Veterans Administration and the passage of Public Law 293 in 1946, provisions were made for a Chief Pharmacist in the Department of Medicine and Surgery and basic educational requirements were established for pharmacists.

The Director of the Pharmacy Service, along with a staff in the Washington office, is responsible for developing overall professional procedures and policies for pharmacy operations. He evaluates the effectiveness and operating efficiency of the pharmacies as a part of the medical care program, ensuring operation in keeping with the principles and practices of the profession of pharmacy.

Training—In-service training is planned and conducted to keep all pharmacists abreast of trends in the field of pharmacy and related technical sciences. Under the present program pharmacists are sent to Institutes on Hospital Pharmacy sponsored by the American Society of Hospital Pharmacists, intra-VA pharmacy conferences are scheduled and held in various localities throughout the United States; Chief Pharmacists from smaller hospitals and clinics are sent for training periods to larger teaching hospitals to benefit from modern trends and developments in professional practices; staff personnel are detailed to other hospitals or clinics for indoctrination periods in administrative and professional procedures, and given opportunities to assume sole responsibility for their application. In-service training programs are subject to continuing review and are changed or adapted to suit special needs or advances in pharmacy and medicine.

Recognizing the need for highly trained specialists in the field of hospital pharmacy, the Veterans Administration conducts a program of hospital pharmacy residency training. The residency is a 2-year combined course established at a hospital in cooperation with the graduate school of a university. It consists of clinical experience in hospital and out-patient pharmacy with assigned duties of the highest professional level including pharmaceutical research. The resident also is given general orientation in hospital administration, and pharmacy's relationship to other professional and administrative services. Approximately half of the resident's time is devoted to hospital and clinic training, and the remainder in attending college classes at the graduate level to satisfy the requirement for the degree of Master of Science or Doctor of Pharmacy (PharmD) degree.

Opportunity is also offered to pharmacy college graduates to train as pharmacy interns in some VA hospitals. During the 1-year program, training and clinical experience under supervision of registered pharmacists is provided. The training program meets the standards for hospital pharmacy internships adopted by the American Society of Hospital Pharmacists. Although given primarily for specialized training in hospital pharmacy, a VA hospital pharmacy internship will meet the practical experience requirements of most State Boards of Pharmacy for registration.

Applications for residencies and internships are made directly to the hospital offering this program. Information on the current programs available may be obtained from the Director, Pharmacy Service, VA Central Office, Washington, D.C. 20420.

To assure uninterrupted professional pharmacy service at all times, a rotating pharmacist program is directed from Central Office. Seven pharmacists are on duty in strategically located hospitals and are on call for temporary assignment to other stations in the general area of their home stations. Availability of professional services thus is assured during periods of emergency sick and vacation leave of regularly assigned pharmacy personnel.

Duties and Responsibilities—Pharmacists perform a full range of professional pharmacy duties and are an integral part of the medical team. Organizationally the Pharmacy Service is at the same level as other professional specialties.

In hospitals and clinics, pharmacists are expected to give indoctrination and refresher training courses. They also prepare lectures and demonstrations for the nursing staff covering topics such as storage of drugs, drug usage, methods of administration, pharmaceutical arithmetic and conversions, percentage solutions, and calculating doses. Topics such as prescription writing, drug usage, posology, and incompatibilities may be assigned for presentation at training sessions of the medical staff. At hospitals with medical residency and intern programs, pharmacists may be called on to prepare lectures for residents and interns as part of the formal training course. Chief pharmacists work with the medical staff in planning and presenting the pharmacy contribution to the teaching situation.

Chief pharmacists serve as secretaries to hospital and clinic committees on therapeutic agents. These committees, usually composed of the Chief of Staff or Clinic Director, as chairman and other designated medical consultants, formulate drug policy, recommend drugs for standard pharmacy stock, and determine which drugs will be added to the formulary and the scope of information to be included.

Pharmacists are responsible for maintaining a working library of standard pharmaceutical references and a current file of pertinent data from professional journals and drug manufacturers' literature.

Guided by general policies established in Central Office, Chief Pharmacists establish procedures, methods, and working schedules for pharmacy operations. The Chief Pharmacist coordinates pharmacy activities with other medical services or clinics. With the co-operation of the personnel office, he selects suitable professional and nonprofessional personnel, initiates promotions, and prepares performance ratings. He is responsible for indoctrinating new personnel and for carrying on a continuous training program for staff pharmacists to keep them informed on new pharmaceutical developments, pharmacy research, and unusual or complex pharmacy problems.

Qualifications—To be eligible for appointment, all applicants must have completed at least a four-year course in pharmacy and have a bachelor's, master's, or doctor's degree from an approved school. The applicant must also be currently registered as a pharmacist in one of the states or territories of the United States or in the District of Columbia. Appointments are made from Civil Service registers established by competitive examinations. The examination consists of rating the applicant on the basis of his education and experience as a registered pharmacist, including the breadth, variety, difficulty and complexity of his work, and his demonstrated ability to supervise.

Appointments—Appointments of registered pharmacists are generally made at the staff pharmacist level, and higher grade vacancies are usually filled by promotion of qualified on-duty VA pharmacists. This provides a maximum of opportunity for career development.

Staff pharmacist positions are generally classified at Grades GS-9 and GS-11, GS-9 being a staff pharmacist with limited responsibilities; it is essentially a training position preparing the employee for the next higher grade level. The GS-11 position applies to a staff pharmacist performing a full range of pharmacy duties as a specialist or generalist.

Chief pharmacist positions are usually classified in Grades GS-11 to GS-14, depending on the extent of the activity and the responsibilities of the position. There are a limited number of administrative positions in Grades GS-14 and GS-15, which are usually filled by promotion of pharmacists within the Veterans Administration.

Benefits—Pharmacists in the Veterans Administration receive numerous benefits afforded by Federal employment, including paid vacations, sick leave pay, low-cost group life insurance, health insurance, and an excellent retirement plan. Salary is based on the standard Federal work week of 40 hours. Table I indicates salary schedules in effect in 1968.

Other Federal Agencies

The Public Health Service supplies pharmaceutical personnel for the Coast Guard and the Bureau of Prisons, and the Navy supplies such personnel for the Marine Corps. Since the medical service for the Marine Corps is supplied by the US Navy, there is no separate medical service corps in the USMC.

Table I—Salaries of Pharmacists in Civil Service

Grade	Entrance salary	Periodic increase	Maximum salary
GS-9	$ 8,462	$282	$11,000
GS-10	9,297	310	12,087
GS-11	10,203	340	13,263
GS-12	12,174	406	15,828
GS-13	14,409	480	18,729
GS-14	16,946	565	22,031

The Bureau of Narcotic and Controlled Drugs of the Department of Justice, the Department of Commerce, and the Internal Revenue Service of the Treasury Department, which deals with problems relating to alcohol, employ pharmacists in various capacities. These include inspectors, laboratory supervisors, and administrative personnel.

The Food and Drug Administration requires pharmacists in its field service, as well as in its main office and laboratories in Washington, D.C. Inspection work in the field includes the tracing of shipments of adulterated and misbranded drugs, preparation of records for enforcement, and prosecution of violations. A considerable amount of the work of the Food and Drug Administration includes education of the professions and industries concerned, on regulatory matters involving the production and distribution of drugs. Pharmacists assist in preparing information, answering correspondence, and addressing meetings of professional and lay groups on the requirements of the Federal Food, Drug and Cosmetic Act.

The Bureau of Narcotic and Controlled Drugs has made a point of employing registered pharmacists in its inspection service since this work requires the background provided by pharmaceutical training. Most of the positions in this service are available in the field rather than in the main office of the Bureau in Washington. They involve not only the inspection of prescription records but also detection of the illicit distribution of narcotic drugs.

State, County, and Municipal Government Agencies

In addition to employment in Federal Government agencies dealing with regulation of the distribution of drugs there are numerous opportunities for similar service with state departments of health, state boards of pharmacy, state bureaus of narcotics, state and county welfare administration departments, and similar agencies where activities such as those described above are carried on at the state and county levels. This applies also to the larger municipalities.

The coordination of municipal, state and federal enforcement procedures with regard to drugs, especially as this pertains to regulation of narcotics, hypnotic drugs such as the barbiturates, and dangerous drugs and poisons, opens a large opportunity for the employment of pharmacists who may be especially interested in regulatory activities. Very often pharmacists who start in federal positions and acquire considerable experience at that level have opportunity to take over administrative functions of a similar nature in state and municipal agencies where coordination is greatly enhanced by the past experience at the Federal level.

The administrative functions of state, county, and local organizations having to do with the enforcement of health and welfare regulations frequently include specific duties that require a background of pharmaceutical training.

Many of these agencies deal with such matters as disease prevention and medical care. A recently increasing function of state governments is the administration of welfare medical care programs. In carrying out this function state and local appropriations are augmented or matched by Federal appropriations to an ever-increasing extent. In such instances pharmacists are frequently employed to supervise the administration of pharmaceutical services in welfare medical care programs, especially those which involve what has become known as "vendor payments" for prescription drugs and pharmaceutical services.

These agencies usually appoint advisory committees consisting of representatives of the various health professions, including pharmacy, to aid in developing and enforcing their programs.

Some pharmacists, as well as other health personnel, are employed by these agencies on a full-time basis and are usually designated as pharmacy advisors or consultants. State welfare agencies which are called on to pay for millions of prescriptions supplied annually to indigent or medically indigent and aging patients at government expense, will employ such consultants on a full- or part-time basis or will create positions under civil service for pharmacists in order to provide for an expert review of the pricing of prescriptions so as to keep them within the range of payment prescribed by the agency.

These pharmacists are expected to give advice on the best methods of reducing drug costs to the welfare agency. They are also expected to work with medical consultants and members of the medical profession in devising such limitations and extension of medical care services as may be indicated.

Government service, while usually not as remunerative as employment in industry, has certain compensations in the form of retirement benefits, medical services, annual and sick leave, and other benefits which constitute attractions. In recent years there has also been a tendency on the part of government agencies to provide time for formal education in various specialties, thus enabling the incumbents of these positions to improve their status.

The Department of Labor as well as the US Civil Service Commission are usually good sources of information for openings in government positions.

7 | Literature

History of American pharmacopeias—official pharmacopeias of the world—official US compendia (USP, NF, and Homeopathic Pharmacopeia)—reference literature of pharmacy, including books, periodicals, and services

This chapter was prepared by

Charles O. Wilson, PhD, *Dean, School of Pharmacy, Oregon State University, Corvallis, Ore. 97331*

Early American literature on materia medica and pharmacy was obtained mostly from Europe, where the ablest physicians of the colonial period were educated. The first pharmaceutical publication in North America was *Electuarium novum Alexipharmacum*, written in 1732 by the Reverend Thomas Harward. In 1734 Benjamin Franklin, the first printer of American medical books, published *Every Man His Own Doctor, or the Poor Planter's Physician*, which prescribed "plain and easy means for persons to cure themselves of all or most of the distempers of this climate, and with very little charge, the medicines being chiefly of the growth and production of this country." The *Lititz Pharmacopœia*, a 32-page pamphlet, was compiled by Dr. William Brown in 1778 for use in the Military Hospital of Washington's Army, but it was not generally applicable since it was restricted to those remedies available during the trying war period. In 1787, immediately after the Revolutionary War, and one year before the Constitution of the United States was ratified, Dr. Schoepf published his book, *Materia Medica Americana Potissimum Regni Vegetabilis*. In it he describes about 400 American medicinal plants which he had studied during the course of his travels throughout North America. In 1808 the Massachusetts Medical Society published for its own use a pharmacopeia written in English with Latin titles; this presentation was a departure from established custom, for previous to that time all similar works had been written in Latin. The first edition of the *Pharmacopœia of the New York Hospital* was published by Dr. Samuel L. Mitchill and Dr. Valentine Seaman in 1816.

Early National Literature

In January, 1817, realizing that previous works were somewhat limited in their use, the farseeing Dr. Lyman Spalding outlined to the New York County Medical Society his plans for the preparation of a national pharmacopœia, to be authorized by all medical societies and medical schools in the United States. Through his efforts a Pharmacopœial Convention was held January 1, 1820, with Dr. Samuel L. Mitchill presiding, and the 1st edition of the *Pharmacopœia of the United States* (USP) was released on December 15, 1820, as the first major step in the creation of an authoritative national literature of pharmacy and medicine. Dr. Spalding prepared the book, which was to be revised decennially, with Latin on the left-hand pages and an English translation on facing pages. The materia medica was divided into two categories: "articles of decided reputation or general use" and "those the claims of which are of a more uncertain kind."

In 1825 the *Journal of the Philadelphia College of Pharmacy*, which became the *American Journal of Pharmacy* in 1835, began publication for the advancement of pharmacy and the promotion of education and research. This was the first American pharmaceutical journal. In the same year the Massachusetts College of Pharmacy prepared the first pharmaceutical library catalog. In 1826 the Philadelphia College of Pharmacy issued *The Druggist's Manual*, a catalog of American and foreign drugs, chemicals, dyes, etc. Between 1828 and 1830 C. S. Rafinesque published his work, *Medical Flora; or Manual of Medical Botany of the United States of North America*, the first dependable book on botany originating in the United States.

The USP Convention of 1830 was called by the President, Dr. S. L. Mitchill, as directed by the 1820 Convention, but, through a misunderstanding, two conventions were finally called, one in New York City and another in Washington, D.C. Both conventions subsequently published a USP of 1830, but only the one which had the authority of the established Washington Convention survived.

In 1830 the Revision Chairman, elected by the Washington Convention, was Dr. Thomas T. Hewson of Philadelphia. He was ably assisted by other Philadelphia physicians, especially Dr. George B. Wood and Dr. Franklin Bache, and also by pharmacists connected with the Philadelphia College of Pharmacy. Among these pharmacists was Daniel B. Smith, President of the College and the first President of the American Pharmaceutical Association.

In 1833 Doctors Wood and Bache published the first edition of the *United States Dispensatory* for the specific purpose of supporting the USP of 1830, as issued by the Washington Convention. This book is discussed on page 62. A number of other dispensatories have been published in this country. The first, the *American Dispensatory* (1806), was prepared by Dr. John Redman Coxe, professor of medicine at the University of Pennsylvania. This book passed through 6 editions, the last of which appeared in 1831. The *National Dispensatory* was first issued in 1879, but it is no longer published.

In New York, Boston, and Philadelphia the colleges of pharmacy cooperated in an unofficial capacity in preparing the USP of 1840, and the name of William Procter, Jr., appeared as an affiliate of the last-named institution. Dr. L. Condict was re-elected President of the Convention and Dr. G. B. Wood was elected Chairman of the Revision Committee. The book was published in 1842, omitting the Latin text, incorporating for the first time a few reagents, and expressing temperatures in degrees Fahrenheit.

Literature: 1850–1900

In 1849 William Procter, Jr., edited Redwood's English translation of Mohr's *Lehrbuch der Pharmaceutischen Technik* under the title *Practical Pharmacy*, but the first truly American textbook on pharmacy was published by Edward Parrish in 1855, under the title *Introduction to Practical Pharmacy*, "a textbook for the student and a guide to the Physician and Pharmaceutist," which passed through five editions, the last appearing in 1884. Professor J. P. Remington was offered the editorship of the 6th edition, but decided instead to publish his own book, *Remington's Practice of Pharmacy* (see below).

During the preparation of the USP of 1850, which became official in 1851, pharmaceutical participation became officially recognized and William Procter, Jr., of the Philadelphia College of Pharmacy, and John Milhau, of the College of Pharmacy of the City of New York, became members of the Revision Committee. Dr. G. B. Wood was again elected Chairman of the Revision Committee, also Convention President. This pharmacopeia admitted for the first time a class of preparations known as fluidextracts, but under this heading were grouped oleoresins, concentrated syrups, and concentrated tinctures.

The Pharmacopœial Convention of 1860 re-elected Dr. G. B. Wood, President, and Dr. F. Bache was elected Chairman of the Revision Committee which included the pharmacists, William Procter, Jr., and Alfred B. Taylor of Philadelphia, Charles T. Carney of Boston, and William S. Thompson of Baltimore; also the physician and pharmaceutical manufacturer, Dr. E. R. Squibb. Professor Parrish of the Philadelphia College of Pharmacy presented at this Convention copies of the *Proceedings of the American Pharmaceutical Association*, which had been published since the founding of the association in 1852. In the 5th edition of the Pharmacopœia (USP of 1860) a strictly alphabetical arrangement by Latin titles was adopted, five grades of the fineness of powders were made official, and resins and collodions were recognized.

The *United States Pharmacopœia* had become a truly national project by 1870. Eight colleges of pharmacy were represented at the Convention held that year. Dr. Joseph Carson, of Philadelphia, was elected President of the Convention and later Chairman of the Revision Committee. The veterans, George B. Wood, William Procter, Jr., Robert Bridges, and Alfred B. Taylor, who had been largely responsible for five revisions, were ready to retire, and F. Bache had died, but C. L. Diehl, A. E. Ebert, Horatio C. Wood, and John M. Maisch, distinguished young men, influenced by the rapidly changing conditions brought about by the Civil War, became active participants. The 6th edition (USP of 1870) was published in 1873. It included tables indicating the relationship of the American system of weights and measures to the metric system, and recognized the following new classes of preparations: chartæ, suppositoria, and glycerita.

During the next decade a committee was appointed by the American Pharmaceutical Association—consisting of Charles Rice, Chairman, Frederick Hoffman, and P. W. Bedford of New York; John M. Maisch, Joseph P. Remington, and Charles Bullock of Philadelphia; G. F. H. Markoe and S. A. D. Sheppard of Boston; John F. Hancock of Baltimore; A. E. Ebert of Chicago; C. L. Diehl of Louisville; E. S. Wayne of Cincinnati; W. H. Crawford of St. Louis; Charles Mohr of Mobile; and E. Painter of San Francisco—to prepare the draft for a new edition. At the 1880 Convention, 11 pharmacy colleges were represented, and the Revision Committee of 25 included 14 pharmacists. Charles Rice, of New York, pharmacist of Bellevue Hospital, was elected Chairman of the Revision Committee for preparing the USP of 1880. As a result the experts so completely modernized the book that the pattern established at that time is followed, in the main, by the pharmacopeias of today. It described botanical drugs as to their physical characteristics, and, when necessary, their chemical properties; it defined each chemical according to its formula, physical properties, and chemical reactions; it provided for purity and identity tests and some assays; it included many descriptions; it expressed temperature in both Fahrenheit and Centigrade degrees; it substituted parts by weight for the apothecary system. Supplements were authorized at this time but were not issued until many decades later.

In the USP of 1880 a large number of the English titles used in former editions were changed, the old vernacular names either being dropped altogether or inserted as synonyms. This advanced step was rendered necessary by the increase in articles used in the materia medica and by a desire for greater accuracy and better methods in nomenclature. Thus the confusion which always existed in different localities concerning the common names of drugs was avoided since the anglicized Latin name was distinctive. Such English names as *Bloodroot, Calabar Bean, Male Fern,* and *Yellow Jasmine,* for instance, were replaced by *Sanguinaria, Physostigma, Aspidium,* and *Gelsemium.* On the other hand, some of the common English names were so fixed by usage that it was not deemed judicious to alter them; besides, a change would often have necessitated the use of a longer and less convenient word. The retention of the English names *Clove, Mustard,* and *Ginger* sufficiently illustrates this.

In 1885 Joseph P. Remington published the first edition of *Remington's Practice of Pharmacy,* "a treatise on the modes of making and dispensing official, unofficial, and extemporaneous preparations, with descriptions of their properties, uses, and doses, intended as a handbook for pharmacists and physicians and a textbook for students." At that time he was Professor of the Theory and Practice of Pharmacy at the Philadelphia College of Pharmacy, Vice-Chairman of the Committee of Revision of the USP and pharmaceutical editor of the *United States Dispensatory.*

In 1888 the American Pharmaceutical Association began publishing the *National Formulary* (NF) to provide standards for those medicinal preparations which were not considered sufficiently important nor of a type suitable for inclusion in the United States Pharmacopœia. The *New York and Brooklyn Formulary* was the forerunner of the NF.

The creation of a responsible executive body in 1880 greatly facilitated subsequent revisions of the USP; experts were engaged to collect and compile criticisms. These *Digests,* compiled in turn by Hans M. Wilder (until 1901), by Florence Yaple and Henry Kraemer (until 1905), by Murray Galt Motter and Martin I. Wilbert (until 1914), by the latter (until 1917), and by A. G. DuMez (until 1924), included the NF after 1905 and during the period from 1909 to 1924 were issued by the US Government as *Bulletins* of the Hygienic Laboratory of the Treasury Department of the United States Public Health Service. From 1926 to 1948 the abstracts appeared in "The Bibliography of Pharmaceutical Research," a section of the *Journal of the American Pharmaceutical Association*. The USP contributed toward the cost.

Horatio C. Wood, Sr., a nephew of George B. Wood, became President of the 1890 Convention. Charles Rice was again elected Chairman and Joseph P. Remington Vice-Chairman of the Committee of Revision composed of 8 physicians and 17 pharmacists. The following changes and additions were among those made in the USP of 1890: Assays for the determination of the active principles of official drugs were provided; optical rotation was added as a physical characteristic; the metric system was introduced for the first time. Two new principles were to be enforced. The introduction into the Pharmacopœia of any substance "which cannot be produced otherwise than under a patented process or which is protected by proprietary rights" was prohibited, and "a definite date, reasonably distant from the actual date of publication when the new Pharmacopœia is intended to go into effect and to supersede the preceding one," must be announced. The 8th edition (USP of 1890) became official January 1, 1894.

USP Since 1900

USP VIII—At the 8th Decennial Convention in 1900, Horatio C. Wood, Sr., was again elected President and Charles Rice was re-elected Chairman of the Revision Committee, which consisted of 18 pharmacists and 7 physicians. Charles Rice died, however, the following year and Joseph P. Remington took his place. Several important changes in the plan of the work were made. The business portion was separated from that of actual revision by creating a Board of Trustees whose duty it was to be responsible for any legal questions which might arise, make contracts, attend to the finances, and place the book on sale. The Convention was also incorporated at that time under a charter issued at Washington, D.C. The USP of 1900, which was published in 1905, adopted average doses, the "Purity Rubric," and 25°C as the standard temperature for specific gravity and solubility statements. The title USP VIII was adopted for the 9th edition to indicate that it was the "8th Revision." A new ruling on scope gave the Committee of Revision authority to admit "any product of nature of known origin; also any synthesized product of definite composition which is in common use by the medical profession, the identity, purity, or strength of which can be determined."

On June 30, 1906, mainly through the efforts of Harvey W. Wiley, Chief Chemist of the Department of Agriculture, the Pure Food and Drugs Act came into effect, establishing the USP and the NF as the legal standards for all medicinal products recognized by these books, whether they are manufactured in this country or imported.

USP IX—At the 9th Decennial Convention in Washington in 1910, Harvey W. Wiley was elected President and Remington was re-elected Chairman of the Committee of Revision, which was increased from 26 to 51 members including the President as an *ex-officio* member. The Convention authorized the formation of an Executive Committee, composed of the 15 chairmen of the Subcommittees. USP IX added for the first time biological assays, biological products, a chapter on diagnostic reagents, a chapter on sterilization, statements of the alcohol percentages of preparations, descriptions of the microscopical characteristics of the official drugs, and a chapter on meth-

ods for analytical determinations. Joseph P. Remington died in 1918 and Charles H. LaWall succeeded him.

USP X—At the 10th Decennial Convention in 1920, Dr. Reid Hunt was elected President and Dr. E. Fullerton Cook was elected Chairman of the Committee of Revision. Every interested organization in the United States participated in this revision and the Pharmacopœial program became enormously involved and elaborate. USP X became official January 1, 1926, and included the first official vitamin assay.

USP XI was prepared by a committee appointed by the National Convention for revising the Pharmacopœia, which met in Washington, D.C., May 13, 1930. Walter A. Bastedo, a physician and former pharmacist, was elected President and Dr. Cook was re-elected Chairman. Fifty-nine medical bodies, 104 incorporated pharmaceutical organizations, and Medical Departments of the Army and Navy, the US Public Health Service, the US Department of Agriculture, the American Medical Association, the American Pharmaceutical Association, the American Chemical Society, the American Dental Association, the Association of American Dairy, Food and Drug Officials, the Association of Official Agricultural Chemists, the National Association of Wholesale Druggists, the National Association of Boards of Pharmacy, the National Association of Retail Druggists, and the American Drug Manufacturers' Association sent delegates to this Convention, which selected from those present 50 members, with the President of the Convention a member *ex-officio*, making the total 51. These were designated as the "General Committee of Revision of the Pharmacopœia of the United States of America."

The convention of 1930 made no change in the organization of the Committee of Revision, and the General Committee, as soon after its election as possible, met, elected officers, and the chairman organized the work of revision, appointing 15 Subcommittees to report upon the several divisions of the work. These Subcommittees were:

1. Scope (Admissions and Deletions)
2. Therapeutics and Pharmacodynamics (Posology)
3. Biological Assays
4. Biological Products and Diagnostic Tests
5. Botany and Pharmacognosy
6. Proximate Assays
7. Inorganic Chemicals
8. Organic Chemicals
9. Reagents and Test Solutions
10. Volatile Oils
11. Extracts, Fluidextracts, and Tinctures
12. Waters, Solutions, Spirits, Syrups, and Elixirs
13. Cerates, Ointments, and Miscellaneous Galenicals
14. Tables, Weights, and Measures
15. Nomenclature

Each Subcommittee organized and elected its own Chairman.

These Subcommittee Chairmen, through appointment by the General Chairman and election by the General Committee and Board of Trustees, formed the Executive Committee of Revision, with the Chairman of the General Committee also as Chairman of the Executive Committee, and the actual work of revision began. According to the Bylaws of the Convention, the "Executive Committee shall execute such orders or resolutions as have been assigned to it by the Convention, the General Committee of Revision, or the Board of Trustees, and have entire charge of the preparation of the manuscript and reading of proof for the revised Pharmacopœia." The General Committee of

Revision represents geographically various parts of the United States, and it is necessary to conduct the revision largely by mail. The Board and Committee remain in office until the next decennial convention, or until their successors are appointed. During the Eleventh Revision it became necessary to obtain the assistance of experts in special fields, and the "USP Vitamin Advisory Board" and the "USP Anti-Anemia Products Advisory Board" were organized. USP XI became official June 1, 1936.

USP XII—At the Pharmacopœial Convention of 1940 Dr. Charles W. Edmunds was elected President (Dr. Cary Eggleston succeeded him on his death in 1941) and Dr. Cook was re-elected Chairman of the Revision Committee. New Advisory Boards were organized for endocrine products, blood substitutes, and sterile products, and Advisory Committees were formed to recommend standards for insulin and glassware. It was decided at this Convention to publish a Pharmacopœia every five years instead of decennially. "In selecting the medicinal substances and preparations for inclusion in the Twelfth Revision, trademark or patent complications which might be involved in some cases have been ignored, the question of therapeutic value only being considered." USP XII became official November 1, 1942.

Since another Pharmacopœial Convention would not be held until 1950, practically the same men who had prepared the last edition prepared USP XIII. A major alteration was made in the titles of the Pharmacopœia; the English title was placed first and a marginal title was included for each monograph and so arranged that all products and preparations of each basic substance were grouped with that substance in an alphabetical arrangement.

Revision of Constitution and Bylaws of the USP Convention—The USP Convention of 1940 authorized the establishment of a committee to revise the Constitution and Bylaws. This committee presented its recommendations to a special meeting of the Convention called for that purpose on April 7, 1942, and as a result several important changes and additions were made in procedures and responsibilities of the Board and the Revision Committee:

1. The Board of Trustees shall maintain headquarters for the business of the Pharmacopœia.
2. At least one year before each Decennial Convention, a Nominating Committee shall be established to select nominees for membership on the Revision Committee of the next decade. These nominees shall be selected from specialists suggested by the medical or pharmaceutical or other organizations represented in the USP Convention.

In all previous revisions the work was directed by a Chairman of the Revision Committee who was elected by the Committee from among its membership at the beginning of each decade. The new Constitution and Bylaws directed the Board of Trustees to elect a "Director of Revision" 6 months prior to each Decennial Convention and a successor should the office become vacant. It also authorized the Board to elect an Assistant to the Director if found necessary, who might also serve as Secretary to the Board of Trustees.

It was believed that these changes in procedure would insure for the direction and membership of the Revision Committee outstanding authorities in a wide variety of sciences essential to the program and also help prevent domination of the Committee's decisions by pressure groups and special interests.

USP XIV—This edition was released in May, 1950, to become official on November 1, 1950. Thus it became the 3rd revision prepared by the Revision Committee elected at the 1940 Convention; also, the diphthong was dropped in the word Pharmacopeia.

The Convention elected 60 specialists to serve as the Committee of Revision. Prior to the Convention Lloyd C. Miller had been elected by the Board of Trustees as the Director of Pharmacopeial Revision in accordance with the provisions outlined in the revised Constitution and Bylaws.

The work of revision was divided among the following 10 Subcommittees (reduced from the former 15):

1. Scope
2. Posology
3. Biologic Assays and Tests
4. Sterile Products
5. Pharmacognosy
6. Alkaloids and Heterocyclic Compounds
7. Aliphatics and Inorganic Compounds
8. Cyclic Compounds
9. External Preparations
10. Internal Preparations

Each member of the Revision Committee serves on one or more of these Subcommittees.

USP XV—This edition was released on July 1, 1955, to become official on December 15, 1955. For the first time, the Latin title was omitted from the official monograph of most drugs. In those instances where the root of a given English title is entirely different from that of the Latin equivalent, the Latin title is given among the official synonyms. This change was made since in most cases the Latin titles of modern drugs are almost identical with the English. There is, furthermore, a definite trend toward the use of English titles in prescription writing and in labeling stock containers in the pharmacy.

The graphic formulas in USP XV were changed in appearance in that hand-drawn formulas were used and all ring structures were depicted in the usual way without showing the carbon and hydrogen atoms as part of the ring. This change greatly simplified the structural formula and is in conformity with general practice in textbooks of chemistry.

The apothecaries system equivalents for the various metric quantities given in dose statements and information on sizes available were no longer given. While it is true that many old drugs such as morphine sulfate are still prescribed in the apothecaries system the Pharmacopeia adheres to the metric system exclusively.

The statements on dose were expanded in USP XV to include the usual dose and the range. Such information is provided as a guide, particularly to the pharmacist who has both a legal and a professional responsibility to make certain that the dosage prescribed is safe.

Another innovation in USP XV was a statement pertaining to the category of the drug. Here, a brief statement is made concerning the major pharmacologic action or use of the drug. In some cases the drug is official as a pharmaceutic necessity. Here, a statement is made listing the preparations in which the substance was used.

USP XVI—This edition was released in March, 1960, to become official October 1, 1960. There were 225 new monographs added and many important changes made in former tests and assays. This volume closely paralleled USP XV as far as the treatment accorded official items was concerned. An innovation was the inclusion of an accepted American Chemical Society (ACS) chemical name as a synonym for all relevant official items. Other minor changes in treatment were also made.

On March 29–30, 1960, the 14th Decennial Convention was held in Washington, D.C. The following officers were elected to serve for the period 1960–1970:

President—Dr. Arthur C. DeGraff
Vice President—Dr. Theodore G. Klumpp
Treasurer—Dr. W. Paul Briggs
Board of Trustees—Dr. Windsor C. Cutting, Dr. Paul L. McLain, Dr. George D. Beal, Dr. Patrick H. Costello, Dr. George F. Archambault, and Dr. Linwood F. Tice.

At a meeting of the Board, Dr. Beal was elected Chairman of the Board and Dr. Adley B. Nichols was elected Secretary of the Board. Dr. Lloyd C. Miller had previously been elected by the retiring Board to serve as Director of Revision for the 1960–1970 decade.

USP XVII—This edition was released in May, 1965, to become official September 1, 1965. It contained 152 new monographs, and a number of the methods of assay were modified in such manner as to be more adequate for purposes of enforcement.

Reference has been made previously to the Spanish editions of the US Pharmacopeia; permission to use the text of the Pharmacopeia is granted upon application to the Chairman of the Board of Trustees under certain regulations which are necessary to guard the copyright. Since the basic objective of the official books of drug standards is to establish uniformity in the quality, purity, and strength of medicinal products, and as they are not published for profit, it has long been an established policy that the more widely the official texts can be made available to students of both medicine and pharmacy through their textbooks, and the official titles known and used by physicians and pharmacists in their practice, the more effectively are the USP and NF performing their functions.

Over 900 substances, including chemicals, crude drugs, and preparations, have been deemed of sufficient importance to merit a place in USP XVII. A number of these substances are not in themselves of therapeutic value but have been admitted as pharmaceutic necessities which are used in manufacturing other official products.

USP XVIII—This edition was made available early in 1970 and became official on September 1, 1970. The number of monographs has been greatly increased over previous editions and totals about 1130. This is an increase from USP XVII of about 350 monographs and accounts for a deletion of about 150 monographs.

No real change in format is recognized except for smaller type, narrower margins, and smaller graphic formulas.

A new quality test (Dissolution Test) was included for tablets that will measure time of solubility of the active ingredient. This is quite different from the disintegration test which is retained. Also, a microbial test is required for tablets to prevent the presence of *Salmonella* and *E. coli*. Attempts are made to provide controls for tablet uniformity as well as content uniformity in an effort to generate better manufacturing procedures.

Official Pharmacopeias of the World

A *Pharmacopeia* (from the Greek *pharmakon,* "a drug or medicine," and *poieo,* "make"), in the modern acceptation of the word, is a book containing a list of medicinal substances, with descriptions, tests, and formulas for preparing the same, selected by some recognized authority. The necessity for legalized standards to define the character, establish the purity, and regulate the strength of medicines is recognized by all civilized nations. Although all of the nations of the globe have not yet formally adopted national standards, in nearly every case where this has not been done the standards of some other country are in use.*

The official pharmacopeias are all issued under the authority of the respective governments, with the exception of the United States Pharmacopeia, which has, however, been accepted by the government and the individual states through the national and state food and drugs acts. Efforts have been made for many years to develop the **International Pharmacopoeia.** A start was made by the establishment of the *International Conference for the Unification of Potent Remedies,* which first met in the city of Brussels in September, 1902, and for a second time in September, 1925. This body in the *protocol* of 1902 agreed upon standards of strength for a number of potent preparations which they requested the various pharmacopeias of the world to adopt. In 1906 representatives from 19 governments met at Brussels and, with certain reservations, formally signed the agreements drawn up in 1902 and also formulated details for further unification. The United States Pharmacopœia (8th Revision) was the first national pharmacopeia to adopt some of these recommendations. Subsequent US Pharmacopeias inserted the Latin title adopted by the International Conference, followed by the letters "PI," below the official title of those preparations which conform to the standards of the protocol. The letters *PI* meant *Protocol Internationale.* The PI titles are now superseded by the titles of the *International Pharmacopoeia* (*Pharmacopoea Internationalis,* abbreviated PhI).

The League of Nations, as recommended by the 1925 Brussels Conference, continued this effort to establish an *International Pharmacopoeia* by appointing, in 1937, a committee of experts to assist in the unification of world pharmacopeias.

The Second World War interrupted this effort, but on the organization of the World Health Organization (WHO) as a Division of the United Nations, the International Pharmacopoeial Committee was re-established. This committee is composed of internationally known specialists in pharmacopeial work and is appointed by the WHO. To assist the Committee, panels of experts on many subjects have also been organized.

The *International Pharmacopoeia* has no legal force in any country unless it has been adopted by the authorities of the country concerned. However, the pharmacopeial committees of all nations have been urged to give consideration to the standards of the *International Pharmacopoeia* and to adopt them in their own Pharmacopœias in so far as they conform to the medical and pharmaceutical needs of their countries so that world uniformity in the strength and purity of the most important medicines will be largely attained.

The first volume of the *International Pharmacopoeia* was completed in 1950 and English, French, and Spanish editions have been published. It is made up chiefly of standards for basic medicinal substances. A second volume containing standards for additional new drugs

---

* Bibliographical information for foreign pharmacopeias which includes publisher and place of publication, also price if the information is available, can be found in the following: "National and International Pharmacopœias, a Checklist," by I. M. Strieby and M. C. Spencer, *Bulletin of the Medical Library Association,* **40,** 153 (April 1952) and, under the same title, a revision by Spencer, *Ibid,* **45,** 410 (July 1957) which includes listing of supplements as well as information on proposed new publications.

and for many tablets and injections was published in 1955. The *Supplementum*, issued in 1959, completed the first edition. It includes a cumulative index of Volumes I and II and of the supplement. A WHO Committee is working on a general revision of the first edition.

Official US Compendia

The ideals of American pharmacy are exemplified by the stated objectives of both the US Pharmacopœial Convention whose Board of Trustees publishes the USP and the American Pharmaceutical Association which publishes the NF.

The objectives of the USP appearing in its certificate of incorporation are stated to be as follows:

"The particular objectives and business of this Association are the encouragement and promotion of the science and art of medicine and pharmacy by selecting by research and experiment and other proper methods, and by naming such materials as may be properly used as medicines and drugs with formulas for their preparation; by establishing one uniform standard and guide for the use of those engaged in the practice of medicine and pharmacy in the United States, whereby the identity, strength, and purity of all such medicines and drugs may be accurately determined, and for other like and similar purposes; and by printing and distributing at suitable intervals such formulas and the results of such and similar selections, names, and determinations among the members of this Association, pharmacists and physicians generally in the United States and others interested in pharmacy and medicine."

The major objective of the NF is to promote the standardization of names and formulas for extensively used dosage forms of drugs not described in the USP. By doing this the NF aids in helping the American Pharmaceutical Association achieve its objectives which are stated to be the following:

"To improve and regulate the drug market by preventing the importation of inferior, adulterated, or deteriorated drugs, and by detecting and exposing home adulterations.

"To improve the science and art of pharmacy by diffusing scientific knowledge among pharmacists and druggists, fostering pharmaceutical literature, developing talent, stimulating discovery and invention, encouraging home production and manufacture in the several departments of the drug business.

"To uphold standards of authority in the education, theory, and practice of pharmacy.

"To create and maintain a standard of professional honesty equal to the amount of our professional knowledge, with a view to the highest good and greatest protection to the public."

Briefly, therefore, the two official compendia have the following basic objectives:

1. To standardize the *names* and *formulas* for extensively used drugs.
2. To provide standards and tests for the *identity, purity*, and *quality* of drugs well established in medical practice within the United States or its possessions.
3. To insure as far as practicable uniformity in *physical properties* and *active constituents*.

The accomplishment of these objectives is insured by establishing suitable requirements and tests for all drugs and preparations included in the USP and NF. See Chapter 36, *Official Requirements and Tests*.

United States Pharmacopeia

That part of the USP devoted to the consideration of the individual official substances constitutes the section on monographs. The content of each monograph is arranged in a definite sequence so that the data follow a uniform pattern. This greatly simplifies the use of the Pharmacopeia, for one can soon learn where to look in the monograph for any information needed. The following is the general order of presentation although individual monographs contain only that information which is pertinent to the particular product: official title, synonyms, chemical formula, definition, purity rubric, description, tests, assay, packaging and storage, available sizes, category, and dose. For certain pharmaceutical products, for example *Cherry Syrup*, a method of manufacture may be given also.

The Official Title—The English title recognized as the official name of the drug or preparation may be a chemical name, a botanical name, a title which indicates the type of dosage form, a name indicative of the source or nature, or a coined word derived usually from an otherwise complex chemical name. When an official product is available under one or more tradenames, the pharmacopeial official name is usually employed by the manufacturer as the "generic" or "nonproprietary" name for the product.

In the case of compounded products, official titles may indicate the principal ingredient, as *Compound Calcium Cyclamate Solution*, but may express the action, as *Hydrophilic Ointment*, or the use, as *Diphtheria Antitoxin*.

Latin titles have been used in most pharmacopeias of the world, including the *International Pharmacopoeia*, and were for several editions used in the USP, in order that similar products might be identified regardless of the language employed in the text. When inorganic salts and botanical drugs made up the bulk of Pharmacopeial entries, Latin titles were easily derived and did represent a useful means of identification. However, as synthetic organic chemicals came into prominence as medicinals, the contrived Latin titles enjoyed less favor and today preference is given to other means of specific identification such as structural formulas.

The names of drugs which are parts of plants have been commonly derived from the Latin botanical name, the latter consisting usually of two words, the first denoting the genus and the second the species to which the plant belongs. *Capsicum frutescens* is the botanical name for the particular variety of capsicum or Cayenne pepper which was formerly official in the Pharmacopeia. Here the generic, or first name, was chosen for the official title, and if no description had followed the title it would be inferred that any part of any plant in the genus "Capsicum" could be officially used for making preparations; but the specific name, "frutescens," limits the use to this species, while the description which followed showed the *part* of the plant which was employed: "the dried, ripe *fruit of Capsicum frutescens* Linné (Fam. Solanaceæ), grown in Africa." NF XI, in which Capsicum was official, added another species, *Capsicum annuum*. The specific name does not begin with a capital letter, except when it has been at some previous time itself a generic name, as in *Atropa Belladonna*, or when it is derived from the name of a person, as in *Garcinia Hanburii*, or when the word is indeclinable, as in *Theobroma Cacao*, or when it is a combination of a noun and an adjective, as in *Xan-*

thoxylum Clava-Herculis. The name of the classifier follows the botanical name, as, *Capsicum frutescens* Linné, and after this the Family to which the plant belongs is indicated in italics, and the whole enclosed in parentheses, as (Fam. *Solanaceæ*).

At the head of each monograph is a *marginal name* which represents the official title of the product arranged as in an index. Monographs thus appear in the alphabetic order of the principal word in the title and related items are more likely to be found adjacent to each other. *Absorbable Surgical Suture* and *Non-absorbable Surgical Suture* are next to each other because of their marginal titles, *Suture, Absorbable Surgical* and *Suture, Nonabsorbable Surgical.* Similarly, *Ristocetin* immediately precedes *Sterile Ristocetin* through employment of the marginal title *Ristocetin, Sterile* for the latter.

Synonyms—Only the official titles of USP and NF drugs are now legally recognized as designations for use in labeling the articles to which they apply. Synonyms, formerly given under official titles, have been deleted in USP XVIII and NF XIII. In the case of organic chemical entities, the systematic chemical name of the substance is usually given, in smaller type below the official title.

In the section on *Nomenclature*, under *General Information and Procedures*, USP XVIII includes a list of "Other Designations of USP Articles," accompanied by the statement that use of formerly official synonyms included in the list does not constitute sanction for their further use.

The Chemical Formula—The USP gives the structural formulas for organic chemicals whenever they have been generally accepted by chemists. It is not intended that they should indicate the purity of the product, but they do indicate the nature of the product and frequently suggest its therapeutic activity. Molecular formulas are given for all chemicals and, in some instances, are helpful in defining the specific product.

Sodium Phosphate is not as precise a term as $Na_2HPO_4.7H_2O$ since there are actually three sodium phosphates. *Magnesium Sulfate* does not always contain the same proportion of water of crystallization, and if the symbolic formula, $MgSO_4.7H_2O$, were not appended to the official title there might be doubt as to which sulfate was intended; the added $7H_2O$, however, accurately defines it.

The Official Definition—The official definition is an essential part of the monograph for any substance which is not a chemical compound and it appears as the first statement in the text portion of the monograph. It is intended to be sufficiently precise as to preclude confusion with any other substance. Purified Cotton, for example, is defined as "the hair of the seed of cultivated varieties of *Gossypium hirsutum* Linné, or of other species of *Gossypium* (Fam. *Malvaceæ*), freed from adhering impurities, deprived of fatty matter, bleached, and sterilized in its final container."

Supplementary to the definition are the official description, the purity rubric, and the prescribed tests for identity, purity, and strength.

For chemical compounds the formula itself generally serves as the definition although, in some cases, a more elaborate statement appears as, for example, "Griseofulvin is a substance produced by the growth of *Penicillium griseofulvum* or by other means. It has a potency equivalent to not less than 900 mcg of $C_{17}H_{17}ClO_6$ per mg, calculated on the anhydrous basis."

The Purity Rubric—This term was first used in USP VIII to indicate the paragraph which limited the quantity of innocuous impurities in chemicals, by stating in terms of percentage the amount of pure substance that must be present. It has been extended to drugs generally and many other articles in later Pharmacopeias. Thus, under *Dapsone* is found the purity rubric as follows: "Dapsone contains not less than 99.0 percent and not more than 101.0 percent of $C_{12}H_{12}N_2O_2S$, calculated on the dried basis." It might seem that a medicinal chemical should contain 100% of the pure product, but practical experience shows that absolute purity is not usually attainable and that minute quantities of harmless impurities do not affect the medicinal value. The purity rubric also makes allowance for such deterioration as may be permissible in certain chemicals and for errors inherent in the assay procedures.

The Official Description—Immediately following the official definition of the substances there appears, in smaller type, what has been termed the *official description*. For drugs, this usually consists of a concise statement of their physical characteristics when entire, and also, in most instances, the structure of the same drug when sectioned or powdered. Concerning chemicals the official description usually includes physical properties such as color, crystalline and other approved forms, odor, taste (if not actively poisonous), and usually the result of exposure to air. It is important for the pharmacist to know whether chemicals are stable or whether they lose or attract moisture. The reaction to litmus or other indicators is sometimes indicated and a melting point may be given.

Solubility—Following the official description is a concise statement concerning the solubility of those substances which are capable of solution. Thus, *Meralluride* is said to be "Slightly soluble in water; soluble in hot water and in glacial acetic acid."

Tests for Identity and Purity—In the USP the tests which establish the identity of a chemical and those which insure the required degree of purity are listed under appropriate headings. Ash limits, to restrict the amount of soil and sand adhering to roots and plants, an occasional identity test, and other means of determining purity or the presence of adulterants have also been appended to vegetable drugs. It is not to be understood that the tests for purity are the final and exclusive indication of quality. The monographs are divided and subheads used only for convenience of reference, and an article to be official must meet every requirement of the text unless specifically exempted as is the case with most solubilities which are given only for the information of physicians and pharmacists.

Assay—The quantitative estimation of chemicals, drugs, and preparations is necessary to fix their value definitely as medicinal agents, and the USP and NF provide assay procedures for most drugs. This work requires skill, knowledge, and experience, and each process requires careful study.

In this text detailed explanations of official assay methods are given in Chapters 36, 37, and 38 of Part V, *Testing and Analysis*.

Packaging and Storage—Under this heading found in many monographs, the USP describes the proper method of packaging and storing the drug to prevent or retard deterioration. Those influences causing deterioration—such as moisture, light, and heat—are guarded against when necessary by the specific directions given. Thus, for *Physostigmine*, the requirement is: "Preserve in tight, light-resistant containers in quantities not exceeding 1 g." Reference is made to the different types of containers and conditions of storage in Chapter 36, *Official Requirements and Tests*.

Available Strengths—For the information of physicians and pharmacists, the USP lists the strengths in which dosage forms such as tablets, capsules, injections, suppositories, and suspensions are generally available.

Category—USP XV was the first revision to provide information on the intended use of each drug. In a single word, or in a brief phrase, is expressed the pharmacological action, the medicinal purpose, or the pharmaceutical use.

Dose—USP VIII was the first to give *average doses* of official drugs. USP XIV altered the terminology and gave *usual doses*. In USP XV the *usual dose* and the *range* appeared for the first time. USP XVIII has continued this valuable information and, for most drugs, provides a *usual dose* and a *usual dose range*. All doses given at the end of monographs for USP or NF drugs in this textbook are the official doses.

National Formulary

The origin of the *National Formulary* dates from 1882 when Charles Rice organized a Committee from New York and Brooklyn to frame a book of formulas for unofficial preparations. The *New York and Brooklyn Formulary* was subsequently enlarged and the joint Committee presented it to the American Pharmaceutical Association in 1885 as the nucleus for the construction of the 1st edition of the NF which appeared in 1888. The 3rd Edition of the NF was made a standard under the Pure Food and Drugs Act, June 30, 1906.

The NF is the property of the American Pharmaceutical Association and its revision is carried out in very much the same way and with the same frequency as the revision of the USP. In effect it serves as a companion to the USP and it has sometimes been suggested that the two volumes should be combined into one. At one time a clear distinction was drawn in the manner of selecting drugs for the two compendia, the USP limiting itself to the most useful and the NF including all other drugs of wide usage. Today both emphasize

effectiveness in the selection of products for inclusion although the USP through long custom, has first option.

In the NF many of the standards of the USP are used; thus, where alcohol, glycerin, syrup, iodine, opium tincture, and other USP drugs and preparations are directed, they must conform in strength and purity to the standards of the USP. The general style and arrangement of the NF monographs are practically identical with those of the USP.

It is important to remember that if a drug or preparation is sold under or by a name recognized in the USP or NF, without qualification, it must not differ from the standards of strength, quality, and purity determined by the tests laid down in either of these books official at the time of the investigation. A drug or preparation, however, is not deemed to be adulterated if it differs from the official standards, provided the manner in which they differ in quality, purity, or strength is clearly stated upon the bottle, box, or container. However, no ingredients directed in formulas may be omitted nor new ingredients added.

The status of the NF makes it desirable that its standards should be given in this book so that the student may not only become familiar with the preparations of both the USP and the NF but also recognize the fact that these books are of equal force before the law.

In both the USP and NF, the standards are intended solely to apply to substances which are used or bought, sold, or dispensed for medicinal purposes. The word *official* as used in this text is intended to refer to those items (and their standards) recognized by USP XVIII and NF XIII.

Homeopathic Pharmacopeia

The *Homeopathic Pharmacopeia* is made available by the American Institute of Homeopathy (1938) to provide standards for drugs used in homeopathic medicine. Techniques are provided for the preparation of drugs, including tinctures, dilutions, triturations, and prescriptions. The area of special pharmaceutic preparations is well covered.

Reference Literature of Pharmacy

Reference Books

In addition to the two official United States compendia described in the preceding section, the pharmacist has need for other sources of basic information. Pharmacy and its related fields of the health professions have become so complex and diversified that no pharmacist can remember all of the data needed in his day-to-day practice. It is essential, therefore, that every pharmacy and pharmaceutical laboratory be equipped with a library containing a variety of information materials, including a number of well-selected reference and textbooks.

Pharmacists who are prepared to supply facts about the nature of a new drug, its pharmacology, side effects, and dosage, as well as the products available, are highly esteemed by physicians and others who have need for such information. Then, too, there are frequent occasions when the physical and chemical properties of a substance, its incompatibilities, or other facts are needed. Access to information sources

and knowing how to use them are of utmost importance. Some useful reference books are described below.

The United States Dispensatory (USD) and Physicians' Pharmacology

The 26th edition (1967) of the Dispensatory, under its new name, is edited by Arthur Osol, Robertson Pratt, and Mark D. Altschule. It is a collection, alphabetically arranged, of articles on individual drugs and of general articles on pharmacologic classes of drugs. Effort is made to describe the pharmacologic actions and therapeutic uses of specific drugs. This volume is smaller than previous editions because of the deletion of hundreds of ineffective drugs and botanicals.

Over the years, it has had many outstanding men as its editors including Horatio C. Wood, Horatio C. Wood, Jr., Joseph P. Remington, and Charles H. LaWall. The editors-in-chief of the 24th and 25th editions were Arthur Osol and George E. Farrar. Those who had USD (1955) were able to bring it up to date by purchasing Volume 2, a small, separately bound volume entitled *New Drug Developments 1960*, edited by Arthur Osol and Robertson Pratt.

British Pharmacopoeia

The *British Pharmacopoeia*, official in Great Britain, provides monographs on drugs and preparations accepted by the General Medical Council. Data and information available is very similar to that in the USP. It is reissued every 5 years.

Pharmacopoea Internationalis

The *International Pharmacopoeia*, published by the World Health Organization, was developed during 1951–1959. There are two volumes with a supplement. This publication supplies standards, strengths, and nomenclature of drugs and is intended for use primarily for countries which have not developed their own pharmacopeia.

Volume I contains monographs for basic chemicals and drugs of plant origin; Volume II contains monographs for medicinal agents with specifications for dosage forms. Both volumes have the usual sections on biologic assay, limit tests, test solutions, and reagents, as well as standards with dosage tables for adults and children. It is available in English, Spanish, and French.

New Drugs (ND)

New Drugs is an annual publication started in 1965 by the American Medical Association. Previous publications related to *New Drugs* were *New and Nonofficial Remedies* (1909–1957) and *New and Nonofficial Drugs* (1958–1964).

New Drugs is an evaluation of drugs and their therapeutic, prophylactic, and diagnostic status by the Council on Drugs of the American Medical Association. The discussions are very comprehensive and are based on available scientific data and reports of investigations.

Pertinent data are gathered and evaluated by the Council on Drugs, which regularly reports its findings in the *Journal of the American Medical Association*.

Each drug is described in a monograph which provides names (nonproprietary and proprietary); chemical or biologic identity; actions and uses, including comparisons with related drugs, limitations, side effects, toxicity, contraindications, etc; dosage; available preparations; and other useful information.

Accepted Dental Remedies

Accepted Dental Remedies has been published annually since 1936 by the American Dental Association. It is concerned with drugs recognized to be of value in dentistry with their dosage forms. The drugs are thoroughly described with indication for use. A formulary useful in dentistry is included.

The Merck Index

This useful reference was first published in 1889. It is now in its 8th (1968) edition. The *Merck Index*, while published by Merck and Co., Inc., is not a manufacturers' buying guide or price catalog but a drug and chemical encyclopedia. In it are listed more than 10,000 descriptions of individual chemicals and drugs, their properties and uses. Structural formulas are shown for hundreds of compounds. More than 30,000 names are listed referring to the chemical descriptions by common, generic, chemical, brand or trade names. Medical and veterinary uses are given for 3500 chemicals. In a sense, the *Merck Index* may be regarded as a dispensatory in abbreviated form. It is widely distributed and used by pharmacists, chemists, and physicians.

Modern Drug Encyclopedia and Therapeutic Index

This is essentially a reference book on proprietary drugs of American manufacture now in its 10th edition (1965). The data given are those supplied by various manufacturers concerning their products. Proprietary drugs are arranged alphabetically with their nature, properties, action, uses, and dose given. The sizes available and the manufacturers are also included. The *Modern Drug Encyclopedia* has many very useful arrangements. For example, all of the proprietary products made by each company are listed together in a special manufacturers' and distributors' index. A therapeutic index groups drugs having similar uses together in an alphabetical arrangement.

Those purchasing this book are supplied regularly with supplements which list new drugs as they are released. Each successive supplement contains a cumulative index covering all previous supplements.

Other Therapeutic Handbooks and Drug Indexes

The *American Drug Index* has been published annually since 1956 by J. B. Lippincott Co. It is an important directory of essential drug information in which products are listed alphabetically with extensive cross-indexing. Names listed are generic or USAN (nonproprietary), brand (proprietary), chemical, USP, NF, ADR and synonyms. Cross references appear from alternate names and from individual drugs to the names of combinations in which they will be found. Data included are generic names, chemical names, manufacturer, pharmaceutical forms, size, dosage and use. The information is accurate and easily located.

Several other drug indexes and therapeutic handbooks, although designed primarily for the use of the physician, are also of value to the pharmacist. While the latter is not trained to diagnose and treat disease, he frequently needs to learn some fact concerning a given disease or its therapy. One of the best known of these is the *Merck Manual of Diagnosis and Therapy*, the 11th edition of which appeared in 1966. This book is divided into three parts: Part I considers diseases grouped into disease entities with the symptoms, diagnoses, etiology, and treatment presented in concise style; Part II is devoted to various medical procedures and practical features such as chapters on diets and ready reference tables; Part III is a comprehensive index of the contents.

Drugs in Current Use, issued annually since 1955 by the Stringer Publ. Co., provides concise statements of the action and use, physical properties, and administration of drugs currently used in clinical medicine. A similar reference is *Current Drug Handbook* (1964–1966), published by Saunders.

In the *Identification Guide for Solid Dosage Forms* [*J. Am. Med. Assoc.*, **182**, 1145–1302 (Dec. 22, 1962)] over 5000 tablets and capsules are assigned code numbers on the basis of their size, shape, color and markings. The code is useful in conjunction with other conclusive tests in identifying products.

The annual publication, *Physicians' Desk References to Pharmaceuticals and Biologicals*, was first made available in 1946. In it drugs are arranged in several sections—the *pink* section contains an alphabetical listing of brand-name products; the *yellow*, a drug, chemical, and pharmacological index to specialties; the *blue*, a therapeutic indications index; and the *white*, a list of major products of manufacturers giving the composition, action, uses, and contraindications of each drug. A quarterly supplement is also published.

Selected List of Reference Books

Accepted Dental Remedies, American Dental Assoc., Chicago.

Principles of Accounting, Prentice-Hall, New York, H. A. Finney and H. E. Miller.

American Drug Index, Lippincott, Philadelphia, C. O. Wilson and T. E. Jones.

American Druggist Blue Book, American Druggist, New York.

American Hospital Formulary Service, American Society of Hospital Pharmacists, Washington, D.C.

American Pharmacy, Lippincott, Philadelphia, J. B. Sprowls.

American Red Cross First Aid Text-Book, McGraw-Hill, New York.

The Art of Compounding, McGraw-Hill, New York, G. L. Jenkins, *et al.*

Biochemistry, Saunders, Philadelphia, A. Cantarow and B. Schepartz.

General Biochemistry, Wiley, New York, J. S. Fruton and S. Simmonds.

Business Law, Uniform Commercial Code Edition, West Publ. Co., St. Paul, Minn., L. Y. Smith and G. G. Roberson.

The Chemical Formulary, Chemical Publ. Co., New York, H. Bennett, ed.

The Chemistry and Manufacture of Cosmetics, Van Nostrand, New York, M. G. DeNavarre.

The Condensed Chemical Dictionary, Reinhold, New York.

Clinical Endocrinology, Little, Brown, Boston, L. Martin.

Clinical Toxicology, Lea & Febiger, Philadelphia, C. H. Thienes and T. J. Haley.

Clinical Toxicology of Commercial Products, Williams & Wilkins, Baltimore, M. N. Gleason, *et al.*

de Haen Nonproprietary Name Index with Therapeutic Guide, Paul deHaen, Inc., New York.

Dental Formulas, Lea & Febiger, Philadelphia, L. I. Grossman.

Dermatologic Medications, Year Book, Chicago, M. R. Lerner and A. B. Lerner.

Drug Topics Red Book, Topics Publ. Co., New York.

Drugs of Choice, Mosby, St. Louis.

Drugs in Current Use, Springer Publ. Co., New York, W. Modell.

Drugs in Our Society, Johns Hopkins Press, Baltimore, P. Talalay, ed.

Textbook of Endocrinology, Saunders, Philadelphia, R. H. Williams.

Facts and Comparisons, E. K. Kastrup, St. Louis.

Handbook of Chemistry, Handbook Publ., Sandusky, Ohio, N. A. Lange, ed.

Handbook of Chemistry and Physics, Chemical Rubber Publ. Co., Cleveland, C. D. Hodgman, ed.

Handbook of Non-Prescription Drugs, American Pharmaceutical Assoc., Washington, D.C., G. B. Griffenhagen, ed.

Kremers and Urdang's History of Pharmacy, Lippincott, Philadelphia, G. Sonnedecker.

The Law of Drugs and Druggists, West Publ. Co., St. Paul, Minn., W. R. Arthur.

Manual of Pharmaceutical Law, Macmillan, New York, W. Pettit.

Dorland's American Illustrated Medical Dictionary, Saunders, Philadelphia.

New Drugs, American Medical Assoc., Chicago.

New Gould Medical Dictionary, McGraw-Hill, New York.

Merck Index, Merck & Co., Inc., Rahway, N.J.

Merck Manual, Merck & Co., Inc., Rahway, N.J.

Merck Veterinary Manual, Merck & Co., Inc., Rahway, N.J.

The Microbial World, Prentice-Hall, New York, R. Y. Stanier, *et al.*

Microbiology, McGraw-Hill, New York, M. J. Pelczar and R. D. Reid.

Modern Drug Encyclopedia, Drug Publications, New York, M. E. Howard, ed.

National Formulary, Mack Publ. Co., Easton, Pa.

Textbook of Organic Medicinal and Pharmaceutical Chemistry, Lippincott, Philadelphia, C. O. Wilson and O. Gisvold, eds.

Pediatric Dermatology, Year Book, Chicago, H. H. Perlman.

Pharmaceutical Calculations, Lea & Febiger, Philadelphia, W. T. Bradley *et al.*

Pharmaceutical and Chemical Synonyms, Excerpta Medica Foundation, New York.

Husa's Pharmaceutical Dispensing, Mack Publ. Co., Easton, Pa., E. W. Martin, ed.

Pharmacognosy, Lea & Febiger, Philadelphia, E. P. Claus and V. E. Tyler.

Textbook of Pharmacognosy, Lippincott, Philadelphia, R. Pratt and H. W. Youngken, Jr.

Pharmacological Basis of Therapeutics, Macmillan, New York, L. Goodman and A. Gilman.

Pharmacology in Medicine, McGraw-Hill, New York, V. A. Drill.

Introduction to Pharmacology, Williams & Wilkins, Baltimore, J. J. Lewis.

Pharmacopeia of the United States, Mack Publ. Co., Easton, Pa.

Pharmacy, a Synthesis of Sciences, Heath, Boston, J. T. Fay, Jr.

PharmIndex, Skyline Publ. Inc., Portland, Ore.

Physical Pharmacy, Lea & Febiger, Philadelphia, A. N. Martin.

Physicians' Desk Reference to Pharmaceutical Specialties and Biologicals, Medical Economics, Inc., Oradell, N.J.

Poisoning, a Guide to Chemical Diagnosis and Treatment, Saunders, Philadelphia, W. F. von Oettingen.

Handbook of Poisoning: Diagnosis and Treatment, Lange Medical Publ., Los Altos, Calif., R. H. Dreisbach.

Prescription Pharmacy, Lippincott, Philadelphia, J. B. Sprowls.

The Profession of Pharmacy, Lippincott, Philadelphia, R. A. Deno *et al.*

Proprietary Names (Trade Names) of Official Drugs, American Pharmaceutical Assoc., Washington, D.C.

Public Relations for the Pharmacist, Lippincott, Philadelphia, W. H. Hall.

Remington's Pharmaceutical Sciences, Mack Publ. Co., Easton, Pa., A. Osol, *et al.*

Retailing: Principles and Methods, R. D. Irwin, Inc., Homewood, Ill., D. J. Duncan and C. F. Phillips.

United States Adopted Names (USAN), United States Pharmacopoeial Convention, Inc., Bethesda, Md.

United States Dispensatory, Lippincott, Philadelphia, A. Osol, *et al.*

Veterinary Drug Encyclopedia, Drug Publ., Inc., New York, H. C. Stephenson and S. G. Mittelstaedt, eds.

Veterinary Applied Pharmacology and Therapeutics, Williams & Wilkins, Baltimore, P. W. Daykin.

A descriptive list of over 1000 books and reference works selected as useful in pharmacy college libraries by faculty members in the member colleges of the American Association of Colleges of Pharmacy was published in the *Am. J. Pharm. Educ.*, **27**, 266–290, 361–421 (1963). An excellent description of foreign books and subscription services dealing with drugs is available in *Drug Information Sources*, compiled by the Pharmaceutical Section, Science-Technology Division, Special Libraries Association, which was published serially in the *American Journal of Pharmacy*, 1957–1958, and available in reprint form. An updated report appears in the same journal beginning in the issue of March-April, 1964.

Serial Abstracts and Indexes

Another type of reference service consists of abstracts and indexes issued on a subscription basis. A relatively inexpensive but particularly important one is *Unlisted Drugs*, issued monthly. It is designed for the identification of experimental drugs under research numbers and for other new products not yet listed in the better known reference compilations. The source of information is always cited. Data are submitted regularly by a number of well-qualified contributors. Both annual and cumulative indexes are issued. (Published since 1949 by the Pharmaceutical Section, ST Division, Special Libraries Association; 31 E. 10th St., New York, N.Y. 10003.) *International Pharmaceutical Abstracts*, published twice a month beginning in 1964 by the American Society of Hospital Pharmacists, provides informative abstracts of articles mostly related to research and development and to professional practice.

Chemical Abstracts and *Biological Abstracts* are important to the student of pharmacy and the need for consulting these may arise occasionally for the practicing pharmacist. Other titles with which both should be familiar are the *Current List of Medical Literature*, published by the National Library of Medicine, now issued as the *Index Medicus*, and the *Index Chemicus*, a monthly index of new chemicals published by the Institute for Scientific Information, 325 Chestnut St., Philadelphia, Pa.

The dental literature is covered by the American Dental Association's *Dental Abstracts* and the *Index to Dental Periodical Literature*.

A recent commercial development is that of *Selective Abstracts, Inc.* with summaries available in five sections, including one on "Drugs" and another on "Cosmetics, Toiletries and Pharmaceuticals." Abstracts are perforated for removal and are accompanied by suggested subject headings for convenience in filing (855 Ave. of the Americas, New York, N.Y.). *Excerpta Medica* is an abstract service in 20 sections each covering a special phase of medicine.

Current Contents, Life Sciences is a service of the Institute for Scientific Information, 325 Chestnut St., Philadelphia, Pa. This is a weekly publication which reproduces the table of contents, in original format, of more than 900 foreign and domestic research journals. *Cambridge Contents* is published monthly by the Cambridge University Press, 32 E. 57th St., New York, N.Y. It is composed of reproductions of the table of contents of recent issues of journals in the biological, medical, and agricultural sciences.

Loose-Leaf and Card Services

Supplementary to the list above are several other types of information sources for the pharmacist. Some of these fall into the category of services. *Facts and Comparisons*, a well-established loose-leaf service, lists drug products in groupings classified broadly according to use. Ingredients are listed in tabular form to facilitate concise comparisons; an annual product index lists all trade, generic, and official names in alphabetical order. Listings of important new products are distributed each month (P.O. Box 8, Baden Station, St. Louis 15, Mo.). *PharmIndex*, also a loose-leaf service available since 1958, is a monthly listing of drug products with midmonthly supplements. It is an excellent source of information because of its prompt-ness, completeness, and up-to-date indexes (Pharm-Index, Box 1029, Federal Station, Portland, Ore.).

Many pharmaceutical manufacturers now routinely distribute to physicians and pharmacists 3×5 cards containing brief statements with use, constituents, toxicity, contraindications, dosage, and form of products, both new and old. A comprehensive card service, offered on a commercial basis, giving product data together with bibliographical references that would lend itself to alphabetical interfiling, may be the next step forward.

Now available is a microfilm service that provides a film every 2 weeks providing practically all pertinent information on over 1600 drug products. These are arranged alphabetically by brand name and are supplied by Micro-Tel Service, Inc., 1209 2nd St., Perry, Iowa 50220. A microfilm reader is necessary.

Sources for Business Information

Since many pharmacists own and operate their own pharmacies, they often have need for business information in addition to that which may be found in the few specific titles mentioned in the section on *Selected List of Reference Books*. Sometimes even a broader coverage of the business field is necessary; at least one or more titles in this category are usually available in the reference department of the local public library. The *Lilly Digest*, published annually since 1931, is a summary, with comment, of the income and expense statements of a large number of cooperating pharmacies (Eli Lilly & Co.).

Closely related to business management is the necessity for maintaining good public relations—in fact, every pharmacist has responsibilities in this area. *Public Relations for the Pharmacist* is one of the titles now available in this field. Exhibits as a public relations media was covered in many issues of the *Journal of the American Pharmaceutical Association* and an annual service is available from the APhA. The *Public Relations Kit*, available annually from the APhA, contains valuable aids for the pharmacist.

US Pharmaceutical Journals

American pharmaceutical journals are published to foster education and research and to promote the utilization of sound business principles in pharmacy and allied fields. They inform the pharmacist of the latest scientific and industrial developments affecting the practice of his profession.

The *American Journal of Pharmacy* is the oldest pharmacy journal in this country. Published originally in 1825 as the *Journal of the Philadelphia College of Pharmacy*, the journal was given its present name in 1835. It is the only scientific and professional journal issued by a college of pharmacy that has survived the vicissitudes of America's growth. Nearly 400 pharmaceutical journals have been published since 1825, but many of these were printed only for short periods and others changed their titles and appearance in rapid succession.

The American Pharmaceutical Association began publishing its *Proceedings* as soon as it was founded in 1852, and in 1906 it started issuing its *Bulletins*. Both of these journals were replaced in 1912 by the *Journal of the American Pharmaceutical Association* which has become undisputed leader of the scientific and professional literature of pharmacy. In order to present the annual report of the progress of pharmacy which had appeared in the *Proceedings*, the *Yearbook of the APhA* was published from 1912 until 1934 and in 1935 "Abstracts" appeared monthly in the *Journal* but were discontinued in 1947. Beginning in 1940 a *Scientific* and a *Practical* edition of the *Journal* were published and in 1961 the Scientific Edition was retitled *The Journal of Pharmaceutical Sciences* and the Practical Edition became simply *The Journal of the American Pharmaceutical Association*.

Several privately owned enterprises have published pharmaceutical journals for many years. The first independent pharmaceutical journal, dating from 1857, was *The American Druggist's Circular* which changed its title in 1906 to *The Druggist Circular*. The pharmaceutical newspaper, *Drug Topics*, which began as the house organ of McKesson and Robbins in 1884, is now published every other week alternating with *Drug Trade News*. In 1940 Drug Topics absorbed The Druggist Circular. *The Interstate Druggist*, which began in 1882 as the *Pharmaceutische Rundschau* with Frederick Hoffman as editor, and several other publications formerly were printed in German or some foreign language. The *Rundschau* became the *Pharmaceutical Review* in 1896. It was edited from then until 1900 by Frederick Hoffman and Edward Kremers, and from 1900 to 1909 by Edward Kremers alone. The latter began publication of the *Pharmaceutical Archives* in 1898 to complete his coverage of pharmacy by printing original papers. From 1909 to 1926 the *Pharmaceutical Review* and the *Archives* were merged with the *Midland Druggist*, and then in 1926 the title was changed to *Interstate Druggist* which ceased publication in 1927. In 1936 the *Archives* again became a separate publication, but it discontinued publication in 1944. *The Oil, Paint and Drug Reporter*, founded in 1871, has absorbed many pharmaceutical journals. This journal, like *Drug and Cosmetic Industry* and *Drug Trade News*, is of interest primarily to pharmaceutical and cosmetic manufacturers.

Another important pharmaceutical journal also began in 1871 under the title *New Remedies, a Quarterly Retrospect of Therapeutics, Pharmacy and Allied Subjects*. It changed its name many times until it eventually became *The American Druggist*.

American Professional Pharmacist, founded in 1934, offers original articles and reviews relating to professional pharmacy and prescription practice. In 1969 its name was changed to Pharmacy Times.

A few independent journals have been accepted as official organs of pharmaceutical associations. Examples of these are the *Rocky Mountain Druggist*, founded in 1888, and the *Southeastern Drug Journal*, founded in 1926. In 1935 the National Association of Boards of Pharmacy began publication of the *NABP Bulletin*, which is issued on an exchange basis.

Many state, county, and city pharmaceutical associations have published journals in an attempt to see that the laws governing the practice of pharmacy are enforced, and to further the professional and commercial interests of their members. The California Pharmaceutical Society published the first state association journal, *The Pacific Pharmacist*, in 1907. It ceased publication in 1919. *The New York State Pharmacist*, which first appeared in 1927, and which is exclusively owned by the association, is an outstanding example of this type of publication.

In 1902 the National Association of Retail Druggists began publishing its *NARD Notes*, the title of which was changed to *NARD Journal* in 1913. In 1937 the American Association of Colleges of Pharmacy published the first issue of the *American Journal of Pharmaceutical Education* as a medium for discussing problems and describing advances in education in pharmacy. Through original articles, reports of committees, and news items in this quarterly journal one can follow developments in American pharmaceutical education. Of value in this connection are the *Proceedings of the Teachers' Conferences* held each year since 1949 with the support of the American Foundation for Pharmaceutical Education.

Lloydia is a quarterly journal of pharmacognosy and allied biological sciences published jointly by the Lloyd Library and Museum and the American Society of Pharmacognosy.

The first journal devoted exclusively to hospital pharmacy practice was started in 1943 and is now issued as the *American Journal of Hospital Pharmacy*. A recent journal is *Hospital Pharmacy*, published by Lippincott.

The *Medical Letter on Drugs and Therapeutics* (305 East 45th St., New York, N.Y. 10017) is a bi-weekly newsletter which provides critical appraisals of new drugs and new clinical experiences with established drugs. *Clin-Alert*, published 3 or 4 times monthly (800 Commonwealth Bldg., Louisville, Ky.), offers abstracts of literature reports of drug reactions.

To satisfy the demand for early information about significant developments in pharmacy certain subscription publications issued as weekly or monthly newsletters (1152 National Press Bldg., Washington 4, D.C.) have come into being and have achieved considerable popularity among those segments of the profession to which they are directed. *F-D-C Reports*, "The Pink Sheet" (weekly), is intended for executives in the drug, cosmetic and related industries. It covers legal, economic, and broad scientific developments. *Weekly Pharmacy Reports*, "The Green Sheet" (weekly), is written primarily for practicing pharmacists with emphasis on matters related to retail distribution. *Drug Research Reports*, "The Blue Sheet" (weekly), and *Medical Research Digest*, "The Gray Sheet" (monthly), cover the areas indicated by their titles and are used by research and management personnel.

House Organs—A number of pharmaceutical companies maintain regular communication with pharmacists, physicians, and other professional personnel through the medium of what are commonly called "house organs." These are publications intended to provide the reader with information of value, thus projecting a good company image. Some appear at monthly intervals, others bimonthly, quarterly, or irregularly. They vary greatly in content and many are intended for rather restricted audiences. Mostly the emphasis is on scientific, technical, or professional articles; reviews and histories are popular.

Other Domestic and Foreign Journals

A great many additional journals of pharmacy and related health fields are available and to the extent that time permits and interest warrants may be utilized by the pharmacist. It is important that he keep abreast of important changes in the closely allied health professions and it is frequently necessary to consult the appropriate specialized publication. Every medical specialty has at least one journal and there are also journals in the various basic medical sciences. For information about medical developments in general, including advances in therapy, the weekly *Journal of the American Medical Association* is valuable to the practicing pharmacist.

The most comprehensive list of serial publications directly concerned with pharmacy is the *World List of Pharmacy Periodicals*, which was published in the *American Journal of Hospital Pharmacy*, **20**, 47–83 (1963).

The Pharmacist's Reference Files

This review of the literature of pharmacy indicates there is not one but many sources to use in order to obtain complete data on the majority of questions asked of the pharmacist. Perhaps electronic equipment will some day be so simple to operate and so low in price that information can be produced quickly, subject to any approach, such as the ingredients or trade name of a product or the name of a manufacturer, or items more difficult to find—literature references, for example. In the meantime, it is suggested that the pharmacist adopt the practice of keeping a 3 × 5-inch card index, recording under appropriate headings all new products, formulas, and developments which come to his attention including his source of information. Cards describing their products, routinely sup-

plied by some manufacturers, can be interfiled with the cards prepared by the pharmacist, as can also some of their "package inserts." Information on new products, published in special sections of some journals of pharmacy, also may be clipped and attached to file cards to save time.

Along with the card index, the pharmacist needs a supplemental file for which he can select and organize carefully the materials he will need when the occasion arises such as government pamphlets; advertising leaflets; special diets; career booklets; professional association constitutions; reprints and clippings of scientific articles; and pictures and photographs of pharmaco-historical significance. As a rule, these informational materials accumulate more quickly than they can be safely weeded. However, much material of this type which might otherwise be overlooked is described in *Copnip List* (published quarterly by the Pharmaceutical Section ST Division, Special Libraries Association). Many informational items will come to the pharmacist unsolicited and some are worth preserving. An excellent example of a pamphlet which should be purchased is the *First Aid Guide*. This is available from the Government Printing Office, Washington, D.C., for 25¢.

8 | Research

The role of research in pharmacy and medicine—research
organizations—laboratory research—clinical research

This chapter was prepared by

Otto K. Behrens, PhD, *Associate Director of Research, and*
Gordon E. Mallett, PhD, *Director of Fermentation Products Research, Eli
Lilly and Company, Indianapolis, Ind. 46206*

*"Take interest I implore you in those sacred dwellings which are
designated by the expressed term, 'laboratories.' Demand that they
be multiplied, that they be adorned; these are the temples of the
future—temples of well being and of happiness. There it is that
humanity grows greater, stronger and better."*

Louis Pasteur

The "temples of the future" to which Pasteur referred have come to a fruition that could not have been
dreamed by that lonely, frustrated pioneer in biologic
experimentation. Koch's primitive kitchen bears no
resemblance to the modern, instrumented laboratory
that today's scientist takes for granted. But the work
that goes on in the laboratories—the investigation of
normal and diseased tissues, the search for agents to
treat or cure disease, the fashioning of new scientific
tools—does indeed help humanity to grow "greater,
stronger and better." In the century since Pasteur's
work, the fundamental research of many individuals
has contributed to the wealth of present-day scientific
knowledge and to the health of the present population
of the world.

The Role of Research in Pharmacy and Medicine

A century ago, pioneer women gathered and dried
herbs for "doctoring"; a housewife zealously guarded
her bag of herbs when her family moved west. Bone-
set tea reduced fevers, peppermint relieved an aching
tooth or a colicky baby, and foxglove was used to revive a failing heart. Even 50 years ago, drug materials were derived only from natural products such as
menthol, from peppermint, used for treatment of
coughs and colds. More recently, chemical research
on the isolation, identification, and synthesis of drugs
has yielded many important drug substances which
are both effective and specific.

Until World War I, most synthetic drugs and chemicals used in the US were discovered and produced in
Europe. When supplies were curtailed by the war, the
impetus was provided for the establishment of an
independent chemical and pharmaceutical industry.
Accordingly, production of chemicals and drugs was
undertaken and was the stimulus for the development
of industrial research. In the following years, the US
pharmaceutical industry made major contributions
through discovery and development of new drugs and
assumed a place of leadership in the world.

Discovery and development of the sulfonamides,
antibiotics, and other anti-infective agents dramatically reduced the death rates from a number of infective
diseases. A large proportion of the deaths from these
diseases occur prior to adulthood; consequently, these
lives are lost before the individuals mature and take
their places in productive activities.

A number of classes of drugs have marked effects on
the quality of life without significantly affecting
longevity. Compounds that control pain are illustrative. The development of reliable oral contraceptive
therapy has made intelligent family planning possible.
Tranquilizers and other central nervous system drugs
have made an important contribution to the control of
mental diseases and the restoration of mental patients
to normal activities.

Many important examples of the impact of drugs on
health and longevity may be cited. Much of the
credit can go to research, along with the development,
production, and distribution facilities of the pharmaceutical industry. Important contributions, particularly in basic research, also originate in academic and
government laboratories. Among the major drugs
discovered and/or developed in the US are insulin,
sulfa drugs, penicillins and broad spectrum antibiotics,
cortisone and other steroid compounds, isoniazid for
the treatment of tuberculosis, diuretics, and the
tranquilizers.

Of the 848 new single-chemical entities introduced
as drugs in the US in the period 1940–1967, the US
pharmaceutical industry originated 483 and shared
credit with other US or foreign originators for the discovery and development of a number of additional
drugs.

These significant contributions to the national
health and welfare have been achieved through effective collaboration of researchers in the biological and
physical sciences. The pharmaceutical industry is an
outstanding example of successful collaboration between scientists of these disciplines.

Chemists and other physical scientists have been
predominantly responsible for synthesis, isolation, and
characterization of medicinal agents. However, the
biological scientists have played an equally essential
role in developing biological assay procedures and
fermentation sources for medicinal agents.

Qualified specialists in many fields—pharmacy,
physics, chemistry, biology, engineering, pharmacology, physiology, medicine, and many others—take
part in the tremendous research effort in pharmaceuticals. Cooperation is a major feature of today's scientific investigations. "Teams" are an essential part of
industrial research, and collaboration in "group projects" wherein graduate students and postdoctoral
fellows pursue various aspects of a problem often is
found in universities; medical research also progresses
more rapidly in cooperative and multidisciplined
groups. The objectives of these research efforts are
many:

To augment present knowledge.
To extend as far as possible information about any known substance, mechanism, or disease.

To discover new methods and materials whose application may be useful.

To develop new methods needed for testing, screening, or studying known materials, diseases, or mechanisms.

To adapt or extend known methods to specific biological, pharmacological, or clinical needs.

To discover, modify, or synthesize drugs specific for treatment of diseases or symptoms, or drugs that will produce certain desired effects.

To study the mode of action of drugs.

To explore the best means of preventing, curing, or ameliorating disease.

Research Organizations

The pharmaceutical industry is a leader among all US industries in the support of research and development. A significant portion of every sales dollar is devoted to drug research activities. For instance, in 1965 companies sponsoring research allocated 10.5% of their US domestic and export sales revenue to research and development (R & D) activities directed toward the discovery and development of human-use and veterinary-use pharmaceuticals and biologicals.

The industry finances almost all (97%) of its research and development with its own funds; no other industry spends as high a percentage of R & D funds for basic and applied research; in addition, it supports the highest ratio of company-financed R & D per industry employee ($1,520).

Research in the pharmaceutical industry has grown from $12 million in 1940 to about $500 million in 1968, and now represents about 20% of the total funds allocated within the nation for medical- and health-related research. Scientists and supporting personnel in industrial R & D activities totaled about 2,000 in 1940 as compared with over 19,000 in 1967.

The academic community has played a vital role in the development of new drugs and will undoubtedly continue in this function. Its role has been in the initial clinical evaluation of new drugs, development of biochemical or physiological rationale for new drug design, basic understanding of disease states, and the training of scientists.

Observations of clinicians often lead to the discovery of new uses for drugs. Chlorpromazine, originally synthesized as an antihistamine, was found to be useful as a tranquilizer. The clinical use of this compound, and of other CNS drugs, has resulted in a marked reduction in the number of the mentally ill needing hospitalization.

Research in the academic community has been supported to a major extent by agencies of the US Government, such as the US Public Health Service, The National Institutes of Health, and The National Science Foundation. The member companies of the pharmaceutical industry also contribute financial support to academic laboratories where research of general or specific interest to the industry is conducted.

Institutes established by Government funds or private endowment—such as Sloan–Kettering Institute, Shrine Children's Hospitals, National Institutes of Health, and the Communicable Disease Center—pursue basic and applied research in many fields related to the public health. Many hospitals also maintain research clinics and/or privately or publicly endowed foundations to pursue causes and treatment of specific diseases, a related group of diseases, diseases endemic to a certain geographic area, or the group of diseases affecting a certain organ of the body (eye, heart, etc). Since research does not depend on the vending of items or services, it is not immediately self-supportive and must necessarily be supported by public as well as private funds.

Laboratory Research

Many scientific disciplines contribute to research in pharmacy and medicine in the laboratories of the university, industry, or government. Among those which play a leading role are the following.

Organic Chemistry—One major area of research in organic chemistry as applied to pharmacy and medicine is the synthesis of new organic compounds having therapeutic value. The second major area is the isolation, structure determination, and synthesis of naturally occurring compounds such as the vitamins, amino acids, alkaloids, and antibiotics. In each case, there is interest in the complex relationships between chemical structure and pharmacologic action.

The search for entirely new chemical structures or entirely new classes of compounds which exhibit physiologic activity is an important, but difficult goal of organic chemical research. When advances are made in basic organic chemistry leading to new classes of compounds, they must be submitted to screening for numerous types of biologic and pharmacologic action. Such basically new compounds open pathways for additional research effort in the expansion of the series and often lead to significant new medicinal products.

The pharmacologic activity of a compound is an involved function of the structure, and very small changes may profoundly modify the pharmacologic

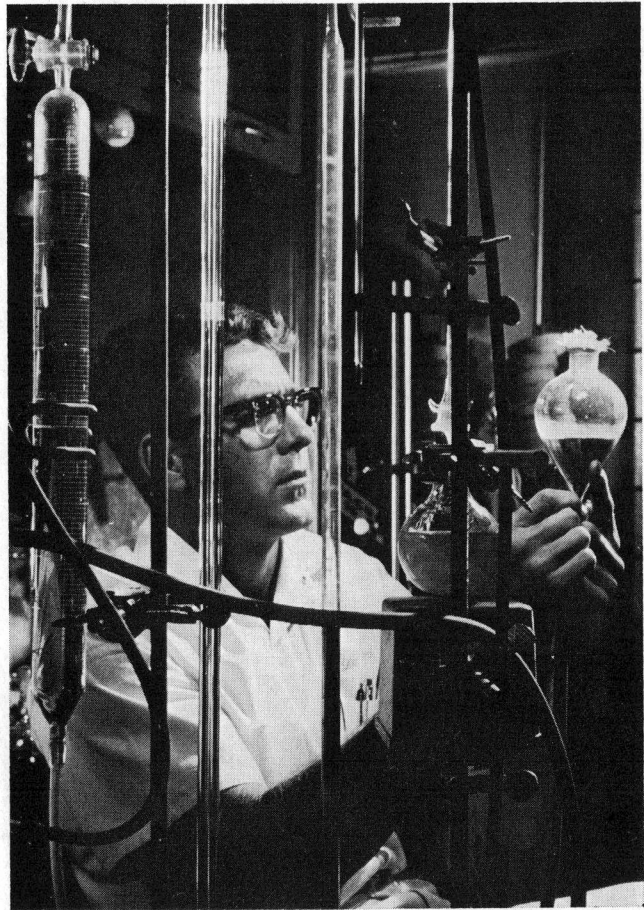

Fig. 17. The synthesis of new organic compounds is conducted by skillful scientists in the search for new therapeutic agents (courtesy, Lilly).

effect. These structural modifications may involve replacing one group with another at a specific point in the molecule, shifting the same group from place to place in the parent molecule, saturating valence bonds, or modifying the acidity or basicity.

Slight changes sometimes completely reverse the action of the compound, as is the case when the terminal methyl group of 1-methylamyl-ethyl-barbituric acid is moved one carbon atom nearer the nucleus to form 1,3-dimethylbutyl-ethyl-barbituric acid. The latter compound produces convulsions and is fatal in small doses. These convulsions can be neutralized and the animal's life saved by a dose of the sedative isomer.

Many of the currently used antispasmodics, anticonvulsants, local anesthetics, non-narcotic analgesics, ataractics, chemotherapeutic agents, and hypnotics have been products of this type of approach.

The determination of the structure of a biologically active molecule provides a twofold benefit to pharmacy and medicine. It makes possible research leading to synthesis and modification of the structure. Changes in structure are accompanied with changes in biologic activity, and occasionally vast improvement is accomplished.

Our present knowledge of adrenal corticosteroids began with the study of the various components in an extract of the adrenal cortex. These were characterized as to structure and studied clinically. Eventually cortisone was synthesized from bile acids. Today, synthetic analogs of cortisone are available which are sometimes superior therapeutically to the naturally occurring steroids.

The tetracyclines are a clinically important group of antibiotics. The first of these, 7-chlorotetracycline, was isolated in 1948 from *Streptomyces aureofaciens*. Shortly thereafter, a group of scientists isolated 5-hydroxytetracycline from *Streptomyces rimosus*, and in 1953 its structure was established. Once the chemical structure of this antibiotic was known, the way was opened for systematic variation of the basic nucleus in order to obtain new drugs with improved properties.

The catalytic removal of chlorine from 7-chlorotetracycline gave tetracycline itself, which proved to be superior to either of the above-mentioned antibiotics, and has displaced them to a considerable extent. Although tetracycline has subsequently been isolated from a *Streptomyces* species, this useful antibiotic is more readily prepared by the semisynthetic method.

Studies on the structure and synthesis of penicillins led to the development of the semisynthetic penicillins and later to cephalosporins. Some of the new compounds have made possible major improvements in antibiotic therapy.

Total synthesis is made possible by knowledge of chemical structures and, in some instances, is important economically in reducing the cost of the drug. Chloramphenicol, which can be obtained from cultures of *Streptomyces Venezuelae*, combats bacteria-produced typhoid dysentery and Rocky Mountain spotted fever. A commercially feasible chemical synthesis has replaced the fermentation process for production of the antibiotic.

Many of the water-soluble vitamins are produced commercially in large amounts by chemical synthesis. In addition, the total synthesis of compounds such as penicillin, tetracycline, and lysergic acid, although not economical, nevertheless represents outstanding contributions to the science of organic chemistry.

Microbiology—Since the discovery and development of penicillin during World War II, the search for new antibiotics among the metabolic products of microorganisms has constituted a major research effort in the pharmaceutical industry. The proved clinical usefulness of several antibiotics in treating many bacterial infections has fully justified this effort.

Microbiologists have searched among a wide variety of fungi and bacteria looking for antibiotic substances.

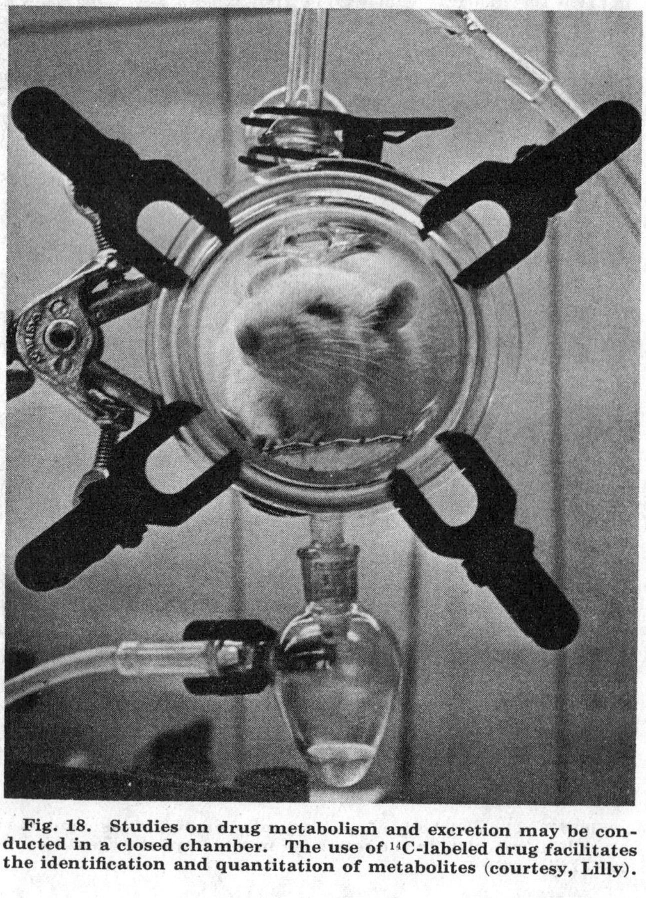

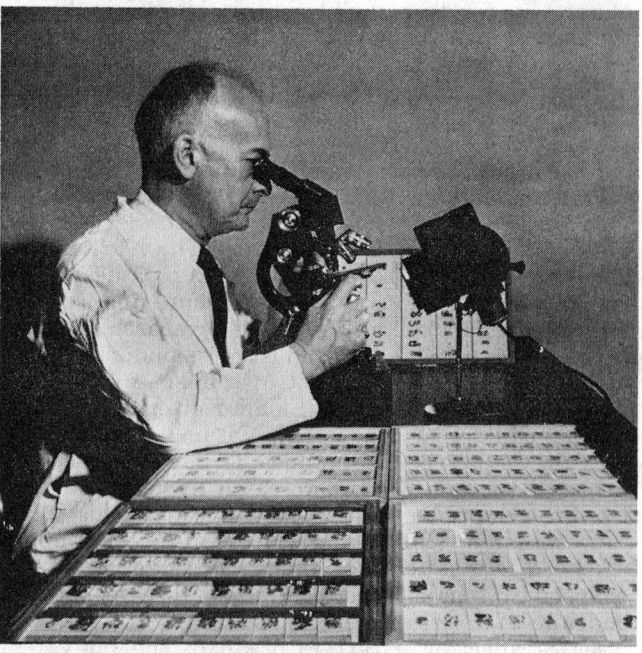

Fig. 18. Studies on drug metabolism and excretion may be conducted in a closed chamber. The use of ^{14}C-labeled drug facilitates the identification and quantitation of metabolites (courtesy, Lilly).

Fig. 19. Chronic toxicity studies include the microscopic examination of many tissue sections in the search for evidence of subtle drug effects (courtesy, Lilly).

In this search, microorganisms from plant tissues, animal sources, the sea, many types of soil, and from many other ecologic niches have been examined. More than 700 antibiotic substances have been detected and at least partially characterized. A combination of microbiological and chemical methods are required to distinguish the new antibiotics from the host of older ones which have already been discovered.

After a culture has been found to produce a new antibiotic, microbiologists then turn their attention to the biosynthesis of the compound, seeking to improve yields in order to produce quantities of the compound for testing and evaluation. An effort is also made to understand biosynthetic pathways, to further improve yields, and to facilitate the biosynthetic production of the isotope-labeled antibiotic for pharmacologic and toxicologic evaluation.

New antibiotics are being evaluated for application in an increasing number of disease conditions. Tests are conducted to determine activity of new antibiotics against a variety of yeasts, molds, and protozoa, as well as against normal and antibiotic-resistant bacterial pathogens. The antibacterial drugs have contributed to major advances in the control of bacterial and other microbial diseases. However, impetus for continued research is provided by problems of drug resistance, patient sensitivity, and the inability to control certain infections.

Microbiologists are concerned not only with the microorganisms which produce antibiotics, but also with the microbial pathogens which the antibiotics are expected to control. The mode of transmission of disease and the pathogenicity, virulence, and invasiveness of the infectious microorganisms are under investigation.

A newly recognized problem in drug resistance involves the transfer of drug resistance among Gram-negative bacteria by means of an episome bearing one or more antibiotic resistance factors. Agents that prevent the emergence of the resistance factor, or that prevent its transfer, may be sought, or future research may be directed toward agents that enhance host resistance.

An integration of microbiologic research and organic chemical research resulted in the production of a series of semisynthetic penicillins and cephalosporins. These antibiotics are chemically modified derivatives of biosynthetically produced antibiotics, which possess improved spectra of action or other advantageous chemical and biological properties.

Biochemistry and Physiology—Research in biochemistry includes investigations on the specific physiologic action of substances affecting the life processes; ie, the mode of action of biologically active compounds. Biochemists are involved in the isolation, purification, and characterization of small and large biologically active molecules.

Biochemistry is concerned also with the underlying biochemical processes which are involved in the wonderfully complex metabolism of living things: the energy-yielding systems, the systems for the synthesis of small molecules, and the processes for the synthesis of proteins, nucleic acids, and other macromolecules. Normal metabolic patterns are determined, and efforts are made to define the abnormal conditions that occur in various disease states.

Biochemists are becoming more concerned with the search for biomedical rationale to guide medicinal chemists in the design of drugs more selective for specific aspects of disease. Knowledge of the structure

and biochemical function of coenzymes has stimulated the chemist to synthesize a large number of analogs of coenzymes, some of which have proved to be useful compounds in the chemotherapy of cancer.

Increasing emphasis is being placed on studies of enzymatic processes such as those related to the biosynthesis of cholesterol, fatty acids, and triglycerides; regulation and control of protein and nucleic acid synthesis; absorption processes; and biochemical mechanisms in central nervous processes.

The increasing sophistication of research demands that an understanding of the molecular bases of diseases emerge as a primary goal. This knowledge will strongly influence both the methodology of testing new drugs and the choice or design of compounds to be tested.

Targets, or receptor locations, where drugs will act will be recognized and, in some instances, may be isolated and characterized. This information will be useful in acquiring new knowledge of the interaction between drugs and their receptor sites and in understanding the requirements for specific spatial orientation of essential structural features of drugs. Drug design will also make provision for those characteristics which will assure absorption, transport to the receptor site, and elimination of the therapeutic agent.

During recent years, the importance of high blood levels of cholesterol and certain other lipids in experimental and clinical atherosclerosis has focused attention on drugs that may influence the metabolic synthesis and disposition of these substances. A few of

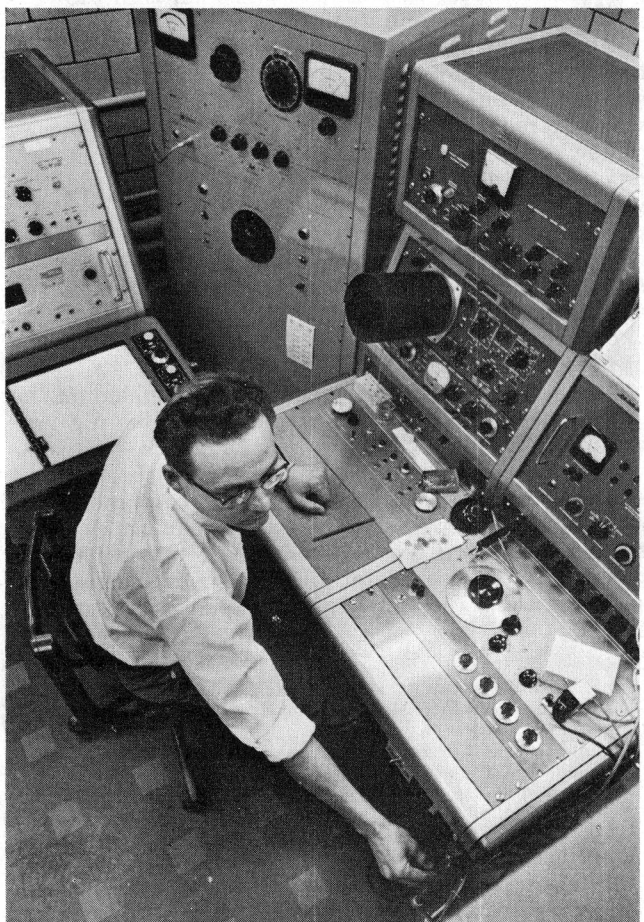

Fig. 20. At this complex control panel, the operator of a nuclear magnetic resonance spectrometer acquires information about the chemical groups in an organic molecule (courtesy, Lilly).

these drugs are beginning to be available, and more may be expected. Many years of careful study may be required before it is possible to demonstrate that such drugs prevent or ameliorate the problems of hardening of the arteries; however, there is some hope that such degeneration may respond to treatment with new drugs.

The acute problems that are associated with atherosclerosis are caused by a formation of thrombi. Two lines of approach are being applied to this problem, and either or both may be productive. Platelet agglutination, the first step in the formation of a clot, is being studied. Some factors that stimulate agglutination are recognized, and compounds may be found to counteract this influence. Studies are also in progress on enzymes that may be capable of dissolving a recently formed clot.

Biochemical investigations on the structure and function of deoxyribonucleic acid (DNA), the genetic code, and the synthesis of nucleic acids and proteins have given us knowledge which has illuminated the paths of scientists interested in virology, immunology, genetics, cancer research, and indeed, all scientists interested in fundamental biological processes.

Physiology, especially reproductive physiology, is of new interest to the industry because of the increasing demand for drugs to regulate fertility and the concern about the effects of drugs on the fetus. Many species of laboratory animals, including subhuman primates, are being used for physiological studies. Reproductive physiologists are urging the use of primates for studies, drawing upon the likelihood of greater similarity in primates and man than, for example, in rodents and man.

Biologic Research on Infectious Diseases—A major objective of biologic research is the design of satisfactory model disease systems in animals that will give reliable predictions of the safety and efficacy of new drugs in humans. Tests for antibiotic activity against bacteria and fungi are done first *in vitro*, after which animal tests using standardized, controlled experimental infections are conducted. The establishment of reliable experimental bacterial infections has facilitated the development of new antibacterial agents. More recently, new methods of establishing experimental fungal infections have led to the discovery of new antifungal compounds.

The search for antiviral agents has depended on the development of both *in vitro* and *in vivo* testing procedures. Development of methodology for propagation and counting of viruses in tissue culture has led to more precise procedures of testing compounds for antiviral activity. Recent research findings, in which some biochemical sequences involved in viral multiplication have been determined, provide insight into several possibilities for drug interference. These include:

1. Interference with viral attachment or penetration of the cell.
2. Interference with viral-induced enzymes responsible for replication of viral nucleic acid.
3. Interference with assembly of viral components.
4. Induction of faulty coding.

An increasing number of antiviral compounds are being discovered. For example, 5-fluorodeoxyuridine is effective in treating herpes of the eye, and isatin thiosemicarbazone has been used against vaccinia. Chemotherapeutic prevention or treatment of more viral diseases may be expected as new antiviral substances are developed.

Tissue culture techniques have made possible the production of large quantities of viruses for vaccine manufacture. This method of culture, which was utilized for the polio and measles vaccines, is now being focused on the study of other viral problems.

New and improved vaccines represent a major objective of biologic research. New separation methods developed in biochemistry and physical chemistry have been applied to the isolation and purification of viruses, and have led to preparation of highly purified and concentrated vaccines. Such vaccines are more effective and produce markedly less side reactions.

Recent research has focused attention on various aspects of immunity other than those concerned with the use of prophylactic vaccines. A number of important diseases such as arthritis and multiple sclerosis appear to be manifestations of autoimmune phenomena. Antibodies appear to be formed against body constituents; these antibodies then combine with the tissue containing the antigen and cause degeneration. For these diseases, suppression of immune phenomena or induction of immune tolerance may be of great importance.

Biologic and immunologic research has also been directed to the problem of cancer. New immunologic and biochemical procedures may throw light on the possible viral etiology of cancer. If this work is successful, and the initiating viruses are determined, vaccines may be developed that would prevent some forms of cancer. The existence of tumor-specific antigens in both virus- and chemically induced tumors, as well as new evidence for host reactions to the tumor, increase the possibility of useful immunologic approaches to cancer.

Pharmacology—Pharmacologic research plays two important roles in its contribution to pharmacy and medicine. The pharmacologist designs and operates model systems for detecting and evaluating the activity of compounds for control of diseases such as those of the central nervous system, the gastrointestinal tract, the cardiovascular bed, the endocrine organs, etc. Following the discovery of a new drug, the dosage, toxicity, mode of action, metabolism, and fate of that drug in the body must be determined.

Whole animals, whole organs, isolated tissue, or purified enzyme systems may be used in modern pharmacology. The classic pharmacologic methods are undergoing rapid changes to more automated and more biochemically oriented methods. The elevation or depression of such important metabolic substances as acetylcholine, histamine, and catecholamines is used as a guide for drug studies. Such biochemical measurements and highly automated methods of recording behavioral responses are employed jointly in the study of CNS drugs.

It is rare to find a potent new drug which does not have side effects in some individuals. The pharmacologist, on the basis of experimental work on a variety of species of laboratory animals, must predict an effective human dose which hopefully will produce a minimum of side effects. He must also be able to tell the physician or the clinical pharmacologist who first uses the drug in humans what form of toxicity might appear, what abnormal conditions in the patient would contraindicate use of the drug, and how other drugs administered simultaneously might affect the recommended dosage schedule.

An important part of pharmacology is the study of drug absorption, distribution, metabolism, and excretion. Whether the drug is unduly concentrated in certain organs must be determined. The fate of the drug must be ascertained; ie, whether it is excreted in the bile or urine, or if the body changes it into some other materials which, in turn, may need to be studied. A necessary preliminary to this type of research is the development by the analytical chemist of exceedingly delicate and accurate methods for measurement of the drug in urine, blood, and other body fluids or tissues.

Toxicology—In order to be certain that a new drug is safe, detailed studies are made of the effects of high doses and of prolonged administration of that drug. The pharmacologist provides acute toxicity data. The toxicologist must then refine the acute toxicity measurement in laboratory animals and begin chronic studies. The latter are conducted in a variety of species, at several dosage levels of the drug, and over periods of time ranging up to two years.

During the test period, animals are observed carefully for all adverse symptoms. At the end of this period, and occasionally during its progress, animals are sacrificed, and their vital tissues, such as liver, heart, kidney, intestine, brain, etc, are removed and studied grossly and microscopically by a competent pathologist.

In addition to gross and microscopic pathology, biochemical and physiologic responses are measured as an indication of liver function, kidney function, endocrine function, etc. During recent years, metabolic investigations have become more sophisticated and have been brought to bear on the comparative effects of drugs on various animals and man. In some instances, the metabolism of drugs or the therapeutic effects of drugs vary from species to species. Such variability can be the basis for differences in toxicity as well as differences in efficacy. For these reasons, increasing emphasis is being given to studies of comparative metabolism in man and animals to determine which laboratory animal handles the drug in a manner similar to man. Selection of that species for extensive toxicity testing should increase confidence that the toxic reactions which may occur in man will have been predicted by the animal tests.

Reproductive studies to determine the potential effects of the new drug on the reproductive processes and on subsequent generations are performed. Teratology studies are done to determine whether or not the new drug affects the fetus. Special toxicity tests have been designed to detect specific toxic reactions, such as nerve damage resulting in hearing loss.

Toxicologic studies are assuming increasing importance in the world of pharmacy and medicine. As knowledge and skills increase, and ability to measure toxic reactions improves, we will be able to assure greater safety and efficacy of new drugs.

Physical Chemistry—Modern research in pharmacy and medicine is supported and expedited by physical instrumentation. Modern instruments make possible the rapid and accurate measurement of physical and chemical properties of molecules. Separation and characterization of molecules sometimes are possible today in a matter of hours or days, whereas only a decade or two ago such work often required days, weeks, or even months.

Examples of the specialized physicochemical methods that are applicable to the research directed at the isolation, characterization, and chemical study of large molecules are the use of the ultracentrifuge and buoyant density techniques, which have been extremely useful in the study of DNA and RNA structure and function. The electron microscope is a valuable in-

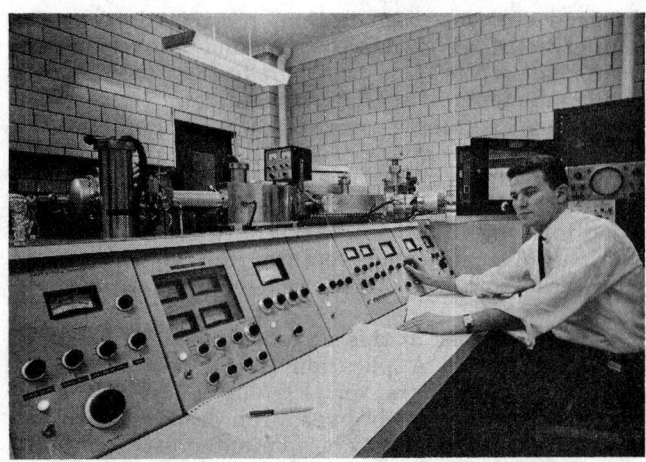

Fig. 21. The console of the mass spectrometer indicates the complexity of this instrument. It is useful in generating information on the molecular weight and empiric formula of organic compounds (courtesy, Lilly).

strument for the study of large nucleic acid or protein molecules, viruses, and organized structures of microorganisms and tissues.

In structure studies in organic chemistry, electrometric titration, polarography, and spectrophotometry in the ultraviolet, visible, or infrared make possible the identification of chemical groups within the molecule.

Nuclear magnetic resonance spectra identify chemical groups and indicate the nature of neighboring chemical groups in the molecule. Mass spectroscopy permits determination of the molecular weight and empiric formula of an organic molecule, and of the major fragments of the molecule. With this information it is often possible to deduce the entire structure of a molecule rapidly and precisely.

X-ray crystallographic analysis enables the physical chemist to determine the precise position of each atom of a molecule as it exists in the crystalline form. Optical rotatory dispersion and circular dichroism techniques are becoming useful in determining the conformation of molecules in solutions.

Physicochemical studies are directed not only at the chemical groups and stereochemical configuration of biologically active molecules, but on a more sophisticated level, calculations are being undertaken which describe molecules in terms of energy and electron distributions, and which approximate the influence of the chemical environment on these distributions.

The spatial and electronic conformation of drugs, and the changes in conformation which occur in various environments, govern the absorption, transport, distribution, and reaction with the receptor site. If description of molecules in these functional terms is achieved, correlation of electronic structure with function may be possible, and the design of safer, specific, and more effective drugs on a rational basis may occur.

Clinical Research

If a compound has desirable activity in an experimental testing system, and appears to be safe upon toxicologic examination, it becomes a candidate for clinical trial.

Two more tasks must be accomplished before clinical trial. First, the pharmaceutical chemist must put the compound in a suitable stable dosage form. The stabilization of a product must preclude physical or chemical change (discoloration, precipitation, or decomposition). The active compound must be available for absorption and transport to the site of action. The components of the pharmaceutical form must be compatible and must provide an elegant product to the physician or the patient.

Because of the many physical forms in which pharmaceuticals are presented, the research necessary is broad in scope, and involves not only the principles of physical pharmacy but requires the application of principles from the allied fields of chemistry and biology.

The second task at this stage is to file an Investigational New Drug Application (IND) with the Food and Drug Administration (FDA). The IND is, in fact, a document which gives a full description of the new drug, where and how it is manufactured, all quality control information and standards, stability, analytical methods, pharmacology, toxicology, documentation of efficacy in animals, the physicians (and their qualifications) who will be doing the clinical studies, and complete protocols of the experiments to be performed.

A new drug is administered to man for the first time by a physician. This investigator is often a professor at a leading medical school and a recognized authority in some special medical area.

The first trial of a drug in man is done with great caution and on a very limited basis. This study, called Phase I, is devoted primarily to ascertaining the safety in the human. When these limits have been established and are found acceptable, the drug is made available to a larger number of practicing specialists for the Phase II study, which is principally concerned with the determination of efficacy.

If, after Phase II, the drug still looks promising, it is distributed more widely to selected practicing physicians in the Phase III study. The purpose at this stage is to secure data from a larger number of patients on efficacy and incidence of side effects.

Finally, before the new drug can be marketed, a New Drug Application (NDA) must be filed with the FDA and approval obtained. The NDA contains most of the information included in the IND, which has been revised and updated, as well as all the results of the clinical studies proving safety and efficacy. Only after FDA approval of the NDA can distribution and marketing of the new drug begin.

The clinical research effort on a new drug represents the culmination of many years of effort by large numbers of scientists of many disciplines and skills. It is the proving ground on which the intelligence, creativity, and perseverance of laboratory researchers comes to fruition. Of the candidate drugs that come to clinical research, only a few survive as safe and effective items to be added to the clinical armamentarium. When this successful conclusion is achieved, the real beneficiary is the recipient of the new drug who may be able to live a longer and more healthful life.

Bibliography

Prescription Drug Industry Fact Book, Pharmaceutical Manufacturers Association, Washington, 1966.
Federation Proc., **28**(1), 160–215 (1969).
Status of Research in Pharmacology and Toxicology, National Institutes of Health, Bethesda, Md., May, 1968.
Chemistry, A New Look, W. A. Benjamin, Inc., New York, 1966.
Baldry, P. E., *The Battle Against Bacteria*, Cambridge, London, 1965.
Stewart, G. T., *The Penicillin Group of Drugs*, Elsevier, New York, 1965.
Davis, B. D., *et al*, *Microbiology*, Hoeber, New York, 1967.
Kohlstaedt, K. G., *Chicago Med.*, **70**(14) (1967).

Part II

PHARMACEUTICS

EDITOR

Alfred N. Martin, PhD, *Dean, School of Pharmacy, Temple University, Philadelphia, Pa. 19140*

9 | Metrology

History of weights and measures—systems of weights and measures—
relationship of various systems—conversion tables—construction and
care of balances—weighing and measuring—density, specific gravity, and
specific volume—definitions—calculations—specific gravity of liquids
and solids (pycnometers, hydrometers, and other instruments)—practical
applications

This chapter was prepared by

Samuel W. Goldstein, PhD, *Executive Secretary, Academy of Pharmaceutical
Sciences, American Pharmaceutical Association, Washington, D.C. 20037*

The first technical operation which the student of
pharmacy must learn is the manipulation of balances
and weights. This entails a study of the various systems of weights and measures, their relationships, and
a mastery of the mathematics involved. This chapter
considers the fundamental principles of metrology
underlying the testing, manufacturing, and compounding of pharmaceutical preparations, under three headings, as listed to the right:

Weights and Measures—an accumulation of facts concerning the
various systems, ancient and modern, with tables of conversion factors and practical equivalents. The relationships among the various
systems of weights and measures are clarified.

Weighing and Measuring—a discussion of the various types of
apparatus and the correct procedures to follow in using and caring
for them.

Specific Gravity and Specific Volume—a consideration of the ratio
of the weight (mass) or volume of one substance to the weight (mass)
or volume of another substance taken as the standard.

Weights and Measures

Weight is a measure of the gravitational force acting
on a body and is directly proportional to its mass. The
latter, being a constant based on inertia, never varies,
whereas weight varies slightly with latitude, altitude,
temperature, and pressure. The effect of these factors
is not usually considered unless very precise weighings
are undertaken.

Measure is the determination of the volume or extent
of a body. Temperature and pressure have a pronounced effect, especially on gases or liquids. These
factors are, therefore, considered when making preparations accurately.

All standard weights and measures in this country
are derived from or based on the United States National Prototype Standards of the Meter and the Kilogram, made of platinum–iridium, in the custody of the
National Bureau of Standards at Washington, D.C.

History of Weights and Measures

A brief outline of the origin of the many systems of
weights and measures may be of service in fixing in the
mind essential distinctions between them. The sense
of the weight of a body cannot be conveyed intelligibly
to the mind unless a means of comparison is chosen.
As weight is the measure of the gravitational force of a
body, so this force is expressed in terms of standards of
resistance, which exactly balance the body and keep it
in equilibrium when used with a mechanical device
constructed for this specific purpose. Such standards
are termed *weights* and the mechanical devices are
called *balances* or *scales*.

The standards which have been chosen by various
nations are arbitrary, and instances are common where
different standards are in use at the same time in the
same country. Many of the ancient standards are
clearly referable to variable parts of the human body,
as nail, foot, span, pace, cubit (length of the forearm),

and fathom or faethm (stretch of the arms). In the
history of metrology three periods may be traced:

1. The *Ancient* period, during which the old classical standards
originated, terminated with the decline of the Roman Empire. It is
interesting to note that the unit of distance used at the present day by
all nations in maritime measurements is the *nautical* or *meridian* mile
or $\frac{1}{60}$ of a degree of the earth's equatorial circumference, and that
this is exactly equal to 1000 Egyptian fathoms or 4000 Egyptian
cubits. These Egyptian measurements, which have persisted for
more than 4000 years, were based on astronomical or meridian
measurements which were imperishably recorded in the great Pyramid of Ghizeh, whose perimeter is exactly 500 of these fathoms, or ½
nautical mile.
2. The *Medieval* period extended to the 16th century. During
this period the old standards were lost, but their names were preserved, and European nations adopted various independent standards.
3. The *Modern* period extends from the 16th century to the present. Since the 17th century the efforts of most enlightened nations
have been directed toward scientific accuracy and simplicity, and
during the present century toward international uniformity.

Historical metrology is also referred to as *Documentary
Metrology*, which is concerned with the study of monu-
ments and records of ancient periods, and *Inductive
Metrology*, which is concerned with the accumulation of
data concerning the measurement of large numbers of
objects which have been referred to as standards but
which have no exact measure except by statutory
regulation.

The English Systems—In Great Britain, in 1266,
the 51st Act of the reign of Henry III declared "that by
the consent of the whole realm of England the measure
of the King was made—that is to say, that an English
silver penny called the sterling, round and without
clipping, shall weigh *thirty-two grains of wheat*, well
dried and gathered out of the middle of the ear; and
twenty pence (pennyweights) do make an ounce and
twelve ounces a pound, and eight pounds do make a
gallon of wine, and eight wine gallons do make a bushel,
which is the eighth of a quarter."

The 16-oz lb (*avoirdupois pound*), undoubtedly of Roman origin, was introduced at the time of the first civilization of the British island. The word "haberdepois," according to Gray, was, however, first used in English laws in 1303. A statute of Edward I (A.D. 1304) states "that every *pound* of money or of *medicines* is of *twenty shillings weight*, but the pound of all other things is *twenty-five shillings weight*. The *ounce of medicines* consists of *twenty pence*, and the *pound* contains *twelve* ounces (the Troy Pound), but in other things the pound contains *fifteen* ounces, in both cases the ounce weighing twenty pence."

These laws unfold the theory of the ancient weights and measures of Great Britain, and reveal the standards, ie, a natural object, grains of wheat; a difference existed then between the Troy and the avoirdupois pound, but the weights now in use are $\frac{1}{16}$ heavier than those of Edward I, owing to the change subsequently made in the value of the coin by the sovereign; in addition to this, the true pennyweight standard was lost, and in the next revision of the weights and measures the present troy and avoirdupois standards were adopted.

The *troy weight* is of still earlier origin. The great fairs of the 8th and 9th centuries were held at several French cities, including Troyes, the gathering place of traders from all countries. Coins were frequently so mutilated that they were sold by weight, and the standard weight of Troyes for selling coin was adopted for precious metals and medicines in all parts of Europe. The troy ounce and the avoirdupois ounce were originally intended to have the same weight, but after the revision it was found that the avoirdupois ounce was lighter by $42\frac{1}{2}$ gr than the troy ounce. The subsequent adoption of troy weight by the London College of Physicians in 1618, on the recommendation of Sir Theodore Turquet de la Mayerne, who compiled their first Pharmacopœia, has entailed upon all apothecaries who are governed by British customs, to this day, the very great inconvenience of buying and selling medicines by one system of weights (the *avoirdupois*) and compounding them by another (the *apothecary* or *troy*).

In the next century efforts were made toward reforming the standards, and the Royal Society, in 1736, began the work, which ended in the preparation, under the direction of the House of Commons, by Mr. Bird, of the standard "yard" and standard "pound" troy in 1760. Copies of these were prepared and no intentional deviation has been made since. In 1816, on account of the growing popularity of the French Metric System, and in view of the desirability of securing a standard which could easily be recovered in case of loss or destruction and which should be commensurable with a simple unit, steps were taken in England to secure these advantages. The labors of English scientists led to the adoption of the *Imperial* measures and standards, which were legalized January 1, 1826, and are now in general use in Great Britain, thus introducing another element of confusion into an already complicated subject.

In this system the *yard* is equivalent to 36 in., and its length was determined by comparison with a pendulum beating seconds of mean time, in a vacuum, at the temperature of 62°F at the level of the sea in the latitude of London, which length was found to be 39.1393 in. The *pound troy* (containing 5760 gr) was determined by comparison with a given measure of distilled water under specified conditions. Thus, a cubic inch of distilled water was weighed with brass weights in air at 62°F, the barometer at 30 in., and it weighed 252.458 gr. The standard for measures of

capacity in Great Britain (either dry or liquid) is the *Imperial gallon*, which contains 10 lb avoir (each 7000 gr) of distilled water weighed in air at 62°F, the barometer standing at 30 in. The *bushel* contains 8 such gal.

Washington, in his first annual message to Congress, January, 1790, recommended the establishment of uniformity in currency, weights, and measures. Action was taken with reference to the currency, and recommendations were made by Jefferson, then Secretary of State, for the adoption of either of the currently used English systems or a decimal system. However, nothing was accomplished until in 1819–1820 when efforts were again made in the United States to secure uniformity in the standards which were in use by the several states. Finally, after a lengthy investigation, the Secretary of the Treasury, on June 14, 1836, was directed by Congress to furnish each state in the Union with a complete set of the revised standards, and thus we have the *troy pound* (5760 gr), the *avoirdupois pound* (7000 gr), and the *yard* (36 in.) all identical with the British standards; but the US *gallon* is quite different, the old wine gallon of 231 cu in., containing 58,372.2 gr of distilled water at its maximum density, weighed in air at 62°F, the barometer standing at 30 in., being retained, while the bushel contained 77.274 lb of water under the same conditions, thus making the dry quart about 16% greater in volume than the liquid quart.

In 1864 the use of the metric measures was legalized in Great Britain, but not made compulsory, and in 1866 the United States followed the same course. *By the United States law of July 28, 1866, all lengths, areas, and cubic measures are derived from the international meter equivalent to 39.37 in.* Since 1893 the United States Office of Standard Weights and Measures has been authorized to derive the yard from the meter, 1 yd equals $\frac{3600}{3937}$ M, *and the customary weights are referred to the kilogram* by Executive order approved April 5, 1893. Capacities were to be based on the equivalent, 1 cu dm equals 1 L, the decimeter being equal to 3.937 in. The gallon still remains at 231 cu in. and the bushel contains 2150.42 cu in. This makes the liquid quart equal to 0.946 L and the dry quart 1.1013 L, while the Imperial quart is 1.1359 L. The customary weights are derived from the international kilogram, based on the value that 1 avoir lb = 453.5924277 Gm and that $\frac{5760}{7000}$ avoir lb equals 1 troy lb.

Avoirdupois weight is in general use in the United States for commercial purposes, including the buying and selling of drugs on the large scale.

The Metric System—The idea of adopting a scientific standard for the basis of metrology, which could be accurately reverified, was suggested by a number of individuals after the Renaissance. Jean Picard, the French astronomer, in the 17th century proposed to take as a unit the length of a pendulum beating 1 sec of time at sea level, at a latitude of 45°.

James Watt, the English inventor in 1783, first suggested the application of decimal notation, and the commensurability of weight, length, and volume. The French National Assembly in 1790 appointed a committee to decide the preferability of the pendulum standard or a terrestrial measure of some kind as a basis for the new system. The committee reported in 1791 in favor of the latter, and commissions were appointed to measure an arc of meridian and to perfect the details of the commensurability of the units and of nomenclature. However, certain inaccuracies were inherent in the early standards and they do not bear to each other the intended exact relationships. The present accepted standards are defined in publications of the National Bureau of Standards.

"In its original conception the meter was the fundamental unit of the metric system, and all units of length and capacity were to be derived directly from the meter which was intended to be equal to one ten-millionth of the earth's quadrant. Furthermore, it was originally planned that the unit of mass, the kilogram, should be identical with the mass of a cubic decimeter of water at its maximum density. At present, however, the units of length and mass are defined independently of these conceptions.

"For all practical purposes calibration of length standards in industry and scientific laboratories is accomplished by comparison with the material standard of length: the distance between two engraved lines on a platinum–iridium bar, the international prototype meter, which is kept at the International Bureau of Weights and Measures.

"The kilogram is independently defined as the mass of a definite platinum-iridium standard, the *International Prototype Kilogram*, which is also kept at the International Bureau of Weights and Measures. The *Liter* is defined as the volume of a kilogram of water, at standard atmospheric pressure, and at the temperature of its maximum density, approximately 4°C. The meter is thus the fundamental unit on which are based all metric standards and measurements of length and area, and of volumes derived from linear measurements.

"Of basic scientific interest is the fact that on October 14, 1960, the 11th General Conference on Weights and Measures, meeting in Paris, adopted a new international definition for the standard of length: the meter is now defined as the length equal to 1,650,763.73 wavelengths of the orange–red light of the krypton-86 isotope. This standard will be used in actual measurements only when extreme accuracy is needed.

"The kilogram is the fundamental unit on which are based all metric standards of mass. The liter is a secondary or derived unit of capacity or volume. The liter is larger by about 27 ppm than the cube of the tenth of the meter, ie, the cu dm—that is, 1 L = 1.000027 cu dm.

"The conversion tables in this publication which involve the relative length of the yard and meter are based upon the relation: 1 M = 39.37 in., contained in the act of Congress of 1866. From this relation it follows that 1 in. = 25.40005 mm (nearly).

"In recent years engineering and industrial interests the world over have urged the adoption of the simpler relation, 1 in. = 25.4 mm exactly, which differs from the preceding value by only 2 ppm. This simpler relation has not as yet been officially adopted by either Great Britain or the United States, but is in wide industrial use."

In the United States, the abbreviation *cc* still persists in general use and is taken as synonymous for the more correct term *ml*. USP IX and NF IV adopted the term *milliliter* with its abbreviated form *mil*, but it proved so unpopular in practice that the following Pharmacopeial Convention directed the return to the older term cubic centimeter (cc). In 1955 USP XV and NF X, however, once again adopted the term milliliter with the abbreviation *ml*.

National jealousies and the natural antipathy to changing established customs interfered greatly with the adoption of the metric system during the early part of the 19th century. At present the metric system is in use in every great country of the world except the United States and Great Britain and in these two countries it is legalized for reference to and definition of other standards and is in exclusive use by nearly all scientists. In the United States the metric system was legalized in 1866, but not made compulsory, and in the same year the international prototype meter and kilogram were adopted as fundamental standards.

The US silver coinage was based upon the metric system, the half dollar being exactly 12½ Gm and the quarter and the dime being of the proportionate weights.

Since 1875 there has been established and maintained an International Bureau of Weights and Measures, with headquarters at Paris. This Bureau is managed by an International Committee on which all civilized countries are represented. One object of the committee is to make and provide prototypes of the Meter and Kilogram for the subscribing nations; approximately 40 such copies have been prepared.

The US prototype standards of both the meter and the kilogram mass, constructed of a platinum–iridium alloy, were brought from Paris in 1890 and are now in the custody of the Bureau of Standards at Washington, D.C. They have been reproduced and distributed by our own government to the various states having bureaus needing such replicas. The original US prototype meter was taken back to Paris in 1957 for reverification and was found to have altered only 3 parts in 100,000,000 after 67 years of use. Thus, there was no demonstrable change within the limits of experimental error.

Adoption of the krypton-86 wavelength of light definition for the meter gives the different countries the means to check their prototype meter bars without returning them to Paris at periodic intervals for comparison with the international meter bar.

Orthography, Pronunciation, and Reading

Orthography—There are two methods of orthography of the metric units in use in the United States; in one of these, the original French, the units are spelled me*tre*, li*tre*, gram*me;* in the other, proposed by the American Metric Bureau, the units are spelled me*ter*, li*ter*, and gram. In the USP and the NF for three decades after the original adoption of the metric system, me*ter* and li*ter* were adopted but the French gram*me* was used. Now official compendia use the spelling gram.

Pronunciation—Meter is pronounced *mee'ter;* liter, *leet'er;* either gram or gramme is pronounced *gram,* not, in two syllables, as sometimes heard, *gram'me;* centimeter should be pronounced *sen'tee-mee-ter,* not *son'tee-mee-ter.* The latter faulty pronunciation is quite common, and is due to confounding the French pronunciation with the English. Either *son-tee-ma'tr* (French) or *sen'tee-mee-ter* (English) would be correct, but to use half of the French and half of the English is obviously improper, and, as the metric system is now Anglicized, the simple English pronunciation is more appropriate.

Reading—Some difficulty is usually experienced by those unfamiliar with the metric system in reading the quantities. In the linear measures in pharmacy centimeters and millimeters are almost exclusively used; thus, 0.05 M would not be read five hundredths of a meter, but 5 centimeters (5 cm); if the millimeter column contains a unit, as in 0.055 M it is read fifty-five millimeters (55 mm), in preference to fifty-five thousandths of a meter.

Fractions of a millimeter must be read decimally, as, 0.0555 M, fifty-five and five-tenths millimeters (55.5 mm). In measures of capacity, cubic centimeters (cc) or milliliters (ml), are used exclusively for quantities of less than a liter, the terms half liter, quarter liter, deciliter, centiliter, milliliter are denoted by 500 ml, 250 ml, 100 ml, 10 ml, 1 ml; with water the milliliter is considered equivalent to a gram. In weight, when the quantity is relatively large, and in commercial transactions, the *kilogram* is abbreviated to *kilo,* pronounced kee-lo; when less than a *kilogram* and not less than a *gram,* the quantity is read with the gram for the unit; 2000 Gm would be read either as two thousand grams or as two kilos, and 543 Gm would be read five hundred and forty-three grams, while 2543 Gm is sometimes read two kilos and five hundred and forty-three grams, although twenty-five hundred and forty-three grams is usually preferred. For quantities below the gram, decigram and centigram are not usually used, but milligram has been regarded as the most convenient unit. With the increase in the use of extremely small doses of very potent drugs and the wide application of more delicate analytical procedures, the term microgram (mcg, μg, or γ), for thousandths of a milligram, is frequently used to designate quantities up to 999 mcg (less than 1.000 mg).

Both the metric and English systems of weights and measures are in use in the United States, and the pharmacist must have a practical knowledge of both. The metric system is gradually replacing the English system in all our calculations and transactions. It has already done so in science and doubtless soon will be accepted and adopted generally.

Weights

The Metric System of Weight

The USP of 1890 adopted the metric system of Weights and Measures to the exclusion of all others except for equivalent dosage statements, and the British Pharmacopeia of 1914 did likewise. In 1944 the Council on Pharmacy and Chemistry of the American Medical Association adopted the Metric system exclusively for use in its *New and Nonofficial Remedies* (NNR). This policy was continued when, in 1957, the name of the Council was changed to Council on Drugs and its publication was renamed *New and Nonofficial Drugs* (NND), and changed in 1965 to *New Drugs* (ND).

The advantages of the metric or decimal system have become more and more readily appreciated, and its simplicity, brevity, and adaptability to everyday needs are now universally conceded. The principal merits are:

1. Every weight and measure bears a *simple relation* to the initial unit, the meter.
2. Every unit is multiplied or divided by the same number (ie, 10) to obtain the various denominations, and increase or decrease is expressed by simply moving the decimal point. It is the system of *decimal progression*, like the system of US coinage. Ten of a lower unit make one of the next higher unit.

$$3.95 \text{ Gm} = \begin{cases} 3 \text{ grams} \\ 9 \text{ decigrams} \\ 5 \text{ centigrams} \end{cases} \qquad \$3.95 = \begin{cases} 3 \text{ dollars} \\ 9 \text{ dimes} \\ 5 \text{ cents} \end{cases}$$

3. The *commensurability* of units of weight, length, and volume. Thus:

```
   10 ml of water weighs.................  10 Gm
   25 ml of water weighs.................  25 Gm
 1000 ml (1 liter) of water weighs..........1000 Gm (1 Kg)
```

4. Its almost universal adoption makes it an *international system*. One alleged disadvantage of the Metric system as compared with the duodecimal system (apothecaries or troy) is the practical indivisibility of 10 by 3.

Table I lists some metric weights. The advantages of this system, mentioned above, are readily apparent.

The prefixes, which indicate multiplication, are of Greek derivation—Deka, 10; Hecto, 100; Kilo, 1000. Myria, 10,000, was a term used in the original system but is not employed in practice. The division of the units is expressed by Latin prefixes—deci, 1/10; centi, 1/100; milli, 1/1000.

Only a few of the most convenient denominations are employed in practical work. Whole numbers from 1 to 1000 are usually expressed in terms of grams while the term Kilo is used as the commercial unit for larger quantities. Quantities between 1 milligram and 1 gram are usually referred to in terms of milligrams;

microgram (mcg) is used in quantitative analysis, biological studies, and for minute dosage statements.

The English Systems of Weight

In the United States both the avoirdupois and apothecaries systems of weight measurement are used in the handling of medicines. In order to avoid confusion the pharmacist must clearly establish in his mind the following facts:

1. The *avoirdupois system* of weight is used by pharmacists *to buy and to sell* all goods other than on prescription.
2. The *apothecary system* is used *to dispense* prescriptions and sometimes to compound medicines.

It must be emphasized that *the pharmacist buys his drugs by avoirdupois and dispenses by apothecary weight.* These two systems differ thus:

1 pound avoirdupois = 7000 gr and is abbreviated lb.
1 pound apothecary = 5760 gr and is abbreviated lb apoth.
1 ounce avoirdupois = 437.5 gr and is abbreviated oz.
1 ounce apothecary = 480 gr and is abbreviated ℥.

The *grain* avoirdupois is exactly the same as the *grain* apothecary. The apothecary pound is therefore 1240 gr *lighter* than the avoirdupois pound, and the apothecary ounce is therefore 42.5 gr *heavier* than the avoirdupois ounce.

The abbreviations of the denominations of apothecary weight are represented by the signs ℥, ounce; ʒ, dram; ℈, scruple; and gr, grain; these have long been in use but may possibly be mistaken for one another in rapid or careless writing. The abbreviations or signs of avoirdupois weight differ from those of apothecary weight, and care should be used not to confound them; they are lb (sometimes written #), pound; oz, ounce; gr, grain. Tables II, III, and IV show three English systems of weight.

Jewelers evaluate precious stones with troy weight, which is very similar to apothecary weight. The apothecary and troy grain, ounce, and pound are identical, but the ounces are subdivided differently. The *carat*, used by jewelers, is equal to 3.168 troy grains or 4 carat grains. When used to express the fineness of gold 1 carat signifies 1/24 part. A 14-carat ring is 14/24 pure gold.

In the United States two systems of liquid measure are in general use—the apothecary (wine) and metric measure.

Because of the proximity of Canada, those who practice in the border states, as well as those pharmacists in the United States who fill British prescriptions, find it necessary to familiarize themselves with Imperial as well as US measure.

Many pharmacists therefore are compelled to be familiar with three systems of liquid measure. In addition, there are two systems of linear measure in use in the United States—English and metric linear measure. The pharmacist must be able to use either one.

Table I—Metric Weight

1 microgram (gamma)	mcg (γ)	=	0.000,001	Gm
1 milligram	mg	=	0.001	Gm
1 centigram	cg	=	0.01	Gm
1 decigram	dg	=	0.1	Gm
1 gram	Gm	=	1.0	Gm
1 Dekagram	Dg	=	10.0	Gm
1 Hectogram	Hg	=	100.0	Gm
1 Kilogram	Kg	=	1000.0	Gm

Note—For a clear picture of the relationships of these units of weight, see the scale drawing on page 82. The abbreviation μg is used for microgram in physics rather than mcg as in pharmacy or γ as in biology.

Table II—Avoirdupois Weight

Pound		Ounces		Grains
lb 1	=	16	=	7000
		oz 1	=	**gr** 437.5

Note—2000 lb = 1 ton and 2240 lb = 1 long ton.

Table III—Apothecary Weight

Pound		Ounces		Drams		Scruples		Grains
lb 1	=	12	=	96	=	288	=	5760
		℥ 1	=	8	=	24	=	480
				ℨ 1	=	3	=	60
						℈ 1	=	**gr** 20

Table IV—Troy Weight

Pound		Ounces		Pennyweights (Pwt)		Grains
lb 1	=	12	=	240	=	5760
		℥ 1	=	20	=	480
				Pwt 1	=	**gr** 24

Note—The abbreviation lb refers to the avoirdupois pound of 7000 gr unless further qualified, as in the headings of Tables III and IV.

Measures

The Metric Systems of Measure

The Metric systems of *linear* and *liquid* measure are used almost exclusively in scientific studies. The pharmacist should be familiar with Tables V and VI.

The English Systems of Measure

The pharmacist must be familiar with the measurement of plasters, bandages, trusses, and many other items found in the modern pharmacy. He experiences no difficulty, however, for the inch, foot, and other common measurements of the English system are used almost exclusively. Only a few items, such as hypodermic needles and catheters, are measured in other systems.

The following facts concerning the US system of liquid measure should be noted:

1. The apothecary fluidounce of distilled water weighs 454.6 gr at 25°C (77°F).
2. The apothecary pint contains 16 fl℥.
3. The US gallon contains 128 fl℥ or 231 cu in. One gallon of distilled water weighs 8.337 avoir lb at 62°F. The US pint therefore weighs 1.04 avoir lb and the pound of distilled water measures only 0.96 pt. *One pound does not measure 1 pt.*

The following facts concerning the Imperial system should be noted:

1. The Imperial fluidounce of distilled water weighs 437.5 gr at 15.6°C (60°F). It therefore weighs 1 avoir oz.
2. The Imperial pint contains 20 fl℥.
3. The Imperial gallon contains 160 fl℥. One gallon of distilled water weighs 10 avoir lb. 16 fl℥ in this system therefore weigh 1 lb avoir.

From the above statements we deduce the following

1. The US fluidounce and minim are larger than the Imperial fluidounce and minim. One US minim or fluidounce equals 1.04 Imperial minims or fluidounces.
2. The Imperial pint and gallon are much larger than the US pint and gallon.

It is, therefore, inaccurate to use measuring devices calibrated in the US system in measuring quantities directed in English prescriptions when the Imperial measure is intended, and, conversely, devices calibrated in the Imperial system should not be used to measure quantities directed in US prescriptions when the US measure is intended. For example, Canadian pharmacists using American graduates should calculate percentage solutions on the basis of 454.6 gr of distilled water to the fluidounce. This is one more argument in favor of adoption internationally by all pharmacists of the metric system of weights and measures.

The Relationships of Weights and of Measures

When the systems of weights and measures in use in this country are studied, the lack of close relation between the different units is at once appreciated. Nevertheless, if the following statements are carefully memorized, many pharmaceutical problems will be greatly simplified.

1. The pharmacist buys merchandise, sells over the counter, weighs himself, calculates postage, etc, by avoirdupois weight which contains *437.5 gr in 1 oz.*
2. He dispenses many prescriptions and compounds many formulas by apothecary weight which contains *480 gr in 1 oz.*
3. One apothecary fluidounce weighs *454.6 gr* at 25°C. Since 480 ♏ weigh 454.6 gr, then 1 ♏ weighs 454.6/480 = 0.95 gr.

1 ♏ does *not* weigh 1 gr
1 fl℥ does *not* weigh 1 oz avoir.

Practical Equivalents

Tables of weights and measures and a table of practical equivalents should be kept in a conspicuous and convenient place in the compounding department, and the following equivalents, which are given with practical accuracy, should be committed to memory. Other equivalents may be calculated from these.

Table V—Metric Linear Measure

1 micromicron	($\mu\mu$)	= 0.000,000,000,001 meter (M)
		(0.001 mμ; 10^{-12}M; 0.01 Ångström unit Å)
1 millimicron	(mμ)	= 0.000,000,001 M
		(0.001 μ; 10^{-9} M; 10 Å)
1 micron	(μ)	= 0.000,001 M
		(0.001 mm.; 10^{-6} M; 10,000 Å)
1 millimeter	(mm)	= 0.001 M
1 centimeter	(cm)	= 0.01 M
1 decimeter	(dm)	= 0.1 M
1 meter	(M)	= 1.0 M
1 dekameter	(Dm)	= 10.0 M
1 hectometer	(Hm)	= 100.0 M
1 kilometer	(Km)	= 1000.0 M

Note—While the meter (M) is observed to be the initial unit, it is seldom necessary to use it in pharmaceutical practice, and the same holds true for a number of the above measures. The micron (μ), millimeter (mm), and the centimeter (cm) are employed in the USP and in the NF in the description of many of the official drugs. Measurements pertaining to spectrophotometric and colorimetric tests and assays of many official drugs are recorded in microns (μ) for infrared and in millimicrons (mμ) for ultraviolet and visible wavelengths of light, respectively.

Table VI—Metric Liquid Measure

1 microliter	(μl)	= 0.000001 L
1 milliliter	(ml)	= 0.001 L
1 centiliter	(cl)	= 0.01 L
1 deciliter	(dl)	= 0.1 L
1 liter	(L)	= 1.0 L
1 dekaliter	(Dl)	= 10.0 L
1 hectoliter	(Hl)	= 100.0 L
1 kiloliter	(Kl)	= 1000.0 L

Note—The Standard of Capacity is the *liter*, which is the volume of 1 Kg of distilled water at its maximum density (approx. 4°C). Microliters (μl) are used to measure volumes of solutions used in chromatographic procedures for the separation and quantitative determination of some USP and NF drugs.

Linear Measure

1 meter	= **39.37 in.**	
1 inch	= **2.54 cm** = **25 mm** (25.4 mm)	
1 micron	= **1/1000 mm** = 10^{-6} m = $1/25{,}000$ in.	

Liquid Measure

1 milliliter	= **16.23** ♏
1 fluidounce	= **30 ml** (29.57 ml)
1 liter	= **33.8 fl℥** (33 fl℥ 391 ♏)
1 pint	= **473 ml** (473.167 ml)
1 gallon	= **3785 ml** (3785.332 ml)

Weight

1 kilogram	= **2.2 lb** (2 lb 3 oz 119.9 gr avoir)
1 pound avoir	= **454 Gm** (453.59 Gm)
1 ounce avoir	= **28 Gm** (28.35 Gm)
1 ounce apoth	= **31 Gm** (31.1 Gm)
1 gram	= **15.432 gr**
1 grain	= **65 mg**

The use of the metric weights and measures in the texts of the USP and the NF, and the tendency on the part of physicians, manufacturers of medicinals, and scientists in general to use the Metric systems, make it necessary for every pharmacist to become familiar with them. An easy method of remembering their relationships to each other and their equivalents in other systems is desirable. In order to aid the pharmacist, therefore, in visualizing the various relationships, Fig. 22 has been prepared.

Approximate Measures

In apportioning doses for a patient the practitioner is usually compelled to order the liquid medicine to be administered in certain quantities that have been established by custom, and estimated as follows:

1 tumblerful	f℥ viii	240 ml
1 teacupful	f℥ iv	120 ml
1 wineglassful	f℥ ii	60 ml
2 tablespoonfuls	f℥ i	30 ml
1 tablespoonful	f℥ iv	15 ml
1 dessertspoonful	f℥ ii	8 ml
1 teaspoonful*	f℥ i	5 ml
½ teaspoonful	f℥ ss	2 ml

Note—1 drop, through a popular error, is considered to be 1 minim. This is incorrect as "drops" are variable. See also page 94.

In almost all cases the modern teacups, tablespoons, dessertspoons, and teaspoons, after careful tests, are found to average 25% greater capacity than the theoretical quantities just given. The physician and the pharmacist should therefore recommend the use of accurately graduated medicine glasses, which may be procured at a trifling cost (Fig. 23).

Approximate Dose Equivalents

For many years the apothecaries' system of weights and measures was widely used by physicians and pharmacists when considering the doses of medicinal substances, and it was customary to translate these apothecaries' doses into relatively exact amounts when the metric equivalents were mentioned. Today, however, a united effort is being made to establish doses primarily in the metric system and to select for these

---

* The volume contained in a teaspoon continues to be a matter of controversy. While many prescribers accept 4 ml as the equivalent of a teaspoonful, the NF and USP consider it to represent 5 ml.

Table VII—English Linear Measure

12 inches	= 1 foot
3 feet	= 1 yard
5½ yards	= 1 rod
320 rods	= 1 mile
3 miles	= 1 league

Note—4 inches equal 1 hand and 6 feet equal 1 fathom.

Table VIII—Apothecary or Wine Measure (US)

Gallon		Pints		Fluidounces		Fluidrams		Minims
Cong 1	=	8	=	128	=	1024	=	61,440
		O. 1	=	16	=	128	=	7.680
				f℥ 1	=	℥ 8	=	480
						f℥ 1	=	♏ 60

Table IX—Imperial Measure (British)

Gallon		Pints		Fluidounces		Fluidrams		Minims
Cong 1	=	8	=	160	=	1280		76,800
		O. 1	=	20	=	160		9,600
				fl℥ 1	=	8	=	480
						fl℥ 1	=	♏ 60

Note—O. is the abbreviation for the Latin word *Octarius;* Cong, for the Latin word *Congius.* The gill, which is ¼ pint, is obsolete, but is occasionally found in old family recipes. 31 US gallons equal 1 barrel.

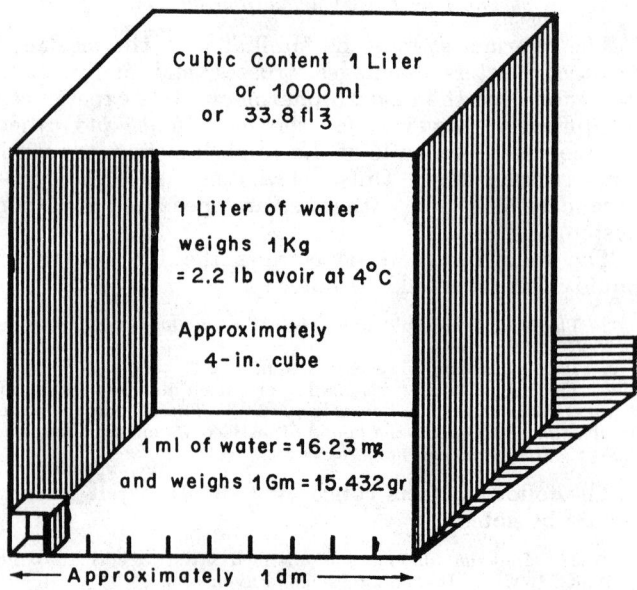

Fig. 22. Metric equivalents. Note: The liter occupies slightly more than a cubic decimeter of water at 4°C. One liter = 1000 ml = 1000.027 cc (see page 79).

Table X—Equivalent Linear Measurements

Unit	in.	mm	μ	mμ	Å	$\mu\mu$	x-u
1 in. (inch)	1	25.4	25,400	2.54×10^7	2.54×10^8	2.54×10^{10}	2.54×10^{11}
1 mm (millimeter)	0.0394	1	1000	10^6	10^7	10^9	10^{10}
1 μ (micron)	3.94×10^{-5}	10^{-3}	1	1000	10,000	10^6	10^{17}
1 mμ (millimicron)	3.94×10^{-8}	10^{-6}	10^{-3}	1	10	1000	10,000
1 Å (angstrom unit)	3.94×10^{-9}	10^{-7}	10^{-4}	0.1	1	100	1000
1 $\mu\mu$ (micromicron)	3.94×10^{-11}	10^{-9}	10^{-6}	10^{-3}	0.01	1	10
1 x-u (seigbahn unit)	3.94×10^{-12}	10^{-10}	10^{-7}	10^{-4}	10^{-3}	0.1	1

doses the metric quantities which produce the desired therapeutic effect, without considering the relation of these metric figures to the corresponding quantities in any other system of weights and measures.

A feature of the renewed effort to establish dose thinking and practice in the metric system was the joint project agreed to in 1950 by the American Medical Association through its Council on Pharmacy and

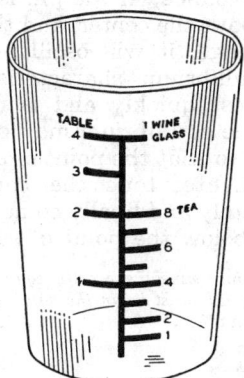

Fig. 23. Medicine glass.

Chemistry, by the USP, and by the NF; the Food and Drug Administration also gave its approval. This consisted of preparing, as an aid to transition from apothecary to metric doses, a table of equivalents for converting quantities in the apothecary systems of liquid measure and of weight to corresponding *approximate* quantities in the metric systems. These were first included in USP XIV and NF IX of 1950. The 1950 revisions

of these compendia also continued to give approximate apothecary doses which appeared only in a secondary place, in parentheses and in small type. The current revisions of the USP, NF, and ND now give only metric doses. The statements and table of approximate equivalents (Table XI) appear also in the current USP and NF.

It is expected that all teaching institutions, hospitals, and pharmaceutical and chemical manufacturers will adopt metric doses as rapidly as possible and that in a short time no one will think of any dose except in metric terms. Practically all of the new medicinal products are marketed with only the metric dose indicated on the labels and accompanying literature.

It should be emphasized that exact alternative formulas in the avoirdupois system of weights and measures are *not* obtained by using approximate equivalents but for the purpose of compounding should be calculated with the use of the conversion tables printed as Tables XII–XV. These give the exact proportionate amounts required to produce an identical formula in the English system. For example, the student will observe that quantities used to make a formula for 1000 ml are frequently converted into quantities required to make 2 pt. Two pints do not equal 1000 ml and therefore all ingredients must be in the same ratio.

If a formula calls for 100 Gm of citric acid in 1000 ml of solution, it forms a 10% *w/v* solution. At 25°C (practical working temperature) 1 oz of water weighs 454.57 gr. Therefore, 2 pt of water weigh $32 \times 454.57 = 14546.24$ gr. A 10% *w/v* solution contains 1454.62 gr or 3 oz avoir 142.1 gr. The USP gives the equivalent as 3 oz avoir 148 gr at 4°C, which is sufficiently accurate for all practical purposes.

Weighing and Measuring

Having studied the several systems of weights and measures, the student can now learn to apply his knowledge to the *weighing* and *measuring* of pharmaceuticals. The former process requires the use of the *balance*, or, for manufacturing purposes, *scales*, and the latter process requires the use of the *measure*, the *graduate*, and the *pipet*. Since the successful performance of many of the operations in pharmacy depends on a thorough knowledge of the principles of the balance and a correct understanding of its care and use, and since weighing is nearly always the preliminary step in any compounding, it will be discussed first.

There is a relativity of accuracy in weighing (or measuring) which must not be overlooked and which may be illustrated by giving consideration to the following graded list: coal, ice, salt, sugar, epsom salt, morphine, strychnine, aconitine, and radium. One of the most important things for the pharmacist to learn is the degree of tolerance or error permissible in weighing or measuring any particular ingredient.

The empiric weighing and measuring methods of the kitchen, embodied in such concepts as a handful, a pinch, or "sweeten to suit your taste," have no place in pharmacy. Accurate work can be accomplished only by means of suitable apparatus.

It is obviously unnecessary to discuss such weighing devices as platform scales, steelyards, crane scales, spring balances, computing scales, or any of the specialized or unusual types not commonly used in the laboratories of professional or industrial pharmacy.

Weighing

In pharmacy, weighing usually refers to the ascertaining of a definite weight of material to be used in compounding a prescription or manufacturing a dosage form.

The *balance* may be defined as an instrument for determining the relative weights of substances, and should be *correctly selected* for the specific task at hand, *skillfully used, carefully protected from injury*, and *periodically checked*, if accurate results are to be obtained. Of even greater importance is its *construction*.

Construction of the Balance

For systematic consideration pharmaceutical balances may be classified as follows: (1) single-beam, equal-arm, (2) unequal arm, (3) compound lever, and (4) torsion.

Single-Beam Equal-Arm Balances—This instrument consists of a metallic lever or beam, divided into two equal arms at the center by a knife edge, on which it is supported. At exactly equal distances from this point of support, and situated in the same plane, are placed the end knife edges; these suspend the pans which carry the substances to be weighed (see *Analytical Balances*, Chapter 37). The principles used in the construction of this balance have been in continuous use from the earliest periods of antiquity. A properly constructed balance of this type should possess the following requirements:

1. When the beam is in a horizontal position, the center of gravity should be slightly below the point of support, or central knife edge, and perpendicular to it.

The relative sensitiveness of the balance depends on the fulfilment of this principle, which may be roughly illustrated by forcing a pin through the center of a circular piece of pasteboard; if the edge of the pasteboard is touched slightly, it does not oscillate at all, but revolves around the center to a degree corresponding to the impulse given it. In this position it illustrates neutral equilibrium. If the pin is removed and inserted at a very short distance above the center, and the edge of the pasteboard touched as before, it will oscillate slowly, corresponding to a very sensitive beam, the point of support being *slightly* above the center of gravity as in the balance; if the pin is again removed and inserted far above the center, and the same impulse imparted to the edge, it will oscillate quickly, illustrating stable equilibrium characteristic of a beam which comes to rest quickly and is not particularly sensitive. Unstable equilibrium may be illustrated by balancing the disk so that the point of support is below the center. The slightest touch then causes it to reverse its position completely and finally come to rest with the center of gravity below the point of support.

2. The end knife edges must be exactly equal distances from the central knife edge; they all must be in the same plane, and the edges absolutely parallel to each other.

Table XI—Metric Doses with Approximate Apothecary Equivalents

These *approximate* dose equivalents in the following table represent the quantities usually prescribed, under identical conditions, by physicians trained, respectively, in the metric or in the apothecary system of weights and measures. In labeling dosage forms in both the metric and the apothecary systems, if one is the approximate equivalent of the other, the approximate figure shall be enclosed in parentheses.

When prepared dosage forms such as tablets, capsules, pills, etc, are prescribed in the metric system, the pharmacist may dispense the corresponding approximate equivalent in the apothecary system, and *vice versa*, as indicated in the following table. For the conversion of specific quantities in a prescription which requires compounding, or in converting a pharmaceutical formula from one system of weights or measures to the other, exact equivalents must be used.

Liquid Measure

Metric ml	Approximate apothecary equivalents	Metric ml	Approximate apothecary equivalents ♏
1000	1 qt	3	45
750	1½ pt	2	30
500	1 pt	1	15
250	8 fl℥	0.75	12
200	7 fl℥	0.6	10
100	3½ fl℥	0.5	8
50	1¾ fl℥	0.3	5
30	1 fl℥	0.25	4
15	4 flʒ	0.2	3
10	2½ flʒ	0.1	1½
8	2 flʒ	0.06	1
5	1¼ flʒ	0.05	⅛
4	1 flʒ	0.03	½

Weight

Metric		Approximate apothecary equivalents	Metric mg	Approximate apothecary equivalents gr
30	Gm	1 ℥	30	½
15	Gm	4 ʒ	25	⅜
10	Gm	2½ ʒ	20	⅓
7.5	Gm	2 ʒ	15	¼
6	Gm	90 gr	12	⅕
5	Gm	75 gr	10	⅙
4	Gm	60 gr (1 ʒ)	8	⅛
3	Gm	45 gr	6	1/10
2	Gm	30 gr (½ ʒ)	5	1/12
1.5	Gm	22 gr	4	1/15
1	Gm	15 gr	3	1/20
0.75	Gm	12 gr	2	1/30
0.6	Gm	10 gr	1.5	1/40
0.5	Gm	7½ gr	1.2	1/50
0.4	Gm	6 gr	1	1/60
0.3	Gm	5 gr	0.8	1/80
0.25	Gm	4 gr	0.6	1/100
0.2	Gm	3 gr	0.5	1/120
0.15	Gm	2½ gr	0.4	1/150
0.12	Gm	2 gr	0.3	1/200
0.1	Gm	1½ gr	0.25	1/250
75	mg	1¼ gr	0.2	1/300
60	mg	1 gr	0.15	1/400
50	mg	¾ gr	0.12	1/500
40	mg	⅔ gr	0.1	1/600

Note—The abbreviation ml for milliliter may be used interchangeably with cc since for all practical purposes they are identical.

Table XII—Converting Metric Quantities to Quantities in Avoirdupois Weight at 25°C

Grams to Grains, etc (Product Measured)

	gr/fl℥		gr, etc/pt		gr, etc/gal		
Gm/L	oz av	gr	oz av	gr	lb av	oz av	gr
1	..	0.45	..	7.3	..	..	58.2
2	.	0.91	..	14.5	..	..	116.4
3	..	1.36	..	21.8	..	..	174.6
4	..	1.82	..	29.1	..	..	232.7
5	..	2.27	..	36.4	..	..	290.9
6	..	2.73	..	43.6	..	..	349.1
7	..	3.18	..	50.9	..	..	407.3
8	..	3.64	..	58.2	..	1	28.0
9	..	4.09	..	65.5	..	1	86.2
10	..	4.55	..	72.7	..	1	144.3
20	.	9.09	..	145.5	..	2	288.7
30	..	13.64	..	218.2	..	3	433.0
40	..	18.18	..	290.9	..	5	139.9
50	..	22.73	..	363.7	..	6	284.2
60	..	27.27	..	436.4	..	7	428.6
70	..	31.82	1	71.6	..	9	135.4
80	..	36.37	1	144.3	..	10	279.8
90	..	40.91	1	217.1	..	11	424.1
100	..	45.46	1	289.8	..	13	131.0
200	..	90.91	3	142.1	1	10	262.0
300	..	136.37	4	431.9	2	7	393.0
400	..	181.83	6	284.2	3	5	86.5
500	..	227.29	8	136.6	4	2	217.5
600	..	272.74	9	426.4	4	15	348.5
700	..	318.20	11	278.7	5	13	42.0
800	..	363.66	13	131.0	6	10	173.0
900	..	409.11	14	420.9	7	7	304.0
1000	1	17.07	16	273.1	8	4	435.0

Example: To make 1 gallon.

Green soap	120 Gm	100 Gm	13 oz	131 gr
		20 Gm	2 oz	289 gr
Camphor	45 Gm	40 Gm	5 oz	140 gr
		5 Gm		291 gr
Oil of rosemary	10 ml	(Table XIII)	1 fl℥	134 ♏
Alcohol	700 ml	"	"5 pt	9 fl℥ 288 ♏
Water, sufficient, to make 1000 ml			or 1 gallon	

Note—It should be particularly noted that the table given above gives conversion figures for use at 25°C, the average temperature of the dispensary. One fluidounce of water weighs 454.6 gr at 25°C. A similar table was printed in the appendix of the USP XIV, but it gave conversion figures for use at 4°C at which temperature 1 fl℥ of water weighs 456.4 gr. For practical purposes the difference between the two tables is negligible.

Table XIII—Converting Metric Quantities to Quantities in Apothecary Measures

ml to ℳ, etc (Product Measured)

ml/L	ℳ/fl℥	ℳ, etc/pt		ℳ, etc/gal		
		fl℥	ℳ	pt	fl℥	ℳ
1	0.48	..	7.68	..	..	61
2	0.96	..	15.36	..	..	123
3	1.44	..	23.04	..	..	184
4	1.92	..	30.72	..	..	246
5	2.40	..	38.40	..	..	307
6	2.88	..	46.09	..	..	369
7	3.36	..	53.76	..	..	430
8	3.84	..	61.44	..	1	12
9	4.32	..	69.12	..	1	73
10	4.80	..	76.80	..	1	134
20	9.60	..	153.60	..	2	269
30	14.40	..	230.40	..	3	403
40	19.20	..	307.20	..	5	58
50	24.00	..	384.00	..	6	192
60	28.80	..	460.80	..	7	326
70	33.60	1	57.60	..	8	461
80	38.40	1	134.40	..	10	115
90	43.20	1	211.20	..	11	250
100	48.00	1	288.00	..	12	384
200	96.00	3	96.00	1	9	288
300	144.00	4	384.00	2	6	192
400	192.00	6	192.00	3	3	96
500	240.00	8	....	4	..	....
600	288.00	9	288.00	4	12	384
700	336.00	11	96.00	5	9	288
800	384.00	12	384.00	6	6	192
900	432.00	14	192.00	7	3	96
1000	480.00	16	....	8	..	...

Example: See under Table XII.

Table XIV—Converting Metric Quantities to Quantities in Apothecary Weights

Parts per 1000 to grains, etc, per pound avoirdupois

Grams per Kilogram	Grains and Apothecaries Ounces per Pound Avoirdupois		Grains and Ounces Avoirdupois per Pound Avoirdupois	
	oz	gr	oz	gr
1	..	7	..	7.0
2	..	14	..	14.0
3	..	21	..	21.0
4	..	28	..	28.0
5	..	35	..	35.0
6	..	42	..	42.0
7	..	49	..	49.0
8	..	56	..	56.0
9	..	63	..	63.0
10	..	70	..	70.0
20	..	140	..	140.0
30	..	210	..	210.0
40	..	280	..	280.0
50	..	350	..	350.0
60	..	420	..	420.0
70	1	10	1	52.5
80	1	80	1	122.5
90	1	150	1	192.5
100	1	220	1	262.5
200	2	440	3	87.5
300	4	180	4	350.0
400	5	400	6	175.0
500	7	140	8	...
600	8	360	9	262.5
700	10	100	11	87.5
800	11	320	12	350.0
900	13	60	14	175.0
1000	14	280	16	...

Example: To make 1 pound avoirdupois.

Camphor Liniment

Camphor..........	200 Gm............	3 oz	87.5 gr
Cottonseed oil......	800 Gm............	12 oz	350.0 gr
To make	1000 Gm	or 1 lb avoir	

It is very apparent that the conditions of a good prescription balance cannot be satisfied if there is inequality in the length of the arms of the beam.   In Fig. 24 the distance from the central knife edge to the one on the left must be exactly the same as the distance from the central knife edge to the one on the right, otherwise unequal weights would be required to establish equilibrium.   If the central knife edge is placed either above or below a line drawn so that it connects the end knife edges, the loading of the pans will either cause the beam to cease oscillating, or will diminish the sensitiveness in proportion to the load.   If the knife edges are not parallel, the weight of a body will not be constant upon every part of the pan, but will be greater if placed near the edge on one side, and correspondingly less at a point directly opposite.

3.   The beam should be inflexible, but as light in weight as possible, and the knife edges in fine balances should bear upon agate planes.

Rigidity of the beam is necessary because any serious deflection caused by a loading of the pans would lower the end knife edges and thus accuracy in weighing would be impossible.   The beam should not be heavier than necessary because the sensitiveness of the balance would be thereby lessened, and to diminish friction which constantly increases with the age and use of a balance, the bearings of the knife edges should be agate planes, which are polished flat pieces of the very hard mineral called agate.

The simplest form in which this principle is utilized is seen in the cheap hand scales which are practically extinct in this country.   The beam is usually of brass, with a steel central knife edge, having a perforation in each end of the beam for the insertion of two wire hooks, to which are attached silken cords for supporting the pans, and, when in use, the beam is suspended from one hand of the operator.   These scales do not comply with the legal requirements for prescription balances.

Unequal-Arm Balances—This type of balance is preferred for laboratory work when large amounts are to be weighed.   The principle upon which these scales are constructed is based on the following law of physics, *"The power is to the weight of resistance in the inverse ratio of the length of the arms of the lever."*   The inequality in the length of the arms of this beam permits the convenient use of movable weights upon the graduated longer arm of the beam, thus dispensing with the use of small weights, which are liable to be lost.   This scale (Fig. 25) is of great advantage in laboratory or manufacturing work because it is particularly adapted for weighing liquids, a sliding tare being set on one beam for the weight of the container, while the other sliding weights can be adjusted at once to the weight of the liquid desired.   These are now to be had with the beams graduated either in the avoirdupois or in the metric system.

Compound-Lever Balances—The principle of the compound lever was first applied in the construction of balances by Robervahl, of Paris, about A.D. 1660.

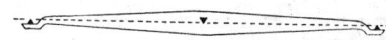

Fig. 24.   Position of knife edges.

It has been skillfully adopted for both prescription balances and the general counter and platform scales. The principal objection to this type of balance, when compared with single-beam balances, consists in the multiplicity of points of contact and suspension, thus necessarily increasing friction and the liability to disarrangement; but their general convenience and improvements in construction have brought them into favor. The principle of the Robervahl compound lever balance, with the arrangement of the levers as utilized in the Troemner prescription balance, is shown in Fig. 29, page 88.

The compound lever type of scale with the working parts enclosed is generally useful for counter and dis-

Table XV—Exact Equivalents of Weights and Measures
Metric, Avoirdupois, and Apothecary

grains	Apothecary oz	Apothecary gr	Avoir. lb	Avoir. oz	Avoir. gr	Metric Weight and Measure, Gm or ml[a]	Fluid oz	Fluid min	fl oz and Fract
15432.4	32	72.4	2	3	119.9	1000	33	391.1	33.815
15360.0	32	...	2	3	47.5	995.311	33	314.9	33.656
15060.5	31	180.5	2	2	185.5	975.906	33	...	33
15046.5	31	166.5	2	2	171.5	975	32	465.3	32.969
14880.0	31	...	2	2	5.0	964.208	32	290.1	32.604
14660.7	30	260.7	2	1	223.2	950	32	59.5	32.124
14604.1	30	204.1	2	1	166.6	946.333	32	...	32
14400.0	30	...	2	..	400.0	933.104	31	265.2	31.553
14274.9	29	354.9	2	..	274.9	925	31	133.7	31.279
14147.8	29	227.8	2	..	147.8	916.700	31	...	31
14000.0	29	80.0	2	..	...	907.185	30	324.6	30.676
13920.0	29	...	1	15	357.5	902.001	30	240.4	30.501
13889.1	28	449.1	1	15	326.6	900	30	207.9	30.433
13691.4	28	251.4	1	15	128.9	887.187	30	...	30
13562.5	28	122.5	1	15	...	878.835	29	344.4	29.718
13503.3	28	63.3	1	14	378.3	875	29	282.2	29.588
13440.0	28	...	1	14	315.0	870.897	29	215.6	29.449
13235.0	27	275.0	1	14	110.0	857.614	29	...	29
13125.0	27	165.0	1	14	...	850.486	28	364.3	28.759
13117.5	27	157.5	1	13	430.0	850	28	356.4	28.742
12960.0	27	...	1	13	272.5	839.794	28	190.8	28.397
12778.6	26	298.6	1	13	91.1	828.041	28	...	28
12731.7	26	251.7	1	13	44.2	825	27	430.6	27.897
12687.5	26	207.5	1	13	...	822.136	27	384.1	27.800
12480.0	26	...	1	12	230.0	808.690	27	165.9	27.346
12345.9	25	345.9	1	12	95.9	800	27	24.9	27.052
12322.3	25	322.3	1	12	72.3	798.469	27	...	27
12250.0	25	250.0	1	12	...	793.787	26	504.0	26.842
12000.0	25	...	1	11	187.5	777.587	26	141.1	26.294
11960.1	24	440.1	1	11	147.6	775	26	99.1	26.206
11865.9	24	345.9	1	11	53.4	768.896	26	...	26
11812.5	24	292.5	1	11	...	765.437	25	423.8	25.883
11574.3	24	54.3	1	10	199.3	750	25	173.3	25.361
11520.0	24	...	1	10	145.0	746.484	25	116.2	25.242
11409.5	23	369.5	1	10	34.5	739.323	25	...	25
11375.0	23	335.0	1	10	...	737.088	24	443.7	24.924
11188.5	23	148.5	1	9	251.0	725	24	247.5	24.516
11040.0	23	...	1	9	102.5	715.380	24	91.4	24.190
10953.1	22	393.1	1	9	15.6	709.750	24	...	24
10937.5	22	377.5	1	9	...	708.738	23	463.6	23.966
10802.6	22	242.6	1	8	302.6	700	23	321.7	23.670
10560.0	22	...	1	8	60.0	684.277	23	66.5	23.139
10500.0	21	420.0	1	8	...	680.389	23	3.4	23.007
10496.7	21	416.7	1	7	434.2	680.177	23	...	23
10416.8	21	336.8	1	7	354.3	675	22	396.0	22.825
10080.0	21	...	1	7	17.5	653.173	22	41.7	22.087
10062.5	20	462.5	1	7	...	652.039	22	23.3	22.049
10040.4	20	440.4	1	6	415.4	650.604	22	...	22
10031.0	20	431.0	1	6	406.0	650	21	470.2	21.980
9645.2	20	45.2	1	6	20.2	625	21	64.4	21.134
9625.0	20	25.0	1	6	...	623.690	21	43.2	21.090
9600.0	20	...	1	5	412.5	622.070	21	16.8	21.035
9584.0	19	464.0	1	5	396.5	621.031	21	...	21
9259.4	19	139.4	1	5	71.9	600	20	138.6	20.289
9187.5	19	67.5	1	5	...	595.340	20	63.0	20.131
9127.6	19	7.6	1	4	377.6	591.458	20	...	20
9120.0	19	...	1	4	370.0	590.966	19	472.0	19.983
8873.6	18	233.6	1	4	123.6	575	19	212.9	19.444
8750.0	18	110.0	1	4	...	566.991	19	82.8	19.173
8671.2	18	31.2	1	3	358.7	561.885	19	...	19
8640.0	18	...	1	3	327.5	559.863	18	447.2	18.932
8487.8	17	327.8	1	3	175.3	550	18	287.1	18.598
8312.5	17	152.5	1	3	...	538.641	18	102.7	18.214
8214.8	17	54.8	1	2	339.8	532.312	18	...	18
8160.0	17	...	1	2	285.0	528.759	17	422.3	17.880
8102.0	16	422.0	1	2	227.0	525	17	361.3	17.753
7875.0	16	195.0	1	2	...	510.291	17	122.5	17.255
7758.5	16	78.5	1	1	321.0	502.739	17	...	17
7716.2	16	36.2	1	1	278.7	500	16	435.6	16.907
7680.0	16	...	1	1	242.5	497.656	16	397.5	16.828
7437.5	15	237.5	1	1	...	481.942	16	142.4	16.297
7330.4	15	130.4	1	..	330.4	475	16	29.8	16.062
7302.1	15	102.1	1	..	302.1	473.167	16	...	16
7200.0	15	...	1	..	200.0	466.552	15	372.6	15.776

grains	Apothecary oz	Apothecary gr	Avoir. lb	Avoir. oz	Avoir. gr	Metric Weight and Measure, Gm or ml[a]	Fluid oz	Fluid min	fl oz and Fract
7000.0	14	280.0	1	..	...	453.592	15	162.3	15.338
6944.6	14	224.6	..	15	382.1	450	15	104.0	15.217
6845.7	14	125.7	..	15	283.2	443.594	15	...	15
6720.0	14	...	..	15	157.5	435.449	14	347.8	14.725
6562.5	13	322.5	..	15	...	425.243	14	182.2	14.379
6558.8	13	318.8	..	14	433.8	425	14	178.2	14.371
6389.3	13	149.3	..	14	264.3	414.021	14	...	14
6240.0	13	...	..	14	115.0	404.345	13	322.9	13.673
6172.9	12	412.9	..	14	47.9	400	13	252.4	13.526
6125.0	12	365.0	..	14	...	396.893	13	202.0	13.421
5932.9	12	172.9	..	13	245.4	384.448	13	...	13
5787.1	12	27.1	..	13	99.6	375	12	326.6	12.681
5760.0	12	...	..	13	72.5	373.242	12	298.1	12.621
5687.5	11	407.5	..	13	...	368.544	12	221.9	12.462
5476.6	11	196.6	..	12	226.6	354.875	12	...	12
5401.3	11	121.3	..	12	151.3	350	11	400.8	11.835
5280.0	11	...	..	12	30.0	342.138	11	273.3	11.569
5250.0	10	450.0	..	12	...	340.194	11	241.7	11.504
5020.2	10	220.2	..	11	207.7	325.302	11	...	11
5015.0	10	215.5	..	11	203.0	325	10	475.1	10.990
4812.5	10	12.5	..	11	...	311.845	10	261.6	10.545
4800.0	10	...	..	10	425.0	311.035	10	248.4	10.518
4629.7	9	309.7	..	10	254.7	300	10	69.3	10.144
4563.8	9	243.8	..	10	188.8	295.729	10	...	10
4375.0	9	55.0	..	10	...	283.495	9	281.4	9.586
4320.0	9	...	..	9	382.5	279.931	9	223.6	9.466
4244.0	8	403.9	..	9	306.4	275	9	143.5	9.299
4107.4	8	267.4	..	9	169.9	266.156	9	...	9
3937.5	8	97.5	..	9	...	255.146	8	301.3	8.628
3858.1	8	18.1	..	8	358.1	250	8	217.8	8.454
3840.0	8	...	..	8	340.0	248.828	8	198.7	8.414
3651.0	7	291.0	..	8	151.0	236.583	8	...	8
3500.0	7	140.0	..	8	...	226.796	7	321.1	7.669
3472.3	7	112.3	..	7	409.8	225	7	292.0	7.608
3360.0	7	...	..	7	297.5	217.724	7	173.9	7.362
3194.7	6	314.7	..	7	132.2	207.010	7	...	7
3086.5	6	206.5	..	7	24.0	200	6	366.2	6.763
3062.5	6	182.5	..	7	...	198.557	6	341.0	6.710
2880.0	6	...	..	6	255.0	186.621	6	149.0	6.311
2738.3	5	338.3	..	6	113.3	177.437	6	...	6
2700.7	5	300.7	..	6	75.7	175	5	440.4	5.918
2625.0	5	225.0	..	6	...	170.097	5	360.9	5.752
2400.0	5	...	..	5	212.5	155.517	5	124.1	5.259
2314.9	4	394.9	..	5	127.4	150	5	34.7	5.072
2281.9	4	361.9	..	5	94.4	147.865	5	...	5
2187.5	4	267.5	..	5	...	141.748	4	380.7	4.793
1929.0	4	9.0	..	4	179.0	125	4	108.9	4.227
1920.0	4	...	..	4	170.0	124.414	4	99.4	4.207
1825.5	3	385.5	..	4	75.5	118.292	4	...	4
1750.0	3	310.0	..	4	...	113.398	3	400.6	3.835
1543.2	3	103.2	..	3	230.7	100	3	183.1	3.381
1440.0	3	...	..	3	127.5	93.310	3	74.5	3.155
1388.9	2	428.9	..	3	76.4	90	3	20.8	3.043
1369.1	2	409.1	..	3	56.6	88.719	3	...	3
1312.5	2	352.5	..	3	...	85.049	2	420.4	2.876
1234.6	2	274.6	..	2	359.6	80	2	338.5	2.705
1157.4	2	197.5	..	2	282.4	75	2	257.3	2.536
1080.3	2	120.3	..	2	205.3	70	2	176.2	2.367
960.0	2	...	..	2	85.0	62.207	2	49.7	2.104
925.9	1	445.9	..	2	50.9	60	2	13.9	2.029
912.8	1	432.8	..	2	37.8	59.146	2	...	2
875.0	1	395.0	..	2	...	56.699	1	440.3	1.917
771.6	1	291.6	..	1	334.1	50	1	331.5	1.691
617.3	1	137.3	..	1	179.8	40	1	169.2	1.353
480.0	1	...	..	1	42.5	31.1035	1	24.9	1.052
463.0	..	...	..	1	25.5	30	1	6.9	1.014
456.380	..	...	..	1	18.88	29.5729	1	...	1
437.5	..	...	..	1	...	28.350	..	460.15	0.959
385.8	..	...	..	..	255.0	25	..	405.78	0.845
308.6	..	...	..	..	...	20	..	324.62	0.676
154.3	..	...	..	..	...	10	..	162.31	0.338
15.4324	..	...	..	..	...	1	..	16.23	0.0338
1	..	...	..	..	...	0.06480	..	1.0517	0.0022
0.9508	..	...	..	..	...	0.06161	..	1	0.0021

[a] *Note*—The abbreviation "ml" for milliliter may be used interchangeably with "cc" for cubic centimeter since they are practically identical. The values given for the relation of weight to measure and *vice versa*, are for water at the temperature of 4°C (39.2°F) *in vacuo*. See page 79.

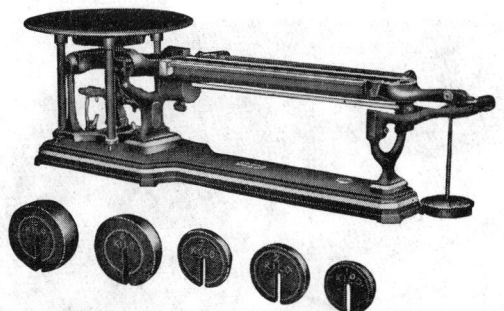
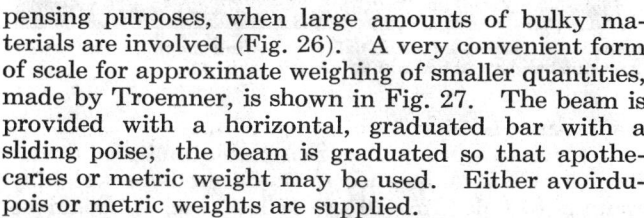

Fig. 25. **Manufacturing laboratory scale and weights** (courtesy, Troemner).

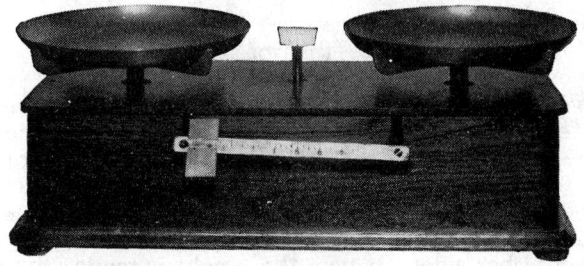

Fig. 26. **Box-type counter scale with graduated beam** (courtesy, Troemner).

pensing purposes, when large amounts of bulky materials are involved (Fig. 26). A very convenient form of scale for approximate weighing of smaller quantities, made by Troemner, is shown in Fig. 27. The beam is provided with a horizontal, graduated bar with a sliding poise; the beam is graduated so that apothecaries or metric weight may be used. Either avoirdupois or metric weights are supplied.

Torsion Balances—A simple illustration of the principle of torsion is afforded by tying a stout piece of cord to a firm support and inserting a lead pencil in the middle of the cord between the strands, at right angles to it. If the free end of the cord is tightly stretched,

and the effort is made to turn the lead pencil over, it will at once be noticed that resistance is offered, and if the pencil is released, it at once flies back to its original position.

Torsion is the term applied to this method of twisting. The principle of supporting the beam of a balance on a tightly stretched wire, with the view of doing away with knife edges and diminishing friction, occupied the attention of inventors for years. In 1882 Prof. Roeder and Dr. Springer contrived an ingenious torsion balance which gave promise of valuable results. Two illustrations of this original balance were shown on page 54 of the first edition of *Remington's Practice of Pharmacy* in 1885. Improvements have greatly in-

Table XV—Continued

From 480 grains down						From 30 grains down			From 5 grains down	
Grains	Metric Weight and Measure, Gm or ml^a	Minims (of Water at 4°C)	Grains	Metric Weight and Measure, Gm or ml^a	Minims (of Water at 4°C)	Grains	Metric Weight and Measure, Gm or ml^a	Minims (of Water at 4°C)	Milligrams (mg)	Grains
480 (1 ʒ)	31.103	504.8	**240 (4 ʒ)**	15.552	252.4	**30 (½ ʒ)**	1.944	31.55	324	5
478.4	**31**	503.2	231.5	**15**	243.5	28.52	1.848	**30**	292	4½
475.4	30.805	**500**	228.2	14.786	**240.0**	23.77	1.540	**25**	259	4
463.0	**30**	486.9	**218.75**	14.175	230.1	20	1.296	21.04	227	3½
			(½ oz av)			19.02	1.232	**20**	194	3
456.4	29.573	**480** (1 fʒ)	216.1	**14**	227.2	15.4324	**1**	16.23	162	2½
									130	2
450	29.160	473.3	**210**	13.608	220.9	15	0.972	15.78	97	1½
447.5	**29**	470.7	200.6	**13**	211.0	14.26	0.924	**15**	65	1
437.5	28.350	460.2	199.7	12.938	**210.0**	14	0.907	14.72		
(1 oz av)						13.31	0.863	**14**	60.7	15/16
432.1	**28**	454.5	185.2	**12**	194.8	13	0.842	13.67	58.3	9/10
427.9	27.725	**450**				12.36	0.801	**13**	56.7	7/8
420 (7 ʒ)	27.216	441.7	**180 (3 ʒ)**	11.664	189.3	12	0.778	12.63	52.6	13/16
416.7	**27**	438.2	171.1	11.090	**180.0**	11.41	0.739	**12**	51.8	4/5
401.2	**26**	422.0	169.8	**11**	178.5	11	0.713	11.57	48.6	3/4
399.3	25.876	**420**	154.3	**10**	162.3	10.46	0.678	**11**	44.5	11/16
390	25.272	410.2	**150**	9.720	157.8				40.5	5/8
385.8	**25**	405.8	142.6	9.242	**150.0**	**10**	0.648	10.52	36.4	9/16
380.3	24.644	**400**	138.9	**9**	146.1	9.51	0.616	**10**	32.4	1/2
370.8	24.028	**390**	123.5	**8**	129.8	**9**	0.583	9.46		
370.4	**24**	389.5				8.56	0.554	**9**	28.3	7/16
360 (6 ʒ)	23.328	378.6	**120 (2 ʒ)**	7.776	126.2	**8**	0.518	8.41	25.9	2/5
354.9	**23**	373.3	114.1	7.393	**120.0**	7.72	**0.5**	8.12	24.3	3/8
342.3	22.180	**360**	**109.375**	7.087	115.0	7.61	0.493	**8**	20.2	5/16
			(½ oz av)			**7**	0.454	7.37	16.2	1/4
339.5	**22**	357.1	108.0	**7**	113.6	6.66	0.431	**7**	12.1	3/16
330	21.384	347.1	**100**	6.480	105.2	6	0.389	6.31	8.1	1/8
324.1	**21**	340.9	95.1	6.161	**100.0**	5.70	0.370	**6**	4.0	1/16
313.8	20.331	**330**	92.6	**6**	97.4				3.2	1/20
308.6	**20**	324.6	**80**	5.184	84.1	**5**	0.324	5.26	2.6	1/25
			77.2	**5**	81.2	4.75	0.308	**5**	2.2	1/30
			76.1	4.929	**80.0**	4	0.259	4.20	1.8	1/36
			61.7	**4**	64.9	3.80	0.246	**4**	1.6	1/40
300 (5 ʒ)	19.440	315.5	**60 (1 ʒ)**	3.888	63.1	**3**	0.194	3.15	1.3	1/50
293.2	**19**	308.4	57.0	3.697	**60.0**	2.85	0.185	**3**	1.1	1/60
285.2	18.483	**300**	**54.6875**	3.544	57.5	**2**	0.130	2.11	1.0	1/64
			(½ oz av)			1.90	0.123	**2**	0.6	1/100
277.8	**18**	292.2	**50**	3.240	52.6	**1**	0.06480	1.0518	0.5	1/128
270	17.496	284.0	47.5	3.081	**50.0**	0.9508	0.06161	**1**	0.4	1/160
262.4	**17**	275.9	46.3	**3**	48.7				0.3	1/210
256.7	16.635	**270**	42.8	2.772	**45.0**				0.2	1/320
246.9	**16**	259.7	**40**	2.592	42.1				0.1	1/640
			38.0	2.464	**40.0**					
			33.3	2.156	**35.0**					
			30.9	**2**	32.5					

^a *Note*—The abbreviation "ml" for milliliter may be used interchangeably with "cc" for cubic centimeter since they are practically identical.

creased its efficiency; the most important difficulty in applying the principle—that of torsional resistance—was overcome by the device of placing a weight just above the center of gravity, torsional resistance having the tendency to keep the beam in a horizontal position, while the elevation of a weight above the center of gravity, by its tendency to produce unstable equilibrium (page 84), exercises an opposite effect—that of inclining the beam to be top-heavy, and therefore to tip on either side. If now the weight is made adjustable, by mounting it upon a perpendicular screw, so that it can be raised or lowered, it is possible to arrange these opposite forces so that one exactly neutralizes the other. In this manner sensitivity is obtained. The torsion principle has been applied to analytical balances and scales designed to carry heavier loads, as well as to prescription balances.

In the torsion prescription balance (Fig. 28) two beams are used, supported on three frames, each of the latter having a flattened metallic band stretched tightly over its edge. Fig. 28 illustrates the skeleton of a Torsion balance with metallic bands stretched tightly around the three trusses or frames. In the prescription balance this mechanism is enclosed as shown in Fig. 30.

The Torsion balance which has a rider beam graduated upon the upper edge from ⅛ to 15 gr and on its lower edge from 0.01 to 1.0 Gm, furnishes a very convenient means of weighing small quantities without having to use small weights. The latest model includes a "damper" to quickly halt the oscillations and a direct-reading dial instead of a rider beam. The Troemner balance also is conveniently constructed. The latest model differs, however, in one respect. The metric scale is now located on the upper edge of the rider beam and the apothecary scale on the lower edge.

The prescription balances may be placed upon a base containing a drawer which can be used for holding weights, powder papers, etc.

Prescription Balances

There are two common types of prescription balances. One type uses the compound lever principle with steel on agate bearings (Fig. 29—Troemner/400 prescription balance). The other type uses the taught wire frame or torsion principle (Fig. 30—Torsion prescription balance). These balances are manufactured to meet the requirements of the National Bureau of Standards Class A and Class B prescription balances. A Class A prescription balance has a maximum maintenance sensitivity of about 6 mg with no load and with a load of 10 Gm on each pan, ie, addition of the 6-mg weight to one pan causes the indicator or the rest point to be shifted not less than one division on the index plate. A Class B balance has a maximum

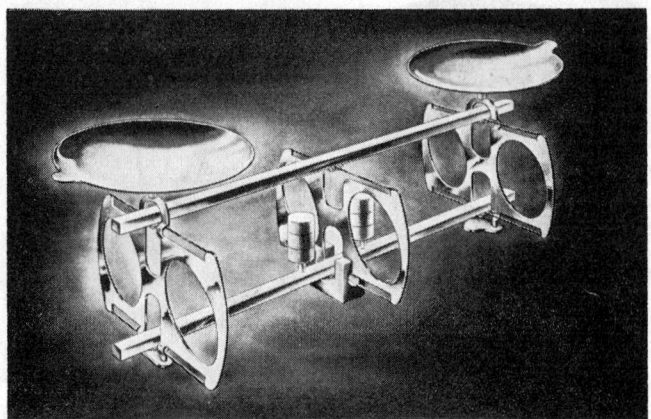

Fig. 28. Skeleton of a Torsion balance showing the three trusses with a metallic band stretched tightly around each.

maintenance sensitivity of about 30 mg.

In order to work within reasonable limits of deviation, the Class A balance must be used for weighing amounts of 0.65 Gm (10 gr) or less, and it should be used for amounts up to 15 to 120 Gm (½ to 4 oz), depending on the stated capacity, and subject to the physical limit of the amount of the material that can be placed upon one pan.

The Class B balance may be used for weighing larger amounts but not for weighing less than 0.65 Gm. The tolerances for the Class B balance are still stringent enough so that weighings of larger amounts on this instrument can be sufficiently accurate. The purpose of having the two types of balances is to make it possible to weigh larger amounts of drugs on a less delicate balance and thus save wear on the more sensitive one; however, the Class A balances now manufactured usually weigh up to 120 Gm without any risk of damage, so that Class B balances are becoming less important. Every prescription department must have a Class A balance. The Class B balance is optional. A Class B balance should be conspicuously marked with the words, "Class B—not to be used in weighing loads of less than 0.65 Gm (10 gr)." Type this on a label and stick it on the front of the balance to remind any operator of the practical limitation of the balance.

Requirements of Prescription Balances—A prescription balance, whether Class A or B, should meet the following general requirements:

1. It should be constructed so as to support its full capacity without developing undue stresses, and should not be thrown out of adjustment by repeated weighings of the capacity load. (The capacity of the balance will be seen on the metal plate attached to the balance.) If the capacity of the balance is not stated, it is assumed

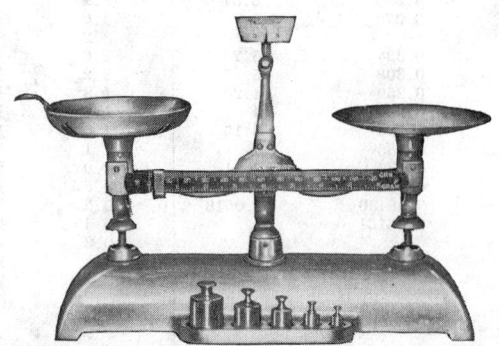

Fig. 27. Scale with graduated parallel beam and sliding poise (courtesy, Troemner).

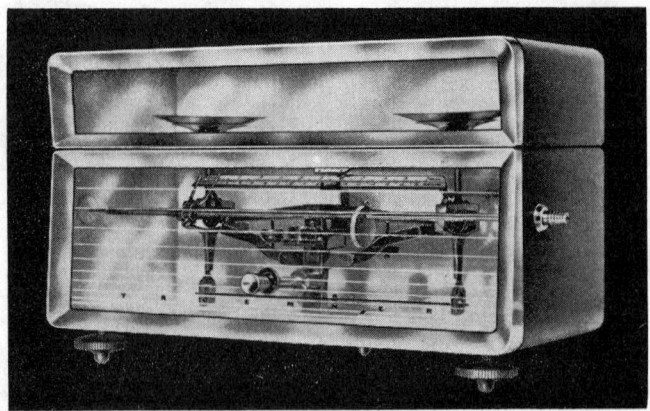

Fig. 29. Troemner/400 prescription balance (courtesy, Troemner).

to be at least 15 Gm (½ oz). The new Class A balances usually have a capacity of 120 Gm (4 oz).

2. The removable pans of a prescription balance should be of equal weight. If the pans show any difference in weight, they should be adjusted. Pans with any appreciable corrosion or wear should be refinished or replaced.

3. A prescription balance should have a leveling device, usually leveling feet or screws, so that the balance can be adjusted to a level position. A balance that does not have these is not entitled to be designated as a prescription balance.

4. The balance that has a rider or poise should have, at the end of the scale, a stop which halts the rider at the "zero" reading. The reading edge of the rider should be parallel to the graduations on the beam.

5. The indicator points, when there are two on the balance, should be sharp, and their ends should not be separated by more than 1 mm (0.04 in.) when the scale is in balance. The distance from the face of the index plate to the indicator pointer or pointers should be small (1 mm or less) to protect the operator against making errors resulting from parallax since it is unlikely that the eye of the operator will be exactly in line with the indicator and the division on the index plate. The indicating elements as well as the lever system of the balance should be protected against drafts. The balance should have a lid which allows a weighing to be made when the lid is closed.

6. A prescription balance must have a mechanical means for arresting the oscillation of the mechanism.

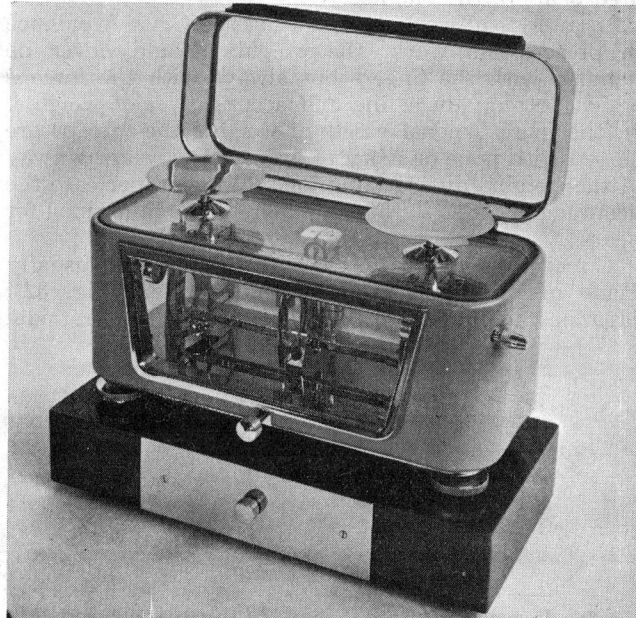

Fig. 30.   Torsion RX-1 prescription balance (courtesy, Torsion).

Testing Balances—Having stated the essential points in the construction of the balance, some of the tests which are always applied by manufacturers before approving a balance will now be described. These tests may be applied by any intelligent and careful person to satisfy himself with regard to the construction and character of a balance, the origin, history, or condition of which is in doubt. The prescription balance, being one of the most delicate and important of the instruments in use by the pharmacist, is selected for illustration.

The following is a simplified statement of the most important tests. Additional tests are carried out by the National Bureau of Standards, by manufacturers, and by local and state testing agencies.

A Class A prescription balance meets the following four basic tests. Use a set of *test weights* and keep the rider on the weighbeam at zero unless directed to change its position.

1. *Sensitivity Requirement*—Level the balance, determine the rest point, place a 6-mg weight on one of the empty pans and again

determine the rest point. Repeat the operation with a 10-Gm weight in the center of each pan. The rest point is shifted not less than one division of the index plate each time the 6-mg weight is added.

2. *Arm Ratio Test*—This test is designed to check the equality of length of both arms of the balance. Determine the rest point of the balance with no weight on the pans. Place in the center of each pan 30 Gm of test weights and determine the rest point. If the second rest point is not the same as the first, place a 20-mg weight on the lighter side; the rest point should move back to the original place on the index plate scale or farther.

3. *Shift Tests*—These tests are designed to check the arm and lever components of the balance.

a. Determine the rest point of the indicator without any weights on the pans.

b. Place one of the 10-Gm weights in the center of the left pan, and place the other 10-Gm weight successively toward the right, left, front, and back side of the right pan, noting the rest point in each case. If in any case the rest point differs from the rest point determined in (a), add the 10-mg weight to the lighter side; this should cause the rest point to shift back to the rest point determined in (a) or farther.

c. Place a 10-Gm weight in the center of the right pan, and place a 10-Gm weight successively toward the right, left, front, and back side of the left pan, noting the rest point in each case. If in any case the rest point is different from that obtained with no weights on the pans, this difference should be overcome by addition of the 10-mg weight to the lighter side.

d. Make a series of observations in which both weights are simultaneously shifted to off-center positions on their pans, both toward the outside, both toward the inside, one toward the outside and the other toward the inside, both toward the back, and so on until all combinations have been checked. If in any case the rest point differs from that obtained with no weights on the pan the addition of the 10-mg weight to the lighter side should overcome this difference.

A balance which does not measure up to these tests *must* be corrected.

4. *Rider and Graduated Beam Tests*—Determine the rest point for the balance with no weight on the pans. Now place on the left pan the 500-mg test weight and move the rider to the 500-mg point on the beam. Now determine the rest point. If it is different from the zero rest point, add a 6-mg weight to the lighter side. This should bring the rest point back to its original position or farther. Repeat this test, using the 1-Gm test weight and moving the rider to the 1-Gm division on the beam. If the rest point is different it should be brought back at least to the zero rest point position by addition of 6 mg to the lighter pan. If the balance does not meet this test, the weighbeam graduations or the rider *must* be corrected.

Protecting Balances—The necessity for protecting the delicate mechanism of a balance is frequently overlooked, notwithstanding the possibility of having a fine apparatus irretrievably ruined by lack of care in using or cleaning it or in protecting it while at rest. The position chosen for the balance or scales should be on a level and firm counter, desk, or table, where it will be subjected to little risk of injury from dampness, dust, or corrosive vapors, and where the knife edges will not be liable to become dulled by jarring or other vibrations.

In the finer class of balances, protection is afforded by enclosing them in glass cases having sash doors in the front and sometimes in the back. They are protected against injury from vibration by a lever for elevating or locking the beam, so that the knife edges are not in contact with any surface whatever. To prevent injury from jarring while the balance is in use, by a weight falling on the pan, or other accident, the finest balances are provided with pan supports, which break the fall and serve the additional purpose of quickly arresting the beam, thus saving time while weighing.

In using a fine prescription balance neither the weights nor the substance that is to be weighed should be placed on the scale pans while the beam is free to oscillate. The desired weight should be placed upon one scale pan (usually the one on the right-hand side) and an amount of the substance to be weighed, approximately the desired weight, placed upon the opposite pan. The beam should be released by means of the lever and if the substance is in excess, the beam should be locked and a small portion removed and the beam again released and the oscillations observed. This procedure should be repeated until the correct amount is obtained. In case of a deficiency of the substance to be weighed the reverse procedure is followed until the correct amount is obtained. With practice this can be done very deftly and very quickly and the sensitiveness of the balance retained for years.

Such balances are often protected against injury from corrosive vapors by having some quicklime (unslaked lime) and some sulfuric acid in separate, open but properly protected, containers within the balance case. This protects from acid and alkaline vapors and also produces dehydration of the air in the case to a certain extent. The quicklime and acid must be frequently renewed to be effective.

Substances which act on metals, such as iodine, corrosive sublimate, etc, and those which are adhesive, such as the extracts, should not be weighed directly upon the scale pans, but upon counterpoised watch crystals, or, if these are not at hand, upon highly glazed paper, care being taken to balance the papers before weighing the substance. In cleaning the scales great care should be exercised; polishing powders should be used sparingly; a portion is very apt to find its way into crevices and elude detection until an attempt is made to adjust the scales, when the increased weight of one of the sides of the beam leads to its discovery. Frequent cleaning with soft leather is generally sufficient to keep a balance in good order; but if through neglect it becomes necessary to use more active measures, some simple polishing powder for the metal work, with soapsuds for nickel plate, and simple brushing for the lacquered brass, is all that is necessary.

As the pans are subjected to more wear and tear than any other part of the balance, it is economical to use *solid* rather than *plated* pans because constant friction wears off the plating and the additional cost for replating soon absorbs the difference in price. Equipped in this way, and with agate bearings, a prescription balance is durable and really cheap because it will remain for a long time fully equal to the most exacting demands. The most expensive, most sensitive, and most accurate type of single-beam, equal-arm balance is the *analytical balance*. This is fully discussed and the balances illustrated in Chapter 37, *Analysis of Medicinals*.

Weights Used in Pharmacy

The weights used by the pharmacist are a very important part of his equipment, and care in their selection and examination is necessary. False economy is particularly to be avoided, as the use of cheap, inaccurate weights must lead ultimately to serious consequences. Prescription weights, so worn that the characters on their faces had disappeared, have been found in use in pharmacies by official inspectors, and, on the contrary, weights have been found with bits of hardened extract and dirt almost entirely obscuring their characters. An unused set of standard weights should be kept on hand, so that at least once a year the weights in daily use can be tested and adjusted or rejected if necessary. The standard weights should be used also when the balance is tested. The set should contain the following weights in a well-fitted box with forceps: two 20-Gm or two 30-Gm, two 10-Gm, one 1-Gm, one 500-mg, one 20-mg, one 10-mg, and one 6-mg weights; all adjusted to NBS tolerances for analytical or Class P weights.

Metric Weights—These may be procured of iron (japanned) for weighing larger quantities. They are preferably hexagonal (Fig. 31) in shape, to distinguish them from the ordinary round avoirdupois weights (Fig. 32). Brass weights are undoubtedly the most convenient type for the pharmacist. They are also supplied in the form of block weights, plainly marked to distinguish them from the avoirdupois weights of similar style. These usually range from 10–1000 Gm.

For prescription purposes, accurate sets ranging from 50 Gm to 10 mg are available. Two inexpensive sets for the use of students are illustrated in Fig. 34 (lower). Other sets are covered as in Fig. 33 and contain forceps.

For analytical purposes, metric weights are almost exclusively used; usually the highest weight is 100 Gm, the lowest 0.001 Gm or 1 mg. The weights, from 1 Gm upward, are of brass, finely lacquered, or of nonmagnetic stainless steel or rhodium-plated bronze. The smaller weights are made of squares of platinum foil, with one corner turned up, to permit them to be easily handled with the forceps. Fractions of a milligram are weighed by means of the rider on the graduated beam of the balance.

In analytical work and in using the Class A balance in prescription work, the weights should never be handled with the fingers but always with the forceps which accompany a fine and accurate set of weights. In the more expensive sets of weights the forceps are tipped with bone or ivory to prevent the wearing away of the weights during handling. With proper care the accuracy of a fine set of weights may be maintained for years.

Common Avoirdupois Weights—These are usually made of iron, and are flat and circular (Fig. 32), japanned to prevent rusting; these form a pyramidal

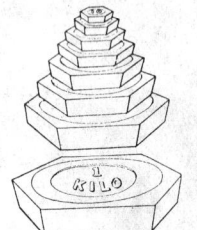

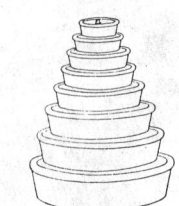

Fig. 31.   Iron metric weights.   **Fig. 32.   Avoirdupois weights.**

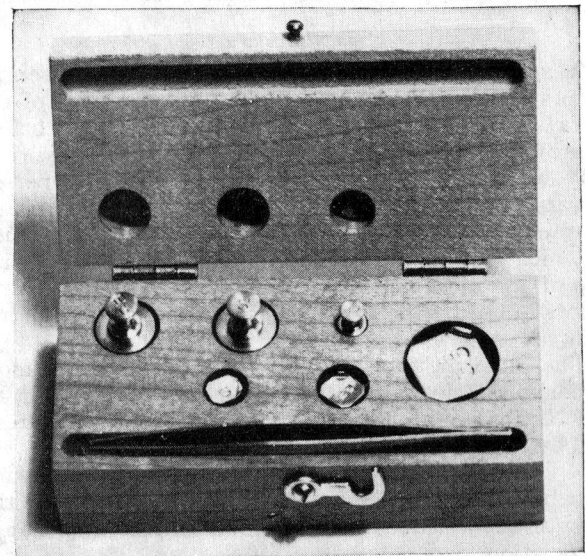

Fig. 33.   Metric standard weights for periodically testing weights in constant use.

pile, and range from ½ oz to 4 lb; they may be adjusted if found to be incorrect by adding to or diminishing the amount of lead which is hammered into a depression in the base of each. These weights are sometimes made of brass in this form, and sometimes of zinc; the latter, however, are brittle and unserviceable. When used for general retail sales, the cylindrical weights, known technically as "block weights," are preferable (Fig. 34). If the block is made of two kinds of wood glued together, to avoid shrinkage, they are very desirable, particularly if each cylindrical hole in the block has been made large enough to hold each weight easily. The advantages of block weights are that the gaps left by missing weights are readily noticed and that the greater surface of the weight is protected from the action of corrosive vapors when not in use.

Apothecary Weights—These may be had either as "block weights" (Fig. 34) or the less desirable flat forms. The round, flat, brass "dram" weights, which have the denomination stamped distinctly on their faces in raised characters, are still used (Fig. 35). These range from 10 to 120 gr in weight. Brass weights of similar shape arranged according to units of the decimal system are also available and are frequently used. The old-fashioned square brass "drachm" weights have passed out of use. The brass foil grain weights are very unsatisfactory and should not be employed because of their liability to corrosion. Undoubtedly the best grain weights are the aluminum wire weights. These are more easily and quickly distinguished from one another than any other form, and there is less likelihood of dangerous mistakes than from the flat weights, where the denomination is stamped on the face, often faintly, and is liable to be obliterated by constant use or by corrosive contact. The number of sides in the wire weights at once gives the denomination (Fig. 36). The aluminum grain weights, cut out of aluminum

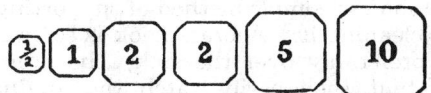

Fig. 37.   Aluminum grain weights.

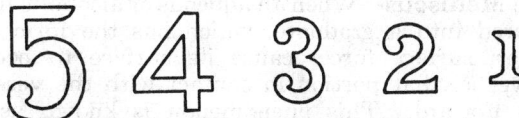

Fig. 38.   Aluminum grain weights.

plates, are preferred to the flat, brass grain weights because they are less liable to corrosive action. They are usually more accurately adjusted; the corners of the weights are clipped, and each weight is usually pressed into a curved form so that it may be picked up easily (Fig. 37).

In still another form of aluminum grain weights the outlines of the arabic numerals themselves are stamped from sheet aluminum (Fig. 38).

Prescription Weights—Too much care cannot be exercised in the selection of weights to be used in compounding prescriptions. The cost of accurate weights is trifling, yet weights have been found by inspectors in this line of investigation which are disgracefully inaccurate. Prescription writing is now taught to medical students in the metric system, and this will lead, in time, to the increased use of metric weights in compounding prescriptions. This is desirable because these weights are made to retain their accuracy and there is less likelihood of error when this system is used.

Measuring

In pharmacy, measuring usually refers to the ascertaining of a definite volume of liquid. Many types of apparatus are used in this operation, depending on the kind and quantity of liquid to be measured and the degree of accuracy required.

Measuring Large Quantities

Glass measures are preferred for measuring liquids, for, although always subject to loss from breakage, they can be adjusted more accurately to indicate the volume. On account of the transparency of glass, the level of the liquid at any height may be seen through the measure, while it is possible to measure accurately with opaque vessels only when they are completely filled.

Glass measuring vessels, larger than 1 liter or 1 quart, are usually in the form of a jar (Fig. 39).

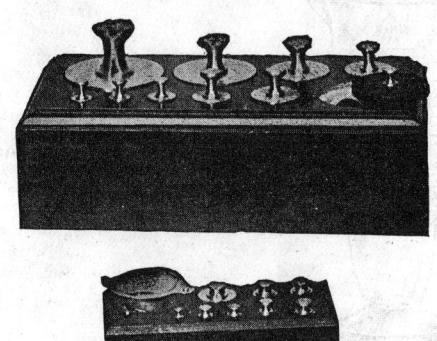

Fig. 34.   Brass weights in wood blocks.

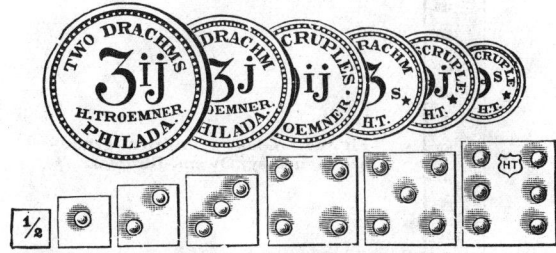

Fig. 35.   Apothecary weights.

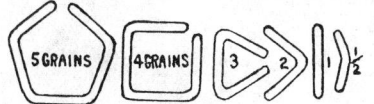

Fig. 36.   Aluminum wire weights.

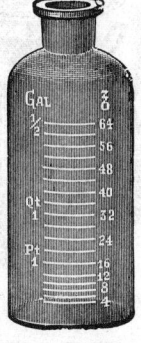

Fig. 39.   Large glass measuring vessel.

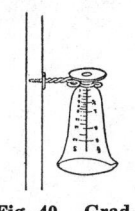

Fig. 40.   Graduate support.

Fig. 40 shows a simple method of supporting a graduate after cleaning it. A brass hook is screwed into an upright, preferably over the sink; the prongs are so adjusted that they easily catch the graduate base. These are usually sold in units containing several metal holders.

The Meniscus—When an aqueous or alcoholic liquid is poured into a graduate, which has the form of a cylinder, surface forces cause its surface to become concave, ie, that portion in contact with the vessel is drawn upward. This phenomenon is known as the formation of a *meniscus* (Fig. 45), and in determining the volume of a liquid *the reading must be made at the bottom of this meniscus*. This regulation has been established by the NBS and all glass measuring vessels are graduated on this basis. Liquids with large contact angles, eg, mercury, form an inverted meniscus, and the reading is then made at the top of the curved surface (see page 308).

In the past most liquid preparations used in the pharmacy were stored in a stock bottle, usually equipped with a glass stopper. When liquids were transferred into a graduate from such a stock bottle, the graduate was taken in the left hand, grasping it securely at its base. The stock bottle was taken in the right hand and the stopper was removed with the free fingers of the left hand. The liquid was poured into the graduate, the stopper replaced, and the stock bottle returned to the counter or shelf.

Today pharmaceutical manufacturers package their liquid preparations in glass or plastic containers (usually pint bottles) equipped with a plastic screw cap. These containers serve as a stock bottle from which liquids may be poured directly into a graduate, thus avoiding a transfer of the liquid from the original container to a stock bottle.

The procedure for pouring liquid from the modern, screw-capped containers follows that which was used with the stock bottle with the exception that the cap is usually removed and placed on the counter while the transfer of liquid is made. While holding the graduate in the left hand, the original container is grasped with the right hand with the label in such a position that, after pouring, any excess of liquid will not soil the label if it should run down the side of the bottle.

The graduate is raised and held so that the graduation point to be read is on a level with the eye, and the liquid is measured. The extension of the graduating mark into a circle which passes entirely around the graduate is an improvement which obviates the necessity of placing the graduate upon a level place, as the corresponding mark upon the opposite side may be seen through the glass and the graduate easily leveled even when held in the hand.

The cap is replaced and the bottle may be returned to the counter or shelf. Finally the liquid is poured into the bottle or mortar, for dispensing or compounding. Notice that the graduations are etched on the glass measure in such a position that the entire operation, including measuring and pouring from the graduate, may be conducted without taking the graduate from the left hand, only tilting it.

Metallic measures nearly cylindrical in shape, but slightly wider at the bottom, are generally used for measuring liquids when the quantity is over a pint. A set of these measures usually consists of five (gallon, half-gallon, quart, pint, and half-pint). Those made of tinned iron, or of the enameled sheet iron called agate ware, are greatly inferior to those made of *tinned copper* or *stainless steel*. Tinned iron measures soon become rusty and, although a protection is afforded if enameled, particles of the enamel chip off and the exposed iron soon contaminates the liquids measured in them. The first cost of copper or stainless steel measures is greater than tinned iron, but they are far more durable. Care must be taken to protect them from blows which will cause dents as these may be serious enough to detract from the accuracy of the measures. Cylindrical metric measures having a diameter just half their height, of tinned copper or *brass*, in sets of 10 (Dekaliter, half-Dekaliter, double liter, liter, half-liter, double deciliter, deciliter, half-deciliter, double centiliter, and centiliter) are obtainable. The most recent metal vessels of this type are of *monel metal*, *pressed molybdenum*, or *stainless steel*. Such containers are relatively expensive but their indifference to corrosion and wear is

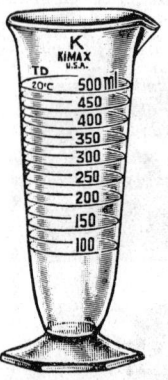

Fig. 43. Glass conical graduate (courtesy, Owens-Illinois).

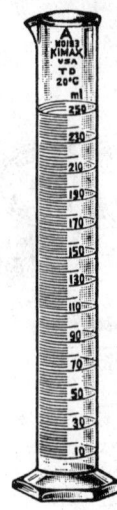

Fig. 44. Glass cylindrical graduate (courtesy, Owens-Illinois).

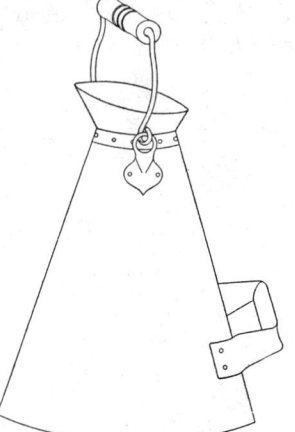

Fig. 41. Special copper measure for alcoholic liquids.

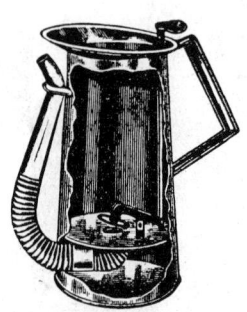

Fig. 42. Measure for oils.

a tremendous advantage. Copper, of course, should not be used, where it is likely to catalyze oxidation.

In Fig. 41 a type of special measure is illustrated. The contracted top prevents spilling and evaporation. Fig. 42 illustrates a form of copper measure much used in measuring oils. The flexible outlet tube permits the delivery of the liquid without danger of spilling.

Graduated Glass Measures—These are nearly always used for quantities of 500 ml or 1 pt or less, and are of 2 forms—*conical* and *cylindrical* (Figs. 43 and 44). The conical graduate is preferred in practical work because of the greater ease with which it can be handled, but cylindrical measures are more accurate because of their uniform and smaller average diameter. In order to explain this point, let us start with a pharmacist who keeps his eyes and, if necessary, his glasses in good condition, and who consistently reads the lower meniscus with a deviation of 1 mm or less from the marks on the graduates (Fig. 45).

While the error in volume caused by a deviation of ±1 mm in reading the meniscus in a graduated cylinder remains constant along the height of the uniform column, the same deviation causes a progressively larger error in a conical graduate because the diameter and, therefore, the volume of the 1-mm column increases along its vertical axis. It is safe to assume that practically all good-grade modern graduates comply with the NBS requirements for internal diameters at stated volumes. The following data are based on actual measurements, using graduates available in 1951.[1]

A deviation of ±1 mm in the meniscus reading will cause an error of approximately 0.5 ml in the measured volume at any mark, on the uniform 100-ml cylinder graduate. At the 10-ml mark on an acceptable blown or pressed glass 125-ml (4-oz) conical graduate, the internal diameter is greater than it is in the 100-ml cylinder; at the 100-ml mark on the conical graduate a deviation of ±1 mm from the mark can cause an error of 1.8 ml. The errors resulting from a ±1-mm deviation at the ascending apothecary markings on the 4-oz conical graduate would be approximately 1.0 ml at 1 oz, 1.7 ml at 2 oz, 1.7 ml at 3 oz, and 1.9 ml at 4 oz.

A more flared type of *pressed glass* or *molded* 100-ml conical graduate presented a larger internal diameter at the 100-ml mark, and a deviation of 1 mm from this mark would result in an error of 2.6 ml.

The above data are based upon the assumption that one can always measure a volume accurately enough to miss the mark by only ±1 mm. This assumption is obviously false. The same individual, exercising the same degree of care, will find it more difficult to adjust a volume of liquid to the 1-mm allowance in some conical graduates than in a uniform cylinder. The curvature at the lower portion and the sloping sides of the conical graduate introduce factors of reflected and refracted light which interfere. The thick pressed-glass graduate reflects lines from the inner surface unless the line is at eye level. The markings of double-scale graduates, with metric and apothecary graduations, set up confusing lines; some laws governing weights and measures forbid their use.

In selecting the graduate for a particular measurement one should use the graduate with a capacity just exceeding the volume of liquid he desires to measure. Data relative to this problem will now be considered. Assume that cylinder graduates are used and that readings average ±1 mm from the volume markings. The measured internal diameter permits the calculation of the volume in 1 mm of the cylinder ($V = \pi r^2 h$). It is desirable for compounding errors to be augmented as little as possible by deviations in measurement. The following example illustrates measuring within 2.5% or within 5% of a given volume. A good 10-ml cylinder with an internal diameter of 1.18 cm would hold 0.109 ml in 1 mm of the column. If this volume represents the 2.5% deviation permitted, the smallest volume that should be measured in the 10-ml cylinder is 4.5 ml. If a deviation of 5% is acceptable, then 2.2 ml should be the smallest volume measured in the 10-ml cylinder.

The important fact revealed here is that either the lower 2.2 ml (22%) or the lower 4.5 ml (45%) of the 10-ml graduate should not be used for measuring. Elimination of the lower markings on graduates was suggested, and in 1955 the NBS specifications for graduates utilized this principle.[2] The NBS Handbook states:

"Effective July 1, 1956 a graduate shall have an initial interval that is not subdivided, equal to not less than one-fifth and not more than one-fourth of the capacity of the graduate."

A composite tabulation (Table XVI) shows the calculated and the assigned blank portions of graduates.

For accurate measurement of volumes less than 1.5 ml a graduated pipet or a graduated dropper could be used (Figs. 46 and 47).

Effect of Liquid and Container—It is most difficult to measure accurately when pouring from a completely filled bottle because of the uneven flow of the liquid. If the graduate being used is clean, the volume can be adjusted by returning any excess to the bottle. After the first portion of the liquid is removed the

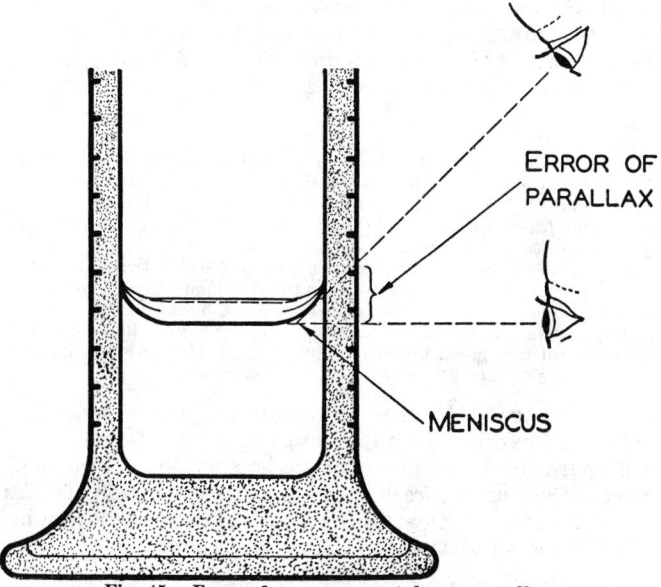

ERROR OF PARALLAX

MENISCUS

Fig. 45.   Error of measurement due to parallax.

Table XVI—Unmarked (Unreliable) Portions of Graduates

| Capacity of graduate, ml | Calculated blanks (1951) | | NBS blanks (1955), ml |
	2.5%[a] allowed, ml	5%[a] allowed, ml	
5	3.0	1.5	1
10	4.4	2.2	2
25	11.8	5.9	5
50	15.8	7.9	10
100	20.9	10.5	20
250	36.3	18.2	50
500	66.5	33.2	100
1000	....	....	200

[a] Calculations by Goldstein and Mattocks[1] based on deviation of ±1 mm from graduation mark and allowable errors of 2.5 and 5%.

shape of the bottle does not influence the ease of pouring to any appreciable extent unless the neck is extremely narrow.

Viscous liquids pour slowly but their accurate measurement is not difficult. Experiments showed that when glycerin is poured into a graduate without letting the liquid run down the inside surface, the precision of measurement can be very high. Naturally, the chance of hitting the inner surface is greater with smaller than with larger graduates. The increase in possible deviation is then caused by the slow movement of the viscous liquid to the desired mark.

Viscous liquids introduce another factor: drainage time. Graduates are calibrated to contain or deliver indicated volumes within specified limits. Aqueous, alcoholic, and hydroalcoholic liquids can be drained from a graduate in ½ min so completely that the delivered and contained volumes are fairly close. When 25 ml of glycerin was measured in the same cleaned and dried cylinders, the received volume measured 23.7 ml after the same time period.

The viscosity factor might be altered when another liquid is to be mixed with the glycerin by measuring and mixing both liquids in a suitable graduate.

Silicone-treated glassware, which is now frequently used, drains completely in a few seconds.

Measuring Small Quantities

For measuring smaller quantities of liquids, graduated glass tubes of much less diameter should be used. The narrower bore permits greater distances between the graduations on the apparatus, and therefore greater accuracy in making the reading is achieved. For example, with a buret (Fig. 48) the pharmaceutical chemist can estimate volumes to the nearest $\frac{1}{100}$ ml.

Pipets (Fig. 46) and similar apparatus are more accurate and convenient than very small graduates, and they are much cleaner to use. The graduations on very small graduates are necessarily in the very small

lowest portion of a comparatively tall measure. Now, if it is desired to measure 1 ml or 10 ♏ of a volatile oil the surface which the oil must traverse when this measure is inverted is so great that probably 20% of the oil will be left adhering to the measure. In those instances of liquid preparations where the smaller liquid is miscible with the larger quantity of diluting liquid, the graduate may be rinsed and this loss recovered, but inconveniences are largely overcome and greater accuracy secured by the use of a pipet.

In administering small quantities of liquids, the very convenient *drop* is almost always used. It should be emphasized that *1 drop is not equivalent to 1 ♏* and that *60 drops are not equivalent to 1 fl dr*. This impression doubtless arose from the fact that 60 ordinary drops of *water* are about equal to 1 fl dr, but the volume of a drop of fluid depends on many factors, including density, temperature, viscosity, surface tension, and the shape and nature of the surface from which it is dropped. Thick viscous liquids, such as the mucilages and the syrups, necessarily produce large drops because the drop adheres to the surface of the glass as long as its weight does not overcome its power of adhesion, while bromine and chloroform—heavy, mobile liquids, having very little adhesion to the dropping surface—produce very small drops, only ⅕ the size of the drop of acacia syrup. The greater the surface tension, the larger will be the drop, and the greater the extent of surface to which the drop adheres, the larger, proportionally, will be the drop.

A "normal" or "standard" drop measure was recommended by the Brussels Conference of 1902 for international adoption. This dropper is recognized in the USP and NF which state:

Medicine Dropper

The pharmacopeial (or National Formulary) medicine dropper is 3 mm in external diameter at its delivery end, and when held vertically delivers 20 drops of water, the total weight of which is between 0.9 Gm and 1.1 Gm (at 25°). In using a medicine dropper, one should keep in mind that few medicinal liquids have the same surface and flow characteristics as water, and therefore the size of drops varies materially from one preparation to another.

When drops are specified on a prescription, the usual custom has been to employ an "eye dropper," but the standard dropper should now be supplied. It is particularly important to use the standard dropper for administering potent medicines when accuracy is required, as in digitalis tincture.

A standard teaspoon has not yet received acceptance. The USP and NF include the following statement describing the current situation:

Teaspoon

Agreement has not been reached on a standard official teaspoon, in spite of the need for such a standard measure in connection with compounding and labeling liquid medicines. For household purposes, an American Standard Teaspoon has been established by the American Standards Association* as containing 4.93 ± 0.24 ml. In view of the almost universal practice of employing teaspoons ordinarily available in the household for the administration of medicine, the teaspoon may be regarded as representing 5 ml.

It must be kept in mind that the actual volume delivered by a teaspoon of any given liquid is related to the latter's viscosity and surface tension, among other influencing factors.

The Human Factor—The human factor of carefulness is of paramount importance in every pharmaceutical operation in which accuracy is essential. The basic necessities for accurate measurement of liquids require (1) accurate technical equipment, (2) careful manipulation, (3) good vision, and (4) a steady hand.

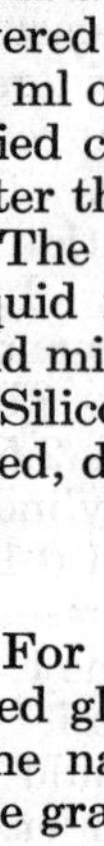

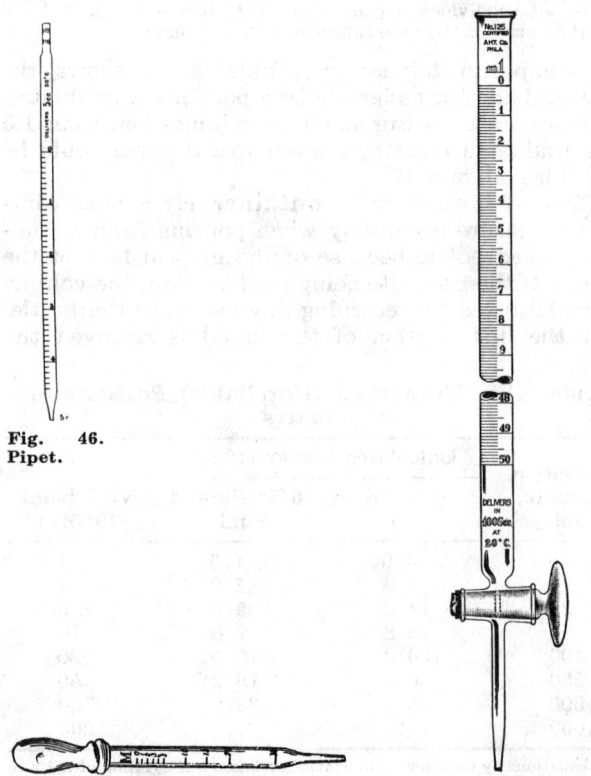

**Fig. 46.
Pipet.**

Fig. 47. Graduated dropper.   **Fig. 48. Glass-valved buret.**

* U.S.A. Standards Institute, 70 E. 45th St., New York, N.Y. 10017.

Density, Specific Gravity, and Specific Volume

Several terms are used to express the mass (weight) of equal volumes of different substances.

Absolute density is the ratio of the mass of an object, determined in or referred to a vacuum, at a specified temperature, to the volume of the object at the same temperature. In metric units this relationship is expressed mathematically as:

$$\frac{\text{mass in grams (in a vacuum)}}{\text{volume in milliliters}} = \text{absolute density}$$

Apparent density differs from absolute density only in that the mass of the object is determined in air, which mass is influenced by the difference in the buoyant effect of air on the object being weighed and on the standard masses (weights) used for comparison (if the object and masses are made of the same material, or have the same density, there will be no difference in the buoyant effect, and the apparent density will be identical with the absolute density).

Relative density is an expression sometimes employed to indicate the mass of 1 ml (not cc, which is very slightly different) of a standard substance, such as water, at a specified temperature, relative to water at 4°C taken as unity. Thus, at 4°C the relative density of water is 1.0000, while its absolute density at the same temperature is 0.999973.* To convert a relative density of water to absolute density, the former should be multiplied by 0.999973.

Specific gravity may be defined as the ratio of the mass of a substance to the mass of an equal volume of another substance taken as the standard. For gases, the standard may be hydrogen or air; for liquids and solids, it is water. From what has been stated, it is obvious that in a determination of specific gravity there will be, in general, a difference in the result if the masses (weights) are determined in air or in vacuum; if determined in, or referred to, a vacuum, the result is a *true specific gravity* (sometimes called *absolute specific gravity*), while if the masses are determined in air, the calculated result is an *apparent specific gravity*. The difference between these specific gravities is, as a rule, very small. A very important variable in specific gravity determinations is temperature, and this is doubly important because both the temperature of the substance under examination and the temperature of the standard may be different. The common practice with regard to the determination of specific gravity is that defined by the USP and NF as follows:

Unless otherwise stated, the specific gravity basis is 25°/25°, ie, the ratio of the weight of a substance in air at 25° to that of an equal volume of water at the same temperature.

But it is not always convenient, or desirable, to determine the weight of both the substance and the water at 25°, or even to determine the weight of the substance at the same temperature as that at which the water is weighed. Thus, the substance may be weighed at 25°, and compared with the weight of an equal volume of water at 4°, in which case the specific gravity is reported as being on a 25°/4° basis; in the case of theobroma oil, which is solid at 25°, the specific gravity is determined on a 100°/25° basis, and for alcohol it is determined on a 15.56°/15.56° basis because many years ago the US Government adopted 60°F (15.56°C) as the temperature at which alcoholometric measurements are to be made in connection with the Government's control of alcoholic liquids.

It is apparent that a completely informative statement of specific gravity must indicate the temperature of the substance under examination, as well as that of the equal volume of water (the temperatures are commonly shown as a ratio, with the temperature of the water always being indicated in the denominator). Furthermore, it should be stated whether the determinations of mass (weight) were made on an "in vacuum" or "in air" basis, in which latter case the material of construction of the weights should also be indicated (since the buoyant effect of air on weights depends on their volume).

Calculations

The heaviest metal known, osmium, has a specific gravity of 22.48. The lightest metal, lithium, has a specific gravity of 0.534. Somewhere between the extremes of 0.534 and 22.48 (at 20°C) will be found the specific gravities of thousands of substances, both liquid and solid, which are of importance in pharmacy. With the exception of mercury and a very few other substances, the specific gravities of liquids lie within the range of 0.5 to 2.0.

The principle underlying the determination of the specific gravity of either a liquid or a solid is the same; it is to find the ratio of the mass (weight) of the substance to that of an equal volume of water.

This may be expressed by a simple relationship:

$$\text{Specific gravity} = \frac{W_s}{W_w}$$

where W_s = weight of substance and W_w = weight of equal volume of water.

Specific Gravity of Liquids

The specific gravity of a liquid may be determined with the aid of a pycnometer (or pipet), a hydrometer, or a Westphal balance.

Pycnometers—The specific gravity bottle (pycnometer) is used for the most accurate determinations of the specific gravity of liquids. Figs. 49 and 50 show two types commonly used. Some are provided with counterpoise weights which exactly balance the empty bottle. In most cases, however, the actual weight of the bottle (called the *tare*) must be previously determined, and this weight subtracted each time a specific gravity is taken. Any flask or container, if it can be accurately weighed and if it has been standardized by weighing the water it contains at the standard temperature, when filled to a mark previously made on the neck, may be used for taking the specific gravity of a liquid.

Sometimes the pycnometer is equipped with a thermometer, so that the weighing may be quickly accomplished when the exact temperature is reached at which the specific gravity is to be taken. The pycnometer should be accurately calibrated under standardized conditions of temperature and pressure. A table for this purpose was provided in the USP XIV.

Similar in principle to the pycnometer is the specific gravity pipet or tube, one form of which is shown in Fig. 58; with such a pipet or tube the liquid under examination is aspirated into the weighed tube to a predetermined point, after which it is again weighed, and

---

* Water attains its maximum absolute density of 0.999973 at 3.98°C.

the specific gravity calculated by dividing into the weight of the liquid the weight of an equal volume of water.

Hydrometers—A hydrometer is an instrument calibrated to indicate the specific gravity of a liquid corresponding to the depth to which the hydrometer sinks in the liquid, this depth being related to the specific gravity of the liquid. The principle of the hydrometer was probably first described by Archimedes and depends on the fact that when a solid body is placed in a liquid in which it is capable of floating, it sinks to a depth where the body has displaced a volume of liquid exactly equal to its own weight. Hydrometers are of two types:

1.   Those in which the weight is constant but the depth of immersion is subject to change.
2.   Those in which the depth of immersion is constant but the weight is subject to change.

The hydrometers in common use are of the first type and of these, two kinds are generally used, one for liquids heavier, the other for those lighter, than water.

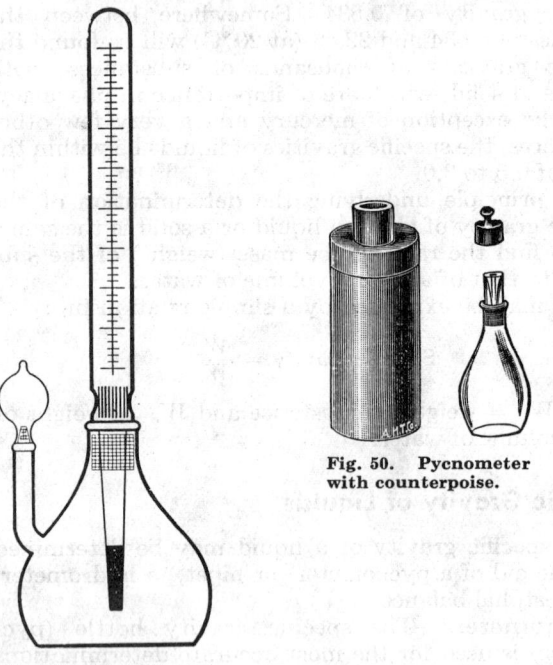

Fig. 50.   Pycnometer with counterpoise.

Fig. 49.   Leach's pycnometer with thermometer.

Most hydrometers are constructed to indicate specific gravity when used at the proper temperature. Earlier hydrometers, used in manufacturing operations conducted by unskilled and uneducated workmen who could not be depended on to understand decimal fractions or observe distinctions based on small decimal differences, but who could be taught to use hydrometers in which an arbitrary scale consisting of whole numbers was employed, were thus calibrated. Many such arbitrary-scale hydrometers have been in use. The most important one is Baumé's. Others of less importance are Twaddell's, Beck's, Sikes', Cartier's, Gay-Lussac's, and Brix's.

Hydrometers of the second type are intended to sink, by the addition of weights, to a given mark on the stem, and thus displace a constant volume of liquid; Fahrenheit's, Nicholson's, Guyton de Morveau's, etc are of this type. These are seldom seen except in physical laboratories or in lecture counter experiments, to illustrate a principle.

Hydrometers of Constant Weight and Variable Depth

Specific Gravity Hydrometers—This form of hydrometer (Fig. 51) is frequently used for accurate measurement of specific gravity over the range of 0.7 to 2. A series of hydrometers, each covering about 0.200 of the range, is required. The range of a hydrometer is determined by the degree to which its bulb is loaded with mercury or shot.

Baumé's Hydrometers—This form was the first one of its type to come into general use, having been originally described by Baumé in his *Éléments de Pharmacie*. Two instruments were used by Baumé, one for liquids heavier than water, the other for liquids lighter than water. The graduations on the stem of Baumé's hydrometer are called degrees. They are entirely arbitrary, and were established in the following manner.

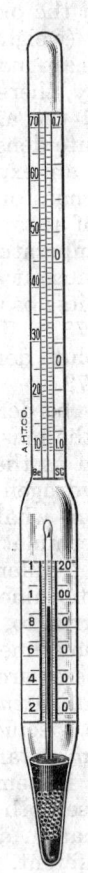

Fig. 51.   Combination specific gravity and Baumé hydrometer (courtesy, Thomas).

The hydrometer to be used for *liquids heavier than water* was prepared by adding sufficient mercury to the lower bulb to cause it to sink in water to a convenient point near the top of the stem; this was marked 0. The instrument was placed in a solution containing 15% by weight of common salt, and the point at which it rested was marked 15. The space between these two points was divided into 15 equal parts, and the scale below was extended by marking off similar spaces.

The hydrometer to be used for *liquids lighter than water* was prepared by placing it in a 10% by weight solution of common salt and loaded so that it floated at a point just above the bulb; this was marked 0. The hydrometer was then transferred to water, the point at which it rested was marked 10, the space between was divided into 10 equal parts, and the scale above was extended by marking off similar spaces.

Formulas are available for converting Baumé's degrees (°Be) into specific gravity by a simple calculation. The following is the formula of the NBS for calculating degrees Baumé from specific gravity:

For liquids heavier than water:

$$°Be = 145 - \frac{145}{\text{sp gr } 60°/60°F}$$

For liquids lighter than water:

$$°Be = \frac{140}{\text{sp gr } 60°/60°F} - 130$$

A close approximation, in which temperature is disregarded, may be obtained from the following formulas for calculating specific gravities from degrees Baumé:

For liquids heavier than water:

$$\text{sp gr} = \frac{145}{145 - °Be}$$

For liquids lighter than water:

$$\text{sp gr} = \frac{140}{130 + °Be}$$

Tables of *Specific Gravities* and *Weight and Volume Relations* were provided in the appendix of the USP XIV, but not in subsequent editions.

The hydrometer cannot be as accurate an instrument for taking specific gravity as the pycnometer or specific gravity bottle. The adhesion of air bubbles to the hydrometer produces a buoyant effect and introduces an error, the liability to variation in the diameter of the stem, and the inaccuracies in the scale lessen the accuracy of hydrometers.

In the illustrations shown in Fig. 53 the arbitrary scales of Baumé are compared with the equivalent specific gravity scales. The scale on the left is for

heavy liquids and that on the right is for light liquids. It is apparent that the graduations of the specific gravity scale gradually increase in size from below upward, the uppermost graduation being nearly four times wider than the lowermost.

Hydrometers are usually floated in the liquid contained in tall, cylindrical, glass jars (Fig. 52); it is imperative that the liquid be at the temperature specified for the measurement. The NBS specifies the manner of reading hydrometers; this is described in Circular No. 16, *The Testing of Hydrometers*, as follows:

In reading the hydrometer scale, the eye is placed slightly below the plane of the surface of the test liquid; it is raised slowly until the surface, seen as an ellipse, becomes a straight line. The point where this line cuts the hydrometer scale should be taken as the reading of the hydrometer.

Special hydrometers have been made for determining the specific gravity of specific liquids, eg, syrups, oils, milk, urine, alcohol, petroleum benzin, ether, vinegar, wine, beer, solutions of silver nitrate, and sea water.

Alcoholometers—These are hydrometers which combine a thermometer with a hydrometer (Fig. 54), the scale commonly indicating the percentage, by volume, of absolute alcohol or degrees proof corresponding to specific gravity.

This instrument cannot be used to determine the alcoholic strength of any liquid containing more than traces of substances other than alcohol and water. For instance, the alcoholic strength of distilled extract of witch hazel, or of hydroalcoholic distillates of any kind, may be directly determined, but not the alcoholic strength of wines or flavoring extracts, which contain other substances besides alcohol and water.

Tralles' hydrometer is an alcoholometer having a centesimal scale. It has been used by the US Government in gauging spirits and at one time was in general use by distillers. Each division of the scale corresponds to a given percentage of pure alcohol, by volume, in the liquor.

Hydrometers of Variable Weight and Constant Depth

Fahrenheit's Hydrometer—This was one of the first instruments of the variable-weight, constant-depth class to come into general use, although Robert Boyle described, in 1675, his "New Essay Instrument," which was very similar to Fahrenheit's hydrometer. It had but a single mark on the stem, which was surmounted by a small-scale pan, and weights were placed on the pan to cause the hydrometer to sink to the mark. As this mark indicated the point at which the instrument would float in water at a given temperature when certain weights were placed on the pan, it follows that when it was immersed in a liquid of different specific gravity, the weights would have to be changed to float the instrument to the fixed mark; the ratio which this weight bore to the weight used for water gave the specific gravity.

Nicholson's Hydrometer—This instrument is similar in principle to Fahrenheit's but is modified so that it can be used for taking the specific gravity of heavy or light solids. Fig. 55 is an illustration of one of the most convenient forms of the instrument, which is usually made of brass. There is a single mark on the stem and a scale pan on the summit. To the lower extremity of the hydrometer two conical cups are attached. Their apexes are joined so as to resemble an hour glass. The lowest cone has several apertures at the top to permit the escape of air when the instrument is immersed. The weight of the hydrometer is usually adjusted so that a fixed weight is needed on the scale pan to float it

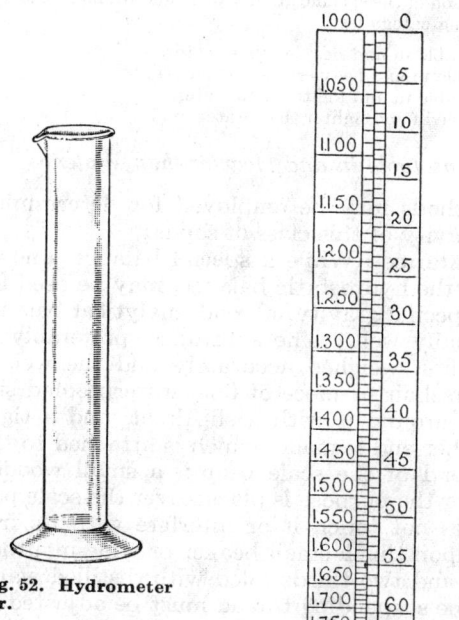

Fig. 52. Hydrometer jar.

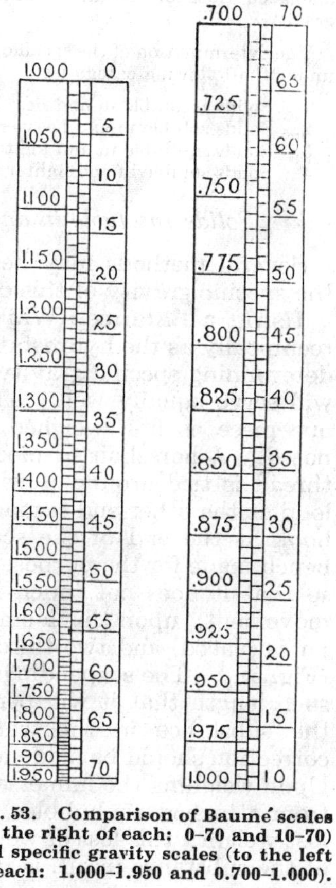

Fig. 53. Comparison of Baumé scales (to the right of each: 0–70 and 10–70) and specific gravity scales (to the left of each: 1.000–1.950 and 0.700–1.000).

to the mark on the stem.   The specific gravity of solid substances is obtained by weighing them first in air, on the upper platform, and then submerged, in the upper cup, and making the necessary calculations from the weights obtained.   The lower cup is used for taking the specific gravity of bodies lighter than water, the weight of the hydrometer keeping the light body submerged when the lower cup is placed over it.   The specific gravity is obtained in the same manner as in the case of bodies heavier than water.

Lovi's Beads—*Specific gravity beads*, as they are also called, have also been used for taking the specific gravity of liquids.   They may be especially useful in operations where a boiling liquid is to be evaporated until it has a given specific gravity, or in mixing liquids of different densities.   They are balloon-shaped hollow globes of glass, of different sizes and weights, having specific gravity figures scratched upon their sides and standardized for use at a definite temperature.   Fig. 56

shows their method of use.   Those heavier than the liquid sink, those lighter float, while the one remaining indifferently suspended indicates the specific gravity of the liquid.   Lovi's beads may be considered as hydrometers which indicate but one specific gravity.

Westphal Specific Gravity Balance

This balance is a very convenient device for taking the specific gravities of liquids (Fig. 57).   The principle of the balance is that a plummet (occupying a volume of about 5 ml) suspended from the beam of the balance is immersed in the liquid to be tested, in which the plummet is subjected to a buoyant effect equivalent to the weight of liquid displaced.   This buoyant effect is measured by placing various weights on the notched beam of the balance to effect submersion of the plummet to a constant reference point.   If the instrument has been calibrated previously with water, the weights that must be added when the plummet is immersed in another liquid are a measure of its specific gravity. Commonly, the weights are a series of riders weighing 5, 0.5, 0.05, and 0.005 Gm, respectively, which may be placed in any one of 10 positions on the notched beam. By using all the weights a specific gravity measurement may be made to the fourth decimal place.

Specific Gravity of Solids

In general, the specific gravity of a solid may be determined by observing the volume of liquid which it displaces when immersed in the liquid, or the apparent loss of weight of the solid while immersed in it.   The displaced volume, or the loss of weight, calculated in terms of the weight of water equivalent to either of these quantities, may be used as follows to calculate specific gravity.

Rule—Divide the weight of the body by the weight of water displaced (loss of weight in water); the quotient is the specific gravity.

The determination of the specific gravity of solids will be considered under the following categories:

1.   Solids insoluble in and heavier than water.
2.   Solids soluble in and heavier than water.
3.   Solids insoluble in and lighter than water.
4.   Solids soluble in and lighter than water.

Solids Insoluble in and Heavier than Water

Several methods may be employed for determining the specific gravity of this class of solids.

Using a Balance—While a special balance, known technically as the hydrostatic balance, may be used for determining specific gravity, a good analytical balance will serve equally well.   The substance, preferably in one piece, is first weighed accurately and the weight noted.   A horsehair or piece of fine, waterproofed silk thread is tied around it with a slip knot, and a tight loop at the other end is made, which is attached to the hook at the end of the scale beam; a small wooden bench made for the purpose is placed over the scale pan so that it does not touch it or interfere with its free movement; upon this a small beaker or wide-mouthed jar is placed, and two-thirds filled with distilled water (Fig. 59).   The suspending thread must be adjusted to such length that it will permit complete immersion of the substance in the water.   (In accurate work a correction should be made for the weight of the thread.) Upon weighing the immersed substance, after freeing it from attached air bubbles, it will be observed to have lost weight; this loss of weight, divided into the weight of the substance in air, is the specific gravity.

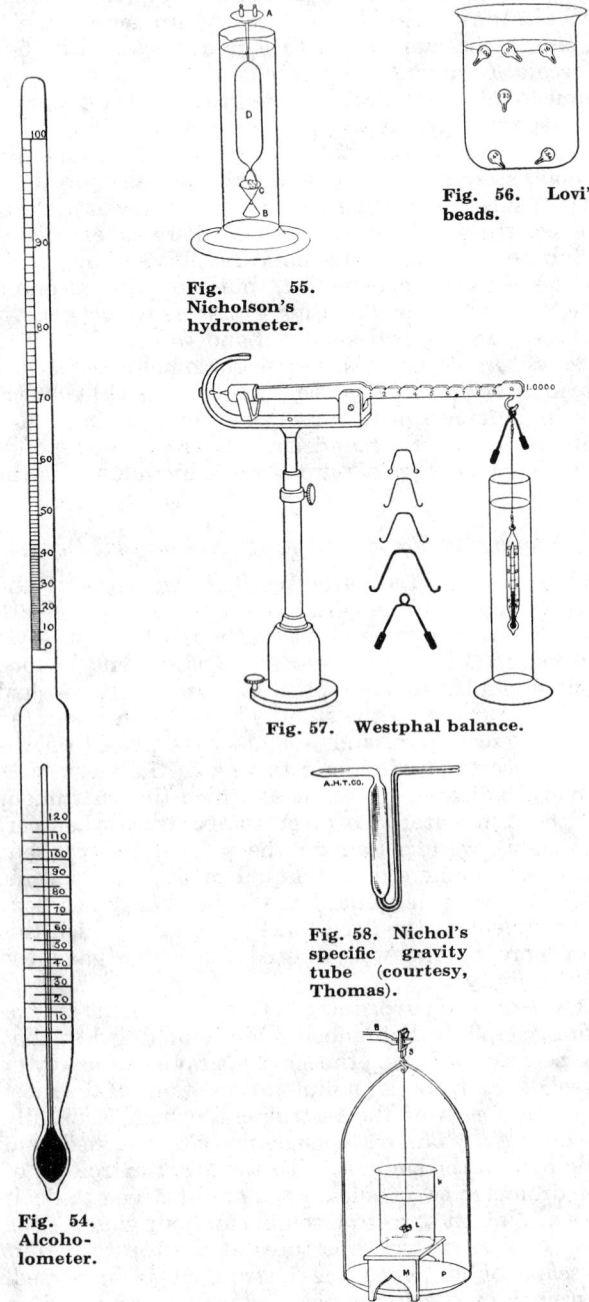

Fig. 56.   Lovi's beads.

Fig. 55. Nicholson's hydrometer.

Fig. 57.   Westphal balance.

Fig. 58. Nichol's specific gravity tube (courtesy, Thomas).

Fig. 54. Alcoholometer.

Fig. 59.   Determining specific gravity with a balance.

Example: 80.45 Gm of copper weigh 71.43 Gm in water. Calculate the specific gravity.

Weight of copper in air........................ 80.45 Gm
Weight of copper in water.................... 71.43 Gm
Loss of weight............................. 9.02 Gm

$$\text{Sp gr of copper} = \frac{80.45}{9.02} = 8.92$$

Using a Specific Gravity Bottle—The specific gravity bottle or pycnometer (Figs. 49 and 50) has already been described. It is particularly adapted to taking specific gravities of solid substances which are in small fragments or even in a much finer state of subdivision. The previously weighed solid material is dropped into the bottle, which is then filled with water at a temperature of 25 °C. The exterior of the bottle is carefully dried and, after the counterpoise (the exact weight of the empty bottle) has been placed on the opposite scale pan, it is weighed. To obtain the *loss of weight* in water of the substance, it is only necessary to deduct the weight of the contents of the bottle (that of the water and the immersed body) from the weight of the body in air, plus that of the water which the bottle holds when full (100 Gm), and divide the weight of the body by its loss of weight in water (weight of water displaced).

Example: A quantity of granular aluminum weighs 10 Gm; when dropped into a 100-Gm bottle, and the bottle filled with water at the proper temperature, the weight of both is 106.2 Gm. Calculate the specific gravity.

Weight of aluminum in air.................... 10.00 Gm
Weight of water held by bottle................ 100.00 Gm
Weight of water and aluminum................ 110.00 Gm
Weight of water and immersed aluminum....... 106.20 Gm
Loss of weight of aluminum in water......... 3.80 Gm

$$\text{Sp gr of aluminum} = \frac{10.00}{3.8} = 2.63$$

The specific gravity of any insoluble powder, eg, calomel and litharge, may be taken in exactly the same way, but care must be observed to agitate the powder with a small quantity of water in the bottle, before adding the rest, to eliminate adhering bubbles of air, which would introduce error.

Using a Graduated Cylinder—Direct measurement of the volume of a solid may be made by observing the volume it displaces when immersed in water (or other suitable liquid) contained in a graduated cylinder. From the density of water at the temperature of observation, the weight of this volume of water may be calculated, and this divided into the weight of the body to give the specific gravity.

Immersion of a Solid in a Transparent Liquid of the Same Density—This method may be applied where the body is small, has a low specific gravity, and is insoluble in the liquid. For example, beeswax may be immersed in a mixture of alcohol and water which is adjusted by the addition of one or the other of these liquids until the mass of wax floats indifferently in the liquid, neither sinking nor rising. The specific gravity of the solid will of course be the same as that of the liquid, which may be determined after removing the wax.

Solids Soluble in and Heavier than Water

A liquid must be selected in which the solid is insoluble, eg, olive oil, petroleum benzin, or turpentine oil, and its specific gravity determined. Subsequently it is used just as if it were water, the object being to find the apparent loss of weight of the substance when immersed in the oil. This having been obtained, the following simple proportion is established: the specific gravity of the oil is to the specific gravity of water, as the loss of weight in the oil is to the loss of weight in water. The specific gravity is then calculated in the usual way.

Example: 20 Gm of citric acid immersed in an oil of specific gravity 0.920 filling a 100-Gm pycnometer to the mark weighs 100.5 Gm. Calculate the specific gravity of the acid.

Weight of citric acid in air.................. 20.0 Gm
Weight of oil held by full pycnometer........... 92.0 Gm
Weight of citric acid and oil................. 112.0 Gm
Weight of oil and immersed acid.............. 100.5 Gm
Weight of oil displaced by acid.............. 11.5 Gm

The oil has a specific gravity of 0.920; therefore the loss of weight in water would be

$$\frac{11.5}{0.920} = 12.5$$

$$\text{Sp gr of acid} = \frac{\text{weight in air}}{\text{weight of water displaced}} = \frac{20.0}{12.5} = 1.60$$

It is obvious that either the balance, specific gravity bottle, or graduated tube can be used in this case.

Solids Insoluble in and Lighter than Water

To determine the specific gravity of this type of substance, a dense insoluble body is attached to the light body to secure immersion of both. Then, if the loss of weight in water of the heavy substance is deducted from the loss of weight in water of both the heavy and the light body, the difference must be the loss of weight in water of the light body alone, and the problem may be solved as before.

Example: A piece of paraffin weighs 17.4 Gm, a piece of brass loses by immersion in water 0.6 Gm, and when the brass is attached to the paraffin, both together lose by immersion in water 20.6 Gm. What is the specific gravity of the paraffin?

Loss in weight of brass plus paraffin............... 20.6 Gm
Loss in weight of brass........................ 0.6 Gm
Loss in weight of paraffin..................... 20.0 Gm
Weight of paraffin............................ 17.4 Gm

$$\text{Sp gr of paraffin} = \frac{17.4}{20.0} = 0.87$$

Solids Soluble in and Lighter than Water

A pycnometer may be used for determining the specific gravity of substances soluble in and lighter than water; the method described for soluble substances heavier than water is employed, but a suitable liquid lighter than the body, and in which it is insoluble, is selected. The proportion used in the calculation is: the specific gravity of the light liquid is to the specific gravity of water, as the loss of weight in the light liquid is to the loss of weight in water.

Some Calculations Involving Specific Gravity

The following relationships and examples illustrate important applications of specific gravity data.

Reducing Metric Fluid Measure to Weight

1 ml of liquid with a sp gr of 1 weighs 1 Gm
1 ml of liquid with a sp gr of x weighs x Gm
Vol. in ml $\times$ sp gr = weight in Gm

Example: What is the weight in Gm of 1 L of chloroform having a sp gr of 1.48?

$$\text{No. of ml} \times \text{sp gr} = \text{weight in Gm}$$
$$1000 \times 1.48 = 1480 \text{ Gm}$$

Reducing Apothecary Fluid Measure to Weight

There is no commensurability of the units between this system and those of avoirdupois or troy weight.

1 fl℥ of water does NOT weigh 1℥
1 ♏ of water does NOT weigh 1 gr
1 fl℥ of water weighs 454.6 gr at 25°C; therefore
1 ♏ of water weighs 454.6 ÷ 480 or 0.95 gr
1 fl℥ of liquid with a sp gr of 1 weighs 454.6 gr
1 fl℥ of liquid with a sp gr of x weighs 454.6 x gr

Any volume in fluidounces may be changed to grains (and thence to larger units) according to the formula:

$$454.6 \times sp\ gr \times number\ of\ fl℥ = wt\ in\ gr$$

Example: Calculate the weight in gr of 1 pt, 1 fl℥, and 4fl ℨ of sulfuric acid with a sp gr of 1.8.

$$1 \text{ pt, } 1 \text{ fl℥, } 4 \text{ fl℥} = 17.5 \text{ fl℥}$$
$$454.6 \times 1.8 \times 17.5 = 14319.9 \text{ gr}$$

The answer may be converted into larger units if desired. Since both the avoirdupois and the apothecary grain are identical, the larger units of either system may be calculated from the above answer.

Since 1 ♏ of water weighs 0.95 gr, the weight in grains of any number of minims of any liquid may be calculated by the following formula.

$$0.95\ gr \times sp\ gr \times number\ of\ ♏ = weight\ in\ gr$$

Reducing Weight to Volume

This process is the reverse of that described above.

$$\text{Vol in ml} = \frac{\text{weight in gm}}{\text{sp gr}}$$

$$\text{Vol in fl℥} = \frac{\text{weight in gr}}{454.6 \times \text{sp gr}}$$

$$\text{Vol in ♏} = \frac{\text{weight in gr}}{0.95 \times \text{sp gr}}$$

Specific Volume

Specific volume is the volume of one substance compared with the volume of an equal weight of another substance selected as the standard, both having the same temperature. The accepted standard is water and, therefore, specific volume is the reciprocal of specific gravity. Specific volume enables one to calculate the volume that a given weight of liquid will occupy.

$$\text{Sp vol} = \frac{\text{volume of a body}}{\text{volume of an equal weight of water}}$$

Note—Because of the reciprocal relationship between specific gravity and specific volume, the one is readily calculated from the other.

$$\text{Sp vol} = \frac{1}{\text{sp gr}} \qquad \text{Sp gr} = \frac{1}{\text{sp vol}}$$

Example 1: 1403 Gm of nitric acid occupies a volume of 1000 ml. What is its specific volume?

Volume of acid.................................... 1000 ml
Volume of an equal weight of water............... 1403 ml*

$$\text{Sp vol} = \frac{1000}{1403} = 0.713$$

Example 2: How many fl℥ are there in 100 oz avoir of nitric acid?

$$100 \text{ oz avoir of water measure } \frac{100 \times 437.5}{454.6} = 96.2 \text{ fl℥}$$

$$\text{Vol. of nitric acid} = 96.2 \times 0.713 = 68.6 \text{ fl℥}$$

References

1. Goldstein, S. W., and Mattocks, A. M., *Professional Equilibrium and Compounding Precision*, American Pharmaceutical Association, Washington, D.C., 1951 (pamphlet).
2. *NBS Handbook*, 44, 2nd ed National Bureau of Standards, Washington, D.C., 1955, pp. 113–116.

---

* The exact volume depends on the temperature, the one used here serving an acceptable approximation.

10 | Calculation

Mathematical principles (significant figures; fractions; exponents, powers, and roots)—logarithms—pharmaceutical problems

This chapter was prepared by

Werner Lowenthal, PhD, *Associate Professor of Pharmacy, School of Pharmacy, Medical College of Virginia, Health Science Division, Virginia Commonwealth University, Richmond, Va. 23219*

Pharmaceutical dispensing and compounding calculations utilize simple arithmetic. The errors that may arise are often due to carelessness, as in improper placing of decimal points, or incorrect conversion from one system of measurement to another, or to uncertainty concerning the system of measurement to be used. Before proceeding with any calculation it is imperative that the problem presented (in a prescription order, formula, etc) be read carefully, the information given and that required be identified, and the procedure to be used in the calculation selected.

Often several steps are necessary to solve problems. Shortcuts should not be taken unless one is certain they are proper. Many problems can be solved by the method of "ratio and proportion," but if the student understands the problem, he may use any method that will give him the correct answer. Many problems can be solved by more than one procedure, and if the student finds a procedure that is more logical to him and gives the correct answer, he should use it. The solutions to sample problems used herein should, therefore, generally be considered suggestive rather than the only way to solve a given type of problem.

Before the student reads this chapter and attempts to solve the problems, he should be thoroughly familiar with, and understand, the information in the preceding chapter on *Metrology* and the concepts of temperature measurement and of density.

Mathematical Principles

A few mathematical principles (eg, common decimal fractions, exponents, powers, and roots, significant figures, and logarithms) will be reviewed; these are areas where students often become careless. Following this, various types of practical pharmaceutical problems that the pharmacist may be required to solve are discussed and solutions are given. Where practical, rules for solving these problems are given. No attempt is made to elaborate on any mathematical theory.

The problems generally consist in determining the quantity or quantities of material(s) required to compound prescription orders properly and make products used to aid the compounding of prescription orders. The materials used to compound prescription orders may be pure or mixtures of substances in varying strengths. The strengths of mixtures may be denoted in different ways. Conversions may be necessary between systems of varying strengths or between different measuring systems. At the end of each section, sample problems are given for the student to solve, the answers to which appear on page 120.

Because of the decreasing importance of the apothecary system, the metric system will be emphasized. Chemicals and preparations most likely will be bought in the avoirdupois or metric systems. Prescription orders are filled in the system indicated on the order, usually the apothecary or metric systems.

The student should become familiar with the terminology used in writing prescription orders such as Latin words and abbreviations used in giving directions to the pharmacist and patient. The prescriber may occasionally use Roman numerals instead of Arabic numerals. Students, therefore, should be familiar with these even if the practice is declining.

Significant Figures

Weighings and measurements can be carried out with only a certain maximum degree of accuracy; the result is always approximate due to the many sources of error such as temperature, limitations of the instruments employed, personal factors, etc. The pharmacist must achieve the greatest accuracy possible with his equipment, but it would be erroneous to claim that he has weighed 1 mg of a solid on a Class A prescription balance, which has a sensibility reciprocal of 6 mg, or that he has measured 76.32 ml of a liquid in a 100-ml graduate, which can be read only to 1 ml. When quantities are written, the numbers should contain only those digits which are "significant" within the precision of the instrument.

Significant figures are digits which have practical meaning. In some instances zeros are significant; in other instances they merely indicate the order of magnitude of the other digits by locating the decimal point. For example, in the measurement 473 ml all the digits are significant, but in the measurement 4730 ml the zero may or may not be significant. In the weight 0.0316 Gm the zeros are not significant but only locate the decimal point. In any result the last significant figure is only approximate, but all preceding figures are accurate. When 473 ml is recorded, it is understood that the measurement had been made within ±0.5 ml or somewhere between 472.5 and 473.5 ml. The student should stop to consider the full implications of this, specifically that the measurement is subject to a maximum error of

$$\frac{0.5}{473} \times 100 = \text{(approx)} \ 0.1\% \text{ or } 1 \text{ part in } 1000$$

A zero in a quantity such as 473.0 ml is a significant figure and implies that the measurement has been made within the limits 472.95 ml and 473.05 ml or with a possible error of

$$\frac{0.05}{473} \times 100 = \text{(approx) } 0.01\% \text{ or } 1 \text{ part in } 10,000$$

Thus, 473 is correct to the nearest ml, 473.0 is correct to the nearest 0.1 ml.

Rules

1. *When adding or subtracting, retain in the sum or remainder no more decimal places than the least number entering into the calculations.* For example:

11.5 Gm		11.50 Gm	
2.65 Gm		2.65 Gm	
3.49 Gm		3.49 Gm	
17.64 Gm		17.64 Gm	
Answer: 17.6 Gm		*Answer:* 17.64 Gm	

In the first column 11.5 Gm was weighed to 0.1 Gm or with an accuracy of ±0.05 Gm. Although the other two weighings were made with an accuracy of ±0.005 Gm, the sum can be expressed properly only to one decimal place.

In the second column 11.50 Gm was weighed to the nearest 0.01 Gm or with an accuracy of ±0.005 Gm. Since all weighings were made with this degree of accuracy, the sum may be stated as in the example, 17.64 Gm.

Retain all figures possible until all the calculations are completed and then retain only the significant figures for the answer. Additions or subtractions involving both large and small quantities, each expressed with maximum significance, are often useless. For example, if one were to add 1.2 and 0.041 Gm, the physical sum would be 1.2 Gm, regardless of the fact that the two numbers add numerically to 1.241. To express the physical sum as 1.241 Gm would convey an erroneous degree of accuracy with which the quantity was known.

2. *When multiplying or dividing, retain in the answer no more significant figures than the least number entering into the calculation.*

The meaning of this rule may be illustrated by the use of equivalents during conversions from one measuring system to another. Table I gives different equivalent values and the number of significant figures to which the answer is correct. Always use an equivalent which will give the desired degree of accuracy. Repeated multiplication of an approximation increases the error progressively; therefore, retain all figures during calculations and drop insignificant figures as the final step.

Table I

Weight, Gm		Equivalent used, gr/Gm		Equivalent weight, gr	Significant figures
4.522	×	15.432	=	69.78	4
4.522	×	15.43	=	69.77	4
4.522	×	15.4	=	69.6	3
4.522	×	15	=	69	2

Fractions

Common Fractions

An example of a common fraction is ⅜. It is read as "three-eights" and indicates three parts divided by eight parts of the same thing. The units with both numbers must be the same. If a pharmacist measures ⅜ of a fluidounce into a graduate, he measures 3 drams, out of 8 drams (a fluidounce contains 8 drams).

The following principles should be applied when using common fractions:

1. The value of a fraction is not altered by multiplying or dividing both numerator and denominator by the same number.
2. Multiplying the numerator or dividing the denominator by a number, multiplies the fraction by that number.
3. Dividing the numerator or multiplying the denominator by a number, divides the fraction by that number.
4. To add or subtract fractions, form fractions with the *lowest common denominator*, perform the arithmetical operation, and reduce to the lowest common denominator.
5. To multiply fractions, multiply all numbers above the line to form the new numerator and multiply all numbers below the line to form the new denominator. Cancel if possible to simplify and reduce to the lowest common denominator.
6. To divide by a fraction, multiply by the reciprocal of the fraction.

Decimal Fractions

Fractions with the power of 10 as denominator are known as *decimal fractions* and are written by omitting the denominator and inserting a decimal point in the numerator as many places from the last number on the right as there are ciphers of 10 in the denominator.

The following principles should be applied when using decimal fractions:

1. When adding or subtracting decimals, keep the decimal points under each other.
2. When multiplying decimals, proceed as with whole numbers, then place the decimal point in the product as many places from the 1st number on the right as the sum of the decimal places in the multiplier and the multiplicand.
3. When dividing by a decimal fraction, move the decimal point to the right, in both divisor and dividend, as many places as it is to the left in the divisor to form a whole number in the divisor; proceed as with whole numbers. The decimal point in the quotient should be placed immediately above the decimal point in the dividend.
4. When converting a common fraction into a decimal fraction, divide the numerator by the denominator and place the decimal point in the correct place.
5. When converting a decimal fraction into a common fraction, place the entire number, as numerator, over the power of 10 containing the same number of ciphers of 10 as there are decimal places. Cancel if possible, to simplify.

Exponents, Powers, and Roots

In the expression $2^4 = 16$, the following names are given to the terms: 16 is called the *power* of the *base* 2, and 4 is the *exponent* of the power. If the exponent is 1, it is usually omitted. The following laws should be recalled:

1. The product of two or more powers of the same base is equal to that base with an exponent equal to the sum of the exponents of the powers; eg, $2^5 \times 2^3 = 2^8$.
2. The quotient of two powers of the same base is equal to that base with an exponent equal to the exponent of the dividend minus the exponent of the divisor; eg, $2^8 \div 2^3 = 2^5$.
3. The power of a power is found by multiplying the exponents; eg, $(2^8)^3 = 2^{24}$.
4. The power of a product equals the product of the powers of the factors; eg, $(2 \times 3 \times 4)^2 = 2^2 \times 3^2 \times 4^2$.
5. The power of a fraction equals the power of the numerator divided by the power of the denominator; eg,

$$\left(\frac{2}{3}\right)^2 = \frac{2^2}{3^2}$$

6. The root of a power is found by dividing the exponent of the power by the index of the root; eg,

$$\sqrt[3]{3^6} = 3^{6/3} = 3^2$$

7. Any number other than 0 with the exponent 0 equals 1; eg, $2^0 = 1$.
8. A number with a negative exponent equals 1 divided by the number with a positive exponent equal in numerical value to the negative exponent; eg,

$$2^{-4} = \frac{1}{2^4}$$

Logarithms

To facilitate the solution of involved and lengthy problems, *logarithms* (*logs*) were invented. Many calculations, which are difficult by ordinary arithmetical processes, are rapidly and easily performed with the aid of logs.

The log of a number is the exponent of the power to which a given base must be raised in order to equal that number. John Napier, of Scotland, who discovered logs over three centuries ago, used the Natural Log Number, $2.71828+$, as the base. Henry Briggs, using Napier's discovery a few years later, introduced 10 as the base, which is the most convenient for practical purposes. Napier's system is called natural logs and Brigg's system is called common logs. In this latter system the natural numbers are regarded as powers of the base 10 and the corresponding exponents are the logs. For example,

$$Y = a^x, \text{ taking logs}$$

$$\log_a Y = X$$

$$8 = 2^3$$

$$\log_2 8 = 3$$

$$100 = 10^2$$

$$\log_{10} 100 = 2$$

$$25 = 10^{1.3979} \text{ or } \log_{10} 25 = 1.3979$$

This reads log to the base 10 of 25 equals 1.3979.

$$2 = 10^{0.3010} \text{ or } \log_{10} 2 = 0.3010$$

Laws and Rules

The following laws, governing the use of logs, are based on the laws of exponents, and hence hold for any log system.

1. The log of a product equals the *sum* of the log of the component numbers; eg, for 25×2.

$$\log (25 \times 2) = \log 25 + \log 2$$
$$= \log 10^{1.3979} + \log 10^{0.3010}$$
$$= 1.3979 + 0.3010 = 1.6989$$

2. The log of a quotient equals the log of the dividend minus the log of the divisor; eg, for $25 \div 2$.

$$\log (25 \div 2) = \log 25 - \log 2 = \log 10^{1.3979} - \log 10^{0.3010}$$
$$= 1.3979 - 0.3010 = 1.0969$$

3. The log of a power of a number equals the log of the number multiplied by the exponent of the power; eg, for $(25)^{12}$.

$$\log (25)^{12} = 12 \log 25 = 12 \times 1.3979 = 16.7748$$

4. The log of a root of a number equals the log of the number divided by the index of the root; eg, for $\sqrt{25}$.

$$\log \sqrt{25} = \frac{\log 25}{2} = \frac{1.3979}{2} = 0.6990$$

The logs of 1, 10, 0.01, etc are integers, but for numbers between these the logs will consist of two parts: an integral part called the characteristic and a fractional part called the mantissa. Thus,

$$10^2 = 100 \qquad \log 100 = 2$$

$$10^1 = 10 \qquad \log 10 = 1$$
$$10^0 = 1 \qquad \log 1 = 0$$
$$10^{-1} = 0.1 \qquad \log 0.1 = -1$$
$$10^{-2} = 0.01 \qquad \log 0.01 = -2$$

The log of a number between 100 and 1000 has 2 for a characteristic plus a fraction, the log of a number between 0.1 and 0.01 has -2 for a characteristic plus a fraction, and so on. The mantissa of a log must always be positive, whereas the characteristic may be either positive or negative.

Every number may be regarded as the product of two numbers, one being 10 with a positive or negative exponent and the other being some number between 1 and 10. For example,

$$760 = 10^2 \times 7.6 = 10^2 \times 10^{0.8808}$$

$$\therefore \log 760 = \log 10^2 + \log 7.6 = 2.8808$$

$$0.076 = 10^{-2} \times 7.6 = 10^{-2} \times 10^{0.8808}$$

$$\therefore \log 0.076 = \log 10^{-2} + \log 7.6 = -2 + 0.8808$$

This is written $\bar{2}.8808$ (or $8.8808 - 10$).

The characteristic is made a positive number by subtracting the -2 from 10 to give a characteristic of $8 \ldots -10$. The -10 is put after the mantissa. From the above explanation the following rules are derived:

1. The characteristic of a number greater than 1 is one unit less than the number of figures to the left of the decimal point; eg, for 1000 the characteristic is 3.
2. The characteristic of a number less than 1 is one unit more than the number of ciphers between the decimal point and the first significant figure; eg, for 0.001 the characteristic is -3.
3. If the characteristic of a log is positive, the integral part of the corresponding number contains one more figure than the number of units in the characteristic; eg, if the characteristic equals 2, the corresponding number lies between 100 and 1000.
4. If the characteristic of a log is negative, the number of zeros between the decimal point and the first significant figure is one less than the number of units in the characteristic; eg, if the characteristic is -2, the corresponding number lies between 0.01 and 0.001.
5. Numbers which are related to each other by some power of 10 possess logs with the same mantissa; eg, log 760 = 2.8808 and log 76 = 1.8808.

Obtaining the Log of a Number

The characteristic of a log is determined readily by inspection of the natural number, but to obtain the mantissa a table of logs must be used. These tables vary in accuracy according to the number of decimal places to which the mantissa is expanded. For most calculations four places are satisfactory.

Under the heading *Natural Numbers* (referred to as N) on the inside front cover, the first two figures of the number are given down the column on the left, while the third figure (from 0 to 9) is given across the top. The mantissa for large numbers or numbers falling between three-place ones may be found by the process of interpolation. For example,

1. Find the log of 273.

Under N find 27 and along the top line find the third number, 3. Across from 27 and under 3 the mantissa for 273 (4362) is found. No interpolation is necessary. By inspection (see Rule 1) the characteristic is 2. Then log 273 = 2 + .4362 = 2.4362.

2. Find the log of 0.08206.

Under N find 82 and along the top find the next number, 0. Now 8206 falls between 820 and 821 ($^6/_{10}$ of the difference). The mantissa for 820 is 9138 and the mantissa for 821 is 9143. The difference between these two mantissas is 5, and $^6/_{10}$ of 5 is 3. The mantissa for 8206 is therefore 9138 + 3 = 9141. By inspection (see Rule 2) the characteristic is -2. Then log 0.08206 = $-2 + 0.9141$ = 8.9141 $- 10$ or $\bar{2}.9141$.

The process of finding a number between two other numbers is known as interpolation. It is based on the assumption that the mantissa varies directly with the number. This is not quite true. Many log tables supply the proportionate parts to facilitate interpolation (see the chart on the right of the log table inside the front cover).

Obtaining the Antilog of a Number

To find the number corresponding to a given log, the reverse procedure of that discussed above is employed. The first step is to find figures corresponding to the mantissa (interpolation may be necessary). The last step is to place the decimal point in the correct position, following Rules 3 and 4. The following examples demonstrate the method:

1. Find the number corresponding to the log 3.8357.

In the log table, 8357 is found across from 68 and under 5. The figures required are therefore 685. Since the characteristic is 3 (Rule 3), the log 3.8357 is the number 6850.

2. Find the number corresponding to the log 0.4351.

In the log table, 4351 is found to fall between 4346 and 4362, the difference being 16. 4351 is 5 units more than 4346 or $^5/_{16}$ of the difference between the two mantissas. The log table gives 272 as the antilog of 4346, to which $^5/_{16}$ or 0.31 must be added. Adding on the 0.3 to the fourth place, the required figures are 2723. Since the characteristic is zero, the required number is 2.723.

Logarithmic Calculations

Representative problems illustrated below show the rapidity and simplicity of calculations with logs.
1. Find the value of 8.52 × 36.4 × 0.0056.

To multiply, add logs of the numbers.

$$\log 8.52 \quad = 0.9304$$
$$\log 36.4 \quad = 1.5611$$
$$\log 0.0056 = \bar{3}.7482$$
$$\log \text{number} = 0.2397$$

To find the natural number corresponding to log number 0.2397, take the antilog.
Answer: antilog 0.2397 = 1.737.

2. Find the fifth root of 0.00475.

To find the *n*th root of a number, divide the log of the number by the index of the root.

$$\log \sqrt[5]{0.00475} = \tfrac{1}{5} \log 0.00475 = \tfrac{1}{5} (\bar{3}.6767) =$$
$$\tfrac{1}{5} (7.6767 - 10) = 1.5353 - 2 \text{ or } \bar{1}.5353$$

To find the natural number corresponding to the log number $\bar{1}.5353$, take the antilog.
Answer: antilog $\bar{1}.5353$ = 0.343.

3. Find the value of

$$\frac{6.062 \times 10^{23}}{0.08206 \times 293.1 \times 760{,}000}$$

Remember: to multiply, add the logs of the numbers; to divide, subtract the logs of the numbers:

log 6.062 = 0.7826	log 0.08206 = $\bar{2}.9141$
log 10^{23} = 23.	log 293.1 = 2.4670
log numerator = 23.7826	log 760,000 = 5.8808
	log denominator = 7.2619

Log value: 23.7826 $-$ 7.2619 = 16.5207.
Answer: antilog 16.5207 = 3.32 × 10^{16}.

4. The pH of a solution is the log of the reciprocal of the hydrogen-ion concentration. If the concentration of [H$^+$] ions in a solution is 2.57 × 10^{-4} Gm-ion/liter, what is the pH?

$$\text{pH} = \log \frac{1}{[\text{H}^+]} = \log \frac{1}{2.57 \times 10^{-4}} = \log \frac{10^4}{2.57}$$

Taking logs,

$$\text{pH} = \log 10^4 - \log 2.57 = 4 - 0.4099 = 3.59$$

Problems

1. The rate of creaming of an emulsion may be calculated by Stokes' law:

$$-V = \frac{2gr^2(d_2 - d_1)}{9\eta}$$

If d_1 = 0.88 Gm/ml, d_2 = 1.32 Gm/ml, g = 980.6 cm/sec^2, r = 10^{-3} cm, and η = 1.14 poise, find the rate, V.

2. The surface tension (S) of a liquid may be found by the Capillary Rise Method using the formula

$$S = \tfrac{1}{2} \, hdgr$$

where h is the height of the liquid in the capillary, d is the density of the liquid, g is the acceleration of gravity, and r is the radius of the capillary. Find S when h = 2.62 cm, d = 2.43 Gm/ml, g = 980.6 cm/sec^2, and r = 0.021 cm.

Pharmaceutical Problems

The student who has knowledge of algebra and has studied the previous sections of this chapter, the theory of weighing and measuring presented in Chapter 9, and Roman numerals and Latin abbreviations used on prescription orders for directions to the pharmacist and patient by the prescriber should have sufficient knowledge to solve the routine problems he may encounter in a pharmacy. The various symbols and abbreviations and their meanings should be well understood. Explanation of practical problems, representative of those one faces in practice, are presented below. Practice problems follow each section and the answers to these problems are found at the end of this chapter (page 120).

To solve each problem properly, the following procedure is suggested:

1. Analyze the problem carefully so that all data are clearly fixed in the mind; determine what is given and what is called for.
2. Select the most direct method of solving the problem. Not all problems can be solved properly in one step. Look up doses, equivalents, and abbreviations when you are not sure.
3. Prove or check the result.

Addition

Review weighing and measuring systems in Chapter 9.

The expression "weighable or measurable quantities" means pounds, ounces, drams, quarts, pints, fluidounces, etc. For example, it is not practical to weigh 300 gr or measure 50 fl oz. These are converted to 5 drams, and 1 qt, 1 pt, 2 fl oz, respectively, which are weighable and measurable quantities. Neither a 300-gr weight nor a 50-fl oz graduate is available.

Rules

1. Add like quantities. If, in the metric system, the quantities are not alike, change to a common unit. For the apothecary or avoirdupois systems, place in columns of like quantities arranged in descending order of magnitude toward the right.
2. In the apothecary or avoirdupois systems, add together the smaller quantities first, then advance to the next higher units in these systems.
3. Always extract the next higher unit, wherever possible, to simplify the answer, which should be stated in weighable or measurable quantities.
4. When adding decimals, keep the decimal points directly under each other.
5. When adding fractions, reduce to the lowest common denominator, add the resulting numerators, and reduce the fraction, if possible, by canceling.

Examples

1. Add 3 Kg, 33 Gm, 433 mg.

Convert to a common unit. The gram is convenient because it is the unit of weight.

3 Kg =	3 × 1000 Gm = 3000	Gm
33 Gm =	33	Gm
433 mg =	433 mg ÷ 1000 = 0.433	Gm
	3033.433	Gm

2. Add 4 pounds, 3 ounces, 1 dram, 59 grains and 5 pounds, 10 ounces, 7 drams, 2 grains (apoth).

℔	℥	ℨ	gr
4	3	1	59
5	10	7	2
9	13	8	61

Explanation:

61 grains = 1 dram + 1 grain (60 gr = 1 ℨ)

Add 1 dram to the next column:

8 + 1 = 9 drams = 1 ounce + 1 dram (8 ℨ = 1 ℥)

Add 1 ounce to the next column:

13 + 1 = 14 ounces = 1 pound + 2 ounces (12 ℥ = 1 ℔)

Add 1 pound to the next column:

9 + 1 = 10 pounds.

Answer: 10 ℔, 2 ℥, 1 ℨ, 1 gr.

3. Add the following volumes: 5 gal, 3 pt, 2 fl oz and 2 pt, 3 fl oz, 4 fl dr.

Write out in proper sequence of the units in the measuring system and arrange the numbers given in the problem under each other. Thus,

gal	pt	fl oz	fl dr
5	3	2	
	2	3	4
5	5	5	4

Note: 5 pt = 2 qt + 1 pt (2 pt = 1 qt).
Answer: 5 gal, 2 qt, 1 pt, 5 fl oz, 4 fl dr.

Problems

1. Add 25 mg, 25 Gm, 210 mg, 2 Kg, 1.75 Gm, 215 mg, 454 Gm, and 30 mg.
2. The following quantities of a drug were removed from a container: 31 Gm, 225 Gm, 855.6 Gm, and 45.4 Gm. What is the total weight removed from the container?
3. What is the weight of powder formed by mixing together 1 ℨ, 175 gr of Drug A, 87.5 gr of Drug B, and 6 ℨ, 55 gr of Drug C? Give the answer in weighable quantities.
4. Add ℥xi, ℨvi, Ɵii, gr xiv and ℥vii, ℨv, Ɵii, gr x. Give the answer in weighable quantities.
5. Each unit of a mixture contains the following drugs: ⅕ gr of Drug M, ¹⁄₉₀ gr of Drug N, ⅙ gr of Drug P, and 2½ gr of Drug Q. What is the total weight of each unit?
6. The inventory card shows the following amounts of a syrup: 3 gal, 2½ qt, 6 pt, 8 fl oz, 19 fl oz. What is the total volume in stock (in measurable quantities)?

Subtraction

Rules

1. Subtract only like quantities. If the quantities are not alike, change to a common unit (metric system) or place in columns of like quantities or units arranged in descending order of magnitude toward the right (avoirdupois and apothecary systems).
2. In the apothecary and avoirdupois systems, begin with the smallest quantities and advance to the largest.
3. When necessary, reduce larger quantities to smaller ones and place in the proper column.
4. Treat common and decimal fractions as indicated under *Addition*.

Examples

1. Subtract 1 pt, 4 fl oz, 6 fl dr from 2 gal.

The problem may be solved as follows: divide 1 gal into 4 qt, leaving 1 gal in its column; divide 1 of the 4 qt into 2 pt, leaving 3 qt; divide 1 pt into 16 fl oz, leaving 1 pt; divide 1 fl oz into 8 fl dr, leaving 15 fl oz.

gal	qt	pt	fl oz	fl dr
1	3	1	15	8
		1	4	6
1	3	0	11	2

Answer: 1 gal, 3 qt, 0 pt, 11 fl oz, 2 fl dr.

2. Subtract 285 ml from 1 liter. Convert to a common unit.

1 liter = 1000 ml	1000 ml
	− 285 ml
	715 ml

Answer: 715 ml.

Problems

1. How much is left in a 5-liter container after the removal of 895 ml?
2. A pharmacist buys 1 oz of Drug C. At intervals he uses the following quantities to compound prescription orders: ℨii, ℨss, Ɵii, 56 gr, and 48 gr. How much of Drug C remains?

3.   A bottle contains 1 pt of a liquid; 8 fl oz and 6 fl dr were removed.   How much of the liquid remains?

4.   A pharmacist buys 5 Gm of a potent drug and at different times dispenses 0.2 Gm, 0.85 Gm, 90 mg, and 150 mg on prescription orders.   How much of the drug remains?

4.   A formula calls for 1 pt, 3 fl oz, 4 fl dr of an oil. How much is required to make 15 times the formula quantity?   Give amounts in measurable quantities.

5.   How many mg are used to make 1500 units, each of which contains 250 mcg of a drug?

Multiplication

Rules

1.   The product has the same denomination as the multiplicand.

2.   If the multiplicand is composed of different denominations in the metric system, form a common unit before multiplying and reduce the product to measurable units.   In the apothecary or avoirdupois systems, arrange the quantities in descending order of magnitude toward the right, and multiply.   Extract the next higher units, beginning with the smallest unit, and place in the proper columns, proceeding to the left.

3.   Multiply fractions and decimals as in any arithmetic problem, and reduce fractional quantities to measurable or weighable units.

Examples

1.   Multiply 4 pt, 7 fl oz, and 3 fl dr by 4.

Begin with the smallest unit, working from right to left. When it becomes necessary, change the product to the next higher unit, writing only the remainder, if there is any, under the unit multiplied as follows:

pt	fl oz	fl dr
4	7	3
		× 4
16	28	12

12 fl dr = 1 fl oz + 4 fl dr remainder

28 fl oz + 1 fl oz = 29 fl oz = 1 pt + 13 fl oz remainder

16 pt + 1 pt = 17 pt = 2 gal + 1 pt remainder

Answer: 2 gal, 1 pt, 13 fl oz, 4 fl dr.

2.   What will be the *total weight* of the ingredients in a prescription order for 25 units, each unit containing 0.4 Gm of Solid F, 0.01 Gm of Solid G, and 5 mg of Solid H?   First, convert to a common unit; eg, grams.

0.4 Gm + 0.01 Gm + 0.005 Gm =

0.415 Gm total weight of 1 unit

0.415 Gm/unit × 25 units =

10.375 Gm total weight of all units

3.   Multiply 22.4 ml by 2.65.

$$\begin{array}{r} 22.4 \text{ ml} \\ \times\ 2.65 \\ \hline 59.36 \text{ ml} \end{array}$$

Problems

1.   Multiply 48.5 ml by 3.24.

2.   A certain preparation is to contain 0.0325 Gm of a chemical in each ml of solution.   How much must be weighed out to make 5 liters of a solution?

3.   How much cod liver oil is necessary to make 2500 capsules, each containing 0.33 ml?

Division

Rules

1.   The quotient always has the same denomination as the dividend.

2.   If the dividend is composed of different denominations, form a common unit in the metric system before dividing and reduce the quotient to weighable or measurable quantities.   In the apothecary or avoirdupois systems arrange as under *Multiplication* and, being division with the largest quantity at the left, convert the remainder, if any, into the next lower units and add to the next column before proceeding with the division.

3.   Treat fractions and decimals as under *Multiplication*.

Examples

1.   Divide 3 liters by 25.

3 liters = 3000 ml

$$\frac{3000 \text{ ml}}{25} = 120 \text{ ml}$$

2.   Divide 10 gal, 3 pt, 8 fl oz by 8.

	gal	pt	fl oz
8 |	10	3	8

$$\frac{10 \text{ gal}}{8} = 1 \text{ gal} + 2 \text{ gal remainder}$$

2 gal = 16 pt

Place 16 pt in the next column.

16 pt + 3 pt = 19 pt

$$\frac{19 \text{ pt}}{8} = 2 \text{ pt} + 3 \text{ pt remainder}$$

3 pt = 48 fl oz

Place 48 fl oz in the next column.

48 fl oz + 8 fl oz = 56 fl oz

$$\frac{56 \text{ fl oz}}{8} = 7 \text{ fl oz}$$

Answer: 1 gal, 2 pt, 7 fl oz or 1 gal, 1 qt, 7 fl oz.

The alternative method is to reduce all quantities to a small unit such as fl oz, divide, and convert to measurable quantities.

(10 gal × 128 fl oz/gal) + (3 pt × 16 fl oz/pt) +

8 fl oz = 1336 fl oz

$$\frac{1336 \text{ fl oz}}{8} = 167 \text{ fl oz}$$

Extract the largest units possible (convert to measurable quantities).

167 fl oz	39 fl oz
− 128 fl oz = 1 gal	− 32 fl oz = 2 pt = 1 qt
39 fl oz remainder	7 fl oz remainder

Answer: 1 gal, 1 qt, 7 fl oz.

3. A pharmacist buys an 8-ounce container of a drug. How many 5-gr capsules can be made from the contents?

a. The pharmacist usually purchases by the avoirdupois system. The first step is to convert ounces to grains.

$$437.5 \text{ gr/oz} \times 8 \text{ oz} = 3500 \text{ gr}$$

b. Since 3500 gr are available and each capsule contains 5 gr, divide the total amount by 5 gr.

$$\frac{3500 \text{ gr}}{5 \text{ gr}} = 700$$

Therefore, 700 5-gr capsules can be made.

Problems

1. How many 65-mg capsules can be made from 50 Gm of a drug?
2. How many 15-minim capsules can be filled from 5 fl oz of an oil?
3. The dose of a drug is 0.1 mg. How many doses are contained in 15 mg of the drug?
4. The dose of a drug is $\frac{1}{150}$ gr. How many doses are obtainable from 1 gr of the drug?
5. How many 325-mg capsules of a drug can be filled from a 454-Gm amount?

Conversion

As long as the student knows the interrelationships of the various units within the different weighing and measuring systems (eg, 20 gr = Ɔ1, 3 Ɔ = 1ʒ, etc; 1000 mg = 1 Gm, etc), there are only three conversions necessary for him to memorize in order to convert between the apoth, avoir, and metric systems. These are:

$$1 \text{ gr (avoir)} = 1 \text{ gr (apoth)}$$

$$15.43 \text{ gr} = 1 \text{ Gm}$$

$$16.23 \text{ ♏} = 1 \text{ ml}$$

Learn them!

With these three conversions the student is able to derive all other necessary conversions.

Review conversions within the apothecary system. Various equalities within the apothecary system may be calculated. The number of grains in a dram, grains in a pound, etc may be calculated as follows:

1.

$$20 \text{ gr/Ɔ} \times 3\text{Ɔ/ʒ} = 60 \text{ gr/ʒ}$$

$$60 \text{ gr/ʒ} \times 8 \text{ ʒ/ʒ} \times 12 \text{ ʒ/℔} = 5760 \text{ gr/℔}$$

Cancel the units. If they do not cancel properly, something has been left out.

2.

$$1 \text{ gr (apoth)} = 1 \text{ gr (avoir)}$$

Since 1 gr (apoth) = 1 gr (avoir), the number of grains in one system equals the number of grains in the other system; eg, 480 gr (apoth) = 480 gr (avoir).

Convert 1 ʒ (apoth) to weighable quantities in the avoir system

$$20 \text{ gr/Ɔ} \times 3 \text{ Ɔ/ʒ} \times 8 \text{ ʒ/ʒ} = 480 \text{ gr/ʒ} \text{ (apoth)}$$

$$480 \text{ gr (apoth)} = 480 \text{ gr (avoir)}$$

$$437.5 \text{ gr} = 1 \text{ oz avoir}$$

$$\begin{array}{r} 480.0 \text{ gr} \\ - \ 437.5 \text{ gr} \\ \hline 42.5 \text{ gr} \end{array}$$

Answer: 1 ʒ (apoth) = 1 oz, 42.5 gr (avoir).

3. Conversions in the metric system are made by moving the decimal point. Moving the decimal point to the right gives a larger number and a smaller unit notation; eg,

$$1.000 \text{ Gm} = 1.000. \text{ mg}$$

Moving the decimal point to the left gives a smaller number and a larger unit notation; eg,

$$1 \text{ Gm} = 0.001. \text{ Kg,}$$

$$1000 \text{ Gm} = 1.000. \text{ Kg}$$

The same procedure is valid for volume measurements in the metric system.

4. Conversions between the apothecary and metric weight systems are based on the fact that 15.43 gr = 1 Gm, which may be restated as 15.43 gr/Gm or 1 Gm/15.43 gr.

a. How many mg equal 1 gr?

$$\frac{1.000 \text{ Gm}}{15.43 \text{ gr}} = 0.0648 \text{ Gm/gr} =$$

$$64.8 \text{ mg/gr or } 64.8 \text{ mg} = 1 \text{ gr}$$

Cancel units.

b. How many grams are in 1 ʒ?

$$\frac{1.000 \text{ Gm}}{15.43 \text{ gr}} \times 480 \text{ gr/ʒ} = 31.1 \text{ Gm/ʒ}$$

c. How many grams are in 1 oz (avoir)? *Remember:* 1 gr (apoth) = 1 gr (avoir).

$$\frac{1.000 \text{ Gm}}{15.43 \text{ gr}} \times 437.5 \text{ gr/oz} = 28.35 \text{ Gm/oz}$$

d. Other weight conversions are then found in a similar manner.

5. Conversions between the apothecary and metric measuring systems are based on the fact that 16.23 ♏ = 1 ml, which may be restated as 16.23 ♏/ml or 1 ml/16.23 ♏.

a. How many ml are in 1 fl oz?

$$60 \text{ ♏/fl dr} \times 8 \text{ fl dr/fl oz} = 480 \text{ ♏/fl oz}$$

$$480 \text{ ♏/fl oz} \times \frac{1 \text{ ml}}{16.23 \text{ ♏}} = 29.57 \text{ ml/fl oz}$$

$$\text{or } 29.57 \text{ ml} = 1 \text{ fl oz}$$

6. *Remember:* 1 Gm = 1 ml = 1 cc for practical purposes, but 1 gr does *not* equal 1 ♏. This means that the student can convert easily between solids and liquids in the metric system but *not* in the apothecary system.

Rules

1. The USP states that for prescription compounding one uses exact equivalents rounded to three (3) significant figures.
2. It may be desirable when multiplying by large numbers to use exact equivalents so that slight errors due to approximation are not magnified.
3. In converting doses the USP uses approximate equivalents. Use USP and NF tables wherever possible.

Examples

1. Convert 1 pt, 4 fl oz into ml.

First, convert into fl oz.

$$16 \text{ fl oz/pt} + 4 \text{ fl oz} = 20 \text{ fl oz}$$

Second, convert fl oz to ml.

$$1 \text{ fl oz} = 29.57 \text{ ml (as calculated above)}$$

$$20 \text{ fl oz} \times 29.57 \text{ ml/fl oz} = 591.4 \text{ ml}$$

Answer: 1 pt, 4 fl oz = 591.4 ml.

2. **What is the weight of 1200 Gm in the apothecary system?**

$$1 \text{ Gm} = 15.43 \text{ gr}$$

$$1200 \text{ Gm} \times 15.43 \text{ gr/Gm} = 18,516 \text{ gr}$$

Convert to weighable quantities.

$$480 \text{ gr} = 1 \text{ ℥}$$

$$480 \text{ gr/℥} \times 38 \text{ ℥} = 18,240 \text{ gr}$$

$$\begin{array}{r} 18,516 \text{ gr} \\ - 18,240 \text{ gr} (38 \text{ ℥}), 38 \text{ ℥} = 3 \text{ ℔}, 2 \text{ ℥} (12 \text{ ℥} = 1 \text{ ℔}) \\ \hline 276 \text{ gr} \end{array}$$

$$\begin{array}{r} - 240 \text{ gr} (60 \text{ gr} = 1 \text{ ʒ}), (4 \text{ ʒ}) \\ \hline 36 \text{ gr} \end{array}$$

Answer: 3 ℔, 2 ℥, 4 ʒ, 36 gr (apoth).

3. **Convert 1 pound (apoth) into grams.**

$$\frac{1 \text{ Gm}}{15.43 \text{ gr}} \times 480 \text{ gr/℥} = 31.11 \text{ Gm/℥}$$

$$1 \text{ ℔} = 12 \text{ ℥}$$

$$12 \text{ ℥} \times 31.11 \text{ Gm/℥} = 373.3 \text{ Gm/℔}$$

4. **Convert 25 gr to grams.**

$$25 \text{ gr} \times \frac{1 \text{ Gm}}{15.43 \text{ gr}} = 1.62 \text{ Gm}$$

5. **Convert 50 grams to grains.**

$$50 \text{ Gm} \times 15.43 \text{ gr/Gm} = 771 \text{ gr}$$

Problems

1. Convert:

   a. 6.50 grains into milligrams.
   b. $\frac{3}{10}$ grain into milligrams.
   c. $3\frac{1}{2}$ apoth ounces into grams.
   d. 2 ʒ into mg.
   e. $3\frac{1}{2}$ avoir ounces into grams.
   f. 1 ℔ into grams.

2. Convert:

   a. 550 Gm into weighable quantities in the avoir system.
   b. 450 mg into grains.
   c. 550 Gm into weighable quantities in the apoth system.
   d. 100 mcg into grains.
   e. 1 Kg into lb (avoir).

3. Convert the following doses into metric weights:

   a. $\frac{1}{100}$ gr.
   b. $\frac{1}{320}$ gr.
   c. $\frac{1}{6}$ gr.
   d. 5 gr.
   e. 20 gr.

4. Convert:

   a. 200 ♏ into ml.
   b. 3 fl dr into ml.
   c. 8 fl oz into ml.
   d. 1 pt into ml.
   e. 5 ♏ into ml.
   f. 0.1 mg into gr.
   g. 5 mg into gr.

5.

   a. How many gr are in 1 ʒ?
   b. How many drams are in 1 ℥?
   c. How many grains are in 1 oz (avoir)?
   d. How many gr are in $\frac{1}{2}$ ℔ (apoth)?
   e. Convert 250 gr to weighable quantities in the apothecary system.

Household Equivalents

Common household equivalents are found on page 81. These are used to interpret the prescriber's instructions to the patient. The teaspoonful is usually indicated by the symbol ʒ or 5 ml, although 1 ʒ does not equal 5 ml. The problem of "the teaspoonful" has been discussed by Morrell and Ordway[1] and Stempel.[2] For the purpose of practical calculations in this chapter, a teaspoonful is equal to 5 ml and 1 ʒ in the directions to the patient on the prescription order means 1 teaspoonful; therefore there are 6 teaspoonful quantities in 1 fluidounce (5 ml × 6 = 30 ml).

For purposes of solving most compounding and dispensing problems, the exact equivalents found on pages 86 and 87 rounded to 3 significant places should be used.

Dosage Calculations

Over the past years various rules for calculating infants' and children's dosages have been devised. All these rules give only approximate dosages because they erroneously assume that the child is a small adult. Some of these rules are still used because as yet no absolute method of calculating an infant's or child's dose has been found. Children are sometimes more susceptible than adults to certain drugs. Doses for infants should be learned where they are known or determined in a book such as the APhA booklet entitled *Usual Doses for Infants and Children*, pharmacology textbooks, or pediatric textbooks. Doses should not be calculated when it is possible to obtain the actual infant's or child's dose.

Rules for Infants' and Children's Doses

1. *Young's Rule* (for children 2 years and older).

$$\frac{\text{Age (yr)}}{\text{Age (yr)} + 12} \times \text{adult dose} = \text{child's dose (approx)}$$

2. *Clark's Rule.*

$$\frac{\text{Weight (lb)}}{150} \times \text{adult dose} = \text{child's dose (approx)}$$

3. *Fried's Rule* (for infants up to 2 years old).

$$\frac{\text{Age (months)}}{150} \times \text{adult dose} = \text{infant's dose (approx)}$$

Rules for Calculating Dosage on Prescription Orders

1. To find the amount of an ingredient/dose in a compound prescription order, divide the total amount of ingredient prescribed by the number of doses.

2. To find the total amount of an ingredient used to compound a prescription order, multiply the amount/dose prescribed by the total number of doses. On prescription orders, when the instructions to the pharmacist includes the expression, D.T.D. No. ... (ie, send ... such doses), it instructs the pharmacist to multiply the dose (amount of drug) stated in the order by the number indicated in the expression, D.T.D. No. ....

3. The *Square Meter Surface Area Method* (see Table III, page 1812) relates the surface area of individuals to dose. It is thought that this may be a more realistic way of relating dosages (see Crawford, *et al*,[3] Talbot, *et al*,[4] Lucey and Driscoll,[5] and Butler and Richie[6]).

$$\frac{\text{Body surface area of child}}{\text{Body surface area of adult}} \times \text{adult dose} =$$

$$\text{child's dose (approx)}$$

The average body surface area for an adult has been given as 1.73 square meters (M^2); hence,

$$\frac{\text{Body surface area of child } (M^2)}{1.73 \ M^2} \times \text{adult dose} =$$

$$\text{child's dose (approx)}$$

The body surface area for individuals may be found in various reference sources such as the previously mentioned APhA booklet, *Usual Doses for Infants and Children*, and in material by Shirkey and Barba.[7] Talbot, *et al*,[4] includes a chart which relates weight to body surface area. Wagner[8] presents a discussion on dosage of drugs.

Many drugs have doses stated as *so much drug/M^2 body surface area* and may be calculated as follows:

$$\text{Amount of drug/}M^2 \times \text{body surface area } (M^2) =$$

$$\text{individual's dose}$$

4. Drug doses are often stated in *mg/Kg body weight* and may be calculated as follows:

$$\text{mg/Kg} \times \text{body weight (Kg)} = \text{individual's dose}$$

5. Drug doses also may be stated in *units;* eg, vitamins A and D, antibiotics, and hormones. This means that a certain quantity of biologic activity of that drug is called 1 unit. When the term unit is used in connection with a drug, the calculations involved are the same as those for more familiar weight or volume notations. The USP often standardizes the unit for such drugs so that the expression "USP Units" is used. This means the units are calculated, based on a USP assay procedure and reference standard.

Examples

1. The adult dose of a drug is 5 gr. What is the dose for a 3-year-old child?

Use Young's Rule:

$$\text{Child's dose (approx)} = \frac{3}{3 + 12} \times 5 \text{ gr} = 1 \text{ gr}$$

2. Determine the dose for each ingredient contained in 1 dose of the following prescription order.

℞

Solid A	300 mg
Solid B	150 mg
Solid C	200 mg

D.T.D. No. 12 M. ft. capsules.

The directions to the pharmacist request him to make and send 12 capsules containing the 3 solids in the amounts indicated. Thus, the dose of each ingredient is as stated in the prescription order.

3. How much of each ingredient is used in compounding the following prescription order?

℞

Drug E	7.2 Gm
Drug F	0.24 Gm
Drug G	1.2 Gm

M. ft. capsules no. 24.

In this prescription order the prescriber requests that 24 capsules be made from the three ingredients. The amounts of the ingredients requested are considerable and drugs usually do not have doses of 7.2 Gm or 1.2 Gm, so that division of the amounts by the number of doses (24) is required. The pharmacist should check a textbook or compendium to confirm the average adult dose.

Drug E: 7.2 Gm ÷ 24 = 0.300 Gm
Drug F: 0.24 Gm ÷ 24 = 0.010 Gm
Drug G: 1.2 Gm ÷ 24 = 0.050 Gm

4. What is the dose for a 40-lb child if the average adult dose of the medicament is 10 mg?

Use Clark's Rule:

$$\text{Child's dose (approx)} = \frac{40}{150} \times 10 \text{ mg} = 2.67 \text{ mg}$$

5. What is the dose for an 8-month-old infant if the average adult dose of a drug is 250 mg?

Use Fried's Rule:

$$\text{Infant's dose (approx)} = \frac{8}{150} \times 250 \text{ mg} = 13.3 \text{ mg}$$

6. If the average adult dose of a drug is 50 mg, what is the dose for a child that has a body surface area equal to 0.57 M^2?

$$\text{Child's dose (approx)} = \frac{0.57}{1.73} \times 50 \text{ mg} = 16.5 \text{ mg}$$

7. A prescription order calls for 10 units of a drug to be taken 3 times a day. How much will the patient have taken after 7 days?

$$10 \text{ units/dose} \times 3 \text{ doses/day} \times 7 \text{ days} = 210 \text{ units}$$

8. If 250 units of an antibiotic weighs 1 mg, how many units are in 15 mg?

$$250 \text{ units/mg} \times 15 \text{ mg} = 3750 \text{ units}$$

Problems

1. Calculate the dose for each ingredient in the following prescription order?

℞

Chemical J	10 mg
Chemical K	50 mg
Chemical L	300 mg

M. ft. capsules D.T.D. No. 14.

2. Calculate the dose of each ingredient in the following prescription order?

℞

Drug Q	10.5 Gm
Drug R	6.3 Gm

Make 21 doses.

3. An 8-fl oz prescription order contains 6 fl dr of a tincture. If 1 teaspoonful 4 times a day is prescribed, how much tincture does the patient take/dose and how much does he take daily?

4. How many 0.3-ml doses are contained in 15 ml of a solution?

5. If 1 mg of a hormone equals 22.5 units, how many mg are required to obtain 1 unit?

6. What is the dose of a drug for a 9-month-old infant if the average adult dose is 25 mg?

7. What is the dose of a drug for a 6-year-old child if the average adult dose is 1½ gr?

8. What is the dose of a drug for a child that weighs 28 lb if the average adult dose is 100 mg?

9. What is the dose of a drug for an individual that has a 1.21 M^2 body surface area? The average adult dose is 400,000 units.

10. What is the dose of a medicament for a child that weighs 66 lb if the dose is stated as 2.5 mg/Kg body weight?

11. What is the dose of a drug for an average adult patient if the dose of the drug is 45 mg/M^2?

12. If a bottle contains 80 units of a drug/ml, how many ml must the patient take to get a 60-unit dose? If the bottle contains 10 ml total volume of the drug solution, how many days' supply will the patient have if he uses 60 units daily?

Remember: It is always better to look up the dose of drugs in textbooks or compendia than to rely on memory or equations.

Reducing and Enlarging Formulas

Rules

1. Determine the total weight or volume of ingredients and convert, if necessary, to the system of the quantities desired. The quantities in the original and new formulas will have the same ratio.

2. To reduce formulas in the metric system, divide by a power of 10 by moving the decimal place to the left the required number of places for each ingredient; to enlarge formulas, multiply by a power of 10 by moving the decimal place to the right the required number of places.

Examples

1. The formula for a syrup is

Drug M	140 Gm
Sucrose	450 Gm
Purified Water, q.s., to make	1000 ml

a. To find the quantities required for 100 ml, move the decimal place to the left since only ⅒, of the original formula quantity is needed.

14.0.	14 Gm
45.0.	45 Gm
100.0.	100 ml

b. What quantities are required to compound 60 ml of the syrup?

The new formula required $^{60}/_{1000}$ or 0.06 parts of the quantities in the original formula (1000 ml). Multiply the original quantities by 0.06 to get the new quantities.

Drug M	0.06 × 140 Gm = 8.4 Gm
Sucrose	0.06 × 450 Gm = 27.0 Gm
Purified Water, to	0.06 × 1000 ml = 60.0 ml

2. Calculate the amounts needed for 100 Gm of antiseptic powder as follows:

Solid A	2 Gm
Solid B	1 Gm
Solid C	7 Gm
Solid D	25 Gm
Solid E	115 Gm
	150 Gm

The original formula calls for a total of 150 Gm and the new one for 100 Gm. Form the following ratio to determine the quantities for the new formula:

$$\frac{100 \text{ Gm}}{150 \text{ Gm}} = 0.667$$

Each ingredient must be multiplied by 0.667 to reduce the original formula of 150 Gm to 100 Gm of finished product.

Solid A	2 Gm × 0.667 = 1.33 Gm
Solid B	1 Gm × 0.667 = 0.667 Gm
Solid C	7 Gm × 0.667 = 4.67 Gm
Solid D	25 Gm × 0.667 = 16.7 Gm
Solid E	115 Gm × 0.667 = 76.7 Gm
	100.067 Gm

3. Prescription orders where the instruction to the pharmacist calls for making a certain number of doses of an ingredient or mixture of several ingredients are a type of formula enlargement. The expression usually used is D.T.D., which means send such doses (see page 1810). Occasionally the prescriber will not use this expression, but inspection of amounts of the ingredients indicates that this is what is desired. For example,

℞

Solid H	50	mg
Solid K	150	mg
Liquid N	0.2	ml

M. ft. capsules, D.T.D. no. 24.

The pharmacist checked the individual doses of the ingredients and found them to be slightly below the average adult dose, confirming that the prescriber wanted the quantities listed to be multiplied by 24.

Ingredients	Amounts		Multiplier	New amounts	
Solid H	50	mg	× 24	1200	mg or 1.2 Gm
Solid K	150	mg	× 24	3600	mg or 3.6 Gm
Liquid N	0.2	ml	× 24	4.8 ml	

Problems

1. The formula for a liquid preparation is

Liquid C	35	ml
Solid B	9	Gm
Liquid R	2.5	ml
Liquid P	20	ml
Purified water, sufficient to make	100	ml

Calculate the quantities of the ingredients to make 2.5 liters.

2. The formula for an ointment is

Solid G	1	℥
Liquid D	30	♏
Solid M	3	℥
Ointment base, sufficient to make	1	℥

Calculate quantities of the ingredients for 2 ℔.

3. How much of each of the 3 solids and how much purified water are needed to properly compound the following prescription order?

℞

Solid N	0.1	mg
Solid Q	2.5	mg
Solid R	150.0	mg
Purified water, q.s., to	5	ml

M. ft. solution, D.T.D. no. 48.

4. How much of each ingredient is required to compound 90 ml of the following product?

Solid S	7.5	Gm
Solid T	25	Gm
Oil C	350	ml
Alcohol	250	ml
Purified water, q.s., to	1000	ml

Density

Density is defined as the mass of a substance per unit volume. It has the units of mass over volume.

Specific gravity is the ratio of the weight of a substance in air to that of an equal volume of water. It does not have any units.

In the metric system both density and specific gravity may be numerically equal, although the density figure has units. In the English system, density and specific gravity are not numerically equal; eg, the density of water is 62.4 lb/ft³ and the specific gravity is 1. This shows the convenience of the metric system. The equations for calculating density, weight, and volume are as follows:

$$Density = \frac{weight}{volume}$$

$$Weight = density \times volume$$

$$Volume = \frac{weight}{density}$$

Given any two variables, the third one can be calculated.

Density and specific gravity are discussed in greater detail in Chapter 9.

The USP states:

"Unless otherwise stated the specific gravity basis is 25°C/25°C (apparent), ie, the ratio of the weight of a substance in air at 25°C to that of an equal volume of water at the same temperature."

Examples

1. A pharmacist weighs out 2 Kg of glycerin (density, 1.25 Gm/ml). What is the volume of the glycerin? Remember to convert to like units; eg, Kg to Gm.

$$Volume = \frac{2000 \ Gm}{1.25 \ Gm/ml} = 1600 \ ml$$

2. What is the weight of 60 ml of oil whose density is 0.9624 Gm/ml?

$$Weight = 60 \ ml \times 0.9624 \ Gm/ml$$

$$= 57.7 \ Gm$$

3. Calculate the weight of 30 ml of sulfuric acid whose density is 1.8 Gm/ml.

$$Weight = 1.8 \ Gm/ml \times 30 \ ml = 54 \ Gm$$

4. If a prescription order requires 25 Gm of concentrated hydrochloric acid (density, 1.18 Gm/ml), what volume should the pharmacist measure?

$$Volume = \frac{25 \ Gm}{1.18 \ Gm/ml} = 21.2 \ ml$$

Problems

1. What is the weight in grams of 1 liter of alcohol (density, 0.816 Gm/ml)?
2. What is the volume (ml) of 1 lb of glycerin whose density is 1.25 Gm/ml?
3. What volume does 65 Gm of an acid whose density is 1.2 Gm/ml occupy?

Ratio and Proportion

This arithmetical procedure often can be used to solve various pharmaceutical compounding and dispensing problems.

A ratio states the relation of one quantity to another and may be written as a common fraction (implying division) or with a colon between the two numbers. For example, three parts compared with four parts is written ¾ or 3:4 and is stated, "three is to four." The ratio is ¾, 3:4, or three is to four. Any units may be substituted for "parts" but the value of the ratio does not change. The units must be the same.

Two equal ratios that are set equal to each other result in an equation which is called a proportion. For example, ¾ = ¹⁵⁄₂₀, 3:4::15:20, or "three is to four as fifteen is to twenty" are ways of writing and stating that 3 and 4 form the same ratio or fraction as 15 and 20.

The first and last terms of a proportion are called the extremes, and the second and third terms are called the means.

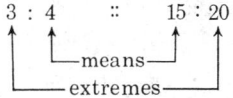

Rules

The following statements are true for any proportion.

1. The product of the means equals the product of the extremes.
2. The product of the means divided by one extreme gives the other extreme.
3. The product of the extremes divided by one mean gives the other mean. Therefore, if any three terms of a proportion are known, the fourth may be found by simple calculation.

In solving problems involving proportions the following procedure may be used.

First—Let the unknown quantity be represented by X and let it be the fourth term.

Second—Let the third term be that number in the question which expresses the same kind of value (unit) as is expected in the answer.

Third—Arrange the remaining two quantities in the same ratio as the third term and X. Thus the first and second terms will express the same kind of values (units) and the third and fourth terms will express the same kind of values. If the answer sought (X) is to be greater than the third term, the second term will be larger than the first, and vice versa.

Fourth—To solve for X, divide the product of the means by the known extreme. Cancel to simplify. Since the first and second terms form a ratio, common factors may be removed without altering the ratio; and since the first and third terms are actually numerators of equal fractions, they can be divided by the same number without changing the proportion.

Example

100 Gm of a drug cost $1.80. How much will 25 Gm cost?

If the three quantities in the problem, namely 100 Gm, $1.80, and 25 Gm are considered, it will be seen readily that 100 Gm bears the same relation to 25 Gm as $1.80 does to the unknown quantity to be calculated. In other words, the quantities and prices form equal ratios. The following proportion can be made:

$$100 \ Gm : 25 \ Gm :: \$1.80 : \$X$$

There are three known terms in the statement and X, the unknown term. Arithmetically the product of the means must equal the product of the extremes. Therefore, if one of the extremes is unknown, it may be calculated by dividing the product of the means by the known extreme.

$$X = \frac{25 \text{ Gm} \times \$1.80}{100 \text{ Gm}} = \$0.45$$

While the proportion is preferably set down as given above, it may be stated in several other ways. These are given below merely to show their relationship to the original form. It may be stated as two equal ratios in equation form:

$$\frac{100 \text{ Gm}}{25 \text{ Gm}} = \frac{\$1.80}{X}$$

Keeping in mind the basic three rules, it is also possible to place the unknown quantity, X, in either the first, second, or third position as long as the relationship of the three known terms is not altered. Thus, the problem may be written as

$$25 \text{ Gm}:100 \text{ Gm}::X:\$1.80 \text{ (Rule 3)}$$

$$\frac{25 \text{ Gm} \times \$1.80}{100 \text{ Gm}} = \$0.45$$

or

$$\$1.80:X::100 \text{ Gm}:25 \text{ Gm} \text{ (Rule 3)}$$

$$\frac{\$1.80 \times 25 \text{ Gm}}{100 \text{ Gm}} = \$0.45$$

or

$$X:\$1.80::25 \text{ Gm}:100 \text{ Gm} \text{ (Rule 2)}$$

$$\frac{\$1.80 \times 25 \text{ Gm}}{100 \text{ Gm}} = \$0.45$$

Obviously, the method of ratio and proportion can be used to solve more involved problems.

Problems

1. If a drug cost $3.00/Gm, how much would 65 mg cost? How much would 5 gr cost?
2. One pound of a chemical costs $7.65. What is the cost of sufficient chemical needed to make 10,000 capsules containing 0.2 Gm of the chemical?

See also the preparation of isotonic solutions by proportion, Chapter 83.

Percentage

Percent, written as %, means per hundred. Fifteen percent is written 15% and means $^{15}/_{100}$, 0.15, or 15 parts in 100 parts. Percent is a type of ratio and has no units. Thus 10% of 1500 tablets is $^{10}/_{100} \times 1500$ tablets = 150 tablets.

To change percent to a fraction the percent number becomes the numerator and 100 is the denominator. To change a fraction to percent, put the fraction in a form having 100 as its denominator; multiply by 100 so that the numerator becomes the percent.

$$\frac{1}{2} = \frac{50}{100}; \quad \frac{50}{100} \times 100 = 50\%$$

$$\frac{1}{8} = \frac{12.5}{100}; \quad \frac{12.5}{100} \times 100 = 12.5\%$$

Calculations involving percentages are continually encountered by pharmacists. He must be familiar, not only with the arithmetical principles, but also with certain compendial interpretations of the different type percentages envolving solutions and mixtures. The USP states:

"Percentage concentrations of solutions are expressed as follows:
"*Percent weight in weight*—(w/w) expresses the number of Gm of a constituent in 100 Gm of solution.

"*Percent weight in volume*—(w/v) expresses the number of Gm of a constituent in 100 ml of solution, and is used regardless of whether water or another liquid is the solvent.
"*Percent volume in volume*—(v/v) expresses the number of ml of a constituent in 100 ml of solution.
"The term *percent* used without qualification means, for mixtures of solids, percent weight in weight; for solutions or suspensions of solids in liquids, percent weight in volume; for solutions of liquids in liquids, percent volume in volume; and for solutions of gases in liquids, percent weight in volume. For example, a 1 percent solution is prepared by dissolving 1 Gm of a solid or 1 ml of a liquid in sufficient of the solvent to make 100 ml of the solution.
"In the dispensing of prescription medications, slight changes in volume owing to variations in room temperature may be disregarded."

Ratio Strength

This is another manner of expressing strength. Such phrases as "1 in 10" are understood to mean that 1 part by volume of a liquid is to be diluted with, or 1 part by weight of a solid dissolved in, sufficient of the solution to make the finished solution 10 parts by volume. For example, a 1:10 solution means 1 ml of a liquid or 1 Gm of a solid dissolved in sufficient solvent to make 10 ml of solution. It can be converted to percent by:

$$1 \text{ Gm}:10 \text{ ml}::X \text{ Gm}:100 \text{ ml}$$

$$X = 10 \text{ Gm in } 100 \text{ ml of solution which is } 10\%$$

The expression "parts per thousand" (eg, 1–5000) always means parts weight in volume when dealing with solutions of solids in liquids and is similar to the above expression. A 1–5000 solution means 1 Gm of solute in sufficient solvent to make 5000 ml of solution. This can be converted to percent by:

$$1 \text{ Gm}:5000 \text{ ml}::X \text{ Gm}:100 \text{ ml}$$

$$X = 0.02 \text{ Gm in } 100 \text{ ml solution which is } 0.02\%$$

The expression "trituration" has two different meanings in pharmacy. One refers to the process of particle-size reduction, commonly by grinding or rubbing in a mortar with the aid of a pestle. The other meaning refers to a dilution of a potent powdered drug with a suitable powdered diluent in a definite proportion by weight. It is the second meaning that is used in this chapter. When a pharmacist refers to a "1 in 10 trituration" he means a mixture of solids composed of 1 Gm of drug plus sufficient diluent (another solid) to make 10 Gm of mixture of *dilution*. In this case the "1 in 10 trituration" is actually a solid dilution of a drug with an inert solid. The strength of a trituration may also be stated as percent *w/w*.

Thus, the term trituration has come to mean a solid dilution of a potent drug with a chemically and physiologically inert solid.

The meanings implied by the USP statements under *Percentage* are illustrated below with a few examples of the three types of percentages.

Weight-in-Volume Percentages

This is the type of percent problem encountered on prescription orders. The preparation of these solutions is very simple if the student will keep in mind that for practical purposes the calculation is made on the basis that 1 ℥ (apoth) of solvent weighs 455 gr, or 1 ml of solvent weighs 1 Gm. The density of the solvent or solution is *not* required in these calculations. The volume occupied by the solute is not considered in *w/v* problems. The volume of the solvent is *not* known because sufficient solvent is added to make a given or known final volume.

Examples

1. Prepare 1 fl oz of a 10% solution.

Since this is a solution of a solid in a liquid, this is a *w/v* solution. Therefore, 455 gr/f℥ is taken as the base.

$$455 \text{ gr/f℥} \times \% \text{ (decimal)} \times \text{no. of f℥} = \text{gr solute}$$

$$455 \text{ gr/f℥} \times 0.10 \times 1 \text{ f℥} = 45.5 \text{ gr solute}$$

45.5 gr. is dissolved in sufficient purified water to make 1 f℥ of solution.

2. How much of a drug is required to compound 4 fl oz of a 3% solution in alcohol?

$$455 \text{ gr/f℥} \times \% \text{ (decimal)} \times \text{no. of f℥} = \text{gr solute}$$

$$455 \text{ gr/f℥} \times 0.03 \times 4 \text{ f℥} = 54.6 \text{ gr drug}$$

It should be emphasized that the percentage of solute is calculated from 455 gr/f℥ of water because this is the only way in which solutions of identical percentage strength can be prepared in both the metric and apothecary systems.

3. How much 0.9% solution of sodium chloride can be made from ½ ℥ of NaCl?

$$480 \text{ gr/℥} \div 2 = 240 \text{ gr in } ½ \text{ ℥}$$

$$455 \text{ gr/f℥} \times \% \text{ (decimal)} \times \text{no. of f℥} = \text{gr solute}$$

$$455 \text{ gr/f℥} \times 0.009 \times Y \text{ f℥} = 240 \text{ gr}$$

$$Y = \frac{240 \text{ gr}}{455 \text{ gr/f℥} \times 0.009} = 58.6 \text{ f℥} = 1 \text{ qt, 1 pt, 10.6 f℥}$$

In the metric system the following equation can be used to calculate the quantity of solute necessary to prepare a given percent *w/v* solution.

$$\text{ml of solution} \times \% \text{ (decimal)} = \text{Gm solute required}$$

4. How many grams of a drug are required to make 120 ml of a 25% solution.

Remember: percent *w/v* is indicated.

$$\text{ml of solution} \times \% \text{ (decimal)} = \text{Gm solute required}$$

$$120 \text{ ml} \times 0.25 = 30 \text{ Gm of drug}$$

5. How would you prepare 480 ml of a 1 in 750 solution of an antiseptic?

Remember: percent *w/v* is indicated.

1 in 750 means 1 Gm of the antiseptic dissolved in sufficient solvent to make 750 ml solution.

By ratio and proportion,

$$1 \text{ Gm}:750 \text{ ml}::U \text{ Gm}:480 \text{ ml}$$

$$U = 1 \text{ Gm} \times 480 \text{ ml}/750 \text{ ml} = 0.640 \text{ Gm antiseptic needed}$$

Dissolve 0.64 Gm of antiseptic in sufficient solvent to make 480 ml solution.

6. How much of a substance is needed to prepare 1 liter of a 1:10,000 solution?

1:10,000 means 1 Gm of a substance in 10,000 ml of solution

$$1 \text{ liter} = 1000 \text{ ml}$$

By ratio and proportion,

$$1 \text{ Gm}:10,000 \text{ ml}::V \text{ Gm}:1000 \text{ ml}$$

$$V = 1 \text{ Gm} \times 1000 \text{ ml}/10,000 \text{ ml} = 0.1 \text{ Gm substance needed}$$

Problems

1. How would you make 3 fl oz of a 12.5% solution?
2. How many liters of a 4% solution can be made from 4 oz of a solid?
3. How many liters of an 8% solution can be made from 500 Gm of a solid?

4. How many grams of a drug are needed to make 4 liters of a 1 in 500 solution?

Weight-in-Weight Percentages

For this type of problem, remember that there are 480 gr in an apothecary ounce (480 gr/℥). Density must be considered in some of these problems. If a weight-in-weight solution is requested on a prescription order, both the solute and solvent must be weighed, or the solute and the solvent may be measured if their densities are taken into consideration in determining the volumes. Since the solutions are made to a given weight, a given volume is not always obtainable; eg, 4 ℥ does *not* equal 4 f ℥ and 100 Gm of solution does *not* equal 100 ml. For the apothecary system, the following equation may be used to calculate the grains of solute required.

$$480 \text{ gr/℥} \times \% \text{ (decimal)} \times \text{no. of ℥} = \text{gr solute required}$$

Examples

1. What weights of solute and solvent are required to make ℥ 2 of a 3% *w/w* solution of a drug in 90% alcohol?

$$480 \text{ gr/℥} \times \% \text{ (decimal)} \times \text{number of ℥}$$
$$= \text{gr solute required}$$

$$480 \text{ gr/℥} \times 0.03 \times 2 \text{ ℥} = 28.8 \text{ gr of drug required}$$

$$480 \text{ gr/℥} \times 2 \text{ ℥} = 960 \text{ gr}$$

$$\begin{array}{r} 960.0 \text{ gr} \\ - 28.8 \text{ gr} \\ \hline 931.2 \text{ gr solvent} \end{array}$$

2. The solubility of boric acid is 1 Gm in 18 ml of water at 25°C. What is the percentage strength, *w/w*, of a saturated solution?

1 Gm of boric acid + 18 ml of water make a saturated solution, 18 ml of water weighs 18 Gm; hence, the weight of solution is 19 Gm. The amount of boric acid present is 1 Gm in 19 Gm solution; therefore, the following proportion can be set up:

$$1 \text{ Gm}:19 \text{ Gm}::X \text{ Gm}:100 \text{ Gm}$$

$$X = 1 \text{ Gm} \times 100 \text{ Gm}/19 \text{ Gm} = 5.26 \text{ Gm}/100 \text{ Gm or } 5.26\%$$

3. How many grams of a chemical are needed to prepare 200 Gm of a 10% *w/w* solution?

10% *w/w* means 10 Gm solute in 100 Gm total solution. If 100 Gm solution contains 10 Gm of solute, there are 90 Gm of solvent (100 Gm solution − 10 Gm solute = 90 Gm solvent). The following proportion may be set up:

$$10 \text{ Gm}:100 \text{ Gm}::M \text{ Gm}:200 \text{ Gm}$$

$$M = 10 \text{ Gm} \times 200 \text{ Gm}/100 \text{ Gm} = 20 \text{ Gm solute needed}$$

4. How would you make 240 ml of a 2% *w/w* solution of a drug in alcohol. The density of alcohol is 0.816 Gm/ml.

a. First, convert 240 ml to weight. *Remember:* alcohol is the solvent and it has a density different from that of water.

$$\text{Density} = \text{weight/volume}$$

$$\text{Weight} = \text{density} \times \text{volume}$$

$$\text{Weight} = 0.816 \text{ Gm/ml} \times 240 \text{ ml} = 195.8 \text{ Gm (196 Gm)}$$

b. 2% *w/w* means 2 Gm solute in 100 Gm solution. In this problem the final weight of solution is not known; 240 ml (196 Gm) of alcohol represents the solvent only. The solvent is 98% *w/w* of the total solution, so that the following proportion may be set up:

$$2 \text{ Gm}:98 \text{ Gm}::N \text{ Gm}:196 \text{ Gm}$$

$$N = 2 \text{ Gm} \times 196 \text{ Gm}/98 \text{ Gm} = 4.00 \text{ Gm}$$

c. Dissolve 4.00 Gm of the drug in 240 ml alcohol. The resulting solution will be 2% *w/w* and have a volume slightly larger than 240 ml because of the volume displacement of the drug.

5. How much of a 5% *w/w* solution can be made from 1 oz avoir of a chemical?

$$480 \text{ gr}/\text{ʒ} \times \% \text{ (decimal)} \times \text{no. of ʒ} = \text{gr of solute}$$

$$1 \text{ oz av} = 437.5 \text{ gr}$$

$$\text{no. of ʒ} = \frac{\text{gr of solute}}{(480 \text{ gr}/\text{ʒ} \times \% \text{ as a decimal fraction})}$$

$$= \frac{437.5 \text{ gr}}{480 \text{ gr}/\text{ʒ} \times 0.05} = 18.2 \text{ ʒ} = 1 \text{ ℔}, 6.2 \text{ ʒ}$$

Compounding problems involving solid preparations (such as mixtures of powder) and semisolid preparations (such as ointments, creams, and suppositories) are also percent *w/w*. For example:

1. How much drug is required to make 2 ʒ of a 10% ointment.

Since this preparation is an ointment, percent *w/w* is indicated.

$$480 \text{ gr}/\text{ʒ} \times \% \text{ (decimal)} \times \text{no. of ʒ} = \text{gr drug}$$

$$480 \text{ gr}/\text{ʒ} \times 0.10 \times 2 \text{ ʒ} = 96 \text{ gr} = 1 \text{ ʒ}, 1 \text{ ϶}, 16 \text{ gr drug}$$

The same procedure could be used for mixtures of powders, suppository masses, etc. Instead of using units in the various measuring systems, quantities can be indicated "by parts" similar to percent *w/v* solutions. The term "parts" can then mean any unit in any measuring system, as long as the units are kept constant. For example:

2.

℞

Solid A.........................	0.5 parts
Powder B........................	3.0 parts
Powder C, q.s., to..............	30 parts

How many Gm of each of the three ingredients are required to make 30 Gm of the product?

Since the product is a mixture of powders, percent *w/w* is indicated· In the above prescription order the total product is 30 parts because Powder C is used to "q.s. to" or "make up to" 30 parts. Therefore, 0.5 Gm of Powder A and 3.0 Gm of Powder B are needed

Powder A...............	0.5 Gm
Powder B...............	+ 3.0 Gm
	3.5 Gm

Total product..........	30.0 Gm	
	− 3.5 Gm	
	26.5 Gm	Powder C needed

3.

℞

Solid D.........................	3.0 parts
Solid E.........................	6.0 parts
Ointment Base Q.................	30.0 parts

How much of each ingredient is needed to make 60 Gm of the ointment?

Solid D.........................	3.0 parts
Solid E.........................	6.0 parts
Base Q..........................	30.0 parts
	39.0 parts total

Since a total of 60 Gm is needed, the following proportions can be made:

$$39 \text{ Parts total in ℞}:60 \text{ Gm total needed}::3.0 \text{ parts}$$

$$\text{Solid D}:X \text{ Gm}$$

$$X = 60 \text{ Gm} \times 3.0 \text{ parts}/39 \text{ parts}$$

$$= 4.62 \text{ Gm Solid D needed}$$

$$39 \text{ Parts}:60 \text{ Gm}::6.0 \text{ parts}:Y \text{ Gm}$$

$$Y = 60 \text{ Gm} \times 6.0 \text{ parts}/39 \text{ parts} = 9.23 \text{ Gm Solid E needed}$$

4.62 Gm Solid D	60.00 Gm	Total
+ 9.23 Gm Solid E	− 13.85 Gm	
13.85 Gm	46.15 Gm	Base Q needed

The amount of ointment base needed can also be calculated by the above ratio and proportion method.

4. What is the percent strength of a salt solution obtained by diluting 100 Gm of a 5% solution to 200 Gm.

a. Since the solutions are expressed by weight, percent *w/w* is indicated. 5% *w/w* means 5 Gm active ingredient plus 95 Gm solvent to make 100 Gm solution.

b. 100 Gm solution is diluted to 200 Gm by the addition of water. The solvent was not stated, so it is assumed to be purified water, and 100 ml of water = 100 Gm.

c. The original 5 Gm active ingredient is now in 200 Gm solution; thus, the following proportion can be set up:

$$5 \text{ Gm}:200 \text{ Gm}::X \text{ Gm}:100 \text{ Gm}$$

$$X = 5 \text{ Gm} \times 100 \text{ Gm}/200 \text{ Gm} = 2.5 \text{ Gm}/100 \text{ Gm} = 2.5\%$$

There is another type of percent *w/w* problem that should be mentioned. This involves compounding *w/w* solutions using the *weight* of 1 fl oz of water. One fl oz of water weighs 455 gr. To solve this type of problem, the density of the final solution must be known. In practice the density of the finished product is usually not known, so that this type of problem has no practical value and will not be illustrated.

Problems

1. How much of the drug and solvent are needed to compound the following prescription order?

℞

Compound A...........................	6% *w/w*
Solvent, q.s., to make...............	4 ʒ

2. How many grams of solute are needed to prepare 240 Gm of a 12% *w/w* solution?

3. How many Kg of a 20% *w/w* solution can be made from 1 Kg of the solute?

4. How would you prepare 120 ml of a glycerin (density, 1.25 Gm/ml) solution that is 3% *w/w* with respect to a drug?

5. How much of each substance is needed to prepare a total of 24 Gm of the following suppository mass?

Compound K...........................	0.3 Gm
Solid H..............................	0.15 Gm
Suppository base, q.s., to...........	2.0 Gm

6. How would you prepare 500 ml of a 15% *w/w* aqueous solution?

7. How much of each of the ingredients is required to make 1 Kg of the following mixture?

Powder P..................	1 part
Powder Q..................	8 parts
Powder R..................	12 parts
Powder S..................	15 parts
	36 parts

Volume-in-Volume Percentages

A direct calculation of percentage from the total volume is made, neglecting slight shrinkages which may occur and making up to the desired volume with the diluent. The following equation is based on the fact that 480 minims = 1 fl oz may be used.

480 ℳ/fl oz × % (decimal) × number of fl oz

$$= \text{minims of drug}$$

Examples

1. How much of a liquid is needed to make 6 fl oz of a hand lotion containing 0.5% v/v of the liquid?

480 ℳ/fl oz × % (decimal) × no. of fl oz = ℳ of drug

480 ℳ/fl oz × 0.005 × 6 fl oz = 14.4 ℳ of liquid needed

Add sufficient lotion to 14.4 ℳ of the liquid to make 6 f ℥ of the product.

2. How much 90% alcohol is required to compound 500 ml of a 10% alcohol mixture? In v/v mixtures, percentage is directly proportional to volume.

a. Since alcohol, a liquid, is mixed with water, percent v/v is indicated. Assume no shrinkage.

b. 500 ml of the 10% solution contains the following amount of alcohol:

$$10 \text{ ml}:100 \text{ ml}::X \text{ ml}:500 \text{ ml}$$

$$X = 10 \text{ ml} \times 500 \text{ ml}/100 \text{ ml} = 50 \text{ ml alcohol}$$

c. 90% alcohol contains 90 ml alcohol in 100 ml solution. 50 ml of pure alcohol is needed; therefore, the following proportion may be set up:

$$90 \text{ ml}:100 \text{ ml}::50 \text{ ml}:Y \text{ ml}$$

$$Y = 100 \text{ ml} \times 50 \text{ ml}/90 \text{ ml} = 55.5 \text{ ml of } 90\% \text{ alcohol needed}$$

Problems

1. How many minims of a liquid are needed to make 4 f℥ of a 12.5% v/v solution?

2. How much purified water should be added to 1 liter of alcohol (95% v/v) to make 50% v/v alcohol?

3. What is the percentage strength, weight in weight, of a liquid made by dissolving 16 Gm of a salt in 30 ml of water?

4. How much drug will be required to prepare 1 fl oz of a 2.5% solution?

5. What is the percentage, weight in weight, of sugar in a syrup made by dissolving 5 Kg of sugar in 8 Kg of water?

6. How many Gm of a drug are required to prepare 120 ml of a 12.5% aqueous solution?

7. How much drug is needed to compound a liter of a 1–2500 aqueous solution?

8. A solution contains 37% of active ingredient. How much of this solution is needed to prepare 480 ml of an aqueous solution containing 2.5% of the active ingredient?

9. How much of a drug is required to make 2 qt of a 1–1200 solution?

Stock Solutions

In order to facilitate the dispensing of certain soluble substances, the pharmacist frequently prepares solutions of high concentration. Portions of these concentrated solutions are diluted to give required solutions of lesser strength. These concentrated solutions are known as stock solutions. This procedure is satisfactory if the substances are stable in solution or if the solutions are to be used before they decompose.

In the case of potent substances, a properly prepared stock solution permits the pharmacist to obtain accurately a quantity of solid which might otherwise be difficult to weigh. In the case of frequently prescribed salt solutions, a stock solution readily provides the required amount of salt without the necessity of weighing and dissolving it everytime.

Stock solutions may be of various concentrations depending on the requirements for use. The stock solutions should be properly labeled and fractional parts needed to make various strengths also may be listed as a further convenience. Typical concentrations might be:

ℳ ml = 1 ml; %; by parts; ratio strength; 100 ml = 1 Gm

There is a type of compounding and dispensing problem that involves the concept of stock solutions. This problem involves the patient diluting a dose from the prescription order to a given volume to obtain a solution of desired concentration.

For example, how many grams of a salt are required to make 90 ml of a stock solution, 5 ml of which makes a 1–3000 solution when diluted to 500 ml?

a. Determine how many Gm are in 500 ml of a 1–3000 solution.

$$1 \text{ Gm}:3000 \text{ ml}::X \text{ Gm}:500 \text{ ml}$$

$$X = 1 \text{ Gm} \times 500 \text{ ml}/3000 \text{ ml} =$$
$$0.167 \text{ Gm salt in 500 ml of 1–3000 solution}$$

b. The 0.167 Gm in the dilute solution came from the 5 ml of the original stock solution (prescription order). The following proportion can be used:

$$0.167 \text{ Gm}:5 \text{ ml}::Y \text{ Gm}:90 \text{ ml}$$

$$Y = 0.167 \text{ Gm} \times 90 \text{ ml}/5 \text{ ml} = 3.01 \text{ Gm salt}$$
needed to make the original 90 ml of stock solution

Problems

1. How much of a drug is needed to compound 120 ml of a prescription order such that when 1 teaspoonful of the solution is diluted to 1 qt, a 1–750 solution results?

2. How many grams of a drug are needed to make 240 ml of a solution of such strength that when 5 ml is diluted to 2 qt, a 1–2500 solution results?

Parts Per Million

An expression that is occasionally used in the compounding of prescription orders is *parts per million* (ppm). This is another way of expressing concentration, particularly concentrations of very dilute preparations. A 1% solution may be expressed as 1 part/100, a 0.1% solution is 0.1 parts/100 or 1 part/1000. A 1 ppm solution contains 1 part of solute/1 million parts of solution; 5 ppm is 5 parts solute/1 million parts solution, and so on. Remember that the two parts must have the same units, except in the metric system where 1Gm = 1 ml of water.

Sodium fluoride is a drug that may be prescribed by a dentist as a preventative for tooth decay in children. It is used only in very dilute solutions due to the drug's toxicity and because only minute quantities are needed.

℞
    Sod. Fluoride, q.s.
    Purified water, q.s. 60 ml
    Make soln. such that when 1 ℥ is diluted to 1 glassful of water a 2 ppm soln. results.
    Sig: 1 ℥ in a glassful of water daily.

The mathematics to solve this compounding problem

is easy once the steps for calculating the answer are outlined. This problem should be worked "backwards."

    a. The amount of NaF needed is not known.
    b. One glassful of water has a volume of 240 ml. The concentration of NaF in 240 ml is 2 ppm.
    c. The NaF solution poured into the glass came from a teaspoonful dose (1 ℥), which is equal to 5 ml.
    d. The 5-ml dose came from the prescription order bottle containing a NaF solution.

Now let us put it in numbers:

    a. 240 ml contains 2 ppm NaF.

$$2 \text{ Gm}:1{,}000{,}000 \text{ ml}::X \text{ Gm}:240 \text{ ml}$$

$$X = 2 \text{ Gm} \times 240 \text{ ml}/1{,}000{,}000 \text{ ml} = 0.00048 \text{ Gm}$$

    b. The 0.00048 Gm NaF in the glass came from the teaspoonful dose; therefore, the teaspoonful (5 ml) contained 0.00048 Gm NaF.
    c. The 5 ml came out of the original prescription order bottle (60 ml).

$$5 \text{ ml}:0.00048 \text{ Gm}::60 \text{ ml}:Y \text{ Gm}$$

$$Y = 0.00048 \text{ Gm} \times 60 \text{ ml}/5 \text{ ml} = 0.00576 \text{ Gm}$$

The pharmacist would weigh out 5.76 mg (actually, he would weigh out a larger quantity and take an aliquot part) and q.s. to 60 ml.

Another variation of this problem is where the prescriber requests the concentration in terms of fluoride ion (F^-). In this case the atomic weight of F^- and molecular weight of NaF are used in the calculation. If the request called for 2 ppm fluoride, the initial calculations would be the same as above and an additional step would be added at the end. The 5.76 mg would now represent the weight of fluoride ion needed. This must be converted to weight of NaF. The molecular weight of NaF is 42 Gm and the atomic weight of fluorine is 19 Gm. The following proportion can be set up:

$$5.76 \text{ mg}:19 \text{ Gm}::Z \text{ mg}:42 \text{ Gm}$$

$$Z = 5.76 \text{ mg} \times 42 \text{ Gm}/19 \text{ Gm} = 12.7 \text{ mg}$$

Problems

1. How many mg of NaF are needed in the following prescription order?

℞
Sodium Fluoride
Purified water, q.s. to 90 ml
M. ft. solution such that when 1 ℥ is dild. to 1 glassful of water a 3 ppm NaF soln. results.

Dilution and Concentration

Stock solutions can be diluted to make a product that has a lower concentration; also, mixtures of powders or semisolids (eg, ointments) can be diluted to give a product of lower concentration of the drug(s). The diluent is an inert solid or semisolid or base which does not contain any of the active ingredients. For example, how much of a diluent must be added to 50 Gm of a 10% ointment to make it a 5% ointment?

1. How many Gm of active ingredient is in 50 Gm of 10% ointment?

$$10 \text{ Gm}:100 \text{ Gm}::V \text{ Gm}:50 \text{ Gm}$$

$$V = 10 \text{ Gm} \times 50 \text{ Gm}/100 \text{ Gm} = 5 \text{ Gm}$$

2. How many Gm of a 5% ointment can be made from 5 Gm of active ingredient?

$$5 \text{ Gm}:100 \text{ Gm}::5 \text{ Gm}:W \text{ Gm}$$

$$W = 100 \text{ Gm} \times 5 \text{ Gm}/5 \text{ Gm} = 100 \text{ Gm}$$

3. How many Gm of base must be added to the 50 Gm of the original 10% ointment?

100 Gm	5% ointment
− 50 Gm	10% ointment
50 Gm	base

The term trituration was used previously to mean a dilute powder mixture of a drug. It is often necessary to further dilute this mixture in order to obtain the required amount of drug. For example, how much of a 1 in 10 trituration of a potent drug contains 200 mg of the drug?

1. A 1 in 10 trituration means 1 Gm of drug in 10 Gm of mixture or 1 Gm of drug plus 9 Gm diluent. *Remember:* mixtures of solids are percent *w/w*. The following proportion can be made:

$$1 \text{ Gm}:10 \text{ Gm}::0.2 \text{ Gm}:T \text{ Gm}$$

$$T = 10 \text{ Gm} \times 0.2 \text{ Gm}/1 \text{ Gm} = 2 \text{ Gm}$$

2. How much diluent must be added to 10 Gm of a 1:100 trituration to make a mixture that contains 1 mg of drug in each 10 Gm of the final mixture?

    a. Determine the amount of drug in 10 Gm of trituration.

$$1 \text{ Gm}:100 \text{ Gm}::M \text{ Gm}:10 \text{ Gm}$$

$$M = 1 \text{ Gm} \times 10 \text{ Gm}/100 \text{ Gm} = 0.1 \text{ Gm}$$

    b. Determine the amount of mixture that can be made from 0.1 Gm (100 mg) of drug.

$$1 \text{ mg}:10 \text{ Gm}::100 \text{ mg}:N \text{ Gm}$$

$$N = 10 \text{ Gm} \times 100 \text{ mg}/1 \text{ mg} = 1000 \text{ Gm}$$

    c. Determine the amount of diluent needed.

1000 Gm	total mixture
− 10 Gm	trituration
990 Gm	diluent

Occasionally it is necessary for a pharmacist to increase the strength of a product. For example, a prescription order calls for 50 Gm of a 10% ointment. The pharmacist only has a 5% ointment and the pure ingredient available. How much of the 5% ointment and the pure ingredient are needed to compound the prescription order?

1. Determine the amount of ingredient needed to compound the prescription order by setting up the following proportion:

$$10 \text{ Gm}:100 \text{ Gm}::Q \text{ Gm}:50 \text{ Gm}$$

$$Q = 10 \text{ Gm} \times 50 \text{ Gm}/100 \text{ Gm} = 5 \text{ Gm}$$

This means that there are 45 Gm (50 Gm − 5 Gm = 45 Gm) of the base (90% of the total).

2. Determine the amount of ingredient in 50 Gm of a 5% ointment by forming the following proportion:

$$5 \text{ Gm}:100 \text{ Gm}::R \text{ Gm}:50 \text{ Gm}$$

$$R = 5 \text{ Gm} \times 50 \text{ Gm}/100 \text{ Gm} = 2.5 \text{ Gm}$$

This means that there are 47.5 Gm of the base.

3. Determine the amount of 5% ointment needed.

$$47.5 \text{ Gm base}:50 \text{ Gm total 5\% ointment}::$$

$$45 \text{ Gm base needed}:S \text{ Gm of 5\% ointment}$$

$$S = 50 \text{ Gm} \times 45 \text{ Gm}/47.5 \text{ Gm} = 47.4 \text{ Gm}$$

4. Determine the amount of active ingredient.

$$
\begin{array}{r}
50.0 \text{ Gm total ointment required} \\
-\ 47.4 \text{ Gm } 5\% \text{ ointment required} \\
\hline
2.6 \text{ Gm active ingredient required}
\end{array}
$$

Mix 2.6 Gm active ingredient with 47.4 Gm of 5% ointment to give 50 Gm of 10% ointment.

Problems

1. The following prescription order was received in a pharmacy. If the only R cream available is a 10% concentration, how much of the 10% cream and how much diluent are required to compound the prescription order?

R

    R Cream 3% . . . . 30 Gm

2. How many grams of a 1:100 trituration contains 100 mcg of the active ingredient?
3. How many grams of a 1:1000 dilution can be made from 1 Gm of a 1:25 trituration?
4. How many grams of a 5% sulfur ointment and pure sulfur are needed to prepare 60 Gm of a 7.5% sulfur ointment?

Mixing Different Strengths

Rules

1. The sum of the products obtained by multiplying a series of quantities by their respective concentrations equals the product obtained by multiplying a concentration by the sum of the quantities. For example, the sum of the products, obtained by multiplying the individual weights or volumes of a series of preparations by the concentration of a given ingredient contained in each preparation, is equal to the product obtained by multiplying the total weight of the series of preparations by the percentage of the given ingredient resulting from a homogeneous mixture of the same series of preparations.
2. When mixing products of varying strengths, the units and type of percent (w/w, w/v, v/v) must be kept constant.

Examples

1. What is the percent of alcohol in a mixture made by mixing 5 liters of 25%, 1 liter of 50%, and 1 liter of 95% alcohol?

a. Determine the total amount of alcohol in the 3 solutions and the total amount of solution (1 liter = 1000 ml). Assume additivity of volumes on mixing.

$$
\begin{array}{r}
25\% \times 5000 \text{ ml} = 1250 \text{ ml} \\
50\% \times 1000 \text{ ml} = 500 \text{ ml} \\
95\% \times 1000 \text{ ml} = 950 \text{ ml} \\
\hline
7000 \text{ ml} \qquad 2700 \text{ ml}
\end{array}
$$

b. Determine the percent of alcohol in the mixture. There is a total of 2700 ml of alcohol in 7000 ml of total solution.

$$2700 \text{ ml}:7000 \text{ ml}::X \text{ ml}:100 \text{ ml}$$

$$X = 2700 \text{ ml} \times 100 \text{ ml}/7000 \text{ ml} = 38.6 \text{ ml}$$

Because 38.6 ml of alcohol are in 100 ml, a 38.6% solution is formed.

2. What is the strength of a mixture obtained by mixing 50 Gm of a 5%, 100 Gm of a 7.5%, and 40 Gm of a 10% ointment?

a.

$$
\begin{array}{r}
5\ \% \times 50 \text{ Gm} = 2.5 \text{ Gm} \\
7.5\% \times 100 \text{ Gm} = 7.5 \text{ Gm} \\
10\ \% \times 40 \text{ Gm} = 4.0 \text{ Gm} \\
\hline
190 \text{ Gm} \qquad 14.0 \text{ Gm}
\end{array}
$$

b. There is a total of 14.0 Gm of active ingredient in 190 Gm of total mixture.

$$14 \text{ Gm}:190 \text{ Gm}::W \text{ Gm}:100 \text{ Gm}$$

$$W = 14 \text{ Gm} \times 100 \text{ Gm}/190 \text{ Gm} = 7.37 \text{ Gm}$$

Since there are 7.37 Gm of active ingredient in 100 Gm of the mixture, a 7.37% preparation results.

Problems

1. What percent of a drug is contained in a mixture of powder consisting of 0.5 Kg, containing 0.038% of a drug, and 10 Kg, containing 0.043% of a drug?
2. What is the strength of a mixture produced by combining the following lots of alcohol: 2 liters of 95%, 2 liters of 50%, and 7 liters of 60% alcohol?
3. What is the percent of drug content in the following mixture: 2 Kg of 3%, 300 Gm of 2.5%, and 500 Gm of 4.2% resin?

Alligation Alternate

Alligation is a rapid method of calculation which is useful to the pharmacist. The name is derived from the Latin *alligatio*, meaning the act of attaching and hence refers to lines drawn during calculation to bind quantities together. This method is used to find the proportions in which substances of different strengths or concentrations must be mixed in order to yield a mixture of desired strength or concentration. When the proportion is found, a calculation may be performed to find the exact amounts of the substances required.

Rules

1. The substance with a higher value than that required is the one with the lower amount.
2. The gain in value or amount of one substance balances the loss in value or amount of another substance.

Examples

1. In what proportion must a preparation containing 10% of drug be mixed with one containing 15% of drug, to produce a mixture of 12% drug strength?

The 10% drug is 2% too weak and the 15% drug is 3% too strong. Therefore, the excess in strength of 3 parts of the stronger can be calculated to just balance the deficiency of 2 parts of the weaker drug. Set up the problem in this manner:

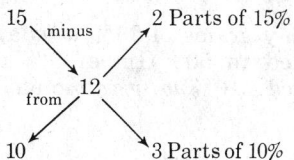

The desired percent or concentration is placed in the center, the lower percentage is placed on the left side below the center, and the higher percentage is placed on the left side above the center. The figure obtained by subtracting 10% from 12% is placed opposite the 15% on the right side and that obtained by subtracting the 12% from 15% is placed opposite the 10% figure on the right side.

Then, mixing 2 parts of 15% drug preparation with 3 parts of 10% drug preparation will produce a drug mixture of the desired 12% strength.

2. In what proportion must 30% alcohol and 95% alcohol be mixed to make 500 ml of 50% alcohol. Set up the problem in the following manner:

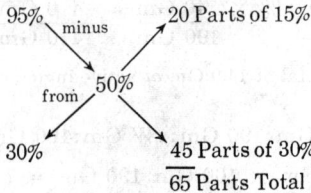

In a total of 65 parts, 20 parts of 95% alcohol + 45 parts of 30% alcohol are needed. Since the total parts is proportional to 500 ml, the following proportion can be made:

$$65 \text{ parts}:500 \text{ ml}::20 \text{ parts}:V \text{ ml}$$

$$V = 500 \text{ ml} \times 20 \text{ parts}/65 \text{ parts} = 154 \text{ ml}$$

The amount of 30% alcohol can be found by a similar proportion, o by subtracting 154 ml from 500 ml:

```
  500 ml   total
- 154 ml   95% alcohol
  346 ml   30% alcohol
```

Thus, when 154 ml of 95% alcohol and 346 ml of 30% alcohol are mixed, 500 ml of 50% alcohol results (assuming there is no contraction in volume on mixing).

3. How many grams of an ointment containing 0.18% of active ingredient must be mixed with 50 grams of an ointment containing 0.14% of active ingredient to make a product containing 0.15% of active ingredient?

a.

```
0.18%              0.01 Parts of 0.18%
        0.15%
0.14%              0.03 Parts of 0.14%
                   0.04 Parts Total
```

b. 0.03 parts is proportional to 50 Gm.

$$0.03 \text{ parts}:50 \text{ Gm}::0.01 \text{ parts}:U \text{ Gm}$$

$$U = 50 \text{ Gm} \times 0.01 \text{ part}/0.03 \text{ part} = 16.7 \text{ Gm}$$

Problems

1. How much of an ointment containing 12% drug, and how much ointment containing 16% drug must be used to make 1 Kg of a product containing 12.5% drug?

2. In what proportion should 50% alcohol and purified water be mixed to make a 35% alcohol solution? (The purified water is 0% alcohol.)

Note: This problem may be solved by a method other than alligation as was shown above.

3. How many grams of 28% *w/w* ammonia water should be added to 500 Gm of 5% *w/w* ammonia water to produce a 10% *w/w* ammonia concentration?

Proof Spirit

The Department of Internal Revenue calculates the strength of pure or absolute alcohol (herein referred to as C_2H_5OH) by means of *proof degrees*. 100 proof spirit contains 50% (by volume) or 42.49% (by weight) of C_2H_5OH, and its specific gravity is 0.93426 at 60°F/60°F. Thus, 2 proof degrees equals 1% (by volume) of C_2H_5OH. One proof gallon is 1 gal of 50%

(by volume) of C_2H_5OH at 15.56°C (60°F). In other words, a proof gallon is a gallon that contains ½ gal of C_2H_5OH. A proof gallon is 100 proof.

The term *10 degrees under proof* (10° u.p.) signifies that 100 volumes of the spirit contains 90 volumes of proof spirit plus 10 volumes of water, and *30 degrees over proof* (30° o.p.) indicates that 100 volumes diluted with water yields 130 volumes of proof spirit. To prepare proof spirit, 50 volumes of C_2H_5OH are mixed with 53.71 volumes of water to allow for the contraction which occurs to yield 100 volumes of product.

The terms *proof strength*, *proof gallon*, *proof spirit*, etc are used so that the tax levied only on the actual quantity of C_2H_5OH contained in any mixture. It is therefore sometimes necessary for the pharmacist to convert alcohol purchased to proof strength to compute tax refunds or convert proof strengths to percent for compounding purposes.

A quantity of solution that contains ½ gal of C_2H_5OH is said to contain 1 proof gal. Proof gallons may be calculated by the following two equations:

$$\text{Proof gal} = \frac{\text{gal} \times \% \, v/v \text{ strength}}{50\% \, v/v}$$

$$\text{Proof gal} = \frac{\text{gal} \times \text{proof strength}}{100 \text{ proof}}$$

The second equation is the same as the first because proof strength is always twice the % *v/v* strength.

With these equations, given any two variables the third can be calculated.

Examples

1. What is the taxable alcohol in 1 pt of Alcohol USP?

$$1 \text{ pt} = \frac{1}{8} \text{ gal} \quad (8 \text{ pt} = 1 \text{ gal})$$

Alcohol USP is 95% *v/v*; therefore,

$$\text{Proof gal} = \frac{\text{gal} \times \% \text{ strength}}{50\%} = \frac{\frac{1}{8} \text{ gal} \times 95\%}{50\%} =$$

$$0.2375 \text{ proof gal}$$

2. How much Diluted Alcohol USP can be made from 1 qt of alcohol labeled ½ proof gallon?

Diluted Alcohol USP is 49% *v/v*; therefore,

$$\text{Proof gal} = \frac{\text{gal} \times \% \text{ strength}}{50\%}$$

$$\frac{1}{2} \text{ proof gal} = \text{gal} \times \frac{49\%}{50\%} = 0.510 \text{ gal}$$

Problems

1. How many proof gallons are there in 1 qt of a preparation that is labeled 75% *v/v* alcohol?

2. How many proof gallons are there in a pint of an elixir that contains 14% alcohol?

3. How much Diluted Alcohol USP can be made from 1 gal of 190 proof alcohol?

Saturated Solutions

Occasionally it is necessary for a pharmacist to make saturated solutions. Solubility in the USP and NF is expressed as the number of milliliters of a solvent that will dissolve 1 Gm of a solid; eg, 1 Gm dissolves in 0.5 ml of water. In other words, if 1 Gm of a solid is dissolved in 0.5 ml of water, a saturated solution results. An example will illustrate this.

How much of a drug is needed to make 120 ml of a saturated solution if 1 Gm of the drug dissolved in 7.5 ml?

The following proportion may be made:

$$1 \text{ Gm}:7.5 \text{ ml}::X \text{ Gm}:120 \text{ ml}$$

$$X = 1 \text{ Gm} \times 120 \text{ ml}/7.5 \text{ ml} = 16 \text{ Gm}$$

When 16 Gm of the drug are dissolved in 120 ml of water, a saturated solution results which has a volume greater than 120 ml because the solid will take up a certain volume. Only 120 ml would be dispensed.

What is the % w/w of the above solution?

$$120 \text{ Gm (ml) solvent} + 16 \text{ Gm solute} = 136 \text{ Gm}$$

of total solution weight. There is 16 Gm of solute in 136 Gm of solution; therefore,

$$16 \text{ Gm}:136 \text{ Gm}::P \text{ Gm}:100 \text{ Gm}$$

$$P = 16 \text{ Gm} \times 100 \text{ Gm}/136 \text{ Gm} = 11.8 \text{ Gm}$$

in 100 Gm of solution; therefore, this is a 11.8% w/w solution.

Problems

1. What is the solubility of a chemical if a saturated solution is 0.5% w/w?
2. How many grams are needed to make 500 ml of a saturated solution if 1 Gm of the solute is soluble in 14 ml of solvent?

Milliequivalents

See Chapter 20 for additional discussion on electrolytic equilibria.

The quantities of electrolytes administered to patients are usually expressed by the term *milliequivalents* (mEq). The reason that weight units (mg, Gm) are not used is that the electrical activity of the ions, which in this instance is important, may be best expressed as mEq.

A mEq is $\frac{1}{1000}$ of an *equivalent* (Eq). An Eq is the weight of a substance which combines with or replaces one Gm-atomic weight of hydrogen. In pharmacy the terms equivalent and equivalent weight (Eq wt) have been used interchangeably. For practical purposes an Eq wt is the weight in grams of an atom or radical divided by the valence of the atom or radical. For example, the Gm-atomic wt of potassium (K) is 39.102 (approx. 39). The Eq wt is calculated by dividing 39 Gm by the valence of K (which is 1), giving 39 Gm/1 = 39 Gm-Eq wt. The mEq of K is the Eq wt divided by 1000. Thus, 39 Gm/1000 = 0.039 Gm = 39 mg. One mEq of K^+ (ion) combines with 1 mEq of Cl^- to give 1 mEq of KCl. The mEq of KCl is 74.5 mg (1 mEq K^+ is 39 mg + mEq Cl^- is 35.5 mg).

Water of hydration contributes to the molecular weight (mol wt) of a compound but *not* to the valence, and the total mol wt is used to calculate mEq.

Examples

1. Calcium (Ca^{2+}) has a Gm-atomic wt of 40.08. What is the mEq wt?

Determine the Eq wt:

$$\text{Gm-atomic wt/valence} = \text{Eq wt}$$

$$40.08 \text{ Gm}/2 = 20.04 \text{ Gm}$$

Determine the mEq wt:

$$\text{Eq wt}/1000 = \text{mEq wt}$$

$$20.04 \text{ Gm}/1000 = 0.02004 \text{ Gm} = 20.04 \text{ mg}$$

2. A solution that contains 409.5 mg of NaCl/100 ml has how many mEq of Na^+ and Cl^-?

$$\text{mEq wt of NaCl} = 58.5 \text{ mg}$$

$$\text{mEq} = \frac{409.5 \text{ mg}}{58.5 \text{ mg/mEq}} = 7 \text{ mEq}$$

of NaCl which dissociates to 7 mEq of Na^+ and 7 mEq of Cl^-.

3. A prescription order calls for a 500 ml solution of potassium sulfate to be made so that it will contain 10 mEq of K^+. How many grams of K_2SO_4 (mol wt: 174 Gm) are needed?

$$\text{Eq wt} = \text{Gm-mol wt/valence}$$

$$\text{Eq wt} = 174 \text{ Gm}/2 = 87 \text{ Gm}$$

$$\text{mEq of } K_2SO_4 = \text{Eq wt}/1000$$

$$\text{mEq of } K_2SO_4 = 87 \text{ Gm}/1000 = 0.087 \text{ Gm} = 87 \text{ mg}$$

1 mEq of K_2SO_4 yields 1 mEq of K^+; 10 mEq of K_2SO_4 yields 10 mEq of K^+:

$$\begin{array}{r} 87 \text{ mg } K_2SO_4/\text{mEq} \\ \times \ 10 \text{ mEq} \\ \hline 870 \text{ mg } K_2SO_4 \end{array}$$

Dissolve 870 mg of K_2SO_4 in sufficient purified water to make 500 ml. This solution will yield 10 mEq of K^+.

4. How many mEq of K^+ are in a 250-mg tablet of potassium phenoxymethyl penicillin (mol wt: 388.49 Gm; valence: 1)?

$$\text{Eq wt} = \text{Gm-mol wt/valence}$$

$$\text{Eq wt} = 388.49 \text{ Gm}/1 = 388.49 \text{ Gm}$$

$$\text{mEq wt} = \text{Eq wt}/1000$$

$$\text{mEq wt} = 388.49 \text{ Gm}/1000 = 0.38849 \text{ Gm} = 388.49 \text{ mg}$$

$$\frac{250 \text{ mg/tablet}}{388.49 \text{ mg/mEq}} = 0.664 \text{ mEq } K^+/\text{tablet}$$

Problems

1. What is the mEq wt of ferrous ion (Fe^{2+}) which has a Gm-atomic wt of 55.85 Gm?
2. What is the mEq wt of sodium phosphate ($Na_2HPO_4 \cdot 7H_2O$)?
3. How many mEq of Na are in 60 ml of an 8% solution of sodium cyclamate (Gm-mol wt: 201.33 Gm; valence: 1)?
4. How many mEq of Ca^{2+} are there in a 600-mg calcium lactate pentahydrate (Gm-mol wt: 308.30 Gm) tablet?

Temperature

Rules

The relationship of Centigrade (C) and Fahrenheit (F) degrees is

$$9(^\circ C) = 5(^\circ F) - 160$$

where °C is the number of degrees Centigrade and °F is the number of degrees Fahrenheit.

Examples

1. Convert 77°F into °C.

$$9(^\circ C) = 5(^\circ F) - 160$$

$$9(^\circ C) = 5(77) - 160$$

$$^\circ C = \frac{385 - 160}{9} = 25^\circ C$$

2. Convert 10°C into °F.

$$9(^\circ C) = 5(^\circ F) - 160$$

$$9(10) = 5(^\circ F) - 160$$

$$\frac{90 + 160}{5} = ^\circ F = 50^\circ F$$

Problems

1. Convert
   a. 30°C into °F
   b. 100°C into °F
   c. 37°C into °F
   d. 120°F into °C

Checking Results

Every calculation which is made in pharmaceutical practice should be verified, preferably by another pharmacist. The first step when checking results is to make certain that the answer is reasonable and of the proper order of magnitude, and that the units are proper.

Addition—Add again in some other order.

Subtraction—The remainder plus the subtrahend should equal the minuend.

Multiplication—Add the digits of the multiplicand repeatedly until a single digit remains. Repeat this procedure for the multiplier and the product. The product of the first number times the second, when reduced to one digit by addition, should equal the third.

$$
\begin{array}{l}
6219 \\
\underline{499} \\
55971 \\
55971 \\
24876 \\
\hline
3103281
\end{array}
$$

$6 + 2 + 1 + 9 = 18 \rightarrow 1 + 8 = 9$
$4 + 9 + 9 = 22 \rightarrow 2 + 2 = 4$ } $\rightarrow 9 \times 4 = 36$
$\rightarrow 3 + 6 = 9$

$3 + 1 + 0 + 3 + 2 + 8 + 1 = 18 \rightarrow 1 + 8 = 9$

Division—Multiply the divisor by the quotient to get the dividend.

References

1. Morrell, C. A., and Ordway, E. M., *Drug Std.*, **22**, 216 (1954).
2. Stempel, E., *J. APhA, Pract. Ed.*, **19**, 548 (1958).
3. Crawford, J. D., *et al, Pediatrics*, **5**, 783 (1950).
4. Talbot, N. B., *et al, Metabolic Homeostasis. A Syllabus for Those Concerned with the Care of Patients*, Harvard Univ. Press, Cambridge, 1959.
5. Lucey, J. F., and Driscoll, T. J., Jr., *Pediatrics*, **24**, 495 (1959).
6. Butler, A. M., and Richie, R. H., *New Engl. J. Med.*, **262**, 903 (1960).
7. Shirkey, H. C., and Barba, W. P., in Nelson, W. E., ed., *Textbook of Pediatrics*, 8th ed., Saunders, Philadelphia, 1964, pp. 209–211.
8. Wagner, J., *Drug Intelligence*, **2**, 144 (1968).

Answers To Problems

Logarithms

1. $V = -0.000084$ cm/sec or -8.4×10^{-5} cm/sec
2. $S = 65.5$ dynes/cm

Addition

1. 2481.23 Gm or 2.48123 Kg
2. 1157 Gm or 1.157 Kg
3. 2 ℥, 3 ℥, 17½ gr
4. 1 ℔, 7 ℥, 4 ʒ, 2 ϶, 4 gr
5. 2 ⁷⁹⁄₉₀ gr
6. 4 gal, 2 qt, 11 fl oz

Subtraction

1. 4105 ml or 4.105 liters
2. 143½ gr
3. 7 fl oz, 2 fl dr
4. 3.71 Gm

Multiplication

1. 157.14 ml
2. 162.5 Gm
3. 825 ml
4. 2 gal, 1 qt, 4 fl oz, 4 fl dr
5. 375,000 mcg or 375 mg

Division

1. 769 capsules + 15-mg remainder
2. 160 capsules
3. 150 doses
4. 150 doses
5. 1396 capsules + 300-mg remainder

Conversions

1. a. 421 mg
   b. 19.4 mg
   c. 109 Gm
   d. 7776 mg
   e. 99.2 Gm
   f. 454 Gm
2. a. 1 lb, 3 oz, 173 gr
   b. 6.94 gr
   c. 1 ℔, 5 ℥, 5 ʒ, 26 gr
   d. 0.00154 gr
   e. 2.2 lb
3. a. 0.648 mg
   b. 0.203 mg
   c. 10.8 mg
   d. 0.325 or 0.324 Gm
   e. 1.299 or 1.296 Gm
4. a. 12.3 ml
   b. 11.1 ml
   c. 237 ml
   d. 473 ml
   e. 0.308 ml
   f. 0.00154 gr
   g. 0.0772 gr
5. a. 480 gr
   b. 8 ʒ
   c. 437½ gr
   d. 2880 gr
   e. 4 ʒ, 10 gr

Dosage Calculation

1. D.T.D. No. 14 means, send 14 such doses. Assuming the doses have been checked, they are for chemicals, J, K, and L (10 mg, 50 mg, and 300 mg, respectively).
2. Drug Q: 0.5 Gm
   Drug R: 0.3 Gm
3. 7.5 ♏/dose; 30 ♏/day
4. 50 doses
5. 0.0444 mg
6. 1.5 mg
7. ½ gr
8. 18.7 mg
9. 280,000 units
10. 75 mg
11. 77.9 mg
12. 0.75 ml contains 60 units; 13⅓-day supply.

Reducing and Enlarging

1. Liquid C   875   ml
   Solid B   225   Gm
   Liquid R   62.5 ml
   Liquid P   500   ml
2. Solid G   24 ʒ or 3 ℥
   Liquid D   720 ♏ or 1 f℥, 4 f ʒ
   Solid M   72 ʒ or 9 ℥
3. Solid N   4.8 mg
   Solid Q   120 mg
   Solid R   7.2 Gm
   Add sufficient purified water to make 240 ml of solution
4. Solid S   6.75 Gm
   Solid T   2.25 Gm
   Oil C   31.5 ml
   Alcohol   22.5 ml

Density

1. 816 Gm
2. 363 ml
3. 54.2 ml

Ratio and Proportion

1. 65 mg costs 19½¢ ($0.20); 5 gr costs 97.4¢ ($0.97)
2. $33.70

Percentage

w/v Solutions

1. Dissolve 171 gr (2 ʒ, 2 ϶, 11 gr) in sufficient solvent to make 3 f℥

2. 2.84 liters
3. 6.25 liters
4. 8 Gm

w/w Products

1. Compound A   115 gr or
1 ʒ, 2 ɘ, 15 gr
    Solvent   3 ʒ, 365 gr
2. 28.8 Gm
3. 5 Kg
4. Dissolve 4.64 Gm of drug in 120 ml (150 Gm) of glycerin
5. Compound K   3.6 Gm
    Solid H   1.8 Gm
    Base   18.6 Gm
6. Dissolve 88.2 Gm of the solute in 500 ml of purified water
    Dispense 500 ml
7. Powder P   27.8 Gm
    Powder Q   222.2 Gm
    Powder R   333.3 Gm
    Powder S   416.7 Gm

Percent (v/v, w/v, and w/w)

1. 240 ♏
2. 900 ml
3. 34.8% w/w
4. 11.4 gr

5. 38.5% w/w
6. 15 Gm
7. 0.4 Gm
8. 32.4 ml of a 37% solution
9. 1.57 Gm

Stock Solutions

1. 30.2 Gm
2. 36.3 Gm

Parts per Million

1. 13 mg

Dilution and Concentration

1. 9 Gm of 10% cream and 21 Gm of diluent (base)
2. 0.01 Gm
3. 40 Gm
4. 58.42 Gm of 5% ointment + 1.58 Gm of sulfur

Mixing Products of Different Strengths

1. 0.0428%
2. 64.6%
3. 3.16%

Alligation Alternate

1. 875 Gm of 12% ointment and 125 Gm of 16% ointment
2. 35 parts of 50% alcohol and 15 parts of purified water
3. 139 Gm of 28% ammonia water

Proof Spirit

1. 0.375 proof gal
2. 0.035 proof gal
3. 1.94 gal

Saturated Solutions

1. 1 Gm in 199 ml
2. 35.7 Gm of solute

Milliequivalents

1. 27.925 mg/mEq
2. 89.3 mg/mEq
3. 23.8 mEq (or 23.9 mEq)
4. 3.9 mEq

Temperature

1. a. 86°F
   b. 212°F
   c. 98.6°F
   d. 48.9°C

II | Statistics

Design of experiment and collection of data—design and conduct of clinical trials—analysis of data collected—interpretation of the analysis—statistics in biological testing

This chapter was prepared by

Lila Knudsen Randolph, * BS, *Mathematical Statistician, Office of the Assistant Commissioner for Planning, US Food and Drug Administration, Washington, D.C. 20025,* and
Joseph L. Ciminera, ScD, *Manager, Statistical Services, Merck Sharp & Dohme Research Laboratories, West Point, Pa. 19486*

In this chapter an attempt will be made to acquaint the student with the nature of the statistical approach as it applies to pharmacy and pharmacological problems, especially biological assay. However, within this division of statistics there are large gaps as yet unexplored and all that is attempted here is an aerial photograph with telescopic views of a few of the most important landmarks. A list of books and articles is given at the end of the chapter as recommended reading for the student who wishes to learn more about this field of statistics.

There are two parts to the definition of the word statistics.

1. Statistics are a collection of data or numbers, such as the number of cases of diabetes per state per year, or the number of capsules in a bottle.
2. Statistics is logic which makes use of mathematics in the science of collecting, analyzing and interpreting data for the purpose of making decisions.

In this chapter we shall deal with the second part of this definition.

Statistics is fundamentally logic and common sense. It is neither a collection of formulas that can be applied to patch up deficiencies in experiments nor a panacea for all the weaknesses of the data. The data cannot be improved simply by applying statistical analysis to them; the resulting analysis is no better than the data themselves. Definite, sweeping conclusions cannot be drawn from a small amount of poor data just because several weeks were spent in making an involved statistical analysis of them.

It is true that there are a great many mathematical formulas in statistics, but logic and reasoning are the true core of this subject. The underlying fundamental ideas in an experiment must be thoroughly investigated. There are different statistical formulas to be used depending on the assumptions made. Each situation must be approached individually, the assumptions set forth, the possible causes of variation enumerated and the problem at hand stated as clearly as possible. Dr. R. A. Fisher, one of the most prominent statisticians in England, has said that a question clearly stated is a problem half solved.

It must be clearly realized at the outset that all nature is inherently variable. One often hears the comparison "as alike as two peas." Actually even peas vary and no two would be *exactly* alike in size, shape color, maturity, blemishes, etc. If an experimenter makes several independent measurements on the length

of a table, no matter how accurately the measurements are made, he will find that they are not all alike.

Statistics recognizes this variability in nature and takes it into account in planning how the data should be gathered. In the analysis of the data gathered, it utilizes this inherent variation by making allowances for it in the interpretation of the results.

The practice of the statistical method may be divided into four parts: (1) design of the experiment, (2) collection of data, (3) analysis of data collected, and (4) interpretation of the analysis. The four parts are inextricably woven together. The plan or design used and the subsequent methods of gathering data under this design to answer the question posed should be considered carefully so as to avoid biases (unintentional or otherwise) that would erroneously influence results; the data then should be analyzed by the proper methods; and an interpretation of the analysis should be made to furnish a sound answer to the question stated. This is the ideal approach. Often, however, the materials already have been gathered before the problem is stated. Even in such cases the interpretation and analysis always should be made with full consideration of any biases that may have entered because of the manner of obtaining the data. In no instance should an interpretation be made without considering the manner of collection.

Design of the Experiment and Collection of Data

Collection of data always involves either the planning or *design of an experiment*, sampling, or complete census. In the collection of data a sample is generally taken except, of course, in such instances as a complete census of the population of the United States. Sometimes a sample is inadvertently taken when it is not the intention to take a sample, as when a questionnaire is sent out to every pharmacist in the state. There will always be some people who do not respond to a questionnaire and anything less than 100% response will constitute a sample.

In the following breakdown according to the type of data sampled, the sampling method is not limited to the field in which the illustration is given. An attempt has been made to give only the broadest type of illustrations in the brief chapter allotted to statistics and yet cover as many types of data as possible.

Questionnaire Type of Response—Suppose questionnaires on the sales of some drug were sent to all the pharmacists in a state and only 50% of the questionnaires were returned; thus only a sample of the pharma-

---

* Deceased.

cists would be taken, and any results tabulated from such a sample would be biased in that those who did not return the questionnaire would not be represented. It has been definitely shown that persons who respond to questionnaires have different characteristics, and possibly different environments, from those who do not respond. In the hypothetical case just mentioned, perhaps sales of the drug were so large that reporting an accurate figure was just too much work, so the questionnaire was left unanswered. Possibly in another community there were no sales of the drug, so the pharmacist did not bother to return the questionnaire. The statistician does not know which is the case. A bias thus enters into the results and the direction and amount of the bias are unknown.

However, there are questionnaire techniques worked out by mathematical statisticians that could have been employed to reduce and sometimes eliminate the bias in the sample of the pharmacists' responses. These same mathematical statisticians have also worked out methods of obtaining not only the average response to the question asked, but also the limits within which the average response might have occurred due to sampling of pharmacists. If only a certain amount of money is available for the survey or questioning there are techniques for obtaining the best design for the limited sampling program with a minimum of error. If, on the other hand, results within certain limits of error are desired regardless of cost, a sampling design can be used which will meet these specifications.

The public opinion polls use certain statistical sampling techniques continuously. These workers have obtained from the Census Bureau and other sources the percentages of men, women, and children in the United States, in various income groups, in certain nationality groups, and in many other types of population groups. Their samples are designed to contain the same proportions in these various groups as are in the population. However, instead of sending questionnaires by mail, interviewers are assigned certain quotas of definite types of people to interview and the interviewers fill out the questionnaire for each person while asking him (or her) the questions.

It is impossible to elaborate fully here on the various methods of sampling such as area sampling, sampling with probability proportionate to size, etc. The purpose is rather to create an awareness to the problems of sampling, and, more important, to show that a design can be used that will give the limits of error of the result for any given expenditure of funds. A few references will be given at the end of this chapter for those interested in this type of sampling. There are other errors in the questionnaire type of response that may introduce bias, such as the way in which the question is stated, the order of the questions, and the actions of the interviewer.

Sampling in the Chemical Laboratory—Gathering data is accomplished in another manner in the laboratory even though it is still sampling. Sampling of the material to be chemically analyzed, sampling of reagents (if any) used, sampling of laboratory personnel used, sampling of conditions in general (such as, possibly, room temperature, room humidity, equipment, etc). Various such factors may contribute some variation to the final results, depending on which factors are important in the method of analysis involved. It has been shown that results differ even from laboratory to laboratory, though sometimes to a very minute extent. However, sampling of the material usually contributes the most variation and this factor usually can be controlled easily.

By way of illustration, several samples may be taken of a large lot of digitalis leaves for the chemical determination of acid-insoluble ash in the lot. In order to represent the lot truly, the samples must be taken from different parts of the lot to insure that every part of the lot is represented in some sample. Naturally, ash determinations from five samples taken from the same part of a lot will probably check each other more closely than if the five samples are taken from entirely different parts of the lot, but the former five samples will not give the best average ash value for the lot. The more heterogeneous the lot, the more effort should be expended in being sure that every part of the lot is represented by a sample. It might be that the leaves having the most ash are in the bottom of the lot; a group of samples all taken from the top then would give too low an estimate for the average ash content of the lot.

Another aspect of sampling in a chemical determination is the sampling of the chemist or chemists who perform the chemical analysis. If a single chemist makes several check determinations on portions taken from the same sample of thoroughly mixed substance, one expects the results to check more closely than if several chemists had made these check determinations. However, the true reproducibility of a method can be indicated only in terms of how closely an analyst at one laboratory can check an analyst at another laboratory on exactly the same material. Thus, due to slight differences in technique, one chemist might always obtain higher results than another chemist. The sampling of chemists might thus have some effect on the results and the method reproducibility.

Sampling in the Biological Laboratory—It should be realized that a biological experiment on, for example, the temperature response of rabbits to pyrogens constitutes a sample of the infinitely possible number of combinations of results that could be obtained from all possible rabbits, laboratories, and technicians. Different breeds of rabbits may give different results. Differences between results from two or more laboratories are usually greater than differences between results obtained by two or more technicians at the same laboratory. Season of the year, temperature, and humidity sometimes cause differences as well as other factors—possibly lack of clarity in the write-up of the method. In biological experimentation the differences between individual animals are likely to be large so that the results of an experiment repeated at the same laboratory may give results different from those obtained the first time. The use of statistical procedures will give an estimate of the amount of variation to be expected under identical conditions. As in the questionnaire problem already mentioned, it is important to know not only the average but also the standard error of that average. Then one can estimate how close is the agreement obtained between results of repetitions of the experiment and just how far off the results might be because of some inherent factor causing variation in the assay.

Frequently, methods are tested for their accuracy and precision by conducting collaborative studies of these methods in several laboratories. Collaborative studies are also made to evaluate a lot of a drug to be used as a reference standard, eg, USP Vitamin D Reference Standard, etc. From such a collaborative study it is necessary to determine what differences can be expected between laboratories. Fig. 60 shows the results of a collaborative assay on a working standard of calcium penicillin[1] plotted according to the potencies obtained from several assays at different laboratories. The

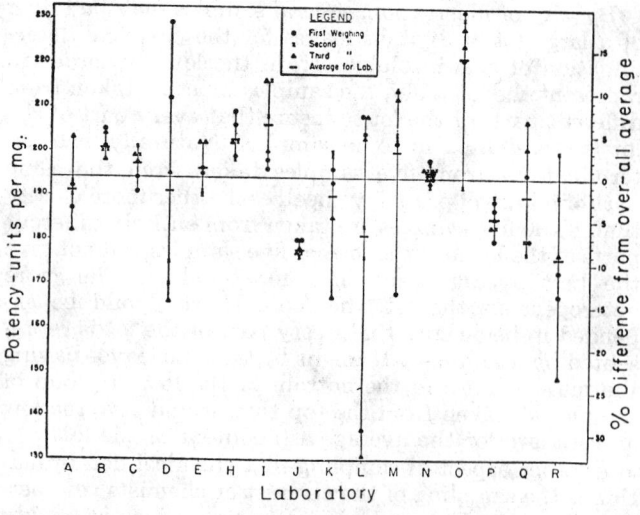

Fig. 60. A chart illustrating the variation between laboratories of collaborative assays on working standard calcium penicillin.

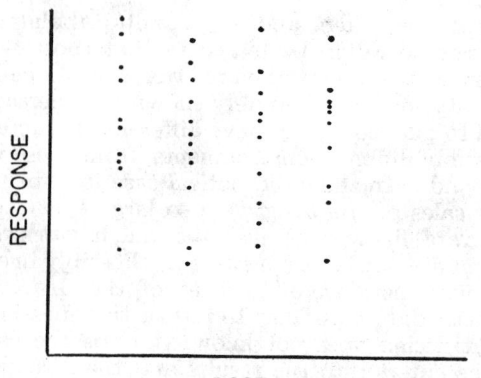

Fig. 62. Partial relationship between dosage and response—a section of Fig. 61 with the dosage scale enlarged.

laboratories are lettered A through R. The average for all the laboratories combined is indicated by the long horizontal line in the center of the chart. Short horizontal lines indicate the averages for each laboratory. Note that some laboratories show very little variation of their individual assay results about the average for that laboratory, eg, laboratory J has an over-all variation of only about 2% as measured on the right-hand scale. However, the average result of that laboratory is almost 10% from the over-all average of all the laboratories. Note also the results from laboratories B, H, I, and P. Compare the variation of the results from laboratory N with that of the results from laboratory L.

Statistics should be used in setting up the design for a single experiment so that biases will not influence the results. This point may be illustrated by an extreme example—something that no experimenter would do. A technician wishes to compare two drugs as to their effects on the growth of rats. He uses 30 rats from a single cage and puts the first 15 rats caught on drug No. 1 and the last 15 caught on drug No. 2. Naturally, the first 15 rats caught are less lively than the last 15 and because they are less lively they very likely differ in size and nervous temperament from the last 15 rats. Thus the results are biased from the very beginning and one drug is "favored" merely by the method of choos-

ing the animals to be used on each drug. Obviously, some method entirely free from subjective influences (unconscious or conscious) should be used. A table of random numbers.[2-4] could be used or a series of numbered metal-edged disks could be shaken and picked out of a hat in some objective manner.

Suppose, for example, one wishes to choose 16 rats, numbered in the order they are taken from the cage, from 1 to 16. Four doses are to be administered. Four consecutively numbered disks are shaken in a container and one selected without looking; then the disks are shaken again and another selected, etc. In this way the order of the doses is randomized. These are labeled a, b, c, and d. Then 16 disks numbered from 1 to 16 are shaken and disks are selected without looking and without replacement. Suppose the first four numbers selected are 12, 2, 15, and 10. Dose a will be given to the twelfth animal chosen from the cage, dose b to the second, dose c to the fifteenth, etc., until all 16 animals have been assigned doses.

Another aspect of sampling in a biological laboratory involves the choice of doses of a drug to be used in an experiment to determine the relationship between dose and response. Usually in administering a single dosage of a drug to a group of animals an average response is noted (the type of response depends on the drug administered). However, there is variation between individual animals. If 10 or 12 different doses are administered to suitably chosen animals, one might obtain a relationship between dosage and response of individual animals as shown in Fig. 61. The larger the dose, the higher the average response elicited. However, if the choosing (sampling) of doses had been such that only the four doses in the central portion of Fig. 61 had been administered, the dosage response relationship would look entirely different as shown in Fig. 62.

In Fig. 61 a very definite relationship between dosage and response is shown, while in Fig. 62, which is part of the same data, there appears to be no relationship merely because the dosages chosen were not far enough apart and did not cover the proper range in order to represent the true picture adequately.

In biological assay it is often advantageous to design the dosage schedule to take advantage of the fact that there is less variation within a litter than between litters, or that there is a trend in the response of a single animal to several consecutive doses of a drug. This can be illustrated by an epinephrine assay wherein a single dog is given 16 consecutive doses, the order of which is determined by a Latin square design. The following pattern illustrates a Latin square:

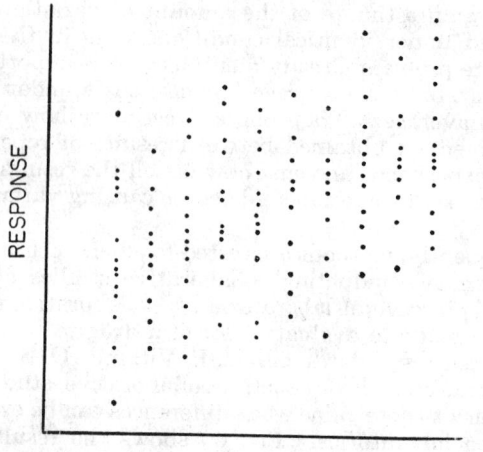

Fig. 61. Typical relationship between dosage and response of individual animals.

```
A    B    C    D
B    C    D    A
C    D    A    B
D    A    B    C
```

Note that each letter occurs only once in each row and each column of the square. A Latin square design was applied to an assay involving two levels of doses of the standard (high and low doses s_H and s_L, respectively), and two levels of doses of the unknown (u_H and u_L). The dosage schedule is given in Table I. In this type of design each dose occurs once in each order of administration (eg, u_H is given first of four doses but once, s_H is given first but once, etc). In this type of assay equal doses of epinephrine given a dog elicit a smaller and smaller rise in blood pressure with each succeeding dose.

In all biological experimentation the design should be planned so that differences in treatment do not coincide with differences in weight, sex, litters, dates of administration, etc. Animals should be assigned to doses at random, and the availability of certain designs should be realized. Fisher[5] has written an excellent book on planning or designing of experiments. He explains fully the various types of designs mentioned here. Another book on design of experiments is by Cochran and Cox.[6] It goes into great detail and gives at least 150 of the most useful experimental designs with complete directions for the analysis of data obtained using any of the designs described therein.

Clinical Type of Data—Certain designs are available for the planning of an experiment or, rather, the purposive sampling involved in setting up an experiment. In the early days of penicillin a clinical experiment on 300 patients was conducted to determine why injections of some penicillins caused pain while others of the same penicillin did not. Data had been gathered hit or miss as penicillin was administered in the hospital. Potency, site of injection, and amount of pain produced were recorded. However, no conclusions could be drawn from the data because the subjective responses of the patients were confounded with the site of injection and the potency. There was no pattern for comparison of responses of the same individual to the different penicillins. A design was set out using a "balanced incomplete block" type of experimental design involving 30 patients with 3 sites of injection for each patient, and the grouping of the commercial penicillin into 6 different concentration levels. The design of the experiment was taken from Table XVII, design No. 1, in the tables by Fisher and Yates,[3] which is given there as:

```
abc    aef    bef
abd    bcf    cde
ace    bde    cdf
adf
```

Since there are only ten groups of letters, this design could be used for ten patients only. However, to increase the precision of the results and also to investi-

gate whether the order of injection affected the pain response, two more groups of ten patients were added making 30 patients in all with three repetitions of the design as given above. The first group of patients received the injection in one order of site of injection (B, T, D), the second group received them in another order (T, D, B), and the third group still another order (D, B, T). Patients were randomized in assigning the set of doses and locations of administration to be used. The manner in which the design was utilized in this experiment is given in Table II, together with the results from each injection on each patient.[7]

The results can be plotted as shown in Fig. 63 and because of the efficient design little formal statistical analysis is necessary for the demonstration of the evident trend. A calculation of averages, as shown by the horizontal lines plotted on the chart, shows that as potency of the penicillin increased the pain produced decreased.

Design and Conduct of Clinical Trials—Proof of efficacy and safety of new drugs or treatments requires testing in human subjects. This is best achieved by carrying out controlled clinical trials. A clinical trial is said to be controlled when it is designed

Table I—Typical Dosage Schedule for Epinephrine Assay

Using a Latin Square Design

	First dose	Second dose	Third dose	Fourth dose
First group	u_L	s_H	s_L	u_H
Second group	s_H	s_L	u_H	u_L
Third group	s_L	u_H	u_L	s_H
Fourth group	u_H	u_L	s_H	s_L

Table II—Balanced Incomplete Block Type of Experimental Design

Showing Site of Injection[a] and Degree of Pain[b]

Patient	a 936 units per mg	b 502 units per mg	c 175 units per mg	d 333 units per mg	e 1127 units per mg	f 711 units per mg
	Order No. 1					
1	B-0	T-3+	D-2+	...	...	...
2	B-3+	T-4+	...	D-3+	...	...
3	B-0	...	T-4+	...	D-2+	...
4	B-0	...	...	T-1+	...	D-2+
5	B-0	...	...	...	T-3+	D-4+
6	...	B-1+	T-2+	...	...	D-2+
7	...	B-0	...	T-2+	D-1+	...
8	...	B-3+	...	...	T-1+	D-2+
9	...	...	B-3+	T-3+	D-2+	...
10	...	...	B-3+	T-4+	...	D-4+
	Order No. 2					
11	T-0	D-2+	B-0	...	...	...
12	T-1+	D-4+	...	B-0	...	...
13	T-1+	...	D-3+	...	B-0	...
14	T-3+	...	...	D-4+	...	B-2+
15	T-1+	...	...	...	D-1+	B-2+
16	...	T-3+	D-3+	...	...	B-2+
17	...	T-2+	...	D-3+	B-0	...
18	...	T-2+	...	...	D-1+	B-1+
19	...	...	T-3+	D-1+	B-0	...
20	...	...	T-3+	D-2+	...	B-1+
	Order No. 3					
21	D-1+	B-0	T-2+	...	...	...
22	D-1+	B-2+	...	T-3+	...	...
23	D-1+	...	B-2+	...	T-1+	...
24	D-1+	...	...	B-3+	...	T-2+
25	D-1+	...	...	...	B-0	T-1+
26	...	D-2+	B-2+	...	...	T-1+
27	...	D-3+	...	B-2+	T-1+	...
28	...	D-2+	...	...	B-0	T-1+
29	...	...	D-2+	B-0	T-0	...
30	...	...	D-4+	B-2+	...	T-2+

[a] B: buttocks; T: triceps; D: deltoid.
[b] 0: no pain; 1+: very slight pain; 2+: slight pain; 3+: moderate pain; 4+: severe pain.

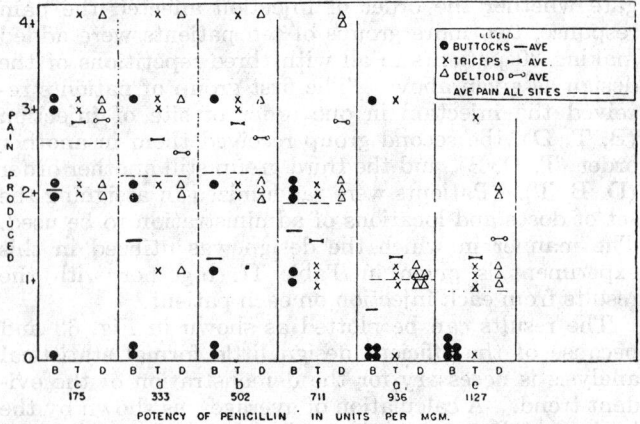

Fig. 63.   Clinical study of relationship of pain produced at site of injection and potency of penicillin sodium.

and carried out in such a manner that the results reflect the true action of the treatments.

The usual procedure is to compare the effects of the treatment with those of a concurrently tested control or placebo. When this is not feasible, drug efficacy may be assessed by testing graded doses of drug and establishing a dosage–response relation. Implicit also is the assurance that the trial includes sufficient and adequate sampling to allow projection of the trial's results to other future patients. The results cannot be projected beyond the types and severity of disease, and the ages and sex of the patients included in the trial.

The distribution among treatments of variables such as age, sex, differences in diagnosis, and initial severity of disease may be controlled by stratification. Where this is not feasible, patients should be assigned to treatments at random, and allowances made for the effects of the variables using suitable statistical methods. A restricted randomization procedure is useful if it is desired to assure about an equal number of patients on all treatment groups as patients enter the trial. This is illustrated below for a completely randomized design in which 15 patients are allocated at random, 5 to each of 3 treatments:

A	B	C
3	1	2
6	5	4
8	9	7
12	10	11
14	13	15

Note that the individual patients in each triad are randomly assigned to one of the three treatments. Another example is shown below for a simple crossover design in which the individual patients in each of five successive pairs are randomly assigned to one of two treatment order groups:

Group	Patient	Period 1	Period 2
	1		
	4		
I	5	A	B
	7		
	10		
	2		
	3		
II	6	B	A
	8		
	9		

The latter design may be more efficient than a completely randomized design since each patient acts as his own control, thus eliminating patient-to-patient

variability. However, this advantage may be offset if drug carryover effects are present, or if the severity of the disease wanes in the second period to the point where treatment differences no longer can be demonstrated.

In order to be certain that the random allocation is strictly followed, and to remove subjective bias on the part of both the patient and the clinical investigator in assessing the effects of the treatments, the clinical trial should be carried out blind. A double-blind trial is one in which neither the patient nor the physician is made aware of the nature of treatment administered.

In order to keep the study blind, all treatments must be put up in identical-appearing dosage forms. This may require a great deal of ingenuity on the part of the pharmacist called upon to prepare such dosage forms, especially with respect to the taste of liquid preparations to be administered orally. In some instances characteristic side effects of the drugs make it impossible to keep a study blind. In these situations we must rely more heavily on objective measures of response, and less on subjective measures.

Federal regulations require that drugs shipped to clinical investigators must be properly labeled with the name of the drug. In order to keep the study blind, a suggested procedure is to use a two-part tear-off label.

One part is glued to the container and reveals only the patient's study number, the period number, and directions for taking the drug; the tear-off part shows the identity of the drug. The name of the drug is overlayed with a water-washable or eraseable ink so as not to reveal the identity of the drug to the physician. This portion of the label is torn off and stapled to the back of the clinical form. The physician is instructed to break the code for an individual patient, if necessary, by washing off or erasing the overlayed ink. However, when this is done, the patient must be considered as a treatment failure.

A less satisfactory procedure, which however does not require an ink overlay, is to have a disinterested individual tear off the identifying portion of the labels before the clinical material is turned over to the clinical investigator. The identifying labels are placed in individual opaque sealed envelopes that are identified only with the patient's study number and the period number.

These then would be handled in the same fashion as the labels with the ink overlay. The unopened envelopes serve as evidence that the study was carried out blind. The physician is instructed to number the patients serially as they enter the trial, and assign them to treatment with the container having the same number, starting with the container for period 1. The drug allocation code is not revealed to the clinician until the study is completed.

To facilitate computerization and statistical evaluation, the results of clinical trials should be recorded on precoded clinical forms. Data pertinent to clinical trials include subjective and objective measures of the course of the disease, laboratory determinations, and adverse reactions.

Subjective measures are exemplified by such determinations as severity of pain, degree of hyperemia, and the patient's or the physician's over-all assessment of the effectiveness of treatment. Blood pressure, body weight, and body temperature are examples of objective measures.

Laboratory determinations usually include such measures as complete blood count, liver function tests, and analyses on urine and stool specimens. The occurrence of adverse effects may be recorded as ascertained by inquiry or as volunteered by the patient. It is informative also to determine the severity as well as the frequency of occurrence of adverse effects, and whether or not the physician feels they were drug related.

Generally, it is more difficult to evaluate clinical data than laboratory animal data. Some of the contributing factors are (1) failure of patients to take the medication as directed, and to report for examination at stated intervals; (2) the use of ancillary or concomitant medications by the patients; and (3) incomplete data caused by patients dropping out of the study for various reasons. These factors are more prevalent among outpatients than among hospitalized patients. A trial secretary can be of great help in assuring the completeness and accuracy of clinical forms.

Analysis of Data Collected

Analysis usually consists of graphing the data, applying some statistical formula or formulas to the data, and drawing inferences from the results. Terminology plays a very important part in statistical method, but unfortunately there is a lack of standardization among various statistical texts. In this text the terminology used will be similar to that given by Youden.[8]

Graphs—There are various types of graphs including:

1. The bar graph or histogram, such as Fig. 67.
2. The "pie chart" in which various sized pieces of pie represent percentages to be compared as part of a whole, sometimes called polar coordinates.
3. A graph in which one variable X is plotted against another variable, sometimes called rectangular coordinates. Since graphing and graphs are well known, the subject need not be elaborated on here. Suffice it to say that it is usually necessary to plot the data, sometimes in several ways before beginning the statistical analysis. The graphic plot can sometimes show the types of analysis to be applied and relationships between various parts of the data.

The Average or Mean—Suppose from a population or universe a sample of n observations is taken as usual in order to determine some of the characteristics of the population. A chemist, for example, may make n determinations on a lot of digitalis leaves in order to be able to estimate the ash content of that lot. The sample of n determinations can be designated by:

$$x_1, x_2, x_3 \ldots x_n$$

The sample mean, $\bar{x}$, can be calculated by:

$$\bar{x} = \frac{x_1 + x_2 + x_3 + \ldots + x_n}{n} = \frac{\Sigma x_i}{n}$$

where i goes from 1 to n.

This sample mean is an estimate of μ, the actual mean of the population or, in this case, the lot of digitalis leaves.

Example I—A series of data on the acid-insoluble ash content of digitalis leaves is given as follows:

4.1	4.4	4.0
4.3	4.2	4.7
4.9	4.6	4.4

$n = 9$. The sum of these 9 values is 39.6.

$$\text{The average} = \bar{x} = \frac{\Sigma x_i}{n} = \frac{39.6}{9} = 4.4$$

This example is given mainly to illustrate the symbols employed.

Fig. 64 is taken from an article by Stearns[9] and illustrates one instance where an average has no meaning.

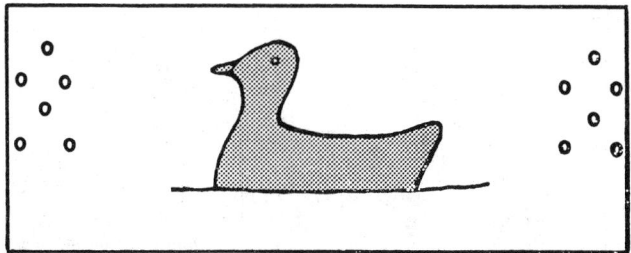

Fig. 64. *On an average the duck was dead.* A hunter fired both barrels of a shotgun at a duck. The first hit 2 ft in front, the second hit 2 ft behind. On an average the duck was dead. What the hunter really wanted was meat on the table. In duck hunting one wants to keep trying until a single shot hits the mark. But in estimating purity by a chemical test the best estimate is usually the average.

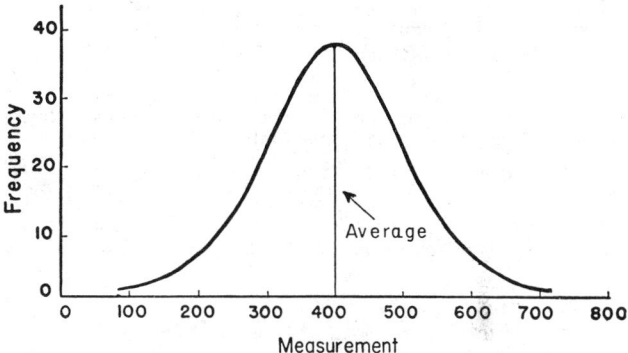

Fig. 65.   The normal probability curve.

Frequency Distributions—There are many types of variation patterns in nature. These patterns are called frequency distributions of data. The most common of these is the normal (or bell-shaped) curve in which most of the observations fall near the average and the greater the distance from the average in either direction the fewer the observations. This is illustrated by the frequency curve shown in Fig. 65. This type of curve is sometimes called the normal curve of error, or *normal probability curve*. Many statistical formulas and interpretations are based on the assumption of a normal frequency curve distribution of data.

Although the normal distribution is the most common, there are many other types of frequency curves such as the *U-shaped curve* for which there is a classic illustration. In getting a distribution of the amount of sunlight for each day over a period of time it was found that many days were entirely sunny and many days were entirely cloudy but that fewer days fell in between these two extremes so that the distribution of amount of sunlight was shaped like a U as shown in Fig. 66. There are also other types of distribution curves such as the *Poisson, binomial, t, Chi-square* distribution, etc.

It is possible to ascertain the distribution of data from a given experiment. It can be approximated roughly by means of a bar chart as shown in the following problem:

Example II—The weights of 50 rats at weaning were as follows:

30 Gm	47 Gm	37 Gm	29 Gm	38 Gm
32	42	32	30	34
34	32	33	37	36
39	33	45	40	35
43	41	35	32	41
36	27	28	35	30
38	28	41	37	34
41	36	32	30	37
31	31	35	28	25
26	49	34	34	33

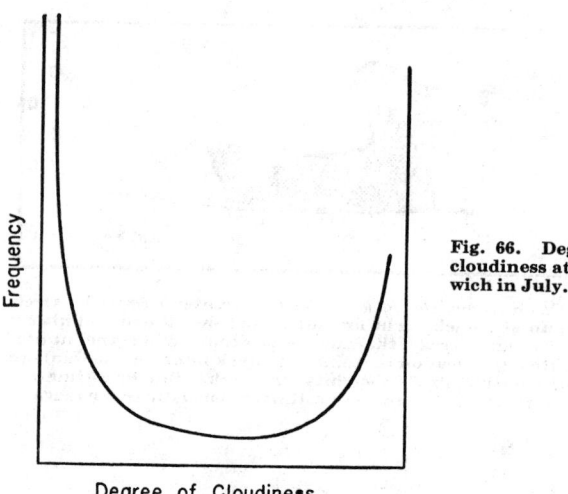

Fig. 66. Degrees of cloudiness at Greenwich in July.

These weights can be assembled in the following groups with the frequency of occurrence in each group tabulated.

Weight group	Frequency
24–25 Gm	1
26–27	2
28–29	4
30–31	6
32–33	8
34–35	9
36–37	7
38–39	3
40–41	5
42–43	2
44–45	1
46–47	1
48–49	1

This can be plotted in the form of a bar chart as shown in Fig. 67.

Measures of Variation—There are statistical formulas for measuring the variation that exists in nature as well as the man-made variation. The simplest measure of variation is the *range*. It is the difference between the highest value and the lowest value in a series of observations. For Example I the range would be $4.9 - 4.0 = 0.9$; for Example II, $49 - 25 = 24$. The range is most valuable in small series of observations usually for n less than 10. Dixon and Massey[4] have an excellent dissertation on the use of the range.

The *standard deviation* is the measure of variation most commonly used. When $n = 2$, the range and the standard deviation are equally as efficient. For n greater than ten, the standard deviation gives a much better estimate of the variation than the range. The

two are quite closely related, especially for sample sizes less than ten. See Table XIII for the average number of standard deviations in the average range.

The standard deviation of the population is usually designated by σ, and the standard deviation of the sample by s where s is an estimate of σ. The standard deviation of a sample is calculated by getting the differences of each observation from the mean and putting them in the following formula:

$$s = \sqrt{\frac{(x_1 - \bar{x})^2 + (x_2 - \bar{x})^2 + (x_3 - \bar{x})^2 + \ldots + (x_n - \bar{x})^2}{n - 1}}$$

The formula can be given in several forms, some of which are easier to calculate:

$$s = \sqrt{\frac{\Sigma(x_i - \bar{x})^2}{n - 1}} = \sqrt{\frac{\Sigma x_i^2 - (\Sigma x_i)^2/n}{n - 1}}$$

Using the data in Example I, $n = 9$, the sum of the nine observations (Σx_i) is 39.6. The sum of the squares of the observations is

$$\Sigma x_i^2 = (4.1)^2 + (4.3)^2 + \ldots + (4.4)^2 = 174.92$$

Putting these values in the formula:

$$s = \sqrt{\frac{\Sigma x_i^2 - (\Sigma x_i)^2/n}{n - 1}}$$

$$s = \sqrt{\frac{174.92 - (39.6)^2/9}{9 - 1}} = \sqrt{\frac{174.92 - 174.24}{8}} = 0.29$$

The $n - 1$ in the denominator of the formula for the standard deviation is called the degrees of freedom, sometimes abbreviated DF, and for the standard deviation is one less than the number of observations.

The standard deviation also can be estimated by using the range as will be shown later. There are tables showing the number of standard deviations contained in the range depending on n, the sample size.

In a normal distribution one standard deviation measured both above and below the population average includes about ⅔ of the number of observations in the whole distribution; two standard deviations measured off on each side of the average includes about 95% of the observations. In fact, tables of the normal probability curve* have been calculated to show the multiple (sometimes fractional) of the standard deviation on either side of the average which would include any desired proportion of the observations (see Fig. 68 and also the bottom line of Table III). It is from such tables and graphs that probabilities can be derived. Note that the title of Fig. 68 is "normal

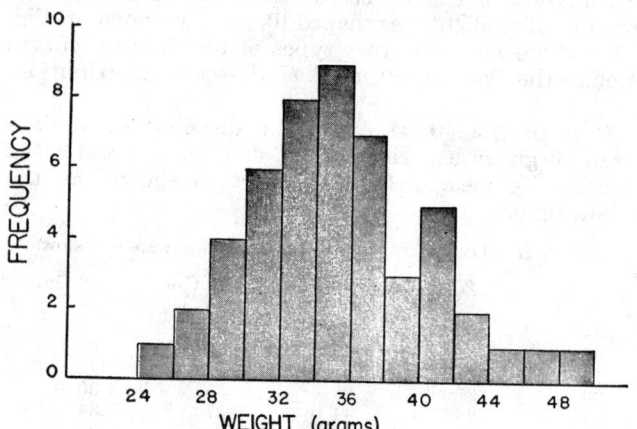

Fig. 67. Bar chart showing frequency distribution of weights of 50 rats at weaning (data in Example II).

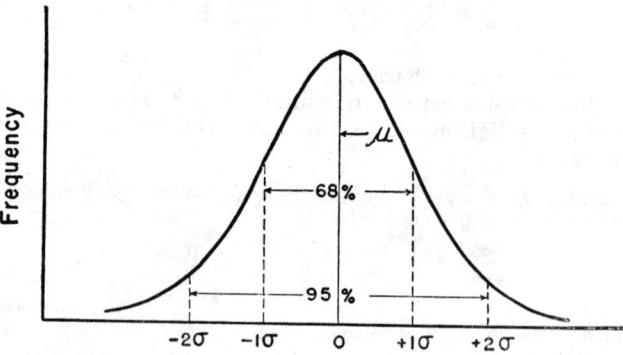

Fig. 68. The normal probability curve showing standard deviation unit around the average.

* One of the most complete tables of this kind can be found in Pearson, K.[10] Other tables can be found in almost any statistical text such as Snedecor, Rider, Fisher, etc (see *Bibliography*), or in Fisher, R. A., and Yates, F.[3]

probability curve," and that the center line at the hump of the curve is the population average, μ. The vertical dotted lines divide the distribution into standard deviation units or sigma (σ) units. (The standard deviation of the infinite parent population is usually denoted by sigma (σ) while the standard deviation of the sample of n observations is denoted by s.) Thus, if 95% of the observations in this distribution are between 2σ above the average and 2σ below the average, only 5% of the observations will be beyond these limits (which are called the 95% confidence limits) and an observation would have a 5% probability of occurrence beyond these limits.

Also, in the bottom line of Table III which applies to an infinitely large sample, the limits indicated by the population average $\pm 2.326\sigma$ (ie, two tails) include all but 2% ($P = 0.02$) of the observations. Only 1% ($P = 0.01$) is *above* $\mu + 2.326\sigma$, using one tail of the distribution. Likewise, 1% ($P = 0.01$) is below the lower limit, $\mu - 2.326\sigma$. Both Fig. 68 and Table III are theoretical distributions. More complete tables of the normal probability distribution are available in statistical texts and books of tables previously referred to.

The standard deviation gives a measure of the variation of *individual observations* around the average. A comparable measure of variation of *averages* of samples about their average is called the *standard error of an*

average. It can be calculated from the standard deviation, s, and the number of observations, n.

$$\text{Standard error of the average} = s_{\bar{x}} = \frac{s}{\sqrt{n}}$$

A short cut (and only approximate) method of estimating the standard error of the average is to divide the range by the number of observations.

$$s_{\bar{x}} = \frac{\text{range}}{n}$$

This method can be used only if n is less than ten.

The square of the standard deviation is called the *variance*. The square of the standard error of the average is called the *variance of the average*. By means of mathematical statistics, it is possible to derive the variance for almost any statistic which can be expressed by a formula. There is not only the variance of an average but also the variance of a weighted average, regression coefficient, etc. Each statistic also has its own distribution about its true value; tables of the normal curve sometimes can be applied to a particular statistic.

Suppose an infinitely large box contains marbles of differing weights with an average weight of 50 Gm and the individual weights of the marbles have a normal distribution and a standard deviation of 9 Gm. If 1000

Table III—The t Table

Distribution of t Giving Both the Two-Sided or Two-Tailed Probability and the One-Sided or One-Tailed Probability According to Degrees of Freedom

				One Tail				
	$P\,0.4$	$P\,0.3$	$P\,0.2$	$P\,0.1$	$P\,0.05$	$P\,0.025$	$P\,0.01$	$P\,0.005$
				Two Tails				
DF	$P\,0.8$	$P\,0.6$	$P\,0.4$	$P\,0.2$	$P\,0.1$	$P\,0.05$	$P\,0.02$	$P\,0.01$
1	0.325	0.727	1.376	3.078	6.314	12.706	31.821	63.657
2	0.289	0.617	1.061	1.886	2.920	4.303	6.965	9.925
3	0.277	0.684	0.978	1.638	2.353	3.182	4.541	5.841
4	0.271	0.569	0.941	1.533	2.132	2.776	3.747	4.604
5	0.267	0.559	0.920	1.476	2.015	2.571	3.365	4.032
6	0.265	0.563	0.906	1.440	1.943	2.447	3.143	3.707
7	0.263	0.549	0.896	1.415	1.895	2.365	2.998	3.499
8	0.262	0.546	0.889	1.397	1.860	2.306	2.896	3.355
9	0.261	0.543	0.883	1.383	1.833	2.262	2.821	3.250
10	0.260	0.542	0.879	1.372	1.812	2.228	2.764	3.169
11	0.260	0.540	0.876	1.363	1.796	2.201	2.718	3.106
12	0.259	0.639	0.873	1.356	1.782	2.179	2.681	3.055
13	0.259	0.538	0.870	1.350	1.771	2.160	2.650	3.012
14	0.258	0.537	0.868	1.345	1.761	3.145	2.624	2.977
15	0.258	0.536	0.866	1.341	1.753	2.131	2.602	2.947
16	0.258	0.535	0.865	1.337	1.746	2.120	2.583	2.921
17	0.257	0.534	0.863	1.333	1.740	2.110	2.567	2.898
18	0.257	0.534	0.862	1.330	1.734	2.101	2.552	2.878
19	0.257	0.533	0.861	1.328	1.729	2.093	2.539	2.861
20	0.257	0.533	0.860	1.325	1.725	2.086	2.528	2.845
21	0.257	0.532	0.859	1.323	1.721	2.080	2.518	2.831
22	0.256	0.532	0.858	1.321	1.717	2.074	2.508	2.819
23	0.256	0.532	0.858	1.319	1.714	2.069	2.500	2.807
24	0.256	0.531	0.857	1.318	1.711	2.064	2.492	2.797
25	0.256	0.631	0.856	1.316	1.708	2.060	2.485	2.787
26	0.256	0.531	0.856	1.315	1.706	2.056	2.479	2.779
27	0.256	0.531	0.855	1.314	1.703	2.052	2.473	2.771
28	0.256	0.530	0.855	1.313	1.701	2.048	2.467	2.763
29	0.256	0.530	0.854	1.311	1.699	2.045	2.462	2.756
30	0.256	0.630	0.854	1.310	1.697	2.042	2.457	2.750
40	0.255	0.529	0.851	1.303	1.684	2.021	2.423	2.704
60	0.254	0.527	0.848	1.296	1.671	2.000	2.390	2.660
120	0.254	0.526	0.845	1.289	1.658	1.980	2.358	2.617
∞	0.253	0.524	0.842	1.282	1.645	1.960	2.326	2.576

Table IV—Confidence Limits for Binomial Distribution[a]

$P = 0.95$ for two limits (both upper and lower)
$P = 0.975$ for only one limit (either upper or lower)

% Fail- ures in sample	Size of sample						
	10	20	30	50	100	250	1000
0	0 31	0 17	0 12	0 07	0 4	0 1	0 0
10	0 45	1 31	2 27	3 22	5 18	7 14	8 12
20	3 56	6 44	8 39	10 34	13 29	15 26	18 23
30	7 65	12 54	15 50	18 44	21 40	24 36	27 33
40	12 74	19 64	23 60	27 55	30 50	34 46	37 43
50	19 81	27 73	31 69	36 64	40 60	44 56	47 53

[a] From McClung, R. M.[11]

samples of 4 marbles each is taken from the box, the average for each of the 1000 samples recorded, and the standard deviation of these averages calculated, this figure would agree very well with the population standard error of the average as calculated from

$$\sigma_{\bar{x}} = \frac{\sigma}{\sqrt{n}} = \frac{9}{\sqrt{4}} = 4.5 \text{ Gm}$$

Also the averages of the 1000 samples of 4 marbles each would be distributed normally about the true average (50 Gm) and have a standard error of the average equal to 4.5 Gm. This means that the averages of about ⅔ of the 1000 samples (about 670) would occur between 50 + 4.5 Gm and 50 − 4.5 Gm (or between 54.5 and 45.5 Gm).

The normal probability tables would apply to the distribution of these averages. About 95% of the averages would occur between the average plus or minus two standard errors of the average. Therefore, beyond these "two sigma" limits on either side of the grand average only about 5% (ie, 100% minus 95%) of the averages will occur. If, sometime in the future, a sample of 4 marbles is drawn from the box the chances are about 5 in 100 or 1 in 20 that the average for this sample will be below 41 Gm or above 59 Gm, ie,

$$50 - 2(4.5) = 41$$
$$50 + 2(4.5) = 59$$

and 1 chance in 100 that the average for this sample will be below 38.4 Gm or above 61.6 Gm, ie,

$$50 - 2.57(4.5) = 38.4$$
$$50 + 2.57(4.5) = 61.6$$

The factors to be used in multiplying the standard error of the average and the probability attached to each factor (eg, 95 or 99%) can be found in any table of the normal probability distribution or normal curve of error as it is sometimes called. This table is usually included in any statistical text or book of statistical tables.[3] The factors are given here in the bottom line of Table III.

Probability—Usually the capital letter P (for probability) is used in statistics to indicate the chances a given result would occur by random sampling from a specific population. If it is found rarely enough (usually $P = 0.05$, 5% of the time, or 1 time in 20), it is considered very unlikely that the sample was taken from that population and it is said to be significantly different.

Confidence Limits—This terminology is used to denote limits around a sample average, $\bar{x}$, that would encompass the true average of the population, μ, a given percentage of the time. These confidence limits are obtained using the standard error of the sample average,

$s_{\bar{x}}$, and a t value (see Table III) corresponding to the degrees of freedom, $n - 1$, and the probability one wishes to associate with the confidence limits.

Upper confidence limit $= \bar{x} + ts_{\bar{x}}$

Lower confidence limit $= \bar{x} - ts_{\bar{x}}$

where $s_{\bar{x}} = s/\sqrt{n}$.

The confidence statement could be written:

$$\bar{x} - ts_{\bar{x}} < \mu < \bar{x} + ts_{\bar{x}}$$

If t corresponds to $P = 0.05$, the population average, μ, lies between these confidence limits 95% of the time; ie, if such intervals are computed in repeated samples of n observations, 95% of such intervals would include μ.

The t distribution is proper when the sample standard deviation is used; then the normal curve of error does not apply. It can be seen, however, that as n increases, the t value approaches the value obtained using the normal distribution.

Suppose, however, that in the example above, the population average, μ, and population standard deviation, σ, were unknown and that instead of 1000 samples of 4, there was only 1 sample of 4;

$$n = 4$$
$$\bar{x} = 50$$
$$s_{\bar{x}} = 4.5$$

and we wish to know the limits within which the true average (μ) of the population would occur 95% of the time. The t table is entered on the row corresponding to the degrees of freedom ($n - 1$ or 3 in this case), and $P = 0.05$ for two tails to obtain $t = 3.182$. Using the equations given for upper and lower confidence limits, we obtain

$$\bar{x} + ts_{\bar{x}} = 50 + 3.182(4.5) = 64.3$$
$$\bar{x} - ts_{\bar{x}} = 50 - 3.182(4.5) = 35.7$$

Thus 95% of the time the confidence limits of 35.7 to 64.3 would include the true average of the box. These limits would be called the confidence limits for $P = 0.95$. Note that these are much larger limits than if knowledge of the standard deviation were based on 1000 samples of 4.

It can also be stated that 2½% of the time the true average will be below the confidence interval, and 2½% of the time above. These are generally referred to as "the tails," and t tables are given for one tail as well as for two tails. Table III is for both two tails and one tail. Note that the probabilities for one tail are just half of those for two tails. Confidence limits can be made smaller by taking a larger sample and thus reducing the size of the standard error of the mean. This is an illustration of how chance operates in sampling procedures because of the inherent variability of nature.

A similar use of sigma limits is applied to biological assays in stating confidence limits for the potency of a drug. In general the probability accompanying the confidence limits indicates the probability that the true figure will be within these limits.

Standard deviations and confidence limits can also be obtained for a percentage. For instance, if questionnaires were sent out to 100 pharmacists asking if they handled a certain new drug, and if 20% of them replied they did and 80% replied they did not, it is possible to calculate or find the confidence limits of that percentage or the limits which would include the true percentage of all pharmacists carrying that drug. The standard deviation could be calculated:

$$s = \sqrt{\frac{pq}{n}} = \sqrt{\frac{0.20(0.80)}{100}} = 0.04$$

where p is the percentage in decimal fractions = 0.20, $q = 1 - p = 0.80$, and n = size of sample = 100.

Thus the 2-sigma limits ($P = 0.95$) would be 12% and 28%. This, however, is an approximation. More accurate confidence limits for percentages have been tabled by Clopper and Pearson, Snedecor, Geigy, and others. A condensed form is given in Table IV where it can be seen that the confidence limits for the example are actually 13 and 29%.

Weighted Average—There are instances where a *grand average* of several averages is desired, such as in collaborative work on a method. The formula given above for the calculation of the average assumes equal weights for all observations. This formula could be used for determining a grand average of several averages if all are determined with the same precision. The precision of an average is dependent on the amount of variation as well as the number of observations and is given by the formula for the *variance of an average*, which is

$$s_{\bar{x}}^2 = \frac{s^2}{n}$$

(*Note*—Variance is the square of the standard deviation and the variance of an average is the square of the standard error of the average.) The more precise an average, the smaller its standard error. Therefore, the *weight* attached to any one average is the reciprocal of the variance of that average.

$$W = \frac{1}{s_{\bar{x}}^2}$$

or the variance may be used instead of the variance of the average.

$$W = \frac{n}{s^2}$$

The formula for the grand average of two averages then becomes

$$\bar{x} = \frac{W_1\bar{x}_1 + W_2\bar{x}_2}{W_1 + W_2}$$

where

$\bar{x}$ = grand average
$\bar{x}_1$ and $\bar{x}_2$ are two individual averages
W_1 and W_2 are weights of $\bar{x}_1$ and $\bar{x}_2$, respectively

This formula can be extended in the same manner for more than two averages:

$$\bar{x} = \frac{\Sigma W_i \bar{x}_i}{\Sigma W_i}$$

where, as before, Σ indicates a summation.

Example III—A few students each made several determinations of the total alkaloids in a single lot of belladonna leaves; however, a different number of determinations was made by each student. The standard deviation was determined for each student's determinations.

Student	n	Average	Std dev
1	10	0.40	0.05
2	5	0.31	0.07
3	4	0.53	0.05
4	7	0.36	0.02

The best estimate of the average total alkaloid content of this lot of belladonna leaves will be given by the weighted average.

Student	n	Average x	Weight W	Product Wx	Product nx
1	10	0.40	4,000	1600	4.00
2	5	0.31	1,020	316	1.55
3	4	0.53	1,000	848	2.12
4	7	0.36	17,500	6300	2.52
Sum	26		24,120	9064	10.19

$$\bar{x} = \frac{\Sigma W_i \bar{x}_i}{\Sigma W_i} = \frac{9064}{24,120} = 0.376$$

If only $\bar{x}$ and n had been given for each student and the variances (also the standard deviations) were assumed to be equal, the weights would be the number of observations and

$$\bar{x} = \frac{\Sigma n_i \bar{x}_i}{\Sigma n_i} = \frac{10.19}{26} = 0.392$$

There are instances where a weighted average is the best to use, and other instances where the actual weights that should be assigned are unknown even though both the number of observations, n, in each group and the standard deviation, s, of these observations is given. The weight in itself should be a measure of the *accuracy*, not the *precision*, of an average. Sometimes it may be that the number of determinations is large because for some reason the analyst suspected that his first results were incorrect and therefore he repeated the determinations. The standard error, although calculated from both n and s does not necessarily give a measure of the *accuracy* of an average; it may give only the *precision*.

Bias, Precision, and Accuracy—The *bias* (or *systematic error*) of a method is indicative of its tendency to measure something other than what was intended, while its *precision* (or *reproducibility*) refers to the agreement among repeated measurements. The comprehensive term, *accuracy*, refers to the closeness of such measurements to the "true" magnitude concerned. In other words, accuracy shows how closely a method measures what it is supposed to measure, while precision shows only how closely many measurements agree. An accurate method of measurement is both precise and unbiased. Given a sample which is known to contain 100 mg of iodine, five determinations by an accurate method might range from 99.5 to 100.5 mg of iodine, while five by an unbiased but imprecise method might range from 95.0 to 105.0 mg. (However, because averages are more precise than individual measurements the average of a large number (eg, 100) of determinations by the second method would be just as accurate as the average of a few (eg, 5) by the first method.) Five measurements made by a biased but precise method might possibly range from 85 to 86 mg of iodine, while five made by a method which is both biased and imprecise might range from 80 to 90 mg. The bias of approximately 15 mg in these last two methods cannot be "averaged out" merely by making additional determinations.

The interrelations of bias, precision, and accuracy are clearly illustrated in Fig. 69 (taken from illustrations by Eisenhart[12] and Stearns[9]). A detailed discussion of these topics is presented by Eisenhart.[12]

Interpretation of the Analysis

There are three types of significance tests that are quite generally used: the t test, χ^2 test, and the F test, or analysis of variance.

The t Test of Significance—If two samples are to be compared to see if they are drawn from the same population, ie, whether they are samples of the same thing or whether they are "significantly" different, the t test can be used as a means of comparison.   (This is the same t we used in calculating confidence limits.) A significant difference means that a real difference *may* exist.   It does not *prove* that it exists, but is an indication that the difference may be real and that the two samples may be drawn from entirely different populations.   (The t test also can be used to compare a sample and a population.)   The formula is:

$$t = \frac{\text{difference}}{\text{standard error of difference}}$$

For calculation purposes we can use

$$t = \frac{\bar{x}_1 - \bar{x}_2}{s} \sqrt{\frac{n_1 n_2}{n_1 + n_2}}$$

where

$\bar{x}_1$ = mean of first sample of n_1 observations
$\bar{x}_2$ = mean of second sample of n_2 observations

and

$$s^2 = \frac{\Sigma x^2{}_{1i} - (\Sigma x_{1i})^2/n_1 + \Sigma x^2{}_{2i} - (\Sigma x_{2i})^2/n_2}{n_1 + n_2 - 2}$$

where

$\Sigma x^2{}_{1i}$ is sum of squares of observations in first sample
Σx_{1i} is sum of observations in first sample
$\Sigma x^2{}_{2i}$ is sum of squares of observations in second sample
Σx_{2i} is sum of observations in second sample
s^2 is the pooled variance of the two samples

Example IV—Suppose one sample of five and one sample of four are taken, respectively, from each of two lots of amobarbital capsules and the milligrams of amobarbital are determined in each capsule and it is desired to determine whether or not there is a significant difference between the two samples.   Do they come from different lots or populations?   It is assumed that there is no difference between them (the null hypothesis), and the probability that they could have been drawn from the same population is found.   If this probability is small enough, there is said to be a "significant" difference.

Sample 1		Sample 2
		9.8
	10.1	9.6
	13.6	10.1
	12.5	11.4
	11.4	9.1
$\Sigma x_{1i} =$	47.6	$\Sigma x_{2i} =$ 50.0
$\Sigma x^2{}_{1i} =$	573.18	$\Sigma x^2{}_{2i} =$ 502.98
$\bar{x}_1 =$	11.90	$\bar{x}_2 =$ 10.00
$n_1 =$	4	$n_2 =$ 5

$$s^2 = \frac{573.18 - (47.6)^2/4 + 502.98 - (50.0)^2/5}{4 + 5 - 2}$$

$$s^2 = \frac{573.18 - 566.44 + 502.98 - 500.00}{7} = \frac{9.72}{7} = 1.3886$$

$$s = 1.18$$

$$t = \frac{\bar{x}_1 - \bar{x}_2}{s} \sqrt{\frac{n_1 n_2}{n_1 + n_2}}$$

$$t = \frac{11.90 - 10.00}{1.18} \sqrt{\frac{4(5)}{4 + 5}}$$

$$t = 1.61(1.49) = 2.40$$

The degrees of freedom involved in the pooled standard deviation are seven, $DF = (n_1 - 1) + (n_2 - 1)$.   In the t table (see Table III), for $P = 0.05$ and $DF = 7$ (two tails) the value of t given is 2.365. The value of t calculated is greater than this.   Therefore, since the probability of these two samples being drawn from the same population is less than 0.05, we conclude that they were drawn from different populations.   (This conclusion may be wrong 5 times in 100.)   It can be stated that there is a significant difference between the two samples.   To determine whether the average of sample one was *greater* than the average of sample two, the "one tail" portion of the t table is

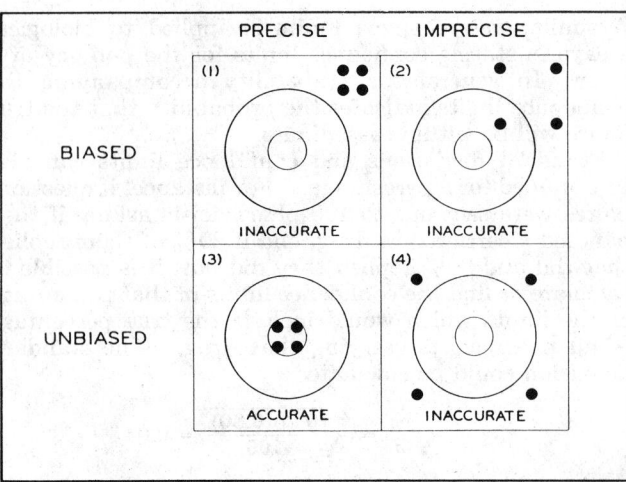

Fig. 69. Diagram illustrating bias, precision, and accuracy. The shots on targets (1) and (2) are biased; in both cases the shots cluster away from the bull's eye. The clusters on targets (3) and (4) are both unbiased; the center of each cluster is on the bull's eye. The shots on targets (1) and (3) are precise; both sets are bunched together. The shots on targets (2) and (4) are widely scattered hence imprecise. Only the shots on target (3) are accurate, ie, precise and unbiased (courtesy, Lilly).

used.   Of course, one must decide before making the test whether one tail or two tails should be used, depending on the question to be answered.

For $DF = 7$ and $P = 0.05$ (one tail) Table III shows $t = 1.895$. Our calculated value of $t = 2.40$ is greater than the tabled value, and we conclude that the average of Sample 1 (11.90) is significantly greater than the average of Sample 2 (10.00).

The standard error of the difference could be estimated crudely using the range:

standard error of difference

$$= \sqrt{\left(\frac{\text{Range}_1}{n_1}\right)^2 + \left(\frac{\text{Range}_2}{n_2}\right)^2}$$

$$= \sqrt{\left(\frac{13.6 - 10.1}{4}\right)^2 + \left(\frac{11.4 - 9.1}{5}\right)^2}$$

$$= \sqrt{(0.875)^2 + (0.460)^2} = 0.986$$

thus, t $= \dfrac{\bar{x}_1 - \bar{x}_2}{\text{standard error of difference}}$

$$= \frac{11.90 - 10.00}{0.986} = 1.93$$

However, now the value of t is smaller than the value from the table, which was 2.365, and we conclude that we have no proof that they were drawn from different populations.

This was an example of a borderline significance test, and the crude estimate of the standard error of the difference may be the cause of the difference between the two tests.   When the significance test is not borderline, the results using the range gives a good approximation to those using the standard deviation, provided n_1 and n_2 are less than 15.

The t test also may be applied to paired (sometimes referred to as correlated) data.   Such data occur when pairs of subjects or test units matched on the basis of certain characteristics (eg, age, sex, etc) are assigned at random, one to each treatment or condition to be tested, or when the same subject or test unit is assigned to each treatment given in random order.   The objective is to remove the inherent variability from test unit to test unit, and thus obtain a more sensitive comparison.   The formula for computational purposes is

$$t = \frac{\bar{d}}{s} \sqrt{n}$$

where

$\bar{d}$ = mean of the differences, $x_1 - x_2$, of the n pairs of observations

$$s^2 = \frac{\Sigma d_i{}^2 - (\Sigma d_i)^2/n}{n - 1}$$

where

$\Sigma d_i{}^2$ = the sum of squares of the n differences
Σd_i = sum of the n differences
n = number of differences or pairs of observations

Example V—Duration of loss of righting reflex (min) was measured in 16 mice following treatment with a barbiturate administered in the morning and the afternoon on two different occasions, the order of giving the morning or the afternoon dose being randomized in each mouse. It was desired to test the null hypothesis that the duration of loss of righting reflex is the same in the morning and the afternoon.

Mouse no.	a.m. x_1	p.m. x_2	Difference $d = x_1 - x_2$
1	75	73	2
2	86	89	-3
3	93	89	4
4	87	79	8
5	91	95	-4
6	87	81	6
7	76	77	-1
8	83	89	-6
9	87	82	5
10	95	91	4
11	91	87	4
12	86	86	0
13	83	78	5
14	76	69	7
15	82	78	4
16	93	88	5

$$\Sigma d_i = 40$$
$$\Sigma d_i{}^2 = 354$$
$$\bar{d} = 2.5$$
$$n = 16$$

$$s^2 = \frac{354 - (40)^2/16}{16 - 1} = \frac{354 - 100}{15} = 16.9333$$

$$s = 4.11$$

$$t = \frac{\bar{d}}{s}\sqrt{n} = \frac{2.5}{4.11}\sqrt{16} = \frac{2.5(4)}{4.11} = 2.43$$

$$DF = n - 1 = 16 - 1 = 15$$

In the t table (see Table III), for $P = 0.05$ and $DF = 15$ (two tails) the value of t given is 2.131. The value of t calculated is greater than this. Therefore, since the probability of the morning and afternoon values being the same is less than 0.05, we conclude that they are different. Apparently, the duration of loss of righting reflex in mice tested on the barbiturate in the morning was longer than when tested in the afternoon.

The Chi-Square Tests of Significance

—The Chi-square test can assume many different forms. In one form it tests agreement between expected frequencies and frequencies observed. Of course, there are many ways of stating what you expect.

$$\chi^2 = \sum \frac{(\text{observed frequency} - \text{expected frequency})^2}{\text{expected frequency}}$$

Example VI—In tossing a coin, 50% tails and 50% heads are expected. Suppose a coin is tossed 40 times and 25 heads and 15 tails are obtained, whereas 20 heads and 20 tails are expected. Is the coin biased or weighted in some way?

Table V—The Chi-Square Table[a]

Probability

DF	$P = 0.20$	$P = 0.10$	$P = 0.05$	$P = 0.01$
1	1.64	2.71	3.84	6.64
2	3.22	4.61	5.99	9.21
3	4.64	6.25	7.82	11.34
4	5.99	7.78	9.49	13.28
5	7.29	9.24	11.07	15.09
6	8.56	10.04	12.59	16.81
7	9.80	12.02	14.07	18.48
8	11.03	13.36	15.51	20.09
9	12.24	14.68	16.92	21.67
10	13.44	15.99	18.31	23.21
20	25.04	28.41	31.41	37.57
30	36.25	40.26	43.77	50.89

[a] Adapted from Fisher, R. A., and Yates, F.[3]

$$\chi^2 = \frac{(25 - 20)^2}{20} + \frac{(15 - 20)^2}{20} = 2.5$$

Again the degrees of freedom associated with χ^2 are one less than the number of categories. Here $\chi^2 = 2.5$ with one degree of freedom. The greater the disagreement between expected and observed, the larger the χ^2. See Table V for probabilities of getting this value or larger. For one degree of freedom the probability of getting a value larger than 2.5 is somewhere between $P = 0.20$ and $P = 0.10$. In order to say that we had a significant departure from the expected values, χ^2 would have to be larger than 3.84 which is the value for $P = 0.05$ at one degree of freedom. A value of χ^2 larger than 6.64 for one degree of freedom would indicate a highly significant ($P = 0.01$) departure from the expected.

Reference is made to sets of tables for determining significance of χ^2 for a fourfold table without any calculations. These tables are self explanatory and were published by Mainland.[13,14] An excellent discussion of χ^2 is given by Dixon and Massey,[15] and a series of articles on χ^2 are given in *Biometrics* (Dec., 1954).

The Chi-square test may be used for comparing two percentages in a 2 × 2 or fourfold contingency table:

Example VII—Following are the survival rates for drug-treated and control pigs with swine dysentery:

Treatment	Survived	Died	Total
Drug	$a = 25$	$b = 14$	$a + b = 39$
Controls	$c = 21$	$d = 22$	$c + d = 43$
Totals	$a + c = 46$	$b + d = 36$	$n = 82$

The survival rates for the drug-treated and control pigs are $p_D = 25/39 = 64\%$ and $p_C = 21/43 = 49\%$, respectively. To test the null hypothesis that there is no difference in the survival rates of drug-treated and control pigs, we calculate

$$\chi^2 = \frac{(|ad - bc| - N/2)^2 N}{(a + b)(c + d)(a + c)(b + d)} =$$

$$\frac{(|25\cdot22 - 14\cdot21| - 82/2)^2 82}{(39)(43)(46)(36)} = 1.36$$

where $|ad - bc|$ is the absolute (ie, positive) difference of $ad - bc$.

The degrees of freedom associated with an $R \times C$ contingency table $= (R - 1)(C - 1)$, so that for a 2 × 2 contingency table we have one degree of freedom. Table V shows that for one degree of freedom the probability of getting a value of χ^2 larger than the calculated value 1.36 is greater than $P = 0.20$. Since P is not equal to or less than 0.05, we conclude that there is insufficient evidence to indicate that the survival rates for the drug-treated and control pigs are different.

The Chi-square test for comparing two correlated percentages for paired data takes a somewhat different form:

Example VIII—Two different types of penicillin were given to each of 22 patients in random order on successive occasions, and the presence or absence of a detectable blood level was determined:

Type I	Type II +	Type II −	Totals
+	$a = 6$	$b = 10$	16
−	$c = 2$	$d = 4$	6
Totals	8	14	22

The percentage of patients with detectable blood levels for the two forms of penicillin are $p_I = 16/22 = 73\%$ and $p_{II} = 8/22 = 36\%$. To test the null hypothesis that there is no difference in the percentage of patients with detectable blood levels for the two forms of penicillin, we calculate

$$\chi^2 = \frac{(|b - c| - 1)^2}{b + c} = \frac{(|10 - 2| - 1)^2}{10 + 2} = \frac{49}{12} = 4.08$$

In Table V, for $P = 0.05$ and $DF = 1$, the value of χ^2 given is 3.84. The value of χ^2 calculated is greater than this. Therefore, since the probability of the percentages for type I and type II penicillin being the same is less than 0.05, we conclude that they are different.

Nonparametric Tests of Significance

—The validity of the t test for comparing two means depends to some extent (especially for small samples) on the assumptions that the two populations sampled are approximately normally distributed and have essentially equal variances. Statistical procedures that do not depend on these assumptions are called nonparametric tests. Three commonly used procedures are the Rank Sum test for unpaired data, and the Signed-Rank Sum and Statistical Sign tests for paired data.

Rank Sum Test of Significance—After the n_1 and n_2 observations are arranged in order of size, the combined values are ranked from 1, for the lowest, to $(n_1 + n_2)$ for the highest, and the sum of the ranks T of the n_1 observations in the smaller sample is computed. Values which are tied are given average ranks. We also calculate $T' = n_1(n_1 + n_2 + 1) - T$, and enter Table VI with n_1, n_2, and T or T', whichever is smaller. If the calculated T (or T') is equal to or less than the tabled value, we reject the null hypothesis at the significance level P.

Example IX—Data were available on the duration of loss of righting reflex (min) for 10 mice given a standard barbiturate and for 11 mice given a test barbiturate:

Standard drug	Rank	Test drug	Rank
96	4.5	0	1
109	8	91	2
126	13	92	3
130	15	96	4.5
130	15	99	6
148	17	103	7
153	18	117	9
158	19	118	10
169	20	119	11
Died	21	120	12
		130	15

$$T = 150.5 \qquad n_2 = 11$$
$$n_1 = 10$$

$$T' = n_1(n_1 + n_2 + 1) - T =$$
$$10(10 + 11 + 1) - 150.5 = 69.5$$

Entering Table VI with $n_1 = 10$, $n_2 = 11$, and $T' = 69.5$, we find that the calculated T' value 69.5 is less than the tabulated value 73 for $P = 0.01$. Therefore, since the probability of the standard drug and test drug values being the same is less than 0.05 (actually, it is less than 0.01), we conclude that they are different. This test compares the medians of the two populations sampled. The median of an ordered set of observations is defined as the middlemost value for an odd number of observations, and as the average of the two middlemost values for an even number of observations. Thus, the median for the standard drug is $(130 + 148)/2 = 139$ and the median for the test drug is 103.

Signed-Rank Sum Test of Significance—The differences between the n paired values are ranked in order of absolute size from 1, for the lowest, to n, for the highest, ignoring zero differences. Tied values are assigned an average rank. After the differences are ranked, the signs of the differences are attached to the ranks, and the sum of the positive ranks and of the negative ranks are obtained. We enter Table VII with n = the number of non-zero differences and the sum T of positive or negative ranks, whichever is smaller. When the calculated T is equal to or less than the tabled T, the null hypothesis is rejected at the significance level P.

Example X—The procedure is illustrated for the data given in Example V:

Differences	Signed-Ranks
2	2
−3	−3
4	6
8	15
−4	−6
6	12.5
−1	−1
−6	−12.5
5	10
4	6
4	6

0	ignore
5	10
7	14
4	6
5	10

Sum of positive ranks = 97.5
Sum of negative ranks = 22.5 = T
$$n = 15$$

Entering Table VII with $n = 15$ and $T = 22.5$, we find that the calculated T value 22.5 is less than the tabulated value 25 for $P = 0.05$. Therefore, since the probability of the morning and afternoon values being the same is less than 0.05, we conclude that they are different.

Statistical Sign Test of Significance—Count the number of positive differences (b) and the number of negative differences (c), ignoring zero differences, and calculate

$$\chi^2 = \frac{(|b - c| - 1)^2}{b + c}$$

where $|b - c|$ is the absolute (ie, positive) difference of $b - c$.

This is referred to the Chi-square table (see Table V) with $DF = 1$, the test being essentially the same as the Chi-square test for correlated percentages illustrated in Example VIII.

Example XI—The procedure is illustrated for the data given in Examples V and X:

$$b = \text{number of positive differences} = 11$$
$$c = \text{number of negative differences} = 4$$
$$\chi^2 = \frac{(|b - c| - 1)^2}{b + c} = \frac{(|11 - 4| - 1)^2}{11 + 4} = \frac{36}{15} = 2.40$$

Table V shows that for one degree of freedom the probability of getting a value of χ^2 larger than the calculated value 2.40 is between $P = 0.10$ and $P = 0.20$. Since P is not equal to or less than 0.05, we conclude that there is insufficient evidence to indicate that the morning and afternoon values are different. This conclusion is not in agreement with that of the t test and the Signed-Rank test. The reason for this is that the Statistical Sign test considers only the sign of the difference and not the magnitude, and thus is a less sensitive test in borderline situations such as this one.

Hotelling's T^2 Test of Significance—This is a multivariate generalization of the t test. For example, if we measure standing and supine, systolic and diastolic blood pressure in two treated groups, we may want a single test of the null hypothesis that the two groups have the same average blood pressures with respect to all four measurements. The procedure is too complex to illustrate and discuss here for other than two variables, and the reader is referred to Hicks[17] for a more detailed discussion of the problem.

Example XII—Sitting systolic and diastolic blood pressure (mm Hg) was measured in 14 patients; in 7 patients after treatment with placebo, and in 7 patients after treatment with an antihypertensive drug. The blood pressure is recorded as systolic/diastolic and is symbolized as S/D.

	$n_1 = 7$ Placebo	$n_2 = 7$ Drug
	150/100	130/90
	180/120	140/100
	140/100	150/100
	180/110	150/110
	180/90	140/90
	190/110	130/90
	170/120	130/90

Variable		
S	$\Sigma S_1 = 1,190$	$\Sigma S_2 = 970$
	$\Sigma S_1^2 = 204,300$	$\Sigma S_2^2 = 134,900$
D	$\Sigma D_1 = 750$	$\Sigma D_2 = 670$
	$\Sigma D_1^2 = 81,100$	$\Sigma D_2^2 = 64,500$
S,D	$\Sigma S_1 D_1 = 127,900$	$\Sigma S_2 D_2 = 93,200$

Table VI—The Rank Sum Table[a]

Values of T or T', Whichever is Smaller, Significant at the 10%, 5%, and 1% Levels

		n_1 (smaller sample)																
n_2	P	4	5	6	7	8	9	10	11	12	13	14	15	16	17	18	19	20
8	0.10	15	23	31	41	51												
	0.05	14	21	29	38	49												
	0.01	11	17	25	34	43												
9	0.10	16	24	33	43	54	66											
	0.05	14	22	31	40	51	62											
	0.01	11	18	26	35	45	56											
10	0.10	17	26	35	45	56	69	82										
	0.05	15	23	32	42	53	65	78										
	0.01	12	19	27	37	47	58	71										
11	0.10	18	27	37	47	59	72	86	100									
	0.05	16	24	34	44	55	68	81	96									
	0.01	12	20	28	38	49	61	73	87									
12	0.10	19	28	38	49	62	75	89	104	120								
	0.05	17	26	35	46	58	71	84	99	115								
	0.01	13	21	30	40	51	63	76	90	105								
13	0.10	20	30	40	52	64	78	92	108	125	142							
	0.05	18	27	37	48	60	73	88	103	119	136							
	0.01	14	22	31	41	53	65	79	93	109	125							
14	0.10	21	31	42	54	67	81	96	112	129	147	166						
	0.05	19	28	38	50	62	76	91	106	123	141	160						
	0.01	14	22	32	43	54	67	81	96	112	129	147						
15	0.10	22	33	44	56	69	84	99	116	133	152	171	192					
	0.05	20	29	40	52	65	79	94	110	127	145	164	184					
	0.01	15	23	33	44	56	69	84	99	115	133	151	171					
16	0.10	24	34	46	58	72	87	103	120	138	156	176	197	219				
	0.05	21	30	42	54	67	82	97	113	131	150	169	190	211				
	0.01	15	24	34	46	58	72	86	102	119	136	155	175	196				
17	0.10	25	35	47	61	75	90	106	123	142	161	182	203	225	249			
	0.05	21	32	43	56	70	84	100	117	135	154	174	195	217	240			
	0.01	16	25	36	47	60	74	89	105	122	140	159	180	201	223			
18	0.10	26	37	49	63	77	93	110	127	146	166	187	208	231	255	280		
	0.05	22	33	45	58	72	87	103	121	139	158	179	200	222	246	270		
	0.01	16	26	37	49	62	76	92	108	125	144	163	184	206	228	252		
19	0.10	27	38	51	65	80	96	113	131	150	171	192	214	237	262	287	313	
	0.05	23	34	46	60	74	90	107	124	143	163	182	205	228	252	277	303	
	0.01	17	27	38	50	64	78	94	111	129	147	168	189	210	234	258	283	
20	0.10	28	40	53	67	83	99	117	135	155	175	197	220	243	268	294	320	348
	0.05	24	35	48	62	77	93	110	128	147	167	188	210	234	258	283	309	337
	0.01	18	28	39	52	66	81	97	114	132	151	172	193	215	239	263	289	315

when $n_1 > 20$ and $n_2 > 20$, significance values are given to a good approximation by
$$n_1(n_1 + n_2 + 1)/2 - z \sqrt{n_1 n_2(n_1 + n_2 + 1)/12}$$
where z is 1.64 for the 10% level, 1.96 for the 5%, and 2.58 for the 1%.

The probability figures given are for a two-tailed test. For a one-tailed test, P is halved.

[a] Adapted from Tate, M. W., and Clelland, R. C.[16]

S $\quad \bar{S}_1 = 1{,}190/7$ $\quad\quad \bar{S}_2 = 970/7$
$\quad\quad = 170.0$ $\quad\quad\quad = 138.6$
$\quad [S_1^2] = 204{,}300 -$ $\quad [S_2^2] = 134{,}900 -$
$\quad\quad\quad (1{,}190)^2/7$ $\quad\quad\quad (970)^2/7$
$\quad\quad = 2000.00$ $\quad\quad\quad = 485.71$

D $\quad \bar{D}_1 = 750/7$ $\quad\quad \bar{D}_2 = 670/7$
$\quad\quad = 107.1$ $\quad\quad\quad = 95.7$
$\quad [D_1^2] = 81{,}100 -$ $\quad [D_2^2] = 64{,}500 -$
$\quad\quad\quad (750)^2/7$ $\quad\quad\quad (670)^2/7$
$\quad\quad = 742.86$ $\quad\quad\quad = 371.43$

S,D $\quad [S_1 D_1] = 127{,}900 -$ $\quad [S_2 D_2] = 93{,}200 -$
$\quad\quad\quad (1{,}190)(750)/7$ $\quad\quad (970)(670)/7$
$\quad\quad = 400.00$ $\quad\quad\quad = 357.14$

t test for systolic blood pressure alone:

$$t = \frac{\bar{S}_1 - \bar{S}_2}{\sqrt{\left(\dfrac{[S_1^2] + [S_2^2]}{n_1 + n_2 - 2}\right)\left(\dfrac{1}{n_1} + \dfrac{1}{n_2}\right)}} =$$

$$\frac{170.0 - 138.6}{\sqrt{\left(\dfrac{2000.00 + 485.71}{7 + 7 - 2}\right)\left(\dfrac{1}{7} + \dfrac{1}{7}\right)}} = 4.08$$

$DF = n = n_1 + n_2 - 2 = 7 + 7 - 2 = 12$

$P < 0.005$

t test for diastolic blood pressure alone:

$$t = \frac{\bar{D}_1 - \bar{D}_2}{\sqrt{\left(\dfrac{[D_1^2] + [D_2^2]}{n_1 + n_2 - 2}\right)\left(\dfrac{1}{n_1} + \dfrac{1}{n_2}\right)}} =$$

$$\frac{107.1 - 95.7}{\sqrt{\left(\dfrac{742.86 + 371.43}{7 + 7 - 2}\right)\left(\dfrac{1}{7} + \dfrac{1}{7}\right)}} = 2.19$$

$DF = n = n_1 + n_2 - 2 = 7 + 7 - 2 = 12$

$0.01 < P < 0.025$

T^2 test for both systolic and diastolic blood pressure:

$$d_1 = \frac{\bar{S}_1 - \bar{S}_2}{\sqrt{\dfrac{1}{n_1} + \dfrac{1}{n_2}}} = \frac{170.0 - 138.6}{\sqrt{\dfrac{1}{7} + \dfrac{1}{7}}} = 58.80$$

$$d_2 = \frac{\bar{D}_1 - \bar{D}_2}{\sqrt{\dfrac{1}{n_1} + \dfrac{1}{n_2}}} = \frac{107.1 - 95.7}{\sqrt{\dfrac{1}{7} + \dfrac{1}{7}}} = 21.35$$

$$a_{11} = \frac{1}{n}\left([S_1^2] + [S_2^2]\right) = \frac{1}{12}(2000.00 + 485.71) = 207.14$$

$$a_{12} = \frac{1}{n}([S_1D_1] + [S_2D_2]) = \frac{1}{12}(400.00 + 357.14) = 63.10$$

$$a_{22} = \frac{1}{n}([D_1^2] + [D_2^2]) = \frac{1}{12}(742.86 + 371.43) = 92.86$$

$$T^2 = \frac{d_1^2 a_{22} - 2d_1d_2a_{12} + d_2^2 a_{11}}{a_{11}a_{22} - a_{12}^2}$$

$$= \frac{(58.80)^2(92.86) - 2(58.80)(21.35)(63.10) + (21.35)^2(207.14)}{(207.14)(92.86) - 3,981.61} = 16.85$$

In order to test the significance of this result, we make use of the fact that

$$F = \left(\frac{n - p + 1}{np}\right)T^2 = \left[\frac{12 - 2 + 1}{(12)(2)}\right](16.85) = 7.72$$

where p = number of variables = 2.

This follows the F distribution with degrees of freedom $f_1 = p = 2$, and $f_2 = n - p + 1 = 11$. We enter the F table (see Table VIII) with $f_1 = 2$, $f_2 = 11$, and $F = 7.72$, and find that the calculated F value 7.72 is larger than the tabulated F value 7.20 for $P = 0.01$. Therefore, since the probability of the average systolic and diastolic blood pressures of the placebo and drug-treated patients being the same is less than 0.05 (actually, it is less than 0.01), we conclude that they are different.

The F Test of Significance—To compare the variances of samples from two populations, we calculate

$$F = s_1^2/s_2^2 \quad \text{with} \quad s_1^2 > s_2^2$$

where

$$s_1^2 = \frac{\Sigma x_{1i}^2 - (\Sigma x_{1i})^2/n_1}{n_1 - 1} = \text{larger variance}$$

$$s_2^2 = \frac{\Sigma x_{2i}^2 - (\Sigma x_{2i})^2/n_2}{n_2 - 1} = \text{smaller variance}$$

To test for significance, the F ratio is referred to the F table (see Table VIII) with $f_1 = n_1 - 1$ and $f_2 = n_2 - 1$ degrees of freedom. The null hypothesis that the two variances are the same is rejected at the $2P$ level of significance.

Example XIII—Two treatments showed the following results:

	A	B
	6	15
	4	4
	3	10
	7	10
	6	5
	4	11
		9
Σx_i	30	64
Σx_i^2	162	668
n_i	6	7
s_i^2	2.40	13.81
f_i	5	6

$$F = s_1^2/s_2^2 = 13.81/2.40 = 5.75$$

$$f_1 = n_1 - 1 = 7 - 1 = 6$$

$$f_2 = n_2 - 1 = 6 - 1 = 5$$

Entering Table VIII with $f_1 = 6$ and $f_2 = 5$ degrees of freedom, we find that the tabulated values of F are 4.95 and 6.98 for $P = 2(0.05) = 0.10$ and $P = 2(0.025) = 0.05$, respectively. Thus, the probability of getting a value of F larger than the calculated value 5.75 is between $P = 0.05$ and $P = 0.10$. Since P is not equal to or less than 0.05, we conclude that there is insufficient evidence to indicate that the two variances are different.

In the test described and exemplified above, both variances were identified as random sampling errors. In some situations (eg, analysis of variance described in Example XV), only one variance can be so identified. The F test then is made by always placing the

Table VII—The Signed-Rank Sum Table[a]

Values of T for Signed-Rank Test, Significant at the 10%, 5%, and 1% Levels

	P		
n	0.10	0.05	0.01
5	0		
6	2	0	
7	3	2	
8	5	3	0
9	8	5	1
10	10	8	3
11	14	10	5
12	17	13	7
13	21	17	9
14	25	21	12
15	30	25	16
16	35	29	19
17	41	34	23
18	47	40	27
19	53	46	32
20	60	52	37
21	67	58	43
22	75	65	49
23	83	73	55
24	91	81	61
25	100	89	68
26	110	97	75
27	120	106	83
28	130	116	91
29	141	126	100
30	152	136	109

when $n > 30$, use

$$T = n(n + 1)/4 - 1 - Z\sqrt{n(n + 1)(2n + 1)/24}$$

where Z is 1.64 for the 10% level, 1.96 for the 5%, and 2.58 for the 1%. The probability figures given are for a two-tailed test. For a one-tailed test, P is halved.

[a] Adapted from Tate, M. W., and Clelland, R. C.[16]

random sampling error in the denominator, regardless of the size of the other variance. We then use the probability values directly from the F table and do not multiply them by 2.

If we desire to compare the variances from paired data, the F test described above would be inappropriate. Instead, we proceed as exemplified below.

Example XIV—A characteristic was measured before and after aging for each of ten items. Is the variability changed with aging?

Item no.	Before aging	After aging
1	8.3	9.3
2	8.4	10.9
3	14.9	13.2
4	14.2	12.8
5	12.5	16.0
6	15.0	15.2
7	17.1	16.8
8	19.2	16.2
9	22.0	17.9
10	18.9	18.9
	$\Sigma x_B = 148.5$	$\Sigma x_A = 147.2$

$$\Sigma x_B^2 = 2,393.81 \qquad \Sigma x_A^2 = 2,252.72$$

$$\Sigma x_A x_B = 2,298.92$$

$$[x_B^2] = 2,393.81 - (148.5)^2/10$$

$$= 188.59$$

$$[x_A^2] = 2,252.72 - (147.2)^2/10$$

$$= 85.94$$

Table VIII—The F Table[a]

10%, 5%, 2.5%, and 1% Points for the Distribution of F

f_2	P	1	2	3	4	5	6	7	8	9	10	20	30	40	60	120	∞
							f_1 Degrees of freedom (for greater mean square)										
5	0.10	4.06	3.78	3.62	3.52	3.45	3.40	3.37	3.34	3.32	3.30	3.21	3.17	3.16	3.14	3.12	3.10
	0.05	6.61	5.79	5.41	5.19	5.05	4.95	4.88	4.82	4.77	4.74	4.56	4.50	4.46	4.43	4.40	4.36
	0.025	10.01	8.43	7.76	7.39	7.15	6.98	6.85	6.76	6.68	6.62	6.33	6.23	6.81	6.12	6.07	6.02
	0.01	16.26	13.27	12.06	11.39	10.97	10.67	10.45	10.27	10.15	10.05	9.55	9.38	9.29	9.20	9.11	9.02
10	0.10	3.28	2.92	2.73	2.61	2.52	2.46	2.41	2.38	2.35	2.32	2.20	2.16	2.13	2.11	2.08	2.06
	0.05	4.96	4.10	3.71	3.48	3.33	3.22	3.14	3.07	3.02	2.98	2.77	2.70	2.66	2.62	2.58	2.54
	0.025	6.94	5.46	4.83	4.47	4.24	4.07	3.95	3.85	3.78	3.72	3.42	3.31	3.26	3.20	3.14	3.08
	0.01	10.04	7.56	6.55	5.99	5.64	5.39	5.21	5.06	4.95	4.85	4.41	4.25	4.17	4.08	4.00	3.91
15	0.10	3.07	2.70	2.49	2.36	2.27	2.21	2.16	2.12	2.09	2.06	1.92	1.87	1.85	1.82	1.79	1.76
	0.05	4.54	3.68	3.29	3.06	2.90	2.79	2.71	2.64	2.59	2.54	2.33	2.25	2.20	2.16	2.11	2.07
	0.025	6.20	4.76	4.15	3.80	3.58	3.41	3.29	3.20	3.12	3.06	2.76	2.64	2.58	2.52	2.46	2.40
	0.01	8.68	6.36	5.42	4.89	4.56	4.32	4.14	4.00	3.89	3.80	3.36	3.20	3.12	3.05	2.96	2.87
20	0.10	2.97	2.59	2.38	2.25	2.16	2.09	2.04	2.00	1.96	1.94	1.79	1.74	1.71	1.68	1.64	1.61
	0.05	4.35	3.49	3.10	2.87	2.71	2.60	2.51	2.45	2.39	2.35	2.12	2.04	1.99	1.95	1.90	1.84
	0.025	5.87	4.46	3.86	3.51	3.29	3.13	3.01	2.91	2.84	2.77	2.46	2.35	2.29	2.22	2.16	2.09
	0.01	8.10	5.85	4.94	4.43	4.10	3.87	3.71	3.56	3.45	3.37	2.94	2.77	2.69	2.61	2.52	2.42
25	0.10	2.92	2.53	2.32	2.18	2.09	2.02	1.97	1.93	1.89	1.87	1.72	1.66	1.63	1.59	1.56	1.52
	0.05	4.24	3.39	2.99	2.76	2.60	2.49	2.40	2.34	2.28	2.24	2.01	1.92	1.87	1.82	1.77	1.71
	0.025	5.69	4.29	3.69	3.35	3.13	2.97	2.85	2.75	2.68	2.61	2.30	2.18	2.12	2.05	1.98	1.91
	0.01	7.77	5.57	4.68	4.18	3.86	3.63	3.46	3.32	3.21	3.13	2.70	2.54	2.45	2.36	2.27	2.17
30	0.10	2.88	2.49	2.28	2.14	2.05	1.98	1.93	1.88	1.85	1.82	1.67	1.61	1.57	1.54	1.50	1.46
	0.05	4.17	3.32	2.92	2.69	2.53	2.42	2.33	2.27	2.21	2.16	1.93	1.84	1.79	1.74	1.68	1.62
	0.025	5.57	4.18	3.59	3.25	3.03	2.87	2.75	2.65	2.57	2.51	2.20	2.07	2.01	1.94	1.87	1.79
	0.01	7.56	5.39	4.51	4.02	3.70	3.47	3.30	3.17	3.06	2.98	2.55	2.38	2.29	2.21	2.11	2.01
40	0.10	2.84	2.44	2.23	2.09	2.00	1.93	1.87	1.83	1.79	1.76	1.61	1.54	1.51	1.47	1.42	1.38
	0.05	4.08	3.23	2.84	2.61	2.45	2.34	2.25	2.18	2.12	2.08	1.84	1.74	1.69	1.64	1.58	1.51
	0.025	5.42	4.05	3.46	3.13	2.90	2.74	2.62	2.53	2.45	2.39	2.07	1.94	1.88	1.80	1.72	1.64
	0.01	7.31	5.18	4.31	3.83	3.51	3.29	3.12	2.99	2.88	2.80	2.37	2.20	2.11	2.02	1.92	1.81
60	0.10	2.79	2.39	2.18	2.04	1.95	1.87	1.82	1.77	1.74	1.71	1.54	1.48	1.44	1.40	1.35	1.29
	0.05	4.00	3.15	2.76	2.53	2.37	2.25	2.17	2.10	2.04	1.99	1.75	1.65	1.59	1.53	1.47	1.39
	0.025	5.29	3.93	3.34	3.01	2.79	2.63	2.51	2.41	2.33	2.27	1.94	1.82	1.74	1.67	1.58	1.48
	0.01	7.08	4.98	4.13	3.65	3.34	3.12	2.95	2.82	2.72	2.63	2.20	2.03	1.93	1.84	1.73	1.60
120	0.10	2.75	2.35	2.13	1.99	1.90	1.82	1.77	1.72	1.68	1.65	1.48	1.41	1.37	1.32	1.26	1.19
	0.05	3.92	3.07	2.68	2.45	2.29	2.18	2.09	2.02	1.96	1.91	1.66	1.55	1.50	1.43	1.35	1.25
	0.025	5.15	3.80	3.23	2.89	2.67	2.52	2.39	2.30	2.22	2.16	1.82	1.69	1.61	1.53	1.43	1.31
	0.01	6.85	4.79	3.95	3.48	3.17	2.96	2.79	2.66	2.56	2.47	2.03	1.86	1.76	1.66	1.53	1.38
∞	0.10	2.71	2.30	2.08	1.94	1.85	1.77	1.72	1.67	1.63	1.60	1.42	1.34	1.30	1.24	1.17	1.00
	0.05	3.84	3.00	2.60	2.37	2.21	2.10	2.01	1.94	1.88	1.83	1.57	1.46	1.39	1.32	1.22	1.00
	0.025	5.02	3.69	3.12	2.79	2.57	2.41	2.29	2.19	2.11	2.05	1.71	1.57	1.48	1.39	1.27	1.00
	0.01	6.64	4.60	3.78	3.32	3.02	2.80	2.64	2.51	2.41	2.32	1.87	1.69	1.59	1.47	1.32	1.00

[a] Adapted from Snedecor, G. W., and Cochran, W. G.,[18] and from Bliss, C. I., and Calhoun, D. W.[19]

$$[x_B x_A] = 2{,}298.92 - (148.5)(147.2)/10$$

$$= 113.00$$

$$t = \frac{([x_B^2] - [x_A^2])\sqrt{n-2}}{2\sqrt{[x_B^2][x_A^2] - [x_B x_A]^2}} =$$

$$\frac{(188.59 - 85.94)\sqrt{8}}{2\sqrt{(188.59)(85.94) - (113.00)^2}} = 2.476$$

$$DF = n - 2 = 10 - 2 = 8$$

In the t table (see Table III), for $P = 0.05$ and $DF = 8$ (two tails), the value of t given is 2.306. The value of t calculated is greater than this. Therefore, since the probability of the variance before and after aging being the same is less than 0.05, we conclude that they are different. Apparently, the variability decreased after aging.

Multiple Comparison Procedures—If three or more samples are to be compared to see if they are all drawn from the same population, the analysis of variance (a sort of multiple t test) can be used as a means of comparison.

Example XV—Groups of three subjects each were given one of ten food regimens and showed the following weight gains (lb):

Analysis of Variance

Source of variation	Degrees of freedom	Sums of squares	Mean squares	F ratio
Among regimens	$t - 1 = 9$	160.54	17.81	8.22
Within regimens	$\Sigma(n_i - 1) = 20$	43.33	$s^2 = 2.17$	
Total	$N - 1 = 29$	203.87		

These are unpaired data, and this type study is referred to as a completely randomized experiment. There are only two sources of variation; the variation among regimens and the variation within regimens, as indicated in the analysis of variance table. The breakdown of the degrees of freedom is self-explanatory. The sums-of-squares are obtained as follows:

$$\text{Total S.S.} = \Sigma x^2 - (\Sigma x)^2/N =$$

$$934 - (148)^2/30 = 203.87$$

$$\text{Among Regimens S.S.} = \frac{(\Sigma x_1)^2}{n_1} + \frac{(\Sigma x_2)^2}{n_2} + \ldots +$$

$$\frac{(\Sigma x_{10})^2}{n_{10}} - \frac{(\Sigma x)^2}{N}$$

$$= \frac{(7)^2}{3} + \frac{(3)^2}{3} + \ldots +$$

Food Regimen

	A	B	C	D	E	F	G	H	I	J	(t = 10 regimens)
	2	1	2	4	9	3	6	7	4	4	
	3	2	4	8	8	8	5	6	4	6	
	2	0	1	7	11	6	6	6	7	6	
											Sums
Σx_i	7	3	7	19	28	17	17	19	15	16	$\Sigma x = 148$
Σx_i^2	17	5	21	129	266	109	97	121	81	88	$\Sigma x^2 = 934$
n_i	3	3	3	3	3	3	3	3	3	3	$N = 30$
$n_i - 1$	2	2	2	2	2	2	2	2	2	2	$\Sigma(n_i - 1) = 20$
$\bar{x}_i$	2.3	1.0	2.3	6.3	9.3	5.7	5.7	6.3	5.0	5.3	

$$\frac{(16)^2}{3} - \frac{(148)^2}{30} = 160.54$$

Within regimens S.S. $= 203.87 - 160.54 = 43.33$

The mean squares are obtained by dividing the sums-of-squares by their corresponding degrees of freedom. The mean square within regimens, s^2, is the pooled variance for the ten samples. Since this is the only variance that can be identified as random sampling error (the mean square among regimens has in addition a component due to the variability among regimens), it becomes the denominator in the F ratio, so that

$$F = \frac{\text{mean square among regimens}}{\text{mean square within regimens}} = \frac{17.81}{2.17} = 8.22$$

To test for significance, the F ratio is referred to the F table (see Table VIII) with $f_1 = t - 1 = 9$ and $f_2 = \Sigma(n_i - 1) = 20$ degrees of freedom. We find that the calculated value 8.22 is larger than the tabulated value 3.45 for $P = 0.01$. Therefore, since the probability of these ten samples being drawn from the same population is less than 0.05 (actually, it is less than 0.01), we conclude that they are not all the same (ie, not all the means are equal).

However, this conclusion in itself is not very helpful. One is generally interested in making multiple comparisons, to determine which means are different from each other and which are not. The general procedure is to list the ranked means from lowest to highest and underline the means which are not statistically significantly different from each other. Sometimes brackets or parentheses are used instead of an underline. The procedure is carried out by calculating a 5% allowance, which is defined as the critical difference between means which allows one to reject the null hypothesis ($\mu_i = \mu_j$) and accept the alternative hypothesis ($\mu_i \neq \mu_j$) for any two sample means $\bar{x}_i$ and $\bar{x}_j$ at $P = 0.05$. To calculate the 5% allowance we need the following:

s^2 = pooled variance from the analysis of variance.

DF = degrees of freedom for the pooled variance from the analysis of variance.

n_i, n_j = the number of observations from which the means $\bar{x}_i$ and $\bar{x}_j$ were determined, respectively.

t = a critical value at $P = 0.05$ which depends upon the DF and the degree of conservatism desired as exemplified by the multiple comparison procedures described below:

Least Significant Difference Procedure—For this method

$$5\% \text{ allowance} = t\sqrt{s^2(1/n_i + 1/n_j)}$$

where t is the value of t from Table III (two tails). This is the least conservative procedure, and assures that the probability that any one comparison is judged to be significant by chance alone is 5%. However, the probability of one or more comparisons being judged significant would be greater than 5%. Applied to the results of Example XV, we have:

$$s^2 = 2.17$$
$$n_i, n_j = 3,3$$
$$DF = 20$$

$t = 2.086$ from Table III for 20 DF and $P = 0.05$ (two tails)

$5\% \text{ allowance} = t\sqrt{s^2(1/n_i + 1/n_j)} =$
$$2.086\sqrt{2.17(1/3 + 1/3)} = 2.51$$

Thus, any two means differing by 2.51 or more are judged to be different.

Ranked Means

B	A,C	I	J	F,G	D,H	E
1.0	2.3	5.0	5.3	5.7	6.3	9.3

or, (BAC) $(IJFGDH)$ (E).

Any two means underscored by the same line (or included in the same parentheses) do not differ statistically at $P = 0.05$.

Any two means *not* underscored by the same line (or *not* included in the same parentheses) are statistically significantly different at $P \leq 0.05$.

Studentized Range Procedure—For this method

$$5\% \text{ allowance} = \frac{Q}{\sqrt{2}}\sqrt{s^2(1/n_i + 1/n_j)}$$

where Q is the Studentized Range value for k treatments from Table IX. This is one of the most conservative procedures, and assures that the probability of one or more comparisons being judged significant by chance alone is 5%. Applied to the results of Example XV, we have:

$Q = 5.01$ from Table IX for $k = 10$ treatments, 20 DF, and $P = 0.05$.

$$5\% \text{ allowance} = \frac{Q}{\sqrt{2}}\sqrt{s^2(1/n_i + 1/n_j)} =$$
$$\frac{5.01}{\sqrt{2}}\sqrt{2.17(1/3 + 1/3)} = 4.26$$

Thus, any two means differing by 4.26 or more are judged to be different.

Ranked Means

B	A,C	I	J	F,G	D,H	E
1.0	2.3	5.0	5.3	5.7	6.3	9.3

or, $(BACI)$ $(ACIJFGDH)$ $(JFGDHE)$.

Duncan's New Multiple Range Procedure—For this method

$$5\% \text{ allowance} = \frac{t_k}{\sqrt{2}}\sqrt{s^2(1/n_i + 1/n_j)}$$

where t_k are values for 2,3, - - - -, k treatments obtained from Table X. The critical values will be A_2, A_3, - - - -, A_k, depending upon how many means are included in the range of ranked means being compared. This is next to the least conservative procedure. Applied to the results of Example XV, we have:

$$5\% \text{ allowance} = \frac{t_k}{\sqrt{2}}\sqrt{s^2(1/n_i + 1/n_j)} =$$
$$\frac{t_k}{\sqrt{2}}\sqrt{2.17(1/3 + 1/3)}$$

Values of t_k from Table X for $k = 2$ to 10 treatments, 20 DF, and $P = 0.05$ give the following allowances:

k	t_k	A_k
2	2.95	2.51
3	3.10	2.64
4	3.18	2.70
5	3.25	2.76
6	3.30	2.81
7	3.34	2.84
8	3.36	2.86
9	3.38	2.87
10	3.40	2.89

Thus, the critical difference between E and B is 2.89 because the range includes ten means; the critical difference between E and H is 2.64 because the range includes three means; etc.

Ranked Means

B	A,C	I	J	F,G	D,H	E
1.0	2.3	5.0	5.3	5.7	6.3	9.3

or, (BAC) $(IJFGDH)$ (E).

Dunnett's Procedure—The three procedures previously described are appropriate when it is desired to compare all possible pairs of means. Dunnett considered the problem when the objective of the study is to

Table IX—The Q Table[a]

Upper 5% Points, Q, in the Studentized Range

DF	2	3	4	5	6	7	8	9	10	11	12	13	14	15	16	17	18	19	20
								k (Number of treatments)											
10	3.15	3.88	4.33	4.66	4.91	5.12	5.30	5.46	5.60	5.72	5.83	5.93	6.03	6.12	6.20	6.27	6.34	6.41	6.47
11	3.11	3.82	4.26	4.58	4.82	5.03	5.20	5.35	5.49	5.61	5.71	5.81	5.90	5.98	6.06	6.14	6.20	6.27	6.33
12	3.08	3.77	4.20	4.51	4.75	4.95	5.12	5.27	5.40	5.51	5.61	5.71	5.80	5.88	5.95	6.02	6.09	6.15	6.21
13	3.06	3.73	4.15	4.46	4.69	4.88	5.05	5.19	5.32	5.43	5.53	5.63	5.71	5.79	5.86	5.93	6.00	6.06	6.11
14	3.03	3.70	4.11	4.41	4.64	4.83	4.99	5.13	5.25	5.36	5.46	5.56	5.64	5.72	5.79	5.86	5.92	5.98	6.03
15	3.01	3.67	4.08	4.37	4.59	4.78	4.94	5.08	5.20	5.31	5.40	5.49	5.57	5.65	5.72	5.79	5.85	5.91	5.96
16	3.00	3.65	4.05	4.34	4.56	4.74	4.90	5.03	5.15	5.26	5.35	5.44	5.52	5.59	5.66	5.73	5.79	5.84	5.90
17	2.98	3.62	4.02	4.31	4.52	4.70	4.86	4.99	5.11	5.21	5.31	5.39	5.47	5.55	5.61	5.68	5.74	5.79	5.84
18	2.97	3.61	4.00	4.28	4.49	4.67	4.83	4.96	5.07	5.17	5.27	5.35	5.43	5.50	5.57	5.63	5.69	5.74	5.79
19	2.96	3.59	3.98	4.26	4.47	4.64	4.79	4.92	5.04	5.14	5.23	5.32	5.39	5.46	5.53	5.59	5.65	5.70	5.75
20	2.95	3.58	3.96	4.24	4.45	4.62	4.77	4.90	5.01	5.11	5.20	5.28	5.36	5.43	5.50	5.56	5.61	5.66	5.71
24	2.92	3.53	3.90	4.17	4.37	4.54	4.68	4.81	4.92	5.01	5.10	5.18	5.25	5.32	5.38	5.44	5.50	5.55	5.59
30	2.89	3.48	3.84	4.11	4.30	4.46	4.60	4.72	4.83	4.92	5.00	5.08	5.15	5.21	5.27	5.33	5.38	5.43	5.48
40	2.86	3.44	3.79	4.04	4.23	4.39	4.52	4.63	4.74	4.82	4.90	4.98	5.05	5.11	5.17	5.22	5.27	5.32	5.36
60	2.83	3.40	3.74	3.98	4.16	4.31	4.44	4.55	4.65	4.73	4.81	4.88	4.94	5.00	5.06	5.11	5.15	5.20	5.24
120	2.80	3.36	3.69	3.92	4.10	4.24	4.36	4.47	4.56	4.64	4.71	4.78	4.84	4.90	4.95	5.00	5.04	5.09	5.13
∞	2.77	3.32	3.63	3.86	4.03	4.17	4.29	4.39	4.47	4.55	4.62	4.68	4.74	4.80	4.84	4.89	4.93	4.97	5.01

[a] Adapted from Snedecor, G. W., and Cochran, W. G.[18]

Table X—The Multiple Range Table[a]

Values of t_k for Duncan's New Multiple Range Test at the 5% Level of Significance

DF	2	3	4	5	6	8	10	14	20
				k (Number of treatments)					
10	3.15	3.29	3.37	3.43	3.46	3.47	3.47	3.47	3.48
12	3.08	3.23	3.33	3.36	3.40	3.44	3.46	3.46	3.48
14	3.03	3.18	3.27	3.33	3.37	3.41	3.44	3.46	3.47
16	3.00	3.15	3.23	3.30	3.34	3.39	3.43	3.45	3.47
18	2.97	3.12	3.21	3.27	3.32	3.37	3.41	3.45	3.47
20	2.95	3.10	3.18	3.25	3.30	3.36	3.40	3.44	3.47
24	2.92	3.07	3.15	3.22	3.28	3.34	3.38	3.44	3.47
30	2.89	3.04	3.12	3.20	3.25	3.32	3.37	3.43	3.47
60	2.83	2.98	3.08	3.14	3.20	3.28	3.33	3.40	3.47
100	2.80	2.95	3.05	3.12	3.18	3.26	3.32	3.40	3.47
∞	2.77	2.92	3.02	3.09	3.15	3.23	3.29	3.38	3.47

[a] Adapted from Duncan, D. B.[20]

compare several treatments with a standard or control, as in a screening procedure. In his method

$$5\% \text{ allowance} = t_D \sqrt{s^2(1/n_i + 1/n_j)}$$

where t_D is Dunnett's t_D value for k treatments (excluding the standard or control) obtained from Table XI. Like the Studentized Range procedure, this is one of the most conservative procedures, and assures that the probability of one or more comparisons between treatments and a standard or control being judged significant by chance alone is 5%. The one-tail values (listed in the tables for $P = 0.10$) are used when the objective of the study is to select only those treatments that have higher (or lower) means than the standard or control; the two-tail values (listed in the table for $P = 0.05$) are used when the objective of the study is to select those treatments that are different from the standard or control. Of course, the decision to carry out a one-tailed or a two-tailed test must be made before the study begins.

In Example XV, suppose J is a standard regimen, and it is desired to determine which regimens show different weight gains from J. We would proceed as follows:

$t_D = 3.07$ from Table XI for $k = 9$ treatments, 20 DF, and

$$P = 0.05 \text{ (two-tails)}$$

$$5\% \text{ allowance} = t_D \sqrt{s^2(1/n_i + 1/n_j)} =$$

$$3.07 \sqrt{2.17 \ (1/3 + 1/3)} = 3.68$$

Thus, any regimen mean that differs from the mean for regimen J by 3.68 or more is judged to be different from J.

Ranked Means

B	A,C	I	J	F,G	D,H	E
1.0	2.3	5.0	5.3	5.7	6.3	9.3

We would conclude that B showed a statistically smaller weight gain than J, that E showed a statistically significantly larger weight gain than J, and that there was insufficient evidence to indicate that the other regimens were different from J.

In the same example, if regimen A is a control group and we knew beforehand that all of the other regimens had to be at least as good as the control or better, it may be desired to select those regimens that are statistically significantly better. We would proceed as follows:

$t_D = 2.60$ from Table XI for $k = 9$ treatments, 20 DF, and

$$P = 0.10 \text{ (this corresponds to a one-tail } P = 0.05)$$

$$5\% \text{ allowance} = t_D \sqrt{s^2(1/n_i + 1/n_j)} =$$

$$2.60 \sqrt{2.17 \ (1/3 + 1/3)} = 3.12$$

Thus, any regimen mean that is larger than the mean for regimen A by 3.12 or more is judged to be better than A.

Ranked Means

B	A,C	I	J	F,G	D,H	E
1.0	2.3	5.0	5.3	5.7	6.3	9.3

We would conclude that F, G, D, H, and E showed a statistically significantly better weight gain than A, and that there is insufficient evidence to indicate that B, C, I, and J were any better than A.

Comparison of Several Variances—The multiple comparison procedures discussed previously can be used also to compare three or more variances. The procedure is illustrated below for data given by Finney,[22] and applying Duncan's New Multiple Range test to an analysis of variance procedure suggested by Levene.[23] The procedure also illustrates the modifications required for Duncan's New Multiple Range test when $n_i \neq n_j$ (ie, unequal number of observations in each sample).

Example XVI—Line test scores (bounded so that they could only vary from 0 to 24) were obtained in groups of rachitic rats given four graded doses of Vitamin D. There was some indication that rats on the lowest and on the highest dose varied less than rats on the two middle doses. Were these differences statistically significant?

Then, these give the critical values R_k:

k	(2)	(3)	(4)
t_k	2.88	3.03	3.11
R_k	3.658	3.848	3.950

The ranked $\bar{Z}_i$ and replication numbers are:

A	D	B	C
1.604	1.924	3.305	4.244
(11)	(9)	(11)	(7)

We next calculate

$$(\bar{Z}_i - \bar{Z}_j)' = (\bar{Z}_i - \bar{Z}_j) \sqrt{2(n_i n_j)/(n_i + n_j)}$$

Thus, for $C - A$, we obtain

$$(C - A)' = (C - A) \sqrt{2(n_i n_j)/(n_i + n_j)} =$$
$$(4.244 - 1.604) \sqrt{2(7)(11)/18} = 7.719$$

Dose

(International units of vitamin D)

	A (0.64)		B (1.28)		C (2.15)		D (4.30)		($t = 4$ doses)
	x	Z	x	Z	x	Z	x	Z	
	2	0.64	4	3.36	8	4.29	14	2.56	
	0	2.64	9	1.64	17	4.71	14	2.56	
	2	0.64	4	3.36	6	6.9	13	3.56	
	4	1.36	13	5.64	14	1.71	19	2.44	
	0	2.64	3	4.36	17	4.71	17	0.44	
	5	2.36	7	0.36	16	3.71	17	0.44	
	3	0.36	4	3.36	8	4.29	20	3.44	
	4	1.36	4	3.36			18	1.44	
	2	0.64	10	2.64			17	0.44	
	6	3.36	12	4.64					
	1	1.64	11	3.64					Sums
Σx_i	29		81		86		149		$N = 38$
n_i	11		11		7		9		
$\bar{x}_i$	2.64		7.36		12.29		16.56		
ΣZ_i		17.64		36.36		29.71		17.32	$\Sigma Z = 101.703$
ΣZ_i^2		38.5456		140.5456		137.4287		46.2224	$\Sigma Z^2 = 362.7423$
$\bar{Z}_i$		1.604		3.305		4.244		1.924	
$n_i - 1$	10		10		6		8		$\Sigma(n_i - 1) = 34$

where

$x_i = $ the individual line test scores
$Z_i = |x_i - \bar{x}_i| = $ the individual absolute (ie, positive) differences between the line test scores in a dose group and the average line test score for that group

An analysis of variance is carried out using the Z's in exactly the same manner as was described in Example XV.

Analysis of variance (Z's)

Source of variation	DF	S.S.	M.S.	F
Among doses	$t - 1 = 3$	39.2967	13.0989	8.12
Within doses	$\Sigma(n_i - 1) = 34$	54.8387	$s^2 = 1.6129$	
Total	$N - 1 = 37$	94.1354		

To test for significance, the F ratio is referred to the F table (see Table VIII) with $f_1 = t - 1 = 3$ and $f_2 = \Sigma(n_i - 1) = 34$ degrees of freedom. We see that the calculated value 8.12 is larger than the tabulated value 4.4 (interpolated from the values 4.51 and 4.31 for f_1, $f_2 = 3{,}30$ and $3{,}40$, respectively) for $P = 0.01$. Therefore, since the probability of these four results being drawn from the same population is less than 0.05 (actually, it is less than 0.01), we conclude that they are not all the same. To apply Duncan's New Multiple Range test, we need

$s = \sqrt{1.6129} = 1.270$
$k = $ number of variances $= 4$
$DF = 34$
$t_k = $ values interpolated from Table X for $k = 2$ to 4 variances, 34 DF, and $P = 0.05$
$R_k = t_k s = $ critical values for ranges of 2 to 4 ranked means.

Similarly, for the other differences we obtain:

$$(D - D)' = 6.510$$
$$(C - B)' = 2.746$$
$$(B - A)' = 5.642$$
$$(B - D)' = 4.345$$
$$(D - A)' = 1.007$$

To test for significance, we compare these to the critical values R_k, as follows:

Test sequences	Result
1. $(C - A)' > R_4$, $(C - D)' > R_3$, $(C - B)' \not> R_2$	(BC)
2. $(B - A)' > R_3$, $(B - D)' > R_2$	
3. $(D - A)' \not> R_2$	(AD)

The final result is:

$$(AD)(BC)$$

The interpretation is that doses A and D have the same variances, doses B and C have the same variances, and doses A and D have smaller variances than doses B and C.

Rejection of Aberrant Observations—It is common practice among chemists and others working in the physical sciences to make observations in duplicate or triplicate. This is usually for the purpose both of obtaining a more accurate result and also detecting mistakes in dilution, weighing, etc. It is quite a common practice to reject the most extreme of the two or three results if it appears to disagree with the others.

Table XI—The t_D Table[a]

Values of t_D for Dunnett's Procedure for Comparing Several Treatments with a Control at the 5% Level of Significance
(Use $P = 0.10$ values for a one-tailed test and $P = 0.05$ values for a two-tailed test)

DF	P	\multicolumn{8}{c}{k (Number of treatments, excluding the control)}							
		2	3	4	5	6	7	8	9
10	0.10	2.15	2.34	2.47	2.56	2.64	2.70	2.76	2.81
	0.05	2.57	2.81	2.97	3.11	3.21	3.31	3.39	3.46
11	0.10	2.13	2.31	2.44	2.53	2.60	2.67	2.72	2.77
	0.05	2.53	2.76	2.92	3.05	3.15	3.24	3.31	3.38
12	0.10	2.11	2.29	2.41	2.50	2.58	2.64	2.69	2.74
	0.05	2.50	2.72	2.88	3.00	3.10	3.18	3.25	3.32
13	0.10	2.09	2.27	2.39	2.48	2.55	2.61	2.66	2.71
	0.05	2.48	2.69	2.84	2.96	3.06	3.14	3.21	3.27
14	0.10	2.08	2.25	2.37	2.46	2.53	2.59	2.64	2.69
	0.05	2.46	2.67	2.81	2.93	3.02	3.10	3.17	3.23
15	0.10	2.07	2.24	2.36	2.44	2.51	2.57	2.62	2.67
	0.05	2.44	2.64	2.79	2.90	2.99	3.07	3.13	3.19
16	0.10	2.06	2.23	2.34	2.43	2.50	2.56	2.61	2.65
	0.05	2.42	2.63	2.77	2.88	2.96	3.04	3.10	3.16
17	0.10	2.05	2.22	2.33	2.42	2.49	2.54	2.59	2.64
	0.05	2.41	2.61	2.75	2.85	2.94	3.01	3.08	3.13
18	0.10	2.04	2.21	2.32	2.41	2.48	2.53	2.58	2.62
	0.05	2.40	2.59	2.73	2.84	2.92	2.99	3.05	3.11
19	0.10	2.03	2.20	2.31	2.40	2.47	2.52	2.57	2.61
	0.05	2.39	2.58	2.72	2.82	2.90	2.97	3.04	3.09
20	0.10	2.03	2.19	2.30	2.39	2.46	2.51	2.56	2.60
	0.05	2.38	2.57	2.70	2.81	2.89	2.96	3.02	3.07
24	0.10	2.01	2.17	2.28	2.36	2.43	2.48	2.53	2.57
	0.05	2.35	2.53	2.66	2.76	2.84	2.91	2.96	3.01
30	0.10	1.99	2.15	2.25	2.33	2.40	2.45	2.50	2.54
	0.05	2.32	2.50	2.62	2.72	2.79	2.86	2.91	2.96
40	0.10	1.97	2.13	2.23	2.31	2.37	2.42	2.47	2.51
	0.05	2.29	2.47	2.58	2.67	2.75	2.81	2.86	2.90
60	0.10	1.95	2.10	2.21	2.28	2.35	2.39	2.44	2.48
	0.05	2.27	2.43	2.55	2.63	2.70	2.76	2.81	2.85
120	0.10	1.93	2.08	2.18	2.26	2.32	2.37	2.41	2.45
	0.05	2.24	2.40	2.51	2.59	2.66	2.71	2.76	2.80
∞	0.10	1.92	2.06	2.16	2.23	2.29	2.34	2.38	2.42
	0.05	2.21	2.37	2.47	2.55	2.62	2.67	2.71	2.75

[a] Adapted from Dunnett, C. W.[21]

Youden[24,25] of the National Bureau of Standards, a chemist as well as a statistician, has made a study of this problem of rejection of observations in an attempt to answer two questions:

1. If the extreme observation of triplicates is always rejected when only normal variation is present, how accurate is the result? Is the average of the two closest observations as good an estimate as the average of all three?
2. By how much should the outlying observation of triplicates differ from the other two in order to be reasonably assured that this difference is due to a blunder rather than normal variation?

He found that by rejection of the outlying observation not only was the variation greatly underestimated but the mean was biased. If a group of 20 samples of three observations each was considered and in each sample the extreme observation was rejected, this operation increased the variation among the averages of the 20 samples.

If one wished to follow a simple rule of rejection[24,25] of observations in samples of three so as to reject not more than 5% of the extreme observations arising from normal variation, a rejection ratio of D/d greater than 20 would be required.

$$D/d = 20$$

where

D = difference between the most extreme observation and its closest neighbor
d = difference between two closest observations

In the USP there is an excellent chapter on the *Design and Analysis of Biological Assays* in which are included some tests for rejection of such observations as may be out of line. Some of the same tests and some others are also given by Dixon and Massey.[26] Two definite criteria are given, one for rejecting single suspect observations in one group and the other for rejecting a whole group of observations when it is suspect as compared with three or more other groups.

To use the first criterion, arrange the observations in the group in order of their magnitude and number them from 1 to n beginning with the supposedly erratic observation, thus

$$y_1, y_2, y_3 \ldots y_n$$

where y_1 is the suspect observation. If there are 3–7 observations in the group, calculate

$$G_1 = \frac{y_2 - y_1}{y_n - y_1}$$

If there are 8–13 observations in the group, and the smallest value seems suspect, again arrange them in order from lowest to highest and calculate

$$G_2 = \frac{y_3 - y_1}{y_{n-1} - y_1}$$

If the largest value is open to suspicion as possibly being aberrant, arrange the observations in order from highest to lowest and number them, always labeling the suspect observation y_1.

If there are 14–24 observations, follow the same procedure, but use the statistic

$$G_3 = \frac{y_3 - y_1}{y_{n-2} - y_1}$$

If the calculated value of G_1, G_2, or G_3 is larger than the tabled value for the desired probability of occurring by chance, it can be assumed that the observation does not truly belong to the group and the observation is rejected. The values of G_1, G_2, and G_3 for a probability $P = 0.01$ that an outlier could occur at either end or $P = 0.02$ that it would occur only at one end is given in the right-hand column of Table XII. This same criterion could be used for testing whether the largest or smallest average in a group of averages differs significantly from the remainder of the averages.

Example XVII—Suppose among the gains in weight of six rats after a feeding experiment one weight was found to be much less than the other five. Can that observation be discarded? The six gains in weight are: 36, 40, 38, 42, 20, and 39.

Rearrange these in order from smallest to largest and label $y_1 \ldots y_6$, where $n = 6$.

y_1	20
y_2	36
y_3	38
y_4	39
y_5	40
y_6	42

$$G_1 = \frac{y_2 - y_1}{y_6 - y_1} = \frac{36 - 20}{42 - 20} = \frac{16}{22} = 0.727$$

Referring to the value of G_1 for $n = 6$ in the table, $G_1 = 0.644$ for $P = 0.01$. Since the calculated value of G_1 is larger than this value, reject the value of 20 and work with the remaining five values.

The second criterion for an aberrant observation as given in the USP compares the variation or range between various groups. It is a test for the homogeneity of the ranges (the range is again the highest value in a group minus the lowest value) and is for the purpose of locating outliers within one group of values. This method and its accompanying table are presented in considerable detail in the USP.

Caution to Be Observed in Interpretation of Results—Again it must be repeated that the purposes and assumptions made in designing the experiment or assay must be kept in mind while interpreting the results. One must not be overwhelmed by the calculations into believing that the use of statistics covers all the weak points in the experiment. As Francis Galton said:

"It is always well to retain a clear geometric view of the facts when we are dealing with statistical problems, which abound with dangerous pitfalls, easily overlooked by the unwary, while they are cantering gaily along upon their arithmetic."

It is unwise to draw sweeping conclusions from one experiment.

Quality-Control Methods—A very short explanation is given here regarding the quality-control methods that were developed primarily by Dr. Walter Shewhart of the Bell Telephone Laboratories. A more complete explanation can be found in two short publications of the American Standards Association[27,28] and many texts, including Dixon and Massey.[29]

The quality-control method for variables involves plotting the data as dots on a graph with the variable measured on the vertical axis and time (hours, days, etc) on the horizontal axis. The "control" is maintained by inserting on the chart the grand average and control limits which have been calculated from accumulated experience and drawn on the chart as parallel horizontal lines as shown in Fig. 70. When all the dots fall within the limits, the results are said to be in a state of "statis-

Table XII—Criteria for Testing Extreme Value

Statistic	n, Number of observations	Critical values
$G_1 = \dfrac{y_2 - y_1}{y_n - y_1}$	3	.976
	4	.846
	5	.729
	6	.644
	7	.586
$G_2 = \dfrac{y_3 - y_1}{y_{n-1} - y_1}$	8	.780
	9	.725
	10	.678
	11	.638
	12	.605
	13	.578
$G_3 = \dfrac{y_3 - y_1}{y_{n-2} - y_1}$	14	.602
	15	.579
	16	.559
	17	.542
	18	.527
	19	.514
	20	.502
	21	.491
	22	.481
	23	.472
	24	.464

tical control." When a dot falls outside the limits, trouble is indicated.

In a control chart usually each dot is an average for a sample consisting of, eg, four observations. The standard error of the average is then calculated for each group of four observations, and an average value for the standard error of the average is obtained. Let us designate this by $s_{\bar{x}}$. The grand average of all the averages plotted is also calculated and is labeled $\bar{x}$. The "3-sigma" control limits used on the control chart can be obtained from:

$$\text{Upper limit} = \bar{x} + 3s_{\bar{x}}$$
$$\text{Lower limit} = \bar{x} - 3s_{\bar{x}}$$

Thus it can be seen that the control chart technique is a graphic means of investigating whether or not the variation exhibited over a very short period of time is the same as the variation that occurs over a long period of time. If the two variations are identical and all of the plotted dots fall within the control limits, the experiments or processes that produced the data are said to be in a state of "statistical control."

It is possible to calculate the control limits by using the range in each group of, eg, four instead of calculating the standard deviation. This is because, on the average, for samples of less than ten, the range and the standard deviation are very closely related. Given the

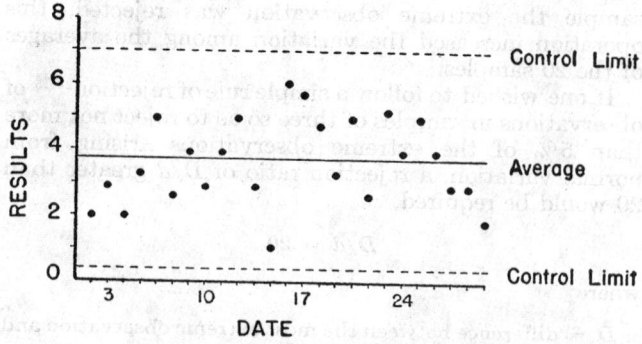

Fig. 70. A typical quality control chart.

Table XIII—Calculation of Standard Deviation from Range

Size of sample (n)	Average number of standard deviations in the average range (d)
2	1.128
3	1.693
4	2.059
5	2.326
6	2.534
7	2.704
8	2.847
9	2.970
10	3.078

Table XIV—Factors for 3-Sigma Limits[a]

Size of sample (n)	Factors for R chart		Factor for X chart
	D_3	D_4	A_2
2	0	3.27	1.880
3	0	2.57	1.023
4	0	2.28	0.729
5	0	2.11	0.577
6	0	2.00	0.483
7	0.08	1.92	0.419
8	0.14	1.86	0.373
9	0.18	1.82	0.337
10	0.22	1.78	0.308

[a] This table contains parts of the tables in Appendix 1 of Z1.3—1958.[27]

number of observations in the sample the standard deviation can be calculated by dividing the range by the appropriate figure given in Table XIII for the size of sample, n. The factors for calculating 3-sigma limits from the range are given as column A_2 in Table XIV.

Control charts using 3-sigma limits can be obtained by the use of figures given in Table XIV. The formulas are as follows:

Upper limit for averages $= \bar{\bar{x}} + A_2\bar{R}$
Lower limit for averages $= \bar{\bar{x}} - A_2\bar{R}$
Upper limit for ranges $= D_4\bar{R}$
Lower limit for ranges $= D_3\bar{R}$
Where $\bar{R} = $ average range

These calculated limits are drawn on the charts as described above.

Example XVIII—A drug manufacturing concern keeps a record of the uniformity of the machine that is filling a given weight of a drug into ampuls. Samples of the finished product are taken at definite time intervals. The data are accumulated and arranged into groups of 4 ampuls according to the order in which they were taken from the filling machine. The average and the range are computed for each group of 4 as given in Table XV according to the time the samples are taken. The resulting quality-control charts are given in Fig. 71.

Control Chart for Fraction Defective—This chart may be applied to results of an inspection that accepts or rejects individual items of a product. The chart is designed with the same objectives in mind as the $\bar{x}$ and $\bar{R}$ charts. Its most effective use is in the improvement of quality, although it also discloses the presence of assignable causes of variation. It provides management with an effective quality history. Fraction defective, p, may be defined as the ratio of the number of defective articles found in any inspection or series of inspections to the total number of articles actually inspected. This is expressed nearly always as a decimal

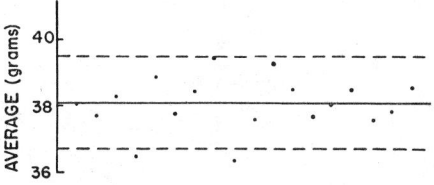

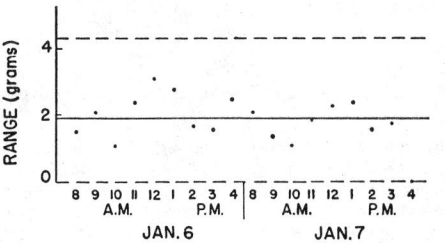

Fig. 71. Quality control charts for data from Table XV.

Table XV—Calculations for a Quality Control Chart

On Averages and Ranges for Samples of 4 from a Filling Machine

Time	Average (gr)	Range (gr)	Time	Average (gr)	Range (gr)
Jan. 6			Jan. 7		
8 am	38.1	1.5	8 am	37.6	2.1
9 am	37.6	2.1	9 am	39.1	1.4
10 am	38.3	1.1	10 am	38.5	1.1
11 am	36.5	2.4	11 am	37.7	1.9
12 M	38.9	3.1	12 M	38.1	2.3
1 pm	37.8	2.8	1 pm	38.5	2.4
2 pm	38.5	1.7	2 pm	37.6	1.6
3 pm	39.4	1.6	3 pm	37.9	1.8
4 pm	36.4	2.5	4 pm	38.6	1.0

Grand average $= \bar{\bar{x}} = 38.1$
Average range $= \bar{R} = 1.9$
Control limits[a] for average $= \bar{\bar{x}} \pm A_2\bar{R} = 38.1 \pm 0.729(1.9)$
Upper limit $= 39.49$
Lower limit $= 36.71$
Control limits[b] for range, are $D_3\bar{R}$ and $D_4\bar{R}$ or 0(1.9) and 2.28(1.9) which equal 0 and 4.33, respectively.

[a] A_2 is the factor for using the range to calculate 3-sigma limits for the average (ie, 3 times the standard error of the average). See Table XIV for $N = 4$.
[b] D_2 and D_4 are the factors for using the range to calculate 3-sigma limits for the range (ie, 3 times the standard error of the range). These values are taken from Table XIV.

fraction (see Fig. 72). The formula for the control limits on a fraction defective chart is

$$\bar{p} \pm 3\sqrt{\frac{\bar{p}(1-\bar{p})}{n}}$$

In the minds of pharmaceutical personnel, defective pieces are usually in the nature of minor blemishes such as scratches on tablets or air bubbles in gelatin capsules. These do not affect the therapeutic quality of the product.

Example XIX—A department head in a capsule department of a large pharmaceutical house keeps a control on the number of defective capsules found in sections (approximately 19,000 capsules are in each section) of large lots of capsules (see Table XVI). In instances where the point plottings fall above the upper control limit this indicates that a greater number of defects are present than one might expect ie, there is lack of statistical control. These sections of production are given special sortings and action is taken at the machine to correct causes of bad quality.

The sample size, n, is 300 capsules from each section and typical data are given in Table XVI.

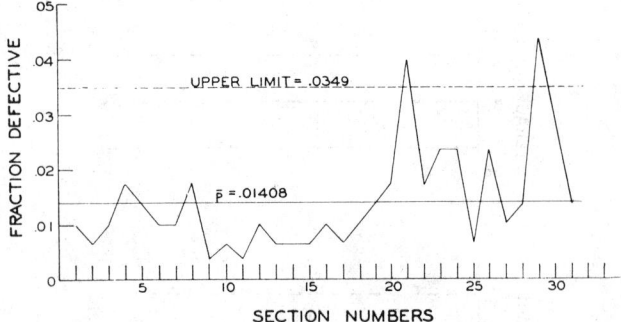

Fig. 72.   Control chart for fraction defective (courtesy, Lilly).

It should be noted that Sections 21 and 29 appear to be out of control. These sections were given 100% sortings. Approximately 4.5% defective capsules were removed from each section.

Another type of chart for attributes can be used that often has advantages over the p chart. If sample sizes are constant, it is convenient to use a control chart for number of defectives or a chart for np. Control limits for this chart are

$$\text{Control limits for } n\bar{p} = n\bar{p} \pm 3\sqrt{n\bar{p}(1 - \bar{p})}$$

Acceptance Sampling—Acceptance sampling has become one of the major fields of statistical quality control. It is used in many phases of manufacturing such as inspection of incoming materials, process inspection at various points in the manufacturing operations, and final inspection of the finished product. Sampling inspection usually is used in lieu of 100% inspection for several reasons; (1) the cost of 100% inspection is prohibitive; (2) 100% inspection is fatiguing and may result in the inspectors making errors; (3) the inspection operation may involve destructive testing; and (4) a statistical sampling plan well applied may give better quality assurance than 100% inspection. In sampling one must consider the laws of probability. There are certain risks involved, namely, the risk of rejecting good quality material and the risk of accepting bad merchandise. Sampling plans can be designed and applied in such a manner as to reduce these risks to a minimum and, over a period of time, give assurance of quality products.

The graph illustrating the performance of a sampling plan (ie, ability to discriminate between acceptable and unacceptable lots) is called an *operating characteristic curve*. For any given quality of submitted material it is possible to determine the probability of acceptance.

Example XX—The following is an example of a *Statistical Sampling Plan.* A pharmaceutical manufacturing company receives empty bottles of a particular size from a supplier in lots of 20,000 bottles each. The drug firm would like the producer to submit material that is 1.0% defective or less most of the time, or specifically 95% of the time. See point A, Fig. 73. However, the pharmaceutical firm has agreed to take one chance in ten of accepting a lot that is 2.6% defective. See point B, Fig. 73.

Table XVI—Data Collected from the Process

Section number	Number defectives	Fraction defective	Section number	Number defectives	Fraction defective
1	3	0.01	17	2	0.0067
2	2	0.0067	18	3	0.01
3	3	0.01	19	4	0.0133
4	5	0.0167	20	5	0.0167
5	4	0.0133	21	12	0.04
6	3	0.01	22	5	0.0167
7	3	0.01	23	7	0.0233
8	5	0.0167	24	7	0.0233
9	1	0.0033	25	2	0.0067
10	2	0.0067	26	7	0.0233
11	1	0.0033	27	3	0.01
12	3	0.01	28	4	0.0133
13	2	0.0067	29	13	0.0433
14	2	0.0067	30	9	0.03
15	2	0.0067	31	4	0.0133
16	3	0.01			

$$\bar{p} = \frac{\text{Total number of defectives}}{\text{Total number inspected}} = \frac{131}{31 \times 300} =$$

$$\frac{131}{9300} = 0.01408$$

$$\text{Control limits for } \bar{p} = \bar{p} \pm 3\sqrt{\frac{\bar{p}(1 - \bar{p})}{n}}$$

$$= 0.01408 \pm 3\sqrt{\frac{0.01408(1 - 0.01408)}{300}}$$

Upper limit = 0.0349
Lower limit = 0

The acceptance sampling plan that complies with these specifications is as follows. Take a random sample of 540 bottles. Inspect the bottles for defectives. If zero to nine bottles are found defective, accept the lot; if ten or more defectives are found, reject the lot. The operating characteristic curve for this plan is illustrated in Fig. 73.

One can also see that using this sampling plan, submitted lots having 0.5% defective will be accepted about 99 times in 100 (probability of acceptance = 0.99) and thus rejected about one time in 100. Submitted lots having 1.75% defective will be accepted 50 times in 100 (probability of acceptance = 0.50) and rejected half the time.

For every sampling plan there is an operating characteristic (OC) curve. In fact there is an OC curve for every standard governing acceptance or rejection of drugs, foods, or materials of any kind. There are OC curves for the manufacturing process and for the inspectional process of every drug in the USP.

In sampling varying sized lots of material having from 50 to 10,000 units in a lot, the size of the sample taken should not be proportional to the size of the lot, or even proportional to the square root of the size of the lot. Fig. 74[30] shows the closely agreeing operating characteristic curves for lot sizes $N = 50$ to $N = 10,000$ and the respective sample sizes $n = 9$, $n = 10$ that should be taken from these lots. If the sample size is to be increased to around 20, Fig. 75[30] shows the lot sizes $N = 50$ to $N = 10,000$ and their respective sample sizes $n = 17$ to $n = 20$ that should be used in order to have the operating characteristic curves relatively constant.

Statistics in Biological Testing

The statistical study of biological investigations or *biometrics* is a well-established tool. A few examples of its application to biological assaying will be presented.

Calculation of a Dosage–Response Curve

It is a well-known fact that the physiological response to a drug varies with the size of the dose given. Many investigators have found that this relationship is usually typified by an S-shaped dosage–response curve, as illustrated in Fig. 76. At a low dosage there is no effect, but as the dosage increases the effect becomes more pronounced until beyond a certain dosage there is no further increase in the effect.

The dosage–response curve is the foundation of much biological experimentation, however there are many different ways of making use of it. Although the dosage–response curve is sigmoid or S-shaped, over a certain range in the center the dosage–response curve sometimes approximates a straight line. The use of some function such as logarithm or square root of the variable instead of the variable itself is called a transformation. There are transformations (changes in scale) that have been used to linearize even greater portions of the dosage–response curve. In these instances when it can be expressed as a straight line, the equation of that line can be calculated easily. The steepness of this line is called the slope and is usually designated by b. The intercept of this line on the vertical axis (y axis) is designated by a. The equation of such a line is then

$$y = a + bx$$

where

$$b = \frac{\Sigma xy - \bar{x}\Sigma y}{\Sigma x^2 - \bar{x}\Sigma x}$$

$$a = \bar{y} - b\bar{x}$$

The term Σxy indicates the sum of the products of x and y. (*Note*—this is entirely different from the product of the sums which would be indicated by $\Sigma x\Sigma y$.) In a vitamin A assay, for instance, the response here is the gain in weight of the rat over a designated period of time after a definitely stated depletion period. For this assay the gain in weight is plotted against the logarithm of the dose to obtain a linear dosage–response curve. In most biological assays the logarithm of the dose is used instead of the dose. Also, the statistical calculations are facilitated if the doses are chosen so that the intervals between the logarithms of the doses are equal.

Example XXI—For determining a dosage–response curve on NF Reference Cod Liver Oil Standard, four dosage levels of this standard are given, one dosage level to each of four groups of rats. There are 12 male rats in each group, representing four male rats from each of 12 litters. The rats conformed to the specifications given in the USP assay for vitamin A. The resulting gains in weight in grams are tabulated as responses* in Table XVII. The four doses used were 0.794, 1.26, 2.00, and 3.17 units daily and their logarithms are 9.9–10, 0.1, 0.3, and 0.5, respectively. (For our purposes we will use 9.9–10 as −0.1.) For each rat the log dose and response are given. There are four rats from each litter. The results are plotted in Fig. 77.

Evaluation of Biological Assays

A biological assay is a means of estimating the strength of a drug (generally by comparison to a standard of the same drug) by using some living organism. There are several types of biological assay, from a statistical viewpoint:

1. Assays which use the direct determination of threshold or lethal dose (eg, USP Digitalis Pigeon Assay).

2. Assays which give a measurable response (eg, gain in weight of rats in a vitamin A assay, or diameter of zone of inhibition in a penicillin assay).

3. Assays which give a "go or no go" (all or none) type of response wherein an individual animal either survives or dies, or an individual object passes or does not pass a set mark (eg, the number of frogs that survive in a digitalis assay, or the number of animals responding in an estrogen assay).

4. Assays which utilize a time factor (eg, the duration of cure of polyneuritis in rats on a vitamin B_1 assay).

In a biological assay the potency of the drug may be measured as a percentage of the standard, or in terms of some established unitage. In recent years it has been increasingly evident that not only should the potency be obtained but also some measure of the reproducibility of the assay such as the standard error of the assay or the confidence limits for the potency. This can be

*For more explicit details see the section on Vitamin A in the chapter on *Biological Testing*.

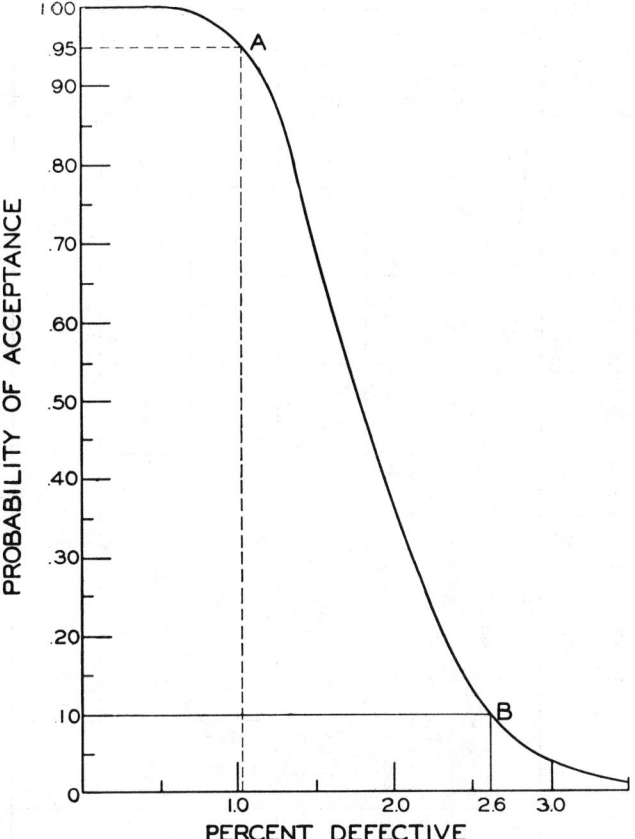

Fig. 73. Operating characteristic curve.

accomplished if the design of the assay is such that it takes into account all the causes of variation within one laboratory.

The calculated error of an assay and the confidence limits for a potency can estimate errors that can be shown to cause variations *within* the assay. Ordinarily, it can neither take into account the errors of weighing and measuring of the material (which are sizable in some assays, notably penicillin), nor can it take into account the differences between materials used in each laboratory, between samples of the lot to be assayed or, most important, between assayists. The assayist *cannot* state, on the basis of the calculated error of the assay, that the lot assayed was, say, 650 ± 20 units per mg. He *can* say that, if he repeated the assay many times under the same conditions using the same "made-up" solutions, this calculated error could be used to estimate the unavoidable variation in his own series of results.

The statistical evaluation of the biological assays as those found in USP XVII is explained by Bliss.[31,32] He explains designs, formulas, and procedures, and gives examples of each assay in which statistical calculations are used in USP XVII. He particularly explains the USP XVII section entitled *Design and Analysis of Biological Assays*.

Direct Determinations of the Threshold Dose

Digitalis Assay—As given in the USP the potency is determined by injecting suitably diluted tincture into suitably selected, randomized, anesthetized pigeons at 5-min intervals until the pigeons die of cardiac arrest. The dilution of the Standard Preparation of Digitalis and the preparation to be assayed shall be such that the estimated fatal dose of each preparation per kg of

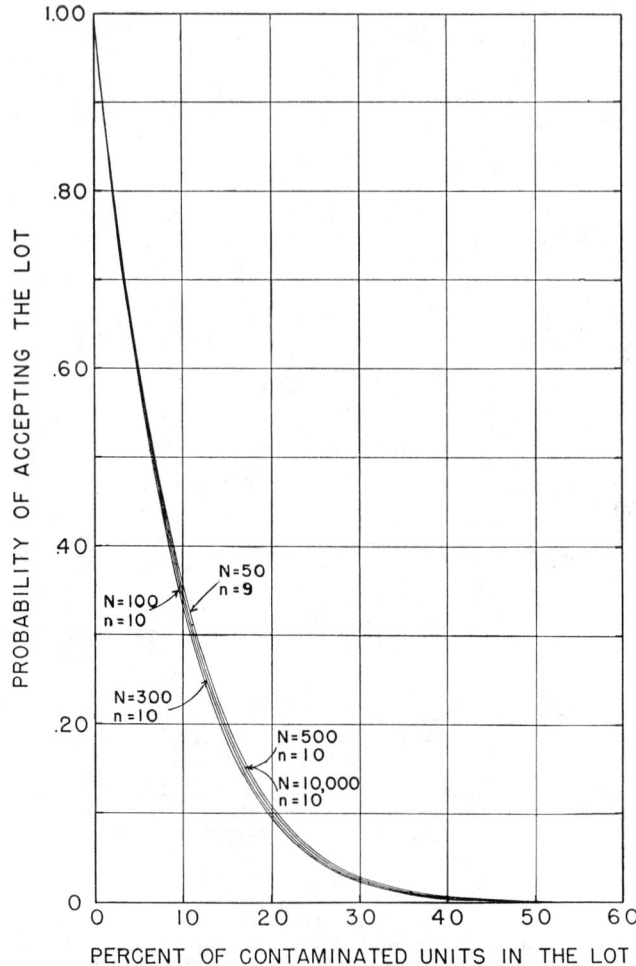

Fig. 74. Operating characteristic curves for several lot sizes (N) and sample size (n) of about 10 units. The lot is passed if there are no contaminated units in the sample tested.[29]

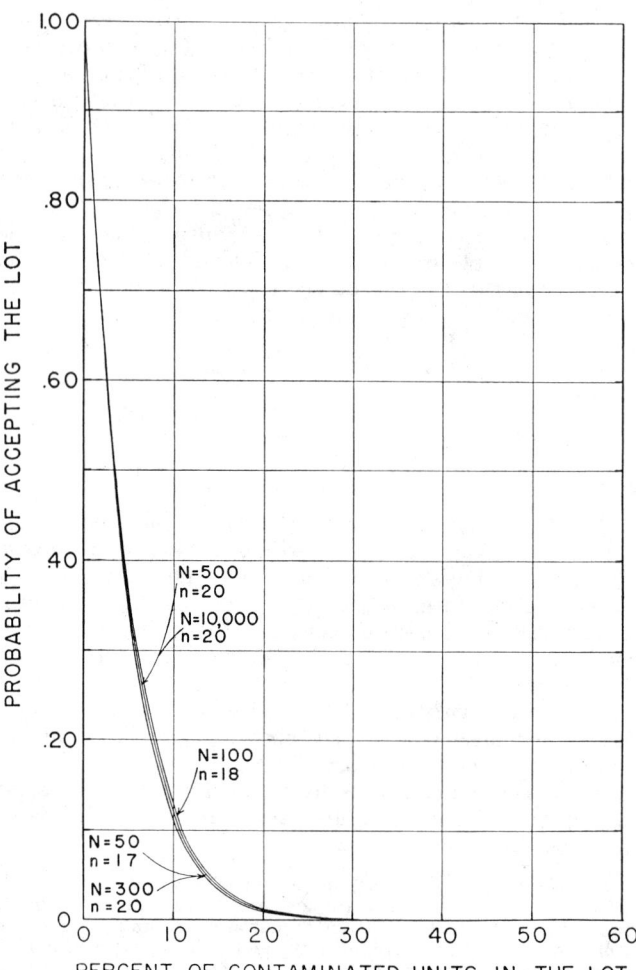

Fig. 75. Operating characteristic curves for several lot sizes (N) and sample size (n) of about 20 units. The lot is passed if there are no contaminated units in the sample tested.[30]

pigeon shall be contained in 15 ml. In the data in Table XVIII the estimated fatal dose of the standard is 0.975 ml. Six pigeons are assigned at random to the standard and six to the unknown. The number of doses (1 ml of the diluted material for each kg of pigeon at 5-min intervals) necessary to produce death in each pigeon is also given. As stated in the USP, the average number of doses for each material must be not less than 13 or greater than 19 to have a valid assay.

To calculate the potency of the preparation assayed in USP Digitalis Units per ml find the average number of doses of the test and standard solutions which were injected and designate these $\bar{v}_u$ and $\bar{v}_s$, respectively.

The potency of the unknown is given by the formula

$$\text{Potency} = P_* = \bar{v}_s R / \bar{v}_u$$

where R is the ratio of the number of ml of standard preparation to the number of ml of assay preparation in 100 ml of their respective test dilutions.

Calculate the square of the standard error of the threshold dose. This is referred to as the error variance since variance is merely the square of the standard deviation.

$$s^2 = \{\Sigma v^2 - T_s^2/f_s - T_u^2/f_u\}/(f_s + f_u - 2)$$

where $T_s = \Sigma v_s$ and $T_u = \Sigma v_u$ and v designates each individual threshold dose.

f_s = number of animals on the standard
f_u = number of animals on the unknown

Notice that the formula for s^2 is merely the pooled variances for the responses to the standard and unknown since the variance for the standard would be

$$s^2 = \frac{\Sigma v_s^2 - (\Sigma v_s)^2/n_s}{n_s - 1}$$

if v_s is used instead of x as on page 128.

The confidence interval is denoted by L in the USP and the value of t used is that corresponding to a probability of $P = 0.05$. The value: potency $+ \frac{1}{2}L$ is the upper confidence limit and the value: potency $- \frac{1}{2}L$ is usually the lower confidence limit. The formula given for L in the USP for the digitalis assay is

$$L = 2\sqrt{(C - 1)(CP_*^2 + R^2 f_u/f_s)}$$

where

$$C = \bar{v}_u^2/(\bar{v}_u^2 - s^2 t^2/f_u)$$

and P_* is the assayed potency in USP units.

If L exceeds 0.30 USP Digitalis Unit, repeat the assay or inject more pigeons with one or both preparations until the confidence interval is 0.30 or less. The confidence limits ($P = 0.05$) for the potency in USP units are:

$$X_{P*} = CP_* \pm \frac{1}{2}L$$

Example XXII—The calculation of the potency and the confidence limits of the assay within one laboratory is given in Table XVIII.

Assays Based on a Dosage–Response Curve

Statistics can best be applied to those assays in which two or more doses of the standard are run simultaneously with two or more doses of the unknown

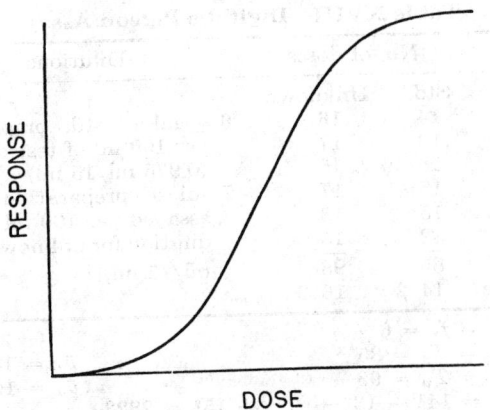

Fig. 76.   A typical dosage-response curve.

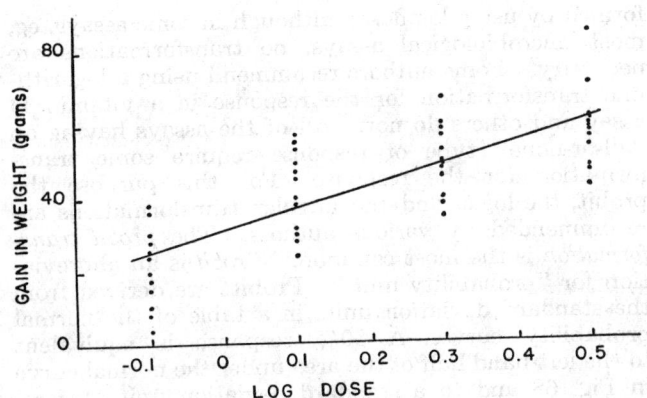

Fig. 77.   Log-dosage-response curve for vitamin A assay (data given in Table XVII).

and the dosage–response curve is calculated from both standard and unknown.

Potency of an unknown is usually calculated as a certain per cent of the standard. It thus can be obtained by getting the antilog of the difference between the logarithms of the doses of the unknown and of a standard having the same response (since a quotient is a difference in terms of logarithms). It has been found that when the logarithm of the dose is plotted against some function of the response the result is a straight line. Much has been written on this subject by various writers. Among the first were Gaddum,[33] Trevan,[34] and Bliss.[35]

It will suffice to say that when the logarithm of the dose is plotted against some function of the response, two parallel straight lines are obtained (as shown in Fig. 78), one for the standard material and one for the assay material (for which a dosage based on an assumed potency was used). Then, since the potency of the unknown is the antilog of the difference between the logarithms of the doses for standard and for unknown,

the potency can be calculated from the horizontal distance between the lines. The parallel lines are usually fitted to the observations by least squares (so called because it mathematically minimizes the sum of the squares of the distances from the observed points to the calculated line). The calculated error of an assay is, then, some quantitative measure of the scatter of the observed points about the lines but depends also on the slope of the lines. At least two assumptions are made in this mathematical reasoning. The first is that the relationship between the log dose and the response is a straight line, and the second is that equal percentage increases in dose of standard and of unknown will give equal increases in response (ie, that the unknown has the same effect as the standard). Both these assumptions should be tested, and no assay run until they are known to be true within the range recommended for the assay.

Various types of transformations have been used for the response in order to make the dosage–response curve linear over most of its range. Dose is usually trans-

Table XVII—Dosage–Response Curve for Vitamin A Assay

Litter no.	Log dose x	Re-sponse y	Log dose x	Re-sponse y	Log dose x	Re-sponse y	Log dose x	Re-sponse y
1	−0.1	4	0.1	24	0.3	35	0.5	43
2	−0.1	24	0.1	55	0.3	46	0.5	60
3	−0.1	18	0.1	45	0.3	50	0.5	58
4	−0.1	8	0.1	30	0.3	38	0.5	54
5	−0.1	15	0.1	28	0.3	48	0.5	47
6	−0.1	28	0.1	40	0.3	57	0.5	62
7	−0.1	36	0.1	49	0.3	49	0.5	57
8	−0.1	38	0.1	53	0.3	67	0.5	85
9	−0.1	30	0.1	57	0.3	59	0.5	71
10	−0.1	20	0.1	47	0.3	60	0.5	59
11	−0.1	25	0.1	38	0.3	53	0.5	62
12	−0.1	10	0.1	31	0.3	40	0.5	48

$$n = 48$$
$$\Sigma x = 9.6$$
$$\Sigma x^2 = 4.32$$
$$\Sigma y = 2061$$
$$\Sigma xy = 557.7$$
$$\bar{x} = 0.2000$$
$$\bar{y} = 42.9375$$

$$\text{Slope} = b = \frac{\Sigma xy - \bar{x}\Sigma y}{\Sigma x^2 - \bar{x}\Sigma x} = \frac{557.7 - 0.2000(2061)}{4.32 - 0.2000(9.6)} = 60.625$$

$$\text{Intercept} = a = \bar{y} - b\bar{x} = 42.9375 - 60.625(0.2000) = 30.8125$$

Equation of dosage–response curve:

$$\text{Response} = 30.8125 + 60.625 \text{ times log dose}$$

formed by using log dose; although in some assays, eg, most microbiological assays, no transformations are necessary. Some authors recommend using a logarithmic transformation for the response in a vitamin D assay and others do not. All of the assays having an "all-or-none" type of response require some transformation for the response. For this purpose the probit, the logit, and the angular transformations are recommended by various authors. The *probit transformation* is the most common. *Probit* is an abbreviation for "probability unit." Probits are derived from the standard deviation units in a table of the normal probability curve. A 50% response is equivalent to the left-hand half of the area under the normal curve in Fig. 68 and to a standard deviation unit of zero. Since probits are obtained by adding 5 to the standard deviation units, a 50% response corresponds to a probit of 5. As can also be seen from Fig. 68, a 16% (½ of the difference between 100% and 68%) response corresponds to a standard deviation unit of about −1 and a probit of approximately 4. A 2.5% response corresponds approximately to a standard deviation unit of −2 and a probit of 3. A 97.5% response corresponds to a standard deviation unit of +2 and a probit of 7 (see Table XIX).

The probit method is essentially a modification of the methods used by Gaddum[33] and Trevan[34]. The logarithm of the dose is used and the response is transformed to probits. There are many refinements that have been made for a very accurate determination of potency and standard error of the assay in using the probit method by Bliss[35] and further outlined by Miller, *et al*,[36] and by Finney.[37] They advocate plotting the empirical probits vs log dose and fitting two parallel straight lines (one for standard and one for unknown) to the points by means of a straightedge. The expected probit for each dose is read from the graph. The corrected probit and the weights to be attached to each observation are read from a series of tables. However, a short cut procedure will be given here using only the empirical probits and their weights in the calculations. The procedure they give from that point on is essentially the same as is given in Example XXIII.

Thyroid Assay—This assay, although not official, serves to illustrate the generalized "least-squares" procedure for estimating the potency and 95% confidence limits for a quantitative graded response assay.

In this assay three graded doses of a standard thyroid preparation and four graded doses of a solubilized test thyroid preparation were given to mice, and the survival time was measured after the mice were placed in airtight containers. For statistical reasons the response was measured as

$$y = \frac{1000}{\text{survival time in minutes}}$$

Actually, six equally spaced log doses of each preparation were tested on an equal number of mice. Data from the original assay were omitted to illustrate the generalized procedure to be used for unbalanced assays.

It can be shown that for the doses selected, the log–dose response lines for the standard and test preparations are linear and parallel within the limits of experimental error of the assay. Accordingly parallel log–dose response lines can be fitted to the data from the equations

$$y_S = \bar{y}_S + b_c(x - \bar{x}_S)$$
$$y_T = \bar{y}_T + b_c(x - \bar{x}_T)$$

Table XVIII—Digitalis Pigeon Assay

No. of doses		Dilutions
Std.	Unknown	
14	16	6½ ml of std. preparation
13	17	per 100 ml of test dilution
16	15	(0.975 ml/15 ml)
15	17	7 ml of preparation to be
15	18	assayed per 100 ml of test
12	15	dilution for unknown (1.05
Sum 85	98	ml/15 ml)
Average 14.2	16.3	

$$f_u = f_s = 6$$
$$\Sigma v_s = T_s = 85 \qquad\qquad \bar{v}_s = 14.2$$
$$\Sigma v_u = T_u = 98 \qquad\qquad \bar{v}_u = 16.3$$
$$\Sigma v^2 = 14^2 + 13^2 + \ldots + 15^2 = 2823$$

$$R = 6\tfrac{1}{2}/7 = 0.928$$
$$\text{Potency} = \bar{v}_s R/\bar{v}_u = 14.2(0.928)/16.3 = 0.808$$

$$\begin{aligned}
s^2 &= \{\Sigma v^2 - T_s^2/f_s - T_u^2/f_u\}/(f_s + f_u - 2)\\
&= \{2823 - (85)^2/6 - (98)^2/6\}/(6 + 6 - 2)\\
&= \{2823 - 1204.17 - 1600.67\}/10 = 1.816
\end{aligned}$$
$$C = \bar{v}_u^2/(\bar{v}_u^2 - s^2 t^2/f_u)$$

From the t table for 10 degrees of freedom and $P = 0.05$ for two tails, $t = 2.228$. Inserting the proper values in the formula for C:

$$\begin{aligned}
C &= (16.3)^2/\{(16.3)^2 - 1.816(2.228)^2/6\}\\
&= 265.69/\{265.69 - 1.5024\} = 1.0057
\end{aligned}$$
$$L = 2\sqrt{(C-1)(CP_*^2 + R^2 f_u/f_s)}$$
$$\begin{aligned}
L &= 2\sqrt{(1.0057 - 1)\{1.0057(0.808)^2 + (0.928)^2(6/6)\}}\\
&= 2\sqrt{0.0057\{0.6566 + 0.8612\}} = 2\sqrt{0.008651}\\
&= 2(0.0930) = 0.1860
\end{aligned}$$

Confidence limits ($P = 0.05$) for the potency in USP units

$$\begin{aligned}
X_{P*} &= CP_* \pm \tfrac{1}{2}L = 1.0057(0.808) \pm \tfrac{1}{2}(0.1860)\\
&= 90.81206 \pm 0.0930\\
X_{P*} &= 0.9056 \text{ and } 0.7196
\end{aligned}$$

where y is response, x is log dose, and b_c is the common slope. The potency of the test preparation relative to the standard is then calculated from

$$R = \text{antilog } M = \text{antilog}\left(\bar{x}_S - \bar{x}_T - \frac{\bar{y}_S - \bar{y}_T}{b_c}\right)$$

The variance, s^2, is generally estimated from the variability "within doses" and the 95% confidence limits are calculated from

$$R_L, R_U = \text{antilog } (M_L, M_U)$$

where

$$M_L, M_U = \bar{x}_S - \bar{x}_T + \left(M - \bar{x}_S + \bar{x}_T \pm\right.$$
$$\left. \frac{t}{b_c}\sqrt{s^2[(1-g)(1/n_S + 1/n_T) + (M - \bar{x}_S + \bar{x}_T)^2/[x^2]]}\right)\Bigg/$$
$$(1-g)$$

The value of t is obtained from a t table for degrees of freedom = $\Sigma(n_1 - 1)$, and g is calculated from

$$g = \frac{t^2 s^2}{b_c^2 [x^2]}$$

A value of $g < 0.05$ may be ignored. As g approaches unity, the assay becomes less valid. A value of $g > 1$ indicates a completely invalid assay due to either too flat a slope, b_c, or to unusually high variability within doses, s^2.

The example given in Table XX shows the calculations of the thyroid assay.

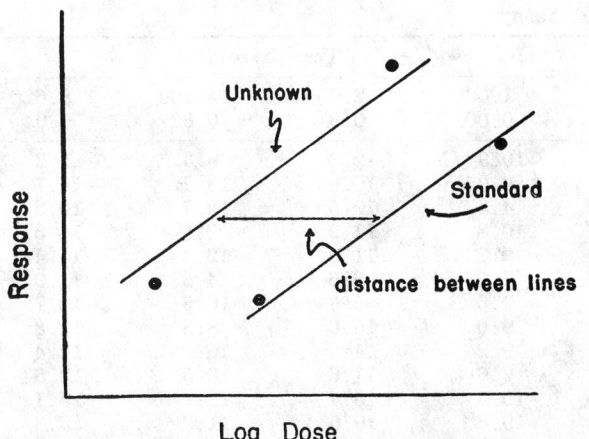

Fig. 78. A graph of the data from a typical assay.

Estrogen Assay—The estrogen assay is described in the chapter on *Biological Testing*. It is one of the "all-or-none" type of assays.

Example XXIII—An example of a 3-level assay is given below demonstrating the application of, first, the probit method to this type of assay, then the angular transformation method. The assay is designed so that the intervals between the log doses are equal on both standard and unknown although the method of calculation given here can be used even if they are not equal.

The data obtained from the assay and the dosages given each group of 16 animals are included with the calculations for the probit method given in Table XXII. Probits and their weights are given in Tables XIX and XXI.

Table XXII gives the generalized form for calculations that can be used even if the number of animals is not equal on all the doses and the differences between consecutive log doses are not equal for standard and unknown. It can also be used on any number of doses although only three doses are used in the example.

Various short cut procedures have been used to shorten the arithmetical calculations for the probit method but these will not be enumerated here. There is another method that has been suggested; namely, the use of the angular transformation instead of the probit transformation.

The *angular transformation* is stated by the formula:

$$p = \sin^2 \theta$$

where p is the percentage response and θ is the transformed value in degrees. See Table XXIII.

The same estrogenic assay can be evaluated by the angular transformation method. A partial table of the angular transformation of proportions to angle is given in Table XXIII. The method of calculation and formulas for a 3-dose assay using this procedure are given in Table XXIV. Note that, in order to use the formulas given in this table, the three-dose assay must be designed so that the number of animals, n, on each dose is the same and the differences between consecutive log doses are equal. In this example, $n = 16$ and the difference between log doses = 0.15.

Here it is assumed that R, the ratio of corresponding doses of standard and unknown, is unity. When this is not the case, the potency must be multiplied by R.

Two-Dose Assay—The following formulas apply to a percentage response assay using the angular transformation in which only two doses are used on each of the standard and the unknown.

$$V = U_H + U_L - S_H - S_L$$
$$W = U_H - U_L + S_H - S_L$$
$$M = \frac{iV}{W}$$

$$\text{Potency} = \text{antilog}\left(2 + \frac{iV}{W}\right)$$

$$\text{Standard error of the assay} = 131.9\,\frac{i(\text{potency})}{W^2\sqrt{n}}\,\sqrt{W^2 + V^2}$$

Four-Dose Assay—The following formulas apply to a percentage response assay using the angular transformation in which four doses are used on each of the standard and the unknown:

$$V = U_L + U_M + U_G + U_H - (S_L + S_M + S_G + S_H)$$
$$W = 3(S_H - S_L + U_H - U_L) + (S_G - S_M + U_G - U_M)$$
$$M = \frac{5iV}{W}$$

$$\text{Potency} = \text{antilog}\left(2 + \frac{5iV}{W}\right)$$

$$\text{Standard error of the assay} = 933\,\frac{i(\text{potency})}{W^2\sqrt{n}}\,\sqrt{W^2 + 5V^2}$$

Insulin Injection Assay—In the USP the assay of Insulin Injection makes use of the twin crossover rabbit test using four equal groups of six or more rabbits each. Two dilutions are made of each of the standard and the unknown. Standard dilution 1 contains 1.0 USP Insulin unit in each ml and Standard dilution 2 contains 2.0 USP Insulin units in each ml. The two sample dilutions contain similar amounts on the basis of the assumed potency. Specific instructions as to choice of animals, feeding schedules, and other details are given. Two injections are given each group of rabbits, the "Second injection being made on the day after the First injection or not more than one week later," according to the following schedule:

Group	First injection	Second injection
1	Standard dilution 2	Sample dilution 1
2	Standard dilution 1	Sample dilution 2
3	Sample dilution 2	Standard dilution 1
4	Sample dilution 1	Standard dilution 2

At 1 hr and 2½ hr from the time of injection, blood samples are obtained from the marginal ear vein. The response in this assay is the sum of the blood sugar concentration at 1 hr and 2½ hr. The "y" values used to calculate the assay results are the individual differences.

Table XIX—Empirical Probits

For Use with Percentage Response in "All-or-None" Assays[a]

%	0	1	2	3	4	5	6	7	8	9
0	...	2.674	2.946	3.119	3.249	3.355	3.445	3.524	3.595	3.659
10	3.718	3.773	3.825	3.874	3.920	3.964	4.006	4.046	4.085	4.122
20	4.158	4.194	4.228	4.261	4.294	4.326	4.357	4.387	4.417	4.447
30	4.476	4.504	4.532	4.560	4.587	4.615	4.642	4.668	4.695	4.721
40	4.747	4.773	4.798	4.824	4.849	4.874	4.900	4.925	4.950	4.975
50	5.000	5.025	5.050	5.075	5.100	5.126	5.151	5.176	5.202	5.227
60	5.253	5.279	5.305	5.332	5.358	5.385	5.413	5.440	5.468	5.496
70	5.524	5.553	5.583	6.513	5.643	5.674	5.706	5.739	5.772	5.806
80	5.842	5.878	5.915	5.954	5.994	6.036	6.080	6.126	6.175	6.227
90	6.282	6.341	6.405	6.476	6.555	6.645	6.751	6.881	7.054	7.326

[a] From Bliss, C. I.[38]

Table XX—Thyroid Assay

	Standard thyroid			Test thyroid			
Dose (mg/mouse)	0.333	0.683	1.400	1.000	2.050	4.200	8.620
log dose, x	−0.48	−0.17	0.15	0.00	0.31	0.62	0.94
	10.0	10.6	13.7	10.9	12.3	9.3	11.2
	9.4	9.9	14.7	9.9	10.6	13.2	14.1
	14.9	12.7	16.4	14.3	10.5	12.7	10.6
	9.1	12.3	11.8	10.8	11.9	12.5	14.5
	11.6	15.2	10.2	9.3	11.8	12.3	15.4
	10.2	16.1	13.7	8.8	8.6	14.3	11.9
	11.9	10.8	14.9	9.6	9.9	10.5	12.7
	12.0	12.3	12.8	9.0	15.6	8.3	12.8
Response, y	13.2	12.3	16.7	9.2	14.5	10.3	11.4
	11.9	13.3	15.2	7.6	11.6	10.5	12.5
	10.5	11.6	9.7	10.2	15.4	11.1	14.1
	11.9	9.7	12.8	10.6	10.5	11.2	13.5
	16.4	15.6	12.7	9.0	11.9	11.0	10.8
	6.5	12.2	12.0	8.7	12.2	13.3	11.4
	10.2	10.0	14.3	7.6	10.1	11.0	11.8
	9.2	11.6	11.6	7.5	8.1	18.5	13.5
	9.3	11.2	9.9	7.8	10.9	14.1	13.3
	9.0	12.7	12.2	10.2	7.1	11.0	11.8
		11.9		11.8	12.2	10.5	14.9
				9.4	9.4	10.0	10.8
				7.8	9.0	11.0	14.9
				8.8	9.5	12.3	14.9
				10.3	9.4	12.0	9.3
				7.9	10.6		
Σy_i	197.2	232.0	235.3	227.0	263.6	270.9	292.1
n_i	18	19	18	24	24	23	23
$\bar{y}_i$	10.96	12.21	13.07	9.46	10.98	11.78	12.70

$$n_S = 55 \qquad n_T = 94$$
$$\Sigma y_S = 664.5 \qquad \Sigma y_T = 1053.6$$
$$\Sigma x_S = -9.17 \qquad \Sigma x_T = 43.32$$
$$\bar{y}_S = 12.08 \qquad \bar{y}_T = 11.21$$
$$\bar{x}_S = -0.167 \qquad \bar{x}_T = 0.461$$
$$N = 149 \qquad \Sigma y = 1718.1$$

$[x^2]_S = 18(-0.48)^2 + 19(-0.17)^2 + 18(0.15)^2 - (-9.17)^2/55 = 3.5724$

$[x^2]_T = 24(0.00)^2 + 24(0.31)^2 + 23(0.62)^2 + 23(0.94)^2 - (43.32)^2/94 = 11.5063$

$[xy]_S = (-0.48)(197.2) + (-0.17)(232.0) + (0.15)(235.3) - (-9.17)(664.5)/55 = 11.9893$

$[xy]_T = (0.00)(227.0) + (0.31)(263.6) + (0.62)(270.9) + (0.94)(292.1) - (43.32)(1053.6)/94 = 38.6953$

$[xy] = [xy]_S + [xy]_T = 11.9893 + 38.6953 = 50.6846$

$[x^2] = [x^2]_S + [x^2]_T = 3.5724 + 11.5063 = 15.0787$

$b_c = [xy]/[x^2] = 50.6846/15.0787 = 3.3613$

$M = \bar{x}_S - \bar{x}_T - \dfrac{\bar{y}_S - \bar{y}_T}{b_c} = -0.167 - 0.461 - \dfrac{12.08 - 11.21}{3.3613}$

$\qquad = -0.887$

Relative potency $= R =$ antilog $M =$ antilog (-0.887)
$\qquad\qquad = $ antilog $(9.113 - 10)$
$\qquad\qquad = 0.13$ or 13% of standard

$[y^2] = (10.0)^2 + (9.4)^2 + \cdots + (9.3)^2 - (1718.1)^2/149 = 742.5980$

$D^2 = \dfrac{(197.2)^2}{18} + \cdots + \dfrac{(292.1)^2}{23} - \dfrac{(1718.1)^2}{149} = 200.6287$

$s^2 = \dfrac{[y^2] - D^2}{\Sigma(n_i - 1)} = \dfrac{742.5980 - 200.6287}{142} = 3.8167$

$g = \dfrac{t^2 s^2}{b_c^2 [x^2]} = \dfrac{(1.98)^2(3.8167)}{(3.3613)^2(15.0787)} = 0.0878$

$M_L, M_U = \bar{x}_S - \bar{x}_T + \left(M - \bar{x}_S + \bar{x}_T \pm \dfrac{t}{b_c}\sqrt{s^2(1-g)(1/n_S + 1/n_T) + (M - \bar{x}_S + \bar{x}_T)^2/[x^2]} \right) \Big/ (1-g)$

$\qquad = -0.628 + \left(-0.259 \pm \dfrac{1.98}{3.3613}\sqrt{3.8167\,[0.9122(1/55 + 1/94) + (-0.259)^2/15.0787]} \right) \Big/ 0.9122$

$\qquad = -0.628 + \dfrac{(-0.259 \pm 0.202)}{0.9122}$

$\qquad = -0.628 - 0.505, \; -0.628 - 0.062$

$\qquad = -1.133, \; -0.690$

$R_L, R_U =$ lower and upper 95% confidence limits
$\qquad = $ antilog $(M_L, M_U) = $ antilog $(-1.133, -0.690)$
$\qquad = $ antilog $(8.867 - 10, \; 9.310 - 10)$
$\qquad = 0.074, \; 0.20$ or 7.4% and 20% of standard

Thus, the solubilized thyroid test preparation is estimated to be 13% as potent as the standard thyroid preparation, with 95% confidence limits of 7.4% and 20%.

Table XXI—Weighting Coefficients for Use with Probits[a]

Probit	Weighting coefficient	Probit
5.0	0.6366	5.0
5.1	0.6343	4.9
5.2	0.6274	4.8
5.3	0.6161	4.7
5.4	0.6005	4.6
5.5	0.5810	4.5
5.6	0.5579	4.4
5.7	0.5316	4.3
5.8	0.5026	4.2
5.9	0.4714	4.1
6.0	0.4386	4.0
6.1	0.4047	3.9
6.2	0.3703	3.8
6.3	0.3359	3.7
6.4	0.3020	3.6
6.5	0.2691	3.5
6.6	0.2375	3.4
6.7	0.2077	3.3
6.8	0.1799	3.2
6.9	0.1554	3.1
7.0	0.1311	3.0
7.1	0.1103	2.9
7.2	0.0918	2.8
7.3	0.0756	2.7
7.4	0.0617	2.6
7.5	0.0498	2.5
7.6	0.0398	2.4
7.7	0.0314	2.3
7.8	0.0246	2.2
7.9	0.0190	2.1

[a] From Bliss, C. I.[38]

Group	Differences	Individual response y	Total response T
1	Standard 2 − Sample 1	y_1	T_1
2	Sample 2 − Standard 1	y_2	T_2
3	Sample 2 − Standard 1	y_3	T_3
4	Standard 2 − Sample 1	y_4	T_4

The number of rabbits in each group is f and

$$T_a = -T_1 + T_2 + T_3 - T_4$$
$$T_b = T_1 + T_2 + T_3 + T_4$$

The logarithm of the relative potency is

$$M' = ci\, T_a/T_b = 0.301\, T_a/T_b$$

The potency in USP units = antilog (M' + log of the assumed potency) where i = the interval in logarithms between successive log doses = log 2 = 0.301 and $c = c' = 1$.

The confidence interval of the log potency M' is determined as given in the USP

$$L = 2\sqrt{(C-1)(CM'^2 + c'i^2)}$$

where $c'i^2$ is equal to 0.09062 since $c' = 1$ and $i = 0.301$ and

$$C = T_b^2/(T_b^2 - s^2t^2N)$$

where t^2 is the square of the value from the t table for $n = 4(f-1)$ degrees of freedom.

$$s^2 = \{\Sigma y^2 - \Sigma T_i^2/f\}/n$$

C is often little greater than unity. The more precise the assay the more nearly C approaches 1.

The upper and lower confidence limits in logarithms at a single laboratory are, respectively:

$$X_M = \log R + CM' + \tfrac{1}{2}L \text{ and } \log R + CM' - \tfrac{1}{2}L$$

where R is assumed potency.

For an insulin assay, if the confidence interval in logarithms is more than 0.1212 (which corresponds to 95% confidence limits of 87 and 115% of the computed potency), the assay should be repeated until the combined data of two or more assays meet this acceptable limit.

Example XXIV—A typical USP XVII Insulin Assay* follows:

S_1 = 1 USP unit per ml
S_2 = 2 USP units per ml
U_1 = 4 mg per 100 ml ⎱ assumed potency equals 25 units
U_2 = 8 mg per 100 ml ⎰ per mg

Dose per rabbit = 0.40 ml in all cases.
Response is sum of blood sugar at 1 hr and 2½ hr
y = response to high dose minus response to low dose

$$T_a = -T_1 + T_2 + T_3 - T_4 = +239 - 113 - 170 + 210 = 166$$
$$T_b = T_1 + T_2 + T_3 + T_4 = -239 - 113 - 170 - 210 = -732$$
$$M' = 0.301\, T_a/T_b = 0.301(166)/-732 = -0.06825$$

log of assumed potency = log 25 = 1.3979
potency in USP units = antilog (M' + log of assumed potency)
$$= \text{antilog}\,(-0.06825 + 1.3979) = 21.4 \text{ units per mg}$$

$N = 24$ and $f = 6$ animals in a group
$t = 2.086$ for $n = 4(f-1)$ or 20 degrees of freedom
$t^2 = 4.351$
$t^2N = 104.424$
$$\Sigma y^2 = (25)^2 + (20)^2 + \ldots + (24)^2 = 25468$$
$$\Sigma T_i^2/f = [(239)^2 + (113)^2 + (170)^2 + (210)^2]/6 = 142890/6 = 23815$$
$$s^2 = \{\Sigma y^2 - \Sigma T_i^2/f\}/n = \{25468 - 23815\}/20 = 82.65$$
$$s^2t^2N = 82.65\,(104.424) = 8630.64$$
$$C = T_b^2/(T_b^2 - s^2t^2N) = (-732)^2/\{(-732)^2 - 8630.64\} = 1.01637$$
$$CM'^2 = 1.01637\,(-0.06825)^2 = 0.00473$$
$$CM'^2 + c'i^2 = 0.00473 + 0.09062 = 0.09535$$
$$L^2/4 = (C-1)(CM'^2 + c'i^2) = 0.01637\,(0.09535) = 0.0015609$$
$$L/2 = \sqrt{0.0015609} = 0.03951$$
$$X_M = \log R + CM' \pm \tfrac{1}{2}L$$

Upper limit $X_M = 1.3979 - 0.06937 + 0.03951 = 1.3680$
Lower limit $X_M = 1.3979 - 0.06937 - 0.03951 = 1.2890$
Then obtaining the antilogarithms of the X_M:

Upper limit = 23.3
Lower limit = 19.4

Thus, the calculated potency is 21.4 units per mg and the upper and lower 95% confidence limits are respectively 23.3 and 19.4 units per mg.

Vitamin D Biological Assay—The NF XII Vitamin D assay is used as an illustration of the calculations involved in bioassay. The following example uses data from a vitamin D assay‡ in which three animals from each of eight litters of rats had been placed at random on the proper diets after the specified depletion procedure. The graded degrees of healing (y = individual response) as found are shown in Table XXVI. Two doses of the standard were used (the highest dose twice the lowest dose) and one dose of the unknown.

This is the Design 2,1 (2 doses of the standard and 1 of the unknown) as shown in the USP (Table 7, page 874) in the section on *Design and Analysis of Biological Assays*, from which it is seen (with slightly different notation):

Design	Row	Factorial coefficients s_1	s_2	u_1	e_i	T_i
2,1	a	−1	−1	2	6	T_a
	b	−1	1	0	2	T_b

For computing	Equation no.	Constant	Value in design 2,1	3,2	4,3
M'	3, 5	c	½	⅚	⁷⁄₆
L	21, 24	c'	¾	25⁄12	49⁄12

*The data in the Insulin Injection Assay example given were kindly furnished by Dr. R. L. Grant, US Food and Drug Administration, Washington, D.C.

‡ The data for the Vitamin D Assay were kindly furnished by Dr. Leo Friedman, US Food and Drug Administration, Washington, D.C.

Table XXII—Probit Method of Calculation

A Three-Dose Assay Having an All-or-None Type of Response

Dose	Log dose x	Re-sponse	%	Probit y	Weight[a] w	wx	wy
			Standard				
8.9	0.95	5/16	31.2	4.51	9.328	8.8616	42.0693
12.6	1.10	8/16	50.0	5.00	10.186	11.2046	50.9300
17.8	1.25	12/16	75.0	5.67	8.632	10.7900	48.9434
			Unknown				
8.9	0.95	2/16	12.5	3.85	6.200	5.8900	23.8700
12.6	1.10	6/16	37.5	4.68	9.808	10.7888	45.9014
17.8	1.25	11/16	68.8	5.49	9.328	11.6600	51.2107

	Standard	Unknown
Σw	28.146	25.336
Σwx	30.8562	28.3388
$\bar{x} = \Sigma wx/\Sigma w$	1.09629	1.11852
Σwy	141.9427	120.9821
$\bar{y} = \Sigma wy/\Sigma w$	5.04309	4.77511
Σwx^2	34.2311	32.0382
Σwxy	157.1681	137.1815
$[wx^2] = \Sigma wx^2 - \bar{x}\Sigma wx$	0.4038	0.3407
$[wxy] = \Sigma wxy - \bar{y}\Sigma wx$	1.5575	1.8606

Combining Standard and Unknown

$$\Sigma[wx^2] = [wx^2]_s + [wx^2]_u = 0.7445$$

$$\Sigma[wxy] = [wxy]_s + [wxy]_u = 3.4181$$

$$b_c = \frac{\Sigma[wxy]}{\Sigma[wx^2]} = 4.5911$$

$$M = \bar{x}_s - \bar{x}_u - \frac{1}{b_c}(\bar{y}_s - \bar{y}_u) = -0.08060$$

$$s_M = \frac{1}{b_c}\sqrt{\frac{1}{\Sigma w_s} + \frac{1}{\Sigma w_u} + \frac{(\bar{y}_s - \bar{y}_u)^2}{b_c\Sigma[wxy]}} = 0.0614$$

$$\text{Potency} = \text{antilog}(2 + M) = 83.1$$

approximate 95% confidence limits for $DF = 4$

$$L_{95} = \text{antilog}\{M \pm ts_M\}$$
$$= \text{antilog}\{-0.0806 \pm 2.78(0.0614)\}$$
$$\text{Lower limit} = \text{antilog}(2 - 0.2513) = 56.1$$
$$\text{Upper limit} = \text{antilog}(2 + 0.0901) = 123.0$$

[a] Weights are from Table XXI times number of animals tested.

In this table are shown the coefficients to be used in multiplying the totals for s_1, s_2, and u_1 (or u) in order to get T_a and T_b. Thus,

$$T_a = 2T_u - T_1 - T_2$$
$$T_b = T_2 - T_1$$

The equation for the log-relative potency of the unknown before adjustment for its assumed potency is

$$M' = ci\, T_a/T_b$$

where $c = \frac{1}{2}$ from the above table and $i = \log$ (high dose/low dose) $= \log 2 = 0.30103$ for this assay.

The equation for the variance as given in the USP is

$$s^2 = \{\Sigma y^2 - \Sigma T_r^2/k - \Sigma T_t^2/f + T^2/N\}/(k-1)(f-1)$$

where k = number of different doses given = 3
f = number of rows (litters) = 8
$N = kf$
T_r = total for each dose
T_t = total for each row (litter)

The confidence limits for the log potency are given in the USP as follows:

$$X_M = \log R + CM' \pm \frac{1}{2}L$$

where R is the ratio of corresponding dose of the standard and of the unknown and where

$$L = 2\sqrt{(C-1)(CM'^2 + c'i^2)}$$

and

$$C = T_b^2/(T_b^2 - e_b fs^2 t^2)$$

where e_b and c' are given in the same table with the factorial co-efficients.

Table XXVII shows a systemized calculation of this assay.

For the Vitamin D Biological Assay, the confidence interval L should not exceed 0.40. Here, $L = 0.2264$. Also, if C is negative, the assay is invalid. Thus the assay yields as the potency of the unknown 109% of the standard with upper and lower 95% confidence limits of 144% and 86%, respectively, of the standard.

Evaluation of a Microbiological Assay—In most microbiological assays it has been found that there is a linear relationship between the *dose* and the response instead of (as in most biological assays) a linear relationship between the *log dose* and the response. Thus instead of fitting two parallel lines to the log-dosage-response data and calculating the potency as the antilogarithm of the horizontal distance between these two lines as in biological assays, in microbiological assays two straight lines are used which intersect at a "common-zero" point and the potency is calculated as the ratio of the slopes of these two lines. See Fig. 79 for

Table XXIII—Angular Transformation

Transformation of Percentages to Angle Theta[a]

%	0	1	2	3	$P = \sin^2 \theta$ 4	5	6	7	8	9
0	0	5.7	8.1	10.0	11.5	12.9	14.2	15.3	16.4	17.5
10	18.4	19.4	20.3	21.1	22.0	22.8	23.6	24.4	25.1	25.8
20	26.6	27.3	28.0	28.7	29.3	30.0	30.7	31.3	31.9	32.6
30	33.2	33.8	34.4	35.1	35.7	36.3	36.9	37.5	38.1	38.6
40	39.2	39.8	40.4	41.0	41.6	42.1	42.7	43.3	43.9	44.4
50	45.0	45.6	46.1	46.7	47.3	47.9	48.4	49.0	49.6	50.2
60	50.8	51.4	51.9	52.5	53.1	53.7	54.3	54.9	55.6	56.2
70	56.8	57.4	58.1	58.7	59.3	60.0	60.7	61.3	62.0	62.7
80	63.4	64.2	64.9	65.6	66.4	67.2	68.0	68.9	69.7	70.6
90	71.6	72.5	73.6	74.7	75.8	77.1	78.5	80.0	81.9	84.3

[a] From Fisher, R. A., and Yates, F.[39]

Table XXIV—Angle Theta Method of Calculation

Three-Dose Assay Having All-or-None Type of Response

Log dose	Response	θ
	Standard	
0.95	5/16	$S_L = 34.0$
1.10	8/16	$S_M = 45.0$
1.25	12/16	$S_H = 60.0$
	Unknown	
0.95	2/16	$U_L = 20.7$
1.10	6/16	$U_M = 37.8$
1.25	11/16	$U_H = 56.0$

n = number of animals on each dose = 16
i = difference between log doses = $1.25 - 1.10$
$\quad = 1.10 - 0.95 = 0.15$
$V = U_H + U_M + U_L - S_H - S_M - S_L = -24.5$
$W = U_H + S_H - U_L - S_L = 61.3$
$M = \dfrac{4iV}{3W} = \dfrac{4(0.15)(-24.5)}{3(61.3)} = -0.079934$
Potency = antilog $(2 + M)$ = antilog (1.920066) = 83.2
$Z = \sqrt{3W^2 + 2V^2} = \sqrt{3(61.3)^2 + 2(24.5)^2} = 111.7$
Standard error of assay = $\dfrac{124.385 \, iZ}{W^2\sqrt{n}}$ (potency) =
$\quad \dfrac{124.385(0.15)111.7}{(61.3)^2\sqrt{16}}(83.2) = 11.5$

Approximate 95% confidence limits for DF = 4
L_{95} = potency $\pm$ t (standard error of assay)
$\quad = 83.2 \pm 2.78 \, (11.5)$
$\qquad\qquad$ Upper limit = 115.2
$\qquad\qquad$ Lower limit = 51.2

Note—The above formulas apply only to a three-dose assay.

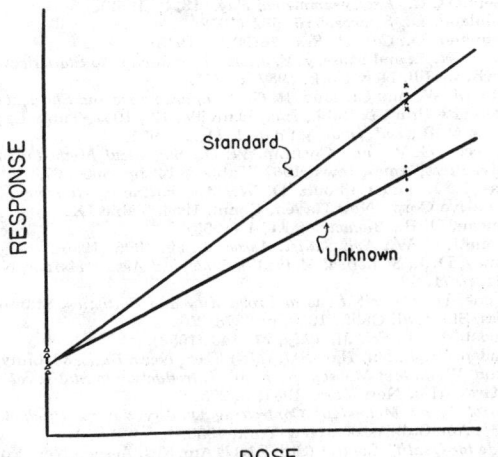

Fig. 79. A typical microbiological vitamin assay. △ indicates responses to blank; × indicates responses to standard; ● indicates responses to unknown.

Table XXV—An Insulin Injection Assay

Group	Rabbit	Response Dilution 2	Dilution 1	y
1	7	122	147	− 25
(S_2 & U_1)	52	81	101	− 20
	62	105	152	− 47
	73	168	213	− 45
	77	87	131	− 44
	80	57	145	− 58
		(650)	(889)	−239 = T_1
2	29	111	124	− 13
(S_1 & U_2)	45	111	134	− 23
	50	121	137	− 16
	72	171	198	− 27
	75	158	177	− 19
	90	177	192	− 15
		(849)	(962)	−113 = T_2
3	30	90	117	− 27
(U_2 & S_1)	47	169	197	− 28
	54	101	130	− 29
	74	158	184	− 26
	78	201	233	− 32
	84	157	185	− 28
		(876)	(1046)	−170 = T_3
4	36	115	139	− 24
(U_1 & S_2)	46	104	151	− 47
	63	151	190	− 39
	66	124	158	− 34
	76	166	208	− 42
	87	140	164	− 24
		(800)	(1010)	−210 = T_4
Total				−732

a graphic illustration of the results of a microbiological assay.

The statistical evaluation of a microbiological assay has been developed by Wood and Finney[40,41] but the calculations are rather complicated as applied to the usual procedure for a microbiological assay and will not be described here. However, one simple type of calculation which they give for a "common-zero 3-dose assay" will be described with a cautioning statement as to its use. When the dose of the standard and the unknown are taken as two arbitrary units of the respective preparations and the same number, n, of tubes (observations) are run on the blank, the standard and the unknown, the formulas for the potency and the standard error of the assay are rather simple. This assay is called a "common-zero 3-dose" assay since the blank is

Table XXVI—Vitamin D Assay

	Response to low dose of standard s_1	Response to high dose of standard s_2	Response to unknown u	Totals T_r
Litter No. 1	1.00	3.75	4.37	9.12
Litter No. 2	2.00	3.37	2.50	7.87
Litter No. 3	2.12	3.75	2.00	7.87
Litter No. 4	3.25	4.50	2.75	10.50
Litter No. 5	2.50	4.50	4.00	11.00
Litter No. 6	1.75	4.00	2.25	8.00
Litter No. 7	2.00	4.50	4.00	10.50
Litter No. 8	1.37	3.37	4.00	8.74
Totals T_t	$T_1 = 15.99$	$T_2 = 31.74$	$T_u = 25.87$	$T = 73.60$

Table XXVII—Vitamin D Assay Calculations

$T_a = 2T_u - T_1 - T_2 = 2(25.87) - 15.99 - 31.74 = 4.01$

$T_b = T_2 - T_1 = 31.74 - 15.99 = 15.75$

$M' = ciT_a/T_b = [0.5(0.30103)4.01]/15.75 = 0.0383$

$R = 1 \therefore M = M'$

$\Sigma y^2 = \Sigma(y_1^2 + y_2^2 + \ldots + y_N^2) = (1.0^2 + 2.0^2 + \ldots + 4.0^2) = 252.8070$

$T^2/N = (73.60)^2/24 = 225.7067$

$\Sigma T_t^2/f = \{(15.99)^2 + (25.87)^2 + (31.74)^2\}/8 = 241.5456$

$\Sigma T_r^2/k = \{(9.12)^2 + (7.87)^2 + \ldots + (8.74)^2\}/3 = 229.6453$

$s^2 = (252.8070 + 225.7067 - 241.5456 - 229.6453)/14 = 0.5231$

$t^2 = 4.601$ using tabled t value for $(k - 1)(f - 1)$ degrees of freedom

$e_b f s^2 t^2 = 2(8)(0.5231)(4.601) = 38.5085$

$C = T_b^2/(T_b^2 - e_b f s^2 t^2) = (15.75)^2/\{(15.75)^2 - 38.5085\} = 1.1838$

$L^2/4 = (C - 1)(CM'^2 + c'i^2) = 0.1838[1.1838(0.0383)^2 + 0.75(0.30103)^2]$
$= 0.1838[0.001736 + 0.067964] = 0.01281$

$L/2 = \sqrt{0.01281} = 0.1132$

$L = 0.2264$

Potency (%) = antilog $(2 + M')$ = antilog $(2 + 0.0383) = 109\%$

$X_M = CM' \pm L/2$

Upper limit $X_M = 1.1838(0.0383) + 0.1132 = 0.1585$

Lower limit $X_M = 1.1838(0.0383) - 0.1132 = 9.9321 - 10$

Obtaining the antilogarithms of the X_M and converting to %
    Upper limit = 144%
    Lower limit = 86%

$$s_B = \frac{R\sqrt{1 - B + B^2}}{D(\bar{y}_s - \bar{y}_0)\sqrt{2n}}$$

There are other designs for microbiological assays which together with the so-called "common-zero 3-point assay design" are given by Wood and Finney.

The range can be used in estimating the standard error of the assay[42] (and also the confidence limits) for other biological assays by substituting the range divided by the appropriate tabled factor (see Table XIII) for the number of standard deviations in the range, given the number of observations, n.

An article by Knudsen[43] explains calculations of potency, standard error of the assay, control chart procedures as used in microbiological assay, and the operating characteristic curves for various types of assay procedures where acceptance or rejection of the lot is based on the results of one to three assays.

common to both dosage–response lines, and the blank, standard, and unknown together constitute three doses.

The uninitiated must exercise great caution in using this type of assay since so many factors in the assay itself may affect one point on the curve and not others. From the point of view of the vitamin assayist, it is safer to run several levels of both standard and unknown.

Let $\bar{y}_0$, $\bar{y}_s$, and $\bar{y}_u$ represent the mean responses to the blank, the standard, and the unknown, respectively. Let R represent the average range in response to each dose, as calculated from the data, and D, the average number of standard deviation units in the range. Then the ratio of the potency of the unknown to the potency of the standard is equal to

$$B = \frac{\bar{y}_u - \bar{y}_0}{\bar{y}_s - \bar{y}_0}$$

and the standard error of the assay is given by

References

1. Welch, H., et al, *J. APhA, Sci. Ed.*, **35**, 102 (1946).
2. Tippett, L. C., *Random Sampling Numbers* (Tracts for Computers No. 15), Cambridge, London, 1927.
3. Fisher, R. A., and Yates, F., *Statistical Tables for Biological, Agricultural, and Medical Research*, Hafner, New York, 1963, Table XXXIII, pp. 134–139.
4. Dixon, W. J., and Massey, F. J., Jr., *Introduction to Statistical Analysis*, McGraw-Hill, New York, 1957, p. 366, Table I.
5. Fisher, R. A., *The Design of Experiments*, 4th ed., Oliver & Boyd, Edinburgh, 1953.
6. Cochran, W. G., and Cox, G. M., *Experimental Designs*, 2nd ed., Wiley, New York, 1957.
7. Herwick, R. P., et al, *J. Am. Med. Assoc.*, **127**, 74 (1945).
8. Youden, W. J., *Statistical Methods for Chemists*, Wiley, New York, 1951.
9. Stearns, E. I., *Chem. Met. Eng.*, **53**, 119 (1946).
10. Pearson, L., ed., *Tables for Statisticians and Biometricians*, Part I, University College, London, 1930.
11. McClung, R. M., *What To Do until the Statistician Comes*, Rocket Div., Naval Ordnance Test Station, Inyokern, Calif.
12. Eisenhart, C., *Photogrammetric Eng.*, **18**, 3 (1952).
13. Mainland, D., *Science*, **116**, 592 (1952).
14. Mainland, D., *Can. J. Res.*, **26**(E), 1 (1948).
15. Dixon, W. J., and Massey, F. J., Jr., *Introduction to Statistical Analysis*, McGraw-Hill, New York, 1957, p. 221.
16. Tate, M. W., and Clelland, R. C., *Nonparametric and Shortcut Statistics*, Interstate Print. & Publ., Inc., Danville, Ill., 1957, Table L, p. 137.
17. Hicks, C. R., *Ind. Quality Control*, **11**, 1 (1955).
18. Snedecor, G. W., and Cochran, W. G., *Statistical Methods*, Iowa State Univ. Press, Ames, Iowa, 1967, Table A-14, pp. 560–567.
19. Bliss, C. I., and Calhoun, D. W., *An Outline of Biometry*, Yale Co-Operative Corp., New Haven, Conn., 1954, Table IX.
20. Duncan, D. B., *Biometrics*, **11**, 1 (1955).
21. Dunnett, C. W., *Am. Statist. Assoc. J.*, **50**, 1096 (1955).
22. Finney, D. J., *Statistical Method in Biological Assay*, Hafner, New York, 1964, p. 71.
23. Levene, H., *Contributions to Probability and Statistics*, Stanford Univ. Press, Stanford, Calif., 1960, pp. 278–292.
24. Youden, W. J., *Sci. Monthly*, **77**, 143 (1953).
25. Youden, W. J., *Ntl. Bur. Std. (US) Tech. News Bull.*, **33** (July) (1949).
26. Dixon, W. J., and Massey, F. J., Jr., *Introduction to Statistical Analysis*, McGraw-Hill, New York, 1957, p. 275.
27. *Control Chart Method of Controlling Quality during Production* (Std. Z1.3), Am. Std. Assoc., New York, 1958.
28. *Guide for Quality Control* (Std. Z1.1), Am. Std. Assoc., New York, 1958.
29. Dixon, W. J., and Massey, F. J., Jr., *Introduction to Statistical Analysis*, McGraw-Hill, New York, 1957, pp. 130, 237.
30. Knudsen, L. F. (now Randolph, L. K.), *J. APhA, Sci. Ed.*, **38**, 332 (1949).

31. Bliss, C. I., *Drug Std.*, **24**, 33 (1956).
32. Bliss, C. I., *Biometrics*, **12** (June) 491 (1956).
33. Gaddum, J. H., *Med. Res. Council Spec. Rept. Ser.*, **183** (1933).
34. Trevan, J. W., *Proc. Roy. Soc. (London) Ser. B*, **101**, 483 (1927).
35. Bliss, C. I., *Ann. Appl. Biol.*, **22**, 134, 307 (1935).
36. Miller, L. C., *et al*, *J. APhA*, **28**, 644 (1939).
37. Finney, D. J., *Probit Analysis*, 2nd ed., Cambridge, London, 1952, p. 65.
38. Bliss, C. I., *Quart. J. Pharm. Pharmacol.*, **11**, 195 (1938).
39. Fisher, R. A., and Yates, F., *Statistical Tables for Biological, Agricultural, and Medical Research*, Oliver & Boyd, Edinburgh, 1963, Table X, pp. 74, 75.
40. Wood, E. C., and Finney, D. J., *Quart. J. Pharm. Pharmacol.*, **19**, 112 (1946).
41. Finney, D. J., *Quart. J. Pharm. Pharmacol.*, **18**, 77 (1945).
42. Randolph, L. K., *J. APhA, Sci. Ed.*, **41**, 438 (1952).
43. Knudsen, L. F. (now Randolph, L. K.), *Ann. NY Acad. Sci.*, **52**, 889 (1950).

Bibliography

Experimental Design

Brownlee, K. A., *Industrial Experimentation*, Chem. Publ. Co., Inc., Brooklyn, 1947.
Cochran, W. C., and Cox, G. M., *Experimental Designs*, 2nd ed., Wiley, New York, 1957.
Finney, D. J., *Experimental Design and Its Statistical Basis*, Univ. Chicago Press, Chicago, 1955.
Fisher, R. A., *Statistical Methods for Research Workers*, 12th ed., Oliver & Boyd, Edinburgh, 1958.
Mainland, D., *The Treatment of Clinical and Laboratory Data*, Oliver & Boyd, Edinburgh, 1938.
Snedecor, G. W., *Statistical Methods: Applied to Experiments in Agriculture and Biology*, 5th ed., Iowa State College Press, Ames, Iowa, 1959.
Steel, J. M., ed., *Methods in Medical Research*, Yearbook, Chicago, 1954.

Statistical Quality Control

Dodge, H. F., and Romig, H. G., *Sampling Inspection Tables*, Wiley, New York, 1951.
Duncan, A. J., *Quality Control and Industrial Statistics*, Richard D. Irwin, Inc., Homewood, Ill., 1953.

Grant, E. L., *Statistical Quality Control*, 2nd ed., McGraw-Hill, New York, 1952.

Sampling

Cochran, W. G., *Sampling Techniques*, Wiley, New York, 1963.
Deming, W. E., *Some Theory of Sampling*, Wiley, New York, 1961.
Hansen, M. H., and Hurwitz, W. H., *Ann. Math. Statist.*, **14**, 333 (1943).
Smith, J. G., and Duncan, A. J., *Fundamentals of Theory of Statistics*, vol. I, McGraw-Hill, New York, 1944, Chaps. II, III.
Yates, F., *Sampling Methods for Censuses and Surveys*, Hafner, New York, 1953.

Biological Assay

Berkson, J., *J. Am. Statist. Assoc.*, **48**, 565 (1953).
Bliss, C. I., and Cattell, M., *Ann. Rev. Physiol.*, **5**, 479 (1943).
Bliss, C. I., *The Statistics of Bioassay with Special Reference to the Vitamins*, Academic, New York, 1952.
Bliss, C. I., *Am. Scientist*, **45**, 449 (1957).
Burn, J. H., *Biological Standardization*, Oxford Univ. Press, New York, 1950.
Finney, D. J., *Statistical Method in Biological Assay*, Hafner, New York, 1952.
Finney, D. J., *Probit Analysis*, 2nd ed., Cambridge, London, 1952.
Mather, K., *Statistics in Biology*, 3rd ed., Interscience, New York, 1947.

General

Armitage, P., *Sequential Medical Trials*, Blackwell Sci. Publ., Oxford, England, 1959.
Bennett, C. A., and Franklin, N. L., *Statistical Analysis in Chemistry and the Chemical Industry*, Wiley, New York, 1954.
Brownlee, K. A., *Statistical Theory and Methods in Science and Engineering*, Wiley, New York, 1960.
Croxton, F. E., and Cowden, D. J., *Applied General Statistics*, Prentice-Hall, New York, 1955.
Davies, O. L., *The Design and Analysis of Industrial Experiments*, Hafner, New York, 1954.
Hoel, P. C., *An Introduction to Mathematical Statistics*, 2nd ed., Wiley, New York, 1962.
Natrella, M. A., ed., *Experimental Statistics* (Ordinance Engineering Design Handbook—ORDP 20-110), June, 1962.

12 | Computer Science

Computer hardware and software—user interaction—applications to information retrieval, clinical data, instruments, and pharmacology

This chapter was prepared by

Paul G. Sanders, MS, *Manager, Applied Mathematics, Abbott Laboratories, North Chicago, Ill. 60064*

One of the byproducts of research spawned in World War II was the electronic computer. While the use of atomic energy marked the end of that war in 1945, the electronic computer has had a much more profound influence on technology and society.

Computer technology is rapidly becoming a factor in such widely diverse areas as journalism, art, politics, production control, and most fields of science. The medical sciences, especially, reflect the pervasive impact of this new technology. Its presence may be noted in the Intensive Care Unit—monitoring an ECG; in the clinical laboratory—returning results *on-line* and feeding the business record computer system for billing; in the psychological laboratory—monitoring and controlling behavioral tests in animals; and in the diagnostic clinic—relieving medical personnel of the tedious chore of taking patient histories.

While these glamorous uses often generate headlines, the greatest use for computers in the health sciences is still as a data transformer and retriever in science and as a recordkeeper in business. Thus, the proof that a new chemical is a safe and effective drug is likely to be based on computer-tabulated data; later, the presence of that drug on the pharmacist's shelf when needed will be assured by a computer-directed distribution system.

The field of computer technology, even when restricted to the pharmaceutical sciences, is too broad for comprehensive treatment in this chapter. The material that follows is divided into the following two sections: Computer Technology and Applications to Biopharmaceutics.

The material is directed to the scientist who has not had extensive experience with computer technology. For this scientist two levels of involvement are open:

1. He may want to use the computer to solve problems in his own research area. He will concentrate on the properties of his problem, spending just enough effort on communicating with computers so that he can use the developments of others.
2. He may choose a stronger level of involvement, becoming expert in those phases of computer technology that are required to solve his problems.

In either case he will need to treat this new tool with respect and understanding. In return he will find that his efforts are rewarded by greatly amplified productivity.

Computer Technology

The modern computer is the latest version in a continuing development chain from many different disciplines. These disciplines are conveniently divided into those concerned with physical construction of the computer (hardware) and those concerned with adapting the hardware to solve problems (software). Hardware will be treated only generally because a detailed treatment of the electronics involved will not aid the new user. Software provides the link between hardware and the aspiring user; hence, it will receive better coverage.

One of the most common ways of specifying computers is by the methods used for producing computations. The best known is the digital computer which operates with *discrete* numbers (by analogy with the counting process associated with our digits). The other type of computer is the *analog*. Here the computing devices operate on *continuously* varying quantities, usually voltages. Computers of both types are in wide use.

Digital Hardware

Coding—Central to the operation of the modern digital computer is the concept of information coding. All such computers use variations of the *binary* number system because of the relative simplicity of designing electronic circuits to handle its elements. Binary numbering systems are built up with elements which can assume only two states. Depending upon the hardware involved, these states may be represented as terms like *off* or *on, zero* or *one, punched* or *not-punched, magnetized* or *not-magnetized,* and *present* or *absent.* All of the digital information storage and processing devices discussed here use some combinations of these two-state devices. Table I shows how the decimal digits 0 through 7 may be represented by a three-element binary number. These elements are referred to as *bits,* from the term, *binary digit.*

The familiar 80-column punched card* uses the bits (punches) in a somewhat different fashion. Fig. 80 shows a standard 80-column card with columns 1 through 64 punched with one of the standard character sets in use. Note that each character occupies 1 column of 12 punch positions. The coding of the

Table I—Binary Representation

Decimal digit	Binary representation[a]
0	0 0 0
1	0 0 1
2	0 1 0
3	0 1 1
4	1 0 0
5	1 0 1
6	1 1 0
7	1 1 1

[a] The digits "0" and "1" represent the two possible states of a binary element (see text). Grouping binary elements into sets of 3 is the basis of the *octal* numbering system since 8 states are possible. Many modern computers use the *hexadecimal* (16 states) system which is based on groups of 4 binary elements.

* Frequently referred to as a Hollerith card, after Herman Hollerith who developed the concept in the late 1800's.

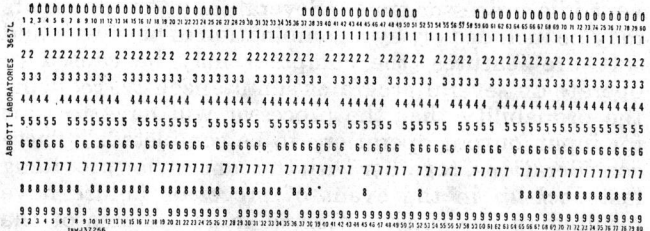

Fig. 80. Eighty-column card. Columns 1 to 64 contain standard punch combinations. Different printed symbols are often substituted for the *special* characters, columns 37 to 64. No symbol is printed over column 37 (which contains no punches and is called a *blank* column) and column 53 which contains punches for which no symbol is assigned. The symbols are present to aid people in identifying and sorting cards, the computer can only read the holes.

digits 0 through 9 is achieved by punching a hole in the row corresponding to the number that is to be coded. Letters are coded by a combination of two punches in a column; some of the *special* characters require three punches. Fig. 81 shows a key punch used for punching required codes in successive columns of a card. The 80 columns are used in groups, called fields, to encode alphabetic and numeric data. The key punch is designed to make punching into specific fields easy. A similar machine, the key verifier, detects errors when data are keyed a second time.

Magnetic tape systems code data into rows of either 7 or 9 bits represented by the presence or absence of magnetized spot in the ferrite coating on the tape. One of the columns on the tape does not carry information but is used for checking purposes against the possibility of dropping a bit due to electronic or mechanical malfunction. Other redundancy checks are often utilized to protect against such errors.

Many different internal codes are used in the processing of information inside the computer. These detailed considerations are important* in the operation and maintenance of the computer, and in the design of systems which must exploit these features for the sake of efficiency. These differences in coding often cause problems when data or programs are transferred from one computer to another. Efforts to standardize codes have improved this situation, but frustrating problems continue to arise.

Data Flow—Fig. 82 contains a simple schematic of the flow of information in a typical computer system. *Input* information (a string of bits) flows through the processor to memory. A program causes the processor to fetch and store the information from memory, modifying it (computing) as it processes. When finished, the information is sent to an *output* device and a new problem is sought. The input stream may

---

* From a computational viewpoint (as opposed to information storage), the most important data coding consideration is the provision of enough bits to insure that answers are free of serious roundoff error. Discussion of this insidious problem has been delayed until after the *Software* section because software may provide solutions to hardware code limitations.

Table II—Typical Input Media for Digital Computers

> 80-column card
> Punched taper tape
> Magnetic tape and disks
> Typewriter keyboard
> Telephone lines (with special adapters)
> Printed forms (optical scanning)
> Voltages and toggle settings from instruments

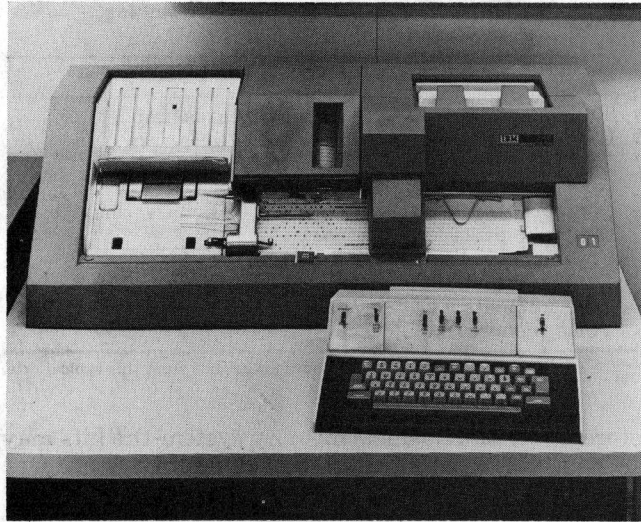

Fig. 81. Keypunch. Cards are fed from the hopper at the upper right through the punching station where holes are punched and symbols printed in successive columns. The punched card continues to the duplicating station where it is read for transmission back to the punch station for card duplication. The punched card is then transferred to the stacker at upper left. The index pointer in the center indicates the column currently being used; the *drum card* above the pointer provides automatic field definition for special formats.

contain *programs* which inform the computer of the procedures for the next job to be accomplished or *data* to be used in the computation. The output stream consists of processed information or information to the programmer and operator about the state of the machine at any time. The processor may be thought of as a *one-step-at-a-time* device that follows the direction of a program of such steps stored in memory.

Input—Information to be processed by computers is originated in many forms. Many different methods of interfacing the computer to the data sources have been constructed. Table II shows the principle input media. All of these are read into the computer by electromechanical devices.

Output—Results of computations must be communicated to people, to other devices, or stored for subsequent computer processing. Table III lists common output media. It will be noticed that many of the *output* media may also be used as *input*. Typical capacities for these devices are included in the table. For instance, the typical capacity of line printers installed in data processing installations is 1000 lines/min. A line of information may contain 144 characters selected from a set of 64 characters which include digits, letters of the alphabet, and *special* characters similar to those shown in Fig. 80.

Memory—The memory is usually the most expensive component of the system. Memory capacity is determined by the number of bits which may be stored in the memory. It may be specified as the number of *characters* of a certain number of bits which may be

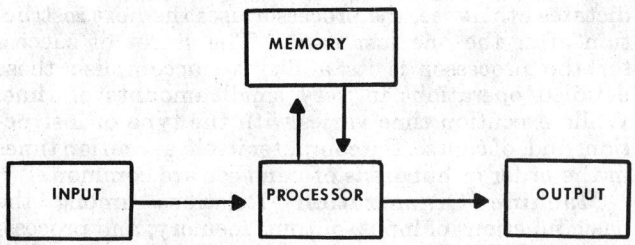

Fig. 82. Information flow in a typical computer system.

Table III—Typical Output Media for Digital Computers

Media	Speed[a]
80-Column cards	400 cards/min
Line printers	1000 lines/min
Teletype-typewriter devices	100 words/min
Graph plotters	
Magnetic tapes	80,000 characters/sec
Magnetic disks	
Cathode ray displays	
Control impulses for other instruments	
Voice reponse	

[a] Actual speeds may vary by an order of magnitude from this typical rate.

stored. Within a single memory system the bits may be collected together in several different ways. One widely used system is based on the number of 8-bit *bytes* contained in the memory. One *byte* can store either 1 alpha-numeric character or 2 decimal digits or it may be looked upon as 8 bits of a larger binary number. Memories of smaller computers are often organized into *words* with a fixed number of bits. Computers with word sizes of 12, 16, 24, and 32 bits are common.

Efficient memory organization requires some computers to have several *levels* of memory differing in speed and cost. Magnetizable ferrite cores are the principal memory device in use; however, small memories of extremely fast circuitry may be included to improve performance.

Memories which are of the order of 100,000 characters are common; large-scale systems exceed that size by an order of magnitude. At the other extreme, memories of only 4,000 words are common in the small, special purpose systems.

Core memories in common use store and retrieve information in approximately 1μ-sec. Special-purpose memories may operate with cycle times of a few hundred nano-sec.

Processors—The function of the processor is to transform data from input to output in accordance with the instructions contained in the program stored in memory. Thus, the processor must perform the following sequence of steps:

1. Obtain instruction word from memory.
2. Decode that word to find out what operation is to be performed and what is the location of information to be processed.
3. Set up the circuitry to accomplish the process.
4. Perform the operation.
5. Determine the address of the next instruction and return to Line 1.

These steps are quite elementary but they are accomplished with such speed that the user or operator is not conscious of their execution. Typical operations performed in this way are shown in Table IV.

As the table shows, the steps may be classified as bookkeeping, computational, branching, and input/output handling. Unless a branching instruction dictates otherwise, the processor uses the next instruction after the one just used. The secret of success for the processor is its ability to accomplish these detailed operations in very small amounts of time. While execution time varies with the type of instruction, and, of course, the computer itself, execution times in the order of hundreds of nano-sec are common.

Machine Organization—Relations among the basic functions of input, output, memory, and processing vary in detail among different systems. Because input/output speeds are usually much slower than processor speeds, various techniques are used to prevent idle processor time. Several input/output units may be included or, by a combination of hardware and software features, the computer may be caused to operate on several programs simultaneously, reducing the probability that the processor will have to wait for input/output operations to be completed. These considerations, together with the concern for providing fast *back-up* in the event of processor failure have resulted in the construction of large systems of the component functions described here. The systems are able to shift workload among the different resource units available so that the operator and the programmer are relieved of concern about these details.

Digital Software

When computers first came into common use it was necessary for the programmer to learn the details of machine operation at the level described in Table IV. For several reasons this proved unacceptable. The chance for mistakes in assembling sequences of detailed steps was large. Training was difficult and the supply of trainees for such exacting work was inadequate. The increasing complexity of the computers made the job harder and harder. Perhaps the most serious problem was that the potential user of computers, scientist or businessman, found it hard to communicate his problem to the programming specialist. The solution to all of these problems turned out to be the computer itself. During the mid 1950's many efforts to use the computer to assist in developing programs for itself were made. This was the beginning of the development of software. This development has been in two directions. One direction was toward the solution of problems indicated in the section on machine organization—the efficient utilization of the computer resources. The noncomputer specialist need not devote time to learning the details of this area. His interface with this software will be concerned with informing the computer of who he is (for accounting purposes) and describing the nature of the job that is to be accomplished. The assignment of the hardware to perform the task is left to this software.

The second direction taken by software development has been to make the job of communicating problem to computer easier for the noncomputer specialist. Three solutions to this need are available:

Table IV—Typical Processor Operations[a]

Operation	Function
Bookkeeping	Fetch a number from memory and store it in register A.
	Store a number contained in a register B at the given address in memory.
Input/output	Read a character from an input device into memory.
	Transmit a character from memory to an output device.
Computational	Multiply the number contained in register A by the number contained in register B leaving the result in register C.
Branching	If the number in a register B is negative, skip the next two instructions in sequence.

[a] The number of different operations (instructions) built into a computer varies from about 8 to several hundred. Some computers are designed so that special instructions may be defined for unusual operations.

general-purpose languages, problem-oriented languages, and problem-oriented consoles.

General-Purpose Languages—Mathematics is the common denominator for the formulation of most problems in the sciences. Here, software has the goal of accepting a problem phrased in a *language* that is as close to mathematics as possible. Four such languages in widespread use are: FORTRAN, ALGOL, BASIC, and PL/I.

Of these, FORTRAN (FORmula TRANslator) is the oldest, and in some senses, the least well developed. ALGOL (ALGOrithmic Language) was developed by an international committee after FORTRAN and other similar languages had been in use for a while. It is in wide use in Europe but has not displaced FORTRAN in the US. BASIC (Beginners All-purpose Symbolic Instruction Code) is one of the younger languages which was developed especially to provide an easy-to-learn language for use with the fast-response time-sharing system at Dartmouth.[1] The language PL/I was announced in 1964 as a major new language for the new IBM line of computers known as System 360. In addition to solving mathematical problems it is intended to be the language of choice for large data processing problems also. Its usage is restricted to the larger systems.

Each of these languages, and others similar to them, have many dialects (idiosyncrasies). Different vendors, and even different computers made by the same vendor, have significant differences in the way that the general-purpose languages work. Nevertheless, these languages have accomplished very much in making it easier for the nonspecialist to communicate his problem to computers and for programs to be shared among different computer systems.

Details of even one of these languages are beyond the scope of this chapter. A potential user should learn the details of the dialect on the system available to him. Fig. 83 contains a short program that performs a familiar computation in FORTRAN.[2,3] By analyzing the steps of this program, the nature of this general purpose language will become clear.

The example we have chosen is the computation of the mean and standard deviation of a sample of 10 numbers. The program uses the following formulas for computing the mean, $\bar{x}$, and the standard deviation, s, of the set of numbers.

$$\bar{x} = \frac{1}{10} \sum_{i=1}^{10} x_i$$

$$s = \sqrt{\frac{\Sigma x_i^2 - (\Sigma x_i)^2/10}{9}}$$

Fig. 84 shows an 80-column card containing 10 numbers whose mean and standard deviation are to be computed. The 10 numbers occupy 10 four-column fields in columns 1 to 40.

Each line in Fig. 84 has a special purpose:

Line 1—*C* indicates that this is a *comment* statement that has no effect on the program other than to describe in writing what is being accomplished.

Line 2—The DIMENSION statement indicates to the computer that it will need to reserve a table of 10 values to be referred to as *X*. The statement causes no computations to be performed; it is known as a *specification* statement.

Line 3 (Together with Line 4)—These statements accomplish the *input* operation. The READ statement, when executed, will cause the 10 data fields from a punched card in the reader to be read and stored in the memory locations reserved for the *X* table in Line 2. By means of the *statement number*, *70*, the READ statement refers to a FORMAT statement (Line 4) which specifies the arrangement of the data in the card. In this case the specification indicates that there are 10 four-column fields to be read from a card. Line 3 is an *executable* statement.

Line 4—A FORMAT statement is another *specification* statement. It supplies information about data fields but is not executed.

Line 5—This is the first example of an *assignment* statement. In this case it causes a value of 0. to be assigned to a variable named *SX*. This variable will be used to build up the sum of values of *X* during the computation.

Line 6—This is another assignment statement that performs a function similar to Line 5 for a variable, *SX*2, which will eventually contain the sum of the squares of the values of *X*.

Line 7—This is a DO statement which controls the flow of the calculation. This statement accomplishes two purposes: (1) it sets up an index value, *I*, that will be used to pick out the values of *X* from the table and (2) it causes the computer to add the successive values of *X* and their squares into *SX* and *SX*2, respectively. This is achieved by causing the statements between Line 7 and Line 9 (which has the statement number of 20) to be repeated 10 times with values of *I* ranging from 1 to 10.

Line 8—This is another assignment statement which causes the values from the *X* table to be successively added to the variable *SX* under control of the DO statement. The statement should be interpreted as "take the current value of *SX*, add the current value of *X* to it, and return the sum to the value of *SX*."

Line 9—This statement contains statement number 20 which indicates that it is the last statement to be effected by the DO in Line 7. It is also an assignment statement and performs a function similar to Line 8 in building up the sum of squares of the *X*'s.

Line 10—This assignment statement evaluates the mean, *XBAR*, by dividing *SX* by 10.

Line 11—This assignment statement computes, from previously determined variables, the standard deviation of the 10 data values. The letters, SQRT,* indicate that the square root of the value of the expression in parenthesis should be extracted. This value is then assigned to the variable *SD*.

Lines 12 and 13—These statements work together to accomplish the *output* operation. Line 12 causes the values computed for *XBAR* and *SD* to be sent to the line printer (indicated by the Number 3 immediately after the left parenthesis) under control of Line 13 which is another FORMAT statement.

```
Line No.
 1        C      FORTRAN MEAN, STANDARD DEVIATION, RPS 69
 2               DIMENSION X(10)
 3               READ(2,70)X
 4            70 FORMAT(10F4.0)
 5               SX=0.
 6               SX2=0.
 7               DO 20 I=1,10
 8               SX=SX+X(I)
 9            20 SX2=SX2+X(I)**2
10               XBAR=SX/10.
11               SD=SQRT((SX2-SX*SX/10.)/9.)
12            30 FORMAT(' MEAN IS',F10.2,2X,'STANDARD DEVIATION IS',F10.2)
13               WRITE(3,30)XBAR,SD
14               CALL EXIT
15               END
```

Fig. 83. Sample FORTRAN program for mean and standard deviation.

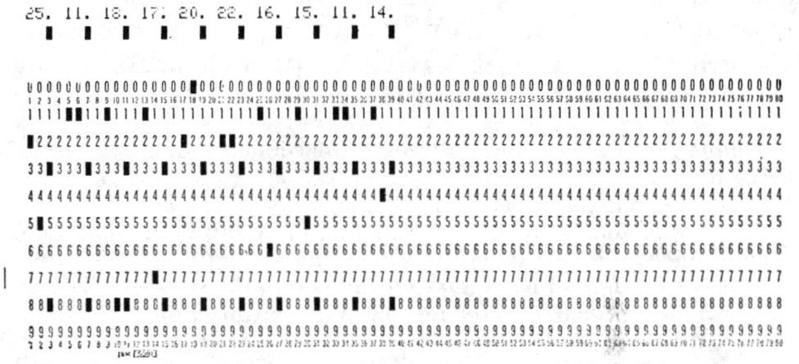

Fig. 84. Input data card for sample program.

*** Besides square roots, FORTRAN systems usually contain subroutines for evaluating logarithms (ALOG), sines (SIN), cosines (COS), arctangents (ATAN), and the absolute value (ABS) of specified arguments. The programmer may define his own subroutines and call them by any name not preempted by others.**

MEAN IS   16.90 STANDARD DEVIATION IS   4.53

Fig. 85. Output of sample program.

Line 13—This FORMAT statement indicates that the program is to print *XBAR* and *SD* on one line with an appropriate annotation. Both the mean and standard deviation are printed as 10 position fields with 2 decimal places indicated by the notation *F10.2*.

Line 14—This statement contains jargon indicating to the computer that the computation is finished and another program may be sought.

Line 15—END indicates to the FORTRAN system that no more FORTRAN statements are to be found.

Fig. 85 contains the output of this program when run using the data of Fig. 84. The statistician who knows FORTRAN could write a program such as this one as fast as he can write the statements on paper. If he had to resort to a lower level language, the time and training required would probably discourage him from successfully completing the program.

Programming in FORTRAN requires the following steps:

1. Define the problem and determine the sequence of steps needed to solve it.
2. Write FORTRAN text.
3. Prepare FORTRAN text on some suitable input medium such as a key punch.
4. Process the FORTRAN text on the computer system. The result of this step is usually *error* messages indicating failure to adhere to the FORTRAN syntax rules.
5. Correct the errors and return to Step 4 until no errors are found.
6. When an error-free processing of the FORTRAN text is achieved, the program is tried with real data for which the answers are known. This may generate a new series of correction steps similar to those in Step 5.
7. When the program finally produces correct answers it is ready for use with real data.*

Note that the programming requires interaction between programmer and the computer. The process of getting the errors out of the program is known as *debugging*. Debugging can be expedited greatly by having fast access to the computer. Almost instantaneous response is achieved in the *time-sharing* systems described in the hardware section.

Problem-Oriented Languages—While the general-purpose languages do much to make problem formulation easier, many scientists do not wish to take the time to master the general-purpose languages. Special-purpose languages have been developed so that specialists need only know the terminology of their profession in order to pose problems to the use computer. Of particular interest to the pharmaceutical scientist would be the digital simulation languages (DSL) which enable digital systems to respond to problems specified for analog systems.

Special Purpose Hardware/Software—The culmination of the trends expressed in software and hardware is the specially designed console which allows the investigator to define and solve his problem concisely.

Such a system for the neuropharmacology laboratory was described at the Spring, 1968, Joint Computer Conference.[4] Here the pharmacologist has an array of previously prepared signal-processing programs available to him at the flick of a switch. Also in this category are the cathode ray tube console systems which allow scientists to explore models with

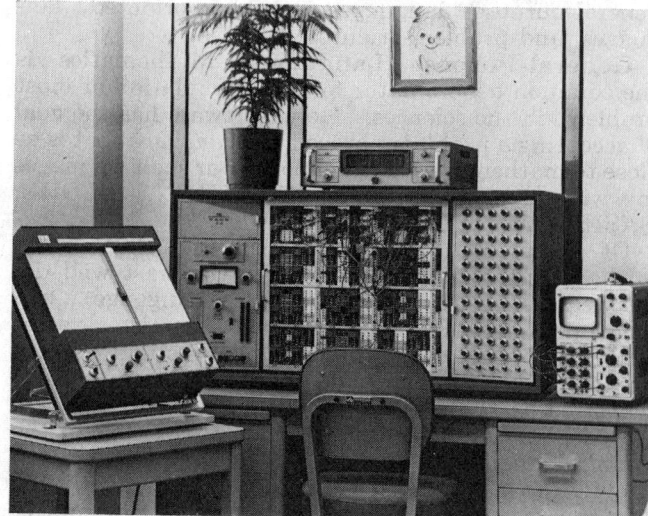

Fig. 86. EAI TR-48 Analog Computer. On the extreme left is the plotter. On the extreme right is the oscilloscope used for dynamic display of simulations. The digital voltmeter on the top of the main computer is used for precise setting of the coefficient potentiometers found on the right panel of the main frame. The left panel contains operating controls.

graphic feedback. While these systems require the least education on the part of the user, they are extremely difficult to develop.

Analog Computers

The analog computer[5] solves problems by constructing an electrical analogy of the problem. Usually the problem must be phrased as a series of differential equations prior to using the analog computer. From these differential equations, a block diagram is drawn which shows the signal flow among the different elements of the computer. Fig. 86 shows a typical small analog computer useful in biological simulations.

Analog computers are essentially parallel systems. That is, they consist of a collection of computing devices all of which operate at once. The relations among the elements are established by removable patch cords and by coefficient potentiometers which may be used to set initial conditions and to attenuate voltages in the course of the computation. Results are plotted on x–y plotters or oscilloscopes. The parameters of a problem may be altered as the problem is being solved.

The capacity of an analog computer is stated in terms of the number of operational amplifiers in the system. The high-gain, dc, chopper-stabilized amplifier is the key to the analog computer function. Fig. 87 illustrates the way in which the amplifier is used. If the element, *F*, in the feedback loop is a resistor the output will be the sum of the input voltages. When *F* is a capacitor, the output of the circuit is the integral, over time, of the sum of the inputs. It is this ability to integrate that gives the analog its ability to solve differential equations.

In pharmaceutical science the analog computer has found its principle uses in modeling drug metabolism and kinetics.[6] It is used heavily in the simulation of dynamic systems such as the cardiovascular system to obtain insight into control characteristics.

Hybrid Computers

The analog computer suffers from the absence of memory and limited ability to take alternate courses based on the progress of the problem. The digital

---

* However, the program may not produce correct answers for *all* data sets because of accumulated roundoff error. For instance, using *regular precision* on an IBM 1800 system, the data set 999.9, 999.8, 999.7, 999.9, 999.8, 999.7, 999.8, 999.9, 999.7, and 999.8 gives *XBAR* = 999.80, and *SD* = 6.84. *XBAR* is correct but *SD* should be 0.08. This particular problem can be resolved by *coding* the data in the program. The moral is "the fact that a program has worked satisfactorily in the past is not sufficient to remove it from suspicion."

computer has ample memory and decision-making capability but its *step-by-step* nature makes it slow at the highly parallel type of problem at which the analog excels. *Hybrid* computers, which contain both analog and digital elements, are being used. The digital subsystem can control the analog subsystems by means of servo-driven potentiometers and switches. The results from the analog subsystem are available to the digital through analog-to-digital converters. Thus, the analog may repetitively solve problems with slightly different parameters under control of the digital until an optimum solution is found.

Time-Sharing

Scientists often need to have the computational power available as a resource in the conduct of their experiments. In early computer systems one had to carry the problem to the computer room and then return for an answer. Sometimes the waiting period was several days. Modern computers can handle input from many devices simultaneously. The ability to transmit programs and data by telephone or direct cable connections has made it possible to move the input/output device out of the computer room and

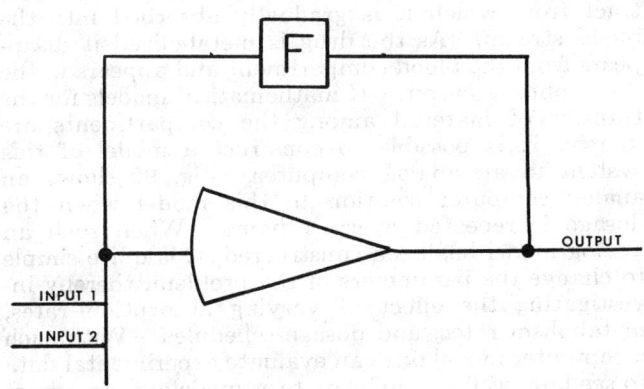

Fig. 87. Amplifier schematic. *F* is the element in the Feedback circuit. When *F* is a resistor, the OUTPUT voltage is proportional to the *sum* of the INPUT voltages. When *F* is a capacitor, the OUTPUT voltage is proportional to the *integral* of the sum of the INPUT voltages over time.

into the user's laboratory. These output devices may range from the relatively slow Teletype (100 words/min) to exceedingly high capacity devices (several hundred lines/min). The consequence is that the scientist can have his own computer terminal at a relatively moderate cost. Hence, he can use the computer interactively, getting fast feedback for problem solution. General- and special-purpose software is provided to speed programming.

Many universities are developing regional networks of such consoles and there are over 40 commercial companies supplying such services. The most common terminal device is the Teletype (Fig. 88). The pioneering system of this kind was at Dartmouth.[1]

The term applied to this use of computers is *time-sharing*. Development of reliable time-sharing systems has greatly increased the adoption of computer techniques by reducing the intellectual and economic overhead associated with starting to use computers and by reducing turnaround time. Time-sharing also has had a profound influence upon both hardware and software. These systems are evolving toward *computer utilities* that will bring the benefits of computers to wider classes of users.

Applications to Biopharmaceutics

Most pharmaceutical scientists will use computers for their potential in expanding research horizons and eliminating tedium. In this context much of the material on hardware and software will be of general interest only. Such scientists will want to exploit work that has already been done in developing computer solutions to common problems. Pioneering in computer applications often interferes with other research!

Because computer science itself is young, and the application to biological problems is even younger, there is not a single well-structured guide to others' experience with computers. Some of the following resources may be helpful in getting started:

1. Colleagues who have experience in computer usage.
2. Contacts through vendors of hardware and software.
3. Libraries of programs maintained either by vendors of hardware, user organizations, or government agencies.
4. The computer installation at ones own institution.
5. Government sponsored research.
6. Books and journals in the scientific fields of study.

In using the programs and systems one must be alert for inconsistencies between claims and the actual performance of a system. A potential user must know his problem, why he needs computation, and what he expects to get from the computer. Constant monitoring of output from ongoing systems is essential since few programs are ever completely free of bugs. The responsible computer scientists endeavors to see that computers are not misused. However, the fundamental responsibility for correct use must lie with the problem formulator. All too often a computer program is used because it is easy to use, not because it will produce the answers that are needed.

Computer application systems may be categorized as *problem solving* and *information handling*. These two categories are not mutually exclusive. In fact, most information-handling systems will contain problem-solving elements. The major distinction lies in

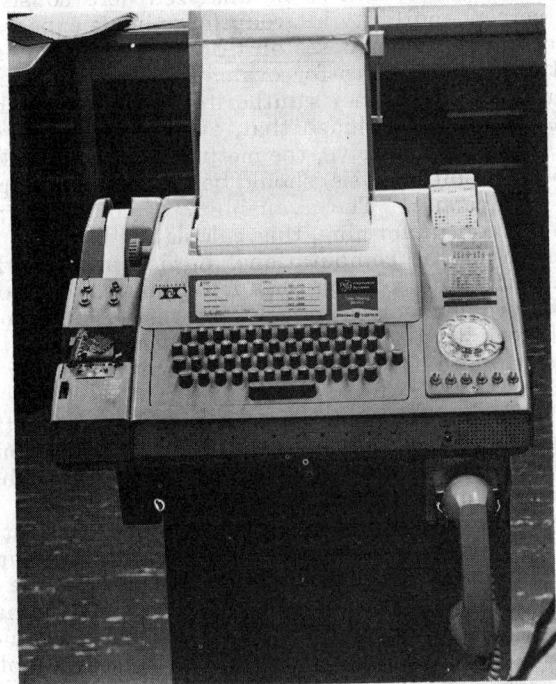

Fig. 88. The Model 33 ASR Teletype. This teletype is used as a terminal for time-sharing computer systems. It may be connected by telephone lines to several different time-sharing computer centers.

Table V—Program Types Available in BMD[7] Series

Class D—Description and tabulation—11 Programs
Class M—Multivariate analysis—7 Programs
Class R—Regression analysis—6 Programs
Class S—Special programs—10 Programs
Class T—Time series analysis—2 Programs
Class V—Variance analysis—8 Programs

that the information-handling systems are in routine, or at least repetitive, operation whereas the problem solving applications are nonrepetitive in nature. For instance, the biologist problem-solver who wants an analysis of variance computed can submit his data to the computer, get the answers back, and (after discussion with a statistician) proceed to write his paper. On the other hand, the behavioral pharmacologist who uses an on-line computer to acquire data and modify his experiments must make provision for handling the information in great detail—storing, retrieving, exception reporting, summarizing, and so on—as well as, if he has time, interpreting the data. The logistics of information handling assume more importance than the evaluation of formulas.

Problem-Solving

Statistics—Chapter 11 outlines the statistical methods that are most useful to the pharmaceutical scientist. Computer programs are available for implementing most of the methods given there and for many others. The most widely used library of such programs has been assembled at UCLA.[7] Table V illustrates the wide variety of programs available. Many university and service bureau computer centers have these programs available for easy use.

The availability of these statistical programs, and the ease with which new ones can be constructed, have contributed greatly to the use of statistical methods in the biological sciences. The evaluation of the median lethal dose, the LD50, provides a good example of the impact of computer methodology in the practice of statistics. The data to be analyzed here consist of the percent mortality in groups of animals exposed to successively higher doses of a drug. Many different statistical techniques for evaluating the LD50 have been used. In Finney's authoritative review[8] of these methods, it is concluded that, even though the computations are extensive, the method of maximum likelihood (probit analysis) should be the method adopted for routine use. The availability of computer programs* for performing this calculation relieves the scientist of the computational burden and provides him with a full solution for a few pennies. Not only is the problem solved quickly and easily, but also all of the validity tests can be routinely performed so that inappropriate use of the technique may be readily detected.

The availability of cheap easy-to-use statistical programs can lead to the inappropriate application of statistical methodology. Computation is no substitute for informed statistical consultation.

Quantum Chemistry—The discipline of quantum chemistry relies even more heavily than statistics upon the computer. The mathematical methods for the determination of electron orbital characteristics have been available for many years. The burden of calculations prevented solution of other than the simplest molecules. Even today's largest, fastest computers

---

* Program BMDO35[7] is an example.

are able to solve only approximate models. Indiana University, through its QCPE program,[9] provides a means of interchanging the programs and techniques in this research community.

The fundamental mathematical operation required is the evaluation of the eigenvalues and eigenvectors (diagonalization) of a matrix whose elements depend on the molecule being studied. The quantum chemist will devote his efforts to interpreting these calculations for the model he is investigating. Programs for several matrix diagonalization[10] methods are already available in FORTRAN from almost any of the general purpose libraries maintained by vendors and computer centers. Thus, when an appropriate method has been found, the chemist need only specify how the procedure is to be used.

Kinetics–Compartmental Analysis—The behavior of pharmaceuticals as they flow among the different *compartments* of a biological system is a fundamental concept in the science of pharmaceutics. Chapters 21 and 42 treat these subjects in detail. Both analog and digital computers are widely used in solving the differential equations which describe these systems.

Fig. 89 shows a simple compartmental model covering the absorption and metabolism of a drug. In this model the drug is introduced into the gastrointestinal tract from which it is gradually absorbed into the blood stream. As the drug is metabolized it disappears from the blood compartment and appears in the metabolite reservoir. If mathematical models for the transfer of material among the compartments are known, it is possible to construct a model of this system in an analog computer. Fig. 90 shows an analog computer solution to this model when the dosage is repeated every 4 hours. When such an analog model has been constructed, it is quite simple to change the parameters of the problem, thereby investigating the effect of varying absorption rates, metabolism rates, and dosage schedules. With such a computer model one can evaluate experimental data to see how well it conforms to a model; then adjust the model to try again. Thus, the analog computer becomes an essential link in developing a thorough understanding of the biological–chemical problem.

Digital computers, also, are very useful in the exploration of these models. They have been used, in effect, to simulate analog computers simulating the physical model. Probably more frequently the approach of the digital computer has been to fit the curves to observed data using the statistical methods of nonlinear least squares. A computer program[11] specifically designed for the model in Fig. 89—with first-order transfer among compartments—finds best-fitting values of absorption rate, metabolism rate, and volume of distribution.

Other Problem-Solving Applications—This list of applications could be continued at some length. In

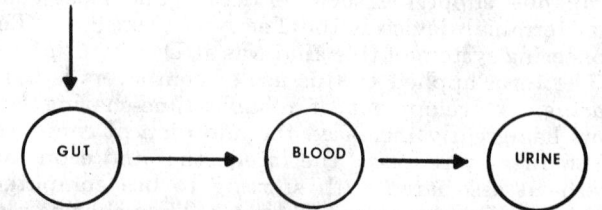

Fig. 89. Compartmental model of drug transport. Drug is introduced into the gastrointestinal tract (GUT) from which it is gradually absorbed into the blood stream (BLOOD). As it is metabolized it disappears from the blood and is excreted (URINE). Different assumptions about the character of the transport among compartments lead to different simulations.

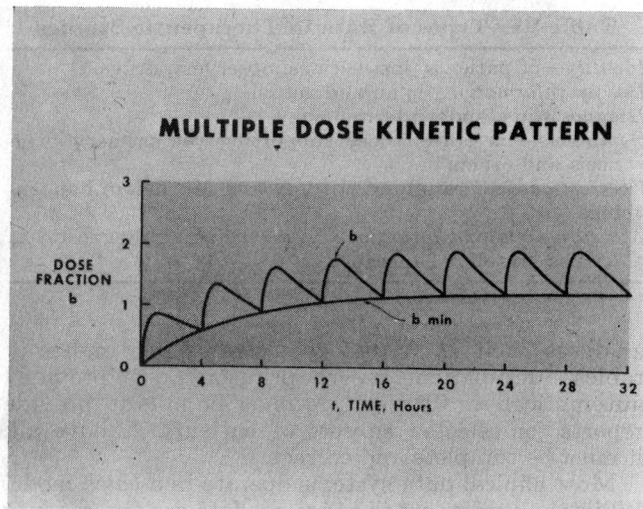

MULTIPLE DOSE KINETIC PATTERN

Fig. 90. Analog computer solution for the model in Fig. 89. First-order kinetics have been assumed (courtesy, Dr. Robert A. Brusenback, Abbott).

fact, most of the disciplines treated in the *Pharmaceutics* section can use computer methods constructively. The mathematical formulations appropriate to these disciplines are to be found in the respective chapters.

Information-Handling Systems

There are two quite distinct types of information-handling systems using computers. The more dynamic system is the one that catches information as it is generated in the laboratory, then processes, stores, and returns results to the laboratory at once. The second type of system may be thought of as the *repository* information file which contains the edited output of the other systems. The first type of system uses smaller, flexible computers which are usually short distances from the laboratories; the latter type usually requires systems with very large memories. For convenience, the first type will be referred to as *laboratory automation* and the second type as *large file*.

Laboratory Automation—The direct linkage of computers to laboratory instruments has required the development of fast, reliable, and responsive systems. Standardized interfaces between the signal generating instrument and the computer have made it economically attractive to link computers to a wide variety of instruments. The problems of laboratory automation are quite similar to the problems of integrating digital computers into process-control systems for large-scale production processes. In both cases systems development is likely to go through a *data-logging* phase in which data are pumped to the computer for storage and analysis with relatively little feedback to the instrument or process. In the next stage of development the computer analyzes the data as it is received and alerts the instrument operator to special problems. At the final stage the computer will actually control the instrument or process without human intervention. Computer systems may be justified economically in any of these configurations.

Significant applications of laboratory automation have been made in analytical chemistry and pharmacology. The applications to analytical chemistry include the direct connection of instruments such as gas chromatographs, mass spectrometers, and automated *wet chemists* by cable and by telephone line to computers. Useful systems range from small computers dedicated to a single kind of instrument up to relatively large systems which can be shared among many different instruments with different signal characteristics. The choice of the best configuration will involve evaluation of such factors as the following:

1. Distance among instruments to be served.
2. Signal characteristics, especially rates.
3. Other computer facilities required.
4. The availability of electronic and computer skills in the organization.

Such systems require communication of experiment design parameters to the computer as well as the actual signal from the instrument. Fig. 91[12] shows a prototype console which invites the scientist to answer the questions necessary to set up an Autoanalyzer® run. The console also provides printed results as they are computed for monitoring in the laboratory. The results are also stored in the computer system for summarization and incorporation into other data files.

The section on *Special-Purpose Hardware and Software* introduced the concept of a neuropharmacology laboratory computer system.[4] That system provides the neuropharmacologist with computer methods for the following problem areas:

1. *Spectral Analysis of EEG Signals*—This technique transforms the EEG signals into a graph which displays the intensity of various frequencies present in the signal. This power spectrum is useful in discriminating among and evaluating changes in EEG's.
2. *Analysis of Evoked Potentials*—Here the shape of a signal is followed after a special stimulus (for instance, a light flash) is applied to the animal. Often many repetitions of the stimulus must be given in order to average out noise in the signal.
3. *Behavioral Experiments with Feedback*—Data are gathered from learning experiments in such a way that the computer can control and modify the problem presented to the animal.

Similar types of application have occurred in other physiological studies. Human subjects as well as animals have been studied. On-line monitoring in the intensive care unit of a hospital may benefit from computer processing.

Large-File Systems—In the course of reaching the market a typical pharmaceutical preparation generates

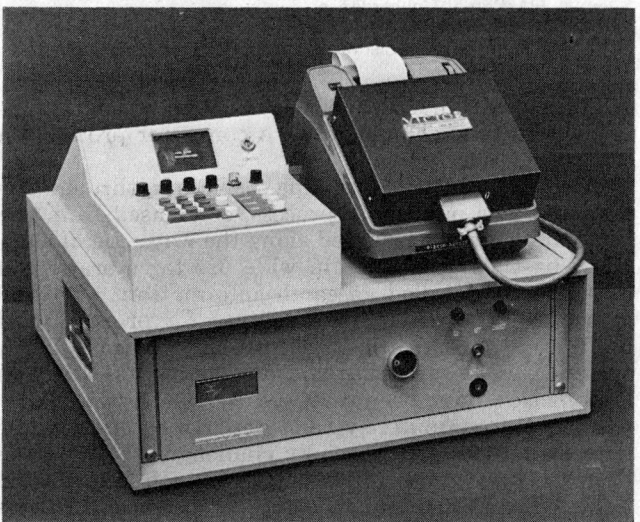

Fig. 91. Laboratory console for computer communication. The keyboard interrupts the computer and is used to provide *set-up* information, including standard curve concentrations, in response to questions produced on the ground glass screen under computer control. The solenoid-operated printer is used to verify set-up information from the computer and to print computed concentrations as they are sent by the computer. A more detailed description of the console may be found in Burns, D. A., and Bass, W. C.[12] (courtesy, Abbott).

a trail of data that is staggering in extent. In the chemistry laboratory its chemical structure and properties are evaluated. As it proceeds, large amounts of information are collected about its behavior in biological systems and its toxicological potential is evaluated in several species. If the picture is still favorable, limited human pharmacology studies are begun. These will be followed by extended therapeutic studies. Even after reaching the market place, reports of adverse experience, new indications, and so on must be added to the file.

Scientists with many different viewpoints will need to be able to assess this data on its own merits and in relation to findings on other pharmaceuticals. The ability of the computer to file, store, select, and retrieve information quickly and precisely is essential to the management of this huge data task. The task is so large that it must be subdivided. The part of the data base which finds its way into the published literature is the subject of three major information services. These are Chemical Abstracts Service, Biological Abstracts, and MEDLARS, maintained by the National Library of Medicine. Each of these organizations is committed to the use of computers as an integral part of their service. The following quotation is from the *Information Services from Chemical Abstracts Service, 1969:*

"The CAS information-handling and publication operations are being converted steadily to computer-based procedures. The ultimate objective is to produce the complete Chemical Abstracts Service through the computer. There is no intention to eliminate printed publications. The aim is to use the computer to prepare a wide range of both printed and machine-readable services from the input of a single data stream and to eliminate duplicate intellectual effort in the provision of these services.

"Currently, four combinations of printed and computer services are available:

1. Printed current-awareness services with computer tapes available.
   a. Chemical–Biological Activities
   b. Chemical Titles
   c. Polymer Science & Technology
2. Machine-readable current-awareness services on computer tape.
   a. Basic Journal Abstracts
   b. CA Condensates (no printed copy)
3. Machine-readable indexes on tape.
   a. CA Patent Concordance
4. Machine-readable library reference and record-keeping tools.
   a. Comprehensive List of Periodicals for Chemistry and Chemical Engineering."

This quotation indicates the extent to which Chemical Abstracts is committed to a computer production control system.

The input to the abstracting services is, through the nature of the publishing process, condensed from the raw data that are gathered along the way. *Local* computer-based systems are in wide use for storage and retrieval of detailed research information. Typical of such local systems are programs for processing of data from therapeutic trials of new drugs. These systems, which are still in a developmental stage in many cases, have been reviewed by Buchanan, *et al.*[13]

From the computer systems design viewpoint, these data structures are especially challenging. Even the best-designed protocols will yield much unexpected data. The system must be able to accept and handle the structured and unstructured information that comes from observing human behavior in the study. Table VI illustrates the complexity of this data. Each of these types of data has its own special requirements. In some cases terminology must be maintained across studies of widely different design. The system must be easy to use. This means that many standard

Table VI—Types of Data in Therapeutic Studies

Identity—of patients, institutions, observers, drugs.
Dosage information—plan and actual
Diagnosis in standard terminology
Symptoms—including those supporting the primary diagnosis and others
Observations—of results of therapy and of random happenings
Measurements and laboratory data—including diagnostic as well as "results of therapy."

analyses such as frequency distributions, multiway tables, and patient record print-outs are provided automatically. The system must be able to provide reports for selected subsets of patients. Above all, it must be complete and correct.

Most clinical data systems operate in a *batch* mode. While the studies are in progress, data are entered into forms which are saved until the end of the study. Then a data editing, coding, and computer file-building operation is done, often taking several weeks. At this point the analysis begins. This requires close cooperation among the team members involved, and many searches of the data base as one search suggests another. Even with the computer based systems described above, there is often a delay of several days in accomplishing each search.

The ideal clinical data system would catch data *on-the-fly* and provide interim analysis on demand. Such a system should produce much higher quality data than the batch system produces because of early detection of erroneous data and failure to adhere to protocols. The full benefit of the computer's potential will be realized when it is fully integrated into the therapeutic study process. Fig. 92 illustrates a data console designed for catching data efficiently at the point of origin in the clinic.

Other local data systems which are vital to pharmaceutical development include:

1. Chemical structure and properties.
2. Biological screening.
3. Toxicologic and pathologic.
4. Quality control, including stability.

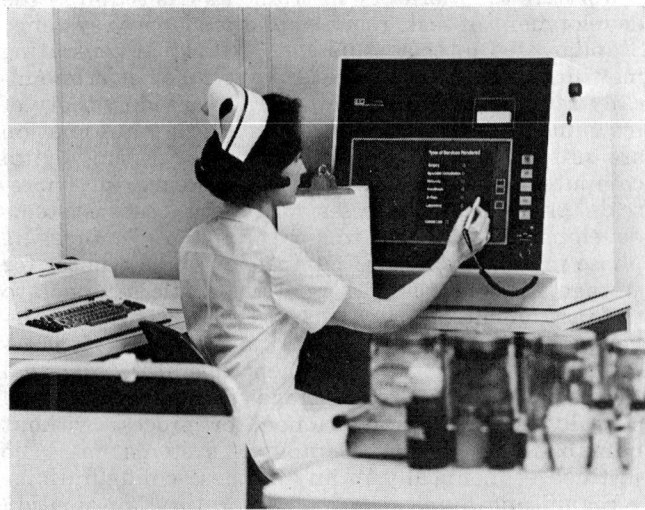

Fig. 92. IBM 2760/2740 communications terminal. Shown in use in a hospital environment, the IBM 2760 provides convenient data entry. The console is split. The right half has a specially designed overlay. The left half can display many different computer selected *forms* for data entry. The typewriter (IBM 2740) may be used for entry of alphanumeric data and for editing messages from the central computer (courtesy, IBM).

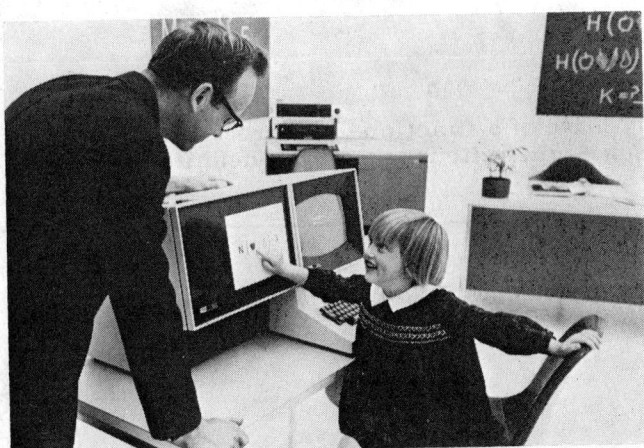

Fig. 93. Computer-assisted instruction. The kindergartner is learning the concept of number from a computer-controlled console. This technology, still in a developmental stage, will do much to amplify the abilities of good teachers (courtesy IBM).

5. Adverse reactions.
6. Market research.
7. Inventory in distribution centers.

Development of computer systems to support such data bases is a major effort, requiring careful identification of all characteristics and disposition of data. It requires a team effort including complete commitment of subject matter experts as well as the information processing professional.

Trends

The preceding edition of this book (published in 1965) did not contain a single reference to "computers." The coverage in this edition indicates the dynamic growth in the computer's impact on the pharmaceutical sciences. This trend is certain to continue. As computer technology is integrated into almost all phases of our society, scenes like that shown in Fig. 93 will become common.

Much of the credit for increased utilization of computers must go to the increased speed, greater reliability, and decreased cost achieved by the breakthrough in solid state electronics. Fig. 94 illustrates this trend. As a result, the application horizon is constantly expanding.

The critical element in securing the advantages offered by computers is the availability of people who can define and implement systems. The pure logic of the computer places unusual stress on the need for communication between the user and the implementer of systems. The attitude of the user–scientist toward the computer is crucial. He must know what he wants, persist until he gets it, report errors and misunderstanding constructively, and sometimes, be patient. In return he will find his output has been greatly amplified.

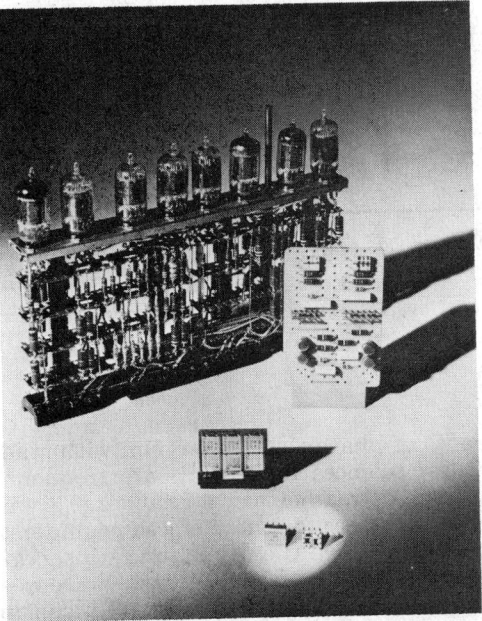

Fig. 94. Computer hardware trends. Three *generations* of computer hardware are shown. The larger circuit board with transistors started to replace vacuum tube circuits in the late 1950's. The smaller solid state circuit board with six circuits replaced the first transistor generation in the mid-1960's. The spotlight shows the finer detail of one of the circuits imbedded in the smaller circuit board. Comparable circuits in future machines would be too small to be seen in this picture (courtesy IBM).

References

1. Kemeny, J. G., and Kurtz, T. E., *Science*, **162** (3850), 223 (Oct. 11, 1968).
2. Organick, E. I., *A FORTRAN IV Primer*, Addison-Wesley, Reading, Mass., 1966.
3. MacCracken, D. D., *A Guide to FORTRAN IV Programming*, Wiley, New York, 1965.
4. Abraham, F. D., *et al*, *AFIPS Conf. Proc.*, **32**, 345 (1968).
5. Truitt, T. D., and Rogers, A. E., *Basics of Analog Computers*, Rider, New York, 1960.
6. Garrett, E. R., *Antibiot. Chemotherapia*, **12**, 227 (1964).
7. Dixon, W. J., ed., *BMD, Biomedical Computer Programs* (Univ. of California Publications in Automatic Computation, No. 2) 1967.
8. Finney, D. J., *Statistical Method in Biological Assay*, Hafner, 1964, Chap. 20.
9. *QCPE, Quantum Chemistry Program Exchange, Catalog and Procedures*, vol. V, Indiana Univ. Chem. Dept., 1969.
10. Ralston, A., and Wilf, H. S., *Mathematical Methods for Digital Computers*, vol. 1, Wiley, New York, 1960.
11. Wiegand, R. G., and Sanders, P. G., *J. Pharmacol. Exptl. Therap.*, **146** (3), 271 (Dec., 1964).
12. Burns, D. A., and Bass, W. C., Abbott Laboratories, North Chicago, Ill., presented to 20th Ann. Pittsburgh Conf., Mar. 3–7, 1969.
13. Buchanan, O. H., *et al*, *Drug Inform. Bull.*, **1** (5), 136 (Oct./Dec., 1967).

Bibliography

Biomedical uses of computers have been reviewed in depth in many places; following are some authoritative references:

McLachlan, G., and Shegog, R. A., ed., *Computers in the Service of Medicine*, vols. I & II, Oxford Univ. Press, London, 1968.
Spencer, W. A., *et al*, *J. Chronic Diseases*, **19**, (Apr., 1966).
Hall, T. L., ed., *Ann. N.Y. Acad. Sci.*, **153** (Art. 2), 389–671 (Nov. 15, 1968).
Whipple, H. E., *N.Y. Acad. Sci.*, **115** (Art. 2), 543–1140 (July 31, 1964).
Ledley, R. S., *Use of Computers in Biology and Medicine*, McGraw-Hill, New York, 1965.
Taylor, T. R., *The Principles of Medical Computing*, Blackwell, Oxford, England, 1967.

13 | Calculus

Functions and their limits—the derivative of a function—the process of differentiation—partial differentiation—indefinite integration—definite integration (and its relationship to summation)

This chapter was prepared by

Edward G. Rippie, PhD, *Professor of Pharmaceutics, College of Pharmacy, University of Minnesota, Minneapolis, Minn.* 55455

Students of pharmacy, in common with students of the natural sciences in general, are frequently concerned with the mathematical analysis of dynamic or kinematic processes for the purpose of understanding the manner in which they function. Observations of such systems often yield data which represent or which must be interpreted in terms of a continuously changing property or component of the system.

This chapter is intended as an introduction to the fundamental concepts and techniques of calculus which are necessary for the adequate mathematical description of systems in such a state of flux. Emphasis will be given to the development of these concepts within a format as uncluttered with formalism and/or complex notation as is possible. For this reason, conditions and limitations required for complete mathematical rigor will be omitted when they do not contribute to a basic understanding of fundamental principles, as they will be applied within the scope of this chapter.

Subjects discussed are limited to those which will be of most use to the undergraduate pharmacy student during his course of study. When greater detail or broader coverage is required, it may be obtained by selective reading from any of the rather large number of excellent calculus texts available.

Functions and Their Limits

The Concept of the Functional Relationship between Variables—Whenever two or more variable quantities are in some way interrelated, such that the value or values any one of them can assume is determined by the values of the others, they are said to be *functions* of each other. Occasionally, the relationships between such variables can be expressed by a mathematical equation or set of equations. These equations then define the functional relationships between the variables and are themselves called *functions*. The equation

$$m = x^2 + 2xy + y^2 \qquad (1)$$

explicitly expresses m as a function of x and y. This equation also can be written symbolically as $m = f(x,y)$, where the right-hand term simply signifies that m is a function of x and y without specifying the exact nature of the relationship.

In this case, however, f is defined by Eq. 1 to denote a particular algebraic expression. If x and y are allowed to take values a and b, respectively, m assumes the value $f(a,b)$. Different functions of x and y may be designated as $g(x,y)$ or $h(x,y)$ to distinguish them from each other. The letters g and h represent no function in particular unless so defined.

In an equation containing n number of variables, any $n - 1$ of them arbitrarily can be assigned numerical values and are called *independent variables*. The value(s) of the remaining variable is thus fixed and it is designated the *dependent variable*.

A function is said to be *single-* or *multiple-valued* depending on the number of values it has for each set of values given the independent variables. Thus, in Eq. 1, m is a single-valued function of x and y. If, however, the equation is solved for x, where $x = m^{1/2} - y$, two values of x result from every positive value of m. x is therefore a double-valued function for $m > 0$, but only a single-valued function of y.

Graphing of Functions—In order to better visualize relationships between variables, it is often desirable to represent them pictorially by means of a *graph*. Graphs drawn in two dimensions can show the mutual behavior pattern of any two variables. While graphs also can be constructed so as to give a three-dimensional perspective, they will not be considered here.

The coordinate system used for construction of a graph is selected arbitrarily and is generally chosen so as to simplify the figure. Since the functions encountered in this chapter are relatively simple, rectangular coordinates will be used unless otherwise stated.

A single point on a graph denotes a value for each of the two variables represented on the axes. Thus, if $y = f(x)$, associated pairs (x,y) can be generated corresponding to values of x and y which satisfy the equation. If the values are plotted on a graph, the resulting points, one for each pair (x,y), lie on a curve which depicts the function.

With the careful selection of a few points, the curve can be sketched without need of calculating points at short intervals over the entire curve. Good choices of points include intercepts (where the curve crosses the axes) and points of discontinuity. Special features such as symmetry and asymptotes are also useful guides.

Example 1—Consider the equation $y = 1/x$. It can be seen that the curve has no intercepts but rather approaches the axes asymptotically. Also, the sign of y is always the same as that of x, indicating that the curve lies within the first and third quadrants of the graph. Consequently, because the point (0,0) does not satisfy the equation, the function must be discontinuous (Fig. 95).

A table of coordinates, as shown in Fig. 95, is a useful aid in the plotting of a graph and reduces the possibility of error.

Increments of Variables and Functions—If an independent variable x is changed by an increment Δx, the variable assumes a new value $x + \Delta x$ which may be either greater or less than before, depending on the sign of Δx. If $y = f(x)$, the dependent variable y will undergo a corresponding change Δy so that $y +$

$\Delta y = f(x + \Delta x)$. While the incremental change Δy is a direct result of the change in x, its magnitude and sign are determined by the functional relationship between x and y, and on the values of x and Δx. Thus

$$\Delta y = f(x + \Delta x) - f(x) \qquad (2)$$

derives from the expression $\Delta y = f(x + \Delta x) - y$.

Example 2—Let $y = x(x - 1) = f(x)$, and calculate the increment Δy when x changes from 1 to 3. In this case, $x = 1$ and $\Delta x = 2$ correspond to the initial value of x and the incremental change in x, respectively. Thus

$$\Delta y = (x + \Delta x)(x + \Delta x - 1) - x(x - 1)$$
$$= \Delta x^2 + 2x\,\Delta x - \Delta x$$

Substituting for x and Δx, Δy is found to be 6. This may also be seen from Fig. 96.

The Concept of the Limit of a Function

—A necessary concept to the understanding of calculus is that of the *limit* (abbreviated lim) of a function. Allow the independent variable x, of a function $y = f(x)$, to assume a sequence of values successively closer to some number a. The dependent variable will then assume a corresponding set of values. The function $f(x)$ is said to approach a limit b as x approaches a, if the absolute difference between $f(x)$ and b can be made arbitrarily small by choosing x sufficiently close in value to a. This is written symbolically as

$$\lim_{x \to a} f(x) = b$$

Although the formal definition of the limit must be modified in some cases, the numbers a and b can take any set of values from $-\infty$ to ∞.

Example 3—Calculate the limit of the function $y = 1 - x^2$ as $x \to 2$. It is apparent in this case that as x assumes values close to 2, y can be made to approach -3; thus

$$\lim_{x \to 2} (1 - x^2) = -3$$

Example 4—Consider again the function $y = 1/x$, discussed in Example 1, and calculate its limit as $x \to 0$. Here, the choice of positive values of x near zero results in large values of y which increase without bound as $x \to 0$. The limit of $1/x$ as $x \to 0$ is thus infinity (∞). If x is allowed to approach zero from negative values, the limit is found to be negative infinity. These results can be written in the form

$$\lim_{x \to 0} (1/x) = \infty; \qquad \lim_{-x \to 0} (1/x) = -\infty$$

and can be visualized from Fig. 95. It is apparent from this discussion that the function $1/x$ is *discontinuous* at the point $x = 0$.

The Properties of Limits

—When finding the limits of relatively complex functions, it is frequently useful to break them down into simpler functions whose limits are more easily calculated. The following rules are necessary for such manipulations and also serve to reinforce the basic concept of a limit.

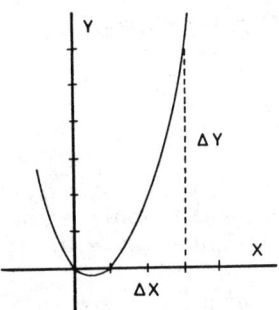

Fig. 96. A plot of the equation $y = x(x - 1) = f(x)$, including the increment Δy when x changes from 1 to 3.

Consider a sequence of functions, $F_1, F_2, F_3, \ldots, F_n$, having a common independent variable x, and which possess limits as x approaches any value in the interval $-\infty \leqslant x \leqslant \infty$.

Rule 1

$$\lim (F_1 + F_2 + \ldots + F_n) = \lim F_1 + \lim F_2 + \ldots + \lim F_n$$

Rule 2

$$\lim (F_1 . F_2 . \ldots . F_n) = \lim F_1 . \lim F_2 . \ldots . \lim F_n$$

Rule 3

$$\lim (F_1/F_2) = \lim F_1/\lim F_2$$

if $F_2 \neq 0$.

Rule 4

$$\lim (F_1{}^r) = (\lim F_1)^r$$

where r may be a fractional number as well as an integer.

Example 5—Evaluate the limit of the function $(x^2 - x + 6)/(x^3 + 1)$ as $x \to 2$. The problem may be simplified by applying Rules 3 and 1 in succession. Thus

$$\lim_{x \to 2} (x^2 - x + 6) \Big/ (x^3 + 1)$$
$$= \lim_{x \to 2} (x^2 - x + 6) \Big/ \lim_{x \to 2} (x^3 + 1)$$
$$= \left[\lim_{x \to 2} (x^2) - \lim_{x \to 2} (x) + \lim_{x \to 2} (6) \right] \Big/ \left[\lim_{x \to 2} (x^3) + \lim_{x \to 2} (1) \right]$$
$$= (4 - 2 + 6)/(8 + 1) = 8/9$$

When Rule 3 is applied to evaluate the limit of a quotient, it may be found that the quotient of limits has the *indeterminate* form 0/0. This result implies that the function is undefined at the limiting value of the independent variable. In spite of this, however, the function may possess a well-defined limit which can be determined if the proper technique is used.

Example 6—Consider the function $(1 - x)/(1 - x^2) = f(x)$. The limit of $f(x)$ as $x \to 1$ can be seen to be indeterminate if computed in the usual way. However, if the function is placed in the form $1/(1 + x)$, the limit can be seen to equal $\frac{1}{2}$.

The concept of the limit of quotients is fundamental to an understanding of calculus, a subject which results in the frequent encounter with indeterminate forms. As will be seen, the problem of indeterminacy is resolved in these cases by defining the limiting behavior in terms of specific functions.

Exercises

1. Given $f(x) = 1 - 3x^2$, calculate $f(1)$, $f(a)$, and $f(b - 1)$.

2. Given $f(y) = y - 1/y$ and $g(x) = x^2$, express $f[g(x)]$ in terms of x.

3. By graphing, show that the curves in Fig. 95 are symmetrical about the lines $y = x$, and $y = -x$.

4. Given $y = 6x - x^2$, calculate Δy if $x = 1$ and $\Delta x = 0.1$.

5. Calculate the following limits:

   a. $\lim_{x \to 1} (x^2 - 3x + 2)$

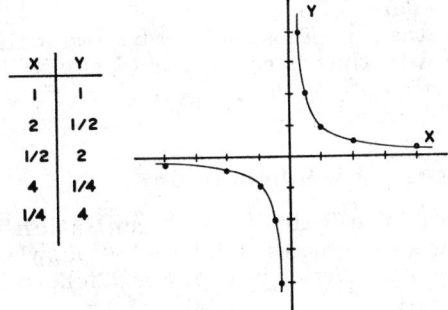

X	Y
1	1
2	1/2
1/2	2
4	1/4
1/4	4

Fig. 95. A plot of the equation $y = 1/x$.

b. $\lim_{x \to 2} [(x^2 - 1)(1 - 1/x)]$

c. $\lim_{x \to 0} [(1 - x)/(3x^2 + 2)]^3$

d. $\lim_{x \to 2} [(3x - 6)/(2 - x)]$

6.   Given $y = 1/x$, calculate $\Delta y / \Delta x$ in terms of x and Δx. What is the limit of this expression for $\Delta y / \Delta x$ when $x = 1$, and $\Delta x = 0$?

The Derivative of a Function

The Derivative as a Limit—The *derivative* of a function $y = f(x)$ is defined formally as the limit of $\Delta y / \Delta x$ as $\Delta x \to 0$. It is apparent that as $\Delta x \to 0$, Δy also approaches zero and that the expression

$$\lim_{\Delta x \to 0} (\Delta y / \Delta x)$$

is in an indeterminate form. When the limit exists, it may be taken out of the indeterminate form by substitution of an expression in x and Δx for the quantity Δy.

Inasmuch as the derivative of a function of x is another related function of x, its value will depend on x. This is implicit in the following notation, which will be used in subsequent work. If $y = f(x)$, the derivative of $f(x)$ with respect to x is

$$dy/dx = \lim_{\Delta x \to 0} (\Delta y / \Delta x) = f'(x) \qquad (3)$$

The mechanism for finding the derivative of a function is simple in principle. Starting with the definition (Eq. 3) it is necessary to first find Δy, in terms of x and Δx, for the particular function under consideration. This is accomplished by means of Eq. 2 so that

$$dy/dx = \lim_{\Delta x \to 0} \left(\frac{f(x + \Delta x) - f(x)}{\Delta x} \right) \qquad (4)$$

After carrying out the necessary algebra to obtain $[f(x + \Delta x) - f(x)]/\Delta x$ explicitly, it only remains to take the limit as $\Delta x \to 0$. The value of the resulting derivative can be obtained for any desired value of x by simple substitution.

Example 7—Find the derivative of y with respect to x, (dy/dx), for the function $y = x^2 - 3x$. What is the value of $f'(x)$ when $x = 2$? Calculating Δy from Eq. 2,

$$\Delta y = (x + \Delta x)^2 - 3(x + \Delta x) - x^2 + 3x$$

$$= 2x\Delta x - 3\Delta x + \Delta x^2$$

Dividing by Δx,

$$\Delta y / \Delta x = 2x - 3 + \Delta x$$

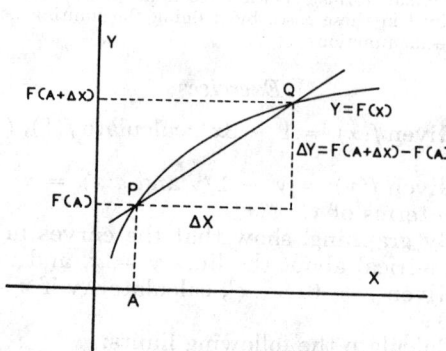

Fig. 97. A portion of the graph of the function $y = f(x)$, where $f(a)$ denotes the derivative of $f(x)$ at a point where $x = a$.

Taking the limit as $\Delta x \to 0$,

$$\lim_{\Delta x \to 0} (\Delta y / \Delta x) = \lim_{\Delta x \to 0} (2x - 3 + \Delta x) = 2x - 3$$

The derivative, dy/dx, is therefore equal to $2x - 3$ for all values of x. The value of the derivative, $f'(x)$, when $x = 2$ is 1.

Graphical Interpretation of the Derivative—The derivative of a function of a single variable, $y = f(x)$, has been defined analytically, in the previous section, as a new function $dy/dx = f'(x)$. The limiting process leading to the derivative can be visualized easily by the use of a graph. Consider the curve in Fig. 97 to represent a portion of the graph of the function $y = f(x)$, and let $f'(a)$ denote the derivative of $f(x)$ at the point where $x = a$. Then by definition,

$$f'(a) = \lim_{\Delta x \to 0} \left(\frac{f(a + \Delta x) - f(a)}{\Delta x} \right)$$

The expression $[f(a + \Delta x) - f(a)]/\Delta x$ represents the slope of a line through the Points P and Q. However, as $\Delta x \to 0$, the Point Q moves down the curve toward P, and the line drawn through P and Q becomes tangential to the curve at Point P. Thus when the limit of $\Delta y / \Delta x$ as $\Delta x \to 0$ is computed for $x = a$, it is numerically equal to the slope of a line tangent to the curve at point P. For this reason the derivative is said to be the slope of the curve, and as a function of x it can be computed for all values* of x.

The Derivative as a Rate of Change—The derivative also may be interpreted physically as the rate of change of one quantity with respect to another. For example, the quotient $\Delta m / \Delta t$ may denote the change in mass of a growing plant over a time interval Δt and therefore represents the average rate of growth for that period. However, the derivative dm/dt is the rate of change of mass at a point in time and represents the instantaneous rate of growth.

The concept of an instantaneous rate of change can be applied to any two variables, one of which changes as a function of the other. Examples of pairs of such related variables which are frequently encountered are distance–time, drug blood level–time, radiation intensity–distance, chemical change–time, and pH as a function of added acid or base.

Exercises

7.   Calculate the derivative of the following functions:

   a. $y = 2x^3 - 5$
   b. $s = t/(1 - t)$
   c. $m = n^5$

8.   Compute the value of dy/dx for Exercise 7a, when $x = 0, 1, -3, a$.

9.   Show that the rate of change of volume of a cube with respect to the length of a side is three times the surface area of one of its sides.

10.   If the rate of loss of drug by degradation from an elixir with time is equal numerically to $\frac{1}{1000}$ the concentration of the drug at any given time, express the rate of loss as a function of concentration.

The Process of Differentiation

Origin of the Rules for Differentiation—As has been shown, the process of differentiation, wherein the derivative of a function is determined, follows logically

---

* Subject to certain limitations not discussed here.

from the formal definition of the derivative, Eq. 4. The procedure, however, can become involved and time consuming even when applied to relatively simple functions. For this reason general rules for differentiation have been developed which greatly simplify matters. These rules arise directly from the application of the methods of the previous section to generalized functions. Tables of several frequently used rules are given and a few of the rules* are derived.

Rule 1—The derivative of the independent variable raised to a constant power n is equal to n times the independent variable to the $n - 1$ power.

Let $y = x^n$, where n is a positive integer. According to Eq. 4,

$$dy/dx = \lim_{\Delta x \to 0} \left(\frac{(x + \Delta x)^n - x^n}{\Delta x} \right)$$

$$= \lim_{\Delta x \to 0} \left(nx^{n-1} + \frac{n(n-1)x^{n-2}\Delta x}{2} + \cdots + \Delta x^{n-1} \right)$$

$$= nx^{n-1}$$

Rule 2—The derivative of a constant times a function is equal to the constant times the derivative of the function.

Let $y = ku = kf(x)$, where k is a constant and $u = f(x)$ is a function of x. According to Eq. 4,

$$dy/dx = \lim_{\Delta x \to 0} \left(\frac{kf(x + \Delta x) - kf(x)}{\Delta x} \right)$$

$$= k \lim_{\Delta x \to 0} \left(\frac{f(x + \Delta x) - f(x)}{\Delta x} \right)$$

$$= kf'(x) = kdu/dx$$

Rule 4—The derivative of the product of two functions is equal to the first function times the derivative of the second function plus the second function times the derivative of the first.

Let $y = u \cdot v$, where $u = f(x)$ and $v = g(x)$. According to Eq. 4,

$$dy/dx = \lim_{\Delta x \to 0} \left(\frac{f(x + \Delta x)g(x + \Delta x) - f(x)g(x)}{\Delta x} \right)$$

$$= \lim_{\Delta x \to 0} \left(\frac{(u + \Delta u)(v + \Delta v) - uv}{\Delta x} \right)$$

$$= \lim_{\Delta x \to 0} \left(\frac{u\,\Delta v + v\,\Delta u + \Delta u\,\Delta v}{\Delta x} \right)$$

$$= u(dv/dx) + v(du/dx)$$

Note: $\lim_{\Delta x \to 0} \left(\frac{\Delta u\,\Delta v}{\Delta x} \right) = \lim_{\Delta x \to 0}(\Delta u) \lim_{\Delta x \to 0} \left(\frac{\Delta v}{\Delta x} \right) = 0$

Rule 6—If y is a function of z, which in turn is a function of x, the derivative of y with respect to x is equal to the product of the derivative of y with respect to z and the derivative of z with respect to x.

Let $y = f(z)$ and $z = g(x)$. If x is changed by an amount Δx, a change in z, Δz, and a change in y, Δy, result. Thus, $\Delta y/\Delta x = (\Delta y/\Delta z)(\Delta z/\Delta x)$.

$$dy/dx = \lim_{\Delta x \to 0}(\Delta y/\Delta x) = \lim_{\Delta x \to 0}(\Delta y/\Delta z)(\Delta z/\Delta x)$$

$$= \lim_{\Delta x \to 0}(\Delta y/\Delta z) \lim_{\Delta x \to 0}(\Delta z/\Delta x)$$

$$= \lim_{\Delta z \to 0}(\Delta y/\Delta z) \lim_{\Delta x \to 0}(\Delta z/\Delta x)$$

$$= (dy/dz)(dz/dx)$$

Higher Order Derivatives—It was shown earlier that the derivative of a function of x is itself, in general, also a function of x. If this *first derivative* is differentiated, a *second derivative* is obtained which is also a function of x. Thus when the process of differentiation is repeated again and again, a succession of higher

---

* While the rules presented are general, the derivations are subject to certain limitations not discussed here.

Table I—Rules for Differentiation[a]

Rule	Function	Derivative
	Primary rules[b]	
1	$y = x^n$	$dy/dx = nx^{n-1}$
2	$y = ku$	$dy/dx = k(du/dx)$
3	$y = u + v$	$dy/dx = du/dx + dv/dx$
4	$y = u \cdot v$	$dy/dx = u(dv/dx) + v(du/dx)$
5	$y = u/v$	$dy/dx = \dfrac{v(du/dx) - u(dv/dx)}{v^2}$
6	$y = f(z),$ $z = g(x)$	$dy/dx = (dy/dz)(dz/dx)$
7	$y = e^u$	$dy/dx = e^u(du/dx)$
8	$y = \ln u$	$dy/dx = (du/dx)/u$
	Secondary rules	
9	$y = k$	$dy/dx = 0$
10	$y = x$	$dy/dx = 1$
11	$y = kx$	$dy/dx = k$
12	$y = u^n$	$dy/dx = nu^{n-1}du/dx$
13	$y = e^x$	$dy/dx = e^x$
14	$y = \ln x$	$dy/dx = 1/x$

[a] Definitions: the variables y, u, and v are functions of x, the independent variable; k and n are constants; e is the base of the natural logarithms, designated by "ln."
[b] Several of these rules are in themselves special cases of more general rules.

order derivatives is obtained, the original function alone determining the number of successive derivatives which may be found. These higher order derivatives are denoted by the following symbols.

1st derivative: $dy/dx = f'(x)$
2nd derivative: $d^2y/dx^2 = f''(x)$
3rd derivative: $d^3y/dx^3 = f'''(x)$
nth derivative: $d^ny/dx^n = f^n(x)$

Example 8—Find all the derivatives of the function $y = x^3 - x + e^x$.

$$dy/dx = 3x^2 - 1 + e^x$$
$$d^2y/dx^2 = 6x + e^x$$
$$d^3y/dx^3 = 6 + e^x$$
$$d^ny/dx^n = e^x \text{ where } n \geqslant 4.$$

It is often desirable to find the high and/or low points of a function analytically and to determine their identity as *maxima* or *minima*. If a function has a lesser value immediately to both sides of a point, that point denotes a *maximum* value of the function. Similarly, a *minimum* exists if the function has a higher value immediately to both sides of a point. Maximum and minimum points do not necessarily represent the greatest or least values taken by the function, and there is no limit to the number of maxima and minima a function can possess.

Both maximum and minimum points are located on the curve where the slope, and hence the first derivative of the function, is equal to zero. This is a necessary but not a sufficient requirement for the existence of maxima or minima points.

The second derivative, which represents the rate of change of slope with distance along the curve, is useful in identifying maxima and minima. As a maximum is approached from small values of the independent variable, the slope decreases, becomes zero, and then becomes negative. Therefore, the second derivative would possess a negative value at a maximum point on the curve. By the same reasoning, the second derivative is positive at a minimum point.

Let $y = f(x)$ possess continuous first and second derivatives. Then if

$$f'(a) = 0, f''(a) < 0; \quad (a,f(a)) \text{ is a maximum point}$$
$$f'(a) = 0, f''(a) > 0; \quad (a,f(a)) \text{ is a minimum point}$$

If the second derivative is equal to zero, the point is neither a maximum nor a minimum but may be a point of inflection at which the line changes its direction of curvature. This will be the case if the third derivative is not zero.

Example 9—Consider the equation $f(x) = x^3/3 + x^2 - 3x + 9$ and find any maxima or minima. These points must satisfy the condition $f'(x) = 0$, and therefore $f'(x) = x^2 + 2x - 3 = (x + 3)(x - 1) = 0$ can occur only when $x = 1, -3$. The second derivative for these values of x will establish their nature. Since $f''(x) = 2x + 2$, when $x = 1$, $f''(1) = 4$ and the point $(1,22/3)$ is a minimum. At the point $(-3,18)$, $f''(-3) = -4$, and the function is at a maximum.

Example 10—Show that the curve $y = 9x^2 - 5$ has no maximum points. It is sufficient to show that d^2y/dx^2 is never negative in value, thereby ruling out the existence of a maximum. Inasmuch as $d^2y/dx^2 = 18$, the proof is complete.

Example 11—Find two numbers x and y whose sum is 10, such that $x^2 + y^2$ is a minimum. Thus,

$$A = x^2 + y^2 = x^2 + (10 - x)^2$$

$$dA/dx = 4x - 20$$

When the first derivative is zero, $x = 5$ and $y = 5$. The second derivative is equal to 4, establishing these values of x and y as those which minimize A.

Exercises

11. Derive Rules 3 and 5 for differentiation.
12. Derive Rules 7 and 8 for differentiation.
13. Derive Rules 9 through 14 for differentiation.
14. Deduce Rules 9 through 14 as special cases of certain of the primary rules listed.
15. Derive a general rule for which Rules 4 and 5 are special cases.
16. Calculate the derivatives of the following functions:

    a. $y = x^3 - 3x + 1/x - 6$
    b. $y = x^{1/2}(1 + x^2)$
    c. $y = e^{x^2}$
    d. $y = \ln (1 + x^2)$

17. If $y = e^z$, $z = 1 - x^2$, calculate dy/dx.
18. Find du/dt if

$$u = (e^{3t} - 3 \ln t)^{5/2}.$$

19. Find all the successive derivatives of the function

$$y = x^5/5 + x^3/3 + x.$$

20. The concentration, C, of a drug in the blood is found to follow the equation

$$C = Dt/(t^2 + 6t + 5)$$

where D is a constant and t is the time in hours. At what time is C a maximum?

21. The volume of a pyramid is equal to $Bh/3$ where B is the area of the base and h is the altitude. If $B + h^2$ is held constant at 300 sq ft, what is the maximum volume that can be occupied by the pyramid?

Partial Differentiation

The Partial Derivative—Differentiation has been defined and discussed thus far only in terms of its application to functions of a single independent variable. The concept of the derivative, however, can be generalized and extended to include functions of several variables.

Whereas a function of a single variable can be visualized as a line in two-dimensional space, a function of two independent variables can be represented by a surface in three-dimensional space. Similarly, functions of $n - 1$ independent variables can be abstractly conceived as "surfaces" in n-dimensional space. If all but one independent variable is held constant, an n-dimensional surface is reduced to a line in two dimensions.

The slope of such a line represents the rate of change of the function with respect to the retained variable, as all the other variables are held at their particular, arbitrarily selected values. This slope may be determined by taking the derivative of the function with respect to the selected variable while holding all the other variables constant.

Such a derivative is termed a *partial derivative* since it represents the rate of change of the function with respect to only a part (one) of the independent variables.

The partial derivative of a function $y = f(x_1, x_2, \ldots, x_k)$, of k independent variables $(x_1, x_2, \ldots, x_k)$, with respect to the variable x_1 is defined as

$$\partial y/\partial x_1$$

$$= \lim_{\Delta x_1 \to 0} \left(\frac{f(x_1 + \Delta x_1, x_2, \ldots, x_k) - f(x_1, x_2, \ldots, x_k)}{\Delta x_1} \right) \quad (5)$$

Example 12—Find the partial derivatives of the function $u = x^3 - 2xy + y^2$ with respect to both x and y. That is, find $\partial u/\partial x$ and $\partial u/\partial y$, where all independent variables are considered as constants except the one with respect to which the derivative is taken. Thus,

$$\partial u/\partial x = 3x^2 - 2y; \quad \partial u/\partial y = -2x + 2y$$

Example 13—The volume of a right circular cylinder is given by the equation $V = \pi r^2 h$, where r is the radius of curvature and h is the height. Find the rate of change of height with respect to radius at constant volume. Expressing the height in terms of r and V,

$$h = \frac{V}{\pi r^2}; \quad \partial h/\partial r = \frac{-2V}{\pi r^3}$$

Total Differentials and Total Derivatives—It was shown previously that if $y = f(x)$, the rate of change of y with respect to x is equal to the derivative, $dy/dx = f'(x)$. Upon rearrangement, $dy = f'(x)\, dx$, where dy is defined as the *differential* of y, and dx as the differential of x. The quantities dx and dy may be intuitively thought of as the "potentials" for change of x and y, respectively.

Consider a lever, as shown in Fig. 98, having arms of length a and b. Let x represent the distance traveled by the tip of the left arm and y that traveled by the right arm. The relationship between x and y is given by the expression $y = bx/a$, and the differential of y is defined by the equation $dy = f'(x)dx = (b/a)dx$. It is clear from Fig. 98 that the "potential" for a change in y is in direct proportion to that for x, and is in the ratio b/a.

The differential of a function of k independent variables $(x_1, x_2, \ldots, x_k)$ is itself a function of the $k\, dx_i$'s and is referred to as the *total differential*. If $y = f(x_1, x_2, \ldots, x_k)$, the total differential of y is defined by the expression

$$dy = \frac{\partial y}{\partial x_1} dx_1 + \frac{\partial y}{\partial x_2} dx_2 + \ldots + \frac{\partial y}{\partial x_k} dx_k \quad (6)$$

Each term of the type $(\partial y/\partial x_i)dx_i$ represents the contribution of the ith independent variable to dy.

Example 14—Find the total differential of $u = xyz$. From Eq. 6, the total differential is given by

$$du = (\partial u/\partial x)dx + (\partial u/\partial y)dy + (\partial u/\partial z)dz$$

Substituting for $\partial u/\partial x$, $\partial u/\partial y$, $\partial u/\partial z$;

$$du = yzdx + xzdy + xydz$$

Let the k variables, x_i, of Eq. 6 not be independent, but rather let them be functions of a single independent variable t. This implies that y is a function of t only and can be expressed in the form $y = g(t)$. While the derivative of y with respect to t then could be computed directly, it is frequently more convenient to calculate dy/dt by a different method.

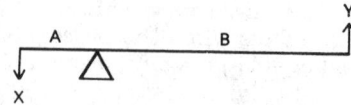

Fig. 98. A lever—A and B: arm lengths; X and Y: distances traveled by the tips of the left and right arms, respectively.

If Eq. 6 is divided through by the differential of t, dy/dt is obtained in the form

$$\frac{dy}{dt} = \frac{\partial y}{\partial x_1} \cdot \frac{dx_1}{dt} + \frac{\partial y}{\partial x_2} \cdot \frac{dx_2}{dt} + \ldots + \frac{\partial y}{\partial x_k} \cdot \frac{dx_k}{dt} \quad (7)$$

and is defined as the *total derivative* of y with respect to t. Eq. 7 therefore permits dy/dt to be calculated without the need to express y explicitly in terms of t.

Example 15—Find the total derivative of y with respect to t for the function $y = u \ln v \, e^z$ where $u = t^2 - 2$, $v = 1/t$, and $z = t^{3/2}$. From Eq. 7,

$$\frac{dy}{dt} = \frac{\partial y}{\partial u}\frac{du}{dt} + \frac{\partial y}{\partial v}\frac{dv}{dt} + \frac{\partial y}{\partial z}\frac{dz}{dt}$$

$$= (\ln v \, e^z)2t - (u \, e^z/v)t^{-2} + (u \ln v \, e^z)(3/2)t^{1/2}$$

$$= -21 \ln t \, e^{t^{3/2}} t - (t^2 - 2) \, e^{t^{3/2}} \, t^{-1}$$

$$- (t^2 - 2) \ln t \, e^{t^{3/2}}(3/2)t^{1/2}$$

Higher Order Partial Derivatives—The first partial derivatives of the function $y = f(x_1, x_2, \ldots, x_k)$ are themselves functions of the variables x_i. As such, they can be differentiated further, to yield higher partial derivatives, without regard to the identity of the variable of the first partial differentiation. Thus, the first partial derivatives $(\partial y/\partial x_1, \partial y/\partial x_2, \ldots, \partial y/\partial x_k)$ yield *second partial derivatives* $(\partial^2 y/\partial x_i \partial x_j$, where i may or may not equal j). Third and higher partial derivatives can be obtained also and are designated by the following notation:

$$\frac{\partial}{\partial x_i}\left(\frac{\partial y}{\partial x_j}\right) = \frac{\partial^2 y}{\partial x_i \partial x_j}$$

$$\frac{\partial}{\partial x_1}\left(\frac{\partial^2 y}{\partial x_i \partial x_j}\right) = \frac{\partial^3 y}{\partial x_1 \partial x_i \partial x_j} \text{ etc}$$

When the given function y and all the partial derivatives up to and including the nth are continuous, the order of differentiation is immaterial in computing the nth partial derivative.[1] This condition is satisfied in most cases encountered in pharmacy.

Example 16—Given the function $u = xy^3 + x^3 y$, calculate $\partial^4 u/\partial x^4$.

$$\partial u/\partial x = y^3 + 3x^2 y$$

$$\partial^2 u/\partial x^2 = 6xy$$

$$\partial^3 u/\partial x^3 = 6y$$

$$\partial^4 u/\partial x^4 = 0$$

Example 17—Given the function $u = x^2 y^2 z^2$, calculate $\partial^3 u/\partial z \partial y \partial x$, and $\partial^3 u/\partial x \partial y \partial z$ and verify their equality.

$$\frac{\partial u}{\partial z} = 2x^2 y^2 z, \quad \frac{\partial^2 u}{\partial y \partial z} = 4x^2 yz, \quad \frac{\partial^3 u}{\partial x \partial y \partial z} = 8xyz$$

$$\frac{\partial u}{\partial x} = 2xy^2 z^2, \quad \frac{\partial^2 u}{\partial y \partial x} = 4xyz^2, \quad \frac{\partial^3 u}{\partial z \partial y \partial x} = 8xyz$$

Exercises

22. Given $u = x^2 + y^2 + z^2$, show that

$$x \frac{\partial u}{\partial x} + y \frac{\partial u}{\partial y} + z \frac{\partial u}{\partial z} = 2u$$

23. Find $\partial u/\partial x$ and $\partial u/\partial y$ if $u = e^{x^2 y^2}$.
24. Calculate the value of $\partial A/\partial u$ when $u = 1$ and $v = 2$ for the function $A = (u^2 v + v^2 u)^2$.
25. Given $M = x^3 y^3$, calculate the numerical value of

$$xy\left(x \frac{\partial^3 M}{\partial x^2 \partial y} + y \frac{\partial^3 M}{\partial x \partial y^2}\right)/9M$$

26. Find the total differential of $u = e^{xyz}$.
27. Derive Eq. 7 from the definitions of the derivative and partial derivative, and independent of Eq. 6.
28. Find the total derivative of the function $u = \ln (xyz)$ if; $x = t$, $y = t^2$, $z = t^3$.
29. Find the total derivative of the function $u = xy^2 z^3$ if; $x = 1/t$, $y = e^t$, $z = \ln t$.
30. Determine the ratio $(\partial^2 u/\partial x^2)/(\partial^2 u/\partial y^2)$ in terms of x and y if $u = (xyz)^{1/2}$.
31. Find all the second partial derivatives of $u = xe^y$.

Indefinite Integration

The Indefinite Integral—The observation that the derivative $dy/dx = f'(x)$ of the function $y = f(x)$ can be found through the application of a formal set of procedures suggests that the inverse also may be true. This process, wherein a function is found when only its derivative is known, is called *integration*.

In particular, the function $f(x) + C$ is defined as the *indefinite integral* of $f'(x)$, where C is the *constant of integration* and where $f'(x)$ is the first derivative of $f(x)$. The term indefinite integral arises from the fact that unless certain information in addition to $f'(x)$ is given, the constant of integration may take on any value whatever.

The process of integration is denoted symbolically as follows:

$$y = \int dy = \int f'(x)dx = f(x) + C \quad (8)$$

The symbol $\int$ is called the integral sign and indicates that the function following it (the integrand) is to be integrated. The differential term to the right of the integrand determines the variable of integration. A useful check on the accuracy of any integration consists of taking the derivative of the integral. The result must equal the integrand.

Basic Rules for Integration—The rules which follow are the result of the definition of integration applied to the rules of differentiation listed in this chapter.

Rule 1

$$\int du = u + C$$

where u is any function and C is an arbitrary constant.
Rule 2

$$\int u^n du = u^{n+1}/(n+1) + C, \text{ if } n \neq -1$$

Rule 3

$$\int ku dx = k \int u dx$$

where u is a function of x and k is a constant.
Rule 4

$$\int (u + v)dx = \int u dx + \int v dx$$

where u and v are functions of x.
Rule 5

$$\int e^u du = e^u + C$$

Rule 6

$$\int du/u = \int d \ln u = \ln u + C$$

Methods of Integration—The method of *integration by parts* is derived directly from Rule 4 for the differentiation of the product of functions.

Given the functions $u(x)$ and $v(x)$, the derivative of the product $u \cdot v$ with respect to x is $d(uv)/dx = u(dv/dx) + v(du/dx)$. Multiplying by dx and rearranging,

$$udv = d(uv) - vdu$$

Integrating both sides,

$$\int udv = uv - \int vdu \qquad (9)$$

Eq. 9 defines the procedure used in this method of integration. It is applied when the integral resulting from the exchange of integrand and differential is easier to integrate than the original integral. That is, when $\int vdu$ is simpler than $\int udv$.

Example 18—Determine $\int xe^x dx$ by the method of parts. Let $x = u$ and $e^x dx = dv$, then it follows that $du = dx$ and $v = e^x$. By substitution into Eq. 9,

$$\int xe^x dx = xe^x - \int e^x dx = xe^x - e^x + C$$

Integrals which do not lend themselves to solution by simple rules or the method of parts can be evaluated frequently by a *change of variable* of integration. That is, a complex integral which is a function of x may be transformed into a simple function of u by the substitution of a suitable function $u(x)$ into the original integral. This method is explained easily by means of an example.

Example 19—Evaluate the integral $\int 2xe^{x^2} dx$. Let $u = x^2$ and substitute into the integral. Since $du = 2xdx$,

$$\int 2xe^{x^2} dx = \int e^u du = e^u + C = e^{x^2} + C$$

Example 20—Evaluate the integral, $\int xdx/(x^2 - 2)$. Let $u = x^2 - 2$, then $du = 2xdx$. Thus,

$$\frac{xdx}{(x^2 - 2)} = \frac{1}{2}\int du/u = \frac{1}{2}\int d \ln u$$

$$= \frac{1}{2} \ln u + C = \frac{1}{2} \ln (x^2 - 2) + C$$

An integral having an integrand in the form of a rational fraction, whose denominator can be factored, is often subject to simplification by *partial fractions*. In this method the original integrand is broken into a sum of fractions whose denominators are factors of the original denominator. Consider the following example.

Example 21—Evaluate the integral, $\int (x - 2)dx/(x^2 - 2x - 3)$. It is necessary to first write the integrand in the partial fractional form as follows:

$$\frac{x - 2}{x^2 - 2x - 3} - \frac{x - 2}{(x + 1)(x - 3)} = \frac{M}{(x + 1)} + \frac{N}{(x - 3)}$$

M and N are constants having values such that the equality is satisfied. Thus, $M(x - 3) + N(x + 1) = x - 2$, since the numerators resulting from the above equation must be equal. Equating coefficients of like powers of x, it may be seen that:

$$M + N = 1; \quad -3M + N = -2$$

Solving these equations simultaneously, M and N are found to equal $\frac{3}{4}$ and $\frac{1}{4}$, respectively. Substituting into the original integral,

$$\int \frac{(x - 2)dx}{x^2 - 2x - 3} = \int \left[\frac{M}{(x + 1)} - \frac{N}{(x - 3)} \right] dx$$

$$= \frac{3}{4} \int \frac{dx}{(x + 1)} + \frac{1}{4} \int \frac{dx}{(x - 3)}$$

$$= \frac{3}{4} \ln (x + 1) + \frac{1}{4} \ln (x - 3) + C$$

The methods of integration presented here represent but a few of those available. They will, however, be adequate for the solution of most of the problems encountered in undergraduate pharmacy.

As mentioned earlier, the constant of integration can be determined if certain information in addition to the integrand is provided. Such information is usually given in the form of *boundary conditions*, which have the effect of fixing the value of C.

Example 22—Determine the integral of $dy/dx = x^2 - x$, if it is known that $y = 0$, if and when $x = 1$. It is first necessary to find the indefinite integral.

$$y = \int (x^2 - x)dx = x^3/3 - x^2/2 + C$$

Applying the boundary conditions to the indefinite integral; when $y = 0$ and $x = 1$,

$$y = 0 = \frac{1}{3} - \frac{1}{2} + C, \therefore C = \frac{1}{6}$$

The desired integral is thus,

$$y = x^3/3 - x^2/2 + \frac{1}{6}$$

Exercises

32. Evaluate the following integrals:

   a. $\int d(x - e^x \ln x)$
   b. $\int (x^7 - x^{-3})^2 d(x^7 - x^{-3})$
   c. $\int 8x^3 dx$
   d. $\int (x^3 + 2x^2 - 7)dx$
   e. $\int 2e^x dx$
   f. $\int dx/(1 + x)$

33. Integrate the following:

   a. $dy/dx = (x - 3)(x + 5)$
   b. $du/dt = e^t - 1/t$

34. Find the following integrals by the method of parts:

   a. $\int x^2 e^x dx$ (*Hint:* apply the method twice in succession)
   b. $\int 7xe^{-2x} dx$
   c. $\int \ln x dx$

35. Evaluate the following integrals by change of variable:

   a. $\int x^2 (x^3 - 1)^{1/2} dx$
   b. $\int (x - 1)(x^2 - 2x)^{-1/2} dx$

36. Evaluate the following integral, $\int x(x^2 - 1)^{-1} dx$, by the method of partial fractions. Check the answer by the method of change of variable.

37. Write and integrate an equation which describes the rate of production of product in the following bimolecular reaction. The starting concentrations of A and B are unequal and that of C is zero.

$$A + B \rightarrow C$$

38. Find y in terms of x for the following.

   a. $dy/dx = e^x$ if $y = 0$ when $x = 0$.
   b. $dy/dx = x^3 + 5$, if $y = 20$ when $x = 2$.

Definite Integration

The Definite Integral—Integrals obtained by reversing the process of differentiation are indefinite to the extent that the values of the constants of integration are unknown. This indeterminacy can be removed either by the application of boundary conditions, as discussed previously, or by taking the difference between two values of the indefinite integral, thereby eliminating the constant of integration. The latter method gives rise directly to the *definite integral*. Consider the indefinite integral of the function $f'(x)$.

$$y = \int f'(x)dx = f(x) + C$$

Let x assume values a and b, and denote the corresponding values of y by y_a and y_b. It then follows that the difference, $y_b - y_a$, is given by

$$y_b - y_a = f(b) - f(a) = \int f'(x) - \int f'(x) \qquad (10)$$
$$\qquad\qquad\qquad\qquad (x = b) \quad (x = a)$$

The last term in Eq. 10 is an integral whose value is completely determined by the function $f(x)$ and by the numbers a and b. For this reason it is termed the definite integral and is denoted by the equation

$$\int_a^b f'(x)dx = \int f'(x)dx - \int f'(x)dx = f(b) - f(a) \qquad (11)$$
$$\qquad\qquad\qquad (x = b) \quad\quad (x = a)$$

This expression provides a link between the concept of the indefinite integral and that of the definite integral. The first term in Eq. 11 denotes the integral of the function $f'(x)$ from the *lower limit of integration, a*, to the *upper limit of integration, b*.

The Relationship of Integration to Summation—One of the most important concepts of integral calculus is that of the relationship of the definite integral to a sum. As will be shown later, this concept may be applied in understanding the calculation of the areas under irregular curves. In general terms, it may be used to compute the sum of the product of a function and infinitesimal increments of its independent variable over a given interval.

Let $f'(x)$ be any continuous and single-valued function in the interval from $x = a$ to $x = b$. Divide the interval $a \leqslant x \leqslant b$ into n segments of length Δx_i, and let x_i be the division point between segments i and $i + 1$. Define the limit L as follows:

$$L = \lim_{\substack{n \to \infty \\ \Delta x_i \to 0}} \sum_{i=1}^{n} f'(x_i)\,\Delta x_i \qquad (12)$$

The mean value theorem of derivatives states[2] that

$$f(q) - f(p) = f'(x_j)\cdot(q - p) \qquad (13)$$

where $f'(x)$ is the derivative of $f(x)$ and where x_j is a suitably chosen point interior to the interval $p \leqslant x \leqslant q$. It is important to point out that while the location of x_j, such that Eq. 13 holds true, will vary depending on $f(x)$ and on the interval $q - p$, x_j will always satisfy the condition $p \leqslant x_j \leqslant q$.

Let p and q represent the initial and final points of the segment Δx_i; that is, let $q - p = \Delta x_i$. Therefore, in the limit as $\Delta x_i \to 0$, $x_j \to x_i$. Eq. 13 thus may be combined with Eq. 12 in the form

$$L = \lim_{\substack{n \to \infty \\ \Delta x_i \to 0}} \sum_{i=1}^{n} f(x_i) - f(x_{i-1})$$

$$= \lim_{\substack{n \to \infty \\ \Delta x_i \to 0}} ([f(x_1) - f(x_0)] + [f(x_2) - f(x_1)] + \cdots$$

$$+ [f(x_n) - f(x_{n-1})])$$

All terms except $f(x_0)$ and $f(x_n)$ cancel in the above sum so that $L = f(x_n) - f(x_0)$. Since $x_0 = a$ and $x_n = b$, this may be written

$$L = f(b) - f(a) \qquad (14)$$

Combining Eqs. 11, 12, and 14, it may be shown that

$$\int_{a}^{b} f'(x)\,dx = \lim_{\substack{n \to \infty \\ \Delta x_i \to 0}} \sum_{i=1}^{n} f'(x_i)\,\Delta x_i \qquad (15)$$

Eq. 15 explicitly defines the relationship between summation and integration. Further, it shows that sums of the kind indicated can be evaluated as definite integrals; this is a distinct advantage in most instances.

Interpretation of the Definite Integral as a Sum—It is often necessary to calculate the area of a region bounded by an irregular line. Such a figure is exemplified by the surface in the xy plane bounded by the curve $y = f'(x)$, the x axis, and the lines $x = a$ and $x = b$. This region can be divided into n segments of width Δx_i and area approximated by $f'(x_i)\Delta x_i$, as shown in Fig. 99. When the areas of the n rectangles are summed, they approximate the area of the figure. An error arises due to the inclusion and/or exclusion of small regions (shown in Fig. 99 in solid black) in the sum. However, in taking the limit of the sum, as the number of rectangles approaches infinity and as their

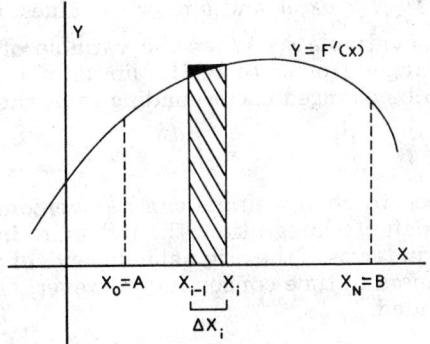

Fig. 99. A plot of the calculation of the area of a region bounded by an irregular line.

width approaches zero, the error vanishes. The area of the figure is thus,

$$\text{Area} = \lim_{\substack{n \to \infty \\ \Delta x_i \to 0}} \sum_{i=1}^{n} f'(x_i)\,\Delta x_i = \int_{a}^{b} f'(x)\,dx$$

It can be seen from this expression that the computation of the given area involves only the evaluation of the definite integral of $f'(x)$ between the limits a and b.

In general terms,* whenever a sum (in the form of the last term of Eq. 15) is encountered, it can be evaluated as a definite integral.

Calculation of Definite Integrals—The following rules regarding the algebra of definite integrals may be deduced directly from either Eq. 11 or Eq. 15 by inspection.

Rule 1

$$\int_{a}^{c} g(x)\,dx = \int_{a}^{b} g(x)\,dx + \int_{b}^{c} g(x)\,dx$$

where a, b, and c are points along the x axis.

Rule 2

$$\int_{a}^{b} kg(x)\,dx = k \int_{a}^{b} g(x)\,dx$$

where k is a constant.

Rule 3

$$\int_{a}^{b} (g(x) + h(x))\,dx = \int_{a}^{b} g(x)\,dx + \int_{a}^{b} h(x)\,dx$$

The general method of evaluation of definite integrals follows from their definition as expressed in Eq 11,

$$\int_{a}^{b} f'(x)\,dx = f(b) - f(a)$$

where $f(x) + C$ is the indefinite integral of $f'(x)$. The problem may be resolved into two stages: (1) finding the indefinite integral of the given integrand and (2) computing the difference in value of the indefinite integral between its upper and lower limits of integration.

A number of methods for accomplishing Step 1 have been presented and discussed. Only one of these, the method of change of variable, need be developed further here. Consider a function $f'(x)$ which is to be integrated following a change in variable such that

$$f'(x) = g'(u)$$

where $u = t(x)$. It should be noted that, in the ex-

---

* Subject to certain limitations not discussed here.

pression $\int_a^b f'(x)dx$, a and b refer to values of the independent variable x. When the variable of integration is changed from x to u, the limits of integration must also be changed corresponding to u, thus

$$\int_a^b f'(x)dx = \int_{t(a)}^{t(b)} g'(u)du$$

The need to change limits can be overcome if, following indefinite integration, the indefinite integral is rewritten in terms of the original independent variable. This is generally time consuming, however, and is not recommended.

Example 23—Rewrite the integral $y = \int_1^2 x(x^2 + 5)^3dx$ with the change of variable $u = x^2 + 5$. Since $du = 2xdx$, $u = 6$ when $x = 1$, and $u = 9$ when $x = 2$, the integral may be transformed as follows:

$$y = \frac{1}{2}\int_1^2 (x^2 + 5)^3 2xdx = \frac{1}{2}\int_6^9 u^3du$$

Step 2 in the evaluation of the definite integral consists of determining the difference $f(b) - f(a)$ in Eq. 11. For convenience of notation, $f(b) - f(a)$ is written $f(x)\big|_a^b$.

Example 24—Complete the evaluation of the integral presented in Example 23.

$$\frac{1}{2}\int_6^9 u^3du = \frac{1}{8}u^4\big|_6^9 = (9^4 - 6^4)/8 = \frac{5265}{8}$$

Example 25—Evaluate the integral, $\int_1^e \ln x\, dx$, by the method of parts. The indefinite integral must be found first. Let $u = \ln x$ and $dv = dx$; then $du = dx/x$ and $v = x$.

$$\int\ln x\, dx = x\ln x - \int dx = x\ln x - x + C$$

$$\int_1^e \ln x\, dx = x\ln x - x\big|_1^e = (e - e) - (0 - 1) = 1$$

Exercises

39. Calculate the area bounded by the curve $y = x^2$, the y axis, and the line $y = 4$, and which lies in the first quadrant.

40. Calculate the value of the following integrals.

a. $\int_1^{10} (1 + \ln x)dx$

b. $\int_1^3 (x^3 - 1)dx$

c. $\int_0^1 xe^{x^2}dx$

d. $\int_1^3 (5 - 3y^2)dy$

41. Calculate a numerical value for t given

$$\int_0^t ydy = 4\int_0^{\ln 3} e^xdx$$

42. Calculate the value of g if

$$2.303\int_{-\infty}^0 e^zdz = \int_g^5 (6 - x)^{-1}dx$$

43. Show that

$$\int_1^5 d\ln a \neq \int_1^5 da/a$$

Answers to Exercises

1. $-2, 1 - 3a^2, -3b^2 + 6b - 2$
2. $x^2 - 1/x^2$
4. 0.39
5. $0, \frac{3}{2}, \frac{1}{8}, -3$
6. $\Delta y/\Delta x = -1/(x^2 + x\Delta x), -1$
7. $6x^2, (1 - t)^{-2}, 5n^4$
8. $0, 6, 54, 6a^2$
10. $d(\text{drug})/dt = -(\text{drug})/1000$
16. $3x^2 - 3 - x^{-2}$,
   $$\frac{(1 + x^2)/2x^{1/2} - 2x^{3/2}}{(1 + x^2)^2},$$
   $2xe^{x^2}$,
   $2x/(1 + x^2)$
17. $dy/dx = e^z(-2x) = -2xe^{1 - x^2}$
18. $(\frac{5}{2})(e^{3t} - 3\ln t)^{3/2}(3e^{3t} - 3t^{-1})$
19. $x^4 + x^2 + 1, 4x^3 + 2x, 12x^2 + 2, 24x, 24, 0\ldots0$
20. $t = 5^{1/2}$ hr
21. $666\frac{2}{3}$ cu ft
23. $2xy^2e^{x^2y^2}, 2x^2ye^{x^2y^2}$
24. 96
25. 4
26. $du = yze^{xyz}dx + xze^{xyz}dy + xye^{xyz}dz$
28. $6/t$
29. $-t^{-2}e^{2t}\ln^3 t + 2t^{-1}e^t\ln^3 t + 3t^{-2}e^{2t}\ln^2 t$
30. y^2/x^2
31. $\partial^2u/\partial x^2 = 0, \partial^2u/\partial y^2 = xe^y, \partial^2u/\partial x\partial y = \partial^2u/\partial y\partial x = e^y$
32. $x - e^x\ln x + C, (x^7 - x^{-3})^3/3 + C, 2x^4 + C, x^4/4 + 2x^3/3 - 7x + C, 2e^x + C, \ln(1 + x) + C$
33. $y = x^3/3 + x^2 - 15x + C, u = e^t - \ln t + C$
34. $x^2e^x - 2xe^x + 2e^x + C, -xe^{-2x}/2 - e^{-2x}/4 + C, x\ln x - x + C$
35. $2(x^3 - 1)^{3/2}/9 + C, (x^2 - 2x)^{1/2}/4 + C$
38. $y = e^x - 1, y = x^4/4 + 5x + 6$
39. $16/3$
40. $23.03, 18, (e - 1)/2, -16$
41. ± 4
42. -4

References

1. Sokolnikoff, I. S., *Advanced Calculus*, McGraw-Hill, New York, 1939, pp. 87–89.
2. Smail, L. L., *Calculus*, Appleton-Century-Crofts, New York, 1949, p. 98.

14 | Matter—Its States and Selected Properties

States and selected properties of matter—distillation—sublimation

This chapter was prepared by

Lloyd Kennon, PhD, *Vice President—Director of Research and Development, Menley and James Laboratories, Philadelphia, Pa. 19101*

The aim of this chapter is to discuss both generalities and specifics, most of which are not explicitly related to dosage forms because the latter will be discussed in other chapters. Some of the principles should be useful to have in mind when dosage forms and their manufacture and processing are studied by the product development pharmacist. It should be noted that due to the range of subjects covered by the chapter title it was necessary to take an eclectic approach in developing mostly qualitative discussions. The goal has been not to produce a difficult in-depth chapter but rather one which presents an overview of the significant states and properties of matter.

Normally, matter exists in one of three states: solid, liquid, or gas, Although it is not pharmaceutically important, two other states of matter exist: one is the plasma state in which matter exists as a hot gaseous cloud of atoms and electrons; the other, a more speculative state which may have only a momentary existence, is one having characteristics of a superdense supermetal. This transient state is produced when material is subjected to very high pressures such as those used to make diamonds by compressing graphite.

To avoid the pitfalls of semantics, there is no need to call attention to other systems of classification, because for all practical purposes it is convenient to think only of the most obvious three states. These states are actually a continuum with two common factors determining the position on the "scale of states."

The first factor is the intensity of intermolecular forces of all kinds: solids have the strongest forces; gases, the weakest. The other common factor is temperature. Obviously, as the temperature of substances is raised, they tend to pass from solid to liquid to gas. When the phrase "as temperature is increased" is used it should be remembered that this is a relative phrase. Even at what is called room temperature, some of the effects of a temperature increase are present because room temperature is far above absolute zero.

As a point of historical interest, note that Lavoisier, the late, great "father of modern chemistry" thought of heat as a type of matter and held already in the 18th century that the three states of aggregation differ only with respect to how much heat they "contain." Although not all are satisfied with this phraseology, the term *enthalpy* (or *heat content*) is still used in thermodynamics.

Thinking further back to the ancient Greek philosophers and their original four elements (earth, air, fire, and water) note again the great significance attached to heat. Although their concepts of the nature of matter were not exactly right, they recognized heat as an integral part of the scheme of things; nothing could be truer. Heat, a vital form of energy, the mirror of molecular motion, is *the* form of energy of greatest importance to mankind.

As alluded to above, there is no clear line of demarcation between the states and selected properties of matter, but the following arbitrary division may make the approach this chapter takes more coherent.

States of Matter

Changes of State

As a solid becomes a liquid and then a gas, heat is absorbed and the enthalpy or heat content increases as the material passes through these phase changes. Thus, the enthalpy of a liquid is greater than that of its solid, and the enthalpy of a gas is greater than that of its liquid, because heat is absorbed when melting and vaporization occur. The *entropy* (a measure of the degree of total molecular randomness) also increases as materials go from solid to liquid to gas.

It is the balance of enthalpy, entropy, and temperature which determines if changes proceed spontaneously or not. Obviously, if systems tend to settle to states of lowest energy, it means that enthalpy and entropy considerations may counteract each other. Much of thermodynamics is concerned with explaining and quantitating the changes which systems undergo.

Latent heat is heat absorbed when a change of state takes place without a temperature change, as when ice turns to water at 0°C. This example is one in which the heat required to produce the change of state is designated the *heat of fusion*. The counterpart, the *heat of vaporization*, is used when a change of state from liquid to gas is involved.

As molecules of a liquid in a closed evacuated container continually leave the surface and go into the free space above it, some molecules return to the surface, depending on their concentration in the vapor. Ultimately, a condition of equilibrium is established, and the rate of escape equals the rate of return. The vapor is then saturated and the pressure is known as the vapor pressure.

Vapor pressure depends on the temperature, but not on the amounts of liquid and vapor as long as equilibrium is established and both liquid and vapor are present. Heat is absorbed in the vaporization process and, therefore, the vapor pressure increases with temperature. As the temperature is raised further, the density of the vapor increases, and that of the liquid decreases. Ultimately, the densities equal each other and liquid and vapor cannot be distinguished. The temperature at which this happens is

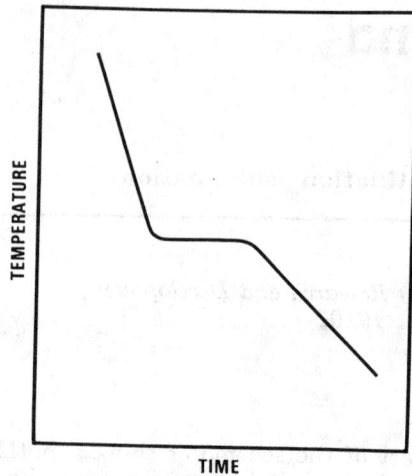

Fig. 100.   A single change of state as shown by a slowing of the cooling rate.

called the critical temperature, and above it there can be no liquid phase.

Solids also have vapor pressures which depend on temperature. When a solid is converted directly into gas, it is said to sublime. Sublimation pressures of solids are much lower than those of liquids at any given temperature. When a solid is transformed directly into a liquid, two types of melting may be distinguished. The first is the crystalline type in which a rigid solid becomes a liquid during which procedure two phases are present; the bulk of the solid or its inner parts are not really changing. The second type is amorphous melting. This involves an intermediate plastic-like condition which envelops the whole mass; the viscosity decreases and a state of liquidity follows. Crystalline melting involves more definite melting points and latent heats than does amorphous melting.

Critical Point

The critical point, by way of a general definition, is expressed as a certain value of temperature or pressure (or molar volume) above which or below which certain physical changes will not take place or certain states of being will not exist. At these points, some properties are constant and are referred to as the critical temperature, pressure, or volume. At the usual critical point, the properties of liquid and gas are identical and the phase diagram curve of P vs T ends. (Phase diagrams will be discussed later.) When a liquid changes to a vapor, increased disorder or randomness and, therefore, increased entropy results. At the critical temperature, the entropy of vaporization is zero as is the enthalpy of vaporization since the gas and liquid are indistinguishable.

Although the gas–liquid critical point is the one most discussed, there are others. Each critical point marks the disappearance of a state. Note that most liquids behave similarly not only at their critical temperatures but also at equal fractions of their critical temperatures. For example, the normal boiling points of many liquids are approximately equal fractions (about 60%) of their critical temperatures (in absolute temperature degrees).

Visualization of Changes of State

This section is to serve as an introduction to the following one entitled *Eutectics*.

When a pure substance cools and is transformed from a liquid to a solid, a graph (Fig. 100) of its (decreasing) temperature vs time is continuous. At the temperature at which solid crystallizes out (that is, the melting point) the cooling curve becomes horizontal. The same is true at the boiling point, the temperature of a liquid at which the continuing application of heat no longer raises the temperature, but rather converts the liquid into vapor; it is the point where the vapor pressure of the liquid (or the sum of its components) equals that of the atmosphere above the liquid.

Increasing the pressure above the liquid or adding solutes, raises the boiling point and *vice versa*. These plateaus observed at certain specific temperatures are due to the release of the heats of fusion or vaporization. Similarly when solutions are cooled, the slope of the cooling curve (Fig. 101) changes when one of the components starts to crystallize out. Although a very horizontal plateau may not be formed as in the case of pure materials, the change in slope indicates precipitation of one of the components. If the same plateaus are formed when binary solutions of varied composition are cooled, it indicates that both components of the binary solution are coming out together. The temperature at which this occurs is the eutectic temperature, and the composition is generally called a eutectic.

Normally, cooling curves *per se* are converted to phase diagrams to facilitate visualization of the interrelationships as phase changes take place. If instead of a minimum point or eutectic, a maximum point is observed, it may indicate that the components are reacting to form a solid compound which can exist in equilibrium with the melt over a range of compositions.

It is undoubtedly true that many unknown phase equilibria exist. Thus when conditions are changed, as for example when a process is scaled up in a manufacturing process, different phase changes may take place and produce different final products. The pharmaceutical use of heterogeneous materials such as waxes and fats certainly provides ample opportunity for these changes to take place.

Distillation phenomena also can be represented in phase diagram form; these are discussed in the section on *Distillation*.

Eutectics

Although many very complex and complicated diagrams, including some three-dimensional models, are needed to characterize certain systems (see Chapter 19, *Solutions and Phase Equilibria*), most interesting to pharmacy are the diagrams (Fig. 102) indicating eutectic formation. This section will only briefly describe this area of technology.

Phase diagrams are constructed by determining the melting points and cooling rates of a series of binary liquid solutions of compositions varying from all A to all B; this will be illustrated shortly—consider first the Fig. 102 phase diagram *per se*. The points where the V-shaped boundary of the melt hit the right and left vertical axes are the melting points of the pure materials. To the left of the base of the V (ie, when solutions rich in A are cooled) solid A separates as the temperature falls; to the right, Solid B separates as shown. Thus, the left arm of the V is the curve which represents the temperature conditions under which various liquid mixtures are in equilibrium with Solid A, and the right arm of the V is that curve which

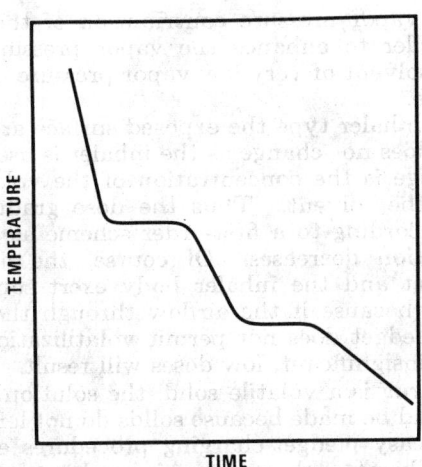

Fig. 101. Two changes of state with resulting temporary decreases in cooling rate.

shows which mixtures are in equilibrium with Solid B.

At the point of the V both Solid A and Solid B are in equilibrium with the liquid; this point, the lowest temperature at which any of the infinite possible combinations of liquid solutions of A and B will freeze (or the lowest melting point of any possible mixture of Solids A and B) is called the eutectic point. Only at this point is the composition of the solid the same as that of the solution from which it is separating; this does *not* necessarily mean that the composition of the eutectic is a chemical compound of A and B. Thus, at the eutectic point, both A and B come out together in a constant proportion.

The eutectic composition is, however, a simple two-phase mixture, but when made *in situ* it has a very fine-grained structure which could impart to it different properties (eg, solubility or gastrointestinal absorption rate) as compared to a gross mixture of the same composition. The structure is very-fine-grained because the crystallization was very intimate since crystals of both phases were formed simultaneously. This is quite a different situation than one in which only one component is separating. It is important to remember that one can be only at one place on a phase diagram at any one time; ie, the diagram describes what a *particular* system is like at a certain temperature, which components are in the liquid and/or solid state, and the proportions of each.

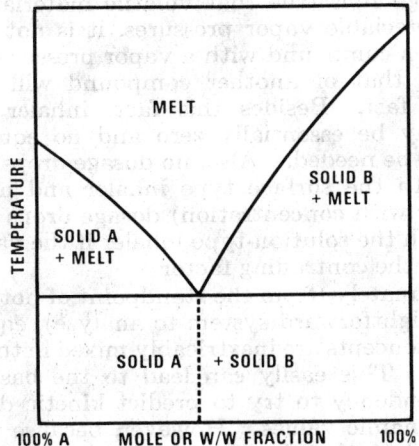

Fig. 102. Simple phase diagram of system showing eutectic point; see text for details.

As mentioned above, the diagrams are constructed from information obtained on the cooling rates of binary solutions. Consider again a cooling curve analysis in which temperature vs time are plotted. The curves change slope to form plateaus when any solid phase separates out; the plateaus tend to become more horizontal as absolute temperatures are lower because the intensity of radiation and conduction are lessened. A final plateau results, of course, when the whole liquid mass (or the last of it) solidifies. Thus, if a molten liquid having a composition lying *between*, eg, pure A and the eutectic were cooled, the following would be observed in a plot of temperature vs time (Fig. 101): first T drops with time; then Solid A will come out of solution, release its heat of fusion, and thus slow the cooling rate to produce the first (upper) plateau; the temperature then starts to drop more sharply again as enough A comes out of solution, and the system changes composition until it contains only the eutectic composition; when the eutectic composition is reached, the second solid (B) also coprecipitates, and the temperature remains constant (lower plateau) until all of the A and B have solidified after which, of course, the temperature will be able to drop further. If the system being

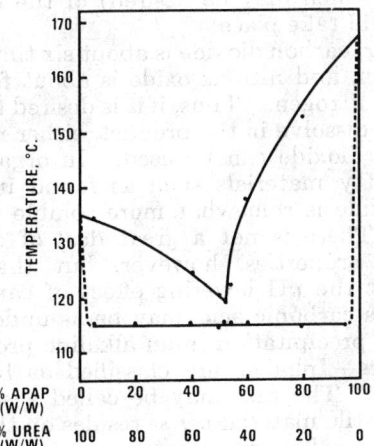

Fig. 103. Phase diagram of the urea:acetaminophen (46%:54%) eutectic melting in the 110°–115°C range (courtesy, Goldberg, et al[2]).

cooled started as the eutectic composition, only the lower break and plateau would be observed; ie, a pure material and a eutectic would have similarly shaped cooling diagrams. This should be clear from the discussion. Note then that a phase diagram can be constructed by studying a number of cooling curves made on a series of mixtures of known composition. To do this, the temperatures at which cooling rate changes are noted are plotted against each particular composition studied. Note that Fig. 102 is idealized in that no solid–solid solution of A and B is formed. If the two components are somewhat soluble in each other, the diagram would differ by having two thin solution areas along the left and right axes; such are partly in evidence in Fig. 103.

Two pharmaceutical examples of eutectic formation are these. The first concerns a mixture of two common antipyretic–analgesic compounds: aspirin and acetaminophen. There has always been some "magic" associated with eutectic formation and, indeed, since such a binary composition does melt at a lower temperature than other combinations, the eutectic probably does have weaker bonding forces if any, and, being very fine grained also, it is more rapidly soluble.

It is known that many drug compounds form eutectics and the aspirin–acetaminophen eutectic (37% APAP by weight) does dissolve more quickly than a simple mixture of the two of the same composition. Since a formed eutectic is created under equilibrium conditions of intimate mixing as noted, the contact of the two compounds is much closer than that achievable by simply mixing the dry powders. The increase in dissolution rate obtained by using the eutectic may result in a greater speed of physiological absorption.

The second example is illustrated in Fig. 103. It was found that urea and acetaminophen formed a eutectic containing approximately 46% urea and 54% APAP (by weight) which melted in the 110°–115°C range.

Gases

Aerosols—Gases *per se* are used directly in dosage forms in the field of aerosols. Although this subject, including the use of the so-called liquefied propellants, is covered elsewhere, note that pressure packs often use nitrogen, nitrous oxide, and carbon dioxide to expel the contents from their containers. The latter two gases are much more soluble in water so that some aeration (which may be desired) of the material discharged will take place.

In water, carbon dioxide is about six times as soluble as nitrogen, and nitrous oxide is about four times as soluble as nitrogen. Thus, if it is desired to have some of the gas dissolve in the product, either nitrous oxide or carbon dioxide can be used. In organic solvents and in fatty materials such as found in emulsions, nitrous oxide is somewhat more soluble than carbon dioxide. There is not a great deal of difference in solubility properties, however, but the possibility exists that the pH lowering effect of carbon dioxide as it forms carbonic acid may be as undesirable as a carbonate precipitation in an alkaline product.

Inhalers—Inhalers are classified as being one of two types. The first may be called a *surface* type; ie, the volatile material *per se* resides on the surface of the pledget. This represents a conventional adsorption situation; it is easy to appreciate the fact that the more surface area the pledget has the greater the surface area of the material exposed to the airflow and the greater the opportunity for volatilization. Hence, a larger or more loosely packed pledget will cause a larger dose to emanate from an inhaler than a smaller or tightly packed pledget.

It is convenient to make this type of inhaler if the volatile material itself is a liquid. The doses produced stay relatively high because the pledget charge is being depleted according to a zero-order scheme (see Chapter 21, *Reaction Kinetics*). This is reasonable because the volatile material has formed a multi-molecular (as distinguished from a monomolecular) layer on the pledget surfaces; thus, even though molecules are stripped off, the surface area and hence the dose remain essentially unchanged. However, as some areas of the pledget are denuded, the total exposed surface area of the volatile material decreases, and so does the dose.

The second inhaler type may be termed a *solution* type; ie, the volatile material is dissolved in a suitable nonvolatile solvent, and this solution is placed on the pledget. The situation may be taken as an example of the operation of Raoult's and Henry's laws, ie, the vapor pressure of the components are proportional in some way to their concentrations. To keep the vapor pressure contribution of the solvent low in order to enhance the vapor pressure of the solute, a solvent of very low vapor pressure is used as the vehicle.

In this inhaler type the exposed surface area of the material does not change as the inhaler is used; what does change is the concentration of the volatile material in the solvent. Thus the dose gradually decreases according to a first-order scheme as the drug concentration decreases. Of course, the nature of the pledget and the inhaler body exert some effect here also, because if the airflow through the inhaler and the pledget does not permit volatilization of the material, insignificant, low doses will result.

If the drug is a volatile solid, the solution type inhaler should be made because solids do not lend themselves to easy pledget-charging procedures even if a volatile solvent such as ether is used to deliver the material to the pledget during manufacturing.

Further amplification and clarification of the surface- and solution-type classification of inhalers might be achieved by considering the existing analogy to chromatographic systems. The surface-type inhaler corresponds to adsorption chromatography with the material being initially adsorbed on a carrier and then desorbed by a passing stream of liquid or gas. The solution-type inhaler corresponds to partition chromatography in which material in a solvent is supported by some medium, partitioned between its original solvent and a passing stream of gas or liquid, and thus removed.

Another point of significance concerns the relationship of the volatile active ingredient to the solvent. An increase in dose should result when the active ingredient is dissolved in solvents which cause it to deviate more positively from Raoult's law. Thus, the less the solute–solvent interaction and the greater the solute–solute interaction, the more pronounced will be the tendency toward volatilization of the solute. Using relative solubility as a gauge of such interaction, one would expect greater doses of a volatile solid from, eg, dibutyl phthalate (if it were less soluble in it) than from benzyl salicylate (if it were more soluble in it) at the same concentrations.

Although it might seem that the vapor pressure of the drug and additives would assume a position of primary importance, this does not appear to be the case. Vapor pressure values represent an equilibrium situation, whereas what is involved in the inhaler cases is a process controlled by factors affecting rates of volatilization.

Although it is true that volatile materials usually have appreciable vapor pressures, it is not generally true that a compound with a vapor pressure value of, eg, twice that of another compound will volatilize twice as fast. Besides this fact, inhaler recovery times may be essentially zero and no equilibration time may be needed. Also, no dosage drops would be noted with the surface type inhaler and no regular (ie, linear with concentration) dosage drops would be noted with the solution-type inhaler if the vapor pressure were the controlling factor.

Unfortunately (from the standpoint of not having a more straightforward system to analyze), equilibrium and rate concepts are inextricably mixed in the present situation. This easily can lead to the basically incorrect tendency to try to predict kinetic data from thermodynamic values. However, because vaporization is relatively unencumbered with entropy and orientation factors, rates of volatilization are often qualitatively proportional to the equilibrium properties of the materials involved.

Equimolar quantities of the following compounds, allowed to evaporate at room temperature under the same conditions, will complete the evaporation process in this order: ether, acetone, chloroform, carbon tetrachloride, ethyl acetate, water. This order corresponds both to the materials' vapor pressures and boiling points.

To further becloud the cause-and-effect relationship, the very magnitude of the numbers (the concentrations in mole fractions) is such that the partial vapor pressure of a volatile solid may increase proportionately with the mole fraction. Hence, although vapor pressure concepts should not be neglected in inhaler development, it is the rates of volatilization which must be controlled or modified. For more information and experimental data on inhalers see Kennon and Gulesich.[1]

Relative Humidity—In the production of effervescent products, one of the most vital factors to be considered is the use of controlled humidity conditions. It is well known that the effective control of humidity is closely related to the success or failure of attempts to produce effervescent products.

It is useful to bring to light some of the facets of this area of technology. Two factors predominate when one views the situation: the effective concentration of water in the air and temperature. In chemical reactions, particularly the kind involved here, the effect of temperature on an equilibrium condition is not very significant when compared to the influence manifested by concentration. Certainly, water of hydration, crystallization, or simple adsorption (which is tenacious at room temperature) does not disappear at temperatures under 100°F. What *is* effective and influential, however, in keeping and increasing such additional moisture on solids is the *concentration* of water in the air.

The concept proposed here is that considerations based purely on relative humidity will probably be unfruitful. For purposes of illustration, note Table I; it shows the amounts of water which are found under conditions encountered during the development of effervescent products.

The following points may be drawn from this information. A 10% relative humidity (RH) at 36°C is equivalent to 25% RH at room temperature. Either of these conditions represents a fairly dry day, but certainly not a very dry day. Therefore, although heating air surely lowers its RH, it probably does not lower the ability of the water in the air to cause trouble. Regardless of the temperature of processing rooms, experience has shown that water concentrations represented by the 72°F, 10–15% RH should not be exceeded if minimum difficulties are desired.

Liquids

The liquid state may be considered an intermediate one entered into as matter goes from solid to gas. Liquids have neither the strong cohesive forces of solids nor the weak ones of gases; hence, they are also intermediate in that they have neither the orderliness of a crystal nor the randomness of a gas. One might then consider a liquid a highly compressed gas or slightly released solid.

Due to the concept of molecular motion, there must be some free space in liquids. Also, if the motion is completely random, some spaces may be larger than others at a particular point in time. Thus, liquids may have holes, and this concept has explained phenomena such as the expansion of volume that materials undergo upon fusion (holes are created), diffusion in liquids, viscosity (movement of holes in the opposite direction of the viscous flow), and density decreases as temperature rises (the solubility of holes increases). It might be said that liquids are solutions of holes in material, whereas gases are solutions of matter in free space.

With respect to fluid mechanics, a fluid can be considered a material which cannot sustain shear forces when in static equilibrium; this is the distinguishing factor separating solids and fluids, the latter of which may be gases or liquids. This movement under the slightest stress is sometimes called "no sideways friction." It can be seen in operation in the case where a sailor standing watch near the gangplank of a docked ship can step on a mooring rope and cause the ship to move toward the dock.

Liquids, just as gases, take the shape of their container, but only the lower part of it as the liquid occupies a definite volume; gases expand to fill their entire container. Intermolecular spaces are greater in a gas than in a liquid so that they can be compressed. Relative to gases, both liquids and solids are quite incompressible. They can be considered already compressed due to the stronger intermolecular forces.

After a fluid is set in motion, it comes to rest because of the internal friction caused by the molecules sliding

Table I—Moisture Content (Gm/m³) Existing at the Conditions Noted

Temperature	Relative humidity (%)			
	10	15	25	40
RT (22°C or 72°F)	1.9	2.9	4.8	7.7
Hot (36°C or 97°F)	4.1	6.2	10.3	16.5

over each other; this resistance to flow is called viscosity and, as is well known, can be quantified. To effect good quantification with viscometers, normal, smooth (laminar or layer) flow is needed. With excessive stirring, at a so-called critical velocity, the fluid becomes turbulent, and instrumental measurements are difficult to effect. As the temperature of fluids increases, viscosity decreases. In general, also, as pressure increases, viscosity increases.

Because fluids have some structure, they may change upon standing so that when one is considering viscous behavior, the recent past history of the sample may have great effects. Thixotropy is the term used for liquids which flow freely if recently stirred, but gel on standing. Solids also flow but more slowly even under minor stresses, including those produced by their own weight. The wavy, bumpy surface of tarred roads, particularly seen on hills, is a result of a flow phenomenon.

Of interest also is the cluster theory of liquids, the main concept being that localized order exists but does not extend to a great distance. One property explained by this visualization is that as the temperature rises, the clusters disintegrate and viscosity decreases; another is that transmitting momentum through a liquid is not due only to molecular movements, but due to the transmissions of elastic waves through the groups of semistationary clusters. It is possible that the cluster theory affords another way of looking at pharmaceutical complexes in solution.

Complexes

As mentioned above, in addition to structure in solvents it is also possible for solutes to create a structure of a sort within the solvent. Thus, it has been shown that benzocaine in water solution with caffeine exhibits a much reduced rate of hydrolysis. In a somewhat similar vein it also has been noted that different salts of the same compound (eg, hydrochloride vs nitrate) may exhibit different stability characteristics. Similarly, it has been shown that saccharin in certain chlorpromazine hydrochloride solutions enhances the light stability of the drug. It appears that such changes are due to the fact that the ionic environment may form a protective molecular "overcoat" or loose ionic atmosphere complex around the drug.

Liquid Crystals

Lipids, when heated, usually do not pass directly from a crystalline to an isotropic structure, but rather they assume intermediate liquid crystal phases. Most interesting pharmaceutically and physiologically is that these structures are, undoubtedly, intimately in-

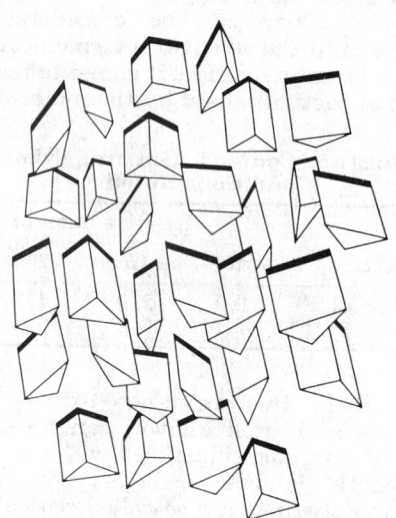

Fig. 104. The nematic phase of a liquid crystal; see text for details (based on Fergason and Brown[3]).

volved in the structure and, hence, the function of membranes and cells.

All biological systems are basically aqueous, and it is particularly in such systems that lyotropic mesomorphism (the formation of liquid crystal phases in the presence of water) takes place. In other words, the lipid phases undergo transformations involving crystal, liquid crystal, and liquid forms, and it is these changes which are mediators of the various physiological absorption, transport, storage, and excretory functions of cells. Many *in vitro* studies of biologically significant lipids have been carried out in attempts to elucidate the mechanisms of their interaction and behavioral properties in aqueous systems.

Liquid crystals differ from solids and gases in that they have some freedom to move and to take on many different shapes while yet maintaining a high degree of order through quite long distances, relatively speaking. In the laboratory, liquid crystals can be prepared from one component by heat treatments (thermotropic systems) or from one or more components by adding controlled amounts of water or

other polar solvents (lyotropic mesomorphism). Note that the only molecules of significance here are asymmetric and have a definite long direction so that their orientation "3-D wise" is essential. This should be remembered throughout the discussion.

For present purposes three types of liquid crystal phases will be described briefly so that at least some appreciation for this particular state of matter may be gained. The phases are generally characterized as being nematic, smectic, or cholesteric.

Nematic molecules (Fig. 104) are set in parallel arrangements and have restricted rotation about at least one axis. The molecules are parallel or nearly so. One might picture this as a long box filled with pencils with the latter being able to roll. Over-all, the system might be considered to be thread or cablelike. Another picture would be that of a group of logs going through a pipe. There is overlap of the pencils or logs somewhat as the cars in an auto race.

The smectic or "two dimensional" crystal (Fig. 105) has its molecules arranged in layers with their long axes essentially normal (ie, at right angles) to the plane of the layers. Their centers of gravity are then mobile in two directions in their plane, and the molecules can rotate about one axis. Over all, one

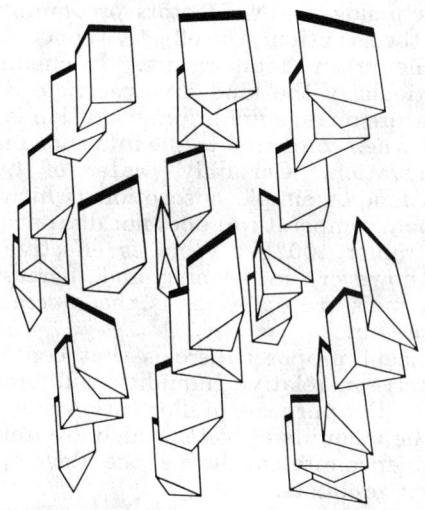

Fig. 105. The smectic liquid crystal phase (based on Fergason and Brown[3]).

could consider the arrangement layerlike with the degree of order just described in each layer.

The smectic arrangement is similar to the nematic in that there is still essentially only one axis of rotation, except in this case there is no overlap. The logs go through the pipe as a member of a group; that is, it would be like a *series* of drag races in which no one wins and all are tied. Each successive group, however, does not follow the same paths as the others; that is, within any one group there may be equal spacings sideways between the long axes or there may not be. Note also that the thickness of the layers is about the same as the length of the molecules.

The cholesteric arrangement (Fig. 106) is to some extent a combination of the nematic and smectic wherein the layers are nematic but, in addition, certain layering formations which resemble the smectic phase are incorporated. In essence, the result is a helical, twisting repetition of the nematic phase which, corkscrewlike, slowly changes head direction (for example, the lead end of the pencil) as one proceeds to examine underlying layers of molecules. The cholesteric arrangement is, *in toto*, much thicker than a smectic layer.

All three structures, as alluded to, are involved in building cells, and each type can (when viewed totally) form curved surfaces, membranes, or any other required micellelike shapes. Some workers constructed cell models utilizing these structures and showed how the mechanics of many cellular functions can be visualized using the known properties of liquid crystals.

The Glassy State

Although glass is usually thought of as a specific, nonconducting, transparent solid, it actually is a *type* of solid matter. It can be considered neither a typical solid nor liquid. The atoms of most solid states are generally structurally strictly ordered, whereas glassy materials are highly disordered. Glasses may, however, have some short-range order just as polymers do. Another characteristic of glasses is that they do not have specific melting points but slowly and gradually become liquids when they are heated. Sometimes glasses are considered supercooled liquids, but this is not strictly accurate.

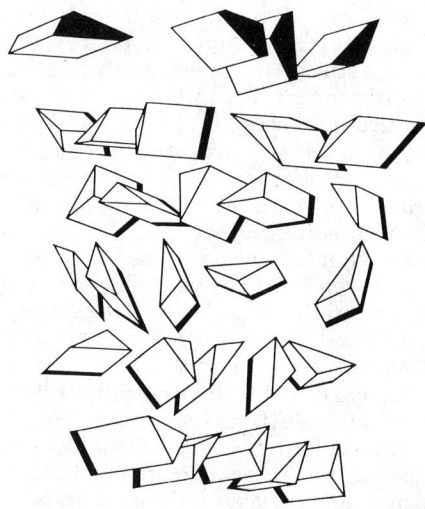

Fig. 106. A 180° turn of the molecules in the cholesteric liquid crystal phase (based on Fergason and Brown[3]).

A graph of volume vs temperature for most substances shows that the volume of a liquid decreases as the crystallization temperature is approached. If solidification is accomplished by crystallization, the volume decreases sharply at the freezing point, after which it continues to decrease gradually depending on its coefficient of thermal expansion. This type of behavior is not exhibited when solidification is followed by glass formation. The uniqueness of the glassy state is evident in its cooling curve. As indicated in Fig. 107, as a glass former is cooled, it does not suddenly undergo a large drop in volume (or density or index of refraction) at any particular temperature or as it passes through the melting point, nor does its volume decrease as rapidly as that of a supercooled liquid although it follows the curve of the latter initially during cooling. With supercooled liquids, the cooling curve is a simple continuation of the liquid curve itself, with no melting or transition points. Atomically, the structure of the glassy state is marked by a random selection of polyhedral molecules considered to be linked together at their corners.

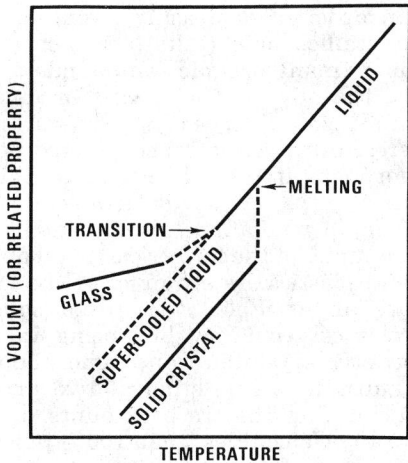

Fig. 107. Composite cooling curve of liquids forming glass, supercooled liquid, and solid crystal states; see text for explanation. For a more detailed discussion, see Dietz.[4]

Certain materials are easy to cast into a glassy state, others can be made glassy with great difficulty, and some, seemingly not at all. At present there seems to be no specific theory to help predict this behavior. Materials which do form glasses seem, however, to have a very high viscosity at their melting point; this inhibits the formation of an ordered structure. In addition, non-glass formers tend to have large energy differences between the ordered form of the solid and the disordered liquid. Thus, the low energy, ordered form of the solid tends to be developed. Obviously, the energetic tendencies here are balanced by entropy factors which tend to favor states of minimum order.

Although the most well-known glass formers are the metal oxides, many other materials can exist in the glassy state; even steel can be so cast if it is very, very quickly cooled. This technique produces glasses as the materials become solid before they have a chance to develop a crystalline structure. With regard to crystal formation, note that in a crystallization process, when concentrated solutions of the material to be crystallized are cooled slowly, larger and more perfect crystals form.

Incomplete or imperfect crystallization, whether due to technique or to the nature of the material itself (for example, natural and synthetic high polymers), often causes the formation of crystallites, glasses, or liquid crystals. Crystallites have no recognizable regular crystal pattern but yet are, in a sense, incipient crystals. Many shapes and arrangements are possible such as globular, rows or clouds of globules, threads, cylinders, or rods.

Solids

The most significant physical property of the solid state is the high degree of order in which substances such as metals and minerals exist. The structure may be crystalline and latticelike or noncrystalline, such as in plastic, glass, or gels which are not latticelike or only partly so. These latter materials do have, however, much more order than liquids and gases. These materials also have, in varying degree, some plastic and elastic properties wherein some resistance to applied stresses exist, but when the stress reaches a certain intensity, either flow or fracture ensues.

Although different classifications exist, four major different types of bonds hold solids together; the stronger bonds impart higher melting points to substances. In order of decreasing strength, the bond types are metallic, ionic (salts), valence (diamond), and molecular (many organic compounds). Thus, in some solids, the atoms or molecules or ions may be arranged in a regularly repeating pattern (crystalline state), whereas other solids are considered noncrystalline or amorphous if they do not have this characteristic of regularity. Although there is some blurring of the division, in general, metals, minerals, rocks, and alloys are examples of the former class and glass, wood, ceramics, and plastics are examples of the latter.

Alloys are an example of a mixed solid having characteristics of regularity but being intermediate between strictly crystalline and amorphous. They are metal substances consisting of two or more elements not counting the trace amounts of materials which make any element less than 100% pure. Alloys are solid solutions of one of two types. In the interstitial type, the smaller solute atoms occupy the interstices between the solvent atoms; the over-all structure is quite like the parent or solvent metal. The other type is the substitutional one and all atoms occupy (ie, contribute to building) a common lattice.

In general, alloys are stronger and harder than purer metals. This is probably due to the fact that both dislocations and the perfectly regular crystal structure of pure metals permit the planes of the crystals to slip over each other. These processes are inhibited in alloys because the resident or solute atoms interact with the dislocations and with the regular sections so that any lattice distortions produced make slipping more difficult.

A process that also depends on the internal structure and possibilities for partial shifting of it is annealing. It is based on the concept that a ductile metal becomes harder and less workable as cold work is done on it. Finally, a point is reached where cracking is imminent. To restore the original ductility, the metal is heated and slowly cooled. The temperatures used just permit the relaxation of the overstrained areas. A visualization might consider this a type of partial recrystallization or atomic rearrangement.

Polymorphism

Polymorphism, the existence of one or more crystalline and/or amorphous forms, is a characteristic of most solid substances. As applied to crystals it refers to the different crystal structures the same chemical compound may have. The various forms also usually have different x-ray diffraction patterns, melting points, and most important pharmaceutically, different solubilities.

Particularly in many cases in which dissolution in the gastrointestinal tract is the rate-limiting factor in absorption, differing solubilities may have a great effect, either good or bad. Different polymorphic forms are produced, depending on such factors as storage temperature, recrystallization solvent *per se*, and the rate of cooling (and hence the rate of crystallization) of the solvent. It appears that all organic materials exist in several polymorphic forms with the number of forms found depending on the effort spent searching! In the field of drugs, polymorphs of such diverse molecules as cortisone and prednisolone to aspirin have been found. As an example of the latter case, two different aspirin polymorphs form depending on whether the material is crystallized from 95% alcohol or *n*-hexane. The two forms have different melting points but most important, the form produced from the hexane dissolves in water much more quickly.

Selected Properties of Matter

Solubility—The solubility of a solid depends on a number of factors. If a solid is placed in a vacuum, volatilization takes place until the sublimation pressure is reached. However, if the evacuated space is replaced with a liquid, generally much more solid dissolves as compared to the amount which sublimes. This is caused by the interaction of the solid's molecules or ions with the solvent. In other words, solvation usually takes place.

Inorganic salts do not dissolve to any great extent in organic solvents such as toluene or carbon tetrachloride because these solvents have minimal dipole moments and so exert no attractive force toward the inorganic salt ions. On the other hand, inorganic salts generally are very soluble in water because the ions become solvated ("hydrated" in this case) by the strongly dipolar water. If the heat evolved by solvation essentially equals the heat absorbed in extracting the molecules or ions out of the solid form, the heat of solution is essentially zero; an example is sodium chloride in water. These solubilities are not altered much by temperature changes.

Many salts exhibit greater solubilities at higher temperatures, particularly those having endothermic heats of solution. The few salts with exothermic heats of solution, in which the energy absorbed in pulling the crystal apart is less than that released by the solvation process, exhibit decreases in solubility as temperature increases.

As is well known, solutes dissolve faster when they are in a finely divided state and thus expose a much larger surface area. In addition to this effect of area, the equilibrium solubility of tiny crystals is actually greater than that of larger ones, just as very tiny droplets of a given liquid have a higher vapor pressure than bulk material. This fact causes small crystals to disappear and large ones to grow larger when they are together in a solvent.

Unreactive gases exhibit some solubility because of the intermolecular attractive forces between themselves and the solvent. Gases with low boiling points have insignificant intermolecular attractions and, therefore, are not very soluble in liquids; solubility and boiling points show good correlation. The presence of other solutes decreases gas solubility in water. This salting-out effect varies with different salts, but a given salt tends to decrease the solubility of different gases to the same relative extent. The usual salting out explanation considers that the water which hydrates the salt is "removed" from the solvent and loses its solvating power. It also can be considered that the water that is oriented around the ions of the salt is thus less able to induce dipoles in the molecules of the gas. Naturally, salting-out phenomena are observed also in the case of liquids and solids dissolved in water or other solvents.

Electric Conductance—Electricity may be conducted in a number of ways, the usual classification being as follows: metallic conductance, in which electrons pass through the crystal lattice; electrolytic conductance, in which mobile ions carry current as they move through solutions; gas conductance, in which the presence of gas ions and electrons permit current to flow; semiconductor conductance, which operates when solids containing ions and ion vacancies carry current. In this case the ion vacancies are called holes and in effect, as the ions shift, the holes move, and thus conductivity is permitted. Superconductivity is manifested by many metals (both pure and alloys) when they are cooled to a point near absolute zero. The phenomenon consists of the metal having a zero electrical resistance.

In solid form, salts are poor conductors but in the fused state, they are excellent ones. Even at temperatures just below their melting points, the ability of salts to conduct becomes much greater, indicating ion mobility. Impurities in salts may also greatly enhance their ability to conduct.

Polarity—Different atoms of a molecule, if they are not identical, have a different affinity for electrons so that when atoms are bonded by electrons, the latter are not shared equally between them. This difference in electron-attracting power or electronegativity causes the bonding electrons to "spend more time" near the atom of higher electronegativity. This creates net positive and negative charges and the molecule is then polar.

In addition to such permanent dipoles, the presence of electric fields or other molecules may enhance or produce a state of polarization. Such polar forces enable molecules to attract and/or repel each other. The electron cloud of different molecules becomes distorted (and the molecule polarized) to greatly different extents depending on the structural makeup of the particular substance.

Density—Density is a property of matter in all its states and is usually measurable; its units or dimensions are given as mass/unit volume. Except for water and gallium, matter in its solid state is denser than in its liquid state, just as liquids are denser than vapors except at the critical point where they are equal.

The density of gases mirrors the magnitude of the intermolecular forces just as the densities of solids are also related to their structure and interatomic distances. Obviously, the density of a gas is more sensitive to changes in temperature and pressure than the densities of liquids or solids. At usual temperatures and pressures of the gaseous state, gas density is about 0.001 that of the liquid or solid state; ie, the molecules must be about ten times as far apart in gases.

The densities of liquids can be an aid in their analysis (eg, USP alcohol tables) and help in monitoring industrial processing where the density changes during the course of the reaction. If two components form a solution with no volume change, the density varies linearly with the relative concentrations. This, too, can be an assay aid. Where there is a volume change, as with alcohol and water, a table based on experimental data must be constructed. Although the density of a saturated vapor increases with a rise in temperature, the density of liquids generally increases as temperature decreases. In general, density increases along with pressure although, understandably, the effect is not linear as materials become less compressible the more they are compressed.

Density should be distinguished from specific gravity. Specific gravity is a unitless number expressing the ratio of a material's density (mass/unit volume) to that of a standard substance; the usual standard is water at 4°C. Because the density of water at 4°C is 1 Gm/cc, the numerical values of a material's specific gravity and density in cgs units are the same.

Surface Tension—Surface tension causes surfaces of liquids to act as films, the familiar floating-needle trick being a demonstration of this fact. This property—also responsible for capillary action, all types of wicking phenomena, and bubble formation—is due to surface forces. The usual units are energy/unit area expressed in ergs/cm^2 or, alternatively, in equivalent units, dynes/cm.

Most simply, it is considered that molecules near a surface are subject to forces of attraction from the main body of the fluid which are not balanced by any from above, hence the skin formation. It is not true that there are no forces from the vapor above, but they are small. When, however, two immisicble fluids are layered one over the other, the forces from above are greater.

The system present is now thought of in terms of having an interfacial tension. The interfacial tension is always less than the difference of the tensions of the individual liquids. It has been shown that this means three pure liquids will not remain in contact each with each other. It is the interfacial tension that is reduced during emulsion formation. As temperature increases, surface tension decreases until at the critical point, a liquid and its vapor are identical and the surface tension drops to zero.

If unimolecular films are put on the surface of solvents, the rates of evaporation are greatly reduced. Monolayers of such materials as stearic acid have been used to conserve water in lakes and reservoirs; plastic chips have seen the same use. An interesting analogy to gases is the fact that some fatty acid films behave like two dimensional gases when they form a film on a surface. The film occupies any given area and the pressure is inversely proportional to the area. The behavior of monolayers is, at times, like that of a gas in the critical region as the film pressure does not depend on the area at a certain pressure which is analogous to the vapor pressure of the two dimensional liquid. Surface tension and monolayers are discussed in more detail in Chapter 22, *Interfacial Phenomena*.

Diffusion—Diffusion, the random molecular motion which transports matter occurs in all materials but, of course, it is much slower in solids. If the medium, not counting the diffusing substance, is homogeneous, the diffusion takes place from regions of higher to lower concentrations. Normally, after a mix is homogeneous and no concentration gradients exist, the diffusion, as distinct from continuous molecular movements, is considered to cease. However, the presence of a temperature gradient may cause partial demixing. This effect, which is more prominent in gases and liquids than in solids, is called, in the case of liquids, the Soret effect.

Apparatus which can be differentially heated can be constructed to utilize this effect and, for example, isotopes can be separated. The heavier molecules congregate near the colder wall, the lighter toward the hotter. Self limiting diffusion reactions may occur when the material through which diffusion or reaction is taking place, changes itself, for example, by oxidizing in the air or tarnishing in an atmosphere containing sulfur or halogens. The products of the reaction form a protective coat for the material.

Although a rigorous treatment of diffusion processes involves complicated mathematics, it might be informative to examine a sample case to illustrate the initial development of a quantitative treatment. Parameters influencing and/or describing diffusion of particles or molecules are their mean velocity, time, and displacement. The latter refers to the distance a particle travels during its zigzaging, colliding movement from time zero to some other time. The mean displacement, in the absence of a concentration gradient is zero because positive and negative displacements cancel each other. Thus, to obtain numerical values for displacement, the mean-square displacement is used. In a process of diffusion where a concentration gradient is being obliterated, the mean-square displacement is a measure of the rate of diffusion; it is, however, time-dependent. To eliminate this dependency, a time-independent factor termed the diffusion coefficient, D, having units of $cm^2\ sec^{-1}$, was introduced. It is related to the mean-square displacement as follows:

$$D = \frac{\text{Mean-square displacement}}{\text{Time} \times 2}$$

As the diffusion process becomes faster, D becomes higher. D is used in the relationship known as Fick's first law, which relates the rate of flow of a diffusing material to the concentration gradient causing the flow:

$$J = -D\left(\frac{dc}{dx}\right)$$

where J is the flux or the amount of material passing perpendicularly through a reference area/unit time. The reference area most pertinent is an imaginary one placed crosswise between the regions of zero or low concentration and the region of high concentration. Then x is the direction of the major flow (as from the bottom to the top of a vertical cylinder) and c is the concentration of the diffusing material. Hence, dc/dx is the rate of change of the concentration in the x direction. Unit analysis indicates that self-consistency is maintained as $J = Gm\ sec^{-1}\ cm^{-2}$.

Adsorption—The attractive forces exerted by the atoms and molecules near the surface of a solid may cause the adsorption of other materials from gas or solution phases of its environment. The forces producing physical adsorption are similar to those which cause gases to condense to form liquids and are of the van der Waals type. The heat evolved is also similar to the heat evolved in gas condensation. The amount of material adsorbed may be many molecular layers thick. When the gas pressure or the concentration of the solute surrounding the solid is decreased, adsorption also decreases.

A different kind of adsorption, also distinguishable, is called chemisorption. It is not readily reversed and usually only unimolecular layers are adsorbed. The heat evolved is larger than that involved in physical adsorption because a type of surface compound is formed. One might consider this situation to be analogous to the familiar formation of complexes in solution.

Distillation

A very important process that involves a change of state—from liquid to vapor and back to liquid—is that of *distillation*.

The term distillation is applied to two types of processes: (1) where a single constituent is vaporized from a solution and subsequently condensed, as in the preparation of distilled water; (2) where vaporization gives rise to a mixture of constituents in the vapor and from which one or more of the substances is to be separated in as pure form as is possible. Some writers prefer to designate the first type of process as evaporation, regardless of the fact that the condensed vapor is the desired product, and to reserve for the second type of process the name distillation.

Two main methods of distillation are practiced. In one the vapor produced by boiling a liquid mixture is separated and condensed in such a way that none of the condensate is returned to the still to come in contact with vapor. In the other a portion of the condensate is returned to the still in such a manner as to effect an intimate "countercurrent" contact with vapor flowing in the direction of the condenser. The former is employed in *simple* distillation, *vacuum* distillation, and *steam* distillation; the latter in *fractional* distillation.

In order to effect a separation of the constituents of a mixture it is essential for the composition of the vapor produced in distillation to differ from that of the liquid from which it emanates. If the composition of both phases is identical, separation of the constituents of a mixture cannot be effected. A brief discussion of the equilibrium relationships between the liquid and vapor phases of several different types of liquid mixtures that may be distilled is presented in the following section.

Theory of Distillation of Mixtures

The boiling point of a simple liquid, ie, a chemical entity, is defined as the temperature at which the vapor pressure of the liquid is equal to the external pressure. The same definition applies to mixtures of liquids, but, unfortunately, there is no generally applicable means of knowing the vapor pressures of mixtures from knowledge of the individual vapor pressures. It follows that, in general, it is not possible with present knowledge to calculate the boiling points of all mixtures from data concerning the components alone. Under these circumstances recourse must be made to experimentally determined values. On the basis of the physical behavior of liquid mixtures it is nevertheless possible to make certain generalizations and classifications. The classifications are these:

1. Mixtures, the components of which are immiscible with each other.
2. Mixtures, the components of which are miscible in all proportions.
3. Mixtures, the components of which are miscible only in certain proportions.

These three classes are treated separately as follows.

Class 1.   Liquids Immiscible with Each Other

1. Each liquid evaporates independently of the other. The vapor pressure of the mixture at any particular temperature is the sum of the vapor pressures of the components for that temperature.

2. From temperature–vapor-pressure tables or graphs it is possible to ascertain the boiling points of such mixtures by summing the vapor pressures of the components all taken at the same temperature and, having done this for a range of temperatures, to read the boiling point from the curve constructed from the temperatures and the calculated vapor pressures. The boiling point is, of course, the temperature at which the vapor pressure equals the external pressure (eg, 760 mm).

3. For a mixture of two components, the ratio of the masses of the components in the condensed vapor will be:

$$\frac{m_A}{m_B} = \frac{p_A M_A}{p_B M_B} \text{ (see footnote*)}$$

where the subscripts represent the different components, m the weight of the liquid in the condensed vapor, p

the vapor pressure of the liquid, and M the molecular weight.

4.   A special case of such mixtures is represented by steam distillation.

Class 2.   Liquids Miscible in All Proportions

These mixtures are subdivided into three groups, depending on the variation of the boiling point with the composition.

1.   The boiling point varies uniformly with the composition of the mixture and is always lower than the boiling point of the least volatile component and greater than that of the most volatile.
2.   The boiling point varies with the composition, but at one particular composition the boiling point has a maximum value, greater than that of the least volatile component.
3.   The boiling point varies with the composition, but at one particular composition the boiling point has a minimum value, less than that of the most volatile component.

In the discussion to follow, mixtures of only two components are treated because of the obvious simplification.   Studies have been made of more complex mixtures and concerning such cases references may be made to monographs on the subject of distillation.

A clearer understanding of the behavior of the several groups of two-component mixtures during distillation may be obtained with the aid of diagrams which show not only the boiling point of all possible mixtures of the two components, but also the composition of the vapor which is in equilibrium with the liquid at the boiling point.   Accordingly, two curves are found in each diagram, the lower one representing the boiling point for any given composition of liquid, the upper indicating the composition of vapor in equilibrium with the liquid.   It will be seen that except for certain mixtures, notably *constant boiling mixtures*, the vapor in equilibrium with a mixed liquid is always of different composition from that of the liquid.   To obtain the composition of vapor in equilibrium with a boiling liquid a horizontal "tie line" should be drawn from the desired point on the liquid curve until it intersects the vapor curve.

The composition of the liquid is here indicated in terms of mole fractions.   In a liquid containing the two components A and B the mole fraction of A, designated N_A, is the number of moles of A divided by the sum of the moles of A and B; mathematically this is expressed as follows:

$$N_A = \frac{n_A}{n_A + n_B}$$

---

* This relationship evolves from the following consideration:
1.   In any given volume of vapor above such a mixture, the following equations hold:

$$p_A = P n_A/(n_A + n_B) \qquad p_B = P n_B/(n_A + n_B)$$

Here P is the total pressure and n is the number of moles contained in the volume chosen.
2.   Dividing the two equations one obtains:

$$p_A/p_B = n_A/n_B$$

3.   By definition of a mole:

$$n_A = m_A/M_A \qquad n_B = m_B/M_B$$

4.   Whence

$$p_A/p_B = m_A M_B/m_B M_A$$

and finally

$$m_A/m_B = p_A M_A/p_B M_B$$

Note that if the molecular weight of B is much smaller than that of A, the proportion of A to B in the distillate will be much greater than the ratio of the corresponding vapor pressures of the two liquids.

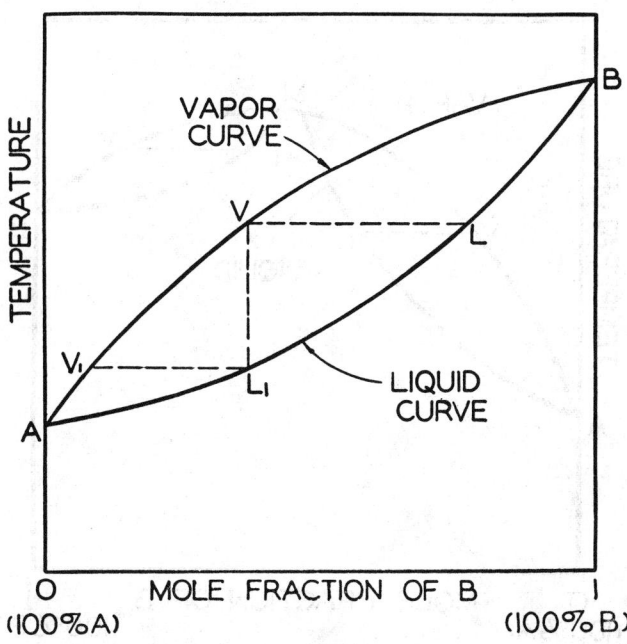

Fig. 108.   **Binary mixture having a regularly increasing boiling point.**

The mole fraction of B is similarly defined:

$$N_B = \frac{n_B}{n_A + n_B}$$

From these equations it is apparent that the sum of the mole fractions of A and B is 1, also that $N_A = 1 - N_B$ and that $N_B = 1 - N_A$.

Group 1—Fig. 108 represents the behavior of various mixtures of liquids A and B, the former having a lower boiling point (since it is more volatile) than the latter. If a liquid having the composition represented by the point L is boiled, the vapor in equilibrium with it will have the composition represented by V; since the vapor is richer in the more volatile substance A, the liquid becomes richer in the less volatile substance B on continued distillation.   The boiling point of the liquid in the distillation chamber rises continuously and eventually pure B is left in the chamber.   If the vapor corresponding to V is condensed to liquid, represented by the vertical line projected from V to L_1, and the condensed liquid redistilled, the new vapor in equilibrium with this liquid will have the composition V_1.   By repeating this process of vaporization and condensation with liquid of composition V_1, which represents what is called fractional distillation, there will eventually be obtained vapor, and liquid, of pure A.   Examples of this group of mixtures are: benzene and toluene; methanol and water;   acetic acid and water.

Group 2—The presence of a maximum in the boiling temperature curve (which corresponds to the development of minimum vapor pressure for that particular composition) is shown by mixtures of two liquids which undergo some kind of interaction, probably of a physical nature.   Since the composition of the mixture having the maximum boiling point rarely, if ever, represents a simple molecular ratio, it seems highly unlikely that a new chemical compound is produced.   The behavior of two-component liquid mixtures exhibiting a maximum boiling point is shown in Fig. 109.   Here again the upper curve represents the composition of the vapor phase, the lower that of the liquid.   At M both liquid and vapor have the same composition;   accordingly, a liquid of composition M distils unchanged and cannot be separated into its components by distillation.   If a

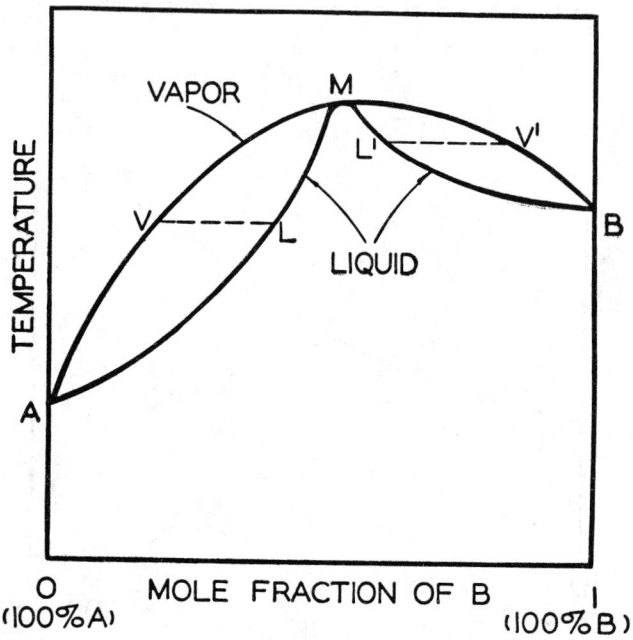

Fig. 109.   Binary mixture having a maximum boiling point.

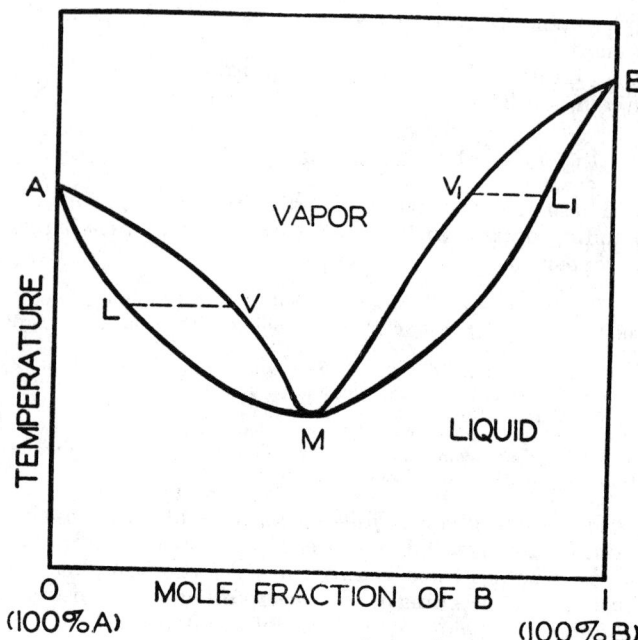

Fig. 110.   Binary mixture having a minimum boiling point.

liquid having the initial composition L is boiled, the vapor will have the composition V; the boiling point of the liquid in the distillation chamber will rise until the concentration M is reached, whereupon the liquid distils unchanged.   If the vapor corresponding to V is condensed and subjected to fractional distillation, it will ultimately yield a distillate of pure A.   Pure B cannot be obtained by the distillation of any mixture having a composition to the left of M.   Similarly, if a liquid of composition L' is boiled, the vapor will have the composition V'; the temperature of the liquid in the distillation chamber will rise until ultimately a liquid of composition M remains in the chamber. Fractional distillation of the condensed vapor V' eventually yields pure B.   Pure A cannot be obtained by distilling any mixture whose composition is to the right of M.

The constant boiling mixture M is often called an *azeotrope* or an *azeotropic mixture*.   That it is not a true chemical compound can be proved by the fact that a change in the external pressure will produce a change in the ratio of the components of this mixture.   Examples of constant boiling mixtures having a maximum boiling point are hydrochloric acid and water, and nitric acid and water.

Group 3—A minimum boiling point (corresponding to the development of maximum vapor pressure at that particular composition) is shown by mixtures of liquids the components of which differ in the degree of intermolecular attraction (the so-called *internal pressure* of the component), in polarity, or in length of hydrocarbon chain or other analogous group, or if one or the other of the components is associated in dimeric or more complex arrangement.   The behavior of two-component liquid mixtures exhibiting a minimum boiling point is shown in Fig. 110.   As in the other diagrams, the upper curve pertains to the vapor phase, the lower to the liquid.   At M the liquid and vapor have the same composition; a liquid of that composition (also called an *azeotrope* or *azeotropic mixture*) may be distilled unchanged, and at constant temperature; there is the important difference, as compared with the corresponding liquid of Group 2, that the former has a minimum boiling point.   If a liquid of initial composition L is

boiled, the vapor in equilibrium with it will have the composition V; distillation of the liquid, which is accompanied by a continuous rise in temperature, will ultimately leave in the chamber a residue of pure A, while fractional distillation of the condensed vapor V will eventually yield a distillate of composition M. Pure B cannot be separated from the mixture.   On the other hand a liquid of composition L_1, which on boiling produces an initial vapor of composition V_1, leaves, ultimately, pure B in the distillation chamber, while fractional distillation of the condensed vapor yields a distillate of composition M.   In this case pure A cannot be obtained by distillation.

A mixture of this type which is of great importance is that of ethyl alcohol and water.   At a concentration of 92.3% by weight of C_2H_5OH, when distilled under 1 atmos of pressure, the minimum boiling point of 78.3°C is observed.   From the above it is apparent why absolute alcohol cannot be obtained by distillation of any hydroalcoholic solution containing less than 92.3% of C_2H_5OH.   Mixtures of isopropyl alcohol and water behave similarly.

Class 3.   *Liquids Miscible in Certain Proportions*

The behavior of mixtures in this class may be better understood with the help of Fig. 111, which is characteristic of many, but not all, members of the class.   In this diagram any mixture whose composition is to the left of X or to the right of Y exists as a single homogeneous liquid; mixtures having a composition between X and Y exist as two homogeneous liquids, one being a saturated solution of A in B, the other a saturated solution of B in A.   If a liquid of composition L is boiled, the vapor in equilibrium with it will be of composition V; on continued distillation the boiling point of the liquid rises and eventually there is left in the chamber pure A, while from the condensed vapor there is ultimately obtained vapor of composition Z, which when condensed separates into two liquids having the compositions X and Y, respectively.   If liquid of composition L' is boiled, the vapor has the composition V'; distillation, which is accompanied by rise in temperature, leaves pure B in the chamber, while fractionation of the vapor V' leads to the same state as before. Distillation of any mixture of immiscible liquids having a composition between X and Y occurs at constant temperature as long as the two liquids are present; the composition of the vapor is in each case represented by Z. If the original liquid mixture has a composition between X and Z, the vapor will be richer in B and the liquid richer in A; eventually a single liquid of composition X is obtained, and from this point on the boiling point rises and the mixture behaves in accordance with curve XA. An original composition of the liquid mixture between Y and Z yields vapor richer in A and liquid richer in B; when the two-liquid mixture reaches the composition Y it becomes one homogeneous liquid whose behavior is depicted by the curve YB.

Fractional Distillation

Distillation of a mixture in which the one component is highly nonvolatile affords a ready method of separation of the components. For instance, it is a simple matter to distil pure water from a water–salt solution, leaving the nonvolatile salt in the still. It is, however, a more difficult task to separate with completeness two components, both of which are relatively volatile. That this can be done, at least in certain instances, is evident from the study of the theory of distillation of mixtures. Using the simplest illustration, it was seen that in the case of mixtures belonging to Class II, Group 1, of which mixtures of methyl alcohol and water are an example, the initial vapors from the mixture contain a higher proportion of methyl alcohol (the more volatile constituent) than is present in the boiling liquid; it was further evident that continued distillation would leave pure water—but not all that was originally present—in the distillation chamber. If the initial vapors were condensed and then redistilled, the new vapors would be still richer in methyl alcohol; repetition of this process of condensation and vaporization would ultimately yield some pure methyl alcohol—but not all of it. So that at least most of the methyl alcohol and the water in the original mixture may be recovered, distillation of the mixture may be performed in such a way as to collect fractions of the distillate,

each fraction representing the portion which distils at a definite interval of temperature. The first and last of these fractions will contain the highest concentration of the more volatile and the less volatile component, respectively. If these fractions are in turn redistilled several times, the net result of the long operation will be a fairly sharp separation of the components of the original mixture.

Numerous devices are available for the convenient collection of fractions (Fig. 112).

Instead of collecting separate fractions of distillate and submitting each of these to further fractional distillation, it is possible to effect the same degree of separation of the components of a mixture by the use of "fractionating columns," of which several laboratory types are shown in Figs. 113 to 116. In these devices a part of the vapor is condensed in the column and, in returning to the vaporizing chamber, comes into intimate contact with rising vapor, ultimately resulting in more or less efficient fractionation of the liquid being distilled. The efficiency of the operation may be further increased by returning a portion of the distillate through the column where it meets ascending vapor and induces further fractionation. That portion of the distillate which is returned to the column is called the *reflux*. Many types of fractionation apparatus are used, ranging in size from the small dimensions of microchemical equipment to diameters of 44 feet and heights of 200 feet for some industrial installations.

Molecular Distillation

In the methods of distillation thus far described, molecules leaving the evaporating surface are very unlikely to reach the condensing surface without being many times deflected from their path by collision with other molecules and often thrown back into the liquid being distilled. By applying a high vacuum in the still the frequency of collisions between molecules is decreased, because the distance a given molecule travels without colliding with another molecule is increased, ie, the "mean free path" of the molecules is lengthened. If, now, the condensing surface is placed so close to the evaporating surface that the

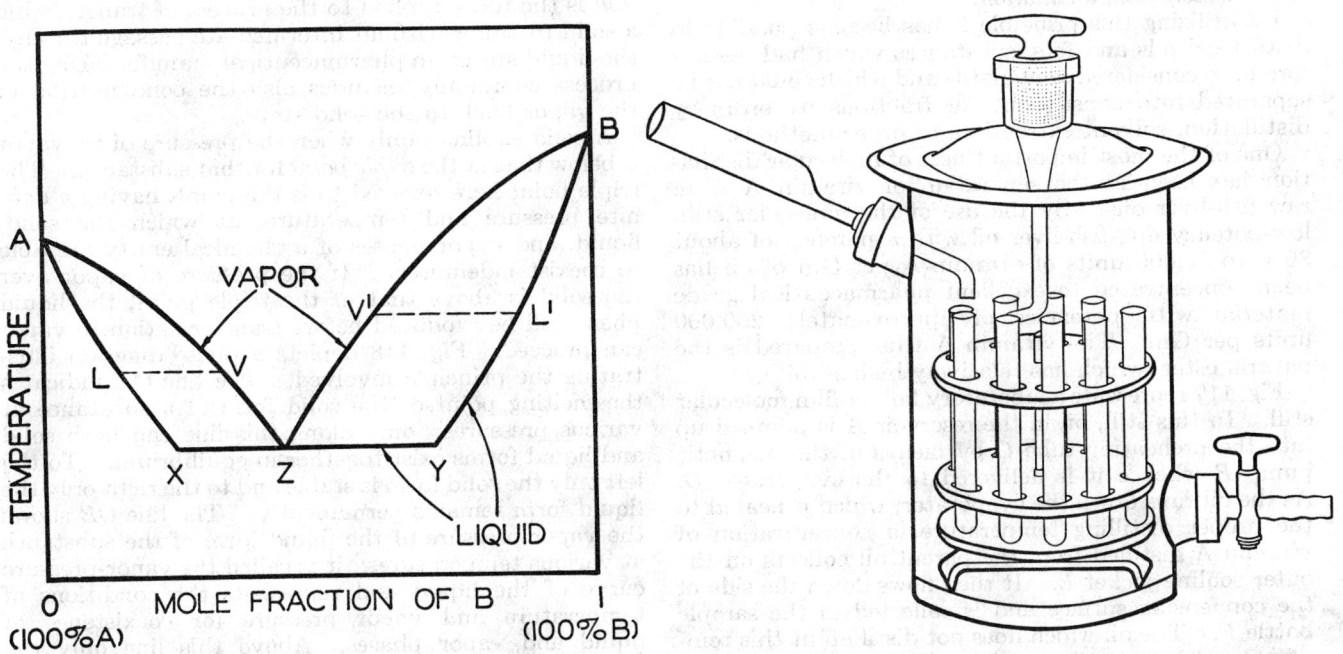

Fig. 111. **Liquids miscible in certain proportions.**   Fig. 112. **Fractional distillate receiver.**

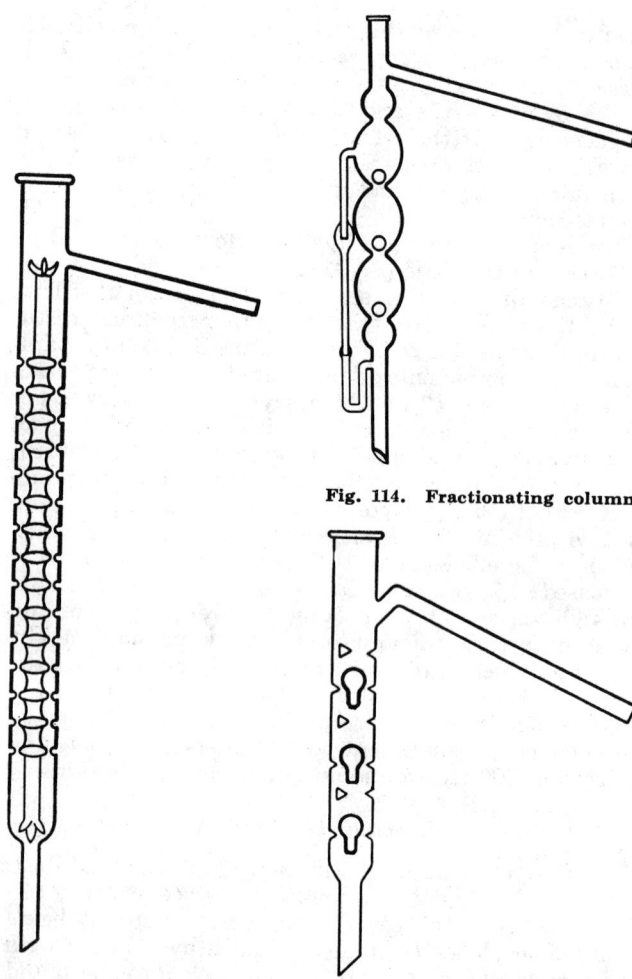

Fig. 113.   Fractionating column.

Fig. 114.   Fractionating column.

Fig. 115.   Fractionating column.

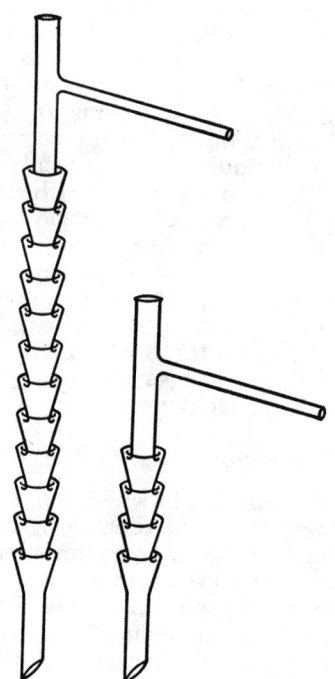

Fig. 116.   Fractionating columns.

distance between the two is less than the mean free path of the molecules being distilled, the process of distillation is most readily carried out, and at the lowest possible temperatures.   This is the principle underlying *molecular distillation* or, as it is better designated, *high-vacuum short-path distillation*.

By utilizing this principle it has become possible to distil fixed oils and fats, substances which had heretofore been considered nonvolatile and which could not be separated into constituents or fractions by ordinary distillation, solvent extraction, or other methods.

One of the most important uses of molecular distillation has been in the separation of vitamin A from raw fish-liver oils.   By the use of the molecular still, low-potency dog fish-liver oil with a potency of about 8000 to 15,000 units of vitamin A per Gm of oil has been concentrated to excellent pharmaceutical grade material with potencies of approximately 200,000 units per Gm.   The vitamin A thus prepared is the natural ester, which has relatively high stability.

Fig. 117 represents a laboratory falling-film molecular still.   In this still, oil in the reservoir A is pumped up into the preheating tube C by means of the magnetic pump B whence it is delivered to the evaporator D. As the oil runs down the evaporator, which is heated to the proper distilling temperature, a concentration of vitamin A distilled from the parent oil collects on the outer cooling jacket E.   It then flows down the side of the condensing surface and is collected in the sample bottle F.   The oil which does not distil off at this temperature collects in the reservoir G where, if its vitamin

content is still significant, it may be returned to reservoir A and recycled.

In commercial operations, molecular distillation of fish-liver oil may be carried out in huge stills which have large rotating plates up to 5 ft in diameter from which the oil is distilled rather than from the heated column shown in the diagram.   Both vitamins A and E can be obtained in this way from fish-liver oil and vegetable oils.

Sublimation

All solids have some tendency to pass directly into the vapor state.   At a given temperature each solid has a definite, though generally small, vapor pressure; the latter increases with rise in temperature.   *Sublimation* is the term applied to the process of transforming a solid to vapor without intermediate passage through the liquid state; in pharmaceutical manufacturing the process commonly includes also the condensation of the vapor back to the solid state.

A solid sublimes only when the pressure of its vapor is below that at the *triple point* for that substance.   The triple point here referred to is the point, having a definite pressure and temperature, at which the solid, liquid, and vapor phases of a chemical entity are able to coexist indefinitely.   If the pressure of vapor over the solid is above that of the triple point, the liquid phase will be produced before transformation to vapor can proceed.   Fig. 118 depicts a phase diagram illustrating the principle involved.   The line OA indicates the melting point of the solid form of a substance at various pressures; only along this line can both solid and liquid forms exist together in equilibrium.   To the left only the solid form is stable and to the right only the liquid form remains permanently.   The line OB shows the vapor pressure of the liquid form of the substance at various temperatures; it is called the vapor-pressure curve of the liquid and represents the conditions of temperature and vapor pressure for coexistence of liquid and vapor phases.   Above this line only the liquid phase exists permanently;   below it only vapor

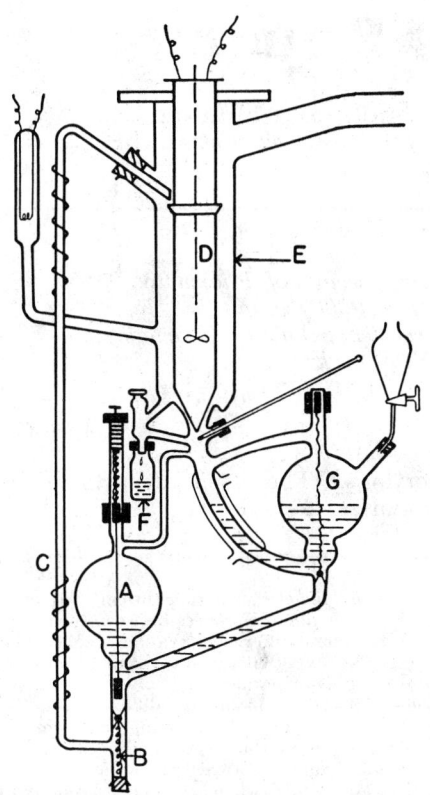

Fig. 117.   Diagram of molecular distillation.

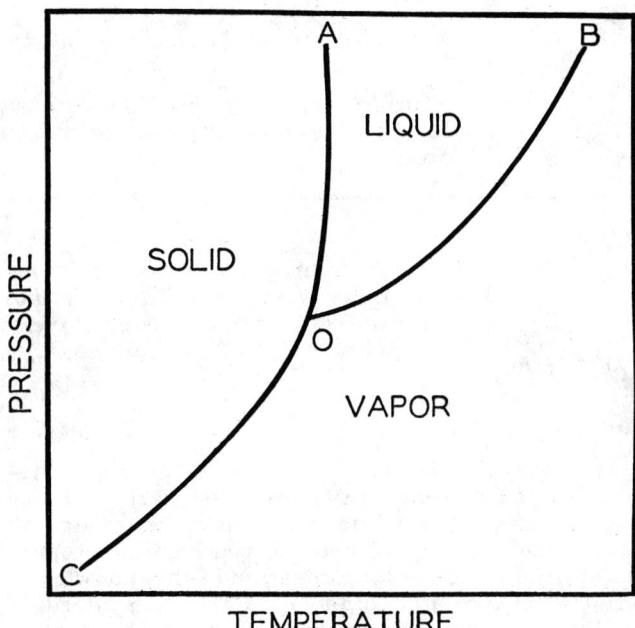

Fig. 118.   Phase diagram to illustrate the principle of sublimation.

occurs.   The line *OC* represents the vapor pressure of the solid at various temperatures; it is designated as the sublimation curve of the solid and represents the conditions of temperature and vapor pressure for the coexistence of solid and vapor phases.   To the left of this line only solid can exist, to the right only the vapor form is stable.   The intersection of the three lines, point *O*, is the triple point.   It is apparent from the diagram that at pressures of vapor below that of the triple point it is possible to pass directly from the vapor to the solid state, and *vice versa*, simply by changing the temperature.   At pressures above the triple point the liquid phase must intervene in transformations between solid and vapor phases, in a closed system.   Since the melting point of a solid is commonly taken at 1 atmos

of pressure, it is evident that if the triple point pressure is less than 1 atmos, fusion of the solid form will occur on heating in a closed vessel; if, on the other hand, the triple point pressure is greater than 1 atmos, the solid form cannot be melted by heating at atmospheric pressure.

In a current of air, however, the conditions are somewhat different; some solids that melt when heated in a closed system now sublime appreciably even at ordinary temperatures because the vapor pressure of the solid does not attain the triple-point pressure.   Thus, camphor, naphthalene, *p*-dichlorobenzene, and iodine, all of which have a triple-point pressure below 1 atmos, will vaporize in a current of air but melt when heated in a closed system.

References

1. Kennon, L., and Gulesich, J. J., *J. Pharm. Sci.*, **51,** 278 (1962).
2. Goldberg, A. H., *et al, J. Pharm. Sci.*, **55,** 482 (1966).
3. Fergason, J. L., and Brown, G. H., *J. Am. Oil Chemists' Soc.*, **45,** 120 (1968).
4. Dietz, E. D., *Sci. Technol.*, 10 (Nov., 1968).

15 | Atomic and Molecular Structure

Atomic structure—molecular structure—intermolecular binding forces—additive physical properties—x-ray crystallographic structural analysis

This chapter was prepared by

Eric J. Lien, PhD, *Assistant Professor of Pharmacy, School of Pharmacy, University of Southern California, Los Angeles, Calif. 90007, and*
Eli Shefter, PhD, *Associate Professor of Pharmaceutics, School of Pharmacy, State University of New York at Buffalo, Buffalo, New York 14214*

The many significant advances in the pharmaceutical sciences in recent years are in large part attributable to the accelerated development of knowledge of the molecular structure and physicochemical properties of drugs, and to the correlation of this knowledge with that of the nature of biological reactions of drugs. In this chapter are discussed fundamental principles of atomic and molecular structure and of certain physicochemical properties which are basically important in the pharmaceutical sciences.

Atomic Structure

Atoms and Elementary Particles—The word atom is derived from the Greek word *atomos*, indivisible; the atoms were believed to be the minute indivisible particles of which all material things were made. The search for the ultimate particle has been a continuous effort since the time of Democritus. Before the discovery of mesons and hyperons, the structure of matter was believed to be much simpler. The nucleus was thought to consist of protons and neutrons, and to form an atom only electrons needed to be added in external shells. Therefore, protons, neutrons, and electrons were considered as the elementary particles.

During the past three decades nuclear physics has progressively probed atoms from their periphery to their center. The search for ultimate units of structure has disclosed the existence of more than 20 subatomic particles. On further study some "elementary particles" are beginning to show that they themselves must have "structure." Some of the subatomic particles known are listed in Table I.

L. de Broglie in 1924 raised the question that if light waves show corpuscular character, should not particles also show wave character? Now it is generally accepted that in the case of a photon there are two fundamental equations to be obeyed: $E = h\nu$ and $E = mc^2$, where E is the energy, h is Planck's constant, ν is the frequency, and c is the speed of light. Combining both equations we have $h\nu = mc^2$ or $\lambda = c/\nu = h/mc = h/p$, where p is the momentum of the photon.

de Broglie proposed that a similar equation should govern the wavelength of the electron wave. It is interesting to note that x-ray diffraction is a good example of the utilization of the wave property of electromagnetic radiation.

Dalton's Atomic Theory—In 1808 Dalton proposed his atomic theory on the basis of three generalizations; namely, the Law of Conservation of Mass, the Law of Definite Proportions, and the Law of Multiple Proportions. The essential parts of the theory can be summarized as follows:

1. All elements are composed of very small, discrete, indivisible particles called atoms.
2. All atoms of any one element are identical. Modern structural theory tells us that electronic differences between the atoms of an element may occur, but these differences arise as a consequence of electronic excitation. The lowest energy state of an atom is more appropriate for purposes of classification.
3. The atoms of no two elements are alike.
4. Atoms undergo no fundamental change in chemical reactions. There are subtle changes in the electronic character of atoms, although this does not change the identity of an atom.
5. Compounds are formed when atoms of two or more different elements combine to form a molecule.
6. In general, atoms combine in simple ratios.

Periodic Table—The periodic classification of the elements is one of the most striking advances in generalizing many isolated facts; moreover, it contributes tremendously to the strength of the atomic theory and extends it to new sets of facts. The periodic table serves as an easily learned summary of almost limitless information about the chemical nature of the elements; it is of prime importance to students of pharmaceutical sciences as well as to students of chemistry.

After the publication of the independent researches of Mendeléeff and Meyer in 1869, the *Periodic Law* was well established. The *Periodic Table* is an arrangement of the elements in accordance with the periodic law (see inside back cover). The present arrangement is essentially the same as that of Mendeléeff, although there are now minor variations due to the incorporation of new elements and modern data. A few terms should be carried in mind for a thorough understanding of the table.

Atomic number (Z) is the positive charge of the nucleus expressed as multiples of the electronic charge e.

Atomic weight is the average weight expressed in atomic weight units of the natural atoms of an element existing as a mixture of isotopes in the same ratio as found in nature. An atomic weight unit, used in chemistry, is exactly $\frac{1}{16}$ the average mass of the oxygen isotopes taken in the same ratio as they occur in nature. One atomic weight unit is equivalent to 1.000272 atomic mass unit.

An *isotope* is one of a group of nuclides of the same element (same Z), having the same number of protons in the nucleus but differing in the number of neutrons, resulting in different mass numbers.

A *nuclide* is any one of the more than 1000 species of atoms and is characterized by the number of protons and neutrons in the nucleus.

Bohr's Theory of Atomic Structure—In 1913 Bohr proposed a theory of atomic structure for the problem of atomic spectra. His picture of the atom had the extranuclear electrons revolving around the nucleus in definite orbits. These orbits were assigned principal quantum numbers 1, 2, 3, ... n, counting outward from the nucleus.

When an electron absorbs a definite increment or quantum of energy, it is promoted to an orbit of higher energy (excited state), and when it falls back to the original orbit, it emits radiation energy. The energy of the various levels in the atom can be related to the frequency of radiation which is emitted from or absorbed by the atom. This relationship is expressed by Eq. (1).

$$\Delta E = E_2 - E_1 = h\nu \qquad (1)$$

where ΔE is the difference of the energy in ergs between two levels, h is Planck's constant (6.624×10^{-27} erg sec), and ν is the frequency. Since the frequency is equivalent to the speed of light c divided by the wavelength, Eq. 1 can be written as

$$\Delta E = hc/\lambda \qquad (2)$$

When the electrons possess the lowest energy possible, the atom is said to be in its *ground state*.

The energy of an electron in an orbit is given by the expression

$$E = \frac{-2\pi^2 Z^2 m e^4}{n^2 h^2} \qquad (3)$$

where Z is the atomic number, m is the mass of the electron (9.1×10^{-28} Gm), e is the charge of the electron in electrostatic units (4.8×10^{-10} esu), n is the principal quantum number, and h is Planck's constant. One can calculate the radiation energy emitted when an electron falls from n_2 orbit to n_1 orbit by Eq. 4

$$E_2 - E_1 = \frac{2\pi^2 Z^2 m e^4}{h^2}\left(\frac{1}{n_1^2} - \frac{1}{n_2^2}\right) \qquad (4)$$

When n_2 is ∞, Eq. 4 gives the energy required for ionization. For example, the ionization potential of the hydrogen atom can be calculated as

$$E_\infty - E_1 =$$

$$\frac{2 \times (3.14)^2 \times (1)^2 \times 9.1 \times 10^{-28} \times (4.8 \times 10^{-10})^4}{(6.624 \times 10^{-27})^2} \times$$

$$\left(\frac{1}{(1)^2} - \frac{1}{(\infty)^2}\right)$$

$$= 2.18 \times 10^{-11} \text{ erg} =$$

$$\frac{2.18 \times 10^{-11} \text{ erg}}{1.60 \times 10^{-12} \text{ erg/electron volt (ev)}}$$

$$= 13.6 \text{ ev}$$

It is interesting to note that the quantum theory is founded on the principle that the energy of an atom or molecule does not change continuously but only by some definite whole number unit of energy referred to as a quantum.

Modern Model of Atomic Structure—After Bohr published his theory, there was a period of intense activity by theoreticians and experimental physicists. Based on mathematical principles and considerable experimental data, a more definite picture of atomic structure emerged. The modern interpretation of the atom is more elaborate than the original idea of

Table I—Subatomic Particles[a]

Group	Particles	Relative mass (electron = 1)	Electric charge	Mean life-time (sec)
Heavy particles	α-Particle (He^{++}, α)	7348	+2	stable
	Triton (T, ^{3}H)	5451	+1	stable
	Deuteron (D, d, ^{2}H)	3674	+1	stable
	Neutron (n)	1837	0	1×10^{-3}
	Proton (p, ^{1}H)	1837	+1	stable
Hyperons	Λ° Particle	~2181	0	2.5×10^{-10}
	$\Sigma^\pm$ Particle	~2326	±1	$\Sigma^+ 0.8 \times 10^{-10}$ $\Sigma^- 1.6 \times 10^{-10}$
	$\Xi^\pm$ Particle	~2580	±1	1.3×10^{-10}
Mesons	K meson (K$^\pm$)	966	±1	1.2×10^{-8}
	K meson (K$^\circ$)	974	0	$10^{-9} - 10^{-10}$
	Pi meson ($\pi^\pm$)	273	±1	2.6×10^{-8}
	Pi meson (π°)	264	0	1.9×10^{-16}
	Mu meson ($\mu^\pm$)	209 ± 2	±1	2.2×10^{-6}
Leptons	Electrons (e$^-$, β^-)	1	−1	stable
	Positron (e$^+$, β^+)	1	+1	stable
	Nutrino (ν)	0.01	0	stable
	Photons (γ)	0	0	stable

[a] For more comprehensive discussions of these particles consult Refs. 1–6.

Bohr. Four quantum numbers are used to describe the energy levels or orbitals of each electron.

The *principal quantum number n* is an approximate measure of the size of the electron cloud; ie, the order of magnitude of the potential energy. It has the values 1, 2, 3, ... 7, corresponding to the K, L, M, ... Q shells of electrons.

The *azimuthal quantum number l* is related to the shape of the electron cloud, indicating whether it is a spherical, dumbbell shaped, or of more complex geometry. It may have values of 0, 1, 2, ... $(n - 1)$, corresponding, respectively, to the terms s, p, d, f, used by spectroscopists. For example, a $4d$ electron would have an n number of 4 and an l value of 2.

The *magnetic quantum number m_l* is related to the orientation of the electron cloud in space. It has values of 0, ± 1, ± 2, ... $\pm l$. For a spherical cloud there is only one orientation. However, the dumbbell-shaped orbital, for example, could be oriented in three different directions corresponding to the x, y, and z axis of a set of Cartesian coordinates.

The *spin quantum number s* (or m_s) gives the orientation of the magnetic component of an electron. There are only two discrete ways an electron can interact with an external magnetic field: like a tiny magnet, it can either line up in the direction of the field or it can orient itself in the opposite direction. The electron's magnetic moment was at first pictured as being due to the rotation of the electron on its axis, and for this reason an electron was said to exhibit spin. The two spin quantum numbers $s = +\frac{1}{2}$ and $s = -\frac{1}{2}$ were used to describe the two observable spin states.

Electronic Configuration of the Elements—Two rules are of extreme importance in the building up of electronic shells of elements (as shown in Fig. 119 and Table II).

The *Pauli exclusion principle* states that an atom cannot exist in a state where two electrons in the same energy level or orbital have the same set of four quantum numbers. This is analogous to the principle in classical physics that no two bodies can be in the same place at the same time. Thus two electrons in the K shell have the same principal, azimuthal, and magnetic quantum numbers ($n = 1$, $l = 0$, $m_l = 0$), and different spin quantum numbers ($s = +\frac{1}{2}$ and $-\frac{1}{2}$).

Hund's rule of maximum multiplicity states that when orbitals are of the same energy electrons distribute themselves one to each orbital so as to maintain parallel spins. For example, oxygen with an atomic number of 8, possesses 8 electrons. Two electrons are in the K shell ($1s^2$), and 6 are in the L shell. In the L shell 2 electrons fill the $2s$ orbitals ($2s^2$) and the remaining 4 fill the $2p$ orbitals ($2p^4$).

According to Hund's rule, 3 electrons occupy $2p_x$, $2p_y$, and $2p_z$ orbitals and spin in the same direction (indicated by the direction of the arrow in Fig. 120); the fourth electron can pair up with any one of these 3 electrons (say $2p_x$). The electronic configuration for oxygen atom can be expressed as $1s^2$ $2s^2$ $2p_x^2$ $2p_y$ $2p_z$.

Molecular Structure

A molecule is the smallest possible quantity of a substance. It is composed of two or more atoms; eg, N_2, O_2, $CHCl_3$, H_2SO_4. There is a chemical bond between atoms when the forces acting between them are strong enough to give an aggregate with sufficient stability to make it convenient for the chemist to consider the aggregate as an independent molecular species. Different types of chemical bonds will be discussed in the following sections.

Covalent Bonds—When two electrons of two atoms are paired and localized in the space between the two atoms, a covalent bond results. The paired electrons (with opposed spins) will then occupy the new molecular orbital encompassing the two atoms. It should be noted that the electron pair held jointly by two atoms is considered to do double duty by completing a stable electronic configuration for each atom.

For instance, in the case of methane, the carbon atom, with its 2 inner electrons and its outer shell of 8 shared electrons, has assumed the stable 10-electron configuration of neon; and the hydrogen atoms have achieved the configuration of helium. Covalent bonds and ionic bonds are found in both organic and inorganic chemistry.

Hybridization of Atomic Orbitals—The ground state of the carbon atom has the electron distribution $1s^2\,2s^2\,2p^2$. Hence it might be expected to be bivalent. However, in all stable compounds carbon is found to have a valence of 4.

To account for this fact, Pauling proposed that the atomic orbitals about an atom may "mix" to form hybrid orbitals. Thus, if one of the $2s$ electrons of carbon is promoted to a $2p$ orbital, the $2s$ and three $2p$ orbitals may merge to form four sp^3 hybrid orbitals containing 1 electron each. This process enables carbon to form four stable covalent bonds instead of only two. The new set of orbitals are called *hybrid atomic orbitals*. They are designated as sp^3, indicating that they are made by mixing one s and three p orbitals. For instance, in methane (CH_4), the four hydrogen atoms lie at the corners of a regular tetrahedron, and

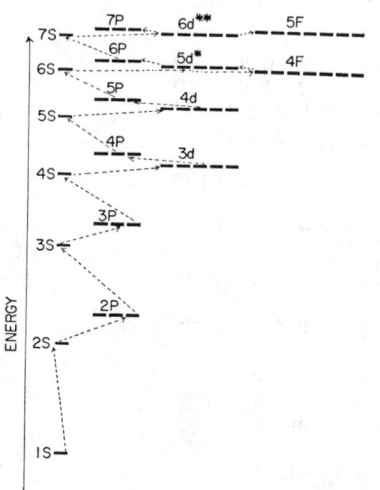

Fig. 119. Atomic energy levels and the order of filling of orbitals: (*) a single $5d$ electron is added before the $4f$ orbitals can be filled; (**) one or more $6d$ electrons must be added before the $5f$ orbitals can be filled.

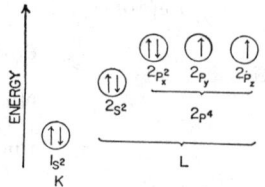

Fig. 120. The electronic configuration of an oxygen atom.

in ethane, (C_2H_6) one CH_3 takes the place of one H in methane (Fig. 121G).

Two other types of hybridizations are useful in describing unsaturated compounds. Mixing an s orbital with two p orbitals gives three equivalent sp^2 hybrids. These *trigonal* orbitals lie in a plane and are symmetrical about axes separated by 120° (Fig. 121E). Hybridization of one s and one p orbital gives a pair of *linear*, or sp, orbitals (Fig. 121F).

Sigma (σ) and Pi (π) Bonds—Covalent bonds may be distinguished by the type of atomic orbitals used in forming the bonds or by the kind of resultant molecular orbitals. The most common covalent bonds are formed from electrons of s and p atomic orbitals. A σ bond results from the overlap of a pair of s orbitals (Fig. 121A); the overlap of an s and a p orbital (Fig. 121B); or the head-on overlap of p orbitals from two atoms (Fig. 121C). The σ bond thus formed is the classical single bond of organic chemistry (Fig. 121G).

When singly occupied p lobes overlap side-by-side, a π bond results (Fig. 121D). This can only take place, however, if a σ bond already exists between the two atoms. A π bond associated with a σ bond is termed a double bond (Fig. 121H).

Furthermore, if the two σ-bonded atoms each have two pairs of singly occupied p lobes oriented properly, they may overlap in four separate zones. Two π bonds now form in addition to the σ bond already present (Fig. 121I). This is the classical triple bond of such substances as acetylene and cyanide ion.

In benzene the six carbon atoms are joined together in a hexagonal plane by bonds involving sp^2 orbitals (Fig. 121E). The molecular orbitals are localized between the nuclei of the carbon atoms in the hexagon. The third sp^2 orbital of each carbon atom overlaps with the s orbitals of the hydrogens to form the C—H bonds in the plane of the molecule. The unhybridized $2p_z$ orbitals of the six carbon atoms extend above and below the plane and overlap to form the nonlocalized π bonds (Fig. 121J).

Interatomic distances decrease appreciably to achieve the overlap needed to form π bonds between atoms. The *bond* distance is characteristic of the atoms involved and the type of bond between them. Table III gives the bond energy and the bond distance for some covalent bonds.

Polar Bonds: Partial Ionic Bond and Ionic Bond—There are many different types of partial ionic bonds between the two extremes of a covalent bond and an ionic bond. The tendency of a pair of atoms to form an ionic or a partial ionic bond is measured by the difference in their abilities to attract an electron, or in their *electronegativities*.

If a molecule acts as if it has a positive and a negative pole (ie, has a partial separation of charge), it is called a dipole. A molecule with dipolar bonds

Table II—Electronic Configurations of Some Elements in Their Ground States

Atomic no.	Elements	1s (K, l=0)	2s (L, l=0)	2p (L, l=1)	3s (M, l=0)	3p (M, l=1)	3d (M, l=2)	4s (N, l=0)	4p (N, l=1)	4d (N, l=2)	4f (N, l=3)
1	H	1									
2	He	2									
3	Li	2	1								
4	Be	2	2								
5	B	2	2	1							
6	C	2	2	2							
7	N	2	2	3							
8	O	2	2	4							
9	F	2	2	5							
10	Ne	2	2	6							
11	Na	*Neon core*			1						
12	Mg				2						
13	Al				2	1					
14	Si				2	2					
15	P				2	3					
16	S				2	4					
17	Cl				2	5					
18	A				2	6					
19	K							1				Beginning of
20	Ca							2				1st long period
21	Sc						1	2			
22	Ti						2	2			
23	V						3	2			
24	Cr						5	1			
25	Mn						5	2				1st transition
26	Fe	*Argon core*					6	2				series
27	Co						7	2			
28	Ni						8	2			
29	Cu						10	1			
30	Zn						10	2			
31	Ga						10	2	1		
32	Ge						10	2	2		
33	As						10	2	3		
34	Se						10	2	4		
35	Br						10	2	5		
36	Kr						10	2	6		

is said to be polar, while an electrically symmetric molecule is designated nonpolar.

The electronegativity values for some common elements are listed in Table IV. The relationship between electronegativity difference and the partial ionic character is shown in Table V.

Dipole Moment—The process by which dipoles arise is known as polarization. The total polarization P can be written as

$$P = P_i + P_o + P_a \qquad (5)$$

The induced or electronic polarization P_i represents the shift of the electron cloud due to the influence of an electric field or an electromagnetic wave such as light. The induced molar polarization P_i can be determined from molar refraction measurements using the D-line of a sodium lamp since the permanent

dipole cannot follow an electromagnetic wave of such high frequency:

$$P_i = \frac{n_D^2 - 1}{n_D^2 + 2} \cdot \frac{M}{d} = R \qquad (6)$$

Eq. 6 is known as the Lorenz–Lorentz equation, where n_D is the refractive index of the liquid measured with the D-line of a sodium lamp, M is the molecular weight, d is the density, and R is the molar refraction.

One can also calculate the induced molar polarization from the electron group refractions given by Smyth,[10] or from the atomic refractivities compiled by Fajans[11] (Table VI). For example, the molar refraction of methyl acetate (CH_3—C—O—CH_3) can be

$$\overset{\|}{\underset{O}{}}$$

calculated as follows:

			Na-D (c.c.)
$3 \times C$	$= 3 \times 2.42$	$=$	7.26
$6 \times H$	$= 6 \times 1.10$	$=$	6.60
$1 \times\, =O$	$= 1 \times 2.21$	$=$	2.21
$1 \times$ —O—	$= 1 \times 1.64$	$=$	1.64
		Total $=$	17.71 (c.c.)

or

$$R = \frac{n_D^2 - 1}{n_D^2 + 2} \cdot \frac{M}{d}$$

$$= \left[\frac{(1.3593)^2 - 1}{(1.3593)^2 + 2}\right] \cdot \left[\frac{74.08}{0.928}\right] \text{(at 20°C)}$$

$$= 17.57 \text{ (c.c.)}$$

An apparent correlation between the activity of chloramphenicol analogs, as determined by microbial kinetics, and the group refraction of their aromatic substituents has been reported.[12]

In Eq. 5 P_o is the orientation polarization due to the permanent dipole, and P_a is the atomic polarization, which may be neglected for practical purposes since it is only 5–10% of P_i. The orientation polar-

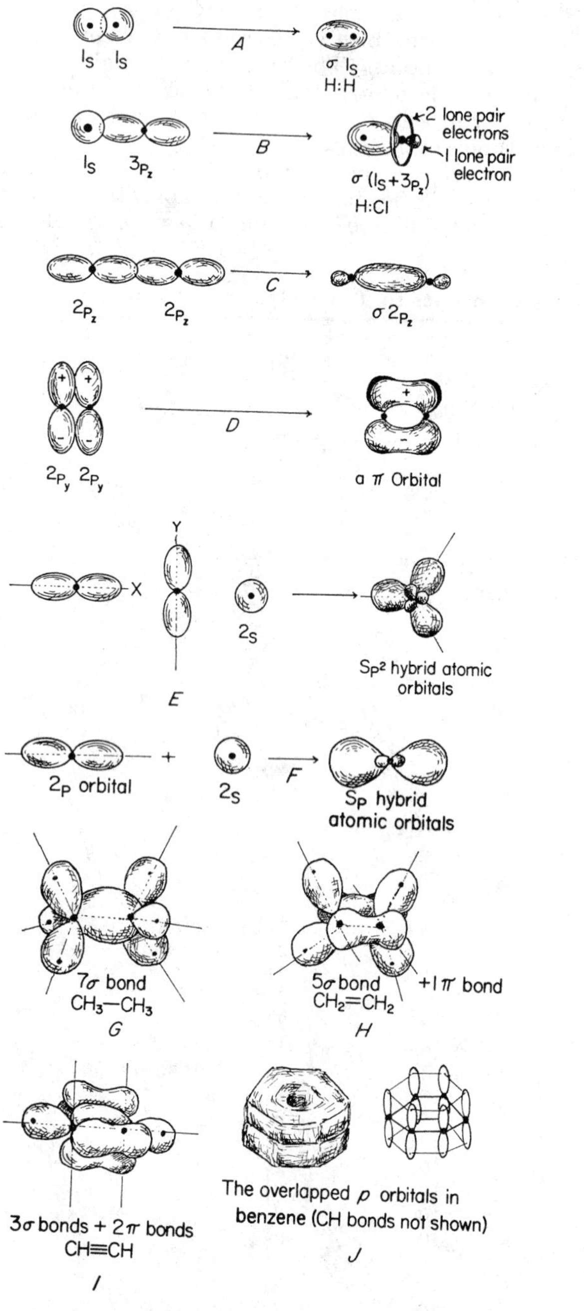

Fig. 121. **Formation of molecular orbitals from the overlap of atomic orbitals.**

Table III—Covalent Bond Energy

Bond	Bond energy, ΔH Kcal/mole	Bond distance, Å
H—H	103.2^a	0.74^c
H—Cl	102.1^a	1.27^c
O—H	109.4^a	0.96^b
N—H	92.2^a	1.01^b
C—H	98.2^a	1.09^b
C—Cl	78^a	1.77^b
Cl—Cl	57.8^a	1.99^c
C—C	80^a	1.54^b
C=C	130^a	1.33^b
C≡C	193^a	1.20^b
C=O	152^b	1.21^b

^{a} From Pitzer.[7]
^{b} From Fieser and Fieser.[8]
^{c} Pauling.[9a]

Table IV—Electronegativity Values for Some Elements^a

F	4.0	I	2.4	Be	1.5
O	3.5	P	2.1	Mg	1.2
N	3.0	H	2.1	Li	1.0
Cl	3.0	B	2.0	Ca	1.0
Br	2.8	Si	1.8	Na	0.9
S	2.5	Sn	1.7	K	0.8
C	2.5	Al	1.5	Cs	0.7

^{a} Adapted from Pauling.[9b]

Table V—The Difference in Electronegativities and Ionic Character of Some Chemical Bonds[a]

Bond	Electronegativity difference, $X_a - X_b$	Partial ionic character, %
C—H	0.4	4
I—Br	0.4	4
I—Cl	0.6	9
O—H	1.4	30
C—F	1.5	44
Si—F	2.2	70
Be—F	2.5	79
K—F	3.2	92

[a] cf, Pauling.[9c]

ization P_o arises from the separation of charges due to the difference in electronegativities of the atoms.

Using an electromagnetic wave of much lower frequency than the frequency of light, such as a radio wave, one can measure the total polarization since the permanent dipole as well as the electron cloud can follow the alternation of direction of the radio wave. In other words one can calculate P from dielectric constant and molar volume (M/d) measurements:

$$P = \frac{\epsilon - 1}{\epsilon + 2} \cdot \frac{M}{d} \quad (7)$$

From Eqs. 5–7, Debye's equation (Eq. 8) for a pure compound, the Clausius-Mossotti equation (Eq. 9), and by neglecting P_a, we have Eq. 10:

$$P = \frac{4}{3} \pi N_A \left(\alpha + \frac{\mu^2}{3kT} \right) \quad (8)$$

$$P_i = \frac{4}{3} \pi N_A \alpha \quad (9)$$

$$P_o = P - P_i = \frac{4}{3} \pi N_A \frac{\mu^2}{3kT} \quad (10)$$

where N_A is Avogadro's number, α is the induced polarizability (a measure of the ease of polarization by an electric field), μ is the dipole moment (esu-cm), k is the Boltzmann constant, and T is the absolute temperature. It should be noted that molar refraction is a molar property and induced polarizability is a molecular property.

Eq. 8 can be written as

$$P = a + b/T \quad (11)$$

where $a = 4\pi N_A \alpha/3 = P_i$, $b = 4\pi N_A \mu^2/9k$. Since Eq. 11 is a linear equation, by plotting values of P at several temperatures (calculated from dielectric constant measurements) vs $1/T$, one can compute α and P_i from the intercept and the permanent dipole moment (μ) of the compound from the slope b. This procedure is usually applied to gases.

For a pure liquid one can obtain the total polarization P according to Eq. 7 and the induced polarization P_i from refractive index and molar volume measurements at a constant temperature (Eq. 6). Regardless of the manner of obtaining P_i, the final equation for the calculation of the dipole moment, usually expressed in Debye units, is the same (Eq. 12). One Debye unit (D) is equivalent to 10^{-18} esu-cm.

$$\mu = \sqrt{\frac{9kb}{4\pi N_A}} = 0.0128 \times 10^{-18} \sqrt{b} =$$

$$0.0128 \times 10^{-18} \sqrt{(P - P_i)T} \text{ (esu-cm)} =$$

$$0.0128 \sqrt{(P - P_i)T} \text{ (Debye units)} \quad (12)$$

There are other equations for calculating dipole moments from measured values of the dielectric constant, refractive index, and density of liquids.[13] However, for pure liquids the results are not very satisfactory. The dipole moment of medicinal substances is usually measured in a nonpolar solvent, eg, benzene, cyclohexane, heptane, or in a solvent with some polarity but without resultant moment, eg, dioxane.

Halverstadt and Kumler[14] suggest using only the results of measurements on dilute solutions in order to eliminate the inaccuracies that arise from treating the solvent in a different way than solutions. For the experimental method and the equation for calculation the student should consult the original paper.

Correlations of biological activity with dipole moment have been reported for the insecticidal activity of chlorphenothane (DDT) isomers,[15] the cholinesterase inhibitory activity of N-alkylsubstituted amides,[16] and the respiratory stimulation activity of cyclic ureas and cyclic thioureas.[17]

When the electronegativities of the bonded atoms are quite different, a formal electron pair bond can no longer exist. The bonding electron pair is now associated exclusively with the more electronegative atom and an *anion* is formed. The atom which has lost its electron becomes positively charged and a *cation* is formed.

Coordinate Covalent Bonds—A coordinate covalent bond is formed when only one atom donates both electrons. For example, the unshared electron pair on the nitrogen atom of an amine can serve to form such a bond with a proton or trimethyl boron:

$$\begin{array}{c} R'' \\ | \\ R'-N: \\ | \\ R \end{array} + H^\oplus \rightarrow \left[\begin{array}{c} R'' \\ | \\ R'-N:H \\ | \\ R \end{array} \right]^\oplus$$

$$\begin{array}{cc} R'' & CH_3 \\ | & | \\ R'-N: & +B-CH_3 \\ | & | \\ R & CH_3 \end{array} \rightarrow \left[\begin{array}{cc} R'' & CH_3 \\ | & | \\ R'-N:B-CH_3 \\ | & | \\ R & CH_3 \end{array} \right]$$

Since the nitrogen suffers a loss of negative charge and the boron atom gains an equivalent negative charge, it is more realistic to depict the complex molecule as:

$$\begin{array}{cc} R'' & CH_3 \\ | & | \\ R'-N^{\delta+}-B^{\delta-}-CH_3 \\ | & | \\ R & CH_3 \end{array}$$

Amine oxides are other examples of coordinate covalent compounds:

$$\begin{array}{cc} R'' & R'' \\ | & | \\ R'-N\rightarrow O \quad \text{or} \quad R'-N^\oplus-O^\ominus \\ | & | \\ R & R \end{array}$$

Because oxygen is far more electronegative than boron (see Table IV), the ionic character of the N-oxide is more pronounced than that of the N—B bond. This is evidenced by the relatively high melting point, high solubility in water, and low solubility in nonpolar solvents of the amine oxides. One can also infer the polar character by a comparison of dipole moments: 6.2 D for KCl (ion pairs), 5.02 D for trimethylamine oxide,

Table VI—Atomic and Group Refractions for Sodium-D Light

Element	Na_D (c.c.)		Na_D (c.c.)
C	2.42	N in	
H	1.10	Aliphatic oximes	3.93
O in OH	1.52	R—CONH₂	2.65
O in ester OR	1.64	R—CONHR′	2.27
O=	2.21	R—CONR′R″	2.71
F	1.22	NO₂ group in	
Cl	5.96	Alkyl nitrates	7.59
Br	8.86	Alkyl nitrites	7.44
I	13.90	Nitroparaffins	6.72
S in SH	7.69	Aromatic nitro	
S in R S	7.97	Compounds	7.30
S in RCNS	7.91	Nitramines	7.51
S in R S	8.11	NO group in	
N in		Nitrites	5.92
Hydroxylamines	2.48	Nitrosamines	5.37
Hydrazines	2.47	Structural units	
RNH₂	2.32	Double bond	1.73
RNHR′	2.49	Triple bond	2.40
RNR′R″	2.84	3-membered ring	0.71
ArNH₂	3.21	4-membered ring	0.48
ArNHR	3.59	Oxirane	
ArNRR′	4.36	Terminal	2.02
R—C≡N	3.05	Non-terminal	1.85
Ar—C≡N	3.79	Conjugation—(cf, Ref. 11)	

and 3.92 D for the trimethylamine–trimethylboron complex.

Chelates—The term chelate (Gk, *chela*, claw) describes this class of compounds appropriately. Chelates consist of a partial ring of atoms which close up by holding a given atom, usually a metal, in a molecular claw. The compounds capable of forming a ring structure with a metal are designated as ligands.

Due to the range of normal bond angles, 5- and 6-member rings are most stable. The 5-membered ring is usually the most stable for a ring of single bonds only, whereas 6-member rings have maximum stability when there are two double bonds in the ring.[18] The copper chelates of glycine (I) and salicylaldehyde (II) and the calcium chelate of ethylenediamine tetraacetic acid (**EDTA, III**) are some examples:

Some biologically important compounds (eg, chlorophyll, hemoglobin, peroxidases, cytochromes, oxidases, ascorbic acid oxidase, tyrosinase, polyphenoloxidase, laccase, phosphatase, carboxylases, insulin, and cyanocobalamin) are naturally occurring chelates. Tetracyclines are also capable of forming chelates with metals. Chelating agents may be used for a number of purposes, such as sequestration of metals, stabiliza-

tion of drug preparations vulnerable to oxidation in the presence of trace of metals, and for the treatment of heavy metal poisoning.

Molecular Bonds—Several classes of compounds contain *intermolecular coordinate covalent bonds*, eg, "sandwich" compounds, charge transfer complexes, and the molecular addition compounds. These types of bonds are referred to as *molecular bonds* for brevity.

Metallocenes—In 1951 Kealy and Pauson accidently discovered ferrocene by oxidizing cyclopentadienemagnesium bromide with anhydrous ferric chloride in ether solution.[19] Ferrocene has aromatic character and is an unusually stable iron-containing orange product with the formula $C_{10}H_{10}Fe$, that melts at 174° and boils at 249°; it is soluble in common organic solvents but insoluble in water. The generally accepted structure of ferrocene was first proposed by Woodward and his co-workers.[20] X-ray and electron diffraction studies have shown that the iron is packed between two parallel cyclopentadienyl rings,[21,22] like a sandwich (**IV**).

The solubility, volatility, and other properties of metallocenes are due to the covalent character of the molecular bonds. This indicates that each cyclopentadienyl ion donates an electron pair to the metal ion. Ferrocene is diamagnetic, hence the six $3d$ electrons of iron are paired up to make available two open $3d$ orbitals. A large number of metallocenes have been prepared and studied since the discovery of ferrocene.

Several different aromatic rings (eg, indene, azulene, benzene, and others) will also form metallocenes. In many metallocenes, CO or NO molecules are found in place of one of the aromatic rings, and the metal may be Cr or Mn, as well as Fe. Metallocenes undergo most of the typical aromatic reactions.[23] Their biological activities would be interesting to explore.

Recent work[24] has opened up a new field of research which combines polyhedral carborane and transition metal chemistry. Several families of polyhedral species are now known in which a transition metal resides in the polyhedral surface (**V, VI**).

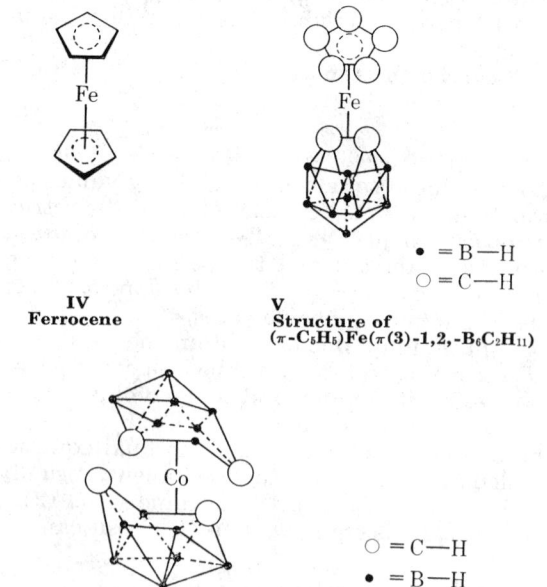

IV
Ferrocene

V
Structure of
$(\pi\text{-}C_5H_5)Fe(\pi(3)\text{-}1,2,\text{-}B_9C_2H_{11})$

● = B—H
○ = C—H

○ = C—H
● = B—H

VI
Structure of the (B₇C₂H₉)₂ CO⁻ ion obtained from B₇C₂H₁₁⁻⁻ and CO⁺⁺

Charge-Transfer Complexes—Certain substances combine in a 1:1 molar ratio to form crystalline

M = Metal ion

I

II

III

addition products. The molecular addition compound is held together by weak forces, such as van der Waals (dipole–dipole, dipole–induced dipole, induced dipole–induced dipole), ion–dipole, and even hydrogen bonds. Polynitroaromatic compounds, such as trinitrobenzene and picric acid, are well known for their ability to form charge-transfer complexes (pi complexes) (VII, VIII).

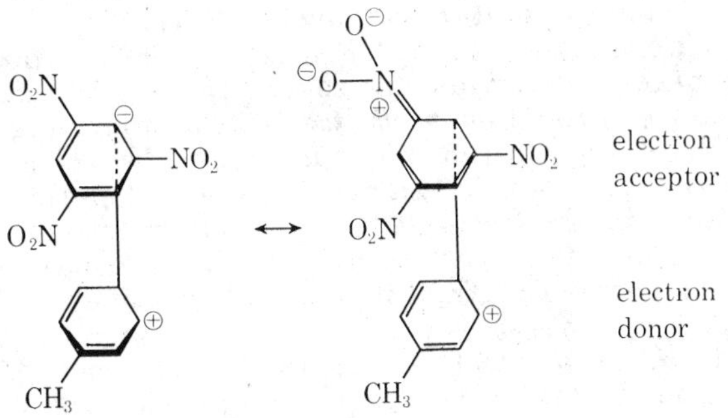

VII
1,3,5-Trinitrobenzene–toluene complex

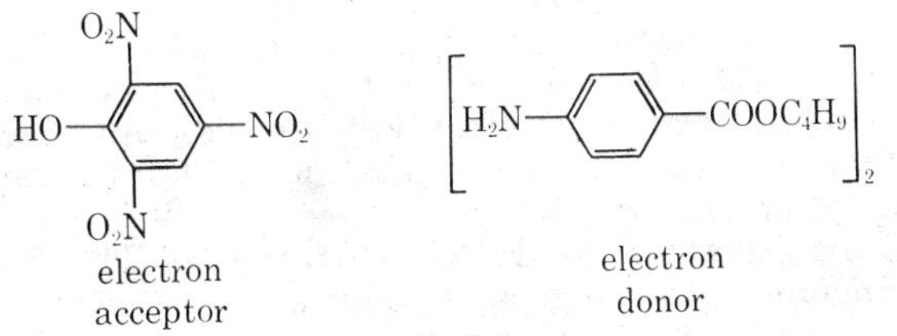

electron acceptor

electron donor

VIII
Butesin picrate

Caffeine complexes with various drugs, such as sodium benzoate, sodium salicylate, sulfonamides, barbiturates[25] and 5-chlorosalicylic acid.[26]

Aromatic Sigma (σ) Bond Complexes—Aromatic compounds react with HCl.AlCl₃ or HF.BF₃ to produce salts that ionize in highly polar nonaqueous solvents, eg, liquid hydrogen fluoride or sulfuric acid:

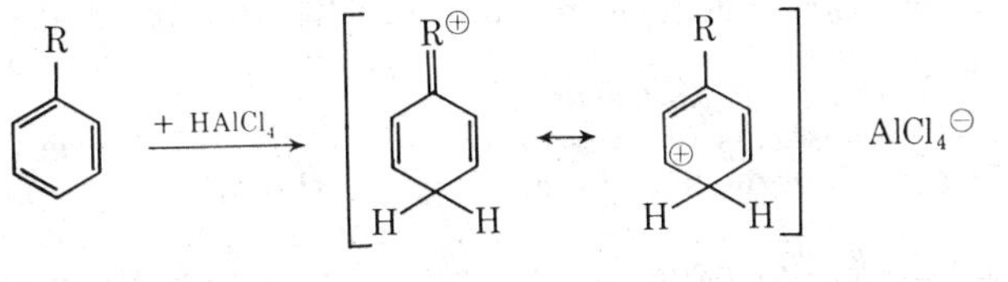

Using NMR spectroscopy Olah and his co-workers[27] detected the *p*-anisonium and the 2,4,6-trimethyl-phenonium ions produced by ionizing β-*p*-anisyl ethyl chloride and β-mesityl ethyl chloride in, respectively, SbF₅—SO₂ at −70° to −60°C:

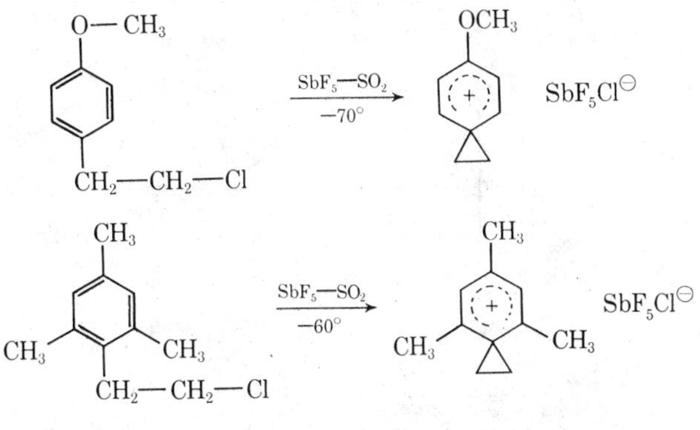

Sigma complexes are molecular complexes resulting from the rupture of a sigma bond (eg, H—AlCl₄,

ArCH₂CH₂—Cl); they also occur in Friedel–Crafts reactions. Since they are reactive toward water, no practical pharmaceutical uses have been made of these complexes.

Stereoisomerism—Early in 1874 van't Hoff envisaged a double bond by joining two tetrahedra at two corners, and correctly predicted that unsymmetrically substituted derivatives of ethylene should exist in two stereochemical forms, or as a pair of *cis* and *trans* isomers. From our previous discussion of σ and π bonds, we know that in an alkene rotation about the σ bond is restricted by the overlap of *p* orbitals comprising the π bond.

The stereoisomerism due to the rigid configuration about a double bond or other rigid structure such as a ring is known as *geometric isomerism*. It is interest-

cis   *trans*

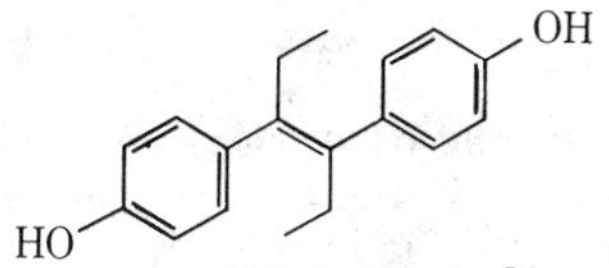

trans-**Diethylstilbestrol**

ing to note that in the case of the synthetic estrogens, the *cis*-isomer of diethylstilbestrol is unstable and has less than one-tenth the activity of the *trans*-isomer.

Due to the presence of symmetry, the type of geometric isomerism occurring in substituted ethylenes is not usually associated with optical activity; some other site in the molecule ordinarily gives rise to optical isomerism.

Another type of geometric isomerism is found in ring compounds, the ring taking the place of the rigid double bond. For example, *trans*-2-phenylcyclopropylamine is more stable than the *cis*-isomer and is a potent monoamine oxidase inhibitor.[28,29]

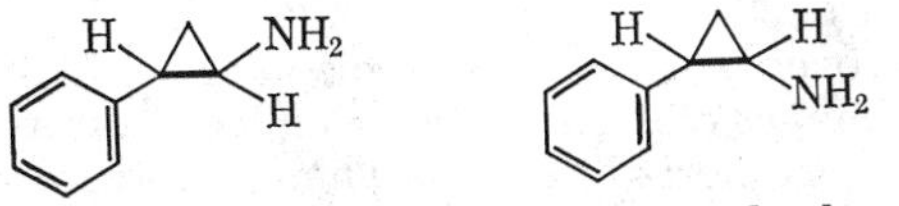

trans-2-**Phenylcyclopropylamine**
(Tranylcypromine)

cis-2-**Phenylcyclopropylamine**

A substance that rotates the plane of polarized light is said to be optically active. *Optical rotation* may be considered as a consequence of the phenomenon of circular double refraction in which a beam of polarized rays is resolved into two circulary polarized rays, one turning clockwise and the other counterclockwise as the beam advances. In an optically active medium these rays have different velocities and on recombination they vibrate in a plane different from that of the incident ray.

The necessary and sufficient condition for a molecule to show optical activity is that the molecule should be dissymmetric; ie, the molecule should not be superimposable with its mirror image. Although many optically active compounds have asymmetric carbon atoms (carbon atoms bearing four different groups), not all compounds possessing asymmetric carbon atoms are optically active. For example, *meso*-tartaric acid has two asymmetric carbon atoms, but it is optically inactive due to the presence of a plane of symmetry within the molecule.

COOH	COOH	COOH
H—C—OH	HO—C—H	H—C—OH
H—C—OH	H—C—OH	HO—C—H
COOH	COOH	COOH
meso-Tartaric acid	D(—)Tartaric acid	L(+)Tartaric acid

Optical isomerism due to restricted rotation (eg, as with *tetra-ortho*-substituted biphenyls and dissymmetric polyphenyls) is well documented in Eliel's book.[30] Atoms other than carbon can serve as a center of asymmetry. For instance, optically active N-oxides, quaternary ammonium compounds, sulfonium and selenonium salts, sulfoxides, and sulfinic esters have been resolved.[31]

Enantiomorphs—Molecules whose mirror images are nonsuperimposable are called enantiomorphs, enantiomers, or optical antipodes. Enantiomorphs have identical physicochemical properties in an optically inactive environment; they rotate the plane of polarized light to the same degree but in opposite directions.

The measurement of optical rotation is useful for the purpose of identifying and/or assaying an optically active substance. The *specific rotation* is defined as:

$$[\alpha]_D^t = \frac{\alpha}{l \cdot (Gm/v)}$$

where D stands for the D-line of sodium vapor lamp, t is the temperature, α is the rotation in degrees, l is the length of the cell in decimeters (1 dm = 10 cm), and Gm/v is the concentration in grams per milliliter.

When equal amounts of *dextro*- and *levo*-isomers are mixed a *racemic modification* arises. They are denoted as (d,l) or $(\pm)$. Racemic modifications occur in most organic syntheses; they also may be obtained by racemization of a pure enantiomer. In a racemic modification the substance in bulk is not optically active, even though the individual molecule is optically active. The over-all rotation is zero due to the cancellation of rotations with equal magnitude but different signs.

Diastereoisomers—Stereoisomers which are not mirror images of each other are called diastereoisomers. Diastereoisomerism exists when a given structural formula has at least two asymmetric atoms:

CHO	CHO	CHO	CHO
H—C—OH	HO—C—H	HO—C—H	H—C—OH
H—C—OH	HO—C—H	H—C—OH	HO—C—H
CH₂OH	CH₂OH	CH₂OH	CH₂OH
(−) Erythrose	(+) Erythrose	(−) Threose	(+) Threose

Enantiomorphs   Enantiomorphs

Diastereoisomers

Optical Rotatory Dispersion (ORD)[32,33]—Optical rotatory dispersion involves the measurement of the angle of optical rotation at various wavelengths. Usually greater rotational angles are obtained at shorter wavelengths. The source of light consists of a xenon arc, and a monochromator to isolate the desired wavelength in the ultraviolet region. A photomultiplier and photometer are used to measure the intensity after the light has passed through the polarimeter.

As the wavelength of the polarized light is varied, the absolute value of rotation may increase continuously, so that the plot of $[\alpha]$ vs λ is a plain curve (Line A, Fig. 122). On the other hand, the rotation may change direction either from left to right or right to left, and show one or more maxima and minima.

The appearance of a maximum and a minimum in a plot of specific rotation vs wavelength is referred to as *single Cotton effect* (Line B, Fig. 122), while the appearance of several maxima and several minima is referred to as a *multiple Cotton effect*. If in approaching the region of the Cotton effect from long wavelengths, one passes first through a maximum and then through a minimum, the Cotton effect is called "positive," but if the minimum is reached first and then the maximum at shorter wavelength, it is called a "negative" Cotton effect.

The Cotton effect is due to the presence of an asymmetric center near a chromophoric group (eg, $C=O$) in the optically active molecule which has unequal absorption of right and left circularly polarized light. ORD is useful for the study of the stereochemistry of natural products,[34] ketosteroids, and for the analysis of randomly coiled and helical configurations of polypeptide chains.[35]

Configuration and Conformation—The spatial arrangement of the groups about a central atom is referred to as the *configuration* of the atom. Three-dimensional models, their projections, or perspective drawings must be used to illustrate the difference between stereoisomers. The particular shape that a molecule assumes by free rotation about single bonds is referred to as its conformation.

It may be thought that an ethane molecule may have an infinite number of conformations because of rotation about the C—C bond; however, only a few conformations are possible which will make the molecular energy a minimum. The conformational preferences of some diastereoisomers have been determined from NMR studies.[36]

For a series of diastereoisomers involving a substituted phenylethyl skeleton, when the alkyl groups attached to each asymmetric center are small (eg, methyl), both *gauche* and *trans* conformers (rotamers) have substantial populations because of the relatively low rotational barriers. Newman projection formulas[37] are used for the illustrations. In these projection formulas, the molecules are viewed from front to

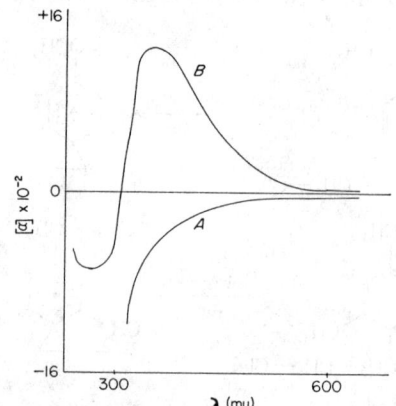

Fig. 122. Rotatory dispersion curves: (A) levorotatory plain curve; (B) positive simple Cotton effect.

back in the direction of the bond linking the asymmetric carbon atoms. In the following formulas, the center of the circle represents C_2 and the circle represents C_3 of 3-phenyl-2-butanol

$$(CH_3 \overset{2}{-} CHOH \overset{3}{-} CH - C_6H_5):$$
$$\underset{CH_3}{|}$$

(gauche)   (gauche)

(trans or anti)   (trans or anti)
Erythro-3-phenyl-   Threo-3-phenyl-
2-butanol   2-butanol

When the alkyl groups are large (eg, isopropyl), steric interactions cause the bulky groups to prefer a *trans* orientation; the vicinal hydrogens are then *trans* in the *erythro* but *gauche* in the *threo* isomers. For a more detailed discussion of potential energy barriers in various systems, the student should consult Eliel's book.[37]

(trans or anti)   (gauche)
2,5-Dimethyl-4-phenyl-3-hexanol

The preferred conformation of serotonin has been calculated using molecular orbital theory.[38] Complementary features of the serotonin receptor have been postulated and the relationship of serotonin in its preferred conformation to the serotonin antagonist, LSD, has been presented as an explanation of LSD's antagonism.

Calculated preferred conformation of serotonin

Intermolecular Binding Forces

An understanding of intermolecular and intramolecular binding forces is very important in many different aspects of pharmaceutical sciences, such as in the manufacture of various preparations, in stability studies, and in the design of new drugs. A knowledge of these forces is not only essential for predicting some physicochemical properties of various dosage forms, but also indispensable for the interpretation of drug action at the molecular level and for structure–activity correlations.

Martin's classification[39] for various types of forces will be used in the following discussion.

Repulsive and Attractive Forces—Intermolecular repulsive forces exist when two dipolar molecules are brought close together "head-to-head" or "tail-to-tail," or when any two molecules are brought so close that their nonbonding electronic clouds interpenetrate. Otherwise, two molecules having opposite charges closer together than the like charges, will attract each other. When the repulsive and the attractive forces are equal, the potential energy of the two molecules is a minimum and an equilibrium will be established. Similar forces may exist in the same molecule (intramolecular) as well as between different molecules. Only intermolecular forces will be discussed here.

Van der Waals Forces—Due to electrostatic attraction, dipolar molecules tend to align themselves with neighboring molecules so that the negative pole of one molecule points towards the positive pole of the next (eg, $\overset{\leftarrow}{O=C<} \ldots \overset{\leftarrow}{:NR_3}$). This type of attraction is known as a *dipole–dipole* interaction and has a force of 1–7 Kcal/mole. Dipole–dipole forces vary inversely as the 4th power of the distance between molecules, $F \propto (1/d^4)$.

The importance of the permanent dipole attractions in the stabilization of an α-helix has been pointed out by Levinthal.[40] The electric dipoles in an α-helix add to one another along the direction of the axis. Two helices that wind in the same direction will, therefore, repel each other and two that wind in opposite directions will attract each other.

Permanent dipoles can induce a transient electric dipole in nonpolar molecules and produce *dipole-induced dipole* or Debye forces. These interactions involve a force of about 1–3 Kcal/mole.

When any two atoms belonging to different molecules are brought sufficiently close together, *induced dipole–induced dipole* or London attractions arise. In this case, the force is about 0.5–1 Kcal/mole. These forces originate from molecular internal vibrations. The temporary dipoles which this vibration creates in the constituent atoms induce dipoles in neighboring atoms of other molecules, and this process results in a net attraction.

This type of force is responsible for the liquefaction of nonpolar gases. London forces vary inversely as the 7th power of the distance between molecules, $F \propto (1/d^7)$.

Hydrogen Bonds—When a hydrogen atom holds two other atoms, a hydrogen bond (hydrogen bridge) is formed. The two bonds attached to the same hydrogen cannot both be covalent bonds. The H-bond must be in part ionic. Indeed, the hydrogen bond is usually formed only between electronegative atoms. In addition, the atoms capable of forming H-bonds have at least one unshared electron pair.

Without hydrogen bonds this world would be much different, since water would boil at a temperature far below 0°C. The surprisingly high boiling point of H_2O (100°) compared to H_2S ($-60.7°$) and H_2Se ($-41.5°$) can be attributed to the higher H-bonding ability of oxygen, which in turn is due to its smaller volume and higher electron density as compared to S and Se.

The most common atoms capable of forming H-bonds are F, O, N, and to a lesser degree Cl and S. There is also some evidence that hydrogen attached to a triply bonded carbon (eg, HCN, HC≡CH, or $CHCl_3$) forms H-bonds. The strength of most H-bonds ranges from 1–7 Kcal/mole:

H-bond	Bond strength (Kcal/mole)
F—H...F	7
O—H...O	4.5–7.6
O—H...N	4–7
C—H...π electrons	2–4
C—H...O	2–3
N—H...O	2–3
N—H...N	1.3

The strength of the H-bond depends on the solvent as well as the state. For instance, the H-bond strength of O—H...O for $(CH_3COOH)_2$ as a vapor is 7.64 Kcal/mole, while that of $(CH_3COOH)_2$ in benzene is 4.85 Kcal/mole. In water the H-bond has been estimated to have an energy of 4.5 Kcal/mole; in ice the bond strength is 6 Kcal/mole. Hydrogen bonding is responsible for the higher boiling point of a carboxylic acid compared with that of its ester. This is due to the fact that in the free acid dimerization can occur by H-bonding, while this is impossible for an ester.

Hydrogen bonding is also responsible for the high solubility of polyhydroxy compounds, such as sugars, in water. During the replication of DNA molecules, hydrogen bonds between base pairs are broken and rematched.

Various physical methods may be used to study H-bonding, such as molecular weight determination, and IR and NMR spectroscopy.

Ion-Dipole and Ion-Induced Dipole Forces—Ion pairs in the solid state have bond strengths comparable to or even stronger than covalent bonds (100–200 vs 50–150 Kcal/mole). However, in a biological system, due to hydration and the large amount of inorganic salts present for ion-exchange, the bond strength would be substantially weakened to the neighborhood of 5 Kcal/mole.[41]

When an ionic bond is reinforced by the simultaneous presence of other forces, such as hydrogen bonding, the bond becomes stronger (10 Kcal/mole for

$$
\begin{array}{ccc}
\text{H} & & \text{O} \\
| & & \text{\textbackslash} \\
—\text{N}^{\oplus} & \ominus \quad \text{C}— \\
\diagup \,\backslash & \diagup \\
\text{H} \quad \text{H} \cdots\cdots \text{O}
\end{array}
).
$$

An ion pair can attract a dipole or induce a dipole in a neighboring nonpolar molecular. The strength of an *ion–dipole* bond (eg, $R_4\overset{\oplus}{N}\ldots:\overset{\leftarrow}{N}R_3$) is about 1–7 Kcal/mole, and that of an *ion–induced* dipole (eg, $\overset{\oplus}{K}—\overset{\ominus}{I}...I—I$) would be somewhat weaker.

Hydrophobic Interactions—The association of nonpolar groups with each other in aqueous solution, arising because of the tendency of water molecule to exclude nonpolar molecules, is known as a hydrophobic interaction, or "hydrophobic bonding." The word hydrophobic is really a misnomer. It implies that the nonpolar molecule dislikes water; in fact, it is water that dislikes the nonpolar molecule.

The formation of hydrophobic bonds is favored because of an entropy effect. Before the formation of a hydrophobic bond, water molecules are arranged in an ordered fashion around exposed nonpolar groups. When hydrophobic interactions occur, the order is disrupted and results in a favorable entropy change. The entropy change is great enough to overcome the enthalpy for the interaction of the nonpolar groups,

and hence the free energy is negative and the process is spontaneous. The strength of hydrophobic interactions has been reported to be 0.37 Kcal/mole per CH_2 group.[42]

A side chain of C_{14} which binds with another nonpolar counterpart would have a bond strength of 5.2 Kcal/mole. This bond, being stronger than an ionic bond or other weak forces in the biological system, may then dominate the mode of binding of a complicated drug molecule. The importance of hydrophobic interactions in stabilizing protein structure, drug–protein binding, transport and storage of drugs, and drug–receptor interaction has been noted in recent years. More practical applications as well as further theoretical study should be expected in the future.

Additive Physical Properties

The division of physical properties into additive, constitutive, and colligative can be found in many textbooks. Additive physical properties depend on the number and kind of atoms in a molecule. Such additivity enables one to calculate many molecular values from a few fundamental constants. The best example is the calculation of molecular weights from atomic weights. The additive nature of molar refractions has been utilized for the calculation of induced polarization (see *Dipole Moment*).

Molar Volume—The term molar volume is self-explaining. It is defined as the molecular weight divided by the density of a liquid (molar volume = MW/d). Using statistical analysis, Exner[43] has shown that the additivity of molar volume is better fulfilled at ordinary temperatures (20°) rather than at the boiling point of each individual substance. This is an interesting result, since from the *Principle of Corresponding States* it might be expected that additivity would hold better at the boiling point.

In the homologous series of nonbranched primary derivatives the accuracy of a calculation of molar volume is relatively good. The deviations increase

Table VII—Some Values of Additive Increments for the Molar Volume Derived from Primary Monosubstituted Aliphatic Derivatives (20°)[a]

CH_2	16.58	COO	19.50
CH_3	31.48	SH	25.81
CH_2=CH—	42.48	S (in methyl sulfides)	10.78
CH≡C—	33.22	—S—S—	27.50
cyclo—C_5H_9	79.17	—NH_2	17.67
cyclo—C_6H_{11}	93.92	=N (in *sec* amines)	7.30
C_6H_5	74.65	≡N (in *tert* amines)	−5.09
1-Naphthyl-	107.32	CN	22.67
2-Naphthyl-	109.52	NO_2	24.51
F	15.11	PO_4	27.43
Cl	22.96	2-Pyridyl	67.66
Br	26.19	3-Pyridyl	66.44
I	32.93	4-Pyridyl	66.35
OH	10.25	2-C_5H_4NCOO—	87.62
O (in ethers)	6.74	3-C_5H_4NCOO—	88.89
—OCH_2O—	29.11	4-C_5H_4NCOO—	89.55
C_6H_5O—	79.20	2-Thienyl	65.58
CHO	25.08	2-C_4H_3SCO—	76.13
CO (in ketones)	10.21	2-C_4H_3SCOO—	87.49
COOH	27.24	C	9.34[b]
H	14.90[b]	5-membered ring	−13.22
Double bond	24.22	6-membered ring	11.17
Triple bond	44.76	(alicyclic)	

[a] Adapted from Exner.[43]
[b] Yielding only correct sums for the groups CH_2 and CH_3.

gradually with polysubstituted derivatives, 1,1-bis derivatives, *ortho* derivatives, and branched isomers; nevertheless, the additive scheme can serve as a first approximation. Table VII summarizes some values of additive increments for the molar volume. The atomic or group volumes may be useful in the estimation of the volume occupied by a molecule or a functional group in designing a new drug, especially when the size or the steric factor is important.

Parachor—The molar parachor is defined as

$$P = M.\gamma^{1/4}/(D\text{-}d)$$

where M is the molecular weight of the liquid, γ is its surface tension, D is the density of the liquid, and d is the density of the saturated vapor. The density of the vapor, since it is small, is generally neglected. This leads to the simpler equation:

$$P = M.\gamma^{1/4}/D$$

The parachor then can be calculated from the experimentally determined quantities γ and D. The surface tension γ has an almost negligible influence on the parachor, because of the exponent $1/4$.

Compilations of parachor values for various atoms and groups are available in the literature.[44,45] However, using statistical criteria Exner[45] has come to the conclusion that the concept of the parachor as a specially defined function of experimental quantities has no reason for existence. The structure problem can be solved on the basis of the molar volume with the same reliability as on the basis of the parachor.

Calculated parachors,[46] solubility parameters, and molar volumes[47] have been used to support the view that the molecular volume of the molecule is quite important in determining the narcotic property of simple organic compounds.

Partition Coefficients and the π Constant—In the early theory of narcosis, lipid solubility was regarded as the most important factor for the inhibition of cell activity. At the beginning of this century Meyer and Overton proposed that narcotic efficiency parallels the coefficient for the partition of a drug between oil and water. Although this theory cannot explain the mechanism of narcotic action, it does explain, at least, the mode of transport to nerve tissues.

It is more logical to use partition coefficients rather than solubility in a single solvent for structure–activity correlations since in a biological system one is dealing with a heterogeneous system rather than a simple solution. Partition coefficients have been used in the study of drug distribution, metabolism, toxicity,[48] and structure–activity correlation.[49]

Collander[50] has shown that the partition coefficients for a given compound in two different solvent systems (eg, ether/water, octanol/water) are related as follows: $\log P_1 = a \log P_2 + b$, where a and b are constants. This suggests that one can use the results from one set of solvents to predict results in a second set.

Hansch's group[51] has systematically extended the use of partition coefficients, measured from octanol/water, to serve as a measure of the ease of random walk of organic molecules through various lipoprotein barriers and/or as a measure of the hydrophobic binding with protein such as bovine serum albumin. From the partition coefficients of a variety of derivatives of the type $X—C_6H_4OCH_2COOH$, $X—C_6H_5$, and $C_6H_5(CH_2)_n—X$, the substituent constants (π) for the aromatic and the aliphatic function (X) have been determined.[52-54]

Table VIII—π Constants for Some Functional Groups[a]

Function	Aromatic system[b]	Aliphatic system
H—	0	0
F—	0.13	−0.17
Cl—	0.76	0.39
Br—	0.94	0.60
I—	1.15	1.00
CH_3—	0.50	0.50
$CH\equiv C$—		0.48
$CH_2=CH$—		0.70
C_2H_5—	1.00	1.00
$(CH_3)C=CH_2$		1.00
$CH_2=CHCH_2$—		1.20
n-C_3H_7—	1.50	1.50
i-C_3H_7—	1.30	1.30
n-C_4H_9—	2.00	2.00
sec-C_4H_9—	1.80	1.80
t-C_4H_9—	1.68	1.68
cyclo-C_3H_5—		1.21
cyclo-C_5H_9—	2.14	2.14
cyclo-C_6H_{11}—	2.51	2.51
C_6H_5—	2.13	2.13
—$(CH_2)_3$—	1.04	
—$(CH_2)_4$—	1.39	
—$(CH)_4$—	1.24	
—CF_3	1.07	
—CH_2OH	−1.03	−0.66
—CH_2COOH	−0.72	−0.76
—COOH	−0.28	−1.26
—$CONH_2$	−1.49	−1.71
—$COOCH_3$	−0.01	−0.27
—$COCH_3$	−0.55	−0.71
—CN	−0.57	−0.84
—OH	−0.67	−1.16
—OCH_3	−0.02	−0.47
—OCH_2COOH	−0.86	
—$OCOCH_3$	−0.64	−0.91
—NH_2	−1.23	−1.19
—$N(CH_3)_2$	−0.18	−0.32
—NO_2	−0.28	−0.82
—$NHCOCH_3$	−0.97	
—$NHCOC_6H_5$	0.72	
—$N=NC_6H_5$	1.69	
—$NHCONH_2$	−1.01	
—$S—CH_3$	0.62	
—SCF_3	1.58	
—SO_2CH_3	−1.26	
—SO_2CF_3	0.93	
—SF_5	1.50	
—SO_2NH_2	−1.82	

[a] Adapted from Refs. 52–55.
[b] From X—C_6H_5 or X—$C_6H_4OCH_2COOH$ system, for different positions in the later system slightly different values were reported in the original paper (Ref. 52). In cases where strong interaction between two functions can occur (eg, in phenol or aniline series), different π values should be used.

The π constant is defined as $\pi = \log P_X - \log P_H$, where P_X is the partition coefficient of a derivative and P_H is that of the parent compound. It is found that, although π varies continuously for a given function depending on its electronic environment, the variation is generally small; it is therefore called additive–constitutive.

The application of the additive–constitutive nature of π constants for the correlation of biological activity with chemical structure has been illustrated for a number of cases.[55-57] Table VIII lists the constants for some important functional groups. One can calculate many log P values from a few constants. The method of calculation can be illustrated with the drug diphenhydramine:

[Chemical structure with annotations:]

$\Sigma\pi = +4.26$ $+0.30$ -0.98 $+0.50$ -0.32

$3.76 = \text{calc} \log P$
$3.40 = \text{obs} \log P$

Good correlation has been reported for the hypnotic action of barbiturates in mice and their $\log P$ values:

$$\text{Activity} = \log 1/C = -0.438 \, (\log P)^2 + 1.579 \log P + 1.926 \quad (13)$$

n	r	s	$\log P_0$
13	0.969	0.098	1.80

In Eq. 13, C represents the moles of drug per kilogram of test animal producing hypnosis in 50% of the animals, n is the number of drugs tested, r is the correlation coefficient, and s is the standard deviation. It is interesting to note that the dependence of activity on $\log P$ is parabolic, and the optimum lipohydrophilic character ($\log P_0$) is not much different from those of alcohols or carbamates (all around 2.0).[58]

A linear relationship between the binding of penicillin derivatives by human serum and the π constant has been reported:[59]

$$\log (B/F) = 0.488 \Sigma\pi - 0.627 \quad \begin{array}{ccc} n & r & s \\ 79 & 0.924 & 0.134 \end{array} \quad (14)$$

In Eq. 14, B/F is the ratio of bound penicillin/free penicillin and $\Sigma\pi$ represents the sum of π values for the attached substituents on the side-chain R—:

[Chemical structure:]

$$R-CONH-CH-CH \overset{S}{\underset{N}{\diagup}} C(CH_3)_2$$
$$\underset{O}{\overset{\|}{C}} \qquad CHCOO^{\ominus}$$

X-ray Crystallographic Structural Analysis

In recent years the number of compounds of medicinal value that have been isolated from plant and animal sources and by purely synthetic means has increased astronomically. In addition to the many compounds isolated, the more sophisticated isolation techniques now available to the chemist have extended his capabilities of exploring biological molecules heretofore thought too complex to understand or investigate. The pharmaceutical chemist is thus faced with the complex task of identifying the chemical structure of a large number of complex materials.

For many of the compounds the chemist may rely on standard spectroscopic methods, ie, IR, UV, NMR, and ORD, together with other chemical measurements to elucidate molecular structure. Newer methods, especially mass spectroscopy, are slowly emerging as useful means of elucidating the structures of complex organic materials. Often these methods can provide only fragmentary evidence about various portions of the molecule, which must be pieced together to get the picture of the whole compound.

One of the most powerful of all techniques, when it can be used, is that of x-ray crystallographic analysis. Using this method, the three-dimensional structure of a molecule can be determined without relying on other chemical information.

The maximum resolution that can be obtained through an ordinary microscope under the most favorable of conditions is of the order of 2000 Å. This limitation is primarily imposed by the wavelength of the light that is utilized. In the more energetic portion of the electromagnetic spectrum, however, other forms of radiation that are capable of giving atomic resolution are found; viz, electron beams, neutrons, and x-rays.

Lenses have been constructed only for the first of these radiations, and at best they have a resolving power of about 6 Å. This resolution is insufficient to measure the distances between atoms, which are of the order of 1.5 Å. It is possible, however, to study the details of molecules without lenses, by means of diffraction experiments. Of the above three radiations, x-rays have proved to be the most useful and fruitful for studying molecular structure, and with the significant advances in computer technology the realm of structure analysis by x-ray diffraction is becoming more accessible to all scientists whose studies involve molecular structure.

The following discussion is primarily concerned with giving a brief survey of crystal structure analysis. A number of texts, which would be useful to the reader who wishes to pursue the subject further, are listed at the conclusion of the article.

Crystalline State

Atoms and molecules tend to organize themselves into their most favorable thermodynamic state, which under certain conditions results in their appearance as crystals. This form is characterized by a highly ordered arrangement of the molecules, associated with which is a three-dimensional periodicity. The repeating three-dimensional patterns, ideally depicted as lattices, are essential for x-ray structural analysis.

The *lattice* consists of an infinite array of points, none of which is distinguishable from the other. In

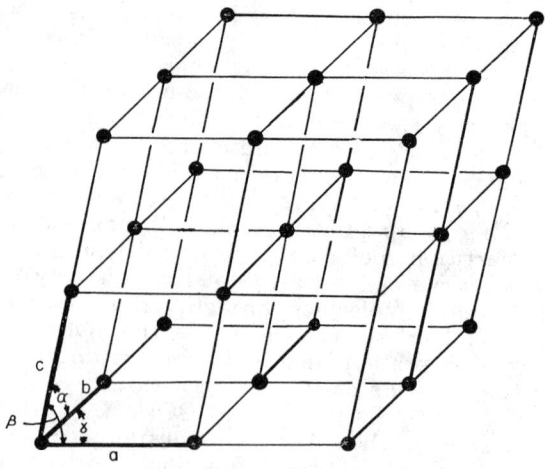

Fig. 123. Lattice network.

Fig. 123, a drawing of such a lattice is shown. It can be seen from this diagram that the points repeat themselves along the three directions labeled a, b, and c. The three unique translations denoted in this figure form a parallelepiped that makes up the basic repeating unit, which is termed the *unit cell*. In general, the unit cell is characterized by the three translational directions and the angles associated with them: α, β, and γ.

Bravais (1848), using geometrical arguments, showed that only 14 possible lattices can be constructed. This means that a similar set of points can be arranged in only 14 different ways in three dimensions. The points in Fig. 123 are aligned in a primitive (P) manner, ie, the unit cell essentially contains one point at each of the eight corners of the cell, each one being shared equally by the eight nearest neighboring cells.

The nonprimitive space lattices contain additional points to the primitive cell and are (1) c-centering (C) with an additional point in the center of the c-faces (defined by the planes parallel to the a and b axis), (2) body-centering (I) with an extra lattice point located at the center of the cell, (3) the face-centered cell (F) which has an additional point at the center of each of the six faces, and (4) the rhombohedral cell (R) which has points displaced along one of the diagonals of the primitive hexagonal cell. The rhombohedral lattice is usually considered to be a subgroup of the hexagonal system.

At this point it should be mentioned that the crystal is an ordered array of molecules or atoms, while the lattice consists only of points. A point, by virtue of its being dimensionless, has no meaningful symmetry associated with it, whereas a molecule may have any degree of symmetry.

Crystals are also classified by the shapes of their unit cells into seven different systems. The rhombohedral class (also referred to as trigonal) is generally considered under the hexagonal system. The various crystal systems together with the possible Bravais lattices associated with them are outlined in Table IX.

The fundamental distinction between these systems is through the symmetries that they possess. The symmetry associated with an isolated object is known as its point symmetry; ie, after a certain operation is performed on the object, it is still indistinguishable from its original appearance. Though there are a large number of symmetry operations, only certain ones are permissible in describing the geometrical shapes of crystals.

The important point symmetry operations are the rotation axes and the rotation–inversion axes. A rotation axis of order n is characterized by a rotation of $2\pi/n$ to bring the object into coincidence with itself. For crystals, n can only equal 1, 2, 3, 4, and 6. The inversion operation (denoted by $\bar{1}$ or i) takes every point x, y, z of the object to the point $-x$, $-y$, $-z$. There are higher order rotation–inversion axes such as $\bar{2}$, $\bar{3}$, $\bar{4}$, and $\bar{6}$, which are characterized by the rotation operation followed by inversion. The $\bar{2}$ operation is commonly symbolized by m (for mirroring).

The ten possible point group operations on crystals can be combined in only 32 different ways. The external symmetry of every crystal must conform with the operations associated with these 32 groups. Since crystals are not always perfectly formed, it is extremely difficult in many instances to discern the actual point group from external morphology. The crystal symmetry may reveal itself by the physical properties of the crystal, such as refractive indices, mechanical properties, conductivity, and thermal expansion.

The distribution of the 32 point groups among the various crystal systems is shown in Table IX together with the Hermann–Mauguin notation for their symmetries.

The repetition of the basic unit throughout the crystal gives rise to translational symmetry operations. In addition to the basic operation of pure translation, there are two other types of operations, namely screw axes and glide planes. The former involves the combined operation of rotation about an axis of order 2, 3, 4, or 6 and translation in the direction of the axis by a fraction (which is a multiple of $\frac{1}{2}$, $\frac{1}{3}$, $\frac{1}{4}$, or $\frac{1}{6}$, respectively) of the primitive translation in that direction.

The glide plane evolves from the combination of reflection across a plane (mirroring) and subsequent translation of a simple fraction of the primitive translation. These translational-symmetry operations, when combined with the point-symmetry of the various crystal systems, give rise to the various space groups. Though it would intuitively seem that there would be a huge number of ways of combining symmetry operations in forming the space groups, it was shown

Table IX

System	Bravais lattices	Unit cell parameters[a]	Point groups
Cubic	P, I, F	$a = b = c$ $\alpha = \beta = \gamma = 90°$	$\bar{4}3$; m3; 43; 43m; m3m
Tetragonal	P, I	$a = b \neq c$ $\alpha = \beta = \gamma = 90°$	4; $\bar{4}$; 4/m; 42; 4m; $\bar{4}2$m; 2/m mm
Hexagonal	P	$a = b \neq c$ $\alpha = \beta = 90°$ $\gamma = 120°$	3; $\bar{3}$; 32; 3m; $\bar{3}$m; 6; $\bar{6}$; 6/m;
Rhombohedral (Trigonal)	R	$a \neq b \neq c$ $\alpha = \beta = \gamma$	62; $\bar{6}$m; 6/m mm; $\bar{6}$m
Orthorhombic	P, C, F	$a \neq b \neq c$ $\alpha = \beta = \gamma = 90$	222; mm; mmm
Monoclinic	P, C	$a \neq b \neq c$ $\alpha = \gamma = 90$ $\beta \neq 90°$	2; m; 2/m
Triclinic	P	$a \neq b \neq c$ $\alpha \neq \beta \neq \gamma \neq 90°$	1; $\bar{1}$

[a] The $\neq$ symbol means *not necessarily equal to.*

independently by Federov and Schonflies in 1890 that there exist only 230 such groups. This was long before the first crystal structure was determined.

Every atomic or molecular arrangement in a crystal will fall into one of these space groups. Whereas the point group may be determined by macroscopic observations, the space groups can be determined only by a detailed examination of the molecular arrangement within the crystal. Volume I of the *International Tables for Crystallography* contains much useful data on these space groups.

X-Ray Diffraction

In 1912 von Laue and two of his students, Friedrich and Knipping, carried out an experiment with x-rays that opened the door to crystallographic structural analysis. They allowed a beam of nonhomogeneous x-rays to pass through a crystal of copper sulfate pentahydrate, and recorded by means of photographic plates, the diffracted x-ray beam. A diagram of the experimental setup is shown in Fig. 124.

The results indicated that x-rays which had been discovered by Roentgen less than two decades earlier had wave characteristics (wavelength: approximately 1 Å). Since a crystal was composed of a regular array of atoms with interatomic separations in the Angstrom (Å) range, they were able to show that the diffraction pattern obtained on the plates was due to the crystal acting as a three-dimensional diffraction grating towards the x-rays.

This discovery led Bragg to make use of x-rays for the study of the internal structures of crystals. He considered that x-rays are reflected from planes of atoms within the crystal lattice. The reflections from a particular family of planes will only occur at a particular angle of incidence and reflection. The essential condition for reflection is diagramed in Fig. 125. In this figure the "crests" of the two incident waves will stay in phase if the thickened portion of the path (as shown in the diagram) of one wave is an integral multiple (n) of the wavelength (λ). The condition for reflection is given by the well-known Bragg equation:

$$n\lambda = 2d \sin \theta.$$

The equation is only satisfied when $n = 1, 2, 3, \ldots$. If n is not a whole number, the waves will destructively interfere with each other and there will be no emergent beam.

In any crystal there are an infinite number of families of planes that can be constructed. These planes are usually denoted by their Miller indices

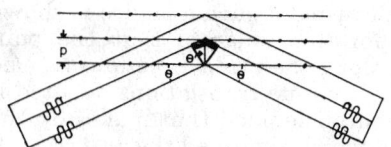

Fig. 125. Bragg condition for reflection.

(hkl), *cf* Fig. 126. These indices are interchangeable with n of the Bragg equation. Since the highest value of θ that is theoretically possible to measure is 90° (reflected beam comes back along the incident beam's path), the number of planes (highest order) that one is capable of orienting in a diffracting position is limited by the wavelength of the radiation utilized.

When monochromatic radiation impinges upon a crystal, a diffraction pattern will occur and this pattern may be recorded on photographic plates. The angle at which the reflected beam meets the film is characteristic of the set of planes that were involved in its diffraction. By orienting the crystal in various directions, many of the planes will come into a position so that the angle of the incident radiation equals the angle of diffraction.

Fig. 127 is a diffraction photograph, in which the crystal has been oscillated about an axis relative to the incident radiation. The various spots on the film arise from reflections from different planes, and each spot can be indexed, according to the Miller indices of the respective plane, by its location on the film. The spacings between the various spots enables one to derive the distances and angles between the primitive translations; ie, the unit cell dimensions.

Structural Analysis

In most cases little information can be obtained from a knowledge of the unit cell dimensions alone. In order to learn about the crystal and molecular structure it is necessary to consider the intensities of the Bragg reflections. We shall consider the case of a one-dimensional crystal so that we may have a better understanding of how differences in the intensities for the various hkl reflections arise, and how they can be utilized to obtain structural information.

A one-dimensional crystal with a repeat unit of a and having 3 scattering points (P, Q, and R) is shown in Fig. 128. The points P and P' scatter in phase at the particular angle of incidence shown, as the Bragg condition for reflection is satisfied.

The amplitude of the diffracted wave is a function of the scattering power at the point. In the case of atoms the scattering is a function of the number of electrons associated with the atom. It also must be realized that atoms are not point scatterers so that the scattering is not the same at different glancing angles (θ). A radial distribution function is usually utilized, since to a good approximation, atoms are spherical.

The points Q and R are displaced from the planes of P and P' by amounts x_1 and x_2, respectively. The

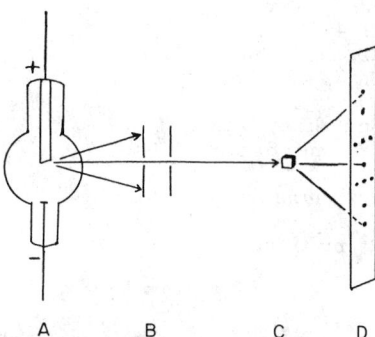

Fig. 124. Diagram of Laue experiment: (*A*) x-ray tube; (*B*) lead slits; (*C*) crystal; (*D*) photographic plate.

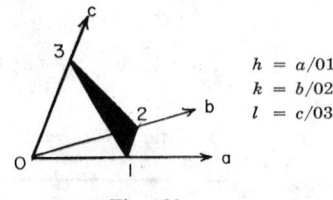

$$h = a/01$$
$$k = b/02$$
$$l = c/03$$

Fig. 126.

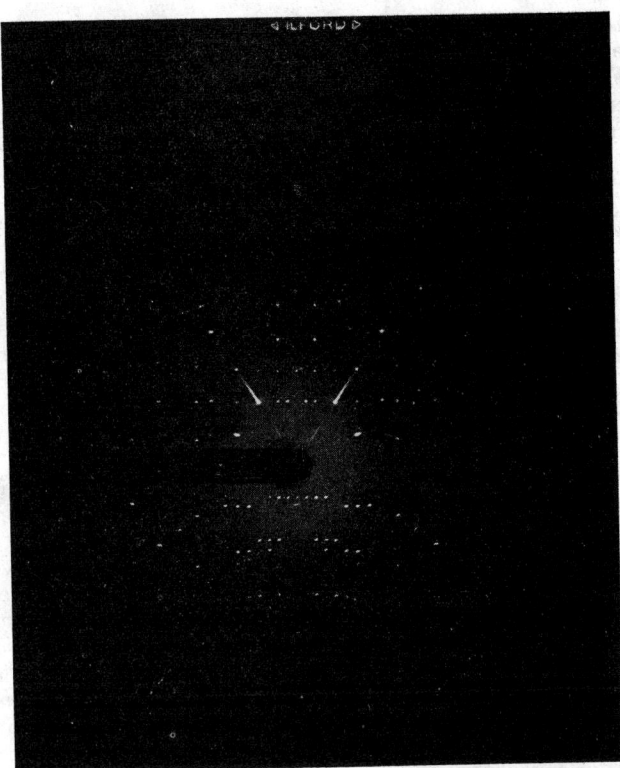

Fig. 127. A 10° oscillation photograph taken about the c axis of a complex between 5-chlorosalicylic acid and caffeine. The most intense reflection is the one having indices 2, 0, 4, which corresponds to the plane containing the complex.

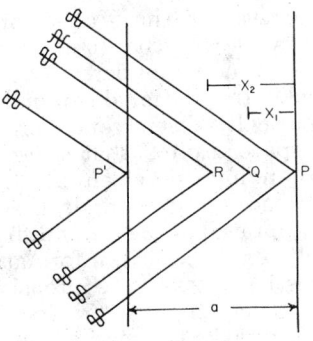

Fig. 128.

The periodic nature of a crystal makes it possible to represent the electron density (scattering matter) in the form of a three-dimensional Fourier series. The series takes the general form of

$$\rho(x,y,z) = \frac{1}{V} \sum_{-\infty}^{\infty} \sum_{-\infty}^{\infty} \sum_{-\infty}^{\infty} F(hkl) \exp\left(-2\pi i(hx + ky + lz)\right)$$

where $\rho(x,y,z)$ is the electron density at the point in the unit cell with the fractional coordinates x, y, and z; V is the volume of the unit cell. The electron density is real throughout the crystal, since the product of the two complex terms (one comes from the structure factor) in the summation gives a real number. The summations are taken over all the values of hkl. In any crystallographic study the intensities of only a limited number of planes can be measured, and one gets series-termination effects, which influence the resolution of the electron density Fourier synthesis.

It is necessary to deduce the phases of the structure factors by some method in order to calculate the electron density at various points in the cell. A typical Fourier synthesis where the phases were determined correctly is shown in Fig. 130. The contours connect points having the same electron density. One can easily analyze the molecular structure by the arrangement and density of the various contours in such a map.

Space Group Analysis—The space group of a crystal can be determined usually by the systematic absences of certain classes of reflections; ie, the intensity of diffraction from particular sets of planes will be zero. These absences arise from the translational symmetry elements that are present in the crystal: screw axes and glide planes. These symmetry elements align the molecules in the lattice in such a way that for certain Bragg planes one series of molecules will be completely out of phase with another. A

diffracted waves from these points will be displaced somewhat relative to the wave from P, and the phase shift of the wave is related to the distance of the atom from the plane. For Q, the wave is shifted by an amount $2\pi hx_1/a$, since the wave does not travel an integral number of wavelengths. It should be noted that a wave function repeats itself every 2π radians.

If, as shown in this figure, x_2 is half of a, the departing wave will be completely out of phase with the one coming from P. The resultant wave will have an amplitude and phase which is the sum of the waves from all the atoms in the unit cell. The analytical expression for the general three-dimensional case is

$$F(hkl) = \sum_{j} f_j \exp[2\pi i(hx_j/a + ky_j/b + lz_j/c)]$$

where the sum is taken over all the atoms (j) in the unit cell. The value of f_j is related to the intrinsic ability of the jth atom to scatter in the direction (hkl). $F(hkl)$ of this equation is a complex vector known as the structure factor which can be represented graphically on an Argand diagram. This vector is shown in Fig. 129 for the one-dimensional case. It is evident from this diagram that the structure factor, which is a vector, has both magnitude and direction. This can be expressed as

$$F(hkl) = |F(hkl)| \exp[i\phi(hkl)]$$

The intensity of any reflection is proportional to $|F(hkl)|^2$ in most cases. The measurement of the intensity of a reflection, therefore, only imparts information on the magnitude of the structure factor and conveys no phase data. Only by knowing the atomic arrangement within the unit cell can the structure factor, $F(hkl)$, be calculated. As a consequence, the positions of the scattering centers in the lattice cannot be obtained directly from intensity data.

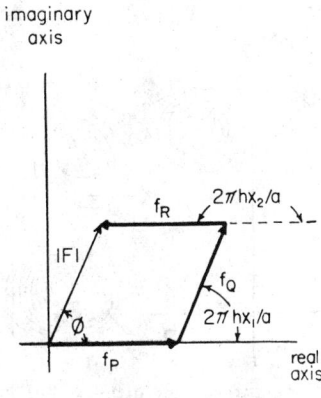

Fig. 129.

2-fold screw axis along the *b* axis, for example, will cause the intensities of the (*oko*) reflections to be zero when *k* is an odd number. The symmetry elements that lack a translational component do not give rise to systematically absent reflections.

There are space groups that differ only in their possession of an inversion center. The distinction between such space groups cannot, therefore, be made from a visual appraisal of the x-ray diffraction pattern. One must rely on chemical information about the molecule, statistical tests on the intensities, or physical measurements (such as pyro- or piezo-electric effects on the crystal) to make the distinction.

The space group can give significant molecular information in many instances. A symmetry element of the lattice may coincide with the molecular symmetry of the compound. Thus valuable structural data would be obtained from the space group symmetry in such a case. Optically active compounds cannot crystallize in space groups containing glide planes or inversion axes. Racemic mixtures will crystallize with any one of these symmetry elements present and are therefore distinguishable from crystals of the pure enantiomorph.

Phase Problem—There are presently no direct methods that are foolproof for calculating the phases of the various reflections directly from their intensities. There is a considerable amount of theoretical work being done along these lines which have shown signs of progress towards this end. Since the direct calculation of phases for all crystal structures is not at hand, the crystallographer must resort to many techniques to overcome the phase problem. A few of the procedures that are currently being used are outlined below.

Patterson Synthesis—In 1934 Patterson showed that a Fourier Synthesis using $|F|^2$ instead of F, for the Fourier coefficients, will yield information about the inter- and intra-atomic vectors. The function exhibits

$$P(U,V,W) = \sum_h \sum_k \sum_l |F|^2 \cos\left(2\pi(hU + kV + lW)\right)$$

maxima at distances (U,V,W) from the origin equal to the distances between pairs of atoms in the unit cell. The relative height of each peak is proportional to the product of the scattering power of the two atoms involved. Within the function there resides all the information needed to obtain the atomic positions in real space. The unscrambling of the data inherent in the function is difficult, even under favorable conditions.

When chemical information about a compound is known, such as the presence of a phenyl ring, the Patterson synthesis can be searched for the vectors which would correspond to this moiety. Patterson searches have been successful in unraveling the structures of some complex molecules, but because of the large number of peaks (vectors) in any map (equal to the square of the number of the atoms in the unit cell), overlap with one another occurs and it is often difficult to separate the various interactions.

In certain instances it is possible to characterize a few of the peaks in the Patterson function as belonging to a particular atom or group of atoms. This information can be utilized with image-seeking functions to deconvolute the Patterson map. Such methods have proved to be very successful, especially when a molecule contains an atom with an atomic number that is at least twice as great as any of the other atoms.

"Heavy" Atom Method—When an element with a much larger atomic number than the other atoms of the molecule is present, the scattering of the x-rays in certain directions will contain a significant contribution from this atom. Since the $|F|^2$'s will be influenced markedly by the presence of such an atom, the vectors in the Patterson function involving this heavy atom will be much higher in magnitude than the others.

It is usually best to have an element whose atomic number squared is at least 25% of the total possible scattering matter (sum of the squares of the atomic numbers of all the atoms in the molecule). It is usually a straightforward process to find the position of such an atom from the vector map. With its position known, a Fourier synthesis with the phases based on the heavy atom position alone will usually show much of the molecule. As more and more of the atoms are located, the phases will be improved and a succession of Fourier maps will resolve the whole structure.

This method is commonly utilized in studies of alkaloids, steroids, and other fairly complex organic structures, where stereochemical and configurational information is of primary importance. The method is not used when accuracy in bond orders is required, as there will be a higher degree of uncertainty in the positions of the lighter atoms when a structure is solved by this method in comparison to one solved without a heavy atom.

Isomorphous Replacement—The requirements that are necessary in order to use this method for phase determination are that one must have a series of crystalline derivatives each containing a different heavy atom, but each of the crystals must have the same crystal structure; ie, same space group and cell dimensions. The method has been used extensively to solve protein structures, where the presence of one heavy atom is not sufficient to dominate the phasing.

The derivatives are commonly made by soaking the crystals of the protein in solutions containing molecular species that diffuse into the crystal and attach themselves to certain residues on the protein surface without altering the basic protein structure. The positions of the heavy atom derivatives are located by calculating a Patterson function with the vectors arising from the native crystals removed (Difference

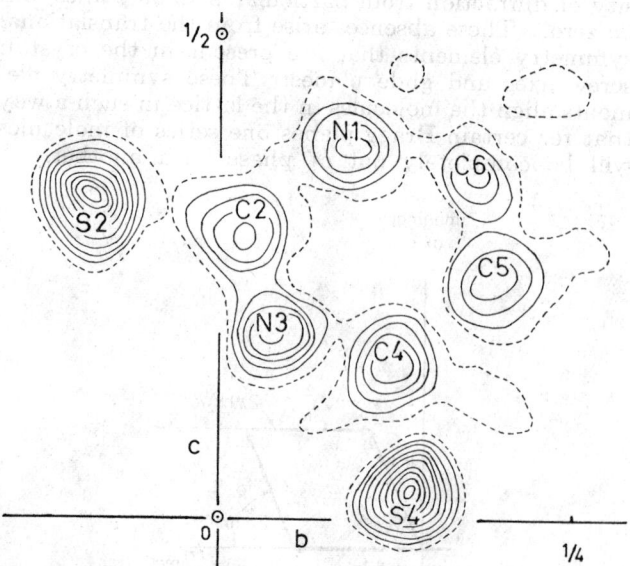

Fig. 130. Fourier synthesis of dithiouracil. The contours are drawn at equal but arbitrary levels of electron density.

Patterson Synthesis). With two or more derivatives it is theoretically possible to obtain the phase angles for the native protein.

Direct Methods—Many attempts have been made to relate phases of the structure factors directly to their magnitudes. In most recent years the statistical methods of Sayre, Hauptman, and Karle have led to equations that presently are being employed with a moderate degree of success. These workers developed a series of equations based on the probability that a certain reflection has a magnitude greater than or less than another reflection whose phase can be arbitrarily assigned.

By application of these equations to various reflections, one can develop the phases of a portion of the diffracted data sufficient to calculate a Fourier synthesis. The method has been applied successfully to complex organic structures, such as reserpine and estriol. The future of this method, which is just beginning to get widespread usage, is very bright.

Methods of Data Collection—In any crystal structure analysis it is necessary to measure both the unit cell parameters and the relative intensities of the various *hkl* reflections for the material. There are two basic approaches that are currently being utilized for the recording of such data; these are photographic and radiation counter techniques.

The photographic methods make use of the fact that a diffracted x-ray beam will darken a film at the point of mutual contact. There are three types of goniometer (camera) designs that are widely used to orient a single crystal relative to the incident radiation such that the intensities of various Bragg planes can be registered on film. These are the Buerger Precession, Weissenberg, and Oscillation cameras. These goniometers move the crystal with respect to the x-ray source so that a large number of planes will come into a diffracting position and thus will be recorded on the film. The reflection from a particular family of planes shows up as a darkened spot on the film; *cf*, the oscillation photograph in Fig. 127.

It is possible to deduce the unit cell parameters and the Miller indices associated with each of the spots by measurement of the Bragg angle for each reflection. The degree of darkening of the spots is proportional to their respective intensities, and are therefore a measure of the relative magnitudes of their squared structure factors. The intensities can be measured either by visual comparison of the blackness of the spot with a standard scale or by using a photometer, which measures the optical density of the spot.

The use of radiation detectors for the measurement of intensity data has been increasing rapidly. The two types of detectors that are commonly used for the detection and measurement of x-rays are the scintillation and proportional counters. These detectors are capable of measuring the intensity of a particular reflection with a higher degree of accuracy than can be obtained using ordinary film methods. The increased accuracy in the intensity data goes hand-in-hand with the ability to derive more highly refined positional and thermal parameters for a molecule.

The goniometers that are used with the detectors are capable also of being automated. The automation is particularly useful in protein crystallography where huge numbers of data must be collected. The two most popular types of goniometers used with radiation detectors are the 4-circle and linear diffractometers. A

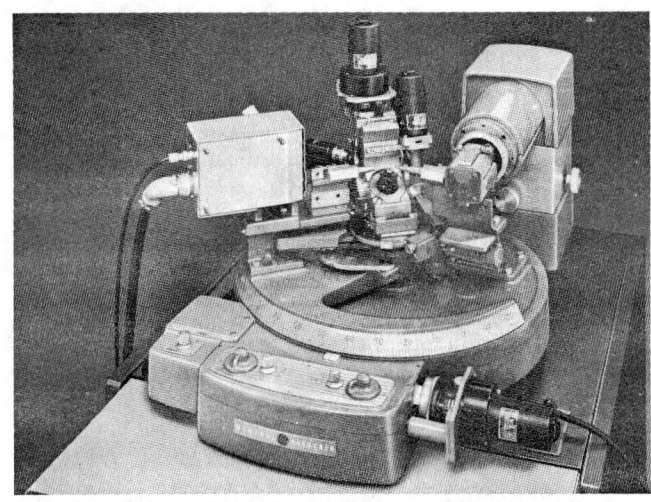

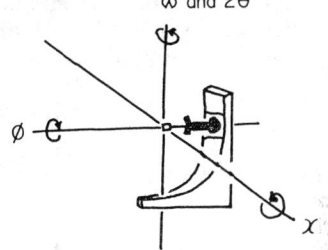

ω and 2θ

Fig. 131. (*A*) An automated 4-circle x-ray diffractometer (courtesy, General Electric); (*B*) the 4 angular motions of the orientor of *A*.

photograph of one of the commercially available 4-circle spectrogoniometers and a diagram of the four angles that can be rotated to place a particular Bragg plane into a diffracting position are shown in Fig. 131. With such an instrument, the data can be collected on a moderately complex compound in less than a few days, and with the nonautomated diffractometer, in a few weeks.

Powder Method—By grinding a crystalline specimen into a fine powder, one is able to produce a sample which would statistically contain very minute crystals oriented in every possible direction. When such a sample is irradiated, a large number of the crystal fragments would have their Bragg planes in the correct orientation for reflection and the various reflections would occur as cones of rays rather than as spots, because of the number of crystallites. The data may be recorded either by photographic or counter techniques. The method is not utilized for structural analysis, except for the simplest of materials (eg, certain elements), but has proved to be useful as a rapid means of identification.

Application of X-Ray Diffraction

Molecular Weight—The measurement of the unit cell parameters provides a means of accurately determining molecular weights of compounds. The density of a crystal can be obtained by means of flotation in a suitable liquid, the density of which is altered by dilution until it matches that of the crystal. The density (Gm/cm^3) is proportional to the molecular weight of the material in the unit cell. The relationship is

$$\text{Mol Wt} = \frac{\text{Density} \times V_{cell} \times N_a}{Z}$$

where N_a is Avogadro's number (6.023×10^{23}) and Z is the number of molecules in the unit cell. The unit cell volume (V_{cell}) can be measured to a very high degree of accuracy. The number of molecules in the unit cell (Z) must be a whole number, with values of 1, 2, 4, and 8 being the most common among organic materials. When there is a high degree of solvation, it is necessary to approximate the amount of liquid bound by another means.

Identification of Materials—Every compound that is crystalline will give a characteristic x-ray diffraction pattern. These patterns can be very useful for identification purposes, and also for quantitative analysis of solid mixtures. They also have been utilized to a great extent by the pharmaceutical industry for the identification and classification of polymorphic and solvated forms of drugs. The powder method is a valuable technique when quick comparisons of different forms are to be made and also when quantitative work is done. An example of such a comparison between the hydrated and anhydrous form of theophylline is shown in Fig. 132.

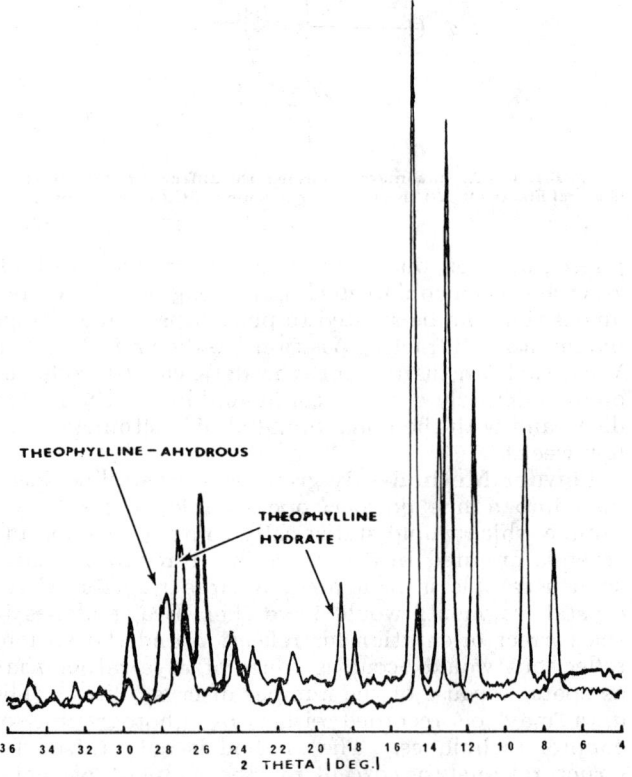

Fig. 132. A tracing of the powder diffraction patterns of theophylline monohydrate and an anhydrous form.

Structure Determination—The body of substances of medicinal value whose structures were primarily elucidated by x-ray diffraction techniques is quite large. They range in molecular size from penicillin, to vitamin B_{12}, on up to the globular proteins. At present the proteins myoglobin, hemoglobin, lysozyme, chymotrypsin, ribonuclease, carboxypeptidase, and papain have had their three-dimensional structure analyzed. The structural determinations, in most instances, have played a major role in uncovering the secrets associated with the biological functions of the various molecules. A photograph of the ribonuclease molecule as determined by the x-ray studies of Kartha, Bello, and Harker is shown in Fig. 133.

There are also large numbers of macromolecules of biological importance which do not form three-dimensional crystals in the usual sense, but will form fibers. The bundles of molecules in the fiber are aligned with respect to one another in a somewhat crystalline manner. These materials give x-ray diffraction patterns that have proved very useful in deriving molecular information. By fitting models to the x-ray pattern, many valuable biological polymers have had their secrets exposed. The best two examples are the α-helices of keratin and the double helix of deoxyribonucleic acid.

Intramolecular Bonding and Configurations—The precise determination of a crystal structure enables the bond lengths and angles between the various atoms to be determined accurately. This information is extremely valuable in the further understanding of how various chemical substituents influence the valence states and configurations of a molecule. With such knowledge, structure–activity relationships that are of fundamental interest to the medicinal chemist have much more depth. The observed bond orders also serve as experimental criteria by which theoretical models can be judged. It is also possible to compare quantum mechanical calculations relating drug interaction with actual observation.

Intramolecular steric effects that tend to distort molecules are easily unraveled by the scrutiny of their structures. It is possible to distinguish between repulsive and attractive effects of substituents. The torsional angles about various bonds are able to be calculated from the atomic positions and are extremely helpful in relating NMR data to structure.

Absolute Configuration—Friedel's Law, which states that the intensity of the hkl reflection equals the intensity of the $-h, -k, -l$ reflection, breaks down under certain conditions. It will not hold when the wavelength of the x-rays is such that the inner shell electrons of one or more atoms of the molecule are excited to a higher energy level. The effect, depending on the wavelength of the x-radiation used, is pronounced for certain atoms of high atomic number. When such an atom is present in a disymmetric compound, the structure factors of the (hkl) and ($-h, -k, -l$) planes can be distinguished.

Bijvoet has shown that the absolute configuration of the molecule can be determined under these conditions. It is quite interesting to note that his study on sodium rubidium D-tartrate established for the

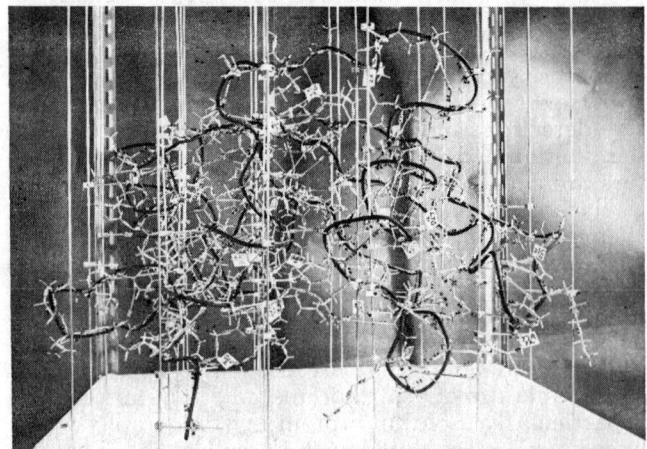

Fig. 133. Model of bovine ribonuclease derived from x-ray data. Snakelike tube marks the backbone of the protein (courtesy, Dr. G. Kartha).

first time that the chemical convention adapted by Fischer turned out to be correct.

References

1. Moore, W. J., *Physical Chemistry*, 3rd ed., Prentice-Hall, Englewood Cliffs, N.J., 1962, pp. 790–816.
2. Daniels, F., and Alberty, R. A., *Physical Chemistry*, 2nd ed., Wiley, New York, 1961, pp. 696–699.
3. Yang, C. N., *Elementary Particles*, Princeton Univ. Press, Princeton, N.J., 1962.
4. Chase, G. D., and Rabinowitz, J. L., *Principles of Radioisotope Methodology*, 3rd rev., Burgess Publ. Co., Minneapolis, 1967.
5. Lapp, R. E., and Andrews, H. L., *Nuclear Radiation Physics*, 3rd ed., Prentice-Hall, Englewood Cliffs, N.J., 1963, p. 258.
6. Mamakrishnan, A., *Elementary Particles and Cosmic Rays*, MacMillan, New York, 1962, p. 221.
7. Pitzer, K. S., *J. Am. Chem. Soc.*, **70**, 2140 (1948).
8. Fieser, L. F., and Fieser, M., *Introduction to Organic Chemistry*, Heath, Boston, 1957, inside back cover.
9. Pauling, L. F., *The Nature of the Chemical Bond*, 3rd ed., Cornell Univ. Press, Ithaca, N.Y., 1960: (a) pp. 225, 226; (b) p. 93; (c) Chap. 3.
10. Smyth, C. P., *Dielectric Behavior and Structure*, McGraw-Hill, New York, 1955, Chap. 14.
11. Fajans, K., *Physical Methods of Organic Chemistry*, vol. 1, part II, 2nd ed., Interscience, New York, 1949, p. 1162.
12. Cammarata, A., *J. Med. Chem.*, **10**, 525 (1967).
13. Murty, C. R. K., *J. Sci. Ind. Res. (India)*, **18B**, 268 (1957).
14. Halverstadt, I. F., and Kumler, W. D., *J. Am. Chem. Soc.*, **64**, 2988 (1942).
15. Martin, A. N., *Physical Pharmacy*, 2nd ed., Lea & Febiger, Philadelphia, 1969, pp. 131, 132.
16. Purcell, W. P., *et al*, *J. Med. Chem.*, **9**, 297 (1965).
17. Lien, E. J., and Kumler, W. D., *J. Med. Chem.*, **11**, 214 (1968).
18. Ferguson, L. N., *The Modern Structural Theory of Organic Chemistry*, Prentice-Hall, Englewood Cliffs, N.J., 1963, pp. 62–88.
19. Kealy, T. J., and Pauson, P. L., *Nature*, **168**, 1039 (1951).
20. Wilkinson, G., *et al*, *J. Am. Chem. Soc.*, **74**, 2125 (1952).
21. Dunitz, J. D., *et al*, *Acta Cryst.* **9**, 373 (1956).
22. Seibold, E. A., and Sutton, L. E., *J. Chem. Phys.* **23**, 1967 (1955).
23. Plesske, K., *Angew. Chem.*, **74**, 301, 347 (1962).
24. Hawthorne, M. F., *Accounts Chem. Res.*, **1**, 281 (1968).
25. Martin, A. N., *Physical Pharmacy*, 2nd ed., Lea & Febiger, Philadelphia, 1969, p. 333.
26. Shefter, E., *J. Pharm. Sci.*, **57**, 1163 (1968).
27. Olah, G. A. *et al*, *J. Am. Chem. Soc.*, **89**, 711 (1967).
28. Burger, A., and Yost, W. L., *J. Am. Chem. Soc.*, **70**, 2198 (1948).
29. Tedeschi, R. E., *et al*, *Proc. Soc. Exptl. Biol. Med.* **102**, 380 (1959).
30. Eliel, E. L., *Stereochemistry of Carbon Compounds*, McGraw-Hill, New York, 1962, pp. 156–179.
31. Noller, C. R., *Chemistry of Organic Compounds*, Saunders, Philadelphia, 1965, pp. 370, 371.
32. Djerassi, C., *Optical Rotatory Dispersion*, McGraw-Hill, New York, 1960.
33. Eliel, E. L., *Stereochemistry of Carbon Compounds*, McGraw-Hill, New York, 1962, pp. 412–433.
34. Snatzke, G., *Angew. Chem.* (Intern. ed., in English), **7**, 14 (1968).
35. Tanford, C., *Physical Chemistry of Macromolecules*, Wiley, New York, 1961, pp. 119–124.
36. Kingsbury, C. A., and Thornton, W. B., *J. Org. Chem.*, **31**, 1000 (1966).
37. Eliel, E. L., *Stereochemistry of Carbon Compounds*, McGraw-Hill, New York, 1962, pp. 23, 124–129.
38. Kier, L. B., *J. Pharm. Sci.*, **57**, 1188 (1968).
39. Martin, A. N., *Physical Pharmacy*, 2nd ed., Lea & Febiger, Philadelphia, 1969, pp. 66–68.
40. Levinthal, C., *Sci. Am.*, **214**, 42 (1956).
41. Albert, A., *Selective Toxicity*, Wiley, New York, 1965, pp. 129, 130.
42. Némethy, G., *Angew. Chem.* (Intern. ed.), **6**, 195 (1967).
43. Exner, O., *Collection Czechoslov. Chem. Commun.*, **32**, 1 (1967).
44. Quayle, O. R., *Chem. Rev.*, **53**, 439 (1953).
45. Exner, O., *Collection Czechlslov. Chem. Commun.*, **32**, 24 (1967).
46. McGowan, J. C., *J. Appl. Chem.* **2**, 323 (1952).
47. Mullins, L. J., *Chem. Rev.*, **54**, 289 (1954).
48. McGowan, J. C., *J. Appl. Chem.*, **4**, 41 (1954).
49. McGowan, J. C., *Nature*, **200**, 1317 (1963).
50. Collander, R., *Acta Chem. Scand.*, **5**, 774 (1951).
51. Hansch, C., *Farmaco*, **23**, 293 (1968).
52. Fujita, T., *et al*, *J. Am. Chem. Soc.*, **86**, 5175 (1964).
53. Iwasa, J., *et al*, *J. Med. Chem.*, **8**, 150 (1965).
54. Hansch, C., and Anderson, S. M., *J. Org. Chem.*, **32**, 2583 (1967).
55. Hansch, C., and Anderson, S. M., *J. Med. Chem.*, **10**, 745 (1967).
56. Lien, E. J., *et al*, *J. Med. Chem.*, **11**, 430 (1968).
57. Hansch, C., *et al*, *Arch. Biochem. Biophys.*, **128**, 319 (1968).
58. Hansch, C., *et al*, *J. Med. Chem.*, **11**, 1 (1968).
59. Bird, A. E., and Marshall, A. C., *Biochem. Pharmacol.* **16**, 2275 (1967).

Bibliography

Buerger, M. J., *Crystal Structure Analysis*, Wiley, New York, 1960.

Buerger, M. J., *Vector Space*, Wiley, New York, 1959.

Nyburg, S. C., *X-ray Structural Analysis of Organic Structures*, Academic, New York, 1961.

Lipson, H., and Cochran, W., *The Determination of Crystal Structures*, G. Bell, London, 1957.

Robertson, J. M., *Organic Crystals and Molecules*, Cornell Univ. Press, Ithaca, N.Y., 1953.

Stout, G. H., and Jensen, L. H., *X-ray Structure Determination, A Practical Guide*, Macmillan, New York, 1968.

International Tables for X-ray Crystallography, vols. I, II, and III, Kynoch Press, Birmingham, 1959, 1952.

Kitaigorodskii, A. I., *Organic Chemical Crystallography* (trans. from Russian ed.), Consultants Bureau, New York, 1961.

16 | Complexation

The concept of complexity—metal complexes—molecular complexes—
no-bond (inclusion) complexes—complex equilibria—ion-exchange
compounds—protein binding of drugs

This chapter was prepared by

Alfonso R. Gennaro, PhD, *Professor of Chemistry, Philadelphia College of
Pharmacy and Science, Philadelphia, Pa. 19104, and*
David E. Guttman, PhD, *Associate Director, Analytical and Physical Chemistry,
Smith Kline and French Laboratories, Philadelphia, Pa. 19101*

In considering the concept of complexity it is unfortunate that a word other than *complex* was not originally or subsequently coined to denote the compounds to be discussed in this chapter. The term *complex* would tend to indicate, especially to the student, a meaning of mysteriousness or even confusion concerning certain properties of these substances. Perhaps this was true at one time since the idea of complexity was originally attributed to those compounds or structures which did not always conform to the classic theories of valency. Thus, even now, complexes or complex compounds, in the broad sense, are considered as those compounds having some deviation from the *normal* concepts of bonding. Yet, many compounds, still referred to as complexes, have been thoroughly studied (eg, coordination compounds), and their structures sufficiently elucidated to no longer classify them as complex. It is, therefore, difficult to delineate the difference between a simple and complex compound, except for the greater number of *common* compounds which adhere to the elementary concepts of bonding.

Complexity, in this definition therefore, has little to do with intricateness of molecular architecture or spatial configuration. What is more complex than the structures of the steroids, proteins, carbohydrates, etc, in the realm of chemistry? Whether these compounds are to be considered *complex* depends entirely on the bonding structure. For example, both cholesterol and digitonin are complicated structures from the standpoint of molecular architecture, but individually would not be considered *complexes* by the chemist. However, the digitonide of cholesterol, formed by mixing alcoholic solutions of each constituent, is known as a complex, since the type of bonding between the individual components is not clearly defined or easily explainable by the usual theories of valency.

Complex compounds are primarily those molecules in which most of the bonding structure can be described by the classic theories of valency between atoms, but one or more of the bonds is somewhat anomalous and therefore *complex*. The complex formed by the association of two molecules of an organic acid in solution consists of atoms held together by normal covalent bonds, shown by a dash between the various elements. However, two molecules of the acid are

$$CH_3-C\underset{O-H\cdots O}{\overset{O\cdots H-O}{\Big\langle\Big\rangle}}C-CH_3$$

joined by *hydrogen bonds*, illustrated as dotted lines,

which are neither covalent, coordinate, nor ionic, but are the result of a *dipole–dipole* attraction between negative oxygen and positive hydrogen.

Such bonds, which create the situation referred to as *complex*, may be of the *ion–dipole, dipole–dipole, dipole-induced dipole*, or even of the *covalent* or *coordinate* type. The term complex is now usually extended to cover a multitude of compounds in which the bonding is simple, intricate, or a combination thereof.

Classification—Classification of complex compounds according to a rigid set of conventions is of necessity a difficult, if not impossible, task. Recently a type of complex compound (*Inclusion Compounds*) has been investigated which is considered a *no-bond* complex. That is, no bonding evidence is available to support the actuality that two or more molecules may form a somewhat stoichiometric combination without the necessity of being joined by some form of adhesive force.

In order to facilitate discussion of complexation some form of classification is required. Two possibilities are suggested and, from the theoretical viewpoint, the type of bonding between the components of the complex offers a simple solution (though difficult to adhere to strictly). Three subdivisions can be included in this classification: *true-bond* types, in which the union between the components can be explained in the classical manner; *weak-bond* types, or those exhibiting attraction due to Van der Waals' forces, hydrogen bonding, etc; and *no-bond* types, which include the inclusion compounds previously mentioned.

From a practical standpoint a classification, not so rigid as the bonding category, which arranges the molecules as to type of complex formed, is more flexible.

Nevertheless, a simple classification is not realistic since some of the compounds discussed will of necessity overlap the aforementioned categories. This chapter will also include a treatment of ion-exchange materials which, in many instances, may not be regarded as complexes. The scope of complexation is of such a magnitude that this chapter is intended to serve mainly to give an insight to the field and will deal primarily with complexation of interest in pharmacy and medicine. The latter portion of this chapter will deal with a specific category of complexation, in which one of the constituents is a proteinlike substance. Protein–drug complexation or "binding" has become a fertile field of investigation in an attempt to elucidate drug action.

The following classification of complex compounds, representing a hybrid arrangement of types of bonds and compounds included in the classification, will be used in this chapter.

Metal Complexes

This category can be subdivided into the inorganic and aromatic types.

Inorganic Complexes—It has long been known that stable "molecular compounds" can be formed by the union of two simple molecules in which the atoms already seem to be exerting their maximum possible valencies. The custom was to indicate the formula for the "molecular compound" by writing the components side by side, eg, $2KI.HgI_2$ or $2KCl.MgCl_2$. However, upon examination of solutions of these "double salts," the former salt was found to yield only three ions, and the latter a total of seven. The formulation of the mercuri compound was then changed to $K_2[HgI_4]$ and the HgI_4^{2-} ion, resulting from the reaction

$$HgI_2 + 2I^- = HgI_4^{2-}$$

was termed a *complex* ion, and the salts *complex* salts. However, analogous ions such as SO_4^{2-} or CrO_4^{2-} are not regarded as complex, again pointing to the somewhat loose definition attributed to this term.

Werner, in 1891, postulated his famous coordination theory, which helped to explain some of the deviations from the classic valency theories for compounds of the above-mentioned type. According to Werner:

1. There are two types of valences: (*a*) primary (ionic) and (*b*) secondary (coordinate).
2. The same type of anion, radical, or molecule may be held by either or both types of valence.
3. For each *central atom* or ion there is a fixed number (*coordination number*) of nonionic valences. The coordinated atoms or groups occupy the *first sphere* or *coordination sphere*. Other atoms are said to be in the *second* or *ionization* sphere.
4. Neutral molecules, as well as ions, may satisfy the nonionic valences.
5. The nonionic valences are directed toward definite positions in space (this explains the existence of stereoisomers of many coordinate complexes). These postulates can be illustrated by the following compound.

> ┌─Central atom
> │ ┌─Ligands(unidentate)
> $[CoCl(NH_3)_5]Cl_2$
> │ └─Ionization sphere
> └─Coordination sphere

In solution this compound will ionize to form $[CoCl(NH_3)_5]^{2+}$ and $2Cl^-$ ions. The chloride ion in the coordination sphere is not precipitated by silver nitrate. The groups which combine with the central atom, by any type of bonding, are known as *ligands*. The type of bonding between the metal and ligand may be electrostatic or covalent. However, whether the bonding is ionic, covalent, or intermediate, the function of the ligand is always that of donating electrons to the central atom. The *coordination number* is the maximum number of atoms or groups which can

Fig. 134.   Unidentate (*a*) and polydentate (*b*) ligands.

combine, in the coordination sphere, with the central atom (usually an even number). Ligands which have more than one electron pair available for coordination with the central ion are said to be bi-, tri-, or poly-*dentate*. In Fig. 134*A* the central atom, M, has a coordination number of 4 and the ligands A, A′, A″, A‴ are *unidentate*, while in Fig. 134*B* ligands A-A′ and A″-A‴ are bidentate.

Compound *A* would be referred to as a metal complex and *B* as a *chelate*. Groups which occupy more than one coordination position in a complex form a ring with the central ion and are termed *chelates* (Greek, *claw*).

Many groups have the ability to coordinate with the central atom, in the following order of decreasing affinity of coordinating groups:

$-O^-$(enolate ion); $-NH_2$(amine); $-N=N-$(azo);

$>N$(ring nitrogen); $-COO^-$(carboxylate ion);

$-O-$(ether); and $-CO-$(carbonyl)

More recently, the *crystal field theory*, originally applied to crystals, has been employed to elucidate the structure of coordination compounds. A complete discussion is beyond the scope of this chapter, but the essence of the theory is that the five *d* orbitals of the central atom, which are of equal energy in the gaseous metal atom, are split by the presence of the electrostatic field due to the ligands, and acquire different energies. Quantitative energy calculations can be made in many cases, and a number of physical and chemical properties can be correlated, such as stability of the complex, magnetic properties, rates and mechanism of reaction, etc.

Perhaps the most familiar members of the nonchelate type of metal complexes (*unidentate ligands*) are: $[Ag(CN)_2]^-$ and $[Cu(CN)_3]^{2-}$ in electrodeposition of silver and copper from aqueous solution; $[Ag(NH_3)_2]^+$ formed in the solution of insoluble silver halides in ammonia; $[Fe(CNS)]^{2+}$ occurring at the end point of the titration with NH_4CNS using ferric alum indicator; use of fluoride or phosphate to form soluble complex with iron; polyphosphates in water-softening to complex calcium and magnesium; gravimetric determination of potassium as the chloroplatinate or cobaltinitrite; and many others.

Chelates—The *chelate* type of metal complex has become of great importance, especially in the pharmaceutical field. Chelation refers to the coordination of a metal with a polydentate ligand (Fig. 134*B*). The complex so formed may result in precipitation of the metal or the formation of a stable, soluble compound. If the ligand forms a stable, water-soluble metal chelate, it is said to be a *sequestering* agent. *Sequestration* (Latin, *sequestrare*, to remove) is the suppression of a property or reaction of a metal without removal of that metal from the system or phase by any process of precipitation or extraction and is usually accomplished by chelation.

Materials such as citric acid have been used to sequester metals in living systems, foods, beverages, and cosmetics for as long as food production has existed.

Metallic complexes of bivalent cations with tartrates and citrates exist in a 1:1 molar ratio of tartrate or citrate to the metal. Salts of citric acid are required to form complexes of the bivalent metals; free citric or tartaric acid will, however, complex trivalent iron, but the ratio of metal to citrate or tartrate is dependent on the acid concentration. The structures of such complexes have been the subject of much study and are still not completely resolved.

Sequestration has two important pharmaceutical uses: in analysis and the removal or deactivation of unwanted ions in solution. Mention has been made of the use of unidentate ligands (fluoride and cyanide ions, etc) as complexing agents, but polydentate agents are much more important for sequestering purposes. One compound, ethylenediaminetetraacetic acid (EDTA), has been studied and employed extensively in

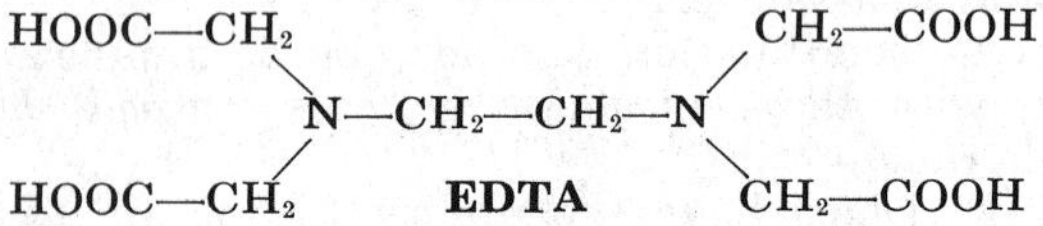

EDTA

the pharmaceutical field. Most of the official drugs containing calcium and the zinc content of zinc stearate are determined by titration with a standard EDTA solution. Several structures for the calcium complex of EDTA have been proposed, such as that depicted below.

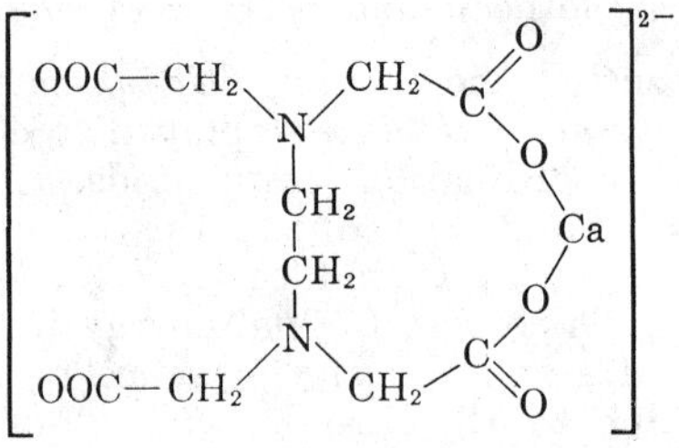

A general term given to the aminopolycarboxylic acids, such as EDTA, is *Complexons*. The following formulas illustrate two such compounds which have not been discussed previously.

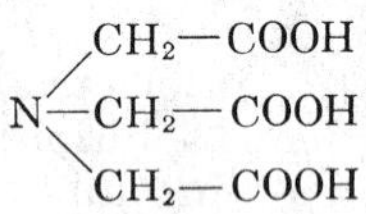

Complexon I
(nitrolotriacetic acid)

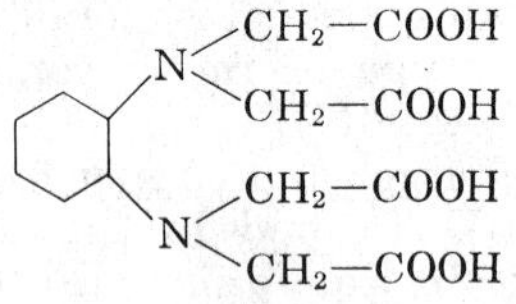

Complexon IV
(1,2-cyclohexylenedinitrolo)-
tetraacetic acid

Complexon II is EDTA and Complexon III or B is the sodium salt of EDTA.

The pharmaceutical applications of EDTA (and other sequestering agents) are infinite; for example, in antibiotic, antihistamine, sulfonamide, epinephrine, anesthetic, and barbiturate preparations to prevent discoloration due to traces of metals; in cosmetic creams or lotions containing unsaturated fatty acids and alcohols to prevent oxidation catalyzed by trace metals; in alkaline bottle-washing compositions to avoid precipitation of metal hydroxides; in the stabilization of ascorbic acid, hydrogen peroxide, gum and resin preparations, formaldehyde, essential oils, folic acid, and hyaluronidase; and as a cleaning agent to retain the efficiency of filters in processes where the filter cloth becomes blocked by precipitation and occlusion of polyvalent metallic salts.

From the medicinal standpoint complexing agents, or the complex itself, have shown promise. Thus,

sequestering agents are used in the treatment of urinary calculi, calciferous corneal deposits, and hypercalcemia. EDTA may be used as an *in vitro* anticoagulant for blood (citrate, oxalate, EDTA, etc, tie up calcium, thus interfering with thrombin formation). In lead poisoning salts of EDTA (and also dimercaprol) form a stable lead chelate which is inert, nontoxic, and rapidly eliminated. EDTA (and other complexing agents) increases the absorption of iron in the gastrointestinal tract. An iron chelate of 8-hydroxyquinoline has antibacterial action. Compounds such as EDTA should not be employed in dentifrices since they may leach calcium from the teeth. Also, the binding of polyvalent metal cations by the tetracyclines has been shown to markedly reduce their efficacy.

Chelation explains some physiological phenomena. One such instance suggests that abnormal (activated) mucoproteins of urine chelate with calcium in solution to form relatively insoluble micelles of colloidal calcium–mucoprotein units as the initial step in the formation of urinary calculi.

Metal chelates are important in analytical pharmacy, as already indicated for EDTA. Dithizone (diphenyl-thiocarbazone) forms colored complexes with many metals and is useful in the estimation of trace quantities of lead and zinc (see Chapter 37, *Analysis of Medicinals*). These two complexes are soluble in carbon tetrachloride or chloroform and can be extracted from aqueous solution, and determined colorimetrically.

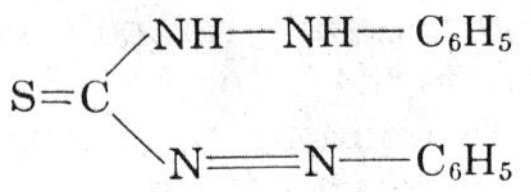

dithizone

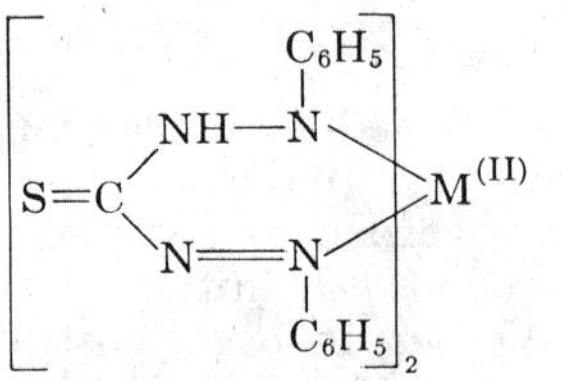

dithizone–divalent
metal complex

The complex of ferrous iron with *o*-phenanthroline or barium diphenylamine sulfonate is used as an indicator in titrations utilizing ceric sulfate. Nickel forms the well-known red complex with dimethylglyoxime. Aluminum and magnesium salts are often precipitated as their 8-hydroxyquinoline complexes.

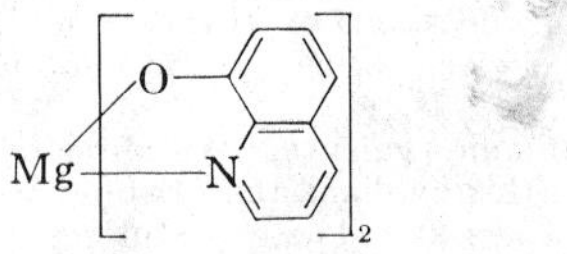

magnesium 8-hydroxyquinoline complex

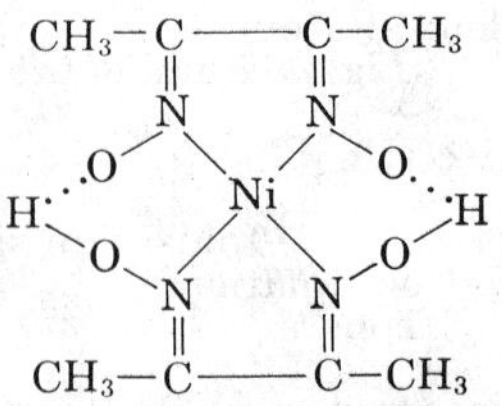

nickel dimethylglyoxime complex

Biological materials are often dependent on formation of metal chelates. The stabilization of insulin with zinc; the enzymatic bond-formation and rupture processes of carbohydrates and nucleoproteins; the iron in heme, magnesium in chlorophyll, and cobalt in vitamin B_{12} are examples of systems in which metal chelate complexes are essential for biologic activity. Many enzymes contain metals which are essential for the activity of the enzyme system. Removal of the metal, or lack of the metal can inactivate the enzyme and therefore trace amounts of copper, cobalt, zinc, manganese, and molybdenum are required in human nutrition. Copper is found associated with the enzyme tyrosinase, cobalt in vitamin B_{12}, zinc in carbonic anhydrase, manganese plays a role in oxidative phosphorylation, and molybdenum occurs in xanthine dehydrogenase.

Olefin Complexes—A third kind of metal complex is known as the olefin type. Perhaps the best known is *ferrocene* or dicyclopentadienyl iron. A single covalent bond appears to link the metal to the plane of each ring. The modern theories of bonding (atomic orbital and molecular orbital) acknowledge the existence of spatially directed valences when two atoms are brought together, this arising because of the engagement of electronic orbits originally separate in each atom. (Refer to Chapter 29, *Organic Pharmaceutical Chemistry* for an extensive discussion of bonding.)

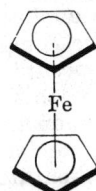

In ferrocene, and other complexes of this nature, one π electron of each ring is used in bonding to the metal atom and the resultant rings now have the $4n + 2$ pi electron configuration $(n = 1)$ and exhibit aromatic character, as evidenced by lack of reaction with maleic anhydride and of certain spectral characteristics. An ionic-type bond is not indicated for ferrocene-like substances as they are nonelectrolytes. Due to the layer structure of the ring-metal complexes they are often referred to as "sandwich" compounds. Many metals also form complexes with straight-chain unsaturation. A complex of platinum with ethylene or styrene is known, and iron, palladium, mercury, silver, iridium complexes are quite stable. Aluminum–olefin complexes are believed to exist but due to the ease of isomerization, polymerization, or cyclization of the olefin, true complexes are difficult to isolate.

Little direct application of the metal–olefin complexes to the pharmaceutical field is in evidence at the present time. However, these complexes are thought to enter into the polymerization of ethylene and propylene to form the well-known polyethylene and polypropylene. The Friedel-Crafts reaction may involve the formation of aluminum chloride–olefin complexes. Many complex-forming metal salts have been found to be effective in the hydration of olefins and gaseous olefins can be extracted from mixtures by saturated solutions of copper (II), silver, mercury (II), and other salts. It is of interest that ferrocene imparts antiknock quality to gasoline, and is said also to potentiate this property of tetraethyl lead.

Molecular Complexes (Addition Compounds)

Complexes formed by the union of two organic molecules by other than covalent bonds generally utilize hydrogen bonds or other electrostatic forces in their formation. For the purpose of this presentation it is expedient to consider such molecular complexes in one of two categories: (1) aromatic complexes; (2) hydrogen-bonded complexes.

Charge-Transfer Complexes—This type of complex functions by sharing of π electrons. The complex-

ing agent, usually a polynitro aromatic hydrocarbon, must by nature be an electron acceptor and, to some degree, be capable of accepting a negative charge from the nucleus of the agent being complexed. Other theories involve the presence of a dipole-induced dipole, dipole–dipole, or ionic complex (a donor molecule shares an electron pair with the acceptor by a process similar to a Lewis acid–base interaction). It is evident that a complete understanding of the bonding structures in these complexes is not clearly defined.

In some cases proof of the existence of such complexes is quite simple to demonstrate. If picric acid is distributed between a chloroform–water mixture and increasing concentrations of an aromatic compound, soluble only in chloroform (such as naphthalene), is added, the concentration of picric acid in the chloroform layer increases and that of the aqueous layer decreases. The picric acid–naphthalene complex which is formed causes an increase in picric acid concentration in the organic phase and further increase of the naphthalene concentration again removes more picric acid from the water layer.

Various physical studies such as solubility measurements, distribution studies, vapor pressure measurements, melting point–composition relationships, spectral characteristics, dipole moment measurements, and viscosity isotherms have been helpful in elucidating the nature of aromatic complexes.

The most common type of aromatic complex exists between the aromatic hydrocarbons and polynitro compounds, usually formed in a 1:1 ratio. Picric acid, styphnic acid, and *sym*-trinitrobenzene form complexes with many polynuclear, aromatic hydrocarbons. The stability of the complex appears to be governed by two factors: the number of electron-attracting groups on the nitro compound and by the ring complexity and presence of electron-releasing groups on the second component. Benzene forms an unstable picrate, whereas naphthalene picrate is very stable. Nitrobenzene does not form a complex with aromatic hydrocarbons but *m*-dinitro- and *sym*-trinitrobenzene do. The presence of methyl or amino groups (electron-releasing) increases the stability of the picrate.

A well-known example of such a complex in use in pharmacy today is Butesin Picrate, a local anesthetic, consisting of a complex of two molecules of butyl *p*-aminobenzoate with one molecule of picric acid.

Butesin Picrate

Hydrogen-Bonded Complexes—A large number of compounds containing the —O—H or —N—H linkage exhibit hydrogen bonding (for a discussion of the hydrogen bond, see under this title on page 256). The most familiar evidence is observed in the abnormalities of such physical constants as boiling point of alcohols, carboxylic acids, and amines. Dimethyl ether and ethanol both have the same molecular formula (C_2H_6O), and hence the same molecular weight, but ethanol boils at a temperature over 100° above that of ether. This phenomenon is easily explained by the presence of hydrogen bonding with ethanol, which increases its *apparent* molecular weight. The hydrogen bond is considered an example of dipole–dipole interaction in which the "positive" hydrogen atoms of one molecule are electrostatically attracted to the "negative" oxygen atoms of a second molecule, thus:

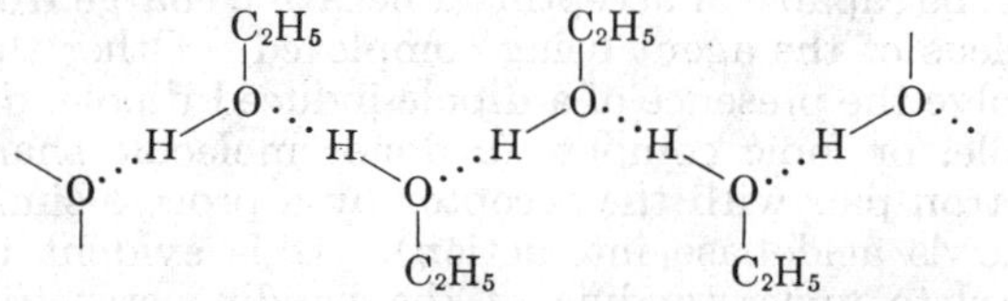

Hydrogen bonds are relatively weak bonds, having about 10% of the strength of an ordinary covalent bond. The solubility of water-soluble organic compounds is achieved by solvation involving hydrogen bond formation.

Complexation will occur only if intermolecular hydrogen bonds are formed since it is equally possible, with compounds such as salicylic acid, for several intramolecular species to exist.

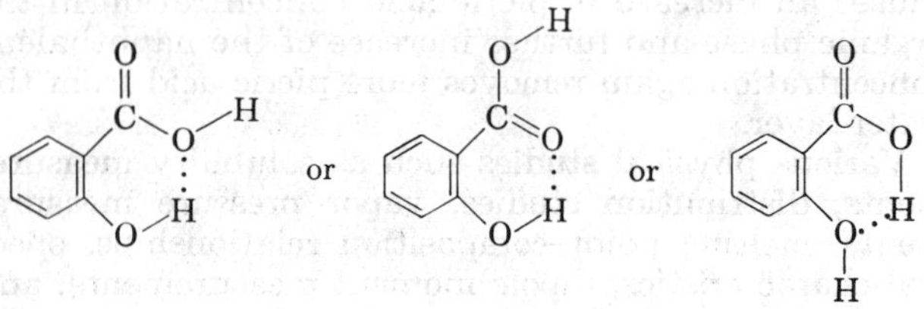

The pharmaceutical literature dealing with hydrogen bonding is extensive, and even a cursory treatment is beyond the range of this chapter. A brief discussion of a few examples of this kind of bonding must suffice.

Saccharin forms water-soluble complexes with theophylline, caffeine, and various amides and phenols. The stability and appearance of pharmaceutical preparations such as aqueous solutions of benzocaine, tetracaine, or procaine are enhanced by the formation of complexes with caffeine. Caffeine is also known to complex, eg, with sulfonamides, p-aminobenzoic acid, and phenobarbital. The complexes aminophylline (theophylline-ethylenediamine), theophylline-sodium acetate, theobromine-sodium salicylate, citrated caffeine, and caffeine-sodium benzoate are well-known medicinal agents. Interaction between the oxygen atom of the carbonyl function of theophylline or caffeine and the hydrogen atom of the acidic second component is thought to be the binding force causing the complex formation. Polyethylene glycols have an affinity for many drugs, including salicylic acid, and p-hydroxy- and p-aminobenzoic acid. Hydrogen bonding between two or more components of a pharmaceutical preparation may give rise to incompatibilities, bring about solubilization, or decrease or increase the activity of an active constituent. For example, the effect of certain nonionic detergents in inhibiting the antiseptic activity of compounds such as hexachlorophene is probably due to complexation.

No-Bond (Inclusion) Complexes

As previously stated, the inclusion compounds or complexes are characterized by the lack of adhesive forces between the components of the complex. They arise from the ability of one compound to spatially enclose another. It is not possible, in most cases, to predict the formation of an inclusion compound between two selected components.

Clathrates—Inclusion compounds, which are formed by the envelopment of a molecule of a "guest" compound in the cage-like hollow space formed by combination of several molecules of the "host" compound,

are known as *clathrates* (Latin, *clathri*, lattice). This type of compound is frequently nonstoichiometric. Clathrates can be depicted by C(M), in which the molecular component M is trapped during the formation of cage C from molecules or other complexes which exist in the same solution with it. One component may be a solid, liquid, or gas retained within the cages of the host; it may be released by dissolving, heating, or grinding the clathrate. Such complexes are usually prepared by crystallization of the host substance from a solution containing the guest component.

In the formation of such a compound four factors are involved: (1) there is no apparent means of linking C and M; (2) component C must be capable of cage formation; (3) M must be replaceable by other molecules that fit into the cages (but not by chemically analogous compounds if their molecules are of unsuited size); (4) the ratio of the cage-forming component C to the number of cavities available to contain M limits the composition, but the composition may vary since not all cavities may be occupied.

Many applications for this novel type of complex have already been demonstrated. Because of the ability of hydroquinone to clathrate inert gases, krypton-85 (radioactive, a β-emitter) can be successfully trapped to provide a solid, easily handled source of the gas. Thiophene can be removed from benzene using Werner complexes as the clathrate host. Synthetic metal-alumino silicates, advertised as "molecular sieves," are available; these materials can be used to store gaseous, volatile, and toxic materials, to dry gases, and to separate gaseous mixtures. It is also possible to "load" the host material of the sieve with substances such as volatile oils, germicidal agents, detergents, and pesticides and provide a convenient, dry material for ease of formulation. The clathrated guest can later be removed by some simple, physical process.

Channel-Lattice Complexes—This type of inclusion complex occurs primarily when the host component crystallizes in such a way as to form channel-like spaces in the crystal lattice. The guest molecule then must be of a shape which will fit into the voids or channels in the lattice. Urea, amylose, the zeolites, and other compounds will complex other materials in this fashion. Since the channels are formed by crystallization of the host, in spring-like spirals, the nature of the guest component is usually limited to long, unbranched, straight-chain compounds. Urea will complex n-octane, but not iso-octane. Choleic acids also function as host components in which the guest components are held in canals situated lengthwise to the crystals. Digitonin–cholesterol complexes are examples of the choleic acid type of complex.

The potential and present applications of the channel-lattice complexes are many. Separation of petroleum products, prevention of oxidation (vitamin A palmitate is successfully complexed with urea and thereby protected), separation of optical isomers (several host compounds have steric features which allow the complexation of only one enantiomorph of a racemic mixture), and many analytical uses are illustrative of such applications. The well-known starch–iodine color has been shown to involve formation of an inclusion compound of iodine in the central channel of the screw-like starch molecule. Other compounds such as the flavones, coumarin, benzophenone, benzamide, and barbituric acid are also capable of giving the blue iodine-addition compound.

Complex Equilibria

Complexing agents, and the complexes formed from them, may have a variety of effects on physiological processes and on the use of medication to influence these processes. They may hinder or promote the efficacy of a drug; they may sustain its action, increase its absorption, protect or increase the stability of a dosage form, or act like a drug by removing toxins deleterious to normal body function.

Certain theories have been advanced advocating that a major portion of drug action occurs through complexation. It is not necessary that a drug be associated with a complexing agent in a dosage form, but it may complex within the body by association with some macromolecular complexing agent such as a protein molecule. In either case the stability of various complexes may be evaluated by assuming the equilibrium

$$\text{drug} + \text{complexing agent} = \text{drug:complex}$$

The stability constant K_s for this equilibrium may be written

$$K_s = \frac{\text{conc of drug:complex}}{\text{drug conc} \times \text{complexing agent conc}}$$

A 1:1 complex, as indicated, is not necessarily the rule, and any stoichiometric relationship may apply. Evaluation of the stability constant involves determination of the molar concentrations of the several terms of the equation by some analytical procedure. It should be evident that knowledge of the relative values of K_s for any one drug, in the systems under investigation, is of utmost importance, as usually only the undissociated drug is physiologically active. Refer to the latter portion of this chapter on *Protein Binding of Drugs*.

Ion-Exchange Compounds

As mentioned previously, ion-exchange phenomena may not correctly be included in a chapter on complexation, but as ion exchange is regarded as both an absorption and adsorption process, there is perhaps some rationale for its inclusion.

Three theories, all of which may be simultaneously applicable, are proposed to explain ion-exchange processes.

1. Crystal-Lattice Theory—If an ionic solid is considered to be completely dissociated, the surface ions are bound to the lattice with a lower binding energy than are internal ions of the same species since the surface ions are not completely surrounded by ions of the opposite charge. When the solid is placed in a polar solvent, extensive solvation of the surface ions further reduces their binding energy with the result that marked dissociation from the lattice occurs. Addition of a foreign electrolyte may then cause an exchange process between the surface ions and those of the same charge of the foreign electrolyte. The ease of replacement at a fixed number of exchange sites is proportional to a number of factors, including the nature of the forces binding the surface ion to the lattice, the charge of the exchange ion, the concentration of exchange ions, the accessibility of lattice ions, the sizes of the two ions, and the solubility effects.

2. Double-Layer Theory—The presence of two rigid charged layers at the surface of the exchanging material is assumed in this theory; the inner layer is fixed, the outer diffuse, with no sharp boundary. The concentration of ions at the diffuse layer is in equilibrium with those in solution. Addition of a foreign ion to the solution upsets the equilibrium and some of the new ions will enter the outer, diffuse layer, by exchange. In the double-layer exchange mechanism the number of exchange sites is not fixed, being dependent both on the concentration of the foreign ion being exchanged and on the pH of the solution.

3. Donnan Membrane Theory—In this theory the interface between the solid, exchange material and liquid is considered a membrane exhibiting an unequal distribution of charges on either side; diffusion through the membrane establishes equilibrium. Disruption of the equilibrium by addition of a foreign electrolyte necessitates a rebalancing, with subsequent exchange of ions through the membrane.

All of the theories are similar, as they require that the exchange must observe the laws of electrical neutrality; they differ in the postulated position and origin of the exchange site. This exchange site is a fixed, nondiffusible, ionic grouping capable of forming an ionic bond with small, diffusible ions of opposite charge.

Modern ion-exchange materials are usually synthetic, being formed from an inert, insoluble polymer of high molecular weight containing suitable ionic groupings as integral parts of the polymer structure. However, such natural materials as clays, zeolites, and ultramarines are still used to advantage. The resins are of the cation-exchange type (formed with acidic groups as part of the polymer) or anionic type (with basic exchange groups). The exchange groups may be of varying degrees of basicity or acidity, selected to suit the intended application. Amino groups are usually the reactive sites of the anion type of exchange resins, while sulfonic acid, carboxylic acid, or phenolic groups are reactive sites in cation exchange resins.

More recently, *electron-exchange* resins have been the subject of study; in these an exchange or transfer of electrons takes place. Several *redox* resins have been prepared which show some promise of utility in removing small quantities of oxidizing agents from water by a process of reduction.

All exchange materials have a finite capacity for exchange which is limited by the number of exchange sites available. After a period of use the exchange process ceases because of the loss of exchange sites; the material then must be regenerated by a reversal of the exchange technique. For example, if a resin is used to soften water through replacement of sodium ions on the resin with calcium or magnesium ions from the water, the process will eventually stop when sodium ions are no longer available. If the resin is now treated with a concentrated solution of sodium ions, reversal of the process occurs, resulting in replacement of calcium by sodium and regeneration of the ion-exchange material.

There are many pharmaceutical and medical uses for ion-exchange materials, besides that of their important use in water conditioning. For example, they are employed in the separation of amino acids obtained from proteins by hydrolysis, and in the purification of alkaloids, vitamins, hormones, serological solutions, and viruses. Potassium penicillin may be converted to the sodium salt and streptomycin sulfate to the chloride by processes of ion exchange.

Ion-exchange resins have been utilized to prepare tablet dosage forms of absorbed drugs that have sustained-release action, the drug being slowly released in the intestine. Several commercial preparations of this type are available. (See Chapter 89, *Prolonged-Action Pharmaceuticals.*)

Some therapeutic applications of ion-exchange compounds include: use as an antacid in peptic ulcer where a weak-base anion exchanger removes acid without adding anything to the gastrointestinal fluid; use of kaolin, a natural ion-exchange material, in diarrhea; removal of body sodium in edema and hypertension with cation exchangers; bulk laxative action of resins that swell in the gastrointestinal tract; removal of waste materials in impaired kidney function; use as an anticoagulant to remove blood calcium; adsorption of bacteria in certain internal infections; use as a drug vehicle, as by the administration of a weak-base ion exchanger simultaneously with *p*-aminosalicylic acid to increase palatability without impairing effectiveness.

Protein Binding of Drugs

It should be recognized by even a beginning student of biochemistry, medicinal chemistry, or pharmacology that fundamental to many biochemical and pharmacologic processes is the ability of specialized functional proteins to interact with lower molecular weight compounds to form complexes known as enzyme–substrate complexes or drug–receptor site complexes. It is known that considerable structural specificity is required for the formation of association products of this type.

Delineation of the structural requirements involved constitutes an important area of biochemical and medicinal chemical research. Such research is especially challenging in view of the difficulties in isolating enzymes in pure form and in characterizing, even qualitatively, the nature of receptor sites which are responsible for drug action.

Perhaps not so widely appreciated by beginning students is that complex formation between small molecules and rather common and widely distributed proteins such as albumins and globulins also occurs to a significant extent.

Protein binding is the term which is generally used in referring to this type of interaction. While the manifestations of protein binding are not as dramatic or as well defined as those resulting from interactions involving enzymes and receptor sites, they can be of importance in drug therapy. For this reason and because of the availability of purified and well-characterized plasma proteins, much attention has been devoted to the study of the binding of drugs and other low molecular weight compounds by plasma proteins, and in particular by albumin.

A large number of publications describing such studies are found in the literature. The studies resulted, either directly or indirectly, from the desire to answer one or more fundamental guideline questions relating to protein binding which were posed by Scatchard, *et al*:[1] "How many? How tightly? Where? Why? What of it?" Thus, many of the reported studies were physical–chemical in nature and were oriented to determining:

1. The maximum number of small molecules which could be bound by a protein molecule.
2. The magnitude of the association constant or constants which characterized the association.
3. The chemical and conformational nature of the binding sites on the protein.
4. The nature of the intermolecular forces which were responsible for interaction.

Other studies attempted to assess the importance of protein binding as it relates to the action and uses of specific drugs.

Mass Law Expressions—Protein binding, like other types of complexation, results from reversible associations and can be described by conventional mass law expressions. It should be recognized, however, that a protein is a macromolecule composed of many hundreds of amino acids linked together to form the primary protein structure.

It is the side-chains of the composite amino acids that possess the functional groups which are responsible for attracting and binding small molecules. For example, epsilon amino groups of certain of the many lysine residues and phenolic hydroxyl groups of some tyrosine residues have been implicated in the binding of a number of drugs by albumin.

It is apparent that many and varied sites, capable of binding, can exist on the same macromolecule. Mass law expressions which are used to treat and interpret data are, therefore, somewhat more complicated than those encountered in more familiar situations such as the ionization of weak electrolytes. Many studies have demonstrated that the sites can be divided into classes with different binding abilities but that, usually, sites within a class possess the same intrinsic affinity for a small molecule. Fundamental studies are designed to gain some idea about the classes of sites involved, the number of sites in a particular class, and the strength of binding to a site.

The simplest case which can be encountered involves a reversible interaction to form a 1:1 protein–small molecule complex; ie,

$$\text{Protein} + \text{Drug} \overset{K}{=} \text{Protein:Drug}$$

The mass law expression, defining this behavior, is

$$K = \frac{(PD)}{(P)(D)} \qquad (1)$$

where K = association constant, (PD) = concentration of the 1:1 complex, (P) = concentration of unbound protein, and (D) = concentration of unbound small molecule.

Experimental methods which are used to study binding behavior usually permit the determination of the concentrations of bound and unbound small molecule. The total concentration of protein is usually known or can be determined readily. It is convenient, for the purpose of data treatment, to define an experimentally determinable quantity, r, as the average number of small molecules bound per mole of protein; ie, for a 1:1 complex,

$$r = \frac{(PD)}{(P)_t} \qquad (2)$$

where $(P)_t$ = total concentration of protein in the binding system. The quantity r can be defined in terms of K and (D) in the following manner:

$$r = \frac{(PD)}{(P) + (PD)} \qquad (3)$$

$$r = \frac{K(P)(D)}{K(P)(D) + (P)} \qquad (4)$$

$$r = \frac{K(D)}{1 + K(D)} \qquad (5)$$

A more complex case is the interaction of a small

molecule species with two sites on the protein. The simplest situation here is that involving two sites which belong to the same class and which behave independently; ie, both sites possess the same intrinsic affinity for the small molecule and the binding of a small molecule to one site does not influence the binding behavior of the remaining site. It should be recognized that three identifiable complexes can result from this situation. For convenience, these can be symbolized by $-PD$, $DP-$, and DPD. Unbound protein is symbolized by $-P-$ to indicate that two sites can participate. Mechanisms and appropriate mass law expressions are

$$-P- + D \overset{K}{=} -PD$$

$$K = \frac{(-PD)}{(-P-)(D)} \tag{6}$$

$$-P- + D \overset{K_1}{=} DP-$$

$$K_1 = \frac{(DP-)}{(-P-)(D)} \tag{7}$$

$$-PD + D \overset{K_2}{=} DPD$$

$$K_2 = \frac{(DPD)}{(-PD)(D)} = \frac{(DPD)}{K(-P-)(D)^2} \tag{8}$$

$$DP- + D \overset{K_3}{=} DPD$$

$$K_3 = \frac{(DPD)}{(DP-)(D)} = \frac{(DPD)}{K_1(-P-)(D)^2} \tag{9}$$

For such a system

$$r = \frac{(-PD) + (DP-) + 2(DPD)}{(-P-) + (-PD) + (DP-) + (DPD)} \tag{10}$$

$$r = \frac{K(-P-)(D) + K_1(-P-)(D) + 2KK_2(-P-)(D)^2}{(-P-) + K(-P-)(D) + K_1(-P-)(D) + KK_2(-P-)(D)^2} \tag{11}$$

$$r = \frac{K(D) + K_1(D) + 2KK_2(D)^2}{1 + K(D) + K_1(D) + KK_2(D)^2} \tag{12}$$

It will be recognized that an equivalent expression is

$$r = \frac{K(D) + K_1(D) + 2K_1K_3(D)^2}{1 + K(D) + K_1(D) + K_1K_3(D)^2} \tag{13}$$

By definition, $K = K_1 = K_2 = K_3$; ie, all sites are equivalent and independent. Therefore, Eqs. 12 and 13 can be written

$$r = \frac{2K(D) + 2K^2(D)^2}{1 + 2K(D) + K^2(D)^2} \tag{14}$$

$$r = \frac{2K(D)(1 + K(D))}{(1 + K(D))^2} \tag{15}$$

$$r = \frac{2K(D)}{1 + K(D)} \tag{16}$$

It can be shown by a similar treatment that if three independent and equivalent sites of the protein can participate in the binding of a small molecule, then

$$r = \frac{3K(D)}{1 + K(D)} \tag{17}$$

In the general case of n equivalent and independent sites,

$$r = \frac{nK(D)}{1 + K(D)} \tag{18}$$

The terms n and K are known as binding parameters with n being the number of sites in a class and K being the intrinsic association constant which characterizes the strength of the binding between the small molecule and a site in the class under consideration.

Suppose, as a further extension, that two entirely different classes of sites exist on the protein molecule and that, as before, all sites are independent and sites within a class are equivalent. A similar treatment can be used to derive an expression for r for this case. It must be recognized, however, that the definition of unbound protein is somewhat different here than in the previous examples of multiple binding. That is, a 1:1 complex, for example, is "seen" as an unbound protein molecule by a small molecule interacting with a site in the class which is not involved in the 1:1 complex but as bound protein by a small molecule interacting with a site which is equivalent to that participating in the 1:1 complex. With this in mind it can be readily shown that

$$r = \frac{n_aK_a(D)}{1 + K_a(D)} + \frac{n_bK_b(D)}{1 + K_b(D)} \tag{19}$$

where n_a = number of binding sites in the "a" class of sites, K_a = intrinsic association constant for the interaction of D with a site in the "a" class, n_b = number of binding sites in the "b" class of sites, and K_b = intrinsic association constant for the interaction of D with a site in the "b" class of sites.

A general expression which describes binding to "i" different classes of sites is

$$r = \sum_{i=1}^{i} \frac{n_iK_i(D)}{1 + K_i(D)} \tag{20}$$

Experimental Methods—A wide variety of experimental methods are available for application to the study of protein binding. Many of the methods are identical to those used for studying other types of complexation. For example, the solubility behavior of a small molecule species in the presence and absence of protein can be studied to assess the degree of interaction. Similarly, the influence of protein on the partitioning behavior of a small molecule between an aqueous phase and an immiscible organic solvent can be investigated. In some cases, binding is manifested by significant changes in the spectral characteristics of a small molecule and such changes can be used to assess the degree to which binding has occurred.

The most commonly used technique for determining the equilibrium between free and bound small molecule in a protein solution is that of equilibrium dialysis. Here, a protein solution is enclosed within a membrane, such as cellophane, which is freely permeable to the small molecule species but which is impermeable to protein and protein complexes. The protein solution, contained within the membrane, is contacted with a solution of the small molecule and the system is gently agitated until equilibrium has been reached. Samples are then withdrawn from the solutions on both sides of the membrane and assayed to determine the concentration of small molecule in each solution. In the absence of binding both solutions will have the same concentration of small molecule. If binding occurs, the protein-containing solution will have a higher concentration of small molecule since both bound and unbound species will be present. Furthermore, the concentration of unbound species will be the same in both solutions. The situation is depicted in Fig. 135. Table I contains data which was obtained in a study of the binding of caffeine by serum albumin[2] and is illustrative of the equilibrium dialysis approach to studying protein binding.

Another widely used technique which is related to equilibrium dialysis is *ultrafiltration*. Here, a solution containing protein and small molecule is filtered, under pressure, through a membrane which is impermeable to the protein and protein complexes. A relatively small volume of filtrate is collected and assayed to yield the concentration of unbound small molecule, and the unfiltered portion is assayed to obtain the total concentration of unbound and bound species. The method is much faster than equilibrium dialysis but involves some uncertainty due to a changing protein concentration during ultrafiltration.

Experimental Results—Many investigators report the results of protein binding studies in terms of the fraction of total small molecule which is present in the bound form. This fraction is usually symbolized by β; ie,

$$\beta = \frac{(D)_b}{(D)_t}$$

where $(D)_b$ = concentration of bound small molecule and $(D)_t$ = total concentration of small molecule in the protein–small molecule system. For example, for the data of Table I:

$$\beta_{\text{caffeine}} = \frac{0.4 \times 10^{-4}}{0.7 \times 10^{-4}} = 0.571$$

which means, of course, that 57.1% of the caffeine in the protein compartment is present in the form of a

protein complex. It should be emphasized, however, that β is not a constant but changes depending on both the concentration of protein and small molecule in the system under study and that a β value does not provide a reflection of the intrinsic affinity of a small molecule for a protein. This can be appreciated readily by considering a binding system in which only one class of sites on the protein participates in the binding. The binding behavior for such a case is described by Eq. 18, which in a slightly different form is

$$\frac{(D)_b}{(P)_t} = \frac{nK(D)}{1 + K(D)}$$

It is instructive to define β in terms of n and K by using Eq. 20. Thus,

$$\beta = \frac{(D)_b}{(D)_t} = \frac{(D)_b}{(D) + (D)_b} \tag{21}$$

$$(D)_b = \frac{nK(D)(P)_t}{1 + K(D)} \tag{22}$$

$$\beta = \frac{\dfrac{nk(D)(P)_t}{1 + K(D)}}{(D) + \dfrac{nK(D)(P)_t}{1 + K(D)}} \tag{23}$$

$$\beta = \frac{nK(D)(P)_t}{(D) + K(D)^2 + nK(D)(P)_t} \tag{24}$$

$$\beta = \frac{1}{1 + \dfrac{(D)}{n(P)_t} + \dfrac{1}{nK(P)_t}} \tag{25}$$

It is apparent from Eq. 25 that β exhibits a dependency on both the protein and small molecule concentrations and can, for the same binding system, vary depending on the design of the experiment. If, for example, a system is studied which contains a relatively low protein concentration and a relatively high small molecule concentration, then a low β value will result. Conversely a high β value would be generated if the protein concentration is large compared to the small molecule concentration.

A much more meaningful and fundamental way to characterize and define binding behavior is by the binding parameters, n and K. A knowledge of these values permits the calculation of β at any protein–small molecule combination. An approach to determining n and K values might be intuitively anticipated by examining Eq. 18, for as (D) becomes very large, r approaches n; ie, the protein becomes saturated

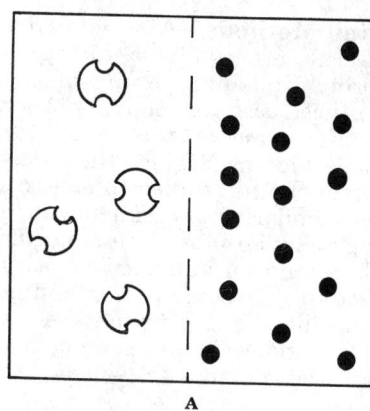

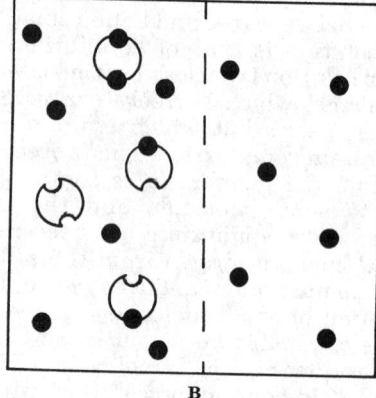

Fig. 135. An equilibrium dialysis experiment. The large open symbols represent protein molecules. The small enclosed circles represent molecules of a low molecular weight compound capable of being protein-bound. *A:* Before equilibration; *B:* after equilibration.

Table I—Results Obtained in a Study of the Binding of Caffeine by Bovine Serum Albumin

	Solution within membrane	Solution outside membrane
Volume	10 ml	10 ml
Concentration of albumin	2.8×10^{-4} M	0
Concentration of caffeine before equilibration	0	1×10^{-4} M
Concentration of caffeine after equilibration	0.7×10^{-4}	0.3×10^{-4}
Concentration of unbound caffeine is, therefore	0.3×10^{-4}	0.3×10^{-4}
Concentration of bound caffeine is, therefore	0.4×10^{-4}	0

$$r = \frac{0.4 \times 10^{-4}}{2.8 \times 10^{-4}} = 0.143$$

with small molecule. Determination of r at very high concentrations of small molecule relative to that of the protein would be expected to yield an estimate of n. With a knowledge of n, K could be determined from studies conducted under concentration conditions well below those resulting in saturation. Unfortunately, this approach is not usually practical or possible because solubility limitations frequently preclude attainment of very high concentrations of many low molecular weight compounds. It is, therefore, necessary to use indirect graphical methods to obtain estimations of n and K. Eq. 18, for example, can be rearranged to the form

$$1/r = 1/nK(D) + 1/n \qquad (26)$$

This form of the binding equation was first proposed by Klotz[3] who suggested that a plot of $1/r$ vs $1/(D)$ should yield, in the case of binding by one class of sites on a protein, a straight line with the ordinate intercept being $1/n$ and the slope, $1/nK$. One disadvantage of the "Klotz plot" is that experimental points obtained at low (D) values are excessively weighted and the plot can mask behaviors that might occur at high values of (D). For example, participation of a second class of sites with a lower K might not be apparent if the data are treated by a Klotz plot. Scatchard,[4] therefore, recommended a different plot based on a different rearrangement of Eq. 18:

$$r/(D) = nK - Kr \qquad (27)$$

A "Scatchard plot" results when $r/(D)$ is plotted as a function of r. In the case of one class of binding sites such a plot should be linear with a slope of $-K$ and extrapolation to the abscissa yields an intercept with the value of n (when $r/(D) = 0$, $r = n$). Furthermore, extrapolation to the ordinate yields an intercept with the value of nK (when $r = 0$, $r/(D) = nK$). Participation of secondary classes of sites is quite apparent when data are presented as a Scatchard plot. Such an occurrence is manifested by marked upward curvature of the plot. It can be shown from Eq. 20 that when more than one class of sites are responsible for binding, curvature should result and that the ordinate and abscissa intercepts are $\Sigma\, nK$ and $\Sigma\, n$.

Frequently it is of interest to evaluate the binding behavior of systems in which the exact nature and concentration of protein components are now known such as, for example, plasma. While, most often, the results of such studies are presented in terms of "fraction bound," more useful methods of data presentation have been suggested.[5-7] These are based on another rearrangement of Eq. 18:

$$\frac{(D)_b}{(D)} = nK(P)_t - K(D) \qquad (28)$$

Binding data can, on this basis, be presented as a plot of $(D)_b/(D)$ vs (D). The plot, which does not require a knowledge of $(P)_t$, is linear if one class of sites are involved in the interaction. Furthermore, the slope of the resulting line is $-K$. Curvature of the plot suggests the participation of more than one protein or multiple classes of sites on a single protein.

Extent of Occurrence—At least two extensive reviews[8,9] are available which emphasize that a host of compounds can undergo interaction with a variety of proteins. Many hundreds of different drugs, for example, have been shown to be bound by whole plasma, albumin, or globulins. Compounds which have been studied include penicillins, tetracyclines, sulfonamides, barbiturates, salicylates, steroids, coumarin anticoagulants, sulfonylureas, local and general anesthetics, various vitamins, hormones, amino acids, natural metabolites, dyes, surfactants, buffer components, and many others. Some substances such as warfarin and certain penicillins are strongly bound while others such as certain barbiturates and chlorpromazine interact rather weakly.

It is suggested that the reader consult the reviews to obtain a quantitative idea of the spectrum of compounds which are known to undergo binding and the spectrum of behaviors that can be encountered.

Significance—Information of both theoretical and practical importance has been derived from studies of protein binding. For example, studies with albumin have provided insights to the nature of the amino acid residues which participate in the binding process, structural characteristics which promote binding, and the intermolecular forces which are responsible for binding. Such information is of significance since it can be extrapolated, to yield a better understanding, at the molecular level, of drug action and enzyme activity.

Of more practical and immediate significance is that nonspecific protein binding in the body can influence the distributional, pharmacologic, and pharmacokinetic properties of drugs. This possibility has a logical basis in view of the inability of proteins and protein complexes to pass through most biological membranes. Thus, the fraction of a dose of drug which is bound by plasma proteins is essentially restricted to the plasma compartment of the body and cannot diffuse to sites of action or metabolism in other compartments.

Verwey and co-workers,[10] for example, developed a method for sampling lymph by cannulation of the peripheral lymphatics of dogs. They then studied, in dogs, the distribution of a number of penicillins between plasma and lymph and demonstrated that the plasma concentrations of penicillin were significantly higher than those found in lymph. They also showed, however, that the concentration of unbound drug was the same in lymph as it was in plasma. Similarly, Kunin[11] showed that with a series of penicillins, as the degree of plasma protein binding decreased, localization of antibiotic in brain, muscle, lung, and heart of rabbits increased.

Martin[12] has provided, by means of a simple model, an excellent quantitative visualization of the potential effects of binding in plasma on drug distribution in the body. His model was essentially that of a large dialysis system at equilibrium; ie, he assumed that drug in the body was distributed into two compartments: plasma with a volume of 3 liters and a second compartment composed of the remaining body water with a volume of 39 liters.

Martin further assumed that binding occurred only in the plasma compartment and resulted from the interaction between albumin, present at a concentration of 5×10^{-4} M, with drug to form nondiffusible 1:1 complexes. As in a dialysis system, unbound drug was considered to be in equilibrium between the two compartments. He then conducted calculations related to the binding of four hypothetical drugs whose interactions with albumin could be characterized by association constants (K) of 10^4, 10^5, 10^6, and 10^7 L mole^{-1}, respectively. For each drug he assumed a concentration of unbound drug (D) and calculated, first, the total concentration of drug in plasma $(D)_t$ by an equation directly derivable from Eq. 25:

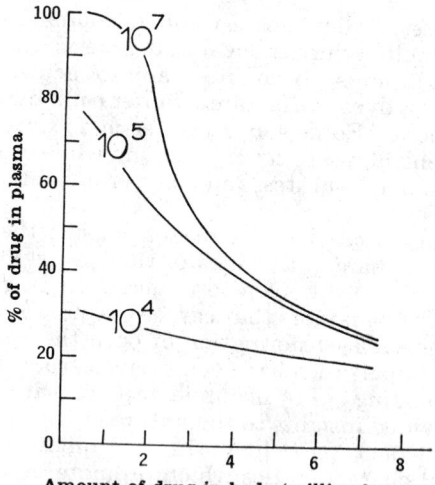

Fig. 136. A plot, based on theoretical considerations, which illustrates the potential influence of plasma-binding on the distribution of drug between plasma and other aqueous compartments in the body. Each curve represents a different value of K (after Martin[12]).

$$(D)_t = (D) \left\{ 1 + \frac{(P)_t}{1/K + (D)} \right\} \qquad (29)$$

He then calculated for each value of (D): (a) the amount of drug in the body = $39(D) + 3(D)_t$; (b) per cent of drug free in the body = $42(D) \times 100/(39(D) + 3(D)_t)$; and (c) per cent of drug in plasma = $3(D)_t \times 100/39(D) + 3(D)_t$. The results of such calculations were presented in graphical form such as those illustrated by Figs. 136 and 137.

It is apparent from these representative theoretical curves that binding can influence drug distribution in the body and that the magnitude of the effect will depend on both the strength of association and the dosage of drug. For example, a strongly bound drug such as that with a K of 10^7 will, at low dosage levels, be concentrated primarily in the plasma compartment. However, at higher dosage levels, the fraction of drug in the plasma will be markedly reduced.

Martin also emphasized another characteristic attributable to the plasma binding of drugs with a high affinity for proteins; that there is a dosage range within which small increases in dose result in relatively large increases in the amount of drug in the body which is not bound. He noted that this behavior can have interesting manifestations on dose–response characteristics and pharmacokinetic properties of such drugs. His treatment additionally emphasizes that binding to plasma proteins will have an appreciable effect on drug distribution only if the strength of binding is quite high. For example, with a drug having a K of 10^4, the "fraction bound" in plasma can be 83.4% but, nevertheless, 73% of the total dose is present in the body in the unbound form.

Martin's model is a highly simplified representation of what might indeed be a complex distributional pattern involving binding to tissue proteins, partitioning into fatty compartments, the unavailability of certain aqueous compartments, etc. Nevertheless, he clearly demonstrates that plasma–protein binding can be an important determinant in drug distribution for some drugs but that for many others it might not be of significance in spite of in vitro demonstrations that interaction occurs to produce a seemingly high "fraction bound."

It is generally considered that protein-bound drug is not pharmacologically active. Rolinson and Sutherland,[13] for example, studied the plasma binding of 17 antibiotics and found that in vitro activity was inversely proportional to the observed extent of binding. Reynolds and Cluff[14] showed that the antipyretic activity of sodium salicylate in rabbits was reduced when albumin was coadministered. Anton[15] demonstrated an inverse correlation between bacteriostatic activity and extent of binding of sulfonamides.

Reversal of this type of drug "inactivation" by the addition of a competitive inhibitor to the binding system has been considered by a number of workers and attempts to evaluate such a possibility, in vitro and in vivo, have been reported. The theoretical basis for this approach can be readily derived, for if a drug, D, and a competitor, C, compete for the same binding site; ie,

$$D + P = PD$$
$$C + P = PC$$

then,

$$r_D = \frac{(D)_b}{(P)_t} = \frac{(PD)}{(P) + (PD) + (PC)}$$
$$= \frac{K_D(D)}{1 + K_D(D) + K_C(C)} \qquad (30)$$

where K_D = association constant for the drug–protein complex, K_C = association constant for the competitor–protein complex, and, (C) = concentration of unbound competitor.

The extent to which D is bound depends on the product $K_C(C)$; the larger the value of $K_C(C)$, the lower the concentration of bound drug in the system.

Anton's[15,16] studies have been frequently cited as an example of this approach to the possible potentiation of the pharmacological activity of a strongly bound drug. He was concerned with the inhibition, in vitro and in vivo, of sulfonamide binding. He demonstrated that phenylbutazone, sulfinpyrazine, ethyl biscoumarate, and iophenoxic acid were effective in displacing protein-bound sulfonamides and that the antibacterial activity of a sulfonamide in the presence of albumin was increased markedly by the presence of a displacing agent. He showed, quite dramatically, that administration of sulfinpyrazone to rats who were dosed with sulfaethylthiadiazole or sulfamethoxypyridazine resulted in a precipitous decline in the total plasma concentration of sulfonamide but an increase in the concentration of unbound drug. Concomitant with this was an increase in the concentration of sulfonamide in tissues.

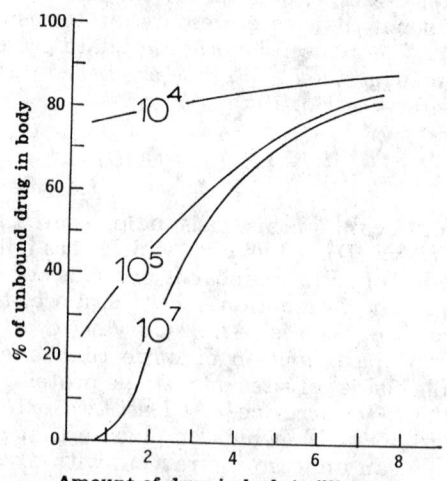

Fig. 137. A plot, based on theoretical considerations, which illustrates the potential influence of plasma-binding on the distribution of drug between bound and unbound forms in the body. Each curve represents a different value of K (after Martin[12]).

Attempts to utilize competitive displacement of bound drug clinically has met with only limited success. Kunin[17] has discussed such studies and noted that the attainment of enhanced clinical activity by displacement might be realized only with difficulty because of the large dosages of competitive inhibitors required and the often limited degree of displacement which may be achieved in man.

Consequences resulting from the displacement by drugs of protein-bound endogenous compounds also have been considered and studied. Bilirubin is an important example since its displacement can result in toxic manifestations in infants and in individuals with impaired bilirubin conjugating mechanisms. Odell[18-20] showed that salicylates and sulfonamides, in concentrations which are encountered clinically, could displace bilirubin and he reviewed the implications of such an event. Similarly, Christensen[21] studied the effect of several benzoates and salicylates on thyroxine binding and has attempted to relate physiologic and toxicologic effects of these drugs to the displacement of bound thyroid hormones.

The influence of protein binding on the time course of drug in the body has been considered by a number of authors. For example, Bennhold[22] showed that the rate of elimination of congo red from patients with depressed albumin levels (0.1 to 0.2% of normal) was approximately 60% more rapid than with normal subjects. Weiner, et al,[23] suggested that the slow biotransformation and negligible kidney elimination of dicoumarol is a result of the high degree of protein binding of this drug. The prolonged blood levels of chlortetracycline were explained by Sirota and Saltzman[24] as being due to protein binding. Kruger-Thiemer, et al,[25] studied the pharmacokinetics of a long-acting sulfonamide, sulfaorthodimethoxine, and showed that its unusual dose-dependent pharmacokinetic behavior could be explained as being due to a high degree of protein binding. Rieder[26] did not observe a correlation between binding parameters and rate of disappearance from plasma or rate of renal excretion for the various sulfonamides which he studied. He pointed out that only when elimination proceeds primarily via glomerular filtration and without significant tubular secretion and reabsorption should binding be anticipated to exert an appreciable effect on the rate of elimination of a drug.

In summary, considerable *in vitro* and *in vivo* evidence is available to indicate that plasma-protein binding can influence the distributional, pharmacologic, and pharmacokinetic properties of drugs. It appears, however, that only in the case of strongly bound drugs, will the manifestations of binding be of practical clinical consequence. A number of important drugs do fall in the category of "strongly bound" and these serve as examples which emphasize the need to consider protein binding in the characterization of drug behavior.

References

1. Scatchard, G. F., et al, in Gurd, F. R. N., ed., *Chemical Specificity in Biological Interactions*, Academic, New York, 1954, pp. 193–220.
2. Eichman, M. L., PhD Thesis, The Ohio State Univ., 1961.
3. Klotz, I. M., *Arch. Biochem.*, **9**, 109 (1946).
4. Scatchard, G. F., *Ann. NY Acad. Sci.*, **51**, 660 (1949).
5. Kruger-Theimer, E., et al, *Congr. Intern. Med. Cibernetica 3°, Napoli, 1964*, 249 (Pub. 1967).
6. Sandberg, A. A., et al, in Nakao, T., et al, eds., *Steriod Dynamics*, Academic, New York, 1966, pp. 33–41.
7. Rosenthal, H. E., *Anal. Biochem.*, **20**, 525 (1967).
8. Goldstein, A., *Pharmacol. Rev.*, **1**, 102 (1949).
9. Meyer, M. C., and Guttman, D. E., *J. Pharm. Sci.*, **57**, 895 (1968).
10. Verwey, W. F., Williams, H. R., and Kalsow, C., *Antimicrobial Agents Chemotherapy*, 476 (1962).
11. Kunin, C. M., *J. Lab. Clin. Med.*, **65**, 406 (1965).
12. Martin, B. K., *Nature*, **207**, 274 (1965).
13. Rolinson, G. N., and Sutherland, R., *Brit. J. Pharmacol.*, **25**, 638 (1965).
14. Reynolds, R. C., and Cluff, L. E., *Bull. Johns Hopkins Hosp.*, **107**, 278 (1960).
15. Anton, A. H., *J. Pharmacol. Exptl. Therap.*, **129**, 282 (1960).
16. Anton, A. H., *J. Pharmacol. Exptl. Therap.*, **134**, 291 (1961).
17. Kunin, C. M., *Clin. Pharmacol. Therap.*, **7**, 180 (1966).
18. Odell, G. B., *Am. J. Diseases Children*, **98**, 624 (1959).
19. Odell, G. B., *J. Clin. Invest.*, **38**, 823 (1959).
20. Odell, G. B., *J. Pediat.*, **55**, 268 (1959).
21. Christensen, L. K., *Acta Pharmacol. Toxicol.*, **16**, 129 (1959).
22. Bennhold, H., in Desgrez, P., and De Traverse, P. M., eds., *Transport Function of Plasma Proteins*, Elsevier, New York, 1965, p. 3.
23. Weiner, M., et al, *J. Pharmacol. Exptl. Therap.*, **99**, 409 (1950).
24. Sirota, J. A., and Saltzman, A., *J. Pharmacol. Exptl. Therap.*, **100**, 210 (1950).
25. Kruger-Thiemer, E., et al, *Antimicrobial Agents Chemotherapy*, 183 (1965).
26. Rieder, J., *Arzneimittel-Forsch.*, **13**, 95 (1963).

17 | Quantum Chemistry

Planck's hypothesis—Bohr atomic theory—wave nature of electrons—
uncertainty principle—Schrödinger wave equation—atomic and
molecular orbitals—bonding and antibonding orbitals—polyatomic
orbitals—hybridization—appendix

This chapter was prepared by

Arthur Cammarata, PhD, *Associate Professor of Physical Medicinal
Chemistry, School of Pharmacy, Temple University, Philadelphia, Pa. 19140*

Quantum theory is concerned with the energetics and interactions of electrons, atoms, and molecules with each other and with electromagnetic radiation. A brilliant achievement of theoretical physics that explains diverse physical and chemical phenomena which had long defied explanation, the quantum approach probably will provide answers also for a diversity of unsolved biological problems. Molecular biology has prepared the way for quantum concepts to be used in the study of biological systems, and the promise of future fruitful achievement through this approach is great.

That many biological phenomena cannot be described in terms of classic chemistry and belong in the domain of quantum mechanics—specifically to quantum biology—has been noted by Albert Szent-Györgyi;[1] he has also suggested that hormones and drugs that produce violent reactions in the body, even though they are chemically inert, may act by influencing electronic excitations at a target site.

Writing on the subject of *Quantum Genetics*, Löwdin[2] calls attention to the fact that protons and electrons obey the laws of quantum mechanics rather than of classic physics. He believes that the protonic and electronic structure of "biologically interesting molecules" has to be treated by quantum chemistry. Among other biologically important quantum concepts is the likelihood that the ultimate cause of spontaneous cancer "is a quantum-mechanical phenomenon associated with two protons changing places over a distance of the order of magnitude of 10^{-8} cm."

In more recent years Pullman and Pullman[3] have applied quantum methods to a number of systems of biochemical interest, and reports are now found in which these methods have indicated probable electronic events that lead to drug response.[4]

Origin of the Quantum Theory

In 1900 the German physicist Max Planck, attempting to explain quantitatively the radiation from a black body, advanced the bold hypothesis that radiation (energy) can be emitted or absorbed only in discrete units, which he called *quanta* (singular, *quantum*). According to Planck, such energy is not a continuous flow of electromagnetic waves; rather, it consists of a stream of individual energy packages (the quanta). Planck assumed that different kinds of radiation carried quanta representing different amounts of energy, the amount for any specific type of quantum being inversely proportional to the wavelength (or directly proportional to the frequency) of the radiation. He proposed the relationship

$$\epsilon = h\nu \qquad (1)$$

where ϵ is the energy of a quantum, ν is the frequency of the radiation in vibrations per second, and h is the proportionality constant called Planck's constant, or the universal constant, with a value of 6.624×10^{-27} erg-sec. This is the fundamental equation of the quantum theory.

Planck's hypothesis explained all the experimental data of radiation, and in 1905 Albert Einstein employed the hypothesis to explain the photoelectric effect. He suggested that light is propagated through space as *photons*, each of which has a quantum of energy equivalent to $h\nu$; when the light is absorbed by a metal, the entire quantum of energy of the photon is given to a single electron in the metal. If the electron acquires sufficient energy as a result of this interaction, it is ejected to initiate a flow of electrons (the photoelectric current).

The quantum hypothesis has developed into a theory that has revolutionized many areas of science and has important applications in many others. For example, it has greatly facilitated the interpretation of spectra, ionization potentials, specific heats, and of diverse photochemical phenomena, to mention only a few of the more prolific areas of investigation.

Bohr Theory of the Atom

Planck's hypothesis enabled Bohr to explain, in 1913, the several series of spectral lines exhibited by hydrogen in the visible region (Balmer series), in the ultraviolet (Lyman series), and in the infrared (Paschen, Brackett, and Pfund series). In these spectra, as in others, the characteristic lines are produced when an electron jumps from one energy level to another; thus, in transferring from a higher energy level E_2 to a lower level E_1, a photon of frequency ν is emitted according to the relationship

$$E_2 - E_1 = \epsilon = h\nu \qquad (2)$$

Bohr assumed first that the electron of a hydrogen atom was restricted to move in orbits corresponding to definite energy levels and, second, that the orbits were limited to those in which the angular momentum of the electron (mvr), is an integral multiple of $h/2\pi$, expressed mathematically as

$$mvr = \frac{nh}{2\pi} \qquad (3)$$

where m is the mass of the electron, v is its velocity, r is the radius of the orbit, h is Planck's constant, and n is an integer (1, 2, 3, 4, etc) which was called the *orbital number*. Equating the centripetal force on the electron moving in an orbit to the force of attraction of the nucleus for the electron (Coulomb's law) affords the relation

$$\text{(centripetal force)} \quad \frac{mv^2}{r} = \frac{Ze^2}{r^2} \quad \text{(force of attraction)} \quad (4)$$

where Z is the atomic number of the nucleus (1 for hydrogen). Substituting in this equation the value of v derived from Eq. 3, the radius of the orbits of the electron of the hydrogen atom may be calculated from

$$r = \frac{n^2 h^2}{4\pi^2 m e^2 Z} \quad (5)$$

Using this equation, the smallest orbit of the electron of a hydrogen atom (when n is 1) is calculated to be 0.529 Å.

The total energy E of the electron is the sum of the kinetic energy E_{kin} and the potential energy E_{pot}. The former is given by

$$E_{kin} = \tfrac{1}{2}mv^2 \quad (6)$$

which is equivalent, from Eq. 4, to

$$E_{kin} = \frac{1}{2}\frac{Ze^2}{r} \quad (7)$$

The potential energy is defined by

$$E_{pot} = \int_\infty^r \frac{Ze^2}{r^2}\,dr = -\frac{Ze^2}{r} \quad (8)$$

The sum is

$$E = \frac{1}{2}\frac{Ze^2}{r} - \frac{Ze^2}{r} = -\frac{Ze^2}{2r} \quad (9)$$

Substituting in Eq. 9 the value of r given by Eq. 5

$$E_n = -\frac{2\pi^2 m Z^2 e^4}{n^2 h^2} \quad (10)$$

which is Bohr's equation for calculating the energy E_n of an electron in an orbit of orbital number n. This equation may be used to calculate the amount of energy emitted when the electron jumps from one orbit to another

$$E_2 - E_1 = \epsilon = h\nu = \frac{2\pi^2 m e^4 Z^2}{h^2}\left(\frac{1}{n_1^2} - \frac{1}{n_2^2}\right) \quad (11)$$

While the Bohr theory accounted precisely for the lines of the hydrogen spectrum and for those of spectra of the ions He^+, Li^{++}, and Be^{+++}, each of which atomic species contains but a single electron, it did not account for all the lines in atoms or ions with many electrons. Also, it did not provide information about the effect of a magnetic field on atomic spectra.

Wave Nature of the Electron

In 1942 a hypothesis of great significance was advanced by Louis de Broglie, namely, that since photons exhibit properties of waves and particles, electrons also may have wave characteristics. He proposed a wavelength, λ, for electrons, defined by the equation

$$\lambda = \frac{h}{mv} \quad (12)$$

where λ is called the de Broglie wavelength, and h, m, and v are defined as in preceding equations. The product mv represents the momentum of the electron.

That electrons actually have wave characteristics was established in 1928, when Davisson and Germer obtained a diffraction pattern by reflecting a beam of electrons off the face of a crystal of nickel. de Broglie wavelengths may be assigned even to macroscopic bodies in motion, but these are too short to be detected. For example, a 45-Gm golf ball with a velocity of 3×10^3 cm/sec has a de Broglie wavelength of only 4.9×10^{-24} Å.

Uncertainty Principle

During the developmental period of the quantum theory, the physicist Werner Heisenberg was considering the problem of measuring both the momentum of an electron and its position in space. With macroscopic objects the principles of classical (Newtonian) mechanics may be used to calculate both momentum and position with considerable exactness, but with microscopic and atomic particles Heisenberg pointed out that unavoidable uncertainty was introduced, this being of such magnitude that the product of uncertainty in the momentum, designated Δmv, and the uncertainty in position, Δx, is approximately equal to h, thus

$$\Delta mv . \Delta x \sim h \quad (13)$$

Eq. 13 is a formulation of *Heisenberg's Uncertainty Principle*, which states that it is impossible to know exactly both the position and momentum of an electron or other small particle. The reason for this is the interaction of the measuring probe with the object being measured and not any defect in the measuring apparatus. Thus, a photon of very short wavelength that might be used to measure the position or velocity of an electron would in the process of measurement impart some of its energy to the electron, changing the velocity of the latter. Such an exchange of energy is called the *Compton effect*. While the same exchange of energy occurs in measuring macroscopic particles, the quantitative effect on the latter is too small to detect. A consequence of the uncertainty principle is that the position of an electron in an atom at a given time cannot be predicted with certainty; only the probability of its occurrence at a given point at a given time may be stated.

The Schrödinger Wave Equation

The foundations of a system of dynamics and mathematics that makes it possible to calculate, among other things, the probability that an electron will be found at a given position relative to the nucleus of an atom were laid, in 1926, by Erwin Schrödinger and Werner Heisenberg. This system, called *wave mechanics* or *quantum mechanics*, is based on a partial differential equation called the Schrödinger wave equation; for a particle of mass m and potential energy V this equation has the form

$$-\frac{h^2}{8\pi^2 m}\left(\frac{\partial^2\psi}{\partial x^2} + \frac{\partial^2\psi}{\partial y^2} + \frac{\partial^2\psi}{\partial z^2}\right) + V\psi = E\psi \quad (14)$$

The quantity ψ is an amplitude-like "wave function" the square of which, ψ^2, is a measure of the probability that the particle, such as an electron, will be found at a point in space defined by the coordinates x, y, and z. The sum of the kinetic energy and the potential energy of the particle is given by E. Only certain values of E, called *eigenvalues* or *characteristic values*, will yield satisfactory solutions of the Schrödinger equation. The forms of ψ thus obtained are called the *eigenfunctions*,

Table I—Permitted Quantum Numbers of Orbital Electrons

Electron state	n	l	m	s	No. of combinations
1s	1	0	0	$+\frac{1}{2}, -\frac{1}{2}$	2
2s	2	0	0	$+\frac{1}{2}, -\frac{1}{2}$	2 } 8
2p	2	1	$+1, 0, -1$	$+\frac{1}{2}, -\frac{1}{2}$	6
3s	3	0	0	$+\frac{1}{2}, -\frac{1}{2}$	2
3p	3	1	$+1, 0, -1$	$+\frac{1}{2}, -\frac{1}{2}$	6 } 18
3d	3	2	$+2, +1, 0, -1, -2$	$+\frac{1}{2}, -\frac{1}{2}$	10
4s	4	0	0	$+\frac{1}{2}, -\frac{1}{2}$	2
4p	4	1	$+1, 0, -1$	$+\frac{1}{2}, -\frac{1}{2}$	6 } 32
4d	4	2	$+2, +1, 0, -1, -2$	$+\frac{1}{2}, -\frac{1}{2}$	10
4f	4	3	$+3, +2, +1, 0, -1, -2, -3$	$+\frac{1}{2}, -\frac{1}{2}$	14

wave functions, or *characteristic functions*. When the particle under consideration is an electron, the specific wave functions are called *orbitals*.

The Schrödinger equation is, apparently, valid also for all subatomic and small atomic systems.

Quantum Numbers

When the Schrödinger equation is applied to hydrogen and other atoms, four numbers, called *quantum numbers*, are required to define the electronic wave functions. These quantum numbers are:

n = *principal quantum number*, which is a function of probable distances of the electron from the nucleus, and which may have values of 1, 2, 3 or any other positive number. Instead of using numbers, the capital letters $K, L, M, N, O,$ and P, are sometimes used to designate n states of 1, 2, 3, 4, 5, and 6, respectively.

l = *angular momentum quantum number*, or *azimuthal quantum number*, which represents the number of nodal surfaces passing through the origin in the three-dimensional vibratory motion of an electron. The values of this number are restricted to integral numbers in the range of 0 to $n - 1$. Instead of using numbers to designate l, the letters $s, p, d,$ and f, corresponding to l values of 0, 1, 2, and 3, respectively, are more generally used.

m = *magnetic quantum number*, which defines the permissible inclinations of precessional motion of an electron in a magnetic field. This quantum number may have integer values from $+l$ to $-l$, including 0.

s = *electron spin number*, expressing the magnetic angular momentum associated with the spinning of an electron. This number can have values only of $+\frac{1}{2}$ and $-\frac{1}{2}$.

Even though the hydrogen atom contains only 1 electron it can have many wave functions, or orbitals, corresponding to different values of n and the allowed values of other quantum numbers. The explanation of this is that while the ground state orbital (that in which an atom is in its normal, or lowest, energy state) of hydrogen is 1s (for $n = 1$, and $l = 0$), the atom may be "excited" to higher energy states, each represented by a different orbital. Solutions of the Schrödinger equation for the hydrogen atom agree exactly with experimental data, but when the equation is applied to atoms with two or more electrons, rigorous solutions are impossible because of the difficulty in evaluating terms which express interaction between electrons. In such cases approximation methods may provide acceptable solutions of the equation.

Pauli Exclusion Principle

While complete and exact solutions of the Schrödinger equation have been obtained only for the hydrogen atom, useful information concerning all elements has been derived from the quantum numbers defined above. These numbers describe the quantum state of each electron in an atom—as a crude analogy the numbers may be thought of as the "address" of an electron in an atom. Every electron, even in the most complex atoms, may be identified by a characteristic set of four quantum numbers and, according to an important generalization enunciated by Wolfgang Pauli, known as the *Exclusion Principle*, no two electrons in an atom can have all four quantum numbers the same. Permitted combinations of quantum numbers for electrons having principal quantum numbers of 1, 2, 3, and 4, corresponding to the $K, L, M,$ and N shells, are given in Table I.

The total number of permitted combinations of quantum numbers, given in the last column of the table, coincides with the number (2, 8, 18, or 32) of elements in the several periods of the periodic table (inside back cover).

Atomic Orbitals

In the section on the *Schrödinger Wave Equation* any specific wave function, ψ, describing the motion of an electron, was called an orbital. An orbital is not to be regarded as an orbit, for it is impossible to describe the path of an electron; the interpretation of ψ has been discussed earlier.

Of several ways to represent pictorially the significance of these orbitals, one very useful method is to show the boundary surface of the square of the angular wave functions, which quantity is proportional to the electron densities. The shape of the boundary surface, however, depends on the value of the quantum number l. In defining this number (see preceding section), it was indicated that it represents the number of nodal surfaces passing through origin in the three-dimensional motion of an electron; values from 0 to $n - 1$ nodal surfaces are permitted for any value of the principal quantum number n. When the value of l is 0, there is no nodal surface, the orbital being spherically symmetrical; such orbitals are called s orbitals. When l is 1, there is one nodal surface, which has three permissible orientations in space; these orbitals are called p orbitals. When l is 2, there are two nodal surfaces with five independent orbitals possible; these are called d orbitals. Pictorial representations of the approximate boundary surface of s, p, and d orbitals are shown in Figs. 138 and 139; the directional characteristics of the different orbitals are evident.

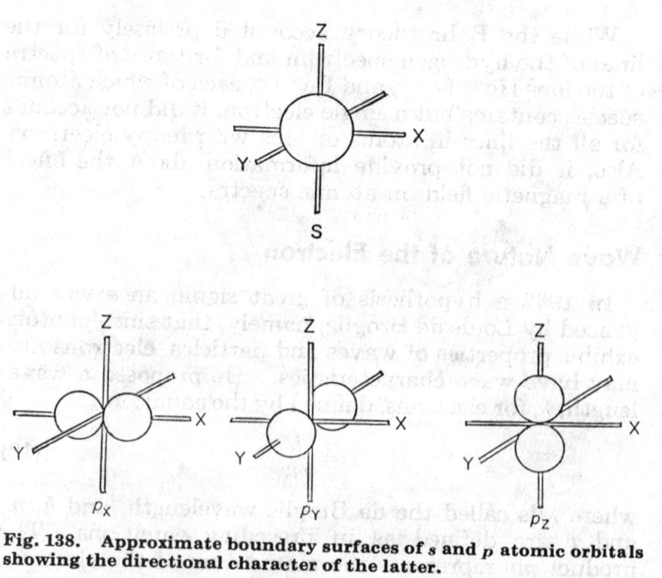

Fig. 138. Approximate boundary surfaces of s and p atomic orbitals showing the directional character of the latter.

In addition to the orbitals represented diagrammatically, there are also *f* orbitals, and even *g* orbitals, but these are too complicated to attempt to diagram.

Molecular Orbitals

An important type of bond between two atoms is that in which a pair of electrons is shared between the atoms; when each atom contributes one of the electrons, the bond is called a normal covalent bond. If the electrons have opposed spins (that is, when the electron spin quantum number, *s*, of one electron is $+\frac{1}{2}$ and of the other $-\frac{1}{2}$), the effect of the pair of electrons is to pull the positively charged nuclei together, the resulting attraction constituting the bond. Except for the fact that quantum theory requires that the electrons comprising the bond have opposed spins, this concept is no different from Lewis' theory of bond formation. When, however, the problem is explored in terms of the orbitals (ψ values) of the electrons forming the bond, certain generalizations of far-reaching utility and applicability may be developed.

To simplify the development of the basic principle it is useful to consider two hydrogen nuclei, A and B,

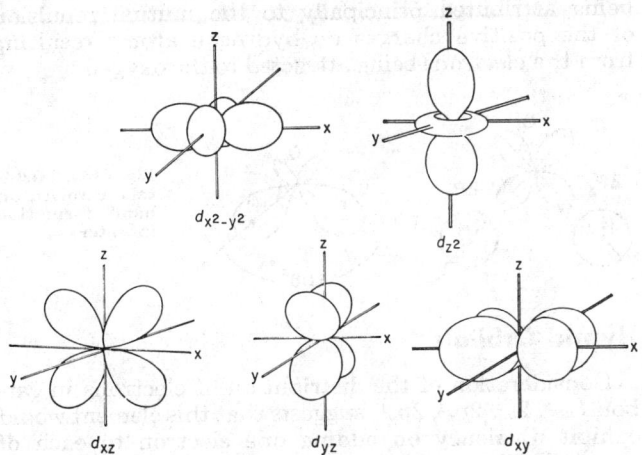

Fig. 139. **Approximate boundary surfaces of the five *d* atomic orbitals.**

brought so close to each other that there is the possibility that a covalent bond may be established when two electrons are placed between the nuclei. The first problem to consider is whether the conditions are right for a bond to form, and thereby to produce a molecule. In approaching the solution of this problem by what is known as *molecular orbital theory*, each electron between the hydrogen nuclei A and B is described by a wave function ψ, called a *molecular orbital*, which is approximated by a linear combination of atomic orbitals (LCAO), as follows

$$\psi = C_A X_A + C_B X_B \tag{15}$$

where X_A is the atomic orbital of the electron about nucleus A if nucleus B were not present, X_B is the atomic orbital of the electron about nucleus B if nucleus A were not present, and C_A and C_B are constants chosen to make the energy between A and B a minimum.

For the second electron a similar equation may be written, and for both electrons the combined wave function is the product of the wave equations for each electron moving in the field of the nuclei A and B. Since the nuclei A and B are symmetrical, the constant C_A in Eq. 15 is equal to $\pm C_B$, so that the allowed molecular orbitals are measured by

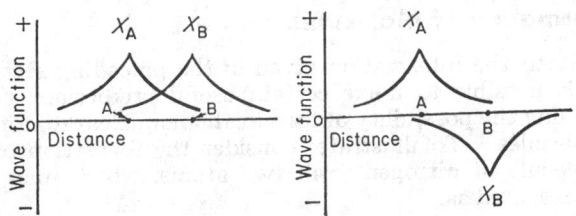

Fig. 140A. **Variation of wave function with distance along nuclear axis.**

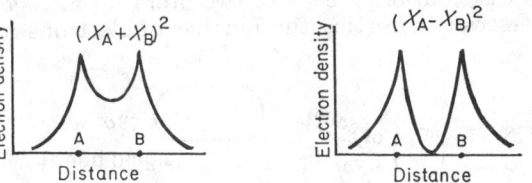

Fig. 140B. **Variation of electron density with distance along nuclear axis.**

$$X_A + X_B \tag{16}$$

and

$$X_A - X_B \tag{17}$$

The variation of the wave functions X_A and X_B with distance along a line connecting the nuclei is represented in Fig. 140*A*.

If the functions $(X_A + X_B)^2$ and $(X_A - X_B)^2$, which measure probable electron density at specified distances, are plotted similarly, the representations in Fig. 140*B* are obtained.

The interpretation of Fig. 140*B* is that the molecular orbital corresponding to $(X_A + X_B)$, in which both atomic orbitals are positive and thus overlap, the electron density builds up between the nuclei and forms a bond. This molecular orbital is called a *bonding orbital*. The orbital corresponding to $(X_A - X_B)$ has, by contrast, an electron density of zero midway between the nuclei; this means that the nuclei are not pulled together, and the molecular orbital is called an *antibonding orbital*.

Bonding and antibonding molecular orbitals or, as they are sometimes called, attractive and repulsive molecular orbitals, are the factors that determine whether or not bonds will form. Which effect, bonding or antibonding, prevails is determined by the relative number of electrons in bonding and antibonding orbitals and on the relative energy values of each type of orbital.

The bonding and antibonding orbitals formed from certain similar *s* and *p* orbitals are shown in Fig. 141; the illustrations show that two important types of bonds arise, designated *sigma* (σ) and *pi* (π), respectively.

A basic distinction between sigma and pi bonds formed from overlapping of *p* orbitals should be noted: A sigma bond is characterized by endwise overlap, while in a pi bond the overlap is sidewise. When multiple bonds are formed by overlap of the *p* orbitals of two atoms it is apparent that if maximum endwise overlap is obtained along the *x* axis, overlap along the *y* and *z* axes can only be sidewise.

The energy of different types of bonding and antibonding orbitals has been determined to increase in the following order:

$$1s\sigma < 1s\sigma^* < 2s\sigma < 2s\sigma^* < 2p_x\sigma < 2p_y\pi =$$
$$2p_z\pi < 2p_y\pi^* = 2p_z\pi^* < 2p_x\sigma^*$$

Formation of Molecules

With the information given in the preceding section it is possible to make certain useful predictions concerning the possibility of forming homonuclear diatomic molecules. To illustrate, consider the formation of a molecule of nitrogen from two atoms, which may be represented as:

$$2N[1s^2 2s^2 2p^3] \rightarrow N_2[(1s\sigma)^2(1s\sigma^*)^2(2s\sigma)^2(2s\sigma^*)^2(2p\sigma)^2(2p\pi)^4]$$

To the left of the arrow is shown, in brackets, the electron distribution of each of two atoms of nitrogen, the superscript indicating the number of electrons in each

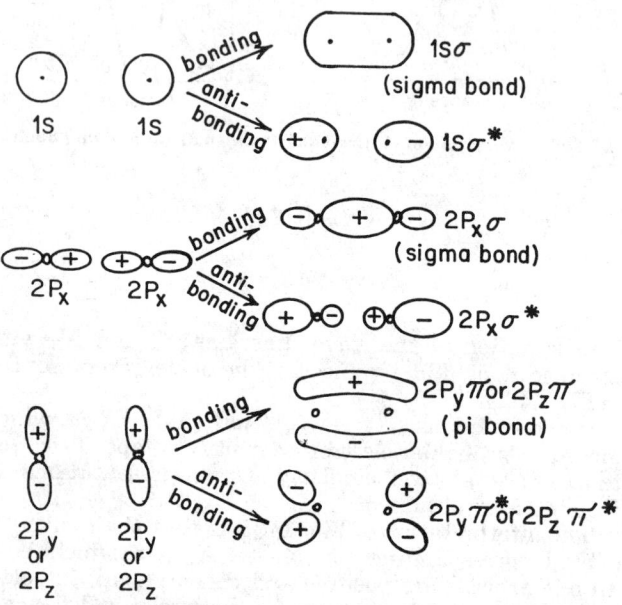

Fig. 141. Bonding and antibonding molecular orbitals formed by linear combination of atomic orbitals. Antibonding orbitals are identified by a superscript asterisk.

atomic orbital (identified as $1s$, $2s$, $2p$); to the right of the arrow is shown the distribution of electrons in bonding and antibonding orbitals. It is evident that ten electrons are in bonding orbitals and four in antibonding orbitals; the net surplus of six bonding electrons results in a triple bond comprised of one sigma bond and two pi bonds, the latter at right angles to each other.

The formation of a molecule of oxygen may be represented as follows:

$$2 O[1s^2 2s^2 2p^4] \rightarrow$$
$$O_2[(1s\sigma)^2(1s\sigma^*)^2(2s\sigma)^2(2s\sigma^*)^2(2p\sigma)^2(2p\pi)^4(2p\pi^*)^2]$$

In this case there is a net surplus of four bonding electrons which form a double bond comprised of a sigma and a pi bond. Because the two $2p\pi^*$ orbitals ($2p_y\pi^*$ and $2p_z\pi^*$) can each hold two electrons, and in molecular oxygen these orbitals are only half filled, the single occupancy results in the electrons having parallel spins, imparting a net magnetic moment to the molecule; this is the reason why oxygen is paramagnetic.

Molecular orbital theory also explains why an element such as helium does not form a diatomic molecule. The explanation is apparent when we write the equation:

$$2He[1s^2] \rightarrow He_2[(1s\sigma)^2(1s\sigma^*)^2]$$

Because the four electrons of the hypothetical helium molecule would be equally divided between a bonding

orbital and an antibonding orbital, there is no net binding force to bring the helium atoms together as a diatomic molecule.

Lithium forms the molecule Li_2 because there is a net surplus of two bonding electrons; beryllium, however, will not form Be_2 because the eight electrons of this hypothetical molecule would be equally divided between bonding and antibonding orbitals and, consequently, no net binding force between the atoms can exist.

Polyatomic Orbitals

Bond formation in polyatomic molecules often involves different types of orbitals. In water, for example, the oxygen atom ($1s^2$, $2s^2$, $2p_x^2$, $2p_y^1$, $2p_z^1$) has two half-filled p orbitals at right angles to each other and each containing only one electron; these can combine with the half-filled $1s$ orbitals of two hydrogen atoms to form two overlapping s-p bonds containing two electrons in each bond. The orbitals involved in bond formation are shown in Fig. 142. Since the p_y and p_z orbitals are at right angles to each other it might be expected that the angle between the two s-p bonds would be 90°. Actually it is 105°, the increase in the angle being attributed principally to the mutual repulsion of the positive charges on hydrogen atoms resulting from the electrons being attracted to the oxygen.

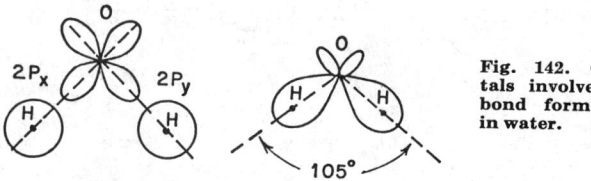

Fig. 142. Orbitals involved in bond formation in water.

Hybrid Orbitals

Consideration of the distribution of electrons in carbon ($1s^2$, $2s^2$, $2p_x^1$, $2p_y^1$) suggests that this element would exhibit divalency on adding one electron to each of the half-filled orbitals; actually, however, carbon commonly forms four covalent bonds. The discrepancy may be explained by assuming that carbon may be "excited" to an energy level permitting one of the $2s$ electrons to be "promoted" into the vacant $2p_z$ orbital, thereby providing four half-filled orbitals which may be expected to form four bonds. In this event three of the bonds, since they involve p orbitals, would be of a different type from the fourth, which involves an s orbital. As the experimental evidence, both physical and chemical, clearly indicates that in molecules of the type of CH_4 all four bonds are equivalent and all inclined at equal angles of 109°28' to each other to form the tetrahedral configuration, the further assumption was made that s and p orbitals undergo a mixing or *hybridization* (a term introduced by Linus Pauling) to give four equivalent bonds and orbitals; this type of hybridization (there are other types) is called *tetrahedral* or sp^3 *hybridization*.

Tetrahedral hybridization is not the only type of hybridization encountered with carbon; two other types, *trigonal* and *digonal*, are important. In trigonal hybridization, one of the p orbitals remains unchanged while the two other p orbitals mix or hybridize with an s orbital to form three equivalent orbitals directed in a single plane at angles of 120° with one another; this is also called sp^2 *hybridization*. Trigonal hybridization is involved in compounds containing the carbon-

carbon double bond. Experimental evidence shows that in ethylene, $H_2C=CH_2$, all six atoms lie in the same plane. The two bonds connecting the hydrogens to each carbon atom and one of the carbon–carbon bonds are equivalent hybrids of the sigma type and are coplanar; the remaining bond, which provides the second linkage between the carbon atoms, is a pi bond which by its sidewise overlap produces regions of high electron density above and below the plane in which the atoms lie. It may be generalized that the carbon–carbon double bond consists of a pair of trigonal sigma orbitals (one originating with each carbon) with a pair of pi orbitals (again one originating with each carbon) above and below the plane of the sigma orbitals.

Digonal hybridization occurs when only one p orbital mixes with an s orbital; this is often referred to as sp *hybridization*. It is involved in the carbon–carbon triple bond, as in acetylene, $HC\equiv CH$, where the hydrogens are linked to carbon by a sigma bond, and the carbons are joined to each other by one sigma bond and two pi bonds formed from the mutually perpendicular unhybridized orbitals. Experimental evidence confirms that the acetylene molecule is linear and possesses axial symmetry. Other triple bonds are similarly formed.

Nonlocalized Molecular Orbitals

In the preceding illustrations and discussions of molecular orbitals it has been possible to localize bonding electrons between specific nuclei. In aromatic and conjugated organic compounds, however, it is not possible to do this. In the case of benzene, the experimental evidence indicates that the carbon atoms lie at the vertices of a regular hexagon, with the hydrogen atoms lying in the same plane; all valence angles are 120°. This means that the carbon atoms are in a state of trigonal or sp^2 hybridization. There remain six electrons, so-called pi electrons, one from each carbon, which form six unhybridized p orbitals extending above and below the plane of the ring. These orbitals can undergo sidewise overlapping to form pi bonds between carbon atoms, but it is implausible to pair the orbitals to assign a specific arrangement of double bonds. According to quantum theory, however, it is not necessary to assign a specific structure or structures for a pi molecular orbital of this type since the electron involved can move around the benzene ring. Thus the six pi electrons are completely delocalized and occupy molecular orbitals which extend above and below all six carbon atoms. This delocalization of electrons corresponds to the concept of resonance of the Kekule structures of benzene.

A number of drug molecules are conjugated or aromatic in nature. The addition of substituents or the replacement of an atom of an aromatic nucleus by a different atom can lead to drastic changes in the general electronic properties of the molecule. For example, caffeine differs from theophylline by a single methyl group; yet, as shown in Fig. 143, the charges on atoms common to each substance are found to differ significantly.[5] The values appearing next to each atom in Fig. 143 may be interpreted as the net accumulation or net decrease in electron density as a result of the atom coming into conjugation with the rest of the molecule.

The charge distribution of molecules may contribute to the formation of molecular association compounds. Such compounds are important as they can conceivably stabilize pharmaceutical preparations. Higuchi

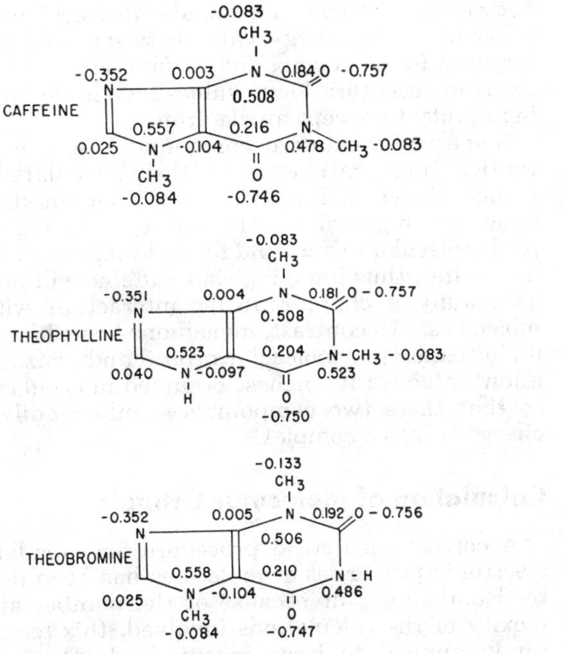

Fig. 143. **Molecular charge distributions arising as a consequence of delocalization.**

and Lachman[6] have shown that the addition of caffeine to benzocaine reduces the rate of hydrolysis of benzocaine. Schnaare and Martin[7] have calculated the electronic distribution in caffeine, A, and benzocaine, B, and, by a comparison of sites of high positive charge on one molecule with low negative charge on the other, it was possible to propose a probable orientation of the benzocaine–caffeine complex (Fig. 144). These considerations suggest that this complex is stabilized by simple electrostatic interactions.

Other influences may also operate in stabilizing intermolecular interactions. One factor to consider is the formation of a *charge-transfer complex*. Charge-transfer is the sharing of electron density between two molecules, one of which is electron-rich, and the other, electron-poor. The electron-deficient molecule is called an *acceptor*, while the electron-rich molecule is called a *donor*. Since each of the molecules involved in the interaction already has its primary valence requirements satisfied, charge-transfer interactions are weak in comparison with covalent bonding between atoms.

The ability of a molecule to participate in a charge-transfer interaction may be estimated using the calculated energy for the outermost molecular orbital which contains electrons or the calculated energy for the innermost molecular orbital which has no electrons. Usually, an energy value between $+0.5$ and 0β is necessary for the compound to function effectively as an electron donor; the lower the value, the

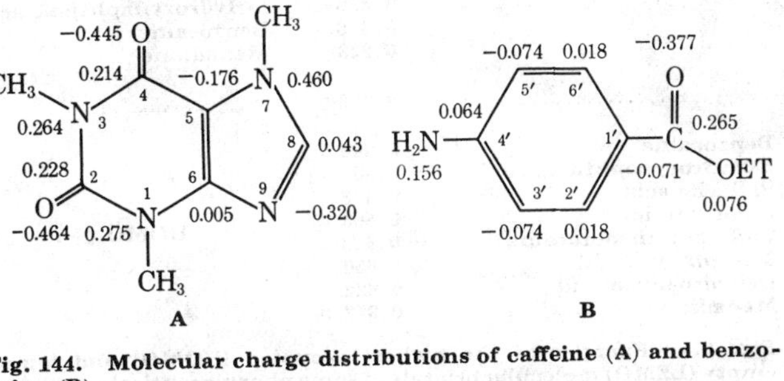

Fig. 144. **Molecular charge distributions of caffeine (A) and benzocaine (B).**

better the molecule can donate an electron. On the other hand, an energy value between -0.5 and 0β is required for the compound to function as an effective electron acceptor; lower values here imply an increasing ability to accept an electron.

Some representative compounds used in pharmaceutical preparations have their calculated energy values[8] shown in Fig. 145. It will be noted that caffeine has a high value for the energy of its highest occupied molecular orbital and for its lowest empty molecular orbital, thus implying that caffeine will not undergo readily a charge-transfer interaction with other molecules. In contrast, menadione has a low value for its lowest empty molecular orbital and benzocaine has a low value for its highest occupied molecular orbital, so that these two compounds should readily form a charge-transfer complex.

Calculation of Molecular Orbitals

A correct theoretical procedure for calculating the electronic properties of molecules has been developed by Roothaan,[9] but because of the number and complexity of the calculations involved, this technique is rarely applied to large organic molecules. A more manageable form of Roothaan's procedure has been presented by Pariser and Parr,[10] who showed that a single approximation, called the *zero differential overlap approximation*, considerably reduces the number of calculations inherent in Roothaan's method. By the use of this approximation, and by determining certain quantities experimentally rather than through calculation, Pariser and Parr[11] and later Pople,[12] provided a basis for molecular orbital methods that are convenient to apply to large molecules.

General Principles

Molecular orbitals are similar to atomic orbitals since each represents the motion of a single electron. However, in contrast to an atomic orbital, where the electron is confined to move about a single nucleus, an electron in a molecular orbital (MO) may move about any of the nuclei associated with a given molecule. For a many-electron molecule, Hartree[13] and Fock[14] showed that the Schrödinger equation for a single electron in the molecule is given by (*cf*, Eq. 14)

$$h\Psi = F\Psi \tag{18}$$

where Ψ is the wave-function describing the molecular orbital and F is the energy of an electron in this orbital. The Hamiltonian h consists of two parts and may be expressed by

$$h = H^c + \bar{V} \tag{19}$$

where the first part H^c is called the *core Hamiltonian* and this operator gives the kinetic energy of an electron travelling about the stationary bare nuclei of a molecule. The second part $\bar{V}$ is the potential energy operator and gives the average repulsion experienced by a single electron due to all of the other electrons in the molecule.

In most MO methods, the MO is written as a linear combination of atomic orbitals (LCAO):

$$\Psi = c_1 X_1 + c_2 X_2 + \ldots + c_n X_n \tag{20}$$

By using an LCAO it is implied that an electron travels about an atom in a molecule in much the same way as when the atom is isolated from the molecule. The coefficients in the LCAO may be considered as representing the fraction of time an electron may be found in a given atomic orbital. Hence, c_1 is the fraction of time an electron may be found in the atomic orbital X_1. The mathematical form for an atomic orbital may be unspecified, as in simple Hückel theory, or it may be taken as similar in form to one of the orbitals of a hydrogen atom, as in the more sophisticated MO theories.

Usually, only the orbitals of an atom which are capable of forming a bond (ie, donate an electron to an orbital of a second atom) are included in the LCAO. These are called the *valence atomic orbitals*. Thus, since the $2s$, $2p_x$, $2p_y$, and $2p_z$ orbitals of carbon may each contain an electron, these orbitals can form a bond (or bonds) with an orbital (or orbitals) of a second atom, so that an LCAO may contain four terms identified with each orbital on a given carbon atom. For example, the LCAO for an ethylene MO could contain eight terms for the orbitals of two carbon atoms and four terms for the $1s$ orbital of four hydrogen atoms.

An entirely equivalent but more easily visualized MO may be constructed using *hybrid orbitals*. By considering the $2p$ orbitals of carbon, for example, as unit vectors, a p-type orbital can be constructed which is directed towards any point in the quadrant formed by adjacent lobes of the $2p_x$, $2p_y$, and $2p_z$ orbitals. The addition of some s-character to this p-type orbital affords a hybrid which is suitable for bonding with an orbital of a second atom. Hybrid orbitals may be represented by the linear combination

$$\text{Hybrid} = g_1(1s) + g_m p_m \tag{21}$$

or, equivalently, by the LCAO

$$\text{Hybrid} = g_1(1s) + g_2(2p_x) + g_3(2p_y) + g_4(2p_z) \tag{22}$$

No matter which representation is used, the coefficients are determined solely by the geometric arrangement of the atoms about the atom whose orbitals are hybridized. For example, a linear bonding arrangement of three atoms could result if the central atom possessed the two hybrid orbitals

$$di = \tfrac{1}{2}(1s) + \tfrac{1}{2}(2p_x)$$

and

$$di = \tfrac{1}{2}(1s) - \tfrac{1}{2}(2p_x)$$

This divalent or digonal type of bonding could result by the "mixing" of equal portions of $1s$ and $2p$ characters to afford two hybrids oriented in opposite directions along the x-axis. A carbon atom in acetylene is

	0.690	Theophylline
	0.688	Theobromine
	0.687	Caffeine
	0.555	Salicylic acid
LEMO (−)	0.546	Dehydroacetic acid
	0.465	Nicotinamide
	0.450	β-Hydroxynaphthoic acid
	0.386	Benzocaine
	0.228	Menadione
....	0.000	....
Benzocaine	0.363	
β-Hydroxynaphthoic acid	0.384	
Salicylic acid	0.438	
Nicotinamide	0.563	
Caffeine; theobromine	0.633	HOMO (+)
Theophylline	0.656	
Dehydroacetic acid	0.822	
Menadione	0.972	

Fig. 145. Energies of the highest occupied (HOMO) and lowest empty (LEMO) molecular orbitals of some pharmaceuticals.

usually thought of as being in this state of hybridization. Trigonal (*tr*) hybrids and tetrahedral (*te*) hybrids may also be constructed from geometric considerations. The student is referred to Coulson[15] for details. A carbon atom in ethylene may be considered as possessing three *tr* hybrids oriented at 120° from each other, and the carbon atom of methane may be said to have four *te* hybrids oriented at 109°28' from each other. In constructing *tr* hybrids, one 2s and two 2p orbitals are required, while the *te* hybrids require one 2s orbital and all three 2p orbitals.

While an atom may possess more than one valence orbital, no two orbitals on the same atom share a common region of space; ie, they do not overlap. The discrete nature of an atomic orbital is expressed by the orthonormalization condition. According to this condition, an atomic orbital is said to be *normalized* when

$$S_{kk} = \int_{-\infty}^{\infty} X'_k X'_k dt = 1 \qquad (23)$$

and it is said to be *orthogonal* to other atomic orbitals when

$$S'_{kj} = \int_{-\infty}^{\infty} X'_k X'_j dt = 0 \qquad (24)$$

Primes are used to designate that the atomic orbitals are on the same atom. The conditions state essentially that if an electron is found in the region of space S_{kk} there is no chance of finding the electron in the region of space S_{kj} between the two atomic orbitals, since the two orbitals do not overlap. The orthonormalization condition applies to hybrid orbitals also, because hybrid orbitals are constructed from valence atomic orbitals.

Similarly, for an electron to be found in the region of space described by an MO, the MO must be normalized:

$$\int_{-\infty}^{\infty} \psi \psi dt = 1 \qquad (25)$$

If the MO is expressed as a LCAO, the normalization condition takes the form

$$\int_{-\infty}^{\infty} (c_1 X_1 + c_2 X_2 + \ldots + c_n X_n) \times$$

$$(c_1 X_1 + c_2 X_2 + \ldots + c_n X_n) dt = 1$$

or, upon expanding and substituting Eq. 23 for appropriate terms,

$$c_1{}^2 + c_2{}^2 + \ldots c_n{}^2 + 2 \sum_{k,j} c_k c_j S_{kj} = 1 \qquad (26)$$

The summation appearing in Eq. 26 gives all of the cross-products resulting from the expansion of Eq. 25. In the summation, the overlap between two atomic orbitals *situated on two different atoms* is defined by

$$S_{kj} = \int_{-\infty}^{\infty} X_k X_j dt \qquad (27)$$

A factor of two appears before the summation since

$$S_{kj} = S_{jk} \qquad (28)$$

because the degree of overlap between two atomic orbitals does not depend on the numbering sequence used to identify the orbitals.

In a number of MO methods it is assumed that there is no overlap between the atomic orbitals of different atoms. By this assumption

$$S_{kj} = S_{jk} = 0 \qquad (29)$$

so that Eq. 26 becomes

$$c_1{}^2 + c_2{}^2 + \ldots + c_n{}^2 = 1 \qquad (30)$$

The assumption of no overlap between orbitals simplifies the calculation for the coefficients in the LCAO and does not ordinarily introduce any great error.

Inspection of Eq. 15 shows that if both sides of the equation are multiplied by ψ, one obtains

$$F \psi \psi = \psi h \psi$$

and an integration performed over all space yields

$$F \int_{-\infty}^{\infty} \psi \psi dt = \int_{-\infty}^{\infty} \psi h \psi dt \qquad (31)$$

The use of Eq. 25 enables the energy to be given as

$$F = \int_{-\infty}^{\infty} \psi h \psi dt \qquad (32)$$

According to the *Variation Principle*, the energy E calculated using an assumed MO (an LCAO, for example) is greater than or equal to the energy F calculated using the true one-electron MO:

$$E \geqslant F \qquad (33)$$

Thus, if an LCAO is to be used as a representation of an MO, it is necessary to obtain the values of the coefficients in the LCAO that will make the energy of an electron in this type MO a minimum. In this way, if an LCAO is a good approximation for a true one-electron MO, the energy calculated will be close to, or equal to, the "true" energy,

$$E \approx F \qquad (34)$$

On the other hand, if the LCAO is not a good approximation, then at least the lowest possible energy for an LCAO–MO will have been obtained:

$$E_m - F = \text{minimum error} \qquad (35)$$

To obtain the minimum energy for an LCAO–MO, the LCAO is substituted into Eq. 31 and the energy is minimized with respect to each of the coefficients in the LCAO. This leads to a set of simultaneous equations known as the secular equations:

$$c_1(H_{11} - ES_{11}) + c_2(H_{12} - ES_{12}) +$$
$$\ldots + c_n(H_{1n} - ES_{1n}) = 0$$

$$c_1(H_{21} - ES_{21}) + c_2(H_{22} - ES_{22}) +$$
$$\ldots + c_n(H_{2n} - ES_{2n}) = 0$$

$$\cdots\cdots\cdots\cdots\cdots\cdots\cdots\cdots\cdots\cdots\cdots\cdots\cdots\cdots$$

$$c_1(H_{n1} - ES_{n1}) + c_2(H_{n2} - ES_{n2}) +$$
$$\ldots + c_n(H_{nn} - ES_{nn}) = 0$$

A physically meaningful solution is obtained only if the coefficients in the simultaneous equations are not all zero, and this is true when the determinant for the terms in the simultaneous equations vanishes, ie,

$$\begin{vmatrix} H_{11} - ES_{11} & H_{12} - ES_{12} & \cdots & H_{1n} - ES_{1n} \\ H_{21} - ES_{21} & H_{22} - ES_{22} & \cdots & H_{2n} - ES_{2n} \\ \cdots\cdots\cdots\cdots\cdots\cdots\cdots\cdots\cdots\cdots \\ H_{n1} - ES_{n1} & H_{n2} - ES_{n2} & \cdots & H_{nn} - ES_{nn} \end{vmatrix} = 0$$

The only new quantities are the terms H_{kk} appearing along the diagonal and the terms H_{kj} and H_{jk} appearing in the off-diagonal parts of these relations. The diagonal terms contain the defined quantity

$$H_{kk} = \int_{-\infty}^{\infty} X_k h X_k dt \qquad (36)$$

which, by comparison with Eq. 32, represents an energy. For the present, each of these terms will be identified as the energy required to remove an electron from the orbital indicated by the subscript; ie, the ionization potential of a valence state atomic orbital. Similarly, noting that the numbering sequence does not affect the energy, the off-diagonal terms are defined by

$$H_{kj} = H_{jk} = \int_{-\infty}^{\infty} X_k h X_j dt \qquad (37)$$

and these represent the energy due to the sharing of an electron between the two orbitals indicated by the subscript.

If it is assumed that there is no overlap between atomic orbitals, then the substitution of Eq. 23 and Eq. 29, enables the simultaneous equations and the associated determinant to be written

$$c_1(H_{11} - E) + c_2 H_{12} + \ldots + c_n H_{1n} = 0$$
$$c_1 H_{21} + c_2(H_{22} - E) + \ldots + c_n H_{2n} = 0$$
$$\cdots\cdots\cdots\cdots\cdots\cdots\cdots\cdots\cdots\cdots\cdots\cdots\cdots$$
$$c_1 H_{n1} + c_2 H_{n2} + \ldots + c_n(H_{nn} - E) = 0$$

and

$$\begin{vmatrix} H_{11} - E & H_{12} & \ldots & H_{1n} \\ H_{21} & H_{22} - E & \ldots & H_{2n} \\ \cdots\cdots & \cdots\cdots & & \cdots \\ H_{n1} & H_{n2} & \ldots & H_{nn} - E \end{vmatrix} = 0$$

The relations which have been developed to this point are totally general and may be used in the calculation of the properties of conjugated and saturated molecules. To illustrate the application of the relations, however, only conjugated systems will be considered. In particular, only the conjugated network formed by parallel $2p_z$ orbitals on each of the atoms in an unsaturated molecule like benzene or ethylene will have its properties calculated. This is the π-approximation, since it applies only to the π-bonded atoms in a planar molecule.

The Hückel Method

Hydrocarbons—In this method the assumptions are made that:

1. Each carbon atom in a conjugated system attracts an electron in its $2p_z$ orbital to an equal extent; ie, $H_{11} = H_{22} = \ldots = H_{nn}$.
2. Only neighboring $2p_z$ orbitals can interact.
3. Overlap can be neglected.

Consider a molecule such as butadiene,

$$\begin{matrix} C & — & C & — & C & — & C \\ 1 & & 2 & & 3 & & 4 \end{matrix}$$

Each carbon atom possesses a $2p_z$ orbital, so that the LCAO–MO is written

$$\Psi = c_1 X_1 + c_2 X_2 + c_3 X_3 + c_4 X_4$$

The determinant for the secular equations can be given immediately by inspection:

$$\begin{vmatrix} H_{11} - E & H_{12} & 0 & 0 \\ H_{12} & H_{11} - E & H_{23} & 0 \\ 0 & H_{23} & H_{11} - E & H_{34} \\ 0 & 0 & H_{34} & H_{11} - E \end{vmatrix} = 0$$

This determinant can be evaluated readily if the assumption is made that an electron can be shared equally between any two neighboring atoms; ie, $H_{12} = H_{23} = H_{34}$. When this assumption is made, each of the terms in the determinant (and the simultaneous equations) when divided by H_{12} lead to the new determinant:

$$\begin{vmatrix} x & 1 & 0 & 0 \\ 1 & x & 1 & 0 \\ 0 & 1 & x & 1 \\ 0 & 0 & 1 & x \end{vmatrix} = 0$$

where for convenience

$$x = \frac{H_{11} - E}{H_{12}} \qquad (38)$$

This determinant is evaluated easily by expanding it in terms of its minors. A minor is the smaller determinant formed by striking out all terms in the column and row intercepting at a given element of the larger determinant. In expanding the determinant in terms of minors, the product of an element and its minor is taken for each of the elements in a given column or row. These are summed alternating the sign as the expansion is made along a column or a row. Thus, for butadiene

$$x \begin{vmatrix} x & 1 & 0 \\ 1 & x & 1 \\ 0 & 1 & x \end{vmatrix} - 1 \begin{vmatrix} 1 & 1 & 0 \\ 0 & x & 1 \\ 0 & 1 & x \end{vmatrix} + 0 \begin{vmatrix} 1 & x & 0 \\ 0 & 1 & 1 \\ 0 & 0 & x \end{vmatrix} - 0 \begin{vmatrix} 1 & x & 1 \\ 0 & 1 & x \\ 0 & 0 & 1 \end{vmatrix} = 0$$

The nonvanishing terms may have their determinants similarly expanded to give

$$x^2 \begin{vmatrix} x & 1 \\ 1 & x \end{vmatrix} - x \begin{vmatrix} 1 & 1 \\ 0 & x \end{vmatrix} - 1 \begin{vmatrix} x & 1 \\ 1 & x \end{vmatrix} = 0$$

Expansions of a two-by-two determinant is simply the product of the diagonal running left to right less the product of the diagonal running right to left. The expanded determinant is therefore

$$x^2(x^2 - 1) - x(x - 0) - 1(x^2 - 1) = 0$$

or

$$x^4 - 3x^2 + 1 = 0$$

By making the substitution $y = x^2$ the expanded determinant is seen to give a quadratic equation:

$$y^2 - 3y + 1 = 0$$

the roots of which are, from the quadratic formula,

$$y = \frac{3 + \sqrt{9 - 4}}{2} = 2.6180 \quad \text{and} \quad y = \frac{3 - \sqrt{9 - 4}}{2} = 0.3820$$

so that

$$x = +1.62, -1.62 \quad \text{and} \quad x = +0.62, -0.62$$

Since, from the previous definition (Eq. 38)

$$E = H_{11} - x H_{12}$$

it is found that an electron in butadiene can have four energies. The available energies are shown in Fig. 146. It shows that an electron which can distribute itself between four conjugated $2p_z$ orbitals may be of either higher or lower energy than when the electron is contained in a $2p_z$ orbital of an isolated atom.

Each $2p_z$ orbital of the butadiene molecule may contain a single electron. Considering the electrons separately, each electron has the same energies available to it in the molecule. Thus, if interelectronic repulsions are neglected, the calculated energies are those for the stable π-system of butadiene, and the electronic configuration for butadiene is that obtained by introducing four electrons into each of the available energy levels in accord with the Aufbau Principle, the Pauli Exclusion Principle, and when appropriate, Hund's Rule. The Aufbau ("building up") Principle states that electrons are placed into the lowest unfilled energy levels; the Pauli Principle states that no two electrons in the same energy level can be of the same spin; and Hund's Rule states that when two or more equal energies make up a level (degenerate energies), each takes on an electron of the same spin until all contain a single electron, and then electrons of opposing spin can occupy the levels.

The total π-energy of a molecule is the sum of the energies associated with each electron. For butadiene each energy level contains two electrons so the total π-energy $E_\pi{}^b$ is

$$E_\pi{}^b = 2E_1 + 2E_2 = 2(H_{11} + 1.62H_{12}) + 2(H_{11} + 0.62H_{12})$$

or

$$E_\pi{}^b = 4H_{11} + 4.48H_{12}$$

If there was no conjugation between atoms 2 and 3 of butadiene, the total π-energy would correspond to that of two ethylene molecules. The determinant for ethylene is

$$\begin{vmatrix} x & 1 \\ 1 & x \end{vmatrix} = 0$$

so that

$$x^2 - 1 = 0$$

and

$$x = \pm 1$$

The total π-energy for one ethylene molecule is

$$E_\pi{}^e = 2E_1 = 2(H_{11} + H_{12})$$

and for two ethylene molecules it is

$$2E_\pi{}^e = 4H_{11} + 4H_{12}$$

The difference D between the calculated total π-energy $E_\pi{}^b$ of butadiene and that for two ethylene molecules represents the extra energy of stabilization due to the conjugation between atoms 2 and 3:

$$D = E_\pi{}^b - 2E_\pi{}^e = (4H_{11} + 4.48) - (4H_{11} + 4H_{12})$$

or

$$D = 0.48H_{12}$$

Since this stabilization is a consequence of electronic delocalization, the difference D is called the *delocalization energy*. It should be noted that H_{12} must be implicitly negative in sign for the delocalization energy to represent a stabilizing influence.

To calculate the coefficients for each LCAO whose energies have been obtained, the simultaneous equations on which the starting determinant was based

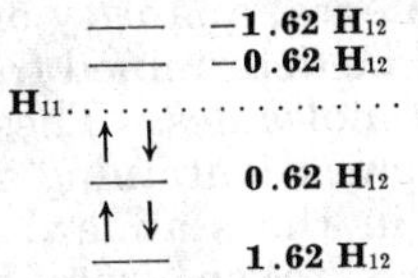

Fig. 146. Filled energy levels of butadiene.

must be solved. This may be done using the method of cofactors which makes use of minors of the initial determinant. The operations involved are

1. Determine the ratio of coefficients according to the relation

$$\frac{c_n}{c_1} = \frac{\text{Minor identified with } c_n}{\text{Minor identified with } c_1}$$

2. Square each of the ratios that have been calculated:

$$\left(\frac{c_n}{c_1}\right)^2$$

3. Sum the squared ratios:

$$\sum \left(\frac{c_n}{c_1}\right)^2$$

4. Take the square root of this sum:

$$\sqrt{\sum \left(\frac{c_n}{c_1}\right)^2}$$

5. Divide each ratio by the square root to obtain the coefficient

$$c_n = \frac{\left(\frac{c_n}{c_1}\right)}{\sqrt{\sum \left(\frac{c_n}{c_1}\right)^2}}$$

The student should satisfy himself by using Eq. 30 to prove the identity given in Step 5.

For butadiene

$$\frac{c_1}{c_1} = 1$$

$$\frac{c_2}{c_1} = \frac{-\begin{vmatrix} 1 & 1 & 0 \\ 0 & x & 1 \\ 0 & 1 & x \end{vmatrix}}{\begin{vmatrix} x & 1 & 0 \\ 1 & x & 1 \\ 0 & 1 & x \end{vmatrix}} = \frac{-(x^2 - 1)}{x^3 - 2x}$$

$$\frac{c_3}{c_1} = \frac{\begin{vmatrix} 1 & x & 0 \\ 0 & 1 & 1 \\ 0 & 0 & x \end{vmatrix}}{x^3 - 2x} = \frac{x}{x^3 - 2x} = \frac{1}{x^2 - 2}$$

$$\frac{c_4}{c_1} = \frac{-\begin{vmatrix} 1 & x & 1 \\ 0 & 1 & x \\ 0 & 0 & 1 \end{vmatrix}}{x^3 - 2x} = \frac{-1}{x^3 - 2x}$$

It should be noted that even-numbered coefficients in the ratio require a negative sign before the minor.

One of the four values of x now may be substituted into the expressions giving the ratios and the coefficients calculated following the steps outlined. This is repeated for each value of x.

The LCAO–MO corresponding to each energy of butadiene thus will be found to be

$$E_4 = H_{11} - 1.62H_{12};$$
$$\Psi_4 = 0.37X_1 - 0.60X_2 + 0.60X_3 - 0.37X_4$$

$$E_3 = H_{11} - 0.62H_{12};$$
$$\Psi_3 = 0.60X_1 - 0.37X_2 - 0.37X_3 + 0.60X_4$$

$$E_2 = H_{11} + 0.62H_{12};$$
$$\Psi_2 = 0.60X_1 + 0.37X_2 - 0.37X_3 - 0.60X_4$$

$$E_1 = H_{11} + 1.62H_{12};$$
$$\Psi_1 = 0.37X_1 + 0.60X_2 + 0.60X_3 + 0.37X_4$$

The low-energy MO's Ψ_1 and Ψ_2 are called *bonding orbitals* since electrons contained in them stabilize a molecule. On the other hand, the high-energy MO's Ψ_3 and Ψ_4 are called *antibonding orbitals* because when an electron is contained in one of these orbitals the molecule becomes destabilized; ie, its total π-energy is decreased. At times a molecule will be found to have an MO whose energy $E = H_{11}$. In this case the MO is called a *nonbonding orbital* because electrons in this orbital neither stabilize nor destabilize the molecule.

The tendency for an electron to remain in an atomic orbital is given by the coefficient in the LCAO, or in stricter terms, by the square of the coefficient, which represents the probability of finding the electron in the atomic orbital. If there are two electrons in the same MO, the probability of finding an electron in a given atomic orbital is doubled; if there is more than one MO containing electrons, the probability is further increased by an amount given by corresponding coefficients in the other MO's. The total probability for finding an electron in a given atomic orbital represents the *charge density* associated with that orbital. Considering only doubly occupied MO's the charge density of an orbital is given by

$$q_k = \sum_{}^{occ} 2c_k{}^2 \qquad (39)$$

where the sum is taken only over the occupied MO's. For butadiene,

$$q_1 = 2(0.37)^2 + 2(0.60)^2 = 1.00$$

$$q_2 = 2(0.60)^2 + 2(0.37)^2 = 1.00$$

$$q_3 = 2(0.60)^2 + 2(-0.37)^2 = 1.00$$

$$q_4 = 2(0.37)^2 + 2(-0.60)^2 = 1.00$$

so that each atomic orbital has a charge density of 1. The *formal charge* of each orbital is the difference between the number of electrons in the isolated orbital and the calculated charge density resulting from the conjugation of this orbital with the other orbitals in a molecule:

$$Q_k = n_k - q_k \qquad (40)$$

A carbon $2p_z$ orbital contains 1 electron in the isolated atom, so that in butadiene

$$Q_1 = Q_2 = Q_3 = Q_4 = 1 - 1.00 = 0$$

ie, according to the Hückel theory, there are no formal charges on any of the atoms of butadiene.

The tendency for an electron to be found between two atomic orbitals is given by the product of the coefficients of the atomic orbitals. When an electron tends to situate itself between two atomic orbitals the atoms containing these orbitals are said to be bonded to each other. Thus, a *bond order* for the bonds in a molecule can be defined by

$$p_{kj} = \sum_{}^{occ} 2c_k c_j \qquad (41)$$

where it is again assumed that each MO is doubly occupied. For butadiene, the bond orders for adjacent pairs of atoms are

$$p_{12} = 2(0.37)(0.60) + 2(0.60)(0.37) = 0.89$$

$$p_{23} = 2(0.60)(0.60) + 2(0.37)(-0.37) = 0.44$$

$$p_{34} = 2(0.60)(0.37) + 2(-0.37)(-0.60) = 0.89$$

The greater values for p_{12} and p_{34} indicate that the terminal bonds of butadiene are stronger than the central bond.

Bond orders may range in value from 0 to 1 corresponding to no bonding between two $2p_z$ orbitals and maximum bonding between two $2p_z$ orbitals, respectively. Negative bond orders may be calculated also, as between atoms 1 and 4 of butadiene:

$$p_{14} = 2(0.37)(03.7) + 2(0.60)(-0.60) = -0.44$$

and this indicates that bond formation between these two atoms is disfavored.

Heteroatomic Systems—The Hückel method when applied to heteroatomic systems is often called the Method of Wheland and Pauling.[17] These workers showed that a conjugated system which includes atoms other than carbon could have its determinant written in a convenient manner such that the effect of the heteroatom could be taken into account without increasing greatly the labor involved in solving the determinant.

In this method all of the assumptions of the Hückel method are maintained, except with regard to a heteroatom. A standard value is assigned to each term in the determinant that refers to a carbon atom or a carbon–carbon bond; ie, the definition is made that

$$\alpha_0 = H_{kk}$$

for a carbon atom and

$$\beta_0 = H_{kj}$$

for a carbon–carbon bond. Values for the diagonal and off-diagonal elements that refer to a heteroatom or a bond involving a heteroatom are then defined in terms of these standard values. Thus,

$$\alpha_0 + h\beta_0 = H_{kk}$$

for a heteroatom and

$$k\beta_0 = H_{kj}$$

for a bond involving a heteroatom, so that for glyoxal

$$\begin{array}{cccc} O & C & C & O \\ 1 & 2 & 3 & 4 \end{array}$$

the determinant becomes

$$\begin{vmatrix} \alpha_0 + h\beta_0 - E & k\beta_0 & 0 & 0 \\ k\beta_0 & \alpha_0 - E & \beta_0 & 0 \\ 0 & \beta_0 & \alpha_0 - E & k\beta_0 \\ 0 & 0 & k\beta_0 & \alpha_0 + h\beta_0 - E \end{vmatrix} = 0$$

By making the definition

$$x = \frac{\alpha_0 - E}{\beta_0}$$

and by dividing each element in the determinant by β_0, there is obtained

$$\begin{vmatrix} x + h & k & 0 & 0 \\ k & x & 1 & 0 \\ 0 & 1 & x & k \\ 0 & 0 & k & x + h \end{vmatrix} = 0$$

Values for h and k are determined by varying them to match some experimental quantity or an experimental quantity that could be determined from the calculated LCAO for standard molecules. These values then are used for other molecules containing a heteroatom similar to that found in the standard molecule. Some representative values taken from Streitwieser[16] are given in Table II. It will be noted that the values

Table II—Parameters for the Wheland and Pauling Method[17]

Atom	h	Bond	k
$\dot{C}$	0	C—C	1
$\dot{O}$	1	C—$\dot{O}$	1
$\ddot{O}$	2	C—$\ddot{O}$	0.8
$\dot{N}$	0.5	C—$\dot{N}$	1
$\ddot{N}$	1.5	C—$\ddot{N}$	0.8

differ depending on whether a heteroatom contains 1 or 2 electrons in its $2p_z$ orbital.

The oxygens of glyoxal are both carbonyl oxygens which contain a single electron in the conjugated $2p_z$ orbital. Thus, using the quantities given in Table II, the determinant becomes

$$\begin{vmatrix} x+1 & 1 & 0 & 0 \\ 1 & x & 1 & 0 \\ 0 & 1 & x & 1 \\ 0 & 0 & 1 & x+1 \end{vmatrix} = 0$$

This determinant can be expanded in terms of its minors, and once the roots of the resulting polynomial are determined, the coefficients appearing in the LCAO of glyoxal are determined following the steps outlined for butadiene. Having determined the coefficients, the charges and bond orders may be determined using Eqs. 39–41.

The Method of Pariser and Parr and Pople

The methods due to Pariser and Parr[11] and Pople,[12] which are called collectively the PPP method, are formally very similar and differ only in the way certain of the parameters are defined and in the respect that as originally written the Pople method was an iterative one while that of Pariser and Parr was not. It is now recognized that both approaches are most fruit-

$$\begin{vmatrix} H_{11}{}^C + K_{11} - E & H_{12}{}^C + J_{12} & J_{13} & J_{14} \\ H_{12}{}^C + J_{12} & H_{22}{}^C + K_{22} - E & H_{23}{}^C + J_{23} & J_{24} \\ J_{13} & H_{23}{}^C + J_{23} & H_{33}{}^C + K_{33} - E & H_{34}{}^C + J_{34} \\ J_{14} & J_{24} & H_{34}{}^C + J_{34} & H_{44}{}^C + K_{44} - E \end{vmatrix} = 0$$

fully applied by iteration to constant charge, in which case the calculated charges are said to be *self-consistent*.

In these methods Eq. 16 is substituted into Eqs. 36 and 37 and the resulting expression is expanded to define the elements in such a manner as to consider the interelectronic repulsions explicitly. It is assumed that there is no overlap between the orbitals of differing atoms so that the terms referring to interelectronic repulsions between overlap regions will disappear. This is the *zero differential overlap approximation*. In this way the diagonal elements of the essential determinant are defined by

$$H_{kk} = H_{kk}{}^C + \tfrac{1}{2}q_k\gamma_{kk} - \sum_{m \neq k} Q_m\gamma_{km} \qquad (42)$$

and the off-diagonal elements by

$$H_{kj} = H_{kj}{}^C - \tfrac{1}{2}p_{kj}\gamma_{kj} \qquad (43)$$

The quantities $H_{kk}{}^C$ and $H_{kj}{}^C$ are interpreted in the same way as in the Hückel method. It is assumed that only neighboring atoms can have a value for $H_{kj}{}^C$, and that these values are characteristic of a given bond. Valence state ionization potentials may be used for $H_{kk}{}^C$. Values for $H_{kj}{}^C$ are determined empirically.

Some representative values for these quantities are given in Table III.

The new quantities γ_{kk} and γ_{kj} represent the repulsion between two electrons situated on the same atom (orbital) and on two different atoms (orbitals), respectively. Ordinarily, the one-center repulsion parameter γ_{kk} is estimated as the difference between the ionization potential I and the electron affinity A of the valence state atom:

$$\gamma_{kk} = I - A \qquad (44)$$

A number of formulas are available for expressing the two-center parameter γ_{kj} in terms of the known one-center values γ_{kk} and γ_{jj}, one being that of Mataga and Nishimoto[19],*

$$\gamma_{kj} = \frac{14.397}{(a^2 + r_{kj}{}^2)^{1/2}}$$

where

$$a = \frac{2 \times 14.397}{\gamma_{kk} + \gamma_{jj}}$$

and r_{kj} is the distance between atom k and j, but a simpler approach due to Pople will be used here. Following Pople, all two-center repulsion parameters will be thought of as given by Coulomb's law for the repulsion between two points of unit charge, so that

$$\gamma_{kj} = \frac{1}{r_{kj}}$$

Thus, if the elements have their relations written more simply as

$$H_{kk} = H_{kk}{}^C + K_{kk}$$

and

$$H_{kj} = H_{kj}{}^C + J_{kj}$$

the determinant for butadiene or for glyoxal would be written

The roots of the determinant will differ depending on the values used for the empirical quantities and the charges and bond orders calculated by the Hückel method for butadiene and for glyoxal.

By choosing benzene as a standard molecule, a comparison can be made between this determinant and those given previously. Each atom of benzene has a charge density q of 1 (thus, a formal charge Q of zero)

Table III—Representative Parameters for the PPP Method

Atom	Ionization potential	Electron affinity	Bond	$H_{kj}{}^C$
C^+	−11.16	0.03	C—C	-2.18^a
C^+	−17.70	2.47	C—$\dot{O}$	-2.76^b
O^{2+}	−32.90	11.37	C—$\ddot{O}$	-2.35^c
N^+	−14.12	1.78	C—$\dot{N}$	-1.68^a
N^{2+}	−26.70	9.26	C—$\ddot{N}$	-1.68^a

a For a bond distance of 1.39 Å.
b For a bond distance of 1.23 Å.
c For a bond distance of 1.36 Å.

* The use of this form of the two-center repulsion integral is illustrated in Martin, *et al.*[20]

and the bond-order for a benzene bond may be set at 0.666 to correspond to its bond distance of 1.39 Å. Thus, the standard elements are

$$\alpha_C = H_C{}^C + \tfrac{1}{2}\gamma_{CC}$$

or

$$\alpha_C = -11.16 + \tfrac{1}{2}(11.16 - 0.03) = -5.60$$

for a benzene carbon atom, and

$$\beta_{CC} = H_{CC}{}^C - \tfrac{1}{2}p_{CC}\gamma_{CC}$$

or

$$\beta_{CC} = -2.18 - \tfrac{1}{2}(0.666)\left(\frac{1}{1.39}\right) = -2.42$$

for a benzene carbon–carbon bond.

The Hückel calculation done previously showed that to a first approximation each atom of butadiene has a charge density of 1. Thus, a PPP calculation could be done using the element defined for a benzene-like atom along the diagonal of the determinant.

On the other hand, the bond-orders for butadiene differ from that of benzene so that the off-diagonal terms referring to neighboring atoms in butadiene may be given, assuming the bond distances are the same as in benzene, by

$$H_{12} = H_{12}{}^C + J_{12} = H_{12}{}^C - \tfrac{1}{2}p_{12}\gamma_{12} =$$
$$-2.18 - \tfrac{1}{2}(0.89)\left(\frac{1}{1.39}\right) = -2.49$$

and

$$H_{23} = H_{23}{}^C + J_{23} = H_{23}{}^C - \tfrac{1}{2}p_{23}\gamma_{23} =$$
$$-2.18 - \tfrac{1}{2}(0.44)\left(\frac{1}{1.39}\right) = -2.33$$

Taken relative to a benzene carbon–carbon bond, these are given equivalently by

$$H_{12} = \frac{-2.49}{-2.42}\beta_{CC} = 1.02\,\beta_{CC}$$

and

$$H_{23} = \frac{-2.33}{-2.42}\beta_{CC} = 0.96\,\beta_{CC}$$

Using the elements deduced, the determinant for the PPP calculation on butadiene takes the form

$$\begin{vmatrix} \alpha_C - E & 1.02\,\beta_{CC} & J_{13} & J_{14} \\ 1.02\,\beta_{CC} & \alpha_C - E & 0.96\,\beta_{CC} & J_{13} \\ J_{13} & 0.96\,\beta_{CC} & \alpha_C - E & 1.02\,\beta_{CC} \\ J_{14} & J_{13} & 1.02\,\beta_{CC} & \alpha_C - E \end{vmatrix} = 0$$

which is similar to the determinant used in the Wheland and Pauling method except for the terms referring to nonnearest neighbors. The latter terms arise because interelectronic repulsions can occur between atoms that are not neighbors.

To evaluate these terms, it must be specified whether cis or trans butadiene is being dealt with, because the distance between the terminal atoms will differ depending on the conformation selected:

$$1C \qquad\qquad C4 \quad 1C$$
$$2C\!-\!C3 \qquad 2C\!-\!C3$$
$$\qquad\qquad\qquad\qquad\quad C4$$

$$\text{s-}cis \qquad\qquad \text{s-}trans$$

Assuming the geometries shown in Fig. 147 for cis and trans butadiene, the properties of a 30°–60° triangle

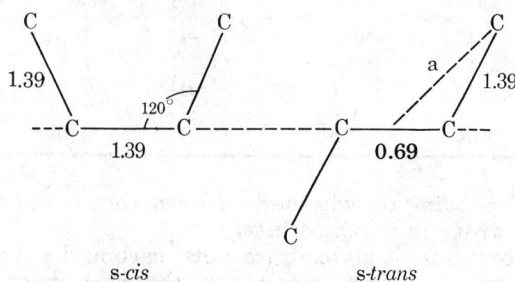

s-cis   s-trans

Fig. 147. Butadiene geometrics.

may be used to arrive at the C_1 to C_4 distance in cis butadiene

$$r_{14} = 1.39 + 2\left(\frac{1.39}{2}\right) = 2.78\ \text{Å}$$

and the Law of Cosines

$$a^2 = b^2 + c^2 - 2bc\cos\theta_{bc}$$

may be used to arrive at the C_1 to C_4 distance in trans butadiene

$$a^2 = \left(\frac{1.39}{2}\right)^2 + (1.39)^2 -$$
$$2\left(\frac{1.39}{2}\right)(1.39)\cos 120° = 3.3810$$

$$r_{14} = 2a = 2(1.83) = 3.66\ \text{Å}$$

In a similar manner, the C_1 to C_3 distance can be determined from the Law of Cosines to give

$$r_{13} = 1.93\ \text{Å}$$

From these distances, and the bond orders calculated for these atoms of butadiene using the Hückel LCAO's, the terms referring to nonneighboring atoms in the determinant are found to be

$$H_{13} = J_{13} = -\tfrac{1}{2}p_{13}\gamma_{13} = -\tfrac{1}{2}(0.00)\left(\frac{1}{1.93}\right) = 0.00$$

and, for cis butadiene

$$H_{14} = J_{14} = -\tfrac{1}{2}p_{14}\gamma_{14} = -\tfrac{1}{2}(-0.44)\left(\frac{1}{2.78}\right) = 0.08$$

while, for trans butadiene

$$H_{14} = J_{14} = -\tfrac{1}{2}(-0.44)\left(\frac{1}{3.66}\right) = 0.06$$

If these are defined relative to a benzene carbon–carbon bond energy, then

$$H_{13} = J_{13} = \frac{0.00}{-2.42}\beta_{CC} = 0.00$$

and for cis and trans butadiene, respectively,

$$H_{14} = J_{14} = \frac{0.08}{-2.42}\beta_{CC} = -0.03\,\beta_{CC}$$

$$H_{14} = J_{14} = \frac{0.06}{-2.42}\beta_{CC} = -0.02\,\beta_{CC}$$

Defining

$$x = \frac{\alpha_C - E}{\beta_{CC}}$$

when all terms in the determinant for *cis* butadiene are divided by β_{CC}, the determinant obtained is

$$\begin{vmatrix} x & 1.02 & 0 & -0.03 \\ 1.02 & x & 0.96 & 0 \\ 0 & 0.96 & x & 1.02 \\ -0.03 & 0 & 1.02 & x \end{vmatrix} = 0$$

The procedures given earlier may be used to evaluate the roots of this determinant and to obtain the coefficients of the new LCAO. From these coefficients, new charges and new bond-orders can be calculated and the elements of new determinant can be determined using these quantities. Repeated calculations are thus possible using the output of one calculation for the input of a second. The calculations are terminated when self-consistency is attained; ie, when the charge densities calculated do not differ by more than, say, 0.0002 between the final two iterations.

In many instances self-consistency is almost attained after the first iteration, so the procedure outlined here may be considered adequate for most purposes.

References

1. Szent-Györgyi, A., *Science*, **124**, 873 (1956).
2. Löwdin, P. O., *Intern. Sci. Tech.*, **17**, 64 (May, 1963).
3. Pullman, B., and Pullman, A., *Quantum Biochemistry*, Interscience, New York, 1963.
4. Cammarata, A., and Stein, R. L., *J. Med. Chem.*, **11**, 829 (1968) and references cited therein.
5. Hata, S., *et al*, *Chem. Pharm. Bull. (Japan)*, **16**, 1 (1968).
6. Higuchi, T., and Lachman, L., *J. Pharm. Sci.*, **44**, 521 (1955).
7. Schnaare, R. S., and Martin, A. N., *J. Pharm. Sci.*, **54**, 1707 (1965).
8. Hata, S., *et al*, *Chem. Pharm. Bull. (Japan)*, **16**, 1 (1968).
9. Roothaan, C. C. J., *Rev. Mod. Phys.*, **23**, 69 (1951).
10. Pariser, P., and Parr, R. G., *J. Chem. Phys.*, **21**, 466 (1953).
11. Pariser, P., and Parr, R. G., *J. Chem. Phys.*, **21**, 767 (1953).
12. Pople, J. A., *Trans. Faraday Soc.*, **49**, 1375 (1953).
13. Hartree, D. R., *Proc. Cambridge Phil. Soc.*, **24**, 89, 111 (1928).
14. Fock, V., *Z. Physik*, **61**, 126 (1930).
15. Coulson, C. A., *Valence*, Oxford Univ. Press, New York, 1961, Chap. VIII.
16. Streitwieser, A., Jr., *Molecular Orbital Theory for Organic Chemists*, Wiley, New York, 1961.
17. Wheland, G. W., and Pauling, J., *J. Am. Chem. Soc.*, **57**, 2086 (1935).
18. Fox, J. L., *et al*, *Biochim. Biophys. Acta*, **109**, 626 (1965).
19. Mataga, N., and Nishimoto, N., *Z. Phys. Chem. (Frankfurt)*, **13**, 140 (1957).
20. Martin, A. N., *et al*, *Physical Pharmacy*, 2nd ed., Lea & Febiger, 1969.

18 | Thermodynamics

Heat—temperature—heat capacity—work—first, second, and third laws of thermodynamics—thermochemistry—heat of formation—Hess's law of heat summation—heat of solution—entropy—reversible processes—free-energy work functions and relationships—chemical potential—Clapeyron and Clausius–Clapeyron equations

This chapter was prepared by

Arthur Cammarata, PhD, *Associate Professor of Physical Medicinal Chemistry, School of Pharmacy, Temple University, Philadelphia, Pa. 19140*

The term *thermodynamics* implies literally an area of science which is concerned with mechanical action produced by heat. From a historical perspective the subject of thermodynamics developed as a consequence of efforts to produce an efficient heat engine, but early in the development it became evident that the concepts of thermodynamics were of much greater generality. It is now recognized, notably through the efforts of Gibbs,[1] that chemical and physical changes can be interpreted in terms of the energy requirements for these processes and that the energy changes accompanying such transformations are predictable through the use of thermodynamic principles. Since pharmaceutical scientists are primarily interested in the energy changes accompanying a chemical or physical conversion, *energetics* is a more descriptive word for the content of this chapter.

Heat—A person can sense whether an object is hot or cold either visually or by contact with the object. A bar of metal removed from a furnace may glow red, and as it cools the color dulls progressively until there is no visual evidence that the bar is still hot. If the bar is touched, however, the resulting sensation indicates immediately whether the bar is hot or cool. If the hot bar of metal is placed in contact with a cooler one, after a short period of time both bars will be found to be equally warm. Heat has been lost from the hot bar and gained by the cold bar, and this transfer of heat stops when the bars are of equivalent warmth; ie, when *thermal equilibrium* is established.

The transfer of heat from one object to another is analogous to a system in which two compartments separated by a porous membrane contain differing levels of water. The compartment having the higher water level loses water to the second compartment until the water level on both sides of the membrane is the same; ie, in this case, until hydrostatic equilibrium is established. Using this analogy, it could be said that a hot substance contains an amount of heat Q_H

which is greater than the amount of heat Q_C contained by a cold substance,

$$Q_H > Q_C \tag{1}$$

For every small increment of heat lost from the hot substance, $-dQ_H$, a corresponding amount of heat must be gained by the cold substance, $+dQ_C$,

$$-dQ_H = +dQ_C \tag{2}$$

When heat is no longer transferred, the two substances are in thermal equilibrium, so that

$$Q_H - \Delta Q_H = Q_C + \Delta Q_C \tag{3}$$

where ΔQ is the total amount of heat that has been transferred. A representation of the conditions suggested by Eqs. 1 to 3 is shown in Fig. 148.

Temperature—While varying amounts of heat may be experienced through the senses, a more accurate measure is needed if quantitative relationships between heat and other forms of energy are to be developed. A measure of heat is called *temperature* and the instrument used in the measurement of temperature is a *thermometer*. To arrive at a graduated indication of the heat of a substance, known as a *temperature scale*, a property of a substance which varies as the substance is heated or cooled may be used. The thermal expansion or contraction of gases and liquids is useful in this regard. The temperature scale used in thermodynamics is derived using a gas thermometer, while liquid thermometers are used in most practical situations. It is seldom realized, however, that the graduations found on a liquid thermometer are based on temperatures determined with a gas thermometer; ie, liquid thermometers are calibrated against a gas thermometer.

Consider an attempt to measure the temperature of a liquid with a thermometer. According to Eq. 3, the heat of the liquid and the heat of the thermometer are the same only after thermal equilibrium has been established. But, in order for thermal equilibrium to be attained, the liquid will have gained or lost an amount of heat ΔQ. This would seem to indicate that the temperature measured by the thermometer is not the true temperature of the liquid. However, if the heat contained by the liquid, Q_L, is very much greater than the amount of heat that has to be exchanged with the thermometer, ΔQ_T, to attain thermal equilibrium

$$Q_L \gg \Delta Q_T \tag{4}$$

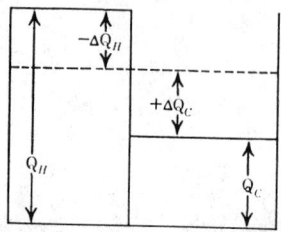

Fig. 148. The conditions preceding (——) and following (- - -) the transfer of heat.

the measured temperature may be considered the true temperature of the liquid.

Thus, introducing Eq. 4 into Eq. 3, when the liquid is initially cooler than the thermometer

$$Q_L = Q_T - \Delta Q_T \qquad (5)$$

and, when the liquid is initially hotter than the thermometer,

$$Q_L = Q_T + \Delta Q_T \qquad (6)$$

The liquid functions as a *heat reservoir* in much the same way as the Atlantic Ocean is a heat reservoir when an ice cube is dropped into it. The ice cube melts, but the ocean is still as warm as it was initially.

Say that a gas thermometer is used in measuring the heat of the liquid. This thermometer may be a cylinder containing a gas, and the pressure of the gas provides an indication of the heat of the liquid. If the liquid is hot, the pressure of the gas is high; if the liquid is cold, the pressure of the gas is low. Because the gas pressure is directly related to the heat of the liquid, one may say that there is a linear relation between the pressure P and the heat of the liquid Q_L,

$$P = aQ_L + b \qquad (7)$$

Since the heat of a substance is said to be given by its temperature, t, it may also be stated that there is a linear relationship between heat and temperature, so that

$$Q_L = ct + d \qquad (8)$$

The substitution of Eq. 8 into Eq. 7 gives the relationship between pressure and temperature:

$$P = kt + I \qquad (9)$$

Hence, as Fig. 149 shows, a plot of P against t is a straight line of slope k having an intercept on the P-axis given by I.

Pressure is measured in units of atmospheres, but to this point no indication has been provided of the units for temperature. Temperature units may be defined by measuring the pressure of the gas when the gas thermometer is immersed in a mixture of ice and water and, subsequently, in boiling water (at sea level). For each pressure reading there is a corresponding temperature, according to Eq. 9, so that at the *boiling point*

$$P_b = kt_b + I \qquad (10)$$

while at the *ice point*

$$P_i = kt_i + I \qquad (11)$$

By taking the difference between Eqs. 10 and 11, a relation is obtained which gives the number of pressure units corresponding to a set number of temperature units between the boiling and ice points of water

$$P_b - P_i = k(t_b - t_i) \qquad (12)$$

Thus, by defining $t_i = 0$ and $t_b = 100$, pressure is related to a temperature scale of 100 units. This is

the centigrade or Celsius scale, and temperatures measured in these units are given the symbol °C. Alternatively, the definition $t_i = 32$ and $t_b = 212$ could be made, in which pressure is related to a temperature scale of 180 units. This is known as the Fahrenheit scale and these units are given the symbol °F.

The Celsius and Fahrenheit temperature scales are related by the equation

$$\frac{°C - 0}{°F - 32} = \frac{100}{180} \qquad (13)$$

so that temperature measured in °F can be converted to °C using Eq. 13 written in the form

$$°C = \frac{5}{9}(°F - 32) \qquad (14)$$

Alternatively, temperature measured in °C can be converted to °F using the equation

$$°F = \frac{9}{5}°C + 32 \qquad (15)$$

A more meaningful temperature scale, from a physical standpoint, is one which would avoid assigning negative heats to substances that are much colder than the ice point of water. Eq. 9 can be used as a basis for constructing a temperature scale fulfilling this requirement by setting the condition that when the pressure is zero the temperature is also zero. This new scale, called the *absolute* temperature scale, is thus based on the relation (Boyle's law)

$$P = kT \qquad (16)$$

in which T is the temperature according to this scale. The absolute temperature scale is also known as the Kelvin scale, and the units are given the symbol °K. Each unit of the Kelvin scale is taken to be equal in magnitude to a Celsius unit, so that interconversions between the two scales are readily accomplished using

$$T(°K) = t(°C) + 273.16 \qquad (17)$$

By international agreement, the terminal constant in Eq. 17 is the number of Celsius units between absolute zero ($T = 0 °K$) and the *triple point* of water, ie, the temperature where water in all its forms (solid, liquid, and gas) at a pressure of 1 atmos. is in a state of equilibrium.

Heat Capacity—It is known from Eq. 3 that in order for two substances, A and B, to come to thermal equilibrium a total amount of heat ΔQ must be transferred between them; ie,

$$-\Delta Q_A = +\Delta Q_B \qquad (18)$$

The heat that is transferred is the difference of the heat content at a stage preceding the heat transfer Q_I and the heat content after thermal equilibrium has been established Q_F. This difference can be determined by a measurement of temperature alone since, by the use of Eq. 8,

$$Q_F - Q_I = C_v(T_F - T_I) \qquad (19)$$

or

$$\Delta Q = C_v \Delta T \qquad (20)$$

The absolute temperature scale is used for reasons already discussed. The constant C_v in Eqs. 19 and 20 is characteristic of a substance and is termed its *heat capacity*. Since the magnitude of this constant

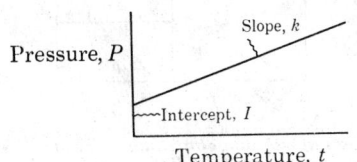

Fig. 149.   **The linear relationship between temperature and pressure.**

is proportional to the quantity of material present, it is convenient to define a heat capacity/unit mass of substance. The unit of mass may be 1 Gm or 1 mole of material. In the former case *specific heat* has been defined; in the latter case *molal heat capacity* has been defined.

The subscript v attached to the constant in Eqs. 19 and 20 designates that the temperature change of a substance is measured under conditions such that the substance underwent no change in volume. A gas contained in a closed cylinder, for example, maintains a constant volume as its temperature is varied, since the walls of the cylinder limit the expansion of the gas. In a large number of instances, however, a change in temperature causes a change in the volume of a material. For example, a glass of water at 70°C (158°F) contains a greater volume of water than when it is at 10°C (50°F). As, under ordinary circumstances, this expansion takes place against the constant pressure of the atmosphere, it is appropriate to ask whether there is a difference between heat capacities determined under conditions of constant volume (C_v) and heat capacities determined under conditions of constant pressure (C_p).

For convenience, consider a closed cubic container containing a gas to have one of its faces in contact with a face of a second cubic vessel containing an equivalent amount of the same gas (Fig. 150). Assume that one of the containers is at a higher temperature than the other, and let the lower temperature container have a movable piston for one of its faces. As heat is transferred to the container of lower temperature, the piston is forced to rise against the constant pressure of the atmosphere due to the thermal expansion of the gas within this container. Hence, when thermal equilibrium is established between the vessels, the container with the movable piston will have the gas confined in a larger volume than it had initially.

Making use of Eq. 18, it may be said that to attain equilibrium an amount of heat given by Eq. 21 has been transferred between the containers.

$$-\Delta Q_v = +\Delta Q_P \qquad (21)$$

However, for the constant-pressure container, a portion of the total heat absorbed was absorbed by the gas and another portion was used in moving the piston against the atmosphere. This may be represented by

$$\Delta Q_P = \Delta Q_p + \Delta Q_w \qquad (22)$$

where ΔQ_p is the heat absorbed by the gas and ΔQ_w is the heat used in moving the piston. Substitution of Eq. 22 into Eq. 21 yields

$$-\Delta Q_v = \Delta Q_p + \Delta Q_w \qquad (23)$$

Since heat capacities refer only to the heat absorbed by a substance, Eq. 20 may be substituted into Eq. 23 to obtain

$$C_v \Delta T = C_p \Delta T + \Delta Q_w \qquad (24)$$

or

$$C_v = C_p + \frac{\Delta Q_w}{\Delta T} \qquad (25)$$

Thus, heat capacities determined at constant volume differ from heat capacities determined at constant pressure by an amount corresponding to the heat absorbed to move against the atmosphere/degree temperature change.

Work—By definition, work W is the force F needed to move an object a given distance, Δs, and the equation relating work to force and distance is

$$W = F \cdot \Delta s \qquad (26)$$

The container discussed in the previous section whose piston moved against a constant pressure was doing work, since the pressure P exerted on the face of the piston has units of force/unit area. Thus, if A is the area of the piston, the work done by the piston is

$$W = P \cdot A \cdot \Delta s \qquad (27)$$

or, recognizing that the change in volume ΔV is given by $A \cdot \Delta s$:

$$W = P \Delta V \qquad (28)$$

Since heat is required to perform this work, it can be said that

$$W = \Delta Q_w \qquad (29)$$

and, therefore,

$$\Delta Q_w = P \Delta V \qquad (30)$$

It should be noted that Eq. 29 is the mathematical form of Joule's statement that heat and *mechanical work* are interconvertible. Mechanical work is the work done on or by a system.

For an ideal gas where

$$PV = nRT \qquad (31)$$

a change in the volume of the gas when the pressure is maintained constant necessarily implies a change in temperature. That is, when there is a volume change of an ideal gas, Eq. 31 can be written

$$P \Delta V = nR \Delta T \qquad (32)$$

when the pressure P and the number of moles of gas n are maintained constant. The quantity R is the gas constant (0.0821 l-atmos./°K-mole, 1.99 cal/°K-mole). Thus, substituting Eq. 32 into Eq. 30, it is found that Eq. 25 may be given by

$$C_v = C_p + nR \qquad (33)$$

For the more general case where the state of a substance (solid, liquid, or gas) does not have to be specified, Eq. 30 can be substituted into Eq. 23 to obtain

$$-\Delta Q_v = \Delta Q_p + P \Delta V \qquad (34)$$

or, from Eq. 28,

$$-\Delta Q_v = \Delta Q_p + W \qquad (35)$$

First Law of Thermodynamics—From the concepts of heat, temperature, and work which have been developed, and which are summarized by Eqs. 34 and 35, the first basic law of thermodynamics can be ob-

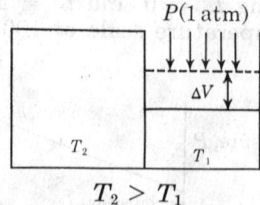

P(1 atm)

ΔV

T_2 T_1

$T_2 > T_1$

Fig. 150. A constant-volume container in contact with a constant-pressure container. The dotted line indicates the position of the movable piston after thermal equilibrium is established between the containers.

tained. In its simplest form, the *first law of thermodynamics* states that *energy may be converted from one form to another, but it cannot be created or destroyed.* Another way of saying this is to state that the first law recognizes the *Law of Conservation of Energy* and deals with all forms of energy as they appear either as heat or work.

Before presenting the mathematical form of the first law, it is suitable at this point to redefine certain of the terms appearing in Eq. 34. For the heat absorbed at constant volume ΔQ_v, a new quantity ΔE, called the *internal energy*, will be defined such that

$$\Delta E = E_F - E_I = \Delta Q_v \qquad (36)$$

In Eq. 36, E_I is the internal energy of a substance at an initial temperature T_I and E_F is the internal energy of the same substance at a second final temperature (where equilibrium may be established) T_F. This new quantity can be determined by a knowledge of heat capacities since the substitution of Eq. 20 into Eq. 36 provides the relation

$$\Delta E = C_v \Delta T \qquad (37)$$

Substituting Eq. 36 into Eq. 34, there is obtained

$$-\Delta E = \Delta Q_p + P\Delta V \qquad (38)$$

which is given equivalently by

$$(E_F - E_I) + P(V_F - V_I) = -\Delta Q_p \qquad (39)$$

Grouping the terms of Eq. 39 yields

$$(E_F + PV_F) - (E_I + PV_I) = -\Delta Q_p \qquad (40)$$

and if another quantity H, called *enthalpy*, is defined by

$$H = E + PV \qquad (41)$$

Eq. 40 can be written

$$\Delta H = H_F - H_I = -\Delta Q_p \qquad (42)$$

Since the negative sign in Eq. 42 signifies a heat loss, a change in sign would designate that heat is being absorbed. Thus, it could be said that enthalpy, defined by

$$\Delta H = H_F - H_I = \Delta Q_p \qquad (43)$$

(note the change in sign), represents heat *absorbed* at constant pressure, and this heat can be obtained from a knowledge of heat capacities using the relation

$$\Delta H = C_p \Delta T \qquad (44)$$

Eqs. 36 and 43 are presented to emphasize that in thermodynamics internal energy and enthalpy are terms used in place of the word heat since these terms specify, by definition, the conditions under which heat is measured.

For the condition where heat is absorbed at constant pressure, Eq. 40 can be written

$$(E_F + PV_F) - (E_I + PV_I) = \Delta H \qquad (45)$$

or, in a form equivalent to Eq. 38,

$$\Delta E = \Delta H - P\Delta V \qquad (46)$$

The *First Law of Thermodynamics* may be obtained by removing the restriction of constant pressure from the right side of Eq. 46,

$$\Delta E = DQ - DW \qquad (47)$$

In Eq. 47, DQ and DW still represent heat and work, respectively, but they are written in this manner to designate that the conditions for their measurement is to be specified before the equation is used. In essence, the reason DQ and DW can remain unspecified is that for any set of conditions one wishes to impose on a given system, the system can always be compared to a second system maintained at a constant volume. One such comparison is made in Fig. 150 for the imposed condition of constant pressure.

In applying the First Law to a given experimental situation, it is necessary to note initially whether the experimental system exchanges heat with or can do work on its surroundings. A material in a perfectly insulated thermos bottle, for example, cannot exchange heat with its surroundings and under these *adiabatic* conditions $DQ = 0$. When heat can be exchanged with the surroundings,

$$DQ = C\Delta T \qquad (48)$$

and a subscript p or v is applied to the molar heat capacity depending on whether the exchange occurs at constant pressure or constant volume.

Work can be done under conditions of constant pressure or constant volume, so that to take into account these two possibilities

$$DW = P\Delta V + V\Delta P \qquad (49)$$

When the pressure is constant $\Delta P = 0$ and

$$DW = P\Delta V \qquad (50)$$

whereas, when the volume is constant $\Delta V = 0$ and

$$DW = V\Delta P \qquad (51)$$

A collapsed metal container caused to return to its original shape by increasing the pressure within it does not have its internal volume changed but yet it does work against the surroundings.

An alternative form for Eq. 49 can be given by assuming that the work is done on or by an ideal gas. By use of the ideal gas law,

$$DW = (nR\Delta T)_p + (nR\Delta T)_v \qquad (52)$$

so that at constant pressure or constant volume

$$DW = nR\Delta T \qquad (53)$$

With Eqs. 48, 49, and, for an ideal gas, 53, the appropriate form of the First Law can be deduced for a variety of experimental conditions. However, in applying these relations care must be taken in recognizing whether the First Law is to refer to a substance or to a process involving the substance. For example, at constant temperature (ie, $\Delta T = 0$) the internal energy of an ideal gas is given by

$$\Delta E = C\Delta T - nR\Delta T \qquad (54)$$

or

$$\Delta E = 0 \qquad (55)$$

If the ideal gas is allowed to expand against a constant pressure while at a constant temperature, then

$$\Delta E = 0 = DQ - DW \qquad (56)$$

or

$$DQ = P\Delta V \qquad (57)$$

In Table I some expressions obtained by the use of the First Law are shown.

Thermochemistry—The study of the heat effects accompanying chemical reactions and certain physical processes such as solution or change of state is called thermochemistry. Thermochemical data are usually obtained by carrying out reactions in calorimeters and measuring the heat absorbed or evolved according to the temperature change of a surrounding weighed amount of water. Heat changes measured in closed calorimeters, where the volume remains constant, correspond to ΔE, while heat changes measured in open calorimeters, where the pressure remains constant, correspond to ΔH. When, during the course of a reaction, there is no change in volume, or only a very small change, $\Delta E = \Delta H$. Thus, it is possible to express thermochemical data in terms of ΔE or ΔH for any specific reaction or process. If the process is *exothermic* (ie, is accompanied by the evolution of heat) ΔE or ΔH has a negative value; conversely, if the process is *endothermic* (ie, is accompanied by the absorption of heat) ΔE or ΔH has a positive value.

Heat of Combustion—The heat evolved when 1 Gm-formula weight of a substance undergoes combustion with oxygen to form water and carbon dioxide is called the *heat of combustion*. The reactants and products of the combustion are considered to be in the form that they would ordinarily be at 25°C and 1 atmos. pressure. These conditions constitute the *standard state* of the substances involved in the reaction. Thus, the combustion of ethanol in an atmosphere of oxygen to afford water and carbon dioxide in an open calorimeter corresponds to the equation

$$C_2H_5OH \ (l) + 3O_2 \ (g) = 2CO_2 \ (g) + 3H_2O \ (l);$$
$$\Delta H^0{}_{298} = -326{,}700 \text{ cal}$$

where the state of the substances, gaseous *g* or liquid *l*, is indicated in parenthesis. Since the substances are in their standard states, the heat measured for the process ΔH has affixed to it a superscript degree sign and a subscript designating the temperature in °K chosen as standard.

Hess's Law of Heat Summation—In 1840 Hess pointed out that the heat absorbed (or evolved) in a given chemical reaction is the same whether it takes place in one step or in several steps. This principle has wide utility, since it provides a means of calculating heat quantities that cannot be determined directly by experiment.

A good illustration of the use of Hess's Law is provided by the calculation of the heat of reaction of carbon (as graphite) when it undergoes combustion to carbon monoxide. This heat of combustion is difficult to measure experimentally because of the complication of the simultaneous formation of carbon dioxide and the incomplete reaction of carbon. It is relatively much easier to measure the heat of combustion of carbon

$$C(graphite) + O_2 \ (g) = CO_2 \ (g); \quad \Delta H^0{}_{298} = -94{,}052 \text{ cal}$$

and of carbon monoxide

$$CO \ (g) + \tfrac{1}{2}O_2 \ (g) = CO_2 \ (g); \quad \Delta H^0{}_{298} = -67{,}636 \text{ cal}$$

and to obtain the desired quantity by subtracting the second equation from the first

$$C(graphite) + \tfrac{1}{2}O_2 \ (g) = CO \ (g); \quad \Delta H^0{}_{298} = -27{,}416 \text{ cal}$$

Heat of Formation—The *heat of formation*, symbolized $\Delta H^0{}_f$, of a substance is the heat evolved when 1 Gm-formula weight of the substance is produced from its constituent elements, the reactants and product being taken as in their standard states. The heat of reaction of carbon and oxygen in forming

Table I—Some Relations Obtained Using the First Law

$$\Delta E = DQ - DW$$

Conditions	Relation
Constant pressure ($\Delta P = 0$)	$\Delta H = C_p \Delta T$
Constant volume ($\Delta V = 0$)	$\Delta E = C_v \Delta T - V \Delta P$
Constant volume; no work ($DW = 0$)	$\Delta E = C_v \Delta T$
Adiabatic ($DQ = 0$)	$\Delta E = -DW$
Constant temperature ($\Delta T = 0$); ideal gas	$\Delta E = 0; \ DQ = DW$
Adiabatic; constant pressure	$\Delta E = -P \Delta V$

carbon dioxide is properly a heat of combustion as well as a heat of formation. In calculating heats of reaction by Hess's Law, one usually obtains the heats of formation of the respective products and reactants from tables (*cf*, Table II) and arrives at the heat of reaction using the relation

$$\Delta H^0 = \Sigma \Delta H^0{}_{f,\text{products}} - \Sigma \Delta H^0{}_{f,\text{reactants}} \quad (58)$$

where Σ designates that the sum of $\Delta H^0{}_f$ for each of the products or the reactants is taken. As an example, consider the calculation of the heat of reaction for the production of acetic acid from methane and carbon dioxide

$$CH_4 \ (g) + CO_2 \ (g) = CH_3CO_2H \ (l)$$

$\Delta H^0{}_f =$	$\Delta H^0{}_f =$	$\Delta H^0{}_f =$
$-17{,}889$	$-94{,}052$	$-116{,}400$
cal	cal	cal

The heat of reaction is found to be

$$\Delta H_0 = (-116{,}400 \text{ cal}) -$$
$$[(-17{,}889 \text{ cal}) + (-94{,}052 \text{ cal})]$$

or

$$\Delta H^0 = -4{,}459 \text{ cal}$$

Thus, if the reaction was to occur as written there would be an evolution of 4,459 cal of heat.

Heat of Solution—When a specified amount, conventionally 1 Gm-formula weight, of a solute is dissolved in a solvent, a quantity of heat called the *heat of solution* is evolved or absorbed. The heat of solution of a given solute–solvent system is generally not constant but varies with the volume of the solvent to which a specified amount of solute is added. Fig. 151 illustrates the variation in the amount of heat evolved when 1 Gm-formula weight of ethanol is added to differing amounts of water.

There are three ways of expressing heats of solution, and each of these may be determined from plots such as is shown in Fig. 151. The *integral heat of solution* is the heat absorbed when 1 Gm-formula weight of solute is dissolved in enough water to form a solution of specified concentration. In Fig. 151, this is the value of ΔH for any given dilution of the alcohol solution. The *differential heat of solution* is the heat

Table II—Heats of Formation for Some Compounds at 25°C

Compound	$\Delta H^0{}_f$, kcal/mole
$H_2O \ (l)$	-68.317
$H_2O \ (g)$	-57.798
$NO \ (g)$	21.600
$CO \ (g)$	-26.415
$CO_2 \ (g)$	-94.052
$CH_4 \ (g)$	-17.889
$C_2H_5O \ (l)$	-66.356
$CH_3CO_2H \ (l)$	-116.4

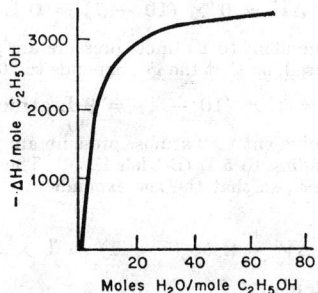

Fig. 151. Integral heat of solution of ethyl alcohol in water (0°C).

absorbed when a quantity of solute so small as to cause no significant change in concentration is added to a solution of a specified concentration. This quantity is obtained from the slope of the curve in Fig. 151 at any specified dilution of the alcohol solution. The *heat of solution at infinite dilution* is the maximum value the heat of solution approaches as the volume of solvent is increased. The practically constant value approached in Fig. 151 gives this quantity for an alcohol solution.

Heats of dilution are obtained from integral heats of solution by taking the difference between the integral heats of solution of two specified concentrations of a solute–solvent system. Compounds that form a hydrate with water have their *heat of hydration* given by the difference between the integral heats of solution of the solvated and nonsolvated solute.

Second Law of Thermodynamics—While all forms of energy can be converted completely into heat, only a fraction of heat energy can be converted into work. The efficiency of this latter conversion is the concern of the Second Law of Thermodynamics. From a theoretical consideration of a reversible cycle of operations performed on a machine whereby heat is converted into work, Carnot (1824) showed that the maximum proportion of work that can be obtained from heat is governed by the following equation, which constitutes a mathematical expression of the Second Law of Thermodynamics.

$$w_{\max} = q_2 \frac{(T_2 - T_1)}{T_2} \qquad (59)$$

In this equation $w_{\max}$ is the maximum work that can be obtained from q_2 units of heat supplied at absolute temperature T_2 to the "boiler" of a hypothetical engine of perfect mechanical efficiency with a "condenser" maintained at absolute temperature T_1. The fraction of heat converted into work—the so-called maximum theoretical efficiency of the process—is expressed by the ratio

$$\frac{w_{\max}}{q_2} = \text{efficiency} \qquad (60)$$

The dependence of this efficiency on the temperature difference $T_2 - T_1$, as well as on the boiler temperature T_2, is illustrated by the following calculations of the maximum work obtainable from 1000 cal of heat supplied to a steam engine operating at (a) a boiler temperature of 100°C and a condenser temperature of 25°C and at (b) a boiler temperature of 150°C (superheated steam) and a condenser temperature of 25°C.

Substituting in Eq. 59:

(a) $\quad w_{\max} = 1000 \dfrac{(373.1 - 298.1)}{373.1} = 201 \text{ cal}$

(b) $\quad w_{\max} = 1000 \dfrac{(423.1 - 298.1)}{423.1} = 295 \text{ cal}$

The greater efficiency of conversion of heat into work when the boiler temperature is high explains why superheated steam (steam under pressure) yields more work than the same amount of heat supplied as steam at a temperature of 100°C. In either case the heat that is not converted to work is retained in the condenser system; none of it is destroyed. If the condenser temperature is reduced, more heat will be converted to work. Thus, if the temperature *could* be maintained continuously at absolute zero—which is, of course, a practical impossibility—all of a given quantity of heat supplied to the boiler could be converted to work.

Entropy—While the total amount of energy (and mass) in the universe is believed to be constant, none of it being created or destroyed, all the chemical and physical processes that occur spontaneously result in a decrease in the proportion of energy that is available for doing work or, conversely, an increase in the proportion of energy that is unavailable for doing work. (The reason why spontaneous processes occur is that the energy of the reacting system is at a higher level than it is when the process is completed.) The possibility is suggested that at some distant time in the future the energy of the universe will be unavailable for doing work because all of it has been degraded to a common level of intensity.

An important thermodynamic quantity that measures the increase in unavailable energy accompanying spontaneous reactions is *entropy*. For a reversible process in which heat DQ_{rev} at absolute temperature T is absorbed by a system (as when a substance changes from one physical state to another), the change in entropy, ΔS, is defined by the relationship

$$\Delta S = \frac{DQ_{\text{rev}}}{T} \qquad (61)$$

This equation may be used to calculate the increase in entropy when a definite amount of water, eg, 1 mole, at a temperature of 100°C, is converted to steam at the same temperature. In this case DQ_{rev} is the amount of heat required to vaporize 18.02 Gm (1 mole) of water, which is 18.02 times 539.7 cal, the latter quantity being the number of calories required to vaporize 1 Gm of water at its normal boiling point. Substituting in Eq. 61:

$$\Delta S = \frac{18.02 \times 539.7}{373.1} = 26.1 \text{ cal/}°K$$

The increase in entropy accompanying the melting of ice at 0°C may be calculated similarly

$$\Delta S = \frac{18.02 \times 79.7}{273.1} = 5.26 \text{ cal/}°K$$

Entropy may be defined as the capacity factor of isothermally unavailable energy; when multiplied by the reference temperature, the product measures the amount of energy unavailable for doing work at the specified temperature. Entropy is sometimes described as being a measure of the randomness, disorder, or "mixed-upness" of a system. In every spontaneous process there is an increase in entropy and hence of the randomness or disorder of the system. To illustrate this aspect of entropy, consider the three states of matter—solid, liquid, and gas. The solid state of any substance represents the highest degree of orderliness of the molecules (or atoms or ions) composing the substance; when it is converted to a liquid by heating, the orderliness of arrangement of the molecules (or atoms or ions) is destroyed and their distribution becomes more random; when the liquid is converted to a gas, there results still greater disorder or mixed-upness of the molecules. The increase in randomness is expressed quantitatively in the examples above for calculating increase in entropy accompanying change of state.

When the temperature of a substance is raised by heating, without changing the state of the substance, the motion of the molecules (or atoms or ions) becomes more disordered, that is, the entropy is increased. To calculate the entropy change, the process may be considered as a series of steps in which an infinitesimal change of temperature, dT, increases entropy by an infinitesimal amount dS, according to the equation

$$dS = \frac{C.dT}{T} \tag{62}$$

where C is the molar heat capacity (essentially the heat absorbed in raising the temperature of 1 mole of the substance through 1°C). The similarity of this equation to Eq. 61 is obvious. In order to apply this equation to a finite process it must be used in its integral form

$$\Delta S = S_2 - S_1 = 2.303 \, C \log \frac{T_2}{T_1} \tag{63}$$

As an example of the application of this equation, the increase in entropy of 1 mole (18.02 Gm) of water when it is heated from 10 to 20°C may be calculated. As the specific heat of water is approximately 1 cal/Gm, it may be assumed that the molar heat capacity of water is 18.02 times the specific heat. The complete calculation is

$$\Delta S = 18.02 \times 2.303 \log \frac{293}{283}$$

$$= 0.62 \text{ cal/°K/mole}$$

Reversible Processes—The concept of a *reversible process*, used in a thermodynamic sense, is quite different from that of a *reversible reaction*, applied to chemical reactions. A reversible process, whether physical or chemical in nature, is one in which a system that has been displaced from equilibrium only minutely by an infinitesimal force may be restored to equilibrium by applying an infinitesimal force in the opposite direction. Any other manner of conducting the process results in more or less irreversibility of the process.

The work obtained by the isothermal expansion of an ideal gas under different conditions of irreversibility may be compared with the work obtained on reversible expansion to illustrate both the distinction between an irreversible and a reversible process and the difference in their respective quantitative effects. Consider 1 liter (L) of an ideal gas, maintained at a constant temperature of 0°C (273.1°K) and at an initial pressure of 10 atmos., enclosed in a cylinder with a weightless, frictionless piston (capable of being locked in position) on which various weights may be placed, the atmosphere above the piston evacuated, and the piston released to permit expansion of the gas. On expansion the gas performs work equivalent to $P.\Delta V$, where P is the *resisting* pressure (produced by the weights on the piston), and ΔV is the increase in volume on expansion. Five different ways of expanding the gas from its initial volume of 1 L to a final volume of 10 L will be considered, and the work obtained in each case calculated.

1. The gas is permitted to expand from 1 L to 10 L without any weights being placed on the piston.

$$w = P.\Delta V = 0 \times (10 - 1) = 0 \text{ L-atmos}.$$

2. Weights equivalent to 1 atmos. pressure are placed on the piston, which is released, so that the gas expands to 10 L.

$$w = 1 \times (10 - 1) = 9 \text{ L-atmos}.$$

3. Weights equivalent to 2 atmos. pressure are placed on the piston, the gas expanding to 5 L (Boyle's law). The weights are then reduced to 1 atmos., so that the gas expands to the final volume of 10 L.

$$w = \Sigma P.\Delta V = 2 \times (5 - 1) + 1 \times (10 - 5)$$

$$= 13 \text{ L-atmos}.$$

4. Weights equivalent to 5 atmos. are placed on the piston, the gas expanding to 2 L; the weights are reduced to 2 atmos., with an expansion of gas to 5 L; finally, the weights are reduced to 1 atmos., with expansion to 10 L.

$$w = \Sigma P.\Delta V = 5 \times (2 - 1) + 2 \times (5 - 2) + 1 \times (10 - 5)$$

$$= 16 \text{ L-atmos}.$$

5. On the basis of the foregoing evidence that the amount of work obtained increases with the load on the piston, it may be deduced that the maximum work will be obtained when the piston load is successively reduced so that it is always infinitesimally less than the pressure of the gas in the cylinder. The process is continued until the infinitesimal increases in volume bring the final volume of gas to 10 L. Such a process is reversible. The total work obtained in the process can be calculated exactly by the expression

$$w_{max} = nRT \int_{V_i}^{V_f} dV/V = 2.303 \, nRT \log \frac{V_f}{V_i}$$

where V_f is the final volume, V_i is the initial volume, and n is the number of moles of gas enclosed in the cylinder (1/2.241). Substituting numerical values

$$w_{max} = \frac{1}{2.241} \times 2.303 \times 0.08205 \times 273.1 \times \log \frac{10}{1}$$

$$= 23.02 \text{ L-atmos}.$$

Free-Energy and Work Functions—What force causes a physical or chemical change to occur spontaneously? Nearly a century ago it was believed that chemical change occurred in the direction of evolution of heat. While this is often true, it is not always the case, for some spontaneous reactions take place with absorption of heat. For systems of constant internal energy (E) and volume, change will occur in the direction in which entropy is increased. But what thermodynamic criteria determine the course of a reaction when temperature and pressure are constant, as is the case with most chemical reactions, or when temperature and volume are constant?

These criteria may be established by introducing two additional thermodynamic quantities: the *Helmholtz free energy* or *work function*, symbolized A (German, *arbeit*, work), and the *Gibbs free energy*, now designated G but formerly (and sometimes still) symbolized by F. Consider the internal energy, E, of a system to consist of a part, A, available for doing work, and the remainder unavailable for performing work, at temperature T. The latter quantity is represented by the product TS (see *Entropy*, page 241). Symbolically,

$$E = A + TS \tag{64}$$

and

$$A = E - TS \tag{65}$$

For systems at constant volume and temperature the driving force of any physical or chemical change resides in the component of the internal energy available for doing work, namely A. The validity of this statement may be developed mathematically as follows. When a system undergoes change, Eq. 65 may be written

$$\Delta A = \Delta E - \Delta(TS) \qquad (66)$$

at constant temperature this becomes

$$\Delta A = \Delta E - T \cdot \Delta S \qquad (67)$$

If for ΔE is substituted its equivalent, $DQ - DW$, from the First Law of Thermodynamics (Eq. 47), we obtain

$$\Delta A = DQ - DW - T \cdot \Delta S \qquad (68)$$

Since, in a reversible process, where maximum work is obtained, $DQ = T \cdot \Delta S$ (Eq. 61), the preceding equation may be simplified to

$$\Delta A = -w_{rev} \qquad (69)$$

or

$$-\Delta A = w_{rev} \qquad (70)$$

This equation indicates that useful work may be obtained when a system undergoes any change in which A at the beginning of the change is greater than A when the change is completed. This decrease of A, as expressed by either Eq. 69 or 70, is a measure both of the capacity of a system to do work and of the driving force impelling the system to undergo spontaneous change in the direction of diminishing its *work capacity* or *function*. For systems at constant temperature and constant volume, a reaction will occur spontaneously only if ΔA has a negative value (or $-\Delta A$ has a positive value), signifying a loss in the capacity of the system to do work.

If a system at constant temperature increases in volume while under constant atmospheric pressure, the capacity of the system for doing work is reduced by an amount equivalent to the work of expansion against the atmosphere. The *net* work that can be obtained is given by

$$w_{net} = w_{rev} - P \cdot \Delta V \qquad (71)$$

Of course, if the volume of the system decreases while it is undergoing a reaction at constant temperature and pressure, the ΔV term is negative, indicating that work equivalent to $P \cdot \Delta V$ is done *on* the system, thereby increasing the capacity of the system for doing work, that is, making w_{net} larger than w_{rev}.

The quantity w_{net} may now be correlated with a thermodynamic function known as *Gibbs free energy*, designated G (or F). This function is formally defined as

$$G = H - TS \qquad (72)$$

Since

$$H = E + PV \qquad (73)$$

$$G = E + PV - TS \qquad (74)$$

When a system undergoes a change at constant pressure and temperature, the change of free energy, designated ΔG, is

$$\Delta G = \Delta E + P \cdot \Delta V - T \cdot \Delta S \qquad (75)$$

Replacing ΔE by $DQ - DW$, and equating $T \cdot \Delta S$ with DQ, we obtain

$$\Delta G = -w_{rev} + P \cdot \Delta V \qquad (76)$$

With signs reversed this becomes

$$-\Delta G = w_{rev} - P \cdot \Delta V \qquad (77)$$

Comparing this with Eq. 71, it is apparent that

$$-\Delta G = w_{net} \qquad (78)$$

For systems at constant pressure and temperature, it is the quantity $-\Delta G$, commonly called the *decrease in free energy* of a process, that measures both the net capacity of a system for doing work and the driving force impelling the system to undergo spontaneous change in the direction of diminishing free energy. If the system undergoes no change in volume, it is obvious that w_{net} equals w_{rev}, and that ΔG and ΔA must be equal.

Some Free-Energy Relationships—Lack of knowledge of absolute values of Gibbs free energy makes it necessary to refer differences in G to some standard state. In dealing with chemical reactions it is convenient to use for reference the *standard free-energy change*, symbolized $\Delta G°$, for a hypothetical reaction in which reactants in their standard states are converted to products in their standard states; the standard state is, commonly, one Gm-mole of substance at 1 atmos. pressure at 25°C.

A very useful equation for calculating the standard free-energy change when the equilibrium constant for a reaction is known is the following:

$$\Delta G° = -2.303RT \log K \qquad (79)$$

Conversely, K may be calculated for any reaction for which $\Delta G°$ is known.

When the standard electromotive force of an electrochemical cell operating reversibly is known, the standard free energy of the chemical reaction occurring in the cell may be calculated by the relationship

$$\Delta G° = -nFE° \qquad (80)$$

where n is the number of electrons transferred in the reaction, F is the faraday (96,500 coulombs), and $E°$ is the standard electromotive force of the cell.

Chemical Potential—In the foregoing discussion of thermodynamic quantities no consideration was given to changes in the number of moles of chemical reactants and products, or exchanges of matter with surroundings; the systems were considered *closed*. In *open systems*, however, cognizance must be taken of changes in free energy (or internal energy) resulting from variations of the number of moles and exchanges of matter with surroundings. This may be done by using a quantity μ, introduced by Gibbs and called by him the chemical potential, which is defined as

$$\mu_1 = \left(\frac{\partial G}{\partial n_1}\right)_{T, P, n_2, n_3, \dots} \qquad (81)$$

This partial differential expression states that the chemical potential of Substance 1 in a mixture of Substances 1, 2, 3, ... is equal to the rate of change in Gibbs free energy of the system with the number of moles n_1 of substance 1 when temperature, pressure, and the number of moles of all other substances in the system are held constant. The product $\mu_1 \cdot dn_1$ then represents the change of free energy produced by dn_1 moles of Substance 1. The summation of such changes for all the different substances in the system, represented as $\Sigma \mu dn$, provides for open systems the necessary correction for changes in free energy resulting from changes in the number of moles of components in the system.

Some Thermodynamic Calculations—The following problems, and their solutions, illustrate the application of the thermodynamic principles discussed in preceding sections.

Problem 1—One mole of liquid water is vaporized reversibly at 100°C and 1 atmos. pressure. The heat of vaporization under these conditions is 539.7 cal/Gm. Calculate DQ, DW, ΔH, ΔE, ΔA, ΔG, and ΔS.

The heat of vaporization per Gm multiplied by the molecular weight represents the heat absorbed in the process; since the process occurs at constant pressure the heat absorbed is ΔQ_p which, according to Eq. 43, is equal to ΔH. Thus

$$\Delta Q_p = \Delta H = 539.7 \times 18.02 = 9725 \text{ cal/mole}$$

The work performed is the increase in volume of the system resulting from vaporization of the water, against a constant pressure of 1 atmos. Then

$$w = P \cdot \Delta V = P(V_{vap} - V_{liq}) \cong P \cdot V_{vap}$$

While the work performed may be calculated using this equation, it is more readily calculated, when the result is to be expressed in calories, as follows:

$$w \cong P \cdot V_{vap} \cong RT = 1.987 \times 373.1 = 741 \text{ cal/mole}$$

$$\Delta E = DQ - DW = \Delta H - P \cdot \Delta V = 9725 - 741 = 8984 \text{ cal/mole}$$

$$\Delta S = \frac{DQ}{T} = \frac{\Delta H}{T} = \frac{9725}{373.1} = 26.0 \text{ cal/°/mole}$$

$$\Delta A = \Delta E - T \cdot \Delta S = 8984 - (373.1 \times 26.0) = -741 \text{ cal/mole}$$

The quantity ΔA may be calculated also from the relationship

$$\Delta A = -w_{rev} = -(741) = -741 \text{ cal/mole}$$

Finally

$$\Delta G = \Delta E + P \cdot \Delta V - T \cdot \Delta S$$
$$= 8984 + 741 - (373.1 \times 26.0) = 0 \text{ cal/mole}$$

Problem 2—The equilibrium constant, K_p, for the reaction $2H_2(g) + O_2(g) \rightarrow 2H_2O(g)$ at 2000° Abs is 1.55×10^7, the partial pressures being expressed in atmospheres. Calculate the standard free-energy change for the reaction, assuming ideal behavior of all the gases.

$$\Delta G° = -RT \ln Kp$$
$$= -2.303 \times 1.987 \times 2000 \log 1.55 \times 10^7$$
$$= -65,800 \text{ cal}$$

Problem 3—The electromotive force of a galvanic cell consisting of a zinc electrode immersed in zinc sulfate solution of unit activity and a copper electrode immersed in cupric sulfate solution of unit activity is 1.100 v, at 25°C. Calculate $\Delta G°$ for the cell reaction

$$Zn + Cu^{++} \rightarrow Zn^{++} + Cu$$

In this reaction two electrons are transferred, hence $n = 2$, and

$$\Delta G° = -2 \times 96,500 \times 1.100 = -212,300 \text{ joules}$$

The calorie equivalent may be calculated from the relationship

$$1 \text{ cal} = 4.184 \text{ joules}$$

or

$$\Delta G° = -\frac{212,300}{4.184} = -50,740 \text{ cal}$$

Miscellaneous Thermodynamic Relationships— The following differential forms of certain equations introduced earlier in this chapter are useful in the study of reversible processes in which the only work done is pressure–volume work.

$$dE = DQ - DW = T \cdot dS - P \cdot dV \tag{82}$$

$$dH = dE + d(PV) = dE + P \cdot dV + V \cdot dP \tag{83}$$

$$dG = dH - d(TS) = dH - T \cdot dS - S \cdot dT \tag{84}$$

From these equations may be obtained, by appropriate substitutions in the equations, the following:

$$dH = V \cdot dP + T \cdot dS \tag{85}$$

$$dG = V \cdot dP - S \cdot dT \tag{86}$$

At constant pressure these become

$$\left(\frac{\partial H}{\partial S}\right)_P = T \tag{87}$$

$$\left(\frac{\partial G}{\partial T}\right)_P = -S \tag{88}$$

At constant temperature equation 86 yields

$$\left(\frac{\partial G}{\partial P}\right)_T = V \tag{89}$$

and for an ideal gas

$$\left(\frac{\partial G}{\partial P}\right)_T = \frac{nRT}{P} \tag{90}$$

rearranging prior to integrating between G_2 at P_2 and G_1 at P_1

$$dG = nRT \frac{dP}{P} \tag{91}$$

then integrating

$$G_2 - G_1 = \Delta G = 2.303 \ nRT \log \frac{P_2}{P_1} \tag{92}$$

Third Law of Thermodynamics—In discussing entropy as a measure of the disorder or randomness of a system it was pointed out that entropy increased (1) with change of state from solid to liquid to gas and (2) with increase of temperature in any given state. The most orderly arrangement of any substance would be expected to be that of a perfect crystal when its temperature is absolute zero; under these conditions the entropy is, according to the Third Law of Thermodynamics, zero. Since it is impossible to reach absolute zero, a better statement of the Law is that the entropy of a perfect crystal approaches zero as the temperature approaches absolute zero. The importance of this law lies in the fact that it provides the basis for calculating absolute values of entropy of pure substances from measurements of their heat capacity; if the absolute entropies and heats of formation of substances are known it is possible to calculate their Gibbs free-energy values and from these to calculate the equilibrium constants for various physical and chemical reactions.

The Clapeyron Equation—An important thermodynamic relationship between the variables of vapor pressure and temperature in any equilibrium between two phases of a substance was developed by Clapeyron in 1834. To derive this equation it is convenient to consider a liquid in equilibrium with its vapor at temperature T and pressure P equal to the vapor pressure of the liquid at the specified temperature. At constant temperature and pressure the Gibbs free energy of the liquid, G_l, must be equal to that of the vapor, G_v:

$$G_l = G_v \tag{93}$$

If the temperature is raised to $T + dT$, the pressure must be increased to $P + dP$ to correspond to the vapor pressure at the higher temperature, to maintain the two phases in equilibrium. The free energy of both liquid and vapor is increased, but since the two phases are in equilibrium, the increase must be the same for both, so that

$$dG_l = dG_v \tag{94}$$

The change of free energy of a pure substance with pressure and temperature being defined by

$$dG = V \cdot dP - S \cdot dT \tag{95}$$

Eq. 94 may be written

$$V_1 . dP - S_1 . dT = V_v . dP - S_v . dT \qquad (96)$$

rearranging

$$\frac{dP}{dT} = \frac{S_v - S_1}{V_v - V_1} \qquad (97)$$

Since Eq. 61 applies,

$$S_v - S_1 = \Delta S = \frac{\Delta H_{vap}}{T} \qquad (98)$$

where ΔH_{vap} is the molar heat of vaporization (the heat absorbed by 1 mole of liquid during vaporization), substitution into Eq. 97 yields

$$\frac{dP}{dT} = \frac{\Delta H_{vap}}{T(V_v - V_1)} \qquad (99)$$

This is the Clapeyron equation, which relates dP/dT, the rate of change of vapor pressure with temperature, to the heat of vaporization of a liquid and to the molar volume of the liquid (V_1) and of the vapor (V_v) at temperature T and pressure equal to the vapor pressure.

The Clapeyron equation is not limited, however, to the equilibrium between a liquid and its vapor in the process of vaporization; it applies, with suitable modifications, to the equilibrium between a solid and a gas phase (as in sublimation), a solid and a liquid phase (as in melting or fusion), and between two crystalline forms, distinguished as 1 and 2, of a solid (as in the transition of one form to the other). The applicable equations are

$$\text{Sublimation} \quad \frac{dP}{dT} = \frac{\Delta H_{sub}}{T(V_v - V_s)} \qquad (100)$$

$$\text{Fusion} \quad \frac{dP}{dT} = \frac{\Delta H_{fus}}{T(V_1 - V_s)} \qquad (101)$$

$$\text{Transition} \quad \frac{dP}{dT} = \frac{\Delta H_{trans}}{T(V_2 - V_1)} \qquad (102)$$

The Clausius–Clapeyron Equation—Clausius placed the Clapeyron equation on a sound thermodynamic basis—dependent on the Second Law of Thermodynamics—and also introduced certain simplifications applicable to the vaporization and sublimation forms of Clapeyron's equation. Clausius assumed that the vapor obeys Boyle's ideal gas law and

that the molar volume of liquid, V_1, or of the solid, V_s, in the sublimation equation, may be neglected in comparison with the volume of a mole of vapor, V_v. Eq. 99 then may be written

$$\frac{dP}{dT} = \frac{P . \Delta H_{vap}}{RT^2} \qquad (103)$$

which is commonly called the Clausius–Clapeyron equation.

This equation is equivalent to

$$\frac{d \ln P}{dT} = \frac{\Delta H_{vap}}{RT^2} \qquad (104)$$

the integral of which is, in Naperian logarithm form

$$\log P = \frac{-\Delta H_{vap}}{2.303 \, RT} + \text{constant} \qquad (105)$$

This integral form of the Clausius–Clapeyron equation indicates that a plot of $\log P$ against $1/T$ yields a straight line, a fact observed some time before the Clausius–Clapeyron equation was known. The slope of the line, $-\Delta H_{vap}/2.303 \, R$, provides a graphical method for calculating ΔH_{vap}. When the equation is integrated between the limits P_2 at T_2 and P_1 at T_1, it becomes

$$\log \frac{P_2}{P_1} = \frac{\Delta H_{vap}(T_2 - T_1)}{2.303 \, RT_2 T_1} \qquad (106)$$

This equation may be used either to calculate the heat of vaporization when the vapor pressure is known at two temperatures (assuming that the heat of vaporization remains constant over the temperature interval), or the vapor pressure at a specified temperature if it is known at another temperature and the heat of vaporization is known and remains constant.

The Clapeyron and the Clausius–Clapeyron equations, in various forms, may be used to calculate a variety of pressure–temperature data, some of which have already been mentioned. The equations are used also to calculate the theoretical value of the molal boiling-point elevation constant and the molal freezing-point depression constant for dilute solutions (see Chapter 19 on *Solutions and Phase Equilibria*, page 264).

References

1. *The Collected Works of J. Willard Gibbs*, Yale Univ. Press, New Haven, Conn., 1928; reprinted 1948.

19 | Solutions and Phase Equilibria

Solutions and solubility—solutions (solids in liquids; liquids in
liquids; and gases in liquids)—molecular structure and solubility—
pharmaceutical solvents—colligative properties of solutions—osmotic-
pressure elevation—vapor-pressure lowering—boiling-point elevation—
freezing-point depression—relationship between osmotic pressure and
vapor-pressure lowering—ideal behavior and deviations from ideal
behavior—activity and activity coefficient—practical applications of
colligative properties

This chapter was prepared by

Theodore D. Sokoloski, PhD, *Associate Professor of Pharmacy, College of
Pharmacy, The Ohio State University, Columbus, Ohio   43210*

Solutions and Solubility

A solution is a chemically and physically homogeneous mixture of two or more substances. The term solution generally denotes a homogeneous mixture that is liquid even though it is possible to have homogeneous mixtures which are solid or gaseous. Thus it is possible to have solutions of solids in liquids, liquids in liquids, gases in liquids, gases in gases, and solids in solids. The first three of these kinds of solutions are most important in pharmacy and ensuing discussions will be concerned primarily with them.

In discussing solutions it is customary to consider them as members of a particular class of dispersions of one substance in another substance. Depending on the size of the dispersed particle they are classified as *true solutions, colloidal solutions,* or *suspensions.* If sugar is dissolved in water, it is supposed that the ultimate sugar particle is of molecular dimensions and that a *true solution* is formed. On the other hand if very fine sand is mixed with water, a *suspension* of comparatively large particles, each consisting of many molecules, is obtained. Between these two extremes lie *colloidal solutions,* the dispersed particles of which are larger than those of true solutions but smaller than the particles present in suspensions. In this chapter only true solutions will be discussed.

It is possible to classify broadly all solutions as one of two types. In the first type, although there may be a lesser or greater interaction between the dispersed substance (the solute) and the dispersing medium (the solvent), the solution phase contains the same chemical entity as found in the solid phase and thus, upon removal of the solvent, the solute is recovered unchanged. One example of this type of solution would be sugar dissolved in water where, in the presence of sugar in excess of its solubility, there is an equilibrium between sugar molecules in the solid phase with sugar molecules in the solution phase. A second example of this kind of a solution would be the dissolving of silver chloride in water. Admittedly, the solubility of this salt in water is small, but it is finite. In this case the solvent contains silver and chloride ions and the solid phase contains the same material. Removal of solvent yields initial solute.

In the second type of solution the solvent contains a compound which is different from that in the solid phase. The difference between the compound in the solid phase and solution is due generally to some chem-ical reaction that has occurred in the solvent. An example of this type of solution would be dissolving aspirin in an aqueous solvent containing some basic material capable of reacting with the acid aspirin. Now the species in solution would not only be undissociated aspirin, but aspirin also as its anion, whereas the species in the solid phase is aspirin in only its undissociated acid form. In this situation, if the solvent were removed part of the substance obtained (the salt of aspirin) would be different from what was initially present in the solid.

Solutions of Solids in Liquids

Reversible Solubility without Chemical Reaction—From the pharmaceutical standpoint solutions of solids in liquids, with or without accompanying chemical reaction in the solvent, are of the greatest importance, and many quantitative data on the behavior and properties of such solutions are available. This discussion will be concerned with definitions of solubility, the rate at which substances go into solution, and with thermodynamic and other factors which control solubility.

Solubility—When an excess of a solid is brought into contact with a liquid, molecules of the former are removed from its surface until equilibrium is established between the molecules leaving the solid and those returning to it. The resulting solution is said to be saturated at the temperature of the experiment, and the extent to which the solute dissolves is referred to as its *solubility.* The extent of solubility of different substances varies from almost imperceptible amounts to relatively large quantities, but for any given solute the solubility has a constant value at constant temperature.

Under certain conditions it is possible to prepare a solution containing a larger amount of solute than is necessary to form a saturated solution. This may occur when a solution is saturated at one temperature, the excess of solid solute removed, and the solution cooled. The solute present in solution, even though it may be less soluble at the lower temperature, does not always separate from the solution and there is produced a *supersaturated solution.* Such solutions, formed by sodium thiosulfate and potassium acetate, for example, may be made to deposit their excess of solute in one of the following ways: (1) by vigorous shaking, (2) by scratching the side of the vessel in contact with the solution, or (3) by introducing into the solution a small crystal of the solute.

Methods of Expressing Solubility—When quantitative data are available, solubilities may be expressed in many ways. For example, the solubility of sodium chloride in water at 25°C may be stated in the following ways:

1. 1 Gm of sodium chloride dissolves in 2.786 ml of water. (An approximation of this method is used by the USP and the NF.)
2. 35.89 Gm of sodium chloride dissolves in 100 ml of water.
3. 100 ml of a saturated solution of sodium chloride in water contains 31.71 Gm of solute.
4. 100 Gm of a saturated solution of sodium chloride in water contains 26.47 Gm of solute.
5. 1 L of a saturated solution of sodium chloride in water contains 5.425 moles of solute. This also may be stated: a saturated solution of sodium chloride in water is 5.425 molar with respect to the solute.

In order to calculate 3 from 1 or 2 it is necessary to know the density of the solution, in this case 1.198 Gm/ml. To calculate 5, the number of grams of solute in 1000 ml of solution (obtained by multiplying the data in (3) by ten) is divided by the molecular weight of sodium chloride, namely, 58.45.

Several other concentration expressions are used. Molality is the number of moles of solute in 1000 Gm of solvent and could be calculated from the data in 4 by subtracting grams of solute from grams of solution to obtain grams of solvent, relating this to 1000 Gm of solvent, and dividing by molecular weight to obtain moles. Mole fraction is the fraction of the total number of moles present which are moles of one component. Mole % may be obtained by multiplying mole fraction by 100. Normality refers to the number of Gm-Eq of solute dissolved in 1000 ml of solution.

In pharmacy, use is made of three concentration expressions. Per cent by weight (% w/w) is the number of grams of solute per 100 Gm of solution and is exemplified by 4 above. Per cent weight in volume (% w/v) is the number of grams of solute per 100 ml of solution and is exemplified by 3 above. Per cent by volume (% v/v) is the number of milliliters of solute in 100 ml of solution, referring to solutions of liquids in liquids. The USP indicates that the term "per cent," when unqualified, means per cent weight in volume for solutions of solids in liquids and per cent by volume for solutions of liquids in liquids.

When in pharmacopeial texts it has not been possible, or in some instances not desirable, to indicate exact solubility, a descriptive term has been used. The following table indicates the meaning of such terms:

Descriptive terms	Parts of solvent for 1 part of solute
Very soluble	Less than 1
Freely soluble	From 1 to 10
Soluble	From 10 to 30
Sparingly soluble	From 30 to 100
Slightly soluble	From 100 to 1000
Very slightly soluble	From 1000 to 10,000
Practically insoluble, or insoluble	More than 10,000

Rate of Solution—It is possible to define quantitatively the rate at which a solute goes into solution. The simplest treatment is based on a model depicted in Fig. 152. A solid particle dispersed in a solvent is surrounded by a thin layer of solvent having a finite thickness, l in cm. The layer is an integral part of the solid and is thus characteristically referred to as the "stagnant layer." This means that regardless of how fast the bulk solution may be stirred the stagnant layer remains a part of the surface of the solid, moving wherever the particle moves. The thickness of this layer may get smaller as stirring of the bulk solution increases, but it is important to recognize that this layer will always have a finite thickness however small it may get.

Using Fick's First Law of Diffusion the rate of solution of the solid can be explained, in the simplest case, as the rate at which a dissolved solute particle diffuses through the stagnant layer to the bulk solution. The driving force behind the movement of the solute molecule through the stagnant layer is the difference in concentration that exists between the concentration of the solute, C_1, in the stagnant layer at the surface of the solid and its concentration, C_2, on the farthest side of the stagnant layer (see *Diffusion in Liquids*, page 261). The greater this difference in concentration $(C_1 - C_2)$, the faster the rate of solution.

According to Fick's Law, the rate of solution is also directly proportional to the area of the solid, A in cm^2, exposed to solvent and inversely proportional to the length of the path through which the dissolved solute molecule must diffuse. Mathematically, then, the rate of solution of the solid is given by

$$\text{Rate of solution} = \frac{DA}{l} (C_1 - C_2) \qquad (1)$$

where D is a proportionality constant called the diffusion coefficient in cm^2/sec. In measuring the rate of solution experimentally, the concentration C_2 is held small compared to C_1 and hence considered to have a negligible effect on the rate. Furthermore, C_1 is most often the saturation solubility of the solute. Hence Eq. 1 is simplified to

$$\text{Rate of solution} = \frac{DA}{l} (\text{saturation solubility}) \qquad (2)$$

Eq. 2 quantitatively explains much of the phenomena commonly observed that affect the rate at which materials dissolve.

1. Small particles go into solution faster than large particles. For a given mass of solute, as we make the particle size smaller, the surface area per unit mass of solid increases and Eq. 2 shows that as area increases, the rate must proportionately increase. Hence, if a pharmacist wishes to increase the rate of solution of a drug, he should decrease its particle size.

2. Stirring a solution increases the rate at which a solid dissolves. This is because the thickness of the stagnant layer depends on how fast the bulk solution is stirred; as stirring rate increases, the length of the diffusional path decreases. Since the rate of solution is inversely proportional to the length of the diffusional path, the faster the solution is stirred, the faster the solute will go into solution. Pharmacists have access to a variety of stirring devices to aid in increasing the dissolution rate of a drug.

3. The more soluble the solute, the faster is its rate of solution. Again, Eq. 2 predicts that the larger the saturation solubility, the faster the rate.

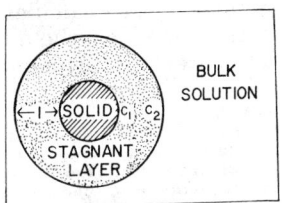

Fig. 152. Physical model representing the dissolution process.

4. With a viscous liquid, the rate of solution is slowed. This is because the diffusion coefficient is inversely proportional to the viscosity of the medium; the more viscous the solvent, the slower the rate of solution.

Energetics of the Solubility Process—Turning from the kinetic aspects of dissolution, this discussion will be concerned with the situation where there is thermodynamic equilibrium between solute in its solid phase* and the solute in solution. As defined earlier, the concentration of solute in solution at equilibrium is the saturation solubility of the substance.

The equilibrium existing between solute molecules in the solid and solute molecules in solution may be treated as any equilibrium. Thus, for a solute A in equilibrium with its solution we can write,

$$A_{(solid)} \rightleftharpoons A_{(solution)}$$

Using the Law of Mass Action we can define an equilibrium constant for this system just as any equilibrium constant may be written. Thus,

$$K_{eq} = \frac{a_{(solution)}}{a_{(solid)}}$$

where a denotes activity† of the solute in each phase. Since the activity of a solid is defined as unity,

$$K_{eq} = a_{(solution)}$$

Because the activity of a compound in dilute solution is closely approximated by its concentration and because in our equilibrium this concentration is the saturation solubility, K_S, we can write

$$K_{eq} = K_S$$

The van't Hoff Reaction Isobar‡ in an ideal† case defines the relationship between an equilibrium constant (here, saturation solubility) and absolute temperature. This relation is

$$\frac{d \log K_S}{dt} = \frac{\Delta H}{2.3RT^2} \tag{3}$$

where $\frac{d \log K_S}{dT}$ is the rate at which $\log K_S$ is changing with a unit change of absolute temperature, T; ΔH is a constant which in this situation is defined as the heat of solution; and R is the gas constant, 1.98 cal/mole/deg. Eq. 3, a differential equation, may be solved to give

$$\log K_S = -\frac{\Delta H}{2.3RT} + J \tag{4}$$

where J is a constant. A more useful form of this equation is

$$\log \frac{K_{S,T_2}}{K_{S,T_1}} = \frac{\Delta H(T_2 - T_1)}{2.3RT_1T_2} \tag{5}$$

where K_{S,T_1} is the saturation solubility at absolute temperature T_1 and K_{S,T_2} is the solubility at temperature T_2. Through the use of Eq. 5, if ΔH and the solubility at one temperature are known, the solubility at any other temperature may be calculated.

It is apparent from Eq. 4 that the quantity ΔH is a very important parameter. Its sign and its magnitude

give important clues as to whether or not a substance may be soluble and whether or not solubility will increase or decrease with temperature change. Since the heat of solution is very significant, discussion will now center about its origin.

Origin of the Heat of Solution§—The mechanism of solubility involves severing of the forces that hold the ions or molecules of a solute together, the separation of molecules of solvent to create a space in the solvent into which the solute can be fitted, and the ultimate response of solute and solvent to whatever forces of interaction may exist between them. In order to sever the force between molecules or ions of solute, energy must be supplied, as is the case also when molecules of solvent are to be separated. If heat is the source of energy it is apparent that both processes require absorption of heat. Solute–solvent interaction, on the other hand, is generally accompanied by evolution of heat since the process occurs spontaneously. In effecting solution there is, accordingly, a heat-absorbing effect and a heat-releasing effect to be considered. Depending on which effect is the greater, solution may be accompanied by a net rise or a net fall of temperature, or there may be no temperature change at all. If there is no, or very little, interaction between solute and solvent, the only effect will be that of absorption of heat to produce the necessary separations of solute and of solvent molecules or ions, and the temperature will fall. If there is sufficient interaction between solute and solvent to liberate an amount of heat in excess of that required to overcome the solute–solute and the solvent–solvent forces, the temperature will rise. If the opposing heat effects are equal, there will be no change of temperature.

The net heat effect may be expressed in terms of *heat of solution*, which may be defined as the quantity of energy evolved (given off) when a definite amount of solute (usually 1 mole) is dissolved in sufficient solvent so that further dilution produces no additional heat effect. The heat of solution may have a positive or a negative value. If the temperature of the solution decreases, the heat of solution is according to the convention of thermodynamics positive (since energy is absorbed rather than given off by the solution), while if the temperature of the solution increases the heat of solution is negative (since energy is given off by the solution).

In general, a large positive value of heat of solution is suggestive of little solute–solvent interaction, while a large negative value implies extensive solute–solvent interaction. It is sometimes stated that the larger the negative value of the heat of solution, the greater the solubility, and that the larger the positive value, the lower the solubility. This statement is based on the premise that heat released by the interaction of solute and solvent supplies energy required for the fundamental process of separating the molecules or ions of the solute one from another. While the statement correlating heat of solution and solubility applies to many solutions, the rule cannot be accepted as one without many deviations. The energy required to separate the molecules or ions of a solute differs for different solutes, and so does the energy which is released as a result of solute–solvent interactions. It is altogether possible that two substances having the same solubility in a particular solvent show large differences in their respective heats of solution, which may even be opposite in sign.

---

* It is assumed that there is an amount of solid material in excess of the amount that can go into solutions; hence a solid phase is always present.

† The concepts of activity and ideality are discussed in Chapter 18, *Thermodynamics*, and later in this chapter under *Colligative Properties of Solutions*.

‡ For a more complete treatment of the van't Hoff Equation, see Martin.[1]

---

§ For an excellent and more complete discussion of the interactions and driving forces underlying the dissolution process, see Higuchi.[2]

Steric Factors—Steric factors may explain some of the deviations observed from the prediction of solubility based on the general rule that a substance will be soluble if it has a negative (or a small positive) heat of solution. Higuchi[2] discusses two types of steric effects that must be considered in the prediction of solubility.

The first of these involves the symmetry of the solute molecule. As an example, a comparison can be made between the solubility of inositol (a symmetrical molecule) and the solubility of citric acid (an unsymmetrical molecule).

The solubility of citric acid is greater than inositol. Yet, on the basis of their heats of solution, inositol should be more soluble. The reason for the higher solubility of citric acid is that although there is no hindrance in the transfer of a citric acid molecule as it goes from the solid phase to the solution phase, when the structurally unsymmetrical citric acid attempts to return to the solid phase from its solution, it must assume an orientation that will allow ready interaction with polar groups already oriented and fixed in the crystal. If it does not have the required orientation, it will not return to the solid but it will remain in solution, thus bringing about a solubility larger than expected on the basis of heat of solution.

On the other hand, the structurally symmetrical inositol, as it leaves the solution phase, can interact with the solid phase without requiring a definite orientation; all orientations are equivalent. Hence, inositol can enter the crystal structure without hindrance and we therefore see no facilitation of its solubility.

In general, then, unsymmetrical molecules tend to be more soluble than symmetrical molecules.

In the second steric effect a hindrance of the transition from solute to solution phase occurs. As an example, a comparison of the solubility of lithium fluoride is made with the solubility of other alkali halides. Lithium fluoride is the least soluble of the alkali halides, yet on the basis of its heat of solution compared with the other salts, it should be the most soluble. The decreased solubility is based on the ability of the very small lithium and fluoride ions to orient water molecules over a considerable distance in the solvent, thus restricting the movement and availability of water. Because of this ordering in the solvent there is a hindrance of the transition of the solid to solution phase with the resultant decrease in solubility.

Effect of Temperature—The solubility of a solid in a liquid is dependent on the temperature, the nature of the solute, and the nature of the solvent. For a given solute and solvent, therefore, the solubility depends on the temperature. If in the process of solution heat is absorbed (as evidenced by a reduction in temperature), the solubility of the solute will be increased by increasing the temperature. Such is the case for most salts, as is shown in Fig. 153. In this figure the solubility of the solute is plotted as ordinate and the temperature as abscissa, and the line joining the experimental points represents the solubility curve for that solute.

If a solute gives off heat during the process of solution (as evidenced by an increase in temperature) its solubility is decreased with increase in temperature. This is the case with calcium hydroxide and, at higher temperatures, with calcium sulfate.* When heat is neither

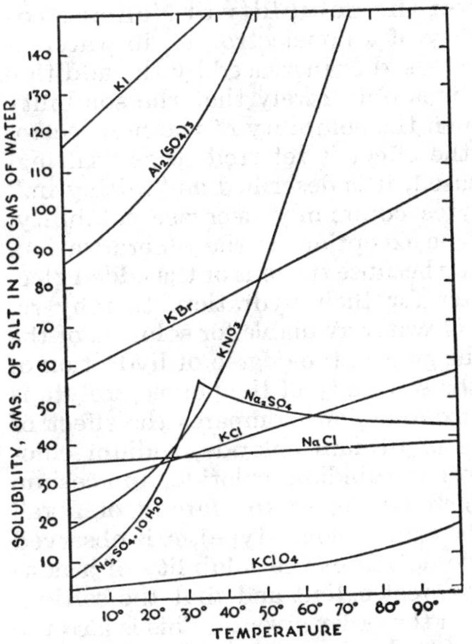

Fig. 153. Effect of heat on solubility (Chapin).

absorbed nor given off, the solubility is not affected by variation of temperature as is nearly the case with sodium chloride.

Solubility curves are usually continuous as long as the chemical composition of the solid phase in contact with the solution remains unchanged, but if there is a transition of the solid phase from one form to another, a break will be found in the curve. Such is the case with $Na_2SO_4.10H_2O$ which dissolves with absorption of heat up to a temperature of 32.4 °C at which point there is a transition of the solid phase to anhydrous sodium sulfate, Na_2SO_4, which dissolves with evolution of heat. This change is evidenced by increased solubility of the hydrated salt up to 32.4 °C, but above this temperature the solubility decreases.

These temperature effects are what would be predicted from Eq. 4. When the heat of solution is negative, signifying that energy is released during dissolution, the relation between $\log K_S$ and $1/T$ is typified in Fig. 154A, where as $1/T$ increases, $\log K_S$ increases. We see that with increasing temperature (T itself actually increases as you go to the left in Fig. 154A) there is a decrease in solubility. On the other hand, when the heat of solution is positive—that is, when heat is absorbed in the solution process—the relation between $\log K_S$ and $1/T$ is typified in Fig. 154B. Here, as temperature increases ($1/T$ decreases), the solubility increases.

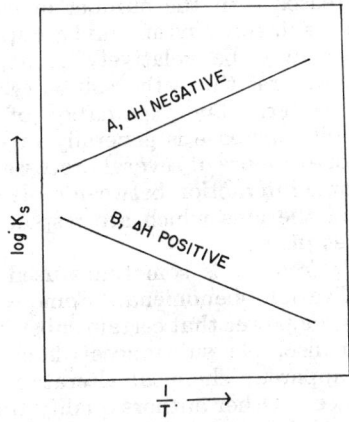

Fig. 154. Typified relationship between the logarithm of the saturation solubility and the reciprocal of the absolute temperature.

---

* Because of the slight solubility of these substances their solubility curves are not included.

Effect of Salts on the Solubility of Nonelectrolytes—The solubility of a nonelectrolyte, in water, is generally either decreased or increased by the addition of an electrolyte; it is only rarely that the solubility is not altered. When the solubility of the nonelectrolyte is decreased, the effect is referred to as "salting-out"; if it is increased, it is described as "salting-in." Inorganic electrolytes commonly decrease solubility, though there are some exceptions to the generalization.

Salting-out occurs because the ions of the added electrolyte require water for their hydration, thereby reducing the amount of water available for solution of the nonelectrolyte. The greater the degree of hydration of the ions the more the solubility of the nonelectrolyte is decreased. If, for example, one compares the effect of equivalent amounts of lithium chloride, sodium chloride, potassium chloride, rubidium chloride, and cesium chloride (all of which belong to the family of alkali metals and are of the same valence type), it is observed that lithium chloride decreases the solubility of a nonelectrolyte to the greatest extent and that the salting-out effect decreases in the order given. This is also the order of the degree of hydration of the cations; lithium ion, being the smallest ion and therefore having the greatest density of positive charge per unit of surface area (see also Table I, *Electronegativity Values*, in this column), is the most extensively hydrated of the cations while cesium ion is hydrated the least. Salting-out is encountered frequently in pharmaceutical operations.

Table I—Electronegativity Values

H 2.1						
Li 1.0	Be 1.5	B 2.0	C 2.5		N 3.0	O 3.5	F 4.0
Na 0.9	Mg 1.2	Al 1.5	Si 1.8		P 2.1	S 2.5	Cl 3.0
K 0.8	Ca 1.0	Sc 1.3	Ti 1.5	Ge 1.8	As 2.0	Se 2.4	Br 2.8
Rb 0.8	Sr 1.0	Y 1.2	Zr 1.4	Sn 1.8	Sb 1.9	Te 2.1	I 2.5
Cs 0.7	Ba 0.9					

Salting-in commonly occurs when either the salts of various organic acids or organic-substituted ammonium salts are added to aqueous solutions of nonelectrolytes. In the first case the solubilizing effect is associated with the anion and in the second with the cation. In both cases the solubility increases as the concentration of added salt is increased. One interesting observation, noted in several experiments, is that the degree of solubilization increases with the number of carbon atoms when the added salt contains an alkyl group. The solubility increase may be relatively great, sometimes amounting to several times the solubility of the nonelectrolyte in water. The explanation of the mechanism of solubility increase is generally unknown; it is possible that one or more of several processes occur. In many cases some interaction between molecules of nonelectrolyte and the ions which are responsible for the salting-in takes place.

The term *hydrotropy* is sometimes used to describe certain solubilization phenomena. Some writers define hydrotropy as the power that certain substances have of making water-insoluble substances dissolve in water without any apparent chemical alteration of the dissolved substance. Other authors qualify this definition by restricting hydrotropy to those systems in which very large amounts of solubilizing agent are added (25–50% or so); this restriction does not appear to be a valid one since the same solubilizing agents increase solubility even at low concentrations, though not to as great an extent as when the concentration is higher. A review of the extensive literature on solubilization has been prepared by Klevens.[3]

Solubility of Solutes Containing Two or More Species—In cases where the solute phase consists of two or more species (as in an inorganic salt), when the solute goes into solution, the solution phase often contains each of these species as discrete entities. For some such substance, AB, we can then write the following for the solution process:

$$AB_{(solid)} \rightleftharpoons A_{(solution)} + B_{(solution)}$$

Since there is an equilibrium between the solute and saturated solution phases, the Law of Mass Action defines an equilibrium constant, K_{eq}:

$$K_{eq} = \frac{a_{A(solution)} \cdot a_{B(solution)}}{a_{AB(solid)}} \tag{6}$$

where $a_{A(solution)}$, $a_{B(solution)}$ and $a_{AB(solid)}$ are the activities of A and B in solution and of AB in the solid phase. Recall from our earlier discussion that the activity of a solid is defined as unity, and that in a dilute solution (eg, where we have a slightly soluble salt), concentrations may be substituted for activities; Eq. 6 then becomes

$$K_{eq} = C_A C_B$$

where C_A and C_B are the concentrations of A and B in solution. K_{eq} in this situation has a special name, the *solubility product*, K_{SP}. Thus,

$$K_{SP} = C_A C_B \tag{7}$$

This equation will hold true theoretically only for slightly soluble salts.

As an example of this type of solution, consider the solubility of silver chloride. We can write for silver chloride

$$K_{SP} = [Ag^+][Cl^-]$$

where the brackets [ ] designate concentrations.

This constant, K_{SP}, is known as the solubility product; at 25°C it has a value of 1.56×10^{-10}, the concentration of silver and chloride ions being expressed in gram-ions (Gm-ions)/L. The same numerical value applies also to solutions of silver chloride containing an excess of either silver or chloride ions. If the silver-ion concentration is increased by the addition of a soluble silver salt, the chloride-ion concentration must decrease until the product of the two concentrations is again numerically equal to the solubility product. In order to effect the decrease in chloride-ion concentration, silver chloride is precipitated and hence its solubility is decreased. In a similar manner an increase in chloride-ion concentration by the addition of a soluble chloride effects a decrease in the silver-ion concentration until the numerical value of the solubility product is attained. Again this decrease in silver-ion concentration is brought about by the precipitation of silver chloride.

The solubility of silver chloride in a saturated aqueous solution of the salt may be calculated by assuming that the concentration of silver ion is the same as the concentration of chloride ion, both expressed in Gm-ions/L, and that the concentration of dissolved silver chloride is numerically the same since each silver chloride molecule gives rise to one silver ion and one chloride ion.   Since

$$[\text{dissolved AgCl}] = [\text{Ag}^+] = [\text{Cl}^-]$$

the solubility of AgCl is equal to $\sqrt{1.56 \times 10^{-10}}$, which is 1.25×10^{-5} Gm-mole per liter.   Multiplying this by the molecular weight of silver chloride (143) we obtain a solubility of approximately 1.8 mg/L.

For a salt of the type PbCl_2 the solubility product expression takes the form

$$[\text{Pb}^{++}][\text{Cl}^-]^2 = K_{SP}$$

while for As_2S_3 it would be

$$[\text{As}^{+++}]^2[\text{S}^-]^3 = K_{SP}$$

Because from the Law of Mass Action we have

$$\text{PbCl}_{2(\text{solid})} \rightleftharpoons \text{Pb}^{++}_{(\text{solution})} + 2\text{Cl}^-_{(\text{solution})}$$

and

$$\text{As}_2\text{S}_{3(\text{solid})} \rightleftharpoons 2\text{As}^{+++}_{(\text{solution})}{}^{3+} + 3\text{S}^-_{(\text{solution})}$$

For further details of methods of using solubility product calculations, the reader is referred to books on qualitative or quantitative analysis, or on physical chemistry.

Recall that the solubility product principle is valid for aqueous solutions of slightly soluble salts, provided the concentration of added salt is not too great. Where the concentrations are high, deviations from the theory occur and these have been explained by assuming that in such solutions the nature of the solvent has been changed.   Frequently deviations may also occur as the result of the formation of complexes between the two salts.   A pharmaceutically important example of increased solubility by virtue of complex-ion formation is seen in the effect of solutions of soluble iodides on mercuric iodide.   According to the solubility product principle it might be expected that soluble iodides would decrease the solubility of mercuric iodide, but because of the formation of the more soluble complex salt K_2HgI_4 which dissociates as follows:

$$\text{K}_2\text{HgI}_4 \rightleftharpoons 2\text{K}^+ + (\text{HgI}_4)^-$$

the iodide ion no longer functions as a common ion.

Practical applications of the solubility product principle are found in qualitative and quantitative analysis whenever an excess of a precipitant is added in order to diminish, by common ion effect, the solubility of the precipitate.

It is possible to formulate some general rules regarding the effect of the addition of soluble salts to slightly soluble salts where the added salt does not have an ion common to the slightly soluble salt.   If the ions of the added soluble salt are not highly hydrated (see *Effect of Salts on the Solubility of Nonelectrolytes*), the solubility product of the slightly soluble salt will increase because the ions of the added salt tend to decrease the interionic attraction between the ions of the slightly soluble salt.   On the other hand, if the ions of the added soluble salt are hydrated, water molecules become less available and the interionic attraction between the ions of the slightly soluble salt increases with a resultant decrease in solubility product.

The effect of temperature is in general what we would expect; increasing the temperature of the solution results in an increase of the solubility product.

Solubility Following a Chemical Reaction— Thus far in this chapter discussion has been concerned with solubility that comes about because of interplay of entirely physical forces.   The dissolution of some substance resulted from overcoming the physical interactions between solute molecules and solvent molecules by the energy produced when a solute molecule interacted physically with a solvent molecule.   The solution process can, however, also be facilitated by a chemical reaction.   Almost always the chemical enhancement of solubility in aqueous systems is due to the formation of a salt following an acid–base reaction.

An alkaloidal base, or any other nitrogenous base of relatively high molecular weight, is generally slightly soluble in water, but if the pH of the medium is reduced by addition of acid, the solubility of the base is increased, considerably so as the pH continues to be reduced.   The reason for this increase in solubility is that the base is converted to a salt, which is relatively soluble in water.   Conversely, the solubility of a salt of an alkaloid or other nitrogenous base is reduced as pH is increased by addition of alkali.

The solubility of slightly soluble acid substances is, on the other hand, increased as the pH is increased by addition of alkali, the reason again being that a salt, relatively soluble in water, is formed.   Examples of acid substances whose solubility is thus increased are acetylsalicylic acid, theophylline, theobromine, the sulfonamides, and the barbiturates.   Conversely, the solubility of salts of the same substances is decreased as the pH decreases.

In the class of inorganic compounds a somewhat similar behavior is observed in many cases.   Tribasic calcium phosphate, $\text{Ca}_3(\text{PO}_4)_2$, for example, is almost insoluble in water, but if an acid is added its solubility increases rapidly with decrease in pH.   This is because hydrogen ions have such a strong affinity for phosphate ions, to form nonionized phosphoric acid, that the calcium phosphate is dissolved in order to release phosphate ions.   Or, stated in another way, the solubilization is an example of a reaction in which a strong acid (which is the source of the hydrogen ions) displaces a weak acid.

In all the examples cited above solubilization occurs as the result of an interaction of the solute with an acid or a base.   Compounds which do not react with either acids or bases are, on the other hand, but slightly if at all influenced in their aqueous solubility by variations of pH.   Such effects as may be observed are generally due to ionic "salt effects."

It is possible to quantitatively analyze solubility following an acid–base reaction by considering solubility as a two-step process.   We will first use as an example an organic acid, designated as *HA*, that is relatively insoluble in water.   Its two-step dissolution can be represented as

$$\text{HA}_{(\text{solid})} \rightleftharpoons \text{HA}_{(\text{solution})}$$

followed by

$$\text{HA}_{(\text{solution})} \rightleftharpoons \text{H}^+_{(\text{solution})} + \text{A}^-_{(\text{solution})}$$

The equilibrium constant for the first step is the solubility of *HA* ($K_S = [HA]_{\text{solution}}$), just as we developed earlier when no chemical reaction took place, and the equilibrium constant for the second step is the dissociation constant of the acid:

$$K_a = \frac{[\text{H}^+][\text{A}^-]}{[\text{HA}]}$$

Since the total amount of compound *in solution* is the sum of nonionized and ionized forms of the acid, we can designate the total solubility $S_{t(HA)}$ as

$$S_{t(HA)} = [\text{HA}] + [\text{A}^-] = [\text{HA}] + K_a \frac{[\text{HA}]}{[\text{H}^+]} \qquad (8)$$

Since $K_S = [HA]$, Eq. 8 becomes

$$S_{t(HA)} = K_S \left(1 + \frac{K_a}{[H^+]} \right) \qquad (9)$$

Eq. 9 is very useful since it equates the total solubility of an acid drug with the hydrogen-ion concentration of the solvent. If the water solubility K_S and the dissociation constant K_a are known, the total solubility of the acid may be calculated at various hydrogen-ion concentrations. Eq. 9 quantitatively shows us how the total solubility of the acid increases as the hydrogen-ion concentration decreases (that is, as the pH increases).

It is possible to develop an equation similar to Eq. 9 for the solubility of a basic drug, B, such as a relatively insoluble nitrogenous base (an alkaloid, for example) at various hydrogen-ion concentrations. The solubility of the base in water may be represented in two steps, as

$$B_{(solid)} \rightleftarrows B_{(solution)}$$
$$B_{(solution)} \rightleftarrows BH^+_{(solution)} + OH^-_{(solution)}$$

Again, if K_S is the solubility of the free base in water and K_b is its dissociation constant,

$$K_b = \frac{[BH^+][OH^-]}{[B]}$$

the total solubility of the base in water $S_{t(B)}$ is given by,

$$S_{t(B)} = [B] + [BH^+] = [B] + \frac{K_b[B]}{[OH^-]} =$$
$$K_S \left(1 + \frac{K_b}{[OH^-]} \right) \quad (10)$$

It is convenient to rewrite Eq. 10 in terms of hydrogen-ion concentration by making use of the dissociation constant for water,

$$K_W = [H^+][OH^-] = 1 \times 10^{-14}$$

Eq. 10 then becomes

$$S_{t(B)} = K_S \left(1 + \frac{K_b}{K_W/[H^+]} \right) = K_S \left(1 + \frac{K_b[H^+]}{K_W} \right) \quad (11)$$

Eq. 11 quantitatively shows how the total solubility of the base increases as the hydrogen-ion concentration of the solvent increases. If K_S and K_b are known, it is possible to calculate the total solubility of a basic drug at various hydrogen-ion concentrations using this equation.

Modes of Effecting Solution of Solids at the Prescription Counter—The method usually employed by the pharmacist when soluble compounds are to be dissolved in water in compounding a prescription is one which requires the use of the mortar and pestle (Chapter 86). The ordinary practice is to crush the substance into fragments in the mortar with the pestle and pour the solvent on it, meanwhile stirring with the pestle until solution is effected. If definite quantities are used, and the whole of the solvent is required to dissolve the given weight of the salt, a portion only of the solvent should be added at first, and when this is saturated the solution is poured off and a fresh portion of solvent added. This operation is repeated until the solid is entirely dissolved; the solutions are then mixed. Other methods of effecting solution are to shake the solid with the liquid in a bottle or flask, or to apply heat to the substances in a suitable vessel. Substances vary greatly in the rate at which they dissolve; some are capable of producing a saturated solution quickly, others require several hours for attainment of saturation. All too often in their haste to prepare a saturated solution pharmacists fail to obtain the required degree of solution of solute.

With hygroscopic substances like pepsin, silver protein compounds, and some others, the best method of effecting solution in water is to place the substance directly upon the surface of the water in which solution is to be effected and then stir vigorously with a glass rod. If the ordinary procedure, such as using a mortar and pestle, is employed with these substances, gummy lumps are formed which are exceedingly difficult to dissolve.

The *solubility* of chemicals and the *miscibility* of liquids are important physical factors for the pharmacist to know, as they often have a bearing on the intelligent and proper filling of prescriptions. Mainly for the information of the pharmacist, the USP and NF give figures to indicate the degree of solubility or miscibility of the various official substances.

Determination of Solubility—For the pharmacist and pharmaceutical chemist the question of solubility is of paramount importance. Not only is it necessary to know solubilities in connection with the preparation and dispensing of medicines, but such information is necessary to effect separation of substances in qualitative and quantitative analysis. Furthermore, the accurate determination of the solubility of a substance is one of the best methods for determining its purity.

The details of the determination of the solubility are markedly affected by the physical and chemical characteristics of the solute and solvent and also by the temperature at which the solubility is to be determined. Accordingly it is not possible to describe a universally applicable method but, in general, the following must be observed in solubility determinations.

1. Purity of both the dissolved substance and the solvent is essential, since impurities in either affect the solubility to a greater or less extent.
2. Constancy of temperature must be accurately maintained during the course of the determination.
3. Complete saturation must be attained.
4. Accurate analysis of the saturated solution and correct expression of the results are imperative.

Consideration should be given also to the varying rates of solution of different compounds, and to the marked effect of the degree of fineness of the particles on the time required for the saturation of the solution.

Many of the solubility data of USP have been determined with regard to the exacting requirements mentioned above.

Method for Determining Solubilities—In brief, this consists in preparing a saturated solution of the given substance and ascertaining, by analysis, the amount present in a definite quantity of the solution. Complete saturation can be attained most readily by constant stirring or agitation by means of a suitable mechanical contrivance. A simple apparatus for this purpose consists of a test tube of medium size fastened upright in a water bath maintained at constant temperature. The solvent and excess of solids are placed in the tube and stirred by means of a motor-driven rotating glass spiral. After a given period of stirring, a definite weight of the clear solution is analyzed and the stirring continued for an additional period of several hours. If analysis shows no increase of dissolved substance after the second period of stirring, the result is to be taken as the solubility at the particular temperature. Details of methods for determining solubilities are described in Bulletin No. 67 of the Hygienic Laboratory, US Public Health Service, and in textbooks on experimental physical chemistry.

Phase Solubility Analysis—The procedure of *Phase Solubility Analysis* is one of the most useful and accurate methods for the determination of the purity of a substance. It involves the application of precise solubility methods to the principle that constancy of solubility, in the same manner as constancy of melting point, indicates that a material is pure or free from foreign admixture. It is important to recognize that the technique can be used to obtain the exact solubility of the pure substance without the necessity for the experimental material itself to be pure.

The method is based on the thermodynamic principles of heterogeneous equilibria which are among the soundest of theoretical concepts of chemistry. Thus it is not dependent on any assumptions regarding kinetics or structure of matter, but applicable to all species of molecules, and is sufficiently sensitive to distinguish between optical isomers unless they be present in the unique ratio of 1:1. The requirements for an analysis are simple since the equipment needed is basic to most laboratories and the quantities of substances required are small.

The standard solubility method consists of five steps:

1. Mixing, in separate systems, increasing amounts of a substance with measured amounts of a solvent.
2. Establishment of equilibrium for each system at identical constant temperature and pressure.
3. Separation of the solid phase from the solutions.
4. Determination of the concentration of the material dissolved in the various solutions.
5. Plotting the concentration of the dissolved material per unit of solvent (*y*-axis, or solution concentration) against the mass of material per unit of solvent (*x*-axis or system concentration).

The solubility method has been established on the sound theoretical principles of the Gibbs phase rule: $F = C - P + 2$, which relates C, the number of components, F, the degrees of freedom (pressure, temperature, and concentration), and P, the phases for a heterogeneous equilibrium. Since solubility analyses are carried out at constant temperature and pressure, a pure solid in solution would show only one degree of

freedom, because only one phase is present at concentrations below saturation. This is represented by section AB in Fig. 155. For a pure solid in a saturated solution at equilibrium (Fig. 155, BC), two phases are present, solid and solution; there is no variation in concentration and thus there are two components, solute and solvent.

The curve ABC of Fig. 155 represents the type of solubility diagram obtained for: (1) a pure material, (2) a solid solution of two or more materials having identical solubilities, or (3) a mixture of two or more materials present in the unique ratio of their solubilities. These latter two cases are rare and often may be detected by a change in solvent system.

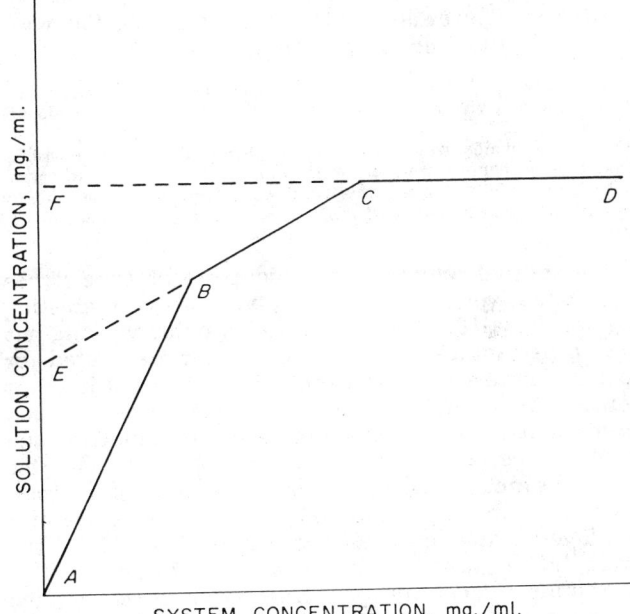

SYSTEM CONCENTRATION, mg./ml.

Fig. 156. Type of solubility curve obtained when a substance contains one impurity.

Section BC of Fig. 155 since it has no slope, usually indicates purity. If, however, this section *does* exhibit a slope, its numerical value is an indication of the amount(s) of impurity present. Point D is the actual solubility of the pure substance.

A representative type of solubility curve which is obtained when a substance contains one impurity is illustrated in Fig. 156. Here, the solution first becomes saturated with one component. In this case there are two phases present: a solution saturated with Component I (usually the major component) containing also some Component II (usually the minor component), and a solid phase of Component I. The one degree of freedom revealed by the slope of the line BC is the concentration of Component II, which is the impurity (usually the minor component). A mixture of *d* and *l* isomers in any ratio other than 1:1 would have such a curve, as would any simple mixtures in which the solubilities are independent of each other.

The section CD indicates that the solvent is saturated with both components of the two-component mixture. Here, three phases are present; the solution saturated with both components and the two solid phases. No variation of concentration is possible, hence no degree of freedom is possible (indicated by the lack of slope of section CD). The distance AE on the ordinate represents the solubility of the major component, and the distance EF the solubility of the minor component.

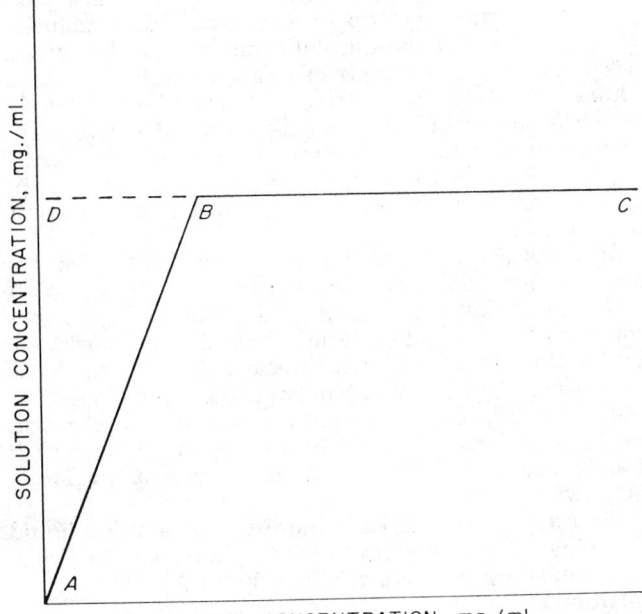

SYSTEM CONCENTRATION, mg./ml.

Fig. 155. Phase solubility diagram for a pure substance.

The fact that the equilibration process is time-consuming, requiring as long as three weeks in certain cases, is offset by the fact that all of the sample can be recovered after a determination. This adds to the general usefulness of the method, particularly in cases where the substance is expensive or difficult to obtain. A use for the method other than the determination of purity or of solubility is to obtain especially pure samples by recovering the solid residues at system concentration corresponding to points on section *BC* in Fig. 156. Thus, the method is useful not only as a quantitative analytical tool, but also as a procedure for purification.

Solutions of Liquids in Liquids

Binary Systems—Under this title the following types of liquid-pairs may be recognized.

1. Those which are completely soluble in each other in all proportions. Examples: alcohol and water; glycerin and water; alcohol and glycerin.
2. Those which are soluble in each other in definite proportions. Examples: phenol and water; ether and water; nicotine and water.
3. Those which are imperceptibly soluble in each other in any proportion. Examples: castor oil and water; liquid petrolatum and water.

The mutual solubility of liquid pairs of type 2 has been extensively studied and found to show interesting regularities. If a series of tubes containing varying but known percentages of phenol and water are heated (or cooled if necessary) just to the point of formation of a homogeneous solution, and the temperatures at such points noted, there will be obtained, upon plotting the results, a curve similar to that in Fig. 157. On this graph the area *A* inside the curve represents the region where mixtures of phenol and water will separate into two layers, while in the shaded region *B* outside of the curve homogeneous solutions will be obtained. The maximum temperature on this curve is called the *critical solution temperature*.

From a study of this graph it is evident that for each temperature up to the critical solution temperature two types of homogeneous mixtures of phenol and water may be obtained. The one type is a solution of phenol in water and the other is a solution of water in phenol. As the temperature is increased, the concentration of

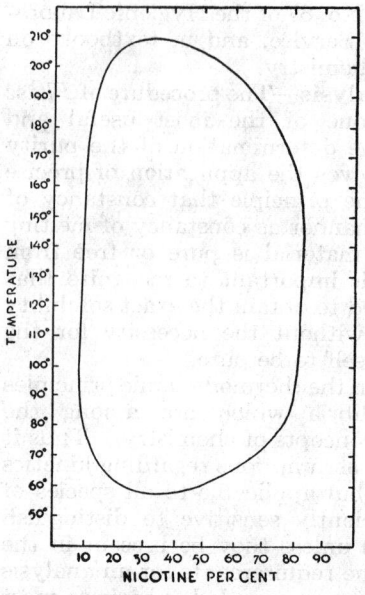

Fig. 158.   Nicotine–water solubility.

phenol in the aqueous solution and the concentration of water in the phenol solution increase until at the critical solution temperature the concentration of phenol in both solutions is identical. This concentration is 34.0% phenol and the temperature is 68.4°C. At any and all temperatures above 68.4°C phenol and water are miscible with each other in all proportions. In pharmacy both types of solutions are frequently encountered, as in the preparation of dilute solutions of phenol in water and the liquefaction of phenol by the addition of 10% water.

In the case of phenol and water the mutual solubility increases with increase in temperature and the critical solution temperature occurs at a relatively high point. In a certain number of cases, however, the mutual solubility increases with decrease in temperature and the critical solution temperature occurs at a relatively low value. Most of the substances which show lower critical solution temperatures are amines, as, for example, triethylamine with water.

In addition to pairs of liquids which show *either* upper or lower critical solution temperatures, there are other pairs which show *both* upper and lower critical solution temperatures and the mutual solubility curve is of the closed type. An example of this type of liquid pair is found in the case of nicotine and water, the curve for which is shown in Fig. 158. Mixtures of nicotine and water represented by points within the curve will separate into two layers, but mixtures represented by points outside of the curve are perfectly miscible with each other.

In a discussion of solutions of liquids in liquids it is evident that the distinction between the terms solute and solvent loses its significance. For example, in a solution of water and glycerin, which shall be considered to be the solute and which the solvent? Again in cases where two liquids are only partially soluble in each other the distinction between solute and solvent might easily be reversed. In such cases the term solvent is usually given to the constituent present in larger quantity.

Ternary Systems—The addition of a third liquid to a binary liquid system to produce a ternary or three-component system can result in several possible combinations.

If the third liquid is soluble in only one of the two original liquids or if its solubility in the two original

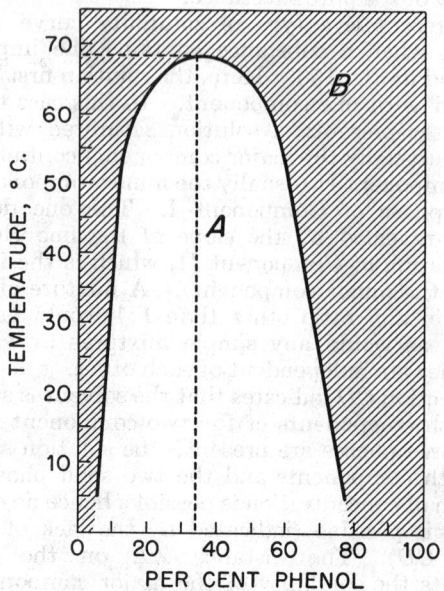

Fig. 157.   Phenol–water solubility.

liquids is markedly different, the mutual solubility of the original pair will be decreased. An upper critical solution temperature will be elevated and a lower critical solution temperature lowered. On the other hand, the addition of a liquid having roughly the same solubility in both components of the original pair will result in an increase in their mutual solubility. An upper critical solution temperature then will be lowered and a lower critical solution temperature elevated.

An equilateral triangle graph may be used to represent the situation in which a third liquid is added to a partially miscible liquid pair, the third liquid being miscible with each member of the original pair. In this type of graph, each side of the triangle represents 0% of one of the components and the apex opposite that side represents 100% of that component. The reader is referred to texts on experimental physical chemistry for details of the construction and use of graphs of this type.

Two other possibilities exist in ternary liquid systems: that in which two components are completely miscible and the third is partially miscible with each, and that in which all combinations of two of the three components are only partially miscible.

Solutions of Gases in Liquids

Nearly all gases are more or less soluble in liquids. One has but to recall the solubility of carbon dioxide, of hydrogen sulfide, and of air in water as common examples of this type of solution.

The amount of gas dissolved in a liquid in general follows **Henry's law,** which states that *the weight of gas dissolved by a given amount of a liquid at a given temperature is proportional to the pressure.* Thus, if the pressure is doubled, twice as much gas will dissolve as at the initial pressure. The extent to which a gas is dissolved in a liquid, at a given temperature, may be expressed in terms of the *solubility coefficient,* which is the volume of gas, measured under the conditions of the experiment, that is absorbed by one volume of the liquid. The degree of solubility is also sometimes expressed in terms of the *absorption coefficient,* which is the volume of gas, reduced to standard conditions, dissolved by one volume of liquid under a pressure of one atmosphere.

Although Henry's law expresses fairly accurately the solubility of slightly soluble gases, it deviates considerably in the case of very soluble gases such as hydrogen chloride and ammonia. Such deviations are most frequently due to chemical interaction of solute and solvent.

The solubility of gases in liquids *decreases* with *rise of temperature* and in general also when salts are added to the solvent, the latter effect being referred to as the "salting-out" of the gas.

Solutions of gases are potentially dangerous when exposed to warm temperatures because of the liberation and expansion of the dissolved gas which may cause the container to burst. Bottles containing such solutions (eg, strong ammonia solution) should be cooled before opening if practicable, and the stopper should be covered with a cloth before attempting its removal.

Molecular Structure and Solubility

The mechanism of the dissolution process has been discussed earlier in this chapter (see *Origin of the Heat of Solution*). We saw that solubility depended, on one hand, on the energy that must be supplied to break the attractive forces between solute molecules and to make space for the solute in the solvent by overcoming the attractive force between solvent molecules and, on the other hand, on the energy produced when a solute molecule interacted with a solvent molecule. The net effect of these energy-requiring and energy-producing interactions determined whether or not a substance was soluble.

The magnitude of the various attractive forces involved between solute, solvent, and solute–solvent molecules may vary greatly. The reason for this is that the molecular structure of the various solutes and solvents determining the interactions possible can themselves vary greatly.*

The solute–solute interaction that must be overcome can vary from the strong ion–ion interaction (as in a salt) to the weaker dipole–dipole interaction (as in nearly all organic medicinals that are not salts) to the weakest induced dipole–induced dipole interaction (as in compounds like naphthalene).

The attractive forces in the solvent that must be overcome are, most frequently, the dipole-dipole interaction (as found in water or in acetone) and the induced dipole–induced dipole interaction (as in liquid petrolatum).

The energy-releasing solute–solvent interactions that must be taken into account may be one of four types. In decreasing energy of interaction these are ion–dipole interactions (eg, a sodium ion interacting with water), dipole–dipole interactions (eg, an organic acid dissolved in water), dipole–induced dipole interaction† (eg, an organic acid dissolved in carbon tetrachloride), and induced dipole–induced dipole interactions (eg, naphthalene dissolved in benzene).

Since the energy-releasing solute–solvent interaction must at least approximate the energy needed to overcome the solute–solute and solvent–solvent interactions, it is apparent why it is not possible to dissolve a salt like sodium chloride in benzene. The interaction between the ions and benzene does not supply enough energy to overcome the interaction between the ions in the solid. On the other hand, the interaction of sodium and chloride ions with water molecules does provide an amount of energy approximating the energy needed to separate the ions in the crystal and the molecules in the solvent.

Our discussion will now focus on solvents available to pharmacists and in particular on the interactions and properties that these solvents have. It is most important that the pharmacist get a real understanding of the possible differences in solubility of a given solute in different solvents since he is most often called on to select a solvent in which the solute is soluble. An understanding of the properties of solvents will allow the intelligent or intuitive selection of suitable solvents.

The solvent–solvent interaction is, in pharmaceutical solvents, always made up of a dipole–dipole interaction (Keesom Force) and an induced dipole–induced dipole interaction (London Force). It is important to keep in mind that both forces are always present; the contribution that each of these forces makes toward the over-all attractive force depends on the structure of the solvent molecule. Some solvents have interactions which predominantly involve the Keesom Force (water, for example), while others are

---

* For a discussion of these effects, see Martin.[4]
† This subject will be discussed later.

predominantly composed of the London Force (chloroform, for example); usually, both forces will be found.

Dipole–Dipole Forces—The unequal sharing of the electron pair between two atoms due to a difference in the electronegativity of the atoms (see Table I) brings about a separation of the positive and negative centers of electricity in the molecule, causing it to become polarized, that is to assume a partial ionic character. The molecule is then said to be a *permanent dipole* and the substance is described as being a *polar compound*.

The greater the difference in the electronegativity of the constituent atoms, the greater the inequality of sharing of the electron pair, the greater the distance between the positive and negative centers of electricity in the molecule, and the more polar the resulting molecule. The character of the bonds being intermediate between those existing in nonpolar compounds and those occurring in ionic salts, it is to be expected that the properties of polar compounds should be intermediate between those of the two other classes. Such is, in fact, generally the case.

Coordinate covalent compounds are all very strongly polar because both of the electrons constituting the bonding pair have been contributed by a donor atom, which in effect loses an electron and becomes positively charged, while the acceptor atom may be considered to gain an electron and become negatively charged.

While, in general, the electronegativity of different kinds of atoms is different, and the expectation is, therefore, that all molecules containing two or more different atoms will be polar, many such molecules are actually nonpolar. Thus, while the electronegativity of chlorine is appreciably different from that of carbon, the molecule of carbon tetrachloride, CCl_4, is nonpolar because the symmetrical arrangement of chlorine atoms about the carbon atom is such as to cancel the effects of the difference in the electronegativity of the constituent atoms. The same is true in the case of methane, CH_4, and for hydrocarbons generally. But the molecules CH_3Cl, CH_2Cl_2, and $CHCl_3$ are definitely polar because of the unsymmetrical distribution of the forces within the molecule. A knowledge of the degree of polarity of various molecules is usually available in the measurement of the *dipole moment*, μ, of the molecules. This quantity is defined as the product of one of the charges on the molecule and the distance between the two average centers of positive and negative electricity. Measurements of the dipole moment of a substance are made, when possible, on the vapor of the substance but when this is not possible a dilute solution of the substance in a nonpolar solvent is employed. A discussion of the experimental methods of determining dipole moments may be found in Daniels, *et al, Experimental Physical Chemistry*, 6th ed., McGraw-Hill, New York, 1962. Table II sets forth the values of the dipole moment for a number of substances.

As was stated previously, the molecules of nonpolar substances are characterized by weak attractions for one another, while molecules of polar substances exhibit a relatively strong attraction which is all the more powerful the greater the dipole moment. The reason for this is readily apparent; the dipoles tend to align themselves so that the opposite charges of two different molecules are adjacent. They affect each other in somewhat the same manner as do two bar magnets the opposite poles of which are adjacent. While thermal agitation tends to break up the alignment or association of the dipoles, there is, nevertheless, a resultant significant intermolecular force present.

Table II—Dipole Moments

Substance	Electrostatic units ($\mu \times 10^{18}$)
Water	1.85
Acetone	2.8
Methyl alcohol	1.68
Ethyl alcohol	1.70
Phenol	1.70
Ethyl ether	1.14
Aniline	1.51
Nitrobenzene	4.19
o-Dinitrobenzene	6.0
m-Dinitrobenzene	3.8
p-Dinitrobenzene	0.3
Benzene	0
Methane	0
Methyl chloride	1.86
Dichloromethane	1.58
Chloroform	1.05
Carbon tetrachloride	0
Carbon monoxide	0.11
Carbon dioxide	0
Oxygen	0
Hydrogen	0
Hydrogen chloride	1.03
Hydrogen bromide	0.78
Hydrogen iodide	0.38
Hydrogen sulfide	0.95
Hydrogen cyanide	2.93
Ammonia	1.49

Induced Dipole–Induced Dipole Forces—It is of interest to inquire at this point what force does exist between the molecules of compounds which are nonpolar, eg, those which have zero dipole moment. If some attractive force did not exist, the molecules could not be expected to cling together, as in the solid and liquid states. Though the attraction is relatively slight, there is a force that arises from momentary polarization of the molecules because of electronic oscillations which are continuously taking place within the molecules. The *temporary dipoles* thus produced induce opposite polarizations in adjacent molecules and the net effect is that there is a small but definite attractive force between the molecules to keep them together in the liquid and solid states. This attraction resulting from mutual polarization is commonly referred to as the London Force and as an induced dipole–induced dipole force.

The Hydrogen Bond—The attraction between oppositely charged ends of two dipoles is accentuated when the positive end of one dipole contains a hydrogen atom and the negative end of the other dipole contains an atom of fluorine, oxygen, or nitrogen. In such instances the nucleus of the hydrogen atom—which is a proton—appears to be able to bind together the negative end of the molecule of which it is a part with the negative end of the adjacent molecule. This may be represented as shown in Fig. 159, adapted from Pauling.[5]

Since the proton is the smallest positively charged atomic particle it can draw together two negatively charged atoms or ions more closely than can any other—and necessarily larger—positively charge particle. Not more than two negative atoms are capable of being attracted at any given instant, as is evident from the

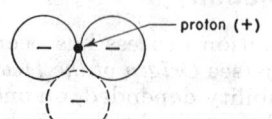

Fig. 159. Hydrogen bonding.

Fig. 159, where a third negative atom is shown to be physically restricted from direct contact with the proton. Water is an excellent example of a substance the molecules of which are associated through the formation of such a bond—called the *hydrogen bond*. An illustration of such bonding in the case of water may be represented as:

$$\begin{array}{ccccc} H & & H & & H \\ | & & | & & | \\ H—O & ---H—O & ---H—O \end{array}$$

in which each dotted line repesents the bond or "bridge" established by the hydrogen of one molecule of water with the oxygen of another molecule of water. It is to be noted that the water molecule is pictured as a bent, rather than as a linear, molecule (H—O—H). This is in accord with the bond angles imposed by the directional character of the bonding orbitals making up the molecule (see Chapter 17). By virtue of its kernel containing six unneutralized protons, not only the valence electrons of the oxygen but also those of the hydrogen atoms are so strongly attracted to the oxygen atom as to make the latter negatively charged, while the rest of the molecule is charged positively.

Table III—Dielectric Constants (at 20 °C)

Hydrogen cyanide	116
Water	80.
Glycerin	46.
Ethylene glycol	41.
Methyl alcohol	33.
Ethyl alcohol	25.
n-Propyl alcohol	22.
Acetone	21.
Aniline	7.0
Chloroform	5.0
Castor oil	4.6
Ethyl ether	4.3
Octyl alcohol	3.4
Olive oil	3.1
Benzene	2.2
Turpentine oil	2.2
Carbon tetrachloride	2.2
Octane	1.9

Originally it was thought that the hydrogen bond was indicative of a bivalent state of hydrogen, but it is now believed that the bond represents a condition in which the hydrogen nucleus vibrates between the negatively charged atoms of the two molecules adjacent to it.

The hydrogen bond is not a strong bond, but it plays an important role in determining the properties of substances in which it occurs. For example, it is primarily responsible for the unusual properties of water. If the substance H_2O followed the course of the related substances H_2Te, H_2Se, and H_2S, in so far as the physical properties of these latter substances are concerned, the freezing point of water would be about $-100\,°C$ and its boiling point about $-80\,°C$. The unexpectedly high values actually observed are attributed to hydrogen bonding between molecules of water; to break such bonds, as for example in vaporizing water in the form of single H_2O molecules during the process of boiling, more energy is required than would be necessary if the water molecules were not linked by hydrogen bonds.

The molecules of at least the low-molecular-weight alcohols are similarly joined by hydrogen bonds to form a latticelike structure.

Another example of the manner in which the hydrogen bond functions is seen in the case of carboxylic acids. Such acids usually exist in dimeric form, the two molecules being joined by hydrogen bonding, which may be depicted as

$$\begin{array}{ccc} & OH------O & \\ RC & & CR \\ & O------HO & \end{array}$$

This tendency is so pronounced in the case of acetic acid that even in the vapor state the substance exists in dimeric aggregation.

Pharmaceutical Solvents

On the basis of the forces of interaction occurring in solvents we may broadly classify solvents as one of three types:

1. *Polar solvents*—those made up of strong dipolar molecules having hydrogen bonding (water and hydrogen peroxide).
2. *Semipolar solvents*—those also made up of strong dipolar molecules but which do not form hydrogen bonds (acetone and amyl alcohol).
3. *Nonpolar solvents*—those made up of molecules having a small or no dipolar character (benzene, vegetable oil, and mineral oil).

Naturally there are many solvents that can fit into more than one of these broad classes; for example, chloroform is a weak dipolar compound but is generally considered nonpolar in character, and glycerin could be considered a polar or semipolar solvent even though it can form hydrogen bonds.

Types

Water—Water is a very unique solvent. Besides being a highly associated liquid, giving rise to its high boiling point, it has another very important property; it has a high dielectric constant. Dielectric constant (ϵ) indicates the effect that a substance has, when it acts as a medium, on the ease with which two oppositely charged ions may be separated. The higher the dielectric constant of a medium, the easier it is to separate two oppositely charged species in that medium. The dielectric constants of a number of liquids are given in Table III. The values listed are relative to a vacuum which by definition has a dielectric constant of unity. According to Coulomb's Law the force of attraction (F) between two oppositely charged ions is

$$F = \frac{Z_1 Z_2}{\epsilon r^2} \qquad (12)$$

where Z_1 and Z_2 are the charges on the ions, r is the distance separating the oppositely charged ions, and ϵ is the dielectric constant of the medium. Eq. 12 indicates that the force of interaction between the oppositely charged ions is inversely proportional to the dielectric constant of the medium. Thus, the interaction force between a sodium and chloride ion in water at a distance r would be $\frac{1}{80}$ that of the same ions in a vacuum separated the same distance. Looking at this example in another way, Coulomb's Law tells us that it is much easier to keep sodium and chloride ions apart in water than in a vacuum. Consider another example: the relative ease with which the ions of sodium chloride may be kept apart the same distance in water as compared to olive oil would stand in the ratio of 80/3.1; that is, it is 80/3.1 times easier to keep these ions apart in water than it is in olive oil. The high solubility of salts in solvents like water and glycerin can be explained on the basis of their high dielectric constant. In general also, the more polar the solvent, the greater its dielectric constant.

There is a very close relationship between dielectric constant and the two types of interactions found in all solvents; that is, the dipole–dipole interaction (Keesom) and the induced dipole–induced dipole interaction (London). The dielectric constant is related to these two forces through a quantity called *total molar polarization*, P, which is a measure of the relative ease with which a charge separation may be made within a molecule. The total molar polarization is given by the equation,*

$$P = \frac{\epsilon - 1}{\epsilon + 2} \cdot \frac{M}{D} \qquad (13)$$

where ϵ is the dielectric constant of the substance, M is the molecular weight, and D is the density of the substance. Total molar polarization is in turn composed of two terms:

$$P = P_\alpha + P_\mu = \tfrac{4}{3}\pi N\alpha + \frac{4}{3}\pi N\left(\frac{\mu^2}{3kT}\right) \qquad (14)$$

where $P_\alpha = \frac{4}{3}\pi N\alpha$ is the contribution due to induced polarization (the London contribution), $P_\mu = \frac{4}{3}\pi N \left(\frac{\mu^2}{3kT}\right)$ is the contribution due to the permanent dipole (the Keesom contribution), N is Avogadro's Number, α is a constant called the polarizability (related to the induced dipole), μ is the dipole moment, k is the Boltzman constant (1.38×10^{-16} erg/mole/deg), and T is the absolute temperature. Grouping all constant terms, it is possible to rewrite Eq. 14 as

$$P = A + B/T$$

and substituting Eq. 13, we get

$$\frac{\epsilon - 1}{\epsilon + 2} \cdot \frac{M}{D} = A + \frac{B}{T} \qquad (15)$$

The first term on the left-hand side of Eq. 15 is the contribution to the dielectric constant of the London Dispersions; it is not temperature dependent. The second term on the left-hand side of the equation is the contribution to the dielectric constant of the Keesom dispersions. This latter contribution is temperature dependent because the contribution from the permanent dipole depends on the dipoles aligning themselves, which tendency is opposed by thermal agitation. Thus, it is apparent from Eq. 15 (and from common sense) that as temperature increases the dielectric constant of dipolar solvents will tend to decrease.

Eq. 15 also tells us that solvents that have large dipole moments tend to have large dielectric constants because of the contribution of the P_μ term. Water, which has a very large dielectric constant, is estimated to have $\tfrac{2}{3}$ of its molecular interaction due to a dipole–dipole interaction and $\tfrac{1}{3}$ due to the induced dipole–induced dipole interaction. On the other hand, compounds such as benzene with a dipole moment of zero will have small dielectric constants since the P_μ term will drop out of Eq. 15.

Alcohols—*Alcohol* itself as a solvent is next in importance to water. It has an important advantage over water in the fact that preparations made with it

keep almost indefinitely, while many aqueous solutions of organic substances soon hydrolyze and become worthless. A further advantage is that growth of microorganisms does not occur in solutions containing alcohol in not too low concentration.

Resins, volatile oils, alkaloids, glycosides, etc are dissolved by alcohol, while many therapeutically inert principles, like gum, albumin, and starch, are insoluble in it, for which reason it is all the more useful as a "selective" solvent. Mixtures of water and alcohol, in proportions varying to suit specific cases, are extensively used. They are often referred to as *hydroalcoholic* solvents or menstrua.

Glycerin is an excellent solvent, although its range is not as extensive as that of water or alcohol. In higher concentrations it has preservative action. It dissolves the fixed alkalies, a large number of salts, and vegetable acids, pepsin, tannin, some active principles of plants, etc, but it also dissolves gum, soluble carbohydrates, starch, etc, and thus its solutions are generally "loaded" with inert constituents. It is also of special value as a simple solvent as in phenol glycerite, or where the major portion of the glycerin is simply added as a preservative and stabilizer of solutions that have been prepared with other solvents (see *Glycerites*).

Propylene glycol, which has been widely used as a substitute for glycerin, is miscible with water, with acetone, and with chloroform in all proportions. It is soluble in ether and will dissolve many essential oils but is immiscible with fixed oils. It is claimed to be as effective as ethyl alcohol in its power of inhibiting mold growth and fermentation.

Isopropyl alcohol possesses solvent properties similar to those of ethyl alcohol, and is used instead of the latter in a number of pharmaceutical manufacturing operations. It has the advantage over ethyl alcohol in that the commonly available product contains not over 1% of water, while ethyl alcohol contains about 5% water, which is often a disadvantage. Isopropyl alcohol is employed in some liniment and lotion formulations. It cannot be taken internally.

General Properties—Low molecular weight and polyhydroxy alcohols form associated structures through hydrogen bonds just as we saw with water. When the carbon atom content of an alcohol rises above five, generally only monomers are then present in the pure solvent. Although alcohols have high dielectric constants compared to other types of solvents, they are small compared to water. As we have seen, the solubility of salts in a solvent should be paralleled by its dielectric constant. That is, as the dielectric constant of a series of solvents increases, the probability of dissolving a salt in the solvent increases. This behavior is observed for the alcohols. Table IV, taken from Higuchi,[3] shows how the solubility of salts follows their dielectric constant.

As mentioned earlier, absolute alcohol is rarely used pharmaceutically in the pure state. However, hydroalcoholic mixtures such as elixirs and spirits are frequently encountered. A very useful generalization is that the dielectric properties of a mixed solvent such as water and alcohol can be approximated as the weighted average of the properties of the pure components. Thus, a mixture of 60% alcohol (by weight) in water should have a dielectric constant approximated by

$$\epsilon_{(mixture)} = 0.6(\epsilon_{(alcohol)}) + 0.4(\epsilon_{(water)})$$

$$\epsilon_{(mixture)} = 0.6(25) + 0.4(80) = 47$$

---

* For further details, see Martin.[6]

Table IV—Solubilities of Potassium Iodide and Sodium Chloride in Several Alcohols and Acetone[a]

Solvent	Gm KI/ 100 Gm solvent	Gm NaCl/ 100 Gm. solvent
Water	148	35.9
Glycerin	...	8.3 (20°C)
Glycol	50	7.1 (30°C)
Methanol	17	1.4
Acetone	2.9	...
Ethanol	1.88	0.065
Propanol	0.44	0.0124
Isopropanol	0.18	0.003
Butanol	0.20	0.005
Pentanol	0.089	0.0018

[a] All measurements at 25°C unless otherwise indicated.

The dielectric constant of 60% alcohol in water is experimentally found to be 43, which is in close agreement with that just calculated. The dielectric constant of glycerin is 46, close to the 60% alcohol mixture. We would, therefore, expect a salt like sodium chloride to have about the same solubility in glycerin as in 60% alcohol. The solubility of sodium chloride in glycerin is 8.3 Gm/100 Gm solvent and in 60% alcohol about 6.3 Gm/100 Gm solvent. This agreement would be even closer if comparisons were made on a volume rather than weight basis. At least qualitatively we can then say that the solubility of a salt in a solvent or a mixed solvent very closely follows the dielectric constant of the medium or, conversely, that the polarity of mixed solvents is paralleled by their dielectric constant based on salt solubility.

Acetone and Related Semipolar Materials—Even though acetone has a very high dipole moment $(2.8 \times 10^{-18}$ esu), as a pure solvent it does not form associated structures. This is evidenced by its low boiling point (57°C) in comparison with the boiling point of the lower molecular weight water (100°C) and ethanol (79°C). The reason why it does not associate is because the positive charge in its dipole does not reside in a hydrogen atom (Fig. 160), precluding the possibility of its forming a hydrogen bond. However, if some substance which is capable of forming hydrogen bounds such as water or alcohol is added to acetone, a very strong interaction through hydrogen bonds will occur (see *Mechanisms of Solvent Action* later in this chapter). Some substances which are semipolar and similar to acetone are aldehydes, low molecular weight esters, other ketones, and nitro-containing compounds.

Nonpolar Solvents—In this class of solvents we find fixed oils such as vegetable oil, petroleum benzin, carbon tetrachloride, benzene, and chloroform. On a relative basis there is a wide range of polarity among these solvents; for example, benzene has no dipole moment while that of chloroform is 1.05×10^{-18} esu. But even the polarity of these compounds normally classified as nonpolar is still in line with the dielectric constant of the solvent. The relation between these quantities is best seen through a quantity called *molar refraction*. The molar refraction,[7] R, of a compound is given by

$$R = \frac{n^2 - 1}{n^2 + 2} \cdot \frac{M}{D} \qquad (16)$$

where n is the refractive index of the liquid, M is its molecular weight, and D is its density. The similarity between Eq. 16 and Eq. 13 is to be noted, and indeed in refractive index measurements using very long wave lengths of light, $n^2 = \epsilon$. Thus, molar refraction under

these conditions approximates total molar polarization. Since in the more nonpolar solvents there is generally no dipole moment, μ, total molar polarization reflects polarization due only to the induced dipoles possible. Thus

$$P_\alpha = \frac{n^2 - 1}{n^2 + 2} \cdot \frac{M}{D} = \frac{\epsilon - 1}{\epsilon + 2} \cdot \frac{M}{D} = \frac{4}{3} \pi N \alpha \qquad (17)$$

It is evident from Eq. 17 that the refractive index of a nonpolar compound reflects its relative polarity. For example, the more polar benzene ($\epsilon = 2.2$) has a higher refractive index, 1.501, than the less polar hexane ($\epsilon = 1.9$), whose refractive index is 1.375.

It should be emphasized again that when a solvent (such as chloroform) has highly electronegative halogen atoms attached to a carbon atom also containing at least one hydrogen atom, such a solvent will be capable of forming strong hydrogen bonds with solutes which are polar in character. Thus, through the formation of such hydrogen bonds such solvents will dissolve polar solutes. For example, it is possible to dissolve alkaloids in chloroform.

Mechanism of Solvent Action

A solvent may function in one or more of several ways. When an ionic salt is dissolved, as by water for example, the process of solution involves separation of the cations and anions of the salt with attendant orientation of molecules of solvent about the ions. Such orientation of solvent molecules about the ions of the solute—a process called *solvation* (*hydration* if the solvent is water)—is possible only when the solvent is highly polar, whereby the dipoles of the solvent are attracted to and held by the ions of the solute. The solvent must also possess the ability to keep the solvated, charged ions apart with a minimum requirement of energy. The role of the dielectric constant in keeping this energy to a minimum has been discussed earlier.

A polar liquid such as water may exhibit solvent action also by virtue of its ability to break a covalent bond in the solute and bring about ionization of the latter. For example, hydrogen chloride dissolves in water and functions as an acid as a result of the following reaction:

$$HCl + H_2O \rightarrow H_3O^+ + Cl^-$$

The ions formed by this preliminary reaction of breaking the covalent bond are subsequently maintained in solution by the same mechanism as in the case of ionic salts.

Still another mechanism by which a polar liquid may act as a solvent is that involved when the solvent and solute are capable of being coupled through hydrogen bond formation. The solubility of the low-molecular-weight alcohols in water, for example, is attributed to the ability of the alcohol molecules to become part of a water–alcohol association complex:

$$\underset{H}{\overset{H}{\mid}}-O-----H-\underset{R}{\overset{R}{\mid}}-O------H-\underset{H}{\overset{H}{\mid}}-O------H-\underset{R}{\overset{R}{\mid}}-O$$

As the molecular weight of the alcohol increases, it

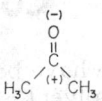

Fig. 160. The charge separation in acetone.

becomes progressively less polar, and less able to compete with water molecules for a place in the latticelike arrangement formed through hydrogen bonding; high-molecular-weight alcohols are, therefore, poorly soluble or insoluble in water. When the number of carbon atoms in a normal alcohol reaches five, solubility in water is materially reduced.

When the number of hydroxyl groups in the alcohol is increased, its solubility in water is generally greatly increased; it is principally, if not entirely, for this reason that such high-molecular-weight compounds as sugars, gums, many glycosides, and such synthetic compounds as the polyethylene glycols are very soluble in water.

The solubility of ethers, aldehydes, ketones, acids, and anhydrides in water—and in other polar solvents—is also largely attributable to the formation of an association complex between solute and solvent by means of the hydrogen bond. While the molecules of ethers, aldehydes and ketones, unlike those of alcohols, are not themselves associated—because of the absence of a hydrogen atom that is capable of forming the characteristic hydrogen bond—the substances are nonetheless more or less polar because of the presence of a strongly electronegative oxygen atom which is capable of association with water through hydrogen bond formation. Acetone, for example, dissolves in water in all likelihood principally because of the following type of reaction:

$$(CH_3)_2CO + H_2O \rightarrow (CH_3)_2CO\cdots H\overset{\displaystyle H}{\underset{\displaystyle |}{-O}}$$

The maximum number of carbon atoms which may be present per molecule while retaining water solubility is approximately the same as with the alcohols.

Since nitrogen is a less electronegative atom than oxygen, when nitrogen has a hydrogen atom attached to it in some compound, we find that such a hydrogen tends to form a weaker hydrogen bond than the hydrogen bond found in a substance like alcohol. Therefore, it is not surprising that such compounds as the amines should be somewhat less soluble in water than their oxygen counterparts, the alcohols. But the mechanism of solubility, however, still depends in a large measure on hydrogen bond formation.

The solvent action of nonpolar liquids involves a somewhat different mechanism. Because they are unable to form dipoles with which to overcome the attractions between ions of an ionic salt, or to break a covalent bond to produce an ionic compound, or to form association complexes with a solute, nonpolar liquids are incapable of dissolving polar compounds. They can only dissolve, in general, other nonpolar substances in which the bonds between molecules are weak. The forces involved are usually of the induced dipole–induced dipole type. Such is the case when one hydrocarbon is dissolved in another, or an oil or a fat is dissolved in petroleum ether. Sometimes it is observed that a polar substance such as alcohol will dissolve in a nonpolar liquid such as benzene. This apparent exception to the preceding generalization may be explained by

Table V—Demonstration of Solubility Rules

Chemical compound	Solubility[a]
Aniline, $C_6H_5NH_2$	28.6
Benzene, C_6H_6	1430
Benzoic acid, C_6H_5COOH	275
Benzyl alcohol, $C_6H_5CH_2OH$	25
n-Butanol, C_4H_9OH	12
tert-Butanol, $(CH_3)_3COH$	Miscible
Carbon tetrachloride, CCl_4	2000
Chloroform, $CHCl_3$	200
Fumaric acid, *trans*-butenedioic acid	150
Hydroquinone, $C_6H_4(OH)_2$	14
Maleic acid, *cis*-butenedioic acid	5
Phenol, C_6H_5OH	15
Pyrocatechol, $C_6H_4(OH)_2$	2.3
Pyrogallol, $C_6H_3(OH)_3$	1.7
Resorcinol, $C_6H_4(OH)_2$	0.9

[a] *Note*—The above solubility table gives number of milliliters of water required to dissolve 1 Gm of solute.

the assumption that the alcohol molecule induces in the benzene molecule a temporary dipole which forms an association complex with the solvent molecules. A binding force of this kind is referred to as a *permanent dipole–induced dipole force*.

Some Useful Generalizations—The preceding discussion indicates that enough is known about the mechanism of solubility to be able to formulate some generalizations concerning this important physical property of substances. Because of the greater importance of organic substances in the field of medicinal chemistry, certain of the more useful generalizations with respect to organic chemicals are presented here in summary form. It should be remembered, however, that the phenomenon of solubility usually involves several variables, and that there may be exceptions to general rules.

One general maxim which holds true in most instances is: *the greater the structural similarity between solute and solvent, the greater the solubility*. Thus phenol is almost insoluble in petroleum benzin but is very soluble in glycerin.

Organic compounds containing polar groups capable of forming hydrogen bonds with water are soluble in water, providing that the molecular weight of the compound is not too great. It is easily demonstrated that the polar groups OH, CHO, COH, CHOH, CH_2OH, COOH, NO_2, CO, NH_2, and SO_3H tend to increase the solubility of an organic compound in water. On the other hand, nonpolar or very weak polar groups, such as the various hydrocarbon radicals, reduce solubility; the greater the number of carbon atoms in the radical, the greater the decrease in solubility. Introduction of halogen atoms into a molecule in general tends to decrease solubility because of increased molecular weight without a proportionate increase in polarity.

The greater the number of polar groups, the greater is the solubility of a compound, provided that the size of the rest of the molecule is not altered; thus pyrogallol is much more soluble in water than is phenol. The *relative positions* of the groups in the molecule also influence solubility; thus, in water, resorcinol (*m*-dihydroxybenzene) is more soluble than pyrocatechol (*o*-dihydroxybenzene), and the latter is more soluble than hydroquinone (*p*-dihydroxybenzene).

Polymers and compounds of high molecular weight are generally insoluble or only very slightly soluble.

High melting points are frequently indicative of low solubility for organic compounds. One reason for high melting points is *association* of molecules; this cohesive force tends to prevent dispersion of the solute in the solvent.

The *cis* form of isomers is more soluble than the *trans* form. See Table V.

Solvation, which is evidence of the existence of a strong attractive force between solute and solvent, enhances the solubility of the solute, providing there is not a marked ordering of the solvent molecules in the solution phase.

Acids, especially strong acids, usually produce water-soluble salts when reacted with nitrogen-containing organic bases.

Colligative Properties of Solutions

Up to this point we have been concerned with dissolving a solute in a solvent. Having brought about the dissolution, the solution, quite naturally, has a number of properties that are different from that of the pure solvent. Of very great importance are the *colligative properties* that a solution possesses.

The colligative properties of a solution are those that depend on the *number* of solute particles in solution, irrespective of whether these are molecules or ions, or large or small.   Ideally, the effect of a solute particle of one species is considered to be the same as that of an entirely different kind of particle, at least in dilute solution.   Practically, there may be differences which may become substantial as the concentration of the solution is increased.

The colligative properties which will be considered in this chapter are:

1. Osmotic pressure.
2. Vapor-pressure lowering.
3. Boiling-point elevation.
4. Freezing-point depression.

Of the four colligative properties, all of which are related, osmotic pressure has the greatest direct importance in the pharmaceutical sciences.   It is the property that largely determines the physiologic acceptability of a variety of solutions used for therapeutic purposes.   As the property of prime importance, it will be considered first.   Afterward the other colligative properties, one of which is much used in pharmacy because it provides an estimate of osmotic pressure, will be studied.

Osmotic-Pressure Elevation

Diffusion in Liquids—Although the property of diffusion is most marked in gaseous systems, it is not limited to such systems.   That molecules or ions in liquid systems possess this same freedom of movement may be demonstrated by carefully placing a layer of water on a concentrated aqueous solution of any salt.   In time it will be observed that the boundary between solvent and solution gradually widens, and eventually the composition of the new solution will become uniform throughout.   This experiment indicates that *substances tend to move or diffuse from regions of higher concentration to regions of lower concentrations* so that differences in concentration eventually disappear.

Osmosis—In carrying out the experiment just described, it is impossible to distinguish between the diffusion of the solute and that of the solvent.   However, by separating the solution and the solvent by means of a membrane that is permeable to the solvent, but not to the solute (or, at most, only slightly permeable to the solute), it is possible to demonstrate visibly the diffusion of solvent into the concentrated solution.   In a similar manner, if two solutions of different concentration are separated by a membrane, the solvent will move from the solution of lower solute concentration to the solution of higher solute concentration.   This diffusion of solvent through a membrane is called *osmosis*.

The phenomenon of osmosis may be visually demonstrated by means of the osmometer shown in Fig. 161.   In this diagram a parchment paper membrane or "diffusion shell," as it is often called, is securely fastened to a long glass tube.   A side tube bearing a stopcock allows solution to be run into the diffusion shell.   To demonstrate osmosis, an aqueous solution of sucrose, or any other suitable solute, is poured into the diffusion shell through the side tube until the level of the solution is above the stopcock, which is then closed.   The diffusion shell is immersed in a jar of water until the level of the solution in the tube is the same as that in the jar.   In a short time the level of the solution in the tube will be seen to rise, sometimes to heights of several feet.   If the experiment is continued, the solution will fall until it is at the same level as the liquid in the jar.   This drop occurs because of the gradual diffusion of sugar molecules from the solution to the solvent, the membrane not being absolutely impermeable to sugar molecules.   In the experiment described here, therefore, the height to which the liquid rises in the tube depends on the difference in rates of diffusion of solvent and solute molecules.   Animal membranes, such as a hog's bladder, for example, function in the same manner as parchment membranes.

Certain artificial membranes have been prepared which are practically impermeable to solute molecules but do permit solvent molecules to pass.   When such membranes, referred to as *semipermeable membranes*, are used in the experiment described above, the solution in the tube rises until the hydrostatic pressure of the column of liquid above the level of the solvent is just sufficient to prevent further osmosis of the solvent.   This *hydrostatic pressure* is numerically equal to the *osmotic pressure* of the solution.

Osmotic Pressure of Nonelectrolytes—From quantitative studies with solutions of varying concentration of a solute that does not ionize, it has been demonstrated that *osmotic pressure is proportional to the concentration of the solute*, ie, twice the concentration of a given nonelectrolyte will produce twice the osmotic pressure in a given solvent.*

Furthermore, the osmotic pressures of solutions of different nonelectrolytes are proportional to the number of molecules in each solution.   Stated in another manner, the osmotic pressures of two solutions of the same molal† concentration are identical.   Thus a solution containing 34.2 Gm of sucrose (mol wt 342) in 1000 Gm of water has the same osmotic pressure as a solution containing 18.0 Gm of anhydrous dextrose (mol wt 180) in 1000 Gm of water.   These solutions are said to be *iso-osmotic* with each other because they have identical osmotic pressures.

A study of the results of osmotic-pressure measurements on different substances led the Dutch chemist Jacobus Henricus van't Hoff, in 1885, to suggest that the solute in a solution may be considered as being analogous to the molecules of a gas and the osmotic pressure as being produced by the bombardment of the semipermeable membrane by the molecules of solute.   According to van't Hoff's theory the osmotic pressure

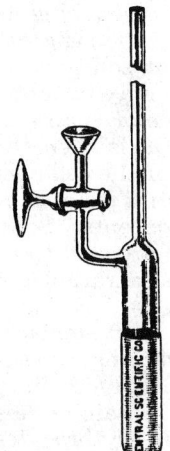

Fig. 161.   Osmometer (courtesy, Central Scientific).

---

* This is not strictly true in solutions of fairly high solute concentration, but does hold quite well for dilute solutions.

† A molal solution is one that contains the mol wt in grams of a given solute in 1000 Gm of solvent.   A 2-molal solution contains twice the gram-molecular weight; a 0.1 molal, 1/10 the gram-molecular weight in 1000 Gm of solvent.

Table VI—Osmotic Pressure of Sucrose Solutions

Conc. (Gm/L), C	Vol. in L in which 1 Gm mole is dissolved, V^a	Pressure in atmos P	P/C	PV
10.00	34.2	0.65	0.065	22.2
20.00	17.1	1.27	0.064	21.7
45.00	7.60	2.91	0.065	22.1
93.75	3.65	6.23	0.067	22.7

^{a} The figures in this column were obtained by calculating the volume of solution in which 342 (mol wt) Gm of sucrose would be dissolved.

of a solution is equal to the pressure which the dissolved substance would exert in the gaseous state if it occupied a volume equal to the volume of the solution. From this it follows that just as in the case of a gas there is a proportionality between pressure and concentration of dissolved substance. This proportionality is well illustrated by the values of the osmotic pressure of solutions of sucrose at 0°C as determined by the Earl of Berkeley and E. G. J. Hartley and shown in Table VI.

In column PV of the foregoing table a quantitative confirmation, at least for fairly dilute solutions, of van't Hoff's oversimplified though useful generalization is shown by the constancy of the values of the product PV. The student will recall that the product of the pressure and the volume of a gas, at constant temperature, is likewise constant (Boyle's law).

Van't Hoff also deduced that the osmotic pressure must be proportional to the absolute temperature, just as in Charles' law for gases, which deduction was confirmed by the experiments of several workers. From this it follows that the equation $PV = nRT$ is valid for dilute solutions of nonelectrolytes just as a similar equation is valid for gases. However, even as Boyle's law does not apply to gases under high pressures and at low temperatures, so van't Hoff's equation for osmotic pressure does not apply in concentrated solutions. For a more thorough discussion of osmotic pressure the student is referred to books on physical chemistry.

Osmotic Pressure of Electrolytes—In discussing the generalizations concerning the osmotic pressure of solutions of nonelectrolytes it was stated that the osmotic pressures of two solutions of the same molal concentration are identical. This generalization, however, cannot be made for solutions of electrolytes, ie, acids, alkalies, and salts.

Van't Hoff pointed out that the osmotic pressures of solutions of electrolytes, particularly of the extensively ionized group, are considerably greater than the osmotic pressures of solutions of nonelectrolytes of the same molal concentration. This anomaly remained unexplained until 1887 when Svante August Arrhenius proposed a hypothesis to account for the abnormal osmotic pressures of solutions of electrolytes. Arrhenius advanced the theory that in aqueous solution, acids, bases, and salts may be considered to be dissociated or ionized into positively and negatively charged particles or ions and that the increased osmotic pressure of such solutions is due to the increased number of particles formed in the process of ionization. For example, sodium chloride is assumed to be ionized as follows:

$$NaCl \rightarrow Na^+ + Cl^-$$

It is evident that each molecule of sodium chloride that is ionized produces two ions and, if sodium chloride is completely ionized, there will be twice as many particles as would be the case if it were not ionized at all. Fur-

thermore, if each ion has the same effect on osmotic pressure as a molecule, it might be expected that the osmotic pressure of the solution would be twice that of a solution containing the same molal concentration of nonionizing substance. Study of osmotic pressure data indicates that in very dilute solutions of salts which yield two ions the pressure is very nearly twice that of solutions of equivalent concentrations of solutes that do not ionize.

For solutions which yield more than two ions as, for example, the following:

$$K_2SO_4 \rightarrow 2K^+ + SO_4^-$$

$$FeCl_3 \rightarrow Fe^{+++} + 3Cl^-$$

it is to be expected that the complete dissociation of the molecules would give rise to osmotic pressures that are three and four times, respectively, the pressure of solutions containing an equivalent quantity of a nonionized solute. Accordingly, the equation $PV = nRT$, which may be employed to calculate the osmotic pressure of a dilute solution of a nonelectrolyte, may also be applied to dilute solutions of electrolytes if it is changed to $PV = inRT$, where the value of i approaches the number of ions produced by the ionization of the strong electrolytes cited in the preceding examples. For weak electrolytes i represents the total number of particles, ions and molecules together, in the solution, divided by the number of molecules that would be present if the solute did not ionize. The experimental evidence indicates that in dilute solutions at least, the osmotic pressures approach the predicted values. It should be emphasized, however, that in more concentrated solutions of electrolytes the deviations from this simple theory are considerable, due to interionic attraction, solvation, and other factors that need not be discussed here. For further information the reader is referred to standard texts on physical chemistry.[8,9]

Biological Aspects of Osmotic Pressure—Osmotic pressure experiments were made as early as 1884 by the Dutch botanist Hugo de Vries in his study of plasmolysis. This term is applied to the contraction of the contents of plant cells placed in solutions of comparatively high osmotic pressure. The phenomenon is caused by the osmosis of water out of the cell through the practically semipermeable membrane surrounding the protoplasm. If suitable cells, for example, the epidermal cells of the leaf of *Tradescanta discolor*, are placed in a solution of higher osmotic pressure than that of the cell contents, water flows out of the cell, causing the contents to draw away from the cell wall. On the other hand, if the cells are placed in solutions of lower osmotic pressure, water enters the cell, producing an expansion which, however, is limited by the rigid cell wall. By immersing cells in a series of solutions of varying solute concentration, a solution may be found in which plasmolysis is barely detectable or is absent. The osmotic pressure of such a solution is then the same, or very nearly the same, as that of the cell contents and it is then said that the solution is *iso-osmotic* or, more exactly, *isotonic* with the cell contents. Solutions of greater concentration than this are said to be *hypertonic* and solutions of lower concentration are said to be *hypotonic*.

Red blood cells or erythrocytes have been similarly studied by immersion into solutions of varying concentration of different solutes. When introduced into water or into sodium chloride solutions containing less than 0.90 Gm of solute per 100 ml, human erythrocytes swell, and often burst, because of the diffusion of water into the cell and the fact that the cell wall is not sufficiently strong to resist the pressure. This phenomenon is referred to as *hemolysis*. If the cells are placed in solutions containing more than 0.90 Gm of sodium chloride per 100 ml, they lose water and shrink. By immersing the cells in a solution containing exactly 0.90 Gm of sodium chloride in 100 ml, no change in the size of the cells is observed; since in this solution the cells maintain their "tone," the solution is said to be *isotonic* with human erythrocytes. For the reasons indicated it is desirable that solutions to be injected into the blood should be made isotonic with erythrocytes. The manner in which this may be done is described in the section on *Isotonic Solutions*.

Distinction Between Iso-osmotic and Isotonic—The terms iso-osmotic and isotonic are not to be considered as being equivalent, although often a solution may be described as being both iso-osmotic and isotonic. If a plant or animal cell is in contact with a solution that has the same osmotic pressure as the cell contents, there will be no net gain or loss of water by either solution *provided* the cell membrane is impermeable to all solutes that are present. Since the volume of the cell contents remains unchanged, the "tone" or normal state of the cell is maintained, and the solution in contact with the cell may be described not only as being iso-osmotic with the solution in the cell but also as being isotonic with it. If, however, one or more of the solutes in contact with the membrane can pass through the latter, it is evident that the volume of the cell contents will change, thus altering the "tone" of the cell; in this case the two solutions may be iso-osmotic, yet not be isotonic.

It is possible that some substances used in an injection dosage form can cause hemolysis of red blood cells, even when their concentrations are such as to produce solutions theoretically iso-osmotic with the cells, because the solutes diffuse through the membrane of the cells. For example, a 1.8% solution of urea has the same osmotic pressure as a 0.9% solution of sodium chloride, but the former solution produces hemolysis of red blood cells; obviously the urea solution is not isotonic with the cells. To determine whether or not a solution is isotonic with erythrocytes, it is necessary to determine the concentration of solute at which the cells retain their normal size and shape. A simple method for doing this was devised by Setnikar and Temelcou,[10] who determined the concentration of a solution at which red blood cells maintained a volume equal to that occupied in an isotonic solution of sodium chloride; the red cell volumes were determined by centrifuging suspensions of them in different solutions, using a hematocrit tube.

Vapor-Pressure Lowering

When a nonvolatile solute is dissolved in a liquid solvent the vapor pressure of the solvent is lowered. This easily can be qualitatively described by visualizing solvent molecules on the surface of the solvent which normally could escape into the vapor being replaced by solute molecules which have little if any vapor pressure of their own. For ideal solutions of nonelectrolytes the vapor pressure of the solution follows Raoult's law,

$$P_A = X_A P_A^\circ \qquad (18)$$

where P_A is the vapor pressure of the solution, P_A° is the vapor pressure of the pure solvent, and X_A is the mole fraction of solvent. This relationship states that

the vapor pressure of the solution is proportional to the number of molecules of solvent in the solution. Rearranging Eq. 18,

$$\frac{P_A^\circ - P_A}{P_A^\circ} = (1 - X_A) = X_B \qquad (19)$$

where X_B is the mole fraction of the solute. This equation states that the lowering of vapor pressure in the solution relative to the vapor pressure of the pure solvent—what is called simply the *relative vapor-pressure lowering*—is equal to the mole fraction of the solute. The *absolute* lowering of vapor pressure of the solution is defined by

$$P_A^\circ - P_A = X_B P_A^\circ \qquad (20)$$

Example—Calculate the lowering of vapor pressure and the vapor pressure, at 20°C, of a solution containing 50 Gm of anhydrous dextrose (mol wt 180.16) in 1000 Gm of water (mol wt 18.02). The vapor pressure of water at 20°C, in absence of air, is 17.535 mm.

First, the lowering of vapor pressure is to be calculated, using Eq. 20, in which X_B is the mole fraction of dextrose, defined by

$$X_B = \frac{n_B}{n_A + n_B}$$

where n_A is the number of moles of solvent and n_B is the number of moles of solute. Substituting numerical values

$$n_B = \frac{50}{180.2} = 0.278$$

$$n_A = \frac{1000}{18.02} = 55.5$$

$$X_B = \frac{0.278}{55.5 + 0.278} = 0.00498$$

the lowering of vapor pressure is

$$P_A^\circ - P_A = 0.00498 \times 17.535$$

$$= 0.0873 \text{ mm}$$

the vapor pressure of the solution is

$$P_A = 17.535 - 0.0873$$

$$= 17.448 \text{ mm}$$

Measurement of Vapor Pressure—The preceding example emphasizes the need for an accurate method of measuring vapor pressure, and especially of small differences of pressure between a solvent and its solutions. Vapor pressure may be determined directly with a suitable manometer or, under certain conditions, by observing the direct depression of the level of mercury in a tube long enough to have an evacuated space above the mercury. A differential manometer, one arm of which is connected to the solution and the other to the solvent, improves the accuracy of measurement. The *isopiestic method*, which is capable of very good precision and accuracy, is based on the principle that if two solutions containing the same solvent are placed side by side in a closed space (preferably evacuated to hasten equilibration), solvent will distil from the solution of higher vapor pressure into the one of lower pressure until both solutions have the same pressure, when they are said to be *isopiestic* (Gr, equal pressure). If the equilibrated solutions are analyzed, and one contains a reference solute of known effect on the vapor pressure of the solvent, it is possible to calculate the vapor pressure of the "unknown" solution.

Boiling-Point Elevation

In consequence of the fact that the vapor pressure of any solution of a nonvolatile solute is less than that of the solvent, the boiling point of the solution—which is the temperature at which the vapor pressure is equal to the applied pressure (commonly 760 mm)—must be higher than that of the solvent. This is clearly evident in Fig. 162.

The relationship between the elevation of boiling point and the concentration of nonvolatile, nonelectrolyte solute may be derived from the Clausius–Clapeyron equation (Eq. 103, page 245), which is

$$\frac{dP}{dT} = \frac{P \cdot H_{vap}}{RT^2} \tag{21}$$

Replacing the differential expression dP/dT by $\Delta P/\Delta T_b$, where ΔP is the lowering of vapor pressure and ΔT_b is the elevation of boiling point, and introducing P_A°, the vapor pressure of the solvent at its boiling point T_0,

$$\frac{\Delta P}{\Delta T_b} = \frac{P_A^\circ \cdot \Delta H_{vap}}{RT_0^2} \tag{22}$$

As the lowering of vapor pressure in an ideal solution is

$$\Delta P = X_B P_A^\circ \tag{23}$$

substitution of this equation into Eq. 22 with rearrangement to provide a solution for ΔT_b gives

$$\Delta T_b = \frac{RT_0^2}{\Delta H_{vap}} X_B \tag{24}$$

This equation may be used to calculate the elevation of boiling point if the concentration of solute is expressed as the mole fraction. A more common expression, however, is in terms of the molality m (the number of Gm moles of solute per 1000 Gm of solvent), which relationship is derived as follows:

$$X_B = \frac{n_B}{n_A + n_B} = \frac{m}{1000/M_A + m} \cong \frac{m}{1000/M_A} \tag{25}$$

In these equations M_A is the molecular weight of the solvent. When the solutions are dilute, so that m is small, it may be neglected in the denominator (but not in the numerator!) to give the approximate equivalent in Eq. 25. Substituting this equivalent into Eq. 24,

$$\Delta T_b = \frac{RT_0^2 M_A m}{1000 \Delta H_{vap}} \tag{26}$$

Grouping the constants into a single term,

$$\Delta T_b = K_b m \tag{27}$$

where

$$K_b = \frac{RT_0^2 M_A}{1000 \Delta H_{vap}} \tag{28}$$

and is called the molal boiling-point elevation constant.

The value of this constant for water, which boils at $373.1^\circ K$, has a heat of vaporization of 539.7 cal/Gm and a molecular weight of 18.02, is

$$K_b = \frac{1.987 \times 373.1^2 \times 18.02}{1000 \times 18.02 \times 539.7} = 0.513^\circ \tag{29}$$

Notwithstanding that K_b is called a molal boiling-point elevation constant, it should not be interpreted as the actual rise of boiling point for a 1-molal solution. Such solutions are generally too concentrated to exhibit the ideal behavior assumed in deriving the equation for calculating the theoretical value of the constant. In dilute solutions, however, the actual boiling-point elevation, *calculated to a 1-molal basis*, approaches the theoretical value, the closer the more dilute the solution.

The elevation of boiling point of a dilute solution of a nonelectrolyte solute may be used to calculate the mol wt of the latter. In a solution containing w_B Gm of solute of M_B in w_A Gm of solvent the molality m is

$$m = \frac{1000 \, w_B}{w_A M_B} \tag{30}$$

substituting this into Eq. 27 and rearranging

$$M_B = \frac{K_b 1000 \, w_B}{w_A \cdot \Delta T_b} \tag{31}$$

The accurate determination of boiling point requires that cognizance be taken of the following potential sources of error: (1) superheating of the liquid; (2) change of concentration of solution as solvent passes into vapor phase; (3) change of boiling point with variation of atmospheric pressure; (4) variation of temperature with position of thermometer or other temperature-measuring device (if placed in vapor above a solution the thermometer measures the boiling point of condensing solvent and not of solution); (5) inaccuracy resulting from use of uncalibrated or improperly calibrated thermometer.

Freezing-Point Depression

The freezing point of a solvent is defined as the temperature at which the solid and liquid forms of the solvent coexist in equilibrium at a fixed external pressure, commonly 1 atmos (760 mm of mercury). At this temperature the solid and liquid forms of the solvent must have the same vapor pressure, for if this were not so the form having the higher vapor pressure would change into that having the lower vapor pressure.

The freezing point of a solution is the temperature at which the solid form of the pure solvent coexists in equilibrium with the solution at a fixed external pressure, again commonly 1 atmos. As the vapor pressure of a solution is lower than that of its solvent, it is obvious that solid solvent and solution cannot coexist at the same temperature as solid solvent and liquid solvent; only at some lower temperature, where solid solvent and solution do have the same vapor pressure, is equilibrium established. A schematic pressure–temperature diagram for water and an aqueous solution, not drawn to scale and exaggerated for the purpose of more effective illustration, shows the equilibrium conditions involved in both freezing-point depression and boiling-point elevation (Fig. 162).

The freezing-point lowering of a solution may be quantitatively predicted for ideal solutions, or dilute

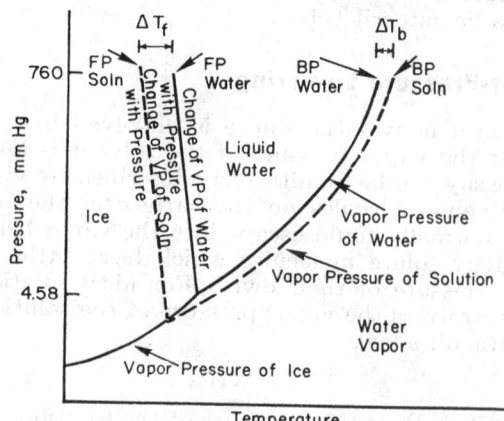

Fig. 162. Vapor-pressure-temperature diagram for water and an aqueous solution, illustrating elevation of boiling point and lowering of freezing point of the latter.

solutions which do not behave ideally, by mathematical operations similar to (though somewhat more complex than) those used in deriving the boiling-point elevation constant. The equation for the freezing point lowering, ΔT_f, is

$$\Delta T_f = \frac{RT_0{}^2 M_A m}{1000 . \Delta H_{fus}} = K_f m \qquad (32)$$

where

$$K_f = \frac{RT_0{}^2 M_A}{1000 . \Delta H_{fus}} \qquad (33)$$

The value of K_f for water, which freezes at 273.1 °K and has a heat of fusion of 79.7 cal/Gm, is

$$K_f = \frac{1.987 \times 273.1^2 \times 18.02}{1000 \times 18.02 \times 79.7} = 1.86° \qquad (34)$$

The molal freezing-point depression constant is not intended to represent the freezing-point depression for a 1-molal solution, which is too concentrated for the premise of ideal behavior to be applicable. In dilute solutions the freezing-point depression, calculated to a 1-molal basis, approaches the theoretical value, the agreement between experiment and theory being the better the more dilute the solution.

The freezing point of a dilute solution of a nonelectrolyte solute may be used, as with the boiling point, to calculate the molecular weight of the solute. The applicable equation is

$$M_B = \frac{K_f 1000 \, w_B}{w_A . \Delta T_f} \qquad (35)$$

The molecular weight of organic substances soluble in molten camphor may be determined by observing the freezing point of a mixture of the substance with camphor. This procedure, called the *Rast method*, utilizes camphor because it has a very large molal freezing-point depression constant, about 40 °C; as the constant may vary with different lots of camphor and with variations of technique, the method should be standardized using a solute of known molecular weight.

Freezing-point determinations have the advantage over boiling-point determinations of greater accuracy and precision by virtue of the larger magnitude of the former; thus, in the case of water the molal freezing-point depression is approximately 3.5 times greater than the molal boiling-point elevation. Potential sources of error in the determination of freezing point include: (1) supercooling of the liquid; (2) increase of concentration of solution if solvent crystallizes out of it; (3) loss of heat by transfer to surrounding freezing bath; (4) liberation of latent heat on crystallization of solid solvent; (5) inaccuracy resulting from use of uncalibrated or improperly calibrated thermometer or other temperature-measuring device.

Reasonably accurate determinations of freezing points may be made by the Beckmann method, which utilizes the Beckmann differential thermometer, which permits temperature readings to ±0.001 °C. The most accurate measurements are obtained by a method in which the difference in temperature between two systems, one of liquid solvent in equilibrium with solid solvent and the other of solution in equilibrium with solid solvent, is determined with a multiple-junction thermocouple and potentiometer.

Relationship Between Osmotic Pressure and Vapor-Pressure Lowering

The lowering of vapor pressure and the development of osmotic pressure in a solution are both manifestations of the basic condition that the free energy of solvent molecules in the pure solvent is greater than the free energy of solvent molecules in the solution. Consequently, solvent molecules will spontaneously transfer, if given an opportunity, from solvent to solution until equilibrium conditions are established. The transfer can take place either through a membrane permeable only to solvent molecules or, if such contact between solvent and solution is not available, by distillation of solvent from pure solvent to solution if access through a vapor phase is provided.

If an experiment is performed with two sets of vessels containing solution and solvent, as illustrated in Fig. 163, differing only in that the long tube of one set has a semipermeable membrane attached to its lower end while the long tube of the other set is permanently sealed at the lower end, in time the same volume of solvent will have transferred to the solution in both cases. For a definite volume, eg, a mole, of solvent transferred to the solution by distillation the change of free energy, ΔG, in the process is

$$\Delta G = RT \ln \frac{P_A}{P_A{}^\circ} \qquad (36)$$

where P_A is the vapor pressure of the solution and $P_A{}^\circ$ is the vapor pressure of the solvent.

For the transfer of the same volume of solvent by osmosis the free energy change is

$$\Delta G = -\bar{V}_A \pi \qquad (37)$$

where $\bar{V}_A$ is the partial molal volume of solvent (the volume of 1 mole of solvent in the solution) and π is the osmotic pressure of the solution. Since the free energy change is the same in both processes

$$-\bar{V}_A \pi = RT \ln \frac{P_A}{P_A{}^\circ} \qquad (38)$$

rearranging

$$\pi = \frac{RT}{\bar{V}_A} \ln \frac{P_A{}^\circ}{P_A} \qquad (39)$$

With this equation the osmotic pressure of a solution may be calculated if its vapor pressure and the partial molal volume of the solvent are known, not only when the solution is sufficiently dilute that Raoult's law is obeyed but also when the concentration is so high as to introduce substantial deviation from the law.

From Eq. 39, which has some resemblance to van't Hoff's empirical equation $\pi V = nRT$ for dilute solutions, the latter equation may be derived as follows.

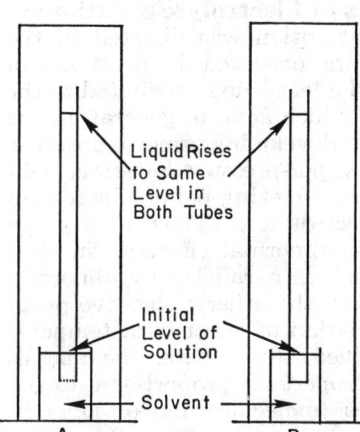

Liquid Rises to Same Level in Both Tubes

Initial Level of Solution

Solvent

A   B

Fig. 163. Transfer of solvent to solution. In Tube A: osmotically, through semipermeable membrane at bottom of tube. In Tube B: by distillation of vapor, into top of tube (bottom of tube is sealed).

If a solution is sufficiently dilute to correspond to Raoult's law

$$P_A = X_A P_A{}^\circ = (1 - X_B)P_A{}^\circ \tag{40}$$

Eq. 39 may be written

$$\pi = -\frac{RT}{\overline{V}_A} \ln (1 - X_B) \tag{41}$$

When X_B is small (as in a dilute solution), the term $-\ln (1 - X_B)$ can be shown to be approximately equal to X_B, so that

$$\pi = \frac{RT}{\overline{V}_A} X_B \tag{42}$$

In dilute solutions the approximations $X_B = n_B/n_A$ (where n_B and n_A are the moles of solute and solvent, respectively) and $\overline{V}_A = V/n_A$ (where V is the volume of solution) may be introduced, yielding

$$\pi V = n_B RT \tag{43}$$

which is van't Hoff's equation.

Ideal Behavior and Deviations from Ideal Behavior

In setting out to derive mathematical expressions for colligative properties such phrases as "for ideal solutions" or "for dilute solutions" were used to indicate the limitations of the expressions. What is an ideal solution? Samuel Glasstone defines it as "one which obeys Raoult's law over the whole range of concentration and at all temperatures" and gives as specific characteristics of such solutions their formation only from constituents which mix in the liquid state without heat change and without volume change. These characteristics reflect the fact that addition of solute to a solvent produces no change in the forces between molecules of the solvent. Thus the molecules have the same "escaping tendency" in the solution as in the pure solvent and the vapor pressure above the solution is proportional to the ratio of the number of solvent molecules in the surface of the solution to the number of the molecules in the surface of the solvent—which is the basis of Raoult's law.

Any change in intermolecular forces produced by mixing the components of a solution may result in deviation from ideality; such a deviation may be expected particularly in solutions containing both a polar and a nonpolar substance. Solutions of electrolytes, except at high dilution, are especially prone to depart from ideal behavior, even though allowance is made for the additional particles that result from ionization. When solute and solvent combine to form solvates, the escaping tendency of the solvent may be reduced in consequence of the reduction in the number of free molecules of solvent; thus, a negative deviation from Raoult's law is introduced. On the other hand, the escaping tendency of the solvent in a solution of nonvolatile solute may be increased because the cohesive forces between molecules of solvent are reduced by the solute; this results in a positive deviation from Raoult's law.

While few solutions exhibit ideal behavior over a wide range of concentration, most solutions behave ideally at least in high dilution, where deviations from Raoult's law are negligible.

Comparison of Colligative Properties—In view of the established interrelationships of the colligative properties of ideal solutions or very dilute real solutions, it is possible to predict by calculation the magnitude of all these properties of such solutions if the concentration of the nonelectrolyte solute is given; also, if the magnitude of one of the properties, say the freezing point, is known for a solution of unspecified concentration, it is possible to calculate the vapor pressure, boiling point and osmotic pressure, provided the solution is ideal or sufficiently dilute to show negligible deviation from ideality. To what upper limit of concentration a nonideal solution remains "sufficiently dilute" to show ideal behavior is difficult to specify; the answer depends at least in part on the degree of agreement expected between experimental and theoretical values. Certainly a 1-molal concentration is much too concentrated for a nonideal solution to show conformance with ideal behavior; even in 0.1-molal concentration deviations are significant and for some purposes may be excessive.

In dealing with colligative properties of solutions that do not behave ideally, caution should be exercised in attempting to predict the magnitude of other colligative properties from one that has been determined experimentally. Earlier an equation was derived for calculating the vapor pressure of a solution from its osmotic pressure, or *vice versa*, this equation being valid even with solutions showing substantial departures from ideal behavior; the equation is limited, however, to comparison of these colligative properties at the same temperature. The degree of deviation from ideal behavior for one colligative property will be exactly the same for another only when the temperature is the same for both. It does not follow that the degree of deviation of the colligative properties of a given nonideal solution will be the same for all the properties since at least two of these (freezing point and boiling point) must be determined at quite different temperatures. While in dilute solutions the intermolecular (and/or interionic) forces and interactions *may* change little over the temperature interval between freezing and boiling, in concentrated solutions the change *may* be marked. In the absence of adequate knowledge about the forces and interactions involved, only by experiment can one establish the magnitude of the colligative properties of other than very dilute nonideal solutions. It is important to keep this in mind in estimating the osmotic pressure of a nonideal solution at body temperature from a freezing point determined some 37 °C lower. While in many cases—possibly the majority of them—such an estimate is warranted by virtue of essential constancy of the various forces and interactions over a wide range of temperature, this is not always the case and the estimate may be significantly inaccurate.

Colligative Properties of Electrolyte Solutions—Earlier in this chapter attention was directed to the increased osmotic pressure observed in solutions of electrolytes, the enhanced effect being attributed to the presence of ions, each of which acts, in general, in the same way as a molecule in developing osmotic pressure. Similar magnification of vapor-pressure lowering, boiling-point elevation, and freezing-point depression occurs in solutions of electrolytes. Thus, at a given constant temperature the abnormal effect of an electrolyte on osmotic pressure is paralleled by abnormal lowering of vapor pressure; the other colligative properties are, subject to variation of effect with temperature, comparably intensified. In general the magnitude of each colligative property is proportional to the total number of particles (molecules and/or ions) in solution.

With strong electrolytes, most of which are commonly assumed to be 100% ionized, the magnitude of effect is determined primarily by the concentration of ions, which concentration may readily be calculated as the product of the molal concentration and the number of ions produced by ionization of each "molecule" (2 ions from such substances as NaCl and $MgSO_4$; 3 from $CaCl_2$ and Na_2SO_4; 4 from $FeCl_3$ and Na_3PO_4; etc). While in *very* dilute solutions the osmotic pressure, vapor-pressure lowering, boiling-point increase, and freezing-point depression of solutions of electrolytes approach values 2, 3, 4, etc times greater (depending on the type of strong electrolyte) than in solutions of the same molality of nonelectrolyte, thus confirming the hypothesis than an ion has the same primary effect as a molecule on colligative properties, two other effects are observed as the concentration of electrolyte is increased. The first effect results in *less* than 2-, 3-, or 4-fold intensification of a colligative property; this reduction is ascribed to interionic attraction between the positively and negatively charged ions, in consequence of which the ions are not completely dissociated from each other and do not exert their full effect in lowering vapor pressure, etc. This deviation generally increases with increasing concentration of electrolyte. The second effect intensifies the colligative properties and is attributed to the attraction of ions for solvent molecules (called solvation or, if water is the solvent, hydration), which holds the solvent in solution and reduces its escaping tendency, with consequent enhancement of the vapor-pressure lowering; solvation may also reduce interionic attraction and thereby further lower the vapor pressure. These factors (and possibly others) combine to effect a progressive reduction in the molal values of colligative properties as the concentration of electrolyte is increased to 0.5 to 1 molal, beyond which the molal quantities either increase, sometimes quite abruptly, or remain almost constant.

Activity and Activity Coefficient

Various mathematical expressions are employed to relate properties of chemical systems (equilibrium constants, colligative properties, pH, etc) to the stoichiometric concentration of one or more molecular, atomic, or ionic species. In deriving such expressions it is either stated or implied that they are valid only as long as intermolecular, interatomic, and/or interionic forces may be ignored or remain constant, under which restriction the system may be expected to behave ideally. But intermolecular, interatomic, and/or interionic forces do exist, and not only do they change as a result of chemical reaction but also they change with variation in the concentration or pressure of the molecules, atoms, or ions under observation. In consequence, mathematical expressions involving stoichiometric concentrations or pressures generally have limited applicability. The conventional concentration terms, while providing a count of molecules, atoms, or ions per unit volume, afford no indication of the physical or chemical activity of the species measured, and it is this activity that determines the physical and chemical properties of the system.

In recognition of this, Gilbert N. Lewis introduced both the quantitative concept and methods for evaluation of activity as a true measure of the physical or chemical activity of molecular, atomic, or ionic species, whether in the state of gas, liquid, or solid, or whether present as a single species or in a mixture. Activity

may be considered loosely as a corrected concentration or pressure which takes into account not only the stoichiometric concentration or pressure but also any intermolecular attractions or repulsions, interactions between solute and solvent in solution, association, and ionization; thus, activity measures the net effectiveness of a chemical species. Because only relative values of activity may be determined, a *standard state* must be chosen for quantitative comparisons to be made; indeed, because activity measurements are needed for many different types of systems several standard states must be selected. The specifications for all these standard states are beyond the scope of this book; they are given in Lewis and Randall, *Thermodynamics*, 2nd ed, 1961, revised by Pitzer and Brewer, McGraw-Hill. It will suffice to mention, since we are concerned mainly with solutions, that the standard state for the solvent is pure solvent, while for the solute it is a hypothetical solution with free energy corresponding to unit molality under conditions of ideal behavior of the solution.

Definitions—The relationship of activity to concentration is measured in terms of the activity coefficient, expressed as

$$m\gamma = a \qquad (44)$$

where m is the molal concentration, γ is the activity coefficient, and a is the activity. The activity coefficient may be variously determined, as by measurement of colligative properties, electromotive force, solubility, distribution coefficients, etc; procedural details are given in Lewis and Randall's work. For a strong electrolyte the *mean ionic activity coefficient*, designated $\gamma_{\pm}$, provides a measure of the deviation of the electrolyte from ideal behavior. The mean ionic activity coefficients of several strong electrolytes at various concentrations, but at constant temperature (25°C), are given in Table VII. It is characteristic of the electrolytes that the coefficients at first decrease with increasing concentration, pass through a minimum, and finally increase with increasing concentration of electrolyte. A partial interpretation of this complex behavior, is given in the preceding section. The variation of activity coefficients with temperature, for several concentrations of solutions of sodium chloride, is given in Table VIII.

Debye-Hückel Theory—In 1923 Debye and Hückel presented a theory for evaluating the activity coefficient of an ion in solution, expressed mathematically by the equation

$$-\ln \gamma_i = \frac{e^3 z_i^2}{(\epsilon kT)^{3/2}} \sqrt{\frac{2\pi N\mu}{1000}} \qquad (45)$$

where

γ_i = activity coefficient of ion species i
e = charge on an electron
z_i = valence of ion i
ϵ = dielectric constant of the medium
k = Boltzman Constant
T = absolute temperature
N = Avogadro number
μ = ionic strength = $\frac{1}{2}\Sigma m_i z_i^2$ (μ is not to be confused with dipole moment used earlier)

Transferring to 10-base logarithms, and substituting the numerical values for the constants, this equation becomes, for water at 25°C,

$$\log \gamma_i = -0.509\, z_i^2 \sqrt{\mu} \qquad (46)$$

and for the mean ionic activity coefficient

$$\log \gamma_{\pm} = -0.509\, z_+ z_- \sqrt{\mu} \qquad (47)$$

where z_+ is the valence of the cation and z_- is the valence of the anion. The significance of the ionic strength, μ, will be discussed in the next section.

The Debye-Hückel theory is a limiting law applicable to very dilute solutions of electrolytes; large deviations are encountered as the ionic strength of the solution increases. Even in dilute solutions deviations occur with electrolytes containing higher valence ions.

Ionic Strength—The usual expressions of concentration—molarity, molality, mole fraction, etc—take no cognizance of the intensity of the electrical field in a solution of a strong electrolyte, which is an important variable in evaluating interionic forces. To take this into account, Lewis and Randall in 1921 proposed its evaluation in terms of ionic strength, μ, defined mathematically as

$$\mu = \frac{1}{2} \sum m_i z_i^2 \qquad (48)$$

where m_i is the molality of ion i, z_i is its valence, and Σ is the summation of the product of molality and the square of the valence of each ion in the solution. Ionic

univalent cation and divalent anion (uni-divalent or 1–2) electrolytes, the ionic strength is in all cases three times the molality. For divalent cation and divalent anion (di-divalent or 2–2) electrolytes the ionic strength is four times the molality. These relationships are evident from the following numerical illustration.

Example—Calculate the ionic strength of 0.1-molal solutions of NaCl, Na$_2$SO$_4$, CaCl$_2$, and MgSO$_4$, respectively. For

$$NaCl \quad \mu = \frac{1}{2}(0.1 \times 1^2 + 0.1 \times 1^2) = 0.1$$
$$Na_2SO_4 \quad \mu = \frac{1}{2}(0.2 \times 1^2 + 0.1 \times 2^2) = 0.3$$
$$CaCl_2 \quad \mu = \frac{1}{2}(0.1 \times 2^2 + 0.2 \times 1^2) = 0.3$$
$$MgSO_4 \quad \mu = \frac{1}{2}(0.1 \times 2^2 + 0.1 \times 2^2) = 0.4$$

Practical Applications of Colligative Properties

One of the most important pharmaceutical applications of colligative properties is in the preparation of isotonic intravenous and isotonic lacrimal solutions, the details of which are discussed in Chapter 83.

Other applications of the colligative properties are found in experimental physiology. One such applica-

Table VII—Mean Ionic Activity Coefficients of Electrolytes at 25°C

Molality	NaCl	KCl	KBr	KI	NaOH	HCl	H$_2$SO$_4$	CaCl$_2$
0.001	0.966	0.965	0.965	0.965	...	0.966	0.830	0.89
0.002	0.953	0.952	0.952	0.951	...	0.952	0.757	0.85
0.005	0.929	0.927	0.927	0.927	...	0.928	0.639	0.79
0.01	0.904	0.901	0.903	0.905	...	0.904	0.544	0.72
0.02	0.875	...	0.872	0.88	...	0.875	0.453	0.66
0.05	0.823	0.815	0.822	0.84	0.818	0.830	0.340	0.57
0.1	0.780	0.769	0.777	0.80	0.766	0.796	0.265	0.52
0.2	0.730	0.719	0.728	0.76	0.727	0.767	0.209	0.47
0.5	0.68	0.651	0.665	0.71	0.693	0.758	0.154	0.52
1.0	0.66	0.606	0.625	0.68	0.679	0.809	0.132	0.71
2.0	0.67	0.576	0.602	0.69	0.698	1.01	0.128	0.79
4.0	0.78	0.579	0.622	0.75	0.888	1.76	0.170	2.93
6.0	0.99	...	...	...	1.28	...	0.257	11.1

Table VIII—Temperature Variation of Mean Ionic Activity Coefficients of Sodium Chloride

Molality	0°	10°	25°	40°	60°	80°	100°
0.1	0.781	0.781	0.778	0.774	0.766	0.757	0.746
0.2	0.731	0.734	0.732	0.728	0.721	0.711	0.698
0.5	0.671	0.677	0.679	0.678	0.671	0.660	0.644
1.0	0.637	0.649	0.656	0.657	0.654	0.641	0.622
2.0	0.630	0.652	0.670	0.678	0.676	0.663	0.641
3.0	0.660	0.691	0.719	0.728	0.726	0.712	0.687
4.0	0.717	0.757	0.791	0.802	1.799	0.777	0.746

strength, being a measure of the intensity of the electrical field in a solution, provides a basis for evaluating electrostatic interaction between ions. It already has been shown that the mean ionic activity coefficient is a function of ionic strength; so also are such diverse phenomena as solubilities of sparingly soluble salts (including proteins), rates of ionic reactions, effects of salts on pH of buffers, electrophoresis of proteins, etc.

The greater effectiveness of ions of higher charge type on a specific property, compared with the effectiveness of the same number of singly charged ions, generally coincides with the ionic strength calculated by Eq. 48. The variation of ionic strength with the valence (charge) of the ions comprising a strong electrolyte should be noted. For electrolytes composed of univalent cations and univalent anions, called uni-univalent or 1–1 electrolytes, the ionic strength is identical with molality. For divalent cation and univalent anion (di-univalent or 2–1) electrolytes, or

tion is in the immersion of tissues in salt solutions, which are isotonic with the fluids of the tissue, in order to prevent changes or injuries that may arise from osmosis.

The colligative properties of solutions also may be used in determining the molecular weight of solutes or, in the case of electrolytes, the extent of ionization. The method of determining molecular weight depends on the fact that each of the colligative properties is altered by a constant value when a definite number of molecules of solute is added to a solvent. For example, in dilute solutions the freezing point of water is lowered at the rate of 1.855°C for each gram molecular weight of a non-electrolyte dissolved in 1000 Gm of water.* The constant 1.855° is commonly called the *molal freezing-*

---

* These constants apply only to solutions that are considerable more dilute than 1 molal; a substantial deviation would be observed if a 1-molal solution were to be used.

point depression of water. To find the molecular weight of a nonelectrolyte, therefore, all that is necessary is to determine the freezing point of a dilute aqueous solution of known concentration of the nonelectrolyte, and, by proportion, to calculate the quantity that would produce, theoretically, a depression of 1.855 °C when 1000 Gm of water is used as solvent. If the substance is insoluble in water, it may be dissolved in another solvent, in which case, however, the freezing-point depression of a solution corresponding to a gram molecular weight of the solute in 1000 Gm of solvent will be some value other than 1.855 °C. In the case of benzene, for example, this value is 5.12 °C; for carbon tetrachloride, it is 2.98 °C; for phenol, 7.27 °C.; and for camphor, about 40°C (see *Freezing-Point Depression*, page 264).

The boiling-point elevation may be used similarly for determining molecular weights. The boiling point of water is raised at the rate of 0.52 °C for each gram molecular weight of solute dissolved in 1000 Gm of water,* the corresponding values for benzene, carbon tetrachloride, and phenol being 2.57 °, 4.88 °, and 3.60 °,

respectively. The observation of vapor-pressure lowering and osmotic pressure likewise may be used to calculate molecular weights.

To determine the extent to which an electrolyte is ionized it is necessary to know its molecular weight, as determined by some other method, and then to measure one of the four colligative properties. The deviation of the results from similar values for nonelectrolytes is then used in calculating the extent of ionization.

---

* See footnote on page 268.

References

1. Martin, A. N., *Physical Pharmacy*, Lea & Febiger, Philadelphia, 1960, p. 640.
2. Higuchi, T., in Lyman, R., *Pharmaceutical Compounding and Dispensing*, Lippincott, Philadelphia, 1949, p. 159.
3. Klevens, H. B., *Chem. Rev.*, **47**, 1 (1950).
4. Martin, A. N., *Physical Pharmacy*, Lea & Febiger, Philadelphia, 1960, p. 42.
5. Pauling, L., *Nature of the Chemical Bond*, 3rd ed., Cornell Univ. Press, Ithaca, N.Y., 1960.
6. Martin, A. N., *Physical Pharmacy*, Lea & Febiger, Philadelphia, 1960, p. 114.
7. Martin, A. N., *Physical Pharmacy*, Lea & Febiger, Philadelphia, 1960, p. 122.
8. Daniels, F., and Alberty, R. A., *Physical Chemistry*, 2nd ed., Wiley, New York, 1961.
9. Glasstone, S., *Textbook of Physical Chemistry*, Van Nostrand, New York, 1946.
10. Setnikar, I., and Temelcou, O., *J. APhA, Sci. Ed.*, **48**, 628 (1959).

20 | Ionic Solutions and Electrolytic Equilibria

Electrolytes—colligative properties—conductivity—modern theories—
acids and bases—ionization of water—pH—species concentration—
proton balance equation—calculations—buffers—determination of pH—
pharmaceutical significance

This chapter was prepared by

Paul J. Niebergall, PhD, *Associate Professor of Pharmacy, Philadelphia
College of Pharmacy and Science, Philadelphia, Pa. 19104*

Electrolytes

In the preceding chapter, attention was directed to the colligative properties of nonelectrolytes, or substances whose aqueous solutions do not conduct electricity. Substances whose aqueous solutions conduct electricity are known as electrolytes, and are typified by inorganic acids, bases, and salts. In addition to the property of electrical conductivity, solutions of electrolytes exhibit anomalous colligative properties.

Colligative Properties

In general, for nonelectrolytes, a given colligative property of two equimolal solutions will be identical. This generalization, however, cannot be made for solutions of electrolytes.

Van't Hoff pointed out that the osmotic pressure of a solution of an electrolyte is considerably greater than the osmotic pressure of a solution of a nonelectrolyte of the same molal concentration. This anomaly remained unexplained until 1887 when Arrhenius proposed a hypothesis which forms the basis for our modern theories of electrolyte solutions.

This theory postulated that when electrolytes are dissolved in water they split up into charged particles known as ions. Each of these ions carries one or more electrical charges, with the total charge on the positive ions (cations) being equal to the total charge on the negative ions (anions). Thus, although a solution may contain charged particles, it remains neutral. The increased osmotic pressure of such solutions is due to the increased number of particles formed in the process of ionization. For example, sodium chloride is assumed to dissociate as follows:

$$Na^+Cl^- \xrightarrow{\text{H}_2\text{O}} Na^+ + Cl^-$$

It is evident that each molecule of sodium chloride that is dissociated produces two ions and, if dissociation is complete, there will be twice as many particles as would be the case if it were not dissociated at all. Furthermore, if each ion has the same effect on osmotic pressure as a molecule, it might be expected that the osmotic pressure of the solution would be twice that of a solution containing the same molal concentration of a nonionizing solute.

Osmotic pressure data indicate that, in very dilute solutions of salts which yield two ions, the pressure is very nearly double that of solutions of equimolal concentrations of nonelectrolytes. Similar magnification of vapor-pressure lowering, boiling-point elevation and freezing-point depression occur in dilute solutions of electrolytes.

Van't Hoff defined a factor i as the ratio of the colligative effect produced by a concentration m of electrolyte, divided by the effect observed for the same concentration of nonelectrolyte, or

$$i = \frac{\pi}{(\pi)_0} = \frac{\Delta P}{(\Delta P)_0} = \frac{\Delta T_b}{(\Delta T_b)_0} = \frac{\Delta T_f}{(\Delta T_f)_0} \tag{1}$$

in which π, ΔP, ΔT_b, and ΔT_f refer to the osmotic pressure, vapor-pressure lowering, boiling-point elevation, and freezing-point depression, respectively, of the electrolyte. The terms $(\pi)_0$, etc refer to the nonelectrolyte of the same concentration. In general, with strong electrolytes (those assumed to be 100% ionized), the van't Hoff factor is equal to the number of ions produced when the electrolyte goes into solution (2 for NaCl and $MgSO_4$, 3 for $CaCl_2$ and Na_2SO_4, 4 for $FeCl_3$ and Na_3PO_4, etc).

In *very* dilute solutions the osmotic pressure, vapor-pressure lowering, boiling-point elevation, and freezing-point depression of solutions of electrolytes approach values 2, 3, 4, or more times greater (depending on the type of strong electrolyte) than in solutions of the same molality of nonelectrolyte, thus confirming the hypothesis that an ion has the same primary effect as a molecule on colligative properties. It bears repeating, however, that two other effects are observed as the concentration of electrolyte is increased.

The first effect results in less than 2-, 3-, or 4-fold intensification of a colligative property; this reduction is ascribed to interionic attraction between the positively and negatively charged ions, in consequence of which the ions are not completely dissociated from each other and do not exert their full effect on vapor pressure and other colligative properties. This deviation generally increases with increasing concentration of electrolyte.

The second effect intensifies the colligative properties and is attributed to the attraction of ions for solvent molecules (called solvation or, if water is the solvent, hydration), which holds the solvent in solution and reduces its escaping tendency, with consequent enhancement of the vapor-pressure lowering; solvation also reduces interionic attraction and thereby further lowers the vapor pressure.

Conductivity

The ability of metals to conduct an electric current results from mobility of electrons in the metals. This type of conductivity is called *metallic* conductance. On the other hand, various chemical compounds— notably acids, bases, and salts—conduct electricity by virtue of ions present or formed, rather than by electrons. This is called *electrolytic* conductance, and the conducting compounds are electrolytes. While the fact that certain electrolytes conduct electricity in the molten state is important, their behavior when dissolved in a solvent, particularly in water, is of greater concern in pharmaceutical science.

The electrical conductivity (or conductance) of a solution of an electrolyte is merely the reciprocal of the resistance of the solution. Hence, to measure conductivity is actually to measure electrical resistance, commonly with a Wheatstone bridge apparatus, and then to *calculate* the conductivity. Fig. 164 is a representation of the component parts of the apparatus. The solution to be measured is placed in a glass or quartz cell having two inert electrodes, commonly made of platinum or gold and coated with spongy platinum to absorb gases, across which passes an alternating current generated by an oscillator at a frequency of about 1000 cps. The reason for using alternating current is to reverse the electrolysis that occurs during flow of current and which would cause polarization of the electrodes and lead to abnormal results. The size of the electrodes and their distance apart may be varied to reduce very high resistance and increase very low resistance in order to increase the accuracy and precision of measurement; thus, solutions of high conductance (low resistance) are measured in cells having small electrodes relatively far apart while solutions of low conductance (high resistance) are measured in cells with large electrodes placed close to each other (electrolytic resistance, like metallic resistance, varies directly with the length of the conducting medium and inversely with its cross-sectional area). The known resistance required for the circuit is provided by a resistance box containing calibrated coils; the balancing of the bridge may be achieved by sliding a contact over a wire of uniform resistance until no (or minimum) current flows through the circuit, as detected either visually with a cathode-ray oscilloscope or audibly with earphones. The resistance, in ohms, is calculated by the simple procedure used in the Wheatstone bridge method; the reciprocal of this is the conductivity, the

units of which are *reciprocal ohms* (also called *mhos*). As the numerical value of the conductivity will vary with the dimensions of the conductance cell, the value must be calculated in terms of *specific conductance, L*, which is the conductance in a cell having electrodes of 1 sq cm cross-sectional area and 1 cm apart. If the dimensions of the cell used in the experiment were known, it would be possible to calculate the specific conductance. But this information is actually not required, because it is possible—and much more convenient—to calibrate a cell by measuring in it the conductivity of a standard solution of known specific conductance and then calculating a "cell constant" which, since it is a function only of the dimensions of the cell, can be used to convert all measurements in that cell to specific conductivity. Solutions of known concentration of pure potassium chloride are used as standard solutions for this purpose.

Equivalent Conductance—In studying the variation of conductance of electrolytes with dilution it is essential to make allowance for the degree of dilution in order that the comparison of conductances may be made for identical amounts of solute. This may be achieved by expressing conductance measurements in terms of *equivalent conductance, Λ*, which is obtained by multiplying the specific conductance, L, by the volume in milliliters, V_e, of solution containing 1 Gm-Eq of solute. Thus

$$\Lambda = LV_e = \frac{1000L}{C} \qquad (2)$$

where C is the concentration of electrolyte in the solution in Gm-Eq/L, ie, the normality of the solution. For example, the equivalent conductance of 0.01 N potassium chloride solution, which has a specific conductance of 0.001413 mho/cm may be calculated in either of the following ways:

$$\Lambda = 0.001413 \times 100,000 = 141.3 \text{ mho cm}^2/\text{Eq}$$

or

$$\Lambda = \frac{1000 \times 0.001413}{0.01} = 141.3$$

Strong and Weak Electrolytes—It is customary to classify electrolytes broadly as *strong electrolytes* and *weak electrolytes*. The former category includes solutions of strong acids, strong bases, and most salts; the latter includes weak acids and bases, primarily organic acids and amines, and a few salts. The usual criterion for distinguishing between strong and weak electrolytes is the extent of ionization; thus, an electrolyte existing entirely or very largely as ions is considered a strong electrolyte, while one that is a mixture of a substantial proportion of molecular species along with ions derived therefrom is a weak electrolyte. For the purposes of this discussion, classification of electrolytes as strong or weak will be on the basis of certain conductance characteristics exhibited in aqueous solution.

The equivalent conductances of a number of electrolytes, at different concentrations, are given in Table I and for certain of these electrolytes again in Fig. 165, where the equivalent conductance is plotted against the square root of concentration. By plotting the data in this manner a linear relationship is observed for strong electrolytes, while a steeply rising curve is noted for weak electrolytes; this difference is a characteristic which distinguishes strong and weak electrolytes. The interpretation of the steep rise in the

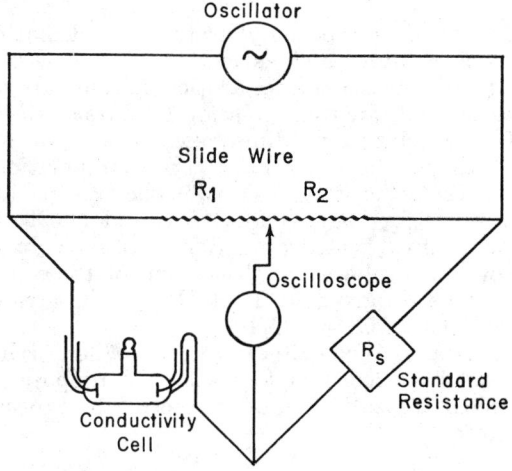

Fig. 164. Alternating current Wheatstone bridge for measuring conductivity.

Table I—Equivalent Conductances at 25°C

Gm-Eq/L	HCl	HAc	NaCl	KCl	NaI	KI	NaAc
Inf. dil.	426.1	390.6[a]	126.5	149.9	126.9	150.3	91.0
0.0005	422.7	67.7	124.5	147.8	125.4	...	89.2
0.001	421.4	49.2	123.7	146.9	124.3	...	88.5
0.005	415.8	22.9	120.6	143.5	121.3	144.4	85.7
0.01	412.0	16.3	118.5	141.3	119.2	142.2	83.8
0.02	407.2	11.6	115.8	138.3	116.7	139.5	81.2
0.05	399.1	7.4	111.1	133.4	112.8	135.0	76.9
0.1	391.3	5.2	106.7	129.0	108.8	131.1	72.8

[a] The equivalent conductance at infinite dilution for acetic acid, a weak electrolyte, was obtained by adding the equivalent conductances of hydrochloric acid and sodium acetate and subtracting that of sodium chloride (see text for explanation).

equivalent conductance of weak electrolytes is that the degree of ionization increases with dilution, becoming complete at infinite dilution; interionic interference effects generally have a minor role in the conductivity of weak electrolytes. With strong electrolytes, which usually are completely ionized, the increase in equivalent conductance results not from increased ionization but rather from diminished ionic interference as the solution is diluted, in consequence of which ions have greater freedom of mobility, ie, increased conductance.

The value of the equivalent conductance extrapolated to infinite dilution (zero concentration), designated by the symbol Λ_0, has special significance. It represents the equivalent conductance of the completely ionized electrolyte when the ions are so far apart that there is no interference with their migration due to interionic interactions. It has been shown, by Kohlrausch, that the equivalent conductance of an electrolyte at infinite dilution is the sum of the equivalent conductances of its component ions at infinite dilution, expressed symbolically as

$$\Lambda_0 = l_0(\text{cation}) + l_0(\text{anion}) \qquad (3)$$

The significance of Kohlrausch's law is that each ion, at infinite dilution, has a characteristic value of conductance that is independent of the conductance of the oppositely charged ion with which it is associated. Thus, if the equivalent conductances of various ions are known, the conductance of any electrolyte may be calculated simply by adding the appropriate ionic conductances. Since the fraction of current carried by cations (*transference number* of the cations) and by anions (transference number of anions) in an electrolyte may be determined readily by experiment, ionic conductances are known. Table II gives the equivalent ionic conductances at infinite dilution of some cations and anions. But it is not necessary to have this information in order to calculate the equivalent conductance of an electrolyte, for Kohlrausch's law permits the latter to be calculated by adding and subtracting values of Λ_0 for appropriate electrolytes. For example, the Λ_0 for acetic acid may be calculated as follows:

$$\Lambda_0(\text{CH}_3\text{COOH}) = \Lambda_0(\text{HCl}) + \Lambda_0(\text{CH}_3\text{COONa}) - \Lambda_0(\text{NaCl})$$

which is equivalent to

$$l_0(\text{H}^+) + l_0(\text{CH}_3\text{COO}^-) = l_0(\text{H}^+) + l_0(\text{Cl}^-) + l_0(\text{Na}^+) + l_0(\text{CH}_3\text{COO}^-) - l_0(\text{Na}^+) - l_0(\text{Cl}^-)$$

This method is especially useful for calculating Λ_0 for weak electrolytes such as acetic acid. As is evident from Fig. 165, the Λ_0 value for acetic acid cannot be determined accurately by extrapolation because of the steep rise of conductance in dilute solutions. For strong electrolytes, on the other hand, the extrapolation can be made very accurately. Thus, in the example above, the Λ_0 values for HCl, CH$_3$COONa and NaCl are all easily determined by extrapolation since the substances are strong electrolytes. Substitution of these extrapolated values, as given in Table II, yields a value of 390.6 for the Λ_0 of CH$_3$COOH.

Ionization of Weak Electrolytes—When Arrhenius introduced his theory of ionization he proposed that the degree of ionization, α, of an electrolyte is measured by the ratio

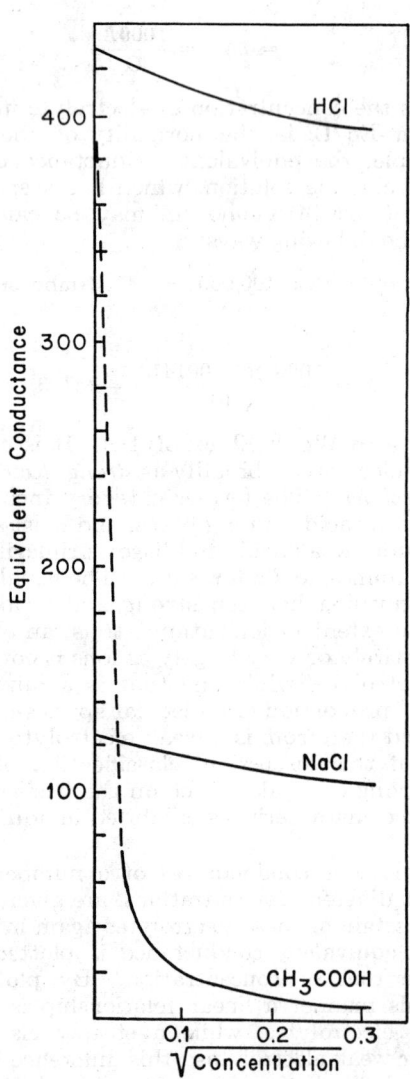

Fig. 165. **Variation of equivalent conductance with square root of concentration.**

$$\alpha = \frac{\Lambda}{\Lambda_0} \qquad (4)$$

where Λ is the equivalent conductance of the electrolyte at any specified concentration of solution and Λ_0 is the equivalent conductance at infinite dilution. As strong electrolytes were not then recognized as being 100% ionized, and interionic interference effects had not been evaluated, he believed the equation to be applicable to both strong and weak electrolytes. Since we now know that apparent variation of ionization of strong electrolytes arises from change of mobility of ions at different concentrations rather than from varying ionization, the equation is not applicable to strong electrolytes; it does provide, however, a generally acceptable approximation of the degree of ionization of weak electrolytes, for which deviations resulting from neglect of activity coefficients and of some change of ionic mobilities with concentration are for most purposes negligible. The following example illustrates the use of the equation to calculate the degree of ionization of a typical weak electrolyte.

Example—Calculate the degree of ionization of $1 \times 10^{-3} N$ acetic acid, the equivalent conductance of which is 48.15 mho cm²/Eq. The equivalent conductance at infinite dilution is 390.6 mho cm²/Eq.

$$\alpha = \frac{48.15}{390.6} = 0.12$$

$$\% \text{ ionization} = 100\alpha = 12\%$$

The degree of dissociation can also be calculated using the van't Hoff factor, i, and the following equation:

$$\alpha = \frac{i-1}{v-1} \tag{5}$$

where v is the number of ions into which the electrolyte dissociates.

Example—A $1.0 \times 10^{-3} N$ solution of acetic acid has a van't Hoff factor equal to 1.12. Calculate the degree of dissociation of the acid at this concentration.

$$\alpha = \frac{i-1}{v-1} = \frac{1.12-1}{2-1} = 0.12$$

This result agrees with that obtained using equivalent conductance and Eq. 4.

Modern Theories

The Arrhenius theory explains why solutions of electrolytes conduct electricity, why they exhibit enhanced colligative properties, and is essentially satisfactory for solutions of weak electrolytes. Several deficiencies, however, do exist when it is applied to solutions of strong electrolytes: it does not explain the failure of strong electrolytes to follow the law of mass action as applied to ionization; discrepancies exist between the degree of ionization calculated from the van't Hoff factor and the conductivity ratio for strong electrolyte solutions having concentrations greater than about 0.5 M.

Table II—Equivalent Ionic Conductivities at Infinite Dilution, at 25°

Cations	l_0	Anions	l_0
H^+	349.8	OH^-	198.0
Li^+	38.7	Cl^-	76.3
Na^+	50.1	Br^-	78.4
K^+	73.5	I^-	76.8
NH_4^+	61.9	Ac^-	40.9
$\frac{1}{2}Ca^{++}$	59.5	$\frac{1}{2}SO_4^-$	79.8
$\frac{1}{2}Mg^{++}$	53.0		

These deficiencies can be explained by the following observations:

1. When molten, strong electrolytes are excellent conductors of electricity. This suggests that these materials are already ionized in the crystalline state. Further support for this is given by x-ray studies of crystals, which indicate that the units comprising the basic lattice structure of strong electrolytes are ions.

2. Arrhenius neglected the fact that ions in solution, being oppositely charged, tend to associate through electrostatic attraction. In solutions of weak electrolytes, the number of ions is not large and it is not surprising that electrostatic attractions do not cause appreciable deviations from theory. In dilute solutions, in which strong electrolytes are assumed to be 100% ionized, the number of ions is large, and interionic attractions become major factors in determining the chemical properties of these solutions. These effects should, and do become more pronounced as the concentration of electrolyte or the valence of the ions is increased.

It is not surprising, therefore, that the Arrhenius theory of partial ionization involving the law of mass action and neglecting ionic charge does not hold for solutions of strong electrolytes. Neutral molecules of strong electrolytes, if they do exist in solution, must arise from interionic attraction rather than from incomplete ionization.

Activity—The significance of activity in relation to electrolytes is treated in Chapter 19, page 267.

Activity Coefficients—The relationship between activity and concentration can be expressed as

$$a = m\gamma \tag{6}$$

where m is the molal concentration, γ is the activity coefficient, and a is the activity. The activity also can be expressed in terms of molar concentration, c, as

$$a = fc \tag{7}$$

where f is the activity coefficient on a molar scale. In dilute solutions (below 0.01 M) the two activity coefficients are identical for all practical purposes.

The activity coefficient may be determined in various ways, such as measurement of colligative properties, electromotive force, solubility, distribution coefficients, etc. For a strong electrolyte, the mean ionic activity coefficient, $\gamma_\pm$ or $f_\pm$, provides a measure of the deviation of the electrolyte from ideal behavior. The mean ionic activity coefficients on a molal basis for several strong electrolytes are given in Table VII, page 268. It is characteristic of the electrolytes that the coefficients at first decrease with increasing concentration, pass through a minimum, and finally increase with increasing concentration of electrolyte. A partial explanation of this complex behavior, which still is incompletely understood, is given in the preceding chapter.

Ionic Strength—As noted in the preceding chapter, the concept of ionic strength, μ, which is a measure of the intensity of the electrical field in a solution, provides a basis for evaluating electrostatic interactions between ions. Ionic strength may be expressed as

$$\mu = \frac{1}{2}\sum c_i z_i^2 \tag{8}$$

where z_1 is the valence of ion i. The mean ionic activity coefficient is a function of ionic strength; so also are such diverse phenomena as solubilities of sparingly soluble substances, rates of ionic reactions, effects of salts on pH of buffers, electrophoresis of proteins, etc.

The greater effectiveness of ions of higher charge type on a specific property, compared with the effectiveness of the same number of singly charged ions, generally coincides with the ionic strength calculated by Eq. 8. The variation of ionic strength with the

Table III—Values of Some Salting-Out Constants for Various Barbiturates at 25°[a]

Barbiturate	KCl	KBr	NaCl	NaBr
Amobarbital	0.168	0.095	0.212	0.143
Aprobarbital	0.136	0.062	0.184	0.120
Barbital	0.092	0.042	0.136	0.088
Phenobarbital	0.092	0.034	0.132	0.078
Vinbarbital	0.125	0.036	0.143	0.096

[a] From Sedam *et al.*[1]

valence (charge) of the ions comprising a strong electrolyte should be noted.

For electrolytes composed of univalent cations and univalent anions (called univalent or 1–1 electrolytes), the ionic strength is identical with molarity. For divalent cation and univalent anion(di-univalent or 2–1) electrolytes, or univalent cation and divalent anion(uni-divalent or 1–2) electrolytes, the ionic strength is three times the molarity. For divalent cation and divalent anion (di-divalent or 2–2) electrolytes, the ionic strength is four times the molarity. These relationships are evident from the following example.

Example—Calculate the ionic strength of 0.1 molar solutions of NaCl, Na$_2$SO$_4$, MgCl$_2$, and MgSO$_4$, respectively. For

$$NaCl \quad \mu = \tfrac{1}{2}\,(0.1 \times 1^2 + 0.1 \times 1^2) = 0.1$$

$$Na_2SO_4 \quad \mu = \tfrac{1}{2}\,(0.2 \times 1^2 + 0.1 \times 2^2) = 0.3$$

$$MgCl_2 \quad \mu = \tfrac{1}{2}\,(0.1 \times 2^2 + 0.2 \times 1^2) = 0.3$$

$$MgSO_4 \quad \mu = \tfrac{1}{2}\,(0.1 \times 2^2 + 0.1 \times 2^2) = 0.4$$

The ionic strength of a solution containing more than one electrolyte is the sum of the ionic strengths of the individual salts comprising the solution. For example, the ionic strength of a solution containing NaCl, Na$_2$SO$_4$, MgCl$_2$ and MgSO$_4$, each at a concentration of 0.1 M would be 1.1.

Debye–Hückel Theory—The Debye-Hückel equations on page 267, applicable only to very dilute solutions (about 0.02 μ), may be extended to somewhat more concentrated solutions (about 0.1 μ) in the simplified form:

$$\log f_i = \frac{-0.51\,z_i^2\sqrt{\mu}}{1 + \sqrt{\mu}} \qquad (9)$$

The mean ionic activity coefficient for aqueous solutions of electrolytes at 25° can be expressed as

$$\log f_\pm = \frac{-0.51\,z_+z_-\sqrt{\mu}}{1 + \sqrt{\mu}} \qquad (10)$$

in which z_+ is the valence of the cation and z_- is the valence of the anion. When the ionic strength of the solution becomes high (approximately 0.3 to 0.5 μ), these equations become inadequate and a linear term in μ is added. This is illustrated for the mean ionic activity coefficient:

$$\log f_\pm = \frac{-0.51\,z_+z_-\sqrt{\mu}}{1 + \sqrt{\mu}} + K_s\mu \qquad (11)$$

in which K_s is a "salting out" constant empirically chosen for each salt. This equation is valid for solutions with ionic strength up to approximately 1.

Salting-Out Effect—The aqueous solubility of a slightly soluble organic substance generally is affected markedly by the addition of an electrolyte. This effect is particularly noticeable when the electrolyte concentration reaches 0.5 M or higher. If the aqueous solution of the organic substance has a dielectric con-

stant lower than that of pure water, its solubility is decreased and the substance is "salted out." The use of high concentrations of electrolytes such as ammonium sulfate or sodium sulfate for the separation of proteins by differential precipitation is perhaps the most striking example of this effect. The aqueous solutions of a few substances such as hydrocyanic acid, glycine, and cystine have a higher dielectric constant than that of pure water, and these substances are "salted in." These phenomena can be expressed empirically as

$$\log S = \log S_0 \pm K_s m \qquad (12)$$

in which S_0 represents the solubility of the organic substance in pure water and S is the solubility in the electrolyte solution. The slope of the straight line obtained by plotting $\log S$ vs m is positive for "salting in" and negative for "salting out." In terms of ionic strength this equation becomes

$$\log S = \log S_0 \pm K_s'\mu \qquad (13)$$

where $K_s' = K_s$ for univalent salts; $K_s' = K_s/3$ for uni-bivalent salts; and $K_s' = K_2/4$ for bivalent salts. The "salting out" constant depends on temperature as well as the nature of both the organic substance and the electrolyte. The effect of electrolyte and of the organic substance can be seen in Table III.[1] In all instances, if the anion is constant, the sodium cation has a greater "salting out" effect than the potassium cation, probably due to the higher charge density of the former. Although the reasoning is less clear, it appears that for a constant cation, chloride anion has a greater effect than bromide anion upon the "salting out" phenomenon.

Acids and Bases

Arrhenius defined an acid as a substance that yields hydrogen ions in aqueous solution and a base as a substance that yields hydroxyl ions in aqueous solution. Except for the fact that hydrogen ions neutralize hydroxyl ions to form water, no complementary relationship between acids and bases (such as that between oxidants and reductants, for example) is evident in Arrhenius' definitions for these substances; rather, their oppositeness of character is emphasized. Moreover, no account is taken of the behavior of acids and bases in nonaqueous solvents. Also, while acidity is associated with so elementary a particle as the proton (hydrogen ion), basicity is attributed to so relatively complex an association of atoms as the hydroxyl ion. It would seem that a simpler concept of a base could be devised.

Proton Concept of Acids and Bases—In pondering the objections to Arrhenius' definitions, Brønsted and Bjerrum in Denmark and Lowry in England developed and in 1923 announced a more satisfactory, and more general, theory of acids and bases. According to this theory an acid is a substance capable of yielding a proton (hydrogen ion), while a base is a substance capable of accepting a proton. This complementary relationship may be expressed by the general equation

$$A \rightleftharpoons H^+ + B$$
$$\text{acid} \qquad \text{base}$$

The pair of substances thus related through mutual ability to gain or lose a proton is called a *conjugate acid–base pair*. Specific examples of such pairs are

Acid		Base
$HCl \rightleftharpoons H^+ + Cl^-$		
$CH_3COOH \rightleftharpoons H^+ + CH_3COO^-$		
$NH_4^+ \rightleftharpoons H^+ + NH_3$		
$HCO_3^- \rightleftharpoons H^+ + CO_3^-$		
$H_2PO_4^- \rightleftharpoons H^+ + HPO_4^-$		
$H_2O \rightleftharpoons H^+ + OH^-$		
$H_3O^+ \rightleftharpoons H^+ + H_2O$		
$Al(H_2O)_6^{+++} \rightleftharpoons H^+ + Al(H_2O)_5OH^{++}$		

It is apparent that not only molecules but also cations and anions may function as acids or bases.

The complementary nature of the acid–base pairs listed is reminiscent of the complementary relationship of pairs of oxidants and reductants where, however, the ability to gain or lose one or more electrons—rather than protons—is the distinguishing characteristic.

Oxidant		Reductant
$Fe^{+++} + e^- \rightleftharpoons Fe^{++}$		
$Na^+ + e^- \rightleftharpoons Na$		
$\frac{1}{2}I_2 + e^- \rightleftharpoons I^-$		

These examples of acid–base pairs and oxidant–reductant pairs represent, however, reactions that are possible in principle only. Ordinarily acids will not release free protons any more than reductants will release free electrons; both protons and electrons, respectively, can only be *transferred* from one substance (an ion, atom, or molecule) to another. Thus, it is a fundamental fact of chemistry that oxidation of one substance will occur only if reduction of another substance occurs simultaneously. Stated in another way, electrons will be released from the reductant (oxidation) only if an oxidant capable of accepting electrons (reduction) is present. For this reason oxidation–reduction reactions must involve two conjugate oxidant–reductant pairs of substances:

$$oxidant_1 + reductant_2 \rightleftharpoons reductant_1 + oxidant_2$$

where subscript 1 represents one conjugate oxidant–reductant pair and subscript 2 represents the other.

Similarly, an acid will not release a proton unless a base capable of accepting it is simultaneously present; this means that any actual manifestation of acid–base behavior must involve interaction between two sets of conjugate acid–base pairs, represented as:

$$A_1 + B_2 \rightleftharpoons B_1 + A_2$$
$$\text{acid}_1 \quad \text{base}_2 \quad \text{base}_1 \quad \text{acid}_2$$

In such a reaction, which is called *protolysis* or a *protolytic reaction*, A_1 and B_1 constitute one conjugate acid–base pair and A_2 and B_2 the other; the proton given up by A_1 (which thereby becomes B_1) is transferred to B_2 (which becomes A_2).

When an acid, such as hydrochloric, is dissolved in water, a protolytic reaction occurs

$$HCl + H_2O \rightleftharpoons Cl^- + H_3O^+$$
$$\text{acid}_1 \quad \text{base}_2 \quad \text{base}_1 \quad \text{acid}_2$$

The ionic species H_3O^+, called *hydronium* or *oxonium* ion, is always formed when an acid is dissolved in water; very often, for purposes of convenience, this is written simply as H^+ and is called hydrogen ion, although the "bare" ion is practically nonexistent in solution.

When a base, eg, ammonia, is dissolved in water the reaction of protolysis is as follows:

$$NH_3 + H_2O \rightleftharpoons NH_4^+ + OH^-$$
$$\text{base}_1 \quad \text{acid}_2 \quad \text{acid}_1 \quad \text{base}_2$$

The proton theory of acid–base function makes the concept of hydrolysis superfluous. When, for example, sodium acetate is dissolved in water, this acid–base interaction occurs.

$$CH_3COO^- + H_2O \rightleftharpoons CH_3COOH + OH^-$$
$$\text{base}_1 \quad \text{acid}_2 \quad \text{acid}_1 \quad \text{base}_2$$

In an aqueous solution of ammonium chloride the reaction is

$$NH_4^+ + H_2O \rightleftharpoons NH_3 + H_3O^+$$
$$\text{acid}_1 \quad \text{base}_2 \quad \text{base}_1 \quad \text{acid}_2$$

Transfer of protons (protolysis) is not limited to dissimilar conjugate acid–base pairs. In the preceding examples H_2O sometimes behaves as an acid and at other times as a base; such an amphoteric substance is called, in Brønsted's terminology, an *amphiprotic substance*.

Electron Pair Concept of Acids and Bases— While the proton concept of acids and bases provides a more general definition for these substances, it does not indicate what the basic reason is for proton transfer, nor does it explain how such substances as sulfur trioxide, boron trichloride, stannic chloride, and carbon dioxide—none of which is capable of donating a proton— can behave as acids. Both deficiencies of the proton theory are avoided in the more inclusive definition of acids and bases proposed by Lewis in 1923. According to Lewis, who in 1916 proposed that sharing of a pair of electrons by two atoms established a bond (covalent) between the atoms, an acid is a substance capable of sharing a pair of electrons made available by another substance called a base, thereby forming a coordinate covalent bond. The base is the substance that donates a share in its electron pair to the acid. The following equation illustrates how Lewis' definitions explain the transfer of a proton (hydrogen ion) to ammonia to form ammonium ion

$$H^+ + \ddot{:}\!N\!:\!H \rightarrow \left[H\!:\!\overset{H}{\underset{H}{\ddot{N}}}\!:\!H \right]^+$$

The reaction of boron trichloride, which according to the Lewis theory is an acid, with ammonia is similar, for the boron lacks an electron pair if it is to attain a stable octet configuration, while ammonia has a pair of electrons which may be shared, thus

$$\overset{Cl}{\underset{Cl}{Cl\!:\!B}} + \ddot{:}\!N\!:\!H \rightarrow \overset{Cl}{\underset{Cl}{Cl\!:\!B}}\!:\!\overset{H}{\underset{H}{\ddot{N}}}\!:\!H$$

Leveling Effect of a Solvent—When the strong acids $HClO_4$, H_2SO_4, HCl, and HNO_3 are dissolved in water the solutions—if they are of identical normality and are not too concentrated—all have about the same hydrogen ion concentration, indicating the acids to be of about the same strength. The reason for this is that each one of the acids undergoes practically complete protolysis in water.

$$HCl + H_2O \rightarrow Cl^- + H_3O^+$$
$$\text{acid}_1 \quad \text{base}_2 \quad \text{base}_1 \quad \text{acid}_2$$

This phenomenon, called the leveling effect of water, occurs whenever the added acid is stronger than hydronium ion; such a reaction manifests the tendency of proton transfer reactions to proceed spontaneously in the direction of forming weaker acid and weaker base.

Since the strongest acid that can exist in an amphiprotic solvent is the conjugate acid form of the solvent, any stronger acid will undergo protolysis to the weaker solvent acid. Since $HClO_4$, H_2SO_4, HCl, and HNO_3 are all stronger acids than hydronium ion, they are converted in water to hydronium ion.

When the strong bases sodium hydride, sodium amide, and sodium ethoxide are dissolved in water, each reacts with water to form sodium hydroxide; these reactions illustrate the leveling effect of water on bases. Since hydroxide ion is the strongest base that can exist in water, any base stronger than hydroxide undergoes protolysis to hydroxide.

Intrinsic differences in the acidity of acids become evident if they are dissolved in a relatively poor proton acceptor such as anhydrous acetic acid. Perchloric acid ($HClO_4$), a strong acid, undergoes practically complete reaction with acetic acid

$$HClO_4 + CH_3COOH \rightarrow ClO_4^- + CH_3COOH_2^+$$

| acid$_1$ | base$_2$ | base$_1$ | acid$_2$ |
| (strong) | (strong) | (weak) | (weak) |

but sulfuric acid and hydrochloric acid behave as weak acids. It is because perchloric acid is a very strong acid when dissolved in glacial acetic acid that it has found many important applications in analytical chemistry as a titrant for a variety of substances which behave as bases in acetic acid (see *Titrimetric Assays Utilizing Nonaqueous Solvents* in the chapter on *Analysis of Medicinals*). Because of its ability to differentiate acidity of different acids, it is called a *differentiating solvent for acids*, this property resulting from its relatively weak proton-acceptor tendency. A solvent that differentiates basicity of different bases must have weak proton-donor tendency; it is called a *differentiating solvent for bases*. Typical of solvents in this category is liquid ammonia. Solvents that have both weak proton-donor and proton-acceptor tendencies are called *aprotic solvents* and may serve as differentiating solvents for both acids and bases; they have little if any action on solutes and serve mainly as inert dispersion media for the solutes. Useful aprotic solvents are benzene, toluene, and hexane.

Strength of Acids and Bases—Acids and bases are commonly classified as strong or weak acids and strong or weak bases according as they are extensively or slightly ionized in aqueous solutions. If, for example, 1 N aqueous solutions of hydrochloric acid and acetic acid are compared, it is found that the former is a better conductor of electricity, reacts much more readily with metals, catalyzes certain reactions more efficiently, and possesses a more acid taste than the latter. Both solutions, however, will neutralize identical amounts of alkali. A similar comparison of 1 N solutions of sodium hydroxide and ammonia reveals the former to be more "active" than the latter, although both solutions will neutralize identical quantities of acid.

The differences in the properties of the two acids is attributed to differences in the concentration of hydrogen (more accurately hydronium) ion, the hydrochloric acid being ionized to a greater extent and therefore containing a higher concentration of hydrogen ion than acetic acid. Similarly, most of the differences between the sodium hydroxide and ammonia solutions are attributed to the higher hydroxyl-ion concentration in the former.

The ionization of incompletely ionized acids may be considered a reversible reaction of the type

$$HA \rightleftharpoons H^+ + A^-$$

where HA is the molecular acid and A^- is its anion. An equilibrium expression based on the law of mass action may be applied to the reaction, thus

$$\frac{[H^+][A^-]}{[HA]} = K_a \tag{14}$$

where K_a is the ionization or dissociation constant, and the brackets signify concentration. For any given acid in any specified solvent and at any constant temperature, K_a remains relatively constant as the concentration of acid is varied, provided the acid is weakly ionized; with increasingly stronger acids, however, progressively larger deviations occur.

Although the strength of an acid is commonly measured in terms of the ionization or dissociation constant defined in Eq. 14, the process of ionization is probably never as simple as shown above. A proton simply will not detach itself from one molecule unless it is simultaneously accepted by another molecule. When an acid is dissolved in water, the latter acts as a base, accepting a proton (Brønsted's definition of a base) by donating a share in a pair of electrons (Lewis' definition of a base). This reaction may be written

$$HA + H_2O \rightleftharpoons A^- + H_3O^+$$

acid$_1$ base$_2$ base$_1$ acid$_2$

Application of the law of mass action to this reaction gives

$$\frac{[H_3O^+][A^-]}{[HA][H_2O]} = K \tag{15}$$

since $[H_2O]$ is a constant this equation may be written

$$\frac{[H_3O^+][A^-]}{[HA]} = K_a \tag{16}$$

This equation is identical with Eq. 14 because $[H_3O^+]$ is numerically equal to $[H^+]$.

Acids which are capable of donating more than one proton are termed polyprotic. The ionization of a polyprotic acid occurs in stages and can be illustrated by considering the equilibria involved in the ionization of phosphoric acid:

$$H_3PO_4 + H_2O \rightleftharpoons H_2PO_4^{-1} + H_3O^+$$
$$H_2PO_4^{-1} + H_2O \rightleftharpoons HPO_4^{-2} + H_3O^+$$
$$HPO_4^{-2} + H_2O \rightleftharpoons PO_4^{-3} + H_3O^+$$

Application of the law of mass action to this series of reactions gives

$$K_1 = \frac{[H_2PO_4^{-1}][H_3O^+]}{[H_3PO_4]} \tag{17}$$

$$K_2 = \frac{[HPO_4^{-2}][H_3O^+]}{[H_2PO_4^{-1}]} \tag{18}$$

$$K_3 = \frac{[PO_4^{-3}][H_3O^+]}{[HPO_4^{-2}]} \tag{19}$$

If the three expressions for the ionization constants are multiplied together, an over-all ionization, K, can be obtained:

$$K = K_1 K_2 K_3 = \frac{[PO_4^{-3}][H_3O^+]^3}{[H_3PO_4]} \tag{20}$$

Each of the successive ionizations is supressed by the hydronium ion formed from preceding stages according to Le Chatelier's principle. The successive dissociation constants always decrease in value, since successive protons must be removed from species that are always more negatively charged. This can be seen from the data in Table IV, in which K_1 for phosphoric

Table IV—Dissociation Constants in Water at 25°

Substance		K
Weak Acids		
Acetic		1.75×10^{-5}
Acetylsalicylic		3.27×10^{-4}
Barbital		1.23×10^{-8}
Barbituric		1.05×10^{-4}
Benzoic		6.30×10^{-5}
Benzyl penicillin		1.74×10^{-3}
Boric	K_1	5.8×10^{-10}
Caffeine		1×10^{-14}
Carbonic	K_1	4.31×10^{-7}
	K_2	4.7×10^{-11}
Citric ($1 . H_2O$)	K_1	7.0×10^{-4}
	K_2	1.8×10^{-5}
	K_3	4.0×10^{-7}
Dichloracetic		5×10^{-2}
Ethylenediaminetetra	K_1	1×10^{-2}
acetic acid (EDTA)	K_2	2.14×10^{-3}
	K_3	6.92×10^{-7}
	K_4	5.5×10^{-11}
Formic		1.77×10^{-4}
Glycerophosphoric	K_1	3.4×10^{-2}
	K_2	6.4×10^{-7}
Glycine	K_1	4.5×10^{-3}
	K_2	1.7×10^{-10}
Lactic		1.39×10^{-4}
Mandelic		4.29×10^{-4}
Monochloracetic		1.4×10^{-3}
Oxalic ($2 . H_2O$)	K_1	5.5×10^{-2}
	K_2	5.3×10^{-5}
Phenobarbital		3.9×10^{-8}
Phenol		1×10^{-10}
Phosphoric	K_1	7.5×10^{-3}
	K_2	6.2×10^{-8}
	K_3	2.1×10^{-13}
Picric		4.2×10^{-1}
Propionic		1.34×10^{-5}
Saccharin		2.5×10^{-2}
Salicylic		1.06×10^{-3}
Succinic	K_1	6.4×10^{-5}
	K_2	2.3×10^{-6}
Sulfadiazine		3.3×10^{-7}
Sulfamerazine		8.7×10^{-8}
Sulfapyridine		3.6×10^{-9}
Sulfathiazole		7.6×10^{-8}
Tartaric	K_1	9.6×10^{-4}
	K_2	4.4×10^{-5}
Weak Bases		
Acetanilid		4.1×10^{-14} (40°)
Ammonia		1.74×10^{-5}
Apomorphine		1.0×10^{-7}
Atropine		4.5×10^{-5}
Benzocaine		6.0×10^{-12}
Caffeine		4.1×10^{-14} (40°)
Cocaine		2.6×10^{-6}
Codeine		9×10^{-7}
Ephedrine		2.3×10^{-5}
Morphine		7.4×10^{-7}
Papaverine		8×10^{-9}
Physostigmine	K_1	7.6×10^{-7}
	K_2	5.7×10^{-13}
Pilocarpine	K_1	7×10^{-8}
	K_2	2×10^{-13}
Procaine		7×10^{-6}
Pyridine		1.4×10^{-9}
Quinine	K_1	1.0×10^{-6}
	K_2	1.3×10^{-10}
Reserpine		4×10^{-8}
Strychnine	K_1	1×10^{-6}
	K_2	2×10^{-12}
Theobromine		4.8×10^{-14} (40°)
Thiourea		1.1×10^{-15}
Urea		1.5×10^{-14}

acid is approximately 100,000 times greater than K_2, which is in turn approximately 100,000 times greater than K_3. Although successive dissociation constants are always smaller, the difference is not always as great as it is for phosphoric acid. Tartaric acid, for example, has $K_1 = 9.12 \times 10^{-4}$ and $K_2 = 4.27 \times 10^{-5}$.

Ionization of a base is best illustrated by using the specific substance NH_3 for an example. Formerly it was customary to explain that NH_3 dissolved in water to form NH_4OH, which underwent ionization

$$NH_4OH \rightleftharpoons NH_4^+ + OH^-$$

The law of mass action was applied to this reaction, thus

$$\frac{[NH_4^+][OH^-]}{[NH_4OH]} = K_b \qquad (21)$$

where K_b is the ionization or dissociation constant of the base. According to Brønsted and Lewis, however, when the base NH_3 is dissolved in water, the latter acts as an acid, donating a proton to NH_3, which accepts it by offering a share in a pair of electrons on the nitrogen atom. This reaction is written

$$\underset{\text{base}}{NH_3} + \underset{\text{acid}}{H_2O} \rightleftharpoons NH_4^+ + OH^-$$

The equilibrium expression for this reaction is

$$\frac{[NH_4^+][OH^-]}{[NH_3][H_2O]} = K \qquad (22)$$

with $[H_2O]$ constant this expression may be written

$$\frac{[NH_4^+][OH^-]}{[NH_3]} = K_b \qquad (23)$$

which is identical with Eq. 21 since $[NH_3]$ is numerically identical with $[NH_4OH]$.

A particularly interesting and useful relationship between the strength of an acid and its conjugate base, or a base and its conjugate acid, exists. For illustration, consider the strength of the base NH_3 and its conjugate acid NH_4^+, in water. The behavior of NH_3 as a base is expressed by

$$NH_3 + H_2O \rightleftharpoons NH_4^+ + OH^-$$

for which the equilibrium, as formulated earlier, is

$$\frac{[NH_4^+][OH^-]}{[NH_3]} = K_b \qquad (24)$$

The behavior of NH_4^+ as an acid is represented by

$$NH_4^+ + H_2O \rightleftharpoons NH_3 + H_3O^+$$

the equilibrium constant for which is

$$\frac{[NH_3][H_3O^+]}{[NH_4^+]} = K_a \qquad (25)$$

Multiplying Eqs. 24 and 25:

$$\frac{[NH_3][H_3O^+][NH_4^+][OH^-]}{[NH_4^+][NH_3]} = K_a . K_b \qquad (26)$$

It is obvious that the product

$$K_a . K_b = K_w \qquad (27)$$

where K_w is the ion product of water as defined in Eq. 35.

The utility of this relationship, which is a general one for any conjugate acid–base pair, is evident from the following deductions: (1) the strength of an acid may be expressed in terms either of K_a or of K_b of its conjugate base, and *vice versa;* (2) the K_a of an acid may be calculated if the K_b of its conjugate base is known, and *vice versa;* (3) the stronger an acid is, the weaker its conjugate base, and *vice versa.*

Bases which are capable of interacting with more than one proton are termed polyacidic, and can be illustrated by the following:

$$PO_4^{-3} + H_2O \rightleftharpoons HPO_4^{-2} + OH^-$$

$$HPO_4^{-2} + H_2O \rightleftharpoons H_2PO_4^{-1} + OH^-$$

$$H_2PO_4^{-1} + H_2O \rightleftharpoons H_3PO_4 + OH^-$$

Applying the law of mass action to this series of reactions, and utilizing the concepts outlined in Eqs. 24–27, it becomes obvious that the relationship between the various K_a and K_b values for phosphoric acid are

$$K_{a1} \times K_{b3} = K_{a2} \times K_{b2} = K_{a3} \times K_{b1} = K_w \quad (28)$$

where K_{a1}, K_{a2}, and K_{a3} refer to the equilibria given by Eqs. 17, 18, and 19, respectively; K_{b1}, K_{b2}, and K_{b3} refer to the reaction of PO_4^{-3}, HPO_4^{-2}, and $H_2PO_4^{-1}$, respectively, with water.

Table IV, page 277, gives the dissociation constants of several weak acids and weak bases, in water, at 25°C. As pointed out previously, strong acids and strong bases do not obey the law of mass action, so that dissociation constants cannot be formulated for these strong electrolytes.

From an inspection of this table it is evident that great variations occur in the strength of weak acids and weak bases. The effect of various substituents on the strength of acids and bases depends on the electronegativity of the substituent atom or radical. For example, the substitution of one chlorine atom into the molecule of acetic acid increases the degree of ionization of the acid; substitution of two chlorine atoms further increases the degree of ionization, and introduction of three chlorine atoms produces a still stronger acid. The explanation of this effect of chlorine is as follows: Acetic acid ionizes primarily because the oxygen atom adjacent to the hydrogen atom of the carboxyl group has a stronger affinity for electrons than has the hydrogen atom; the result is that when acetic acid is dissolved in water the polar molecules of the latter have a stronger affinity for the hydrogen of acetic acid than has the latter. The acetic acid ionizes as a consequence of this difference in affinities. When an atom of chlorine is introduced into the acetic acid molecule, forming $CH_2ClCOOH$, the electrons in the molecule are very strongly attracted to the chlorine because of its relatively high electronegativity; the bond between the hydrogen and the oxygen in the carboxyl group is thereby weakened and the degree of ionization increased. Introduction of two, or of three, chlorine atoms further weakens the bond and increases the strength of the acid. On the other hand, substitution of chlorine into the molecule of ammonia reduces the strength of the base because of its decreased affinity for hydrogen ion.

Determination of Dissociation Constants—The determination of the dissociation or ionization constant of a weak acid or a weak base may be performed in various ways. One method is based on the determination of the *degree of ionization* by measuring the conductance of a solution of the acid or base (see discussion under *Ionization of Weak Electrolytes*, page 272). The procedure for calculating the ionization constant for an acid is as follows. Starting with the equation for ionization of the weak acid HA in water

$$HA + H_2O \rightarrow H_3O^+ + A^-$$

the ionization constant is defined by

$$\frac{[H_3O^+][A^-]}{[HA]} = K_a \quad (29)$$

if the molar concentration of the acid is designated c and its degree of ionization α, we may write

$$\frac{(\alpha c)(\alpha c)}{(1 - \alpha)c} = K_a \quad (30)$$

or

$$\frac{\alpha^2 c}{1 - \alpha} = K_a \quad (31)$$

Since α is measured by the ratio Λ/Λ_0, where Λ is the equivalent conductance of the electrolyte at concentration c, and Λ_0 is the equivalent conductance of the same electrolyte at infinite dilution, we may substitute for α the conductance ratio and obtain

$$\frac{\Lambda^2 c}{\Lambda_0(\Lambda_0 - \Lambda)} = K_a \quad (32)$$

When the degree of ionization is small, an acceptable approximation to Eq. 32 is

$$\frac{\Lambda^2 c}{\Lambda_0^2} = K_a \quad (33)$$

Another method for determining the ionization constant of a weak acid in aqueous solution is based on the measurement of the hydronium-ion concentration of a solution containing equimolar concentrations of the acid and a strong-base salt of the acid. The principle of this method is evident from inspection of Eq. 29; when equimolar concentrations of HA (the acid) and A^- (the salt) are present, the ionization constant K_a is numerically equal to the hydrogen-ion concentration (also, the pK_a of the acid is equal to the pH of the solution). Instead of preparing a solution containing equimolar concentrations of acid and salt, the same information may be obtained by measuring the hydronium-ion concentration (or pH) of the acid at the point of half neutralization during a quantitative titration with strong alkali.

The preceding methods may be used also to determine the ionization constant of a base employing, of course, the appropriate equations. Whether used for acids or bases, however, the procedures are valid only to the extent that it may be assumed that conventional concentration units measure the activity of the ionic and molecular species involved; this assumption limits the utility of the methods to dilute solutions. Even so, these methods serve to give acceptable values of dissociation constants in many cases.

Ionization of Water

Although it is a poor conductor of electricity, pure water does ionize through a process known as *autoprotolysis*, in the following manner:

$$2H_2O \rightleftharpoons H_3O^+ + OH^-$$

Application of the law of mass action to this reaction gives the following:

$$\frac{[H_3O^+][OH^-]}{[H_2O]^2} = K \quad (34)$$

where K is the equilibrium constant for the reaction.

Since the concentration of H_2O (molecular water) is very much greater than either the hydronium-ion or hydroxyl-ion concentrations, it can be considered to be constant and can be combined with K to give a new constant, K:, known as the *ion product* of water, and Eq. 34 becomes

$$[H_3O^+][OH^-] = K_w \qquad (35)$$

The numerical value of K_w varies with temperature; at $25°$ it is approximately equal to 1×10^{-14}.

Since the autoprotolysis of pure water yields one hydronium ion for each hydroxyl ion produced, $[H_3O^+]$ must be equal to $[OH^-]$. At $25°$ each has a value of 1×10^{-7} moles/liter ($1 \times 10^{-7} \times 1 \times 10^{-7} = K_w = 1 \times 10^{-14}$). A solution in which $[H_3O^+]$ is equal to $[OH^-]$ is termed a *neutral* solution.

If an acid is added to water, the hydronium-ion concentration will be increased and the equilibrium between hydronium and hydroxyl ions will be *momentarily* disturbed. To restore equilibrium, some of the hydroxyl ions, originally present in the water, will combine with a *part* of the added hydronium ions to form nonionized water molecules until the product of the concentrations of the two ions has been reduced to 10^{-14}. When equilibrium is again restored, the concentrations of the two ions will no longer be equal. If, for example, the hydronium-ion concentration is $1 \times 10^{-3} N$ when equilibrium is established, the concentration of hydroxyl ion will be 1×10^{-11} (the product of the two concentrations being equal to 10^{-14}). Since $[H_3O^+]$ is much greater than $[OH^-]$, the solution is said to be *acid* or *acidic*.

In a similar manner, the addition of an alkali to pure water momentarily disturbs the equilibrium between hydronium and hydroxyl ions; to restore equilibrium, some of the hydronium ions originally present in the water will combine with part of the added hydroxyl ions to form nonionized water molecules. The process continues until the product of the hydronium- and hydroxyl-ion concentrations is again equal to 10^{-14}. Assuming that the final hydroxyl-ion concentration is $1 \times 10^{-4} N$, the concentration of hydronium ion in the solution will be 1×10^{-10}. Since $[OH^-]$ is much greater than $[H_3O^+]$, the solution is said to be *basic* or *alkaline*.

pH

The numerical values of hydronium-ion concentration may vary enormously; for a normal solution of a strong acid the value is nearly 1, while for a normal solution of a strong base it is approximately 1×10^{-14}; ie, a variation of 100,000,000,000,000 between these two limits. Because of the inconvenience of dealing with numbers that vary so greatly, Sorenson, in 1909, proposed that hydronium-ion concentration be expressed in terms of the logarithm (log) of its reciprocal. To this value he assigned the symbol pH. Mathematically it is written

$$pH = \log \frac{1}{[H_3O^+]} \qquad (36)$$

and since the logarithm of 1 is zero, the equation may also be written

$$pH = -\log[H_3O^+] \qquad (37)$$

from which it is evident that pH may also be defined as the negative logarithm of the hydronium-ion concentration. In general, this type of notation is used to indicate the negative logarithm of the term that is preceded by the "p," which gives rise to the following:

$$pOH = -\log[OH^-] \qquad (38)$$

$$pK = -\log K \qquad (39)$$

Thus, taking logarithms of Eqs. 27 and 35 gives

$$pK_a + pK_b = pK_w \qquad (40)$$

$$pH + pOH = pK_w \qquad (41)$$

The relationship of pH to hydronium-ion and hydroxyl-ion concentrations may be seen in Table V.

The following examples illustrate the conversion from exponential to "p" notation:

1. Calculate the pH corresponding to a hydronium-ion concentration of 1×10^{-4} Gm-ion/L.

Solution:

$$pH = \log \frac{1}{1 \times 10^{-4}}$$
$$= \log 10,000 \text{ or } \log (1 \times 10^{+4})$$
$$\log (1 \times 10^{+4}) = +4$$
$$pH = 4$$

2. Calculate the pH corresponding to a hydronium-ion concentration of $0.000036 N$ (or Gm-ion/L.) (*Note*—This is more frequently written as a number multiplied by a power of 10, thus, 3.6×10^{-5} for 0.000036.)

Solution:

$$pH = \log \frac{1}{3.6 \times 10^{-5}}$$
$$= \log 28,000 \text{ or } \log (2.8 \times 10^{+4})$$
$$\log (2.8 \times 10^{+4}) = \log 2.8 + \log 10^{+4}$$
$$\log 2.8 = +0.44$$
$$\log 10^{+4} = +4.00$$
$$pH = 4.44$$

This problem may also be solved as follows:

$$pH = -\log (3.6 \times 10^{-5})$$
$$\log 3.6 = +0.56$$
$$\log 10^{-5} = -5.00$$
$$\overline{-4.44} = \log (3.6 \times 10^{-5})$$
$$pH = -(-4.44) = +4.44 = 4.44$$

Table V—Hydronium-Ion and Hydroxyl-Ion Concentrations

	pH	Normality in terms of hydronium ion	Normality in terms of hydroxyl ion
	0	1	10^{-14}
	1	10^{-1}	10^{-13}
Increasing acidity	2	10^{-2}	10^{-12}
	3	10^{-3}	10^{-11}
	4	10^{-4}	10^{-10}
	5	10^{-5}	10^{-9}
	6	10^{-6}	10^{-8}
Neutral point	7	10^{-7}	10^{-7}
	8	10^{-8}	10^{-6}
	9	10^{-9}	10^{-5}
Increasing alkalinity	10	10^{-10}	10^{-4}
	11	10^{-11}	10^{-3}
	12	10^{-12}	10^{-2}
	13	10^{-13}	10^{-1}
	14	10^{-14}	1

The following examples illustrate the conversion of "p" notation to exponential notation:

1. Calculate the hydronium-ion concentration corresponding to a pH of 4.44.

Solution:

$$pH = \log \frac{1}{[H_3O^+]}$$

$$4.44 = \log \frac{1}{[H_3O^+]}$$

$$\frac{1}{[H_3O^+]} = \text{antilog of } 4.44 = 28{,}000 \text{ (rounded off)}$$

$$[H_3O^+] = \frac{1}{28{,}000} = 0.000036 \text{ or } 3.6 \times 10^{-5}$$

This calculation may also be made as follows:

$$+4.44 = -\log [H_3O^+]$$
$$\text{or} \quad -4.44 = +\log [H_3O^+]$$

In finding the antilog of -4.44 it should be kept in mind that the mantissa (the number to the right of the decimal point) of a log to the base 10 (the common or Briggsian logarithm base) is *always positive* but that the characteristic (the number to the left of the decimal point) may be *positive* or *negative*. As the entire log -4.44 is negative, it is obvious that we cannot look up the antilog of -0.44. However, the number -4.44 may also be written $(-5.00 + 0.56)$ or, as more often written, $\bar{5}.56$, where the bar across the characteristic indicates that it alone is negative, while the rest of the number is positive. Looking up the antilog of 0.56 we find it to be 3.6 and as the antilog of -5.00 is 10^{-5}, it follows that the hydronium-ion concentration must be 3.6×10^{-5}.

2. Calculate the hydronium-ion concentration corresponding to a pH of 10.17.

Solution:

$$10.17 = -\log [H_3O^+]$$
$$-10.17 = \log [H_3O^+]$$
$$-10.17 = (-11.00 + 0.83) = \bar{11}.83$$

The antilog of $0.83 = 6.8$
The antilog of $-11.00 = 10^{-11}$
The hydronium-ion concentration is therefore $6.8 \times 10^{-11} N$.

In the section on acid–base equilibria it was shown that the hydronium-ion concentration of pure water, at 25°C, is $1 \times 10^{-7} N$, corresponding to a pH of 7.* This figure is, therefore, designated as the neutral point and all values below a pH of 7 represent acidities, the smaller the number, the greater the acidity. Values above 7 represent alkalinities, the larger the number the greater the alkalinity. The pH scale usually runs from 0 to 14, but mathematically there is no reason why negative numbers or numbers above 14 should not be used. In practice, however, such values are never encountered because solutions which might be expected to have such values are too concentrated to be extensively ionized or the interionic attraction is so great as to materially reduce ionic activity.

It should be strongly emphasized that the generalizations stated concerning neutrality, acidity, and alkalinity hold exactly only when: (1) the solvent is water; (2) the temperature is 25°C; and (3) there are no other factors to cause deviation from the simply formulated equilibria underlying the definition of pH given in the preceding discussion.

Species Concentration

When a weak acid, H_nA, is added to water, $n + 1$ species including the unionized acid can exist. After

---

* The pH of the purest water obtainable, so-called "superconductivity" water is 7.0 when the measurement is carefully made under conditions to exclude carbon dioxide and prevent errors inherent in the measuring technique (such as acidity or alkalinity of the indicator). Upon agitating this water in the presence of carbon dioxide in the atmosphere the value drops rapidly to 5.7, which is the pH value of nearly all distilled waters that have been exposed to the atmosphere for even a short time.

equilibrium is established, the sum of the concentrations of all species must be equal to C_a, the stoichiometric (added) concentration of acid. Thus, for a triprotic acid H_3A:

$$C_a = [H_3A] + [H_2A^{-1}] + [HA^{-2}] + [A^{-3}] \quad (42)$$

In addition, the concentrations of all acidic and basic species in solution vary with pH, and can be represented solely in terms of equilibrium constants and the hydronium-ion concentration. These relationships may be expressed[2] as in Eqs. 33 and 44:

$$[H_nA] = [H_3O^+]^n C_a/D \quad (43)$$

$$[H_{n-j}A^{-i}] = [H_3O^+]^{n-i} K_1 \ldots K_i C_a/D \quad (44)$$

in which n represents the total number of dissociable hydrogens in the parent acid, j is the number of protons dissociated, C_a is the stoichiometric concentration of acid, and K represents the acid dissociation constants. The term D is a power series in $[H_3O^+]$ and K, starting with $[H_3O^+]$ raised to the nth power. The last term is the product of all the dissociation constants. The intermediate terms can be generated from the last term by substituting $[H_3O^+]$ for K_n to obtain the next to last term, then substituting $[H_3O^+]$ for K_{n-1} to obtain the next term, etc, until the first term is reached. The following examples show the denominator, D, to be used for various types of acids:

$$H_3A : D = [H_3O^+]^3 + K_1[H_3O^+]^2 +$$
$$K_1K_2[H_3O^+] + K_1K_2K_3 \quad (45)$$

$$H_2A : D = [H_3O^+]^2 + K_1[H_3O^+] + K_1K_2 \quad (46)$$

$$HA : D = [H_3O^+] + K_a \quad (47)$$

The numerator, in all instances, is C_a multiplied by the term from the denominator that has $[H_3O^+]$ raised to the $n - j$ power. Thus, for diprotic acids such as carbonic, succinic, tartaric, etc,

$$[H_2A] = \frac{[H_3O^+]^2 C_a}{[H_3O^+]^2 + K_1[H_3O^+] + K_1K_2} \quad (48)$$

$$[HA^{-1}] = \frac{K_1[H_3O^+]C_a}{[H_3O^+]^2 + K_1[H_3O^+] + K_1K_2} \quad (49)$$

$$[A^{-2}] = \frac{K_1K_2C_a}{[H_3O^+]^2 + K_1[H_3O^+] + K_1K_2} \quad (50)$$

Example—Calculate the concentrations of all succinic acid species in a $1.0 \times 10^{-3} M$ solution of succinic acid at pH 6.0. Assume that $K_1 = 6.4 \times 10^{-5}$ and $K_2 = 2.3 \times 10^{-6}$.

Eqs. 48–50 have the same denominator, D, which can be calculated as follows:

$$D = [H_3O^+]^2 + K_1[H_3O^+] + K_1K_2$$
$$= 1.0 \times 10^{-12} + 6.4 \times 10^{-5} \times 1.0 \times 10^{-6} + 6.4 \times$$
$$10^{-5} \times 2.3 \times 10^{-6}$$
$$= 1.0 \times 10^{-12} + 6.4 \times 10^{-11} + 14.7 \times 10^{-11}$$
$$= 21.2 \times 10^{-11}$$

Therefore,

$$[H_2A] = \frac{[H_3O^+]^2 C_a}{D} =$$
$$\frac{1.0 \times 10^{-12} \times 1.0 \times 10^{-3}}{21.2 \times 10^{-11}} = 4.7 \times 10^{-6} M$$

$$[HA^{-1}] = \frac{K_1[H_3O^+]C_a}{D} =$$
$$\frac{6.4 \times 10^{-11} \times 1.0 \times 10^{-3}}{21.2 \times 10^{-11}} = 3.0 \times 10^{-4} M$$

$$[A^{-2}] = \frac{K_1 K_2 C_a}{D} =$$

$$\frac{14.7 \times 10^{-11} \times 1.0 \times 10^{-3}}{21.2 \times 10^{-11}} = 6.9 \times 10^{-4} \, M$$

Proton Balance Equation

In the Brønsted–Lowry system the total number of protons released by acidic species must equal the total number of protons consumed by basic species. This results in a very useful relationship known as the proton balance equation (PBE), in which the sum of the concentration terms for species that form by proton consumption is equated to the sum of the concentration terms for species that are formed by the release of protons. The PBE forms the basis of a unified approach to pH calculations, since it is an exact accounting of all proton transfers occurring in solution.

When HCl is added to water, for example, it dissociates yielding one Cl^- for each proton released. Thus, Cl^- is a species formed by the release of a proton. In the same solution, and actually in all aqueous solutions,

$$2H_2O \rightleftharpoons H_3O^+ + OH^-$$

where H_3O^+ is formed by proton consumption and OH^- is formed by proton release. Thus, the PBE is

$$[H_3O^+] = [OH^-] + [Cl^-] \tag{51}$$

In general, the PBE can be formed in the following manner:

1. Start with the species added to water.
2. Place all species that can form when protons are released on the right side of the equation.
3. Place all species that can form when protons are consumed on the left side of the equation.
4. Add $[H_3O^+]$ to the left side of the equation and $[OH^-]$ to the right side of the equation. These result from the interaction of two molecules of water as shown above.

Example—When H_3PO_4 is added to water, the species $H_2PO_4^{-1}$ forms with the release of one proton, HPO_4^{-2} forms with the release of 2 protons, and PO_4^{3-} forms with the release of 3 protons to give the following PBE:

$$[H_3O^+] = [OH^-] + [H_2PO_4^{-1}] +$$
$$2[HPO_4^{-1}] + 3[PO_4^{-3}] \tag{52}$$

Example—When Na_2HPO_4 is added to water, it dissociates into $2 \, Na^+$ and $1 \, HPO_4^{-2}$. The sodium ion is neglected in the PBE since it is not formed from the release or consumption of protons. The species HPO_4^{2-}, however, may react with water to give $H_2PO_4^{-1}$ with the consumption of 1 proton, H_3PO_4 with the consumption of 2 protons, and PO_4^{-3} with the release of 1 proton to give the following PBE:

$$[H_3O^+] + [H_2PO_4^{-1}] + 2[H_3PO_4] =$$
$$[OH^-] + [PO_4^{-3}] \tag{53}$$

Calculations

The pH of solutions of acids, bases, and salts may be calculated using the concepts presented in the preceding sections.

Strong Acids or Bases

When a strong acid such as HCl is added to water, the following reactions occur:

$$HCl + H_2O \rightarrow H_3O^+ + Cl^-$$

$$2H_2O \rightleftharpoons H_3O^+ + OH^-$$

The proton balance equation for this system would be

$$[H_3O^+] = [OH^-] + [Cl^-] \tag{54}$$

In most instances ($C_a > 4.5 \times 10^{-7} \, M$) the $[OH^-]$ would be negligible[3] compared to the $[Cl^-]$ and the equation simplifies to

$$[H_3O^+] = [Cl^-] = C_a \tag{55}$$

Thus, the hydronium-ion concentration of a solution of a strong acid would be equal to the stoichiometric concentration of the acid. This would be anticipated, since strong acids are generally assumed to be 100% ionized.

In a similar manner the hydroxyl-ion concentration for a solution of a strong base such as NaOH would be

$$[OH^-] = [Na^+] = C_b \tag{56}$$

The pH of a 0.005 M solution of HCl is therefore calculated as follows:

$$pH = -\log 0.005 = 2.30$$

and the pH of a 0.005 M solution of NaOH would be

$$pOH = -\log 0.005 = 2.30$$

$$pH = pK_w - pOH = 14.00 - 2.30 = 11.70$$

Weak Acids or Bases

If a weak acid, HA, is added to water, it will equilibrate with its conjugate base, A^-, as follows:

$$HA + H_2O \rightleftharpoons H_3O^+ + A^-$$

Accounting for the ionization of water gives the following proton balance equation for this system:

$$[H_3O^+] = [OH^-] + [A^-] \tag{57}$$

The concentration of A^- as a function of hydronium-ion concentration can be obtained as shown previously to give

$$[H_3O^+] = [OH^-] + \frac{K_a C_a}{[H_3O^+] + K_a} \tag{58}$$

Algebraic simplification yields

$$[H_3O^+] = K_a \frac{(C_a - [H_3O^+] + [OH^-])}{([H_3O^+] - [OH^-])} \tag{59}$$

In most instances for solutions of weak acids, $[H_3O^+] \gg [OH^-]$ and the equation simplifies to give

$$[H_3O^+]^2 + K_a[H_3O^+] - K_a C_a = 0 \tag{60}$$

This is a quadratic equation* which yields

$$[H_3O^+] = \frac{-K_a + \sqrt{K_a^2 + 4K_a C_a}}{2} \tag{61}$$

since $[H_3O^+]$ can never be negative. Furthermore, if $[H_3O^+]$ is less than 5% of C_a, Eq. 60 is simplified further to give

$$[H_3O^+] = \sqrt{K_a C_a} \tag{62}$$

It is generally preferable to use the simplest equation to calculate $[H_3O^+]$. However, when $[H_3O^+]$ is calculated, it must be compared to C_a in order to determine whether the assumption $C_a \gg [H_3O^+]$ is valid.

---

* The general solution to a quadratic equation of the form

$$aX^2 + bX + c = 0$$

is

$$X = -b \pm \frac{\sqrt{b^2 - 4ac}}{2a}$$

If the assumption is not valid, the quadratic equation should be used.

Example—Calculate the pH of a 5.00×10^{-5} M solution of a weak acid having a $K_a = 1.90 \times 10^{-5}$.

$$[H_3O^+] = \sqrt{K_aC_a}$$

$$= 1.90 \times 10^{-5} \times 5.00 \times 10^{-5}$$

$$= 3.08 \times 10^{-5} \, M$$

Since $C_a[(5.00 \times 10^{-5} M)]$ is not much greater than $[H_3O^+]$, the quadratic equation (Eq. 61) should be used:

$$[H_3O^+] = \frac{-1.90 \times 10^{-5} + \sqrt{(1.90 \times 10^{-5})^2 + 4(1.90 \times 10^{-5} \times 5.00 \times 10^{-5})}}{2}$$

$$= 2.26 \times 10^{-5} \, M$$

$$pH = -\log (2.26 \times 10^{-5}) = 4.65$$

Note that the assumption $[H_3O^+] \gg [OH^-]$ is valid. The hydronium-ion concentration calculated from Eq. 62 has a relative error of 36% when compared to the correct value obtained from Eq. 61.

When a salt obtained from a strong acid and a weak base—ie, ammonium chloride, morphine sulfate, pilocarpine HCl, etc—is dissolved in water, it dissociates as follows:

$$BH^+X^- \xrightarrow{\text{H}_2\text{O}} BH^+ + X^-$$

in which BH^+ is the protonated form of the base B, and X^- is the anion of a strong acid. Since X^- is the anion of a strong acid, it is too weak a base to undergo any further reaction with water. The protonated base, however, can act as a weak acid to give

$$BH^+ + H_2O \rightleftharpoons B + H_3O^+$$

Thus Eqs. 61 and 62 are valid with C_a being equal to the concentration of the salt in solution. If K_a for the protonated base is not available, it can be obtained by dividing K_b for the base B, into K_w.

Example—Calculate the pH of a 0.026 M solution of ammonium chloride. Assume that K_b for ammonia is 1.74×10^{-5} and K_w is 1.00×10^{-14}:

$$K_a = \frac{K_w}{K_b} = \frac{1.00 \times 10^{-14}}{1.74 \times 10^{-5}} = 5.75 \times 10^{-10}$$

$$[H_3O^+] = \sqrt{K_aC_a}$$

$$= \sqrt{5.75 \times 10^{-10} \times 2.6 \times 10^{-2}}$$

$$= 3.87 \times 10^{-6} \, M$$

$$pH = -\log (3.87 \times 10^{-6}) = 5.41$$

Since C_a is much greater than $[H_3O^+]$ and $[H_3O^+]$ is much greater than $[OH^-]$, the assumptions are valid and the value calculated for pH is sufficiently accurate.

Weak Bases

When a weak base, B, is dissolved in water it ionizes to give the conjugate acid as follows:

$$B + H_2O \rightleftharpoons BH^+ + OH^-$$

The proton balance equation for this system is

$$[BH^+] + [H_3O^+] = [OH^-] \tag{63}$$

Substituting $[BH^+]$ as a function of hydronium concentration and simplifying, in the same manner as shown for a weak acid, gives

$$[OH^-] = K_b \frac{(C_b - [OH^-] + [H_3O^+])}{([OH^-] - [H_3O^+])} \tag{64}$$

If $[OH^-] \gg [H_3O^+]$, as is generally true,

$$[OH^-]^2 + K_b[OH^-] - K_bC_b = 0 \tag{65}$$

which is a quadratic with the following solution

$$[OH^-] = \frac{-K_b + \sqrt{K_b^2 + 4K_bC_b}}{2} \tag{66}$$

If $C_b \gg [OH^-]$, the quadratic equation simplifies to

$$[OH^-] = \sqrt{K_bC_b} \tag{67}$$

Once $[OH^-]$ is calculated, it can be converted to pOH, which can be subtracted from pK_w to give pH.

Example—Calculate the pH of a 4.50×10^{-2} M solution of a weak base having $K_b = 2.00 \times 10^{-4}$. Assume that $K_w = 1.00 \times 10^{-14}$:

$$[OH^-] = \sqrt{K_bC_b}$$

$$= \sqrt{2.00 \times 10^{-4} \times 4.50 \times 10^{-2}}$$

$$= \sqrt{9.00 \times 10^{-6}} = 3.00 \times 10^{-3} \, M$$

Both assumptions are valid:

$$pOH = -\log 3.00 \times 10^{-3} = 2.52$$

$$pH = 14.00 - 2.52 = 11.48$$

When salts obtained from strong bases and weak acids —ie, sodium acetate, sodium sulfathiazole, sodium benzoate, etc—are dissolved in water, they dissociate as follows:

$$Na^+A^- \xrightarrow{\text{H}_2\text{O}} Na^+ + A^-$$

in which A^- is the conjugate base of the weak acid, HA. The Na^+ undergoes no further reaction with water. The A^-, however, acts as a weak base to give

$$A^- + H_2O \rightleftharpoons HA + OH^-$$

Thus, Eqs. 66 and 67 are valid with C_b being equal to the concentration of the salt in solution. The value for K_b can be obtained by dividing K_a for the conjugate acid, HA, into K_w.

Example—Calculate the pH of a 0.05 M solution of sodium acetate. Assume K_a for acetic acid is equal to 1.75×10^{-5} and $K_w = 1.00 \times 10^{-14}$:

$$K_b = \frac{K_w}{K_a} = \frac{1.00 \times 10^{-14}}{1.75 \times 10^{-5}}$$

$$= 5.71 \times 10^{-10}$$

$$OH^- = \sqrt{K_bC_b} = \sqrt{5.71 \times 10^{-10} \times 5.0 \times 10^{-2}}$$

$$= 5.34 \times 10^{-6} \, M$$

Both assumptions are valid.

$$pOH = -\log (5.34 \times 10^{-6}) = 5.27$$

$$pH = 14.00 - 5.27 = 8.73$$

Ampholytes

Substances such as $NaHCO_3$ and NaH_2PO_4 are termed *ampholytes*, and are capable of functioning both as acids and bases. When an ampholyte of the type NaHA is dissolved in water, the following series of reactions can occur:

$$Na^+HA^- \xrightarrow{H_2O} Na^+ + HA^-$$

$$HA^- + H_2O \rightleftharpoons A^{-2} + H_3O^+$$

$$HA^- + H_2O \rightleftharpoons H_2A + OH^-$$

$$2H_2O \rightleftharpoons H_3O^+ + OH^-$$

The total proton balance equation for the system is

$$[H_3O^+] + [H_2A] = [OH^-] + [A^{-2}] \qquad (68)$$

Substituting both $[H_2A]$ and $[A^{-2}]$ as a function of $[H_3O^+]$ (see Eqs. 48 and 50), yields

$$[H_3O^+] + \frac{[H_3O^+]^2 \, C_s}{[H_3O^+]^2 + K_1[H_3O^+] + K_1K_2} =$$
$$\frac{K_w}{[H_3O^+]} + \frac{K_1K_2C_s}{[H_3O^+]^2 + K_1[H_3O^+] + K_1K_2}$$

This gives a fourth-order equation in $[H_3O^+]$, which can be simplified using certain judicious assumptions to

$$[H_3O^+] = \sqrt{\frac{K_1K_2C_s}{K_1 + C_s}} \qquad (69)$$

In most instances, $C_s \gg K_1$ and the equation further simplifies to

$$[H_3O^+] = \sqrt{K_1K_2} \qquad (70)$$

and $[H_3O^+]$ becomes independent of the concentration of the salt. A special property of ampholytes is that the concentration of the species HA^{-1} is at a maximum at the pH corresponding to Eq. 70.

When the simplest amino acid, glycine hydrochloride, is dissolved in water, it acts as a diprotic acid and ionizes as follows:

$$^+NH_3CH_2COOH + H_2O \rightleftharpoons {}^+NH_3CH_2COO^- + H_3O^+$$

$$^+NH_3CH_2COO^- + H_2O \rightleftharpoons NH_2CH_2COO^- + H_3O^+$$

The form, $^+NH_3CH_2COO^-$, is an ampholyte since it can also act as a weak base as follows:

$$^+NH_3CH_2COO^- + H_2O \rightleftharpoons {}^+NH_3CH_2COOH + OH^-$$

This type of substance, which carries both a charged acidic and a charged basic moiety on the same molecule is termed a *zwitter ion*, and since the two charges balance each other, the molecule acts essentially as a neutral molecule. The pH at which the *zwitter-ion* concentration is at a maximum is known as the isoelectric point, which can be calculated from Eq. 70.

On the acid side of the isoelectric point, amino acids and proteins are cationic and incompatible with anionic materials such as the naturally occurring gums used as suspending and/or emulsifying agents. On the alkaline side of the isoelectric point, amino acids and proteins are anionic and incompatible with cationic materials such as benzalkonium chloride.

Salts of Weak Acids and Weak Bases

When a salt such as ammonium acetate (which is derived from a weak acid and a weak base) is dissolved in water, it undergoes the following reactions:

$$BH^+A^- \xrightarrow{H_2O} BH^+ + A^-$$

$$BH^+ + H_2O \rightleftharpoons B + H_3O^+$$

$$A^- + H_2O \rightleftharpoons HA + OH^-$$

The total PBE for this system is

$$[H_3O^+] + [HA] = [OH^-] + [B] \qquad (71)$$

Replacing $[HA]$ and $[B]$ as a function of $[H_3O^+]$, gives

$$[H_3O^+] + \frac{[H_3O^+]C_s}{[H_3O^+] + K_a} = [OH^-] + \frac{K_a'C_s}{[H_3O^+] + K_a'} \qquad (72)$$

in which C_s is the concentration of salt; K_a is the ionization constant of the conjugate acid formed from the reaction between A^- and water; and K_a' is the ionization constant for the protonated base, BH^+. In general, $[H_3O^+]$, $[OH^-]$, K_a, and K_a' are usually smaller than C_s and the equation simplifies to

$$[H_3O^+] = \sqrt{K_aK_a'} \qquad (73)$$

Example—Calculate the pH of a 0.01 M solution of ammonium acetate. The ammonium ion has a K_a equal to 5.75×10^{-10}, which represents K_a' in Eq. 73. Acetic acid has a K_a of 1.75×10^{-5}, which represents K_a in Eq. 73:

$$[H_3O^+] = \sqrt{1.75 \times 10^{-5} \times 5.75 \times 10^{-10}}$$

$$= 1.05 \times 10^{-7}$$

$$pH = -\log (1.05 \times 10^{-7}) = 6.98$$

Note that all of the assumptions are valid.

Buffers

The terms *buffer*, *buffer solution*, and *buffered solution* when used with reference to hydrogen-ion concentration or pH, refer to the ability of a system, particularly an aqueous solution, to resist change of pH on adding acid or alkali, or on diluting it with solvent.

If acid or base is added to water, the pH of the latter is changed markedly, for water has no ability to resist change of pH; it is completely devoid of buffer action. Even a very weak acid such as carbon dioxide changes the pH of water, decreasing it from 7 to 5.7 when the small concentration of carbon dioxide present in air is equilibrated with pure water. This extreme susceptibility of distilled water to change of pH on adding very small amounts of acid or base is often of great concern in pharmaceutical operations. Solutions of neutral salts such as sodium chloride similarly lack ability to resist change of pH on adding acid or base; such solutions are called unbuffered.

Characteristic of buffered solutions (such as are listed in Table VI), which undergo small changes of pH on addition of acid or base, is the presence either of a weak acid and a salt of the weak acid, or a weak base and a salt of the weak base. An example of the former system is acetic acid and sodium acetate; of the latter, ammonium hydroxide and ammonium chloride. From the proton concept of acids and bases discussed earlier it is apparent that such buffer action involves a conjugate acid–base pair in the solution; it will be recalled that acetate ion is the conjugate base of acetic acid, and that ammonium ion is the conjugate acid of ammonia (the principal constituent of what is commonly called ammonium hydroxide).

The mechanism of action of the acetic acid–sodium acetate buffer pair is that the acid, which exists largely in molecular (nonionized) form, combines with hydroxyl ion that may be added to form acetate ion and water, thus

$$CH_3COOH + OH^- \rightarrow CH_3COO^- + H_2O$$

while the acetate ion, which is a base, combines with hydrogen (more exactly hydronium) ion that may be added to form essentially nonionized acetic acid and water, represented as

$$CH_3COO^- + H_3O^+ \rightarrow CH_3COOH + H_2O$$

As will be illustrated later by an example, the change of pH is slight as long as the amount of hydronium or hydroxyl ion added does not exceed the capacity of the buffer system to neutralize it.

The ammonia–ammonium chloride pair functions as a buffer because the ammonia combines with hydronium ion that may be added to form ammonium ion and water, thus

$$NH_3 + H_3O^+ \rightarrow NH_4^+ + H_2O$$

Table VI—Buffer Mixtures of USP XVII (Clark and Lubs)

Hydrochloric Acid Buffer[a]

pH			
1.2	85.0 ml $M/5$ HCl	50 ml $M/5$ KCl	Dilute to 200 ml
1.3	67.2 ml $M/5$ HCl	50 ml $M/5$ KCl	Dilute to 200 ml
1.4	53.2 ml $M/5$ HCl	50 ml $M/5$ KCl	Dilute to 200 ml
1.5	41.4 ml $M/5$ HCl	50 ml $M/5$ KCl	Dilute to 200 ml
1.6	32.4 ml $M/5$ HCl	50 ml $M/5$ KCl	Dilute to 200 ml
1.7	26.0 ml $M/5$ HCl	50 ml $M/5$ KCl	Dilute to 200 ml
1.8	20.4 ml $M/5$ HCl	50 ml $M/5$ KCl	Dilute to 200 ml
1.9	16.2 ml $M/5$ HCl	50 ml $M/5$ KCl	Dilute to 200 ml
2.0	13.0 ml $M/5$ HCl	50 ml $M/5$ KCl	Dilute to 200 ml
2.1	10.2 ml $M/5$ HCl	50 ml $M/5$ KCl	Dilute to 200 ml
2.2	7.8 ml $M/5$ HCl	50 ml $M/5$ KCl	Dilute to 200 ml

Acid Phthalate Buffer

pH			
2.2	50 ml $M/5$ KHPhthalate	49.5 ml $M/5$ HCl	Dilute to 200 ml
2.4	50 ml $M/5$ KHPhthalate	42.2 ml $M/5$ HCl	Dilute to 200 ml
2.6	50 ml $M/5$ KHPhthalate	35.4 ml $M/5$ HCl	Dilute to 200 ml
2.8	50 ml $M/5$ KHPhthalate	28.9 ml $M/5$ HCl	Dilute to 200 ml
3.0	50 ml $M/5$ KHPhthalate	22.3 ml $M/5$ HCl	Dilute to 200 ml
3.2	50 ml $M/5$ KHPhthalate	15.7 ml $M/5$ HCl	Dilute to 200 ml
3.4	50 ml $M/5$ KHPhthalate	10.4 ml $M/5$ HCl	Dilute to 200 ml
3.6	50 ml $M/5$ KHPhthalate	6.3 ml $M/5$ HCl	Dilute to 200 ml
3.8	50 ml $M/5$ KHPhthalate	2.9 ml $M/5$ HCl	Dilute to 200 ml
4.0	50 ml $M/5$ KHPhthalate	0.1 ml $M/5$ HCl	Dilute to 200 ml

Neutralized Phthalate Buffer

pH			
4.2	50 ml $M/5$ KHPhthalate	3.0 ml $M/5$ NaOH	Dilute to 200 ml
4.4	50 ml $M/5$ KHPhthalate	6.6 ml $M/5$ NaOH	Dilute to 200 ml
4.6	50 ml $M/5$ KHPhthalate	11.1 ml $M/5$ NaOH	Dilute to 200 ml
4.8	50 ml M/5 KHPhthalate	16.5 ml $M/5$ NaOH	Dilute to 200 ml
5.0	50 ml $M/5$ KHPhthalate	22.6 ml $M/5$ NaOH	Dilute to 200 ml
5.2	50 ml $M/5$ KHPhthalate	28.8 ml $M/5$ NaOH	Dilute to 200 ml
5.4	50 ml $M/5$ KHPhthalate	34.1 ml $M/5$ NaOH	Dilute to 200 ml
5.6	50 ml $M/5$ KHPhthalate	38.8 ml $M/5$ NaOH	Dilute to 200 ml
5.8	50 ml $M/5$ KHPhthalate	42.3 ml $M/5$ NaOH	Dilute to 200 ml

Phosphate Buffer

pH			
5.8	50 ml $M/5$ KH_2PO_4	3.6 ml $M/5$ NaOH	Dilute to 200 ml
6.0	50 ml $M/5$ KH_2PO_4	5.6 ml $M/5$ NaOH	Dilute to 200 ml
6.2	50 ml $M/5$ KH_2PO_4	8.1 ml $M/5$ NaOH	Dilute to 200 ml
6.4	50 ml $M/5$ KH_2PO_4	11.6 ml $M/5$ NaOH	Dilute to 200 ml
6.6	50 ml $M/5$ KH_2PO_4	16.4 ml $M/5$ NaOH	Dilute to 200 ml
6.8	50 ml $M/5$ KH_2PO_4	22.4 ml $M/5$ NaOH	Dilute to 200 ml
7.0	50 ml $M/5$ KH_2PO_4	29.1 ml $M/5$ NaOH	Dilute to 200 ml
7.2	50 ml $M/5$ KH_2PO_4	34.7 ml $M/5$ NaOH	Dilute to 200 ml
7.4	50 ml $M/5$ KH_2PO_4	39.1 ml $M/5$ NaOH	Dilute to 200 ml
7.6	50 ml $M/5$ KH_2PO_4	42.4 ml $M/5$ NaOH	Dilute to 200 ml
7.8	50 ml $M/5$ KH_2PO_4	44.5 ml $M/5$ NaOH	Dilute to 200 ml
8.0	50 ml $M/5$ KH_2PO_4	46.1 ml $M/5$ NaOH	Dilute to 200 ml

Alkaline Borate Buffer

pH			
8.0	50 ml $M/5$ H_3BO_3, $M/5$ KCl	3.9 ml $M/5$ NaOH	Dilute to 200 ml
8.2	50 ml $M/5$ H_3BO_3, $M/5$ KCl	6.0 ml $M/5$ NaOH	Dilute to 200 ml
8.4	50 ml $M/5$ H_3BO_3, $M/5$ KCl	8.6 ml $M/5$ NaOH	Dilute to 200 ml
8.6	50 ml $M/5$ H_3BO_3, $M/5$ KCl	11.8 ml $M/5$ NaOH	Dilute to 200 ml
8.8	50 ml $M/5$ H_3BO_3, $M/5$ KCl	15.8 ml $M/5$ NaOH	Dilute to 200 ml
9.0	50 ml $M/5$ H_3BO_3, $M/5$ KCl	20.8 ml $M/5$ NaOH	Dilute to 200 ml
9.2	50 ml $M/5$ H_3BO_3, $M/5$ KCl	26.4 ml $M/5$ NaOH	Dilute to 200 ml
9.4	50 ml $M/5$ H_3BO_3, $M/5$ KCl	32.1 ml $M/5$ NaOH	Dilute to 200 ml
9.6	50 ml $M/5$ H_3BO_3, $M/5$ KCl	36.9 ml $M/5$ NaOH	Dilute to 200 ml
9.8	50 ml $M/5$ H_3BO_3, $M/5$ KCl	40.6 ml $M/5$ NaOH	Dilute to 200 ml
10.0	50 ml $M/5$ H_3BO_3, $M/5$ KCl	43.7 ml $M/5$ NaOH	Dilute to 200 ml

[a] These "buffer" solutions function by virtue of the fact that the high concentration of hydrogen ion is only very slightly affected by moderate additions of either acid or base. The potassium chloride has no role as a buffer.

and ammonium ion, which is an acid, combines with added hydroxyl ion to form ammonia and water, as

$$NH_4^+ + OH^- \rightarrow NH_3 + H_2O$$

Again, the change of pH is slight if the amount of added hydronium or hydroxyl ion is not in excess of the capacity of the system to neutralize it.

Besides these two general types of buffers, a third appears to exist. This is the buffer system composed of two salts, as monobasic potassium phosphate, KH_2PO_4, and dibasic potassium phosphate, K_2HPO_4. This is not, however, a new type of buffer; it is actually a weak-acid–conjugate-base buffer in which an ion, $H_2PO_4^-$, serves as the weak acid, and HPO_4^{-2} is its conjugate base. When hydroxyl ion is added to this buffer the following reaction takes place:

$$H_2PO_4^- + OH^- \rightarrow HPO_4^- + H_2O$$

and when hydronium ion is added the following occurs:

$$HPO_4^- + H_3O^+ \rightarrow H_2PO_4^- + H_2O$$

It is apparent that the mechanism of action of this type of buffer is essentially the same as that of the weak-acid–conjugate-base buffer composed of acetic acid and sodium acetate.

Calculations—A buffer system composed of a conjugate acid–base pair, NaA − HA (such as sodium acetate and acetic acid) would have a PBE of

$$[H_3O^+] + [HA] = [OH^-] + [A^-] \tag{74}$$

Replacing [HA] and [A$^-$] as a function of hydronium-ion concentration, gives

$$[H_3O^+] + \frac{[H_3O^+]C_b}{[H_3O^+] + K_a} = [OH^-] + \frac{K_aC_a}{[H_3O^+] + K_a} \tag{75}$$

where C_b is the concentration of the salt, NaA, and C_a is the concentration of the weak acid, HA. This equation can be rearranged to give

$$[H_3O^+] = K_a \frac{(C_a - [H_3O^+] + [OH^-])}{(C_b + [H_3O^+] - [OH^-])} \tag{76}$$

In general, both C_a and C_b are much greater than $[H_3O^+]$, which is in turn much greater than $[OH^-]$, and the equation simplifies to

$$[H_3O^+] = \frac{K_aC_a}{C_b} \tag{77}$$

or, expressed in terms of pH, as

$$pH = pK_a + \log \frac{C_b}{C_a} \tag{78}$$

This equation is generally called the Henderson–Hasselbalch equation.

This equation applies to all buffer systems formed from a single conjugate acid–base pair, regardless of the nature of the salts. For example, it applies equally well to the following buffer systems: ammonia–ammonium chloride; monosodium phosphate–disodium phosphate; phenobarbital–sodium phenobarbital; etc. In the ammonia–ammonium chloride system, ammonia is obviously the base and the ammonium ion is the acid (C_a equal to the concentration of the salt); in the phosphate system, monosodium phosphate is the acid and disodium phosphate is the base; in the phenobarbital buffer system, phenobarbital is the acid and the phenobarbiturate anion is the base (C_b equal to the concentration of sodium phenobarbital).

As an example of the application of this equation, the pH of a buffer solution containing acetic acid and sodium acetate, each in 0.1 M concentration, may be calculated. The K_a of acetic acid, as defined above, is 1.8×10^{-5}, at 25 °C.

Solution:

First, the pK_a of acetic acid is calculated:

$$\begin{aligned} pK_a &= -\log K_a = -\log 1.8 \times 10^{-5} \\ &= -\log 1.8 - \log 10^{-5} \\ &= -0.26 - (-5) = +4.74 \end{aligned}$$

Substituting this value into Eq. 78,

$$pH = \log \frac{0.1}{0.1} + 4.74 = +4.74$$

The Henderson–Hasselbalch equation predicts that any solutions containing the same molar concentration of acetic acid as of sodium acetate will have the same pH. Thus, a solution of 0.01 M concentration of each will have the same pH, 4.74, as one of 0.1 M concentration of each component. Actually, there will be some difference in the pH of the solutions, for the *activity coefficient* of the components varies with concentration; for most practical purposes, however, the approximate values of pH calculated by the Henderson–Hasselbalch equation are satisfactory. It should be pointed out, however, that the buffer of higher concentration of each component will have a much greater capacity for neutralizing added acid or base; this point will be discussed further under *Buffer Capacity*.

The Henderson–Hasselbalch equation is useful also for calculating the ratio of molar concentrations of a buffer system required to produce a solution of specific pH. As an example, suppose that an acetic acid–sodium acetate buffer of pH 4.5 is to be prepared. What ratio of the buffer components should be used?

Solution:

Rearranging Eq. 78, which is used to calculate the pH of weak acid-salt type buffers, we obtain

$$\log \frac{[\text{base}]}{[\text{acid}]} = pH - pK_a$$

$$= 4.5 - 4.76 = -0.24 = (9.76 - 10)$$

$$\frac{[\text{base}]}{[\text{acid}]} = \text{antilog of } (9.76 - 10) = 0.575$$

The interpretation of this result is that the *proportion* of sodium acetate to acetic acid should be 0.575 mole of the former to 1 mole of the latter to produce a pH of 4.5. A solution containing 0.0575 mole of sodium acetate and 0.1 mole of acetic acid per liter would meet this requirement, as would also one containing 0.00575 mole of sodium acetate and 0.01 mole of acetic acid per liter. The actual concentration selected would depend chiefly on the desired buffer capacity.

Buffer Capacity—The ability of a buffer solution to resist changes in pH upon addition of acid or alkali may be measured in terms of *buffer capacity*. In the preceding discussion of buffers, we have seen that, in a general way, the concentration of acid in a weak-acid–conjugate-base buffer determines the capacity to "neutralize" added base, while the concentration of salt of the weak acid determines the capacity to neutralize added acid. Similarly, in a weak-base–conjugate-acid buffer the concentration of the weak base establishes the buffer capacity toward added acid, while the concentration of the conjugate acid of the weak base determines the capacity toward added base. When the buffer is equimolar in the concentrations of weak acid and conjugate base, or of weak base and conjugate acid, it has equal buffer capacity toward added strong acid or strong base.

Donald D. Van Slyke, the biochemist, introduced a quantitative expression for evaluating buffer capacity. This may be defined as the amount, in gram-equivalents (Gm-Eq) per liter, of strong acid or strong base, required to be added to a solution to change its pH by 1 unit; a solution has a buffer capacity of 1 when 1 L requires 1 Gm-Eq of strong base or acid to change the pH 1 unit (in practice, considerably smaller increments are measured, the expressed as the ratio of acid or base added to the change of pH produced). From this definition it is apparent that the smaller the pH change in a solution caused by the addition of a specified quantity of acid or alkali, the greater is the buffer capacity of the solution.

The following numerical examples illustrate certain basic principles and calculations concerning buffer action and buffer capacity.

Example 1—What is the change of pH on adding 0.01 moles of NaOH to 1 L of 0.10 M acetic acid?

(a) Calculate the pH of a 0.10 molar solution of acetic acid:

$$[H_3O^+] = \sqrt{K_a C_a} = 1.75 \times 10^{-4} \times 1.0 \times 10^{-1} = 1.33 \times 10^{-3}$$

$$pH = -\log 1.33 \times 10^{-3} = 2.88$$

(b) On adding 0.01 moles of NaOH to a liter of this solution, 0.01 moles of acetic acid are converted to 0.01 moles of sodium acetate, thereby decreasing C_a to 0.09 M, and $C_b = 1.0 \times 10^{-2}$ M. Use of the Henderson–Hasselbalch equation gives

$$pH = 4.76 + \log \frac{0.01}{0.09} = 4.76 - 0.95 = 3.81$$

The pH change is, therefore, 0.93 units. The buffer capacity as defined above is calculated to be

$$\frac{\text{moles of NaOH added}}{\text{change in pH}} = 0.011$$

Example 2—What is the change of pH on adding 0.1 mole of NaOH to 1 L of buffer solution 0.1 M in acetic acid and 0.1 M in sodium acetate?

(a) The pH of the buffer solution before adding NaOH is

$$pH = \log \frac{[\text{base}]}{[\text{acid}]} + pK_a$$

$$= \log \frac{0.1}{0.1} + 4.76 = 4.76$$

(b) On adding 0.01 mole of NaOH per liter to this buffer solution, 0.01 mole of acetic acid is converted to 0.01 mole of sodium acetate, thereby decreasing the concentration of acid to 0.09 M and increasing the concentration of base to 0.11 M. The pH is calculated as follows:

$$pH = \log \frac{0.11}{0.09} + 4.76$$

$$= 0.086 + 4.76 = 4.85$$

The change of pH in this case is only 0.09 unit, about $\frac{1}{10}$ the change in the preceding example. The buffer capacity is calculated as

$$\frac{\text{moles of NaOH added}}{\text{change of pH}} = \frac{0.01}{0.09} = 0.11$$

Thus the buffer capacity of the acetic acid–sodium acetate buffer solution is approximately 10 times that of the acetic acid solution.

As is in part evident from the preceding examples, and may be further evidenced by calculations of pH changes in other systems, the degree of buffer action, and therefore the buffer capacity, are dependent on the kind and concentration of the buffer components, the pH region involved, and the kind of acid or alkali added.

Strong Acids and Bases as "Buffers"—In the foregoing discussion, buffer action was attributed to systems of (1) weak acids and their conjugate bases, (2) weak bases and their conjugate acids, and (3) certain acid-base pairs which can function in the manner either of (1) or (2).

The ability to resist change in pH on adding acid or alkali is possessed also by relatively concentrated solutions of strong acids and strong bases. If to 1 L of pure water having a pH of 7.0 is added 1 ml of 0.01 M hydrochloric acid, the pH is reduced to about 5.0. If the same volume of the acid is added to 1 L of 0.001 M hydrochloric acid, which has a pH of about 3, the hydronium-ion concentration is increased only about 1% and the pH is reduced hardly at all. The nature of this buffer action is quite different from that of the true buffer solutions. The very simple explanation is that when 1 ml of 0.01 M HCl, which represents 0.00001 Gm-Eq of hydronium ions, is added to the 0.0000001 Gm-Eq of hydronium ions in 1 L of pure water, the hydronium-ion concentration is increased 100-fold (equivalent to 2 pH units), but when the same amount is added to the 0.001 Gm-Eq of hydronium ions in 1 L of 0.001 M HCl, the increase is only 1/100 the concentration already present. Similarly, if 1 ml of 0.01 M NaOH is added to 1 L of pure water, the pH is increased to 9, while if the same volume is added to 1 L of 0.001 molar NaOH, the pH is increased almost immeasurably.

In general, solutions of strong acids of pH 3 or less, and solutions of strong bases of pH 11 or more, exhibit this kind of buffer action by virtue of the relatively high concentration of hydronium or hydroxyl ions present. The USP includes among its *Standard Buffer Solutions* a series of hydrochloric acid buffers, covering the pH range 1.2 to 2.2, which also contain potassium chloride; the salt does not participate in the buffering mechanism, as is the case with salts of weak acids, instead it serves as a nonreactive constituent required to maintain the proper electrolyte environment of the solutions.

Solutions for Preparing Official Buffers—The USP lists the following:

1. *Hydrochloric Acid, 0.2 M, and Sodium Hydroxide, 0.2 M*—Prepare and standardize.
2. *Potassium Biphthalate, 0.2 M*—Dissolve 40.846 Gm of potassium biphthalate ($KHC_6H_4[COO]_2$) in water, and dilute to 1000 ml.
3. *Potassium Phosphate, Monobasic, 0.2 M*—Dissolve 27.218 Gm of monobasic potassium phosphate (KH_2PO_4) in water, and dilute to 1000 ml.
4. *Boric Acid and Potassium Chloride, 0.2 M*—Dissolve 12.366 Gm of boric acid (H_3BO_3) and 14.911 Gm of potassium chloride (KCl) in water, and dilute to 1000 ml.
5. *Potassium Chloride, 0.2 M*—Dissolve 14.911 Gm of potassium chloride (KCl) in water, and dilute to 1000 ml.
6. *Phosphate Buffers*—In addition to the above buffer solutions, the USP provides directions for preparing several phosphate buffers (*0.1 M*, pH 4.5; *0.05 M*, pH 6.0; *1%*, pH 6.0; *0.1 M*, pH 7.9) for use in microbial assays.

The pH of buffer solutions varies with temperature as shown in Table VII.

Determination of pH

Colorimetry

One of the most extensively used methods for the determination of pH consists in adding an appropriate indicator to the solution to be tested and comparing the resultant color with the colors of a series of solutions of known containing the same indicator.

The function of the indicator in this determination depends upon the fact that its color changes with pH

Table VII—Variation in pH with Temperature

Temperature °C	0.1 M Hydrochloric acid pH	0.05 M Phthalate pH	0.025 M Phosphate pH	0.01 M Borate pH
0	1.10	4.01	6.98	9.46
10	1.10	4.00	6.92	9.33
15	1.10	4.00	6.90	9.27
20	1.10	4.00	6.88	9.22
25	1.10	4.01	6.86	9.18
30	1.10	4.01	6.85	9.14
40	1.10	4.03	6.84	9.07
50	1.11	4.06	6.83	9.01
60	1.11	4.10	6.84	8.96

within certain limits. According to a commonly accepted theory, indicators are either weak acids or weak bases which in ionized form possess one color and in molecular form possess another color.

The ionization of a weak acid type of indicator may be illustrated by the following reaction, in which HIn is the conventional abbreviation for the complex molecule of the indicator which exists in acid form, and In$^-$ is the abbreviation for the complex ion which exists in basic form:

$$HIn + H_2O \rightleftharpoons H_3O^+ + In^-$$

According to the theory, the molecules of HIn have one color, say red, and the ions of In$^-$ have another color, say yellow. The relative proportion of HIn and In$^-$ is determined by the pH of the solution in which the indicator is placed. When the solution is quite acid, the red color of the HIn molecules predominates, obscuring the yellow color of the relatively few In$^-$ ions which are also present. When the solution is sufficiently alkaline, the yellow color of In$^-$ ions predominates, obscuring the red color of the few HIn molecules that must also be in the solution. But in a certain pH range there will be a blend of various proportions of red and yellow forms of the indicator as the latter undergoes a transition from a predominantly red to a predominantly yellow solution, or *vice versa*. This pH range is referred to as the *transition interval* of the indicator, or as its *pH range;* it is the range in which an indicator is useful for colorimetric determination of pH. The transition interval of an indicator may be approximately calculated from the ionization constant of the indicator, which is defined for an acid-type indicator by the expression

$$\frac{[H_3O^+][In^-]}{[HIn]} = K_i \tag{79}$$

or

$$\frac{[H_3O^+][\text{basic form}]}{[\text{acid form}]} = K_i \tag{80}$$

rearranging

$$[H_3O^+] = K_i \frac{[\text{acid form}]}{[\text{basic form}]} \tag{81}$$

from which may be derived

$$-\log [H_3O^+] = -\log K_i + \log \frac{[\text{basic form}]}{[\text{acid form}]} \tag{82}$$

or

$$pH = pK_i + \log \frac{[\text{basic form}]}{[\text{acid form}]} \tag{83}$$

While discernible differences in the color of a mixture of acid and basic forms of an indicator vary with different indicators, in general color changes apparent to the eye occur only when the ratio of the two indicator forms varies within the range of 10 parts of basic form to 1 part of acid form as one limit to 1 part of basic form to 10 parts of acid form as the other. When the ratio of acid to basic form of an indicator exceeds 10, the color is so predominantly that of the acid form that further increase in the proportion of the acid form produces no discernible change of color; conversely, when the ratio of basic to acid form exceeds 10, the color is so predominantly that of the basic form that further increase in the proportion of the basic form is not discernible. These ratio limits correspond to

$$pH = pK_i + \log \frac{10}{1} = pK_i + 1$$

and

$$pH = pK_i + \log \frac{1}{10} = pK_i - 1$$

or

$$pH = pK_i \pm 1$$

From this it is obvious why the transition interval of an indicator is approximately 2 pH units. It should be recognized, however, that the interval for a specific indicator may be greater or less than 2 pH units, depending on the ease of detecting variation of color with variation in the proportion of acid and basic forms of the indicator.

pH Indicators—Most indicators are of the two-color type, ie, are changed from one color to another by the addition of acid or alkali. Phenolphthalein exhibits only one color—the pink color of its alkaline form—but the general indicator theory is still applicable, the only difference being that the acid form of the indicator is colorless.

A partial list of indicators, with their transition intervals and colors corresponding to the limits of the interval, is given in Table VIII.

Preparation—Solutions of indicators of the basic type and of the phthaleins are prepared by dissolving them in alcohol. In preparing solutions of indicators containing an acid group, this group must be neutralized first with sodium hydroxide. The procedure is as follows:

One-tenth (0.100) Gm of the indicator is triturated in an agate mortar with the volume of 0.02 N sodium hydroxide specified in the above table, or with its equivalent. When the indicator has dissolved, the solution is diluted with carbon-dioxide-free distilled water to make 200 ml (0.05%).

These solutions must be protected from light in amber-colored stoppered bottles.

Colorimetric Comparison Sets—These contain, in sealed ampuls, buffer solutions to which have been added appropriate indicators. Each set of buffer solutions generally covers a range of 1.6 pH units in intervals of 0.2 of a unit, corresponding to the useful transition interval of the indicator employed. The number of sets required depends on the reaction of the solutions being tested. Where a certain type of solution is continuously being tested, one or two sets of buffer standards will suffice. Fig. 166 shows a set of such solutions marketed by the LaMotte Chemical Products Co., Baltimore, Md. A convenient apparatus, known as the Roulette Comparator, contains openings for inserting the buffer solutions of three sets and by means of a lamp in the center of the comparator provides for the direct comparison of solutions under uniform illumination. This apparatus is shown in Fig. 167 and is also made by LaMotte.

Instead of comparing the solutions to be tested with standard buffer solutions it is also possible to make colorimetric determinations without the use of buffer solutions. This determination depends on the fact that any color of an indicator within the range of its transition interval may be matched by distributing a constant number of drops of indicator between two solutions, one of which is acid enough to transform all of the indicator into the acid color, the other being sufficiently alkaline to transform the indicator completely to the alkaline form. Test tubes may be used for the test. Examined transversely through the two tubes the color produced will be found to depend on the relative distribution of the indicator. This method, known as the *Gillespie Drop Ratio* method for determining hydrogen-ion concentration, is described in detail

in books on physical chemistry. The matching of indicator color may also be performed by the use of a special hydrogen-ion colorimeter permitting different depths of solutions containing the acid and alkaline forms, respectively, of indicator to be superimposed and the resultant color observed.

Indicators

In the determination of an unknown pH value a suitable indicator first must be found. Only indicators which show an intermediate color between the extreme acid and alkaline colors can be used.

The first step in the choice of a suitable indicator is the determination of the approximate pH value of the solution under investigation. A few simple tests will usually supply the necessary information. Add a drop or two of phenolphthalein TS to a small portion of the solution. If the indicator remains colorless, the pH of the solution is less than 8.4. A second test is conducted in the same manner, using methyl orange TS as the

Table VIII—pH Indicators

Indicator		Range		Preparation
Methyl violet	yellow	0.1–1.5	blue	0.25 Gm in 100 ml water
Metacresol purple	red	0.5–2.5	yellow	0.10 Gm in 13.6 ml N/50 NaOH; water to 200 ml
Thymol blue	red	1.2–2.8	yellow	0.10 Gm in 10.75 ml N/50 NaOH; water to 200 ml
Tropaeolin OO	red	1.3–3.0	yellow	0.10 Gm in 100 ml water
Methyl violet	blue	1.5–3.2	violet	0.25 Gm in 100 ml water
Methyl yellow	red	2.9–4.0	yellow	0.10 Gm in 200 ml alcohol
Bromophenol blue	yellow	3.0–4.6	blue	0.10 Gm in 7.45 ml N/50 NaOH; water to 200 ml
Congo red	blue	3.0–5.2	red	0.10 Gm in 100 ml water
Methyl orange	red	3.0–4.4	yellow	0.10 Gm in 100 ml water
Bromocresol green	yellow	3.8–5.4	blue	0.10 Gm in 7.15 ml N/50 NaOH; water to 200 ml
Methyl red	red	4.2–6.2	yellow	0.10 Gm in 18.6 ml N/50 NaOH; water to 200 ml
Litmus	red	4.5–8.3	blue	0.5 Gm in 100 ml water
Chlorophenol red	yellow	5.0–6.6	red	0.10 Gm in 11.8 ml N/50 NaOH; water to 200 ml
Bromocresol purple	yellow	5.2–6.8	purple	0.10 Gm in 9.25 ml N/50 NaOH; water to 200 ml
Bromothymol blue	yellow	6.0–7.6	blue	0.10 Gm in 8.0 ml N/50 NaOH; water to 200 ml
Phenol red	yellow	6.8–8.4	red	0.10 Gm in 14.20 ml N/50 NaOH; water to 200 ml
Cresol red	yellow	7.2–8.8	red	0.10 Gm in 13.1 ml N/50 NaOH; water to 200 ml
Thymol blue	yellow	8.0–9.6	blue	0.10 Gm in 10.75 ml N/50 NaOH; water to 200 ml
Phenol-phgthalein	colorless	8.2–10	red	1 Gm in 100 ml alcohol
Indiro camine	blue	11.6–14.0	yellow	0.25 Gm in 100 ml 50% alcohol

indicator. If the solution assumes the alkaline color (yellow), the pH of the solution is greater than 4.4 and lies somewhere between 4.4 and 8.4. A few more tests with methyl red (pH interval 4.2–6.3), bromothymol blue (6.0–7.6), and phenol red (6.8–8.4) will give a close enough approximation of the pH value to show which indicator may be successfully used in the determination.

Instead of approximating the pH of the liquid with indicator solutions, the spot method, using indicator papers, may be substituted. Also, by using a universal indicator in place of the several indicator solutions suggested above, some time may be saved.

When the approximate pH value has been determined and a suitable indicator chosen, a 2- to 10-ml portion of the unknown solution (depending on the amount of the liquid available), is transferred to a hard, resistant glass test tube approximately 15 cm long with a 1.5-cm bore, and a measured amount of the indicator solution added. As a rule, 0.1 to 0.2 ml of the indicator solution per 10 ml of the solution being tested constitutes a proper indicator concentration. This amount should be added from a 1-ml pipet graduated to 0.01 ml.

Transfer from 4 to 6 portions of the buffer solutions, the pH values of which overlap that of the unknown solution, to test tubes and treat in exactly the same way as the solution being analyzed. The same amounts of indicator must be added to the unknown and to the buffer solutions. It is essential that all of the test tubes used be of the same dimensions and of the same type of glass as already indicated. The color of the unknown solution is then compared with the colors of the buffer solutions and the pH value of the solution thus determined.

In judging the colors, observe them against a white background with the light transmitted through the whole length of the tube. A suitable colorimeter also may be used. A sufficient number of reference solutions must be taken so that the color of the unknown falls between two of the series, differing by not more than 0.2 pH. The pH of the unknown can thus be easily approximated to within 0.1 and with practice to 0.05.

The dissociation constants of indicators hold for aqueous solutions only. Alcohol changes this value and therefore for alcoholic solutions a correction factor must be used.

A special word of caution is necessary concerning the interpretation of pH values observed for unbuffered liquids such as distilled water and isotonic sodium chloride solution. In general, the observed pH will not be the true pH of the liquid unless the pH of the indicator solution employed in the test is the same as that of the liquid being tested. If the indicator has a pH higher than that of the liquid, the observed pH will be higher than the correct value; if the indicator has a lower pH, the reverse will be true. The error may amount to more than 1 pH unit on either side of the correct value. Whether or not an indicator solution is more acid or more alkaline than the liquid under test may be determined by adding a small amount of the indicator solution, say 5 drops, to 10 ml of liquid and then finding a buffer solution which will produce a color match when the same amount of indicator is added to the latter. Following this observation, 5 drops more of the indicator solution are added to both the liquid and the buffer; if the colors no longer match the indicator is either more acid or more alkaline than the liquid under test, its reaction being apparent from observation of the direction of the color change (whether toward the acid or alkaline side). A portion of the indicator solution is then adjusted by addition of a small amount of a dilute solution of an acid or alkali, as the case may be, until a color match obtained when 5 drops of indicator are added is not altered by the addition of 5 more drops of indicator. Obviously, fresh portions of test liquid and buffer solution must be employed each time the reaction of the indicator is altered. When, finally, the indicator solution has the same pH as the liquid under test, the former is said to be *isohydric* with the latter. For further information concerning this procedure, see Kolthoff and Kameda.[4]

Potentiometry

Electrometric methods for the determination of pH are based on the fact that the difference of electrical potential between two suitable electrodes dipping into a solution containing hydronium ions depends on the concentration (or activity) of the latter. Development of a potential difference is not a specific property of hydronium ions; a solution of any ion will develop a potential proportional to the concentration of that ion if a suitable pair of electrodes is placed in the solution.

The relationship between the potential difference and concentration of an ion in equilibrium with the electrodes may be derived as follows. When a metal is immersed into a solution of one of its salts, there is a tendency for the metal to go into solution in the form of ions. This tendency is spoken of as the *solution pressure* of the metal and is comparable to the tendency of sugar molecules, for example, to dissolve in water. The metallic ions in solution tend, on the other hand, to be-

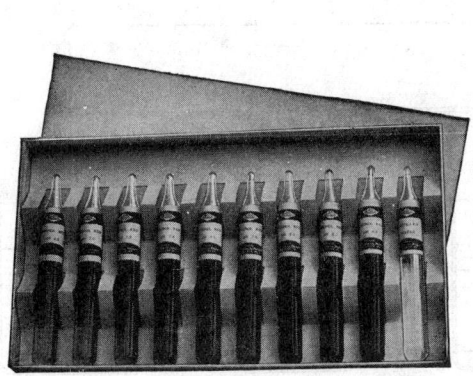

Fig. 166. **Colorimetric standards.**

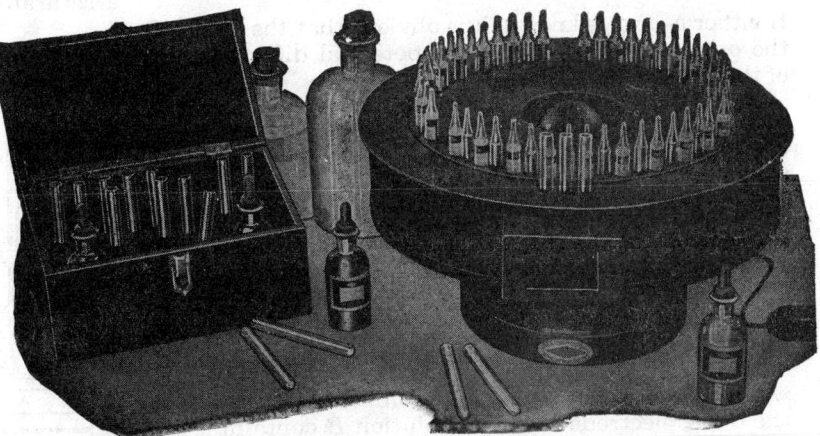

Fig. 167. **Roulette comparator for pH determination.**

come discharged by forming atoms, this effect being proportional to the *osmotic pressure* of the ions. In order for an atom of a metal to go into solution as a positive ion, electrons, equal in number to the charge on the ion, must be left behind on the metal electrode with the result that the latter becomes negatively charged. The positively charged ions in solution, however, may become discharged as atoms by taking up electrons from the metal electrode. Depending on which effect predominates, the electrical charge on the electrode will be either positive or negative and may be quantitatively expressed by the following equation proposed by H. W Nernst in 1889:

$$E = \frac{RT}{nF} \ln \frac{p}{P} \tag{84}$$

where

E = potential difference or electromotive force
R = the gas constant = 8.316 joules
T = absolute temperature
n = valence of the ion
F = the Faraday of electricity = 96,500 coulombs
p = osmotic pressure of the ions
P = solution pressure of the metal

Inasmuch as it is impossible to measure the potential difference between one electrode and a solution with any degree of certainty, it is customary to use two electrodes and to measure the potential difference between them. If two electrodes both of the same metal are separately immersed in solutions containing ions of that metal, at osmotic pressure p_1 and p_2, respectively, and connected by means of a tube containing a nonreacting salt solution (a so-called "salt-bridge"), the potential developed across the two electrodes will be equal to the difference between the potential differences of the individual electrodes, thus

$$E = E_1 - E_2 = \frac{RT}{nF} \ln \frac{p_1}{P_1} - \frac{RT}{nF} \ln \frac{p_2}{P_2} \tag{85}$$

Since both electrodes are of the same metal $P_1 = P_2$ and the equation may be simplified to

$$E = \frac{RT}{nF} \ln p_1 - \frac{RT}{nF} \ln p_2 = \frac{RT}{nF} \ln \frac{p_1}{p_2} \tag{86}$$

In place of osmotic pressures it is permissible, for dilute solutions, to substitute the concentrations c_1 and c_2 which were found (see Chapter 19, page 261) to be proportional to p_1 and p_2. The equation then becomes

$$E = \frac{RT}{nF} \ln \frac{c_1}{c_2} \tag{87}$$

If either c_1 or c_2 is known, it is obvious that the value of the other may be found if the potential difference, E, of this cell can be measured.

For the determination of hydronium-ion concentration, or pH an electrode at which an equilibrium between hydrogen gas and hydronium ion can be established must be used in place of metallic electrodes. Such an electrode may be made by electrolytically coating a strip of platinum, or other noble metal, with platinum black and saturating the latter with pure hydrogen gas. This device then functions as a *hydrogen electrode*. Two such electrodes may then be set up as shown in Fig. 168.

In this diagram one electrode dips into solution A which is of known hydronium-ion concentration and the other electrode dips into solution B containing an unknown concentration of hydrogen ion. The two

electrodes and solutions, sometimes called half-cells, are then connected by a bridge of neutral salt solution which has no significant effect on the solutions which it connects. The potential difference across the two electrodes is measured by means of a potentiometer P. If the concentration, c_1, of hydronium ion in solution A is one normal, Eq. 87 simplifies to

$$E = \frac{RT}{nF} \ln \frac{1}{c_2} \tag{88}$$

or in terms of Briggsian logarithms,

$$E = 2.303 \frac{RT}{nF} \log_{10} \frac{1}{c_2} \tag{89}$$

If for $\log_{10} 1/c_2$ there is substituted its equivalent pH, the equation becomes

$$E = 2.303 \frac{RT}{nF} \text{pH} \tag{90}$$

and finally by substituting numerical values for R, n, and F, and assuming the temperature to be 20 °C, the following simple relationship is derived:

$$E = 0.0581 \text{ pH} \quad \text{or} \quad \text{pH} = \frac{E}{0.0581} \tag{91}$$

The hydrogen electrode dipping into a solution of known hydronium-ion concentration, called the *reference electrode*, may be replaced by a calomel electrode, one type of which is shown in Fig. 169. The elements of a calomel electrode are mercury and calomel in an aqueous solution of potassium chloride; the potential of this electrode is constant, regardless of the hydronium-ion concentration of the solution into which it dips. The potential depends on the equilibrium which is set up between mercury and mercurous ions from the calomel, but the concentration of the latter is governed, according to the solubility product principle, by the concentration of chloride ions which are mainly derived from the potassium chloride in the solution. Therefore the potential of this electrode varies with the concentration of potassium chloride in the electrolyte.

Because the calomel electrode always indicates voltages which are higher, by a constant value, than those obtained when the normal hydrogen electrode chain shown in Fig. 168 is used, it is necessary to subtract, from the observed voltage, the voltage due to the calomel electrode itself. As the magnitude of this voltage depends on the concentration of potassium chloride in the calomel electrode electrolyte, it is necessary to know the concentration of the former. For most purposes a saturated potassium chloride solution is used which

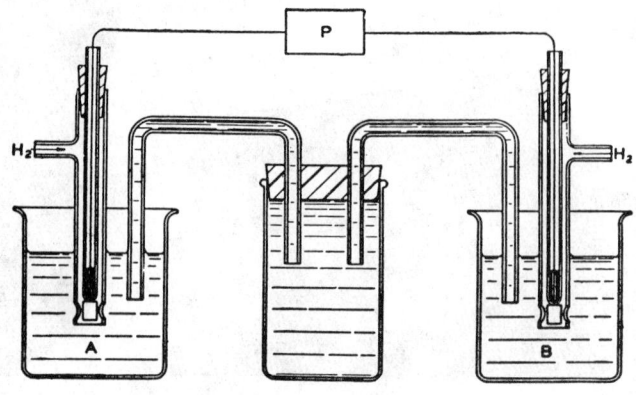

Fig. 168.   Hydrogen-ion concentration chain.

has a potential difference of 0.2488 v. Accordingly, before using Eq. 91 for the calculation of pH from the the voltage of a cell made up of a calomel and a hydrogen electrode dipping into the solution to be tested, 0.2488 v must be subtracted from the observed potential difference. Expressed mathematically, Eq. 92 is used for calculating pH from the potential difference of such a cell.

$$pH = \frac{E - 0.2488}{0.0581} \qquad (92)$$

In measuring the potential difference between the electrodes, it is imperative that very little current be drawn from the cell, for with current flowing the voltage changes, owing to polarization effects at the electrode. Because of this it is not possible to make accurate measurements with a voltmeter which requires appreciable current to operate it. In its place is used a potentiometer which does not draw a current from the cell being measured or, as in most potentiometers in use today, electronic amplification of the voltage developed at the electrodes is effected.

There are many limitations to the use of the hydrogen electrode. For example, it cannot be used in solutions containing strong oxidants such as ferric iron, dichromates, nitric acid, peroxide, and chlorine or reductants such as sulfurous acid and hydrogen sulfide. It is also affected by the presence of organic compounds which are fairly easily reduced. Furthermore, the hydrogen electrode cannot be successfully used in solutions containing cations that fall below hydrogen in the electrochemical series. Erratic results are also obtained in the measurement of unbuffered solutions unless special precautions are taken. Moreover, hydrogen electrodes are troublesome to prepare and maintain. Since other electrodes, more convenient to use, are now available, the hydrogen electrode is today rarely used. Nevertheless, the hydrogen electrode is the ultimate standard for pH measurements.

To avoid some of the difficulties with the hydrogen electrode, the *quinhydrone* electrode was introduced and was popular for a long time, particularly for measurements of acid solutions. The unusual feature of this electrode is that it consists of a piece of gold or platinum wire or foil dipping into the solution to be tested, in which has been dissolved a small quantity of quinhydrone. A calomel electrode may be used for reference, just as in determinations with the hydrogen electrode.

Quinhydrone consists of an equimolecular mixture of quinone and hydroquinone; the relationship between these substances and hydrogen-ion concentration is as follows:

Quinone + 2 hydrogen ions + 2 electrons ⇌ hydroquinone

In a solution containing hydrogen ions the potential of the quinhydrone electrode is logarithmically related to hydronium-ion concentration if the ratio of the hydroquinone concentration to that of quinone is constant and practically equal to one. This ratio is maintained in an acid solution containing an excess of quinhydrone and measurements may be made quickly and accurately however, quinhydrone cannot be used in solutions more alkaline than pH 8.

An electrode which, because of its simplicity of operation and freedom from contamination or change of the solution being tested, has replaced both the hydrogen and quinhydrone electrodes is the glass electrode. It functions by virtue of the fact that when a thin membrane of a special composition of glass separates two solutions of different pH there is developed across the membrane a potential difference which depends on the pH of both solutions. If the pH of one of the solutions is known, the other may be calculated from the voltage measurement. In practice the glass electrode usually consists of a bulb of the special glass fused to the end of a tube of ordinary glass. Inside the bulb is placed a solution of known pH, in contact with an internal silver–silver chloride or other electrode; this glass electrode and another reference electrode are immersed in the solution to be tested and the potential difference is measured. A potentiometer providing electronic amplification of the small current produced is employed; the modern instruments available permit reading the pH directly and provide also for compensation of variations due to temperature in the range of $0 - 50\,^{\circ}C$ and to the small but variable asymmetry potential inherent in the glass electrode. See Fig. 170.

Pharmaceutical Significance

In the broad realm of knowledge concerning the preparation and action of drugs few, if any, variables are so important as pH. For the purpose of this presentation, four principal types of pH-dependence of drug systems will be discussed: (1) solubility, (2) stability, (3) activity, and (4) absorption.

Drug Solubility

If a salt, NaA, is added to water to give a concentration, C_s, the following reactions occur:

$$Na^+A^- \xrightarrow{\ H_2O\ } Na^+ + A^-$$

$$A^- + H_2O \rightleftharpoons HA + OH^-$$

If the pH of the solution is lowered, more of the A^- would be converted to the unionized acid, HA, in accordance with Le Chatelier's principle. Eventually a pH will be obtained, below which the amount of HA formed exceeds its aqueous solubility, S_0, and the acid will precipitate from solution. This pH, below which precipitation occurs, can be designated as pH_p. At this point, at which the amount of HA formed just

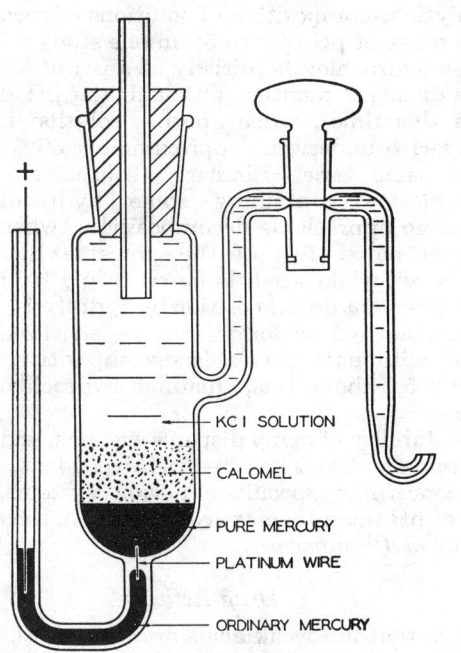

Fig. 169. Calomel electrode.

KC l SOLUTION

CALOMEL

PURE MERCURY

PLATINUM WIRE

ORDINARY MERCURY

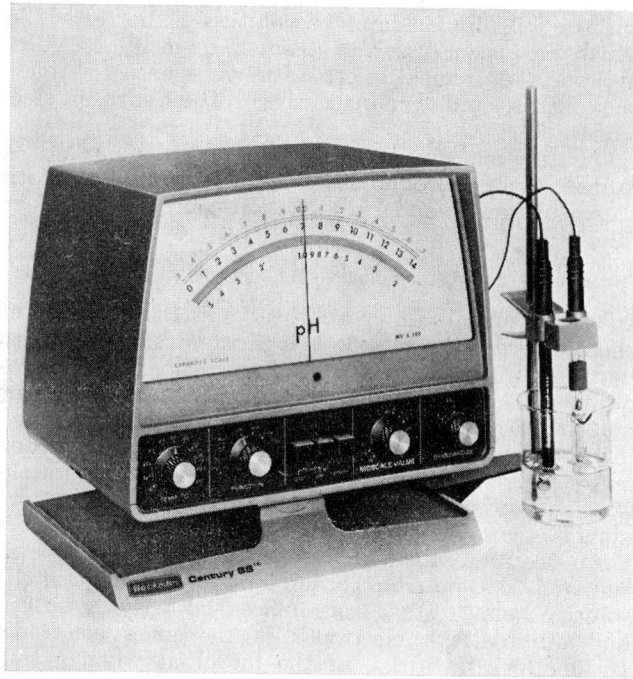

Fig. 170.   Beckman solid state pH meter.

equals S_0, a mass balance on the total amount of drug in solution yields

$$C_s = [HA] + [A^-] = S_0 + [A^-] \qquad (93)$$

Replacing $[A^-]$ as a function of hydronium-ion concentration gives

$$C_s = S_0 + \frac{K_a C_s}{[H_3O^+]_p + K_a} \qquad (94)$$

where K_a is the ionization constant for the conjugate acid, HA, and $[H_3O^+]_p$ refers to the hydronium-ion concentration above which precipitation will occur. This equation can be rearranged to give

$$[H_3O^+]_p = K_a \frac{S_0}{C_s - S_0} \qquad (95)$$

Taking logarithms, gives

$$pH_p = pK_a + \log \frac{C_s - S_0}{S_0} \qquad (96)$$

Thus, the pH below which precipitation occurs can be seen to be a function of the amount of salt added initially, the pK_a and the solubility of the free acid formed from the salt.

The analogous equation for salts of weak bases and strong acids (such as pilocarpine HCl, cocaine HCl, codeine phosphate, etc) would be

$$pH_p = pK_a + \log \frac{S_0}{C_s - S_0} \qquad (97)$$

in which pK_a refers to the protonated form of the weak base.

Example—Below what pH will free phenobarbital begin to precipitate from a solution initially containing 1.3 Gm of sodium phenobarbital/100 ml at 25°. The molar solubility of phenobarbital is 0.0050 and its pK_a is 7.41. The molecular weight of sodium phenobarbital is 254.

The molar concentration of salt initially added is

$$C_s = \frac{Gm/liter}{mol\ wt} = \frac{13}{254} = 0.041\ M$$

$$pH_p = 7.41 + \log \frac{0.051 - 0.005}{0.005}$$

$$= 7.41 + 0.96 = 8.37$$

Example—Above what pH will free cocaine begin to precipitate from a solution initially containing 0.0294 moles/liter? The pK_b of cocaine is 5.59, and its molar solubility is 5.60×10^{-3}.

$$pK_a = pK_w - pK_a = 14.00 - 5.59 = 8.41$$

$$pH_p = 8.41 + \log \frac{0.0056}{0.0294 - 0.0056}$$

$$= 8.41 + (-0.63) = 7.78$$

Drug Stability

One of the most diversified and fruitful areas of study is the investigation of the effect of hydrogen-ion concentration on the stability, or in more general terms the reactivity, of pharmaceutical systems. The evidence for enhanced stability of systems when these are maintained within a narrow range of pH, as well as of progressively decreasing stability as the pH departs from the optimum range, is abundant. Stability (or instability) of a system may result from gain or loss of a proton (hydrogen ion) by a substrate molecule—often accompanied by an electronic rearrangement—which reduces (or increases) the reactivity of the molecule. Instability results when the substance desired to remain unchanged is converted to one or more other, unwanted, substances. In aqueous solution, instability may arise through the catalytic effect of acids or bases, the former by transferring a proton to the substrate molecule, the latter by accepting a proton.

Specific illustrations of the effect of hydrogen-ion concentration on the stability of medicinals are myriad; only a few will be given here, these being chosen to show the importance of pH adjustment of solutions that require sterilization. Morphine solutions are not decomposed during 60-min exposure at a temperature of 100 °C if the pH is less than 5.5; neutral and alkaline solutions, however, are highly unstable. Minimum hydrolytic decomposition of solutions of cocaine occurs in the range of pH of 2 to 5; in one study a solution of cocaine hydrochloride initially at a pH of 5.7 remained stable during 2 months (although the pH dropped to 4.2 in this time), while another solution buffered to about pH 6 underwent approximately 30% hydrolysis in the same time. Similarly, solutions of procaine hydrochloride containing some hydrochloric acid showed no appreciable decomposition; when dissolved in water alone, 5% of the procaine hydrochloride hydrolyzed, while when buffered to pH 6.5 from 19 to 35% underwent decomposition by hydrolysis. Solutions of thiamine hydrochloride may be sterilized by autoclaving without appreciable decomposition if the pH is below 5; above this, thiamine hydrochloride is unstable.

The stability of many disperse systems, and especially of certain emulsions, is often pH-dependent. Information concerning specific emulsion systems, and the effect of pH upon them, may be found in the chapter on *Interfacial Phenomena*.

Drug Activity

Drugs that are weak acids or weak bases, and hence may exist in ionized or nonionized form (or a mixture of both), may be active in one form but not in the other; often such drugs have an optimum pH range for maximum activity.   Thus, mandelic acid, benzoic acid, and salicylic acid have pronounced antibacterial activity in nonionized form but have practically no such activity in ionized form; accordingly, these substances require an acid environment to function effectively as antibacterial agents.   For example, sodium benzoate is effective as a preservative in 4% concentration at pH 7.0, in 0.06 to 0.1% concentration at pH 3.5 to 4.0, and in 0.02 to 0.03% concentration at pH 2.3 to 2.4. Other antibacterial agents, on the other hand, are active principally if not entirely in cationic form; included in this category are the acridines and quaternary ammonium compounds.

Drug Absorption

The degree of ionization and lipoid solubility of a drug are two important factors that determine rate of absorption of drugs from the gastrointestinal tract and, indeed, their passage through cellular membranes generally.   Drugs that are weak organic acids or bases, and which in nonionized form are soluble in lipids, are absorbed through cellular membranes by virtue, apparently, of the lipoidal nature of the membranes. Completely ionized drugs, on the other hand, are absorbed poorly, if at all.   Rates of absorption of a variety of drugs are related to their ionization constants and in many cases may be quantitatively predicted on the basis of this relationship.   Thus, not only the degree of the acidic or basic character of a drug but consequently also the pH of the physiological medium (gastric or intestinal fluid, plasma, cerebrospinal fluid, etc) in which a drug is dissolved or dispersed—since this pH determines the extent to which the drug will be converted to ionic or nonionic form—become important parameters of drug absorption.   Further information concerning factors influencing drug absorption is given in Chapter 42, *Drug Absorption, Action, and Disposition.*

References

1. Sedam, R. L., *et al*, *J. Pharm. Sci.*, **54**, 215 (1965).
2. Niebergall, P. J., *Am. J. Pharmacy*, **138**, 232 (1966).
3. Freiser, H., and Fernando, Q., *Ionic Equilibria in Analytical Chemistry*, Wiley, New York, 1966, p. 49.
4. Kolthoff, I. M., and Kameda, T. *J., Am. Chem. Soc.*, **53**, 825 (1931).

21 | Reaction Kinetics

Reaction rate—reaction order—effects of temperature and reaction
medium on reaction rate—acid-base catalysis—drug decomposition
reactions—drug stabilization—stability testing

This chapter was prepared by

Harry B. Kostenbauder, PhD, *Assistant Dean for Research, College of
Pharmacy, University of Kentucky, Lexington, Ky. 40506*

Reaction kinetics is the study of rate of chemical change and the way in which this rate is influenced by conditions of concentration of reactants, products, and other chemical species which may be present, and by factors such as solvent, pressure, and temperature. Reaction kinetics permits formulation of models for the intermediate steps through which reactants are converted to other chemical compounds, and is a powerful tool in elucidation of mechanisms by which chemical reactions proceed. In application to pharmaceutics, such information permits a rational approach to stabilization of drug products and prediction of shelf-life and optimum storage conditions.

The treatment presented in this chapter is intended as a general introduction to the subject of reaction kinetics. A comprehensive review of experimental approaches and interpretation of data, and a compilation of information relative to studies on pharmaceuticals, has been published by Garrett.[1]

Reaction Rate and Reaction Order

The rate of a reaction is the velocity with which a reactant or reactants undergo chemical change. The first quantitative study of a rate of reaction was performed in 1850 by Wilhelmy, who observed the velocity of hydrolysis (inversion) of sucrose to glucose and fructose in aqueous solution, under the catalytic influence of acid. The equation for the over-all reaction is:

$$C_{12}H_{22}O_{11} + H_2O \rightarrow C_6H_{12}O_6 + C_6H_{12}O_6$$
$$\text{Sucrose} \qquad\qquad \text{Glucose} \qquad \text{Fructose}$$

The rate at which the concentration of sucrose, designated c, decreases with time, t, was found to be proportional to the concentration of unhydrolyzed sucrose. The change may be expressed in the notation of calculus by the differential equation

$$- dc/dt = k.c \qquad (1)$$

where $-dc/dt$ is the velocity (rate) with which the concentration of sucrose *decreases* (the minus sign indicates a decrease) as it undergoes hydrolysis, and k is a constant called the *velocity constant* or *rate constant*.

The term *reaction order* refers to the way in which concentration of a reactant, or reactants, influences the rate of a chemical reaction.

First-Order Reactions—When the rate of a reaction is proportional to the first power of the concentration of a reactant and may be expressed mathematically in the form of Eq. 1, the reaction is said to be first-order with respect to the reactant.

The hydrolysis of sucrose is not strictly first-order since the rate varies also with the concentration of water. The amount of water required for hydrolysis of sucrose is so small, however, relative to the large quantity present, that there is no significant change in the concentration of water; for practical purposes, therefore, the concentration of water is constant.

It may be noted here that the rate constant k for the hydrolysis of sucrose increases with the hydrogen-ion concentration of the medium because of the catalytic effect of hydrogen ion on the reaction.

Eq. 1 may be written

$$\frac{dc}{c} = -k.dt \qquad (2)$$

which, on integration, yields in natural logarithm form

$$\ln c = -k.t + \text{constant} \qquad (3)$$

or in common logarithm form

$$\log c = -\frac{t}{2.303} + \text{constant} \qquad (4)$$

Both Eqs. 3 and 4 will be recognized as producing straight lines if $\ln c$ or $\log c$ is plotted against t; this is an identifying characteristic of reactions in which the rate of reaction is proportional to the concentration of a single reactant, that is, of a *first-order reaction* (see Fig. 171). The rate constant k may be readily calculated from the slope of the line, which is $-k/2.303$.

Concentration is usually expressed in moles/liter and time in seconds, although other convenient units may be employed. The rate constant, k, for a first-order reaction has units of reciprocal time (time^{-1}).

If Eq. 4 is integrated between the limits of concentration c_0 at the beginning of the reaction when time is zero and when the concentration is c at a later time t, Eq. 5 is obtained

$$\log \frac{c_0}{c} = \frac{k}{2.303} t \qquad (5)$$

which on rearrangement becomes

$$k = \frac{2.303}{t} \log \frac{c_0}{c} \qquad (6)$$

A modification of this equation, in which a is the initial amount of reactant and x is the amount that has reacted in time t, is

$$k = \frac{2.303}{t} \log \frac{a}{a-x} \qquad (7)$$

Eq. 6 may be used to calculate k for first-order reactions when both the concentration at the beginning of the reaction (c_0) and at elapsed time t are known. Sometimes c_0 is either not known or is not a suitable reference concentration, in which cases the concentrations c_1 at time t_1 and c_2 at a later time t_2 are used to calculate k by the following modification of the preceding equation

$$k = \frac{2.303}{t_2 - t_1} \log \frac{c_1}{c_2} \qquad (8)$$

A useful exponential form of Eq. 6, when the latter is written in natural logarithm notation, is

$$c = c_0 e^{-kt} \qquad (9)$$

Although reaction rates may be quantitatively expressed in terms of numerical values of k, for many purposes a more useful expression is in terms of the *half-life* of a reaction, which is the time, $t_{1/2}$, required for half of the substance (reactant) to undergo reaction. Writing Eq. 6 in the form

$$k = \frac{2.303}{t_{1/2}} \log \frac{c_0}{c_0/2} = \frac{0.693}{t_{1/2}} \qquad (10)$$

it is apparent that

$$t_{1/2} = \frac{0.693}{k} \qquad (11)$$

From Eq. 11 it is obvious that, for first-order reactions, a constant time interval is required for disappearance of one-half of the substance present at the beginning of the interval, irrespective of the concentration of the substance. Thus, in a first-order reaction, 50% of an initial amount of reactant remains after the first half-life period, 25% after the second, 12.5% after the third, and so on.

It can also be shown by an expression similar to Eq. 10 that the time interval required for loss of *any*

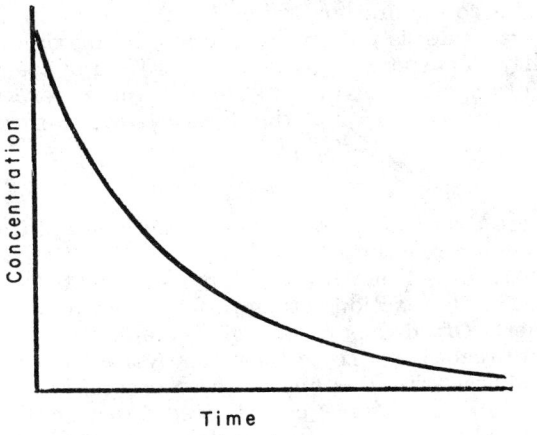

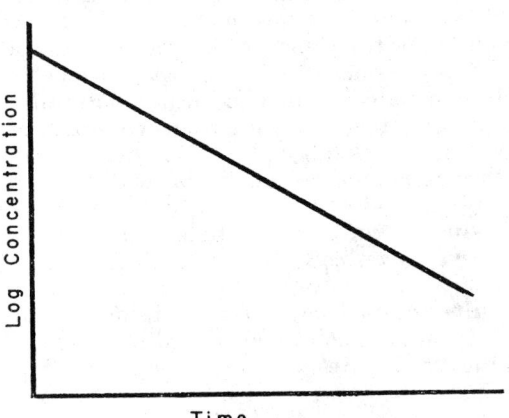

Fig. 171. **A first-order reaction.** *Top:* concentration vs time plot; *bottom:* log concentration vs time plot.

specified fraction of the reactant will be constant irrespective of the concentration of reactant. Thus, a term sometimes used in studies of drug stability is the time required for loss of 10% of the original concentration, or time required for concentration to decrease to 90% of the original concentration. This interval is referred to as $t_{0.90}$.

It is apparent also that an infinite period of time would be required for all of the substance to undergo reaction. It is thus impossible to measure first-order reaction rates to completion of the reaction, and plots such as those of Fig. 171 can not be extrapolated to zero concentration. It might be noted, however, that if a first-order reaction is followed through 10 half-lives, less than 0.1% of the original concentration of reactant remains. In practical studies of rate of reaction it is common to study the change of concentration with time through two or three half-life periods.

First-order rate processes are not restricted to chemical reactions. The passive diffusion of drugs across biological membranes, and processes of drug absorption, distribution, metabolism, and excretion can often be shown to occur at rates proportional to the concentration of drug and thus be described as first-order rate processes. Rate of growth of microorganisms and rate of killing or inactivation of microorganisms by heat or chemical agents are usually first-order processes.

Second-Order Reactions—A second-order reaction is one in which the experimentally determined rate of reaction is found to be proportional to the concentration of each of two reactants or to the second power of the concentration of one reactant. If substances A and B undergo reaction at a rate proportional to the concentration of each (c_A and c_B, respectively) we may write

$$-\frac{dc_A}{dt} = -\frac{dc_B}{dt} = k \cdot c_A c_B \qquad (12)$$

If a and b represent the molar concentrations of A and B at the start of the reaction, and x is the number of moles of each which has reacted at time t the reaction rate, dx/dt, may be expressed as

$$\frac{dx}{dt} = k(a - x)(b - x) \qquad (13)$$

If the initial concentrations of A and B are equal, Eq. 13 simplifies to

$$\frac{dx}{dt} = k(a - x)^2 \qquad (14)$$

On integration

$$\frac{1}{(a - x)} = k \cdot t + \text{constant} \qquad (15)$$

The constant may be evaluated by substituting 0 for x when $t = 0$, so that

$$k = \frac{1}{t} \cdot \frac{x}{a(a - x)} \qquad (16)$$

If the initial concentrations of A and B are not equal, integration of Eq. 13, by partial fractions, and evaluation of the integration constant, gives

$$k = \frac{2.303}{t(a - b)} \log \frac{b(a - x)}{a(b - x)} \qquad (17)$$

A reaction is second-order if on substitution of the required analytical data into Eq. 16 or 17 (whichever applies) constant values of k at different times of reaction are obtained. Alternatively, a plot of $x/a(a - x)$ vs t

(see Eq. 16) will result in a straight line when a equals b in a second-order reaction; when a is not equal to b a plot of log $b(a - x)/a(b - x)$ vs t (see Eq. 17) will give the straight line, if the reaction is second-order.

An example of a second-order reaction in which two reactants are involved is the saponification of an ester, such as ethyl acetate, in alkaline solution.

$$CH_3COOC_2H_5 + OH^- \rightarrow CH_3COO^- + C_2H_5OH$$

The course of this reaction may be followed by determining by titration, at specified times, the decrease in concentration of hydroxide ions as these are consumed in the reaction.

When only one reactant is involved in a second-order reaction, Eqs. 14, 15 and 16 apply. A reaction of this type is the decomposition of hydrogen iodide, which in the gaseous state undergoes the reaction

$$2HI \rightarrow H_2 + I_2$$

The reaction rate in this case is expressed by

$$-\frac{dc_{HI}}{dt} = k . c_{HI}^2 \qquad (18)$$

The half-life of a second-order reaction has significance only when a single reactant or when two reactants, each at the same initial concentration, are involved. In both these cases the time, $t_{1/2}$, required for half of the reactant or reactants (at equal concentration) to undergo reaction may be calculated from Eq. 15 to be

$$t_{1/2} = \frac{1}{ka} \qquad (19)$$

It is obvious that while the half-life for a first-order reaction (see Eq. 11) is independent of the concentration of the reactant, it varies inversely as the initial concentration of reactant in a second-order reaction.

First- and second-order reactions are by far the most common types of rate processes encountered in consideration of drug stability. If a reaction is of higher order than first-order, it is often convenient to adjust experimental conditions so that the concentrations of all but one of the reactants remains constant throughout the experiment. If, for example, the concentration of hydroxide ion in the saponification of an ester is in great excess of the concentration of ester, or if a buffer system is employed to control hydroxide-ion concentration, then the concentration of hydroxide ion is essentially invariant throughout the course of the experiment.

The observed rate of the reaction therefore depends only on the changing concentration of the ester, and the reaction is said to be *apparent first-order* or *pseudo first-order*. The apparent first-order rate constant thus obtained is $k(OH^-)$ and, of course, is different for each hydroxide-ion concentration. The actual rate constant, k, can be obtained easily by dividing the experimentally determined apparent first-order rate constant, $k(OH^-)$, by the concentration of hydroxide ion maintained throughout the study.

In the study of complex reactions, it is often desirable to use this approach of maintaining the concentration of all but one of the reactants constant to facilitate determination of the dependency of reaction rate on each of the reactants in turn.

Third-Order Reactions—A third-order reaction is one in which the experimentally determined rate of reaction is found to be proportional to the concentration of each of three reactants, or proportional to the concentration of one of two reactants and to the second power of the concentration of the other, or proportional

to the third power of the concentration of a single reactant. Third-order reactions are very rare.

For the case of a reaction between one molecule each of A, B, and C, at molar concentrations a, b, and c, respectively, the rate equation is

$$-\frac{dc_A}{dt} = -\frac{dc_B}{dt} = -\frac{dc_C}{dt} = k . c_A c_B c_C \qquad (20)$$

Using the notation of Eq. 13, this becomes

$$\frac{dx}{dt} = k(a - x)(b - x)(c - x) \qquad (21)$$

When $a = b = c$

$$\frac{dx}{dt} = k(a - x)^3 \qquad (22)$$

On integration

$$\frac{1}{2(a - x)^2} = k . t + \text{constant} \qquad (23)$$

Evaluating the constant by substituting 0 for x when $t = 0$, we obtain

$$k = \frac{1}{2t} \left[\frac{1}{(a - x)^2} - \frac{1}{a^2} \right] \qquad (24)$$

Zero-Order Reactions—In some reactions the rate is independent of the concentration of reactant or reactants, and such reactions are termed *zero-order* reactions. Photochemical reactions—in which the rate-determining factor is the light intensity, rather than the concentration of reactant—are examples of reactions which may be found to be zero-order. In such cases the rate is expressed as

$$-dc/dt = k \qquad (25)$$

If a compound for which decomposition in solution is first-order is present in excess of its maximum solubility (a suspension), the concentration of reactant in solution will be invariant so long as there is excess solid reactant present, and the observed reaction rate will be of the form of Eq. 26

$$-dc/dt = k . c_s \qquad (26)$$

where c_s is a constant. Such reactions are *apparent zero-order* reactions.

Complex Reactions—Many chemical reactions are not simple reactions of zero-, first-, second-, or third-order. Often they consist of a combination of two or more reactions; sometimes the over-all reaction can be characterized as one of these orders, but the rate equation may be a complicated function involving first-, second-, or third-order intermediate steps. Experiment may indicate a reaction order which is nonintegral, or fractional, when reactions are complex. Nevertheless, concentrations of the various reactants usually can be controlled to permit determination of the order of a reaction with respect to each reactant, and by this means integral reaction order with respect to each component can be established.

Among complicating factors that may be involved in the kinetic study of a complex reaction are *simultaneous reactions*, *consecutive reactions*, and *opposing reactions*.

Simultaneous Reactions—Consider a substance, A, that is simultaneously converted into B and C, each at characteristic rates:

$$A \xrightarrow{k_1} B$$

$$A \xrightarrow{k_2} C$$

The equation for rate of disappearance of A is the first-order equation

$$-\frac{dc_A}{dt} = k_1 c_A + k_2 c_A = (k_1 + k_2)c_A \qquad (27)$$

On integration and arrangement in exponential form we obtain

$$c_A = c_{A0}e^{-(k_1+k_2)t} \qquad (28)$$

where c_{A0} is the initial concentration of A at $t = 0$ and c_A is the concentration at time t.

The equation for rate of formation of B is given by

$$\frac{dc_B}{dt} = k_1 c_A = k_1 c_{A0} e^{-(k_1+k_2)t} \qquad (29)$$

Integrating and arranging in exponential form

$$c_B = -\frac{k_1 c_{A0}}{(k_1 + k_2)} e^{-(k_1+k_2)t} + \text{constant} \qquad (30)$$

setting $c_B = 0$ when $t = 0$

$$\text{constant} = \frac{k_1 c_{A0}}{(k_1 + k_2)} \qquad (31)$$

then

$$c_B = \frac{k_1 c_{A0}}{(k_1 + k_2)} [1 - e^{-(k_1+k_2)t}] \qquad (32)$$

since $c_A + c_B + c_C = c_{A0}$ (initial concentration of A) it follows that

$$c_C = \frac{k_2 c_{A0}}{(k_1 + k_2)} [1 - e^{-(k_1+k_2)t}] \qquad (33)$$

Inspection of Eqs. 32 and 33 shows that the fraction of A ultimately converted to B (at infinite time) is $k_1/(k_1 + k_2)$; the fraction converted to C is $k_2/(k_1 + k_2)$.

Consecutive Reactions—If two first-order reactions occur consecutively, thus

$$A \xrightarrow{k_1} B \xrightarrow{k_2} C$$

the rate equations for each substance are

$$-\frac{dc_A}{dt} = k_1 c_A \qquad (34)$$

$$-\frac{dc_B}{dt} = -k_1 c_A + k_2 c_B \qquad (35)$$

$$\frac{dc_C}{dt} = k_2 c_B \qquad (36)$$

If at $t = 0$ we set $c_A = c_{A0}$, $c_B = 0$, and $c_C = 0$, Eq. 33 on integration and arrangement in exponential form becomes

$$c_A = c_{A0}e^{-k_1 t} \qquad (37)$$

substituting for c_A in Eq. 35 and integrating

$$c_B = \frac{k_1 c_{A0}}{(k_2 - k_1)} [e^{-k_1 t} - e^{-k_2 t}] \qquad (38)$$

since $c_A + c_B + c_C = c_{A0}$ (initial concentration of A)

$$c_C = c_{A0}\left[1 + \frac{1}{(k_1 - k_2)} (k_2 e^{-k_1 t} - k_1 e^{-k_2 t})\right] \qquad (39)$$

Opposing Reactions—The rate equation for an opposing (reversible) first-order reaction, represented by

$$A \underset{k_2}{\overset{k_1}{\rightleftharpoons}} B$$

may be expressed thus

$$\frac{dc_A}{dt} = -k_1 c_A + k_2 c_B \qquad (40)$$

At equilibrium the velocity of the forward reaction, $k_1 c_A$, is equal to the velocity of the reverse reaction, $k_2 c_B$, and $dc_A/dt = 0$. If the initial concentration of A is designated c_{A0}, and the concentrations of A and B at equilibrium are c_{Ae} and c_{Be}, respectively, then

$$\frac{c_{Be}}{c_{Ae}} = \frac{c_{A0} - c_{Ae}}{c_{Ae}} = \frac{k_1}{k_2} = K \qquad (41)$$

where K is the equilibrium constant of the reaction.

Effects on Reaction Rate

Temperature

The application of heat to increase the rate of a chemical reaction is a common laboratory procedure. The rate of most solvolytic reactions of pharmaceuticals is increased roughly 2- to 3-fold by a 10°C increase in temperature in the vicinity of room temperature.

Arrhenius noted, in 1889, that the variation with temperature of the rate constant of chemical reactions could be expressed by the equation

$$k = se^{-E_a/RT} \qquad (42)$$

where E_a is the Arrhenius *activation energy* (the difference between the average energy of reactive molecules and the average energy of all molecules), $e^{-E_a/RT}$ is the Boltzmann factor which represents the fraction of molecules having the energy E_a, s is a constant called the frequency factor, R is the gas constant (1.987 cal/°K.-mole), and T is the absolute temperature.

In logarithmic form the Arrhenius equation becomes

$$\log k = \log s - \frac{E_a}{2.303\,RT} \qquad (43)$$

If this equation is valid—and it is for a large number of reactions—a straight line is obtained on plotting $\log k$ against the reciprocal of the absolute temperature. E_a may be calculated from the slope of the line, which is $-E_a/2.303\,R$; the intercept on the $\log k$ axis is $\log s$ (see Fig. 172).

On differentiating the natural logarithm form of Eq. 43 with respect to temperature

$$\frac{d \ln k}{dT} = \frac{E_a}{RT^2} \qquad (44)$$

and on integration between the limits k_2 and k_1 at temperatures T_2 and T_1

$$\log \frac{k_2}{k_1} = \frac{E_a}{2.303R} \left(\frac{T_2 - T_1}{T_1 T_2}\right) \qquad (45)$$

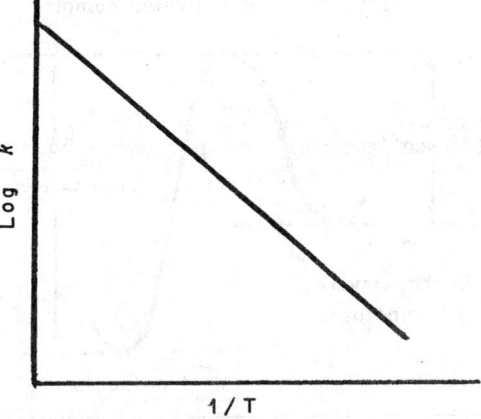

Fig. 172. **Variation of rate constant with temperature, illustrating the applicability of Arrhenius equation.**

which equation makes it possible to calculate E_a for a reaction when the rate constants are known at two temperatures or to calculate the rate constant at one temperature if E_a and the rate constant at another temperature are known.

Most solvolytic reactions of pharmaceuticals exhibit activation energies in the range of 8 to 20 Kcal/mole. Using Eq. 45 and the appropriate activation energy one can readily calculate that a reaction having an activation energy of 8 Kcal/mole would show an increase of approximately 1.5-fold in k for a temperature increase from 25° to 35°C; a reaction having an activation energy of 20 Kcal/mole would show an increase of 3.0-fold in k for a similar temperature increase.

When two molecules undergo chemical interaction, it is reasonable to suppose that they must first come close enough to each other to effect a "collision" and then, if conditions are right, undergo a rearrangement of certain electrons to form the bonds characteristic of new molecules. This means that while "collision" is a prerequisite for interaction, not all collisions lead to chemical change. If all collisions did lead to reaction, all chemical reactions would occur with great rapidity since collision frequencies are very high. The explanation is that the colliding molecules must possess at least the amount of energy E_a before reaction can occur. This energy, called the activation energy, must be sufficient to overcome the mutual repulsion of the interacting molecules and enable them to approach each other close enough to effect certain bond ruptures and simultaneously establish new bonds characteristic of the products. The greater this energy requirement is, the smaller the proportion of colliding molecules that will have the necessary energy, and the slower will be the reaction.

In the Arrhenius equation, s is a factor related to frequency of collisions, and $e^{-E_a/RT}$ is the probability that at temperature T a collision will occur with sufficient energy to provide a "successful" collision.

It would appear that in the reaction

$$A + B \rightleftharpoons [AB]^* \rightarrow \text{products}$$

there is an activated complex or transition state, represented by $[AB]^*$, which is not a complex in the usual sense but involves a critical intermediate geometric configuration in which the bonds of the reactants are weakened and the bonds of the products begin to form; if the complex has sufficient energy to effect the changes,

the reaction proceeds; if it has not, it reverts to the state of the separate reactants.

The question arises as to the significance of energy of activation in first-order reactions, where only one kind of molecule undergoes chemical change and collision with, or close proximity to, a molecule of different species is not involved. Here again only those molecules that possess energy equal to the activation energy can react. Molecules can acquire the added energy by collisions of the proper kind; hence collisions do play an important role also in reactions involving a single molecular species.

The concept of energy of activation, in relationship to the energy of the reactants and of the products, is illustrated in Fig. 173.

Other Effects

Specific Acid and Specific Base Catalysis—The term *specific acid catalysis* refers to catalysis by the hydrated proton or hydrogen ion, and *specific base catalysis* refers to catalysis by the hydroxide ion.

If the rate of hydrolysis of an ester such as ethyl acetate is studied at constant pH in a strongly buffered solution, the rate of disappearance of intact ester will be an apparent first-order reaction. If the reaction is studied in solutions buffered at several different pH values in a sufficiently acid pH region, a different apparent first-order rate constant will be observed for each pH value.

The observed rate depends on the concentration of both the ester and hydrogen ion and is actually a second-order reaction, although at a constant hydrogen-ion concentration it is an apparent first-order reaction.

$$k_{observed} = k_1(\text{H}^+) \qquad (46)$$

The observed apparent first-order rate constant determined in buffered solution is therefore proportional to hydrogen-ion concentration. The variation in observed rate constant with pH can be illustrated by taking logarithms of Eq. 46.

$$\log k_{observed} = \log k_1 + \log (\text{H}^+) \qquad (47)$$

$$\log k_{observed} = \log k_1 - \text{pH} \qquad (48)$$

Thus a plot of logarithm $k_{observed}$ vs pH should be linear with a slope of -1.

Similarly, if the same hydrolysis reaction is studied in buffered solution at several pH values in a sufficiently alkaline region of the pH scale, the observed apparent first-order rate constants will be found to vary with hydroxide-ion concentration.

$$k_{observed} = k_2(\text{OH}^-) \qquad (49)$$

$$\log k_{observed} = \log k_2 + \log (\text{OH}^-) = \log k_2 + \log \frac{K_w}{(\text{H}^+)} \qquad (50)$$

$$\log k_{observed} = \log k_2 + \log K_w + \text{pH} \qquad (51)$$

A plot of logarithm $k_{observed}$ vs pH would be a straight line with a slope of $+1$.

The complete rate expression for hydrolysis of the compound described above at all pH values would therefore be

$$-dc/dt = [k_1(\text{H}^+) + k_2(\text{OH}^-)]c \qquad (52)$$

At any specified pH value

$$k_{observed} = k_1(\text{H}^+) + k_2(\text{OH}^-) \qquad (53)$$

The complete logarithm $k_{observed}$ vs pH profile would

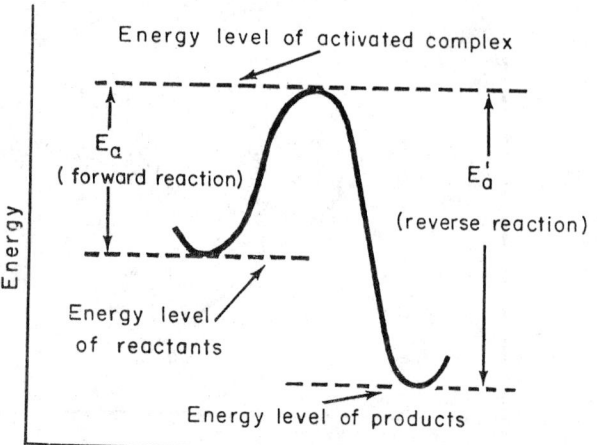

Fig. 173.   Relation between activation energy and energy levels of reactants, products, and activated complex.

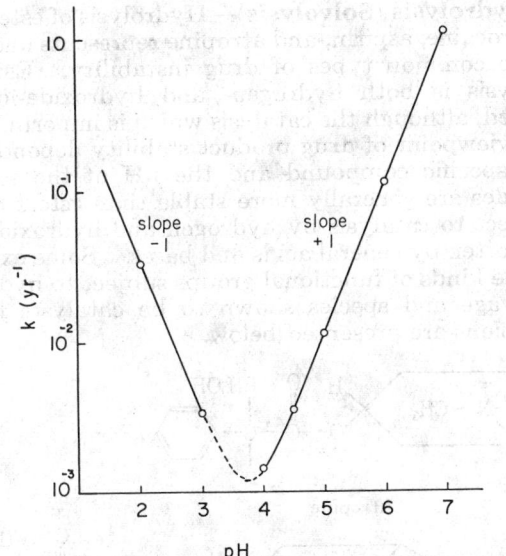

Fig. 174. **Apparent first-order rate of hydrolysis of atropine as a function of pH at 30°C. The reaction is an illustration of specific hydrogen- and hydroxide-ion catalysis (courtesy, data, Kondritzer and Zvirblis[2]).**

be similar to that illustrated in Fig. 174 for the hydrogen-ion- and hydroxide-ion- (specific acid and specific base) catalyzed hydrolysis of the ester, atropine.[2] The pH at which the minimum rate of hydrolysis is observed is a function of the relative magnitude of the specific rate constants k_1 and k_2.

In the atropine example the minimum rate of hydrolysis is at pH 3.7. If for a specific chemical species $k_1 = k_2$, the expected minimum rate of reaction for that species would be expected to occur at pH 7 (for a temperature of 25°C, at which $pK_w = 14$, and $(H^+) = (OH^-)$ at pH 7.0).

At pH values below the minimum in the plot of logarithm $k_{observed}$ vs pH, the hydrogen-ion-catalyzed reaction is much more significant than the hydroxide-ion-catalyzed reaction, and the plot has a slope of -1. At pH values above the minimum in the plot, the hydroxide-ion-catalyzed reaction is the much more important reaction and the plot has a slope of $+1$.

If a reaction is catalyzed not only by hydrogen ion and hydroxide ion, but also by the solvent (also called the uncatalyzed reaction), the logarithm $k_{observed}$ vs pH plot might appear as in Fig. 175, indicating a flat region where the rate of reaction is apparently not pH dependent. In this region the solvent reaction is much more important than that of either the hydrogen ion or hydroxide ion. The apparent first-order rate constant for such a reaction is

$$k_{observed} = k_0 + k_1(H^+) + k_2(OH^-) \qquad (54)$$

For compounds which are weak acids or weak bases, and can therefore exist in both ionized and nonionized species, the pH rate profiles become more complex. Often both the ionized and nonionized species are subject to decomposition and catalysis by hydrogen and hydroxide ion, but each of the drug species may react at a different rate. For example, hydrolysis of the weakly basic drug procaine can be represented by the following reactions:[3]

$$-dc/dt = k_1(OH^-)(Pr) + k_2(OH^-)(PrH^+) \qquad (55)$$

where Pr is the nonionized procaine molecule and PrH^+ is the protonated form. The concentration of each species can be related to the total procaine concentration by the relationships:

$$(Pr) = \frac{(OH^-)}{K_b + (OH^-)} \cdot \text{Total Procaine};$$

$$(PrH^+) = \frac{K_b}{K_b + (OH^-)} \cdot \text{Total Procaine} \qquad (56)$$

where K_b is the classical dissociation constant for the weak base procaine.

The complete rate expression for procaine hydrolysis is therefore, from Eqs. 55 and 56,

$$-dc/dt = \left[\frac{k_1(OH^-)^2}{K_b + (OH^-)} + \frac{k_2(OH^-)K_b}{K_b + (OH^-)} \right] c \qquad (57)$$

The pH dependency of procaine hydrolysis is illustrated graphically in Fig. 176 by a plot of logarithm $k_{observed}$ vs pOH for the pH region 7–13.

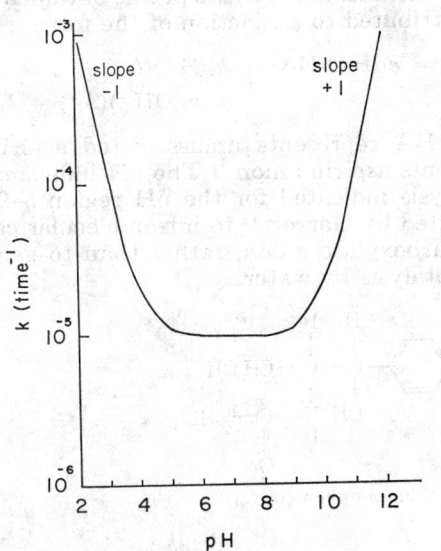

Fig. 175. **Apparent first-order rate of decomposition as a function of pH for a hypothetical case where $k_{H^+} = k_{OH^-} = 1 \times 10^{-1}$, $k_0 = 1 \times 10^{-5}$. The uncatalyzed reaction predominates in the pH region 5–9.**

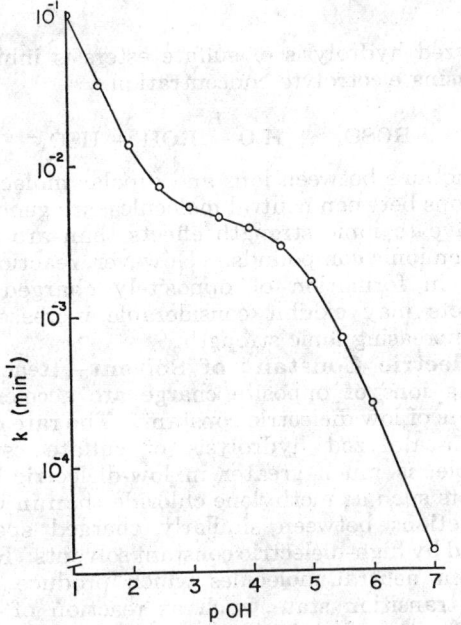

Fig. 176. **Apparent first-order rate of hydrolysis of procaine as a function of hydroxide-ion concentration at 40°C (courtesy, Higuchi, et al[3]).**

General Acid and General Base Catalysis—Acid and base catalysis is not restricted to hydrogen ion and hydroxide ion. Undissociated acids and bases can often be demonstrated to produce a catalytic effect, and in some instances metal ions and various anions can serve as catalysts.

Inversion of sucrose in acetate buffer is catalyzed by hydrogen ion, hydroxide ion, acetate ion, and undissociated acetic acid. Also, the rate of barbiturate hydrolysis in ammonia buffers is increased by increasing buffer concentration at constant pH as a result of catalysis by NH_3.[4] Hydrolysis of the amide function of chloramphenicol exhibits, in addition to solvent and specific acid–base catalysis, general acid–base catalysis in phosphate and citrate buffers.[5,6] General acid–base catalysis is to be anticipated if there is evidence of a significant solvent catalysis as illustrated in the pH-rate profile of Fig. 175.

Ionic Strength—In general the effects of increasing concentrations of electrolytes on reaction rate can be predicted by consideration of the influence of ionic strength on interionic attraction. The Debye–Hückel equation[7] may be used to demonstrate that increased ionic strength would be expected to decrease rate of reaction involving interaction between oppositely charged ions, and increase rate of reaction between similarly charged ions. Thus, the hydrogen-ion-

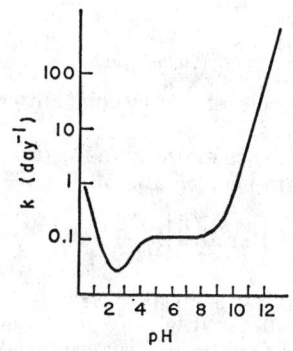

Fig. 177. Apparent first-order rate of hydrolysis of aspirin as a function of pH at 17°C (courtesy, Edwards[11]).

catalyzed hydrolysis of sulfate esters is inhibited by increasing electrolyte concentration.[8]

$$ROSO_3^- + H_2O \xrightarrow{H^+} ROH + HSO_4^-$$

Reactions between ions and dipolar molecules, and reactions between neutral molecules, are generally less sensitive to ionic strength effects than are reactions between ionic compounds. However, reactions which result in formation of oppositely charged ions as products may exhibit considerable increase in rate with increasing ionic strength.

Dielectric Constant of Solvent—Reactions involving ions of opposite charge are accelerated by solvents of low dielectric constant. The rate of hydrogen-ion-catalyzed hydrolysis of sulfate esters, for example, is much greater in low-dielectric constant solvents such as methylene chloride than in water.[9]

Reactions between similarly charged species are favored by high-dielectric constant solvents. Reactions between neutral molecules which produce a highly polar transition state, such as reaction of triethylamine with ethyl iodide to produce a quaternary ammonium salt,[10] will also be enhanced by high-dielectric constant solvents.

Hydrolysis (Solvolysis)—Hydrolysis of esters such as procaine, aspirin, and atropine represents one of the more common types of drug instability. Ester hydrolysis is both hydrogen- and hydroxide-ion catalyzed, although the catalysis which is important from the viewpoint of drug product stability depends upon the specific compound and the pH of the solution. Amides are generally more stable than esters but are subject to catalysis by hydrogen and hydroxide ions, and often by general acids and bases. Some examples of the kinds of functional groups subject to hydrolytic cleavage and species shown to be catalysts for the reactions are presented below.

Atropine

Hydrolysis of the ester function of atropine is typical of ester hydrolysis in that the only important reactions are catalysis by hydrogen ion and hydroxide ion.[2] Figure 174 illustrates a pH-rate profile which might be considered typical for such a reaction. Below pH 3 the principal reaction is hydrogen-ion-catalyzed hydrolysis of the protonated form of atropine. Above pH 5 the principal reaction is hydroxide-ion-catalyzed hydrolysis of the same species. Maximum stability at 30° is at pH 3.7.

Aspirin

Hydrolytic cleavage of aspirin to salicylic acid and acetic acid was studied by Edwards,[11] who obtained the interesting pH-rate profile reproduced in Fig. 177. The unusual pH-rate profile obtained for aspirin was attributed to a reaction of the form

$$-dc/dt = k_1(H^+)(HA) + k_2(H^+)(A^-) +$$
$$k_3(OH^-)(A^-) + k_0(A^-) \quad (58)$$

where HA represents undissociated aspirin and A^- represents aspirin anion. The pH-independent anion hydrolysis indicated for the pH region 5–9 has been attributed by Garrett[12] to intramolecular catalysis by orthocarboxylate anion, rather than to general acid–base catalysis by water.

Chloramphenicol

Chloramphenicol decomposition below pH 7 proceeds primarily through hydrolytic cleavage of the amide function.[6]   The reaction may be represented as

$$-dc/dt = [k_0 + k_1(H^+) + k_2(OH^-) +$$
$$k_{HB}(HB) + k_B(B)]c \quad (59)$$

In addition to hydrogen- and hydroxide-ion catalysis there is an uncatalyzed (or water) reaction, and there may be general acid–base catalysis, represented above by the buffer species HB and B. In general, rate of hydroxide-ion-catalyzed hydrolysis of amides is greater than rate of hydronium-ion-catalyzed hydrolysis.

$$(CH_3)_2C(OH).CCl_3 \rightarrow 3Cl^- + (CH_3)_2CO + CO +$$
Chlorobutanol $(CH_3)_2C(OH).COOH$

The over-all reaction for decomposition of chlorobutanol in aqueous solution is represented above. The reaction is solvent and specific hydroxide-ion catalyzed and the rate of decomposition is not significant below pH 4.[13]

$$-dc/dt = [k_0 + k_1(OH^-)]c \quad (60)$$

Barbiturate hydrolysis involves hydroxide-ion attack on both the undissociated acid and the ionized species. Hydrogen-ion-catalyzed hydrolysis is not observed in the pH range of interest in pharmaceutical products.

$$-dc/dt = k_1(OH^-)(HP) + k_2(OH^-)(P^-) \quad (61)$$

Modest buffer catalysis has been observed in ammonia buffers.[4,14] Cleavage of the ring system leads to loss of pharmacologic activity, with further decomposition of the initial acyclic products.

The decomposition of penicillin in aqueous solution was first studied in detail by Broderson.[15–18] Hydrolysis is catalyzed by hydrogen ion,[15] solvent,[15] hydroxide ion,[19] and certain buffer species.[19] Maximum stability in aqueous solution is at about pH 7.[18]

Racemization—The acid-catalyzed racemization of epinephrine,[20] with loss of characteristic pharmacologic activity of epinephrine, is illustrative of an additional type of drug decomposition which may be encountered.

Oxidation—Compounds such as phenols, aromatic amines, aldehydes, ethers, and unsaturated aliphatic compounds are subject to oxidation upon exposure to air or oxidizing chemicals. Epinephrine, ascorbic acid, phenothiazines, and vitamin A are examples of important pharmaceutical products which are readily oxidized.

Of particular concern are oxidations which occur when solutions are exposed to atmospheric oxygen. Such reactions are termed autoxidation (or self-oxidation) and are complex reactions which proceed via what is termed a free-radical mechanism. A free radical is a highly unstable (highly reactive) species containing an unpaired electron. Autoxidation reactions are autocatalytic in that free-radical reactions generate additional free radicals, causing a chain reaction. A technique utilized to protect pharmaceuticals susceptible to autoxidation is to include in the formulation agents which will react readily with free radicals, but which will terminate the chain-propagation either by forming relatively stable radicals (resonance stabilized) or by forming products which do not include additional free radicals.

Photochemical Decomposition—Numerous dyes and drugs are subject to photochemical decomposition. Light-catalyzed oxidations and reductions of photo-excited species are common, and are often mechanistically complex reactions involving free-radical intermediates. Pharmaceuticals such as riboflavin[21] and phenothiazines[22] are examples of common drugs which are extremely light sensitive.

Interaction between Components—Because drugs are often combined in solution with buffers, antioxidants, flavoring agents, antimicrobial preservatives, and other drugs, potential interaction between components of a formulation must be considered in pharmaceutical formulation development. Some obvious interactions, such as possibility of reaction of a drug having a primary amino function with an aldehyde such as vanillin to produce a Schiff base can be predicted, but a number of interesting, less-well-recognized, reactions have been encountered.

In addition to buffer species acting as general acid–base catalysts, as previously indicated, some buffer species undergo specific interactions with drug molecules to form new chemical compounds. Higuchi and Miki[23] observed formation of amides, in aqueous solution, between amines such as benzocaine and buffers such as citric acid.

Cannell[24] observed reaction of the aromatic amino function of procaine with glucose to form procaine N-glycoside. Goto, et al,[25] noted reaction of phenylethylamine with dehydroacetic acid to form a Schiff base-type compound. Schwartz[26,27] observed catalysis of penicillin hydrolysis by catechols.

Higuchi and Schroeter[28] demonstrated that bisulfite, an agent commonly employed to protect epinephrine against oxidative decomposition, is capable of inducing epinephrine degradation through attack on the optically active side chain.

$$HO-\underset{HO}{\bigcirc}-\underset{\underset{OH}{|}}{CH}-CH_2-NHCH_3 \ + \ SO_3^= \ \longrightarrow$$

$$HO-\underset{HO}{\bigcirc}-\underset{\underset{SO_3H}{|}}{CH}-CH_2-NHCH_3$$

Scheindlin[29] demonstrated that although a solution of folic acid alone is stable to light, a combination of riboflavin and folic acid showed rapid loss of folic acid through formation of a coupled oxidation–reduction system in which riboflavin was photoreduced with folic acid being utilized as reducing substrate and being itself irreversibly oxidized. In the dark and in the presence of oxygen, the riboflavin was regenerated, and when the solution was again irradiated the cycle was repeated with further destruction of folic acid. The riboflavin is termed a *photosensitizer* in this reaction and would cause the decomposition not only of folic acid but also of ascorbic acid or any other easily oxidized substrate.

The presence of micellar surfactants and certain high-molecular-weight polymers commonly employed in pharmaceuticals also has been shown to lead to decreased drug stability in some cases. Both nonionic and anionic surfactants, as well as polymers such as polyvinylpyrrolidone, accelerate the photodecomposition of riboflavin in aqueous solution.[19] Nonionic surfactants are capable also of increasing the rate of hydrolysis of sulfate esters which may be incorporated in or on the micellar surface.[30]

Drug Stabilization

Some drug decomposition reactions, such as photolytic and oxidative reactions, are relatively easy to avoid by protection of components from light to protect against photodecomposition or exclusion of oxygen and use of chain-terminating reagents or free-radical scavengers to terminate free-radical mediated reactions. Solvolysis reactions, however, can not be stopped by such procedures, but several techniques may be employed to retard reactions sufficiently to permit formulation of a suitable drug product. The following approaches may be useful in attempts to retard solvolytic reactions.

Selection of Optimum pH, Buffer, and Solvent —Consideration of the mechanism of the reaction and the way in which the reaction rate is influenced by pH, buffer species, and solvent permits selection of the optimum conditions for drug stability. Often, however, ideal conditions for maximum stability may be unacceptable from the viewpoint of pharmaceutically acceptable formulation or therapeutic efficacy, and it may be necessary to prepare a formulation with conditions less than optimum for stability of the drug. If a suitable compromise between conditions for maximum stability and conditions for a pharmaceutically acceptable formulation can not be achieved, techniques such as those described below may be useful in retarding solvolysis reactions.

Specific Complexing Agents—The technique of stabilization by formation of complexes in solution was introduced by Higuchi and Lachman,[31] who demonstrated that the rate of hydrolysis of the ester function of benzocaine was significantly retarded in the presence of caffeine, a reagent with which the benzocaine formed a soluble complex. It was further demonstrated that in these systems the complexed drug did not hydrolyze at all, and that the observed rate of hydrolysis could be ascribed to the concentration of the free or uncomplexed drug which was in equilibrium with the drug complex.

Riegelman and Fischer[32] demonstrated that boric acid chelation of the catechol function of epinephrine stabilizes epinephrine against attack by bisulfite and sulfite.

Surfactants—Riegelman[33] demonstrated that the incorporation of benzocaine into surfactant micelles could significantly retard the rate of ester hydrolysis. Nonionic and anionic surfactants retarded the hydroxide-ion-catalyzed hydrolysis, but cationic surfactants somewhat increased the rate of hydroxide-ion-catalyzed hydrolysis. Similar observations have been reported for a number of drugs which are sufficiently lipophilic to be solubilized by surfactant micelles.

Suspensions—If the solubility of a labile drug is reduced, and the drug prepared in a suspension form, the rate at which the drug degrades will be related only to the concentration of drug in solution, rather than to the total concentration of drug in the product. Thus Swintosky, *et al*,[34, 35] were able to demonstrate that penicillin G procaine suspensions degraded at a rate proportional to the low concentration of penicillin in solution. Since the penicillin in solution was in equilibrium with excess solid penicillin G procaine, the penicillin concentration in solution was constant and the observed order of reaction was apparent zero-order.

Stability Testing of Pharmaceutical Products

If a product is sufficiently stable to be marketed, it would require relatively long storage at room temperature, or actual temperature at which it will be stored prior to ultimate use, to permit observation of the rate at which the product degrades under normal storage conditions.

To avoid this undesirable delay in evaluating potential formulations, the manufacturer attempts to predict stability under conditions of room temperature, or actual storage conditions, through use of data for rate of decomposition obtained at several elevated temperatures. This prediction is accomplished through use of an Arrhenius plot to predict from high-temperature data the rate of product breakdown to be expected at actual storage conditions. The methods[36] and facilities[37, 38] for accomplishing these predictions have been reviewed and will not be discussed here.

Prediction based on data obtained at elevated temperature is generally satisfactory for solution dosage forms. Success is more uncertain when non-homogeneous products are involved. Suspensions of drugs may not provide linear Arrhenius plots because there is often the possibility that the solid phase which exists at elevated temperature may not be the same solid phase which exists at room temperature, and differences in solubility of the several solid phases which may exist can invalidate the usual Arrhenius plots.

Such difficulties should be anticipated when polymorphic crystal forms or several different solvates are known to exist. Also, when solid dosage forms such as tablets are subjected to high temperatures, changes in the quantity of moisture in the product may greatly influence the stability of the product.

Arrhenius plots also suffer limitations in application to reactions which have relatively low activation energies, and therefore are not greatly accelerated by increase in temperature. While it is usually desirable to determine drug stability by analyzing samples for the amount of intact drug remaining—in instances where there is very little drug decomposition, and particularly when it is not convenient to accelerate the reaction by increasing temperature—it is sometimes advantageous to determine initial reaction rates from determination of amount of reaction product formed.

For example, if the concentration of a drug decreased from 100% to 98% during the course of study, the determination of the rate of reaction would be based on a concentration change of only 2% in the assay results. However, if 0.1% of the product of reaction could be detected, then product formed in the same reaction could be followed from 0.1% to 2%, and the determination of the reaction rate based on reaction product concentration would be based on a 20-fold difference in assay value.

Such an approach can only be utilized, however, if the reaction is sufficiently characterized to assure that the quantity of product determined can be properly related to the extent of drug decomposition.

Since manufacturers are most interested in the time required to produce just a few per cent breakdown in their product, it is not uncommon for them to employ terminology such as $t_{.90}$ or $t_{.95}$, which is the time required for the drug to decompose to 90% or 95%, respectively, of original potency. This terminology is completely analogous to the terminology $t_{1/2}$, or $t_{.50}$, used to represent the half-life period.

An Arrhenius-type plot, analogous to that illustrated in Fig. 172, can be obtained by plotting logarithm of time required for the specified fractional decomposition vs reciprocal of absolute temperature. The time required for the product to decrease in potency to 90% of original potency at room temperature then can be obtained directly from the plot.

While manufacturers wish to be able to predict the stability of formulations to storage conditions, and utilize accelerated stability testing to achieve these predictions, they also maintain products under actual storage conditions to assure that actual stability under storage conditions agrees with the prediction of the accelerated testing.

References

1. Garrett, E. R., in Bean, H. S., *et al*, *Advances in Pharmaceutical Sciences*, vol. 2, Academic, New York and London, 1967, pp. 2–94.
2. Kondritzer, A. A., and Zvirblis, P., *J. APhA, Sci. Ed.*, **46**, 531 (1957).
3. Higuchi, T., *et al*, *J. APhA, Sci. Ed.*, **39**, 405 (1950).
4. Goyan, J. E., *et al*, *J. APhA, Sci. Ed.*, **49**, 627 (1960).
5. Higuchi, T., *et al*, *J. APhA, Sci. Ed.*, **43**, 129 (1954).
6. Higuchi, T., and Marcus, A. D., *J. APhA, Sci. Ed.*, **43**, 530 (1954).
7. Frost, A. A., and Pearson, R. G., *Kinetics and Mechanism*, 2nd ed., Wiley, New York, 1961, p. 150.
8. Kurz, J. L., *J. Phys. Chem.*, **66**, 2239 (1962).
9. Burstein, S., and Lieberman, S., *J. Am. Chem. Soc.*, **80**, 5235 (1958).
10. Menschutkin, N., *Z. Physik. Chem. (Leipzig)*, **6**, 41 (1890).
11. Edwards, L. J., *Trans. Faraday Soc.*, **46**, 723 (1950).
12. Garrett, E. R., *J. Am. Chem. Soc.*, **79**, 3401 (1957).
13. Nair, A. D., and Lach, J. L., *J. APhA, Sci. Ed.*, **48**, 390 (1959).
14. Tishler, F., *et al*, *J. Pharm. Sci.*, **51**, 214 (1962).
15. Broderson, R., *Acta Chem. Scand.*, **1**, 403 (1947).
16. Broderson, R., *Acta Pharmacol. Toxicol.*, **3**, 345 (1947).
17. Broderson, R., *Kgl. Danske Videnskab. Selskab Mat.-fys. Medd.*, **24**, 14 (1948).
18. Broderson, R., *Inactivation of Penicillin in Aqueous Solution*, Munksgaard, Copenhagen, 1949.
19. Finholt, P., *et al*, *J. Pharm. Sci.*, **54**, 387 (1965).
20. Schroeter, L. C., and Higuchi, T., *J. APhA, Sci. Ed.*, **47**, 426 (1958).
21. Kostenbauder, H. B., *et al*, *J. Pharm. Sci.*, **54**, 1243 (1965).
22. Felmeister, A., and Discher, C. A., *J. Pharm. Sci.*, **53**, 756 (1964).
23. Higuchi, T., and Miki, T., *J. Am. Chem. Soc.*, **83**, 3899 (1961).
24. Cannell, J. S., *J. Pharm. Pharmacol.*, **3**, 741 (1951).
25. Goto, S., *J. Pharm. Sci.*, **56**, 579 (1967).
26. Schwartz, M. A., *J. Pharm. Sci.*, **53**, 1433 (1964).
27. Schwartz, M. A., *J. Pharm. Sci.*, **54**, 1308 (1965).
28. Higuchi, T., and Schroeter, L. C., *J. APhA, Sci. Ed.*, **48**, 535 (1959).
29. Scheindlin, S., *Drug Cosmetic Ind.*, **83**, 46 (1958).
30. Motsavage, V. A., and Kostenbader, H. B., *J. Colloid Sci.*, **18**, 603 (1963).
31. Higuchi, T., and Lachman, L., *J. APhA, Sci. Ed.*, **44**, 521 (1955).
32. Riegelman, S., and Fischer, E. Z., *J. Pharm. Sci.*, **51**, 206 (1962).
33. Riegelman, S., *J. APhA, Sci. Ed.*, **49**, 339 (1960).
34. Swintosky, J. V., *et al*, *J. APhA, Sci. Ed.*, **45**, 34 (1956).
35. Swintosky, J. V., *et al*, *J. APhA, Sci. Ed.*, **45**, 37 (1956).
36. Garrett, E. R., *J. Pharm. Sci.*, **51**, 811 (1962).
37. Lachman, L., and Cooper, J., *J. APhA, Sci. Ed.*, **48**, 226 (1959).
38. Lachman, L., and Cooper, J., *J. APhA, Sci. Ed.*, **48**, 233 (1959).

22 | Interfacial Phenomena

Interfacial forces and energetics—adhesional and cohesional forces—
wetting phenomena—capillarity—pressure differences across curved
surfaces—monomolecular surface films—micelle formation—
solubilization in micellar solutions—adsorption on solid surfaces—
surface-active agents

This chapter was prepared by

George Zografi, PhD, *Associate Professor, College of Pharmacy, University
of Michigan, Ann Arbor, Mich. 48104*

The study of interfacial phenomena is concerned
with the properties of molecules situated at or very
near the boundary between immiscible phases,
generally called the interface or the interfacial region.
In systems of pharmaceutical and medicinal interest
the number of situations where multiphase systems,
and thus interfaces, occur is quite great.

Consider, as examples, the variety of heterogeneous dosage forms such as suspensions (solid dispersed in liquid), emulsions (liquid in liquid), foams
(vapor in liquid or solid), and powders (solid in solid),
as well as the contact of drug molecules with various
interfaces during transport from the dosage form,
passage through biologic membranes, and accumulation at the cellular site of activity.

Interfacial Forces and Energetics

In the bulk portion of each phase, molecules are
attracted to one another equally in all directions, such
that no resultant forces are acting on any one molecule.
The strength of these forces determines whether a
substance exists as a vapor, liquid, or solid at a
particular temperature and pressure.

At the boundary between phases, however, molecules are acted upon unequally since they are in contact with other molecules exhibiting different forces
of attraction. For example, the primary intermolecular forces in water are due to hydrogen bonds,
whereas those responsible for intermolecular bonding
in hydrocarbon liquids, such as mineral oil, are due
primarily to the London dispersion forces.

Since, in such systems, the forces between like
molecules usually are greater than between unlike
molecules (hence the immiscibility), these unequal
forces will be greater in a direction normal to the
interface and toward each bulk phase. For interfaces
containing mobile molecules, as with liquids, these
unequal forces produce a tendency for molecules to
reduce the area of contact by leaving the interface,
resulting in an increased intermolecular distance in
the interface at equilibrium.

Any attempt to reverse this process by increasing
the area of contact between phases causes the interface to resist expansion and to behave as though it
is under a tension everywhere in a tangential direction.
The force of this tension per unit length of interface
generally is called the interfacial tension, except when
dealing with the air–liquid interface, where the terms
surface and surface tension are used.

To illustrate the presence of a tension in the interface, consider an experiment where a circular metal
frame, with a looped piece of thread loosely tied to it,
is dipped into a liquid. When removed and exposed
to the air, a film of liquid will be stretched entirely
across the circular frame, as when one uses such a
frame to blow soap bubbles. Under these conditions
(Fig. 178A), the thread will remain collapsed. If
now a heated needle is used to puncture and remove
the liquid film from within the loop (Fig. 178B), the
loop will spontaneously stretch into a circular shape.

The result of this experiment demonstrates the
spontaneous reduction of interfacial contact between
air and the liquid remaining and, indeed, that a tension
causing the loop to remain extended exists parallel to
the interface. The circular shape of the loop indicates
that the tension in the plane of the interface exists at
right angles or normal to every part of the looped
thread. The total force on the entire loop divided by
the circumference of the circle, therefore, represents
the tension per unit distance of surface, or the surface tension.

Just as work is required to extend a spring under
tension, work should be required to reverse the
process seen in Figs. 178A and B, thus bringing more
molecules to the interface. This may be seen quantitatively by considering an experiment where tension
and work may be measured directly. Assume that we
have a rectangular wire with one movable side (Fig.
179). Assume further that by dipping this wire into
a liquid, a film of liquid will form within the frame
when it is removed and exposed to the air. As seen
earlier in Fig. 178B, since it comes in contact with air,
the liquid surface will tend to contract with a force,
F, as molecules leave the surface for the bulk. To
keep the movable side in equilibrium, an equal force
must be applied to oppose this tension in the surface.
We then may define the surface tension, γ, of the
liquid as $F/2l$, where $2l$ is the distance of surface over
which F is operating ($2l$ since there are two surfaces,
top and bottom). If the surface is expanded by a
very small distance, Δx, one can then estimate that
the work done is:

$$W = F\Delta x \qquad (1)$$

and, therefore,

$$W = \gamma 2l \Delta x \qquad (2)$$

Since

$$\Delta A = 2l \Delta x \qquad (3)$$

where ΔA is the change in area due to the expansion
of the surface, we may conclude that

$$W = \gamma \Delta A \qquad (4)$$

Thus, the work required to create a unit area of surface, known as the surface free energy/unit area, is equivalent to the surface tension of a liquid system, and the greater the area of interfacial contact between phases, the greater the free-energy increase for the total system. Since a prime requisite for equilibrium is that the free energy of a system be at a minimum, it is not surprising to observe that phases in contact tend to reduce area of contact spontaneously.

Liquids, being mobile, may assume spherical shapes (smallest interfacial area for a given volume), as when ejected from an orifice into air or when dispersed into another immiscible liquid. If a large number of drops are formed, further reduction in area can occur by having the drops coalesce, as when a foam collapses or when the liquid phases making up an emulsion separate.

Surface tension is expressed in units of dynes/cm, while surface free energy is expressed in ergs/cm². Since an erg is a dyne-cm, both sets of units of course are equivalent.

Values for the surface tension of a variety of liquids are given in Table I, while interfacial tension values for various liquids against water are given in Table II. Other combinations of immiscible phases could be given but most heterogeneous systems encountered in pharmacy usually contain water so that emphasis only will be given to aqueous systems.

Values for these tensions are expressed for a particular temperature. Since an increased temperature increases the thermal energy of molecules, the work required to bring molecules to the interface should be less, and thus the surface and interfacial tension will be reduced. For example, the surface tension of water at 0°C is 76.5 dynes/cm and 63.5 dynes/cm at 75°C. As would be expected from the discussion so far, the relative values for surface tension should reflect the nature of intermolecular forces present; hence, the relatively large values for mercury (metallic bonds) and water (hydrogen bonds), and the lower values for benzene, chloroform, carbon tetrachloride, and the n-alkanes.

Benzene with π electrons exhibits a higher surface tension than the alkanes of comparable molecular weight, but increasing the molecular weight of the alkanes (and hence intermolecular attraction) increases their surface tension closer to that of benzene. The lower values for the more nonpolar substances, perfluoroheptane and liquid N₂, demonstrate this point even more strongly.

Values of interfacial tension should reflect the differences in chemical structure of the two phases involved; the greater the tendency to interact, the less the interfacial tension. The 20-dynes/cm difference between air–water tension and that at the octane–water interface reflects the small but significant interaction between octane molecules and water molecules at the interface. This is seen also in Table II, by

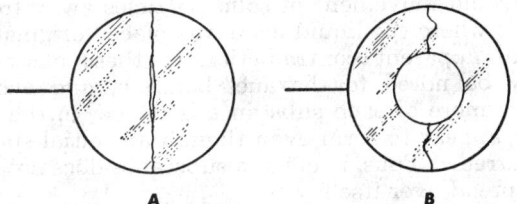

Fig. 178. A circular wire frame with a loop of thread loosely tied to it: (A) a liquid film on the wire frame with a loop in it; (B) the film inside the loop is broken (courtesy, Semat[1]).

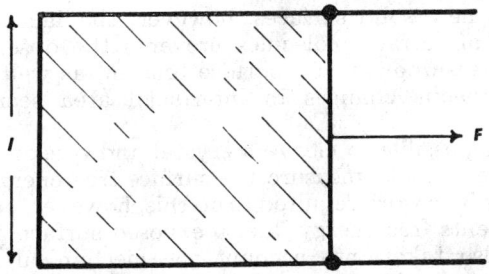

Fig. 179. A movable wire frame containing a film of liquid being expanded with a force, F.

comparing values for octane and octanol, oleic acid and the alkanes, or chloroform and carbon tetrachloride.

In each case the presence of chemical groups capable of hydrogen bonding with water markedly reduces the interfacial tension, presumably by satisfying the unbalanced forces at the interface. These observations strongly suggest that molecules at an interface arrange themselves or orient so as to minimize differences between bulk phases.

That this occurs even at the air–liquid interface is seen when one notes the relatively low surface-tension values of very different chemical structures such as the n-alkanes, octanol, oleic acid, benzene, and chloroform. Presumably, in each case, the similar nonpolar groups are oriented toward the air with any polar groups oriented away toward the bulk phase. This tendency for molecules to orient at an interface is a basic factor in interfacial phenomena and will be discussed more fully in succeeding sections.

The strong intermolecular forces existing in solids lead to relatively large values for the work required to

Table I—Surface Tension of Various Liquids at 20°C

Substance	Surface tension, dynes/cm
Mercury	476
Water	72.8
Glycerin	63.4
Oleic acid	32.5
Benzene	28.9
Chloroform	27.1
Carbon tetrachloride	26.8
n-Octanol	26.5
Hexadecane	27.4
Dodecane	25.4
Decane	23.9
Octane	21.8
Heptane	19.7
Hexane	18.0
Perfluoroheptane	11.0
Nitrogen (at 75°K)	9.4

Table II—Interfacial Tension of Various Liquids against Water at 20°C

Substance	Interfacial tension, dynes/cm
Decane	52.3
Octane	51.7
Hexane	50.8
Carbon tetrachloride	45.0
Chloroform	32.8
Benzene	35.0
Mercury	428
Oleic acid	15.6
n-Octanol	8.51

create new solid surfaces, however, the lack of mobility of surface molecules prevents the observation and measurement of a surface tension, as well as the spontaneous changes in interfacial area seen with liquids.

It is possible to cleave a crystal and to expose new surface so as to measure the surface free energy/unit area. The work required to do this, however, not only represents free energy due to exposed surface groups, but also takes into account the mechanical energy associated with the crystal (ie, plastic and elastic deformation and strain energies due to crystal imperfections).

Also contributing to the complexity of a solid surface is the heterogeneous behavior due to the exposure of different crystal faces, each having a different surface free energy/unit area. Surface roughness and porosity also will add to the difficulty of interpreting the surface behavior of solids.

The properties of molecules at the vapor–solid and liquid–solid interfaces will be discussed in later sections, but based upon the complexities discussed above, any definitive discussion of solid-surface energetics must be limited until more fundamental information is available.

Adhesional and Cohesional Forces

Of prime importance to those dealing with heterogeneous systems is the question of how two phases will behave when brought in contact with each other. It is well known, for instance, that some liquids, when placed in contact with other liquid or solid surfaces, will remain retracted in the form of a drop (known as a lens), while other liquids may exhibit a tendency to spread and cover the surface of this liquid or solid.

Based upon concepts developed to this point, it is apparent that the individual phases will exhibit a tendency to minimize the area of contact with other phases, thus leading to phase separation. On the other hand, the tendency for interaction between molecules at the new interface will offset this to some extent and give rise to the spontaneous spreading of one substance over the other.

In essence, therefore, phase affinity is increased as the forces of attraction between different phases (adhesional forces) become greater than the forces of attraction between molecules of the same phase (cohesional forces). If these adhesional forces become great enough, miscibility will occur and the interface will disappear, so that the present discussion is concerned only with systems of limited phase affinity.

A convenient approach used to express these forces quantitatively involves the use of the terms, work of adhesion and work of cohesion.

The work of adhesion, W_a, is defined as the energy per cm² required to separate two phases at their boundary and is equal but opposite in sign to the free energy/cm² released when the interface is formed. In an analogous manner the work of cohesion for a pure substance, W_c, is the work/cm² required to produce two new surfaces, as when separating different phases, but now both surfaces contain the same molecules. This is equal and opposite in sign to the free energy/cm² released when the same two pure liquid surfaces are brought together and eliminated.

By convention, when the work of adhesion between two substances, A and B, exceeds the work of cohesion for one substance, eg, B, spontaneous spreading of B over the surface of A should occur with a net loss of free energy equal to the difference between W_a and W_c. If W_c exceeds W_a, no spontaneous spreading of B over A can occur. The difference between W_a and W_c is known as the spreading coefficient, S; thus, only when S is positive will spreading occur.

The values for W_a and W_c (and hence S) may be expressed in terms of surface and interfacial tensions, when one considers that upon separation of two phases, A and B, γ_{AB} ergs of interfacial free energy/cm² (interfacial tension) are lost, but that γ_A and γ_B ergs/cm² of energy (surface tensions of A and B) are gained; upon separation of bulk phase molecules in an analogous manner, $2\gamma_A$ or $2\gamma_B$ ergs/cm² will be gained. Thus,

$$W_a = \gamma_A + \gamma_B - \gamma_{AB} \tag{5}$$

and

$$W_c = 2\gamma_A \text{ or } 2\gamma_B \tag{6}$$

For B spreading on the surface of A, therefore,

$$S_B = \gamma_A + \gamma_B - \gamma_{AB} - 2\gamma_B \tag{7}$$

or

$$S_B = \gamma_A - (\gamma_B + \gamma_{AB}) \tag{8}$$

Utilizing Eq. 8 and values of surface and interfacial tension given in Tables I and II, S can be calculated for three representative substances—decane, benzene, and oleic acid—on water at 20°.

Decane: $S = 72.8 - (23.9 + 52.3) = -3.4$

Benzene: $S = 72.8 - (28.9 + 35.0) = 8.9$

Oleic Acid: $S = 72.8 - (32.5 + 15.6) = 24.7$

As expected, relatively nonpolar substances such as decane exhibit negative values of S, whereas the more polar materials yield positive values; the greater the polarity of the molecule, the more positive the value of S. The importance of the cohesive energy of the spreading liquid may be noted also by comparing the spreading coefficients for hexane on water and water on hexane:

$$S_{H/W} = 72.8 - (18.0 + 50.8) = 4.0$$

$$S_{W/H} = 18.0 - (72.8 + 50.8) = -105.6$$

Here, despite the fact that both liquids are the same, the high cohesion and air–liquid tension of water prevents spreading on the low-energy hexane surface, while the very low value for hexane allows spreading on the water surface. This also is seen when comparing the positive spreading coefficient of hexane to the negative value for decane on water.

To see whether spreading does or does not occur, a powder such as talc or charcoal can be sprinkled over the surface of water such that it floats; then, a drop of each liquid is placed on this surface. As predicted, decane will remain as an intact drop, while hexane, benzene, and oleic acid will spread out, as shown by the rapid movement of solid particles away from the point where the liquid drop was placed originally.

An apparent contradiction to these observations may be noted for hexane, benzene, and oleic acid when more of each substance is added, in that lenses now appear to form even though an initial spreading occurred. Thus, in effect a substance does not appear to spread over itself.

It is now established that the spreading substance forms a monomolecular film which creates a new surface having a lower surface free energy than pure water. This arises because of the apparent orientation of the molecules in such a film so that their most hydrophobic portion is oriented towards the spreading phase. It is the lack of affinity between this exposed portion of the spread molecule and the polar portion of the remaining molecules which prevents further spreading.

This may be seen by calculating a final spreading coefficient where the new surface tension of water plus monomolecular film is used. For example, the presence of benzene reduces the surface tension of water to 62.2 dynes/cm so that the final spreading coefficient, S_F, is

$$S_F = 62.2 - (28.9 + 35.0) = -1.7$$

The lack of spreading exhibited by oleic acid should be reflected in an even more negative final spreading coefficient, since the very polar carboxyl groups should have very little affinity for the exposed alkyl chain of the oleic acid film. Spreading so as to form a second layer with polar groups exposed to the air would also seem very unlikely, thus leading to the formation of a lens.

Wetting Phenomena

In the experiment described above it was shown that talc or charcoal sprinkled onto the surface of water float despite the fact that their density is much greater than that of water. In order for immersion of the solid to occur, the liquid must displace air and spread over the surface of the solid; when liquids cannot spread over a solid surface spontaneously, we say that the solid is not wetted.

An important parameter which reflects the degree of wetting is the angle which the liquid makes with the solid surface at the point of contact (Fig. 180).[2] By convention, when wetting is complete, the contact angle is zero; in nonwetting situations it theoretically can increase to a value of 180°, where a spherical droplet makes contact with solid at only one point. The macroscopic roughness of a surface, which increases the surface area of the solid, can change the contact angle such that[3]

$$\cos \theta' = r \cos \theta, \tag{9}$$

where θ is the expected angle for a smooth surface, θ' for the actual rough surface, and r is the ratio of the true area to the apparent area assuming smoothness. Since r is generally greater than one, when θ is greater than 90°, θ' will be greater than θ; however, when θ is less than 90°, θ' will be less than θ. Thus roughening a surface increases contact angle if the angle is ordinarily greater than 90°, but decreases it if the angle is ordinarily less than 90°.

Table III—Contact Angle on Paraffin and Nylon for Various Liquids of Differing Surface Tension

Substance	Surface tension, dynes/cm	Contact angle Paraffin	Nylon
Water	72.8	130°	70°
Glycerin	63.4	96°	60°
Formamide	58.2	91°	50°
Methylene iodide	50.8	66°	41°
α-Bromonaphthalene	44.6	47°	16°
tert-Butylnaphthalene	33.7	38°	spreads
Benzene	28.9	24°	"
Dodecane	25.4	17°	"
Decane	23.9	7°	"
Nonane	22.9	spreads	"

In order to express contact angle in terms of solid–liquid–air equilibria, one can balance forces parallel to the solid surface at the point of contact between all three phases (Fig. 180), as expressed in the Young equation[4]:

$$\gamma_{SV} = \gamma_{SL} + \gamma_{LV} \cos \theta \tag{10}$$

where γ_{SV}, γ_{SL}, and γ_{LV} represent the surface free energy/unit area of the solid–air, solid–liquid, and liquid–air interfaces, respectively. Although difficult to use quantitatively because of uncertainties with γ_{SV} and γ_{SL} measurements, conceptually the equation is useful because it shows that the loss of free energy due to elimination of the air–solid interface by wetting is offset by the increased solid–liquid and liquid–air area of contact as the drop spreads out.

The $\gamma_{LV} \cos \theta$ term arises as the horizontal vectorial component of the force acting along the surface of the drop, as represented by γ_{LV}. Factors tending to reduce γ_{LV} and γ_{SL}, therefore, will favor wetting, while the greater the value of γ_{SV} the greater chance for wetting to occur. This is seen in Table III for the wetting of a low-energy surface, paraffin (hydrocarbon), and a higher energy surface, nylon, (polyhexamethylene adipamide). Here, the lower the surface tension of a liquid, the smaller the contact angle on a given solid, and the more polar the solid, the smaller the contact angle with the same liquid. That the air–solid term (γ_{SV}) and the air–liquid tension (γ_{LV}) are usually more significant than the affinity between solid and liquid (γ_{SL}) is demonstrated nicely when one considers that hexane and other hydrocarbons readily wet polar solid surfaces, whereas water and other polar liquids do not readily wet hydrocarbon solid surfaces, despite similar solid–liquid interaction forces.

The significance of the γ_{SV} and γ_{LV} terms was first developed quantitatively by Zisman[2] when he plotted $\cos \theta$ vs the surface tension of a series of liquids and found that a linear relationship, only dependent on the solid, was obtained. When such plots are extrapolated to $\cos \theta$ equal to one or a zero contact angle, a value of surface tension required to just cause wetting is obtained. Doing this for a number of solids, it was shown that this surface tension (known as the critical surface tension, γ_c) parallels expected solid surface energy γ_{SV}; the lower γ_c, the more nonpolar the surface.

Table IV indicates some of these γ_c values for different surface groups, indicating such a trend. Thus, water with a surface tension of about 72 dynes/cm will not wet polyethylene ($\gamma_c = 31$ dynes/cm), but heptane with a surface tension of about 20 dynes/cm

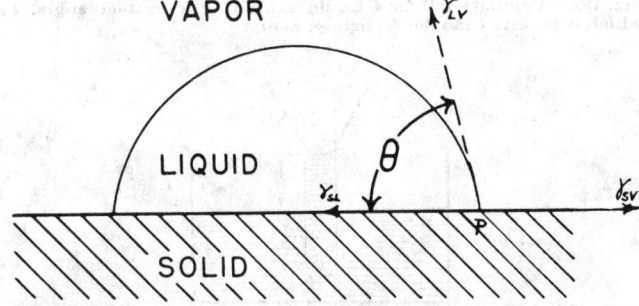

VAPOR

LIQUID

SOLID

Fig. 180. Forces acting on a nonwetting liquid drop exhibiting a contact angle of θ (courtesy, Zisman[2]).

Table IV—Critical Surface Tensions of Various Polymeric Solids

Polymeric Solid	γ_c, Dynes/cm at 20°C
Polymethacrylic ester of ϕ'-octanol	10.6
Polyhexafluoropropylene	16.2
Polytetrafluoroethylene	18.5
Polytrifluoroethylene	22
Poly(vinylidene fluoride)	25
Poly(vinyl fluoride)	28
Polyethylene	31
Polytrifluorochloroethylene	31
Polystyrene	33
Poly(vinyl alcohol)	37
Poly(methyl methacrylate)	39
Poly(vinyl chloride)	39
Poly(vinylidene chloride)	40
Poly(ethylene terephthalate)	43
Poly(hexamethylene adipamide)	46
Starch Polymers	40–45

will. Likewise, Teflon (polytetrafluoroethylene) ($\gamma_c = 19$) is not wetted by heptane but is wetted by perfluoroheptane with a surface tension of 11 dynes/cm.

One complication associated with the wetting of high-energy surfaces is the lack of wetting after the initial formation of a monomolecular film by the spreading substance. As in the case of oleic acid spreading on the surface of water, the remaining liquid retracts because of the low-energy surface produced by the oriented film. This phenomenon, often called autophobic behavior, is an important factor in many systems of pharmaceutical interest since many solids, expected to be wetted easily by water, may be rendered hydrophobic if other molecules dissolved in the water can form these monomolecular films at the solid surface. Wetting phenomena in the presence of dissolved molecules will be discussed more fully in a later section.

Capillarity

Because water shows a strong tendency to spread out over a polar surface such as clean glass (contact angle 0°), one would expect to observe the meniscus which forms when water is contained in a glass vessel such as a pipet or buret. This behavior is accentuated dramatically if a fine-bore capillary tube is placed into the liquid (Fig. 181); not only will the wetting of the glass produce a more highly curved meniscus, but the level of the liquid in the tube will be appreciably higher than the level of the water in the beaker.

The spontaneous movement of a liquid into a capillary or narrow tube due to surface forces is defined as capillarity and is responsible for a number of important processes involving the penetration of liquids into porous solids. In contrast to water in contact

with glass, if the same capillary is placed into mercury (contact angle on glass: 130°), not only will the meniscus be inverted (see Fig. 182), but the level of the mercury in the capillary will be lower than in the beaker. In this case one does not expect mercury or other *nonwetting* liquids to easily penetrate pores unless external forces are applied.

To quantitate the factors giving rise to the phenomenon of capillarity, let us consider the case of a liquid which rises to a height, h, above the bulk liquid in a capillary having a radius, r. If (shown as in Fig. 181) the contact angle of water on glass is zero, a force, F, will act upward and vertically along the circle of liquid–glass contact. Based upon the definition of surface tension this force will be equal to the surface tension, γ, multiplied by the circumference of the circle, $2\pi r$. Thus,

$$F = \gamma 2\pi r \qquad (11)$$

This force upward must support the column of water, and since the mass, m, of the column is equal to the density, d, multiplied by the volume of the column, $\pi r^2 h$, the force W opposing the movement upward will be

$$W = mg = \pi r^2 dgh \qquad (12)$$

where g is the gravity constant.

Equating the two forces at equilibrium gives

$$\pi r^2 dgh = \gamma 2\pi r \qquad (13)$$

so that

$$h = \frac{2\gamma}{rdg} \qquad (14)$$

Thus, the greater the surface tension and the finer the capillary radius, the greater the rise of liquid in the capillary.

If the contact angle of liquid is not zero (as shown in Fig. 183), the same relationship may be developed, except the vertical component of F which opposes the weight of the column is $F \cos \theta$ and, therefore,

$$h = \frac{2\gamma \cos \theta}{rdg} \qquad (15)$$

This indicates the very important fact that if θ is less

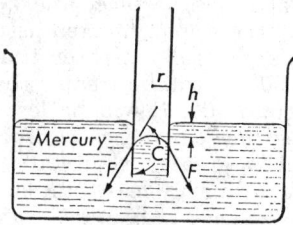

Fig. 182. Capillary fall for a liquid exhibiting a contact angle, C, which is greater than 90° (courtesy, Semat[1]).

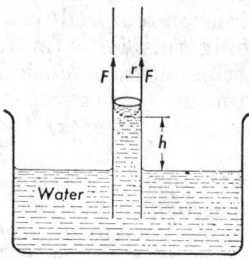

Fig. 181. Capillary rise for a liquid exhibiting zero contact angle (courtesy, Semat[1]).

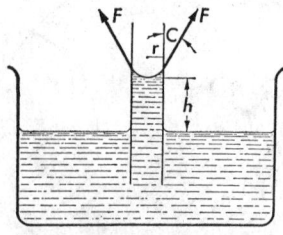

Fig. 183. Capillary rise for a liquid exhibiting a contact angle, C, which is greater than zero but less than 90° (courtesy, Semat[1]).

Table V—Ratio of Observed Vapor Pressure to Expected Vapor Pressure of Water at 25 °C with Varying Droplet Size

$P/P_0{}^a$	Droplet size, μ
1.001	1
1.01	0.1
1.1	0.01
2.0	0.005
3.0	0.001
4.2	0.00065
5.2	0.00060

a P is the observed vapor pressure and P_0 is the expected value for "bulk" water.

than 90°, but greater than 0°, the value of h will decrease with increasing contact angle, until at 90° ($\cos \theta = 0$), $h = 0$. Above 90°, values of h will be negative, as indicated in Fig. 182 for mercury. Thus, based on these equations we may conclude that capillarity will occur spontaneously even if the contact angle is greater than zero, but it will not occur at all if the contact angle becomes 90° or more.

Pressure Differences across Curved Surfaces

From the preceding discussion of capillarity another important concept follows. In order for the liquid in a capillary to rise it must develop a higher pressure than the lower level of the liquid in the beaker. However, since the system is open to the atmosphere, both surfaces are in equilibrium with the atmospheric pressure, P_0. In order to be raised above the level of liquid in the beaker and produce a hydrostatic pressure equal to hgd, the pressure just below the liquid meniscus, in the capillary, P_1, must be less than P_0 by hgd, and therefore,

$$P_0 - P_1 = hgd \qquad (16)$$

Since, according to Eq. 15,

$$h = \frac{2\gamma \cos \theta}{rgd}$$

then

$$P_0 - P_1 = \frac{2\gamma \cos \theta}{r} \qquad (17)$$

For a contact angle of zero, where the radius of the capillary is the radius of the hemisphere making up the meniscus,

$$P_0 - P_1 = \frac{2\gamma}{r} \qquad (18)$$

The consequences of this relationship (known as the Laplace equation) are important for any curved surface when r becomes very small and γ is relatively significant. For example, a spherical droplet of air formed in a bulk liquid and having a radius, r, will have a greater pressure on the inner concave surface than on the convex side, as expressed in Eq. 18.

A more familiar situation is the example of very fine water droplets making up cloud formations. If one measures the vapor pressure of water at such surfaces, one finds that the smaller the value of r, the greater the vapor pressure, due to the greater pressure on the concave side of the liquid–drop surface. Thus, the energy required to produce condensation at any atmospheric pressure is greater than would be necessary at a plane surface, and condensation of the fine droplets is retarded. The ratio of vapor pressure

observed to vapor pressure of water normally observed is given in Table V as a function of particle radius, r. This same behavior may be seen when measuring the solubility of very fine solid particles, since both vapor pressure and solubility are measures of escaping tendency. Indeed, the equilibrium solubility of extremely small particles has been shown to be greater than the usual value noted for coarser particles; the greater the surface energy and smaller the particles, the greater this effect.[5]

Monomolecular Surface Films

Insoluble Films

It was suggested above that molecules exhibiting a tendency to spread out at an interface might be expected to orient so as to reduce the interfacial free energy produced by the presence of the interface. Direct evidence for molecular orientation has been obtained from studies dealing with the spreading on water of insoluble polar substances containing long hydrocarbon chains; eg, fatty acids.

In the late 19th century Pockels and Rayleigh[6,7] showed that a very small amount of olive or castor oil—when placed on the surface of water—spread out, as discussed above. If the amount of material was less than could physically cover the entire surface only a slight reduction in the surface tension of water was noted. However, if the surface was compressed between barriers, as shown in Fig. 184,[8] the surface tension was reduced considerably.

Devaux[9] extended the use of this technique by dissolving small amounts of solid in volatile solvents and dropping the solution onto a water surface. After assisting the water-insoluble molecules to spread, the solvent evaporated, leaving a surface film containing a known amount of solute.

Compression and measurement of surface tension indicated that a maximum reduction of surface was reached when the number of molecules/unit area was reduced to a value corresponding to complete coverage of the surface. This suggested that a monomolecular film forms and that surface tension is reduced upon compression because contact between air and water is reduced by the presence of the film molecules. Beyond the point of closest packing the film apparently collapses very much as a layer of corks floating on water would be disrupted when laterally compressed beyond the point of initial physical contact.

Using a refined quantitative technique based on these studies, Langmuir spread films of pure fatty acids, alcohols, and esters on the surface of water.[10] Comparing a series of saturated fatty acids, differing only in chain length, he found that the area/molecule at collapse was independent of chain length, corresponding to the cross-sectional area of a molecule oriented in a vertical position. These values along with those obtained for other substances are given in Table VI. Note that tristearin exhibits a value

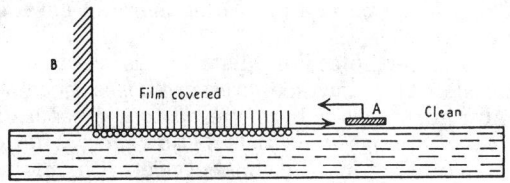

Fig. 184. Insoluble monomolecular film compressed between a fixed barrier, B, and a movable barrier, A (courtesy, Osipow[8]).

approximately three times as great as stearic acid, confirming the expected type of orientation.

Calculation of molecular length for these compounds by dividing the collapse area into the total volume of substance spread gives values (Table VI) which reflect the vertical orientation proposed; the longer the chain length, the greater the molecular length. An interesting exception to this picture is the case when double bonds are present in the alkyl chain. Note that oleic acid and triolein give cross-sectional areas which are greater than expected and molecular lengths which are less than expected.

Langmuir suggested that the polar double bonds in the hydrocarbon chain retain contact with water so that (eg, in oleic acid) methylene groups between the double bond and the carboxyl group remain oriented horizontally on the water surface, while those 8 alkyl groups beyond the double bond assume a vertical orientation. The reduction in the length of oleic acid (Table VI) to about half that of stearic acid is in keeping with this concept.

Thus, we see that each portion of a molecule contributes to its orientation at an interface such that polar groups prefer to remain in close contact with water while nonpolar portions orient away toward the more nonpolar air.

Table VI—Cross-Sectional Areas and Molecular Lengths from Studies of Monomolecular Films[10]

Substance	Formula	Cross-section, $Å^2$	Length/carbon atom, $Å$
Palmitic acid	$C_{15}H_{31}COOH$	21	1.50
Stearic acid	$C_{17}H_{35}COOH$	22	1.39
Cerotic acid	$C_{25}H_{51}COOH$	25	1.20
Tristearin	$(C_{18}H_{35}O_2)_3C_3H_5$	66	1.32
Oleic acid	$C_{17}H_{33}COOH$	46	0.62
Triolein	$(C_{18}H_{33}O_2)_3C_3H_5$	126	0.69
Cetylpalmitate	$C_{15}H_{31}COOC_{16}H_{33}$	23	2.56
Myricyl alcohol	$C_{30}H_{61}OH$	27	1.37

In addition to the evidence for molecular orientation, Langmuir's work with surface films revealed that each substance exhibits film properties which reflect the interactions between molecules in the surface film. This is best seen by plotting the difference in surface tension of the clean surface, γ_0, and that of the surface covered with the film, γ, vs the area/molecule, A, produced by film compression (total area ÷ the number of molecules). The difference in surface tension is called the surface pressure, π, and thus,

$$\pi = \gamma_0 - \gamma. \quad (19)$$

Fig. 185 depicts such a plot for a typical fatty acid monomolecular film. At areas greater than 50 $Å^2$/molecule the molecules are far apart and do not cover enough surface to reduce the surface tension of the clean surface to any extent and thus the lack of appreciable surface pressure. Since the molecules in the film are quite free to move laterally in the surface, they are said to be in a two-dimensional "gaseous" or "vapor" state.

As the intermolecular distance is reduced upon compression, the surface pressure rises because the air–water surface is being covered to a greater extent. The rate of change in π with A, however, will depend on the extent of interaction between film molecules; the greater the rate of change, the more "condensed" the state of the film.

In Fig. 185, from 50 $Å^2$ to 30 $Å^2$/molecule, the curve shows a steady increase in π, representative of a two-dimensional "liquid" film, where the molecules become more restricted in their freedom of movement because of interactions. Below 30 $Å^2$/molecule the increase in π occurs over a narrow range of A, characteristic of closest packing and a two-dimensional "solid" film.

The extent of molecular interaction in the film also can be ascertained by measuring the surface viscosity, just as one might measure the viscosity or consistency of a three-dimensional gas, liquid, or solid.[11] Surface viscosity represents the resistance to movement exhibited by surface-film molecules under the influence of a force tangential to the interface. In effect, one measures the flow of one oriented molecule past another and, therefore, the resistance produced by interaction between film molecules.

Any factor tending to increase polarity or bulkiness of the molecule—such as increased charge, number of polar groups, reduction in chain length, or the introduction of aromatic rings, side chains, and double bonds—should reduce molecular interactions, while the longer the alkyl chain and the less bulky the polar group, the closer the molecules can approach and the stronger the extent of interaction in the film. Both the change in π with A and surface viscosity values at any area/molecule reflect these expected effects.

Soluble Films and Adsorption from Solution

If a fatty acid exhibits highly "gaseous" film behavior on an aqueous surface, we should expect a relatively small change in π with A over a considerable range of compression. Indeed, for short-chain compounds—eg, lauric acid (12 carbons) and decanoic acid—not only is the change in π small with decreasing A but at a point just before the expected closest packing area the surface pressure becomes constant without any collapse.

If lauric acid is converted to the laurate ion, or if a shorter chain acid such as octanoic acid is used, spreading on water and compression of the surface produces no increase in π; the more polar the molecule (hence, the more "gaseous" the film), the higher the area/molecule where a constant surface pressure occurs.

This behavior may be explained by assuming that polar molecules form monomolecular films when spread on water but that, upon compression, they are caused to enter the aqueous bulk solution rather than to remain as an intact insoluble film. The constant surface pressure with increased compression arises because a constant number of molecules/unit area

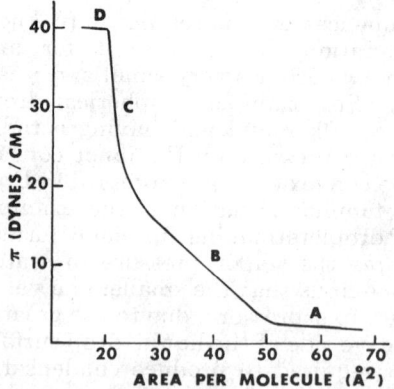

Fig. 185. A surface pressure–area curve for an insoluble monomolecular film: Region A, "gaseous" film; Region B, "liquid" film; Region C, "solid" film; Region D, film collapse.

remain at the surface in equilibrium with dissolved molecules. The extent of such behavior will be greater for substances exhibiting weaker intermolecular interaction and greater water solubility.

Starting from the other direction, it can be shown that short-chain acids and alcohols (when dissolved in water) reduce the surface tension of water, thus producing a surface pressure, just as with insoluble films. That dissolved molecules are accumulating at the interface in the form of a monomolecular film is suggested from the similarity in behavior to systems where slightly soluble molecules are spread on the surface. For example, compressing the surface of a solution containing "surface-active" molecules has no effect on the initial surface pressure, whereas increasing bulk-solution concentration tends to increase surface pressure, presumably by shifting the equilibrium between surface and bulk molecules.

At this point we may ask, why should water-soluble molecules leave an aqueous phase and accumulate or "adsorb" at an air–solution interface? Since any process will occur spontaneously if it results in a net loss in free energy, such must be the case for the process of adsorption.

A number of factors will produce such a favorable change in free energy. First, the presence of the oriented monomolecular film reduces the surface free energy of the air–water interface. Second, the hydrophobic group on the molecule is in a lower state of energy at the interface, where it no longer is as surrounded by water molecules, than when it is in the bulk-solution phase. Increased interaction between film molecules also will contribute to this process.

A further reduction in free energy occurs upon adsorption because of the gain in entropy associated with a change in water structure. Water molecules, in the presence of dissolved alkyl chains are more highly organized or "ice-like" than they are as a pure bulk phase; hence, the entropy of such structured water is lower than that of bulk water.[12]

The process of adsorption requires that the "ice-like" structure "melt" as the chains go to the interface and, thus, an increase in the entropy of water occurs. The adsorption of molecules dissolved in oil can occur but it is not influenced by water structure changes and, hence, only the first factors mentioned are important here.

It is very rare that significant adsorption can occur at the hydrocarbon–air interface since little loss in free energy can occur by bringing hydrocarbon chains with polar groups attached to this interface; however, at oil–water interfaces the polar portions of the molecule can interact with water at the interface, leading to significant adsorption.

Thus, whereas water-soluble fatty acid salts are adsorbed from water to air–water and oil–water interfaces, their undissociated counterparts, the free fatty acids, which are water insoluble, form insoluble films at the air–water interface, are not adsorbed from oil solution to an oil–air interface, but show significant adsorption at the oil–water interface when dissolved in oil.

Since soluble or adsorbed films cannot be compressed, there is no simple direct way to estimate the number of molecules/unit area coming to the surface under a given set of conditions. For relatively simple systems it is possible to estimate this value by application of the Gibbs equation,[13] which relates surface concentration to the surface-tension change produced at different solute activities. The derivation of this equation is beyond the scope of this discussion, but it arises from a classical thermodynamic treatment of the change in free energy when molecules concentrate at the boundary between two phases. The equation may be expressed as

$$\Gamma = -\frac{a}{RT}\frac{d\gamma}{da} \qquad (20)$$

where Γ is the moles of solute adsorbed/unit area; R is the gas constant; T is the absolute temperature; and $d\gamma$ is the change in surface tension with a change in solute activity, da, at activity, a. For dilute solutions of nonelectrolytes, or for electrolytes when the Debye–Hückel equation for activity coefficient is applicable, the value of a may be replaced by solute concentration, c. Since the term dc/c is equal to $d\ln c$, the Gibbs equation is often written as

$$\Gamma = -\frac{1}{RT}\frac{d\gamma}{d\ln c} \qquad (21)$$

In this way the slope of a plot of γ vs $\ln c$ multiplied by $1/RT$ should give Γ at a particular value of c. Fig. 186 depicts typical plots for a series of water-soluble surface-active agents differing only in the alkyl chain length. Note the reduction of surface tension that

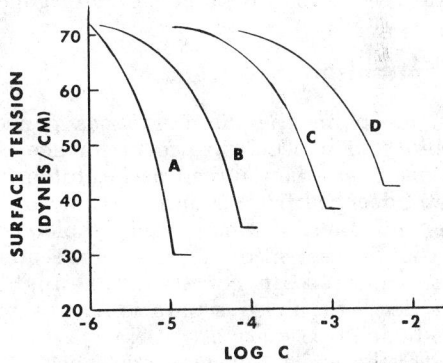

Fig. 186. The effect of increasing chain length on the surface activity of a surfactant at the air–aqueous solution interface (each figure depicted to differ by two methylene groups with *A*, the longest chain, and *D*, the shortest).

occurs at lower concentrations, the greater the alkyl chain length. Also, note the greater slope for the longer chain length compound.

It should be stressed that the uncertainty of solute activity in most cases really limits the applicability of the Gibbs equation as a quantitative means of estimating surface concentration, and that other more direct means are often required. One approach of counting radioactively tagged compounds at the surface has been developed and should prove fruitful for studying many organic compounds whose solute activity is greatly influenced by solution conditions.[14]

Mixed Films

It would seem reasonable to expect that the properties of a surface film could be varied greatly if a mixture of surface-active agents were in the film. As an example, consider that a mixture of short- and long-chain fatty acids would be expected to show a degree of "condensation" varying from the "gaseous" state, when the short-chain substance is used in high amount, to a highly condensed state when the longer chain substance predominates. Thus, each component in such a case would operate independently by bringing a proportional amount of film behavior to the system.

More often, the ingredients of a surface film do not behave independently but, rather, interact to produce a new surface film. An obvious example would be the combination of organic amines and acids which are oppositely charged and would be expected to interact strongly.

In addition to such polar-group interactions, chain–chain interaction will strongly favor mixed condensed films. An important example of such a case occurs when a long-chain alcohol is introduced along with an ionized long-chain substance. Together the molecules form a highly condensed film despite the presence of a high number of like charges. Presumably this occurs as seen in Fig. 187, by arranging the molecules so that ionic groups alternate with alcohol groups; however, if chain–chain interactions are not strong, the ionic species often will be displaced by the more nonpolar unionized species and "desorb" into the bulk solution.

On the other hand, sometimes the more soluble surface-active agent produces surface pressures in excess of the collapse pressure of the insoluble film and displaces it from the surface. This is an important concept because it is the underlying principle behind cell lysis by surface-active agents and some drugs, and behind the important process of detergency.

Micelle Formation

Up to this point the discussion has concentrated on the ability of molecules to form surface monomolecular films, first when spread as insoluble films and then when adsorbed from solution at an air–water or oil–water interface. When such molecules have reached the concentration of maximum adsorption, any further increase in concentration might be expected to lead to phase separation as a means of further reducing free energy.

Before this happens, however, one more mechanism for free energy reduction is possible, namely the aggregation of single molecules (monomers) into small soluble units known as micelles. Micelles in water may consist of 50–150 molecules oriented in a near-spherical structure such that the polar groups are oriented towards the water while the nonpolar groups are oriented in toward one another (Fig. 188A). Likewise, in nonaqueous solvents the presence of the polar group on a surfactant will result in the formation of a micelle with nonpolar portions of each monomer exposed to the solvent and the polar groups isolated within the micelle (Fig. 188B).

Geometric considerations associated with packing polar groups into a micelle interior tends to limit the size of such micelles to a rather low number of monomers, usually less than 30. In a sense, therefore, in the former case we have a hydrocarbon core (like an oil droplet) dispersed in an aqueous environment, but maintained in a dissolved state by a "shield" of polar groups; in the latter case, a highly polar "phase" is dispersed in a nonpolar solvent, protected by a shield of nonpolar groups.

It is important to look at micelles in this manner since this helps to explain how micellar solutions can solubilize substances not ordinarily soluble in a particular solvent.

It should be stressed at this point that micelle formation, although not an interfacial effect, occurs with molecules which exhibit interfacial activity. Therefore, whenever handling surfactants, the possibility of micelle formation must be considered.

If micelle formation is a bulk-solution property of the molecule, we should expect any number of solution properties to change when micelles form. For example, aggregation from monomer to a unit of 50 molecules should produce a marked change in colligative properties, refractive index, density, or electrical conductance (if the monomers are ionized).

That this is so is seen in Fig. 189[15] where a variety of properties all seem to change abruptly over a very narrow range of concentration, known as the *critical micelle concentration* (cmc). Since micelles do not exhibit the ability to lower surface tension, the abrupt cessation of surface-tension lowering at higher concentrations noted in Fig. 186 also may be used as a measure of the cmc.

Since the forces causing molecules to form micelles are essentially the same as those causing adsorption, we should expect changes in the hydrocarbon and the polar portions of these molecules to influence significantly the cmc. As with adsorption, increasing the chain length should facilitate transfer from an aqueous phase to the micellar form, thus producing a decrease in the cmc of micelles forming in water. This is shown in Table VII.

The steric nature of the hydrocarbon chains is important also, since the chains must come together inside the micelle. Thus, branched chains, ring systems, and double bonds tend to raise the cmc. In water, increased polarity of the polar portion (hence, greater interaction with water) will retard micelle formation. For this reason ionized surfactants will have higher cmc values than unionized substances with equivalent hydrophobic groups.

An additional retarding factor due to ionic polar groups is the repulsion of like-charged groups caused by close contact in the micelle. Neutral electrolytes and specific counter-ions of opposite charge tend to screen these repulsive effects and lower the cmc, as do nonionic molecules capable of forming mixed micelles.

In nonpolar solvents the formation of micelles also is influenced by chemical structure, but in this case the more polar the group, the lower the cmc, and the longer the hydrocarbon chain, the higher the cmc.

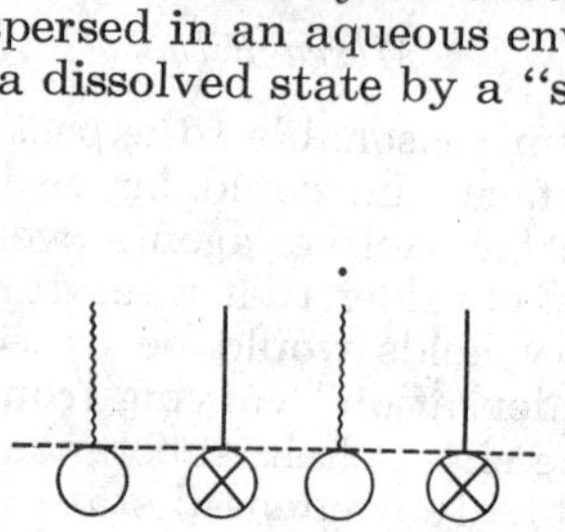

Fig. 187. A mixed monomolecular film. ⊗: a long-chain ion; ○: a long-chain nonionic compound.

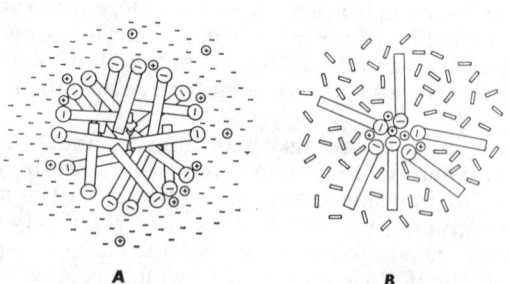

A   **B**

Fig. 188. Micellar structure: *A:* in aqueous solution; *B:* in nonaqueous solution (courtesy, Sprowles and Beal[15]).

Table VII—Critical Micelle Concentration of Various Typical Surfactants in Water

Substance	Temperature, °C	cmc. (M/L)
Octyl sulfate	40°	0.136
Dodecyl sulfate	40°	0.0086
Tetradecyl sulfate	40°	0.0024
Hexadecyl sulfate	40°	0.00058
Octadecyl sulfate	40°	0.00017
Potassium stearate	50°	0.00045
Potassium oleate	50°	0.0012
Potassium laurate	25°	0.0125
Dodecyl sulfate	25°	0.008
Dodecyl sulfonate	25°	0.009
p-Dodecylbenzene sulfonate	30°	0.00119
Dodecylamine HCl	25°	0.014
Dodecyltrimethylammonium Cl	25°	0.016
Dodecylglucoside	25°	0.00019
Dodecyl-polyoxyethylene (6)	25°	0.000087
Di-(2-ethylhexyl)sodium sulfosuccinate	25°	0.0124

More important in these systems are the geometric considerations associated with packing molecules such that polar groups are isolated from the solvent. Apparently short, bulky chains, containing rings and branched chains, are preferable since compounds such as the oil-soluble dialkylsulfosuccinates and dialkylarylsulfonates appear to be excellent in this regard.

One important aspect of micelle formation centers on the question of what happens as the concentration of the surface-active agent is increased well above the cmc. Although exact details go beyond the scope of this chapter, a few general statements should be worthwhile.

Based upon techniques used to estimate the size and shape of polymers, it appears that just beyond the cmc micelles increase in number but remain as spheres of constant size. Increasing total concentration, however, eventually produces changes in size and shape as well as some intermicellar interaction before phase separation occurs. Since some of the more concentrated micellar solutions exhibit a high

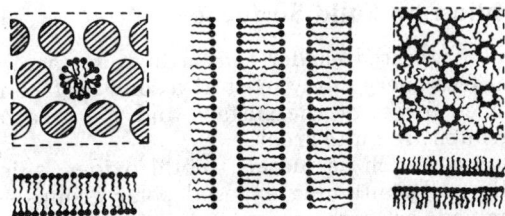

Fig. 190. Some mesophases exhibited by surfactants in concentrated solution. *Left:* hexagonal arrangement of long cylinders with polar groups out; *center:* lamellar array of parallel double layers separated by water; *right:* hexagonal arrangement of long cylinders with polar groups facing inward to water core (courtesy, Winsor[17]).

degree of organization, much like crystalline solids (Fig. 190),[16] these systems are often called mesophases or lyotropic liquid crystals.[17] The investigation of such systems is of some biologic and medicinal interest since many organized cellular structures such as biologic membranes are believed to be lipid, protein, or carbohydrate mesophases. Micellar and mesophase solutions also have been shown to influence the rate of chemical reactions, very much as membranes influence many important enzymatic processes.

Solubilization in Micellar Solutions

It was stated above that micelles may be thought of as separate phases dispersed throughout a second phase of distinctly opposite polarity, yet in solution because of the similarity between exposed chemical groups and the solvent. It is reasonable to expect, therefore, that very water-insoluble substances such as hydrocarbons might be able to partition into the interior of a micelle in water, or that water can be dissolved in the interior of a nonaqueous micelle. Two major mechanisms by which water-insoluble substances may be dissolved by micelles are depicted in Fig. 191.[18]

The first mechanism occurs when very nonpolar molecules, such as hydrocarbons, dissolve in the interior of the micelle (Fig. 191A) and is limited by the alkyl chain length and over-all dimensions of the micelle. Solubilization by means of this mechanism initially occurs just at the cmc of the surfactant, so that this is often a means of determining cmc.

The second mechanism occurs when the insoluble substance is capable of forming a mixed micelle (Fig. 191B) with the surfactant, thus forming a new micelle with a reduced cmc.

Since so many organic molecules such as drugs have polar and nonpolar portions, this mechanism would seem to be the one which occurs most widely in systems of pharmaceutical interest. Further comment on solubilization will be made after discussing some specific surfactant systems in a later section.

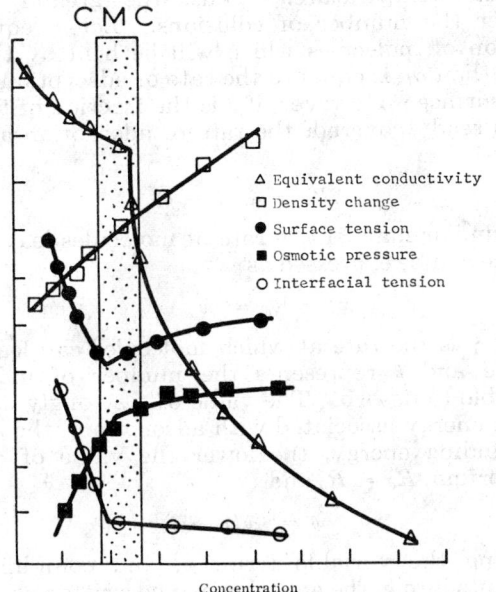

Fig. 189. The abrupt change in various physical–chemical properties exhibited by a surfactant when the critical micelle concentration is reached (courtesy, Sprowles and Beal[15]).

△ Equivalent conductivity
□ Density change
● Surface tension
■ Osmotic pressure
○ Interfacial tension

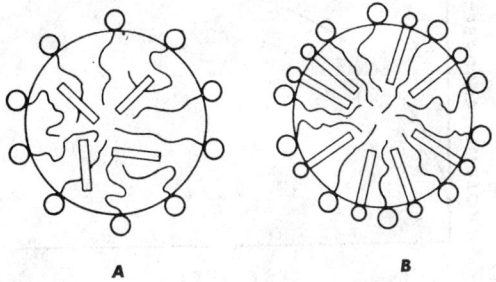

Fig. 191. Mechanisms for micellar solubilization of a water-insoluble substance. *A:* within the hydrocarbon core of the micelle; *B:* formation of a mixed micelle (courtesy, Shinoda[18]).

Adsorption on Solid Surfaces

It was suggested earlier that a high surface or interfacial free energy may exist at a solid surface if the unbalanced forces at the surface and the area of exposed groups are quite great.

Substances such as metals, metal oxides, silicates, and salts—all containing exposed polar groups—may be classified as high-energy or hydrophilic solids; nonpolar solids such as carbon, sulfur, polyethylene, or Teflon (polytetrafluoroethylene) may be classified as low-energy or hydrophobic solids. Whereas liquids satisfy their unbalanced surface forces by changes in shape or by adsorption from solutions, pure solids (which exhibit no surface mobility) must rely on reaction with molecules either in the vapor state or in a solution which comes in contact with the solid surface.

Vapor adsorption, although appearing to have only limited applicability to pharmaceutical systems, is the simplest model of how solids reduce their surface free energy and, hence, it is useful as a basis for understanding the more complex interfacial phenomena associated with solids.

Depending on the chemical nature of the adsorbent (solid) and the adsorbate (vapor), the strength of interaction between the two species may vary from strong specific chemical bonding to interactions produced by the weaker more nonspecific London dispersion forces. Ordinarily, these latter forces are those responsible for the condensation of relatively nonpolar substances such as N_2, O_2, CO_2, or hydrocarbons.

When chemical reaction occurs, the process is called chemisorption; when dispersion forces predominate, the term physical adsorption is used. Physical adsorption occurs at temperatures approaching the liquefaction temperature of the vapor, whereas, for chemisorption, temperatures depend on the particular reaction involved.

In order to study the adsorption of vapors onto solid surfaces one must measure the amount of gas adsorbed/unit area or unit mass of solid, at different pressures of gas. Since such studies usually are conducted at constant temperature, plots of volume adsorbed vs pressure are referred to as adsorption isotherms. If the physical or chemical adsorption process is monomolecular, the adsorption isotherm should look like that shown in Fig. 192. Note the significant increase in adsorption with increasing pressure, followed by a leveling off. This leveling off is due either to a saturation of available specific chemical groups, as in chemisorption, or to the entire available surface being covered by physically adsorbed

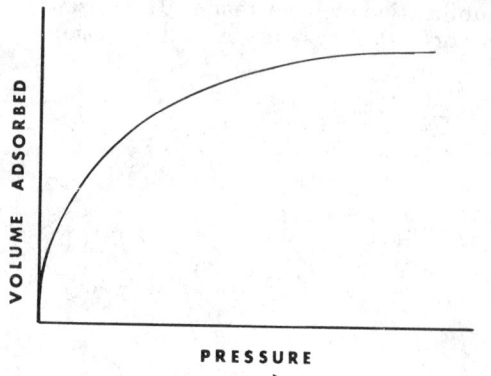

Fig. 192. The adsorption of vapor onto a solid surface when adsorption approaches a limiting monomolecular layer.

molecules. Often in the latter case, after adsorption levels off, a marked increase in adsorption occurs, presumably due to multilayered adsorption. In this case vapor molecules essentially condense upon themselves as the liquefaction pressure of the vapor is approached.

In order to have some quantitative understanding of the adsorption process and to be able to compare different systems, two factors must be evaluated; it is important to know (1) what the capacity of the solid is or what the maximum amount of adsorption is under a given set of conditions and (2) what the affinity of a given substance is for the solid surface or how readily does it adsorb for a given amount of pressure? In effect, this second term is the equilibrium constant for the process.

A significant development along these lines was introduced by Langmuir[19] when he proposed his theory of monomolecular adsorption. He postulated that for adsorption to occur a solid must contain uniform adsorption sites, each capable of holding a gas molecule. Molecules colliding with the surface may bounce off elastically or they may remain in contact for a period of time. It is this contact over a period of time that Langmuir termed adsorption.

Two major assumptions were made in deriving the equation: (1) only those molecules striking an empty site can be adsorbed, hence, only monomolecular adsorption occurs, and (2) the forces of interaction between adsorbed molecules are negligible and, therefore, the probability of a molecule adsorbing onto or desorbing from any site is independent of the surrounding sites.

The derivation of the equation is based upon the relationship between the rate of adsorption and desorption, since at equilibrium the two rates must be equal. Let μ equal the number of molecules striking each sq cm of surface/sec. From the kinetic theory of gases

$$\mu = \frac{p}{(2\pi mkT)^{1/2}} \tag{22}$$

where p is the gas pressure, m is the mass of the molecule, k is the Boltzmann gas constant, and T is the absolute temperature. Thus, the greater p, the greater the number of collisions. Let α equal the fraction of molecules which will be held by the surface; then $\alpha\mu$ is equal to the rate of adsorption on the bare surface. However, if θ is the fraction of the surface already covered, the rate of adsorption actually will be

$$R_a = \alpha\mu(1 - \theta) \tag{23}$$

In a similar manner the rate of molecules leaving the surface can be expressed as

$$R_d = \gamma\theta \tag{24}$$

where γ is the rate at which molecules can leave the surface and θ represents the number of molecules available to desorb. The value of γ strongly depends on the energy associated with adsorption; the greater the binding energy, the lower the value of γ. At equilibrium, $R_a = R_d$ and

$$\gamma\theta = \alpha\mu(1 - \theta) \tag{25}$$

Isolating the variable term, p, and combining all constants into k, the equation can be written as

$$\theta = \frac{kp}{1 + kp} \tag{26}$$

and, since θ may be expressed as

$$\theta = \frac{V_a}{V_m} \qquad (27)$$

where V_a is the volume of gas adsorbed and V_m is the volume of gas covering all of the sites, Eq. 26 may be written as

$$V_a = \frac{V_m k p}{1 + kp} \qquad (28)$$

A test of fit to this equation can be made by expressing it in linear form:

$$\frac{p}{V_a} = \frac{1}{V_m k} + \frac{p}{V_m} \qquad (29)$$

The value of k is, in effect, the equilibrium constant and may be used to compare affinities of different substances for the solid surface. The value of V_m is valuable since it indicates the maximum number of sites available for adsorption. In the case of physical adsorption the maximum number of sites is actually the total surface area of the solid and, therefore, the value of V_m can be used to estimate surface area if the volume and area/molecule of vapor are known.

Since physical adsorption most often involves some multilayered adsorption, an extension of the Langmuir equation, derived by Brunauer, et al.[20] has been found to fit the data more correctly. The equation is too involved to derive here, but as an extension of the Langmuir equation it allows for the determination of V_m. The most widely used vapor for this purpose is nitrogen, which adsorbs nonspecifically on most solids near its boiling point at $-195°C$ and appears to occupy about $16 Å^2$/molecule on a solid surface.

Adsorption onto solid surfaces by molecules dissolved in solution may occur if the dissolved molecules and the solid surface have chemical groups capable of interacting. Nonspecific adsorption also will occur if the solute is surface-active to begin with, and if the surface area of the solid is quite high. Except for a few reported cases, most adsorption from solution is monomolecular rather than multilayered as with vapors.

Adsorption from solution is usually more complex than gas adsorption because of the solvent and other components which may be in solution; these other components can compete for the solid surface. Adsorption from solution may be measured by separating solid and solution and either estimating the amount of adsorbate adhering to the solid or the loss in concentration of adsorbate from solution.

In view of the possibility of solvent adsorption, the latter approach really only gives an apparent adsorption. For example, if solvent adsorption is great enough, it is possible to end up with an increased concentration of solute after contact with the solid; here, the term negative adsorption is used.

Solvent not only influences adsorption by competing for the surface but, as discussed in connection with adsorption at liquid surfaces, the solvent will determine the escaping tendency of a solute; eg, the more polar the molecule, the less the adsorption that occurs from water. It is difficult to predict these effects but, in general, the more chemically unlike the solute and solvent and the more alike the solid surface groups and solute, the greater the extent of adsorption.

Despite such complexities, the affinity and capacity for adsorption may be obtained if the Langmuir equation is applicable and, in particular, for systems showing some tendency for chemisorption the Langmuir equation has proved quite useful. Suffice it to say whenever solutions containing drugs or surface-active agents are in contact with insoluble solids, the possibility of some type of solute adsorption must be considered.

Surface-Active Agents

Throughout the discussion so far, examples of surface-active agents (surfactants) have been restricted primarily to fatty acids and their salts. It has been shown that both a hydrophobic portion (alkyl chain) and a hydrophilic portion (carboxyl and carboxylate groups) are required for their surface activity, the relative degree of polarity determining the tendency to accumulate at interfaces or to form micelles. It now becomes important to look at some of the specific types of surfactants available and to see what structural features are required for different pharmaceutical applications.

The classification of surfactants is quite arbitrary, but one based on chemical structure appears best as a means of introducing the topic. It is generally convenient to categorize surfactants according to their polar portions since the nonpolar portion is usually made up of alkyl or aryl groups. The major polar groups found in most surfactants may be divided as follows: (1) anionic, (2) cationic, (3) amphoteric, and (4) nonionic. As we shall see, the last group is the largest and most widely used for pharmaceutical systems, so that it will be emphasized in the discussion that follows.

Types

Anionic Agents—The most commonly used anionic surfactants are those containing carboxylate, sulfonate, and sulfate ions. Those containing carboxylate ions are known as soaps and are generally prepared by the saponification of natural fatty acid glycerides in alkaline solution. The most common cations associated with soaps are sodium, potassium, ammonium, and triethanolamine, while the chain length of the fatty acids ranges from 12 to 18.

The degree of water solubility is greatly influenced by the length of the alkyl chain and the presence of double bonds. For example, sodium stearate is quite insoluble in water at room temperature, whereas sodium oleate under the same conditions is quite water soluble.

Multivalent ions, such as calcium and magnesium, produced marked water insolubility, even at lower alkyl chain lengths; thus, soaps are not useful in hard water which is high in content of these ions. Soaps, being salts of weak acids, are subject also to hydrolysis and the formation of free acid plus hydroxide ion, particularly when in more concentrated solution.

To offset some of the disadvantages of soaps, a number of long alkyl chain sulfonates, as well as alkyl aryl sulfonates such as sodium dodecylbenzene sulfonate, may be used; the sulfonate ion is less subject to hydrolysis and precipitation in the presence of multivalent ions. A popular group of sulfonates, widely used in pharmaceutical systems, are the dialkyl sodium sulfosuccinates, particularly di-(2-ethylhexyl) sodium sulfosuccinate, best known as Aerosol OT. This compound is unique in that it is both oil and water soluble and hence forms micelles in both phases. It reduces surface and interfacial tension to extremely low values and acts as an excellent wetting agent in many types of solid dosage forms.

A number of alkyl sulfates are available as surfactants, but by far the most popular member of this group is sodium lauryl sulfate, which is widely used as an emulsifier and solubilizer in pharmaceutical systems. Unlike the sulfonates, sulfates are susceptible to hydrolysis which leads to the formation of the long-chain alcohol, so that pH control is most important for sulfate solutions.

Cationic Agents—A number of long-chain cations, such as amine salts and quaternary ammonium salts, are often used as surface-active agents when dissolved in water; however, their use in pharmaceutical preparations is limited to that of antimicrobial preservation rather than as surfactants. This arises because the cations adsorb so readily at cell membrane structures in a nonspecific manner, leading to cell lysis (eg, hemolysis), as do anionics to a lesser extent. It is in this way that they act to destroy bacteria and fungi.

Since anionic and nonionic agents are not as effective as preservatives, one must conclude that the positive charge of these compounds is important; however, the extent of surface activity has been shown to determine the amount of material needed for a given amount of preservation.[21] Quaternary ammonium salts are preferable to free amine salts since they are not subject to effect by pH in any way; however, the presence of organic anions such as dyes and natural polyelectrolytes is an important source of incompatibility and such a combination should be avoided.

Amphoteric Agents—The major group of molecules falling into this category are those containing carboxylate or phosphate groups as the anion and amino or quaternary ammonium groups as the cation. The former group is represented by various polypeptides, proteins, and the alkyl betaines, while the latter group consist of natural phospholipids such as the lecithins and cephalins. In general, long-chain amphoterics which exist in solution in zwitterionic form are more surface active than ionic surfactants having the same hydrophobic group since in effect the oppositely charged ions are neutralized. However, when compared to nonionics, they appear somewhere between ionic and nonionic.

Nonionic Agents—The major class of compounds used in pharmaceutical systems are the nonionic surfactants since their advantages with respect to compatability, stability, and potential toxicity are quite significant. It is convenient to divide these compounds into those that are relatively water insoluble and those that are quite water soluble.

The major type of compounds making up this first group are the long-chain fatty acids and their water-insoluble derivatives. These include (1) fatty alcohols such as lauryl, cetyl (16 carbons), and stearyl alcohols; (2) glyceryl esters such as the naturally occurring mono-, di-, and triglycerides; and (3) fatty acid esters of fatty alcohols and other alcohols such as propylene glycol, polyethylene glycol, sorbitan, sucrose, and cholesterol. Included also in this general class of nonionic water-insoluble compounds are the free steroidal alcohols such as cholesterol.

To increase the water solubility of these compounds and to form the second group of nonionic agents, polyoxyethylene groups are added through an ether linkage with one of their alcohol groups. The list of derivatives available is much too long to cover completely, but a few general categories will be given.

The most widely used compounds are the polyoxyethylene sorbitan fatty acid esters which are found in both internal and external pharmaceutical formulations. Closely related compounds include polyoxyethylene glyceryl, and steroidal esters, as well as the comparable polyoxypropylene esters. It is also possible to have a direct ether linkage with the hydrophobic group as with a polyoxyethylene–stearyl ether or a polyoxyethylene–alkyl phenol. These ethers offer advantages since, unlike the esters, they are quite resistant to acidic or alkaline hydrolysis.

Besides the classification of surfactants according to their polar portion, it is useful to have a method that categorizes them in a manner that reflects their interfacial activity and their ability to function as wetting agents, emulsifiers, solubilizers, etc. Since variation in the relative polarity or nonpolarity of a surfactant significantly influences its interfacial behavior, some measure of polarity or nonpolarity should be useful as a means of classification.

One such approach assigns a hydrophile–lipophile balance number (HLB) for each surfactant[22] and, although developed by a commercial supplier of one group of surfactants, the method has received widespread application. The HLB value, as originally conceived for nonionic surfactants, is merely the percentage weight of the hydrophilic group divided by five in order to reduce the range of values. On a molar basis, therefore, a 100% hydrophilic molecule (polyethylene glycol) would have a value of 20.

Thus, as seen in Table VIII, variation in polyoxyethylene chain length increases polarity and, hence, the HLB value; at constant polar chain length, an increase in alkyl chain length or number of fatty acid groups decreases polarity and the HLB value. One immediate advantage of this system is that to a first approximation one can compare any chemical type of surfactant to another type when both polar and nonpolar groups are different.

HLB values for nonionics are calculatable on the basis of the proportion of polyoxyethylene chain present; however, in order to determine values for other types of surfactants it is necessary to compare physical chemical properties reflecting polarity with those surfactants having known HLB values. Relationships between HLB and phenomena such as water solubility, interfacial tension, and dielectric constant have been used in this regard. Those surfactants exhibiting values greater than 20 (sodium lauryl sulfate and cetyl ethyl morpholinium ethosulfate in Table VIII) demonstrate hydrophilic behavior in excess of the polyoxyethylene group alone.

Surfactant Drugs

Many drugs in aqueous solution exhibit the ability to lower surface tension and to form micelles. The variety of chemical species demonstrating such behavior is indicated in Table IX.

Some of these agents, like the cationic surfactants, can cause cell lysis and, indeed, this is the mechanism by which some antibiotics work. Other substances act to influence various cellular processes in a more specific manner and it is not as clear how their surface behavior influences their action. Consider, however, that the cell is made up of a variety of organelles which, in turn, contain a significant number of organized lipid and protein membranes. Such cell organelles include the nucleus, the mitochondrion, and the endoplasmic reticulum.

Lysosomes and synaptic vesicles, believed to be the site of action for many drugs, are also membranous in nature. Either by affecting permeability of sub-stances through these membranes or by interfering with the enzymatic reactions occuring there, the ad-sorption or accumulation of drug molecules at mem-brane surfaces could be a major aspect of their phar-macologic activity. An excellent review of this topic is suggested for the interested reader.[23]

Table VIII—Calculated or Determined HLB Values of Some Surfactants Used in Pharmaceuticals

Chemical designation	HLB
Sorbitan trioleate	1.8
Sorbitan tristearate	2.1
Propylene glycol monostearate	3.4
Sorbitan sesquioleate	3.7
Glycerol monostearate, non-self-emulsifying	3.8
Sorbitan monooleate	4.3
Propylene glycol monolaurate	4.5
Sorbitan monostearate	4.7
Diethylene glycol monostearate	4.7
Glycerol monostearate, self-emulsifying	5.5
Diethylene glycol monolaurate	6.1
Sorbitan monopalmitate	6.7
Sorbitan monolaurate	8.6
Polyoxyethylene (4) lauryl ether	9.5
Polyoxyethylene (4) sorbitan monostearate	9.6
Polyoxyethylene (2) sorbitan monooleate	10.0
Polyoxyethylene (20) sorbitan tristearate	10.5
Polyoxyethylene (4) sorbitan trioleate	11.0
Polyoxyethylene glycol 400 monooleate	11.4
Polyoxyethylene glycol 400 monostearate	11.6
Triethanolamine oleate	12.0
Polyoxyethylene (9) nonyl phenol	13.0
Polyethylene glycol 400 monolaurate	13.1
Polyoxyethylene (4) sorbitan monolaurate	13.3
Polyoxyethylene (20) sorbitan monostearate	14.9
Polyoxyethylene (20) sorbitan monooleate	15.0
Polyoxyethylene (20) stearyl ether	15.3
Polyoxyethylene (20) oleyl ether	15.4
Polyoxyethylene (20) sorbitan monopalmitate	15.6
Polyoxyethylene (20) cetyl ether	15.7
Polyoxyethylene (30) stearate	16.0
Polyoxyethylene (40) stearate	16.9
Sodium oleate	18.0
Polyoxyethylene (100) stearate	18.8
Potassium oleate	20.0
Cetyl ethyl morpholinium ethosulfate	25–30
Sodium lauryl sulfate	Approx 40

Table IX—Various Drugs Shown to Have Surface Activity

I. Tranquilizers and antidepressants
   a. Phenothiazines
   b. Reserpine
   c. Chlordiazepoxide

II. Local anesthetics
   a. Nupercaine
   b. Tetracaine
   c. Procaine
   d. Cinchocaines

III. Antibiotics and antibacterials
   a. Acridines
   b. Phenols
   c. Quaternary ammonium salts
   d. Penicillins
   e. Streptomycin
   f. Tyrocidin
   g. Polymyxin B
   h. Polyenes

IV. Miscellaneous
   a. Barbiturates
   b. Vitamin A
   c. Progesterone
   d. Veratrum alkaloids

Pharmaceutical Application

The specific use of surfactants in a very practical pharmaceutical formulation and manufacturing prob-lems will be discussed in later chapters dealing with these topics. Emphasis here will be placed on the three major pharmaceutical uses of surfactants as wetting, solubilizing, and emulsifying agents. The latter topic will be covered briefly since emulsions will receive detailed attention in Chapter 24.

Wetting Agents—As described in the section deal-ing with wetting by pure liquids, many solids will not be wetted if their critical surface tension is exceeded by the surface tension of the liquid. Thus water with a value of 72 dynes/cm will not wet polyethylene with a critical surface tension of 31 dynes/cm.

Based on this concept we should expect a good wet-ting agent to be one which reduces the surface tension of a liquid to a value below the solid critical surface tension. This was confirmed in a study concerned with the wetting of polyethylene and Teflon ($\gamma_c = 19$ dynes/cm) by aqueous solutions of various sur-factants.[24]

Only those surfactants able to reduce the surface tension of water below 30 dynes/cm were able to wet polyethylene, while no surfactant with hydrocarbon groups could reach the critical surface tension of Teflon. In view of this, we may conclude that one requirement for a wetting agent is that it exhibits the ability to reduce surface tension to relatively low values before micelle formation occurs.

Aerosol OT and some of the polyoxyethylene non-ionics are good wetting agents, presumably because of their irregular molecular shape which makes it diffi-cult to pack into micelles. In this way, relatively high concentrations of monomer are available for adsorption at the air–water interface.

It is generally considered that surfactants act pri-marily by reducing γ_{SL} upon adsorption at the solid–liquid interface; however, this is not that simple a concept. If a surfactant adsorbs on the surface of a solid with polar groups oriented towards the aqueous solution, the surface should appear more polar, thus increasing the apparent critical surface tension of a solid and producing wetting.

As a general rule, however, adsorption onto solid surfaces often occurs with polar groups attracted to the solid and the hydrocarbon groups oriented towards the aqueous solution. For example, aqueous solutions of long chain amines, despite their low surface tensions do not wet glass or silica below their cmc, whereas pure water does.

Since glass is negatively charged, the cationic amines should adsorb as shown in Fig. 193.[25] If, however, the concentration of surfactant is raised near to or above its cmc, a bimolecular layer with polar groups ex-posed to the aqueous solution occurs and cationic amine solutions wet glass; this provides the polar surface required for aqueous wetting.

Another complication occurs when surfactant ad-sorbs since this reduces the bulk concentration of the advancing liquid drop, which in turn may raise the air–liquid surface tension to a value above the solid

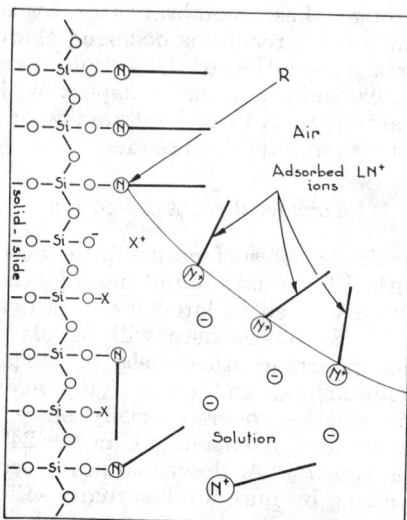

Fig. 193. The adsorption of a cationic surfactant, LN^+, onto a negatively charged silica or glass surface, exposing a hydrophobic surface as the solid is exposed to air (courtesy, Ter-Minassian-Saraga[25]).

critical surface tension. We, therefore, may conclude that the best wetting agents to use produce low air–liquid surface tension and are not readily adsorbed by the solid.

Solubilizing Agents—The use of micellar solutions to solubilize drugs is a most important application of surfactants. Not only can the amount of drug in solution be increased, but its biologic availability and chemical stability also may be influenced greatly. Since micelles are required for solubilization, a relatively low cmc and large micellar size is required for maximum efficiency, with regard to moles of drug solubilized/mole of surfactant.

Table X illustrates the solubilizing behavior of various surfactants for the hormone estrone.[27] Note in particular the significant concentration differences for the various surfactants and the variation in solubilization efficiency with alkyl chain length. In order to maintain a relatively high concentration of micelles with long hydrophobic chains, it is not surprising that all of these compounds are quite water soluble with high HLB values; thus, as a rule, good solubilizers have HLB values above 15.

The role of the polar group is also important when polyoxyethylene nonionic surfactants are used since the ethylene oxide units may act as a site of drug

Table X—Micellar Solubilization Capacities of Surfactants for Estrone[26]

Surfactant	Concentration range, M	Temp., °C	Moles estrone/ mole micellar substance
Sodium caprylate	0.45–0.9	40	0.0038
Sodium caprate	0.13–0.4	40	0.0070
Sodium laurate	0.025–0.23	40	0.011
Sodium myristate	0.006–0.10	40	0.021
Sodium oleate	0.002–0.35	40	0.019
Sodium lauryl sulfate	0.004–0.15	40	0.014
Sodium cholate	0.09–0.23	20	0.0042
Sodium desoxycholate	0.007–0.36	20	0.0021
Sodium dehydrocholate	0.45–0.72	20	0.0022
Aerosol OT	0.002–0.05	40	0.0051
Tetradecyltrimethyl ammonium bromide	0.005–0.08	20	0.022
Hexadecylpyridinium chloride	0.001–0.1	20	0.031
Tween 20	0.002–0.15	20	0.0062
Tween 60	0.0008–0.11	20	0.012

interaction. Solubilization of water and water-soluble substances in nonpolar liquids is of more limited interest in pharmacy, but such systems are of potential use in fluorocarbon aerosol propellants or in nonaqueous cosmetic solutions. Excellent examples of useful surfactants in this regard are the short-chain polyoxyethylene alkylphenols and Aerosol OT.

The variety of agents used as solubilizers in pharmacy is quite great, so that a recent review is suggested for a more detailed discussion of this topic.[27]

Emulsifying Agents—The main interfacial requirement of surfactants as emulsifiers, both for o/w and w/o emulsions, is that they accumulate at an oil–water interface, form relatively condensed surface films, and prevent droplet coalescence. The commonly discussed function of being able to reduce interfacial tension appears to be of secondary importance since many polymers and solids will form barriers at oil–water interfaces without markedly reducing interfacial tension.

The surface coverage of ionized surfactants is limited by the repulsive forces of like-charged groups, so that used alone they do not make very stable emulsions. For the same reason, namely a lack of film condensation, polyoxyethylene nonionics alone are not very good emulsifiers. In this case the bulkiness of the ethylene oxide chains, particularly when heavily hydrated, reduce surface coverage.

In both cases surface coverage may be increased by forming mixed films which are more condensed and have a higher surface viscosity. For example, sodium lauryl sulfate combined with lauryl alcohol or cholesterol produces films with high surface viscosity and good emulsifying properties. Combinations of oil-soluble and water-soluble nonionics also seem to increase emulsifying efficiency as compared to the individual surfactants.

This topic will be discussed more fully in a subsequent chapter, so that at this point it will be sufficient to say that the state and surface viscosity of any emulsifier film should be one factor in its choice for pharmaceutical emulsions.

References

1. Semat, H., *Fundamentals of Physics*, 3rd ed., Holt-Rinehart-Winston, New York, 1957.
2. Zisman, W. A., *Advan. Chem. Ser.*, **43**, 1 (1964).
3. Wenzel, R. N., *Ind. Eng. Chem.*, **28**, 988 (1936).
4. Adamson, A. W., *Physical Chemistry of Surfaces*, 2nd ed., Interscience, New York, 1967, p. 352.
5. Adamson, A. W., *Physical Chemistry of Surfaces*, 2nd ed., Interscience, New York, 1967, p. 346.
6. Pockels, A., *Nature*, **43**, 437 (1891).
7. Rayleigh, Lord, *Phil. Mag.*, **48**, 331 (1899).
8. Osipow, L. I., *Surface Chemistry: Theory and Industrial Applications*, Reinhold, New York, 1962.
9. Devaux, H., *J. Phys. Radium*, **699**, 891 (1912).
10. Langmuir, I., *J. Am. Chem. Soc.*, **39**, 1848 (1917).
11. Joly, M., in Danielli, J. F., *et al*, eds., *Recent Progress in Surface Science*, Academic, New York, 1964, p. 1.
12. Némethy, G., *Angew. Chem. Intern. Ed. Engl.*, **6**, 195 (1967).
13. Gibbs, J. W., *The Collected Works of J. W. Gibbs*, vol. I, Longmans-Green, New York, 1931, p. 219.
14. Salley, D. J., *et al*, *Proc. Roy. Soc.* (*London*) *Ser. A*, **203**, 42 (1950).
15. Sprowles, J. B., and Beal, H. M., eds., *American Pharmacy*, 6th ed., Lippincott, Philadelphia, 1966.
16. Hutchinson, E., and Shinoda, K., in Shinoda, K., ed., *Solvent Properties of Surfactant Solutions*, Marcel Dekker, Inc., New York, 1967, p. 222.
17. Winsor, P. A., *Chem. Rev.*, **68**, 1 (1968).
18. Shinoda, K., *et al*, *Colloidal Surfactants: Some Physico-Chemical Properties*, Academic, New York, 1963.
19. Langmuir, I., *J. Am. Chem. Soc.*, **40**, 1361 (1918).
20. Brunauer, S., *et al*, *J. Am. Chem. Soc.*, **60**, 309 (1938).
21. Weiner, N. D., *et al*, *J. Pharm. Pharmacol.*, **17**, 350 (1965).
22. Griffin, W. C., *J. Soc. Cosmetic Chemists*, **1**, 311 (1949).
23. Florence, A. T., *Advan. Colloid Interface Sci.*, **2**, 115 (1968).
24. Bernett, M. K., and Zisman, W. A., *J. Phys. Chem.*, **63**, 1241 (1959).
25. Ter-Minassian-Saraga, L., *Advan. Chem. Ser.*, **43**, 232 (1964).
26. Sjöblom, L., in Shinoda, K., ed., *Solvent Properties of Surfactant Solutions*, Marcel Dekker, Inc., New York, 1967, p. 222.
27. Sjöblom, L., in Shinoda, K., ed., *Solvent Properties of Surfactant Solutions*, Marcel Dekker, Inc., New York, 1967, p. 189.

23 | Colloidal Dispersions

Classes of colloidal systems—adsorption—lyophobic and lyophilic
systems—purification of sols—properties of colloids

This chapter was prepared by

Louis A. Reber, PhD, *Director of Graduate Studies, Philadelphia College
of Pharmacy and Science, Philadelphia, Pa. 19104*

While engaged in a comprehensive study of the
phenomena underlying diffusion, Thomas Graham, in
1850, published a paper which is regarded as the first
on colloid chemistry. He pointed out that, of the
many substances investigated by him, it was possible to
set up two different classes based on their relative rates
of diffusion through water and through certain membranes. In one class he placed those substances that
diffused readily and rapidly through an aqueous
medium. Because these were all crystalline in nature
(such as the inorganic salts) he assigned the name
crystalloids to them. The second class included those
substances such as gelatin, starch, and gums which diffused much more slowly; these he termed *colloids*
(*Greek,* glue) because they were indicative of the glue-
like nature of the substances to which this name is
applied.

Subsequent work by Graham, and by other investigators, has modified this original distinction between
crystalloids and colloids to the point where they are no
longer considered to be two separate *classes* of substances. The term "colloid" is now properly applied
to a certain state of matter, having a certain set of properties peculiar to it and by which it may be recognized.
These properties are developed when the individual particles of the substance fall within a certain size range.
They will be discussed in greater detail in later sections.
It should be pointed out, however, that a substance
cannot be cataloged as a colloid or a "noncolloid"
merely by virtue of its chemical nature. One and the
same substance may be colloidal under one set of conditions, and not under another. Even such definitely a
crystalline material as sodium chloride has been obtained in a gelatinous, colloidal condition, while such
typically colloidal materials as gelatin and albumin have
been crystallized.

Definitions and Classes of Colloidal Systems—It
has been mentioned that a substance is said to be colloidal when its particles fall within a certain size range.
Colloidal particles are intermediate in size between
molecules, atoms, and ions on the one hand, and matter
in mass on the other. The limits of the colloidal range
are indefinite; they extend from about 1 mμ to about
500 mμ (1 mμ = one-millionth of a millimeter). Particle size, however, is not the only criterion for establishing the colloidal state; in addition a colloidal system
possesses other characteristics, peculiar to it, by which
it may be recognized. Colloidal particles usually consist of aggregates containing many molecules, yet
typically colloidal substances such as albumin may
exist in water dispersions as single molecules.

When two different substances are mixed together so
that they mingle intimately, there is obtained what is
called a two-component system, of which the individual
substances are the *components*. When one component
is distributed more or less uniformly throughout the

second, the first component is called the *dispersed
phase* or *disperse phase* and the second is called the *dispersion medium* or *continuous phase*. Such a system,
consisting of two (or more) components, is known as a
dispersion. The individual particles of the disperse
phase may vary in size all the way from the smallest
molecules or ions, through particles of colloidal dimensions, to particles large enough to be visible to the unaided eye. The dispersions are correspondingly classified as *molecular dispersions* (true solutions), *colloidal
dispersions*, and *coarse dispersions* (suspensions).

The true solutions may be referred to more precisely
as *micromolecular* dispersions and colloidal dispersions
as *macromolecular* dispersions in which the individual
particles are macromolecules of large size and molecular weight. In the latter group are included many
protein molecules such as pepsin, insulin, and albumin
having molecular weights from about 17,000 to
about 70,000; protein particles consisting of single
molecules of molecular weight over a million have
been identified.

It has been suggested that the number of atoms in
the dispersed particle (which may be a single molecule
or an aggregate of many molecules) be used in defining the colloidal state. On this basis colloidal
particles contain from 10^3 to 10^9 individual atoms.

The components of a dispersion may exist in any of
the three states of matter (solid, liquid, or gas). A component in any of these states may be dispersed in a
medium in any of these states. This makes possible
nine different classes of dispersions based on the state of
aggregation of the components. All of these may be
colloidal dispersions with the exception of a gas dispersed in a second gas. Since all gases mingle mo-
lecularly with each other, mixtures of gases are true
solutions. The remaining eight classes of colloidal
dispersions and examples of each are listed in Table I.

Certain terms have come into common use to describe different types of colloidal dispersions. *Sol* is a
general term used for dispersions of solids in liquid,
solid, or gaseous media; more often it is used for dispersions of solids in liquids, the so-called *colloidal solutions*. Prefixes are used to designate the dispersion
medium, eg, *hydrosol, alcosol,* and *benzosol*. Dispersions of either solids or liquids in gases are called *aerosols*. *Emulsions* are dispersions of liquids in liquids
(or, rarely, liquids in solids).

There are some colloidal dispersions which under
proper conditions of concentration and temperature
set to a solid or semisolid. In such a state they are
known as *gels;* they owe their rigidity to an intertwin-
ing network which traps and holds firmly the dispersion
medium. Many gels may become fluid as a result of
agitation and then resume their gel structure if allowed
to remain undisturbed for a period of time. This phenomenon is known as *thixotropy* (page 367).

Table I—Types of Colloidal Systems

Dispersion medium	Dispersed phase	Examples
Gas	Liquid	Mists, fogs
Gas	Solid	Smokes, volcanic dust
Liquid	Gas	Foams
Liquid	Liquid	Emulsions
Liquid	Solid	Suspensions
Solid	Gas	Solid foams
Solid	Liquid	Solid emulsions
Solid	Solid	Solid suspensions

A broad classification of colloidal systems which is especially useful is that based on the degree of attraction between the dispersed phase and dispersion medium. If the degree of attraction is small, the system is designated as a *lyophobic* colloid; if the mutual attraction is great, the system is *lyophilic*. In those cases where water is the dispersion medium, the terms *hydrophobic* and *hydrophilic*, respectively, may be substituted. Lyophobic colloids are also called *irreversible colloids* or *suspensoids*, while lyophilic colloids are known as *reversible colloids* or *emulsoids*. A single substance may form a lyophobic system with one dispersion medium and a lyophilic system with another. For example, starch is lyophobic in alcohol and lyophilic in water, whereas rubber is lyophobic in water and lyophilic in benzene. Lyophilic colloidal systems are easily prepared due to the affinity between the phases; lyophobic systems are more difficult to prepare and are less stable.

Physical Properties and Particle Size—The remarkable change in properties which occurs when comparatively large particles of matter are subdivided until the particles are of colloidal dimensions is due to the increased contribution of surface properties to the over-all behavior of the material. This, in turn, is due to an enormous increase in the *specific surface* (ratio of surface area to volume) which accompanies the process of subdivision. How pronounced this is may be judged from the following example. If a cube, 1 cm on edge, is repeatedly subdivided into smaller cubes until each of the latter is 1 mμ on edge (of colloidal dimensions), the total surface area will increase from 6 sq cm to 6000 sq m (more than an acre), and the specific surface will increase from 6 to 60 million (10 million times). It is no wonder that those properties which reside in all surfaces and which may play a subordinate role in determining the behavior of large particles should become of major importance in the properties of matter in the colloidal state.

As the surface area increases there is a corresponding increase in surface energy. In an attempt to decrease this energy, small particles or drops tend to group together and thus bring about a decrease in surface area. From this viewpoint, colloidal dispersions may be considered as innately unstable, showing a tendency to flocculate.

Among the properties which are affected by the large increase in specific surface are some which are usually considered fixed and constant. It is somewhat surprising to learn that certain materials, when sufficiently finely divided, show an increase in *solubility*, an increase in *vapor pressure*, and a decrease in *melting point*. Another property intimately associated with particle size is *color*. Finely divided antimony trisulfide is yellow, changing toward red as the particle size increases. The same is true of arsenic trisulfide. Colloidal sols vary in color as the size of the dispersed particles increases. Sols of metallic gold show a variety of colors ranging from brilliant red (containing very small particles) through shades of purple to blue (containing coarser particles). Sols of sulfur have been obtained which exhibit colors changing in the order yellow, red, blue, purple, green, and brown as the particle size increases.

Many important properties of colloidal dispersions depend on the particle shape as well as on size. For example, particles which are *spherical* or *globular* in shape confer upon their dispersions lower viscosities than do long, threadlike particles, while the latter show a greater tendency to set into semisolid jellies. Hemoglobin is an example of a spherical colloid, while fibrin is a so-called linear colloid.

The phenomenon known as *adsorption* is probably the most important result of the tremendous surface exhibited by matter in the colloidal state. Since the properties of colloids are greatly influenced by adsorption, the next section will be devoted to a consideration of the basic principles underlying this phenomenon.

Adsorption

The process of *adsorption* involves the concentration or accumulation of a gas, liquid, or solid on the surface of a liquid or solid with which it is in contact. The substance being adsorbed may be in the pure state, or may be adsorbed from solution. The adsorbing material is called the *adsorbent;* the substance which accumulates on its surface is called the *adsorbate.* Adsorption is a surface phenomenon; molecules (or ions) in the surface have unbalanced attractive forces which are responsible for adsorption. *Absorption* differs from adsorption in that it involves a penetration of one substance into another so that a molecular intermingling results. The process of solution is an example of absorption. It has been suggested that the term *sorption* be used instead of "adsorption" or "absorption" since it is often true that adsorption on a surface is followed by absorption and condensation in capillaries and crevices. Indeed, it is frequently difficult to distinguish the two processes. In those cases where they are distinct and unequivocal, there is an advantage in retaining the separate designations.

Adsorption may occur at a liquid or solid surface in contact with air (or some other gas) or the second phase may be another liquid or solid. The boundary layer, where two phases meet, is in general spoken of as an *interface;* the term surface is usually reserved for phase boundaries which involve air or another gas. Adsorption may (and usually does) occur at any type of interface. When a solution is one of the phases at an interface, both the solute and the solvent are adsorbed. When the solute is adsorbed to a relatively greater extent, it is termed *positive adsorption; negative adsorption* is the preferential adsorption of the solvent relative to the solute. A solution decreases in concentration as a result of positive (and increases as a result of negative) adsorption.

A thorough discussion of adsorption is beyond the scope of this book, but some of the more important principles may be mentioned. An outstanding characteristic of the process is that it is highly specific. The extent to which any substance is adsorbed, even under identical conditions, depends on the physical and chemical nature of both the adsorbent and adsorbate. Thus, activated charcoal adsorbs nitrogen, oxygen, and argon from air at 100 °C, but not neon and helium. At −185 °C, neon is adsorbed very strongly, but helium is not. By methods based on selective adsorption, separation and purification of these and other gases have been accomplished.

All types of adsorption are markedly affected by changes in temperature and pressure (or concentration). The extent of adsorption is always greater at lower temperatures.   In the adsorption of many gases a decrease from $0\,°C$ to the temperature of liquid air results in a tenfold (or more) increase in the amount of gas adsorbed. Although the temperature range is more limited, a similar effect is observed in adsorption from solutions. The greater the pressure of a gas, the greater its adsorption. The relationship between amount of adsorption and pressure is expressed by the following equation, due to Freundlich:

$$x/m = kp^{1/n}$$

This equation relates the amount of gas adsorbed (x) by m Gm of adsorbent with the gas pressure (p) at constant temperature; k and n are constants. A graph constructed by plotting the quantity x/m as the ordinate and p as the abscissa is known as an *adsorption isotherm* (Fig. 194).

In its logarithmic form Freundlich's equation is

$$\log x/m = \log k + 1/n \log p$$

If one plots data for the adsorption of a gas at constant temperature for a series of pressures, making $\log x/m$ the ordinate and $\log p$ the abscissa, a straight line will be obtained if the equation fits the data (Fig. 195). From such a plot the constants k and n may be evaluated. Freundlich's equation may also be used to relate the amount of adsorption of a solute from solution as a function of its concentration. The equation then takes the form

$$x/m = kc^{1/n}$$

in which the solute concentration (c) has replaced the gas pressure (p) and all other symbols retain their original significance. As in the case of gaseous adsorption, by taking logarithms of each side, an equation is obtained which yields a linear plot and permits evaluation of the constants. Freundlich's equation describes satisfactorily the approximate quantitative behavior of most cases of adsorption. It fails, however, over a wide range of pressures (or concentrations) and is especially inaccurate at high pressures (or concentrations). Whereas the equation predicts continuously increasing adsorption with increasing pressure, experiment indicates a leveling off at the point where the adsorbent becomes saturated. Other equations have been developed which are more satisfactory in explaining the quantitative aspects of adsorption. Moreover, they have the advantage over the empiric Freundlich equation in that they propose a mechanism of adsorption and their constants have fundamental significance.

Langmuir developed an equation which is somewhat more satisfactory than that of Freundlich.   It is based on the view that the adsorbent surface possesses a fixed number of active sites or centers, each capable of adsorbing a single molecule of gas (or solute). When every active site has an attached molecule, the adsorbent is saturated and its surface is covered with an adsorbed monolayer (a layer one molecule thick). Langmuir's equation may be written as follows:

$$x/m = \frac{abp}{1 + bp}$$

or rearranged to the linear form:

$$\frac{p}{x/m} = \frac{1}{ab} + \frac{p}{a}$$

If $p/x/m$ is plotted against p, a straight line is obtained from which the constants a and b may be evaluated.   In applying Langmuir's Adsorption Isotherm to adsorption from solution, p (the pressure of the gas) is replaced by c (the concentration of the solution).

Both the Freundlich and the Langmuir equations have limited application and there are many instances of adsorption, especially at high pressures (or from concentrated solutions), which are not adequately explained. Gases at high pressure appear to form adsorption layers many molecules thick and exhibit behavior quite different from the typical low-pressure isotherm (Fig. 194). Theories and equations for multilayer adsorption have been developed which deal more or less successfully with high-pressure adsorption of gases.

An important development of these concepts has led to one of the most satisfactory methods for determining surface area and particle size of powders.   It is known as the Brunauer, Emmett, and Teller (BET) method and involves measurement of the volume of nitrogen adsorbed by the powder in an evacuated bulb at a series of pressures.

It is, perhaps, easiest to visualize the process of adsorption occurring at the surface of a solid where it comes in contact with a gas or a solution. Thus, we can easily picture silica gel or activated alumina adsorbing water vapor or activated charcoal adsorbing coloring matter from a solution. It is somewhat more difficult to realize, however, that in a simple solution, with no added adsorbent, the process of adsorption occurs. The site of adsorption is the surface of the solution in contact with air; adsorption occurs whenever this surface layer is of different concentration than the solution proper. The extent to which adsorption occurs depends on the concentration, surface tension, and temperature of the solution according to Gibbs' adsorption equation:

$$a = -(c/RT).d\gamma/dc$$

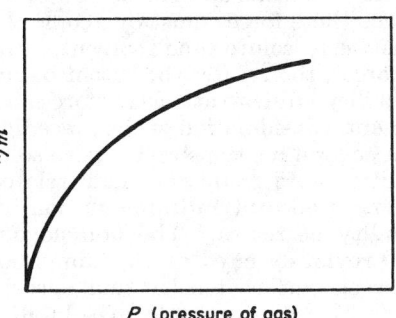

Fig. 194. A typical adsorption isotherm for a gas adsorbed on a solid.

x/m

P (pressure of gas)

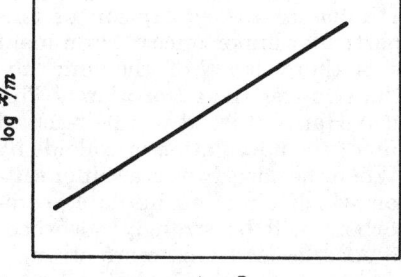

Fig. 195. A typical logarithmic plot of adsorption of a gas on a solid.

$\log x/m$

$\log P$

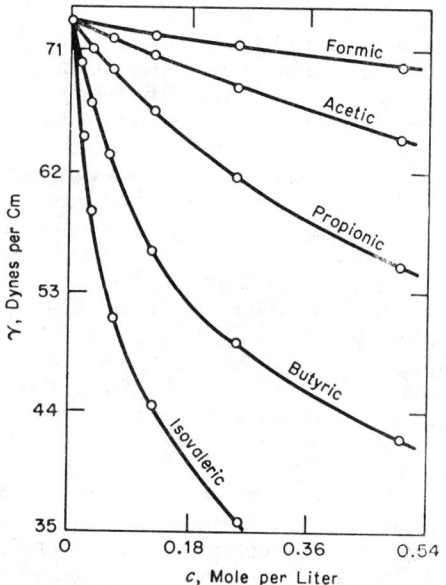

Fig. 196. The relation of surface tension and concentration for solutions of fatty acids (courtesy, Weiser).

In this equation a is the amount of solute adsorbed per sq cm of surface, c is the molarity of the solution, R is the molar gas constant, T is the absolute temperature, and $d\gamma/dc$ is the rate of change of the surface tension with concentration. Consideration of this equation leads to the conclusion that substances which lower surface tension are adsorbed and become concentrated at the surface of a solution; those substances which raise the surface tension of a solution are squeezed out of the surface layer and are negatively adsorbed. The validity of Gibbs' equation has been established, at least qualitatively, by analysis of the surface layers of solutions and comparison with their bulk concentrations.

The relationship between surface tension and adsorption at the solution–air interface is also apparent at a solution–solid adsorbent interface. Thus, there is a parallelism between the effectiveness of a solute in lowering the surface tension of a solution and the ex-

tent to which that solute is adsorbed. The homologous series of fatty acids demonstrates this relationship. Each succeeding member in the series of fatty acids (formic, acetic, propionic, etc) is increasingly effective in lowering the surface tension of water (Fig. 196). It is also true that activated charcoal will adsorb increasing amounts of these fatty acids from water solution as the molecular weight increases (Fig. 197).

This regularity in behavior has been formulated as Traube's Rule, which states that the adsorption of organic compounds from aqueous solution increases regularly as the molecular weight increases in an homologous series. The rule is limited in application, and instances of an actual reversal of this behavior have been observed.

The quantitative dependence of surface tension of a solution on the concentration of the solution is also given by Freundlich's equation in a slightly modified form:

$$\Delta\gamma = kc^{1/n}$$

In this equation, $\Delta\gamma$ is the change in surface tension (surface tension of solvent minus surface tension of solution), c is the molar concentration, and k and n are constants which may be evaluated as previously mentioned.

It is difficult, and sometimes dangerous, to attempt to make completely general statements concerning the controlling factors in the process of adsorption. The statements which follow should be considered as guiding principles only. The effects of temperature, pressure, and concentration have already been discussed. The adsorption of gases on solids is due to physical forces of attraction between them. These forces are likely to be greater as the dissymmetry and complexity of the gas molecules increase. The same properties are involved in the liquefaction of gases, and the adsorbability of gases usually parallels the ease of liquefaction. Thus, such physical constants as boiling point, critical temperature, latent heat of vaporization, the constant a of van der Waals' equation, all of which are related to the ease of liquefaction, may be used to predict the relative extent of adsorption. The adsorption of substances from solution is due to physical forces of attraction between the solute particles and the adsorbent. In order for adsorption to occur these forces must overcome the attractive forces between solute and solvent; the weaker these latter forces, the greater the extent of adsorption. Since solubility is due to attractive forces between solute and solvent, consideration of the preceding statements leads to a general relationship between solubility and adsorbability. In a group of similar, related compounds the extent of adsorption from solution increases as the solubility decreases. The homologous series of fatty acids previously cited as an example of the relationship between surface tension and adsorbability (Fig. 196) serves as an example of solubility effects as well since solubility of these compounds in water decreases with increasing molecular weight.

The factors which influence the adsorption of ions from solution are of particular importance. Prominent among these factors is the valence of the ion; the higher the valence, the stronger the adsorption. This is known as the Schulze–Hardy rule; it will be referred to again in a discussion of the flocculation of colloids by adsorption of ions. When the adsorbent is a salt or salt-like compound, an ion which forms an insoluble compound with the adsorbent will be strongly adsorbed. Thus, barium sulfate adsorbs lead ions more strongly than magnesium; lead sulfate is less soluble than mag-

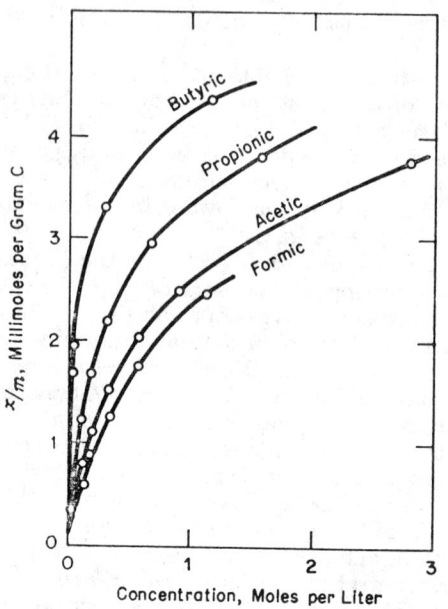

Fig. 197. The relation between adsorption and molecular weight of fatty acids (courtesy, Weiser).

nesium sulfate. This also serves to explain the strong adsorption of common ions by an ionic precipitate; a highly insoluble compound is formed which, moreover, fits perfectly into the crystal lattice of the precipitate.

This very brief discussion of the important phenomenon of adsorption will be concluded by mentioning a few of its applications. Activated charcoal is used in gas masks to adsorb poisonous gases. Charcoal has been used to liquefy gases, obtain extremely high vacua, separate gas mixtures, and purify gases. Activated alumina (aluminum oxide, Al_2O_3) and silica gel (silicon dioxide, SiO_2) are two other important adsorbents. Both are excellent adsorbents for water vapor and are used for drying gases. They are capable also of adsorbing many organic vapors and are used to recover valuable solvents such as alcohol, ether, benzene, and acetone in several industrial processes. Many substances become chemically reactive when adsorbed; this is the basis for the use of adsorbents such as alumina as contact catalysts. Lubrication is an example of adsorption of liquids on solids; adhesives are adsorbed by the surfaces which they hold together. Paints and other protective coatings are adsorbed on the surfaces they cover; agricultural sprays are effective only if they are adsorbed and spread over the surfaces to which they are applied. The process of dyeing textiles involves either direct adsorption of the dye on the fibers or indirectly through *mordants*, which are themselves held on the fibers by adsorption. The hydrous oxides of the heavy metals (aluminum, iron, chromium, tin) are useful mordants. The combination, by adsorption, of the mordant and dye, is known as a *lake*. The adsorption of electrolytes from solution is frequently encountered in analytical chemistry. Sometimes adsorption is to be avoided, as in the contamination of precipitates obtained in gravimetric analysis. There are other occasions when adsorption is desired and controlled, as in the use of adsorption indicators in precipitation titrations. The increasingly important techniques of chromatography (on columns of adsorbents or on filter paper) and of ion exchange make use of selective adsorption of solutes.

Among substances which are pharmaceutically and medically important because of their adsorptive powers are charcoal, kaolin, and fuller's earth. Medicinal (activated) charcoal removes strychnine sulfate so effectively from solution that Mayer's reagent produces no precipitate when added to the filtered solution. Kaolin and other clays have been reported to adsorb strongly the toxic products released by the bacteria responsible for many intestinal disorders and because of this property have found extensive use in the treatment of gastrointestinal diseases. Insulin has been purified by adsorption on charcoal, removing the impurities by washing, and finally removing the insulin by washing with a suitable liquid. The process of removing an adsorbed substance is known as *desorption* or *elution;* the liquid used for this purpose is the *eluant,* and the resulting solution is the *eluate.*

This very incomplete recital of the varied applications of adsorption should serve to indicate the importance of the subject and to awaken an interest in further study.

Colloidal Systems—Lyophobic and Lyophilic

The meaning of these terms has already been explained (page 320); as can be seen from Table II, the two types of colloidal systems differ radically in their properties. For this reason, in the following discussions it will be convenient to treat lyophobic systems first, and then to describe lyophilic systems, pointing out the similarities and differences between the two.

Substances in the colloidal condition are in a state of subdivision intermediate between the molecular dispersion of true solutions and the coarse dispersion of suspensions. Accordingly, the colloidal state may be achieved by the aggregation of molecules until the particles are of colloidal dimensions (*condensation methods*) or by the disintegration of materials in mass into colloidal particles (*dispersion methods*).

Condensation methods usually involve starting with substances in true solution and causing a chemical or physical change which would ordinarily produce a precipitate. However, by a careful control of conditions it is possible to halt the growth of particles short of the formation of a precipitate, and to produce and maintain a colloidal dispersion. The conditions favorable to the formation of colloids will be discussed briefly. The process of precipitation is pictured as taking place in two stages: the first, in which molecules (or ions) condense to form invisible nuclei; the second, a period in which the nuclei grow until they are large enough to precipitate. The size of the particles produced is governed by the ratio of the rates at which these two processes take place. The greater the ratio, the smaller the particles. Any factors which favor the formation of nuclei at the expense of the growth of particles will favor the formation of a relatively large number of very small particles which may remain in colloidal dispersion. Important in this connection is the supersaturation of the solution.

When a chemical (or physical) change occurs in a solution which produces a quantity (Q) of an insoluble substance, the solution momentarily is supersaturated. The absolute supersaturation of the solution is the amount of insoluble material which cannot remain in solution at equilibrium and is denoted by ($Q - L$) where L is the equilibrium solubility.

The rate of particle growth is proportional to the absolute supersaturation. Relative supersaturation, defined as the ratio of the absolute supersaturation to the solubility (or $Q - L/L$) is the prime determinant of rate of nucleus formation. This is often referred to as the "Von Weimarn Ratio" in recognition of the pioneer investigations of this German scientist.

Table II—Properties of Lyophobic and Lyophilic Sols

Property	Lyophobic sols	Lyophilic sols
Behavior toward electrolytes	Stabilized by small amount; slight excess causes coagulation	May be stable in absence of electrolytes; requires high concentration for coagulation
Reversibility	Upon evaporation of dispersion medium, residue not easily redispersed	Upon evaporation of dispersion medium, residue is easily redispersed
Tyndall effect	Intense	Diffuse
Electrical charge	Essential to stability, not readily changed	Not essential to stability, readily changed by adjusting pH
Viscosity	Similar to that of dispersion medium	Greater than dispersion medium; markedly affected by changes in temperature or concentration

In 1914 he performed experiments designed to determine the effect of concentration on the particle size and character of barium sulfate, and was able to produce a variety of forms from coarse, crystalline particles by slow precipitation from dilute solutions all the way to clear jellies representing colloidal dispersions of minute particles. The latter were formed instantaneously when concentrated solutions of the reactants were mixed.

Solubility and concentration are not the only important factors. Particle size is affected also by the total *amount* of dissolved material and by the *viscosity* of the medium. As a result, it is not unusual to find that small particles of colloidal dimensions are produced from extremely dilute as well as from extremely concentrated solutions, while particles of larger size are produced from solutions of intermediate, moderate concentrations.

The *temperature* of the medium is a significant factor in determining particle size. An increase in temperature increases both the rate of nucleus formation and the rate of particle growth. It also usually results in an increased solubility, thus decreasing supersaturation. The total effect is therefore complex and differs in individual cases. Substances of moderate solubility usually form relatively large particles from hot solution due to increase in solubility. Extremely insoluble materials, however, behave in the opposite fashion; the increase in rate of nucleus formation overshadows the slight solubility increase, and smaller particles result at higher temperatures. The formation of a dispersion of hydrated ferric oxide from hot solution is an example.

Even when conditions are ideal for the production of a colloidal dispersion, the primary particles may cling together (*agglomerate*), grow in size, and eventually precipitate unless other precautions are taken. One very important factor is the kind and concentration of electrolytes formed as byproducts. It is, therefore, important to keep this factor in mind in choosing a chemical reaction suitable for the production of a colloidal dispersion. For example, arsenous sulfide can be produced by either of the following reactions:

$$2AsCl_3 + 3H_2S = As_2S_3 + 6HCl$$
$$As_2O_3 + 3H_2S = As_2S_3 + 3H_2O$$

The first will result in a precipitate because the hydrochloric acid causes the agglomeration of the arsenous sulfide particles; the second reaction forms a colloidal dispersion of arsenous sulfide which is stabilized by hydrogen sulfide. The absence of electrolytes permits the formation of a reasonably permanent colloid. Additional examples of reactions in which colloids are produced in the absence of electrolytes are:

$$5HI + HIO_3 = 3I_2 + 3H_2O$$
$$2H_2S + SO_2 = 3S + 2H_2O$$

Frequently, it is impossible to find a satisfactory reaction which produces only nonelectrolytes. In that case, a weak electrolyte as a byproduct is preferable to a strong electrolyte. For example, a sol of mercuric sulfide is produced in the first but not the second of the following reactions:

$$Hg(CN)_2 + H_2S = HgS + 2HCN$$
$$HgCl_2 + H_2S = HgS + 2HCl$$

When a strong electrolyte is produced in the reaction, its charge type is important in determining whether or not a colloid is produced. For example, hydrolysis of ferric chloride produces a temporary sol of hydrous ferric oxide:

$$2FeCl_3 + 6H_2O = Fe_2O_3.3H_2O + 6HCl$$

The chloride ion eventually causes coagulation of the sol. Hydrolysis of ferric sulfate, however, fails to produce a sol:

$$Fe_2(SO_4)_3 + 6H_2O = Fe_2O_3.3H_2O + 3H_2SO_4$$

This is so because the sulfate ion is much more effective in causing the precipitation of the colloidal particles.

Hydrolysis is the reaction most often used to prepare hydrous oxide sols. Among the sols prepared in this manner are the hydrous oxides of iron, aluminum, chromium, tin, and silicon. They also may be prepared by the addition of ammonium hydroxide to such salts as ferric or aluminum chloride, or by adding hydrochloric acid to aluminates, stannates, or silicates. Products obtained in this way are unstable and must be purified by dialysis to remove the electrolyte impurities.

Sols of the metals (gold, platinum, silver) are usually prepared by treatment of a metallic salt with a suitable reducing agent. Some examples are:

$$2HAuCl_4 + 3H_2O_2 = 2Au + 8HCl + 3O_2$$
$$2HAuCl_4 + 3HCHO + 11KOH = 2Au + 3HCOOK + 8KCl + 8H_2O$$
$$HAuCl_4 + P + 3H_2O = Au + H_3PO_3 + 4HCl$$
$$Ag_2O + H_2 = 2Ag + H_2O$$

The color of gold sols varies with the size of the particles; those containing the smallest particles are pink or red, while blue or purple sols consist of larger particles of gold. A sol known as "purple of Cassius" is obtained when a solution of chlorauric acid is reduced by stannous chloride; the particles contain both gold and stannic oxide.

Condensation methods of preparing sols sometimes depend on physical, rather than chemical, changes. Thus, sols may be produced by solvent replacement. Colloidal dispersions of sulfur and of phosphorus are formed when alcoholic solutions of the elements are poured into water. Alcoholic solutions of resinous materials (rosin, mastic, benzoin) form sols when mixed with water. Silver iodide is appreciably soluble in concentrated potassium iodide solution, as is silver chloride in concentrated hydrochloric acid; upon dilution with water, sols of the respective silver halides are produced. Sols are formed by rapid cooling of vapors; dispersions of sulfur or selenium result when hot vapors are passed through water. Hydrosols of metals such as gold, platinum, and silver may be prepared electrically. Two thick wires of the desired metal are placed in water (or a suitable solution) and an electric arc is struck between them. Either a direct (Bredig's method) or an alternating (Svedberg's method) current arc may be used. The metal is believed to first vaporize and then condense as a colloidal dispersion.

Dispersion methods of preparing sols require the disintegration of materials in mass into particles of colloidal dimensions and subsequent suspension in a suitable medium. The simplest method would appear to be grinding in a mortar, but this is effective only to a very limited extent. The degree of dispersion attainable is not very great; the particles so produced are coarse and considerably larger than colloidal dimensions. Furthermore, very fine particles tend to cling together so that even prolonged grinding is ineffective. Better results may be obtained by grinding coarse particles in the presence of a liquid in a *colloid mill*. The mixture is introduced into the colloid mill where it passes between a rotating and a stationary disk which are separated by carefully controlled distances of the order of thousandths of an inch. The rotating disk travels at high speed and by its shearing effect produces dispersions approaching the colloidal range. These dispersions usually require the addition of protective agents such as gums or gelatin in order to make them stable. Emulsions are also prepared in this manner; for illustration of various types of colloid mills and a further discussion of this subject, see Chapters 24 and 80.

Sols may be prepared by *peptization*, a term used to describe a rather complex process. A general definition may be the formation of a colloidal dispersion by the action of a solvent. It would be desirable, however, to distinguish two types of peptization. The first occurs when a substance goes into colloidal dispersion essentially spontaneously (when brought into contact with a suitable solvent) by a process involving extensive solvation. Such a process is essentially the formation of a solution; albumin and water and gelatin and warm water form sols in a manner very much like the dissolving of sugar in water. The second type of peptization involves the bringing of precipitated substances into colloidal dispersion either by providing a peptizing agent or by removing a flocculating agent.

Electrolytes very often function as both peptizing agents (at low concentrations) and as flocculating agents (at high concentrations). Particles of a precipitate may adsorb selectively the ions of an electrolyte, acquire a charge, and pass into the colloidal state. A dispersion of charged colloidal particles, on the other hand, will attract and adsorb additional ions from the surrounding medium, reducing the charge on the particles, causing flocculation and the formation of a precipitate. Such a precipitate may be peptized (returned to the sol state) if the adsorbed electrolyte is removed by prolonged washing. Thus, aluminum hydroxide (better, hydrous aluminum oxide) goes through a colloidal stage when precipitated by ammonium hydroxide and ammonium chloride. The latter aids in the flocculation of the colloid. If the precipitate is washed with pure water, it gradually reverts to the colloidal state as the excess ammonium chloride is removed. In gravimetric analysis, where this is to be avoided, ammonium chloride is added to the wash liquid to prevent loss of the precipitate. Lyophilic colloids may also act as peptizing agents. When added to a precipitate consisting of fine particles which have been flocculated, they are adsorbed by these particles and cause them to return to a colloidal dispersion. There is evidence that the lyophilic substance forms a protective, monomolecular layer on the surface of the lyophobic particles; from this action derives the designation "protective colloid" applied to such materials. Peptization by this mechanism is exhibited in the action of soap solution on finely divided charcoal. If a suspension of charcoal is filtered, the particles are retained on the filter paper. If a soap solution is now poured through the paper, the carbon particles will be peptized and pass through. The action of protective colloids is best known in increasing the stability of suspensions or lyophobic dispersions and will be referred to again.

Irradiation with ultrasonic waves is capable of producing many interesting effects, among them the formation of colloidal dispersions. Disks made of quartz connected to a high-frequency electrical generator produce high-frequency intense mechanical oscillations in the ultrasonic range. Frequencies in the range of 20,000 to 200,000 cps (and higher) are used to produce dispersions of precipitates and of minute droplets of liquids of colloidal size, forming emulsions of such materials as oil, benzene, and mercury in water. Dispersions of liquid droplets in gases also have been prepared in this manner. Other effects of ultrasonic energy include disruption of bacteria and other small organisms, liquefaction of gels, and reduction of viscosity of certain solutions of high polymers; it is even used as the basis of a mechanical cleaning device. It is of interest also to point out that ultrasonic waves of low intensity are capable of destroying colloidal dispersions presumably by increasing the motion of suspended particles causing more frequent and more violent collisions between them.

Purification of Sols by Dialysis and Ultrafiltration

Many lyophobic sols contain, in addition to colloidally dispersed particles, more or less material in true solution. The latter may be undesirable for any of a number of reasons; electrolyte impurities are especially so because they will eventually cause the flocculation of the sol. Substances in true solution may be separated from those in colloidal dispersion by means of dialysis or ultrafiltration.

Dialysis is based upon the fact that colloidal particles do not diffuse, or at most very slowly, through membranes of parchment, cellophane, collodion, or certain animal tissues, while particles of molecular or ionic dimensions diffuse relatively rapidly. The procedure employed by Graham, in his early studies on colloids, was quite simple (Fig. 198). The sol to be dialyzed is placed in a wide cylindrical tube, closed with parchment paper, and immersed in a larger vessel containing water. The diffusible material in the sol gradually passes through the membrane into the water, which is periodically changed. Efficiency and speed of dialysis are determined by several factors; modifications of Graham's dialytic cell have been made in an effort to control these factors to best advantage. Dialysis is hastened by: (1) increase in surface of sol exposed to membrane; (2) increase in temperature; (3) electrical potential across the membrane; and (4) maximum concentration difference of dissolved substances across the membrane. Thimbles and tubes (sausage casing) permit a large exposed surface of membrane; the sol, the water, or both may be stirred or kept moving; either or both may be heated; *electrodialysis* is carried out in a three-compartment vessel with electrodes in the outer compartments containing water and the sol in the center compartment. A typical apparatus is shown in Fig. 199; application of electrical potential causes cations to migrate to the negative electrode compartment and

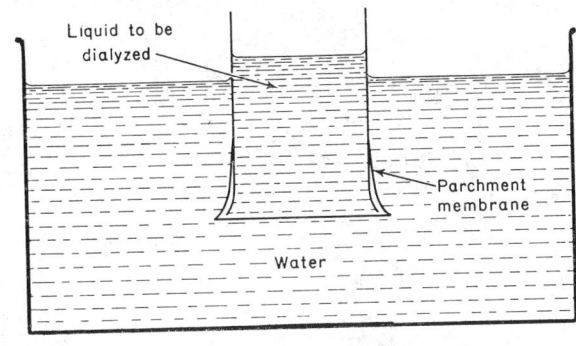

Fig. 198. Dialytic cell similar to that used by Graham (courtesy, Hartman).

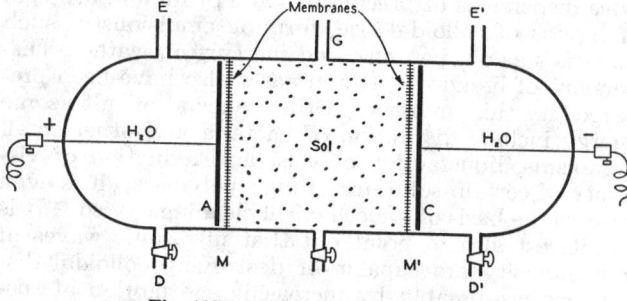

Fig. 199.   Electrodialysis apparatus.

anions to move to the positive electrode compartment, in both of which running water ultimately removes the electrolyte. Other types of dialysis equipment are shown in Figs. 200 and 201.

Ultrafiltration is an extension of the usual process of filtration to the separation of colloidal particles from those of molecular dimensions found in true solution. Ordinary filtering media are, of course, not suitable since colloidal particles pass through without difficulty. For use in ultrafiltration, filter paper or cloth may be impregnated with nitrocellulose or with gelatin hardened with formaldehyde. Ultrafilter membranes of graded porosity are made by varying the ratio of alcohol to ether in the nitrocellulose solution and by controlling the degree of drying. The most impermeable membranes (ie, those which will retain the smallest particles) are made from collodions containing the smallest proportion of alcohol and by more prolonged drying. The collodion may be deposited in the pores of unglazed porcelain vessels; the ultrafilter then possesses the strength and rigidity to withstand pressure or suction used to hasten ultrafiltration. An applied electromotive force will also speed up the process in the same manner as electrodialysis. Such a process is called *electroultrafiltration* (Fig. 202). Another type of ultrafiltration apparatus is shown in Fig. 203.

Both dialysis and ultrafiltration are very useful tools in the laboratory and in commercial processes. Most lyophobic sols must be dialyzed to remove dissolved electrolytes if they are to be stable. Ultrafiltration serves to concentrate sols since both solvent and dissolved impurities are separated from the dispersed particles. Ultrafilters of graded pore size are used to determine particle size in colloidal dispersions. By the addition of fresh solvent and a repetition of the ultrafiltration, a pure, stable sol may be obtained. The preparation of many biological products such as antitoxins and purified globulins involves removal of electrolytes which have been added in the course of isolation and purification. Both dialysis and ultrafiltration are used for this purpose and in laboratory studies of the properties of biochemical systems. *Dialyzed iron* is a colloidal dispersion of hydrated ferric oxide which has been freed of electrolyte impurities by dialysis.

Properties of Colloids

Electric Charge—Colloidal particles dispersed in a liquid medium are either single, large molecules of high molecular weight (*macromolecules*) or aggregates of smaller molecules. In either case they nearly always possess an electric charge which is responsible in large degree for their stability. Electrostatic repulsion, which occurs when particles of like charge approach each other, operates against the formation of larger particles and eventual flocculation.

The charge on the particle may be acquired by selective adsorption of ions from the surrounding medium. The electrolyte which furnishes these ions is known as the *stabilizing electrolyte*. Ions of one charge type are strongly adsorbed in a layer firmly attached to the colloidal particle and give the particle its charge. These ions are the *potential determining ions*. The ions

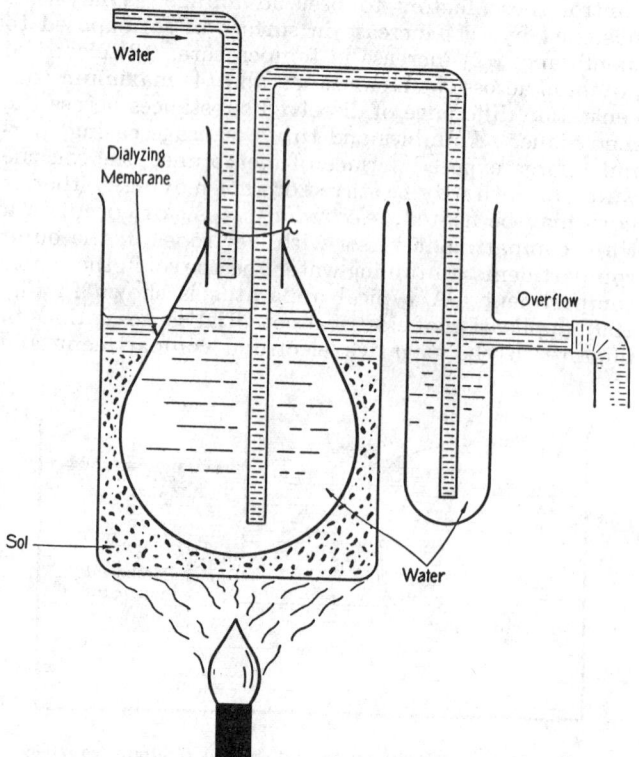

Fig. 200.   Neidle dialyzer.

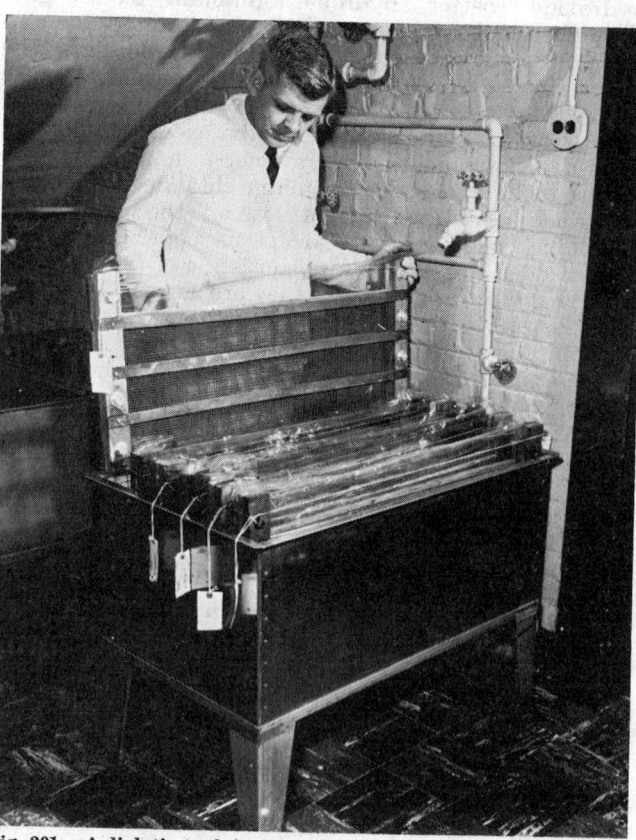

Fig. 201.   A dialytic tank in operation at the Greenfield Biological Laboratories (courtesy, Lilly).

of opposite charge are attracted to the vicinity of the charged particle and form a second, more diffuse, layer. These ions are called the *counter ions*. The entire particle is electrically neutral but is surrounded by a double layer of adsorbed ions within which there is a charge separation. For example, a silver iodide sol may be prepared by the addition of silver nitrate solution to an excess of hydriodic acid. Each particle in such a sol consists of many molecules of silver iodide, whose surface has become negatively charged by the strong adsorption of iodide ions. The negative particles now attract hydrogen ions to their immediate vicinity. In this example hydriodic acid is the stabilizing electrolyte, iodide ion is the potential determining ion, and hydrogen ion is the counter ion. In Table III is represented the structure of certain colloidal dispersions frequently encountered.

A particle may become charged as a result of dissociation of groups or molecules of which it is composed. Thus, the dissociation of carboxyl groups on the surface of a particle will produce a negative particle having hydrogen ions in the diffuse, outer portion of the double layer. Particles may consist of aggregates of molecules containing groups capable of a high degree of dissociation (such as the soaps and other detergents). Dispersions of such particles show a high conductance due to the large number of charges and the resulting high charge-to-mass ratio.

In the case of lyophobic sols, the electric charge of the particle is essential for stability because two particles of similar charge will repel each other and will not unite to form larger particles (will not precipitate). Particles in a lyophilic sol, however, may or may not have an electric charge and yet be stable. Hydration and charge contribute to the stability of hydrophilic sols; of the two, hydration is the more important. For example, gelatin particles in the presence of water swell up and adsorb a large amount of solvent; gelatin is *peptized* by warm water. Such a sol is stable whether or not the particles have an electric charge; the existence and sign of the charge depends on the pH of the medium.

Gelatin, and other proteins, are amphoteric in nature; they have both acidic and basic properties. When its acidic properties predominate, it is negatively charged; when it acts as a base, it is positively charged. At a certain, rather definite pH value a protein shows acidic and basic properties to the same degree; this is called the *isoelectric point* of the protein and here it is uncharged. Most lyophilic colloids (casein is a notable exception) are not coagulated even when brought

Table III—Structure of Colloidal Dispersions

Nature of particle	Charge	Stabilizing electrolyte
Silver iodide	−	Hydrogen iodide
Silver iodide	+	Silver nitrate
Arsenous sulfide	−	Hydrogen sulfide
Hydrated ferric oxide	+	Ferric chloride
Sulfur	−	Polythionic acids
Silver	−	Silver hydroxide

to their isoelectric point. Thus electric charge is not essential to the stability of such colloids; such a charge, however, does contribute to stability, and lyophilic colloids are always least stable at the isoelectric point.

At lower (more acid) pH values, protein particles are positively charged, and at higher (more alkaline) pH values they are negatively charged. The presence of electric charges on colloidal particles will cause them to move in the dispersion medium under the influence of an applied electric field. This motion is known as *electrophoresis*, and is entirely analogous to the movement of ions during the electrolysis of a solution. The particles move toward the electrode of opposite charge; their speed depends, among other things, on the magnitude of their charge. Electrophoresis studies are, therefore, an important method of determining the sign and magnitude of the charge on colloidal particles (known as the *electrokinetic potential* or *zeta potential*).

In addition, electrophoresis is a valuable tool in the separation and purification of mixtures of proteins and other substances. In the *moving boundary* method the protein mixture is carefully layered over with a buffer and, under influence of the electric potential, the proteins move at varying velocities into the buffer. The amount and location of each component is determined by measurements of refractive index in this boundary layer.

Another technique is known as *zone electrophoresis* and involves migration of charged particles under influence of electric potential on a porous supporting medium such as cellulose acetate, and gels of starch,

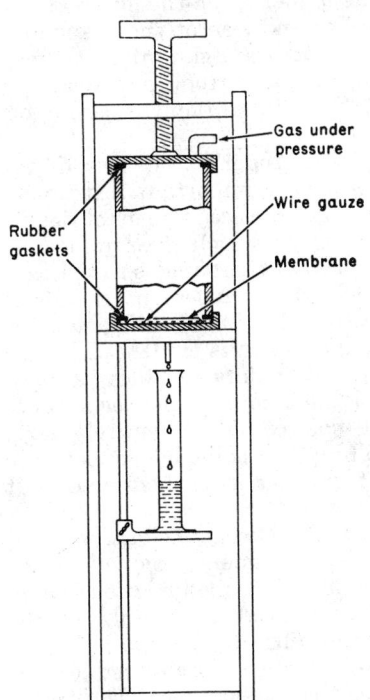

Fig. 203. Ultrafiltration at high pressure (courtesy, Weiser).

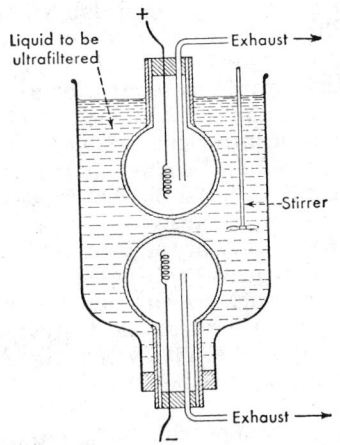

Fig. 202. An electroultrafiltration assembly at reduced pressure. (courtesy, Hartman).

agar, polyacrylamide, and filter paper. The latter forms the basis of the widely used technique of *paper electrophoresis*. Useful clinical procedures have been developed utilizing zone electrophoresis in the examination of blood serum. Abnormalities in the composition of serum protein are of value in the diagnosis of certain pathologic states.

Additional information on these techniques may be found in the chapter on *Chromatography*, page 678.

Optical Properties—Particles of colloidal dimensions, suspended in a transparent medium, scatter and, to a certain extent, polarize light which falls upon them. As a result, if a beam of light is passed through a colloidal dispersion, the path of the beam is visible. In a true solution the light beam would be invisible; the solution is said to be "optically empty." This behavior of colloids was extensively studied by Tyndall and is called the *Tyndall phenomenon;* the illuminated light path is known as the *Tyndall cone* or *Tyndall beam*. Certain characteristics of the phenomenon were investigated by Rayleigh and formulated in an equation which bears his name; the intensity was found to depend on several factors. It is more intense the greater the difference between the index of refraction of the two phases. As a result, lyophobic systems exhibit most intense Tyndall effects; certain lyophilic systems show little or no effect. One should not, therefore, rely upon the Tyndall phenomenon as a test to determine whether a given dispersion is a true solution or a colloidal dispersion.

According to the Rayleigh equation, the intensity of the Tyndall beam is inversely proportional to the fourth power of the wavelength of the incident light. As a result, when a colloidal dispersion is illuminated by white light, the various components are scattered to varying degrees, those of shorter wavelength to a greater degree than the longer waves. This causes the scattered light to be richer in light towards the blue end of the spectrum, and accounts for the bluish color ("Tyndall blue") frequently noted. The blue color of the sky is believed to result from this source.

Another relationship which derives from the Rayleigh equation is the dependence of the intensity of the light upon the number and size of the suspended particles. Measurements of this light intensity may therefore be used as an analytical tool, and form the basis of an analytical technique known as nephelometry.

The Tyndall phenomenon underlies the use of the *ultramicroscope*, which is a very important instrument for the study of colloids. In practice, a beam of light is transmitted through a solution which is examined by means of a microscope placed at right angles to the path of the beam. With such an arrangement no direct light enters the microscope but light diffracted by colloidal particles in the dispersion is evidenced by the appearance of small glittering dots or lines of light against an otherwise dark background. In the absence of colloidal particles the field of view is entirely dark. The points of light exhibited by colloidal particles do not represent images of the particles themselves but rather the light which they scatter.

The ultramicroscope was devised by Zsigmondy and Siedentopf in 1903; this instrument, known as the "slit" ultramicroscope, and other modifications more recently introduced, have proved invaluable in the study of colloids. Using an ultramicroscope it is possible to detect (but not see) particles having a diameter as small as 5 mμ, whereas the smallest particle directly observable by a microscope has a diameter of about 100 mμ. Although the size of the light spot in the microscopic field bears no relation to the size of the particle, it is possible to count the number of particles in a known volume and, with the knowledge of the mass and the density of the particles, to calculate the diameter of each particle if it is assumed that they are spheres.

The spots of light seen in the dark field of the ultramicroscope usually exhibit zigzag motion, the smaller the particle the more rapid being the motion. This phenomenon, which has frequently been observed even with ordinary microscopes, was first correctly interpreted in 1827, by the English botanist, Robert Brown, after whom the motion has been called *Brownian movement*. The present view regarding the cause of the motion is a development of Brown's original explanation and holds that the movement is due to the bombardment of the suspended particles by the molecules of the suspending medium. It is believed that this fact may also contribute to the permanency of colloidal suspension.

Stability—An important consideration in the study and application of colloids is their stability. As has been mentioned, lyophobic colloids owe their stability principally to the presence of an electric charge on the particles. If this charge is removed, or reduced below a critical value, the colloidal particles cling together and rapid coagulation or precipitation occurs. This reduction of charge on the colloidal particles is usually accomplished by the addition of an electrolyte, and certain generalizations concerning the effect of electrolytes may be mentioned. Most important is the influence of charge type and valence of the ions of the added electrolyte. Their effect is summed up in the *Schulze-Hardy Rule* which states, first, that the effectiveness of an electrolyte is determined primarily by the nature of the ion opposite in charge to the colloidal particle and, second, as the valence of this ion increases, the effectiveness of the electrolyte increases markedly. For example, in the precipitation of a negative arsenous sulfide sol by electrolytes, the nature of the cation is important, while the anion plays a subordinate role. The higher the valence of the cation, the more effective the salt is in bringing about precipitation. In one series of experiments aluminum chloride was found to be about ten times as effective as magnesium chloride, and 500 times as effective as sodium chloride. In the precipitation of a positive sol (such as hydrous ferric oxide) the nature of the anion is most important; sodium phosphate, sulfate, and chloride should be in that order of decreasing effectiveness. Lyophilic colloids owe their stability to both solvation (hydration) and electric charge; as a result, they are usually more stable than lyophobic colloids. In order to coagulate a lyophilic colloid both the protective sheath of solvent surrounding the particle and the electric charge must be removed. To accomplish this with electrolytes alone, much higher concentrations are needed than for the coagulation of lyophobic colloids. It is significant that valence is a subordinate factor in determining the effectiveness of an electrolyte in this process; more important is the ability of the ions to bind water. The process is spoken of as "salting-out." Instead, a dehydrating agent (such as alcohol or acetone) may be used in conjunction with an electrolyte; in this case, low concentrations of electrolyte, comparable to those used in coagulating lyophobic colloids, will be found adequate.

When two lyophobic colloids are mixed, their behavior depends on their charge and relative amounts. If of the same charge type, little or no interaction occurs. If of the opposite charge type, mutual coagulation occurs when the sols are mixed in certain proportions, while an excess of one sol produces a mixed sol whose charge is that of the one present in excess. Thus, in mixing positive ferric oxide sol with negative arsenous sulfide, certain proportions give a precipitate, excess ferric oxide a positive, and excess arsenous sulfide, a negative, mixed sol.

Two hydrophilic sols may mutually coagulate each other. Under certain conditions the dispersed particles separate in the form of liquid droplets. This phenomenon is termed *coacervation*, and the liquid droplets are called *coacervates*. For example, positive gelatin sol will form a coacervate with a gum acacia (negative) sol. The coacervate may be caused to redisperse by the addition of a suitable electrolyte.

Certain protein sols (eg, albumin) coagulate when heated. Heat causes *denaturation* (intramolecular rearrangement) of the protein; this is followed by flocculation and coagulation. It is interesting to point out that flocculation can be prevented by shifting the protein from its isoelectric point. Thus, egg albumin, heated with dilute acid, is denatured but remains clear and does not coagulate. Flocculation and coagulation do occur, however, when sufficient base is added to return the protein to its isoelectric point.

When a hydrophilic colloid is added to a hydrophobic system in sufficient amount, the hydrophobic particles become coated with hydrophilic material and take on some of the properties of the hydrophilic particles. The hydrophobic system is now much more stable toward electrolytes; it is protected from their action, and the hydrophilic substance is called a *protective colloid*. The protective action of various hydrophilic materials is measured by their *gold number;* this is defined as the number of milligrams of material which, when added to 10 ml of red gold sol just fails to prevent the change in color from red to blue on the addition of 1 ml of 10% sodium chloride solution. Typical gold numbers, which are measures of the relative protective action,

are: gelatin, 0.005; gum arabic, 0.15; dextrin, 6.2; potato starch, 25; sodium oleate, about 2. The lower the gold number, the higher the protective or stabilizing action. Since this protective action may be different for different hydrophobic materials, an alternative test, similar in principle but using a colloidal dye (congo rubin), has been introduced.

Lange's gold sol reaction is a clinical test useful in the diagnosis of certain types of syphilis. The test depends on the fact that normal spinal fluid, mixed with a gold sol, contains proteins which protect against the coagulating effect of sodium chloride, whereas spinal fluid from syphilitic cases fails to prevent coagulation and accordingly produces a color curve diagnostic of the disease.

In pharmacy there are numerous examples of this protective action of certain colloids. All of the silver protein preparations owe their stability to the action of colloidal proteins which are added to protect the colloidal silver oxide or other silver compound formed in the manufacturing process. Similarly, colloidal silver iodide is protected by the addition of gelatin. Agar, acacia, bentonite, tragacanth, and similar substances exert protective action and at least partly for this reason are often used to hold in suspension insoluble medicaments prescribed in liquid form. However, such insoluble substances are usually present in comparatively large particles and much of the value of the suspending material depends upon the increased viscosity of the dispersion medium which delays sedimentation. If the large particles are further subdivided, the stability of the suspension will be improved even more.

Bibliography

Adamson, A. W., *The Physical Chemistry of Surfaces*, Interscience, New York, 1960.

Jirgensons, B., and Straumanis, M. E., *Colloid Chemistry*, 2nd ed., Macmillan, New York, 1962.

Mysels, K. J., *Introduction to Colloid Chemistry*, Interscience, New York, 1959.

Shaw, D. J., *Introduction to Colloid and Surface Chemistry*, Butterworths, London, 1966.

24 | Coarse Dispersions

Suspensions (interfacial properties—settling—formulation)—emulsions (formation and breakdown of dispersed liquid droplets—the emulsifying agent—preparation—stability)

This chapter was prepared by

James Swarbrick, PhD, *Professor, and Chairman, Division of Pharmaceutics, School of Pharmacy, University of Connecticut, Storrs, Conn. 06268*

For the purposes of the present chapter a dispersed system will be regarded as a two-phase system in which one phase is distributed as particles or droplets in the second, continuous, phase. Since each phase can exist in the solid, liquid, or gaseous state, there are nine possible combinations. However, since gases are miscible in all proportions, in reality there are but eight combinations. This chapter will be restricted to a discussion of those solid–liquid and liquid–liquid dispersions of coarse particles which are of pharmaceutical significance, namely suspensions and emulsions. Frequently, in these systems the dispersed phase is also referred to as the discontinuous or internal phase, while the continuous phase is termed the external phase or dispersion medium.

All dispersions may be classified into three groups on the basis of the size of the dispersed particles. Chapter 23 considers one such group—colloidal dispersions—in which the size of the dispersed particles ranged from approximately 10 Å to 0.5 μ. Molecular dispersions, the second group in the classification, are discussed in Chapters 19 and 20. The remaining group consists of those dispersions in which the particle size exceeds 0.5 μ. These *coarse dispersions* are the subject of the present chapter. A knowledge of coarse dispersions is important to the pharmacist since both pharmaceutical suspensions (solid–liquid dispersions) and emulsions (liquid–liquid dispersions) fall into this category and comprise a large segment of dispensing operations.

Suspensions

A pharmaceutical suspension may be defined as a coarse dispersion containing finely divided insoluble material suspended in a liquid medium. Since some products are occasionally prepared in a dry form, to be placed in suspension at the time of dispensing by the addition of an appropriate vehicle, this definition should be extended to include these products.

There are certain criteria that a well-formulated suspension should meet. The dispersed particles should be of such a size that they do not settle rapidly in the container. However, in the event that sedimentation occurs, the sediment must not form a hard cake. Rather, it must be capable of redispersion with a minimum effort on the part of the patient. Additionally, the product should be easy to pour, pleasant to take, and resistant to microbial attack.

The two major problem areas associated with suspensions are (1) settling of the dispersed particles and (2) caking of these particles in the sediment so as to resist redispersion. Much of the following discussion will deal with the factors that influence these processes and the ways in which they can be minimized.

Interfacial Properties

When considering the interfacial properties of dispersed particles, two factors must be taken into account, regardless of whether the dispersed phase is solid or liquid. The first relates to an increase in the free energy of the surface as the particle size is reduced and the specific surface increased. The second deals with the presence of an electrical charge on the surface of the dispersed particles.

Surface Free Energy—When solid and liquid materials are reduced in size, they tend to agglomerate or stick together. This clumping, which can occur in either air or a liquid medium, is an attempt by the particles to reduce the excess surface free energy of the system. The increase in surface free energy is related to the increase in surface area produced when the particle size is decreased. It may be expressed as follows:

$$\Delta F = \gamma \Delta A \tag{1}$$

where ΔF is the increase in surface free energy in ergs, ΔA is the increase in surface area in cm^2, and γ is the interfacial tension, in dynes/cm, between the dispersed particle or droplet and the dispersion medium. The smaller is ΔF, the more thermodynamically stable is the suspension of particles. A reduction in ΔF often is effected by the addition of a wetting agent which is adsorbed at the interface between the particle and the vehicle, thereby reducing the interfacial tension. Unfortunately, while the particles remain dispersed, or deflocculated, and settle relatively slowly, they can form a hard cake at the bottom of the container when they eventually settle. Such a sediment can be extremely difficult to redisperse. In recent years the approach adopted in suspension formulation has been to reduce ΔF by reducing ΔA.[1,2] The suspension is deliberately formulated so that the particles form loose aggregates, or flocs, which settle rapidly. However, because of their highly porous nature, the flocs do not pack tightly at the bottom of the container. Rather, they form a loose mass that can be redistributed with the minimum of agitation.

The formulation of suspensions is frequently, therefore, a compromise between (1) keeping the particles in suspension for as long as possible, and having them cake when they finally do settle, or (2) deliberately forming agglomerates which, while settling rapidly, are easy to redisperse.

Surface Potential—As has been discussed in detail in the previous chapters dealing with interfacial phenomena (Chapter 22) and colloidal dispersions (Chapter 23), both attractive and repulsive forces exist between particles in a liquid medium. The balance achieved between these opposing forces determines whether or not two particles approaching each other actually make contact or are repulsed at a certain distance of separation. The attractive forces are van der Waal's forces of the London dispersion type. The repulsive forces arise from the presence of an electrical potential relative to the surrounding medium. Usually, the particles acquire a charge as a result of (1) ionization of the molecules at the surface, (2) adsorption of ions by the particles from the surrounding liquid, or (3) a difference in the dielectric constants of the continuous phase and the dispersed particles.

Much of the theoretical work on electrical surface potentials in dispersed systems has been carried out on lyophobic colloids;[3,4] however, the theories developed in this area have been applied to suspensions and emulsions. It is recommended that the reader, at this point, refer to the detailed discussion on surface potential and the concepts of the diffuse double layer and zeta-potential presented on pages 326 and 355. A knowledge of these principles is vital to an understanding of the stability of coarse dispersions.

Flocculation and Deflocculation—Zeta-potential is a measurable indication of the potential existing at the surface of a particle. When the zeta-potential is high, the repulsive electrical forces between two particles exceed the attractive London forces. Accordingly, the particles are dispersed and are said to be *deflocculated*. Even when brought close together by random motion or agitation, deflocculated particles resist collision due to their high surface potential.

The addition of a preferentially adsorbed ion, whose charge is opposite in sign to that on the particle, tends to neutralize the surface potential and leads to a progressive lowering of the zeta-potential. At some concentration of the added ion the electrical forces of repulsion are lowered sufficiently that the forces of attraction predominate. Under these conditions the particles may approach each other more closely and form loose aggregates, termed flocs. Such a system is said to be *flocculated*.

The continued addition of the flocculating agent can, however, reverse the above process, if enough is added to cause the zeta-potential to increase sufficiently in the opposite direction. Thus, the adsorption of anions onto positively charged deflocculated particles in suspension will lead to flocculation when the zeta-potential is reduced enough. The addition of more anions can eventually generate a net negative charge on the particles. When this has achieved the required magnitude, deflocculation may occur again. The only difference from the starting system is that the net charge on the particles in their deflocculated state is negative rather than positive. Some of the major differences between suspensions of flocculated and deflocculated particles are presented in Table I.

Settling

In order to control the settling of dispersed material in suspension, the pharmacist must be aware of the factors involved. He must, for example, have an appreciation of those physical factors which will affect the rate of sedimentation of particles under ideal conditions. This knowledge then may be applied to a typical pharmaceutical suspension which likely will contain a heterogeneous dispersion of nonspherical particles. He must be familiar also with the effect flocculation will have on the structure and volume of the sediment. Finally, he must be aware of the various coefficients used to express the amount of flocculation in the system.

Sedimentation Rate

The rate at which particles in a suspension sediment is related to the size and density of the particles and the viscosity of the suspension medium. In addition, Brownian movement may exert a significant effect, as will the absence or presence of flocculation in the system.

Stokes' Law—The velocity of sedimentation of a uniform collection of spherical particles is governed by Stokes' law, which may be expressed as follows:

$$v = \frac{d^2(p_1 - p_2)g}{18\eta} \qquad (2)$$

where v is the terminal velocity in cm/sec, d is the diameter of the particles in cm, p_1 and p_2 are the densities of the dispersed phase and the dispersion medium, respectively, g is the acceleration due to gravity, and η is the Newtonian viscosity of the dispersion medium in poises. Stokes' law holds only if the downward

Table I—Properties of Flocculated and Deflocculated Particles in Suspension

Deflocculated	Flocculated
1. Particles exist in suspension as separate entities.	Particles form loose aggregates.
2. Rate of sedimentation is slow, since each particle settles separately and particle size is minimal.	Rate of sedimentation is high, since particles settle as a floc, which is a collection of particles.
3. A sediment is formed slowly.	A sediment is formed rapidly.
4. The sediment eventually becomes very closely packed, due to weight of upper layers of sedimenting material. Repulsive forces between particles are overcome and a hard cake is formed which is difficult, if not impossible, to redisperse.	The sediment is loosely packed and possesses a scaffold like structure. Particles do not bond tightly to each other and a hard, dense cake does not form. The sediment is easy to redisperse, so as to reform the original suspension.
5. The suspension has a pleasing appearance, since the suspended material remains suspended for a relatively long time. The supernatant also remains cloudy, even when settling is apparent.	The suspension is somewhat unsightly, due to rapid sedimentation and the presence of an obvious, clear supernatant region. This can be minimized if the volume of sediment is made large. Ideally, volume of sediment should encompass the volume of the suspension.

motion of the particles is not sufficiently rapid to cause turbulence.

While conditions in a pharmaceutical suspension may not be in strict accord with those laid down for Stokes' law, Eq. 2 provides those factors that can be expected to influence the rate of settling. Thus, sedimentation will be reduced by decreasing the particle size, provided the particles are kept in a deflocculated state. The rate of sedimentation will be an inverse function of the viscosity of the dispersion medium. This provides one of the most frequently used approaches to formulating a stable suspension. However, too high a viscosity is not desirable, especially if the suspending medium is Newtonian rather than shear-thinning (see Chapter 26), since it then becomes difficult to redisperse material which has settled. It also may be inconvenient to remove a viscous suspension from its container.

According to Stokes' law, the rate of sedimentation will be reduced if the difference in the densities of the dispersed particles and the continuous phase can be decreased. This is rarely possible in practice, and will not be discussed further.

Brownian Movement—When the size of particles undergoing sedimentation is reduced to approximately 2μ, random Brownian movement is observed and the rate of sedimentation departs markedly from the theoretical predictions of Stokes' law. The actual

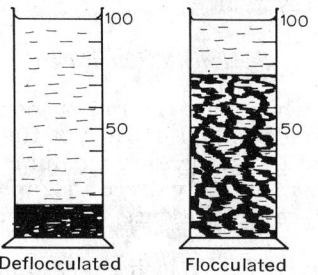

Fig. 204. Sedimentation parameters of suspensions. Deflocculated suspension: $F_\infty = 0.15$. Flocculated suspension: $F = 0.75$; $\beta = 5.0$.

size at which Brownian movement becomes significant depends on the density of the particle as well as the viscosity of the dispersion medium. However, at the lower limit of the coarse-size range, the dispersed particles may remain suspended for a prolonged period of time due to this phenomenon.

Effect of Flocculation—In a deflocculated system containing a distribution of particle sizes, the larger particles naturally settle faster than the smaller particles. The very small particles remain suspended for a considerable length of time, with the result that no distinct boundary is formed between the supernatant and the sediment. Even when a sediment becomes discernible, the supernatant remains cloudy due to these small particles, held in suspension as a result of Brownian movement.

When the same system is flocculated (in a manner to be discussed later), two effects are immediately apparent. First, the flocs tend to fall together so that a distinct boundary between the sediment and the supernatant is readily observed; second, the supernatant is clear, showing that the very fine particles have been incorporated into the flocs. The initial rate of settling in flocculated systems is determined by the size of the flocs and the porosity of the aggregated mass. Under these circumstances it is perhaps better to use the term *subsidence*, rather than sedimentation.[2]

Quantitative Expressions of Sedimentation and Flocculation

Frequently, the pharmacist needs to be able to assess a formulation in terms of the amount of flocculation in the suspension and to compare this with that found in other formulations. The two parameters commonly used for this purpose are outlined below.

Sedimentation Volume—The *sedimentation volume*, F, is the ratio of the equilibrium volume of the sediment, V_u, to the total volume of the suspension, V_0. Thus,

$$F = V_u/V_0 \qquad (3)$$

As the value of F, which normally ranges from 0 to 1, increases, the volume of suspension that appears occupied by the sediment increases. In the system where $F = 0.75$, for example, 75% of the total volume in the container is apparently occupied by the loose, porous flocs forming the sediment. This is illustrated in Fig. 204. Obviously, in a particular suspension, if F can be made to approach closer to unity, the product becomes more acceptable, since the volume of supernatant (undoubtedly regarded as unsightly) is being progressively reduced. When $F = 1$, no sediment is apparent even though the system is flocculated. This is the ideal suspension for, under these conditions, no sedimentation will occur. Caking also will be absent. Furthermore, the suspension is esthetically pleasing, there being no visible, clear supernatant.

Degree of Flocculation—A better parameter for comparing flocculated systems is the *degree of flocculation*, β, which relates the sedimentation volume of the flocculated suspension, F, to the sedimentation volume of the suspension when deflocculated, F_∞. It is expressed as

$$\beta = F/F_\infty \qquad (4)$$

The degree of flocculation is, therefore, an expression of the increased sediment volume resulting from flocculation. If, for example, β has a value of 5.0 (Fig. 204), this means that the volume of sediment in the flocculated system is five times that in the deflocculated state. The flocs are quite porous and the desirable scaffoldlike structure is present. If a second flocculated formulation results in a value for β of say 6.5, this latter suspension obviously is preferred, if the aim is to produce as flocculated a product as possible. On the other hand, as β approaches unity, the theoretical minimum value, the degree of flocculation in the system is being reduced.

Formulation

A pharmacist concerned with the formulation of a suspension possessing optimal physical stability can adopt one of several approaches. Essentially, these depend on whether the particles in suspension are to be flocculated or remain deflocculated. The first approach involves the use of a structured vehicle to keep deflocculated particles in suspension; the second depends on controlled flocculation as a means of preventing cake formation. Ideally, the third, a combination of the two previous methods, results in a product with optimum stability properties.

The first prerequisite in formulating a suspension is to ensure that the particles are adequately wetted and form a uniform dispersion. The particles are invariably deflocculated at this stage. If controlled flocculation is desired in the product, this is achieved following dispersion. Such a suspension could constitute the final product, if the sedimentation volume F were close to 1. However, the formulator may wish to prepare a suspension in which deflocculated particles are suspended in a structured vehicle. Alternatively, he may wish to incorporate a structured vehicle into a flocculated suspension to capitalize on the optimum properties of both the controlled flocculation and structured vehicle approaches. The several schemes are illustrated in Fig. 205.

Dispersion of Particles—The first step in preparing a suspension is to ensure that the particles are adequately dispersed in and wetted by the dispersion medium. This can be a problem with lyophobic particles that are poorly wetted by the vehicle alone. Because the vehicle is usually aqueous, the materials causing the most trouble are hydrophobic in nature.

Wetting agents act by lowering the contact angle between the surface of the particle and the wetting liquid. Surface-active agents commonly are used as wetting agents; maximum efficiency is obtained when the HLB value lies within the range of 7–9.[5] A concentrated solution of the wetting agent in the vehicle may be used to prepare a slurry of the powder; this is diluted with the required amount of vehicle. Alcohol and glycerin may be used sometimes in the initial stages to disperse the particles, thereby allowing the vehicle to penetrate the powder mass.

Only the minimum amount of wetting agent should be used, compatible with producing an adequate dispersion of the particles. Excessive amounts may lead to foaming or impart an undesirable taste or odor to the product. Invariably, as a result of wetting, the dispersed particles in the vehicle are deflocculated.

Structured Vehicles—Structured vehicles are generally aqueous solutions of polymeric materials such as the hydrocolloids. They function as viscosity-imparting or suspending agents and, as such, reduce the rate of sedimentation of dispersed particles. This is a direct result of Stokes' law (Eq. 2), which shows that the rate of sedimentation is inversely proportional to the viscosity of the dispersion medium. It should be noted that Stokes' law applies strictly only to Newtonian fluids; the great majority of suspending agents used in practice are non-Newtonian.

The rheological properties of suspending agents are considered elsewhere (Chapter 26). Ideally, these form pseudoplastic or plastic systems which undergo shear-thinning. Some degree of thixotropy is also desirable. Non-Newtonian materials of this type are preferred over Newtonian systems because, if the particles eventually settle to the bottom of the container, their redispersion is facilitated by the vehicle thinning when shaken. When the shaking is discontinued, the vehicle regains its original consistency and the redispersed particles are held suspended. This process of redispersion, facilitated by a shear-thinning vehicle, presupposes that the deflocculated particles have not yet formed a cake. If sedimentation and packing have proceeded to the point where considerable caking has occurred, redispersion is virtually impossible.

Most suspending agents used in pharmacy are hydrocolloids which are usually negatively charged in aqueous solution. Typical examples are methylcellulose, carboxymethylcellulose, acacia, bentonite, and Carbopol (*Goodrich*). The concentration employed will depend on the desired consistency of the

suspension which, in turn, will relate to the size and density of the suspended particles.

Controlled Flocculation—When using this approach, the formulator takes the deflocculated, wetted dispersion of particles and attempts to bring about flocculation. This is achieved by the addition of a flocculating agent; most commonly, these are either electrolytes, polymers, or surfactants. The aim is to *control* flocculation by adding that amount of flocculating agent which results in the maximum sedimentation volume.

Electrolytes are probably the most widely used flocculating agents. They act by reducing the electrical forces of repulsion between particles, thereby allowing the particles to form the loose flocs so characteristic of a flocculated suspension. Since the ability of particles to come together and form a floc depends on their surface charge, zeta-potential measurements on the suspension as an electrolyte is added provide valuable information as to the extent of flocculation in the system.

This principle is illustrated by reference to the following example, taken from the work of Haines and Martin.[6] Particles of sulfamerazine in water bear a negative charge. The serial addition of a suitable electrolyte, such as aluminum chloride, causes a progressive reduction in the zeta-potential of the particles. This is due to the preferential adsorption of the trivalent aluminum cation. Eventually, the zeta-potential will reach zero and then become positive as the addition of $AlCl_3$ is continued.

If sedimentation studies are run simultaneously on suspensions containing the same range of $AlCl_3$ concentrations, a relationship is observed between the sedimentation volume, F, the presence or absence of caking, and the zeta-potential of the particles. The situation is illustrated in Fig. 206. It is apparent that in order to obtain a flocculated, noncaking suspension with the maximum sedimentation volume, the zeta-potential must be controlled so as to lie within a certain range. This is achieved by the judicious use of an electrolyte.

An exactly comparable situation is observed when a negative ion such as $PO_4{}^{-3}$ is added to a suspension of positively charged particles such as bismuth sub-

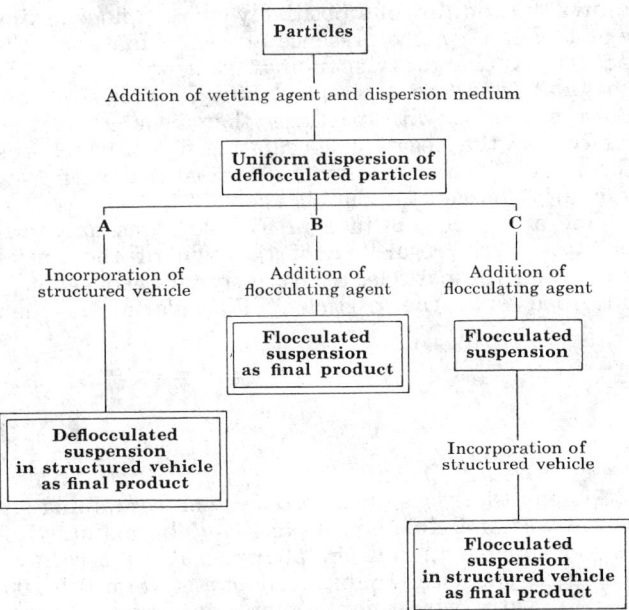

Fig. 205. **Alternative approaches to the formulation of suspensions.**

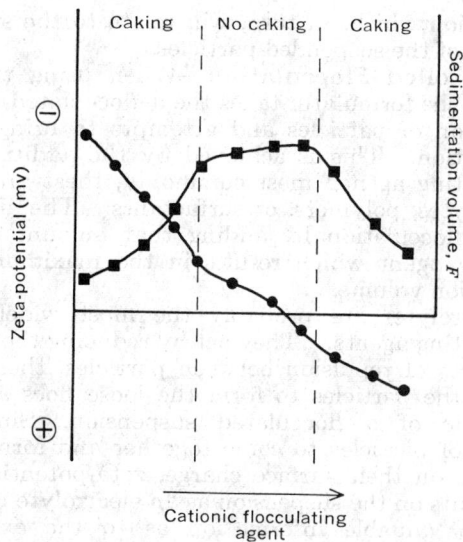

Fig. 206. Typical relationship between caking, zeta-potential, and sedimentation volume, as a positively charged flocculating agent is added to a suspension of negatively charged particles. ●: zeta-potential; ■: sedimentation volume.

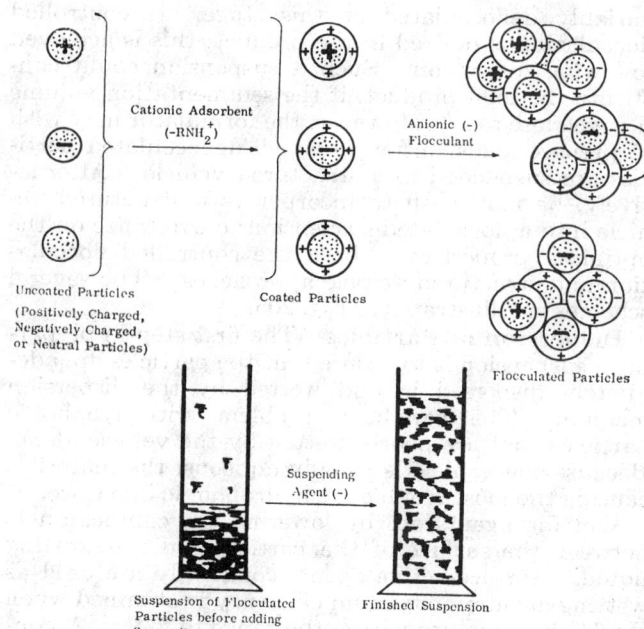

Fig. 207. Sequence of steps involved in the preparation of a stable suspension, regardless of the initial charge on the particles (courtesy, Martin and Swarbrick[7]).

nitrate. Ionic and nonionic surfactants and lyophilic polymers also have been used to flocculate particles in suspension.[2]

Flocculation in Structured Vehicles—The ideal formulation for a suspension would seem to be when flocculated particles are supported in a structured vehicle. The advantages of such a combination, in view of the previous discussion, should be obvious to the reader.

As shown in Fig. 205 (under C), the process involves dispersion of the particles and their subsequent flocculation. Finally, a lyophilic polymer is added to form the structured vehicle. In developing the formulation, care must be taken to ensure the absence of any incompatibility between the flocculating agent and the polymer used for the structured vehicle. A limitation is introduced here, in that virtually all the structured vehicles in common use are hydrophilic colloids, and these carry a negative charge. This means that an incompatibility arises if the charge on the particles is originally negative. Flocculation in this instance requires the addition of a positively charged flocculating agent or ion; in the presence of such a material, the negatively charged suspending agent will invariably coagulate and lose its suspendability. This situation does not arise with particles that bear a positive charge, as the negative flocculating agent which the formulator must employ is compatible with the similarly charged suspending agent.

One approach, outlined in Fig. 207, has universal utility. Here, regardless of the sign of the initial charge on the particle, a positively charged agent is adsorbed onto the particles. Flocculation is then brought about by means of an anionic flocculant which is compatible with the hydrophilic colloid used to keep the flocs in suspension.

Preparation of Suspensions—The small-scale preparation of suspensions may be readily undertaken by the practicing pharmacist with the minimum of equipment. It is probably true to say that any suspension will only be as good as the initial dispersion of the particles. This preliminary step is best carried out, therefore, by trituration in a mortar, the wetting agent being added in small increments to the powder. Once the particles have been wetted adequately, the slurry may be transferred to the final container. The next step depends on whether the deflocculated particles are to be suspended in a structured vehicle, flocculated, or flocculated and then suspended. Regardless of which of the alternative procedures outlined in Fig. 205 is employed, the various manipulations can be carried out easily in the bottle, especially if an aqueous solution of the suspending agent has been prepared beforehand.

If the structured vehicle has a high consistency, it may be advisable to leave the slurry in the mortar and add the suspending agent there. Gentle trituration ensures complete dispersion of the powder throughout the vehicle. The final product is then transferred to the container.

For a detailed discussion of the methods used in the large-scale production of suspensions, see the relevant section in Chapter 80.

Emulsions

An emulsion is a dispersed system containing at least two immiscible liquid phases. The majority of conventional emulsions in pharmaceutical use have dispersed particles ranging in diameter from 0.1–100 μ. As with suspensions, emulsions are thermodynamically unstable as a result of the excess free energy associated with the surface of the droplets. The dispersed droplets, therefore, strive to come together and reduce the surface area. In addition to this flocculation effect, also observed with suspensions, the dispersed particles can coalesce, or fuse, and this can result in the eventual destruction of the emulsion.

In order to minimize this effect a third component, the *emulsifying agent*, is added to the system to improve its stability. The choice of emulsifying agent is critical to the preparation of an emulsion possessing optimum stability. The efficiency of present-day emulsifiers permits the preparation of emulsions which are stable for many months and even years, even though they are thermodynamically unstable.

Emulsions have been used medicinally since at least the beginning of the 17th century. However, only in the past few decades has our knowledge of emulsion systems improved and a scientific approach to emulsification been adopted. Even so, it should not be assumed that all research into emulsions has been undertaken or that universal agreement exists as to some of the principles of emulsion science.

Emulsions are widely used in pharmacy and medicine, and emulsified materials can possess advantages not observed when formulated in other dosage forms. Thus, certain medicinal agents having an objectionable taste have been made more palatable for oral administration when formulated in an emulsion. The principles of emulsification have been applied extensively in the formulation of dermatological creams and lotions. In these, and cosmetic preparations also, the skilled formulator can prepare systems that are greasy or nongreasy, smooth or abrasive, and solid, semisolid, or liquid in consistency. The process of penetration into the skin can be facilitated if the formulator designs an emulsion that is shear-thinning. Intravenous emulsions of contrast media have been developed to assist the physician in undertaking x-ray examinations of the body organs while exposing the patient to the minimum of radiation. Considerable attention has been directed towards the use of sterile, stable intravenous emulsions containing fat, carbohydrate, and vitamins all in one preparation. Such products are administered to patients unable to assimilate these vital materials by the normal oral route.

It is apparent that the use of emulsions in pharmacy will continue in the foreseeable future, especially as the area of emulsion science continues to grow. Emulsions offer potential in the design of systems capable of giving controlled rates of drug release and of affording protection to drugs susceptible to oxidation or hydrolysis. There is still a need for well-characterized dermatological products with reproducible properties, regardless of whether these products are antibacterial, sustained-release, protective, or emollient lotions, creams, or ointments. The principle of emulsification is involved in an increasing number of aerosol products and it seems most likely that, as the use of such products expands, this trend will continue.

The pharmacist must be familiar with the types of emulsions and the properties and theories underlying their preparation and stability; such is the purpose of the remainder of this chapter. For a presentation of the various methods used to achieve emulsification, see Chapter 80.

Emulsion Type and Means of Detection

For an emulsion to be stable it must contain at least three components; namely, the dispersed phase, the dispersion medium, and the emulsifying agent. Invariably, one of the two immiscible liquids is aqueous while the second is an oil. Whether the aqueous or the oil phase becomes the dispersed phase depends primarily on the emulsifying agent used and the relative amounts of the two liquid phases. Emulsions can be classified depending on which liquid forms the dispersed phase. Hence, an emulsion in which the oil is dispersed as droplets throughout the aqueous phase is termed an oil-in-water, O/W, emulsion. On the other hand, when water is the dispersed phase and an oil the dispersion medium, the emulsion is of the water-in-oil, W/O, type. Most pharmaceutical emulsions designed for oral administration are of the O/W type; emulsified lotions and creams are either O/W or W/O, depending on their use. Butter and salad creams are W/O emulsions.

On theoretical grounds the volume of the dispersed phase can constitute up to approximately 75% of the total volume of the emulsion. However, the assumptions on which this figure is based (namely, that the droplets are rigid spheres of uniform size) are not realized in practice. Accordingly, the volume of the dispersed phase can exceed this value. There comes a point, however, at which the volume of continuous phase is insufficient to contain the dispersed phase. Either the emulsion breaks, or it inverts, whereupon the internal phase now becomes the continuous phase, and *vice versa*. This change in type with increasing phase volume is frequently accompanied by a marked change in viscosity. Other factors involved in inversion are mentioned later.

It is important for the pharmacist to know the type of emulsion he has prepared or is dealing with, since this can affect its properties and performance. Unfortunately, the several methods available can give incorrect results, and so the type of emulsion determined by one method should always be confirmed by means of a second method.

Dilution Test—This method depends on the fact that it is possible to add more of the continuous phase of an emulsion without causing any incompatibility. In essence, the emulsion is being "diluted" with its own vehicle. However, if an attempt is made to add more of the dispersed phase, it does not blend in with the emulsion and an obvious incompatibility results. Thus, an O/W emulsion can be diluted with water and a W/O emulsion with oil. When oil is added to an O/W emulsion or water to a W/O emulsion, the additive is not incorporated into the emulsion and separation is apparent. The test is greatly improved if the addition of the water or oil is observed microscopically.

Conductivity Test—An emulsion in which the continuous phase is aqueous can be expected to possess a much higher conductivity than an emulsion in which the continuous phase is an oil. Accordingly, it frequently happens that when a pair of electrodes, connected to a lamp and an electrical source, are dipped into an O/W emulsion, the lamp lights due to passage of a current between the two electrodes. If the lamp does not light, it is assumed that the system is W/O. Unfortunately, some O/W emulsions have a low conductivity while the conductivity of W/O emulsions increases with the concentration of the dispersed phase. Erroneous conclusions as to the emulsion type can therefore arise when this test is applied to some emulsions.

Dye-Solubility Test—The knowledge that a water-soluble dye will dissolve in the aqueous phase of an emulsion while an oil-soluble dye will be taken up by the oil phase provides a third means of determining emulsion type. In general, a small amount of, say, a water-soluble dye is placed on a microscope slide and a drop of emulsion is added. If microscopic examination shows that the dye has been taken up by the continuous phase, we are dealing with an O/W emulsion. If the dye has not stained the continuous phase, the test is repeated using a small amount of an oil-soluble dye. Coloring of the continuous phase confirms that the emulsion is of the W/O type.

Formation and Breakdown of Dispersed Liquid Droplets

An emulsion exists as the result of two competing processes; namely, the dispersion of one liquid throughout another as droplets and the combination of these droplets to reform the initial bulk liquids. The first process increases the free energy of the system, while the second works to reduce the free energy. Accordingly, the second process is spontaneous and continues until breakdown is complete; ie, the bulk phases are reformed.

It is of little use to form a well-dispersed emulsion if it quickly breaks down. Similarly, unless adequate attention is given to achieving an optimum dispersion, the stability of an emulsion system may be compromised from the start. Therefore, in order to optimize emulsification it is necessary to promote dispersion of the bulk liquids and minimize the reverse process. The first process is brought about by well-designed and well-operated machinery, capable of producing a fine dispersion of droplets in a relatively short period of time. Such equipment is discussed in Chapter 80. The second process, in which the bulk phases are reformed, is minimized by utilizing those parameters which influence the stability of the emulsion once it is formed. It is these parameters that will be discussed later.

Dispersion Process To Form Droplets—Consider two immiscible liquid phases in a test tube. The heavier phase lies below the second liquid and the system is thermodynamically stable. In order to disperse one liquid as droplets within the other, the interface between the two liquids must be disturbed to a sufficient degree so that "fingers" or threads of one liquid pass into the second liquid, and *vice versa*. These threads are unstable, and become varicosed or beaded. The beads separate and become spherical, as illustrated in Fig. 208. Depending on the agitation or the shear rate used, larger droplets are also deformed to give small threads, which in turn produce smaller drops. For a particular method of agitation producing a given rate of shear, a point is reached when the number of drops being formed increases to such an extent that the number of collisions between drops resulting in coalescence becomes significant.

The time of agitation is important. Under normal conditions, the mean size of droplets decreases rapidly in the first few seconds of agitation. The limiting size range is generally reached within 1 to 5 min,[8] and results from the number of droplets coalescing being equivalent to the number of new droplets being formed. It is uneconomical to continue agitation any further.

The liquids may be agitated or sheared by several means. Shaking is commonly employed, especially when the components are of low viscosity. Interestingly, it has been found that intermittent shaking, with rest periods between shakes, is frequently more efficient than continued shaking. A plausible explanation of this phenomenon, based on the mechanism of threading described above, is that the short time interval between shakes allows the thread which is forced across the interface time to break down into drops which are then isolated in the opposite phase. Continuous, rapid agitation tends to hinder this breakdown to form drops. A mortar and pestle is employed frequently in the extemporaneous preparation of emulsions. It is not a very efficient technique and is not used on a large scale. Improved dispersions are achieved by the use of high-speed mixers, blenders, colloid mills and homogenizers. Ultrasonic techniques also have been employed and are described in Chapter 80.

The phenomenon of spontaneous emulsification, as the name implies, occurs without any external agitation. There is, however, an internal agitation arising from certain physicochemical processes that affect the interface between the two bulk liquids. For a description of this process, the reader is referred to the text by Davies and Rideal.[9]

Coalescence of Droplets—Coalescence is a process distinct from flocculation (aggregation), which commonly precedes it. While flocculation is the clumping together of particles, coalescence is the fusing of the agglomerates into a larger drop, or drops. Coalescence is usually rapid when two immiscible liquids are shaken together, since there is no large energy barrier to prevent fusion of drops and reformation of the original bulk phases. When an emulsifying agent is added to the system, flocculation still may occur but coalescence is reduced to an extent depending on the efficacy of the emulsifying agent to form a stable, coherent interfacial film. It is therefore possible to prepare emulsions that are flocculated, yet which do not coalesce.[10] In addition to the interfacial film around the droplets acting as a mechanical barrier, the drops also are prevented from coalescing by the presence of a thin layer of continuous phase between particles clumped together.[11]

Davies[12] showed the importance of coalescence rates in determining emulsion type; this work is discussed in more detail on page 342.

The Emulsifying Agent

The process of coalescence can be reduced to insignificant levels by the addition of a third com-

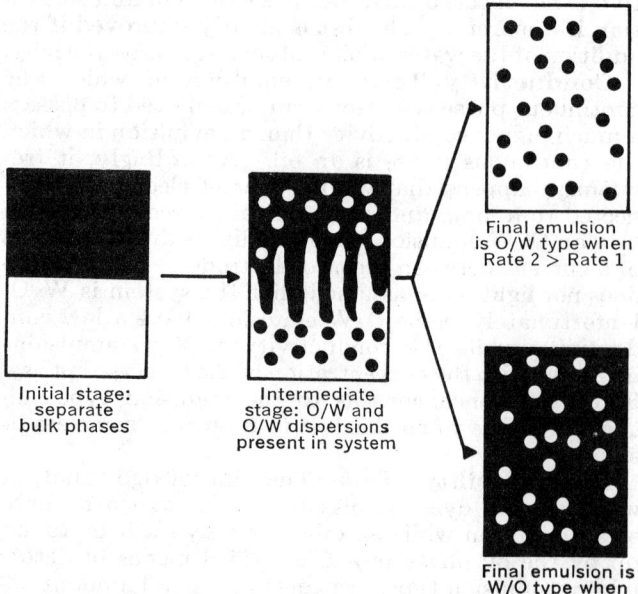

Initial stage: separate bulk phases

Intermediate stage: O/W and O/W dispersions present in system

Final emulsion is O/W type when Rate 2 > Rate 1

Final emulsion is W/O type when Rate 1 > Rate 2

Fig. 208. Effect of rate of coalescence on emulsion type. Rate 1: O/W coalescence rate; Rate 2: W/O coalescence rate. ●: oil; ○: water.

ponent—the emulsifying agent or emulsifier. The proper choice of emulsifying agent is frequently critical in developing a successful emulsion. It is necessary that the pharmacist be aware of (1) the desirable properties of emulsifying agents, (2) how different emulsifiers act to optimize emulsion stability, and (3) how the type and physical properties of the emulsion can be affected by the emulsifying agent.

Desirable Properties

According to Cobb[13] some of the desirable properties of an emulsifying agent are that it should (1) be surface active and reduce surface tension to below 10 dynes/cm, (2) be adsorbed quickly around the dispersed drops as a condensed, nonadherent film which will prevent coalescence, (3) impart to the droplets an adequate electrical potential so that mutual repulsion occurs, (4) increase the viscosity of the emulsion, and (5) be effective in a reasonably low concentration. Not all emulsifying agents possess these properties to the same degree; in fact, not every good emulsifier necessarily possesses all these properties. Further, there is no one "ideal" emulsifying agent because the desirable properties of an emulsifier depend, in part, on the properties of the two immiscible phases in the particular system under consideration.

Interfacial Tension—Lowering of interfacial tension is one way in which the increased surface free energy associated with the formation of droplets, and hence surface area, in an emulsion can be reduced (Eq. 1). Assuming the droplets to be spherical, it can be shown that

$$\Delta F = \frac{6\gamma V}{d} \qquad (5)$$

where V is the volume of dispersed phase in ml and d is the mean diameter of the particles. In order to disperse 100 ml of oil as 1 μ (10^{-4}-cm) droplets in water when $\gamma_{o/w} = 50$ dynes/cm, requires an energy input of

$$\Delta F = \frac{6 \times 50 \times 100}{1 \times 10^{-4}} = 30 \times 10^7 \text{ ergs}$$

$$= 30 \text{ joules or } 30/4.184 = 7.2 \text{ cal}$$

The system attempts to lose this excess surface free energy to its surroundings by coalescence of the droplets. These grow in size and decrease in number until one large drop (the original bulk phase) is formed. This has minimum surface area in contact with the second phase and the surface free energy is now at a minimum. However, an emulsifying agent which is adsorbed as a monolayer at an interface lowers surface tension in accordance with Gibbs' law:

$$\Gamma = -\frac{c}{RT} \cdot \frac{d\gamma}{dc} \qquad (6)$$

where Γ is the surface excess in moles/cm² and $d\gamma/dc$ is the change in surface tension with amphiphile concentration at the bulk-phase concentration c, in moles/liter, R is the gas constant, and T is the temperature in °A. Accordingly, the surface free energy can be lowered by the addition of a surface-active material which causes a reduction in surface tension.

In the above example the addition of an emulsifier that will reduce γ from 50 to 5 dynes/cm will reduce the surface free energy from 7.2 to around 0.7 cal. Likewise, if the interfacial tension is reduced to 0.5 dynes/cm, a common occurrence, the original surface free energy is reduced a hundredfold.

While the above calculations are an oversimplification of the total energies involved in emulsification, they do serve to show that a reduction of interfacial tension by the addition of an emulsifying agent can serve to preserve the surface area generated during the dispersion process.

Film Formation—The major requirement of a potential emulsifying agent is that it readily form a film around each droplet of dispersed material. The main purpose of this film—which can be a monolayer, a multilayer, or a collection of small particles adsorbed at the interface—is to form a barrier which prevents the coalescence of droplets that come into contact with one another. For the film to be an efficient barrier, it should not thin out and rupture when it is sandwiched between two droplets. If broken, the film should have the capacity to reform rapidly. The film should, therefore, possess some degree of surface elasticity, which will assist in preserving its integrity.

Electrical Potential—The origin of an electrical potential at the surface of a droplet is discussed in detail in Chapters 23 and 25. Insofar as emulsions are concerned, the presence of a well-developed charge on the droplet surface is significant in promoting stability by causing repulsion between approaching drops. This potential is likely to be greater when an ionized emulsifying agent is employed.

Emulsion Rheology—According to Sherman[14,15] the emulsifying agent can affect the rheologic behavior of an emulsion in several ways. These, and the various ways in which the other components of an emulsion can influence rheologic behavior, are shown in Table II. Space does not permit discussion of all these individual points; the interested reader should consult the original articles. Suffice it to say that the rheology of emulsions has not received as much attention as that given to other dispersed systems. This is due, most probably, to the fact that emulsions are difficult

Table II—Factors Influencing Emulsion Viscosity[a]

1. Internal phase
   a. Volume concentration (ϕ); hydrodynamic interaction between globules; flocculation, leading to formation of globule aggregates.
   b. Viscosity (η_1); deformation of globules in shear.
   c. Globule size, and size distribution, technique used to prepare emulsion; interfacial tension between the two liquid phases: globule behavior in shear; interaction with continuous phase; globule interaction.
   d. Chemical constitution.
2. Continuous phase
   a. Viscosity (η_0), and other rheological properties.
   b. Chemical constitution, polarity, pH; potential energy of interaction between globules.
   c. Electrolyte concentration if polar medium.
3. Emulsifying agent
   a. Chemical constitution; potential energy of interaction between globules.
   b. Concentration, and solubility in internal and continuous phases; emulsion type; emulsion inversion; solubilization of liquid phases in micelles.
   c. Thickness of film adsorbed around globules, and its rheological properties, deformation of globules in shear; fluid circulation within globules.
   d. Electroviscous effect.
4. Additional stabilizing agents
   Pigments, hydrocolloids, hydrous oxides; effect on rheologic properties of liquid phases, and interfacial boundary region.

[a] From: Sherman.[14]

systems to study: the droplets of the internal phase are deformable under shear and this can affect their rheology. Additionally, the adsorbed layer of emulsifier affects the interactions between adjacent droplets and also between a droplet and the continuous phase. It is not surprising that the literature contains conflicting reports as to the effect of one parameter or another on emulsion rheology.

Concentration of Emulsifier—Since the main objective of an emulsifying agent is to form a condensed film around the droplets of the dispersed phase, the concentration of emulsifier present must be sufficient for the task. An inadequate concentration will do little to prevent coalescence. Apart from a possible increase in viscosity, there is little advantage in having a large excess present either; indeed, it may produce such undesirable effects as excessive foaming. Rowe[16] found that increasing the emulsifier concentration above an optimum level achieves very little in terms of increased stability. However, he did find that the median particle diameter was decreased as the concentration of emulsifying agent was raised. In practice the aim is to use the minimum amount consistent with producing a satisfactory emulsion.

It frequently helps to have some idea of the amount of emulsifier required to form a condensed film, one molecule thick, around each droplet. Suppose we wish to emulsify 50 Gm of an oil, density = 1.0, in 50 Gm of water. The desired particle diameter is 1 μ. Thus,

Particle diameter = $1 \mu = 1 \times 10^{-4}$ cm

Volume of particle = $\dfrac{\pi d^3}{6} = 0.524 \times 10^{-12}$ cm^3

Total number of particles in 50 Gm =

$$\frac{50}{0.524 \times 10^{-12}} = 95.5 \times 10^{12}$$

Surface area of each particle = $\pi d^2 = 3.142 \times 10^{-8}$ cm^2

Total surface area = $3.142 \times 10^{-8} \times 95.5 \times 10^{12} =$

$$300 \times 10^4 \text{ cm}^2$$

If the area each molecule occupies at the oil/water interface is 30Å^2 (30 $\times$ 10^{-16} cm^2), we require

$$\frac{300 \times 10^4}{30 \times 10^{16}} = 1 \times 10^{21} \text{ molecules}$$

A typical emulsifying agent might have a molecular weight of 1000. Thus, the required weight is

$$\frac{1000 \times 10^{21}}{6.023 \times 10^{23}} = 1.66 \text{ Gm}$$

To emulsify 10 Gm of oil would require 0.33 Gm of the emulsifying agent, etc. While the approach is an oversimplification of the problem, it does at least allow the formulator to make a reasonable estimate of the required concentration of emulsifier.

Mechanism of Action

Emulsifying agents may be classified in accordance with the type of film they form at the interface between the two phases. Such a classification is summarized in Table III.

Monomolecular Films—Those surface-active agents which are capable of stabilizing an emulsion do so by forming a monolayer of adsorbed molecules or ions at the oil/water interface (Fig. 209). In accordance with Gibbs' law (Eq. 6) the presence of an interfacial excess necessitates a reduction in interfacial tension. This results in a more stable emulsion because of a proportional reduction in the surface free energy. Of itself, this reduction is probably not the main factor promoting stability. More significant is the fact that the droplets are surrounded now by a coherent monolayer which prevents coalescence between approaching droplets. If the emulsifier forming the monolayer is ionized, the presence of strongly charged and mutually repelling droplets increases the stability of the system. With unionized, nonionic surface-active agents, the particles may still carry a charge; this is not due to ionization but arises from adsorption of a specific ion or ions from solution.

Multimolecular Films—Hydrated lyophilic colloids form multimolecular films around droplets of dispersed oil[17] (Fig. 209). Although these agents have been used widely in pharmacy, their use has declined in recent years because of the large number of synthetic surface-active agents available which possess well-marked emulsifying properties. While these hydrophilic colloids are adsorbed at an interface (and can be regarded therefore as "surface active"), they do not cause an appreciable lowering in surface tension. Rather, their efficiency depends on their ability to form strong, coherent multimolecular films. These act as a coating around the droplets and render them highly resistant to coalescence, even in the absence of a well-developed surface potential. Furthermore, any hydrocolloid not adsorbed at the interface serves to increase the viscosity of the continuous aqueous phase; this enhances emulsion stability.

Solid Particle Films—Small solid particles that are wetted to some degree by both aqueous and nonaqueous liquid phases act as emulsifying agents. If the particles are too hydrophilic, they remain in the

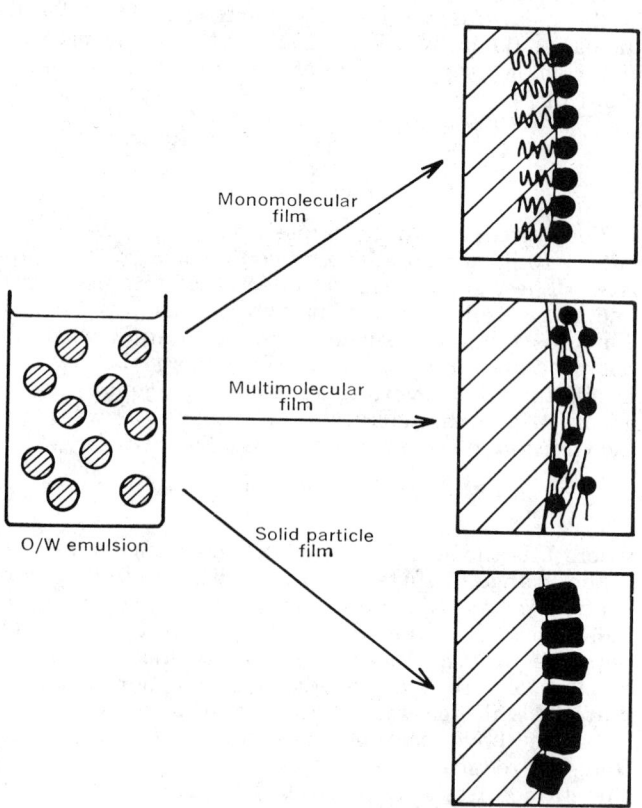

Fig. 209. Types of films formed by emulsifying agents at the oil/water interface. Orientations are shown for O/W emulsions. ▨: oil; ☐: water.

Table III—Mechanism of Action of Emulsifying Agents

Type of film	Example	Mechanism
Monomolecular	Potassium laurate Polyoxyethylene sorbitan monooleate	Coherent, flexible film formed by surface-active agents. These agents also lower interfacial tension markedly, and this contributes to stability of emulsion. Are widely used, especially the nonionic type. Depending on the particular agent(s) chosen, can prepare O/W or W/O emulsions.
Multimolecular	Acacia Gelatin	Strong, rigid film formed, mostly by hydrocolloids which produce O/W emulsions. Interfacial tension is not reduced to any degree; stability due mainly to strength of interfacial film.
Solid Particle	Bentonite Graphite Magnesium hydroxide	Film formed by solid particles that are small in size compared to the droplet of dispersed phase. Particles must be wetted by both phases to some extent in order to remain at the interface and form a stable film. Can form either O/W or W/O emulsions, depending on method of preparation.

aqueous phase; if too hydrophobic, they are dispersed completely in the oil phase. A second requirement is that the particles are small in relation to the droplets of the dispersed phase (Fig. 209).

Chemical Types

We have seen in the previous section that emulsifying agents act by forming an interfacial film around the dispersed droplets which may be either monomolecular, multimolecular, or consist of solid particles. The present section is concerned with classifying emulsifying agents in terms of their chemical structure. There is some correlation between the two classifications. For example, the majority of emulsifiers forming monomolecular films are synthetic, organic materials. Most of the emulsifiers that form multimolecular films are obtained from natural sources and are organic. A third group is composed of solid particles, invariably inorganic, that form films composed of finely divided solid particles.

Accordingly, the classification adopted divides emulsifying agents into *synthetic, natural, and finely dispersed solids* (Table IV). A fourth group, the *auxiliary materials* (Table V), are weak emulsifiers. The lists of agents are designed to illustrate the various types available; they are not meant to be exhaustive.

Synthetic Emulsifying Agents—This group of surface-active agents which act as emulsifiers may be subdivided into anionic, cationic, and nonionic, depending on the charge possessed by the surfactant.

Anionics—In this group the surfactant ion bears a negative charge. *Soaps* are widely used amphiphilic salts formed from various fatty acids containing, preferably, from 12 to 18 carbon atoms. Alkali soaps, such as the potassium, sodium, and ammonium salts of lauric and oleic acid, are soluble in water and are good O/W emulsifying agents. They do, however, have a disagreeable taste and are irritant to the gastrointestinal tract; this limits them to emulsions prepared for external use. Potassium laurate, a typical example, has the structure:

$$CH_3(CH_2)_{10}CH_2COO^- \quad K^+$$

Solutions of alkali soaps have a high pH; they start to precipitate out of solution below pH 10 because the unionized fatty acid is now formed, and this has a low aqueous solubility. Further, the free fatty acid is ineffective as an emulsifier and so emulsions formed from alkali soaps are not stable at pH values less than about 10.

The calcium, magnesium, and aluminum salts of fatty acids, often termed the metallic soaps, are water

insoluble and result in W/O emulsions. As with the alkali soaps, they are restricted to external emulsions such as liniments and creams.

Another class of soaps are those salts formed from a fatty acid and an organic amine such as triethanolamine. While these O/W emulsifiers are also limited to external preparations, their alkalinity is considerably less than that of the alkali soaps and they are active as emulsifiers down to around pH 8. These agents are less irritating than the alkali soaps.

Frequently, soaps of organic amines are prepared *in situ*. In this process the triethanolamine is added to the aqueous phase while the fatty acid is dissolved in the oil phase. When the two phases are mixed, triethanolamine stearate is formed at the interface between the two phases, the very place where it is required.

Sulfated alcohols are neutralized sulfuric acid esters of such fatty alcohols as lauryl and cetyl alcohol. These compounds are an important group of pharmaceutical surfactants. They are used chiefly as wetting agents, although they do have some value as emulsifiers, particularly when used in conjunction with an auxiliary agent. Probably the most frequently used compound is sodium lauryl sulfate:

$$CH_3(CH_2)_{10}CH_2OSO_3^- \quad Na^+$$

Sulfonates are a class of compounds in which the sulfur atom is connected directly to the carbon atom, giving the general formula

$$CH_3(CH_2)_nCH_2SO_3^- \quad Na^+$$

Sulfonates have a higher tolerance to calcium ions and do not hydrolyze as readily as the sulfates. A widely used surfactant of this type is sodium dioctyl sulfosuccinate.

Cationics—The surface activity in this group resides in the positively charged cation. While not used as widely as the anionic or nonionic types of synthetic emulsifiers, these compounds are valuable since they have marked bactericidal properties. This makes them desirable in emulsified anti-infective products such as skin lotions and creams. The pH of an emulsion prepared with a cationic emulsifier lies in the pH 4–6 range. Since this includes the normal pH of the skin, cationic emulsifiers are advantageous in this regard also.

Cationic agents are weak emulsifiers and are generally formulated with a stabilizing or auxiliary emulsifying agent such as cetostearyl alcohol. The only group of cationic agents used extensively as emulsifying agents are the *quaternary ammonium compounds*.

Table IV—Classification of Emulsifying Agents

Type	Type of film	Examples

Synthetic (surface-active agents)	Monomolecular	*Anionic:*
		  Soaps
		    Potassium laurate
		    Triethanolamine stearate
		  Sulfates
		    Sodium lauryl sulfate
		    Alkyl polyoxyethylene sulfates
		  Sulfonates
		    Dioctyl sodium sulfosuccinate
		Cationic:
		  Quaternary ammonium compounds
		    Cetyltrimethylammonium bromide
		    Lauryldimethylbenzyl ammonium
		      chloride
		Nonionic:
		  Polyoxyethylene fatty alcohol ethers
		  Sorbitan fatty acid esters
		  Polyoxyethylene sorbitan fatty acid esters

Natural	Multimolecular	*Hydrophilic colloids:*
		  Acacia
		  Gelatin

	Monomolecular	Lecithin Cholesterol

Finely divided solids	Solid particle	*Colloidal clays:*
		  Bentonite
		  Veegum
		Metallic hydroxides:
		  Magnesium hydroxide

An example is cetyltrimethylammonium bromide:

$$CH_3(CH_2)_{14}CH_2N^+(CH_3)_3 \quad Br^-$$

Cationic emulsifiers should not be used in the same formulation with anionic emulsifiers as they will interact. While the incompatibility may not be immediately apparent as a precipitate, virtually all of the desired antibacterial activity will have been lost.

Nonionics—These undissociated surfactants find widespread use as emulsifying agents when they possess the proper balance of hydrophilic and lipophilic groups within the molecule. Their popularity is based on the fact that, unlike the anionic and cationic types, nonionic emulsifiers are not susceptible to pH changes and the presence of electrolytes. The number of nonionic agents available is legion; the most frequently used are the glyceryl esters, polyoxyethylene glycol esters and ethers, and the sorbitan fatty acid esters and their polyoxyethylene derivatives.

A *glyceryl ester*, such as glyceryl monostearate, is too lipophilic to serve as a good emulsifier; it is widely used as an auxiliary agent (Table V) and has the formula

$$CH_2OOC_{17}H_{35}$$
$$|$$
$$CHOH$$
$$|$$
$$CH_2OH$$

Sorbitan fatty acid esters, such as sorbitan monopalmitate (Span 40, *Atlas*),

are nonionic oil-soluble emulsifiers that promote W/O emulsions. The *polyoxyethylene sorbitan fatty acid esters*, such as polyoxyethylene sorbitan monopalmitate (Tween 40, *Atlas*),

are hydrophilic water-soluble derivatives that favor O/W emulsions.

Polyoxyethylene glycol esters, such as the monostearate,

$$C_{17}H_{35}COO(CH_2OCH_2)_nH$$

are widely used also.

Very frequently, the best results are obtained from blends of nonionic emulsifiers. Thus, an O/W emulsifier such as Tween 40 customarily will be used in an emulsion with a W/O emulsifier such as Span 40. When blended properly, the nonionics produce fine-textured stable emulsions.

Natural Emulsifying Agents—Of the numerous emulsifying agents derived from natural (ie, plant and animal) sources, consideration will be given only to acacia, gelatin, lecithin, and cholesterol. Many other natural materials are only sufficiently active to function as auxiliary emulsifying agents or stabilizers.

While acacia and gelatin form interfacial multilayers, lecithin and cholesterol form monomolecular layers at the oil/water interface. These latter agents, whose behavior is closer to that of the synthetic surface-active agents, are used primarily in the preparation of emulsified ointments and ointment bases.

Acacia is a carbohydrate gum that finds wide application in pharmaceutical emulsions for internal use, particularly those prepared extemporaneously. The gum, available in granular and powdered form, is soluble in water and forms O/W emulsions. In addition to being both colorless and odorless, the

Table V—Auxiliary Emulsifying Agents[a]

Product	Source and composition	Principal use
Agar	Dried colloid substance from certain algae containing a polygalactose sulfate and other constituents	Hydrophilic thickening agent and stabilizer for O/W emulsions
Bentonite	Colloidal hydrated aluminum silicate	Hydrophilic thickening agent and stabilizer for O/W and W/O lotions and creams
Cetyl alcohol	Chiefly $C_{16}H_{33}OH$	Lipophilic thickening agent and stabilizer for O/W lotions and ointments
Chondrus	Dried bleached seaweed	Hydrophilic thickening agent and stabilizer for O/W emulsions; weak O/W emulsifier
Glyceryl monostearate	$C_{17}H_{35}COOCH_2CHOHCH_2OH$	Lipophilic thickening agent and stabilizer for O/W lotions and ointments
Magnesium hydroxide	$Mg(OH)_2$	Hydrophilic stabilizer for O/W emulsions
Methylcellulose	Series of methyl esters of cellulose	Hydrophilic thickening agent and stabilizer for O/W emulsions; weak O/W emulsifier
Pectin	Purified carbohydrate extracted from the inner rind of citrus fruits and apple pomace	Hydrophilic thickening agent and stabilizer for O/W emulsions; weak O/W emulsifier
Silica gel	Hydrous oxide of silica	Hydrophilic stabilizer used in the preparation of ointments
Sodium alginate	The sodium salt of alginic acid, a purified carbohydrate extracted from giant kelp	Hydrophilic thickening agent and stabilizer for O/W emulsions
Sodium carboxy-methylcellulose	Sodium salt of the carboxymethyl esters of cellulose	Hydrophilic thickening agent and stabilizer for O/W emulsions
Spermaceti	Waxy substance from the head of the sperm whale, containing cetyl palmitate	Lipophilic thickening agent and stabilizer for O/W and W/O ointments
Stearic acid	A mixture of solid acids from fats, chiefly stearic and palmitic	Lipophilic thickening agent and stabilizer for O/W lotions and ointments. Forms a true emulsifier when reacted with an alkali
Stearyl alcohol	Chiefly $C_{17}H_{35}OH$	Lipophilic thickening agent and stabilizer for O/W lotions and ointments
Tragacanth	Dried gummy exudation from species of *Astrogalus*, containing a soluble portion and an insoluble portion that swells in water	Hydrophilic thickening agent and stabilizer for O/W emulsions; weak O/W emulsifier
Veegum	Colloidal magnesium aluminum silicate	Hydrophilic thickening agent and stabilizer for O/W lotions and creams

[a] From: Martin and Swarbrick.[7]

consistency of an aqueous solution of this gum is such that it helps retard creaming of the dispersed droplets. Emulsions prepared with acacia are stable over a wide pH range. Because it is a carbohydrate it is necessary to preserve acacia emulsions against microbial attack by the use of a suitable preservative. The gum can be precipitated from aqueous solution by the addition of high concentrations of electrolytes or solvents less polar than water, such as alcohol. The preparation of emulsions using acacia as the emulsifying agent is described on page 346.

Gelatin, a protein, has been used for many years as an emulsifying agent. Only in recent years has the relationship between its amphoteric nature and emulsifying properties become apparent, specifically of the isoelectric point of the material (the pH at which the net charge on the molecule is zero) and the minimum solubility at this pH. Gelatin can have two isoelectric points, depending on the method of preparation. So-called Type A gelatin, derived from an acid-treated precursor, has an isoelectric point of between pH 7 and 9. Type B gelatin, obtained from an alkali-treated precursor, has an isoelectric point of approximately pH 5. Type A gelatin acts best as an emulsifier around pH 3, where it is positively charged; on the other hand, Type B gelatin is best used around pH 8, where it is negatively charged. The question as to whether the gelatin is positively or negatively charged is fundamental to the stability of the emulsion when other charged emulsifying agents are present. In order to avoid an incompatibility, all emulsifying agents should carry the same sign. Thus, if gums (such as tragacanth, acacia, and agar) which are negatively charged are to be used with gelatin, Type B material should be used at an alkaline pH. Under these conditions the gelatin is similarly negatively charged.

Lecithin is a phospholipid which, because of its strongly hydrophilic nature, produces O/W emulsions. It is liable to microbial attack and tends to darken on storage. While it is the chief emulsifying agent present in egg yolk, it is rarely used alone as an emulsifier.

Cholesterol is a major constituent of wool alcohols, obtained by the saponification and fractionation of wool fat. It is cholesterol that gives wool fat its capacity to absorb water and form a W/O emulsion.

Finely Dispersed Solids—This group of emulsifiers forms particulate films around the dispersed droplets and produces emulsions which, while coarse-grained, have considerable physical stability. It appears possible that any solid can act as an emulsifying agent of this type, provided it is reduced to a sufficiently fine powder. In practice the two groups of compounds used most frequently are the colloidal clays and the metallic hydroxides.

Several *colloidal clays* find application in pharmaceutical emulsions; the most frequently used are bentonite, a colloidal aluminum silicate, and Veegum (*Vanderbilt*), a colloidal magnesium aluminum silicate.

Bentonite is a white to gray, odorless, and tasteless powder that swells in the presence of water to form a translucent suspension with a pH of around 9. Depending on the sequence of mixing it is possible to prepare both O/W and W/O emulsions. When an O/W emulsion is desired, the bentonite is first dispersed in water and allowed to hydrate so as to form a magma. The oil phase is then added gradually with constant trituration. Since the aqueous phase is always in excess, the O/W emulsion type is favored. To prepare a W/O emulsion, the bentonite is first dispersed in oil; the water is then added gradually.

While Veegum is used as a solid particle emulsifying agent, it is employed most extensively as a stabilizer in cosmetic lotions and creams. Concentrations of less than 1% Veegum will stabilize an emulsion containing anionic or nonionic emulsifying agents.

Two insoluble *metallic hydroxides*, namely magnesium and aluminum hydroxides, have some utility as pharmaceutical emulsifiers. Magnesium hydroxide has been used to emulsify liquid paraffin while some forms of aluminum hydroxide have been employed as emulsifiers for such materials as benzyl benzoate. Quite often, these emulsifiers are present in an emulsion because of their pharmacologic properties rather than their emulgent properties.

Auxiliary Emulsifying Agents—Included under this heading are those compounds which are normally incapable themselves of forming stable emulsions. Their main value lies in their ability to function as thickening agents and thereby help stabilize the emulsion. Thus, tragacanth or agar is sometimes combined with acacia to increase the consistency of the aqueous phase of an O/W emulsion. These, and other such agents in common use, are listed in Table V.

Emulsifying Agents and Emulsion Type

For a molecule, ion, colloid, or particle to be active as an emulsifying agent, it must have some affinity for the interface between the dispersed phase and the dispersion medium. With the mono- and multilayer films the emulsifier is in solution and, therefore, must be soluble to some extent in one or both of the phases. At the same time it must not be overly soluble in either phase, otherwise it will remain in the bulk of that phase and not be adsorbed at the interface. This balanced affinity for the two phases also must be evident with finely divided solid particles used as emulsifying agents. If their affinity, as evidenced by the degree to which they are wetted, is either predominantly hydrophilic or hydrophobic, they will not function as effective wetting agents.

The great majority of the work on the relation between emulsifier and emulsion type has been concerned with surface-active agents that form interfacial monolayers. The present discussion, therefore, will concentrate on this class of agents.

Bancroft's Rule—A great deal of the work on emulsions carried out in the early part of the 20th century has very little significance today. However, an observation by Bancroft[18] in 1913 is still valid. Bancroft recognized that the phase in which the emulsifier was most soluble formed the continuous phase of the emulsion. No explanation of any consequence was offered at the time. Recent work (see page 343) has provided a theoretical basis for this rule.

Hydrophile–Lipophile Balance—As the emulsifier becomes more hydrophilic, its solubility in water increases and the more likely is the formation of an O/W emulsion. Conversely, W/O emulsions are favored with the more lipophilic emulsifiers. This led to the concept that the type of emulsion is related to the balance between hydrophilic and lipophilic solution tendencies of the surface-active emulsifying agent.

Table VI—Relationship between HLB Range and Surfactant Application

HLB range	Use
0–3	Antifoaming agents
4–6	W/O emulsifying agents
7–9	Wetting agents
8–18	O/W emulsifying agents
13–15	Detergents
10–18	Solubilizing agents

As described in Chapter 22, surface-active agents are *amphiphiles* in which the molecule or ion contains both hydrophilic and lipophilic portions. Griffin[5] developed a scale based on the balance between these two opposing tendencies. This so-called *HLB scale* is a numerical scale, extending from 1 to approximately 50. The more hydrophilic surfactants have high HLB numbers (in excess of 10), while surfactants with HLB numbers from 1 to 10 are considered to be lipophilic. Surfactants with a proper balance in their hydrophilic and lipophilic affinities are effective emulsifying agents since they tend to concentrate at the oil/water interface. The relationship between HLB values and the application of the surface-active agent is shown in Table VI. Some commonly used emulsifiers and their HLB numbers are listed in Table VII.[19] The utility of the HLB system in rationalizing the choice of emulsifying agents when formulating an emulsion will be discussed in a later section.

Rate of Coalescence and Emulsion Type—Recent work by Davies[12] indicated that the type of emulsion produced in systems prepared by shaking is controlled by the relative coalescence rates of oil droplets dispersed in the oil. Thus, when a mixture of oil and water is shaken together with an emulsifying agent, a multiple dispersion is produced initially which contains oil dispersed in water and water dispersed in oil (Fig. 208). The type of the final emulsion which results depends on whether the water droplets or the oil droplets coalesce more rapidly. If the O/W coalescence rate (Rate 1) is much greater than the W/O coalescence rate (Rate 2), a W/O emulsion is formed since the dispersed water droplets are more stable than the dispersed oil droplets. Conversely, if Rate 2 is significantly faster than Rate 1, the final emulsion is an O/W dispersion because the oil droplets are more stable.

According to Davies, the rate at which oil globules coalesce when dispersed in water is given by the expression

$$\text{Rate 1} = C_1 e^{-W_1/RT} \tag{7}$$

The term C_1 is a collision factor which is directly proportional to the phase volume of the oil relative to the water, and is an inverse function of the viscosity of the continuous phase (water). W_1 relates to an energy barrier that must be overcome before coalescence can take place. This energy barrier is made up of several contributing factors. First, it depends on the electrical potential of the dispersed oil droplets, since this affects repulsion. Second, with an O/W emulsion the hydrated layer surrounding the polar portion of emulsifying agent must be broken down before coalescence can occur. This hydrated layer is probably around 10 Å thick with a consistency of butter. Finally, the total energy barrier depends on the fraction of the interface covered by the emulsifying agent.

Eq. 8 describes the rate of coalescence of water

globules dispersed in oil, namely

$$\text{Rate } 2 = C_2 e^{-W_2/RT} \qquad (8)$$

Here, the collision factor C_2 is a function of the water/oil phase volume ratio divided by the viscosity of the oil phase. The energy barrier W_2 is, as before, related to the fraction of the interface covered by the surface-active agent. Another contributing factor is the number of $-CH_2-$ groups in the emulsifying agent; the longer the alkyl chain of the emulsifier, the greater the gap that has to be bridged if one water droplet is to combine with a second drop.

Davies[12] showed that the HLB concept is related to the distribution characteristics of the emulsifying agent between the two immiscible phases. An emulsifier with an HLB of less than 7 will be preferentially soluble in the oil phase and will favor formation of a W/O emulsion. Surfactants with an HLB value in excess of 7 will be distributed in favor of the aqueous phase and will promote O/W emulsions. As a result, the rule founded empirically by Bancroft in 1913 has been related to the recent concept of HLB and the even more recent interpretation of coalescence rates of O/W and W/O emulsions.

Preparation of Emulsions

Several factors must be taken into account in the successful preparation and formulation of emulsified products. Usually, the type of emulsion (i.e., O/W or W/O) is specified; if not, it probably will be implied from the anticipated use of the product. The formulator's attention is focused primarily on the selection of the emulsifying agent, or agents, necessary to achieve a satisfactory product. With experience, he should be able to select an effective emulsifier with the minimum of experimentation. At the same time, he has to take steps to ensure that no incompatibilities occur between the various emulsifiers and the several components commonly present in pharmaceutical emulsions. Finally, the pharmacist must be able to prepare the product in such a way as not to prejudice his formulation. This requires not only a knowledge of the available methods of small-scale preparation, but a possession of the necessary practical skills.

Selection of Emulsifying Agents

The selection of the emulsifying agent, or agents, is of prime importance in the successful formulation of an emulsion. In addition to its emulsifying properties, the pharmacist must ensure that the material chosen is nontoxic and that the taste, odor, and chemical stability are compatible with the product. Thus, an emulsifying agent which is entirely suitable for inclusion in a skin cream may be wholly unacceptable in the formulation of an oral preparation due to its potential toxicity. This consideration is

Table VII—Approximate HLB Values for a Number of Surfactants[a]

Generic or chemical name	Trademark	HLB
Sorbitan trioleate	Span 85,[b] Arlacel 85[b]	1.8
Polyoxyethylene sorbitol beeswax	Atlas G-1706[b]	2.0
Sorbitan tristearate	Span 65[b]	2.1
Ethylene glycol fatty acid ester	Emcol EO-50[c]	2.7
Propylene glycol monostearate (pure)		3.4
Sorbitan sesquioleate	Arlacel C[b]	3.7
Glycerol monostearate	Atmul 67,[b] Atmul 84,[b] Tegin 515,[d] Aldo 33,[e] pure form	3.8
Sorbitan mono-oleate	Span 80[b]	4.3
Propylene glycol monolaurate	Atlas G-917,[b] Atlas G-3851[b]	4.5
Sorbitan monostearate	Arlacel 60[b]	4.7
Glyceryl monostearate (self-emulsifying)	Aldo 28,[e] Tegin[d]	5.5
Diethylene glycol monolaurate (soap-free)	Atlas G-2124[b]	6.1
Sorbitan monopalmitate	Span 40,[b] Arlacel 40[b]	6.7
Acacia		8.0
Polyoxyethylene mannitol dioleate	Atlas G-2800[b]	8.0
Sorbitan monolaurate	Span 20,[b] Arlacel 20[b]	8.6
Polyoxyethylene lauryl ether	Brij 30[b]	9.5
Gelatin		9.8
Methocel 15		10.5
Polyoxyethylene monostearate	Myrj 45[b]	11.1
Polyethylene glycol 400 monostearate	S-541l[e]	11.6
Triethanolamine oleate		12.0
Polyoxyethylene alkyl phenol	Igepal CA-630[f]	12.8
Polyoxyethylene alkyl aryl ether	Atlas G-1690[b]	13.0
Tragacanth		13.2
Polyoxyethylene sorbitan monolaurate	Tween 21[b]	13.3
Polyoxyethylene castor oil	Atlas G-1794[b]	13.3
Polyoxyethylene sorbitan monostearate	Tween 60[b]	14.9
Polyoxyethylene sorbitan monooleate	Tween 80[b]	15.0
Polyoxyethylene monostearate	Myrj 49[b]	15.0
Polyoxyethylene sorbitan monopalmitate	Tween 40[b]	15.6
Polyoxyethylene monostearate	Myrj 51[b]	16.0
Polyoxyethylene sorbitan monolaurate	Tween 20[b]	16.7
Polyoxyethylene lauryl ether	Brij 35[b]	16.9
Polyoxyethylene monostearate	Myrj 52[b]	16.9
Sodium oleate		18.0
Sodium lauryl sulfate		40.0

[a] From: Martin.[19]
[b] Atlas.
[c] Emulsol.
[d] Goldschmidt.
[e] Glycol.
[f] Gen. Aniline.

most important when formulating intravenous emulsions.

The HLB System—Until the 1950's the selection of emulsifiers for a product was quite literally a trial-and-error procedure. With the increasing number of available emulsifiers, particularly the nonionics, the problem was compounded and the number of combinations became legion. The work of Griffin[5,20] provided a logical means of selecting emulsifying agents. Griffin's method, based on the balance between the hydrophilic and lipophilic portions of the emulsifying agent, is now widely used and has come to be known as the *HLB system*. It is used most in the rational selection of combinations of nonionic emulsifiers, and we shall limit our discussion accordingly.

In the HLB system the surface-active agent is assigned a number; the higher the number, the more hydrophilic the agent. The actual number has no significance, except as a means of ranking the surfactants. This ranking was based on extensive experimentation, as a result of which Griffin was able to assign an application to the surfactant based on its HLB number (Table VI). Herein lies the utility of the HLB system. If an O/W emulsion is required, the formulator should use emulsifiers with an HLB in the range of 8–18. Emulsifiers with HLB values in the range of 3–6 are given consideration when a W/O emulsion is desired. Some typical examples are given in Table VII.

Another factor is the presence or absence of any polarity in the material being emulsified, since this will affect the polarity required in the emulsifier. Again, as a result of extensive experimentation, Griffin evolved a series of "required HLB" values; i.e., the HLB value required by a particular material if it is to be emulsified effectively. Some values for oils and related materials are contained in Table VIII. Naturally, the required HLB value differs depending on whether the final emulsion is O/W or W/O. In order to prepare an O/W emulsion of liquid petrolatum, the emulsifier should have an HLB value close to 10.5; on the other hand, if a W/O emulsion with liquid petrolatum as the continuous phase is desired, the emulsifier HLB should approximate 4.

Fundamental to the utility of the HLB concept is the fact that the HLB values are algebraically additive. Thus, by using a surfactant with a low HLB with one having a high HLB it is possible to prepare blends having HLB values intermediate between those of the two individual emulsifiers. Naturally, one should not use emulsifiers that are incompatible. Assuming, for the moment, that the required HLB of the oil phase and the type of emulsion desired are known, the formulator chooses two emulsifying agents, one with an HLB value above and the second with an HLB value below that required by the oil. These are blended to give a mixture of the correct HLB. The following formula should serve as an example.

O/W Emulsion

Liquid petrolatum (HLB 10.5)................. 50 Gm
Emulsifying agents........................ 5 Gm
  Span 80 (HLB 4.3)
  Tween 80 (HLB 15.0)
Water, q.s................................ 100 Gm

By simple algebra it can be shown that 4.5 parts by weight of Span 80 blended with 6.2 parts by weight of Tween 80 will result in a mixed emulsifying agent having the required HLB of 10.5. Since the formula calls for 5 Gm, the required weights are 2.1 Gm Span 80 and 2.9 Gm Tween 80. The oil-soluble Span is dissolved in the oil and heated to 75°; the water-soluble Tween is added to the aqueous phase which is raised to 70°. At this point the oil phase is mixed with the aqueous phase and the whole stirred continuously until cool.

The formulator is not restricted to Span 80 and Tween 80 to produce a blend with an HLB of 10.5. Table IX shows the various proportions required, using four other pairs of emulsifying agents, to form a blend of HLB 10.5. When carrying out preliminary investigations with a particular material to be emulsified, it is advisable to try several pairs of emulsifying agents. Based on an evaluation of the emulsions produced, it should be possible to choose the best combination.

Occasionally, the required HLB of the oil may not be known, in which case it becomes necessary to determine this parameter. Various blends are prepared to give a wide range of HLB mixtures and emulsions are prepared in a standardized manner. The HLB of the blend used to emulsify the best product, selected on the basis of physical stability, is taken to be the required HLB of the oil. The experiment should be repeated using another combination of emulsifiers to confirm the value of the required HLB of the oil to within, say, ±1 HLB unit.

It should be apparent that this technique can be employed also to calculate the HLB of a new emulsifying agent. Here, an oil of known required HLB is used together with an emulsifying agent of known HLB. The latter is combined with the unknown emulsifier in known proportions and a series of emulsions is made. Let us suppose that the required HLB of the oil was 11 and that the known emulsifier had an HLB of 4.3. Further, let us assume that, in the best emulsion prepared, the ratio of known emulsifier to unknown emulsifier was 40/60. Therefore, the HLB of the unknown agent is

$$(0.40 \times 4.3) + (0.60 \times U) = 11$$

or

$$U = \frac{(11 - 1.72)}{0.60} = 15.5$$

There are other methods for finding the HLB value of a new surface-active agent. Griffin[20] developed simple equations which can be used to obtain an estimate with certain compounds. Ross and co-workers[21] have shown that the ability of a compound to spread at a surface is related to its HLB. In another approach Gorman and Hall[22] observed a linear relation between HLB and the logarithm of the dielectric constant for a number of nonionic surfactants. An approach worthy of note has been de-

Table VIII—Required HLB Values for Some Common Emulsion Ingredients

Substance	W/O	O/W
Acid, stearic	...	17
Alcohol, cetyl	...	13
Lanolin, anhydrous	8	15
Oil, cottonseed	...	7.5
mineral oil, light	4	10–12
mineral oil, heavy	4	10.5
Wax, beeswax	5	10–16
microcrystalline	...	9.5
paraffin	...	9

Table IX—Nonionic Blends having HLB Values of 10.5

Surfactant blend[a]	HLB	Required amounts (%) to give HLB = 10.5
Span 65	2.1	34.4
Tween 60	14.9	65.6
Arlacel 60	4.7	43.2
Tween 60	14.9	56.8
Span 40	6.7	57.3
Tween 40	15.6	42.7
Arlacel C	3.7	48.5
Brij 35	16.9	51.5

[a] Atlas.

Table X—HLB Group Numbers[a]

	Group number
Hydrophilic groups	
—SO$_4$'Na$^+$	38.7
—COO'K$^+$	21.1
—COO'Na$^+$	19.1
N (tertiary amine)	9.4
Ester (sorbitan ring)	6.8
Ester (free)	2.4
—COOH	2.1
Hydroxyl (free)	1.9
—O—	1.3
Hydroxyl (sorbitan ring)	0.5
Lipophilic groups	
—CH—	
—CH$_2$—	
CH$_3$—	−0.475
=CH—	
Derived groups	
—(CH$_2$—CH$_2$—O)—	+0.33
—(CH$_2$—CH$_2$—CH$_2$—O)—	−0.15

[a] From: Davies.[12]

veloped by Davies[12] and is related to his studies on the relative rates of coalescence of O/W and W/O emulsions (page 342). According to Davies, hydrophilic groups on the surfactant molecule make a positive contribution to the HLB number, whereas lipophilic groups exert a negative effect. Davies calculated these contributions and termed them HLB Group Numbers (Table X). Provided the molecular structure of the surfactant is known, one simply adds the various group numbers in accordance with the following formula:

$$HLB = \Sigma(\text{hydrophilic group numbers}) -$$
$$m(\text{group number/ —CH}_2\text{— group}) + 7$$

where m is the number of —CH$_2$— groups present in the surfactant. Very good agreement is found between the HLB values calculated in this manner and those obtained by Griffin.

Several devices are available to the formulator to aid him in determining the exact amount of each emulsifying agent needed to prepare a blend of a particular HLB. One such aid is shown in Fig. 210. A line is drawn between the HLB values of the two emulsifiers to be used. The graph is then entered from either side at the level of the required HLB and the point of interception determined. The intercept on the baseline gives the necessary percentage of the hydrophilic emulsifier. By difference, the percentage lipophilic emulsifier required can be determined. An ingenious device called *The HLB Surfactant Selector* (Fig. 211) is also available.

Finally, a word of caution regarding the use of the HLB system. Experience has shown that, depending on the specific techniques used to determine the HLB, the values may differ by as much as 4 or 5 units. This may necessitate running several series of emulsions before a reasonably good HLB value is achieved. In formulating an emulsion, blends of emulsifiers with HLB values to either side of that required by the oil should be used whenever possible, since the conditions in different formulations may favor a slightly higher or lower HLB number.

The observant reader will have already realized that the HLB system gives no information as to the *amount* of emulsifier required. Having once determined the correct blend, the formulator must prepare another series of emulsions, all at the same HLB, but containing increasing concentrations of the emulsifier blend. Usually, the minimum concentration giving the desired degree of physical stability is chosen.

Mixed Emulsifying Agents—Emulsifying agents are frequently used in combination since a better emulsion is usually obtained. This enhancement may be due to several reasons, one or more of which may be operative in any one system. Thus, the use of a blend or mixture of emulsifiers may (1) produce the required hydrophile–lipophile balance in the emulsifier, (2) enhance the stability and cohesiveness of the interfacial film, and (3) affect the consistency and feel of the product.[7]

The first point has been considered in detail in the previous discussion of the HLB system.

With regard to the second point, the use of mixed emulsifiers to produce stable interfacial films, and hence stable emulsions, was first rationalized by Schulman and Cockbain.[23] These workers showed that combinations of certain amphiphiles formed stable films at the air/water interface. It was postulated that the complex formed by these two materials

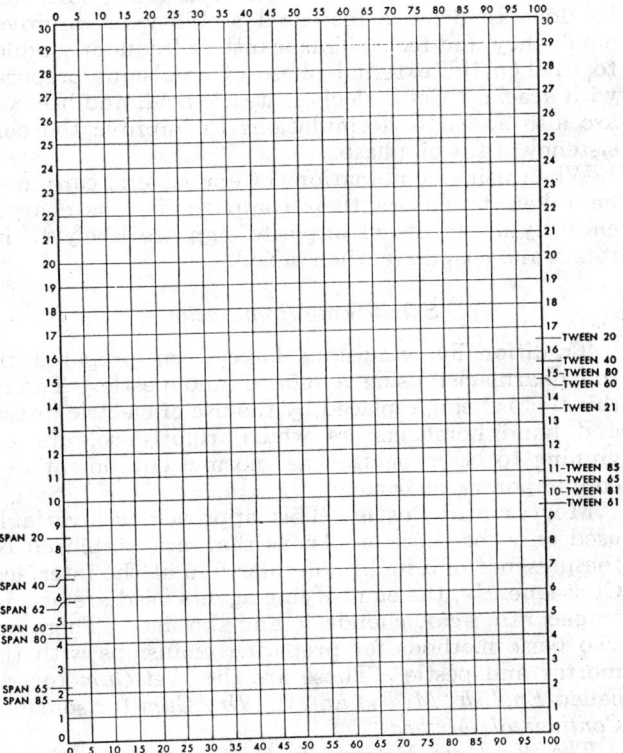

Fig. 210. Atlas HLB Computing Chart for combinations of surface-active agents.

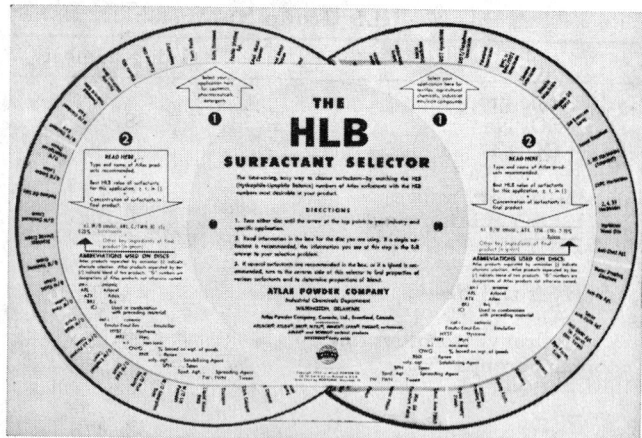

Fig. 211.   The HLB surfactant selector (courtesy, Atlas).

(one, oil-soluble; the other, water-soluble) at the air/-water interface was also present at the O/W interface. This interfacial complex was held to be responsible for the improved stability. For example, sodium cetyl sulfate, a moderately good O/W emulsifier, and elaidyl alcohol or cholesterol, both stabilizers for W/O emulsions, show evidence of an interaction at the air/water interface. Furthermore, an O/W emulsion prepared with sodium cetyl sulfate and elaidyl alcohol is much more stable than an emulsion prepared with sodium cetyl sulfate alone.

Elaidyl alcohol is the *trans* isomer. When oleyl alcohol, the *cis* isomer, is used with sodium cetyl sulfate, there is no evidence of complex formation at the air/water interface. Significantly, this combination does not produce a stable O/W emulsion either. Such a finding strongly suggests that a high degree of molecular alignment is necessary at the O/W interface to form a stable emulsion.

Finally, some materials are added primarily to increase the consistency of the emulsion. This may be done to achieve increased stability or improved emolliency and feel. Tragacanth is frequently added to thicken the external phase of emulsions prepared with acacia. Cetyl alcohol, stearic acid, and beeswax are also added to formulations to improve the consistency of the oil phase.

When using combinations of emulsifiers, care must be taken to ensure their compatibility, as charged emulsifying agents of opposite sign are likely to interact and coagulate when mixed.

Small-Scale Preparation

Traditionally, emulsions have been prepared by the pharmacist using a mortar and pestle. Today, this tool is being replaced by the use of electric mixers and hand homogenizers which, rightly so, are beginning to be recognized as normal equipment in a contemporary pharmacy.

Mortar and Pestle—This approach is invariably used only for those emulsions that are stabilized by the presence of a multimolecular film at the interface. Consequently, the emulsifying agents used are acacia, tragacanth, agar, chondrus, and the like. There are two basic methods for preparing emulsions with the mortar and pestle. These are the *Wet Gum* (or so-called *English) Method* and the *Dry Gum* (or so-called *Continental) Method.*

The Wet Gum Method—In this method the emulsifying agent is placed in the mortar and dispersed in water to form a mucilage. The oil is added in small amounts with continuous trituration, each portion of the oil being emulsified before adding the next increment.   Acacia is the most frequently used emulsifying agent when preparing emulsions with the mortar and pestle.   When emulsifying a fixed oil, the optimum ratio of oil:water:acacia to prepare the initial emulsion is 4:2:1.   Thus, the preparation of 60 ml of a 40% cod liver oil emulsion requires the following:

Cod liver oil	24 Gm
Acacia	6 Gm
Water, q.s.	60 ml

The acacia mucilage is formed by adding 12 ml of water to the 6 Gm of acacia in the mortar and triturating.   The 24 Gm of oil is added in increments of 1–2 Gm and dispersed. The product at this stage is known as the *primary emulsion,* or *nucleus.* The primary emulsion should be triturated for at least 5 min, after which sufficient water is added to produce a final volume of 60 ml.

The preparation of the primary emulsion is critical to the stability and appearance of the final product. The presence of the characteristic "cracking" sound as the primary emulsion is being triturated with the pestle is generally the best index of success. If the primary emulsion becomes too thin during its preparation, it is impossible to emulsify any additional oil. A fresh mucilage should be prepared, to which it may be possible to add the first emulsion. However, it may be necessary to start over with the whole preparation. If the primary emulsion becomes too thick to absorb the oil, a small amount of oil may be added to regain the correct consistency.

The wet gum method is tedious and requires considerable skill in order to ensure repeated success on the part of the pharmacist. It is for these reasons that most pharmacists prefer to use the dry gum method.

The Dry Gum Method—Here, the gum is added to the oil, rather than the water as with the wet gum method. Again, the approach is to prepare a primary emulsion from which the final product can be obtained by dilution with the continuous phase. If the emulsifier is acacia and a fixed oil is to be emulsified, the ratio of oil:water:gum is again 4:2:1.

In order to prepare the 40% cod liver oil emulsion, mentioned previously, by the dry gum method, the 24 Gm of oil is placed in a dry mortar. The acacia, as a fine powder, is added to the oil and dispersed thoroughly by gentle trituration; 12 ml of water is added at one time and the whole triturated vigorously until the primary emulsion is formed. A "cracking" sound during this latter stage of preparation again indicates that the formation of the primary emulsion is proceeding satisfactorily. Dilution with the continuous phase (i.e., water) can then proceed as above.

Provided dispersion of the acacia in the oil is adequate, the dry gum method can almost be guaranteed to produce an acceptable emulsion. Because there is no incremental addition of one of the components, the preparation of an emulsion by this method is rapid.

With both methods the oil:water:gum ratio may vary, depending on the type of oil to be emulsified and the emulsifying agent used. The usual ratios for tragacanth and acacia are shown in Table XI.

Other Methods—The preparation of emulsions by both the wet and dry gum methods can be carried out in a bottle rather than a mortar and pestle. In the wet gum method the mucilage is placed in a bottle, a small amount of oil is added, the bottle is capped and

Table XI—Usual Ratios of Oil, Water, and Gum Used to Produce Emulsions

System	Acacia	Tragacanth
Fixed oils (excluding liquid petrolatum and linseed oil)	4	40
Water	2	20
Gum	1	1
Volatile oils, plus liquid petrolatum and linseed oil	2–3	20–30
Water	2	20
Gum	1	1

shaken to disperse the oil, more oil is added, and the shaking is repeated. This process is continued until all the oil has been incorporated. In the dry gum method the oil is placed in a dry bottle and the emulsifier is added; following dispersion of the emulsifier by gentle shaking, the amount of water necessary to form the primary emulsion is added at one time and the bottle is shaken until emulsification of the contents is achieved.

An increasing number of emulsions are being formulated with synthetic emulsifying agents, especially of the nonionic type. The components in such a formulation are separated into those that are oil soluble and those that are water soluble. These are dissolved in their respective solvents by heating to about 70–75°. When solution is complete, the two phases are mixed and the product is stirred until cool. This method, which requires nothing more than two beakers, a thermometer, and a source of heat, is necessarily used in the preparation of emulsions containing waxes and other high-melting-point materials that must be melted before they can be dispersed in the emulsion. The relatively simple methodology involved in the use of synthetic surfactant-type emulsifiers is one factor which has led to their widespread use in emulsion preparation. This, in turn, has led to a decline in the use of the natural emulsifying agents.

Hand homogenizers and blenders are being used more widely by practicing pharmacists for preparing emulsions. With hand homogenizers an initial rough emulsion is formed by trituration in a mortar or shaking in a bottle. The rough emulsion is then passed several times through the homogenizer. A reduction in particle size is achieved as the material is forced through a narrow aperture under pressure. A satisfactory product invariably results from the use of a hand homogenizer and overcomes any deficiencies in technique. Should the homogenizer fail to produce an adequate product, the formulation, rather than the technique, should be suspected.

For a discussion of the techniques and equipment used in the manufacture of emulsions, see Chapter 80, *Solutions, Emulsions, and Suspensions.*

Stability of Emulsions

There are several criteria which must be met in a well-formulated emulsion. Probably the most important and most readily apparent requirement is that the emulsion possess adequate physical stability; without this, any emulsion soon will revert back to two separate bulk phases. In addition, if the emulsified product is to have some antimicrobial activity (e.g., a medicated lotion), care must be taken to ensure that the formulation possesses the required degree of activity. Frequently, a compound exhibits a lower antimicrobial activity in an emulsion than, say, in a solution. Generally, this is because of partitioning effects between the oil and water phases, which cause a lowering of the "effective" concentration of the active agent. Finally, the chemical stability of the various components of the emulsion should receive some attention, since such materials may be more prone to degradation in the emulsified state than when they exist as a bulk phase.

In the present discussion, detailed consideration will be limited to the question of physical stability. Reviews of this topic have been published by Garrett[24] and Kitchener and Mussellwhite.[25] For information on the effect that emulsification can have on the biologic activity and chemical stability of materials in emulsions, see Wedderburn,[26] Burt,[27] and Swarbrick.[28]

The physical stability of an emulsion depends on many factors, some of which have been discussed. Thus, the various properties of an emulsifying agent (see page 337) are all considered desirable because each makes a contribution to the physical stability of the emulsion.

The three major phenomena associated with physical stability are (1) the upward or downward movement of dispersed droplets relative to the continuous phase, termed *creaming* or *sedimentation*, respectively; (2) the aggregation and possible coalescence of the dispersed droplets to reform the separate, bulk phases; and (3) inversion, in which an O/W emulsion inverts to become a W/O emulsion, and *vice versa.*

Creaming and Sedimentation—Creaming is the upward movement of dispersed droplets relative to the continuous phase, while sedimentation, the reverse process, is the downward movement of particles. In any one emulsion either one process or the other takes place, depending on the densities of the disperse and continuous phases. For the purposes of this discussion we shall imagine the emulsion to be an O/W system in which the oil has a density less than that of water. Creaming will therefore take place. This concentrating of dispersed phase towards the top of the emulsion means that the system is no longer homogeneous. This is undesirable in a pharmaceutical product where homogeneity is essential for the administration of the correct and uniform dose. Furthermore, creaming, or sedimentation, brings the particles closer together and may facilitate the more serious problem of coalescence. For these reasons creaming or sedimentation should be minimized.

As was introduced on page 331, the rate at which a spherical droplet or particle sediments in a liquid is governed by Stokes' law (Eq. 2). While there have been other equations developed for bulk systems,[29] Stokes' equation is still useful since it points out the factors that influence the rate of sedimentation or creaming. These are the diameter of the suspended droplets, the viscosity of the suspending medium, and the difference in densities between the dispersed phase and the dispersion medium.

Usually, only the use of the first two factors is feasible in affecting creaming or sedimentation, although a few successful attempts have been made to equalize the densities of the oil and aqueous phases, to reduce the rate of movement to zero. Reduction of particle size contributes greatly towards overcoming or minimizing creaming, since the rate of movement is a square-root function of the particle diameter. There are, however, technical difficulties in reducing the diameter of droplets to below about 0.1 μ. The most frequently used approach is to raise the viscosity of the continuous phase, although this can be done only to the extent that the emulsion still can be removed from its container and spread or administered conveniently.

Aggregation and Coalescence—Even though creaming and sedimentation are undesirable, they do not necessarily result in the breakdown of the emulsion, since the dispersed droplets retain their individuality. Furthermore, the droplets can be redispersed with mild agitation. More serious to the stability of an emulsion are the processes of aggregation and coalescence. In aggregation (flocculation) the dispersed droplets come together but do not fuse. Coalescence, the complete fusion of droplets, leads to a decrease in the number of droplets and the ultimate separation of the two immiscible phases. Aggregation precedes coalescence in emulsions; however, coalescence does not necessarily follow from aggregation, as was shown by Higuchi, *et al.*[10] Aggregation is, to some extent, reversible. While not as serious as coalescence, it will accelerate creaming or sedimentation, since the aggregate behaves as a single drop.

While aggregation is related to the electrical potential on the droplets, coalescence depends on the structural properties of the interfacial film. In an emulsion stabilized with surfactant-type emulsifiers forming monomolecular films, coalescence is opposed by the elasticity and cohesiveness of the films sandwiched between the two droplets. In spite of the fact that two droplets may be touching, they will not fuse until the interposed films thin out and eventually rupture. Multilayer and solid-particle films confer on the emulsion a high degree of resistance to coalescence, due to their mechanical strength. More detailed discussion of this important aspect of physical stability may be found elsewhere.[24,25,30]

Particle-size analysis can reveal the tendency of an emulsion to aggregate and coalesce long before any visible signs of instability are apparent. The methods available have been reviewed by Groves and Freshwater.[31]

Inversion—An emulsion is said to invert when it changes from an O/W to a W/O emulsion, or *vice versa*. Inversion sometimes can be brought about by the addition of an electrolyte or by changing the phase–volume ratio. For example, an O/W emulsion having sodium stearate as the emulsifier can be inverted by the addition of calcium chloride, because the calcium stearate formed is a lipophilic emulsifier and favors the formation of a W/O product.

Salisbury, *et al*,[32] have studied the effect of phase volume on inversion. For their particular system the the presence of less than 45% water led to the formation of a W/O emulsion. Whenever the concentration of water exceeded 45%, an O/W product was formed. These, and other studies on inversion have been summarized by Becher.[30]

Inversion often can be seen when an emulsion, prepared by heating and mixing the two phases, is being cooled. This takes place presumably because of the temperature-dependent changes in the solubilities of the emulsifying agents.

Little quantitative work has been carried out on the process of inversion; nevertheless, it would appear that the effect can be minimized by using the proper emulsifying agent in an adequate concentration. Wherever possible, the volume of the dispersed phase should not exceed 50% of the total volume of the emulsion.

References

1. Martin, A. N., *J. Pharm. Sci.*, **50**, 513 (1961).
2. Heistand, E. N., *J. Pharm. Sci.*, **53**, 1 (1964).
3. Derjaguin, B. V., and Landau, L., *Acta Phys.-Chim. URSS.*, **14**, 633 (1941).
4. Verwey, E. J. W., and Overbeek, J. Th.G., *Theory of Stability of Lyophilic Colloids*, Elsevier, New York, 1948.
5. Griffin, W. C., *J. Soc. Cosmetic Chem.*, **1**, 311 (1949).
6. Haines, B. A., and Martin, A. N., *J. Pharm. Sci.*, **50**, 228, 753, 756 (1961).
7. Martin, A. N., and Swarbrick, J., in *American Pharmacy*, 6th ed., Lippincott, Philadelphia, 1966, Chap. 8.
8. Gopal, E. S. R., in *Emulsion Science*, Academic, New York, 1968, p. 18.
9. Davies, J. T., and Rideal, E. K., *Interfacial Phenomena*, Academic, New York, 1963, p. 359, *et seq.*
10. Higuchi, W. I., *et al*, *J. Pharm. Sci.*, **51**, 683 (1962).
11. Sumner, C. G., *Chem. Ind.*, 1066 (1960).
12. Davies, J. T., *Proc. Intern. Congr. Surface Activity, 2nd, London*, **1**, 426, (1957).
13. Cobb, R. M. K., in *Emulsion Technology*, Chem. Publ. Co., Brooklyn, 1946, p. 13.
14. Sherman, P., in *Emulsion Science*, Academic, New York, 1968, Chap. 4.
15. Sherman, P., *Rheology of Emulsions*, Macmillan, New York, 1963, p. 73.
16. Rowe, E. L., *J. Pharm. Sci.*, **54**, 260 (1965).
17. Serrallach, J. A., *et al*, *Ind. Eng. Chem.*, **25**, 816 (1933).
18. Bancroft, W. D., *J. Phys. Chem.*, **17**, 514 (1913).
19. Martin E. W., ed., *Husa's Pharmaceutical Dispensing*, 6th ed., Mack Publ. Co., Easton Pa., 1966, p. 234.
20. Griffin, W. C., *J. Soc. Cosmetic Chem.*, **5**, 249 (1954).
21. Ross, S., *et al*, *J. Phys. Chem.*, **63**, 1681 (1959).
22. Gorman, W. G., and Hall, G. D., *J. Pharm. Sci.*, **52**, 442 (1963).
23. Schulman, J. H., and Cockbain, E. G., *Trans. Faraday Soc.*, **36**, 651, 661 (1940).
24. Garrett, E. R., *J. Pharm. Sci.*, **54**, 1557 (1965).
25. Kitchener, J. A., and Mussellwhite, P. R., in *Emulsion Science*, Academic, New York, 1968, Chap. 2.
26. Wedderburn, D. L., in *Advances in Pharmaceutical Sciences*, vol. 1, Academic, London, 1964, pp. 195–268.
27. Burt, B. W., *J. Soc. Cosmetic Chem.*, **16**, 465 (1965).
28. Swarbrick, J., *J. Soc. Cosmetic Chem.*, **19**, 187 (1968).
29. Greenwald, H. L., *J. Soc. Cosmetic Chem.*, **6**, 164 (1955).
30. Becher, P., *Emulsions: Theory and Practice*, 2nd ed., Reinhold, New York, 1965, Chap. 5.
31. Groves, M. J., and Freshwater, D. C., *J. Pharm. Sci.*, **57**, 1273 (1968).
32. Salisbury, R., *et al*, *J. APhA, Sci. Ed.*, **43**, 117 (1954).

25 | Particle Phenomena

Intermolecular forces—particle-particle interactions—flow behavior of powders—particle-particle interactions in liquid systems—flocculation kinetics

This chapter was prepared by

William I. Higuchi, PhD, *Professor of Pharmacy, and*
Anthony P. Simonelli, PhD, *Associate Professor of Pharmacy, College of Pharmacy, University of Michigan, Ann Arbor, Mich. 48104*

The understanding of particle phenomena is important in many areas of pharmaceutics and biopharmaceutics. In the formulation and manufacture of dosage forms such as powders, capsules, tablets, suspensions, emulsions, and aerosols, knowledge of particle technology is essential. Also, it is becoming increasingly important to consider such factors as the particle size and the degree of deaggregation in drug utilization by the patient.

Our understanding of particle-particle interactions and particle phenomena in general is based largely upon our knowledge of basic interatomic and intermolecular forces. Today physical chemistry has evolved to a point where the relevant relationships involving such interaction forces have been well established.

Intermolecular Forces

All interactions involving molecules and ions and aggregates of molecules and ions include both attractive and repulsive forces. These forces depend upon the nature of species, the distance of separation, the orientation of the molecules, and the nature of the medium.

Ion–Ion Electrostatic Interactions—The interionic interaction of two polarizable ions (see Fig. 212) obeys the following laws:

$$\text{Energy} = E = \frac{q_1 q_2}{\epsilon r} \tag{1}$$

and

$$\text{Force} = F = -\frac{q_1 q_2}{\epsilon r^2} \tag{2}$$

where q_1 and q_2 are the charges on ion 1 and 2, respectively, r is the distance of separation of the ions, and ϵ is the dielectric constant of the medium. As can be

seen, if q_1 and q_2 are of the same sign, the force, F, is negative and therefore repulsive in nature. On the other hand, if the charges are of opposite sign, the interaction is attractive. It should be noted that the distance dependence for this situation is inversely proportional to the first power in r for E and second power for F. This difference in the distance dependence results from the fact that

$$E = \int_{-\infty}^{r} F dr \tag{3}$$

which states that the energy is equal to the work, W, of bringing together the two ions from infinity to a distance r from each other.

An example calculation for sodium chloride can be used to illustrate the magnitude of the ion–ion interaction. For the sodium chloride molecule in the vapor state, r is about 2.5×10^{-8} cm, $q_{Na^+} = -q_{Cl^-} =$ electronic charge $= 4.8 \times 10^{-10}$ esu (electrostatic units), and the dielectric constant may be assumed to be unity. Therefore,

$$W = \frac{(4.8 \times 10^{-10})^2}{2.5 \times 10^{-8}} \approx 10^{-11} \text{ ergs/ion pair}$$

or

$$W = 120,000 \text{ cal/mole}$$

since

$$\text{cal/mole} = \frac{(\text{ergs/molecule}) N_0}{4.18 \times 10^7 \text{ ergs/cal}}$$

The value for the work, W, represents the amount of work required to separate one mole of sodium chloride molecules in the vapor state into one mole of sodium and one mole of chloride ions.

Other Electrostatic Interactions—In addition to the ion–ion interaction other electrostatic interactions may be possible involving ions, dipoles, and induced dipoles.

A permanent dipole moment exists in a molecule when the "center of gravity" of the negative charges does not coincide with that for the positive charges.

The field of an ion or permanent dipole temporarily may polarize molecules which may not have a permanent dipole. When this occurs, the resulting polarization leads to an induced dipole in the molecule.

Various pair combinations of ions, permanent dipoles, and induced dipoles give rise to higher order electrostatic interactions such as the ion–dipole, the ion–induced dipole, the dipole–dipole, and dipole–induced dipole. These interactions are weaker and generally more short range than the ion–ion interaction, the distance dependence for the energies

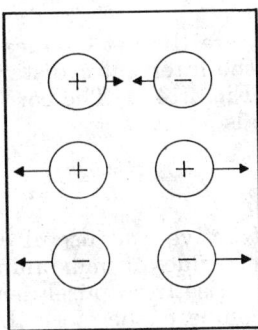

Fig. 212. Interionic interactions of two polarizable ions. Like charges repel and unlike charges attract.

Table I—Distance Dependence of Various Electrostatic Interactions

Type interaction	Distance Dependence	
	Force	Energy
Ion–ion	$1/r^2$	$1/r$
Ion–dipole	$1/r^3$	$1/r^2$
Dipole–dipole	$1/r^4$	$1/r^3$
Dipole–induced dipole	$1/r^7$	$1/r^6$
London dispersion forces	$1/r^7$	$1/r^6$

ranging from r^{-2} to r^{-6} (see Table I). Furthermore, all of these interactions usually are directionally dependent.

Hydrogen-Bonding—A hydrogen atom attached to an electronegative atom such as oxygen or nitrogen effectively produces a dipole with a highly exposed positive end. As a result, the proton end can participate in unusually strong dipole–dipole interactions with other strongly electronegative centers. Each water molecule has two such hydrogen-bonding protons and therefore water molecules in liquid water and ice are highly associated. The hydrogen-bonding capabilities of water also partially explain its unusually good solvating ability for other polar molecules.

London Dispersion Forces—These attractive forces arise from the fact that at any given instant the electron distribution around an atomic nucleus may not be symmetrical and consequently this leads to the formation of a temporary dipole moment. Such temporary dipoles in neighboring atoms are correlated so as to produce an effective induced dipole–induced dipole interaction.

The characteristics of the dispersion forces are that they are approximately additive, they are not directionally dependent, and they follow the $1/r^6$ dependence in energy. As will be seen later, the London Forces, along with hydrogen-bonding forces, are generally the most important in describing the intermolecular and the interparticulate behavior of nonionic compounds in solutions and dispersions.

Born Repulsive Forces—If molecules or ions are brought very close together, the outer electron clouds of the atoms will begin to overlap. This gives rise to a mutual repulsive force that increases very rapidly

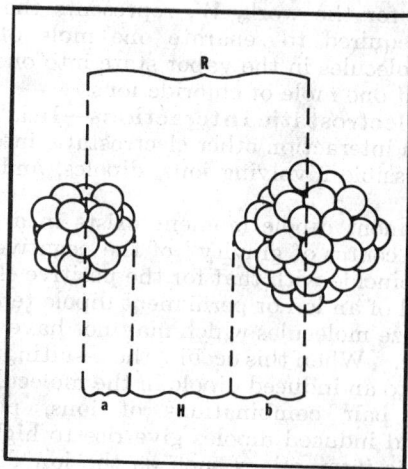

Fig. 213. Parameters used to describe the interactions between particles where a and b are the particle radii of the particles involved, R is the intercenter distance of separation of the two particles, and H is the distance of separation between the two surfaces of the interacting particles.

($\sim 1/r^{12}$) as the atoms are brought closer together such as one might expect when two hard rubber balls touch and are pressed together.

Particle–Particle Interactions

The interaction between particles may be analyzed by the same type of forces responsible for interatomic and intermolecular interactions. Let us consider first the interaction of two arbitrary particles as shown in Fig. 213.

The kinds of interactions contributing to the particle–particle binding energies are:

1. The various electrostatic contributions (attractive and repulsive).
2. The London dispersion forces between the atoms of one particle with those in the other (attractive).
3. The covalent bonds (attractive).
4. The Born repulsion forces.

The latter two can contribute only when the two particles are touching.

A rigorous quantitative treatment of the above contributions to particle–particle binding is beyond the scope of this text. However, considerable insight into the magnitude, nature, and the applications of these forces can be gained by "order of magnitude" theoretical calculations using approximate theories and simplified models.

Charge–Charge Interactions—Let us examine the possibility of electrostatic interactions between two particles, A and B (see Fig. 214). While contributions from charge–dipole, charge–induced dipole, and dipole–dipole interactions between an atom, ion, or molecule of one particle and that in the other may occur, generally these are probably of much less importance than the charge–charge interactions. Therefore, as a first approximation let us consider only the charge–charge forces between the two particles.

The energy of coulombic interaction may be written as the summation of Eq. 1 (assuming $\epsilon = 1$) over all possible ion–pair combinations between the two particles; ie,

$$E = \sum_{i=1}^{M} \sum_{j=1}^{N} \frac{q_i q_j}{r_{ij}} \qquad (4)$$

where q_i is the charge on the ith ion in Particle A which contains M ions, q_j is the charge on the jth ion in Particle B which contains N ions, and r_{ij} is the distance between ions i and j. If it is assumed that the particles are spheres and that charges on each sphere are uniformly distributed, Eq. 4 simply reduces to

$$E = \frac{Q_A Q_B}{R} \qquad (5)$$

where Q_A and Q_B are the net charges on Particles A and B and R is the intercenter distance between the two spheres (see Fig. 214). The corresponding equation for the force is

$$F = \frac{-Q_A Q_B}{R^2} \qquad (6)$$

It is both instructive and useful at this point to examine the magnitude of maximum energies and forces that might arise from purely electrostatic contributions and compare them to the gravitational forces on the particles. The maximum charge on a given particle in air is limited by the electric breakdown field of about 60 esu, which corresponds to a charge of

$$Q = 60a^2 \qquad (7)$$

where a is the radius of the sphere.

Table II tabulates the results of calculations for E and F based on Eqs. 5–7 for different-sized particles. It must be kept in mind that these values represent the *maximum* electrostatic interaction limited by surface electrical discharge in air.

It can be noted that for small particles, electrostatic effects may be important. For example, two 1 μ particles with the same maximum charge may repel each other with a force that is 10,000 times greater than the gravitational force. Thus, for example, these calculations explain why certain dry powders that become charged during trituration in the mortar defy the laws of gravity. Interestingly, as the particle size is reduced, this phenomenon increases in accordance with the predictions of Table II, which shows that the relative importance of the electrostatic force as compared to the gravitational force should increase with decreasing particle size.

London Dispersion Forces—The London dispersion force contribution to the particle–particle interaction may be estimated by summing the attraction over all possible atom pair combinations between the two particles (see Fig. 215). Thus, we may write

$$E = \sum_{i=1}^{M} \sum_{j=1}^{N} \epsilon_{ij} \qquad (8)$$

or

$$E = \sum_{i=1}^{M} \sum_{j=1}^{N} \frac{k_{ij}}{r_{ij}} \qquad (9)$$

where k_{ij}, the London constant, is characteristic of the atom pair involved and is a function of the polarizabilities and the ionization energies of the atoms.

In case of two equal-sized spheres of the same substance the summations in Eq. 9 may be transformed to double integrals and the following equation is obtained for energy:

$$E = \frac{-A}{6} \left[\frac{2a^2}{R^2 - 4a^2} + \frac{2a^2}{R^2} + \ln\left(\frac{R^2 - 4a^2}{R^2} \right) \right] \qquad (10)$$

where $A = \pi^2 n^2 k$, n is the number of atoms/cm³, k is the London dispersion force constant, R is the particle–particle intercenter distance, and a is the radius of the sphere. A more rigorous equation may be deduced which takes into account the so-called "retardation effect," but it would not significantly contribute to the present discussion.

Table II—Maximum** Electrostatic Energy and Force of Interaction between Uniformly Charged Spheres Near Contact**[a] **($R \simeq 2a$ and Field = 60 esu) as a Function of Particle Size**[b]

Radius (cm)	Electrostatic		Gravitational force (dynes)
	Energy (ergs)	Force (dynes)	
10^{-4} (1 μ)	1.8×10^{-9}	9×10^{-6}	4.1×10^{-9}
10^{-3}	1.8×10^{-6}	9×10^{-4}	4.1×10^{-6}
10^{-2}	1.8×10^{-3}	9×10^{-2}	4.1×10^{-3}
10^{-1} (1 mm)	1.8	9	4.1
1	1.8×10^{3}	9×10^{2}	4.1×10^{3}

[a] For these calculations the particles are assumed to be touching. These values approximately apply for particles not touching if distances of separation are not comparable to the particle radius.
[b] Density of 1 is assumed.

It is worthwhile to present the limiting forms of Eq. 10. First, when R is much greater than $2a$ (ie, when the intercenter distance is large compared to the sphere diameter), one can show that the energy and force would be inversely proportional to the 6th and 7th power of R, respectively. On the other hand, when the closest distance, H, between the surfaces of the two spheres is much smaller than the sphere radius, one can show that

$$E = \frac{-Aa}{12H} \qquad (11)$$

and

$$F = \frac{Aa}{12H^2} \qquad (12)$$

where $H = R - 2a$ and $H <<< a$ (see Fig. 213).

In order to gain an appreciation for the magnitude of the London attraction between two particles one can compute the energies and forces using Eqs. 11 and 12 employing the appropriate values for A. Table III gives a list of A values. These may be used in the present calculations. As can be seen from the A values, the London forces do not differ too greatly among materials with widely differing properties. The results of using Eqs. 11 and 12 and an A value of 10^{-12} ergs are presented in Table IV for two distances of separation, 5×10^{-8} and 5×10^{-7} cm. For other A values the reader may make the appropriate adjustments using Table III information. The H value of 5×10^{-8} should be a reasonable limiting distance of closest approach (within a factor of two) for two atoms involved in the contact of the two macroscopic spheres.

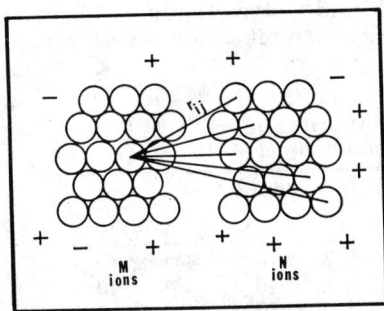

Fig. 214. Electrostatic interactions between two particles containing M_i and N_j ions, respectively. The distance r_{ij} is the distance between the ith ion of one particle with the jth atom of the other particle.

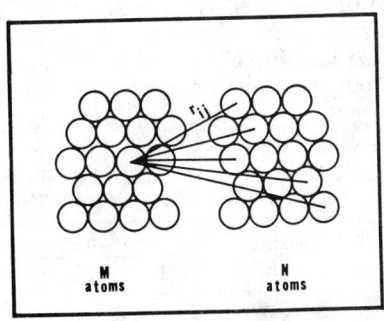

Fig. 215. The London dispersion force contribution to the particle–particle interaction. This may be estimated by summing the attraction over all possible atom-pair combinations between the two particles. The above illustrates the interaction of the ith atom of one particle with j atoms of the other particles where j is 1, 2, 3, 4, 5, etc.

Table III—Tabulation of A Values[a]

Material	$A \times 10^{12}$ ergs
H$_2$O	0.31
Paraffin	0.35
Polyethylene	0.50
Polystyrene	0.63
Fe	1.4
Graphite	1.6
Silica	1.8
Rutile	2.1
Mercury	2.9

[a] Taken from Fowkes, F. M. (see *Bibliography*).

An examination of the results presented in Tables II and IV reveals several important relationships. First, as was the case with electrostatic interactions, London forces decrease much more slowly than the gravitational forces with decreasing particle size. Thus, as can be seen at a distance of separation of 5 Å, 1 μ particles exhibit London attractive forces that are approximately one million times stronger than gravity, but 1-mm particles have approximately the same forces. For this reason fine particles tend to be "stickier" than coarse particles.

Secondly, the London attractive forces decrease more slowly than the electrostatic forces with decreasing particle size. Thus, a tenfold decrease in particle size corresponds to only a tenfold decrease in the London forces but to a 100-fold decrease in electrostatic forces. Thus, for 1 μ particles or smaller, it is likely that London forces are always more important than electrostatic forces when the particles are near contact. However, as the distance of separation is increased, the electrostatic forces remain relatively constant while the London forces decrease rapidly. For example, as the distance of separation is changed from 5 to 50 Å, the London forces are decreased by a factor of a hundred while the electrostatic forces for all particles in Table II essentially remain constant. Thus, electrostatics may play an important role in the flow behavior of powders in which the particles are separated sufficiently during handling; eg, during mixing operations. However, once the powder particles are sufficiently packed, London forces should dominate.

It appears that the above relationships have not always been adequately emphasized in the literature. Texts which discuss electrostatic and London forces limit their discussion to molecular interactions in solutions and in solid crystals and do not apply them to solid particulate interactions. This leaves the impression that London forces are only important in the absence of electrostatic forces, which is obviously not true in solid particle–particle interactions.

Nonspherical Particles—The above discussion was restricted to uniform spheres which do not gener-

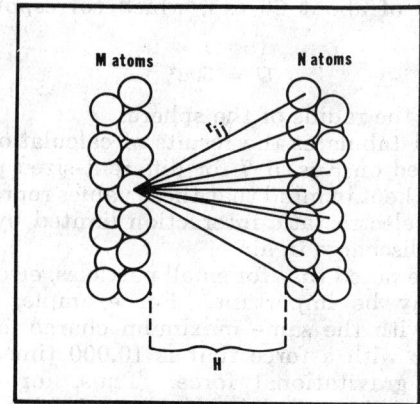

Fig. 216. The interaction of two particles based on the flat-plate model.

ally represent real powders. Real powder particles are also subject to both plastic and elastic deformation which would provide larger areas of contact between them. The actual situation for powders would be expected to lie somewhere between the interaction between uniform spheres and that for parallel plates and is much more complicated than either of the above cases. Thus, for example, the interaction of two contacting cubes, in contrast to that for two spheres, also depends upon their relative orientation (face to face, face to edge, corner to face, edge to edge, etc). In addition to the mutual orientation and shape effects for real powders, one must consider the particle-size distribution and the important factor of whether or not the particle is deformable (plastic and/or elastic) under the prevailing conditions.

It would be beyond the scope of this text to attempt detailed considerations of the above factors. However, in order to gain an appreciation for the magnitudes of the possible London force interactions between real powder particles it is helpful to examine the limiting case of the two interacting flat plates (see Fig. 216).

For two parallel flat surfaces separated by a distance, H, the equations for the London Force interacting energy and force/unit area are

$$E = \frac{-A}{12\pi H^2} \tag{13}$$

and

$$F = \frac{+A}{6\pi H^3} \tag{14}$$

Table V tabulates the results of calculations for the same two distances of separation used in Table IV for comparison purposes.

Tables IV and V show that suitably oriented cubical particles may exhibit interactions several orders of

Table IV—London–van der Waal Energies and Forces for Spheres as a Function of Particle Size (assuming $A = 10^{-12}$)[a]

Radius (cm)	Energy (ergs)		Force (dynes)		
	$H = 5$ Å	$H = 50$ Å	$H = 5$ Å	$H = 50$ Å	Gravity
10^{-5}	1.7×10^{-11}	1.7×10^{-12}	3.3×10^{-4}	3.3×10^{-6}	4.1×10^{-12}
10^{-4}	1.7×10^{-10}	1.7×10^{-11}	3.3×10^{-3}	3.3×10^{-5}	4.1×10^{-9}
10^{-3}	1.7×10^{-9}	1.7×10^{-10}	3.3×10^{-2}	3.3×10^{-4}	4.1×10^{-6}
10^{-2}	1.7×10^{-8}	1.7×10^{-9}	3.3×10^{-1}	3.3×10^{-3}	4.1×10^{-3}
10^{-1}	1.7×10^{-7}	1.7×10^{-8}	3.3	3.3×10^{-2}	4.1

[a] Average thermal energy $= kT = 4 \times 10^{-14}$ ergs.

Table V—London–van der Waal Energies and Forces for Parallel Plates[a] as a Function of Contact Area (assuming $A = 10^{-12}$)

Area (cm²)	Energy (ergs)		Force (dynes)	
	H = 5 Å	H = 50 Å	H = 5 Å	H = 50 Å
10^{-12}	1×10^{-11}	1×10^{-13}	5×10^{-4}	5×10^{-7}
10^{-10}	1×10^{-9}	1×10^{-11}	5×10^{-2}	5×10^{-5}
10^{-8}	1×10^{-7}	1×10^{-9}	5	5×10^{-3}

[a] Forces and energies are applicable to cubes with a linear dimension of the square root of the area listed.

magnitude greater than those for rigid spheres of the same size.

Flow Behavior of Powders

The understanding of the flow behavior of bulk powder is extremely complex as there are many factors which must be considered. While the above discussion shows that the London attractive forces between particles are rather sensitive to shape and mutual orientation, it can be shown that the electrostatic forces between two particles are not very dependent upon these factors. Therefore, Eqs. 5 and 6 should approximately describe the energy and force between two nonspherical particles where R represents the distance of separation of the electrical centers of gravity for the two particles. The development presented in the previous sections of this chapter, however, may be used as a basis for semiquantitatively describing many aspects of powder-flow behavior.

As would be expected, the flow properties of powders are principally functions of the interparticulate interactions. Therefore, any factor contributing to enhancing or diminishing the interparticulate interaction should substantially influence the bulk behavior.

True Area of Contact—One of the most important of the above factors is the true area of contact between particles. This was clearly illustrated by the comparison of the results given in Tables IV and V, which showed that for two particles the face-to-face interaction of two cubes is orders of magnitude greater than the interaction between comparable spheres when the closest distance of approach between the surfaces is the same. Thus, it would be expected that any means used to increase the effective contact area should result in enhanced attraction between particles.

For this reason powder materials that undergo plastic deformation under the conditions prevailing in the powder bed should be expected to exhibit poorer powder flow due to increased interactions. This can be illustrated best with soft materials such as waxes which exhibit poor powder-flow characteristics. Nonplastic–elastic materials (glass powder) which may be classified as hard and brittle generally show much less stickiness and therefore good flow behavior.

Even for nonplastic materials the flow characteristics may show wide variations if other factors are present which may influence the true area of contact. As an example, the effect of humidity can be cited. Moisture may lead to capillary condensation at the points of contact between particles (see Fig. 217). The resulting liquid film effectively can increase the true area of contact between the particles by many orders of magnitudes. Similarly, other impurities such as residue remaining from solvents used during crystallization may have the same effects.

The effect of humidity upon the flow behavior of a powder is demonstrated in Fig. 218. At low MgO

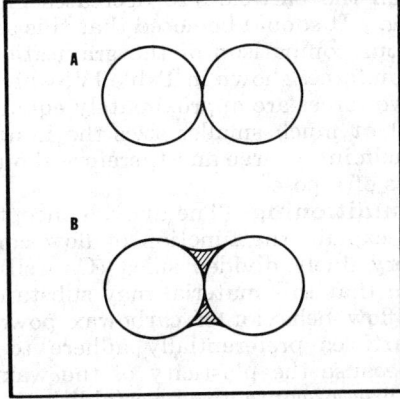

Fig. 217. The effect of humidity on the true area of contact. *A*: The Contact of two particles under conditions of low humidity; *B*: the increase in the true area of contact when capillary condensation occurs at the point of contact under conditions of high humidity. ▨ = H_2O.

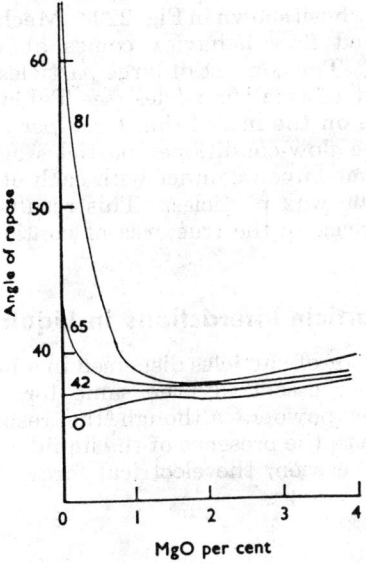

Fig. 218. The angle of repose of sucrose (100 μ) and mixtures with magnesium oxide at relative humidities of 0, 42, 65, and 81% (courtesy, Craik and Miller[1]).

concentrations and high humidities it can be seen that the sucrose powder exhibits a large angle of repose which is inversely related to powder flowability.

Particle-Size Effects—The flow behavior of a powder is related to its tensile strength, which is the force necessary to pull apart a unit cross-sectional area of powder, and is given by

$$\text{Tensile strength} = \frac{\alpha F}{a^2} \qquad (15)$$

where F is the particle–particle force of interaction, a is the effective radius of powder particles, and α is a function of the average coordination number and the porosity of the powder bed. The coordination number is the number of contacts of a given particle with surrounding particles. For a bed of spheres involving London Forces, F is given by Eq. 12 which gives a first-order dependence on a. Substitution of Eq. 12 for F in Eq. 15 shows that the tensile strength is inversely proportional to the particle size. As a result, the finer the particle size, the poorer the powder flow. This particle-size dependence upon powder flowability is demonstrated in Fig. 219, where it can be seen that for a large number of materials the flowability becomes poorer when the particle size decreases much below about 100 μ.   It should be noted that this agrees very well with our comparison of the gravitational forces with London forces shown in Table IV, which predicts that the two forces are approximately equal at 100 to 1000 μ, but at much smaller sizes the London forces are overwhelmingly large and therefore should lead to large angles of repose.

Flow Conditioning—The above concepts may be utilized to explain the function of flow conditioners such as very finely divided silica (Cabosil).   It has been shown that this material may substantially improve the flow behavior of carbowax powder.   The Cabosil particles preferentially adhere to the wax particles because the plasticity of the wax allows a larger true area of contact to be established than upon contact with another Cabosil particle.   As a result, contact between the wax particles is prevented.   In its place contact between the flow conditioner particles is established.   This is shown by the electron micrographs of carbowax 6000 particles in the presence and absence of Cabosil shown in Fig. 220.   Mechanistically, this improved flow behavior comes about for two reasons: (1) The contact of large particles is replaced by a contact of small particles (see Table IV for the effect of size on the interaction force *per se*).   (2) In addition, the flow-conditioner particles are not plastically deformed upon contact with each other as contrasted to the wax particles.   This results in a substantial decrease in the true area of contact (see Fig. 221).

Particle–Particle Interactions in Liquid Systems

The behavior of particles dispersed in a liquid media are subject to essentially the same forces as those described for powders although the results can be different due to the presence of the liquid.   For example, as will be seen, the electrical forces in aqueous

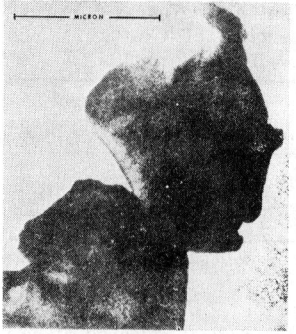
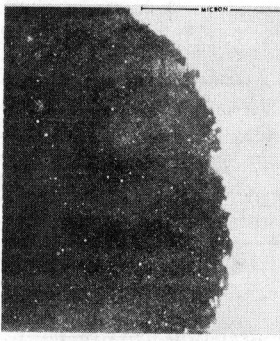

Fig. 220.   Electron micrographs of a Carbowax 6000 particle (*left*) and a Carbowax 6000 particle coated with Cabosil (*right*) (courtesy, Nash, *et al*[2]).

media between particles can play a more important role than in powders under certain conditions.

Effect of Charges—A solid particle or a droplet of an immiscible liquid in a liquid may be electrically charged because an excess of ions of one sign may be present at the interface.   The charge-conferring ions may be a constituent of the particle itself, impurity ions from the external-phase liquid, or surfactant ions preferentially adsorbed at the interface.

The particle charge gives rise to a surface potential, ψ_0, at the surface of the particle (see Fig. 222).   The potential will drop to zero at some distance away from the surface depending on the concentration of the counter-ions in the external-phase bulk.   The region in which the influence of the surface charge is appreciable is called the electrical double-layer region.

The double layer may be visualized as being made up of two parts.   The specific adsorption of counter-ions in the Stern Layer comprises the first part, the thickness of which is the order of ionic dimensions. The potential drop across this region is $\psi_0 - \psi_\delta$. The second part is called the diffuse double layer across which the potential drop is ψ_δ.   The thickness of the diffuse double layer is given by the Debye-Hückel quantity $1/K$.

$$1/K = \left(\frac{\epsilon kT}{4\pi e^2 \Sigma n_i z_i^2} \right)^{1/2} \qquad (16)$$

where ϵ is the dielectric constant in the diffuse double-layer region, k is the Boltzmann constant, e is the electronic charge, n_i is the bulk concentration of ion i, and z_i is its valence.

According to Eq. 16 a 1% aqueous sodium chloride solution at room temperature gives $1/K = 8$Å, a 0.01% solution gives $1/K = 80$Å, a 1×10^{-4}% solution gives $1/K = 800$ Å, etc.   These calculations show that the electrical influence among particles in

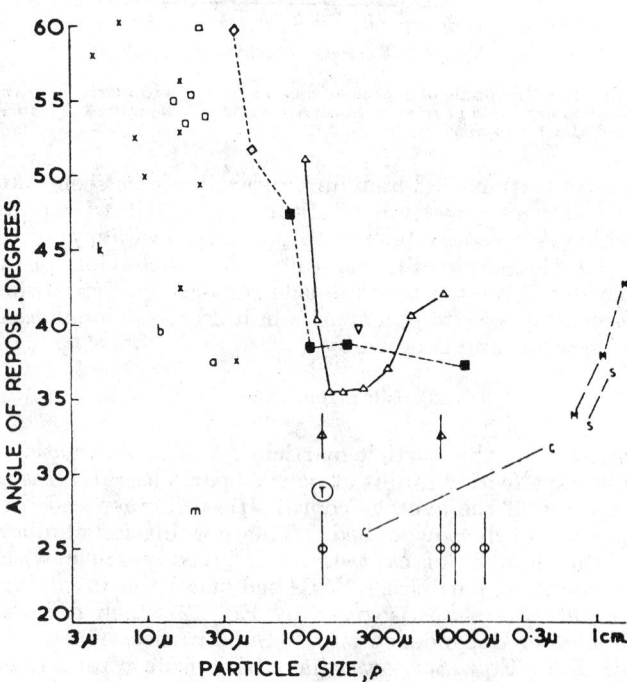

Fig. 219.   Angle of repose for materials of different particle sizes. ϕ: Glass spheres and lead shot, G: glass beads, S: steel ball bearings, M: alumina spheres, ■: Pentremawr coal, ◇: Pentremawr coal, △: silica sand, ⊤: glass spheres, ▽: silver sand, m: microspheres (25–50 μ), k: refined kaolin, x: ground limestone, □: Gypsum, a: Flue dust, b: chance mud (courtesy, Ref. 2).

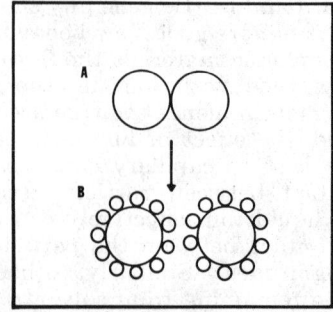

Fig. 221.   Model illustrating the mechanism of flow conditioners. *A*: The contact of two large particles; *B*: the addition of a flow conditioner to the system. If small particles are 100 times smaller, the force and energy of attraction is also 100 times smaller.

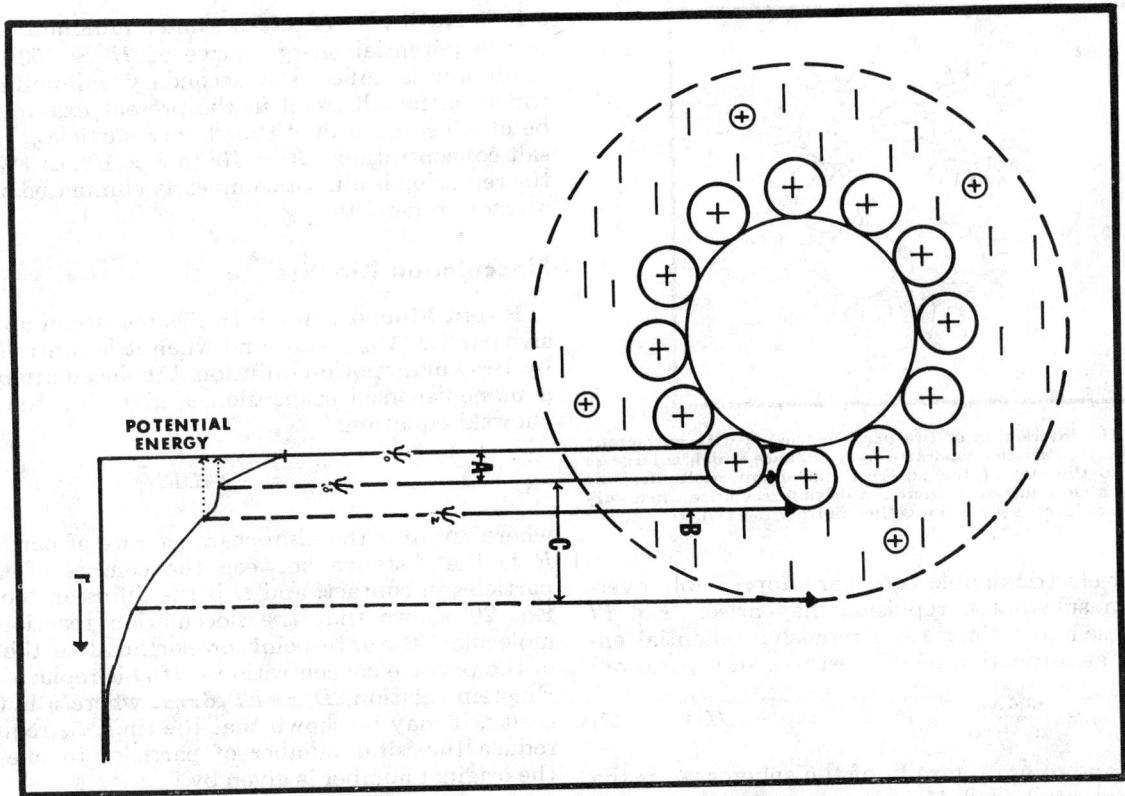

Fig. 222.   The electrical double layer and the symbols used to describe the potential at various points.   A: The Stern layer, B: the plane of shear, and C: the sphere of influence of the diffuse double layer.

aqueous media is relatively short range compared to that involving powder particles which, as predicted by Eqs. 1 and 2, extend to distances the order of particle dimensions.

In nonpolar media n, the bulk ionic concentration, is usually very small.   Therefore, $1/K$ values of the order of centimeters are sometimes encountered, and in such cases the distances of electrical influence approach those encountered in powders.   This frequently leads to the "electrostatic" problems in such systems.   Antistatic agents are helpful in these situations by reducing $1/K$ and by relieving the buildup of charge.

Eq. 16 also shows that polyvalent counter-ions are much more effective than monovalent ions in reducing the double-layer thickness.   A 2–2 electrolyte is about four times more effective than a 1–1 electrolyte in reducing the diffuse double-layer thickness.

Zeta-Potential—When a charged particle suspended in a liquid is placed in an electrical field, it will migrate towards the electrode with the opposite charge.   The ions in the Stern Layer and the bound solvent molecules are also carried along with the particle.   Thus, the plane of shear (see Fig. 222) is very close to the Stern Layer but slightly farther away from the particle surface.   While the exact relationship between the zeta-potential, ψ_z, and ψ_δ is not clear, it is generally supposed that ψ_δ and ψ_z are of the same order of magnitude, the latter being slightly smaller.   If, in addition, ψ_0 is small ($\gtrsim 50$ mv) and there is little special counter-ion-binding tendencies at the interface, the zeta-potential will also reflect the ψ_0 value and the changes in it.

As will be seen in the next section, when electrical repulsion is present, the flocculation behavior of suspensions and emulsions strongly depends upon the surface charge on the particles which is reflected in the

magnitude of ψ_z.   Generally when ψ_z is the order of 25 mv or less, the system becomes kinetically unstable to flocculation and aggregation or coalescence may take place.

Particle–Particle Interactions—According to the theory of the stability of lyophobic colloids a number of forces are at play in determining the over-all interaction among particles.   Consideration of these interaction forces is helpful in the understanding of the dispersion process as well as of the aggregation and coalescence behavior of dispersed particles.   At relatively large distances of separation ($\gtrsim 10$Å) the primary forces are the London dispersion forces of attraction and the electrical repulsive forces resulting from the interaction of the diffuse double layers of the particles.   The electrolyte flocculation behavior of suspensions and emulsions is frequently attributed to the interplay of the electrical and the dispersion forces.

Other forces of repulsion should also be considered, particularly at close distances of approach between the particles.   These are the repulsive contributions due to the surfactant molecules themselves, arising from steric hinderance (see Fig. 223).   Particles at very close distances of approach may be kept apart by this mechanism and by the resistance of the adsorbed agents from being displaced (desorbed) from the interface.   When surfactant desorption is involved, work must be done against those same forces that are responsible for the interfacial-tension lowering.   Barriers to particle–particle (and/or droplet coalescence) are also set up by adsorption of polymers and finely divided solids.   Lyophilic polymers often provide thick films ($\gtrsim 100$Å) that effectively prevent close approach of the particles.

Diffuse Double-Layer Repulsion—When two spherical particles of the same size are close enough so

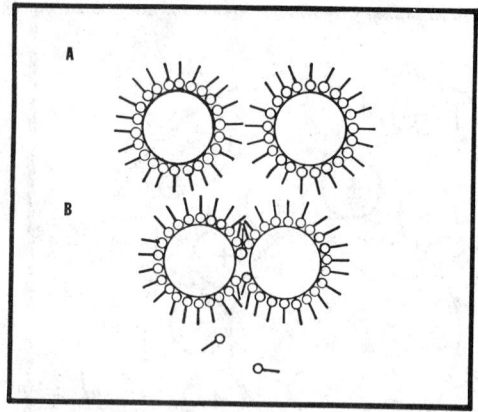

Fig. 223. The interaction of two particles coated with surfactant molecules. A: Particles separated by a distance which is large as compared to the size of the adsorbed surfactant molecules; B: particles at a close distance where repulsive forces arise when surfactant molecules are squeezed together and/or desorbed.

that their electric double layers are appreciably overlapping, a substantial repulsion may arise. Eq. 17 may be used to estimate the repulsive potential energy, V_R, as a function of the distance of separation:

$$V_R = \frac{\epsilon a_1 a_2 \psi_0^2}{(a_1 + a_2)} + \ln\left[1 - \exp(-KH)\right] \quad (17)$$

where a_1 and a_2 are the radii of the spheres, ψ_0 is the surface potential, and H is the shortest distance of separation between the surfaces of the spheres. Eq. 17 was derived for the case in which the double-layer thickness, $1/K$, is small compared to the radius of the smaller particle. This generally would be a good assumption for most situations in which water is the continuous phase and for particle sizes down to *ca* 100Å. The equation is only applicable for small ψ_0 values, *viz* $\psi_0 \gtrsim 25$ mv. If larger ψ_0 values are involved, it may be more appropriate to substitute ψ_δ for ψ_0 in Eq. 17.

London Dispersion Forces of Attraction—As previously stated, the London dispersion forces are generally regarded as short range and relatively weak. However, considering the small number of molecules in a suspension particle or an emulsion droplet, one finds that the aggregate attraction between two particles may be significant even at surface separation distances (H) the order of 100Å.

Eq. 18 gives the attraction energy between two spheres according to theory:

$$V_A = -\frac{A' a_1 a_2}{6(a_1 + a_2)} \frac{\lambda}{\lambda H + 3.54 \pi H^2} \quad (18)$$

where λ is the London wavelength, usually taken as 10^{-5} cm, and A' is the effective Hamaker's constant.

Total Interaction—The net interaction of two spherical particles considering only the London Forces of attraction and the electrical repulsion is given by combining V_A and V_R from Eqs. 17 and 18:

$$V_{\text{Total}} = V_A + V_R \quad (19)$$

Fig. 224 shows plots for V_{Total} for two particles employing Eq. 19 and $a_1 = a_2 = 0.10$ μ at different ionic strengths in water. At low ionic strengths where $1/K$ is large (see Eq. 16), electrical repulsion dominates at most distances, and V_{Total} is positive for all distances beyond the first few Angstroms. At this point the maximum potential, V_{max}, is large, ~ 25 kT. As the salt concentration is increased ($K = 4 \times 10^6$, *ca*

0.10% NaCl), V_{max} decreases and a minimum develops in the potential energy curve at $H \simeq 150$Å. This minimum is called the secondary minimum, V_{min}, which, although small in the present example, could be of substantial depth for larger particles. At high salt concentrations ($K = 10^7$ to 2×10^7, *ca* 1% NaCl) the repulsion is almost completely eliminated and only attraction persists.

Flocculation Kinetics

Rapid Flocculation—In the absence of any repulsive barrier ($V_{\text{Total}} = 0$) and when it is controlled only by Brownian motion diffusion, the flocculation rate of a monodispersed suspension is given by the Smoluchowski equation:

$$\frac{dN}{dt} = -4\pi DRN^2 \quad (20)$$

where dN/dt is the disappearance rate of particles/cc, R is the distance between the centers of the two particles in contact, and D is the diffusion coefficient. Eq. 20 shows that the flocculation reaction is bimolecular, the rate being proportional to the square of the particle concentration. If D is replaced by the Einstein relation, $D = kT/6\pi\eta a$, where η is the viscosity, it may be shown that the time, $t_{1/2}$ required to reduce the total number of particles to one-half of the original number is given by

$$t_{1/2} = \frac{3\eta}{4kTN} \quad (21)$$

In water ($\eta = 0.01$) at 25°C for a 0.1% (by volume) suspension of spheres with $a = 1.0 \times 10^{-5}$ cm, $t_{1/2} \simeq 1$ sec.

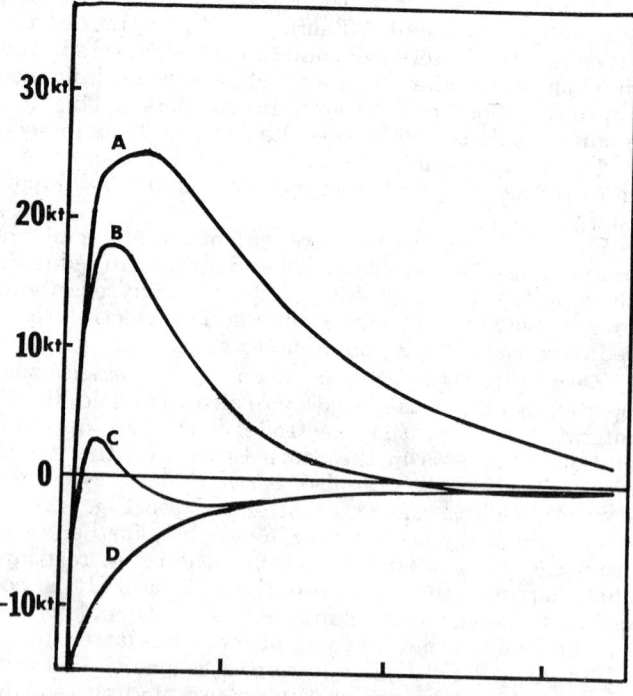

INTERPARTICLE DISTANCE (ANGSTROMS)

Fig. 224. The net interaction of two spherical particles considering only the London forces of attraction and electrical repulsion (kt units) as a function of the interparticle distance (Å) for two equally sized particles of 0.1 μ. A: $K = 2 \times 10^6$, B: $K = 4 \times 10^6$, C: $K = 10^7$, and D: $K \geq 2 \times 10^7$. The peaks represent the maximum potential, $V_{t\,\text{max}}$. These calculations used the following values: $A = 10^{-12}$ ergs, $\psi_0 = 25$ mv, and $\lambda = 10^{-5}$ cm.

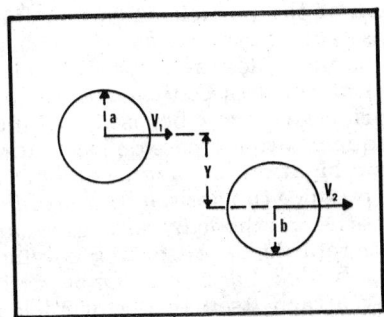

Fig. 225. The influence of shear upon aggregation rate. If $V_1 > V_2$, collision will occur. Also, any other particle whose center is within the target area $4\pi a^2$ will collide if its velocity is less than Particle 1. The velocity gradient, G, is given by $(V_1 - V_2)/Y$; V_1 is the velocity of Molecule 1 and V_2 is the velocity of Molecule 2.

It is well known that agitation promotes flocculation but appears to have little influence in the initial stages of the flocculation. In the simplest case (see Fig. 225) consider the particles in a laminar shear field with a velocity gradient, G, so that other particles are swept into the sphere of action of a central particle. The increase in the flocculation rate is evident when the collisions caused by the movement of the liquid and by Brownian motion are added. By comparing the probability of laminar shear collision, J, with the probability of Brownian collision, I,

$$J/I = \frac{\eta a^3 G}{2kT} \qquad (22)$$

the measure of the relative contributions of these types of motions to flocculation is found. Table VI shows that for small colloidal particles collisions caused by agitation are few compared to that caused by

Table VI—Rapid Flocculation of Spherical Particles by Brownian Motion and by Laminar Shear[a]

Radius (μ)	Brownian motion only ($t_{1/2}$)	Brownian and laminar shear motions	
		$G(\text{sec}^{-1})$	J/I
0.05	0.4 sec	100	1/1000
		1,000	1/10
		10,000	1
0.5	400 sec	100	10/1
5.0	111 hr	100	1000/1

[a] Concentration of particles is 0.1% in water at 25°C.

Brownian motion unless the shear gradient is very high. It also shows the transition between the region of colloidal dispersions, where Brownian motion is predominant, and the region of suspensions, where agitation may govern flocculation.

Slow Flocculation (Energy Barrier)—When an energy barrier such as the electrical one discussed in the previous section is present, the flocculation rates may be much smaller than those predicted by Eq. 20. When shear effects in the medium are negligible, one may write

$$G_{12} = \frac{2kT}{3\eta W_{12}}\left(\frac{1}{a_1} + \frac{1}{a_2}\right)(a_1 + a_2)N_1N_2 \qquad (23)$$

where G_{12} is the sticking rate of two particles of radii a_1 and a_2 with concentrations of N_1 and N_2, respectively. The factor W_{12} accounts for the energy barrier and is given by

$$W_{12} = 2\int_2^\infty \exp(V_{\text{Total}}/kT)\,\frac{ds}{S^2} \qquad (24)$$

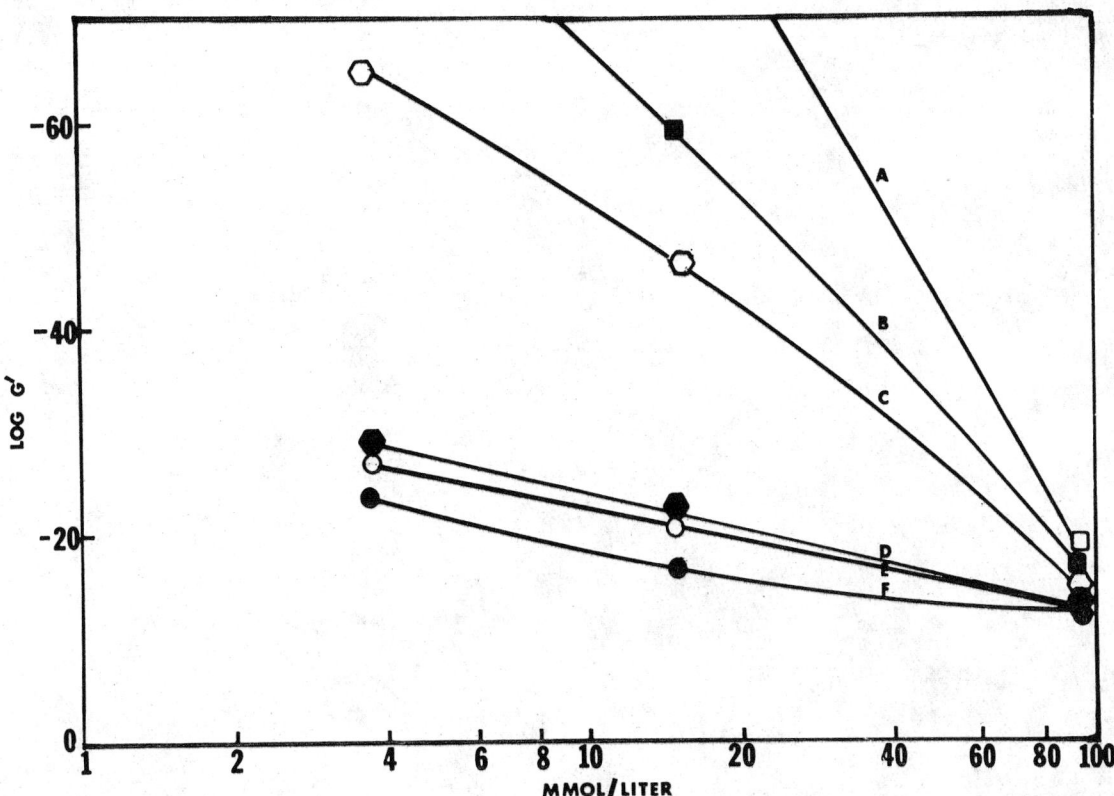

Fig. 226. The calculated rates of aggregation of 0.1 μ, 0.5 μ, and 1 μ particles with themselves and with larger particles as a function of concentration of a 1–1 electrolyte in solution. ψ_0 is 25 mv and A' is 1×10^{-13} ergs. A: 1.0/1.0μ; B: 0.5/1.0μ; C: 0.5/0.5μ; D: 0.1/1.0μ; E: 0.1/0.5μ; F: 0.1/0.1μ.

where $S = 2R/(a_1 + a_2)$, R is the intercenter distance between the two particles, and V_{Total} is the potential energy function.

When V_{Total} is primarily the result of the diffuse double-layer repulsion and the London attraction, V_{Total} may be expressed by Eqs. 17 and 18 for aqueous media.

Fig. 226 gives the results of calculation with Eqs. 17–19, 23, and 24. The quantity G' is defined by

$$G' = \frac{G_{12}}{N_1 N_2} = \frac{2kT}{3\eta W_{12}} \left(\frac{1}{a_1} + \frac{1}{a_2} \right) (a_1 + a_2) \qquad (25)$$

It can be seen how electrolyte concentration may markedly increase the preference for the aggregation (or coalescence) of small particles with each other or with large particles. Thus, when $K \simeq 2$ to 4×10^6 for $\psi_0 \simeq 25$ mv, it can be seen (Fig. 226) that the rate of aggregation (or coalescence) of 0.1-μ particles with itself or larger particles may be 10 to 30 orders of magnitude greater than that for two 0.5-μ particles.

Controlled Flocculation—Controlled flocculation may provide a means for obtaining a noncaking suspension. This concept is based on the observation that an initially peptized suspension tends to form a dense compact. Such a sediment is difficult to redisperse and it eventually becomes a very hard cake. Controlled flocculation with loosely bonded particles gives a porous sediment that can be dispersed easily.

One of the various methods employed to induce controlled flocculation of a peptized suspension is electrolyte flocculation. The theory that applies to this process has been discussed above. A good noncaking suspension may be produced if the particle charge is maintained low and/or the electrolyte controlled at a sufficiently high level. Ionic surfactants may be employed to induce flocculation by neutralization of the particle surface charges. Addition of excess surfactants leads to a charge reversal which may be more desirable for controlled flocculation because of the less critical nature in this case. Nonionic surfactants may be used to influence flocculation, frequently to increase deflocculation. Thus, a suitable combination of ionics, nonionics, and electrolytes can produce the desired degree of flocculation.

There are other methods by which flocculation may be induced or retarded. Adsorbing polymers may be employed to bridge particles. One portion of the polymer may attach itself to one particle, while the other portion may attach itself to another. The flocculation of calcium phosphate suspensions by many organic polymers is explained by this mechanism. On the other hand, suspensions can be deflocculated by polymers if conditions are such (eg, long agitation times) that adsorption of all segments of a polymer molecule onto one particle is favored. In this case thick interfacial films are obtained that deflocculate the suspension by the steric hindrance mechanism (protective colloid).

Bibliography

Hiestand, E. N., *J. Pharm. Sci.*, **55**, 1325 (1966).
Fowkes, F. M., in Gushee, D. E., ed., *Chemistry and Physics of Interfaces*, Am. Chem. Soc., Washington, D.C., 1965, Chap. 1.
Ho, N. F. H., and Higuchi, W. I., *J. Pharm. Sci.*, **57**, 436 (1968).
Nash, J. H., *et al*, *Ind. Eng. Chem. Prod. Res. Develop.*, **4**, 140 (1965).
Orr, C., Jr., *Particulate Technology*, Macmillan, New York, 1966.
Rumpf, H., in Knepper, W. A., ed., *Agglomeration*, Interscience, New York, 1962, pp. 379–418.
Kruyt, H. R., *Colloid Science*, vol. I, Elsevier, New York, 1952.
Higuchi, W. I., *et al*, *Theory of Dispersion Techniques*, Lea & Febiger, Philadelphia, 1970.

References

1. Craik, D. J., and Miller, B. F., *J. Pharm. Pharmacol.*, **10**, 136T (1958).
2. *Powders in Industry* (SCI Monograph No. 14), Gordon & Breach Sci. Publ., New York, 1963, p. 153.
3. Nash, J. H., *et al*, *Ind. Eng. Chem. Prod. Res. Develop.*, **4**, 140 (1965).

26 | Rheology

Newtonian flow—plastic flow—pseudoplastic flow—dilatant flow—
methods for measuring viscosity—effects of temperature and
concentration on viscosity—polymer solutions—thixotropy—
pharmaceutical applications

This chapter was prepared by

Grafton D. Chase, PhD, *Professor of Chemistry, Philadelphia College of
Pharmacy and Science, Philadelphia, Pa. 19104*

Rheology is that branch of Physics which deals with the flow of matter. The *viscosity* of fluids (gases or liquids) has been defined as the resistance to the movement of molecules, a movement usually described as flow. There are many types of flow, many basic theories on the nature of flow and, unfortunately, few actual materials which adhere strictly to these theories. To be sure, the subject of rheology is rather complicated but, in spite of certain shortcomings in this relatively new field of science, an application of certain basic principles to pharmacy can be made advantageously.

Types of Flow

Various types of flow have been described. *Newtonian (simple) flow* represents an ideal situation in which the flow of a fluid conforms to Newton's basic equation. If the flow characteristics do not conform to the Newton equation, the material is said to be *non-Newtonian (complex)*. Non-Newtonian materials exhibit several distinct and identifiable types of nonideal behavior which are known as *plastic flow, pseudoplastic flow, dilatant flow,* and *thixotropic flow*. These are described in the following paragraphs.

Newtonian Flow—Newtonian or viscous flow is the most simple of all types of flow. Sir Isaac Newton assumed that the rate of shear, customarily written as a differential, dv/dr, where v is the velocity and r is the distance between the planes enclosing the fluid, is directly proportional to the tangential shearing force or stress, F, and expressed this relation mathematically as

$$F = \eta \, dv/dr$$

or

$$\eta = \frac{F}{dv/dr} = \frac{\text{shearing force}}{\text{shearing rate}}$$

where the proportionality constant, η, is the coefficient of viscosity. Its unit is the *poise* or dyne-sec/cm², and is defined (see Fig. 227) as the tangential force (F)

required to maintain a relative velocity of 1 cm/sec between two planes (A and B) 1 cm² in area and 1 cm apart. However, a more useful unit of viscosity is the *centipoise*, a centipoise being 0.01 of a poise.

Newtonian flow is the *ideal* type of flow. It is ideal in the same sense that a gas is "ideal" if it obeys exactly the relation $PV = nRT$. Similarly, a fluid is "ideal" if it obeys the relation $F = \eta dv/dr$. Such an ideal liquid is called a *Newtonian (simple) liquid*. There is reason to believe that such a liquid does not exist but certainly, to within the accuracy of most measuring instruments, this condition of flow is exemplified by most solvents, eg, water, alcohol, benzene, etc, mixtures of solvents, and true solutions. Fluids which are not true solutions, such as suspensions, "solutions" of the so-called water-soluble gums, eg, tragacanth, methylcellulose, etc, emulsions, and certain other fluids containing high-molecular-weight substances do not belong to this category.

Newtonian flow is portrayed graphically in Fig. 228 N where dv/dr, the rate of shear, is plotted vs F, the shearing stress. It will be noted that the graph consists of a straight line passing through the origin. The direct proportionality assumed by Newton is thereby illustrated. This same information is demonstrated in a different manner (Fig. 230N) which emphasizes the independence of viscosity of Newtonian fluids from the rate of shear. The practical importance of this independence of viscosity from shearing rate lies in the fact that different methods for measuring the viscosity of Newtonians can be used and then directly compared accurately. No anomalies are observed.

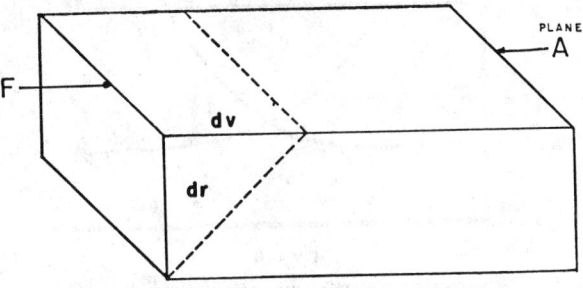

Fig. 227. Newtonian model of flow.

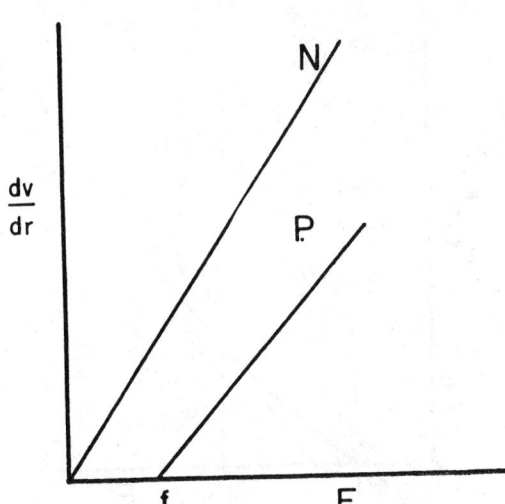

Fig. 228. Graphic portrayal of Newtonian flow (N) and the curve described by the Bingham equation (P) obtained by plotting rate of shear vs shearing stress.

Plastic Flow—As mentioned, certain fluids such as solutions of the water-soluble gums, or apparently any fluid other than pure solvents and true solutions, do not conform to Newton's equation. All such fluids have been called "non-Newtonian fluids" or "generalized Newtonian fluids." In non-Newtonian flow it appears as though certain forces which oppose the flow of the fluid, in addition to the force defined by Newton's coefficient of viscosity, also must be overcome in order to produce flow. To account for this new characteristic, Bingham introduced a modification of Newton's equation and coined the term "plastic flow." In Bingham's equation

$$u(F - f) = dv/dr$$

u is the mobility and is comparable to the "fluidity" $(1/\eta)$ of Newtonian liquids; f is called the "yield value," and was first used by Bingham and Green in 1918.

The *yield value* or *yield stress* is the shearing stress f (expressed in dynes/cm), which must be exceeded before flow will occur. If a material tends to remain deformed, even after the shearing force is again reduced to a value less than the yield value, it is said to possess *plasticity*. On the other hand a material is said to possess *elasticity* if it tends to regain its original shape when the shearing force is removed.

Fig. 228P represents the curve described by the Bingham equation, a straight line intercepting the force axis at f, the yield value. In practice the lower portion of the curve for plastic flow is not straight but tends to bend toward the origin as in Fig. 229. This deviation between theory and observation appears to be a weakness of the Bingham equation, but it can be shown that it is due, at least in part, to the nature of the viscometer itself. An additional complication has been introduced by this lower bending of the curve in that it has given rise to three, rather than to one, yield values. These are shown in Fig. 229 and have been designated f_l, the lower or true yield value; f_B, the Bingham yield value which is the intercept of the extrapolated upper portion of the curve with the force axis; and f_h, the higher yield value.

Unlike the case of Newtonians, the observed value of viscosity (apparent viscosity or consistency) is not a constant but changes with the rate of shear. This dependence of apparent viscosity on the rate of shear, and hence on the method of measurement, is illustrated in Fig. 230P. Because many pharmaceutical prepara-

tions are non-Newtonian this fact is of great importance. Therefore "one point" methods, ie, methods consisting only of an observation at a single rate of shear, are usually meaningless. For a proper evaluation of a non-Newtonian fluid the entire viscosity-shear rate curve must be considered.

Pseudoplastic Flow—All types of non-Newtonian flow are not accurately described by Bingham's equation. Pseudoplastic flow has been described as a type of flow wherein no true yield value exists and the lower portion of the curve approaches the origin of the graph instead of some specific yield value. Fig. 231PP illustrates pseudoplastic flow. Actually some question exists as to whether there is any difference between plastic flow and pseudoplastic flow in consequence of the basic question raised by some investigators regarding the very existence of a yield value. They have referred to this as the yield value myth. Nevertheless, until more definite information is available, it will be found convenient to assume, at least, that a yield value, in particular the Bingham yield value, does exist.

Dilatant Flow—Osborn Reynolds first recognized dilatant materials in 1885. Materials of this type have a consistency curve which is concave toward the force axis (see Fig. 231D) and the curve appears to pass through the origin in most cases. In a sense, this type of flow is the opposite of plastic flow in that the viscosity increases with the rate of shear instead of decreasing as in the case of plastic flow. Fig. 230D illustrates the change of viscosity with shearing rate. One frequently observes dilatancy with heavy suspensions such as paints where the fluid appears to become much thicker when rapidly stirred. Dilatancy is presumably caused by an increase in effective volume of certain types of dispersed particles when a system is subjected to a shearing stress. If this is the case, the observed increase in consistency can be explained by the Einstein equation (page 367), which relates viscosity to the concentration of the dispersed phase.

Thixotropic Flow—When a thixotropic material is sheared, a reversible breakdown of its structure occurs. The result is a decrease in the consistency of the material. If allowed to remain undisturbed, the structure of the material recovers in time. This buildup of structure is accompanied by a corresponding increase in consistency. Thixotropic flow is a type of non-Newtonian flow similar to plastic flow in that both exhibit a yield value. In fact, there is a distinct possibility that plastic

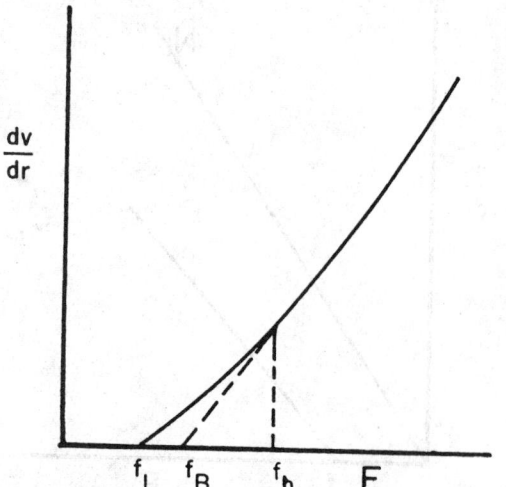

Fig. 229. The curve described by the Bingham equation is a straight line, while the curve measured by experiment tends to bend toward the origin at the lower end as illustrated.

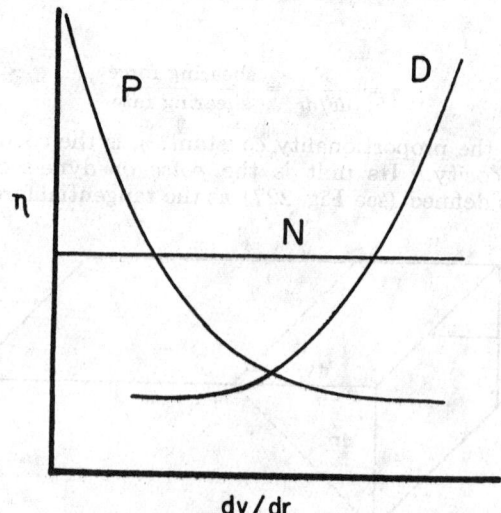

Fig. 230. Illustration of dependence of apparent viscosity on rate of shear.

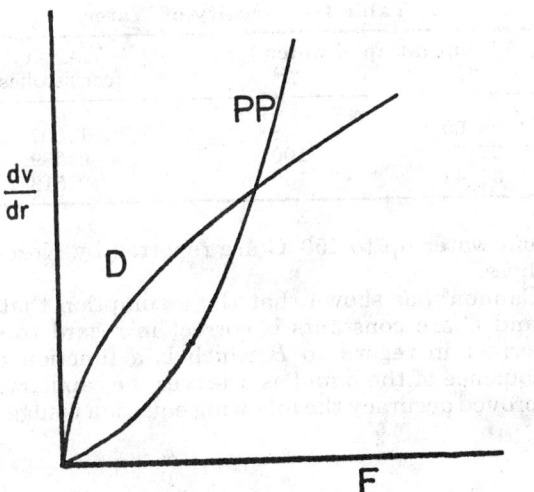

Fig. 231.   Curves illustrating pseudoplastic and dilatant flow.

flow merely represents a special case of thixotropic flow; that is, the case where the recovery of structure is very rapid.   Because of its special importance thixotropy is discussed in detail on page 367.

Models of Flow

Mechanical models,[1] devised to illustrate various modes of flow, are constructed of three basic components, either singly or in combination.   These components are represented by (1) a dashpot, (2) a block sliding on a surface, and (3) a spring.   Each mode of flow is associated with a specific type of body.

A *Newton body* is one which exhibits Newtonian flow, ie, simple or viscous flow, as illustrated in Fig. 228N. It is represented by a dashpot—a cylinder filled with oil into which is inserted a loosely fitting piston.   The piston moves at a rate proportional to the applied force. When the force is removed the piston remains stationary.

A *Saint-Venant body* exhibits true plastic flow and is represented by a block or weight resting on a flat surface.   The weight will not move until the applied force overcomes starting friction—the analog of yield value— between the block and the surface.   When the force is removed, the block remains stationary.   It is assumed that sliding friction is negligible, a force in excess of the yield value thus causing the weight to move at an ever increasing velocity.   Such a body is theoretical; it

must be used in combination with other bodies to illustrate a practical system.

A *Bingham body* exhibits a behavior expressed by the Bingham equation $u(F-f) = dv/dr$.   This is the plastic flow shown in Fig. 228P.   The model consists of a Newton body and a Saint-Venant body in parallel combination.   No motion will occur in the system until the applied force is in excess of the yield value, ie, in excess of that required to move the block.   Then the system will move at a rate proportional to the applied force in excess of the yield force and will be regulated by the motion of the piston through the oil in the cylinder of the Newton body.

A *Hooke body*, represented by a helical spring, exhibits perfect elasticity.   The deformation of a Hooke body is proportional to the stress.   Unlike the Newton and Saint-Venant bodies, when the stress is removed, the Hooke body will return to its original form.

Still other models of flow have been designed, eg, the Kelvin body and the Maxwell body, to explain the behavior of various unique rheological systems.

Methods for Measuring Viscosity

Numerous methods have been devised for measuring viscosity[2] but, except for a few miscellaneous methods, they may be classified as one of several types.   These are the capillary, rotational, oscillational, and falling-sphere methods.   *Capillary methods* are perhaps most generally used.   They are particularly useful for measuring the viscosity of comparatively fluid Newtonian liquids although a few adaptations such as the capillary tube plastometer have been designed specifically for the study of non-Newtonian materials.   Equations such as that derived by Buckingham[3] to describe viscosity curves obtained when plastics flow through capillary tubes do not check too well with the experimental data. *Rotational methods* find extensive industrial use for control purposes.   The Stormer and MacMichael viscometers (Figs. 242, 243) rank among the better known commercial instruments.   Again, as with capillary-type instruments, the behavior of Newtonian fluids has been accurately and thoroughly worked out and has been confirmed by experiment.   To describe the curve obtained for plastics in rotational viscometers Reiner and Riwlin[4] have developed an equation which applies to the upper, supposedly linear portion of the curve.   Williamson[5] has developed an empirical relationship for the lower portion.   *Oscillational methods* are similar in theory to rotational methods, the main difference being that the bob, suspended by means of a torsion wire, oscillates back and forth instead of rotating in one direction only.   Viscosity is calculated from the observed values of period, inertia, and decrement of amplitude.   *Falling-sphere methods* are based on the rate of fall through the liquid of a sphere of known size and density or upon the rate of ascent of an air bubble. Substitution of these measured values into Stokes' equation permits a ready calculation of the viscosity.

Any of these methods can be used interchangeably for measuring the viscosity of Newtonian fluids, but in view of the foregoing discussion on the different types of flow *all methods must be used judiciously when the material being investigated is non-Newtonian.   In general, commercial viscometers having "precalibrated" scales give correct readings only with Newtonian fluids.*   This is so because of the manner in which the "viscosity" of non-Newtonian fluids depends on, and hence changes with, the rate of shear produced by the particular viscometer used.

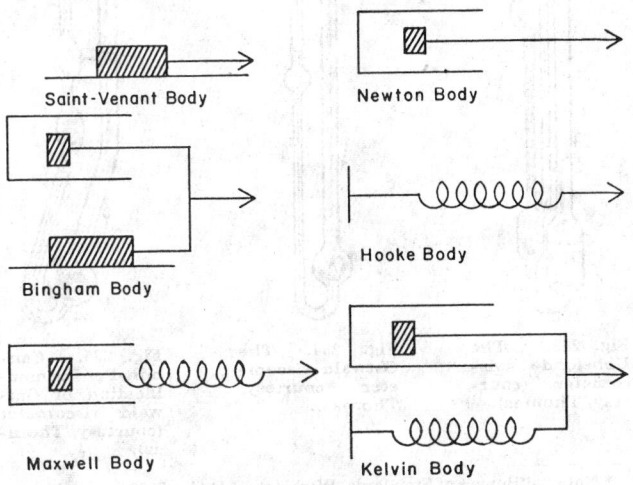

Fig. 232.   Models of flow.

Capillary Methods—Poiseuille was the first to derive the expression for the viscous flow of liquids through capillary tubes, *viz*:

$$\eta = \pi p r^4 t / 8vl$$

which relates the coefficient of viscosity, η, with the volume v of the liquid flowing through the tube in time t under a driving force or pressure p; r is the radius and l the length of the tube. This is a fundamental equation. However, the experimental determination of absolute viscosity using the Poiseuille equation *per se* is a difficult task. The measurement of *relative viscosity*, the ratio of the viscosity of some liquid to the viscosity of a standard liquid such as water, is a comparatively simple procedure and usually adequate for most purposes. If desired, the absolute viscosity then can be calculated from the relative viscosity if the absolute viscosity of the standard liquid is known. In practice the *Ubbelohde viscometer* (Fig. 233), the *Ostwald viscometer* (Fig. 234), or the *Cannon-Fenske modification* of the Ostwald viscometer (Fig. 235) are frequently used. To use one of the latter type, the viscometer is inverted and the tip of the narrow, graduated tube immersed in the liquid; suction is applied to the larger tube to draw the liquid up to the upper graduation; the viscometer is returned to its normal position. This measuring procedure assures that the same volume of liquid is used for all measurements, thereby eliminating loading errors arising from different driving head levels. Pressure is now applied to the larger tube to force the liquid up above the upper mark in the graduated tube. Both tubes are opened to the air and the efflux time between the two graduations is measured by means of a stop watch. If the same volume of standard and unknown liquids is used, then the efflux times will be proportional to the driving force, ie,

$$\frac{\eta_1}{\eta_2} = \frac{\rho_1 t_1}{\rho_2 t_2}$$

where η_1 and η_2, ρ_1 and ρ_2, and t_1 and t_2 are the viscosities, densities, and times of efflux, respectively, for the two liquids.

It is frequently more convenient to use *kinematic viscosity* when using capillary methods. Kinematic viscosity is uncorrected for density and is related to the absolute viscosity by the expression

$$\nu = \eta / \rho$$

where ν is the kinematic viscosity in stokes, η is the absolute viscosity in poises, and ρ is the density. For the measurement of kinematic viscosity the Ostwald viscometer (Fig. 234) or a similar instrument can be used. The commonly used expression relating kinematic viscosity with efflux time is

$$\nu = Ct - B/t$$

where t is the efflux time and B and C are assumed to be constants. The term B/t is called the kinetic energy correction and should be small compared to the term Ct for a well-designed viscometer.[6] In the case of viscometers having small diameter capillaries the constants are conveniently evaluated by standardizing the viscometer with water. The efflux time for water is determined at several different temperatures. Using the values for the viscosity of water as established by the American Society for Testing Materials[7] (see Table I), the simultaneous solution of the above equation using data for two different temperatures will provide values for the constants B and C. Viscosity data for

Table I—Viscosity of Water

| Temperature of water | | Viscosity |
°C	°F	(centistokes)
20.00	68	1.007
37.78	100	0.689
54.44	130	0.518

liquid water up to 150°C are reported by Korosi and Fabuss.[8]

Cannon[6] has shown that the assumption that both B and C are constants is correct in regard to C but incorrect in regard to B which is a function of the turbulence of the liquid as it leaves the capillary. For improved accuracy the following equation is suggested:

$$\nu = \frac{\eta}{\rho} = Ct - \frac{E}{t^2}$$

The constants C and E are determined experimentally as were B and C above.

Viscometers having large-bore capillaries are best standardized using standard oils available from the National Bureau of Standards* or from the Cannon Instrument Company.† Calibrating liquids, capillary tube viscometers and calibration methods are described by Hardy.[9] The Ostwald-type viscometer as modified by Cannon and Fenske is available in several capillary sizes in order to cover a wider range of viscosity. They are available in standard sizes (see Table II).

A great variety of other capillary-type viscometers is available.[10] These include the *Cannon-Fenske Viscometer—Reverse Flow Type for Opaque Liquids*, the *FitzSimons Viscometer*, the *Zeitfuchs Viscometer for Transparent Liquids*, the *Zeitfuchs Cross-Arm Viscometer*, the *Lantz-Zeitfuchs Type Reverse Flow Viscometer*, the *SIL Viscometer*, and the *Atlantic Viscometer*.

The *Dudley Viscosity Pipet* (Fig. 238) is an ingeniously simple device using the capillary principle. It consists essentially of a standard transfer pipet but having a calibration mark on the lower stem in addition to one on the stem above the bulb. It is normally filled by mouth suction, and the time required for the liquid to drain from one calibration mark to the other is the efflux time. Calibrated against water or other stan-

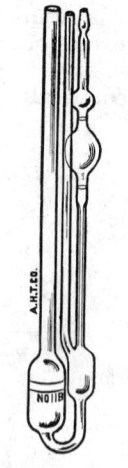 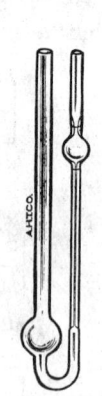 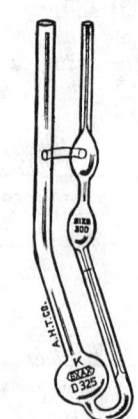

| Fig. 233. The Ubbelohde viscometer (courtesy, Thomas). | Fig. 234. The Ostwald viscometer (courtesy, Thomas). | Fig. 235. Cannon-Fenske modification of Ostwald viscometer (courtesy, Thomas). |

* National Bureau of Standards, Washington, D.C. 20234.
† Cannon Instrument Co., Box 812, University Park, Pa. 16802.

dard liquids, this viscometer is useful for measuring kinematic viscosity.

Other viscometers used in a manner similar to the capillary-tube method but which are designed for use in a manner referred to more accurately as orifice methods have been used for some time for the measurement of kinematic viscosity. Of these, the *Ford cup* (Fig. 237) may well find applications for control purposes in the pharmaceutical industry. It consists of a brass cylindrical cup with a cone-shaped bottom having a calibrated orifice (available in different sizes) at the apex of the cone. The volume of the cup is slightly in excess of 100 ml. It is normally used by closing the orifice with the index finger while the cup is filled level with the top. The time required for 100 ml of the liquid to run into a graduated cylinder is the efflux time.

The *Zahn cup* type viscometer (Fig. 236) is useful for the control of viscosity in manufacturing processes. It is similar to the Ford cup but is attached to a long handle. To make a reading, the cup is lifted out of the liquid and as it leaves the surface a stop watch is started. When the stream flowing from the orifice suddenly breaks, the time is noted. Using a calibration curve the viscosity in centistokes can be estimated from Zahn seconds but such conversion does not give consistently accurate results when applied to liquids of vastly differing properties.

Other orifice-type viscometers such as the *Engler* (Fig. 239), *Saybolt* (Fig. 240), and *Scott* (Fig. 241) have found considerable use by the petroleum industry. Methods using these instruments are well established and readily available.[11]

Rotational Methods—Rotational viscometers consist of a cylindrical cup to contain the sample under test and a bob, centered on the same axis as the cup, usually suspended by a fine torsion wire at such a height that the lower portion of the bob is immersed in the liquid. In some instruments, such as the MacMichael (Fig. 242), the cup is rotated by a driving mechanism and the torque, induced on the bob through the liquid, is read from a scale fastened directly to the bob. In other instruments, such as the Stormer viscometer (Fig. 243), the cup is stationary and the bob is made to rotate in the liquid. However, regardless of whether it is the bob or the cup which is made to rotate, the basic mode of action is the same in that there is a relative

Table II—Viscometer Capillary Sizes

Modified Ostwald viscometer	Efflux time sec	Capillary diameter mm	Approx. viscosity range Centistokes	Saybolt Univ. sec
Series 50	300–1500	0.40–0.45	0.8–3	
100	200–700	0.60–0.65	2–10	35–65
200	100–700	0.97–1.03	10–70	60–325
300	100–700	1.20–1.30	25–175	120–800
400	100–700	1.80–1.90	120–850	550–4000
500	100–700	2.70–2.90	800–5600	3600–25,000

motion between the bob and the cup producing a shearing action on the liquid contained between them. The viscosity of the liquid is related to the dimensions of the viscometer by the equation

$$\eta = T/4\pi\omega h(1/R_b^2 - 1/R_c^2)$$

where T is the torque required to produce a rotational velocity of ω radians/sec in a viscometer having a bob of radius R_b cm immersed in the liquid to a depth of h cm, the liquid being contained in a cup of radius R_c, cm. It is obvious that this equation is somewhat limited for general use in its present form. In addition to its being applicable only to Newtonian liquids, it is normally somewhat difficult to measure the value of T. Furthermore, it is normally necessary to correct for the "end effects" produced by the action of the liquid on the end of the bob immersed in the liquid. Generally, it is easier to lump all of these factors together into one constant, k, the instrument constant, which can be evaluated readily by standardizing the instrument against liquids of known viscosity. The working form of such an equation depends upon the type of instrument used and hence will be discussed separately under the description of the instruments.

The mechanical energy required to maintain the spindle rotating is converted into heat energy in the fluid. While at low shear rates, the resultant temperature rise is negligible, when operating rotational viscometers at high shear rates, it is necessary to consider such temperature effects.[12]

The *MacMichael viscometer* (Fig. 242) consists of a bob or spindle suspended from a torsion wire of fixed length which is attached at the top of the instrument. The

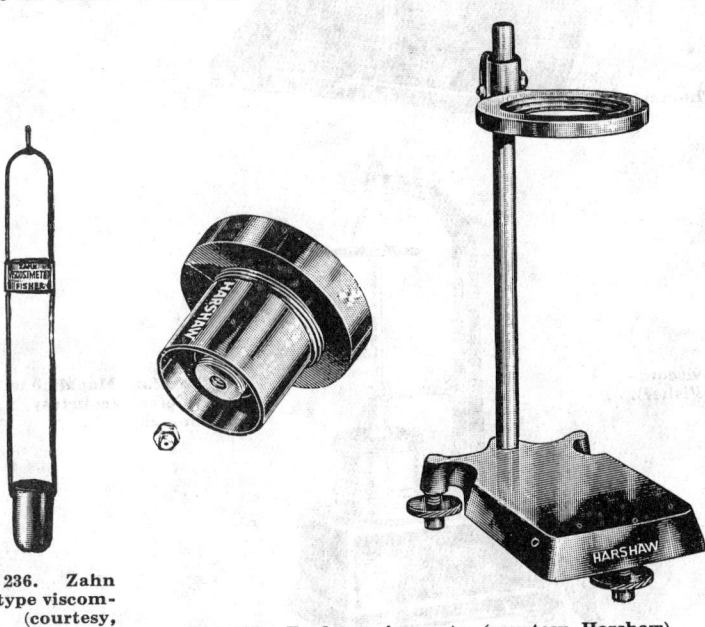

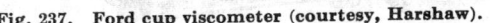

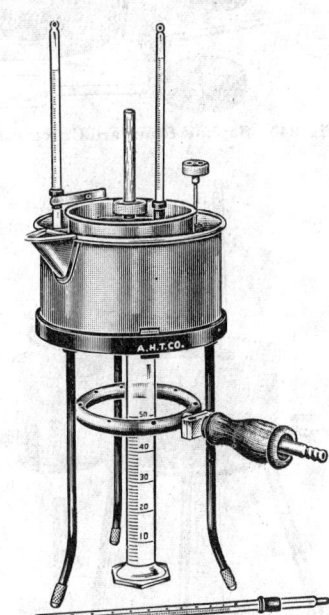

Fig. 236. Zahn cup type viscometer (courtesy, Fisher).

Fig. 237. Ford cup viscometer (courtesy, Harshaw).

Fig. 238. Dudley viscosity pipet (courtesy, Fisher).

Fig. 239. Engler viscometer (courtesy, Thomas).

material to be tested is placed in a cup which is revolved on a motor-driven platform. The amount of twist imparted to the wire depends on the viscosity of the material and is read on a graduated disk attached to the spindle. The readings are in arbitrary degrees, one "degree" being $\frac{1}{300}$ of a circle. The cup is placed within a larger cup equipped with a heating coil which serves as a bath. By using different wire gages it is possible to measure a wide range of viscosities. The speed of the rotating platform and hence the speed of rotation of the cup is adjustable by means of a governor from about 10 to 40 rpm. The bobs are available in three diameters and the cups in two different diameters and, being interchangeable, provide a rather large working range of viscosity. To convert the MacMichael degrees, M, to viscosity, an equation of the following form is used:

$$\eta = kM/rpm$$

The instrument constant, k, is most easily evaluated by standardizing the viscometer with a liquid of known viscosity.

A modification[13] of the MacMichael viscometer, described in a publication of the ASTM, provides for control of temperature which is not possible with the unmodified instrument.

The *Stormer viscometer* (Fig. 242) is likewise a rotational viscometer, but it has a stationary cup and a rotating bob. To measure viscosity with this instrument it is necessary to determine the time required for a definite number of revolutions of the rotating cylinder or other type rotor which has been immersed in the sample placed in the cup. The rotor is driven by a falling weight through a series of gears and a revolution counter attached to the spindle tallies the total number of turns of the spindle. A particular temperature is maintained by means of a water or oil bath. *Relative viscosity* is obtained by dividing the time required for the rotor to make a specified number of revolutions in the material under examination by the time required for the cylinder to make the same number of revolutions in distilled water or other reference liquid, using the identical procedure, at the same temperature, and using the same weight. If the absolute viscosity of the standard is known, the absolute viscosity of the unknown can be calculated. One disadvantage of the Stormer viscometer is that it is frequently necessary to make a correction for the friction of the gear system, particularly when working with liquids of low viscosity.

The *Fisher Electroviscometer* (Fig. 244) and the *Brookfield Synchro-Lectric Viscometer* (Fig. 245) are directly

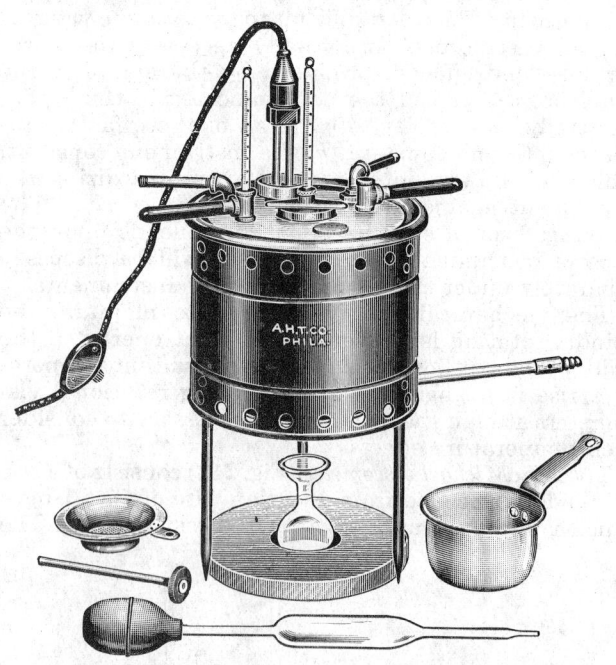

Fig. 240. **Saybolt Standard Universal viscometer (courtesy, Thomas).**

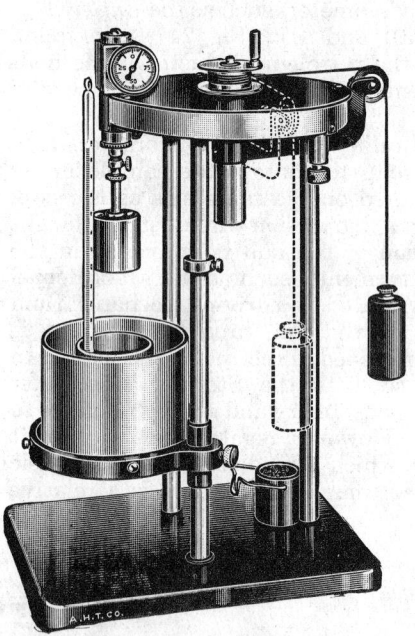

Fig. 242. **Stormer viscometer (courtesy, Thomas).**

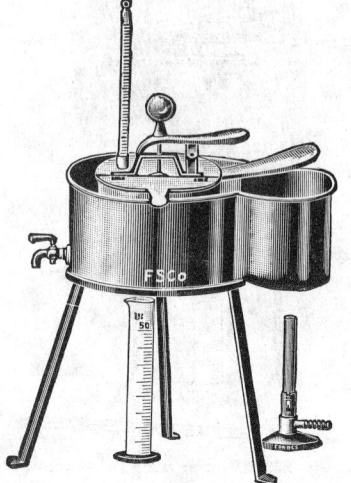

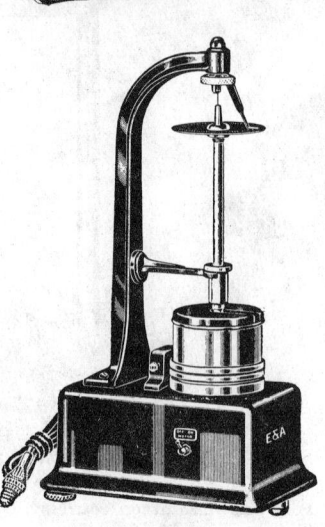

Fig. 241. **Scott viscometer (courtesy, Fisher).**

Fig. 243. **MacMichael viscometer (courtesy, Thomas).**

calibrated in centipoises when used with Newtonian materials. Both instruments are designed to cover a wide range of viscosity in a series of different ranges. Operating on rotational principles, the Brookfield viscometer permits viscosity determinations of Newtonian materials in the range from one to 32,000,000 centipoises. The torque on a spindle rotating at constant speed is measured by a calibrated spring. Dial readings are in centipoises but normally must be multiplied by a correction factor which is a function both of the angular velocity and the spindle used. The Brookfield Helipath stand, shown in Fig. 245, when used in conjunction with a Brookfield viscometer, permits testing plastic materials by slowly lowering the spindle into new layers, a feature useful in studies of thixotropic materials. The motor-drive stand lowers the spindle through the material so that measurements on nonflowing substances such as gels, pastes, greases, etc may be made.

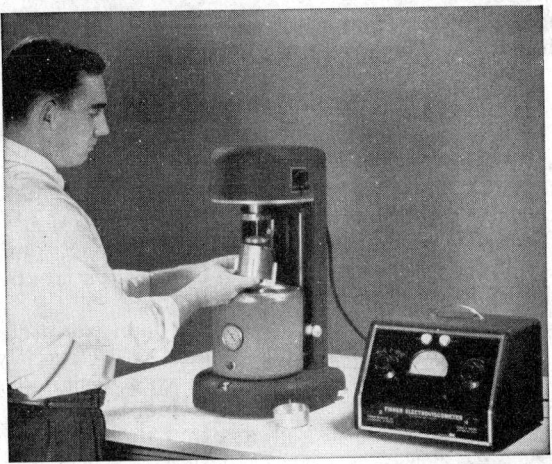

Fig. 244. Fisher electroviscometer (courtesy, Fisher).

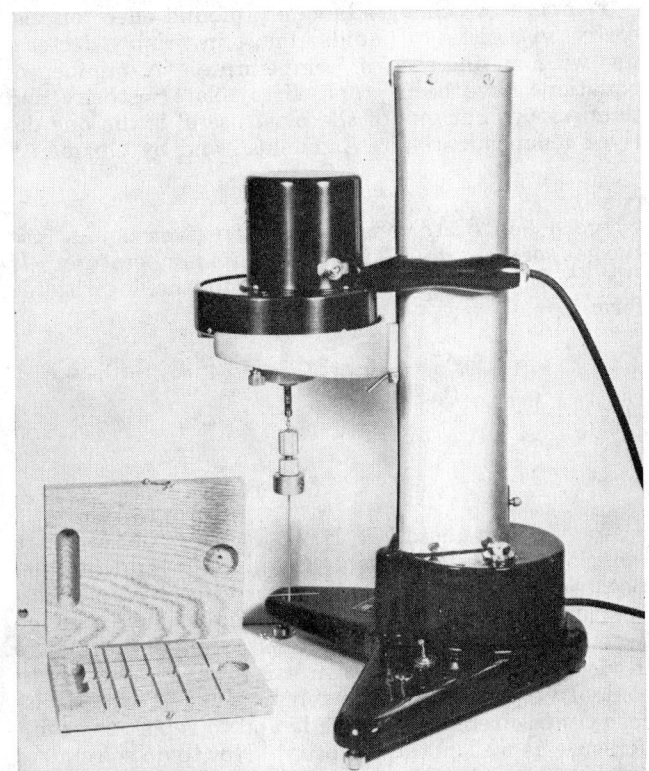

Fig. 245. Brookfield Synchro-Lectric viscometer and Helipath stand (courtesy, Brookfield).

It should be noted, however, that although this type of viscometer is calibrated, the data obtained with non-Newtonian materials require special interpretation, as discussed previously under *Types of Flow*. Several methods[14-17] have been suggested for the interpretation of data for non-Newtonian systems where the data have been obtained by use of a Brookfield viscometer.

Other commercially available rotational viscometers of potential interest in pharmacy include the Haake Rotovisco (Brinkmann*), the Contraves Viscometer (Fecker*), and the Ferranti Portable Viscometer (Will*). Commercial viscometers have been modified and others specially made to meet particular requirements of high shear rate,[18] high pressure,[19] increased sensitivity through scale expansion,[20] measurements on samples of rapidly settling suspensions,[21] and versatility through automation and readout.[22]

Falling-Sphere Methods—Falling-sphere methods are particularly useful for measuring the viscosity of viscous liquids. They consist essentially of introducing a small sphere of some suitable material such as steel, glass, or plastic, beneath the surface of the liquid and observing the rate at which the sphere falls through the liquid under the influence of gravity. The liquid should be contained in a tall glass cylinder having two marks a given distance apart. For the measurement of *relative viscosity* this is all that is required. Since the distance traversed by the sphere is the same for all measurements, the time required for the sphere to fall between the two marks is proportional to the viscosity and hence

$$\eta_1/\eta_2 = t_1/t_2$$

assuming that the densities of the liquids being compared are equal. If the densities of the liquids differ then the relationship becomes

$$\eta_1/\eta_2 = t_1(\rho_1 - \rho_2)/t_2(\rho_1 - \rho_3)$$

where ρ_1 is the density of the sphere and ρ_2 and ρ_3 are the densities of the two liquids.

If it is desired to measure the *absolute viscosity* use is made of Stokes' equation

$$\eta = 2gr^2(\rho_1 - \rho_2)/9V$$

where g is the gravitational constant, r the radius of the sphere in cm, ρ_1 the density of the sphere in Gm/cc and ρ_2 the density of the liquid, and V is the velocity of the sphere in cm/sec per second. This form of Stokes' equation is applicable to a solid sphere falling through a liquid or gas, to a drop of liquid falling through a gas, or to a drop of liquid, eg, oil, falling or rising through a liquid. The method is capable of accurate measurements if suitable corrections are made. Primarily, this equation is based on the assumption that the liquid is infinite in extent and not bounded by the walls of the container. The Landenburg corrections[23] for the container are sufficiently accurate for most purposes and apply to a cylindrical container of radius R and height H. Applying these corrections, Stokes' equation becomes

$$\eta = \frac{2gr^2(\rho_1 - \rho_2)}{9V(1 - 2.4r/R)(1 - 3.1r/H)}$$

It is also necessary to be sure to use a sphere of proper size and density so that its velocity is not excessive. At high velocities the flow of the liquid around the sphere becomes turbulent and beyond this point erratic results will be obtained.

If used with non-Newtonian systems, it is necessary to separate Stokes' equation into the components of shearing force, F, and shearing rate, dv/dr, if a thorough analysis of the data is to be performed. Lamb[24] has shown that the maximum velocity gradient, dv/dr, at the equator of the sphere, as the sphere falls through an infinite liquid, is given by

$$dv/dr = (\rho_1 - \rho_2)gr/3\eta$$

but since shearing force, $F = \eta\, dv/dr$, it follows that

$$F = (\rho_1 - \rho_2)gr/3$$

In practice, where the dimensions of the liquid are defined by the size of the containing cylinder, the shear rate must be corrected for the wall and end effects.

$$dv/dr = 2r/3V(1 - 2.4r/R)(1 - 3.1r/H)$$

Falling-sphere equipment is available from certain suppliers of chemical apparatus, but in general the equipment required can be assembled easily from standard materials found in most laboratories.[25-28] A de-

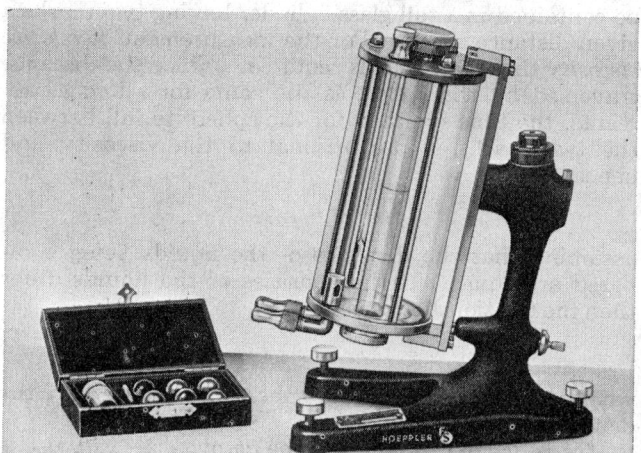

Fig. 246. The Hoeppler precision viscometer (courtesy, Sargent).

sirable refinement is to enclose the fall tube in a water jacket through which water can be circulated from a constant temperature bath by a small pump.

Rising bubble methods for measuring viscosity are based also on Stokes' equation. It will be noted that the term $(\rho_1 - \rho_2)$ becomes negative indicating that the sphere is rising rather than falling. Excellent results have been obtained using air bubbles or droplets of oil. The main difficulty with this method is in measuring the radius of the droplets. Oil droplets can be measured by removing them from the column as they near the top of the liquid using a dropper. They can then be transferred, along with some of the solution, to a microscope slide having a depression and the size of the droplet determined with an ocular micrometer in the eyepiece of the microscope.

A *"rising sphere"* instrument has been described by McVean and Mattocks.[29] As a stainless steel sphere, suspended by a very fine wire, is pulled upward through the liquid, stress is recorded as a function of strain. Data obtained through the use of this instrument are very informative. In addition to the advantages of the falling-sphere method, this method has the added advantage that the velocity of the sphere can be varied at will—even reduced to zero if desired—thus permitting measurements on the system as a function of time.

Measurement of recovery time, for example, is possible with the rising sphere instrument.

The rising sphere apparatus was modified by McVean and Goyan[30] by placing the fluid sample in the core of an electromagnet. Static yield values were obtained by variation of the electromagnetic field. The device has been called an *electromagnetoyieldometer*. In another modification of this instrument[31] the ball is replaced by a cylinder. An advantage claimed for the rising cylinder rheometer is the ability to make measurements at very low shear rates.

The *Hoeppler viscometer* is similar to a falling-sphere viscometer except that the fall tube is on an incline and the sphere is allowed to roll down the side of the tube. This has the advantage that the velocity of the sphere is reduced. By using the same sphere for all measurements, the error introduced by the wall effect will be constant and thus relative results can be obtained. See Fig. 246.

For a given combination of ball and tube, the viscosity can be calculated from the relation

$$\eta = K(\rho_1 - \rho_2)t$$

The constant K is evaluated by the use of a standard liquid of known viscosity η and density ρ_2 and a sphere of density ρ_1. Hubbard and Brown[32] carried out a systematic experimental calibration and dimensional analysis of a rolling-ball viscometer. Lewis[33] derived the calibration curve through a theoretical treatment of the hydrodynamics of viscous liquids.

The rolling-ball viscometer has been adopted for high-pressure viscosity measurements.[34] Recently an instrument was described[35] which was designed specifically for high-pressure measurements of viscosity on electrolytic fluids as well as other fluids.

Effect of Temperature on Viscosity

Temperature changes have a profound effect on viscosity, viscosities of liquids almost invariably decreasing with an increase in temperature. A number of equations have been proposed to relate viscosity and temperature but one of the most useful is the one derived independently by Arrhenius[36] and by Guzmán,[37]

$$\eta = Ae^{B/RT}$$

where A and B are constants for the given liquid, R is the gas constant, and P is the absolute temperature. If the above equation is converted to the logarithmic form

$$\log \eta = \frac{B}{2.30R} \times \frac{1}{T} + \log A$$

or

$$\log \eta = a + \frac{b}{T}$$

where $a = \log A$ and $b = B/2.30R$, it can be seen that the plot of the log η vs $1/T$ will be a straight line. Because the relationship between viscosity and temperature is exponential, an extremely small change in temperature can produce an extremely large change in viscosity. For this reason it is always necessary to control very carefully the temperature at which viscosity measurements are made and to report the temperature as well as the viscosity. Not to do so renders the value for viscosity valueless.

The viscosities of a few liquids at different temperatures are given in Table III.

Table III—Viscosity in Centipoises				
	0°C	25°C	50°C	75°C
Water	1.793	0.895	0.549	0.380
Benzene	0.90	0.61	0.44	...
Ethanol	1.79	1.09	0.698	...

Influence of Concentration of the Dispersed Phase

Emulsions and suspensions are found to have a viscosity greater than that of the external phase. This increase in viscosity can be explained on the basis of the interference to flow produced by the particles of the dispersed phase. For very dilute dispersions this increase in viscosity can be expressed mathematically by the Einstein equation

$$\eta = \eta_0(1 + 2.5C_v)$$

where η is the viscosity of the dispersion, η_0 the viscosity of the solvent or dispersing medium, and C_v is the volume concentration of the dispersed phase. Since Einstein derived this equation on the assumptions that the system was very dilute so that there would be no influence of one dispersed particle on another and also that the dispersed particles were perfect spheres, if applied to a system not conforming to these assumptions, the results may be expected to deviate from the calculated values. Many modifications of the Einstein equation have been proposed to extend its use to higher concentrations, but the following one has received rather general use:

$$\eta = \eta_0(1 + 2.5C_v + 14.1C_v{}^2)$$

The Einstein equation applies equally well for dilute "true" solutions in which case the "dispersed phase" consists of ions or of single molecules rather than of agglomerates of molecules.

A notable difference is observed with colloidal systems between the viscosity of lyophilic and lyophobic dispersions. With the former (eg, gelatin sol) a large increase in viscosity is observed over that of the dispersion medium. With the latter (eg, colloidal gold sol) only minor increases in viscosity over that of the dispersion medium are observed. This can be explained by assuming that many solvent molecules adhere to the lyophilic solute molecules, probably through hydrogen bonding, thus producing a considerable increase in the effective volume of the solute and hence a corresponding increase in C_v, the volume concentration.

Arrhenius has likewise proposed an equation showing that the viscosity of dispersions varies logarithmically with the concentration:

$$\eta = \eta_0 e^{kc}$$

Again it has been shown that this equation, too, is valid only at moderate concentrations.

Viscosity of Polymer Solutions

If η is the viscosity of a solution of concentration C (expressed in grams of solute per 100 ml of solution) and η_0 is that of the pure solvent, then the *specific viscosity*, η_{sp} as defined by Staudinger is

$$\eta_{sp} = (\eta - \eta_0)/\eta_0 = \eta/\eta_0 - 1 = \eta_r - 1$$

where η_r is the *relative viscosity* and is defined as η/η_0. The specific viscosity is of interest because it is a measure of the relative thickening of the solvent due to the presence of the dissolved polymer.

A rearrangement of the Einstein equation gives

$$\eta_r = \eta/\eta_0 = 1 + 2.5C_v$$

and therefore

$$\eta_{sp} = 2.5C_v$$

indicating that the specific viscosity should be directly proportional to the concentration of the solution. When this equation is extended to apply at higher concentrations it becomes

$$\eta_{sp} = 2.5C_v + 14.1C_v{}^2$$

or

$$\eta_{sp} = AC + BC^2$$

By introducing the *reduced viscosity*, η_{sp}/C, the equation for a straight line is obtained:

$$\eta_{red} = A + BC$$

where A is the intercept and B is the slope. For most polymer solutions this equation holds for concentrations up to about 1 per cent. The significance of A was first pointed out by Kraemer who called it the *intrinsic viscosity* (η). Using the intrinsic viscosity and the relationship between A and B as determined from the values of the coefficient 2.5 and 14.1, a general equation of the following form is obtained

$$\eta_{red} = (\eta) + k(\eta)^2C$$

where (η), the intrinsic viscosity, corresponds to the coefficient A in the above equation and can be evaluated by plotting the reduced viscosity against the concentration. Extrapolation to zero concentration gives a value for (η).

For solutions of long-chain molecules the intrinsic viscosity is related to the average molecular weight of the dissolved substance by an expression proposed by Mark[38] and Houwink:[39]

$$(\eta) = K\overline{M}^a$$

where K and a are constants for a given series of long-chain compounds. An equation of this form, with a equal to unity, was suggested empirically by Staudinger. Later investigations have shown that for some series of compounds the actual value for a is somewhat less than unity. Graphs on log-log paper show the relationship between intrinsic viscosity and degree of polymerization.

Thixotropy

The term "thixotropy" was coined by Peterfi[40] and Freundlich.[41] Literally meaning "to change by touch," it is defined by some authorities as a reversible, isothermal sol–gel formation. The phenomenon may not be so dramatic as is suggested by the term "reversible sol–gel formation" but implies the property of decreasing consistency (thinning) of a material as it is subjected to a shearing stress followed by an increase of consistency (thickening) when the stress is removed. Let us consider a practical example of this phenomenon in which a rather extreme case is illustrated. A dispersion of small solid particles in a liquid results in the formation of a rigid gel when the mixture is at rest. On shaking this same mixture, the gel becomes a mobile liquid, called a sol. If the mixture is allowed to rest for a period of time, a rigid gel once again forms.

Characteristic of thixotropy, this reversible sol–gel formation occurs without any temperature change. It should be remembered, however, that the gel which forms in a thixotropic system is not necessarily a solid gel but may be a non-Newtonian of varying fluidity.

Blood plasma and colloidal suspensions of ferric oxide were some of the materials originally described as being thixotropic. Today we realize that dispersions of certain natural minerals such as bentonite, attapulgite, and hectorite and many alkaline earth salts as well as solutions of the so-called "water-soluble gums" including tragacanth, acacia, sodium carboxymethylcellulose, methylcellulose, and others exhibit thixotropy under proper conditions. Practical illustrations are found also in some paints, quicksand, in drilling muds, an important factor in petroleum oil field development, and in many emulsions and suspensions.

Theories—Although various theories have been proposed through the years, thixotropic structure has never been completely explained. Hauser[42] proposed a theory of thixotropy concerning the shape of thixotropic particles, stating that it is characteristic of anisometric (having unsymmetrical parts) particles and the gel setting a result of orientation of the particles. Other workers have observed that anisotropic (having different properties when tested along the axes) particles give greater degrees of thixotropy than anisometric particles. Smaller-sized particles tend to give higher degrees of thixotropy. Electrolytes are not absolutely essential for thixotropy although their presence may influence the degree. Pryce-Jones,[43] working with paints, stated that four factors were concerned with thixotropy: concentration of pigment, degree of wetting of pigment, presence of soap, and presence of water. Hydrogen-ion concentration has been shown to have an influence on thixotropy.[44] Heller,[45] reporting on the thixotropic state of ferric oxide sols, stated that thixotropy depended on the rate of germ (centers of gelation) formation, rate of germ growth into elementary gels (geloids), and the rate at which these geloids associate. He therefore brought in the factor of time for thixotropic formation. By means of dilatometric measurements[46] a volume change of about 2.4×10^{-4} % was observed during the sol–gel–sol transition of a sodium bentonite suspension, the gel occupying a slightly greater volume than the sol. A progressive buildup, during gelation, of a water structure less dense than in the sol, is proposed.

One popular theory suggests that electrical forces on the surfaces of the particles are responsible for thixotropic phenomena. These forces allow each particle to act in a manner similar to magnets each of which has a north and south pole. Such charged particles are referred to as dipoles. Particles become oriented in a manner whereby oppositely charged poles face each other. At this stage a gel structure results. The gel buildup is not immediate because of a varying degree of dipole alignment of the particles; therefore, the gel formation is not instantaneous but there are varying time lags until the process is completed. This arrangement may be disturbed by agitation, resulting in particles being torn loose and tumbling over each other; ie, a sol is formed. Fig. 247 illustrates Green's scheme for the explanation of the electrical theory.[47]

In 1943 Englehardt[48] explained thixotropy as the result of various factors which include a relationship between Winkler number (time for thixotropic gel to set) and a hardness test, the total potential of attractive and repulsive forces between particles, the polarity of the medium, and the presence of flat particles rather than spheres.

Pryce-Jones[43] has stated: "It may be safely assumed that at the present time no theory can explain the behavior of thixotropic systems or can predict the type of flow resulting from a dispersion of a given volume of fine particles in a fluid. Nevertheless, from the theoretical work completed thus far, it may be said that the following factors are criteria in causing and producing thixotropic systems: particle size and shape orientation of the particles, the distance between particles or the concentration of the mixture, elasticity and yield value of the gel, the type solvent present, the dielectric constant or the dipole moment of the gel, presence of electrolytes and repulsive forces, the degree of wetting of the substance, pH of the medium, time, and the diameter and shape of the container."

Measurement—A "single-point" viscosity measurement cannot be used to characterize thixotropic and other non-Newtonian materials. A viscometer must be used which permits measurement of shearing stress at different rates of shear. The fundamental problem with non-Newtonian fluids lies in their inability to sustain shear without altering the very property one is trying to measure.[49] It is for this reason that the falling-sphere method is most nearly ideal for non-Newtonian measurements since the fluid is undisturbed until the very instant the sphere passes. With capillary and rotational methods there is a continual shearing of the entire fluid.

One method which has been found useful for obtaining empirical data relating the relative degree of thixotropy of different materials employs a rotational viscometer. Preferably, a rotational viscometer is used which is equipped with an automatic control to first increase the rate of shear linearly with time and then to decrease the rate of shear linearly with time. It is convenient if the viscometer is equipped also with an automatic recording device. Such an instrument is described by Samyn and Mattocks.[22] With a viscometer of this type one is able to measure a useful index of thixotropic breakdown and thixotropic buildup of a system. The data, when plotted, produce a *thixotropic hysteresis loop* (Fig. 248).

Manually controlled rotational viscometers may be used but usually with some sacrifice of accuracy and versatility. To obtain data from which the upcurve (thixotropic breakdown) of this loop can be plotted, the shearing stress is measured for each value of the shear rate as the shear rate is increased a given and regular amount at equal time intervals. This procedure is continued until a given (or maximum) shearing rate is attained. Then, without interruption, the process is reversed. That is, the shear rate is incrementally

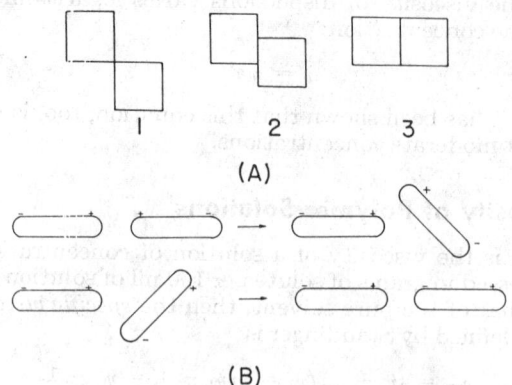

(A)

(B)

Fig. 247.   Green's scheme for the explanation of the electrical force theory. A shows thixotropic bonds of different strength. B shows time lag in a thixotropic system.

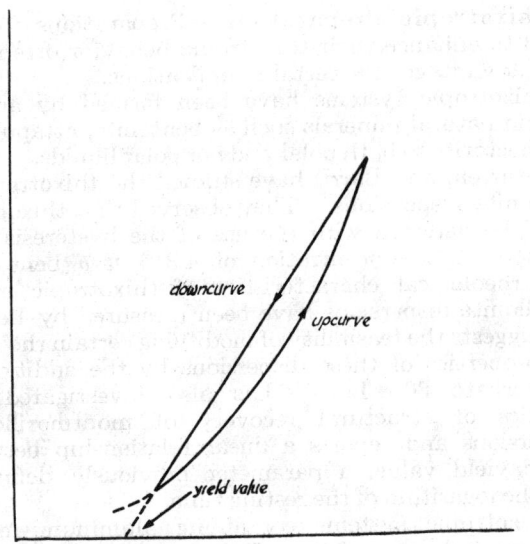

Fig. 248.   Thixotropic hysteresis loop.

decreased at regular time intervals. Measurement of the shearing stress for each value of shearing rate provides the data from which the downcurve (thixotropic buildup) can be plotted. If the rate of thixotropic buildup is slow, the downcurve will be a straight line. The upcurve and downcurve produce a closed geometric figure known as the hysteresis loop. The relative degree of thixotropy exhibited by similar systems may be estimated empirically by a comparison of the areas of these hysteresis loops.

Capillary viscometers also can be used with fluids exhibiting anomalous flow. Some of the problems encountered with such systems are discussed by Calderwood, et al.[50] A three-level capillary viscometer was designed by Honig and Singleterry[51] for the study of non-Newtonian flow in sealed systems. Non-Newtonian systems are described by a pair of constants, one describing the consistency level of the systems under specified shearing conditions and the other characterizing the deviation from Newtonian flow.

Application of Rheology to Pharmacy

Emulsions and Suspensions—In the formulation of emulsions and suspensions it is important that the dispersing medium be sufficiently viscous to retard separation. Water-soluble gums and other suspending agents are frequently employed for this purpose. Their rheological behavior and suspending efficiency can be measured by means of the Stokes equation (page 365):

$$V = \frac{2gr^2(\rho_1 - \rho_2)}{9\eta}$$

which shows that the rate at which a dispersed particle will rise or settle (ignoring the influence of other dispersed particles) is inversely proportional to the viscosity of the dispersing phase. The advantage of a viscous preparation is therefore readily apparent. If the product is made sufficiently viscous, no separation of the dispersed phase will occur at all. In practice, however, fluid products are frequently desired. The objective in such cases is to formulate a preparation which appears very viscous to a small particle and which at the same time appears fluid with respect to ease of pouring. The answer is to be found with non-Newtonian systems.

If a system behaves in a Newtonian fashion, the viscosity is invariant with shear force. The viscosity will therefore appear the same to the particle as it does with respect to pouring. It has been shown that this does not represent optimal conditions. On the other hand plastic and pseudoplastic systems, especially if thixotropic, are quite useful since the observed viscosity appears very great for small shearing forces (of the magnitude exhibited by a small dispersed particle) while at the same time appears relatively low at greater values of shearing force (of the magnitude represented by pouring the preparation). These points are illustrated in Fig. 249. Substance A gives a rather steep curve, being very viscous at low rates of shear and very fluid at high rates of shear, actually crossing the curves for B and C. Curve C represents a Newtonian liquid such as glycerin. Most methods for measuring viscosity use relatively great shear forces and would therefore indicate C to be the best suspending agent by virtue of its high viscosity and A to be the poorest. In reality, however, the reverse would be true because the particles in the dispersion exert only a very low shearing force and hence should be evaluated from the relative positions of the left sides of the graphs.

Higuchi[52] calls attention to other limitations to a theoretical evaluation of creaming and sedimentation rates and mentions especially the influence of one particle on another in a concentrated dispersed phase. The effect of thixotropy on the suspension ability of dispersing media has been reported by Foernzler, et al.[53] while Knoechel and Wurster[54] have investigated the stability of emulsions of various viscosities.

Concentration of the dispersed phase not only complicates the calculation of sedimentation and creaming rates[52] but influences the viscosity of the emulsion or suspension itself (cf page 367). The influence on viscosity of oil emulsions stabilized with methylcellulose has been investigated by Sheth, et al.[55] It is also well known that identical formulations will exhibit different flow properties if they have received different treatments such as degree of homogenization. A study of such effects is reported by Simon, et al.[56]

Among the many factors which influence the stability of oil-in-water emulsions are temperature, gravitational or centrifugal force, coalescence, density differences, properties of the dispersed oil, viscosity, surface tension, concentration, aging, and time. These factors have been the subject of reviews by Garrett.[57,58] The effects of aging and surfactant concentration on the

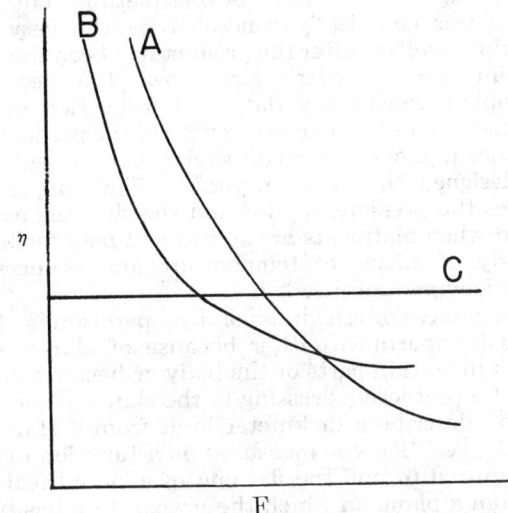

Fig. 249.   Effect of shearing rate on viscosity.

rheology and droplet-size distribution of nonaqueous emulsions have also been discussed by Hamill, *et al.*[59] Special reports are also available on the emulsifying and rheological properties of carrageenin and acacia[60] and a new polysaccharide gum[61] as well as on the rheological properties of various dermatological lotions.[62]

Several groups of investigators[63–66] have measured the rheological properties of a variety of suspending agents. They have attempted to relate the apparent viscosity, the concentration, and the suspending action of these agents in various systems. Martin[67] reviewed the formulation of suspensions from a physical chemical approach while Samyn[68] discussed the industrial approach to suspension formulation. The importance of rheological properties is illustrated. The effect of flocculation on suspension stability and the relationship of viscosity to flocculation rate also have been the subjects of several reports and reviews.[67,69–73] Bujake[74] measured the flow properties of concentrated calcium phosphate suspensions and attempted to correlate the effect of electrolytes on the viscosity of calcium phosphate–water systems with sedimentation volume data.

Ointments and Creams—Kostenbauder and Martin[75] studied the rheological properties of ointments and creams in an effort to evaluate the "true consistency" of these products. They have shown that the consistency can be interpreted fully only by inspection of the consistency curve of each system which is obtained by the plotting of rheological data.

Since these preparations are non-Newtonians, their rheological properties will be influenced by the rate of shear. The products may be sheared or worked on by spreading on the skin, rubbing it with a spatula, and processing in a mill; thus the consistency may vary.

Petrolatum has been shown to possess thixotropy although not of the rapid sol–gel type demonstrated by more fluid dispersions.[76] Heating petrolatum to its melting point, however, permits arrangement of the crystal network so that the product, after cooling, again exhibits the initial thixotropic condition. The addition of wax to petrolatum results in an increase in the plastic viscosity, yield value, and thixotropy of the petrolatum. These values are reduced upon the addition of liquid petrolatum to petrolatum. The addition of increasing concentrations of water to hydrophilic petrolatum caused a decrease in yield value and an increase in plastic viscosity and thixotropy of the base. Hydrophilic Ointment, USP was found to have a plastic viscosity higher than that of petrolatum, but this property was completely concealed by the very low yield value resulting after the product had been sheared. This ointment, in particular, shows the necessity for complete consistency data and inspection of the consistency curve for characterization of the product.

A device to measure the consistency of ointments has been designed by Havemeyer.[77] The apparatus simulates the pressure applied and the shearing action involved when ointments are spread and may facilitate the study of effects of temperature and changes in formulation upon consistency.

The tackiness or stickiness of a preparation is often of special importance either because of skin-to-skin adhesion in certain parts of the body or because of adhesion of a protective dressing to the skin. Wood and Lapham[78] describe a tackmeter built from a Harvard Trip balance. Tack is measured as a function of the force required to pull the flat end of a cylindrical pin away from a plane on which the preparation has been applied.

Thixotropic Preparations—Preparations formulated to enhance their thixotropic behavior often present advantages for certain applications.

Thixotropic systems have been formed by adding certain natural minerals such as bentonite, attapulgite, and hectorite to both polar and nonpolar liquids.

Bernstein and Barr[79] have studied the thixotropy of bentonite suspensions. They observed that thixotropy could be detected with the use of the hysteresis loop method at a concentration of 4.3% *w/v* bentonite. The rheological characteristics of thixotropic montmorillonite dispersions have been measured by Levy.[80] He suggests the feasibility of modifying certain rheological properties of these dispersions by the addition of polysorbate 80. Levy[81] has also investigated the kinetics of structural recovery of montmorillonite dispersions and reports a linear relationship between static yield value, a parameter previously defined,[80] and the logarithm of the resting time.

Thixotropic systems containing aluminum monostearate and some of the celluloses have also been reported. They may be formed also by reacting various substances together chemically and then properly treating their resultants. Thixotropic mixtures have been prepared by Schneiderwirth and Wilcox[44] by reacting aqueous solutions of alkaline earth metal salts of phosphates, carbonates, and silicates. They prepared a mixture of calcium and magnesium phosphates and carbonates which exhibited thixotropy by reacting a solution of calcium and magnesium chloride with a solution of sodium carbonate and phosphate. Particle size and shape were influenced by the temperature at which the reaction took place; agitation and rate of flow at which the solutions were combined were also of importance. The solutions were prepared in concentrations close to the saturation point and approximately stoichiometric quantities of the reacting chemicals were used. This system exhibited thixotropy at a pH range 5–5.5, citric acid being used to obtain this pH. It was found that the pH range of thixotropic behavior could be broadened considerably, and thixotropy in general enhanced when carbohydrates such as lactose and dextrose, or hexahydric alcohols such as sorbitol or mannitol, were added to the alkaline earth mineral gels and dissolved therein. Thus thixotropy was obtained within a pH range of from 4 to above 10.

Thixotropy may be utilized advantageously in the preparation of liquid suspensions. By preparing thixotropic suspensions, it is possible to minimize or completely eliminate sedimentation and coagulation of the insoluble substances in such preparations because of gelling. If sedimentation of the suspended substances is minimized, the substances will not settle to the bottom of the container and uniform dosage is brought about more simply by agitation of the preparation so that it will flow. Where thixotropic oral mixtures are taken by the patient, it will be found that they have less of a gritty and unpleasant taste than would be the case with a regular suspension. Preparations of high concentration may also be prepared which are in the state of gel when at rest but pour easily upon agitation.

Another useful aspect of thixotropy is that substances which are susceptible to decomposition, such as the vitamins, are found to be stable for longer periods of time in thixotropic preparations. This is understandable when one considers that such substances are in a state of complete rest, imprisoned in a solid gel in the presence of a stabilizing agent usually present in the formulation.

Still another application of thixotropy was reported by Ober, *et al.*[82] By controlling the rheological properties of procaine penicillin G suspensions, they have been able to obtain a prolonged therapeutic response. After injection into muscle tissue, the suspensions formed deposits which behaved as solid matter because stress exerted by the surrounding muscle tissue was not in excess of the yield value. On the other hand, no difficulty was encountered in the process of injection because the suspensions became quite fluid under the stress applied by the barrel of the syringe.

Stability of Water-Soluble Gums—The stability of solutions of various water-soluble gums has been the subject of several investigations. These include the measurement of viscosity changes of sodium alginate solution after freezing and thawing,[83] the aging stability of Veegum suspensions,[84] of tragacanth solutions[85] and of hydroxyethyl cellulose solutions,[86] as well as the aging stability of certain other hydrophilic polymers[87,88] including sodium alginate and carboxymethylcellulose.

References

1. Reiner, M., *Deformation and Flow*, H. K. Lewis & Co., Ltd., London, 1949.
2. *ASTM Proc.*, **51**, 441 (1951).
3. Buckingham, *ASTM Proc.*, **21**, 1154 (1921).
4. Reiner and Riwlin, *Kolloid-Z.*, **43**, 1 (1927).
5. Williamson, R. V., *Ind. Eng. Chem.*, **21**, 1108 (1929).
6. Cannon, M. R., *et al*, *Anal. Chem.*, **32**, 355 (1960).
7. *ASTM D 445-46T* (Standard on Petroleum Products and Lubricants), Am. Soc. Testing Mater., Philadelphia.
8. Korosi, A., and Fabuss, B. M., *Anal. Chem.*, **40**, 157 (1968).
9. Hardy, R. C., *Natl. Bur. Std. (US) Monograph*, **55** (Dec., 26, 1962).
10. *ASTM D 445-53T*, Am. Soc. Testing Mater., Philadelphia.
11. *ASTM D 88-56* (Standard Method of Test for Saybolt Viscosity), Am. Soc. Testing Mater., Philadelphia.
12. Mill, C. C., and Gates, E. R., *Anal. Chem.*, **25**, 1390 (1953).
13. *ASTM D 115*, Am. Soc. Testing Mater., Philadelphia.
14. Bowles, R. L., *et al*, *Mod. Plastics*, **32**, 142 (1955).
15. Runikis, J. O., *et al*, *J. APhA, Sci. Ed.*, **47**, 758 (1958).
16. Back, A. L., *Rubber Age (NY)*, **77**, 639 (1959).
17. Wood, J. H., *et al*, *J. Pharm. Sci.*, **52**, 296 (1963).
18. Barber, E. M., *et al*, *Anal. Chem.*, **27**, 425 (1955).
19. Reamer, H. H., *et al*, *Anal. Chem.*, **31**, 1422 (1959).
20. Zimmerman, E., *Anal. Chem.*, **39**, 1305 (1967).
21. Bhattacharya, A., and Roy, A., *Anal. Chem.*, **27**, 1287 (1955).
22. Samyn, J. C., and Mattocks, A. M., *J. APhA, Sci. Ed.*, **46**, 310 (1957).
23. Landenburg, R., *Ann. Physik*, **23**, 447 (1907).
24. Lamb, H., *Hydrodynamics*, Cambridge, London, 1906.
25. Malm, C. J., *et al*, *Anal. Chem.*, **22**, 656 (1950).
26. Roy, A. S., *Anal. Chem.*, **33**, 1426 (1961).
27. Lim, W. K., *et al*, *Anal. Chem.*, **36**, 2482 (1964).
28. Seibert, E. E., *et al*, *Anal. Chem.*, **37**, 613 (1965).
29. McVean, D. E., and Mattocks, A. M., *J. Pharm. Sci.*, **50**, 785 (1961),
30. McVean, D. E., and Goyan, J. E., *J. Pharm. Sci.*, **53**, 438 (1964).
31. McVean, D. E., and Goyan, J. E., *J. Pharm. Sci.*, **53**, 557 (1964).
32. Hubbard, R. M., and Brown, G. G., *Ind. Eng. Chem., Anal. Ed.*, **15**, 212 (1943).
33. Lewis, H. W., *Anal. Chem.*, **25**, 507 (1953).
34. Horne, R. A., and Johnson, D. S., *J. Phys. Chem.*, **70**, 2182 (1962).
35. Stanley, E. M., and Batten, R. C., *Anal. Chem.*, **40**, 1751 (1968).
36. Arrhenius, *Medd. Kgl. Velenskapsakad Nobel-Inst.*, **2** (8), 1–34 (1912).
37. Guzmán, *Anales Real Soc. Espan. Fis Quim.*, **11**, 353 (1913).
38. Mark, H., *Der feste Körper*, Herzel, Leipzig, 1938, p. 103.
39. Houwink, R., *J. Prakt. Chem.*, **155**, 241 (1940).
40. Peterfi, *Arch. Entwicklungsmech. Organ.*, **112**, 660 (1927).
41. Freundlich, H., *Thixotropy*, Actualites Scientifiques et Industrielles, N. 267, Hermann et Cie, Paris, 1935.
42. Hauser, E. A., *J. Rheol.*, **2**, 5 (1931).
43. Pryce-Jones, J., *J. Oil Colour Chemists' Assoc.*, **17**, 305 (1934).
44. Schneiderwirth, H. J., and Wilcox, P. W., *J. APhA, Sci. Ed.*, **36**, 402 (1947).
45. Heller, W., *Compt. Rend.*, **202**, 1507 (1936).
46. Anderson, D. M., *et al*, *Science*, **141**, 1040 (1963).
47. Green, H., *Industrial Rheology and Rheological Structure*, Wiley, New York, 1949, pp. 48–62.
48. Englehardt, W., *Kolloid-Z.*, **102**, 217 (1943).
49. McKennell, R., *Anal. Chem.*, **32**, 1458 (1960).
50. Calderwood, G. F. N., *et al*, *Anal. Chem.*, **25**, 935 (1953).
51. Honig, J. G., and Singleterry, C. R., *Anal. Chem.*, **26**, 677 (1954).
52. Higuchi, T., *J. APhA, Sci. Ed.*, **47**, 657 (1958).
53. Foernzler, E. C., *et al*, *J. APhA, Sci. Ed.*, **49**, 249 (1960).
54. Knoechel, E. L., and Wurster, D. E., *J. APhA, Sci. Ed.*, **48**, 1 (1959).
55. Sheth, B. B., *et al*, *J. Pharm. Sci.*, **51**, 265 (1962).
56. Simon, T. H., *et al*, *J. Pharm. Sci.*, **50**, 880 (1961).
57. Garrett, E. R., *J. Pharm. Sci.*, **51**, 35 (1962).
58. Garrett, E. R., *J. Pharm. Sci.*, **54**, 1557 (1965).
59. Hamill, R. D., and Petersen, R. V., *J. Pharm. Sci.*, **55**, 1268 (1966).
60. Fitzgerald, B. W., and Skauen, D. M., *J. APhA, Sci. Ed.*, **44**, 358 (1955).
61. Araujo, O. E., *J. Pharm. Sci.*, **56**, 1141 (1967).
62. Setnikar, I., *et al*, *J. Pharm. Sci.*, **57**, 671 (1968).
63. Kabre, S. P., *et al*, *J. Pharm. Sci.*, **53**, 492 (1964).
64. Kabre, S. P., *et al*, *J. Pharm. Sci.*, **53**, 495 (1964).
65. Storz, G. K., *et al*, *J. Pharm. Sci.*, **54**, 85 (1965).
66. Lesshafft, C. T., *J. Pharm. Sci.*, **55**, 1371 (1966).
67. Martin, A. N., *J. Pharm. Sci.*, **50**, 513 (1961).
68. Samyn, J. C., *J. Pharm. Sci.*, **50**, 517 (1961).
69. Stanko, G. L., and DeKay, H. G., *J. APhA, Sci. Ed.*, **47**, 104 (1958).
70. Heistand, E. N., *J. Pharm. Sci.*, **53**, 1 (1964).
71. Higuchi, W. I., *et al*, *J. Pharm. Sci.*, **54**, 510 (1965).
72. Matthews, B. A., and Rhodes, C. T., *J. Pharm. Sci.*, **57**, 569 (1968).
73. Barr, M., *J. APhA*, NS4, 180 (1964).
74. Bujake, J. E., *J. Pharm. Sci.*, **54**, 1599 (1965).
75. Kostenbauder, H. B., and Martin, A. N., *J. APhA, Sci. Ed.*, **43**, 401 (1954).
76. Boylan, J. C., *J. Pharm. Sci.*, **55**, 710 (1966).
77. Havemeyer, R. N., *J. APhA, Sci. Ed.*, **45**, 121 (1956).
78. Wood, J. H., and Lapham, E. A., *J. Pharm. Sci.*, **52**, 825 (1963).
79. Bernstein, H., and Barr, M., *J. APhA, Sci. Ed.*, **44**, 375 (1955).
80. Levy, G., *J. Pharm. Sci.*, **51**, 947 (1962).
81. Levy, G., *J. Pharm. Sci.*, **51**, 952 (1962).
82. Ober, S. S., *et al*, *J. APhA, Sci. Ed.*, **47**, 667 (1958).
83. Schwarz, T. W., and Levy, G., *J. APhA, Sci. Ed.*, **46**, 562 (1957).
84. Wood, J. H., *et al*, *J. Pharm. Sci.*, **52**, 354 (1963).
85. Levy, G., and Schwarz, T. W., *J. APhA, Sci. Ed.*, **47**, 451 (1958).
86. Powell, D. R., *et al*, *J. Pharm. Sci.*, **55**, 601 (1966).
87. Levy, G., and Schwarz, T. W., *J. APhA, Sci. Ed.*, **47**, 455 (1958),
88. Levy, G., *J. Pharm. Sci.*, **50**, 429 (1961),

27 | Separation

Countercurrent distribution—centrifugation—filtration—clarification and decoloration—lotion, decantation, and colation—expression—precipitation—separation of immiscible liquids—specialized separation techniques

This chapter was prepared by

Adelbert M. Knevel, PhD, *Professor of Medicinal Chemistry, School of Pharmacy and Pharmacal Sciences, Purdue University, Lafayette, Ind.   47907*

Separation may be defined as an operation which brings about the isolation and purification of a single chemical constituent or a group of chemical constituents. Many medicinal agents require some degree of purification before being incorporated into desirable dosage forms. The analysis of pharmaceutical preparations many times requires the separation of the chief constituent from other formulation constituents before quantitative measurement can be made.

While the problems of separation are the concern chiefly of pharmaceutical manufacturers, at times they may be encountered also by the pharmacist in his prescription laboratory or in the hospital pharmacy, so that all pharmacists should have knowledge of the principles underlying, and the techniques employed, in the basic processes of separation.

The processes of separation may be divided into two general categories—simple and complex—depending on the complexity of the method used.

Simple processes bring about separation of constituents through a single mechanical manipulation. Some examples of this type are the use of (1) a separatory funnel or pipette to separate two immiscible liquids such as water and ether; (2) a distillation process to separate two miscible liquids such as benzene and chloroform; (3) a garbling process to separate solids: and (4) centrifugation, filtration, and expression processes to separate solids from liquids.

Processes in this category are limited usually to separations of relatively simple mixtures or solutions.

Complex processes require the formation of a second phase by the addition of either a solid, liquid, or gas plus mechanical manipulation in order to bring about an effective separation. One example is the separation of acetylsalicylic acid from salicylic acid. In this mixture, salicylic acid is considered to be an impurity and, in order to separate the impurity from the desired constituent, a suitable solvent is added as a second phase to the mixture for the purpose of recrystallizing the acetylsalicylic acid. The contaminant remains in solution and is removed in the filtrate during the filtration process.

Fig. 250 shows the operations of separation for *complex mixtures* and is based on a separation scheme prepared by Harris[1] for the separation prior to analysis. The material of interest and the impurities are present initially as a solid, liquid, or gas (designated *Initial Phase*). The addition of a second phase—solid, liquid, or gas—is required with the object of effecting a separation in such a manner that one phase will contain the material of interest and the other, the impurities. There are nine major types of separation involving many processes shown. Certain of these processes will be covered in some detail here. Discus-

sions covering other pharmaceutical separations are found in such chapters as Complexation, Gases, Liquids, and Solids, Colloidal Dispersions, Particle Phenomena, Chromatography, and Extraction and Extractives.

Countercurrent Distribution

Countercurrent distribution (CCD) may be defined as a series of liquid–liquid extractions (immiscible solvents) conducted in a multiple-tube apparatus in which one phase is permitted to advance to the next tube in the series independently of the other phase.[2] The separation of the components in the mixture depends upon the distribution coefficients of each of the components, volume of the solvents used, and number of transfers taken.

Some important applications of CCD in the pharmaceutical sciences are (1) the isolation and purification of chemicals and biochemicals which might otherwise be damaged by the extremes of temperature or pH which occur during the separation processes, (2) the separation of a crude plant extract into its various alkaloidal fractions as a preparative step, (3) the determination of purity and homogeneity of chemicals and medicinal agents, and (4) the characterization of substances extracted from biochemical systems in

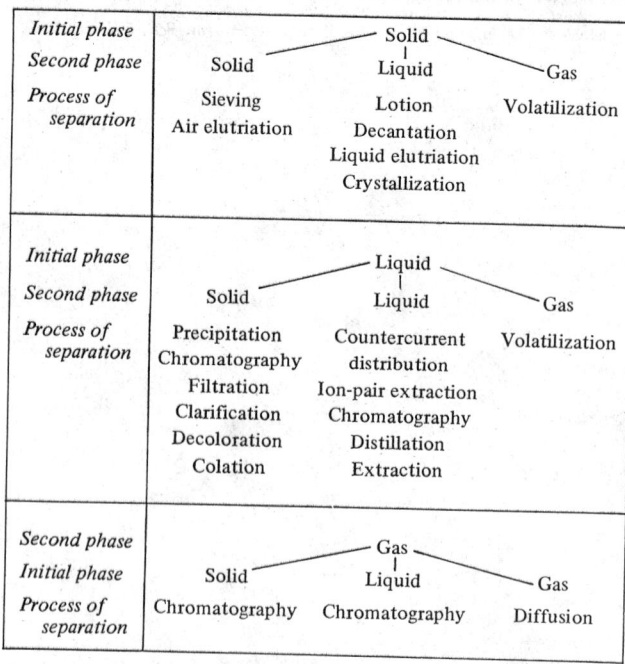

Initial phase		Solid	
Second phase	Solid	Liquid	Gas
Process of separation	Sieving Air elutriation	Lotion Decantation Liquid elutriation Crystallization	Volatilization
Initial phase		Liquid	
Second phase	Solid	Liquid	Gas
Process of separation	Precipitation Chromatography Filtration Clarification Decoloration Colation	Countercurrent distribution Ion-pair extraction Chromatography Distillation Extraction	Volatilization
Second phase		Gas	
Initial phase	Solid	Liquid	Gas
Process of separation	Chromatography	Chromatography	Diffusion

Fig. 250.   Separation involving complex processes.

studies determining the metabolic or biologic disposition of drugs.

Separation using CCD is based upon Nernst's Law. According to this law, if two practically immiscible solvents are in contact with each other and a substance which is soluble in each is added, the substance distributes itself in such a way that at equilibrium and at a given temperature the ratio of the concentrations of the two solutions is a constant. Strictly speaking, it is the activity ratio rather than the concentration ratio which remains constant. For most purposes, however, concentration values give satisfactory approximations.

When the ratio of concentrations expresses a distribution value for a single chemical species, the constant is designated as a partition coefficient or distribution coefficient, K, and may be expressed mathematically as

$$K = C_u/C_l \tag{1}$$

In this expression C_u and C_l represent concentrations in the upper and lower phases, respectively.

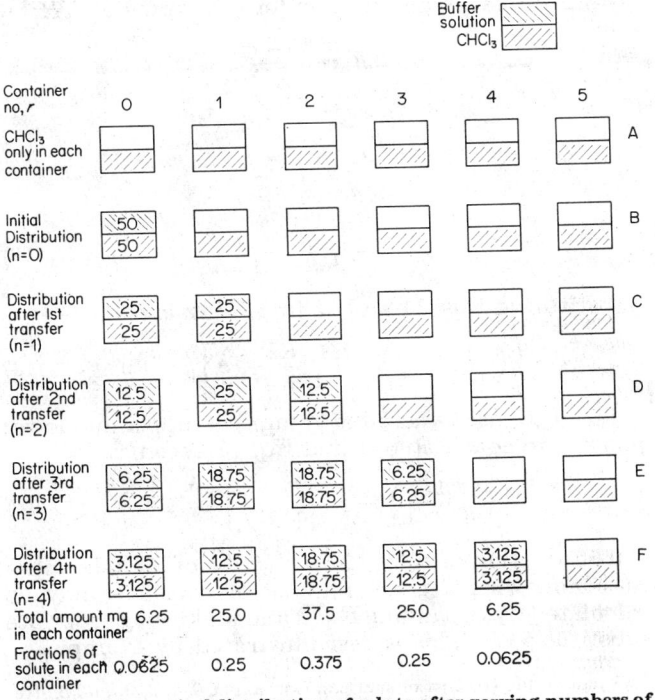

Fig. 251. Theoretical distribution of solute after varying numbers of transfer.

There is no accepted convention to date and the distribution coefficient could just as well be expressed as the reciprocal of Eq. 1, C_l/C_u.

In actual practice one deals with and measures total analytical concentrations and hence more than one chemical species is usually present in each phase. Rogers[3] has called this type of distribution the partition ratio and has defined it mathematically as $K_p = C_u/C_l$ where C_u and C_l represent total analytical concentrations of the chemical in the upper and lower phases, respectively. An example would be the distribution of benzoic acid between benzene and water. In the aqueous phase, benzoic acid would be present both in the ionized (A^-) and unionized form (HA). In benzene, benzoic acid would be present in the unionized form (HA) and in the dimerized form $(HA)_2$. The ratio expressing total benzoic acid in the organic phase and total benzoic acid in the aqueous phase is

called the partition ratio or the apparent distribution coefficient, K_p.

Although the purpose of using CCD is to bring about the separation of two or more substances, the basic principles of operation are best introduced by first considering the distribution pattern of a single solute.

First, assume that the solute under consideration has a distribution coefficient of unity when distributed between chloroform and buffer solution and that there are no deviations from Nernst's law of distribution due to molecular associations, dissociation, ionization, or chemical reactions.

Next, consider six containers such as 250-ml glass-stoppered Erlenmeyer flasks, each holding 50 ml of chloroform (lower phase) as shown in Fig. 251 (Row A). Add to container No. 0 100 mg of solute under consideration dissolved in 50 ml of buffer solution and shake until equilibrium has been established. Because equal volumes of solvent are used and the distribution coefficient of solute in these two solvents is unity, the solute at equilibrium will distribute itself in such a way that one-half is found in each of the upper and lower phases (Row B). Since 100 mg was originally present, 50 mg will be found in both layers of Container 0 (Row B).

Now, transfer the upper phase of Container 0 holding 50 mg of solute to Container 1 (Row B) and add fresh buffer solution to Container 0 (Row B). Shake both containers until equilibrium has been established. At equilibrium the quantity of solute in each phase of Containers 0 and 1 (Row C) will be 25 mg.

Next, transfer the upper phase of Container 1 (Row C) to Container 2 (Row C), and the upper phase of Container 0 (Row C) to Container 1. Add fresh buffer solution to Container 0 (Row C) and shake all three containers until equilibrium has been established. At equilibrium the quantity of solute (25 mg) in Container 2 (Row D) will have distributed itself so that one-half (12.5 mg) is in the upper phase and one-half (12.5 mg) is in the lower phase. Since 25 mg of solute was transferred to Container 1 from Container 0, 25 mg of solute will be present in each phase of Container 1 (Row D). The quantity (25 mg) of solute in Container 0 will distribute itself between the chloroform layer and freshly added buffer solution so that one-half (12.5 mg) will be present in each layer (Row D).

Continue this general procedure of transferring the upper phases of Containers 0, 1, and 2 to Containers 1, 2, and 3, respectively; then add fresh buffer to Container 0. Shake the four flasks until equilibrium is established. A distribution is obtained as shown in Row E. Continuing in a like manner will give a distribution as shown in Row F. A plot of the fraction (f) of solute in each container vs container number is shown in Fig. 252. The significance of this curve is that distribution of the solute shows a peak with the maximum quantity (fraction of solute) located in a specified container. In this case it is Container 2.

Fig. 252 illustrates the distribution of a solute after only four transfers. In actual practice between 8 and 200 containers or tubes are usually used in multiple extractions of this kind. The tubes are connected in series in a train and are rocked simultaneously rather than individually in order to bring about distribution of solutes between the two phases. The device also permits the transfer of upper phases to the next tube in series in one operation. A device of this type is shown in Fig. 253 and is called a countercurrent distribution apparatus.

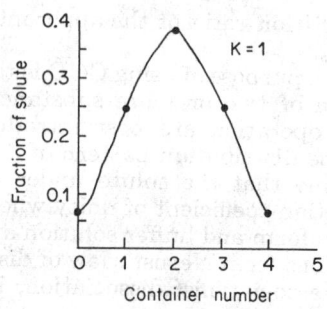

Fig. 252.   Distribution of solute after four transfers.

To study the distribution of a given solute after passage through a CCD apparatus containing many tubes, it is convenient to derive an equation which describes this distribution mathematically. For this purpose it is first necessary to recognize that the distribution may be expressed in terms of a binomial equation:

$$(q + p)^n = 1.0 \qquad (2)$$

where p and q represent the fraction of solute in the upper and lower phases, respectively, and n represents the number of transfers.

The terms p and q are related to the distribution coefficient, K, as follows:

$$p = \frac{\text{amount of solute in upper phase}}{\text{total solute}} = \frac{C_u V_u}{C_u V_u + C_l V_l} \qquad (3)$$

$$q = \frac{\text{amount of solute in lower phase}}{\text{total solute}} = \frac{C_l V_l}{C_u V_u + C_l V_l} \qquad (4)$$

where the subscript u and l represent upper and lower phases, respectively, C represents the concentration of solute in a given phase, and V represents volume of a given phase.

Dividing Eq. 3 by Eq. 4 gives

$$\frac{p}{q} = \frac{C_u V_u}{C_l V_l} \qquad (5)$$

Substituting K for C_u/C_l and R for the ratio of volumes, V_u/V_l, of solvent taken gives

$$\frac{p}{q} = KR \qquad (6)$$

Since p and q represent fractions of solute distributed

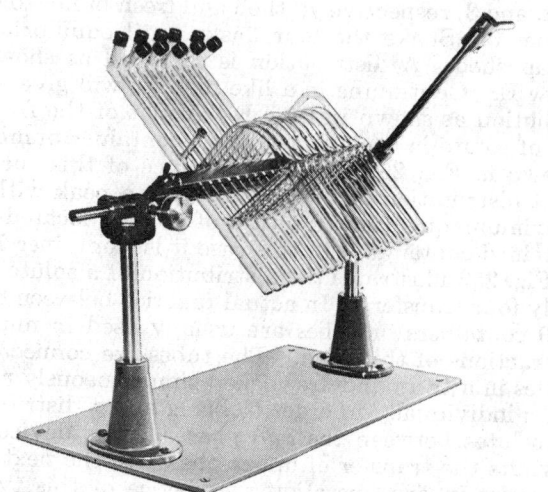

Fig. 253.   Poly-Stage Fractionator, a countercurrent distribution apparatus (courtesy, Pope).

in each phase, then at all times the sum is equal to unity.

$$q + p = 1.0 \qquad (7)$$

Rearranging Eq. 7 gives

$$q = 1 - p \qquad (8)$$

and

$$p = 1 - q \qquad (9)$$

Substituting Eq. 8 into Eq. 6 gives

$$KR = \frac{p}{1 - p} \qquad (10)$$

Rearranging and solving for p in terms of KR gives

$$KR - KRp = p$$

$$KR = p + KRp$$

$$KR = p(1 + KR)$$

$$p = \frac{KR}{1 + KR} \qquad (11)$$

In a similar manner, solve for q in terms of KR:

$$KR = \frac{1 - q}{q}$$

$$KRq = 1 - q$$

$$KRq + q = 1$$

$$q(KR + 1) = 1$$

$$q = \frac{1}{KR + 1} \qquad (12)$$

Substituting Eqs. 11 and 12 into Eq. 2 gives

$$\left[\left(\frac{1}{KR + 1} \right) + \left(\frac{KR}{1 + KR} \right) \right]^n = 1.0 \qquad (13)$$

In those cases where the volumes of upper and lower phases are equal, $R = 1$ and Eq. 13 becomes

$$\left[\left(\frac{1}{K + 1} \right) + \left(\frac{K}{1 + K} \right) \right]^n = 1.0 \qquad (14)$$

The fraction of solute in each tube of a CCD apparatus following a given number of transfers may be calculated by expanding Eq. 2 and making appropriate substitutions. This is best illustrated by example.

Calculate the fraction of solute in Containers 0, 1, 2, 3, and 4 after four transfers are made in a CCD apparatus using equal volumes of upper and lower phases. The K value for the solute in the solvent system is 1.0.

$$(q + p)^4 = 1q^4 + 4pq^3 + 6p^2q^2 + 4p^3q + 1p^4$$

Tube no.	0	1	2	3	4
Fraction solute/tube	0.0625	0.25	0.375	0.25	0.0625

Each term of the expanded binomial equation corresponds to a specific tube number. To determine the fraction of solute present in each tube, one simply solves for the corresponding term in the binomial equation as follows: Using Eqs. 11 and 12, determine the values for p and q. The fraction of solute in the desired tube is then calculated by substituting the appropriate values into the binomial term which corresponds to that tube: Tube $3 = 4p^3q = (4) (0.5)^3 (0.5) = 0.25$. This method of determining the fraction of solute in each tube becomes tedious when the number of tubes and transfers becomes large. However, any single term in the binomial expansion may be solved using Eq. 15:

$$f_{n,r} = \frac{n!}{r! \, (n - r)!} \, p^r q^{(n-r)} \qquad (15)$$

where n represents the number of transfers, r represents the specific

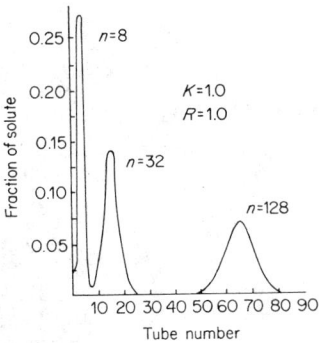

Fig. 254. Distribution of solute after varying numbers of transfers.

tube number, and $f_{n,r}$ represents the fraction of solute in the rth tube after n transfers. To determine the tube number which contains the maximum amount of solute, Eq. 16 is used:

$$r_{\max} = np \qquad (16)$$

Eq. 15 also may be written in terms of K and R as follows:

$$f_{n,r} = \frac{n!}{r!\,(n-r)!}\left(\frac{1}{1+KR}\right)^n (KR)^r \qquad (17)$$

Either equation may be used to calculate the fraction of solute present in a particular tube. The use of Eqs. 15, 16, and 17 will be illustrated as follows:

Calculate $r_{\max}$ and the fraction of solute in Containers 0, 1, 2, 3, and 4 after four transfers are made in a CCD apparatus using equal volumes of upper and lower phase. The K value for the solute in the solvent system is 1.0.

$$r_{\max} = (4)(0.5) = 2$$

(Tube 2 contains maximum quantity of solute.)

$$f_{4,3} = \frac{4!}{3!\,(4-3)!}\,(0.5)^3(0.5)^1 = 0.25$$

By Eq. 17:

$$f_{4,3} = \frac{4!}{3!\,(4-3)!}\left[\frac{1}{1+1}\right]^4 (1)^3 = 0.25$$

By similar calculations the fraction of solute in Tubes 0, 1, 2, and 4 are found to equal

$$f_{4,0} = 0.0625$$

$$f_{4,1} = 0.25$$

$$f_{4,2} = 0.375$$

$$f_{4,4} = 0.0625$$

When a large number of transfers (>50) are made and K is near unity it is more convenient to use a Gaussian treatment[3] to calculate the fraction of solute in a particular tube. The appropriate equations are:

$$y_x = \frac{1.00}{\sqrt{2\pi nKR/(KR+1)^2}} \cdot$$

$$\exp\left\{-\left(\frac{x^2}{2nKR/(KR+1)^2}\right)\right\} \qquad (18)$$

$$r_{\max} = \frac{nKR}{KR+1} \qquad (19)$$

where y_x represents the fraction of solute with distribution coefficient K in the tube that is x distant from the peak tube; e is the base of the natural logarithm ($\pi = 3.14$); K, R, and n are terms which have been previously defined; and $r_{\max}$ represents the number of the tube containing the maximum amount of solute.

The use of these equations will be illustrated in the following example.

Calculate the fraction of solute in the peak tube, y_0, and six neighboring tubes (y_1, y_{-1}, y_2, y_{-2}, y_3, and y_{-3}) in a 100-transfer experiment in which K for the solute and R for the solvent ratio equal unity.

1. Locate the *number* of the tube (peak tube) containing the maximum fraction of solute using Eq. 19.

$$r_{\max} = \frac{nKR}{KR+1} = \frac{(100)(1)(1)}{(1)(1)+1} = 50$$

2. Determine the fraction of solute in peak tube designated $r_{\max}$ or y_0. To facilitate calculations, first solve for $\dfrac{2nKR}{(KR+1)^2}$, then substitute its value, 50, in this case and the corresponding value of x in Eq. 18.

$$y_0 = \frac{1.00}{\sqrt{3.14 \times 50}} \cdot e^0 = 0.0798$$

3. The fraction of solute in the neighboring tubes are then determined as follows:

Tubes 51 and 49; $y_1 = y_{-1} = y_0 e^{-1/50} =$

$$0.0798 \cdot e^{-0.02} = 0.0782$$

Tubes 52 and 48; $y_2 = y_{-2} = y_0 e^{-4/50} =$

$$0.0798 \cdot e^{-0.08} = 0.0737$$

Tubes 53 and 47; $y_3 = y_{-3} = y_0 e^{-9/50} =$

$$0.0798 \cdot e^{-0.18} = 0.0667$$

Distribution curves may be prepared from hypothetical data using Eqs. 15–19 or from a computer program utilizing these equations. Fig. 254 illustrates a series of curves for a solute in which $K = 1.0$ and $R = 1.0$ following 8, 32, and 128 transfers. It is interesting to observe that as the number of transfers increases, the amplitude of the curve decreases and the solute spreads through more and more tubes.

At first thought, this would seem undesirable, but the significant point is that the fraction of vessels containing solute after 128 transfers is now much less than after 10 transfers. Therefore, two solutes with different but similar K values can be separated in 128 transfers because each solute occupies a smaller fraction of total tubes. If this separation were attempted with 10 to 20 transfers, both solutes would occupy nearly all of the tubes and no separation would be obtained.

Fig. 252 illustrates the distribution patterns obtained in a 16-transfer experiment for solutes having different distribution coefficients. Under no circumstances can a separation be obtained if the distribution coefficients of the solutes are equal.

The procedure of operation which has been considered thus far is known as the *fundamental procedure*. Here the solute is distributed through a specified number of tubes and nothing is withdrawn from the system until the entire operation is completed. Then

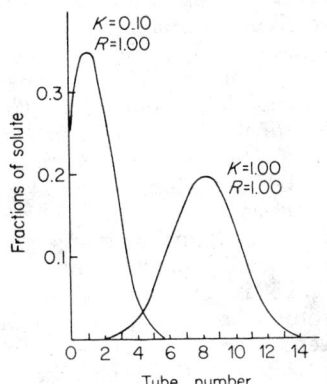

Fig. 255. Distribution of two solutes with different K values.

the tube contents are withdrawn and analyzed for the purpose of determining solute concentrations or the solutes are withdrawn simply for the purpose of isolating them from a mixture.

Another procedure of operation which is of interest primarily due to its analogy to elution chromatography is known as *end withdrawal*. In this operation the fundamental procedure is followed for a predetermined number of transfers as previously described. Then the upper phase only of the last tube in the train is collected. All other upper phases are advanced to the next tube in succession and after equilibration the upper phase of the last tube, n, is again collected. This process is continued until all upper phases have passed through n tubes containing lower phase.

In elution chromatography, as previously stated, the analogy is similar. However, fresh upper phase is added continuously to the first "tube" (called a "plate" in elution chromatography) until the solute travels a desired distance.

In summary, the degree of separation of two or more solutes using CCD depends upon the distribution coefficients of the solutes, nature and volume of the solvents used, and number of transfers taken.

Another application of CCD is the determination of the purity of a sample using a graphical approach.[4] The following equation is relevant.

$$\left[\log D - \log \left(\frac{n!}{r! \ (n-r)!} \right) \right] =$$
$$\log D_t - n \log (K+1) + r \log K \quad (20)$$

where D is the amount of solute in a given tube (r) expressed in any convenient units (weight, absorbance, etc), D_t is the total amount of solute in all tubes of the distribution, n is the number of transfers in the distribution, and K is the distribution coefficient in which equal volumes of solvent are used.

Eq. 20 may be treated as an equation for a straight line ($y = mx + b$):

$$\left[\log D - \log \left(\frac{n!}{r! \ (n-r)!} \right) \right] \text{ vs } r \quad (21)$$

A plot of the terms within the brackets along the y-axis vs r along the x-axis yields a single straight line for a pure sample. The slope of the line is $\log K$. If there are more than one straight-line regions, each section represents one component that has been isolated. As before, the slope of the line is equal to $\log K$.

When one of the straight-line regions is extrapolated to $r = 0$, the value for $\log D_t - n \log (K+1)$ is obtained from which the total amount, D_t, of a given component in the original sample is obtained. Sections of the plot which are curved correspond to unresolved mixtures of two or more components.

CCD also is used widely as an adjunct in the analytical determination of medicinal agents in biologic disposition studies. Way and Afifi[5] studied the biologic disposition of methotrimeprazine and employed CCD and partition behavior at varying pH values to characterize the UV-absorbing material extracted from the carcasses of mice.

In biologic studies of this type an eight-plate transfer separation is usually carried out. The apparatus as shown in Fig. 253 is very convenient for this purpose but is not absolutely necessary. Separations may be conducted in separatory funnels, centrifuge bottles, or other similar materials. The use of the CCD principle in a biologic disposition study is illustrated in the following example.

Table I

Tube no.	Absorbance A_r	Fraction of solute/tube	
		Exptl $f_r = A_r/A_t$	Calc
0	0.012	0.0034	0.0032
1	0.116	0.033	0.027
2	0.352	0.099	0.099
3	0.720	0.202	0.208
4	0.960	0.27	0.27
5	0.800	0.23	0.23
6	0.420	0.12	0.12
7	0.152	0.043	0.036
8	0.020	0.006	0.005
	A_t 3.552		

Suppose we are interested in determining if a UV absorbing material extracted from a biologic sample (brain, blood, etc) of an experimental animal previously administered a given amine-type drug is the same material as the product originally administered.

Comparing UV spectra usually is not sufficient for identification purposes because molecular alterations of the original compound may give an almost identical UV spectrum. Hence, the extracted material is distributed in an eight-plate transfer apparatus using two suitable solvents such as cyclohexane and phosphate buffer. (The two solvents should be saturated with each other before they are used in the distribution study; this can be accomplished readily by first placing both solvents in a large separatory funnel and shaking intermittently for 8 hours.)

After the distribution is completed a sufficient amount of dilute NaOH solution is added to each tube to render the aqueous phase alkaline. Under these conditions practically all of the amine base partitions into the organic phase. An aliquot of the organic phase is taken from each tube and analyzed spectrometrically and from this data the fraction of amine in each tube is calculated and recorded as shown in Table I. A graph (Fig. 256) is prepared by drawing a smooth curve through the points obtained by plotting the fraction of each tube vs the tube number. This curve is designated the experimental curve and from it one obtains, by inspection, the value, r_{max}, on the x-axis which corresponds to the maximum of the curve. This value does not necessarily have to be a whole number. Using Eq. 19, the distribution coeffi-

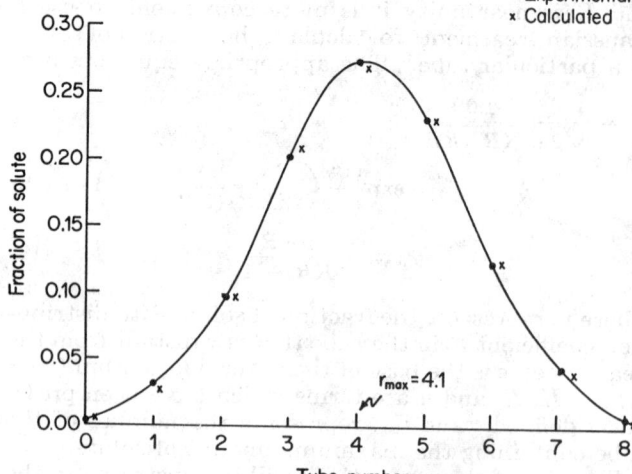

Fig. 256. **Experimental and calculated curves of extracted medicinal agent.**

cient is determined and the fraction of solute in each tube may be calculated using Eq. 17. Both equations have been repeated here for convenience.

$$f_{n,r} = \frac{n!}{r!\,(n-r)!} \left(\frac{1}{1+KR}\right)^n (KR)^r \qquad (17)$$

$$r_{max} = \frac{nKR}{KR+1} \qquad (19)$$

It can be shown that in an eight-plate transfer system the fraction of solute in a given tube is related to the $(r-1)$th tube by the following equation:

$$f_r = FKf_{r-1} \qquad (22)$$

where $F = (n+1-r)/r$.

If the apparatus is such that the lower phase is transferred from tube to tube, the following equation is used:

$$f_r = F'(1/K)f_{r+1} \qquad (23)$$

where

$$F' = \frac{(r+1)}{(n-r)} \qquad (24)$$

Assume that the absorbance values listed in Table I were obtained in an eight-plate transfer system in which the upper phase was transferred. From Fig. 256, the maximum value obtained by inspection of the x-axis is found to equal 4.1. Rearranging Eq. 19 and solving for K gives

$$K = \frac{r_{max}}{(n-r_{max})} = \frac{4.1}{(8-4.1)} = 1.05$$

The fraction of solute in Tube 0 is found by using the following equation:

$$f_0 = \left[\frac{1}{K+1}\right]^n = \left[\frac{1}{1.05+1}\right]^8 = (0.488)^8 = 0.0032$$

Using Eq. 22 the fraction of solute in Tubes 1 through 8 are found to equal

$$
\begin{aligned}
f_1 &= FKf_0 = (8)(1.05)(0.0032) = 0.027\\
f_2 &= FKf_{r-1} = FKf_{2-1} = FKf_1 =\\
&\quad (7/2)(1.05)(0.027) = 0.099\\
f_3 &= FKf_2 = (6/3)(1.05)(0.099) = 0.208\\
f_4 &= FKf_3 = (5/4)(1.05)(0.208) = 0.274\\
f_5 &= FKf_4 = (4/5)(1.05)(0.274) = 0.231\\
f_6 &= FKf_5 = (3/6)(1.05)(0.231) = 0.121\\
f_7 &= FKf_6 = (2/7)(1.05)(0.121) = 0.036\\
f_8 &= FKf_7 = (1/8)(1.05)(0.036) = 0.005
\end{aligned}
$$

These calculated values are then plotted on the same graph as that used for the experimental values (Fig. 256). A comparison of the two sets of data in Fig. 256 indicates that the substance extracted from the biologic sample is a single compound. If two or more substances had been present, deviations of the data would have been observed.

In order to identify the compound in the extracted material, distribution ratios of authentic medicinal agent in an organic solvent–water system at various pH values of the aqueous phase are compared to those obtained from the extracted substance recovered from sacrificed animals receiving the original drug. Detailed instructions for this portion of the study may be obtained from the work of Way and Afifi.[5]

Centrifugation

A large number of separations may be accomplished with the centrifuge. This instrument consists essentially of a container in which a mixture of solid and liquid, or of two liquids, is rotated at high speeds so that the mixture is separated into its constituent parts by the action of centrifugal force. A solid or liquid, mixed with a liquid of lesser density, may be separated since the substance of higher specific gravity is thrown outward with greater force and therefore will be impelled to the bottom of the container leaving a clear supernatant layer of pure liquid.

Centrifugation is particularly useful when separation by ordinary filtration is difficult, eg, in separating a highly viscous mixture. Separations may be accomplished more rapidly in a centrifuge than under the action of gravity. In addition, the degree of separation which is attainable may be greater since the forces available are of a far higher order of magnitude. The centrifuge has become a valuable analytical tool, particularly in biochemical and bacteriological research. It has wide application in pharmaceutical laboratories and its use as a means of predicting emulsion stability has been suggested recently.

Two basic types of centrifuges are available: *sedimentation* and *filtration*. The *sedimentation type* of centrifuge depends on differences in the densities of the two or more phases comprising the mixture. The efficiency of the process depends on the velocity of rotation to which the mixture is subjected.

Sedimentation Centrifuges

The design of the bottle centrifuge and the disc centrifuge are based on the sedimentation principle (ie, separation by density difference).

Bottle Centrifuge—This type of centrifuge (Fig. 257) consists of a vertical spindle that rotates the containers in a horizontal plane and is commonly used to separate materials of different densities. Separation in a centrifugal field is brought about because denser particles in a mixture require greater forces to hold them in a circular path of a given radius than lighter particles. Thus, the lighter particles are displaced toward the axis of the centrifuge by the heavier particles. During the centrifugation of blood, for example, a speed of 3000 rpm is required to separate blood corpuscles from serum. If the radius of the centrifuge is assumed to be 10 cm, the acceleration, a, acting on a particle can be approximated to be 10^6 cm/sec^2, or about 1000 times the acceleration due to gravity (g):

$$
\left[
\begin{aligned}
&a = 4\pi^2 N^2 r = \frac{4(3.14)^2(3000)^2(10)}{3600} = 10^6 \text{ cm/sec}^2\\[4pt]
&N = \text{revolutions/sec}; \quad r = \text{radius in cm}\\[4pt]
&\frac{10^6 \text{ cm/sec}^2}{10^3 \text{ cm/sec}^2} = 1000 \ (g)\\[4pt]
&10^3 \text{ cm/sec}^2 = \text{approximate acceleration due to gravity}
\end{aligned}
\right]
$$

Under these conditions the blood corpuscles eventually migrate under the influence of centrifugal force to the tip of the centrifuge tube.

The fundamental equation relevant to centrifugation is Newton's second law of motion which may be expressed mathematically as follows:

$$F = ma \qquad (25)$$

where F is the force in dynes, m is the mass in Gm, and a is the acceleration in cm/sec^2.

It can be shown[6] that angular velocity and linear or tangential velocity are related by the following equation:

$$v = \omega r \qquad (26)$$

and

$$\omega = 2\pi N \qquad (27)$$

where v is the tangential velocity, ω is the angular velocity, N is the number of rps, and r is the radius in cm.

Further, it can be shown that centripetal (centrifugal) acceleration is related to tangential velocity and radius by the following equation:

$$a = v^2/r \qquad (28)$$

Squaring Eq. 26 and substituting into Eq. 28 gives

$$a = r^2\omega^2/r = r\omega^2 \qquad (29)$$

Substituting Eq. 27 into Eq. 29 gives

$$a = r(2\pi N)^2 = 4\pi^2 N^2 r \qquad (30)$$

Finally, substituting Eq. 30 into Eq. 25 gives

$$F = 4\pi^2 N^2 rm \qquad (31)$$

In order to express force in Gm rather than in dynes, the right side of Eq. 31 is divided by g, the acceleration due to gravity:

$$F' = 4\pi^2 N^2 rm/g \qquad (32)$$

where F' is the force in Gm. As a convenience, N is expressed in rpm rather than rps. Substituting numerical values into Eq. 32 as indicated gives

$$F' = 4(3.14)^2 N^2 rm/(980.7)(60)^2 = 0.00001117 rN^2 m \qquad (33)$$

Eq. 33 is frequently found in reference texts and is used primarily as a basis to design centrifuges.

An equation which is especially useful when centrifuges are to be compared without regard to the physical characteristics of a particle or its surrounding fluid, is obtained by dividing both sides of Eq. 33 by m:

$$a = F'/m = 0.00001117 rN^2 \qquad (34)$$

The separation of particles in a liquid medium depends on the nature of the medium. A solid particle settling under the influence of acceleration due to gravity in a liquid phase accelerates until a constant terminal velocity is reached. The terminal velocity is known as the settling velocity of the particle and is described mathematically by Stokes' Law.[7] It can be shown that Stokes' law can be extended to those cases where settling takes place in a centrifugal field:

$$v_s = v_g \frac{\omega^2 r}{g} \qquad (35)$$

where v_s is the settling velocity of a particle in a centrifugal field, v_g is the settling velocity of a particle in a gravitational field (Stokes' law), ω is the angular velocity of the particle in the settling zone, and r is the radius at which the settling velocity is determined.

Consider a solid particle at an initial position in a liquid medium and a distance r from the axis of rotation. Under these conditions

$$v_s = dr/dt \qquad (36)$$

Substituting Eq. 36 into Eq. 35 gives

$$dr/dt = v_g \frac{\omega^2 r}{g} \qquad (37)$$

Rearranging and integrating between limits gives

$$\int_r^{rc} \frac{dr}{r} = \int_0^t v_g \frac{\omega^2 r}{g}\, dt \qquad (38)$$

$$\ln \frac{r_c}{r} = v_g \frac{\omega^2 t}{g} \qquad (39)$$

where r_c is the distance between the surface of the sedimented cake in the tip of the tube and the axis of rotation and t is the time during which the particle is subjected to centrifugal acceleration while the particle travels the distance from r to r_c. Eq. 39 shows that if centrifuging conditions for a given suspension are to be compared in different centrifuges, the speed, bottle size, centrifuge dimensions, and centrifuging time must be taken into consideration. Ambler and Keith[7] and Lavanchy and Keith[8] mathematically describe approaches which should be taken for this purpose.

Disc Centrifuge—This unit basically consists of a stack of thinly spaced discs situated within a cylindrical bowl. The discs serve to reduce the settling distance from the depth of the liquid to the distance between the disc surfaces. Thus, small amounts of solids of fine particle size may be deposited rapidly on the discs in an efficient and continuous manner. The De Laval Separator Co., Poughkeepsie, N.Y., makes available a number of models of disc-type centrifuges.

The principle of operation of a disc centrifuge may be more clearly understood by reference to Fig. 258. This diagram represents a concept of the De Laval Model 65 "Uni-Matic." The feed material containing oil, water, and solids is fed in at the top inlet (A).

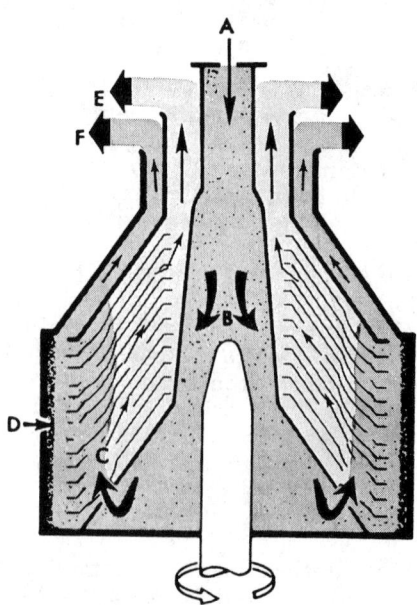

Fig. 258. Operation of disc bowl centrifuge.

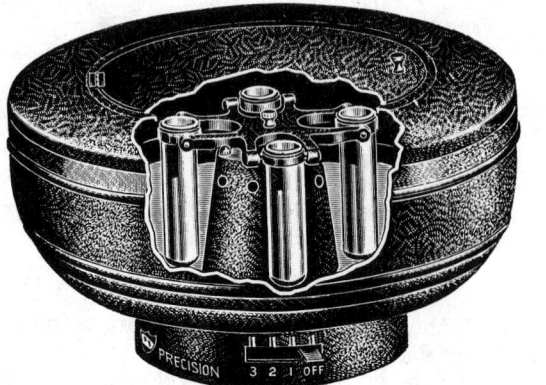

Fig. 257. Covered laboratory centrifuge (courtesy, Precision).

The mixture travels down the inlet tube (B) into the centrifuge bowl. The bowl speed is usually about 60,000 rpm, an optimum efficiency speed which generates a force of greater than 10,000 times the force of gravity.

The mixture is forced upward through the holes in the intermediate discs (C) and into the spaces between them. This is where centrifugal action separates the mixture immediately into the heavy and light phases (oil, water, and solids). The solids are thrown directly to the bowl wall (D). The oil, with its lighter density, is displaced inward and travels upward through the space around the inlet tube to the light phase discharge (E). The heavy phase, thrown outward by centrifugal force, is displaced by incoming feed material and travels upward along the outer edge of the bowl to the heavy phase discharge (F).

Filtration Methods

Whereas the sedimentation centrifuge may be used for separating both solid–liquid and liquid–liquid mixtures, the use of the filtration centrifuge is restricted to the former system. The filtration centrifuge is similar in principle to the sedimentation type but rather than containers it possesses a porous wall through which the liquid phase may pass but upon which the solid phase is retained. An example is the *basket centrifuge* (Fig. 259). Analogous to filtration, this process requires consideration of the flow of liquid through the solid bed which accumulates on the porous plate.

Continuous Centrifuges

These machines are commonly used in industry for the separation of mother liquor from crystals, the clarification of liquids, and a number of other large-scale operations. Several mechanical principles have been applied to produce a variety of continuous centrifuges.

Tubular Centrifuge—For a given force acting on a material in a centrifuge, the stress in the walls of the basket is lowest when the radius of the basket is small. The supercentrifuge (Fig. 260) consists of a basket with a 4-in. diameter and which is up to $3\frac{1}{2}$ ft in length. Mixtures are subjected to a separating force as high as 62,000 times the force of gravity.

The liquid to be centrifuged is fed by either gravity or pressure to the feed tube at the bottom of the unit. By means of the feed nozzle, the mixture is introduced into the rotor. The rotor may attain speeds up to 60,000 rpm. The large centrifugal force generated by this high speed acts in a direction perpendicular to the axis of rotation.

Under the influence of this centrifugal force, separation takes place. Solids present in the liquid are deposited against the walls of the rotor. Discharge of the two separated liquids takes place through separate discharge ports at the top of the rotor.

The Ultracentrifuge—When extremely fine solid matter must be separated from a liquid, eg, in colloid research, the ultracentrifuge is employed. In this instrument a relatively small rotor is operated at speeds exceeding 100,000 rpm and forces up to one million times gravity are exerted. High speeds are attained with air or oil turbines and bearings lubricated with a film of compressed air. Friction heat may be minimized by the use of high vacuum.

By placing the colloidal dispersion in specially constructed cells and spinning them in the ultracentrifuge, it is possible to separate the dispersed phase from the continuous phase rather rapidly. To aid the investigator, optical attachments may be employed to photograph the settling while the centrifuge is in operation.

Only small batches of material can be handled in these instruments during a single run. Ultracentrifuges are employed in the determination of particle size and molecular weight of polymeric and other high-molecular-weight materials such as proteins and nucleic acids by direct or indirect observation of the rate of separation of particles in solution or suspension.

Filtration

Filtration is the process of separating liquids from solids with the purpose of obtaining optically transparent liquids. This is accomplished by the intervention of a porous substance, called the *filter* or the *filtering medium*. The liquid which has passed through the filter is called the *filtrate*.

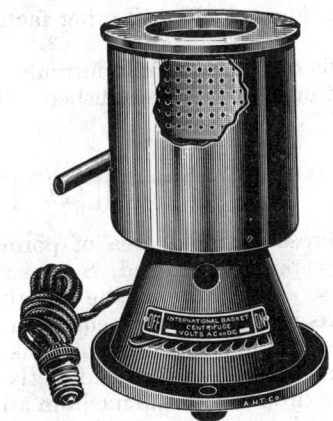

Fig. 259. Laboratory centrifuge (courtesy, Thomas).

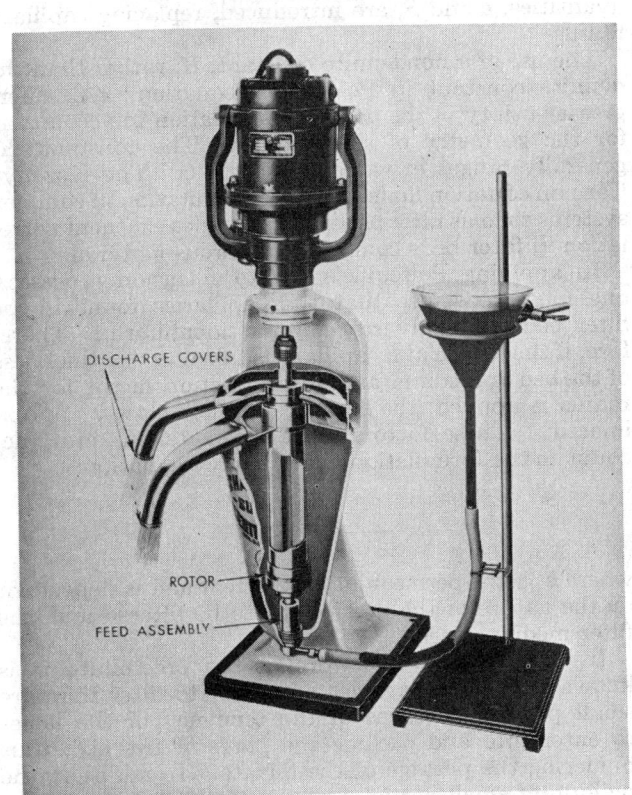

Fig. 260. Sharples laboratory supercentrifuge.

Mathematics of Filtration

In 1842 Poiseuille proposed a relationship for streamlined flow of liquids under pressure through capillaries. This equation in its simplified form is represented by

$$V = \frac{\pi \Delta p r^4}{8L\eta}$$

where V = flow velocity, r = capillary radius, L = capillary length, η = viscosity of the fluid, and Δp = pressure differential at the two ends of the capillary.

The modified Poiseuille equation has been shown to be valid for liquid flow through sand, glass beads, and various porous media. It represents the foundation for all mathematical models of filtration which were subsequently developed. Of critical importance in this equation is the powerful effect of capillary radius, ie, by reducing it to ⅛ its size, the pressure differential must be increased more then 4000 times in order to obtain the same flow velocity, all other factors remaining constant.

On the basis of the Poiseuille formula, the Kozeny–Carman relationship was established. This may be expressed as

$$V = \left[\frac{e^3}{KS^2(1-e)^2}\right]\left[\frac{A\Delta pg}{\eta L}\right]$$

where A = cross-sectional area of porous bed (filter medium), e = porosity of bed, S = surface area of medium, K = constant, and the remaining symbols are the same as in the Poiseuille equation.

The Kozeny–Carman relationship, like Poiseuille's law, states that the rate of flow is directly proportional to the pressure drop across the medium and to the area of the bed, and inversely proportional to the viscosity of the liquid and the thickness of the bed. To characterize the material composing the bed, two new quantities, e and S, are introduced, replacing capillary radius.

The use of a nondefinite constant, K, rather than the definite constant in Poiseuille's equation, $\pi/8$, offers greater utility in the use of this equation in accounting for the geometry of the medium. The constant, K, generally ranges in value from 3 to 6. The Kozeny–Carman equation finds its greatest limitation in complex systems such as filter paper but provides excellent correlation in filter beds composed of porous material.

In applying Poiseuille's law to filtration processes, one must recognize that the capillaries found in the filter bed are highly irregular and nonuniform. Therefore, if the length of a capillary is taken as the thickness of the bed or medium and the correction factor for the radius is applied, the flow rate is more closely approximated. These factors have been taken into account in the formulation of the Darcy equation:

$$V = \frac{k\Delta p}{L\eta}$$

where k = the permeability coefficient and is dependent on the nature of the precipitate to be filtered and the filter medium itself.

In considering the nature of the precipitate it is known that large particles are easier to filter than are small particles because of the tendency of the latter to enter into and occlude the pores of the bed, thus hindering the passage of the filtrate. In addition, the buildup of small particles on the filter tends to form a nonporous, densely packed bed which also resists passage of the filtrate.

Filtering Media

The filtering medium, whether a filter paper, synthetic fiber, or porous bed of glass, sand, or stone, is composed of countless channels which impart *porosity* to the medium. Almost without exception these channels or pores are nonuniform and possess a rather tortuous nature.

The mechanism of filtration basically involves a two-step process: (1) the filter medium itself resists the flow of solid material while permitting the passage of liquid and (2) during the course of the filtration the suspended, solid material builds up on the filter medium and therby forms a *filter bed* which acts a second, and often more efficient, filter medium.

The ability of a filter medium to eliminate solid matter from a liquid is termed *retention*. It must be borne in mind that the filtration process must compromise retention with filtration rate, ie, the speed at which the purified liquid (the filtrate) is recovered. To illustrate this point, it will be noted that a slab of marble will most effectively retain the solid material contained in a suspension; unfortunately, it would require a few centuries to collect the purified filtrate.

Both the retentive ability of a filter medium and filtration rate of a liquid through the medium are dependent on the porosity of the medium. Each factor, however, is influenced significantly by the following: (1) the viscosity of the liquid, (2) the proportion of solid matter in the liquid, and (3) the size, shape, and physical nature of the suspended solids.

The flow of a liquid through a filter bed follows the same basic rules that govern the flow of any liquid through a medium offering resistance. The flow rate through the medium will vary directly with the area of the medium, as well as the pressure drop or driving force across the bed.

$$\text{Rate of flow} \propto \frac{(\text{driving force})(\text{cross-sectional area})}{\text{resistance}}$$

The flow rate is retarded by the viscosity of the liquid being filtered and by any obstruction to flow. These obstructions include the resistance of the filter medium itself and the second filter bed or filter cake which builds up on the medium at a rate dependent on the solids content of the liquid. The resistance offered by the medium itself will not vary significantly during the filtration process. It is dependent on the thickness of the medium as well as its porosity. The resistance of the filter cake, on the other hand, is not constant and generally increases continuously during the operation. The resistance offered by the cake is dependent both on its thickness and physical nature. The thickness of the cake is dictated by the amount of filtrate passing through the filter and on the solids content of the liquid. The physical nature of the cake, ie, whether it is loose, compacted, coarse, fine, granular or gelatinous, determines whether or not it will readily allow the flow of liquid.

Paper Filters—Paper filters are the most useful filters for the community pharmacist and are employed in all operations requiring clarification. The solid materials are separated more completely by filtration through high quality paper filters than through strainers because the pores of the paper are smaller. In addition, the large number of these pores allows for a relatively rapid filtration rate. The paper used for this purpose is especially prepared, and is termed *filter paper*. It is manufactured on a large scale and can be had of excellent quality. Unlike a strainer, it is rarely used

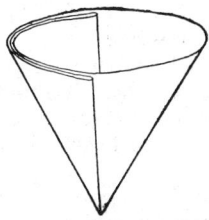

Fig. 261.   Plain filter.

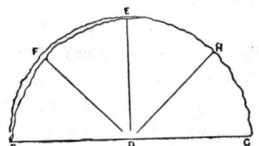

Fig. 262.   Folding plaited filter.

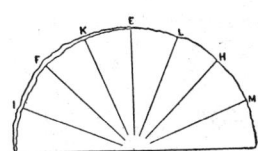

Fig. 263.   Folding plaited filter.

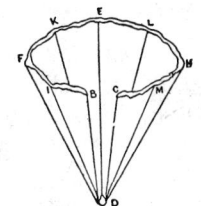

Fig. 264.   Folding plaited filter.

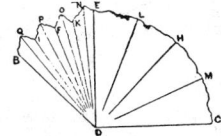

Fig. 265.   Folding plaited filter.

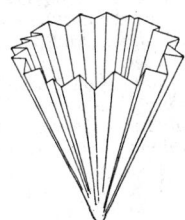

Fig. 266.   Plaited filter.

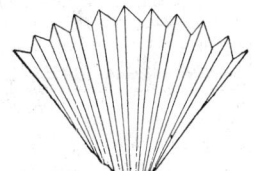

Fig. 267.   Plaited filter parallel folds.

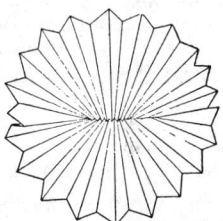

Fig. 268.   Plaited filter, inside view.

more than once; its cost is so trifling, and it is so easily ruptured when wet, that it is not worthwhile to attempt to save filters for subsequent use. Filter paper is generally supplied in two forms—large, square sheets and circular sheets available in a number of different sizes. The former is used for large-scale filtration processes. The pharmacist generally uses circular sheets.

The filtering medium must always be regarded as a possible source of contamination to the finished solution. Thus, for all pharmaceutical operations a high-quality filter paper must be used.

Methods of Folding Filtering Paper—Filter papers are used in two ways—*plain* and *plaited*.

Plain Filter—This is the form of filter used by the analytical chemist and preferred when precipitates are to be collected (Fig. 261); it is made by doubling a circular sheet of filtering paper upon itself, and folding this directly in the middle, so that, when opened, four equal divisions or sectors appear. The filter is used by separating one of the sectors from the other three, and placing the cone formed into a funnel; the liquid is poured on the filter and the process of filtration commences. The advantages of the plain filter are (1) simplicity and rapidity in folding and (2) in collecting precipitates, only ½ of the surface of the filter (two sectors) is in contact with the moist precipitate, which is often closely adherent, and therefore ½ of the surface has to be washed free when the precipitate is collected. In some cases there may be a disadvantage in the use of the plain filter in that the unequal rate of flow, caused by the tendency of the three folds to attract the liquid to the side of the funnel on which they rest, results in the precipitate not being uniformly washed. If the sides of the funnel have an angle of 60°, the plain filter made as described will fit the funnel properly; but it frequently happens that the angles of funnels vary, and if an ordinary plain filter is placed in a funnel not having an angle of 60°, a portion of the filter is left unsupported and the weight of the liquid may rupture the moist paper. This difficulty may be overcome by making a fresh crease in the outside fold of the plain filter; if this is made to the right of the original crease of the 60° filter, and the inside fold pushed around a corresponding distance, a filter having a smaller angle is produced, while if the fresh crease is made to the left of the original crease, a larger angled filter may be made.

Plaited Filter—This may well be called the "pharmacist's filter," for it is the form largely used in ordinary filtering operations. It is advantageous in that it produces a much faster filtration rate than the plain filter since the effective filtration surface is considerably increased. Figs. 262 to 268 show the progressive steps in the folding of a plaited filter. It is made by folding a circular sheet of filtering paper twice, as in making a plain filter. The edge *BD* (Fig. 262) is then laid on *ED*, and the crease *FD* is formed; in like manner *CD* is laid on *ED*, and *HD* is formed. Then *BD* is laid on *FD*, and *ID* is formed, and by rolling over the fold

in the same direction once more until *FD* is laid on *ED*, the crease *KD* is made (Fig. 263). In the same way *CD* is laid on *HD* and *HD* upon *ED*, and it will be noticed that the folded semicircle has been creased into eight equal spaces, and that the direction of each crease is the same, so that if the paper is lifted it will appear as shown in Fig. 264.

The next step is to fold each one of these spaces *back on itself* (Fig. 265). *BD* is laid on *FD*, and *BD* is turned upward and back until it is laid on *ID*. This makes the crease *QD*, which is the first fold in the opposite direction. Taking both folds between the forefingers and thumbs of both hands, the edges *BD* and *ID* are folded upward and back on *FD*, and the crease *PD* is formed; these three edges, *BD*, *ID*, and *FD*, are taken all together and folded back on *KD*, and the crease *OD* is formed, and so on, each space in turn being folded back in the opposite direction until the last one is reached. The folded filter is held at the apex with the left hand on a table or flat counter, pressed and smoothed out with the right hand in order to emphasize the folds. It should be placed in the funnel, while still unopened, to see whether it needs trimming; if the edges of the filter project above the top of the funnel, the filter must be removed and the edges must be cut off neatly so that the entire filter may be placed inside of the funnel.

General Considerations

1. In folding a filter, care should be observed not to extend the creases entirely to the apex, but to end them at a distance of about half an inch from it, because the point at which all the creases converge would be thereby so weakened that the weight of the liquid may rupture the filter. When the filter has been plaited and the creases emphasized by pressure, it is then carefully opened, placed in a dry funnel, and pressed firmly into place so that the point enters the throat of the funnel. The speed of filtration is markedly increased if

this precaution is carefully observed. When a filter is carelessly placed in the funnel, it forms a bag at the apex, which readily breaks, or clings to the sides of the funnel, which reduces the filtration rate.

2. The filter in the funnel should be moistened with the liquid to be filtered or with a liquid corresponding to the solvent employed. This promotes a more rapid filtration. Washing the filter with the appropriate solvent also insures reduced contamination.

3. When a filter paper must withstand a high degree of pressure, eg, a large volume of solution, vacuum, etc, a double filter may be used. In analytical operations the apex of the filter is usually supported by means of a small cone made of perforated sheet platinum. The apex is always the weakest, the most exposed, and yet the most important part of the filter.

4. In pouring the liquid into the filter, the stream should never be delivered directly on the apex, but on one of the sides so that the force of the stream will be dispersed before the weakest point, ie, the apex, is reached.

5. The filter should be entirely within the funnel. If the edges of the paper project above the funnel, waste from evaporation of volatile liquids and from the increased and unnecessary sorption due to the excess of filter paper ensues. In addition, an untidy and careless habit is encouraged.

6. If the receiving vessel is small, the tip of the funnel should touch its side so that the filtrate will trickle down its inside edge. By this expedient splashing will be avoided (Fig. 269).

7. In filtering into a bottle, care should be taken to leave sufficient space between the neck of the funnel and the mouth of the bottle for the escape of air. If this precaution is ignored, the air pressure within the bottle will act to retard or stop the filtration flow. In addition, the end of the funnel should project below the lowest part of the neck of the bottle (Fig. 270). If the diameter of the end of the funnel is too large to permit this, or if it is only half inserted, the filtrate will be apt to fill the intervening space and flow over the side of the bottle.

Membrane Filters

Membrane Filters—These filter media are produced from pure cellulose or cellulose derivatives and have an extremely uniform micropore structure as well as an exceptionally smooth surface. The integral structure contains no fibers or particles which can work loose and contaminate a filtrate. This is a particular advantage in the filtration of ophthalmic solutions. The presence of these fibers is difficult to prevent when using many other filter media, including paper filters.

The efficiency of membrane filters is due to the uniform pore system which functions like a highly effective sieve. The pore size, of different types of these filters, ranges from 10 mμ to 10 μ. All particles in liquids or gases which are larger than the pore of a given filter are retained on the surface. The thickness of these membrane filters range from 50 to 200 μ.

The pores which penetrate these filters pass directly through the entire thickness of the membrane, with a minimum of crosslinkage. Porosity or pore volume is estimated as 80% of the total filter volume. The high porosity of these filters, coupled with the "straight-through" configuration of the pores, results in flow rates through membrane filters which are at least 40 times faster than flow rates through conventional filter media which possess the same particle size retention capabilities.

Two major producers of these filters are the Millipore Filter Corp., Bedford, Mass., and Carl Schleicher & Schuell Co., Keene, N.H. The membrane filters are available as circular discs of varying diameter. Different types are available for use in the filtration of either aqueous and nonaqueous liquids. The discs are generally used in conjunction with specialized holders of either metal or glass composition. Because of the minute pore size these filters are almost always used with vacuum techniques.

In addition to their obvious utility in routine filtration processes on both a laboratory and industrial scale, these filters have been used for a wide range of purposes, including chemical analysis, microbiological analysis, and bacterial filtration. The latter process provides an economical and rapid method for sterilizing heat-labile material (see Chapter 81, *Sterilization*).

Other Filtering Media—Many devices have been advanced to replace filter paper, which has many disadvantages, particularly for large-scale operations. A great many variations of filtering processes, each designed to fit the needs of special cases, are found in the modern pharmaceutical laboratory. The filter press, the centrifugal filter, the vacuum filter, the sand-bed filter, the charcoal filter, paper–pulp filter, and porous procelain filter, are all examples of specialized filtration methods. Each one of these possesses some advantageous quality, and it is the experience of the laboratory operators that guides them in their selection of appropriate filtering devices. Reference is made later in the text to many of these special large-scale filters.

However, it would not be inappropriate to refer briefly to special filtering devices which may be useful in the laboratory or at the prescription counter.

Cotton Filters—A small pledget of absorbent cotton, loosely inserted in the neck of a funnel, adequately serves to remove large particles of extraneous material from a clear liquid. Although this properly might be termed colation, the cotton can also be used to serve as a fairly efficient filter. It is sometimes necessary to return the liquid a number of times to secure perfect transparency. This should be remembered in filtering ophthalmic solutions through cotton, when small detached filaments are carried through on initial filtration.

Asbestos and Glass-Wool Filters—When solutions of highly reactive chemicals, such as strong acids, are to be filtered, filter paper cannot be used. In its place either asbestos or glass wool may be used as one uses absorbent cotton for filtering. These two substances are resistant to ordinary chemical action and when properly packed into the neck of a funnel constitute very effective filtering media.

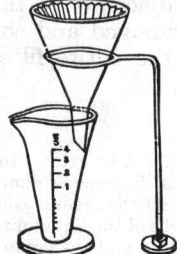

Fig. 269. Arrangement of funnel in filtration.

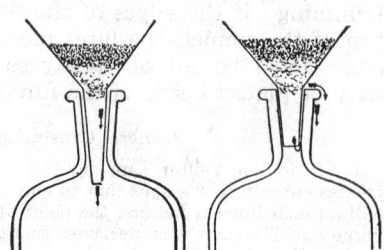

Fig. 270. Filtering into a bottle.

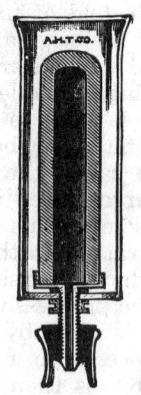

Fig. 271. Candle filter, Berkefeld type (courtesy, Thomas).

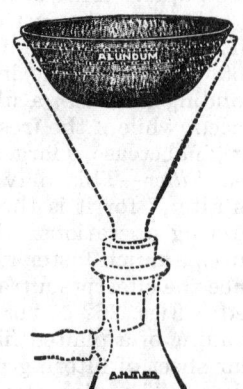

Fig. 272. Alundum filter (courtesy, Thomas).

Stoneware Filters—For small- and large-scale filtrations many patented varieties of porous stoneware filters are available. These are highly effective for some purposes, their special advantage being that they may be cleaned by igniting them to red heat, thus destroying organic matter, or by treating them with strong acids, to which they are highly resistant.

Bacterial Filters—Filtration as a method of removing bacteria from a liquid is a very important process, particularly for the sterilization of solutions containing heat-sensitive medicaments. There are several types of bacteriaproof filters available; in one type of filter the filtering agent is a hollow cylinder or candle made of unglazed porous porcelain or of diatomaceous earth, eg, the Berkefeld or Chamberland filter (Fig. 271); in another type, specially prepared asbestos films resembling filter pads are used, eg, the Seitz filter (see chapters on *Sterilization* and *Parenteral Solutions*). By necessity, all of these units require the application of a vacuum.

Alundum Filter—This type of filter is made of an aluminum silicate in the form of dishes or crucibles and replaces the Gooch crucible for collecting the finest precipitates (Fig. 272).

Sand Filters—This type of filter is used in large-scale operations, as in the municipal purification of drinking water. A large bed of properly proportioned layers of sand, stone, and gravel constitutes the filter through which the great bulk of water passes on its path to purification. These filters are materially aided in their water-purifying efficiency by the action of bacteria present in the filter bed.

Sintered Glass Filters—These filters have as the filtering medium a flat or convex plate consisting of particles of Jena glass powdered and sifted to produce granules of uniform size which are molded together. These plates are fused into glass apparatus of any required shape (Fig. 273). These filters vary in porosity, depending on the size of the granules used in the plate. They are very useful in the filtration of solutions such as those intended for parenteral injection. A vacuum attachment is necessary to facilitate the passage of the liquid through the filter plate (see Chapter 81, *Sterilization*).

Funnels

Funnels, formerly called *tunnels*, are conical-shaped utensils intended to facilitate the pouring of liquids into narrow-mouthed vessels. They are also widely used in Pharmacy for supporting filter media. Funnels may be made of copper, tinned copper, tinned iron, iron, aluminum, hard rubber, porcelain, stainless steel, polyethylene, glass, or any other material which serves this specific purpose. Metallic funnels have an ad-

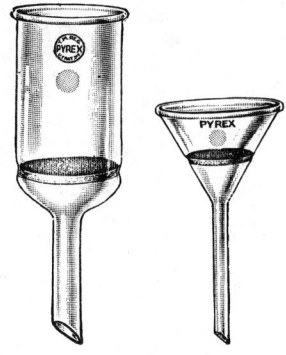

Fig. 273.   Sintered glass filters.

vantage in point of durability as compared to porcelain and glass, but they are chemically sensitive to a number of materials and are more difficult to clean.

The triangle formed by the sides of the funnel and the line joining them should be equilateral (Fig. 274), the angles each being 60°. A funnel having this shape will provide maximum support for a plain filter prepared in the usual way. Funnels are frequently fluted, grooved, or ribbed for the purpose of facilitating the downward flow of the filtrate (Fig. 275). Wire frames, either fixed or folding, are sometimes arranged in a funnel with the same object. These aids are of dubious utility.

Copper funnels, though superior to those made from iron, have a very limited use except for transferring hydroalcoholic solutions of vegetable drugs. They may never be used for acid or alkaline liquids.

Hard rubber funnels are light in weight, and are not very easily broken (Fig. 276). They are resistant to most chemicals and with ordinary care will display high durability. They lack one advantage of those made from glass, however, in the absence of transparency.

Enameled steel funnels are made from seamless steel with their surface entirely covered with white enamel which resists the action of most chemical substances.

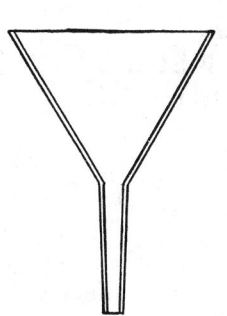

Fig. 274.   Plain funnel.

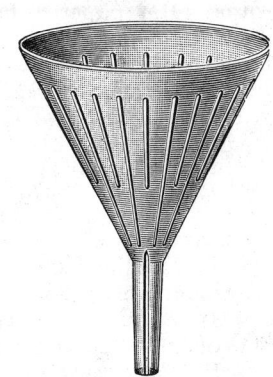

Fig. 275.   Ribbed funnel.

If carefully used, they serve many purposes. The greatest objection to their use arises from the brittleness of the enamel, which is apt to chip off if the funnel is dropped on the floor or subjected to a blow. At the point where the neck of the funnel is joined to the body, the enamel coating is so thin that by constant use it is soon chipped off; the exposed iron quickly rusts, and the neck breaks off. Tinned iron funnels, once frequently used, were popular because of their cheapness, but it is quite possible for a pharmacist to ruin in one operation a preparation worth ten times the cost of the funnel by filtering it through a tinned iron funnel and allowing it to come in contact with the iron exposed by the wearing off of the tinned surface.

Polyethylene funnels (Fig. 277) are made from a flexible, lightweight plastic with a reinforced rim. They are unbreakable in ordinary use. These funnels are suitable for use at room temperature with most strong acids and alkalies as well as concentrated hydrogen peroxide, but they are attacked by bromine, carbon bisulfide, and concentrated nitric acid.

Funnels made from a number of plastic materials are available and have become quite popular. A distinct disadvantage of some of these materials is their relatively great ability to adsorb a wide range of chemical substances. This drawback may result in a loss of active ingredients and a source of future contamination.

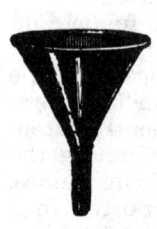

Fig. 276. Hard rubber funnel.

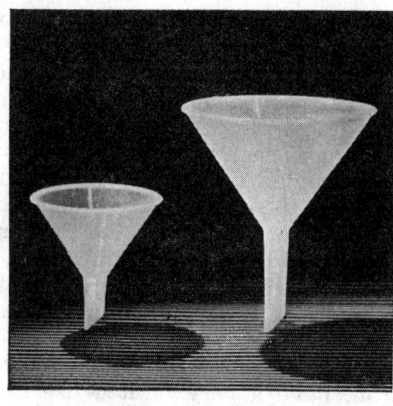

Fig. 277. Polyethylene funnels (courtesy, Thomas).

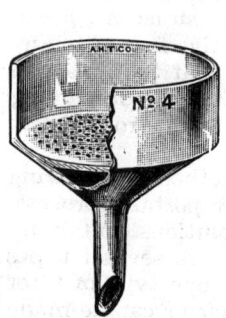

Fig. 280. Büchner funnel (courtesy, Thomas).

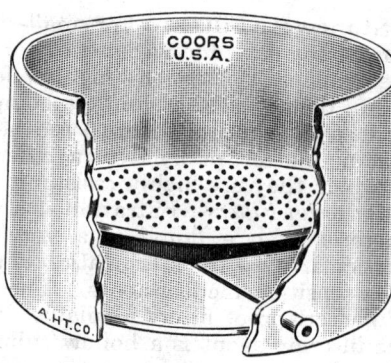

Fig. 281. Büchner table-top funnel (courtesy, Thomas).

Fig. 278 shows a funnel stand useful for filtering operations in the laboratory or at the prescription counter. Fig. 279 shows a ring stand with a horseshoe base which permits containers for filtrates to be placed close to the stand.

The *Büchner* type of funnel (Fig. 280) is largely used today in pharmaceutical laboratories. A piece of round filter paper is laid on the perforated porcelain diaphragm and the filtration conducted. This funnel is especially applicable to vacuum filtration (see *Vacuum Filtration*, page 385). The funnel illustrated in Fig. 281 has a removable perforated plate to facilitate cleaning and is of the table-top type.

Filtration Methods

Continuous Filtration—Most of the expedients used in continuous washing (page 389) are applicable to continuous filtration.

Filtration of Volatile Liquids—It is evident that the ordinary methods of filtering liquids will not be practical for very volatile liquids because of the loss through evaporation and the liability to explosion, in the case of flammable volatile liquids. Funnels must be covered, the receiving vessel must be closed, and provision made for the escape of the confined air in the receiving vessel. The following method is quite useful. A rubber cover, perforated to admit a tube, is placed on top of the funnel, and connection between the bottle and funnel is effected as shown in Fig. 282.

Among many other devices to obviate the use of open funnels, from which excess evaporation is liable to occur, especially in the filtration of alcoholic liquids, is the type of filter shown in Fig. 283. It requires but a moment to renew the filtering sheets. There are no rubber gaskets or wire screens, just a top and bottom plate which are easily cleaned, and any grade of filter paper may be used. It is substantial, compact, easily handled, and portable.

A quart, a gallon, or hundreds of gallons can be filtered through this apparatus. All parts of the filter that are in contact with the liquid are made of bronze and when so desired may be heavily plated with a noncorrosive metal.

Aids to Filtration—It has long been known that the addition of an insoluble adsorbent powder to a liquid prior to its filtration greatly increases the efficiency of the process. Purified talc, siliceous earth (kieselguhr), clays, charcoal, paper pulp, chalk, magnesium carbonate, bentonite, silica gel, etc, have been used for this purpose. There are also commercial compounds, such as *filter-cel*, which are so used.

It must not be overlooked, however, that powdered substances employed for such purposes must be insoluble and inert and not all of those in the foregoing list are applicable for general filtration.

Talc is nonadsorbent to materials in solution and is a chemically inert medium for filtering any liquid, provided it has been purified for this purpose and it is not the impalpably fine variety which will pass through the filter paper.

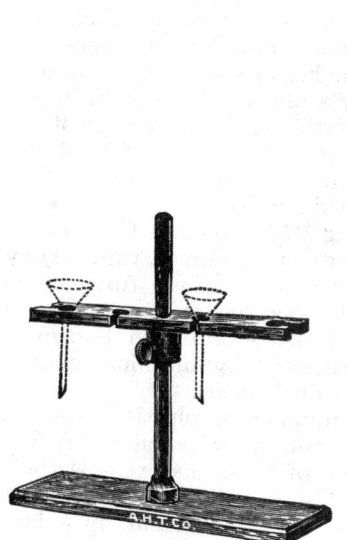

Fig. 278. Funnel stand.

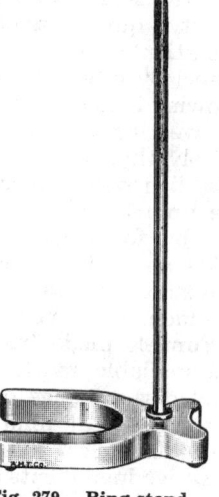

Fig. 279. Ring stand.

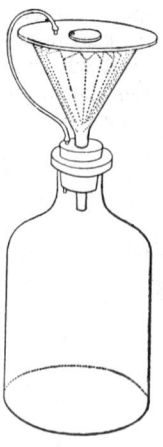

Fig. 282. Filtration of volatile liquids.

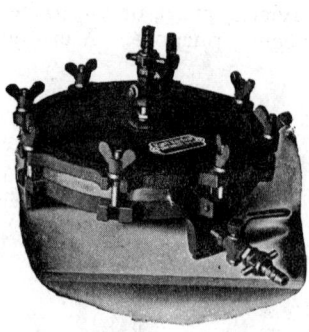

Fig. 283. Filter apparatus for volatile liquids.

Kieselguhr is almost pure silica (SiO_2). It is as applicable as talc for general filtration purposes, with no danger of removing active constituents by adsorption.

Siliceous earths or *clays*, such as fuller's earth or kaolin when in the hydrated form, which occurs when they are brought into contact with aqueous liquids, are safe for general use only in filtering fixed oils. Liquids containing coloring matter or alkaloidal principles must not be filtered through these media, for adsorption of both color and alkaloids occurs and the filtrate is altered in composition.

Charcoals, as a rule, possess adsorptive properties not only toward color but for many active constituents of medicinal preparations, eg, alkaloids and glycosides.

Consequently, charcoal should never be used as a filtering medium unless the removal of such constituents is desirable.

Chalk and *magnesium carbonate* readily react with acids and possess a finite solubility in water and aqueous fluids, with the production of alkalinity in the filtrate. This is particularly true of magnesium carbonate; the degree of alkalinity imparted to the filtrate is sufficiently great to cause precipitation of alkaloids. Either of these media, when added to an alkaloidal preparation prior to filtration, will precipitate and remove all of the alkaloidal constituents. Neither is suitable for general use.

Hot Filtration—The appearance of many solid or semisolid products may be improved by filtering them while molten. Thus, yellow wax is frequently full of mechanical impurities; ordinary straining will not remove these, but by the application of heat it may be filtered through paper and thoroughly purified. Jellies, benzoinated lard, petrolatum, cerates, ointments, etc, also may be filtered in the molten state. The most convenient apparatuses for hot filtration are shown in Figs. 284 and 285. They are especially useful for filtering hot saturated solutions to speed filtration and prevent clogging of the filter with crystallized solute.

Rapid Filtering Apparatus—Much attention has been given to methods for increasing the rapidity of filtration. This may be accomplished by introducing pressure upon the filter or by creating a vacuum in the receiving vessel.

Vacuum Filtration—One of the first practical efforts made to create a vacuum to aid filtration was by means of the Bunsen pump. Its action depends on the principle that a column of water descending through a tube from a height is capable of carrying with it the air contained in a lateral tube, if the latter is properly placed. This form of aspirator is practicable where water pressure is available.

Pumps Acting by Water Pressure—The variety of aspirator or vacuum pumps which operate under the influence of water pressure are all based on the same principle. The following are selected for illustration from the great variety in use. Fig. 286 shows Chapman's vacuum pump. Valve *a* prevents the water from flowing into the bottle which carries the filter when the pressure of water ceases or is reduced. Fig. 287 illustrates Richard's pump, largely used in analytical laboratories for hastening filtration. The zigzag form of the tube serves the same purpose as the projection in the lower portion of the outlet tube of the Chapman pump, ie, to break the direction of the solid stream of flowing water and assist in drawing the air from the bottle.

Fig. 288 shows a very efficient form of filter pump capable of exhausting a 1-gallon vessel, to produce a 29.5-inch vacuum in 10 minutes with a 10-pound water pressure.

On a larger scale the vacuum for filtration is produced by one of the many types of vacuum pumps now available. An excellent type for laboratory use is shown in Fig. 289. The pump should be protected from vapors by placing a suitable vapor trap between the

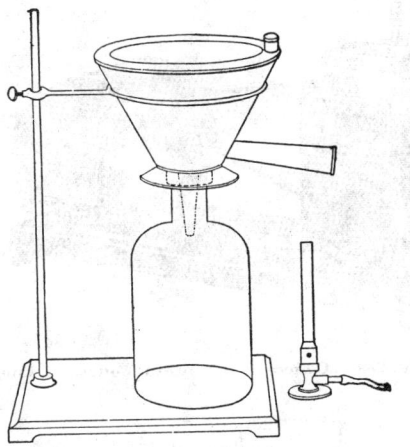

Fig. 284. **Jacketed hot water funnel.**

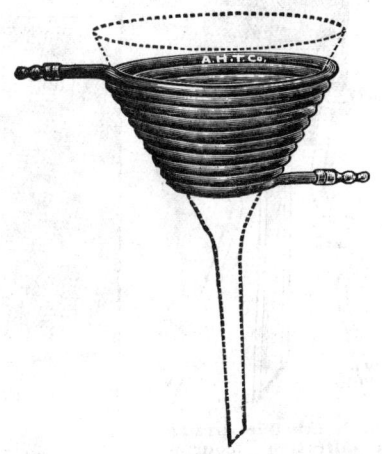

Fig. 285. **Funnel in coil (courtesy, Thomas).**

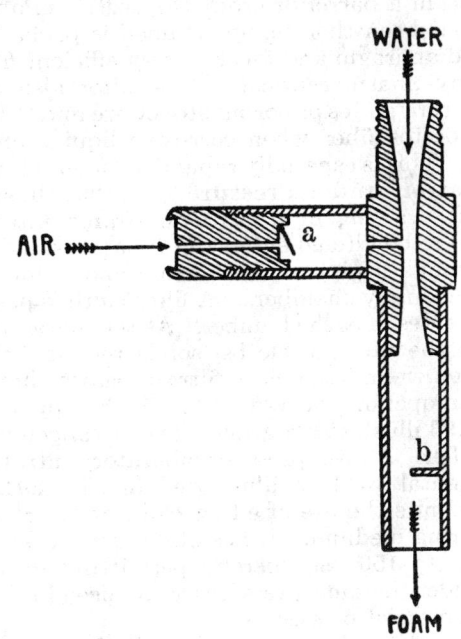

Fig. 286. **Chapman's pump.**

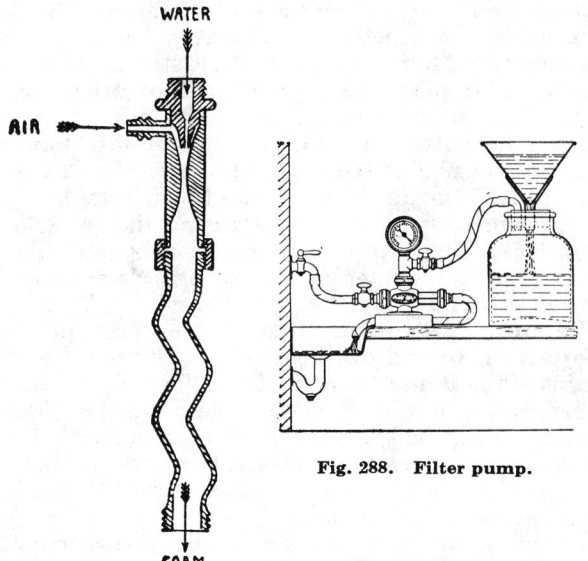

Fig. 287. Richard's pump.

Fig. 288. Filter pump.

filter unit and the pump. The trap is usually cooled to very low temperatures by means of dry ice and acetone when very high vacuum is needed.

In assembling a filtering apparatus using the vacuum principle, it is necessary that there be no leaks in the connections from the filter to the aspirator. If filter paper is used in connection therewith, a plainly folded paper must be used and its tip must be protected against breakage by reinforcing it with a filter paper support or some other device. A Büchner filter may also be used employing a specially strong filter paper.

In analytical work it is customary to use the Gooch crucible and flask (Fig. 290) for rapid filtration. The flask, of especially thick glass, is provided with a side tube which is connected with the vacuum pump. The perforated crucible bottom is converted into a filter bed of the required thickness by means of a layer of asbestos fibers prepared by pouring on the porcelain base.

The principle of vacuum filtration is also applied on a large scale through the use of a perforated diaphragm arranged in a barrel or crock (Fig. 291). Paper pulp which has been thoroughly steamed is packed on the porous diaphragm and forms a very efficient filter bed for many pharmaceuticals. The filter also may be formed from plates of porous stoneware and "chinked" with asbestos fiber when corrosive liquids are to be filtered. This is especially rapid if a vacuum is applied.

Filtration under Pressure—Fig. 292 illustrates a sectional drawing of a plate-and-frame filter press. Material to be filtered enters the apparatus under pressure through a pipe at the bottom and is forced into one of the many chambers. A filter cloth is positioned on both sides of each chamber. As the material passes through the filtering cloths, solids remain behind in the chamber and the clear filtrate passes through an out of an opening located on top of the apparatus.

Fig. 293 illustrates a gravity feed arrangement with bottle filler. A filter press for laboratory filtration and experimental work is illustrated in Fig. 294. This press permits the use of either cloth or filter paper as the filtering medium. It is suitable for working pressures up to 150 psi, thereby permitting tests to be made under the same pressures as are used in the large-size commercial presses.

Another type of pressure filter designed for large-scale filtration is shown in Fig. 295.

Rotary-drum vacuum filters are widely used in the pharmaceutical industry, especially in the preparation of antibiotics by the fermentation process. In this type of filtration a perforated drum, wrapped with a cloth or other suitable substance holding a filter medium, is partially immersed in a tank holding the material to be filtered (Fig. 296).

The drum is rotated through the slurry of material and a vacuum within the drum draws the material into and through the filter medium. During this step of the process the filtrate is taken into the drum and collected, while the solid material remains deposited on the outer surface of the drum. This material is then removed by a scraper in the last step of the operating cycle, just before the rotating drum repeats another cycle.

Filter discs (Fig. 297) usually employ asbestos and cellulose as the filtering medium and require no additional material such as talc or kieselguhr. The asbestos discs are obtainable in various grades suitable for filtering a variety of liquid, even oils or syrups, and also can be procured of a quality suitable for the removal of bacteria.

The filter discs may be used repeatedly for the same kind of liquid if removed from the filter and dried between operations. They retain their form and strength even though repeatedly used. They are discarded when plugged sufficiently to reduce the filtration rate significantly. Filters of much greater capacity with multiple discs are obtainable.

Some discs are composed of dozens of layers of filter fibers. Fibers on the top (rough) side of each disc are

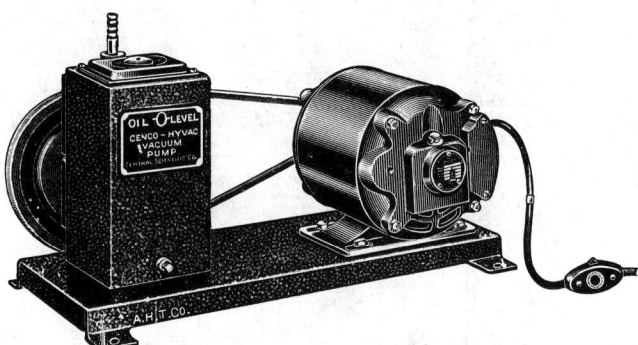

Fig. 289. Cenco-Hyvac pump (courtesy, Thomas).

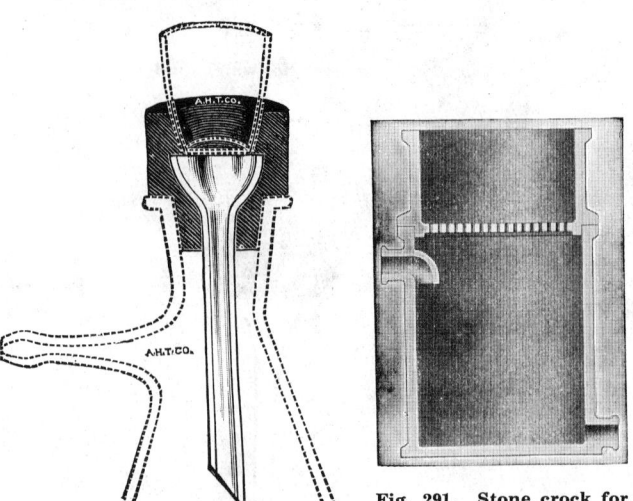

Fig. 290. Gooch crucible arranged for vacuum filtration (courtesy, Thomas).

Fig. 291. Stone crock for filtration.

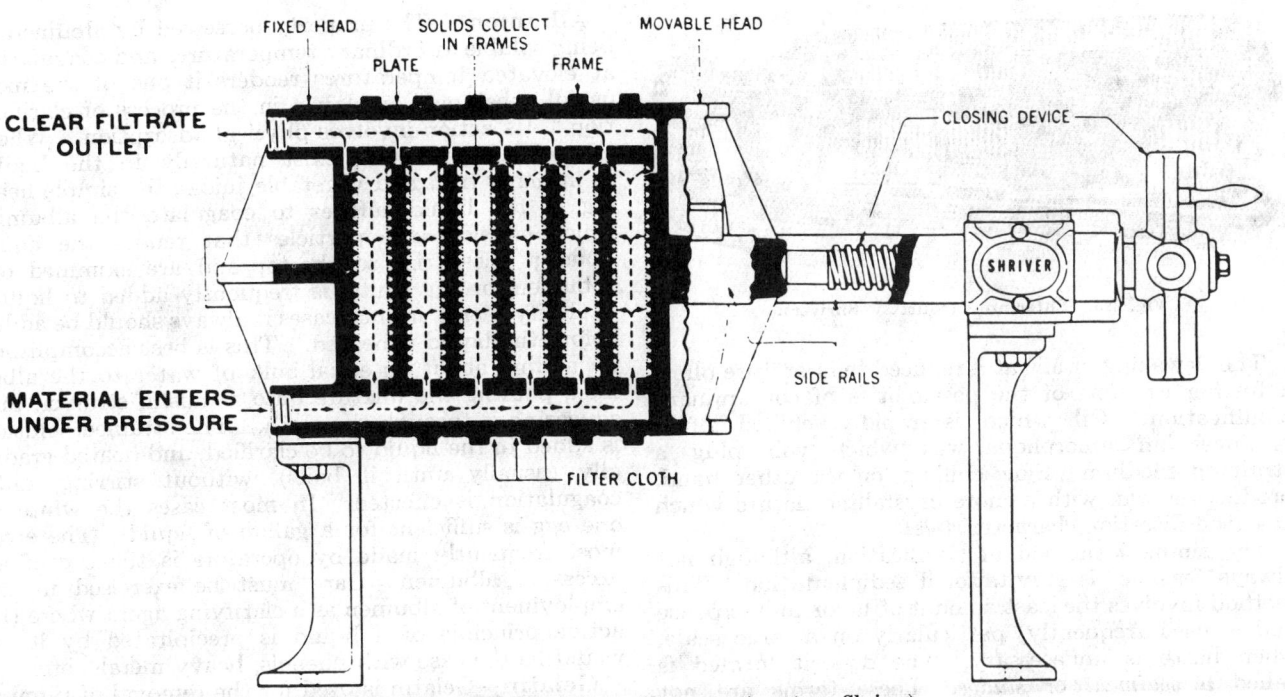

FIXED HEAD   SOLIDS COLLECT IN FRAMES   MOVABLE HEAD
PLATE   FRAME
CLEAR FILTRATE OUTLET
CLOSING DEVICE
SHRIVER
SIDE RAILS
MATERIAL ENTERS UNDER PRESSURE
FILTER CLOTH

Fig. 292.   A plate-and-frame filter press (courtesy, Shriver).

long and loosely matted. Each succeeding layer contains shorter and more closely packed fibers.

The loose layers catch coarse particles of foreign matter, while each additional layer stops finer particles as they penetrate the disc. The final result is a clarified solution, free from all foreign particles and cloudiness.

The progressive density of filter discs prevents their rapid clogging in the manner of filter paper, blotting paper, cardboard, or porous stone. Fig. 298 illustrates an Alsop filter connected to a "Centri-Poise" pump, a special centrifugal type which is compact and efficient, with no metal-to-metal contacts, thus eliminating wear from abrasives or dirt.

Clarification and Decoloration

Clarification

Clarification is the process by which finely divided solids and colloidal materials are separated from liquids without the use of filters. The process is employed to remove suspended oil from aqueous solutions, eg, as in aromatic waters, and for the removal of undesirable solids which interfere with the transparency of such natural products as honey and fruit juices.

Clarification is generally resorted to when the contaminating material is finely subdivided, amorphous, or colloidal in nature and tends to plug a filtration medium rapidly. A number of methods are available to handle this difficult problem.

When the solids are not of a granular or free-filtering nature, it may be possible to improve the characteristics of the suspended solids. This may involve varying the temperature or pH of the medium. When a viscid liquid is heated, its viscosity and specific gravity are decreased and particles which are suspended in it will separate. Those particles which are more dense than the liquid will fall to the bottom, while those which are less dense will rise to the surface. In the latter case the minute bubbles of steam formed in the heating process become enveloped in the viscid particles, rise through their buoyancy, and a scum is formed which may be separated readily. The process formerly official for the clarification of honey is an illustration of the use of heat in this connection.

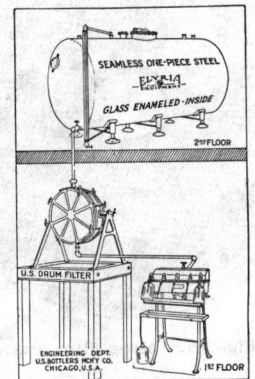

Fig. 293.   Filter with gravity feed.

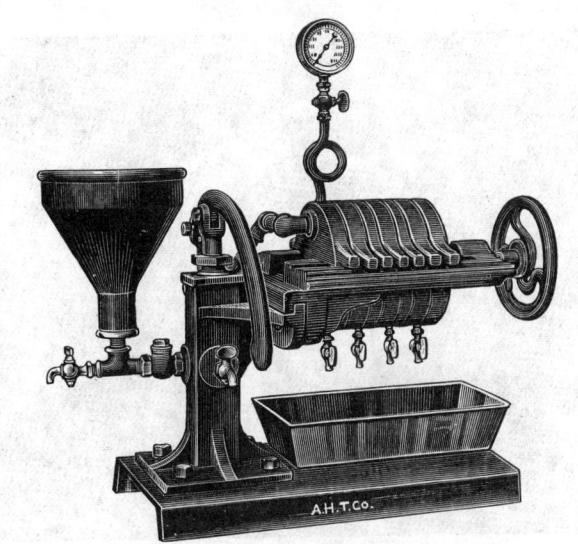

Fig. 294.   Filter press (courtesy, Thomas).

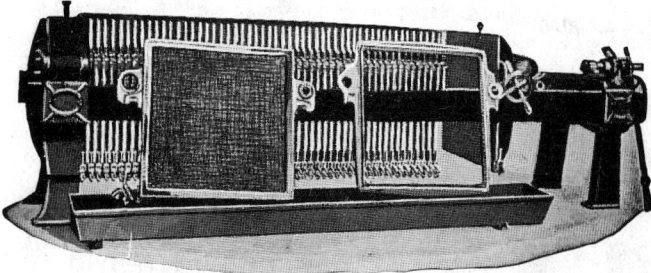

Fig. 295.   Filter press (courtesy, Shriver).

The dewaxing of oils at a reduced temperature offers a further example of the possibilities of contaminant modification. Oil which is rapidly chilled often produces an amorphous wax which will plug a straining medium. Slow chilling, on the other hand, produces a wax with a more crystalline nature which has good filtration characteristics.

The simplest method of clarification, although not always feasible, is gravitational sedimentation. This method involves the least amount of labor and expense and is used frequently, particularly on a large scale, when haste is unnecessary. The deposit formed is called a *sediment* or *sludge*. These terms are not synonymous with *precipitate*. A sediment is solid matter separated merely by the action of gravity from a liquid in which it has been suspended. A precipitate, on the other hand, is solid matter separated from a previously clear solution by physical or chemical change. Fixed oils are usually clarified by gravitational sedimentation; in vegetable oils the sediment consists principally of albuminous and gummy substances, cellular tissue, and water, all of which have been separated with the oil during the expression process.

The clarification process is generally carried out by adding a clarifying agent such as paper, pulp, talc, infusorial earth, as well as a number of other materials to the turbid liquid. These agents usually act to reduce turbidity by physical adsorption of the contaminating material, although a large number of specific, physical–chemical coagulants are also in use. After the addition of the clarifying agent the mixture is agitated and the agents, along with the adsorbed impurities, are removed by filtration or any other suitable means. A number of clarifying agents are of sufficient interest to warrant further discussion.

Albumen*—The property possessed by albumen of being soluble at ordinary temperatures and coagulating at elevated temperatures renders it one of the most useful substances employed in the process of clarification. Its action involves physical adsorption. Where albuminous principles exist naturally in the liquid, as in many fruit and vegetable juices, the simple heating of the liquid suffices to coagulate the albumin, which envelops the particles that render the liquid cloudy; these rise to the top and are skimmed off. Albumen, or egg white, is frequently added to liquids to clarify them; in such cases it always should be added before the liquid is heated. This is best accomplished by adding about an equal bulk of water to the albumen, pouring the mixture onto a muslin strainer, and squeezing it through the cloth. The strained solution is added to the liquid to be clarified, and heated gradually (usually until it boils), without stirring, until coagulation is effected. In most cases the white of one egg is sufficient for a gallon of liquid. The error most frequently made by operators is the use of an excess of albumen. Care must be exercised in the employment of albumen as a clarifying agent where the active principle of a liquid is precipitated by it, as would be the case with phenols, heavy metals, etc.

Gelatin—Gelatin is used for the removal of tannins as well as for the removal of turbidity arising from other sources. Its action depends on the fact that gelatin forms an insoluble compound with tannin which is the basis of leather. Gelatin is used by adding a 1 or 2% hot-water solution to the liquid and allowing it to stand. After a short time a flocculent precipitate forms which enmeshes the particles responsible for the turbidity. The insoluble compound which forms must be strained or filtered out. An ounce of gelatin will suffice for clarifying a barrel of wine, and it is the preferred medium for this purpose. In the gelatin clarification of liquids which do not contain tannins, the principle involved is one of colloid neutralization. The positive gelatin neutralizes the negatively charged particles responsible for turbidity, thus making their agglomeration and sedimentation possible.

Synthetic Coagulants—These materials are used extensively in the purification of water and in sewage control. Almost all of the earlier synthetic organic coagulants were anionic or nonionic polyamides. At present a great deal of attention is being given to the development of cationic materials, the majority of which to date have been polyamines. These com-

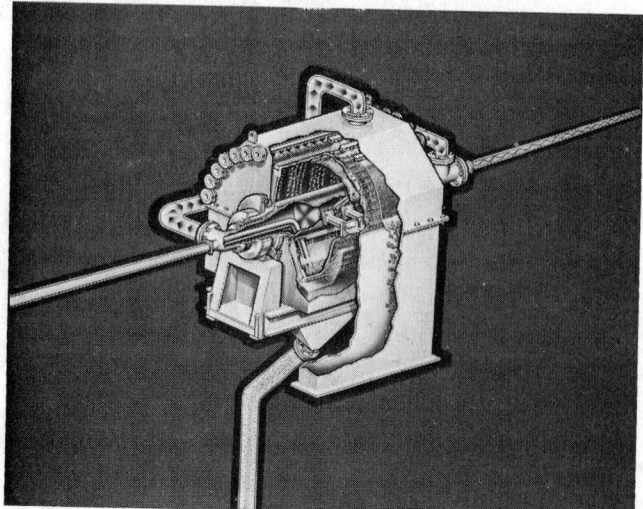

Fig. 296.   Rotary filter (courtesy, Bird Machine).

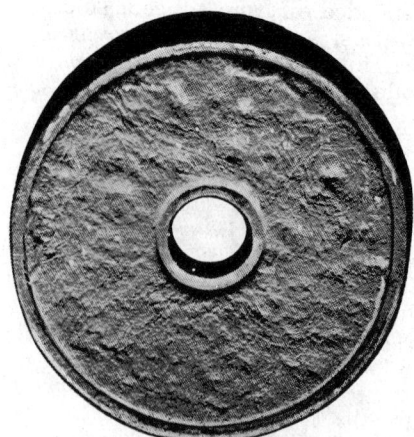

Fig. 297.   Alsop filter disk.

* Egg *albumen* consists chiefly of the protein *albumin*.

pounds act by a coagulation mechanism which is based on the relationship of *zeta potential*, the electrokinetic charge that surrounds suspended particulate matter, to colloidal stability.

Zeta potential is predominantly electronegative on colloidal or near-colloidal solids suspended in raw water and sewage. This charge is strong enough to cause significant mutual repulsion of the particles, and to prevent their agglomeration and gravitational sedimentation. The cationic polyelectrolytes act to neutralize the negative charges, thereby permitting coagulation of the solids.

Due to the high cost of these cationic polyamines they are generally used in combination with the less efficient but far less costly inorganic coagulants such as alum and ferric sulfate, which act in a similar manner.

Decoloration

Decoloration or decolorization, as it is sometimes called, is the process of depriving solutions of color by the use of an appropriate adsorptive medium. In many respects it is closely related to the clarification process. Decoloration is used for the removal of coloring matter from a number of raw materials, both natural and synthetic, and from many finished products.

Animal Charcoal, or bone black, is produced by heating bones in closed vessels out of contact with air and grinding the resultant charred mass. It is generally preferred in decolorizing operations and is the most widely used decolorizing medium.

Animal charcoal varies greatly in its decolorizing power. Purified animal charcoal is not as powerful a decolorizer as the crude animal charcoal from which it is made. The inorganic matter (calcium salts) present in crude animal charcoal is capable of causing contamination of some solutions, particularly those which are acid, and it is sometimes necessary to use purified animal charcoal even though it possesses a lower degree of efficiency. The animal charcoal which possesses the greatest efficiency as a decolorizer is produced by carbonizing dried blood.

Wood Charcoal possesses much less decolorizing power than animal charcoal. The selective removal of color by certain charcoals and clays is an adsorption phenomenon, the principle of which is discussed in the chapter on *Colloidal Dispersions*, page 320.

Activated Charcoal, otherwise known as activated carbon, is made from various organic substances and as a final treatment it has its adsorptive powers increased by heating in an atmosphere of some inert gas or by some other process which serves to increase its effective surface area. For most decolorizing operations utilized by the pharmacist on a small scale, the solutions, melted fats, oils, etc, can be poured directly on the animal charcoal which is placed in a funnel and prevented from passing through by the insertion of a plug of absorbent cotton. It may also be arranged in an ordinary percolator and the cold liquid percolated through the charcoal. At times it is satisfactory simply to shake the charcoal with the liquid and subsequently filter, as is done with clays when they are used as decolorizing media. Generally, however, the deeper the layer of charcoal through which the liquid must pass, the greater the efficiency of the operation.

Clays are used as decolorizing agents by mixing them intimately with the liquid to be decolorized and, after allowing them to stand for a time, filtering to remove the clay. Among the most widely used clay decolorizers

are kaolin, bentonite, and fuller's earth. Materials such as calcium and magnesium carbonate and phosphate have also been employed but because of their alkaline nature they are incompatible with acidic solutions. They impart sufficient alkalinity to a liquid to cause undesirable reactions such as precipitation of alkaloids from aqueous solutions of their salts. The mechanism of color removal by clays is also due to the adsorption phenomenon cited previously.

Both charcoal and clay adsorb a number of active medicinal principles, eg, aloin, tannin, quinine, morphine, and strychnine. Charcoal has even been used as an antidote for alkaloid poisoning. Thus, these materials should always be used with discrimination in decoloration processes for it may be found that in striving to improve or restore the appearance of a preparation by reducing the color, its potency has been diminished. It has been demonstrated that many of the clays, including kaolin and fuller's earth, even when simply shaken with alkaloid solutions, completely remove the active principles from solution. These substances should therefore never be used as filtering or clarifying agents for alkaloidal preparations.

Lotion, Decantation, and Colation

Lotion

Lotion (displacement washing) is the process by which soluble impurities are removed from insoluble material by the addition of a suitable washing solvent. The wash liquid is usually separated from the purified solid by decantation or filtration. The process of lotion is found in the preparation of a number of official products including Precipitated Calcium Carbonate USP, Tribasic Calcium Phosphate NF, and Magnesium Phosphate NF. An expedient method of adding the washing solvent to the solid in a fine, controlled spray, is by the use of wash bottles. The polyethylene wash bottle (Fig. 299) is most convenient for this purpose.

Continuous Washing—The use of the wash bottle is limited to small operations. A simple method of automatically supplying the wash liquid in larger quantities is shown in Fig. 300. This requires attention

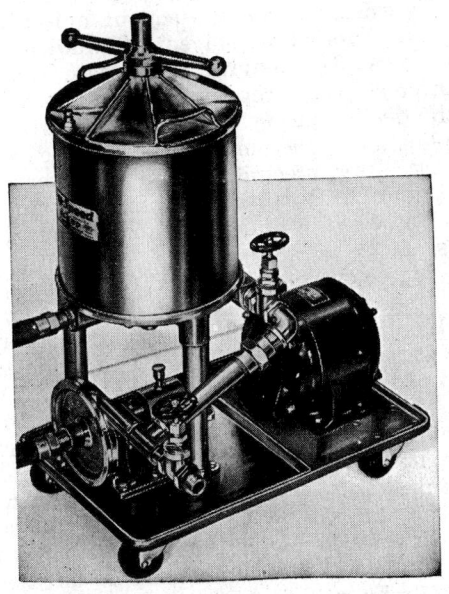

Fig. 298. Alsop filter connected to a Centri-Poise pump.

from the operator only at the beginning of the operation. The inverted bottle containing the washing solvent is furnished with a perforated stopper and a short glass tube. All that is necessary is to fill the bottle and adjust it over the funnel so that the end of the tube is at the height at which the level of liquid in the funnel is to be maintained. On tilting the bottle slightly (if the tube selected is not too narrow in diameter) the liquid runs into the funnel until it rises to the orifice of the tube, whereupon the flow ceases. As the liquid gradually passes through the solid substance in the funnel, the level falls below the orifice, bubbles of air pass through the tube into the bottle, the liquid once more flows, and the operation continues until the upper bottle is empty. Many elaborate methods of continuous washing have been suggested, but the simple apparatus just described is quite satisfactory if a tube of proper diameter has been selected, that is, one of such size that the force of capillary attraction will not be strong enough to prevent the passage of air.

Decantation

The simplest method available for the separation of a solid from its soluble impurities is the technique

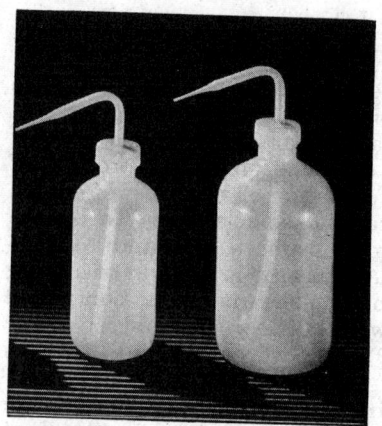

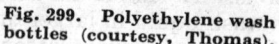

Fig. 299.   Polyethylene wash bottles (courtesy, Thomas).

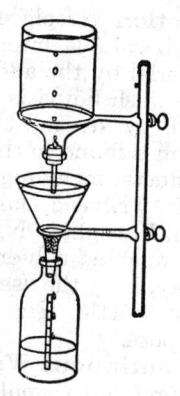

Fig. 300.   Continuous washing.

of decantation. This method involves the following steps: (1) washing and subsequent agitation of the solid with an appropriate solvent, (2) allowing the solid to settle, and (3) removing the supernatant solvent. These three steps are repeated as often as required to attain the desired purity of the solid. This method is also applicable to the simple separation of solids and liquids, eg, after precipitation of a material from a mother liquor. Decantation provides an efficient method for washing magmas and other gelatinous products.

Some degree of skill is required to effectively decant liquids. It is most convenient to decant from a lipped vessel which is not filled to capacity. In addition, the use of a stirring rod is suggested as a guide to steady the hand of the operator.

When dealing with large quantities of materials, it is often more expedient to utilize a *siphon* for removal of supernatant liquid rather than a pouring technique. In its simplest form the siphon is a U tube with one arm longer than the other. The siphon may be started in one of two ways, either by filling the entire tube with supernatant liquid and immersing it as depicted in Fig. 301, or by applying suction at D. The distance CD is greater than AB and the rate of flow of super-

natant liquid from A to D is proportional to the difference in length between AB and CD.

Colation

Colation, or straining (L, *colare*, to strain), is the process of separating a solid from a fluid by pouring the mixture on a cloth or porous substance which will permit the fluid to pass through, but will retain the solid. This operation is frequently used for separating sediment or mechanical impurities of various kinds from liquids.

Colation should not be considered as a separate process but simply as a crude form of filtration, with larger pores in the straining medium than are usually employed for filtration.

The essential apparatus is a straining medium (*colatorium*) and a strainer support or frame (*tenaculum*). The straining medium is usually a cloth material such as flannel, muslin, wool, or cheesecloth. The material should be colorless and washed before use.

Fabrics, particularly those of cotton, are usually treated or impregnated with a material called *sizing* to improve their appearance and quality for certain purposes. For use as a strainer, the fabric must be free of sizing as it causes contamination. Many

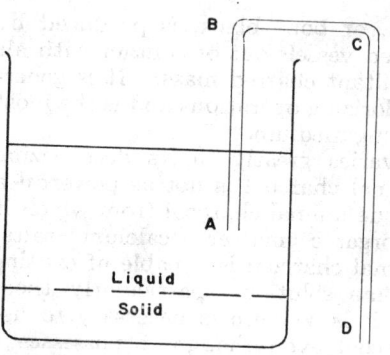

Fig. 301.   Siphon principle.

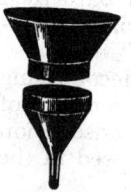

Fig. 302.   Hard rubber strainer.

different substances are used for sizing, some being soluble in cold water, others only in hot water. The proper method for their removal, therefore, is first to soak the fabric for a few hours in cold *distilled water*, rinse thoroughly and cover with *distilled water*, boil for a few minutes, finally rinsing well in distilled water to remove the last traces of the gelatin, albumin, glue, or starch which may have been present in the sizing.

Highly corrosive liquids cannot, of course, be strained through any medium composed of animal or vegetable fibers. In such cases glass wool or an asbestos mat may be used.

Colation in Smaller Operations—When solid particles are to be separated from liquids in the operations of the dispensing counter, several methods may be used. One of the most convenient is to insert a plug of absorbent cotton in the neck of a funnel and pass the liquid through. A popular piece of apparatus for this purpose is shown in Fig. 302. It is a two-piece funnel made of hard rubber. A piece of muslin can easily be placed between the two sections, providing a quick and convenient means of straining preparations at the prescription counter.

Expression

Expression is a process of *forcibly* separating liquids from solids. A number of mechanical principles have been recognized in the operation of expression: namely, the use of the spiral twist press, the screw press, the roller press, the filter press, and the hydraulic press.

Spiral Twist Press—The principle of this press is best and most practically illustrated in the usual process of manually expressing a substance contained in a cloth.

Screw Press—This is the most useful of all forms for pharmaceutical work where great force is not desired. There are two kinds of screw presses: (1) single-screw presses; (2) double-screw presses. Each of these forms may be subdivided into those in which the position of the screw or screws is *vertical* and those in which the position of the screw or screws is *horizontal*.

The single-screw press is generally operated in a vertical position with a lever or a combination of levers. It is the simplest kind of press; properly constructed, it is very satisfactory for small-scale manufacturing operations. The screw should have a square-faced thread, and be well made. The plunger should be disconnected from the end of the screw or else move freely around it. The parts of the press which come in direct contact with the material to be pressed should be constructed of inert material.

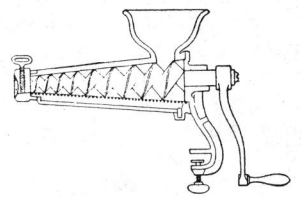

Fig. 303. Horizontal screw press.

Fig. 303 represents a horizontal-screw press. It consists essentially of a tapering case with a hopper on the upper side at its large end and a strong screw fitting closely to the inner surface, the thread of which diminishes in size as the screw becomes smaller. Along the under side of the cylinder is formed a channel adapted to receive a perforated brass plate. The latter has a transverse concavity corresponding to that of the inner surface of the cylinder and the perforations allow the escape of the expressed fluids into the channel or gutter beneath, from which it escapes by a proper outlet.

A large-scale screw press, termed an *expeller*, is illustrated in Fig. 304. The *Anderson Expeller* consists primarily of a hopper feeding into a warming jacket where a crude drug may be warmed if necessary. The drug then drops through a vertical worm on one in a horizontal position and from there is forced, by the action of the horizontal worm, against a friction cone which can be adjusted to exert a predetermined amount of pressure. Exhausted marc coming over the cone is in the form of a hard cake and contains but 5 to 10% of solvent. The disadvantage of the expeller lies in the fact that material passing through it must be of an oily, fatty, or self-lubricating nature. The pressure in front of the cone, required for the expression process, is built up between the worm and barrel bars, thereby causing considerable friction. The advantages lie in the fact that little menstruum or solvent is lost, extrac-

tion is rapid, and unskilled labor can be utilized in the process.

Roller Press—This is used for the large-scale pressing of oily seeds, fatty substances, etc. Its principle is demonstrated in the well-known clothes wringer, which serves as a very efficient press for many substances. Care must be taken to apply the force gradually to the bag containing the material to be pressed, and not to use it on substances which will be corrosive to the rubber rollers.

Hydrostatic or Hydraulic Press—Of the presses heretofore mentioned, each has some special advantage of use, but each also has some objectionable feature. The spiral twist is not powerful and its action is limited. The screw presses have friction with which to contend. The friction of a screw increases with the intensity of the pressure applied, and when a certain limit is reached all further force applied is wasted, and if persisted in, involves the destruction of the press. The roller press is very limited in its action. The hydraulic press is expensive, but after the first cost it is the most econom-

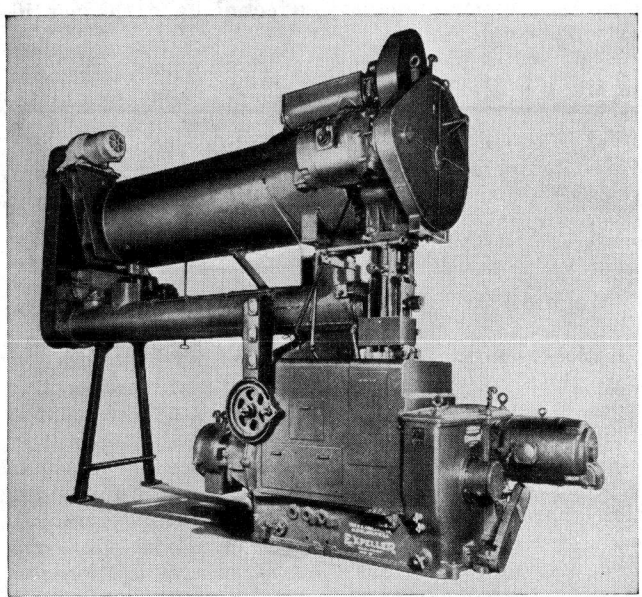

Fig. 304. Anderson Expeller for removing vegetable oils by expression.

ical because the greatest power is obtained at the expense of the least labor. The principle of a hydraulic press is based on the fact that pressure exerted upon an enclosed liquid is transmitted equally in all directions. By construction, a hydraulic press makes possible the achievement of tremendous pressures.

The following rules should be observed in operating presses:

1. All moving parts of the press should be well lubricated before attempting expression.
2. Pressure should be *gradually* increased; sudden strains should always be avoided. If this precaution is neglected, either the press cloth or press bag will burst, the finer solid particles will be forced through the meshes, or breakage of press plates or press will result.
3. To secure optimum results, the pressure should be unrelaxed but intermittent. After apparently reaching the limit of compression, no further increase in pressure should be exerted. If the pressure is maintained constant, it will be found that in a short time further pressure may be applied and more liquid separated. In this way, by alternately exerting pressure and resting, the utmost limit of the power of the press may be gradually reached without undue strain. Screw presses have more ability to maintain pressure than hydraulic presses: the valves of the latter frequently leak to a slight extent, and the pressure has to be continually renewed.

Precipitation

Precipitation is the process of separating solid particles from a previously clear liquid, ie, a solution, by physical or chemical changes. The separated solid is termed a *precipitate;* the cause of precipitation, the *precipitant;* and the liquid which remains in the vessel above the precipitate, the supernatant liquid.

The Object of Precipitation—In pharmacy, precipitation may be useful for many purposes. It provides a convenient method of obtaining solid substances in the form of fine particles, eg, the precipitation of calcium carbonate (precipitated chalk). White Lotion USP provides an example of a preparation prepared by precipitation, ie, by mixing aqueous solutions of zinc sulfate and sulfurated potash to form an insoluble, finely divided zinc sulfide, free sulfur, and various polysulfides.

Precipitation was widely used in analytical chemistry in a large number of quantitative, gravimetric analyses, but it is generally being replaced by more rapid, instrumental techniques. Nevertheless, precipitation is still a rather important qualitative technique for the identification of compounds.

One of the most important uses of precipitation is in the purification of solids. The process as applied to purification is termed *recrystallization.* The impure solid is usually dissolved in a suitable solvent at elevated temperatures. On cooling, the bulk of the impurities remain solubilized while the purified solid product precipitates. This procedure is repeated as many times as necessary, utilizing a number of solvents if required.

Mechanism of Precipitation—All precipitation phenomena, physical or chemical, are based on simple solution chemistry. A solid has a finite solubility in any given solvent under given environmental conditions of temperature, pH, etc. When this concentration is exceeded, either one of two conditions will be observed; spontaneous precipitation or the state of *supersaturation.* The latter is a nonequilibrium condition characterized by retention of solute by the solvent, in amounts in excess of the maximum solubility. The nonequilibrium observed in supersaturation will eventually give way to precipitation of the excess solid. This, however, may require a great deal of time. The process may be hastened by *nucleation.* This is simply an induced crystallization and may be achieved by scratching the inner side of the container or by adding a seed crystal of the expected precipitate. The exact mechanism of nucleation is extremely complex and not completely understood.

Method of Effecting Precipitation—Precipitation may be produced in several ways. If solutions containing albuminous matter are heated, a flocculent precipitate of coagulated albumin will be produced. Similarly, if solutions of silver salts are exposed to light, precipitation will take place. Precipitation will usually occur when a hot saturated solution of an amorphous substance is allowed to cool, or when a liquid in which the dissolved substance is insoluble is added to a solution of that substance, as when alcohol is added to acacia mucilage, or if water is added to an alcoholic solution of a resinous substance, eg, coal tar solution. Precipitation in the form of fine crystalline granules usually takes place when alcohol is added to concentrated solutions of chemical salts. This phenomenon is known as *salting-out.* It is due to a stronger solvent–precipitant attraction than solvent–solute interaction. Thus, solvent concentration about the original

solute is effectively decreased to a value below the minimum level and precipitation occurs.

One of the most important methods of effecting precipitation is by chemical precipitation. The familiar precipitate in the bottom of a container of calcium hydroxide solution is due to the reaction of calcium hydroxide with dissolved carbon dioxide, which gives rise to the insoluble calcium carbonate.

Manner of Conducting Precipitation—If two solutions are used, and it is known that they contain the exact molecular quantity of solutes to react completely without leaving an excess of one or the other, the rapidity with which the substances are mixed is immaterial, although the physical character of the precipitate is sometimes affected by the speed of the reaction. When this is not the case, however, and the precipitant is to be added until precipitation is complete, it is necessary to proceed with caution. The precipitant is added gradually and where acid or alkaline solutions are used litmus paper is useful in indicating the approach of an excess. In other cases the precipitate may be allowed to sediment and the precipitant slowly dropped into the clear supernatant liquid until it is observed that further addition is without effect. Ammonia water is one of the most useful alkaline precipitants because an excess is noticed at once by the odor produced.

Factors Affecting the Physical Nature of Precipitates—Hot, concentrated solutions usually produce coarse precipitates, and such precipitates are more readily washed from adherent contaminating salts than those which are light and bulky.

An additional advantage is that these coarse precipitates occupy less space, and consequently their use in solid medication is facilitated. An example of this is found in the manufacture and use of the heavy and light magnesium carbonates. The former is used in solid dosage forms while, the use of the latter is restricted to liquid, suspension products.

In many cases of precipitation the order of mixing the ingredients may be disregarded and either component may be looked on as the precipitant. This is not always the case, however, and it is particularly not true of precipitates caused by mixing solutions of iron salts with solutions of carbonates or hydroxides. In this case the proper procedure is to pour the solution of the iron salt into the solution of the carbonate or hydroxide in order that the latter may be in excess at all stages of the operation. If the reverse of this procedure is done, the first portions of the precipitate are partly composed of basic salts of iron which remain as contaminants.

Whenever a doubt exists as to the order of mixing, a safe rule to follow is to use the electropositive element or group of the desired precipitate. Thus, in precipitating lead sulfate the solution of the lead compound is added to the one containing the sulfate. In forming a precipitate with a hydroxide always try to keep the hydroxide in excess to the end of the operation.

Collecting and Washing Precipitates—In small operations precipitates are collected on plain filters or in a Büchner apparatus on a flat fiber. The special advantages of such filters have already been mentioned. It is frequently necessary to digest a very fine precipitate for some time in water before it may be retained on a filter. In such a process the small particles slowly dissolve and build up on the larger, causing a gradual transition to larger particles. In the washing of a precipitate it is frequently necessary that the wash water contain some electrolyte such as hydrochloric acid or ammonia water, inasmuch as continued washing with pure water might so completely remove all adsorbed salts from the precipitate that it would be peptized to the form of a colloidal solution which would allow it to pass through the filter. The advantage of an electrolyte such as hydrochloric acid or ammonia water is that after washing it may be removed easily by heating. The electrolyte chosen should not react with the precipitate or tend to dissolve it. In some instances a saturated solution of the precipitate is used as the washing solution. This prevents loss of the precipitate due to solvent action.

Separation of Immiscible Liquids

The separation of liquids which are mutually soluble is usually effected by distillation, if one or both of the liquids are volatile. The separation of liquids which are immisicible is generally a simpler process.

Separations of this kind are necessary in (1) analytical procedures, (2) manufacturing operations, (3) distillation of volatile oils, and (4) accidental contaminations and admixtures.

Pipet—This instrument, which is usually employed for accurately measuring small volumes of liquids, has other uses as well. It consists of a narrow tube with its lower end drawn out to a capillary orifice. To increase its capacity, the diameter of the middle portion is often increased, or a bulb, either globular or elongated, is blown in it near the top. Small amounts of liquids floating on the surface of other liquids usually may be separated by the careful use of a pipet. The lower orifice is dipped into the liquid that is to be separated, and suction is applied by some means at the upper end; the liquid rises, fills the bulb, and if the end of the moistened forefinger is applied to the top, the liquid may be transferred to a more appropriate receptacle. Figs. 305 and 306 show two forms of the instrument. In a modification of these, a rubber bulb is attached to the pipet. A medicine dropper may be used for very small quantities. When the bulb is pressed, the air is partially expelled; if the tip of the pipet is then inserted in the liquid and the pressure is relaxed, the liquid will rise, and it may be transferred to another vessel.

Glass Syringe—This instrument is useful in collecting a small quantity of oil floating on top of a liquid contained in a beaker or open vessel. The removal of a very small quantity of supernatant liquid may be accomplished with the aid of a hypodermic syringe (see Chapter 99, *Health Accessories*). The pipet filler

(Fig. 307), while not primarily intended to separate immiscible liquids, is worthy of mention. It makes possible very accurate pipetting without the use of the mouth. One type consists basically of a rubber bulb, glass pipet tube, and a controlled plunger which is adjustable by means of a slotted volume selector and a vernier adjustment which may be quickly fixed to deliver accurately a specified volume of a liquid.

Separatory Funnel—This piece of apparatus is used to facilitate the separation of immiscible liquids. The mixed liquid is poured into the funnel, which is kept at rest until separation takes place, and the lower liquid is allowed to run off by opening the stopcock. With careful use, liquids can be separated with great accuracy in this way. Where the liquid is valuable or very volatile, as with some of the oils, the closed separatory funnels, such as the pear-shaped separator (Fig. 308), which can be stoppered securely and evaporation prevented, are preferred. In assay processes, when immiscible liquids are to be separated, this latter form is preferred because the narrowing of the lower portion makes the line of demarcation between the liquids more readily observed. These funnels are now available with Teflon stopcocks. This self-lubricating plastic obviates the need for lubricating grease, which is often a source of contamination. In addition, Teflon is impervious to all solvents normally used in pharmaceutical processes and the frequent freezing problem encountered with glass stopcocks is completely removed. The Ultramax separatory funnel (Fig. 309) provides an example of this useful feature.

Florentine Receiver—The separation of volatile oils from the water which accompanies them during steam distillation is a very important part of their manufacturing process. Where the volatile oil is lighter than water, the principle shown in Fig. 310 may be used. The oil and water collect in the glass receiver

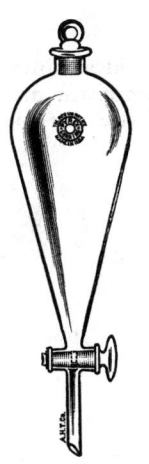

Fig. 308. Pear-shaped separatory funnel.

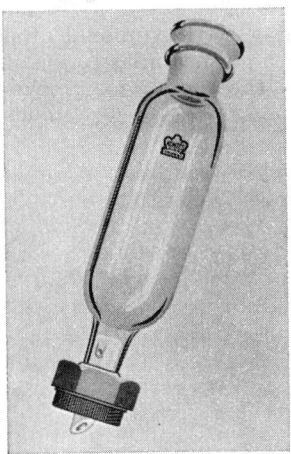

Fig. 309. Ultramax cylindrical separatory funnel (courtesy, Kontes).

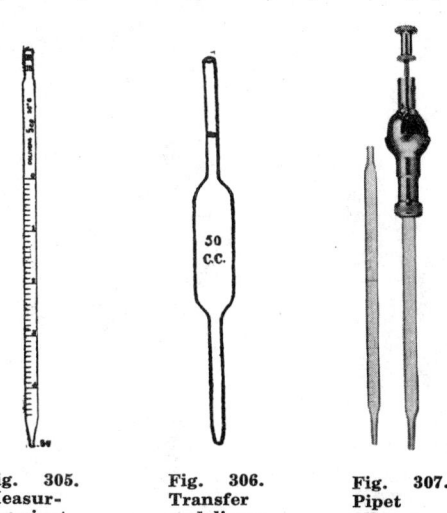

Fig. 305. Measuring pipet.

Fig. 306. Transfer or delivery pipet.

Fig. 307. Pipet filler.

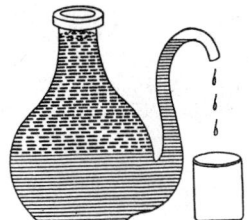

Fig. 310. Florentine receiver.

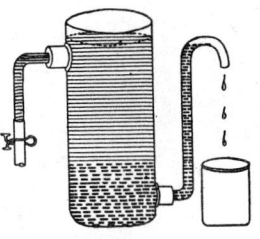

Fig. 311. Receiver for light or heavy oils.

during distillation, the oil floating on the top, while the water ascends the bent tube from the bottom; further addition of distillate causes the water to overflow from the side tube. The reverse action is produced in the receiver for light or heavy oils (Fig. 311), in which either a lighter or a heavier fraction may be collected continuously.

Specialized Separation Techniques

Diffusion Phenomena

Diffusion is the spontaneous penetration of one substance into another under the potential of concentration gradient. Simply stated, material will tend to move from a region of higher concentration to one of lower concentration. The driving force or potential of such a process may be enhanced by the application of an electric field.

If the two regions of concentration noted are separated by a selective membrane, certain species will diffuse through the membrane, while other molecular species will be held back. When this selectivity is dictated by the porosity of the membrane, the process is termed *dialysis*. Dialysis is used principally for the separation of small molecules and ions contained in a mixture with colloidal material. The latter substances diffuse with difficulty or not at all. Materials such as gums, starch, albumin, and proteins fall into this colloidal, nondiffusible category.

The rate of diffusion across a semipermeable membrane is directly proportional to the concentration gradient between the two surfaces of the membrane and to the area of the membrane but inversely proportional to the membrane thickness. These factors are expressed in Fick's law of diffusion:

$$\frac{dS}{dt} = \frac{kA(C_i - C_0)}{h}$$

where S = the amount of substance diffused at time t, k = a permeability constant, A = the membrane area, h = the membrane thickness, ds/dt = the diffusion rate, C_i = concentration on one side, and C_0 = concentration on the other side of the membrane.

Gel Filtration

Gel filtration is a rather new fractionation procedure in which separation is based on molecular size. The phenomenon of "molecular sieving" is an essential factor in gel filtration. The major breakthrough in this field was the introduction of cross-linked dextran gels. They are commercially available from A.B. Pharmacia, Uppsala, Sweden (tradename: *Sephadex*).

The principle by which dextran gels operate as molecular sieves is rather complex. The gel-forming particles are allowed to hydrate and swell in an aqueous solvent. Solute molecules penetrate the gel matrix to an extent which is dependent on the steric relationship existing between the molecular structure of the gel itself and that of the solute. Therefore, the shape and size of the solute molecules largely dictate their distribution between the gel particles and the interstitial solvent between the particles.

The following procedure is generally prescribed for the use of dextran gels. The solution containing the solutes to be separated is allowed to enter one end of a column packed with dextran gel which has been allowed to hydrate and swell in a suitable solvent. On washing the column with a solvent, the components of the mixture migrate at different rates and eventually appear in the filtrate in the order of increasing molecular size.

References

1. Harris, W. E., Lecturer, National Science Foundation Short Course on Theory of Chromatography, Drew Univ., Madison, N.J., 1968.
2. Craig, L. C., and Craig, D., in Weissberger, A., *Technique of Organic Chemistry*, vol. III, part 1, 2nd ed., Interscience, New York, 1956, Chap. II.
3. Rogers, L. B., in Kolthoff, I. M., and Elving, P. J., *Treatise on Analytical Chemistry*, vol. 2, part 1, Interscience, New York, 1961, Chap. 22.
4. *Organic Chemical Bulletin*, vol. 32, no. 3, Eastman Kodak Co., Rochester, N.Y., 1960.
5. Way, E., and Afifi, A. M., *J. Pharm. Sci.*, **56**, 720 (1967).
6. Glathart, J. L., *Foley's College Physics*, 4th ed., Blakiston, Philadelphia, 1947, pp. 74, 75.
7. Weissberger, A., *Technique of Organic Chemistry*, vol. III, part 1, 2nd ed., Interscience, New York, 1956, Chap. IV.
8. Mark, H. F., et al, *Kirk–Othmer Encyclopedia of Chemical Technology*, vol. 4, 2nd ed., Interscience, New York, 1964, pp. 710–758.

art
III

PHARMACEUTICAL CHEMISTRY

EDITORS

Clarence T. Van Meter, PhD, *Project Director, Office of Engineering Research, University of Pennsylvania, Philadelphia, Pa. 19104*

Alfonso R. Gennaro, PhD, *Professor of Chemistry, Philadelphia College of Pharmacy and Science, Philadelphia, Pa. 19104*

28 | Inorganic Pharmaceutical Chemistry

The elements—fundamental atomic features—atomic bonds—molecular orbitals—additional bond types—bond types and compound properties—nomenclature—current activities—hydrogen and its oxides—the elements of the individual periodic groups and their pharmaceutical uses

This chapter was prepared by

Clarence T. Van Meter, PhD, *Project Director, Office of Engineering Research, University of Pennsylvania, Philadelphia, Pa. 19104, and*
Alfonso R. Gennaro, PhD, *Professor of Chemistry, Philadelphia College of Pharmacy and Science, Philadelphia, Pa. 19104*

Brief reflection on the total spectrum of operations which constitute pharmacy reveals at once the important position of basic and applied chemistry among the sciences and technologies represented, and this becomes abundantly evident on examination of the contents of the curricula of modern schools of pharmacy. The basic courses in chemistry are usually pursued as parts of pre-pharmacy education, and the knowledge thus gained is applied later, as it becomes appropriate, in the various pharmaceutical courses.

Since *Remington's Pharmaceutical Sciences* is designed to function in the latter area, it is inappropriate to treat in detail of the basic material of chemistry. However, inasmuch as the properties of pharmaceutical chemicals, like the properties of all applied chemicals, are referable to composition and structure, it is pertinent here to review briefly the more fundamental aspects of atomic structure and the various interatomic and intermolecular forces involved in the formation of different structural types of compounds. Although the general principles involved apply throughout the total field of chemistry, the subject matter is divided into the two classic areas: inorganic chemistry (this chapter) and organic chemistry (the next chapter).

The Elements

The identity of 103 elements has been established. With the exception of technetium (At. No. 43), promethium (At. No. 61), and all 11 elements of At. No. greater than 92, all have been isolated from natural sources. An element of At. No. 104 has been reported. Tentatively named dubnium, it is currently under investigation and is expected to emulate hafnium in its properties.

About half of the elements are so rare that they are of little, if any, practical importance. A modern form of the *Periodic Table* (Chart) of the elements is presented on the inside back cover of this text. The ordering of the cells in the chart reflects that the properties of elements are periodic functions of atomic number (*Periodic Law*), and some detailed information is packed in each cell for convenient future reference. Additional information is provided in the several tables which appear later in this chapter where the elements are subdivided into families (*Periodic Groups*) for further treatment.

The following elements are official in one or more forms: aluminum, helium, iodine, nitrogen, oxygen, and sulfur.

Isotopes of nearly all elements are known. Some occur naturally and others are produced artificially. Many are unstable, ie, radioactive. Isotopes of various elements are highly useful in the elucidation of diverse biological, pharmacological, and medical problems, and some find therapeutic application. As of early 1968, the United States Adopted Name Council had assigned nonproprietary names to 76 radioactive pharmaceuticals which, collectively, represented 26 individual isotopes [*J. Am. Med. Assoc.,* **203**(9), 780(Feb. 26, 1968)]. Specific radioactive isotopes represented in official preparations include ^{198}Au, ^{57}Co, ^{60}Co, ^{51}Cr, ^{197}Hg, ^{203}Hg, ^{125}I, ^{131}I, ^{22}Na, and ^{32}P. Isotopes of many elements may be purchased through the US Atomic Energy Commission. For detailed discussion of isotopes, see Chapters 33–35.

Fundamental Atomic Features

While all atoms are composed of the same kinds of subatomic particles, each known element has certain distinct characteristics which make it different from all the rest. Conversely, certain traits have been observed which indicate a definite kinship among several elements, allowing them to be arranged in groups, ie, the *Periodic Table.*

Although the Periodic Table highlights gross differences and similarities among the elements as individual entities, it tells little about the tendency of the elements to combine with each other in the formation of *compounds.* Certain general features concerning the structure of atoms can be utilized to predict the following: (a) the affinity of one atom for another, (b) the kind or type of *bond* which will unite two or more atoms to form a molecule, and (c) the stability and certain other properties of the resulting compound.

Although many subatomic particles have been discovered during recent decades, only the nucleus and extranuclear electrons are of interest here. Every high school chemistry student is familiar with the classic concept of the atom—a nuclear "sun" and "planetary" electrons. Those electrons farthest removed from the nucleus are termed *valence* electrons and are intimately associated with the formation of bonds between elements. However, the valence electrons do not operate independently of the rest of the atom, but are markedly influenced by the nucleus and other *orbital* electrons.

For example, the energy required to completely remove the most loosely bound electron from a neutral atom of an element to form a positive *ion* is called the (*first*) *ionization potential* of that element. If all valence electrons behaved only as their charge and mass attributes (their own unique characteristics), the ionization potential would be similar for every element. It is well known that the converse is true. Those elements which have relatively small ionization potentials (easily form positive ions) are known as *metals*, while the *nonmetals* have little tendency to form positive ions and have relatively large ionization potentials.

It should be evident that the amount of energy needed to pry the valence electron loose is proportional to the degree of attraction between this electron and the parent atom. Many factors influence the ease or difficulty with which this electron is lost. In general, the greater the nuclear charge, the greater the attraction for the extranuclear electrons. Also, the smaller the *atomic radius* (the closer the outermost electrons to the nucleus), the more energy is necessary to remove these electrons. The attraction of an atom for its valence electrons is termed the *electronegativity* of the element. Metals, in general, have low electronegativities (actually they are *electropositive*), while nonmetals (especially the halogens) have high electronegativities.

Atomic Bonds

A relationship can be seen to exist between electronegativity, ionization potential, valence, and the various bonds formed between atoms. Several years ago Pauling indicated that the two principal types of bonds known to cement atoms into molecules could not be sharply defined as *ionic* or *covalent*. If a molecule behaved such that it appeared that an actual transfer of electrons occurred during compound formation, then an ionic bond joining the atoms in question was indicated. For a covalent bond, or sharing of valence electrons, other characteristics of the compound were evident. However, many compounds considered to be covalent were shown to have some ionic character and *vice versa*. Therefore, many shades of gradation from truly ionic to truly covalent exist.

It is assumed that all bonds are principally covalent with more or less associated ionic character. A compound such as sodium chloride is said to be ionic or *polar*. It is formed by a transfer of an electron from sodium to chlorine. Sodium chloride is a polar molecule since the centers of positive and negative charge are not coincidental, as they are in neutral atoms. This is an extreme case in which the sodium ion is completely positive and the chloride ion completely negative. The "covalent" bond, which occurs between atoms of extremely different electronegativities (metal + halogen), is predominantly polar (has mostly *ionic character*). The other extreme exists between atoms of similar electronegativities, exemplified in particular by the hydrogen molecule. Since both atoms of the molecule are of exactly equal electronegativity, the bond is completely covalent (no ionic character).

Covalent bonding is considered as the sharing of an electron pair between two atoms, each atom supplying one electron to the bond. It is also known that one atom may furnish both electrons to form the bond and this is termed *coordinate covalence*. The formation of the ammonium ion from ammonia (with an unshared electron pair) and a proton illustrates this concept.

Once formed, a coordinate bond is indistinguishable from an ordinary covalent bond.

Molecular Orbitals

Thus far, the bonding or valence electrons have been considered as occupying definite positions (*orbitals*) in each atom (*atomic orbitals*). Once a bond has been formed and a molecule results, the bonding electrons are no longer restricted to their original atomic orbitals, but are free to roam over the entire molecule in what are known as *molecular orbitals*. Molecular orbitals are produced by the *overlap* of two or more atomic orbitals.

Molecular orbitals are somewhat similar to their predecessors, the atomic orbitals, in that they are regions about the several nuclei of a molecule in which the electrons are most likely to be found. They are *volumes of probability*. While it is theoretically possible for an electron to exist anywhere in the volume of space surrounding the nuclei, there are certain regions of maximum electron density and the probability of an electron being found in this region is great. When two atomic orbitals overlap (bond), two molecular orbitals are produced—a *bonding orbital* and an *antibonding orbital*. Only the bonding orbital is pertinent to this discussion, but a more complete treatment can be found in Chapter 17, *Quantum Chemistry*.

The shape of a molecular orbital can be approximated from the shapes of the individual atomic orbitals which formed the bond. If a bond is produced from *s* electrons, which occupy roughly spherical orbitals, the resultant bond appears as two spheres pushed together very much like two rubber balls slightly pushed into one another. A union of *s* atomic orbitals is said to give *sigma* (σ) bonds or orbitals. For *p* orbitals, two possibilities for bonding or overlap exist. The atomic orbitals are dumbbell shaped and can overlap coaxially (end on end) to give a resultant orbital which looks very much like a paper wrapper twisted about a party favor. This is also a *sigma* bond. The overlap can also occur side-by-side, each end of the dumbbell fusing with its counterpart on the other atom, to yield an orbital resembling two spheres just touching. This latter bond is composed of *pi* (π) orbitals.

Additional Bond Types

Other types of bonds are known and are often simply combinations of the three previously mentioned: ionic, covalent, or coordinate. Hydrogen bonding or *bridging* (see Chapter 19, *Solutions and Phase Equilibria*), *clathrates* and *chelates* (see Chapter 16, *Complexation*), and *metallic* and *intermetallic* bonds are examples of other kinds of bonds, but these usually exist between atoms of preformed molecules. These types of bonds are commonly formed by attraction between dissimilar ends of dipoles and are much weaker energetically than bonds formed by overlap of atomic orbitals.

Bond Types and Compound Properties

Certain generalizations can be deduced regarding the characteristics of compounds produced by the union of two or more atoms incorporating the bond types previously discussed. Ionic compounds are typified as being high-melting water-soluble crystalline

Table I—Miscellaneous Inorganic Syllables

Prefixes

bi-   in addition to its numerical significance as in mercury *bi*chloride, *bi*- is often used to denote a simple acid salt as in sodium *bi*carbonate and sodium *bi*phosphate.

holo-   denotes the completely hydrated form of an acid as in *holo*phosphoric acid, H_5PO_5. See also ortho- below.

hydro-   indicates a binary compound of hydrogen as in *hydro*chloric acid (HCl), *hydro*sulfuric acid (H_2S), etc. Becomes *hydr*- in cases where the next letter is a vowel as in *hydr*iodic acid (HI).

hypo-   indicates lowest state of oxidation of a non-metal or metalloid characteristic of a series of oxy-acids, as in *hypo*chlorous acid (HClO) and *hypo*nitrous acid (HNO).

iso-   indicates an isomeric form as in *iso*cyanic acid (HNCO) as distinguished from cyanic acid (HOCN).

meta-   indicates in general a low hydrated form of an acid; specifically, an acid resulting by the removal of one molecule of water from one molecule of an *ortho*-acid, as in *meta*phosphoric acid (HPO_3) and *meta*odric acid (HBO_2).

ortho-   as commonly used, indicates the highest hydrated form of an oxy-acid which is stable under ordinary conditions as in *ortho*phosphoric acid (H_3PO_4); frequently used to indicate *maximum* hydration state of an oxyacid as in *ortho*carbonic acid (H_4CO_4) and *ortho*stannic acid (H_4SnO_4).

oxy-   occasionally used to indicate a basic salt as in bismuth *oxy*chloride (BiOCl).

para-   sometimes employed to indicate a hydrated form of an acid as in *para*periodic acid, $H_3IO_5(HIO_4.H_2O)$.

per-   indicates a high state of oxidation as in the case of chlorine in *per*chloric acid, $HClO_4$, and of manganese in *per*manganic acid, $HMnO_4$; also used to denote the —O—O— structure as in *per*oxides, *per*borates, etc.

peroxy-   indicates presence of peroxide (—O—O—) (or peroxo-)   group as in *peroxy* (or *peroxo*)monosulfuric acid, $HO.SO_2.O.OH$.

poly-   rarely used in inorganic nomenclature except to refer qualitatively to more than one atom or group as in potassium *poly*sulfide (K_2S_x), *poly*silicates, *poly*metaphosphates, etc.

proto-   indicates lowest oxidative state in a series of compounds as in nitrogen *proto*xide (N_2O) or mercury *proto*iodide (Hg_2I_2). Rarely employed nowadays.

pyro-   indicates loss of water; specifically refers to an acid which results from the loss of one molecule of water from between two molecules of an ortho-acid as in *pyro*phosphoric acid, $H_4P_2O_7$ ($2H_3PO_4$ less H_2O).

sub-   indicates low state of valence as in mercury *sub*oxide, Hg_2O; rarely employed in this sense. Frequently employed to indicate a basic salt as in bismuth *sub*nitrate.

super-   rarely used; indicates "highest state" as in *super*oxide (peroxide) and *super*phosphate (dihydrogen phosphate).

thio-   indicates substitution of an oxygen atom by a sulfur atom, as in sodium *thio*sulfate, $Na_2S_2O_3$.

Suffixes

-ate   indicates the salt of an acid the name of which ends in *-ic*, as in sodium sulf*ate*, calcium phosph*ate*, etc.

-ic   indicates a higher valence state as in ferr*ic* chloride, cupr*ic* oxide, sulfur*ic* acid, etc.

-ide   indicates binary compound as in hydrogen chlor*ide*, calcium brom*ide*, sodium phosph*ide*, etc.

-ite   indicates the salt of an acid the name of which ends in *-ous*, as in sodium sulf*ite*.

-ous   indicates a lower valence state as in ferr*ous* chloride, cupr*ous* oxide, nitr*ous* acid, etc.

-yl   indicates an oxyacid minus its OH groups as in carbon*yl*, $=C=O$, nitros*yl*, $—N=O$, etc; also used to indicate a basic salt as in bismuth*yl* chloride, BiOCl.

---

materials while covalent compounds are low-melting materials with limited water solubility. The *transition metals*, with their valence electrons in more than one *shell* (orbit), exhibit colored ions in solution and many of their compounds are *paramagnetic* (move under the influence of a magnetic field). Other properties of molecules can be ascertained simply by a knowledge of the bondings which exist among the constituent atoms.

Nomenclature

The great advances in chemistry during the past several decades have made necessary constant revision in systems of nomenclature designed to give more precise information with respect to the composition of chemical compounds. Thus, whereas such names as oil of vitriol, lunar caustic, calcined magnesia, and soda ash served a useful purpose at one time, they must be looked upon today as trivial and it is pleasing to observe that they are gradually passing into a well-deserved state of oblivion. The need for better nomenclature did not become apparent overnight; instead, it was experienced gradually over the years as chemical knowledge accumulated. The natural result of this process was that various systems of naming compounds have been developed from time to time. Certain systems

appealed to some chemists and different systems found favor with others, with the net result that parts of many systems constitute the commonly used nomenclature of today.

Prior to elucidation of the structure of coordination complexes, the problem was handled reasonably satisfactorily through the continuing invention and utilization of non-numerical prefixes and suffixes and the employment of Latin or Greek numerical prefixes. In general, the main function of these syllables was to indicate the oxidation states of elements of variable valence, although some were intended to connote other structural characteristics. A list of the non-numerical syllables commonly employed in naming inorganic compounds is provided in Table I. Many are not part of modern precise nomenclature, and most of those which are have restricted meaning and application. However, in their former sense shown here, they are encountered frequently in commercial, technical, and scientific literature.

The brilliant researches of Werner, in which he taught of primary and secondary valence characteristics, focused sharp attention on the need for developing a more precise systematic scheme of nomenclature. Recognizing this need, the International Union of Pure and Applied Chemistry established a Commission on the Nomenclature of Inorganic Chemistry which drafted its first comprehensive set of Rules in 1938. These were published in 1940 and became known as the "1940 Rules." Through further experience, these rules were gradually revised and amplified, and the completely rewritten rules were presented in the 1957 Report of the Commission as the Definitive Rules for Nomenclature of Inorganic Chemistry. This report is published in *J. Am. Chem. Soc.*, **82**, 5523 (1960) and reprints are available through Chemical Abstracts Service. A further revision and elaboration of the 1957 Rules is currently in process.

Collectively, the 1957 Rules comprise a system which not only discriminates conveniently among the various types of inorganic compounds but also provides a unique name for each individual compound and accommodates various classes of compounds (such as metal coordination complexes in which one or more of the ligands contain carbon) which bridge the gap between the classical realms of inorganic and organic chemistry. The system is not rigid in the sense that it allows continued use of various terms, such as sulfate, nitrite, etc., which, through decades of actual usage, are recognized as unambiguous. Comprehensive treatment of the system as it pertains to indexing methods employed in *Chemical Abstracts* will be found in the Introduction to the *Subject Index of Chemical Abstracts*, **56** (1962), reprints of which are available through Chemical Abstracts Service. From the standpoint of nomenclature, the treatment of inorganic groups and radicals (Appendix II) and that of anions (Appendix III) in these Chemical Abstracts reprints are especially helpful. An extensive revision of the Chemical Abstracts nomenclature and indexing methods covering both inorganic and organic chemistry was undertaken in 1966 and is summarized in the Combined Introductions to the *Indexes*, **66** (1967).

Current Activities

Progress in probing the intimacies of chemical bondings is reflected in an increased understanding of the composition and the physical and chemical characteristics of compounds, and such progress in the inorganic field has been nothing short of dramatic during the last quarter-century. Knowledge concerning the fine structure of atoms has increased greatly and, through application of advanced electron theory, this provides ready insight into the actual mechanisms of interatomic and intermolecular bondings. Indeed, modern theory often permits prediction of physical and chemical characteristics prior to actual observation.

As various authors have remarked, the net result of these advances is that the field of inorganic chemistry is currently in a state of vigorous renaissance, both from the standpoint of research and application. Diverse phenomena hitherto poorly, if at all, explicable now rest on firmly established scientific principles, and a highly impressive body of literature is rapidly accumulating. Texts dealing with specific segments of the total field are becoming available at a greatly increased rate, and comprehensive works of reference treating the entire field are undergoing extensive revision. The periodical literature is also increasing as illustrated by the relatively new American Chemical Society journal, *Inorganic Chemistry*. Since its inception in 1962, this journal has evolved from quarterly to monthly publication and now amounts to about 2000 pages per year. Each issue contains about 30 papers dealing with active research in inorganic chemistry.

The Periodic Groups of Elements

Presented in the following sections of this chapter are brief discussions of the families of related elements disclosed by the ordering of the Periodic Table. The presentation is severely restricted to some general types of information since the details are readily available from various chemistry texts and handbooks. Tables are provided which list some of the more important characteristics of the elements in each family. Within each group, the elements pertinent to pharmacy are identified, and the brief discussion of each is concluded with a disclosure of the nature of its pharmaceutical applications. Consonant with the general plan of this text, however, detailed information on official compounds is presented at other locations where the monographs are treated under their appropriate pharmacologic categories. (For the precise locations, consult the general index under the respective monograph titles.) With the continuing advances in chemotherapy through the employment of synthetic organic chemicals, the use of inorganic medicinals in the US has gradually declined during the past few decades, and this has been reflected in the change in contents of the official compendia.

Hydrogen and Its Oxides

Hydrogen—H = 1.00797; At. No. 1

In combined form, hydrogen occurs abundantly, particularly as water and in organic combination in animal and vegetable tissues. It is manufactured by several processes, among the more important of which are:

1. The interaction of superheated steam with red-hot iron.
2. Electrolysis of water.
3. Separation from water gas (a mixture of hydrogen and carbon monoxide produced by passing steam over coke at about 1000°C).
4. Interaction of ferrosilicon (an alloy or compound or iron and silicon) with sodium hydroxide solution.
5. Hydrolysis of metallic hydrides.

In the pure state the element hydrogen is a color-less, odorless, and tasteless gas. At 0°C and 1 atmos pressure, one liter weighs 0.08987 Gm. Specific gravity (air = 1.00), 0.06947; critical temperature, −240°C; critical pressure, 12.8 atmos; boiling point of liquid hydrogen, −253°C; melting point of solid hydrogen, −259°C. Sparingly soluble in water (about 1.8 ml in 100 ml H_2O at 15°C). Diffuses more rapidly than any other gas. Absorbed by many metals (one volume of palladium black will absorb nearly 900 volumes of hydrogen), probably partly through formation of metal hydride.

Hydrogen functions chemically only by completion of its 1s orbital. This is nearly always accomplished through the exercising of a single covalence. In the case of the hydrides of highly electropositive metals, however, the accomplishment is through electron transfer, the hydrogen thus functioning in anionic capacity.

In some of the covalent compounds, eg, hydrogen chloride, the bond is sufficiently polar as to permit dissociation, in the presence of water or various other polar solvents, into the solvated proton and the anion characteristic of the compound. Failure to take the solvent into account gives rise to the illusion that the hydrogen alone is functioning in cationic capacity.

In the case of molecules consisting of hydrogen bonded to an atom small in size but high in electronegativity, the pair of shared electrons is sufficiently strongly attracted to the negative atom to impart a residual positive charge on the hydrogen. This charge, which is primarily electrostatic in character, is often strong enough to cause additional bonding between the hydrogen and a second electronegative atom which may be in the same molecule or a neighboring one. This is the so-called *hydrogen bond* or *hydrogen bridge*. For further discussion see page 256.

Hydrogen is frequently allowed to occupy two positions in the Periodic Chart. Placement in Group I-A reflects the presence of a single electron in its valence orbit, and placement in Group VII-A reflects its capability of filling that orbit through the acquisition of one electron (ie, formation of hydride ion).

Chemically, *molecular* hydrogen is relatively inactive under ordinary conditions of temperature and pressure. It unites very slowly with oxygen at ordinary temperature, but in the presence of suitably prepared catalysts such as platinum or palladium, the reaction proceeds with sufficient velocity to cause explosive ignition. Pure hydrogen burns in air with a light-blue flame to form water. This reaction is applied industrially in the oxyhydrogen torch to yield a flame having a temperature in the neighborhood of 2500 °C. Hydrogen combines directly with the halogens to produce the familiar hydrogen halides. The reaction with iodine requires catalysis. Under the influence of catalysts it combines also with nitrogen to yield ammonia. At a high temperature it reduces the oxides of iron and those of lesser active metals. In the presence of suitable catalysts, hydrogen effectively reduces various organic linkages; eg, —C≡C— and —CH=CH— to —CH$_2$—CH$_2$, =CO to =CH(OH), —C≡N to —CH$_2$NH$_2$, and many others.

Atomic hydrogen, in which the element exists primarily in the atomic, rather than the molecular, form, is extremely reactive. It may be produced by passing molecular hydrogen through an electric arc. Atomic hydrogen is very unstable as is reflected by the fact that reconversion to the molecular form is accompanied with the liberation of about 98,000 cal/Gm-mole of hydrogen formed. Application of this is made in atomic hydrogen welding torches in which atomic hydrogen first forms molecular hydrogen which then burns to form water, the over-all process producing temperatures on the order of 5000 °C. Atomic hydrogen is a very energetic reducing agent. It converts many metals and nonmetals into their hydrides. It readily reduces oxides and certain salts of many metals to the free metals, and it can effect many organic hydrogenations. In conducting all such reactions the atomic hydrogen, because of its short half-life, must be generated in intimate contact with the substance to be reduced.

The term *nascent hydrogen* refers to hydrogen produced in a liquid environment containing also the substance to be reduced. This increases the efficiency of the reduction by affording an increased opportunity for the hydrogen to react with the substance rather than merely combine with itself to form relatively inactive molecular hydrogen. Many synthetic and analytic reductive operations utilize nascent hydrogen.

Pharmaceutical Uses—Hydrogen is not employed as a therapeutic agent. In some of its active reducing forms, it is used as a reactant in synthetic and analytic operations. Its oxide (water), in various states of purity, and its peroxide (3% solution) are official, and it is the element common to all official acids. It is also present in various other compounds such as ammonia, ammonium salts, sodium hydroxide, hydrates, etc.

Isotopes of Hydrogen

Three isotopic forms of hydrogen have been prepared. They are protium ^1_1H; deuterium ^2_1D; and tritium ^3_1T. Hydrogen from natural sources consists of more than 99.8% protium, and thus the observed properties of ordinary hydrogen are primarily those of protium.

Deuterium—Deuterium occurs in nature. It may be isolated from liquid hydrogen by fractional distillation or by electrolysis of deuterium oxide (see *Heavy Water*, page 402).

The physical constants for deuterium are significantly different from those of protium, but in its chemical reactions, deuterium emulates protium, forming compounds with analogous formulas such as *deuterium oxide*, D$_2$O; *deuterium chloride*, DCl; *deuteroammonia*, ND$_3$; and *deuteromethane*, CD$_4$. In general, velocities of reactions involving deuterium are lower than velocities of analogous reactions involving protium. The cation from deuterium, D$^+$, is called *deuteron* just as that from protium, H$^+$, is termed *proton*.

Deuterium is employed as a bombarding agent in the form of deuteron to effect certain nuclear reactions and as a tracer in pharmacological investigations. As an example of the former, bombardment of sodium with deuterons yields radioactive sodium according to the following nuclear equation:

$$^{23}_{11}Na + ^2_1D \rightarrow ^{24}_{11}Na + ^1_1H$$

As an example of the latter, substitution of protium by deuterium has yielded useful information relative to fat metabolism.

Tritium—Tritium has been estimated to occur in nature to the meager extent of about 7 atoms in 10^{18} atoms of ordinary hydrogen. However, its natural occurrence has not been completely established. Its preparation is therefore exclusively synthetic. Among other methods, it may be produced by bombarding beryllium with deuterons.

$$^9_4Be + ^2_1D \rightarrow ^3_1T + ^8_4Be$$

Tritium is radioactive and has a half-life of about 12 years. It emits beta particles as shown below, forming an isotope of helium:

$$^3_1T \rightarrow ^3_2He + e^-$$

Hydrogen Oxides

Hydrogen oxides of pharmaceutical importance are ordinary water (usually represented by the formula H$_2$O), deuterium oxide (heavy water, D$_2$O), and hydrogen peroxide (H$_2$O$_2$).

Water

About three-quarters of the earth's surface is covered with liquid water. In vapor form, water is also an important constituent of the earth's atmosphere. In combined form, water also occurs abundantly in minerals such as in gypsum ($CaSO_4.2H_2O$). In addition, water occurs in animal and vegetable tissues. As examples, it constitutes some 70% of the human body and over 90% of such vegetables as cucumbers and watermelons.

Naturally occurring waters frequently contain dissolved mineral substances indigenous to the region in which they are found. Such waters are variously described as mineral waters, alkaline waters, carbonated waters, chalybeate waters, lithia waters, saline waters, sulfur waters, siliceous waters, etc., appropriate to their mineral content. Owners of springs or other sources of such waters often claim fanciful therapeutic effects for their products but, in general, these claims have not been adequately demonstrated.

Potable Water—Potable water is water which is fit to drink. Since water dissolves a part of nearly everything with which it comes in contact, absolutely pure water does not occur in nature.

The water for drinking and domestic purposes is generally supplied by rivers, lakes, wells, and springs. Such waters commonly contain salts of calcium, iron, magnesium, potassium, and sodium; organic matter from falling leaves and twigs; and traces of carbon dioxide, oxygen, nitrogen, ammonia, and other gases from the atmosphere. There is also a variety of suspended matter in natural water, such as fine particles of clay, sand, microscopic organisms including bacteria, and fragments of vegetation.

Supplying potable water is one of the most important operations in civilized communities. The over-all process involves (1) removal of insoluble matter through appropriate coagulating, settling, and filtering processes; (2) destruction of pathogenic microorganisms by aeration and chlorination or other methods; (3) improvement of palatability through aeration and filtration through charcoal. In some regions where the water is excessively hard, softening is effected by partial chemical removal of dissolved calcium, magnesium, and iron by precipitation or by reaction with ion-exchange resins. In order to assure an adequate provision of the essential element, fluorine, fluoridation is frequently effected by the introduction of fluosilicates. Standards for potable water are issued by the US Public Health Service.

On a small scale, water may be purified (rendered free of microorganisms) by boiling for 15–20 min or by treatment with a chlorinating agent such as *Halazone* (page 1179) or *Succinchlorimide* (page 1194).

The greatly increased utilization of detergents during the past few years for household cleaning and various industrial purposes has created serious water pollution problems in many localities. This is caused by various chemical types of detergents which are not destroyed either by natural microorganisms or by existing water purification methods, with the result that their concentration in the water is gradually, but continuously, increasing. In some European countries the problem has become so acute that legislation has been enacted requiring that any marketed detergent must be not less than 90% biodegradable, ie, capable of destruction by natural microorganisms. Similar legislation is under consideration in the United States.

Pharmaceutical Uses—Primarily because of its solvent powers and physiological inertness, water is an extremely important pharmaceutical agent. It is official in four different states of purity and the uses are presented under the separate monographs.

Deuterium Oxide (Heavy Water), $D_2O = 20.03$

Because of its relationship to ordinary water this deuterium compound has been studied intensively. It occurs to the extent of only a few parts per million in ordinary water. In its properties, it differs significantly from ordinary water; as examples under 1 atmos pressure, D_2O freezes at 3.82°C, boils at 101.4° C, and has a specific gravity of approximately 1.10 at 25°C. Other physical constants such as critical temperatures, critical pressure, coefficient of viscosity, surface tension, ion-product, etc, also differ from those for H_2O.

Chemically, D_2O resembles H_2O in its reactions but is generally less reactive. Metallic oxides react to form deuteroxides ($K_2O + D_2O \rightarrow 2KOD$); nonmetallic oxides react to form deuteroacids ($SO_3 + D_2O \rightarrow D_2SO_4$). Interaction with magnesium nitride produces deuteroammonia, ND_3; and with calcium carbide produces deuteroacetylene, C_2D_2. Deuterates (also called deuterohydrates) form readily and have formulas analogous to hydrates as in $CuSO_4.5D_2O$ and $NaSO_4.10D_2O$.

Deuterium oxide is prepared by the electrolysis of ordinary water which consists preponderantly of H_2O with only traces of D_2O. H_2O is much more readily electrolyzed than D_2O with the result that after several hundred thousand volumes of ordinary water have been concentrated through electrolysis to less than one volume, the residual water consists largely of D_2O.

Deuterium oxide has no known therapeutic applications. However, it has been used widely as a research tool in biological and pharmacological investigations. It is commercially available in large quantities and finds use as a moderator in nuclear reactors.

Hydrogen Peroxide—$H_2O_2 = 34.01$

Anhydrous hydrogen peroxide contains 47.0% by weight of available oxygen. It is offered commercially as aqueous solutions containing from 3 to 90% H_2O_2 by weight.

Hydrogen peroxide solutions are prepared by metathesizing barium peroxide with phosphoric acid and by electrolysis of ammonium persulfate. Concentration is effected by distillation.

Description—Concentrated hydrogen peroxide is a colorless, caustic liquid with a bitter taste. (*Caution—Do not taste undiluted.*) It is very unstable and can only be distilled in a high vacuum. The strength of hydrogen peroxide is frequently designated according to the volume of active oxygen it yields. Each 1% by weight is equivalent to about 3.3% by volume; thus: 100 volume hydrogen peroxide corresponds to 30%; 30 volume to 9%; and 10 volume to 3% by weight.

Stability—Pure concentrated (30% or stronger) solutions of hydrogen peroxide are quite stable. The commercial products, however, rapidly deteriorate in the absence of a preservative. A number of such preservatives have been used or proposed, but acetanilid is the one most generally used. The presence of small quantities of mineral acids also aids in the stabilization, but with too much acid the stability is so great that the solution is impaired for use as an antiseptic since it fails to liberate nascent oxygen. Alkalies, on the other hand, rapidly decompose solutions of hydrogen peroxide with the liberation of oxygen.

Storage—In small packages, solutions of hydrogen peroxide are always kept in tight, light-resistant bottles and preferably not above 35°C. To insure greater stability the inside of the bottles should be as free as possible from rough points as these promote decomposition.

Pharmaceutical Uses—Solution of hydrogen peroxide (or *"dioxide"* as it is sometimes *incorrectly* termed) is an energetic oxidizing agent by virtue of the nascent oxygen it readily yields, and its medicinal, as well as industrial, uses are based on this property. It is an effective, albeit transient, germicide and de-odorant, and its liberation of gaseous oxygen provides an additional cleansing action on open wounds. It is used extensively as a hair bleach and has been suggested as an effective oxidizing antidote for phosphorus and cyanide poisonings. Strong solutions injure tissue and must be handled with care.

Elements of Group 0

This group, *the inert elements*, consists of helium neon, argon, krypton, xenon, and radon. Each is characterized by the important structural feature that the outermost orbit is populated s^2p^6. Since all electrons are paired and bonding orbitals are absent, the extreme stability (chemical inertness) of the group is not unexpected and is reflected in terms of peak ionization potentials and various other characteristics. Under unusual reaction conditions, there is some evidence that these inert elements may be caused to form hydrates and to unite with hydrogen and various metals. In general, such "compounds" are quite unstable under ambient conditions. To the contrary, some relatively stable fluorides, eg, XeF_2, XeF_4, and XeF_6, and a crystalline sodium perxenate are known. However, in comparison with other elements, those of Group Zero are still logically and usefully classed as chemically inert. In contrast with hydrogen, oxygen, and other diatomic gases, the molecules of inert elements in the gaseous state are monatomic.

Physically, all elements of Group Zero are colorless, odorless gases under ordinary conditions of temperature and pressure. They vary widely in atomic mass and atomic volume, and these differences are reflected in the values of their physical constants (see Table II).

At the time Mendeléeff constructed his original periodic table, the inert elements were unknown and thus no spaces were provided for them. With their later discovery, however, it became apparent both from the standpoints of atomic structure and properties that these elements fitted nicely into Mendeléeff's arrangement and explained the transition in properties from decidedly electronegative elements such as the halogens to pronounced electropositive elements such as the alkali metals.

Chronology of Group Zero Elements

1785—Cavendish demonstrated the presence of nonreactive substances in air.

1868—Janssen discovered an unknown element in the sun's spectrum. Frankland and Lockyer named the new element **helium** (Greek, *sun*).

1889—Hildebrand isolated an inert gas from the mineral cleveite.

1894—Rayleigh demonstrated that the density of nitrogen isolated from air was significantly greater than the density of nitrogen prepared by chemical processes from pure nitrogen compounds. Further research in collaboration with Ramsay resulted in the isolation of **argon** (Greek, *inert*).

1898—Ramsay and Travers isolated **neon** (Gr, *new*) by fractional distillation of impure liquid argon prepared from air. Soon afterward, these same researchers isolated **krypton** (Greek, *hidden*) and **xenon** (Greek, *stranger*) from the fraction of liquid air remaining after all of the more volatile constituents had distilled.

1901—Dorn discovered **radon,** the only radioactive member of the Group Zero elements. It is formed from radium by emission of an alpha particle:

$$^{226}_{88}Ra \rightarrow {}^{228}_{86}Rn + {}^{4}_{2}He$$

1907—Cady and McFarland isolated helium from natural gases. **Thoron** (from thorium) and **actinon** (from actinium) are isotopes of radon.

All Group Zero elements except radon occur in the atmosphere. With the exception of argon, the quantities are very minute as shown in Table II. Helium also occurs in certain natural gases such as those in southwestern United States, and entrapped in radioactive minerals such as monazite.

Argon, neon, krypton, and xenon are produced commercially from liquid air by fractionation processes. Helium is produced by similar methods starting with natural gases relatively rich in this element. Radon is produced during the natural decay of radium.

Pharmaceutical Uses—Helium is the only member of the inert family having therapeutic applications. Because of its lightness, an "artificial air" composed of 20% oxygen with helium alleviates difficult respiration.

Krypton and xenon have been investigated for possible use as anesthetics, but the sparsity with which these elements occur in nature imposes severe limitations on any conjectured use.

Radon has been used instead of radium in the treatment of certain types of cancer. Sealed tubes containing the element are imbedded in the tissues to be treated. Both radium and radon emit alpha particles in the first stage of their radioactive decay.

Table II—Some Characteristics of Group 0 Elements

Symbol	He	Ne	Ar	Kr	Xe	Rn
Atomic number	2	10	18	36	54	86
Atomic weight	4.0026	20.179	39.948	83.80	131.30	[222][a]
Density (Gm/L at 0°C and 1 atmos)	0.178	0.900	1.78	3.71	5.85	9.73
Atomic radius (Å)	0.93	1.31	1.74	1.89	2.09	2.14
Orbital electrons	s^2	$s^22s^22p^6$	$[Ne]3s^23p^6$	$[Ar]3d^{10}4s^24p^6$	$[Kr]4d^{10}5s^25p^6$	$[Xe]4f^{14}5d^{10}6s^26p^6$
Melting point (°K)	0.9	24	84	104	133	202
Boiling point (°K)	4.2	27	87	121	164	211
Critical temperature (°K)	5.2	44	151	120	290	378
Critical pressure (atmos)	2.3	27	48	54	58	62
% by volume in air	5×10^{-4}	15×10^{-4}	0.94	11×10^{-5}	9×10^{-6}	

[a] Mass number of the isotope of longest known half-life.

Elements of Group I

All elements in Group I are characterized by the presence of only one electron in an outermost s orbital. They divide into two distinct groups according to their total electronic arrangements, and this is reflected in their locations in the periodic table.

Group I-A elements include lithium, sodium, potassium, rubidium, cesium, and francium. Except for the small lithium atom, the common structural denominator is an $(n - 1)p^6ns^1$ orbital population. Francium is distinguished from the other members of the group through its natural radioactivity.

Group I-B elements include copper, silver, and gold, and the orbital population common to all is an $(n - 1)d^{10}ns^1$.

Elements of Group I-A

Commonly referred to as the *alkali metals*, this group comprises the most active of all metallic elements, the reactivity increasing with increasing atomic number. As might be expected from their low electronegativities and orbital populations, they function only with an electropositive valence of one, yielding general types of compounds such as oxides, M_2O (wherein M represents one atom of any element of the group); peroxides, M_2O_2; hydroxides, MOH; halides, MX; sulfates, M_2SO_4; hydrides, MH; etc. Because of their high order of chemical reactivity, these metals occur terrestrially only in combined form; mineral forms include primarily halides, sulfates, and complex silicates. Alkali metal salts of common inorganic and organic acids are colorless (white in powder or granular form) and, with few exceptions, are readily soluble in water.

Some of the more important characteristics of the alkali metals are presented in Table III.

Lithium, sodium, and potassium are the only members of this group having any pharmaceutical pertinence, and further treatment is confined to them. For reasons given later, compounds containing the alkali-like ion *ammonium* are described immediately following the section dealing with potassium compounds.

Lithium—Li = 6.939 (At. No. 3)

Lithium occurs widely in nature, chiefly in the form of silicates and phosphates, and usually is associated with other metals, particularly potassium, sodium, aluminum, iron, and manganese. Common minerals include *petalite*, *lepidolite*, *amblygonite*, and *spodumene*. Like potassium and sodium, lithium is commonly prepared by electrolysis of its fused chloride. Lithium salts often differ decidedly from corresponding salts of other alkali metals. Thus, the carbonate, fluoride, and phosphates are only slightly soluble.

Pharmaceutical Uses—Certain lithium salts were introduced for the treatment of gout, rheumatism, and related maladies when it was found that lithium urate was quite soluble. However, because lithium urate reacts with physiologically abundant sodium and potassium ions to precipitate the less soluble urates of these metals, employment of lithium salts in treatment of the above-mentioned maladies is of no therapeutic advantage. The actions of lithium salts in which therapeutic application is inherent to the anionic portion of the compound are similar to those of the corresponding sodium and potassium compounds. However, because of the relatively *toxic* character of the lithium ion, as revealed during recent years with dietary salt substitutes, continuance of such use of lithium compounds is unjustifiable. While there are no official lithium compounds, they have found some use in the treatment of psychiatric disorders.

Sodium—Na = 22.9898 (At. No. 11)

From the standpoint of isolation of the free metal, the most important sodium mineral is sodium chloride. It occurs in solid deposits (*rock salt*) from which it is mined, and also in solution in sea water and certain inland lakes. Other important naturally occurring sodium compounds include sodium nitrate (*Chile saltpeter*, formerly a very important source of nitrate), sodium aluminum fluoride (*cryolite*, important as a source of aluminum), and sodium tetraborate (*borax*, important as a source of boron). Metallic sodium is prepared today primarily by electrolysis of fused sodium chloride conducted under carefully controlled conditions. Chlorine is an important byproduct of the operation.

Table III—Elements of Group 1-A

Element	Lithium	Sodium	Potassium	Rubidium	Cesium	Francium
Symbol	Li	Na	K	Rb	Cs	Fr
Atomic number	3	11	19	37	55	87
Atomic weight	6.939	22.9898	39.102	85.47	132.905	[223]^a
Atomic radius (Å)	1.34	1.54	1.96	2.11	2.25	...
Ionic (crystal) radius (Å) (for coordination number 6)	0.60(+1)	0.95(+1)	1.33(+1)	1.48(+1)	1.69(+1)	1.76(+1)
Electronegativity (Pauling scale)	1.0	0.9	0.8	0.8	0.7	0.7
Orbital electrons	[He]2s^1	[Ne]3s^1	[Ar]4s^1	[Kr]5s^1	[Xe]5s^1	[Rn]7s^1
Isotopes, natural (mass numbers)	6, 7	23	39, 40, 41	85, 87	133	223
Specific gravity (20°C)	0.54	0.97	0.86	1.53	1.90	
Melting temperature (°C)	180	98	64	39	28	
Boiling temperature (°C)	1336	883	758	700	670	
Abundance (% of earth's crust)	6.5×10^{-3}	2.8	2.6	3.1×10^{-2}	7×10^{-4}	

^{a} Mass number of the isotope of longest known half-life.

Table IV—Elements of Group 1-B

Element	Copper	Silver	Gold
Symbol	Cu	Ag	Au
Atomic number	29	47	79
Atomic weight	63.546	107.868	196.967
Atomic radius (Å)	1.38	1.53	1.50
Ionic (crystal) radii (Å)	0.96(+1)	1.26(+1)	1.37(+1)
(for coordination number 6)	0.69(+2)	0.89(+2)	0.85(+3)
Electronegativity (Pauling scale)	1.9	1.9	2.4
Orbital electrons	$[Ar]3d^{10}$-$4s^1$	$[Kr]4d^{10}$-$5s^1$	$[Xe]4f^{14}$-$5d^{10}6s^1$
Isotopes, natural (mass numbers)	63, 65	107, 109	197
Specific gravity (20°C)	8.92	10.5	19.3
Melting temperature (°C)	1083	960	1063
Boiling temperature (°C)	2310	1950	2600
Abundance (% of earth's crust)	10^{-4}	10^{-8}	10^{-9}

Pharmaceutical Uses—Sodium compounds are widely used in pharmacy and medicine for various purposes. With few exceptions, however, such as sodium chloride (electrolyte replenisher), sodium phosphate (cathartic), etc, the therapeutic activity is referable to the anionic component of the compound. In general, sodium and potassium salts exert similar therapeutic actions, and which type of salt is used often depends on geographic availability, cost, or physical characteristics. Because of their propensity to promote retention of water in tissues, sodium salts are used with caution in the treatment of cardiac and renal conditions in which edema is an important part of the syndrome.

Sodium is very commonly the cation of choice to optimize the pharmaceutical utility of organic medicaments, eg, sodium methiodal, sodium phenobarbital, sodium carboxymethylcellulose, sodium citrate, etc.

The artificial radioactive isotopes of sodium, ^{22}Na and ^{24}Na, have been employed in various pharmacological investigations as tracers and as possible diagnostic and curative therapeutic agents. See Chapter 34.

Potassium—K = 39.102 (At. No. 19)

Important potassium minerals include *sylvite* [KCl], *carnallite* [KCl.MgCl$_2$.6H$_2$O], *kainite* [K$_2$SO$_4$.MgSO$_4$.-MgCl$_2$.6H$_2$O], and *polyhalite* [K$_2$SO$_4$.MgSO$_4$.2CaSO$_4$.-2H$_2$O]. Other commercial sources of potassium include potash derived from ashes of beet sugar residues and from *suint*, the residue obtained by evaporating the water used to scour the fleece of sheep. Commercial preparation is by electrolysis of the fused chloride.

Pharmaceutical Uses—As with sodium, compounds of potassium generally find employment in medicine due to their anionic component. Potassium chloride is a notable exception in its employment as an ingredient of electrolyte replenishers. Potassium is the alkali metal cation indigenous to intracellular fluids. Because they are frequently more readily purified by crystallization techniques and are much less prone to crystallize in hydrated form from aqueous solution, potassium salts are often preferred to their sodium analogs. Some drugs, eg, hydrochlorothiazide, promote potassium excretion to an extent requiring auxiliary, dietary or medicamentary intake of potassium. The ^{42}K artificial radioactive isotope has been employed in investigations relative to mineral metabolism and adrenal physiology.

Ammonia and Ammonium Compounds

Ammonia [NH$_3$] coordinates readily with proton to form the ammonium ion [NH$_4$]$^+$. This ion displays many of the properties of alkali metal ions, and it is because of this that ammonium is frequently referred to as a hypothetical alkali metal. It forms an amalgam with mercury and forms salts which show striking resemblances to potassium and rubidium salts with which they are commonly isomorphous. The relationship even extends to solubilities as evidenced by the general water-solubility of ammonium salts of common inorganic and organic acids, and the low water-solubility of such salts as the bitartrate, chloroplatinate, and perchlorate.

Because of these relationships, ammonia and inorganic ammonium compounds are treated at this place in the text. However, it should be remembered that despite close resemblances to alkali metals, ammonium is actually a union of nitrogen and hydrogen; and this makes for important differences between ammonium compounds and corresponding compounds of true alkali metals. Thus, ammonium hydroxide is feebly basic in comparison with true alkali metal hydroxides. Susceptibility to thermal decomposition constitutes another marked point of difference. As examples, the carbonate decomposes at ordinary temperature, the chloride dissociates very appreciably at about 300°C into ammonia and hydrogen chloride, and the nitrate decomposes explosively at only relatively slightly elevated temperature.

Formerly the only source of ammonia and its salts was the gaseous byproduct from the coking of coal for metallurgical operations or for the production of illuminating gas. Nowadays, most is produced synthetically from nitrogen of the air, either by direct union of the nitrogen and hydrogen at a temperature between 500° and 700° and a pressure of 200 atmos in the presence of a catalyst (*Haber* process and variations), or by the *cyanamide* process in which calcium cyanamide is interacted with superheated steam.

Aqueous solutions of ammonia exhibit alkaline reaction, and have other properties similar to those of solutions of the alkali hydroxides. This has been attributed to ammonium hydroxide [NH$_4$OH] formed by combination of NH$_3$ with water and, although there is little ammonium hydroxide present, ammonia water is often referred to and labeled as a solution of ammonium hydroxide.

Liquid ammonia is an excellent solvent for a great

variety of compounds. In this respect, it is second only to water. Like water, it is a typical ionizing solvent, and this makes possible the use of liquid ammonia as a medium for conducting many different kinds of reactions. Extensive experimentation in this field has focused sharp attention on the need for extending theoretical chemical considerations to other than water systems.

In commerce, ammonia is available, either in the form of aqueous solutions of varying concentration, or as anhydrous ammonia furnished in the liquefied form in metal cylinders. The ammonia in household use contains 10% NH_3 and is also known as 16° *ammonia*.

Pharmaceutical Uses—In the form of an aqueous solution, ammonia is used in various pharmaceutical processes as a mild alkalizer. It is often preferred to the fixed alkalies because of its volatility, any excess being readily detected by the odor and readily removed by heat.

Ammonium salts commonly used therapeutically include the carbonate, chloride, and bromide. The carbonate (actually a mixture of the bicarbonate and the carbamate) liberates ammonia copiously which, on inhalation, acts as a reflex stimulant. The bromide is used as a central depressant, and the chloride as a systemic acidifier. The latter also enhances the diuresis of organic mercurials. Both the chloride and carbonate are common ingredients in expectorant preparations.

Elements of Group 1-B

Commonly referred to as the *coinage metals*, these elements have been employed for centuries as monetary wealth standards and in the fabrication of coins. In order of increasing atomic number, the group comprises copper, silver, and gold. As with Group I-A metals, negative oxidation states are nonexistent.

In sharp contrast with the alkali metals, the coinage metals are relatively hard, melt at high temperatures, occur in nature both in the free and combined states, are much less reactive chemically, and are relatively stable on exposure to air under ordinary conditions. In addition, the coinage metals exhibit variable valence, form complex (coordination) compounds, and their cations are readily reducible to the metallic state. Each is known to function in the three oxidation states ($+1$, $+2$, and $+3$), but $+1$ is most characteristic of silver, $+2$ of copper, and $+3$ of gold. The hydroxides and many of the simple salts are practically insoluble in water. Colored compounds are numerous.

A summary of important characteristics of Group I-B elements is presented in Table IV. This is followed by further brief treatment of the individual elements and their pharmaceutical applications.

Copper—Cu = 63.546 (At. No. 29)

Copper occurs naturally in the elementary state, but chiefly in combination. Important minerals include *chalcocite* (Cu_2S), *chalcopyrite* ($CuFeS_2$), and *cuprite* (Cu_2O). Copper is obtained from ores in which it occurs natively by melting operations in the presence of a suitable flux. Most commercial copper is obtained through processing sulfide ores which involves complicated roasting and reduction operations.

Of the monovalent copper compounds, cuprous oxide [Cu_2O], known commercially as red copper oxide, and cuprous chloride [Cu_2Cl_2], are the ones most frequently used. Practically all cuprous salts are insoluble or only slightly soluble in water. Of the cupric compounds, the oxide [CuO] and the sulfate [$CuSO_4$] are the most important.

Pharmaceutical Uses—Copper compounds have limited therapeutic application. The relative ease of reduction of the cupric ion to form colored insoluble compounds finds important diagnostic uses, eg, determination of glucose in blood and urine. The only official copper compound is Cupric Sulfate, which is offered as an astringent and emetic. Small quantities of copper may enhance physiological utiliza-

tion of iron and are thus often present in hematopoietic preparations. Various copper compounds find commercial application as algaecides, fungicides, and insecticides. The artificial radioactive ^{64}Cu isotope has been employed in mineral metabolism studies.

Silver—Ag = 107.868 (At. No. 47)

Silver is found in nature in the metallic state, and as the sulfide (*argentite* or *silver glance*) and the chloride (*horn-silver*). The sulfide is frequently associated with lead sulfide (*galena*) and considerable quantities of silver are derived from this source. The metallurgy of silver is complicated primarily because of difficulties associated with separating it from other metals with which it commonly occurs, often in trace quantities; amalgamation, cyanidation, and reduction processes are commonly employed.

With the exception of the nitrate and fluoride, most common salts of silver are insoluble or only slightly soluble in water. Nearly all silver salts are darkened to a greater or lesser degree by sunlight. Many silver salts of the inorganic acids, as well as the oxide, react with and dissolve in ammonia water; the iodide and sulfide, however, are important exceptions.

Pharmaceutical Uses—Silver compounds are employed in medical practice to provide local astringent, caustic, or germicidal action. In general, these actions result from the ability of silver ion to precipitate protein. Prior to the advent of the modern synthetic organic germicides, various preparations containing silver or silver compounds in colloidal solution were widely employed, primarily topically, as antiseptics. A present day survivor is Mild Silver Protein. The ready reducibility of silver ion to elementary silver gives rise to various instability problems and incompatibilities which degrade its pharmaceutical utility.

Gold—Au = 196.967 (At. No. 79)

Gold generally occurs in the free state as veins in quartz, and in river sands which have resulted from disintegration of gold-bearing rock. It is also found in small amounts in many pyritic and other sulfide and telluride ores. Because of its relatively high specific gravity, gold is often isolated by purely physical methods such as flotation. Amalgamation, cyanidation, and reduction processes are also employed to win the last traces of the precious metal from its ores.

In its lower oxidation state, gold yields *aurous* compounds such as AuCl. In the tripositive state, it yields *auric* compounds such as $AuCl_3$. In general, *aurous* compounds are less soluble than their *auric* analogues. *Auric* compounds readily undergo thermal decomposition to yield *aurous* compounds; the latter, in turn, usually succumb at higher temperatures to liberate the free metal. Gold shows a decided tendency to enter into complexes in which it functions anionically, eg, chlorauric acid ($HAuCl_4$), gold sodium thiosulfate [$Na_3Au(S_2O_3)_2$], etc. Auric hydroxide is amphoteric. In its weakly acidic capacity, it forms aurates of the *meta* variety; eg, $NaAuO_2$.

Pharmaceutical Uses—Because of its precious and noble character, gold has been investigated extensively down through the ages with respect to possible application as a therapeutic agent for the curing of various human ills. Results, however, have been disappointing. At the present time, gold compounds are occasionally employed in the treatment of lupus erythematosus and rheumatoid arthritis. Administration is by intravenous injection since absorption from the gastrointestinal tract is poor. Gold compounds are toxic; dimercaprol is an effective antidote.

The radioactive isotope, [198]Au, is employed therapeutically in the treatment of certain malignancies. See Chapter 34.

A solution of colloidal gold is used to determine the protective power of colloids. The *Gold Number* (Zsigmondy), an index of the protective power of colloids, is the number of milligrams of protective colloid which just fails to prevent the change in color of 10 ml of gold hydrosol from red to blue upon the addition of 1 ml of a 10% solution of sodium chloride. Some typical gold numbers are:

Gelatin	0.005–0.01	Tragacanth	2.0
Casein	0.01	Dextrins	6.0–20.0
Acacia	0.15 –0.5	Starch	25.0

Elements of Group II

Each element in this group is characterized by the presence of two electrons in an outermost *s* orbital. Group II-A elements include beryllium, magnesium, calcium, strontium, barium, and radium. Except for the small beryllium atom, each displays an $(n-1)p^6ns^2$ electron configuration, and each represents an element of Group I-A to which has been added one proton in the nucleus and one electron in the outermost electron orbit. Group II-B elements comprise zinc, cadmium, and mercury. Each displays an $(n-1)d^{10}ns^2$ electron configuration and bears the same structural relationship to an element of Group I-B as II-A elements do to those of I-A. Because of certain physical and chemical properties, some authors treat beryllium and magnesium with Group II-B elements. Because of its natural radioactivity, radium is commonly treated separately; such procedure is followed in this text. See Chapter 33.

Elements of Group II-A

These elements, like those of Group I-A, are strictly metallic. They function uniformly with a +2 oxidation state yielding compounds having the following general type formulas wherein M represents one atom of any of the group: oxides, MO; peroxides, MO_2; hydroxides, $M(OH)_2$; halides, MX_2; sulfates, MSO_4; hydrides, MH_2; etc. Relationships among calcium, strontium, and barium are particularly striking, and this has resulted in grouping these elements under the common heading of *alkaline earth elements*. Radium is sometimes included in the same grouping, but because of its natural radioactivity, it is usually treated separately.

As with the alkali metals, elements of Group II-A, because of their high order of chemical reactivity, do not occur free in nature. Carbonate, sulfate, and phosphate minerals occur relatively abundantly. The oxides are not reducible by treatment with carbon at high temperature; thus, liberation of the metals is commonly effected by electrolysis of the fused chlorides.

Beryllium and magnesium resemble Group II-B elements in many respects. The relative insolubility of their hydroxides and the relative solubility of their sulfates are cited as examples. They differ, however, from Group II-B elements in that they are light metals (specific gravity is less than 5); their oxides do not yield the free metal when treated thermally with carbon; and they do not enter into complex ion formations. Beryllium oxide is amphoteric and, in this respect, resembles boron and aluminum.

Calcium, strontium, and barium react readily with water under ordinary conditions to form hydroxides with the simultaneous evolution of hydrogen. Although relatively insoluble in comparison with hydroxides of the alkali metals, hydroxides of alkaline earth metals are nevertheless strongly basic. Carbonates, sulfates, phosphates, and fluorides are quite insoluble. These differences are important analytically.

Some of the more important properties of the elements of Group II-A are listed in Table V.

Beryllium—Be = 9.0122 (At. No. 4)

Beryllium occurs primarily as silicates, alone or in combination with other metals. The principal source of the element is the mineral *beryl* [$Al_2Be_3Si_6O_{18}$]. The metal is prepared commercially by electrolysis of fused potassium beryllium fluoride [K_2BeF_4].

Pharmaceutical Uses—Neither beryllium nor its compounds find application as therapeutic agents. Experiences associated with metallurgical operations and with use of compounds of the element in the fluorescent lighting industry have demonstrated conclusively that beryllium is a very toxic metal. Occurrences of severe granulomatous lesions of the skin, mucous membranes, and lungs following exposure are recorded in the literature. Exposure may result through external cuts or abrasions, or through inhalation of dust during metallurgical or fabrication operations. Inhalation exposure leads directly to lung

Table V—Elements of Group II-A

Element	Beryllium	Magnesium	Calcium	Strontium	Barium	Radium
Symbol	Be	Mg	Ca	Sr	Ba	Ra
Atomic number	4	12	20	38	56	88
Atomic weight	9.0122	24.305	40.08	87.62	137.34	[226][a]
Atomic radius (Å)	0.90	1.30	1.74	1.92	1.98	...
Ionic (crystal) radius (Å) (for coordination number 6)	0.31(+2)	0.65(+2)	0.99(+2)	1.13(+2)	1.35(+2)	1.40(+2)
Electronegativity (Pauling scale)	1.5	1.2	1.0	1.0	0.9	0.9
Orbital electrons	[He]2s^2	[Ne]3s^2	[Ar]4s^2	[Kr]5s^2	[Xe]6s^2	[Rn]7s^2
Isotopes, natural (mass numbers)	9	24, 25, 26	40, 42, 43, 44, 46, 48	84, 86, 87, 88	130, 132, 134, 135, 136, 137, 138	226
Specific gravity (20°C)	1.86	1.75	1.55	2.6	3.6	5.0
Melting temperature (°C)	1280	651	851	800	850	960
Boiling temperature (°C)	1500	1107	1487	1366	1537	1140
Abundance (% of earth's crust)	6×10^{-4}	2.1	3.6	0.03	0.025	1.3×10^{-10}

[a] Mass number of the isotope of longest known half-life.

damage, usually referred to as a type of chemical pneumonitis. Symptoms of beryllium intoxication are frequently long delayed and chronic and proceed from brief exposures. Aurintricarboxylic acid (ammonium salt = aluminon) has been suggested as an antidote.

Magnesium—Mg = 24.305 (At. No. 12)

Magnesium is a relatively abundant element and occurs widely distributed. Some of the more important minerals are *magnesite* [MgCO$_3$], *dolomite* [MgCO$_3$.CaCO$_3$], *carnallite* [KCl.MgCl$_2$.6H$_2$O], *kieserite* [MgSO$_4$.H$_2$O], and *brucite* [Mg(OH)$_2$]. It also occurs abundantly in the form of silicates such as *talc*, *soapstone*, *meerschaum*, and many varieties of *asbestos*. The metal is produced primarily by electrolytic processes, particularly by electrolysis of the fused chloride. The chloride is commonly obtained from underground brines and sea water.

Chemically, magnesium is quite active. Dry air does not attack it but exposure to moist air results in the slow formation of a coating of basic carbonate. The metal ignites readily in air burning with a flame rich in actinic rays to form a mixture of magnesium oxide [MgO] and magnesium nitride [Mg$_3$N$_2$]. The powdered metal decomposes water at elevated temperatures to form magnesium hydroxide with the simultaneous evolution of hydrogen. It readily displaces hydrogen from dilute mineral acids but is insoluble in alkali hydroxide solutions (an important point of difference from zinc and aluminum).

Pharmaceutical Uses—Magnesium compounds are employed for a variety of purposes in therapeutics. Of the inorganic compounds, the oxide, hydroxide, carbonate, phosphate, and trisilicate are offered as gastric antacids, the hydroxide and sulfate as cathartics, and the sulfate, via intramuscular or intravenous injection, as an anticonvulsant. A concentrated solution of the sulfate is often applied topically for its anti-inflammatory action. Toxic manifestations following magnesium administration are relatively rare. Calcium gluconate given intravenously is an effective antidote. The artificial radioactive ^{27}Mg isotope has been employed in research involving photosynthesis.

Calcium—Ca = 40.08 (At. No. 20)

Calcium occurs abundantly in nature. Important minerals include *marble*, *limestone*, and *chalk*, each of which is a form of calcium carbonate [CaCO$_3$]; *gypsum* and *selenite*, forms of calcium sulfate [CaSO$_4$.2H$_2$O]; *apatite*, [3Ca$_3$(PO$_4$)$_2$.CaF$_2$]; *phosphate rock* [Ca$_3$(PO$_4$)$_2$]; and *fluorspar* [CaF$_2$]. Silicate minerals are also common. The phosphate is the most important inorganic constituent of bones and teeth. Commercially, the free metal is obtained by electrolysis of the fused chloride.

Although much less reactive chemically than the alkali metals, calcium is a relatively reactive metal. Heated in air, it forms a mixture of calcium oxide and calcium nitride. It decomposes water slowly at ordinary temperatures forming calcium hydroxide with the simultaneous liberation of hydrogen. Soluble calcium salts undergo metathesis with soluble *borates*, *carbonates*, *citrates*, *oxalates*, *phosphates*, *sulfates*, and *tartrates* to yield insoluble calcium compounds; this propensity often leads to pharmaceutical incompatibilities.

Pharmaceutical Uses—Calcium compounds are widely and extensively used, and are indispensable to life, industry, and civilized economy. Calcium is essential for biologic processes and nutrition. It constitutes nearly 40% of ashed bones. Therapeutic categories represented by official inorganic compounds include: antacid (carbonate and tribasic phosphate), astringent (hydroxide), and calcium replenisher (chloride and dibasic phosphate).

Calcium is frequently the cation of choice to carry a therapeutically active anion, eg, calcium aminosalicylate, calcium cyclobarbital, etc. In some instances this is referable to better physical characteristics of the calcium compound; in others it is a deliberate attempt to avoid unnecessary intake of sodium. The artificial radioactive ^{45}Ca isotope has been employed in studies involving mineral metabolism.

Strontium—Sr = 87.62 (At. No. 38)

The chief minerals of strontium are *celestite* [SrSO$_4$] and *strontianite* [SrCO$_3$]. The metal may be prepared by electrolysis of the fused chloride. In its chemical and physical properties, strontium strongly resembles calcium, except that it is somewhat more reactive chemically. With respect to water solubility, strontium salts resemble in general those of calcium and barium. As to be expected, there are slight differences in degree of solubility among alkaline earth compounds. Such differences occasionally assume analytical importance such as in the case of the hydroxides and sulfates.

Pharmaceutical Uses—The therapeutic properties of strontium compounds are attributable to their anionic components, strontium merely serving as a carrier of the ion. There is no evidence of superiority over calcium and sodium compounds. Artificial radioactive isotopes of strontium have been used in connection with studies involving bone physiology. Strontium cannot function as a physiologic replacement for calcium. There are no official strontium compounds.

Barium—Ba = 137.34 (At. No. 56)

The most important mineral of barium is *barite*, also known as *barytes* and *heavy spar*, a form of barium sulfate [$BaSO_4$]. Of secondary importance is the mineral *witherite*, a form of barium carbonate [$BaCO_3$]. Commercially, barium is produced either by electrolysis of the fused chloride or by electrolysis of an aqueous solution of the chloride using a mercury cathode.

Chemically, barium is the most active of the calcium-strontium-barium triad of elements. It reacts readily with water at ordinary temperature to form barium hydroxide with the simultaneous liberation of hydrogen. Barium hydroxide is a strong base and because of this and its solubility characteristics, it often finds useful application in analytic and synthetic operations. The barium ion is colorless; thus simple barium salts such as the chloride and the nitrate are white. Color may be imparted due to the anionic component of the salt, for example, yellow barium chromate.

Pharmaceutical Uses—With the exception of barium sulfate, which finds considerable use as a radiopaque substance in diagnostic explorations of the gastrointestinal tract, barium compounds are seldom employed as medicinal agents. In sharp contrast with calcium and strontium, barium ion is highly toxic. *All barium compounds which are soluble either in water or in dilute acid are poisonous.* The most readily available antidote for barium poisoning is magnesium sulfate (Epsom Salt). Artificial radioactive isotopes of barium have been employed in pharmacological investigations involving absorption, distribution, and excretion.

Elements of Group II-B

This group is sometimes referred to as the *zinc family of elements*, but family relationships are not strong. Each member has an outer electron arrangement of $(n-1)d^{10}ns^2$. Zinc and cadmium function exclusively in the +2 oxidation state; mercury, however, performs in both the +1 and +2 states. All form oxides of the type MO (wherein M represents one atom of any member of the group); halides of the type MX_2; sulfates of the type MSO_4; etc. In its univalent capacity, mercury forms an additional series of compounds exemplified by Hg_2O, Hg_2Cl_2, and Hg_2SO_4. All participate generously, as the central atom, in the formation of coordination complexes.

Zinc and cadmium occur only in the combined state. Sulfide, carbonate, and silicate minerals predominate. The two elements are often associated in the same mineral. Although small quantities of mercury occur free in nature, the only important occurrence of this element is as the sulfide.

With respect to physical and chemical properties, zinc and cadmium differ decidedly from mercury. The former are solids at ordinary temperature and function as base metals (combine with oxygen below red heat); mercury, on the other hand, is liquid at ordinary temperatures and emulates the noble metals (ie, does not combine with oxygen below red heat and liberates

Table VI—Elements of Group II-B

Element	Zinc	Cadmium	Mercury
Symbol	Zn	Cd	Hg
Atomic number	30	48	80
Atomic weight	65.37	112.40	200.59
Atomic radius (Å)	1.31	1.48	1.49
Ionic (crystal) radii (Å) (for coordination number 6)	0.74(+2)	0.97(+2)	1.27(+1) 1.10(+2)
Electronegativity (Pauling scale)	1.6	1.7	1.9
Orbital electrons	[Ar]$3d^{10}$-$4s^2$	[Kr]$4d^{10}$-$5s^2$	[Xe]$4f^{14}$-$5d^{10}6s^2$
Isotopes, natural (mass numbers)	64, 66, 67, 68, 70	106, 108, 110, 111, 112, 113, 114, 116	196, 198, 199, 200, 201, 202, 204
Specific gravity (20°C)	7.14	8.64	13.46
Melting temperature °C	419	321	−38.9
Boiling temperature °C	907	767	357
Abundance (% of earth's crust)	1.3×10^{-2}	1.5×10^{-5}	ca 10^{-6}

oxygen readily from its oxides on heating). Zinc and cadmium react readily with dilute hydrochloric acid, but mercury does not. All react easily with moderately dilute nitric acid. Zinc oxide is amphoteric. A summary of some of the more important characteristics is presented in Table VI.

Zinc—Zn = 65.37 (At. No. 30)

The most important zinc mineral is *zinc blende*, also known as *sphalerite* and *black jack*, a crystalline and metallic appearing form of zinc sulfide [ZnS]. Zinc minerals of lesser importance include *Smithsonite*, a form of zinc carbonate [$ZnCO_3$]; *calamine*, an impure zinc orthosilicate [$Zn_2SiO_4.H_2O$]; *zincite*, a form of zinc oxide [ZnO]; and *Franklinite*, a mineral which contains both iron and manganese in addition to zinc. Current production methods involve conversion of the zinc in an ore to zinc oxide (by heating in the case of zinc carbonate ores and by roasting in the case of zinc sulfide ores) followed by thermal reduction of the oxide with carbon.

Zinc is stable in dry air at ordinary temperatures. On heating in air to about 500°, it burns with a characteristic bluish white flame to form zinc oxide. Continued exposure to moist air at ordinary temperature results in the gradual formation of a coating of basic carbonate. Zinc powder and dust react with hot water to form the oxide with evolution of hydrogen. Pure zinc reacts very slowly with dilute mineral acids, but commercial zinc usually reacts readily because of the presences of traces of impurities. Zinc also reacts with strong alkalies such as sodium hydroxide to form zincates in which the zinc functions anionically; eg, sodium zincate [Na_2ZnO_2]. Zinc ion is colorless and thus zinc salts are white unless the anionic component imparts color such as in zinc chromate.

Pharmaceutical Uses—Elementary zinc finds no direct therapeutic applications. Zinc oxide in various forms is employed topically as an astringent and protectant, zinc chloride is used as an astringent and desensitizer for dentin, zinc sulfate is a popular ophthalmic astringent, and zinc peroxide is an oxidizing type of topical anti-infective. Zinc compounds which are soluble in water or in gastric fluid are poisonous. The most readily available antidote is sodium bicarbonate (baking soda). Artificial radioactive isotopes of zinc have been employed in studies of mineral metabolism.

Cadmium—Cd = 112.40 (At. No. 48)

Cadmium occurs in nature only in combined form, commonly associated with zinc. It is produced commercially primarily as a byproduct in the smelting of zinc ores. It is obtained first in the form of its oxide which is subsequently reduced thermally with carbon to produce the free metal.

Cadmium slowly tarnishes on exposure to air and burns on strong heating in air to form the brown oxide, CdO. It is slowly soluble in hydrochloric acid, but

readily dissolves in dilute nitric acid. The metal is relatively unaffected by cold sulfuric acid, but heating with the concentrated acid slowly converts it to the sulfate. Cadmium oxide functions exclusively in basic capacity.

Pharmaceutical Uses—Neither elemental cadmium nor any of its salts find therapeutic applications. There are no official cadmium compounds.

Mercury—Hg = 200.59 (At. No. 80)

Mercury occurs in small, unimportant quantities in the free state, but the principal source of mercury is *cinnabar*, which is mercuric sulfide [HgS]. Ores of mercury of low quality must be concentrated by flotation prior to extraction of the mercury. The concentrate is then roasted in air whereby the sulfur in the ore is converted to sulfur dioxide and the mercury is liberated and distilled.

When pure, mercury does not tarnish in the air at ordinary temperatures. It forms amalgams with many metals. Iron is an important exception. The metal combines with sulfur at ordinary temperature, forming black mercuric sulfide. It is not attacked by hydrochloric or cold sulfuric acids, but is converted to sulfate by hot concentrated sulfuric acid, and readily dissolves in moderately dilute nitric acid, especially on warming.

Pharmaceutical Uses—In former years, metallic mercury was important therapeutically as a cathartic and parasiticide. Today, however, it has been largely replaced for such purposes by more efficacious and less toxic medicaments. Compounds of mercury are employed in modern therapy primarily for their diuretic, germicidal, and antiluetic actions, and many of these compounds are organic, eg, meralluride, nitromersol, etc. Modern inorganic survivors include calomel (a cathartic), mercury bichloride (a disinfectant), yellow mercuric oxide (an ophthalmic antibacterial), and ammoniated mercury (a topical and ophthalmic anti-infective). The radioactive nuclides, ^{197}Hg and ^{203}Hg, function in diagnostic capacity. See Chapter 34.

Mercury metal is poisonous, and prolonged inhalation even of minute amounts of mercury volatilized from it at room temperature may be fatal. If mercury is spilled in poorly ventilated rooms, it should not be allowed to remain there for any length of time.

With the exception of the sulfide, all common mercury salts are poisonous. The best antidote for mercury poisoning, particularly for the bichloride, is *Sodium Formaldehyde Sulfoxylate* (page 1318).

Egg albumen may be used in emergency if the poisoning is discovered shortly after ingestion. The white of one egg should be administered for each 250 mg of mercuric chloride ingested. Emesis should be induced promptly thereafter.

Elements of Group III

This group in the periodic classification includes a total of 36 elements which, on the basis of electronic structure, subdivide quite disproportionately into the 5 elements comprising Group III-A and the 31 elements comprising Group III-B. (See the *Periodic Chart of the Elements* on the back cover.)

Elements of Group III-A include boron, aluminum, gallium, indium, and thallium. Each of these elements is characterized by the presence of an ns^2np^1 valence shell of electrons and also by the fact that subsequent increases in atomic number soon lead in each instance to an element of group zero without altering the population of the inner electron orbits.

Elements of Group III-B include scandium, yttrium and the lanthanide and actinide series of elements. Each is characterized structurally by the presence of an ns^2 valence shell of electrons and also by the fact that it constitutes the first step in a lengthy succession of electron additions to inner orbitals during the Periodic architectural process.

The *lanthanide series* is commonly referred to as the *rare earth elements*. It includes lanthanum, cerium, praseodymium, neodymium, promethium, samarium, europium, gadolinium, terbium, dysprosium, holmium, erbium, thulium, ytterbium, and lutetium. The *actinide series* includes actinium, thorium, protactinium, uranium, neptunium, plutonium, americium, curium, berkelium, californium, einsteinium, fermium, mendelevium, nobelium, and lawrencium. The elements following uranium are often referred to as the *transuranium elements*.

The naturally occurring members of the actinide series are treated, along with other radioactive elements, in Chapter 33. Except for the employment of certain ceric salts as analytical reagents, the other members of Group III-B are of no pharmaceutical interest and are not treated further. Common oxidation states are recorded in the Periodic Chart.

Elements of Group III-A

As is to be expected from the ns^2np^1 electron structure, each element in this group functions with a positive valence of three, forming oxides of the type M_2O_3, halides of the type MX_3, sulfates of the type $M_2(SO_4)_3$, etc. With increasing atomic weight, there is an increasing tendency on the part of these elements to function also in the $1+$ oxidation state. This tendency reaches its peak with thallium which forms the two very distinct thallous and thallic series of compounds.

The trivalent state is largely achieved by these elements through covalence. This results in the formation of compounds in which Group III-A elements contain (through sharing) only six electrons in the outermost orbit—two electrons short of the number required for the stable structure of an inert element. Such compounds are frequently described as being "electron-deficient" and are characterized by their propensity to form complexes through coordination with electron-rich compounds or through hydrogen bonding. Thus, even the simple hydrides of these elements do not show the formula MH_3 which might be expected, but exist instead as polymers such as M_2H_6, etc.

Group III-A elements are not found free in nature. They are isolated by various processes which ultimately involve reduction of boron trioxide.

With regard to chemical characteristics, boron is decidedly nonmetallic, aluminum is amphoteric, and the three remaining elements, gallium, indium, and thallium, are decidedly metallic. Some of the more important characteristics are presented in Table VII. Boron, aluminum, and thallium are the only elements in this group of pharmaceutical interest, and therefore further treatment in this text will be limited to these three.

Boron—B = 10.811 (At. No. 5)

The more important minerals of boron are *tincal* [$Na_2B_4O_7.10H_2O$], *boracite* [$2Mg_3B_8O_{15}.MgCl_2$], *borocalcite* [$CaB_4O_7.6H_2O$], and *boronatrocalcite* or *ulexite* [$Na_2B_4O_7.2CaB_4O_7.18H_2O$]. Boron may be obtained by heating the trioxide with metallic aluminum or magnesium.

Boron combines directly with fluorine, chlorine, and bromine, and at high temperature with oxygen, nitrogen, and carbon. It is scarcely affected by the halogen hydracids but is acted upon by acids which can attack through oxidation. Several oxyacids (or salts thereof) are known, most prominent among which are *orthoboric* [H_3BO_3], (*poly*)*metaboric* [$(HBO_2)_n$], *tetraboric* [$H_2B_4O_7$], and *peroxyboric* (*perboric*) [HBO_3]. Ammonium and alkali borates are soluble in water. Borates of other metals are slightly soluble or almost insoluble in water, but all borates are readily decomposed by diluted mineral acids.

The size, electron configuration, and intermediate electronegativity of the boron atom render its total chemistry quite complex, and features relative to the structural intimacies of various types of boron compounds are in process of elucidation. Advanced texts devoted exclusively to the subject are available. In many of the types of compounds, the boron atom emulates the behavior of a 4-covalent atom although it contains but three valence electrons. Structures displaying hydrogen bridges are numerous, and a veritable universe of open and closed carbon–boron chain compounds is gradually emerging.

Pharmaceutical Uses—Boric acid in various dosage forms is employed as a topical anti-infective and ophthalmic irrigant. Sodium borate is bacterio-

Table VII—Elements of Group III-A

Element	Boron	Aluminum	Gallium	Indium	Thallium
Symbol	B	Al	Ga	In	Tl
Atomic number	5	13	31	49	81
Atomic weight	10.811	26.9815	69.72	114.82	204.37
Atomic radius (Å)	0.82	1.18	1.26	1.44	1.48
Ionic (crystal) radii (Å)			1.48(+1)	1.32(+1)	1.40(+1)
(for coordination number 6)	0.20(+3)	0.50(+3)	0.62(+3)	0.81(+3)	0.95(+3)
Electronegativity (Pauling scale)	2.0	1.5	1.6	1.7	1.8
Orbital electrons	[He]2s²-2p¹	[Ne]3s²-3p¹	[Ar]3d¹⁰-4s²4p¹	[Kr]4d¹⁰-5s²5p¹	[Xe]4f¹⁴-5d¹⁰6s²-6p¹
Isotopes, natural (mass numbers)	10, 11	27	69, 71	113, 115	203, 205
Specific gravity (20°C)	2.4	2.70	5.93	7.29	11.9
Melting temperature (°C)	2300	660	29.8	155	304
Boiling temperature (°C)	2550	2270	2070	1450	1457
Abundance (% of earth's crust)	3×10^{-4}	8.13	1.5×10^{-3}	10^{-5}	ca 10^{-4}

static and is a frequent ingredient of cold creams, eye washes, and mouth washes. Neither boric acid nor the borates are germicides. Sodium perborate is an oxidizing type of local anti-infective.

Boric acid readily undergoes esterification with glycerin, propylene glycol, and various other polyhydroxy compounds. Some of the resulting compounds are fairly strong acids and are utilized in the volumetric determination of boric acid.

Boric acid and borates are toxic either by ingestion or by absorption through nonintact skin. As a result of indiscriminate use or confusion with other substances, numerous fatalities have occurred, especially with boric acid, and this has led to the institution of rigid controls over the substance in nurseries and dispensaries. There is no effective chemical antidote; treatment of poisoning is symptomatic and supportive.

Aluminum—Al = 26.9815 (At. No. 13)

Aluminum is the most abundant of all metals and the third most abundant element, being exceeded in natural occurrence only by oxygen and silicon. In so far as isolation of elementary aluminum is concerned, the only important ores are *bauxite* [approximate composition: $Al_2O_3.2H_2O$] and *cryolite* [$3NaF.-AlF_3$]. Aluminum is prepared commercially by electrolysis of purified aluminum oxide dissolved in a molten mixture of sodium, calcium, and aluminum fluorides. The purified oxide is prepared from bauxite, and the sodium and aluminum fluorides are obtained from cryolite.

Aluminum oxidizes superficially in moist air forming a tightly adhering, protective layer of aluminum oxide. The metal reacts readily with diluted hydrochloric or sulfuric acid but is resistant to attack by nitric or acetic acid. It reacts readily with aqueous solutions of the fixed alkalies with evolution of hydrogen and formation of aluminate ion. The common compounds of aluminum are white.

Pharmaceutical Uses—In paste form, aluminum powder is employed topically as a protective. Among aluminum inorganic compounds, the hydroxide and phosphate find extensive use in various dosage forms as gastric antacids; aluminum sulfate, in the form of alum, is an astringent; and kaolin, a hydrated aluminum silicate, is an adsorbent and demulcent. Basic aluminum chloride is a popular ingredient in astringent, antiperspirant, and deodorant cosmetic preparations. Bentonite, another naturally occurring hydrated aluminum silicate, is useful as a suspending agent.

Thallium—Tl = 204.37 (At. No. 81)

Thallium occurs in nature primarily as sulfides and selenides, usually in combination with other metals. Its principal source is as a contaminant of iron pyrites.

Thallium compounds are not employed in medicine. They are highly toxic percutaneously as well as by ingestion. The element is mentioned here only because the salts are sometimes present in commercial rodenticidal preparations, and the use of these has often proved fatal. The employment of thallium compounds in depilatory preparations has also produced disastrous results. Intravenous administration of sodium iodide followed by sodium thiosulfate is reportedly the best antidotal treatment that can be used.

Elements of Group IV

The elements of Group IV subdivide into Group IV-A, in which the common structural feature is an ns^2np^2 disposition of outer orbit electrons, and Group IV-B, in which the valence electron distribution is $(n-1)d^2ns^2$. In the absence of other considerations, oxidation states $+2$ and $+4$ are thus expectable with all members of the Group. In general, the Group IV-A elements are the more familiar.

Elements of Group IV-A

Group IV-A elements include carbon, silicon, germanium, tin, and lead. Containing four electrons in the outermost orbit, each represents a half-way stage in the architecture toward an inert (Group Zero) element, and this imparts some rather characteristic chemistry to the group. The $+2$ oxidation state is rarely encountered with carbon but becomes increasingly apparent with increasing atomic size and is strongly evident with tin and lead. In both the $+2$ and $+4$ oxidation states, the bonding in compounds is essentially covalent, the 4-covalent state being achieved by a shift in the outer electron arrangement from s^2p^2 to sp^3. Except possibly for carbides and silicides of strongly electropositive metals, achievement of negative oxidation states through electron gain is unknown. Carbon is exclusively nonmetallic, and metallic properties begin to appear with silicon and become quite characteristic of tin and lead. The oxides of carbon and silicon are acidic while those of the other elements in the group are amphoteric. Table VIII summarizes some of the more important characteristics of the group. The combined features (electron disposition, atomic size, and electronegativity) of the carbon atom suffice to render the chemistry of carbon very unique, and this is the basis for the classical subdivision of the total field of chemistry into the inorganic and organic subfields. For further discussion, see Chapter 29.

Carbon—C = 12.01115 (At. No. 6)

Carbon occurs widely distributed in nature in numerous forms. In the free state, it occurs as *diamond, graphite,* coal, peat, lignite, etc. In the combined state, it is a constituent of all naturally occurring organic substances, eg, hydrocarbons, carbohydrates, proteins, alkaloids, etc, and it also occurs as various carbonate minerals, eg, limestone, magnesite, siderite, etc. The free element is produced in various forms, eg, charcoals, lampblacks, coke, etc,

Table VIII—Elements of Group IV-A

Element	Carbon	Silicon	Germanium	Tin	Lead
Symbol	C	Si	Ge	Sn	Pb
Atomic number	6	14	32	50	82
Atomic weight	12.01115	28.086	72.59	118.69	207.19
Atomic radius (Å)	0.77	1.11	1.22	1.41	1.47
Ionic (crystal) radii (Å)	2.60(−4)	2.71(−4)	0.93(+2)	1.12(+2)	1.20(+2)
(for coordination number 6)	0.15(+4)	0.41(+4)	0.53(+4)	0.71(+4)	0.84(+4)
Electronegativity (Pauling scale)	2.5	1.8	1.8	1.8	1.8
Orbital electrons	$[He]2s^2\text{-}2p^2$	$[Ne]3s^2\text{-}3p^2$	$[Ar]3d^{10}\text{-}4s^24p^2$	$[Kr]4d^{10}\text{-}5s^25p^2$	$[Xe]4f^{14}\text{-}5d^{10}6s^26p^2$
Isotopes, natural (mass numbers)	12, 13	28, 29, 30	70, 72, 73, 74, 76	112, 114, 115, 116, 117, 118, 119, 120, 122, 124	204, 206, 207, 208
Specific gravity (20°C)	3.51 (diamond)	2.4 (amorphous)	5.36	7.31 (white tin)	11.34
	2.22 (graphite)	2.3 (crystalline)		5.75 (gray tin)	
Melting temperature (°C)	ca 3600	1420	959	232	328
Boiling temperature (°C)	ca 3500 (sublimes)	ca 2600	ca 2700	ca 2260	ca 1620
Abundance (% of earth's crust)	3.2×10^{-2}	27.7	7×10^{-4}	4×10^{-3}	1.0×10^{-3}

by heating organic materials to high temperature with minimal access to air.

Carbon does not readily combine with hydrogen, but at a temperature of about 300° and under great pressure the two elements unite to form a mixture of hydrocarbons similar to petroleum. At elevated temperatures, carbon combines directly with oxygen to produce CO or CO_2 depending on available oxygen supply.

Carbon monoxide is a *very poisonous*, odorless gas. It burns in the air with a blue flame forming carbon dioxide. It is only slightly soluble in water. It is one of the waste products of the internal combustion engine, such as the automobile engine, and is the cause of death, known as *petro mortis*, in those who inhale the combustion gases in a confined space where a gas or gasoline engine is running. The carbon monoxide combines with the hemoglobin of the blood forming methemoglobin which is more stable than oxyhemoglobin and the hemoglobin thus loses its power to function in the oxygen-carbon dioxide interchange.

Carbon dioxide is produced commercially by several processes. Unlike carbon monoxide, it is not toxic by reason of interaction with hemoglobin. It is toxic, however, through suffocation if its inspiration occurs at the expense of sufficient oxygen inhalation.

Under appropriate conditions, carbon forms various other binary compounds such as cyanogen $[(CN)_2]$, carbon disulfide, carbon tetrachloride, and numerous carbides and hydrocarbons. The important inorganic acids of carbon are carbonic $[H_2CO_3]$, percarbonic (peroxydicarbonic) $[H_2C_2O_6]$, and the pseudobinary acid, hydrocyanic $[HCN]$. All are relatively feeble as acids and are available primarily in the form of salts.

Pharmaceutical Uses—Carbon dioxide, usually in concentrations ranging from 5 to 7½% in oxygen, is an effective respiratory stimulant which is applied in the treatment of asphyxia and various other conditions requiring hyperventilation. The slightly soluble carbonates or basic carbonates of calcium, magnesium, and aluminum find extensive use as gastric antacids. Sodium bicarbonate is also effective but its action is systemic as well as gastric. The normal

carbonates of sodium and potassium are too strongly alkaline for such employment. Potassium bicarbonate is used as a source of potassium ion in electrolyte replenishers. Bismuth subcarbonate is an astringent and protective which adheres well to cutaneous and membranous surfaces and is therefore widely employed in lotions and ointments for external use. Ammonium carbonate is an effective reflex stimulant by virtue of its release of ammonia for inhalation. It is also employed as an expectorant.

Silicon—Si = 28.086 (At. No. 14)

Next to oxygen, silicon is the most abundant element on earth. It does not occur free in nature, but its compounds with oxygen and other elements are present everywhere. *Sand, agate, quartz,* and *opal* are forms of silicon dioxide. *Kaolin* (clay), *asbestos, bentonite, pumice, talc,* and *meerschaum* consist chiefly of aluminum, calcium, or magnesium silicates. Many other silicate minerals occur in nature. Silicon may be prepared by heating silicon dioxide with an excess of powdered magnesium metal, then extracting the magnesium oxide and the excess of magnesium with diluted hydrochloric acid.

Silicon unites in the cold or on heating with the halogens, forming a variety of silicon halides. The *tetrahalides* are hydrolyzed by water, forming *silicic acid* and the corresponding halogen hydracids.

Silicon forms one well-known oxide, *silicon dioxide* $[SiO_2]$, commonly known as *silica*. It occurs abundantly in nature in both amorphous and crystalline forms, eg, sand, quartz, onyx, etc. Pure silica is white. It is insoluble in water and in acids, but is readily attacked by hydrofluoric acid, forming gaseous *silicon tetrafluoride.* Finely powdered silicon dioxide slowly dissolves in fixed alkali hydroxides upon heating, forming the alkali *silicates*. The alkali silicates may be obtained also by fusing powdered silica with an excess of alkali carbonates.

Silicon forms numerous silicic acids, eg, *orthosilicic acid* $[H_4SiO_4]$, *disilicic acid* $[H_6Si_2O_7]$, and *metasilicic acid* $[H_2SiO_3]$, and various of these occur in nature in the form of silicates. Except for the alkali salts, silicates are insoluble in water or acids, but they are all readily attacked by warm hydrofluoric acid, preferably in the presence of some sulfuric acid. Under these conditions the silicon is converted into gaseous silicon tetrafluoride.

Silica gels are amorphous forms of polysilicic acids prepared from inorganic or organic orthosilicates by various hydrolytic processes. Structurally, they may be looked upon as condensation polymers of orthosilicic acid. They are available in various commercial grades of hydration and porosity and find applications as gas adsorbents, desiccants, thickeners, and gelling agents.

The close relationship between carbon and silicon has prompted considerable research during the past two decades in that phase of silicon chemistry trivially referred to as the organic chemistry of silicon. The compounds involved are analogs of carbon compounds in which silicon functions in place of one or more of the carbon atoms. Simple members such as *silane* [SiH_4], *silanol* [SiH_3OH], *disiloxane* [$H_3Si—O—SiH_3$], etc have long been known. The present interest is in more complex compounds which contain both carbon and silicon. The *silicones (alkylsiloxanes)* are condensation polymers of various types of alkylsilanols and represent one type of research in the field which is currently finding extensive commercial application. For further discussion, see page 768.

Silicosis is a lung disease caused by dust of silica or silicates accumulating in the lungs. Workers in stone quarries, or in other industries where sand or other silicate dusts are prevalent, are prone to contract this disease. Measures to prevent this disease have been published by the US Bureau of Mines.

Pharmaceutical Uses—The various types of applications of silica gels have been mentioned above. All official inorganic silicon compounds are complex insoluble silicates and, with the exception of magnesium trisilicate, occur naturally.

Magnesium trisilicate is actually a mixture of magnesium oxide and silica, each in various states of hydration, prepared by precipitation involving a soluble silicate and a soluble magnesium salt. Its effectiveness as an antacid is practically exclusively referable to its magnesium oxide content. The silicic acid component contributes protective action through its good adhering quality. The trisilicate is also employed as a suspending agent.

Among the natural silicates, kaolin and bentonite are hydrous aluminum silicates. Suitable grades of the former have long been employed for their adsorbent and demulcent properties; bentonite is recognized officially as a suspending agent. Talc is a hydrous magnesium silicate which is useful in various ways as a dusting powder. Pumice is a complex aluminum potassium sodium silicate of volcanic origin. Its inertness and hardness make it useful as a filtering medium, a dispersing agent, and an abrasive. Its official category of use is as a dental abrasive.

Tin—Sn = 118.69 (At. No. 50)

Tin occurs in nature as stannic oxide [SnO_2], primarily in the minerals known as *cassiterite* or *tinstone*. The metal is prepared by reducing the refined dioxide with carbon.

Massive tin is stable in air, but in powdered form it oxidizes in air, especially in the presence of moisture. It is slowly soluble in cold hydrochloric acid, in dilute nitric acid, or in hot, moderately diluted sulfuric acid; it readily dissolves in concentrated hydrochloric acid. Strong nitric acid converts it into insoluble metastannic acid. It is also slowly soluble in cold, and more readily in hot, solutions of the caustic alkalies.

Tin functions generously in both the +2 and +4 oxidation states. The stannous ion is a powerful and much used reducing agent. The fundamental tin anions are stannite [SnO_2^{2-}] and stannate [SnO_3^{2-}].

Pharmaceutical Uses—The only official tin compound is stannous fluoride [tin(II) fluoride] applied topically as a dental prophylactic. Experimental evidence demonstrates the superiority of this fluoride over other soluble fluorides for this kind of application. The ready susceptibility of stannous fluoride to oxidative and hydrolytic decomposition causes problems in the preparation and storage of suitable dosage forms. Various tin dioxide [tin(IV) oxide] preparations have been used externally for their germicidal effect, particularly against staphylococcal organisms which are often resistant to various other germicides.

Lead—Pb = 207.19 (At. No. 82)

Lead occurs in nature in the form of several minerals. Native lead sulfide, *galena* or *galenite*, is practically the

Table IX—Elements of Group IV-B

Element	Titanium	Zirconium	Hafnium
Symbol	Ti	Zr	Hf
Atomic number	22	40	72
Atomic weight	47.90	91.22	178.49
Atomic radius (Å)	1.36	1.48	1.44
Ionic (crystal) radii (Å)	0.90(+2)	...	...
(for coordination number 6)	0.68(+4)	0.80(+4)	0.81(+4)
Electronegativity (Pauling scale)	1.5	1.4	1.3
Orbital electrons	[Ar]3d²-4s²	[Kr]4d²-5s²	[Xe]4f¹⁴-5d²6s²
Isotopes, natural (mass numbers)	46, 47, 48, 49, 50	90, 91, 92, 94, 96	174, 176, 177, 178, 179, 180
Specific gravity (20°C)	4.43	6.49	13.3
Melting temperature (°C)	1730	1860	2230
Boiling temperature (°C)	above 3000	above 2900	above 3200
Abundance (% of earth's crust)	0.44	0.022	4.5×10^{-4}

only ore from which lead is obtained. The metal is produced by roasting lead sulfide in a reverberatory furnace until a part of the sulfide is changed into lead oxide and lead sulfate. The air supply is then cut off, the temperature increased, and the following reaction takes place:

$$2PbS + PbSO_4 + 2PbO \rightarrow 5Pb + 3SO_2$$

Lead is practically unaffected by cold hydrochloric, hydrofluoric, or sulfuric acid, or by cold concentrated nitric acid, but it is attacked by almost all acids when heated. It is readily dissolved by diluted nitric acid and also by acetic acid in the presence of air. Lead is attacked by the caustic alkalies and their carbonates.

Like tin, lead functions in both the +2 and +4 oxidation states, but the +2 lead state is much less susceptible to oxidation than the +2 tin analog. The fundamental lead anions are analogous to those of tin, ie, plumbite [$PbO_2{}^{2-}$] and plumbate [$PbO_3{}^{2-}$].

Pharmaceutical Uses—Lead compounds have no important medicinal applications at present. Lead ion precipitates protein and this action was responsible for its former official recognition, in the form of organic salts, as an astringent for application to intact cutaneous surfaces. Due to the toxicity of lead, however, the use of these substances has gradually been abandoned.

Lead compounds are poisonous via ingestion, inhalation, or percutaneous absorption. Lead is cumulative in the body and thus the poisoning may be of the acute or chronic types. Sodium and magnesium sulfates are commonly available chemical antidotes for poisoning by ingestion. Calcium disodium edetate administered intravenously renders lead in the blood physiologically inert via complexation.

Elements of Group IV-B

A detailed treatment of the elements of Group IV-B (titanium, zirconium, and hafnium) is not presented in this textbook because of their minor pharmaceutical importance. Although comparatively inert at ordinary temperatures, all react readily at high temperatures with oxygen, sulfur, water vapor, and other substances. The +4 oxidation state is common to all members, yielding oxides of the type MO_2 and chlorides of the type MCl_4. Titanium also forms two well-defined series of compounds in which it functions in +2, and +3 states. All elements of this group possess amphoteric characteristics, and all occur in nature in combined states. They may be produced in the elementary state by reducing their chlorides with magnesium at elevated temperatures. Titanium and zirconium are discussed briefly in the following sections. Hafnium occurs in relatively small quantities and has not been exploited for pharmaceutical or other purposes. It will, therefore, not be considered further. Some of its more characteristic properties, however, are included in Table IX.

Titanium—Ti = 47.90 (At. No. 22)

Titanium occurs either as the dioxide, as in *rutile* and *brookite*, or in the form of *titanates*, eg, *perovskite* [$CaTiO_3$] or *ilmenite* [$FeTiO_3$].

Titanium is soluble in dilute mineral acids with the liberation of hydrogen. Similar to salts of iron and aluminum, titanium salts are hydrolyzed by boiling with large quantities of water, forming metatitanic acid [$TiO(OH)_2$].

Titanium forms four oxides [TiO, Ti_2O_3, TiO_2, and TiO_3] and salts corresponding to the three lower oxides. The most important titanium compound is the dioxide, which is official. The soluble salts of divalent and trivalent titanium are violet colored and are powerful reducing agents.

Pharmaceutical Uses—The only official titanium compound is the dioxide [TiO_2] and its category of use is that of a solar ray protectant. As such, it is a popular ingredient in various lotions and creams for the prevention of undesirable effects from exposure to sunlight. This action is the result of its high covering power as a white pigment which is a consequence of its high refractive index.

Zirconium—Zr = 91.22 (At. No. 40)

Zirconium occurs largely as a silicate [$ZrSiO_4$] called *zircon* which constitutes the principal source of the metal and its compounds.

Zirconium is attacked only slowly by acids, except hydrofluoric in which it dissolves readily in the cold. The element functions primarily in the +4 oxidation state. Like the other metals in Group IV-B, zirconium performs in both cationic and anionic capacities. The fundamental anionic species is zirconate (IV) [$ZrO_3{}^{2-}$].

Zirconium carbonate and oxide, in various hydrous states, are used as antipruritics for dermatitis caused by contact poisons, such as poison ivy, and in minor skin irritations. Basic zirconium chlorides of varying composition frequently appear as the main ingredients of antiperspirant and deodorant preparations. In general, the mechanism involved in all of these zirconium applications is believed to be complexation of the truly causative agent with hydrous forms of zirconium dioxide. There are no official zirconium compounds.

Elements of Group V

The elements of Group V subdivide into two groups. The common structural feature among the Group V-A members is an ns^2np^3 outer orbit electron population. Due to the architectural irregularity observed with niobium, a similar common structural feature is absent in Group V-B, being $(n-1)d^3ns^2$ in the case of vanadium and tantalum but $(n-1)d^4ns^1$ in the case of niobium. Nevertheless, theoretical considerations predict that the +5 oxidation state is common to all Group V elements.

Elements of Group V-A

Group V-A elements include nitrogen, phosphorus, arsenic, antimony, and bismuth. The group displays strikingly regular gradations in properties ranging all the way from the exclusively non-metallic nitrogen to the almost exclusively metallic bismuth.

Oxidation states of +3 and +5 are common to all members of the group, thus yielding oxides of the types M_2O_3 and M_2O_5, halides of the types MX_3 and MX_5, etc. Bismuth functions primarily in the +3 state. All members except bismuth also function in the −3 oxidation state. Simplest hydrides are of the covalent MH_3 type and are characterized by an unshared pair of electrons which permits compound formation through electron pair donation. The ability to function in elementary cationic capacity becomes evident with the higher atomic number members.

The oxides of nitrogen and phosphorus are exclusively acidic. Those of arsenic and antimony are definitely amphoteric but are sufficiently acidic in character that most authors classify these elements with the non-metals. The common oxide of bismuth, Bi_2O_3, is basic; the lesser important pentoxide is acidic. Some of the more characteristic properties of these elements are presented in Table X.

Nitrogen occurs free in the atmosphere and also combined, as in nitrates and many organic compounds. Phosphorus always occurs combined, usually as phosphates. Arsenic and antimony occur free in trace amounts but usually in combined form as sulfides. Bismuth, however, occurs primarily in the free state.

Nitrogen is conveniently prepared by fractional distillation of liquid air. Phosphorus, arsenic, antimony, and bismuth may be produced in the elementary state by thermal reduction of their oxides with carbon. Native bismuth is often obtained by simple fusion since it melts at a comparatively low temperature.

Nitrogen—N = 14.0067 (At. No. 7)

Nitrogen constitutes about 78% of the earth's atmosphere. In combined form, it is invariably a part of all plants and animals. As sodium nitrate it occurs in large deposits in Chile; formerly, these deposits constituted the exclusive source of nitric acid and all nitrates for many years. Industrially, nitrogen is prepared today primarily by the fractional distillation of liquefied air.

Nitrogen is a colorless, tasteless, and odorless, inert gas. It is nonflammable and does not support combustion. Due to its stable triple-bond structure, the N_2 molecule shows little activity toward other elements, but at the temperature of the electric arc it combines with oxygen forming nitric oxide, which can be converted into nitrates or nitrites. In the presence of metallic catalysts and at great pressure and elevated temperature, it combines with hydrogen to form ammonia.

Nitrogen forms several oxides: *nitrous oxide* [N_2O] also known as nitrogen monoxide, *nitric oxide* [NO], *nitrogen trioxide* or *nitrous anhydride* [N_2O_3], *nitrogen dioxide* or *tetroxide* [NO_2 or N_2O_4], and *nitrogen pentoxide* or *nitric anhydride* [N_2O_5]. Several oxyacids are known, often only in the form of salts, the most important of which are *nitrous acid* [HNO_2] and *nitric acid* [HNO_3].

Pharmaceutical Uses—Although therapeutically inactive, elementary nitrogen is employed pharmaceutically as an inert atmosphere in various ampuls and other containers of substances which would be adversely affected by air. Nitrous oxide is an inhalatory general anesthetic. Sodium nitrite is official as an antidote to cyanide poisoning; it is also a vasodilator but is slower acting than the organic nitrite and nitrate esters commonly used for this purpose. Potassium nitrate is one of the most potent of the diuretic potassium compounds. Bismuth subnitrate is often employed for its astringent, adsorbent, and protective actions. Silver nitrate functions as an astringent, caustic, and germicide. Nitrite ion is toxic through its interaction with hemoglobin to form methemoglobin. Nitrate ion is reducible to nitrite in the intestine and may thus also elicit methemoglobinemia.

Phosphorus—P = 30.9738 (At. No. 15)

Phosphorus occurs in nature in the form of phosphates, chiefly of aluminum in the mineral *wavellite* [$4AlPO_4 . 2Al(OH)_3 . 9H_2O$]; of calcium in the minerals *apatite* [$Ca_3(PO_4)_2$ with some $CaCl_2$ or CaF_2], and *phosphorite* [$Ca_3(PO_4)_2$], and of iron in *vivianite* [$Fe_3(PO_4)_2$.-

Table X—Elements of Group V-A

Element	Nitrogen	Phosphorus	Arsenic	Antimony	Bismuth
Symbol	N	P	As	Sb	Bi
Atomic number	7	15	33	51	83
Atomic weight	14.0067	30.9738	74.9216	121.75	208.980
Atomic radius (Å)	0.75	1.06	1.19	1.38	1.46
Ionic (crystal) radii (Å)	1.71(−3)	2.12(−3)	2.22(−3)	2.45(−3)	1.20(+3)
(for coordination number 6)	0.11(+5)	0.34(+5)	0.47(+5)	0.62(+5)	0.74(+5)
Electronegativity (Pauling scale)	3.0	2.1	2.0	1.9	1.9
Orbital electrons	[He]$2s^2$-$2p^3$	[Ne]$3s^2$-$3p^3$	[Ar]$3d^{10}$-$4s^24p^3$	[Kr]$4d^{10}$-$5s^25p^3$	[Xe]$4f^{14}$-$5d^{10}6s^2$-$6p^3$
Isotopes, natural (mass numbers)	14, 15	31	75	121, 123	209
Specific gravity of solid (20°C)	0.88 (at −210°C)	1.82 (white P) 2.20 (red P)	5.7 ("metallic" As)	6.6 ("metallic" Sb)	9.8
Melting temperature (°C)	−210	44 (white P) 590 (red P, 43 atmos)	814 ("metallic" As, 36 atmos)	630 ("metallic" Sb)	271
Boiling temperature (°C)	−196	281 (white P)	615 (sublimes)	1380	1450
Abundance (% of earth's crust)	4.6×10^{-8}	0.12	5×10^{-4}	1×10^{-4}	2×10^{-5}

8H$_2$O]. The calcium phosphate minerals are the principal source. Phosphorus is now generally prepared by heating a mixture consisting of phosphatic minerals, coke, and quartz sand to a high temperature in an electric furnace.

Phosphorus exists in two common allotropic forms, yellow or colorless, and red or amorphous. *Yellow Phosphorus*, also known as *white phosphorus*, has a distinctive, disagreeable ozone-like odor. When exposed to the air it emits white fumes which are luminous in the dark and have an odor resembling garlic. On longer exposure to the air, or when heated at about 50° it ignites spontaneously. Yellow phosphorus is almost insoluble in water, but is soluble in chloroform, benzene, or carbon disulfide. It is poisonous.

Red Phosphorus—Red Phosphorus is a brown to red powder. It is nonpoisonous, nonflammable in air, except at high temperatures, and is nonluminous. It is insoluble in any common solvent.

Phosphorus forms compounds with hydrogen known as *phosphines* some of which ignite spontaneously in the air. It also combines with metals forming *phosphides*.

Phosphorus readily combines with chlorine giving rise to *phosphorus trichloride* [PCl$_3$], *phosphorus pentachloride* [PCl$_5$], and *phosphorus oxychloride* [POCl$_3$]. It forms similar compounds with bromine. Sulfides of phosphorus result from heating red phosphorus with sulfur in the proper proportions.

With oxygen, phosphorus forms two important oxides: *phosphorus trioxide* or *phosphorous anhydride* [P$_2$O$_3$] and *phosphorus pentoxide* or *phosphoric anhydride* [P$_2$O$_5$]. Phosphorus yields a number of oxyacids, the more important of which are *orthophosphoric acid* [H$_3$PO$_4$], *pyrophosphoric acid* [H$_4$P$_2$O$_7$], *metaphosphoric acid* [HPO$_3$], *phosphorous acid* [H$_3$PO$_3$], and *hypophosphorous acid* [HPH$_2$O$_2$].

Pharmaceutical Uses—The use of inorganic phosphorus compounds in modern medicine is restricted primarily to the orthophosphates. The tribasic calcium, magnesium, and aluminum phosphates find extensive use as gastric antacids. Dibasic sodium phosphate is the active ingredient in various saline cathartic preparations. Monobasic alkali phosphates are effective urinary acidifiers. Phosphoric acid and hypophosphorous acid are official as pharmaceutical necessities, not for any therapeutic actions in their own right, and monobasic potassium phosphate is a useful buffering agent. The radioactive isotope, ^{32}P, is employed therapeutically (see Chapter 34).

Phosphorus is one of the essential elements for plant and animal life. A complex basic calcium phosphate constitutes the main inorganic component of human bones and teeth. Dihydrogen phosphate and monohydrogen phosphate ions circulate in body fluids and play important roles in the metabolism of various organic materials, eg, carbohydrates.

Arsenic—As = 74.9216 (At. No. 33)

The most important minerals containing arsenic are *realgar* [As$_2$S$_2$], *orpiment* [As$_2$S$_3$], and *arsenopyrite* (*Mispickel*) [FeAsS]. Elementary arsenic may be prepared from arsenopyrite by heating in the absence of air. The arsenic sublimes leaving a residue of ferrous sulfide.

When heated with air (oxygen) arsenic forms *arsenic trioxide*. It is not attacked by cold hydrochloric or sulfuric acid; it is oxidized to *arsenic trioxide* by hot dilute nitric acid and by hot concentrated sulfuric acid; hot concentrated nitric acid oxidizes it to *arsenic acid*. In the trivalent state arsenic functions both as a base-forming and as an acid-forming element. The metal combines readily with free halogens to form the trihalide salts. In the pentavalent state arsenic functions primarily as an acid-forming element. As with phosphorus, arsenic functions in numerous anionic capacities, the more familiar of which are *arsenite* [AsO$_3$$^{3-}$], *arsenate* [AsO$_4$$^{3-}$], and their thio analogs.

Pharmaceutical Uses—Inorganic arsenic compounds are rarely employed in modern medicine and there are no longer any such official compounds. Arsenic trioxide and potassium arsenite were the last to disappear from the official compendia and were used as alteratives, tonics, and antileukemics.

Arsenic compounds are poisonous. A mixture of freshly precipitated ferric hydroxide and magnesium hydroxide has long been employed as an orally administered antidote, provided the poison is still in the gastrointestinal tract. For absorbed arsenic, dimercaprol by intravenous injection is effective.

Antimony—Sb = 121.75 (At. No. 51)

Antimony is found in nature in the free state; the principal source, however, is the sulfide (called *antimonite* or *stibnite*). It is manufactured by reducing its oxide with carbon.

Antimony is unaffected by cold dilute acids, but is attacked by hot concentrated sulfuric acid, and when finely divided, it dissolves in hot concentrated hydrochloric acid. It is soluble in aqua regia. Nitric acid converts it into antimonous or antimonic oxides, depending on conditions.

Antimony is trivalent and pentavalent. In both of the valences it functions as a base-forming and an acid-forming element. As an acid-forming element, antimony forms a variety of *antimonites* and *antimonates*.

Pharmaceutical Uses—Antimony elicits anthelmintic, emetic, and expectorant actions, but the compounds employed nowadays are organic in character. There are no official inorganic antimony compounds. Antimony toxicity resembles that of arsenic and is also treatable with intravenous dimercaprol.

Bismuth—Bi = 208.980 (At. No. 83)

Bismuth occurs in nature both in the free and combined states. The most important minerals are *bismite* (*bismuth ocher*) [hydrated Bi$_2$O$_3$], *bismutite* [a hydrated basic carbonate], and *bismuthinite* or *bismuth glance* [Bi$_2$S$_3$]. The free element may be prepared from the ore bismuthinite by heating in the presence of carbon or iron.

Bismuth is insoluble in hydrochloric or cold sulfuric acid and in solutions of alkali hydroxides, but dissolves in moderately diluted nitric acid. With the exception of *sodium bismuthate* [NaBiO$_3$], in which the bismuth functions anionically in the +5 oxidation state, the important bismuth compounds of commerce are of the Bi^{3+} cationic variety. Basic (bismuthyl) compounds are common.

Pharmaceutical Uses—Basic bismuth salts are employed internally for their astringent, mild germicidal, and antacid properties. They are also used externally, in the form of ointments, dusting powders, and lotions, to provide astringent and protective actions. The most popular representatives are the subcarbonate and the subnitrate. Like arsenic and antimony, soluble bismuth compounds are poisonous, and intravenous dimercaprol is an effective antidote.

Elements of Group V-B

The elements of Group V-B (vanadium, niobium, and tantalum) are of little pharmaceutical importance and will be treated but briefly.

As with Group IV-B elements, these are relatively unreactive; they do, however, combine at elevated temperature with oxygen, carbon, sulfur, halogens, nitrogen, etc. All function in the +5 oxidation state, yielding oxides of the type M_2O_5 which are preponderantly acidic. Vanadium and niobium also function commonly in the +3 state, and vanadium forms well-defined series of compounds in which it functions in the +2 and +4 states.

In their important ores, these elements occur in a combined state and are usually associated with minerals of other elements. They may be isolated in the free state by thermal reduction methods employing carbon, hydrogen, sodium, etc as the reducing agent; and also by electrolysis of fused double fluorides such as K_2TaF_7. Some of the more important characteristics of these elements are presented in Table XI.

Vanadium—V = 50.942 (At. No. 23)

Vanadium is obtained commercially from the mineral *Chileite*, a sulfide of vanadium, *vanadinite*, which is a double salt of lead vanadate and lead chloride $[Pb_5Cl(VO_4)_3]$, and *carnotite*, a vanadate of uranium and potassium.

The metal is not affected by hydrochloric or cold sulfuric acid, but is slowly attacked by the latter acid when hot. It is readily attacked and dissolved by nitric acid.

The lower oxides of vanadium are basic and form salts with strong acids. Most of these salts are basic salts containing the *vanadyl* group VO^{+2}, such as vanadyl chloride, $VOCl_2$. In its pentavalent capacity it gives *vanadium pentoxide* $[V_2O_5]$, the anhydride of the well-known *vanadic acid* $[H_3VO_4]$. The latter, like phosphoric acid, exists also in the form of *ortho-*, *meta-*, and *pyro*-vandates.

There are no official vanadium compounds.

Tantalum—Ta = 180.948 (At. No. 73)

Tantalum occurs in various minerals, such as tantalite and columbite, practically always in association with niobium. The metal is not attacked by acids including nitrohydrochloric acid, but is slowly attacked by hydrofluoric acid, with the evolution of hydrogen. It is not affected by solutions of alkali hydroxides, but by fusion with alkali hydroxides it is converted into alkali tantalates. The best known and most readily producible compounds of this element are the *tantalates*, which are salts of *metatantalic acid* $[HTaO_3]$. The alkali salts of the several tantalic acids are soluble in water.

Pharmaceutical Uses—Tantalum is unaffected by body fluids, and, in sheet form, is used in surgical repair of bones, muscles, and nerve tissues. Muscle tissue will attach itself to tantalum as though it were bone. Powdered tantalum oxide has been shown to exert a very favorable epithelizing action upon damaged tissue. Soon after applying it to third degree burns and painful wounds, a crust quickly forms and pain ceases. There are no official tantalum compounds.

Elements of Group VI

The elements of Group VI subdivide into Group VI-A, members of which have in common an outer orbit electron configuration of ns^2np^4, and Group VI-B, members of which do not have a common outer electron configuration, being $(n-1)d^5ns^1$ with chromium and molybdenum but $(n-1)d^4ns^2$ with tungsten. All of these configurations, however, suggest functioning in the +6 oxidation state, and, with the exception of oxygen, this is commonly observed with all members of Group VI.

Elements of Group VI-A

Group VI-A elements include oxygen, sulfur, selenium, tellurium, and polonium. Relationships among them are pronounced, but there are also pronounced property differences which distinguish oxygen and polonium from the intermediate triad of elements. Oxygen is exclusively nonmetallic in character while polonium is exclusively metallic; the other members show both characteristics, the metalic variety increasing with increasing atomic number. Polonium is further distinguished by its natural radioactivity.

The sulfur-selenium-tellurium triad displays especially strong family relationships. Although there are quantitative differences, each functions generally in the −2, +4, and +6 oxidation states, thus forming many analogous series of compounds. Allotropic varieties of each element in the triad are numerous. Some of the more important characteristic properties of Group VI-A elements are presented in Table XII. Oxygen and sulfur are the only members having pharmaceutical pertinence.

Oxygen—O = 15.9994 (At. No. 8)

In a free form, oxygen constitutes about one-fifth by weight of air. In combined form, it constitutes about seven-eighths by weight of water and important fractional parts by weight of minerals such as $CaCO_3$,

Table XI—Elements of Group V-B

Element	Vanadium	Niobium	Tantalum
Symbol	V	Nb	Ta
Atomic number	23	41	73
Atomic weight	50.942	92.906	180.948
Atomic radius (Å)	1.22	1.34	1.34
Ionic (crystal) radii (Å)	0.74(+3)	. . .	. . .
(for coordination number 6)	0.59(+5)	0.70(+5)	0.73(+5)
Electronegativity (Pauling scale)	1.6	1.6	1.5
Orbital electrons	$[Ar]3d^3$-$4s^2$	$[Kr]4d^4$-$5s^1$	$[Xe]4f^{14}$-$5d^36s^2$
Isotopes, natural (mass numbers)	51	93	181
Specific gravity of solid (20°C)	6.07	8.57	16.7
Melting temperature (°C)	1710	1950	3030
Boiling temperature (°C)	3000 (?)	3300 (?)	5300 (?)
Abundance (% of earth's crust)	1.5×10^{-2}	2.4×10^{-3}	2.1×10^{-4}

MnO_2, Fe_2O_3, etc. The most important industrial method for preparing oxygen involves physical separation from air. The air is first liquefied by cooling to a very low temperature under high pressure. When *liquid air* is allowed to evaporate under controlled conditions, the nitrogen and some of the rarer gases escape first because of their greater volatility, and the gas that comes off last is nearly pure oxygen.

Chemically, oxygen is very reactive, combining directly under appropriate conditions with all elements except mercury, silver, gold, and members of the platinum family. It is electronegative with respect to all elements except fluorine. The oxides of typically nonmetallic elements are acidic, while those of typical metals are basic. The oxides of many elements, eg, antimony and tellurium, are amphoteric, and elements in which this dual characteristic is pronounced are often referred to as metalloids.

Ozone $[O_3]$, an allotropic form of oxygen, is a powerful oxidizing agent. Ozonized air (air treated so as to convert a few per cent of its oxygen into ozone) is used in various disinfecting and bleaching operations.

Isotopes of oxygen have been prepared and introduced into specific molecules as tracer elements. The "average oxygen atom" represented by the mixture of oxygen isotopes occurring in nature was the standard for all chemical atomic weights for nearly a century. It was replaced by the most abundant natural isotope of carbon, ^{12}C, as of 1 January 1962.

Pharmaceutical Uses—Oxygen is employed as a therapeutic gas in the treatment of a variety of conditions in which hypoxia is a feature of the syndrome. The applications of oxides, peroxides, and hydroxides are mentioned in this chapter as they become appropriate to the elements functioning in positive oxidation states in these compounds. Oxygen is automatically present in all oxyacids and their salts, and in all hydrated compounds.

Table XII—Elements of Group VI-A

Element	Oxygen	Sulfur	Selenium	Tellurium	Polonium
Symbol	O	S	Se	Te	Po
Atomic number	8	16	34	52	84
Atomic weight	15.9994	32.064	78.96	127.60	$[210]^a$
Atomic radius (Å)	0.73	1.02	1.16	1.35	1.53
Ionic (crystal) radii (Å)	1.40(−2)	1.84(−2)	1.98(−2)	2.21(−2)	. . .
(for coordination number 6)	0.09(+6)	0.29(+6)	0.42(+6)	0.56(+6)	0.67(+6)
Electronegativity (Pauling scale)	3.5	2.5	2.4	2.1	2.0
Orbital electrons	$[He]2s^2$-$2p^4$	$[Ne]3s^2$-$3p^4$	$[Ar]3d^{10}$-$4s^24p^4$	$[Kr]4d^{10}$-$5s^25p^4$	$[Xe]4f^{14}$-$5d^{10}6s^2$-$6p^4$
Isotopes, natural (mass numbers)	16, 17, 18	32, 33, 34, 36	74, 76, 77, 78, 80, 82	120, 122, 123, 124, 125, 126, 128, 130	$[210]^a$
Specific gravity of solid (20°C)	1.14 (liquid at −183°C)	2.07 (rhombic) 1.96 (monoclinic)	4.80 (gray) 4.50 (monoclinic)	0.24 (metallic)	
Melting temperature (°C)	−219	113 (rhombic) 120 (monoclinic)	217 (gray)	450 (metallic)	
Boiling temperature (°C)	−183	445	688	1390	
Abundance (% of earth's crust)	46.6	0.052	1×10^{-7}	1×10^{-7}	1×10^{-14}

^{a} Mass number of best known isotope.

Sulfur—S = 32.064 (At. No. 16)

Sulfur is found in the free state in Sicily and the United States and is prepared almost exclusively from these native deposits by mining operations.

In combination with metals as *sulfides* and *sulfates*, sulfur is widely and abundantly distributed in nature. Many of the important metals, eg, antimony, bismuth, lead, mercury, molybdenum, and zinc are smelted from their sulfide ores.

Sulfur exists in several crystalline forms and also in an amorphous form. The most stable is the *rhombic* sulfur in which form it occurs in nature. It ignites in the air at about 250°, burning to *sulfur dioxide* [SO_2] which has a characteristic choking odor. It dissolves on heating in solutions of alkali or alkaline earth hydroxides forming a *polysulfide* and *thiosulfate*. It dissolves readily in solutions of ammonium and alkali monosulfides forming the corresponding *polysulfides*. Nitric acid and chlorine or bromine, in the presence of water, oxidize it to *sulfuric acid*. In the presence of alkali hydroxides, it is readily oxidized to *sulfate* by hydrogen peroxide.

Sulfur functions in various anionic capacities prominent among which are: sulfide [S^{2-}], polysulfide [S_n^{2-}], sulfoxylate [SO_2^{2-}], dithionite [$S_2O_4^{2-}$], sulfite [SO_3^{2-}], sulfate [SO_4^{2-}], thiosulfate [$S_2O_3^{2-}$], tetrathionate [$S_4O_6^{2-}$], pyrosulfate [$S_2O_7^{2-}$], sulfamate [$SO_3NH_2^{1-}$], and peroxydisulfate [$S_2O_8^{2-}$].

Pharmaceutical Uses—Elementary sulfur is employed in various dosage forms, eg, ointments, creams, lotions, dusting powders, etc., for its germicidal, fungicidal, and keratolytic actions. Soluble sulfides and polysulfides find application as external parasiticides and in the treatment of certain dermatitic conditions, eg, acne. Zinc sulfide, freshly prepared as in White Lotion, provides external astringent and protective properties. Selenium disulfide in the form of suspensions, ointments, gels, etc., is an effective antiseborrheic.

Sulfur dioxide and its related salts, sodium bisulfite [$NaHSO_3$] and sodium metabisulfite [$Na_2S_2O_5$], are frequently introduced into pharmaceutical preparations as antioxidants, preservatives, and stabilizers. Sodium thiosulfate is officially recognized as an antidote to cyanide. It is also antidotal to iodine and is used to combat certain parasitic skin infections. Gold sodium thiosulfate is an injectable antirheumatic.

Several metal sulfates are official but with the exception of sodium sulfate (a saline cathartic) and barium sulfate (a gastrointestinal radiopaque medium), the applications are more appropriately ascribed to the metal and these sulfates are therefore distributed accordingly in this chapter.

Selenium—Se = 78.96 (At. No. 34)

Tellurium—Te = 127.60 (At. No. 52)

These are nonmetallic elements, chemically related to oxygen and sulfur. They occur to some extent in nature in the free state but primarily in combination with metals in the form of *selenides* and *tellurides*.

Like sulfur, both of these elements are acid-forming, giving rise to selenious and tellurous acids [H_2SeO_3 and H_2TeO_3], and to selenic and telluric acids [H_2SeO_4 and $(H_2TeO_4)_n$].

Selenium and tellurium are insoluble in water and in hydrochloric acid. They are oxidized by nitric acid to selenium dioxide and to telluric acid, respectively. They dissolve with oxidation in sulfuric acid and are dissolved by solutions at the fixed alkali hydroxides or sulfides. Like sulfur, both elements exist in allotropic forms.

In general, the types of compounds formed by selenium and tellurium are analogous to those of sulfur. Observed differences are largely those to be expected in terms of relative atomic size and electronegativity.

Pharmaceutical Uses—The only official selenium compound is Selenium Sulfide (selenium disulfide) [SeS_2] used as an antiseborrheic agent. There are no recognized applications of tellurium compounds.

Elements of Group VI-B

Although of limited direct therapeutic application, compounds of the elements of Group VI-B (chromium, molybdenum, and tungsten) are important in synthetic and analytical pharmaceutical operations. Relatively stable at ordinary temperature, all of these metals react readily at elevated temperature with carbon, nitrogen, oxygen, sulfur, and the halogens.

Oxidation states are multiple, ranging from +2 to +6, as illustrated respectively by chlorides of the MCl_2 type and oxides of the MO_3 type. In the lowest state, functioning is primarily metallic; in the highest valency state, functioning is primarily non-metallic.

Elements of this group occur in important quantities only in combined forms. Chromium occurs primarily as chromites and chromates of such metals as iron and lead. Molybdenum occurs in the form of sulfides and as molybdates of iron and lead. Tungsten occurs as complex tungstates of iron, manganese, lead, calcium, and copper. Isolation of any of these elements in the free state is readily accomplished by thermal reductive processes utilizing carbon, hydrogen, sodium, or other reducing agents. Electrolytic processes are also employed. A summary of some of the more important characteristics of these elements is presented in Table XIII.

Chromium—Cr = 51.996 (At. No. 24)

Chromium occurs in nature primarily as the chrome iron ore, *chromite* ($FeO \cdot Cr_2O_3$). Chromium *metal* may be prepared by heating chromic oxide [Cr_2O_3] with carbon in the electric furnace, or by the aluminothermic process whereby chromium oxide is reduced by finely powdered aluminum when they are mixed and ignited.

Chromium is soluble in diluted hydrochloric or sulfuric acid, but is insoluble in nitric acid. It is attacked by the caustic alkalies as well as by their carbonates.

Chromium functions in +2, +3, and +6 valence states. In the first two valences it acts as a base-forming element, yielding *chromous* and *chromic* salts, respectively. The chromous salts are usually white or nearly so. Chromic salts are green or violet-red.

In the hexavalent state it is an acid-forming element and functions in many anionic capacities. Most prominent among these are the chromate(VI) [$CrO_4{}^{2-}$] and the dichromate(VI) [$Cr_2O_7{}^{2-}$] ions. The alkali and ammonium chromates and dichromates are freely soluble in water. Of the alkaline earth chromates the barium salt is the least soluble. Lead chromate is one of the most insoluble salts known.

Pharmaceutical Uses—There are no official inorganic chromium compounds containing natural chromium. Certain salts of the radioactive isotope, ^{51}Cr, are employed as a biological tracer in certain hematological procedures. See Chapter 34.

Molybdenum—Mo = 95.94 (At. No. 42)

Molybdenum occurs as the minerals *wulfenite*, which is lead molybdate [$PbMoO_4$], *powelite*, which

molybdates are insoluble either in water or in dilute acids.

There are no official molybdenum compounds. Complex molybdophosphate anions serve useful analytical purposes.

Tungsten—W = 183.85 (At. No. 74)

The most common tungsten ores are *wolframite*, which is iron tungstate [$FeWO_4$], and *scheelite*, which is calcium tungstate [$CaWO_4$]. The free metal is isolated by reducing its oxide thermally with carbon, hydrogen or aluminum.

Tungsten is scarcely attacked by the single mineral acids, but is dissolved readily by a mixture of nitric and hydrofluoric acids. The powdered metal dis-

Table XIII—Elements of Group VI-B

Element	Chromium	Molybdenum	Tungsten
Symbol	Cr	Mo	W
Atomic number	24	42	74
Atomic weight	51.996	95.94	183.85
Atomic radius (Å)	1.17	1.29	1.30
Ionic (crystal) radii	0.69(+3)	0.68(+4)	0.70(+4)
(Å) (for coordination number 6)	0.52(+6)	0.62(+6)	0.62(+6)
Electronegativity (Pauling scale)	1.6	1.8	1.7
Orbital electrons	[Ar]3d^5-4s^1	[Kr]4d^5-5s^1	[Xe]4f^{14}-5d^{4}6s^2
Isotopes, natural (mass numbers)	50, 52, 53, 54	92, 94, 95, 96, 97, 98, 100	180, 182, 183, 184, 186
Specific gravity of solid (20°C)	7.19	10.2	19.3
Melting temperature (°C)	1900	2620	3370
Boiling temperature (°C)	2480 (?)	4800 (?)	5900 (?)
Abundance (% of earth's crust)	2×10^{-2}	ca 5×10^{-4}	ca 5×10^{-4}

is a mixture of calcium molybdate and calcium tungstate, and *molybdenite*, the disulfide [MoS_2]. The metal is usually prepared commercially by reducing its oxide with carbon in the electric furnace.

Molybdenum is not affected by halogen hydracids but is attacked by hot concentrated sulfuric acid. Nitric or nitrohydrochloric acid oxidizes it to the trioxide.

Molybdenum functions in the +2, +3, and +6 valence states. Its best known and most frequently used compounds are derived from molybdenum trioxide [MoO_3], which functions as an acid anhydride and gives rise to the molybdate [$MoO_4{}^{2-}$] ion as the best known among a sizeable family of anions. Except for the alkali salts, which are soluble, most

solves also in boiling fixed alkali hydroxide solutions with the evolution of hydrogen and the formation of a tungstate.

The important valence state of tungsten is +6. Salts in which tungsten functions as the cation are but little known, but the tungstates, especially calcium and sodium tungstates, are widely used. As with molybdenum, tungsten participates in various anions, but the most common one is tungstate(VI) [$WO_4{}^{2-}$]. The alkali tungstates are readily soluble in water, but the tungstates of most other metals are insoluble.

There are no official tungsten compounds. Similarly with molybdenum, complex tungstophosphate anions play useful analytical roles.

Elements of Group VII

The elements of Group VII subdivide into Group VII-A, members of which have in common an outer orbit electron configuration of ns^2np^5, and Group VII-B, members of which have in common an $(n-1)$-d^5ns^2 outer electron configuration. Theoretically,

each configuration suggests functioning in a +7 oxidation state, and, with the exception of the simplest member, fluorine, such functioning is observed with all members of Group VII. Astatine, technetium, and rhenium are relatively unfamiliar elements.

Elements of Group VII-A

Group VII-A elements (the halogens) include fluorine, chlorine, bromine, iodine, and astatine. Each is but one proton and one planetary electron short of the structure of an inert (Group 0) element. As in Group VI-A, relationships among these elements are pronounced, and there are outstanding differences which distinguish the smallest and largest elements of the group from the intermediate triad. Fluorine functions exclusively in the negative oxidation state. Astatine is primarily a synthetic radioactive element; it resembles iodine but is more metallic, is of no pharmaceutical import, and is not remarked on further.

Fluorine, chlorine, bromine, and iodine all function in the −1 oxidation state, yielding hydrides of the type HX and metal salts of the types MX, MX_2, etc. Chlorine, bromine, and iodine function in the +1, +3, +5, and +7 states, yielding oxides of the types X_2O, X_2O_3, X_2O_5, and X_2O_7.

The tendency of halogens to function like metals is so slight that these elements are commonly considered to be exclusively nonmetallic. All hydrogen halides display some degree of electrovalency, the tendency increasing through the series HF, HCl, HBr, and HI. Oxides of chlorine, bromine, and iodine are exclusively acidic.

Because of their high chemical reactivity, the halogen elements occur terrestrially only in combined form, usually as halides. Commercial preparation of the free elements is usually effected either through specially designed electrolytic processes or through methods involving halide ion oxidation.

The halogens constitute an important group of elements from a pharmaceutical viewpoint. Some of their more fundamental characteristics are presented in Table XIV.

Fluorine—F = 18.9984 (At. No. 9)

Prominent fluorine minerals include *fluorite* or *fluorspar* [CaF_2], *cryolite* [Na_3AlF_6], and *fluor-apatite* [$CaF_2 \cdot 3Ca_3(PO_4)_2$]. The free element may be obtained by the electrolysis of fused potassium bifluoride [KF.HF].

Fluorine is the most reactive of the electronegative elements. With the exception of gold and platinum it attacks all metals at ordinary temperatures, and combines directly with all nonmetals, excepting oxygen, chlorine, nitrogen, and the rare gases. It decomposes water forming hydrogen fluoride and oxygen and ozone. By indirect methods, fluorine may be caused to unite with oxygen to form binary compounds such as O_2F_2 and OF_2. The small size of the fluorine atom coupled with its high electronegativity cause it to appear frequently as a ligand in complex ions, such as tetrafluoroborate [BF_4^{1-}], hexafluorosilicate [SiF_6^{2-}], hexafluoroarsenate(V) [AsF_6^{1-}], etc.

Fluorine in drinking water, when present in excessive amounts, has been found to be the cause of the mottled appearance of the enamel of the teeth, thus presenting a public health problem. On the other hand, amounts of fluorine in the water insufficient to produce mottled enamel are said to render teeth less susceptible to dental caries. Excessive amounts of fluorine in water, it has recently been reported, can be removed by passing the water through ion exchange resins treated with a solution of an aluminum salt.

Pharmaceutical Uses—Fluorine is a physiologically essential element. Calcium fluoride, in the form of a complex with basic calcium phosphate, is a normal constituent of bones and teeth. Sodium fluoride is official for use as a fluoridating agent for drinking water and as a topically applied dental prophylactic to lessen susceptibility to caries. Stannous fluoride is also official for the latter purpose and is reportedly the fluoride of choice for such use.

Chlorine—Cl = 35.453 (At. No. 17)

Chlorine is found in large quantities combined with alkali metals and magnesium as chlorides which compose the largest portion of the solid constituents of sea water. Sodium chloride is also found as rock-salt in large deposits in various localities. The element is isolated by electrolysis of a solution of sodium chloride contained in a specially constructed cell.

Chlorine is a greenish yellow gas having a very suffocating odor. It is soluble in water to approximately 0.4%; it is more soluble in water at lower temperatures. Its aqueous solutions deteriorate on keeping or on exposure to light, forming hydrogen chloride and oxygen.

Chlorine is an extremely energetic element. It

Table XIV—Elements of Group VII-A

Element	Fluorine	Chlorine	Bromine	Iodine	Astatine
Symbol	F	Cl	Br	I	At
Atomic number	9	17	35	53	85
Atomic weight	18.9984	35.453	79.904	126.9044	[210][a]
Atomic radius (Å)	0.72	0.99	1.14	1.33	...
Ionic (crystal) radii (Å) (for coordination number 6)	1.36(−1) 0.07(+7)	1.81(−1) 0.26(+7)	1.95(−1) 0.39(+7)	2.16(−1) 0.50(+7)	... 0.62(+7)
Electronegativity (Pauling scale)	4.0	3.0	2.8	2.5	2.2
Orbital electrons	[He]2s²2p⁵	[Ne]3s²3p⁵	[Ar]3d¹⁰4s²4p⁵	[Kr]4d¹⁰5s²5p⁵	[Xe]4f¹⁴5d¹⁰6s²-6p⁵
Isotopes, natural (mass numbers)	19	25, 37	79, 81	127	215, 216, 218
Specific gravity of solid	1.3	1.9	3.4 (3.11 liquid)	4.9	...
Melting temperature (°C)	−223	−102	−7.3	114	...
Boiling temperature (°C)	−187	−35	59	183	...
Abundance (% of earth's crust)	8×10^{-2}	3×10^{-2}	1.6×10^{-4}	3×10^{-5}	...

[a] Mass number of the isotope of longest known half-life.

attacks practically all metals, forming chlorides, and combines vigorously with hydrogen at elevated temperatures, or at room temperature in the presence of an activator (charcoal, etc), forming hydrogen chloride gas and generating much heat during the combination. Chlorine combines indirectly with oxygen forming several oxides: chlorine monoxide $[Cl_2O]$, chlorine dioxide $[ClO_2]$, chlorine hexoxide $[Cl_2O_6]$, and chlorine heptoxide $[Cl_2O_7]$. These are related to the following acids: hypochlorous acid $[HClO]$, chlorous acid $[HClO_2]$, chloric acid $[HClO_3]$, and perchloric acid $[HClO_4]$ which, except the last, are not known in the pure state. Salts of all of the acids, however, are well known and find considerable use.

Pharmaceutical Uses—Hydrochloric acid is a pharmaceutical necessity for purposes such as neutralizing, stabilizing, or solubilizing other substances. In diluted form, it is an effective gastric acidifier but other compounds more readily amenable to administration are usually preferred. Sodium, potassium, and calcium chlorides are employed as electrolyte replenishers; the first is also the sole ingredient of physiological salt solution. A strong solution of sodium chloride is emetic. Ammonium chloride is an expectorant and a systemic acidifying agent. The chloride ion is frequently the carrier of choice for other metal cations such as those of zinc, aluminum, and mercury, but with these the medicinal value is referable to the metal rather than the chloride.

Sodium hypochlorite solutions are effectively germicidal and deodorizing due to the oxidizing power of the hypochlorite ion and, in sufficiently dilute form, are used in a variety of conditions for topical application. The hypochlorite ion is rapidly reduced by organic matter in general. Potassium chlorate is weakly antiseptic but is still occasionally present in mouth washes, vaginal douches, and other local cleansing preparations.

Bromine—Br = 79.904 (At. No. 35)

The important minerals of bromine are the bromides of sodium, potassium, calcium, and magnesium which occur in important quantities in sea water, salt brines, and certain mineral deposits such as at Stassfurt, Germany. Sea water contains on the order of 70 ppm. $MgBr_2$ and domestic salt brines contain bromides equivalent to on the order of 1300 ppm of bromine. Commercial production of bromine is by electrolysis of the concentrated sea water or brine.

Bromine is a dark reddish brown, fuming liquid of a suffocating odor. The fumes are highly irritating to the mucous membranes and they burn and blister the skin. It attacks all metals and organic tissue. In its general chemistry, bromine resembles chlorine with slight differences referable to comparative sizes of the two atoms and their electronegativities.

Pharmaceutical Uses—Bromine is a powerful caustic and germicide but is not employed as a medicinal agent. It is a common chemical reagent, however, and is official as such. The *utmost care* should be exercised in handling bromine; the vapor not only attacks the eyes and nostrils, but renders the air irrespirable. If exposed to the vapors of bromine, the part should be washed with a solution of sodium bicarbonate. All work with bromine should be carried on under ideal conditions of ventilation.

Caution—Bromine containers should be opened only after they have been thoroughly cooled.

In proper dosage, the bromide ion provides central depressant action, and potassium, sodium, and ammonium bromides are the salts commonly employed today. Excessive continued dosage may elicit brominism, a toxic condition characterized by skin eruptions, headache, sleeplessness, and loss of strength.

Iodine—I = 126.9044 (At. No. 53)

Iodine does not occur free in nature. In combination as iodides, it is found in the ashes of certain marine algae or weeds. Until recently, the most important source of iodine was crude Chile saltpeter. It occurs there primarily as sodium iodate to the extent of about 0.8%. Recently it has been found in the brine of oil wells, and this source now furnishes a considerable portion of the iodine requirements of this country as well as of Russia. Iodine is prepared (a) from the iodide in the ashes of seaweed by chlorination, (b) from the iodate in Chile saltpeter by reduction with sulfite ion, and (c) from the iodide in oil well brines by oxidation with chlorine or nitrite ion.

Iodine is a highly reactive element, although less so than bromine or chlorine. With due allowance for its larger size and lesser electronegativity, the chemistry of iodine is analogous to that of bromine and chlorine. The iodide ion is especially prone to oxidation, and iodine functions in numerous anionic capacities. It attacks most metals, forming iodides. It does not readily combine with hydrogen except in the presence of a suitable catalyst.

Pharmaceutical Uses—Solutions of elemental iodine are highly effective, locally acting germicides. These solutions usually contain potassium or sodium iodide to enhance the solubility of the iodine through the formation of polyiodide ion. Iodine is essential for proper thyroid functioning and is physiologically utilized either in the elemental form or in the form of iodide ion as in potassium or sodium iodide. In proper dosage, iodide ion exerts expectorant action; examples are hydrogen iodide (as Hydriodic Acid Syrup NF XII) and Potassium Iodide USP.

Elementary iodine is toxic. Cornstarch and sodium thiosulfate are effective chemical antidotes. The radioactive isotopes, ^{125}I and ^{131}I, have various diagnostic and therapeutic applications. See Chapter 34.

Elements of Group VII-B

Group VII-B elements include manganese, technetium, and rhenium. As somewhat of an analogy with the elements of VII-A, each is characterized by being one proton and one planetary electron short of the structure of a transition element in Group VIII.

Pharmaceutically, manganese is the only important element in this group and detailed discussion will be limited to it. Technetium (from Greek *technetos*, meaning artificial) was so named because it was the first element produced artificially; it was recognized among the decay products of neutron or deuteron-bombarded molybdenum. Later, it was shown to be present in large amounts among the products resulting from uranium 235 fission. Rhenium is a very rare element and

Table XV—Elements of Group VII-B

Element	Manganese	Technetium	Rhenium
Symbol	Mn	Te	Re
Atomic number	25	43	75
Atomic weight	54.9380	[99][a]	186.2
Atomic radius (Å)	1.16	...	1.27
Ionic (crystal) radii (Å)	0.80(+2)	...	0.72(+4)
(for coordination number 6)	0.47(+6)	0.56(+7)	0.56(+7)
Electronegativity (Pauling scale)	1.5	1.9	1.9
Orbital electrons	$[Ar]3d^5 4s^2$	$[Kr]4d^5 5s^2$	$[Xe]4f^{14}$- $5d^5 6s^2$
Isotopes, natural (mass numbers)	55	none	185, 187
Specific gravity of solid (20 °C)	7.21	11.5	21
Melting temperature (°C)	1260		3140
Boiling temperature (°C)	1900		
Abundance (% of earth's crust)	0.1	zero (?)	1×10^{-7}

[a] Mass number of best known isotope.

finds little technical applications. Alone and in combination with other metals, it has been employed as a catalyst to encourage dehydrogenation reactions.

Oxidation states of these elements are multiple. Manganese forms well-defined compounds in which it functions in positive states of 2, 3, 4, 6, and 7; observed positive states of technetium are 6 and 7; reported positive states of rhenium are 3, 4, 5, 6, and 7. All elements in this group are decidedly metallic in appearance, but amphoteric characteristics are abundantly evident as demonstrated by the existence of anions such as manganate $[MnO_4^{2-}]$, permanganate $[MnO_4^{1-}]$, perrhenate $[ReO_4^{1-}]$, etc. A summary of some of the more important characteristics of Group VII-B elements is presented in Table XV.

Manganese—Mn = 54.9380 (At. No. 25)

Manganese occurs in nature chiefly in the form of its oxides—*pyrolusite*, which is a manganese dioxide $[MnO_2]$, *hausmannite* or mangano-manganic oxide $[Mn_3O_4]$, and *braunite* $[3Mn_2O_3 \cdot MnSiO_3]$. The free metal is obtained by reducing the dioxide with carbon, aluminum, or magnesium, and by electrolytic processes.

Manganese slowly decomposes hot water with the evolution of hydrogen and is dissolved by dilute acids. It is a rather unique element in that it can function in an unusual number of oxidation states. Most important are those compounds in which it displays a positive valence of 2, 4, 6, and 7. Respective examples of such compounds are *manganous sulfate* $[MnSO_4]$, *manganese dioxide* $[MnO_2]$, *potassium manganate* $[K_2MnO_4]$, and *potassium permanganate* $[KMnO_4]$. Hydrated manganous salts are pink in color, anhydrous manganous salts are usually white, manganates are green, and permanganates form solutions which are characteristically deep purple violet.

Pharmaceutical Uses—The only official manganese compound is potassium permanganate. Categorized officially as a local anti-infective of the oxidizing type, it is also an astringent and powerful deodorant and cleanser. It is applied in the form of dilute (0.01–1%) solutions. Gastric lavage with dilute solutions is antidotal for various alkaloids and other toxic substances which have been ingested in small amounts and which are destroyed by oxidation. Manganese is frequently present is mineral supplements and in hematopoietic preparations, but its value in such products has yet to be demonstrated.

Elements of Group VIII

The elements of Group VIII are commonly referred to as the *transition elements*. Modern treatment suggests that all elements involving preferential filling of inner electron orbits with increase of atomic number might well be considered transition elements. According to this concept, the first series of transition elements begins with scandium and ends with nickel; the second series begins with yttrium and ends with palladium; the third series begins with lanthanum and ends with platinum; and the fourth and final series begins with actinium and extends through all the rest of the known elements. All elements of B groups become transition elements by this definition. See the *Periodic Chart of the Elements* on the back cover.

In this chapter, however, the term transition elements is used in its more restrictive sense and refers exclusively to those elements which fall automatically between the elements of Group VII-B and the elements of Group I-B when arranged in order of increasing atomic number. Such treatment preserves the useful similarity of arrangement between elements of Group VIII and those of Group Zero, since the latter fall between the elements of Group VII-A and the elements of Group I-A.

Treatment in this fashion limits the transition elements to three triads occurring in the three long periods of the periodic chart. The first triad is encountered immediately following manganese and includes iron, cobalt, and nickel. The second triad follows technetium and includes ruthenium, rhodium, and palladium. The third triad follows rhenium and includes osmium, iridium, and platinum. These transition elements are definitely metallic but all do function in anionic, as well as cationic, capacities. All participate readily in the formation of coordination complexes.

The First Triad of Group VIII

This triad consists of the familiar elements iron, cobalt, and nickel. They are frequently referred to as the *ferrous metals*. There is little resemblance between the properties of the elements of this triad and those of the elements of the second and third transition triads.

The important valencies are plus two and plus three, thus giving rise to oxides of the MO and M_2O_3 types and halides of the MX_2 and MX_3 types. In the free and metal(II) ion states, these elements are important reducing agents. The metal(III) state has useful oxidizing potential.

Iron, cobalt, and nickel all occur in the free state in meteorites. In the earth's crust, iron is usually found in the form of oxides, sulfides, and carbonate. Nickel and cobalt are found in the form of simple and mixed sulfides and arsenides; these two elements often occur associated. Oxides of all three elements are thermally reducible with carbon or hydrogen to yield the free metals. Important characteristics are presented in Table XVI.

Iron—Fe = 55.847 (At. No. 26)

Iron is widely distributed in nature, occurring primarily in combination with other elements. The oxides of iron, *magnetite* [Fe_3O_4] and *hematite* [Fe_2O_3], constitute the most important iron ores. Iron sulfides, *pyrites* and *marcasite* [FeS_2], are also abundant but they are less suitable for the extraction of the metal. On a commercial scale, iron is prepared by heating its oxide ores with a mixture of coke and limestone in a specially constructed furnace known as a blast furnace. A current of preheated air is caused to pass upward through the furnace whereby carbon monoxide is formed which reduces the iron oxide to metallic iron. The calcium carbonate functions as a flux to combine with the siliceous gangue to form a fusible calcium aluminum silicate slag.

Iron functions in divalent and trivalent capacities forming respectively ferrous and ferric compounds. Ferrous salts are usually green in the hydrated state and white when anhydrous. Ferric salts are usually yellow to brown in the hydrated state but vary in color when rendered anhydrous. Aqueous solutions of both ferrous and ferric salts are acid because of hydrolysis.

Chemically, iron is quite an active metal. On exposure to moist air, it is slowly oxidized to a hydrated ferric oxide. Strongly heated in air, iron burns to ferroso-ferric oxide [Fe_3O_4]. Treated in the red-hot state with superheated steam, it yields the same oxide with simultaneous liberation of hydrogen. It displaces hydrogen from even relatively weak acids forming ferrous salts. If the acid employed is also an oxidizing agent and if it is employed under conditions which will permit it to exercise its oxidizing capacity, a ferric salt results. If iron is immersed in fuming nitric acid for a brief period and then rinsed with water, it assumes a *passive state* in which it does not react with such reagents as dilute acids, copper sulfate, etc. This is presumed to be due to the formation of a protective coating of Fe_3O_4. Nickel, cobalt, chromium, molybdenum, tungsten, and vanadium may also be caused to assume a passive state.

Ferrous and ferric ions form soluble coordination complexes with many agents such as *ammonium salts*, *citrates*, *tartrates*, *amines*, *sugar*, and *glycerin*, which protect the iron from precipitation by the usual iron precipitants. Examples of such complexes are iron and ammonium citrate, ferric citrochloride (tincture), ferric glycerophosphate, and soluble ferric phosphate. Complexes of ferrous iron are less easily oxidized than ferrous iron itself.

Pharmaceutical Uses—Reduced iron and various iron salts are generously employed in medicine as hematinics in the treatment of iron deficiency anemias and as a source of iron in mineral supplement preparations. The only surviving official inorganic representative is Ferrous Sulfate. The ferric ion is astringent and preparations of ferric salts for such use were formerly recognized. Various iron oxides and hydrous oxides are employed as pigments in cosmetics.

Cobalt—Co = 58.9332 (At. No. 27)

Cobalt is usually found associated with arsenical ores in *cobaltite* [$CoAs_2 \cdot CoS_2$] and *smaltite* [$CoAs_2$]. Some cobalt is usually present in nickel ores and vice versa. The free metal is isolated from its oxide by thermal reduction with aluminum, carbon, or hydrogen.

Cobalt is a gray, magnetic metal. It is very slowly attacked by cold hydrochloric or sulfuric acid, but dissolves readily in diluted nitric acid.

The more important cobalt salts of commerce are of the cobalt(II) variety. Most contain water of hydration and are red in color. When rendered anhydrous, they are bluish. The red color of solutions of the soluble salts is changed to blue by the addition of an excess of concentrated hydrochloric acid. The halogen salts, the nitrate, and the sulfate are freely soluble in water and, with the exception of the sulfate, are also soluble in alcohol.

Pharmaceutical Uses—There is some evidence that the presence of traces of cobalt may catalyze the physiological utilization of iron. This has led to the introduction of medicinal specialty products containing iron in association with cobalt designed for use in the treatment of iron deficiency anemias. Cobalt is present in the cyanocobalamin molecule (Vitamin

Table XVI—Elements of the First Triad of Group VIII

Element	Iron	Cobalt	Nickel
Symbol	Fe	Co	Ni
Atomic number	26	27	28
Atomic weight	55.847	58.9332	58.71
Atomic radius (Å)	1.16	1.15	1.15
Ionic (crystal)	0.76(+2)	0.78(+2)	0.78(+2)
radii (Å) (for coordination number 6)	0.64(+3)	0.63(+3)	0.62(+3)
Electronegativity (Pauling scale)	1.8	1.8	1.8
Orbital electrons	[Ar]3d^6-4s^2	[Ar]3d^{7}4s^2	[Ar]3d^8-4s^2
Isotopes, natural (mass numbers)	54, 56, 57, 58	59	58, 60 61, 62, 64
Specific gravity of solid (20°C)	7.9	8.7	8.9
Melting temperature (°C)	1540	1490	1450
Boiling temperature (°C)	2740	2900	2730
Abundance (% of earth's crust)	5	2.3×10^{-3}	8×10^{-3}

B_{12}). There are no official inorganic cobalt compounds.

The radioactive isotopes, [57]Co and ^{60}Co, are used diagnostically and therapeutically. See Chapter 34.

Nickel—Ni = 58.71 (At. No. 28)

The principal source of nickel is the magnetic iron *pyrites* (or *nickeliferous pyrrhotite*) in the province of Ontario, Canada. It is also a constituent of the mineral *garnierite* (or *genthite*), a hydrated double silicate of nickel and magnesium, as well as of the mineral *niccolite*, a nickel arsenide. From its sulfide ores, nickel is produced by roasting the ore in air to form nickel oxide, reducing the oxide thermally with carbon or carbon monoxide to form volatile nickel carbonyl, and thermally decomposing the carbonyl.

Nickel is slowly attacked by hydrochloric or diluted sulfuric acid and is readily dissolved by diluted nitric acid.

The nickel(II) salts predominate commercially. They usually contain water of hydration and are green in color. The halogen salts, the nitrate, and the sulfate are freely soluble in water and, with the exception of the sulfate, they are also soluble in alcohol. Neither nickel nor any of its compounds find important applications as therapeutic agents. There are no official nickel compounds.

The Second and Third Triads of Group VIII

These six elements are usually treated together under the designation *platinum metals*. Member elements are ruthenium, rhodium, palladium, osmium, iridium, and platinum. One of their most distinguishing properties is that, with the exception of osmium, they do not combine with oxygen below a red heat. The three elements, mercury, gold, and silver, behave similarly, and it is for this reason that all nine elements are often referred to as the *noble metals*. In contrast, other metals which do form oxides below a red heat are commonly termed *base metals*.

The platinum metals function in various oxidation states, the more important being 3, 4, 6, and 8 for Ru; 3 for Rh; 2 and 4 for Pd; 3, 4, 6, and 8 for Os; 3 and 4 for Ir; and 2 and 4 for Pt. The various members occur primarily in the elemental state, and are commonly found associated. Isolation of any one of these elements in the elementary state from a pure compound is usually relatively simple; heat alone often suffices to liberate the metal, especially from oxide combination. This is a reflection of the nobility and general chemical inertness of the entire group. However, separation of the individual metals from ores in which they occur associated is usually an involved operation. Physically and chemically, the platinum elements are definitely metallic, even though they frequently function in anionic states.

These elements are often employed in important catalytic operations. Presented in Table XVII are some of their more important characteristics. Further treatment in this text will be confined to palladium, osmium, and platinum.

Palladium—Pd = 106.4 (At. No. 46)

In contradistinction to the other platinum group metals, palladium metal dissolves slowly in nitric acid, forming palladous nitrate. Finely powdered palladium metal has the very characteristic property of being able to absorb about 700 times its own volume of hydrogen and consequently exerts a very strong catalytic effect. The common commercial compounds are of the palladium(II) type.

There are no official palladium compounds.

Osmium—Os = 190.2 (At. No. 76)

This element is invariably associated with platinum ores. Unlike the other metals of the platinum group, it is oxidized by heating it in air, forming the very

Table XVII—Elements of the Second and Third Triads of Group VIII

Element	Ruthenium	Rhodium	Palladium	Osmium	Iridium	Platinum
Symbol	Ru	Rh	Pd	Os	Ir	Pt
Atomic number	44	45	46	76	77	78
Atomic weight	101.07	102.905	106.4	190.2	192.2	195.09
Atomic radius (Å)	1.24	1.24	1.27	1.25	1.26	1.29
Ionic (crystal) radii (Å) (for coordination number 6)	0.69(+3) 0.65(+4)	0.68(+3) ...	0.80(+2) 0.65(+4)	0.88(+4) 0.69(+6)	0.68(+4) ...	0.80(+2) 0.65(+4)
Electronegativity (Pauling scale)	2.2	2.2	2.2	2.2	2.2	2.2
Orbital electrons	[Kr]$4d^75s^1$	[Kr]$4d^85s^1$	[Kr]$4d^{10}5s^0$	[Xe]$4f^{14}5d^66s^2$	[Xe]$4f^{14}5d^76s^2$	[Xe]$4f^{14}5d^{10}6s^0$
Isotopes, natural (mass numbers)	96, 98, 99, 100, 101, 102, 104	103	102, 104, 105, 106, 108, 110	183, 186, 187, 188, 189, 190, 192	191, 193	192, 194, 195, 196, 198
Specific gravity of solid (20°C)	12.43	12.42	12.03	22.70	22.64	21.45
Melting temperature (°C)	1950	1966	1555	2500	2450	1770
Boiling temperature (°C)	>2700	>2500	2200	>5300	>4800	4300
Abundance (% of earth's crust)	(present)	1×10^{-7}	1×10^{-6}	(present)	1×10^{-7}	5×10^{-7}

poisonous osmium tetroxide, known also as *osmic acid* [OsO$_4$]. Osmium is insoluble in acids at ordinary temperatures and is scarcely attacked by nitrohydrochloric acid. It is made soluble by fusion with sodium peroxide or by burning in air to form osmium tetroxide.

Osmium compounds, other than the tetroxide, have very little use and have not been studied extensively. There are no official osmium compounds.

Platinum—Pt = 195.09 (At. No. 78)

Platinum is found in nature exclusively in the free state, but frequently in association with other metals of the platinum group such as palladium, rhodium, and ruthenium.

Platinum is insoluble in single acids, but slowly attacked and dissolved by nitrohydrochloric acid or by the halogens in the presence of water. Platinum-(II) salts are usually insoluble in water, but form readily soluble double salts with the alkali and alkaline earth metals. Platinum(IV) salts are usually very soluble in water. Ammonium or potassium salts of chloroplatinic acid [H$_2$PtCl$_6$] are only slightly soluble in water.

Platinum double salts, especially the cyanides such as barium and potassium platinocyanides, are used in radiography for making X-ray screens.

Neither platinum nor any of its compounds find therapeutic use. There are no official platinum compounds.

29 | Organic Pharmaceutical Chemistry

The uniqueness of carbon—organic compounds (types, nomenclature, literature, and natural sources)—organic pharmaceuticals and their classification

This chapter was prepared by

Clarence T. Van Meter, PhD, *Project Director, Office of Engineering Research, University of Pennsylvania, Philadelphia, Pa. 19104, and*
Alfonso R. Gennaro, PhD, *Professor of Chemistry, Philadelphia College of Pharmacy and Science, Philadelphia, Pa. 19104*

The fact that upwards of 90% of all known chemical compounds contain carbon is a direct consequence of the unique structural characteristics of the carbon atom. In an empirical way this has long been recognized, but satisfactory scientific reasons for it, especially in terms of modern electron theory, have been established only within relatively recent times. One prominent result has been the evolution of modern logic in support of the classic subdivision of the total field of chemistry into the two areas, inorganic and organic.

It is not the purpose of this text to provide a basic treatment of organic chemistry. Readers are expected to have pursued the usual basic courses in organic chemistry and to be cognizant of the various advanced texts and other readily available works of reference. Accordingly, the remainder of this chapter is restricted primarily to a brief presentation of the structural features of the carbon atom and the various kinds of bonding it exercises in the formation of compounds, followed by a listing of the more prominent structural types of compounds and an exposition of the major chemical classes of official (USP and NF) pharmaceuticals. Detailed treatment of the individual pharmaceuticals is provided at other locations in the text; refer to the index.

The Uniqueness of Carbon

In the previous chapter, reference was made to types of bonds which could exist between atoms and to the effects of bond types on the properties of these compounds. Since organic chemistry is concerned mainly with carbon and its compounds, closer attention is warranted to the kinds of bonds exhibited by the carbon atom.

Carbon (and, to a much lesser extent, boron and beryllium) is in a special class. Although only the twelfth most abundant element on earth, its compounds far outnumber those of the remainder of the periodic table *combined*. The exact number of existing carbon compounds is probably unknown and the theoretical number is infinite. For example, the number of known hydrides of carbon is about 2300, while the next most prolific member (boron) of this period in the periodic table can boast of only seven! This uniqueness stems from the simple fact that carbon is capable of bonding with itself in many unusual modes.

Carbon Bonds

Ordinarily, carbon is said to exhibit a valence of four. Thus it can combine with four other monovalent atoms or groups or with four other carbon atoms in a linear or cyclic fashion with or without branching, or any combination thereof:

Also, carbon atoms can unite to each other or to other atoms such as nitrogen, oxygen, or sulfur by means of multiple bonds. To compound the situation further, the structural diagrams just presented are not flat objects, but are three dimensional. For example, a six-membered carbon ring may have several configurations, such as:

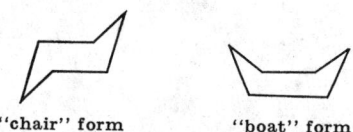

"chair" form   "boat" form

This feature alone could essentially double the number of compounds of this type.

Hybridization—What is so unusual about the constitution of the carbon atom which allows so many diverse compounds? Simply stated, the reason is *hybridization*, and a review of the electronic configuration of the atom is required to explain what hybridization is and how it is attained. The extranuclear configuration of an isolated carbon atom is $1s^2 2s^2 2p_x^1 2p_y^1 2p_z^0$ which means that there are two electrons in the 1s level, two in the 2s level, and two in the 2p level, but since the two 2p electrons reside in different subshells (p_x and p_y) they are unpaired (see

Chapter 17, *Quantum Chemistry*). Since only unpaired valence electrons are capable of bonding, it would be expected that carbon should exhibit a valence of two. However, in every instance (except for possibly carbon monoxide) carbon combines with four univalent atoms or groups.

Bond formation is a stabilizing (exothermic) process and there is a tendency to form as many bonds as possible, even if the resulting molecular orbitals bear little resemblance to the atomic orbitals which exist in the isolated or *ground* state of an atom. A carbon atom must be elevated or *excited* (energetically) to assume a valence state of four and to do this four unpaired electrons must be created. This feat can be accomplished by promoting one electron from the 2s level to the vacant $2p_z$ level and thus the resulting extranuclear electronic configuration becomes $1s^2 2s^1 2p_x^1 2p_y^1 2p_z^1$. More than enough energy is available during the process of bond formation to excite the 2s electron. Four unpaired electrons are now available for bonding purposes.

It might now be expected that carbon could form two different types of bonds, viz, three bonds of a type using p orbitals $(2p_x, 2p_y, 2p_z)$ and a fourth bond utilizing the 2s orbital. This is contrary to known fact—all four bonds are equivalent so far as bond energy and bond length are concerned.

The simplest two-dimensional picture of such a carbon atom, as noted in the diagram of the molecule dichloromethane, CH_2Cl_2, would be as in *A*:

$$\begin{array}{cc} \text{Cl} & \text{Cl} \\ | & | \\ \text{H}-\text{C}-\text{Cl} & \text{H}-\text{C}-\text{H} \\ | & | \\ \text{H} & \text{Cl} \\ \textbf{A} & \textbf{B} \end{array}$$

However, it can readily be observed that if the molecule was flat, it should exist in the two isomeric forms, *A* and *B*. Since only one dichloromethane is known (and for other, more convincing, reasons) the structure as depicted is spatially incorrect. In 1874 LeBel and van't Hoff demonstrated, using the concept of stereoisomerism, that a carbon atom assumes a *tetrahedral* configuration. That is, each covalent bond is directed to a corner of a regular tetrahedron:

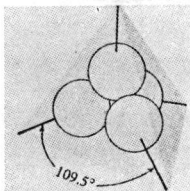

To more clearly illustrate the three-dimensional aspect of this arrangement, the usual two-dimensional diagram is better shown as follows:

* Adapted from Nebergall, W. H., *et al*, *College Chemistry*, Raytheon, Boston, 1968.

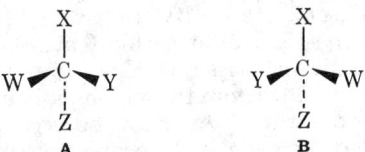

in which a solid line is understood to be in the plane of the paper, a broken line extends behind the plane, and solid arrowheads extend in front of the plane. Study of the many kinds of three-dimensional organic models is very beneficial in the understanding of this concept. A cursory look at such models (or the diagram) indicates that *A* and *B* are not identical (not superimposable) but are in reality isomers. This situation is known as *stereoisomerism* and the phenomenon essentially doubles the number of possible compounds of this particular type.

Since the resultant bonds are comprised of three p and one s electron and are neither of the spherical s or linear p configuration, but some combination thereof, they are said to be *hybridized*. This *tetrahedral* or sp^3 hybridization can be explained by the tendency for unshared electrons to get as far from each other as possible (Pauli *exclusion* principle) and for four bonds the tetrahedral configuration satisfies this requirement. Covalent bonds, beside having characteristic bond length and energy, are also associated with direction in space.

Another peculiarity is associated with carbon-to-carbon bonding. Beside the aforementioned tetrahedral or sp^3 hybridization, two other possibilities are known to occur in the bonding of two carbon atoms; trigonal or sp^2 and linear (digonal) or sp hybridization.

Alkenes are examples of the sp^2 type, the hybrid orbitals being directed toward the corners of an equilateral triangle. This permits the hybrid orbitals to be as far removed from each other as possible. An unhybridized p orbital also exists perpendicular to the plane of the sp^2 orbitals:*

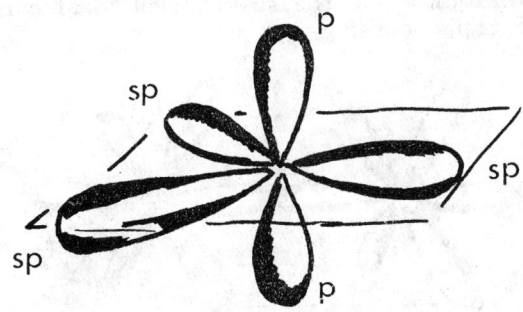

The union of two carbon atoms of this type produces a multiple bond, involving two electron pairs (a *double bond*), shown at the bottom of this page.* Overlap of the sp^2 orbitals forms a sigma (σ) bond and the p orbital overlap produces a pi (π) bond. A carbon-carbon double bond is not composed of two similar bonds, as might be interpreted from the usual notation of $C=C$, which is used. Each bond is a

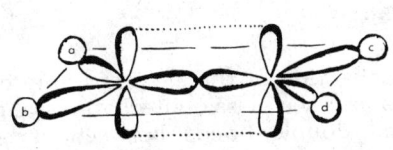

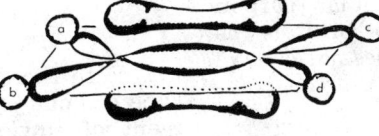

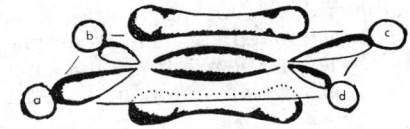

distinct and separate entity and many physical and chemical properties confirm this feature. All of the sigma bonds lie in the same plane, but the pi bonds project above and below the plane as is evident from the previous diagram. As might be expected, because of the added "cementing" properties of the extra electrons, the carbon atoms of a multiple bond are held more closely. Thus the carbon-carbon bond distance for a double bond is 1.34 Å in ethylene compared to 1.54 Å for the single carbon-carbon bond of ethane.

Another interesting situation occurs due to the configuration of the sigma-pi double bond. Reference to the above illustration of the completed molecule shows that groups *a*, *b*, *c*, and *d* are in the same plane and, by reversing the two substituent groups at either end of the molecule (as in *B* and *C*), we have now generated an isomer; a *geometric* isomer. Again, this phenomenon leads to a doubling of the number of compounds of this particular type.

A third variety of hybridization which exists involves the coalition of one s and one p electron (sp). The resulting two sp orbitals produced are directed axially, 180° apart and 90° removed from the plane of the unhybridized p orbitals:*

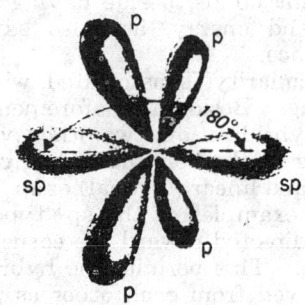

A combination of two carbon atoms exhibiting sp hybridization along the sp axis will yield carbon-carbon triple bonds:*

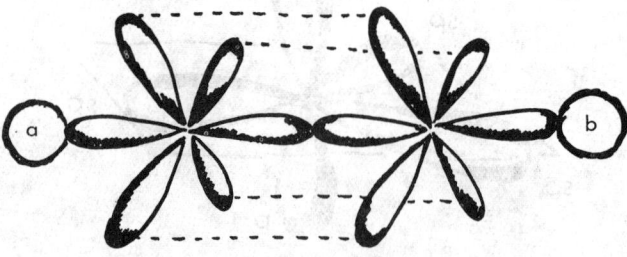

The p orbitals from a cylindrical sheath about the sigma bond. For a carbon-carbon triple bond the interatomic distance is smaller than a single or double bond, being 1.20 Å. Isomerism (geometric or stereoisomerism) is not possible with a triple bond as the substituents, a and b, are located axially.

Delocalization—Benzene represents a large series of compounds exhibiting a kind of bonding which is perhaps as unique and different from the usual carbon-carbon bond types as is carbon from the rest of the periodic table. Although the six annular carbon atoms are bonded to each other via sp² orbitals (as with ethylene), the resultant molecule does not behave as an unsaturated compound. Although the com-

pound is depicted as having a conjugate system of three double bonds (*B*, *C*, and *D*):

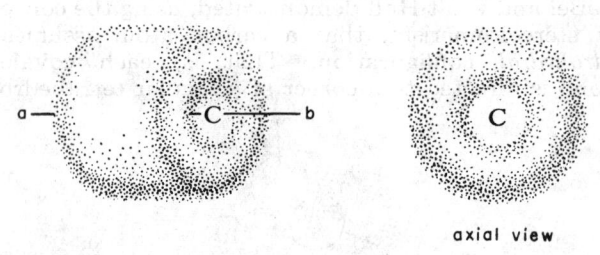

the benzene molecule does not behave chemically like a simple conjugated diene. Reactions normally occur by substitution of a hydrogen atom rather than the expected addition to the double bond. Also two simple disubstitution products would be expected:

However, only one disubstitution product is known. Benzene, therefore, must exhibit an entirely different kind of bonding than those previously discussed. It is believed that the p orbitals, above and below the plane of the benzene ring, overlap in *both* directions and each electron can participate in several bonds. The ability of the pi electrons to be active in joining several atoms results in stronger bonds and a more stable molecule. This phenomenon of *delocalization*

axial view

of electrons results in a delocalization or *resonance* energy of stability.

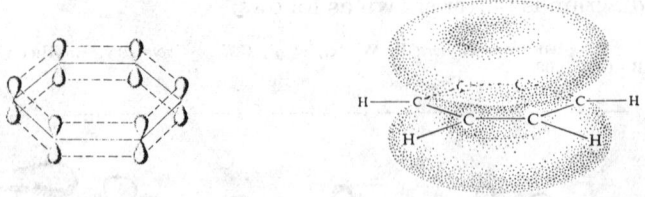

Due to the delocalization of the electrons only one type of bond exists and the classic alternate arrangement of single and double bonds between carbon atoms of the benzene molecule is misleading and incorrect. The carbon-carbon bond distance for benzene is 1.39 Å, lying between the single- and double-bond interatomic distance. The term *delocalization* better describes the resultant molecular orbital picture of benzene, rather than the concept of resonance. The term *resonance* may imply a rapid alternation between two or among several structural forms, which is totally incorrect.

Delocalization (resonance) stabilization is evident for many organic compounds which contain multiple bonds. Just as a lowering of energy results from the formation of molecular orbitals whereby electrons are associated with two positive nuclei, a further lowering results if a molecular orbital is formed by utilizing several nuclei. This *extra* energy lowering increases the stability of a compound and the net energy difference derived from summing bond energies and that of the heat of combustion of the molecule is termed resonance or delocalization energy. Several types of organic compounds, other than benzene, exhibit the delocalization phenomenon:

$$\left[R-C\begin{smallmatrix}O \\ \\ O\end{smallmatrix} \right]^- \qquad CH_2{=}{=}CH{-}{-}CH{=}{=}CH_2$$

carboxylate ion   1,3-Butadiene

Delocalization accounts for the stability of *aromatic* compounds such as naphthalene, anthracene, pyridine, pyrimidine, thiophene, furan, etc. *Aromaticity* has become synonymous with the unusual stability and chemical behavior of benzene-like compounds. A quantum mechanical treatment of cyclic, conjugated systems indicates that aromaticity exists in those rings associated with $(4n + 2)$ pi electrons, where n is an integer. Thus rings having 6, 10 or 14π electrons may be aromatic (if they are planar), while those of 4, 8 or 12π electrons cannot. While the supporting mathematical theory is beyond the scope of this chapter, chemical evidence easily suggests that compounds such as pyridine, thiophene, or furan do behave as benzene, while cyclooctatetraene—although a cyclic, conjugate system—behaves merely as a typical conjugated alkene and does not show the exceptional stability of an aromatic compound.

Carbon-Heteroatom Bonds

Practically all of the foregoing material pertains to the structure of a carbon-to-carbon or carbon-to-hydrogen bond. A majority of the compounds normally included in the area of organic chemistry also contain *heteroatoms* (atoms other than carbon and hydrogen) and the mode of bonding between carbon and the heteroatoms is of great importance. A rigorous treatment of this subject is well outside the limits of this chapter but several general observations are in order. Carbon forms a typical sigma bond with the univalent nonmetals (halogens) and with other electronegative polyvalent elements such as oxygen, nitrogen, sulfur, and phosphorus. Because of the differing electronegativities of the atoms on either side of the sigma bond, the bond is not entirely symmetrical and the slightly uneven distribution of bonding electrons causes an asymmetry leading to increased values of dipole moments with increased difference is electronegativities.

Multiple bonds can also exist between the polyvalent elements and carbon. Typical of this group is the carbonyl function ($=C=O$), an example of sp^2 hybridization. The carbon atom is joined to two other atoms and the oxygen atom by sigma bonds; the remaining p orbital of the carbon overlaps a p orbital of oxygen to form a typical π bond. Thus carbon and oxygen are joined by a double bond. Each of the three sigma bonds radiating from the carbon atom is at an angle of 120°, and the carbonyl portion and the two atoms to which it is attached lie in the same plane.

The electrons of the carbonyl double bond join two elements of quite different electronegativity and hence are not shared equally; the electron cloud being pulled more strongly toward the electronegative oxygen atom. As the π electrons are of a lower energy than sigma electrons, they are more easily influenced by the electronegative oxygen atom. This effect is much more pronounced with multiple bonds than for a single (sigma) bond and results in the occurrence of a permanent polarity. Therefore, aldehydes and ketones (which contain the carbonyl function) exhibit fairly large dipole moments (2.3–2.75 D) because of the polarity of the carbonyl group as shown below. A lower-case delta (δ) indicates that a *fractional* charge of appropriate sign resides on the designated atoms:

$$\overset{\delta^+}{R{-}\underset{\underset{R}{|}}{C}}{=}\overset{\delta^-}{O}$$

The structure of the carbonyl group largely determines the physical and chemical properties of aldehydes and ketones. Similar analogies can be drawn for carbon to sulfur and carbon to nitrogen multiple bonds.

Although carbon usually bonds to other elements by covalent-type linkages, several examples of ionic type bonds are known (carbanion $R_3C{:}^-$ and carbonium ion R_3C^+), but these are very short lived and are primarily useful in explaining the *mechanism* of various organic reactions via intermediates of transient existence.

Noncarbon Bonds

The magnitude of the number of organic compounds is not due solely to the intricacies shown in carbon-to-carbon and carbon-to-heteroatom bonds. The electronegative elements, especially nitrogen and oxygen, impart their individualities such that a carbon-to-oxygen or carbon-to-nitrogen bond can participate in new types of bonds not previously discussed. As an example, the *hydrogen bond* or *bridge* can cause intermolecular association which can lead to an apparent increase in molecular weight or is the reason for a drug binding to certain sites of activity. Formation of *chelates, clathrates,* coordination complexes, etc. also extend the number of compounds which would be possible if only classic types of bonding existed between elements. Chapter 16, *Complexation,* deals in depth with the concepts mentioned in this paragraph, and the reader is referred there for more information.

Table I—Types of Organic Compounds

Acetals
R.C(H or R)(OR)₂
CH₃CH(OCH₃)₂
acetaldehyde dimethyl acetal
(1,1-dimethoxyethane)
(CH₃)₂C(OC₂H₅)₂
acetone diethyl acetal
(2,2-diethoxypropane)

Acid Anhydrides
1. Of Monocarboxylic Acids
R.C(:O).O.(O:)C.R
(CH₃CO)₂O
acetic (acid) anhydride

2. Of Dicarboxylic Acids
$\overline{\text{R.C(:O).O.O.C(:O)}}$
CH₂CH₂CO.O.CO
succinic (acid) anhydride

Acid Halides (Acyl Halides)
R.C(:O).X
CH₃COCl
acetyl chloride

Acids (Carboxylic) (other acids are listed under their characteristic names, eg, Sulfonic Acids, Nitrolic Acids, etc)
R.C(:O)OH
CH₃COOH
acetic acid

Acyloins (α-Hydroxy Ketones)
R.CO.CH(OH).R or H
CH₃COCH(OH)CH₃
acetoin
CH₃CH₂COCH(OH)CH₃
propiononin
C₆H₅COCH(OH)C₆H₅
benzoin

Alcoholates (Alkoxides)
R.O. Metal
where R is aliphatic or alicyclic
C₂H₅ONa
sodium ethyl alcoholate
sodium ethylate
sodium ethoxide

Alcohols
R.OH
where R is aliphatic or alicyclic
C₂H₅OH
ethyl alcohol
CH₂(CH₂)₄CHOH
cyclohexyl alcohol

Aldehydes
R.CH:O
CH₃CHO
acetaldehyde

Alkoxides (see Alcoholates)
Alkylhalosilanes
R.(SiH₂)n.X
where one or more H's may be substituted by additional R's or X's
CH₃SiH₂Cl
methylchlorosilane

Alkylselenium Halides
R₂SeX₂
(C₂H₅)₂SeBr₂
diethylselenium dibromide
RSeX₃
CH₃SeBr₃
methylselenium tribromide

Alkylsilanes
R.(SiH₂)n.H
where one or more H's may be substituted by additional R's
CH₃SiH₃
methylsilane
C₂H₅SiH₂SiH₂C₂H₅
sym-diethyldisilane

Alkylsilanols
Types here illustrated are limited to derivatives of silane; ie, (mono)-silane, SiH₄. There are similar derivatives of the di-, tri-, etc, silanes.
R.SiH₂.OH   R.SiH(OH)₂   R.Si(OH)₃
alkylsilanols   alkylsilanediols   alkylsilanetriols
R₂SiH.OH   R₂Si(OH)₂
dialkylsilanols   dialkylsilanediols
R₃Si.OH
trialkylsilanols

Alkylsiloxanes
Various linear and cyclic types. (see Silicones, page 768). A common linear type consisting of condensation polymers of dialkyl-silanediols is shown.
HO.(SiR₂.O)n.SiR₂OH

Amic Acids
R[C(:O)NH₂][C(:O)OH]
CH₂(CONH₂)(COOH)
malonamic acid

Amides
R.C(:O).NH₂
CH₃CONH₂
acetamide

Amidines
R.C(:NH).NH₂
CH₃C(NH)NH₂
acetamidine

Amines
R.N(H or R)(H or R)
R.NH₂ types = Amino Compounds
CH₃NH₂
methylamine or aminomethane
(C₂H₅)₂NH
diethylamine
CH₃N(C₂H₅)C₃H₇
methylethylpropylamine

Amino Acids
R(NH₂).C(:O)OH
CH₂(NH₂)COOH
aminoacetic acid

Ammonium Derivatives
[RH₃Ṅ]X̄
where X = OH or a salt anion and any or all H's may be R's. If N is a ring member, specific "ium" nomenclature is employed to denote the heterocycle.
[(CH₃)₃Ṅ]Ī
tetramethylammonium iodide
[(C₆H₅)₂ṄH₂]C̄l
diphenylammonium chloride
(diphenylamine hydrochloride)
[CH:CH.CH:CH.CH:Ṅ(CH₃)]B̄r
1-methylpyridinium bromide

Anilic Acids
R[C(:O)NHR'][C(:O)OH]
where R' = phenyl or substituted phenyl
CH₂(CONHC₆H₅).CH₂COOH
succinanilic acid

Anilides
R.C(:O).NHR'
where NHR' is derived from aniline
CH₃CONHC₆H₅
acetanilide

Note—If .NHR' is derived from:

from:	Compounds are termed:
toluidine	toluidides
xylidine	xylidides
anisidine	anisidides
phenetidine	phenetidides

Anils (Schiff bases)
RCH:NR
C₆H₅CH:NC₆H₅
N-Benzylideneaniline

Arsenoso Compounds
R.As.O
C₆H₅AsO
arsenosobenzene

Arsine Oxides
R₃As:O
(CH₃)₃AsO
trimethylarsine oxide

Arsines
R.As(H or R)(H or R)
R.AsH₂ types = Arsino Compounds
CH₃AsH₂
methylarsine or arsinomethane
(CH₃)₂AsH
dimethylarsine
(CH₃)₃As
trimethylarsine

Arsinic Acids
R₂(or RH)As(:O)OH
(CH₃)₂AsOOH
dimethylarsinic acid

Arsinous Acids
R₂(or RH)As.OH
(CH₃)₂AsOH
dimethylarsinous acid

Arso Compounds
R.As(:O)₂
C₆H₅AsO₂
arsobenzene

Arsonic Acids
R.As(:O)(OH)₂
CH₃AsO(OH)₂
methanearsonic acid or methylarsonic acid

Arsonium Compounds
[RH₃As⁺]X̄
where X = OH or a salt anion and any or all H's may be R's
[(CH₃)₄As]C̄l
tetramethylarsonium chloride

Arsonous Acids
R.As(OH)₂
CH₃As(OH)₂
methanearsonous acid or methylarsenous acid

Azides (Acyl Azides)
R.C(:O).N:Ṅ:N̄
CH₃CO.N:Ṅ:N̄
acetyl azide

Azido Compounds
R.N:Ṅ:N̄
C₂H₅.N:Ṅ:N̄
azidoethane

Azines
R₂C:N.N:CR₂
(CH₃)₂C:NN:C(CH₃)₂
acetone azine

Azo Compounds
R.N:N.R
C₆H₅N:NC₆H₅
azobenzene

Azoxy Compounds
R.N:N(:O).R
C₆H₅N:N(O)C₆H₅
azoxybenzene

Benzils (Aromatic α-Diketones)
R.C(:O).C(:O).R
where R is aromatic
p-CH₃C₆H₄COCOC₆H₄CH₃-p
p,p'-dimethylbenzil

Benzoins (Aromatic α-Hydroxy Ketones)
R.CH(OH).C(:O).R
where R is aromatic
p-CH₃C₆H₄CH(OH)COC₆H₄CH₃-p
p,p'-dimethylbenzoin or p-toluoin

Betaines
R₃Ṅ.R.C(:O).Ō
(CH₃)₃ṄCH₂CH₂COO⁻
β-alanine, trimethylbetaine

Borates (see Esters)
Borines
R.B(H or R)(H or R)
B(CH₃)₃
trimethylborine

Borinic Acids
R₂BOH
(C₆H₅)₂BOH
diphenylborinic acid

Boronic Acids
R.B(OH)₂
CH₃B(OH)₂
methaneboronic acid

"Boron Oxides" (Borinic Acid Anhydrides) (Trivial Name)
(R₂B)O
[(C₂H₅)₂B]₂O
bis(diethylboron) oxide
diethylborinic acid anhydride

Carbonates (see Esters)
Carbylamines (Isocyanides; Isonitriles)
R.N:C
C₆H₅NC
phenyl {carbylamine, isocyanide, or isonitrile

Cyanates
R.O.C:N
C₆H₅OCN
phenyl cyanate

Cyanides (see Nitriles)
Cyanohydrins
R.C(CN)(OH)(H or R)
CH₃C(CN)(OH)CH₃
acetone cyanohydrin

Diazoamino Compounds (Triazene Derivatives)
R.N:N.NH.R
C₆H₅N:NNHC₆H₅
diazoaminobenzene or 1,3-diphenyltriazene

Diazo Compounds
Type A R.N:N.X
where X = OH or a salt anion
C₆H₅N:NCl
benzenediazochloride
Type B R.N:N.O Metal (diazoates)
C₆H₅N:NONa
sodium benzenediazoate

Table I—Continued

Type C C(H or R)(H or R):$\overset{\cdot\cdot}{N}$:$\overset{\cdot\cdot}{N}$ CH$_2$:$\overset{+}{N}$:$\overset{\cdot\cdot}{N}$
diazomethane

Diazonium Compounds
[R.$\overset{+}{N}$(:N)]$\bar{X}$
where X = OH or a salt anion [C$_6$H$_5$$\overset{+}{N}$(:N)]$\bar{O}$H
benzenediazonium hydroxide

Diboranes
R.BH$_2$.BH$_3$
One to four of the H's may be replaced by R's (CH$_3$)$_2$BHBH(CH$_3$)$_2$
sym-tetramethyldiborane

Epoxy Compounds
CH$_2$.(CH$_2$)n.CH$_2$.O
where n = zero or greater and any or all H's may be R's CH$_2$CH$_2$O
epoxyethane
CH$_3$CHCH$_2$CH(CH$_3$)O
2,4-epoxypenthane

Esters (of Carboxylic Acids)
R.C(:O).OR CH$_3$COOC$_2$H$_5$
ethyl acetate

Esters (of Inorganic Oxy Acids)
The listing here is intentionally limited to esters of the more important oxy acids of nitrogen, phosphorus, sulfur, boron, silicon, and carbon. In each instance, the type formula shown is for the ester which results from the replacement of all acidic H's by R's. Where more than one R is present, acid esters (ie, esters still containing one or more unreplaced H's) are possible.

Nitrates	N(:O)$_2$OR	C$_2$H$_5$NO$_3$ ethyl nitrate
Nitrites	N(:O)OR	C$_2$H$_5$ONO ethyl nitrite
(Ortho)phosphates	P(:O)(OR)$_3$	(C$_2$H$_5$)$_3$PO$_4$ ethyl phosphate
Metaphosphates	P(:O)$_2$OR	C$_2$H$_5$PO$_3$ ethyl metaphosphate
Pyrophosphates	(RO)$_2$(O:)P.-O.P(:O)(OR)$_2$	(C$_2$H$_5$)$_4$P$_2$O$_7$ ethyl pyrophosphate

(Ortho)phosphites P(OR)$_3$ (C$_2$H$_5$)$_3$PO$_3$ ethyl phosphite
(Structure in doubt. More likely R.P(:O)(OR)$_2$; ie, that of dialkyl alkylphosphonates. *Cf* Phosphonic Acids.)
Hypophosphites HP(OH)(OR) C$_2$H$_5$H$_2$PO$_2$ ethyl hypophosphite
(Structure in doubt. More likely H$_2$P(:O)OR; ie, that of alkyl phosphinates. *Cf* Phosphinic Acids.)

Sulfates	S(:O)$_2$(OR)$_2$	(C$_2$H$_5$)$_2$SO$_4$, ethyl sulfate
Sulfites	S(:O)(OR)$_2$	(C$_2$H$_5$)$_2$SO$_3$, ethyl sulfite
Orthoborates	B(OR)$_3$	(C$_2$H$_5$)$_3$BO$_3$, ethyl orthoborate
Metaborates	B(:O)OR	C$_2$H$_5$BO$_2$, ethyl metaborate
Orthosilicates	Si(OR)$_4$	(C$_2$H$_5$)$_4$SiO$_4$, ethyl orthosilicate
Metasilicates	Si(:O)(OR)$_2$	(C$_2$H$_5$)$_2$SiO$_3$, ethyl metasilicate
Orthocarbonates	C(OR)$_4$	(C$_2$H$_5$)$_4$CO$_4$, ethyl orthocarbonate
Carbonates	C(:O)(OR)$_2$	(C$_2$H$_5$)$_2$CO$_3$, ethyl carbonate

Ethers
R.O.R. CH$_3$OC$_2$H$_5$
ethyl methyl ether

Fluorophosphates (see Phosphorofluoridates)

Glycerides
ROCO.CH$_2$.CH(OCOR).CH$_2$.-OCOR C$_3$H$_5$(C$_2$H$_3$O$_2$)$_3$ or (CH$_3$COO)$_3$-C$_3$H$_5$
glyceryl triacetate or triacetin

Glycerophosphates (see page 462)

Glycols
HOCH$_2$.(CH$_2$)n.CH$_2$OH CH$_2$(OH)CH$_2$OH
ethylene glycol

where n = zero or greater
CH$_2$(OH)CH$_2$CH$_2$OH
trimethylene glycol

Guanidino Compounds—see page 460

Haloalkylsilanes
XR.(SiH$_2$)n.H ClCH$_2$SiH$_3$
where one or more of the H's in R may be substituted by additional X's and one or more of silicon hydrogens may be substituted by additional .RX groups chloromethylsilane

Halohydrins
CH$_2$X.CH$_2$OH
where either or both of the CH$_2$'s may be CHR or CR$_2$ CH$_2$ClCH$_2$OH
ethylene chlorohydrin

Hemiacetals
R.C(H or R)(OR)(OH) CH$_3$CH(OC$_2$H$_5$)OH
acetaldehyde ethyl hemiacetal (1-ethoxyethanol)

Hydrazides
R.C(:O).NH.NH$_2$ CH$_3$CONHNH$_2$
acetic acid hydrazide

Hydrazines
R.N(H or R).N(H or R)(H or R) C$_6$H$_5$NHNH$_2$
phenylhydrazine

Hydrazones
R$_2$(or RH)C:N.NH$_2$ (CH$_3$)$_2$C:NNH$_2$
acetone hydrazone
C$_6$H$_5$CH:NNH$_2$
benzaldehyde hydrazone

Hydrocarbon Halides (Alkyl, Alkylene, Alkylidene, Alkenyl, Aryl, Arylene, etc. Halides)
RX*n*
when n = valence of R CH$_3$Cl
methyl chloride
CH$_2$:CHBr
vinyl bromide
CH$_3$CHCl$_2$
ethylidene chloride
C$_6$H$_5$I
phenyl iodide

Hydrosulfamines
N-Derivatives RH(or R$_2$)N.S.H C$_6$H$_5$NHSH
N-phenylhydrosulfamine

Hydroxamic Acids
R.C(:NOH)OH CH$_3$CH$_2$C(:NOH)OH
propionohydroxamic acid

Hydroxy Acids
R(OH).C.(:O)OH CH$_3$CH(OH)COOH
α-hydroxypropionic acid or lactic acid

Hypophosphites (see Esters)

Imides (Carboximides)
R.C(:O).N(H or R).C:O CH$_2$CH$_2$CONHCO
succinimide
1,2-ethanedicarboximide

Imidic Acids
R.C(:NH)OH CH$_3$C(:NH)OH
acetimidic acid

Imines
R:NH CH$_3$CH$_2$:NH
ethylideneimine
CH$_2$CH$_2$NH
ethyleneimine

Iodonium Compounds
[R$_2$$\overset{+}{I}$]$\bar{X}$
where X = OH or a salt anion [(C$_6$H$_5$)$_2$I]$\bar{B}$r
diphenyliodonium bromide

Iodoso Compounds
R.I:O C$_6$H$_5$IO
iodosobenzene

Iodoxy Compounds
R.I(:O)$_2$ C$_6$H$_5$IO$_2$
iodoxybenzene

Isocyanates
R.N:C:O C$_6$H$_5$NCO
phenyl isocyanate

Isocyanide Dichlorides (Imidocarbonyl Chlorides)
R.N:CCl$_2$ C$_2$H$_5$NCCl$_2$
ethyl isocyanide dichloride
ethylimidocarbonyl chloride

Isocyanides (see Carbylamines)
Isonitriles (see Carbylamines)
Isothiocyanates (Isosulfocyanates; Thiocarbimides; Mustard Oils)
R.N:C:S CH$_3$NCS
methyl isothiocyanate, etc.

Ketals
R$_2$C.(OR)$_2$
(Commonly treated as acetals, q.v. above) (CH$_3$)$_2$C(OC$_2$H$_5$)$_2$
acetone diethylketal (2,2-diethoxypropane)

Ketenes
R.C(H or R):C:O (CH$_3$)$_2$C:C:O
dimethyl ketene

Keto Acids (monobasic)
H(CH$_2$)n.C.(:O).(CH$_2$)n.C.(:O)-OH
where n = zero or greater and any or all H's may be R's. May also be polybasic. CH$_3$COCH$_2$COOH
β-ketobutyric acid or acetoacetic acid
HOOCCH$_2$COCOOH
ketosuccinic acid or oxalacetic acid

Ketones
R.C(:O).R
where R's are aliphatic or alicyclic. If one or both R's are aromatic, compounds are termed Phenones. CH$_3$COC$_2$H$_5$
ethyl methyl ketone

Lactams
CH$_2$.(CH$_2$)n.C(:O).NH
where n = 2 in γ-lactams and 3 in δ-lactams and any or all H's may be R's. CH$_2$CH$_2$CH$_2$CH$_2$CONH
δ-aminovalerolactam (2-piperidone)

Lactides
CH$_2$C(:O).O.CH$_2$.C(:O).O
where any or all of the H's may be R's CH$_3$CHCO.O.CH(CH$_3$)COO
α-hydroxypropionic acid lactide "lactide"

Lactims
as per lactams except
.C(:O).NH becomes .C(OH):N CH$_2$CH$_2$CH$_2$CH$_2$C(OH):N
δ-aminovalerolactim

Lactones
CH$_2$(CH$_2$)n.C.(:O).O
where n = 2 in γ-lactones and 3 in δ-lactones and any or all H's may be R's CH$_2$CH$_2$CH$_2$CH$_2$COO
δ-valerolactone

Mercaptals
R.CH(SR)$_2$ CH$_3$CH(SC$_2$H$_5$)$_2$
acetaldehyde diethylmercaptal

Mercaptans (see Thiols)
Mercaptides
R.S. Metal C$_2$H$_5$SNa
sodium ethyl mercaptide

Mercaptoles
R$_2$C(.SR)$_2$ (CH$_3$)$_2$C(SC$_2$H$_5$)$_2$
acetone diethylmercaptole

Morpholides
R.C(:O).N.CH$_2$.CH$_2$.O.CH$_2$.CH$_2$ CH$_3$CONCH$_2$CH$_2$OCH$_2$CH$_2$
acetmorpholide (4-acetylmorpholine)

Nitrates (see Esters)
Nitriles (Cyanides; Carbonitriles)
R.C:N CH$_3$CH$_2$CN
propionitrile
ethyl cyanide
ethanecarbonitrile

Nitrites (see Esters)
Nitro Compounds
R.N(:O)$_2$ CH$_3$NO$_2$
nitromethane
C$_6$H$_5$NO$_2$
nitrobenzene

Nitrolic Acids
R.C(:NOH).NO$_2$ CH$_3$C(:NOH)NO$_2$
acetnitrolic acid

Nitroso Compounds
R.N:O C$_6$H$_5$NO
nitrosobenzene

Nitrosolic Acids
R.C(:NOH).NO CH$_3$C(:NOH)NO
acetnitrosolic acid

Table I—Continued

Organometallic (Metallo-organic) Compounds
Note—Restricted here to compounds having a direct metal-carbon linkage.
Commonest types are:
  MR_v and $R_{(v-1)}MX$ $(C_2H_5)_4Pb$
  where M = *metal functioning with*   tetraethyl lead
    valence v
  R = *univalent unsubsti-* CH_3MgBr
    tuted, or, substi-   methylmagnesium bromide
    tuted, hydrocarbon
    radical
  X = *univalent anion* $C_6H_5HgNO_3$
    phenylmercuric nitrate
    $(CH_3)_3SnOH$
    trimethylstannic hydroxide
    Ag_2C_2
    silver acetylide

Osazones [Bis(phenylhydrazones)]
  (H or R).C(:N.NHPh).C- $C_6H_5C(:NNHPh)C(:NNHPh)C_6H_5$
  (:N.NHPh).(R or H)   benzil osazone
  where Ph = phenyl   [Benzil bis(phenylhydrazone)]

Oximes
  R.C(H or R):NOH $CH_3CH:NOH$
    acetaldoxime
    $(CH_3)_2C:NOH$
    dimethylketoxime
    (acetone oxime)

Oxoboryl Compounds
  R.B:O C_6H_5BO
    oxoborylbenzene

Oxo Compounds (see Aldehydes, Ketones, Quinones, Keto Acid)

Oxonium Salts

1. Noncyclic $[R_2H\overset{+}{O}]\bar{X}$ $[(CH_3)_2H\overset{+}{O}]\bar{Cl}$
  where X = *salt anion*   dimethyloxonium chloride

2. Cyclic $[R:\overset{+}{O}]\bar{X}$ $[\overline{C(CH_3):CH.C(CH_3):CH.C(CH_3):}$
    $\overset{\lceil}{O}]ClO_4^-$
  where X = *salt anion*   2,4,6-trimethylpyrilium perchlorate

Ozonides
  $\overset{\lceil-O-\rceil}{R.CH.O.O.CH.R}$ $\overset{\lceil-O-\rceil}{CH_3CH.O.O.CHCH_3}$
    2-butene ozonide

Peptides (Polypeptides)
  $NH_2[.R.C(:O).NH]n.R.C(:O)OH$ $NH_2(CH_2CONH)_2CH_2COOH$
    glycine tripeptides
    glycyl-glycyl-glycine

Peroxides
  R.O.O.(R or H) $C_2H_5O.OC_2H_5$
    ethyl peroxide

Peroxy Acids
  R.C(:O)O.OH $CH_3CO.O.OH$
    peroxyacetic acid

Phenolates (Phenoxides)
  R.O. Metal C_6H_5ONa
  where R is aromatic   sodium phenolate
    sodium phenoxide

Phenols
  R.OH $p\text{-}CH_3C_6H_4OH$
  where R is aromatic p-methylphenol
    (p-cresol)

Phenones (see Ketones)
Phenoxides (see Phenolates)
Phosphates (see Esters)
Phosphine Imides
  $R_3P:NH$ $(CH_3)_3PNH$
    P,P,P-trimethylphosphine imide

Phosphine Oxides
  $R_3P:O$ $(CH_3)_3PO$
    trimethylphosphine oxide

Phosphines
  R.P(H or R)(H or R) CH_3PH_2
  $R.PH_2$ types = Phosphino   methylphosphine or phosphino-
  Compounds   methane
    $(C_2H_5)_2PH$
    diethylphosphine
    $CH_3P(C_2H_5)C_3H_7$
    methylethylpropylphosphine

Phosphinic Acids
  $R_2(\text{or } RH)P(:O)OH$ $(CH_3)_2POOH$
    dimethylphosphinic acid

Phosphinic Halides
  $R_2(\text{or } RH)P(:O)X$ $(CH_3)_2POCl$
    dimethylphosphinic chloride

Phosphinous Acids
  $R_2(\text{or } RH)P.OH$ $(CH_3)_2POH$
    dimethylphosphinous acid

Phosphinous Halides [Di(or mono)-alkylhalophosphines]
  $R_2(\text{or } RH)P.X$ $C_2H_5.P(CH_3)Cl$
    ethylmethylphosphinous chloride

Phosphites (see Esters)
Phospho Compounds
  $R.P(:O)_2$ $C_6H_5PO_2$
    phosphobenzene

Phosphonic Acids
  $R.P(:O)(OH)_2$ $CH_3PO(OH)_2$
    methylphosphonic acid or
    methanephosphonic acid

Phosphonic Dihalides
  $R.P(:O)X_2$ CH_3POCl_2
    methylphosphonic dichloride or
    methanephosphonic dichloride

Phosphonium Compounds
  $[RH_3\overset{+}{P}]\bar{X}$ $[(CH_3)_4\overset{+}{P}]\bar{I}$
  where X = OH or a salt anion and   tetramethylphosphonium iodide
  any or all H's may be R's

Phosphonous Acids
  $R.P(OH)_2$ $CH_3P(OH)_2$
    methylphosphonous acid or
    methanephosphonous acid

Phosphonous Dihalides (Alkyldihalophosphines)
  $R.PX_2$ CH_3PCl_2
    methyldichlorophosphine or
    methylphosphonous dichloride

Phosphorofluoridates (Fluorophosphates)
  $F.P(:O)(OR)_2$ $FPO[OCH(CH_3)_2]$
    diisopropyl phosphorofluoridate
    diisopropyl fluorophosphate

Phosphoroso Compounds
  R.P:O C_6H_5PO
    phosphorosobenzene

Phosphorus Compounds (General)
  In addition to the compounds in this listing, phosphorus forms a very large number of types of compounds containing direct linkages between the phosphorus and halogens, cyanogen, nitrogen, and sulfur. Many of these contain also phosphorus-oxygen linkages. For a comprehensive presentation of organic compounds containing phosphorus, see the report entitled *Organic Compounds Containing Phosphorus*, which is available from Chemical Abstracts Service.

Phthaleins, simplest type only (see page 455)
  $\overline{R.C(R'OH)_2.O.CO}$ $\overline{m\text{-}C_6H_4.C(.p\text{-}C_6H_4OH)_2.O.CO}$
  where R is o-phenylene, R' is p-   phenolphthalein
  phenylene, and either or both may
  be substituted.

Piperidides
  $\overline{R.C(:O).N.CH_2CH_2.CH_2.CH_2.CH_2}$ $\overline{CH_3CONCH_2CH_2CH_2CH_2CH_2}$
    acetpiperidide
    (1-acetylpiperidine)

Polyborane Derivatives
  Embraces numerous types of $B_2H_2(CH_3)_4$
  compounds which consist of   tetramethyldiborane(6)
  a polyborane, such as Dibor- $B_{10}H_{13}(COOH)$
  ane(6) [B_2H_6], Decaborane(14)   decaborane(14)carboxylic acid
  [$B_{10}H_{14}$], with one or more of
  the H atoms replaced by a
  carbon-containing group.

Quaternary Ammonium Compounds
  $[R_4\overset{+}{N}]\bar{X}$ $[(CH_3)_4\overset{+}{N}]\bar{Cl}$
  where X = OH or a salt anion   tetramethylammonium chloride

Quinones
  O:R:O $p\text{-}O:C_6H_4:O$
  where R is a quinonoid cycle p-benzoquinone

Salts (Metal)   Formulas as per acids except that the acidic H's are replaced by metal equivalent.

Selenides (Seleno Ethers)
  R.Se.R $(CH_3)_2Se$
    (di)methyl selenide
    dimethyl selenoether

Seleninic Acids
  R.Se(:O)OH C_2H_5SeOOH
    ethaneseleninic acid

Seleno Acids
  R.C(:O)SeH CH_3COSeH
    selenoacetic acid

Selenocyanates
  R.SeCN C_6H_5SeCN
    phenyl selenocyanate

Seleno Ketones
  R.C(:Se).R $(CH_3)_2CSe$
    dimethyl selenoketone
    selenoacetone

Selenols (Acid Selenides)
  R.SeH C_2H_5SeH
    ethaneselenol
    ethyl acid selenide

Selenones
  $R.Se(:O)_2.R$ $(CH_3)_2SeO_2$
    dimethyl selenone

Selenonic Acids
  $R.Se(:O)_2OH$ $C_6H_5SeO_2OH$
    benzeneselenonic acid

Selenonium Compounds
  $[R_3\overset{+}{Se}]\bar{X}$ $[(C_2H_5)_3\overset{+}{Se}]\bar{Br}$
  where X = OH or a salt anion   triethylselenonium bromide

Selenoxides
  R.Se(:O).R $(C_2H_5)_2SeO$
    (di)ethyl selenoxide

Semicarbazones
  R.C(H or R):N.NH.CO.NH₂ $(CH_3)_2C:NNHCONH_2$
    acetone semicarbazone

Silicates (see Esters)
Silicon Compounds (General)
  Because of its position in Group IV of the Periodic Table, it is not surprising that silicon enters freely into organic-type chemical combinations. Like carbon, although to a much lesser extent, silicon forms stable chain compounds containing —Si.Si— linkages. Compounds which contain hydrogen as the only other element are termed silanes: eg, SiH_4, silane (silicane, silicomethane); Si_2H_6, disilane (disilicoethane); and Si_3H_8, trisilane. Cyclosilanes, $SiH_2.(SiH_2)_n.SiH_2$ are also well known. These silicon-hydrogen compounds are analogous to the alkanes and cycloalkanes in the carbon family of compounds. They form various types of derivatives; eg, SiH_3OH, $H_2Si(:O)$, $HSi(:O)OH$, $HOSiH_2.SiH_2OH$, $SiHCl_3$, $H_2Si: NH$, $(SiH_2)_3N$, etc. These formulas are completely analogous to carbon compounds. Silicon also shows a strong tendency to form stable chain compounds containing —Si.O.Si— linkages; these are the siloxanes: eg, $H_3Si.O.SiH_3$, disiloxane; $H_3Si.O.SiH_2.O.SiH_3$, trisiloxane; etc. Analogous compounds containing imino instead of oxygen, are also well known. These are the silazanes: eg, $H_3Si.NH.SiH_3$, disilazane; $H_3Si.NH.SiH_2.NH.SiH_3$, trisilazane; etc.
  It will be noted that none of the above types of compounds contain carbon, and in this sense, they are not organic compounds. However,

Table I—Continued

alkyl derivatives of these, which are very numerous, are organic in the same sense as alkyl derivatives of hydrogen compounds of other elements such as nitrogen and sulfur. Since the alkyl groups in the derivatives may also contain substituent functional groups, it is readily apparent that there are a great many types of organic silicon compounds. Only a few of the better known types are included in this listing.

Siliconic Acids
  Ortho form $R.Si(OH)_3$ $CH_3Si(OH)_3$
  methaneorthosiliconic acid (methylsilanetriol)

  Meta form $R.Si(:O)(OH)$ C_6H_5SiOOH
  benzene(meta)siliconic acid

Silylalkanols (silicoalcohols)
  Alcohols in which one (or more) of the C.H hydrogens is replaced by silyl ($.SiH_3$) or substituted silyl groups. In contrast to the silanols compounds of this type contain hydroxyl in true organic combination. There are many subtypes. $(C_2H_5)_3Si.CH_2.CH_2OH$ β-triethylsilylethanol

Stibine Oxides
  $R_3Sb:O$ $(CH_3)_3SbO$
  trimethylstibine oxide

Stibines
  $R.Sb(H\ or\ R)(H\ or\ R)$ $(CH_3)_3Sb$
  $R.SbH_2$ types = Stibino   trimethylstibine
  Compounds $C_6H_5SbH_2$
  stibinobenzene

Stibinic Acids
  $R_2(or\ RH)Sb(:O)OH$ $(CH_3)_2SbOOH$
  dimethylstibinic acid

Stibinous Acids
  $R_2(or\ RH)Sb.OH$ $(CH_3)_2SbOH$
  dimethylstibinous acid

Stibo Compounds
  $R.Sb(:O)_2$ $C_6H_5SbO_2$
  stibobenzene

Stibonic Acids
  $R.Sb(:O)(OH)_2$ $C_6H_5SbO(OH)_2$
  benzenestibonic acid or phenylstibonic acid

Stibonium Compounds
  $[R_4\overset{+}{Sb}]\overline{X}$ $[(C_6H_5)_4\overset{+}{Sb}]\overline{I}$
  where X = OH or a salt anion and   tetraphenylstibonium iodide
  any or all H's may be R's

Stibonous Acids
  $R.Sb(OH)_2$ $CH_3Sb(OH)_2$
  methanestibonous acid or methylstibonous acid

Stiboso Compounds
  $R.Sb:O$ C_6H_5SbO
  stibosobenzene

Sulfamic Acids
  $RNH(or\ R_2N).SO_2.OH$ CH_3NHSO_2OH
  methanesulfamic acid
  $(C_2H_5)_2NSO_2OH$
  diethylsulfamic acid

Sulfates (see Esters)
Sulfenamides
  $R.S.NH_2$ $C_6H_5SNH_2$
  benzenesulfenamide

Sulfenic Acids
  $R.S.OH$ C_6H_5SOH
  benzenesulfenic acid

Sulfenyl Halides
  $R.S.X$ C_6H_5SCl
  benzenesulfenyl chloride

Sulfides (Thio Ethers)
  $R.S.R.$ $(CH_3)_2S$
  (di)methyl sulfide
  (di)methyl thioether

Sulfimides
  $R.CO.NH.SO_2$ $o\text{-}C_6H_4CONHSO_2$
  o-benzosulfimide

Sulfinamides
  $R.S(:O).NH_2$ $C_6H_5SONH_2$
  benzenesulfinamide

Sulfinic Acids
  $R.S(:O)OH$ C_6H_5SOOH
  benzenesulfinic acid

Sulfinyl Halides
  $R.S(:O).X$ C_6H_5SOCl
  benzenesulfinyl chloride

Sulfites (see Esters)
Sulfonamides
  $R.S(:O)_2.NH_2$ $C_6H_5SO_2NH_2$
  benzenesulfonamide

Sulfones
  $R.S(:O)_2.R$ $(C_2H_5)_2SO_2$
  diethyl sulfone

Sulfonic Acids
  $R.S(:O)_2OH$ $C_6H_5SO_2OH$
  benzenesulfonic acid

Sulfonium Compounds
  $[R_3\overset{+}{S}]\overline{X}$ where X is OH or a salt $[(CH_3)_3\overset{+}{S}]\overline{I}$
  anion. If S is a ring member,   trimethylsulfonium iodide
  specific "ium" nomenclature is $[\overline{CH_2.CH_2.CH_2.CH_2.CH_2.S}]^+$
  employed to denote the heterocycle.
  $(C_2H_5)]PtCl_6$
  1-ethylhexahydrothiapyrylium chloroplatinate

Sulfonyl Halides
  $R.S(:O)_2.X$ $C_6H_5SO_2Cl$
  benzenesulfonyl chloride

Sulfoxides
  $R.S(:O).R$ $(C_2H_5)_2SO$
  diethyl sulfoxide

Sultams
  Analogous to Lactams, qv
  with $.S(:O)_2.$ replacing $.C(:O).$

Sultones
  Analogous to Lactones, qv
  with $.S(:O)_2.$ replacing $C.(:O).$

Tellinic Acids
  $R.Te(:O)OH$ C_2H_5TeOOH
  ethanetellinic acid

Tellonic Acids
  $R.Te(:O)_2OH$ $C_6H_5TeO_2OH$
  benzenetellonic acid

Tellurides (Telluro Ethers)
  $R.Te.R$ $(CH_3)_2Te$
  (di)methyl telluride
  dimethyl telluroether

Telluro Ketones
  $R.C(:Te).R$ $(CH_3)_2CTe$
  dimethyl telluroketone
  telluroacetone

Tellurols (Acid Tellurides)
  $R.TeH$ C_2H_5TeH
  ethanetellurol
  ethyl acid telluride

Tellurones
  $R.Te(:O)_2.R$ $(CH_3)_2TeO_2$
  dimethyl tellurone

Telluronium Compounds
  $[R_3\overset{+}{Te}]\overline{X}$ $[(C_2H_5)_3\overset{+}{Te}]\overline{Br}$
  where X is OH or a salt anion   triethyltelluronium bromide

Telluroxides
  $R.Te(:O).R$ $(C_2H_5)_2TeO$
  (di)ethyl telluroxide

Thetins
  $R_2\overset{+}{S}.CH_2.C(:O).\overline{O}$ $(CH_3)_2\overset{+}{S}CH_2COO^-$
  S,S-dimethylthetin

Thio Acids
  1. Thiolic $R.C(:O).SH$ CH_3COSH
  thioloacetic acid
  ethanethiolic acid
  2. Thionic $R.C(:S).OH$ CH_3CSOH
  thionoacetic acid
  ethanethionic acid
  3. Thionothiolic $R.C(:S).SH$ CH_3CSSH
  (Dithioic)   thionothioloacetic acid
  ethanedithioic acid

Thio Aldehydes
  $R.CH.S$ CH_2CHS
  thioacetaldehyde

Thiocyanates (Sulfocyanates; Rhodanates)
  $R.S.C:N$ C_6H_5SCN
Thio Ethers (see Sulfides)
Thiols (Mercaptans; Acid Sulfides; Hydrosulfides; Sulfhydryl Compounds)   phenyl thiocyanate, etc.
  $R.SH$ C_2H_5SH
  ethanethiol
  ethyl $\{$ mercaptan / acid sulfide / hydrosulfide
  sulfhydrylethane

Thiones (Thio Ketones)
  $R.C(:S).R$ CH_3CSCH_3
  propanethione
  dimethyl thioketone

Thionium Compounds (see Sulfonium Compounds)
Thioureides-Ureides (qv) with the urea oxygen replaced by sulfur.
Ureides, simplest types only (see page 460)
  acyclic $R.CO.NH.CO.NH.(H$ $CH_3CONHCONH_2$
  or CO.R)
  acetic acid ureide (acetylurea)

  cyclic $\overline{R.CO.NH.CO.NH.CO}$ $\overline{CH_2CONHCONHCO}$
  malonic acid ureide (malonylurea)

Urethans (Carbamate esters)
  $NH_2.C(:O).OR$ $NH_2COOC_2H_5$
  (ethyl) urethan
  (ethyl carbamate)

Table II—Chemical Classification of Types of Compounds in Table I

Nitrogen
  Amic Acids
  Amides
  Amidines
  Amines
  Amino Acids
  Ammonium Derivatives
  Anilic Acids
  Anilides
  Anils (Schiff Bases)
  Azides (Acyl Azides)
  Azido Compounds
  Azines
  Azo Compounds
  Azoxy Compounds
  Betaines
  Carbylamines
  Cyanates
  Cyanides
  Cyanohydrins
  Diazo Compounds
  Diazoamino Compounds
  Diazonium Compounds
  Guanidino Compounds
  Hydrazides
  Hydrazines
  Hydrazones
  Hydrosulfamines
  Hydroxamic Acids
  Imides (Carboximides)
  Imidic Acids
  Imines
  Isocyanates
  Isocyanide Dichlorides
  Isocyanides
  Isonitriles
  Isothiocyanates
  Lactams
  Lactims
  Morpholides
  Nitrate Esters
  Nitriles
  Nitrite Esters
  Nitro Compounds
  Nitrolic Acids
  Nitroso Compounds
  Nitrosolic Acids
  Osazones
  Oximes
  Peptides
  Piperidides
  Polyborane Derivatives
  Quaternary Ammonium Compounds
  Selenocyanates
  Semicarbazones
  Sulfamic Acids
  Sulfenamides
  Sulfimides
  Sulfonamides
  Sultams
  Thiocyanates (Sulfocyanates; Rhodanates)
  Thioureides
  Ureides
  Urethans (Carbamate Esters)
Phosphorus
  Fluorophosphates
  Glycerophosphates
  Hypophosphite Esters
  Phosphate Esters
  Phosphine Imides
  Phosphine Oxides
  Phosphines
  Phosphinic Acids
  Phosphinic Halides
  Phosphinous Acids

Phosphinous Halides
Phosphite Esters
Phospho Compounds
Phosphonic Acids
Phosphonic Dihalides
Phosphonium Compounds
Phosphonous Acids
Phosphonous Dihalides
Phosphorofluoridates
Phosphoroso Compounds
Phosphorus Compounds (General)
Arsenic
  Arsenoso Compounds
  Arsine Oxides
  Arsines
  Arsinic Acids
  Arsinous Acids
  Arso Compounds
  Arsonic Acids
  Arsonium Compounds
  Arsonous Acids
Antimony
  Stibine Oxides
  Stibines
  Stibinic Acids
  Stibinous Acids
  Stibo Compounds
  Stibonic Acids
  Stibonium Compounds
  Stibonous Acids
  Stiboso Compounds
Oxygen
  Acetals
  Acid Anhydrides
  Acids (Carboxylic)
  Acyloins
  Alcoholates
  Alcohols
  Aldehydes
  Alkoxides
  Benzils
  Benzoins
  Carbonate Esters
  Epoxy Compounds
  Esters (Carboxylic)
  Esters of Inorganic Oxy Acids
  Glycerides
  Glycerophosphates
  Glycols
  Hemiacetals
  Hydroxy Acids
  Ketals
  Ketenes
  Keto Acids
  Ketones
  Lactides
  Lactones
  Oxo Compounds
  Oxonium Salts
  Ozonides
  Peroxides
  Peroxy Acids
  Phenolates
  Phenols
  Phenones
  Phenoxides
  Phthaleins
  Quinones
  Salts (Metal)
Sulfur
  Hydrosulfamines
  Isothiocyanates
  Mercaptals
  Mercaptans

Table II—Continued

Mercaptides	Alkylselenium Halides
Mercaptoles	Haloalkylsilanes
Sulfamic Acids	Halohydrins
Sulfate Esters	Hydrocarbon Halides
Sulfenamides	Isocyanide Dichlorides
Sulfenic Acids	Iodonium Compounds
Sulfenyl Halides	Iodoso Compounds
Sulfides	Iodoxy Compounds
Sulfimides	Phosphinic Halides
Sulfinamides	Phosphinous Halides
Sulfinic Acids	Phosphonic Dihalides
Sulfinyl Halides	Phosphonous Dihalides
Sulfite Esters	Phosphorofluoridates
Sulfonamides	Sulfenyl Halides
Sulfones	Sulfinyl Halides
Sulfonic Acids	Sulfonyl Halides
Sulfonium Compounds	Boron
Sulfonyl Halides	Borate Esters
Sulfoxides	Borines
Sultams	Borinic Acids
Sultones	Boronic Acids
Thetins	Boron Oxides
Thio Acids	Diboranes
Thio Aldehydes	Oxoboryl Compounds
Thiocyanates	Silicon
Thio Ethers	Alkylhalosilanes
Thiols	Alkylsilanes
Thiones	Alkylsilanols
Thionium Compounds	Alkylsiloxanes
Thioureides	Haloalkylsilanes
Selenium	Silicate Esters
Alkyl Selenium Halides	Silicon Compounds (General)
Selenides	Siliconic Acids
Seleninic Acids	Silylalkanols
Seleno Acids	Metals
Selenocyanates	Alcoholates (Alkoxides)
Seleno Ketones	Mercaptides
Selenols	Organometallic (Metallo-organic Compounds)
Selenones	Phenolates (Phenoxides)
Selenonic Acids	Salts (Metal)
Selenonium Compounds	Ionic Compounds
Selenoxides	Ammonium Derivatives
Tellurium	Arsonium Compounds
Tellinic Acids	Diazonium Compounds
Tellonic Acids	Iodonium Compounds
Tellurides	Oxonium Compounds
Telluro Ketones	Phosphonium Compounds
Tellurols	Quaternary Ammonium Compounds
Tellurones	Selenonium Compounds
Telluronium Compounds	Stibonium Compounds
Telluroxides	Sulfonium Compounds
Halogens	Telluronium Compounds
Acid Halides	Thionium Compounds (see Sulfonium Compounds)
Alkylhalosilanes	

Types of Organic Compounds

A comprehensive understanding of organic chemistry would be extremely difficult were it not for the fact that the hundreds of thousands of known compounds fall conveniently into a very much smaller number of general types based on molecular structure. Similarities and differences among the physical and chemical properties of the diverse compounds thus become more apparent and understandable, and this is useful both in providing explanations for observed phenomena and in making predictions for possible applications of compounds known and compounds projected for synthesis.

Organic compounds may be classified into types in many ways, the desired intricacy of any particular scheme being dependent upon the purpose of performing the classification. Thus, for one purpose it may suffice to construct a single broad class of hydroxy compounds, while for other purposes it is desirable to subdivide this broad class into alcohols and phenols and perhaps even subdivide these further into subclasses of alcohols and phenols. It is appropriate here, for purposes of convenient reference, to list those types of compounds most commonly encountered in the systematic study of organic chemistry and to display their general (type) formulas. The types of compounds which are especially pertinent to pharmacy are treated in greater detail later in the chapter, where examples of official drugs belonging to each class are also provided.

To enhance utility as a reference tool, the listing in

Table I is alphabetical rather than by any chemical classification scheme. Prefatorily, the following explanatory notes are provided.

Unless otherwise specified, the formulas shown are for compounds containing only one of the particular functional group involved. Formulas for compounds containing more than one of the same functional group can easily be derived.

Naturally occurring classes of compounds such as carbohydrates, proteins, alkaloids, glycosides, and lipids are not treated as types of compounds in this classification. A separate, more detailed presentation of these is provided in Chapter 30.

Although a few heterocyclic types such as imines (azacyclic), anhydrides of dibasic acids (oxacyclic), lactides (dioxacyclic), etc. automatically enter into the listing, it will be observed that parent heterocycles in general (eg, thiophene, pyridine, dioxane, etc) are not included. Heterocycles represented in official drugs are listed later in the chapter.

In type formulas such as in the Table, the symbol R is conventionally employed to denote a hydrocarbon radical. Unless otherwise specified it may be aliphatic, alicyclic, or aromatic, and its valence varies to satisfy the requirements of its attachment to the rest of the molecule. The degree of saturation in R does not enter into the scheme. When a formula contains more than one R, the radicals may be either identical or different. In a few instances, it is possible that even if two monovalent R's are replaceable by a single divalent R the same type of compound is retained; eg, aliphatic ketones (R.CO.R) and cyclic ketones (R.CO).

The type formulas assume a useful broader meaning if R instead of being restricted to designate only a *hydrocarbon* radical, is permitted to (1) be a residue from a heterocycle and (2) carry substituent groups. The latter automatically extends the listing to embrace polyfunctional compounds, but it also introduces the complicating feature of order of precedence of functional groups. This matter is discussed later in the chapter.

Wherever it has been deemed appropriate in the interest of precise portrayal of structure, oxygen atoms in the type formulas are placed in parentheses as (:O). No differentiation is made between a double covalent binding (=O) and a coordinate covalent binding (→O).

Unless otherwise specified, the symbol X stands for a member of the halogen family.

In addition to the type formulas, one or more specific examples of each type of compound is also provided, showing how the formulas usually appear in somewhat condensed form and illustrating the manner in which the type names become parts of individual compound names. However, it should be remembered that, although correct, such names are not always the preferred names in modern nomenclature practice.

Table II provides a chemical classification of the types of compounds listed in Table I in terms of the heteroelements (elements other than carbon and hydrogen) they contain. Examples: amines appear in the list under nitrogen, thiols under sulfur, and thiocyanates under *both* nitrogen and sulfur. Because of its prevalence, an exception is made in the case of oxygen where the listing is restricted to types of compounds in which oxygen is the *only* heteroelement. Example: nitro compounds are listed under nitrogen but *not* under oxygen. The concluding category (Ionic Compounds) of the Table lists those types of compounds which are commonly structured as disconnected cations and anions. These types of compounds are also distributed among the preceding categories of the Table on the basis of the heteroelement characteristic of the cation. The anionic portions are, of course, of variable composition. The listings in all categories of the Table are alphabetical.

Nomenclature of Organic Compounds

In the early decades of organic chemistry, newly discovered compounds were commonly provided with names which indicated either the source or some outstanding property of the compound. Thus, marsh gas, wood alcohol, benzoic acid, cadaverine, morphine, chlorophyll, and thousands of other similar names were invented. As more and more compounds were isolated or synthesized, it became apparent, however, that some systematic manner of naming organic compounds in terms of their structure would have to be devised. Early systems of nomenclature, while adequate for the period in which they were invented, soon required modification as the number of known compounds increased. The result has been that the system (or rather the combination of systems) now in use represents an evolution spreading over several decades.

That a truly effective system of nomenclature is bound to be very complex is obvious when one reflects that it must not only discriminate, unequivocally, among the approximately three million compounds already known, but must also allow adequate provision for encompassing new compounds which are being synthesized at a rate of about 75,000 per year. Fundamentally, therefore, such discrimination means that each specific name coined through the system must account for (1) the quantitative elementary composition (molecular formula) and (2) all of the structural features for one, and only one, specific compound.

The IUPAC and CAS Systems of Nomenclature

Of the various comprehensive systems proposed and used to varying extents, the two most widely used and most thoroughly updated through revision and enlargement are those devised by the International Union of Pure and Applied Chemistry (IUPAC) and the Chemical Abstracts Service (CAS). Each of these systems represents an implementation of the rules devised by the IUPAC Commission on the Reform of the Nomenclature of Organic Chemistry, which has been actively and continuously engaged in the subject for the past four decades. The two systems are identical in most respects. The CAS system intentionally departs from that of IUPAC wherever such departure contributes to the main purpose of Chemical Abstracts, ie, indexing the world's chemical literature. Recognizing the desirability of compatibility of the two systems, however, CAS identifies each such departure and displays the alternative IUPAC treatment.

It is obviously inappropriate and space-prohibitive to include in this text a discussion of the multiplicity of details in either of these two systems. Suffice it to state that, from a structural viewpoint, each system must adequately describe for each compound the following:

Composition and configuration of the carbon skeleton.
Interruptions of the carbon skeleton by heteroatoms.
State of hydrogenation of the skeleton.
Presence and location of substituents, ie, atoms or groups of atoms (radicals) functioning in place of hydrogen.
Features of stereoisomerism.

For the reader desirous of the details of the systems, reference is made to the continuing series of reports issued by the IUPAC Commission on the Nomenclature of Organic Chemistry and to the CAS publication entitled *The Naming and Indexing of Chemical Compounds from Chemical Abstracts*. The latter, which first appeared as an introduction to the Subject Index of Vol. 56 of *Chemical Abstracts*, recently underwent very extensive revision and enlargement and was concluded by CAS in 1969. The Introduction to the Subject Index of Vol. 66 provides a useful summary treatment. Reference is also made to the American Chemical Society publication, *The Ring Index*, for a very detailed systematic presentation of closed-chain systems identified through literature up to 1964.

Three general features common to both systems deserve special comment, *viz*, the employment of trivial names, the order of precedence of functional groups, and permissive ambiguity.

Trivial Names—By a trivial name is meant one which, *per se*, does not rigidly describe a compound in terms of the absolute structure notations embodied in the system, but which has earned worldwide recognition as being specific for that compound. Acetic acid (for ethanoic acid), purine (for $7H$-imidazo[4,5-d]pyrimidine), and pregnane (for $10\beta,13\beta$-dimethyl-17β - ethyl - $9\alpha,14\alpha,5\beta,8\beta$ - perhydrocyclopenta[a]-phenanthrene)are common examples. Without allowing for the judicious employment of such trivial names, any scheme of nomenclature would be hopelessly complex and of little, if any, practical utility. On the other hand, the wholesale indiscriminate admission of trivial names to a system is equally disastrous. Arriving at a satisfactory compromise between these two extremes obviously requires detailed deliberation, and the compromise position taken by IUPAC has also been adopted by CAS, *ie*, trivial names admitted by IUPAC are also those admitted by CAS.

Precedence Order of Functional Groups—An order of precedence (priority) of functional groups is necessary in order to manage, systematically, polyfunctional compounds. As a simple example, in the absence of a systematic method, the compound CH_2-$(NH_2)CH_2CH_2OH$ could be named either as an aminopropanol or as an hydroxypropylamine. But in the order of precedence, hydroxyl is higher than amino and, since the system requires that only the function of highest priority shall be represented by the suffix part of the name, the systematic name becomes 3-amino-1-propanol. The order of precedence of functional groups is clearly prescribed (see Table I of the Introduction to the Subject Index of *Chemical Abstracts*, Vol. 66) and is identical in both the IUPAC and CAS systems.

Permissive Ambiguity—Ambiguity (lack of complete structural specificity) is permissive to the extent that it reflects structural features of a compound which either are unknown or have not yet been incorporated into the system. Prohibition of such ambiguity would disallow the cataloging of a very significant percentage of known compounds, especially among those which involve features of stereoisomerism.

Nomenclature Practice of USP and NF

Lack of adherence to the principles of systematic nomenclature, in both the commercial and academic worlds, has led to a multiplicity in the types of chemical names in actual use. It is not at all unusual to find a specific compound referred to by several different names, each of which is chemically correct. This, of course, creates a very confused state which, if it persists in the indexing literature, often renders searching via nomenclature extremely difficult and, not infrequently, impossible. It is for this reason that, wherever possible, *Chemical Abstracts* translates

an author's nonsystematic nomenclature into its CAS equivalent.

Recognizing the advantages of adhering to a standard system of nomenclature, the USP and NF a few revisions ago elected to adopt names preferred by CAS. The principle of operation is simply that either the title or one of the subtitles of an official chemical must be the currently preferred CAS name. It is well to observe that the structural relationships established on the basis of principal functional group may automatically hide relationships involving functional groups of lesser priority. Thus, for example, Amphetamine is named as a derivative of phenethylamine, whereas Hydroxyamphetamine becomes a derivative of phenol; similarly, Sulfamerazine is named as a derivative of sulfanilamide, whereas Phthalylsulfacetamide becomes a derivative of phthalanilic acid.

Chemical Syllables

In addition to whatever numbers, numerical syllables, and individual Greek and English letters are required, systematic chemical names consist of a collection of syllables each of which carries a chemical connotation of some sort. Many, such as chloro-, hydroxy-, methyl-, etc, clearly indicate specific elements or radicals, and the more important of these are included in the list of radicals in Table V.

Many others, such as andro- (Gr., man), tauro- (Latin, bull), neo- (Gr. new), and pseudo- or ψ (Greek, false), are of no chemical significance from a structural viewpoint, but are often very useful in forming the so-called trivial or common names for complex molecules such as androsterone, taurocholic acid, neoantergan, pseudoglobulin, etc, the correct chemical names for which would often be extremely cumbersome. Because of their lack of structural chemical significance, however, these will not be discussed further here.

The third group of these syllables consist of miscellaneous prefixes and suffixes and is of sufficient importance to warrant abbreviated treatment, because, like those of the first group, these have structural significance and often constitute a necessary part of systematic chemical names. A list of the more commonly encountered ones of this group is provided in Tables III and IV. Many of these have multiple meanings, and the definitions given herein represent the commonest sense in which they are used in organic chemistry. Those shown in italics are commonly used in italicized form and/or enclosed in parentheses when used in organic nomenclature. It must also be remembered that the precise meanings shown here do not always apply to trivial names. Thus, for example, the meaning of -ene or of -ylene does not apply to acetylene; similarly, the meaning of -ol does not apply to benzol. Caution must always be exercised in attempting to attach significance to the various parts of such common names.

The systematic treatment of cyclic systems utilizes a generous miscellany of syllables with specific meanings. For listings and explanations of these, consult the *Ring Index*.

Radicals in Organic Chemistry

Through the concept and utilization of radicals, a logical and very helpful classification of the huge number of organic compounds is possible. Furthermore, a knowledge of the chemical properties of the

Table III—Prefixes

a- (or *adj-*)   Abbreviation for *adjacent* (see *vic-*)

ald- (or *aldo-*)   refers to *aldehyde*, as aldoxime and aldohexose

allo-   signifies a *close* (usually isomeric) *relationship*, as allocholesterol (coprostenol) is an isomer of cholesterol

anhydro-   denotes *abstraction of water*, as anhydrohydroxyprogesterone

anti-   equivalent to *trans*, qv, in certain —C=N geometric isomers, eg, *anti*-benzaldoxime

apo-   usually signifies *formation from the compound* whose name is attached, as apomorphine may be formed (produced) from morphine

ar-   abbreviation for *aromatic*, as aryl

as-   abbreviation for *asymmetric*

bis-   used instead of di-, meaning *two*, before complex expressions, as in bis(*m*-nitrophenyl)-

cis-   refers to that *geometric isomer* in which the two groups are on the *same* side, as *cis*-butenedioic acid, $\begin{array}{l}\text{CHCOOH}\\\|\\\text{CHCOOH}\end{array}$

cyclo-   indicates a *cyclic* structure, as cyclopropane

d-   see *dextro-*

D-   signifies a *structural relationship* to D-glyceraldehyde without any reference to direction of optical rotation, as D-glucose

de- (or *des-*)   denotes *removal of something*, as hydrogen in dehydrocholic acid, and oxygen in desoxyephedrine

Δ (the capital Greek letter *delta*)   used to indicate, or focus attention on, *double bonds*, as in Δ²-butene [CH₃.CH:CH.CH₃]

dehydro-   see *de-*

desoxy-   see *de-*

dextro- [or *d-* or (+)-]   signifies *dextrorotatory* form, as *d*-glucose

dl- (or *d,l-*)   see *racemic*

E and *Z*   descriptors used to distinguish stereoisomers differing in the spatial distribution of groups about a doubly-bound atom pair. *E* signifies that the group of higher priority (by the Cahn–Ingold–Prelog sequence) on one of the atoms and the group of higher priority on the other atom are on opposite sides of the double bond. *Z* signifies that these higher priority groups are on the same side of the double bond. For further discussion, see *J. Am. Chem. Soc.*, **90**, 509 (1968). Examples:

(*E*)-3-methyl-2-pentenoic acid

(*Z*)-3-methyl-2-pentenoic acid

epi- (or *ep-*)   connotes a *difference in steric configuration*, as epicholesterol is the 3α-hydroxy epimer of cholesterol; also used to signify a bridge, as in epichlorohydrin and 1,3-epoxybutane.

epoxy-   see *epi-*

gem-   refers to *two groups attached to the same carbon atom*, as the *gem*-dimethyl grouping in 2,2-dimethylpropane and in camphor

hetero-   means *different*, or *not all the same*, as in heterocyclic

hom- (or *homo-*)   indicates a *homolog* of another compound, as homatropine

hydro- (or *hydr-*)   refers to *hydrogen*, as hexahydrobenzene and hydracrylic acid

hypo-   signifies a *lower state of oxidation* in relation to another compound, as hypoxanthine

i-   abbreviation for *inactive* (see *racemic*); sometimes used instead of iso- (qv)

iso- (rarely, *i-*)   denotes an *isomer* of another compound, as isobutane and isopropyl alcohol

ket- (or *keto-*)   refers to *ketone*, as ketoxime or ketohexose

levo [or *l-* or (−)-]   signifies *levorotatory* form, as *l*-ephedrine

L-   signifies a *structural relationship* to L-glyceraldehyde without any reference to direction of optical rotation, as L-glucose

m-   see *meta-*

meso-   signifies *optical inactivity due to internal compensation*, as mesotartaric acid

meta- (or *m-*)   indicates the *1,3- positions in benzene*, as in *m*-dihydroxybenzene

n-   abbreviation for *normal*, as *n*-butanol

N-   refers to *nitrogen*, as in *N*-methylaniline, indicating that the methyl group is attached to the nitrogen.

nor-   indicates a *relationship, usually through alkylation or isomerization*, between the compound whose name carries the prefix and the compound whose name does not. Examples: ephedrine is an *N*-methylated norephedrine; camphane is a trimethylated norcamphane; and leucine (2-amino-4-methylpentanoic acid) is an isomer of the normal form represented by norleucine (2-amino-hexanoic acid).

o-   see *ortho-*

ortho- (or *o-*)   signifies the *1,2- positions in benzene*, as in *o*-hydroxybenzoic acid

oxo-   denotes an *oxygen* atom with both bonds attached to the *same* atom as in aldehydes and ketones

oxy- (or *-oxy*)   denotes an —O— configuration, in *contrast* to an oxo- (=O) configuration, as in hydroxybenzene and ethoxyethane (ethyl ether)

p-   see *para-*

para- (or *p-*)   signifies the *1,4- positions in benzene*, as in *p*-aminobenzoic acid

per-   signifies *maximum state of substitution or addition*, as in perchloroethane, C_2Cl_6; perchloroethylene, $Cl_2C:CCl_2$; perhydrobenzene, C_6H_{12}. Sometimes used synonymously with peroxy, qv

peroxy-   indicates *presence of the peroxide grouping*, as in peroxyacetic acid, CH₃.CO.O.OH.

poly-   indicates a *union of several* identical molecules or molecular fragments, as in polymers and polysaccharides

R and *S*   notations used in the Cahn–Ingold–Prelog convention to describe configuration about an asymmetric center. The system utilizes a set of rules to establish a priority rating for the substituent

Table III—Continued

	groups around a center and the rating is then applied to the structure to describe the configuration. Unlike the D-L system, the convention does not involve comparisons with reference compounds. For further discussion, see *J. Chem. Educ.*, **41**, 116 (Mar., 1964).	*t-*	doxime see *tert-*
racemic [or dl- or i- or (±)-]	signifies *optical inactivity due to equimolecular mixture of d- and l- forms*	*tert-* (or *t-*)	abbreviation for *tertiary*, as in *tert*-butyl alcohol and *tert*-amines
s-	see *sym-*	tetrakis-	used instead of tetra, meaning *four*, before complex expressions (see bis-)
S and *R*	see *R* and *S*	*trans-* (or *anti-*)	refers to that *geometric isomer* in which the two groups are on *opposite* sides, as
sec-	abbreviation for *secondary*, as in *sec*-butyl alcohol and *sec*-amines		
sub-	denotes a *basic salt*, as in aluminum sub-acetate		$$\begin{array}{c} CHCOOH \\ \parallel \\ HOOCCH \end{array}$$ *trans*-butenedioic acid,
sym- (or *s-*)	abbreviation for *symmetrical*, as in *sym*-dichloroethane, $ClCH_2.CH_2Cl$; specifically signifies the 1,3,5 positions in benzene, as in *sym*-trinitrobenzene	tris-	used instead of tri-, meaning *three*, before complex expressions (see bis-)
		uns-	see *unsym-*
		unsym- (or *uns-*)	abbreviation for *unsymmetrical*, as in *unsym*-dichloroethane, $CH_3.CHCl_2$; specifically signifies the 1,2,4 positions in benzene, as in *unsym*-trihydroxybenzene
syn-	equivalent to *cis*, qv, in certain —C═N geometric isomers, eg, *syn*-benzal-	*v-*	see *vic-*
		vic- (or *v-* or *adj-* or *a-*)	signifies the 1,2,3 *positions in benzene* as *vic*-trimethylbenzene
		Z and *E*	see *E* and *Z*

Table IV—Suffixes

-al	indicates an *aldehyde*, as methanal, HCHO
-ane	indicates *saturated hydrocarbon or saturated heterocycle* as ethane, androstane, and furane
-ase	characteristic ending for *enzymes*, as zymase, amylase, polypeptidase, etc
-ate	characteristic ending for *salts and esters of acids* ending in -ic, as acetate, phosphate, etc
-ene	denotes *one double bond*, as ethene, butadiene, etc (see also -*ylene*)
-ine	characteristic ending for various *basic nitrogen compounds such as amines and alkaloids*, as histamine, epinephrine, morphine, etc
-ite	characteristic ending for *salts and esters of acids* ending in -ous, as phosphite, nitrite, etc
-oic	refers to the —COOH *group*, as in ethanoic, benzoic, etc, acids
-ol	characteristic ending for *alcohols, phenols, naphthols, etc*, as in ethanol, cyclohexanol, etc
-one	indicates a *ketone*, as in propanone, acetophenone, etc
-osan	generic ending for *polysaccharides*, as pentosans, hexosans, etc
-ose	characteristic *carbohydrate* ending, especially for *sugars*, as dextrose, sucrose, etc
-oside	generic ending for *glycosides*, as glucoside, rhamnoside, etc
-oyl	characteristic ending for *acyl* radicals, as ethanoyl (for acetyl), carbamoyl, etc
-yl	indicates a *radical*, especially a *univalent hydrocarbon radical*, as methyl, phenyl, etc
-ylene	signifies a *bivalent hydrocarbon radical* with the free bonds on *different* carbon atoms, as in ethylene —$[CH_2.CH_2—]$ and *o*-phenylene ; used also to indicate a *double bond* in olefin hydrocarbons, as in ethylene $[CH_2:CH_2]$
-ylidene	signifies a *bivalent hydrocarbon radical* with the free bonds on the *same* carbon atom, as in ethylidene $[CH_3.CH═]$ and benzylidene
-yne	denotes *one triple bond*, as in ethyne [CH:CH], ethynyl [CH:C—], etc

individual radicals commonly makes possible either a prediction or an explanation of the chemical properties of compounds because, in general, the chemical properties of a compound are completely or partly the combined properties of the radicals present in the molecule.

Several hundred different radicals have been recognized, named, and classified. A comprehensive list ordered by both names and formulas is periodically published as part of the annual subject index to *Chemical Abstracts*. The most recent list appears in the index for Vol. 66, p. 28I *et seq.*

For purposes of convenient reference, a list of radicals frequently encountered in pharmaceutical chemistry is provided in Table V (page 444). Classification into chemical types has been sacrificed in favor of an alphabetical arrangement. Included in the list are many inorganic radicals which are frequently present in organic combination.

Chemical Notation Systems

The complexity and cumbersomeness of modern organic chemical nomenclature has encouraged attempts to develop "shorthand expressions" variously referred to as notations, ciphers, codes, and alphamerics which, for certain purposes, would be more convenient to use than the chemical names. Several systems have been proposed,* the best known of which are those of Dyson (considered for adoption by IUPAC)[1] and Wiswesser.[2] In general, these involve assigning chemical meanings to the characters usually available on, or readily adapted to, a standard typewriter keyboard and devising rules for their use in constructing the notations. Final assessment of the over-all utility of notations has yet to be made; they are particularly appealing because their brevity (in comparison with descriptive chemical nomenclature as illustrated in Table VI, page 446) greatly increases storage efficiency in printed indexes and in machine memories. In addition, they automatically avoid the troublesome "trivial name feature" encountered in

---

* The National Academy of Sciences-National Research Council Publication No. 1150 entitled *Survey of Chemical Notation Systems* (1964) provides a comprehensive review of the history and present state of development of the various systems.

practical nomenclature. However, they are not pronounceable words and do not eliminate the need for descriptive chemical nomenclature in the written and spoken word.

Several of these notations have been found useful for retrieving compounds on a structural basis from relatively small, usually specialized files of compounds stored in digital computers in the same notations. The extent to which techniques for accomplishing such retrieval may be usefully applied to a file comprising the universe of chemical compounds is the subject of considerable interest and debate.

Special typewriters have been devised whereby structural formulas may be coded directly on punched tape and also stored in the memory of a digital computer in the form of a matrix which can be searched at any future time on an atom-by-atom basis. This technique permits retrieval of compounds on a highly intimate structural basis which need not involve either nomenclature or the above mentioned notations, but does involve computer programs. Auxiliary devices exist for regenerating the actual structural formulas of retrieved compounds either by actual printout or by display on a cathode-ray tube.

Organic Chemical Literature

The constantly accelerating rate of research and development during the last four decades has created severe literature problems, not only in the areas of basic chemistry but also in the numerous other areas of science and technology where chemical information is primarily applied rather than generated. The history of Chemical Abstracts illustrates the magnitude of this so-called "information explosion." Commencing in 1906, it required 32 years for CA to produce its first million abstracts (1938), but only 17 years for the second million (1955), 8 years for the third million (1963), and 6 years for the fourth million (1969).

Today's volume of chemical literature is so great that many libraries, some even of relatively recent construction, simply do not have enough shelf space to accommodate it and have resorted to microfilming. More important is the fact that selective retrieval of information from the literature has become an extremely arduous task. As a consequence, various industrial, academic, and governmental institutions

(several pharmaceutical firms actually pioneered the effort) have developed computerized systems of storage and retrieval of those kinds of chemical information pertinent to their interests. Participating governmental agencies include the Food and Drug Administration, National Library of Medicine, National Science Foundation, US Patent Office, National Aeronautics & Space Administration, and various elements of the Department of Defense. With support from the National Science Foundation, Chemical Abstracts Service has been engaged for several years in computerizing its extensive files and plans to process all of its information via computer by 1972. An experimental computer search system was made available in 1969 which probes connection table representations of structural formulas and furnishes Chemical Abstracts references to compounds contained in a registry numbering in excess of one million compounds and to which compounds are being added at a rate of 5000 per week. Arrangements exist whereby customers may either purchase the magnetic tapes and conduct their own searches or purchase the search service from CAS. The Institute for Scientific Information (ISI) in Philadelphia has also computerized its abstract journal, *Index Chemicus*, has put more than one million compounds in its registry, and is adding new compounds at a rate of about 150,000 per year. Computer programs are available to customers which provide the capability to search and retrieve on the basis of either structural features via the Wiswesser notation, or properties, applications, and bibliographic information.

The huge continuing flood of published literature has also severely taxed the abilities of abstracting services to keep current. The magnitude of the task is illustrated by *Chemical Abstracts* experience which shows that the approximate number of papers and patents abstracted increased from 50,000 in 1950 to 120,000 in 1959 and to 230,000 in 1968. The lag between publication of original articles and that of their abstracts has been sufficiently severe to foster the production of various so-called "current awareness tools" and specialty publications such as *Index Chemicus* and *Current Contents* of ISI and *Chemical Titles*, *Chemical-Biological Activities* (CBAC), *Polymer Science and Technology* (POST), *Basic Journal Abstracts* (BJA), and *CA Condensates* of CAS. These are also computer-based services.

Natural Sources of Organic Compounds

Many different kinds of organic compounds occur abundantly and are widely distributed in the plant and animal kingdoms. Examples include: carbohydrates (sugars, starches, and celluloses), proteins, fats and fixed oils, essential oils, alkaloids, glycosides, sterols and steroids, enzymes, vitamins, hormones, antibiotics, fruit acids, vegetable flavors and colors, toxins and antitoxins, etc. Some of these classes such as the carbohydrates and proteins have distinguishing chemical characteristics and are grouped together and treated from a chemical viewpoint in separate sections of Chapter 30, page 469. Other classes such as the vitamins and hormones do not have common chemical denominators, and the individual compounds in these classes are therefore not grouped together on a chemical basis. Instead, they are distributed through the text according to their pharmacology. Consult the general index for their locations.

Natural gas, petroleum, and bituminous coal also occur abundantly in nature, and these, too, originate from plant and animal material. Natural gas consists largely of methane and is used extensively as a fuel. Large quantities are also consumed in the manufacture of carbon blacks, eg, lampblack, which find extensive use as pigments and fillers for rubber and plastics.

Petroleum and bituminous coal are two of man's prime sources of native organic compounds.

Petroleum

Petroleum consists essentially of a mixture of hydrocarbons; the nature of the hydrocarbons, however, differs decidedly according to the source. Pennsylvania oil consists almost entirely of saturated aliphatic hydrocarbons. On the other hand, the oil from Caucasia, usually referred to as *Russian oil*, contains large quantities of cycloparaffin hydrocarbons (naphthenes). Also, in contrast to the Pennsylvania oil, the oil of California contains a considerable proportion of unsaturated hydrocarbons. A variety of aromatic hydrocarbons is also present in most petroleums. Among those usually present are benzene, toluene, and certain of the cumenes. Borneo crude oil has an unusually high content of aromatics, about 40 per cent.

The crude petroleum is separated into the marketable fractions—*petroleum benzin* (petroleum ether, ligroin), *gasoline, kerosene* (coal oil), *naphtha, lubricating oils*, etc, by fractional distillation. The distillation is carried out in wrought-iron retorts at gradually rising temperatures up to about 320°, whereby all the volatile ingredients are distilled leaving from 5 to 10% of a solid or semisolid residue. The several fractions are further purified by filtration through fuller's earth or by treatment with sulfuric acid, or both. The residue yields *petroleum jelly* (*petrolatum*) and *petroleum coke* or *asphalt*.

Owing to the enormous demand for *gasoline*, the distillation of petroleum is now carried out by the so-called "cracking process." In this process the oil is distilled in the presence of a catalyst which causes the high-molecular, high-boiling hydrocarbons to break up into smaller and lower-boiling hydrocarbons, and thereby yielding a greater proportion of gasoline. With this process about 75% gasoline is obtained against 2% or so obtained by normal distillation. The "cracking process" also causes the formation of large quantities of the unsaturated gaseous hydrocarbons such as *ethylene, propylene*, and *butylene* which are used as raw materials for the manufacture of such important chemicals as ethylene glycol, isopropyl alcohol, and butyl alcohol. Considerable quantities of ethyl alcohol are now produced from ethylene by absorbing the hydrocarbon in sulfuric acid and distilling after the addition of water. Ether is a side product in this process of making alcohol, and part of the ether consumed in this country is derived from this source.

Coal and Coal Tar

Coal is fossil fuel, which is found in the earth at various depths, and which has been formed by the decomposition of prehistoric cellulose and lignin, under the changing influences of moisture, temperature, and pressure to which it has been subjected.

Anthracite (hard) coal is used primarily as a fuel. It contains relatively much more carbon and much less hydrogen than bituminous (soft) coal. When bituminous coal is destructively distilled (distilled in the dry state without access to air), an exceedingly important group of fractions and products is obtained. The initial separation is into gas, coal tar, and coke. The gas consists principally of hydrogen and methane with relatively small quantities of unsaturated hydrocarbons, carbon monoxide, hydrogen sulfide, carbon disulfide, cyanogen, and ammonia. The last two are commonly recovered and serve as commercial sources for the manufacture of ammonium compounds and cyanides. After removal of the sulfur compounds, the residual gas mixture is marketed as a fuel and an illuminant.

Coal tar is a by-product of the coking of coal for the steel and illuminating gas industries. Some idea of the complexity of the tar is apparent from the fact that well over 200 chemical compounds have been isolated from it, and the tar serves as the commercial source of nearly 50 of these. Indeed, one of the important benefits which will accrue from the commercial development of nuclear energy is that it will permit man to conserve his fast dwindling coal supplies so that they may be used as a source of important chemicals rather than merely as a fuel.

When coal tar is subjected to fractional distillation, a number of valuable commercial products are obtained directly from it. These are termed *coal tar fractions*. The substances of value which are produced by chemical reactions, using these coal tar fractions as the starting point, are called *coal tar derivatives*. Some substances not actually existing in coal tar (but actually prepared from compounds which are present in the tar) are so frequently used in the manufacture of related synthetic products that they are known as *coal tar intermediates*. The term *coal tar product* has been loosely and indefinitely applied to any member of these groups. The first fractions obtained in the distillation of coal tar are complex mixtures in themselves and are called *light oils, middle* or *carbolic oils, heavy* or *creosote oils*, and *anthracene oils;* a nonvolatile residue called pitch remains in the still.

Each of these fractions is subjected to redistillation and the simple products are separated from each other by various chemical and physical methods. Ammonium sulfate is obtained from the aqueous portions of the distillate from coal and a small additional amount is separated from the coal tar itself. Among the fractions of the light oils are *carbon disulfide, pentane, hexane, acetonitrile, benzene, toluene, xylene, cumene*, and other hydrocarbons of the paraffin and benzene series.

From the middle oils are obtained *naphthalene, phenols*, and *cresols*. The heavy oils yield *naphthalene, dinaphthalene, methylnaphthalene, xylenol, naphthol*, and *paraffins*. The "heavy oil" finds its principal use as a timber preservative, as wood when impregnated with this material under pressure resists decay and is known as *creosoted lumber*.

The anthracene oils contain a small amount of phenol, but the main constituent, *anthracene*, is one of the most valuable of all the coal tar fractions. There are also present small amounts of *methylanthracene, phenanthrene, diphenyl, naphthalene, pyrene, retene, carbazol, pyridine, quinoline*, and *aniline*.

The coal tar industry, meaning the industry in which coal tar is used as a starting point, is one of the most important of the chemical industries. It links together the production of synthetic medicines, of artificial dyes and colors, of cosmetics, and of munitions.

Other Sources

In addition to coal, various other complex substances of organic origin yield mixtures of organic compounds when subjected to destructive distillation. Prominent among these other substances are wood, waste cereal products, and bones.

Wood yields first a mixture of gases (principally carbon monoxide, carbon dioxide, hydrogen, and methane), then the liquid wood tar, and finally the residue of charcoal. The composition and relative quantities of these products vary with the kind of wood that is used and the conditions under which the distillation is conducted.

Nothing of commercial value is separated from the gases; the mixture is commonly used as augmentative fuel to heat the wood. The wood tar may be subjected to fractional distillation to yield an aqueous liquid (*pyroligneous acid*) and a tarry liquid. The aqueous liquid contains acetic acid and other low molecular

Table V—Organic Radicals[a]

acetamido	CH_3CONH-
acetate	CH_3COO-
acetonyl	CH_3COCH_2-
acetoxy	see *acetate*
acetyl	CH_3CO-
acridinyl	$C_{13}H_8N-$
acyl	generic term signifying an acid minus its OH group or groups as *acetyl*, CH_3CO-, and *carbonyl*, $=CO$
adipoyl	$-CO(CH_2)CO-$
alanyl	$CH_3CH(NH_2)CO-$
alkoxy	generic term signifying a radical consisting of an alkyl joined to oxygen as *methoxy*, CH_3O-, and *ethoxy*, C_2H_5O-
alkyl	generic term signifying a saturated hydrocarbon radical with a valence of one as *methyl*, CH_3-, and *ethyl*, C_2H_5-
alkylamino	generic term signifying $RNH-$ wherein R is an *alkyl*
allyl	$CH_2{:}CH.CH_2-$
amide (amido)	$-CONH_2$
amidino	$H_2NC(:NH)-$
amine (amino)	$-NH_2$
aminoacetate	$H_2NCH_2.COO-$
aminobenzoate	$H_2NC_6H_4COO-$ (*o-, m-,* and *p-* isomers)
n-amyl (amyl)	see pentyl
tert-amyl	see *tert*-pentyl
anilino	C_6H_5NH-
anthryl	$C_{14}H_9-$, from anthracene
arseno	$-As{:}As-$
arsenoso	$-AsO-$
arsinico	$=As(O)OH$
arsino	$-AsH_2$
arso	$-AsO_2$
arsono	$-AsO(OH)_2$
aryl	generic term signifying an aromatic hydrocarbon radical as phenyl, [structure], *o.*tolyl [structure], etc.
auro	$Au-$
azido	$-N{=}\overset{+}{N}{=}\overset{-}{N}$
azo	$-N{:}N-$
azoxy	$-N(O)N-$
benzal	see benzylidene
benzamido	C_6H_5CONH-
benzenesulfonamido	$C_6H_5SO_2NH-$
benzenesulfonyl	$C_6H_5SO_2-$
benzhydryl	see diphenylmethyl
benzoate	C_6H_5COO-
benzoyloxy (benzoxy)	see *benzoate*
benzoyl	C_6H_5CO-
benzyl	$C_6H_5CH_2-$
benzylidene	$C_6H_5CH=$
biphenylyl	$C_6H_5C_6H_4-$ (3 isomers)
bisulfide	$-SH$; see *thiol*
bisulfate	$HOSO_2O-$ or HSO_4-
bisulfite	$HOSOO-$ or HSO_3-
borate (orthoborate)	$B{-}O-$ or BO_3-
bromo (bromide)	$Br-$
n-butyl (butyl)	$CH_2(CH_2)_3-$
sec-butyl	$CH_3CH_2CH(CH_3)-$
tert-butyl	$(CH_3)_3C-$
butyrate	$CH_3.CH_2.CH_2.COO-$
cacodyl	see *dimethylarsino*
carbamate	H_2NCOO-
carbamoyl	H_2NCO-
carbethoxy	see *ethoxycarbonyl*
carbomethoxy	see *methoxycarbonyl*
carbonyl	$=CO$
carboxyl (carboxy)	$-COOH$
cetyl	see *hexadecyl*
chloro (chloride)	$Cl-$
chloromercuri	$ClHg-$
cinnamoyl	$C_6H_5CH{:}CHCO-$
cinnamyl	$C_6H_5CH{:}CHCH_2-$
citrate	$-OOC.CH_2.C(OH)(COO-).CH_2.COO-$ or $C_6H_5O_7^{\equiv}$
cresyl	$CH_3C_6H_4O-$ (3 isomers); also used to designate *ar*-hydroxytolyls $(HO)(CH_3)C_6H_3-$
cyanato (cyanate)	$N{\equiv}C{-}O-$
cyano (cyanide)	$-CN$
cyclohexyl	$C_6H_{11}-$
cyclopentyl	C_6H_9-
cyclopropyl	C_3H_5-
n-decyl (decyl)	$CH_3(CH_2)_9-$ or $C_{10}H_{21}-$
dialkylamino	R_2N- wherein R's are *alkyls*
diazo	$-N{:}N-$ or $-N(:N)-$
diazoamino	$-N{=}N{-}NH-$
diazonium	$\overset{+}{N}(:N)-$
dimethylamino	$(CH_3)_2N-$
dimethylarsino	$(CH_3)_2As-$
diphenylmethyl	$(C_6H_5)_2CH-$
dodecyl	$CH_3(CH_2)_{11}-$
epoxy	$-O-$ oxygen united to two different atoms already united in some other way
ethenyl	see *vinyl*
ethoxy	C_2H_5O-
ethoxycarbonyl	$C_2H_5OC(O)-$
ethyl	C_2H_5-
ethylamino	C_2H_5NH-
ethylene	$-CH_2.CH_2-$
ethylenedioxy	$-OCH_2CH_2O-$
ethylidene	$CH_3.CH=$
ethylthio	CH_3CH_2S-
ethynyl	$CH{:}C-$
fluoro (fluoride)	$F-$
fluorophosphate	see *phosphorofluoridate*
formamido	$HC(:O)NH-$
formate	$HCOO-$ or CHO_2-
formyl	$-CHO$
furfuryl	$O.CH{:}CH.CH{:}C.CH_2-$ (two isomers, but used unqualified to refer specifically to the 2-form)
furfurylidene	$O.CH{:}CH.CH{:}C.CH=$ (two isomers, but used unqualified to refer specifically to the 2-form)
furyl	C_4H_3O- (2 isomers)
glucosyl	$C_6H_{11}O_5-$
glyceryl	$-CH_2.CH-.CH_2-$ or $C_3H_5{\equiv}$
glycinate	NH_2CH_2COO-
glycyl	NH_2CH_2CO-
guanidino	$H_2NC(:NH)NH-$
hexadecyl	$CH_3(CH)_{15}-$
hexamethylene	$-CH_2(CH_2)_4CH_2-$
n-heptyl (heptyl)	$CH_3(CH_2)_6-$
n-hexyl (hexyl)	$CH_3(CH_2)_5-$ or $C_6H_{13}-$
hydrazino	H_2NNH-
hydrazo	$-NH.NH-$
hydroxy (hydroxyl)	$-OH$
hydroxyamino	$HONH-$
hydroxyimino	$HON=$
hydroxymethyl (methylol)	$HOCH_2-$

Table V—Continued

Term	Definition
imide	$=NH$, as in succinimide
imino	$HN=$
indolyl	C_8H_6N- (several isomers)
iodo (iodide)	$I-$
isoamyl	see *isopentyl*
isobutyl	$(CH_3)_2.CH_2.CH_2-$
isocyanato (isocyanate)	$O=C=N-$
isocyano (isocyanide)	$-NO$
isonitrile	see *isocyano*
isopentyl	$(CH_3)_2.CH_2.CH_2.CH_2-$
isopropoxy	$(CH_3)_2CHO-$
isopropyl	$(CH_3)_2CH-$
isothiocyano (isothiocyanato, isothiocyanate)	$-NCS$
keto	see *oxo*
lactate	$CH_3.CH(OH).COO-$ or $C_3H_5O_3$-
malonyl	$-CO.CH_2.CO-$
mandelate	$C_6H_5.CH(OH).COO-$
menthyl	$C_{10}H_{19}$ (several isomers)
mercapto (mercaptan)	$-SH$; see *thiol*
mercuri	$-Hg-$
mesityl	$2,4,6-(CH_3)_3C_6H_2-$
methenyl	see *methylidyne*
methoxy	CH_3O-
methoxycarbonyl	CH_3OCO-
methoxyphenyl	$CH_3OC_6H_4-$ *o, m, p* forms
methyl	CH_3-
methylene	$CH_2=$
methylenedioxy	$-OCH_2O-$
methylidyne	$CH\equiv$
methylol	see *hydroxymethyl*
methylsulfonyl	CH_3SO_2-
methylthio	CH_3S-
morpholino	$\overline{CH_2.CH_2.O.CH_2.CH_2.N}-$
naphthyl	$C_{10}H_7-$ (from naphthalene; α and β isomers)
neopentyl	$(CH_3)_3CCH_2-$
nitramino	O_2NNH-
nitrate	$-ONO_2$
nitrile	see *cyano*
nitrilo	$\equiv N$
nitrite	$-ONO$
nitro	$-NO_2$
nitroso	$-NO$
n-nonyl (nonyl)	$CH_3(CH_2)_8-$
n-octyl (octyl)	$CH_3(CH_2)_7-$
oleate	$CH_3(CH_2)_7CH:CH(CH_2)_7COO-$ or $C_{18}H_{33}O_2-$
oxalyl	$-CO.CO-$
oxalate	$-OOC.COO-$ or $C_2O_4=$
oxo	$O=$
oxy	$-O-$ as a connective
palmitate	$CH_3(CH_2)_{14}COO-$ or $C_{16}H_{31}O_2-$
pentyl	$CH_3(CH_2)_3CH_2-$
tert-pentyl	$CH_3CH_2C(CH_3)_2-$ (1,1-dimethylpropyl)
perchlorate	O_3Cl-O-
perchloryl	O_3Cl-
peroxy	$-O-O-$
phenethyl	$C_6H_5CH_2CH_2-$
phenoxy	C_6H_5O-
phenyl	C_6H_5-
phenylene	$C_6H_4=$ (o-, m- and p-isomers)
phenylsulfonyl	see *benzenesulfonyl*
phosphate (orthophosphate)	$O=P\begin{smallmatrix}/O-\\-O-\\\backslash O-\end{smallmatrix}$ or $PO_4\equiv$
phosphino	H_2P-
phosphono	$(HO)_2OP-$
phospho	$-PO_2$
phosphoro	$-P:P-$
phosphorofluoridate	$F-P\begin{smallmatrix}O\;\;O-\\\parallel\\\;\;\;\;O-\end{smallmatrix}$
phosphoroso	$-PO$
phthalate	$o-C_6H_4(COO-)_2$
phthalidyl	$o-\overline{C_6H_4.CO.O.CH}-$
phthaloyl	$o-C_6H_4(CO-)_2$
picrate	$2,4,6-(NO_2)_3C_6H_2O-$
piperidino	$\overline{CH_2.CH_2.CH_2.CH_2.CH_2.N}-$
piperidyl	2,3 or $4-C_5H_{10}N-$
pivaloyl	$(CH_3)_3CCO-$
propenyl	$CH_3.CH:CH-$
propionate	$CH_3.CH_2.COO-$ or $C_3H_5O_2-$
propionyl	$CH_3.CH_2.CO-$
propoxy	$CH_3.CH_2.CH_2O-$
n-propyl (propyl)	$CH_3.CH_2.CH_2-$
propylene	$CH_3.CH-.CH_2-$
pteroyl	$C_{14}H_{11}N_6O_2-$
pyranyl	C_5H_5O- (3 isomers)
pyrazolidinyl	$C_3H_7N_2-$ (isomers)
pyridyl	C_5H_4N- (3 isomers)
pyrimidinyl (pyrimidyl)	$C_4H_3N_2-$ (3 isomers)
quinolyl	C_9H_6N (isomers)
salicyl	$o-C_6H_4(OH)CO-$
salicylate	$o-C_6H_4(OH)COO-$ or $C_7H_5O_3-$
silyl	$-SiH_3$
stearate	$CH_3(CH_2)_{16}COO-$ or $C_{18}H_{35}O_2-$
stibo	O_2Sb-
styryl	$C_6H_5CH:CH-$
succinate	$-OOC.CH_2.CH_2.COO-$ or $C_4H_4O_4=$
succinyl	$-OC.CH_2.CH_2.CO-$
sulfamoyl	H_2NSO_2-
sulfanilamido	$p-H_2NC_6H_4SO_2NH-$
sulfanilyl	$p-H_2NC_6H_4SO_2-$
sulfate	$-OSO_2O-$ or SO_4^-
sulfhydryl	see *thiol*
sulfide	$-S-$; characteristic of thioethers as *ethyl sulfide* (ethyl thioether), $C_2H_5-S-C_2H_5$
sulfinyl	$-SO-$
sulfite	$-OSOO-$ or $SO_3=$
sulfo	see *sulfonic acid*
sulfonamido	$-SO_2NH-$
sulfonate	$-SO_2O-$
sulfone	see *sulfonyl*
sulfonic acid	$-SO_2OH$
sulfonyl (sulfone)	$=SO_2$
sulfoxide	see *sulfinyl*
sulfuryl	see *sulfonyl*
tetradecyl	$CH_3(CH_2)_{12}CH_2-$
tetramethylene	$-CH_2(CH_2)_2CH_2-$
tartrate	$-OOC.CH(OH).CH(OH).COO-$ or $C_4H_4O_6^-$
tetrazolyl	CHN_4- (isomers)
thenyl	$C_4H_3S.CH_2-$ (2 isomers)
thiazolyl	C_3H_2NS- (3 isomers)
thienyl	C_4H_3S- (2 isomers)
thio	see *sulfide*
thiocarbonyl	$=CS$
thiocyano (thiocyanato, thiocyanate)	$-SCN$
thiol (thiolo)	$-SH$
thionyl	see *sulfinyl*
toloxy (tolyloxy)	$CH_3C_6H_4O-$ (o-, m-, and p-isomers)

Table V—Continued

tolyl	$CH_3C_6H_4$— (o-, m-, and p-isomers)	valerate	$CH_3(CH_2)_3COO$— or $C_5H_9O_2$—
tolylsulfonyl	$CH_3C_6H_4SO_2$— o, m, p forms	vinyl	$CH_2:CH$—
tosyl	= tolylsulfonyl, qv	xanthenyl	
trimethylene	—$CH_2CH_2CH_2$—	(xanthyl)	$C_{13}H_9O$—(5 isomers)
trityl	$(C_6H_5)_3C$—	xenyl	see biphenylyl
ureido	H_2NCONH—	xylyl	$(CH_3)_2C_6H_3$—(6 isomers)

a Anionic radicals have slightly different names than given here when present as ligands. Examples: acetate vs acetato; nitrite vs nitrito; thiol vs thiolo.

weight aliphatic acids along with acetone, methanol, furfural, and methylamine. It was formerly an important commercial source of methanol (hence the name *wood alcohol*), acetone, and acetic acid, but these are all manufactured today by cheaper, more efficient processes. The tarry liquid consists essentially of a mixture of aromatic hydrocarbons and phenolic compounds. A fraction containing about 50% of guaiacol and creosol along with numerous other phenols constitutes the *creosote* of commerce. The viscid residue from the wood tar is commonly called *black pitch*. Wood (or vegetable) charcoal is an important article of commerce.

Various waste cereal products such as corn cobs and oat hulls are relatively rich in pentosans and thus serve as the prime source of the commercially important aldehyde, furfural. The waste products are heated with sulfuric acid, whereby the pentosans are hydrolyzed to pentoses which then undergo dehydration. The resulting furfural is widely used in the solvent, paint and varnish, and plastics industries, and in the synthesis of furane derivatives.

Destructive distillation of bone yields a liquid (*bone oil* or *Dippel's oil*) which contains many azacyclic bases prominent among which are pyrrole, pyridine, and quinoline.

Organic Pharmaceuticals

The contrast between the drugs of today and those of yesterday is a dramatic one in several respects. Only a half-century ago, man relied almost exclusively on nature to produce the organic drugs he needed, and the contributions of pharmacy were confined largely to the preparation of extracts, tinctures, and other dosage forms of the crude drugs and to the isolation of active principles, especially alkaloids and glycosides. Synthetics began to appear at a noticeably accelerated rate in the 1920's, and this is generally attributed to the very large expansion of the American chemical industry fostered by World War I. Many observers view the advent of the sulfa drugs in the early 1930's as marking the beginning of the modern era of synthetic drugs.

The great majority of today's new basic drugs are distinct organic chemical compounds. Most of these are products of synthetic organic chemistry, although some, such as reserpine, ACTH, and most of the antibiotics, are products of natural origin. Even with drugs of the latter group, however, the chemist has played a very important role in devising processes to produce them economically not only in the large quantities required but also in a sufficient state of purity. He has also succeeded in the deliberate chemical alteration of these naturally occurring compounds and produced derivatives which are either more potent or superior in some other respect, eg, dehydrocholic acid, dihydroergotamine, fluorocorticosteroids, semisynthetic penicillins, methyltestosterone, etc.

Such molecular modification of known pharmacodynamic compounds, both natural and synthetic, constitutes one of the main kinds of research effort in the field of chemotherapy. While it is true that such effort frequently results in cluttering the market with drugs which are not superior to those being imitated, nevertheless a critical review of the results achieved over the past quarter century provides abundant evidence that the effort yields a gratifying percentage of new, highly beneficial drugs.[3] Many of the new admissions to the official compendia are of such genesis.

The tremendous successes achieved in the commercial production of antibiotics have caused chemists and microbiologists to team up and explore further the possibility of utilizing the "services" of certain organisms in the "synthesis" of organic compounds. This is especially pertinent to complex compounds which are difficultly prepared by the methods commonly described as synthetic organic. Impressive accomplishments are accumulating. For example, several delicate chemical operations such as specific dehydrogenations, hydroxylations, side-chain cleavages, etc, on various steroidal molecules can now be performed microbiologically, and research designed to produce certain alkaloids by artificial culture of appropriate fungi under carefully controlled conditions is in progress. Petroleum companies are displaying greatly increased research interest in microbial synthesis utilizing hydrocarbons as the substrate, and early results (*Chem. Eng. News*, Jan. 13, 1964) point to marked advances in fermentation technology with high potential for commercial application. The well-known usefulness of microorganisms for the selective preparation of enantiomorphs rather than racemates is also finding increasing commercial application.

Considerable initial research is also proceeding with the so-called *tissue culture techniques* whereby dispersed animal or vegetable tissues may bring about chemical synthesis from nutrient compounds contained in specially prepared substrates. As an example, pro-

Table VI—Illustrations of Notation Brevity

Descriptive name (Chemical Abstracts)	Dyson notation	Wiswesser notation
1-chloro-3-methylbutane	C_4C2Ch4	G2Y
p-aminobenzoic acid	B6CXLN4	ZR-DVQ
1-naphthalenemethanol	$B6_2CQ3$	L66J-BLQ

gesterone has been produced by cultures of cells obtained from an abnormal growth of human embryonic tissue. Such total syntheses are of especial interest in connection with highly complex compounds such as the various pituitary hormones (see page 956), which are either very difficult or impossible to synthesize by known chemical methods, and for which nature does not provide close chemical relatives which might serve as convenient precursors.

Biological methods such as the above seem destined to become considerably important in the commercial production of organic compounds, many of which will undoubtedly emerge as pharmaceuticals.

Fig. 312 portrays the trend toward the use of pure organic chemicals as official medicaments. The curve is based on actual counts of monographs contained in all issues of the USP starting with the prototype (1820) and extending through the USP XVIII (1970). The counts include both natural and synthetic compounds, and they are net; ie, the count for each revision reflects not only the new admissions to that revision but also deletions of drugs contained in the previous revision. The counts are also minimal in that different salts of a given acid (or base) are *not* considered as separate drugs except in cases where the difference is significantly reflected in therapeutic application.

A few examples of drugs (or types of drugs) of unusual significance are tabulated below the curve and identified with the USP's to which they were first admitted. Synthetics having a specific pharmaceutical flavor began to appear about 1870; they were largely of German origin and continued to be so until about 1920 when, as a result of World War I, the US chemical industry was born. The French disclosure (1935) of sulfanilamide as the therapeutic moiety of Prontosil gave unprecedented impetus to the quest for synthetics, as reflected in the change in slope of the curve, and it was during the early years of this period that the American pharmaceutical industry took a commanding lead among the world's discoverers and producers of drugs—a lead which continues to this day. A 1964 study[4] disclosed that US companies originated 61% of the 587 new single entity chemical drugs which appeared as prescription items on the domestic market during the 1941–1963 period.

Such activity is rather dramatically reflected in revisions of the official US drug compendia. The revision committees and panel specialists usually find it necessary to review and evaluate about five times as many candidate drugs to identify the roughly 20% which satisfy the criteria for admission to the compendia. The history of NF X (1955) through NF XII (1965) is particularly revealing. During this brief period, 729 articles were deleted and 803 new drugs were added, resulting in an almost complete transition in the NF population.

With the increasing rate of appearance of new and improved drugs, the average life expectancy of a synthetic drug is gradually decreasing. A logical corollary is that, with the passing of time, new admissions to the official compendia will come more into balance with deletions with the result that the slope of the curve in Fig. 312 will decrease. This can be expected to continue until the next major breakthrough in pharmaceutical research such as, perhaps, the discovery of effective chemotherapy for the treatment of viral diseases, cancer, circulatory disorders, etc.

With the increasing application of pure organic chemicals as medicinal agents, the need for simple vegetable drugs (ie, crude drugs, oils, and resins and other exudates) gradually declined. Thus, whereas nearly 70% of the single entity drugs of USP I (1830) were of this type, USP X (1926) contained only about 37% and USP XVII (1965) contained but about 10%. The only crude vegetable drugs still accorded USP status due to their therapeutic actions are Belladonna (anticholinergic), Cascara (cathartic), Digitalis (cardiotonic), Ipecac (emetic), and Opium (antiperistaltic ingredient of Paregoric).

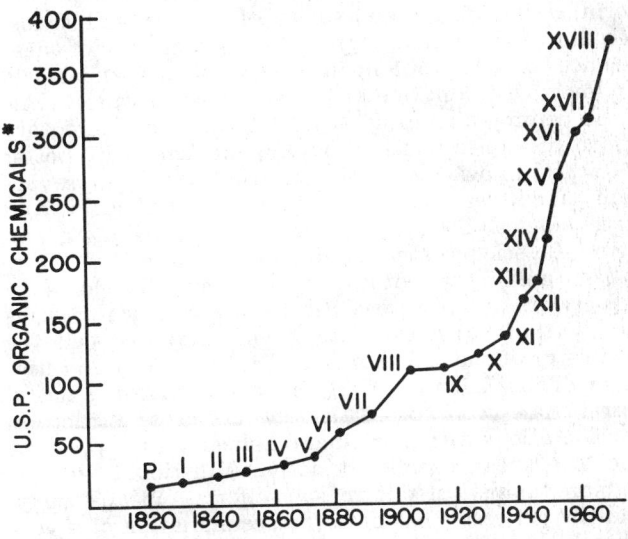

USP	Examples
I	Morphine; Quinine.
II	Strychnine.
III	Chloroform; Glycerin.
IV	Atropine; Ether.
V	Phenol.
VI	Apomorphine.
VII	Acetanilid.
VIII	Ethyl Chloride; Cocaine.
IX	Arsphenamine; Benzocaine; Phenolphthalein.
X	Aspirin; Barbituric Acids; Synthetic Hormones (Epinephrine; Thyroxin).
XI	Sulfa Drugs (Sulfanilamide; Sulfapyridine); Vitamins (Ascorbic Acid; Thiamine Hydrochloride).
XII	Estrone; Estradiol; Diethylstilbestrol; Menadione.
XIII	Penicillin Sodium; Benzalkonium Chloride; Testosterone; Thiopental; Progesterone; Digitoxin; Digoxin.
XIV	Antihistaminics (Tripelennamine; Diphenhydramine); Meperidine; Oxytocin; Folic Acid; Tubocurarine; Bishydroxycoumarin.
XV	Cortisone; Tetracycline; Desoxycorticosterone; Chlorpromazine; Methantheline Bromide; Prednisone; Reserpine; Radiopharmaceuticals.
XVI	Chlorothiazide; Morphinan Derivatives; Erythromycin; Tolbutamide; Antineoplastics; Ion-Exchange Resins; Semisynthetic Penicillins.
XVII	Griseofulvin; Spironolactone; Dexamethasone; Cyclophosphamide; Sulfinpyrazone.
XVIII	Allopurinol; Ethionamide; Idoxuridine; Penicillamine; Pralidoxime Chloride; Tolnaftate; Vinblastine; Vincristine.

Fig. 312.

* Up to USP XVI, the data for this curve were supplied by Dr. George D. Beal of Merritt Island, Florida, to whom American pharmacy is greatly indebted for many years of valuable, devoted service in broad areas of USP and NF activity involving drug development and standardization.

Dr. Beal has engaged in a comprehensive study of drugs admitted to USP's, and the countings represented on the curve were made largely from his compilation entitled *Organic Chemicals of the United States Pharmacopeia*.

Chemical and Pharmacological Classifications

During the early years of the modern era of synthetic organic pharmaceuticals, it was common practice to classify these new drugs on a chemical basis. This was logical not only because they were fundamentally the products of chemical research but also because the sciences of pharmacology and biochemistry were still in their early stages of development. Indeed, the ever-increasing need for more precise knowledge concerning the efficacy and safety of new drugs has fostered, to a significant degree, the rapid growth of these sciences to their present impressive status, and it will undoubtedly continue to do so in the future. The most comforting result is that these complementary efforts are continuously providing medicine with better tools and knowledge to the end that effective prevention and treatment of human physiological and psychological ills are constantly becoming more and more of a science and less and less of an art.

The guiding hypothesis underlying all efforts to classify organic pharmaceuticals on a chemical basis is simply that some correlation will exist between the chemistry of the compounds and their actions and uses as medicinal agents. Early efforts to discover useful correlations were based largely on gross structural considerations with particular emphasis on the presence and location of chemically active (functional) groups. In more sophisticated form, such efforts continue today, and the net result has been the accumulation of a very large body of knowledge on the broad subject of drug action. This knowledge strengthens materially the belief that the pharmacodynamics of drugs will ultimately be explicable in terms of their chemical characteristics; but it also points indisputably to the fact that a complete understanding of the mechanisms of drug actions is a long way in the future and that it will involve much more information than presently can be visualized from structural formulas and molecular models.

It is not the purpose of this chapter either to review the past accomplishments or to describe the present state of the pharmacological and biochemical sciences. Pertinent topics from these sciences are discussed in following chapters in which important drugs are presented on a pharmacologic basis. For more detailed discussion, other treatises constructed primarily to serve the above-mentioned purposes must be consulted. Further treatment in this chapter will of necessity be limited to some general observations.

It has become clear that the pharmacological actions of drugs must be viewed as functions of the *total* molecules. For example, all barbituric acids contain the malonylurea fragment, but the relative actions of the different barbiturates vary widely with respect to quantitativeness, onset time, and duration, depending upon substituents at the 1, 3, and 5 positions (see page 1078). The official sulfa drugs provide another example. The antibacterial portion common to all sulfas is the parent compound sulfanilamide, but chemical alterations at the N^1 and N^4 positions produce derivatives which differ importantly in their actions and chemotherapeutic applications.

Dependence of pharmacological activity on *total* molecular structure is commonly evident with drugs which are polyfunctional from a chemical viewpoint. The sulfa drugs provide a good example of this also; elimination of either the amino or sulfonamido portions, or even a change in their relative positions, results in loss of bacteriostatic activity. Similarly, aspirin loses its analgetic action if either its carboxyl or acetoxy group is completely removed or if the relation of these groups is other than *ortho*.

Similar dependence is common in the area of stereochemistry. Thus, the *trans* form of diethylstilbestrol is estrogenically potent whereas the *cis* form is not. This is reminiscent of the α and β forms of estradiol, the latter being about ten times as potent as the former. As an example involving diastereoisomers, one might cite the widely different mydriatic and pressor potencies of ephedrine and pseudoephedrine. Similar differences in physiological activity are also commonly observed between enantiomorphs. Thus, the D and L ephedrines differ markedly in mydriatic and pressor potencies; the D forms of the α-aminoacids are vastly inferior to the L forms as nutrients; and (−)-epinephrine is more than 20 times as potent a sympathomimetic as the (+)-form.

It must be clearly understood that the examples cited above are not isolated cases. Quite to the contrary, such experience is common in the broad field of drug action, and, as mentioned earlier, the search for useful drugs often consists of intentionally varying the molecular structure around a portion known to be important with respect to physiological activity. Such, for example, has been the continuing state of research effort with derivatives containing the cyclopentaphenanthrene (steroid) nucleus.

When one reflects on the large number of industrial and institutional laboratories engaged in some aspect of biochemical or pharmacological research, it is not surprising that numerous molecular patterns of possible drug action have been catalogued, and these often constitute integral parts of screening programs for testing new synthetics for possible therapeutic utility. These patterns are of varying degrees of firmness, many being hardly more than speculations, while others are quite well established. Some, such as with the barbiturates and sulfas cited previously, involve molecular fragments which impart specified types of actions. Others involve structural alterations designed to enhance an existing therapeutic utility by increasing potency, decreasing toxicity, eliminating undesirable side-reactions, and by advantageously changing onset and duration times of action. Relatively simple chemical alterations such as halogenation, esterification, etherification, sulfonation, hydrogenation, dehydrogenation, alkylation, acylation, etc, often produce derivatives which are superior drugs in comparison to their parent compounds. However, the effects of any one operation are often very variable from one class of parent compounds to another; thus, extrapolations from experiences with one type of drug to expectations with other types are extremely hazardous.

In an attempt to obtain more useful information relating chemical structure and physiological activity, numerous investigations have been conducted in which correlations were sought between activity and measured physical and chemical properties such as dissociation constants, distribution coefficients, spectral characteristics, dipole moments, resonance energy, oxidation-reduction potentials, etc. These endeavors have disclosed some interesting correlations but, in general, like the relations between activity and structure, they are firm only for limited series of closely related compounds.

The interesting concept of *isosterism* has also developed from these efforts. *Isosteres* may be defined as compounds having identical (or very similar) sizes, shapes, molecular weights, and distributions of electrons. Theory holds that such strong similarity should bring about similarities in physiological activity, and such similarities have been demonstrated with many pairs of compounds. It has been suggested, for example, that the estrogenic activity of diethylstilbestrol and certain other nonsteroidal synthetic estrogens (see page 992) is the result of isosteric resemblance to the natural estrogen β-estradiol.

Of possibly even greater importance has been the observation that isosteres are frequently biologically antagonistic. The broad hypothesis that knowledge concerning such antagonism can lead to the discovery of drugs which will be useful because of their effects on metabolic and hormonal processes is currently finding considerable pursuit in pharmaceutical research. Impressive success has been achieved in the field of anovulatory (fertility control) agents and to a lesser extent in the field of antineoplastic agents.

From the preceding material, it is clear that difficulties are encountered whenever one attempts to classify organic drugs on a chemical basis and obtain a system which simultaneously separates these drugs on a pharmacologic basis. As will be seen in subsequent parts of this text, drugs which fall into the same chemical category often display, collectively, quite a number of different actions; and conversely, drugs of widely different chemical characteristics frequently provide the same kind of action when used as medicinal agents. Since, from a practical viewpoint, these agents are important because of the actions they provide (irrespective of their chemical composition), their monographs are presented in the subsequent chapters on a pharmacologic basis.

Chemical Classification of Official Organic Pharmaceuticals

The remainder of this chapter is devoted to a chemical classification of the official—USP and NF—organic pharmaceuticals. The different classes of compounds are presented in the same order that they are commonly encountered in a systematic study of organic chemistry. Official heterocyclic compounds are classified also on the basis of the composition of their nuclei.

Space permits only very brief mention of some of the more important characteristics of each class. The general pattern of information provided for each of the classes is as follows:

1. Further discussion, where necessary (beyond that provided in Table I, page 432), pertaining to structure and nomenclature.
2. Methods of synthesis.
3. Selected characteristic properties.
4. Examples of official compounds containing the functional group characteristic of the class.

With regard to methods of synthesis and chemical properties, it is very important to understand that the information provided is *general* in character. The size and type of hydrocarbon radical attached to a functional group and the presence of additional (identical or different) functional groups often brings about decided alterations in electron distribution within molecules; and these alterations often exert profound effects on synthesizability and reactivity.

Wherever it is deemed necessary, the examples of official compounds are divided into categories based usually on the number of *kinds* of functional groups present. The divisions commonly used are *monofunctional* (contain only *one kind* of functional group) and *polyfunctional* (contain *more than one kind* of functional group). In instances where a class embraces a large number of compounds (eg, alcohols, esters, amines, etc), the division into categories is more elaborate.

It is obvious that monofunctional compounds present no classification problem. Polyfunctional compounds do, however, because with these it is immediately apparent that rigid classification (relegating each compound to one selected chemical class) is a matter requiring arbitrary decisions on the part of the classifier with respect to which functional group shall take precedence.

The official set of rules provided in systematic organic nomenclature which prescribes such precedence is not commonly employed in reporting through the primary literatures, and this has resulted in mixed, often confusing, practices in chemical publications.

The need for decision on the basis of functional group precedence can be avoided through multiple listings of each polyfunctional according to *all* functional groups present. As a single example, Ephedrine, which is simultaneously both an alcohol and an amine, need not be labeled specifically as either, being considered instead both as a polyfunctional containing the alcohol function and as a polyfunctional containing the amine function. This procedure often serves much better the varied interests of pharmacy.

Economic limitations on space prohibit such a multiple-listing system in comprehensive works of reference. Thus, the reference of greatest importance to American and many other chemists, *Chemical Abstracts*, long ago found it necessary to establish a priority list of functional groups for the purpose of concise, useful indexing of polyfunctionals. Commonly referred to as the "Order of Precedence of Functions," this list has experienced increasing acceptance among chemists. Because of the great value of *Chemical Abstracts* as a "key to the world's chemical literature," the following brief description of its treatment of polyfunctional compounds is provided.

As to be expected, the complete list (see *Chemical Abstracts*, Vol. 66, pp. 26I–27I) is lengthy. However, arranged in order of decreasing procedence, the entries in the *Chemical Abstracts* list which serve for most cases are: *"Onium" Compounds* (compounds containing an ammonium-type organic cation such as tetramethylammonium, pyridinium, and quinolinium; other organic cations such as oxonium, phosphonium, arsonium, carbonium, etc); *Acids* (carboxylic, sulfonic, phosphonic, arsonic, sulfinic, etc); *Acid Halide; Amide; Imide; Amidine; Nitrile; Isocyanide; Aldehyde; Ketone* and *Quinone; Alcohol; Phenol; Thiol; Amine; Imine; Ether; Sulfide, Sulfoxide*, and *Sulfone*.

The general rule for applying this listing (either for cataloguing new compounds or for locating old ones already in the literature of *Chemical Abstracts*) is as follows: The preferred *chemical entry* is chosen so that the compound is treated as a member of that class of compounds characterized by the functional group appearing first in the listing. Example: Ephedrine, $C_6H_5 \cdot CH(OH) \cdot CH(CH_3) \cdot NHCH_3$, contains both the alcohol and amine functions; the former takes precedence and, therefore, the compound is treated as a derivative of benzyl alcohol rather than as a derivative of phenethylamine, thus giving as the preferred *chemical entry* Benzyl Alcohol, α-[1-(methylamino)ethyl], rather than Phenethylamine, β-hydroxy-N,α-dimethyl. *Note*—Special attention is called to the important fact that the preferred *chemical entry* is very often *not* employed by *Chemical Abstracts* as the *main entry* (the entry with which references to the literature are associated). Instead, firmly established non-chemical names (*trivial names*) are employed. Such is the case, for example, with Ephedrine used in the previous illustration.

It will be observed that the *Chemical Abstracts* list is restricted to represent functional groups which appear in chemical names either as suffixes or terminal words. Thus, such familiar functional group designations as halo (chloro, bromo, iodo), azo, nitro, arsenoso, and various others of lesser importance are not included in the list because they appear in the names of compounds as prefixes or intermediate syllables. In other words, *Chemical Abstracts* treats halo, azo, nitro, arsenoso, and these other compounds as substituted derivatives of hydrocarbons rather than as separate classes of compounds. For pharmaceutical purposes, however, it is desirable to treat these as separate classes, and they are, therefore, presented as such in the ensuing classification.

To enhance further pharmaceutical utility, the ensuing classification also provides separate treatment for various types of compounds such as Amino Acids, Hydroxy Acids, Salts, Esters, Lactones, Phthaleins, Ureides, and Metallo-Organic Compounds. Carbohydrates, Glycosides, Proteins, Alkaloids, and Steroids are also presented as separate classes.

It will be observed that although unsaturated carbon-to-carbon linkages commonly function as spots of chemical reactivity, nevertheless they play no part in functional group classification schemes. Where it becomes pertinent (eg, in the cyclic ketones and cyclic ethers), special attention is called to those instances in which the carbon or other principal atom of the functional group is in cyclic union. With the latter (noncarbon) type, cross references to the subsequent classification of official heterocycles are provided.

Wherever possible, without doing violence to the classification, the examples provided cite only that portion of the official title which denotes the part of the compound containing the functional group under discussion; eg, under the *Amines*, Amphetamine rather than Amphetamine Sulfate or Phosphate; and under the *Ketones*, Hydrocodone rather than Hydrocodone Bitartrate.

Hydrocarbons

From the standpoint of systematic organic chemistry, the hydrocarbons are the parents of all organic compounds; ie, all other organic compounds *may be looked upon* as having been derived from hydrocarbons through appropriate actual or hypothetical substitution reactions.

Fundamentally, the hydrocarbons subdivide conveniently into the two types: *acyclic* (aliphatic) and *cyclic*. The cyclic type further subdivides into *aromatic* (*benzenoid*) and *alicyclic*. Various combination types are also represented; eg, styrene is partly acyclic (the vinyl side-chain) and partly aromatic (the benzene residue).

The parent *heterocycles*—ie, furan, pyridine, nortropane, etc—may be looked upon as hydrocarbons in which the carbon closed chain is interrupted by one or more heteroatoms.

The important natural sources of hydrocarbons are petroleum, coal, and certain essential (volatile) oils of plant origin. The essential oils contain hydrocarbons of the *terpene* class and are further discussed in Chapter 30, page 502. Petroleum consists largely of a mixture of aliphatic hydrocarbons and naphthenes, although varieties from some geographic sources contain also considerable quantities of aromatic hydrocarbons. The hydrocarbons from coal are primarily aromatic; they are not present in the coal as such, but are produced by pyrolysis. Petroleum may be made to yield aromatic hydrocarbons by high-temperature catalytic dehydrogenation processes. Conversely, coal may be caused to yield aliphatic and alicyclic hydrocarbons by high-temperature, high-pressure catalytic hydrogenation.

Preparation of hydrocarbons by synthesis is often necessary if it is desirable to produce a pure individual member. Some of the general methods of synthesis involve *dehalogenation* of alkyl halides with active metals, *hydrolysis* of alkyl magnesium halides, *pyrolytic and electrolytic decarboxylation* of (elimination of CO_2 from) carboxylic acids, *aluminum chloride-catalyzed elimination* of HCl between aromatic hydrocarbons and alkyl halides, *reduction* of ketones by various methods including catalytic hydrogenation, *dehydration* of alcohols, and *removal of hydrogen halide* from halogenated hydrocarbons.

Ethylene and Cyclopropane are the only official individual hydrocarbons. Official hydrocarbon mixtures include Mineral Oil and the Petrolatums.

Halogen Derivatives

Monofunctional members contain only C, H, and one or more halogen atoms. Many are important in their own right as industrial chemicals. As a class, however, their importance resides in their ease of production and their ready susceptibility to further chemical treatment to yield other types of compounds such as alcohols, amines, nitriles, etc.

Halogen derivatives are often prepared directly from hydrocarbons through appropriate substitution or addition reactions with halogens or halogen hydracids. They are also commonly produced by reacting hydroxy compounds (alcohols and phenols) with halogen hydracids or with reactive halogen compounds such as the phosphorus and sulfur halides and oxyhalides.

Many official drugs contain a halogen function and most of these are polyfunctional. In some instances, eg, Iopanoic Acid and Tribromoethanol, the presence of the halogen is essential for the physiological action. In others, eg, Chlorobutanol, Chlorpheniramine, Chlordiazepoxide, Chlorpromazine, Dexamethasone, etc, the halogen potentiates or otherwise enhances a physiological action inherent to the nonhalogenated parent compound.

Examples of Monofunctional Halogen Derivatives—Gamma Benzene Hexachloride, Dichlorotetrafluoroethane, Halothane, Iodoform, Tetrachloroethylene.

Examples of Polyfunctional Halogen Derivatives—Brompheniramine, Chlortetracycline, Fluroxene, Hydroxyzine, Propyliodone, Tribromoethanol.

Certain other compounds, such as Halazone and Isoflurophate, also contain halogen but as part of a larger functional group.

Alcohols

Alcohols are hydroxy derivatives of hydrocarbons, with the important stipulation that the C atoms to which the OH groups are attached must be aliphatic or alicyclic in character; ie, *not* aromatic. They are *primary*, *secondary*, or *tertiary*, depending on whether the carbinol carbon atom is bonded, respectively, to two, one, or zero hydrogen atoms. They are *mono-hydric*, *dihydric*, *trihydric*, etc, according to the number of hydroxyls present. Dihydric alcohols are often termed *glycols;* eg, ethanediol is ethylene glycol.

Cyclopropanol $[\overline{CH_2 . CH_2 . CHOH}]$ is the simplest cyclic alcohol (it is automatically secondary); benzyl alcohol $[C_6H_5CH_2OH]$ is the simplest aromatic alcohol. Examples of cyclic alcohols important pharmaceutically are menthol and estradiol.

Alcohols may be produced by: saponification of esters (including hydrocarbon halides); reduction of aldehydes, ketones, and esters; and hydrolysis of the addition compounds formed between alkyl magnesium halides and aldehydes, ketones, and carboxylic esters. Individual alcohols are often manufactured commercially by special processes; eg, methanol by catalytic hydrogenation of carbon monoxide, ethanol by fermentation of carbohydrates, etc.

The most important chemical characteristic of alcohols is their behavior on oxidation. Primary alcohols yield aldehydes as their first oxidation products, whereas secondary alcohols yield ketones; tertiary alcohols undergo intramolecular degradation on oxidation due to lack of *alpha*-hydrogen. Other prominent chemical properties of alcohols include: intramolecular dehydration to yield unsaturated hydrocarbons; intermolecular dehydration to yield ethers: condensation with ammonia to yield amines, and with acids to yield esters; and reaction with active metals to form the highly reactive *alcoholates* (*alkoxides*).

Examples of Monofunctional Alcohols—Alcohol, Benzyl Alcohol, Cholesterol, Glycerin, Propylene Glycol, Sorbitol, Terpin Hydrate.

Examples of Polyfunctional Alcohols—Chlorobutanol, Ephedrine, Estradiol, Hydrocortisone, Methyltestosterone, Morphine, Polyethylene Glycols, Triethanolamine.

Also containing the alcohol function are (1) those *Hydroxy Acids*, page 453 (and their *Salts* and *Esters*) in which the OH is in aliphatic union and (2) the *Carbohydrates*, page 452.

Phenols

Like the alcohols, these are hydroxy derivatives of hydrocarbons; but in the phenols the OH groups are attached *directly* to an aromatic nucleus, eg, benzene, naphthalene, anthracene, etc. This structural difference imparts decidedly acidic properties to the phenols with the result that they form salts (*phenolates* or *phenoxides*) with strong bases, whereas alcohols do not.

By strict meaning, the term phenol refers to hydroxy derivatives of benzene (phene is an old name for benzene), but in modern usage it is a general term embracing hydroxy derivatives of other aromatic hydrocarbons as well. These latter phenols are also commonly designated by specific terms to indicate the parent hydrocarbon; eg, naphthols (hydroxy derivatives of naphthalene), phenanthrols (hydroxy derivatives of phenanthrene), etc.

Hydroxy derivatives of pyridine, quinoline, and other heterocycles of aromatic character display phenolic characteristics, but they are not usually termed phenols.

Methods frequently employed to make phenolic compounds are: saponification of aryl halides (more difficult than with alkyl halides); diazotization of primary arylamines followed by thermal decomposition of the resulting diazonium compound; and fusion of aromatic sulfonic acids with strong bases.

Phenols are readily etherified by such reagents as alkyl iodides and dialkyl sulfates, and esterified by acyl halides and acid anhydrides. They are easily oxidized, frequently proceeding through polyhydric stages to quinones. Conversion to amines is often accomplished by heating with ammonia under pressure, and to hydrocarbons by heating with zinc dust. The presence of phenolic hydroxyl facilitates further substitution of hydrogens in the aromatic ring by halogens, nitro, sulfonic acid, and other groups.

Examples of Monofunctional Phenols—Anthralin, Diethylstilbestrol, Phenol, Resorcinol, Alpha Tocopherol.

Examples of Polyfunctional Phenols—Acetaminophen, Epinephrine, Folic Acid, Levallorphan, Nalorphine, Salicylamide, Tubocurarine Chloride, Vanillin.

Pyridoxine, Bishydroxycoumarin, and Warfarin exemplify compounds which contain hydroxyl and display phenolic characteristics, but which are not, strictly speaking, phenols.

Also containing the phenol function are those *Hydroxy Acids* such as salicylic (and their *Salts* and *Esters*) in which the OH is in aromatic union.

Ethers

Ethers $[R—O—R']$ may be regarded as anhydrides of alcohols or phenols. They are *simple* if the R's are identical, as in diethyl ether; and *mixed* if the R's are different, as in ethyl methyl ether. The so-called *cyclic ethers* are an additional type having the general formula $R—\overline{O}$. These are actually heterocyclic compounds and are commonly named either as such or as *epoxy* compounds. Example: $\overline{CH_2 . CH_2 . CH_2 . CH_2 . O}$ is tetrahydrofuran or 1,4-epoxybutane.

Ethers may be conveniently prepared by reacting alkoxides or phenoxides with alkyl iodides or dialkyl sulfates; also by reacting alkyl acid sulfates with alcohols. Some ethers, eg, diethyl ether, are formed when the vapor of the corresponding alcohol is passed at high temperature over aluminum oxide.

The ether linkage is characterized by high chemical inertness, and it is often partly because of this that ethers find generous use as solvents. The linkage is split by refluxing with strong hydrogen iodide solution yielding alkyl iodide. Certain cyclic ethers, notably ethylene oxide, are highly reactive due to ring instability.

Examples of Monofunctional Ethers—Anethole, Ether, Vinyl Ether.

Examples of Polyfunctional Ethers—Benztropine, Codeine, Erythromycin, Flurothyl, Phenoxymethyl Penicillin, Phenacaine, Polyethylene Glycols, Reserpine, Sulfadimethoxine.

Examples of ethers in which the oxygen is entirely in cyclic union are provided under the oxacyclic heterocycles listed later in this chapter.

Aldehydes

Aldehydes $[R . CHO]$ are the first oxidation products of primary alcohols.

In instances where the corresponding primary alcohols are available, aldehydes are commonly prepared from them by carefully controlled oxidation. Other well-known methods include catalytic reduction of acyl chlorides and pyrolysis of calcium salts of carboxylic acids mixed with calcium formate. Individual aldehydes are often made by special processes; eg, acetaldehyde by catalytic hydration of acetylene, and benzaldehyde by the chromyl chloride oxidation of toluene. Several processes are available for formylation of aromatic rings.

Aldehydes are among the most reactive organic compounds. Many, eg, formaldehyde and acetaldehyde, are so highly reactive that they readily polymerize. All are very susceptible to oxidation (exposure to air is often sufficient), forming the corresponding acids. Thus, aldehydes readily reduce such reagents as Tollen's, Fehling's and Benedict's. Several of the characteristic reactions involve rupture of the C=O linkage. Reaction with various reducing agents thus results in the formation of primary alcohols. Similarly, HCN adds to produce α-hydroxynitriles; $NaHSO_3$ also adds mole for mole to form readily crystallizable solids; NH_3 adds to give α-hydroxyamines which usually polymerize. Condensation reactions resulting in replacement of the carbonyl oxygen atom are also characteristic. Such condensation with alcohols produces acetals; with mercaptans produces mercaptals; and with hydroxylamine, hydrazine, and semicarbazide produces respectively oximes, hydrazones, and semicarbazones. Under the influence of alkali, many aldehydes, especially the aromatics, undergo self-oxidation-reduction to produce equimolar quantities of the corresponding alcohol and acid.

Examples of Monofunctional Aldehydes—Benzaldehyde, Formaldehyde, Paraldehyde (trimer of acetaldehyde).

Examples of Polyfunctional Aldehydes—Chloral Hydrate, Nifuroxime (oxime of 5-nitro-2-furaldehyde), Pralidoxime Chloride (oxime of 2-formyl-1-methylpyridinium chloride), Streptomycin, Vanillin.

Ketones

Ketones [R.CO.R'] are the first oxidation products of secondary alcohols; thus, they are isomeric with aldehydes. In *simple* ketones the radicals are identical; in *mixed* ketones, they are different. The so-called *cyclic ketones* comprise an additional type in which the C of the =CO group is part of a cycle, thus giving them the general formula R.C=O. *Example:* cyclohexanone $CH_2(CH_2)_4CO$. Ketones in which one of the R's is a benzene residue are often called *phenones;* similarly, if a naphthalene residue, *naphthones.*

Usual methods for synthesizing ketones include: oxidation of secondary alcohols; pyrolysis of metal salts of carboxylic acids; hydrolysis of addition complexes formed between alkyl magnesium halides and acid chlorides, esters, or nitriles; and hydrolysis of β-keto acids. Aromatic ketones are synthesized smoothly through the aluminum chloride-catalyzed reaction between aromatic hydrocarbons and acid chlorides.

On reduction, ketones give rise to secondary alcohols. Due to the lack of hydrogen in the =CO group, oxidation is much more difficult than with aldehydes; moreover, it is a more drastic type of oxidation resulting in fission of the ketone molecule and conversion of its

fragments into a mixture of acids. For the same reason, ketones, unlike aldehydes, are not prone to polymerization. Ketone reactions with hydrogen cyanide, alcohols, mercaptans, hydroxylamine, hydrazine, and semicarbazide are similar to those of aldehydes (qv). Acetone, other aliphatic ketones in which one of the R's is methyl, and "cyclic" ketones having up to 8 carbon atoms yield addition products with $NaHSO_3$ as per aldehydes; but acetophenone and other aromatic ketones do not. Ammonia forms condensation products.

Examples of Monofunctional Ketones—Acetone, Anisindione, Camphor, Diphenadione, Methyl Isobutyl Ketone, Progesterone.

Examples of Polyfunctional Ketones—Betamethasone, Estrone, Griseofulvin, Hydrocodone, Methadone, Propiomazine, Testosterone, Warfarin.

Fluocinolone and Triamcinolone Acetonides are examples of acetals of the reference ketone, acetone.

Quinones

Quinones may be looked upon as oxidation products of o- or p-dihydroxy derivatives of aromatic hydrocarbons. The oxidation consists of removal of the two phenolic hydrogens, thus producing, theoretically, an aromatic peroxide which, through rearrangement, assumes the structure of an unsaturated alicyclic diketone. Quinones are derivable from various aromatic ring systems; eg, benzoquinones from benzene, naphthoquinones from naphthalene, anthraquinones from anthracene, etc.

Quinones are commonly prepared by the carefully controlled oxidation of phenols, aminophenols, or amines. They are readily reducible to dihydric phenols, and they display various other properties also characteristic of ketones, eg, formation of oximes and imines, and reaction with Grignard reagents to produce tertiary alcohols. The presence of the unsaturated alicyclic nucleus is abundantly evident through numerous addition reactions with such agents as halogens, amines, mercaptans, etc. The oxidation-reduction relation between hydroquinone and quinone is used for the convenient, potentiometric measurement of hydrogen ion concentration (see page 291).

The quinones are colored compounds, and many naturally occurring principles such as alizarin in the root of the madder plant and muscarufin in the skin of the common poisonous mushroom have been characterized as quinones or quinone derivatives. The quinonoid grouping is the characteristic chromophore of the triphenylmethane, indophenol, indamine, azine, and certain other classes of dyes.

Example of a Monofunctional Quinone—Phytonadione.

Examples of Polyfunctional Quinones—Danthron, Menadione Sodium Bisulfite.

Carbohydrates

Included in this category of compounds are the aliphatic polyhydroxy aldehydes and polyhydroxy ketones along with their condensation polymers. They are discussed and further classified in Chapter 30, page 469.

Examples of Official Items which are either carbohydrates, manufactured carbohydrate derivatives, or natural products useful because of their carbohydrate or carbohydrate derivative content—Dextrose, Cellulose, Methylcellulose, Plantago Seed, Sodium Alginate, Sucrose, Starch, Tragacanth.

Aurothioglucose, Meglumine Diatrizoate, and Sodium Glucosulfone are examples of synthetics which contain a carbohydrate (D-glucose) moiety. Carbohydrate residues are always present in glycosides (see Chapter 30) and are frequently present in antibiotics (eg, erythromycin, kanamycin, novobiocin, streptomycin, etc) and in various other biologically active substances (eg, enzymes, coenzymes, glycoproteins, vitamins, etc).

Glycosides

Glycosides are compounds formed by condensation of sugars with other organic molecules containing hydroxyl (occasionally sulfhydryl) groups. The pharmaceutically important ones are of natural origin.

Glycosides are discussed in Chapter 30.

Various crude drugs—eg, aloe, cascara, rhubarb, etc—contain glycosides as active principles. Also, various antibiotics and other biologically active substances contain carbohydrate residues in glycosidic union but are not commonly classed as glycosides.

Examples of Glycosides—Deslanoside, Digitoxin, Digoxin, Lanatoside C, Ouabain.

Carboxylic Acids

There are many types of organic acids. Those included under this heading are acids because they contain the *carboxyl* (—COOH) group, thus distinguishing them from sulfonic, phosphonic, and other types of acids. Carboxyl represents the highest oxidative state of organic carbon; further oxidation produces CO_2.

Carboxylic acids are produced readily from esters by saponification, and this method is of great practical moment since esters occur abundantly in nature. Other important methods of synthesis include: oxidation of primary alcohols and aldehydes; hydrolysis of nitriles; and hydrolysis of acyloxy magnesium halides formed by the addition of CO_2 to Grignard reagents.

The extent of ionization of carboxylic acids varies considerably depending upon the number of carboxyls and the size and type of the hydrocarbon radical. In general, however, these acids are much less dissociated than the ionically strong mineral acids such as hydrochloric, nitric, and sulfuric. Substitutions in the hydrocarbon radical often exert a pronounced effect on the ionization; for example, trichloroacetic acid and *o*-nitrobenzoic acid are much more highly ionized than their unsubstituted parent acids.

The more important chemical characteristics of acids are: reaction with bases or other alkalies to produce salts; condensation with alcohols and phenols to form esters; interaction with phosphorus halides to make acid halides; dehydration to produce acid anhydrides; and condensation with ammonia to form acid amides. The presence of carboxyl increases the chemical reactivity of certain hydrogen atoms in the hydrocarbon radical portion of the acid; this is observed especially with the α- and β-hydrogens in the aliphatics and with the *m*-hydrogens in benzene.

The acid chlorides and acid anhydrides mentioned in the previous paragraph are highly reactive chemicals. They react with water to regenerate their respective acids. They are often employed in syntheses to effect acylation; eg, they react with alcohols and phenols to produce esters, and with ammonia (or primary and secondary amines) to form acid amides (or *N*-alkylated amides). Through appropriate Grignard and Friedel-Crafts reactions, the acid halides and anhydrides also serve as starting compounds for the synthesis of ketones. Acid chlorides are readily hydrogenated catalytically to yield aldehydes; they also react readily with anhydrous salts of carboxylic acids to form acid anhydrides. There are no official monographs on either acid halides or acid anhydrides. Cantharidin, the active constituent of cantharides, is an acid anhydride, and acetyl chloride and acetic anhydride are official reagents.

The inner acid anhydrides of polyacids are actually heterocyclic compounds and are often named as such; eg, maleic anhydride, $\overline{CO.CH{:}CH.CO.O}$, is 2,5-dihydro-2,5-furandione.

Examples of Monofunctional Carboxylic Acids—Acetic, Benzoic, Nicotinic, Oleic, Undecylenic.

Examples of Polyfunctional Carboxylic Acids—Aspirin, Dehydrocholic, Halazone, the Penicillins, Phthalylsulfacetamide, Trichloroacetic. The hydroxy acids and amino acids, which are treated separately below, also belong to this general class.

Hydroxy Acids

As the name implies, these are compounds containing one or more hydroxyl groups and one or more carboxyl groups. The OH group may be alcoholic, as in lactic acid, or phenolic, as in salicylic acid. Hydroxy derivatives of acids other than carboxylic acids are not included.

Some general methods for synthesizing hydroxy acids are: saponification of halogen substituted acids; catalytic hydration of unsaturated acids; controlled oxidation of polyhydric alcohols and saccharides; hydrolysis of hydroxy nitriles; thermal decomposition of diazotized amino acids; and addition of CO_2 to phenols.

The general chemical properties of hydroxy acids are those to be expected of acids plus those of alcohols or phenols (qv). Specific dehydration reactions of interest: α-OH acids yield cyclic diesters (*cf*, lactides, page 433); β-OH acids yield unsaturated acids; γ-and δ-OH acids yield lactones (see later section in this chapter).

Examples of Hydroxy Acids (all are inherently at least bifunctional)—Aminosalicylic, Oxidized Cellulose, Citric, Lactic, Salicylic.

Lactones

Broadly, lactones are inner esters (often termed inner anhydrides) of hydroxy acids. However, for reasons of ease of formation, stability, and natural occurrence, the definition is commonly limited to include the inner esters of only the γ- and δ-hydroxy acids, and further treatment here will be confined to these.

The γ-lactones are very readily formed from their corresponding acids. Indeed, the stability of the tetrahydrofuran (C_4O) ring is so great that synthetic operations designed to yield γ-hydroxy acids (eg, saponification of the γ-halo acids) produce the lactones instead. Even in aqueous solution, the γ-hydroxy acids undergo dehydration to produce equilibrium mixtures consisting mostly of lactone. The ease of formation of the γ-lactones is further illustrated by the ease with which Δ^3-alkenecarboxylic acids rearrange to lactones under the influence of sulfuric acid. In general, the δ-lactones are producible by the same methods as the γ-lactones, except that the reaction conditions are made more drastic to provide good yields.

The important reactions of lactones are those which result in rupture of the ring structure. These are: hydrolysis by alkali to produce salts of the corresponding hydroxy acids; ammonolysis to form hydroxy amides; reaction with concentrated halogen acids to produce halogenated acids; and hydrogenation to give hydroxy aldehydes. The γ-lactones are more resistant to these reactions than their δ-analogs.

Lactones are true heterocyclic compounds and they are often named as such. For example, γ-butyro-

lactone, $\overline{CH_2CH_2CH_2CO.O}$ is 2-tetrahydrofuranone.

Examples of lactones (all are polyfunctional)—Ascorbic Acid, Bishydroxycoumarin, Deslanoside, Erythromycin, Noscapine, Ouabain, Pilocarpine, Spironolactone.

Amino Acids and Lactams

For the purpose of this classification, amino acids are carboxylic acids which contain an amino (NH_2) group attached to any carbon atom in the radical that is attached to carboxyl. The amino group may thus be attached to an aliphatic, alicyclic, or aromatic moiety; the aliphatic variety is by far the most important, and further group discussion here is directed primarily to this class.

The biologic importance of amino acids has led to the discovery of many methods for their preparation. Some of the general synthetic methods are: ammonolysis of halogen-substituted acids; interaction of halogen-substituted acids with potassium phthalimide, followed by hydrolysis; and condensation of cyanohydrins with ammonia followed by hydrolysis of the resulting amino nitriles. Amino acids containing amino in aromatic union are conveniently prepared by complete hydrogenation of the corresponding nitro compounds.

Amino acids display chemical properties characteristic of amines and carboxylic acids. Thus, for example, they may be caused to react with nitrous acid to yield hydroxy acids; also, they form typical salts and esters. Formaldehyde condenses readily with the amino group to yield analytically important N-methylene derivatives. The amino acids undergo dehydration reactions precisely analogous to those of hydroxy acids (qv); the γ- and δ-aminoacids thus give rise to lactams which also exist in the tautomeric lactim form (see page 433). Being true heterocycles, the lactams are often named as such; eg, γ-aminobutyrolactam,

$\overline{NHCH_2CH_2CH_2CO}$ is also called 2-pyrrolidinone.

Of great importance is the amphoteric nature of the amino acids; the presence of both carboxyl and amino groups permits simultaneous acidic and basic ionizations, each governed by its own dissociation constant. High pH environment favors release of proton by carboxyl; conversely, low pH favors acceptance of proton by amino. At some intermediate pH, called the *isoelectric point*, the two potentials are equal and the molecule exists only as the *zwitterion* (also called an inner salt and a dipolar ion) which, because its net electric charge is zero, will not migrate in either direction in an electrolytic cell. Illustrating with amino-

acetic acid:

$$\overset{+}{H_3}NCH_2COOH \underset{OH^-}{\overset{H^+}{\rightleftharpoons}} \overset{+}{H_3}NCH_2COO^- \underset{OH^-}{\overset{H^+}{\rightleftharpoons}} H_2NCH_2COO^-$$

| amino acid cation at pH 2.35, cation-zwitterion concentrations equal | zwitterion pH 6.1 | amino acid anion at pH 9.78, anion-zwitterion concentrations equal |

The isoelectric point is a function of the *total* structure of an amino acid; thus each acid is characterized by its own value, and this is applied in separating mixtures of amino acids. The technique is especially valuable in protein chemistry because, like amino acids, proteins also contain amino and carboxyl groups and thus exist as zwitterion complexes at their isoelectric points.

The α-amino acids are the fundamental structural units of proteins, and further treatment of them is therefore presented in the section of Chapter 30 devoted to proteins.

Examples of Amino Acids (all are inherently at least bifunctional)—Aminoacetic, Aminohippuric, Aminosalicylic, Folic, Iopanoic, Methionine.

Examples of Lactams—Methyprylon, the Penicillins

(the 2-oxoazetidine, portion of the heterosystem is a residue of a β-lactam).

Proteins

From a chemical viewpoint, the term protein is commonly employed to embrace the following substances: (1) naturally occurring condensation polymers of α-aminoacids and of derivatives of these acids; (2) naturally occurring conjugates of these polymers with other (non-protein) substances; and (3) products formed from naturally occurring proteins by hydrolytic and coagulative processes. Proteins are discussed and further classified in Chapter 30.

Examples of Official Articles Commonly Categorized as Proteins—Serum Albumin, Fibrinogen, Gelatin, Protamine, Protein Hydrolysate.

Many other official items are, or contain, proteins but are usually placed in more specific use-categories. These include *enzymes* (eg, Hyaluronidase, Pancreatin, Pepsin, and Trypsin); *some hormones* (eg, Insulin and certain of the pituitary hormones); *various biological products* (eg, antigens, antitoxins, toxins, toxoids, sera, vaccines, blood, plasma, and plasma fractions); *surgical sutures* (gut and silk); Zinc Gelatin, and the *silver protein* bacteriostat, Mild Silver Protein. Colistin (and its derivative, Sodium Colistimethate), Oxytocin, and Vasopressin are polypeptides.

Salts

The salts of carboxylic acids have the H of the —COOH replaced with a metal or with ammonium or a substituted ammonium.

The soluble metallic salts are prepared by neutralization of acids with the proper base or alkali; insoluble ones are produced from soluble salts by metathesis with other salts, eg, zinc stearate by mixing solutions of sodium stearate and zinc sulfate. The ammonium and substituted ammonium salts are commonly produced by treating the acid directly with ammonia or the appropriate amine or amine derivative.

Salts of carboxylic acids liberate their acids upon treatment with strong mineral acids. The alkali and alkaline-earth metal salts of monofunctional acids are frequently used to synthesize hydrocarbons (page 450), aldehydes (page 452), ketones (page 452), and esters (this page); the ammonium salts are often dehydrated to produce amides (page 459) and nitriles (page 459).

The following examples of official salts is confined to metal and ammonium salts of carboxylic and noncarboxylic acids. Salts of organic bases (ie, substituted ammonium salts such as Ergotamine Tartrate, Phentolamine Mesylate, Ephedrine Sulfate, etc, of which there are a great number official) are *not* included; instead, these are classified in this chapter on the more useful basis of the functional groups contained in the respective organic bases.

In many instances the metal functions merely as the carrier of the medicinally active anionic portion of the salt. In some, however, such as Ferrous Gluconate and Aluminum Subacetate, the metal is responsible for the therapeutic action.

Examples of Salts of

A. Monofunctional Carboxylic Acids—Aluminum Subacetate, Ferrous Fumarate, Magnesium Stearate, Potassium Sorbate, Sodium Acetate, Zinc Undecylenate.

B. Hydroxy Carboxylic Acids—Aluminum Aspirin, Antimony Potassium Tartrate, Calcium Aminosalicylate, Calcium Pantothenate, Magnesium Citrate, Sodium Carboxymethylcellulose.

C. Amino Carboxylic Acids—Calcium Aminosalicylate, Dihydroxyaluminum Aminoacetate, Methotrexate, Sodium Liothyronine.

D. Polyfunctional Carboxylic Acids (other than *B* and *C* above)—Chloramphenicol Sodium Succinate, Disodium Edetate, Gold Sodium Thiomalate, Sodium Dehydrocholate, Sodium Mercaptomerin, Sodium and Potassium Penicillins.

E. Noncarboxylic Acids—Calcium Cyclamate, Dexamethasone Sodium Phosphate, Menadione Sodium Bisulfite, Sodium Lauryl Sulfate, Sodium Sulfoxone, and the sulfonic acids treated in a following section of this chapter.

Metal derivatives of compounds not treated systematically as acids (eg, ureides, phthaleins, sulfimides, sulfonamides, etc) are not included in the above. Instead, they are exemplified at other places in this chapter under their more specific designations.

Esters

Esters are condensation products of acids with alcohols or phenols. The acid may be organic, as in ethyl acetate, or inorganic, as in ethyl nitrite. Esters of binary acids are commonly treated and classified under other headings; eg, those of the halogen hydracids under alkyl, alkylene, etc, halides; those of hydrosulfuric acid (H_2S) under thiols and thio ethers; etc.

Esters of organic acids occur abundantly in nature and thus are important natural sources of alcohols and acids. Two large groups of these naturally occurring esters have common names. They are the:

(1) *Fats* (and *Fixed Oils*), which are glyceryl esters of medium and high molecular weight fatty acids; and

(2) *Waxes*, which are esters of high molecular weight monohydric alcohols and high molecular weight fatty acids. Both groups are discussed in Chapter 30.

Esters are generally prepared by reacting (esterifying) the alcohol or phenol with the appropriate acid, acid anhydride, or acid chloride, the choice of reagent depending largely on the reactivity of the hydroxy compound. They are also sometimes prepared by reacting salts with alkylating agents such as alkyl halides and dialkyl sulfates.

The characteristic and most important chemical property of all esters is their ability to undergo hydrolysis (saponification) to yield their alcohol and acid components. The hydrolysis is usually conducted in the presence of acid or alkali to hasten it. Esters vary widely with respect to the readiness with which they hydrolyze. Some, such as the waxes, are quite resistant.

Esters may be reacted with Grignard reagents to yield ketones and tertiary alcohols. The β-ketonic esters, eg, ethyl acetoacetate (acetoacetic ester), $CH_3 \cdot CO \cdot CH_2COOC_2H_5$, are highly reactive and are, therefore, important in synthetic operations.

Examples of

A. Esters and Partial Esters of Inorganic Acids—Amyl Nitrite, Dexamethasone Sodium Phosphate, Echothiophate Iodide, Neostigmine Methylsulfate, Pentaerythritol Tetranitrate, Stibophen. Also *Halogen Derivatives* (page 450), *Thiols* (page 461), and *Thio Ethers* (page 461).

B. Monofunctional Esters of Carboxylic Acids—Alpha Tocopheryl Acetate, Benzyl Benzoate, Estradiol Dipropionate. Also *Fixed Oils and Fats* and *Waxes* (Chapter 30).

C. Esters of Hydroxy Acids—Atropine, Ethyl Biscoumacetate, Methylparaben, Penthienate Bromide, Polysorbate, Scopolamine.

D. Esters of Amino (NH_2) *Acids*—Benzocaine, Carbachol, Ethinamate, Meprobamate, Urethan.

E. Polyfunctional Esters of Carboxylic Acids (other than *C* and *D* above)—Acetylsalicylic Acid, Erythromycin Ethylcarbonate, Glyceryl Monostearate, Hydrocortisone Acetate, Methacholine Bromide, Methylprednisolone Sodium Succinate, Polyoxyl 40 Stearate, Propoxyphene, Reserpine.

F. Esters of Noncarboxylic Acids—Busulfan, Spironolactone.

Phthaleins

Phthaleins (page 434) are products resulting from the condensation of two molecules of a phenol with one molecule of phthalic anhydride. The primary condensation involves the *p*-hydrogen atoms in the phenol molecules and one of the oxo oxygens in the anhydride. When the phenol is polyhydric, secondary condensations may occur between the phenolic hydroxyls, eg, fluorescein. The phthaleins represent a specific class of γ-lactones.

Either the phenol or the phthalic anhydride may carry additional functional groups, usually halogens and nitro. An important sub-class, the so-called sulfonphthaleins, involves utilization of *o*-sulfobenzoic anhydride instead of phthalic anhydride. These represent a specific class of γ-sultones.

The fundamental reaction involved in the preparation of all phthaleins is thermal condensation of the appropriate anhydride with the appropriate phenol. When desired, halogen and nitro groups are introduced via the usual substitution reactions. If such substitutions are desired in the anhydride portion of the phthalein, they are effected prior to the condensation (see Sodium Sulfobromophthalein, page 1310); but if desired in the phenol portion, they are often conveniently effected after the condensation.

Phthaleins produced from unsubstituted phthalic anhydride and unsubstituted monohydric phenols are colorless; the others are usually colored. The most important property of all phthaleins is that they undergo a change in color over critical pH intervals. The change in color is referable to a shift from a benzenoid structure to a quinonoid structure during "salt" formation as illustrated below for phenol phthalein. The color changes are reversible and occur over

| colorless | pH transition interval 8.3–10.0 | red |

pH transition intervals which are narrow and which differ for different phthaleins. These properties make many of the phthaleins useful as indicators in volumetric analysis and in the colorimetric estimation of pH, and several of them are therefore official as reagents (see page 604).

Examples of Phthaleins—Phenolphthalein, Phenolsulfonphthalein, Sodium Fluorescein, Sodium Sulfobromophthalein.

Steroids

From a chemical viewpoint, the members of this class of compounds are all related through the cyclic nuclei they contain and not through any functional group common to all. Each member contains a partly or completely hydrogenated 17H-cyclopenta-[a]phenanthrene nucleus. Steroids which contain alcoholic hydroxyl as the only kind of functional group are commonly referred to as sterols.

The commercially important sterols are isolated from natural sources and the polyfunctional steroids are presently prepared by partial synthesis starting with these sterols or with other, naturally occurring polyfunctional steroids. However, total synthesis of certain polyfunctional steroids has been accomplished and is reported to be commercially feasible. Steroids are discussed further in Chapter 30.

Examples of Sterols—Cholesterol, Sitosterols. Cholecalciferol, Dihydrotachysterol, and Ergocalciferol are usually classed with the sterols even though, in these, the carbocyclic nucleus has been ruptured.

Examples of Other Steroids—Cortisone, Dehydrocholic Acid, Deslanoside, Digitoxin, Estradiol, Prednisolone, Progesterone, Testosterone.

Nitro Compounds

These are usually represented by the type formula $R.NO_2$, although the actual constitution is that of a resonance hybrid between the two forms $R.N(:O)(\rightarrow O)$ and $R.N(\rightarrow O)(:O)$. Nitro compounds must be distinguished sharply from the organic nitrites, $R.O.NO$, with which they are isomeric, and the organic nitrates, $R.O.NO_2$. The latter are often referred to

erroneously as nitro compounds; eg, glyceryl trinitrate is commonly called nitroglycerin. In contrast to nitro compounds, both the nitrites and nitrates are true esters and are thus saponifiable. Because of their ease of production and their usefulness as intermediates in syntheses, aromatic nitro compounds are more important than nitro aliphatics and alicyclics.

Aromatic hydrocarbons readily yield nitro compounds by treatment with concentrated nitric acid, usually in the presence of sulfuric acid which, through its dehydrating action, facilitates the condensation. The process is usually termed *nitration*. When necessary, the reaction atmosphere is made more strenuous through the employment of the fuming varieties of the acids. Aromatic hydrocarbon derivatives often nitrate with great ease; eg, phenol reacts readily with diluted nitric acid to yield a mixture of o- and p-nitrophenols. Until relatively recent times, all nitro compounds from aliphatic and alicyclic hydrocarbons were prepared indirectly by metathesizing the corresponding chlorohydrocarbons with silver nitrite. This process yields a mixture of nitroalkane and alkyl nitrite. Today, however, nitromethane and some other low molecular weight nitroalkanes are produced industrially by high temperature vapor phase nitration.

Complete reduction of nitro compounds results in the formation of primary amines; it can be accomplished readily in the presence of acid with reducing agents such as stannous chloride and metals. This reduction is especially useful for the preparation of aromatic amines which then serve as the starting compounds in many synthetic processes.

Reduction of nitro to amino represents the over-all change from the maximum oxidation state of organic nitrogen to the maximum reduction state. As is to be expected, there are several intermediate reduction stages which can be reached through milder, controlled reductive operations. Many such procedures have been developed. Monomolecular intermediate reduction products include the nitroso compounds, $R.N:O$, and the hydroxylamine derivatives, $R.NHOH$. Dimolecular intermediate reduction products include the azoxy, azo, and hydrazo compounds.

The presence of the strongly negative nitro group activates hydrogen atoms and substituent groups in certain positions in the nitro compounds. Thus, for example, nitrobenzene readily undergoes disproportionation under the influence of alkali to yield o- and p-nitrophenol along with other products. Similarly, the chlorine atoms in o- and p- nitrochlorobenzene are easily saponifiable, even with such a weak alkali as sodium carbonate, to yield the corresponding nitrophenols. Such potentiated activities are often used to advantage in preparative chemistry.

In the aliphatic nitro compounds, the α-hydrogens are highly activated, and explorations in this field during the last decade have led to the commercial availability of many types of compounds, some useful as solvents, others as intermediates in syntheses. As a single example, nitromethane, having three α-hydrogens, readily enters into addition with formaldehyde to yield the mono-, di-, and trimethylolnitromethanes (nitroalcohols), $CH_{3-n}(CH_2OH)_nNO_2$, which are easily reducible to the reactive methylolamines (aminoalcohols). Primary and secondary aliphatic nitro compounds, ie, RCH_2NO_2 and R_2CHNO_2, dissolve readily in alkali by virtue of tautomeric shift to the *aci*-form, $RH(or R_2)C:N(O)OH$. Lacking α-hydrogen, neither the tertiary aliphatic nor the monofunctional aromatic nitro compounds are alkali-soluble.

The nitro group is often toxiphoric and is seldom present in drugs designed to elicit systemic effects.

Examples of Nitro Compounds (all are polyfunctional) —Chloramphenicol, Nifuroxime, Nitrofurantoin, Nitromersol.

Amines

Amines may be defined as derivatives of ammonia in which one or more of the NH_3 hydrogens is replaced by a hydrocarbon radical. The radicals may be aliphatic, alicyclic, aromatic, or derived from a heterocycle. Amines are termed *primary* if they conform to the general formula RNH_2; *secondary*, if to R_2NH; and *tertiary*, if to R_3N. They are also classified according to the number of nitrogen atoms in the molecule; ie, *monamines* (eg, ethylamine, $C_2H_5NH_2$); *diamines* (eg, ethylenediamine, $NH_2CH_2CH_2NH_2$); or *triamines* (eg, diethylenetriamine or 2,2'-diaminodiethylamine, $NH_2CH_2CH_2NHCH_2CH_2NH_2$). The nitrogens in *polyamines* may be mixed primary, secondary, and tertiary in character as in 1,4-dimethyldiethylenetriamine $NH_2CH_2CH_2N(CH_3)CH_2CH_2N-HCH_3$.

The classical method of synthesizing aliphatic amines is by alkylation of ammonia with alkyl halides. However, multiple alkylation occurs, leading to a mixture of products which are often difficultly separable; hence, the method is seldom employed for practical preparation.

A variety of methods, including catalytic hydrogenation techniques, have been devised whereby nitro compounds, nitriles, amides, oximes, and certain other nitrogen compounds can be reduced to amines. Through the judicious selection of starting compounds, some of these methods afford the opportunity to produce primary, secondary, or tertiary amines as desired. For example, reduction of amides of the $RCONH_2$, $RCONHR$, and $RCONR_2$ types by means of lithium aluminum hydride gives primary, secondary, and tertiary amines, respectively. The reduction of nitro compounds to primary amines is especially important in the aromatic series because nitration is often a convenient entering chemical wedge into aromatic hydrocarbons.

Primary amines are also often produced from amides by treatment with hypohalites and by hydrolysis of *N*-alkylphthalimides, which are readily formed by reacting potassium phthalimide with alkylhalides. Secondary and tertiary amines are often produced from primary amines by suitable alkylation methods, and certain specific amines are often prepared industrially by special processes; eg, the ethanolamines from ethylene oxide and ammonia.

The most characteristic chemical property of amines is their ability to unite with acids to form salts. As in the case of NH_3, the N atoms in amines contain a lone pair of unshared electrons which renders them capable of accepting proton, thus functioning as bases. The resulting substituted ammonium salts are often referred to as "onium compounds" and represented as illustrated in the following:

$$[(CH_3)_2\overset{+}{N}H_2]\bar{C}l$$
dimethylammonium chloride

$$[(CH_3)_2\overset{+}{N}H_2]_2SO_4^{2-}$$
dimethylammonium sulfate

Onium compounds in which the charged N atom is in a cycle are frequently named by the IUPAC procedure whereby the final "e" (if any) in the name of the base is changed to "ium" and then the name of the anion is added. Thus, pyridine forms pyridinium salts, pyrrole forms pyrrolium salts, etc.

For purposes of indexing and automated storage and retrieval, it is convenient to structure and name these salts as addition compounds consisting of the amine (or other basic compound) united to the acid. Chemical Abstracts, USP, NF, and USAN treat the compounds in this fashion, whereby the two compounds above, for example, would become:

$$(CH_3)_2NH.HCl$$
dimethylamine hydrochloride

$$[(CH_3)_2NH]_2.H_2SO_4$$
dimethylamine sulfate(2:1)

In this text, all compounds of this type are structured by the former of the above procedures but named according to the latter. In some compounds which contain more than one N atom in the basic moiety, one cannot with certainty assign the positive charge to one particular N. With these, the charged structure is represented by $[Base \overset{+}{H}]_n$ Anion as in the following example:

$$[H_2NCH_2CHNH_2 \quad \overset{+}{H}]\bar{C}l$$
$$|$$
$$CH_3$$
1,2-propanediamine monohydrochloride

The reactions of typical aliphatic and aromatic amines with nitrous acid are of synthetic and analytic importance. Primary amines react, through the intermediate formation of diazonium compounds, to liberate nitrogen and form hydroxy compounds. In the case of the aliphatics, the alcohols formed are not directly related to the starting amines and other products also form; consequently, the reaction is of little synthetic value. The yield of nitrogen, however, is quantitative, and the reaction thus has significant analytical utility. The intermediate diazo compounds are of considerable importance in aromatic synthesis, convenient well-established methods being available for converting them into hydrocarbons, aryl halides, phenols, phenol ethers, nitriles, amides, carboxylic acids, and azo and hydrazo compounds.

Secondary aliphatic and aromatic amines react with nitrous acid to form yellow, difficultly soluble, *N*-nitrosamines, R.N.NO. Aliphatic tertiary amines are stable toward nitrous acid, while the aromatics undergo ring nitrosation.

Primary and secondary amines react with acid halides and acid anhydrides to produce mono and dialkylated amides, respectively. Tertiary amines are easily oxidized to the amine oxides, $R_3N \rightarrow O$, in which the lone remaining pair of N electrons is coordinated with oxygen.

Examples of

A. *Monofunctional Amines*—Amphetamine, Benzathine (in Benzathine Penicillin G), Benzphetamine, Mecamylamine, Pheniramine, Promazine, Tuaminoheptane.

B. *Amine Derivatives of Alcohols and Phenols*— Cyclopentolate, Ephedrine, Hydroxyamphetamine, Monoethanolamine, Thiamine.

C. *Amino Acids*—See page 454.

D. *Amino Acids, Esters of*—See page 455.

E. *Amino Acids, Salts of*—See page 455.

F. Amine Derivatives of Amides (with and without other functional groups)—Chlortetracycline, Dibucaine, Folic Acid, Methotrexate, Tryparsamide.

G. Amine Derivatives of Sulfonamides—Sulfacetamide, Sulfadiazine, Sulfamethoxazole, Sulfisoxazole.

H. Polyfunctional Amines (other than *B* through *G* above)—Aminophylline, Chlordiazepoxide, Cyclophosphamide, Disodium Edetate, Methadone, Methoxamine, Oxophenarsine, Quinacrine, Streptomycin.

Many heterocyclic compounds, including the alkaloids, contain $=$N— or —NH—(or —NR—) in the ring and therefore display properties of amines although they are not classified as such here. They are, however, exemplified in Table VII, page 465, on the basis of heterocyclic rings present. *Synthetic* heterocycles having nuclei of the $\overline{C.C_n.NH}$(or R) type are presented also in the following section on *Imines*.

Imines

Of the R:NH type of imine wherein R is an aliphatic or cyclic radical of the alkylidene type, the only one involved in official drugs is methyleneimine, $CH_2:NH$. However, quite a number of official drugs contain saturated or unsaturated residues from the cyclic polymethyleneimines (often referred to as cyclic imines) which may be represented by the formula $\overline{CH_2(CH_2)_nNH}$.

The simplest of these cyclic imines is ethyleneimine (aziridine), $\overline{CH_2CH_2NH}$ which, due to ring strain, is a highly reactive chemical. As the number of C atoms in the ring increases, however, this reactivity subsides. The result is that these higher members display essentially the properties of secondary amines and are, indeed, often considered as such.

These cyclic imines are true heterocyclic compounds, and they and their derivatives are often so named.

For example, tetramethyleneimine, $\overline{CH_2CH_2CH_2\text{-}CH_2NH}$ is the familiar pyrrolidine. They are readily produced by cyclization of the corresponding amino alcohols through appropriate dehydration procedures. Like the amines, qv, they add acids to form (-iminium) salts, and the imino hydrogen is readily alkylable to give *N*-alkyl derivatives which resemble chemically the tertiary amines.

Examples of Compounds Containing the Imine Function

A. Derivatives of Methyleneimine—Nitrofurantoin, Nitrofurazone.

B. Derivatives of Monocyclic Imines—Alphaprodine, Diphemanil, Eucatropine, Guanethidine, Meperidine, Pyrvinium Pamoate, Sodium Iodomethamate, Triethylenemelamine, Triprolidine.

C. Imine Derivatives Containing Fused Ring Systems—Apomorphine, Dextromethorphan, Homatropine, Sodium Indigotindisulfonate, Thiabendazole.

Note—This display is limited to *synthetic* compounds. In the case of the cyclic imine derivatives, it is further limited to those containing nuclei of the $\overline{C.C_n.NH}$ (or R) type, present as such or as part of a fused ring system. Various additional official compounds containing more complex heterocyclic nuclei could also be classed as imine derivatives, but these are presented elsewhere in more specific categories. Several naturally occurring alkaloids, also not exemplified here, have imine fragments in their molecules. Of the above, all except Diphemanil and Triethylenemelamine are polyfunctional.

Hydrazines

This term is restricted in this classification to refer only to alkyl and aryl derivatives of hydrazine. The only official representative is of the $RHN.NH_2$ type, members of which are frequently designated specifically as hydrazino compounds. Where R is aromatic, this type is usually conveniently synthesized from the corresponding diazonium chloride by reduction with sodium sulfite. Phenylhydrazine, $C_6H_5NH.NH_2$, readily undergoes condensation with aldehydes and ketones to yield hydrazones which are useful for identification purposes (page 452).

Example of a Hydrazine—Hydralazine (monofunctional).

The semicarbazones (page 460) may be looked upon as 2-carbamoyl derivatives of 1-alkylidenehydrazines.

Quaternary Ammonium Compounds

The general formula commonly given for this type of compound, $\left[R_4\overset{+}{N}\right]$ (where X = hydroxyl in the *bases* and an anion in the *salts*) is too restrictive in that it embraces only the simplest (tetraalkyl) type, eg, tetramethylammonium, compounds. The fundamental characteristic is that the N atom is attached directly to C atoms by 4 bonds, and it is obvious that this can be achieved without involving 4 alkyls. Especially important are the types in which the quaternary N is a member of a cycle such as $\left[R.CH_2\overset{+}{N}R_2\right]$, eg, dialkylpiperidinium; and $\left[R.CH:\overset{+}{N}R\right]$, eg, alkylpyridinium. The tetraalkyl types are named as substituted ammonium compounds; eg, $\left[(CH_3)_4\overset{+}{N}\right]\overline{C}l$ is tetramethylammonium chloride. The cyclic types are named to indicate the particular heterocycle; eg, $\left[CH:CH.CH:CH.CH:\overset{+}{N}.CH_3\right]\overline{I}$ is methylpyridinium iodide.

The electron configuration in quaternary ammonium compounds is similar to that in ammonium compounds; ie, the unshared pair of electrons on the N atom of a tertiary amine accepts a carbonium-type ion. The ionic character is usually emphasized by the employment of brackets and charge signs, eg, $\left[(CH_3)_4\overset{+}{N}\right]\overline{B}r$.

Quaternary ammonium *salts* form readily when tertiary amines are brought into contact with inorganic esters. The reaction is one of direct chemical union, and the esters most frequently employed are the alkyl halides and the dialkyl sulfates. Quaternary ammonium *bases* are readily formed from the corresponding halides by interaction with moist silver oxide (AgOH). The base may then be reacted with various acidic substances to prepare salts not otherwise readily producible.

Quaternary ammonium salts differ importantly from the salts of primary, secondary, and tertiary amines with respect to their reaction with bases. Whereas the amine salts liberate the amine, the quaternary ammonium salts, containing no ammonium hydrogen, cannot react similarly. Instead, an equilibrium mixture containing the quaternary base is produced. For preparative purposes, the equilibrium is shifted in favor of the quaternary base by using a halide salt and AgOH. The quaternary ammonium bases rival the fixed alkali hydroxides in extent of ionic dissociation; in addition, they readily absorb carbon dioxide, attack glass, and are crystalline, usually deliquescent solids.

A quaternary ammonium base which contains a hydrogen *beta* to the nitrogen pyrolyzes to yield an unsaturated hydrocarbon which discloses the identity of the radical containing the hydrogen. This reaction is applied in a procedure (exhaustive methylation) which is very useful in elucidating structures and other features of azacyclic compounds, especially alkaloids.

Examples of Quaternary Ammonium Compounds (Salts)

Monofunctional—Benzalkonium Chloride (mixture).

Polyfunctional—Bethanechol Chloride, Cetylpyridinium Chloride, Denatonium Benzoate, Gallamine Triethiodide, Homatropine Methylbromide, Indocyanine Green, Methylrosaniline Chloride (mixture), Neostigmine Methylsulfate, Tubocurarine Chloride.

Azo Compounds

Only the aromatic members of this R—N=N—R' class of compounds are of sufficient importance to warrant discussion here. The simplest member is azobenzene, $C_6H_5.N:N.C_6H_5$, but such monofunctional azo compounds find little commercial application. Very important, however, are derivatives of these containing one or more amino, alkylated amino, nitro, or phenolic hydroxyl groups. These comprise the so-called azo dyes, certain of which, eg, methyl orange, are also useful as indicators (see page 604).

Symmetrical (identical R's) monofunctional azo compounds are easily prepared by reducing the corresponding nitro compounds with sodium amalgam or sodium stannite. The azo dyes are prepared by diazotizing (treating the appropriate arylamine with sodium nitrite in the presence of excess hydrochloric acid) followed by coupling (condensing) the resulting diazonium compound with the appropriate amine or phenol.

Azo compounds oxidize easily with agents such as hydrogen peroxide and peroxyacetic acid to form azoxy compounds. More drastic oxidation yields nitro compounds. Under controlled reduction with zinc dust and alkali, azo compounds are convertible into hydrazo compounds. Further reduction results in fission, forming two amine molecules. The hydrazo compounds readily undergo isomerization under the influence of strong mineral acids to yield commercially important benzidine-type compounds; eg, hydrazobenzene, C_6H_5-NH.NHC$_6$H$_5$, yields p,p'-diaminobiphenyl (benzidine), $4,4'$-$H_2NC_6H_4.C_6H_4NH_2$.

Examples of Polyfunctional Azo Compounds—Amaranth, Evans Blue.

Amides

The amides are acyl derivatives of ammonia. Some authors prefer the name acid amides. Only the primary type (one acyl group, general formula: RCO-NH$_2$) are sufficiently important to warrant discussion. *N*-alkylated derivatives of primary amides (RCONHR and RCONR$_2$) are frequently encountered; eg, the *N*-phenyl derivatives (RCONHC$_6$H$_5$) comprise the anilides.

From a hydration viewpoint, the amides occupy a midposition between nitriles and ammonium salts of carboxylic acids (RCN $\xrightarrow{H_2O}$ RCONH$_2$ $\xrightarrow{H_2O}$ RCOONH$_4$). It is understandable, therefore, that amides are producible by thermal dehydration of the ammonium salts, and by controlled hydration of nitriles with

strong sulfuric acid. Amines are also prepared conveniently by the ammonolysis of carboxylic esters, acid halides, and acid anhydrides. Utilization of amines instead of ammonia in these processes results in the formation of the *N*-alkylated amides.

The most important chemical properties of the amides are the following. Heating with mineral acids causes hydration to the carboxylic acid. Alkalies also cause hydration, forming the alkali salt of the acid and liberating ammonia. Dehydration with P$_2$O$_5$ produces nitriles. Interaction with nitrous acid forms the free carboxylic acid with the liberation of nitrogen. The reaction with hypohalites constitutes an important method for the preparation of primary amines.

Examples of Monofunctional Amides—Diethyltoluamide, Niacinamide, Nikethamide, Pyrazinamide, Urea.

Examples of Polyfunctional Amides—Acetaminophen, Acetazolamide, Colchicine, Cyanocobalamin, Ergonovine, Meglumine Iothalamate, Mercaptomerin, the Penicillins, Prilocaine, Salicylanilide, Tetracycline, Tryparsamide.

The *Ureides* (page 460) are sometimes treated as amide derivatives.

Imides

The diamides of dicarboxylic acids, $R(CONH_2)_2$, are prone to lose ammonia on strong heating, resulting in the formation of imides, $\overline{R.CO.NH.CO}$. The imido hydrogen is acidic, thus the imides form well defined salts with alkalies; it is also readily substituted by chlorine and bromine, thus forming the strongly oxidizing *N*-haloimides, eg, *N*-chlorosuccinimide.

Examples of Imides—Ethosuximide, Glutethimide, Methsuximide, Phenelzine, Phensuximide.

Hydrazides

This term is commonly restricted to refer to the *mono*acyl derivatives of hydrazine; ie, compounds of the type RCO.NHNH$_2$ (eg, acetic acid hydrazide or acetohydrazide, CH$_3$CO.NHNH$_2$). Hydrazides are thus closely related to the primary amides (*mono*acyl derivatives of *ammonia*). Hydrazine derivatives containing more than one acyl group are commonly named as acylated hydrazines; eg, CH$_3$CO.NHNH.-COCH$_3$ is 1,2-diacetylhydrazine.

Hydrazides are conveniently prepared by hydrazolysis of esters, the procedure being simply to heat a mixture of the ester and 40% aqueous hydrazine hydrate. The reaction is analogous to the ammonolysis of esters to produce amides.

Hydrazides are useful for the synthesis of aromatic aldehydes. The aromatic hydrazide is first converted into a diacylated hydrazine by interaction with benzene (or toluene) sulfonyl chloride, and this is then heated with sodium carbonate in ethylene glycol.

Treatment of hydrazides with nitrous acid (often termed diazotization, *cf* primary amines, page 457) yields the relatively unstable acyl azides, R.CO.-$\overline{N.N:N}$, which find application in the synthesis of isocyanates, urethanes, and primary amines.

Examples of Hydrazides—Isoniazid, Isocarboxazid. Other compounds such as Phenylbutazone and Sulfinpyrazone may be looked upon as acylated hydrazine derivatives.

Amidines

These may be looked upon as iminoamides. The simplest members are thus $R.C(:NH).NH_2$. Substituted amidines (one or more of the N-H's replaced) are common; eg. N-methyl-N,N'-diphenylbenzamidine, $C_6H_5C(:NC_6H_5)N(CH_3)(C_6H_5)$.

One fruitful method for synthesizing amidines consists of ammonolyzing esters of imino acids (also known as imino ethers); the required esters may be obtained by causing alcohols to undergo addition to nitriles. The use of amines instead of ammonia in the above process yields N-alkylated derivatives. Amidines may be produced by several other methods. One which permits the convenient preparation of the N,N-disubstituted type consists of condensing a substituted amide with a primary amine by refluxing a PCl_3 solution of the reactants.

Unlike the amides, the amidines are strongly basic and form easily crystallizable, stable salts in which the acid adds to the amidine as in the salts derived from ammonia and amines. As is to be expected, the amidines are susceptible to hydrolysis with the ultimate formation of carboxylic acids. By means of appropriate condensation reactions, eg, with β-diketones, amidines find application in the synthesis of pyrimidine derivatives.

Examples of Polyfunctional Amidines—Hydroxystilbamidine, Phenacaine.

Guanidino Compounds

The presence of the guanidino (sometimes called guanido) group, $NH_2C(:NH)NH$—, in the amino acids creatine and arginine, and the presence of a guanidino residue in folic acid and in the purine base guanine (contained in certain nucleic acids) are indicative of the importance of the group in certain metabolic processes, and this has encouraged research interest in the guanidino series of compounds $[R.NHC:(NH)NH_2]$. One method of producing them consists of condensing the appropriate amine with 2-methyl-2-thiopseudourea whereby methanethiol is eliminated.

Examples of Guanidino Compounds—Guanethidine, Streptomycin. Phenformin is a related biguanide derivative.

Some compounds containing the *guanyl* group $[—C(:NH)NH_2]$ have been found useful as specific antimicrobials (eg, propamidine as a trypanosomicide), but these are actually amidines.

Semicarbazones

Semicarbazones $RHC(or R_2C):N.NH.CONH_2$ are condensation products of carbonyl compounds (aldehydes and ketones) with semicarbazide, $H_2NNHCONH_2$. They usually form readily (some require a few days) upon treating an alcoholic or dilute acetic acid solution of the aldehyde or ketone with a concentrated solution of semicarbazide hydrochloride, followed by the addition of solid potassium acetate.

The semicarbazones are well defined crystalline compounds. They are difficultly soluble in water, have sharp melting points, and liberate the carbonyl compound readily on proton catalyzed hydrolysis. Because of these properties, the semicarbazones find extensive application in the isolation, identification, stabilization, and purification of aldehydes and ketones.

Example of a Semicarbazone—Nitrofurazone.

Ureides

The ureides comprise a variety of compounds, the common structural characteristic of which is that they contain a urea residue attached to an acyl group. This means that they must contain the group $R.CO.NH.CO.NH$—. They are sometimes broadly defined as acylated ureas.

Acyclic ureides are relatively simple and are of two types, *viz*, the *monoureides* ($RCO.NHCONH_2$), and the *acyclic diureides* ($RCO.NHCONH.COR$).

Only the two most important types of cyclic ureides will be described. One type represents a double condensation of one molecule of a dibasic carboxylic acid with one molecule of urea. Those derived from saturated acids thus have the general formula $\overline{CH_2(CH_2)_nCO.NHCONH.CO}$ in which any or all of the H's may be R's. *Note*—these are actually *diureides* (each urea N is in acyl union). The barbituric acids belong to this class of cyclic ureides.

The other important type of cyclic ureide represents a double condensation of one molecule of a hydroxy acid and one molecule of urea. Members derived from saturated hydroxy acids thus have the general formula, $\overline{CH_2(CH_2)_nCO.NHCONH}$ (H's may be R's), and in these it will be observed that only one of the urea N's is in acyl union. Hydantoin is a ureide of this type, the hydroxy acid involved being glycolic.

On close inspection, many oxygen derivatives of diazacyclic compounds may be looked upon as cyclic ureides and, indeed, are often referred to as such in the literature. For example, $2,4,6(1H,3H,5H)$-pyrimidinetrione and its alkylated derivatives comprise the familiar barbituric acids mentioned previously. Other important examples include the imidazolidinedione derivatives allantoin and hydantoin, and the xanthine (2,6-purinedione) derivatives theophylline, theobromine, and caffeine.

Acyclic and the simpler cyclic ureides are conveniently prepared from urea by treatment with the required acid halide or anhydride. Several processes have been devised for synthesis of the substituted barbituric acid type of ureide; a common procedure is described under *Barbital*, page 1080. Many of the complex ureides such as allantoin, theophylline, uric acid, etc. are either obtained from natural sources or are produced by minor chemical alterations of related compounds of natural origin.

Ureides are weakly acidic and form well defined salts with strong bases. Weak acids (even CO_2) will reverse the reaction and liberate the free ureide. Completely N-alkylated ureides, eg. caffeine, contain no —CONH— group and, therefore, cannot form salts with bases.

Examples of Compounds Containing a Ureide Function

A. *Acyclic*—Meralluride. Chlorpropamide and Tolbutamide are acyclic ureides of sulfonic acids.

B. *Cyclic*—All barbituric acids [eg, Amobarbital, Mephobarbital, Phenobarbital, Vinbarbital] and barbiturates [eg, Sodium Pentobarbital, Sodium Thiamylal (a thioureide)]. Others include, eg, Caffeine, Diphenylhydantoin, Fluorouracil, Idoxuridine, Nitrofurantoin, Riboflavin, Theobromine, Theophylline, Thioguanine.

The Thioureides are included under *Organic Sulfur Compounds* in a later section. Carbarsone (a ureido compound but not a ureide) is included later under *Arsonic Acids*.

Urethans

This is a trivial generic name for the esters of carbamic acid, thus the general formula $H_2N.CO.OR$. Members are easily prepared by ammonolysis of the corresponding chloroformate, $RO.CO.Cl$; by alcoholysis (using the corresponding alcohol) of carbamoyl chloride, H_2NCOCl; and by condensing urea with the corresponding alcohol.

As is to be expected from their structure, the urethans display properties reminiscent of esters and amides. Thus, complete hydroxyl catalyzed hydrolysis liberates the alcohol and produces ammonia and carbonate, and reaction with nitrous acid yields the alcohol, nitrogen, and carbon dioxide.

Examples of Urethans—Bethanecol Chloride, Ethinamate, Meprobamate, Neostigmine, Physostigmine, Urethan.

Alkaloids

Alkaloids are nitrogenous principles which occur abundantly in the plant kingdom. They are practically always azacyclic and are basic in character. In pharmacy, the definition is now frequently extended so that it embraces not only the true (naturally occurring) alkaloids, but also medicinally useful derivatives formed from them by relatively slight alterations in their structures. These derivatives, eg, apomorphine, nalorphine, etc, are sometimes referred to as "synthetic alkaloids."

Alkaloids are discussed in general in the following chapter.

Heterocycles represented in official alkaloids are included in the display of heterocycles in a later section of this chapter.

Examples of Alkaloids—Atropine, Caffeine, Codeine, Ergonovine, Quinine, Reserpine, Tubocurarine.

Examples of Synthetic Alkaloids—Apomorphine, Dimethyl Tubocurarine, Ethylmorphine, Nalorphine, Rescinnamine. The completely synthetic morphinan derivatives, *viz*, Levallorphan, etc, are also included in this group by some authors.

Organic Sulfur Compounds

There are several types of official organic sulfur compounds. The thiols, thio ethers, sulfonium compounds, and thioureides are sulfur analogues of corresponding oxygen compounds. The others are distinctively sulfur compounds and do not have oxygen analogs. Treatment here must necessarily be very limited and is devoted primarily to an exposition of structural and chemical relationships and a display of official representatives of each type.

Thiols or Mercaptans—These sulfhydryl compounds are the sulfur analogs of alcohols and phenols. They may also be looked upon as acid esters (bisulfides). A general method of synthesis involves heating the corresponding bromo compound with potassium bisulfide. The thiols are weakly acidic and dissolve readily in NaOH solution, forming R.S.Na compounds (*mercaptides*, page 433), the sulfur analogues of alkoxides and phenoxides. Mild oxidizing agents such as iodine convert mercaptans into dialkyl disulfides (RS.SR), while strong oxidants such as nitric acid convert them into sulfonic acids.

Examples of Thiols—Dimercaprol, Mercaptopurine, Methimazole, Monothioglycerol, Penicillamine, Thioguanine.

Examples of Mercaptides—Aurothioglucose, Gold Sodium Thiomalate, Sodium Mercaptomerin, Sodium Thiamylal, Sodium Thiopental, Thimerosal.

Thio Ethers—These are actually the diesters of hydrosulfuric acid (H_2S) and are frequently named as such (sulfides). They are conveniently prepared from alkali mercaptides by interaction with alkali alkylsulfates. Similar to tertiary amines, thio ethers undergo addition with alkyl halides. The resulting sulfonium salts (page 435) ionize readily and react readily with AgOH to form sulfonium bases which, like the quaternary ammonium bases, rival NaOH in ionic dissociation. Under mild oxidative conditions (eg, dilute HNO_3), the alkyl sulfides give rise to sulfoxides, R_2SO; more drastic oxidation (eg, with $KMnO_4$) results in sulfones, R_2SO_2. Cyclic thio ethers are well known and are commonly named as heterocycles; eg, $\overline{CH_2CH_2\text{-}}$ $\overline{CH_2CH_2S}$ is tetrahydrothiophene or thiacyclopentane.

Examples—Bithionol, Methionine, and Thiethylperazine contain noncyclic thio ether linkages. The thiacyclics are represented under their appropriate parent heterocycles in Table VII, page 465.

Sulfonium Compounds—See the discussion of thio ethers (this page).

Examples—Azure A Dye (in Azuresin), Methylene Blue, Trimethaphan Camsylate. The sulfonium sulfur is part of a heterocycle in each instance.

Sulfones—See the discussion of thio ethers (this page).

Examples—Dapsone, Sodium Glucosulfone, Sodium Sulfoxone, Sulfinpyrazone. Each is polyfunctional. Phenolsulfonphthalein may be looked upon as a cyclic sulfone derived from 2,1(3H)-benzoxathiole, but it is more revealingly classed as a type of phthalein (see page 455). Similarly, Saccharin may be considered as a sulfone derivative of 1,2-benzisothiazole, but its properties are more evident if it is classed as a sulfimide (see later in this section).

Sulfonic Acids—It is in this type of compound, RSO_2OH, that sulfur achieves its maximum state of oxidation in organic combination. R may be aliphatic, alicyclic, or aromatic, but from the standpoint of usefulness in synthetic chemistry, the aromatic sulfonic acids are by far the most important. Sulfonic acids may be prepared by various processes. The aliphatics and alicyclics result conveniently by the oxidation of mercaptans with nitric acid. The aromatics are usually prepared by direct condensation of aromatic hydrocarbons with sulfuric acid; the process is termed *sulfonation* and is analogous to the nitration of aromatic hydrocarbons with nitric acid.

All sulfonic acids react readily with alkalies to form salts (sulfonates). The alkali metal sulfonates are usually quite soluble in water, and thus introduction of either the $-SO_3Na$ or $-SO_3K$ is often resorted to in order to solubilize otherwise insoluble organic compounds. All sulfonic acids react with PCl_5 to form the highly reactive sulfonyl chlorides, RSO_2Cl, which are widely used in the synthesis of derivatives such as the sulfonamides, sulfinic acids, and mercaptans.

The aromatic sulfonic acids often serve as the starting points in aromatic syntheses, thus resembling the halides in the aliphatic and alicyclic series. Of particular importance are their conversion into phenols by fusion with NaOH and into nitriles by dry distillation with NaCN. Nitriles find extensive application in the synthesis of carboxylic acids and primary amines.

Examples (Sulfonate Salts or Esters)—Amaranth,

Benztropine Mesylate, Busulfan, Hydroxystilbamidine Isethionate, Prochlorperazine Edisylate, Sodium Methiodal, Sodium Suramin, Stibophen.

Sulfonamides—Monofunctional sulfonamides, ie, RSO_2NH_2, are readily produced in good yield from sulfonyl chlorides by interaction with ammonia. If amines are used instead of ammonia, *N*-alkylated sulfonamides result. The sulfonamides are readily crystallizable and melt sharply; they are therefore useful for identifying sulfonic acids which commonly melt with decomposition over relatively wide temperature ranges. Sulfonamides and their *N*-monoalkyl derivatives dissolve readily in NaOH solution, forming salts of the type $RSO_2N(H$ or $R)Na$. The amido hydrogens are easily susceptible to chlorination by treatment with chlorine and alkali (or with hypochlorite) yielding the so-called sulfonchloramides, (eg, chloramine-T), which are strong oxidizing agents.

The sulfonamides found initial therapeutic application as antibacterial agents and were popularly referred to as *sulfa drugs*. Continuing research, however, has yielded other sulfonamide drugs which, collectively, elicit a variety of other therapeutic actions, eg, hypoglycemic, diuretic, antihypertensive, and uricosuric actions. The official *antibacterial* sulfonamides are characterized structurally by the presence of the *para* —$NH.C_6H_4.SO_2NH$— fragment of the parent compound, sulfanilamide.

Examples—Acetazolamide, Benzthiazide, Chlorothiazide, Furosemide, Probenecid, Sulfadiazine, Tolbutamide. Halazone is an *N*-chlorosulfonamide.

Sulfamic Acids—These are derivatives of sulfamic acid, $NH_2.SO_2.OH$, with one or both of the amido hydrogens replaced by hydrocarbon radicals. They are easily prepared by interacting chlorosulfonic acid with the appropriate amine. The hydroxylic hydrogen is strongly acidic.

Examples—Calcium and Sodium Cyclamates.

Sulfimides—These may be considered as a subclass of imides in which one of the CO groups is replaced by SO_2, thus giving the general formula $\overline{R.CO.NH.SO_2.}$ As with the imides, the imido hydrogen is acidic.

Examples—Saccharin and its calcium and sodium derivatives.

Sulfinic Acids—These bear the same relationship to sulfurous acid as the sulfonic acids do to sulfuric acid, thus giving the general formula, $R.SO(OH)$, frequently written as RSO_2H. Sulfinic acids are readily prepared by reducing the corresponding sulfonyl chlorides with zinc dust and water. They are acidic (salts are sulfinates), but decidedly less so than the sulfonic acids. They are readily susceptible to air oxidation, and they are oxidized at once by agents such as chlorine and iodine to the sulfonic state.

Examples—Sodium Sulfoxylate, Sodium Sulfoxone.

Sultams—Several compounds of this general class (page 435) have recently achieved prominence in chemotherapy. They are usually named as *S*-dioxides of the corresponding thiacyclic compounds. A popular method of synthesis effects ring closure through condensation of an appropriately substituted *o*-aminosulfonamide with formic acid (see *Chlorothiazide*, page 945).

Examples—Bendroflumethiazide, Chlorothiazide, Cyclothiazide, Hydrochlorothiazide, Polythiazide.

Thioureides—These are ureides (see page 460) in which the urea oxygen is replaced with sulfur. All of the four official members are cyclic. Two (Thiamylal and Thiopental) are diureides, more specifically thio-

barbiturates. The other two are uracil derivatives, contain only one acyl ureide linkage, and represent double condensation products of thiourea with β-hydroxyacrylic acid or its appropriate β-alkyl derivative. Like the ureides, qv, the official thioureides are acidic and form well-defined salts.

Examples—Methylthiouracil, Propylthiouracil, Sodium Thiamylal, Sodium Thiopental.

Esters of Inorganic Sulfur Acids—The thiols (bisulfides) and thio ethers have been presented earlier, and the total and partial esters of the sulfur oxyacids were included in the section on *Esters* (page 455).

Other Sulfur Compounds—Ethionamide is a thiocarbamide, Tolnaftate is an ester of an *N*-substituted thio aminoacid, and Acetohexamide may be looked upon as an *N*-substituted acyclic ureide of a sulfonic acid. Sulfur compounds which also contain phosphorus, arsenic, or antimony are included in their appropriate following sections.

Organic Phosphorus Compounds

Although there are many types of organic phosphorus compounds (a partial listing is provided in Table I), few have found application as drugs.

Phosphates—Examples of this class are Dexamethasone Sodium Phosphate and Menadiol Sodium Diphosphate. Each is an ester-salt of the ROPO-$(ONa)_2$, type, the salt moiety functioning to enhance water solubility.

Glycerophosphates—These are metallic salts of the dibasic glycerophosphoric acid, which is the monoglyceride of orthophosphoric acid, $CH_2(OH).CH(OH).$-$OPO(OH)_2$. Thus, they are esters and salts at the same time. The acid is prepared by direct esterification from glycerin and phosphoric acid. Salts may be prepared from the acid by neutralization with appropriate alkalies (eg, the sodium, calcium, and magnesium salts, qv), or from calcium glycerophosphate by metathesis (eg, the sodium and ferric salts, qv). Many metals, eg, Ca, Mn, Fe, etc, which form insoluble phosphates produce soluble glycerophosphates through chelation. Boiling solutions of glycerophosphates with alkali saponifies the ester linkage yielding glycerin and a phosphate. Heated dry, glycerophosphates liberated flammable vapors having a pungent odor (acrolein). Calcium, ferric, manganese, and sodium glycerophosphates were official for several decades prior to 1960.

Phosphorofluoridates—These have the general formula $F.PO(OR)_2$. They are the diesters of phosphorofluoridic acid, $F.PO(OH)_2$. The acid is also frequently referred to by its older name, fluorophosphoric acid, whereby the esters become fluorophosphates. Saponification affects the P-F linkage as well as the P.OR ester linkages, thus yielding fluoride, phosphate, and the organic hydroxy compound. For further discussion see page 904 where the official representative, Isoflurophate, is presented.

Various types of organic phosphorus compounds are potent anticholinesterases; ie, they inactivate the enzyme, cholinesterase, and thus inhibit the transmission of nerve impulses across cholinergic synapses. Examples, in addition to Isoflurophate, include tetraethyl pyrophosphate (TEPP), octamethylpyrophosphoramide (OMPA), and diethyl *p*-nitrophenyl phosphorothionate (Parathion). Several such compounds have been investigated for possible value as parasympathomimetic agents (see page 902) and as insecticides and pesticides (see page 1287). Some of the more potent members, eg, ethyl dimethylphosphoramidocyanidate (Tabun), $PO[(CH_3)_2N][CN][OC_2H_5]$ and isopropyl methylphosphonofluoridate (Sarin), CH_3-$PO[F][OCH(CH_3)_2]$, are of military interest as nerve gases.

Other Phosphorus Compounds—Thiotepa is the tris(1-aziridinyl) derivative of phosphine sulfide $[PH_3(S)]$.

Echothiophate Iodide is the methiodide of the S-[2-(dimethylamino)ethyl] O,O-diethyl ester of phosphorothioic acid $[PO(OH)_2SH]$.

Cyclophosphamide is a phosphine oxide type of derivative of the completely hydrogenated form of the heterocycle, 2H-1,3,2-oxazaphosphorine $O \cdot PH \cdot N : CH \cdot CH : CH$. It may be looked upon as a derivative of the intramolecular ester of N-(3-hydroxypropyl)phosphorodiamidic acid $[(HO)PO(NH_2)$-$(NHCH_2CH_2CH_2OH)]$.

Organic Arsenic, Antimony, and Bismuth Compounds

Official compounds in this broad category are frequently treated along with organic compounds containing mercury and gold under trivial and often misleading headings such as metal organic compounds. Actually, each of these compounds drops into logical, much more meaningful, positions in the orderly arrangement of organic compounds on the basis of functional groups; the following brief presentation is designed primarily to disclose such categorization.

Arsenoso Compounds—These R.As:O compounds (page 432) are analogous to the nitroso compounds in the nitrogen series. Instead of being named as arsenoso compounds, eg, arsenosobenzene, they are often named as alkylarsenic oxides and as alkyl arsinoxides. Arsenoso compounds are often conveniently prepared by reducing the corresponding arsonic acids with SO_2 in the presence of HI. Oxidizing agents readily convert the arsenic in arsenoso compounds into its maximum oxidative state.

The only *official arsenoso compound* is Oxophenarsine (2-amino-4-arsenosophenol) Hydrochloride.

Arsonic Acids—These are the arsenic analogues of the phosphonic acids. They may be looked upon as orthoarsenic acid with *one* of its OH groups replaced with a hydrocarbon radical; ie, R.As(:O)(OH)_2. Either the name of the hydrocarbon or the name of its radical is used in naming the acids; eg, C_6H_5AsO-$(OH)_2$ is known both as benzenearsonic acid and phenylarsonic acid. Arsonic acids are frequently prepared by *arsonation;* ie, heating the parent hydrocarbon (or derivative) directly with concentrated orthoarsenic acid. They also result when diazonium salts are reacted with sodium arsenite in the presence of alkali and cuprous chloride. The salts of arsonic acids are termed arsonates.

Examples of marketed pharmaceuticals in this class include the arsonic acid, Carbarsone, and the arsonates Tryparsamide, Drocarbil (an arecolinium salt), and Glycobiarsol (a bismuthyl salt).

Arsinic Acids—Like the arsonic acids, these are also derivatives of orthoarsenic acid, but in this case *two* of the OH groups are replaced with hydrocarbon radicals, thus giving the general formula, $R_2As(:O)OH$. The best-known is dimethylarsinic acid, $(CH_3)_2AsO_2H$, usually called cacodylic acid. Similarly, its salts, the dimethylarsinates, are commonly referred to as caco-

dylates. Cacodylic acid is easily produced from cacodyl oxide $[(CH_3)_2AsOAs(CH_3)_2]$ by oxidation with mercuric oxide in the presence of water. Cacodyl oxide is prepared from a mixture of arsenic trioxide and potassium acetate by dry distillation. Cacodylic acid is a weak acid and is readily reducible, eg, with hypophosphorous acid, forming cacodyl (tetramethyldiarsine). Sodium and ferric cacodylates were official for many years prior to 1960.

Arsonous Acids—These are the arsonic acids minus the oxo oxygen, ie, R.As(OH)_2. The only official representative is Melarsoprol, which is a cyclic ester of a substituted dithiobenzenearsonous acid. Dithiobenzenearsonous acid is $C_6H_5.As(SH)_2$.

Antimony Compounds—Antimony Potassium Tartrate is a basic antimony (antimonyl) salt and is classified under the salts of hydroxy carboxylic acids (page 455). Stibophen is a substituted o-phenylene phenyl orthostibnite ester and is classified under the *Esters of Inorganic Acids* (page 455). Being an ester, it is readily susceptible to saponification, and the liberated stibnite ion is easily oxidized (eg, with iodine) to stibnate.

Bismuth Compounds—Glycobiarsol, the only **official organic bismuth compound**, is the bismuthyl salt of p-(hydroxyacetamido)benzenearsonic acid and has been classified previously in this section under the *Arsonic Acids*.

Metallo-Organic (or Organometallic) Compounds

The characteristic feature of these compounds is a direct bond between carbon and the metal. Examples of the simpler types are provided on page 434. In those of the metal alkyl type, the character of the bond varies with different metals, being significantly ionic with Group IA and IIA metals and primarily nonionic with other metals. Thus, sodium methyl ionizes to give Na^+ and the carbanion CH_3^-, ie, $H : \overset{H}{\underset{H}{C}} : ^-$, whereas lead tetraethyl is typically covalent and does not display the characteristics of lead ion. Those of the RMX type in which X is an anion other than OH display saltlike characteristics due to ionization at the M-X linkage. For the same reason, those of the RMOH type are typical bases.

The simple metallo-organic compounds are commonly named by designating the radicals and the metal present. Thus, $Zn(CH_3)_2$ is dimethylzinc (or zinc dimethyl) and C_2H_5MgBr is ethyl magnesium bromide. In the case of polyfunctional, mercury-containing types, however, the radical containing the mercury is often named as a substituent group; eg, o-hydroxyphenyl mercuric chloride is usually known under the name o-chloromercuriphenol. Other examples will be encountered in some of the official mercurials (page 939, *et seq*).

From a preparative viewpoint in chemistry, the RMX type of metallo-organic compound finds many applications. Predominantly valuable in many kinds of organic syntheses are the highly reactive alkyl magnesium halides (Grignard reagents) and to a lesser extent the corresponding zinc compounds. These RMX types are usually prepared by causing the metal to react directly with the corresponding alkyl halide. Various methods have been devised for preparing compounds of the metal alkyl type. One method having wide utility consists of heating a mixture of the appropriate Grignard reagent and a halide of the required metal; eg, $3C_2H_5MgCl + AlCl_3 \rightarrow Al(C_2H_5)_3 + 3MgCl_2$. Basic research interest in various types of organometallic compounds is currently high and there are strong indications that important commercial applications will be forthcoming.

All of the official metallo-organic compounds are mercury compounds. Some authors include various official compounds of arsenic, antimony, bismuth, and gold in this category; but with these, either the metal is not in true metalloorganic combination (no direct metal to carbon linkage), or, in the case of arsenic, the compounds are preferably classified on the basis of functional groups in accordance with established International and American chemical practice.

The introduction of mercury (*mercuration*) into aromatic compounds is often effected by heating a solution of the compound with mercuric acetate, whereby direct substitution of hydrogen by the acetoxymercuri radical occurs. Mercuric acetate also can be made to participate readily in addition reactions to olefinic double bonds, thus introducing the mercury in aliphatic union. For specific examples, refer to the discussions in this text of the preparation of the official mercurials.

Examples of marketed pharmaceuticals in this class include Chloromerodrin, Meralluride, Merbromin, Mercaptomerin, Mercurophylline, Nitromersol, Phenylmercuric Acetate, Phenylmercuric Nitrate, and Thimerosal.

Heterocycles Present in Official Pharmaceuticals

Many important biochemical compounds and drugs of *natural* origin contain heterocyclic ring structures. Numerous examples occur, eg, among the carbohydrates, essential amino acids, vitamins, alkaloids, glycosides, antibiotics, etc. The presence of heterocyclic structures in such diverse types of compounds is strongly indicative of the profound effects such structures exert on physiological activity, and recognition of this is abundantly reflected in efforts to find useful *synthetic* drugs. Examples include researches leading to a wide variety of modern drugs such as Chlordiazepoxide (tranquilizer), Methazolamide (carbonic anhydrase inhibitor), Guanethidine (antihypertensive), Stanozolol (anabolic) Dapsone (leprostatic), Cyclophosphamide and Thiotepa (antineoplastics), Hydrochlorothiazide (diuretic and antihypertensive), Imipramine (antidepressant), Lucanthone (antischistosomal), and many others.

As to be expected, this trend in research finds reflection in the changing character of the contents of official drug compendia. Thus, whereas only about 16% of the organic chemical drugs* in USP XII (1942) were synthetic heterocyclics, about 31% of those in USP XVI (1960) were in this category; a survey discloses that this percentage is about 50 for new drugs scheduled for admission to USP XVIII and NF XIII (1970).

Intensive research in diverse heteroareas will continue to yield new medicinal agents, and Table VII (page 465) is designed to portray the spectrum of heterocycles presently represented in USP and NF drugs. The classification is patterned after that employed in *The Ring Index*[5] and in *Chemical Abstracts*.[6] The rings are presented in the order of increasing complexity. The bold-face figures show the total number of atoms in the rings, and the number of bold-face figures shows the number of rings present in the systems. As an example, the notation 5, 6 indicates a system composed of two rings, one of which contains five atoms while the other one contains six atoms. The formulas such as C_3NS-C_6 portray the kind and number of atoms present in the ring or rings. Associated with each of these formulas are the graphic formulas and *Ring Index* names† of the individual heterocycles, and, *in italics*, one or two examples of official drugs (or the portions of them) containing these heterocycles.

Structures and numbering schemes‡ are according to *The Ring Index* and thus do not portray any inherent features of stereospecificity.[5] It will be observed that some of the names for the heterocycles are trivial (eg, pyrimidine, nortropane, etc) while others are rigidly systematic. Trivial names are employed in the table wherever advisable; ie, wherever, through continued use, they have become recognized by chemists (as reflected by *IUPAC* adoption and *Chemical Abstracts* indexing) as denoting the structures to which they refer. In all other instances, systematic names must be used in order to distinguish between the heterocycle of interest and its isomeric forms.

Presentation is exclusively on the basis of the *most complex ring "system"* containing the hetero atom or atoms, the term "system" meaning either a single ring or a combination of rings of the fused, bridged, or spiro types. For example, quinine is presented *only* as a quinoline derivative and *not* also as a pyridine derivative, even though quinoline is a benzopyridine. Similarly, theophylline is presented *only* as a purine derivative and *not* as either a pyrimidine or an imidazole derivative, even though purine is an imidazopyrimidine.

In a complete presentation of this type, drugs containing two or more *separate* hetero ring systems would appear under each of the systems; eg, chlorothen would emerge both as a thiophene derivative and as a pyridine derivative.

Wherever possible, only that portion of the official title is used which embraces the heterocycle; eg, phenindamine instead of Phenindamine Tartrate and thiamine instead of Thiamine Hydrochloride.

References

1. *Rules for I.U.P.A.C. Notation for Organic Compounds*, Wiley, New York, 1961.

---

* Therapeutic organic compounds identified in the USP either by structural formula or by chemical name.

† Heterocyclic structures are often actually or theoretically produced by relatively simple chemical operations such as condensation and dehydrogenation on aliphatic structures. Because of this, many authors prefer to name such heterocycles in a manner designed to disclose the relationship to the aliphatics rather than employ *The Ring Index* nomenclature used in this table. The situation has already been illustrated with the following types of compounds of interest to pharmacy: inner acid anhydrides (page 453), cyclic ethers (page 451) and thio ethers (page 461), imides (page 459), imines (page 458), lactams (page 454), lactones (page 453), and ureides (page 460).

‡ Extreme caution must be exercised in interpreting position numbers as given in the names of compounds in different texts and works of reference. The situation often arises in which two different numbering schemes, through long continued usage, have become firmly established for a particular ring system; and this leads to different numbers in an otherwise identical pair of names for a given compound. Also, authors of texts frequently indulge in the reprehensible practice of inventing their own pet numbering schemes.

2. Smith, E. G., *The Wiswesser Line-Formula Chemical Notation*, McGraw-Hill, New York, 1968.
3. For a detailed discussion, see the published papers presented during the *Symposia on Influence of Molecular Modification in Drug Design* conducted by the Division of Medicinal Chemistry of the American Chemical Society, New York, Sept. 9–13, 1963.
4. "Compilation of New Drugs, 1941–1963," *Am. Profess. Pharmacist*, **30**, (1964).
5. *The Ring Index*, 2nd ed, American Chemical Society, Washington, D.C., 1960; Supplement I, 1963; Supplement II, 1964; Supplement III, 1965.
6. *Chemical Abstracts*, Vol. 68, Index of Ring Systems.

Table VII—Heterocycles in Official Drugs

3 C_2N

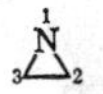

Aziridine
Examples: *Thiotepa; Triethylenemelamine.*

5 C_2AsS_2

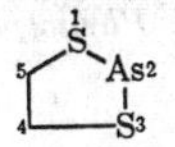

Dithiarsolane
Example: *Melarsoprol.*

C_2N_2S

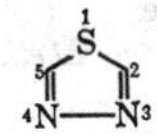

1,3,4-Thiadiazole
Examples: *Acetazolamide; Sulfamethizole.*

C_2N_2S

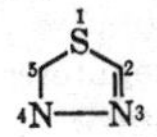

1,3,4-Thiadiazoline
Example: *Methazolamide.*

C_3NO

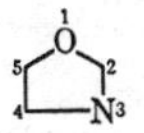

Oxazolidine
Example: *Paramethadione.*

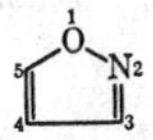

Isoxazole
Examples: *Isocarboxazid; Sulfisoxazole.*

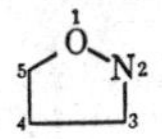

Isoxazolidine
Example: *Cycloserine.*

C_3NS

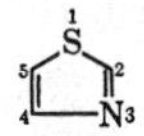

Thiazole
Examples: *Thiabendazole; Thiamine.*

C_3N_2

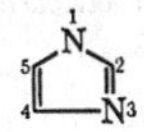

Imidazole
Examples: *Histamine; Pilocarpine.*

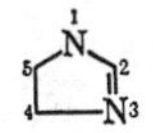

2-Imidazoline
Examples: *Antazoline; Phentolamine.*

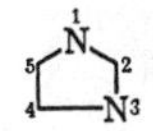

Imidazolidine
Examples: *Diphenylhydantoin; Nitrofurantoin.*

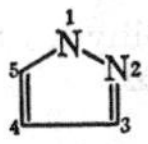

Pyrazole
Example: *Betazole.*

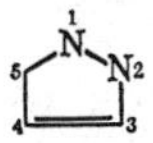

3-Pyrazoline
Example: *Antipyrine.*

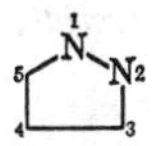

Pyrazolidine
Examples: *Phenylbutazone; Sulfinpyrazone.*

C_4N

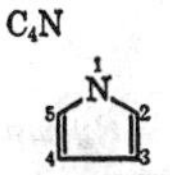

Pyrrole
Example: *Pyrvinium Pamoate.*

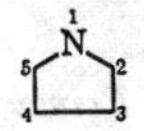

Pyrrolidine
Examples: *Methsuximide; Pyrrobutamine.*

C_4O

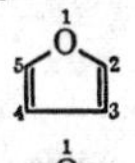

Furan
Examples: *Nitrofurantoin; Nitrofurazone.*

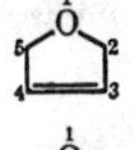

2,5-Dihydrofuran
Examples: *Ascorbic acid; Digitoxin.*

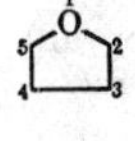

Tetrahydrofuran
Examples: *Streptomycin; Sucrose.*

C_4S

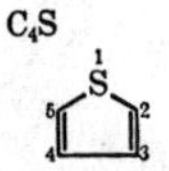

Thiophene
Examples: *Chlorothen; Methapyrilene.*

6 C_3NOP

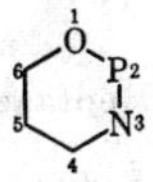

Tetrahydro-2*H*-1,3,2-oxazaphosphorine
Example: *Cyclophosphamide.*

C_3N_3

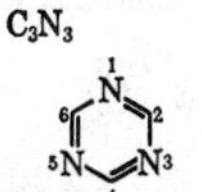

s-Triazine
Examples: *Melarsoprol; Triethylenemelamine.*

C_3O_3

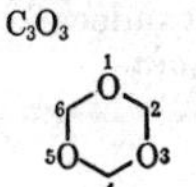

s-Trioxane
Example: *Paraldehyde.*

C_4NO

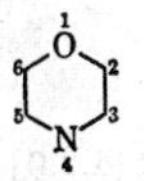

Morpholine
Examples: *Phenmetrazine; Pramoxine.*

C_4N_2

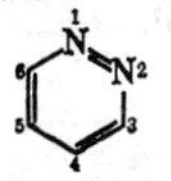

Pyridazine
Example: *Sulfamethoxypyridazine.*

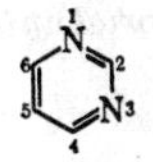

Pyrimidine
Examples: *Pyrimethamine; Sulfadiazine.*

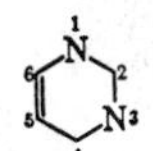

1,2,3,4-Tetrahydropyrimidine
Examples: *Idoxuridine; Propylthiouracil.*
1,4,5,6-tetrahydro form
Example: *Oxyphencyclimine.*

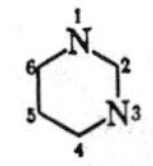

Hexahydropyrimidine
Examples: *All barbituric and thiobarbituric acids; Primidone.*

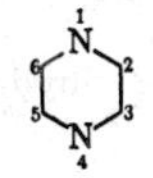

Piperazine; Hexahydropyrazine
Examples: *Chlorcyclizine; Prochlorperazine.*

C_5N

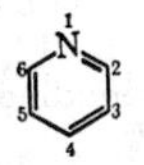

Pyridine
Examples: *Cetylpyridinium Chloride; Niacinamide; Tripelennamine.*

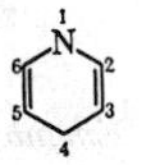

1,4-Dihydropyridine (4*H*-Pyridine)
Example: *Propyliodone.*

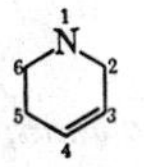

1,2,5,6-Tetrahydropyridine
Examples: *Arecoline; Drocarbil.*

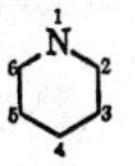

Piperidine; Hexahydropyridine
Examples: *Alphaprodine; Glutethimide; Meperidine.*

C_5O

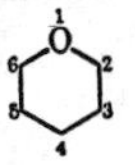

Tetrahydropyran
Examples: *Lactose; Streptomycin.*

Table VII—Continued

7 C₆N

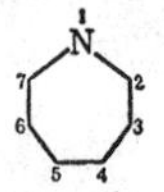

Hexahydroazepine
Example: *Ethoheptazine.*

8 C₇N

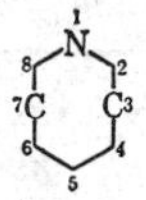

Octahydroazocine
Example: *Guanethidine Sulfate.*

14 C₁₃O

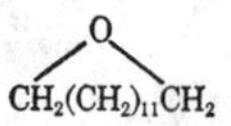

CH₂(CH₂)₁₁CH₂

Oxacyclotetradecane
Example: *Erythromycin.*

24 C₁₈N₈

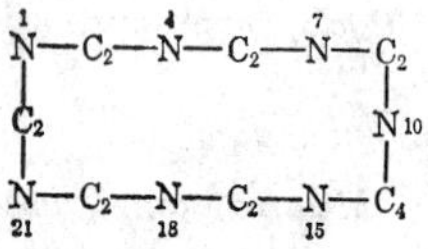

1, 4, 7, 10, 15, 18, 21-Heptaazacyclo-
tricosane
Examples: *Colistin; Sodium Colistimethate.*

3,14 C₂O-C₁₃O

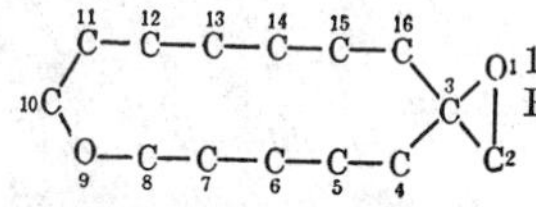

1,9-Dioxaspiro[2.13]hexadecane
Example: *Oleandomycin.*

4,5 C₃N-C₃NS

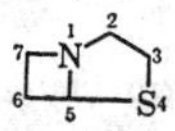

4-Thia-1-azabicyclo[3.2.0]heptane
Example: *Penicillins.*

4,6 C₂HgO-C₆

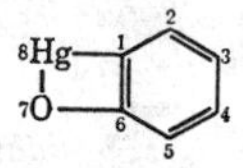

7-Oxa-8-mercurabicyclo[4.2.0]-1, 3, 5-
octatriene
Example: *Nitromersol.*

C₃N-C₄NS

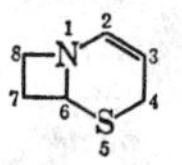

5-Thia-1-azabicyclo[4.2.0]oct-2-ene
Example: *Sodium Cephalothin.*

5,6 C₂O₂Sb-C₅

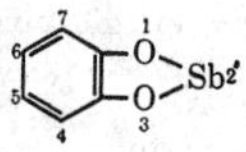

1,3,2-Benzodioxastibole
Example: *Stibophen.*

C₃NS-C₆

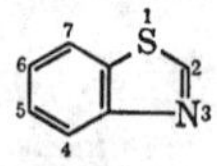

Benzothiazole
Example: *Ethoxzolamide.*

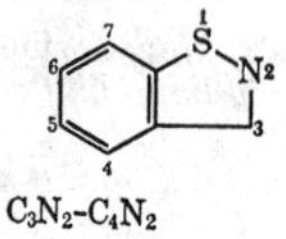

1,2-Benzisothiazole, 2,3-dihydro form
Example: *Saccharin.*

C₃N₂-C₄N₂

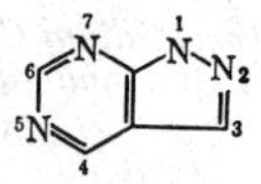

1H-Pyrazolo[3,4-d]pyrimidine
Example: *Allopurinol.*

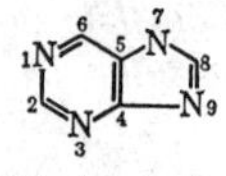

Purine
Examples: *Caffeine; Dimenhydrinate.*

C₃N₂-C₆

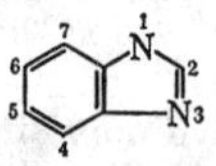

Benzimidazole
Examples: *Cyanocobalamin; Thiabendazole.*

C₃OS-C₆

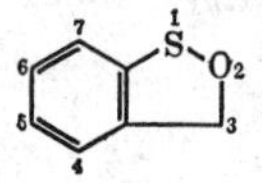

3H-2,1-Benzoxathiole
Example: *Phenolsulfonphthalein.*

C₄N-C₅N

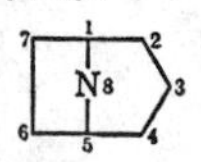

Nortropane
Examples: *Atropine; Cocaine.*

C₄N-C₆

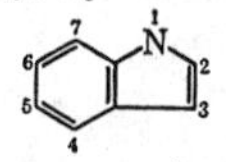

Indole
Example: *Indomethacin.*

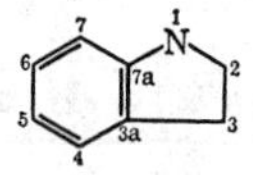

Indoline
Example: *Sodium Indigotindisulfonate.*

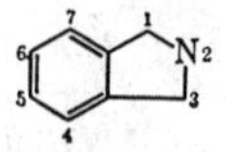

Isoindoline
Example: *Chlorthalidone.*

C₄O-C₆

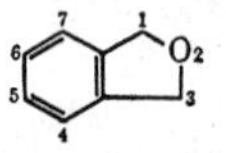

Phthalan
Examples: *Noscapine; Phenolphthalein.*

C₅-C₅N

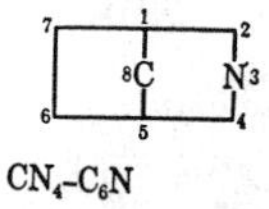

3-Azabicyclo[3.2.1]octane
Example: *Trimethidinium Methosulfate.*

5,7 CN₄-C₆N

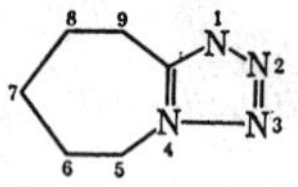

6,7,8,9-Tetrahydro-5H-azepotetrazole
Example: *Pentylenetetrazole.*

6,6 C₃N₂S-C₆

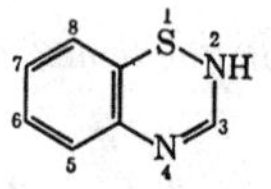

2H-1,2,4-Benzothiadiazine
Examples: *Benzthiazide; Chlorothiazide.*

3,4-dihydro form
Examples: *Hydrochlorothiazide; Polythiazide.*

C₄N₂-C₄N₂

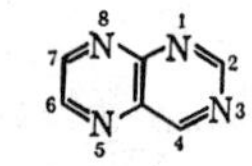

Pteridine
Examples: *Folic Acid; Methotrexate.*
5,6,7,8-Tetrahydro form
Example: *Leucovorin.*

C₄N₂-C₆

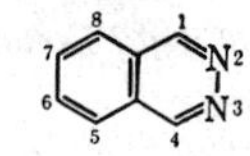

Phthalazine
Example: *Hydralazine.*

C₅N-C₅N

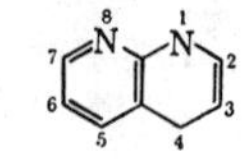

1,8-Naphthyridine, 1,4-dihydro form
Example: *Nalidixic Acid.*

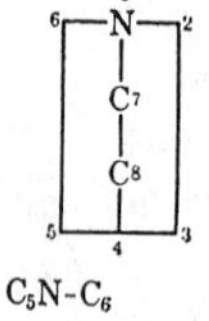

Quinuclidine
Examples: *Clidinium Bromide; Quinine.*

C₅N-C₆

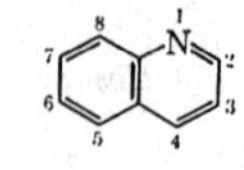

Quinoline
Examples: *Chloroquine; Pyrvinium
Pamoate; Quinine.*

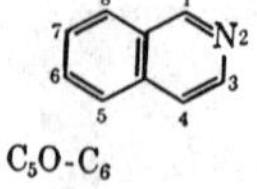

Isoquinoline
Examples: *Papaverine; Primaquine.*
1,2,3,4-Tetrahydro form
Example: *Emetine.*

C₅O-C₆

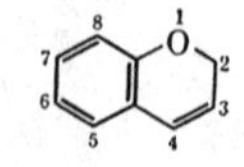

2H-1-Benzopyran
Examples: *Bishydroxycoumarin; Warfarin.*

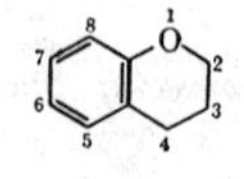

Chroman (Dihydrobenzopyran)
Example: *Alpha Tocopherol.*

Table VII—Continued

6,7   C$_6$-C$_5$N$_2$

2-Oxabicyclo[2.2.2]octane
Example: *Eucalyptol.*

3*H*-1,4-Benzodiazepine
Example: *Chlordiazepoxide.*

2*H*-1,4-Benzodiazepine, 1,3-dihydro form
Examples: *Oxazepam; Diazepam.*

3,5,6   C$_2$O-C$_4$N-C$_5$N

3-Oxa-9-azatricyclo[3.3.1.0^{2,4}]nonane
Examples: *Methscopolamine Bromide; Scopolamine.*

5,5,5   C$_3$N$_2$-C$_4$S-C$_4$S

Imidazo[4,5-c]thieno[1,2-a]thiolium
Example: *Trimethaphan Camsylate.*

5,5,6   C$_3$NO-C$_4$N-C$_4$N$_2$

8*H*-Oxazolo[3,2-a]pyrrolo[2,1-c]-pyrazine, perhydro form
Example: *Ergotamine.*

C$_4$N-C$_4$N-C$_6$

Pyrrolo[2,3-b]indole, 1,2,3,3a,8,8a-hexahydro form
Example: *Physostigmine.*

5,6,6   C$_3$O$_2$-C$_5$N-C$_6$

1,3-Dioxolo[4,5-g]isoquinoline, 5,6,7,8-tetrahydro form
Example: *Noscapine.*

C$_4$N-C$_6$-C$_6$

1*H*-Benz[e]indolium
Example: *Indocyanine Green.*

7*H*-Furo[3,2-g][1]benzopyran
Example: *Trioxsalen.*

C$_4$O-C$_6$-C$_6$

Spiro[benzofuran - 2(3*H*),1' - [2] - cyclohexene]
Example: *Griseofulvin.*

C$_5$-C$_5$N-C$_6$

1*H*-Indeno[2,1-c]pyridine, 1,2,3,4-tetrahydro form
Example: *Phenindamine.*

6,6,6   C$_3$N$_3$-C$_3$N$_3$-C$_3$N$_3$

Hexamethylenetetramine
Example: *Methenamine.*

C$_4$NO-C$_6$-C$_6$

3*H*-Phenoxazine
Example: *Dactinomycin.*

C$_4$NS-C$_6$-C$_6$

Phenothiazine
Examples: *Chlorpromazine; Prochlorperazine.*

C$_4$N$_2$-C$_4$N$_2$-C$_6$

Phenazathionium
Examples: *Azure A Dye (in Azuresin);* Methylene Blue.

C$_5$N-C$_5$N-C$_6$

Benzo[g]pteridine, 2,3,4,10-tetrahydro form
Example: *Riboflavin.*

C$_5$N-C$_6$-C$_6$

2*H*-Benzo[a]quinolizine, 1,3,4,6,7,11b-hexahydro form
Example: *Emetine.*

Acridine
Example: *Quinacrine.*

2,6-Methano-3-benzazocine, 1,2,3,4,5,-6-hexahydro form
Example: *Phenazocine.*

C$_2$O-C$_6$-C$_6$

Xanthene
Example: *Methantheline; Propantheline.*

3*H*-Isoxanthene
Examples: *Fluorescein Sodium; Rose Bengal Sodium.*

C$_5$S-C$_6$-C$_6$

Thioxanthene
Examples: *Chlorprothixene; Lucanthone.*

6,6,7   C$_6$-C$_6$-C$_5$N

10,11-Dihydro-5*H*-dibenz[b,f]azepine
Examples: *Desipramine; Imipramine.*

5,6,6,6   C$_4$N-C$_5$N-C$_6$-C$_6$

Indolo[4,3-fg]quinoline 4,6,6a,7,8,9-hexahydro form
Examples: *Ergonovine; Ergotamine.*

C$_5$-C$_5$O-C$_6$-C$_6$

2-Oxa-5-androstane*
Example: *Oxandrolone.*

5,6,6,9   C$_4$N-C$_5$N-C$_6$-C$_8$N

10*H*-3,7-Methanoazacycloundecino-[5,4-b]indole, 1,2,4,5,6,7,8,9-octahydro form
Examples: *Vinblastine; Vincristine.*

6,6,6,6   C$_5$N-C$_6$-C$_6$-C$_6$

4*H*-Dibenzo[de,g]quinoline, 5,6,6a,7-tetrahydro form
Example: *Apomorphine.*

2*H* - 10,4a-Iminoethanophenanthrene, *cis*-1,3,4,9,10,10a-hexahydro form; morphinan
Examples: *Dextromethorphan; Levorphanol.*

---

* Alternative name and numbering shown. See Ring Index No. 4760 for IUPAC presentation.

Table VII—Continued

5,5,5,5,15 $C_4N-C_4N-C_4N-C_4N-C_{11}N_4$

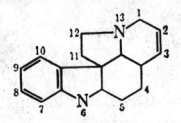

Corrin
Example: *Cyanocobalamin*

5,5,6,6,6 $C_3N_2-C_5-C_6-C_6-C_6$

Androstano[3,2-*c*]pyrazol*
Example: *Stanozolol.*

$C_4N-C_4N-C_5N-C_6-C_6$

1*H*-Indolizino[8,1-*cd*]carbazole,
3a,4,5,5a,6,11,12,13a-octahydro
form
Examples: *Vinblastine; Vincristine.*

_____

* Alternative name and numbering shown.   See Ring Index No. 5557 for
IUPAC presentation.

5,6,6,6,6 $C_4N-C_5N-C_5N-C_6-C_6$

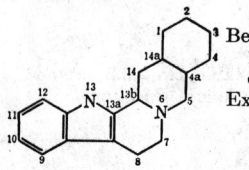

Benz[*g*]indolo[2,3-*a*]quinolizine,
1,2,3,4,4a,5,7,8,13,13b,14,14a-do-
decahydro form
Examples: *Reserpine; Syrosingopine*

$C_4O-C_5N-C_6-C_6-C_6$

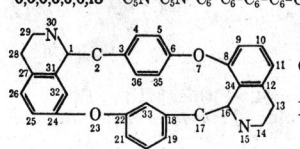

4a*H* - 8,9*c* - Iminoethanophenanthro
[4,5-*bcd*]furan
5,7a,8,9-Tetrahydro form
Examples: *Codeine; Morphine; Nal
orphine.*
5,6,7,7a,8,9-Hexahydro form (rin
marked A saturated)
Examples: *Hydrocodone;   Hydro
morphone.*

6,6,6,6,6,6,18 $C_5N-C_5N-C_6-C_6-C_6-C_6-C_{16}O_2$

Octahydro form of Ring Index No
7408.
Example: *Tubocurarine.*

30 | Natural Products

Carbohydrates—glycosides—lipids (fixed oils, fats, waxes, and sterols)—
proteins—alkaloids—volatile oils—plant exudates

This chapter was prepared by

Clarence T. Van Meter, PhD, *Project Director, Office of Engineering Research,
University of Pennsylvania, Philadelphia, Pa. 19104, and*
Alfonso R. Gennaro, PhD, *Professor of Chemistry, Philadelphia College of
Pharmacy and Science, Philadelphia, Pa. 19104*

This chapter provides a discussion of the fundamental characteristics of the following, essentially
chemical, classes of naturally occurring products.

1. Carbohydrates
2. Glycosides
3. Lipids (Fixed Oils, Fats, Waxes, Sterols, and Phospholipids)
4. Proteins
5. Alkaloids
6. Volatile Oils
7. Plant Exudates (Resins, Oleoresins, Gum Resins, and Balsams)

Each class yields official drugs, examples of which
are provided at the conclusion of each section. The
treatment of all individual monographs is presented at
appropriate places elsewhere in the text, the distribution being on a pharmacological basis.

For the location of other classes of natural products, eg, hormones, vitamins, enzymes, antibiotics,
etc, consult the general index.

Carbohydrates

Composition

This important class of organic compounds embraces
(1) aliphatic polyhydric alcohols in which either the
primary alcohol function has been oxidized to aldehyde or the secondary alcohol function has been
oxidized to ketone, and (2) condensation polymers of
these partially oxidized polyalcohols. The fundamental structural units are thus the aldehyde-alcohols
and ketone-alcohols which constitute (1). These are
frequently termed *monosaccharides** (sometimes simply *saccharides*) and are subclassified into *aldoses* and
ketoses according to whether they contain the aldehyde or the ketone group. The condensation polymers which constitute (2) are sometimes referred to as
saccharide anhydrides; they are subclassified into
disaccharides, *trisaccharides*, etc according to the number of monosaccharide units present. The term *polysaccharide* is used differently by different authors, some
using it broadly to embrace all of the polymers including the disaccharides, and others restricting it variously so as to exclude the *di-* and sometimes also the
tri- and *tetra*saccharides. The *di-*, *tri-*, and up to
about the *deca*saccharides are sometimes grouped
under the term *oligo*saccharides (oligo, of Greek
origin, meaning a few).

The term *sugar* is also used with various meanings.
It is sometimes employed synonymously with the
term carbohydrate. Probably more conventionally, it
is used to refer only to those carbohydrates which are
soluble and have a sweet taste; and nutritionists
frequently restrict it to mean carbohydrates which are
physiologically assimilable. The monosaccharides are
sometimes termed *simple sugars*.

Early analytical chemists recognized the few carbo-

hydrates known then as hydrates of carbon [ie,
$C_n(H_2O)_{n'}$], thus the term carbohydrate (from the
French, *hydrate de carbone*). Many carbohydrates
known today, however, do not correspond to such
simple algebraic representation.

Classification and Structure

Space permits scarcely more than a statement of the
essential features of this complex, fascinating subject,
elucidation of which constitutes a brilliant chapter in
organic chemistry.

Monosaccharides are classified first into *dioses*,
trioses, *tetroses*, etc, according to the number of carbon
atoms they contain. This is also the number of
oxygen atoms in the case of the common, important
carbohydrates; and no further treatment will be given
to carbohydrates in which this identicalness does not
exist. The terms diose, etc, are frequently combined
with aldose or ketose to give a more completely descriptive name. Thus, xylose is an *aldopentose* (contains the aldehyde function and a total of five carbon
atoms); similarly, fructose is a *ketohexose* (contains
the ketone function and a total of six carbon atoms).

The simplest aldose is the diose, glycolaldehyde.
All of the more complex aldoses may be predicted and
visualized by inserting additional —CH(OH)— groups
in the glycolaldehyde formula, one at a time, and
always adjacent to the terminal CH_2OH group, thus
passing successively through trioses, tetroses, etc.
The scheme is shown in Table I, the intermediate
—CH(OH)— groups being represented by horizontal
lines drawn to the side to which the OH group is
attached. It will be observed that, starting with the
aldotrioses, the insertion of each —CH(OH)— group
automatically introduces an asymmetric carbon atom,
thus giving rise to an increasing number of stereo-

---

* The syllable "ose" is often used instead of "ide" in saccharide names.

isomers. The enantiomorphs of each stereoisomeric pair are distinguished by the *configurational* notation D and L, referring respectively to whether the OH of the last inserted —CH(OH)— is on the right or left of the vertical axis when the formulas are drawn as shown in the Table. It is important to remember that the D and L notations have nothing to do with direction of optical rotation, and also that the actual demonstration of whether a given stereoisomer is D or L is a matter of laboratory experimentation.

The simplest ketose is the triose, dihydroxyacetone. The scheme in Table I depicts the more complex members in the same manner described above for the aldoses.

Cyclic Structures

Measurements of various characteristics (propensity to function as reductants, ability to form acetal derivatives, mutarotation, etc) have demonstrated conclusively that the open-chain formulas shown above do not represent the true structure of at least the higher monosaccharides, the pentoses and hexoses. Rather, the structures are cyclic (variously termed "ring," "oxide," or "lactone-type" structures) and may be looked upon as internal hemiacetals (page 432) involving the carbonyl oxygen atom and one of the alcoholic hydroxyls. Although such a reaction can involve any of the hydroxyl groups, theoretical considerations suggest that the γ- and δ-hydroxyl groups are more ideally situated to participate in the cyclization, thus giving rise to furanose (contain the furan ring) and pyranose (contain the pyran ring) structures. Experimental evidence indicates that the hexoses, in their normal monosaccharide states, exist largely in the pyranose form.

Thus, for example, the open-chain formula (A) for D-glucose gives way to the corresponding cyclic structures (B):

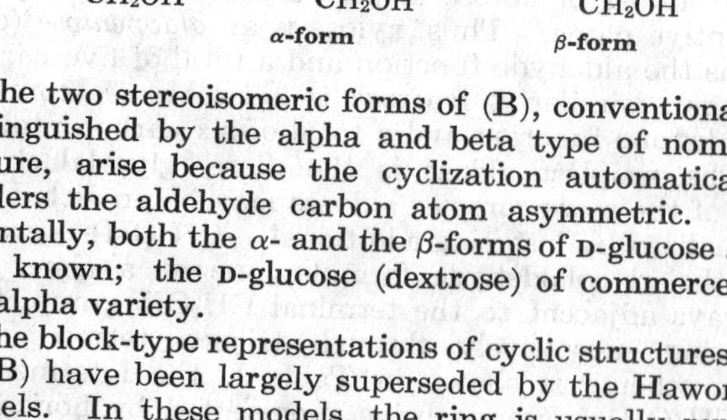

The two stereoisomeric forms of (B), conventionally distinguished by the alpha and beta type of nomenclature, arise because the cyclization automatically renders the aldehyde carbon atom asymmetric. Incidentally, both the α- and the β-forms of D-glucose are well known; the D-glucose (dextrose) of commerce is the alpha variety.

The block-type representations of cyclic structures as in (B) have been largely superseded by the Haworth models. In these models, the ring is usually *represented* as planar, and disposition of hydrogen atoms and substituents is portrayed by vertical assignment upward and downward from the ring plane. Haworth models for some selected hexoses are shown below along with the conventional ring numbering. For comparison, both the furanose and pyranose structures are shown for α-D-glucose.

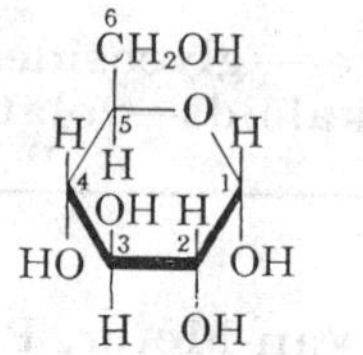

α-D-Glucose (α-D-Glucopyranose)   α-D-Glucose (α-D-Glucofuranose)

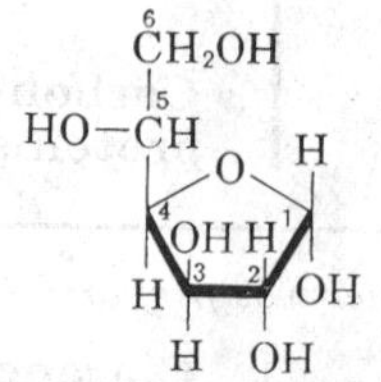

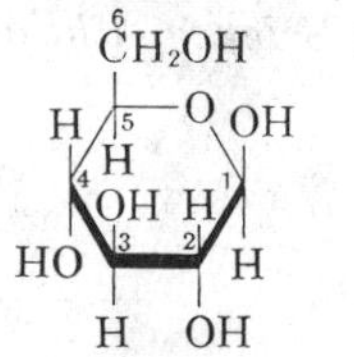

β-D-Glucose (β-D-Glucopyranose)   α-D-Fructose (α-D-Fructopyranose)

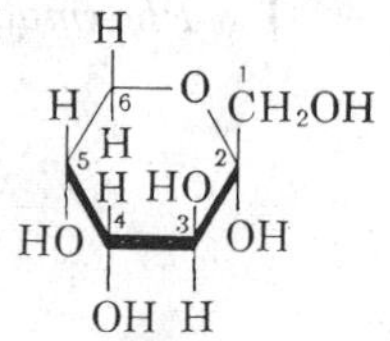

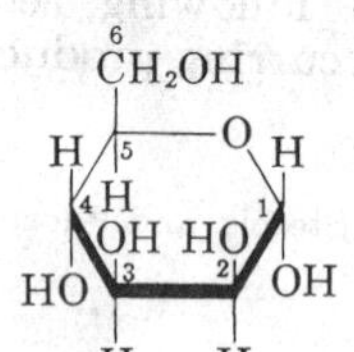

α-D-Galactose (α-D-Galactopyranose)   α-D-Mannose (α-D-Mannopyranose)

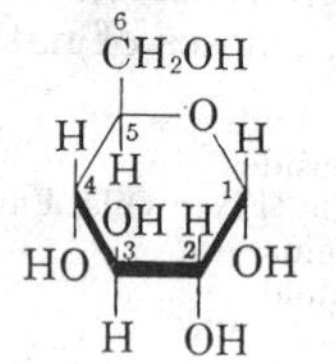

The structures and descriptive names of the four best-known disaccharides are shown below. It will be observed that the descriptive [bracketed] names identify

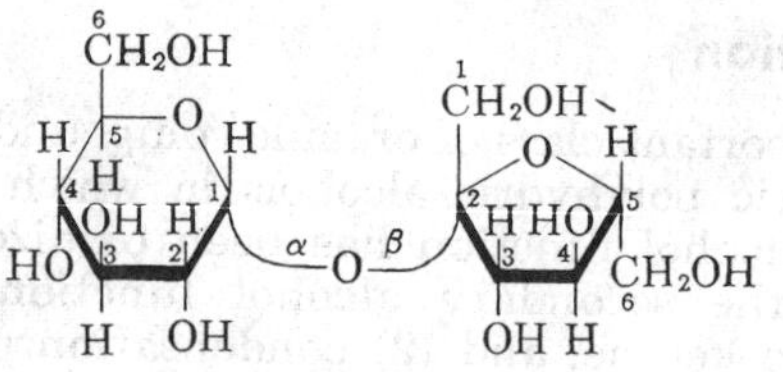

Sucrose
[α-D-Glucopyranosyl-β-D-fructofuranoside]

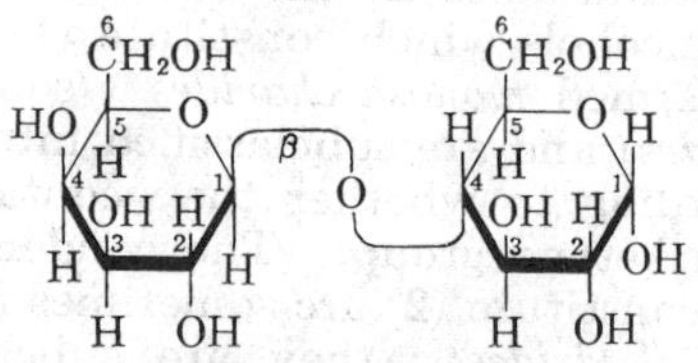

Lactose (α-Lactose)
[4-O-β-D-Galactopyranosyl-α-D-glucopyranose]

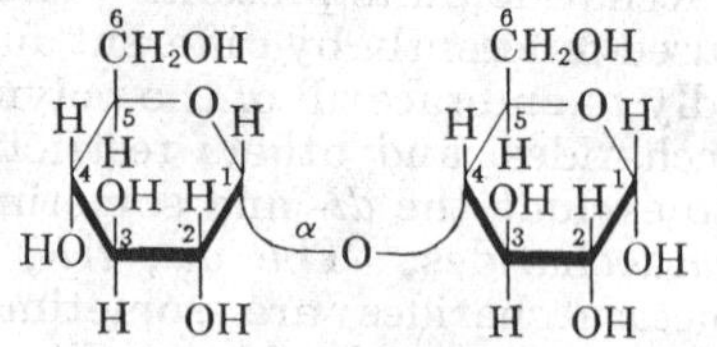

Maltose
[4-O-α-D-Glucopyranosyl-α-D-glucopyranose]

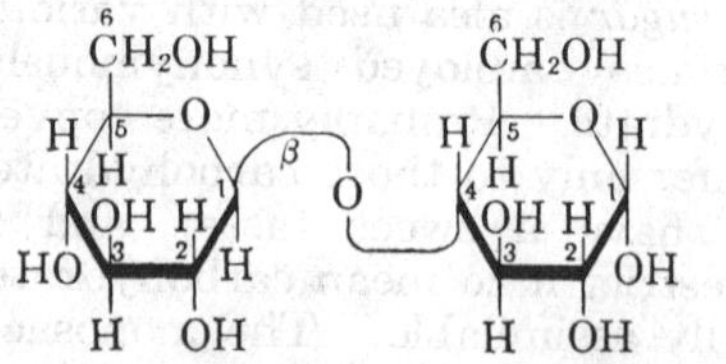

Cellobiose
[4-O-β-D-Glucopyranosyl-β-D-glucopyranose]

precisely the location of the terminals of the oxygen bridge joining the two monosaccharide residues.

It will also be observed that the completely descriptive names are cumbersome and consequently

Table 1—Monosaccharides*

Aldoses

Diose	Trioses	Tetroses	Pentoses	Hexoses
Glycolaldehyde (Parent molecule of the Aldoses)‡				
	D-Glyceraldehyde	D-Erythrose	D-Ribose	D-Allose
				L-Talose
			D-Ribose	D-Gulose
			L-Lyxose	L-Mannose
		L-Threose	L-Lyxose	D-Glucose
			D-Xylose	L-Idose
				D-Galactose
		D-Threose	L-Arabinose	L-Altrose
				D-Altrose
			D-Arabinose	L-Galactose
				D-Idose
		L-Erythrose	L-Xylose	L-Glucose
				D-Mannose
			D-Lyxose	L-Gulose
	L-Glyceraldehyde			D-Talose
			L-Ribose	L-Allose

Ketoses†

Triose	Tetroses	Pentoses	Hexoses
Dihydroxyacetone (Parent molecule of the ketoses) §			
	D-Erythrulose	D-Ribulose	D-Psicose
			L-Tagatose
		L-Xyloketose	D-Sorbose
			D-Fructose
	L-Erythrulose	D-Xyloketose	L-Fructose
			L-Sorbose
		L-Ribulose	D-Tagatose
			L-Psicose

* Scheme is terminated with hexoses although some higher members are known.

† Scheme is limited to 2-ketohexoses. Other ketoses are not usually treated in carbohydrate chemistry.

‡ In all aldose representations, the vertical line stands for $\overset{CHO}{\underset{CH_2OH}{|}}$.

Thus, for example, the representation $\vdash$ for D-Glyceraldehyde actually portrays $\overset{CHO}{\underset{CH_2OH}{H-C-OH}}$; the representation $\dashv$ for L-Threose

actually portrays $\overset{CHO}{\underset{CH_2OH}{HO-C-H}}$; etc.

§ In all ketose representations, the symbol $\models O$ stands for $\overset{CH_2OH}{\underset{CH_2OH}{CO}}$.

Thus, for example, the representation $\models O$ for D-Erythrulose actually

portrays $\overset{CH_2OH}{\underset{CH_2OH}{C=O}}$: the representation $\models O$ for L-Xyloketose

actually portrays $\overset{CH_2OH}{\underset{CH_2OH}{HO-C-H}}$: etc.

find little use in ordinary chemical practice. Recognizing this, both IUPAC and Chemical Abstracts admit the commonly used trivial names. A pamphlet describing the detailed rules for the systematic nomenclature of carbohydrates and their derivatives is available through Chemical Abstracts Service.

The naturally occurring polysaccharides (eg, the starches, cellulose, glycogen, and inulin), although all classed generally as high molecular weight condensation polymers of monosaccharides, vary considerably among themselves in size and structure. Thus, inulin appears to be a relatively small polymer composed of some 30 fructose (fructofuranose) units, whereas cellulose appears to be a relatively large polymer probably containing not less than 1000 glucopyranose units. In some polysaccharides, eg, cellulose, the evidence is strong that the polymers are purely linear; in others, eg, glycogen, a satisfactory explanation for observed experimental data requires that considerable branching occur along the chain. Polysaccharides are often classified on the basis of their monomers; eg, hexosans are polymers of hexoses, and pentosans are polymers of pentoses. Such classification is also frequently rendered specific; eg, cellulose is a glucosan (the hexose unit is D-glucose), and inulin is a fructosan (the hexose unit is D-fructose).

Physical Properties

The common monosaccharides, *viz*, the pentoses and hexoses, are white, crystalline solids which usually melt rather sharply but with simultaneous decomposition. They are readily soluble in water, much less soluble in methanol and ethanol, and relatively insoluble in ether. The common disaccharides, all hexabioses, also display these characteristics. However, the higher polysaccharides—eg, starch, cellulose, and inulin—are amorphous, do not melt sharply, and are much less water-soluble. The soluble, lower molecular weight carbohydrates are characterized by a sweet taste, but the relative sweetness varies considerably. Thus, lactose is only about one-sixth, maltose about one-third, and glucose about three-fourths as sweet as sucrose; fructose, on the other hand, is about 1.7 times as sweet as sucrose.

All carbohydrates are optically active, and their specific rotations serve as useful identification tags. Many display the phenomenon of *mutarotation*—a continuing change in the value of the rotation until a final fixed value is attained. The classic example is that of α-D-glucose, a freshly prepared aqueous solution of which has an $[\alpha]_D^{20°C}$ of $+113°$, but which gradually changes to a final value of $+52°$. Elucidation of this phenomenon constitutes one of the high points in structural carbohydrate chemistry. It has been demonstrated abundantly that such changes in rotation are referable to structural shifts, and that the final value is quantitatively characteristic of the components present in the equilibrium mixture. In the case of glucose, for example, the final rotation value is that to be expected of an equilibrium mixture containing both the α and the β forms of D-glucose. The attainment of the equilibrium state is hastened by proton and by hydroxyl, hundreds of times more so by the latter.

Chemical Properties

The chemical properties of the carbohydrates are, in general, those to be expected on the basis of their structural features previously described. Treatment here is necessarily limited to a brief mention of the more characteristic reactions.

Reduction—Aldoses and ketoses are readily reduced (sodium amalgam, catalytic hydrogenation, and electrolytic processes) to the corresponding polyhydric alcohols; eg, D-glucose → D-sorbitol, D-mannose → D-mannitol. A ketose automatically gives rise to an epimeric pair of alcohols due to the asymmetrization of the carbonyl carbon atom; eg, D-fructose → D-mannitol and D-sorbitol.

Oxidation—Oxidation of aldoses and ketoses results in the formation of acids. Depending upon the severity of the oxidative procedure, an aldose gives rise to one of three types of acids, *viz: onic* acids (eg, gluconic, in which the CHO has been oxidized to COOH); *uronic* acids (eg, glucuronic, in which the CHO remains unaltered and the terminal CH_2OH has been oxidized to COOH); and the *saccharic* acids (eg, glucosaccharic, which are dibasic and in which both the CHO and the terminal CH_2OH have been oxidized to COOH). Ketoses are more resistant to oxidation, and when they do succumb, they split, as might be expected, to produce a mixture of acids; eg, nitric acid oxidizes fructose to give a mixture of tartaric and glycollic acids.

Carbonyl Condensation Reactions—Both aldoses and ketoses undergo the typical carbonyl condensation reactions with various aldehyde and ketone reagents such as hydroxylamine (to form oximes) and hydrazines (to form, initially, hydrazones). See pages 451 and 452.

The oxime reaction is of analytical interest in the Wohl degradation, whereby the number of —CH(OH)— groups in an aldose may be decreased by one for each performance of the degradation reaction.

The reactions with phenylhydrazine are of especial interest. The initial condensation products (phenylhydrazones, page 458) are generally water-soluble and difficult to crystallize. However, more of the reagent quickly oxidizes an adjacent —CH(OH)— group to —CO— and the latter condenses readily with more phenylhydrazine to yield the relatively insoluble, crystalline osazones (phenylosazones, page 434).

Because of their mode of formation, crystalline structure, and sharp melting points, the osazones play important roles in the identification and structural elucidation of the carbohydrates. Osazones are formed not only by the monosaccharides but also by those polysaccharides such as lactose and maltose which, like the monosaccharides, contain the required potential carbonyl function sometimes referred to as a "free sugar group"; ie, a $\overset{\overset{\displaystyle O}{\vert}}{CH(OH).CH(OH)}$— group. Since it does not contain this group, sucrose, for example does not form an osazone.

Reaction with Oxidizing Cations—All monosaccharides, and all disaccharides and polysaccharides which contain a free sugar group (see above), readily undergo oxidation under the influence of various metal ions such as Cu^{2+}, Bi^{3+}, and Hg^{2+} in the presence of alkali. The reaction with Cu^{2+} is applied in various tests (see Fehling's and Benedict's solutions) for the so-called reducing sugars. In these copper tests, the reduction product of the Cu^{2+} (yellow cuprous hydroxide, $Cu_2(OH)_2$, or red cuprous oxide, Cu_2O) is the substance observed and measured. Of the common disaccharides, sucrose is distinguished by its lack of ability to reduce Cu^{2+}.

Cyanohydrin Formation—Both aldoses and ketoses undergo addition with HCN to form cyanohydrin derivatives (pages 432 and 452). The reaction has particular significance in the Kiliani synthesis, whereby the number of —CH(OH)— groups in an aldose can be increased by one for each performance of the synthesis.

Reaction with Alkalies—Under the influence of strong alkali, carbohydrates commonly behave as weak acids and form salts, eg, glucosates, sucrates, etc. The reaction is often represented as involving first a tautomerization yielding an acidic enediol structure, —C(OH):C(OH)—. Like the alcoholates (alkoxides) and phenolates (phenoxides), these salts are highly hydrolyzed and readily surrender their base portions to even such weak acids as CO_2.

Etherification and Esterification Reactions—All carbohydrates are susceptible to these operations, and the extent to which they succumb provides important evidence with respect to their structure. Thus, glucose yields a pentamethyl ether and a pentaacetate, sucrose yields similar octa derivatives, etc. The reaction conditions are those to be expected from the alcoholic nature of the hydroxyl groups (page 451). Glycosides (page 474) comprise a special class of the ether derivatives. Among the inorganic esters, the nitrates and phosphates are especially well known. Certain phosphate esters of glucose and fructose are intimately involved in the physiologic use of carbohydrates.

Hydrolysis—All polysaccharides are hydrolyzable. Indeed, it is through such cleavage that much of the knowledge concerning the monosaccharide composition of these polymers is disclosed. The hydrolysis is proton-catalyzed and is often conducted by refluxing an acidified aqueous solution of the polymer. Nature provides many enzymes (eg, amylases, cellulases, sucrases, glucosidases, maltases, invertase, etc) which also catalyze the hydrolysis. Quite commonly these enzymes show high specificity, not only with respect to the polysaccharides they hydrolyze but also with respect to the linkages they cleave. Nature's enzymic methods for synthesizing and utilizing carbohydrates are most intriguing, and much remains to be done if man is to integrate the bits of information he has accumulated on the subject into a pattern having maximum predictive value for presently unknown applications.

Fermentation—With respect to carbohydrates, this term, in its broadest sense, embraces all reactions which are brought about by the action of microorganisms (fungi, bacteria, etc). Thousands of such reactions are known, but the mechanisms are usually incompletely understood except that, in general, they are referable to enzymes elaborated by the organism. Among the best understood are the interactions of various yeasts with certain D-monosaccharides to yield alcohol. The commercial production of various other organic compounds (eg, *n*-butyl alcohol from the action of *Clostridium acetobutylicum* on starch, citric acid from the action of fungi of the *Aspergillus niger* group on sucrose, and L-sorbose from the action of *Acetobacter suboxydans* on D-sorbitol) represent additional applications of fermentation processes. The fermentability of carbohydrates under various conditions has proved a useful tool in carbohydrate classification, and intimate categorization of fermentation characteristics may someday make possible a better understanding of diverse phenomena associated with the cause and cure of disease.

Occurrence

Carbohydrates occur abundantly in nature. Indeed, it has been estimated that more carbohydratic material occurs naturally than all other organic material combined. While they are preponderantly important in the vegetable kingdom, carbohydrates also occur generously and play very important biologic roles in the animal world. The naturally occurring carbohydrates are almost exclusively pentosic and hexosic. In order to accomplish her needs, nature engages generously both in the condensation of monosaccharides to produce polysaccharides and in the reverse hydrolytic operation. In attempting to unlock nature's secrets, man's efforts to date have been directed very largely toward the hydrolysis of polysaccharides as nature provides them.

Glucose and fructose are the only monosaccharides which occur in the free state to any important extent. They are present in the juices of many ripe fruits. Among the disaccharides, only sucrose (cane or beet sugar) and lactose (milk sugar) occur in important quantities. Prominent, naturally occurring, hexosan polysaccharides include cellulose (the primary structural material in the vegetable world), starch (the primary carbohydrate reserve in the vegetable world), and glycogen, often dubbed animal starch (the primary carbohydrate reserve in the animal world). Pentosan polysaccharides occur abundantly in cereal straws and beans, eg, corn cobs; they are distinguished by the fact that they yield the industrially important furfural upon suitable treatment with sulfuric acid.

Carbohydrate derivatives (chemical combinations with noncarbohydratic substances or carbohydrates slightly altered chemically) occur plentifully in nature. The role of monosaccharide phosphate esters in physiological utilization has already been mentioned. A special class of derivatives, the *glycosides*, are discussed in the next section. Other classes include the *gums*, *pectins*, *mucilages*, *glycoproteins*, and *glycolipids* (*cerebrosides*). Chitin, a condensation polymer of *N*-acetyl-D-glucosamine (contains NH_2 instead of OH in the 2 position) comprises the skeletal material of crabs, lobsters, and insects of the arthropoda class. This same acetylglucosamine is also present in hyaluronic acid, an important constituent of connective tissue. Many bacteria have been shown to elaborate complex carbohydratic materials, and some are known to have immunologic import.

Official Carbohydrates

Examples of official articles in the various classes of carbohydrates follow.

Monosaccharides—Dextrose; Fructose; and Glucose, Liquid (mixture).

Disaccharides—Lactose; and Sucrose.

Polysaccharides—Dextran; Starch; and Cotton.

Natural Products (other than the above and which are important because of their carbohydrate or carbohydrate derivative content)—Acacia; Agar; Pectin; Plantago Seed; and Tragacanth.

Carbohydrate Derivatives (other than the above) —Aurothioglucose; Cellulose, Oxidized; Cellulose Acetate Phthalate; Ethylcellulose; Hydroxypropyl Methylcellulose; Methylcellulose; Pyroxylin; Sodium Alginate; Sodium Carboxymethylcellulose; and Sucrose Octaacetate.

Carbohydrate residues are essential components of glycosides (this page) and are frequently present in antibiotics (eg, erythromycin, streptomycin, novobiocin, etc) and in various other biologically active substances (eg, enzymes, coenzymes, glycoproteins, vitamins, etc).

Glycosides

Glycosides may be defined broadly as condensation products of sugars with various kinds of organic hydroxy (occasionally thiol) compounds, with the added restriction that the OH of the hemiacetal portion of the carbohydrate must participate in the condensation. It is obvious that the polysaccharides are also encompassed in this broad definition; and, indeed, some authors treat polysaccharides as a subclass (*holosides*) of the glycosides. In this text, however, the term glycoside is reserved to embrace products resulting from condensation of a sugar molecule with a nonsugar entity. Some authors refer to these glycosides as *heterosides* in contradistinction to the holosides. The nonsugar portion is termed an *aglycone* (or *aglycon*), or a *genin*. From a structural viewpoint, the glycosides may be looked upon as internal acetals (see below).

The most characteristic chemical property of the glycosides is their susceptibility to hydrolysis, whereby they yield their sugar and nonsugar moieties. Indeed, it is through identification of the hydrolytic decomposition products that the composition of glycosides is commonly revealed. In general, the hydrolysis is energetically catalyzed by proton and is commonly brought about in the laboratory by digestion with dilute acid. Nature produces many enzymes which also catalyze the hydrolysis; these are often quite specific in their actions. The enzymes frequently occur in the same plant along with the glycosides, but usually in different cells. When the structure of the plant is destroyed by grinding or other means, the enzyme contacts the glycoside and soon exerts its hydrolytic action. It is, therefore, necessary to destroy any enzymes which are present before attempting to isolate glycosidal constituents.

Classification—In modern terminology, the glycosides are usually classified according to the identity of their sugar moiety. Thus, in glucosides, the sugar moiety is glucose; in fructosides, it is fructose; in galactosides, it is galactose; etc. In older literature, the term *glucoside* is used in a generic sense and is then synonymous with the modern term *glycoside*.

Classification according to the complexity of the sugar moiety is frequently employed; ie, *monosides* if the sugar is a monosaccharide, *biosides* if a disaccharide, *triosides*, etc. Total classification on the basis of the aglycones, while feasible, is intricate because of the large variety of aglycones; however, with certain classes of glycosides, eg, the cardiotonics, such subclassification is occasionally encountered in the literature.

The fundamental feature of systematic glycoside nomenclature is that the terminal "e" in the name of the sugar is changed to "ide." However, with increasing complexity of the glycoside, systematic names soon become quite cumbersome and are seldom employed in common practice. Both the IUPAC and Chemical Abstracts systems therefore admit the commonly used trivial names.

Occurrence—Glycosides are widely distributed in the plant kingdom. Many fruits and other parts (eg, seeds, barks, and leaves) of plants contain them. The pigments of flowers (anthocyanins) are of glycosidic character. Glycosides of animal origin are relatively rare. The aglycones of the majority of glycosides are of cyclic, and frequently of aromatic, structure. Steroidal aglycones are very common.

Many naturally occurring compounds which are not usually classed among the glycosides actually contain glycosidic linkages in their structures. Examples include novobiocin and streptomycin among the antibiotics, solanine and various other alkaloids (glucoalkaloids), nucleosides (consist of a purine or pyrimidine base linked with D-ribose or D-2-deoxyribose), etc.

Table II portrays a number of common glycosides selected partly on the basis of pharmaceutical interest and partly because they display a variety of aglycones and sugars.

Structure of Glycosides—Two series of stereoisomeric glycosides are known, the α- and β-glycosides. Taking the methyl-D-glucosides as a simple example, they are represented by the following formulas:

α-Methyl-D-glucoside   **β-Methyl-D-glucoside**

The glycosidic linkage is formed by dehydration involving a hydroxyl group of the aglycone (methanol here) and the hydroxyl group on the hemiacetal carbon of the sugar, thus forming an acetal type of structure (see page 432). If the OR (in the above case, OCH_3) group is in the same steric sense as the CH_2OH group on C^5, the glycoside configuration is designated β; if in the opposite steric sense, it is designated as α. For an illustration of how this relationship is reflected in the Haworth-type formulas, see amygdalin, a typical β glycoside, below. The great majority of naturally occurring glycosides are of the β variety.

The same enzyme is often able to hydrolyze different glycosides, but the α- and β-stereoisomers of the same glycoside are usually not hydrolyzed by the same enzyme. *Emulsin*, for instance, has been found to hydrolyze all β-glycosides and, therefore, those glycosides which are attacked by emulsin are regarded as β-glycosides. Maltase hydrolyzes only α-glycoside.

The sugar in a large number of glycosides is D-glucose, hence the former designation "glucosides," but many important glycosides contain other sugar moieties as, for example:

D-*Glucose* is the sugar constituent of arbutin, salicin, and sinigrin.
Galactose is found in the digitalis glycoside, digitonin.
D-*Arabinose* is found in α-hederin, helleborein, and barbaloin.
Digitoxose is found in digitoxin and other digitalis glycosides.
Cymarose is the sugar of the glycoside cymarin found in several species of *Apocynum*.
Rhamnose occurs in baptisin, hesperidin, frangulin, ouabain, quercitrin, rutin, and xanthorhamnin.

The carbohydrate in condensation union with the aglycone is frequently a di- or polysaccharide, eg, amygdalin, digitoxin, and rutin (see Table II). In many instances it is possible, under carefully controlled hydrolysis, to cleave only a portion of the aglycone moiety of the natural (*primary*) glycoside, thus yielding a derived substance which is still glycosidic. Amygdalin, for example, hydrolyzes under the influence of the enzyme amygdalase to yield glucose and prunasin (see Table II). Such derived glycosides are often referred to as *secondary* glycosides.

The synthesis of amygdalin was announced in 1924. It has the structure shown below.

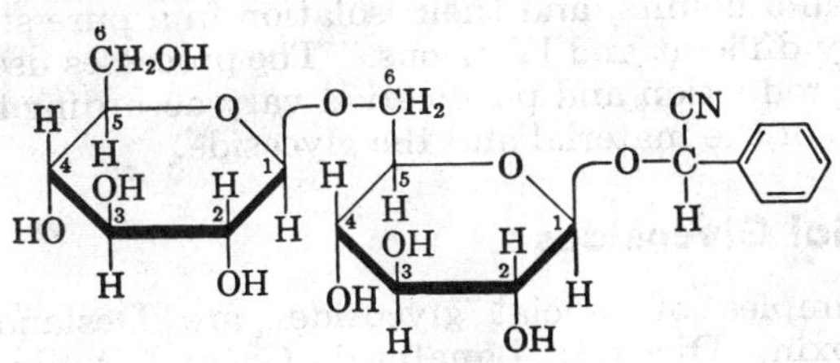

Amygdalin

The glycosidic linkage is considered to be β since it is hydrolyzed by emulsin; therefore, the formula is written as shown above with the linking oxygen on the same side of the plane of the ring as the CH_2OH group on C^5. This compound, like all other glycosides, contains several asymmetric carbon atoms and is optically active. In this instance the aglycone is also optically active due to the asymmetric carbon to which the phenyl, nitrile, hydrogen, and gentiobiose residue are attached. Salicin is another β-glycoside (see next page).

There are no simple identifying tests for glycosides. The ultimate test involves characterization of the

Table II—Selected Glycosides

Names and molecular formulas[a]	Sources[b]	Aglycone (Genin)	Sugar moieties[c]
Amygdalin $C_{20}H_{27}NO_{11}$	Seeds of *Amygdalaceae*, *Drupaceae*, and *Pomaceae*; principally from almonds	D-Mandelonitrile → Benzaldehyde + HCN	Gentiobiose → 2 D-Glucose
Arbutin (Ursin) $C_{12}H_{16}O_7$	Leaves of plants of the *Ericaceae and Rosaceae*	Hydroquinone	D-Glucose
Coniferin (Abietin; Laricin) $C_{16}H_{22}O_8$	Plants of the *Coniferae*, eg, pine, spruce, and fir	Coniferyl alcohol [4-Hydroxy-3-methoxycinnamyl alcohol]	D-Glucose
Cymarin $C_{30}H_{44}O_9$	Various species of *Apocynum*	Strophanthidin (a steroid)	Cymarose (3-Methyldigitoxose)
Daphnin $C_{15}H_{16}O_9$	Barks and flowers of varieties of *Daphne*	7,8-Dihydroxycoumarin	D-Glucose
Digitoxin $C_{41}H_{64}O_{13}$	Leaves of *Digitalis purpurea* and *Digitalis lanata*	Digitoxigenin (a steroid)	3 Digitoxose (Digitoxose is a 2,6-bis-desoxyaldohexose)
Digoxin $C_{41}H_{64}O_{14}$	Leaves of *Digitalis lanata* or *Digitalis orientalis*	Digoxigenin (12-Hydroxydigitoxigenin) (a steroid)	3 Digitoxose
Frangulin $C_{21}H_{20}O_9$	Seeds and barks of various species of *Rhamnus*, especially alder buckthorn	4,5,7-Trihydroxy-2-methyl-anthraquinone	Rhamnose
Lanatoside A $C_{49}H_{76}O_{19}$	Leaves of *Digitalis lanata*	Digitoxigenin (a steroid)	2 Digitoxose + Acetyl-digitoxose + D-Glucose
Lanatoside B $C_{49}H_{76}O_{20}$	Leaves of *Digitalis lanata*	Gitoxigenin (16-hydroxydigitoxigenin) (a steroid)	2 Digitoxose + Acetyl-digitoxose + D-Glucose
Lanatoside C $C_{49}H_{76}O_{20}$	Leaves of *Digitalis lanata*	Digoxigenin (a steroid)	2 Digitoxose + Acetyl-digitoxose + D-Glucose
Ouabain (G-strophanthin) $C_{29}H_{44}O_{12}$	Seeds of *Strophanthus gratus* and several varieties of *Acokanthera*	Ouabagenin (a steroid)	Rhamnose
Phlorizin (Phlorhizin; Phloridzin) $C_{21}H_{24}O_{10}$	Roots and leaves of various plants of the *Rosaceae*	Phloretin [β-(p-Hydroxyphenyl)-2,4,6-trihydroxypropiophenone]	D-Glucose
Prunasin $C_{14}H_{17}NO_6$	Various parts of many *Prunus* plants	D-Mandelonitrile → Benzaldehyde + HCN	D-Glucose
Rutin (Melin, Eldrin, and others) $C_{27}H_{30}O_{16}$	Occurs in many plants. Chief source is the buckwheat plant, *Fagopyrum esculentum*	Quercetin [3,3',4',5,7-pentahydroxyflavone]	Rutinose → L-Rhamnose + D-Glucose
Salicin $C_{13}H_{18}O_7$	Various *Salix* and *Populus* plants, especially from the bark	Saligenin [o-Hydroxybenzyl Alcohol]	D-Glucose
Scillaren A $C_{36}H_{52}O_{13}$	Bulbs of *Urginea maritima*	Scillaridin A (a steroid)	Scillabiose → L-Rhamnose + D-Glucose
Sinigrin (Potassium Myronate) $C_{10}H_{16}KNO_9S_2$	Seeds of *Brassica nigra*, *Brassica juncea*, and other plants of the *Cruciferae*	$CH_2:CH.CH_2.N:C(SH).OSO_3K$ → $CH_2:CH.CH_2.NCS + KHSO_4$	D-Glucose
K-Strophanthin-β $C_{36}H_{54}O_{14}$	Seeds of *Strophanthus Kombé*	Strophanthidin (a steroid)	Strophanthobiose → cymarose + D-Glucose

[a] Shown for the anhydrous forms. As isolated, many glycosides are hydrated.
[b] Typical and well-known, but not exclusive.
[c] Produced on complete hydrolysis or as otherwise indicated.

Salicin

hydrolytic cleavage products. Methods for the detection of glycosides and for their quantitative determination involve the estimation of reducing sugars before and after hydrolysis by boiling with dilute acids, or by the action of enzymes.

Saponins—The saponins are a group of amorphous, colloidal glycosides, which are readily soluble in water and which produce a froth when the aqueous solution is agitated. They are excellent emulsifying agents and the aqueous solutions of some of them were formerly used as detergents to replace soap (see *Quillaja*). They are acrid in taste and in powder form cause sneezing. Many conform to the general formula $C_nH_{2n-8}O_{10}$.

The aglycones, usually prepared by acid-catalyzed hydrolysis, are usually termed *sapogenins*. Two general types are well known, *viz, steroid* as in digitonin and *triterpenoid* as in aesculin.

Many of the saponins are markedly toxic. These are called *sapotoxins*. Saponins usually exert a powerful hemolytic action on red blood corpuscles. They have been used as fish poisons.

The saponins are widely distributed in the botanical kingdom. The commercial product *saponin* is prepared from the yucca plant or from Quillaja.

Properties—The greater portion of the known glyco-sides, when pure, are colorless or white, optically active, and soluble in alcohol or in diluted alcohol. They are extracted from the plant material by water, alcohol, or a mixture of the two. The glycosides occur in the plant in small amounts, and their isolation in a pure state is usually difficult and laborious. The processes used for their production and purification vary according to the nature of the material and the glycoside.

Official Glycosides

Examples of official glycosides are Deslanoside; Digitoxin; Digoxin; Lanatoside C; and Ouabain.

The physiological actions of many drugs of plant origin are referable to glycosidal constituents. Examples include aloe, cascara, digitalis, gentian, rhubarb, sarsaparilla, senna, squill, strophanthus, taraxacum, viburnum, wild cherry and many others.

The wide spectrum of physiological actions exerted by these drugs invites scientific curiosity; and maximally useful elucidation of the mysteries associated with the occurrence and composition of the glycosides they contain (as these may relate to their possible therapeutic value) awaits disclosure. It is interesting to note that various plant products formerly of empiric importance as pharmaceuticals are now recognized to contain aglycones which are related to modern synthetics having impressive therapeutic significance. As a single example, dioscorea, one of the Mexican yams, formerly used as a crude drug in the treatment of various rheumatic disorders, contains the sapogen diosgenin which is conveniently convertible chemically into cortisone.

Lipids

The lipids, known also as *lipins* or *lipoids*, are the fat and fat-like substances which occur in plants and animals. Like the carbohydrates and proteins, the lipids constitute a very important group of organic substances from the standpoint of physiological utilization. Unlike the carbohydrates and proteins, the lipids comprise a rather heterogeneous group of substances in terms of chemical composition. They are grouped together primarily on the basis of solubility characteristics; in general, they are soluble in the usual fat solvents such as ether and chloroform and are insoluble in water. The lipids may be divided into five classes according to their chemical structure:

1. **Fixed Oils and Fats**—esters of glycerol and fatty acids. An example is olive oil. Fixed oils which are solid at ordinary temperatures are commonly called *fats*. An example is lard.

2. **Waxes**—esters of high molecular weight, monohydric alcohols, and high molecular weight fatty acids. An example is spermaceti.

3. **Sterols**—alcohols containing the cyclopentaphenanthrene (steroid) nucleus (see page 479). Typical examples include the familiar cholesterol and ergosterol.

4. **Phospholipids (Phosphatides)**—esters consisting of glycerol in combination with fatty acids, phosphoric acid, and certain nitrogenous compounds. Pharmaceutically, the most important members of this group are the lecithins.

5. **Glycolipids (Cerebrosides)**—substances isolated from the brain and from various other sources which on hydrolysis yield fatty acids, galactose, and the nitrogenous compound *sphingosine* (2-amino-4-octadecene-1,3-diol). Examples are phrenosin and kerasin. Because the sugar moiety is practically always galactose, the glycolipids are sometimes referred to as galactolipids. At present, the glycolipids have no pharmaceutical applications and will not be further discussed.

Fixed Oils and Fats

Fixed oils and fats are mixtures of glyceryl esters of the so-called high fatty acids, ie, the higher molecular weight aliphatic acids, especially palmitic, stearic, and oleic acids. The individual glyceryl esters themselves are frequently referred to as *glycerides*.

The difference in consistency between fixed oils and fats is caused by the relative proportions of liquid and solid glyceryl esters present. Fixed oils contain relatively high quantities of liquid glycerides, such as glyceryl oleate, whereas fats are relatively rich in solid glycerides such as glyceryl stearate. Glycerides of unsaturated fatty acids have lower melting points than those of saturated acids with the same number of carbon atoms.

Fixed oils are to be distinguished sharply from volatile oils. Physically, the former are nonvolatile under ordinary conditions (hence the name *fixed* oils), in contradistinction to the latter which, as the name implies, are volatile. From the standpoint of composition, the volatile oils differ greatly one from the other; but, as a group, they differ from fixed oils in that they do not contain glyceryl esters.

Preparation—Most of the fixed oils and fats are obtained by *expression* from the plant or animal tissues in which they occur. Generally the material is first ground and subsequently submitted to hydraulic pressure, and to heat when necessary.

The oils as obtained by the first expression usually are of the highest commercial value, as, for example, olive oil where the first pressings are called *virgin olive oil*, but sometimes the expressed oil from plant tissues is crude in its character and requires subsequent purification, as in the case of cottonseed oil. Fixed oils and fats are frequently bleached by treatment with fuller's earth or similar clays, and subsequent filtration.

Some few oils for technical purposes are not obtained by expression but are extracted from the plant tissues by means of *volatile solvents* which are later recovered. Animal fats and oils are usually separated from the tissues by the process known as *rendering* which consists in heating the tissues until the fat melts and separates mechanically.

Analytical Characteristics—The analytical factors of greater importance in identifying fixed oils and in judging of their quality are the *Iodine value* (page 588), *Saponification value* (page 588), *Refractive index* (page 594), and *Acid value* (page 588). The specific gravity, color, odor, and congealing point are of little value. Some oils, such as cottonseed oil and sesame oil, are identifiable by specific tests, but the identification of a fixed oil is only inferentially possible as a rule, after taking many physical and chemical factors into account.

Properties—Fixed oils and fats are rather distinctive in their physical properties. They are greasy to the touch and leave a permanent oily stain upon filter paper. They are all lighter than water and insoluble therein, but are soluble in ether, chloroform, and some other water-immiscible solvents. A few of them, such as castor oil, are soluble in alcohol. When purified, they are nearly colorless and of a bland odor and taste with very little distinctiveness. The yellow color of fats is usually due to the presence of carotene, one of the provitamins A.

When heated moderately, fats liquefy and oils become thinner. When heated strongly, they undergo decomposition with the production of acrid, flammable vapors; and when ignited, they burn with a sooty flame. The acridity of an overheated fixed oil or fat is due largely to the formation of *acrolein* (*propenal*).

The property common to all fats and fixed oils is their propensity to undergo hydrolysis to yield glycerol and the fatty acids representative of the fat or oil. Uncatalyzed, the reaction proceeds very slowly; it is therefore commonly accelerated by employing high temperatures and high pressures and by the presence of either acids or alkalies. If alkalies are employed, the liberated acids are automatically converted into their corresponding metallic salts. Since such salts are commonly referred to as soaps, the alkali-catalyzed hydrolysis of fats and fixed oils is frequently referred to as *saponification*. The term is also frequently used to refer to hydrolysis of all kinds of esters, regardless of how accomplished. Many naturally occurring enzymes also catalyze fat and fixed oil hydrolysis. Such enzymes are termed *lipases*. Steapsin of the human pancreatic juice is an important example.

Constituents—Three glycerides, *olein, palmitin,* and *stearin,* are common to many fixed oils.

Olein is *glyceryl trioleate* [$C_3H_5(C_{18}H_{33}O_2)_3$], a liquid at ordinary temperature. It is the predominating constituent in expressed almond oil, in lard oil, and in many of the more fluid animal oils and those of vegetable origin. It is separated and purified by cold expression, the other constituents being retained by their lack of fluidity at low temperatures.

Palmitin is *glyceryl tripalmitate* [$C_3H_5(C_{16}H_{31}O_2)_3$]. It is a solid at ordinary temperature (m. p. 60°). It predominates in palm oil and coconut oil.

Stearin is *glyceryl tristearate* [$C_3H_5(C_{18}H_{35}O_2)_3$]. Its melting point is 71°. It predominates in many of the solid fats and may be separated by expression under controlled temperature conditions, which removes the olein and palmitin.

Olein, and glyceryl esters of other unsaturated acids, may be converted into stearin by *hydrogenation* in the presence of a catalyst such as finely divided nickel. Liquid oils such as cottonseed, soybean, and peanut are often commercially transformed (hardened) by this process into solid fats. The proprietary cooking fat, *Crisco*, is a well-known example. Through partial hydrogenation, the consistency of such hardened oils may be varied between wide limits.

The glycerides in a fixed oil may be *simple* or *mixed*. In simple glycerides, such as olein, palmitin, and stearin, all three fatty acid groups are identical. In the more frequently encountered mixed glycerides more than one fatty acid is present. Because of the many possible combinations in the mixed glycerides, different fats having entirely different physical properties often show the same chemical analysis. The following formula illustrates a mixed glyceride:

$$C_{15}H_{31}COOCH_2 \quad \alpha'$$
$$C_{17}H_{35}COOCH \quad \beta$$
$$C_{17}H_{33}COOCH_2 \quad \alpha$$

α-Oleo-α′,β-palmitostearin
(or 1-oleo-3-palmito-2-stearin)

Mono-, di-, and triglycerides, containing, respectively, one, two, or three molecules of fatty acid esterified with one molecule of glycerol, have been prepared synthetically, but only triglycerides occur commonly in nature.

Table III above lists the formulas and some important sources of the more common saturated and unsaturated acids occurring in natural fats. There are approximately 50 of these, and except for isovaleric acid (the only odd-numbered fatty acid) which is found in the blubbers of the dolphin and the porpoise, and a few of the rarer acids, such as hydnocarpic (cyclic acid from Chaulmoogra Oil) and tuberculostearic (branched chain acid found in the tubercle bacillus), the natural fatty acids are nearly all straight-chain and contain an even number of carbon atoms (C_4 to C_{26}).

Of all the fatty acids, stearic, palmitic, and oleic are the most widely distributed. Stearic acid is found mostly in animal fats, but it is occasionally an important constituent in vegetable oils. The saturated fatty acids lower than C_{12} are found in the milk of mammals, although butter fat contains all of the even-numbered fatty acids from C_4 to C_{18} as well as olein.

Oils and fats, when subjected to pressure at certain temperatures, can be fractionated to some extent into the glycerides composing it. On aging, fixed oils often develop a precipitate of stearin which will reliquefy on warming.

In the days before artificial refrigeration the oils expressed in the summer (at a higher temperature), when the stearin was kept in solution to a greater ex-

Table III—Fatty Acids

Name	Formula	Mol. wt.	Source
Butyric	$CH_3—(CH_2)_2—COOH$	88	Butter fat
Caproic	$CH_3—(CH_2)_4—COOH$	116	Butter fat, goat's milk, coconut oil
Caprylic	$CH_3—(CH_2)_6—COOH$	144	Coconut oil, butter fat, palm oil butter
Capric	$CH_3—(CH_2)_8—COOH$	172	Butter fat, coconut oil
Lauric	$CH_3—(CH_2)_{10}—COOH$	200	Coconut oil, palm kernel oil
Myristic	$CH_3—(CH_2)_{12}—COOH$	228	Nutmeg oil, butter fat
Palmitic	$CH_3—(CH_2)_{14}—COOH$	256	Palm oil, nearly all fats
Stearic	$CH_3—(CH_2)_{16}—COOH$	284	Beef, mutton tallow
Arachidic	$CH_3—(CH_2)_{18}—COOH$	313	Peanut oil
Behenic	$CH_3—(CH_2)_{20}—COOH$	341	Ben oil
Lignoceric	$CH_3—(CH_2)_{22}—COOH$	369	Phospholipids
Oleic	$CH_3—(CH_2)_7—\overset{cis}{CH}=CH—(CH_2)_7—COOH$	282	Olive oil, almond oil, peanut oil, corn oil
Linoleic acid	$CH_3(CH_2)_4\overset{cis}{CH}=CHCH_2\overset{cis}{CH}=CH—(CH_2)_7COOH$	280	Cottonseed oil, peanut oil, linseed oil, safflower oil, corn oil
Linolenic acid	$CH_3CH_2\overset{cis}{CH}=CHCH_2\overset{cis}{CH}=CHCH_2\overset{cis}{CH}=CH(CH_2)_7COOH$	278	Linseed oil, seed fats

Table IV—Fixed Oils

Fixed oil	Iodine value	Saponification value
Almond Oil, Expressed	95–105	190–200
Castor Oil	83– 88	179–185
Coconut Oil	7– 10	251–262
Corn Oil	112–128	187–193
Cottonseed Oil	109–116	190–198
Linseed Oil	Not less than 170	187–195
Olive Oil	79– 88	190–195
Palm Oil	49– 57	196–205
Peanut Oil	88– 98	186–194
Persic Oil	90–108	185–195
Safflower Oil	122–141	188–203
Sesame Oil	103–115	188–193

tent, were found to deposit the stearin much more readily than those oils that were pressed in the winter (at a lower temperature), and "*summer pressed*" and "*winter pressed*" were commercial designations which still obtain, although at the present time it is a matter of temperature control at the time of pressing, irrespective of the season.

Drying and Nondrying Oils—Fixed oils are classified into *drying* and *nondrying* oils. The former when exposed to the air undergo oxidation with the formation of a tough hard film. Linseed oil is an example of the class of drying oils which find their greatest use in the manufacture of paints and varnishes. The nondrying oils when exposed to the air remain sticky to the touch for an indefinite period and therefore cannot be used in paints and varnishes. Olive oil and expressed almond oil are examples of nondrying oils. The drying quality is caused by the presence of unsaturated fatty acids of a distinctive character such as linoleic and linolenic acids.

Table IV lists the iodine and saponification values for some common fixed oils. The iodine value gives an indication of the amount of unsaturated fatty acids present and the saponification value varies with the length of the fatty acid chains. Thus these two values are specified when a definite degree of unsaturation and a definite molecular weight range for the fatty acids in oils are desired.

Uses—Fats and fixed oils contain certain unsaturated fatty acids which are essential foods. Their absence in the human diet has produced eczematous skin conditions, and in experimental animals has resulted in scaly skin, emaciation, necrosis, and premature death. Experimental evidence exists to support the view that fats such as safflower oil which are rich in linoleic and possibly other unsaturated acids *may* play an important role in the mobilization and utilization of food cholesterol, provided dietary fat intake is suitably controlled. This is of particular nutritional and medical interest in connection with possibly preventing and correcting the hypercholesterolemia which is commonly observed in atherosclerosis. Certain oils, such as those of peanut and sesame, are used extensively as solvents in the preparation of intramuscular injections. A few oils have medicinal actions in their own right—eg, castor oil as a cathartic, cod liver oil as an antirachitic, and olive oil as an emollient. Chaulmoogra oil was formerly used in the treatment of leprosy.

Salts of several of the fatty acids are fungicidal. Other derivatives of glycerides are soaps and various related surface-active compounds which are employed as detergents and germicides.

Waxes

Waxes, like fixed oils and fats, are esters of fatty acids. They differ, however, in that the alcohol represented is *not* glycerol. In place of this trihydric alcohol is found one of the sterols (this page) or one of the higher, even-numbered, monohydric alcohols from C_{16} to C_{36}.

Waxes often contain these alcohols and fatty acids (C_{24} to C_{36}) in free state, and some of the waxes obtained from plants also contain paraffin hydrocarbons. The esters in waxes are usually much more resistant to saponification than the glycerides of fats and fixed oils.

In the body are found waxes containing sterols, the concentrations of which vary widely when the body is diseased. Excessive quantities of cholesterol, for example, are present in diabetes, obstructive jaundice, and hypothyroidism. The fact that the tubercle bacillus has been shown to contain a wax may prove to have some significance. Wool fat obtained from the wool of sheep consists of cholesterol esters and related substances, and this "fat" is therefore chemically a wax. Other examples of naturally occurring waxes include Beeswax (contains myricyl palmitate, $C_{30}H_{61}C_{16}H_{31}O_2$, as a predominant constituent) and sperm oil (contains cetyl palmitate, $C_{16}H_{33}C_{16}H_{31}O_2$, as a predominant constituent).

Various waxes find extensive commercial application as ingredients of polishes and lubricants and in the manufacture of candles. The pharmaceutical applications of waxes involve primarily the preparations of lotions and ointments with desired physical characteristics.

Sterols

The sterols are alcohols structurally related to the *steroids*, those naturally occurring compounds, obtained from plants and animals, which contain the partly or completely hydrogenated 17*H*-cyclopenta-[*a*]phenanthrene nucleus. In addition to the sterols, the steroids include various other substances, such as compounds of adrenal origin, certain alkaloids, antirachitic vitamins, bile acids, cardiac glycosides, saponins, sex hormones, and toad poisons. The general formula for the basic structure of these compounds may be *represented* as follows. In actual conformation, however, the structure is not planar.

General steroid formula

The rings are conventionally lettered and numbered as indicated, and the Greek letter Δ is often used to indicate the location of any double bonds. Since usually one or more rings are completely saturated, several centers of asymmetry are present; this, plus restricted rotations due to ring fusions, results in rather complex stereochemical relationships. In the naturally occurring compounds, substitutions in the rings occur most frequently on C^3, C^7, and C^{11}.

Following the more or less standard convention, the direction of projection from the plane of the ring system of substituting groups located at centers of asymmetry is commonly indicated by use of the letters α and β. An α-substituting group is viewed as projecting beneath the ring plane and is represented by a broken line; a β-substituting group is viewed as projecting above the ring plane and is represented by a solid line. See the examples provided below.

The prefixes *cis* and *trans* are also often employed (but *not* in standardized nomenclature) to distinguish the α- and β-members of a pair of compounds which are otherwise stereochemically identical. However, this requires the selection of a substituting group to serve as a reference point in the steroid molecule, and a "rule" frequently used is that the nearest angular (branching off of a ring) methyl group is so selected. In the case of the sterols, for example, the angular methyl group nearest to the 3-hydroxyl group is the one at C^{10} and is represented as having the β-configuration; thus the 3-β-hydroxycholestane becomes *cis*-3-hydroxycholestane, and the 3-α-hydroxycholestane becomes *trans*-3-hydroxycholestane. Most naturally occurring sterols have the 3-hydroxyl group in the β, or *cis*, position. The prefix *epi* is often employed to designate specifically the corresponding epimers in which this OH is α, or *trans;* eg, epicholesterol and epicoprosterol.

Classification of Steroids—Different investigators use slightly different methods of classifying the steroids. One method is to divide them into five classes according to the type of substituent group at carbon 17, ie, group R. For a detailed discussion which is beyond the scope of this text see Burger, *Medicinal Chemistry*, vol II, Wiley, New York, 1961, p. 586 *et seq.* A classification commonly used is as follows:

1. *Sterols*—R is an aliphatic side chain. They contain one or more OH groups attached in alicyclic linkage.
2. *Sex Hormones*—C^{17} bears a ketonic or hydroxyl group and frequently carries a two-carbon side chain. See page 988.
3. *Cardiac Glycosides*—R is a lactone ring. The glycosides also contain sugars linked through oxygen in other parts of the molecule. Hydrolysis yields this sugar and the *cardiac aglycone*. See page 858.
4. *Bile Acids*—R is a five-carbon side chain terminating in a carboxylic acid group. The bile acids are treated in Chapter 44, page 794.
5. *Sapogenins*—R contains an oxacyclic (ethereal) ring system.

Further discussion of steroids is limited in this chapter to the sterols. Justification for this limitation resides primarily in the lipoidal characteristics of the sterols as evidenced by (1) their distribution in nature, especially the distribution in body tissues; and (2) their solubility characteristics. It is to be noted also that the sterols are important, naturally occurring compounds which serve as the starting points in the commercial synthesis of various other steroidal compounds. Indeed, the many advances in pharmaceutical application of diverse types of steroids over the past decade have encouraged intensive investigation into the occurrence, isolation, and possible utilization of natural sterols for such synthesis.

Description and Properties of Sterols

The parent hydrocarbon of natural sterols is cholestane which exists in two forms depending on the configuration of the hydrogen atom at C^5. These are drawn below and labeled with their standard (IUPAC) names and, in parentheses, their trivial names:

5α-Cholestane
(Cholestane)

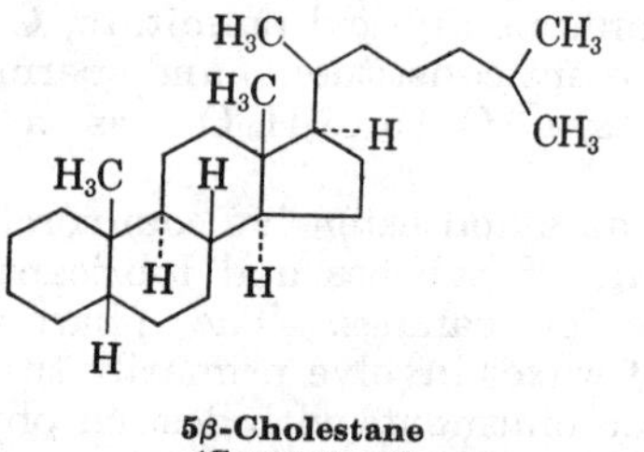

5β-Cholestane
(Coprostane)

The characteristic function of natural sterols is the 3-hydroxyl in *beta* orientation. Thus, 5α-cholestan-3β-ol and 5β-cholestan-3β-ol are commonly looked upon as the parent sterols. Other sterols are often named as derivatives of them although most have commonly accepted trivial names such as cholesterol, ergosterol, stigmasterol, etc. These parent sterols are shown below along with their various names. The two cholesterols are also illustrated. In trivial notation, the prefix *epi-* is employed to denote the unnatural *alpha* orientation of the 3-hydroxyl. Note that in the cholest-5-enols, there is no H at C^5 and thus no α or β accompanies the numeral 5.

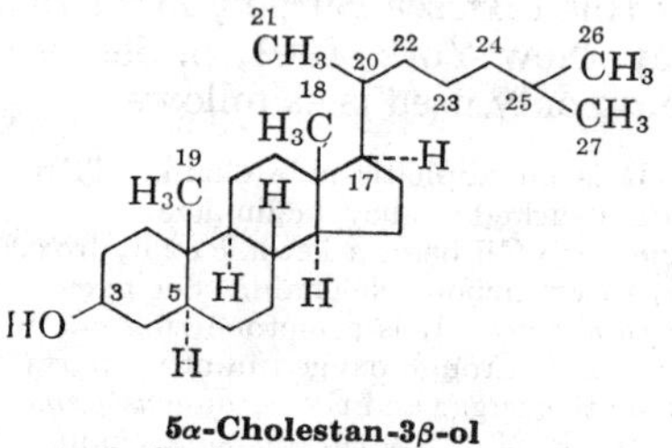

5α-Cholestan-3β-ol
3β-Hydroxy-5α-cholestane
(Cholestanol)

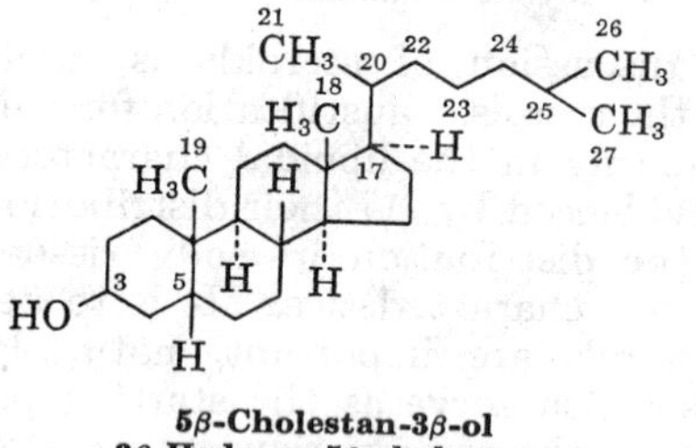

5β-Cholestan-3β-ol
3β-Hydroxy-5β-cholestane
(Coprostanol)

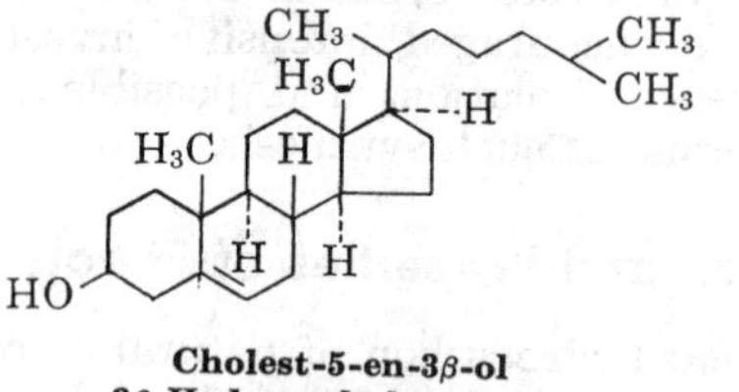

Cholest-5-en-3β-ol
3β-Hydroxycholest-5-ene
Δ⁵-Cholesten-3β-ol
3β-Hydroxy-Δ⁵-cholestene
(Cholesterol)

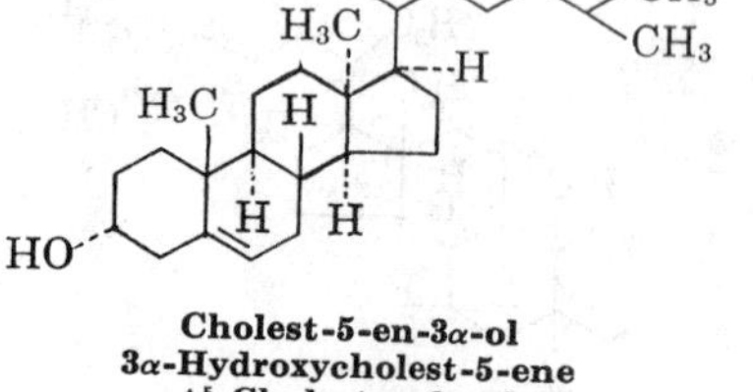

Cholest-5-en-3α-ol
3α-Hydroxycholest-5-ene
Δ⁵-Cholesten-3α-ol
3α-Hydroxy-Δ⁵-cholestene
(Epicholesterol)

Sterols occur abundantly in nature and often constitute a sizable fraction of the total unsaponifiable portion of lipoidal extractive matter from animal and vegetable tissue.

Sterols are often classified on the basis of their occurrence as follows:

Class Name	Origin	Examples
Zoösterols	Animal	Cholesterol
		Pregnanediol
		Coprosterol
Phytosterols	Plant	Stigmasterol
		Sitosterol(s)
Mycosterols	Yeasts and Fungi	Zymosterol
		Ergosterol

Most natural sterols contain the single functional alcoholic hydroxyl at the C^3-position. The pregnanediols, containing an additional C^{20}-hydroxyl, constitute an important class of exceptions. The pregnanediols are exceptional also in that they contain only a two-carbon chain at C^{17}, whereas most of the others contain an eight-, or higher-, carbon chain at the same point.

In their pure state, the sterols are white, crystalline compounds, commonly distinguishable from each other by means of their melting points and optical rotations. They are generally insoluble in water but are readily soluble in lipid solvents such as hydrocarbons, ethers, ketones, chlorinated hydrocarbons, carbon disulfide, etc. The difference in solubility in cold and hot alcohol often renders crystallization from alcohol a useful purification procedure.

The common chemical properties of the naturally occurring sterols are largely referable to the presence of secondary alcohol functions, especially the one common to all at the C^3-position, and to points of unsaturation which occur most commonly at C^5, C^7, and C^{22}. Thus, at the carbinol locations, properly regulated oxidation produces ketone derivatives and suitable esterification and etherification procedures yield expected ester and ether derivatives. For example, cholesterol is readily oxidized to yield the corresponding 3-ketone (cholestenone, or, more descriptively, cholest-5-ene-3-one). Also it reacts readily with aryl halides and other esterificants to yield various esters, eg, cholesterol acetate, palmitate, etc, and with alkyl halides and dialkyl sulfates to yield ethers. The usual types of addition reactions (eg, with hydrogen, hydrogen halides, and halogens) as well as various oxidative cleavages are commonly evident at the locations of alicyclic or aliphatic unsaturation. Cholesterol, for example, is readily hydrogenated to yield dihydrocholesterol and readily adds halogens to produce the so-called cholesterol dihalides (5,6-dihalocholestan-3-ols). Special attention is called to the fact that even such simple chemical operations as the above very commonly result in the creation of new possibilities for the formation of stereoisomeric modifications. As a single example, the dihydrocholesterol cited previously as a hydrogenation product of cholesterol exists in two forms which differ with respect to whether the added H at C^5 is in α or β configuration (see cholestanol and coprostanol formulas, this page). The stereochemical considerations constitute collectively one of the most perplexing problems associated with the physiological production and utilization of all steroid compounds.

Several empirical color reactions have been developed which are useful in steroid chemistry for purposes of identification. Most prominently cited are the Salkowski, Liebermann-Burchard, and Rosenheim reactions. For discussions of these, consult reference texts in biochemistry.

The 3β-hydroxysteroids readily form sparingly soluble molecular complexes with the glycoside digitonin. These complexes are commonly referred to as *digitonides*, and they find extensive application in various research operations involving isolation and characterization of the individual steroids.

Several sterols undergo intramolecular rearrangement under the influence of controlled ultraviolet radiation resulting in compounds which display antirachitic (vitamin D) activity. Thus, for example, ergosterol, a mycosterol occurring abundantly in yeast and ergot, is readily converted in good yield to ergocalciferol (vitamin D₂). The structure shown below emphasizes the locus of scission of the cyclic nucleus. The structure provided on page 1016 better portrays the stereoisomerism associated with the conjugate double bond feature.

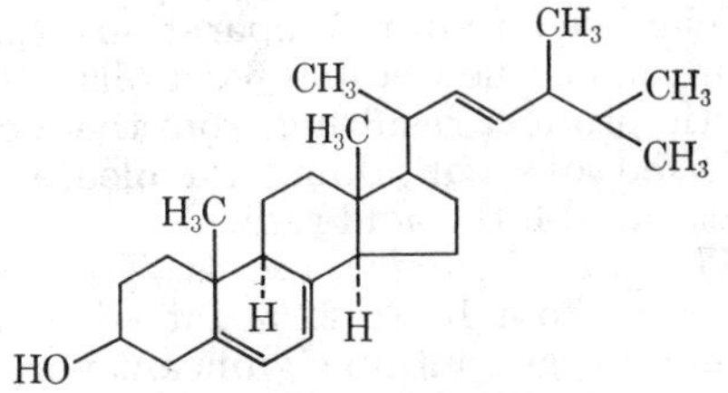

Ergosterol
5,7,22-Ergostatrien-3β-ol

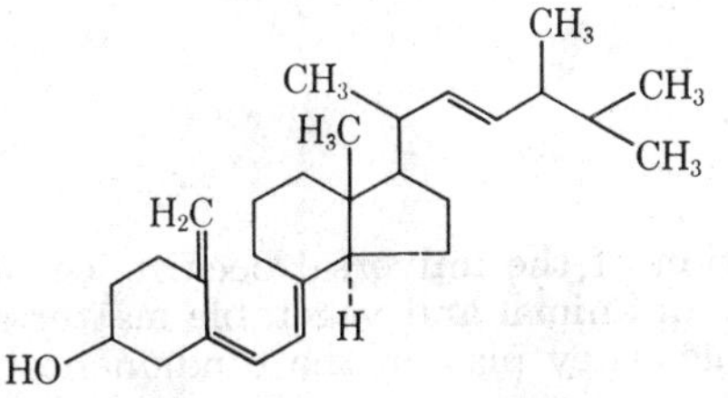

Ergocalciferol (vitamin D₂)
9,10-Seco-5,7,22-ergostatrien-3β-o

Phospholipids (Phosphatides)

The *phospholipids* (phosphatides) include all lipoidal constituents which contain phosphorus in their molecules; they appear to be essential components of every plant and animal cell. They have been divided into (1) lecithins, (2) cephalins, and (3) sphingomyelins. The chemical composition in all cases is revealed through quantitative measurement of the products resulting from hydrolysis under various conditions. The only phospholipids with pharmaceutical applications are the lecithins.

The Lecithins—When completely hydrolyzed, each molecule of a lecithin yields two molecules of fatty acid, and one molecule each of glycerol, phosphoric acid, and a basic nitrogenous compound (usually choline).

The fatty acids obtained from lecithins on hydrolysis are usually oleic, palmitic, and stearic. The phosphoric acid may be attached to the glycerol in either an α- or the β-position, forming *α-glycerophosphoric acid* or *β-glycerophosphoric acid*, respectively, and producing the corresponding series of lecithins which are known as α- and β-lecithins. The representations below are in

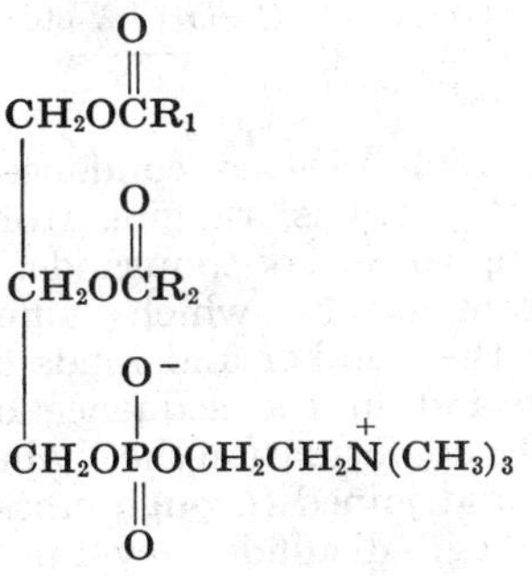

α-Lecithin 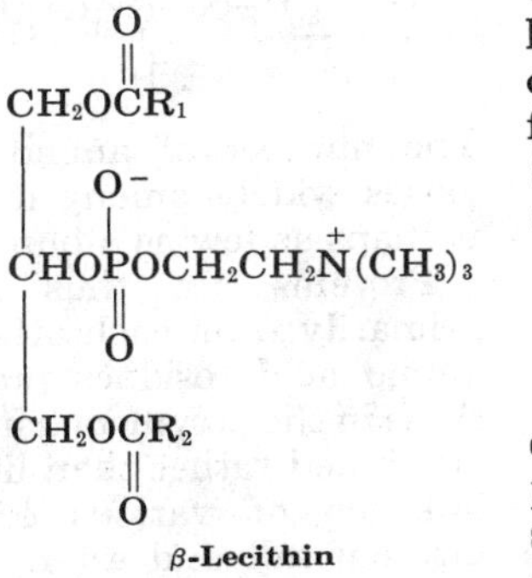   **β-Lecithin**

the *zwitterion* (internal salt) form. Each series of lecithins may differ in the fatty acids attached to the glycerol. The naturally occurring lecithins are of the α-variety.

Choline, a very strong base, is a member of the vitamin B complex (page 1026). It functions in the body to prevent accumulation of fat in the liver and also, as the acetylated derivative *acetylcholine*, is released at the parasympathetic nerve endings when these nerves are stimulated and thus controls the transmission of impulses across cholinergic synapses.

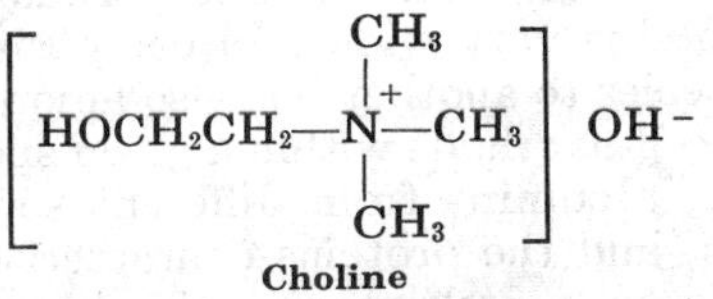

Choline

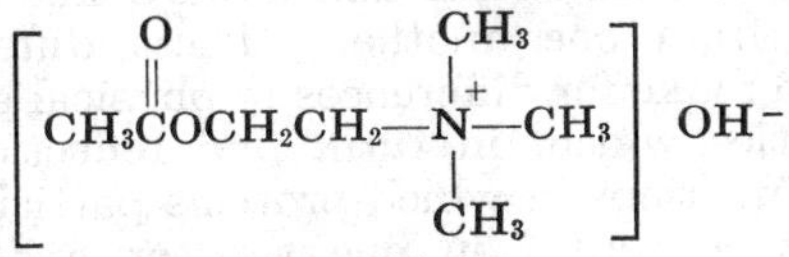

Acetylcholine

Commercially lecithin is obtained by extraction processes from egg yolk, brain tissue, or soybeans. *Ovolecithin* (*vitellin*) from eggs and *vegilecithin* from soybeans as well as purified lecithin from calves brains are used as emulsifiers, antioxidants, and stabilizers in foods and pharmaceutical preparations. Lecithins oxidize readily on exposure to air and, simultaneously, darken in color.

The Cephalins—Cephalins, which are associated with the process of blood clotting, are closely related to lecithin in structure and are known to be essential constituents of various body tissues. They differ from lecithins in that choline is replaced by *cholamine* (ethanolamine), *serine* (page 483), or *meso-inositol* (page 1029).

$HOCH_2CH_2NH_2$ $HOCH_2CH(NH_2)COOH$
Cholamine   **Serine**

The Sphingomyelins—When completely hydrolyzed, a sphingomyelin yields a fatty acid, phosphoric acid, choline, and a second nitrogenous substance, *sphingosine*, which is the unsaturated amino alcohol, 2-amino-4-octadecene-1,3-diol [$CH_3 \cdot (CH_2)_{12}$-$CH:CH \cdot CH(OH) \cdot CH(NH_2) \cdot CH_2OH$]. Sphingomyelins are found closely associated with the lecithins and cephalins in the phospholipid fraction of the brain tissue.

Official Lipids

Examples of official articles in the various classes of lipids follow.

Fixed Oils—Almond Oil; Castor Oil; Cod Liver Oil; Corn Oil; Cottonseed Oil; Olive Oil; Peanut Oil; Persic Oil; and Sesame Oil.

The official oleovitamin preparations (page 1021) also contain unspecified edible fixed oils. Iodized oil is a synthetic product resulting from the iodination of vegetable fixed oils containing an oleate radical or other unsaturated fatty acid radicals.

Fats—The only official fat is Theobroma Oil. Cocoa contains from 10 to 22% fat (theobroma oil). Various crude drugs contain significant percentages of fat, but this is incidental and their official status is not a consequence of their fat content. Crude drugs are usually defatted prior to preparing extracts.

Waxes—Carnauba Wax; Spermaceti; Lanolin; Wax, White; and Wax, Yellow.

Sterols—The only official sterols are Cholesterol and Sitosterols. Ergocalciferol and various other activated sterols are sometimes classed with the sterols although they are actually sterol derivatives (see page 481).

Proteins

Recognition of the universal occurrence of proteins in all forms of animal and vegetable matter and of the intimate roles they play in the fundamental processes of tissue formation, regeneration, and function has won for this class of substances the distinction of being the primary component of all living matter—hence the term protein, of Greek origin, meaning *first*. In sharp contrast with carbohydrates and fats which are also essential for life and which function primarily as energy sources, proteins vary widely in composition not only from one species to another but also among the various tissues and cellular fluids within a given species. Thus, for example, albumins from different sources vary in composition, and the proteins characteristic of human epithelial tissue, muscle, brain, kidney, and other tissues differ from one another. These differences in composition make for differences in physical and chemical properties which, in turn, find reflection in the diverse biofunctions in which proteins participate.

Scientists concerned in one way or another with bioactivity problems have long recognized that satisfactory elucidation of biophenomena in general depends very largely on the ability to fathom the mysteries of protein physics and chemistry. Working with the tools and techniques available prior to about 1940, progress, although important, was slow and almost exclusively analytical. In sharp contrast, the discovery and application of new methodologies have rendered subsequent progress, both analytical and synthetic, little short of phenomenal; and these advances are generously reflected in various technologies, especially in pharmacology and biochemistry.

Occurrence and Isolation

Although proteins are present in all living matter, important differences in distribution are clearly evident. With plants, in which the structural parts are essentially carbohydratic, protein concentration is usually very much higher in the seed than in any of the other plant parts. No similar gross variation is observed in the animal world, but different tissues vary considerably in their approximate percentage protein contents, eg, skin, 27; skeletal muscle, 21; brain, 11; adipose tissue, 5.

Insoluble proteins are usually isolated simply by removing contaminating material by means of a suitable array of solvents. Debridement is often facilitated through the appropriate use of enzymes. Soluble proteins are usually obtained first as crude extracts in aqueous solutions from which, after subjecting to dialysis to remove contaminating solutes, the protein is obtained either through precipitation by means of salt solutions or organic solvents or through lyophilization techniques.

As first isolated, proteins are frequently mixtures. Separation into individual components was formerly accomplished only by means of tedious fractional precipitation operations, but is nowadays achieved much more conveniently and completely through chromatographic procedures using ion exchange resins and various cellulose derivatives.

Composition and Structure

All proteins contain carbon, hydrogen, oxygen, and nitrogen. Sulfur is also generally present, phosphorus frequently, and other elements, eg, iodine, copper, iron, and zinc, occasionally. Nitrogen is the distinguishing element. It constitutes approximately 16% of most proteins and thus leads to the rough factor 6.25 generally employed for converting protein nitrogen found by analysis to protein.

The fundamental structural units of proteins are α-amino acids, about 20 of which are known to participate prominently in protein formation. All except the simplest one, glycine, are capable of existing in both D and L configurations but proteins contain only the L-enantiomorphs. The actual protein molecule consists of long chain polymers which may be looked upon as having resulted from condensation of the amino acids thus producing amide (commonly called peptide) linkages:

The number of amino acid molecules so condensed varies widely among different proteins, ranging from perhaps as few as a hundred up to tens of thousands.

Proteins are thus macromolecules which differ primarily from each other in the number and kinds of amino acid residues present and in the sequence of these in the polymer chain. In conformation the chains are folded rather than linear and joined through cross-linkages of various kinds, eg, disulfide (cystine), internal salt and ester, and hydrogen bonds. Molecular configuration ranges from globular to fibrous, and the existence of coiled (helix) structures has been demonstrated. As with other kinds of macromolecules, molecular weights are less meaningful than usual. Determined by various methods, eg, diffusion, sedimentation, viscosity, x-ray analysis, Tyndallization, ultracentrifugation, electron microscopy, etc, values for different proteins range from about 10^4 up to about 10^7; and the value found for a given protein often varies with the method used.

Collectively, these features of structural variability permit the ready conclusion that the number of *theo-*

retical proteins is very large indeed. They also point up the wide range in stereodisposition of chemically functional groups, and the current view is that specificity in biofunction is referable to such disposition. For these and other reasons, specialists in protein technology are presently applying all of the appropriate advanced techniques and instrumentations to probe more deeply into these many structural features.

Amino Acid Content and Sequence

Those amino acids which have been definitely established as prominent protein components are listed in Table V. Several additional ones, eg, diiodotyrosine, hydroxylysine, et al, known to be present in a few pro-

teins, are not included. The conventional classification into neutral, acidic, and basic refers to the ratio of carboxyl groups and basic nitrogen atoms in the molecule. Approximate isoelectric pH ranges for the three groups are, respectively, 5.0–6.4, 2.9–3.2, and 7.6–10.8. Provided in the listing are common name, conventional (IUPAC) abbreviation, chemical name, and structural formula.

The two fundamental problems involved in the elucidation of the composition of a protein are (1) quantitative assay of the individual amino acids present and (2) determination of the sequence of all amino acid residues in the chain. Each is a highly specialized field of endeavor. Prior to the advent of modern techniques based on selective adsorption, ion exchange, chromatography, electrophoresis, counter current dis-

Table V—Prominent Protein Amino Acids

Neutral Aliphatic
Glycine Gly
  aminoacetic acid $CH_2(NH_2)COOH$
Alanine Ala
  2-aminopropionic acid $CH_3CH(NH_2)COOH$
Serine Ser
  2-amino-3-hydroxypropionic acid $CH_2(OH)CH(NH_2)COOH$
Threonine Thr
  2-amino-3-hydroxybutyric acid $CH_3CH(OH)CH(NH_2)COOH$
Valine Val
  2-amino-3-methylbutyric acid $CH_3CH(CH_3)CH(NH_2)COOH$
Leucine Leu
  2-amino-4-methylvaleric acid $CH_3CH(CH_3)CH_2CH(NH_2)COOH$
Isoleucine Ile
  2-amino-3-methylvaleric acid $CH_3CH_2CH(CH_3)CH(NH_2)COOH$

Neutral Thioaliphatic
Cysteine Cys
  2-amino-3-mercaptopropionic acid $CH_2(SH)CH(NH_2)COOH$

Cystine Cys Cys
  3,3′-dithiodi(2-aminopropionic acid) $[-SCH_2CH(NH_2)COOH]_2$
Methionine Met
  2-amino-4-methylthiobutyric acid $CH_2(SCH_3)CH_2CH(NH_2)COOH$

Neutral Aromatic
Phenylalanine Phe
  2-amino-3-phenylpropionic acid
Tyrosine Tyr
  2-amino-3(p-hydroxyphenyl)propionic acid

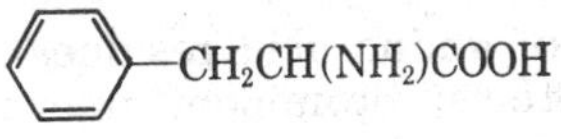

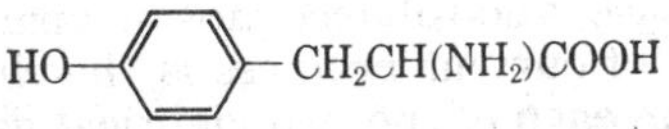

Neutral Heterocyclic
Proline Pro
  2-pyrrolidinecarboxylic acid

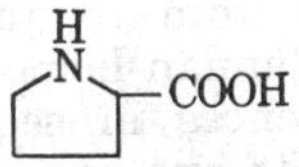

Hydroxyproline 4 Hyp
  4-hydroxy-2-pyrrolidinecarboxylic acid

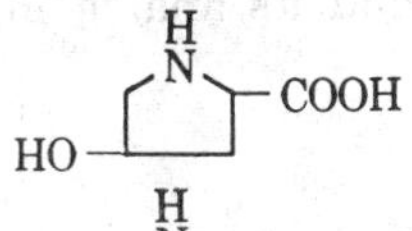

Tryptophan Trp
  α-aminoindole-3-propionic acid

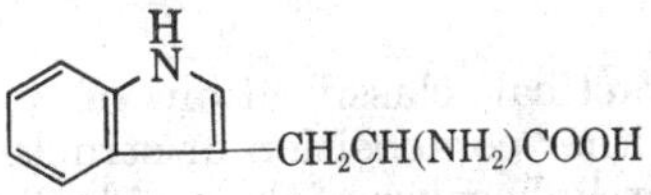

Acidic
Aspartic Acid Asp
  aminosuccinic acid $HOOCCH_2CH(NH_2)COOH$
Glutamic Acid Glu
  2-aminoglutaric acid $HOOCCH_2CH_2CH(NH_2)COOH$

Basic
Histidine His
  α-aminoimidazole-4-propionic acid

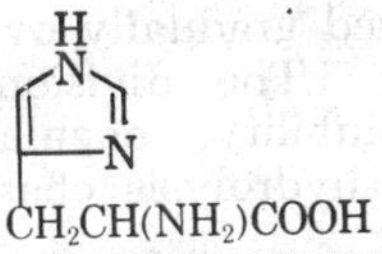

Lysine Lys
  2,6-diaminohexanoic acid $CH_2(NH_2)CH_2CH_2CH_2CH(NH_2)COOH$
Arginine Arg
  2-amino-5-guanidinovaleric acid $NH_2C(:NH)NH-CH_2CH_2CH_2CH(NH_2)COOH$

Table VI—Amino Acid Composition of Selected Proteins[a]

	Gelatins	Milk:* mixed proteins	Casein	Serum albumin*	γ-Globulin	Hemo-globin: horse	Insulin	Clostridium botulinum toxin
Alanine	9.2	...	3.0	6.2	...	7.4	4.5	3.9
Arginine	8.8	4.2	4.1	6.0	4.8	3.7	3.1	4.6
Aspartic Acid	6.3	...	7.1	10.3	8.8	10.6	6.8	20.1
Cystine	0.1	1.0	0.3	6.5	3.1	1.0	12.5	0.8
Glutamic Acid	11.7	21.5	22.4	17.0	11.8	8.2	18.6	15.6
Glycine	30.5	2.3	2.7	2.0	4.2	5.6	4.3	1.4
Histidine	0.7	2.8	3.1	4.0	2.5	8.7	4.9	1.0
Hydroxyproline	14.5	...	0	0	0?	0?	0?	...
Isoleucine	1.9	7.5	6.1	3.0	2.7	0?	2.8	11.9
Leucine	3.2	11.0	9.2	12.0	9.3	15.2	13.2	10.3
Lysine	5.1	8.7	8.2	12.7	8.1	8.5	2.5	7.7
Methionine	0.9	3.2	3.4	1.3	1.1	1.0	0	1.1
Phenylalanine	2.1	5.5	5.0	7.0	4.6	7.7	8.1	1.2
Proline	16.3	...	11.3	5.1	8.1	8.5	2.5	2.6
Serine	3.8	4.3	6.3	7.0	11.4	5.8	5.2	4.4
Threonine	2.2	4.7	4.9	7.1	8.4	4.4	2.1	8.5
Tyrosine	0.7	6.0	6.3	5.5	6.8	3.0	13.0	13.5
Tryptophan	0	1.5	1.2	1.0	2.9	1.7	0	1.9
Valine	3.1	7.0	7.2	6.0	9.7	9.0	7.8	5.3

[a] The data in this table were taken from a more comprehensive table in Hawk, P. B., *et al*, *Practical Physiological Chemistry*, 13th ed., Blakiston, New York, 1954, with the kind permission of the publishers. All values are in Gm/100 Gm of protein except those marked * which are in Gm/16 Gm total nitrogen.

tribution, isotope dilution, nutritional requirements of microorganisms, *et al*, progress was discouragingly slow. That it is excitingly rapid today is abundantly evident from reports appearing regularly in the various literatures of biochemistry.

The amino acid composition of various selected proteins is presented in Table VI. In view of the diverse analytical methods employed, slight variations in reported values are expectable and are encountered in the literature. With simple (nonconjugated) proteins, the total mass of the amino acids exceeds the mass of the source protein because of the water which becomes fixed during hydrolytic cleavage of the peptide linkages.

The precise sequence of amino acid residues is now known for only a few proteins; prominent among these are insulin, ribonuclease, and tobacco mosaic virus. A noteworthy example of current progress is the elucidation of the sequence in each of the two identical gamma chains (each contains 146 residues from 18 different amino acids) of the globin in fetal human hemoglobin and the identification of 39 differences in sequence between each of these chains and its analog in adult human hemoglobin.

Classification

A satisfactory practical classification of proteins on the sole basis of either composition or structure has not been achieved, partly because of their wide diversity and partly because of incomplete knowledge. Classifications in terms of occurrence and function are frequently encountered in the literature but these are designed for special purposes and usually do not embrace the total protein field. A classification having some practical utility has evolved gradually over the years and is presented below. The division into classes is based primarily on solubility, coagulability, conjugation, denaturation, and hydrolysis characteristics.

1. **Simple proteins** are naturally occurring proteins which yield only alpha-amino acids or their derivatives on hydrolysis. They may be of several types and include:

(a) *Albumins*, which are soluble in water and coagulated by heat, eg, ovalbumin in egg white and serum albumin in blood.

(b) *Globulins*, which are insoluble in water but soluble in dilute salt solutions and coagulable by heat, eg, serum globulin in blood.

(c) *Glutelins*, which are insoluble in water or dilute salt solution but soluble in dilute acid and alkali, eg, glutenin in wheat.

(d) *Prolamines*, which are insoluble in neutral solutions but soluble in 80% alcohol, eg, zein in corn and gliadin in wheat.

(e) *Albuminoids*, which are dissolved only by boiling in strong acids, eg, keratins in hair and horny tissue, elastins in tendons and arteries, and collagens in skin and tendons.

(f) *Histones*, which are basic in reaction, soluble in water but insoluble in dilute ammonia, and difficultly heat-coagulable, eg, thymus histone and hemoglobin.

(g) *Protamines*, which are strongly basic in reaction and soluble in water, dilute acid, and ammonia, eg, salmin and sturin in fish sperm. They precipitate many other proteins.

2. **Conjugated proteins** are those proteins which are combined in nature with some nonprotein substance. They are classified according to the nature of the prosthetic (nonprotein) group. The classes, which are not mutually exclusive, include:

(a) *Phosphoproteins*—contain a phosphoric acid moiety as the prosthetic group, eg, casein in milk and ovovitellin in egg yolk.

(b) *Nucleoprotein*—the nonprotein portion is a nucleic acid, eg, nuclein in cell nuclei.

(c) *Glycoproteins*—simple proteins united to a carbohydrate group, eg, mucins in vitreous humor and saliva.

(d) *Chromoproteins*—contain a colored prosthetic group, eg, hemoglobin in blood, and flavoproteins.

(e) *Lipoproteins*—proteins in combination with lipid materials such as sterols, fatty acids, lecithin, etc.

(f) *Metalloproteins*—the prosthetic group contains a metal, eg, enzymes such as tyrosinase, arginase, and xanthine oxidase.

3. **Derived proteins** are substances formed from simple or conjugated proteins by various means such as the action of heat, acids, alkalies, water, enzymes, alcohol, radiant energy, and mechanical shock. They differ in one or more respects from the proteins from which they are formed; and, in general, the extent of this difference, as reflected by changes in various physical and chemical properties, constitutes the basis for the classification described below.

Primary derived proteins are commonly referred to as *denatured proteins*. They differ only slightly from the proteins from which they are derived, probably only in conformation, with the peptide linkages remaining pretty much intact. They are subdivided as follows:

(a) *Proteans*—These are insoluble substances formed during the early stages of the action of water, enzymes, or dilute acid on the original protein. They sometimes result merely from mechanical agitation of a solution of protein. Examples are fibrin from fibrinogen and myrosan from myosin.

(b) *Metaproteins*—These are substances formed during the early stages of protein hydrolysis by means of acid or alkali. In general, they are easily soluble in dilute acids and alkalies; this is indicative of some hydrolytic cleavage of the peptide linkages in the original protein. They are insoluble in neutral solvents and, like most natural proteins, are coagulable. Examples are the acid and alkali albuminates.

(c) *Coagulated proteins*—These are insoluble substances formed from proteins usually by the action of heat or alcohol. They may also be produced from protein solutions by actinic irradiation, by mechanical shock, or by the application of high pressure. Coagulated egg albumin and cooked meat are familiar examples.

Secondary derived proteins are substances formed during the progressive hydrolysis of proteins; thus, in comparison with the primary derived proteins, they differ much more decidedly from their original proteins. Secondary derived proteins cover a very wide range of molecular weights, the weight in each case depending upon the extent of the hydrolytic cleavage of the original protein. They are subclassified into the following broad categories:

(a) *Proteoses*—These constitute the highest molecular weight group and thus represent the least hydrolyzed state of the original protein. They are generally more readily soluble in water than the original protein, and they are of sufficiently reduced complexity as to be noncoagulable by heat. Saturation of their aqueous solutions with ammonium sulfate causes them to precipitate.

(b) *Peptones*—These are lower in molecular weight than the proteoses and thus represent a more degraded hydrolytic state of the original protein. Like the proteoses, they are readily soluble in water and noncoagulable by heat. Due to their lesser molecular complexity, they are not precipitated (salted out) from aqueous solution by saturation with ammonium sulfate. They are precipitated as complexes, however, by phosphotungstic acid.

(c) *Peptides*—These are very small hydrolytic fragments of their original proteins. They contain from 2 to possibly 20 or so amino acids joined via amide linkages, and are commonly subdivided into di-, tri-, etc, peptides according to the number of amino acid residues they contain. Collectively, the higher members are often termed *polypeptides*. Various individual peptides have been isolated from protein hydrolysates. Many have also been synthesized, eg, oxytocin, *qv*, page 953. The peptides are readily soluble in water. They are noncoagulable by heat and are not precipitated from their solutions by saturation with ammonium sulfate.

Physical and Chemical Properties

In general, pure proteins are relatively odorless and tasteless. In their normal biologic environment, they are highly hydrated. Color varies. On heating, they decompose with or without simultaneous liquefaction, and emit the characteristic odor of singed hair. They vary greatly in their solubilities in such solvents as water, salt solutions, monohydric and polyhydric alcohols, and dilute acids and bases, forming colloidal solutions from which heat often precipitates the protein in coagulated form. Precipitation in unaltered form is frequently accomplished by means of salt solutions, eg, sodium chloride and ammonium sulfate, and by diluted ethanol. Many proteins have been obtained in crystalline form but, unlike in the case of crystalline substances in general, this is not necessarily evidence of homogeneity since some have been further resolved into two or more components through chromatographic, electrophoretic, and other procedures.

Although the exceptional vulnerability of proteins in general to chemical attack often requires careful control of reaction conditions, nevertheless their chemical characteristics are quite in accord with those to be expected from the functional groups present. Thus, the amide groups are readily hydrolyzable under the catalytic influence of acids, alkalies, and enzymes. Terminal amino groups are readily convertible to hydroxyl by treatment with nitrous acid and are susceptible to alkylation, acylation, hydroxymethylation with formaldehyde, etc, and free carboxyl groups are neutralizable and esterifiable.

Containing many carboxyls and amino-type nitrogens (β-lactoglobulin, for example, is reported to contain 59 of the former and 38 of the latter), proteins may be viewed as multiple zwitterion (see page 454) complexes. Each has its characteristic isoelectric point, ie, that pH at which the protein is electrically neutral, is equally capable of donating or accepting proton, and exhibits minimal solubility, electrical conductivity, osmotic pressure and viscosity.

Numerous other reactions are referable to functional specificities of the individual amino acid residues. Thus, the phenolic moiety of tyrosine is readily nitrated and will also couple with diazo compounds to yield colored azo derivatives; similarly, the thiol group in cysteine enables reaction with nitroprusside. Most of the numerous color tests of protein chemistry find ready explanation in terms of well known interactions between such functional groups and the reagents.

Synthesis

Historically, synthesis is a logical sequel to structure elucidation of organic compounds and, although extremely formidable problems are encountered with proteins due to their miscellaneous features of chemical vulnerability, nevertheless impressive achievements are being reported. Numerous highly versatile methods of synthesis have been developed since 1903 when Fischer reported his classis synthesis of an unnatural polypeptide containing 3 leucine and 15 glycine residues. Among the more recently announced achievements are (1) the total synthesis of β-corticotropin (a 39-unit peptide containing 15 different amino acid residues in specific sequence) which is completely identical in all respects, including bioactivity, with swine ACTH; and (2) the separate synthesis of the sheep insulin-A chain (21 units, 10 different amino acids) and of what appears to be the B chain (30 units, 15 different amino acids) followed by uniting them chemically to produce an insulin moiety which, even in crude form, displays definite, although slight, insulin bioactivity.

As recently as 1950, such achievements were considered hopeless. Today they portend dramatic accomplishments which will add greatly to man's knowledge of biofunctioning and thus give rise to many new types of highly effective, specific drugs.

Tests for Proteins and Amino Acids—In addition to the modern chromatographic, electrophoretic, and other procedures mentioned previously, many older test methods still find useful application. The hydrolysis of protein yields amino acids which, on treatment with *nitrous acid*, liberate nitrogen. This reaction along with other techniques forms the basis of Van Slyke's nitrogen distribution method which has important uses in clinical chemistry. Amino acids and the free amino groups in proteins react with ninhydrin. The presence of peptide linkages can be shown by means of the *Biuret* test. Numerous color tests are available for individual amino acids, including the *Ehrlich* and *Hopkins-Cole* tests for tryptophan, the *Sakaguchi* test for arginine, the *nitroprusside* test for cystine and cysteine, the *Millon* test for tyrosine, the *xanthroproteic* test for tyrosine and phenylalanine, the

Pauly diazo test for histidine and tyrosine, and the *basic lead* test for the sulfur-containing acids.

Precipitates are formed with amino acids on the addition of various reagents such as heavy metal salts, and certain acids such as picric, phosphotungstic, trichloroacetic, or sulfosalicylic acids. Simple tests for certain proteins are based on precipitation with heat or acid.

Specific Proteins and Peptides—Proteins and peptides vary greatly in biological activity and exhibit widely different and specific properties. No more than mere mention can be made of examples of some of the more important groups of these substances. Each group represents a distinct and important biochemical field in which current research is greatly expanding our fund of knowledge.

Several *hormones* are peptides. *Insulin* is a protein, the amino acid sequence of which is well known. *Thyroxine* is an amino acid which is important in regulating metabolism. The amino acid contents of *oxytocin* and *vasopressin*, two posterior pituitary hormones having quite distinct functions, are quite similar. The structure of each is known and they have been synthesized (see page 959).

Certain *antibiotics* such as bacitracin, polymyxin, tyrocidin, gramicidin, subtilin, actinomycin, and colistin represent another group of peptides with distinctive biological properties.

Table VII—Recommended Intakes of Essential Amino Acids for Man[a]

Amino acid	Daily intake, Gm.
Leucine	2.2
Isoleucine	1.4
Lysine	1.6
Methionine	2.2
Phenylalanine	2.2
Threonine	1.0
Tryptophan	0.5
Valine	1.6

[a] From Rose, W. C., *Chem. Eng. News* **30**, 2385 (1952).

By a variety of techniques it has been found possible to identify different *hemoglobins* (eg, A, F, S, C, D, E). It has been shown that these various types are inherited. Some are associated with disease conditions of the blood.

Some of the most important protein substances are the *enzymes* which are involved in the metabolism of food constituents. See page 1049.

The field of immunology is based on the relations of substances now known to be proteins or composed largely of protein. Resistance to disease may be either natural or acquired. In natural resistance, the *phagocytes* of an individual with adequate nutrition quickly destroy invading organisms. In prolonged protein deficiency there is a scarcity of phagocytes and their precursors in the mesenchymal tissues (spleen, bone marrow, and lymphoid tissues). In acquired resistance, since *pathogenic microorganisms* are proteins foreign to the body, they activate the antibody system within the tissues. *Antibodies* appear to be modified serum globulins which are extremely specific in their reaction and in their immunizing effect. Normal antibody production has been shown to be affected by prolonged protein deficiency. *Gamma globulin*, a fraction of serum protein, is prophylactic against measles and has been shown to provide some protection against infectious hepatitis and poliomyelitis.

Many *toxins* also are proteins, the chemical nature of which furnishes little clue to their mode of action which varies markedly. On a per mole basis many are several orders of magnitude more toxic than any other kind of toxic substance. Some toxins are produced by organisms which cause infections in the host such as diphtheria and scarlet fever. Others, such as the toxin produced by *Cl. botulinum* in spoiled food, act directly when ingested. Since toxins are antigens it is possible to immunize animals against their toxic effect, eg, against tetanus.

Amino acids such as glycine and cysteine have important roles in detoxification mechanisms. They are important in maintaining normal liver function.

Uses for Amino Acids and Proteins

Nutrition—Some living systems, like the plants, can manufacture all of the amino acids which they require from dietary inorganic nitrogen, carbon and water. Others, like certain bacteria, can manufacture several amino acids from a single amino acid. Man, on the other hand, can manufacture only a portion of the amino acids he requires to meet the needs for maintenance and growth. Those amino acids which are not synthesized in adequate amounts and must therefore be supplied in the diet have been called "essential" by Rose. The amino acids which are considered to be essential for an adult man are leucine, isoleucine, lysine, methionine, phenylalanine, threonine, tryptophan, and valine. The intakes of these amino acids recommended by Rose for man are shown in Table VII. These amounts are double the actual minimum daily requirements (amounts demonstrated as necessary to maintain human nitrogen equilibrium, ie, balance between dietary nitrogen intake and excreta nitrogen) as found by Rose but other workers have felt that they are still too low and should be two to four times as great.

While it is of fundamental interest to know the amino acid requirements of individuals, from a practical standpoint it is also important to know if an individual is obtaining an adequate amount of protein in his diet. The allowances recommended by the Food and Nutrition Board of the National Research Council can be used as an indication of adequacy and are given in Table VIII. As would be expected, the figures indicate an increased requirement for growth, pregnancy, and lactation.

Not all proteins possess the same nutritive value. For maintenance in the human it has been shown that, if egg white is given a value of 100, whole egg has a value of 103, beef 74, casein 75, peanut flour 62, and wheat gluten 46. The variation in value is caused largely by the amino acid composition of the protein. The addition of a specified amino acid or acids to some proteins has been found to improve their nutritive value. Similarly one protein may be used to supplement another. Cereal proteins with a deficiency in lysine may be supplemented to advantage with proteins from animal sources or with lysine itself.

Several methods have been proposed for evaluating the nutritive value of proteins. One of the most common is that of determining the ability of the protein to promote growth in the rat. From the ratio of the gain in body weight of the rat to the weight of protein consumed, the protein efficiency ratio for that particular protein is calculated. The biological value of protein may also be obtained from nitrogen balance determinations. In this method the biological value is taken as the percentage of the absorbed nitrogen (nitrogen intake minus fecal nitrogen of dietary origin) that is not eliminated in the urine. It has been demonstrated that a close relationship usually exists between the growth-promoting method and the nitrogen balance procedure.

Another method for the assay of the nutritive value of proteins in rats is based on the fact that the amount of labile cytoplasm present in the liver depends on the quantity and quality of protein fed. It has been shown, however, that the ability of a given protein to regenerate liver protein is not necessarily correlated to the biological value of that protein. In the rat repletion method rats which have been maintained on a diet low in protein for 3 weeks are fed the protein being examined for a 10-day period and the gain in body weight is recorded. The amino acid composition of a protein has been used also as an indication of its nutritive value. This technique has shown considerable promise in adult human nutrition, although it is pointed out that food proteins may undergo certain changes, especially under the influence of heat, that may impair their nutritive value without disturbing the amino acid composition as ordinarily determined.

It is well established that excessive heating of a protein may result in a pronounced change in its nutritive value and that the protein content alone of a food is not necessarily a good index of its value in protein nutrition. The nutritive value of the protein of the soybean and other legumes improves with moderate heating, while overheating reverses this effect. There appear to be constituents in the raw leguminous protein which inhibit utilization of the protein; these are destroyed by the heating process resulting in an apparent increased value. Cereal proteins, on the other hand, have been shown to decrease in nutritive value upon heating. In studies on the biological value of the proteins of ready-to-eat cereal breakfast foods, it was found that the ratio of gain in body weight to protein consumed is depressed by two-thirds by the "gun explosion" of an oats-corn-rye mixture and by three-fourths by the "gun explosion" of oats alone. Thus the nutritive value of the protein of the final product may bear little relation to that of the original food. The biological values of the proteins of peanut meal, sunflower seed meal, and cottonseed flour have been found to be decreased by heating.

The application of moist heat to meat proteins does not appear to lower their nutritive value. The average digestibilities of protein for raw and roast beef and the average biological values are similar and there are no grounds for presuming that the roasting modifies the nutritive value of the protein for growing rats.

Damage by dry heat in the absence of carbohydrates appears to result in the production of a new lysine linkage which is either not digestible by enzymes or is digested at too slow a rate to be of value. Under conditions of moist heat and the presence of reducing substances the destruction of some of the amino acids may be responsible for the reduction in nutritive value. It should be pointed out that the danger of reducing the nutritive value of the proteins in a good diet by heat processing, commonly found in home-cooking techniques, is not great and little destruction takes place in the kitchen.

The metabolism of a protein may be said to involve all the changes which occur in that protein during ingestion, digestion, absorption, transport, storage, utilization, synthesis, conversion to carbohydrate and fat, breakdown, and excretion. Digestion of the protein begins in the stomach and continues in the intestine under the influence of proteolytic enzymes until it is broken down into amino acids and peptides. These are absorbed and carried to the liver from whence they are distributed to the various tissues requiring them. Many of the amino acids will be used in the synthesis of tissue proteins or will become a part of special proteins such as enzymes, hormones, and hemoglobin. Other amino acids will be deaminated; the nitrogenous portion is converted primarily to urea and the remainder of the molecule is converted to carbohydrate or fat. While there does not appear to be widespread storage of protein in the body as there is of fat, nevertheless, the body does reserve some protein for use during periods of dietary protein insufficiency.

Contrary to earlier theories, it has been established by the use of ^{15}N-labeled amino acids that tissue proteins even in a mature animal are labile and are undergoing continual breakdown and synthesis. There is an equilibrium between proteins, amino acids, and decomposition products which permits the animal to accommodate itself more readily to changing environment, food supply, stress, etc. The basis of this equilibrium

Table VIII—Recommended Daily Allowances for Protein[a]

	Age, years	Weight, Kg	Protein, Gm
Men	18–75	70	70
Women	18–75	58	53
		Pregnant[b]	78
		Lactating	98
Infants[c]	0–1	8	Kg × 2.5
Children[d]	1–3	13	32
	3–6	18	40
	6–9	24	52
Boys[d]	9–12	33	60
	12–15	45	75
	15–18	61	85
Girls[d]	9–12	33	55
	12–15	47	62
	15–18	53	58

[a] From *Recommended Daily Dietary Allowances*, National Academy of Science, Washington, D.C., revised 1963.
[b] 2nd and 3rd trimester.
[c] Protein allowances per Kg for infants are considered to decrease progressively from birth.
[d] Entries represent allowances for the midpoint of the specified age periods, ie, line for children 1–3 is for age 2 years (24 months); 3–6 is for age 4½ years (54 months); etc.

lies in the lability of the peptide bond. The rate of amino acid exchange varies with the tissues; the turnover in liver and plasma accounts for 41% of the total exchange in man. In mammals nitrogen is excreted primarily as urea. It has been estimated that about 1 Gm of free amino acids and 2 Gm of conjugated amino acids are excreted per day.

Clinical Uses—Adequate protein nutrition requires the intake of sufficient protein to meet daily requirements. This protein must be of the necessary "quality," ie, supply the essential amino acids. Protein deficiency thus may be caused by a reduced intake, or the use of low-quality protein. Obviously, the actual intake of protein may be influenced by factors such as high excretion in conditions of kidney damage or blood loss, or an increased requirement associated with thyrotoxicosis or high fever. Symptoms of deficiency include loss of weight, nutritional edema, and skin changes and are associated with such conditions as nephrosis, sprue, and colitis. Deficiency may result also in a reduced resistance to infection since an adequate protein intake is necessary for the formation of phagocytes, leucocytes, and antibodies. Stress, such as brought on by accidental or surgical trauma, pregnancy, and lactation may also cause a deficiency of amino acids and greater intakes of protein are required in these conditions. The disease Kwashiorkor has been shown to respond to adequate supplies of proteins.

For the treatment of protein deficiency several types of products are available. High protein natural foods should be used where possible. Protein concentrates such as skim milk powder to which may be added casein and lactalbumin are also available. Where the bulk of high protein foods is undesirable or where the patient is unable to digest whole protein, hydrolysates may be indicated. They have the disadvantage in many instances of being unpalatable, but are particularly useful in tube feeding. Daily doses of 150 Gm protein or more are usually prescribed. There is some evidence that orally administered protein hydrolysates may be superior to whole protein in ulcer therapy.

Parenteral preparations are useful where the gastrointestinal tract cannot be used and when rapid restoration of reserves is important. They have also been found helpful in maintaining adequate nutrition in cases of food allergy where it may be impossible for the patient to consume a normal diet. Losses of hemoglobin caused by hemorrhage may be replaced by whole blood or plasma tranfusions. With the addition of protein hydrolysates to electrolytes, glucose, and vitamins it is possible to maintain a patient in good nutrition for considerable time without the use of the gastrointestinal tract.

Individual amino acids have not been widely used in clinical medicine for where there is protein deficiency several amino acids are usually concerned. Methionine has been used as a lipotropic agent in some preparations.

Protein Hydrolysates—Protein hydrolysates may be prepared by the action of an acid, a base, or an appropriate enzyme. Acid hydrolysis of proteins ordinarily results in the complete destruction of tryptophan and also presents the difficulty of removing the acid from the products of hydrolysis. Alkaline hydrolysis is of no practical use as it leads to the destruction of some and the racemization of most amino acids. The most suitable method of preparing a protein hydrolysate for oral administration is by enzymic digestion. However, enzymic hydrolysates often possess a disagreeable taste which must be masked for acceptable palatability.

There are some commercial protein hydrolysates which are recommended for oral administration. None of these preparations is highly palatable, although lactalbumin hydrolysates are claimed to be the least objectionable. Attempts to mask this unpleasant taste by adding flavoring materials or by diluting the hydrolysate with carbohydrate have met with varying success. The oral route, if it is available for the administration of proteins, is to be preferred to the intravenous route.

By the intravenous route, it is seldom possible to give more than the equivalent of 75 Gm of protein per day together with glucose. If hydrolysates are injected too quickly, nausea and sometimes vomiting may lead to less efficient use of the amino acids. Because of the difficulty of infusing sufficient protein, it is generally agreed that it is not possible to make good the requirements of the protein-depleted organism entirely by intravenous injection. It is not wise to give fluid containing more than 5% protein hydrolysate and 5 percent glucose.

Biological assay of protein hydrolysates to determine their nutritional adequacy will also supply evidence of the absence of acute or toxic factors. Protein hydrolysates for parenteral use must be sterile, nonpyrogenic, and well tolerated. They must also be nonantigenic to preclude the likelihood of possibly fatal anaphylactic shock which might ensue on subsequent administration to a previously sensitized individual.

Official Proteins

Examples of the various types of official protein materials have been provided on page 454.

Alkaloids

Sertürner's paper, in 1817, "Morphis, a New Salt-forming Substance, and Meconic Acid, as the Chief Constituents of Opium," opened a new era of discovery in organic plant chemistry. His isolation of the first alkaloid was soon followed by the isolation of narcotine by Robiquet and strychnine by Pelletier and Caventou. These basic compounds were at first called vegetable alkalies, but were later renamed alkaloids, meaning alkali-like. It is of special interest to note that many of the most important alkaloids were discovered by pharmacists.

Alkaloids, as the active principles of many plants, were isolated and announced in rapid succession by various investigators. That the effort continues today is abundantly evident from the literature. For example, the Subject Index to Vol. 65 of Chemical Abstracts, which covers the period July–December, 1966, lists more than 300 references under the main entry "Alkaloids" alone. The most recent comprehensive survey[1] shows that a total of 1932 individual compounds have been reported as alkaloids by the investigators who isolated them from various genera of 158 botanical families. A few are obtained from Cryptogams (flowerless plants), but the majority are extracted from the Phanerogams (flowering plants), most of them being from dicotyledons. In this connection, it is interesting to note that phytochemists estimate that less than 5% of the known flowering plants have been investigated for possible alkaloid content.

Notwithstanding the many extremely valuable synthetic medicinal and antibiotic agents that have been added to the list of weapons against disease, the alkaloids still constitute an indispensable and most potent group of substances for the treatment and mitigation of functional disturbances and relief from suffering. It is for this reason that some of the larger pharmaceutical firms maintain continuing programs for the pharmacologic screening of alkaloids, both new and old. Reserpine, much valued today for its antihypertensive and psychotherapeutic actions, emerged from such a program in the 1950's; and an intensive current effort with the *Vinca* (*catharanthus*) alkaloids has already yielded some oncolytic drugs of value in the treatment of certain types of cancer.

Alkaloids are largely derived from plants although a

few are found in the living animal body and others result from decomposition of dead animal tissue. The term *leucomaines* is sometimes applied to those from living animal tissues and *ptomaines* to the products of decomposition in dead animal tissues. When found in plants they occur in nearly all of the organs, and several theories, each of which has supporting facts, have been advanced concerning both the mode and purpose of their formation.

A few alkaloids have been made synthetically and there are also a number of synthetic drugs of an alkaloidal character which do not occur in nature. Distinction should be made between *total synthesis*, in which the end product is the result of chemical processes which employ only materials that can be built up from the elements (carbon, hydrogen, oxygen, etc), and *partial synthesis* in which the end product is produced from a naturally occurring complex substance which is already closely related structurally to the desired end product (eg, the synthesis of ergonovine from lysergic acid).

In their native environment, alkaloids usually exist in the form of salts, frequently of the simple organic acids such as lactic, malic, tartaric, and citric. Unusual, often distinctive acids are also encountered, eg, quinic with cinchona and meconic with opium alkaloids. In addition to their basic nitrogen moiety, alkaloids usually contain one or more chemically functional groups. Thus, cocaine contains two ester functions, quinine contains both the secondary alcohol and aromatic methoxy functions, ergonovine contains a substituted amide function, etc. Some alkaloids, eg, solanine and tomatine, actually occur as glycosides.

Classification—Alkaloids may be classified in a variety of ways, eg, according to source, chemical structure, pharmacologic action, etc. Any attempt at comprehensive chemotaxononic classification is far beyond the scope of concern in this text; for such treatment, consult the continuing encyclopedic work of Manske which now encompasses 11 volumes.[2] A partial classification which includes most of the more

important pharmaceutical alkaloids is presented in Table IX. As in all such condensed classifications, caution must be exercised in interpreting the entries under "Nucleus." Different hydrogenated forms of a given nucleus are often present in different alkaloids, eg, nicotine contains pyridine whereas piperine contains hexahydropyridine (piperidine). Also, some alkaloids contain more than one nucleus, eg, quinine contains both quinoline and quinuclidine. In many instances, the nucleus shown in the table is merely the best known fragment of the total fused ring system actually present in the alkaloid. Thus, for example, while it is true that each of the ergot alkaloids contains an indole ring in its nucleus, actually the indole is but a fragment of the fused tetracyclic ring system, indolo-[4,3-*fg*]quinoline, which constitutes the total nucleus. The complete heteronuclei represented in official alkaloids are included in the display of heterocycles in Table VII, page 465.

Properties—The more important characteristic features of alkaloids are the following:

1. In addition to carbon and hydrogen they all contain nitrogen and generally also oxygen. The nitrogen, which is usually contained in whole or in part in the heteronucleus, confers the alkali-like properties to alkaloids.
2. Most of the nonvolatile alkaloids are solid; the volatile ones are mainly liquid and these often contain no oxygen.
3. They are mainly crystallizable, though a few are amorphous. Some, eg, nicotine, are liquid (as the free alkaloid) under ordinary conditions.
4. They are generally white though berberine is yellow and sanguinarine, itself colorless, yields red salts.
5. They are either insoluble or sparingly soluble in water (with a few exceptions, such as colchicine) but soluble in alcohol, chloroform, benzene, some in ether, and a few in petroleum benzin. Their salts behave conversely in the matter of solubility.
6. Most of them are physiologically active, some being extremely poisonous. In the majority of instances they are the medicinally important substances of the plants from which they are derived.
7. Alkaloids unite with acids to form substituted ammonium salts. The stability of these salts toward hydrolysis varies with the basic strength of the alkaloid and the nature of the acid used. With the exception of the xanthine group, most common alkaloids have pK values less than 7. The alkaloids are freed from their salts by the addition of alkali.

Table IX—A Partial Classification of Alkaloids

Nucleus	Plant genera	Alkaloids
Benzazulene	Aconitum, Delphinium	Aconitine, delphinine, delsoline
Imidazole	Pilocarpus	Pilocarpine, pilocarpidine, pilosine, *pseudo*pilocarpine, *pseudo*jaborine, *iso*pilocarpine
Indole	Peganum, Psilocybe, Stropharia, Evodia, Corynanthe, Claviceps, Physostigma, Strychnos, Rauwolfia	Brucine, ergonovine, ergotamine, harmine, physostigmine, psilocybin, reserpine, strychnine, yohimbine
Isoquinoline	Hydrastis, Papaver, Corydalis, Berberis, Chondodendron, Ipecacuanha, Sanguinaria	Anhalonine, bebeerine, berberine, cephaëline, codeine, corydaline, cotarnine chloride, emetine, erythramine, erythroidine, hydrastine, menispermine, morphine, papaverine, sanguinarine, tubocurarine chloride
Phenylalkylamine	Ephedra, Lophophora	Ephedrine
Purine	Guarana, Cola, Coffea, Thea, Theobroma	Caffeine,[a] theobromine,[a] theophylline[a]
Pyridine	Anabasis, Areca, Conium, Lobelia, Piper, Punica, Ricinus, Nicotiana	Anabasine, aphylline, arecaidine, arecoline, coniine, guvacine, lobeline, nicotine, pelletierine, piperine, ricinine, trigonelline
Quinoline	Cinchona, Cusparia	Cinchonine, cinchonidine, cusparine, ethylhydrocupreine, quinacrine, quinine, quinidine
Quinolizine	Anagyris, Laburnum, Lupinus, Sophora	Anagyrine, cytisine, lupanine, lupinine, matrine, sparteine
Steroidal[b]	Solanum, Veratrum, Lycopersicon, Holarrhena, Schoenocaulon	Cevadine, cevine, conessine, jervine, rubijervine, solanidine, solanine, tomatidine, veratramine, veratridine
Tropane	Erythroxylon, Atropa, Datura, Hyoscyamus, Scopola	Atropine, benzoylecgonine, cocaine, eucatropine, homatropine, hygrine, hyoscyamine, scopolamine

[a] Some authors do not classify these relatively feebly basic compounds as alkaloids.
[b] Various nuclei are represented in this group. In general, they have some resemblance to the steroid (cyclopentaphenanthrene) nucleus.

8. In addition to its basic character, a given alkaloid displays all of the chemical properties predictable on the basis of its chemically functional groups.

9. They are precipitated by one or more of the following reagents; with some they form definite chemical compounds which are used for their identification: mercuric-potassium iodide (Mayer's reagent); potassium-cadmium iodide (Marme's reagent); potassium-bismuth iodide (Dragendorff's reagent); phosphomolybdic acid (Sonnenschein's reagent); a solution of iodine with potassium iodide (Wagner's reagent); phosphotungstic acid (Scheibler's reagent); gold chloride; tannic acid; and picric acid.

10. Alkaloids display all expectable types of stereoisomerism. Most contain one or more centers of asymmetry thus giving rise to enantiomorphic and diastereoisomeric structures. Variations in nuclear conformation are also often possible. The pharmacologic and therapeutic actions of alkaloids are usually highly stereospecific.

Identification—Various kinds of tests have been devised to identify known alkaloids. Their effective use, however, usually requires some relevant knowledge of the history of the sample under examination. In general, these tests involve combinations of two or more of the following: melting points of the alkaloid and at least one of its salts or other derivatives, specific rotation, solubility in various solvents, color reactions with specified reagents, and microscopic examination of the crystals obtained by the action of suitable precipitants under controlled conditions.

Closely related alkaloids such as morphine and codeine do not differ sufficiently in their absorption of ultraviolet light to permit differentiation on the basis of their respective spectrograms. However, the infra-red spectrum of an alkaloid is individual and if a reference graph has been reported identification can be made with certainty.

Preparation—The isolation of alkaloids on a commercial scale is highly specialized. It requires skill and many years of experience to establish an alkaloid production process on an economic basis. In many instances commercial production requires large-scale operations similar to the methods employed in proximate assaying (see page 617).

In a representative type of process the crude milled drug is moistened with an aqueous alkali such as sodium carbonate, sodium bicarbonate or lime—to liberate the alkaloids from their salts—and percolated with benzene, ether, or some other suitable water-immiscible solvent. The solvent layer is extracted with dilute acid to convert the alkaloids into salts and to bring them into the aqueous phase. The free alkaloids, substantially without other plant materials, are precipitated by the addition of alkali and then separated by appropriate means. The operations involved are based on the physical as well as the chemical properties of the alkaloids sought. Purification is usually accomplished by the crystallization of the alkaloidal salts, but distillation and other procedures are also employed.

In some cases, when the alkaloidal content of a drug is low, and large volumes of dilute aqueous solutions are obtained, it is of advantage to adsorb the alkaloids on ion-exchange resins (page 677). If the several alkaloids adsorbed on a resin differ sufficiently in basicity, it may be possible to affect at least a partial separation of the alkaloids in the course of the elution from the resin.

Separation of alkaloids of very similar physical and chemical properties is often accomplished by various chromatographic techniques (page 675) and also by counter current distribution. In one of the simpler procedures, a nonaqueous solution of the mixture of alkaloids is passed down slowly through a column of activated adsorbent such as alumina, silica gel, etc. The alkaloids are held in discrete zones on the adsorbent; the solvent passes through. A series of eluting solvents (which may be mixtures of two or more solvents) is then passed through the column to desorb the alkaloids one at a time. The individual alkaloids are then collected in separate fractions. If the zones are not visible by ordinary light they may sometimes be made apparent by ultraviolet light; if neither method is useful, it is necessary to collect numerous fractions of the eluate and to determine by analytic means the order in which the alkaloids are being removed and the point at which one alkaloid has been removed and the next one appears.

An excellent example of the problems encountered and of some of the modern techniques employed in the separation of a complex mixture of alkaloids is provided by the review[3] of researches on the *Vinca* alkaloids.

Synthesis—This section briefly presents significant aspects of the very active and diverse roles synthetic organic chemistry is playing in the alkaloid field.

On the one hand, the total synthesis of a complex alkaloid, eg, strychnine (page 1161), even though it has no probable future practical manufacturing importance, is recognized as a monumental achievement; on the other hand, the emergence of what seemed like a simple effective substitute for morphine (methadone) caused a flurry of activity in laboratories throughout the world and resulted in the publication of hundreds of individual chemical research reports and the results of numerous pharmacological investigations. Each type of development will undoubtedly continue to affect the status of alkaloidal drugs.

Total syntheses are usually undertaken with the purely scientific objective of adding to our knowledge. The molecular structure of an alkaloid is deduced from experiments in which (1) the identity of its chemically functional groups is established, and (2) the alkaloid is degraded to simpler fragments. The nature of these functional groups and of the fragments and their own reactions lead to a hypothesis concerning the structure of the original material.* This hypothesis is expressed in the form of a written structural formula or other model, which must adequately explain the chemical and physicochemical properties (spectra, x-ray analysis, nuclear magnetic resonance, etc) of the alkaloid. Final confirmation of the hypothesis can come only from a total synthesis which, step by step, employs unequivocal reactions and at each stage in the build-up produces intermediates of proved structure.

Since the final products usually have several asymmetric centers, syntheses are further complicated by the requirement that they proceed through stages which will lead to the product with a stereochemical configuration corresponding to that of the natural product. This requirement imposes the need for inventing at appropriate steps stereospecific means for proceeding to the next step or, alternatively, for choosing at a given step, from among a mixture of intermediate products, only the one which is suitable for the further transformations contemplated.

The achievement of a total synthesis is a result of imagination, intellect, and experimental skill. Whether the methods that are used to reach the objective will lend themselves to technological exploitation is usually not germane to the issue. It is, therefore, often very unlikely that total chemical synthesis will compete economically with the processes for deriving the more complex alkaloids from natural sources.†

---

* The review article on Vinca alkaloids provides a good illustration of structural elucidation.

† It is conceivable that a combination of chemical and biological means (use of enzymes, etc) may in certain cases lead to practical synthesis of alkaloids, but this is not true total synthesis.

However, the outlook for synthetic analogs of and substitutes for alkaloids is different. Procaine has already displaced cocaine to a notable extent; similarly for many uses the synthetic quinolines are replacing quinine, and synthetic morphinan derivatives are replacing some opium alkaloids. From the long-range point of view it appears likely that many of the naturally occurring alkaloids currently in use will eventually be at least partly supplanted by synthetic products.

Whatever role an alkaloid plays in the physiology of a plant the *therapeutic use* discovered for the alkaloid is certainly not part of its botanical function. A particular alkaloid is, therefore, not necessarily the best drug of its pharmacologic class.

Using the structural formula of an alkaloid as a prototype, efforts have been made to determine the *pharmacodynamically* important portion of the molecule, that is, the structural arrangement of atoms or groups mostly responsible for the main physiological action of the compound. Once this has been determined (often quite empirically), synthetic variants of the fundamental structure are prepared and tested until a single compound, or family of compounds, is found which offers greatest promise for further study.

The structural resemblance among several alkaloids and their respective analogs or substitutes can be seen from the tables presented throughout this chapter.* It will also be noted that in some cases large sections of the alkaloidal molecule are not reproduced in the synthetic molecule because they are not fundamentally involved in the physiological effect produced. Very often, also, the complicated stereochemistry of the natural product is not followed in detail in the construction of the synthetic product; morphine has several centers of asymmetry whereas meperidine has only one.

Speculations concerning the *biogenesis* of alkaloids have had fruitful results in increasing our understanding of nature and in stimulating the invention of novel synthetic processes. A biogenetic theory attempts to deduce how the plant, using intermediates known to be present in it, and known conditions of temperature, pH, etc ("physiological conditions"), is able to elaborate a whole group of alkaloids and sometimes several chemical classes of alkaloids. An effort may then be made to reproduce these conditions *in vitro*.

The building blocks of the alkaloids are presumed to be the amino acids and their metabolic degradation products. Formaldehyde sources (eg, glyoxylic and formic acids) are also available, and biological processes of deamination, decarboxylation, and oxidation are operative. How the plant effects the synthesis is best determined by a study of the plant chemistry itself, but *in vitro* experiments often provide strong clues.

In one of the earliest trials at syntheses under "physiological conditions," Schöpf and his co-workers[4] were able to prepare lobelanine in high yield by keeping a mixture of benzoylacetic acid, methylamine hydrochloride, and glutaric dialdehyde at pH 4 and 25° for 8 hours.

As another example, Robinson synthesized tropinone (which on electrolytic reduction yields tropine) by allowing an aqueous solution of succinaldehyde, acetone, and methylamine to stand for 30 minutes.

It was later shown[4] that the yield reaches a maximum (85–90%) at 25° and pH 5–7.

Robinson's views on the relationship between the benzylisoquinoline group of opium alkaloids and the morphine group found confirmation in Grewe's synthesis[5] of the morphinan ring system from an octahydro-1-benzyl-2-methylisoquinoline (although this was not achieved under "physiological conditions"):

N-Methyl-morphinan

Incompatibilities—Most alkaloids are soluble in alcohol and other organic solvents and insoluble in water; they react with acids to form salts which usually are soluble in water and only slightly soluble in alcohol. The addition of a *base*, therefore, to an aqueous solution of an alkaloidal salt, will generally precipitate the free alkaloid. In the same manner, *alkaline salts* such as the *acetates, carbonates, citrates, benzoates, salicylates*, and *basic phosphates* of sodium, potassium, and ammonium will precipitate the free alkaloid from such a solution, or, in some instances, will convert it to a less soluble salt.

Among the so-called "alkaloid precipitants" several may appear in prescription practice. *Iodine, picric acid, tannic acid, potassium mercuric iodide*, and *mercuric chloride* form insoluble compounds with most alkaloids. An occasional difficulty arises from the use of a galenical made from a tannin-containing drug. Frequently, a very small amount of alcohol will suffice to prevent these precipitations.

Many of the alkaloids are soluble in liquid petrolatum, while the salts are generally insoluble. Other alkaloids can be rendered soluble in liquid petrolatum by conversion to the oleates.

As a general rule, alkaloids are incompatible with *oxidizing agents*, some undergoing oxidation readily on exposure to air. Various antioxidants such as sodium metabisulfite and sodium sulfite are effective in retarding this deterioration. Oxidation is more rapid in alkaline solution and buffers which maintain the solution at a pH designed to retard it are commonly used. The hydrolysis of ester and glycosidic alkaloids is pH-catalyzed.

Classification

Alkaloids may be classified in a variety of ways, eg, on a botanical, or chemical, or pharmacological, etc.

---

* Often in the past this resemblance was noted only after the therapeutic effectiveness of a synthetic had been discovered. At the present time more and more alkaloid substitutes are "tailor-made" by design.

basis. Various systems are employed depending upon the nature of the primary interests of the various authors. Each system has its advantages and disadvantages, and a realistic appraisal of the present situation points to the firm conclusion that much more needs to be learned about the occurrence, composition, and physiological actions of the alkaloids before a comprehensive classification having maximum practical utility can be produced. The usual chemical classifications take into account the cyclic nuclei and the number, locations, and types of substituent functional groups; and, while it is abundantly evident that these classifications have led to the charting of research paths which have yielded very useful synthetic drugs, nevertheless it is equally clear that the present state of correlation between pharmacologic actions and various features of molecular architecture leaves much to be desired. This has led to a current revival of interest in the various stereochemical aspects of alkaloids in an attempt to resolve the many anomalies, and expectations are high that sufficiently intensive investigation in this area of endeavor will yield useful information.

For the purpose of the abbreviated presentation in this chapter, the alkaloids are classified under the headings enumerated below. Miscellaneous alkaloids not belonging to any of these classes are treated at other locations in the text. Consult the index for precise locations.

1. Opium Alkaloids
2. Cinchona Alkaloids
3. Tropane Alkaloids
4. Xanthine Alkaloids
5. Ergot Alkaloids
6. Rauwolfia Alkaloids
7. Veratrum Alkaloids
8. Vinca Alkaloids
9. Miscellaneous Alkaloids

It will be observed that this classification is partly botanical and partly chemical. To some extent, the groupings also reflect similarities in therapeutic application.

Special attention is called to the fact that the following display is limited strictly to natural alkaloids and derivatives of these which may be produced by effecting relatively simple chemical operations. Deliberately avoided in this section has been any attempt to include synthetic compounds such as (1) meperidine, methadone, and the several synthetic morphinan derivatives which are often included in other texts in the opium group; (2) chloroquine, hydroxychloroquine, and other synthetic antimalarials which are often presented with alkaloids of the cinchona group; (3) eucatropine, procaine, and various other synthetics often presented with alkaloids of the tropane group; etc. It should also be recalled that many crude drugs, eg, hydrastis, aconite, etc., which are not included in this chapter, owe their therapeutic effectiveness to their alkaloid content. Monographs dealing with all of the official alkaloids and their derivatives and related synthetics are distributed throughout the text on a pharmacologic basis. (Consult the general index.)

Structural Formulas and Nomenclature

The structural formulas for all alkaloids in this text are presented in the style adopted by Chemical Abstracts commencing with the Subject Index to Vol. 66. This style portrays the alkaloids in what has been termed their "absolute configuration," ie, portrays the stereochemistry of all asymmetric centers, and is employed whenever the stereochemical configuration is definitive and can be expressed unambiguously by the Cahn–Ingold–Prelog sequence convention.[6]

In its new treatment of alkaloids, Chemical Abstracts frequently abandons the systematic (Ring Index) names in favor of stereospecific trivial names such as aporphine, morphinan, yohimban, etc. It frequently also departs from Ring Index orientation and numbering in favor of schemes more commonly used in the reporting literature. As to be expected, these differences in orientation and numbering are also reflected in differences in nomenclature and thus complicate further literature searches and structural comparisons of compounds. The preferred Chemical Abstracts names for all official alkaloids and alkaloid salts are provided as subtitles to the monograph captions at other locations in the text.

For a detailed discussion of the Chemical Abstracts method of naming, structuring, and indexing alkaloids, see the Introduction to the Vol. 66 Subject Index of Chemical Abstracts.

Opium Alkaloids

Opium is official as such, and its monograph, along with monographs on various official items containing it, are presented on page 1121, et seq.

The many alkaloids obtained from the opium poppy, *Papaver somniferum*, are often divided into the following five approximate chemical "groups": (1) *Benzylisoquinoline*, (2) *Phenanthrene*, (3) *Tetrahydroisoquinoline*, (4) *Cryptopine*, and (5) *Alkaloids of Unknown Structure*, and the classification shown in Table XI is on this basis. An additional group is provided to accommodate the important semisynthetic derivatives of morphine and codeine. The specific heteronuclei present are identified by footnotes; the number in parentheses following the name is the Ring Index (2nd ed) number.

It will be observed that the pharmaceutically important alkaloids displayed in Table X derive from the so-called benzylisoquinoline and phenanthrene groups. Ginsburg[7] has produced a recent treatment of various selected topics dealing with opium alkaloids.

The parent heterocycle of the phenanthrene group of alkaloids is 4a*H*-8,9c-iminoethanophenanthro[4,5-*bcd*]furan. In the hexahydro state characteristic of codeine and morphine, its Ring Index (IUPAC) orientation and numbering are shown below. The specific stereoisomer present in these alkaloids is shown at the right in Chemical Abstracts style which treats it as a 4,5α-epoxy morphinan and numbers it by the familiar Cahn–Robinson sequence.

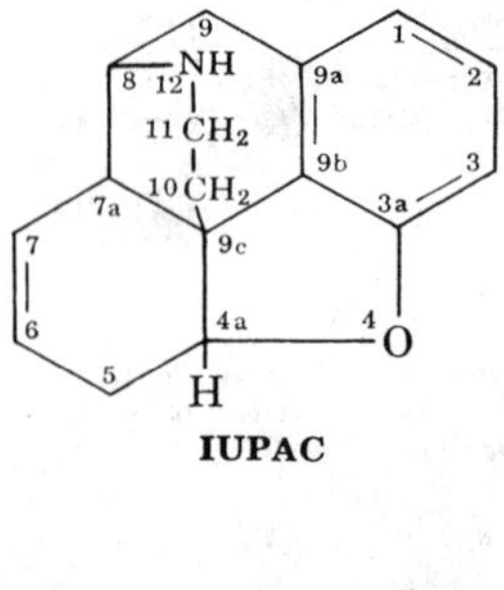

IUPAC 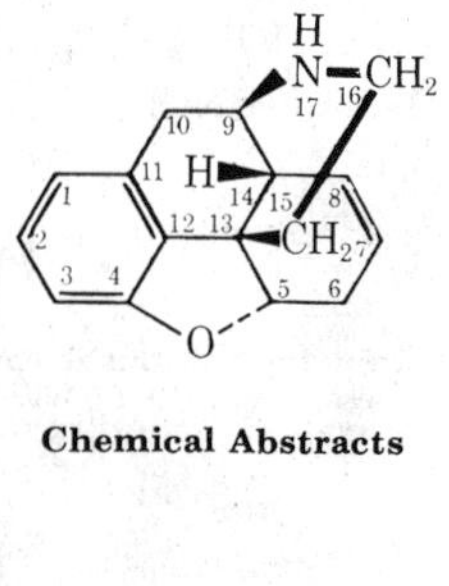   **Chemical Abstracts**

Table X—Opium Alkaloids and Derivatives

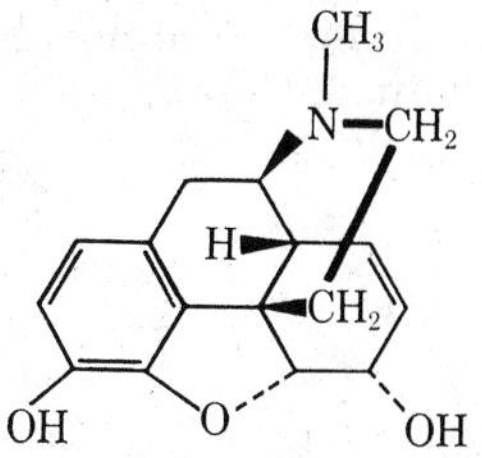

Morphine

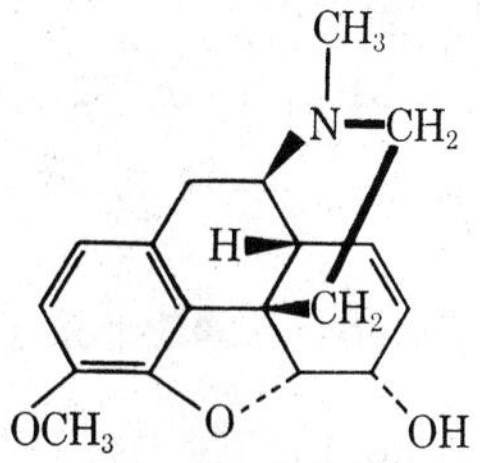

Codeine

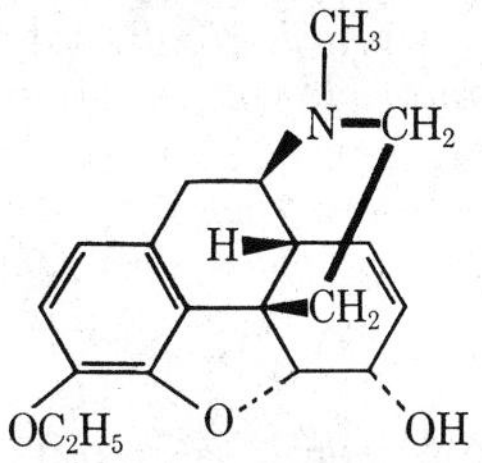

Ethylmorphine

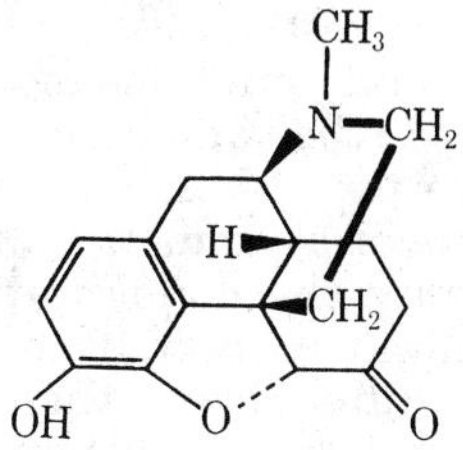

Hydromorphone

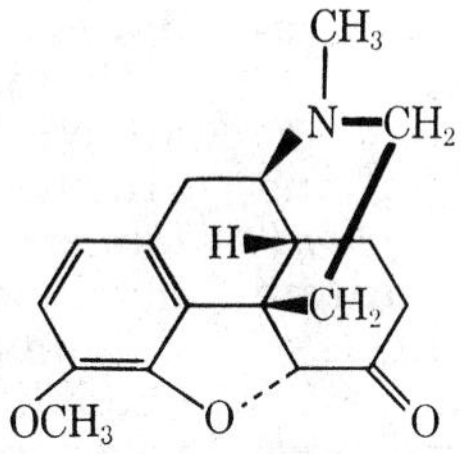

Hydrocodone

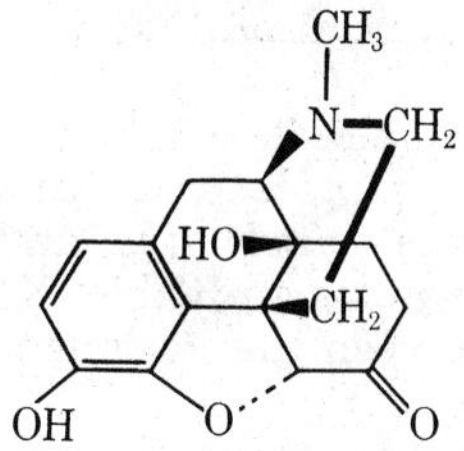

Oxymorphone

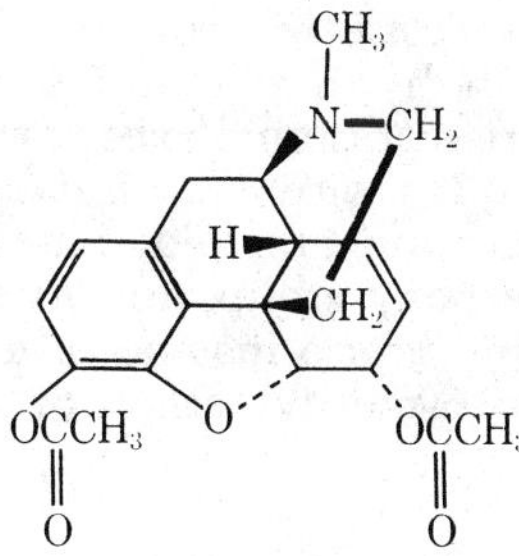

Heroin

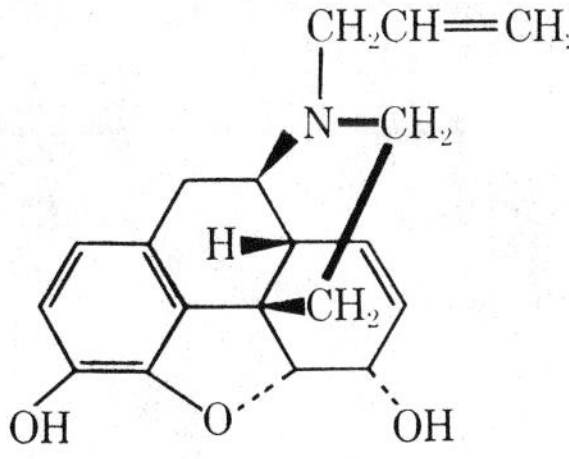

Nalorphine

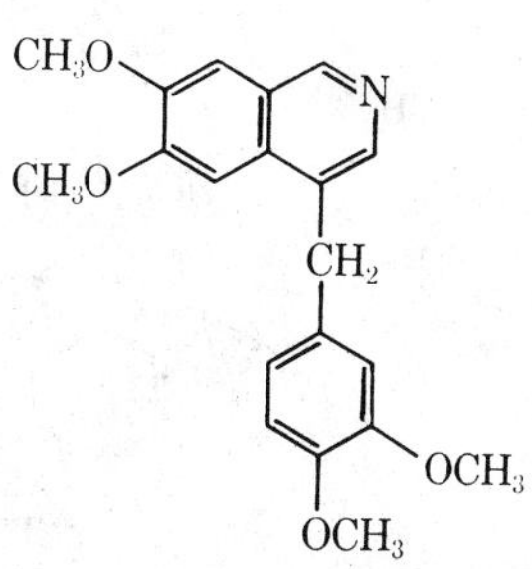

Papaverine

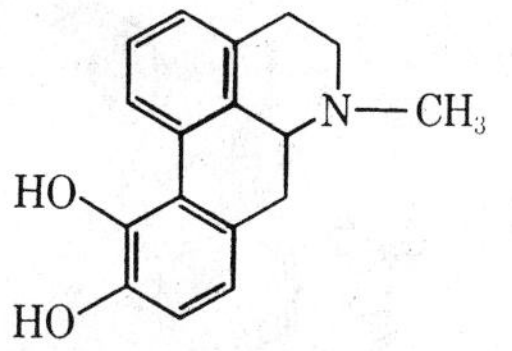

Apomorphine

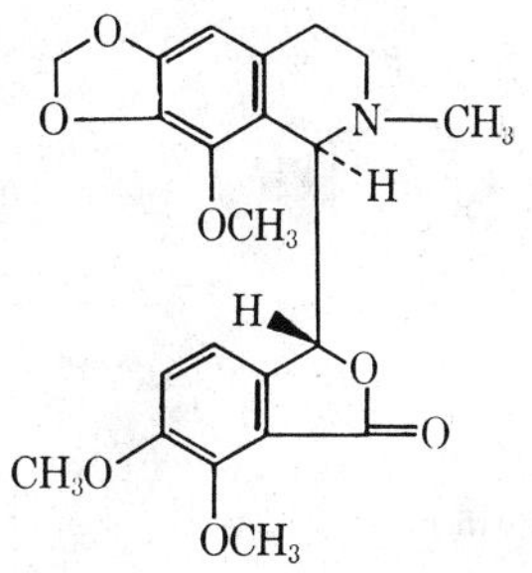

Noscapine (*l*-Narcotine)

Table XI—Classification of Opium Alkaloids

Benzylisoquinoline Group

Codamine [$C_{20}H_{25}NO_4$][d]

Gnoscopine [$C_{22}H_{23}NO_7$][e,b]

Laudanidine [$C_{20}H_{25}NO_4$][d]

dl-Laudanine [$C_{20}H_{25}NO_4$][d]

Laudanosine [$C_{21}H_{27}NO_4$][d]

Narceine [$C_{23}H_{27}NO_8$][a]

Narcotoline [$C_{21}H_{21}NO_7$][e,b]

l-Narcotine [$C_{22}H_{23}NO_7$][e,b]

Oxynarcotine [$C_{22}H_{23}NO_8$][e,b]

Papaverine [$C_{20}H_{21}NO_4$][c]

Xanthaline [$C_{20}H_{19}NO_5$][c]

Phenanthrene Group

Codeine [$C_{18}H_{21}NO_3$][h]

Morphine [$C_{17}H_{19}NO_3$][h]

ψ-Morphine [($C_{17}H_{18}NO_3$)$_2$][h]

Neopine [$C_{18}H_{21}NO_3$][g]

Thebaine [$C_{19}H_{21}NO_3$][f]

Tetrahydroisoquinoline Group

Hydrocotarnine [$C_{12}H_{15}NO_3$][e]

Cryptopine Group

Cryptopine [$C_{21}H_{23}NO_5$][i]

Protopine [$C_{20}H_{19}NO_5$][j]

Alkaloids of Unknown Structure

Aporeine [$C_{18}H_{16}NO_2$]

Lanthopine [$C_{23}H_{25}NO_4$]

Meconidine [$C_{21}H_{23}NO_4$]

Papaveramine [$C_{21}H_{25}NO_6$]

Rhœadine [$C_{21}H_{21}NO_6$]

Derivatives of Natural Alkaloids

Apomorphine[k]

Hydrocodone (dihydro-codeinone)

Hydromorphone (dihydro-morphinone)

Dionine (ethylmorphine)

Heroin (diacetylmorphine)

Metopon (methyldihydro-morphinone)

Nalorphine (N-allylnor-morphine)

Oxymorphone

---

[a] 2,3-dihydrobenzofuran (coumaran). (1328)

[b] 1,3-dihydroisobenzofuran (phthalan). (1330)

[c] isoquinoline. (1708)

[d] 1,2,3,4-tetrahydroisoquinoline. (1708)

[e] 5,6,7,8-tetrahydro-1,3-dioxolo[4,5-*g*]isoquinoline. (2810)

[f] 8,9-dihydro-4a*H*-8,9c-iminoethanophenanthro[4,5-*bcd*]furan. (5922)

[g] 5,6,8,9-tetrahydro-4a*H*-8,9c-iminoethanophenanthro[4,5-*bcd*]furan. (5922))

[h] 5,7a,8,9-tetrahydro-4a*H*-8,9c-iminoethanophenanthro[4,5-*bcd*]furan. (5922

[i] 6,7,12,13,14,15-hexahydrobenzo[*e*]-1,3-dioxolo[4,5-*l*][2]benzazecine. (4874)

[j] 4,5,6,7,13,14-hexahydrobis[1,3]benzodioxolo[4,5-*c*:5′,6′*g*]azecine. (5777)

[k] 4*H*-dibenzo[*de*,*g*]quinoline. (5171)

Official Opium Alkaloids and Derivatives

Opium alkaloids and derivatives, official as such and/or as salts, include: Apomorphine; Codeine; Ethylmorphine; Hydrocodone; Hydromorphone; Morphine; Nalorphine; Noscapine; Oxymorphone; and Papaverine.

Cinchona Alkaloids

There are more than twenty alkaloids obtainable from the bark of various species of *Cinchona* and *Remijia* (*Cuprea*) and many of these are convertible by chemical processes into closely related, useful, synthetic derivatives.

The most important alkaloids of cinchona are the pair of diastereoisomers, *quinine* and *quinidine*, and their 6-demethoxy analogs, *cinchonine* and *cinchonidine*. The structural formulas in Table XII indicate the close relationships between the various members of this group of alkaloids.

Examination of the formulas of these compounds shows that they all contain a *quinoline* ring attached through a hydroxymethylene group to a *quinuclidine* ring.

Quinuclidine   Quinoline

By altering the side chains attached to these rings and by esterifying and/or oxidizing the alcohol group, a large number of compounds have been produced and investigated.

Quinine and quinidine both have a *methoxy* group attached to the quinoline ring and a *vinyl* group attached to the quinuclidine ring. Each has the same four centers of asymmetry, but the diastereoisomerism involves only the configurations at the carbinol and 2-quinuclidine carbon atoms. Cinchonine and cinchonidine differ from these two alkaloids in that they do not have a methoxy group on the quinoline ring. Quinidine and cinchonine are dextrorotatory whereas quinine and cinchonidine are levorotatory. *Hydroquinine*, obtained from quinine by reduction with hydrogen and a catalyst, has the same structure as quinine except the vinyl group is reduced to an ethyl group. *Cupreine*, another naturally occurring cinchona alkaloid, has an OH group in place of the methoxy group, and *hydrocupreine* is cupreine with an ethyl group instead of a vinyl group. Thus quinine is the 6-methyl ether of cupreine and hydroquinine is

Table XII—Cinchona Alkaloids and Derivatives

Quinine	Quinidine	Cinchonine
Cinchonidine	Hydroquinine	Quinine Ethylcarbonate
Cupreine	Hydrocupreine	Ethylhydrocupreine

the corresponding ether of hydrocupreine. Quinine was first synthesized in 1944 by Woodward and Doering but the process is too costly for commercial use.

The salts of the alkaloids are typical onium salts, ie, the hydrogen of the acid attaches itself to the tertiary nitrogen atom forming a substituted ammonium radical which forms an ionic compound with the negative radical of the acid. Since there are two nitrogen atoms present in the molecules of the cinchona alkaloids it is possible to form salts containing one or two equivalents of acid, eg, mono- and di-hydrochlorides.

Identification—Quinine and its diastereoisomer, quinidine, are characterized (1) by the blue fluorescence of their solutions in dilute sulfuric or other oxy-acids and (2) by the *thalleioquin reaction*. The addition of 2 drops of bromine TS to 5 ml of a saturated solution of quinine or quinidine or a 1:1000 solution of their salts, followed by 1 ml of ammonia TS produces an emerald green color due to the formation of thalleioquin. They are differentiated by their optical rotations and by their behavior toward alkali tartrate. In neutral or slightly acid solutions quinine is precipitated by this reagent, while quinidine is not. On the other hand, quinidine in moderately dilute solution is precipitated by soluble iodides but quinine is not affected. The same differences are exhibited by cinchonidine and its diastereoisomer cinchonine; the former is levorotatory and, like quinine, it is precipitated by alkali tartrates while cinchonine is unaffected by the reagent and is dextrorotatory.

Cinchona

[Cinchona Bark; Peruvian Bark]

Cinchona is the dried bark of the stem or of the root of *Cinchona succirubra* Pavon et Klotzsch or its hybrids, known in commerce as Red Cinchona, or of *Cinchona Ledgeriana* (Howard) Moens et Trimen, *Cinchona Calisaya* Weddell or hybrids of these with other species of *Cinchona*, known in commerce as Calisaya Bark or as Yellow Cinchona (Fam, *Rubriaceæ*).

Cinchona yields 5% of the alkaloids of Cinchona. The crude drug is no longer official.

History—This drug derives its name from the Countess of Cinchon, who was instrumental in introducing it into European medical practice in 1640. It was also called Jesuit's Bark in recognition of the fact that it was used by the members of this ecclesiastical order in treating fever and ague. Its adoption as a valuable official remedy followed the purchase by Louis XIV, in 1680, of the secret of a proprietary remedy sold by an English apothecary's clerk named Robert Talbor, which contained cinchona as a basis. The romance of Cinchona has been published in various books and is well worth perusal.

Constituents—The alkaloids listed below have been isolated from cinchona barks. Some of these are found in only one kind of bark, as cupreine, and some are doubtless "split products"—that is, not existing naturally in the bark, but the result of the action of chemical agents upon it.

Quinine, $C_{20}H_{24}N_2O_2$
Quinidine, $C_{20}H_{24}N_2O_2$
Cinchonine, $C_{19}H_{22}N_2O$
Cinchonidine, $C_{19}H_{22}N_2O$
Quinamine, $C_{19}H_{24}N_2O$
Conquinamine, $C_{19}H_{24}N_2O_2$
Homoquinine, $C_{39}H_{46}N_4O_4$
Cinchonamine, $C_{19}H_{24}N_2O$
Paytine, $C_{21}H_{24}N_2O.H_2O$
Homocinchonidine, $C_{19}H_{22}N_2O$
Cusconine, $C_{23}H_{26}N_2O_4$
Cusconidine, $C_{23}H_{26}N_2O_4$
Concusconine, $C_{22}H_{26}N_2O_4$
Aricine, $C_{23}H_{26}N_2O_4$
Paricine, $C_{16}H_{18}N_2O$
Hydroquinine, $C_{20}H_{26}N_2O_2$
Hydroquinidine, $C_{20}H_{26}N_2O_2$
Cinchotine, $C_{19}H_{24}N_2O$
Hydrocinchonine, $C_{19}H_{24}N_2O$
Hydrocinchonidine, $C_{19}H_{24}N_2O$
Diquinidine, $C_{40}H_{46}N_4O_3$
Cupreine, $C_{19}H_{22}N_2O_2$

The acids present in Cinchona are *quinic acid*, (*hexahydro-1,3,4,5-tetrahydroxybenzoic acid*), *quinotannic acid*, and *quinovic acid* (*3β-hydroxyurs-12-ene-27,28-dioic acid*). Also present are α-quinovin (a glycoside), *cinchona-red*, other coloring matter and a volatile oil.

The quinine and total alkaloid content is highest in bark from cultivated cinchona. In bark from the uncultivated plant cinchonine and cinchonidine predominate. Java bark, representing highly cultivated cinchona, contains 7 to 10% of total alkaloids of which about 70% is quinine.

Quinine, quinidine, cinchonine, and cinchonidine are the most important alkaloids found in cinchona and are frequently referred to as the "*crystallizable cinchona alkaloids.*" Cinchonidine, cinchonine, and quinidine are usually spoken of as the "minor cinchona alkaloids." The noncrystalline residue remaining after the removal of the crystallizable alkaloids is known as *quinoidine*.

Uses—Cinchona is little used in modern therapeutics in the United States, but is elsewhere employed as a cheap substitute for quinine. It shares the *antimalarial*, *antipyretic*, and *analgetic* actions of quinine, but the alkaloidal salts are to be preferred to the galenical preparations.

One of the principal difficulties in preserving galenical preparations of cinchona arises from the alteration and precipitation which the cinchotannic acid and its compounds undergo upon keeping. Glycerin has proved to be very useful by dissolving and holding these in solution, and hence it is present in nearly all of the preparations.

Dose—*Usual*, 1 Gm.

Veterinary Dose—*Horses* and *Cattle*, **4 to 8 Gm**; *Dogs*, **300 mg to 1 Gm.**

Official Cinchona Alkaloids

Cinchona alkaloids official as such and/or salts, include: Quinidine and Quinine.

Tropane Alkaloids

The Tropane alkaloids will be considered under two headings: (1) Atropine and Related Alkaloids and (2) Cocaine.

They are grouped together because all are formally derivatives of tropane.

$$CH_2—CH——CH_2$$

Tropane

Atropine and Related Alkaloids

The alkaloids of the atropine group (Table XIII) are closely related chemically. Most of the natural alkaloids are esters of *mandelic acid* or *tropic acid* with *tropine** or *scopine*. For example, atropine is the

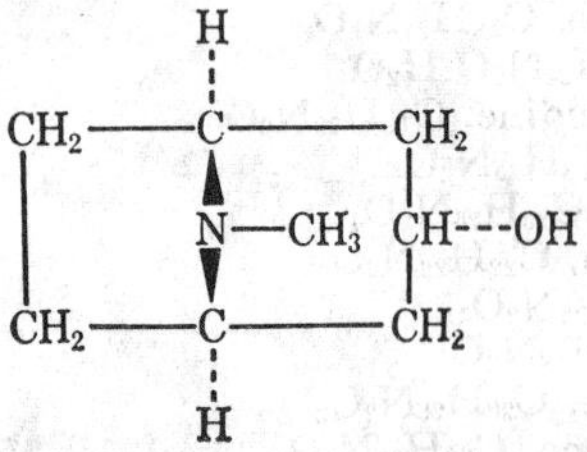

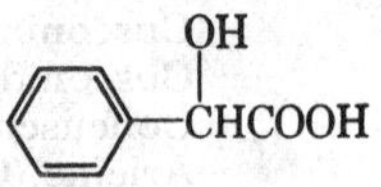

Tropine (1αH,5αH-Tropan-3α-ol)   **Mandelic Acid**

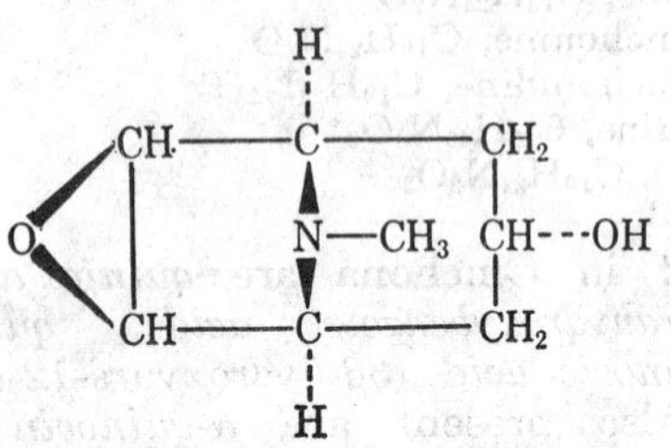

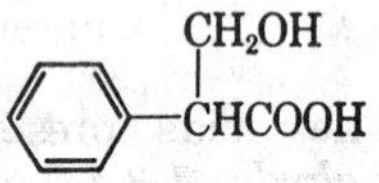

Scopine (6β,7β-Epoxy-1αH,5αH-tropan-3α-ol)   **Tropic Acid**

racemic variety of tropine tropate, hyoscyamine is the levorotatory enantiomorph of the same compound, and scopolamine is scopine tropate. Scopine is epoxytropine, the only difference being the 6,7-oxygen bridge. It is therefore to be expected that these three alkaloids give similar color reactions. Eumydrine is also closely related; it is 8-methylatropinium nitrate, a quaternary ammonium salt. Homatropine is tropine mandelate and Novatropine is the 8-methylhomatropinium bromide. Benztropine is the benzhydryl ester of tropine. See Table XIII.

Belladonna (see page 916), hyoscyamus, and stramonium yield mydriatic alkaloids, characteristic of the *Solanaceæ* Family. There are also many other plants of this group which are being used largely in the manufacture of the various alkaloids. The distribution of alkaloids in the most important plants is shown in Table XIV.

Atropine rarely occurs as such in any of the plants, but is always the product of the racemization of the levo-isomeride, hyoscyamine, which is converted into atropine by the action of weak alkalies. This racemization involves the conversion of the (−)-tropic acid moiety of hyoscyamine to (±)-tropic acid.

Table XIV—Distribution of Solanaceous Alkaloids

Plant	Part yielding alkaloid	Per cent of total alkaloid	Most important alkaloids
Atropa belladonna	Leaves	0.15 −0.6	Hyoscyamine
	Root	0.1 −0.7	Hyoscyamine
	Seeds	About 0.8	Hyoscyamine
Datura metel	Leaves	0.25 −0.55	Scopolamine (Hyoscine)
Datura stramonium	Leaves	0.2 −0.45	Hyoscyamine
	Seeds	0.2 −0.5	Hyoscyamine
Duboisia myoporoides	Seeds	0.2 −0.5	Hyoscine and hyoscyamine
Hyoscyamus muticus	Leaves	1 −1.4	Hyoscyamine
Hyoscyamus niger	Leaves	0.045−0.08	Hyoscyamine
	Tops	0.07 −0.10	Hyoscine

* Esters of tropine are called tropeines; eg, tropine mandelate is mandelyltropeine.

In this country stramonium is the principal source of the hyoscyamine used in the manufacture of atropine. Scopolamine (hyoscine) is produced to a large extent from *Datura Metel* as well as from the mother liquors

Table XIII—Atropine and Related Alkaloids and Derivatives

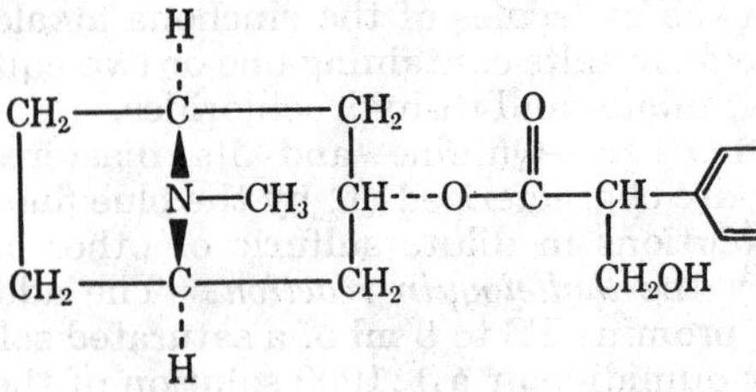

Atropine (Tropine (±)-Tropate)
Hyoscyamine (Tropine (−)-Tropate)

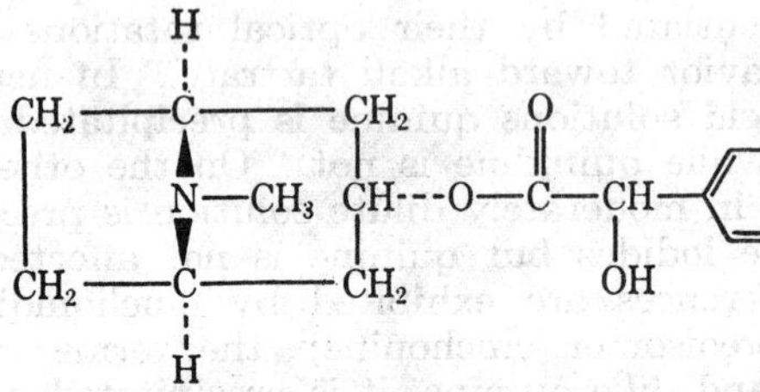

Homatropine

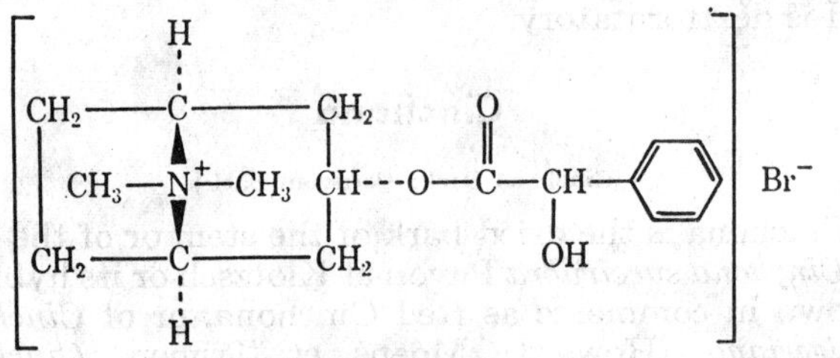

Novatropine
(Homatropine Methylbromide)

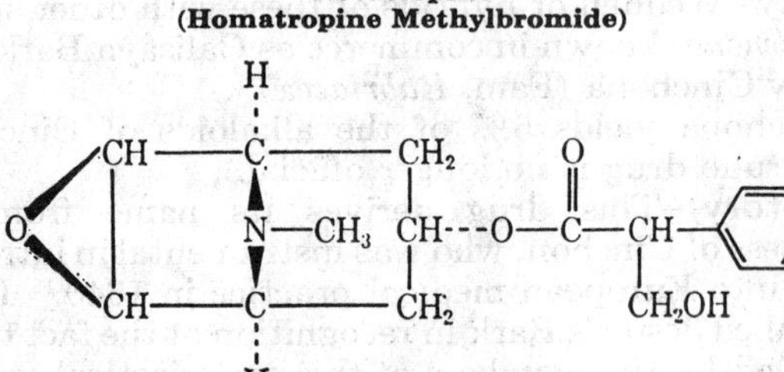

Scopolamine
(6β,7β-Epoxyhyoscyamine)

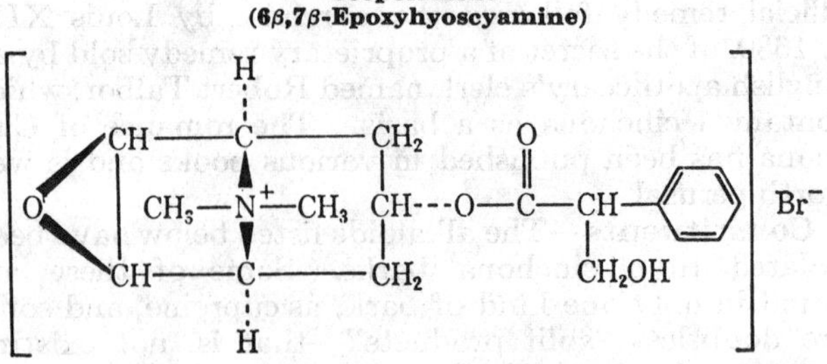

Methscopolamine Bromide

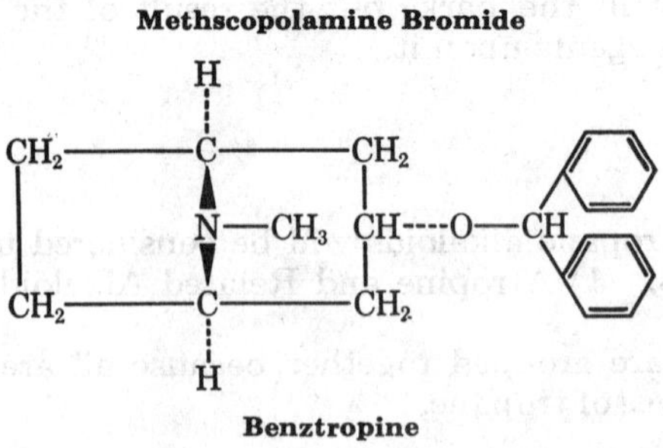

Benztropine

Table XV—Ecgonine Derivatives

R	R'	Name of derivative
H	H	Ecgonine
CH_3	C_6H_5CO (benzoyl)	Cocaine
H	CH_3	Methylecgonine
H	$C_6H_5CH=CHCO$ (cinnamoyl)	Cinnamoylecgonine
H	C_6H_5CO	Benzoylecgonine

remaining after crystallization of the hyoscyamine. Other alkaloids of lesser importance present in various members of the *Solaneceæ* include *atropamine, belladonnine, meteloidine,* and several others.

Atropine, as well as a number of other tropeines which do not occur naturally, have been prepared by total synthesis. Of the several classical syntheses of tropine the most interesting is that due to Robinson.[8] See page 491. Variations of this process are employed commercially. Racemic tropic acid has also been synthesized and resolved.

The most characteristic physiological property of the Solanaceous alkaloids is their mydriatic effect (dilation of the pupil of the eye). This property is the basis for the most sensitive test for their identification. As little as one drop of a 1 in 25,000 solution will cause a distinct dilation of the pupil of a cat's eye.

Cocaine and Related Alkaloids

The cocaine group of tropane alkaloids is distinguished chemically from the atropine group by the presence of carboxyl (or esterified carboxyl) at the 2β-position and by the β-configuration (instead of α) of

the 3-ester function. They thus become derivatives of ecgonine (3β-hydroxy-$1\alpha H,5\alpha H$-tropan-2β-carboxylic acid). Their general structural formula and the specific structure of the only official member, cocaine, are shown below.

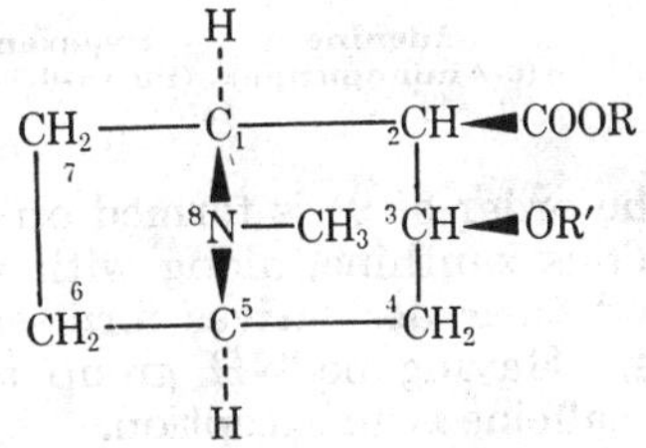

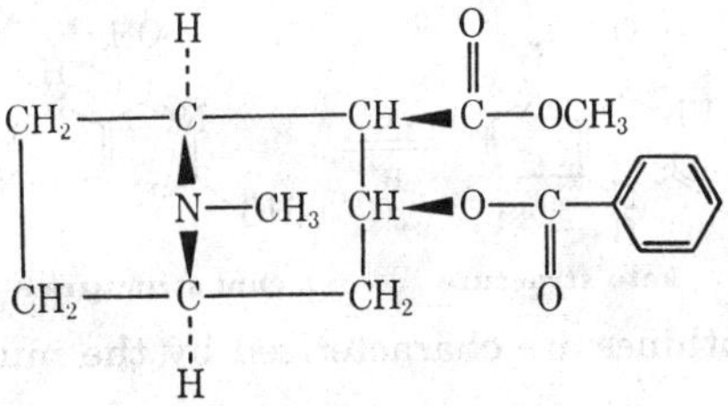

Table XV portrays the identities of R and R' for the common ecgonine derivatives. For further discussion, see Cocaine, page 1067.

Official Tropane Alkaloids and Derivatives

Tropane alkaloids and derivatives, official as such and/or as salts, include: Atropine; Benztropine; Cocaine; Homatropine; Homatropine Methylbromide; Hyoscyamine; Scopolamine; and Methscopolamine Bromide.

Xanthine Alkaloids

The important medicinal alkaloids of this group, *viz,* theophylline, theobromine, and caffeine, are methylated xanthines. Their structural relationships are portrayed in Table XVI. The parent molecule of each one is purine.

Many textbooks still retain the old "box formula" presentations which are of course equivalent. For example, the xanthine structure is also represented by:

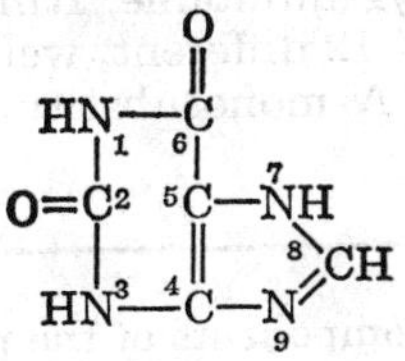

Other bases closely related to purine are *hypoxanthine, adenine,* and *guanine,* all of which are normally found in animal tissues. The last two bases are constituents

of nucleic acids and nucleoproteins which are found in cell nuclei, and hypoxanthine is produced in the body during the first stage of adenine oxidation. Further oxidation yields *xanthine,* then *uric acid.* In man the end product of protein metabolism is *urea.* In certain animals the end product is *allantoin* (page 498), formed by further oxidation of uric acid. The structures of these compounds are illustrated at the top of page 498. The oxygen-containing compounds are depicted here in keto form but they are often shown in texts in enol form as illustrated below with xanthine. The enol forms are often named specifically to reflect the hydroxyl groups, eg, purine-2,6,8-triol or 2,6,8-trioxypurine for uric acid.

Properties—The xanthines are very weak bases, having pK_b's of the order of 13–14. They form salts with the stronger acids which, of course, are readily hydrolyzed. By tautomeric shift of hydrogen from nitrogen to keto oxygen (enolization) a weakly acidic

Table XVI—Xanthine Alkaloids

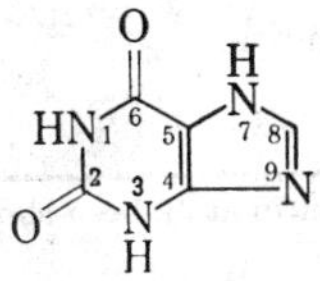

| Xanthine (Purine-2,6($1H,3H$)-dione) | Theophylline (1,3-Dimethylxanthine) | Theobromine (3,7-Dimethylxanthine) | Caffeine (1,3,7-Trimethylxanthine) |

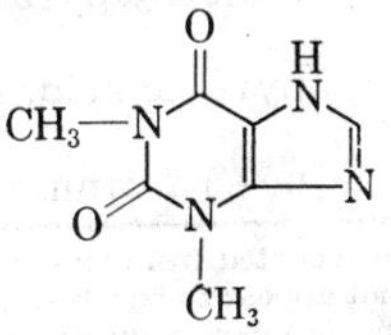

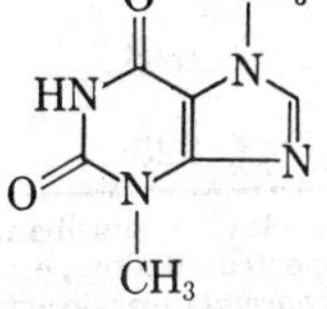

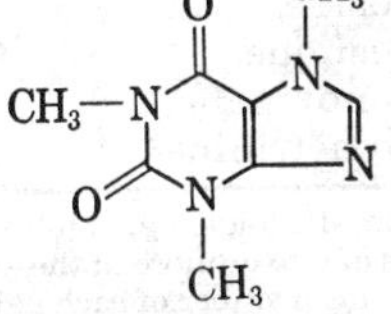

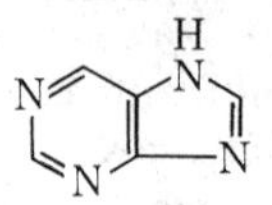

Purine 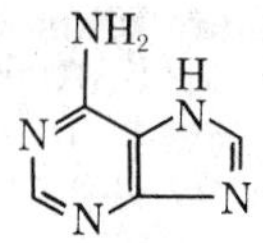   Adenine (6-Aminopurine) 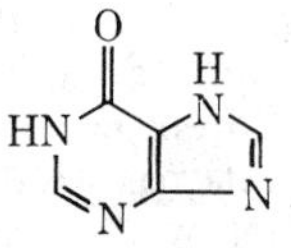   Hypoxanthine (Purin-6(1H)-one) 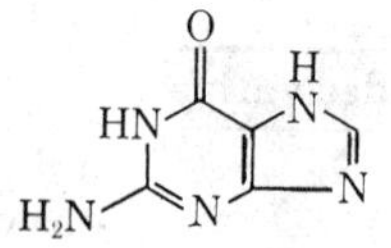   Guanine (2-Aminopurin-6(1H)-one) 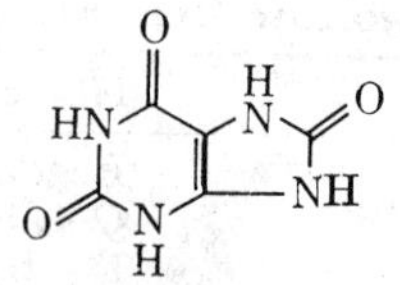   Uric Acid (Purine-2,6,8(1H,3H,9H)-trione) 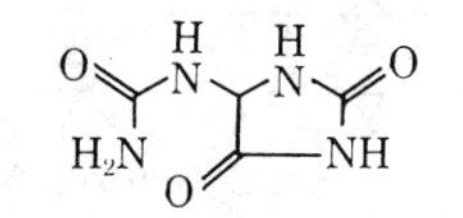   Allantoin (5-Ureidohydantoin)

H (pK_a's of the order of 9) is formed on the resulting OH group. Thus xanthine, along with various other oxopurines, and their derivatives form salts with the stronger bases. Having no NH group to participate in enolization, caffeine is an exception.

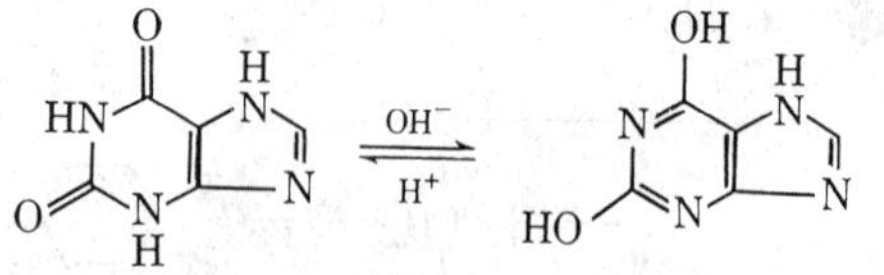

keto structure   enol structure

The xanthines are characterized by the murexide re-

action which involves evaporating a nitric acid solution of the test sample to dryness and treating the residue with ammonia whereupon a purplish-red color develops. The color is due to the formation of murexide, an ammonium salt of purpuric acid. Uric acid and various other purine derivatives also respond to the test.

Official Xanthine Alkaloids and Derivatives

Xanthine alkaloids and derivatives, official as such and/or as salts, include: Aminophylline [Theophylline Ethylenediamine Compound (2:1)]; Caffeine; and Theophylline.

Ergot Alkaloids

Ergot

Ergot is a morbid growth formed when the fungus, *Claviceps purpurea*, develops on various plants of the Gramineae (grass) and Cyperaceae (sedge) families such as rye, wheat, oats, barley, and rice. If the infestation of the plant occurs naturally, the resulting ergot is called *natural* ergot; if the infestation is brought about artificially, ie, wholly or partly by man through intention, the resulting ergot is referred to in the trade as *cultivated* ergot. Ergots from different plants vary in composition and they are thus not medicinally equivalent. It is for this reason that rye is stipulated as the source of the official ergot. Considerable research has been conducted in an attempt to produce ergot (or its equivalent from an alkaloid viewpoint) by microbiologic processes similar to those employed in the production of various antibiotics. For a further discussion of previously official ergot, see page 953.

Constituents—Ergot has been referred to as a veritable storehouse of chemicals. In addition to many alkaloids, it contains various carbohydrates, glycerides, sterols (eg, ergosterol and fungisterol), amino acids

(eg, histidine, leucine, and tyrosine), amines (eg, histamine and tyramine), quaternary ammonium compounds (eg, choline and betaine), and coloring principles. The lysergic acid group of alkaloids are the important medicinal constituents, and further treatment here is confined to them. They are all substituted amide derivatives of lysergic acid, which is shown below along with the official compounds and the important, but unofficial, diethylamide.

An understanding of the ergot alkaloids requires a knowledge of the isomerism of lysergic acid which exists in two diastereoisomeric forms depending on the spatial configuration of the carboxyl group relative to that of the 5β-hydrogen. In the *normal* lysergic acid (commonly called lysergic acid) this relative configuration is of the *cis* variety (carboxyl in β-configuration); in the *isolysergic acid*, it is of the *trans* type (carboxyl in α-configuration). Chemical Abstracts treats lysergic and isolysergic acid compounds as derivatives of ergoline which is the 4,6,6aβ,7,8,9,10,10aα-octahydro form of indolo[4,3-*fg*]quinoline, Ring Index No. 4550.

Ergot has yielded 12 different, well-defined alkaloids, each of which is an *N*-monosubstituted amide of either

Table XVII—The Ergot Alkaloids[a]

Alkaloid[b]	Formula	Mol. wt.	Specific rotation[c]	Organic components of the peptide moiety[d]
Ergocristine			−183	
Ergocristinine	$C_{35}H_{39}N_5O_5$	609	+366	dimethylpyruvic acid, D-proline, L-phenylalanine
Ergotamine			−160	
Ergotaminine	$C_{33}H_{35}N_5O_5$	581	+369	pyruvic acid, D-proline, L-phenylalanine
Ergocryptine			−187	
Ergocryptinine	$C_{32}H_{41}N_5O_5$	576	+408	dimethylpyruvic acid, D-proline, L-leucine
Ergocornine			−188	
Ergocorninine	$C_{31}H_{39}N_5O_5$	562	+409	dimethylpyruvic acid, D-proline, L-valine
Ergosine			−161	
Ergosinine	$C_{30}H_{37}N_5O_5$	548	+420	pyruvic acid, D-proline, L-leucine
Ergonovine[e]			−16	
Ergometrinine	$C_{19}H_{23}N_3O_2$	325	+416	L(+)-2-amino-1-propanol

[a] Other alkaloids, eg, ergotoxine, ergotinine, ergoclavine, sensibamine, etc, have been reported from time to time, but have ultimately been shown to be mixtures of two or more of the above. Another reported alkaloid, ergomonamine, does not appear to be a lysergic acid derivative.
[b] The *-ine* member of each pair is a derivative of *normal* lysergic acid; the *-inine* member is a derivative of *isolysergic acid*.
[c] Values are from The *Merck Index*, 8th ed. All values are in reference to solutions in chloroform except for ergonovine which is in pyridine.
[d] As revealed through hydrolytic cleavage.
[e] Other names: for ergonovine-ergobasine and ergometrine; for ergometrinine-ergobasinine.

the normal or the isolysergic acids. The substituting

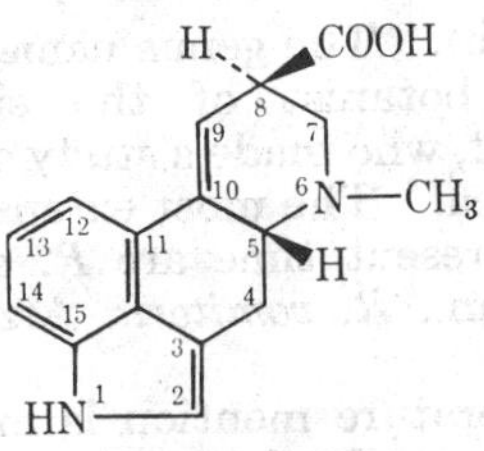

Lysergic Acid
(9,10-Didehydro-6-methylergoline-8β-carboxylic Acid)

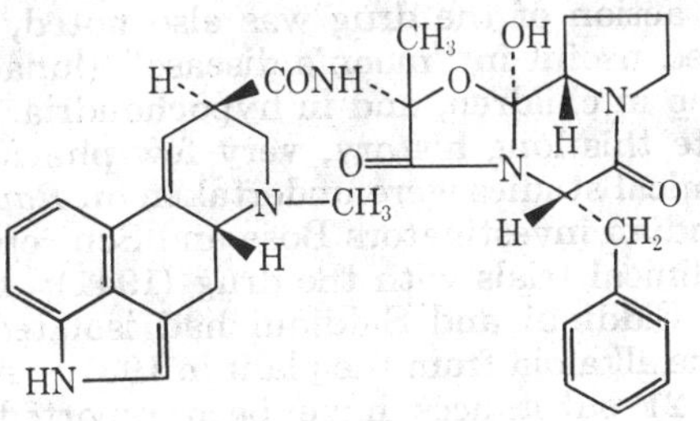

Ergotamine

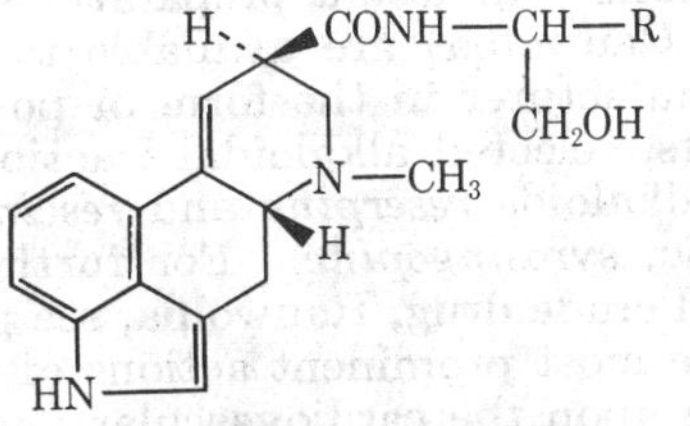

Ergonovine — R = CH₃
Methylergonovine — R = CH₂CH₃

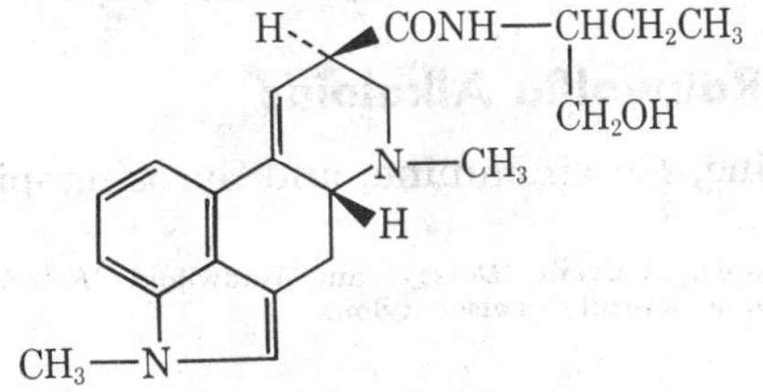

Methysergide

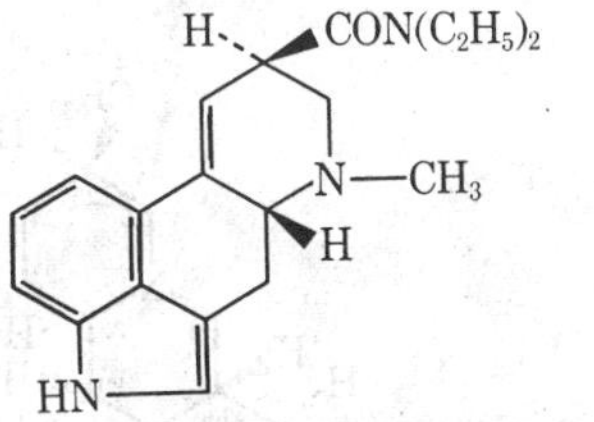

N,N-Diethyllysergamide (LSD)

group on the amide nitrogen is commonly referred to as the *peptide moiety* of the alkaloid because it always contains one or more peptide (amide) linkages. The 12 alkaloids divide into 6 pairs which differ from each other with respect to the composition of their peptide moieties. The 2 members of each pair differ from each other with regard to whether the lysergic acid moiety is the normal or iso variety. The members related to the normal acid are conventionally designated by the suffix *-ine;* and those related to the iso acid by *-inine.* The former are much more active physiologically than the latter. They are also levorotatory, whereas the latter are dextrorotatory, but, as indicated above and as is apparent from Table XVII, the members of any given pair are not enantiomorphs. The *-ine* member of a pair may be converted into its *-inine* isomer by refluxing its methanolic solution or by treatment with

alcoholic alkali; the reverse conversion may be effected by refluxing an acetic acid solution of the *-inine* isomer or by treating it with alcoholic phosphoric acid.

The important ergot alkaloids are summarized in Table XVII. Much of the knowledge concerning their composition and structure resulted from the researches of Jacobs and Craig of New York, who first demonstrated that lysergic acid was a common moiety, and to the long continued investigations of Stoll and Hofmann of Basle, Switzerland. Various color reactions characterisitic of the alkaloids, such as the Keller test (blue color with acetic acid-ferric chloride-sulfuric acid reagent) and the Van Urk test (blue color with *p*-dimethylaminobenzaldehyde reagent), are referable to the lysergic acid component.

Ergonovine, simpler by far than any of the other ergot alkaloids, is commercially available both as the natural alkaloid and as a synthetic compound (see page 951). The crude lysergic acid required for the synthesis is readily prepared by subjecting the total ergot alkaloid fraction to alkaline hydrolysis and then acidifying. Lysergic acid itself has been synthesized starting with the commercially available coal tar derivative, indole-3-propionic acid, but the synthesis is lengthy and the present cost is unfavorable. A microbiologic synthesis utilizing *Claviceps paspali* and suitable for relatively large scale manufacture has been patented.

Methylergonovine is not a natural ergot alkaloid. It is synthesized from lysergic acid by the same procedure as that employed for *Ergonovine* (see page 951) except that (+)-2-amino-1-butanol is used to furnish the peptide moiety.

Methysergide, another unnatural alkaloid, is the 4-methyl homologue of methylergonovine.

***N,N*-Diethyl-lysergamide,** a compound of considerable interest, does not occur in nature. The physiologically active isomer is the (+)-enantiomorph of the *N,N*-diethylamide of normal lysergic acid and is commonly referred to as LSD-25 or simply LSD. Methods for its synthesis from lysergic acid have been developed. In normal subjects, LSD elicits a temporary combination of physiological and psychological effects which collectively mimic syndromes characteristic of psychotic states, eg, schizophrenia. Because of this action, speculation often occurs in the public press relative to the possible use of the compound as a nonlethal chemical warfare agent. LSD has been the subject of intense clinical investigation during the past five years. There are no established therapeutic applications at present, but it has found some application as a diagnostic tool in psychiatry (see page 1119) and as a tool in the rapid developing field of psychopharmacology. Discovery of the psychotogenic activity of LSD has led to extensive research with various types of lysergic acid derivatives. It has also given rise to serious social problems.

Dihydro analogs of lysergic acid and its derivatives form readily by catalytic hydrogenation, the addition occurring at the expense of the 9:10 double bond. Such hydrogenation of the ergot alkaloids results in marked changes in their physiological actions (see *Dihydroergotamine,* page 953). Dihydro-LSD is relatively devoid of psychotogenic action.

Official Ergot Alkaloids

Ergot alkaloids, official as salts, include: Ergonovine; Ergotamine; Methylergonovine (synthetic); and Methysergide (synthetic).

Rauwolfia Alkaloids

Reserpine, obtained from several *Rauwolfia* species, was the first alkaloid of this group to be officially recognized. Interest in the remarkable therapeutic properties of these powerful agents became so keen that reserpine alkaloid, injection, and tablets were admitted to the USP XV by Supplement (1959). Rescinnamine soon followed, NF XI (1960), and Syrosingopine gained NF XII recognition (1965).

The general structure of these three alkaloids is shown below. Chemical Abstracts uses the familiar Barger, Scholz numbering. It will be observed that they are all esters of methyl reserpate, the only difference being in the identity of the acyl represented in the ester group at locus 18 of the heteronucleus. By the Chemical Abstracts system, methyl reserpate is the methyl ester of 18β-hydroxy-11,17α-dimethoxy-3β,-20α-yohimban-16β-carboxylic acid. Yohimban is the 4aβ,13bα,14aα stereoisomer of the 1,2,3,4,4a,5,7,8,-13,13b,14,14a-dodecahydro form of Ring Index No. 5874, benz[*g*]indolo[2,3-*a*]quinolizine. Reserpine and Rescinnamine occur naturally; Syrosingopine is synthetic.

Alkaloid	Acyl
Reserpine	3,4,5-trimethoxybenzoyl
Rescinnamine	3,4,5-trimethoxycinnamoyl
Syrosingopine	carbethoxysyringoyl

History—The genus *Rauwolfia*, natural order *Apocyanaceæ*, contains almost fifty species which grow in tropical and semitropical regions (India, Burma, Ceylon, Java, etc). The genus name honors a German physician and botanist of the sixteenth century, Leonard Rauwolf, who made a study of medicinal plants in Asia and Africa. The most extensively investigated species at the present time are *R. serpentina* Benth., *R. canescens* Linn., *R. vomitoria* Afzel, and *R. heterophylla*, Roem.

In ancient literature mention is made of the use of *Rauwolfia* as a remedy for snake bites and scorpion stings, as a febrifuge, and as a cure for dysentery. The sedative action of the drug was also noted, for it was considered useful in "moon's disease" (lunacy), to induce sleep in children, and in hypochondria.

Despite this long history, very few pharmacological and chemical studies were undertaken on *Rauwolfia* until the Indian investigators Bose and Sen reported successful clinical trials with the drug (1941); the Indian chemists Siddiqui and Siddiqui had isolated the first crystalline alkaloid from the plant in 1931. At present, at least 21 substances have been reported from *R. Serpentina* alone. These are listed in Table XVIII.

Preparations—*Rauwolfia* preparations (known collectively as Rauwolfia) are available to the pharmaceutical manufacturer in the form of powdered whole root, extracts, selected alkaloidal fractions,* the pure crystalline alkaloids *reserpine* and *rescinnamine*, and the synthetic, *syrosingopine*. For further discussion of the official crude drug, Rauwolfia, see page 912.

Uses—The most prominent actions of the rauwolfia alkaloids are upon the cardiovascular and central nervous systems. They are widely employed as *antihypertensive agents* and as *adjuncts in psychotherapy*.

Official Rauwolfia Alkaloids

Reserpine, Rescinnamine, and Syrosingopine.

---

* For example, Rauvera (*Dorsey*) and Rauwiloid (*Riker*) contain the fraction known generically as alseroxylon.

Veratrum Alkaloids

The veratrum alkaloids are derived from 12 known species of *Veratrum*, the more important of which are *viride*, *album*, *sabadilla*, and *grandiflorum*. The alkaloids may be divided into two groups for which Fieser[9] has proposed the designations *jerveratrum* and *ceveratrum*. Practically all of the alkamines (alkaloids lysed of ester or glucose moieties) of both groups are polyhydroxylated $C_{27}N$ fused polycyclics which, because they bear some resemblance to the steroid nucleus and also carry the 3β-OH characteristic of natural sterols, are often termed steroidal. In the jerveratrum group, the alkamines contain only 2 or 3 oxygens and the alkaloids consist either of the free alkamine, eg, *jervine* and *rubijervine*, or of the alkamine in D-glucosidic union, eg, *veratrosine*. In the ceveratrum group, the alkamines contain from 7 to 9 oxygens and the alkaloids consist of ester of the alkamines. The jerveratrum group is devoid of therapeutic activity and further treatment is therefore confined to the ceveratrum group.

The alkamines of the ceveratrum alkaloids are all polyhydroxy derivatives of 4,9-epoxycevane which is shown below in Chemical Abstracts orientation and numbering. It is an epoxytrimethyl derivative of a stereospecific hydrogenated form of Ring Index Parent No. 11363.

Ceveratrum nucleus

Many published papers portray an alternate orientation and numbering.

The relationship among the four alkamines is apparent from the following:

Alkamine	Type of polyol	Location of hydroxyl groups
Veracevine $C_{27}H_{43}NO_8$	heptol	3β,4β,12,14,16β,17,20
Germine $C_{27}H_{43}NO_8$	heptol	3β,4β,7α,14,15α,16β,20
Protoverine $C_{27}H_{43}NO_9$	octol	3β,4β,6α,7α,14,15α,16β,20
Zygadenine $C_{27}H_{43}NO_7$	hexol	3β,4β,14,15α,16β,20

Table XVIII—Alkaloids from R. Serpentina[c]

Ajmaline	$C_{20}H_{26}N_2O_2$
Ajmalicine	$C_{21}H_{24}N_2O_3$
Ajmalinine	$C_{20}H_{26}N_2O_3$
Isoajmaline	$C_{20}H_{26}N_2O_2$
Neoajmaline	$C_{20}H_{26}N_2O_2$
Raubasine	$C_{21}H_{25}N_2O_3$
Raubasinine	$C_{22}H_{26}N_2O_4$
Rauhimbine[a]	$C_{21}H_{26}N_2O_3$
Raupine	$C_{20}H_{26}N_2O_3$
Rauwolfine	$C_{20}H_{26}N_2O_3$
Rauwolfinine	$C_{19}H_{26}N_2O_2$
Rescinnamine	$C_{35}H_{42}N_2O_9$
Reserpine	$C_{33}H_{40}N_2O_9$
Reserpinine	$C_{22}H_{26}N_2O_4$
Sarpagine	$C_{19}H_{22}N_2O_2$
Serpine	$C_{21}H_{26}N_2O_3$
Serpinine	. . . . . .
Serpentine	$C_{21}H_{22}N_2O_3$
Serpentinine	$C_{20}H_{20}N_2O_5$
Yohimbine	$C_{21}H_{26}N_2O_3$
Allo-Yohimbine	$C_{21}H_{26}N_2O_3$
delta-Yohimbine[b]	$C_{21}H_{24}N_2O_3$

[a] Same as corynanthine.
[b] Same as ajmalicine.
[c] Molecular formulas are from Reference No.[1] *op cit.*

The alkamines can be obtained by subjecting their ester-alkaloids to mild alkaline hydrolysis. In contrast to the ester-alkaloids, the alkamines are relatively devoid of pharmacologic activity.

A partial listing of the ceveratrum alkaloids is presented in Table XIX. Listed also are the alkamines along with their loci of esterification and the acids involved. For a complete listing of all veratrum alkaloids (both jerveratrum and ceveratrum groups), consult the Morgan and Barltrop reference.[10] Kupchan and associates have conducted research-in-depth on the intimate chemistry of veratrum alkaloids. Under the general title *Veratrum Alkaloids*, their findings have been reported in a lengthy series of papers which, although published in various journals, can be located readily through the *Author Index* to *Chemical Abstracts*.[11]

Uses—Certain Veratrum alkaloids and alkaloid mixtures find some use as antihypertensive agents. For further discussion, see *Veratrum Alkaloids*, page 850. The crude drug, Veratrum Viride, was official for many years prior to 1960. Neither it nor any of the Veratrum alkaloids is currently official.

Table XIX—Composition of Selected Ceveratrum Alkaloids

Alkaloid	Molecular formula	Alkamine	Esterification loci[a]	Acid — Name	Acid — Structure
Cevadine	$C_{32}H_{49}NO_9$	Veracevine[b]	3	*cis*-2-methyl-2-butenoic (angelic)	CH_3H $\|$ $\|$ $CH_3C{=}CCOOH$
Germerine	$C_{37}H_{59}NO_{11}$	Germine	3 7	(+)-2-hydroxy-2-methylbutyric D-(−)-2-methylbutyric	CH_3 $\|$ CH_3CH_2CCOOH CH_3 OH $\|$ $\|$ CH_3CH_2CCOOH
Veratridine	$C_{36}H_{51}NO_{11}$	Veracevine[b]	3	3,4-dimethoxybenzoic (veratric)	$CH_3O{-}\!\!\bigcirc\!\!{-}COOH$ OCH_3
Protoveratrine A[c]	$C_{41}H_{63}NO_{14}$	Protoverine	3 5 and 6 7	(+)-2-hydroxy-2-methylbutyric acetic D-(−)-2-methylbutyric	CH_3 $\|$ CH_3CH_2CCOOH $\|$ OH CH_3COOH CH_3 $\|$ CH_3CH_2CCOOH
Protoveratrine B[c]	$C_{41}H_{63}NO_{15}$	Protoverine	3 5 and 6 7	(+)-*threo*-2,3-dihydroxy-2-methylbutyric as per Protoverine A as per Protoverine A	H OH $\|$ $\|$ $CH_3{-}C{-}C{-}COOH$ $\|$ $\|$ OH CH_3

[a] Numbering is in the IUPAC-notation described previously.
[b] Formerly thought to be cevine (the 3α-hydroxy analog of veracevine), but subsequent investigation disclosed cevine to be an artifact deduced from failure to recognize a rearrangement which occurred during degradative operations.
[c] Protoveratrines A and B were formerly thought to be only one alkaloid, protoveratrine. See Kloks, M. V., *et al*, *J. Am. Chem. Soc.*, **74,** 5107 (1952) and Nash, H. A., and Brooker, R. M., *Ibid*, **75,** 1942 (1953).

Vinca Alkaloids

Pharmacological inquiries during the late 1950's into the purported antihyperglycemic activity of principles contained in the apocynaceous plant, *Vinca rosae* Linn., led to the initial discovery that two of the alkaloidal constituents, vincaleukoblastine and leurosine, possessed certain demonstrable kinds of oncolytic (antitumor) activity. The same inquiries provided evidence of the presence of other alkaloids having similar activity, and pursuit of this lead bore fruit in the later discovery of leurocristine and leurosidine.

The over-all result of these discoveries has been that the plant has been the subject, during the past decade, of one of the most intensive phytochemical studies on record. Upwards of 50 different alkaloids have been demonstrated to be present, and more than half of these are recognized as new chemical compounds. The complete structure has been determined for some of the new ones while with others it is still in process of elucidation.

The therapeutic efficacy of vincaleukoblastine and leurocristine has been sufficiently established to accord them official status in the USP in the form of their (1:1) sulfates as antineoplastic agents. The structures of these two closely related alkaloids are portrayed below. The four-ring heterosystem is a stereospecific hydrogenated form of 10H-3,7-methano-azacycloundecino[5,4-b]indole, Ring Index No. 13276, and the five-ring system is a similar form of 1H-indolizino[8,1-cd]carbazole, Ring Index No. 11065. Leurosine and leurosidine are under clinical investigation. Generic names have been adopted for all four of these alkaloids by the USAN Council. In the order of their appearance in this paragraph, the respective USAN names are Vinblastine, Vincristine, Vinleurosine, and Vinrosidine.

The costliness of vinblastine and vincristine has provided increased interest in producing them synthetically. The five-ring indoline system is known to be available from other natural alkaloid sources, so effort at present is concentrated on synthesizing the four-ring indole system in suitably substituted form for coupling with the indoline moiety. Results to

In Vinblastine (vincaleukoblastine), R = CH₃
In Vincristine (leurocristine), R = CHO

date are encouraging.

An excellent review of the accomplishments during the first seven years of intense research on the Vinca alkaloids is provided, along with an extensive bibliography, in *J. Pharm. Sci.*, **51**, 707 (1962). For further discussion of the official articles, see the monographs on Vinblastine Sulfate and Vincristine Sulfate at other locations in this text.

Official Vinca Alkaloids

Vinblastine and Vincristine.

Miscellaneous Alkaloids

Several official and unofficial alkaloids, eg, Arecoline, Colchicine, Dimethyl Tubocurarine Iodide, Emetine, Ephedrine, Physostigmine, Pilocarpine, Tubocurarine, etc., do not fall within the classes of alkaloids presented in this chapter. For locations of discussions of these, consult the general index.

Volatile Oils

Volatile oils, or *essential oils*, are found in various plant organs and tissues. In some countries they are called *olea ætherea*. In some instances they are called *Essences*, a name which conflicts with our ordinary use of that word which designates an alcoholic solution of a volatile oil. In Germany they are called *ätherische öle* or *flüctige öle*; in France they are called *huiles essentielles* or *huiles volatiles*; in Italy they are called *olii distillati* or *olii volatiti*; and in Spain they are called *aceites volátiles*, *aceites esenciales*, or *aceites etéreos*. They usually constitute the savory and odorous principles of the plants in which they exist, and they either pre-exist in the tissues or are produced by the reaction of certain constituents when the tissues are brought into contact with water. Volatile oils are sometimes formed through destructive distillation, as the oils of tar and of amber, these being occasionally referred to as *pyrolea*.

The Constituents of Volatile Oils

In some volatile oils, as thyme, a separation into a solid and a liquid portion occurs on standing in the cold. The solid portion is frequently known by the name *stearoptene*, and the liquid portion is called *eleoptene*. Some of the stearoptenes are of commercial importance (examples: thymol, camphor, menthol). The eleop-

tenes are often used as adulterants of volatile oils (examples: oil of camphor and dementholized oil of peppermint).

The following groups of compounds occur in the volatile oils: hydrocarbons, alcohols, acids, esters, aldehydes, ketones, phenols and phenol ethers, lactones, and various nitrogen and sulfur organic compounds.

The hydrocarbons of chief importance are the *terpenes* ($C_{10}H_{16}$) and the *sesquiterpenes* ($C_{15}H_{24}$; literally, "one and one-half terpenes"). The terpenes have the formula C_nH_{2n-4} and can occur theoretically in the following configurations: (1) three double bonds and no cycle, eg, *myrcene* (found in myrcia oil) and *ocimene* (found in the volatile oil from the leaves of *Ocimum gratissimum*); (2) two double bonds and one cycle, eg, *limonene* (of widespread occurrence, but especially in the citrus oils); (3) one double bond and two cycles, eg, either *α-pinene* or *β-pinene* (the first of which is of very widespread occurrence; together, these two terpenes comprise at least 90% of the bulk of turpentine oil); and (4) three cycles. No examples are known of terpenes having the last structure.

The sesquiterpenes have the formula C_nH_{2n-6} and can therefore theoretically occur in an even more varied configuration. Although a number of examples of this group of hydrocarbons have been isolated, in many instances the structure is not definitely known. Among those of known structure may be mentioned *zingiberene* (from ginger oil) and *bisabolene* (from Bisabol myrrh oil).

Hydrocarbons other than the terpene types are sometimes present. An example is the saturated hydrocarbon, *n*-heptane (C_7H_{16}), which occurs in the volatile oil obtained from the oleoresin of *Pinus Sabiniana* and *P. Jeffreyi* and from the fruits of *Pittosporum resiniferum* (the so-called "petroleum nuts" of a tree growing in the Philippines).

The terpenes and sesquiterpenes in general are practically insoluble in water, but soluble in alcohol, ether, chloroform, benzene, petroleum benzin, and the fixed and volatile oils.

Many of the essential oils, however, owe their character and their value to constituents other than hydrocarbons. Among these will be found organic *acids*, such as acetic, benzoic, cinnamic, phenylacetic, etc; *alcohols* like benzyl alcohol, borneol, cinnamyl alcohol, citronellol, geraniol, linalool, menthol, phenylethyl alcohol, terpineol, etc; *aldehydes* such as anisic aldehyde, cinnamic aldehyde, benzaldehyde, citral, piperonal or heliotropin, salicylic aldehyde, vanillin, etc; *ketones* like carvone, camphor, thujone, pulegone, etc; *esters* such as bornyl acetate, methyl salicylate, benzyl benzoate, geranyl acetate, linalyl acetate, etc; *phenols* such as thymol, carvacrol, chavicol, etc; *phenol ethers* like anethol, eugenol, safrol, etc; and many other more complex compounds, such as coumarin, indol, etc. Many of these products are found in flower oils and are used in the production of synthetic perfumes.

It is beyond the scope of this book to attempt an exhaustive presentation of the chemistry of the numerous constituents occurring in the volatile oils. In the case of those compounds which are official, the structural formulas are given in the respective monographs. In certain other instances, substances such as *carvone*, *borneol*, and *linalyl acetate* are mentioned in the official text; and since their structures are not provided, a few of the more important of these are displayed below.

Terpenes

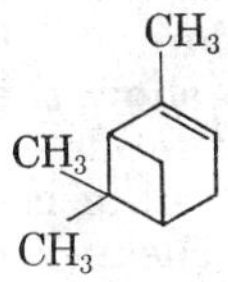

α-Pinene

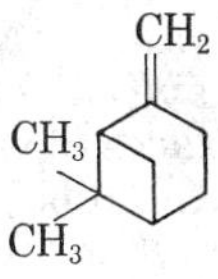

β-Pinene

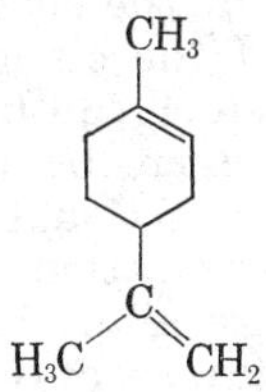

Limonene

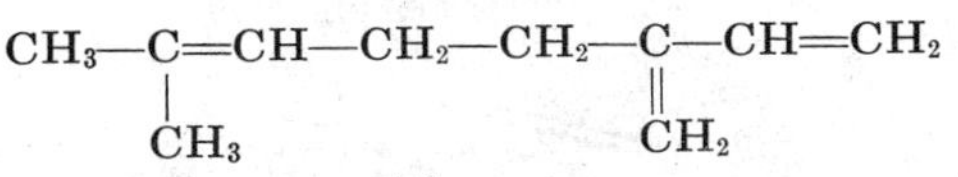

$$CH_3-C=CH-CH_2-CH_2-C-CH=CH_2$$
$$\qquad\quad |CH_3 \qquad\qquad\qquad ||CH_2$$

Myrcene

Alcohols

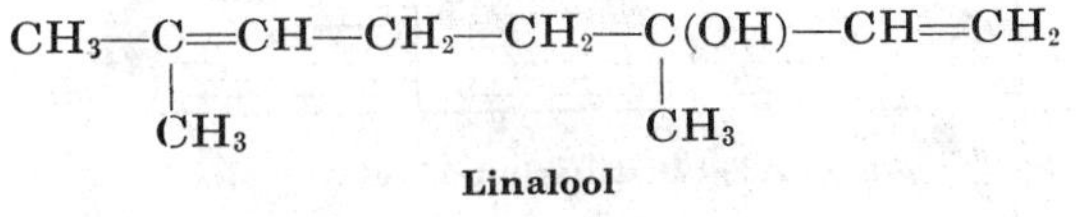

$$CH_3-C=CH-CH_2-CH_2-C(OH)-CH=CH_2$$
$$\qquad\quad |CH_3 \qquad\qquad\qquad\quad |CH_3$$

Linalool

$$CH_3-C=CH-CH_2-CH_2-CH-CH_2-CH_2OH$$
$$\qquad\quad |CH_3 \qquad\qquad\qquad\quad |CH_3$$

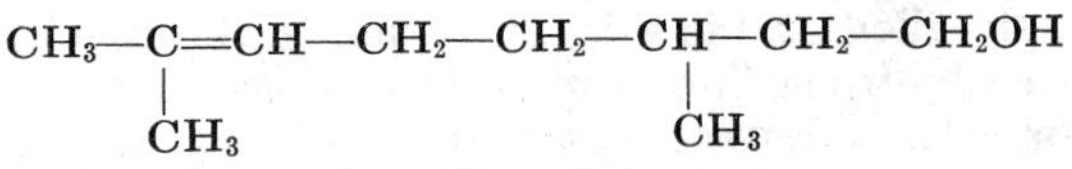

Citronellol

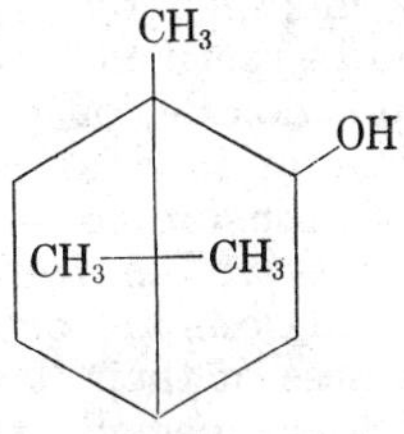

Borneol

Aldehydes

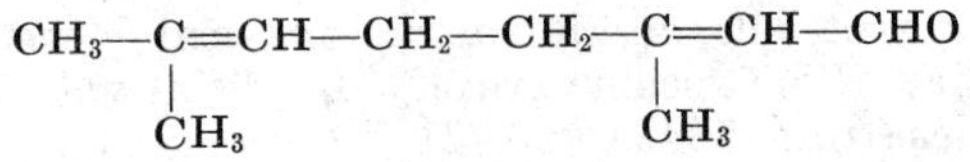

$$CH_3-C=CH-CH_2-CH_2-C=CH-CHO$$
$$\qquad\quad |CH_3 \qquad\qquad\qquad |CH_3$$

Citral
(*cis*-Neral)
(*trans*-Geranial)

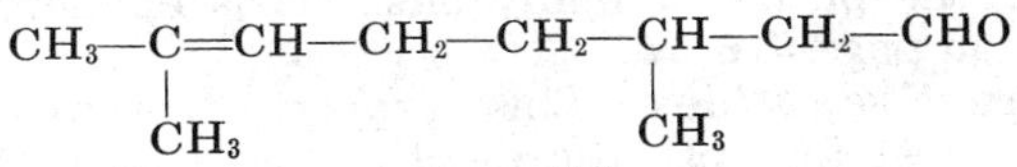

$$CH_3-C=CH-CH_2-CH_2-CH-CH_2-CHO$$
$$\qquad\quad |CH_3 \qquad\qquad\qquad\quad |CH_3$$

Citronellal

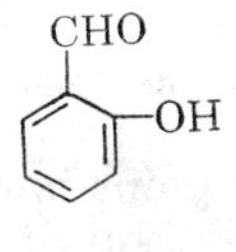

Salicylaldehyde 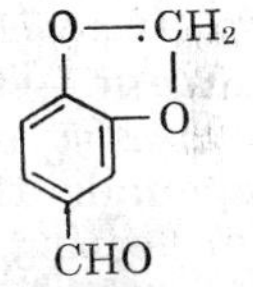   Heliotropin (Piperonal)

Ketones

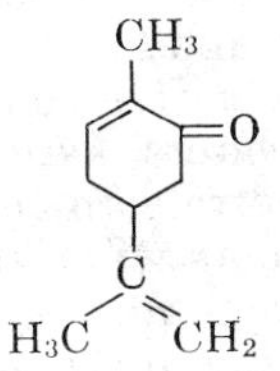

Carvone 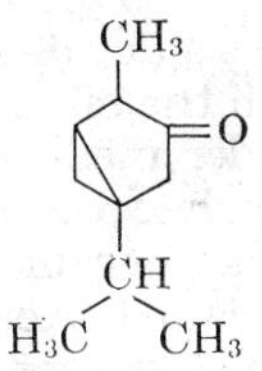   Thujone 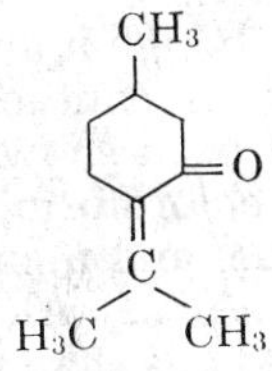   Pulegone

Phenols and Phenol Ethers

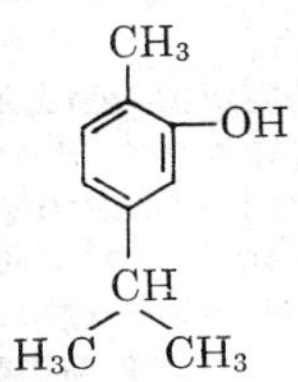

Carvacrol 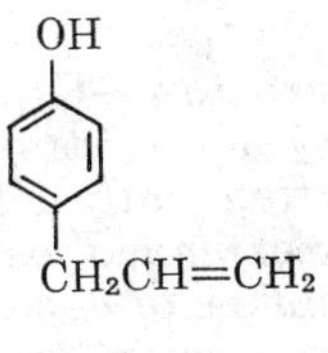   Chavicol

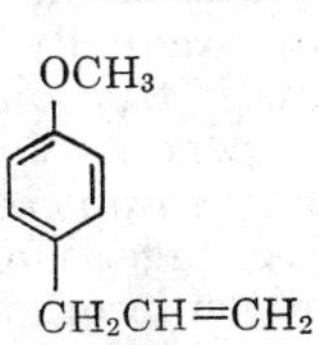

O-Methylchavicol 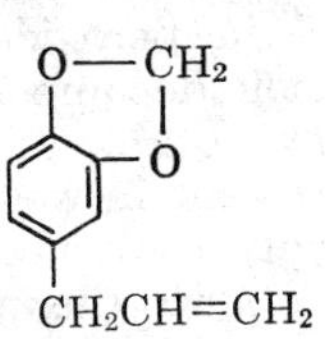   Safrol

Properties of Volatile Oils

Color—Most of the volatile oils are colorless when pure and fresh, or can be made colorless by redistillation. Upon exposure to the air they acquire various colors, becoming green, as in oil of wormwood; yellow, as in oil of peppermint; red, as in oil of origanum; brown, as in oil of cinnamon. The blue color of oil of chamomile is an inherent property of the oil even when freshly distilled and is said to be due to the highly unsaturated hydrocarbon *chamazulene* ($C_{15}H_{18}$).

Odor—The odors of volatile oils are extremely variable. It is their most characteristic feature. The odor of an oil is sensibly modified by exposure to the air. Oil of turpentine may be rectified by redistillation in an atmosphere of carbon dioxide, or *in vacuo*, so that it will be almost odorless, or have an agreeable, fragrant odor. A very slight exposure to the air is sufficient, however, to restore the well-known unpleasant odor. Other terpene-containing oils are quickly oxidized and the delicacy and fineness of their flavor and odor seriously impaired. This is especially true of orange and lemon oils.

Taste—The tastes of volatile oils are almost as variable as their odors. Some are sweet, others have a mild, pungent, hot, acrid, caustic, or burning taste.

Density—The specific gravity of official volatile oils also varies (from 0.842 to 1.172). The majority of them are lighter than water.

Optical Activity—This property is used in determining the purity of many oils. It is explained at length on page 616.

Refractive Index—This property serves as a delicate test for both the identity and purity of oils and fats. It is explained under *Refractometry and Interferometry* (page 710).

Boiling Range—Owing to the fact that most volatile oils consist of complex mixtures of many types of compounds, the boiling point is of small significance. On heating in a distillation apparatus, the fraction having the lowest boiling point distils first; then the temperature rises until the boiling point of the next higher boiling fraction is reached; and so on.

Solubilities—Water is a poor solvent for volatile oils, although it acquires a decided odor and flavor when brought in contact with the oil in a finely divided state, as has been shown under medicated waters. Alcohol, ether, chloroform, glacial acetic acid, petroleum benzin, benzene, and many other organic solvents will dissolve volatile oils. Alcohol is a better solvent for the oxygenated oils than for the terpenes. Many of the official oils are required to meet specific solubility tests in 70, 80, or 95% alcohol. Volatile oils freely dissolve fixed oils, fats, resins, camphors, and usually sulfur and phosphorus.

Deterioration—Exposure to light and air impairs the quality and destroys the fragrance of volatile oils. Peroxides frequently develop in oils containing terpenes, and, after extended exposure, the oils thicken and become resinified, or deposit crystalline compounds. The whitening of corks, inserted for a long time in bottles containing certain volatile oils, is due to the bleaching action of the peroxides which are gradually produced during their decomposition. This is true only of oils containing notable amounts of terpenes. Volatile oils should be kept in well-filled, tightly stoppered, amber-colored bottles, in a cool place. A suggestion has been made to replace the air with nitrogen in original packages to prevent oxidation. Storage in tin cans causes pronounced deterioration in odor and the development of color.

Volatile oils do not deteriorate so readily when mixed with alcohol, and it is the practice of some pharmacists to preserve them in this manner. Fixed oils, when present to the extent of 5 or 10%, have a remarkable preserving power, even upon such easily decomposed oils as those of the citrus family. In using oils so preserved allowance must be made for the dilution. It should be kept in mind also that if fixed oil is present,

difficulties may arise in the manufacture of certain preparations.

Action of Acids, Alkalies, Etc—Nitric acid, if strong, decomposes volatile oils with great rapidity. Iodine reacts with some oils with explosive violence. Alkalies affect volatile oils containing esters or phenolic compounds, as the oils from lavender, gaultheria, clove, thyme, etc.

Terpeneless and Sesquiterpeneless Oils—Certain of the volatile oils are available commercially in a form known as *terpeneless oils* and *sesquiterpeneless oils*. In the first type, only the terpenes have been removed; in the latter, both the terpenes and sesquiterpenes have been eliminated. This procedure involves distillation under high vacuum, washing with dilute alcohol (in which the oxygenated constituents are soluble, but not the hydrocarbons), elimination of the plant waxes, and other processes held secret by the various producers.

Terpeneless and sesquiterpeneless oils are much more expensive than the original oils, but they possess certain advantages which render them very useful. They have much higher flavoring and odoriferous properties than ordinary oils, in some instances up to 35 or 40 times as much. Because the portion of the original oil which is least stable towards oxidation has been removed, the resulting product maintains its characteristic odor and taste for a much greater time. The deterpenated oils have a much greater solubility in low-proof alcohol than the ordinary type, a factor of importance in the manufacture of toilet waters and soft beverages.

Adulterations—The volatile oils are costly enough to tempt the cupidity of some manufacturers of these products. A fixed oil is sometimes used to adulterate the volatile oil. This adulteration may be detected by dropping the suspected oil on a piece of filter paper. The stain of a pure volatile oil is not permanent. By slightly heating the volatile oil it should vaporize; if fixed oil is present, the stain remains after the odor has disappeared. Alcohol may be detected by shaking the mixed oil in a graduated tube with glycerin or water. The volume of the oil will be diminished, and that of the water or glycerin correspondingly increased, in proportion to the amount of alcohol present. This test is not susceptible of fine determination, because of a slight solubility of volatile oils in water and in mixtures of alcohol and water. Metallic sodium, calcium chloride, aniline red have all been used to show the presence of alcohol and traces of water in volatile oils. The adulteration of volatile oils by the addition of cheaper grades of the same oil, or by using a cheaper oil having a similar odor, is sometimes practiced. The only reliable test here is the use of the senses of smell and taste applied to dilutions of the oil in various media. By practice, the sense of smell can be highly developed by the pharmacist, perfumer, or analyst. The optical rotation, the index of refraction, the specific gravity, the iodine value, the saponification value, the acid value, and the ester value are all useful constants, wherever appropriate, for the purpose of detecting adulterations. The detection of adulterations in volatile oils is difficult,

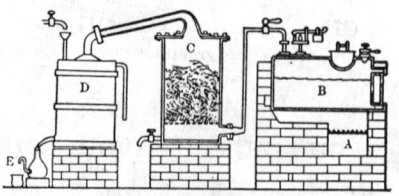

Fig. 513.   Distillation of volatile oils

and as a rule those who practice this nefarious art are very skillful. Stipulation of several physical characteristics of a volatile oil often eliminates the need for a USP or NF assay. In some instances, eg, clove oil, assays for valuable constituents are provided.

Preparation of Volatile Oils

Volatile oils are generally obtained from plants by the following methods: (1) distillation with steam; (2) distillation *per se;* (3) expression; (4) extraction.

1. Distillation with Steam—This is the method most frequently employed. The general procedure is as follows: Place the substance from which the oil is to be extracted into a still (see *Distillation*, page 184), and add enough water to cover it; then distil by a regulated heat into a large condenser. Separate the distilled oil from the water which comes over with it.

The substances from which the volatile oils are extracted may be employed in either the recent or the dried state. Certain flowers, however, such as orange flowers and roses, must be used fresh, or preserved with salt or by means of glycerin, as they afford little or no oil after desiccation. Dried substances, such as sandalwood, clove, cinnamon bark, etc, before being submitted to distillation, require to be macerated in water until they are thoroughly penetrated by this fluid; and, to facilitate the action of the water, it is necessary, when of a hard or tough consistency, that they should be properly comminuted.

The water which is added to the substance to be distilled answers the double purpose of preventing the decomposition of the vegetable matter by regulating the temperature, and of facilitating the volatilization of the oil, which, though in most instances it readily rises with the vapor of boiling water, requires, when distilled alone, a considerably higher temperature, and is at the same time liable to be partly decomposed. Some oils, however, will not ascend readily with steam at 100°C, and in the distillation of these it is customary to use water saturated with common salt, which raises the boiling point to about 108°C. Other oils, again, may be volatilized with water at a temperature below the boiling point and may be distilled with the aid of a partial vacuum. To prevent injury from heat, it has been recommended to suspend the substance containing the oil in a basket, or to place it upon a perforated shelf, in the upper part of the still, so that it may be penetrated by the steam without being in direct contact with the water. Steam can be very conveniently applied for this purpose by causing it to pass through a coil of tube, of an inch or three-quarters of an inch bore, placed in the bottom of a common still. In some instances it is desirable to conduct the steam immediately into the still near the bottom, by which the contents are kept in a state of brisk ebullition. The distillation of volatile oils is now conducted on a large scale with enormous stills. (For description and illustrations see Gildemeister and Hoffmann, *The Volatile Oils*, translated from the German by Prof. Edward Kremers. For a more recent treatise, the reader is referred to the series of volumes titled *The Essential Oils* by Dr. Ernest Guenther.[12])

The quantity of water added is of importance. Too large an amount causes loss by holding the oil in solution when the mixed vapors are condensed. On the contrary, if the quantity is too small, there will be danger of the substance in the still adhering to the sides of the vessel and thus becoming burnt. A wire cage will be found useful in this connection. Where the yield of oil is very small, the process of *cohobation* is applicable; this consists in repeatedly returning the aqueous portion of the distillate to the still, the water in this way becoming supersaturated, and the yield of oil increased. Fig. 513 illustrates one method of distilling volatile oils from plants. *A* shows the fire box, *B* the steam boiler, *C* the tank containing the plant on the slat or perforated bottom, *D* the condenser, and *E* the Florentine flask used as the receiver.

2. Distillation *per se*—By this is meant the distillation of certain bodies without the use of water (*per se,* "by itself"). This is done in the cases of certain oleoresins, copaiba, etc, water not being required in the process, and always being difficult to separate from the distillate.

3. Expression (see page 391)—This method is very limited in its application and generally produces the most fragrant products, because there are very few volatile oils whose aroma is not injuriously affected by the action of heat. The volatile oils of the Citrus family (orange, lemon, bergamot, and lime) are generally obtained by expressing the rind of the fresh fruit. These are usually known as "hand pressed." Three methods are practiced: (1) the sponge process; (2) the écuelle method; and (3) the machine process.

In the *sponge process* the rind is removed from the fruit, and, after dipping in water, is pressed by hand, the oil collecting in a shallow bowl from which it is transferred to a larger container for separation.

In the *écuelle method* the fruit is rolled about in hollow bowls, the walls of which are covered with spikes. The oil cells are punctured and the oil which exudes is collected in the hollow handle.

In the *machine process* either the sponge or the écuelle processes are adapted to machines which perform the operation on a larger scale. The machine process, as practiced by the California Fruit Growers Exchange, is conducted as follows:

The fruit, after being washed, is conveyed mechanically to crushers, which reduce the whole fruit to a pulp. The pulpy mass passes over a system of heavy, horizontal rollers where it is thinned out. Solid particles adhere to the cylinders and are removed by scraping. The liquid portion consists of an emulsion of the volatile oil in the juice of the fruit.

The liquid portion is then centrifuged in a battery of Sharples centrifuges. It is important that the oil and juice must not remain in contact with each other for a great length of time, because the citral would partially dissolve in the juice, resulting in a loss of this valuable constituent, and further because citral is quite easily converted to *p*-cymene by the action of acids in the presence of water.

The press residues of the crushed fruit are subjected to steam distillation in order to recover additional volatile oil. This product is sold separately, since it is not as fine a grade as the cold-pressed oil.

4. Extraction—Some volatile oils are so readily decomposed that they are dissociated by distillation, or exist in such minute traces as to make their commercial production impracticable. In such cases the odorous principle may be extracted by some form of solution or absorption. This may be effected by maceration, digestion, percolation with an appropriate immiscible solvent, enfleurage, or extraction with a volatile solvent.

Maceration—In obtaining volatile oils by maceration, the odorous portions of the plant (generally fragrant flowers) are allowed to remain in contact with a bland, inodorous, fixed oil or fat; the oil or fat absorbs the odor, and after a certain length of time the oil is strained

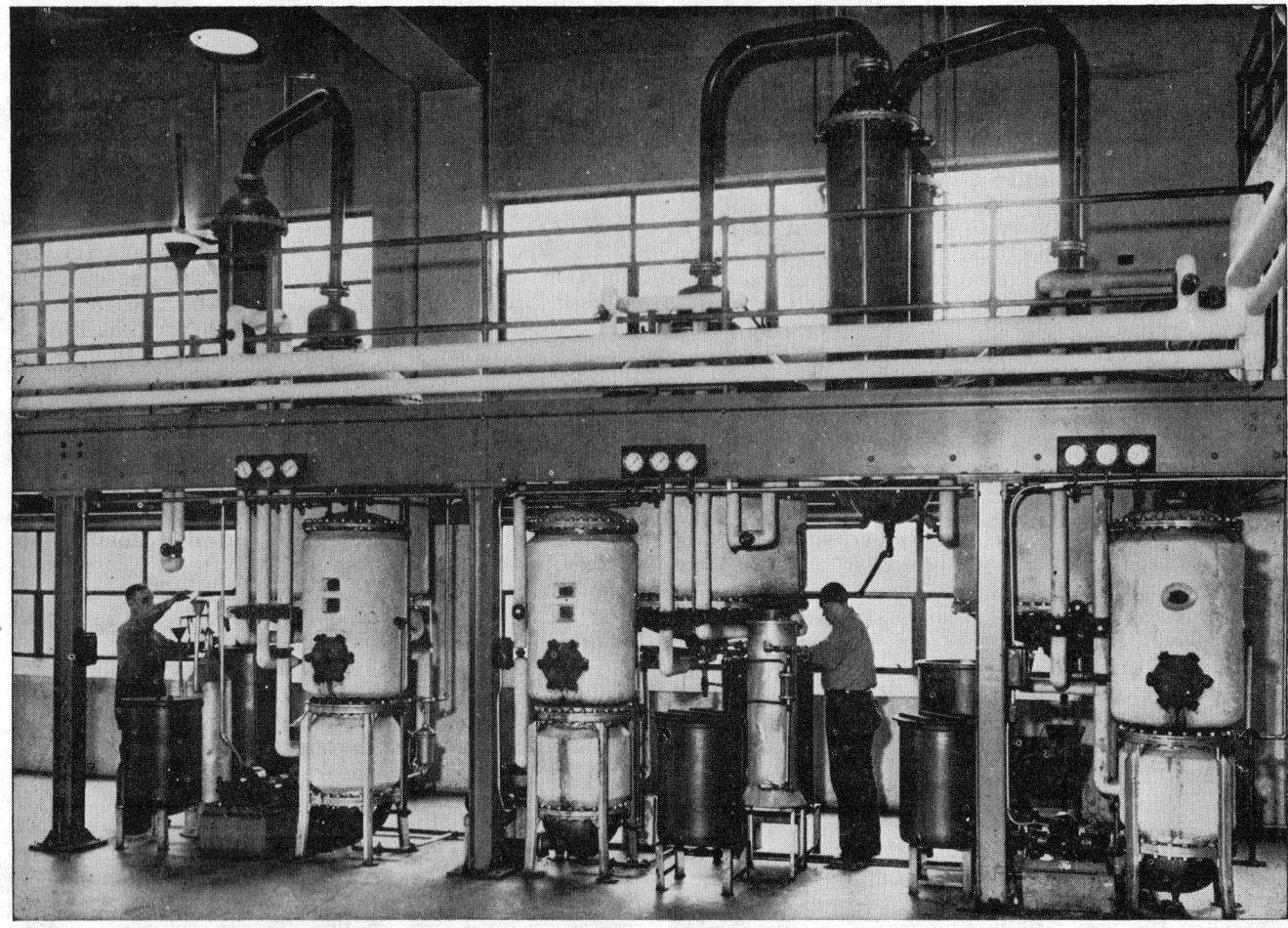

Fig. 514. A battery of three essential oil stills in operation in a large modern volatile oil plant. The equipment provides for distillation under reduced pressure to prevent excessive heating (courtesy, Fritzche).

and is subsequently used in the manufacture of perfumes in a manner similar to pomades. The flowers extracted by this method are chiefly cassie, rose, violet, orange flowers, narcissus, and lily of the valley.

Digestion—This process is similar to maceration, except that a moderate heat is employed, by the use of a salt bath, to aid in the extraction.

Enfleurage was at one time largely used for extracting the odors of very delicate flowers. It is a cold process, and consists in spreading a thin layer of purified inodorous fat (a mixture of beef tallow 40% and lard 60%) upon both sides of sheets of glass, held in frames, known as a *chassis*. These resemble an ordinary window sash, with one pane of glass in each. The flowers, deprived of calices, are spread lightly upon the surface of the fat, and a number of chassis thus prepared is arranged in tiers so that the flowers are between layers of fat. The whole is left undisturbed for a time varying from 12 hours to four days. The flowers continue to live for a period of time varying from one to several days, giving off their volatile oil. The length of time that the flowers remain on the chassis is variable: 24 hours for jasmine, 48 hours for jonquil, and 72 hours for tuberose. The resulting fatty product impregnated with the floral odor is called a "pomade." When strong pomades are desired, the flowers are replaced daily by fresh lots, as long as the absorption continues, the old flowers being removed by the use of a vacuum. The fat is usually exposed thirty times. The pomades are known commercially as Nos. 6, 12, 18, 24, and 36, the numbers indicating the relative strength. The ab-

sorbed volatile products are then obtained from the pomade by washing in pure alcohol in an appropriate mixing device. The alcohol dissolves out the floral oils, and usually also a trace of the fat, but this trace may be separated by subjecting it to a cold atmosphere in a refrigerator, when the congealed fat can be filtered out. The enfleurage process is used for jasmine, tuberose, cassie, rose, violet, jonquil, lily of the valley, orange flowers, and a few others. It has been observed that jasmine and tuberose give good yields only with the enfleurage process. On the other hand, rose, cassie, and violet can be treated equally well with warm fat or volatile solvents.

The pomades are mostly imported from Grasse, France, but their use today is very limited, having been largely replaced by *concretes* and *absolutes*.

Percolation with Volatile Solvents—The chief solvent employed is a highly purified petroleum benzin of a specific gravity of 0.650. The solvent is allowed to flow through the flowers which are arranged on trays in the apparatus. The extraction requires about 8 hours. This process is used for rose, Parma and Victoria violets, orange blossom, cassie, mignonette, and occasionally for carnation, lily of the valley, heliotrope, and a few others. The volatile solvent is then removed by vacuum distillation and the resulting product is known as a *concrete*.

These concretes contain the plant or flower waxes, which are removed by dissolving the odorous portion in strong alcohol and separating the insoluble waxes by filtration. Small quantities of alcohol-soluble waxes are removed by chilling to −20°C; the resulting products are known as *absolutes*. These products, although very costly, are largely used in perfumery, their great odor value making their employment economically possible.

Synthetic Perfumery

Many of the constituents of volatile oils, already enumerated, and other alcohols, aldehydes, ketones, esters, etc, are now manufactured synthetically for use in perfumery. This has become an extensive business and requires a comprehensive knowledge of organic

synthesis and methods for the purification of the resulting compounds.

Official Volatile Oils

Volatile oils *official as such* include: Anise; Caraway; Cinnamon; Clove; Coriander; Eucalyptus; Fennel; Lavender; Lemon; Myristica; Orange; Orange Flower; Peppermint; Pine Needle; and Spearmint.

Some of the crude drugs from which the above oils are derived are also official.

Plant Exudates

Plant exudates, for purposes of classification in this textbook, comprise naturally occurring, solid or semisolid, chemically complex mixtures of vegetable origin, such as balsams, gums, oleoresins, and resins. The proportion of their constituents may vary with the climate, season of the year, and other factors. Those plant principles which can be isolated in the pure state and which can be characterized structurally by chemical and physical methods, eg, alkaloids, carbohydrates, glycosides, and vitamins, are considered at other locations under their appropriate headings.

Resins—These are natural or induced solid or semisolid exudations from plants or from insects feeding on plants. They are characterized by being insoluble in water, mostly soluble in alcohol or ether, often uncrystallizable, and softening or melting at a moderate heat. They range in specific gravity from 0.90 to 1.25. Ignited in the air they burn with a smoky flame. They are usually the oxidized terpenes of the volatile oils of plants, and, owing to their insolubility in water, have little taste; they show no uniformity of chemical composition; some of them are acids, and combine with alkalies, forming "soaps" as in the case of common rosin.

Resins, when pure, are usually transparent; when they contain water, they are opaque, and no longer hard and brittle. They are nonconductors of electricity, but when rubbed they become negatively electrified.

A clear distinction must be made between *natural resins* and *prepared resins*. A natural resin is one which occurs as an exudation. The formerly official Mastic is an example. A prepared resin may be made by exhausting a drug, which owes its activity to resinous constituents, with alcohol, pouring the concentrated alcoholic percolate into an excess of water, collecting, washing, and drying the precipitate. The resins of podophyllum, jalap, etc (pages 778 and 798) are examples of this class. A prepared resin may also be derived from a natural oleoresin by driving off the volatile oil by heat. Rosin NF is an example of this class.

Careful distinction must also be made between the above classes of resins and a large class of so-called synthetic resins. The latter are polymeric substances which are readily formed either by condensation or by addition from readily available common chemicals. Thus, as examples, phenol and formaldehyde interact initially to produce o- and p- hydroxybenzyl alcohols which then condense to yield a large series of phenolformaldehyde (Bakelite) resins; methyl methacrylate and various other acrylic acid derivatives, on the other hand, polymerize exclusively by addition at the expense

of their olefinic unsaturation to yield a large series of methacrylic (Lucite, Plexiglas, etc) resins. These and many other synthetic resins constituent the foundation of the modern plastics industry. In addition, many of them have proved to be valuable tools in diverse kinds of operations requiring control of certain ion concentrations in the environment in which they are placed (see page 677). A few, eg, Carbacrylamine Resins (page 950) and the official Azuresin and Sodium Polystyrene Sulfonate (see index) have found useful diagnostic and therapeutic applications.

Oleoresins—Natural oleoresins are mixtures of volatile oils and resin, generally obtained by incising trunks of trees in which they are found. Turpentine and Copaiba are natural oleoresins formerly recognized by the NF.

A distinction must be made also between the natural and prepared oleoresins. The *prepared oleoresins* are concentrated liquid preparations made by percolating drugs, naturally containing both volatile oil and resin, with an appropriate solvent, ie, acetone, ether, or alcohol, and concentrating the percolate until the solvent has been dissipated. The formerly official Aspidium, Capsicum, and Ginger oleoresins are examples.

Gum Resins—These are natural mixtures of gum and resin, usually obtained as exudations from plants, as the formerly official Myrrh and Gamboge.

Balsams—These are resinous substances containing benzoic or cinnamic acids or their esters, as Tolu Balsam USP, Peruvian Balsam NF, etc.

Much faulty nomenclature occurs in the ordinary trade designations for many plant exudates. The word *gum* is frequently the one most misapplied as in *gum thus* for turpentine oleoresin, *gum guaiac* for resin of guaiac, *gum asafetida* for oleo-gum-resin of asafetida. The word *balsam* is also wrongly applied to certain oleoresins, such as Copaiba and Canada Turpentine, neither of which contains any of the constituents characteristic of balsams.

Acacia (Gum Arabic) and Tragacanth (Gum Tragacanth) are classed in this text as natural carbohydrate derivatives.

Official Plant Exudates

This listing is limited to *natural* and *prepared* exudates which are official as such. Official crude drugs (eg, Podophyllum, etc) from which some of the exudates are derived are not included. In this connection, it should also be remembered that some official crude drugs other than those which yield official exudates (eg, Eriodictyon) contain significant percentages of resin, oleoresin, etc.

Resins: Podophyllum Resin; Rosin.

Balsams: Benzoin; Peruvian Balsam; Storax;
Tolu Balsam.

References

1. Williaman, J. J., and Schubert, B. G., *Alkaloid-Bearing Plants and Their Contained Alkaloids*, Tech. Bull. No. 1234, US Dept. of Agriculture, Washington, D. C., 1961.
2. Manske, R. H. F., *The Alkaloids*, 11 vols, Academic Press, New York, 1950–1965.
3. Svoboda, G. H., *et al*, *J. Pharm. Sci.*, **51,** 707 (1962).
4. Schöpf, C., and Lehmann, G., *Ann.*, **518,** 1 (1935).
5. Grewe, R., *Naturwissenschaften*, **33,** 333 (1946).
6. Cahn, R. S., *J. Chem. Educ.*, **41,** 116–125 (1964).
7. Ginsburg, D., *The Opium Alkaloids*, Wiley, New York, 1962.
8. Robinson, *J. Chem. Soc.* (London), 762 (1917).
9. Fieser, L. F., and Fieser, M., *Steroids*, Reinhold, New York, 1959, p. 867.
10. Morgan, K. J., and Barltrop, J. A., *Quart. Rev.* (*London*) **12,** 34–60 (1958).
11. Example: Kupchan, S. M., *et al*, "Veratrum Alkaloids (XLIX)," *Author Index, Chemical Abstracts*, **57,** 554 (1962).
12. Guenther, E., *The Essential Oils*, 6 vols, Van Nostrand, New York, 1949–1952.

31 | Drug Nomenclature – United States Adopted Names

Types of drug names—the USAN Council—procedure for selecting a USAN—guiding principles for coining a USAN—basic requirements of a USAN—International Nonproprietary Names—dissemination of nomenclature information

This chapter was prepared by

Mary Celeste Alessandri, * BA, *Downers Grove, Ill. 60515, and*
Joseph B. Jerome, * PhD, *Secretary, United States Adopted Names Council, Chicago, Ill. 60610*

Within recent years advances have been made in many disciplines at such an accelerated rate that the processing of available information has become somewhat of a discipline in its own right. Processing of information includes such subspecialties as collection, collation, abstracting, storage, retrieval, and dissemination.

One area in which it sometimes seems that information has gotten ahead of those seeking it is that involving drugs. The sheer numbers of new potential drug entities that have been researched in the past 20 years have made the task of monitoring the literature a formidable one.

If one considers that a given drug may be known by a chemical name, one or more code numbers, a trivial designation, a formally selected nonproprietary name, and two or three trademarks, plus any variations on these that exist in other countries, it will become apparent that a meaningful nonproprietary nomenclature system is essential to the efficient use of drug information.

Such a nomenclature system has been developed, and a discussion of its accomplishments and its problems, as well as its history, scope, functions, and operation is the subject of this chapter.

Types of Drug Names

The term "drug nomenclature" indicates several types of names for drugs, each having its own function.

For compounds of known composition, the first name to be applied is generally the *chemical name.* This is a systematically derived name which provides complete and accurate chemical identification. For those substances which are of animal or plant origin, scientific identification of the source is given in terms of *technical biochemical, botanical, or zoological names.* Although in either case these designations are scientifically precise, they tend to be very long, unwieldy, and not generally useful to the physician, pharmacist, and others in related fields.

Since chemical names are not suitable for routine use, a potential drug often acquires a *code designation* as a convenient reference for those working with it during laboratory investigation. This kind of nomenclature is generally of two types: (1) a letter and number combination (eg, SH 567) in which the letter(s) generally refers to the laboratory involved and the number is often arbitrarily assigned and (2) a letter combination (eg, IDU) which is usually derived from portions of the chemical name.

Although code designations are usually considered simply a convenient "shop label" and are generally meant to be discarded when a more appropriate name is selected, many of them find their way into the literature when published reports on early investigative work appear prior to the selection of a nonproprietary name. These code designations must, therefore, be considered as a part of drug nomenclature. Again, however, they cannot be considered acceptable for general usage since, in themselves, they provide no identification of the compound to which they refer. Also, with arbitrarily selected number codes, errors are difficult to detect and, therefore, occur more frequently.

In some instances *trivial names* are assigned (usually by individual researchers working on the drugs) to new compounds during early investigative stages. These are complete names and may be of the type one could loosely call a generic or nonproprietary name. Nomenclature agencies strongly discourage the use of such trivial names, since they are generally coined in a haphazard manner with little concern for the availability (ie, freedom from conflict with established names) of the term used or for the relationship which may exist between the new compound and an older established drug.

If a drug has come through the successive research stages and appears to be heading for the market, a *trademark* is assigned; this very often designates not the drug itself, but rather a formulation and its manufacturer.

Trademarks are the legal possessions of their owners and cannot be used in a public sense. Moreover, when a given drug is manufactured by more than one firm, each may market its specific formulation under its own trademark. Scientific considerations are also significant. Trademarks are selected for their brevity, catchiness, and ease of retention or recall. They often fail to indicate the chemical and pharmacological relations that may exist between individual drugs.

Although each type of name mentioned has a specific purpose, none fulfils the need of those in the health professions for a single, simple, informative designation

---

* The material in this chapter is based on an earlier work by the authors.[1]

which is freely available for public use. The *nonproprietary name* is intended to fill this specific need. It is concise, meaningful, and available. The nonproprietary name has also been called a generic name, but this term is inaccurate. In this discussion the term nonproprietary name is restricted to those names that have been selected through a formal process of adoption carried out between a manufacturer and a nomenclature agency; this artificial restriction will help differentiate such names from the trivial names coined without having been considered by a nomenclature agency.

The USAN Council

In the US the nomenclature agency responsible for the selection of appropriate nonproprietary names for drugs is the United States Adopted Names (USAN) Council. This expert committee on drug nomenclature is jointly sponsored by the American Medical Association (AMA), the United States Pharmacopeial Convention, and the American Pharmaceutical Association (APhA). Tracing the involvement of these sponsoring agencies in nomenclature selection provides a good history of the practice in this country and is a guide to the evolution of the USAN Council to its present status.

The *United States Pharmacopeia* (USP) has been supplying standards for pharmaceutical preparations since the first edition appeared in 1820. In its concern for the selection of titles for compendium monographs the USP was among the first to recognize the need for a standardized system of drug nomenclature and to take significant action in that direction.

Publication of a second compendium, the *National Formulary* (NF), was begun by the APhA in 1888; thus, in this way, this organization also became concerned not only with establishing standards for those drugs admitted to the NF but also with providing nonproprietary names for them.

Current policies regarding admission of any drug to the compendia require proved therapeutic merit of the drug entity; prior to 1960, the NF required extensive use as a criterion for admission. Thus, new products are almost automatically excluded from the compendia and are thereby removed from their sphere of nomenclature activity.

As the number of new pharmaceutical products increased during this century, the need for providing appropriate nonproprietary names for new compounds became increasingly apparent. This gap was filled, to some extent, by the AMA's Council on Pharmacy and Chemistry (now known as the Council on Drugs).

In 1910 the Council began a nomenclature program to provide names for use in its publications, for those drugs that were available under two different trademarks, and in the early 1940's the Council began to require a nonproprietary name for every active compound included in its publications. However, large numbers of drug products were not the subjects of either Council or compendia monographs. These compounds were known by their chemical names or by trivial names selected by the manufacturers.

As drugs, nomenclature, medicine, and pharmacy became more sophisticated, still another need was recognized. Each new drug needed a nonproprietary name selected early in its history; moreover, it was apparent that such names must be systematically selected to assure their appropriateness in the over-all nomenclature picture and must be acceptable to the USP, the NF, the AMA, and the manufacturer.

A significant step toward this goal was taken in June, 1961, with the formation of the AMA–USP Nomenclature Committee. Any names adopted by this Committee were deemed automatically acceptable as potential compendia monograph titles, and the term USAN (United States Adopted Name) was coined to designate those drug names so adopted. Although actively participating in the program from its inception, the publisher of the NF, the APhA, did not become a full sponsor until January, 1964, and at this time the name of the group was changed to the USAN Council.

It is advisable here to consider the role of the federal government in nonproprietary nomenclature, both historically and currently.

In 1906 the government legally recognized the significance of the work being done by the USP and the NF by declaring these publications "official" compendia of the US. Since that time monograph titles have had the status of official nonproprietary names.

The 1938 Food, Drug and Cosmetic Act stipulated that "the common or usual name" (the official name or the nonproprietary name established either by the Council on Pharmacy and Chemistry or by use) should be used on the labeling; in the absence of such a name (or until a name attained this status) a chemical name should be used.

The Drug Amendments of 1962 replaced the "common or usual" terminology with the more meaningful requirement that nonproprietary names must be "simple and useful." For the first time the Commissioner of the Food and Drug Administration (FDA) was given the authority (acting for the Secretary of Health, Education and Welfare) to designate an official name if he determined that such action was necessary or desirable.

Although the FDA and the USAN Council had operated in effective liaison for some time, it became clear early in 1967 that a more formal cooperative effort in the development of nonproprietary nomenclature would be of value. This realization resulted in an agreement (effective in June, 1967) between the sponsors of the USAN Council and the FDA: the latter would appoint a member to the USAN Council and agree to accept any name on which the Council is unanimous as the established or official name.

The reorganization agreement reserved the right of the Commissioner of the FDA to select the official name in those instances in which the USAN Council cannot reach unanimous agreement. Also, it should be noted that adoption of USAN as "official names" by the FDA does not follow automatically but is accomplished by publication in the *Federal Register*. The USAN Council program remains a privately conducted effort by agencies dedicated to serving the public welfare.

It is emphasized that the adoption of a nonproprietary name does not imply that the article is being offered for either clinical use or investigation; furthermore, its adoption is independent of clinical evaluation or acceptance by the medical profession, by the FDA, or by the USAN Council sponsors of any specific brand(s) of the drug to which the name applies.

The USAN Council, then, under its present organization, is sponsored by the AMA, the APhA, and the USP; it is a five-member group, with one member appointed by each sponsor, one member-at-large who must be approved by all three sponsors, and one member from the FDA.

Council members for 1969 were Windsor C. Cutting, MD, Chairman; Durward F. Dodgen, MS; Lloyd C. Miller, PhD; Ralph G. Smith, MD, PhD; and Lauren A. Woods, MD, PhD. The Council staff, provided by the AMA, is headed by Joseph B. Jerome, PhD, Assistant Director of the AMA Department of Drugs. For a number of years Kurt Loening, PhD, of Chemical Abstracts Services, Clarence Van Meter, PhD, and John J. Hefferren, PhD have provided expert special services to the USAN Council on essentially every negotiation.

The Council operates primarily through correspondence, with meetings held twice a year to discuss policy matters.

It must be anticipated that, on occasion, difficulties will arise over the adoption or proposed adoption of a particular name. In the majority of such cases, the Council and the interested manufacturer(s) can, in time, work out acceptable solutions. A USAN Review Board has been established as a last resource to handle those situations when the normal procedures fail. The services of this Board have been requested in only two cases (as of January, 1969).

Members of the Review Board for 1969 were Raymond D. McMurray, LLB, Chairman; Carl A. Dragstedt, MD; George P. Hager, PhD; Ovid O. Meyer, MD; Linwood F. Tice, DSc; and Arthur G. Zupko, PhD. At the time of any appeal to the Board, representatives of the firms involved in the specific case can participate in the deliberations but exercise no voting privileges.

The primary functions of the USAN Council are:

1. To negotiate with pharmaceutical manufacturers in the selection of meaningful and distinctive nonproprietary names for new drug entities.
2. To publicize the adopted names, the guiding principles used in devising these names, and the procedures involved in their adoption.
3. To cooperate with other national and international agencies, particularly the World Health Organization (WHO), in standardizing, as much as possible, the nonproprietary nomenclature for drugs.

Procedure for Selecting a USAN

A proposal for a USAN originates usually from a firm or an individual who has developed a substance of potential therapeutic usefulness to the point where there is a distinct possibility of its being marketed in the US. Occasionally, the initiative is taken by the USAN Council in the form of a request to parties interested in a substance for which a nonproprietary name appears to be lacking.

Proposals are expected to conform to the established Guiding Principles (*vide infra*) and to be reasonably free from conflict with other names, including both trademarks and nonproprietary names. When the initial screening of the proposals suggests that they fail to conform or that they appear to conflict, the USAN Council Secretary offers suggestions with a view to expediting the selection process.

Each proposal should be accompanied by a statement covering as much as possible of the following information:

1. The chemical structure.
2. The chemical name (preferably the *Chemical Abstracts* index name).
3. Any code designation(s) by which the substance may have been known in the course of its testing and development.
4. The source (if it is a product of natural origin) or such other descriptive characteristics as will distinguish it adequately.

5. The kind of pharmacologic activity or therapeutic usefulness claimed for it.
6. Any trademark(s) that may have been applied to it.

This information, supplemented by the results of searches conducted by the Secretary, is referred to the Council members, whose views then are exchanged until a tentative decision can be submitted to the sponsor for comment. It should be emphasized that although the Council can ascertain the preferred chemical nomenclature for a structure claimed for any compound of definite composition, the Council is not in a position to confirm the structure or the claims for pharmacologic activity.

When general agreement has been reached on a name and often even earlier, the latter is published in the *Trademark Bulletin* of the Pharmaceutical Manufacturers Association as a "Proposed USAN." This informs those who have access to the Bulletin of the Council's intention to adopt the name and serves as an invitation for comments or protests within 30 days following its publication. No disclosure of the name of the manufacturer or of the chemical nature of the substance appears in these Bulletin statements.

At the same time the same information is referred to Chemical Abstracts Service and to the USA Standards Association for review of the proposed names as to freedom from conflict with existing names.

If the compound concerned is a dental or veterinary drug, an antibiotic, or a biochemical, the proposed name and other nomenclature information (without manufacturer identification) is referred, as appropriate, to the American Dental Association, the American Veterinary Medical Association, the American Society for Microbiology, or the Office of Biochemical Nomenclature for review and comment.

The above screening procedures are necessary since nonproprietary names that appear to be rather well established with members of a research group with specialized interests may be unavailable (usually because of conflict with established names) for selection as a USAN; the USAN Council does not desire to adopt as a USAN a designation that would infringe on the valid rights of legally established trademarks or would produce confusion with similar nonproprietary names for compounds that differ significantly in chemical structure and pharmacologic activity.

As a result of its experience in the above reviews of proposed names, the Nomenclature Committee of the American Society for Microbiology has recommended that the USAN Council set forth more definite requirements for the format of submission of names to the USAN Council to include:

1. A pertinent bibliography illustrative of the synthesis or biosynthesis and chemistry, including especially items having a bearing on the proposed name.
2. Any names that have been applied to this substance previously with pertinent bibliographic references.
3. Names of other drug(s) or likely drugs that have closely similar or identical names with pertinent bibliographic references.
4. The reason the name chosen is deemed an appropriate name for the drug in question, in the light of the guiding principles enumerated by the USAN Council.

The USAN Council endorses the above recommendation since, with this information available, the selection of better nonproprietary names appears more certain.

If the sponsor consents, and in any case if the name and/or nomenclature information has been published elsewhere, the tentatively adopted USAN is then submitted for consideration to several cooperating agencies. These agencies include the WHO, the British Pharmacopoeia Commission, the French Codex Commission, and the Nordic Pharmacopoeia Council, as well as the USP, the NF, and the FDA.

If no objections are raised by the cooperating agencies, adoption is considered final, the USAN is published in the *Journal of the American Medical Association,* and proof copies are distributed to the American pharmaceutical press (see *Dissemination of Nomenclature Information,* page 516).

Several bound publications, such as the *American Drug Index,* the *Modern Drug Encyclopedia,* and *The Merck Index* give special attention to the USAN.

Despite the efforts to give notice of the proposed adoption of a USAN in the early stages and to exercise care in avoiding conflicts with established names, objections sometimes arise rather late. All valid objections receive conscientious attention from the Council.

Guiding Principles for Coining a USAN

A USAN is a nonproprietary name selected according to the following principles, the primary purpose of which is to assure consistency in the choice of names of maximal usefulness. As a guidelines, the principles take into account practical considerations, such as the existence of trademarks, and the fact that the intended uses of the substances for which names are being selected may change. Therefore, the principles are flexible and may be revised in the light of experience.

General Rules

1. A nonproprietary name should be useful primarily to health practitioners, especially physicians, dentists, veterinarians, pharmacists, and nurses.

   a. The principal criterion for judging a name's usefulness is suitability, including safety, for use in the routine processes of ordering, dispensing, and administering drugs throughout the US.

   b. A second criterion is the name's suitability for use in educational programs for students of these health professions.

2. Attributes that contribute to usefulness are simplicity (both brevity and ease of pronunciation) and those qualities that lend euphony and enhance ready recognition and recall. The essential criterion of simplicity is the ease with which the name is used by personnel trained in the above-mentioned professions.

   a. The name for the active moiety of a drug should be a single word, preferably of not more than four syllables.

   b. The name for the active moiety may be modified by a single term, preferably of not more than three syllables, to show a chemical modification (eg, the chemical formation of cortisone acetate from cortisone).

   c. Only under compelling circumstances is a name acceptable with more than one modifying term (eg, pharmaceuticals containing radioactive isotopes).

   d. Acronyms, initials, condensed words, symbols, and numerals may be acceptable in otherwise appropriate terminology (eg, methyldopa, ibufenac, and dextran 40).

3. A name should reflect pharmacologic, chemical, or other characteristics and relationships of actual practical value to the users.

   a. A common syllable or simple word element (a "stem") should be incorporated in the names of all members of a group of drugs when useful common characteristics can thus be indicated (eg, similarity of pharmacologic action) (see Tables II and III). When pharmacologic similarity is found in drugs of distinctly different chemical nature, the stems should differ (eg, reserpine, promazine).

   b. Characteristically different terminology is sometimes necessary for specific drugs or groups (eg, insulin I 131, dextran 40).

4. A nonproprietary drug name should be free from conflict with other nonproprietary names or with trademarks, and should be such that it is neither confusing nor misleading.

5. Preference should be given to the choice of a name of established usage, provided it conforms reasonably well to these principles.

Specific Rules

1. Esters, salts, chelates, and complexes ordinarily require a two-word name to indicate the inactive as well as the active portion.

2. The preferred order for the name of an inorganic salt is cation–anion (eg, sodium bromide). The same order is preferred for well-known salts of simple organic acids (eg, sodium lactate, magnesium citrate, potassium acetate). However, for most organic compounds, the pharmacologically active portion should be named first (eg, oxacillin sodium, codeine phosphate).

3. A name for a salt or ester should in general be derived from the pharmacologically active moiety or corresponding acid (eg, acetic acid, sodium acetate, ethyl acetate). When a non-acid suffix is used, as is customary in the penicillin series, a salt should be named without modification of the parent acid name (eg, oxacillin, oxacillin sodium). Names for different salts or esters of the same active moiety should differ only in the name of the inactive portion (eg, estradiol enanthate, estradiol undecylenate); exceptions are permissible when both parts of the salt or ester possess pharmacologic activity (eg, aminophylline, prednazate).

4. A name for a quaternary ammonium substance should designate the cation and anion appropriately and separately (eg, octonium bromide, not octonine methylbromide).

5. A name for a complex of two or more components should indicate the composition by means of separate words, the last of which bears the suffix "*-ex*" (eg, bisacodyl tannex).

Table I—Examples of Accepted Symbols, Abbreviations, and Contractions

Cations	
Aluminum	Al
Ammonium	Am
Calcium	Cal or Ca
Magnesium	Mag or Mg
Potassium	Pot or K
Sodium	Sod or Na

Non-carboxylate Anions	
Bichloride	Biclor
Bromide	Brom or Br
Carbonate	Carb
Chloride	Clor or Cl
Hydroxide	Drox
Nitrate	Nit
Phosphate	Phos
Sulfonate	Sylate

Carboxylate Anions	
Acetate	Acet
Benzoate	Benz
Bitartrate	Bitart
Carbamate	Carbam
Citrate	Cit
Diacetate	Diacet
Dipropionate	Diprop
Gluconate	Gluc
Lactate	Lac
Maleate	Mal
Monoacetate	Monacet
Propionate	Prop
Tartrate	Tart

Hydrohalides	
Hydrobromide	Hybrom or HBr
Hydrochloride	Hyclor or HCl

6. A name for a drug containing a radioactive atom should be constructed in the following pattern: tolpovidone I 131; rose bengal sodium I 131; cyanocobalamin Co 60; potassium bromide Br 82.[2]

7. It is recognized that for some purposes, such as in labeling, in advertising, or in package inserts, the use of standard chemical symbols and abbreviations of certain radicals may be desirable, and such usage is considered acceptable. Examples are shown in Table I.

Preferred Spelling

1. The use of an isolated letter or number, or hyphenation, should be restricted to those groups of substances for which such usage fulfils a clearly demonstrable purpose.

2. To facilitate translation and pronunciation, "f" preferably should be used instead of "ph," "t" instead of "th," and "e" instead of "ae" or "oe." The World Health Organization also recommends that the letters "h" and "y" be avoided as much as possible so that nonproprietary names can be spelled identically in various languages.

3. Syllables such as "methylhydro" and "chlor" preferably should be condensed (eg, to "medro" and "clo").

Preferred Construction

Group relationships in a name preferably should be shown by use of the syllables (stems) listed in Tables II and III; conversely, use of the stem for other than the appropriate group should be avoided. When conflict arises, the stem conveying the most information should be used.

Basic Requirements of a USAN

An examination of nonproprietary names for drugs currently in use is likely to result in an inaccurate evaluation of present nomenclature activities. Many of these names were coined prior to the adoption of present nomenclature procedures and principles; indeed, many of these names made obvious the need for the action that has been taken by the USAN Council. Current names, then, reflect a mixture of new and old nomenclature practices.

There are three basic requirements for the selection of a good nonproprietary name:

1. These names must be relatively simple.
2. They must not conflict with any previously established drug name, either trademark or nonproprietary.
3. They should indicate a chemical or pharmacologic relationship to established drugs, if such exists.

In many instances poorly named drugs are due to the early practice of condensing the full chemical name into a chemically oriented nonproprietary name. At the time this practice came into being the chemistry of most drugs was not too complex. With advancing chemical complexity of drug entities, however, nonproprietary names so derived became increasingly long and difficult to spell, pronounce, and remember.

In addition to the problems caused by the complexity of the word itself, chemically derived names have been aptly criticized because they fail to provide useful information to anyone but a pharmaceutical chemist. (Although his need is recognized, he has the more scientific and accurate chemical nomenclature to serve his purpose.)

Nonproprietary nomenclature is intended primarily for physicians, pharmacists, and those in related health professions. A physician is not too concerned with the sometimes subtle structural manipulation of molecules which produce a potential new drug. He is more properly concerned with the understanding of the drug's pharmacological and therapeutic properties. Therefore, it must be emphasized again that nonproprietary names should be coined in such a way as to

Table II—Group Relationships: Listing by Category

Categories	Syllables
alkaloids and organic bases	-ine
amines, quaternary	-ium
anabolic steroids	bol-; or -bol-
analgesics (meperidine series)	-eridine
androgens	-andr-; or -stan-; or -ster-
anesthetics, local	-caine
anorexiants	-orex
antibiotics: cephalosporanic acid derivatives	ceph-
antibiotics: *Streptomyces* strains	-mycin
antibiotics: tetracycline derivatives	-cycline
anticholinesterases (neostigmine type)	-stigmine
anticoagulants (cumarin type)	-arol
anticoagulants, polysulfonic	-apol-
anticonvulsants, hydantoin	-toin
antimicrobial acridine derivatives	-crine
antimicrobial sulfonamides	sulfa-
antineoplastics (nucleotoxic)	mito-
barbituric acid derivatives	-barb
cortisone derivatives	-cort-
curare-like drugs	-curine
dibenzazepine compounds (imipramine type—straight side chain)	-pramine
diuretics: sulfamoylbenzoic acid derivatives	-pamide
diuretics: thiazide derivatives	-thiazide
estrogens	-estr-
hypoglycemics, oral {guanidine	-formin
sulfonamide}	gly-
iodine-containing contrast media	io-
mercurials	-mer-
5-nitrofuran derivatives	nifur-
N-alkylnormorphine derivatives that are morphine antagonists	nal-
penicillins: 6-aminopenicillanic acid derivatives	-cillin
progestogens	-gest-
Rauwolfia alkaloid derivatives	-serpine
steroids that are acetonide derivatives	-olide
tranquilizers (propanediol and pentanediol series)	-bamate

Table III—Group Relationships: Listing by Syllables[a]

Syllables	Categories
-andr-; or -stan-; or -ster-	androgens
-apol-	polysulfonic anticoagulants
-arol	anticoagulants (cumarin type)
-bamate	tranquilizers (propanediol and pentanediol series)
-barb	barbituric acid derivatives
bol-; or -bol-	anabolic steroids
-caine	local anesthetics
ceph-	antibiotics: cephalosporanic acid derivatives
-cillin	penicillins: 6-aminopenicillanic acid derivatives
-cort-	cortisone derivatives
-crine	antimicrobial acridine derivatives
-curine	curare-like drugs
-cycline	antibiotics: tetracycline derivatives
-eridine	analgesics (meperidine series)
-estr-	estrogens
-formin	guanidine oral hypoglycemics
-gest-	progestogens
gly-	sulfonamide oral hypoglycemics
-ine	alkaloids and organic bases
io-	iodine-containing contrast media
-ium	quaternary amines
-mer-	mercurials
mito-	nucleotoxic, antineoplastic agents
-mycin	antibiotics: *Streptomyces* strains
nal-	*N*-alkylnormorphine derivatives that are morphine antagonists
nifur-	5-nitrofuran derivatives
-olide	steroids that are acetonide derivatives
-orex	anorexiants
-pamide	diuretics: sulfamoylbenzoic acid derivatives
-pramine	dibenzazepine compounds (imipramine type—straight side chain)
-serpine	*Rauwolfia* alkaloid derivatives
-stigmine	anticholinesterases (neostigmine type)
sulfa-	antimicrobial sulfonamides
-thiazide	diuretics: thiazide derivatives
-toin	hydantoin anticonvulsants

[a] Recommended prefixes and suffixes are of the form gly- and -barb, respectively.

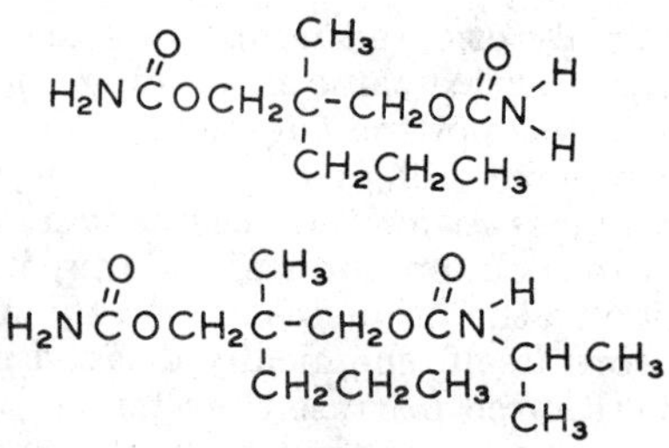

Fig. 315. Meprobamate (top) and carisoprodol (bottom) are closely related chemically and pharmacologically; the assigned names, however, do not indicate this relationship.

be most useful to, and usable by, their primary users: those in the health professions.

A well-coined nonproprietary name should be distinctive. Repetitious use of chemical prefixes is to be avoided; how many hundreds of drug names begin with di-, meth-, chlor-, oxy-, and phen-? By abandoning strict adherence to chemical antecedents, names can be made not only simpler but more unique.

There is, however, a more important aspect to be considered in the selection of distinctive nonproprietary names. For obvious reasons of safety, as well as for legal reasons, in some cases, names for drugs must be distinctive enough so they do not conflict with other established drug names. The USAN Council takes great care in its screening procedure to limit the possibility of conflict between a name under consideration and any established trademark or nonproprietary name.

In addition to utilizing the expertise of Council members in this area, the Council staff maintains extensive files on nonproprietary names and, to a lesser extent, on trademarks in use in this country and throughout the world. Moreover, manufacturers are requested to conduct the standard legal searches to help clear names which appear likely to be adopted.

The USAN Council also publishes proposed USAN, along with the therapeutic claim made for the drug, in the *Trademark Bulletin*. These lists should be consulted by the legal, trademark, and scientific staffs of the pharmaceutical manufacturers so that any existing objections can be referred to the USAN Council prior to formal adoption of a proposed name as a USAN.

Proposed USAN are also circulated to a number of nomenclature agencies in other countries, as well

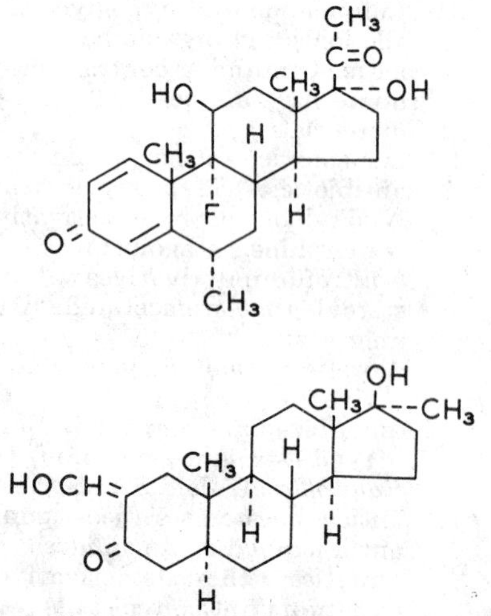

as to the WHO, in order to ferret out possible objection or conflict. Obviously, every effort is made to assure a conflict-free choice on the part of the USAN Council.

It seems reasonable that similar precautions should be taken by pharmaceutical manufacturers in the selection of trademarks for their drug products. In fact, the task should be simpler, since trademarks need only be simple and distinctive and need not necessarily be meaningful.

Unfortunately such is not always the case. A glance at any representative sampling of nonproprietary names and their corresponding trademarks will reveal several instances where the trademark, coined after the adoption of the nonproprietary name, differs only slightly from the nonproprietary name and often incorporates the syllable(s) recommended in the Council's Guiding Principles for the particular category of drug involved.

This type of trademark frequently acts as a bar to the subsequent adoption of appropriate nonproprietary names for closely related drugs. It also has the disadvantage (to the manufacturer) of obviously diluting the value of his trademark. For these reasons, the USAN Council condemns this unimaginative approach to trademark selection.

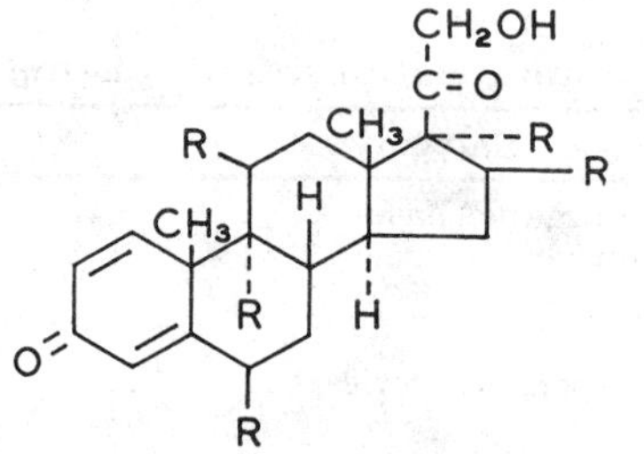

Fig. 317. The "R" groups indicate the positions on the glucocorticoid nucleus where the principal variations occur. Such variations give rise to the subseries in which the suffix *-olone* or *-sone* is used in the subseries stem—eg, *-cinolone* (triamcinolone, fluocinolone); *-cortolone* (clocortolone, flucortolone); *-methasone* (betamethasone, flumethasone); *-cortisone* (cortisone, hydrocortisone).

In order to assign meaningful nonproprietary names to new drug compounds it is necessary to indicate through the name any relationship that exists between the new entity and established drugs. Conversely, inappropriate names suggesting nonexisting relationships are to be avoided. The USAN Council has made use of standardized suffixes, prefixes or stem syllables to apply to particular classes of drugs. The recommended list of these syllables (see Tables II and III) is revised and updated regularly to keep pace with the changing chemical and pharmacologic nature of new drugs.

Again, a random survey of names for drugs currently in use will show a mixture of "old" and "new" nomenclature practices. In fact, such a survey, presented below, should effectively illustrate the principles behind the newer nomenclature approach.

Figure 315 presents a pair of compounds named some years ago, meprobamate and carisoprodol, that are related both chemically and pharmacologically; despite these similarities, the drugs have dissimilar names.

The opposite situation is illustrated in Fig. 316; the relationship between fluorometholone and oxymetholone begins and ends with the fact that both compounds are steroids. This class of compounds, however, is so

Fig. 316. Illustrative of poor practice in nomenclature are the compounds fluorometholone (top) and oxymetholone (bottom). The compounds are not as closely related as the names suggest.

large and so diverse that ring structure alone is hardly sufficient to warrant the use of a common stem (-metholone).

The steroids are, in fact, typical of several large groups of compounds which (within each group) exhibit somewhat similar chemical and pharmacologic properties. Because of diversity within the group, however, it is desirable to establish subseries of names based on the nature of the substituent groups present and on the placement of such substituents. In recent years the USAN Council has increasingly developed this principle, which is typified by the examples in Figs. 317 and 318.

Figure 317 depicts a basic glucocorticoid structure (glucocorticoids in themselves being a division of the broader category of steroids) in which the "R" groups indicate the positions at which the principal differences in the subseries occur. There is no common suffix for the entire glucocorticoid series, but the suffixes -olone and -sone are indicative of this series and are used in the stems of the various subseries.

The phenothiazine tranquilizers are a large series of drugs built on the nucleus shown in Fig. 318. The side chain variations that determine which suffix is to be used are also shown, along with examples of some names in each subseries. Since nuclear substitution

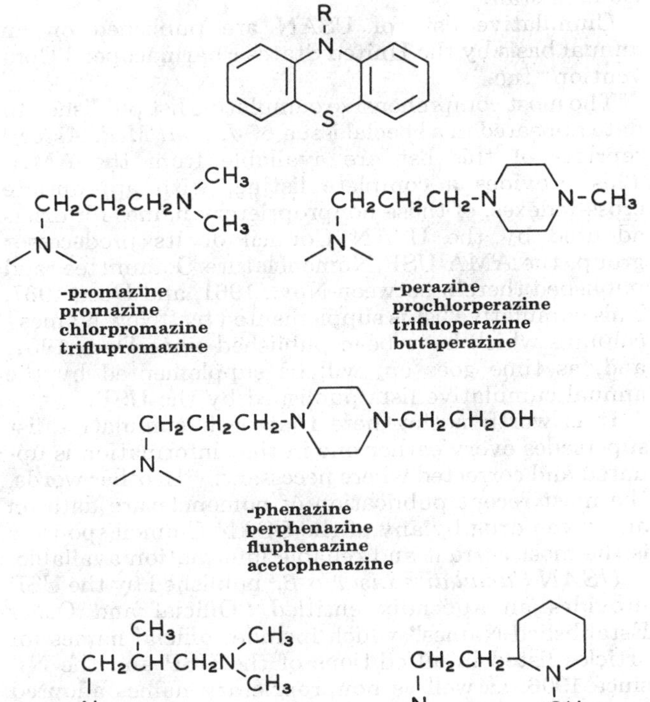

Fig. 318. The nucleus of phenothiazine tranquilizers and side-chain variations.

has not influenced the selection of the distinguishing suffixes (but on occasion has been used to provide a prefix), the figure neglects nuclear substitution. The suffix -azine is common to each of the five more specific suffixes of the various subseries illustrated and thus helps to exhibit the broad relationship among all these drugs.

The use of common stems to indicate particular classes of drugs is constantly re-examined by the USAN Council. The development of nomenclature

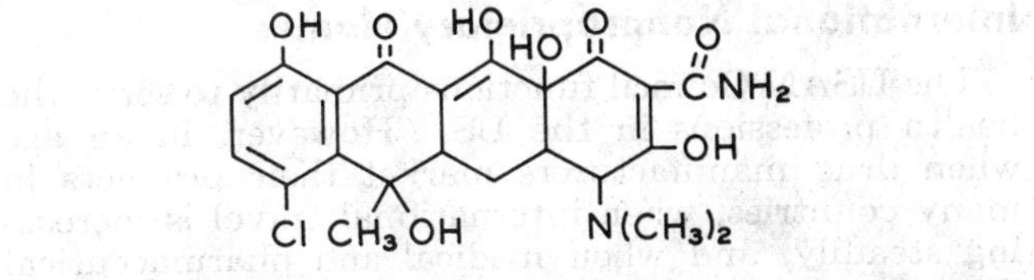

Fig. 319. Chlortetracycline; other names in this series include rolitetracycline, meclocycline, amicycline, and the newly adopted demeclocycline which replaces the earlier designation, demethylchlortetracycline.

for the tetracycline series of drugs (see Fig. 319) demonstrates the review and revision processes by which the Council's principles are assessed in order to assure their validity in the light of current nomenclature thought.

The first drugs in this series were chlortetracycline and oxytetracycline, both of which can be chemically converted to the parent compound, tetracycline. Further research led to still another variant, demethylchlortetracycline, which, in keeping with the standard practice of the time, was named in strict accordance with its chemical derivation.

The next member of this series to come to negotiation was characterized by a distinctive pyrrolidine group and, following traditional patterns, the name might have become pyrrolidinotetracycline. Instead, the first step was taken toward simplifying names in this series by shortening the prefix and the resulting name became rolitetracycline. The next step was to drop the syllables "tetra" from the suffixes of newer nonproprietary names for drugs in this group thus yielding simpler and more useful designations. Examples of such designations are amicycline, sancycline, and doxycycline.

Although it is a very difficult thing to do, occasionally the need and the opportunity arises to go back and change the poorly coined name of a well-established drug. Such is the case with the above-mentioned drug, demethylchlortetracycline. The name of this compound, which is commercially available as the hydrochloride salt, has been changed to demeclocycline hydrochloride. Because the compound is the subject of an NF monograph, this change will become official in 1970.

Chlorothiazide (Fig. 320) and the early related compounds which followed it were assigned chemically derived nonproprietary names. The -thiazide stem, while chemically oriented, came to have a pharmacologic significance to medical scientists, indicating to them a group of diuretic and antihypertensive drugs. This stem, then, has been retained in the names of all drugs in this group, although excessive dependence on chemical antecedents (as exemplified in the name hydroflumethiazide) has given way to simpler names such as althiazide and polythiazide.

These few examples serve as a guide to the direction of the Council's thought as it seeks to provide appropriate and meaningful nonproprietary names for drugs which are, at the same time, relatively simple and useful to members of the medical and related health professions.

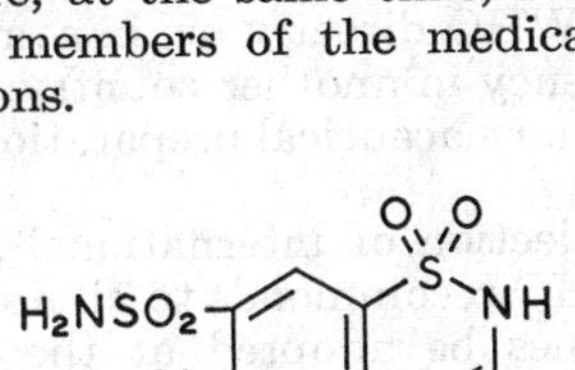

Fig. 320. Chlorothiazide; other drugs in this diuretic and anti-hypertensive series are hydrochlorothiazide, bendroflumethiazide, polythiazide, and althiazide.

International Nonproprietary Names

The USAN Council functions primarily to serve the health professions in the US. However, in an age when drug manufacturers market their products in many countries, when international travel is increasing steadily, and when medical and pharmaceutical literature is read widely around the world, the need for cooperation regarding nomenclature among the major drug-producing countries is clearly evident.

In addition to the USAN Council in the United States, national nomenclature agencies exist in Great Britain, France, Italy, Japan, the Nordic countries, and the Union of Soviet Socialist Republics.[3] These agencies operate at varying levels of national authority and cooperate with pharmaceutical manufacturers within their national areas in the selection of appropriate nonproprietary names.

The agencies maintain liaison with one another in an effort to secure the wide adoption of the most appropriate designation for each drug. The natural concern of each of these groups is with the drugs that are currently being synthesized, isolated, investigated, produced, or marketed in its own national area. Because such activity for any specific drug rarely, if ever, occurs simultaneously throughout the world, the need for the different national agencies to act on a nonproprietary name for a particular drug will vary in time.

The national agencies of the US, Great Britain, and France have set up procedures, with the knowledge and consent of the manufacturers involved, which circulate the names proposed for adoption, along with the pertinent chemical data, to the other agencies with a request that they be reviewed for appropriateness, availability, and the possible existence of another nationally adopted designation for the specific drug. If no valid objection to the proposed name is received, it can be assumed that the name then adopted will receive primary consideration by the other agencies if and when the drug becomes of interest elsewhere.

To prevent the confusion which arises when several nonproprietary names are used for a single drug, either in the same country or in several different countries, the WHO has assumed the responsibility of coordinating existing nomenclature efforts at the international level.

Through its Committee on Nonproprietary Names, whose members are drawn primarily from representatives of the national nomenclature agencies, the WHO has developed a procedure and guiding principles for the selection of International Nonproprietary Names (INN). Where national nomenclature agencies exist, they usually act as agents for national manufacturers by referring their selected designations (usually prior to national adoption) to the WHO with the request that these be considered for selection as international nonproprietary names.

A manufacturer located in a country without a national agency can direct his request for a nonproprietary name to WHO directly or, in some instances, to an existing agency in another country, preferably one in which the pharmaceutical preparation is likely to be marketed.

After the selection of international nonproprietary names, the WHO recommends to all its member states that such names be adopted at the national level. Formal adoption in accordance with national practice is necessary to provide review of the suitability of the international name for national use and leads to orderly documentation of nomenclature data.

Although it is not possible to have one name in use throughout the world for every given drug, increased national and international cooperation is providing an ever-expanding number of international nonproprietary names which serve as fundamental communication tools to the health professions around the world.

Dissemination of Nomenclature Information

The fact that nonproprietary names for drugs are being selected with ever-increasing thought and skill means little if these names are not brought to the attention of and used by those for whom they are intended. To accomplish this the USAN Council and its sponsors have developed a publication program to disseminate nomenclature information.

The Council publishes a monthly "New Names" column in the *Journal of the American Medical Association*. Proof copies of this column are distributed widely to the American pharmaceutical press for republication either in full or in part, with the result that the USAN quickly receives wide publicity.

Since this journal is the original source of publication of this information, it must be considered the most authoritative. In addition, reprints of the these columns are available on request from the USAN Council staff.

Cumulative lists of USAN are published on an annual basis by the United States Pharmacopeial Convention, Inc.

The most comprehensive cumulative list published to date appeared in a special issue of *J. Am. Med. Assoc;*[4] reprints of this list are available from the AMA. This provides a complete listing, with appropriate cross-indexes, of those nonproprietary names for drugs adopted by the USAN Council or its predecessor group, the AMA-USP Nomenclature Committee, and published therein between Nov., 1961, and Dec., 1967. This cumulative list is supplemented by "New Names" columns which have been published since Dec., 1967, and, as time goes on, will be supplemented by the annual cumulative lists published by the USP.

It is worth noting here that each cumulative list supersedes every earlier one in that information is updated and corrected where necessary. In other words, the most recent publication of nomenclature data on any given drug by any of the USAN Council sponsors is the most current and reliable information available.

USAN Cumulative List No. 6,[5] published by the USP provides an appendix entitled "Official and Other Established Names" which includes official names for articles listed in all editions of the USP and the NF since 1906, as well as nonproprietary names adopted by the AMA Council on Drugs since 1950.

Many other reference books on drugs include nomenclature information in varying degrees of reliability. This particular subject has been well treated by Feldmann.[6]

Although the advances made in drug nomenclature have been significant, the task ahead does not diminish, but grows increasingly complex. It remains the aim and the hope of the USAN Council to continue to provide an effective service in this field.

References

1. Alessandri, M. C., and Jerome, J. B., *J. APhA*, NS6, 584 (1966).
2. *J. Am. Med. Assoc.*, **184**, 228 (1963).
3. Alessandri, M. C., and Jerome, J. B., *J. Am. Med. Assoc.*, **192**, 405 (1965).
4. *J. Am. Med. Assoc.*, **203**, 659 (1968).
5. *United States Adopted Names (USAN)*, No. 6, United States Pharmacopeial Convention, Inc., Bethesda, Md., 1968.
6. Feldmann, E. G., *J. APhA*, NS6, 582 (1966).

32 | Structure-Activity Relationship and Drug Design

Chemotherapy—biologic factors—physicochemical factors—theories of drug action—drug design—molecular modification—isomerism

This chapter was prepared by

Murray Zanger, PhD, *Associate Professor of Chemistry,*
Philadelphia College of Pharmacy and Science, Philadelphia, Pa. 19104, and
Alfonso R. Gennaro, PhD, *Professor of Chemistry,*
Philadelphia College of Pharmacy and Science, Philadelphia, Pa. 19104

For many centuries man has utilized chemical agents in the treatment of specific diseases. About the year 1500 Carpensis employed mercury compounds in the treatment of syphilis. Cinchona bark (quinine), to combat malaria, was known in the middle of the 17th century. Nicolaier introduced methenamine, as a urinary antiseptic, about 1895. None of these medicaments resulted from an organized, planned research program, utilizing pharmacologic and biochemical data obtained from the screening of known molecules. Rather, they were the end-products of many years of empirical testing procedures.

In 1909 Ehrlich introduced his "magic bullet" of arsphenamine (salvarsan), derived as a consequence of a carefully thought out series of experiments. The romanticism involved in the discovery of "606" has been widely publicized and popularized. Trypan red, a coal-tar dye, had been found to selectively stain the causative organism of syphilis, but not the host animal. Ehrlich reasoned that by incorporating toxic materials (one of which was arsenic) into the Trypan red molecule, he could perhaps design a substance which was selectively toxic to the syphilis-causing organism.

Following Ehrlich's success, Germany was a pioneer in drug research. Plasmochin in the year 1924 and Atabrine in 1930 were synthesized as antimalarials. In the late 1930's the sulfonamides began their remarkable career as bacteriostatic agents and about 1940 the first antibiotic, penicillin, was introduced, from England.

It should be noted that all of the medicinal agents mentioned are antibacterial in nature. Because of the protracted efforts of the 19th-century microbiologists, many of the bacterial agents which caused the common, easily diagnosed, human diseases had been identified and could be cultured, studied, and the effect of chemical agents noted. Ehrlich had a target, therefore, for which to fashion his bullet. Such is not the case today, for many human afflictions. Cancer, heart, and mental diseases go unchecked primarily because the causative agent, the "target," is unknown. In the first quarter of this century pharmacology and chemotherapy were infants, not to mature until World War II provided the impetus. Only in the past 30 years have the biological sciences become sufficiently quantitative so that the more subtle and sophisticated human ailments could be studied and the effects of therapeutic agents evaluated.

Chemotherapy

Chemotherapy is the use of chemical agents in the treatment of disease. A very simple, succinct definition, but extremely difficult to reduce to practice. The problem, briefly stated, is to find a chemical entity or entities which can be administered to the body, transported to the desired site, perform its function, and then be metabolized and excreted without producing too many side effects or causing untoward toxicity. It is to this end that a study of the architecture of a chemical substance, in relation to its physiologic activity, is directed.

Certain organic structures or functional groups are known to possess or enhance certain biologic activities when incorporated in organic molecules. Table I[1] shows the diversity of activities attributed to the many groups illustrated. It is apparent that the assignment of a specific type of activity to any single functional group is virtually impossible. It is not then possible to construct a medicinal substance by selecting a biologically inert organic substance and append those functional groups which should impart the desired qualities to the molecule.

The enormity of the problem of drug design begins to become evident. Because of the many biologic activities possessed by a single functional group, the medicinal chemist is confronted with the enigma of nonspecificity. If the drug is not specific it must entertain a degree of toxicity by interference with normal metabolic processes along with the abnormal, disease-causing process. Nonspecificity is only one of a multitude of factors which greatly influence the activity of a drug and because of the large number of variables encountered, it is often surprising that any success is achieved in the attempt to "tailor-make" a drug molecule.

In designing a drug to have a distinctive activity in the treatment of specific disease conditions, several approaches are currently pursued. Perhaps the most common approach (although not necessarily the most productive) is a quasi-empirical method, whereby the chemist and pharmacologist work quite closely. For example, it has been shown (Table I) that organic compounds with both amino and ester functions exhibit local anesthetic activity. The chemist may then synthesize several types of molecules possessing these functional groups and the pharmacologist deter-

Table I—Activities Associated with Certain Structural Units[a]

Chemical group	Type structures	Drug example or prototype	Activity
Acetals (see also *Ethers*)	$R_2C-O-CH_2CH\ CH_2NR_2$ $\quad\quad\quad\overline{O}$	Glyketal Febrifugine Paraldehyde	Anticholinergic Antimalarial Hypnotic
Acids	RCOOH	Propionic acid	Fungistatic
	RCHOHCOOH	Chaulmoogric acid Mandelic acid Salicylic acid Salicylates Aspirin	Mycobacteriostatic Bacteriostatic Keratolytic Antirheumatic Antipyretic
	$RCH(NH_2)COOH$	Amino acids Thyroxine	Nutritional Antimitotic Hormonal
Alcohols (see also *Carbohydrates*)	ROH, where R is simple or complex	Benzyl alcohol 3-Pyridylmethanol Ethanol 2-Propanol Vitamins A and E, pyridoxine, thiamine, riboflavin Choline	Local anesthetic Vasodilator Sedative Anticonvulsant Vitamins Transmethylation
Amides (see also *Amidines; Imides; Sulfamides; Ureides; Semicarbazides; Thioamides*)	RCONHR $ArCONH(CH_2)_nNR_2$ $ArNHCOCH_2NR_2$ heterocyclic-$CONR_2$ Cyclic peptides Cyclic imides Polyfunctional amides	Phenacetin Procainamide Lidocaine Nikethamide LSD ACTH, insulin Oxytocin Polymyxin Barbiturates Idoxuridine Hydantoins Phensuximide Chloramphenicol Tetracycline Colchicine Angiotensin Amide	Analgesic Cardiotonic Local anesthetic Analeptic Psychotomimetic Hormonal Antibiotic Hypnotic Antiviral Anticonvulsant Antibiotic Antimitotic Hypertensive
Amidines (see also *Amides; Guanidines*)	$RC(NH_2)=NH$	Phenacine Hydroxystilbamidine	Local anesthetic Trypanocidal
Amines	ArCHOH—CHR—NHR $CH_3(CH_2)_nCH(NH_2)CH_3$ $R_2N(CH_2)_nNR_2$ $R_2CHO(CH_2)_nNR_2$ Carbocyclic-NH_2 Heterocyclic-$NH(CH_2)_nNR_2$ $H_2NArCOOR$ $R_2NCH_2CH_2Cl$ $RN(CH_2CH_2Cl)_2$ RNHCl	Phenethylamine Epinephrine Amphetamine Tuaminoheptane Tripelennamine Diphenhydramine Chlorpheniramine Oxyphencyclimine Methadone Amantadine Primaquine Lucanthone Benzocaine Phenoxybenzamine Nitrogen Mustards Chloramines	Pressor Vasoconstrictor CNS stimulant Vasoconstrictor Antihistamine Antispasmodic Analgesic Antiviral Antimalarial Antischistosomal Local anesthetic Adrenergic block Antineoplastic Antiseptics
Amino alcohols	$ArCHOH(CH_2)_nNR_2$	Acetylcholine Levarterenol Ephedrine Quinine	Cholinergic Pressor CNS stimulant Vasoconstrictor Antimalarial
Amino ethers	$R-O-CH_2CH_2NR_2$	Dimethisoquine Benzodioxanes Phenoxybenzamine Methoxyphenamine Dimenhydrinate	Local anesthetic Antihistamine Sympatholytic Sympathomimetic Antinauseant
Amino ketones	$Ar_2C(COR)(CH_2)_nNR_2$ Cyclic ketone	Methadone Tetracyclines	Analgesic Antibiotic
Ammonium compounds (quaternary)	R_4N^+ $R_3\overset{+}{N}CH_2CH_2OCOR$ $ArCH_2\overset{+}{N}(CH_3)_2-R$ (long)	Tetraethylammonium Decamethonium Hexamethonium Neostigmine Methantheline Benzethonium	Vasodilator Neuromuscular block Hypotensive Anticholinesterase Anticholinergic Antiseptic
Carbohydrates (see also *Alcohols*)	$R(CHOH)_nCHO$	ATP Lactulose Riboflavin Streptomycin	High-energy phosphate Cathartic Vitamin Antibiotic

Table I—Continued

Chemical group	Type structures	Drug example or prototype	Activity
Dyestuffs	Azo dyes Triphenylmethane type Phthaleins Pyronine type	Evans Blue Gentian Violet Phenolphthalein Fluorescein	Diagnostic Antibacterial Cathartic Diagnostic
Enols, enediols	$\begin{array}{c} R \\ | \\ C-OH \\ \| \\ C-R \\ | \\ R \end{array}$ and $\begin{array}{c} R-C-OH \\ \| \\ R-C-OH \end{array}$	Ascorbic Acid Tetracycline	Vitamin Antibiotic
Esters	$RSO_2O(CH_2)_nOSO_2R$ $RONO_2$ $H_2NArCOOR$ $ArCOO(CH_2)_nNR_2$ Alicyclic aminoester Heterocyclic aminoester	Busulfan Nitroglycerin Benzocaine Procaine Cocaine Scopolamine Meperidine	Antineoplastic Vasodilator Local anesthetic Cholinergic block Analgesic
Ethers (see also *Pyrones*)	R_2O Epoxide Ar—O—R Ar—O—Ar $ArOCH_2CH_2NR_2$ $Ar_2CHOCH_2CH_2NR_2$	Ethyl ether Vinyl ether Ethylene oxide Scopolamine Codeine Mephenesin Morphine Papaverine Streptomycin Thyroxine Dimethisoquine Diphenhydramine	Anesthetic Fumigant Cholinergic block Antitussive Muscle relaxant Analgesic Vasodilator Antibiotic Hormonal Local anesthetic Antihistamine
Guanidines (see also *Amides; Amidines*)	$RNHC(=NH)NHR$	Streptomycin Guanethidine Sulfaguanidine	Antibiotic Hypotensive Bacteriostatic
Halogen compounds	RCl CCl_4 $CHCl_3$ Br_3CCH_2OH $CHCl{=}CCl_2$ Cl_3CCHO Cyclic-Cl CHI_3 $HOArCl_n$ $RNHCl, RSO_2NHCl$ Aryl iodinated compounds Fluorinated steroids	Ethyl chloride Carbon tetrachloride Chloroform Tribromoethanol Trichloroethylene Chloral DDT, BHC Iodoform Hexachlorophene Halazone Iopanoic acid Dexamethasone	Local anesthetic Anthelmintic Anesthetic Hypnotic Parasiticide Antiseptic Anti-infective Disinfectant Radiopaque Glucocorticoids
Hydrocarbons		Cyclopropane Ethylene	Anesthetic
Ketones (see also *Pyrones*)	$ArCOR$ $Ar(CO)_2$ $(HOAr)_2CO$	Acetophenone Diphenadione Camphor Ketonic steroids Dioxybenzone	Sedative Anticoagulant External analgesic Anti-inflammatory, hormonal Ultraviolet screen
Lactones (see also *Esters*)		Ascorbic acid Bishydroxycoumarin Digitoxin Phenolphthalein Pilocarpine Santonin Tetracyclines	Vitamin Anticoagulant Cardiotonic Cathartic Cholinergic Anthelmintic Antibiotic
Mercaptans		Dimercaprol Methimazole	Chelating agent Antithyroid
Mercurials		Thimerosal Meralluride	Antiseptic Diuretic
Nitro compounds	$ArNO_2$	Chloramphenicol Nitrofurans Nitrocresols Nitrostyrenes	Antibiotic Coccidicidal Bactericidal Weight reducing Fungistatic
Oximes	R—CH=NOH	Pralidoxime	Cholinesterase reactivator
Phenols	ArOH	Amodiaquine Cresols Estradiol, diethylstilbestrol Guaiacol Hexylresorcinol Hydroxymorphinans	Antimalarial Antiseptic Estrogenic Expectorant Anthelmintic Analgesic

Table I—Continued

Chemical group	Type structures	Drug example or prototype	Activity
Phosphorus compounds	$R_2N(RO)P(O)NHR$ $(R_2N)_3P(S)$ $(R_2N)_2P(O)NHCOOR$ $R_3\overset{+}{N}(CH_2)_nSP(O)(OR)_2$ $F{-}P(O)(OR)_2$	Cyclophosphamide Thiotepa Uredepa Echothiophate Isofluorophate	Antineoplastic Anticholinesterase
Pyrones (see also *Ethers; Ketones; Lactones*)		Kojic acid Khellin Bishydroxycoumarin Lucanthone	Antibiotic Cardiovascular Anticoagulant Schistosomicidal
Quinones (see also *Ketones*)		Emodin Vitamin K Menadione	Cathartic Coagulant
Semicarbazones	$ArCH{=}NHNHCONH_2$	Nitrofurazone	Bacteriostatic
Thiosemicarbazones	$ArCH{=}NHNHCSNH_2$	Thiacetazone Methisazone	Tuberculostatic Antiviral
Silicones	$R_3SiO(R_2SiO)_nSiR_3$	Simethicone	Antiflatulent
Stilbenes	$RArC{=}CArR$	Hydroxystilbamidine Diethylstilbestrol	Trypanocidal Fungicidal Estrogenic
Sulfonamides	H_2NArSO_2NHR $ArSO_2NHCONHR$	Sulfonamide drugs Acetazolamide Tolbutamide	Bacteriostatic Diuretic Hypoglycemic
Sulfonimides		Saccharin	Sweetening agent
Sulfones	R_2SO_2 Ar_2SO_2	Sulfonal Dapsone Sulfinpyrazone	Hypnotic Leprostatic Uricosuric
Thioureas and Ureides (see also *Thiosemicarbazones*)	$RNHCSNHR'$	Thiourea Thiouracil α-Naphthylthiourea Thiobarbiturates	Antithyroidal Anticoagulant Hypnotic
Ureas	$RNHCONHR'$	Urea Diethylcarbamazine Suramin	Diuretic Filaricide Trypanocidal
Ureides (see also *Amides*)	$RNHCONHCOR'$ ┊---------------------┊	Barbiturates Hydantoins Theophylline	Hypnotic Anticonvulsant Diuretic
Urethans (Carbamates) (see also *Amides*)	$ROCONH_2$ $ROCONR_2$ Dithiocarbamates Metal dithiocarbamates	Meprobamate Ethinamate Novobiocin Neostigmine Trimethadione Disulfiram Thiram	Muscle relaxant Hypnotic Antibiotic Anticholinesterase Anticonvulsant Alcoholism Antifungal

[a] Adapted from a drug prototype listing by Burger.[1]

mines the relative activity of each compound. Usually the activities are referred to a standard medicinal agent—a known local anesthetic, in this case.

Or, in generally screening random compounds, the pharmacologist may uncover an interesting biologic activity and communicate his findings to the chemist. Then, the chemist utilizes the pharmacologic information to alter his original molecules, again giving the new compounds over to further testing. The pharmacologist, of course, must have previously developed reliable testing procedures.

Some of the synthetic compounds will probably show greater activity than others and the chemist, in conjunction with the pharmacologist, then evaluates the results and decides in what manner he might possibly modify the organic molecule to enhance a desired effect—or perhaps to subdue an undesirable one. This sequence of synthesis—test—synthesis—test may proceed for a number of cycles, until a new medicinal is born, or until the futility of the project is realized and a new route selected. Such an empirical process

is slow, requiring months and even years to attain even partial fruition.

One often forgotten aspect of biologic activity is that we become intensely concerned with the action of the drug on the body and seldom pay much attention to the action of the body on the drug! Since the drug is subject to a variety of biochemical reactions, it is important that the chemist is cognizant of the biochemical fate of the drug. Thus, another method of investigation involves the detection and structure determination of metabolites of known, biologically active agents. During the metabolic process, biotransformation may yield a metabolite of a drug which retains activity and, in fact, may even be superior to the parent compound. Prontosil forming sulfanilamide, chloral hydrate yielding trichloroethanol, phenacetin going to *p*-acetamidophenol, oleandomycin yielding the triacetyl derivative (TAO), and zoxazolamine forming chlorzoxazone are several examples of this phenomenon (see Fig. 321). By identifying, synthesizing, and pharmacologically testing excreted metabolites, the reactive portion of a molecule often can be ascertained.

Yet another line of research is employed whereby currently used drugs can be improved or modified. The concept of *Drug Latentiation* has been promulgated by Harper. It involves the chemical modification of a known biologically active compound to form a new substance, which upon *in vivo* enzymatic attack will liberate the parent compound. Several reasons for accomplishing the latentiation process are: to modify duration of action; to modify transportation and distribution of the drug in the body; to reduce toxicity; and to overcome difficulties encountered in pharmaceutical formulation procedures or in the dosage form itself.

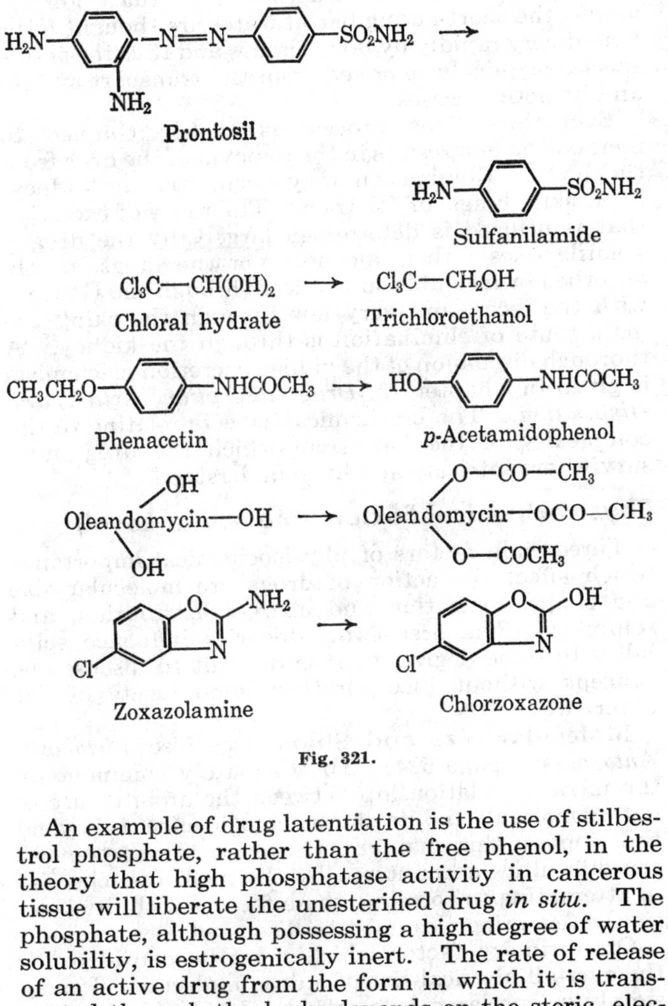

Fig. 321.

An example of drug latentiation is the use of stilbestrol phosphate, rather than the free phenol, in the theory that high phosphatase activity in cancerous tissue will liberate the unesterified drug *in situ*. The phosphate, although possessing a high degree of water solubility, is estrogenically inert. The rate of release of an active drug from the form in which it is transported through the body depends on the steric, electronic, and configurational aspects of X (Fig. 322). If the active drug is an ester, as in *a*, *b*, or *d*, the rate of release of the alcohol depends upon the nature of X. That the rate of enzymatic hydrolysis is influenced by electronic factors has been amply demonstrated. Numerous other examples could be cited to substantiate the feasibility of drug latentiation.

Still another approach to drug design has progressed tremendously with the advent of the computer era. If it were possible to evaluate and assess the manner in which all (or at least, the important) of the factors affect the efficacy of a drug and relate these factors to the complex biosystem through which the drug must survive in order to be efficaceous, then, perhaps, one could intelligently construct a molecule which would

be effective in the treatment of a specific disease state. This goal has never been attained, but enormous gains have been made and it is not improbable that success will be forthcoming in the near future. Later, in this chapter, a more detailed discussion will be given on the use of a mathematical model to correlate chemical with biologic activity.

Structural organic formulas are a very poor means of representing the physical, chemical, or biologic properties of a molecule. Structural formulas merely depict the way the various atoms are strung together to form what is known as a *molecule*. Drugs which are strikingly similar in structure may demonstrate widely differing pharmacologic properties, while two drugs of apparently different structure can exhibit almost identical activity. Reference to Table I easily confirms these facts. There are many factors other than simple structural variation that have an effect on the activity of a drug.

In order to more fully appreciate these factors it is important to review the biologic and physicochemical aspects associated with or which have an effect on drug activity.

Biologic Factors

Absorption—The preferred route of administration of a drug is by the oral route, which means the medicament must be absorbed into the body, via the mouth, stomach, or intestinal tract. Immediately that a drug is exposed to the gastrointestinal tract it becomes prey for the variety of enzymes and mucins contained therein. Hydrolytic peptidases, esterases, carbohydrases, etc begin to attack those functional groups which are susceptible. Mucins tend to bind several compounds (eg, quaternary amines) and the alkaline earth ions (Ca^{2+}, etc) effectively remove those drugs capable of forming insoluble chelates (eg, tetracyclines).

Obviously, pH is also of import; some substances (eg, penicillin) are rapidly hydrolyzed at the low pH of the stomach, while many carboxylic acid salts are precipitated as the free acid. It is well known that drugs are most effectively absorbed in a nonionized form. The more completely ionized a drug is, the greater proportion of it passes through the body unabsorbed. Also, to effect maximum absorption it is necessary that the drug be in solution. Thus, if it is desired that a drug exert its effect in the urogenital tract, high solubility is a requisite. To be effective in the GI system, low solubility must be "built-in."

Finally, the exact mechanism by which a drug is absorbed is unknown. It is not simply the passage of

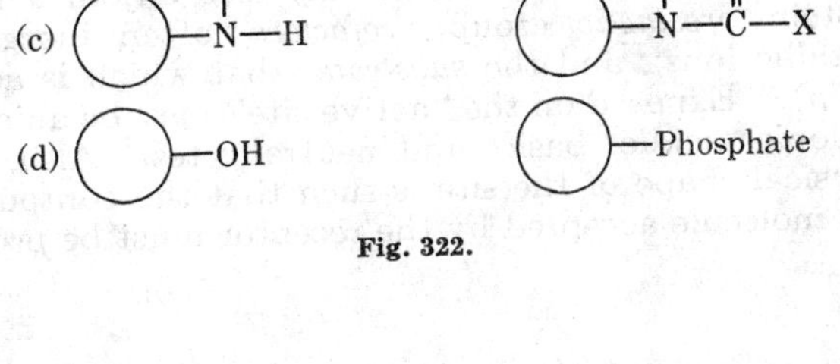

Fig. 322.

a molecule through a membrane, as in osmosis. Many biochemical reactions occur at the absorption interface, which again influences the survival rate of a drug. That much of the drug does not survive the digestive tract is demonstrated by the fact that in many cases a smaller parenteral dose is required for the same drug than if administered orally.

Transport—Quite often a drug is not administered directly at the required site, but if taken orally or parenterally, the drug must be carried to the desired location (as well as other, undesirable areas) by the blood. Due to size and weight factors, it is probable that most drugs, once absorbed into the bloodstream, are not very soluble and are carried along as a protein–drug complex (see Chapter 16, *Complexation*), conjugated to one of the plasma protein fractions. This binding of drug to protein must be of sufficient strength to prevent excess loss of the drug by excretion, but not so strong that adequate, unbound drug to maintain reasonable and effective tissue levels cannot be attained.

Metabolism and Biotransformation—Once the drug molecule has divested itself of the transport mechanism and has entered the various body tissues, it is again bound to protein—ie, tissue protein. It may be misleading to construe a high tissue level (concentration) of a drug to mean that the tissue is also the primary site of action. A great affinity for a drug molecule may occur at a nonactive site and serve to deplete the concentration of the drug in the transport system. With the tissue-bound drug the degradative process of catabolism is initiated by the tissue enzymes, especially those of the liver. In the liver microsomes the oxidative processes of *N*- and *O*-dealkylation, side-chain hydroxylation, sulfoxide formation, and deamination of primary amines occur. Also, other metabolic processes of ester and amide hydrolysis, reduction of nitro and azo compounds, formation of glucuronides from phenols, alcohols, acids and free amines, etc alter the structure of the parent drug molecule. Although not occurring in the liver, other metabolic enzymes convert phenols to ether sulfates, amines to acyl derivatives, and acids to glycine conjugates.

In the over-all metabolic process, drugs are progressively converted to compounds of increasing polarity until they can be excreted readily by the kidneys. By this *polarization process*, the drug is removed from the body and the concentration at the active sites is thereby reduced. For this reason also the chemist attempting to design a drug molecule must take cognizance of the chemical changes in the drug which occur during metabolism.

Reactions at Active Sites (see *Antimetabolites*, page 524)—Ehrlich first introduced the concept that a drug must first combine with a *receptor* (active site) in order to be effective. A receptor is considered to be some cellular substance upon which a drug acts to produce its desired (or undesired) effect. It is believed that enzymes are the primary receptors and drug action is a consequence of the influence of the drug on the enzyme. An enzyme system is composed of: a *coenzyme*, usually non-protein in nature; an *apoenzyme* (the protein portion) which may also enjoin a non-protein *prosthetic* group; *cofactors*, often inorganic metallic ions; and the *substrate* (that which is acted upon). Exposed on the "active site" may be anionic, cationic, acidic, basic, and neutral sites. Also, the physical shape of the site is such that the contour of the molecule accepted by the receptor must be proper

to insure a "fit" (see *Molecular Size and Shape* under *Physicochemical Factors*). Beyond this point little concrete evidence is available to validate the theoretical excursions into the theory of drug action.

Binding and Storage (see Chapter 16, *Complexation*)—Mention was made previously of the fact that mucins and proteins bind drugs. That is, some form of molecular adhesion causes the drug to be coupled with protein substances and other macromolecules. If the binding force is strong, the drug may combine quickly with the macromolecule and be thus removed from the transport system, metabolized, and excreted. Besides complexation to macromolecules, storage can also occur by dissolution in the body lipids or chelation by bony tissue, etc. In any case, the location and degree of storage is a factor influencing the potency, toxicity, and duration of action of a drug. For example, the short-acting barbiturates are thought to be bound very rapidly by body tissues and thus the active species is quickly removed from the transport system and its action ceases.

Excretion—This process is closely coupled to metabolism and results in the removal of the drug from the body. Elimination may occur via the kidney, liver, skin, lungs, or GI tract. The route of excretion that is utilized is determined largely by the drug—volatile ones (ether, alcohol) via the lungs, poorly absorbed or insoluble substances through the GI tract with the feces, and very few through the skin; the main route of elimination is through the kidney. A thorough discussion of the kidney excretion mechanism is given in Chapter 42, *Drug Absorption*, *Action*, and *Disposition*. The biochemical aspects relating to the complexity of the biosystem which the drug must survive are intricate and little understood.

Physicochemical Factors (Molecular Level)

Three main factors of physicochemical importance which affect the action of drugs are molecular size and shape, ionization and charge distribution, and solubility. The first two categories influence solubility to some degree, so it is difficult to discuss one concept without incorporating some facets of the other two.

Molecular Size and Shape (see also *Metabolite Antagonism*, page 524)—To adequately comment on the intricate relationship between the architecture of a drug molecule and its pharmacologic effect is beyond the scope of this chapter. However, to comprehend the difficulties encountered by the medicinal chemist in attempting to correlate these factors with drug design, a few principles must be discussed.

One primary factor which must be considered is the over-all physical size of a drug molecule. It may simply be too large to be effectively absorbed, transported, and transferred through the cellular membranes to elicit a reaction. For this reason the chemist cannot indiscriminantely concoct a drug molecule by "throwing together" functional groups in order to enhance or subdue a certain biologic effect. The molecule may become unwieldy and could not be readily utilized in a biologic system.

Previously, the concept of the *receptor* was discussed and it was considered as the cell component with which the drug combines to initiate a response. How the drug and receptor coalesce depends to a large extent on the architecture of both the drug molecule and receptor site. Ehrlich described it as a "lock and key" theory—each drug molecule must be the proper "key" to fit the receptor "lock."

It is postulated that for a drug (or any substrate) to effectively combine with a receptor (usually an enzyme), besides having the proper conformation, an attachment must occur at three separate sites. Thus, what may appear to be a relatively minor defect in the configuration or conformation of a drug, such as the opposite antipode of a stereoisomeric substance, may have appreciable effect on the extent of activity. A typical example is shown in Fig. 323[2] for the epinephrine molecule. Thus, there must be a mutual melding of drug and receptor and a mutual adaptation so far as shape and charge distribution are concerned. To further illustrate the point, the antihistamine, chlorpheniramine, was (and still is) employed for many years before it was discovered that the (+) isomer, dexchlorpheniramine (as the maleate), has about twice the potency of the racemate and a wider margin of safety.

Ionization, Charge Distribution, and Solubility—Lipid-soluble drugs usually cross cellular boundaries by dissolving in or interacting with the lipid membranes and diffusing across into the intracellular aqueous phase. Most drugs are weak organic electrolytes, present in equilibrium between two forms, of which only the nonionized form possesses lipid solubility. In general, therefore, water-soluble compounds

$$AH \rightleftharpoons A^- + H^+$$
nonionized drug   ionized drug

which are either completely ionized or have lipid-insoluble nonionized forms are poorly absorbed. Quaternary amines and streptomycin are fully ionized

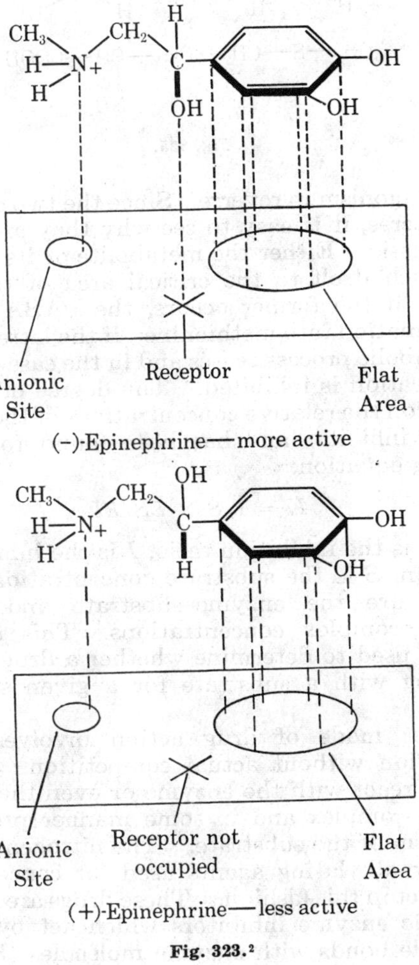

Anionic Site   Receptor   Flat Area

(−)-Epinephrine—more active

Anionic Site   Receptor not occupied   Flat Area

(+)-Epinephrine—less active

Fig. 323.[2]

and not absorbed to a great extent. At biologic pH values many sulfonamides exist in the nonionic form but are not absorbed well due to lipid insolubility.

Solubility characteristics of an effective drug must be optimized. If too soluble, rapid excretion via the kidneys results, or blood levels remain high and tissue levels low; if very insoluble, absorption does not occur and excretion is facilitated by the GI route.

Thus, it should be evident, that all of the nuances of molecular structure—interatomic distance, geometric and stereochemical conformation, rigidity and flexibility, and charge distribution—are factors that require attention in the over-all consideration of drug design.

All of the foregoing data have been presented to emphasize the many kinds of attrition a medicinal agent must survive in order to reach the active site. If it is successful in avoiding the biochemical hazards, it is further required that its physical and electronic makeup be acceptable to the active site for a reaction to take place. To endeavor to design a drug to perform a specific function, each of these factors (and, no doubt, some as yet unrecognized) must be considered. It also should be noted that although the scientist is cognizant of the existence of these biochemical and physicochemical "roadblocks," so little is known about their fundamental influence on drug substances that the design of drugs is still largely based on empirical concepts.

Theories of Drug Action

Through the years numerous theories have been advanced which, with limited success, have been able to correlate drug activity with some physical parameter. One of the earliest hypotheses which attempted to define a mechanism of drug action was the Meyer–Overton Narcosis Theory. Working independently, both men in 1901 observed that, for general anesthetics, activity was related to the lipid/water partition coefficient; cyclopropane with a coefficient of 65 was far more effective than nitrous oxide with a value of 2.2. The Meyer–Overton Theory, however, as an explanation of drug action, suffers from several deficiencies. For one, all true anesthetics are inert chemical compounds, but numerous inert compounds possess no anesthetic activity. More fundamentally, the theory does not really explain how anesthesia is produced in the organism. One will find for the most part that the other theories attempting to explain drug action are also severely limited and usually apply only to specific classes of drugs. The subject of drug activity is so complex that most theories must seem naive in their attempt to unravel its intricacies.

In more recent times, workers such as Tolstoouhov have used physicochemical characteristics to define drug activity and drug action. As has been correctly indicated, structural modification of drugs is often a fruitless means for obtaining new active compounds. Thousands of compounds of a given structural type may be synthesized and found to be less active or inactive when compared to the parent compound. The physicochemical approach depends upon the dissociation constants of a drug and its relationship to the isoelectric point of the tissues or organisms with which it is supposed to interact. The theory might be likened to an acid–base reaction. If at the pH of the blood, a given drug is too weakly basic to react with an acidic site in the biosystem, its activity will be minimal. If a modification of the drug increases its basicity, activity will increase. Tolstoouhov has been able to show good correlation of activity vs pK_b for several series of drugs, the active drugs lying within a narrow range of dissociation constants. Among a group of 19 sulfonamide compounds, only those which have a pK_b in the range 11.66–12.36 were active. Unfortunately, Tolstoouhov's results have been questioned recently, especially the validity of his pK_b measurements. However, the physicochemical mechanisms should not be discounted entirely. One feature of this approach is its complete disregard of chemical isosterism; widely differing structural types exhibit activity when their physicochemical characteristics fall within the critical range.

Most other theories of drug action have evolved from the concept of drug–receptor interactions (see *Reactions at Active Sites*). Receptors are usually thought of as enzymes or other proteins vital to the life process. In a viable biosystem a variety of substrates are known to be metabolized through the intervention of enzyme systems. A large proportion of drugs are believed to act by altering the ability of the substrate to interact with the enzyme or receptor. Without attempting to be comprehensive, extensions of the drug–receptor concept will be discussed which have some experimental verification. The theory of *Metabolite Antagonism* is one which has gained great currency. An antimetabolite can function in one of several ways; it can complex with a metabolite and thus effectively remove it from the biochemical cycle; in a similar fashion it can inactivate a metabolite by forming a compound with it; and finally it can, through structural or functional group similarity, compete with a metabolite by blocking a site on an enzyme at which the metabolite ordinarily reacts. This latter mechanism, *enzyme inhibition*, has probably been studied by pharmacologists more than any other single mechanism. In its most up-to-date version the theory postulates that on the surface of the enzyme there are sites of particular conformation, spacing, and chemical affinity such that only a molecule which has a shape which mirror-images the enzyme surface and has the correct chemical groups can interact with the enzyme.

The receptor surface of acetyl cholinesterase has been studied, and some of the dimensional and functional group properties of this enzyme are depicted in Fig. 324. By modifying the structure of acetylcholine, the distance between the receptor sites has been determined, and by altering the substituent parts of the acetylcholine molecule, the chemical nature of the receptor sites has been ascertained. Amine (—NH₂), sulfhydryl (—SH) and hydroxyl (—OH) are the most common substituents, both on the drug and receptor molecules, through which interactions take place. The spacing, arrangement, and polarity of the binding sites on the receptor surface might be

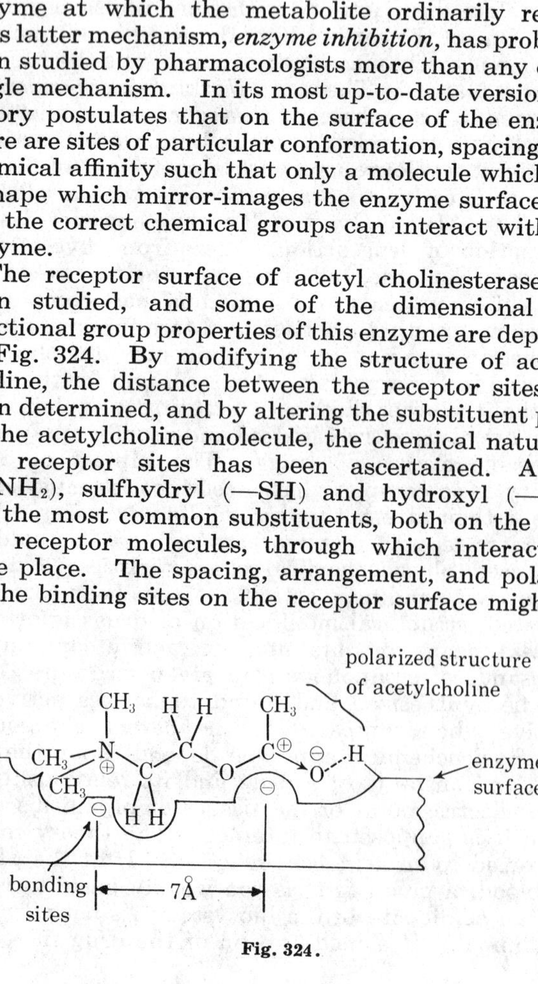

likened to a "lock" and the substrate or drug which interacts with it must fit these sites in order for reaction to occur.

This "lock-and-key" theory would explain, then, why molecules which structurally resemble a metabolite can act pharmacologically by substituting for the metabolite and thus effectively block any further reactions. Two molecules of approximately the same size and shape are called isosteres, and the synthesis of isosteres of known metabolites is one approach to the discovery of new pharmocodynamic agents. Sometimes, however, the chemist is fooled and a synthetic *isostere* (see *Isosterism* under *Molecular Modification*) instead of being antagonistic actually mimics the action of the natural compound. The synthetic Vitamins K are good examples of this type of action.

The classic examples of metabolite antagonism by a drug are sulfanilamide and its derivatives. In work carried out by Woods, sulfanilamide was shown to be antagonistic to *p*-aminobenzoic acid (PABA), a biologic precursor of methionine (Fig. 325). A fascinating feature of these studies was the demonstration that PABA would reverse the effect of sulfanilamide on a bacterial culture, an example of metab-

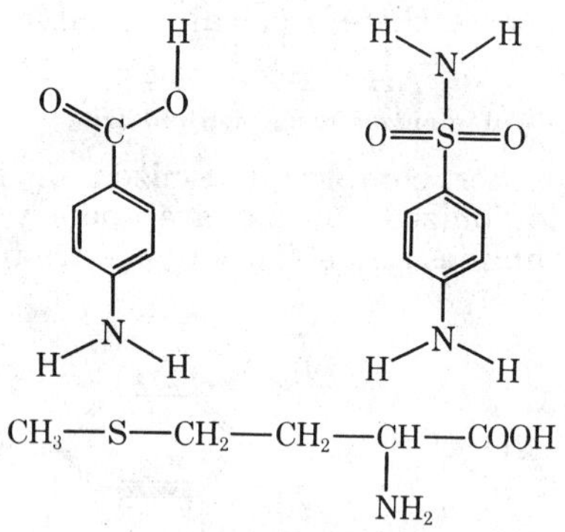

Fig. 325.

olite antagonism in reverse. Since the two compounds are isosteres, it is easy to see why they are mutually antagonistic. Either the metabolite or its antagonist can attach itself to the critical area of the enzyme surface; if the former occurs, the PABA begins its transformation into methionine; if the latter happens, the metabolic process ceases and in the case of bacteria multiplication is inhibited. The degree of inhibition depends on the relative concentrations of the substrate and the inhibitor and has been found to obey the following equation:

$$K = I/S \times ES/EI$$

where K is the inhibition ratio, I is the inhibitor concentration, S is the substrate concentration, and ES and EI are the enzyme–substrate and enzyme–inhibitor complex concentrations. This expression has been used to determine whether a drug is in fact competing with a substrate for a given site on an enzyme.

Another mode of drug action involves enzyme deactivation without actual competition. Here the drug can react with the enzyme or even the enzyme–substrate complex and in some manner prevent the metabolism of the substrate. The nitrogen mustards and other alkylating agents used for cancer chemotherapy act in this fashion. These drugs are relatively nonspecific enzyme inhibitors which act by forming irreversible bonds with enzyme molecules (Fig. 326).

Fig. 324.

In doing so they may not necessarily block a particular site but rather many active sites and in this way inactivate the enzyme.

Another explanation which has been advanced is the *Molecular Perturbation Theory*. It has been well established in recent years that living proteins (enzymes included) assume specific shapes or conformations in an organism. In these conformations certain functional groups are exposed and are spatially related to other groups, thus producing the active sites at which the substrate can attach. However, suppose that a noncompetitive drug could bond to an enzyme in such a way as to distort the enzyme surface. The active site would no longer have the same shape or spacings between its bonding groups and the substrate "key" would no longer fit its enzyme "lock." The enzyme, in effect, would have been chemically denatured. Reactions which alter receptor conformation are called *allosteric*. It has been previously mentioned that an antimetabolite can compete with a substrate for an enzyme. Some drugs, however, may act by actual substitution and incorporation into a macromolecule. In this fashion, rather than inactivating an enzyme, they may actually form a new enzyme-like molecule with either no activity or altered activity.

The above discussion has centered largely around mechanisms of drug action involving enzymic processes. Since metabolic pathways are so complex, there are available numerous ways of altering or inhibiting them. Another, albeit poorly understood, aspect of drug action involves the transport of vital ions or metabolites. The movement of molecules either into or out of a cell or across a synapse is an important aspect in the biochemical process. Simple diffusion often is not adequate for the demands of an organism. Thus, there are available other mechanisms of transport which transcend simple diffusion both as to rate and even direction of movement across a membrane. Certain drugs, such as the local anesthetics, appear to act by affecting membrane permeability. Since the structures of these compounds are so dissimilar chemically, it is believed that their action does not involve receptor sites and is probably physicochemical in nature. It also has been demonstrated that sodium, potassium, and calcium ion transport is affected by the administration of various compounds, but how the diffusion rate is changed is not understood. Several tentative explanations of these phenomena have been offered, including membrane depolarization and ion competition, but a really detailed and substantiated mechanism is still forthcoming.

As intimated in the beginning of this section, the mechanisms of drug action remain a fruitful area of investigation. This discussion is merely a brief survey of some of the pathways, which have some experimental basis, through which chemical compounds are assumed to act in a biologic environment. Most of the theories propounded are questioned by certain investigators and among scientists in this field there are all too few areas of general agreement.

A long-standing goal of workers in the area of structure–activity correlation has been the development of a quantitative means of determining the relative activities of a series of compounds. The Meyer–Overton theory was an early attempt at such a correlation. In the field of theoretical chemistry, Hammett was the first to demonstrate the predictability of the pK_a values of substituted benzoic acids as a function of the various substituents attached to the ring, and their abilities to either donate or withdraw electrons from the carboxyl group. He was then able to extend these results to other reactions and other series of compounds using the same substituent constants he had derived from the benzoic acid series. In his equation,

$$\log k/k_0 = \rho\sigma$$

where k is the rate constant for the substituted acid, k_0 is the rate constant for the unsubstituted acid, ρ is the reaction constant, and σ is the substituent constant. Later work led to substituent constants in which the electronic effect is separated into inductive and resonance terms and, in the Taft equation, a term E_s is defined as a measure of the steric requirements of a substituent.

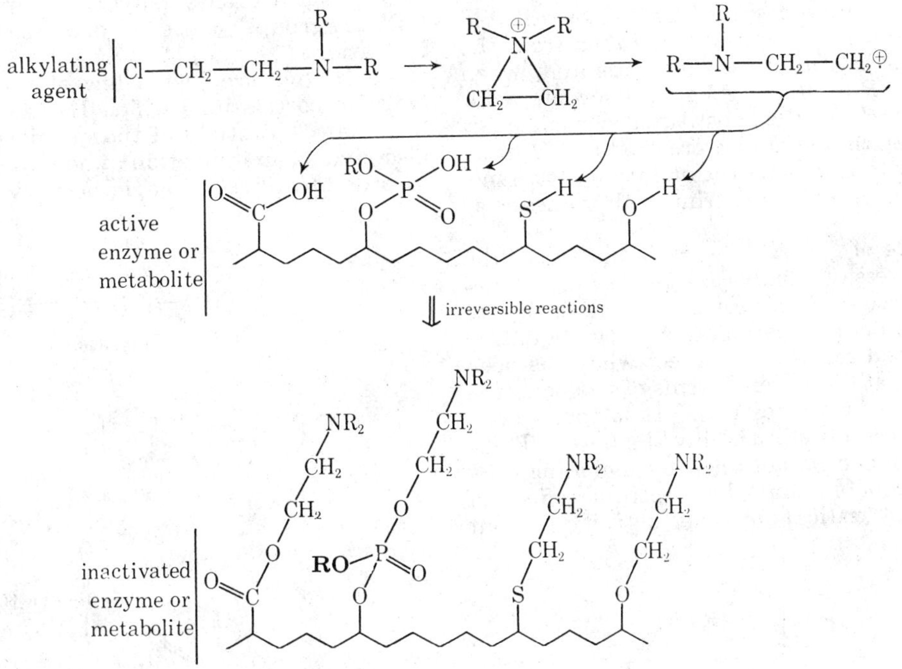

Fig. 326.

In more recent times there have been numerous attempts to mathematically correlate molecular structure with drug activity. Many of these attempts were destined to fail because they grossly oversimplified what we now know as a very complex problem, even more so than "simple" chemical reactivity. Others have had moderate success within narrow limits of drug type, but a universal equation has yet to find expression.

One of the most successful investigators in this field is Hansch who has derived a general equation based on linear free energy considerations. Inherent in his equation is the ability to incorporate parameters which encompass the full range of known biologic requirements for drug activity. Among these are terms for biologic transport, drug/enzyme binding energies, substituent effects (both electronic and steric), and electron densities of possible active sites on the drug molecule.

The most general form of the Hansch equation is usually written

$$\log 1/C = -a(\log P)^2 + b \log P + \rho\sigma + c$$

Activity is expressed as $1/C$, where C is the concentration of a drug required to elicit a given response. P is the octanol/water partition coefficient and is a measure of the hydrophobic bonding power of the drug. Its magnitude is indicative of the ability of a drug to move through biologic systems. ρ is the Hammett reaction constant which is characteristic of a given molecular type. σ is the Hammett substituent constant which is a measure of the electronic effect on the rate of reaction.

The equation is also expressed

$$\log 1/C = -a\pi^2 + b\pi + \rho\sigma + c$$

where $\pi = \log P_x - \log P_H$, P_x is the partition coefficient of the substituted molecule, and P_H is the partition coefficient of the parent unsubstituted molecule. The particular benefit of the new term π is the observation by Hansch that π-values are additive and thus numerous partition coefficients can be calculated without the necessity of synthesizing and measuring P_x of the actual compound. An example was the calculation of P_x values for a series of substituted benzeneboronic acids. π values were taken from the known series of substituted benzoic acids and, when added to the log P_H value for benzeneboronic acid, gave values of log P_x for the substituted boronic acids (Fig. 327). When these values were used in a Hansch equation predicting drug penetration into brain tissue, excellent correlation with experimental values was obtained.

Another feature of Hansch's work is his use of the technique of regression analysis. In seeking structure-activity correlation it is often not necessary to include all of the defined parameters in the equation in order to get good results. In effect what has been done is to fit the data to several forms of the equation using the method of least squares. It is then determined which equation is statistically the best. Thus, if good correlation can be obtained by including only π-values, it is probable that the electronic effect of substituents is not critical for drug activity in that

series. Postulates as to specific drug mechanisms can thus be made when activity dependence, or lack thereof, is found for a given parameter. Further expansions of the equation also permit mechanistic considerations to be formulated. The $\rho\sigma$ term (actually a log k term) can be expanded to include a steric parameter (E_s) or electron density parameters for various parts of a molecule. Thus, if inclusion of a steric substituent constant leads to improved correlation, the steric requirements of the drug/enzyme interaction can be better understood. Several examples are given below for derived equations in which excellent correlation with experimental results is found when one or more parameters are omitted.

For the antibacterial effects on Gram-negative bacteria of a series of diguanidines of structure shown in Fig. 328, the equation

$$\log 1/C = -0.081\pi^2 + 1.483\pi - 1.578$$

predicts quantitative activity very accurately. Substituent effects here are neglected since molecular modification involves only a change in the number of methylene groups.

For the antibacterial activity of substituted phenols of structure of Fig. 329, the equation

$$\log 1/C = 0.684 \log P - 0.921\sigma + 0.268$$

best fits the data. It would seem here that substituents which donate electrons ($-\sigma$ values) would have the highest activity, but in the series studied these compounds have relatively small values of log P and this offsets much of the substituent effect. Thus, the most active compounds were those which had the best balance between partition coefficient and electronic effect.

Phosphonate esters are known to inhibit cholinesterase. In the series of compounds of Fig. 330, the equation which gave the best correlation was

$$\log K = 0.152\pi - 1.684\sigma^* + 4.053 E_s + 7.212$$

where K is the inhibition constant, σ^* is the substituent constant for aliphatic systems, and E_s is the Taft steric constant. Here is a series in which steric effect of the substituents plays an important role. The bulkier groups cause a decrease in cholinesterase inhibition.

The above are just a few of the many structure-activity correlations which Hansch has been able to formulate. A study of those equations of best fit can also give us an indication of how to modify a structure in order to affect biologic activity. Thus, in deter-

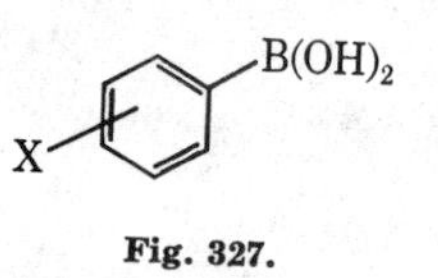

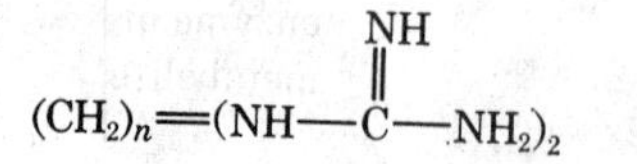

Fig. 328.

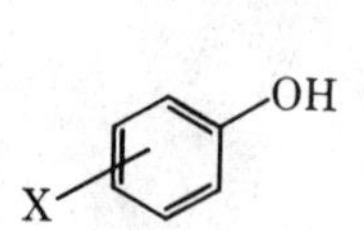

Fig. 329.

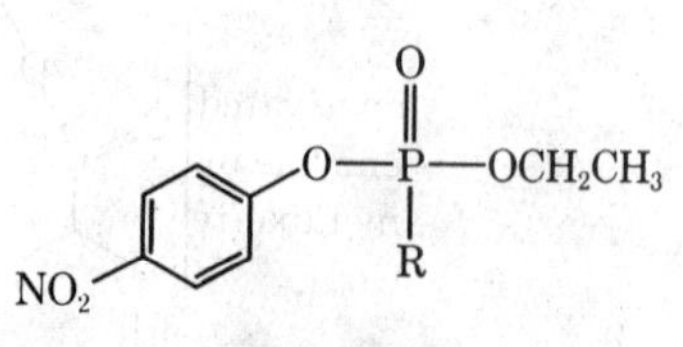

Fig. 330.

Fig. 327.

mining the relative sweetness of the derivatives of 2-amino-4-nitrobenzene, electron-releasing groups were found to increase the sweetness. Also in a study of thyroxine derivatives, it was predicted (and substantiated) that the replacement of iodine by a *t*-butyl group should lead to a more active molecule. To date, the Hansch equation is the most ambitious attempt to explain drug activity in terms of structural variations. That the equation fails to accurately correlate structure/activity in some systems only indicates that there are still some parameters, perhaps unknown, which should be incorporated.

A relatively recent approach, and one which should assume increasing importance in the future, involves molecular orbital calculations for various atoms in a drug molecule. This approach is exemplified by the work of Pullman and Pullman and of Holland. Essentially, drug activity is correlated to the electron densities of one or more atoms in the molecule. The carcinogenic activity of various polycyclic aromatic hydrocarbons was in this way related to the electron densities of two regions in the molecules. Efforts along these lines are important because (1) they can indicate which atoms or groups are the active sites for drug/receptor interactions, (2) they give some idea as to the spacings between reactive sites and collaterally picture the geometry and structural features of the receptor surface, and (3) one can study how molecular modification alters the electron density (hence activity) of drug molecules. These workers admit that their efforts have certain shortcomings, namely that they ignore other parameters of drug activity such as biologic transportation, steric interactions or inhibitions, and other physical factors. Nevertheless, this area of investigation can offer much in terms of understanding drug/receptor binding on a submolecular level.

There has been a great deal of other work using statistical methods to define structure–activity relationships. Free and Wilson, and Kopecky among others have been active along lines somewhat similar to the efforts of Hansch. All of these investigators have sought to further the assault upon that lofty goal, a quantitative structure–activity relationship of universal application. In summary, there follows a listing of some of the parameters which have been found to correlate with drug activity in specific cases:

> solubility, partition coefficients, R_f values
> Hammett (substituent) constants
> Taft (steric) constants
> infrared and ultraviolet data
> pK_a values
> molecular orbital (MO) electron density calculations
> polarographic half-wave potentials
> oxidation–reduction potentials
> nuclear magnetic resonance chemical shifts
> surface activity
> dipole moments
> electronic polarizability

Drug Design

Literally volumes have been written on the subject of drug design and yet ideal drugs remain to be synthesized. Even aspirin, which might lay claim to the title, cannot be tolerated by certain individuals, and it is also contraindicated by people on anticoagulant drugs and, of course, by patients with ulcers. In spite of the fact that our arsenal of effective drugs is ever expanding and ever improving, the goal is still the ideal drug. One must now consider those aspects of

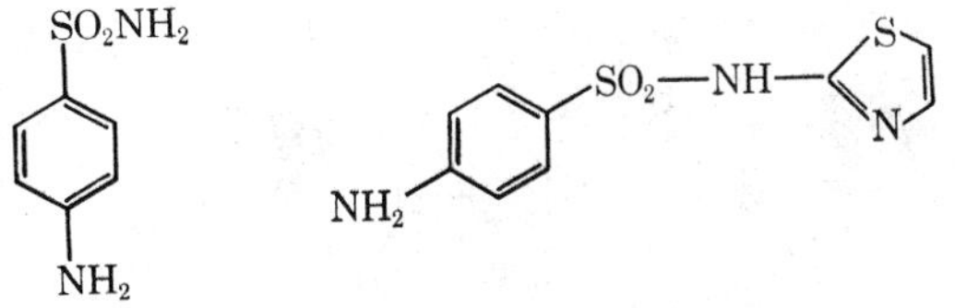

Fig. 331.

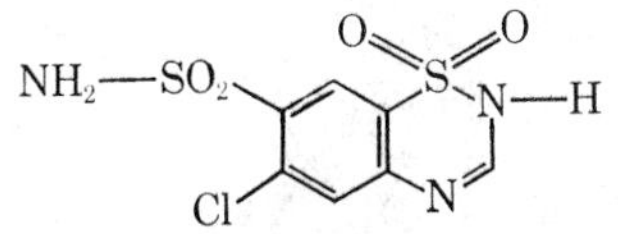

Fig. 332.

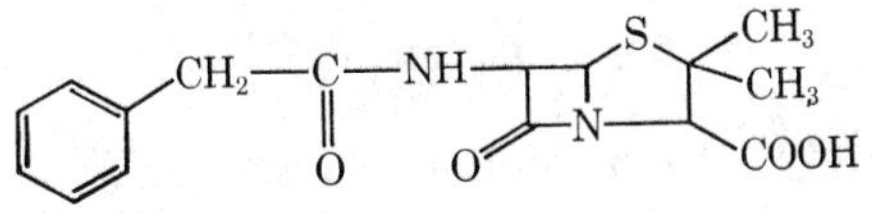

Fig. 333.

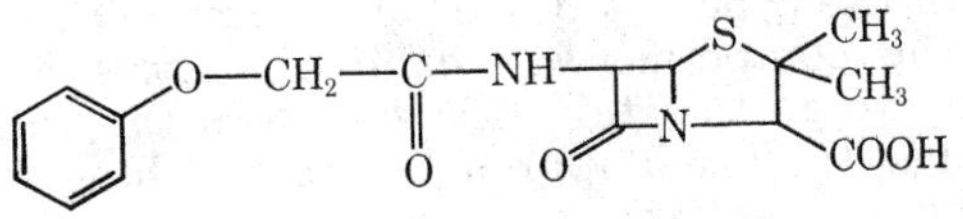

Fig. 334.

drug action which one seeks to modify by creating new pharmacodynamic agents.

Potency—A known drug may not have a maximal effect at optimum dose. That is, if the therapeutic ratio of a drug or its biologic spectrum is too narrow, a more potent compound should be sought. The first sulfonamide, sulfanilamide, Fig. 331A, has been supplanted by a host of more effective sulfonamides. By modifying the sulfanilamide structure sulfathiazole (Fig. 331B) was synthesized, probably the most effective agent (even though the most toxic) in this class of compounds.

Specificity—One of the banes and curses of drug action is its lack of specificity. No drug acts exclusively on one biochemical system and, if a drug is utilized for a specific action, one must often put up with secondary or side effects. If these effects are too deleterious, they may seriously hamper the utility of the drug and may necessitate redesigning the molecular structure to accentuate the positive and eliminate the negative effects. The early antihistamines produced severe drowsiness. Molecular modification has lessened but not eliminated this problem. On the other hand, side effects have often led to new types of drugs. By redesigning the molecule it may be possible to create a new compound in which the secondary effect becomes the primary one. Sulfanilamide exhibited side effects which led to the development of diuretics, exemplified by chlorothiazide (Fig. 332).

Physiologic Factors—Certain drugs have shown activity *in vitro* and exhibited diminished activity when used *in vivo*. Absorption, distribution, elimination, and detoxification—any of these factors may be the cause. Penicillin G (Fig. 333), a potent antibiotic, when taken orally is severely degraded by stomach acids. Modification of this structure to Penicillin V (Fig. 334) led to a compound of comparable potency, identical antibacterial spectrum, but very resistant to acid hydrolysis. In the area of barbiturate sedatives, hexobarbital (Fig. 335) has a very short onset of action and its action is of short duration. A structural modification gives phenobarbital (Fig. 336), whose sedative effect may last up to 12 hours.

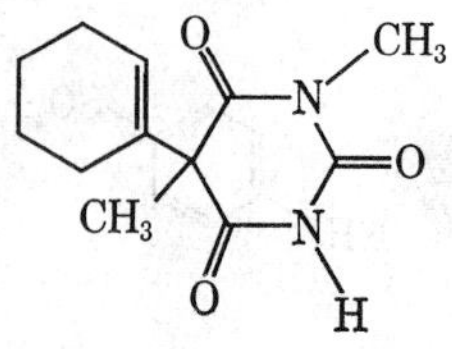

Fig. 335.

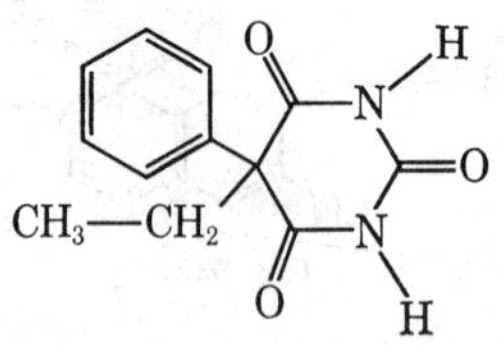

Fig. 336.

Fig. 337.

Fig. 338.

Fig. 339.

Fig. 340.

Ultimately, the medicinal chemist may be able to depict the structure of an as yet unsynthesized molecule, and by making certain *a priori* assumptions, predict both the type and degree of pharmacologic action which the compound will exhibit. There is still a long way to go to attain this goal. In the search for new drugs, the usual approach is to first have in mind some known active compound and then attempt various structural modifications in the hope of either altering or attenuating its known biologic activity. The only alternative to this is a random screening of all organic compounds, across a broad spectrum of possible actions—a monumental and wasteful technique. Molecular modification, too, could verge on the infinite were it not for guidelines which have been established by several generations of investigators.

There are several sources from which we may derive the original structure–activity reference point in our quest for new compounds. Originally, all prototypes came from nature. The adrenergic phenethylamines all derive from ephedrine (Fig. 337), a naturally occurring compound whose use in medicine goes back some 5000 years. Over the years, however, numerous compounds have been synthesized which exhibit some pharmacologic response. Some were developed from biologic sources, others by exploiting secondary effects of known compounds, and still others by pure luck or serendipity. In any event, we now have a considerable supply of compounds and their modifications which can serve to stimulate and direct our efforts to develop improved drugs (see Table I). The following is a brief description of some of the ways in which an active molecule can be modified to alter and improve its action.

Molecular Modification

Isosterism—When two or more molecules have approximately the same size and shape, they are said to be isosteric. Inherent in this definition are certain qualifications which may or may not apply, depending on how the term is used. The molecules should have the same number and type of bonds and they should be isoelectric. Electron density, resonance energy, and dipole moment should also be similar. In Table II are listed some isosteric equivalents which have been utilized by various chemists.

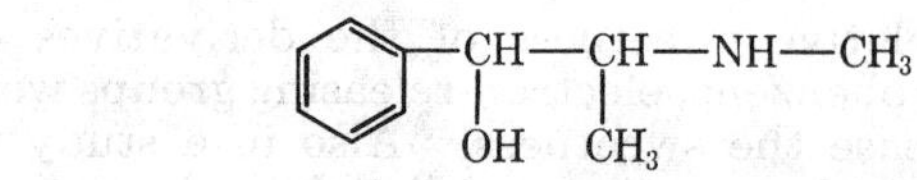

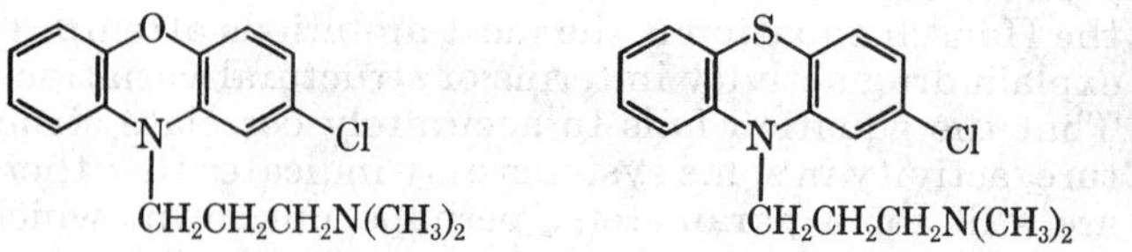

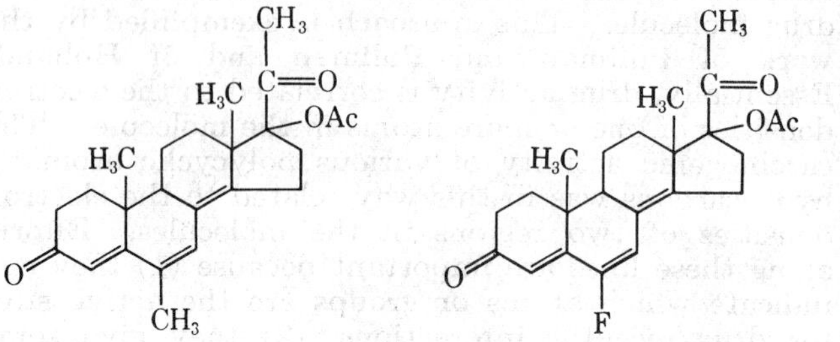

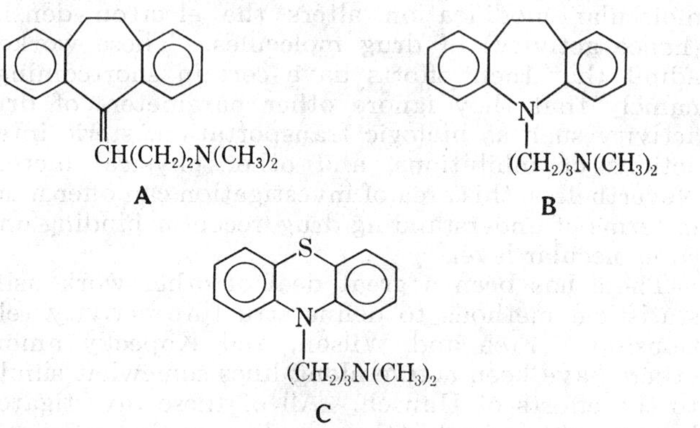

The following are some examples of isosteres. In the first pair of compounds the oxygen isostere (Fig. 338A) of chlorpromazine (Fig. 338B) has only $\frac{1}{10}$ of its tranquilizing activity. In the second pair of compounds the replacement of the CH_3-group in 6-dehydromethylpregnone (Fig. 339A) with a fluorine atom leads to the more active ovulation inhibitor 6-dehydrofluoropregnone (Fig. 339B). A final example of isosteric replacement shows the evolution of amitriptyline (Fig. 340A) from imipramine (Fig.

Table II—Isosteric Equivalents

—N=	to	—CH=					—S—	to	—CH=CH—	to	—CH₂—CH₂—	to	—O—
—O—	to	—NH—	to	—CH₂—			—F	to	—H				
—F	to	—OH	to	—NH₂	to	—CH₃	—N—CH₂—			to			
									—CH=CH—				

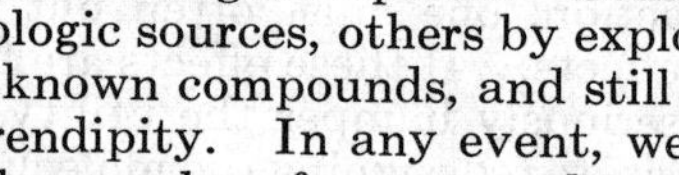

40B) which in turn derived from promazine (Fig. 40C). All three drugs have antidepressant and sedative properties even though the heteroatoms of the original phenothiazine (promazine) have evolved into the nonheterocyclic amitriptyline.

Group Substitution—There are two basic ways to modify a drug using group substitution. The first involves changing the type or position of a substituent, usually attached to a ring portion of a molecule. The second method requires that a basic portion of the molecule be kept constant while the remainder can be modified quite extensively. The synthetic penicillins typify both types of approach. One of the naturally occurring antibiotics is penicillin G (Fig. 333). Chemical studies determined that 6-aminopenicillanic acid (6-APA) (Fig. 341) was the penicillin nucleus and that a variety of synthetic "penicillins" could be synthesized using this nucleus in combination with a variety of carboxyl-containing compounds. Many semisynthetic penicillins were also made by introducing ring-substituted phenylacetamide precursors into the natural fermentation process. By these means the following penicillin varieties have been synthesized (Fig. 342).

In this series the basic penicillin structure has been maintained but a variety of ring substituents have been introduced which by their electronic effects alter both the activity and specificity of the compounds. Another "substituted" penicillin is ampicillin (Fig. 343) where modification involves the introduction of an amino group at the benzyl carbon atom. Synthetic penicillins which are therapeutically useful and those in which the phenylacetyl moiety has been com-

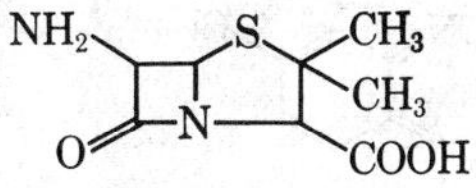

Fig. 345.

Fig. 341.   APA.

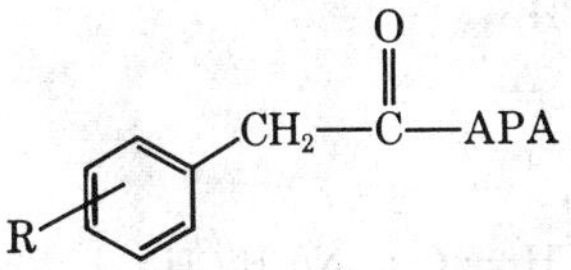

Fig. 342.

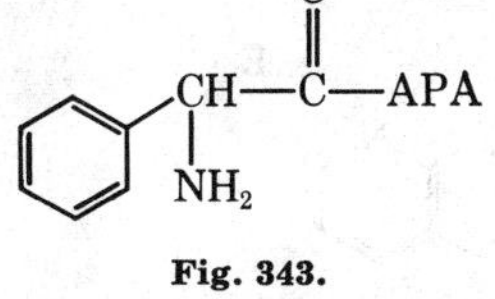

Fig. 343.

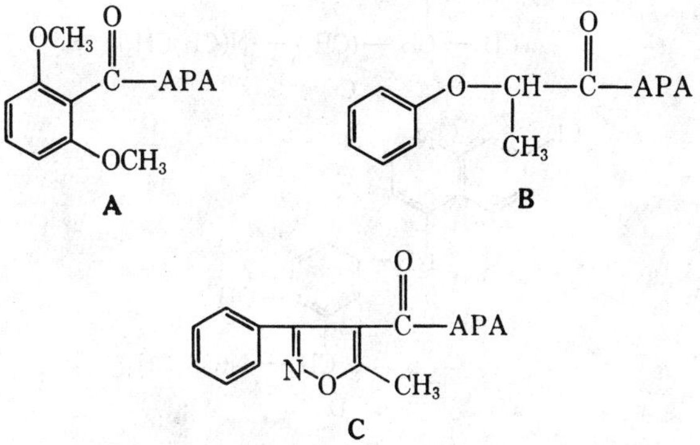

Fig. 344.   A: **methicillin**;   B: D(−)**phenethicillin**;   C: **oxacillin**.

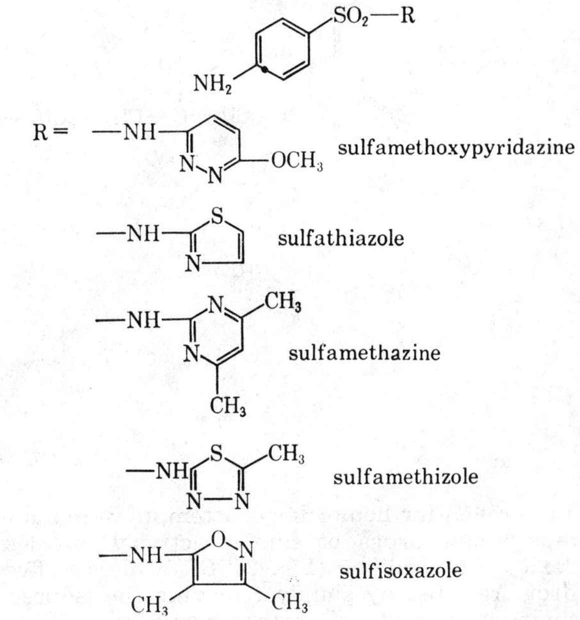

Fig. 346.

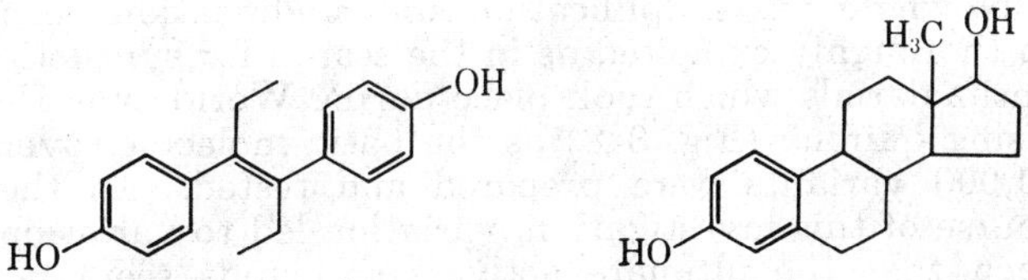

pletely changed are pictured in Fig. 344A, B, and C. These drugs were prepared by acylating 6-APA. The "nucleus" concept of drug modification is also amply demonstrated by the sulfonamides. With these drugs, the parent compound sulfanilamide is also the nucleus and modification is effected by replacement of the NH₂— group by a large variety of heterocyclic amines. Some of the important drugs developed by this technique are shown in Fig. 345. These few compounds illustrate the variety of heterocyclic amines which have been utilized. Literally thousands of modifications of sulfanilamide have been prepared, only a few of which have become important in medicine.

Simplification—Often, when a naturally occurring pharmacodynamic agent has finally had its structure elucidated, the molecule is one of great complexity. Total synthesis or synthetic modifications of the basic molecule may prove difficult or expensive. It is then usually through a long and tedious period of trial and error that the chemist attempts to delineate those portions of the structure which determine the activity and to incorporate them in a less complex molecule. Without a doubt, the most spectacular example of simplification must be diethylstilbestrol (Fig. 346A). This potent estrogen evolved, via a painstaking synthetic excursion, from estradiol (Fig. 346B). Unless the structure of diethylstilbestrol is depicted as shown in Fig. 346A, the simplification is so complete that one could fail to see the similarity which actually exists between the two compounds.

The natural vitamins K are naphthoquinone derivatives bearing a methyl group and a side chain consisting of several isoprene related units (Fig. 347A). When it was shown that these compounds were

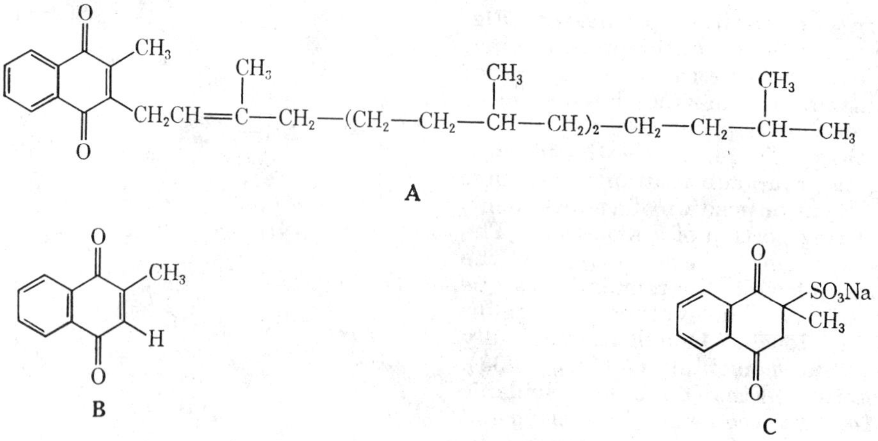

Fig. 347. A: vitamin K₁.

useful in preventing hemorrhage, attempts were made to prepare new drugs of similar activity but less complexity. Menadione (Fig. 347B), a highly effective drug, resulted by simply removing the isoprene side-chain completely. A further modification led to a water-soluble anticoagulant, menadione sodium bisulfite (Fig. 347C).

Nowhere has simplification and modification been so thoroughly exploited as in the search for synthetic antimalarials which took place during World War II. Using quinine (Fig. 348) as the basic molecule, over 14,000 variants were prepared and tested. In the course of this investigation, variation led to variation such that the ultimate active compounds seem remote indeed from the quinuclidine–quinoline composite from which they were derived. Without attempting to describe the synthetic progressions which led to them, the following are representative of the many "quinine inspired" drugs which were developed. (Fig. 349A–D). It is rather discouraging to note that in spite of this vast effort, today still other compounds to combat new drug-resistant malarial parasite strains are being sought.

Isomerism—Molecular modification also can be achieved by preparing compounds which are isomeric with the drug model. These isomers may be of two basic types: positional and steric. Chart I shows examples of some of the different sub-categories of isomers which have been utilized in the search for improved drugs.

Orthoform (Fig. 350A), a local analgetic, led to Orthoform New (Fig. 350B), an isomer whose synthesis proved somewhat easier. In the barbiturate family of drugs, pentobarbital (Fig. 351A) and amobarbital (Fig. 351B) differ only in the type of 5-carbon side-chain which they bear, but the former has a short duration of action while the latter is of intermediate duration. Betaine ester (Fig. 352A) and acetylcholine (Fig. 352B) are isomeric esters with the functional groups reversed. Both are about equal in their cholinergic activity.

Optical isomerism often leads to striking differences in pharmacologic activity. Estradiol (Fig. 346B) exists in two geometric forms. The *beta*-compound has been shown to be far more active than the *alpha*-isomer. When chlorine is added to benzene, nine benzene hexachloride cis/trans isomers (Fig. 353B) can be formed. Only one isomer, the *gamma* form (Fig. 353A), is useful as an insecticide. Since this compound comprises only 10–15% of the reaction product, activity is lessened considerably unless the active isomer is separated. Enantiomerism may produce even more remarkable variations in activity since, to the uninitiated, the isomers are indistinguishable. Chlorpheniramine, a potent antihistamine (Fig. 345) can exist in

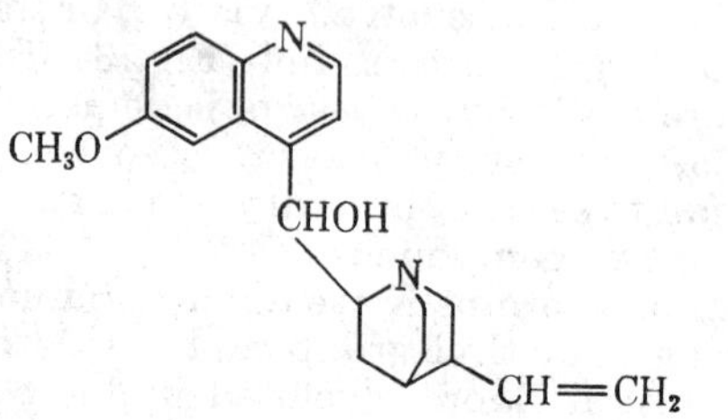

Fig. 348.

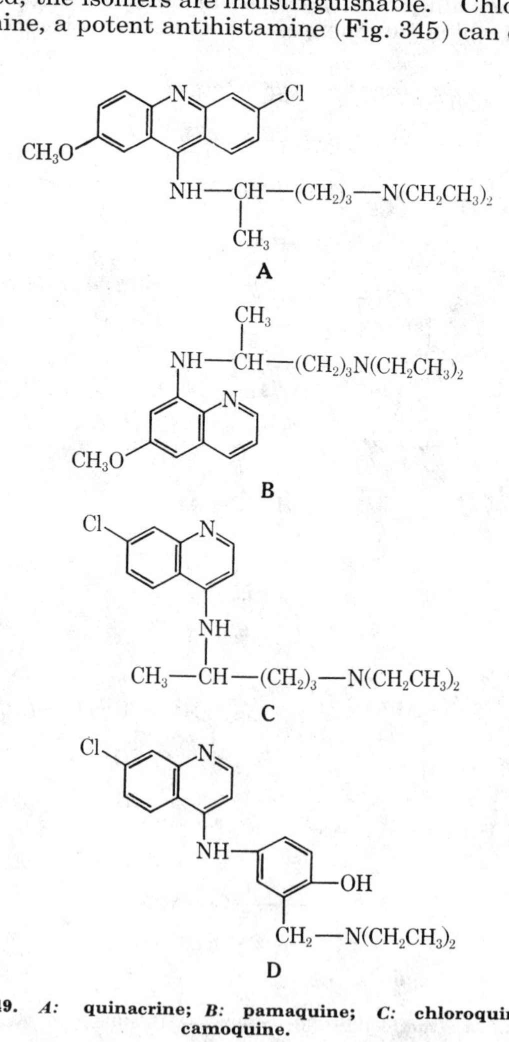

Fig. 349. A: quinacrine; B: pamaquine; C: chloroquine; D: camoquine.

(+) or (−) forms. Tests have shown that the (+)-isomer is more active and exhibits fewer undesirable side effects than its enantiomer. Quinine (Fig. 348) and quinidine are also enantiomers, the latter being dextrorotatory. Here too, mirror image isomerism leads to gross differences in activity. Quinidine finds application as a cardiac suppressant while quinine exhibits a broad spectrum of medicinal uses ranging from antipyretic to anesthetic.

Drug design then applies numerous principles, extensive syntheses, comprehensive pharmacologic testing, and the experience and insight to minimize the

Chart 1—Structural Modification through Isomer Syntheses

A. Positional isomers

1. Position isomers

Fig. 350.

2. Chain isomers

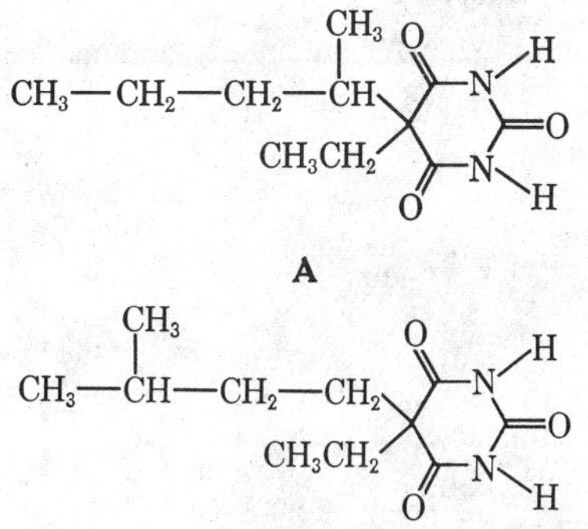

Fig. 351.

3. Functional group isomers

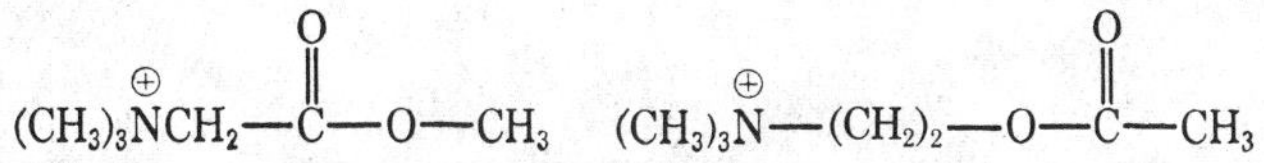

Fig. 352.

B. Stereo isomers

1. Geometric isomers

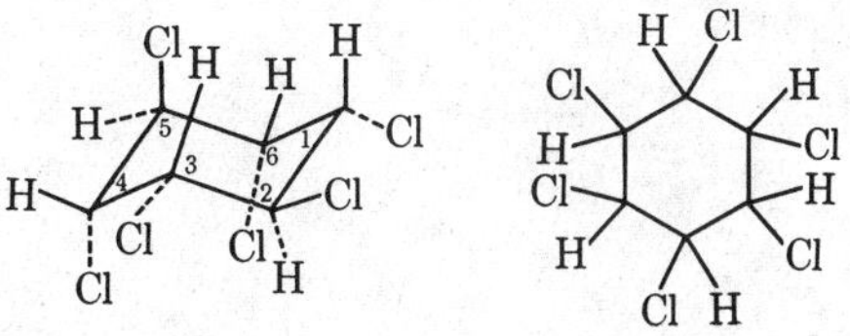

Fig. 353.

2. Enantiomers

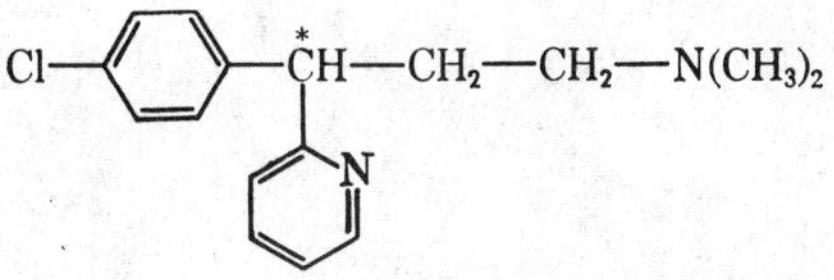

Fig. 354.

* = asymmetric carbon atom

effort required to evolve a new active molecule. It must be remembered, however, that with all of our background experience and theories, new drugs of superior action and specificity are still discovered infrequently. Were it not for the efforts of countless scientists even these drugs might still not be available.

References

1. Burger, A., *J. Chem. Educ.*, **35,** 142 (1958).
2. Wilson, C. O., and Gisvold, O., *Organic Chemistry in Pharmacy*, 5th ed., Lippincott, Philadelphia, 1966.

Bibliography

Holland, W. C., *et al*, *Introduction to Molecular Pharmacology*, Macmillan, New York, 1964.

Binns, T. B., *Absorption and Distribution of Drugs*, Williams & Wilkins, Baltimore, 1964.

Goldstein, A., *et al*, *Principles of Drug Action*, Harper & Rowe, New York 1968.

"Molecular Modification in Drug Design," *Advan. Chem. Ser.*, **45** (1964).

Stuart, D. M., "Drug Metabolism," *Pharm Index*, **10**(9A), 3–8 (1968); *Ibid* **10**(10A), 4–16 (1968).

Gill, E. W., "Drug Receptor Interactions," *Progr. Med. Chem.*, **4,** 39–85 (1965).

Harper, N. J., "Drug Latentiation," *J. Med. Chem.*, **12,** 467–500 (1969).

Mautner, H. G., "The Molecular Basis for Drug Action," *Pharmacol. Rev.* **19,** 107–139 (1967).

Burger, A., *Medicinal Chemistry*, 2nd ed., Interscience, New York, 1960.

Ann. Rev. Pharmacol., **6** (1966).

Schueler, F. W., *Chemobiodynamics and Drug Design*, McGraw-Hill, New York, 1960.

Ariens, E. J., *Physicochemical Aspects of Drug Action*, Pergamon, New York, 1968.

Tolstoouhov, A. V., *Ionic Interpretation of Drug Action in Chemotherapeutic Research*, Chemical Publ. Co., New York, 1955.

Part IV

RADIOISOTOPES in PHARMACY and MEDICINE

EDITOR

Grafton D. Chase, PhD, *Professor of Chemistry,*
Philadelphia College of Pharmacy and Science, Philadelphia, Pa. 19104

33 | Fundamentals of Radioisotopes

Particles and waves—atoms and nuclei—production of radioisotopes—natural radioactivity—radioactive decay—instruments for radiation measurement—techniques of radiation measurement—characterization of radioactive substances—characterization of radiation—x-rays

This chapter was prepared by

Grafton D. Chase, PhD, *Professor of Chemistry, Philadelphia College of Pharmacy and Science, Philadelphia, Pa. 19104*

For years the alchemist sought the secret of *transmutation* without success. Today this nuclear process, which converts one element into another, is commonplace. Yet, our knowledge of nuclear processes is of recent origin. It was not until 1896 that Becquerel observed the fogging of his photographic plates by a uranium salt. His observation aroused the curiosity of the Curies concerning the uranium ore, pitchblende, from which they isolated the elements polonium and radium. Research in the next few years by the Curies, Becquerel, Schmidt, Debierne, and others soon resulted in the discovery and isolation of still other new elements from uranium and thorium ores. These elements, too, were found to fog photographic plates.

It was known that the fogging of photographic plates was caused by some sort of radiation. By 1899 Rutherford concluded that this radiation was of two types, which he called *alpha* and *beta*. The next year P. Curie and Villard observed a third, very penetrating, type of radiation which was called *gamma*. The *theory of radioactive disintegration* was proposed by Rutherford and Soddy in 1903. They suggested that atoms of radioactive elements undergo spontaneous emission of alpha and beta particles with the formation of atoms of a new element. These deductions, which today we know to be correct, were amazing when one considers the status of atomic knowledge of that day. The *electron*, later found to be physically identical with the beta particle, had been discovered by J. J. Thomson in 1897, but the alpha particle was not identified as a positively charged helium nucleus until 1909. That Rutherford and Royds should identify the alpha particle as a helium nucleus in 1909 is also remarkable, for it was not until 1911 that Rutherford performed his famous experiment which enabled him to propose the

nuclear theory, *viz*, that the positive charge of an atom is concentrated in a centrally located *nucleus* rather than being interspersed with the negatively charged electrons. Two years later Bohr published his theory of atomic structure, based upon Rutherford's nuclear theory and the quantum theory of Max Planck. The same year (1913) Soddy proposed the name *isotope* (*Greek*, same place), for Aston had just separated two isotopes of neon by fractional diffusion in confirmation of J. J. Thomson's discovery of these two forms of neon in 1912.

Rutherford was unquestionably the foremost nuclear scientist of his time. It was he who also observed the first *artificial transmutation* in 1919. This he achieved by bombarding nitrogen with alpha particles, the nitrogen being converted into an isotope of oxygen with a mass of 17. It is regrettable that he should have died in 1937 believing that nuclear power would never be achieved, because it was achieved only five year later when Fermi built the first nuclear reactor in Chicago.

Constructive research on the nucleus of the atom has not only resulted in the means to harness this tremendous power for the production of electricity and other forms of useful energy but has also provided scientists with more than 1300 different species of atoms. These find innumerable applications in industry, medicine, pharmacy, agriculture, and all other fields and disciplines where the atom is used for the benefit of mankind.

Particles and Waves

Elementary Particles—Electrons, protons, and neutrons constitute the basic building blocks of atoms, both stable and radioactive atoms. The *electron* is the smallest of these three particles. Its mass, m_e, is 9.1091×10^{-28} Gm. For simplicity, the mass of the electron, m_e, is used as a unit of mass. Thus, the mass of the proton is $1836\ m_e$ and that of the neutron is $1838\ m_e$. Also, for simplicity, the electron is assigned a charge of -1. Thus the charge of the proton is $+1$ and that of the neutron is zero. Although the mass and charge of each of these particles are known with a high degree of accuracy, the size of each is known only approximately. It is in the order of 10^{-13} cm. Size, when applied to such small objects, does not have the customary significance because of inherent uncertainties introduced by the very nature of the measurement to determine size.

The *neutrino* is a very unusual particle. Its existence was suggested by Pauli in 1934 and was confirmed by experiment in 1957. It has zero charge and,

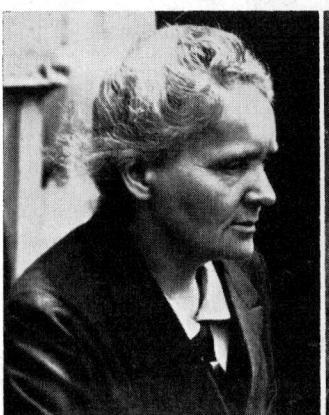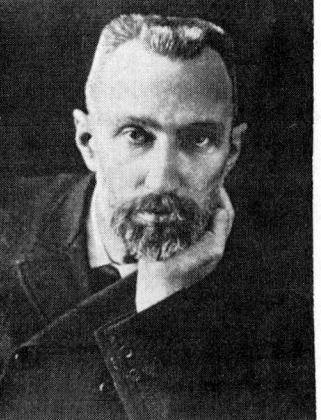

Fig. 355. Madame and Pierre Curie.

Table I—Particles of Nature

Particle	Symbol	Charge	Mass[a]
Negatron (Negative beta)	e^- (β^-)	-1	1
Positron (Positive beta)	e^+ (β^+)	$+1$	1
Proton	p	$+1$	1836
Neutron	n	0	1837
Alpha	α	$+2$	7346
Neutrino	ν	0	0
Gamma ray[b] (a photon)	γ	0	0

[a] Mass is expressed in electron masses.
[b] Although gamma rays are electromagnetic radiation, they do possess particulate properties.

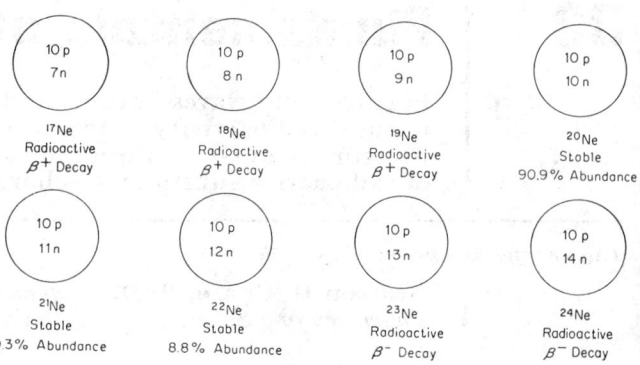

Fig. 357.   Isotopes of neon.

if it has any mass at all, its mass is less than 1/1000 that of the electron. Yet, this particle plays a very important role in beta decay (see page 537).

Particles with mass equal to or less than that of the electron are called *leptons*. Leptons include the electron, positron, and neutrino. Particles found within the nucleus are known as *nucleons* and include the proton and neutron. *Mesons* are those particles with mass greater than that of a lepton but less than that of a nucleon. *Hyperons* have a mass greater than the nucleons. Although mesons and hyperons play an important role in nuclear science, a detailed knowledge of these particles is not essential to an understanding of other topics in this chapter.

Radiation from Radioactive Nuclei—Three types of radiation are most frequently emitted from radioactive nuclei. These are alpha, beta, and gamma radiations.

Alpha particles, which constitute alpha radiation, are compound particles consisting of two protons and two neutrons. Thus, the alpha particle is identical with the helium nucleus; that is, a helium atom less two electrons. As an alpha particle loses energy, its velocity decreases. It then attracts electrons to its *K-shell* and becomes an ordinary helium atom. The *range* of alpha particles in air is about 5 cm, and less than 100 microns in tissue.

Beta radiation is of two types because there are two kinds of electrons, the *negative electron*, or *negatron*, which has been discussed previously, and the *positive electron*, or *positron*. The positron is identical with the negatron in all respects except for its charge of +1 instead of −1. The positron is also known as the *antiparticle* of the electron. When these electrons are emitted from radioactive nuclei, they are called *beta particles*. Thus, the two particles β^- and β^+ are the same as e^- and e^+, respectively, except for their origin. Beta particles may have a range of over 10 feet in air and up to about 1 mm in tissue.

Gamma radiation is basically different from alpha and beta radiation. Gamma radiation is electromagnetic, whereas alpha and beta radiation is particulate. Gamma rays are radiated as photons or quanta of energy at a velocity, c, of 3.0×10^{10} cm/sec. Gamma radiation differs from x-rays, ultraviolet rays, visible light, etc., only in wave length (or frequency), as illustrated in Fig. 356. Gamma rays are the most pene-

trating of all types of radiation emitted by radioisotopes (except neutrinos) and can easily pass through more than a foot of tissue or several inches of lead.

Atoms and Nuclei

Atomic Structure—A neutral atom consists of a positively charged nucleus (composed of protons and neutrons) with which are associated orbital electrons. The number of orbital electrons is equal to the number of protons in the nucleus, and the number of protons in the nucleus defines the *atomic number*, Z. The *neutron number*, N, is the number of neutrons in the nucleus, and the *mass number*, A, is equal to the sum of the protons and neutrons. Thus, A = Z + N.

The radius of an atom is approximately 10^{-8} cm or 1 Ångstrom unit. The nucleus is roughly 1/100,000 the size of the atom. For example, the radius of the oxygen nucleus is about 3×10^{-13} cm, and that of the lead nucleus is about 7×10^{-13} cm. To gain some appreciation of the smallness of the nucleus, let us suppose that the oxygen nucleus is magnified until it appears to be the size of a golf ball. The golf ball, similarly magnified, would appear to have a diameter of about 100 million miles, or roughly the distance from the earth to the sun.

Atoms are quite "empty." The nucleus and orbital electrons occupy but a very small fraction of space in matter. Further, most of the mass of matter is concentrated in the nucleus, which has a density of 2.4×10^{14} Gm/cc. Thus 1 cc of the substance of which nuclei are made would weigh over 200 million tons. It is with this very unusual material of the nucleus that we are concerned in nuclear reactions and radioactivity.

Nuclides and Isotopes—In 1912 J. J. Thomson developed an analytical process known as "positive ray analysis" by which he could measure the mass of particles such as atoms. When he attempted to determine the mass of the neon atom, two lines appeared on the screen of his apparatus, indicating two types of neon atoms with masses of 20 and 22, respectively. Thus, by means of a process which was the forerunner of mass spectrometry, Thomson demonstrated the existence of nuclei possessing the same number of protons (and, hence, of the same chemical element) but a different number of neutrons (and, hence, of different mass). Soddy later called these *isotopes*.

The atomic number, Z, of neon is 10. From the relationship A = Z + N, we can deduce that the difference between these two forms of neon lies in the number of neutrons, N, in the nucleus.

$$A = 20 = 10 + N \qquad \therefore N = 10$$
$$A = 22 = 10 + N \qquad \therefore N = 12$$

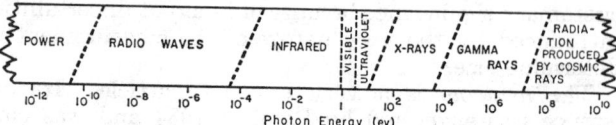

Fig. 356.   Electromagnetic spectrum.

Today at least eight isotopes of neon are known. These are illustrated in Fig. 357.

Isotopes are species of *nuclides* which possess the same number of protons but a different number of neutrons. That is, isotopes are nuclides of the same chemical element and, therefore, have the same chemical properties but differ in mass. They may also differ in stability. Certain mass numbers may represent stable nuclei, whereas other mass numbers may represent radioactive nuclei. A *nuclide* is any one of the more than 1390 known species of atoms characterized by the number of protons and the number of neutrons in the nucleus. Nuclides which have the same mass are called *isobars*. Nuclides which possess the same number of neutrons are called *isotones*. Consider the nuclides illustrated in Fig. 358, ^{1}H, ^{2}H (deuterium), and ^{3}H (tritium) are isotopes; ^{3}He and ^{4}He are isotopes also. On the other hand, ^{3}H and ^{3}He are isobars, and ^{3}H and ^{4}He are isotones.

Nuclear Equations—The nuclear equation expressing the first artificial transmutation observed by Rutherford is expressed by the notation:

$$^{14}_{7}N + ^{4}_{2}He \rightarrow ^{1}_{1}H + ^{17}_{8}O$$

In this reaction, nitrogen of mass 14 is bombarded with a helium nucleus of mass 4 (ie, an alpha particle) to produce oxygen of mass 17 and a proton. In writing the symbol for a nuclide, the atomic number is written as a subscript preceding the symbol for the

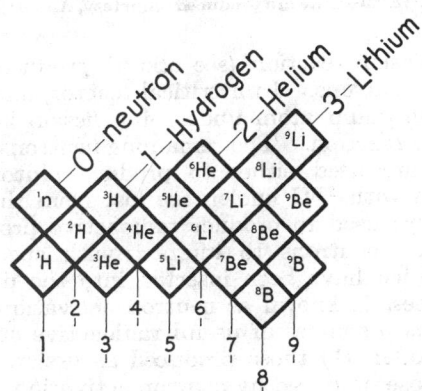

Fig. 358.   Chart of nuclides-to mass number 9.

element, and the mass number is written as a superscript. Thus the symbol $^{14}_{7}N$ describes the nitrogen nucleus whose atomic number, Z, is 7 and whose mass, A, is 14.

It will be noted that nuclear equations must balance. Thus, the sum of the masses on the left (14 + 4 = 18) must equal the sum of the masses on the right (1 + 17 = 18). Also, the sum of the atomic numbers on the left (7 + 2 = 9) must equal the sum of the atomic numbers on the right (1 + 8 = 9). This same reaction may also be represented by a "short-hand" notation.

$$^{14}N(\alpha, p)^{17}O$$

Nuclear Reactions—Nuclear reactions may be either spontaneous or induced. An element which undergoes a spontaneous nuclear reaction is said to be *radioactive*. Such elements are radioactive because the configuration of protons and neutrons in the nucleus produces an unstable structure. During the process of spontaneous decay the ratio of neutrons to protons changes. After one or more decay processes a stable nucleus is formed.

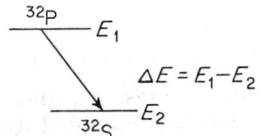

Fig. 359.   Energy-level diagram for decay of phosphorus-32.

Alpha decay is illustrated by the decay of polonium-210 to lead-206:

$$^{210}_{84}Po \rightarrow ^{4}_{2}He + ^{206}_{82}Pb$$

In this example, the nucleus of lead-206, which contains 82 protons and 124 neutrons is stable and does not undergo further decay. The majority of nuclides which undergo alpha decay have atomic numbers greater than 82.

Beta decay is illustrated by the decay of phosphorus-32 to sulfur-32:

$$^{32}_{15}P \rightarrow ^{32}_{16}S + \beta^{-} + \nu$$

Note that the atomic number of the *daughter*, sulfur-32, is greater than that of the *parent*, phosphorus-32. In this process a new proton has been produced, but because there is no change in the mass number, a neutron has been lost. This is explained by the *particle reaction*,

$$^{1}_{0}n \rightarrow ^{1}_{1}p + e^{-} + \nu$$

which shows the decay of a neutron into a proton, a negative electron, and a neutrino. Note also the change in the ratio of neutrons to protons as the phosphorus-32 decays to stable sulfur-32.

The beta particles emitted during the decay of a given radioactive species do not all possess the same energy but are emitted with a continuous energy distribution extending from zero to a specific maximum value, E_{max}. That this should be, posed an enigma for some time. The decay of phosphorus-32 of energy E_1 to sulfur-32 of energy E_2 should be associated with the release of energy equal to ΔE, where $\Delta E = E_1 - E_2$ (Fig. 359). A new particle, the *neutrino*, was postulated to explain the energy change not associated with the beta particle. Thus, the sum of the energies of the beta particle and its associated neutrino is equal to ΔE or E_{max} (Fig. 360).

If the ratio of neutrons to protons is too *low* for stability, a nucleus may decay by *positron emission* (ie, *positron decay*):

$$^{11}_{6}C \rightarrow ^{11}_{5}B + \beta^{+} + \nu$$

In this instance the particle reaction which illustrates

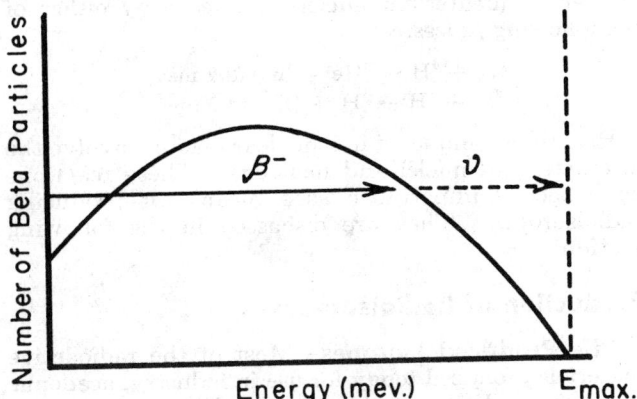

Fig. 360.   Typical beta spectrum.

the change is

$$_1^1p \rightarrow _0^1n + e^+ + \nu$$

Again no change in mass number occurs, but the decay of ^{11}C to ^{11}B is accompanied by the change of a proton into a neutron. The energies of the positrons extend from zero to E_{max} in a manner similar to the energy distribution of negative beta particles. Again the neutrino is required to account for the balance of the energy.

If insufficient energy is available for positron emission, the neutron–proton ratio is sometimes increased to a stable condition by a process known as *electron capture*. In this process, an orbital electron is captured by the nucleus. An example is the decay of ^7Be to ^7Li:

$$_4^7Be + e^-(K) \rightarrow _3^7Li$$

The corresponding particle reaction is

$$e^- + _1^1p \rightarrow _0^1n$$

Electron capture has also been called *K-capture* because the electron captured in the process is usually from the K shell. However, the electron may come from the L or M shell instead.

Fission is a radioactive process in which a relatively heavy nucleus splits into two new nuclei of nearly equal size with the simultaneous emission of two or three neutrons. Fission may be spontaneous, but normally the reaction is induced by bombardment of the parent nucleus with a neutron,

$$^{235}U + _0^1n \rightarrow X + Y + 2.5\ n$$

where X and Y are fission products (new nuclei) with a value of Z between about 30 and 65. Fission reactions may be self-sustaining. For each neutron consumed, an average of 2.5 new neutrons are produced which may initiate the fission of other nuclei. Such a reaction is called a *chain reaction*. If at least one of the 2.5 neutrons produced is used to sustain the reaction, the reaction is said to be *critical*. This is the reaction which occurs in the uranium bomb, as well as in the *atomic reactor*.

Fusion results when two light nuclei are caused to collide with sufficient energy. This energy must be supplied by high temperatures, ie, millions of degrees. To date such reactions have not been sustained for more than a fraction of a second. When controlled fusion reactions become a reality, the world will be assured of an ample supply of power for many thousands of years. The energy theoretically available from the deuterium found in ordinary water is 150 times greater than would result from burning an equal volume of oil. Deuterons (deuterium nuclei) can react by either of the following processes:

$$_1^2H + _1^2H \rightarrow _2^3He + _0^1n \quad (3.2\ mev)$$
$$_1^2H + _1^2H \rightarrow _1^3H + _1^1H \quad (4.0\ mev)$$

Reactions conducted in a nuclear reactor involve the interaction of nuclei and neutrons. These reactions have special importance as a means for producing radioisotopes. They are discussed in the following section.

Production of Radioisotopes

Pile-Produced Isotopes—Most of the radioactive materials produced today for use in industry, academic research, medicine, etc, are prepared in a nuclear pile (nuclear reactor). See Fig. 361. In the reactor the

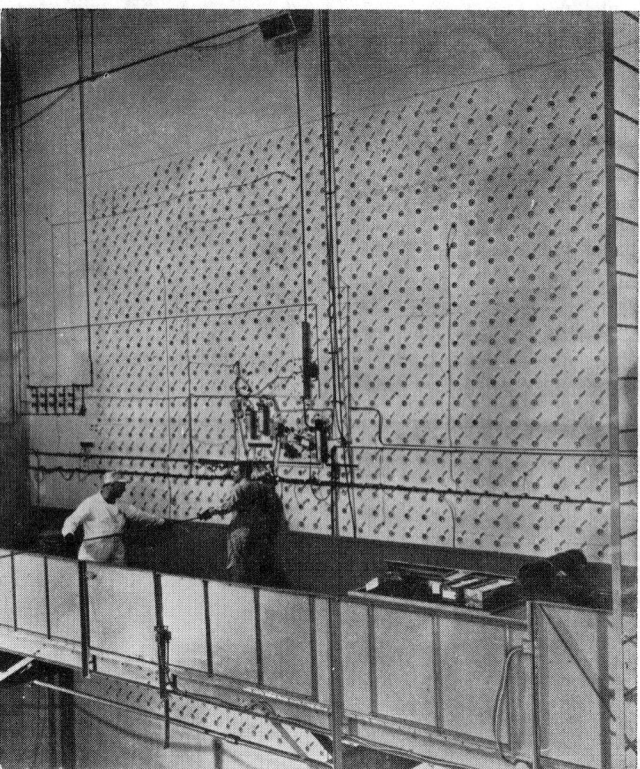

Fig. 361. Oak Ridge nuclear reactor in which most of the radioisotopes used in medicine are produced (courtesy, Abbott).

uranium fission reaction (see above) produces a large supply of neutrons. In a critical reactor, one neutron for each uranium atom undergoing fission is used to sustain the reaction. The remaining neutrons (one and one-half) are used either to produce plutonium by interaction with ^{238}U nuclei, are lost from the critical mass, or are used to produce radioactive products by causing the neutrons to interact with specific substances which have been inserted into the pile. The latter process is known as neutron activation. Thus, there are two sources of useful radioactive substances from the pile: (1) those produced as fission products and (2) those produced by neutron activation.

The following reactions illustrate but one of many combinations of fission reactions which are possible.

$$_{92}^{238}U + _0^1n \rightarrow _{50}^{131}Sn + _{42}^{106}Mo + _0^1n + _0^1n$$

The ^{131}Sn and the ^{106}Mo are very radioactive and have very short half-lives. They immediately decay by a series of beta decay processes:

$$_{50}^{131}Sn \rightarrow _{51}^{131}Sb \rightarrow _{52}^{131}Te \rightarrow _{53}^{131}I$$
$$_{42}^{106}Mo \rightarrow _{43}^{106}Tc \rightarrow _{44}^{106}Ru \rightarrow _{45}^{106}Rh$$

Both ^{131}I and ^{106}Ru are available commercially as fission-produced isotopes. Before use, however, they must be separated chemically from a large number of other fission-produced radioisotopes. For many of the isotopes produced by fission, separation is too difficult or costly; thus, the majority of radioactive compounds are prepared by neutron activation.

Neutron activation may result either from simple neutron capture or from a transmutation process. For example, radioactive phosphorus (^{32}P) can be prepared from stable phosphorus (^{31}P) by *neutron capture*:

$$_{15}^{31}P + _0^1n \rightarrow _{15}^{32}P + \gamma$$

The disadvantage of this method is that the radio-

Table II—Radioisotope Generators

Parent isotope	Half-life		Daughter isotope	Half-life		Mode of decay
^{68}Ge	250	d	^{68}Ga	68	m	β^+
^{87}Y	80	h	^{87m}Sr	2.8	h	I.T.
^{90}Sr	28	y	^{90}Y	64	h	β^-
^{99}Mo	67	h	^{99m}Tc	6.0	h	I.T.
^{113}Sn	118	d	^{113m}In	1.7	h	I.T.
^{132}Te	3.2	d	^{132}I	2.3	h	β^-
^{137}Cs	30	y	^{137m}Ba	2.6	m	I.T.
^{144}Ce	285	d	^{144}Pr	17.3	m	β^-

active phosphorus (^{32}P) is highly diluted with stable ^{31}P. ^{32}P of low specific activity can be used for certain purposes, such as the investigation of phosphate fertilizers, but would be less useful for many biological and medical applications.

Radioactive phosphorus can be made by *transmutation* if high specific activities are required.

$$^{32}_{16}S + ^1_0n \rightarrow ^{32}_{15}P + ^1_1p$$

In this case the radioactive phosphorus can be separated from the unreacted sulfur by chemical procedures. Where ^{32}P is made from ^{31}P such chemical separations are not practical. Transmutation is useful for the preparation of many radioactive nuclides, especially those of low atomic number. As the atomic number increases, "n,γ" reactions are favored over "n,p" reactions. Thus, cobalt-60 is produced by the reaction ^{59}Co(n,γ)^{60}Co because the reaction ^{60}Ni(n,p) ^{60}Co does not occur with sufficient frequency to make the process commercially feasible.

Cyclotron-Produced Isotopes—Certain radioisotopes are cyclotron-produced. The cyclotron and similar *particle accelerators* can be used only with charged particles such as electrons, protons, deuterons, etc. because the operation of such machines depends upon the interaction of magnetic and/or electrostatic fields with the charge (either + or −) of the particle undergoing acceleration. When the particles have been accelerated to a high velocity, even approaching the velocity of light and representing enormous energies, they are caused to strike a target containing the atoms to be bombarded. Sodium-22 is prepared in this way by the interaction of high-velocity deuterons with magnesium. The nuclear equation is

$$^{24}Mg(d,\alpha)^{22}Na$$

Radioisotope Generators—Where clinical tests require that a radioisotope be administered internally, it is advantageous to use an isotope with a short half-life to minimize the radiation dose received by the patient. But it is evident that the shorter the half-life, the greater will be the problem of supply. One answer to this problem is the *radioisotope generator* or *"radioisotopic cow."* A radioisotope generator or cow is an ion-exchange column containing a resin or alumina upon which has been absorbed a long-lived parent nuclide. Radioactive decay of the long-lived parent results in the production of a short-lived radioactive daughter nuclide which is eluted or "milked" from the column by means of an appropriate eluant. Characteristics of a number of parent–daughter systems which have been used in radioisotope generators will be found in Table II.

Natural Radioactivity

If it were not for the naturally occurring radioisotopes, there would be no artificially produced isotopes except those produced in the cyclotron and other particle accelerators, for without naturally occurring radioisotopes, there could be no atomic reactor. The natural radioisotopes include all elements with an atomic number greater than 83, several with atomic numbers of 81 to 83 (isotopes of thallium, lead, and bismuth) and a few isotopes of the lighter elements with atomic numbers less than 81 (^{3}H, ^{14}C, ^{40}K, ^{87}Rb, ^{115}In, ^{138}La, ^{144}Nd, ^{147}Sm, ^{176}Lu, ^{187}Re, and ^{190}Pt).

Some of the heavier radioactive elements disintegrate in a definite known sequence until stable nuclear configurations are achieved. Four such sequences or radioactive series have been established, of which the uranium (or uranium-radium) series is the best known. It commences with uranium-238, passes through a

Table III—Uranium Disintegration Series

Old Name	Element	Atomic Wt.	Atomic No.	Radiation[a]	Range, cm in air of α	Energy in mev	Half-life
Uranium I	Uranium	238	92	α(e$^-$, γ)	2.7	4.2	4.51×10^9 years
Uranium X$_1$	Thorium	234	90	(β)γ	...	0.10	24.1 days
Uranium X$_2$	Protoactinium	234	91	...	...	1.3	1.18 min
Uranium II	Protoactinium	234	91	α(e$^-$, γ)	3.3	4.7	2.48×10^5 years
Ionium	Thorium	230	90	α(e$^-$, γ)	3.2	4.6	7.6×10^4 years
Radium	Radium	226	88	α(γ)	3.4	4.8	1620 years
Radon	Radon	222	86	α	4.2	5.5	3.82 days
Radium A	Polonium	218	84	α(β)	4.7	6.0	3.05 min
Radium B	Lead	214	82	β(γ)	...	0.6	26.8 min
Radium C	Bismuth	214	83	β(γ)	...	1.65	19.7 min
Radium C'	Polonium	214	84	α	7.0	7.7	1.6×10^{-4} sec
Radium C''	Thallium	210	81	β	...	1.8	1.32 min
Radium D	Lead	210	82	β	...	0.023	22 years
Radium E	Bismuth	210	83	β	...	1.17	5.0 days
Radium F	Polonium	210	84	α(γ)	4.0	5.4	138 days
Radium G	Lead	206	82	Inactive	...	...	Stable

[a] e: internal-conversion electrons.

series of decay processes ending with stable radium G (lead-206). Table III shows the uranium series. The mass of each member of this series is given by the expression $4n + 2$ in which n is a whole number. Thus, this relation serves to characterize the uranium-238 series. The actinium series, which has uranium-235 as the parent nuclide, is characterized by the relation $4n + 3$, and the thorium series, which begins with thorium-232 and ends with lead-208, by $4n$. The last series to be discovered, the $4n + 1$ series, is unique in that its members are artificially radioactive. Its initial member is the synthetic element curium-241.

Radium—Ra = 226.02 (At. no. 88)

History and Occurrence—The word Radium is from the Latin *radius* which means *ray*. The name is appropriate to the active emanations from this element. Radium was first obtained in 1911 by Mme. Curie and Debierne by electrolysis of a solution of radium chloride.

A salt of radium had been isolated 13 years earlier by M. and Mme. Curie in 1898 from the ore pitchblende, obtained from North Bohemia. This was an extension of work instituted by Henri Becquerel in 1896. The latter worker, a Frenchman, is credited with the discovery of radioactivity as a result of his work with uranium potassium sulfate which he found to produce blackening of a photographic plate. From several tons of pitchblende Madame Curie extracted a material possessing considerably more activity than uranium. This substance she named *Polonium*, after her native country Poland. During December, 1898, she finally isolated radium from the same ore. Weight for weight it was found to be approximately two million times more active than uranium.

Today radium is produced primarily from *carnotite* and *pitchblende*. These ores are found chiefly in the Belgian Congo, and in the Great Bear Lake region of Canada. Until 1925 most of the world supply of radium was obtained from the mineral carnotite, which was mined in Colorado and Utah. The cost of one gram of radium at that time was about $100,000. The Belgian Congo deposits were discovered in that year, however, and product costs were lowered soon thereafter. However, even as late as 1954 the price remained $20,000 per Gm (1 Gm = 1 curie). The current price of cobalt-60 producing an equivalent amount of radiation is approximately $2 plus handling charges. For this very obvious reason, radium has in many ways been supplanted by artificially produced radioactive substances. See previous sections of this chapter.

Description—A bright, white metal which immediately darkens upon exposure to the air. Its physical constants are given on page 539. It has a valence of 2. Its half-life is 1620 years. 1 Gm of radium produces 1×10^{-4} ml of radon per day. Radium salts color a flame a carmine-red.

Uses—Radium is marketed commercially as the bromide. One of its chief industrial uses has been in the production of luminous paints, used extensively in painting instrument dials. The use of such paints on the dials of wrist watches and clocks for domestic use is subject to criticism as a needless source of additional radiation for the human race.

It has enjoyed wide popularity in the medical field as a source of radiation in treating cancer. It is generally used in the form of radium needles for vaginal application in treatment of cancer of the cervix, and to a lesser degree in the treatment of certain malignant lesions of the oral cavity.

A radioactive gas called *radon* is continuously discharged from radium and can be collected and sealed in small tubes of glass. These are popularly known as *radon seeds* and, though not used nearly as extensively with the advent of more convenient and accurately controlled methods employing artificially radioactive substances, they may be implanted directly in cancer tissue which is not surgically removable. Radon is chemically an inert gas related to xenon, neon, argon, etc., and has a short half-life of only 3.8 days. Hence, seeds so implanted in tissue cease to emit gamma radiation after a relatively short period, decaying to lead-210 with a 22-year half-life. Although the lead-210 (Radium D) and its daughters are radioactive, they emit principally beta and alpha radiation.

When radium *needles* are used, care must be taken to remove them after the proper dose has been administered. Further, care must be exercised with radium because of the ease with which it is taken up by the circulation and deposited in bone (being in the calcium group, the metabolism is similar thereto). This could have disastrous consequences, as shown by the production of osteogenic sarcomas and anemias in watch dial factory workers who have been poisoned by moistening radium-contaminated paint brushes with their tongues. It is interesting that radiation which has the property to *destroy* certain cancers is also capable of *causing* similar growths.

Caution—Radium is an extremely hazardous material and must be handled only by properly protected and adequately trained personnel.

Unofficial Inorganic Radium Compounds and Ores

Carnotite, Potassium Uranovanadate [$K_2O.2U_2O_3.V_2O_5.3H_2O$].

Pitchblende, Uraninite [$UO_3.UO_2$, PbO, etc]—is a complex, variable uranate of lead, thorium and certain rare earths.

Radium Bromide [$RaBr_2$]—The commercial salt is usually mixed with barium bromide. White or slightly brownish crystals. *Uses:* see *Radium* above.

Radium Chloride [$RaCl_2$]—The commercial salt is usually mixed with barium chloride. White or slightly brownish crystals. *Uses:* see *Radium* above.

Radium Nitrate [$Ra(NO_3)_2$]—Crystals. Soluble 13.9 Gm per 100 ml of water at 20°. *Uses:* see *Radium* above.

Radium Sulfate [$RaSO_4$]—White powder, usually mixed with barium sulfate. Less soluble in water and acids than barium sulfate. *Uses:* see *Radium* above.

Thorium—Th = 232.04 (At. no. 90)

History and Occurrence—The name *thorium* was given this element by its discoverer, Berzelius, in honor of the ancient Scandinavian god *Thor*. It occurs in the minerals *thorite* [$ThSiO_4$] and *thorianite*, which contains about 70% of ThO_2 and about 10% of uranium dioxide. Its principal source in the United States is *monazite sand* in which it occurs as phosphate to the extent of 3 to 9%.

Description—A white to grayish white metal, having a specific gravity of 11.2 and melting at 1845°. It is scarcely attacked by hydrochloric or nitric acids but is dissolved by nitrohydrochloric acid and converted to sulfate by heating with sulfuric acid.

Thorium is radioactive, yielding a number of disintegration products, the most important of which is *mesothorium*. Due to the fact that thorium has such a high atomic number (90) its insoluble compounds, particularly the oxide or hydroxide, are good absorbers of X-rays. For this reason suspensions of thorium compounds were used to diagnose diseases of the renal pelvis and the urinary tract.

Thorium is tetravalent and its oxide [ThO_2] occurs as the mineral *thoria*. It was used orally or rectally as a contrast medium in roentgenography, and is a constituent in the electron-emitting elements of radio tubes. It was formerly an important constituent of incandescent gas mantles.

Thorium has many properties in common with the alkaline earths as well as the iron–aluminum group. With potassium sulfate it forms a *thorium alum* which is only very slightly soluble in water.

Uses—All thorium compounds are extremely hazardous if used internally, if not from their chemical toxicity, certainly from the radiation which is emitted. Thorium compounds are retained by the body almost indefinitely. Coupled with the long half-life of thorium, a serious radiation hazard results. Of particular note, thorium dioxide has been employed as a contrast medium in roentgenography, especially for the visualization of blood vessels. It was injected intravenously and produced few immediate toxic effects. However, this agent was retained in the body. Fibrosis of the liver, kidney, spleen, and lymph nodes has been attributed to its persistent radioactivity. The element is now important as a source of fissionable material. Neutron bombardment of thorium-232 yields the fissionable isotope, uranium-233.

Unofficial Inorganic Thorium Compounds

Thorium Chloride [$ThCl_4$]—White crystals. Soluble in water or alcohol.

Thorium Nitrate [$Th(NO_3)_4$]—White crystals soluble in water. Used as a reagent in the determination of fluorine.

Thorium Oxide, Thorium Dioxide [ThO_2]—This is the most important thorium compound. It is a white, heavy, infusible crystalline powder. When heated it is incandescent. Specific gravity, 9.7. *Uses:* Formerly used in incandescent gas mantles and as a contrast medium in roentgenography.

Thorium Sulfate [$Th(SO_4)_2.xH_2O$]—Colorless or white crystals. Soluble in about 70 parts cold water and 15 parts hot water; insoluble in alcohol.

Uranium—U = 238.03 (At. no. 92)

History and Occurrence—*Uranium* was named by its discoverer, Klaproth, in 1789, in honor of the planet *Uranus*. It was first isolated in an elemental state by Peligot, in 1841. The principal sources of uranium and its compounds are the minerals *uranite* and *pitchblende*, found in Czechoslovakia, and *carnotite*, which is potassium uranovanadate. Radioactivity was discovered in 1891 by Becquerel when he observed that uranium salts affected a photographic plate just as X-rays did. In 1898 and 1899 Madame Curie and her husband, Professor Curie, showed that these properties were not due to the presence of uranium but to another substance to which they gave the name radium.

Description—A silvery white and fairly hard metal, but not as hard as steel. Its specific gravity is 18.7, it melts at about 1850°, and it is soluble in the strong mineral acids.

It has two valences, IV and VI, and forms two oxides, the dioxide [UO_2] and the trioxide [UO_3]. The salts derived from tetravalent uranium are termed *uranous;* those containing hexavalent uranium are usually basic salts containing the divalent *uranyl* group, UO_2^{++}, such as uranyl nitrate, $UO_2(NO_3)_2$. Uranyl salts are often referred to simply as uranium salts; for example, uranyl nitrate is often called simply uranium nitrate.

Uranous salts are green, while uranyl salts are yellow with a green fluorescence. Uranyl compounds, except the oxides, phosphate, sulfide, and uranates, are soluble in water.

Uses—Uranyl compounds were used in the manufacture of glass to produce a greenish yellow fluorescent glass known as *uranium glass* or "vaseline" glass. They have also been used for making a black pigment for china painting, and to some extent as intensifiers in photography. Government curtailments and restrictions now prohibit the use of uranium in glass and pottery. The most recent use of uranium metal is in the production of *radioactive isotopes* in the atomic pile.

Caution—Uranium is an extremely hazardous material and must be handled only by properly protected and adequately trained personnel.

Unofficial Inorganic Uranium Compounds

Uranium Chloride, Uranyl Chloride [$UO_2Cl_2.H_2O$]— Yellow deliquescent crystals. Very soluble in water; also soluble in alcohol and ether.

Uranium Dioxide, Uranous Oxide [UO_2]—A brown to black powder; insoluble in water or dilute acids; soluble in concentrated acids.

Uranium Nitrate, Uranyl Nitrate [$UO_2(NO_3)_2$]—This salt was official in USP IX. Yellow, odorless, radioactive crystals, melting at about 60°. Very soluble in water; freely soluble in alcohol. The nitrate is the principal uranium salt of commerce. *Uses:* a reagent in analytical chemistry. Formerly used to a small extent medicinally, but this use was abandoned as it is too dangerous.

Uranium Sulfate, Uranyl Sulfate [$UO_2SO_4.3H_2O$]—Yellow crystals or crystalline masses. It is freely soluble in water, soluble in alcohol.

Radioactive Decay

Statistics—Unstable nuclei which undergo a spontaneous nuclear reaction are said to be radioactive. If a single radioactive atom could be separated for observation, there would be no way to predict at which moment decay of its nucleus would occur. If, however, a large number of similar radioactive atoms are considered, it then becomes possible to predict how many will decay within a certain interval of time. This problem can be understood if a comparison is made to the similar situation existing with life insurance. Although the insuring company cannot predict when a particular policy holder will die, the fraction of a large group of policy holders who will die within a given time interval can be predicted. The larger the group considered, the more accurate the prediction can be. Such is the case with nuclei; the greater the number of nuclei considered, the more accurate the measurement of decay rate.

The need to recognize the influence of random decay upon analytical results is extremely important. The significance is illustrated by the statistical analysis which follows. The following example will illustrate the use of this information as well as demonstrate the importance of statistics.

If the total observed number of decaying atoms is	There is a 50% chance that the error will be greater than	Or a 50% chance that the observed result is in error by more than
30	3.68	12.27%
50	4.77	9.54%
100	6.74	6.74%
500	15.07	3.01%
1000	21.31	2.13%
5000	47.60	0.95%
10000	67.40	0.67%
30000	116.74	0.39%

Assume that a radioactive sample is decaying at the rate of exactly 500 atoms per minute. If the number of decaying atoms during each of 10 different 1-minute intervals were measured, for five of these intervals the data would lie between 500 − 15.07 and 500 + 15.07 or between 485 and 515. Data for the other 50 per cent of the measurements will fall either below 485 or above 515. Such variations, if truly of a statistical nature, should not be interpreted as indicating faulty equipment, faulty technique, or inaccurately calibrated samples. An increase in counting time to record a greater number of decay processes will result in an increase in counting accuracy. The chapter on *Statistics*, page 122, should be consulted for further details.

Fundamental Decay Law—*Decay rate* is the time rate at which atoms undergo radioactive disintegration.

It is expressed by $-dN/dt$, where $-dN$ is the change in the number of atoms, N, and dt is the change in the time, t. The negative sign merely indicates that the number of atoms is decreasing in time. The rate of decay $(-dN/dt)$ is proportional to the number of atoms, N, present at any time, t. Thus,

$$-dN/dt = \lambda N$$

where λ is a proportionality constant usually called the *decay constant*. The decay of radioactive atoms is therefore a first-order reaction. Integration of the equation above results in the useful relation

$$\ln \frac{N_t}{N_0} = -\lambda t$$

where N_0 is the number of atoms present at zero time and N_t is the number of atoms present at time t. This relation is sometimes more conveniently used in the exponential form

$$N_t = N_0 e^{-\lambda t}$$

This relation is illustrated graphically in Fig. 362. The rate of decay, $-dN/dt$, is sometimes called the *activity* and is represented by the symbol, A. Since the activity, A, is proportional to the number of atoms, N, the following useful relations can also be derived.

$$\ln \frac{A_t}{A_0} = -\lambda t \quad \text{or} \quad A_t = A_0 e^{-\lambda t}$$

The *absolute activity* is usually expressed as disintegrations per second (d/s or dps) or disintegrations per minute (d/m or dpm). The *observed activity*, which is less than the absolute activity by a factor equal to the efficiency of the counting system, is expressed in counts per second (c/s or cps) or in counts per minute (c/m or cpm).

The *half-life* of a radioactive species is the time required for one-half of a given number of atoms to decay. The half-life, $t_{1/2}$ is related to the disintegration constant, λ, by the equation:

$$t_{1/2} = 0.693/\lambda$$

Units of Radioactivity—One Gm of radium was selected as the unit of radioactivity and was called the *Curie*. It has been extremely difficult to measure the absolute decay rate (dps) of a curie of radium, although the average of many measurements, using a variety of methods, is approximately 3.7×10^{10} dps. In view of these discrepancies, the International Radium Standards Commission has recommended the use of the arbitrary value 3.7×10^{10} until the third significant figure is agreed upon. Although originally defined in

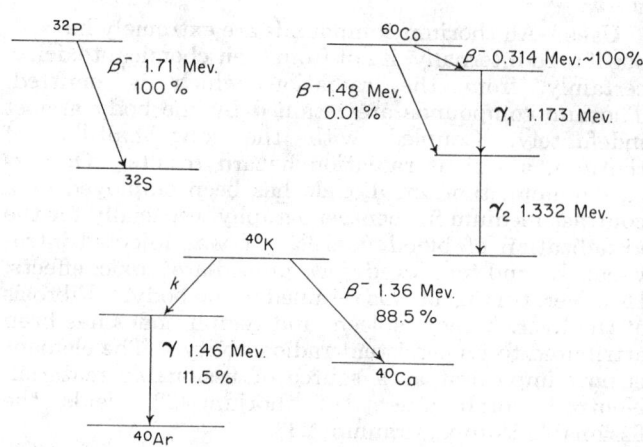

Fig. 363. Modes of decay. Radioactive atoms may decay by any one of numerous processes. Beta decay is shown by an arrow slanting to the right, electron or k-capture by an arrow slanting to the left, and gamma emission by a vertical arrow.

terms of radium, the curie is now used as a standard for the disintegration rate of any radioisotope. For example, 1 curie of carbon-14 means that amount of carbon-14 necessary to provide 3.7×10^{10} disintegrating atoms/sec.

$$1 \text{ millicurie (mCi)} = 10^{-3} \text{ curie}$$
$$1 \text{ microcurie (μCi)} = 10^{-6} \text{ curie}$$

Modes of Radioactive Decay—When it is desired to measure the absolute decay rate of a particular nuclear species, it is necessary to establish its mode of decay in order to determine the relationship of the number of particles or gamma rays emitted to the number of atoms actually undergoing decay. The mode of decay is often represented by an energy-level diagram (see Fig. 363). Three different modes of decay are illustrated. The first illustrates the simple beta decay of phosphorus-32. In this instance, each decaying atom of ^{32}P emits one beta particle. Thus, if the number of beta particles is measured, the number of decaying atoms is also known. The decay of an atom of cobalt-60 also results in the emission of a single beta particle but, in addition, two gamma rays are also emitted. Thus, if the decay rate is measured by counting the number of beta particles emitted, a 1:1 ratio exists. If, on the other hand, the decay rate is determined from the number of gamma rays emitted, it must be remembered that the number of decaying atoms is equal to only one-half the number of gamma rays. In the third example, the decay of 113 atoms of ^{40}K results in the emission of only 100 beta particles. The other 13 atoms decay by electron capture. Thus, a microcurie of ^{40}K does not emit 3.7×10^4 beta particles per second, but only $100/113 \times 3.7 \times 10^4$ beta particles.

Units of Radiation and Dosage—Equal quantities (ie, the same number of microcuries or millicuries) of different radioactive species will not produce equal quantities of radiation, nor will equal quantities produce equal doses of radiation. The fundamental reasons for this fact are explained above. Although equal quantities (millicuries) of different radioactive atoms represent equal numbers of atoms decaying per unit of time, the mode of decay must be considered. The number, type, and energy of the radiation emitted is indicated by the decay scheme. These parameters must be known if units of radioactivity are to be related to units of radiation and dosage.

Roentgen—The roentgen is a unit of *X- or gamma* radiation. (It is *not* a unit of alpha or beta radiation.)

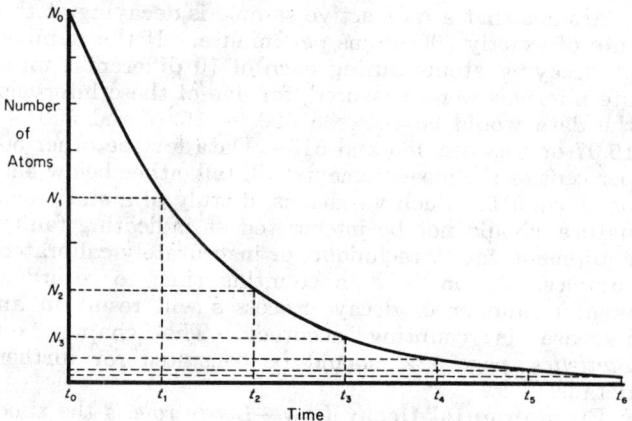

Fig. 362. Radioactive decay curve.

The roentgen is defined as that quantity of X- or gamma radiation which will produce one electrostatic unit of charge in 1 cc of air. While the roentgen is useful for calibrating sources and for measuring the dose in air, the energy dissipated by one roentgen of radiation in air will not be the same as that dissipated in muscle tissue. The *roentgen-equivalent-physical* (*rep*) and the *roentgen-equivalent-man* (*rem*) have been used as units of tissue dose but have now been largely replaced by the *RAD*. The dose is one *RAD* if the energy lost by ionization is 100 ergs/Gm of tissue.

Units of radioactivity (eg, millicuries) may be related to dose rate (eg, milliroentgens per hour) by the following expression.

$$mr/hr = \frac{\Gamma C}{d^2}$$

C is the number of millicuries of radioactive material, d is the distance to the radioactive source, and values of Γ in milliroentgens per millicurie per hour at one centimeter for several radioisotopes are listed below.

Radioisotope	Γ
Cobalt-60	12,800
Gold-198	2,350
Iodine-131	2,200
Iron-59	6,100
Radium	8,400
Sodium-24	18,400

These values of Γ are for the gamma component of the radiation only. For pure alpha and beta emitters, the value of Γ is zero. This includes ^{3}H, ^{14}C, ^{32}P, ^{35}S, ^{45}Ca, and ^{90}Sr.

Suppose we wish to calculate the dose rate received from 10 mg of radium at a distance of 100 cm. By definition, 1 Gm of radium = 1 curie and, hence, 10 mg of radium = 10 millicuries. Thus,

$$\text{Dose rate} = \frac{(8400)(10)}{100^2} = 8.4 \text{ mr/hr (at 100 cm)}$$

and the dose received at a distance of 100 cm from a source of 10 mg of radium over a period of, say, 10 hours would be 8.4 × 10 = 84 milliroentgens.

Instruments for Radiation Measurement

When a radioactive atom decays it emits a particle or electromagnetic radiation or both, depending upon the mode of decay of the nucleus. It is the radiation resulting from the decay of atoms which is detected by the radiation measuring equipment. Various types of radiation detection instruments have been designed, each especially adapted for the detection of a particular type of radiation. If radiation is to be detected with efficiency, the type of radiation must be known and the detector selected accordingly.

Geiger–Müller Counters—The Geiger–Müller counter (Geiger counter or G–M counter) is perhaps the best known of all radiation detectors. It is particularly efficient for the detection of beta particles. It consists of a cylinder of stainless steel, or of glass, silvered on the inner surface, which serves not only as the body of the tube but as the cathode as well. A fine wire, mounted coaxially, is the anode. The space within the cylinder, and hence between the anode and cathode, is filled with a special gas mixture. Radiation passing through the gas causes atoms of gas to ionize. If a

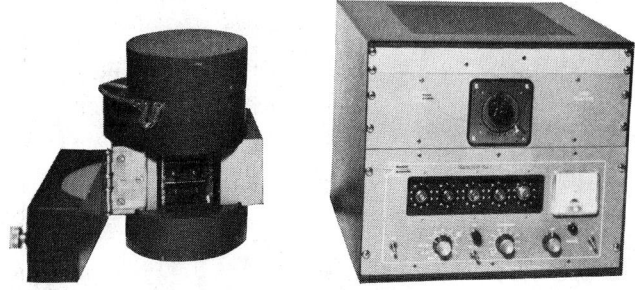

Fig. 364. Scaler and vertical shield for Geiger tube and sample (courtesy, Baird-Atomic).

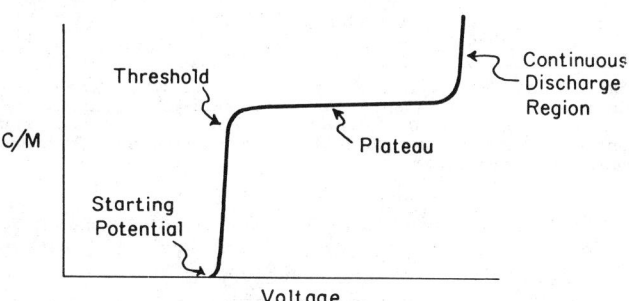

Fig. 365. Characteristic curve for Geiger-Müller tube.

high voltage, usually 800–1300 volts, is maintained between the electrodes, the electrons and the positively charged ions of gas produced by this ionization process are thus attracted to and collected by the anode and cathode, respectively. The passage of these ions through the Geiger tube constitutes a flow of current. Each particle of radiation causes a brief flow or pulse of current to flow. Each pulse, representing the passage of a particle through the tube is then recorded by a device such as a scaler to accumulate and indicate the total number of pulses.

Radiation enters a Geiger tube through a very thin section of the outer wall known as a "window." In the *end-window* type of tube, radiation enters through the end of the tube. In the *side-window* type, the side of the tube is made extremely thin to allow the passage of radiation.

To measure the characteristics of a Geiger tube, a radioactive source is placed near the tube. The voltage applied to the tube is then increased by increments, and the observed activity for each voltage setting is recorded and plotted vs the voltage. The result is a characteristic plateau curve. Below a particular voltage, the *threshold voltage*, no activity is recorded. At the threshold the observed activity increases sharply and then levels off. The level part of the curve is known as the *plateau*. If the voltage is further increased indiscriminately, the tube will go into *continuous discharge* and may be destroyed. The proper operating potential for the tube is normally in the lower region of the plateau. See Figs. 364 and 365.

Proportional Counters—The basic construction of the proportional counter is similar to that of the Geiger–Müller counter but modified by changing the gas composition and the shape of one or both of the electrodes. The construction of one type of proportional counter is illustrated by the cross section in Fig. 366. Here the anode is in the form of a small loop and the cathode is hemispherical rather than cylindrical.

The purpose of the proportional counter is to distinguish between alpha and beta particles. If a radioactive source emitting both alpha and beta particles

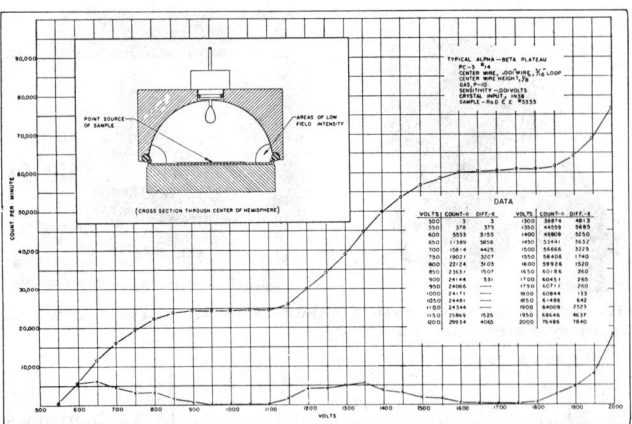

Fig. 366. *A:* **Cross section of a proportional counter. The center wire is in the form of a loop. The construction of the counter provides 2 π geometry. *B:* Characteristic curve for a proportional counter. The presence of both the α and β plateaus is illustrated (courtesy, Nuclear Measurements).**

is placed in the chamber, and the voltage applied to the chamber slowly increased, the observed activity in counts per minute will increase as shown in the graph of Fig. 366. In this instance, at about 1000 volts, only alpha particles are detected. The flat section of the curve in this region is known as the *alpha plateau.* At about 1800 volts both alpha and beta particles are detected by the instrument. This section of the curve is known as the *beta plateau.*

Ionization Chambers—Any two conducting surfaces separated by a small distance behave as an electric capacitor. The surfaces may be two flat plates or may consist of a wire mounted inside a hollow metal cylinder. If a potential source is connected between the plates momentarily, the capacitor will be charged. Ionizing radiation passing between the plates will discharge the capacitor. The rate at which discharge occurs is a measure of the radiation intensity. The extent to which discharge has occurred is a measure of the quantity of radiation.

Many types of ionization chambers are available. The classical gold-leaf electroscope is the oldest and best known. Refinements of the electroscope are found in the Landsverk and Lauritsen instruments, and in pocket chambers used for personnel protection. A research version of the ionization chamber, illustrated in Fig. 367, employs a vibrating reed electrometer to

measure the potential developed across the chamber. Ion chambers are also useful for routine calibration of isotope shipments. One such unit is shown in Fig. 368.

Scintillation Counters—When radiation strikes certain substances known as *phosphors* or *fluors*, a flash of light is produced. One of the oldest and simplest instruments employed for the detection of radiation by this process is the *spinthariscope.* In the spinthariscope flashes of light, produced by the radiation as it strikes a fluorescent screen, are observed by the naked eye. It is possible to measure alpha, beta, gamma, and other types of radiation with scintillation detectors if the detector is suitably modified for the type of radiation to be measured.

Because gamma rays are very penetrating, the phosphor used is a crystal of sodium iodide. The high density of sodium iodide favors the absorption of gamma radiation within the crystal, and this feature, coupled with the ability of the sodium iodide to fluoresce, results in a high gamma detection efficiency. Sodium iodide crystals usually contain about 1% of thallium to enhance the degree of fluorescence. See Fig. 369.

Gamma radiation passes through a thin light-tight window of aluminum and enters the NaI(Tl) crystal where it produces a small flash of visible light. The crystal is optically coupled to a photomultiplier tube which in turn detects the flash of light and converts it into an electrical impulse. This electrical impulse is then recorded directly by means of a scaler, or pulses may first be amplified and then sorted according to their respective amplitudes before being recorded. This sorting process is accomplished by means of a *pulse-height analyzer* or *pulse-height discriminator.* By the use of such a device it is possible to measure the energy of the gamma rays striking the sodium iodide crystal.

The *liquid scintillation counter* (see Fig. 370), a modification of the scintillation instrument described previously, is used to measure beta radiation, especially beta radiation of low energy such as that emitted by tritium, carbon-14 and sulfur-35. In place of a solid crystal of sodium iodide one uses a liquid phosphor. A commonly used liquid scintillator has the following composition.

PPO	(2,5-diphenyloxazole)	3 Gm
POPOP	(2,2'-paraphenylene bis 5-phenyloxazole)	100 mg
Toluene		1000 ml

The radioactive sample is dissolved or suspended directly in about 20 ml or more of this toluene solution in a special vial. The vial containing sample and liquid scintillator is positioned in front of a photomultiplier tube so that each flash of light, produced as a beta particle emitted by the radioactive sample passes through the phosphor, will be detected. Because the beta particle energies in this case are very low, the amplitudes of the corresponding light flashes will also be small, which in turn necessitates a considerable degree of electrical amplification of the pulses. The result is an increase in the number of noise pulses observed. It is common practice, therefore, to place the detector in a deep-freeze at a temperature of about −5° C to reduce the number of noise pulses produced.

Accessory Equipment—Various instruments must be used in conjunction with the detectors described above. A *scaler* such as that illustrated in Fig. 364, is the most commonly used device for recording and indicating the total number of impulses produced by Geiger–Müller, proportional, and scintillation counters. A scaler is simply an electronic adding machine. Most scalers also provide a source of high voltage for the

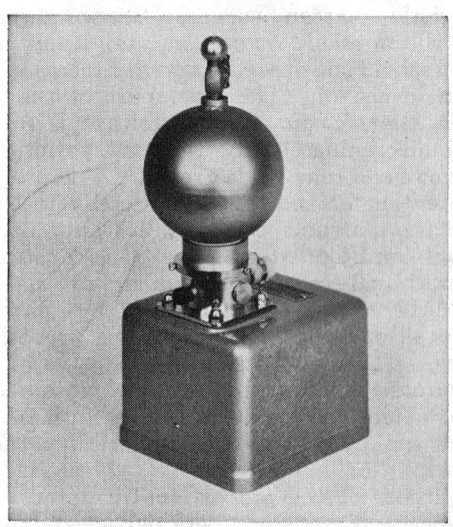

Fig. 367. Cary vibrating-reed electrometer and ionization chambers (courtesy, Applied Physics).

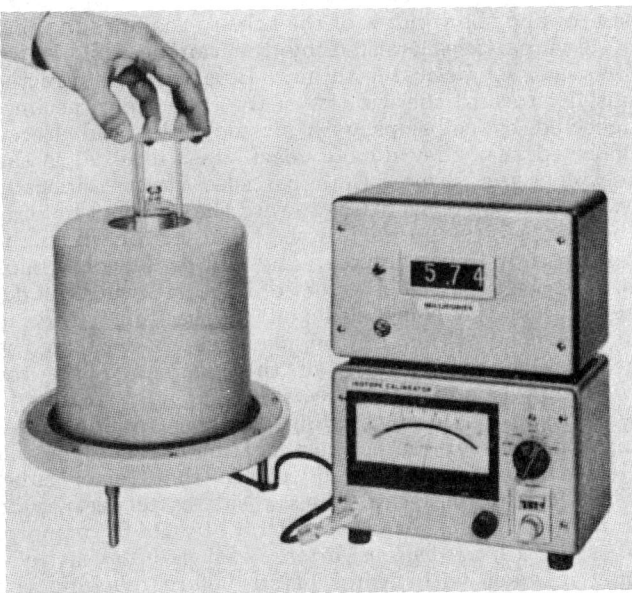

Fig. 368. The Calibrator (courtesy, Nuclear Associates).

operation of the detector, although the high voltage supply may be a separate unit. In addition, an electronic timer or stop-watch must be employed to measure the time during which a given number of pulses is accumulated.

While a scaler, in a sense, corresponds to the odometer of the automobile, indicating "how far you have traveled," a rate meter corresponds to the speedometer in that, like the speedometer, it tells you "how fast you are getting there." Rate meters are calibrated directly in "counts per minute" or "counts per second"; thus a timer is not required as an accessory to a rate meter. Rate meters commonly contain a high voltage supply for the operation of the detector. Rate meters, generally, are also equipped with an output jack which enables them to be connected to a recorder. In this way it is possible to record the activity of a sample as a function of time.

Techniques of Radiation Measurement

Sample Preparation—Before a measurement of radioactivity can be made the sample must be suitably mounted so that it can be placed in position beneath a G–M counter both accurately and reproducibly. Several techniques have been developed for this purpose.

Card mounts have been employed for many years. An aluminum or plastic card is used, in the center of which is cut a 1 inch-diameter hole. A piece of thin plastic film is fastened to the card by strips of cellophane tape. The card is then placed flat on the table with the plastic film on the bottom. The sample is measured onto the film in the center of the hole and dried. If desired, a similar film can be fastened to the opposite side of the card as a cover with the sample protectively sandwiched between the two plastic films. Card mounts provide the advantage that they cause a minimum of scattering of radiation.

Planchet mounts are very convenient, reproducible, and relatively inexpensive. A planchet is a little cup in which the sample can be measured. Planchets made of glass, plastic, and various metals, are available in a variety of shapes and sizes.

Micropipets are available in sizes ranging from 1 microliter (0.001 ml, also called a lambda) to 500 μl. These pipets are made "to contain," rather than "to deliver," the indicated volume. Hence, they should be rinsed and the rinse liquid added to the measured sample. Remote pipeting techniques are necessary for handling high radioactive solutions. Devices for this purpose are available commercially.

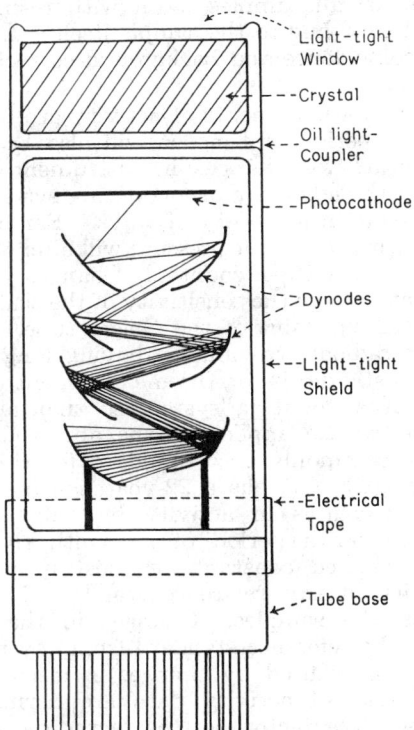

Fig. 369. Cross section of a crystal scintillation detector.

Light-tight Window
Crystal
Oil light-Coupler
Photocathode
Dynodes
Light-tight Shield
Electrical Tape
Tube base

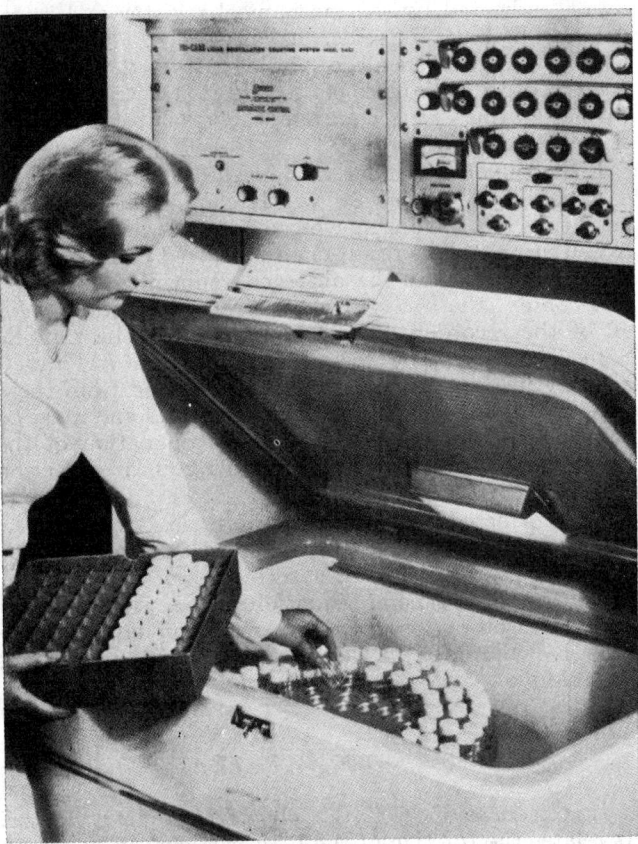

Fig. 370. Liquid-scintillation counter for the measurement of tritium and carbon-14 (courtesy, Packard Instrument).

Such devices increase the distance between the radioactive material and the operator and also permit the convenient use of massive shielding. Mouth suction should never be used in the radioisotope laboratory. A variety of devices are available for applying suction to a pipet. For micropipets, a small (number 00 or smaller) one-hole rubber stopper is inserted on the end of a 1-ml syringe. When the upper end of the pipet is inserted in the opposite end of the stopper, filling of the pipet can be controlled easily with one hand. An excellent pipetting device for this purpose is the Clay-Adams pipeter, which has a screw type control. Larger pipets, from 2 ml to 100 ml, are easily manipulated with the aid of a pipeting device such as the Propipetter.

Drying of samples is accomplished efficiently with an infrared lamp held simply by a clamp and ringstand above the sample.

Relation of Observed Activity to True Activity— The measurement of radiation may be performed with one of two basic objectives in mind; namely, (1) to determine the absolute disintegration rate of a sample or (2) to make only a relative comparison of the activity of one sample with respect to the activity of another. When relative comparisons are made, a knowledge of the absolute disintegration rate need not be known.

Consider the determination of the absolute disintegration rate, $-dN/dt$. Although it is assumed that absolute activities would normally be determined by methods to be mentioned later, the method of *defined geometry* serves to illustrate the many parameters of measurement which must be considered. Let us suppose the radioactivity of a sample has been measured with a Geiger tube and scaler. The sample was placed, for example, on the second shelf of the sample holder, the scaler was properly adjusted and used, and the count, indicated by the mechanical register and interpolation lights of the scaler, has been recorded. What, now, is the relationship of the activity, A, which has been recorded (in counts per second) to the true activity (disintegrations per second), ie, the absolute disintegration rate, dN/dt?

First, the observed activity or counting rate must be corrected for *coincidence*, which compensates for the dead time or time during which the tube was insensitive to radiation. This results in a corrected counting rate slightly higher than the observed counting rate.

Secondly, the *background* must be subtracted. Not all of the recorded counts are caused by the sample. Some are caused by cosmic radiation, natural radioactivity in the building, etc. All radiation from these outside sources constitutes the background and must be subtracted from the gross count. Application of the coincidence correction and the background correction gives the corrected net count.

The corrected net count of the sample, c/s, may now be related to the absolute disintegration rate of the sample, d/s, by applying a series of geometrical corrections. The general equation for a simple beta-emitting isotope, assuming all radiation entering the sensitive volume of the Geiger tube produces an ionizing event, follows:

$$d/s = \frac{c/s}{G.F_a.F_b.F_h.F_s.F_w}$$

In this relation, G is the physical geometry factor. It relates the fraction of the beta particles emitted in a direction included by the solid angle formed by the sample and the window of the tube to the total number of beta particles emitted by the sample. F_a is the *forescattering factor* due to air. Beta particles directed initially toward the window of the tube are sometimes deflected by collisions with air molecules and are so deflected that they do not reach the tube. F_b is the *backscattering factor*. Beta particles directed initially away from the Geiger tube toward the planchet holding the sample will interact with the atoms of which the sample support is composed and will be deflected back toward the tube. The extent of backscattering will depend upon the composition of the backing material, ie, the composition of the planchet, as well as the geometrical arrangement of the sample. F_h is the *sidescattering factor* and corrects for the degree to which beta particles, colliding with the atoms composing the walls of the support holding the sample and Geiger tube, are deflected toward the Geiger tube. The effects of backscattering and sidescattering may be to increase the observed count rate by 100% or more. F_2 is the *self-absorption factor*. Just as beta particles may interact with atoms of air before reaching the Geiger tube (*factor F_a*), they may also interact with atoms of the radioactive sample itself. Self-absorption errors are not significant if the radioactive sample is very thin, but if the sample has any thickness whatever, especially if the beta particles are not especially energetic as in the case of carbon-14 and sulfur-35, the self-absorption correction may be considerable, even exceeding that caused by scattering. Finally, F_w is the factor for absorption by air and the window of the Geiger tube.

Relative Measurements of Activity—If it is desired to make only a relative comparison of the activities of two or more radioactive samples (of the same radioactive isotope), the procedure is considerably simplified. Fortunately, many of the measurements made of radioactivity fall into this category. Where relative results only are desired, it is necessary to observe one basic precaution. That is, one must reproduce faithfully the exact geometry and counting conditions for all samples, both with respect to the equipment used and to the sample itself. In addition, both the coincidence and background corrections must be employed.

If relative measurements of activity are to be made over a long period of time, it will also be necessary to compensate for changes in instrument efficiency. Changes in the efficiency of a counting system may be brought about in a variety of ways. For example, a change in temperature or pressure will alter the characteristics of the Geiger counter. Changes in the line voltage may change the sensitivity of the scaler, as well as the operating point of the Geiger tube. Prepared mounts of radioactive samples having long half-lives are used as standards for the measurement of relative efficiency of a counting system so that appropriate corrections can be applied to the observed counting rate. One commonly used standard for this purpose is Radium-DEF. It has a 22-year half-life and consequently decreases in activity by only about 3% per year. Over a period of a month the activity can be considered constant for most measurements. The activity of this reference standard is measured along with the samples. Changes in the observed activity of the reference standard from day to day are assumed to be caused by changes in instrument efficiency. Thus, all activity data are normalized by multiplying by a factor, ie, the factor by which the Ra-DEF activity must be multiplied to correct it to the observed activity on the day selected as the reference time.

Coincidence Loss—The coincidence loss is the loss of register of events caused by their occurring within a span of time too short to be resolved by an electronic circuit. It is also referred to as the *dead-time loss*, *counting loss*, or *resolving-time loss*. The correction applied is termed the *coincidence correction*. In a Geiger tube, a beta particle entering the sensitive volume initiates a chain of events which requires a finite time (approximately 100 to 300 μsec) to complete. If, during this interval, a second beta particle enters the Geiger tube, it will not be observed, and the result is an error in the observed counting rate. The greater the counting rate, the greater the probability of such a loss, and the greater the counting error. For a dead time of about 300 μsec this loss amounts to $\frac{1}{2}$ of 1% per 1000 counts/min. Thus, if the observed counting rate is 10,000 counts/min the loss is 5%, at 20,000 counts/min it is 10%, and at 50,000 counts/min it is 25%. Resolving time can be measured by the method of paired sources.

Method of Paired Sources—Two radioactive sources are prepared on identical mounts, each having about the same activity (about 10,000 counts/min). The activity of each source is carefully determined individually and then combined, identical geometry and backscattering being maintained throughout all measurements. The resolving time, T, is then calculated from the relation

$$T = \frac{n_1 + n_2 - n_{1,2}}{2n_1n_2}$$

in which n_1, n_2, n_b = activities of samples 1 and 2 and the background, respectively, and $n_{1,2}$ = activity of the combined samples.

The activity corrected for coincidence may be obtained from the equation

$$N = \frac{n}{1 - nT}$$

in which

N = activity corrected for coincidence
n = uncorrected activity
T = resolving time

Calibration Methods—The calibration of radioactive samples entails the determination of the absolute decay rate, $-dN/dt$, or the determination of the number of radioactive atoms, N. These quantities are related by

$$-dN/dt = \lambda N$$

If two of these terms are known, the third can be calculated. The determination of any two of these terms serves as the basis for all radioactive standardizations. If the decay constant is known or is calculated from a known value of half-life ($\lambda = 0.693/t_{1/2}$), there then remains only one term to be evaluated.

Primary standardization methods are not generally useful as routine calibration procedures in most laboratories, such methods being rather complex and tedious and usually requiring very specialized equipment. It is better, from a practical point of view, to leave primary standardization to laboratories such as those of the National Bureau of Standards. These laboratories, in turn, supply *secondary standards* for distribution to other laboratories throughout the world.

The term "secondary standard" implies a standard which has been calibrated with the use of a primary standard for reference. Secondary standards are available from a number of manufacturers, as well as from the National Bureau of Standards. They are classified as alpha, beta, or gamma standards. Several types are available within each classification. The standard may be prepared from the *same* isotope as the unknown or the standard may be prepared from a *different* isotope than the unknown. *Simulated reference sources* are of the second type. For each classification and type of standard used, attention must be paid to the instrumentation required, the usefulness of the particular standard, and its limitations.

Standards of Same Isotope—When a radioactive standard is prepared from the same isotope as that to be measured, only three simple precautions are required to secure reliable results. These are: (1) readings must be made with the standard in the same position as that at which readings are made on the sample, (2) the sample must be uniformly distributed over approximately the same geometrical area as the standard, and (3) the sample must be supported on a layer of material identical with that supporting the standard, or at least one producing the same backscattering effect. In other words, a relative comparison of the activities is made (see page 546).

Standards of long-lived isotopes (Fig. 371) are available from a number of manufacturers. The problems of preparation and distribution contingent on a short half-life are, of course, not true of these long-lived standards which may be kept on hand in the laboratory and require only a simple calculation for the determination of their current activity.

Standards of Different Isotope—Short-lived radioactive reference sources are available only periodically and retain a useful amount of activity for only a short time. If it is necessary to calibrate such isotopes at other times, one must resort to the use of standards prepared from long-lived isotopes. These standards will, of course, consist of different nuclear species than the unknowns to be calibrated. One such reference is the Radium-DEF beta ray standard. Formerly available only from the National Bureau of Standards, they may now be obtained from several suppliers.

One type of Radium-DEF standard consists of an electrolytic deposit of lead containing Ra-D in the form of PbO_2 on the palladium surface of a palladium-clad silver disk. The silver backing provides saturation backscattering of the beta particles so that beta sources compared with these standards should have similar mountings. The beta spectra of the standard and unknown will undoubtedly differ. If the beta energy distributions are not identical, and they will not be, a different degree of absorption by the air and window

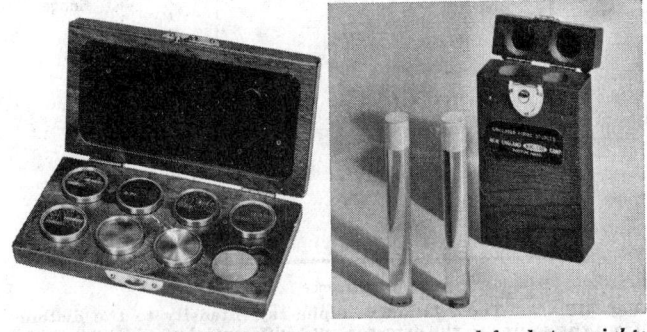

Fig. 371. Beta and gamma reference sources; *left:* beta; *right:* gamma (courtesy, New England Nuclear).

will occur; hence, the ratio of the radiation detected to that emitted by each source will not be the same, and an error will be introduced into the measurement. A correction for air and window absorption must therefore be applied. To correct for air and window absorption, absorption curves must be plotted for each source using calibrated aluminum absorbers. These absorption curves are then extrapolated to zero absorber thickness.

*Routine Calibration of Millicurie Quantities—*Standard ion chambers are commercially available for the routine calibration of millicurie sources by technicians. One of these called The Calibrator is illustrated in Fig. 368. It is a well-type ion chamber with both an analog and an optional digital readout which displays the sample activity directly in millicuries or in microcuries. The instrument has been calibrated for over 15 gamma emitting isotopes of medical importance. Selection of the proper setting of the calibration control compensates for differences in the value of the specific gamma ray constant. Applications of calibrators of this sort include checking the activity of ^{131}I shipments and the output of ^{99m}Tc generators or "cows."

Autoradiography—A method of detecting radioactivity that is especially useful in physiological studies of plants and animals is the autoradiographic technique, which may be illustrated by the following example. A radioactive substance is administered to an animal and after sufficient time has elapsed for localization in a given tissue, a bit of that tissue is removed and imbedded in paraffin. Very thin slices are then made with a microtome and these sections are placed in close contact with a photographic emulsion in a darkroom. The radioactive atoms which were collected by the cells in question continue to emit particles which have the same ability to darken a photographic emulsion as does light. Hence, after sufficient exposure time the emulsion is developed and fixed in the routine photographic fashion. By examination under a microscope it is then possible to correlate areas of darkening in the photographic emulsion with cell groups in the tissue and to determine, among other things, the rate at which the radioactive substance was metabolized and also the extent to which it was localized in the tissues studied.

Characterization of Radioactive Substances

Chemical substances are identifiable on the basis of their chemical and physical properties. If a substance is radioactive, it may also be necessary to establish the type or types of radioactive elements present. This may be accomplished by the measurement of certain radiological properties. The properties generally found useful for identification are (1) the half-life of the nuclear species and (2) the type and energy of the radiation emitted.

Half-Life—The most direct approach to the measurement of half-life involves the periodic measurement of the activity of the radioactive substance. An amount of the unknown radioactive material, calculated to give an activity of approximately 10,000 counts per minute, is placed in a planchet or other type of mount in such a way that loss of the sample will not occur from volatilization. All measurements of activity are then made on this same sample, special care being taken to reproduce the geometry for all observations of activity. Corrections for background, dead time, and instrument efficiency are applied to the data which are subsequently plotted on semilogarithmic graph paper. If a single nuclear species is present, the plot of these data will be a straight line.

If two or more independently decaying isotopes are present, the slope of the decay curve will not be constant. If this is the case, it may be necessary to separate the nuclear species by means of a suitable radiochemical separation technique. Various techniques which may be employed for this purpose are chromatography, ion exchange, precipitation and coprecipitation techniques, electrodeposition, solvent extraction, distillation, etc. The purpose of separating a mixture of nuclides prior to identification is to simplify the interpretation of data.

Characterization of Radiation

The identification of the type of radiation (ie, alpha, beta, gamma, etc) rests largely upon the interpretation of measurements of the interaction of the radiation with matter or with electric or magnetic fields. For example, the interaction of radiation with a magnetic field will yield a knowledge of the nature of the electrical charge of the radiation. Positively

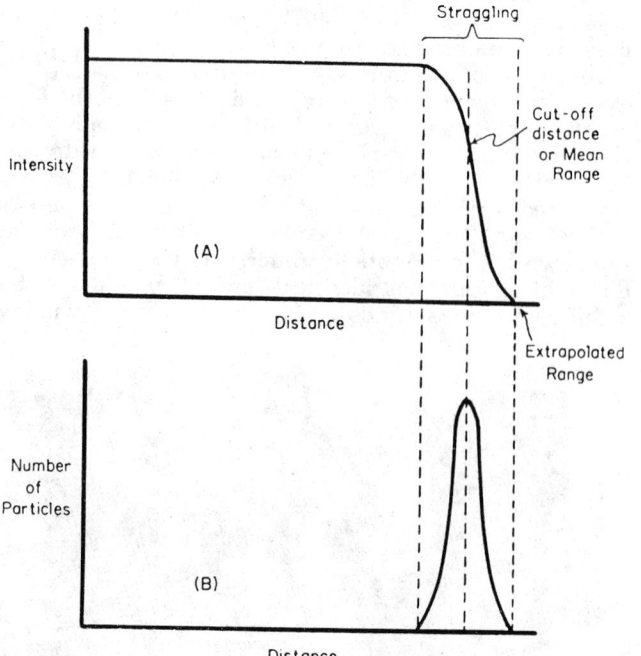

Fig. 372. *A:* The relation of alpha-ray intensity to the distance from the source to the detector. *B:* Differential of curve (*A*), which further illustrates the range distribution of alpha particles.

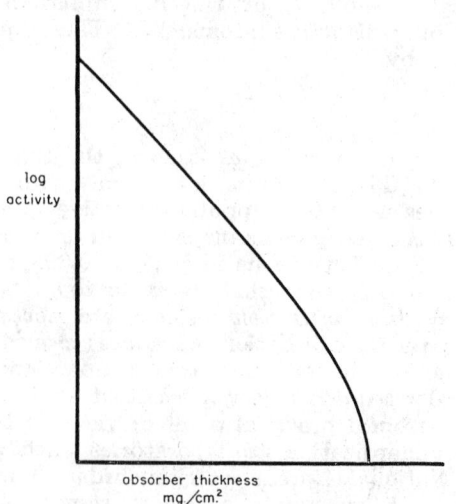

Fig. 373. Beta-particle absorption curve.

charged alpha particles and positrons are deflected in one direction, negative electrons in the opposite direction, and gamma rays are not influenced at all by a magnetic field.

Range of Radiation—A relatively simple and reliable method for the identification of the most common types of radiation is through the measurement of the range of the radiation. For this purpose, calibrated mica, aluminum, and lead absorbers are used. Absorption of radiation depends upon the *thickness* of the absorbing material and upon the *density* of the absorbing material. Absorbers are therefore calibrated in terms of the product of their thickness (cm) and their density (Gm/cm^3 or mg/cm^3), the unit of absorber thickness, therefore, being Gm/cm^2 or $mg/cm.^2$ For radiation range measurements, appropriate absorbers are interposed between the radioactive sample and the detector. The observed relation between activity and absorber thickness is not only characteristic of the type of radiation but can also be utilized to calculate the radiation energy.

Alpha Particles are easily absorbed by an absorber thickness of about 5 or 6 mg/cm^2 or less. An absorber of this thickness is approximately equivalent to one or two sheets of paper. The range of alpha particles, even in air, is only a few centimeters and in aluminum and tissue less than about 100 microns. Calibrated mica absorbers are generally used to determine the range of alpha particles. Alpha radiation is characterized by a sharp decrease in activity as the absorber thickness exceeds a specific value. Because all alpha particles from a given radioactive source are monoenergetic one would anticipate that all alpha particles would have the same range, and this is nearly so. The monoenergetic nature of alpha particles thus accounts for the shape of the absorption curve illustrated in Fig. 372.

Beta particles are more penetrating than alpha particles, yet, they are less penetrating than gamma radiation. When aluminum absorbers of increasing thickness are interposed between the beta source and the detector, the activity is observed to decrease in a more gradual manner. Whereas alpha particles are monoenergetic, beta particles are not. The less energetic particles are thus stopped by relatively thin absorbers, whereas much thicker absorbers are required to stop the more energetic beta particles. If the logarithm of the observed activity is plotted versus the absorber thickness, a nearly linear relationship is obtained over a portion of the curve. See Fig. 373. Lack of linearity, though disconcerting, does not prevent the utilization of the slope of such a plot for the identification of a radioactive species. If the curve is assumed to be linear, then

$$A = A_0 e^{-\mu x}$$

or

$$\mu = \frac{2.30 \ (\log A_1 - \log A_2)}{x_1 - x_2}$$

where

μ = the absorption coefficient
A_1 = the observed activity with an absorber of thickness x_1
A_2 = the observed activity with an absorber of thickness x_2

In this case it should be remembered that μ is not a true absorption coefficient since it is not constant over the entire range of data. If, however, an un-

known and known are compared over the same range of absorber thicknesses, the value of this measurement becomes evident.

Gamma radiation is the most penetrating radiation of all. Thus, lead absorbers are most frequently used to study its penetration characteristics, although aluminum absorbers are also useful. The absorption of gamma radiation is essentially logarithmic. That is to say, by analogy with visible light absorption, gamma radiation obeys Beer's law. Thus, the relation

$$\mu = \frac{2.30 \ (\log A_1 - \log A_2)}{x_1 - x_2}$$

can be used with less precaution but still not without regard for the effects caused by scattered radiation. Lead shields about the detector and the sample housing also scatter large amounts of radiation, and it is therefore necessary to consider such geometry variables.

Of the several absorption coefficients which have been defined, two are of particular importance here. These are the *linear absorption coefficient* and the *mass absorption coefficient*. If μ is the linear absorption coefficient (units $= cm^{-1}$), then the mass absorption coefficient (units $= cm^2/Gm$ or cm^2/mg) is defined by μ/ρ where ρ is the density of the absorber either in Gm/cm^3 or in $mg/cm.^3$

Of interest, too, if the half-thickness or half-value-layer (HVL) defined as the thickness of absorber required to reduce the intensity of a beam of gamma radiation to one half the initial value. The half-thickness, $x_{1/2}$ is related to the linear absorption coefficient

$$x_{1/2} = 0.693/\mu$$

Energy of Radiation—Radiation energy and radiation range are related. Thus, one approach to the determination of radiation energy is to determine the range and then apply the appropriate relation between range and energy. For alpha particles it is found that the energy in *mev* is approximately equal, numerically, to the air range of the alpha particles in centimeters. For greater accuracy a graph of the range-energy relation should be consulted.[1]

In the case of beta particles where energy values vary continuously from zero to a particular maximum energy, E_{max}, only the maximum energy is of particular interest and is calculated from the maximum range of the beta particles. Here, the measurement of the maximum range presents a special problem, for although one could presumably measure the maximum range merely by increasing the absorber thickness until that thickness is used which results in a sample activity equal to background, such an approach is not practical. As absorber thickness is increased, the time required for an observation of activity would of necessity have to be increased also. The increase in counting time would have to be excessive in order to attain statistically significant results. To overcome this difficulty the method of Feather[2,3] may be employed in which the beta particle range of the unknown nuclide is compared with that of a known. By a process of extrapolation the true range of the unknown is obtained. It is then only necessary to apply the relation

$$E = 1.85 \ R + 0.245$$

to obtain the value of E_{max} for the unknown beta emitter. This relation is valid except for relatively small values of range or energy ($R > 300 \ mg/cm^2$).

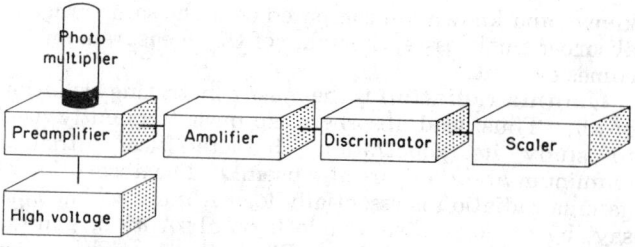

Fig. 374. Basic Gamma Ray Scintillation Spectrometer (courtesy Baird-Atomic, from a handbook, *Scintillation Spectrometry*).

Gamma radiation energies can be obtained from values of half-thickness (the half-value-layer) or the absorption coefficient by reference to the appropriate table or graph,[3] but it is more expedient to use a gamma ray spectrometer. A basic gamma ray spectrometer consists of a scintillation detector (NaI crystal and photomultiplier tube), preamplifier, amplifier, pulse height analyzer (discriminator), and scaler (or ratemeter and recorder). See Fig. 374. Its operation depends upon the production of a flash of light in the NaI crystal of the detector, the intensity of which is proportional to the gamma ray energy absorbed in the crystal. The photomultiplier tube, in turn, produces an electric pulse proportional in amplitude to the intensity of the flash of light produced in the crystal and, hence, proportional also to the gamma ray energy. If these pulses are linearly amplified, proportionality is maintained and the pulses become of sufficient amplitude or voltage that they can be sorted electronically according to their voltage. This process is referred to as discrimination or pulse height analysis. It is thereby possible to measure the number of gamma rays which lie between a particular range of energies (wavelengths or frequencies) and to record this number on a scaler. If, on the other hand, the scaler is replaced by a ratemeter and recorder, and if the pulse height analyzer is made to scan the range of pulse heights at a given rate, it is possible to record a gamma ray spectrum directly. Such a spectrum is shown in Fig. 375.

X-Rays

X-rays were discovered in the fall of 1895 by Wilhelm Konrad Roentgen, Professor of Physics at Würzburg University in Bavaria. Professor Roentgen realized the medical importance of his discovery when, during his investigation, he saw the bones of his hand clearly outlined on a fluorescent screen. After a thorough study of this new phenomenon he telegraphed his findings to the London Medical Society, which was then in session, and the world had its first news of this important discovery.

Production of X-rays—X-rays are produced by applying a large direct-current voltage across an evacuated tube. The positive terminal of the high voltage is connected to a target which is generally made of some metal with a high melting point such as tungsten or molybdenum, or of a metal with a high coefficient of conductivity of heat, such as copper. The negative terminal is connected to the cathode, which in the modern x-ray tubes consists of a heated filament. It has been found that a heated filament is a copious source of electrons. The electrons are accelerated toward the positively charged target, and strike it with a velocity which depends upon the voltage applied across the x-ray tube. The energy, and therefore the velocity, with which the electrons strike the target is given by the following equation:

$$\tfrac{1}{2}mv^2 = Ve$$

$\tfrac{1}{2} mv^2$ is the kinetic energy of the electron, m is its mass, v is its velocity, and e is its charge, while V represents the voltage applied across the x-ray tube (Fig. 376).

If the applied voltage is above the threshold voltage, and if the accelerated electrons have sufficient energy to penetrate the atoms composing the target of the tube, x-rays are emitted from the target and travel in all directions from it. X-rays are electromagnetic in nature, and therefore behave like visible light waves except that they are much shorter in wavelength. This means they travel with the velocity of light, can be reflected, refracted, polarized, and absorbed as are light waves.

Absorption of X-rays—The penetrating power of x-rays depends on two things, first the voltage applied across the x-ray tube, and, second, the absorbing ability of the material through which they pass. The higher the voltage across the tube the more penetrating is the x-radiation given off. Very penetrating or deep therapy radiation is produced by applying 100,000 volts or more across the tube, while soft easily absorbed rays are produced by 20,000 volts or less. Many hospitals in this country are now using up to 1,000,000-volt radiation, and there is a tendency to use even higher voltages in an attempt to concentrate radiation effectively within deeply situated cancers while sparing the overlying normal tissues.

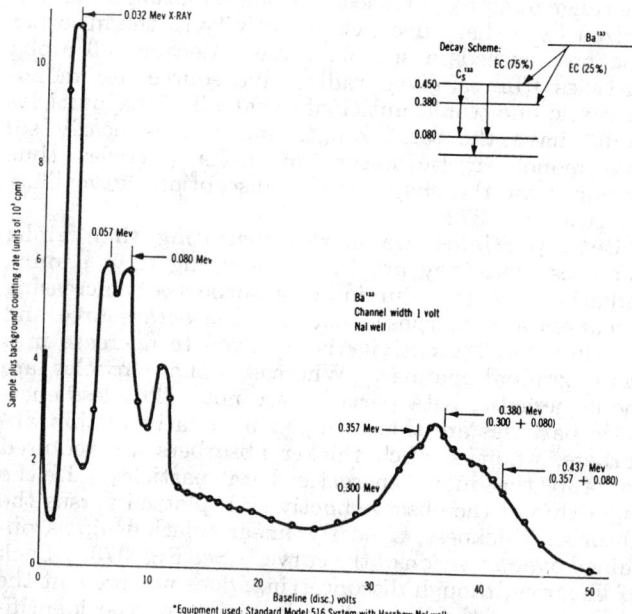

Fig. 375. Differential gamma-ray spectrum of barium-133 (courtesy, Baird-Atomic, from a handbook, *Scintillation Spectrometry*).

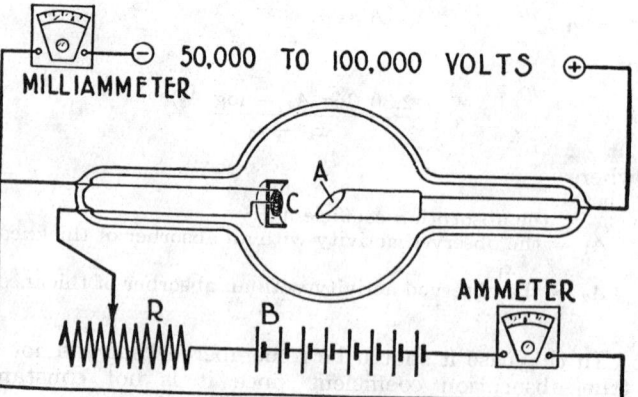

Fig. 376. X-ray tube connected in circuit.

The absorbing ability of a material for x-rays depends upon its atomic weight. It is for this reason that barium in the form of barium sulfate is used as an absorbing material to study the intestinal tract. Iodine-containing compounds and oils also are widely used as "contrast media" in outlining arteries, ureters, kidneys, gall bladder, etc. Both of these materials have a high coefficient of absorption for x-rays because of their high molecular weights. For a given wave length of x-rays and for a given absorbing material such as lead, for example, the absorption of x-rays by a thickness, t, is determined by the following equation:

$$I = I_0 e^{-ut}$$

where I_0 represents the original intensity, I the intensity after passing through a thickness t, e the Naperian base, and u the coefficient of absorption for the material through which it passes.

References

1. Aron, Hoffman, and Williams, US Atomic Energy Comm. Rept. AECU-663 (1951).
2. N. Feather, *Proc. Cambridge Phil. Soc.*, **34**, 599 (1938).
3. L. E. Glendenin, *Nucleonics*, **2**, 12 (1948).

34 | Medical Applications of Radioisotopes

Medical applications of isotopes (therapeutic and diagnostic)—
establishment of a medical radioisotope program—roentgenography—
official and unofficial radiopharmaceuticals

This chapter was prepared by

Grafton D. Chase, PhD, *Professor of Chemistry, Philadelphia College of Pharmacy and Science, Philadelphia, Pa. 19104*

Radium has the distinction of being the first radio-isotope used in medicine, having been employed as early as 1901. This nuclide was the most important medical radioisotope in use up to about 1946 when artificially produced radioisotopes became available in quantity. Since that date, growth in the medical applications of radioisotopes has been very rapid as their usefulness has become more and more apparent in diagnosis, therapy, and medical research and as greater numbers of physicians and other scientific personnel have been trained in their use. Current medical procedures employ more than a dozen radioisotopes in a wide variety of chemical and physical forms.

Radioisotopes are used in medicine in two different ways. They may be used (1) as radiation sources or (2) as radioactive tracers. As *radiation sources* their principal role is in therapy. Here, the choice of the isotope for a given application is governed largely by the properties of the radiation required for treatment; type and energy of the radiation and range in tissues are prime considerations. Except in special cases, the chemical properties or chemical form of a given isotope are relatively unimportant.

As a *radioactive tracer* the chemical identity and form of the nuclide are most important since, with but few exceptions, the tracer must be isotopic with the element being traced or must otherwise be capable of being incorporated as a part of a particular molecule. The nature of the radiation emitted by a tracer radioisotope is important primarily from the standpoint of its ease of detection. Radioactive tracers are used in medicine principally for diagnostic purposes.

Where radioisotopes are used as external sources or as sealed sources implanted in a tissue, the dose is terminated by removal of the source. When they are administered internally as an unsealed source, the dose administered to the patient, either deliberately in therapy or incidentally in diagnosis, cannot be terminated at will by removal of the source. In therapeutic applications the total dose must be calculated from a knowledge of the effective half-life of the isotope, the type and energy of the radiation emitted, and the concentration of the isotope in the tissue.

When radioisotopes are used for diagnosis, the radiation dose delivered to the patient is maintained at as low a level as possible. This is accomplished through the judicious choice of isotope for the best combination of minimum half-life, minimum retention in the body, and minimum quantity of isotope which will permit its detection and accurate measurement. Accordingly, certain isotopes, such as, ^{90}Sr, ^{226}Ra, and many others, are never used as unsealed, internal sources or tracers. In order to reduce the radiation dose to the population there is a trend toward the use of shorter lived isotopes, when available, for diagnostic purposes. It is for this reason that ^{57}Co and ^{58}Co are often used in place of ^{60}Co, where possible, in diagnostic procedures.

Therapeutic Applications of Isotopes

For therapy, isotopes are used as radiation sources, not as tracers. These sources may be used either externally or internally. Their use may be summarized as follows:

External sources
    Teletherapy sources—^{60}Co, ^{137}Cs
    Surface sources—^{90}Sr, ^{32}P
Internal sources
    Infusion—^{198}Au
    Interstitial implant—^{192}Ir
    Selectively absorbed or concentrated—^{32}P, ^{131}I

The therapeutic area of clinical chemistry is basically justified by the fact that radioactive material, when present in a tissue or organ in sufficient quantity, will produce emanation capable of destroying existing cells and preventing the formation of new tissue. For this reason isotopic therapy is generally applied only to those diseases in which there exists extensive cellular metabolic malfunction or to those conditions in which an organ or tissue produces physiological harm through overactivity.

Radiotherapy, involving internal sources, is largely confined to treatment with four different radioisotopes:

1. *Gold Au 198,* introduced as a colloidal gold suspension into a fluid-containing serous cavity, will initially diffuse rapidly throughout the fluid; it will then localize on the surface of the cavity as large aggregates of precipitate. Used in this way, it has found wide and successful use in the treatment of peritoneal and pleural effusions associated with malignant tumors in those cases in which fluid has accumulated in the abdomen or chest without the presence of large masses or of severe constitutional effects from the tumor. The tumor itself is generally destroyed only superficially or not at all. A side effect of radiation sickness has been noted occasionally, more frequently in intraperitoneal than in intrapleural administration.[1] See Fig. 377.

^{198}Au has been used experimentally in the treatment of prostate and cervix uterine carcinoma and bladder tumors. The evaluation of results is as yet incomplete.[2-4]

2. *Iridium Ir 192 Seed Ribbons,* consisting of ^{192}Ir seeds spaced at intervals along a nylon ribbon, are used for removable interstitial implant therapy of tumors. The procedure is a surgical one which must be conducted in an operating room.

3. *Sodium Phosphate P 32* may be used in the treatment of polycythemia vera to decrease the rate of formation of the erythrocytes. Since ^{32}P is metabolized in a manner similar to naturally occurring phos-

phorus, the isotope is readily distributed to all tissues and is concentrated in those tissues where proliferation is most rapid. Thus cancerous tissues concentrate the greatest amount of the isotope. A large dose of ^{32}P—3 to 5 millicuries—will concentrate in the bone marrow but will suppress erythrogenesis only partially. In severe cases of polycythemia a phlebotomy is necessary in conjunction with ^{32}P therapy.

^{32}P may also be utilized in the treatment of chronic granulocytic leukemia. This treatment, however, cannot achieve a cure, but can serve only to alleviate the symptoms of the disease. When ^{32}P is used in conjunction with local x-ray treatment, some phases of the disease may be controlled in the earlier stages.

Radiophosphorus rarely induces a side effect of radiation sickness, but excessive doses can result in serious effects on the hematopoietic system.[5]

4. *Sodium Iodide I 131* has several therapeutic applications. In cases of hyperthyroidism, therapeutic doses of ^{131}I will destroy thyroid tissue by means of radiation produced from within the gland. This procedure provides a more desirable mode of therapy than external roentgen-ray treatment since there is less radiation danger to the surrounding tissues.

^{131}I is used along the same lines in the management of euthyroid cardiac disease including congestive heart failure and angina pectoris. The control of cardiac disease is based on the ability of the isotope to reduce thyroid activity by radiation thyroidectomy, thereby lowering the total metabolic rate of the body and thereby reducing the stress on the heart. Dosage ranges from 10 to 25 millicuries, given as a single dose or extended over a period of a few weeks.

Some cases of thyroid carcinoma with metastases may respond to ^{131}I therapy. Dosage must be regulated carefully in treatment of hyperthyroidism since too large a dose may induce hypothyroidism.[6]

Diagnostic Applications of Isotopes

For diagnosis, isotopes are used as radioactive tracers and not as radiation sources. If results are to be meaningful, the tagged substances must be handled by the body in a manner similar to that of the untagged substance.

Radioisotope studies may be divided into four categories. These are: (1) isotope dilution; (2) rate of isotope transfer; (3) rate of isotope disappearance; and (4) degree of isotope concentration, or metabolic rate.

1. *Isotope Dilution.* The principles of isotope dilution are discussed in Chapter 33. The clinical application of this technique is illustrated by its use for the measurement of blood volume. The more popular procedure uses radio-iodinated human serum albumin injected intravenously.[7,8] Ten minutes after injection, a time sufficient to allow adequate mixing of the labeled albumin in the intravascular pool, yet not long enough for metabolic activity or seepage into extravascular pools to occur, a blood sample is withdrawn. The blood volume is calculated from the measured decrease in radioactivity of the injected sample upon its dilution by the blood. Red blood cell volume and plasma volume are related to the blood volume by the peripheral venous hematocrit. RBC volumes can also be determined by the use of cells labeled with ^{51}Cr in the form of sodium chromate.

Radioactive hydrogen ^{3}H in the form of tritiated water can be used to determine total body water.[9] Total body potassium, sodium and chloride, usually

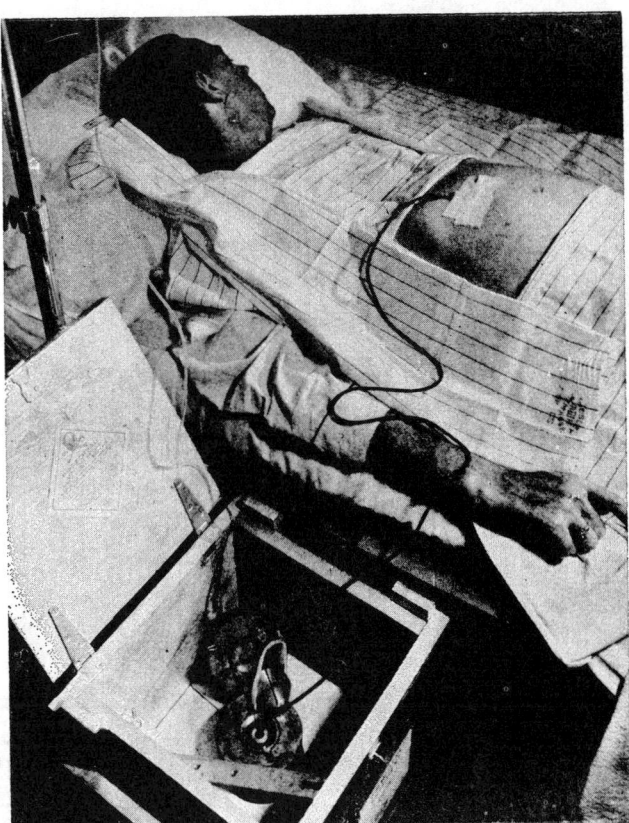

Fig. 377. Hospitalized cancer patient is treated with a solution of radioactive gold. Radioactivity retards the formation of fluid in the peritoneal cavity which bloats the abdomen. Though not a cure, treatment relieves distress and reduces need of tapping and draining (courtesy, Abbott).

referred to as "spaces," can be determined by the use of the radioactive isotopes of these elements.[10-12] In the case of chloride, ^{82}Br is usually used instead of ^{36}Cl because of the long half-life of the latter.[13]

2. *Rate of Isotope Transfer.* In these procedures, a labeled substance is injected into one part of the vascular system and the time required for its arrival at another part is determined. This technique has been used widely to determine circulation times, especially in the extremities. ^{24}Na is well suited for this purpose, since it has a short half-life, is a normal body constituent, is not selectively absorbed by any tissue and is readily detected.[14,15]

An extension of these methods has been used in the measurement of cardiac output. The passage of a radioisotope through the heart and lungs, following intravenous injection, can be recorded either by assay of serial arterial blood samples or by external counting over the heart. It is important that the radioactive material does not diffuse into the tissues during the studies. Radio-iodinated serum albumin has been found most satisfactory; measurements are possible with as little as 25 microcuries injected intravenously.[16,17]

3. *Rate of Isotope Disappearance.* The rate at which an isotope disappears from a tissue into which it has been injected is a measure of the circulation in that tissue. This test has been used successfully to determine the extent of circulation in tubed skin grafts in plastic surgery.[18,19] A small amount of an isotope, eg, radiosodium chloride, is injected directly into the tissue. The disappearance rate of the isotope is measured by means of a counter placed directly over the site of injection.

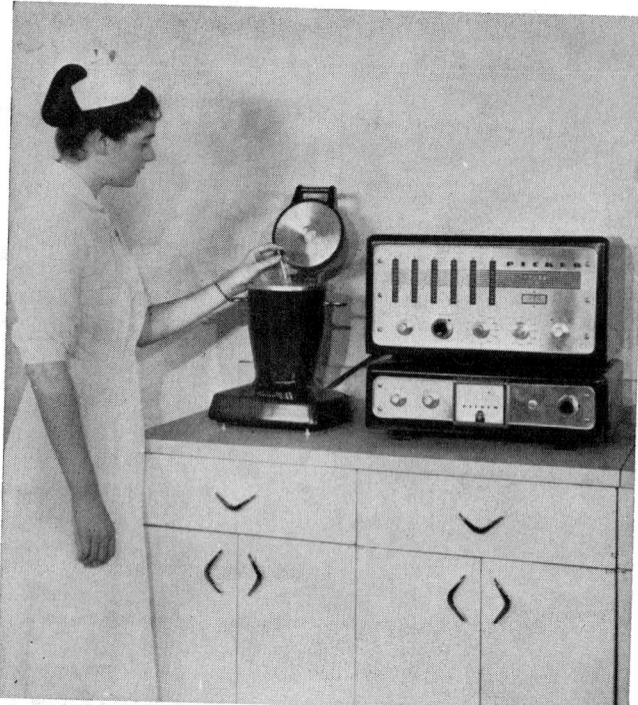

Fig. 378. A well-type scintillation counter is employed to assay small quantities of gamma emitters in liquids (courtesy, Picker X-Ray).

The RBC destruction mechanism and RBC half-life are measured by means of a disappearance-rate technique. If erythrocytes are labeled *in vitro* with ^{51}Cr and then re-injected, the fate of the tagged cells can be followed by assay of serial blood samples taken every two or three days for at least two weeks. See Fig. 378. Since the labeled cell group contains cells of all ages, only a mean survival time can be determined for these cells. The rate of decrease in circulating ^{51}Cr is approximately exponential and can thus be characterized by a half-clearance-time. The normal RBC half-life is about 26 days. This study is a valuable aid in the diagnosis of hemolytic anemias. See Fig. 379.

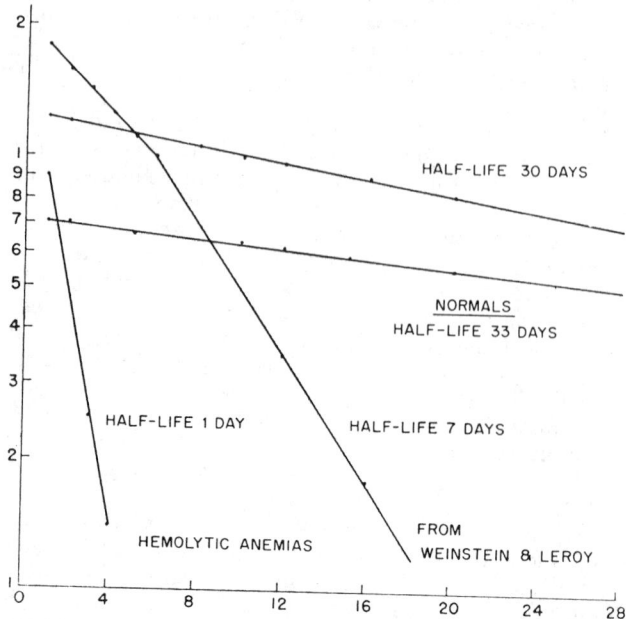

Fig. 379. Red-cell tagging with ^{51}Cr permits a direct determination of erythrocyte life in anemic patients (courtesy, Picker X-Ray).

Gastrointestinal bleeding can be detected and measured by the use of red cells tagged with chromium 51.[20-24] This procedure can be performed concurrently with the red-cell-survival study mentioned above. Gastrointestinal bleeding will be manifest by the appearance of radioactivity in the stools and, in severe cases, by a decrease in the blood-cell survival time. From quantitative measurements of blood and stool activities, the volume of blood in the stool can be calculated. A loss of up to 2 ml of blood per day is considered normal.

4. *Isotope Concentration or Metabolic Rate.* Most of the more familiar radioisotope studies are in this category. The concentration of a particular radioisotope in normal or abnormal tissue or in an organ provides data from which the function of the tissue or the metabolic condition of the organ can be evaluated.

Several studies of thyroid function can be carried out with the aid of radioactive ^{131}I. These studies include: (a) the rate of deposition of iodine in the gland *in vivo;* (b) the total accumulation of iodine in the gland within a specified period of time; and (c) the output of thyroid hormone into which radioactive iodine has been incorporated.

Because the thyroid has such an avidity for iodine, precautions must be taken to prevent exposure to or ingestion of even small amounts of iodine by the patient if valid results are to be obtained. Treatments to be avoided include the external application of iodine, ingestion of iodine-containing medicaments (may influence thyroid uptake for weeks), the use of x-ray contrast media containing organic iodine compounds (these may produce an effect on the thyroid for months), and myelography and bronchography (these may have a permanent effect). The radio-iodine thyroid uptake may, in addition, be lowered by such substances as thyroid preparations, antithyroid drugs, thiocyanate and perchlorate, corticotropin and corticosteroids, phenylbutazone, sulfonamides and *p*-aminosalicylic acid, arsenic, lead, and mercury. Malabsorption syndromes and renal disease will also lower thyroid uptake.

The thyroid gland concentrates inorganic iodide from the blood and converts it to thyroxine, the thyroid hormone, through the action of a peroxidase enzyme. When a thyroid gland is relatively "iodine starved," ie, receiving no more iodine than is found in the normal diet, the administration of a small dose of radioactive iodine results in a portion of the dose being retained by the thyroid while the remainder of the radioactive isotope is excreted in the urine. The amount of radioactive iodine retained by the thyroid is an index of thyroid function.

For *thyroid uptake* the most commonly employed technique[25-32] involves the oral administration of from 5 to 25 microcuries of Na^{131}I followed by a measure of the radioactivity of the thyroid after the elapse of a given time. An identical sample of sodium iodide I 131 is set aside as a standard. After the elapse of, say, 24 hours, the radioactivity of the thyroid is determined with a gamma-sensitive detector and the activity compared to that of the standard when measured under *identical conditions of geometry.* See Fig. 380.

The radiation emitted from the patient consists of at least three components:

1. Direct radiation from the thyroid—0.36 mev primaries of ^{131}I plus a small amount of radiation of lower energy.
2. Scattered radiation, resulting especially from Compton interactions of the primary radiation with neck tissue.
3. Radiation from parts of the body other than the thyroid.

Error from the third source is normally small after 24 hours and accounts for only 2 to 3% of the observed radiation. Compton scattering, however, may represent 20 to 30% of the observed radiation. If the *surroundings* of the standard ^{131}I and the thyroid are different, the measurements will be in error as a consequence of the difference in the extent of Compton scattering. A "phantom neck" is sometimes employed with the standard to produce deliberately Compton scattering equivalent to that produced by the patient's neck tissues. It has also been shown that a sheet of lead, $\frac{1}{32}$-inch thick, placed in front of the detector, will remove a large percentage of this low energy, scattered radiation while at the same time removing only a small amount of the high-energy, direct radiation. A spectrometer may also be used to eliminate scattered radiation through pulse-height analysis.

While the problems of measurement mentioned above result in an increase in the amount of observed radiation, absorption of radiation by the tissues of the neck tend to decrease the observed activity. Absorption errors are difficult to estimate but may generally be reduced in magnitude by using a phantom neck.

The normal range for iodine uptake is about 10 to 40% in 24 hours. Uptakes from 10 to 15% and from 35 to 45% may be considered borderline. An uptake exceeding 50% is highly suggestive of hyperthyroidism while an uptake of less than 15% may usually be interpreted as indicating myxedema.

The use of radioiodine is contraindicated during the second and third trimesters of pregnancy. The fetal thyroid is sufficiently developed at 12 to 14 weeks to pick up iodine from the maternal circulation. Even a tracer dose given to the mother may be sufficient to inhibit or injure the fetal thyroid.

Two mechanisms compete for the iodine circulating in the body: (1) uptake by the thyroid and (2) urinary excretion. The amount of iodine excreted by the kidneys is inversely related to the amount fixed by the thyroid. Urinary excretion may therefore be used as indirect measure of thyroid function.[33-38]

An advantage in the use of urinary ^{131}I output over the measure of thyroid uptake rests in the ability to reproduce the counting geometry more accurately. A second advantage is that the patient need not be present when radioactivity measurements are performed. This method has two disadvantages, however, which may introduce serious errors. First, it is necessary to collect a reliable urine specimen. Loss of urine will yield low results. Secondly, accuracy of the test is contingent upon normal kidney function.

With a hyperfunctioning thyroid, generally less than 30% of the dose will appear in the urine in 24 hours; with a hypofunctioning gland, over 80% will usually appear. The normal range is approximately 40 to 70%. Theoretically, the iodine uptake plus the urinary excretion should equal about 90% of the dose.

The *thyroid clearance* test measures the rate of clearance of ^{131}I from the plasma. First, a small amount of the isotope is given intravenously, then the rate of uptake over the thyroid gland is measured for 30 minutes. At the end of this time the urinary excretion of ^{131}I is measured. The iodine collected by the thyroid per minute is divided by the average plasma concentration of [131]I (μCi/ml) during the elapsed time. The result is thyroid clearance in ml per minute. The normal clearance is about 25 ml per minute. In hyperthyroidism the value may rise to 250 ml per minute while for hypothyroidism the clearance may fall to 2 ml per minute.

The *protein-bound iodine conversion ratio* is a measure of thyroid activity. It is the fraction of inorganic iodide converted to thyroid hormone and bound to the plasma proteins in 24 hours.[39-47]

Assimilated inorganic iodine is concentrated in the thyroid gland where it is converted, in part, to thyroxine. Upon release from the thyroid, the thyroxine is found to be reversibly bound with the serum protein. Treatment of the serum or plasma with trichloroacetic acid (TCA), for example, causes the protein to precipitate. Protein-bound iodine will be found in this precipitate. If, on the other hand, the serum or plasma is passed through a suitable ion-exchange column, inorganic iodine will be retained on the column while the protein-bound fraction passes on through.

The conversion ratio is an expression of the fraction, usually indicated as per cent, of radioiodine in the blood that is protein bound to the total iodine present in the serum or plasma at a given time—2, 4, 6, 12, 24 or 72 hours—after administration of the dose.

In humans an oral dose of 50 μCi of Na[131]I has been found satisfactory for euthyroid patients although only 25 μCi need be used if exophthalmic goiter is indicated and as much as 100 μCi may be required in cases of myxedema.

Current procedures for the determination of the PBI conversion ratio are essentially the same except for the step involving the separation of the protein-bound and the inorganic iodide. The procedure may be outlined as follows:

1. Administration of the dose.
2. Wait for a predetermined period of time.
3. Collection of blood sample.
4. Determination of the activity of an aliquot of the serum or plasma.
5. Separation of the protein fraction from the inorganic fraction.
6. Determination of the activity of the protein fraction.
7. Calculation of the ratio—organic PBI[131]/total plasma I[131].

Normal values are usually in the range of 13 to 42% with hypothyroidism being indicated by values below and hyperthyroidism by values above these limits.

Thyroid activity can be measured by two *in vitro* methods in which ^{131}I in the form of labeled *triiodothyronine* (T-3) is bound to the red cells or to plasma proteins. The first of these is the Hamolsky T-3 RBC uptake[48] which measures the percentage of T-3 absorbed on the surface of the cells. The uptake is increased in hyperthyroidism and decreased in hypo-

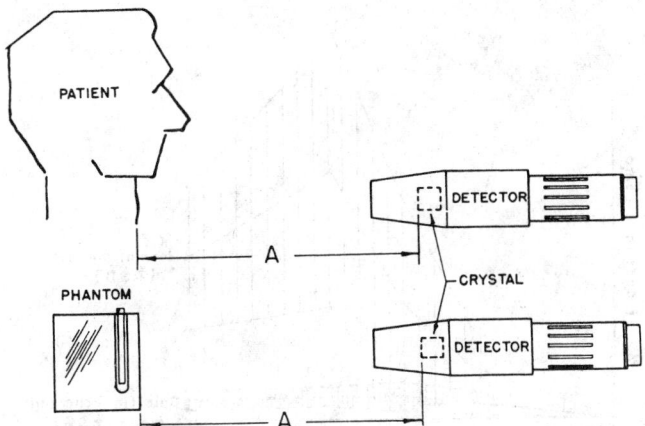

Fig. 380. **In practice, thyroid uptake is measured by intercomparison of the activity of the standard ^{131}I capsules (or source) in a phantom with the activity in the patient's thyroid (courtesy, Picker X-Ray).**

thyroidism. Simplified methods have been developed.[49] A newly developed Sephadex method[50] determines the capacity of plasma proteins for binding with labeled T-3. A high capacity of plasma proteins indicates hypothyroidism; a low capacity indicates hyperthyroidism. In contrast to *in vivo* studies with ^{131}I, test results with T-3 are but little affected by exogenous iodines or iodides, anxiety, hypertension, congestive heart failure and polycythemia.

The *Shilling Test* is useful for the detection of pernicious anemia and for its differentiation from other macrocytic anemias.[51-59]

In a normal individual, over 50% of an oral dose of vitamin B_{12} is absorbed through the walls of the gastrointestinal tract. This absorption only occurs in the presence of the intrinsic factor of Castle with which the vitamin must presumably combine in order to pass through the intestinal walls. (The biochemical defect in pernicious anemia is the failure of the gastric mucosa to elaborate intrinsic factor.) By means of ^{60}Co-labeled vitamin B_{12} it has been shown that over half of an oral dose soon appears in the blood. Normally only a small amount of activity appears in the urine, but if a large "flushing" dose (1000 mcg) of vitamin B_{12} is given parenterally within an hour after the tagged oral dose, the renal threshold is exceeded and radioactivity is observed in the urine.

In the pernicious anemia patient, there is a deficiency of intrinsic factor which causes poor absorption of the vitamin and most of the ingested B_{12} will therefore be found in the feces. The degree of absorption or of fecal excretion can be measured by the use of labeled vitamin B_{12}.

Other anemias, such as those associated with sprue and idiopathic steatorrhea, are also accompanied by a decrease in vitamin B_{12} absorption. They may be differentiated from pernicious anemia through the oral administration of intrinsic factor. A marked increase in vitamin B_{12} absorption results in the pernicious anemia patient but not in the case of sprue and other malabsorption syndromes.

In order to reduce the radiation dose received by the patient, while at the same time improving the available sensitivity of the test, cobalt-57 and cobalt-58 have recently been used instead of cobalt-60 as the radioactive tag for vitamin B_{12} (cyanocobalamin).

If plasma iron is labeled by intravenous injection of Ferrous Citrate Fe 59, it is possible to obtain a comprehensive evaluation of the *kinetics of iron metabolism*.[60-68] Among the parameters which can be measured are:

1. plasma iron clearance half-time
2. plasma volume
3. hematocrit
4. blood volume
5. red cell iron incorporation
6. daily iron clearance, (plasma iron turnover; plasma iron transport rate)
7. daily hemoglobin formation
8. per cent daily hemoglobin replacement

The iron turnover, from the catabolism of hemoglobin, can be estimated in the following way. The average blood volume of a normal adult is about 5000 ml. The hemoglobin content is about 15 Gm per 100 ml of blood or about 750 Gm per person. Iron represents 0.334% of hemoglobin. The hemoglobin iron content per person is, therefore, about 2.6 Gm. If the nominal life of a red cell is 110 to 125 days, then approximately 21 to 24 mg of iron per day is released through the catabolism of red cells. The plasma iron level is from 2 to 3 mg while the amount of iron ex-

creted amounts to only about 1 mg per day. Hence the plasma iron turnover rate must be of the order of six to eight times, or more, per day.

[14]C has been used in many metabolic studies such as those involving cholesterol and steroids. The use of radiocarbon and other radioisotopes for intermediary metabolism studies is for the most part experimental.[69,70] Limitations on the usefulness of tagging should be considered for accurate measurement.[71]

Oils and fats are composed almost entirely of glycerides—esters of glycerin and fatty acids. Before absorption can occur through the intestinal wall these esters must be hydrolyzed by the action of pancreatic lipase. Following absorption, the fatty acids and glycerin recombine to form neutral triglycerides for distribution throughout the body.

Studies of the *absorption of orally administered radioactive fats and fatty acids* provide useful clinical information in certain disorders of the gastrointestinal tract. Although much of the earlier work was done by measurement of fecal excretion of the labeled fat, more recent studies have shown that the determination of blood levels of radioactivity is an easier and more accurate procedure.

Fats can be labeled with carbon-14 or with iodine, either ^{131}I or [125]I. An iodine tag is introduced into the fat molecule by iodination of one of the unsaturated fatty acids, eg, oleic acid. The iodine tag alters the chemical composition of the fat and causes some minor changes in the absorption rate when compared to a carbon-14-labeled fat, but the small difference does not decrease the value of the test as an empiric measure of fat absorption. See Fig. 381.

The plasma lipid radioiodine level rises over a six hour period to about 12% of the administered dose. The normal level is above 8%. In the case of sprue, pancreatitis, etc, the plasma level is much lower. Fecal radioactivity may also be calculated. The normal individual excretes less than 2% of the administered labeled fat in the 48 hours following injection.[72-76] The rate of gastric emptying and gastrointestinal mobility will influence excretion and absorption patterns. In malabsorption states plasma levels are lower and fecal excretion is increased. Abnormal patterns have been described in individuals with coronary artery disease.[77,78]

Liver function is measured by intravenous injection of radioiodinated ^{131}I rose bengal and external counting over the area of the liver. Normally radioactivity over the liver reaches a peak 15 to 20 minutes after injection

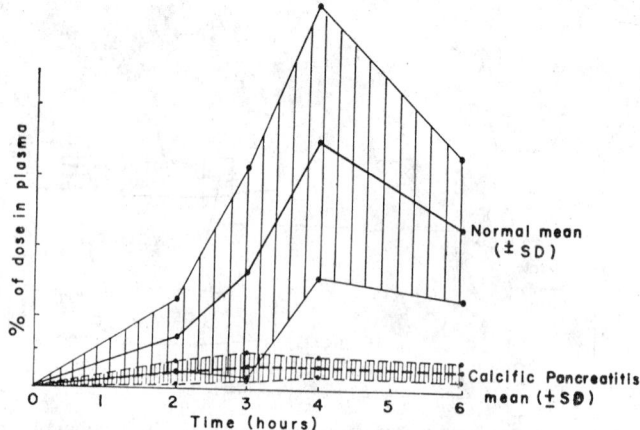

Fig. 381. The use of triolein (^{131}I) offers a rapid method for the determination of the cause of fat malabsorption (courtesy, Picker X-Ray).

and falls off gradually as excretion takes place.   In liver disease there is a decreased uptake of the dye by the liver.   In biliary obstruction the uptake remains normal in the absence of parenchymal involvement, but the excretion rate is diminished.[79]   Liver function has also been studied by measurement of the rate of excretion of various labeled radioactive materials such as iodipamide.[80]

In certain types of hemolytic anemias, red cells disappear rapidly from the blood stream, being trapped and eventually destroyed by the spleen.   The extent of RBC uptake by the spleen can be determined by tagging the cells *in vitro* with ^{51}Cr, re-injecting them intravenously, counting externally over the spleen and liver and calculating the ratio of spleen:liver radioactivity.   A high ratio, associated with decreased RBC survival, may indicate the need for a splenectomy.[81]

The renal function test was introduced by Winter and co-workers[82-86] in 1956.   In their original work they used iodopyracet.   However, 10 to 15% of this compound is excreted through the liver.   One of the best materials now known is sodium *o*-iodohippurate tagged with either ^{131}I or ^{125}I.   Nordyke and Tubis[87,88] report this compound to be excreted rapidly and exclusively by the kidney thereby increasing the accuracy of the test and at the same time reducing the time required to perform the test.   The isotope is given intravenously and excretion from the renal area is measured externally by means of a pair of radiation detectors.   The radioactivity of each kidney is recorded graphically to provide a pattern of the renal function. See Fig. 382.

^{32}P has been used in attempts to detect and localize gastrointestinal, gastrourinary, pulmonary, and breast tumors, but the results have not been too favorable. ^{32}P has been of value in the detection and delineation of eye tumors.[89,90]   Experiments have been undertaken recently to localize prostatic metastases and lesions by use of ^{32}P.   The isotope is administered orally and the radioactive uptake by the prostate is determined by means of an internal radiation detector.   In the field of brain tumors the isotope may be administered preoperatively and at surgery the marginal limit of the

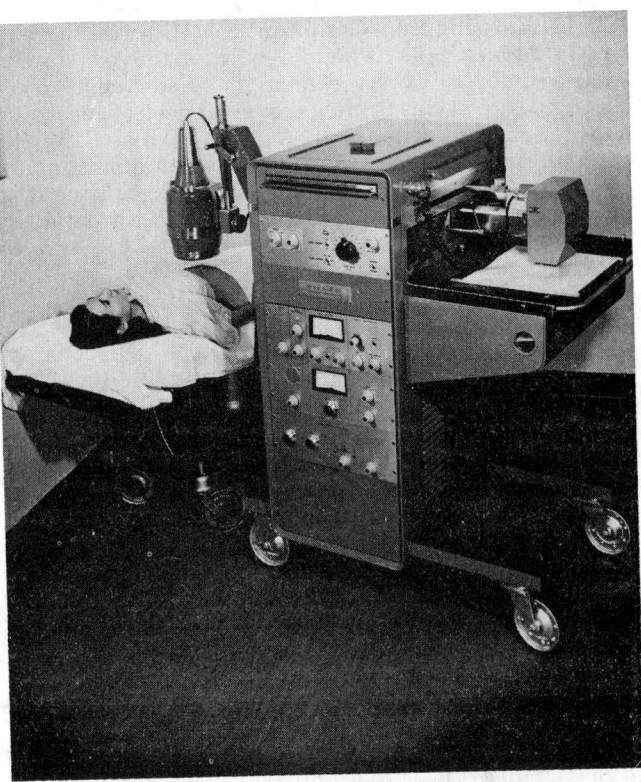

Fig. 383.   Medical scanner used to visualize tissues and organs in which a diagnostic dose of a radioactively tagged compound has concentrated (courtesy, Picker X-Ray).

tumor may be delineated by the use of detectors in the brain.[91]

Scanning Techniques—In recent years scanning techniques have developed rapidly and are now among the most useful tools in diagnostic medicine.   By means of scanning, tissues and organs can be visualized and such visualization facilitates the detection of abnormalities in their function.   In general, a scanning technique consists of (1) administration of a radioactively tagged compound, (2) concentration of the compound in the organ or tissues concerned, and (3) scanning of the region of the organ to prepare a "contour" map of the radioactivity relating the concentration of radioactivity and its physical location. A typical scanner for this purpose is shown in Fig. 383. Organs which have been mapped by such techniques with particular success include the lungs, kidneys, thyroid, liver, heart, spleen, and brain.

For detection of the tagged compound to be possible, the radiation emitted by the tagging nuclide must be sufficiently penetrating to pass through tissues so it can reach a detector located outside the body.   For this reason, gamma-emitting nuclides must normally be used.   (In the interest of minimizing the radiation dose to the patient there should be no alpha component in the radiation and preferably no beta component.   In addition, the gamma component should be no "harder" than necessary and the half-lives, both biologic and radiologic, should be as short as convenient.)   A list of medically important isotopes and their properties is found in Table I.

One of the first detectors to be used for scanning was the thallium-activated sodium iodide NaI(Tl) crystal detector, collimated by means of lead shielding to make it directional.   Collimation was improved electronically by means of a pulse-height analyzer adjusted to the photopeak of the tagging nuclide.

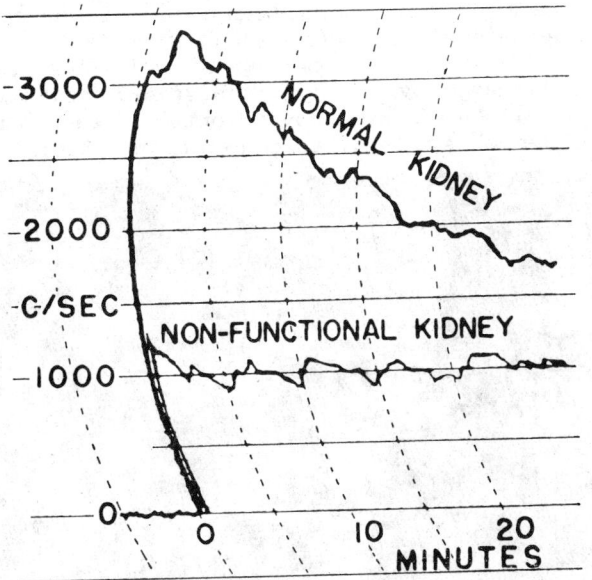

Fig. 382.   Kidney function is studied graphically with *Iodopyracet Injection* which has been labeled with radioactive iodine (courtesy, Picker X-Ray).

Problems arising from Compton scattering are thereby largely eliminated. The detector is moved slowly, back and forth, over the area to be scanned. Synchronously, a stylus is moved over a sheet of recording paper. Pulses produced by gamma rays striking the detector are stored electronically. Accumulation of a given number of pulses triggers the stylus causing it to make a mark on the recording paper. The greater the radioactivity, the more closely spaced the marks or dots will be. The result is a *dot scan* (Fig. 384A).

Attempts to improve delineation of organs and of "hot" or "cold" spots within organs led to the development of methods by means of which contrast could be increased. One method uses photographic recording. The intensity of a tiny light is modulated by the rate of radiation detection. The light is made to move over a sheet of photographic film synchronously with the motion of the sodium iodide detector over the patient. Development of the film results in the *photoscan*. Contrast can be controlled not only by applying a bias potential to the light bulb but also by appropriate selection of the film. A typical photoscan is seen in Fig. 384B.

Color scanning[92] represents another approach to improved contrast. In one instrument eight colored typewriter ribbons are employed, ranging through the spectrum from violet to red. The ribbon struck by the stylus is selected by the count rate. A dot scan is produced in which "hot" areas are recorded by red dots and the "coolest" areas by violet dots. Quantitative information on the concentration of tagged compound in various regions of the organ is obtained readily from the recording color.

An important disadvantage of single-detector systems, such as those described above, lies in the time required to complete a scan. It is often inconvenient or even impossible for an ill patient to remain immobile long enough to prepare a dot or photoscan. A natural solution to this problem is the use of multiple-detector systems. Hindel and Gilson[93] describe the *Dynapix*, a system in which the detector consists of 10 parallel sodium iodide crystals coupled through light pipes to 10 photomultiplier tubes. The system combines improved detection geometry with data processing and storage. Because data are stored on magnetic tape, worthless scans can be replayed, after resetting controls, to produce useful scans in which the delineation of anatomical details has been optimized.

The *scintillation camera*, also known as the *radiation camera* or *gamma camera*, is a nonscanning device. Two types are available. One, developed by Anger, et al[94-96] consists of a single sodium iodide crystal 11½ inches in diameter which is viewed by an array of 19 photomultiplier tubes. Scintillations produced in the crystal are displayed on an oscilloscope as flashes of light that correspond in position with the original image in the scintillation crystal. Images are projected from the radioactive tissue onto the crystal either by pinhole collimation of the radiation or by multichannel collimation. Multichannel collimators consist of a lead block penetrated by a honeycomblike network of holes. The image appearing on the oscilloscope screen is recorded photographically. The time required to obtain a useful image by means of the scintillation camera is only about ¹⁄₁₀ that required for scanning.

The second type of scintillation camera is the Autofluoroscope (see Fig. 385) developed by Bender and Blau.[97,98] Instead of one large crystal, an array of several hundred crystals is used in combination with multichannel collimation. Each crystal is coupled through light pipes to a rank-and-file system of photocells so that pulses appearing in a particular pair of photocells uniquely identifies a particular crystal. Displayed on an oscilloscope, the image can be recorded photographically. Information can also be stored in a magnetic memory for future analysis to optimize contrast. Because scintillation cameras are so fast, dynamic processes can be observed. For example, serial photographs have been prepared showing heart and kidney function.

For many years Sodium Iodide I 131 has been used for thyroid scanning (see Fig. 384B). Through its use one can demonstrate the presence or absence of "hot" or "cold" nodules, which is helpful information in deciding what course of treatment should be followed. Parathyroid tumors have been shown to concentrate Selenomethionine Se 75 to a small extent and its use with external scanning has been helpful in some cases for detecting the presence of such a tumor.

A variety of radioactive substances has been used for liver scanning. Both Sodium Rose Bengal I 131 and Gold Au 198 are removed from circulation by the Kupffer-cell system, thus concentrating these com-

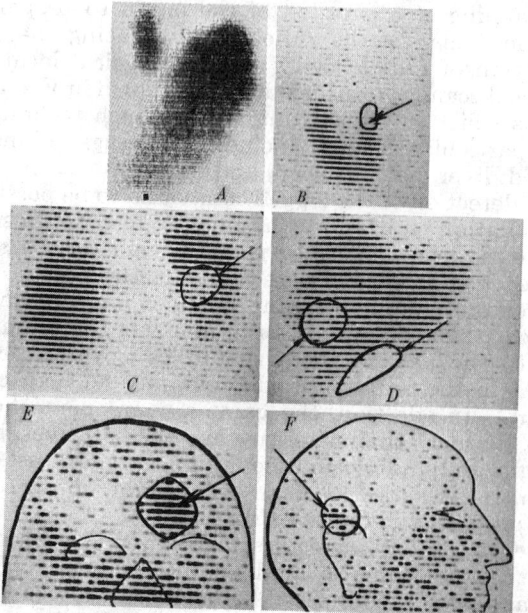

Fig. 384. Typical scans. *A:* Dot scan of thyroid (courtesy, Picker X-Ray); *B:* photoscan of thyroid; *C:* photoscan of kidney; *D:* photoscan of liver; *E* and *F:* photoscans of brain. Arrows point to malignancies.

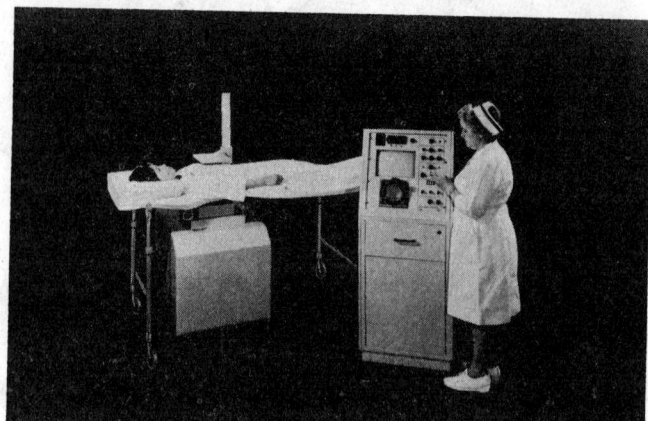

Fig. 385. The Autofluoroscope, a scintillation camera for rapid visualization of the distribution of gamma-emitting radioisotopes within the human body (courtesy, Baird-Atomic).

Table I—Properties of Frequently Used Medical Isotopes

Isotope	Radiological half-life	Beta energies[a] (mev)	Gamma energies (mev)
^{2}H	stable	. . .	. . .
^{3}H	12.26 years	0.018(100%)	. . .
^{14}C	5770 years	0.156(100%)	. . .
^{22}Na	2.58 years	β^+0.54(89%), EC(11%)	1.28(100%), 0.51[b]
^{24}Na	15.0 hours	1.39(100%)	1.37(100%), 2.75(100%)
^{32}P	14.3 days	1.71(100%)	. . .
^{35}S	86.7 days	0.168(100%)	. . .
^{42}K	12.4 hours	3.53(82%), 2.01(18%)	1.52(18%)
^{45}Ca	165 days	0.25(100%)	. . .
^{47}Ca-^{47}Sc	4.5 days	0.66(83%), 1.96(17%)	1.31(16%)
(Daughter ^{47}Sc)	3.4 days	0.44(74%), 0.60(26%)	0.16(74%)
^{51}Cr	27.8 days	EC(100%)	0.32(8%)
^{59}Fe	45 days	0.46(54%), 0.27(46%)	1.10(57%), 1.29(43%), 0.19(2.8%)
^{57}Co	267 days	EC(100%)	0.122(93%), 0.137(7%)
^{58}Co	71 days	β^+0.48(14%), EC(86%)	0.81(100%), 0.51[b]
^{60}Co	5.24 years	0.31(100%)	1.17(100%), 1.33(100%)
^{64}Cu	12.9 hours	EC(43%), 0.57(38%), β^+0.66(19%)	0.51[b]
^{65}Zn	245 days	EC(98.5%), β^+0.325 (1.5%)	1.11(45%), 0.51[b]
^{74}As	18 days	1.36(17%), 0.69(16%), β^+0.90(26%), EC(38%)	0.60(63%), 0.64(16%), 0.51[b]
^{75}Se	120 days	EC (100%)	0.265(71%), 0.136(24%), 0.405(14%), 0.077(14%), 0.098(6%), 0.281(5%)
^{82}Br	36 hours	0.44(100%)	0.78(87%), 0.55(70%), 0.62(43%), 1.04(30%), 0.70(29%), 1.32(28%), 0.83(26%), 1.48(18%)
^{85}Kr	10.26 years	0.67(99+%)	0.052(0.65%)
^{86}Rb	18.7 days	1.77(91%), 0.7(9%)	1.08(9%)
^{85}Sr	65 days	EC(100%)	0.514(100%)
^{90}Sr-^{90}Y	28 years	0.54(100%)	. . .
(Daughter ^{90}Y)	64.2 hours	2.26(100%)	. . .
^{99m}Tc	5.997 hours	. . .	I.T. 0.002(98.6%), 0.140 (98.6%), 0.142(1.4%)
^{125}I	57.4 days	EC	0.035 (7%), IC(93%)
^{131}I	8.08 days	0.61(87%), 0.33(9%), 0.25(3%)	0.36(80%), 0.64(9%), 0.28(5%), 0.72(3%)
^{192}Ir	74 days	0.67(48%), 0.53(41%), 0.26(7%), EC(3.5%)	0.296(29%), 0.31(28%), 0.60(11%), 0.61(7%), 0.48(6%), 0.59(6%)
^{198}Au	64.8 hours	0.97(99%), 0.28(1%)	0.411(96%), 0.674(1%)
^{197}Hg	65 hours	EC(100%)	0.077(19.3%), 0.091 (0.5%)
^{203}Hg	47 days	0.21(100%)	0.279(83%), IC(17%)
^{226}Ra	1620 years	α4.78(94.3%), α4.59(5.7%)	0.187(4%)
(^{226}Ra daughters)		Many	Many

[a] Unless otherwise specified, the energies given are for negatrons.
[b] Annihilation radiation from positron emission.
Events occurring in less than 1% of the decays have been omitted.

pounds in the liver. Not only can the general outline of the liver be observed by external scanning but it is also possible to show the presence of nodules (Fig. 384D). Recently Technetium Sulfide Tc 99m has gained favor for liver visualization since it combines several advantages over iodine and gold-tagged compounds; namely, (1) a lower dose is delivered to the patient (^{99m}Tc emits only a 140 kev gamma ray and has a physical half-life of only 6 hours) and (2) increased clarity and resolution of the scan is obtained since the radiation is easily collimated.

Visualization of the pancreas is complicated by the presence of the liver. Selenomethionine Se 75 is concentrated by the pancreas but it is also concentrated by the liver which overlies and obscures it. On the other hand, Blau and Manske[99] found the pancreatic concentration to be 8 or 9 times that of the liver in dogs. It is helpful, first, to make a liver scan to outline the liver with Gold Au 198 several days prior to the pancreatic scan, the pancreas thereby being more easily identified. Another approach utilizes a double tracer technique. One of the other labeled compounds taken up by the liver is administered simultaneously with Selenomethionine Se 75. Then, through pulse-height analysis, it is possible to subtract the contribution from the liver electronically leaving only the image of the pancreas.

A technique for visualization of the spleen is based on the function of this organ to remove damaged red cells from circulation. If red cells (tagged by means of Sodium Chromate Cr 51) are heated, they can be converted to spherocytes or spherical fragments without significant release of hemoglobin. These cells are quickly taken up by the spleen allowing it to be identified by scanning.

Iodinated I 131 Serum Albumin Aggregated is used to visualize the pulmonary vasculature through lung scanning.[100] The particles of radioactive albumin concentrate selectively in those regions of the lung possessing an adequate blood supply where they are apparently trapped for a short time by the narrow capillaries. The aggregate remains in the lungs long enough to complete a scan. In time they break down to smaller particles and are carried by the blood to the liver where they are phagocytized by the Kupffer cells.

Numerous radioactive compounds have been used for cerebral tumor detection (see Fig. 384*E* and *F*). Iodinated I 131 Serum Albumin has found extensive use for years, but there are reports[101] that Chlormerodrin Hg 203 is faster and gives sharper definition in the scans. Chlormerodrin Hg 197 has replaced the [203]Hg compound largely because the dose to the patient is less with the latter. Chlormerodrin is also used for kidney scanning. For brain tumor detection a dose of meralluride is usually given first to minimize renal uptake of the labeled chlormerodrin.[102] One of the latest techniques for brain tumor localization employs Sodium Pertechnetate Tc 99m which is readily available from a "cow." Other compounds used for brain scans include Sodium Arsenate As 74, Povidone I 131, and Povidone I 125.

Kidney scans have been useful for demonstrating both normal and abnormal renal function (see Fig. 384*C*). Compounds used for this purpose include Sodium Iodohippurate I 131, Sodium Iodohippurate I 125, Chlormerodrin Hg 203, and Chlormerodrin Hg 197. Other applications of scanning techniques include the use of Strontium Chloride Sr 85 for bone scanning and ^{99m}Tc-labeled human serum albumin for placental location.

Establishment of a Medical Radioisotope Program

Types of Programs—There are two types of clinical radioisotope programs:

1. Institutional program sponsored by a medical organization or hospital and carried out under the guidance of a medical isotope committee, and
2. Private medical practice programs.

Among the latter, a distinction may be made between private practice programs confined primarily to the use of radioactive materials in a private office and private practice programs where the materials are used within a medical facility. For radiological safety it is advisable that patients receiving a dose of more than 30 microcuries of radioactive material be hospitalized. In most cases physicians have found it desirable to carry out their treatments within a hospital rather than in their private offices. The responsibility still remains with the individual physician, however, the hospital merely providing the facilities.

A number of publications are available which are of great value to institutions organizing a radioisotopes program.[103-106]

Personnel—Radioactive compounds used in humans for therapy and diagnosis are radioactive drugs and should be treated as such. The administration of any drug, including radioactive ones, to humans, must be supervised by a physician specially trained in their use. Thus to organize a medical radioisotope program there

must be at least one qualified physician. His training must be ample to satisfy the AEC that he can use the radioactive material properly and safely for the particular procedure proposed. Suggested minimum experience requirements for the physician for specific diagnostic and therapeutic procedures have been published by the AEC.

The organization of an isotope committee is highly recommended. Membership on the committee may include physicians, physicists, chemists, pharmacists, business administrators or others as required for the proper functioning of the committee. One member of the isotope committee should be designated as *Health Officer*. His specific responsibility is to see that all radioisotopes are handled with minimum hazard to personnel and that all regulations governing the use of radioisotopes are observed.

Program—One of the first duties of the isotope committee is to outline the radioisotope program for the hospital. Although hospital programs may differ one from the other, they all have certain common problems. Some of the subjects to be considered by the committee are:

Diagnostic or therapeutic procedures to be performed
Facilities and work areas required (treatment room, laboratory, counting area, etc)
Instrumentation (selection, cost)
Licensure and reports (AEC, state, city)
Records (licenses, isotopes ordered and received, disposition of isotopes, patients' records, personnel safety records)
Isotopes (procurement, storage, waste disposal)

Facilities and Work Area—An isotope storage area, a laboratory for the manipulation of isotopes and the preparation of prescribed dosage forms, a counting area for calibration of the dose, and a treatment room are among the facilities and work areas which should be considered. With the availability of precalibrated dosage forms of most radiopharmaceuticals, elaborate facilities are not required for many diagnostic procedures. An existing, standard chemical laboratory will normally provide all necessary facilities for the preparation and handling of small amounts of radioactive drugs.

In some hospitals radiopharmaceuticals are dispensed by the hospital pharmacist.[107] Nonradioactive pharmaceuticals, including stable forms of most of the radiopharmaceuticals listed in Table I, have been dispensed by the pharmacist for years. Adding the property of radioactivity to these substances modifies them but does not cause them to be less of a drug than they were before. It therefore seems quite logical that these products be dispensed by the hospital pharmacist where he has taken the initiative to acquire the necessary knowledge and training.

In the selection of the counting area, the location of x-ray equipment and other radiation sources must be considered lest the background in the counting area be erratic or excessively high.

Instrumentation—The majority of clinical studies and analyses can be performed with the aid of but a few different types of radiation detection equipment. Of these the scintillation detector will usually be found most useful.

Because the 24-hour radioiodide thyroid uptake is one of the routine clinical procedures most commonly employed, the instruments necessary to carry out this study may be considered essential equipment for a clinical radioisotope laboratory. The necessary components of the system are an adjustable gamma scintillation probe attached to a scaler equipped with an elapsed-time clock. With this system the uptake of gamma-emitting isotopes can be measured in any organ of the body. The uptake of ^{131}I by the thyroid and the uptake of ^{51}Cr-labeled red blood cells by the spleen are examples of techniques possible with this basic equipment.

Use of a scintillation counter is greatly enhanced by a pulse-height analyzer. The resulting spectrometer can be "tuned" to a particular isotope. Such a system not only allows the detection of one isotope in the presence of others but also permits the use of a smaller amount of radioactive material in a diagnostic procedure because of the significant reduction in background and the improved statistics resulting therefrom. A further advantage to the use of a spectrometer, again resulting from the possible high selectivity or "tuning" effect, is the resulting discrimination against Compton scattered radiation which could otherwise cause serious errors in the measurements, especially should changes in the counting geometry occur. With a gamma-ray spectrometer, studies utilizing ^{51}Cr, ^{59}Fe, ^{60}Co, ^{131}I, and ^{137}Cs, as well as other isotopes, may be performed.

For the *in vitro* counting of gamma-emitting isotopes such as those above, a well-type detector will provide detection efficiencies as high as 60% or more. Accordingly, the addition of a well counter to the basic scintillation system, or better, to a scintillation spectrometer system, will provide the necessary instrumentation for performing numerous other diagnostic procedures. Included are blood volume measurements as well as other isotope dilution techniques, RBC survival time, test of gastrointestinal bleeding, PBI conversion ratio, triiodothyronine *in vitro* uptake studies, Schilling test, fat absorption, and others.

Measurements to determine the relative concentration of an isotope throughout an organ can be accomplished by means of scintillation scanning. A scintillation probe moving evenly and uniformly over the radioactive site detects differences in activity concentrated in the organ. The impulses detected by the probe are amplified and made to modulate a small beam of light which is directed onto a sheet of x-ray film. Since the detector and the light are connected mechanically, visible evidence of the pattern of radiation concentration in the area under examination is produced in the form of a photoscan. Dense regions in the scan, produced by greater exposure to the light, are indicative of regions of high activity. During the recording of the film scan, a mechanical dot scan can also be produced by means of a stylus which transmits the pattern of activity detection to a sheet of electrically sensitive paper. Variations in activity may be observed throughout the scanning procedure by means of a rate meter and an audio signal. A scintillation scanner such as this permits accurate mapping of radioactivity uptake in such organs as the thyroid, brain, liver, kidneys, spleen, and cardiac blood pool.[108,109]

Renal function may be evaluated by means of radioactive renograms. A useful instrument for this study is a dual-probe kidney scintillation scanner. By the intravenous administration of ^{131}I-labeled hippuric acid and the use of a scintillation probe positioned directly over each kidney, radioactivity of each kidney may be recorded by means of a dual rate meter and a dual recorder.

Licensure and Reports—Until recently all users of radioisotopes in the United States were required to obtain a license for their use from the Atomic Energy Commission. This is still true in most states. Application for license may be made on forms 313 and 313A which are available from the Division of Licensing and Regulation, US Atomic Energy Commission, Washington 25, D.C.

Effective March 26, 1962, the Commonwealth of Kentucky assumed certain of the Atomic Energy Commission's regulatory authority in that state. Individuals or organizations desiring to use radioisotopes in Kentucky should contact the State Commissioner of Health, Frankfort, Ky. Similar agreements have been made with the State of Mississippi, effective July 1, 1962, and the State of California, effective September 1, 1962. Similar agreements for state regulation have been made with Alabama, Arizona, Arkansas, Colorado, Florida, Kansas, Louisiana, Nebraska, New Hampshire, New York, North Carolina, Oregon, Tennessee, Texas, Washington, and, effective October 1, 1968, with Idaho.

While the above state programs replace AEC regulations, most states have radiation control programs which supplement those of the AEC. State regulations frequently require registration of radiation sources. Similar registration is desirable with the local municipality, especially with fire and police officials, even though not always required.

Roentgenography

Diagnostic Use—In addition to the diagnostic use of x-rays in the examination of broken and carious bones, the teeth, the gums, and the sinuses, there are many other useful applications. X-rays can be used diagnostically in conjunction with materials which have the ability to absorb them strongly. The x-ray absorbing ability of a material depends on its atomic weight. The higher the atomic weight, the better it will absorb x-rays, all other things being equal. The reason the bones of the body absorb x-rays better than the flesh and muscle is that they are largely composed of calcium, phosphorus, etc, which have higher atomic weights than hydrogen, oxygen, carbon, and nitrogen, which to a large measure are found in the rest of the body.

Therefore, for x-ray diagnostic use, it is desirable to find materials of high atomic number in a form which will have no ill effects on the body. Where liquids are desired, some form of iodine and thorium have proved useful, while the nontoxic forms of barium are used when an emulsion or a suspension is called for. Thorium-containing compounds are no longer considered to be safe for these purposes, however, since they are retained in tissues for years and have been responsible for the formation of cancers and sarcomas. Table II shows a partial list of some of these materials now in common use for x-ray diagnostic purposes.

X-rays can also be used to examine the normal functions of parts or organs of the body. For example, they can be used to "see" the action of the muscles, the joints, the diaphragm, and the heart. They can also be used diagnostically in the case of pregnancy. Not only is it possible to tell whether or not the fetus is growing and developing properly, but it is possible to tell whether a cephalic or breech delivery is to be expected. X-rays also will clearly show whether the fetus is a singlet, a doublet, or a triplet. Such applications must of course be used with discretion.

Therapeutic Uses—The major use for x-ray therapy is in treatment of *cancer*. Many superficial lesions can be completely cured and for them x-ray therapy is the treatment of choice. However, malignant tumors lying deeper in the body are not regularly cured, though their growth may be halted and they may even regress strik-

Table II—Compounds Used in Roentgenography

Part of body to be examined	Diagnostic opaques
Head	Lipiodol
Paranasal Sinuses	Iodochlorol
Salivary Glands	Brominol
Pharynx	Rugar
Esophagus	Barium Sulfate
	Skiabaryt
Respiratory System	Lipiodol
Bronchus	Iodochlorol
Cavities	Brominol
Fistulas	
Circulatory System	Diodrast
Skull	Neo-Iopax
Arms	
Legs	
Hands	
Feet	
Digestive System	Rugar
Esophagus	Barium Sulfate
Stomach	Skiabaryt
Duodenum	Gelobarin
Intestines	
Gall Bladder	Priodax
	Stipolac
	Iso-Iodeikon
	Iodeikon
	Telepaque
Urinary Tract	Diodrast
	Hippuran
	Iodochlorol Emulsion
	Neo-Iopax
	Skiodan
	Urokon
Obstetrical	Skiodan
Genital Organs	Iodochlorol
Pregnancies	Lipiodol
	Brominol
	Hippuran
	Neo-Iopax
Spinal Cord	Iodized Oil
	Pantopaque

ingly, only to return after weeks, months, or years. X-rays are also often used to advantage before the surgical removal of some cancers, particularly of the lower bowel or the uterus, to assist in curing infections which would otherwise complicate healing after surgery. A number of other afflictions are often treated with x-rays. Some controversy exists regarding the advisability of these applications, however, since the possibility of tumor induction years later always exists. It has been shown that the incidence of leukemia (a form of cancer) is higher in radiotherapists than in the population at large.

Dosage—Quite often, as in the treatment of superficial skin cancers, etc, x-ray therapists may deliver between 2000 and 6000 roentgens (see page 542 for definition of roentgen).

It has been found that the intermittent application of fractions of the total ultimate dose produce better therapeutic results with less damage to surrounding normal tissue. Hence, treatment may be prolonged for as long as three or four weeks with the administration of from 50 to 200 roentgens per day. Ordinarily when doses in this range are employed, changes occur in the skin which are suggestive of ordinary thermal burns. However, these are not burns in the strict sense of the word, and simply indicate that sufficient dosage has been administered. Treatment of these x-ray "reactions" consists simply in keeping the area clean and free from infection, and applying a local anesthetic cream.

Other Applications—In addition to their diagnostic and therapeutic use x-rays have a wide range of applications of interest to the physician, the pharmacist, and the chemist. In the first place x-rays have been used extensively to examine the structure of atoms, molecules, and crystals, and to determine the forces and actions which are going on within the atom, molecule, or crystal. In recent years this method has opened up new frontiers which are of considerable importance and interest to the manufacturing and pharmaceutical chemist. For example, the crystal structures of such simple chemicals as sodium chloride, potassium chloride, and calcium carbonate have long been known, but recently the crystal structures of many complex materials such as insulin, oxalic acid, and glass have been elucidated by x-ray analysis.

Detecting Adulteration—X-rays have a practical application in the packaging of food and drug products. Many companies now examine their packaged products with x-rays to make sure that they are in perfect condition before they are released to the public. Another practical application of x-rays is the examination of bales of crude drugs as they are bought from the grower. The addition of lead pipes or plates or other metallic parts for illegitimate weighting purposes can be easily detected without opening or disturbing the original bale.

Since postal and customs inspectors now use x-rays for examining mail, packages containingun developed film should be plainly marked or the film may be exposed to x-rays and spoiled.

Official Radiopharmaceuticals

Iodinated I 125 Serum Albumin USP

[Risa-125 (*Abbott*);   Radio-Iodinated (I-125) Serum Albumin (Human) (*Nuclear Consultants*)]

Radiological Constants for ^{125}I

Half-Life:	60 days
Radiations:	Beta..........None
	Gamma........0.035 mev (7%), IC (93%)
	Other.........0.027 mev—Te X-rays
	EC (100%)

Iodinated I 125 Serum Albumin is a sterile, buffered, isotonic solution prepared to contain not less than 10 mg of radio-iodinated normal human serum albumin per ml, and adjusted to provide not more than 1 milli-curie of radioactivity per ml. It is derived by mild iodination of normal human serum albumin with the use of radioactive iodide (^{124}I) to introduce not more than 1 Gm-atom of iodine for each Gm-molecule (60,000 Gm) of albumin.

Iodinated I 125 Serum Albumin contains 95.0–105.0% of the labeled amount of ^{124}I as iodide expressed in microcuries or in millicuries per ml at the time indicated in the labeling. Other chemical forms of radioactivity do not exceed 3.0% of the total radioactivity. Its production and distribution are subject to federal regulations (see *Biologics*, page 1425, and *Radioactivity*, page 535).

Caution—In making dosage calculations, correct for

radioactive decay. *The radioactive half-life of* ^{125}I *is* 60 days.

Description—Clear, colorless to slightly yellow solution. Upon standing both the Albumin and the glass container may darken as a result of the effects of the radiation.

Uses—The uses of Iodinated I 131 Serum Albumin this page) are generally pertinent to Iodinated I 125 Serum Albumin also. The compounds differ in the isotopic tag used.

There are several advantages to the use of Iodine-125 as a tag over the use of Iodine-131. The shelf life of ^{125}I-tagged compounds is greater owing to the longer radiological half-life of the isotope and, because ^{125}I emits no beta radiation and its gamma radiation is relatively "soft," the radiation dose is minimal. The resulting decrease in radioautolysis of the tracer compound further increases its shelf life. Of even greater importance is the decrease in the dose delivered to the patient. Collimation of the radiation is also simpler so it is possible to obtain greater resolution. Shielding problems and the protection of personnel are likewise simplified.

Dose—*Usual, intravenous,* **5 to 60 microcuries.**

Dosage Forms—Solution USP: in such sizes as may be requested by the physician.

Iodinated I 131 Serum Albumin USP

[Radio-iodinated (I^{131}) Serum Albumin (Human); Albumotope (*Squibb*); Risa (*Abbott*)]

Radiological Constants for ^{131}I

Half-Life:[110] 8.08 days
Radiations: Beta.................0.608 mev (87.2%)
Gamma.............0.364 mev (80.0%)

Iodinated I 131 Serum Albumin is a sterile, buffered, isotonic solution prepared to contain at least 10 mg of radio-iodinated normal human serum albumin per ml, and adjusted to provide not more than 1 millicurie of radioactivity per ml. It is derived by mild iodination of normal human serum albumin with the use of radioactive iodide (^{131}I) to introduce not more than 1 Gm-atom of iodine for each 1 Gm-molecule (60,000 Gm) of albumin.

Iodinated I 131 Serum Albumin contains 95.0–105.0% of the labeled amount of ^{131}I as iodide, expressed in microcuries or in millicuries per ml at the time indicated in the labeling. Other chemical forms of radioactivity do not exceed 3.0% of the total radioactivity. Other radionuclides are absent. Its production and distribution are subject to federal regulations (see *Biologics*, page 1425, and *Radioactivity*, page 535).

Caution—In making dosage calculations, correct for radioactive decay. The radioactive half-life of ^{131}I *is 8.08 days.*

Preparation—Iodination is usually carried out at 10°C, in a slightly alkaline medium, by the dropwise addition or very dilute hypochlorite to a mixture of iodide and the protein. Unbound iodide is removed by an ion-exchange column and the product is sterilized by a Seitz filtration.

Description—A clear, colorless to slightly yellow solution. Upon standing, both the solution and the glass container may darken as a result of the effects of the radiation. The pH is between 7.0 and 8.5.

Uses—Iodinated I 131 serum albumin (human) is used as a diagnostic aid in the determination of blood or plasma volumes, circulation times or cardiac output, and as an adjunct to other diagnostic procedures in the detection and localization of brain tumors. Although available evidence indicates that the immunologic nature of human serum albumin is not altered by iodination with radio-iodine, it is possible that patients receiving subsequent doses of this radioactive iodine compound may exhibit allergic reactions.

Dose—*Usual, intravenous,* **5 to 60 microcuries.**

Dosage Forms—Solution USP: in such sizes as may be requested by the physician.

Chlormerodrin Hg 197 Injection USP

[Chloro(2-methoxy-3-ureidopropyl)mercury-^{197}Hg; Chlormerodrin Hg-197 (*Nuclear Consultants & Squibb*); Neohydrin-197 (*Abbott*)]

Radiological Constants for ^{197}Hg

Half-Life: 65 hours
Radiations: Beta.................None
Gamma.............0.077 mev (19.3%),
0.091 mev (0.5%)
Other.................EC

Chlormerodrin Hg 197 Injection is a sterile solution containing chlormerodrin ($C_5H_{11}Cl^{197}HgN_2O_2$) in which a portion of the molecules contain radioactive mercury (^{197}Hg) in the molecular structure. ^{197}Hg is produced by the neutron bombardment of enriched ^{196}Hg.

Chlormerodrin Hg 197 Injection contains 90.0–110.0% of the labeled amount of ^{197}Hg as chlormerodrin expressed in microcuries or millicuries at the time indicated in the labeling. Other chemical forms of radioactivity do not exceed 5.0% of the total radioactivity.

Caution—In making dosage calculations, correct for radioactive decay. The radioactive half-life of ^{197}Hg *is 65 hours.*

For the structure and preparation of Chlormerodrin, see page 939.

Description—Clear, colorless solution. The pH is between 7.0 and 8.5.

Uses—Chlormerodrin Hg 197 and Chlormerodrin Hg 203 are radioactively tagged compounds useful for scanning the brain for suspected lesions and the kidneys for anatomical and functional abnormalities. In the brain chlormerodrin concentrates in neoplastic lesions. That which remains in the circulation is rapidly cleared by the kidneys. For brain scans Chlormerodrin Hg 203 provides several advantages over the use of Iodinated I 131 Serum Albumin in that it delivers less than half the radiation dose and, because of its rapid clearance from the circulation, a high tumor-to-background activity is achieved in about 4 hours, thereby permitting the scan to be made sooner after administration of the tracer dose. In addition it has a longer shelf life and, because the radiation is more easily collimated, better resolution is obtained in the scans. A further reduction in radiation dose to the patient is provided through the use of Chlormerodrin Hg 197.

Dose—*Usual, intravenous,* for *brain scanning,* **10 microcuries** per **Kg** of body weight, for a maximum total of about 700 microcuries.

Dosage Forms—Injection USP: in such sizes as may be requested by the physician.

Chlormerodrin Hg 203 Injection USP

[Chloro(2-methoxy-3-ureidopropyl)mercury-203Hg; Chlormerodrin Hg-203 (Nuclear Consultants; Squibb); Neohydrin-203 (Abbott)]

Radiological Constants for ^{203}Hg

Half-Life: 46.6 days
Radiations: Beta.........0.21 mev (100%)
                 Gamma......0.279 mev (83%), IC (17%)

Chlormerodrin Hg 203 Injection is a sterile solution containing chlormerodrin ($C_5H_{11}Cl^{203}HgN_2O_2$) in which a portion of the molecules contain radioactive mercury (^{203}Hg) in the molecular structure. ^{203}Hg is produced by the neutron bombardment of enriched ^{202}Hg.

Chlormerodrin Hg 203 Injection contains 90.0–110.0% of the labeled amount of ^{203}Hg as chlormerodrin expressed in microcuries or millicuries at the time indicated in the labeling. Other chemical forms of radioactivity do not exceed 5.0% of the total radioactivity.

Caution—In making dosage calculations, correct for radioactive decay. The radioactive half-life of ^{203}Hg is 46.6 days.

For the structure and preparation of Chlormerodrin, see page 939.

Description—Clear, colorless solution.

Uses—See *Chlormerodrin Hg 197.*
Dose—*Usual, intravenous,* for *brain scanning,* **10 microcuries** per **Kg** of body weight, for a maximum total of about 700 microcuries.

Cyanocobalamin Co 57 Capsules USP

[Cobalt-57 Tagged Vitamin B-12 (*Nuclear Consultants*); Rubotope 57 (*Squibb*); Racobalamin 57 (*Abbott*)]

Radiological Constants for ^{57}Co

Half-Life: 270 days
Radiations: Beta...............None
                 Gamma............0.122 mev, 0.014 mev, 0.137 mev

Cyanocobalamin Co 57 Capsules contain cyanocobalamin in which a portion of the molecules contain radioactive cobalt (^{57}Co) in the molecular structure ($C_{63}H_{88}{}^{57}CoN_{14}O_{14}P$). Each Capsule contains 90.0–110.0% of the labeled amount of Co 57 as cyanocobalamin expressed in microcuries at the time indicated in the labeling. The cyanocobalamin content is 90.0–110.0% of the labeled amount. The specific activity is not less than 0.5 microcurie per mcg of cyanocobalamin. Other radionuclides are absent.

Caution—In making dosage calculations, correct for radioactive decay. The radioactive half-life of Co 57 is 270 days.

For the structure of Cyanocobalamin, see page 1034; its preparation is given on page 1037.

Description—May contain a small, rectangular solid or solids, or may appear empty.

Uses—See *Cyanocobalamin Co 60 Solution,* page 564.
Dose—*Usual,* the equivalent of **0.5** to **1 microcurie.**
Dosage Forms—Capsules USP: in such sizes as may be requested by the physician.

Cyanocobalamin Co 57 Solution USP

[Cobalt-57 Tagged Vitamin B-12 (*Nuclear Consultants*); Rubotope 57 (*Squibb*); Racobalamin 57 (*Abbott*)]

Note—For the *Radiological Constants of Co 57,* see *Cyanocobalamin Co 57 Capsules* (this page).

Cyanocobalamin Co 57 Solution is a solution suitable for oral administration, containing cyanocobalamin in which a portion of the molecules contain radioactive cobalt (Co 57) in the molecular structure ($C_{63}H_{88}{}^{57}Co-N_{14}O_{14}P$).

Cyanocobalamin Co 57 Solution contains 90.0–110.0% of the labeled amount of Co 57 as cyanocobalamin expressed in microcuries at the time indicated in the labeling. The cyanocobalamin content is 90.0–110.0% of the labeled amount. The specific activity is not less than 0.5 microcurie per mcg of cyanocobalamin. Other radionuclides are absent. Cyanocobalamin Co 57 Solution contains a suitable bacteriostatic agent.

Caution—In making dosage calculations, correct for radioactive decay. The radioactive half-life of Co 57 is 270 days.

For the structure of Cyanocobalamin, see page 1034; its preparation is given on page 1037.

Description—Clear, colorless to pink solution. The pH is between 4.0 and 5.5.

Dose—See *Cyanocobalamin Co 57 Capsules.*
Dosage Forms—Solution USP: in such sizes as may be requested by the physician.

Cyanocobalamin Co 60 Capsules NF

Note—For the *Radiological Constants* of ^{60}Co, see *Cyanocobalamin Co 60 Solution* (this page).

Cyanocobalamin Co 60 Capsules contain cyanocobalamin in which a portion of the molecules contain radioactive cobalt (^{60}Co) in the molecular structure ($C_{63}H_{88}{}^{60}CoN_{14}O_{14}P$). Cyanocobalamin Co 60 Capsules contain 90.0–110.0% of the labeled amount of ^{60}Co as cyanocobalamin expressed in microcuries at the time indicated in the labeling. The cyanocobalamin content is 90.0–110.0% of the labeled amount. The specific activity is not less than 0.5 microcurie per mcg of cyanocobalamin. Other radionuclides are absent.

Caution—In making dosage calculations, correct for radioactive decay. The radioactive half-life of ^{60}Co is 5.27 years.

For the structure of Cyanocobalamin, see page 1034; its preparation is given on page 1037.

Description—May contain a small, rectangular solid, or may appear empty.

Uses—See *Cyanocobalamin Co 60 Solution.*
Dose—The equivalent of **0.5 to 1 microcurie;** *usual,* **0.5 to 2 mcg,** containing not more than 1 microcurie.
Dosage Forms—Capsules NF: in such sizes as may be requested by the physician.

Cyanocobalamin Co 60 Solution NF

[Radiocyanocobalamin (^{60}Co) Solution; Racobalamin 60 (*Abbott*); Rubrotope 60 (*Squibb*) Cobalt-60 Tagged Vitamin B-12 (*Nuclear Consultants*)]

Radiological Constants for ^{60}Co

Half-Life: 5.27 years
Radiations: Beta...............0.306 mev
                 Gamma............1.17 mev, 1.33 mev

Cyanocobalamin Co 60 Solution is a solution suitable for oral administration, containing cyanocobalamin in which a portion of the molecules contain radioactive cobalt (^{60}Co) in the molecular structure ($C_{63}H_{88}{}^{60}Co-N_{14}O_{14}P$).

Cyanocobalamin Co 60 Solution contains 90.0–110.0% of the labeled amount of ^{60}Co as cyanocobalamin expressed in microcuries at the time indicated in the labeling. The cyanocobalamin content is 90.0–110.0% of the labeled amount. The amount of cobalt 60 as cyanocobalamin is not more than 1 microcurie per ml. The specific activity is not less than 0.5 microcurie per mcg of cyanocobalamin. Other radionuclides are absent. Cyanocobalamin Co 60 Solution contains a suitable bacteriostatic agent.

Caution—In making dosage calculations, correct for radioactive decay. The radioactive half-life of ^{60}Co is 5.27 years.

For the structure of Cyanocobalamin, see page 1034.

Preparation—Cyanocobalamin, tagged with radioactive cobalt, is prepared by the growth of the organism *Lactobacillus leichmannii*, in the presence of radioactive cobalt salts and purified by a complex system of extractions. Since absorption from the gastrointestinal tract is markedly dependent on the specific activity, this should be kept as constant as possible, preferably in the range of 600 to 1000 μCi per mg of vitamin B$_{12}$. This is not difficult in the case of the ^{60}Co product because of the long half-life of the isotope.

Description—Clear, colorless to pink solution. The pH is between 4.0 and 5.5.

Uses—Cyanocobalamin Co 60 solution, ^{60}Co-labeled vitamin B$_{12}$, is used to study the absorption and deposition of vitamin B$_{12}$ in normal individuals and in patients with megaloblastic anemias. Since the normal human intestine can absorb significant amounts of the usually ingested quantities of vitamin B$_{12}$ only in the presence of the intrinsic factor, radiocyanocobalamin solution is useful in the diagnosis of pernicious anemia, a clinical condition characterized by a marked deficiency or absence of this factor. Three different tests, using the orally administered radioactive substance, have been used for the estimation of intrinsic factor activity: (1) the estimation of the unabsorbed tracer in the stool, (2) the measurement of the radiation emanating from the liver, and (3) the determination of urinary radioactivity following a large parenteral dose of nonradioactive vitamin B$_{12}$. The first test requires the analysis of total fecal collections for 5 to 10 days; the second necessitates repeated body surface counts using a scintillation counter; and the third directly quantitates, in terms of the administered vitamin B$_{12}$-^{60}Co, the radioactivity in a 24-hour urine sample. Although the half-life of ^{60}Co is 5.24 years, recent evidence suggests that cyanocobalamin Co 60 solution is subject to decomposition on storage. Therefore, it appears advisable to retest stocks for radiochemical purity at intervals of 1 month or less.

Dose—See *Cyanocobalamin Co 60 Capsules*.

Dosage Forms—Solution NF: in such sizes as may be directed by the physician.

Gold Au 198 Injection USP

[Radiogold Solution USP XVI; Sterile Radioactive Gold Colloid; Sterile Radiogold (Au^{198}) Colloid; Aurcoloid-198, Auroscan-198 (*Abbott*); Aureotope (*Squibb*)]

Radiological Constants for ^{198}Au

Half-Life:[111] 65 hours
Radiations:[112] Beta..............0.97 mev (99%)
Gamma............0.411 mev (96.1%)

Gold Au 198 Injection is a sterile, pyrogen-free, colloidal solution of radioactive gold (^{198}Au) stabilized by the addition of gelatin and suitable reducing agents. It contains 90.0–110.0% of the labeled amount of ^{198}Au as colloidal gold expressed in millicuries per ml at the time indicated in the labeling. Other chemical forms of radioactivity and other radionuclides are absent.

Caution—In making dosage calculations, correct for radioactive decay. The radioactive half-life of ^{198}Au is 2.70 days.

Description—It is a deep cherry-red, colloidal solution. The colloidal particle size ranges from 0.002 μ to 0.2 μ. Upon standing, both the Solution and the glass container may darken as a result of the effects of the radiation. The pH is between 4.3 and 6.3.

Use—Radiogold Solution is used as a *neoplastic suppressant*.

Administration is carried out by allowing a flow of saline from a conventional infusion system to pass through the bottle in which the colloid has been shipped. If the exit needle, leading to the body cavity, is at the bottom of the container, all activity can be transferred with a minimum of exposure to the operators. A silver-coated gold colloid has been studied and found effective, but it does not seem to have met with wide acceptance.

Dose—*Usual*, by *intracavitary injection*, **35 to 150 millicuries** as antineoplastic; *intravenous*, for *liver scanning*, **1 to 5 microcuries** per **Kg** of body weight.

Dosage Forms—Injection USP: in such volume as may be ordered for the individual needs of the patient.

Sodium Chromate Cr 51 Injection USP

[Sterile Radioactive Chromium Solution; Sterile Sodium Radiochromate (^{51}Cr) Solution; Rachromate (*Abbott*); Chromitope Sodium (*Squibb*)]

Radiological Constants for ^{51}Cr

Half-Life: 27.8 days
Radiations: Beta..............none
Gamma^{113}..........0.32 mev ($\sim$8%)
Other..............EC (emits 5 kev x-rays)

Sodium Chromate Cr 51 Injection is a sterile solution of radioactive chromium (^{51}Cr) processed in the form of sodium chromate in water for injection. For those uses where an isotonic solution is required, sodium chloride may be added in appropriate amounts as provided under *Injections*, page 1519. Chromium 51 is produced by the neutron bombardment of enriched chromium 50.

Sodium Chromate Cr 51 Injection contains 90.0–110.0% of the labeled amount of ^{51}Cr as sodium chromate expressed in millicuries at the time indicated in the labeling. The sodium chromate content is 90.0–110.0% of the labeled amount. The specific activity is not less than 40 millicuries per mg of sodium chromate at the time of standardization. Other chemical forms of radioactivity do not exceed 10.0% of the total radioactivity. Other radionuclides are absent.

Caution—In making dosage calculations, correct for radioactive decay and the quantity of chromium. The half-life of ^{51}Cr is 27.8 days.

Description—It is a clear, slightly yellow solution. The pH is between 7.5 and 8.5.

Uses—Sodium chromate Cr 51 is used as a biological tracer to measure circulating red cell volume, red cell survival time, and whole blood volume (red cell mass and plasma volume). To tag erythrocytes, a sample of the patient's blood or of donor blood is mixed with a solution of sodium chromate Cr 51 and allowed to remain until the isotope diffuses into cells (15 to 60 minutes). Once inside the cell, the bivalent chromate anion (CrO_4^{-2}) is reduced to the trivalent chromic cation (Cr^{+3}), which firmly associates with the globin portion of the cell contents. The unbound chromium (in the plasma) is either reduced with ascorbic acid or removed by washing the cells. The treated blood or suspension of cells is then injected into the circulation, time allowed for complete *in vivo* mixing, and samples taken for scintillation counting. Red cell or whole blood volume is estimated by the radioisotope dilution method. Normal mean values for whole blood volume obtained by the isotope method are 65.6 ± 5.95 ml per Kg of body weight.

Such tagged cells also provide an excellent means of studying red cell disappearance, as in hemolytic anemias and gastrointestinal bleeding. Platelets may also be labeled, though less effectively. For such purposes, it is essential that the specific activity be high—at least 5 to 15 mc per mg. Such a solution, prepared by the peroxide oxidation of $CrCl_3$, is essentially colorless.

For greatest tagging efficiency, sterile vials are available containing a special formula ACD solution. The blood and chromate are added directly to these vials wherein tagging takes place.

For those uses where chromic chloride is required, it may be easily secured by the addition of ascorbic acid to the above mentioned chromate solution.

Sodium radiochromate (^{51}Cr) has not been shown to produce any significant deleterious effects on normal erythrocytes.

The usual dose given below is mixed with 40 or 50 ml of whole blood withdrawn from the patient or from a compatible donor.

Dose—*Intravenous*, the equivalent of **10 to 200 microcuries**; *usual*, the equivalent of **50 microcuries**.

Dosage Forms—Injection USP: in such sizes as may be requested by the physician.

Sodium Iodide I 125 Solution USP

[Iodotope I-125 (*Squibb*); Sodium Iodide I 125 (*Abbott; Nuclear Consultants*)]

Note—For the *Radiological Constants of* ^{125}I, see *Iodinated I 125 Serum Albumin* (page 562).

Sodium Iodide I 125 Solution is a solution suitable for either oral or intravenous administration, containing radioactive iodide (^{125}I) processed in the form of sodium iodide from the neutron bombardment of xenon gas in such a manner that it is essentially carrier-free. Sodium Iodide I 125 Solution contains 90.0–110.0% of the labeled amount of ^{125}I as iodide expressed in microcuries or millicuries at the time indicated in the labeling. Other forms of radioactivity do not exceed 5.0% of the total radioactivity.

Caution—*In making dosage calculations, correct for radioactive decay. The radioactive half-life of* ^{125}I *is 60 days.*

Description—Clear, colorless solution. Upon standing, both the Solution and the glass container may darken as a result of the effects of the radiation.

Uses—Sodium Iodide I 125 Solution is used as a *diagnostic aid* in determining *thyroid function*.

Dose—*Usual, oral, diagnostic*, the equivalent of **50 to 100 microcuries**.

Dosage Forms—Solution USP: in such volumes as may be requested by the physician.

Sodium Iodide I 131 Capsules USP

[Radioactive Iodine Capsules]

Note—For the *Radiological Constants of* ^{131}I, see *Iodinated I 131 Serum Albumin* (page 563).

Sodium Iodide I 131 Capsules contain radioactive iodine (^{131}I) processed in the form of sodium iodide from products of uranium fission or the neutron bombardment of tellurium in such manner that it is essentially carrier-free and contains only minute amounts of naturally-occurring iodine 127.

Each Capsule contains 90.0–110.0% of the labeled amount of ^{131}I as iodide expressed in microcuries or in millicuries at the time indicated in the labeling. The activity of each Capsule is 97.0–103.0% of the mean activity of the individual Capsules in the lot. Other chemical forms of radioactivity do not exceed 5.0% of the total radioactivity. Other radionuclides are absent.

Caution—*In making dosage calculations, correct for radioactive decay. The half-life of* ^{131}I *is 8.08 days (see above).*

Preparation—These are prepared by the evaporation of an alcoholic solution of carrier-free iodide on the interior wall of a gelatin capsule. The activity remains firmly attached and, especially if the unit is sealed, capsules provide an extremely convenient and safe way of handling and administering both diagnostic and therapeutic doses of radioiodide.

Description—They may contain a small amount of solid or solids, or may appear empty.

Uses—See *Sodium Iodide I 131 Solution*.

Dose—*Usual, oral* or *intravenous, diagnostic*, the equivalent of **1 to 100 microcuries**; *therapeutic*, the equivalent of **1 to 200 millicuries**.

Dosage Forms—Capsules USP: in such sizes as may be directed by the physician.

Sodium Iodide I 131 Solution USP

[Radioactive Iodine Solution; Sodium Radio-iodide (I^{131}) Solution (USP XV) Oriodide-131, Theriodide-131 (*Abbott*); Iodotope I-131, Iodotope Therapeutic (*Squibb*)]

Note—For the *Radiological Constants of* ^{131}I, see *Iodinated I 131 Serum Albumin* (page 563).

Sodium Iodide I 131 Solution is a solution suitable for either oral or intravenous administration, containing radioactive iodine (^{131}I) processed in the form of sodium iodide from the products of uranium fission or the neutron bombardment of tellurium in such manner that it is essentially carrier-free and contains only minute amounts of naturally-occurring iodine 127.

Sodium Iodide I 131 Solution contains 90.0–110.0% of the labeled amount of ^{131}I as iodide expressed in microcuries or millicuries at the time indicated in the labeling. Other chemical forms of radioactivity do not exceed 5.0% of the total radioactivity. Other radionuclides are absent.

Caution—*In making dosage calculations, correct for radioactive decay. The radioactive half-life of* ^{131}I *is 8.08 days.*

Description—It is a clear, colorless solution. Upon standing, both the solution and the glass container may darken as a result of the effects of the radiation. The pH is between 7.5 and 9.0.

Uses—Sodium Iodide I 131 Solution is used as a *diagnostic aid* in determining thyroid function and as a *neoplastic suppressant*.

Dose—See *Sodium Iodide I 131 Capsules.*

Dosage Forms—Solution USP: in such volumes as may be requested by the physician.

Sodium Iodohippurate I 131 Injection USP

[Sodium *o*-Iodohippurate-[131]I Injection; Hipputope (*Squibb*) Hippuran-131 (*Abbott*); Hippuran I 131 (*Nuclear Consultants*)]

Note—For the *Radiological Constants of* [131]I see *Iodinated I 131 Serum Albumin* (page 563).

CONHCH$_2$COONa
I

Sodium Iodohippurate I 131 Injection is a sterile solution containing sodium *o*-iodohippurate in which a portion of the molecules contain radioactive iodine (^{131}I) in the molecular structure ($C_9H_7{}^{131}INNaO_3$).

Sodium Iodohippurate I 131 Injection contains 90.0–110.0% of the labeled amount of ^{131}I as sodium iodohippurate expressed in microcuries or millicuries at the time indicated in the labeling. Other chemical forms of radioactivity do not exceed 3.0% of the total radioactivity. Other radionuclides are absent.

Caution—In making dosage calculations, correct for radioactive decay. The radioactive half-life of ^{131}I is 8.08 days.

Preparation—*o*-Iodobenzoyl chloride-^{131}I is condensed with glycine with the aid of a dehydrochlorinating agent and the resulting *o*-iodohippuric acid is reacted with sodium hydroxide.

Description—Clear, colorless solution. The pH is between 7.0 and 8.5.

Uses—The excretion of certain compounds is almost entirely by way of the kidneys. If both kidneys are functioning properly, each should excrete approximately 50% of these compounds or any other substance with a blood concentration in excess of the renal threshold. The performance of the kidneys can be determined by injection of a radioactive compound which is quickly and exclusively excreted by the kidneys. The radioactive tag is selected from those nuclides which emit gamma radiation to permit external detection of the isotope. The relative concentration of the tagged compound in each kidney can then be measured by means of two identical crystal scintillation detectors, one being positioned over each kidney. Renal malfunction is indicated if the measured activities are unequal.

Dose—*Usual, intravenous, diagnostic*, the equivalent of **2 to 35 microcuries.**

Dosage Forms—Injection USP: in such volumes as may be requested by the physician.

Sodium Phosphate P 32 Solution USP

[Radioactive Phosphorus Solution; Sodium Radio-phosphate (P^{32}) Solution (USP XV); Phosphotope (*Squibb*)]

Radiological Constants for ^{32}P

Half-Life:	14.3 days
Radiations:	Beta.........................1.71 mev
	Gamma.......................none

Sodium Phosphate P 32 Solution is a solution suitable for either oral or intravenous administration, containing radioactive phosphorus (^{32}P) processed in the form of sodium phosphate from the neutron bombardment of elemental sulfur. Inactive sodium phosphate may be added during the processing.

Sodium Phosphate P 32 Solution contains 90.0–110.0% of the labeled amount of ^{32}P as phosphate expressed in microcuries or millicuries at the time indicated in the labeling. Other chemical forms of radioactivity are absent.

Caution—In making dosage calculations, correct for radioactivity decay. The radioactive half-life of ^{32}P is 14.3 days.

Description—Clear, colorless solution. Upon standing, both the Solution and the glass container may darken as a result of the effects of the radiation. The pH is between 5 and 6.

Uses—Sodium Phosphate P 32 Solution is used as a *neoplastic* and *polycythemic suppressant* and as a *diagnostic aid*.

Dose—*Usual, oral or intravenous, diagnostic*, the equivalent of **250 microcuries to 1 millicurie;** *therapeutic*, the equivalent of **1 to 12 millicuries.**

Dosage Forms—Solution USP: in such volumes as may be requested by the physician.

Sodium Rose Bengal I 131 Injection USP

[Disodium 4,5,6,7-Tetrachloro-2′,4′,5′,7′-tetraiodofluorescein-[131]I Injection; Robengatope (*Squibb*)]

Note—For the *Radiological Constants of* [131]I see *Iodinated I 131 Serum Albumin* (page 563).

Sodium Rose Bengal I 131 Injection is a sterile solution containing sodium rose bengal in which a portion of the molecules contain radioactive iodine (^{131}I) in the molecular structure ($C_{20}H_2Cl_4{}^{131}I_4Na_2O_5$). It may contain a suitable buffer.

Sodium Rose Bengal I 131 Injection contains 90.0–110.0% of the labeled amount of ^{131}I as sodium rose bengal expressed in microcuries or millicuries at the time indicated in the labeling. The sodium rose bengal content is 90.0–110.0% of the labeled amount. Other chemical forms of radioactivity do not exceed 10.0% of the total radioactivity. Other radionuclides are absent.

Caution—In making dosage calculations, correct for radioactive decay. The radioactive half-life of ^{131}I is 8.08 days.

Preparation—Sodium Rose Bengal may be prepared by the thermal condensation of tetrachlorophthalic anhydride with 2,4-diiodoresorcinol and reacting the resulting phthalein with sodium hydroxide.

Description—Clear, deep-red solution. The pH is between 7.0 and 8.5.

Uses—Sodium Rose Bengal I 131 Injection is used as a *diagnostic aid* (*liver function*).

Dose—*Intravenous*, the equivalent of **10 to 200 microcuries;** *usual*, the equivalent of **150 microcuries.**

Dosage Forms—Injection USP: in such volumes as may be requested by the physician.

Unofficial Radiopharmaceuticals

Chromic Phosphate P 32

[Chromic Phosphate P 32 Suspension, Chromic Phosphate P 32 (*Abbott*); Chromphosphotope (*Squibb*); Phosphocol (*Nuclear Consultants*)]

Note—For the *radiological constants of* ^{32}P, see *Sodium Phosphate P 32 Solution USP* (page 567).

Chromic Phosphate P 32 is supplied as a sterile suspension of $Cr^{32}PO_4$ in a suitable vehicle. The suspension is grayish-green to brownish-green in color.

Uses—Chromic Phosphate P 32 is used as a neoplastic suppressant and has given best results for the palliative treatment of pleural and peritoneal effusions. For this purpose it has largely replaced Gold Au 198 Solution. Because ^{32}P emits no gamma component in its radiation (other than Bremsstrahlung), the hazard to personnel is greatly reduced. In addition, the dose delivered per millicurie during an effective half-life period is about 10 times greater for ^{32}P than for ^{198}Au. Relatively smaller doses of ^{32}P can therefore be used, the usual dose being about 5 millicuries intrapleurally and about 10 millicuries intraperitoneally.

Cobalt Co 60 and Iridium Ir 192 Sources

[Actaloy Wire Sources (*Abbott*); Iriditope (*Squibb*)]

Radiological Constants for ^{60}Co

Note—See *Cyanocobalamin Co 60 Solution* (page 564).

Radiological Constants for ^{192}Ir

Half-Life: 74.37 days
Radiations: Beta[114]......0.673 mev (48%), 0.537 mev (41%)

Gamma[114]...0.316 mev (80%), 0.468 mev (51%), 0.296 mev (29%), 0.308 mev (28%), 0.605 mev (11%), 0.613 mev (7%), 0.484 mev (6%), 0.589 mev (6%)

Other.......EC

Cobalt-60 has replaced radium, which is relatively expensive, for many radiation uses of the latter element. The use of cobalt-60 in alloys rather than the pure metal has increased the physical stability, making quite feasible its incorporation in sealed cells to fit various applicators. The 1.17 and 1.3 mev gamma radiation is fully the equivalent of radium in biological effectiveness.

Iridium-192 provides a softer radiation, i.e., less penetrating; the radioactive source is enclosed in nylon for interstitial use.

Insulin I 125 and Insulin I 131

[Insulin I 125 (*Nuclear Consultants*); Inusay-125 (*Abbott*)]
[Insulin I 131 (*Abbott; Nuclear Consultants*); Inusay-131 (*Abbott*)]

Note—For the *Radiological Constants of* ^{125}I, see *Iodinated I 125 Serum Albumin* (page 562). For the *Radiological Constants of* ^{131}I, see *Iodinated I 131 Serum Albumin* (page 563).

Insulin I 125 and Insulin I 131 are insulin containing a radioactive tag of ^{125}I and ^{131}I, respectively. The radioactive insulins are prepared by mild iodination with high-specific-activity radioactive iodine. Iodination is followed by purification of the product by means of dialysis, ion-exchange and other processes. It is assumed that the addition of radioactive iodine occurs on available tyrosine moieties.

Radioactive insulin is used for the *in vitro* assay of circulating insulin, either free or bound. If prepared for use in humans, radioactively tagged insulin can also be used to study insulin kinetics including plasma disappearance.

Iron-59 as Ferric Chloride Fe 59, Ferrous Citrate Fe 59, or Ferrous Sulfate Fe 59

[Ferric Chloride Fe 59 (*Abbott*); Fe-59 Ferric Chloride (*Nuclear Consultants*)]
[Ferrous Citrate Fe 59 (*Abbott*); Fe-59 Ferrous Citrate (*Nuclear Consultants*); Ferrutope (*Squibb*)]
[Ferrous Sulfate Fe 59 (*Abbott*); Fe-59 Ferrous Sulfate (*Nuclear Consultants*)]

Radiological Constants for ^{59}Fe

Half-Life: 45.1 days
Radiations:[115]   Beta......0.462 mev (54%), 0.271 mev (46%)

Gamma...0.191 mev, 1.098 mev, 1.289 mev

Ferrous citrate is especially useful in that it may be administered directly into the blood stream where it reacts with the metal-binding globulin normally present in excess, thus avoiding the isolation and *in vitro* tagging of that protein. The rate of disappearance of iron-59 from the blood, the rate of reincorporation into red cells, and the intermediate storage in the reticuloendothelial system may all be followed by appropriate gamma counting techniques.

Uses—Iron-59, in the form of ferrous citrate, ferrous sulfate, or ferric chloride, is used in ferrokinetic studies of iron absorption and turnover rates.

Oleic Acid I 125, Oleic Acid I 131, Triolein I 125, and Triolein I 131

[Oleotope I-125 (*Squibb*); Oleic Acid I 125 (*Nuclear Consultants*)]
[Raoleic Acid-131 (*Abbott*); Oleotope and Oleotope Diagnostic (*Squibb*); Oleic Acid I 131 (*Nuclear Consultants*)]
[Triolein I 125 (*Nuclear Consultants*)]
[Raolin-131 (*Abbott*); Triolein I 131 (*Nuclear Consultants*); Trioleotope (*Squibb*)]

Radiological Constants for ^{125}I

Note—See *Iodinated I 125 Serum Albumin* (page 562).

Radiological Constants for ^{131}I

Note—See *Iodinated I 131 Serum Albumin* (page 563).

Iodinated triolein is prepared by the action of iodine monochloride on the highly purified fat, triolein, in a carbon tetrachloride solution. After removal of the solvent, and also any "free iodide," it is diluted with peanut oil to an activity of about 1 mc per ml. The iodine bond is relatively stable in the digestive tract, but is liberated as the molecule is metabolized in the blood stream and tissues.

Iodinated oleic acid is prepared in a similar manner and has similar properties.

Uses—These are used as diagnostic agents for measuring fat absorption in suspected pancreatic disease or other gastrointestinal dysfunction. The use of these agents is based on the fact that the triolein, requiring pancreatic lipase for hydrolysis prior to passage through the gastrointestinal wall, is not absorbed in cases of pancreatitis and cystic fibrosis, while the free acid, not requiring such hydrolysis, is taken up in the normal fashion. The assay for extent of absorption

Table III—Unofficial Radiopharmaceuticals

Nonproprietary name	Available forms
Calcium Chloride Ca 45	Calcium Chloride Ca 45 (*Abbott; Nuclear Consultants*)
Calcium Chloride Ca 47	Calcium Chloride Ca 47 (*Abbott*)
Cesium Chloride Cs 131	Cescan-131 (*Abbott*)
Chromated Cr 51 Serum Albumin	Chromalbin (Squibb)
Chromic Chloride Cr 51	Chromic Chloride Cr 51 (*Abbott; Nuclear Consultants*); Chromitope Chloride (*Squibb*)
Chromic Phosphate Cr 51	
Chromic Phosphate P 32	Chromphosphotope (*Squibb*); Chromic Phosphate P 32 (*Abbott*); Phosphocol (*Nuclear Consultants*)
Cobalt Co 60	Actaloy Wire Sources (*Abbott*)
Cobaltous Chloride Co 57	Cobaltous Chloride Co 57 (*Abbott*); Cobatope-57 (*Squibb*)
Cobaltous Chloride Co 60	Cobatope-60 (*Squibb*)
Cupric Acetate Cu 64	Cupric Acetate Cu 64 (*Abbott*)
Deuterium Oxide	Deuterium Oxide (*Abbott*)
Diohippuric Acid I 125	
Diohippuric Acid I 131	
Diotyrosine I 131	Diotyrosine I 131 (*Abbott*)
Ethiodized Oil I 131	Ethiodol-131 (*Abbott*)
Ferric Chloride Fe 59	Ferric Chloride Fe 59 (*Abbott*); Fe-59 Ferric Chloride (*Nuclear Consultants*)
Ferrous Citrate Fe 59	Ferrous Citrate Fe 59 (*Abbott*); Fe-59 Ferrous Citrate (*Nuclear Consultants*); Ferrutope (*Squibb*)
Ferrous Sulfate Fe 59	Ferrous Sulfate Fe 59 (*Abbott*); Fe-59 Ferrous Sulfate (*Nuclear Consultants*)
Insulin I 125	Insulin I 125 (*Nuclear Consultants*); Inusay-125 (*Abbott*)
Insulin I 131	Insulin I 131 (*Abbott; Nuclear Consultants*); Inusay-131 (*Abbott*)
Iodinated I 131 Serum Albumin Aggregated	Albumotope-LS and Albumotope-H (*Squibb*); Aggregated Radioiodinated (I 131) Albumin (Human) (*Nuclear Consultants*)
Iodoantipyrine I 131	Iodoantipyrine I 131 (*Abbott; Nuclear Consultants*)
Iodopyracet I 125	
Iodopyracet I 131	Diodrast-131 (*Abbott*); Diodrast, Iodopyracet I 131 (*Nuclear Consultants*)
Iotyrosine I 131	Iotyrosine I 131 (*Abbott*)
Iridium Ir 192	Iriditope (*Squibb*)
Krypton Clathrate Kr 85	
Liothyronine I 125	Lyothyronine I 125 (*Nuclear Consultants*)
Liothyronine I 131	Triomet-131 (*Abbott*); Tri-Thyrotope (*Squibb*); Liothyronine I 131 (*Nuclear Consultants*)
Merisoprol Hg 197	Merprane (*Squibb*)
Merisoprol Acetate Hg 197	MHP Acetate Hg 197 (*Nuclear Consultants*)
Merisoprol Acetate Hg 203	MHP Acetate Hg 203 (*Nuclear Consultants*)
Oleic Acid I 125	Oleotope I-125 (*Squibb*); Oleic Acid I 125 (*Nuclear Consultants*)
Oleic Acid I 131	Raoleic Acid-131 (*Abbott*): Oleotope, Oleotope Diagnostic (*Squibb*); Oleic Acid I 131 (*Nuclear Consultants*)
Polymetaphosphate P 32	Polymetaphosphate P 32 (*Nuclear Consultants*)
Potassium Chloride K 42	Potassium Chloride K 42 (*Abbott*)
Povidone I 125	
Povidone I 131	
Rubidium Chloride Rb 86	Rubidium Chloride Rb 86 (*Abbott; Nuclear Consultants*)
Selenomethionine Se 75	Sethotope (*Squibb*); Selenomethionine Se 75 (*Nuclear Consultants*)
Sodium Arsenate As 74	Sodium Arsenate As 74 (*Abbott*)
Sodium Chloride Na 22	Sodium Chloride Na 22 (*Abbott; Nuclear Consultants*)
Sodium Diatrizoate I 125	Hypaque (*Nuclear Consultants*)
Sodium Diatrizoate I 131	Radio-Renografin (*Squibb*); Hypaque (*Nuclear Consultants*); Hypaque-131 Sodium (*Abbott*)
Sodium Iodide I 125	Iodotope I-125 (*Squibb*); Sodium Iodide I 125 (*Abbott; Nuclear Consultants*)
Sodium Iodipamide I 131	Radio-Cholografin (*Squibb*)
Sodium Iodohippurate I 125	Hipputope I-125 (*Squibb*); Hippuran-125 (*Abbott*); Hippuran I 125 (*Nuclear Consultants*)
Sodium Iothalamate I 125	Glofil-125 (*Abbott*)
Sodium Iothalamate I 131	Glofil-131 (*Abbott*)
Sodium Pertechnetate Tc 99m	Sodium Pertechnetate Tc 99m (*Nuclear Consultants*)
Sodium Rose Bengal I 125	Rose Bengal Sodium I 125 (*Abbott*); Rose Bengal I 125 (*Nuclear Consultants*); Robengatope I-125 (*Squibb*)
Sodium Sulfate S 35	Sodium Sulfate S 35 (*Abbott*)
Strontium Chloride Sr 85	Strontium Chloride Sr 85 (*Abbott; Nuclear Consultants*)
Strontium Nitrate Sr 85	Strotope (*Squibb*); Strontium Nitrate Sr 85 (*Nuclear Consultants*)
Technetium Tc 99m	Technetope (*Squibb*); TechneKow Tc 99m (*Nuclear Consultants*)
Thyroxine I 125	Thyroxine I 125 (*Nuclear Consultants*)
Thyroxine I 131	Thyroxine I 131 (*Abbott; Nuclear Consultants*); Thyroxine (*Squibb*)
Tolpovidone I 131	Raovin-131 (*Abbott*)
Triolein I 125	Triolein I 125 (*Nuclear Consultants*)
Triolein I 131	Raolein-131 (*Abbott*); Triolein I 131 (*Nuclear Consultants*); Trioleotope (*Squibb*)
Tritiated Water	Tritiated Water (*Abbott*); Tritiotope (*Squibb*)
Zinc Chloride Zn 65	Zinc Chloride Zn 65 (*Nuclear Consultants*)

may be made on blood samples taken 2 to 8 hours after administration, or on 24 to 36-hour stool samples.

Liothyronine I 131

[T-3; Triomet (*Abbott*); Tri-Thyrotope (*Squibb*); Liothyronine I 131 (*Nuclear Consultants*)]

Note—For the *Radiological Constants of* ^{131}I, see *Iodinated I 131 Serum Albumin* (page 563).

Liothyronine I 131 ($C_{15}H_{12}{}^{131}I_3NNaO_4$), commonly called T-3, is prepared by the exchange of crystalline synthetic hormone with ^{131}I under carefully controlled conditions. Since such reactions always result in a mixture of products, purification must be effected by column and/or paper strip chromatography.

Due to the high specific activity required, radiation damage can easily take place. This is in part prevented by the use of propylene glycol (50%) as a solvent. Packages should be refrigerated or even frozen during storage, and should not be used longer than two weeks.

For the structure of Liothyronine, see *Sodium Liothyronine*, page 985.

Uses—These tagged hormones are used in studies of metabolism. In one such study red cell uptake of T-3 is used as a test for thyroid function.

Sodium Chloride Na 22 Injection

[Sodium Chloride Na 22 (*Abbott; Nuclear Consultants*)]

Radiological Constants for ^{22}Na

Half-Life: 2.58 years
Radiations: Beta............β^+ 0.54 (89%)
             Gamma..........1.28 (100%), 0.51
                            (annihilation radiation)
             Other...........EC (11%)

Uses—Sodium 22 is cyclotron produced by bombarding magnesium-24 with deuterons. The reaction is $^{24}Mg(d,\alpha)^{22}Na$. While the use of sodium-24 has certain advantages over the use of sodium-22 in medicine, its half-life of only 15 hours creates problems of supply and the usual tracer dose of sodium-22 is well within the accepted tolerance level.

Because sodium-22 emits positrons it can be detected readily by coincidence counting methods which combine the advantages of low background activity with high resolution.

Sodium Chloride Na 22 has been used for the determination of "circulation times," "the sodium space," and "total exchangeable sodium."

Sodium Iodide I 125 Capsules

[Iodotope I-125 (*Squibb*); Sodium Iodide I 125 (*Abbott; Nuclear Consultants*)]

Note—For the *Radiological Constants of* ^{125}I, see *Iodinated I 125 Serum Albumin* (*page 562*).

Sodium Iodide I 125 Capsules contain radioactive iodine (^{125}I) processed in the form of sodium iodide from the neutron bombardment of xenon 124 in such manner that it is essentially carrier-free. Each capsule contains 90.0–110.0% of the labeled amount of ^{125}I as iodide expressed in microcuries or in millicuries per ml at the time indicated in the labeling. Other forms of radioactivity do not exceed 5.0% of the total radioactivity.

Description—May contain a small solid or solids, or may appear empty.

Uses and **Dose**—See *Sodium Iodide I 125 Solution*, page 563.

Sodium Iodide (^{131}I) Injection BP

Note—For the *Radiological Constants of* ^{131}I, see *Iodinated I 131 Serum Albumin* (page 563).

This is a sterile solution which complies with the tests for Sodium (^{131}I) Solution BP for identity and purity. Because it is sterile it can be used for intravenous administration.

Sodium Pertechnetate Tc 99m and Technetium Tc 99m

[Sodium Pertechnetate Tc 99m; TechneKow Tc 99m (*Nuclear Consultants*); Technetope (*Squibb*); Pertgen-99m (*Abbott*)]

Radiological Constants for ^{99m}Tc

Half-Life: 5.997 hours
Radiations: Beta............None
             Gamma........IT, 0.002 (98.6%), 0.140
                         (98.6%), 0.142 (1.4%)

Technetium 99m is obtained by elution of a generator or "cow" containing Molybdenum-99 (half-life: 67 hours). Decay of ^{99}Mo results in the buildup of its daughter, ^{99m}Tc, at a rate which permits eluting the generator about once a day.

Generators are usually sterilized by the manufacturer so a sterile, pyrogen-free solution of sodium pertechnetate Tc 99m can be obtained by means of asceptic elution. Prior to use, the sodium pertechnetate Tc 99m solution should be assayed. Cobalt-57 standards are usually used for this purpose since the 123 kev and 137 kev photopeaks of ^{57}Co are of nearly the same energy as the 140 kev and 142 kev photopeaks of ^{99m}Tc.

^{99m}Tc is an almost ideal isotope for medical applications. Its half-life is long enough to allow completion of diagnostic procedures using it yet short enough that the radiation dose to the patient is minimal. Lack of a beta component in the radiation further decreases the dose delivered to the patient. Because greater activities can therefore be used scanning time can be reduced accordingly. The 140 kev gamma energy is weak enough that good collimation is readily achieved yet hard enough to penetrate tissue so deep organ scanning is possible.

The chemistry of technetium is similar to that of other members of Group VIIB, manganese and rhenium. The pertechnetate $TcO_4{}^{-1}$ resembles iodine in that it is taken up by the thyroid. To reduce thyroid uptake of ^{99m}Tc a protective dose of potassium perchlorate is often administered.

Sodium pertechnetate Tc 99m has been used for the detection and location of cranial lesions. As the sulfide, ^{99m}Tc has also been used for liver visualization.

Sodium Phosphate (^{32}P) Injection BP

Note—For the *Radiological Constants of* ^{32}P, see *Sodium Phosphate P 32 Solution* (page 567).

This is a sterile solution of sodium phosphate P-32 in saline solution isotonic with blood. The solution contains added phosphate as a carrier but the specific activity is not less than 1 mc per mg of phosphate ion. Specifications are given for its identification by means of the beta ray absorption curve and for its radiochemical purity using a descending chromatographic technique. It is administered in the treatment of polycythemia vera by intravenous injection. The initial dose is 5 mc which may be followed by a dose of 3 mc in 3 months according to the needs of the patient.

Thyroxine I 125 and Thyroxine I 131

[Thyroxine I 125 (*Nuclear Consultants*)]
[Thyroxine I 131 (*Abbott; Nuclear Consultants*); Thyroxine (*Squibb*)]

Note—For the *Radiological Constants of* ^{125}I, see *Iodinated I 125 Serum Albumin* (page 562). For the *Radiological Constants of* ^{131}I, see *Iodinated I 131 Serum Albumin* (page 563).

For the structure of Thyroxine, see page 986.

Thyroxine, labeled with either ^{125}I or ^{131}I is chemically synthesized L-thyroxine ($C_{15}H_{11}I_4NO_4$) which has been tagged with radioactive iodine in the 3' position.

Labeled thyroxine is used to study the metabolism of endogenous thyroxine and supplements other tests of thyroid function. Following administration of a tracer dose, serial blood samples are measured for radioactivity. When data are plotted on semilogarithmic paper the disappearance half-time, calculated from the curve, provides useful information on thyroid function.

Radioactively labeled thyroxine is also used to measure thyroxine-binding protein capacity. When incubated with a small amount of the patients serum, endogenous and tagged thyroxine will exchange and equilibrate. Separated by electrophoresis, the extent of binding can be determined by measuring the radioactivity of the bound and unbound thyroxine fractions.

References

1. *Technical Data Sheet, Bull. A-7839*, E. R. Squibb & Sons, New York, Apr. 1962.
2. Flocks, R. H., *et al*, in Hahn, P. F., ed, *Therapeutic Use of Artificial Radioisotopes*, Wiley, New York, 1956.
3. Sherman, A. I., in Hahn, P. F., ed, *Therapeutic Use of Artificial Radioisotopes*, Wiley, New York, 1956.
4. Nelson, C., *Southern Med. J.*, **48**, 245 (Mar., 1955).
5. *Technical Data Sheet, Bull. A-8097*, E. R. Squibb & Sons, New York, June, 1962.
6. *Technical Data Sheet, Bull. A-8096*, E. R. Squibb & Sons, New York, June, 1962.
7. Fields, T., *et al*, *J. Lab. Clin. Med.*, **43**, 332 (1954).
8. Erickson, J. R., *et al*, *Science*, **118**, 595 (1953).
9. Prentice, T. C., *et al*, *J. Clin. Invest.*, **31**, 412 (1951).
10. Forbes, G. B., and Perley, A., *J. Clin. Invest.*, **30**, 558 (1951).
11. Corsa, L., Jr., *et al*, *J. Clin. Invest.*, **29**, 1280 (1950).
12. Robinson, C. V., *et al*, *J. Clin. Invest.*, **34**, 134 (1955).
13. Wallace, G. B., and Brodie, B. B., *J. Pharmacol. Exptl. Therap.*, **65**, 214 (1939).
14. Wright, H. P., *et al*, *J. Obstet. Gynaecol. Brit. Empire*, **56**, 36 (1949).
15. Quimby, E. H., *Am. J. Roentgenol.*, **75**, 1068 (1956).
16. MacIntyre, W. J., *et al*, *Radiology*, **59**, 849 (1952).
17. Huff, R. L., *et al*, *J. Clin. Invest.*, **33**, 944 (1954).
18. Conway, H., *et al*, *Proc. Soc. Exptl. Biol. Med.*, **77**, 348 (1951).
19. Kiehn, C. L., *et al*, *A. M. A. Arch. Surg.*, **65**, 477 (1951).
20. Bannerman, R. M., *Brit. Med. J.*, **II**, 1032 (1957).
21. Ebaugh, F. G., Jr., *et al*, *Am. J. Med.*, **25**, 169 (1958).
22. Jones, H. C. H., *Brit. Med. J.*, **I**, 493 (1958).
23. Owen, C. S., Jr., *et al*, *J. Lab. Clin. Med.*, **44**, 238 (1954).
24. Roche, M., *et al*, *J. Clin. Invest.*, **36**, 1183 (1957).
25. Hertz, S., *et al*, *Proc. Soc. Exptl. Biol. Med.*, **38**, 510 (1938).
26. Hamilton, J. G., and Solely, M. H., *Am. J. Physiol.*, **127**, 557 (1939); **131**, 135 (1940).
27. Oddie, T. H., *Brit. J. Radiol.*, **22**, 261 (1949).
28. Luellen, T. J., *et al*, *J. Clin. Invest.*, **28**, 207 (1949).
29. Riggs, D. S., *Pharmacol. Rev.*, **4**, 284 (1952).
30. Hare, E. H., and Haigh, C. P., *Clin. Sci.*, **14**, 441 (1955).
31. Bishopric, G. A., *et al*, *J. Clin. Endocrinol. Metab.*, **15**, 592 (1955).
32. Rall, J. E., *Am. J. Med.*, **20**, 719 (1956).
33. Keating, F. R., Jr., *et al*, *J. Clin. Invest.*, **26**, 1138 (1947).
34. Childs, D. S., Jr., *et al*, *J. Clin. Invest.*, **29**, 726 (1950).
35. Perry, W. F., and Hughes, J. F. S., *J. Clin. Invest.*, **34**, 454 (1952).
36. Berson, S. A., *et al*, *J. Clin. Invest.*, **31**, 141 (1952).
37. Fraser, R., *et al*, *Quart. J. Med.*, **22**, 99 (1953).
38. Hlad, C. J., Jr., and Bricker, N. S., *J. Clin. Endocrinol. Metab.*, **14**, 1939 (1954).
39. Clark, D. E., *et al*, *Surgery*, **26**, 331 (1949).
40. Harsha, W. N., *J. Clin. Endocrinol.*, **11**, 1524 (1951).
41. Sheline, G. E., *et al*, *J. Clin. Endocrinol.*, **11**, 91 (1951).
42. Scott, K. G., and Reilly, W. A., *Metab. Clin. Exptl.*, **3**, 506 (1954).
43. Van Middleworth, L., *et al*, *J. Clin. Endocrinol. Metab.*, **14**, 1056 (1954).
44. Paley, K. R., *et al*, *J. Clin. Endocrinol. Metab.*, **15**, 995 (1955).
45. Clarke, K. H., and Sherriff, E. V., *Med. J. Australia*, **II**, 89 (1955).
46. Fields, T., *et al*, *J. Lab. Clin. Med.*, **47**, 333 (1956).
47. Zieve, L., *et al*, *J. Lab. Clin. Med.*, **47**, 663 (1956).
48. Hamolsky, M. M., *et al*, *J. Clin. Endocrinol. Metab.*, **17**, 33 (1957). **19**, 103 (1959); **19**, 92 (1959).
49. Shapiro, B., and Rabinowitz, J. L., *J. Nucl. Med.*, **3**, 417 (1962).
50. Rabinowitz, J. L., and Shapiro, B., *J. Nucl. Med.*, **3**, 181 (1962).
51. Schilling, R. F., *J. Lab. Clin. Med.*, **42**, 860 (1953).
52. Schilling, R. F., *et al*, *J. Lab. Clin. Med.*, **45**, 926 (1955).
53. Krevans, J. R., *et al*, *J. Chronic Diseases*, **3**, 234 (1956).
54. Meyer, L. M., *et al*, *Proc. Soc. Exptl. Biol. Med.*, **91**, 129 (1956).
55. Rath, C. E., *et al*, *Blood*, **11**, 96 (1956).
56. Reisner, E. H., Jr., *Am. J. Clin. Nutr.*, **4**, 134 (1956).
57. Arias, I. M., *et al*, *New Engl. J. Med.*, **255**, 164 (1956).
58. Goldberg, S. R., *et al*, *J. Lab. Clin. Med.*, **49**, 582 (1957).
59. Grasbeck, R., *et al*, *Proc. Soc. Exptl. Biol. Med.*, **97**, 780 (1958).
60. Dubach, R., *et al*, *J. Lab. Clin. Med.*, **31**, 1201 (1946).
61. Finch, C. A., *et al*, *Blood*, **4**, 905 (1949).
62. Huff, R. L., *et al*, *J. Clin. Invest.*, **29**, 1041 (1950).
63. Loeffler, R. K., *et al*, *Proc. Soc. Exptl. Biol. Med*, **88**, 441 (1955).
64. Spencer, R. P., *et al*, *Am. J. Clin. Pathol.*, **28**, 123 (1957).
65. Bothwell, T. H., *et al*, *Blood*, **12**, 409 (1957).
66. Finch, C. A., *et al*, *Blood*, **11**, 807 (1956).
67. Teng, C. T., *et al*, *Am. J. Roentgenol.*, **84**, 687 (1960).
68. Pollycove, M., and Mortimer, R., *J. Clin. Invest.*, **40**, 753 (1961).
69. LeRoy, G. V., *Ann. Internal Med.*, **42**, 239 (1955).
70. Rabinowitz, J. L., *et al*, *Proc. Soc. Exptl. Biol. Med.*, **105**, 241 (1960).
71. Rabinowitz, J. L., *et al*, *Biochim. Biophys. Acta*, **27**, 544 (1958).
72. Stanley, M. M., and Thannhauser, S. J., *J. Lab. Clin. Med.*, **34**, 1634 (1949).
73. Ruffin, J. N., *et al*, *New Engl. J. Med.*, **255**, 595 (1956).
74. Maln, J. R., *et al*, *Proc. Soc. Exptl. Biol. Med.*, **92**, 471 (1956).
75. Beres, P., *et al*, *Gastroenterology*, **32**, 1 (1957).
76. Berkowitz, D., *et al*, *Ann. Internal Med.*, **50**, 247 (1959).
77. Likoff, W., *et al*, *Circulation*, **18**, 1118 (1958).
78. Seller, R. H., *et al*, *Am. J. Med.*, **27**, 231 (1959).
79. Taplin, G. V., *et al*, *J. Lab. Clin. Med.*, **45**, 665 (1955).
80. Taplin, G. V., *et al*, *J. Lab. Clin. Med.*, **48**, 886 (1956).
81. Schloesser, L. L., *et al*, *J. Clin. Invest.*, **36**, 1470 (1957).
82. Winter, C. C., *J. Urol.*, **76**, 182 (1956).
83. Taplin, G. V., *et al*, *J. Lab. Clin. Med.*, **48**, 886 (1956).
84. Winter, C. C., and Taplin, G. V., *J. Urol.*, **79**, 573 (1958).
85. Winter, C. C., *Am. J. Roentgenol.*, **82**, 862 (1959).
86. Serratto, M., *et al*, *A. M. A. Arch. Internal. Med.*, **103**, 851 (1959).
87. Nordyke, R. A., *et al*, *Clin. Res.*, **8**, 116 (1960).
88. Tubis, M., *et al.*, *Proc. Soc. Exptl. Biol. Med.*, **103**, 497 (1960).
89. Friedell, H. L., *et al*, *Am. J. Ophthalmol.*, **33**, 525 (1950).
90. Dunphy, E. B., *et al*, *Am. J. Ophthalmol.*, **37**, 45 (1954).
91. Selverstone, B., and White, J. C., *Am. J. Surg.*, **134**, 387 (1951).
92. Hine, G. J., *J. Nuclear Med.*, **4**, 439 (1964).
93. Hindel, R., and Gilson, A. J., *Nucleonics*, **25**(3), 52 (1967).
94. Anger, H. O., *Nucleonics*, **21**(10), 56 (1963).
95. Anger, H. O., *J. Nuclear Med.*, **5**, 515 (1964).
96. Anger, H. O., *et al*, *Nucleonics*, **23**(1), 57 (1965).
97. Bender, M. A., and Blau, M., *J. Nuclear Med.*, **1**, 105 (1960).
98. Bender, M. A., and Blau, M., *Nucleonics*, **21**(10), 52 (1963).
99. Blau, M., and Manske, R. F., *J. Nuclear Med.*, **2**, 102 (1961).
100. Taplin, G. V., *et al*, *J. Nuclear Med.*, **5**, 259 (1964).
101. Feindel, W., *et al*, *J. Nuclear Med.*, **4**, 195 (1963).
102. Wagner, H. N., Jr., *et al*, *J. Am. Med. Assoc.*, **174**, 162 (1960).
103. *The Medical Use of Radioisotopes: Recommendations and Requirements* by the Atomic Energy Commission, Isotopes Extension, Division of Civilian Application, US Atomic Energy Commission, Oak Ridge, Tenn., February, 1957.
104. *Starting an Isotope Unit*, Abbott Laboratories, North Chicago, Ill., 1960.
105. *Radioisotopes in Medicine: A General Guide for Physicians and Hospital Personnel*, Abbott Laboratories, North Chicago, Ill., rev. July, 1961.
106. *Handbook of Rules for Administration of Radioactive Materials to Patients*, M. D. Anderson Hospital and Tumor Institute, Texas Medical Center, Houston, Tex. Reproduced and distributed through special permission by E. R. Squibb & Sons, New York, 1959.
107. Latiolais, C. J., *et al*, *Bull. Am. Soc. Hosp. Pharm.*, **12**, 372 (1955).
108. Wagner, H. N., Jr., *et al*, *J. Am. Med. Assoc.*, **174**, 162 (1960).
109. *Bull. N-5261*, Picker X-Ray Corp., White Plains, N.Y.
110. Seliger, H. H., *et al*, *Phys. Rev.*, **90**, 443 (1953).
111. Ball, R. E., and Yaffe, L., *Can. J. Phys.*, **32**, 416 (1954).
112. Brosi, A. R., *et al*, *Phys. Rev.*, **84**, 586 (1951).
113. Lyon, W. S., *Phys. Rev.*, **87**, 1126 (1952).
114. Baggerly, L. L., *et al*, *Phys. Rev.*, **100**, 1364 (1955).
115. Metzger, F. R., *Phys. Rev.*, **88**, 1360 (1952).

Bibliography

Behrens, C. P., *Atomic Medicine*, 3rd ed., Williams & Wilkins, Baltimore, 1959.

Beierwaltes, W. H., *et al*, *Clinical Use of Radioisotopes*, Saunders, Philadelphia, 1957.

Blahd, W. H., *et al*, *Practice of Nuclear Medicine*, Thomas, Springfield, Ill., 1959.

Burnazyan, A. E., *et al*, *Radiation Medicine*, Pergamon, New York, 1964.

Fields, T., and Seed, L., *Clinical Use of Radioisotopes*, Year Book, Chicago, 1960.

Hahn, P. F., *Therapeutic Use of Artificial Radioisotopes*, Wiley, New York, 1960.

International Atomic Energy Agency, *Medical Uses of Ca*[47] Tech. Rept. #32, International Publications, Inc., New York, 1965.

International Atomic Energy Agency, *Medical Radioisotope Scanning*, International Publications, Inc., New York, 1965.

Lajtha, L. A., *The Use of Isotopes in Haematology*, Blackwells, Oxford, 1961.

Low-Beer, B. V. A., *Clinical Use of Radioactive Isotopes*, Thomas, Springfield, Ill., 1950.

Owen, C., *Diagnostic Use of Radioisotopes*, Thomas, Springfield, Ill., 1959.

Quimby, E. H., *et al*, *Radioactive Isotopes in Clinical Practice*, Lea & Febiger, Philadelphia, 1958.

Quimby, E. H., and Feitelberg, S., *Radioactive Isotopes in Medicine and Biology*, Lea & Febiger, Philadelphia, 1963.

Silver, S., *Radioactive Isotopes in Medicine and Biology*, Lea & Febiger, Philadelphia, 1962.

Veall, N., and Vetter, H., *Radioisotope Techniques in Clinical Research and Diagnosis*, Butterworths, London, 1958.

Winter, C. C., *Radioisotope Renography*, Williams & Wilkins, Baltimore, 1963.

35 | Nonmedical Applications of Radioisotopes

Modes of use, areas of use, and production of radioactive pharmaceuticals

This chapter was prepared by

Grafton D. Chase, PhD, *Professor of Chemistry, Philadelphia College of Pharmacy and Science, Philadelphia, Pa. 19104*

The availability of large quantities of radioisotopes as by-products of the operation of nuclear reactors has resulted in the development of many nonmedical uses since the first shipment of a radioisotope to a non-government laboratory by the United States Atomic Energy Commission (AEC) in August 1946. There are now more than a thousand industrial uses for radioisotopes, and the savings effected thereby are estimated at hundreds of millions of dollars annually.

The extent to which radioisotopes are now used may be judged by a comparison of the total amount of processed radioisotopes shipped by the Oak Ridge National Laboratory of AEC, this being 222,708 curies in 1959 and 3,118,116 curies for the first 11 months of 1967. Domestic sales of radioisotopes, radiochemicals, and radiopharmaceuticals for 1968 (including the value of AEC-supplied radioisotopes purchased by private companies for further processing) are estimated to amount to a total of $22–$28 million, of which $12–$15 million is for radiopharmaceuticals.

Modes of Use

The general industrial applications of radioisotopes can be classified into categories: (1) *tracer applications*, (2) the use of radioactive materials as *radiation sources*. The specific applications seem to be limited only by the imagination and ingenuity of the user. A third category of importance to pharmacy is the production of radioactive pharmaceuticals.

Tracer Applications

As the word "tracer" suggests, applications in this category employ the radioactive atom as a tag or label by means of which an object may be traced, located, or identified at a later time. The radioisotope, in this particular application, merely serves as a new, extremely small and useful tag. The objects tagged radioactively may be atoms or such larger entities as molecules, bacteria, mosquitoes, or even a packing box. Objects into which a tracer has been incorporated are said to be tagged or labeled. Hence, we speak of tagged molecules (or labeled molecules), tagged mosquitoes, etc.

When used as a tracer, the radioactive material or radioactively tagged object may be introduced during a manufacturing process and its pathway through the manufacturing process may then be followed by the use of radiation detection instruments. As indicated, the physical size of the tracer or tagged material may extend over a considerable range, from single atoms to an encapsulated source of rather large physical dimensions. The radioactive tag may further consist of any one of more than 100 nuclides whose radiological constants make them suitable for tracer applications. In this respect, tracers are also classified as being *isotopic* if a radioactive element is being used to trace the same stable element, or *nonisotopic* if any convenient and suitable radioactive element is used as a tracer in applications where the exact chemical nature of the radioelement is not critical.

It is sometimes necessary to describe the location (or change of location) of tracers or, more specifically of their *physical location* or *chemical location*. Physical location refers to the position of the radioisotope in space. Chemical location refers to the location of the radioactive atom or tagged group of atoms in a molecule. The latter usage is important, for example, in the elucidation of reaction mechanisms.

Radioisotopes as Radiation Sources

When used as a radiation source, it is the type and energy of radiation emitted which is of importance, rather than the chemical properties of the isotope. In this respect, applications of radiation can be divided conveniently into two general categories: (1) those in which an effect of matter on radiation is utilized and (2) those in which an effect of radiation on matter is involved.

Effects of Matter on Radiation—The first category, applying an effect of matter on radiation, involves the attenuation or absorption of radiation and the scattering phenomena of radiation. Typical applications include density and thickness gages, interface detection, radiography, and certain analytical applications. The size of the radioactive source may vary from a few microcuries to a curie or more. Rather delicate and ingenious instrumentation is employed for these applications.

When alpha, beta, or gamma radiation impinges upon matter (a sheet of paper, an aluminum foil, etc), it interacts with the charged particles of which the matter is composed. These interactions result in an energy loss associated with a decrease in the velocity of alpha and beta particles or, in the case of gamma radiation, in a decrease in frequency or the complete absorption of a particular photon. Scattering of the radiation also occurs, especially in the case of beta and gamma radiations. These processes, described in Chapter 33, page 548, may be utilized to elucidate the nature of the scattering material.

Effects of Radiation on Matter—The second category, utilizing an effect of radiation on matter, is illustrated by such typical examples as static elimination, promotion of chemical reactions, sterilization, etc. The source size may be as small as a few microcuries (static eliminators), but more often it exceeds a curie and is frequently in the kilocurie range. Massive shielding is usually required.

When radiation interacts with matter, a great variety of chemical and biological effects occur. Most of the observed effects can be attributed to the ionizing action of radiation. When electrons are stripped from gas molecules, the ions which result conduct an electric current and hence will discharge static

573

charges. In other cases the ions so produced promote a variety of chemical reactions, some to advantage, others to disadvantage. The disruption of valence electrons may cause large molecules to degrade, or conversely, the molecules so activated may polymerize. In biological systems chromosomes may be split or toxic compounds may be produced within an organism in sufficient concentration to cause the death of the organism.

Areas of Use

Radioisotopes are now used by the pharmaceutical industry in nearly all phases of drug production—in basic research, product development, production, and in process and quality control. The following examples are typical and illustrate the radioisotope in the role of a tracer or as a radiation source.

Basic Research

The development of new drugs must be based on a sound knowledge of normal human physiology. Thousands of references may be found to the use of radioisotopes in the study of metabolic pathways and other physiological phenomena. A knowledge of abnormal physiology is also important if the action produced by a drug is to be recognized and evaluated. Because research in these areas has been so very extensive it would not be practical to attempt a survey for this book.

As new drugs are produced, their pharmacologic activity, fate in the body, and excretion rate must be measured. To do this the drug is prepared with an isotopic label. It is administered to an animal by injection, orally, or other suitable route, after which the animal may be placed in a metabolism cage which allows collection of urine, feces, and sometimes the exhaled air as well. Assuming a known amount of a carbon-14-labeled drug was administered in the dose, measurement of carbon-14 in the urine, feces, in the carbon dioxide in the breath, as well as in specific organs of the sacrificed animal, provides knowledge concerning the physical location of the isotopic tag (as either the original labeled compound or as a metabolite) and the rate of its elimination. On the other hand the metabolic pathway is elucidated primarily by use of chromatography and other suitable separation techniques which aid in the identification of any new radioactively tagged compounds produced as metabolic products of the administered drug.

Product Development

Once the activity of a drug has been established and it has been found free of objectionable side effects, the manufacturer must formulate the drug into a product which is pleasant for the patient and which releases the drug where and when needed. Also the product must have a reasonable shelf-life. Among the topics to be considered are drug absorption by tissues, penetration into tissues, permeability through tissues or membranes, and release of the drug from a formulation, as well as product stability. In addition a technique known as activation may be found useful in the course of product development.

Absorption, Penetration, and Permeability—Lark-Horowitz and Leng[1] were probably the first to report on the use of a radioisotope for the solution of a pharmaceutical problem. Using Sodium-24 as a label they developed a method for testing enteric coatings. Incorporated in a tablet the sodium was released as the coating dissolved. Release was followed by measuring the radioactivity of the released sodium-24 in the hand or other extremity. Absorption from sublingual tablets was studied by Katz and Barr.[2] They incorporated iodine-131-labeled sodium iodide in the tablets and measured the extent of uptake by observing the level of radioactivity in the tail of the test animal. The kinetics of rectal absorption has been the subject of a study by Riegelman and Crowell[3] in which a collimated counter positioned over the rectum was used to measure the rate of decrease of activity from the rectum. Peterson, et al[4] performed similar experiments, also using iodine-131. For the evaluation of certain sustained-release preparations Nash and Crabtree[5] used tritiated d-desoxy-ephedrine. In measuring the release of this compound from cation-exchange resins they used a liquid-scintillation counter to determine blood levels of the tritiated product. In an interesting double experiment Montgomery, et al,[6] measured the sustained release of carbon-14-labeled aspirin and of chlorine-36-labeled phenylephrine hydrochloride simultaneously in simulated gastric fluid by dual-channel liquid-scintillation counting.

Radioactive tracers have been used extensively for determining the release of medication from ointment bases. Patel, et al,[7] and Barker, et al,[8] have studied the release of medicaments into agar plates. Although similar, in some respects, to the standard method for measuring the bacteriostatic effect of an incorporated medicament, the isotopic method enables the quantitation of drug released into the agar. The influence of surfactants on the release of ions from ointment bases has been investigated by Stark, et al,[9] using radioactive mercury and iodine while Ruggiero, et al,[10] have developed a chick embryo technique for evaluation of the absorption of radioactive iodide from ointment bases. Experimental results are also given for a number of preparations.[11]

Sorby and Plein[12] studied the absorption of mercury-203 labeled ammoniated mercury by applying the ointment to the intact skin of rats and measuring the activity in the kidneys. In a similar experiment Hupf, et al,[13] measured the percutaneous absorption of carbon-14-labeled salicylic acid by observing the blood radioactivity.

The effects of astringents and antiperspirants on the permeability of frog skin have been the subject of several investigations.[14,15] The variety of applications to product development is further illustrated by the report of Gerding, et al,[16] who describe a method for the evaluation of insect repellants by measuring the retention of the carbon-14-labeled compounds on the skin of horses and of Clark and Swartz,[17] who describe a method for determining the absorption of water in pharmaceutical closures by use of tritium-labeled water.

Product Stability—The evaluation of shelf-life is inherently difficult because the need is to compress time. To avoid this problem one can use a sensitive means to detect very small changes in the product. By extrapolation one can estimate stability. Because radioisotopes are capable of detection in miniscule quantities, they often supply the means to the solution of such problems.

Changes in dispersed systems are often not visible and are equally difficult to detect by standard analytical methods. To measure the creaming rate of emulsions Appino, et al,[18] developed a radioisotopic method. Sodium radioiodide was used to label the aqueous phase and iodobenzene (I^{131}) was used to label the oil phase. Emulsions were tested by placing them in vertical glass tubes. Radioactivity was measured at both the top and bottom ends of the tube. From these activities a radioisotopic creaming rate was calculated. The method is said to require less time and to be more sensitive than previous methods for measuring creaming rate.

Vitamin B-12 stability in multivitamin mixtures was investigated by Rosenblum and Woodbury.[19] They used vitamin B-12 labeled with cobalt-60 by fermentation synthesis. Following extraction the activity of the vitamin could be measured directly in the mixture.

Activation—Machine parts such as bearings and pistons, which are particularly prone to wear, may produce the malfunction of the apparatus. Redesign or proper lubrication may prevent machine failure if the degree of friction wear were known but if one must depend upon chemical analysis of lubricants to determine the amount of metal worn from the moving part, many days of operation are required before detectable quantities of metal appear in the lubricant. This problem may be resolved as follows. Machine parts, irradiated by neutrons in an atomic pile, become radioactive. As these parts wear, the metal appearing in the lubricant is radioactive and is quite readily detectable at extremely low concentrations; the test requires only minutes or hours, rather than days or weeks. Such methods have become routine with numerous oil companies for testing lubricating oils.[20] The method is so sensitive that the rate of engine wear can be measured at different temperatures as the engine "warms up." This technique not only has the advantage of speed but also permits different lubricants to be compared in the same engine under identical conditions of wear. One large oil company using radioactive piston rings to study lubrication-wear problems in diesel and gasoline engines estimates it obtained more information in 4 years for the expenditure of $35,000 than it could have obtained without the tracer technique by spending $1 million over a period of 60 years.[21]

Product Production

Radioisotopes are sometimes used as a necessary component in a production process to bring about a desired change in a product. In some instances the radioisotope may actually be essential to the formation of the product. In such cases radioisotopes are used as radiation sources, not as tracers. In general, sources of gamma radiation have been found most useful. Combining the need for a substantial half-life with the need for gamma radiation leads to the selection of such isotopes as cobalt-60 and cesium-137. These materials are available in large quantities at relatively low cost.

Radiation-Induced Chemical Reactions—The utilization of radiation to promote chemical reactions is still more or less in the state of a laboratory curiosity, but it is perhaps in this field that the greatest potential for future development is to be found. One of the major problems yet to be overcome is production cost. Thus, there is now no advantage in producing a product by radiation-induced reactions which can be produced by standard chemical means. Complete agreement still has not been reached on the potential value of irradiation as a processing technique[22-27] for other than high-value products such as pharmaceuticals and other medical supplies.[28]

If the induced reaction is between thermodynamically unstable compounds, is autocatalytic, or proceeds by chain induction, only a moderate amount of radiation is required. If, on the other hand, radiation energy is required for each reacting molecule, billions of roentgens are required.

The yield of a radiation-induced reaction is expressed in terms of the "G value," which is defined as the number of molecules produced or converted per 100 electron volts (ev) of energy absorbed. Thus, if the bond energy is 25 ev (the approximate value for a C—H bond), then $G = 4$. The G value for the oxidation of Fe(II) to Fe(III) in air-saturated dilute sulfuric acid is 15.5 (i.e., 100/15.5, or about 6.5 ev, is required per atom of Fe oxidized). The greater the value of G, the less the amount of radiation required to induce the reaction. An increase in molecular weight has a similar effect.

AEC contracts have been granted to study the direct fixation of atmospheric nitrogen by means of radiation-induced reactions.[24] A reactor designed for this purpose would produce about 2 tons of nitric acid per Gm of uranium-235. The oxidation of sulfur dioxide to sulfur trioxide, and the production of ammonia from nitrogen and hydrogen also look like promising applications. Unsaturated compounds have been made to undergo polymerization reactions. Irradiated lubricating oils increase in viscosity as a result of the predominance of condensation reactions over degradation reactions. Fatty acids generally decarboxylate under irradiation. For compounds not easily produced by standard means, radiation holds some promise. Such is the case with fluorine-substituted benzenes.

The field of polymerization has received a great deal of emphasis. Radiation offers no advantage in many cases, but radiation crosslinking of polymers after fabrication may produce new products with improved properties. For example, products fabricated of polyethylene show improved properties at high temperature. Irradiated polyethylene bottles may be subjected to heat sterilization. Carbon-filled polyethylene also shows improved properties after irradiation[29] and is less prone to changes in shape at high temperature.

It is commonly known that radiation produces color changes in glass. In a rather unique application, diamonds are colored to order (green, blue-green, or brown) by controlled irradiation processes.[30]

Irradiation Sterilization—Development of processes for irradiation sterilization have received the greatest emphasis in two fields, namely, foods and pharmaceuticals, including biological materials. This method of sterilization is particularly attractive for products which are heat sensitive. Irradiation sterilization seems to hold special possibilities in the pharmaceutical field[28,31] but is not without its disadvantages.

The main advantages of irradiation sterilization may be summarized as follows. Radiation sterilizes without the need of heat. Gamma radiation permits immediate penetration of a product, whereas heat transfer may be slow. In some cases a radiation sterilization process is less critical than heat sterilization, and sterilization can be conducted continuously on sealed packages.

The main disadvantages of irradiation sterilization are threefold. Detrimental changes often occur in the product during irradiation, the process is potentially hazardous to personnel, and the cost is presently greater than that for heat or chemical sterilization. Upjohn* was perhaps the first to market an irradiation-sterilized product. In 1955 they manufactured eye ointments which were sterilized by radiation.

---

* See page 2023.

These contained neomycin and hydrocortisone, alone and in combination.

A major step forward in this field was made by Ethicon* which introduced irradiation sterilization of sutures (with high-energy electrons) in 1958. Formerly, sutures were heat sterilized and aseptically packaged. The temperature had to be controlled to within 3%. Irradiation sterilization dosage can be increased 40% with no harm to the product. Silk, catgut, and nylon sutures may be processed in this manner, but cotton sutures are degraded by the radiation. Sterilization of catgut sutures with a Van de Graaff accelerator was reported by Dunn, et al.[32]

Cotton and gauze products are difficult to sterilize in bulk by steam. These products may be sterilized by gamma radiation, but there is some tendency for them to be degraded. However, advantages cited for the radiation sterilization[33] of bulk medical supplies such as bandages, cotton, and gauze include:

1. Ability of gamma rays to penetrate large masses of the material without inducing radioactivity in the product itself.
2. Complete sterilization, even of tightly packed pallet loads of product in tightly sealed containers.
3. Freedom to use continuous rather than batch sterilization processes.
4. Freedom to use moisture-proof packaging not possible when steam sterilization is used.

The survival curve of irradiated organisms is exponential. Sterility is generally assumed when, by extrapolation, it is computed that the surviving concentration of bacteria is 10^{-11} per ml or 1 bacterium per 10^{11} ml. The amount of radiation required to attain this state of sterility depends on the nature of the bacteria, the nature of the product, and the original concentration of organisms but, as a guide, may be assumed to be about 10^6 rads. Thus, a product must withstand this dose if the method is to be useful.

Antibiotics in powder form generally withstand doses of 2×10^6 rads but show degradation at about 2×10^7 rads. In aqueous solution they are much less stable.

Enzymes in dilute solutions are inactivated by relatively small doses of radiation but require large doses (up to 10^7 rads) for inactivation if present in their natural habitat, eg, vegetables and meat. Irradiation inactivation of enzymes does not, therefore, hold promise as a practical process at present. The behavior of enzymes on irradiation is similar to that of other substances consisting of large molecules, such as vitamins.

Vitamin stability towards ionizing radiation (x-rays and cathode rays) has been the subject of numerous investigations.[34-39] Other pharmaceutical products have also been investigated for radiation stability.[40-43] Several generalizations may be drawn from data in these reports. The rate of radiation degradation of vitamins, as well as of most other chemical substances, is essentially first order. In dilute solutions the rate of degradation is greater, in terms of per cent of solute destroyed, than in more concentrated

solutions. The presence of other chemical substances, such as those found in the natural environment of the vitamin, decreases the rate of radiation destruction. For example ascorbic acid is more stable in orange juice than in distilled water solution.

The sensitivity of various substances to radiation is conveniently expressed in terms of *inactivation dose* and *specific inactivation dose*. The inactivation dose, D_0, is the amount of radiation (in roentgens) required to destroy 63% of the solute.* However, the inactivation dose, D_0, is a function of the solute concentration, C. If sensitivity is expressed as specific activation dose D_0/C, a value independent of concentration is obtained. For x- or gamma-radiation, the units of D_0/C are roentgens/Gm/ml if D_0 is expressed in roentgens and concentration, C, in Gm/ml. General ranges of specific inactivation dose for a few substances are given in Table I.

Process Control

Difficult problems in the control of industrial processes often can be solved or more easily accomplished by use of radioisotopes. Applications in process control may require the use of a radioisotope just on occasion, such as in the detection of leaks or when testing for the uniformity of distribution of ingredients in a mixing process. On the other hand application may require the use of an isotope for around-the-clock monitoring of a process. Thickness and density gages, liquid-level controls, and package monitors are examples of the latter type of application. Monitoring devices normally require the use of radioisotopes with reasonably long half-lives so that replacement of the source or frequent calibration of the instrument is not necessary.

Liquid Flow Through Pipes—The transportation of liquids over great distances, through pipes, is a common practice, especially in the petroleum industry. A radioactive tracer, injected at the interface between two different liquids being pumped consecutively through the same pipe, will enable the identification and location of the interface at any subsequent point. On occasion, especially over relatively short distances, a "go-devil" may be used to separate the two liquids. In this case, the radioactive source is encapsulated in the "go-devil." Radiation detectors placed near the pipe are then used to indicate the passage of the interface past a given position. Such a tracer must emit gamma radiation in order that it can be detected through a steel pipe. "Go-devils" are also used to clean pipelines, but occasionally they become stuck within the pipe. If they are radioactive, they can be located quite easily and the necessary measures taken to remove them.

If the radioactive tracer is to be injected directly into the fluid, then, in addition to emitting penetrating gamma radiation, it must also be soluble in the fluid. Isotopes which have been utilized for this purpose

Table I

Substance	Approximate range for specific inactivation dose[a] (D_0/C)
Niacin	8×10^9 to 4×10^{11}
Riboflavin	2×10^9 to 9×10^9
Ascorbic acid	2×10^8 to 4×10^9
Amino acids	1×10^9 to 1×10^{10}
PABA	5×10^9 to 2×10^{10}

[a] Values selected from Refs. 44 to 49.

* The significance of selecting a value of 63% is seen from the following derivation. If the rate of destruction is that of a first-order reaction, then the concentration, C, at time, t, is given by:

$$C = C_0 e^{-kt}$$

where C_0 is the initial concentration, e is the base of natural logarithms, and k is the reaction rate constant. When the product of k and t is unity ($kt = 1$), then

$$C = C_0 e^{-1} = \frac{C_0}{e} = 0.37\, C_0$$

Thus, when $kt = 1$, the concentration of substance remaining is equal to 37% of the original concentration (for 63% has been destroyed).

include antimony-124, lanthanum-140, and barium-140. These isotopes have half-lives sufficiently long to be useful for the intended purpose, yet sufficiently short that they will decay to a negligible quantity in a few weeks. As the fluids are pumped through miles of pipe, a certain degree of mixing occurs at the interface. The radioactive tracer is also used to indicate the extent of such mixing.[44]

Leak Detection—It can be very troublesome to find a leak in a pipeline. One method for the location of the leak involves pumping a radioactive solution, under pressure, through the pipe. The pipe is cleaned by pumping a rinse solution through it. The leak is located by detection of the radioactive residues which will be found about the pipe at the location of the leak. An aqueous solution of sodium-24 as Na-HCO$_3$, for example, has been found useful for this purpose. Leaks in tanks may be detected and located in a similar manner by the use of a radioactive gas such as tritium which, after suitable dilution with air or other gas, is pumped into the tank under pressure. One can "smell" the leak with a device such as a sensitive, continuous-flow ionization chamber.

Activation Analysis—Neutron activation in an atomic reactor, or with any one of several smaller neutron sources now available commercially, makes possible a very sensitive method of analysis.[45–51] In this method the sample to be analyzed is subjected to neutron bombardment, whereupon the various chemical elements in the sample become radioactive. The extent to which a particular chemical element will become radioactive depends on the neutron flux density, the nuclear cross section, and the irradiation time of the sample. If the element for which the analysis is made is present in trace amounts only, and this is often the case, a measured quantity of stable isotope is added to allow a chemical separation to be performed. From a measurement of the radioactivity of the isolated element the quantity present in the original sample can be calculated. For the benefit of laboratories for which the purchase of a neutron source is not feasible, activation analysis service is now offered by a number of companies.[52] A special application for activation analysis of particular merit has been reported by Phillips Petroleum.[53] By the use of a Cockcroft–Walton accelerator, deuterons are made to strike a target of ZrT$_4$. A nuclear reaction of the deuterons with the tritium produces neutrons. In turn, these neutrons are used to activate oxygen and from the radioactivity induced in the oxygen the quantity of this element is measured nondestructively at 2-minute intervals.

Test of Dehydration Process—The efficiency of a process involving the dehydration of various products is measured with the aid of radioactive water. Either deuterated water (heavy water) or tritiated water is added to the product before dehydration. Moisture remaining in the product after dehydration is estimated from the amount of residual radioactivity. Although this technique appears to be straightforward, certain precautions must be observed. Deuterated water is not radioactive and must be measured with special techniques. Tritiated water is radioactive but tritium, too, requires special techniques such as liquid-scintillation counting or gas-phase counting for its measurement. Tritium also exhibits a considerable isotope effect because of its large mass compared to that of ordinary hydrogen. This effect causes tritiated water to react or evaporate at a slower rate than ordinary water. Finally, the exchange of tritium (or

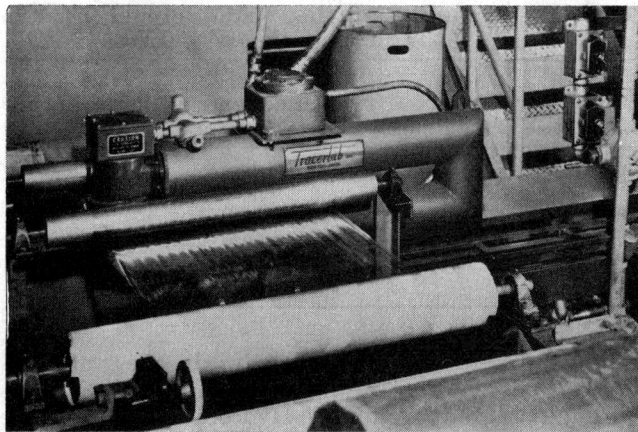

Fig. 386. Beta-ray gage installation at Permacel Tape Corp. used to monitor the thickness of plastic film (courtesy, Tracerlabs).

deuterium) from labeled water with ordinary hydrogen in the product may occur. This loss of label by exchange can cause serious errors in the data.

Thickness Gages—Beta-ray gages and gamma-ray gages for the continuous measurement of the thickness of paper or metal sheets are the most extensively used of all instruments. One type of thickness gage (Fig. 386) measures the transmission of beta or gamma rays from a radioactive source through a material to a detector on the opposite side. It will be recalled from Chapter 33, page 548, that the attenuation of beta and gamma rays is a function of both the absorber thickness and the absorber density. The relation is very nearly logarithmic. Thus, if the density of the absorbing material remains constant, the intensity of the radiation reaching the detector will be a function of the thickness of the absorbing material.

Beta particle thickness gages are useful for measurements from about 0.1 to 1000 mg/cm^2. For the greatest accuracy a beta source should be selected such that approximately 50% of the beta particles are absorbed by the material under measurement. Beta-emitting isotopes commonly employed for this purpose are given in Table II. These sources have been selected for long half-life and purity of beta emission.

If greater thicknesses are to be measured, gamma sources are employed. Gamma sources frequently used for this purpose are listed in Table III.

In a unique application of the principle of transmission gages the thickness of the walls of hard gelatin capsules was determined. A chlorine-36 source was mounted in the tip of a stainless steel capsule dipping pin.[54] With a capsule placed on the pin, beta-particle transmission was measured with an anthracene crystal scintillator.

Thickness gages may also operate on the basis of backscattering of beta particles[55] rather than on their absorption. Backscattering is a function of density and atomic number. This type of thickness gage is

Table II—Beta-Emitting Radioisotopes Used in Thickness Gages

Isotope	Half-life	Maximum energy (mev)	Maximum range mg/cm^2	Useful range mg/cm^2
^{63}Ni	85 y	0.067	6.7	0.1–1
^{35}S	87 d	0.167	31	0.5–5
^{147}Pm	2.6 y	0.223	49	1–15
^{204}Tl	4.0 y	0.765	300	10–150
^{90}Sr + ^{90}Y	28 y	2.24	1000	50–600

Table III—Gamma-Emitting Radioisotopes Used in Thickness Gages

Isotope	Half-life		Gamma energy (mev)	Half value layer (inches of iron)
^{55}Fe	2.9	y	0.006	0.0005
^{170}Tm	127	d	0.07	0.04
^{75}Se	127	d	0.07 to 0.4	. . .
^{192}Ir	74	d	0.14 to 0.61	. . .
^{137}Cs + ^{137}Ba	33	y	0.66	0.65
^{60}Co	5.3	y	1.17, 1.33	0.90

especially useful for measuring the thickness of coatings such as zinc galvanizing or paint.

Density Measurement—Hydrometers, too, have been replaced by the radioisotope[56] for the control of processes requiring a continuous and nondestructive method for measuring density. Similar to absorption thickness gages, operation of the absorption density gage also depends on both the thickness and density of the sample. The operation differs from that of the thickness gage in that sample thickness instead of density is maintained constant. Radiation gages have been developed to measure the density of liquid flowing through a pipe. A radiation source is placed on one side of the pipe and a detector on the other. In this way the source-to-detector distance and sample thickness are held constant. Instruments of this type usually employ a second source and a second detector as a standard. The working and standard detectors are connected in a balanced circuit such as a bridge circuit. Such an arrangement has the advantage of greater stability, automatic correction for decay of the isotope, and the special feature, if desired, of scale expansion.

Liquid-Level Control—If a gamma source and a detector are placed at the same level but on opposite sides of a pipe or tank, the accurate control of liquid level is possible. See Fig. 387. Even a very small movement of the liquid level will produce large changes in the detector output because of the great difference in absorption of gamma rays between the gas and liquid phases. If an indication of liquid level over a range is desired, the source and detector are arranged as shown in Fig. 388.

These same instruments can be used to indicate the level of an interface between two immiscible liquids. Thus, the vapor phase in the above examples is replaced by a liquid such as oil. Unless the gamma-ray absorption is very nearly the same in the two phases, a high degree of accuracy is possible.

Package Monitoring—The same basic principle that applies to density and thickness gaging can also be applied to package monitoring if suitably modified or redesigned equipment is employed. A radioactive source and a detector, located one on either side of the conveyor belt, provide the means for continuous monitoring of fill, which may be coupled with a device for automatic rejection of under or overfilled containers. To insure that the packages are properly located between the source and detector at the time of measurement, a location system using a light beam and photocell may be employed.

Gamma-Ray Scattering Gages—Devices based on gamma-ray scattering have found numerous applications. Scattering measurements are made with the source and detector on the same side of the sample. The extent of scattering into the detector depends on the nature of the sample and its thickness. Thus, if the composition of the sample is constant, its thickness can be measured. Gamma-ray thickness gages are useful for measuring the thickness of metal sheets and castings when only one side of the sample is accessible. Similarly, gamma scattering gages can be used to detect corrosion in pipes from the outside.

Static Elimination—Electrostatic charges which collect on various materials may constitute a severe fire hazard, a shock nuisance to personnel, or may otherwise disrupt a manufacturing process. Frequently, such charges can be dissipated through ionization of the air by radiation. The specific ionization of alpha particles is about 1000-fold greater than the specific ionization of beta particles which, in turn, is approximately 1000-fold greater than the specific ionization of gamma radiation. The radioisotope of choice is, therefore, an alpha-emitting nuclide if it is necessary only to ionize air for a relatively short distance (about 5 cm) from the source. If air ionization over greater distances is required, a beta-emitting nuclide must be used. Polonium-210 is often used as a pure alpha source. In use, such a pure alpha source constitutes no external radiation hazard but represents a potentially serious hazard if ingested. Beta radiation from bismuth-210 (in secular equilibrium with lead-210 and polonium-210) may be used for static elimination up to nearly a foot from the source. Simultaneously polonium-210 alpha particles are available, and both bismuth-210 and polonium-210 have an apparent half-life equal to that of lead-210 (about 22 years). Gamma radiation is rarely used for static elimination.

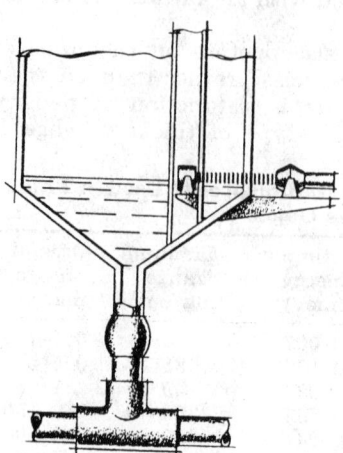

Fig. 387. Predetermined level gage. A small source of radiation is placed inside or outside a tank. A scintillation detector is placed outside of one side on the same horizontal line with the desired level. When material is interposed between the source and the detector, the reading from the gage decreases (courtesy, Radiation Counter).

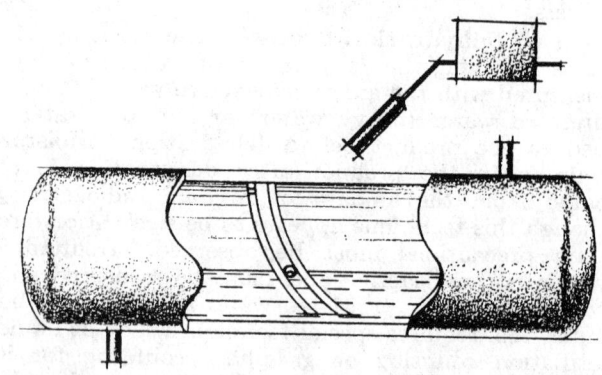

Fig. 388. Continuous liquid-level gage. A small source of radioactivity is enclosed in a float which follows the liquid level. Appropriate guides inside the tank direct this float along a predetermined path so as to give the desired results of linearity and accuracy. A scintillation detector situated outside the tank detects the radiation emitted by the source in the float (courtesy, Radiation Counter).

Quality Control

Efficiency of Bacterial Filters—In this application bacteria are grown in media containing a radioactive metabolite. In this way they become radioactively tagged. Retention of the bacteria on the filter or their passage through the filter is measured with a suitable radiation detection instrument. Although simple in theory, it is necessary to ascertain that the radioactive tag is not lost from the bacteria. It is equally necessary to wash the bacteria thoroughly after tagging them to free them from excess radioactive media.

Isotope Dilution—For the analytical determination of a substance which is difficult to separate quantitatively from a mixture, the isotope dilution method[57,58] is indispensable. The technique consists of:

1. Addition of a known amount of radioactively labeled compound to the unknown mixture. The labeled compound must be chemically identical with the substance to be measured. It is thoroughly mixed with the unknown to obtain a uniform distribution.
2. Suitable treatment of the mixture to isolate the same compound in pure form. It is essential that the isolated compound be pure, but it is not necessary to separate all of the compound from the mixture.
3. Determination of the isotope content of the isolated portion of the compound. The mass, M, of the inactive compound present in the original mixture is then calculated from the relation

$$M = M'[(S'/S) - 1]$$

where M' is the mass and S' is the specific activity of the isotopically labeled compound added and S is the specific activity of the portion of the compound isolated from the mixture. In essence, the radioisotope has provided here a means for computing per cent recovery.

Hydrogen/Carbon Ratio—At least two basic methods employing radioisotopes are available for the measurement of the ratio of hydrogen to carbon in a hydrocarbon. The first of these methods[59] depends on the absorption of beta particles in the hydrocarbon, as well as a knowledge of the sample density. The attenuation of beta particles by matter depends on the number of electrons encountered in the sample. Hydrogen has more electrons per unit weight than any other element. It has, in fact, about twice as many electrons per unit weight as carbon and, consequently, absorbs approximately twice as many electrons per unit weight as carbon. From these two measurements (the beta particle attenuation and the density) the H/C ratio is calculated.

The second method utilizes the degree of backscattering of beta particles in conjunction with a density measurement. In one method[60] beta particles from a 20 mCi ^{90}Sr source are caused to strike the sample in which they are scattered. Those scattered through nearly 90° are measured with an ionization chamber and electrometer. After applying a density correction to the electrometer reading, the carbon–hydrogen ratio is obtained by reference to a calibration chart.

Gamma Radiography—The first known use of a radioisotope for radiography was the experiment of Becquerel in 1896.[61] Further work by Tenney[62] promoted the use of gamma-emitting radioisotopes to replace x-ray tubes as a source of penetrating radiation, and their use today in gamma radiography of metals is a well-established inspection process. The percentage of flaw-free castings manufactured has undoubtedly increased through the use of ^{60}Co, ^{192}Ir, ^{170}Th, ^{137}Cs, and other isotopes.

In principle, gamma radiography consists of placing a gamma-emitting radioisotope on one side of a casting, or object, whose internal structure is to be photographed, and a sheet of x-ray film, suitably protected from light in a cassette, on the opposite side. After exposure for a calculated time the film is developed.

In selecting the proper gamma-emitting isotope, consideration must be given not only to half-life but especially to gamma-ray energy. If very thick castings are to be examined, very hard gamma rays such as those from sodium-24 or lanthanum-40 are used, but these isotopes have relatively short half-lives. Cobalt-60 and tantalum-182 emit gamma radiation which is not quite so hard, but these sources provide the advantage of longer half-life. Iridium-192, and cesium-137 are excellent sources of softer radiation suitable for the examination of thin sections and thulium-170 is the best available source of very soft gamma radiation. Details of this technique, including methods for computing exposure times, have been published.[63–66]

Autoradiography—Yagoda[67] and Boyd[68] describe numerous applications for a very useful technique known as autoradiography (sometimes called radioautography). A photographic emulsion, often in the form of x-ray film, replaces the Geiger tube as the radiation detector. A distinct advantage of an emulsion over the Geiger tube is the increase in resolving power possible when necessary to pinpoint the location of a radioactive tracer. Whereas a Geiger tube may be able to resolve two sources a few millimeters apart (or to locate a single source to within a few millimeters), autoradiography can extend the resolution to a fraction of a micron.

In this technique a photographic emulsion is exposed by placing it in contact with a radioactive object for a calculated length of time and is then developed. The exact location of the radioactivity is indicated by a blackening of the film caused by the alpha, beta, or gamma radiation in much the same way that light causes the film to blacken. During exposure the film must, of course, be protected from light.

In one application a radioactive metal is used in the production of an alloy. If a mirror-smooth face is prepared on a sample of the resulting alloy, contact with a photographic film will result in an autoradiogram from which it is possible to determine if the metal was evenly distributed throughout the alloy; frequently certain structures and crystalline patterns within the alloy may be discerned.

Extensive use of this technique is made in the biological sciences. For example, it is possible to determine the site of deposition of phosphorus or calcium in bones, or fluorine in teeth, and of metabolites in plant tissues. The resolving power possible with autoradiography is illustrated by an experiment in which the location of radioactive nucleosides was determined within the chromosome.[69]

Public Health and Other Fields

Control of Insects, Mold, and Fungus—A new approach[70] to the control of insects is to release tremendous numbers of males of the species which have been rendered infertile by exposure to radiation as pupae. If the males are otherwise healthy, compete successfully for the females, and if the females mate only once, the entire insect population should be eliminated in a short time. Insects controlled by this method must be capable of collection and breeding under laboratory conditions. It is also necessary to determine the critical dosage of radiation which will result in sterilization but not in death of the insect. It is also necessary to know the mating habits of the insect. This technique was used with success to eliminate the screwworm fly from the Dutch island of Curacao in the Caribbean in 1955, and from Florida in 1958.

Radioisotopic tagging has been useful for elucidating the role of arthropods in the epidemiology of diseases.[71] Dispersal and flight-range studies on mosquitoes, houseflies, and other insects[72-74] have been made by tagging the insects with ^{32}P or other radioactive substances. The tagged insects are released and later recaptured. Such studies show the average dispersal of flies to be between 5 and 10 Km, whereas mosquitoes generally disperse over a somewhat less extensive area. Labeled cockroaches[75] released in sewer manholes indicated no movement in the sewage system in 8½ weeks. Experiments by Jenkins[76] showed large amounts of radioactivity in dragonflies, damsel flies, caddis flies, and other insects after making radioactive mosquitoes available to them. The usefulness of these insects for mosquito control was thereby demonstrated.

The effectiveness of insecticides can be demonstrated, also, by tagging DDT, parathion, pyrethrins, lead arsenite, and other insecticides with suitable isotopes. In this connection ^{14}C, ^{35}Cl, ^{35}S, ^{74}As, and other isotopes have been used.

In another application of the interaction of radiation with matter, optical instruments subject to destruction by mold growth were coated with polonium-210, a radium lacquer, or a radium foil.[77] A marked decrease in the rate of mold formation was observed with treated instruments.

Production of New Biological Species—Two new plant varieties produced by radiation, a bush navy bean and an improved peanut variety, have been released to plant breeders. New varieties of numerous other fruits and vegetables have been produced, including disease-resistant varieties. Mutant varieties of medicinal plants open an entirely new field for investigation.

Production of Radioactive Pharmaceuticals

Radioactive compounds are prepared by over 50 individual manufacturers and a great variety of these radioactively labeled compounds is now available. Over 500 carbon-14-labeled compounds alone are manufactured. Most of these radioactive products are for research purposes and are generally called radioactive chemicals. But some are radioactive pharmaceuticals, intended for human use, and must therefore conform to the applicable drug standards.

Except for a few cyclotron-produced radioisotopes, all are produced in a nuclear reactor or pile. The reactor at the Oak Ridge National Laboratory (ORNL) supplies the major portion of isotopes used in the United States, although some are obtained from Canada and elsewhere. The unstable nature of isotopes usually necessitates procurement from a nearby source with prompt delivery. Some of these isotopes are fission products which have been chemically separated from other fission products by the original producer, eg, ORNL. Others contain radioactive elements prepared by neutron reactions with stable isotopes. In either case the resulting compounds are normally not of medicinal grade at this point even though they have undergone a rigorous purification process and are generally better than 99% pure. When received in bulk by the pharmaceutical manufacturer they must be further processed to assure (1) chemical and radiological purity, (2) conversion to the proper chemical form, and

(3) proper dilution, and sterility and freedom from pyrogens, where required, before they are distributed to the hospital or physician. As an example, a few of the considerations necessary in the production of Sodium Iodide I[131] USP (Capsules or Solution) are discussed.

A very thorough discussion of the problems and techniques involved in the preparation of radioactive chemicals for clinical use is found in a publication by Briner.[78]

Iodine-131 is separated and shipped by ORNL as the sodium salt. Upon receipt by the manufacturer it is first assayed to determine the quantity present. Iodine-131 which may be present as iodate must then be converted to iodide to conform to USP specifications. (Radioactive iodine administered to a patient as iodate would certainly result in an incorrect diagnosis or faulty therapy.) It is then necessary to check by means of paper chromatography that the iodate has been reduced. Dilutions of the stock solution are now prepared, and the concentration of the activity is measured by beta and gamma counting. Final tests must also be made of the purity of the preparation. These tests include a measurement of the absorption coefficient by the use of aluminum absorbers and the preparation of a gamma-ray spectrum to determine if activities other than iodine-131 are present. Having ascertained the strength and radiochemical purity of the preparation, it is now sealed into ampuls if for parenteral use or measured into screwcap bottles if for oral use. If intended for parenteral use, it must be sterilized and the additional precaution of pyrogen testing must be taken.

The manufacturing area for radiopharmaceuticals may more nearly resemble a chemical laboratory than a pharmaceutical manufacturing department. Fig. 389 illustrates one section of the Abbott Laboratories' production area. Here, cleanliness and orderliness are of prime importance. Larger quantities of radioactive materials are handled in "hot cells" or "caves" such as that illustrated in Fig. 390. In the hot cell all operations are conducted remotely, and the operator is protected from radiation by shielding on all sides, including the top and bottom of the cave.

For convenience certain radiopharmaceuticals are prepared in a variety of dosage forms. Capsules, in

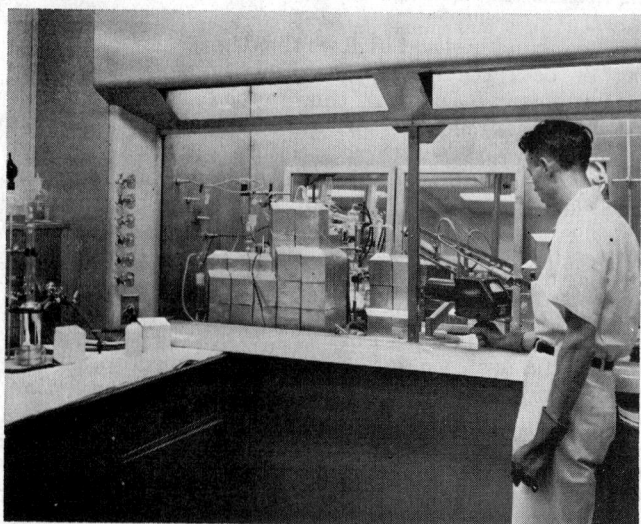

Fig. 389. Production of radioactive pharmaceuticals. Radioisotopes for medical use must be processed to meet requirements for purity, potency, and sterility. Lead bricks protect lab workers from rays. Mirrors at rear of hood provide view of operations which must be conducted by means of mechanical "hands" remotely controlled (courtesy, Abbott).

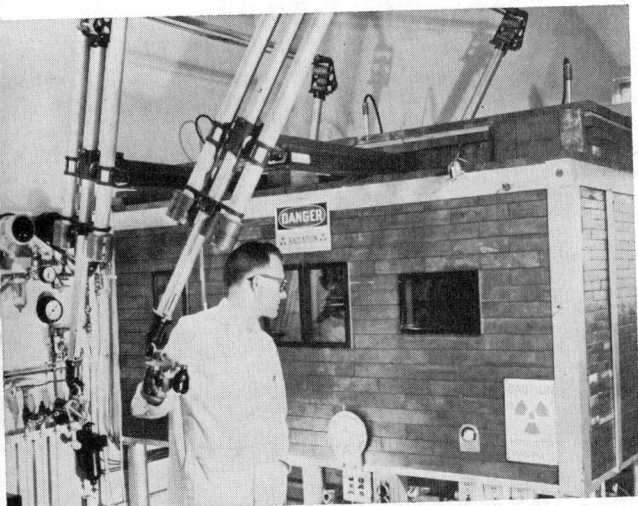

Fig. 390. Radioactive drugs are manufactured in a "cave" behind 4-inch walls and leaded windows. Hot materials are handled with remote-controlled manipulators to avoid contamination from drug's radioactivity (courtesy, Squibb).

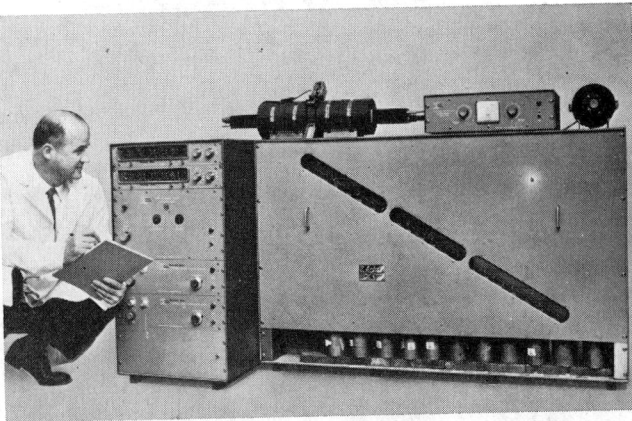

Fig. 391. Automatic radioactive-capsule device measures and sorts capsules according to their radioactivity and drops them into marked lead cups (courtesy, Squibb).

particular, have found widespread usage, especially for sodium radioiodide-131, which is widely used for measuring thyroid activity. It is necessary for the manufacturer to check the activity of each capsule to assure that all capsules in a given shipment contain the same amount of radioactivity. Fig. 391 illustrates a machine specifically designed to do this job. It measures and sorts capsules according to their radioactivity and drops them into marked lead cups.

References

1. Lark-Horowitz, K., and Leng, H. R., *J. APhA, Sci. Ed.*, **31**, 99 (1942).
2. Katz, M., and Barr, M., *J. APhA, Sci. Ed.*, **44**, 476 (1955).
3. Riegelman, S., and Crowell, W., *J. APhA, Sci. Ed.*, **47**, 115 (1958).
4. Peterson, C., *et al*, *J. APhA, Sci. Ed.*, **42**, 73 (1953).
5. Nash, and Crabtree, R., *J. APhA, Sci. Ed.*, **50**, 134 (1961).
6. Montgomery, K. O., *et al*, *J. Pharm. Sci.*, **53**, 340 (1964).
7. Patel, K., *et al*, *J. Pharm. Sci.*, **50**, 300 (1961).
8. Barker, D. Y., *et al*, *J. APhA, Sci. Ed.*, **45**, 601 (1956).
9. Stark, J., *et al*, *J. APhA, Sci. Ed.*, **47**, 223 (1958).
10. Ruggiero, J. S., and Skauen, D. M., *J. Pharm. Sci.*, **51**, 233 (1962).
11. Ruggiero, J. S., and Skauen, D. M., *J. Pharm. Sci.*, **51**, 235 (1962).
12. Sorby, D., and Plein, E., *J. APhA, Sci. Ed.*, **48**, 308 (1959).
13. Hupf, H., Chase, G., and Barr, M., paper presented before the Scientific Section of the APhA, Washington, D.C., 1960.
14. Lux, R., and Christian, J. E., *J. APhA, Sci. Ed.*, **40**, 160 (1951).
15. Urakami, C., and Christian, J. E., *J. APhA, Sci. Ed.*, **42**, 179 (1953).
16. Gerding, P., *et al*, *J. APhA, Sci. Ed.*, **44**, 574 (1955).
17. Clark, G. S., and Swartz, H. A., *J. Pharm. Sci.*, **52**, 999 (1963).
18. Appino, J. B., *et al*, *J. Pharm. Sci.*, **51**, 254 (1962).
19. Rosenblum, C., and Woodbury, D., *J. APhA, Sci. Ed.*, **41**, 368 (1952).
20. Pinotti, P. L., *et al*, *Quart. Transcript Soc. Automotive Engines*, **3**, 634 (1949).
21. *Chem. Eng. News*, **34**, 919 (Feb. 27, 1956).
22. *Chem. Eng. News*, **30**, 647 (Feb. 18, 1952).
23. *Chem. Eng. News*, **34**, 920 (Feb. 27, 1956).
24. *Chem. Eng. News*, **37**, 46 (Aug. 10, 1959).
25. *Chem. Eng. News*, **37**, 48 (Sept. 7, 1959).
26. *Chem. Eng. News*, **37**, 42 (Dec. 21, 1959).
27. *Chem. Eng. News*, **37**, 34 (Dec. 28, 1959).
28. *Radiation—A Tool for Industry*, USAEC, Y3. At7:22/ALI-52, USGPO, Washington, D.C., 1959.
29. *Chem. Eng. News*, **33**, 509 (Nov. 21, 1955).
30. *Chem. Ind.* (London), 923 (Sept. 8, 1956).
31. Proctor, B. E., and Goldblith, S. A., *A Critical Evaluation of the Literature Pertaining to the Application of Ionizing Radiations to the Food and Pharmaceutical Fields*, Mass. Inst. of Tech., Cambridge, 1952.
32. Dunn, C. G., *et al*, *J. Appl. Phys.*, **19**, 605 (1948).
33. Brownell, L. E., and Bulmer, J. J., *1st Intern. Conf. Peaceful Uses At. Energy, Geneva*, 1955.
34. Anderson, R. S., and Harrison, B., *J. Gen. Physiol.*, **27**, 69 (1943).
35. Proctor, B. E., and Goldblith, S. A., *Nucleonics*, **3** (2), 32 (1948).
36. Proctor, B. E., and Goldblith, S. A., *Nucleonics*, **5** (3), 56 (1949).
37. Goldblith, S. A., and Proctor, B. E., *Nucleonics*, **5** (2), 50 (1949).
38. Goldblith, S. A., *et al*, *J. Biol. Chem.*, **179**, 1163 (1949).
39. Corson, M., *et al*, *Arch. Biochem. Biophys.*, **33**, 263 (1951).
40. Controulis, J., *et al*, *J. APhA, Sci. Ed.*, **43**, 65 (1954).
41. Laug, E. P., *J. APhA, Sci. Ed.*, **45**, 357 (1956).
42. Colovos, G. C., and Churchill, B. W., *J. APhA, Sci. Ed.*, **46**, 580 (1957).
43. Prusak, L. P., and Sciarrone, B. J., *J. Pharm. Sci.*, **52**, 546 (1963).
44. Hull, D. E., and Kent, J. W., *Ind. Eng. Chem.*, **44**, 2745 (1952).
45. Meinke, W. W., and Anderson, R. E., *Anal. Chem.*, **25**, 778 (1953).
46. *Chem. Eng. News*, **37**, 40 (Nov. 9, 1959).
47. Atkins, D. H. F., and Smalls, A. A., *Advan. Inorg. Chem. Radiochem.*, **1**, 315 (1959).
48. Guinn, V. P., and Wagner, C. D., *Anal. Chem.*, **32**, 317 (1960).
49. Vacik, J. P., and Christian, J. E., *J. Pharm. Sci.*, **50**, 225 (1961).
50. Wainerdi, R. E., *Nucleonics*, **22**, No. 2, 57 (Feb. 1964).
51. Tuckerman, M. M., *et al*, *J. Pharm. Sci.*, **53**, 983 (1964).
52. Buyers Guide Issue, *Nucleonics* (Nov. of each year).
53. *Chem. Eng. News*, **38**, 58 (Apr. 11, 1960).
54. Peck, G. E., *et al*, *J. Pharm. Sci.*, **53**, 607 (1964).
55. Carlin, J. R., *Rubber Age*, **66**, 173 (1949).
56. Schreiber, A. P., *Nucleonics*, **2**, No. 1, 33 (1948).
57. Yankwich, P. E., *Anal. Chem.*, **21**, 318 (1949).
58. Rosenblum, C., *Anal. Chem.*, **29**, 1740 (1957).
59. Jacobs, R. B., and Lewis, L. G., *Oil Gas J.*, **52**, 128 (1953).
60. Gray, R. G., *et al*, *Anal. Chem.*, **31**, 2065 (1959).
61. Becquerel, H., *Compt. Rend.*, **122**, 420 (1896).
62. Tenney, G. H., *Nondestructive Testing*, **6**, 7 (1948).
63. Eastwood, W. S., *Proc. Intern. Conf. Peaceful Uses At. Energy, Geneva*, **15**, 177 (1956).
64. Brook, B., *et al*, *Proc. 2nd United Nations Intern. Conf. Peaceful Uses At. Energy*, **19**, 219 (1958).
65. Morrison, A., *Nucleonics*, **5**, 19 (1949).
66. Dick, C. M., *Welding J.*, **36**, 456 (1957).
67. Yagoda, H., *Radioactive Measurements with Nuclear Emulsions*, Wiley, New York, 1949.
68. Boyd, G. A., *Autoradiography in Biology and Medicine*, Academic, New York, 1955.
69. Taylor, J. H., *Proc. Symp. Advan. Tracer Appl. Tritium*, New England Nuclear Corp., Boston, 1959, p. 38.
70. Bushland, R. C., and Hopkins, D. E., *J. Econ. Entomol.*, **46** (4), 648 (1953).
71. Jenkins, D. W., *Intern. Conf. Peaceful Uses At. Energy*, A/Conf. 8/P./224 (June 28, 1955).
72. Quaterman, K. D., *et al*, *J. Econ. Entomol.*, **48**, 30 (1955).
73. Provost, M. W., *Mosquito News*, **12**, 174 (1952).
74. Schoof, H. F., and Siverly, R. E., *J. Econ. Entomol.*, **47**, 830 (1954).
75. Schoof, H. F., and Siverly, R. E., *Am. J. Trop. Med. Hyg.*, **3**, 367 (1954).
76. Jenkins, D. W., *Exptl. Parasitol.*, **3**, 474 (1954).
77. Berk, S., and Teitell, L., *Ind. Eng. Chem.*, **46**, 778 (1954).
78. Briner, W. H., *Am. J. Hosp. Pharm.*, **20**, (1963).

Bibliography

Bradford, R. J., ed., *Radioisotopes in Industry*, Reinhold, New York, 1953.
Crowther, J. G., *Nuclear Energy in Industry*, Pitman, New York, 1956.
Desrosier, N. W., and Rosestock, H. M., *Radiation Technology in Food, Agriculture and Biology*, Avi, Westport, Conn., 1960.
Dick, W. E., *Atomic Energy in Agriculture*, Philosophical Library, New York, 1957.
Extermann, R. C., ed., *The Peaceful Uses of Atomic Energy* (12 vols.), Pergamon, New York, 1958.
Hughes, D. J., *On Nuclear Energy: Its Potential for Peacetime Uses*, Harvard Univ. Press, Cambridge, 1957.
International Atomic Energy Agency, Radioisotope Applications in Industry. A Survey, Intern. Publ., New York, 1964.
Klineberg, O., ed., *Social Implications of the Peaceful Uses of Nuclear Energy*, Intern. Publ., New York, 1965.
Luntz, J. D., *Handbook of Radioisotope Applications*, Nucleonics, New York, 1956.
Mann, M., *Peacetime Uses of Atomic Energy*, Crowell, New York, 1957.
McMahon, J. J., and Berman, A., *Radioisotopes in Industry*, Natl. Ind. Conf. Board, New York, 1959.
Rochlin, R. S., and Schultz, W. W., *Radioisotopes for Industry*, Reinhold, New York, 1959.
Shilling, C. W., *Radiation: Use and Control in Industrial Applications*, Grune & Stratton, New York, 1960.
Woodbury, D. O., *Atoms for Peace*, Dodd–Meade, New York, 1955.

TESTING and ANALYSIS

EDITOR

Alfonso R. Gennaro, PhD, *Professor of Chemistry,*
Philadelphia College of Pharmacy and Science, Philadelphia, Pa. 19104

A summary of the general notices, tests, and processes of the United States Pharmacopeia and the National Formulary which provide a basis for drug standardization

This chapter was prepared by

Alfonso R. Gennaro, PhD, *Professor of Chemistry, Philadelphia College of Pharmacy and Science, Philadelphia, Pa. 19104*

The United States Pharmacopeia and the National Formulary provide certain "General Notices Applying to Standards, Tests and Assays" and, in the appendices of the respective books, the "General Tests, Processes and Apparatus" pertaining to official substances. Certain of these notices, and such tests, processes and apparatus as are of general application, are included and/or described in this chapter, usually in an abstracted form which explains the underlying principle. Under no circumstances are the explanatory and interpretative statements in this chapter to be considered the equivalent of corresponding statements in the official texts, which should be consulted for complete and exact specifications.

General Notices of the USP and NF

The following material is selected and abstracted from the General Notices of the USP and NF. See also page 602.

Deviations Permitted

Ingredients and Processes—Certain deviations in the manufacture of an official preparation are permitted so long as the finished material conforms to the official standards. Reference should be made to the official compendia for detailed specifications.

Percentage of Alcohol—All statements of percentages of alcohol refer to percentage, by volume, of C_2H_5OH at 15.56°.

Denatured Alcohol—If alcohol is used in the manufacture of an official preparation, but does not remain in the finished product (eg, alcohol in tablet granulations), alcohol denatured with benzene, methanol or acetone may be used but the finished product must conform to the official standards.

Capsules and Tablets—Capsules and tablets may be manufactured with suitable diluents, colors, lubricants, and adhesives, such as starches, lactose, sucrose, and other innocuous materials. Capsules, and tablet coatings, may be colored with an official article or a color certified as suitable for coloring drugs under the terms of the Federal Food, Drug and Cosmetic Act.

Ointments and Suppositories—In official ointments and suppositories, the proportions of the substances constituting the base may be varied to maintain a suitable consistency under different climatic conditions, provided the proportion of active ingredients is not varied.

Tolerances—The minimum purity limits specified for official articles are established with a view to the use of the latter as drugs. Such limits do not bar the use of lots of an article which more nearly approach 100% purity nor do they constitute a basis for a claim that such lots "exceed" the official requirements.

The tolerances stated for preparations and dosage forms allow for assay error, for unavoidable variations in compounding, and for deterioration to an extent considered insignificant under practical conditions. In compounding preparations and dosage forms, the quantity of each ingredient used shall be not less than 100% of that called for in the formula or of the amount declared on the label.

Added Substances—Unless otherwise specified in the individual monograph, suitable substances may be added to a pharmacopeial article or preparation to enhance its permanency or usefulness. Such substances may be regarded as suitable only if they are non-toxic and harmless in the amounts administered and do not interfere with the therapeutic efficacy of the article or preparation or with the tests and assays prescribed for determining compliance with the pharmacopeial standards.

Packaging, Storage, Labeling, and Preservation

Containers—The *container* is the device which holds the drug and which is or may be in direct contact with the drug. The *immediate container* is that which is in direct contact with the drug at all times. The *closure* is a part of the container. The container does not interact physically or chemically with the drug that it holds so as to alter the strength, quality, or purity of the drug beyond the official requirements. Types of *containers* specified as: *Well-Closed, Tight, Hermetic, Light-Resistant, Single-Dose* and *Multiple-Dose* are described in detail in the USP.

Storage Temperature—These are defined as follows:
Cold—Any temperature not exceeding 8° (46°F). A refrigerator is a cold place in which the temperature is held between 2° and 8° (36° and 46°F).
Cool—Any temperature between 8° and 15° (46° and 59°F). Articles for which storage in a cold place is indicated can also be stored in a refrigerator, unless otherwise indicated.
Room Temperature—The temperature prevailing in a working area. Controlled Room Temperature is maintained thermostatically between 15° and 30° (59° and 86°F)
Excessive Heat—The expression "excessive heat" designates temperatures above 40° (104°F).
Protection from Freezing—Where, in addition to the risk of breakage of the container, unintentional freezing subjects a product to loss of strength or potency, or to destructive alteration of the dosage form, the container label bears appropriate notice to protect from freezing.
Storage of Biologics—Because biologics are usually stored in mechanically operated refrigerators, occasionally they are frozen. Provided the container remains intact, such freezing does not affect the potency of the product unless the labeling indicates to the contrary.

Bulk Packages—Unless otherwise specified in the monograph, bulk packages from importers, manufacturers, or wholesale distributors are exempt from the storage requirements when the products are intended for manufacture or for subsequent repackaging for the dispenser or retail distributor.

Nonspecific Storage Conditions—Where no specific storage conditions are stated it is to be understood that the storage conditions include protection from water, freezing and excessive heat.

Labeling—Shipping containers, unless such containers are also essentially the immediate containers or the outside of the retail package, are exempt from the official labeling requirements.

Amount of Ingredient per Dosage Unit—Official articles in capsule, tablet or other unit dosage forms shall be labeled to express the quantity of each therapeutically active ingredient container in each such unit.

Labeling Vitamin-Containing Products—The vitamin content of official preparations shall be stated on the label in metric units. The amounts of vitamins A and D may be stated also in USP Units.

Quantities of vitamin A declared in metric units refer to the equivalent amounts of vitamin A alcohol (retinol).

Special Tablets—The label of any form of Tablet intended for administration other than by swallowing intact bears a prominent indication of the manner in which it is to be used. If enteric coated, the label must so state.

Expiration Date—The monographs on several official articles, particularly those which are biologic in origin, require that the label bear an expiration date which generally indicates the time beyond which the article may not have the required potency, provided the prescribed storage conditions have been maintained.

Tests and Assays

Apparatus—A specification for a definite size or type of container or apparatus in a test or assay is given solely as a recommendation except with respect to volumetric flasks or other exact measuring, weighing, classifying, or sorting devices.

Where an instrument for physical measurement, such as a spectrophotometer, is specified in a test or assay by its distinctive name, another instrument of equivalent or greater sensitivity or accuracy may be used.

Where use of a centrifuge is specified, the directions are predicated upon the use of an apparatus having an effective radius of about 20 cm, and driven at a speed effecting clarification of the supernatant layer within 15 minutes.

Extraction Apparatus—Where a separator is directed to be used for separating immiscible solvents used to extract a drug principle, a suitable centrifuge, with appropriate transfer devices, may be used instead. Continuous extraction with hot or cold solvents may replace use of separators where it is demonstrated that the extraction is complete and does not cause deterioration of drug principles.

Steam Bath—Where the use of a steam bath is directed, exposure to actively flowing steam or the heat of vigorously boiling water, or to another form of regulated heat, corresponding in temperature to that of flowing steam, may be used. Where the term *water bath* is still used without a qualifying statement as to the temperature, a bath of vigorously boiling water is to be used.

Foreign Substances—Tests for the presence of foreign substances are provided to limit such substances to amounts which are unobjectionable under conditions in which the medicinal agent is customarily employed.

Unofficial Methods for Detecting Added Foreign Substances—While one of the primary objects of the USP and NF is to assure the user of official medicinal substances of their identity, strength, quality, and purity, it is manifestly impossible to include in each monograph a test for every impurity or adulterant that might be present. Tests suitable for detecting impurities, the presence of which is inconsistent with good pharmaceutical practice, may be employed in addition to the tests provided.

Procedures—The strength and quality of articles or preparations for which assay processes are provided, and the limit of other substances in official drugs, are to be determined by the prescribed procedures, including the general tests.

In stating the appropriate quantities to be taken for assays, the word "about" is used to indicate that a quantity within 10 per cent of the specified amount is satisfactory. However, the quantity taken is accurately determined and the assay result is based upon this exact weight or volume.

Where it is directed, in the assay of Tablets, to "weigh and finely powder not less than" a given number, usually 20, of the Tablets, it is intended that a counted number of tablets shall be weighed, and reduced to a fine powder representative of the whole Tablets. The portion of the powdered tablets taken for assay is, in turn, weighed accurately.

Tests and assays in which the substance is directed to be dried previously may be performed on the undried substance and the results calculated on the dry basis, provided a *Loss on drying* or *Water* test is given in the monograph.

Desiccator—The term "in a desiccator" specifies the use of a tightly closed container of suitable size and design which maintains an atmosphere of low moisture content by means of a suitable desiccant in effective condition, such as anhydrous calcium chloride, magnesium perchlorate, phosphorus pentoxide, or silica gel.

Drying to Constant Weight—The specification "dried to constant weight" means that the drying shall be continued until two consecutive weighings do not differ by more than 0.5 mg/Gm of substance taken, the second weighing following an additional hour of drying.

Indicators—Where the use of a test solution as an indicator is specified in a test or assay, 3 drops of the solution shall be added, unless otherwise directed.

Logarithms—Logarithms used in the assays are to the base 10.

Negligible—This term indicates a quantity not exceeding 0.5 mg.

Odorless—The term "odorless" in the *Description* applies to examination, after exposure to the air for 15 minutes, of a freshly opened package of the article, for packages containing not more than 25 Gm or, for larger packages, of a portion of about 25 Gm of the article that has been quickly removed from its package to an open evaporating dish of about 100-ml capacity.

Pressure Measurements—The term "mm of mercury" used with respect to measurements of blood pressure, pressure within an apparatus, or atmospheric pressure refers to the use of a suitable manometer or barometer calibrated in terms of the pressure exerted by a column of mercury of the stated height.

Purified Water—Where water is called for in tests and assays, Purified Water (page 1338) is to be used.

Solutions—Unless otherwise specified in the individual monograph, all solutions are prepared with purified water. An expression such as "(1 in 10)" means that 1 part *by volume* of a liquid is to be diluted with, or 1 part *by weight* of a solid is to be dissolved in, sufficient of the diluent or solvent to make the volume of the finished solution 10 parts *by volume*. When normalities or molarities of solutions are specified in an assay, other suitable standardized solutions may be used provided allowance is made for the difference in concentration.

Specific Gravity—Unless otherwise stated, the specific gravity basis is 25°/25°, i.e., the ratio of the weight of a substance in air at 25° to that of an equal volume of water at the same temperature. See page 95.

Temperatures—Unless otherwise specified, all temperatures in the USP and NF are expressed in centigrade degrees. All measurements are made at 25° unless otherwise directed.

With respect to sterilization processes involving the use of steam under pressure, the stated temperature are those at the exhaust line of the autoclave when the steam has completely replaced the air.

Time Limit—In conducting the limit tests for impurities (chloride, iron, etc), 5 minutes shall be allowed for the reaction to take place unless otherwise specified.

Vacuum—The term "in vacuum" specifies exposure to a pressure of less than 20 mm of mercury.

Water and Loss on Drying—A distinction is made in providing limit tests for volatile matter that may be adsorbed or present as water of hydration. Where available data indicate that water is the only volatile substance present, the test is given under the heading *Water* with directions for a titrimetric estimation or a determination of loss on drying.

Where it is less certain that the loss on drying of an article is actually water, or where the loss is known to represent loss of organic solvents, etc, the test is given under the heading *Loss on drying*.

Solubility—Official articles, when brought into solution, may show slight physical impurities, such as fragments of filter paper, fibers, and dust particles, unless excluded by definite tests in the individual monograph.

Units of Potency

For those antibiotic, pharmacodynamic, and endocrine preparations as well as most of the serums, toxins, vaccines, and related products, for which it is still necessary to express the potency in terms of units by reference to a suitable working standard (usually a USP or NF Reference Standard), the individual monographs refer to USP or NF Units of activity. Without exception, these units are equivalent to the corresponding international units, where such exist, and to the units of activity established by the Food and Drug Administration in the case of antibiotics, and by the National Institutes of Health in the case of biological products.

The potency of some antibiotics is defined in terms of mcg or mg of the parent drug, even though the antibiotic concerned may be in the form of a salt, ester or other chemical combination.

Vegetable and Animal Drugs

Vegetable and Animal Drugs—The official requirements apply to vegetable and animal drugs as they enter commerce; however, lots of such drugs intended solely for the manufacture or isolation of volatile oils, alkaloids, glycosides, or other active principles may depart from such requirements.

Foreign Matter—Vegetable and animal drugs are to be as free as reasonably practicable from molds, insects and other animal contamination, and from animal excreta. They shall show no abnormal discoloration, abnormal odor, sliminess, or evidence of deterioration.

The amount of foreign inorganic matter in vegetable or animal drugs, estimated as *Acid-insoluble ash*, shall not exceed 2% of the weight of the drug, unless otherwise specified in the individual monograph.

Vegetable drugs are to be freed of stones, dust, lumps of dirt, and other foreign inorganic matter that can be separated by mechanical means before grinding or powdering.

In commerce it is seldom possible to obtain vegetable drugs in a state of absolute purity, and some adherent or admixed, innocuous, foreign matter is usually not detrimental. No poisonous, dangerous, or otherwise noxious foreign substance, however, may be present. Foreign organic matter includes any part of the plant not specified as constituting the drug.

Preservation—Vegetable or animal substances may be protected from insect infestation by means of a suitable fumigant, such as chloroform, carbon tetrachloride, or methyl bromide.

General Tests and Processes

The appendices of the USP and NF contain much information bearing on official procedures and specifications. Some of this information is included in various other chapters of this book. Hereunder are described general tests and processes which are of general analytical interest. Certain other information, notable examples of which are standards for official reagents and formulas for test solutions, is not included; reference should be made to the USP and NF for such standards and formulas.

General Information and Procedures

Reference Standards*

To a greater extent than heretofore, reference standards are called upon in the official assays. Originally introduced for the biological assays of USP X, the use of reference standards has been extended to the point where they are now required for many other assays as well. A set of six standards is provided for checking the reliability of apparatus used for melting-point determinations.

With a view to preventing confusion in clinical research or as a possible first step in pharmacopeial standardization, reference standards or substances are provided occasionally for endocrine or enzyme activity in advance of the actual pharmacopeial admission of a product representing that activity. Such products are designated as "substances" if they are heterogeneous in nature and if the prospect of their assuming pharmacopeial status is fairly remote; however, heterogeneous substances may be designated as "reference standards" if they are the counterparts of international standards. Among such standards at present are the eight "essential" amino acids and preparations of the thyrotropic hormone and of the growth hormone.

Also provided, on the same basis as the reference standards, but under the immediate supervision of the USP Steroid Advisory Board, is a group of products known as the USP Steroid Substances. These are pure specimens of steroids suitably diluted with an inert diluent for use in the chromatographic identification of steroids. A total of 72 such reference substances is now available.

Negative Control Plastic specimens are also available from USP to be used as controls in the testing of plastic containers intended for use with injectable materials.

The release of USP Reference Standards and USP Reference Substances is authorized by the USP Board of Trustees upon recommendation by the USP Reference Standards Committee which plans, supervises, and finally passes upon the suitability of each lot. The critical characteristics of the specimens selected for the standard are usually determined independently in three or more laboratories, generally including the federal regulatory agencies of both the United States and Canada.

Suitable standards for radioactive substances (^{60}Co, ^{51}Cr, ^{198}Au, ^{131}I, and ^{32}P) can be obtained from commercial sources.

A similar program to provide international standards is maintained by the World Health Organization (WHO), a unit of the United Nations. The WHO program is concerned mainly with standards for serums, toxins, vaccines, endocrine extracts, and vitamins. As a rule, an International Standard is no longer provided once the substance responsible for its characteristic activity has been isolated, identified, and made readily available. The USP Reference Standards Committee collaborates very closely with the WHO in order not only to insure that the differences in the actual units of potency will be minimized, but also in certain cases to arrange for physical identity of the respective reference standards.

* Reference Standards and Steroid Substances may be obtained from USP Reference Standards, 4630 Montgomery Ave., Washington, D.C. 20014. Reference Standards listed in the NF may be obtained from the Chairman of the Committee on NF, American Pharmaceutical Association, 2215 Constitution Ave., N.W., Washington, D.C. 20037.

Vegetable and Animal Drugs, Methods for Sampling and Analysis

Sampling—Specific directions are indicated in the official compendia for obtaining an *official*, representative sample. The amount taken for a sample is dependent upon such factors as: size of component parts, total weight of material being sampled, etc.

Foreign Organic Matter in Whole Vegetable Drugs—This determination is made by noting the difference in weight of a portion of the *official sample* subsequent to mechanical removal of the foreign matter.

Preparation of Vegetable or Animal Drugs for Analysis—A representative portion of the *official sample* is ground, sieved, and mixed thoroughly before analysis.

Total Ash in Vegetable Drugs—Ash is determined by incineration of a sample of the ground drug. A carbon-free ash must be obtained, either directly, or by the use of water extraction of the ash, or by ignition of the charred ash with alcohol.

Acid-insoluble Ash in Vegetable Drugs—The ash obtained as indicated in the preceding paragraph is extracted with diluted hydrochloric acid and the change in weight noted.

Moisture—Moisture is determined by simply determining the loss in weight of a dried sample, if no other volatile constituents are present. If volatile components are known to occur in the drug, the *Toluene Distillation Method* (page 595) must be employed.

Extractives

Alcohol-soluble Extractive—A sample of the drug is extracted in a *Soxhlet Extraction Apparatus*, with alcohol, and the weight difference of the dried residue noted. Moisture is also determined by the *Toluene Distillation Method* (page 595) and the loss of weight of the sample, calculated on a dry basis, is the *Alcohol-soluble Extractive*.

Diluted Alcohol-soluble Extractive—A sample of the drug is extracted with diluted alcohol by agitation and an aliquot of the extracting solution is evaporated to dryness and weighed.

Solvent Hexane-soluble Extractive—A sample of the drug is extracted with solvent hexane for 20 hours, in a continuous extraction apparatus, and the residue obtained on evaporation of the solvent weighed.

Non-volatile Ether-soluble Extractive—Proceed as directed under *Volatile Ether-soluble Extractive* (next paragraph).

Volatile Ether-soluble Extractive—Proceed as under *Solvent Hexane-soluble Extractive* (above) but using absolute ether. The residue is dried to constant weight at 105°.

Water-soluble Extractive—Proceed as directed under *Diluted Alcohol-soluble Extractive* above, using water instead of diluted alcohol.

Volatile Oil Determination—The drug is distilled with steam into a graduated receiver constructed to return excess water to the distilling flask. The oil volume is measured and the volume of oil per 100 Gm of drug calculated. Different receivers are employed for oils which are heavier or lighter than water. If considerable starch or mucilage is present in the drug it is first extracted with alcohol or ether to remove the oil, the extract is evaporated, the residue mixed with sawdust and then subjected to steam distillation.

Chemical Tests and Assays

In addition to the more specific tests and assays included in the official monographs there are a number of tests and assays which are more general in nature. Because of the frequency with which they occur, they are described in this chapter and cross references are made from the monographs to which they apply. Not all of the tests and assays are included (eg, Epinephrine, Choline, Thiamine, etc) since these procedures are included in Chapter 37, *Analysis of Medicinals*. Resumés of the official directions are given below.

Alkali Salts of Organic Acids

A weighed quantity of the salt is ignited to sodium carbonate and digested with excess standard sulfuric acid, filtered, and the excess acid titrated with standard alkali using methyl orange indicator. This assay is not applicable for alkali salts of organic acids which contain sulfur or halogens.

Arsenic Test

This test is a variation of the time-honored *Gutzeit* procedure. The arsenic test apparatus (Fig. 392) consists of a generator flask (*a*) which contains sulfuric acid, potassium iodide, stannous chloride, granulated zinc, and the sample. Hydrogen gas, formed by the zinc and acid serves both to aid in the reduction of arsenic to arsine and to carry the arsine gas into the absorber tube (*e*). The scrubber unit (*c*) contains cotton moistened with lead acetate solution to absorb any hydrogen sulfide formed during the reduction. After passing through the scrubber, the arsine gas flows into the absorber tube (*e*) which contains silver diethyldithiocarbamate TS, and a red color is produced. The absorbance of the red color is measured at 525 mμ and compared to a standard.

Antimony, sulfites, sulfides, thiosulfates, or other compounds which form stibine or hydrogen sulfide, under the conditions of the test, interfere. Excessive darkening of the lead acetate scrubber may necessitate repetition of the test on a portion of the sample which is first oxidized with nitric acid.

Cobalamin Assay—Radiotracer Method

By means of solvent extraction and column chromatography, a quantity of pure cobalamin is isolated from the preparation being assayed. The quantity isolated is measured spectrophotometrically against standard cyanocobalamin. The efficiency of the extraction process (which may vary from sample to sample) is determined by an isotope dilution technique utilizing a sample of cyanocobalamin tagged with ^{60}Co. Thus from the efficiency of the extraction and from the quantity isolated from the original sample, the amount of Cobalamin in the preparation is calculated.

Content Uniformity

Most dosage forms, other than liquids, creams, or lotions, which contain 50 mg or less of an active ingredient are subject to a *content uniformity* test. From a selection of 30 individual dosage units (tablets, capsules, containers, etc), 10 units are individually assayed and all 10 units must fall within the limits of 85% to 115% of the mean of the tolerances specified in the rubric definition in the official monograph.

If one, but not more than one, result falls outside these limits, the contents of the remaining 20 dosage units is individually assayed. The requirements are met if not more than one of the 30 results is outside the 85% to 115% limit.

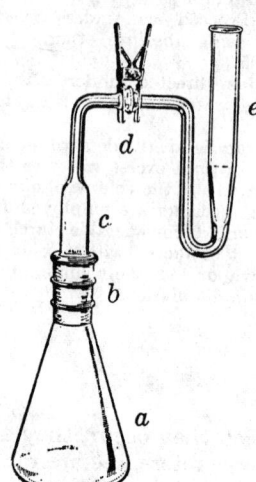

Fig. 392. Arsenic test apparatus consisting of an arsine generator (a) fitted with a scrubber unit (c) and an absorber tube (e), with standard-taper or ground-glass ball-and-socket joints (b and d) between the units.

Fats and Fixed Oils

The following definitions and general procedures apply to fixed oils, fats, waxes, resins, balsams, and similar substances.

Preparation of Sample—If the sample is turbid or a solid at room temperature, it may be warmed and/or filtered to insure homogeneity before sampling.

Specific Gravity—Determination of the specific gravity is accomplished at 25°, unless otherwise specified (eg, for a solid), in a pycnometer fitted with a capillary stopper. The pycnometer is weighed empty, filled with sample at the specified temperature and also filled with water at 25°. The quotient of the weight of the sample divided by the weight of water is the specific gravity at the temperature of observation referred to water at 25°.

Melting Temperature—The melting temperature is determined as directed for substances of *Class II* (see page 594).

Solidification Temperature of Fatty Acids (Frequently referred to as the "titer").

Free fatty acids are obtained from the sample of oil or fat by saponification with a glycerol-potassium hydroxide mixture followed by dilution with water and acidification. The separated fatty acids are washed to remove mineral acid and dried. A type V thermometer is suspended in a tube containing the fatty acids and the temperature adjusted to 15° to 20° above the expected reading while stirring with the thermometer. After allowing the thermometer to hang quietly the maximum constant reading attained by the mercury column is the solidification temperature.

Free Fatty Acids—The acidity in the Pharmacopeia is usually expressed as the number of ml of 0.1N alkali required to neutralize the free acids in 10 Gm of substance. Acidity is frequently expressed as the *Acid Value* which is the number of mg. of potassium hydroxide required to neutralize the free acids in 1 Gm of the substance. To determine these values a solution of the sample in neutralized alcohol is titrated with 0.1N sodium hydroxide using phenolphthalein TS as the indicator.

Acetyl Value of Fatty Acids—This is the number of mg. of potassium hydroxide required to neutralize the acetic acid obtained by the saponification of 1 Gm of acetylated fatty acids.

In this procedure the fatty acids are acetylated with acetic anhydride, and the purified acetylated acids saponified to determine the saponification value.

Determine the acid value, expressed in mg of potassium hydroxide per Gm of acid and calculate the acetyl value, A, by the following formula:

$$A = \frac{S - F}{1 - 0.00075S}$$

A is the acetyl value of the free fatty acids.

S is the saponification value of the acetylated fatty acids.

F is the acid value of the original fatty acids expressed as mg of potassium hydroxide required to neutralize 1 Gm of fatty acids.

Ester Value—The Ester Value is the number of mg of potassium hydroxide required to saponify the esters in 1 Gm of the substance. If the *Saponification Value* and the *Acid Value* have been determined, the difference between these two represents the Ester Value.

A sample of the fat or oil, in neutral alcohol, is first titrated to a phenolphthalein end-point with alkali, to neutralize the free acids, and then saponified with excess alcoholic potassium hydroxide. The excess alkali is titrated with standard hydrochloric acid and a blank run on the alcoholic hydroxide. The *Ester Value* is computed from the volume of standard acid consumed.

Iodine Value (*Hanus method*)—The Iodine Value represents the number of Gm of iodine absorbed, under the prescribed conditions, by 100 Gm of the substance.

Hanus Solution (iodine monobromide in glacial acetic acid) is allowed to react with a sample of fat or oil and the excess determined by addition of potassium iodide, liberating iodine, which is titrated with standard thiosulfate, using starch as the indicator. A blank determination is conducted on the Hanus Solution. The volume of 0.1N thiosulfate equivalent to the sample, multiplied by 1.269 and divided by the sample weight, is the *Iodine Value*.

Note—If more than half of the iodobromide TS is absorbed by the portion of the substance taken, repeat the determination, using a smaller portion of the substance under examination.

Saponification Value—The Saponification Value is the number of mg of potassium hydroxide required to neutralize the free acids and saponify the esters contained in 1 Gm of the substance.

The sample is saponified with a measured excess of alcoholic potassium hydroxide and the excess determined by titration to a phenolphthalein end-point with 0.5N hydrochloric acid. A blank on the alcoholic alkali is also run.

If the oil has been saturated with carbon dioxide for the purpose of preservation, expose it in a shallow dish in a vacuum desiccator for 24 hours before weighing the samples.

Unsaponifiable Matter—The term, Unsaponifiable Matter, in oils or fats, refers to those substances that are not saponifiable by alkali hydroxides but are soluble in the ordinary fat solvents.

The sample is saponified with alcoholic potassium hydroxide and the alcohol evaporated. The residue is dissolved in water and the aqueous solution extracted with ether, the ether solution washed until neutral and evaporated. The weight of the dried residue represents Unsaponifiable Matter.

Water and Sediment in Fatty Oils—Centrifugation of benzene solutions of the sample under specified conditions, in graduated conical tubes, yields a water-sediment layer in the bottom of the tube. The sum of the volumes of combined water and sediment represents the percentage, by volume, of water and sediment in the oil.

Heavy Metals Test

This test is provided to demonstrate that the content of metallic impurities that are colored by hydrogen sulfide does not exceed the *Heavy metals* limit given in the individual monograph in terms of the parts (by weight) of lead per million parts of the test substance, as revealed by a parallel comparison with a standard lead solution.

Method I is for the simpler and colorless substances, while Method II is for colored substances and those which by virtue of their complex nature interfere with the precipitation of heavy metals by sulfide.

For Method I, direct comparison of the prepared test solution and a lead standard containing the limit specified in the individual monograph, in Nessler tubes containing hydrogen sulfide TS, is made. The test solution must be no darker than the standard tube.

In Method II, the sample is first ignited with nitric and sulfuric acids, neutralized and filtered before proceeding as in Method I. The treatment removes any colored substances which interfere with the test.

Procedure for Volatile Oils

Shake 10 ml of the oil with an equal volume of water to which 1 drop of hydrochloric acid has been added, and pass hydrogen sulfide through the mixture until it is saturated: no darkening in color is produced in either the oil or the water.

Hydroxypropoxy Determination

Hydroxypropoxyl groups, $(OCH_2CHOHCH_3)$, are determined in a specialized apparatus (see the official NF method). The sample is oxidized with chromium trioxide in a flask through which is passed a stream of nitrogen and into which water is added dropwise. Acetic acid is formed and distilled into a receiver in which it is titrated with standard alkali to a phenolphthalein end point. A blank determination is run on the reagents. Each ml of 0.02N sodium hydroxide, equivalent to the acetic acid distilled, is equal to 1.5 mg of (OC_3H_6-OH).

Identification Tests

Under this heading are placed tests which are frequently specified in USP and NF monographs.

When identification problems arise the chemist should turn to the original literature, i.e., the USP or NF for items official in those books, and use the identification tests provided therein with discretion and in the light of his own knowledge and experience. Absolute identification of an unknown is possible only by using the official identification tests in conjunction with elemental analyses, the preparation of derivatives with recorded physical properties, and the application of other appropriate methodology.*

With the advent of infrared spectrophotometric identity tests included in many of the official monographs (page 601), rapid, conclusive identification of many substances is easily accomplished by comparison of the spectrum of the material in question with the spectrum of an official Reference Standard.

Limit Tests

Chloride—A solution of the substance and a specified volume of 0.02N hydrochloric acid, in different cylinders, are each treated with nitric acid and silver nitrate. The turbidity produced in the sample should not exceed that of the standard.

Sulfate—This test is similar to the *chloride* limit test substituting barium chloride for the silver nitrate and using sulfuric acid (0.02N) as a standard.

Lead—A solution of the sample and *Standard Lead Solution* is treated with *Dithizone* in chloroform to produce the characteristic violet color of the lead complex (see page 211). The color of the sample should be no deeper shade of violet than that of the standard.

Mercury—The NF provides a limit test for mercury in *Danthron* (page 797). The drug is refluxed with nitric and sulfuric acids, to destroy all organic matter, and the resulting solution titrated with a standard dithizone solution in the presence of hydroxylamine hydrochloride.

Selenium—Much of the sulfur now used commercially comes from lower grade deposits and may have appreciable amounts of selenium associated with it. For this reason the official compendia have incorporated a selenium limit test for many organic pharmaceuticals which contain a large percentage of sulfur and which are used over long periods of time; eg, Tolbutamide.

The test involves decomposition of the sample by the *Oxygen Flask Combustion* method, using 0.5N nitric acid as the absorbing liquid. After adjustment of pH, a solution of 2,3-dinitronaphthalene is added, the mixture extracted with cyclohexane, and the absorbance of the extract determined at 380 mμ. A blank and standard are run concomitantly.

Methoxy Determination

In this procedure the methoxy groups of the sample are hydrolyzed with hydriodic acid to yield methyl iodide which is carried by a stream of carbon dioxide through a red phosphorus suspension in cadmium sulfate solution to absorb any free iodine or hydrogen sulfide. The methyl iodide is absorbed in a bromine-acetic acid solution which liberates iodine monobromide. Excess bromine in the receiver oxidizes the IBr to iodic acid, to which is added potassium iodide, and the liberated iodine titrated with thiosulfate. A blank is performed on the reagents. Each ml of 0.1N sodium thiosulfate is equivalent to 0.517 mg of (OCH_3). Specialized apparatus is required and reference to the official procedure should be made for exact specifications.

Nitrogen Determination

Kjeldahl Method

The following procedure may be employed for many organic compounds containing nitrogen which will yield ammonia on digestion with sulfuric acid and subsequent alkalinization with fixed base. It may *not* be used, however, for certain alkaloids and other nitrogen-containing compounds which resist complete decomposition with sulfuric acid.

The general procedure for the Kjeldahl method involves the digestion of the sample with a mixture of sulfuric acid and potassium sulfate with copper sulfate as a catalyst. The sulfuric acid-potassium sulfate mixture has a higher boiling point than the acid alone and facilitates decomposition of the sample. Copper or mercury salts have been found to catalyze the digestion of the sample. After conversion of the organic nitrogen to ammonium sulfate, alkali is added and the liberated ammonia distilled. A reagent blank is usually run concurrently.

The sample, weighed by difference or directly on a sheet of nitrogen free paper, is mixed with the acid, sulfate, and catalyst in a Kjeldahl flask and heated, gently at first until the frothing subsides, and then strongly. The reaction mixture is black at first, due to charring, finally becoming almost colorless (or pale blue-green if a copper salt catalyst is used). After cooling, water is added and the flask arranged for distillation using a bubble trap. Excess concentrated sodium hydroxide and a few pieces of "mossy" zinc (to minimize "bumping") are added to the flask and the mixture, distilled through the condenser, fitted with a delivery tube dipping below the surface of the liquid in the receiver (see summary of the official methods below).

If nitrites or nitrates are known to be present, salicylic acid or benzoic acid is added to the initial digestion mixture to aid in the reduction of the nitrite or nitrate function to ammonia.

Method I (Macro Procedure)

The official method is essentially that as outlined above. A 500-ml Kjeldahl flask is employed and an approximately 1 Gm. sample is used. The condenser delivery tube dips below the surface of an excess of 0.5N sulfuric acid which is partially neutralized by the distilled ammonia. Methyl red-methylene blue TS is used as the indicator and the excess acid titrated with 0.5N sodium hydroxide solution. A blank determination is run, omitting only the sample, and the necessary correction made. Each ml of 0.5N acid consumed is equivalent to 7.004 mg of nitrogen in the weight of sample taken.

Method II (Semi-micro Procedure)

This method also follows the general procedure outlined previously except that the sample weight is of the order of 50 mg taken to contain about 5 mg of nitrogen. After digestion and alkalinization steam is passed through the digestion flask to assist in removal of the

---

* See, for example, such references as Shriner, Fuson, and Curtin, *The Systematic Identification of Organic Compounds*, and Huntress and Milliken, *Identification of Pure Organic Compounds*, both published by Wiley, New York.

ammonia. Saturated boric acid is used in the receiver and the distilled ammonia is directly titrated with standard alkali (0.02N) using methyl red as the indicator.

For detailed directions as to the performance of the above methods reference should be made to the USP.

Nitrogenous Bases

Identification—The base is liberated from the salt (either from the bulk or dosage form) with dilute sodium hydroxide, the organic layer dried, and the infrared spectrum determined at 7–15μ. Comparison of the spectrum with a standard run in similar fashion serves to identify the base.

Assay—After liberation of the base as above, it is extracted into ether solution, then back into dilute sulfuric acid, and the absorbance in the ultraviolet region determined at the wavelength specified in the monograph. A standard is carried through the procedure concomitantly.

Oxygen Flask Combustion

This method is provided as the preparatory step in the determination of bromine, chlorine, iodine, and sulfur in many organic compounds. The procedure converts covalent halogen and sulfur into soluble ionic products which are then analyzed as directed in the individual monographs. The sample is weighed on a piece of halide free filter paper (or in a gelatin capsule if liquid) and placed in a platinum holder attached to a glass stopper. An absorbing solution, dependent upon the element being analyzed, is placed in a thick walled iodine flask and the flask filled with oxygen. A small paper fuse strip protruding from the platinum holder is ignited and the stopper immediately placed in the flask. When the combustion is complete the flask is shaken to dissolve the products of combustion and the solution treated as indicated in the monograph.

Because of the possibility of shattering the flask during combustion, a special type of stopper is available whereby the ignition can be performed electrically while keeping the flask behind a safety shield.

Readily Carbonizable Substances Test

The sample is stirred into a volume of 95% sulfuric acid which causes carbonization to take place. Matching fluids, consisting of solutions of specified volumes of cobaltous chloride, ferric chloride and cupric sulfate, are prepared and compared with the unknown under similar conditions.

Residue on Ignition

A sample of the material is ignited at the lowest possible temperature, moistened with sulfuric acid and reignited until any carbonaceous material is completely consumed. The weight of the residue is noted. For *Non-Volatile Residue*, the sulfuric acid treatment is omitted.

Rosin Test

In testing for rosin as an adulterant in resins, gum resins, and balsams, the powdered sample is extracted with solvent hexane, filtered and the filtrate shaken with dilute cupric acetate solution: the hexane layer should not show a green color.

Steroid Assay (Total Steroids Assay, USP)

The general method for the assay of steroid materials in pharmaceutical preparations involves the formation of a color with blue tetrazolium TS and tetramethylammonium hydroxide TS, using a suitably prepared sample. The intensity of the color is determined spectrophotometrically at 525 mμ and the concentration calculated by comparison with the absorbance of a reference standard steroid treated similarly.

Steroid Chromatographic Purity (NF)

Known as the Single Steroid Assay (USP). In both the USP and NF procedures a sample and standard are chromatographed, using the thin-layer technique, on silica gel. After development, the proper bands are located under UV light, marked and removed by scraping. The adsorbed steroid is then removed by extraction with alcohol. In the NF procedure the absorptivities in the UV region of the standard and sample are compared directly. For the USP procedure the blue tetrazolium method for the *Steroid Assay* (above) is employed.

Zinc Determination

Zinc is determined in a manner similar to that for lead (page 589) using dithizone. The color of the sample is compared with that of a zinc standard in a spectrophotometer at 530 mμ.

Physical Tests and Determinations

Alcohol Determination

Alcohol is distilled from a water-diluted sample, recovering about 2 ml less than the original sample volume. The specific gravity of the distillate is determined at 25° and the percentage of alcohol calculated from the Alcoholometric Table (Table I). Frothing and/or bumping of the sample being distilled may be minimized by acidification with a nonvolatile acid, or other means, and by the addition of "boiling stones." Samples containing glycerin should be diluted so as to contain at least 50% water. If iodine is present it must be reduced with zinc or sodium thiosulfate and sodium hydroxide.

Volatile substances must be removed by extraction of the sample, diluted with saturated sodium chloride solution, with petroleum benzin. Free ammonia, other volatile bases or volatile acids must be neutralized before distillation of the sample.

An alternative procedure using gas–liquid chromatography (page 672) is also employed whereby the ratio of the peak areas of the sample to a standard alcohol dilution is used to calculate the alcohol content. Acetone is used as an internal standard.

Boiling or Distilling Range or Temperature

Method I

This method is used for liquids for which the permissible boiling range is 5° or less. The sample is distilled, in a specified type of apparatus, and the initial temperature noted when the first drops of distillate have been collected.

The final or upper temperature is that reading when the last liquid evaporates from the bottom of the distilling flask. The distillation is conducted so as to collect about 4 to 5 ml/minute.

Method II

This method is used for liquids for which the permissible range in boiling temperature exceeds 5°.

The procedure is conducted as in *Method I*, except that a measured volume (usually 100 ml) of the sample is distilled and the *volume* of the distillate coming over between the temperature limits specified in the monograph is noted.

Chloroform Determination

The NF provides detailed descriptions of the apparatus and procedure prescribed for the determination of chloroform in mixtures with alcohol or with alcohol and water.

Congealing Range or Temperature

The congealing temperature of a solid is frequently referred to in commerce as the "melting temperature," although its determination involves solidification or congealation from the molten state upon controlled cooling. With respect to fatty acids, it is spoken of as the "titer." See *Solidification Temperature of Fatty Acids*, page 588.

The determination is conducted in a test tube fitted with a cork stopper carrying a suitable, short range thermometer (USP, page 844) in the center and a wire loop stirrer, passing through the cork off center, surrounding the thermometer, which is manipulated by raising and lowering the exposed wire. The sample is melted and placed in the test tube, the stopper inserted and the whole placed in a water bath, consisting of two concentric containers, at a temperature 4° or 5° below the expected congealing point of the sample. The outside container is equipped with a Type I thermometer. The

Table I—Alcoholometric Table (By Weight)[a]

By wt	By vol at 15.56°C.	at $\frac{25°}{25°}$	at $\frac{15.56°}{15.56°}$	By wt	By vol at 15.56°C.	at $\frac{25°}{25°}$	at $\frac{15.56°}{15.56°}$
	Percentage of C_2H_5OH	Specific gravity in air			Percentage of C_2H_5OH	Specific gravity in air	
0	0.00	1.0000	1.0000				
1	1.26	0.9981	0.9981	51	58.84	0.9102	0.9159
2	2.51	0.9963	0.9963	52	59.85	0.9079	0.9137
3	3.76	0.9945	0.9945	53	60.85	0.9056	0.9114
4	5.00	0.9927	0.9928	54	61.85	0.9033	0.9092
5	6.24	0.9911	0.9912	55	62.84	0.9010	0.9069
6	7.48	0.9894	0.9896	56	63.82	0.8987	0.9046
7	8.71	0.9879	0.9881	57	64.80	0.8964	0.9024
8	9.94	0.9863	0.9867	58	65.77	0.8941	0.9001
9	11.17	0.9848	0.9852	59	66.73	0.8918	0.8978
10	12.39	0.9833	0.9839	60	67.69	0.8895	0.8955
11	13.61	0.9818	0.9825	61	68.64	0.8871	0.8932
12	14.83	0.9804	0.9812	62	69.59	0.8848	0.8909
13	16.05	0.9789	0.9799	63	70.52	0.8824	0.8886
14	17.26	0.9776	0.9787	64	71.46	0.8801	0.8862
15	18.47	0.9762	0.9774	65	72.38	0.8777	0.8839
16	19.68	0.9748	0.9763	66	73.30	0.8753	0.8815
17	20.88	0.9734	0.9751	67	74.21	0.8729	0.8792
18	22.08	0.9720	0.9738	68	75.12	0.8706	0.8768
19	23.28	0.9706	0.9726	69	76.02	0.8682	0.8745
20	24.47	0.9692	0.9714	70	76.91	0.8658	0.8721
21	25.66	0.9677	0.9701	71	77.79	0.8634	0.8697
22	26.85	0.9663	0.9688	72	78.67	0.8609	0.8673
23	28.03	0.9648	0.9675	73	79.54	0.8585	0.8649
24	29.21	0.9633	0.9662	74	80.41	0.8561	0.8625
25	30.39	0.9617	0.9648	75	81.27	0.8537	0.8601
26	31.56	0.9601	0.9635	76	82.12	0.8512	0.8576
27	32.72	0.9585	0.9620	77	82.97	0.8488	0.8552
28	33.88	0.9568	0.9605	78	83.81	0.8463	0.8528
29	35.03	0.9551	0.9590	79	84.64	0.8439	0.8503
30	36.18	0.9534	0.9574	80	85.46	0.8414	0.8479
31	37.32	0.9516	0.9558	81	86.28	0.8389	0.8454
32	38.46	0.9498	0.9541	82	87.08	0.8364	0.8429
33	39.59	0.9480	0.9524	83	87.89	0.8339	0.8404
34	40.72	0.9461	0.9506	84	88.68	0.8314	0.8379
35	41.83	0.9442	0.9488	85	89.46	0.8288	0.8354
36	42.94	0.9422	0.9470	86	90.24	0.8263	0.8328
37	44.05	0.9402	0.9451	87	91.01	0.8237	0.8303
38	45.15	0.9382	0.9342	88	91.77	0.8211	0.8276
39	46.24	0.9362	0.9412	89	92.52	0.8184	0.8250
40	47.33	0.9341	0.9392	90	93.25	0.8158	0.8224
41	48.41	0.9320	0.9372	91	93.98	0.8131	0.8197
42	49.48	0.9299	0.9352	92	94.70	0.8104	0.8170
43	50.55	0.9278	0.9331	93	95.41	0.8076	0.8142
44	51.61	0.9256	0.9310	94	96.10	0.8048	0.8114
45	52.66	0.9235	0.9289	95	96.79	0.8020	0.8086
46	53.71	0.9213	0.9268	96	97.46	0.7992	0.8057
47	54.75	0.9191	0.9246	97	98.12	0.7962	0.8028
48	55.78	0.9169	0.9225	98	98.76	0.7932	0.7988
49	56.81	0.9147	0.9203	99	99.39	0.7902	0.7967
50	57.83	0.9124	0.1981	100	100.00	0.7871	0.7936

[a] Based upon data appearing in *Natl. Bur. Std.* (US) *Tech. News Bull.*, **9**, 424, 425 (1925).

Table I—Alcoholometric Table (By Volume)[a]

Percentage of C_2H_5OH		Specific gravity in air		Percentage of C_2H_5OH		Specific gravity in air	
By vol at 15.56°C.	By wt	at $\frac{25°}{25°}$	at $\frac{15.56°}{15.56°}$	By vol at 15.56°C.	By wt	at $\frac{25°}{25°}$	at $\frac{15.56°}{15.56°}$
0	0.00	1.0000	1.0000				
1	0.80	0.9985	0.9985	51	43.43	0.9269	0.9322
2	1.59	0.9970	0.9970	52	44.37	0.9248	0.9302
3	2.39	0.9956	0.9956	53	45.33	0.9228	0.9282
4	3.19	0.9941	0.9942	54	46.28	0.9207	0.9262
5	4.00	0.9927	0.9928	55	47.25	0.9185	0.9241
6	4.80	0.9914	0.9915	56	48.21	0.9164	0.9220
7	5.61	0.9901	0.9902	57	49.19	0.9142	0.9199
8	6.42	0.9888	0.9890	58	50.17	0.9120	0.9177
9	7.23	0.9875	0.9878	59	51.15	0.9098	0.9155
10	8.05	0.9862	0.9866	60	52.15	0.9076	0.9133
11	8.86	0.9850	0.9854	61	53.15	0.9053	0.9111
12	9.68	0.9838	0.9843	62	54.15	0.9030	0.9088
13	10.50	0.9826	0.9832	63	55.17	0.9006	0.9065
14	11.32	0.9814	0.9821	64	56.18	0.8983	0.9042
15	12.14	0.9802	0.9810	65	57.21	0.8959	0.9019
16	12.96	0.9790	0.9800	66	58.24	0.8936	0.8995
17	13.79	0.9778	0.9789	67	59.28	0.8911	0.8972
18	14.61	0.9767	0.9779	68	60.33	0.8887	0.8948
19	15.44	0.9756	0.9769	69	61.38	0.8862	0.8923
20	16.27	0.9744	0.9759	70	62.44	0.8837	0.8899
21	17.10	0.9733	0.9749	71	63.51	0.8812	0.8874
22	17.93	0.9721	0.9739	72	64.59	0.8787	0.8848
23	18.77	0.9710	0.9729	73	65.67	0.8761	0.8823
24	19.60	0.9698	0.9719	74	66.77	0.8735	0.8797
25	20.44	0.9685	0.9708	75	67.87	0.8709	0.8771
26	21.29	0.9673	0.9697	76	68.98	0.8682	0.8745
27	22.13	0.9661	0.9687	77	70.10	0.8655	0.8718
28	22.97	0.9648	0.9676	78	71.23	0.8628	0.8691
29	23.82	0.9635	0.9664	79	72.38	0.8600	0.8664
30	24.67	0.9622	0.9653	80	73.53	0.8572	0.8636
31	25.52	0.9609	0.9641	81	74.69	0.8544	0.8608
32	26.38	0.9595	0.9629	82	75.86	0.8516	0.8580
33	27.24	0.9581	0.9617	83	77.04	0.8487	0.8551
34	28.10	0.9567	0.9604	84	78.23	0.8458	0.8522
35	28.97	0.9552	0.9590	85	79.44	0.8428	0.8493
36	29.84	0.9537	0.9576	86	80.66	0.8397	0.8462
37	30.72	0.9521	0.9562	87	81.90	0.8367	0.8432
38	31.60	0.9506	0.9548	88	83.14	0.8335	0.8401
39	32.48	0.9489	0.9533	89	84.41	0.8303	0.8369
40	33.36	0.9473	0.9517	90	85.69	0.8271	0.8336
41	34.25	0.9456	0.9501	91	86.99	0.8237	0.8303
42	35.15	0.9439	0.9485	92	88.31	0.8202	0.8268
43	36.05	0.9421	0.9469	93	89.65	0.8167	0.8233
44	36.96	0.9403	0.9452	94	91.03	0.8130	0.8196
45	37.87	0.9385	0.9434	95	92.42	0.8092	0.8158
46	38.78	0.9366	0.9417	96	93.85	0.8053	0.8118
47	39.70	0.9348	0.9399	97	95.32	0.8011	0.8077
48	40.62	0.9328	0.9380	98	96.82	0.7968	0.8033
49	41.55	0.9309	0.9361	99	98.38	0.7921	0.7986
50	42.49	0.9289	0.9342	100	100.00	0.7871	0.7936

[a] Based upon data appearing in *Natl. Bur. Std.* (US) *Tech. News Bull.*, **9**, 424, 425 (1925).

Table II—Thermometric Equivalents[a]

Fahrenheit to Centigrade Scales

$$(F° - 32) \times \tfrac{5}{9} = C°$$

F	C	F	C	F	C	F	C
0	−17.78	52	11.11	101	38.33	152	66.67
1	−17.22	53	11.67	102	38.89	153	67.22
2	−16.67	54	12.22	103	39.44	154	67.78
3	−16.11	55	12.78	104	40.	155	68.33
4	−15.56	56	13.33	105	40.56	156	68.89
5	−15.	57	13.89	106	41.11	157	69.44
6	−14.44	58	14.44	107	41.67	158	70.
7	−13.89	59	15.	108	42.22	159	70.56
8	−13.33	60	15.56	109	42.78	160	71.11
9	−12.78	61	16.11	110	43.33	161	71.67
10	−12.22	62	16.67	111	43.89	162	72.22
12	−11.11	63	17.22	112	44.44	163	72.78
14	−10.	64	17.78	113	45.	164	73.33
16	−8.89	65	18.33	114	45.56	165	73.89
18	−7.78	66	18.89	115	46.11	166	74.44
20	−6.67	67	19.44	116	46.67	167	75.
22	−5.56	68	20.	117	47.22	168	75.56
24	−4.44	69	20.56	118	47.78	169	76.11
26	−3.33	70	21.11	119	48.33	170	76.67
28	−2.22	71	21.67	120	48.89	171	77.22
29	−1.67	72	22.22	121	49.44	172	77.78
30	−1.11	73	22.78	122	50.	173	78.33
31	−0.56	74	23.33	123	50.56	174	78.89
32	0.	75	23.89	124	51.11	175	79.44
33	0.56	76	24.44	125	51.67	176	80.
34	1.11	77	25.	126	52.22	177	80.56
35	1.67	78	25.56	127	52.78	178	81.11
36	2.22	79	26.11	128	53.33	179	81.67
37	2.78	80	26.67	129	53.89	180	82.22
38	3.33	81	27.22	130	54.44	181	82.78
39	3.89	82	27.78	131	55.	182	83.33
40	4.44	83	28.33	132	55.56	183	83.89
41	5.	84	28.89	133	56.11	184	84.44
42	5.56	85	29.44	134	56.67	185	85.
43	6.11	86	30.	135	57.22	186	85.56
44	6.67	87	30.56	136	57.78	187	86.11
45	7.22	88	31.11	137	58.33	188	86.67
46	7.78	89	31.67	138	58.89	189	87.22
47	8.33	90	32.22	139	59.44	190	87.78
48	8.89	91	32.78	140	60.	191	88.33
50	10.	92	33.33	141	60.56	192	88.89
		93	33.89	142	61.11	193	89.44
		94	34.44	143	61.67	194	90.
		95	35.	144	62.22	195	90.56
		96	35.56	145	62.78	196	91.11
		97	36.11	146	63.33	197	91.67
		98	36.67	147	63.89	198	92.22
		99	37.22	148	64.44	199	92.78
		100	37.78	149	65.	200	93.33
				150	65.56		

Centigrade to Fahrenheit Scales

$$\tfrac{9}{5}\,C° + 32 = F°$$

C	F	C	F	C	F	C	F	C	F
−20	−4.0	21	69.8	61	141.8	101	213.8	141	285.8
−19	−2.2	22	71.6	62	143.6	102	215.6	142	287.6
−18	−0.4	23	73.4	63	145.4	103	217.4	143	289.4
−17	1.4	24	75.2	64	147.2	104	219.2	144	291.2
−16	3.2	25	77.	65	149.	105	221.	145	293.
−15	5.	26	78.8	66	150.8	106	222.8	146	294.8
−14	6.8	27	80.6	67	152.6	107	224.6	147	296.6
−13	8.6	28	82.4	68	154.4	108	226.4	148	298.4
−12	10.4	29	84.2	69	156.2	109	228.2	149	300.2
−11	12.2	30	86.	70	158.	110	230.	150	302.
−10	14.	31	87.8	71	159.8	111	231.8	151	303.8
−9	15.8	32	89.6	72	161.6	112	233.6	152	305.6
−8	17.6	33	91.4	73	163.4	113	235.4	153	307.4
−7	19.4	34	93.2	74	165.2	114	237.2	154	309.2
−6	21.2	35	95.	75	167.	115	239.	155	311.
−5	23.	36	96.8	76	168.8	116	240.8	156	312.8
−4	24.8	37	98.6	77	170.6	117	242.6	157	314.6
−3	26.6	38	100.4	78	172.4	118	244.4	158	316.4
−2	28.4	39	102.2	79	174.2	119	246.2	159	318.2
−1	30.2	40	104.	80	176.	120	248.	160	320.
0	32.	41	105.8	81	177.8	121	249.8	161	321.8
1	33.8	42	107.6	82	179.6	122	251.6	162	323.6
2	35.6	43	109.4	83	181.4	123	253.4	163	325.4
3	37.4	44	111.2	84	183.2	124	255.2	164	327.2
4	39.2	45	113.	85	185.	125	257.	165	329.
5	41.	46	114.8	86	186.8	126	258.8	166	330.8
6	42.8	47	116.6	87	188.6	127	260.6	167	332.6
7	44.6	48	118.4	88	190.4	128	262.4	168	334.4
8	46.4	49	120.2	89	192.2	129	264.2	169	336.2
9	48.2	50	122.	90	194.	130	266.	170	338.
10	50.	51	123.8	91	195.8	131	267.8	171	339.8
11	51.8	52	125.6	92	197.6	132	269.6	172	341.6
12	53.6	53	127.4	93	199.4	133	271.4	173	343.4
13	55.4	54	129.2	94	201.2	134	273.2	174	345.2
14	57.2	55	131.	95	203.	135	275.	175	347.
15	59.	56	132.8	96	204.8	136	276.8	176	348.8
16	60.8	57	134.6	97	206.6	137	278.6	177	350.6
17	62.6	58	136.4	98	208.4	138	280.4	178	352.4
18	64.4	59	138.2	99	210.2	139	282.2	179	354.2
19	66.2	60	140.	100	212.	140	284.	180	356.
20	68.								

[a] F represents Fahrenheit degrees and C represents Centigrade degrees.

temperature of the sample is noted every 30 seconds, while stirring continuously. The temperature falls gradually, becomes constant, and finally again falls gradually. This constant reading or plateau of the "cooling curve" so determined is noted as the congealing temperature. Constant stirring is required to prevent supercooling and a resulting deviation from the normal temperature pattern.

Containers—Glass

Light Transmission

To determine the transmissive properties of glass used for container purposes a clean sample of the glass, of a specified thickness is placed in a suitable spectrophotometer and a curve, plotting transmission vs wave length (spectral transmission curve), is obtained. The characteristics of the container material are obtained from this curve in the ultraviolet visible and very near infrared regions of the spectrum. (See the USP for additional details.)

Chemical Resistance

The following tests are designed to determine the resistance of various types of glass to acid or alkaline attack. The degree of attack is determined by the amount of alkali released from the glass under the influence of the attacking medium under the conditions specified. This quantity of alkali is extremely small in the case of the more resistant glasses, thus calling for particular attention to all details of the tests. All equipment used in these tests should be of high quality and precision and the tests should be carried out in a laboratory relatively free from fumes and excessive dust. The USP and NF provide detailed descriptions of the apparatus and reagents used in the *Powdered Glass Test and Water Attack at 121°.*

Four types of glass are listed which are characterized by the degree of resistance to attack by the chemical agents used. They are: Type I, Highly resistant, usually borosilicate; Types II, III, and NP, soda lime glasses of varying resistance.

Containers—Plastic

Certain biological and chemical test procedures are performed on plastic materials intended for use as containers for parenteral dosage forms. Several extracting agents—such as polyethylene glycol 400, sesame or cottonseed oil, or isotonic sodium chloride solution—are used to remove any soluble materials from the plastic and the extracts are utilized in animal toxicity studies.

Chemical tests are concerned only with aqueous extracts and on these are determined the nonvolatile residue, residue on ignition, heavy metals, and reaction toward acid and base.

Rubber Closures for Injections

Biological and chemical tests similar to those described for plastic containers are applied also to rubber.

Freezing Point

The freezing point of a substance is defined as that temperature, approached by cooling a liquid, at which the solid phase is in equilibrium with the liquid phase. If supercooling does not take place, this is the lowest temperature remaining constant for a short period of time. In the presence of supercooling this point is the highest temperature remaining constant for a short period of time during the solidification of a substance from its molten state.

NF XII (page 454) provided elaborate details for *Freezing point of phenothiazine.* See also *congealing range* (NF, page 794) and the *NF Comm. Bull.,* 12, 47 (1944).

Loss on Drying

A sample of the material is heated at the temperature specified in the monograph and the loss in weight noted as *Loss on drying.* If the substance melts at a lower temperature than that specified it is usually heated at a point 5° to 10° below the specified temperature, for a period of time, and finally dried at the indicated temperature.

Melting Range or Temperature

For pharmacopeial purposes, the melting range or temperature of a solid is defined as those points of temperature within which, or the point at which the solid coalesces and is completely melted, when determined as directed below. Any apparatus or method capable of equal accuracy may be used. The accuracy may be checked by the use of one or more of the six USP Melting Point Reference Standards (USP, page 823).

Five procedures for the determination of melting range or temperature are given herein, varying in accordance with the nature of the substance. When no class is designated in the monograph, the procedure for *Class I* is to be used.

The material must be in a finely divided state (for Class I and Ia) and dried as specified in the monograph, or dried over sulfuric acid if drying is not specifically indicated. Continuous stirring of the bath liquid is required to insure equilibrium conditions at all times.

The procedure known as the mixed-melting point determination whereby the melting range of a solid under test is compared with that of an intimate mixture of equal parts of the solid and an authentic specimen of it may be used as a confirmatory identification test. Agreement of the observations on the original and the mixture constitutes reliable evidence of chemical identity.

Apparatus—The melting range apparatus consists of a glass container for a bath of colorless fluid, a suitable stirring device, an accurate thermometer (see USP, page 844), and a controlled source of heat. The bath fluid is selected with a view to the temperature required, but light paraffin is used generally and certain liquid silicones are well adapted to the higher temperature ranges. The fluid is deep enough to permit immersion of the thermometer to its specified immersion depth so that the bulb is still about 2 cm above the bottom of the bath. The heat may be supplied by an open flame or electrically. The capillary tube is about 10 cm long and 0.8 to 1.2 mm in internal diameter with walls, 0.2 to 0.3 mm in thickness.

The thermometer is preferably Type I or Type II (see USP, page 844), selected for the desired range or temperature.

Procedure for Class I—A glass capillary, of specified dimensions, closed at one end, is charged with the sample, packing it into the closed end. The capillary is attached to the thermometer, with the sample end of the capillary adjacent to the thermometer bulb, and the combination inserted into the heating bath, at a temperature about 30° below the expected melting point. Heating of the bath is continued at a rate of about 3° per minute to within 3° of the indicated melting point, then at the rate of 1° to 2° per minute. The point at which the sample is observed to collapse against the side of the capillary is noted as the beginning of the melting range, and the point at which the sample becomes liquid throughout is defined as the end of melting.

Procedure for Class Ia—Prepare the sample and charge the capillary glass tube as directed for Class I. Heat the bath until a temperature 10 ± 1° below the expected melting range is reached, then introduce the charged tube, and heat at a rate of rise 3 ± 0.5° per minute until melting is complete. Record the melting range as for Class I.

Procedure for Class Ib—Without previously powdering the cooled sample, it is charged into a capillary, dried in a vacuum desiccator and then the open end of the capillary sealed. The melting range is determined as directed under *Class Ia.*

Procedure for Class II—A melted sample is drawn into a capillary, open at both ends, cooled, and the open capillary attached to the thermometer and the melting range determined as indicated for *Class I,* except that the rate of temperature rises is decreased to 0.5° to 1.0° per minute when within 5° of the expected melting temperature. The temperature at which the sample rises in the capillary is noted as the melting temperature.

Procedure for Class III—A layer of the sample is formed on the bulb of a Type III thermometer, by a specified procedure, and the thermometer is placed in a water bath at 16°. The temperature of the bath is gradually increased and temperature at which the first drop of sample falls from the thermometer bulb is noted. This determination must be repeated several times, on a freshly melted sample, and an average taken.

Phase Solubility Analysis

This physical method for determining the purity of a substance depends on the precise measurement of its solubility in a suitable solvent. A detailed description of the method is given in Chapter 19, *Solutions and Phase Equilibria.*

Refractive Index

The refractive index (n) of a transparent substance is the ratio of the velocity of light in air to its velocity in that material under like conditions. It is equal to the ratio of the sine of the angle of incidence made by a ray in air to the sine of the angle of refraction made by the ray in the material being tested. This physical constant is used as a means for identification of, and detection of impurities in volatile oils. The Abbé refractometer measures the range of indices of the official materials for which these values are given. Other refractometers of equal or greater accuracy may be employed at the discretion of the operator.

Water Determination

Many pharmacopeial drugs are either hydrates or contain water in absorbed form. As a result, the determination of the water content is important in demonstrating compliance with the official standards. Generally, one of the three methods given below is called for in the individual monograph, depending upon the nature of the article. In rare cases, a choice is allowed between two methods. When the article contains water of hydration, the Karl Fischer Method or the Toluene Distillation Method is specified, and the requirement is given under the heading, *Water*.

The heading, *Loss on Drying*, is used in those cases where the loss sustained on heating may not be entirely water.

I—Karl Fischer (Titrimetric) Method

The Karl Fischer titrimetric determination of water depends upon the fact that a solution of sulfur dioxide and iodine in pyridine and methanol reacts with water quantitatively. The entire operation requires rigid exclusion of atmospheric moisture.

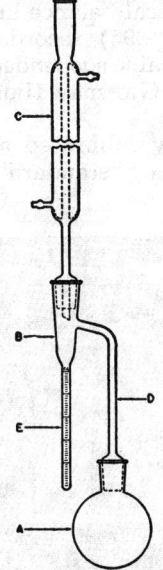

Fig. 393.   Toluene moisture apparatus.

In colorless solutions, the end-point of the titration may be determined electrometrically or visually by a change from a canary yellow to an amber color. In colored solutions the end-point is obscured and is best determined electrometrically. For this purpose, the required apparatus embodies a simple electrical circuit which serves to pass 5 to 10 microamperes of direct current at a 1.5-volt potential between a pair of platinum electrodes immersed in the solution to be titrated. An ordinary pH meter will serve this purpose nicely. At the end-point of the titration a slight excess of the reagent increases the flow of current to between 50 and 150 microamperes for 30 seconds or longer, depending upon the solution being titrated. The time is shortest for substances which react with the reagent.

Apparatus—Any apparatus may be used which provides for adequate exclusion of atmospheric moisture and determination of the end-point. Commercially available apparatus generally comprises a closed system consisting of one or two automatic burets and a tightly covered titration vessel fitted with the necessary electrodes and a magnetic stirrer. The air in the system is kept dry with a desiccant such as phosphorus pentoxide, anhydrous granular calcium chloride, or silica gel. The latter may contain an indicator to reveal its state of hydration.

Karl Fischer Reagent—The reagent is prepared by mixing a solution of sulfur dioxide in pyridine and methanol with a solution of iodine in pyridine. Each ml of the prepared reagent should be equivalent to about 5 mg of water. A prepared, stabilized reagent is commercially available. Standardization is effected by titrating a standard solution of water in anhydrous methanol or by the use of sodium tartrate dihydrate as a primary standard.

Procedure—Unless otherwise specified, add about 25 ml of methanol to the titration flask and titrate to the end-point with the *Karl Fischer Reagent*, disregarding the volume consumed, since it does not enter into the calculations. Weigh or measure sufficient sample to contain preferably 10 to 50 mg of water, and quickly transfer it to the titration flask. Stir vigorously, and again titrate with the *Karl Fischer Reagent*. The water content of the sample, in mg, is given by the formula $S \times F$, in which S is the volume of reagent used to titrate the sample, and F is the water equivalence factor defined above.

II—Toluene Distillation (Volumetric) Method

By the use of the apparatus shown in Fig. 393 water may be determined by volume measurement. The sample and toluene are placed in flask A and the mixture distilled. Toluene and water form an azeotropic mixture and codistil into the condenser C and the cooled vapors, after condensation, fall back into the receiver B. Water, being of greater density than toluene, falls to the graduated portion E and the volume read directly. Care must be taken to insure that any water droplets adhering to B or C are washed into E.

III—Gravimetric Method

Procedure for Chemicals—Proceed as directed in the individual monograph, preparing the chemical as directed under *Loss on Drying*, USP, page 935.

Procedure for Biologicals—Proceed as directed in the individual monograph.

Procedure for Vegetable Drugs—Place about 10 Gm of the drug, prepared as directed (USP, page 837) and accurately weighed, in a tared evaporating dish. Dry at 105° for 5 hours, and weigh. Continue the drying and weighing at 1-hour intervals until the difference between two successive weighings corresponds to not more than 0.25%.

IV—Dew-point Method

At very low concentrations the amount of water vapor in a system may be determined by noting the temperature at which a dew or mist forms when the system is suddenly cooled under adiabatic expansion following release of compression (similar to a Wilson cloud chamber). Reference to calibrated charts gives the water content of the vapor.

V—Electrolytic Hygrometer Method

For extremely low concentrations of water the principle of selective electrolysis of water can be employed and the amount of electric current required is a measure of the water content.

37 | Analysis of Medicinals

Analytical balances—sources of information—specialized analytical methods and equipment—official physical and chemical assays

This chapter was prepared by

Alfonso R. Gennaro, PhD, *Professor of Chemistry,*
Philadelphia College of Pharmacy and Science, Philadelphia, Pa.   19104

From the time of the early apothecaries, who worked with meager equipment in small laboratories, pharmacists have made important contributions in the field of medicinal chemistry, both in discovering or isolating new therapeutic agents and in developing methods for standardizing and controlling medicinals.   Today such activity is rarely a function of the prescription laboratory, but in manufacturing laboratories pharmacists often perform physical and chemical analyses either in the course of developing dosage forms of new products or in the control of standard products.   In small laboratories the responsibility for performing analyses may be delegated entirely to pharmacist staff members. But whether or not a pharmacist may have occasion to conduct analyses, he should at least understand the basic principles involved in the standardization and control of the medicinal agents he dispenses.

Analytical Balances

Equipment of a very modest character may be used in the initial stages of the development of an analytical department, and as the need develops and opportunities occur a more complete laboratory can be built up in which work of the most complex type may be performed.   The manufacturing pharmacist's first duty, of course, is in the direction of the maintenance of quality and purity in such items of his own stock as are likely to deviate from the standards, especially those which are apt to change on account of deterioration.

It is assumed that there will be available a balance which is sensitive enough to serve for certain analytical procedures, particularly those involving the preparation of volumetric solutions for making titrimetric determinations such as apply to a number of commonly used preparations, reagents, and test solutions which should be frequently tested and adjusted if necessary.

An analytical balance differs from a high-class prescription balance in the matter of sensitiveness; a satisfactory analytical balance is sensitive to the tenth of a milligram and should never be used for weighing a total load of more than 100 Gm at one time.

Modern analytical balances are constructed with extraordinary care and accuracy.   They are usually provided with leveling devices, with levers for arresting the motion of the balance and with magnetic damping devices so as to expedite weighing.   The beam of an analytical balance is graduated (sometimes on both sides of the center of the beam) and equipped with a platinum wire rider, which is manipulated by a sliding adjustable lever.   The fractions of a milligram are weighed by means of this rider, which may be quickly transferred to any portion of the beam.   A. H. Thomas and Henry Troemner and Co., of Philadelphia, list many analytical balances (Figs. 394, and 395)

The type of analytical balance known as the Chainomatic balance (Fig. 395) records fractional weights by means of an adjustable suspended chain, and individual weights under 1 Gm may thus be dispensed with entirely.

A set of accurately calibrated analytical weights is used with the regular or "standard" analytical balance.

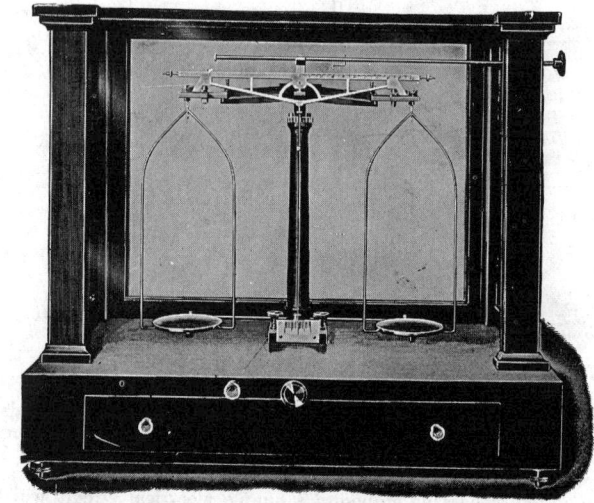

Fig. 394.   Troemner analytical balance.

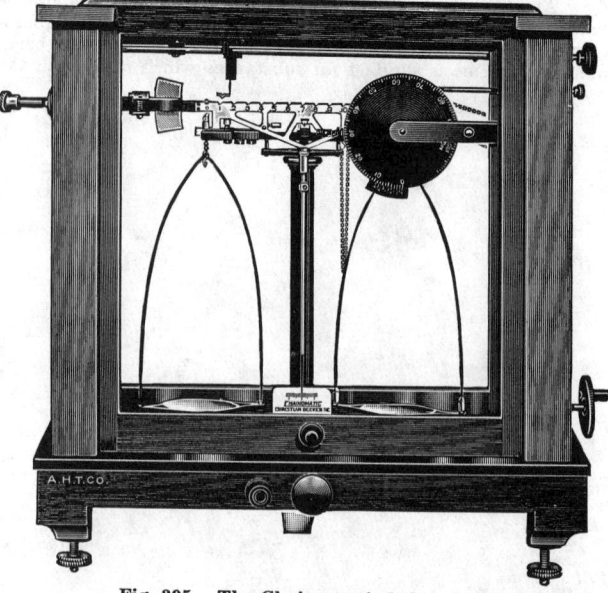

Fig. 395.   The Chainomatic balance.

These should never be left uncovered when not in use and the individual weights should always be handled with the forceps accompanying the set (Fig. 396). Tolerances for analytical weights are published in a circular available from the US Government Printing Office.[1]

The single pan balance, eg, the Mettler (Fig. 397), has all but replaced the two-pan balance. This type of balance does not require any extra weights and is entirely self-contained. The balance is always under constant load, since to determine the weight of an object, weights are removed from the single pan to restore equilibrium. Removal of the weights is accomplished by knobs on the front panel and the amount removed is registered on a dial. Fractions of

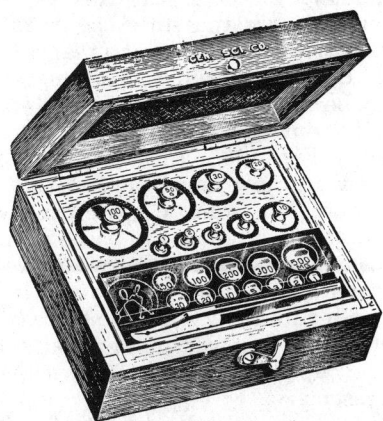

Fig. 396.   Analytical balance weights.

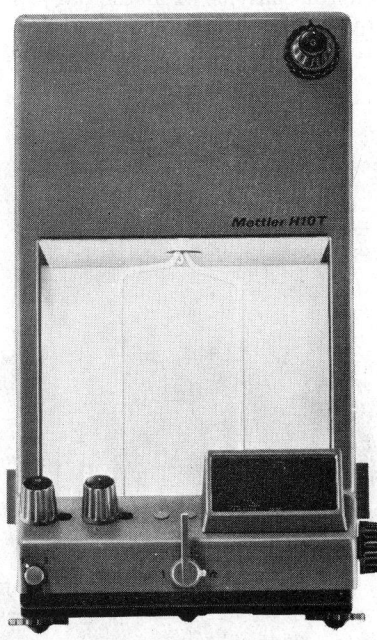

Fig. 397. Mettler digital balance model H10T (courtesy, Will Scientific, Inc.).

mass less than 0.1 Gm are read from a screen on which is focused the image produced by an optical lever. Weighings can be performed with high accuracy very rapidly. As the pan is always under constant load there is little change in sensitivity.

Other types of balances utilize electrical systems; one of these is the Cahn Electrobalance (Fig. 398). It is of the null type (as are all those previously described), but the restoring torque is not applied by adding or removing weights but rather by varying a current applied to a coil in a magnetic field, the pointer being attached to the coil. The great advantage of the electromagnetic principle is the freedom from drift or change in sensitivity. The balance can be operated remotely but has a great disadvantage in its low maximum capacity (*ca.* 0.1–1 Gm).

Several manufacturers have recently developed balances which can continuously record variations in weight with time.

Sources of Information

The works of reference needed in an analytical laboratory depend entirely upon the scope of work. For pharmaceutical testing of official substances, the USP and NF, of course, are given primary consideration. Among the indispensable adjuncts of the analyst's library are the latest editions of the following works:

Clarke, E. G. C., *Isolation and Identification of Drugs*, The Pharmaceutical Press, London, 1969.
Connors, K. A., *Textbook of Pharmaceutical Analysis*, Wiley, New York, 1967.
Feigl, F., *Spot Tests in Organic Analysis*, 7th ed., Elsevier, The Netherlands, 1966.
Food and Chemicals Codex, National Academy of Sciences Publ. 1046, Washington, D. C., 1966.

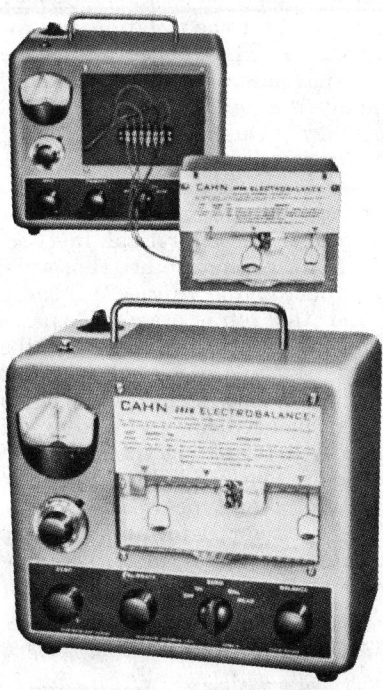

Fig. 398.   Cahn electrobalance (courtesy, Will Scientific, Inc.).

Gearien, J. E., and Grabowski, B. F., *Methods of Drug Analysis*, Lea & Febiger, Phila., 1969.
Higuchi, T., and Brochmann-Hanssen, E., *Pharmaceutical Analysis*, Interscience, New York, 1961.
Jenkins, G. L., *et al*, *Quantitative Pharmaceutical Chemistry*, 6th ed., McGraw-Hill, New York, 1967.
Kingzett, C. T., *Chemical Encyclopedia*, 9th ed., Van Nostrand, Princeton, N. J., 1967.
Kolthoff, I. M., *et al*, *Volumetric Analysis* (3 vols.), Interscience, New York, 1957.
Merck Index, 8th ed., Merck & Co., Inc., Rahway, N. J., 1968.
Rosin, J., *Reagent Chemicals and Standards*, 5th ed., Van Nostrand-Reinhold, New York, 1967.
Schwarzenbach, G., *Complexometric Titrations*, Interscience, New York, 1957.
Scott, W. W., *et al*, *Standard Methods of Chemical Analysis* (3 vols.), 6th ed., Van Nostrand, Princeton, N. J., 1966.
Siggia, S., *Quantitative Analysis via Functional Groups*, Wiley, New York, 1963.

Many valuable publications may be obtained from the various departments of the United States Government.

Specialized Analytical Methods and Equipment

In the following section some important analytical methods used by large manufacturing concerns are discussed. The average pharmacist, of course, cannot afford to purchase the expensive apparatus generally required, but he should at least be familiar with the type of analyses conducted with each instrument.

A large proportion of the medicinal products of today are still being assayed by the time-honored procedures of gravimetric and titrimetric analysis, although here, too, the use of high-precision projection-reading balances that are magnetically damped and the microburet have considerably improved these classical procedures.

A wide diversity in the types of technique has always been characteristic of assay methods for pharmaceutical products. Simple distillations are very useful in determining the alcohol content of liquids (Fig. 399), in the analysis of proteins (Fig. 400), and in the determination of certain alkaloids that are volatile in a current of steam. Fractional distillations have for a long time provided suitable methods for the analytical separation of constituents in volatile liquids. An important milestone was reached in the development of a quantitative method for the isolation and measurement of gaseous nitrogen. This procedure has been particularly useful in determining amino acids. Combustion methods of analysis have now been improved to a high degree of efficiency. Quantitative microanalytical, and even ultramicroanalytical, methods have made it possible to determine very small amounts of substances, both inorganic and organic.

Familiar examples of analytical methods that are purely physical in their nature are those which involve the use of the microscope (Fig. 401), the polarimeter (Fig. 402), and the refractometer (page 711). The identity and relative purity of many substances are often determined by microscopical examination. The polarimeter, which is also referred to as the polariscope, has long been recognized for its usefulness in assaying certain liquids by determining their ability to bend or rotate the plane of polarized light. Both the Abbé and the immersion or dipping types of refractometer are now quite generally used for determining the purity of a substance on the basis of its refractive index.

The determination of the moisture content in various substances involves several types of analytical measurement. These methods include drying in a desiccator or in a heated oven, either under ordinary atmospheric conditions or in vacuum under reduced pressure. An innovation is the "moisture balance" in which the sample pan is directly heated by an infrared lamp, thus eliminating removal of the sample from the balance. Other procedures involve distillation of vegetable drugs with toluene or with benzene, then noting the volume of water that separates in a graduated tube containing the distillate. A more specific and convenient procedure for determining water in many substances is the Karl Fischer titrimetric method. In this procedure, the water is quantitatively measured by titration under anhydrous conditions by the use of a reagent containing iodine, sulfur dioxide, pyridine, and methanol. The end-point may be detected visually, or preferably by the use of the electrometric and automatic titration assembly shown in Fig. 403. Electrical methods for determining water are now being applied to a variety of industrial products, in some cases during continuous processing operations. These are based upon the principle that if a substance is placed between two condenser plates, the capacitance will vary with the dielectric constant of the medium between the plates. Since the dielectric constant of water is greater than that of other substances, the capacitance will vary with the amount of moisture present.

The determination and adjustment of pH or hydrogen ion concentration has become an important function in the control analysis of medicinal products. For a discussion of methods of determining pH see the chapter on *Ionic Solutions and Electrolytic Equilibria* (page 270).

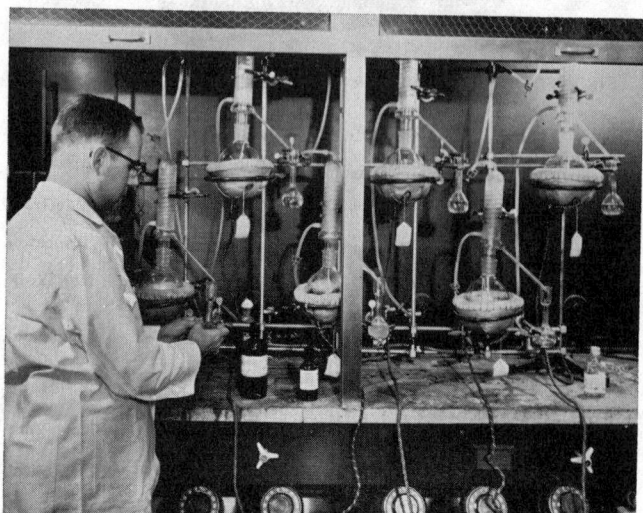

Fig. 399. Preliminary distillations in the determination of alcohol (courtesy, Lilly).

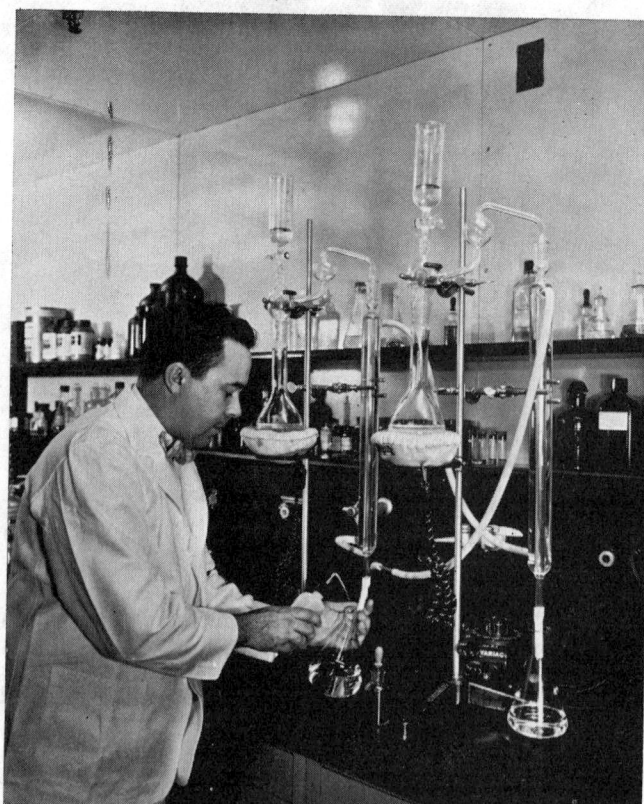

Fig. 400. The Kjeldahl distillations for the determination of nitrogen (courtesy, Lilly).

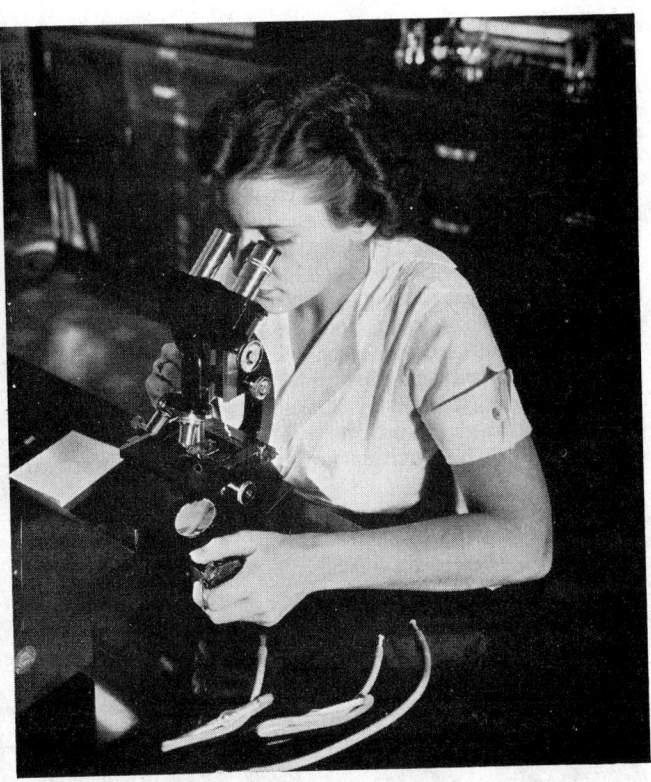

Fig. 401. The microscope is used to make blood-cell counts, examine bacteria, identify crystals, and observe other microscopic bodies.

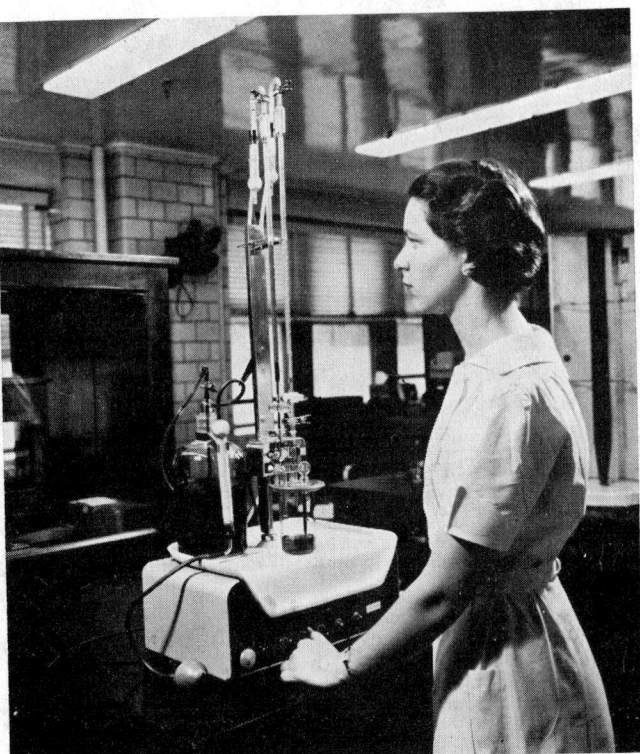

Fig. 403. The Beckman Karl Fischer assembly for the determination of water (courtesy, Lilly).

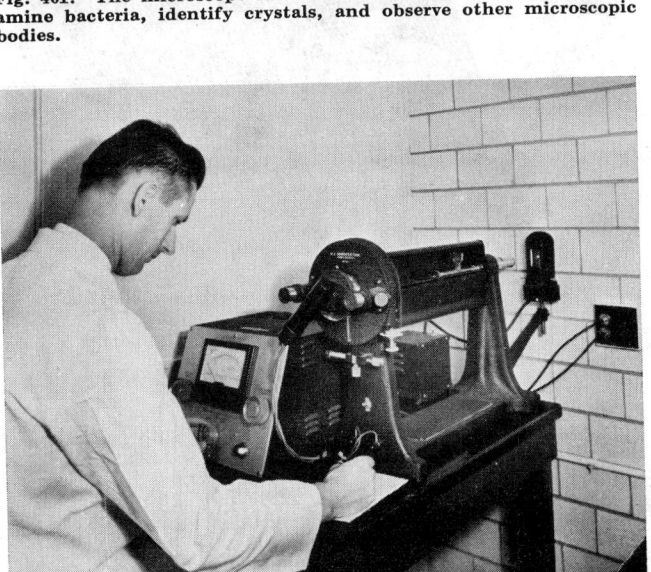

Fig. 402. The photoelectric polarimeter for determining angular rotations (courtesy, Lilly).

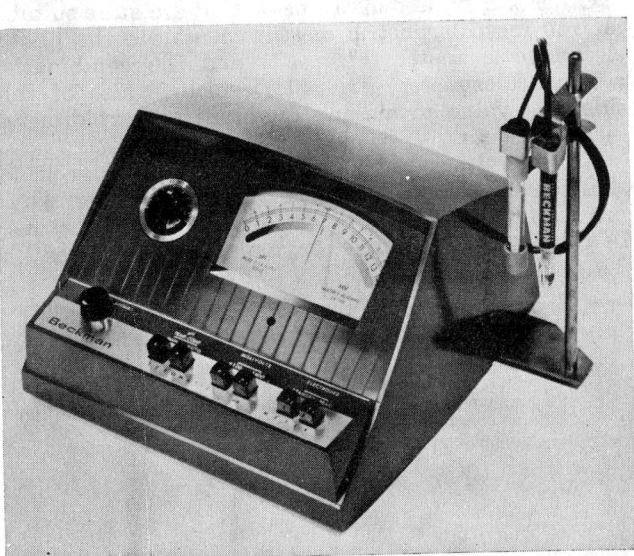

Fig. 404. Beckman zeromatic pH meter (courtesy, Will Scientific, Inc.).

Chromatographic methods of analysis (Fig. 405) represent an interesting type of approach to the problem of making analytical separations. These methods, based upon differential adsorption in a countercurrent process, are described in the chapter on *Chromatography* (page 670).

Vapor phase or "gas" chromatography is also an extremely useful qualitative and quantitative tool in modern analysis. In this process a small sample (on the order of microliters) of a liquid or a gas is volatilized in a stream of an inert gas (hydrogen or helium) and passed through a long, heated column containing adsorbent material. The separated fractions are detected by electronic methods and the effluent gases can be chilled to recover the separate fractions (see Fig. 406).

The photoelectric spectrophotometer has become an especially useful instrument for analysis, since it enables the analyst to seek the answers to his analytical problems with "eyes" that see not only in the visible range, but throughout the electromagnetic spectrum. The analytical possibilities in this direction can be more readily understood when one considers that the ultimate molecules and atoms that make up a material transmit, absorb, and scatter radiation according to their individual natures. Assay methods based upon absorption in the ultraviolet, infrared and visible portions of the spectrum are extensively used. The principles underlying such determinations are discussed in the chapter on *Instrumental Methods of Analysis* (page 694). A widely used spectrophotometer suitable for

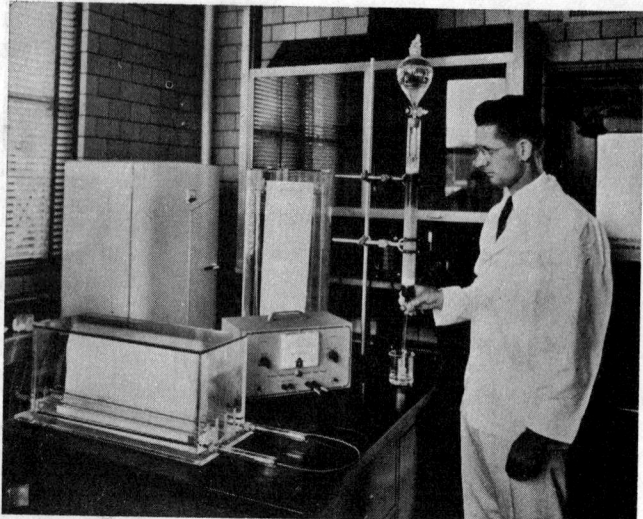

Fig. 405. Chromatographic and ion-exchange separation methods in preparing the sample for quantitative measurements (courtesy, Lilly).

measurements in the visible and ultraviolet regions of the spectrum is shown in Fig. 409. In some spectrophotometric analytical procedures a colorless substance required to be analyzed is converted to a derivative having color, the intensity of the color being measured in a suitable spectrophotometer and compared with that developed by a known amount of a "reference standard" grade of the same substance.

Other widely used instruments that are quite suitable for routine colorimetric measurements are the photoelectric colorimeter (Fig. 407) and the combination nephelo-colorimeter (Fig. 408) which is also of considerable value in making quantitative turbidimetric measurements.

Not the least important of photoelectric cell instruments is the one known as fluorophotometer, which provides for the measurement of fluorescence that may be present in the sample, or, more frequently, may be

developed in the sample. This method provides a means of evaluating the potency of a large group of pharmaceutical products, as, for example, those containing thiamine hydrochloride. A solution in which the thiamine has been quantitatively converted into thiochrome is placed in the fluorophotometer where it is caused to fluoresce upon exposure to light. This fluorescence activates the photocell and the intensity is indicated on the scale of the attached galvanometer. A comparison of the observed readings with those obtained on standard control samples which have been prepared and observed under exactly the same conditions serves as a basis upon which the potency of the unknown vitamin sample can be readily calculated.

At the opposite end of the electromagnetic spectrum are the infrared radiations. These are known as the heat rays and their utilization marks another important

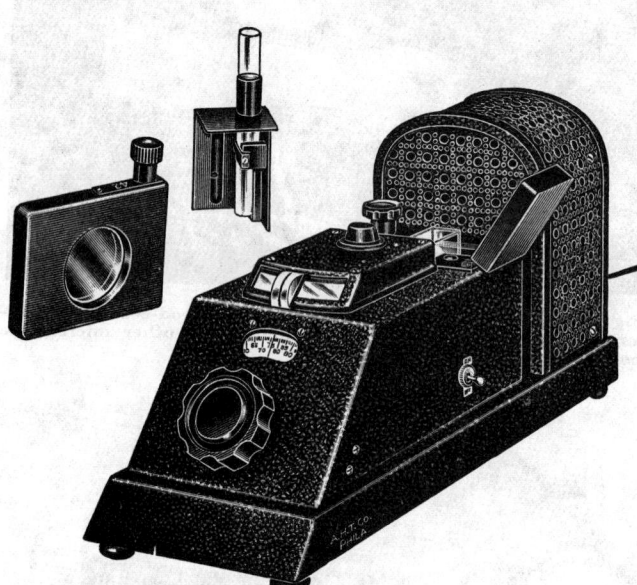

Fig. 407.   Klett–Summerson photoelectric colorimeter.

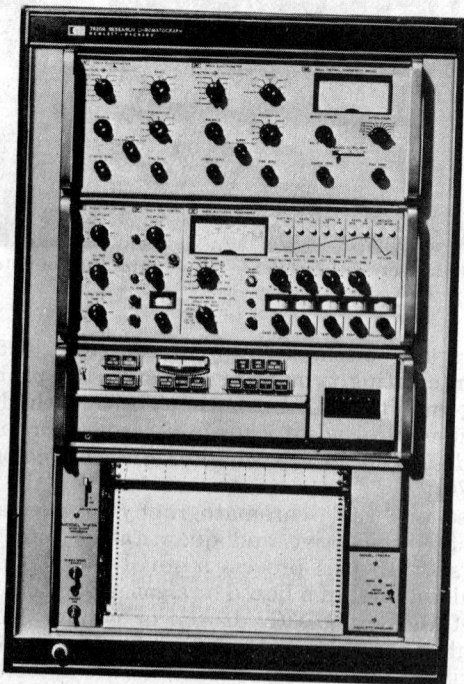

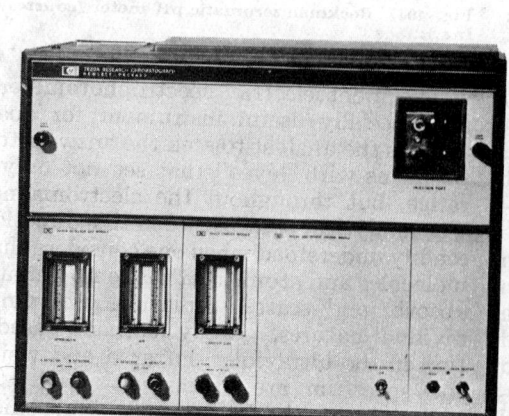

Fig. 406.   Hewlett-Packard gas chromatograph Series 7620A fully equipped with two electrometers, TC bridge, six temperature controllers, multilevel oven temperature programmer, subambient control module, and electronic digital integrator (courtesy, Avondale).

contribution to analytical research. Infrared spectrophotometry involves placing the sample in a cell which is traversed by the radiation from a hot globar element. The transmitted radiation on passing into the spectrophotometer is dispersed into a spectrum by a prism made of a crystal of sodium chloride. The spectrum is scanned by a bolometer, an instrument capable of detecting exceedingly small changes in temperature, and with the aid of an electronic amplifier radiation intensity thus measured is registered by a pen type recorder. Many recording analytical infrared spectrophotometers (page 702) are now available. An important application of infrared spectrophotometry in the USP and NF is in the "fingerprinting" of organic compounds, by which means they may be identified. Thus, the essential similarity of the infrared spectra of prednisone and an extract of prednisone tablets (Fig. 410) serves to identify the latter.

The spectrograph has long been recognized as a very useful analytical instrument, since it enables the analyst

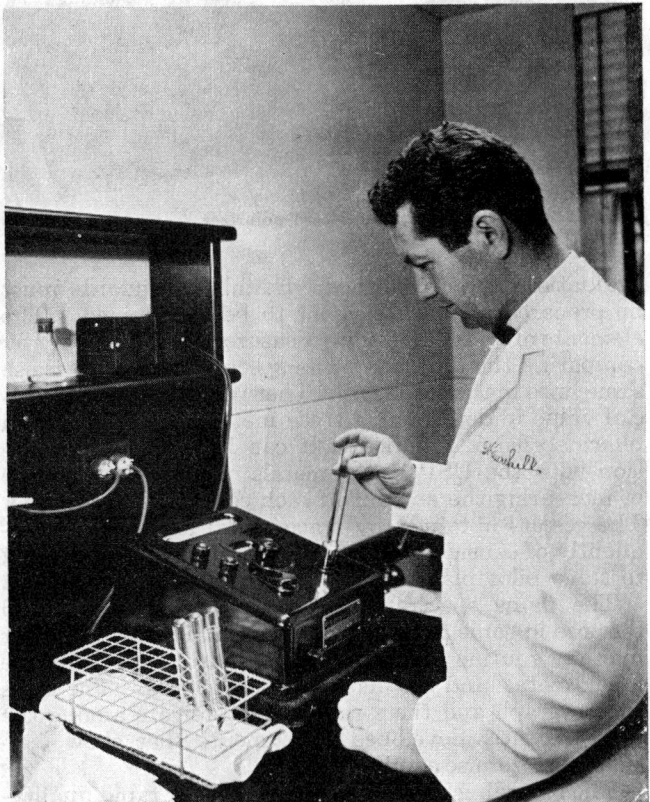

Fig. 408. Nephelo-colorimeter (Coleman) for making turbidimetric and colorimetric determinations (courtesy, Lilly).

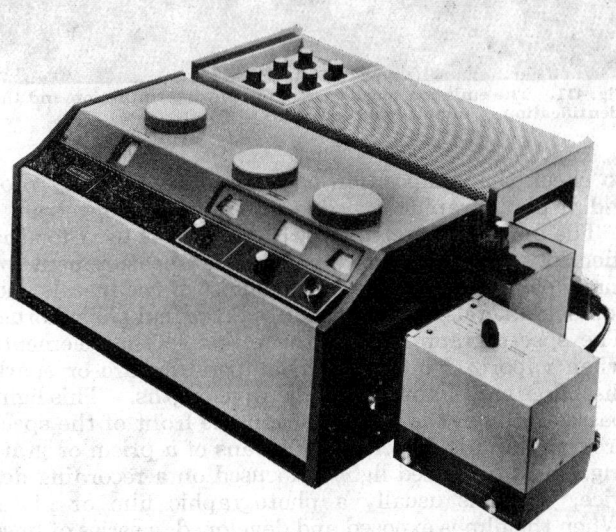

Fig. 409. DU-2 ultraviolet spectrophotometer with ac power (courtesy, Beckman).

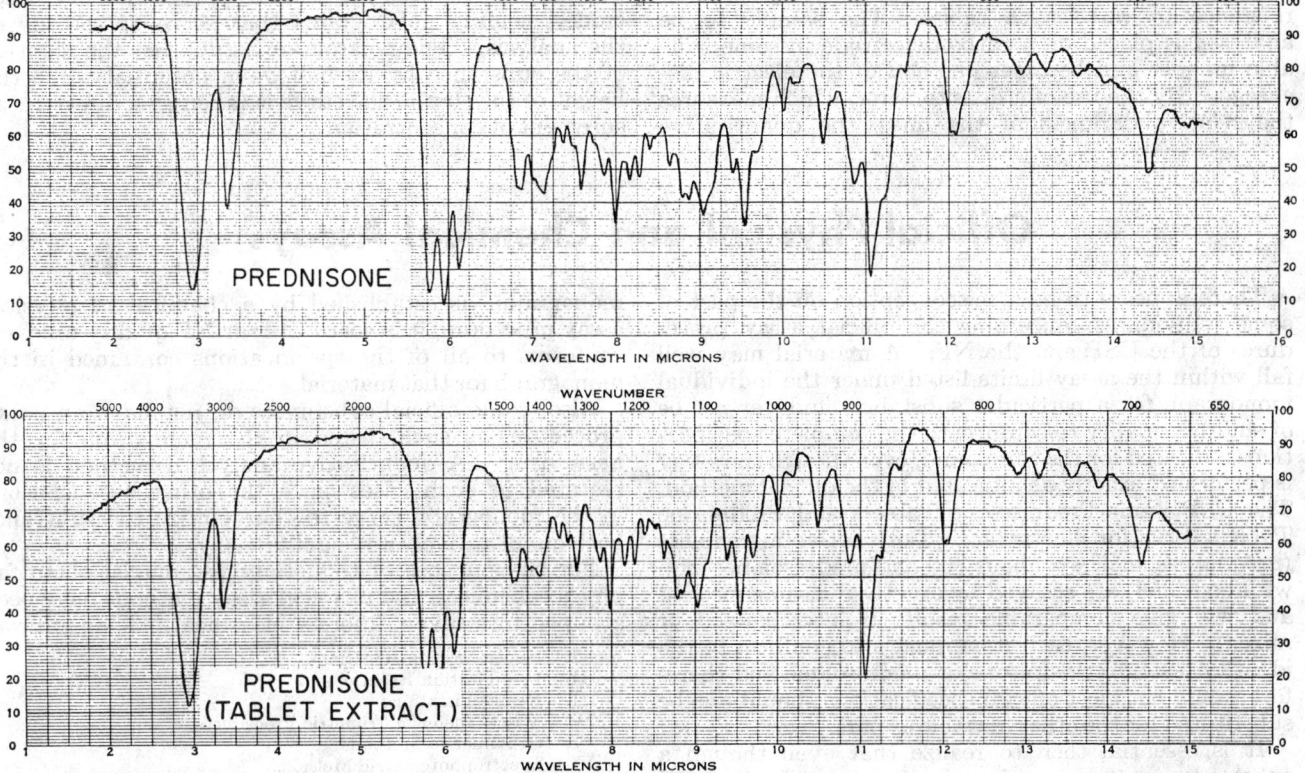

Fig. 410. Infrared spectra of prednisone and tablet extract (courtesy, Phila. College of Pharmacy and Science).

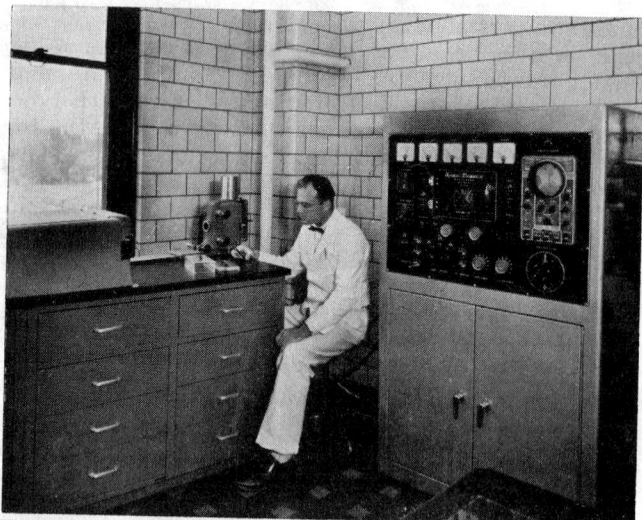

Fig. 411. The emission spectrograph for the determination and the identification of metals (courtesy, Lilly).

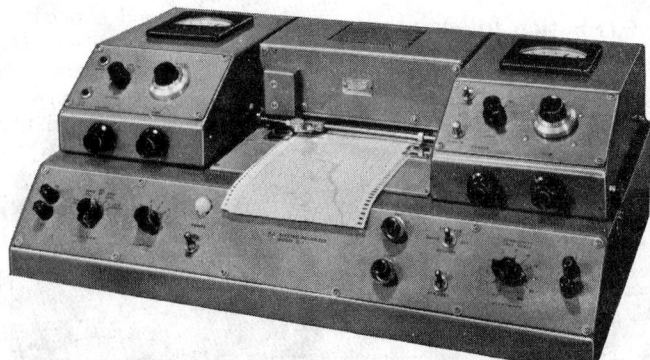

Fig. 412. American Optical electro-polarizer (courtesy, Will Scientific, Inc.).

to check the composition of many substances by providing photographic records of their emission spectra.

The emission spectrograph (Fig. 411) is used for the identification and the quantitative measurement of many elements. These include most of the metals and some nonmetals, such as boron, silicon, and phosphorus. The spectrograph utilizes the principle that elements when vaporized into a high temperature arc or spark discharge emit light in definite wavelengths. This light passes through the narrow slit in the front of the spectrograph and is dispersed by means of a prism or grating. The dispersed light is focused on a recording device, which is usually a photographic film or plate. When the film is exposed and developed, a series of lines or spectra appear. These lines are images of the slit and correspond to different wavelengths of light. By determining the wavelengths of the lines the various elements present in the sample may be determined by reference to wavelength tables. The sample to be analyzed is placed on a carbon electrode in some suitable manner and becomes one end of the electric discharge. By the use of a densitometer, which measures the relative darkness of the lines, the quantitative

evaluation is accomplished. Suitable standards must be prepared for each element to be determined. The elements of an unknown are measured quantitatively by comparing the darkness of its spectral lines with those same lines in the standard. The spectrograph is of special value in determining trace metal contamination in pharmaceutical products. It can be used in conjunction with the USP heavy metals test for the purpose of measuring the amount of each contaminating metal. The results obtained by trace metal analysis are frequently of considerable value in research and in helping to solve pilot plant, processing, and control problems.

The flame spectrophotometer now serves a useful purpose in some industrial and hospital laboratories for making routine determinations, particularly of the alkali metals and the alkaline earth metals. The mass spectrograph and the x-ray photometer are among the more recently developed instruments that show considerable promise as analytical tools.

The recording polarograph provides for rapid qualitative and quantitative analyses by automatic recording of current-voltage curves (Fig. 412). In the operation of this instrument reducible ions and organic compounds are reduced at the dropping mercury electrode, yielding polarograms that serve as records of the analysis. The polarogram establishes the identity of the substance by its half-wave potential while the height of the step in the curve is taken as a direct measurement of concentration.

Official Physical and Chemical Assays

There appears to be a misconception on the part of some individuals concerning the official assay procedures of the USP and the NF. A material may well fall within the assay limits listed under the individual monograph for a particular substance, and yet *not* be of suitable quality to conform to the complete specifications indicated for the compound, even though the assay is performed exactly as indicated in the official method. The USP items Prednisolone Tablets and Prednisone Tablets serve for illustration. Both active ingredients (prednisone, mol. wt. about 360 and prednisolone, mol. wt. about 358) are assayed by exactly the same method and will give comparable results if interchanged or mixed. However, each item must also conform to the identity tests for prednisone or prednisolone and therefore would *not* meet official specifications should one be substituted for the other in whole or part.

It is essential then to realize that even though a substance meets the purity specifications of an official

monograph, as established by a chemical or physical assay procedure, it is *not* of USP or NF quality unless it conforms to all of the specifications contained in the monograph for that material.

Also, some official substances do not have an assay procedure, as such, listed in the monograph for the basic drug. A quantitative analytical method is not required in such cases since the other specifications in the monograph serve to characterize the substance both quantitatively and qualitatively.

For the purpose of this study the official chemical, physicochemical, and physical assay methods have been grouped into seven different classifications, as follows:

   I.   Neutralization Reactions
  II. Precipitation Reactions
 III. Redox Titrations
 IV. Miscellaneous Titrimetric Procedures
  V. Gravimetric Methods
 VI. Spectrophotometric Methods
VII. Other Methods.

Classification I through IV are titrimetric methods. The seven classifications are further divided into 44 categories, which may be further subdivided. At the end of this chapter is a complete categorized index (page 603) for all USP and NF drugs which are assayed by chemical or physical means. Refer to the footnotes at the bottom of page 619 for directions on the use of the index.

Titrimetric Assay Methods

The titrimetric assay procedure is the one most frequently encountered by the pharmaceutical chemist in the standardization of official products. Every titrimetric assay is based on the determination of the volume of a solution of known strength required to complete a chemical reaction with the substance being analyzed. Such a solution is called a *standard solution* or a *volumetric solution* and is sometimes referred to by means of the abbreviation "VS."

Indicators for Determining End-Points

It is imperative to avoid the error of using an insufficient amount of a volumetric solution, thus failing to complete a reaction, and it is equally necessary to guard against overstepping a reaction by adding

Table I—Indicators, Color Developing Reagents, Etc[a]

AAP	4-aminoantipyrine		MDB	metadinitrobenzene
ACBD	4-amino-6-chloro-1,3-benzenedisulfonamide (diazotized)		MeO	methyl orange
			MeR	methyl red, TS
ACT	ammonium cobaltothiocyanate		MeY	methyl yellow (p-dimethylaminoazobenzene)
AM	ammonium molybdate		MRB	methyl red—methylene blue, TS
AN	alpha-naphthol		MV	methyl violet, TS
AP	alkaline picrate, TS			
AS	ammonium molybdate and stannous chloride		Nb	alpha-naphtholbenzein
AT	ammonium thiocyanate		NBP	meta-nitrobenzaldehyde and perchloric acid
AV	azoviolet		NiB	Nile blue hydrochloride
BcB	bromocresol blue		ON	oxidized nitroprusside solution
BcG	bromocresol green		ONA	ortho-nitroaniline
BcP	bromocresol purple		Op	ortho-phenanthroline, TS
BM	Bratton—Marshall reagent; N-(1-naphthyl)ethylenediamine added to the diazotized solution		PA	picric acid
			PAN	1-(2-pyridylazo)-2-naphthol
BnF	beta-naphthoquinone sulfonate—formaldehyde		PC	potassium chromate, TS
BpB	bromophenol blue		PDA	(see methyl yellow, MeY)
BPy	2,2'-bipyridine		PDB	para-dimethylaminobenzaldehyde
BT	blue tetrazolium		PdC	palladium chloride
BtB	bromothymol blue		PDS	phenoldisulfonic acid
			PH	phenylhydrazine hydrochloride
CAN	ceric ammonium nitrate, TS		Phth	phenolphthalein
C–S	cyanogen bromide—sulfanilic acid		Poten	potentiometric determination of the end-point
CRTB	cresol red—thymol blue, TS		PR	phenol red
CrV	crystal violet, TS		PTC	potassium thiocyanate
DbC	2,6-dibromoquinone chlorimide		QR	Quinaldine red
DP	diphenylamine, TS			
DNP	2,4-dinitrophenylhydrazine		R	Reinecke's salt
DT	dithizone, TS			
			SC	antimony trichloride and acetylchloride
EBT	eriochrome black T		SK	sodium nitroprusside—potassium ferrocyanide
EY	eosin Y, TS		SM	sulfuric acid in methanol
			SN	sodium nitrite in acid solution
FAS	ferric ammonium sulfate, TS		SaO	Safranin O
FC	ferric chloride, acid, TS		SP	sulfonated phenol and cobalt nitrite
FCiT	ferrocitrate reagent		SPI	starch-potassium iodide, TS, or paper
FCP	Folin-Ciocalteau-Phenol, TS		St	starch, TS
FCU	ferric chloride—urea			
FDP	ferric chloride and 2,2'-bipyridine		TB	thymol blue
FH	ferric chloride and hydroxylamine		TBP	tetrabromophenolphthalein, TS
FET	ferrous tartrate reagent		TBPE	tetrabromophenolphthalein, ethyl ester, TS
			TP	thymolphthalein
HDA	hexanitrodiphenylamine		TTC	triphenyltetrazolium chloride
HNB	hydroxynaphthol blue			
			UV	ultraviolet radiation
IN	isoniazid reagent			
IP	iron-phenol reagent		VS	vanadyl sulfate
MAG	malachite green, TS		Xan	xanthydrol
MeB	methylene blue			

[a] These are coded in the third column of the *Assay Index*, page 619. They are usually employed as solutions and quite often are the official Test Solutions (TS).

too much of the volumetric solution. To meet this situation an interesting group of chemicals known as *Indicators* is used. These are substances that show when the endpoint of a reaction has been reached, either by a change in color or by the formation of a precipitate.

Indicator Solutions

Solutions of indicators which are used for volumetric determinations are referred to as Test Solutions, abbreviated TS, and those used for determination of hydrogen ion concentration are termed pH Indicators.

The indicators used for colorimetric pH determinations are either weakly acid or weakly basic. However, most of the indicators used for this purpose, such as the phthaleins and sulfonated phthaleins, behave like weak acids.

The usual concentration of the indicator solution is 0.05%. From 0.1 to 0.2 ml of the indicator solution is generally used for 10 ml of the liquid being examined.

Solutions of indicators of the basic type and of the phthaleins are prepared by dissolving them in alcohol. In preparing solutions of indicators containing an acid group, this group must first be neutralized with sodium hydroxide.

Unless otherwise stated each acid-base indicator solution is so adjusted that when 0.15 ml of the indicator solution is added to 25 ml of carbon dioxide-free water, 0.25 ml of 0.02N acid or alkali, respectively, will develop the characteristic color changes.

The solutions should be kept in glass-stoppered bottles, and protected from light.

Indicators for Reactions Involving Neutralization

In the USP indicators are used either to indicate the completion of a chemical reaction in volumetric analyses or to indicate the hydrogen ion concentration (pH) of solutions.

Most of the indicators for acid-base titrations and for pH measurement are acidic. They contain a carboxyl, a sulfonic, or a phenolic group. In many instances the same indicator is applicable either to acid-base titrations or to pH measurements, the difference being only in the preparation of the indicator solution. The following are the pH indicators of the Pharmacopeia; in each case Test Solutions (TS) of the following indicators are used.

Bromocresol Green (*Bromocresol Blue: Tetrabromo-m-cresolsulfonphthalein*)—Transition interval: from pH 3.8 to 5.4. Color change: from yellow to blue.

Bromocresol Purple (*Dibromo-o-cresolsulfonphthalein*)—Transition interval: from pH 5.2 to 6.8. Color change: from yellow to purple. This solution and the next two are satisfactory in the titration of weak bases.

Bromophenol Blue (*Tetrabromophenolsulfonphthalein*)—Transition interval: from pH 3.0 to 4.6. Color change: from yellow to blue.

Bromothymol Blue (*Dibromothymolsulfonphthalein*)—Transition interval: from pH 6.0 to 7.6. Color change: from yellow to blue.

Cresol Red (*o-Cresolsulfonphthalein*)—Transition interval: from pH 7.2 to 8.8. Color change: from yellow to blue.

Cresol Red-Thymol Blue TS—Transition interval: from 7.7 to 9.1. Color change: from yellow to violet.

Methyl Orange (*Helianthin* or *Tropæolin D*)—The sodium salt of dimethylaminoazobenzene sulfonic acid or dimethylaminoazobenzene sodium sulfonate. Transition interval: from pH 3.1 to 4.4. Color change: from pink to red. Useful in the titration of weak bases.

Methyl Red (*Dimethylaminoazobenzene-o-carboxylic acid; o-carboxylbenzene-azodimethylaniline*)—Transition interval: from pH 4.2 to 6.3. Color change: from red to yellow. Useful in the titration of weak bases.

Methyl Red-Methylene Blue TS—Transition interval: from 4.8 to 6.2. Color change: from red-violet to green.

Methyl Yellow (*p-Dimethylaminoazobenzene*)—Transition interval: from pH 2.4 to 4.0. Color change: red to yellow.

Phenolphthalein—Use *Phenolphthalein USP*—Transition interval: from pH 8.3 to 10. Color change: from colorless to red. Useful in the titration of acids with strong bases.

Phenol Red—Use *Phenolsulfonphthalein USP*. Transition interval: from pH 6.8 to 8.4. Color change: from yellow to red.

Quinaldine Red (*5-Dimethylamino-2-styrylquinolinium iodide*)—Transition interval: pH 1.4 to 3.2. Color change: colorless to red.

Thymol Blue (*Thymolsulfonphthalein*)—*Acid*—Transition interval: from pH 1.2 to 2.8. Color change: from red to yellow. *Alkaline*—Transition interval: from pH 8 to 9.6. Color change: from yellow to blue.

Thymolphthalein—Transition interval: pH 9.3 to 10.5. Color change: colorless to blue.

Indicators for Reactions Involving Precipitation

Eosin Y (Sodium Tetrabromofluorescein) TS.

Ferric Ammonium Sulfate Test Solution—8% in water. This indicator, which is well known as *Ferric Alum*, is generally used when titrating with standard ammonium thiocyanate in the presence of silver nitrate. A red color of the ferric thiocyanate complex forms immediately when the silver thiocyanate has been completely precipitated.

Potassium Chromate Test Solution—10% in water. This indicator gives a red precipitate of silver chromate in a neutral or slightly alkaline solution, after silver halides have been completely precipitated by titration with standard silver nitrate.

Tetrabromophenolphthalein TS.

Tetrabromophenolphthalein, Ethyl Ester TS.

Indicators for Nonaqueous Titrations

Azo-violet.

Crystal Violet (TS)—1% in glacial acetic acid.

Malachite Green—Use Malachite Green TS.

Methyl Red—Use Methyl Red TS.

Methyl Violet—Use Methyl Violet TS.

α-Naptholbenzein—(4-[α-(4-hydroxy-1-naphthyl)benzylidene]-1-(4H)-naphthalenone).

Phenol Red—Use Phenol Red TS.

Quinaldine Red—Use Quinaldine Red TS.

Thymol Blue—Use Thymol Blue TS.

Indicators for Complexometric Titrations

Diphenylamine TS.

Dithizone (*Diphenylthiocarbazone*) **TS.**

Eriochrome Black T—0.05% aqueous solution (should be freshly prepared but can be stabilized).

Hydroxynaphthol Blue.

Murexide (*Acid Ammonium Purpurate*)—Used as a powder; usually mixed with an inert carrier (potassium sulfate) to facilitate handling.

Naphthol Green TS.

1-(2-Pyridylazo)-2-naphthol.

Indicators for Reactions Involving Changes in Valence

Free Iodine—Iodine serves as its own indicator in those assays where it is liberated and determined volumetrically by titration with standard potassium iodate. The end-point is shown by the disappearance of a violet color from the chloroform which is agitated with the mixture being titrated for the purpose of dissolving and concentrating the iodine.

Methyl Orange TS.—Used in conjunction with potassium bromate titrations; the color of the indicator is discharged by excess reagent.

Ortho-phenanthroline Test Solution—1.5% in 1.5% ferrous sulfate solution. The ferrous sulfate solution must be prepared immediately before dissolving the ortho-phenanthroline. Preserve the solution in well-closed containers. This is the indicator of choice in titrations involving the use of standard ceric sulfate. The color changes from red to pale green as the slightest excess of ceric sulfate is added to the oxidized solution.

Oxalic Acid Volumetric Solution—This standard solution generally functions without the use of an indicator inasmuch as most of the reactions in which it takes part depend upon the decolorization of the potassium permanganate, as explained in the following paragraph.

Potassium Permanganate Volumetric Solution—This highly colored solution is decolorized upon being reduced in those titrations where it is used as an oxidizing agent. The nature of this color change makes it unnecessary to add an indicator.

Potassium Thiocyanate—Used in conjunction with ferric chloride volumetric solution; forms a red ion at the end point.

Starch Iodide Paste Test Solution—Approximately 5% suspension of potato starch in 0.75% potassium iodide with zinc chloride preservative.

Starch iodide paste test solution must show a definite blue streak when a glass rod, dipped in a mixture of 1 ml of tenth-molar sodium nitrite, 500 ml of water, and 10 ml of hydrochloric acid, is streaked on a smear of the paste.

Starch-Potassium Iodide Test Solution—0.5% KI in Starch TS. Must be freshly prepared.

Starch Test Solution—A 0.5% suspension of arrowroot starch in water. This test solution must be freshly prepared. It is added to accentuate the color change in a titration as free iodine is produced or as it is caused to disappear. The blue color yielded by starch in the presence of free iodine is quite well known.

Indicator Papers

Strong, white filter paper is treated with hydrochloric acid and washed with water until the washings no longer show an acid reaction to methyl red. It is then treated with ammonia TS and again washed with water, until the washings are no longer alkaline toward phenolphthalein. It is then thoroughly dried.

The dry paper is then saturated with the proper strength indicator solution and carefully dried. The drying is accomplished by suspending the paper in a room free from acid or alkali fumes.

The papers so prepared are kept in glass-stoppered bottles, carefully protected from light and moisture.

Lead Acetate Test Paper— Prepared from lead acetate TS.

Litmus Paper, Blue—Usually in the form of strips about 50 mm in length and 6 mm in width.

Litmus Paper, Red—Usually in the form of strips about 50 mm in length and 6 mm in width.

Mercuric Bromide Test Paper—Prepared from alcoholic mercuric bromide TS.

Phenolphthalein Paper—Prepared from a 0.1% solution of phenolphthalein in diluted alcohol.

Potassium Iodate-Starch Paper—Impregnate strips of white filter paper with a solution prepared by mixing a 5% solution of potassium iodate with an equal volume of freshly prepared starch TS.

Starch Iodate Paper—Impregnate strips of white filter paper with a mixture of equal volumes of starch TS and potassium iodate solution (1 in 20).

Starch Iodide Paper—Impregnate strips of white filter paper with a solution of 500 mg of potassium iodide in 100 ml of freshly prepared starch TS.

Turmeric Paper—Impregnate strips of white filter paper with turmeric solution prepared as directed in the USP.

Potentiometric Determination of End-Points

The detection of the end-point in titrimetric assays by use of colorimetric indicators may sometimes be difficult, especially if the solution being titrated is colored or turbid. In some instances titration to the equivalence or true end-point is essential, which requirement is not conveniently met when an indicator is employed. In such cases the end-point may be indicated potentiometrically, most commonly employing a potentiometer calibrated in millivolts. The potentiometric determination of end-points depends upon the fact that in most titrations the potential across two suitable electrodes immersed in the solution being titrated undergoes a sharp change at the true end-point (equivalence point), this corresponding to the point where an indicator undergoes marked change of color. In some titrations neither the change of color nor the change of potential is sharp at the end-point, in which case titration to a predetermined voltage or voltage deflection is necessary; since it is generally more convenient to do this potentiometrically, rather than colorimetrically, this electrical method is employed. Suitable electrodes, such as a combination of glass and calomel electrodes, undergo no reaction with the solution being titrated or with the titrant; they serve only as a means of *detecting* the end-point.

It may be pointed out here that the change of other electrical properties, such as resistance or the amount of current flowing in a solution being titrated, may be utilized to indicate the end-point in a titration. The general term *electrometric titrations* is sometimes applied to such titrations; specific titrations in this category are referred to as *amperometric*, *conductometric*, and *high-frequency* titrations.

Classification of Titrimetric Assays

The first 27 categories deal with titrimetric assay methods and include neutralization, precipitation, redox, and nonaqueous procedures.

Titrimetric Procedures

I. Neutralization Reactions

1. Direct Titration of an Acid by Base

In this category a free acid is titrated directly using the method indicated in the monograph to determine the end-point.

NF Items

Boric Acid—The use of glycerin increases the acid strength of the boric acid so that it behaves as a monobasic acid according to the equation

$$H_3BO_3 + NaOH = NaBO_2 + 2H_2O$$

Caffeine, Citrated—citric acid content.

Calcium Saccharin—on treatment with mineral acid, free saccharin is liberated, extracted with ether, the solvent removed, and the residual saccharin titrated.

Oxyphenbutazone—even though a phenol, it is sufficiently strong to be titrated directly.

Potassium Phosphate—See *Sodium Phosphate*, below.

Sodium Phosphate—treatment of the salt with hydrochloric acid liberates phosphoric acid and the end-point is determined potentiometrically from pH readings. Only one hydrogen of phosphoric acid is titrated in this procedure.

Sulfur, Sublimed—sulfur is oxidized to sulfuric acid by the Oxygen Flask technique, then titrated.

Undecylenic Acid Ointment, Compound—for undecylenic acid. Hydrochloric acid is added to liberate the organic acid, extract with ether, evaporate, and titrate the residual undecylenic acid.

Zinc Undecylenate—the free acid is liberated from the salt with hydrochloric acid and treated as the *Ointment*, above.

USP Items

Aluminum Acetate Solution—for acetic acid, after distillation.

Aluminum Subacetate Solution—for acetic acid, after distillation.

Cellulose Acetate Phthalate—phthalyl content.

Methenamine Mandelate—for mandelic acid.

Orange Syrup—citric acid content.

Storax—acid value.

Sulfinpyrazone (and Tablets)—the sulfonyl group (—SO$_2$—) makes the alpha-hydrogen sufficiently acid so that it may react with base.

Sulfur—see *Sulfur, Sublimed, NF*, above.

Tolu Balsam—acid value.

2. Titration of a Liberated Acid by a Base

USP Items

Cellulose, Oxidized—the sample is shaken with calcium acetate solution, to exchange calcium ion for hydrogen ion of the free carboxyl groups. The liberated hydrogen ion is then titrated with standard base.

Lemon Oil—the aldehydes of the oil react with hydroxylammonium chloride to form the oxime, liberating free hydrochloric acid, which is titrated and the aldehyde content calculated as citral:

$$RCH{=}O + HONH_3Cl = RCH{=}NOH + HCl + H_2O$$

Orange Oil—see *Lemon Oil*, above; results calculated as decanal.

3. Sorenson Formol Titration

NF Item

Meprobamate Oral Suspension—after hydrolysis of the ester.

USP Items

Meprobamate (and Injection and Tablets)—after hydrolysis.

Protein Hydrolysate Injection—for alpha-amino nitrogen.

In each case the free amino acid is treated with formaldehyde to form the methylimino or methylol derivative, reducing the basicity of the amino group so that the free carboxyl group may be titrated.

$$R{-}CH(NH_2)COOH + HCHO =$$
$$R{-}CH(NHCH_2OH)COOH \text{ or } RCH(N{=}CH_2)COOH$$

4. Residual Titration of Excess Base after Interaction with Acid

In this type of assay a measured excess of standard base is added to the prepared sample and the excess titrated with standard acid. Quite often a blank titration is performed, whereby the same volume of base, which was added to the sample, is titrated with standard acid. The difference in the volume of titrant used for the blank and sample is the volume of titrant equivalent to the sample.

NF Items

Aluminum Phosphate Gel
Calcium Phosphate, Tribasic
Chloral Betaine
Magnesium Phosphate
Methenamine and Sodium Biphosphate Tablets—for sodium biphosphate.

USP Items

Anticoagulant Citrate Phosphate Dextrose Solution—for phosphate.
Chloral Hydrate
Chloral Hydrate Capsules and Syrup

All of the above phosphates are assayed by first precipitating ammonium phosphomolybdate from a dilute nitric acid solution of the sample:

$$AlPO_4 + 12(NH_4)_2MoO_4 + 24HNO_3 =$$
$$(NH_4)_3PO_4.12MoO_3 + 21NH_4NO_3 + Al(NO_3)_3 + 12H_2O$$

The precipitated yellow molybdate is filtered, washed free of adhering nitric acid, and dissolved in an excess of standard alkali:

$$(NH_4)_3PO_4.12MoO_3 + 23NaOH = 11Na_2MoO_4 +$$
$$NaNH_4HPO_4 + (NH_4)_2MoO_4 + 11H_2O$$

Excess standard alkali is then titrated with standard acid.

The chloral containing compounds are treated with excess standard sodium hydroxide which hydrolyzes the chloral to chloroform and sodium formate. Excess base is titrated with standard acid.

$$CCl_3CHO.H_2O + NaOH = CHCl_3 + HCOONa + H_2O$$

With Chloral Hydrate Syrup a correction must be made for original acidity by a preliminary titration of the sample, with base.

5. Direct Titration of Base by Acid

NF Items

Levopropoxyphene Napsylate—the sample is passed through an anion-exchange resin and the eluate, containing hydroxyl ion which was exchanged for the 2-naphthalenesulfonic acid, is titrated by acid.
Oxtriphylline—for choline, using MeB.
Triethylenemelamine—sodium thiosulfate reacts with each ethyleneimine group to liberate one equivalent of alkali, which is then titrated with standard acid.

$$-N{\Large\langle}\genfrac{}{}{0pt}{}{CH_2}{CH_2} + Na_2S_2O_3 + H_2O =$$
$$-NHCH_2CH_2S_2O_3Na + NaOH$$

Tromethamine for Injection—for tromethamine using BcP.

USP Items

Aminophylline (and Injection and Tablets)—for ethylenediamine using MeO.
Anticoagulant Citrate Dextrose Solution—for citric acid with Phth.
Anticoagulant Citrate Phosphate Dextrose Solution—for citric acid with Phth.
Potassium Hydroxide—for potassium hydroxide using Phth and for potassium carbonate content using MeO.
Thiotepa—see *Trimethylenemelamine*, above.

6. Titration of Volatile Bases after Distillation

Compounds in this category are usually hydrolyzed by boiling with strong alkali and the ammonia or amines formed are distilled into excess standard acid or into a saturated boric acid solution. In either case, the excess standard acid is titrated with standard base, or the ammonia-boric acid complex titrated with acid, methyl red being the indicator for either method. If the nitrogen content only is determined, the Kjeldahl procedure is used (see Chapter 36, *Official Requirements and Tests*).

NF Items

Ichthammol—for ammonia; make alkaline and distil into excess standard acid.
Methenamine and Sodium Biphosphate Tablets—as for *Ichthammol*, for methenamine content.
Phensuximide Oral Suspension—methylamine distilled.
Urethan Tablets—nitrogen content by Kjeldahl.

USP Items

Calcium Pantothenate—nitrogen content by Kjeldahl.
Glucagon—nitrogen content by Kjeldahl.
Neostigmine Methylsulfate—dimethylamine distilled.

Paramethadione (and Capsules and Solution)—methylamine distilled.
Pyrazinamide—amide hydrolyzed and ammonia distilled.

7. Titration of Metal Salts with Acid

USP Item

Caffeine and Sodium Benzoate Injection—the caffeine is extracted with chloroform, ether is added to the residual aqueous solution and the mixture titrated with acid, shaking vigorously. As free benzoic acid is liberated by titration with hydrochloric acid it is immediately extracted into the ether phase. As the end-point is exceeded, excess titrant causes the indicator (MeO) to change.

8. Residual Titration of Excess Acid after Interaction with Base

For this category a basic substance is treated with a measured excess of standard acid and the excess acid titrated with standard base.

NF Items

Ammonia Spirit, Aromatic—for the total ammonia assay, the sample is boiled with excess standard acid and the excess titrated with sodium hydroxide. The ammonium carbonate is converted into an equivalent amount of sodium carbonate.
Pyrrocaine Hydrochloride and Epinephrine Injection—for pyrrocaine (MeR and BcB).

USP Item

Magnesium Trisilicate (and Tablets)—for magnesium oxide (MeO).

9. Residual Titration of Excess Acid following Liberation of a Base by a Stronger Base

Assays of this kind are also applied to extractions made of vegetable drugs containing alkaloidal principles and to the pharmaceutical preparations obtained from them. These determinations are considered in Category 38, *Proximate Assays*.

All of the assays are based upon the principle that the relatively weak organic bases are readily displaced from their salts by the action of a stronger base, such as sodium hydroxide, sodium carbonate, or ammonium hydroxide. The last compound is more generally employed for the liberation of the alkaloids from their salts. The liberated free bases are then extracted into an organic solvent (ether or chloroform) and the separated organic phase evaporated.

NF Item

Morphine and Atropine Sulfates Tablets—for morphine (MeR).

10. Titration of Carbonate Residues from Ignited Salts

In general the ignition of an alkali metal salt of a carboxylic acid forms sodium carbonate, carbon dioxide, and water as exemplified by sodium citrate:

$$2Na_3C_6H_5O_7 + 9O_2 = 3Na_2CO_3 + 9CO_2 + 5H_2O$$

Excess standard acid is added to the ignition residue and the excess titrated with base. The volume of standard acid consumed is multiplied by the appropriate conversion factor to determine the amount of alkali salt in the sample taken.

NF Items

Magnesium Citrate Solution—for citric acid (Phth), after precipitation of calcium citrate and ignition of the filtered salt.
Potassic Saline Injection, Lactated—lactate content.

USP Items

Anticoagulant Citrate Dextrose Solution—for sodium citrate (Phth).
Anticoagulant Citrate Phosphate Dextrose Solution—for sodium citrate (Phth).
Ringer's Injection, Lactated—for sodium lactate (MeO).

11a. Residual Titration Involving Saponification of an Ester

In general esters are determined by a saponification procedure which involves boiling the sample in excess standard alcoholic alkali, which acts as a mutual solvent. The excess free alkali is determined with standard acid. A blank is usually run on the same volume of alkali used for the saponification procedure.

NF Items

Alcohol, Rubbing—for sucrose octaacetate.
Oxandrolone—the ester is present in *lactone* form.
Tybamate (and Capsules)—sodium methoxide solution is used to effect the saponification.
Urethan—sodium methoxide solution used for saponification.

Cellulose Acetate Phthalate—acetyl content.
Peppermint Oil—for total menthol content. The free menthol is first acetylated with acetic anhydride to form the ester, menthyl acetate. After purification, to remove excess acetic acid and water, the ester is subjected to the saponification procedure.
Polyoxyl 40 Stearate—saponification value.
Polysorbate 80—saponification value.
Storax—saponification value.
Tolu Balsam—saponification value.

11b. Residual Titration following an Acylation Reaction

The general method involves the treatment of an alcohol with an acylating reagent, usually acetic anhydride or phthalic anhydride in pyridine. Any excess anhydride remaining after the esterification reaction is converted to the free acid with water, and the acid titrated with standard base. A blank is usually run employing all the reagents except the sample. The difference in titer between the blank and the sample is the volume of base equivalent to the alcohol content of the sample taken.

NF Item

Polyethylene Glycol 300 and 1540—for average molecular weight, using phthalic anhydride in pyridine.

11c. Residual Titration following the Hydrolysis of Alkoxyl Groups

A previously neutralized sample is saponified with excess standard base and the excess determined in the usual manner.

NF Items

Hydroxypropyl Methylcellulose—for hydroxypropoxyl groups.
Pectin—for methoxyl groups.

II. Precipitation Reactions

12a. Titration of Liberated Nitric Acid

In assays of this type silver nitrate reacts with the substance being assayed, to form an insoluble silver derivative, simultaneously releasing an equivalent amount of nitric acid which is titrated with standard alkali.

NF Items

Ethinamate (and Tablets)—an acetylenic hydrogen reacts with silver nitrate.
Oxtriphylline—for theophylline. The solution from the choline assay is treated with silver nitrate and the above method followed.

12b. Direct Titration of a Theophylline–Silver Complex

The theophylline-silver complex is separated by filtration, dissolved in nitric acid and the liberated silver ion titrated with thiocyanate (FAS indicator).

USP Item

Aminophylline Suppositories—for theophylline.

12c. Residual Titration of a Theophylline–Silver Complex

For this category the insoluble silver complex is precipitated from an ammoniacal solution of the sample by warming with excess standard silver nitrate. After filtration, the excess silver ion is determined in the filtrate by titration with thiocyanate (FAS indicator).

USP Items

Aminophylline Injection and Tablets—for theophylline.
Dimenhydrinate (and Tablets)—for 8-chlorotheophylline.

12d. Direct Titration of Halogen

These assays may involve the conversion of organic halogen to halide ion (if covalently bound), before titration. Silver nitrate is the titrant in all cases.

NF Items

Calcium Ipodate (and Oral Suspension)—after reduction with zinc and alkali to liberate iodide.
Methyclothiazide—after release of chloride with methanolic KOH.
Povidone–Iodine—for total iodine after reduction with bisulfite.
Pipobroman (and Tablets)—after hydrolysis with KOH.
Ringer's Solution—for chloride (FAS).
Sodium Ipodate (and Capsules)—after reduction with zinc.

USP Items

Iopanoic Acid—after treatment with zinc and alkali.
Meglumine Diatrizoate ⎫
Meglumine Iodipamide ⎬ after hydrolysis with base.
Meglumine Iothalamate ⎭
Sodium Diatrizoate Injection—after treatment with zinc and alkali.
Sodium Iodipamide Injection—after treatment with zinc and alkali.
Sodium Lauryl Sulfate—for sodium chloride (PC).

12e. Residual Titration of Halogen

Excess standard silver nitrate is added to a solution of the prepared sample, containing ionic halogen. The excess silver nitrate is then titrated with standard ammonium thiocyanate. This method has long been known as the Volhard procedure. Nitrobenzene is added, in the titration involving silver chloride, to prevent its interaction with thiocyanate. Ferric Alum (FAS) is the usual indicator. Quite often the ionic halogen must be liberated from the organic compound.

NF Items

Chlorotrianisene—after treatment with sodium metal.
Potassic Saline Injection, Lactated—for chloride.
Sodium Chloride and Dextrose Tablets—for sodium chloride.
Tribromoethanol (and Solution)—after hydrolysis with base.

USP Items

Chlorobutanol—after hydrolysis with base.
Chlorophenothane—after treatment with sodium and isopropyl alcohol.
Dextrose and Sodium Chloride Injection—for sodium chloride.
Mannitol and Sodium Chloride Injection—for sodium chloride.
Ringer's Injection—for sodium chloride.
Ringer's Injection, Lactated—for sodium chloride.

13a. Direct Titrations with Thiocyanate

Silver ion or mercury(II) ion is titrated directly with thiocyanate. In the first instance insoluble silver thiocyanate is formed during the titration reaction and for mercury, the unionized mercury(II) thiocyanate is produced. Ferric Alum (FAS) is the usual indicator.

NF Items

Calcium Benzoylpas—p-benzamidosalicylic acid is precipitated as the silver salt with excess standard silver nitrate and the excess titrated with thiocyanate.
Silver Protein, Mild—after digestion with nitric acid.

III. Redox Titrations

14a. Titrations Involving Direct Oxidation with Ceric Sulfate

Ceric sulfate is of value in titrating iron(II) salts in mixtures that contain excipients or diluents which have a reducing action on permanganate, but have no effect on ceric sulfate. The equation which applies is:

$$2FeSO_4 + 2Ce(SO_4)_2 = Fe_2(SO_4)_3 + Ce_2(SO_4)_3$$

NF Items

Menadione (and Tablets)—after reduction with zinc and acid.
Menadione Sodium Bisulfite (and Injection)—the Menadione preparations are first reduced with zinc and acid to menadiol, which is then reoxidized during the titration.
Vitamin E—for alpha-tocopherol acid succinate and acetate (FDP).

USP Item

Homatropine Hydrobromide (and Ophthalmic Solution)—after hydrolysis with base; the liberated mandelic acid is oxidized by the titrant.

14b. Residual Titration with Ceric Sulfate

Excess standard ceric sulfate is added to the sample and the excess is titrated with standard ferric ammonium sulfate.

Ringer's Injection and Ringer's Injection, Lactated—for potassium chloride. Potassium is precipitated as the cobaltinitrite, which is separated, washed, and dried. It is then dissolved and oxidized in an excess of standard ceric sulfate. The excess ceric ion is titrated with ferric ammonium sulfate (Op). The equation which applies is

$$K_2NaCo(NO_2)_6 + 6O = 2KNO_3 + NaNO_3 + Co(NO_3)_3$$

15a. Direct Titration with Potassium Permanganate

The sample is directly oxidized by the permanganate titrant. No indicator is required as a slight excess of permanganate imparts a distinct pink color to the solution.

NF Item

Calcium Phosphate, Dibasic—after precipitation of calcium oxalate. The oxalate is dissolved in acid and the oxalic acid titrated with permanganate.

$$5H_2C_2O_4 + 2KMnO_4 + 3H_2SO_4 =$$
$$K_2SO_4 + 2MnSO_4 + 10CO_2 + 8H_2O$$

USP Item

Cherry Juice—for malic acid; calcium oxalate is precipitated, collected, dissolved in acid, and titrated.

15b.

In this category excess ferric ammonium sulfate is added to the sample and the iron is reduced to iron(II), which is then titrated with permanganate.

USP Item

Titanium Dioxide—the sample is dissolved in a mixture of ammonium sulfate and sulfuric acid, reduced with zinc amalgam, and treated with excess ferric ammonium sulfate. Iron(III) is reduced by titanium(III) and the permanganate titration applied.

15c. Residual Titration Utilizing Oxalic Acid and Permanganate

USP Items

Potassium Permanganate—excess standard oxalic acid is caused to react with a warm, acidified solution of the sample. The excess oxalic acid is then titrated with permanganate.

Sodium Nitrite—nitrite is first oxidized to nitrate with excess standard permanganate and the unconsumed permanganate is reduced with excess oxalic acid. Finally, the excess oxalic acid is titrated with more standard permanganate.

16a. Dichlorophenol–Indophenol Titration

The titration with standard dichlorophenol-indophenol brings about an oxidation of the ascorbic acid while the volumetric solution also serves as its own indicator. During the titration the blue color of the standard dichlorophenol-indophenol is discharged by the reducing action of the ascorbic acid until the end-point is reached. This is indicated by the appearance of a permanent reddish color which is imparted to the mixture upon adding the slightest excess of dichlorophenol-indophenol. The reaction is explained as follows:

2,6-dichlorophenolindophenol
(blue in alkaline,
red in acid solution)

reduced indicator
(colorless)

16b. Sodium Tetraphenylboron Titration

Quaternary ammonium salts are capable of forming chloroform-soluble compounds with bromophenol blue as indicated below:

| bromophenol | quaternary | | chloroform- |
| blue | salt | | soluble product |

The product is extracted from alkaline solutions into chloroform. Titration with sodium tetraphenylboron removes the quaternary salt from the product, discharging the color from the chloroform layer. In this assay the quaternary salt and bromophenol blue, in a mixture of chloroform and water, is titrated with the sodium tetraphenylboron solution.

16c. Assays Involving Diphasic Amine–Surfactant Titration

NF Items

Benzphetamine Hydrochloride Tablets—see A, below.
Dicyclomine Hydrochloride Capsules and Syrup—see A, below.
Dioctyl Calcium Sulfosuccinate (and Solution)—see B, below (TBA).
Dioctyl Calcium Sulfosuccinate Capsules—see A, below; the Assay
    Preparation is employed as the titrant.
Methylbenzethonium Chloride Powder—see A, below.
Valethamate Bromide Injection—see A, below.

USP Items

Dioctyl Sodium Sulfosuccinate (and Capsules and Tablets)—see B, below (CAC).

A. In this type of assay the amine salt is dissolved in chloroform, indicator added and the mixture shaken. The indicator dissolves in the organic phase. Titration of this two phase system (with adequate shaking) with a surfactant solution, such as sodium lauryl sulfate, produces a water-soluble complex between amine and surfactant. As the end-point is exceeded the excess surfactant reacts with the basic dye (in the organic layer) and the indicator color changes from pale yellow to red(MeY) or blue(BpB). Standardization of the titrant is effected using a pure sample of the substance being assayed as the standard.

B. In this modification the surfactant is the substance being assayed and is added to the chloroform–water–indicator mixture. The titration is now performed utilizing a solution of a quaternary amine (cetalkonium chloride–CAC or tetrabutylammonium iodide–TBA) and the end point is reached when the color *disappears* from the chloroform layer.

17a. Direct Titration with Titanium Trichloride

These titrations depend upon the reduction of the colored sample and subsequent discharge of the color at the end-point.

17b. Residual Titration with Titanium Trichloride

The sample is heated with excess standard titanium trichloride, in an inert atmosphere. Excess reagent is determined by titration with ferric ammonium sulfate; thiocyanate ion, as the indicator, gives the familiar red end-point.

Titrations for Iodine Utilizing Sodium Thiosulfate

18a. Titration of Iodine Liberated from Potassium Iodide

Assays in this category involve the addition of the substance being assayed to an acidified solution of potassium iodide as exemplified by the equation with cupric sulfate:

$$2CuSO_4 + 4KI = 2CuI + I_2 + 2K_2SO_4$$

The liberated iodine is titrated with thiosulfate, starch being employed as the indicator:

$$I_2 + 2Na_2S_2O_3 = 2NaI + Na_2S_4O_6$$

In many cases the sample requires an initial special treatment.

NF Items

Ethylcellulose—for ethoxyl; *Methoxy Determination*, page 589.
Hydroxypropyl Methylcellulose—for methoxyl; see *Ethylcellulose*, above.
Iodized Oil—see *A*, below.
Selenium Sulfide (and Detergent Suspension)—after treatment with fuming nitric acid to form selenous acid. Potassium iodide then reduces the selenium, liberating iodine.

$$H_2SeO_3 + 4KI + 4H^+ = Se + 2I_2 + 4K^+ + 3H_2O$$

Sodium Dextrothyroxine—see *A*, below.
Sodium Dextrothyroxine Tablets—see *B*, below

USP Items

Diodohydroxyquin (and Tablets)—see *A*, below.
Ethiodized oil—see *A*, below.
Ferrous Fumarate Tablets—the sample is decomposed with nitric acid. Addition of KI to the iron(III) solution, causes reduction of the iron and liberation of free iodine, which is titrated with thiosulfate.
Iophendylate Injection—see *A*, below.
Methylcellulose—methoxyl; see *Ethylcellulose*, above.
Propyliodone (and Dosage Forms)—see *A*, below.
Sodium Levothyroxine—see *A*, below.
Sodium Levothyroxine Tablets—see *B*, below.
Sodium Liothyronine—see *A*, below.
Sodium Liothyronine Tablets—see *B*, below.
Thyroid (and Tablets)—see *B*, below.
A. The items in this category are initially decomposed using the *Oxygen Flask Method* (page 590), and the sample is treated with bromine, etc, as directed for *B*, below
B. The sample is fused with potassium carbonate, acidified, and oxidized with bromine to form iodate and bromide ion. The solution is boiled to expel bromine; phenol or formic acid is added to scavenge any remaining halogen; then KI is added and the iodate ion liberates free iodine which is titrated.

18b. Titrations with Potassium Iodate

When potassium iodate solution is titrated into an acidified solution of an alkali metal iodide, free iodine is liberated according to the following equation:

$$5KI + KIO_3 + 6HCl = 6KCl + 3I_2 + 3H_2O$$

When this step of the reaction is complete, and if a sufficiently high concentration of hydrochloric acid is present, the liberated iodine is converted into iodine monochloride, as is shown by:

$$KIO_3 + 2I_2 + 6HCl = KCl + 5ICl + 3H_2O$$

or combining both reactions:

$$KIO_3 + 2KI + 6HCl = 3KCl + 3ICl + 3H_2O$$

The end-point of this titration is shown by the disappearance of the iodine color from a few ml of chloroform added to act as an indicator.

NF Items

Hydralazine Hydrochloride Injection and Tablets—the hydrazino group of hydralazine is oxidized by the potassium iodate to nitrogen and is replaced by a hydroxyl group on the phthalazine ring in accordance with the following equation:

hydralazine

$$KCl + ICl + \text{[structure]} + N_2 + 2H_2O$$

1-phthalazinol

Iodine Ampuls and Solution—for sodium iodide: free iodine is first reduced by titration with arsenite.
Stannous Fluoride—for tin(II); in HCl solution, KI is added and iodide is converted to iodine, which is titrated with iodate.

USP Items

Iodine Solution, Strong—for potassium iodide; as for *Iodine Ampuls*, above.
Iodine Tincture—for sodium iodide; as for *Iodine Ampuls*, above.

18c. Reaction of KI with Excess Periodate

USP Items

Mannitol (and Injection)—an acidified solution of the prepared sample is heated with periodate and acid, oxidizing the mannitol as follows:

$$C_6H_{14}O_6 + 5HIO_4 = 2HCHO + 4HCOOH + 5HIO_3 + H_2O$$

The excess periodate and the iodate formed in the reaction react with KI to liberate iodine:

$$HIO_3 + HIO_4 + 12HI = 7I_2 + 7H_2O$$

A blank is performed and the difference in the volumes of thiosulfate titrant is equivalent to the mannitol in the sample.

Mannitol and Sodium Chloride Injection—for mannitol, as above.

18d. Direct Titration of Iodine with Thiosulfate

No preliminary preparation of the sample is necessary, as the iodine is present in the free state.

NF Item

Povidone–Iodine—for available iodine.

18e. Residual Titration of Iodine following Dichromate Precipitation

These assays are based on the insolubility of the dichromate precipitated from an aqueous solution of the sample on the addition of excess standard potassium dichromate. After removal of the precipitate the excess dichromate in the filtrate is determined by adding excess KI, which liberates free iodine and is titrated with thiosulfate.

$$Cr_2O_7^{2-} + 14H^+ + 6I^- = 3I_2 + 2Cr^{3+} + 7H_2O$$

18f. Residual Titration of Excess Standard Iodine

A sample of the assay material is oxidized or converted to a periodide or iodine substitution product with standard iodine and the excess iodine determined by titration with thiosulfate.

NF Item

Antipyrine—forms an insoluble monoiodo-substitution product.

USP Items

Methionine (and Capsules and Tablets)—the sample is converted to a periodide in which one molecule of methionine combines with one molecule of iodine.
Methenamine Mandelate—for methenamine; which is hydrolyzed to formaldehyde. The formaldehyde reacts with a modified Nessler's reagent to yield metallic mercury; this is oxidized by excess standard iodine to mercury II and the excess iodine titrated with thiosulfate.
Isoniazid (and Injection, Syrup, and Tablets)—the hydrazide is oxidized by iodine according to the equation

$$C_5H_4NCONHNH_2 + 2I_2 + 4NaHCO_3 =$$
$$N_2 + C_5H_4NCOOH + 4NaI + 4CO_2 + 3H_2O$$

Phenelzine Sulfate (and Tablets)—the hydrazine is oxidized by iodine as is indicated by the equation

$$C_6H_5CH_2CH_2NHNH_2 \cdot H_2SO_4 + 2I_2 + 5NaHCO_3 =$$
$$C_6H_5CH_2CH_2I + 3NaI + Na_2SO_4 + 5CO_2 + 5H_2O + N_2$$

19. Iodimetric Determination of Phenols

In these assays the precipitation of a bromophenol derivative is brought about by adding standard bromine solution to a solution of the sample. Hydrochloric acid is then added to liberate free bromine from the standard bromine solution:

$$5KBr + KBrO_3 + 6HCl = 6KCl + 3Br_2 + 3H_2O$$

The free bromine immediately reacts with the phenolic substance according to the following equation, using phenol as an example:

$$C_6H_5OH + 3Br_2 = C_6H_2Br_3OH + 3HBr$$

Potassium iodide is then added and the excess bromine liberates free iodine:

$$2KI + Br_2 = 2KBr + I_2$$

and it is titrated with thiosulfate. A blank is run on the same quantity of reagents, omitting the sample.

20a. Direct Titration with Standard Iodine

The sample is titrated directly, Starch TS usually being employed as the indicator.

NF Item

Carbarsone (and Dosage Forms)—the sample is first subjected to an acid digestion and reduction of the arsenic to the trivalent form. The resulting arsenite is then titrated:

$$Na_2HAsO_3 + I_2 + H_2O = Na_2HAsO_4 + 2HI$$

Added sodium carbonate reacts with the HI formed to prevent reversal of the reaction.

USP Items

Ascorbic Acid—a direct titration. If ascorbic acid is present in a multiple vitamin preparation, the procedure of Category 16 is employed.

Echothiophate Iodide (and Echothiophate Iodide for Ophthalmic Solution)—The ester is first hydrolyzed with base to yield the free mercaptan, which is then oxidized, by titration with iodine, to the disulfide. Any free mercaptan in the original sample is corrected for by a preliminary titration. The following equations apply:

$$[(C_2H_5)_2(PO)—S—CH_2CH_2N(CH_3)_3]^+I^- + H_2O =$$
Echothiophate
$$[HSCH_2CH_2N(CH_3)_3]^+I^- + (C_2H_5)_2(PO)OH$$

$$2[HSCH_2CH_2N(CH_3)_3]^+I^- + I_2 =$$
mercaptan
$$2[—SCH_2CH_2N(CH_3)_3^+]I^- + 2HI$$

Sulfur Dioxide—upon absorption in sodium hydroxide the bisulfite ion is produced and then titrated with iodine.

20b. Residual Titration of Excess Thiosulfate with Iodine

USP Items

Mechlorethamine Hydrochloride and Mechlorethamine Hydrochloride for Injection—thiosulfate reacts with the active chlorine atoms according to the equation

$$CH_3N(CH_2CH_2Cl)_2.HCl + NaHCO_3 + 2Na_2S_2O_3 =$$
$$CH_3N(CH_2CH_2S_2O_3Na)_2 + 3NaCl + CO_2 + H_2O$$

21. Direct Titration of Iodine with Arsenite

Free or liberated iodine is titrated with a standard sodium arsenite solution according to the equation indicated under category 20a.

USP Items

Iodine (and Ampuls and Solution)—for iodine.
Iodine Solution, Strong—for free iodine.
Iodine Tincture—for free iodine.
Sorbitol and Sorbitol Solution—after chromatographic separation, the sample is treated as indicated for *Mannitol* under Category 18c, except sodium arsenite is used as a titrant.

22. Direct Titration with Ferric Chloride

USP Item

Sodium Fluoride—the sample is titrated with iron(III) chloride employing thiocyanate as the indicator. The ion $(FeF_6)^{3-}$ is formed.

23. Direct Titration with Standard Bromine

USP Item

Thymol—a warm solution of the sample is titrated to produce a bromo-derivative, analogous to the determination of phenols in Category 19. However, an excess is not employed, since methyl

orange is used as an indicator and the color is bleached as the equivalence point is exceeded.

24. Direct Titration with Potassium Ferricyanide

NF Items

Methyprylon (and Capsules and Tablets)—in this assay the ferricyanide oxidizes the diketopiperidine ring effecting the loss of 2 atoms of hydrogen; 2 moles of ferricyanide are consumed per mole of methyprylon. The end-point is determined potentiometrically

methyprylon → **dehydro derivative**

25. Titrations Involving Sodium Nitrite Solution

Most of the compounds in this group, being primary aromatic amines or derivatives which may be converted to such amines, are capable of undergoing quantitative diazotization of the amino group substituted on the aromatic ring, as illustrated by the following equation utilizing *p*-aminobenzoic acid.

$$H_2NC_6H_4COOH + NaNO_2 + 2HCl \rightarrow$$
$$ClN_2C_6H_4COOH + NaCl + 2H_2O$$

The titration with sodium nitrite is performed in a solution containing crushed ice, to prevent decomposition of the diazonium salt, until a drop of the titrated solution produces an immediate blue color with starch iodide paste used as an external indicator.

Sulfonamides in which the reactive amino group is acylated must be subjected to preliminary hydrolysis to release the free amine form of the sulfonamide prior to diazotization.

NF Items

Procaine and Tetracaine Hydrochlorides and Levarterenol Bitartrate Injection—for procaine (SPI); and, for tetracaine after removal as the thiocyanate (SPI).
Procaine and Tetracaine Hydrochlorides and Levonordefrin Injection—for procaine and tetracaine, as above.
Procaine, Tetracaine, and Phenylephrine Hydrochlorides Injection—for procaine and tetracaine, as above.
Propoxyphene and Procaine Hydrochlorides and Levonordefrin Injection—for procaine.
Sodium Cyclamate and Sodium Saccharin Solution and Tablets—for cyclamate (SPI).
Sulfacetamide, Sulfadiazine, and Sulfamerazine Suspension (and Tablets)—potentiometric titration for sulfacetamide after removal of the diazine and merazine by precipitation with acid (SPI).

USP Items

Primaquine Phosphate (and Tablets)—this substance contains a secondary amino group and nitrosation rather than diazotization occurs, the =NH group being converted to =N—NO (N-nitroso).
Trisulfapyrimidines Oral Suspension (and Tablets)—assay for total sulfapyrimidines.

IV. Miscellaneous Titrimetric Methods

Complexometric Titrations

26a. Direct with Ethylenediaminetetracetic Acid (EDTA)

EDTA complexes with many polyvalent metals to form an undissociated chelate (see Chapter 16, *Complexation*). A buffered solution of the sample is titrated with EDTA (as the disodium salt). The indicator used is a dye which forms a weak chelate with the assay material. As the end-point is passed, the color changes when the indicator–metal complex is completely destroyed.

NF Item

Magaldrate (and Oral Suspension and Tablets)—for magnesium oxide (EBT).

USP Items

Alumina and Magnesia Oral Suspension (and Tablets)—for magnesium hydroxide, using ammonium hydroxide and ammonium chloride buffer (EBT).

Calcium Disodium Edetate (and Injection)—mercury (II) nitrate is the titrant.
Calcium Pantothenate (and Tablets)—calcium content.
Calcium Pantothenate, Racemic—calcium content.
Disodium Edetate (and Injection)—primary standard calcium carbonate, after suitable preparation, is titrated with a solution of the assay preparation.
Magnesia and Alumina Oral Suspension (and Tablets)—for magnesium oxide (EBT).

26b.   Residual Titration Involving EDTA

To assay for aluminum in many combinations containing both magnesium and aluminum a residual method is employed. Excess EDTA is added to a suitably buffered sample and the excess determined by titration with standard zinc sulfate solution. By use of proper buffers and masking agents (weak complexing materials) it is often possible to determine mixtures of calcium and aluminum, calcium and magnesium, or zinc and aluminum without preliminary separation.

NF Item

Magaldrate (and Oral Suspension and Tablets)—for aluminum oxide (DT).

USP Items

Alumina and Magnesia Oral Suspension (and Tablets)—for aluminum oxide (DT).
Aluminum Acetate Solution—for aluminum oxide (DT).
Aluminum Subacetate Solution—for aluminum oxide (DT).
Magnesia and Alumina Oral Suspension (and Tablets)—for aluminum oxide (DT).

26c.   Miscellaneous Complexometric Methods

Penicillamine (and Capsules)—direct titration with mercury (II) acetate; penicillamine is an excellent complexing agent and readily combines with mercury. As the end-point is passed, excess titrant forms the violet mercury–dithizone complex.

Titrimetric Assays Utilizing Nonaqueous Solvents

Titrimetric methods employing nonaqueous solvents are now extensively used for the assay of certain materials which cannot be easily titrated in aqueous systems. As is explained in the chapter on *Ionic Solutions and Electrolytic Equilibria*, page 270, water is a leveling solvent and many weak acids or bases do not give a sufficiently sharp break in the titration curve to evidence a distinct end-point. However, in a nonaqueous solvent, such as glacial acetic acid, weak organic bases and their salts can be titrated with an acetic acid solution of perchloric acid. While the strongest acid available in aqueous medium is the

hydronium ion, H_3O^+, in acetic acid the proton of perchloric acid forms the acetonium ion, $CH_3C(OH)_2^+$, an extremely strong acid.

$$CH_3COOH + HClO_4 = CH_3C(OH)_2^+ + ClO_4^-$$

The reaction between the acetonium ion and an amine (a weak base) is illustrated by the following equation, forming the ammonium ion and acetic acid.

$$CH_3C(OH)_2^+ + RNH_2 = CH_3COOH + RNH_3^+$$

No difficulty is experienced in the titration of amine salts other than salts of halogen acids. In the latter case mercury (II) acetate is added to form undissociated mercury (II) halide, thus preventing interference by the halogen acid which would be liberated in its absence.

Weak organic acids, such as carboxylic acids, phenols, barbiturates, sulfonamides or enols may also be titrated in nonaqueous medium using a strong base. These include the sodium or lithium salts of methanol or ethanol and the reaction is of the ordinary neutralization type, as illustrated below for an organic acid with sodium ethoxide.

$$RCOOH + C_2H_5ONa = RCOONa + C_2H_5OH$$

In both types of titration, acid or base, the end point may be determined with indicators or potentiometrically as depicted in the accompanying chart (Table II) taken from the USP.

27a.

NF Items

Chloral Betaine—for betaine (Nb).
Diphenoxylate Hydrochloride and Atropine Sulfate Solution—for diphenoxylate (poten.).
Ephedrine Sulfate Tablets—ephedrine base is separated and titrated.
Isobucaine Hydrochloride and Epinephrine Injection—for isobucaine (MeR).
Meperidine Hydrochloride Syrup—the free base is liberated, extracted into chloroform, and titrated.
Mepivacaine Hydrochloride and Levonordefrin Injection—for mepivacaine (MeR).
Meprylcaine Hydrochloride and Epinephrine Injection—for meprylcaine (CrV).
Potassium Acetate—titration of a salt of a carboxylic acid.
Potassium Sodium Tartrate—see *Potassium Acetate*.
Potassium Sorbate—see *Potassium Acetate*.
Terpin Hydrate and Codeine Elixir—for codeine (MeR).
Trimethobenzamide Hydrochloride and Benzocaine Suppositories—for trimethobenzamide (CrV).

USP Items

Dimenhydrinate—for diphenhydramine (poten.).
Niacinamide—for the pure substance only; in combination as in Hexavitamin or Decavitamin preparations, use the method for *Niacinamide Injection*.

27b.   Titration of Acidic Substances

A strong base is used to titrate very weak acids. Special precautions must be employed to exclude atmospheric carbon dioxide which interferes with the titration. The titrants used are indicated as a suffix number to the category. For example, Acetohexamide is in Category 27b-2; the number 2 indicating sodium methoxide solution as the titrant.
Titrants employed:
1—Lithium methoxide solution.
2—Sodium methoxide solution.
3—Tetrabutylammonium hydroxide solution.
4—Tributylethylammonium hydroxide solution.

V.   Gravimetric Assay Methods

In gravimetric methods of analysis the assay results are generally obtained either by determining the weight of a substance in the sample, or the weight of

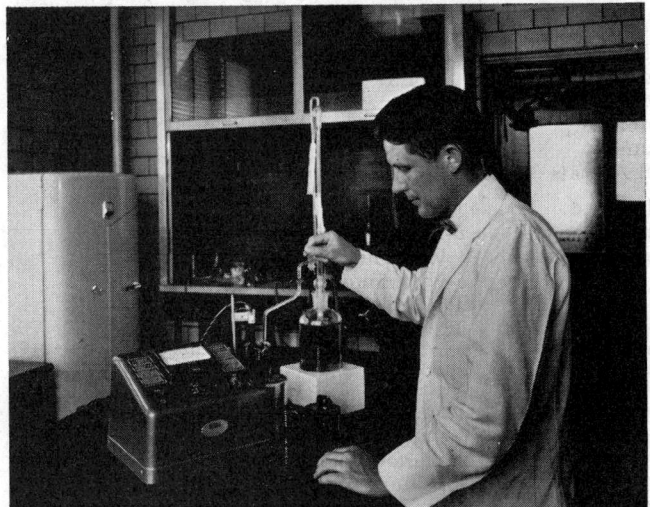

Fig. 413.   Essential apparatus for making titrations in nonaqueous solvents (courtesy, Lilly).

some other substance derived from the sample, the equivalent weight of which serves as the basis for calculating the result. The separation of the substance ultimately weighed is frequently accomplished by purely physical methods. On the other hand, there are many instances in which it is necessary to utilize a chemical reaction in order to convert the substance to a corresponding amount of some other substance which can be separated, purified, and weighed. The various types of official gravimetric assays may be conveniently grouped into the following categories for discussion.

28. Weighing the Active Ingredient after Separation

The active principle is separated, dried, and weighed.

NF Items

Caffeine, Citrated—for caffeine.

Estrone Injection—an elaborate purification procedure is involved whereby the estrone is converted to a water-soluble derivative using trimethylacethydrazide ammonium chloride (Girard's reagent for carbonyl compounds); the aqueous extract contains only ketonic material as the reagent reacts only with carbonyl compounds. The aqueous extract is then decomposed with acid to regenerate estrone, which is extracted into chloroform, the solvent removed, and the residue weighed.

Silicon Dioxide, Colloidal—silica is determined by difference; the sample is weighed before and after treatment with hydrofluoric acid, which converts silica into the volatile silicon tetrafluoride. The difference in weight represents the silica content of the sample.

Zinc–Eugenol Cement—for rosin by loss in weight after chloroform extraction.

USP Items

Caffeine and Sodium Benzoate Injection—for caffeine, after solution of the sodium benzoate in water.

Collodion–pyroxylin is precipitated by water, dried, and weighed.

Storax—the sample is saponified with alcoholic base, acidified, extracted with ether, and the solvent removed to give cinnamic acid, which is weighed.

29. Weighing of the Residue after Ignition of the Sample

NF Items

Aluminum Aspirin—ignite to aluminum oxide.

Zinc–Eugenol Cement—for total zinc, as the oxide.

Zinc Oxide Paste with Salicylic Acid—for total zinc, as the oxide.

USP Items

Aluminum Monostearate—as aluminum oxide.

Bismuth Subcarbonate—as bismuth sesquioxide.

30. Precipitation and Weighing of a Derivative of the Active Ingredient

NF Items

Camphorated Parachlorophenol—for para-chlorophenol; silver chloride is precipitated after liberation of chloride ion by oxidation with hot permanganate. For camphor; as the 2,4-dinitrophenylhydrazone.

Dihydroxyaluminum Sodium Carbonate—for carbon dioxide; on treatment with acid, CO_2 is liberated and absorbed on carbon dioxide absorbent and the increase in weight noted.

Ichthammol—for total sulfur as barium sulfate after oxidation with nitric acid and perchlorate.

Magnesium Citrate Solution—for MgO as the 8-hydroxyquinolate.

Papaverine Injection (and Tablets)—as the free base.

Pentylenetetrazol—as the phosphotungstate.

Phenacaine Hydrochloride—as the free base.

Phenolphthalein Tablets—as the tetraiodo derivative.

Phentolamine Hydrochloride (and Tablets)—as the trichloroacetate salt.

Potash, Sulfurated—as copper (II) sulfide.

Progesterone Suspension, Sterile—as the 2,4-dinitrophenylhydrazone.

Quinine Hydrochloride Injection—as the free base.

Sitosterols (and Suspension)—for total sterols as the digitonide.

Sodium Butabarbital (and Capsules and Elixir)—as the free acid.

Sodium Cyclamate and Sodium Saccharin Solution (and Tablets)—for saccharin; as $BaSO_4$, after extraction with ether from the acidified solution, evaporation of the solvent, and fusion of the residue with K_2CO_3.

Sodium Phosphate Solution—$MgNH_4PO_4$ is precipitated and ignited to magnesium pyrophosphate, $Mg_2P_2O_7$.

Sodium Thiamylal for Injection—as the free acid.

Sodium Vinbarbital for Injection—as the free acid.

Trimethidinium Methosulfate (and Tablets)—as the chloroplatinate.

Undecylenic Acid Ointment, Compound—for zinc undecylenate; the sample is digested with a nitric–sulfuric acid mixture, neutralized and the zinc precipitated as the 8-hydroxyquinolate.

USP Items

Aurothioglucose (and Injection)—gold is precipitated and weighed.

Barium Sulfate—the sample is fused with sodium carbonate and barium chromate precipitated and weighed.

Betazole Hydrochloride (and Injection)—as the phosphotungstate.

Bethanechol Chloride Injection (and Tablets)—tetraphenylboron derivative.

Gold Sodium Thiomalate (and Injection)—gold precipitated and weighed.

Table II—Solvent Systems for Nonaqueous Titrations

Type of solvent	Acidic (for titration of bases and their salts)	Relatively neutral (for titration of bases)	Basic (for titration of acids)
Solvent[a]	Glacial Acetic Acid Acetic Anhydride Formic Acid Propionic Acid Sulfuryl chloride	Acetonitrile Alcohols Benzene Chlorobenzene Chloroform Dioxane Ethyl Acetate	n-Butylamine Dimethylformamide Ethylenediamine Pyridine Morpholine
Indicator	Crystal Violet Methyl Red Thymol Blue α-Naphtholbenzein Quinaldine Red Malachite Green	Methyl Red Methyl Orange α-Naphtholbenzein	Azo Violet p-Hydroxyazobenzene o-Nitroaniline Thymol Blue Thymolphthalein
Electrodes	Glass-silver-silver chloride Glass-calomel Mercury-Mercuric acetate	Calomel-silver-silver chloride Glass-calomel	Antimony-antimony Antimony-calomel Antimony-glass Platinum-Calomel

[a] Relatively neutral solvents of low dielectric constant such as benzene, chloroform, or dioxane may be used in conjunction with any acidic or basic solvent in order to increase the sensitivity of the titration end-points.

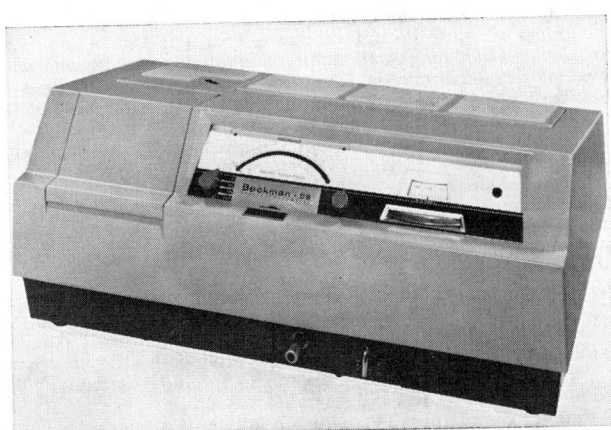

Fig. 414. Beckman model DB spectrophotometer.

Histamine Phosphate—as the 1:1 salt with nitranilic acid (2,5-dihydroxy-3,6-dinitro-p-benzoquinone).
Hydroxyamphetamine Hydrobromide Ophthalmic Solution—as the diacetyl derivative.
Magnesia Tablets—as the 8-hydroxyquinolate.
Magnesium Trisilicate (and Tablets)—as silicon dioxide.
Meralluride (and Injection)—as mercury (II) sulfide.
Piperazine Citrate (and Tablets)—as the picrate.
Raspberry Juice—for citric acid: the sample is treated with magnesium oxide, which dissolves forming magnesium citrate. Excess MgO is filtered and magnesium is determined in the filtrate as magnesium ammonium phosphate which is ignited to the pyrophosphate. The weight of pyrophosphate multiplied by 1.259 represents the weight of citric acid in the volume of juice taken for a sample.
Sodium Amobarbital—as the free acid.
Sodium Diphenylhydantoin (and Capsules and Sterile)—as the free acid.
Sodium Fluorescein (and Ophthalmic Solution)—as fluorescein.
Sodium Lauryl Sulfate—for sodium sulfate; as $BaSO_4$. For unsulfated alcohols; the sample is extracted with hexane, the solvent evaporated, and the residue weighed. The unsulfated alcohols are nonpolar and therefore soluble in hexane. For total alcohols; the sample is hydrolyzed with HCl to liberate the free alcohols which are extracted into ether, the solvent removed, and the residue weighed. In each case the appropriate gravimetric factor is multiplied by the residue weight to determine the quantity of assayed material in the portion of sample taken.
Sodium Mercaptomerin (and Injection and Sterile)—as mercury (II) sulfide.
Sodium Phenobarbital (and all Dosage Forms)—as the free acid.
Sodium Pentobarbital (and all Dosage Forms)—as the free acid.
Sodium Secobarbital (and Sterile)—as the free acid.
Sulfur Ointment—the sample is oxidized with nitric acid to convert sulfur to sulfate, which is precipitated and weighed as barium sulfate.

VI. Spectrophotometric Methods

Photometric analysis depends upon the measurement of the amount of light absorbed by a solution (*spectrophotometry*), or by a suspension (*turbidimetry*), or the amount of light scattered by a suspension (*nephelometry*), or the intensity of the light emitted by an element when subjected to high temperatures (*flame photometry*). These measurements are usually made with the aid of photoelectric instruments (pages 600 and 601). The measurement of light in the visible region (*colorimetry*) may be accomplished photoelectrically with the aid of a photoelectric colorimeter or spectrophotometer or less accurately by visual comparison with color standards.

Spectrophotometry involves the measurement of the ability of a dissolved substance to absorb electromagnetic radiation of definite and narrow wavelength ranges. These absorptions are measured at wavelengths that are generally characteristic of the chemical composition of the dissolved absorbing substance. Absorption measurements made at several wavelengths enable the analyst to identify the dissolved substance,

as well as determine its concentration. In the official assays of this type practically all of the absorption measurements are made within the visible and the ultraviolet ranges of the spectrum. The unit of measurement generally used is the millimicron (mμ), which is the millionth part of a millimeter. See Chapter 41, *Instrumental Methods of Analysis*, for a more detailed treatment.

Radiant energy waves that are of importance to spectrophotometry range from 200 to 400 mμ in the ultraviolet, from 400 to 750 mμ in the visible range, and from 750 to 25,000 mμ in the near infrared and infrared regions. These measurements are made by the use of several models of spectrophotometers (see Fig. 414 and page 601) that are commercially available. Their essential parts include a source of radiant energy, a dispersing device with a slit for selecting the desired wavelength band, a cell for the sample, and a photometer for indicating the intensity of the transmitted radiation. The relatively large number of spectrophotometric assays that are now officially described in the USP and in the NF testifies to the widespread development and general acceptance of the analytical methods that belong in this category.

31a. Colorimetric Assays

Under this heading, perhaps more correctly termed *spectrophotometric colorimetry*, are considered those assays that depend upon the development of color or upon the color of the substance being assayed. The absorbances are accordingly measured at wavelengths that are within the visible range of the spectrum. These colorimetric assays generally consist of adding a reagent to the assay preparation or to the substance being tested, in order to produce a color which is compared with that of a standard preparation that has been prepared simultaneously and contains approximately an equal quantity of a reference standard. When the absorbance of a frequently assayed substance has been found to conform to Beer's law over a reasonable range of concentration, it is considered permissible to utilize a standard curve, prepared with the respective USP reference standard, for interpolation of the data obtained with the assay preparation.

In some instances characteristic colors are developed in *flame photometers* by subjecting an inorganic element or its compound in solution to an intensely hot flame. The intensity of the colors (radiations) is compared photoelectrically in a suitable spectrophotometer with standard solutions containing the same element.

The various models of available spectrophotometers are suitable for making these colorimetric measurements. Photoelectric colorimeters of the filter type, in which the light absorption is measured by sensitive photoelectric cells, are also largely used for making these determinations and several of them are commercially available (see Fig. 407, page 600).

Steroid Assay (†31a)

Those compounds for which the category number is daggered (eg, †31a) are determined by the *Assay for Total Steroids* in Chapter 36, *Official Requirements and Tests*, page 590.

Dye-Complex Method (‡31a)

Those compounds which exhibit the double-daggered entry (‡31a) are assayed by the following technique. As was indicated under Category 16b, quaternary salts and many amines are capable of forming chloroform-soluble complexes with indicators, such as bromophenol blue. The usual procedure is to shake a mixture of the assay preparation, chloroform, and a buffer containing the indicator. The dye-complex partitions into the organic layer, which is separated, filtered to remove any adhering aqueous phase and the absorbance determined. The indicator listed under Column 3 is the dye employed to form the complex.

NF Items

If a three-digit number followed by a letter code is given, this indicates the analytical wavelength and color developing reagent employed.
Antipyrine and Benzocaine Solution—for benzocaine; 550, BM.
Cobalamin Concentrate—see *Cobalamin Assay—Radiotracer Method*, page 588; 361 and 550.
Diethylstilbestrol Dipropionate Tablets—after saponification.
Diphenoxylate Hydrochloride and Atropine Sulfate Solution (and Tablets)—for atropine; 515, PDB.

Ergotamine Tartrate and Caffeine Suppositories (and Tablets)—for ergotamine; 515, PDB.

Iodochlorhydroxyquin and Hydrocortisone Cream (and Lotion, and Ointment)—for hydrocortisone; 525, BT.

Isobucaine Hydrochloride and Epinephrine Injection—for epinephrine; 530, FCiT.

Mepivacaine Hydrochloride and Levonordefrin Injection—for levonordefrin; 530, FCiT.

Meprylcaine Hydrochloride and Epinephrine Injection—for epinephrine; 530, FCiT.

Metabutethamine Hydrochloride and Epinephrine Injection—for epinephrine; 530, FCiT.

Procaine and Phenylephrine Hydrochlorides Injection—for phenylephrine; 500, AAP.

Procaine and Tetracaine Hydrochlorides and Levarterenol Bitartrate Injection—for levarterenol; 530, FCiT.

Procaine and Tetracaine Hydrochlorides and Levonordefrin Injection—for levonordefrin; 530, FCiT.

Procaine Hydrochloride and Levonordefrin Injection—for levonordefrin; 530, FCiT.

Procaine, Tetracaine, and Phenylephrine Hydrochlorides Injection—for phenylephrine; 500, AAP.

Procaine and Propoxycaine Hydrochlorides and Levarterenol Bitartrate Injection—for levarterenol; 530, FCiT.

Propoxycaine and Procaine Hydrochlorides and Levonordefrin Injection—for levonordefrin; 530, FCiT.

Pyrrocaine Hydrochloride and Epinephrine Injection—for epinephrine; 530, FCiT.

Stannous Fluoride—for fluoride; 590; a zirconium-dye lake is bleached by fluoride ion.

Sulfacetamide, Sulfadiazine, and Sulfamerazine Suspension (and Tablets)—for sulfadiazine and sulfamerazine. The sample is chromatographed on paper, the diazine and merazine spots cut out (after spraying a reference strip to locate the spots), dissolved in water, diazotized with nitrous acid, and coupled with Bratton–Marshall (BM) reagent to produce a red color measured at 525 mμ.

Sulfadiazine and Sulfamerazine Tablets—as for *Sulfacetamide, Sulfadiazine, and Sulfamerazine*, above.

Terpin Hydrate and Dextromethorphan Hydrobromide Elixir—for dextromethorphan; 420, BcG.

Trimethobenzamide Hydrochloride and Benzocaine Suppositories—for benzocaine; 540, BM.

Vitamin E—for non-alpha-tocopheryl acetates and non-alpha-tocopherols; 540, SN.

USP Items

Polyethylene Glycol 400—ethylene and diethylene-glycols limit; 525, CAN.

Trisulfapyrimidines Oral Suspension and Tablets—for sulfadiazine, sulfamerazine, and sulfamethazine employing the method indicated for *Sulfacetamide, Sulfadiazine, and Sulfamerazine*, above.

31b. Spectrophotometric Assays in the Ultraviolet

Spectrophotometric assays in which the absorbances are directly measured in the ultraviolet range are described in the official monographs for the substances that are listed below.

Applied to solutions, spectrophotometry is more specific than colorimetry because the absorption depends upon wavelength in a complicated manner that is generally characteristic of the chemical composition of the absorbing substance. Measurement of absorption at several wavelengths may permit identification of the solute as well as the determination of its concentration. Tests of this kind are made usually on solutions, rarely on pure liquids or solids.

Solvents used for dilution usually require special purification which is often exacting and different from the requirements for other uses. Some assays direct that blank runs be made on the solvent and reagents used to obtain a correction for their inherent absorbances.

Spectrophotometers used in official assays must be carefully calibrated with the aid of standard glasses or standard solutions.[2]

Lambert's and Beer's Laws—Lambert in 1760 postulated that for a fixed pathlength through a given substance, the ratio of the intensities of the transmitted and incident light is independent of the intensity of the incident light. This empirical law has been found experimentally to be accurately followed by practically all substances under extreme ranges of conditions. Lambert also pointed out that layers of the same thickness of the same substance absorb the same fraction of the incident light. If the mathematical statement of Lambert's laws is integrated, the law for the dependence of the absorption ratio on pathlength can be derived:

$$I/I_o = e^{-kl}$$

where I is the intensity of the transmitted light, I_0 is the intensity of the incident light, l is the length of the path, and k is a constant characteristic of the substance.

For most solutions, the constant k is approximately proportional to the mass of solute in unit volume of solution; this is known as *Beer's law*. Thus, for practical purposes, the absorptivity of a substance, as defined below, is a constant with respect to changes in concentration and/or length of the light path, with the result that concentration may be determined photometrically.

Terminology—There is some nonuniformity of terminology employed in spectrophotometry. The following definitions and symbols are designated as official:

Transmittance: I/I_o. The ratio of the transmitted light intensity to the incident light intensity. Symbol: T.

Absorbance: $-\log T$. The negative logarithm of the transmittance. Symbol: A.

Concentration: Where related to spectrophotometry, concentrations are expressed in Gm of solute per liter of solution. Symbol: c.

Absorptivity: The absorbance of a solution containing 1 Gm per 100 ml contained in a cell having an absorption path of 1 cm. Symbol: a. This is identical with the term "Specific Absorbancy" defined in USP XIV, for which the symbol was $E_{1\,cm}^{1\%}$.

Reference Standards—In practically all cases a Reference Standard (USP or NF) is used in conjunction with the sample under assay. The standard preparation is prepared and observed in the same manner as the test specimen. The purpose of this specification is to avoid any errors due to wavelength or slit width variation among various spectrophotometers, as well as to avoid errors arising from differences in transmittance and placement of cells.

A three-digit number in parenthesis is the analytical wavelength.

NF Items

Aluminum Aspirin—for aspirin.

Angiotensin Amide (and Injection)—the difference in absorbance of an alkaline and acidic sample and standard preparation (tyrosine) is determined. As the phenolic group is the only pH sensitive chromophore, this technique yields more specific results than a simple one-point determination.

Antipyrine and Benzocaine Solution—for antipyrine (266).

Aspirin, Phenacetin and Caffeine Tablets—for caffeine (276), phenacetin (285), and aspirin (280 and 310).

Cobalamin Concentrate—see *Cobalamin Assay, Radiotracer Method*, page 588.

Codeine Phosphate, Aspirin, Phenacetin, and Caffeine Tablets—for caffeine (276), phenacetin (285), and aspirin (280 and 310), after chromatographic separation.

Cod Liver Oil—for vitamin A (at 310, 325 and 334); before and after catalytic hydrogenation. Hydrogenation reduces the conjugated unsaturated chromophore, removing the absorption due to this moiety.

Ergotamine Tartrate and Caffeine Suppositories and Tablets—for caffeine (276).

Ethinyl Estradiol and Dimethisterone Tablets—for dimethisterone (380-IN).

Furazolidone and Nifuroxime Powder (and Suppositories)—for furazolidone (367) and nifuroxime (341) after chromatographic separation.

Metabutethamine Hydrochloride and Epinephrine Injection—for metabutethamine (315).

Pentazocine Lactate Injection—the sample is passed through a cationic-exchange column and eluted with methanolic–hydrochloric acid.

Procaine and Phenylephrine Hydrochlorides Injection—for procaine (272).

Procaine Hydrochloride and Levonordefrin Injection—for procaine (272).

Procaine and Propoxycaine Hydrochlorides and Levarterenol Injection—for procaine (272) and propoxycaine (296) as a binary system.

Propoxycaine and Procaine Hydrochlorides and Levonordefrin Injection—for propoxycaine (300).

Theophylline, Ephedrine Hydrochloride, and Phenobarbital Tablets—for theophylline (275), ephedrine (257), and phenobarbital (240) after chromatographic separation.

USP Items

Amitriptyline Hydrochloride Injection—after oxidation with periodate and permanganate.

Benztropine Mesylate Tablets—after treatment with dichromate.

Cholestyramine Resin—for exchange capacity of sodium glycocholate. The absorbance of a solution of sodium glycocholate standard is compared to the absorbance of an equivalent volume of solution which has been in contact with a weighed quantity of resin.

Dexamethasone Sodium Phosphate (and Injection)—after treatment with phosphatase as directed for *Hydrocortisone Sodium Phosphate*, below.

Hydrocortisone Sodium Phosphate—the phosphate group is removed with a phosphatase enzyme and the resulting hydrocortisone extracted into methylene chloride and the absorbance determined. Hydrocortisone is employed as the reference standard.

Meralluride (and Injection)—for theophylline (242 and 272).

Prednisolone Sodium Phosphate (and Injection and Ophthalmic Solution)—as for *Hydrocortisone Sodium Phosphate*, above.

31c. Infrared Assays

The quantitative estimation of compounds by infrared methods is quite similar to the techniques employed in the ultraviolet and visible regions. However, due to the difficulties involved in measuring the absolute absorbance at a particular absorbance maximum, the "baseline" technique is often utilized. In this method a synthetic "baseline" is constructed between the minima at the sides of the absorption maximum and a vertical line, intersecting the peak of the maximum, is erected perpendicular to the abscissa. The length of the vertical line, measured from the intersection of the synthetic base line and the peak of the absorption maximum is used as the absorbance in quantitative calculations, as illustrated in Fig. 415.

In some cases, due to sampling difficulties, it is advantageous to employ an *internal standard*, as is done with Cyclophosphamide USP. In this assay ferric thiocyanate (which exhibits a sharp maximum at 4.9 μ) is mixed with the Cyclophosphamide Reference Standard (and the sample) and three concentrations of this mixture are used to plot a standard curve; the ratio of the absorbance at 9.5 μ (the analytical peak for Cyclophosphamide) to the absorbance at 4.9 μ being plotted against concentration. The samples are dispersed in a potassium bromide pellet for this assay. In the actual assay procedure the same ratio is calculated and the concentration of Cyclophosphamide determined from the standard curve.

For a further discussion of the theory involved in infrared absorption, see Chapter 41, *Instrumental Methods of Analysis*.

NF Items

Iodochlorhydroxyquin and Hydrocortisone Cream (and Lotion, and Ointment)—at 14.4 and 14.9 μ for iodochlorhydroxyquin.
Propoxyphene Hydrochloride and Aspirin Capsules—for propoxyphene at 5.80 μ, after extraction from an alkaline solution with chloroform. The aqueous layer is retained, saponified, acidified, extracted with chloroform, and aspirin determined as salicylic acid at 6.02 μ.
Sitosterols—for unsaturated sterols at 9.52 μ.

31d. Assays Involving Flame Photometry

This method deals with the emission of energy of a particular wavelength when a dilute solution of a metallic ion is sprayed into a colorless flame. The intensity of the emitted radiation is determined by a suitable spectrophotometer and compared to standards. Sodium, at 588 mμ, and potassium, at 766 mμ, are determined by this technique for the official substances indicated below.

NF Items

Potassic Saline Injection, Lactated
Ringer's Solution
Tromethamine for Injection

USP Items

Protein Hydrolysate Injection
Sodium Polystyrene Sulfonate—for sodium content and potassium exchange capacity. For the latter assay, the concentration of a dilute KCl solution is determined before and after equilibration with the cation-exchange resin sample. The decrease in potassium concentration is a measure of the exchange capacity.

31e. Fluorophotometric Assay Methods

Riboflavin in official vitamin preparations is quantitatively assayed by measuring its degree of fluorescence in ultraviolet light. Thiamine is also assayed by a fluorophotometric method, the principal

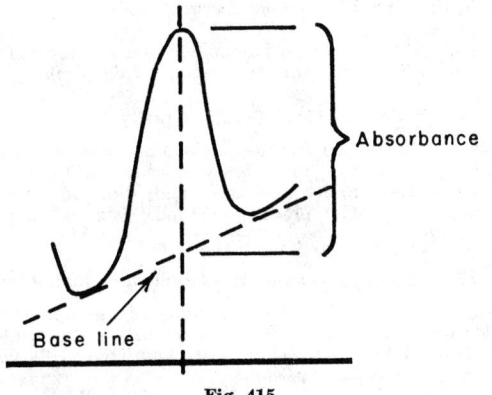

Fig. 415.

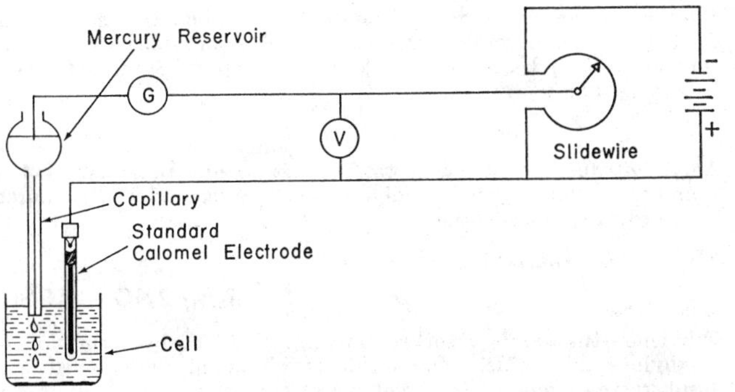

difference from the riboflavin assay being that thiamine is first oxidized to thiochrome, the fluorescence of which is quantitatively measured in isobutyl alcohol solution. The intensity of fluorescence is measured at right angles to the incident monochromatic radiation in an instrument known as a fluorophotometer (described on page 709), or in certain spectrophotometers equipped with the required accessories. Quantitative evaluation of the fluorescence data is achieved through comparison with similar data obtained with solutions containing known amounts of reference standard thiamine hydrochloride.

Multivitamin preparations and Dried Yeast are assayed also for riboflavin and thiamine by this procedure.

31f. Atomic Absorption Analysis

This technique is similar to flame photometry except that the photometer determines the decrease in intensity of a beam of energy passed through a flame in which the metallic ion under test is sprayed. The incident radiation is generated by a lamp, the cathode of which is fabricated from the same metal as the ions of the solution being assayed. See Chapter 41 for a detailed discussion. Thimerosal NF and its Dosage Forms are assayed, based upon the mercury content, by this procedure.

32. Polarographic Analysis

Quantitative polarographic methods of analysis are specified for several official substances. The polarograph (Fig. 412, page 602) in its simplest form is diagrammed in Fig. 416. A slidewire in parallel with a fixed source of low-voltage direct current, is connected in series with the reservoir of a *dropping mercury electrode* and a standard calomel electrode, both dipping into the solution to be analyzed. Rotation of the slidewire allows a variable voltage to be applied to the cell, while the applied voltage and the resulting current are measured by voltmeter V and galvanometer G, respectively. In modern recording instruments the slidewire is mechanically rotated in synchronism with the time base of an automatic recording device so that the applied voltage corresponds to the abscissa. The current is amplified electronically and activates the recording pen along the ordinate scale of the recording chart to produce a polarogram as shown in Fig. 417. The jagged appearance of the curve is due to the rapid increase in current as the size of the mercury drop increases before it drops. A new drop begins to form, repeating the process.

The *diffusion current* (i_d) is proportional to the concentration of the electro-active species under test while the *half-wave potential* ($E_{1/2}$) is characteristic of the kind of electro-active species and is independent of concentration. In the official assay methods the diffusion current of a sample and a reference standard solution is measured under identical conditions and the concentration of the sample is calculated from the ratio of the sample to reference standard diffusion currents.

A complete review of the theory of polarography is beyond the scope of this chapter, and a more complete discussion can be found in Chapter 41.

NF Items

Dienestrol Cream and Tablets—the excipients are first removed by formation of a urea complex (see Chapter 16, *Complexation*) and column chromatography.

VII. Other Methods

33. Gasometric Assay Methods

Gasometric methods of analysis depend upon the measurement of the volume of a gas liberated under the conditions that are described in the assay, or of the decrease in volume of a gas when a suitable reagent is used to remove one of the gases present. There are six official items in which the purity of the substance is determined by

Fig. 416. Polarograph.

the measurement of a gas. These determinations are usually conducted in a gas buret or nitrometer, which is provided with a two-way stopcock and a two-way outlet and is properly connected with a balancing tube.

NF Items

Amyl Nitrite—the sample is treated with acidic potassium iodide and the volume of nitric oxide liberated is measured in a gas buret, according to the equation

$$2KI + 2C_5H_{11}ONO + H_2SO_4 =$$
$$2C_5H_{11}OH + I_2 + 2NO + K_2SO_4$$

Ethylene—the gas is absorbed into bromine TS, by formation of ethylene dibromide. The residual volume of undissolved gas, subtracted from the total volume of the sample is a measure of the purity.

USP Items

Carbon Dioxide—the sample is absorbed in 50% potassium hydroxide and the volume of residual gas measured, as for Ethylene NF.

Cyclopropane—the sample is absorbed by concentrated sulfuric acid and the residual volume measured, as for Ethylene NF.

Nitrogen—the gas sample is exposed to the action of an ammoniacal copper solution, which removes oxygen. The residual gas volume is nitrogen.

Oxygen—same method as for Nitrogen, but the residual volume is a measure of the impurities present.

34. Assays Involving Volumetric Measurements

Those assays that depend upon the separation and the measurement of oily or aqueous immiscible layers will now be considered. In general, these volumetric measurements are made possible as the result of processes that involve solvent separations, steam distillations, or chemical changes, in which an important constituent of the official substance (ie, volatile oil), such as an aldehyde, a ketone, or a phenol, is purposely converted to a water-soluble substance. In the latter case, the volume of residual oil is measured and the assay result is then determined by difference.

NF Items

Caraway Oil—the ketone, carvone, is converted into a water-soluble bisulfite addition compound and the residual oily volume measured.

Cinnamon—for volatile oil content; by steam distillation and measurement of the volume of insoluble oily layer.

Cresol Solution, Saponated—for cresol; kerosene is added, the mixture distilled, and the distillate extracted with 50% H_2SO_4, then with a measured volume of 15% NaOH. Cresol dissolves in the alkali and the increase in volume of the sodium hydroxide solution represents the volume of cresol in the sample.

Peppermint Spirit—for mixed oils; the oils are separated in a Babcock bottle after first mixing and centrifuging with kerosene and an acidified, saturated calcium chloride solution. A correction in the measured volume is made for the kerosene used.

Spearmint Oil—for carvone, as for Caraway Oil.

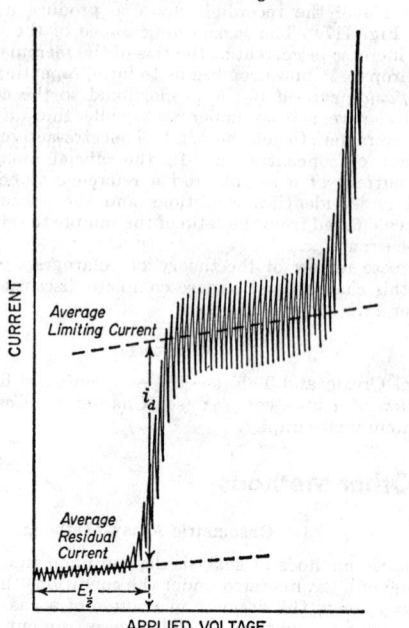

Fig. 417. Typical polarogram (courtesy, USP XVIII, p. 817).

USP Items

Cinnamon Oil—for aldehydes; as for Caraway Oil.

Clove Oil—for phenolic substances; the phenols are converted into water-soluble phenolates by sodium hydroxide and the residual, insoluble oil volume measured.

Orange Spirit, Compound—for mixed oils; as for Peppermint Spirit.

Tetrachloroethylene Capsules—the sample is distilled with glycerin in a toluene moisture apparatus and volume of the lower layer of the distillate measured.

35a. Assays Depending upon Measurement of Optical Rotation

Many organic substances, or their solutions, have the property of rotating the plane of polarized light either to the right or to the left and this property is referred to as the optical activity, or the optical rotation, of that substance. The measurement of this rotatory power serves as the basis for determining the purity, as well as the identity, of a number of official substances since the optical activity is a function of their chemical constitution, as well as their concentration. When the rotation is to the right the dissolved substance is said to be dextrorotatory, while levorotatory substances are those which rotate the plane of polarized light to the left. The extent of observed rotation is measured and expressed in terms of degrees and the instrument used in making these measurements is called a polariscope or polarimeter (see Fig. 402, page 599).

The term *optical rotation* when used in the official monographs refers to *angular rotation* and this represents the number of degrees a substance, or its solution, under specified conditions of concentration, temperature, and length of the tube, will rotate the plane of polarization.

The *specific rotation*, [α], of a liquid is defined as the angular rotation in degrees through which the plane of polarization of polarized monochromatic light is rotated by passage through 1 decimeter (100 mm) of the liquid, calculated on the basis of a specific gravity of 1. In the case of solutions of an optically active substance the specific rotation is calculated on the basis of a concentration of 1 Gm of solute in 1 ml of solution.

For calculating the specific rotatory power of an optically active liquid substance, or the solution of an optically active solid, the following formulas apply generally.

$$\text{For liquid substances, } [\alpha]_D^t = \frac{a}{ld} \quad \text{For solutions, } [\alpha]_D^t = \frac{100a}{lpd}$$
$$\text{or } [\alpha]_D^t = \frac{100a}{lc}$$

a = the observed rotation in degrees of the liquid at a temperature t, using a sodium light;

l = the length of the tube in decimeters;

d = the specific gravity of the liquid or solution at the temperature of observation;

p = the concentration of the solution expressed as the number of Gm of active substance in 100 Gm of solution;

c = the concentration of the solution expressed as the number of Gm of active substances in 100 ml. of solution.

t = temperature of measurement.

D = D line of sodium (light source).

NF Item

Sodium Chloride and Dextrose Tablets—for dextrose.

USP Items

Anticoagulant Citrate Dextrose Solution—for dextrose.

Anticoagulant Citrate Phosphate Dextrose Solution—for dextrose.

Dextrose and Sodium Chloride Injection—for dextrose.

Epinephrine (and all Dosage Forms)—rotation of the triacetyl derivative.

Epinephrine Bitartrate Ophthalmic Solution—as for Epinephrine.

Levallorphan Bitartrate Injection—as for Epinephrine.

35b. Specific Gravity

Many substances are mixtures of several compounds and can have varied composition. A simple assay procedure will not establish the purity or efficacy of such a material and, therefore, they are quite often characterized by physical methods, one of which may be specific gravity.

35c. Assays Involving Measurement of Radioactivity

In this type of assay, the radioactivity of a sample and of a calibrated radioactive standard are determined at the same time and under identical geometric conditions, as outlined in Part IV, Radioisotopes in Pharmacy and Medicine.

The radiochemical purity of many official radioactive substances is determined by first chromatographing the substance on a paper strip and determining the radioactive distribution on the developed chromatogram.

36. Assays Involving Chromatographic Separation

With many of the dosage forms (and occasionally the pure material) it is necessary to remove the substance being assayed from contaminants which may interfere with the assay. A variety of chromatographic and ion exchange techniques are available and a thorough discussion can be found in Chapter 40, *Chromatography*.

Isopropamide Iodide Tablets NF
Pralidoxime Chloride Tablets USP

Both of the above use ion-exchange techniques for separation.

37. The Assay of Enzyme-Containing Substances

The official enzymatic assays depend upon the ability of enzymes (page 1049) to catalyze reactions of a certain type under the conditions that are described in the assay. Those enzymes that bring about the conversion of starch into water-soluble sugars are known as diastatic enzymes. Other official enzyme-containing substances are those that digest proteins and peptides, changing them into peptones and eventually amino acids. These are called proteolytic enzymes. A third type of enzyme encountered in the official assays is the one which causes or prevents the coagulation of serum. In all of these assays the enzymatic activity of the sample is determined by comparison with that of a reference standard.

NF Items

Chymotrypsin—a dilute hydrochloride solution of the sample is incubated with buffered N-acetyl-L-tyrosine ethyl ester in a spectrophotometer cell with the instrument set at 237 $m\mu$. The change in absorbance with respect to time is noted. One NF Chymotrypsin unit is the activity causing a change in absorbance of 0.0075/minute under the conditions of the assay.
Hyaluronidase for Injection—hyaluronidase activity is assayed on the basis of the ability of preparations of the enzyme to decrease the turbidity of colloidal suspensions of a substrate consisting of potassium hyaluronate and protein *in vitro*. Assay preparations are compared to a reference standard and calculation of potency is based on measurements of the absorbance of solutions containing hyaluronidase, potassium hyaluronate, hydrolyzed gelatin, phosphate buffer, and serum.
Pancreatin—the *starch digestive power* is determined on a prepared sample by testing its quantitative ability to hydrolyze starch to the extent that no blue or reddish color develops upon the addition of iodine. The *casein digestive power* is determined by placing a suitably prepared casein solution in each of two tubes. To one tube is added a 20% solution of Pancreatin and to the other tube is added a similar amount of Pancreatin Reference Standard. Both tubes are diluted and incubated at 40° for 1 hour. The addition of alcoholic acetic acid solution produces no more haze in the tube containing Pancreatin than in that containing the Reference Standard, indicating that the proteolytic activity of the former is at least as great as that of the latter.
Trypsin—the method is similar to that used for *Chymotrypsin;* N-benzoyl-L-arginine ethyl ester hydrochloride is the substrate measured at a wavelength of 253 $m\mu$. One NF Trypsin unit is the activity causing a change in absorbance of 0.003/minute under the conditions of the assay.

USP Items

Protamine Sulfate (and Injection)—the activity of Protamine Sulfate Injection is assayed on the basis of its ability to nullify the anticoagulant action of sodium heparin *in vitro*. Varying concentrations of sodium heparin are added to a series of test tubes containing uniform amounts of citrated sheep plasma, calcium chloride–thromboplastin solution, and Protamine Sulfate Injection. Calculation of potency is based on that amount of sodium heparin which results in a clotting time most nearly approaching the clotting time observed in a control tube.
Sodium Heparin (and Injection)—the anticoagulant activity of Sodium Heparin is determined by its ability to inhibit the clotting of sheep plasma *in vitro*. Assay preparations are compared to a reference standard and calculation of potency is based on determinations of the extent of clotting which has occurred 1 hour after addition of heparin and calcium chloride to samples of citrated plasma.

38. Proximate Assays

At one time the extensive use of vegetable drugs, extracts and other galenicals in pharmacy required that the analyst be concerned with a great many *proximate assays*. Currently, due to the majority of more specific, well defined medicinals, usually of synthetic origin, in common use, the proximate assay is required to a lesser degree. By proximate assay is meant the determination of the amount of any

organic constituent which may be present in any vegetable drug or plant to which its value or therapeutic activity is attributed. The separations are dependent mainly on the use of a variety of solvents selected after elaborate and painstaking research. Acid and alkali solutions, chloroform, ether, alcohol and many other organic solvents play an important role in proximate assays.

Although largely associated with the alkaloidal content of vegetable drugs, proximate assays also include the determination of alcohol-soluble, ether-soluble or water-soluble constituents of various drugs by solvent extraction.

The officially described proximate assays that involve weighing the dried residue obtained upon evaporating a complete solvent extraction of the drug are listed as follows:

NF Item	Official Standards
Vanilla	Not less than 12% of diluted alcohol-soluble extractive

USP Items	Official Standards
Aloe	Not less than 50% of water-soluble extractive
Benzoin	Not less than 75% of alcohol-soluble extractive from Sumatra Benzoin and not less than 90% of alcohol-soluble extractive from Siam Benzoin
Cacao	Not less than 10% nor more than 22% of nonvolatile ether-soluble extractive
Podophyllum	Not less than 5% of Podophyllum resin by alcohol–chloroform extraction

39. Alkaloidal Drug Assays

Alkaloidal assays present the most important application of proximate assay methods with which the pharmaceutical chemist has to deal. Quantitative experiments must necessarily be done with great care and in conducting proximate assays of alkaloidal drugs particular attention must be paid to all details. The alkaloidal substances to be separated are organic chemical compounds which are difficult to extract from the drug. They are present in comparatively small quantities and in many cases are easily destroyed by improper manipulation.

These assays are conducted largely through the use of immiscible solvents, such as chloroform, ether, amyl alcohol, etc, except where the properties of the alkaloid sought necessitate a special method, as for morphine in opium. Advantage is taken of the fact that the free alkaloids are practically insoluble in water (except colchicine, ephedrine, sparteine, nicotine, and a few others), whereas they are very soluble in one or more of the immiscible solvents such as chloroform, ether, etc. The salts of the alkaloids behave in the reverse manner, being practically insoluble in the immiscible solvents and soluble in water. There are several exceptions, such as the salts of caffeine, theobromine, colchicine, etc, which bases are feebly basic and the salts of which hydrolyze readily with the liberation of the free alkaloid.

Three general steps are required for the separation and estimation of alkaloids in vegetable drugs:

1. Extraction of the drug.
2. Subsequent separation and purification of the alkaloid.
3. Determination of the amount of alkaloid obtained, either by the gravimetric or the titrimetric method.

Extraction of the Crude Drug

After reduction to proper fineness by grinding, the drug may be "defatted" by extraction with petroleum benzine, or directly treated with a solvent to extract the active constituent. Depending on the alkaloid present the drug is treated in one of the following methods:

1. Extraction with an organic solvent, after addition of ammonia to insure the complete liberation of the basic alkaloid (belladonna and ipecac).
2. Extraction with water (morphine in opium).
3. Extraction with acidulated water, if the alkaloid is present as such or in the form of weakly combined organic salts.

The extraction procedure is usually accomplished by use of separatory funnels (separators) with mechanical agitation or in a Soxhlet extraction apparatus.

The assay processes for extracts, fluidextracts, tinctures and powdered extracts of an alkaloidal drug are in general similar to those described for the crude drug. *Powdered and pilular extracts* are usually liquefied by the use of an appropriate solvent and then extracted directly. *Fluidextracts* are often diluted with water and *tinctures* are concentrated to a small volume by means of a preliminary evaporation. After the mixture is made alkaline it is extracted, directly, with the most suitable solvent.

Automatic Extraction Apparatus—The need for an automatic extraction apparatus for use in the assay of alkaloidal galenicals prompted the design of an improved apparatus. The simple type is easily constructed, requires only a small amount of solvent and practically no attention, and gives a clear extraction in one operation.

In the simple type of apparatus (Fig. 418) the same jacket, condenser, and boiling flask are used for light and heavy solvents. For light solvents the funnel tube containing very small openings at its lower end, is used in the jacket, as shown in *B*. For heavy solvents, as shown in *A*, the wide tube open at both ends is used. The manner in which the extractors function is shown by the illustrations.

In both cases the extracting solvent is continuously returned to the boiling flask and reused. In *A*, the chloroform returns to the boiling flask under the bottom and around the inner jacket, whereas in *B*, the nonaqueous layer is always on top and is returned by overflow.

Separation and Purification of the Alkaloid

The extract of the crude drug or galenical usually contains impurities which may interfere with the ultimate method of assay. Especially in the case of extraction with immiscible solvents, whereby oils, tannins and soluble coloring matter can obscure the end-point in a titration or add to the weight of a gravimetric method. For these reasons purification of the alkaloidal extract is accomplished by: crystallization, as in the case of morphine in opium; removal of associated alkaloids by chemical methods; or by use of immiscible solvents. This latter method is most often employed and involves repeated extraction of the alkaloid from aqueous and organic solvent. For example, the original organic solvent extract containing the basic alkaloid is shaken with dilute acid, thus transferring the alkaloid to the aqueous layer due to the formation of the more polar acid salt. The aqueous acid layer is then made basic with ammonia (or a stronger base if required) and again extracted into an immiscible organic solvent as the free base. This process is repeated until the alkaloid is sufficiently pure for the final assay.

Estimation of the Alkaloid

Final determination of the alkaloid is accomplished by either a quantitative gravimetric or volumetric procedure, the latter method being preferred. In the gravimetric method all, or a portion, of the solution containing the extract is carefully evaporated to dryness in a tared container, the increase in weight of the container is then the weight (or some fraction thereof, if an aliquot was used) of the alkaloid in the sample.

In the volumetric method the solvent is carefully evaporated to a small volume and an excess of standard acid plus a small amount of alcohol is added and the evaporation continued. The residual method is resorted to, and the acid added before complete removal of solvent so that the alkaloid is converted to the salt since some of the alkaloids are fairly volatile in the form of the free base.

For examples of both the gravimetric and volumetric procedures in the estimation of alkaloids see pages 606 and 612, this chapter.

40. Miscellaneous Assay Methods

NF Items

Phenazopyridine Hydrochloride Tablets—a coulometric determination (see Chapter 41, page 721). Each coulomb is equivalent to 646.9 mcg of phenazopyridine.
Sulfisoxazole and Phenazopyridine Hydrochloride Tablets—for phenazopyridine as above.
Yeast (Dried and Tablets)—assayed for the following (method reference in parenthesis); Niacin (31a), riboflavin(31e), protein Kjeldahl(6), and thiamine(31e).

USP Items

Estrogens, Conjugated (and Esterified and Dosage Forms)—the sample is chromatographed, eluted, hydrolyzed with hot HCl to deconjugate, and extracted into benzene. *Total conjugated estrogens* are determined in this benzene solution at 525 mµ (IP). For *sodium equilin sulfate*, the benzene solution is evaporated and the residue treated with trimethylacethydrazide ammonium chloride (Girard's reagent) to form the substituted hydrazone of the ketone group of estrone. This derivative is water-soluble and the aqueous solution is extracted with chloroform to remove non-ketonic substances. The aqueous solution of the derivative is then hydrolyzed with sulfuric acid to regenerate the ketone and estrone is determined at 635 mµ (31a, SP). For *sodium estrone sulfate* the original benzene extract is evaporated and the residue determined by Method 31a (IP).
Mecamylamine—phase solubility analysis. Portions of the sample representing from 50 to 250 mg of the substance are equilibrated with isopropyl alcohol and the solution concentrations determined. From a plot of solution vs system concentrations the purity may be established from the slope of the resulting line (see Chapter 19).

41. Biological Assays

Substances in this category either do not list a chemical or physical assay method under the individual monograph or require a biological procedure. If a biological assay is stipulated a detailed treatment will be found in Chapter 38, *Biological Testing*.

Many of the materials included in this category require batch certification by either the Food and Drug Administration or the National Institutes of Health.

42. Gas Chromatographic Methods

A comprehensive treatment of the theory and technique of this method can be found in Chapter 40, *Chromatography*.

NF Items

Codeine Phosphate, Aspirin, Phenacetin, and Caffeine Tablets—for codeine, using Propoxyphene Hydrochloride USP as an internal standard.
Hyoscyamine Sulfate Tablets—using anthracene as an internal standard.
Morphine and Atropine Sulfates Tablets—for atropine using anthracene as an internal standard.
Sodium Secobarbital and Sodium Amobarbital Capsules—for both substances using aprobarbital as an internal standard.
Terpin Hydrate and Codeine Elixir—for terpin hydrate.
Terpin Hydrate and Dextromethorphan Elixir—for terpin hydrate.

USP Items

Nitrous Oxide—compare to a standard helium–air mixture.
Stearic Acid—converted to the methyl ester with methanol–boron trifluoride before chromatographing.
Stearyl Alcohol—determined as is, in methanol.

43. Multivitamin Preparations

Assay categories are given in parenthesis.
Hexavitamin Capsules and Tablets NF—for vitamin A, vitamin D, ascorbic acid, niacinamide, thiamine hydrochloride and riboflavin; all as for *Decavitamins*, below.
Decavitamin Capsules and Tablets USP—for vitamin A(31a), vitamin D (see Chapter 36), ascorbic acid(16), calcium pantothenate (see Chapter 38), cyanocobalamin (see Chapter 38), niacinamide (31a), pyridoxine hydrochloride (as for the Injection, 31a), riboflavin(31e), and thiamine hydrochloride(31e).

44. Fixed Oils

The fixed oils (corn, cottonseed, olive, etc) are largely composed of mixtures of fatty acid esters and it is possible that each component has a relatively wide concentration limit without sacrificing the quality of the oil. It is for this reason that a single-substance assay is of little value and many parameters are necessary to stipulate the quality of the oil. Some of the many kinds of tests performed on the materials in this category are: saponification value, acid number, acetyl value, iodine number, specific gravity, melting range of fatty acids, etc.

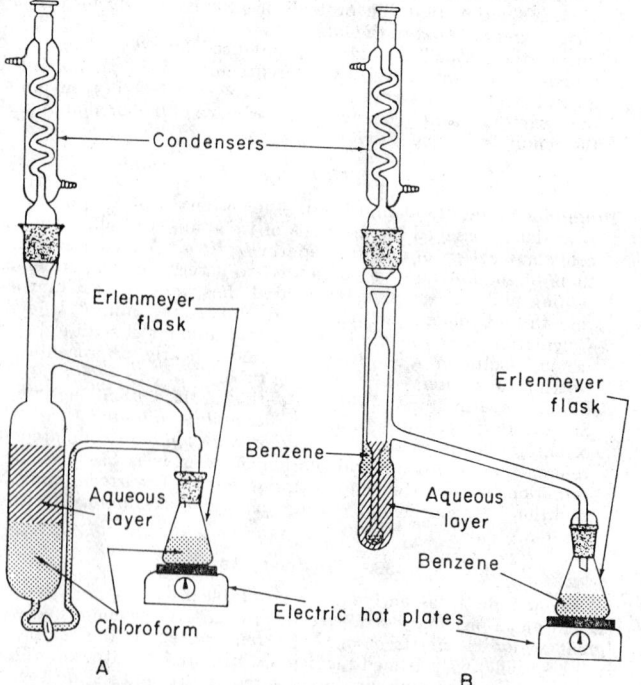

Fig. 418. Automatic extraction apparatus for alkaloids.

References

1. *Design and Test of Standards of Mass*, Circular No. 3, US Bureau of Standards, Washington, D.C.; available from US Government Printing Office, Washington, D.C. 20402.

2. Standards for Checking the Calibration of Spectrophotometers (200–1000 mμ), Letter Circular LC-1017, Jan., 1955, National Bureau of Standards, Washington, D.C. 20234.

Table III—Assay Index

NF Drugs

	Assay category[a]	Analytical wavelength[b]	Indicator[c]		Assay category[a]	Analytical wavelength[b]	Indicator[c]
Acetaminophen	31b	249		Bendroflumethiazide	*27b-1		TB
Elixir	31b, 36	249		Tablets	31a	515	BM
Tablets	31b	249		Benzaldehyde	2		BpB
Acetic Acid, Diluted	1		Phth	Elixir, Compound	None		
Acetohexamide	*27b-2		TB	Benzestrol	31a	750	MP
Tablets	31b	249		Tablets	31a	750	MP
Acetone	None			Benzethonium Chloride	16b		BpB
Acetophenazine Maleate	27a		CrV	Solution	16b		BpB
Tablets	31b	278		Benzocaine	25		SPI
Acetyldigitoxin	31b	217		Ointment	25		Poten
Tablets	31a	485	AP	Benzonatate	11a		BtB
Acetyl Sulfisoxazole	25		Poten	Capsules	31a	500	FeH
Oral Suspension	25		Poten	Benzphetamine Hydrochloride	27a		CrV
Alcohol, Rubbing	*11a, 31b	410		Tablets	*16c		MeY
Almond Oil	44			Benzthiazide	31b	283	
Alphaprodine Hydrochloride	27a		CrV	Tablets	31b	295	
Injection	27a		MeR	Benzyl Alcohol	None		
Alum	26b		DT	Benzyl Benzoate Lotion	11a		Phth
Aluminum Aspirin	*29, 31b	278, 308		Betamethasone	†31a	525	BT
Tablets	31b	278, 308		Cream	31a	485	TTC
Aluminum Chloride	26b		DT	Tablets	‡31a	525	BT
Aluminum Phosphate Gel	4		Phth	Betamethasone Acetate	†31a	525	BT
Alverine Citrate	27a		MeR	Betamethasone Sodium			
Tablets	27a		MeR	Phosphate	31b	241	
Amantadine Hydrochloride	27a		CrV	and Betamethasone	†31a	525	for the acetate
Capsules	27a		CrV	Acetate Injection	31b	241	for the phosphate
Syrup	27a		CrV	Betamethasone Valerate	†31a	525	BT
Ambenonium Chloride	27a		CrV	Cream	†31a	525	BT
Tablets	31b, 36	271		Biperiden	27a		CrV
Aminoacetic Acid	27a		CrV	Biperiden Hydrochloride	27a		CrV
Solution, Sterile	3		Phth	Tablets	‡31a	408	BcP
Aminocaproic Acid	27a		CrV	Biperiden Lactate Injection	‡31a	408	BcP
Injection	27a		CrV	Bisacodyl	27a		Nb
Tablets	27a		CrV	Suppositories	31b	263	
Ammonia Solution, Strong	8		MeR	Tablets	31b	309	
Ammonia Spirit, Aromatic	8		MeR, MeO	Bishydroxycoumarin			
Ammonium Carbonate	8		MeO	Capsules	31b	309	
Amobarbital Elixir	30	Amobarbital		Bismuth, Milk of	29		Bi₂O₃
Amodiaquine Hydrochloride	31b	342		Bismuth Subnitrate	29		Bi₂O₃
Tablets	31b	342		Boric Acid	*1		Phth
Amphetamine Sulfate	31b, 36	257		Bromodiphenhydramine			
Injection	31b, 36	257		Hydrochloride	27a		CrV
Tablets	31b, 36	257		Capsules	8, 36		MeR
Amyl Nitrite	*33			Elixir	8, 36		MeR
Amylene Hydrate	None			Brompheniramine Maleate	27a		CrV
Angiotensin Amide	*31b	294		Elixir	27a		CrV
for Injection	*31b	294		Tablets	31b	263	
Anileridine	27a		CrV	Butalbital	1		Tp
Injection	31a	560	BM	Butethamine Hydrochloride	31b	290	
Anileridine Hydrochloride	27a		Nb-MV	and Epinephrine Injection	31b	290	Butethamine
Tablets	31a	560	BM		31a	530	Epinephrine–FCiT
Anisindione	*27b-3		Poten	Butyl Aminobenzoate	20		SIP
Tablets	31b	289					
Antazoline Phosphate	27a		Poten	Caffeine, Citrated	*1, *28		
Ophthalmic Solution	31b	242		Tablets	28	Caffeine	
Anthralin	31b	354, 432		Calcium Aminosalicylate	20		Poten
Ointment	31b	354, 432		Capsules	20		Poten
Antipyrine	18f		St	Tablets	20		Poten
and Benzocaine Solution	*31a, *31b			Calcium Benzoylpas	13a		FAS
Apomorphine Hydrochloride	9		MeR	Tablets	31b	274	
Tablets	9		MeR	Calcium Carbonate Tablets	26a		HNB
Aprobarbital	27b		TB	Calcium Cyclamate	20		SIP
Elixir	23		Poten	and Calcium Saccharin	20	Cyclamate	SIP
Ascorbyl Palmitate	20			Solution	31b	266	Saccharin
Aspirin Capsules	31b, 36	280		and Calcium Saccharin	20	Cyclamate	SIP
Aspirin, Phenacetin and				Tablets	31b	266	Saccharin
Caffeine Tablets	*31b, 36			Calcium Ipodate	*12d		EY
Atropine	27a		CrV	for Oral Suspension	12d		EY
Azuresin	31a	690	None	Calcium Lactate	26a		HNB
				Tablets	26a		HNB
Belladonna Extract	39			Calcium Phosphate, Dibasic	*15a		
Belladonna Leaf Fluidextract	39			Tribasic	*4		Phth

[a] *Assay Category*—A total of 44 categories, several of which are further subdivided, are utilized to facilitate location of an analytical procedure for each of the monograph substances listed in USP XVIII or NF XIII, if the method is chemical or physical in nature. Those items for which no assay is specified, are biological in nature, or are certified by The Federal Food and Drug Association or National Institutes of Health.

To find an assay method for a particular NF or USP item locate the monograph title in the Index. The Assay Category column indicates the number of the category and reference to the specified category (pages 605 to 618) will yield the desired information. If a category number is preceded by an asterisk, dagger, or double-dagger, more information is given for this specific item under the designated category.

If category Number 30 is specified, the succeeding two columns are not utilized as specified under superscripts b and c below, but the name of the weighed derivative is indicated.

[b] *Analytical Wavelength*—If the Category 31 is listed in the first column, then column two specifies the corresponding analytical wavelength. If Category 32 is specified, the figures in column two indicate the voltage employed for the polarographic determination.

[c] *Indicator*—This column should also be headed *Color Developing Reagents*. The coded entries are listed in Table II with their decoded connotations.

Table III—Continued

	Assay category[a]	Analytical wavelength[b]	Indicator[c]
Calcium Saccharin	*1		Phth
Calcium Stearate	26a		HNB
Calcium Sulfate	26a		HNB
Camphor Spirit	30	Dinitrophenylhydrazone	
Camphorated Para-chlorophenol	*30		
Caraway Oil	*34		
Carbarsone	*20a		St
Capsules	*20a		St
Tablets	*20a		St
Carbetapentane Citrate	27a		QR
Carbinoxamine Maleate	27a		CrV
Elixir	27a		CrV
Tablets	27a		CrV
Carbol-Fuchsin Solution	None		
Carphenazine Maleate	31a	490	PdC
Tablets	31a	490	PdC
Cetyl Alcohol	11b		Phth
Cetylpyridinium Chloride	16b		BpB
Solution	16b		BpB
Chloral Betaine	*4, *27a		Phth, Nb
Tablets	4		Phth
Chlorcyclizine Hydrochloride	27a		CrV
Tablets	31b	261	
Chlordiazepoxide	27a		MeR
Tablets	31b	311	
Chlormadinone Acetate and Mestranol Tablets	31b	285	
	31b	285—Chlormadinone	
	31a	545, SM—Mestranol	
Chlormerodrin	30	HgS	
Tablets	30	HgS	
Chloroform	None		
Chloroprocaine Hydrochloride	27a		Poten
Injection	31b	278	
Chlorothen Citrate	27a		Poten
Tablets	31b	313	
Chlorothiazide	27b		TB
Tablets	32	—	
Oral Suspension	31b	292	
Chlorotrianisene	*12e		FAS
Capsules	31b, 36	310	
Chlorpheniramine Maleate Injection	31b	264	
Chlorprothixene	27a		MeR
Tablets	31b	324	
Chymotrypsin	*37	273	
Sterile	*37	273	
Injection	*37	273	
Cinnamon	*34		Nb
Clidinium Bromide	27a		Poten
Clofibrate	31b, 36	226	
Capsules	31b, 36	226	
Cobalamin Concentrate	*31a, b, 35c		
Cocaine	27a		CrV
Cocaine Hydrochloride Tablets	9		MeR
Codeine	8		MeR
Codeine Phosphate, Aspirin, Phenacetin, and Caffeine Tablets	*31b, 36, *42		
Codeine Sulfate	27a		Poten
Tablets	9		MeR
Cod Liver Oil	*31b, *41		
Nondestearinated	*31b, *41		
Cresol	None		
Solution, Saponated	*34		
Cupric Sulfate	18a		St
Cyanocobalamin Co 60 Capsules	35c		
Solution	35c		
Cyclopentamine Hydrochloride	27a		CrV
Injection	9		MeR
Solution	9		MeR
Cyclothiazide	*27b-2		ONA
Tablets	31b	271	
Cycrimine Hydrochloride	27a		CrV
Tablets	‡31a	405	BcP
Cyproheptadine Hydrochloride	27a		CrV
Syrup	‡31a	405	BcP
Tablets	31b, 36	286	
Danthron	31a	432	None
Tablets	31a	432	None
Dehydrocholic Acid	1		Phth
Tablets	1		Phth
Denatonium Benzoate	27a		CrV
Desipramine Hydrochloride	27a		Poten
Capsules	31b	252	
Tablets	31b	251	
Desoxycorticosterone Acetate Pellets	†31a	525	BT
Desoxycorticosterone Pivalate	†31a	525	BT

	Assay category[a]	Analytical wavelength[b]	Indicator[c]
Suspension, Sterile	31b, 36	241	
Dexamethasone Aerosol	†31a	525	BT
Elixir	†31a	525	BT
Dexamethasone Sodium Phosphate Cream	31a	410	PH
Ophthalmic Ointment	31a	410	PH
Ophthalmic Solution	31a	410	PH
Dexbrompheniramine Maleate	27a		CrV
Tablets	31b	264	
Dexchlorpheniramine Maleate	27a		CrV
Syrup	31b	265	
Tablets	31b	265	
Dextriferron Injection	31a	510	BPy
Dextroamphetamine Phosphate	31b, 36	257	
Tablets	31b, 36	257	
Dextromethorphan Hydrobromide	27a		CrV
Syrup	31b	278	
Diazepam	27a		NiB
Injection	31b	368	
Tablets	31b	285	
Dibucaine	27a		CrV
Cream	31b	247	
Ointment	31b	247	
Dichlorodifluoromethane	None		
Dichlorotetrafluoroethane	None		
Dicyclomine Hydrochloride	27a		CrV
Capsules	*16c		MeY
Syrup	*16c		MeY
Dienestrol	30	Diacetate	
Cream	*32, 36		
Tablets	*32, 36		
Diethylpropion Hydrochloride	31b	253	
Tablets	31b	253	
Diethylstilbestrol Dipropionate	30	Diethylstilbestrol	
Tablets	*31a	520	VS
Digitalis Capsules	41		
Digitoxin Injection	31a, 36	495	AP
Dihydroxyaluminum Aminoacetate	26b		DT
Magma	26b		DT
Tablets	26b		DT
Dihydroxyaluminum Sodium Carbonate	*26b, *30		DT
Tablets	26b		DT
Dimethindene Maleate	27a		Nb
Syrup	31b	263	
Tablets	31b	258	
Dimethisoquin Hydrochloride	31b	328, 360	
Lotion	31b	328, 360	
Ointment	31b	328, 360	
Dimethisterone	31b	242	
Dimethyl Tubocurarine Iodide	31b	280	
Injection	41		
Dioctyl Calcium Sulfosuccinate	*16c		BpB
Capsules	*16c		BpB
Solution	*16c		BpB
Syrup	‡31a	650	MeB
Diphemanil Methylsulfate	‡31a	412	BpB
Injection	‡31a	412	BpB
Tablets	‡31a	412	BpB
Diphenadione	31b	289	
Tablets	31b	289	
Diphenylhydantoin Oral Suspension	27b		AV
Diphenoxylate Hydrochloride and Atropine Sulfate	27a		Poten
Solution	*27a, *31a		
and Atropine Sulfate Tablets	*27a, *31a		
Doxapram Hydrochloride	27a		CrV
Injection	31b	258	
Dromostanolone Propionate	31c	5.9	
Injection	31c, 36	5.9	
Dydrogesterone	31a	420	IN
Tablets	31a	420	IN
Ephedrine	8		MeR
Ephedrine Hydrochloride	27a		MeR
Ephedrine Sulfate and Phenobarbital Capsules	27a	Ephedrine	MeR
	27b	Phenobarbital	TB
Ephedrine Sulfate Tablets	*27a		MeR
Ergotamine Tartrate and Caffeine Suppositories	*31a, *31b, 36		
Tablets	*31a, *31b, 36		
Erythrityl Tetranitrate	31a	405	PDS
Tablets	31a	405	PDS
Estradiol	31a	525	IP
Injection, Aqueous	31a	525	IP
Pellets	31a	525	IP
Tablets	31a	525	IP

Table III—Continued

	Assay category[a]	Analytical wavelength[b]	Indicator[c]
Estradiol Benzoate	31a, 36	525	IP
Injection	31a, 36	525	IP
Estradiol Cypionate	31a	510	IP
Injection	31a	510	IP
Estradiol Dipropionate	31a	500	ACBD
Injection	31a	500	ACBD
Estrone	31b	280	
Injection	*28		
Ethamivan	31a	660	FCP
Injection	31a	660	FCP
Ethchlorvynol	12a		MRB
Capsules	12a		MRB
Ethinamate	*12a		MRB
Tablets	12a		MRB
Ethinyl Estradiol and Dimethisterone Tablets	*31a, *31b		
Ethisterone	31b	241	
Tablets	31b	241	
Ethoheptazine Citrate	27a		CrV
Tablets	27a		CrV
Ethyl Acetate	11a		Phth
Ethyl Biscoumacetate	1		MeR
Tablets	1		MeR
Ethyl Chloride	None		
Ethylcellulose	*18a		St
Ethylene	*33		
Ethylmorphine Hydrochloride	27a		CrV
Ethyl Vanillin	27b		TB
Eucalyptus Oil	44		
Ferrous Gluconate	14a		Op
Tablets	14a		Op
Ferrous Sulfate Syrup	14a		Op
Fluocinolone Acetonide	†31a	525	BT
Fluorometholone	31a	410	IN
Cream	31a	410	IN
Fluphenazine Enanthate	27a		CrV
Injection	27a		CrV
Fluphenazine Hydrochloride	27a		CrV
Injection	31b	255	
Tablets	31a	480	PdC
Fluprednisolone	†31a	525	BT
Tablets	†31a	525	BT
Fluradrenolide	31a	520	BT
Cream	31a	520	BT
Ointment	31a	520	BT
Flurothyl	42		
Fluroxene	42		
Fructose	35a		
and Sodium Chloride	35a	Fructose	
Injection	12e	NaCl	FAS
Fuchsin, Basic	None		
Furazolidone	31b	367	
and Nifuroxime Powder	*31b, 36		
and Nifuroxime Suppositories	*31b, 36		
Gitalin	31a, 36	531	Xan
Tablets	31a	495	PA
Glutamic Acid Hydrochloride	1		BtB
Capsules	1		BtB
Glutethimide	31b	257	
Tablets	31b, 36	257	
Glycerin Suppositories	None		
Glyceryl Guaiacolate	31b	275.5	
Syrup	31b	275.5	
Glyceryl Monostearate	None		
Glycobiarsol	25		SIP
Tablets	25		SIP
Glycopyrrolate	27a		CrV
Tablets	‡31a	410	BcP
Haloperidol	27a		Nb
Solution	31b	245	
Tablets	31b	245	
Hexavitamin Capsules	*43		
Tablets	*43		
Hexylcaine Hydrochloride	31b	232	
Injection	31b, 36	275	
Solution	31b, 36	275	
Hexylresorcinol	19		St
Pills	19		St
Homatropine Methylbromide	27a		CrV
Tablets	31a	525	R
Hyaluronidase for Injection	*37		
Hydralazine Hydrochloride	*18b		
Injection	*18b		
Tablets	31b	260	
Hydrochloric Acid, Diluted	1		MeR
Hydrocortisone Lotion	31a	525	BT
Hydroflumethiazide	31b	273	
Tablets	31b, 36	273	
Hydromorphone Hydro-chloride	27a		CrV
Injection	31a	440	SN
Tablets	31a	440	SN
Hydroquinone	14a		DP
Cream	14a		DP
Hydroxypropyl Methyl-cellulose	*11c, *18a		
Hydroxyzine Hydrochloride	27a		QR
Syrup	27a		QR
Tablets	27a		QR
Hydroxyzine Pamoate	27a		QR
Capsules	31b	232	
Oral Suspension	31b	232	
Hyoscyamine Hydrobromide	27a		CrV
Hyoscyamine Sulfate	27a		Poten
Tablets	*42		
Hypophosphorous Acid	1		Phth
Ichthammol	*6, *30		
Indomethacin	1		Phth
Capsules	31b		318
Iodine Ampuls	*18b, *21		
Solution	*18b, *21		
Iodized Oil	*18a		
Iodochlorhydroxyquin and Hydrocortisone Cream	*31a, *31c		
Lotion	*31a, *31c		
Ointment	*31a, *31c		
Iodochlorhydroxyquin Powder, Compound	31b	267	
Tablets	30	Copper derivative	
Iodoform	12e		FAS
Iodopyracet Injection	12d		TBPE
Iron Dextran Injection	31a	510	BPy
Isobucaine Hydrochloride	27a		CrV
and Epinephrine Injection	*27a, *31a		
Isocarboxazid	25		Poten
Tablets	31a	420	AM
Isoflurophate Ophthalmic Ointment	31a	710	AS
Isopropamide Iodide	27a		CrV
Tablets	31b, *36	258, 280	
Isopropyl Alcohol	None		
Isopropyl Rubbing Alcohol	35b		
Isoproterenol Sulfate Aerosol	31a	530	FCiT
Isoxsuprine Hydrochloride	31b	269, 300	
Tablets	31b	269, 300	
Lanatoside C	31a	490	AP
Tablets	31a	490	AP
Lavender Oil	11a		Phth
Levonordefrin	27a		CrV
Levopropoxyphene Napsylate	*5, 36		Poten
Capsules	31c	5.8	
Levorphanol Tartrate	27a		MeR
Injection	27a		MeR
Tablets	27a		MeR
Magaldrate	*26a, *26b		
Oral Suspension	*26a, *26b		
Tablets	*26a, *26b		
Magnesium Carbonate	8		MeO
Magnesium Citrate Solution	*10, *30		
Magnesium Hydroxide	8		MeR
Magnesium Phosphate	*4		
Menadiol Sodium Diphos-phate Tablets	14a		Poten
Menadione	*14a		Op
Injection	31a	635	DNP
Tablets	*14a		
Menadione Sodium Bisulfite	*14a		
Injection	*14a		
Mepenzolate Bromide	27a		Poten
Tablets	31a	620	ACT
Meperidine Hydrochloride Syrup	*27a		CrV
Mephobarbital	*27b-1		TP
Tablets	28		
Mepivacaine Hydrochloride	27a		CrV
Injection	27a		MeR
and Levonordefrin Injection	*27a, *31a		
Meprobamate Oral Suspension	*3		Phth
Meprylcaine Hydrochloride	9		MeR
and Epinephrine Injection	*27a, *31a		
Mercuric Oxide, Yellow	13b		FAS
Ointment	13b		FAS
Metabutethamine Hydro-chloride	31b	315	
and Epinephrine Injection	*31a, *31b		

Table III—Continued

	Assay category[a]	Analytical wavelength[b]	Indicator[c]
Methacholine Bromide	27a		CrV
Tablets	27a		CrV
Methacholine Chloride	27a		CrV
Sterile	27a		CrV
Methandrostenolone	31b	245	
Tablets	31b	245	
Methantheline Bromide	27a		CrV
Tablets	31b	282	
Methapyrilene Hydrochloride	27a		Poten
Capsules	31b	313	
Tablets	31b	313	
Metharbital	31b	244	
Tablets	31b	244	
Methdilazine	31b	275	
Tablets	31a	460	PdC
Methdilazine Hydrochloride	31b	252, 275	
Syrup	31a	460	PdC
Tablets	31a	460	PdC
Methenamine	8		MeR
Tablets	8		MeR
and Sodium Biphosphate Tablets	*4, *6		
Methionine	*18f		St
Capsules	*18f		St
Tablets	*18f		St
Methocarbamol	31c	5.78	
Injection	31c	5.78	
Tablets	31c	5.78	
Methotrimeprazine	27a		CrV
Injection	31a		BcG
Methoxyflurane	42		
Methscopamine Bromide	27a		CrV
Methscopolamine Bromide			
Injection	‡31a	420	BtB
Tablets	‡31a	420	BtB
Methsuximide	31b	247	
Capsules	31b	247	
Methyclothiazide	*12d		Poten
Tablets	32		
Methylbenzethonium Chloride	23		
Powder	*16c		SaO
Methyl Isobutyl Ketone	None		
Methylprednisolone	†31a	525	BT
Tablets	†31a	525	BT
Methylprednisolone Acetate	†31a	525	BT
Suspension, Sterile	†31a	525	BT
Methylprednisolone Sodium Succinate	†31a	525	BT
for Injection	†31a	525	BT
Methyltestosterone	31b	241	
Tablets	31b	241	
Methylthiouracil	*27b-2		TB
Methyprylon	*24		Poten
Capsules	*24		Poten
Tablets	*24		Poten
Methysergide Maleate	27a		CrV
Tablets	31b	322	
Monobenzone	30	Acetyl derivative	
Lotion	30	Acetyl derivative	
Ointment	30	Acetyl derivative	
Monoethanolamine	5		MeR
Morphine and Atropine Sulfates Tablets	*9, *42		
Myristica Oil	44		
Nalidixic Acid	*27b		TP
Tablets	31b	258	
Nandrolone Decanoate	31a	380	IN
Injection	31a, 36	380	IN
Nandrolone Phenpropionate	31a	380	IN
Injection	31a	380	IN
Naphazoline Hydrochloride	9		MeR
Solution	31b	280	
Niacin	1		Phth
Injection	31a	450	C-S
Tablets	31a	450	C-S
Nialamide	31a	440	AM
Tablets	31a	440	AM
Nifuroxime	31b	341	
Nikethamide	27a		CrV
Injection	6		MeR
Nitrofurazone	31b	375	
Cream	31b	285	
Ointment	31b, 36	375	
Solution	31b, 36	375	
Nitromersol	*13b		FAS
Solution	*13b		FAS
Tincture	*13b		FAS
Norethandrolone	31a	380	
Tablets	31a	380	
Norethindrone Acetate	31b	240	
Tablets	31b	240	
Norethindrone Tablets	31b	240	
Nortriptyline Hydrochloride	27a		CrV
Capsules	31b	239	
Noscapine	27a		CrV
Nylidrin Hydrochloride	27a		CrV
Injection	27a		MeR
Tablets	27a		MeR
Octoxynol	None		
Oleovitamin A and D	43		
Capsules	43		
Orphenadrine Citrate	27a		CrV
Oxandrolone	*11a		Phth
Tablets	31c, 36	5.78	
Oxazepam	*27b-3		Poten
Capsules	31b	229	
Oxtriphylline	*5, *12a		
Tablets	31b, 36	277	
Oxymetazoline Hydrochloride	27a		CrV
Solution	31b	279	
Oxymetholone	31b	315	
Tablets	31b	315	
Oxymorphone Hydrochloride	27a		MV
Injection	31b	282	
Tablets	31b	282	
Oxyphenbutazone	*1		BtB
Tablets	31b	254	
Oxyphencyclimine Hydrochloride	27a		QR
Tablets	31b	239	
Pancreatin	*37		
Papaverine Hydrochloride	27a		CrV
Injection	*30		
Tablets	*30		
Parachlorophenol	19		
Paramethasone Acetate	31a	405	IN
Tablets	31c	6.04	
Pargyline Hydrochloride	27a		Poten
Tablets	27a		Poten
Pectin	11c		
Pentaerythritol Tetranitrate	31a	409	PDS
Tablets	31a	409	PDS
Pentazocine Lactate	27a		CrV
Injection	*31b	278	
Penthienate Bromide	27a		CrV
Tablets	31b	238	
Pentylenetetrazol	*30		
Injection	31c	10.05	
Peppermint Spirit	*34		
Perphenazine	27a		CrV
Injection	31b	254	
Tablets	31b	254	
Persic Oil	44		
Phenacaine Hydrochloride	*30		
Phenazopyridine Hydrochloride	31b	387	
Tablets	*40		
Phenindamine Tartrate	27a		CrV
Tablets	31b	260	
Phenmetrazine Hydrochloride	12d		Poten
Tablets	31b	256	
Phenolphthalein	18f		St
Tablets	*30		
Phenprocoumon	1		Poten
Tablets	31b	311	
Phensuximide	31b	258	
Capsules	31b	258	
Oral Suspension	*6		MeR-MeB
Phentolamine Hydrochloride	*30		
Tablets	*30		
Phenylethyl Alcohol	None		
Phenylmercuric Acetate	*13b		FAS
Phenylmercuric Nitrate	*13b		FAS
Phenylpropanolamine Hydrochloride	27a		CrV
Phosphoric Acid	1		TP
Diluted	1		TP
Phthalylsulfacetamide	25		Poten
Tablets	25		Poten
Phthalylsulfathiazole	25		SPI
Tablets	25		SPI
Picrotoxin	None		
Injection	28		
Piminodine Esylate	27a		CrV
Injection	27a		CrV
Tablets	27a		CrV
Pine Needle Oil	11a		Phth
Pipobroman	*12d		Poten
Tablets	*12d		Poten
Polyethylene Glycol 300	*11b		Phth
1540	*11b		Phth
Polythiazide	31b	268	
Tablets	31b, 36	268	
Posterior Pituitary	41		
Injection	41		

Table III—Continued

	Assay category[a]	Analytical wavelength[b]	Indicator[c]
Potash, Sulfurated	*30		
Potassic Saline Injection, Lactated	*10, *12e, *31d		
Potassium Acetate	*27a		CrV
Potassium Citrate	27a		CrV
Potassium Gluconate	31d	767	
Elixir	31d	767	
Tablets	31d	767	
Potassium Guaiacolsulfonate	31b	279.5	
Potassium Iodide Solution	23		
Potassium Phosphate, Monobasic	*1		Poten
Potassium Sodium Tartrate	*27a		CrV
Potassium Sorbate	*27a		CrV
Potassium Warfarin	31b	308	
Tablets	31b	307	
Povidone	None		
Povidone-Iodine	*12d, *18d		
Aerosol	18d		St
Solution	18d		St
Pramoxine Hydrochloride	27a		CrV
Cream	27a		CrV
Jelly	31b	286	
Prednisolone Succinate	1		Poten
Prednisolone Sodium Succinate for Injection	†31a	525	BT
Prilocaine Hydrochloride	27a		CrV
Injection	27a		CrV
Procaine and Phenylephrine Hydrochlorides Injection	*31a, *31b		
Procaine and Tetracaine Hydrochlorides and Levarterenol Bitartrate Injection	*25, *31a		
Procaine and Tetracaine Hydrochlorides and Levonordefrin Injection	*25, 31a		
Procaine Hydrochloride and Levonordefrin Injection	*31a, *31b		
Procaine, Tetracaine, and Phenylephrine Hydrochlorides Injection	*25, *31a		
Procaine and Propoxycaine Hydrochlorides and Levarterenol Bitartrate Injection	*31a, *31b		
Prochlorperazine	27b		CrV
Suppositories	31b	254	
Progesterone	31b	241	
Injection	*30		
Suspension, Sterile	28		
Tablets	28		
Promazine Hydrochloride	31b	301	
Injection	31b	301	
Syrup	31b	301	
Tablets	31b	301	
Propiomazine Hydrochloride	31a	465	PdC
Injection	31a	465	PdC
Propoxycaine Hydrochloride	25		SPI
Injection	31b	303	
Propoxycaine and Procaine Hydrochlorides and Levonordefrin Injection	*25, *31a, *31b		
Propoxyphene Hydrochloride and Aspirin Capsules	*31c		
Propylhexedrine	5		MeR
Inhalant	8		MeR
Pseudoephedrine Hydrochloride	27a		CrV
Syrup	27a		CrV
Tablets	31b	257	
Pyrilamine Maleate	27a		CrV
Tablets	31b	315	
Pyrrobutamine Phosphate	27a		CrV
Tablets	31b	226	
Pyrrocaine Hydrochloride	27a		CrV
and Epinephrine Injection	*8, *31a		
Quinine Dihydrochloride	32		
Injection	*30		
Rauwolfia Serpentina	31a	390	SN
Powdered	31a	390	SN
Tablets	31a	390	SN
Rescinnamine	31a	390	SN
Tablets	31a	390	SN
Resorcinol Monoacetate	None		
Resorcinol Ointment, Compound	None		
Ringer's Solution	*12e, *31d		
Salicylamide	*27b-2		TB
Suspension	31b	302	

	Assay category[a]	Analytical wavelength[b]	Indicator
Tablets	*27b		TB
Salicylanilide	*27b		TB
Selenium Sulfide	*18a		St
Detergent Suspension	*18a		St
Silicon Dioxide, Colloidal	*28		
Silver Protein, Mild	*13a		FAS
Sitosterols	*30, *31c		
Suspension	*30		
Sodium Acetate	27a		CrV
Sodium Alginate	None		
Sodium Biphosphate	1		Phth
Sodium Butabarbital	*30		
Capsules	*30		
Elixir	*30		
Tablets	31b	240	
Sodium Carboxymethylcellulose Tablets	27a		CrV
Sodium Citrate Solution, Anticoagulant	27a		CrV
Sodium Chloride and Dextrose Tablets	*12e, *35a		
Sodium Chlorothiazide for Injection	31b	292	
Sodium Cyclamate and Sodium Saccharin Solution	25		SPI
and Sodium Saccharin Solution	*25, *30		
and Sodium Saccharin Tablets	*25, *30		
Sodium Dehydrocholate Injection	2		TB
Sodium Dextrothyroxine	*18a		St
Tablets	*18a		St
Sodium Hypochlorite Solution	18a		St
Diluted	18a		St
Sodium Ipodate	*12d		TBPE
Capsules	*12d		TBPE
Sodium Methiodal	*12d		TBPE
Injection	*12d		TBPE
Sodium Methohexital for Injection	31b	247	
Sodium Phosphate	*1		Poten
Dried	*1		Poten
Effervescent	None		
Solution	*30		
Sodium Propionate	27a		CrV
Sodium Saccharin	2		Phth
Tablets	31b	269	
Sodium Secobarbital and Sodium Amobarbital Capsules	*42		
Sodium Thiamylal for Injection	*30		
Sodium Vinbarbital Injection	*30		
Sorbic Acid	1		Phth
Spearmint Oil	*34		
Stannous Fluoride	*18b, *31a		
Stanozolol	27a		CrV
Tablets	31b	380	NBP
Sucrose Octaacetate	11a		Phth
Sulfacetamide	25		Poten
Tablets	25		Poten
Sulfacetamide, Sulfadiazine and Sulfamerazine Suspension	*25, *31a, *36		
Tablets	*25, *31a, *36		
Sulfadiazine and Sulfamerazine Tablets	31a, 36	525	BM
Sulfadimethoxine	25		Poten
Oral Suspension	25		Poten
Tablets	25		Poten
Sulfaethidole	25		SPI
Sulfamerazine Tablets	25		SPI
Sulfamethizole	25		Poten
Suspension	25		Poten
Tablets	25		Poten
Sulfamethoxazole	25		Poten
Oral Suspension	25		Poten
Tablets	25		Poten
Sulfisoxazole and Phenazopyridine Hydrochloride Tablets	*31a, *40		
Sulfur, Sublimed	*1		Phth
Syrosingopine	31a	390	SN
Tablets	31a	390	SN
Tartaric Acid	1		Phth
Terpin Hydrate	42		
Elixir	42		
and Codeine Elixir	*27a, *42		
and Dextromethorphan Elixir	‡31a, *42		
Testosterone	31b	241	
Pellets	31b	241	

Table III—Continued

	Assay category[a]	Analytical wavelength[b]	Indicator[c]		Assay category[a]	Analytical wavelength[b]	Indicator[c]
Suspension, Sterile	31b	241		Trimeprazine Tartrate	27a		CrV
Tetracaine	25		SPI	Syrup	31b	251, 276	
Ophthalmic Ointment	31b	310		Tablets	31b	251, 276	
Tetrahydrozoline Hydrochloride	27a		QR	Trimethadione Tablets	6		MeR
Ophthalmic Solution	‡31a	415	BpB	Trimethidinium Methosulfate	*30		
Solution	31a	570	ON	Tablets	*30		
Theophylline, Ephedrine Hydrochloride, and Phenobarbital Tablets	*31b, 36			Trimethobenzamide Hydrochloride	27a		QR
Theophylline Tablets	12c		FAS	Capsules	31b	258	
Theophylline Sodium Acetate	12c		FAS	Injection	31b	258	
Tablets	12c		FAS	and Benzocaine Suppositories	*27a, *31a		
Theophylline Sodium Glycinate	12c		FAS	Trioxsalen	31b	252	
Tablets	12c		FAS	Tablets	31b	252	
Thiethylperazine Maleate	27a		CrV	Triprolidine Hydrochloride	27a		CrV
Tablets	31b	267		Tablets	31c	12.13	
Thihexinol Methylbromide	27a		CrV	Tromethamine	5		BcP
Thimerosal	31f	253.65		for Injection	*5, *31d		
Aerosol	31f	253.65		Trypsin	*37		
Solution	31f	253.65		Tuaminoheptane Sulfate	6		MeR
Tincture	31f	253.65		Solution	6		MeR
Thioguanine	31b	348		Tybamate	*11a		Phth
Tablets	31b	348		Capsules	*11a		Phth
Thiopropazate Hydrochloride	27a		Poten				
Tablets	27a		Poten	Undecylenic Acid	1		Phth
Tranylcypromine Sulfate	27a		Poten	Ointment, Compound	*1, *30		
Tablets	31b	271, 285		Urethan	*11a		Phth
Triacetin	11a		Phth	Tablets	*6		MeR
Aerosol	11a		Phth				
Cream	11a		Phth	Valethamate Bromide	27a		Poten
Powder	11a		Phth	Injection	*16c		MeY
Triamcinolone Acetonide Aerosol	†31a	525	BT	Vanilla	*38		
Triamcinolone Diacetate	†31a	525	BT	Vinbarbital	5		TP
Suspension, Sterile	†31a	525	BT	Capsules	5		TP
Syrup	‡31a	525	BT	Vinyl Ether	None		
Tribromoethanol	*12e		FAS	Vitamin E	*14a, *31a		
Solution	*12e		FAS				
Trichlormethiazide	27b-3		PR	White Lotion	None		
Tablets	31b	267					
Trichlormonofluoromethane	None			Xylometazoline Hydrochloride	27a		Nb
Triclobisonium Chloride	27a		CrV	Solution	31a		SK
Cream	‡31a	415	BtB				
Ointment	‡31a	415	BtB	Yeast, Dried	*40		
Tridihexethyl Chloride	27a		TB	Tablets	*40		
Tablets	‡31a	415	BcP				
Triethylenemelamine	*1		Phth	Zinc-Eugenol Cement	*28, *29		
Tablets	*1		Phth	Zinc Oxide Paste with Salicylic Acid	*29		
Trifluoperazine Hydrochloride	27a		CrV	Zinc Undecylenate	*1		Phth
Injection	31b	255, 278					
Tablets	31b	255, 278					
Triflupromazine Hydrochloride	27a		CrV				
Tablets	31b	255					

USP Drugs

	Assay category[a]	Analytical wavelength[b]	Indicator[c]		Assay category[a]	Analytical wavelength[b]	Indicator[c]
Acetazolamide	31c	7.38		Amitriptyline Hydrochloride	27a		CrV
Tablets	32			Injection	*31b	265	
Acetic Acid	1		Phth	Tablets	31b	239	
Glacial	1		Phth	Ammonium Chloride	12e		FAS
Albumin, Iodinated I 125				Injection	6		MeR
Serum	35c			Tablets	6		MeR
I 131	35c			Amobarbital	*27b-2		TB
Alcohol, Diluted	35b			Tablets	31b	239	
Allopurinol	31b	250		Anethole	None		
Tablets	31b	250		Anise Oil	44		
Aloe	38			Anticoagulant Citrate Dextrose Solution	*5, *10, *35a		
Alumina and Magnesia Oral Suspension	*26a, *26b			Anticoagulant Citrate Phosphate Dextrose Solution	*4, *5, *10, *35a		
Tablets	*26a, *26b			Anticoagulant Heparin Solution	*40		
Aluminum Acetate Solution	*1, *26b			Antimony Potassium Tartrate	20a		St
Aluminum Hydroxide Gel	26b			Ascorbic Acid	*20a		St
Gel, Dried	26b			Injection	16a		None
Tablets	26b			Tablets	16a		None
Aluminum Monostearate	*29			Aspirin	11a		Phth
Aluminum Subacetate Solution	*1, *26b			Suppositories	31b, 36	280	
Aluminum Sulfate	26b			Tablets	31b, 36	280	
Amaranth	17a		None	Atropine Sulfate	27a		Poten
Solution	17a		None	Injection	9		MeR
Aminohippuric Acid	25		Poten	Ophthalmic Solution	31b	257	
Aminophylline	*5, *12c			Tablets	9		MeR
Injection	*5, *12c			Aurothioglucose	*30		
Suppositories	*12c			Injection	*30		
Tablets	*5, *12c						
Aminosalicylic Acid	25		Poten				
Tablets	25		Poten				

Table III—Continued

	Assay category[a]	Analytical wavelength[b]	Indicator[c]		Assay category[a]	Analytical wavelength[b]	Indicator[c]
Barium Sulfate	*30			Syrup	None		
Belladonna Leaf	9, *39		MeR	Clove Oil	*34		
Belladonna Tincture	9, *39		MeR	Cocaine Hydrochloride	27a		QR
Benzalkonium Chloride	18b		CHCl₃	Cocoa	*38		
Solution	18b		CHCl₃	Syrup	None		
Benzene Hexachloride,				Codeine Phosphate	27a		Poten
Gamma	12e		FAS	Injection	9		MeR
Cream	12e		FAS	Tablets	9		MeR
Lotion	12e		FAS	Colchicine	None		
Benzoic Acid	1		Phth	Tablets	28		
Benzoin	*38			Collodion	*28		
Tincture, Compound	None			Coriander Oil	44		
Benztropine Mesylate	27a		MeR	Corn Oil	44		
Injection	31b	258		Corticotropin Injection	41		
Tablets	*31b	247		Repository	41		
Benzyl Benzoate	11a		Phth	Corticotropin Zinc Hydroxide			
Betazole Hydrochloride	*30			Suspension, Sterile	41		
Injection	*30			Cortisone Acetate	†31a	525	BT
Bethanechol Chloride	27a		CrV	Ophthalmic Suspension	†31a	525	BT
Injection	*30			Sterile Suspension	†31a	525	BT
Tablets	*30			Tablets	†31a	525	BT
Bishydroxycoumarin	28			Cottonseed Oil	44		
Tablets	31b	309		Cyanocobalamin	31b	361	
Bismuth Subcarbonate	*29			Injection	31b	361	
Busulfan	2		Phth	Co 57 Capsules	35c		
Tablets	2		Phth	Co 57 Solution	35c		
Butylparaben	11a		BtB	Cyclizine Hydrochloride	27a		Poten
				Tablets	31b	264	
Caffeine	27a		Poten	Cyclopentolate Hydrochloride	9		MeR
and Sodium Benzoate				Ophthalmic Solution	9		MeR
Injection	*7, *28			Cyclophosphamide	31c	9.5	
Calamine	8		MeO	for Injection	31c	9.5	
Lotion	None			Tablets	31c	9.5	
Lotion, Phenolated	None			Cyclopropane	*33		
Calcium Carbonate,							
Precipitated	26a		HNB	Dapsone	25		Poten
Calcium Chloride	26a		HNB	Tablets	25		Poten
Calcium Disodium Edetate	*26a		DT	Decavitamin Capsules	*43		
Injection	*26a		DT	Tablets	*43		
Calcium Gluconate	26a		HNB	Demecarium Bromide	27a		CrV
Injection	26a		HNB	Ophthalmic Solution	31a	292	
Tablets	26a		HNB	Deslanoside	31a	590	FC
Calcium Hydroxide	26a		HNB	Injection	31a	590	FC
Solution	5		Phth	Desoxycorticosterone Acetate	†31a	525	BT
Calcium Pantothenate	*6, *26a, *41			Injection	†31a	525	BT
Tablets	*26a, *41			Dexamethasone	†31a	525	BT
Calcium Pantothenate,				Tablets	†31a	525	BT
Racemic	*26a, 41			Dexamethasone Sodium			
Camphor	None			Phosphate	*31b	236	
Carbachol	27a		CrV	Dextroamphetamine Sulfate	9		MeR
Ophthalmic Solution	31a	525	R	Elixir	31b, 36	257	
Carbon Dioxide	*33			Tablets	31b, 36	257	
Castor Oil	44			Dextrose	35a		
Cellulose, Oxidized	*2		Phth	Injection	35a		
Cellulose Acetate Phthalate	*1, *11a		Phth	and Sodium Chloride In-			
Cherry Juice	*15a		None	jection	*12e, *35a		
Cherry Syrup	None			Dibucaine Hydrochloride	27a		CrV
Chloral Hydrate	*4		Phth	Injection	31b	247	
Capsules	*4		Phth	Dichlorphenamide	*27b-2		TP
Syrup	*4		Phth	Tablets	32	−1.65	
Chlorambucil	1		Phth	Diethylcarbamazine Citrate	27a		CrV
Tablets	31b	301		Syrup	27a		TB
Chlordiazepoxide Hydro-				Tablets	27a		TB
chloride	27a		CrV	Diethylstilbestrol	31a	418	UV
Capsules	31b	245		Injection	31a	418	UV
for Injection	31b	245		Suppositories	31a	418	UV
Chlormerodrin Hg 197	35c			Tablets	31a	418	UV
Hg 203	35c			Diethyltoluamide	31c	14.1, 14.4	
Chlorobutanol	*12e		FAS	Solution	31c	14.1, 14.4	
Chlorophenothane	12e		FAS	Digitalis	41		
Chloroquine	27a		CrV	Powdered	41		
Chloroquine Hydrochloride				Tablets	41		
Injection	31b	343		Digitoxin	31a, 36	495	PA
Chloroquine Phosphate	31b	343		Tablets	31a, 36	495	PA
Tablets	31b	343		Digoxin	31a	620	MDB
Chlorpheniramine Maleate	27a		CrV	Elixir	31a	590	FC
Elixir	31b	264		Injection	31a	590	FC
Tablets	31b	264		Tablets	31a	590	FC
Chlorpromazine	27a		CrV	Dihydrotachysterol	None		
Chlorpromazine Hydro-				Diiodohydroxyquin	*18a		St
chloride	27a		Poten	Tablets	*18a		St
Injection	31b	254, 277		Dimenhydrinate	*12c, *27a		
Syrup	31b	254, 277		Syrup	8		MeR
Tablets	31b	254, 277		Tablets	12c		FAS
Chlorpropamide	31b	232		Dimercaprol	20		None
Tablets	31b	232		Injection	20		None
Chlorthalidone	31b	275		Dioctyl Sodium Sulfo-			
Tablets	31b	275		succinate	*16c		BpB
Cholecalciferol	None			Capsules	*16c		BpB
Cholesterol	None			Tablets	*16c		BpB
Cholestyramine Resin	*31b	318		Diphenhydramine Hydro-			
Chromic Phosphate P 32	35c			chloride	27a		CrV
Cinnamon Oil	*34			Capsules	31b	258	
Citric Acid	1		Phth	Elixir	31b	258	

Table III—Continued

	Assay category[a]	Analytical wavelength[b]	Indicator[c]		Assay category[a]	Analytical wavelength[b]	Indicator[c]
Injection	31b	258		Injection	41		
Diphenylhydantoin	*27b		AV	for Injection	41		
Capsules	27b		AV	Guanethidine Sulfate	31a	500	SK
Tablets	27b		AV	Tablets	31a	500	SK
Disodium Edetate	*26a		HNB				
Injection	*26a		HNB	Halazone	18a		St
Dyclonine Hydrochloride	27a		CrV	Tablets for Solution	18a		St
Solution	27a		CrV	Halothane	None		
				Helium	None		
Echothiophate Iodide	*20a		Poten	Hexachlorophene	1		Poten
for Ophthalmic Solution	*20a		Poten	Liquid Soap	31b	312	
Edrophonium Chloride	27a		QR	Histamine Phosphate	*30		
Injection	31b	273		Injection	31a	460	BNF
Emetine Hydrochloride	9		MeR	Homatropine Hydrobromide	*14a		Op
Injection	9		MeR	Ophthalmic Solution	*14a		Op
Ephedrine Sulfate	27a		MeR	Hydrochloric Acid	1		MeR
Capsules	27a		MeR	Hydrochlorothiazide	27b-2		AV
Injection	27a		MeR	Tablets	32	−1.90	
Solution	27a		MeR	Hydrocodone Bitartrate	9		MeR
Syrup	27a		MeR	Syrup	9		MeR
Epinephrine	27a		CrV	Tablets	9		MeR
Inhalation	*35a			Hydrocortisone	†31a	525	BT
Injection	*35a			Cream	†31a	525	BT
Solution	*35a			Ointment	†31a	525	BT
Sterile Suspension	*35a			Tablets	†31a	525	BT
Epinephrine Bitartrate	27a		CrV	Hydrocortisone Acetate	†31a	525	BT
Ophthalmic Solution	*35a			Ointment	†31a	525	BT
Ergocalciferol	None			Ophthalmic Ointment	†31a	525	BT
Capsules	31a	500, 550	SC	Ophthalmic Suspension	†31a	525	BT
Solution	31a	500, 550	SC	Suspension, Sterile	†31a	525	BT
Ergonovine Maleate	9		BpB	Hydrocortisone Sodium			
Injection	31a	550	PDB	Phosphate	*31b	238	
Tablets	31a	550	PDB	Injection	31a	525	BT
Ergotamine Tartrate	27a		CrV	Hydrocortisone Sodium			
Injection	31a, 36	550	PDB	Succinate	†31a	525	BT
Suppositories	31a	550	PDB	for Injection	†31a	525	BT
Tablets	31a	550	PDB	Hydrogen Peroxide Solution	15a		None
Estradiol Valerate	None			Hydroxyamphetamine			
Injection	31b	300		Hydrobromide	27a		CrV
Estrogens, Conjugated	*40			Ophthalmic Solution	*30		
Injection	*40			Hydroxychloroquine Sulfate	31b	243	
Tablets	*40			Tablets	31b	243	
Estrogens, Esterified	*40			Hydroxyprogesterone			
Tablets	*40			Caproate	None		
Ethacrynic Acid	19		St	Injection	31b, 36	380	IN
Tablets	19		St	Hydroxystilbamidine			
Ether	None			Isethionate	31b	344	
Ethinyl Estradiol	31a	538	SM	Sterile	31b	344	
Tablets	31a	538	SM				
Ethiodized Oil	*18a		St	Idoxuridine	*27b-2		TB
Ethionamide	31b	290		Ophthalmic Ointment	31b, 36	283	
Tablets	31b	290		Ophthalmic Solution	31b, 36	283	
Ethohexadiol	11b		CRTB	Imipramine Hydrochloride	27a		CrV
Ethosuximide	*27b-2		AV	Injection	31b	250	
Capsules	*27b-2		AV	Tablets	31b	250	
Ethoxzolamide	31b	299		Indocyanine Green	31a	785	None
Tablets	31b	299		Sterile	31a	785	None
Ethylenediamine	5		BpB	Insulin Injection	41		
Ethylparaben	11a		BtB	Insulin, Globin Zinc,			
Ethynodiol Diacetate	31b	236		Injection	41		
Eucatropine Hydrochloride	9		MeR	Insulin, Isophane, Suspension	41		
Eugenol	44			Insulin Zinc Suspension	41		
Evans Blue	31a	610	None	Extended	41		
Injection	31a	610	None	Prompt	41		
				Insulin, Zinc, Protamine,			
Fennel Oil	44			Suspension	41		
Ferrous Fumarate	14a		Op	Iodine	18b		St
Tablets	*18a		St	Solution, Strong	*18b, *21		
Ferrous Sulfate	15a		None	Tincture	*18b, *21		
Tablets	14a		Op	Iodochlorhydroxyquin	31c	14.4, 14.9	
Dried	15a		None	Cream	31c	14.4, 14.9	
Fluorouracil	27b-3		TB	Ointment	31c	14.4, 14.9	
Injection	31b	266		Suppositories	31c	14.4, 14.9	
Fluoxymesterone	†31a	525	BT	Iopanoic Acid	*12d		TBP
Tablets	†31a	525	BT	Tablets	1		TB
Folic Acid	31a	550	BM	Iophendylate Injection	*18a		
Injection	31a	550	BM	Ipecac	9, 39		MeR
Tablets	31a	550	BM	Powdered	9, 39		MeR
Furosemide	1		BtB	Syrup	9, 39		MeR
Tablets	31b	274		Iron Dextran Injection	31a	510	BPy
				Iron Sorbitex Injection	31a	510	BPy
Gallamine Triethiodide	27a		BpB	Isoflurophate Ophthalmic			
Injection	‡31a	416	BcG	Solution	31a	710	AS
Gentian Violet	17b		AT	Isoniazid	18f		St
Solution	17b		AT	Injection	18f		St
Glucagon	*6		MeR	Syrup	18f		St
for Injection	41			Tablets	18f		St
Glucose, Liquid	None			Isoproterenol Hydrochloride	31b	279	
Glycerin	None			Inhalation	31b, 36	278	
Gold Au 198 Solution	35c			Injection	31b, 36	278	
Gold Sodium Thiomalate	*30			Tablets	31b, 36	278	
Injection	*30			Isoproterenol Sulfate	27a		CrV
Gonadotropin, Chorionic	41			Inhalation	31b, 36	278	

Table III—Continued

	Assay category[a]	Analytical wavelength[b]	Indicator[c]		Assay category[a]	Analytical wavelength[b]	Indicator[c]
Lactic Acid	4		Phth	Methylene Blue	31a	663	None
Lactose	None			Injection	31a	663	None
Lanolin	44			Methylergonovine Maleate	31a	555	PDB
Anhydrous	44			Injection	31a	555	PDB
Lemon Oil	*2		Poten	Tablets	31a	555	PDB
Levallorphan Tartrate	27a		Poten	Methylparaben	11a		BtB
Injection	‡31a	420	BcG	Methylphenidate Hydro-			
Levarterenol Bitartrate	27a		CrV	chloride	27a		Nb
Injection	*35a			for Injection	27a		Nb
Lidocaine	8		BgM	Tablets	27a		Nb
Ointment	9		Poten	Metronidazole	27a		MaG
Lidocaine Hydrochloride	9		Poten	Suppositories	27a		MaG
Injection	9		Poten	Tablets	27a		MaG
Jelly	9		Poten	Metyrapone	31b	260	
Lucanthone Hydrochloride	31b	256		Tablets	31a	450	DNP
Tablets	31b	256		Morphine Injection	8		MeR
				Morphine Sulfate	*27b-2		PR
Magnesia, Milk of	8		MeR	Tablets	8		MeR
Magnesia Tablets	*30						
Magnesia and Alumina Oral				Nalorphine Hydrochloride	31b	285	
Suspension	*26a		DT	Injection	31b	285, 310	
Tablets	*26a		DT	Neostigmine Bromide	27a		CrV
Magnesium Oxide	8		MeO	Tablets	31a	420	HDA
Magnesium Stearate	8		MeO	Neostigmine Methylsulfate	*6		MeR
Magnesium Sulfate	26a		EBT	Injection	31a	420	HDA
Injection	26a		EBT	Niacinamide	*27a		CrV
Magnesium Trisilicate	*8, *30			Injection	31a	450	CnS
Tablets	*8, *30			Tablets	31a	450	CnS
Mannitol	18c		St	Nitrofurantoin	31b	367	
Injection	18c		St	Oral Suspension	32	−0.60	
and Sodium Chloride				Tablets	32	−0.60	
Injection	*12e, *18c			Nitrogen	33		
Mecamylamine Hydro-				Nitroglycerin Tablets	31a	410	PDS
chloride	*40			Nitrous Oxide	*42		
Tablets	8		MeR	Norethindrone	31b	240	
Mechlorethamine Hydro-				Norethynodrel	31b	240	
chloride	*20b		St				
for Injection	*20b		St	Oleic Acid (Acid Value)	1		Phth
Meclizine Hydrochloride	27a		QR	Olive Oil	44		
Tablets	27a		QR	Opium	*39		
Medroxyprogesterone Acetate	31b	380	IN	Powdered	*39		
Suspension, Sterile	31b	380	IN	Orange Oil	*2		Poten
Tablets	31b	380	IN	Orange Spirit, Compound	*34		
Meglumine	5		MeR	Orange Syrup	*1		Phth
Diatrizoate Injection	*12d		TBPE	Ouabain	31a, 36	495	PA
Iodipamide Injection	*12d		Poten	Injection	31a, 36	495	PA
Iothalamate Injection	*12d		Poten	Oxygen	*33		
Melphalan	*12d		Poten	Oxytocin Injection	41		
Tablets	31b	260					
Menadiol Sodium				Paraldehyde	None		
Diphosphate	14a		Poten	Sterile	None		
Injection	14a		Poten	Paramethadione	*6		MeR
Menthol	None			Capsules	*6		MeR
Meperidine Hydrochloride	27a		CrV	Solution	*6		MeR
Injection	27a		CrV	Parathyroid Injection	41		
Tablets	27a		CrV	Paregoric	31b, 36	285	
Mephentermine Sulfate	27a		Nb	Peanut Oil	44		
Injection	27a		Nb	Penicillamine	*26c		DT
Tablets	27a		Nb	Capsules	*26c		DT
Meprobamate	*3		Phth	Peppermint Oil	*11a, *11b		Phth
Injection	*3		Phth	Phenacetin	31b	250	
Tablets	*3		Phth	Tablets	28		
Meralluride	*30, *31b			Phenelzine Sulfate	*18f		St
Injection	*30, *31b			Tablets	*18f		St
Mercaptopurine	*27b-2		TB	Phenformin Hydrochloride	31a	565	AN
Tablets	31b	325		Tablets	31b	233	
Mercury, Ammoniated	*13b		FAS	Phenobarbital	1		Poten
Ointment	*30			Elixir	31b	240	
Mestranol	31a	545	SM	Tablets	31b	240	
Metaraminol Bitartrate	27a		CrV	Phenol	*19		St
Injection	31b	272		Liquefied	*19		St
Methadone Hydrochloride	27a		CrV	Phenolsulfonphthalein	31a	559	None
Injection	9		MeR	Injection	31a	559	None
Tablets	9		MeR	Phentolamine Mesylate	31b	278	
Methamphetamine Hydro-				for Injection	31b	278	
chloride	27a		CrV	Phenylbutazone	1		Phth
Tablets	31b	257		Tablets	*27b-3		Poten
Methazolamide	31b	258		Phenylephrine Hydrochloride	19		St
Tablets	32	−1.62		Injection	31b, 36	271	
Methenamine Mandelate	*1, *18f			Ophthalmic Solution	31b, 36	271	
Oral Suspension	1		Phth	Solution	31b, 36	271	
Tablets	*18f			Physostigmine	27a		Poten
Methimazole	12a		BtB	Physostigmine Salicylate	27a		Poten
Tablets	12a		BtB	Physostigmine Sulfate	27a		Poten
Methotrexate	31b, 36	306		Phytonadione	None		
for Injection	31b, 36	306		Injection	31b, 36	248	
Tablets	31b, 36	306		Tablets	31b, 36	248	
Methoxamine Hydrochloride	27a		CrV	Pilocarpine Hydrochloride	27a		CrV
Injection	9		MeR	Ophthalmic Solution	31a	500	FH
Methyl Salicylate	11a		Phth	Pilocarpine Nitrate	27a		Poten
Methylcellulose	*18a			Ophthalmic Solution	31a	500	FH
Methyldopa	27a		CrV	Piperazine Citrate	27a		CrV
Tablets	31a	520	FeT	Syrup	*30		
Methyldopate Hydrochloride	27a		CrV				
Injection	31a	520	FeT				

Table III—Continued

	Assay category[a]	Analytical wavelength[b]	Indicator[c]
Tablets	*30		
Podophyllum	*38		
Polyethylene Glycol 400	*11b, *31a		
4000	*11b		Phth
Polyoxyl 40 Stearate	*11a		Phth
Polysorbate 80	*11a		Phth
Potassium Aminosalicylate	25		Poten
Tablets	25		Poten
Potassium Bicarbonate	5		MeO
Potassium Chloride	12e		FAS
Injection	12e		FAS
Tablets	12e		FAS
Potassium Hydroxide	*5		MeO
Potassium Iodide	23		CHCl₃
Potassium Permanganate	*15c		None
Tablets for Solution	*15c		None
Pralidoxime Chloride	31b	293	
Sterile	31b	293	
Tablets	31b, *36	293	
Prednisolone	†31a	525	BT
Tablets	†31a	525	BT
Prednisolone Acetate	†31a	525	BT
Suspension, Sterile	†31a	525	BT
Prednisolone Sodium Phosphate	*31b	241	
Injection	*31b	241	
Ophthalmic Solution	*31b	241	
Prednisone	†31a	525	BT
Tablets	†31a	525	BT
Primaquine Phosphate	*25		SPI
Tablets	*25		SPI
Primidone	31b	257	
Oral Suspension	31b, 36	257	
Tablets	31b, 36	257	
Probenecid	1		Phth
Tablets	31b	257	
Procainamide Hydrochloride	27a		CrV
Capsules	25		SPI
Injection	27a		CrV
Procaine Hydrochloride	25		SPI
Injection	31b	280	
Sterile	25		SPI
Prochlorperazine Edisylate	27a		CrV
Injection	31b	254, 278	
Syrup	31b	254, 278	
Prochlorperazine Maleate	27a		Poten
Tablets	31b	254, 278	
Promethazine Hydrochloride	27a		CrV
Injection	31b	298	
Syrup	31b	298	
Tablets	31b, 36	298	
Propantheline Bromide	27a		Poten
for Injection	27a		Poten
Tablets	27a		Poten
Proparacaine Hydrochloride	27a		CrV
Ophthalmic Solution	31b	310	
Propoxyphene Hydrochloride	27a		CrV
Capsules	31c	5.80	
Propylene Glycol	None		
Propyliodone	*18a		
Suspension, Sterile	*18a		
Suspension in Oil, Sterile	*18a		
Propylparaben	11a		BtB
Propylthiouracil	12a		BtB
Tablets	12a		BtB
Protamine Sulfate	*37		
Injection	*37		
for Injection	*37		
Protein Hydrolysate Injection	*31d		
Pyrazinamide	*6		MeR
Tablets	31b	268	
Pyridostigmine Bromide	27a		QR
Syrup	‡31a	415	BcG
Tablets	31b	269	
Pyridoxine Hydrochloride	27a		CrV
Injection	31a	650	DcC
Tablets	31a	650	DcC
Pyrimethamine	27a		QR
Tablets	31b	273	
Pyrvinium Pamoate	31a	508	None
Oral Suspension	31a, 36	516	None
Tablets	31a, 36	516	None
Quinacrine Hydrochloride	27a		CrV
Tablets	31a	525	None
Quinethazone	*27b-4		Poten
Tablets	31c	7.45	
Quinidine Gluconate	27a		MaG
Injection	31b, 36	352	
Quinidine Sulfate	27a		MaG
Capsules	27a		Nb
Tablets	27a		Nb
Quinine Sulfate	27a		MaG

	Assay category[a]	Analytical wavelength[b]	Indicator[c]
Capsules	27a		Nb
Tablets	27a		Nb
Raspberry Juice	*30		
Reserpine	31a	390	SN
Injection	31a	390	SN
Tablets	31a	390	SN
Resorcinol	19		St
Riboflavin	31e	460	
Injection	31e	460	
Tablets	31e	460	
Ringer's Injection	*12e, *14b, *26a		
Lactated	*10, *12e, *14b, *26a		
Saccharin	1		Phth
Salicylic Acid	1		Phth
Collodion	1		BtB
Plaster	19		St
Scopolamine Hydrobromide	27a		CrV
Injection	8		MeR
Tablets	8		MeR
Secobarbital	27b-2		TB
Elixir	31b	240	
Sesame Oil	44		
Silver Nitrate	13a		FAS
Ophthalmic Solution	13a		FAS
Toughened	13a		FAS
Sodium Acetazolamide, Sterile	32	−0.70	
Sodium Aminohippurate Injection	25		SPI
Sodium Aminosalicylate	25		Poten
Tablets	25		Poten
Sodium Amobarbital	*30		
Capsules	31b	239	
Sterile	*30		
Sodium Ascorbate	20		St
Sodium Benzoate	27a		CrV
Sodium Bicarbonate	5		MeO
Injection	5		MeO
Tablets	5		MeO
Sodium Bisulfite	18f		St
Sodium Borate	5		MeO
Sodium Carbonate	5		MeO
Sodium Carboxymethylcellulose	27a		Poten
Sodium Chloride	12e		FAS
Injection	12e		FAS
Injection, Bacteriostatic	12e		FAS
Solution	12e		FAS
Tablets	12e		FAS
Sodium Chromate Cr 51 Injection	31b, 35c	370	
Sodium Citrate	27a		Poten
Sodium Diatrizoate Injection	12d		TBPE
Sodium Diphenylhydantoin	*30		
Capsules	*30		
Sterile	*30		
Sodium Ethacrynate for Injection	19		St
Sodium Fluorescein	*30		
Ophthalmic Solution	*30		
Sodium Fluoride	*22		PTC
Sodium Glucosulfone Injection	*25		SPI
Sodium Heparin	*37		
Injection	*37		
Sodium Hydroxide	5		MeO
Sodium Indigotindisulfonate	17		None
Injection	17		None
Sodium Iodide	23		CHCl₃
I 125 Capsules	35c		
I 125 Solution	35c		
I 131 Capsules	35c		
I 131 Solution	35c		
Sodium Iodipamide Injection	*12d		TBPE
Sodium Iodohippurate I 131 Injection	35c		
Sodium Iothalamate Injection	12d		Poten
Sodium Lactate Injection	27a		CrV
Sodium Lauryl Sulfate	*12d, *30		
Sodium Levothyroxine	18a		St
Tablets	18a		St
Sodium Liothyronine	18a		St
Tablets	18a		St
Sodium Mercaptomerin	*30		
Injection	*30		
Sterile	*30		
Sodium Morrhuate Injection	8		MeO
Sodium Nitrite	*15c		None
Sodium Pentobarbital	*30		
Capsules	*30		

Table III—Continued

	Assay category[a]	Analytical wavelength[b]	Indicator
Elixir	*30		
Injection	*30		
Sodium Phenobarbital	*30		
Injection	*30		
Sterile	*30		
Sodium Phosphate P 32			
Solution	35c		
Sodium Polystyrene			
Sulfonate	*31d		
Sodium Rose Bengal I 131			
Injection	31a, 35c	550	None
Sodium Salicylate	27a		CrV
Tablets	7		BtB
Sodium Secobarbital	*30		
Capsules	31b	241	
Sterile	*30		
Sodium Sulfacetamide	25		SPI
Ophthalmic Ointment	25		SPI
Ophthalmic Solution	25		SPI
Sodium Sulfadiazine	25		SPI
Injection	25		SPI
Sodium Sulfobromophthalein	31a	580	Na$_2$CO$_3$
Injection	31a	580	Na$_2$CO$_3$
Sodium Sulfoxone	31a	560	BM
Tablets	31a	560	BM
Sodium Thiopental	31b	304	
for Injection	31b	304	
Sodium Thiosulfate	20		St
Injection	20		St
Sodium Tolbutamide	31b	263	
Sterile	31b	263	
Sodium Warfarin	31b	308	
for Injection	31b	308	
Tablets	31b	307	
Sorbitol	*21, 36		St
Solution	*21, 36		St
Spironolactone	31b	238	
Tablets	31b	238	
Stearic Acid	*42		
Stearyl Alcohol	*42		
Stibophen	20a		St
Injection	20a		St
Storax	*1, *11a, *28		
Succinylcholine Chloride	27a		CrV
Injection	11a		BtB
Sterile	27a		CrV
Succinylsulfathiazole	25		SPI
Tablets	25		SPI
Sucrose	None		
Sulfadiazine	25		SPI
Tablets	25		SPI
Sulfamerazine	25		SPI
Sulfamethazine	25		SPI
Sulfapyridine	25		SPI
Tablets	25		SPI
Sulfinpyrazone	*1		Phth
Tablets	*1		Phth
Sulfisoxazole	*27b-2		TB
Tablets	*27b-2		TB
Sulfur Dioxide	*20a		St
Sulfur, Precipitated	*1		Phth
Sulfur Ointment	*30		
Testosterone Cypionate	*31a	380	IN
Injection	‡31a, 36	380	IN
Testosterone Enanthate	*31a	380	IN
Injection	‡31a, 36	380	IN
Testosterone Propionate	31a	380	IN
Injection	‡31a, 36	380	IN
Tetracaine Hydrochloride	25		SPI
Injection	31b	310	
Sterile	31b	310	
Tetrachloroethylene	None		
Capsules	*34		
Theobroma Oil	44		
Theophylline	12c		FAS
Thiabendazole	27a		CrV
Oral Suspension	31b	302	

	Assay category[a]	Analytical wavelength[b]	Indicator[c]
Thiamine Hydrochloride	*31e		
Injection	*31e		
Tablets	*31e		
Thiamine Mononitrate	*31e		
Thioridazine Hydrochloride	27a		Poten
Solution	31b	265	
Tablets	31b	265	
Thiotepa	*5		Phth
for Injection	31c	10.75	
Thymol	*23		MeO
Thyroid	*18a		St
Tablets	*18a		St
Titanium Dioxide	*15b		
Tolazamide	1		Phth
Tablets	31b	262	
Tolbutamide	1		Phth
for Injection	31b	263	
Tablets	31b	263	
Tolnaftate	31b	257	
Cream	31b	260	
Solution	31b	260	
Tolu Balsam	*1, *11a		Phth
Triamcinolone	31b, 36	238	
Tablets	†31a	520	BT
Triamcinolone Acetonide	31b, 36	238	
Cream	†31a	520	BT
Ointment	†31a	520	BT
Suspension, Sterile	†31a	520	BT
Triamterene	27a		Poten
Capsules	31b	357.5	
Trichloroacetic Acid	1		Phth
Trichloroethylene	None		
Triethanolamine	5		MeR
Trihexyphenidyl Hydro-			
chloride	27a		TB
Elixir	‡31a	408	BcP
Tablets	‡31a	408	BcP
Trimethadione	6		MeR
Capsules	6		MeR
Solution	6		MeR
Trimethaphan Camsylate	27a		Poten
Injection	‡31a	420	BcG
Tripelennamine Citrate	27a		CrV
Elixir	31b	313	
Tripelennamine Hydro-			
chloride	27a		CrV
Injection	31b	313	
Tablets	31b	313	
Trisulfapyrimidines Oral			
Suspension	*25, *31a, 36		
Tablets	*25, *31a, 36		
Tropicamide	27a		CrV
Ophthalmic Solution	31b	253	
Tubocurarine Chloride	31b	280	
Injection	41		
Urea	6		MeR
Sterile	6		MeR
Vanillin	31b	308	
Vasopressin Injection	41		
Vinblastine Sulfate	31b	267	
for Injection	31b	267	
Vincristine Sulfate	31b	267	
for Injection	31b	267	
Vitamin A	31b	310, 325, 334	
Capsules	31b	310, 325, 334	
Zinc Chloride	26a		EBT
Zinc Gelatin	None		
Zinc Oxide	8		MeO
Ointment	26a		EBT
Paste	26a		EBT
Zinc Stearate	26a		EBT
Zinc Sulfate	26a		EBT
Ophthalmic Solution	26a		PAN

38 | Biological Testing

Bioassay procedures—animal assays—microbial assays—biological tests

This chapter was prepared by

G. Victor Rossi, PhD, *Professor of Pharmacology, Philadelphia College of Pharmacy and Science, Philadelphia, Pa. 19104*

Biological Testing includes the quantitative assay of drugs by biological methods as well as the application of qualitative biological tests. Such testing utilizes intact animals, animal preparations, isolated living tissues, or microorganisms. The quantitative assays are considered in this chapter under the headings *Animal Assays* and *Microbial Assays*. The official qualitative tests are considered in the section on *Biological Tests*. Major emphasis is directed toward the quantitative assays; many of the qualitative tests are only briefly discussed.

The majority of currently available therapeutic agents are substances of known chemical composition which can be assayed by quantitative chemical or physical analyses. There remains, however, a limited number of useful drugs which cannot be assayed satisfactorily by chemical or physical means. Such drugs, which are primarily of natural origin, are assayed by biological methods. Biological standardization procedures are generally less precise, more time-consuming, and more expensive to conduct than ordinary chemical assays; therefore, they are generally reserved for use mainly:

1. If the chemical identity of the active principle has not been fully elucidated, eg, parathyroid hormone.
2. If no adequate chemical assay has been devised for the active principle, although its chemical structure has been established, eg, insulin.
3. If the drug is composed of a complex mixture of substances of varying structure and activity, eg, digitalis, posterior pituitary.
4. If purification of the crude drug, sufficient for the performance of a chemical assay, is not possible or practical, eg, the separation of vitamin D from certain irradiated oils.
5. If the chemical assay is not a valid indication of biological activity, due, for example, to lack of differentiation between active and inactive isomers.

There are several situations in which factors such as specificity, sensitivity, or practicality dictate the use of a biological rather than a chemical assay procedure.

A chemical assay quantitatively determines the amount of a specific compound or structural moiety present in a given sample. On the basis of the established concentration, an assumption is made relative to the biological activity of the sample. In contrast, a biological assay measures the actual biological activity of a given sample, which may represent the algebraic sum of the interaction of numerous chemical and physical-chemical factors. For example, the data obtained from a chemical assay may not provide information concerning the contribution to the net biological activity of trace amounts of substances which do not influence the chemical analysis. Such substances may produce qualitative variations in biological activity which may be responsible for unexpected side-effects or toxic reactions. Furthermore, the augmentory or inhibitory influence of variations in the physical state of the active principle is not reflected in the results of a chemical assay. The safety, efficacy, and dependability of dosage of modern drugs are contingent upon standardization, and biological assays must be employed in some instances even though the chemical identities of the active principles in the preparation may be known. Each new revision of the USP and NF witnesses the replacement of several biological assays by chemical or physical procedures as improved techniques are developed.

Animals

As animals are an important "unknown" factor in most biological assays the need for their proper selection and adequate care thereafter is self-evident. Most laboratories seek a reliable source of animals which can supply their needs from colonies maintained for this purpose. Institutions engaged in the breeding of animals for laboratory use are to be found in most sections of the country; some make a specialty of offering only one species, such as the rat. Others may breed several species, including the rat, mouse, guinea pig (cavy), or the hamster, and in addition offer more than one strain. In any one test it is desirable to use animals of only one strain. Actually bioassayists may adopt a specified strain for all work of a particular type. In this manner experience is gained as to the normal variation that is to be expected. For some assays a specific sex must be employed, ie, estrogenic tests; in other assays either sex may be used but the effect that sex may play in the response should not be overlooked. The male rat, for instance, has a faster growth rate than the female; therefore indiscriminate use of both males and females in a rat growth test should be avoided. Differences in the response of sexes may extend into other categories, eg, response toward toxic materials.

Cats and dogs must be obtained from dealers in laboratory animals who are licensed under the federal Laboratory Animal Welfare Act of 1966 (P.L. 89-544).

Federal Regulations—Public Law 89-544 (the Animal Welfare Act), enacted by Congress on August 24, 1966 gave the US Department of Agriculture authority to promote standards governing the humane handling, care, treatment, and transportation of dogs, cats, guinea pigs, hamsters, rabbits, and nonhuman primates. Minimum standards concerning housing, feeding, watering, sanitation, ventilation, shelter, separation by species, and adequate veterinary care were published in 1967.[1]

Research facilities that use and dealers that supply dogs or cats, and which are required by the law to be registered (research facilities) or licensed (dealers), are subject to the regulations. During actual performance of research or experimentation the regulations do not apply. The premises of dealers and research facilities are subject to periodic inspection by a Veterinarian in Charge in each state.

In addition to the federal regulations, the Institute

of Laboratory Animal Resources has prepared an informative guide[2] which details specific suggestions and recommendations for operating an animal facility in optimum condition.

Bioassay Procedures

Bioassays are conducted by determining the amount of a preparation of unknown potency required to produce a definite effect on suitable test animals or organs under standard conditions. Originally, the results of such tests were expressed as "animal units"; for example, a *cat unit* of digitalis was the amount of a preparation per kilogram of cat necessary to produce death. Statistical studies by Magnus and others demonstrated the unreliability of this procedure, for animals vary greatly in their sensitivity to a given preparation as a result of differences in heredity, age, diet, surroundings, and so forth.

Reference Standards—To minimize the source of error resulting from animal variation, standard reference preparations are used in certain bioassay procedures. The principle of the standard consists of testing successively the unknown and standard preparations on two groups of similar animals, or in some cases (eg, epinephrine, posterior pituitary) on the same animal or organ. The amount of the unknown preparation required to produce an effect equal to that produced by a certain amount of the standard will be inversely proportional to their relative potencies. The potency of the unknown can therefore be expressed as a percentage of that of the standard by employing a simple formula:

$$\text{Potency of unknown} = \frac{\text{Dose of standard}}{\text{Dose of unknown}} \times 100 = \%$$

In many instances reliable results cannot be obtained by this simple calculation. Therefore, in some assays it is necessary to adopt more precise methods of calculating potency based upon observations of relative but not necessarily equal effects. Likewise, methods of computation have been devised to determine the statistical reliability of the results. These procedures are discussed in Chapter 11, *Statistics*, page 122. The section on *General Tests* in the USP also presents a detailed consideration of factors germane to the *Design and Analysis of Biological Assays*.

Reference standards, for use in the several assays in which they are required, are available as a service from the USP Revision Committee, 4630 Montgomery Ave., Bethesda, Md. 20014, or from the NF Revision Committee, 2215 Constitution Ave., N.W., Washington, D.C. 20037. They are standardized in terms of such corresponding International Standards as may exist. Those preparations which are generally called Reference Substances, while not required in official assays, serve as a common base of reference where needed.

Disadvantages of Bioassays—Biological assays leave much to be desired in several respects. Although some are extremely sensitive in detecting small differences in concentration, their quantitative accuracy usually falls considerably below that obtainable with most chemical analyses. The techniques and interpretations involved can often vary with different operators in spite of the rigid requirements specified by the official publications, and hence there is a considerable subjective element present. Furthermore, the effect measured in the test animals is often not that which the drug is intended to produce in treating patients. The importance of this discrepancy was formerly minimized, but recent studies have shown that when several active principles are present in a crude drug, those producing the maximal therapeutic effect are not necessarily the ones chiefly responsible for the action measured in the assay. As a result, samples found to be of equal strength by assay may show different potencies when employed clinically. An example of this situation is found in the discussion on digitalis.

Classification of Bioassay Procedures—Bioassays are classified in three groups according to whether the effect produced is all or none (as death), graded (as rise in blood pressure), or is characterized by developing in a measured period of time (as the curative response to thiamine). It should be noted that in all three types, with few exceptions, the calculations of potency are based on the sizes of doses necessary to produce approximately equal effects and not on the intensities of the responses. Furthermore, *the results derived from all are quantitative* in that the potency of the unknown is expressed in terms of the standard.

Animal Assays

In the following section biological assay procedures involving the use of intact animals, animal preparations, or isolated, surviving, animal tissues or organs are considered. The presentation is restricted largely to the general principles and basic experimental approaches involved in each of several representative types of biological assay methods. For complete details of the official procedures the reader is directed to the corresponding monographs in the current USP or NF.

Digitaloid Drugs

The digitaloid group of drugs includes Digitalis (the dried leaf of *Digitalis purpurea*), which is used medicinally as the powdered material, as the tincture prepared from the powdered leaf, or in the form of capsules or tablets. These products of natural origin contain, in addition to the cardioactive glycoside *digitoxin* and *gitoxin*, a saponin-like glycoside, termed *digitonin*, largely devoid of the cardiac effects of Digitalis, and a complex mixture of constituents including digitoflavin, digitophyllin, lipids, carbohydrates, and other nonspecific plant components. Although the cardiotonic glycosides are similar in chemical structure and pharmacodynamic activity, they differ markedly in potency, efficiency of gastrointestinal absorption, speed of onset, and duration of action. Furthermore, there is considerable variation among different lots of crude drug in respect to the total active glycoside content and the relative concentration of each active principle.

It is apparent that *chemical* assay procedures, such as the determination of total glycosides or total aglycones, cannot adequately measure the pharmacodynamic activity of the crude drug or galenical preparation of

Digitalis. Such drugs, composed of a complex mixture of substances of varying structure and activity, must be subjected to a *biological* assay.

As a rule, it is desirable that the parameters of a biological assay simulate, as closely as practicable, the conditions generally associated with clinical usage of the drug in question. In this respect the currently employed biological assay procedure for Digitalis has several disadvantages and limitations. For example, the preparation to be assayed is given by fractional, intermittent, intravenous injection, whereas in the treatment of patients with cardiac disorders digitaloid drugs are most often administered orally. The assay procedure does not, therefore, take into consideration variations in clinical effectiveness among different members of this medicinal group which may be attributable to differences in the rate and completeness of absorption from the gastrointestinal tract. Furthermore, the calculation of potency is based on the amount of drug required to produce death of the test animal due to cardiac arrest. Thus the end-point of the assay corresponds to a toxic rather than a therapeutically desirable event. However, it may be claimed that the toxic effects of Digitalis on the heart constitute extensions of the cardiodynamic changes which are beneficial in certain cardiac disorders. Because of the limitations of the pigeon method many attempts have been made to develop more satisfactory bioassay procedures. None of the alternatives devised to date has any impelling advantage over the current USP method.

Separation and identification of the active principles of crude drugs having characteristic digitalis-like effects on the heart has resulted in the availability, for therapeutic use, of products consisting essentially of a single relatively pure cardiotonic glycoside. These additional members of the digitaloid group of drugs include Acetyldigitoxin, Deslanoside, Digoxin, and Lanatoside C (all of which are derived from *Digitalis lanata*), Digitoxin (a glycosidal constituent of both *Digitalis purpurea* and *Digitalis lanata*), and Ouabain (a glycoside obtained from the seeds of *Strophanthus gratus*). Preparations containing these glycosides are assayed quantitatively by colorimetric methods described in Chapter 37, *Analysis of Medicinals*, page 596. Chemical assay procedures enable precise determination of the amount of glycoside present in a particular dosage formulation. However, it must be emphasized that the response to digitaloid drugs varies considerably among cardiac patients. A "clinical assay" must, therefore, be performed with each patient regardless of whether the digitaloid preparation being used was standardized on the basis of a chemical or biological assay procedure.

The USP Pigeon Method

Preparations Assayed by the Pigeon Method— This assay is official for the following preparations of the USP: *Digitalis, Powdered Digitalis*, and *Digitalis Tablets; Digitalis Capsules* NF are assayed by the same method.

Standards—The above preparations are assayed against the USP Digitalis Reference Standard, 100 mg of which represents one USP Digitalis Unit. A standard preparation in the form of a tincture is prepared by weighing accurately and rapidly the contents of one container of the Reference Standard, transferring the contents to a hard-glass, glass-stoppered container, and adding 10.0 ml of menstruum (4 parts ethanol, 1 part water by volume) per Gm of powder. The mixture is shaken continuously for 22 to 26 hours at a temperature of 20° to 30°. It is then immediately centrifuged and the supernatant liquid is decanted into a hard-glass bottle which is tightly stoppered and refrigerated until used. The material is termed "Standard preparation" and may be used as an assay standard for a period of 30 days.

Preparation of Samples for Assay—The U.S. Pharmacopeia and National Formulary give specific directions under each preparation for the potency requirements and methods to be used in preparing the material for assay. In general, preparations of digitalis leaf are treated in the same manner as the reference material, using a sufficiently large sample, adding a quantity of menstruum expected to correspond to 1.0 ml per USP Digitalis Unit, and carrying out a similar extraction. Capsules containing digitalis suspended in water-immiscible media (ie, fats and oils) are subjected to a preliminary extraction with solvent hexane. The alcoholic extractions may be used for assay at any time within 30 days of preparation. On the day of the test, the standard preparation and the preparation to be assayed are diluted with isotonic sodium chloride solution so that 15 ml contains the estimated fatal dose per kilogram of pigeon (approximately 0.86 to 1.0 USP Digitalis Unit). With some preparations it is essential that final dilution for the assay be made just before use, for upon standing precipitation may occur.

Assay Procedure—Specific directions are given in the USP for *Digitalis* and in the NF for *Digitalis Capsules*. Groups of at least 6 pigeons must be employed for the Standard preparation and for the preparation to be assayed. The pigeons used should be adults which are not emaciated or grossly diseased, and should be of sufficiently uniform size that the heaviest is less than twice the weight of the lightest, and the average weights of the two groups do not differ by more than 30%. Food is withheld for 16 to 28 hours prior to assay. Each pigeon is immobilized on a holder which is shaped in the form of a cross, the upright about 12 inches in length and the cross arm 14 inches. The wings are individually, but firmly immobilized by tying to adjacent cross arms and the legs by tying to the upright. The pigeon is then lightly anesthetized with ether, and the alar vein is exposed. A cannula, attached by a short length of rubber tubing to a small-bore calibrated buret containing the diluted preparation, is inserted into the vein and firmly tied in place. Before insertion, all air bubbles must be expressed from the apparatus. It is important that anesthesia be kept in the first or analgetic stage throughout the assay, as indicated by the absence of pain, but with retention of the corneal and pupillary reflexes, and some degree of muscular tension. A deeper stage of anesthesia may augment the toxic effects of the preparation being injected and thereby give false results. One ml of dilution per Kg pigeon is rapidly injected, and this dose is repeated at 5-minute intervals until the bird dies of cardiac arrest. Death is usually accompanied by a closer lie of the feathers and complete flaccidity of all the skeletal muscles. Although no specific instruction is given concerning a final injection when death occurs simultaneously, it is advisable to disregard it, inasmuch as digitalis acts relatively slowly and the earlier doses are more significant in contributing to the lethal effect than are the later ones.

The average number of doses of each preparation necessary to produce death must be between 13 and 19, and the lowest dose shall not differ by more than 4 doses from the highest dose, otherwise the data are to be regarded as preliminary and the series repeated, using an adjusted dilution. The assay must be completed within a period of 30 days.

The mathematical procedures for the calculation of potency are detailed in the USP monograph for *Digitalis* and the NF monograph for *Digitalis Capsules*. Because of the variability inherent in biological assays, the potency of *Powdered Digitalis*, *Digitalis Tablets*, and *Digitalis Capsules* is considered satisfactory if it is equivalent to not less than 85.0% and not more than 120.0% of labeled potency.

Because of the relatively large permissible variation, two Digitalis preparations labeled identically as to potency may actually differ considerably from each other in this respect.

Epinephrine

Epinephrine is prepared both by extraction of the natural product from the medulla of adrenal glands of domestic animals, where it exists solely in the highly active levorotatory form, and synthetically, where racemic mixtures of the levo- and less active dextrorotatory isomers are obtained. Epinephrine obtained from natural sources contains varying amounts of norepinephrine (levarterenol), which differs chemically from epinephrine only by the absence of the terminal methyl group.

Neither the formerly official (USP XIV) biological assay nor the current USP chemical assay for epinephrine differentiates between epinephrine and norepinephrine; however, the small amounts of the latter which may be present in epinephrine obtained from natural sources do not materially influence the biological response to such preparations.

The formerly official (USP XIV) assay for epinephrine is described briefly because it illustrates the basic approach to the biological determination of pressor activity. Furthermore, the current USP and NF direct that certain medicinals obtained from natural sources be assayed for pressor substances on the basis of this type of bioassay procedure.

Standard—A standard solution is prepared by dissolving 91 mg of USP Epinephrine Bitartrate Reference Standard (equivalent to 50 mg of epinephrine base) in 10 ml of freshly prepared sodium bisulfite solution (1 in 150) and diluting to 50 ml with distilled water. This 1 in 1000 standard solution is stored in tightly-stoppered, hard-glass containers in a dark, refrigerated place. It may be used for assay for a period of 6 months unless any discoloration or precipitate appears, in which case it is discarded.

Assay Procedure—A medium-sized healthy dog is anesthetized deeply enough to prevent any muscular movements. For this purpose 35 mg of pentobarbital per Kg may be given intravenously or intraperitoneally, and followed by a smaller dose if necessary. The trachea is exposed and cannulated so that artificial respiration can be administered conveniently in the advent of respiratory failure. If the room temperature is below 25°C it is directed that the animal be protected against excess loss of body heat. The carotid artery, which lies alongside the trachea in the carotid sheath together with the sympatheticovagus nerve and internal jugular vein, is exposed and cannulated. The cannula is connected to a suitable pressure measuring and recording device, using an anticoagulant solution in the connecting tube, such as heparin in isotonic sodium chloride solution, which will not affect the blood pressure if it diffuses back into the general circulation. A femoral vein is then exposed and an injection of 0.1 ml of a 1% aqueous solution of atropine sulfate per Kg is given. This is done for the purpose of blocking the vagal cardioinhibitory mechanism; otherwise each rise in blood pressure following an injection of epinephrine will be complicated by a reflex tachycardia which diminishes the accuracy of the assay. Vagal paralysis is tested for by the intravenous injection of 0.1 ml/Kg of a 0.01% freshly prepared aqueous solution of acetylcholine chloride. If the latter injection produces any fall in blood pressure, atropinization is incomplete, and subsequent doses of half the original dose of atropine should be given until the dose of acetylcholine chloride elicits no fall.

The standard solution of Reference Epinephrine and the preparation to be assayed are diluted with isotonic sodium chloride solution so that the intravenous injection of 0.5 to 1.5 ml of each dilution of the standard produces a rise in blood pressure equivalent to 30 to 60 mm of mercury and of the unknown 30 to 60 mm. During the course of the assay, any dilution which develops even a trace of pink color must be discarded.

The dog is then tested for sensitivity and uniformity of response by making alternate injections into the femoral vein of two doses of the test dilution of the standard solution which differ in amount by no more than 20% of the smaller and which produce rises in blood pressure of between 30 and 60 mm of mercury. A constant interval of 5 minutes should be allowed between injections, or longer if the blood pressure does not return to approximately the original level in this period. After two or more injections of each dose have been made alternately, the rises in blood pressure are measured to the nearest millimeter, and the average rise and the maximal difference in rises produced by each dose are calculated. If the two average rises differ by at least 5 mm, and this difference is at least twice the maximal difference in the rises produced by each dose, the animal is considered satisfactory. Otherwise, it must be discarded.

The actual assay may now be undertaken by giving at regular intervals alternate injections of the dilutions of the standard and preparation to be assayed in such a fashion that their relative potencies can be calculated statistically. This is done by keeping the dose of the standard constant unless the sensitivity of the animal changes, in which case the dose is increased or decreased so as to give a rise in blood pressure of between 30 and 50 mm of mercury. The intervening doses of the assayed preparation are varied at random so as to obtain the following responses: 2 responses approximately one-fifth less than, 2 approximately equal to, and 2 approximately one-fifth greater than the responses to the immediately adjacent doses of standard. If the high dose of the unknown has been properly selected the maximum rise will not materially exceed 60 mm. The kymograph record of a typical assay is reproduced in Fig. 419.

Recording Mercury Manometer—A specially constructed manometer is described in the USP XVII, page 824, for recording blood pressure during biological assays. A drawing and dimensions are also provided.

Calculation of Results—The calculation of the potency of an epinephrine assay and of the standard error of the assay are detailed in *Remington's Pharmaceutical Sciences*, 13th ed., 1965, p. 142.

Insulin

Insulin is a hormone secreted by *beta* cells of the islet tissue of the pancreas. Structurally, insulin is composed of two polypeptide chains (A and B) having a total molecular weight of approximately 6000. The

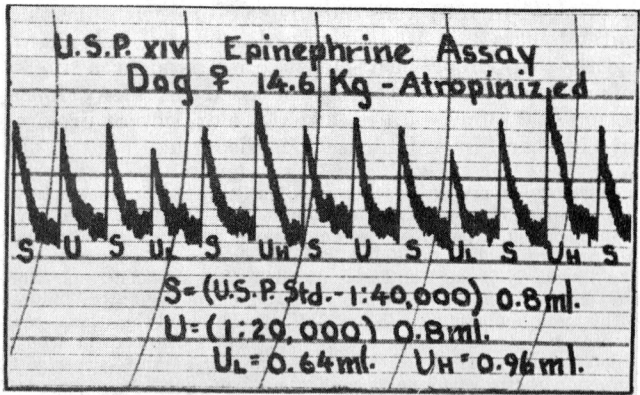

Fig. 419. Kymograph record (ink recording) of blood pressure response in epinephrine assay (courtesy, LaWall & Harrisson).

A chain, comprising 21 amino acids, is linked by two disulfide (—S—S—) bridges to the B chain, composed of 30 amino acids. Although there are some variations in the amino acid sequence and immunological specificity of insulins isolated from different animal species, they have fundamentally similar biological activities.

Since the isolation of insulin by Banting and Best in 1922, the hormone has constituted the keystone of the therapeutic control of diabetes mellitus. Insulin used for medicinal purposes is prepared by extraction of the pancreas obtained from domestic animals. Accurate standardization of insulin preparations is essential inasmuch as discrepancies in the order of 10% from the required dose may result in severe adverse reactions in the diabetic patient. Inadequate insulin replacement therapy may be associated with the appearance of any of the characteristic symptoms of diabetes mellitus including ketoacidosis and diabetic coma; overdosage may result in marked hypoglycemic reactions.

Insulin Zinc Suspension USP, *Extended Insulin Zinc Suspension USP*, and *Prompt Insulin Zinc Suspension USP* are not subject to biological assay, whereas *Insulin Injection USP*, *Isophane Insulin Suspension USP*, *Protamine Zinc Insulin Suspension USP*, and *Globin Zinc Insulin Injection USP* are standardized on the basis of biological assay. Briefly the assay is based on a comparison between the potencies of the unknown and the standard preparation in lowering the blood sugar level of intact rabbits following subcutaneous injection.

In addition to the quantitative bioassay procedures a qualitative identification test, which also depends on hypoglycemic activity, is described for these preparations. The test is performed by demonstrating that the convulsions induced in rabbits by subcutaneous injection of high doses of the preparation are relieved by the intravenous injection of dextrose solution (refer to the section on *Identification Tests*, page 644).

Insulin preparations are subject to the regulations of the Federal Food, Drug and Cosmetic Act, which requires certification by the Food and Drug Administration (FDA) of each lot marketed. Many of the tests and criteria employed by the FDA follow closely those specified by the USP. In addition to the biological assays, certain chemical and bacteriological tests must be performed to meet the requirements for certification by the FDA. The Act (particularly Section 506) and regulations thereunder should be consulted for specific details concerning the steps that must be followed in obtaining such certification.

Insulin Injection USP is available as solutions containing 40, 80, 100, and 500 USP Insulin Units per ml. Globin Zinc Insulin Injection and Protamine, Isophane, and Insulin Zinc Suspensions provide either 40 or 80 units/ml. A variation of not more than 5% from the labeled potency is permitted. The assays are described separately below. For details in respect to the official method of determining blood sugar and the preparation of certain reagents used in the assays, reference should be made to the monographs of the seven preparations in the USP.

Insulin Injection

Standard—The activity of the USP Zinc-Insulin Crystals Reference Standard is stated on the label in terms of USP Insulin Units/mg. A Standard solution containing 40 units/ml is prepared by dissolving an appropriate amount of the crystals in an aqueous solution of phenol or cresol (0.1 to 0.25% *w/v*) and glycerin (1.4 to 1.8% *w/v*) plus sufficient hydrochloric acid to bring the pH of the final solution to between 2.5 and 3.5. It should be stored in a cold place above freezing temperature and may be used for 6 months from the time of preparation. At the time of the assay two dilutions of the standard solution are made which contain 1.0 and 2.0 units/ml, respectively, using as the diluent a solution similar to that prepared above in respect to phenol or cresol and glycerin contents and final pH. On the basis of assumed potency, two dilutions of the preparation to be assayed are prepared in the same manner as the standard dilutions. The dose of the dilutions to be injected is selected on the basis of trial or experience so that the volume of the dilution injected will be between 0.30 and 0.50 ml. For each animal the volume of the standard dilution should be the same as that of the sample dilution.

Assay Procedure—Healthy rabbits weighing at least 1.8 Kg should be kept in the laboratory under standard conditions for at least a week. On the day preceding the assay, approximately 20 hours before the assay is to be conducted, each rabbit is provided with an amount of food which will be consumed within 6 hours. The same schedule is followed before each test day. During the actual assay all food and water is withheld until after the final blood samples are taken. In order to minimize the error introduced by individual variation, the assay is conducted along the lines of a cross-over test, ie, the response of each animal to both standard and unknown is determined. This is accomplished by arbitrarily dividing the rabbits into 4 groups containing not less than six rabbits each, and making injections according to the following schedule, with an interval of not more than 1 week between injections. It is important that the rabbits be kept in individual cages during each assay and that all unnecessary excitement be avoided, since the latter may produce an epinephrine hyperglycemia which will distort the results accordingly. Bleeding is best accomplished by placing the animal in a specially constructed box which permits only the head to protrude. A small artery clip is placed proximally over the marginal ear vein and dilation may be enhanced by lightly rubbing the surface with a xylol-soaked cotton pledget. The vein is quickly punctured with a sharp number 20 needle or pointed scalpel blade and slightly more than 1 ml of blood is allowed to run directly into a small test tube containing about 3 mg of sodium oxalate. Hemorrhage is stopped by removing the clip and applying light pressure over the site of puncture. Blood sugar determinations are conducted preferably by a procedure that depends on the reduction of ferricyanide and that may be automated (see USP for details).

Plan of Injections

Group	First injection	Second injection (not more than 1 week later)
1	Standard dilution 2	Sample dilution 1
2	Standard dilution 1	Sample dilution 2
3	Sample dilution 2	Standard dilution 1
4	Sample dilution 1	Standard dilution 2

After collecting the control samples, the rabbits are injected subcutaneously in accordance with the above schedule. Blood samples are again taken at 1 and 2½ hours after injection. If the blood sugar values indicate that the dose used for the standard is satisfactory, the assay is repeated not more than one week later, using the dilution schedule for the second injection.

Calculation of Potency—The data observed in a typical assay, the calculation of potency, and of the confidence limit is given in the chapter on *Statistics*.

Protamine Zinc Insulin Suspension

Both Protamine Insulin Suspension and Globin Zinc Insulin Injection are assayed by modifications of the method used for Insulin Injection; the chief differences in the procedures are introduced to take into account the slower onset and greater prolongation of hypoglycemia which they produce.

Standard—A Standard suspension is extemporaneously prepared from USP Zinc-Insulin Crystals Reference Standard, USP Protamine Reference Standard, zinc oxide, hydrochloric acid and dibasic sodium phosphate, glycerin, and phenol or cresol in accordance with the specific directions given in the USP. The final suspension should have a reaction of between pH 7.2 and 7.5 and should contain either 40 or 80 USP Insulin Units/ml according to the potency of the preparation to be assayed. It may be used on the third day and up to 6 months thereafter.

Preparation of Sample for Assay—Neither the standard, prepared as described above, nor the unknown sample is diluted for injection. Each rabbit receives the same volume of standard as of unknown in the crossover test.

Assay Procedure—The same directions apply here as in the assay of Insulin Injection in respect to the rabbits used, the starvation period prior to the assay, the use of individual cages, the size of the dose selected, the techniques of injection and blood sampling, and the determination of blood sugar values. Otherwise, there are several important differences in the assay procedure. The rabbits are divided into two similar groups of at least 6 each; after initial blood samples have been taken, one group is injected subcutaneously with the Standard preparation, the other with the assumed same dosage of unknown. The dose of Standard used should be such that it produces an average fall in blood sugar at the time of the final bleeding to 70 to 95% of the average initial value, but does not cause convulsions in more than 25% of the rabbits. Following injection, at least 3 blood samples are taken at intervals of 1½ to 3 hours, extending over a total period of at least 9 hours. One week later the groups are reversed and the animals which originally received the Standard are injected with the same volumes of the unknown preparation and *vice versa*. A similar series of blood samples is taken at intervals equivalent to those used previously.

Calculation of Results—The blood sugar concentrations of all rabbits are averaged for each interval at the time when the standard was injected. Similar averages are obtained for each bleeding period at the time of the administration of the unknown preparation and the latter averages are subtracted from the equivalent ones found for the standard. If the following criteria are met, the unknown preparation is considered to be of satisfactory potency:

1. The difference between each pair of averages so obtained must be no greater than ±6 mg/100 ml, with the exception of the final samples where the averages may differ by as much as 8.
2. When the differences are averaged (excluding the preinjection values), taking into account the sign of each, the figure obtained must not exceed ±3.

Globin Zinc Insulin Injection

The assay procedure and potency requirements are identical with those for Protamine Zinc Insulin Injection with the exception of certain minor details. The Standard preparation of globin zinc insulin is prepared with USP Globin Reference Standard in place of

the Protamine, and is adjusted to a final pH of 3.4 to 3.8. The dose selected should produce the same fall in blood sugar (to 70 to 95% of the initial value) at 6 to 8 hours after injection, the same number of blood samples are taken over a period of not less than 9 hours. In the calculation of results, the average values obtained up to and including 5 hours after injection must not differ by more than 6 mg/100 ml, and at subsequent bleeding times by not more than 8 mg/100 ml.

Isophane Insulin Suspension

The biological assay of Isophane Insulin Suspension is conducted in a manner similar to that indicated for Insulin Injection with the exception of the several modifications set forth below. In this assay the preparation is first centrifuged and the assay conducted on the supernatant liquid. Two dilutions of the standard solution are made containing 0.1 and 0.2 USP Insulin Units/ml respectively. Two sample dilutions are made employing the same diluents and which may be expected to contain 0.5 and 1.0 USP Insulin Units/-ml assuming that the supernatant liquid contains the maximum limit of free insulin activity. Each group in the assay may consist of three rabbits.

Glucagon

Glucagon, which has also been referred to by the cumbersome but biochemically descriptive designation *hyperglycemic glycogenolytic factor* (HGF), is a polypeptide hormone secreted by the alpha cells of the pancreatic islets of Langerhans. It is obtained commercially from the pancreas glands of domestic animals used for food by man. Glucagon for Injection USP is a mixture of the hydrochlorides of glucagon with one or more suitable, dry diluents.

Parenteral administration of glucagon in persons with adequate hepatic glycogen stores elicits a prompt elevation of the blood-sugar level. This reaction constitutes the basis of the primary therapeutic indication (ie, termination of hypoglycemic coma) and biological assay of Glucagon for Injection.

The bioassay of Glucagon for Injection fundamentally involves comparison of the blood-sugar elevation induced in healthy, fasted, anesthetized cats by intravenous injection of alternating doses of suitable dilutions of the test sample and USP Glucagon Reference Standard. Specific procedures relating to preparation of assay dilutions of test sample and reference standard, sequence of injection and blood sampling, and calculation of potency are detailed in the USP.

Parathyroid

The parathyroid hormone plays an important physiological role in the regulation of calcium metabolism. Although the precise amino acid sequence has not been elucidated as yet, the biologically active principle of the parathyroid gland appears to be a low-molecular-weight (about 9000) protein.

The only official parathyroid preparation, *Parathyroid Injection* USP, is prepared from an aqueous extract of the parathyroid glands of domestic animals, and possesses a potency of not less than 100 USP. Parathyroid Units/ml. By definition, 100 units produces an average rise in the serum calcium of normal dogs of 1 mg/100 ml within 16 to 18 hours after subcutaneous administration.

Assay Procedure and Potency Calculation—The official method for the determination of serum calcium in the assay is to be found under Parathyroid Injection in the USP.

At least 10 mature, healthy male dogs which must weigh between 8 and 16 Kg, no two differing by more than 5 Kg, are used in the assay. They should be maintained under similar dietary and environmental conditions and should be trained for venipuncture. The latter condition is particularly important inasmuch as excessive excitement at the time when blood samples are taken will in itself cause a rise in serum calcium. The site of puncture is a matter of personal preference; the external jugular and superficial fore and hind leg veins have all been found satisfactory. A clean, dry syringe with a sharp-pointed number 22 needle should be used. While hemostasis is maintained by light pressure applied proximally, a sample of at least 10 ml should be withdrawn under a minimum of negative pressure so as to avoid hemolysis. It is immediately transferred to a centrifuge tube, allowed to clot, and the clot freed from the side of the tube with a glass rod. After centrifuging and removing the clear supernatant serum, its calcium content is determined as directed.

By preliminary trial a dose of the preparation is selected which is expected to produce a rise in serum calcium of between 2.0 and 5.0 mg/100 ml in the dogs used. It should be noted that the assay may not be repeated with a given animal without a lapse of at least 4 weeks since the previous assay. After taking control blood samples, each dog is injected subcutaneously with the selected dose, and 16 to 18 hours later a second series of samples is obtained. If the average rise in serum calcium for the entire group of dogs is not less than 1.0 mg/100 ml serum/ml of preparation injected, the potency of the material is satisfactory.

Posterior Pituitary

Extracts of the posterior lobe of the neurohypophysis when injected into responsive animals, may exert a variety of pharmacodynamic effects including a rise in blood pressure, contraction of uterine smooth muscle, (oxytocic effect), an increased renal tubular reabsorption of water (antidiuresis), and milk-ejection (galactorrhea) in the lactating mammary gland. Although there is no conclusive agreement on the number of different hormones elaborated by the neurohypophysis, two distinct active principles have been separated from extracts of this structure (Kamm and associates, 1928). These are *oxytocin*, which possesses primarily oxytocic and galactorrheic activities, and *vasopressin*, which exhibits predominantly pressor and antidiuretic activities. Both of these principles are octapeptides; the amino acid sequences of these fractions obtained from several animal species have been determined and corresponding octapeptide amides have been synthesized.

Posterior Pituitary (powder) and Posterior Pituitary Injection, which are prepared from the posterior lobe of the pituitary gland of domestic animals, contain oxytocic and vasopressor principles in varying amounts.

Each mg of Posterior Pituitary NF possesses an oxytocic activity equivalent to 1 USP Posterior Pituitary Unit,* the permissible lower limit of assayed potency being 0.85 Unit/mg. Although the standardization of Posterior Pituitary is based on *oxytocin* content, the major therapeutic use of this preparation (ie, control of diabetes insipidus) depends primarily on the *vasopressin* (antidiuretic hormone) content.

Each ml of Posterior Pituitary Injection NF possesses an oxytocic activity equivalent to 10 USP Posterior Pituitary Units (permissible range, 8.5 to 12 Units), and not less than 5 Units of vasopressin. Since the separate fractions (oxytocin and vasopressin) are available in purified form, Posterior Pituitary Injection, which represents a mixture of the active principles, is used relatively infrequently.

Oxytocin Injection USP possesses, in each ml, an oxytocic activity equivalent to 10 USP Posterior Pituitary Units (permissible range of assayed potency is 8.5 to 12 Units). Oxytocin Injection is subject to a maximum allowable limit of pressor activity, corresponding to not more than 0.02 USP Posterior Pituitary Unit for each USP Unit of oxytocic activity found in the assay.

Each ml of Vasopressin Injection USP possesses a pressor activity equivalent to 20 USP Posterior Pituitary Units, the permissible lower and upper limits being 17 and 24 Units, respectively. The oxytocic activity of Vasopressin Injection may not exceed that which corresponds to 1.2 USP Posterior Pituitary Units for each 20 USP Units of pressor activity found in the assay.

The oxytocic activity of Posterior Pituitary and Posterior Pituitary Injection was formerly assayed on the basis of contractions induced in the isolated guinea pig uterus. Although unrelated to the therapeutic objective of oxytotic agents, the transient decrease in blood pressure elicited in the anesthetized chicken by intravenous injection of posterior pituitary extracts provides a criterion for biological assay which is more reproducible, convenient, and specific for oxytocin. The *Chicken Vasodepressor Method* constitutes the current assay for the primary biological activity of Posterior Pituitary NF, Posterior Pituitary Injection USP, and Oxytocin Injection USP. However, due to interference with the vasodepressor assay by a predominance of pressor substances, the small but permissible amount of oxytocic activity in Vasopressin Injection USP is determined on the basis of the *Guinea-Pig Uterus Method*.

The potency of Vasopressin Injection USP is standardized on the basis of the *Rat Vasopressor Method*. Briefly the assay involves measurement of the blood-pressure elevation produced by intravenous injection of the hormone preparation in anesthetized male rats previously treated with phenoxybenzamine (Dibenzyline—SK&F). Replacement therapy in the treatment of diabetes insipidus constitutes the major use of Vasopressin (Injection and Tannate). Since pressor and antidiuretic activities are properties of the same molecule, potency may be determined on the basis of blood-pressure-elevating (ie, vasopressor) activity, although the inappropriately named *vasopressin* is no longer recommended for use as a *pressor* agent. The small but permissible limit of pressor activity in Oxytocin Injection USP is determined also by the *Rat Vasopressor Method*.

Standard—USP Posterior Pituitary Reference Standard is used for all of the potency assays and limiting tests cited above. A standard reference solution is prepared by heating with continuous, gentle shaking in a boiling water bath for 5 minutes, a 250-ml flask containing 50 to 100 mg, accurately weighed, of USP Posterior Pituitary Reference Standard and 1 ml of dilute glacial acetic acid (1 in 400) for each mg of powder. The flask is cooled with running water, the contents are filtered and the filtrate is sealed in hard-glass ampuls which are then heated in flowing steam for 20 minutes on each of three successive days. This stock solution, which is equivalent to 2 Units of oxytocic activity and 1.75 Units of vasopressin activity/ml, is stored in a refrigerator and may be used for as long as 6 months. On the day of the assay a primary test dilution is prepared by adding sufficient isotonic sodium chloride solution to a measured volume of stock solution so that the resulting standard preparation contains a known activity in the range of 0.1 to

---

* One USP Posterior Pituitary Unit represents the potency of 0.5 mg of USP Posterior Pituitary Reference Standard.

0.4 USP Posterior Pituitary Units/ml, the concentration being indicated by the determination of the sensitivity of the animal preparation.

Preparation of Samples for Assay—Posterior Pituitary is prepared for assay by placing about 50 mg, accurately weighed, in a 250-ml flask and proceeding as described in preparation of the Standard solution. The filtrate is used in the assay. At the time of assay the unknown preparation is diluted to suitable concentrations with isotonic sodium chloride solution.

The Chicken Vasodepressor Method

Assay Procedure—A young adult chicken weighing between 1 and 2.5 Kg (White Leghorns have been found satisfactory) is anesthetized by the intravenous injection of approximately 180 mg of sodium phenobarbital/Kg and prepared for kymographic recording of the blood pressure by means of a mercury manometer of thin bore or a standardized aneroid manometer so adjusted that each mm change represents no more than 2 mm of mercury. The pressure is recorded from the ischiatic (popliteal) artery which is cannulated by a medium bore needle, after tying off the afferent branches for about 2 cm; 8.5% sodium citrate is a suitable anticoagulant for filling the recording system. Injections are made via the crural or brachial vein.

The standard solution is 0.2 Unit/ml and the trial dose of dilution producing a precipitous, evanescent fall in blood pressure of 20 to 40 mm of mercury is determined. If the dose required to produce this effect falls outside the limits of 0.15 and 0.50 ml at any time during the test, the dilution must be adjusted accordingly. This constant dose of the standard dilution is given several times at intervals of 1.5 to 5 minutes; if the intensity of response begins to decrease, the animal must be discarded.

The comparison between the preparation to be assayed and the standard is now undertaken. The former is diluted with isotonic saline solution to the same approximate potency as the standard dilution. At this point the selected dose of the standard dilution is given and repeated at regular intervals of 3 to 10 minutes thereafter. At the mid-point (1.5 to 5 minutes) of the time interval between successive, equal doses of the standard preparation, one of two doses of the assay solution is injected. These doses are selected on the basis of the assumed potency so that their geometric mean corresponds approximately to the dose of the standard solution and the lesser of the two doses is expected to produce a response approximately one-fifth less than that of the standard solution. Thus, three or more sets of four doses are given in which each set consists of the low and high doses of the assay solution and two doses of the standard solution. The low and high doses are randomized within each set. The calculation of potency of the assayed preparation and the confidence limits of the assay are detailed in the NF.

The Rat Vasopressor Method

Assay Procedure—About 18 hours prior to the assay a male rat weighing 275 to 325 Gm is injected intravenously with a solution of phenoxybenzamine hydrochloride, 10 ml/Kg of body weight. The solution is made by dissolving 5 mg of phenoxybenzamine hydrochloride in 0.1 ml of alcohol, acidifying with one drop of hydrochloric acid, and diluting to 5 ml with saline TS.

Solutions of the standard and assay preparations are prepared in saline TS to represent 0.2 USP Posterior Pituitary Units/ml. On the day of the assay the rat is anesthetized and the trachea cannulated for artificial respiration. Blood pressure is recorded from the carotid artery using a mercury manometer and a solution of heparin sodium (1000 units/ml) in the cannula. Injections of the standard and assay dilutions are made through a cannula in either a femoral or jugular vein.

The dose of the standard solution which produces consistent blood pressure elevations of 20 to 70 mm of mercury when injected at intervals of 12 to 15 minutes is determined by trial. From these observations two doses (S_1 and S_2) are selected which are in the ratio of approximately 2 to 3. After a similar trial two doses (U_1 and U_2) of the assay preparation are selected. The doses are injected in random pairs. The sequence of doses within each pair is as follows:

Pair 1. S_2, U_1
Pair 2. S_1, U_2
Pair 3. U_2, S_1
Pair 4. U_1, S_2

Calculation of Potency—The calculation of potency of the assayed preparation and the confidence limits of the assay are detailed in the USP.

The Guinea-Pig Uterus Method

Assay Procedure—The apparatus employed consists principally of a water bath in which are fixed the fluid reservoir and an isolated organ chamber of approximately 100-ml capacity; the bath is maintained constant to 0.1°C at a temperature between 37° and 38°C by a suitable thermostatically controlled heater and motor-driven stirring device. In suspending the uterine horn in the chamber, the upper end is connected with an isotonic writing lever which records the contractions on a moving kymograph paper. The lower end of the horn can be fixed conveniently to an adjustable oxygen inlet tube by means of a small platinum hook fused into the latter. If several chambers are placed in the bath, as many determinations can be run simultaneously. The bathing fluid used is Locke-Ringer's solution. It is convenient to prepare a 20-fold stock concentrate of the chlorides of this solution. This concentrate can be diluted and the proper amount of glucose and sodium bicarbonate added at the time of setting up the assay.

A healthy virgin female guinea pig not in estrus, weighing between 175 and 350 Gm, is decapitated, the uterus removed and divided into two horns by saggital bisection and a horn suspended in the chamber for recording contractions as described above. Oxygen is bubbled through the chamber continuously, and the tension on the muscle lever is adjusted so as to induce maximal relaxation without over-stretching. It may require as long as an hour for complete relaxation to take place, at which time spontaneous contractions should be minimal. A dose of the standard solution, diluted with 0.9% sodium chloride solution so that 0.5 ml will produce a submaximal contraction (about 1:1000 dilution), is then "injected" into the chamber and the response observed. If the lever does not rise to the peak of contraction within 2 or 3 minutes, it indicates that the tension on the organ is probably too great and appropriate adjustment should be made. Once the official assay has been started, the tension must be left unchanged. After the peak of contraction is reached, the lever should begin to fall rapidly. When it has come down sufficiently to clearly indicate that it has passed the peak, the fluid in the chamber is quickly flushed out and fresh Locke-Ringer's solution admitted from the reservoir in the same bath. A strip should continue to relax until it reaches the same base line, when another "injection" of the drug is introduced into the chamber. After the uterine horn has been found to respond uniformly to submaximal doses of the standard, the activity of the unknown preparation should be estimated by finding the amount of the dilution, prepared in accordance with the aforementioned directions, which produces a rise slightly less than that elicited by a given dose of standard. When this is known, an official assay is attempted and must consist of the following: four submaximal, approximately equal contractions produced by alternate doses of constant amounts of standard and unknown, followed by a third dose of standard, 25% greater than that given previously (Fig. 420). If the difference between the contractions produced by the two equal doses of the Standard is less than half the difference between the lower of these contractions and the contraction produced by the 25% increased dose of standard, the former are considered submaximal. If the responses to the preparation to be assayed do not exceed those following the standard, and the equivalence conforms with the maximum limit stated above, the oxytocic requirement is met.

In spite of the apparent simplicity of the procedure, it sometimes requires several attempts before a satisfactory assay is obtained, because of the variable responses given by many uterine horn preparations.

Adrenal Cortex Injection

Adrenal Cortex Injection is a sterile solution in alcohol and water for injection containing a mixture of the endocrine principles derived from the cortex of adrenal glands of healthy domestic animals used for food by man. The multiple physiologic properties of the adrenal cortical steroids provide the basis for various biological assay procedures. One of the principal metabolic actions of the glucocorticoids was adopted as the criterion for the biological assay of Adrenal Cortex Injection, namely the ability to promote the formation of liver glycogen in the fasting adrenalectomized rat. This method is well standardized, has a high degree of reproducibility and adequate sensitivity. The standard employed in this assay is USP Hydrocortisone Reference Standard.

Adrenal Cortex Injection is no longer recognized in the official compendia, however the standardization procedure (based on that detailed in the NF XII) is

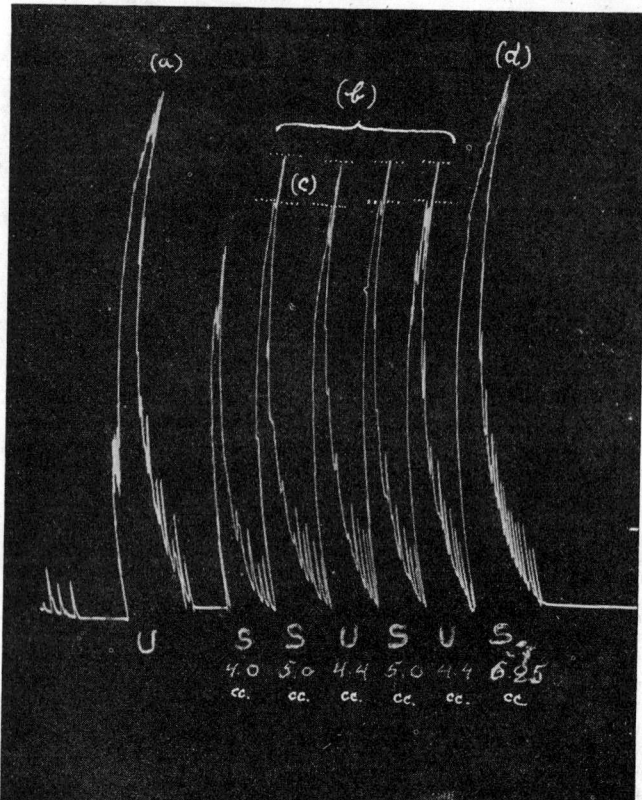

Fig. 420. Pituitary assay tracing using isolated guinea-pig uterus for oxytocic activity: (*a*) **experimental contractions;** (*b*) **4 assay contractions, alternate doses of standard and unknown;** (*c*) **washing contraction, not taken into consideration;** (*d*) **final dose of standard 25% greater than previous dose, to prove uterus is working under its ceiling response (courtesy, LaWall & Harrisson).**

described briefly inasmuch as it represents a pharmacologic assay procedure coupled with a chemical quantitation of an endogenous substrate (ie, glycogen).

Assay Procedure—A stock solution of USP Hydrocortisone Reference Standard is prepared in alcoholic saline TS to contain 100 mcg of hydrocortisone in each ml. From this solution a dilution is prepared with saline TS so that the amount of USP Hydrocortisone Reference Standard in 4.0 ml may be expected to result in an average increase in liver glycogen of approximately 70 mg. A second dilution is prepared by diluting 3 volumes of the first dilution with 2 volumes of saline TS. The alcohol concentration of the sample to be assayed is reduced to 5% or less and two dilutions are prepared in the manner described for the reference standard.

The NF directs that strains of albino rats of proved sensitivity and response to hydrocortisone be utilized in this assay. Sources of laboratory animals have been mentioned earlier in this chapter. Male rats weighing between 140 and 160 Gm each are selected and under ether anesthesia are bilaterally adrenalectomized via the lumbar route. The animals are marked for identification, weighed, and placed on a high protein diet with sodium chloride solution (1 to 100) as drinking water. On the fourth day after adrenalectomy food is withheld and on the fifth day, before injections are started, the saline drinking water is removed. The rats are again weighed and any animal showing a gain or loss in weight of greater than 20% of his original weight is discarded. On the fifth day after adrenalectomy the rats are assembled at random into four or more groups of at least five rats each having equal numbers in the groups assigned to the two test dilutions of each preparation. Each rat is injected subcutaneously with 1.0 ml of the assigned test dilution and using different sites for each injection, the injection is repeated 2, 4, and 6 hours later.

Within 1.5 to 2.5 hours after the last injection the rats are anesthetized with phenobarbital sodium and the entire liver of each animal is excised and digested in hot potassium hydroxide solution. The glycogen content of the liver of each rat is determined by a titration procedure.

Diet for Assay—This diet is prepared by mixing the constituents in the order listed, followed by storage in a tight container until used. The compositions of the diet and the salt mixture used in the diet are specified in the NF XII.

Corticotropin

Corticotropin Injection is a sterile preparation of the principle or principles derived from the anterior lobe of the pituitary of mammals used for food by man, which exert a tropic influence on the adrenal cortex.

Corticotropin acts on the cortex of the adrenal gland to stimulate the secretion of adrenocortical steroid hormones, predominantly hydrocortisone. Secretory activity is reflected by a reduction in the concentration of ascorbic acid in the adrenal gland. The USP biological assay is essentially that devised by Sayers and his associates[3] and is based on the extent of depletion of ascorbic acid in the adrenal glands of the hypophysectomized rat.

Corticotropin Injection labeled for intramuscular or subcutaneous administration is biologically assayed by a method (described in subsequent paragraphs) involving *subcutaneous* injection into the test animal. The procedure for the assay of the potency of Corticotropin Injection labeled for intravenous administration only is similar to the above except that the preparation is injected *intravenously* into the test animal. Corticotropin Injection may be labeled for administration either subcutaneously or intramuscularly or intravenously provided the ratio of the observed potency by *subcutaneous* assay and that by *intravenous* assay is not less than 0.80 and not more than 1.25.

Repository Corticotropin Injection is corticotropin in a solution of partially hydrolyzed gelatin. The gelatin menstruum retards the absorption of corticotropin at the site of intramuscular injection thereby prolonging the period of therapeutic effectiveness. The biological assay of Repository Corticotropin Injection is identical with that specified in the *subcutaneous* method for Corticotropin Injection.

Sterile Corticotropin Zinc Hydroxide Suspension represents corticotropin adsorbed on a suspension of zinc hydroxide. Following intramuscular administration, the absorption of the preparation is delayed in comparison to Corticotropin Injection. In preparation for biological assay, sufficient 0.1 N hydrochloric acid is added to Sterile Corticotropin Zinc Hydroxide Suspension to effect complete solution. Using this solution, the assay is identical with that specified in the *subcutaneous* method under Corticotropin Injection.

Assay (Subcutaneous Method) Procedure—The standard preparation is made by dissolving sufficient USP Corticotropin Reference Standard in 2.5 ml gelatin TS to make a concentration of 2.0 USP Corticotropin Units/ml. Then using gelatin TS as a diluent, three standard dilutions are made so that the respective concentrations of corticotropin constitute a geometric series such as 1:2:4 or 1:3:9 and so that the quantity of corticotropin in each 0.5 ml lies within the range of 10 to 300 milliunits. The assay preparation is prepared in the same manner and concentrations corresponding to those of the standard.

Healthy rats of the same but either sex are anesthetized with ether and the hypophysis exposed to permit removal by means of gentle suction through a fine-tipped glass tube. Between 16 and 48 hours after the operation six equally-sized groups of rats weighing 80 to 180 Gm are selected. The number of rats selected for each group must be in multiples of 6 and no rat may be more than 30% heavier than the lightest. One of the six test dilutions (3 standard, 3 assay) is assigned at random to each group.

All rats are injected subcutaneously with their assigned test dilutions and returned to their cages. Three hours after the injection the animals are anesthetized and their adrenal glands removed taking care to free the glands of adhering tissue. Each pair of glands is promptly weighed to the nearest 0.1 mg. The weighed glands from each rat are placed in separate 8-ml portions of metaphosphoric acid solution (1 in 40) to preserve and extract the ascorbic acid, then comminuted by a suitable method such as grinding with a portion of washed sand. The determination of ascorbic acid is carried out by the procedure specified in the USP.

The observed concentration of ascorbic acid in the adrenal glands of each rat is tabulated and the potency calculated on the basis of dosage-response lines.

The assay for the injections intended for intravenous use is conducted along similar lines except that saline TS is used in preparing the test dilutions. In addition the quantity of hormone in each 0.5 ml is reduced to 1 to 10 milli-units. All rats are injected intravenously and sacrificed 1 hour later for the removal of the adrenal glands.

The USP specifies an upper limit on the permissible vasopressin activity of Corticotropin Injection and Repository Corticotropin Injection; the *Rat Vasopressor Method*, described in the section on *Posterior Pituitary*, is employed for determination of this activity.

Estrogenic Substances

A large number of naturally occurring and synthetic compounds possessing estrogenic activity are described in Chapter 55, *Hormones*, page 955. Among the estrogenic substances included in the USP are: Conjugated Estrogens, Diethylstilbestrol, Estradiol Valerate, and Ethinyl Estradiol. Those recognized in the NF include: Benzestrol, Chlorotrianisene, Diethylstilbestrol Dipropionate, Estradiol, Estradiol Benzoate, Estradiol Cypionate, Estradiol Dipropionate, and Estrone. All of these estrogenic compounds, in the different dosage forms in which they are available, are assayed by chemical or spectrophotometric methods. Many of the bioassay procedures employed in the evaluation of the biological activity of estrogenic substances are based on changes in the vaginal mucosa of spayed (ovariectomized) rats induced by injection of the test material. No official bioassay for estrogenic activity is now recognized; a description of a representative assay is presented here as an example of an "all-or-none" (quantal) type of biological assay.

Reference Standards—There are two International Standards, Crystalline International Standard Estrone (10,000 International Estrone Units/mg) and Estradiol Benzoate (10,000 International Estradiol Benzoate Units/mg). Equivalent Reference Standards are prepared and distributed by the US Pharmacopeia Revision Committee. These two standards are used for comparison of the potencies of free and esterified preparations, respectively. Potencies are often referred to in Rat Units, one Rat Unit of Estrone being equivalent to approximately 10 International Units (1000 Rat Units/mg) and one Rat Unit of Estradiol Benzoate to approximately 1.67 International Units (6000 Rat Units/mg).

Assay Procedure—Healthy female rats raised under similar conditions are examined for normal estrus at approximately 8 weeks of age. This is done by taking a vaginal smear, using a cotton-covered toothpick or micro-pipet, and staining with methylene blue or hematoxylin-eosin. In anestrus, the only cells observed are leukocytes and occasional nucleated epithelial cells. During estrus, cornified epithelial cells predominate, with only occasional nucleated epithelial cells and leukocytes appearing rarely. Immediately before and after estrus, all gradations between these two pictures are seen. As the estrus cycle in rats is approximately one week, normal animals should show the typical changes of estrus if smears are taken daily for this period. All animals which appear normal are then ovariectomized under ether anesthesia, using aseptic technique. As each ovary is removed, a portion of the uterus as well as the attached Fallopian tube are removed to prevent regeneration. After ovariectomy, daily smears are again taken for two weeks. Animals showing estrus at this time are discarded.

A weighed amount of the appropriate Reference Standard is dissolved in alcohol and measured amounts of this solution are added to corn oil to give the desired final concentration. The oily solution is then heated to evaporate off the alcohol. Each animal is given one or two priming doses of 2 to 3 mcg (20 to 30 IU) of standard estrone in 0.2 ml by subcutaneous injection in the abdominal region. Smears are taken at periods of 48, 56, and 64 hours (in some instances also at 52 and 72 hours) after injection and only animals showing a positive response (estrus) at one or more of these times are used. A week is allowed to elapse between each priming dose.

The assay is performed one week following the priming dose or doses. Three dose levels, each employing 10 to 20 rats, are used for both standard and unknown, choosing middle-dose levels calculated to produce a 50% response (0.8 to 1.5 mcg of estrone or 0.16 to 0.22 mcg of estradiol benzoate). The actual response of the animals to the standard will vary with the season, the strain of animal, and the interpretation of the investigator. A second dose calculated to give a response under 20% and a third dose to give a response greater than 80%, constitute with the middle dose the three-dose levels. For con-

venience of statistical calculation and uniformity of response it is desirable to have all the doses in uniform logarithmic spacing. The same diluent is used for the unknown as for the standard, and the doses are given subcutaneously in two equal parts at approximately 7-hour intervals. At 48, 56, and 64 hours after the first injection, smears are taken and read.

Some laboratories also observe readings at 52 and 72 hr. With products where the action is prolonged or delayed (ie, Estradiol Benzoate) the 72-hour and even a 76-hour reading is desirable. All rats showing estrus, as described above, in any one smear are counted as positive; those showing anestrus in all smears are recorded as negative. For greater precision, the cross-over test should be performed one week later; the animals originally receiving the standard then receive the unknown and *vice versa*.

Animals can be used for successive assays at weekly intervals for a total of about 16 assays. In weeks that assays are not performed, priming doses of 1.5 to 2.0 mcg of standard estrone should be given.

Calculation of Potency and Standard Error—The treatment of data obtained in a typical three-level assay is presented in Chapter 11, *Statistics*, page 122, wherein both the probit method and angle Theta method of calculating potency and standard error are detailed. The calculations applicable to 2-dose and 4-dose assays are also presented in this section.

Testosterone

The biological assay described in this section is based upon the increase in weight of the seminal vesicles ("androgen-dependent" tissue) of castrated rats subsequent to the injection of the drug. This assay is considered here because of its representative nature, although Testosterone Cypionate USP, Testosterone Enanthate USP, Testosterone Propionate USP, Testosterone NF, and Methyltestosterone NF are assayed by chemical methods.

Preparation of Solutions for Assay—Testosterone Propionate Stock Solution is prepared by dissolving approximately 10 mg of USP Testosterone Propionate Reference Standard, accurately weighed, in 50 ml of alcohol. It is stored under refrigeration in a paraffin-sealed, glass-stoppered flask. A Testosterone Propionate Standard Solution is made up at the time of assay by adding an appropriate quantity of the stock solution to a portion of vegetable oil, measured by a calibrated syringe, mixing thoroughly, and removing the alcohol under a vacuum while heating on a water bath. The Testosterone Propionate content of the standard solution should be such that 0.2 ml administered to rats, as described below, will result in an increase in weight of the seminal vesicles to approximately 22 mg. A diluted Testosterone Propionate Standard Solution containing one-quarter of the Testosterone Propionate concentration of the standard solution is similarly prepared. Two dilutions in oil of the preparation to be assayed are made which correspond to the Testosterone contents of the standard dilutions, on the basis of the assumed potency. The four dilutions are designated as S_h, S_l, U_l, and U_h, respectively, the subscript letters signifying high and low doses.

Preparation of Animals—Inasmuch as approximately 40 castrated rats are required in conducting the assay, at least 60 should be prepared to assure sufficient survivors, and to allow for the injection of additional animals if necessary. At least two weeks prior to assay, the testes are removed from healthy male rats approximately 28 days old. Ether anesthesia is most satisfactory, and can be administered dropwise, using a gauze-covered wire mesh. Aseptic technique should be employed insofar as possible, ie, sterilizing the instruments, and painting the operative field with diluted iodine solution which is then removed with alcohol.

Assay Procedure—The castrated rats are divided into 4 approximately equal groups of about 10 each (the largest group must not exceed the smallest by more than 10%) and each group is administered one of the 4 dilutions described above. Every animal receives the same volume of dilution (0.20 ml), half of which is injected into the muscles of each hind leg; 72 hours after injection the animals are sacrificed and the sex glands exposed by a lower midline incision through the abdominal wall. The seminal vesicles consist of a pair of hook-shaped convoluted glands surrounding the bladder, along with the coagulating glands which lie along their concavities in the same capsules, and the two pairs of prostate glands. The connective tissue, connecting the tips of the seminal vesicles with the coagulating glands, is broken with 2 pairs of fine forceps, and the capsules are stripped off, carrying the coagulating glands with them. After dissecting away the prostate glands, each seminal vesicle is pinched off where it joins the ejaculatory duct, the 2 glands are washed with isotonic saline solution, blotted with filter paper, and their combined weight is taken to the nearest 0.5 mg as rapidly as possible.

Calculation of Potency and Standard Error—The sum of the weights of the seminal vesicles is obtained for each of the four injected groups, and the resulting figures are substituted for the symbols S_h, S_l, U_h, and U_l in the following equations:

$$V = U_h - S_h + U_l - S_l$$
$$W = U_h + S_h - U_l - S_l$$

$$P = \text{antilog} \frac{iV}{W}$$

$$i = \log_{10} \text{ of the ratio } \frac{\text{high dose}}{\text{low dose}}$$

$$\text{Potency (in mg/ml)} = P \times \text{Assumed potency of Assayed Preparation (in mg/ml)}$$

$$\text{Standard Error of the Assay (in mg/ml)} = \frac{1.15 \text{ Potency } iR}{kW} \sqrt{N\left(1 + \frac{V^2}{W^2}\right)}$$

R = the sum of the ranges of the weights, obtained by subtracting the smallest from the largest weights of the seminal vesicles, in each group, and adding the four differences.

N = the average number of rats in each group. The value of k is dependent upon N, and is obtained from the following table:

N	8	9	10	11	12	13	14
k	2.85	2.97	3.08	3.18	3.26	3.34	3.40
N		15	16	17	18	19	20
k		3.48	3.52	3.58	3.64	3.68	3.74

The assay is considered satisfactory if the standard error is no greater than 15% of the figure obtained for the potency. If it exceeds this limit, the assay must be repeated or a sufficient additional number of rats injected with both preparations to bring the error below the accepted maximum.

The potency obtained from the assay must not vary by more than 15% of the labeled potency to meet the requirements formerly provided by the USP XIV.

Tubocurarine Chloride Injection

Tubocurarine, typical of the *curariform drugs*, is a valuable adjuvant to general anesthesia because of the muscular relaxation it produces by depression of transmission at the neuromuscular junction. Since doses slightly in excess of the desired amount can result in respiratory paralysis, its accurate assay is of extreme importance. The alkaloid has been isolated in pure form and can be assayed chemically in this state. However, similar substances of variable pharmacological potency are often present and consequently a biological assay is necessary. Biological assay of the skeletal muscle paralyzing activity of Tubocurarine Chloride Injection is based on the amount required to produce temporary paralysis of the neck muscles, or "head drop," when administered by fractional, inter-mittent intravenous injection into unanesthetized rabbits.

Preparation of Solutions—A Standard Solution of USP Tubocurarine Chloride Reference Standard is prepared containing 0.30 mg/ml of distilled water, and is stored in a tight container in the cold. It can be used within 90 days of preparation. The preparation to be assayed is diluted with distilled water to approximately the same strength according to the expected potency.

Assay Procedure—The assay requires a total of at least 16 healthy rabbits weighing between 1.5 and 4.0 Kg, but of sufficient uniformity that the heaviest is not more than twice the weight of the lightest. The rabbits must have been kept on a uniform, unrestricted diet for at least one week prior to assay without weight loss. They may be used as often as once a day for assay, and if a period of 7 days has elapsed since any animal was last used, it must be primed by giving a "head-drop" dose.

The rabbits are divided into 2 equal groups, distributed between the standard and unknown preparations, and restrained in the prone position by tying down the legs. The assigned solution is injected by means of a hypodermic needle, inserted into the marginal ear vein and attached to the ear by means of adhesive tape, and connected through flexible tubing to a small-bore calibrated buret. Each animal receives 0.1 ml every 15 seconds. Doses must be given uniformly as the destruction and excretion rates of tubocurarine are rapid. "Head-drop" is manifested by the inability of the animal to lift its head in response to a light tap on the back, or to raise the head when it is placed on one cheek by the operator. Any animal which struggles vigorously during the procedure must be replaced. On the following day, a cross-over test is performed, in which rabbits, previously having received the standard, are given the unknown preparation, and *vice versa*.

Calculation of Potency—The calculation of the potency of the assayed preparation and determination of the confidence interval of the assay are detailed in the USP.

The assay for Dimethyl Tubocurarine Iodide Injection NF is similar to that outlined for Tubocurarine Chloride Injection, except that the standard solution for the former assay is prepared from NF Dimethyl Tubocurarine Iodide Reference Standard.

Vitamins

Chemical or spectrophotometric assay procedures are specified for all preparations of vitamin A and vitamin B_1 (thiamine) in the USP and NF, and all preparations containing vitamin D in the USP. The NF retains a biological assay for determination of vitamin D activity of Cod Liver Oil, Nondestearinated Cod Liver Oil, and Oleovitamin A and D. Descriptions of the formerly official biological assay methods for vitamins A and B_1 will be found in *Remington's Pharmaceutical Sciences*, 13th ed., pp. 1600–1602. Details of the biological method for the assay of vitamin D are presented in the section on General Tests of the NF, and were reviewed in *Remington's Pharmaceutical Sciences*, 13th ed., pp. 1602–1604.

Microbial Assays

As previously noted in this chapter, *biological assay* refers to measurement of the relative potency or activity of compounds by determining the amount required to produce a stipulated effect on a suitable test animal or organ under standard conditions. The experimental animals mentioned in specific test procedures described in the previous section include mice, rats, guinea pigs, rabbits, cats, dogs, and pigeons. In its broadest sense, however, a biological assay may involve observations or measurements of effects obtained in any form of living matter, plant or animal. The term *microbial* (contraction of microbiological) *assay* designates a type of biological assay, specifically, a biological assay performed with *microorganisms*, eg, bacteria, yeasts, and molds.

The principles involved in microbial assays are in general those which apply to assays utilizing higher forms of plant or animal life. One notable difference involves the relative size of the experimental population. In a typical bioassay procedure the response of each individual test animal is noted and the results obtained with a series of animals is subjected to statistical analysis to calculate mean activity, standard error, etc. In a typical microbial assay each evaluation is performed with a culture of microorganisms and the measurement represents the average response of an extremely large population of test organisms. In the case of most bioassays a linear relationship exists between the *log dose* and the response, whereas in most microbial assays there is a linear relationship between the *dose* and the response (within certain limits). The importance of this relationship in the evaluation of microbial assays is considered in Chapter 11, *Statistics*, page 148.

Vitamins

Microbiological procedures are available for the assay of Calcium Pantothenate, Niacinamide, and Vitamin B_{12} activity of Cyanocobalamin Co 57 Solution and Capsules, and Cyanocobalamin Co 60 Solution and Capsules.

A fundamental requirement in a microbial assay for the activity of a vitamin or amino acid (factor) is the inability of the test organism to synthesize the factor being assayed. Furthermore, the test organism must require the factor in question for normal growth, and should be sensitive to very small amounts of the required factor. For such microbial assays special media are prepared which are nutritionally complete in all respects except for the factor under study. Control tubes containing the suitable media inoculated with the test species exhibit no, or only minimal, growth. If the basic requirements specified above are satisfied, the growth response of the test organism is, within limits, proportional to the amount of factor added to the medium.

The extent of the growth response may be determined either turbidimetrically, spectrophotometrically, or by titration of the acid produced. The turbidity of the culture is proportional to the amount of microbial growth; the development of acidity also reflects quantitatively the growth response. Sufficient levels of reference standard are included to enable construction of a curve of response for each assay. The activity of an assay dilution is determined by interpolation from the standard curve.

Niacin or Niacinamide

The techniques and procedures used in the microbiological assay for niacin are common to many of the microbiological methods and a description of the niacin method will serve to give the pattern generally employed.

The Microorganism—In the case of niacin there has been adequate demonstration that the assay organisms employed metabolize only the forms of niacin that are available to the animal. The fact that some organisms are more limited than the animal in their ability to utilize niacin derivatives serves as basis for differentiating such compounds in biological materials. For example, *Lactobacillus plantarum* is able to utilize, in addition to the free niacin, niacinamide, nicotinuric acid, cozymase, and niacinamide nucleoside.

Although a number of microorganisms require niacin for their metabolic processes, and are unable to synthesize it for themselves, the acid-forming organism

L. plantarum is most widely used for assay purposes. It is nonpathogenic, easy to culture, and is affected to only a limited degree by stimulatory or inhibitory substances normally found in foods or pharmaceutical preparations containing niacin. It may be grown on a simple stab-culture medium containing gelatin, yeast extract, and glucose, and is cultured for use in the assay tubes by direct transfer to the liquid medium consisting of the basal assay medium containing an optimum amount of added niacin.

One important advantage of microbiological procedures is that only a minute quantity of a vitamin is needed to give a measurable response. For example, the range of niacin added to the series of standard tubes is 0.05 to 0.5 mcg/tube. Thus the niacin content of extremely small amounts of biological materials may be readily measured. Modifications utilizing microanalytical apparatus, and a lower range of vitamin additions have been described for blood and tissue analysis.

The Test Solution—The first step in the assay procedure is the preparation of the test solution of the material to be assayed. If the sample is a dry or semisolid material, the niacin is extracted by heating the sample in a measured volume of normal H_2SO_4 in an autoclave for 30 minutes. Liquid preparations are autoclaved 30 minutes after addition of the H_2SO_4 to give a concentration of one-normal. Although niacin is soluble in water, certain precursors, found particularly in cereals, are unavailable to the test organism unless hydrolyzed. Either acid or alkali is equally effective for the extraction but acid is preferred, owing to the possibility of hydrolysis of trigonelline in alkaline solution. Preparation of the test solution is completed by neutralizing with strong NaOH solution, then diluting to a volume that contains 0.1 mcg of niacin per ml. Further purification of the test solution is not ordinarily important since *L. plantarum* is relatively unaffected by substances that inhibit or stimulate other test organisms.

The Medium—The basal medium employed in a niacin assay is simple to prepare (see the NF XII) and with properly treated casein hydrolysate is otherwise nutritionally complete. A medium suitable for use in the assay of amino acids is prepared by replacement of the casein hydrolysate with an amino acid mixture, omitting in each instance the acid under assay. Both dehydrated complete media and dehydrated casein hydrolysates are available commercially and appear to be entirely satisfactory for assay purposes.

Details of the microbial assay procedure for niacin (including preparation of standard niacin solution, spectrophotometric determination of cell density, and calculation of the niacin content of the test samples) are specified in the section on General Tests of the NF.

Calcium Pantothenate

In the USP assay of Calcium Pantothenate, the turbidimetric procedure is followed, using *Lactobacillus plantarum*.

Vitamin B_{12} Activity

Determination of vitamin B_{12} activity requires special treatment of the material to be assayed in order that the vitamin may be made available to the test organism, which, in this case, is a culture of *Lactobacillus leichmannii*. The basal medium used is quite complex, being prepared as a mixture in solution, of a great variety of essential nutritional components. To one set of tubes containing this medium are added measured amounts of the material to be assayed, and to a corresponding second set are added measured amounts of the Standard Cyanocobalamin Solution. The tubes are inoculated with a small amount of culture of the test organism and then incubated. The extent of growth which has occurred is measured by determining light transmittance by means of a spectrophotometer. A concentration-response curve is drawn by plotting the transmittance for each level of the Standard Cyanocobalamin Solution against the concentrations in the respective tubes in terms of millimicrograms. The amount of vitamin B_{12} contained in the test solution is determined by proper interpolation of the observed values on the standard curve.

Antibiotics

The term antibiotic, as used in the USP and NF, designates a medicinal preparation containing a significant quantity of a chemical substance that is produced by a microorganism or artificially by synthesis and that has the capacity to inhibit or destroy microorganisms in dilute solution. Under the terms of the Federal Food, Drug and Cosmetic Act of 1938, as amended by Public Law 87–781, all antibiotics intended for use in man are subject to production and testing controls under federal supervision, including batch certification prior to distribution. For the purposes of administering the certification program, standards of potency and purity for antibiotics are established by the Food and Drug Administration in the form of regulations published from time to time in the *Federal Register*.

Since all of the antibiotics recognized in the USP and NF are subject to the provisions of the regulations, the latter determine the official standards. The federal regulations governing all aspects of antibiotic testing are extremely detailed and subject to periodic amendment; they should be consulted with regard to prescribed methods for the assay of individual antibiotics and their preparations.

In evaluation of the potency of antibiotic substances the measured effect is inhibition of the "growth" of a suitable strain of microorganisms, ie, prevention of the multiplication of the test organisms. The procedures employed in microbial assay of antibiotics may be divided into two broad classifications: The *Cylinder-Plate Method* and the *Turbidimetric Method*.

Cylinder-Plate Method

The Cylinder-Plate (Cup) Assay of antibiotic potency is based on measurement of the diameter of zones of microbial growth inhibition surrounding cylinders (cups) containing various dilutions of test compound, which are placed on the surface of a solid nutrient medium previously inoculated with a culture of a suitable organism. Inhibition produced by the test compound is compared with that produced by known concentrations of a Reference Standard.

Turbidimetric Method

The Turbidimetric Assay of antibiotic potency is based on inhibition of microbial growth as indicated by measurement of the turbidity (transmittance) of suspensions of a suitable microorganism in a fluid medium to which have been added graded amounts of the test compound. Changes in transmittance produced by the test compound are compared with those produced by known concentrations of reference material.

Biological Tests

In the following sections of this chapter are discussed those biological tests each of which has as its objective the qualitative determination of a specific characteristic of a biological product or of the container in which it is supplied (eg, transfusion assemblies). These tests are designed to determine with a high degree of certainty the absence or presence of a type of activity (antibacterial activity, pressor activity, etc), or quality (non-antigenicity, toxicity, etc), or constituent (depressor substances, pyrogen, etc). Animals are employed in some tests and microorganisms in others.

Several biological tests are reviewed in other parts of this text, eg, *Requirements for Injections, Sterility Tests*, etc. The tests below are arranged alphabetically.

Absorption from Injection Site

It is necessary to ascertain that the colloidal complex of ferric hydroxide and dextran (ie, Iron Dextran Injection) is absorbed essentially completely from intramuscular sites of injection. This is determined by injecting, in a precisely specified manner, a dose of 0.4 ml of Iron Dextran Injection per Kg of body weight, into the musculature of one leg of each of two rabbits. Seven days after the injection the animals are sacrificed, the injected area is dissected and examined grossly. The muscle tissue should evidence only slight discoloration; there should be no heavy black deposit of unabsorbed iron compounds.

Antibacterial Tests

Antiseptics, Disinfectants, Fungicides, and Germicides are tested for antibacterial activity by procedures specified in official *Methods of Analysis* of the Association of Official Analytical Chemists.

The terminology associated with antiseptic, germicide, etc. formerly was conflicting, but with the passage of the Food, Drug and Cosmetic Act of 1938 the meaning of these words has become more definite and unless label claims alter the meaning they may be defined as follows:

Antiseptic—The Federal Food, Drug and Cosmetic Act states: "The representation of a drug, in its labeling, as an antiseptic shall be considered to be a representation that it is a germicide, except in the case of a drug purporting to be, or represented as, an antiseptic for inhibitory use as a wet dressing, ointment, dusting powder, or such other use as involves prolonged contact with the body."

The term thus has in the main become limited to products employed upon living tissue and it may mean either a bactericide (germicide) or bacteriostatic agent depending upon the application, use, or directions.

Bactericide—An agent that kills both pathogenic and nonpathogenic bacteria.

Bacteriostat—An agent that prevents the growth or multiplication of both pathogenic and nonpathogenic bacteria.

Disinfectant—An agent which in the broad sense kills pathogenic microorganisms (viruses, rickettsiae, bacteria, yeasts, fungi). The term is probably more properly restricted to products which are commonly used to disinfect inanimate objects, and may by labeling be further restricted to pathogenic organisms.

Fungicide—An agent that kills both pathogenic and nonpathogenic fungi.

Fungistat—An agent which prevents the growth or multiplication of both pathogenic and nonpathogenic fungi.

Germicide—An agent which kills both pathogenic and nonpathogenic microorganisms, but it is often limited to the former. It is used to describe an agent for use on either animate or inanimate matter.

Current editions of the USP and NF do not include any preparations of the types defined above to which antibacterial tests are applied. Descriptions of the phenol coefficient test and other antimicrobial testing procedures will be found in *Remington's Pharmaceutical Sciences*, 13th ed., pp. 1608–1609.

Antigenic Value

A test for antigenic value is required for the official preparations containing toxoids. These preparations include *Diphtheria Toxoid*, *Tetanus Toxoid*, the combination of these two, the combination of these two with pertussis vaccine, and the *alum precipitated* and *aluminum hydroxide adsorbed* toxoids alone or in the same combinations.

For the plain toxoids, the test is performed by injecting subcutaneously a specified number of healthy guinea pigs, each meeting specified weight requirements, with a specified fraction of the total immunizing dose of the toxoid, and then, not more than 6 weeks later, subcutaneously injecting each animal with 10 MLD's of the specific test toxin. Not less than 80% of the animals survive for at least 10 days.

For the alum precipitated and the aluminum hydroxide adsorbed toxoids, no challenge is made, at the end of the period allowed for the development of antibodies, with toxin. Instead, the antitoxin content of the pooled sera obtained from the test animals is determined in reference to the NIH Standard Diphtheria Antitoxin. It should be not less than 2 units/ml.

Antimicrobial Agents

For those products that require the presence of an effective level of antimicrobial activity, the USP specifies several tests in order to demonstrate that the content of agent(s) present agrees with the amount claimed on the label and that this amount is sufficient to afford an adequate degree of activity. These tests and standards apply only to the product in the original, unopened container in which it was distributed by the producer. The tests depend upon the use of an inoculum consisting of a relatively large number of the specified microorganisms (*Candida albicans, Aspergillus niger, Escherichia coli, Pseudomonas aeruginosa* and *Staphylococcus aureus*) with a view to overcoming possible bacteriostatic or fungistatic effect of the agent under consideration. The section on General Tests of the USP should be consulted for details of the performance and interpretation of tests for the content and effectiveness of antimicrobial agents.

Bacterial Content

Under the title *Microbial Limit Tests*, the USP provides tests for estimating the number of viable aerobic microorganisms present and for determining freedom from certain microbial species in pharmaceutical articles of all kinds, from raw materials to finished forms.

Procedures for conducting tests for *Total Aerobic Microbial Count, Staphylococcus aureus, Pseudomonas aeruginosa, Salmonella* species, and *Escherichia coli* are given, as are also morphological characteristics of specific organisms cultured in various media, and formulas for 14 media. Special directions for preparing solutions of gelatin for microbial limit tests are also provided.

The value of these tests depends largely on the adequacy of a demonstration that test samples to which they are applied do not of themselves inhibit the multiplication, under the test conditions, of microorganisms that may be present. For this reason, samples to be tested should be inoculated with viable cultures of the aforementioned four microorganisms, prior to making tests for their presence, to determine if the samples have any inhibitory effect on the microorganisms.

For sampling, the USP directs that three 10-ml or 10-Gm samples, each of which represents a composite of 1-ml or 1-Gm portions taken from not less than 10 individual finished packages or from each of not more than 10 containers of bulk material shall be used.

Doubtful results are directed to be confirmed, for any of the procedures outlined, by performing retests on 25-Gm samples, rather than on the 10-Gm samples specified for the original test.

The term "growth" as used in these tests has the special meaning of denoting "the presence and presumed proliferation of viable microorganisms."

Bacteriological Purity Tests

Water USP and Purified Water USP are required to meet the regulations of the USPHS for potable water with respect to bacteriological purity.

Biological Adequacy Test

This test is designed to establish the nutritional completeness of *Protein Hydrolysate Injection* with regard to its content of essential amino acids.

This assay is comprised of several steps which may be divided as follows:

Step	Diet	Duration, days	Effect
A	Depletion diet and water	12	Loss in weight
B	Depletion diet and control nitrogen supplement in water	3	Gain in weight
C	Depletion diet and water	3	Loss in weight
D	Depletion diet and sample under test in water	5	Gain in weight

For the depletion and control periods a group of not less than 6 male rats 2 to 4 months of age and weighing between 190 and 225 Gm is selected and placed in individual cages. The animals are allowed free access to water and the *Depletion Diet* for 12 days, as this diet is deficient in total nitrogen and the essential amino acid requirements of the rat, the animals will decline in weight. At the end of this period the rats are weighed and any rat which weighs more than 90% of its starting weight is discarded.

All drinking water is removed from the cages and for the next 3 days a *Control Nitrogen Supplement* mixture is offered instead. This mixture is administered in a quantity equivalent to 0.12 Gm of nitrogen per rat per day, diluted to 20 ml, and offered at the same time each morning either in a dish suitable for preventing spillage or in a reservoir fitted with a drinking tube. The depletion diet, which is essentially nitrogen free, is continued during the period the animals are receiving the control nitrogen supplement. On the third day each rat is weighed. Animals which have not consumed all of the control nitrogen supplement are discarded.

For the next 3 days the control nitrogen supplement is replaced with water and the rats continued on the depletion diet without nitrogen supplement. The rats are again weighed and any which have not lost weight since the previous weighing are discarded.

For the actual test a group of not less than six rats is assembled which have completed the depletion and control periods. The weight of each rat is determined and recorded as the starting weight. The rats are maintained for 5 days on the depletion diet with a daily supplement of 20 ml of a solution containing the Protein Hydrolysate Injection being tested, in an amount equivalent to 0.12 Gm of nitrogen, offered each morning in the same manner as the control nitrogen supplement was previously offered. Water is withheld for at least 2 hours prior to offering the supplement and for 4 hours afterward. Then if the supplement has been consumed, water may be offered *ad libitum*.

On the afternoon of the fifth day, each rat is again weighed and the respective final and starting weights compared. Not more than one rat of a group of six used in the test or two rats in a group of ten should fail to gain or maintain their weight during the test if the preparation is to be considered to have met the USP requirements.

The compositions of the Depletion Diet and Control Nitrogen Supplement, together with the details of their preparation, are given in the USP.

Biological Indicators

Biological indicators serve to demonstrate the adequacy of a sterilization process. Viable cultures of various types of microorganisms are either incorporated into representative units of the product to be sterilized, or if this is not practicable (ie, solids), the cultures are added to a suitable model of the unit to be subjected to sterilization. Details of procedure for various classes of products, and the interpretation of the observations are to be found in the section on General Tests of the NF.

Depressor Substances

A few pharmaceuticals of natural origin, as well as some of synthetic origin, contain small but significant amounts of histamine-like depressor substances. The following USP products are required to meet the official test for depressor substances: Chloramphenicol, Chloramphenicol Sodium Succinate, Sterile Chloramphenicol Sodium Succinate, Lincomycin Hydrochloride, Lincomycin Hydrochloride Injection, Sodium Colistimethate, Streptomycin Sulfate, Streptomycin Sulfate Injection, Tetracycline Hydrochloride for Injection,

Sterile Tetracycline Hydrochloride, Viomycin Sulfate, and Sterile Viomycin Sulfate. As it is impractical to carry purification of these to such a point as to remove completely the "histamine bodies," a limit as to the amount of such activity that may be present is established by a biological test.

The USP Depressor Substance Test is conducted in an adult cat anesthetized with phenobarbital sodium (150 mg/Kg, intraperitoneally) and prepared for recording of blood pressure in a manner similar to that described for the dog in the section on the assay of epinephrine. The sensitivity of the animal is determined by injecting successively, at uniform intervals of not less than 5 minutes, doses of histamine dihydrochloride solution (equivalent to 1.0 microgram of histamine base/ml) representing 0.05, 0.1, and 0.15 microgram of histamine base/Kg of test animal. The middle dose is repeated several times to insure uniformity of response; if this is not satisfactory, the cat must be discarded. To an animal whose sensitivity has been established in this manner, two injections of a dilution in saline TS of the substances under test (concentration of the dilution is specified in the individual monograph) are then interposed between additional injections of 0.1 microgram/Kg of histamine base, maintaining the same time interval. If the average fall in blood pressure following injection of the test dilution is not greater than that obtained with 0.1 microgram/Kg of histamine base, the substance under test is considered satisfactory in respect to maximum depressor activity.

Identification Tests

Identity tests which depend on biological reactions are included in the USP and NF for official tablets or injections containing *Atropine Sulfate*, for official injections containing *Insulin*, and for the ophthalmic ointment and ophthalmic solution containing *Isoflurophate*. These tests are relatively sensitive and specific.

Atropine—A sufficient number of tablets, or volume of injection, to represent 0.6 to 1 mg of atropine sulfate is dissolved in 10 ml of water and the solution is filtered. When 1 drop of the filtrate is instilled into a cat's eye, dilation of the pupil is apparent within 2 hours.

Insulin—Six rabbits, from which food has been withheld for the previous 18 to 24 hours and which weigh between 1.8 and 2.2 Kg each, are used for the test. A quantity of Insulin Injection which causes convulsions in at least three of the animals is injected subcutaneously into each. Immediately after convulsions occur in an animal, 5 ml of a 50% solution of dextrose is injected intravenously into that animal. The convulsions should be relieved and at least four of the animals should remain alive for at least 3 days. This identification test is specified in the monographs on Insulin Injection. All Insulin Suspensions must be acidified before administration to dissolve the suspended protein.

Isoflurophate—The identification test for Isoflurophate Ophthalmic Ointment and Ophthalmic Solution, based on its mitotic activity, is made by placing about 100 mg of the ointment (0.1 ml of the solution) in the right eye of each of 3 rabbits. A positive identification is indicated by an average diameter of the pupils of the treated eyes at least 2 mm smaller than the average diameter of the untreated eyes. The conjunctivas of the treated eyes should show not more than a slight reddening which disappears within 4 hours.

NIH Tests

All biological products for the parenteral prevention, diagnosis, or treatment of disease in man must meet specified tests (such as those for stability, safety, toxicity, sterility, and potency) and other requirements of the Division of Biologics Standards of the National Institutes of Health. Included among such products are the *Antitoxins, Blood Products, Toxins, Toxoids, Vaccines, Polyvalent Crotaline Antivenin*, and *Tuberculins*.

Nonantigenicity Test

This test is applied to *Protein Hydrolysate Injection*. Because of their cost, mixtures of pure amino acids for parenteral administration are not yet generally available. The preparations presently on the market consist of acid or enzymatic hydrolysates of suitable proteins such as casein, lactalbumin, plasma, or fibrin.

The problem of providing an adequate intake of nitrogen by means of intravenously administered protein hydrolysates is complicated by various untoward reactions. Nausea and vomiting, venous thrombosis, and edema of the extremity in which the injection is made may occur if the rate of injection and concentration of protein are excessive. Although relatively infrequent, other untoward reactions which may occur are hyperpyrexia, urticaria, and angioneurotic edema. The last-mentioned reactions may be related to allergic phenomena and the US Pharmacopeia requires that this preparation must be nonantigenic when tested in guinea pigs. In addition to this

test and others carried out for all injections, the preparation is tested for the biological adequacy of the proteins it contains. This test is carried out in protein-deficient rats in which the criterion for adequacy is the gain in weight when protein is restored in the form of the test preparation. See *Biological Adequacy Test*, page 643.

Nonantigenicity Test—A sensitizing solution is prepared by selection of a suitable quantity of the protein identical in nature and quality with that from which the hydrolysate was prepared and subjecting it to the same hydrolytic process used in the manufacture. However, in this preparation, the time of hydrolysis is reduced to one-third.

Six ml of the sensitizing solution is injected intraperitoneally into healthy, male guinea pigs weighing between 420 and 480 Gm on the second, fourth, and sixth days of each of two successive weeks. Not less than 30 days and not more than 37 days after the last sensitizing dose the animals may be used. Animals not used during the 7-day period may be resensitized by injecting intraperitoneally a booster dose of 6 ml of the sensitizing solution. Resensitized animals may be used not less than 9 days and not more than 16 days after the injection of the booster dose.

The actual test for antigenicity is conducted by injecting intravenously, 3 ml of Protein Hydrolysate Injection, at the rate of 2 ml/minute, using a 5-ml syringe fitted with a 27 gauge needle, into a dorsal vein of the penis of each of five guinea pigs sensitized as mentioned above. During the injection and the following 15 minutes, the animals are observed for any of the following symptoms: (1) licking the nose or rubbing the nose with the forefeet; (2) ruffing of the fur; (3) weakness or diminished tone; (4) labored and depressed breathing; (5) sneezing or coughing (three or more times); (6) retching. For an acceptable preparation none of the injected animals may show more than one of the symptoms just mentioned and no animal may show rales, convulsions, prostration, or death.

In case none of the test animals show any of the listed symptoms, the sensitivity of the animals is proved by injecting one of them with the original sensitizing solution in the same dosage and rate as the assay preparation. In this case the animal should show positive signs of anaphylaxis such as rales, convulsions, prostration, and/or death in addition to one or more of the reaction symptoms.

Potency Tests

USP XVII provided tests for potency for *Diphtheria Diagnostic Toxin* and *Influenza Virus Vaccine*.

Diphtheria Diagnostic Toxin—At least 5 healthy guinea pigs, each weighing 225 to 275 Gm, are used for the test. Into each is injected subcutaneously 5 ml (containing 1 MLD) of toxin. No animals should survive and at least three-fourths should die between 72 and 96 hours after the toxin was injected.

Influenza Virus Vaccine—The potency of each lot of Influenza Virus Vaccine is determined by its power to stimulate the formation of specific virus-neutralizing antibodies in mice. For practical purposes, the potency is expressed, in the labeling, in terms of the chicken red-cell agglutination titer (as "CAA units" in each ml).

Smallpox Vaccine—Doses of the vaccine representing dilutions of specified concentrations are applied to denuded and lightly scarified areas of the skin of rabbits weighing 2.25 to 2.75 Kg. The lesions produced should equal or exceed those produced by a Smallpox Vaccine meeting the specifications established by the National Institutes of Health (including trial administration to human subjects) and applied in an identical manner.

Pyrogen Test

Parenteral solutions are officially tested for the presence of pyrogens by a biological test in which the "fever" response of rabbits is used as the criteria.

The USP and NF direct that most parenteral products be tested for pyrogens, as indicated in the individual monographs. The official test follows.

The pyrogen test is designed for products that can be tolerated by the test rabbit in a dose of 10 ml/Kg. For products requiring a slower rate of injection, or a dose smaller than 10 ml/Kg, or for those requiring dilution or adjustment of pH, or the addition of pyrogen-free sodium chloride to render them isotonic, the additional directions given in the individual monograph must be followed.

Temperature Recording—An accurate clinical thermometer which has been tested to determine the time necessary to reach the maximum reading, or any other temperature-recording device of equal sensitivity, may be used for this test. The device is inserted into the rectum of the rabbit to a depth of not less than 7.5 cm and sufficient time allowed to reach a maximum temperature before taking the reading (see Fig. 421).

Test Animal—Healthy, mature rabbits are used which weigh not less than 1500 Gm each and which have maintained their weight for at least 1 week under the environmental conditions specified for these tests. The rabbits are housed individually in an area of uniform temperature (±3°) and free of disturbances likely to excite them. Rabbits which have been used for previous pyrogen tests must have a rest period of at least 48 hours before reuse if the sample under test was non-pyrogenic. If the sample was adjudged pyrogenic, the rest period must be at least 2 weeks. For animals which have not been used in any tests for the previous 2 weeks, a sham test is conducted for conditioning. The actual injection of a solution is omitted in the sham test.

Procedure—The test is conducted in the area where the animals are housed or under similar environmental conditions. On the day of the test all food is withheld from the rabbits until after completion of the test. Access to water may be allowed. The "control temperature" of each animal is determined and in any one test only those animals are used in which the control temperatures do not differ more than 1° from each other. Any animal with a temperature greater than 39.8° is excluded from the tests.

Syringes, needles, and glassware used for the test may be rendered free of pyrogens by heating at 250° for not less than 30 minutes or any other suitable method. The sample to be tested is warmed to approximately 37° prior to injection.

Except where specifically stated otherwise, the test sample is injected into an ear vein of each of 3 rabbits 30 minutes subsequent to the determination of the control temperature. A dosage of 10 ml/Kg of body weight is specified. The temperature is again determined at 1, 2, and 3 hours subsequent to the injection.

The test is positive if each rabbit shows an individual rise in temperature of 0.6° or more above its respective control temperature or if the sum of the three temperature rises exceeds 1.4°. If 1 or 2 rabbits show a temperature rise of 0.6° or more, or if the sum of the temperature rises exceeds 1.4°, the test must be repeated using 5 other rabbits. The test is positive if 4 or more of the 8 rabbits show individual rises in temperature of 0.6°, or if the sum of the eight temperature rises exceeds 3.7°.

Testing for the presence of pyrogens by manufacturers of parenteral solutions is carried out on an extensive scale for which specialized equipment is often developed.

Purified pyrogenic materials also have their useful application: they are employed to cause febrile reactions in animals which are then used to evaluate antipyretic agents.

Safety Test

The USP directs that the safety of *Iron Dextran Injection* be determined on the basis of acute toxicity following intravenous injection of specified doses of the solution in mice.

Salmonella Test

Screening tests for Salmonella contamination of powders; filled gelatin capsules; greasy, oily, or fatty samples; animal feed; swabs; environmental samples; frozen animal glands; liquid products; water; bile; gelatin; thyroid related products (powder or tablets); and dried yeast are described in detail under General Tests in the NF. Methods of sampling the various types of preparations, and isolation and presumptive identification procedures for Salmonella are provided.

Sterility Tests

All injections and other products to be used parenterally, including certain crystalline or powdered solids, all surgical dressings and related materials, sutures, antibiotics, ophthalmic solutions, and other items used for administering parenteral materials must be sterile. Refer to Chapter 81, *Sterilization*.

Toxicity Tests

Diphtheria Toxoid—Inject, subcutaneously, not fewer than 4 healthy guinea pigs each weighing between 300 and 400 Gm with a volume of Diphtheria Toxoid that is at least 5 times the intended human immunizing dose but not less than 2 ml. To comply with the requirements of this test, no local or general symptoms of diphtheria toxin poisoning should appear within 30 days.

Rubber Closures—The NF directs that specially prepared extracts of rubber closures for injectables be subjected to (1) an *acute systemic toxicity test* based on gross toxicity and mortality following intraperitoneal and intravenous injection of the extracts in mice and (2) an *intracutaneous reactivity test* based on tissue reactions (erythema, edema, necrosis) at sites of intracutaneous injection of the extracts in albino rabbits.

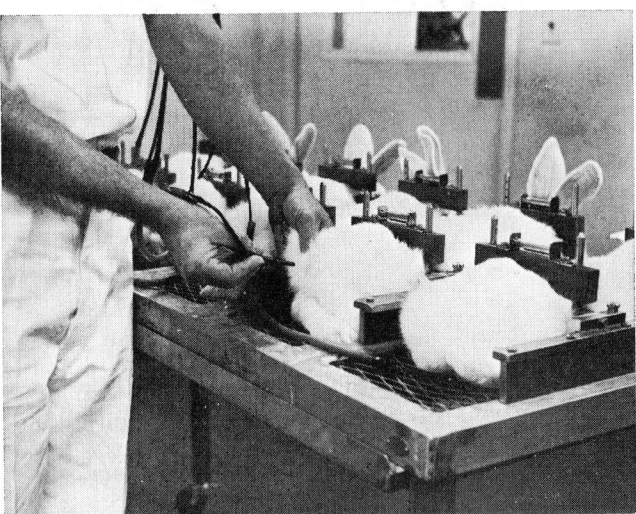

Fig. 421. Insertion of Foxboro Resistance Thermometer Bulb used in recording rectal temperature of rabbits (courtesy, Upjohn).

Tetanus Toxoid—Inject, subcutaneously, not fewer than 4 healthy guinea pigs each weighing between 300 and 400 Gm with a volume of Tetanus Toxoid that is at least 5 times the greatest intended individual human immunizing dose but not less than 2 ml. No symptoms of tetanus toxin poisoning should appear within 21 days.

Transfusion and Infusion Assemblies

The safety and efficacy of several pharmacopeial preparations depend upon the satisfactory character of the equipment by which they are given intravenously in relatively large volumes. Therefore the following tests are provided for transfusion and infusion assemblies of tubing for application to representative samples from each sterilizer charge of the assemblies.

Sterility—Not less than ten assemblies are selected from various levels of the sterilizer chamber. The lumen of each is flushed with 10 ml of Fluid Thioglycollate Medium (USP); the effluent is incubated at 30° to 32° for 7 days. Needles which may be supplied separately with such assemblies are either immersed in sufficient Fluid Thioglycollate Medium to cover them or flushed with 10 ml of medium. Culture time and temperature are the same as for a complete assembly. Following incubation the cultures are examined for the presence of viable organisms. If growth is found, the test may be repeated to rule out laboratory contamination by using twice the number of samples. The samples for retest must also be representative of the sterilizer load. If repeat tests confirm the presence of contamination, the materials do not meet the requirements for sterility.

Pyrogens—The test for pyrogens is conducted by passing 40-ml portions of sterile, pyrogen-free saline TS through the lumen of not less than ten assemblies at a flow rate of approximately 10 ml/minute. The effluent is then pooled and tested for the presence of pyrogens as indicated in the USP.

Safety—In this test each assembly from a representative sample is filled as completely as practicable with sterile saline TS and clamped securely on each end. The filled assembly is then completely immersed in water and heated at not less than 85° for 1 hour. At the end of this treatment the contents of the assembly are drained and diluted to 250 ml with sterile saline TS. Five healthy mice weighing between 17 and 23 Gm are each injected intravenously with 0.5 ml of the solution so prepared. The animals are examined at the end of 4, 24, and 48 hours for symptoms of toxicity. If any of the animals show gross signs of toxicity or die, the test is repeated using 5 unused mice weighing 19 to 21 Gm each. In the repeat test all animals must survive for 48 hours.

References

1. Agr. Res. Serv., Dept. of Agr., *Federal Register*, **32**, 3270–3282 (1967).
2. *Guide for Laboratory Animal Facilities and Care* (USPHS Publ. 1024), 3rd ed. (rev.), Natl. Res. Council, Inst. of Lab. Animal Resources, Washington, D.C., 1968.
3. Sayers, M. A., "Assay of Adrenocorticotrophic Hormone by Adrenal Ascorbic Acid Depletion Method," *Endocrinology*, **42**, 379 (1948).

39 | Clinical Analysis

Hematology—blood-bank technology—techniques of analysis—microbiology—serology

This chapter was prepared by

Robert D. Smyth, MSc, *Manager, Department of Biological Chemistry, Research Division, William H. Rorer, Inc., Fort Washington, Pa. 19034*

Characterization and quantitation of the various components of blood, urine, and other body fluids is the primary function of the clinical laboratory. The major divisions of clinical analysis are clinical biochemistry, hematology, blood-bank technology, histopathology, and microbiology. Accurate diagnosis of disease and determination of a potential therapeutic regimen are frequently based on the laboratory analysis of blood, urine, feces, gastric secretions, or cerebrospinal fluid. Modern medical practice is tending toward greater reliance on laboratory results as definitive measures of pathologic or normal states.

Advances in instrumentation and technology have resulted in the development of highly accurate and specific methodology for the analysis of body fluids. The pharmacist should familiarize himself with the basic principles involved in sample collection, analysis, and diagnostic significance of the various clinical parameters. The role of the pharmacist in community health necessitates his comprehension of the biochemical nature and diagnostic value of clinical laboratory procedures.

Hematology

Determination of the morphologic, physiologic, and pathologic aspects of peripheral blood and the blood-forming organs (hematopoietic system) is a function of the hematology laboratory. The various phases of hematology[1] may be categorized as follows: (1) analysis of cellular elements, and specific biochemical and physiological parameters of peripheral blood and the hematopoietic system; (2) blood-coagulation analysis; and (3) blood-bank technology.

Peripheral blood is a biphasic liquid tissue system of cellular elements suspended in a liquid plasma phase. The cellular phase comprises about 45% of the blood volume and contains erythrocytes (red blood cells), leukocytes (white blood cells), and thrombocytes (platelets). The plasma phase is primarily water (90–92%) with about 7% protein.

Hematologic analysis of blood is primarily concerned with enumeration and differentiation of the various cellular elements. Analysis of the hematopoietic system (eg, bone marrow) determines the status of blood-cell precursors in the tissues. Determination of specific biochemical (hemoglobin) and physiologic (blood volume, blood-cell distribution) blood parameters are observed in a complete evaluation of the hematopoietic system. The normal hematologic values in the adult, newborn, and 10-year-old are presented in Table I.

Erythrocytes and Hemoglobin—The erythrocytic system is the mature erythrocytes in peripheral blood and their precursors in red bone marrow. The normal erythrocyte (normocyte) is a flexible, elastic, biconcave, enucleated structure with a mean diameter of 7.3 μ and a thickness in the range of 2.2 μ. The chemical constituents of the red blood cell include water (63%), lipids (0.5%), glucose (0.8%), minerals (0.7%), non-hemoglobin protein (0.9%), methemoglobin (0.5%), and hemoglobin (33.6%).

The stroma of insoluble material which remains after red-cell disruption (hemolysis) constitutes 2–5% of the wet cell weight; it is primarily protein (40–60%) and lipid (10–12%). The stroma proteins include stromatin (a fibrous or structural protein) and elinin (a fraction associated with A, B, and O blood-group substances). The lipid fractions include phosphatides (lecithin, cephalin, and sphingomyelin) with some cholesterol, cholesterol esters, neutral fats, cerebrosides, and glycolipid.

The red cell membrane, a dynamic component of the cell, is associated with energy metabolism in the maintenance of the permeability characteristics of the cell to various cations (Na^+, K^+) and anions (Cl^-, HCO_3^-). The primary function of the erythocyte is oxygen transport by combination with reduced hemoglobin to form oxyhemoglobin.

Hemoglobin, a conjugated protein with an approximate molecular weight of 67,000, contains four heme groups and globin. Heme, which constitutes about 4% of the weight of the molecule, is a metal

Table I—Normal Hematological Values in Man

	Normal value	Normal range of values
Erythrocytes (cu mm $\times 10^6$)		
Male	5.4	4.6–6.2
Female	4.8	4.2–5.6
Reticulocytes (cu mm $\times 10^3$)	50	10–100
Hemoglobin (Gm%)		
Male	16.0	14.0–18.0
Female	14.0	12.0–16.0
Hematocrit (%)		
Male	47.0	40.0–54.0
Female	42.0	37.0–47.0
Mean corpuscular volume (μ^3)	87	82–92
Mean corpuscular hemoglobin (μ mcg)	29	27–31
Mean corpuscular hemoglobin concentration (%)	34	32–36
Mean corpuscular diameter (μ)	7.3	6.7–7.7
Leukocytes (cu mm $\times 10^3$)	7.0	5.0–10.0
Leukocyte differential (%)		
Neutrophils	63	57–67
Eosinophils	1	1–3
Basophils	1	0–1
Lymphocytes	30	25–33
Monocytes	5	3–7
Platelets (cu mm $\times 10^5$)	3.0	1.4–6.0

complex consisting of an iron atom in the center of a porphyrin structure. The globin group consists of two pairs of polypeptide chains. In the intact cell, hemoglobin is constantly shifting from the functional, reduced state to an oxidized, ferric hemoglobin (methemoglobin). Sufficient reduced hemoglobin supplies are maintained by the enzyme methemoglobin reductase. The hemoglobin molecule is functional only in the reduced state as to capability for oxygenation with four molecules of oxygen to form oxyhemoglobin.

The precursors of erythrocytes, as found in erythropoietic system (red bone marrow), are classified as to degree of nucleation and characteristics of cytoplasmic constituents. The sequence of erythrocyte formation in bone marrow based on gradual denucleation of the cell, generation of the chromatin structure, and changes in nucleolar structure and cytoplasmic constituents, is as follows: rubriblast → prorubricyte → rubricyte → metarubricyte → basophilic erythrocyte → erythrocyte.

The first four types are nucleated and are normally seen only in bone marrow. In normal erythrocyte formation these immature bone marrow cells are designated as *normoblastic* or *normocytic*. In pernicious anemia and related conditions, these immature cells become abnormally large and are designated *megaloblastic* or *megalocytic*. In iron-deficiency anemia, these cells become abnormally small and are designated normoblastic or normocytic— of the iron-deficiency type.

Erythrocytes may be enumerated by either visual[2] or electronic procedures.[3,4] In the visual procedures a measured quantity of blood is diluted with a fluid which is isotonic with blood and which will prevent its coagulation. The diluted blood is then placed in a counting chamber (hemocytometer) and the number of cells in a circumscribed area is enumerated microscopically. Hayem's solution (sodium sulfate, 2.5 Gm; sodium chloride, 0.25 Gm; mercuric chloride, 0.25 Gm; distilled water, 100 ml), Toison's fluid (sodium sulfate, 8 Gm; sodium chloride, 1 Gm; methyl violet, 0.025 Gm; glycerine, 30 ml; distilled water, 180 ml), and 0.9% sodium chloride are used as diluting fluids.

The over-all error of this method is about 8%. A greater degree of accuracy and reproducibility can be achieved by erythrocyte enumeration in an electronic counting apparatus; eg, "Coulter Counter" or "Fisher Autocytometer." The Coulter method determines the number and size of particles suspended in an electrically conductive liquid. The blood cells traverse a small aperture and so displace electrolyte as to produce a change in resistance between electrodes; the magnitude of the voltage pulse is proportional to cell volume, and the resultant pulses are then amplified, scaled, and automatically counted.

In the Fisher Autocytometer (Fig. 422), the cells pass through an illuminated counting chamber. Each cell reflects a pulse of light from the source lamp to a photomultiplier tube which in turn converts them into electrical pulses of varying duration and intensity. These pulses are then amplified to uniform size and duration, integrated, and automatically totalized. In addition to increased speed of counting, the over-all error of the electronic procedures is reduced to about 1%.

The *hematocrit value* is a measure of the erythrocyte portion of blood. A sample of blood is placed in a graduated hematocrit or heparinized capillary tube, centrifuged, and the volume of packed red cells (hematocrit value) determined. The centrifuged sample in the hematocrit tube appears as a red

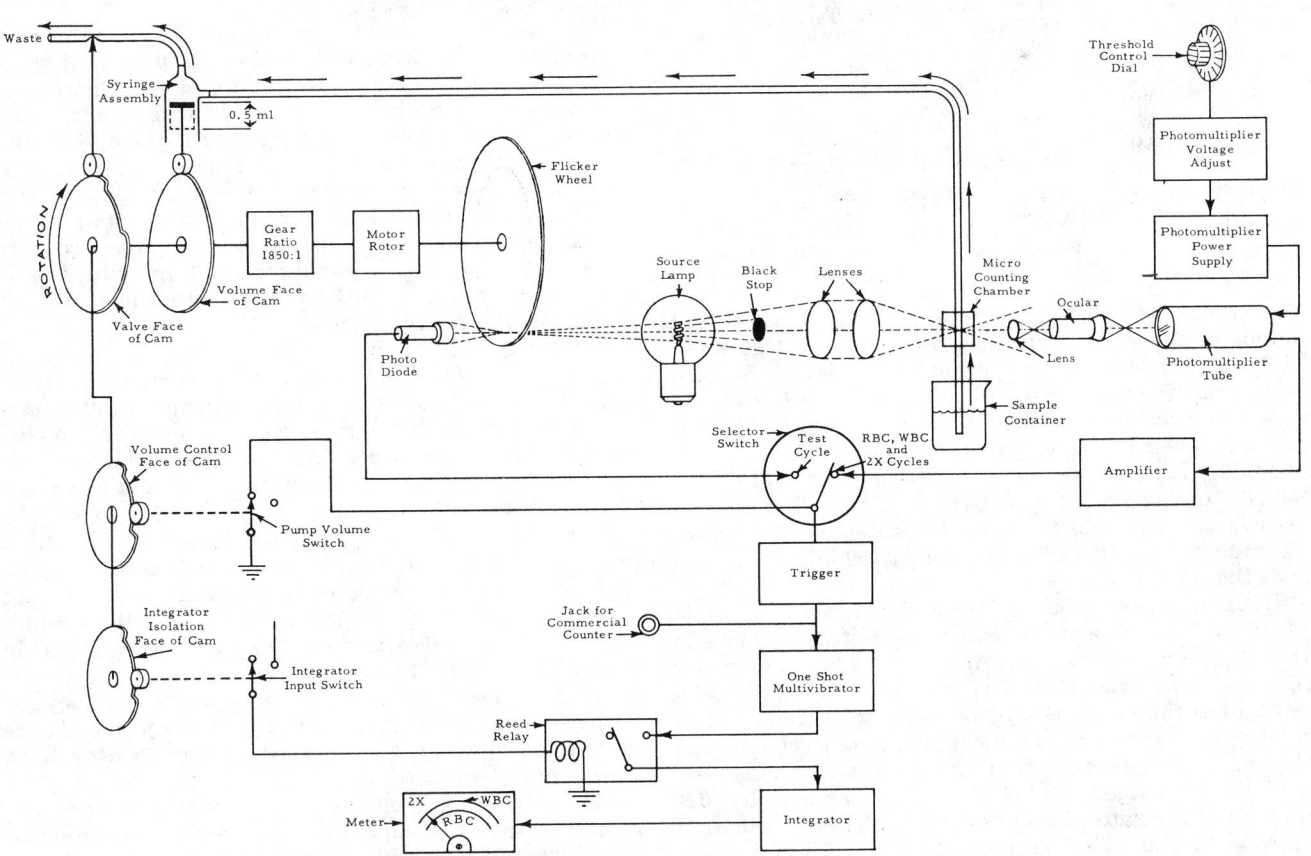

Fig. 422. **Autocytometer—an automatic cell-counting apparatus (courtesy, Fisher).**

layer of packed erythrocytes over which is found a gray layer of packed leukocytes and platelets, and a supernatant plasma phase. The hematocrit value is an index of the number and size of the red cells.

The *hemoglobin* concentration is measured spectrophotometrically after lysis of whole blood and conversion of hemoglobin to hematin, oxyhemoglobin, or cyanmethemoglobin.[5,6] The addition of strong base (NaOH) to pH 10 converts oxyhemoglobin, carboxyhemglobin, and methemoglobin to hematin, which can be estimated photometrically. Weak base (Na_2CO_3 or NH_4OH) converts hemoglobin to oxyhemoglobin for analysis.

Total hemoglobin is also measured by conversion to cyanmethemoglobin by alkaline potassium cyanide–potassium ferricyanide reagent. Hemoglobin standards certified by the Clinical Standards Committee of the College of American Pathologists are used in the above procedures, and all results are expressed as "Gm hemoglobin per 100 ml blood."

Differences in the structural sequence of amino acids in the peptide portion of the hemoglobin molecules are responsible for different types of hemoglobin. Based on characteristic mobility of the hemoglobin proteins in an electric field (electrophoresis) on starch, paper, cellulose acetate, agar, or acrylamide gel media, many hemoglobin types have been recognized.[7] Types, P, F, and A-A₄ are found in normal blood. Sickle cell anemia and erythroblastic anemia (thalassemia) are blood diseases associated with abnormal hemoglobin types; eg, Types S and C, respectively.

Erythrocyte count, hemoglobin content, and hematocrit value are used for the determination of various blood indices in the diagnosis and treatment of anemia. These measurements are:

Mean corpuscular volume [MCV (μ^3)] =

$$\frac{\text{Hematocrit (\%)} \times 10}{\text{Erythrocyte count (millions/cu mm)}}$$

$$\frac{\text{Mean corpuscular hemoglobin}}{\text{MCH } (\mu\text{mcg})} =$$

$$\frac{\text{Hemoglobin (Gm/100 ml)} \times 10}{\text{Erythrocyte count (millions/cu mm)}}$$

$$\frac{\text{Mean corpuscular hemoglobin concentration}}{\text{MCHC (\%)}} =$$

$$\frac{\text{Hemoglobin (Gm/100 ml)} \times 100}{\text{Hematocrit (\%)}}$$

Anemias are classified as to red cell volume and hemoglobin concentration. *Macrocytic* (large cell: MCV > 94), *normocytic* (normal cell: MCV, 82–92), or *microcytic* (small cell: MCV < 80) are the classifications according to cell volume. Cellular hemoglobin concentration categorizes the cells as to *hyperchromic* (MCHC > 38), *normochromic* (MCHC: 32–36), or *hypochromic* (MCHC < 30). The anemia associated with chronic blood loss is of the hypochromic microcytic type, whereas pernicious anemia is of the macrocytic type.

Determinations of the suspension stability of whole blood and erythrocyte fragility are useful adjuncts in the diagnosis of various diseases. The *erythrocyte sedimentation rate* (ESR)[2] is an estimate of the suspension stability of red blood cells in plasma; it is related to the number and size of the red cells and to the relative concentration of plasma proteins, especially fibrinogen. This test is performed by determining the rate of sedimentation of blood cells in a standard tube. Normal blood ESR is 0–15 mm/hour. Increases are found in acute generalized infections

and inflammatory conditions such as rheumatoid arthritis. The *erythrocyte fragility test*[8] is based on resistance of cells to hemolysis in decreasing concentrations of hypotonic saline. Increased osmotic fragility of the red cells is associated with various types of hemolytic anemia; increased resistance has been observed in the presence of jaundice and thalassemia.

An inherited deficiency of the enzyme, glucose-6-phosphate dehydrogenase (G-6-PD), in erythrocytes is the basis of a screening procedure for detection of susceptibility to drug-induced or nonspherocytic hemolytic anemia. G-6-PD deficiency is found predominantly in Mediterranean peoples, Southeast Asians, Africans, and American negroes. The enzyme can be quantitated spectrophotometrically by measuring the rate of reduction of triphosphopyridine nucleotide (TPN) in the presence of G-6-P. Presumptive screening tests based on reduced glutathione (GSH) content of blood before and after incubation with acetylphenylhydrazine are also used.[9]

Leukocytes—Mature leukocytes in peripheral blood and their precursors in bone marrow is the leukocytic system. Various types of leukocytes are found in normal blood. Differentiation of the lymphocytic, monocytic, and granulocytic leukocyte types is based on cell size, and morphologic characteristics of the nucleus and cytoplasm.

The primary function of leukocytes is the development of the various defensive and reparative processes in inflammatory and immune response mechanisms. Migration of leukocytes to microorganisms in blood or tissues (chemotaxis) is associated with the release of biochemical substances from foreign particles or injured tissue. The leukocyte (macrophage) then engulfs and destroys the foreign substance by the process of phagocytosis.

The chemical composition of the leukocyte includes water (82%), nucleoprotein, phospholipids, and trace minerals. Enzyme content, glycogen, and histamine levels vary in the different types of white cells. Deficiency in enzymes associated with glycolytic metabolism (hexokinase) and increases in phosphomonoester hydrolases (alkaline phosphatase) have been observed in leukocytes of patients with certain types of leukemia. Specific leukocytes are primary sources of blood histamine, which is stored in cytoplasmic granules, and subsequently released in the development of the inflammatory process.

The precursors of leukocytes are found in bone marrow and are classified according to degree of cytoplasmic granulation, dye-affinity of the granules, and shape of the nucleus (Schilling, Arneth, or Cooke–Ponder Classification). As undifferentiated cells (myeloblasts) mature, metachromatic granules appear in the cytoplasm (granulocytes).

In the *basophilic* and *eosinophilic* leukocytes, these granules develop an affinity for a basic dye or acidic dye, respectively; those cells whose granules do not stain are called *neutrophils*. As the cells acquire mobility, the nuclei undergo progressive changes in shape, from round to multilobular forms, and are designated *myelocytes*, and *band* or *segmented* leukocytes. In peripheral blood the mature granulocytic cells are designated *polymorphonuclear leukocytes—neutrophilic*, *eosinophilic*, or *basophilic*.

The other types of white cells normally observed in peripheral blood have no granules as to size and shape into the *monocyte* and *lymphocyte* which is formed in lymphoid tissue.

Leukocytes are enumerated by procedures similar to those utilized for erythrocytes. In the visual procedures,[2] the blood is diluted with a fluid (3% *v/v* acetic acid) which lyses the red cells, and total leukocyte count is determined microscopically. Eosinophils may also be differentially analyzed by use of a diluting fluid which renders the red cells nonrefractile and invisible, and lyses the base-labile leukocytes, leaving the base-stable eosinophils intact. A suitable diluting fluid for this purpose is Pilot's Fluid (propylene glycol, 50 ml; distilled water, 40 ml; 1% phloxine, 10 ml; 10% sodium carbonate, 1 ml; and heparin sodium, 100 units). Electronic procedures[3,4] are similar to those used for erythrocytes with the added advantage of speed, accuracy, and reproducibility.

A differential count[9] of the leukocytes will provide information as to the relative numbers of each type (Fig. 423). A thin film of blood is prepared on a microscope slide, stained with a polychromatic preparation such as Wright's or Giemsa's stain, and analyzed microscopically. Wright's stain contains polychromed methylene blue and eosin dyes; the erythrocytes are stained pink; the nuclei of the leukocytes, purplish-blue; neutrophilic granules, violet-pink; eosinophilic granules, red; basophilic granules, blue; and platelets, blue.

The normal adult leukocyte value is 5,000 to 10,000 cells/cu mm. Values greater than 10,000 (leukocytosis) are encountered in the newborn infant, young children, after violent exercise, convulsive seizures of epilepsy, leukemia, and cancer. Values of less than 5,000 (*leukopenia*) are observed in certain microbial infections (eg, typhoid fever, measles, malaria, septicemia), cirrhosis of the liver, chronic anemias, and radiation injury.

Polymorphonuclear neutrophilic leukocytes (neutrophils, "polys") normally comprise 62% (50–67%) of the total leukocyte count. These cells are irregular in shape (10–15 μ in diameter) and usually contain a multilobated nucleus with fine, lightly stained cytoplasmic granules. An immature or juvenile form of neutrophil, with a band-shaped nonsegmented nucleus constitutes 3–5% of peripheral blood leukocytes. Increases in the relative percentage of these cells (neutrophilia) is observed in acute microbial infections (eg, meningitis, smallpox, poliomyelitis), metabolic disorders (diabetic acidosis, gout), drug intoxication (digitalis, epinephrine), vaccination, coronary thrombosis, and malignant neoplasms.

Polymorphonuclear eosinophilic leukocytes (eosinophils) normally comprise about 1–3% of total circulating white blood cells. In appearance they are similar to the neutrophil with the exception of large, redstained cytoplasmic granules. Eosinophilia has been observed in certain skin diseases (psoriasis, eczema), parasitic infestations (pork round worm—trichinosis), certain hypersensitivity reactions, scarlet fever, and pernicious anemia.

Polymorphonuclear basophilic leukocytes (basophils) possess large cytoplasmic granules which stain a deep blue. These cells, which are primary sources of blood heparin and histamine constitute less than 1.0% of the leukocytes. Basophilic leukocytosis is seen in chronic myelocytic leukemia, hemolytic anemia, and Hodgkin's disease. Basophilic leukopenia occurs following radiation or therapy with glucocorticoids.

Lymphocytes are formed in lymphoid tissue (lymph glands, spleen). Cell diameter ranges from 7–10 μ to 10–18 μ. They have a round, or slightly indented, deeply stained nucleus and normally comprise 25–33%

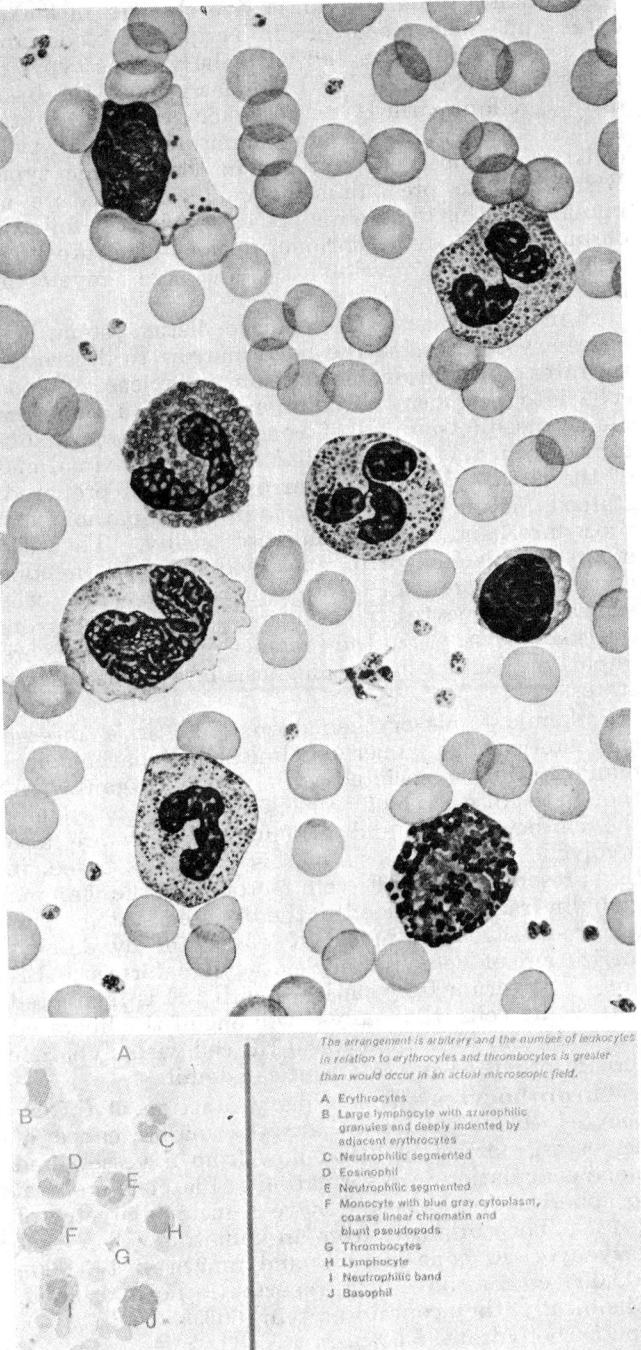

Fig. 423. Cell types found in smears of peripheral blood from normal individuals (courtesy, Abbott).

of the leukocytes. Lymphocytosis is seen in infectious mononucleosis, lymphocytic leukemia, rickets, and in most conditions associated with neutrophilic leukopenia (neutropenia).

Monocytes constitute 3–7% of the leukocytes. They are larger (12–20 μ) than the other leukocytes and possess an abundant, pale, bluish-violet-stained cytoplasm with a fine, reticulated chromatin structure in the nucleus. The monocytes (macrophages) phagocytize bacteria, parasitic protozoa, foreign particles, and even erythrocytes. Monocytosis is seen in certain microbial infections (tuberculosis, typhus, malaria), Hodgkin's disease, and monocytic leukemia.

As qualitative and quantitative changes in leukocytes and their precursors in peripheral blood and body tissue are associated with the various types of leukemia, this disease has been classified on the basis of the predominating type of leukocyte. Leukocytes in acute leukemia are more immature ("blast"-type cells) than those encountered in the chronic type. Based on the predominating cell type (mature or immature), this disease may be categorized as follows: chronic lymphocytic, chronic myelocytic, acute lymphoblastic, acute myeloblastic, and acute myelo- or histiomonocytic.

In many diseases of the hematopoietic system, it is necessary to examine the bone marrow to determine the rates of formation, maturation, and release of blood cells into peripheral circulation. Using a puncture biopsy needle, samples of bone marrow may be obtained from the sternum, iliac crest, or proximal end of the tibia. Smears of marrow are then prepared, stained (Wright's stain or specialized histopathological procedure), and examined microscopically. The ratio of myeloid leukocyte to nucleated red cells in bone marrow, the presence of abnormal (*nonmyeloid*) cells such as lymphocytes, the number of platelet precursors (*megakaryocytes*), and the presence of focal lesions are important factors in the diagnosis of various disease states.

Systemic lupus erythematosus (LE) is a disease characterized by numerous clinical and pathological manifestations associated with various organs. Although the disease chiefly affects the lymphatic system, the cardiac, renal, and articular systems are also involved. The diagnosis of this disease is based on the presence of a LE cell factor[10] in the gamma globulin fraction of blood in the diseased state. This factor dissolves the nuclei of leukocytes by depolymerization of deoxyribonucleic acid to form the LE body. If serum from patients with LE is incubated with white cells, the "polys" will engulf the liberated LE body and form the typical LE cell with a characteristic progressive loss of nuclear detail.

Thrombocytes—The primary function of thrombocytes (blood platelets) are the maintainance of hemostasis (arrest of blood flow from a vessel) and blood coagulation (clot formation). Platelets are oval to spherical in shape and have a mean diameter of $2-4 \mu$. They originate from an immature cell (megakaryocyte) in bone marrow and ranges of 140,000–600,000/cu mm have been reported in normal blood. Chemically, they contain protein (60%), lipid (15%), and carbohydrate (8.5%).

Adhesiveness, aggregation, and agglutination are the principal physical properties of platelets responsible for hemostasis and coagulation reactions. As of the present time, there is no satisfactory method for enumeration of blood platelets. The size and physical properties of the platelet seriously deter the development of accurate and reproducible methodology.

Indirect methods[11] of analysis are based on the proportion of platelets to erythrocytes in a stained blood smear. Blood samples obtained directly from the skin puncture are diluted with an anticoagulant fluid which will simultaneously stain the platelets. The ratio of platelets to red cells is then determined microscopically and the number calculated from the predetermined red cell count.

In the direct procedures[12] a sample of blood is obtained by venipuncture, placed in a siliconized tube, diluted, and subsequently analyzed by counting the platelets in a microscopic counting chamber using conventional or phase microscopy apparatus. Suitable diluting fluids are the Rees–Ecker Fluid (sodium citrate, 3.8 Gm; formaldehyde, 0.22 ml; brilliant cresyl blue, 0.05 Gm; water, qs 100 ml) and Brecher Fluid (1% ammonium oxalate). Persistent increases in platelet count (thrombocythemia or piastrinemia) have been observed in chronic myelocytic leukemia and splenic atrophy. Acute or temporary increases in platelet values (thrombocytosis) are seen in trauma and asphyxiation.

Thrombocytopenia or a decrease in platelets to values less than 60,000/cu mm occurs in various purpuras or hemorrhagic states (idiopathic or symptomatic thrombocytopenic purpura). Leukemia, extensive burns, splenic disorders, and agents such as quinidine, sulfonamides, and hydrochlorothiazide have been implicated in the etiology of symptomatic thrombocytopenia. Decreases in platelet count are also accompanied by morphologic changes in the size, shape, and cytoplasmic granulation of these cells.

Reticulocytes—In normal peripheral blood 0.5–1.5% of the erythrocytes possess a fine reticulum on the cytoplasm. In blood smears prepared with Wright's, Giemsa, or other Romanowsky methods, basophilic stippling of the erythrocyte occurs in lead poisoning (plumbism). This is not to be confused with the basophilic staining of the reticulocyte which can only be seen when cells are stained by supravital procedures (mixture of dyes with wet blood prior to preparation of air-dried blood smear). The observed granular filaments or reticulum of this immature erythrocyte are a result of endoplasmic coagulation by lipophilic dyes used in the supravital procedures. Reticulocytes are enumerated by supravital staining of fresh blood[13] with an anticoagulant–dye solution.

In indirect counting methods a thin film of the blood–dye mixture is prepared on a microscope slide, counterstained with Wright's stain, and the reticulocytes enumerated in proportion to a predetermined erythrocyte count. In direct procedures[14] reticulocytes are enumerated in wet films without counterstaining. Suitable dyes are brilliant cresyl blue, new methylene blue and Janus green. These methods are subject to high counting error.

An increase in the number of reticulocytes is an index of accelerated hematopoiesis and is observed in acute hemorrhage or adequate therapeutic management of iron-deficiency or pernicious anemia. In cases of chronic blood loss or bone marrow depression, a decrease in reticulocytes is seen.

Blood Volume and Erythropoietic Mechanisms—The mean red cell mass in normal males is 30.3 ml/Kg and the average plasma volume is 41.1 ml/Kg. The determination of these blood-volume parameters is based on the dilution of an intravenously injected indicator substance by the individual's blood volume. Dyes[15] (Evans Blue) and radioisotopes[16] (^{32}P, ^{51}Cr, ^{131}I) are accurate indicators. In the latter technique, radioiodine-tagged human serum albumin (RISA) is administered intravenously; after 10 min, a sample of blood is removed and analyzed in a scintillation well counter. The dilution of injected RISA by blood is equated to the activity of a RISA standard preparation and blood volume is thus calculated. Blood volume and red cell mass is reduced in hemorrhage and increased in polycythemia vera and certain types of leukemia.

The specific determination of *red cell volume* is accurately estimated by tagging the erythrocytes with ^{51}Cr *in vitro* or ^{59}Fe *in vivo*. These isotopes are incorporated into the hemoglobin of the erythrocytes and subsequent isotope dilution in blood also can be used for calculation of red cell mass. In hemolytic anemia there is a decrease in the normal life span (108–120 days) of the erythrocyte as indicated by a decreased survival time of ^{51}Cr-tagged red cells in blood.

Studies with ^{59}Fe have demonstrated a prolonged plasma iron turnover time (normal, 0.46–0.75 mg/Kg/day) in aplastic anemia. The metabolic defect in pernicious anemia, characterized by inadequate gastrointestinal (GI) absorption of vitamin B_{12}, is readily diagnosed by monitoring urinary radioactivity following oral administration of cyanocobalamin-^{60}Co with and without intrinsic factor.[17] The per cent recovery of the isotope in normal patients is 3–25% and in pernicious anemia 0–2.5%.

^{51}Cr-tagged erythrocytes are also used in studying the effects of various compounds, such as salicylates, on GI bleeding. The patient's blood cells are tagged with ^{51}Cr and the agent under test is administered. If GI bleeding occurs, there is an increase in ^{51}Cr content of fecal samples as a result of blood loss into the lumen of the GI tract.

Blood Coagulation—*Hemostasis*, the arrest of blood flow from a vessel, is regulated by extravascular (muscle, skin, and subcutaneous tissue), vascular (blood vessels), and intravascular (blood-coagulation) mechanisms. This discussion will be limited to those processes related to the blood-coagulation mechanism. When blood is allowed to clot, the free-flowing liquid is converted into a firm cell clot surrounded by serum. If an anticoagulant is added to blood, coagulation does not occur and the blood cells are suspended in a liquid phase–plasma. The clotting mechanism involves three stages: (1) formation of plasma *thromboplastin*, (2) conversion of *prothrombin* to *thrombin*, and (3) conversion of *fibrinogen* to *fibrin*.[18]

The International Committee on Nomenclature of Blood Clotting Factors[19] has numerically designated the blood-coagulation factors (Table II). Fibrinogen and Factors V and VIII are absent in normal blood serum as a result of the clotting process. The adsorption characteristics of certain blood-coagulation factors on calcium phosphate or barium sulfate is used in the differential analysis of specific factors.

In Stage 1 of the coagulation process, the contact of injured tissue with blood results in the activation of Factor XII, which reacts with calcium, PTA, PTC, AHF, and Factors III, V, and X to yield intrinsic or blood thromboplastin. This stage is normally completed in 3–5 min. Extrinsic or tissue thromboplastin is rapidly (<12 sec) formed in various tissues in the

body such as lung and brain in the presence of calcium and Factors V, VII, and X. In Stage 2 thromboplastin catalyzes the conversion of prothrombin to thrombin (8–15 sec) in the presence of Factors V, VII, and X and calcium. In stage 3 the thrombin rapidly converts fibrinogen into fibrin. The fibrin then forms a network of fibers which traps red cells and thus forms the blood clot.

Blood contains natural inhibitors of coagulation such as antithrombin, heparin, and antithromboplastin. The dissolution of blood clots occurs by action of blood proteolytic enzyme—plasmin or fibrinolysin. Plasmin is formed from its precursor, plasminogen, after activation by tissue and body fluids or substances of bacterial origin (streptokinase).

The routine tests performed in the coagulation laboratory are indices of vascular function (blood in contact with tissue factors) or intrinsic clotting mechanisms. The determination of *bleeding time* or *capillary fragility* are estimates of blood coagulation in the presence of platelets and tissue or vascular factors. In the Ivy method for determination of *capillary bleeding time*,[20] a blood-pressure cuff is placed on the forearm and inflated to 40 mm Hg; a puncture wound is made and the time required for bleeding to stop is noted. The normal bleeding time, as determined by this method, is 1–9 min. The *capillary fragility* or *tourniquet test*[21] is based on the incidence of petechiae (small red marks) formation produced by an inflated blood-pressure cuff over a 5-min period. Normally, a few tiny petechiae may appear.

Analysis of the *intrinsic coagulation mechanism* is concerned with determination of levels of the specific clotting factors in whole blood. In preliminary studies of a suspected hemorrhagic disorder, determination of *coagulation time, clot retraction, platelet count, bleeding time*, and *petechiae formation* are usually performed.

In the Lee–White procedure,[20] the coagulation time of whole blood is determined in regular or siliconized tubes. Normal values are 8.5–15 min in glass and 19–60 min in siliconized tubes. Siliconization of glassware prevents platelet aggregation and thus delays coagulation. The samples used in the analysis of coagulation time are then inspected at 0.5, 1, 2, 4, and 24 hr after clotting to determine the time required for various phases of clot retraction. The tubes are also observed for evidence of clot lysis or dissolution. The clot will normally start to retract in 30 min, completely retract within 24 hr, and will show no evidence of lysis over a 72-hr period.

Prolonged bleeding times and positive tourniquet tests are seen in thrombocytopenic purpura. Prolonged coagulation times are associated with hemophilia, hypofibrinogenemia, and Factor IX deficiency. Abnormalities in any of the above tests indicate the requirements for further coagulation studies.

The *prothrombin time test* is a measure of the levels of prothrombin complex (Factors II, V, VII, and X) and an index of the capacity of plasma to form thrombin. In the "One Stage" test,[22] the plasma sample is mixed with calcium chloride and tissue thromboplastin, and the time required for fibrin-clot formation is determined. Results are compared with a normal plasma control, and the prothrombin time is reported either in seconds or as per cent prothrombin calculated from a standard activity curve.

A modification[23] (*prothrombin–proconvertin procedure*) of this technique using a 1:10 dilution of both patient and control plasma in the presence of prothrombin-free plasma as a source of Factors I and V,

Table II—Blood-Coagulation Factors

Factor	Synonym
I	Fibrinogen
II	Prothrombin
III	Thromboplastin (tissue)
IV	Calcium
V	Labile factor, plasma accelerator
VI	Globulin, proaccelerin
VII	Stable factor, co-thromboplastin, proconvertin
VIII	Antihemophilic factor (AHF), thromboplastinogen
IX	Christmas factor, plasma thromboplastin component (PTC)
X	Stuart–Prower factor
XI	Plasma thromboplastin antecedent (PTA)
XII	Hageman factor
XIII	Fibrin-stabilizing factor (FSF)

is a more sensitive index of specific deficiencies in prothrombin, Factor VII, and Factor X.

Owren's *thrombotest*,[24] as performed on whole blood, is sensitive to changes in both extravascular and intravascular clotting mechanisms, including Factor IX. The dosage of anticoagulant drugs, such as Dicumarol, are adjusted in accordance with prothrombin time determinations; patients are usually maintained within a therapeutic range of 10–20% prothrombin activity (normal range, 80–130%). Reduced prothrombin levels, with prolonged prothrombin times, are observed in vitamin K deficiency, hemorrhagic disease of the newborn, excessive anticoagulant therapy, and liver disease.

The *prothrombin consumption test*[22] is an index of the efficiency of conversion of prothrombin to thrombin in the coagulation process. The blood sample is allowed to clot under standardized conditions and then the quantity of prothrombin complex removed in the serum is determined in the presence of extrinsic fibrinogen. At least 80% of the prothrombin is normally consumed. Reduced consumption of prothrombin (<80%) is observed in coagulation deficiencies (hemophilia) related to thromboplastin generation.

Other types of coagulation tests detect deficiencies in *thromboplastin generation mechanism*. The *thromboplastin generation time test*[25] (TGT) provides a means of detecting specific deficiencies of Factors V, VIII, IX, X, XI, or XII. In the initial phase of this procedure the clotting time of the patient's adsorbed plasma is determined in the presence of a standardized platelet factor reagent, calcium chloride, plasma substrate reagent (Factors I, II, and V), and the patient's serum. If the clotting time is abnormal (>16 sec), further tests are performed with the patient's plasma or serum. Adsorption of the plasma sample on barium sulfate removes Factors II, VII, IX, and X and facilitates differentiation of a Factor IX–X from V–VIII deficiency in the thromboplastin generation mechanism. Thromboplastin generation is reduced in hemophilia and thrombocytopenia.

The *activated partial thromboplastin time test*[26] (PTT) is based on the observation that hemophilic plasma has a normal clotting time in the presence of a complete thromboplastin (extrinsic-saline extract of brain tissue), as used in prothrombin determinations, but will give a markedly prolonged clotting time with an incomplete thromboplastin (cephalin). Cephalin is a thromboplastic, ether-soluble phospholipid factor with plateletlike activity. In this test the clotting time of the patient's plasma is determined in the presence of calcium chloride and activated cephalin. This test is used primarily to detect deficiencies in Stage I of the coagulation mechanism and is rather sensitive to changes in Factors VIII and IX, as seen in classical hemophilia, and Factor IX deficiency (Hemophilia B or Christmas Disease).

In Stage 3 of the coagulation process, the presence of adequate levels of fibrinogen and thrombin is critical. *Fibrinogen levels*[27] are analyzed semiquantitatively by determining the clotting time of a diluted plasma sample in the presence of extrinsic thromboplastin. This test is basically independent of prothrombin levels. Fibrinogen concentrations of 125 mg% or greater are adequate; deficiencies (hypofibrinogenemia) have been observed in liver disease, carcinomatosis, and in certain complications of pregnancy.

Deficiencies in the clotting mechanisms can usually be partially and temporarily corrected by transfusion of normal blood or plasma. When this fails, the presence of *circulating anticoagulants* (antithrombin, antithromboplastins, heparin) must be considered. Circulating anticoagulants[20] are detected by determining the effect of normal plasma on the clotting time (*recalcification time*) of the patient's oxalated plasma in the presence of calcium chloride. If the addition of the normal plasma does not shorten the prolonged recalcification time, a circulating anticoagulant state can be reported.

Since the end-point of all coagulation tests is the conversion of fibrinogen to fibrin, it is vital that the analyst rigidly standardize his concepts of fibrin formation in visual recording procedures. The use of mechanical instrumentation in the detection of clot formation has significantly increased the standardization, accuracy, and reproducibility of coagulation procedures. These instruments measure and record the process of fibrin formation via increased turbidity[28] (coagulogram) or changes in electrical conductance[29] in the reaction mixtures.

The process of blood coagulation, analysis of coagulation factors, and interpretation of results is a highly complex system. The coagulation laboratory and the physician function together in the diagnosis and treatment of coagulation-deficiency diseases.

Blood-Bank Technology

Blood-bank technology in the modern laboratory is part of the blood-transfusion service. As blood for transfusion is a biologically active therapeutic substance, a complete analysis of its chemical and biologic characteristics is vital to the assurance of successful therapeutic effects. The transfusion service is responsible for:

1. Reception and examination of the donor.
2. Collection, processing, and storage of the blood.
3. Typing of recipient and donor for ABO and Rh blood-group factors.
4. Compatibility (crossmatching) testing before transfusion.
5. Issuance of blood for transfusion.
6. Evaluation of transfusion complications.
7. Performance of special serologic tests pertinent to blood groups and other factors.

In this section a discussion of pertinent factors[30]–[32] related to the various phases of the transfusion service will be presented.

Reception and Examination of the Donor—A complete registry[33] of prospective donors should be maintained, with specific reference to age, sex, weight, address, occupation, and telephone number. Donors should preferably be between the ages of 21 and 60 and should weigh no less than 110 lb. The donor may be rejected on the basis of previous or active incidence of certain microbial diseases (recurrent malaria, syphilis, infectious or homologous serum hepatitis, tuberculosis), bleeding abnormalities, convulsions, allergic syndromes, skin or heart diseases, diabetes, drug addiction, cancer, or blood-pressure abnormalities (acceptable blood pressure: >100/50 and <200/100; pulse rate: 60/120/min).

A period of at least 8 weeks should have elapsed since blood was withdrawn and the blood hemoglobin level should be 12.5–13.5 Gm% or greater. Serum bilirubin and transaminase levels should also be evaluated in donors with previous incidence of jaundice. Levels of glucose-6-phosphate dehydrogenase should be determined in suspected cases of hemolytic anemia.

Table III—Blood-Group Systems

Blood group	Agglutinogen in cell	Agglutinin in serum	Reaction[a] with anti-A serum	Reaction[a] with anti-B serum	Frequency (%) in caucasians
A	A	Anti-B	+	−	41
B	B	Anti-A	−	+	10
AB	AB	None	+	+	4
O	None	Anti-A and B	−	−	45

[a] Agglutination.

Collecting, Processing, and Storage of the Blood—A tourniquet is applied to the arm of the donor to occlude the venous return, the skin area is sterilized, and the blood is collected by venipuncture (phlebotomy). NIH Formula A or B [ACD(Acid–Citrate–Dextrose) or ACD-phosphate] solutions are used as anticoagulants in the sterile blood-collecting containers. Evacuated containers may be of regular or siliconized glass; if blood is collected by gravity feed, glass or plastic collection apparatus is used.

The preservation of the red cells in blood is improved by complete removal of trapped air in the blood-collection apparatus, rapid cooling after collection, and storage at 4°C. Properly collected whole blood is usually stable for 21 days at 1°–6°C. Deterioration of whole blood is related to increased cellular fragility and decreased glucose utilization. Although leukocytes are not well preserved, platelet deterioration and loss of associated factors (Factors V and VIII) are minimal in siliconized-glass or plastic containers.

Blood also may be processed into plasma or red cell components by centrifugation. *Plasmapheresis* is the process whereby plasma is separated from donor blood by centrifugation and the packed red cells reinfused into the same donor within 4 hr after separation of plasma.

ABO Blood-Group Classification—Human red cells can be classified into various groups or types on the basis of reactivity of certain blood factors (*agglutinogens*) located on the erythrocyte membrane. The Landsteiner system (Table III) for the four blood groups is based on the presence or absence of either A or B agglutinogen on the cell surface (Group A, B, AB, or O, respectively).

Serum does not contain the antibody (*agglutinin*) for the antigen present in an individual's own red cells. The clumping or agglutination of the red cells by reaction of agglutinogen with agglutinin is utilized in blood-grouping techniques. In certain instances hemolysin antibodies, present in serum containing anti-A or anti-B agglutinins, cause the disruption of cells and release of hemoglobin (hemolysis).

Human blood cells are grouped by two separate reactions: cellular or "front" grouping and serum or "reverse" grouping. The blood group is ordinarily determined by testing an individual's red cells with standardized anti-A or anti-B serum (certified by Div. of Biological Standards, NIH). Confirmation of the blood group (reverse typing) is accomplished by analysis of an individual's agglutinin titer. In this procedure the individual's serum is heated at 56°C for 10 min to destroy hemolysins, and then mixed with known subgroup A_1 or B_1 human red (Rh negative) cells in the agglutination test. These two tests should be in agreement prior to release of blood for transfusion.

Although human blood cells of Group B react uniformly with Anti-B serum, Group A and AB cells show a wide range of reactivity with Anti-A or Anti-A_1B serum. These blood groups may be further categorized into Subgroups A_1A_2, A_1B, A_2B and A_x on the basis of their reaction with absorbed Anti-A (Anti-A_1) and Anti-AB (Group O) serum.

As the human blood cell contains many antigens with rather complex biochemical structures, the blood factors have been further classified into various subsystems. The Kell (K), Lutheran (Lu), Lewis (Le), Duffy (Fy), Kidd (Jk), MNS, Sutter (Js), Diego (Di), and P blood-factor systems are based on the detection of a specific antigen on or within the red cell by means of specific antibody (isohemagglutinin) reactions. Some of these factors (eg, Kidd, Kell, and Lewis) have been involved in transfusion reactions.

The Rh–Hr System and Antihuman Globulin Test—The presence or absence of Rh_0 agglutinogen in human blood is of prime importance in transfusion reactions, paternity disputes, and isosensitization phenomena. There are eight blood Rh phenotypes which are determined by their reaction with three specific serum agglutinins (Anti-Rh_0, Anti-rh′, and Anti-rh″): rh, rh′, rh″, rh′rh″, Rh_0, Rh_0′, Rh_0″, Rh_0′Rh_0″. The rh groups do not contain the Rh_0 factor on the cell surface and are designated "Rh-negative."

The absence of the Rh antigen in about 15% of the population does not preclude the presence of other factors; the use of specific antisera (Anti-hr′ and Anti-hr″) has demonstrated the existence of the Hr factors (Hr_0, hr′, hr″). For example, the Rh-negative cell—rh″—possesses rh″hr′Hr_0 antigens.

The Rh antibodies are either *saline agglutinins* (complete) or *"blocking" antibodies* (incomplete). The latter type, which is routinely used in Rh testing procedures, is produced more commonly, and in higher titer in the human. It will not agglutinate saline suspensions of normal Rh-positive red cells except in the presence of a high concentration of albumin, serum, or conglutinin (AB serum with albumin) at a temperature of 35–37°C.

In Rh testing procedures, a sample of blood (oxalated or heparinized) or a suspension of cells in serum or albumin is mixed with Anti-Rh_0 serum on a slide or in a tube at 37–47°C. The presence of clumping indicates that the blood possesses Rh_0 antigen. Confirmation of an Rh-negative test may be performed by retesting with Anti-rh′Rh_0rh″ serum.

In Rh testing procedures, red cells from patients with acquired hemolytic anemia are partially coated with human autoantibody, and cells from erythroblastotic infants are coated with maternal antibody globulins and may be falsely clumped by Rh typing serum containing a high protein concentration. The use of the saline agglutinin antisera in combination with a saline suspension of the patient's cells will usually verify the results of previous testing procedures.

Anti-Rh antibodies are not present in normal human serum. Such antibodies may be acquired via isosensitization. The transfusion of Rh-positive blood to an Rh-negative recipient, or transfer of Rh antigen through the placental barrier will result in formation of antibodies to Rh agglutinogens not present in the cells of the recipient or mother, respectively.

Hemolytic blood-transfusion reactions and hemolytic disease of the newborn (erythroblastosis fetalis) involve *isosensitization phenomena* usually related to the Rh_0 antigen. If an expectant mother is Rh-negative and the father Rh-positive, the Rh genotype of the father should be determined. If the father is homozygous, the erythrocytes will contain a pair of Rh_0 factors and the offspring will inherit the Rh_0 factor; if he is heterozygous, one Rh_0 and one Hr_0 factor will be present and his offspring may or may not inherit the factor.

If the fetus is Rh-positive, the mother may be sensitized to the Rh antigen and in subsequent pregnancies, the development of high titers of Anti-Rh antibodies will result in hemolytic disease of the fetus. These antibodies enter the fetal circulation via the placental barrier, coat the red cells of the fetus, and cause excessive erythrocyte destruction, icterus (jaundice), hydrops fetalis (edema), or congenital anemia of the newborn.

The *Coomb's antiglobulin test* is a method of detecting the blocking-type antibodies which are attached to red cell antigens associated with isosensitization phenomena. This type of antibody is present in the globulin fraction of blood serum.

In the "direct" test procedure a saline suspension of the individual's washed red cells is mixed with anti-human globulin antiserum; presence of agglutination is indicative of the combination of human antibody with antigen on the red cell.

An "indirect" procedure is utilized to demonstrate the presence of blocking antibody in the serum of pregnant Rh-negative women and in transfusion reactions. In this procedure the patient's serum is incubated with a suspension of Group O Rh-positive red cells; the cells are washed and then antihuman globulin antiserum is added to detect the coating of the red cells with antibody globulin from the patient's serum by agglutination phenomena. If agglutination occurs in the first part of the procedure, a saline agglutinin is also present.

Compatibility Testing—Crossmatching procedures are designed to detect incompatibilities in the blood of donors and recipient. These incompatibilities are usually related to blood-group Rh–Hr antibodies. For each transfusion, a *major* and *minor crossmatch* should be performed.

In the major test a saline suspension of the donor's cells are mixed with the recipient's serum; the minor test includes the donor's serum and the recipient's cells, usually in the presence of 15–20% albumin. Complete saline crossmatches are also performed to detect antibodies inhibited by high protein concentrations. The presence of agglutination or hemolysis at room temperature indicates incompatibility. The major side of the reaction should be repeated at 45–50°C with and without albumin.

The indirect antihuman globulin procedure is also performed with recipient's serum and donor's cells (major side) and the donor's serum and recipient's cells (minor side). The use of proteolytic enzymes (bromelain, papain, or trypsin) enhances the agglutination of red cells by low-titer or weakly reacting Rh–Hr antibodies. The red cells used in the indirect Coombs test are treated with the enzyme prior to absorption of antibodies and addition of antiglobulin reagent.

The usual crossmatching techniques involve (1) a room temperature procedure, preferably with the addition of albumin; (2) a high-protein procedure with heat; and (3) an antiglobulin procedure.

The presence of nonspecific *autoantibodies, cold agglutinins,* and *bacteriogenic agglutination* sometimes complicate the crossmatching procedure. If the recipient's serum reacts more strongly with his own cells than with the donor's, then autoantibodies should be suspected. Cold agglutinins will usually agglutinate all blood, regardless of type, at low temperatures, but will not react at 37°C. Agglutination as a result of bacterial contamination of blood is called panagglutination.

Issuance of Blood and Evaluation of Transfusion Reactions—Whole blood, red cell suspensions, plasma, and platelet-rich plasma are products of the transfusion service. Transfusion reactions are related to antibody phenomena or transmission of disease. The hemolytic reaction resulting from transfusion of incompatible cells is the most serious problem. Transfusion of microbially contaminated blood can result in pyrogenic reaction or transmission of infectious diseases such as malaria, syphilis, and infectious hepatitis. Allergic reactions (urticaria, asthmatic seizures), circulatory overload, and embolic complications (blood clot or air emboli) also may be encountered. The transfusion service is an integral unit in the evaluation of such complications.

Techniques of Analysis

This section will describe the principles of the procedures used in the analyses of various substances in blood, plasma, or urine. The significance of such tests in clinical diagnosis will be presented briefly. A complete description of the physiologic and pharmacologic aspects of the blood constituents can be found in the references.

Blood

Collection of Blood and Preparation for Chemical Analysis[34]—Using aseptic technique, a blood sample is obtained by venipuncture and usually placed in evacuated glass tubes.[35] If serum is desired, the blood sample is allowed to clot and the serum is separated by centrifugation. When whole blood or plasma is to be used in the analysis, an anticoagulant is added to the collecting tube.

The following concentrations of specific anticoagulants are routinely used per 10 ml blood; lithium, potassium or sodium oxalate (15–25 mg), sodium citrate (40–60 mg), sodium fluoride (35–45 mg), heparin sodium (2 mg), disodium or tripotassium ethylenediaminetetracetate (EDTA—Na_2 or K_3—10–30 mg) or ACD-Formula B Solution (1.0 ml).

Heparin prevents blood coagulation by inhibiting thrombin-catalyzed conversion of fibrinogen to fibrin. The other anticoagulants either precipitate blood calcium or convert ionized calcium into a nonionized form which cannot function in the coagulation reaction. Heparin and EDTA do not significantly alter the cellular elements of blood. Sodium fluoride and thymol are used as preservatives or enzyme inhibitors to prevent deterioration of various substances in the blood sample.

The separation of plasma or serum, and chemical analysis, are usually performed as soon as possible after collection of the sample. The addition of polystyrene granules to the blood sample prior to centrifugation facilitates the isolation of serum or plasma.[36] Changes in the ratio of CO_2, chloride, and electrolytes in cells and plasma, glycolytic conversion of glucose to lactic acid, hydrolysis of ester phosphate to free inorganic phosphate, bacterial conversion of urea to ammonia, and conversion of pyruvate to lactate are examples of changes that can occur in contaminated, improperly preserved, or unrefrigerated blood specimens.

The first stage in many of the chemical determinations is the removal of blood protein and preparation of *protein-free blood filtrate*. The protein is precipitated with tungstic acid, trichloroacetic acid, zinc hydroxide, or organic solvents such as alcohol and acetone, and then filtered or centrifuged to remove the protein coagulum. Tungstic acid precipitation is performed by mixing 1 volume of blood or 2 volumes of plasma with 9 volumes of stabilized tungstic acid reagent. The filtrate obtained in this procedure should be in the pH range 3.0—5.1 to assure adequate removal of proteins (<2 mg% in filtrate).[37]

The "Somogyi" filtrate is prepared by mixing 1 volume of blood with 5 volumes of water, 2 volumes of 5% zinc sulfate and 2 volumes of 0.3 N barium hydroxide.[38] The barium sulfate is precipitated and the zinc hydroxide, formed in the reaction, precipitates the blood proteins. This filtrate is free of reducing substances other than glucose. Trichloracetic acid (10%), in a ratio of 9:1 with blood, yields greater volumes of filtrate due to a more complete formation of protein agglomerates.

Blood Glucose—Methods for the determination of blood glucose are based on the utilization of glucose as a reducing agent and on the enzymatic oxidation of glucose to gluconic acid. In the Folin–Wu technique glucose is determined in a protein-free blood filtrate by reduction of alkaline cupric sulfate and subsequent reaction with a phosphomolybdic[39] or arsenomolybdic acid reagent to form a blue complex which can be estimated colorimetrically.

The Nelson–Somogyi[40] method uses a protein-free blood filtrate prepared with zinc hydroxide to remove the majority of interfering reducing substances other than glucose. The presence of a terminal aldehyde in the glucose molecule is the basis of a colorimetric determination with phenolic hydroxyl reagents (phenol in aqueous methyl salicylate or phosphorylated 1,3-dihydroxybenzene) in the presence of strong sulfuric acid and heat.[41]

In the previous techniques interfering substances such as lactose, galactose, and glutathione are measured and the value is reported in the nonspecific term "sugar." Enzymatic determination with glucose oxidase[42] is the only test that measures true blood glucose. Blood glucose is converted to gluconic acid and hydrogen peroxide by glucose oxidase; the peroxide is then estimated by iodimetric procedures or by reaction with o-dianisidine and peroxidase.

Another enzymatic procedure utilizes the hexokinase-catalyzed conversion of glucose to glucose-6-phosphate (G-6-P) and then to 6-phosphogluconate and TPNH in the presence of TPN and G-6-P dehydrogenase. The TPNH thus formed is equivalent to the amount of glucose present and is estimated at 340 or 366 mμ with a spectrophotometer.

Normal fasting blood-sugar values for adults are 80–120 mg/100 ml; true glucose is 65–100 mg/100 ml. When the blood sugar value exceeds 120 (hyperglycemia), diabetes mellitus should be suspected. The effect of ingested carbohydrate on blood sugar can be determined by the *glucose tolerance test*[1,43]; 100 Gm of glucose, in water or a flavored beverage, are administered orally and blood- and urine-sugar determinations are performed at hourly intervals for 3 hr. Values above 160 at 1 hr and 110 mg/100 ml at 2 hr are abnormal. The renal threshold for glucose is 180–200 mg/100 ml of blood, and sugar should not appear in the urine of normal subjects in the tolerance test.

Hyperglycemia and decreased glucose tolerance are seen in diabetes mellitus (to 500 mg/100 ml), and hyperactivity of the adrenals, pituitary, and thyroid glands. Hypoglycemia, with a blood-sugar value of <60 mg/100 ml and increased glucose tolerance, is encountered in insulin overdosage, glucagon deficiencies, and hypoactivity of various endocrine glands. Intravenous glucose tolerance studies are used in order to circumvent defective absorption of glucose in the gastrointestinal tract; eg, steatorrhoea.

The β cells of pancreatic islet tissue secrete insulin and the α cells secrete glucagon, a substance antagonistic to insulin and having a hyperglycemic effect. In *glucagon tolerance studies*[1] the effect of parenteral administration of glucagon on blood-sugar values is useful in the diagnosis of pancreatic and hepatic function. *Insulin and tolbutamide tolerance studies*[1] are used in the diagnosis of endocrine disorders, differentiation of insulin-resistant diabetics, and determination of functional hypoglycemia and islet cell tumors.

Galactosemia,[44] the presence of galactose in blood, is due to an inborn error of galactose metabolism; deficiencies in galactokinase or galactose-1-phosphate uridyl transferase result in inadequate galactose metabolism. Deficiencies in lactose-metabolizing enzymes (lactase) have been associated with gastrointestinal diseases.

Lactic acid[1] is a product of glucose metabolism; it is readily converted into pyruvic acid and reduced diphosphopyridine nucleotide (DPNH) by lactic dehydrogenase (LDH) in the presence of diphosphopyridine nucleotide (DPN).

Blood lactic acid is estimated by reaction with LDH to form pyruvate and DPNH; the DPNH level is analyzed spectrophotometrically at 340 mμ and is a function of lactic acid concentration. It is elevated (>20 mg/100 ml) following exercise, anesthesia, and certain types of acidosis. The lactate/pyruvate blood ratio should be calculated in order to determine the presence of excess lactic acid in blood in acidosis, thiamine deficiency, and decompensated heart disease.

Blood pyruvic acid is analyzed by the reverse procedure; ie, conversion of pyruvate to lactate in the presence of LDH and DPNH. Normal blood pyruvic acid ranges from 0.6–1.3 mg/100 ml.

Nonprotein Nitrogen Compounds—Nonprotein nitrogen (NPN) refers to all nitrogen-containing compounds in biologic fluids exclusive of protein. This includes nitrogen from amino acids, low-molecular-weight peptides, urea, nucleotides, uric acid, creatinine, creatine, and ammonia. Blood NPN is usually determined by digestion of protein-free blood filtrate with sulfuric acid in the presence of a catalyst (SeO$_2$) to convert nitrogen to ammonium sulfate; the excess acid is then neutralized and ammonia determined by Nesslerization[2] or reaction with alkaline hypochlorite.

The normal blood NPN is 25–45 mg/100 ml (48% urea N, 14% amino acid N, 4% creatine N, 1% creatinine N, 3.0% uric acid N, and 30% residual N). In renal damage, NPN is elevated to values ranging from 60–500 mg/100 ml (*azotemia*). As variations in NPN mainly reflect alterations in blood urea nitrogen (BUN), urea determinations are preferred as a guide to kidney function.

The primary pathway of nitrogen metabolism in man is the synthesis of urea from ammonia in the liver and then rapid renal excretion of urea. In renal disease (nephritis) the excretion of urea is diminished and blood NPN and BUN are increased. In BUN procedures urea is enzymatically converted to ammonia by urease; the ammonia is then determined by Nesslerization,[1] reaction with phenol–alkaline hypochlorite,[45] aeration into standard acid and subsequent titration, or reaction with salicylate–nitroprusside reagent at pH 11.8–12.0 in the presence of alkaline dichloroisocyanurate to form a green chromogen which can be estimated colorimetrically.[46] Direct chemical determinations of urea are based on reaction with 2,3-butanedione in an acid medium (Fearon reaction).

BUN is increased in chronic and acute nephritis, metallic poisoning, and cardiac failure; reduced levels occur in rapid dehydration or following diuresis. In severe liver damage due to diminished urea formation, an increase in blood ammonia and decrease in BUN is observed. Urine urea output (6–17 Gm/day) is an index of *glomerular filtration rate* (GFR) and kidney function. Increased dietary protein and gastrointestinal hemorrhage will increase urine urea.

The *nitrogen balance* represents the balance between nitrogen input or produced (N_{in}) and nitrogen excreted (N_{out}); in normal individuals $N_{in} = N_{out}$. N_{out} is regulated by renal GFR; in renal disease GFR is decreased, $N_{in} > N_{out}$, and BUN is increased. The rate of urinary excretion of parenterally administered dyes (phenolsulfophthalein), inulin sodium, *p*-aminohippurate, and mannitol are sensitive indices of GFR in *renal clearance studies*.[1]

Creatine (methylguanidoacetic acid) and creatinine (creatine anhydride) are involved in the physiology of muscle contraction. Creatine is an intracellular source of high-energy phosphate bonds via the reaction of creatine phosphate and creatine kinase. Creatinine is the waste product of creatine metabolism and is the normally excreted compound.

Blood creatinine[47] is determined by reaction with alkaline picrate to form a red chromogen. These values usually represent 20–30% non-creatinine-interfering substances. Absolute determinations can be made by absorption of creatinine from protein-free blood filtrates on aluminum silicate prior to the final determination. Creatine is determined after hydrolytic conversion to creatinine with boiling picric or hydrochloric acid.

Renal clearance of endogenous creatinine is related to GFR and is normally 1–2 Gm/day (creatinine coefficient = 20–26 mg/Kg/24 hr). Normal blood creatinine is 1–2 mg/100 ml; creatine, 2–7 mg/100 ml. Higher values (5 mg/100 ml) indicate glomerular damage.

Uric acid is a catabolite of purine metabolism as derived from nucleic acids or nucleotide cofactors. Direct methods for determination of uric acid involve reaction with alkaline phosphotungstic acid[47] to form a "tungsten blue," which is estimated colorimetrically. In another method alcoholic NaOH is added to a protein-free filtrate to eliminate interfering reducing substances (ascorbic acid, glutathione) prior to reduction of uric acid with acid copper chelate to form a cupric chromogen complex.[48]

In indirect procedures uric acid is hydrolyzed by the enzyme urease; the decrease in absorbency at 290–293 mμ is a function of initial concentrations of uric acid.[1] The normal blood value is 1.5–6.0 mg/100 ml. It is elevated in renal disease, in gout due to increased metabolic pools of uric acid, and in leukemia as a result of increased turnover of cellular nucleoprotein.

Amino acid determinations in blood are performed by conventional ninhydrin techniques or reaction with alkaline β-naphthoquinone-4-sulfonate.[47] Normal plasma values range from 3.9–7.8 mg/100 ml. A variety of metabolic disorders may be detected by analysis of increased levels of specific amino acids in urine or blood. Total urine amino acids are determined by formol titration; formaldehyde reacts with basic amino groups and thus permits subsequent titration of the acidic groups of the amino acids. Daily excretion of amino acid nitrogen ranges from 100–400 mg, constituting 1–2% of total urine nitrogen.

Identification and quantitation of specific amino acids in blood and urine is accomplished by chromatographic and electrophoretic separation of electrolytically desalted blood or urine samples. Two-dimensional chromatography in phenol and butanol–acetic acid solvents provides excellent separation of the amino acids.

The chromatograms are developed with ninhydrin reagent and quantitated by colorimetric estimation of the spots in a densiometric scanning apparatus. Phenylalanine and tyrosine may be detected as a blue spot by spraying with sodium bicarbonate; homocystine as a pink spot with mercuric nitrate; cystine with an iodoplatinate reagent. Abnormal amino acid metabolism[49–51] (*aminoacidopathies*) usually results in the presence of abnormal quantities of specific amino acids in the urine (aminoaciduria).

The aminoacidurias are divided into two main groups:

1. *Primary overflow aminoaciduria* in which blood amino acids are elevated [phenylketonuria (PKU), Maple Syrup Urine disease (MSUD), tyrosinosis, and alkaptonuria].
2. Aminoacidurias characterized by elevated amino acid urine levels with normal blood levels (*transport diseases* with a defect in the kidney tubule—eg, Cystinuria—and "no threshold" aminoaciduria in which the kidney has no mechanism for reabsorbing the amino acid involved—eg, homocystinuria).

PKU, a disease characterized by mental deficiency, is associated with the presence of phenylpyruvic acid in the urine and elevated serum phenylalanine levels due to an hereditary deficiency of hepatic phenylalanine hydroxylase which converts phenylalanine to tyrosine. Serum phenylalanine determinations are based on the fluorescence of a complex with ninhydrin and copper in the presence of L-leucyl-L-alanine.

MSUD is characterized by the odor of the urine and is rapidly fatal to infants. It is associated with a deficiency in the oxidative decarboxylation of α-keto acids leading to an accumulation of both the keto and amino acids in the blood and urine (valine, leucine, isoleucine).

Alkaptonuria is a rare, hereditary disease in which homogentisic acid cannot be further metabolized due to a lack of homogentisic acid oxidase. This causes homogentisic aciduria, ochronosis, and arthritis.

In Hartnup disease indole and tryptophane appear in the urine due to defective renal and intestinal absorption of tryptophane. Tryptophane is an intermediary metabolite in the synthesis of serotonin (5-hydroxytryptamine) and 5-hydroxyindole acetic acid (HIAA). Excessive production of serotonin and the presence of its HIAA metabolite in urine is associated with metastatic carcinoid tumors. HIAA is measured after removal of interfering keto acids with dinitrophenylhydrazine, extraction, and estimation with nitrosonaphthol reagent.[47,52] Normal values are less than 10 mg/24-hr urine specimen.

Proteins—The plasma proteins (albumins, globulins, and fibrinogen) are concerned with nutrition, electrolyte and acid–base balance, transport mechanisms, coagulation, immunity, and enzymatic action. Total plasma proteins may be determined by Kjeldahl, Nesslerization, or biuret procedures. The latter technique is based on the reaction of -CONH- groups joined by carbon or nitrogen linkages in protein with alkaline copper sulfate to yield the biuret complex which can be estimated colorimetrically.

The *albumin–globulin* (A/G) *ratio* is determined by the biuret method after precipitation of the globulins with a sodium sulfate–sulfite reagent. The normal range is 5.5–8.0 Gm% total protein with an A/G ratio of 1.4–2.4. Changes in total protein and A/G ratio occur in kidney and liver disease, hemorrhage, dehydration, rheumatoid arthritis, and multiple myeloma.

The physiochemical properties of the plasma proteins —molecular weight (68,000–300,000) and isoelectric point (pH of minimum solubility and ionic neutrality) —provide the basis for the electrophoretic separation of plasma proteins (Fig. 424). The plasma sample is spotted on a paper or cellulose acetate strip, or in a polyacrylamide gel ("Disc" electrophoresis) at pH 8.6.

At this pH the proteins are electroanionic and, under the influence of electric current, will migrate to the anode at a rate dependent on their isoelectric point. The strips are then stained with a protein dye (Bromophenol blue, Amidoschwarz, Ponceau S), and the concentrations of the various proteins are estimated colorimetrically.

The normal ranges for the major proteins are (in Gm%): albumin, 3.8–5.0; total globulin, 2.0–3.9; α_1-globulin, 0.1–0.5; α_2-globulin, 0.5–0.9; β-globulin, 0.5–1.2; γ-globulin, 0.7–1.6.[53]

Enzymes[54–58]—Enzymes are proteins whose biologic function is the catalysis of chemical reactions in living systems. Enzymes combine with the substances on which they act (substrate) to form an enzyme-substrate complex which is then converted to a reaction product and liberated enzyme which continues its catalytic function.

Serum enzymes are intracellular in origin and are elevated in hyperactivity, disease, or injury to cardiac, hepatic, pancreatic, muscle, bone, or malignant tissue. As the specific tissue involved will determine the type of enzyme that will be elevated, such determinations are valuable diagnostic tools in the differentiation of various pathologic states.

Enzymes are named and classified according to the type of reaction that they catalyze, and to their substrate specificities. Enzyme activity is usually expressed in "International Units" (IU) which is related to the μ moles substrate converted per minute per liter at 25°C. See Chapter 57 for a more complete discussion of enzymes.

Transferases are enzymes that catalyze the transfer of amino or phosphate groups from one compound to another. Serum glutamic–oxaloacetic (GOT) and glutamic–pyruvic (GPT) transaminases are important enzymes in clinical diagnosis. These enzymes catalyze the transfer of the amino group from glutamic acid to keto acids (oxaloacetic or pyruvic) to form aspartic and α-ketoglutaric acids with GOT, and alanine and α-ketoglutaric acid with GPT.

Colorimetric methods of determination are based on estimation of substrate concentrations (oxaloacetic or pyruvic acid) with dinitrophenylhydrazine, or reaction products (α-ketoglutaric acid) by coupling with 6-benzamido-4-methoxy-*m*-toluidinediazonium chloride.

Spectrophotometric and fluorometric methods of analysis are based on the reaction of substrate with reduced nicotinoyl adenine dinucleotide (NADH$_2$) in the presence of malic dehydrogenase (GOT) or lactic dehydrogenase (GPT) to form NAD; final NADH$_2$ concentration in the reaction mixture is a function of initial enzyme activity.

Normal SGOT and SGPT levels are 2–19 IU. GOT is present in large amounts in liver, cardiac, and skeletal muscle, whereas GPT is primarily found in liver tissue. SGOT is elevated in myocardial infarction and Duchenne muscular dystrophy; SGOT and SGPT are increased in liver disease, acute toxic or viral hepatitis, infectious mononucleosis, obstructive jaundice, and hepatic cirrhosis.

Creatinine phosphokinase (CPK) is a transaminase found in skeletal and cardiac tisue. It catalyzes the transfer of phosphate groups from creatine phosphate

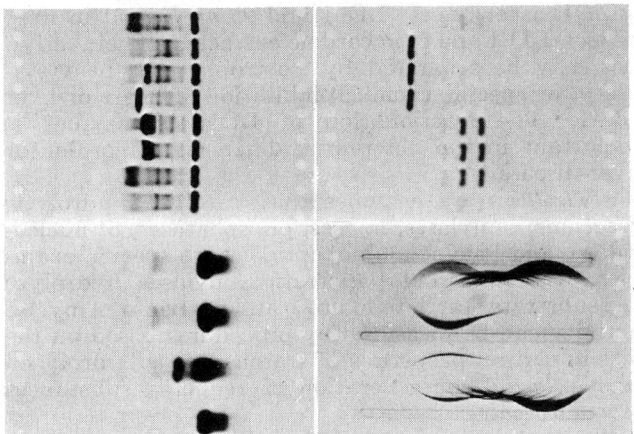

Fig. 424. Electrophoretic separation of serum proteins, isoenzymes, hemoglobins, and immune plasma protein (courtesy, Spinco).

to adenosine diphosphate (ADP) to form adenosine triphosphate (ATP). Normal serum levels are 44–66 IU; it is elevated in myocardial infarction and Duchenne muscular dystrophy but remains at normal levels in liver disease.

Ornithine transcarbamylase (OTC) in serum is the only enzyme of the urea cycle which has been used in the clinical investigation of liver disease. It catalyzes the conversion of ornithine to citrulline. The normal serum value is 0–0.40 IU.

Dehydrogenases are enzymes that catalyze hydrogen transfer in cellular oxidation processes. Lactic (LDH), α-hydroxybutyric (HBDH), malic (MDH), isocitric (ICDH), and sorbitol (SDH) dehydrogenase are of diagnostic importance in myocardial and liver disease.

LDH catalyzes the conversion of pyruvic to lactic acid in the presence of DPNH. The activity may be estimated colorimetrically by formation of the pyruvic acid hydrazone with 2,6-dinitrophenylhydrazine; spectrophotometric or fluorimetric estimation of DPNH is also used to estimate enzyme activity. The normal serum LDH value is <240 IU. LDH is increased to a much greater extent (700–2000 IU) and for a more prolonged period than SGOT or CPK in myocardial infarction; it is also increased to varying degrees in certain types of hepatic disease, disseminated malignancies, and muscular dystrophy.

HBD reduces α-ketobutyric acid to α-hydroxybutyric acid in the presence of $NADH_2$; estimation of the α-keto acid via hydrazone formation is the basis of activity measurements. The normal serum HBD level is <140 IU; it is elevated in myocardial infarction.

MDH and SDH, in the presence of DPN, catalyze the conversion of malate or sorbitol to oxaloacetate or fructose, respectively. They are of diagnostic value in myocardial infarction (MDH > 48 IU) and acute liver injury (SDH > 96 IU).

ICDH oxidizes isocitrate, in the presence of TPN or DPN, to α-keto glutarate; it is elevated (>5.0 IU) in acute hepatitis.

Recent advances in protein chemistry and technical methodology have fractionated enzymes, previously thought to be homogeneous, into heterogenous moieties. These multiple molecular forms of enzymes (*isoenzymes*) have similar substrate specificity but different biophysical properties. LDH, MDH, phosphatases, and leucine aminopeptidase are actually isoenzymes.

LDH isoenzymes (LD 1 and 2) are found in liver tissue; LD 4 and 5, in cardiac extracts. Their activities may be separated by electrophoresis, heat stability, or specific chemical inhibition of heart or liver LDH. The fractionation of LDH isoenzymes is important in the differential diagnosis of cardiac or liver disease.

Hydrolases are enzymes that catalyze hydrolytic reactions; amylases, lipases, phosphatases, 5'-nucleotidase, and leucine aminopeptidase are specific examples. Salivary and pancreatic amylases hydrolyze the substrate starch to maltose and dextrins. Amylase activity can be measured by procedures based on the loss in certain properties of starch as it is hydrolyzed (*amyloclastic*), or generation of reducing substances (*saccharogenic*).

The amyloclastic methods utilize the decrease in viscosity and turbidity of hydrolyzed starch substrates, or the reaction of starch with iodine for the method of estimation. The saccharogenic methods determine the reaction products (reducing sugars) by previously described methodology. The normal serum level is 140 IU; elevations are noted in acute pancreatitis, acute abdominal conditions (perforated peptic ulcer, common bile duct obstruction), and salivary gland disease.

Lipases catalyze the conversion of triglycerides to glycerol and fatty acids. Clinical determinations are based on titrimetric analysis of fatty acids liberated from an emulsified olive oil substrate. Serum lipase is increased in pancreatic carcinoma.

Phosphatases catalyze the hydrolysis of orthophosphoric acid esters and are classified according to pH of optimal activity into alkaline (pH > 7) or acid (pH < 7) phosphatases. Activity (alkaline, pH 8–10; acid, pH 4–6) is measured with phenylphosphate, glycerophosphate, *p*-nitrophenylphosphate, or thymolphthalein monophosphate substrates.

With the latter two chromogenic substrates, the amount of *p*-nitrophenol or thymolphthalein liberated by phosphatase hydrolysis is estimated colorimetrically in an alkaline medium. With glycerophosphate or phenylphosphate substrate, the liberated phosphorus is determined by molybdenum blue formation with phosphomolybdic-phosphotungstic acids; phenol may also be estimated with 4-aminoantipyrine or Folin-Ciocalteau reagent.

Acid phosphatase activity may be differentiated by the use of inhibitors in the assay mixture; formaldehyde has no effect on acid phosphatase of prostatic origin, but it inhibits other acid phosphatases, while tartrate is a selective inhibitor of the prostatic enzyme.

Normal values for *alkaline phosphatase* activity depend on the substrate used; they are elevated in bone and liver disease. *Acid phosphatase* is of primary diagnostic value in prostatic malignancy.

The enzyme 5'-nucleotidase is an alkaline phosphomonoesterase that hydrolyzes nucleotides with a phosphate radical attached to the 5'-position of the pentose (eg, adenosine monophosphate). The normal serum value is 17 IU; it is elevated in posthepatic obstructive jaundice.

Leucine amino peptidase is an exopeptidase which hydrolyzes the peptide bond adjacent to a free amino group. It liberates amino acids from the *N*-terminal group of proteins and polypeptides. Activity is determined by spectrophotometric estimation following hydrolysis of the amide bond of a leucinamide substrate at 238 mμ. A fluorimetric determination of naphthylamine liberated from a leucyl-β-naphthylamide substrate has also been utilized. The normal value is 15–60 IU; it is elevated in the last trimester of pregnancy, hepatic biliary disease, and pancreatic carcinoma.

Lyases are enzymes which split C–C bonds without group transfer. Aldolase is a glycolic lyase which catalyzes the reversible splitting of fructose-1,6-diphosphate to form dihydroxyacetone phosphate and glyceraldehyde-3-phosphate. In estimation of activity the triose phosphate reaction products are hydrolyzed with alkali and the resultant trioses are reacted with 2,4-dinitrophenylhydrazine to form chromogenic hydrazones for colorimetric analysis. The normal value is <7.2 IU; it is elevated in muscular dystrophy, polymyositis, and acute hepatitis.

Lipids—The major classes of blood lipids[59] are: fatty acids, cholesterol, triglycerides, phospholipids, sphingoglycolipids, and lipoproteins.

Cholesterol,[47] a sterol molecule, is an essential substance in steroid hormone synthesis by the adrenal cortex and bile acid production in the liver. It exists in blood as the free sterol and as cholesterol esters of fatty acids.

In the determination of *total cholesterol* the serum is extracted with an alcohol–ether mixture and the cholesterol estimated colorimetrically after reaction with acetic anhydride–sulfuric acid reagent (Liebermann–Buchard reaction). Precipitation of free cholesterol with digitonin will differentiate free from esterified cholesterol. Chromatographic separation of cholesterol from its esters on alumina, silicic acid, or magnesium silicate columns with organic solvents has also been used.

Gas chromatographic procedures[60] have resulted in separation and quantitation of cholesterol, its metabolites, and precursors; this is a type of partition chromatography in which a volatilized sample is partitioned between a liquid stationary phase and a mobile gas phase. The normal total serum cholesterol level is 150–240 mg/100 ml; it is increased in nephrosis, diabetes mellitus, and myxedema and decreased in hyperthyroidism and hepatic disease. Free cholesterol forms 20–40% and the ester fraction 60–80% of the total cholesterol.

Phospholipids[61] are "compound" or "heterolipids" in which one of the hydroxyl groups of glycerol is in an ester linkage with phosphoric acid which is, in turn, esterified with a nitrogenous base. Lecithin and cephalin (phosphatidylethanolamine) are clinically important members of this class.

These serum lipids are extracted into an alcohol–ether mixture, digested with sulfuric acid–hydrogen peroxide, and the liberated phosphorus determined by previously described colorimetric techniques. The normal lipid phosphorus is 6–11 mg/100 ml; about one-half is lecithin. The average ratio of cholesterol to lipid phosphorus when cholesterol is normal is 21. Phospholipid changes are usually associated with cholesterol changes.

Sphingoglycolipids differ from lecithin and cephalin as they contain two nitrogenous bases (choline and sphingosine) per molecule. They are primarily found in brain tissue (eg, sphingomyelin, galactolipin).

The blood fatty acids[47,61] occur in esterified (EFA) and nonesterified (NEFA) forms. *Total lipid* (triglyceride) is determined on alcohol–ether extracts of whole blood; the triglycerides in the extract are hydrolyzed to glycerol and fatty acids. The glycerol liberated by hydrolysis is oxidized with periodate to formaldehyde, and the latter is measured colorimetrically after reaction with chromotropic acid; glycerol can also be determined fluorometrically after condensation with o-aminophenol and subsequent oxidation to 8-hydroxyquinoline. Fatty acids in the hydrolysate may be directly determined by titration with NaOH. *EFA* analyses are based on the reaction of alkaline hydroxylamine with esters of fatty acids to form hydroxamic acids which produce a red color with ferric chloride.

Gas chromatographic procedures have been used to quantitate the various fatty acids; ie, palmitic, stearic, oleic, linoleic, and linolenic acids. Mono-, di-, and triglycerides can also be separated into classes by column or thin-layer chromatography, and infrared spectroscopy.[62] The total fatty acids of plasma range from 200–450 mg/100 ml in the fasting state; they are derived from glycerides, neutral fats (0–150 mg/100 ml), cholesterol esters, phospholipids, and sphingolipids. An increase in neutral fat will produce a milky appearance of serum or plasma (hyperlipemia).

Lipoproteins[63] are lipid-conjugated proteins that migrate electrophoretically with the α_1–β_1 plasma globulin fractions and are designated α_1- and β_1-lipoprotein. The lipid constituents are primarily cholesterol esters and phospholipids. Electrophoretic separation of plasma, followed by staining with fat-soluble dyes (eg, Oil Red O, Sudan Black) and densiometric quantitation of the various bands, is the usual analytical procedure. Low-density β-lipoprotein also may be semiquantitated by reaction with specific anti-β-lipoprotein sera to form an antigen–antibody precipitate. The α-fraction constitutes 20–35% of the total lipoprotein; it is proportionally decreased in atherosclerosis, hypothyroidism, and nephrosis. The α–β-lipoprotein:cholesterol ratio is lower than normal (0.44) in conditions known to result in susceptibility to heart disease; eg, nephrosis (0.05) and diabetes (0.25).

Steroids and Related Substances—17-Ketosteroids (17-KS)[64] are derived from adrenal and, in the male, testicular function. The principal urinary steroid metabolites in this group of androgens are epi-, dehydroepi-, and androsterone in the free form, and as conjugates of glucuronates, sulfates, or acetates. Their determination in urine involves acid hydrolysis of the conjugates, extraction with organic solvent, reaction with alkaline m-dinitrobenzene (Zimmerman reaction), and colorimetric estimation of the chromogen. The normal urine values are: male, 9–24 mg/day; female, 5–17 mg/day. Decreased excretion is seen in hypoactive disease of the pituitary, gonads, and adrenals.

17-Hydroxycorticosteroids,[64] mineralocorticoids, and glucocorticoids are produced by the adrenal cortex. The most important members of this class are cortisone and cortisol; the urinary metabolites are tetrahydro- and allotetrahydrocortisol, cortol, cortolone, and tetrahydrocortisol. The determination involves pretreatment of the urine with borohydride to reduce the 17-KS to alcohols, followed by mild oxidation with acidic sodium bismuthate to convert 17-ketogenic steroids to 17-KS and final estimation with Zimmerman reagents. The normal urine values are: male, 8–25 mg/day; female, 5–18 mg/day.

Plasma glucocorticoids can be estimated colorimetrically by the reaction of the steroidal dihydroxyacetone group with a phenylhydrazine sulfuric acid reagent, or by fluorometric procedures. Normal plasma level is 5–20 mcg/100 ml. It is decreased in adrenal, thyroid, and pituitary insufficiency.

Pregnanediol[1] is derived from progesterone, the hormone secreted by the corpus luteum and placenta. In the analysis of urine the pregnanediol glucuronide is acid hydrolyzed, extracted with toluene, oxidized with permanganate, chromatographed on alumina, and the isolated diacetate derivative estimated colorimetrically after reaction with sulfuric acid. Fluctuations in urine levels are associated with the menstrual cycle, pregnancy, and corpus luteum cysts.

The natural estrogens[47] are 17β-estradiol, estrone, and estriol. In the determination, after acid hydrolysis and ether extraction of the urine, the estrogens are methylated with dimethyl sulfate and chromatographically separated prior to reaction with guinolsulfuric acid to yield a red chromogen for colorimetric analysis. The normal estrogen output is 4–60 mcg/24 hr in the female and up to 25 mcg in the male. Estrogen deficiency can be related to ovarian failure and pituitary deficiency.

The anterior pituitary secretes three substances (*gonadotropins*) which govern gonadal activity: follicle-stimulating hormone (FSH), luteinizing hormone (LH), and luteotropin (LTH). The gonadotropins are glycoproteins. Bioassay methods are used to determine gonadotrophic activity. After fractionation and isolation, the urine extract is assayed in test animals as to follicular growth of the ovaries in hypophysectomized animals or increase in testicular, ovarian, or uterine weight.

The presence of human chorionic gonadotropin (HCG) in urine is the basis of an immunologic test to detect pregnancy.[65]

In the presence of HCG antiserum, tanned sheep erythrocytes sensitized with HCG will agglutinate; when HCG is in the urine, inhibition of the red cell–antibody reaction occurs. This *in vitro* test compares favorably with the standard *in vivo* toad or rat ovarian hyperemia test for pregnancy. HCG also has been quantitated in serum by the immunologic method.

Human growth hormone and insulin are endocrine protein secretions which are of diagnostic value in growth rate studies and diabetes. They are best quantitated by bioassay or by immunologic procedures with ^{131}I-antigen preparations.

Epinephrine and norepinephrine are biologically active catecholamines derived from the adrenal medulla and sympathetic nerve endings. Total catecholamines are measured in blood and urine after fractionation on alumina or ion-exchange columns, oxidation at pH 3.5 or 6.0, and subsequent fluorimetric analysis. Urine catecholamines are increased to >350 mcg/24 hr in adrenal medullary tissue tumors (pheochromocytoma). The normal plasma level is 2.1–6.5 mcg/liter with about 80% as norepinephrine.

Vanillylmandelic acid (VMA) is the urine metabolite of these two catecholamines. Its quantity in urine reflects the endogenous secretion of catecholamines. VMA can be determined colorimetrically, after extraction of the urine with ethylacetate, and diazotization with p-nitroaniline and ethanolamine in the presence of carbonate ion. The normal output is 0–12 mg/24 hr.

Bilirubin,[1] a tetrapyrrol which is synthesized from hemoglobin, normally occurs in low concentration in the blood. In the bile it is present as the water-soluble conjugated glucuronide. The reduction of bilirubin in the intestine yields urobilinogen which is, in turn, oxidized to a brown pigment—urobilin.

Serum bilirubin is determined by coupling with diazotized sulfanilic acid to form azobilirubin for colorimetric analysis. The *direct* or *conjugated bilirubin* test is performed in aqueous media; the *indirect* or *free bilirubin* analysis is performed in methanol or caffeine–sodium benzoate solution. Normal values in serum are: direct, 0–0.3 mg/100 ml; total, 0–1.5 mg/100 ml.

Clinical jaundice is a yellowing of the tissues associated with hyperbilirubinemia; in hemolytic disease of the newborn due to Rh and ABD incompatibilities, indirect serum bilirubin is elevated, whereas acute hepatitis results in increases in the direct type.

Electrolytes—The normal plasma electrolyte level is 154 mEq/liter of cations and 154 mEq/liter of anions.

The osmotic effects of chloride, sodium, and potassium are important in the maintenance of normal muscle contraction and water distribution between cells, plasma, and interstitial fluid.

Sodium and potassium serum concentrations are readily measured by flame photometry[47] or atomic absorption spectroscopy.[66] The latter technique is similar to emission-flame photometry, except that it measures energy as it is absorbed by atoms rather than as it is emitted by atoms. Both techniques are based on the characteristic absorption or emission wavelengths of the cations.

Chloride levels in serum or urine are determined by titration with acid mercuric nitrate solution in the presence of 5-diphenylcarbazone indicator.[67] It also may be determined potentiometrically with a silver–silver chloride pH electrode assembly. The normal serum values are 135–155 mEq Na/liter, 3.9–5.6 mEq K/liter, and 95–106 mEq Cl/liter; urine levels are 150–197 mEq Na/day, 20–64 mEq K/day, and 180–270 mEq K (as NaCl)/day.

Serum sodium, potassium, and chloride are increased in adrenal cortical insufficiency, renal and cardiac failure, anuria, and dehydration; decreases occur in alimentary tract diseases associated with diarrhea and vomiting, or increased renal electrolyte excretion (diuretic therapy).

The determination of excess chloride (>50 mEq/liter) in the perspiration of patients with pancreatic cystic fibrosis is an accurate diagnostic tool. Perspiration is stimulated by placing the subject's hand in a plastic bag for 15–20 min or, preferably, by an iontophoresis technique in which pilocarpine nitrate ions are transported through small areas of the skin to produce local perspiration.[68] The chloride content may be quantitated with silver nitrate–potassium chromate-impregnated papers or by conductivity measurements with selective ion electrodes.

Bicarbonate, phosphates, sodium, potassium, and chloride concentrations are related to maintenance of acid–base balance in the body. The pH of the blood reflects the state of the acid–base balance and is mathematically related to HCO_3 concentration and partial pressure CO_2(pCO_2) in blood by the Henderson–Hasselbalch equation

$$pH = 6.01 + \frac{\log(HCO_3)}{0.0308 \times pCO_2}$$

Blood pH, as measured electrometrically, has a normal range of 7.36–7.40 for venous samples and 7.38–7.42 for arterial samples. The pCO_2 level[69] in blood is determined by measuring the pH of the blood at three different pCO_2 concentrations—one native to the blood and the other two obtained by equilibration with gas mixtures of known pCO_2. Blood bicarbonate levels also may be determined by measuring the amount of acid neutralized by plasma or serum and pCO_2 calculated by the above equation. The role of oxygen and hemoglobin in respiration has been discussed previously.

Blood oxygen (pO_2) and per cent oxygen saturation is measured by a polarographic method; the blood sample is placed in a chamber and separated from a combined platinum and silver–silver chloride electrode by a polypropylene membrane. By diffusion through the membrane, equilibrium is established between the pO_2 of the blood and a film of solution in contact with the electrode. A current, which is proportional to blood pO_2, is generated after application of a polarizing voltage.

In respiratory acidosis, blood pH and chloride are decreased, whereas pCO_2 is increased; in metabolic acidosis, pH and pCO_2 are decreased.

Calcium and phosphorus are important minerals in the processes of bone calcification, nerve irritability, muscle contraction, and blood coagulation. Calcium is present in plasma as an ultrafilterable (ionic and nonionic) form, and a protein-bound fraction. Blood phosphorus consists of inorganic phosphorus, organic ester phosphates (G-6-P, ATP), and phospholipids.

Serum and urine calcium levels are routinely determined by titration with EDTA using a fluorescent calcein indicator. Interference from magnesium and phosphates is eliminated by addition of KOH to the titration mixture.[70] Other methods are based on the precipitation of calcium oxalate and subsequent titration with potassium permanganate. As with all cations, calcium can be determined by emission- or absorption-flame photometry.

Inorganic phosphorus levels are determined by reaction with acid molybdate reagent to form phosphomolybdic acid which, in turn, is reduced with aminonaphtholsulfonic acid or p-dimethylaminophenol sulfate to give a blue complex which is estimated colorimetrically. Normal serum levels are: 2.5–4.5 mg P/100 ml, 9–11 mg Ca/100 ml.

Calcium is decreased and phosphorus is increased in hypoparathyroidism; an opposite effect is seen in hyperactivity of this gland. In rickets and osteomalacia, both elements are decreased.

Copper, magnesium, zinc, and iron are trace elements in blood. They are readily quantitated by flame photometric or colorimetric techniques.

Organ Function Tests—Analysis of various blood constituents, and determination of metabolic excretion rates of administered compounds are parameters associated with *in situ* activity of various organs. Organ function studies are performed in diseases associated with the liver, kidney, parathyroid, thyroid, and pituitary gland, gastrointestinal tract, pancreas, and adrenals. Many of the analyses used in such evaluations have been described in other sections of this chapter.

Tests for hepatic function[1] are based on pigment (bilirubin) and carbohydrate metabolism (galactose tolerance test), plasma protein changes (cephalin flocculation test and A/G ratio), abnormal fat metabolism, detoxification mechanisms (hippuric acid synthesis), excretion of injected substances (bromsulfophthalein–BSP–dye), prothrombin formation, and enzyme levels.

Diseases of the liver are due to cellular alterations (hepatocellular) or obstructions to the flow of bile (obstructive jaundice). Hepatocellular liver disease can be of the chronic (postnecrotic cirrhosis, carcinoma) or acute (viral hepatitis, alcoholism, toxin induced) types.

The liver ordinarily converts galactose to glucose-1-phosphate (G-1-P) and then to G-6-P. In the *galactose tolerance test*,[71] galactose is administered intravenously (0.5 Gm/Kg) and the amount appearing in the blood is quantitated as a reducing sugar after treatment of the plasma with glucose oxidase to destroy blood glucose. The normal individual will have <10.0 mg galactose/100 ml blood within 2 hr after administration.

The *cephalin flocculation test* is based on the flocculation of cephalin-emulsified cholesterol by γ-globulin. In normal serum an albumin-like protein will inhibit this reaction; in hepatic diseases, which produce abnormal γ-globulin or reduced albumin levels, the flocculation will occur.

The detoxification mechanisms of the liver can be evaluated by intravenous administration of sodium benzoate and estimation of the benzoic acid metabolite, hippuric acid, in the urine. In hepatoparenchymal disease, a reduced capacity of the liver to form hippuric acid by conjugation of glycine and benzoic acid is observed.

The ability of the liver to excrete an injected dye is determined in the *BSP test;* the serum is analyzed for dye concentration at a suitable time interval after IV administration of 2–5 mg BSP/Kg. Radioiodinated (^{131}I) Rose Bengal dye has also been used in dye-excretion studies with isotopic estimation of urine dye levels.

The enzymes SGOT, SGPT, LDH, CPK, MDH, SDH, and alkaline phosphatase are valuable diagnostic tools in liver disease. In the icteric stage of infectious viral hepatitis, increases in serum and urine bilirubin, SGOT, SGPT, alkaline phosphatase, cephalin flocculation, and plasma globulin occur. In chronic inflammatory liver diseases, changes in the enzymes and proteins also occur.

Kidney function tests[47,72] are based on the determination of blood nonprotein nitrogenous substances (urea, uric acid, and creatinine), blood acid–base balance, and the clearance of administered compounds in the urine. Most clearance studies are performed with dyes (phenol sulfophthalein) or substances that are not resorbed by the renal tubules (inulin, mannitol, or sodium *p*-aminohippurate). These substances are administered intravenously and the rate of urine clearance is estimated by analysis of the urine (see the sections on *Nonprotein Nitrogen Compounds* and *Electrolytes*).

Sodium iodohippurate (^{131}I), which is almost completely extracted from the blood on a single passage through the kidney, also has been used in renal function studies[73]; a *renogram* or isotopic scan of both kidneys is performed. The test is primarily useful as a comparison of kidney function between kidneys of the same patient.

The primary function of the thyroid is the synthesis of thyroxine. The thyroid gland converts ingested iodide to iodine which, in turn, is stored in the gland after combination with the tyrosine of thyroglobulin (TBG).

Under the influence of pituitary thyroid-stimulating hormone (TSH), TBG releases thyroxine (T_4) and triiodothyronine (T_3) into the circulation. T_4 is strongly bound to plasma protein and is the primary source of plasma *protein-bound iodine* (PBI) or *butanol-extractable iodine* (BEI).

The uptake of orally administered Na^{131}I preparations by the thyroid gland can be estimated by isotopic scanning of the gland 24 hr after ^{131}I administration and is a good index of glandular function (hyperactive, >50% uptake; hypoactive, <15%).

TBG determinations involve the addition of T_4–^{131}I to serum, electrophoretic separation of proteins, and radiometric determination of ^{131}I in the TBG fraction (normal = 12–20 mcg T_3 uptake/100 ml).

PBI determinations[74] are based on precipitation of protein-bound thyroxine, removal of inorganic iodine by basic- or anion-exchange chromatography, alkaline incineration to convert thyroxine to inorganic iodide, and finally, quantitation of iodide by reaction with arsenous acid and ceric ammonium sulfate.

The BEI determination is only an index of the globulin-bound iodine as butanol precipitates albumin. (Normal PBI is 4–8 mcg/100 ml; BEI, 3.2–6.4 mcg/100 ml.)

The *PBI conversion ratio* is an estimate of the rate of conversion of inorganic iodide to PBI. Radioiodide (^{131}I) is administered to the subject; after 24 hr, a sample of blood is obtained and the ^{131}I to PB^{131}I is estimated by radiochromatographic procedures with ion-exchange resins (normal conversion, 13–42%).

An *in vitro* procedure for evaluation of thyroxine has many advantages over techniques which involve administration of ^{131}I to a subject. In hyperthyroidism the primary binding sites are nearly saturated; the *in vitro* uptake of T_3–^{131}I added to plasma samples is an index of thyroid function. In the T_3 *test*,[75] T_3–^{131}I is mixed with the plasma sample in the presence of a resin sponge. If the plasma protein binding sites are saturated, the concentration of radioactivity in the resin sponge will be increased (normal, 25–35% uptake). In hyperthyroidism increases in PBI, BEI, T_3 uptake, PBI conversion, and ^{131}I-thyroid uptake occur.

Parathyroid[76] and *pancreatic function* studies were discussed under "calcium–phosphorus (electrolyte)" and "blood-sugar" determinations, respectively.

Adrenocortical function is evaluated by estimation of urinary 17-ketosteroids and 17-hydroxycorticosteroids (androgen and corticosteroid metabolism), serum electrolytes (aldosterone metabolism) and blood adrenocorticotrophic hormone (ACTH) levels.

The intravenous administration of ACTH and subsequent determination of urinary ketosteroids is a reliable estimation of adrenocortical function. In hypoactive states (Addison's disease) there is an insignificant rise in urine ketosteroids and no change in urine corticoid content following ACTH administration. In adrenocortical hyperfunction there is an increase in urinary 17-ketosteroids, 17-hydroxycorticoids, and plasma ACTH and no change in serum potassium and pCO_2 following administration of the pituitary suppressant—dexamethasone.

In adrenomedullary hyperfunction (pheochromocytoma), there is an elevated 24-hr output of urinary catecholamines and VMA. The principles of the assay methods for adrenal and pituitary function were previously described in the section on *Steroids and Related Substances*.

Automated Blood Analysis—Within the past decade several automated systems have been introduced in the clinical laboratory for routine blood-chemistry determinations. The most popular system is the Technicon Autoanalyzer (Fig. 425).

Samples are pumped into a flowing reagent stream with a peristaltic-action pump which permits separation of reagents by an air interphase. The samples are automatically dialyzed, filtered, or centrifuged prior to addition of reagent and spectrophotometric analysis. The results may be channeled into a computer data-processing system for automatic calculation and final reporting of data.

Commercially available testing systems for determination of routine blood-chemistry parameters are available. These systems contain complete reagent sets, accessories, and necessary instrumentation.

Ultramicro analytical systems are extremely valuable in pediatric blood-chemistry determinations where the volume of blood sample is small.[77] The advantages of automation are: rapid results, reduced costs, greater efficiency, and accuracy.

The use of prepackaged reagent kits has become increasingly popular in the clinical laboratory. Enzymes, sugar, BUN, protein, uric acid, PBI, sterols, steroids, and electrolyte reagent kits are some of the tests available from reputable suppliers. Standards of known concentration should always be carried through the analytical blood procedures. Versatol, Enzatrol (Warner-Chilcott), Hyland Lab control serum, and Lab-Trol and Patho-Trol (Dade Reagents) are some of the reliable standards for use in such determinations. The manufacture of certified clinical laboratory reagents and standards is now under the supervision of the Biological Section of the Pharmaceutical Manufacturers Association, and the American Association of Clinical Chemists.[78]

Urine

The regulation of the internal environment of the blood and tissues by the kidneys involves three processes:

1. Removal of blood-plasma water and its dissolved substances by glomerulofiltration.
2. Selective tubular reabsorption of substances necessary to maintain the internal environment.
3. Secretory excretion of metabolic products and foreign substances.

Excretory function, electrolyte and water homeostasis, and regulation of body pH are the most important components of renal function.[79] Urea, phosphates, sulfates, ammonium, and creatinine are classified as "no-threshold" substances and appear in the urine whenever they are present in any quantity in the plasma. They are not reabsorbed by the tubular epithelium. Sodium chloride, dextrose, and amino acids are excreted in the urine only when their plasma concentrations exceed a threshold level. Reabsorption of these substances occurs in the tubules.

Kidney disease (nephritis) may be classified, according to mode of onset, into acute glomerulonephritis and chronic nephritis. Acute glomerulonephritis usually follows a streptococcal infection and is characterized by inflammatory renal lesions. The chronic group includes nephrosis, which is anatomically characterized by degenerative lesions of the renal tubular parenchyma.

The determination of urinary nitrogenous substances and electrolytes, renal function, and blood pH was presented in an earlier section. The determinations most commonly performed in routine urinalysis are: volume, pH, color, odor, turbidity, specific gravity, protein, glucose (reducing substances), acetone (ketone bodies), occult blood, bilirubin, and microscopic examination of the sediment.

The method used for collection of the urine will depend on the substances to be analyzed.[35] For routine urinalysis the morning urine specimen is usually collected in a clean container, preferably sterile and disposable. Contamination from feces and vaginal discharges must be avoided. Refrigeration will preserve the urine for a few hours. If a 24-hr specimen

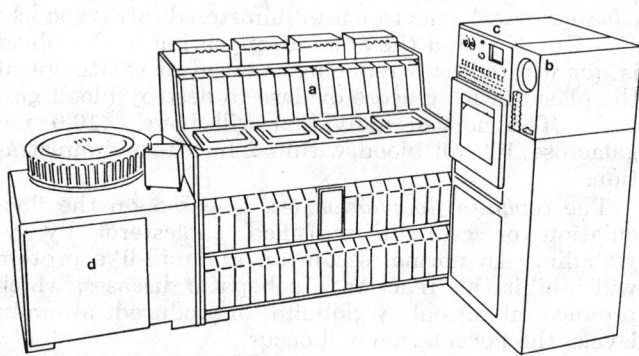

Fig. 425.   Technicon SMA 12/60 Autoanalyzer—*a:* 12 separate plug-in analytical cartridges; *b:* oscilloscope phasing display; *c:* completely electronic programmer; *d:* console with built-in refrigerator for working recent storage. This equipment performs sequential analysis of unmeasured serum samples for 12 selected biochemical parameters at the rate of 60/hour (courtesy, Technicon).

must be collected, or if the sample is to be shipped to a laboratory, a suitable preservative (eg, formalin, thymol, methenamine, or toluene) should be added. Refrigeration, toluene, or hydrochloric acid are used in the preservation of urine specimens for steroidal hormone and enzyme assay.

Appearance—Freshly voided urine is normally clear and transparent unless it is obtained shortly after a meal containing high concentrations of protein or vegetables. On standing, a slight cloudiness due to deposition of small quantities of mucus–nucleoprotein may occur. Normal acid urines may develop a precipitate of pinkish amorphous urates or colorless calcium oxalate crystals, whereas amorphous and crystalline phosphates can normally appear in alkaline urine. Abnormal quantities of epithelial cells, leukocytes, and mucus will result in cloudiness, even in freshly voided urine specimens.

Volume and Specific Gravity—The normal urine output is 0.5–1.5 liters/day, with a total solids content of 20–60 Gm/day and a specific gravity of 1.008–1.030. The total solids content is about 40% inorganic electrolytes (chloride, sulfates, and phosphates of sodium, potassium, calcium, ammonium, and magnesium) and 60% organic compounds (urea, uric acid, creatinine, hippuric acid, purine and xanthine bases, amino acids, conjugated ether sulfates, disulfide or sulfhydryl compounds, oxalic acid, urinary pigments, vitamins, and hormones). Creatinine is the only substance in the daily urine output whose concentration is fairly constant. The levels of the other constituents and the urinary volume are related to weight, diet, metabolic activity, renal function, and fluid intake.

The *total solid content* and *specific gravity* of the urine is related to the ability of the kidney to concentrate or dilute urine. Specific gravity determinations are performed by hydrometric (urinometer), refractometric, or by photoelectric procedures. The refractometric methods simultaneously determine specific gravity and total solids in a precalibrated instrument.

Diabetes, diuretic therapy, and pituitary disease result in an increase in daily urine output (polyuria). Decreased volume (oliguria) or complete suppression of urination (anuria) occurs in acute renal inflammatory and toxemic conditions.

Specific gravity is increased in dehydration and other disease states associated with an oliguria; in diabetes mellitus, nephritis, and glomerulonephritis, it is increased due to increased concentrations of chemicals in the urine.

The determination of the urine *osmolality* (855–1355 mOsmol/Kg) is a unique measure of the summation effect of all the particles in solution.[80] It is determined by comparing the freezing point of urine with that of a NaCl solution of known osmotic pressure, and has the advantage of not depending on concentration or refractive index.

pH—The normal urine pH is 5.0–7.5. The first morning urine specimen is more acidic than those collected during the day. Changes in pH are associated with electrolyte disturbances, dehydration, and diabetic, metabolic, or respiratory acidosis. The pH of the urine may be determined electrometrically, or with a test paper impregnated with methyl red–bromthymol blue indicator.[81] The titratable acidity of the normal urine ranges between 20–40 mEq/day.

Color—The color of freshly voided urine varies from faint straw to definite yellow, depending on the water concentration. The color of normal urine is due to the pigment urochrome, which is probably a urobilin–urobilinogen–peptide complex. Pale urine samples occur in polyuric conditions such as diabetes and chronic nephritis.

The occurrence of abnormal pigments will significantly change urine color: bilirubin and bile pigment—greenish yellow; blood oxyhemoglobin—red; blood methemoglobin—brownish black; porphyrins—reddish color.

The color of urine should not change significantly on standing at room temperature. Diet (anthocyanin red pigment of beets), drugs (methylene blue, pyridium, and phenolphthalein) and phenol poisoning will also alter the color of urine. The presence of melanogen or homogentisic acid (alkoptonuria) in the urine will cause the urine to change to a brownish black color on standing. This is due to the conversion of melanogen to melanin or homogentisic acid to a chromogenic substance, respectively.

Odor—The normal aromatic odor of freshly voided urine is due to *urinod* and volatile organic acids. Unpreserved nonsterile urine samples will develop an ammoniacal odor on standing, due to bacterial decomposition. The presence of a putrid odor in a fresh specimen is a result of bacterial action on urinary mucus and albumin. A fruity odor due to acetone or ketones may be present in diabetic urine. The presence of keto and amino acids (allo-isoleucine) in the urine of infants with "Maple Syrup" urine disease (MSUD) imparts a maple syrup odor to the urine.

Protein—Proteins are found in the urine (proteinuria, albuminuria) in various pathologic conditions and also in healthy young adults (functional albuminuria). Plasma proteins, hemoglobin, methemoglobin, abnormal Bence–Jones' protein, and proteins (nucleo-, phospho-, and glycoproteins) derived from leukocytes and mucus may be present in the urine in nephritis, nephrosis, lesions of the urinary tract, gastrointestinal dehydration, and renal congestion.

Qualitative urine protein tests are based on the coagulation of protein by nitric acid, acidification and heat, or sulfosalicylic acid. Protein is also detected with a paper strip[81] impregnated with tetrabromophenol blue indicator and citrate buffer; the change in color of the indicator from yellow to green is related to the concentration of albumin or globulin in the urine. Highly alkaline urines may give false positive reactions with the strips. The lower limit of sensitivity of these tests is about 20 mg protein/100 ml.

Globulins may be differentiated from albumins by conventional electrophoretic techniques or by testing the urine for protein after removal of the globulins by precipitation with one-half saturated ammonium sulfate. Mucus can be distinguished from protein by being precipitated with excess acetic acid in the cold.

In multiple myeloma of the bone, the abnormal *Bence–Jones' protein* appears in the urine. Whereas albumin and globulin begin to precipitate between 60–70°C, this abnormal protein starts to precipitate at 40–60°C and redissolves as the temperature approaches the boiling point. Sulfosalicylic acid will precipitate the Bence–Jones protein, but subsequent heating will redissolve it. Urine proteins may be quantitated by the techniques used for serum proteins (normal output <100 mg/day; proteinuria, >1.0 Gm/day).

Reducing Substances—The presence of glucose in the urine (glycosuria) is associated with hyperglycemic (diabetes, hyperthyroidism, hyperadrenalism, hyperpituitarism) and normoglycemic (renal glycosuria with a low threshold, normal pregnancy) states. Reducing sugars such as lactose, fructose, and galactose are present in the urine due to dietary conditions or congenital defects in their metabolism (galactosemia).

The usual qualitative tests are sensitive to glucose and reducing substances. The detection of reducing substances by reaction with alkaline copper solutions (Fehling's or Benedict's test, Clinitest (*Ames*) tablets)[82] to form a reddish yellow cuprous oxide precipitate is sensitive to 0.1% concentrations.

True glucose can be determined by testing the urine with a reagent strip impregnated with a mixture of glucose oxidase, catalyst, and chromogen; this test is sensitive to the 0.01% level. The presence of glucose, fructose, or glucuronates in urine may be established by formation of phenylglucosazone crystals on reaction of acidified urine with phenylhydrazine.

Galactose may be identified by selective formation of an *o*-tolylgalactohydrazone. Lactose and maltose will form a violet chromogen on heating with alkaline methylamine. Pentoses may be identified by formation of a green chromogen on reaction with acidified orcinol. The presence of fructose in the urine is established by the development of a red-colored compound after conversion to furfuraldehyde and reaction with resorcinol (Seliwanoff test).

The identification of reducing hexoses, pentoses,

and disaccharides in the urine can be accomplished by paper or thin-layer chromatography. The developing solvent may be ethylacetate–pyridine–water or a two-dimensional system of butanol–acetic acid–water and phenol. The chromatograms are sprayed with benzidine, ammoniacal silver nitrate, or aniline hydrogen oxalate reagent for detection of hexoses and pentoses; naphthoresorcinol, for ketoses; and phloroglucinol, for pentoses.

Urine sugars may be quantitated by chemical or enzymatic techniques used for blood-sugar determinations. Ascorbic acid, salicylates, homogentisic acid, glucuronides, and excess quantities of uric acid or creatinine will interfere with many of these tests.

Ketones—Ketonuria may result from conditions such as carbohydrate deprivation, digestive disturbances, ketogenic diets, hepatic damage, and diabetic ketoacidosis.

The ketones—acetone and diacetic acid—are detected by formation of a red, acid-stable ferropentocyanide complex in the presence of alkaline sodium nitroprusside,[81] or a red chromogen after reaction with ferric chloride. The latter test is specific for diacetic acid and for acetone. The qualitative tests are not sensitive to β-hydroxybutyric acid, which comprises the greater part of the "acetone bodies" causing diabetic acidosis. The qualitative nitroprusside test is sensitive to 5–10 mg acetoacetic acid/100 ml and is less sensitive to acetone.

Total ketone bodies may be quantitated by gas-chromatographic procedures, or by gravimetric determination of acetone–mercuric sulfate–sulfuric acid precipitate before and after oxidation of β-hydroxybutyric acid to diacetic acid and then to acetone. In normal urine less than 50 mg acetone is excreted daily, while in the diabetic urine values of 10–50 Gm/liter may be found.

The presence of phenylketone in the urine may be established by the conventional chemical and chromatographic procedures previously described. Screening procedures with a test strip[81] impregnated with ferric ammonium sulfate, magnesium ion, and cyclohexylsulfamic acid buffer will detect >8 mg of phenylpyruvic acid/100 ml. The detection of phenylketonuria in the early weeks of life is important in the prevention of the induced mental deficiency (phenylpyruvic oligophrenia).

Bilirubin—The presence of bilirubin in the urine is often the first warning of biliary obstruction, hepatic parenchymatous disease, or hepatitis. A positive urine bilirubin with negative urine urobilinogen rules out hemolytic jaundice and indicates hepatic obstruction, hepatitis, or cirrhosis.

Ictotest (*Ames*) tablets[81] are used in screening of blood or urine for bilirubin. The urine is added to a cellulose asbestos mat, a tablet is then placed on the moistened area, and water is added; the reaction of bilirubin with a stabilized *p*-nitrobenzene-diazonium *p*-toluenesulfonate–sulfosalicylic acid mixture produces a purple color within 30 sec.

Bile pigments may also be detected in urine by the presence of a greenish yellow foam on shaking the specimen, or development of a varied-colored biliverdin–bilicyanin complex after oxidation with nitric acid.

Urobilinogen and urobilin are determined after conversion of urobilinogen to urobilin by acid iodine reagent; the development of greenish fluorescence on the addition of zinc acetate, due to formation of zinc urobilin, or the development of a red color on heating with *p*-dimethylaminobenzaldehyde (Ehrlich's test), are the usual qualitative tests. Urobilinogen values are high in hemolytic jaundice and low in obstructive jaundice. Urinary bilirubin is normally <0.1 mg/100 ml and corresponds to the lower limits of sensitivity of the qualitative tests.

Hemoglobin—The presence in the urine of hemoglobin (hemoglobinuria) or intact erythrocytes (hematuria) is indicative of intravascular damage or renal lesions. Free hemoglobin or that resulting from the hemolysis of intact cells by the test reagents is usually detected with *o*-toluidine or benzidine. Hemoglobin, at an acid pH, catalyzes the oxidation of *o*-toluidine or benzidine by peroxide to form a blue color. False positive results due to the presence of mucus or pus cells may be eliminated by heating the urine prior to the test.

Microscopic Examination—In the diagnosis of renal disease an accurate interpretation of the microscopic examination of the urine is one of the most valuable tests.[83] The urinary sediments can be classified into *unorganized* (chemical substances) and *organized* (cells and casts) constituents (Fig. 426). The normal *sediment volume* is 0–0.02 mg/100 ml at pH 5.5.

The urine is centrifuged and the precipitate prepared for microscopic analysis. In an alkaline urine amorphous or crystalline ammonium–magnesium phosphates, calcium carbonate or oxalate crystals, and ammonium urate may occur normally. Amorphous or crystalline urates, uric acid, and calcium oxalates are normally seen in acid urines. The presence of tyrosine, leucine, or cystine crystals is associated with various diseases. Chemical crystals are identified by solubility in acid and/or alkali, colorimetric reactions, and crystalline structure.

A quantitative estimate (*Addis Count*) of organized sediments—such as casts, red and white blood cells, and epithelial cells—is used to follow the course of renal disease. The presence of large numbers of renal epithelial cells indicates excess desquamation of the urinary tract and the site of the origin is indicated by the cell morphology.

Casts are proteinaceous cylindroid bodies of renal parenchymal origin, molded in the tubules, and subsequently found in the urine. They are classified as to their microscopic appearance. Hyaline casts are pale and cylindrical and do not contain any cells. Epithelial, blood, and leukocyte casts occur in tubular damage and are characterized by the presence of nucleated epithelial cells or blood cells. Granular and fatty casts contain products of degeneration of the tubular cells.

Mucus fibers or cylindroids, spermatozoa, bacteria, parasites, and other cellular debris also may be found in normal urine.

Calculi[1,84]—Knowledge of the composition of renal and bladder calculi ("stones") is essential in the planning of the therapeutic regimen in such diseases. Mixed calcium phosphate and oxalate stones form predominantly in alkaline urines, while uric acid calculi are generally associated with acid urines. Hyperexcretion of one of the calculi components, pH, renal blockage, and the presence of foreign objects in the urinary tract are the most probable causal factors in the formation of renal calculi. Cysteine, cholesterol, and bile salts are minor components of the calculi. The chemical content of the stones is established by routine qualitative analysis for calcium, magnesium, ammonium, phosphate, carbonate, and oxalate ions, and subsequent confirmation by optical crystallographic methods, x-ray diffraction, and infrared spectroscopy.

Feces

Normal feces consists of undigested food remnants, products of digestion, bacteria, and secretions of the gastrointestinal tract. *Macroscopic, chemical,* and *microscopic* determinations are routinely performed. The normal quantity of feces is about 200 Gm/day. The brown color is due to the reduction of bilirubin to urobilinogen and then to urobilin (strecobilin); bilirubin is not normally present in feces, but biliverdin (a component of meconium) is excreted during the first days of life. Bilirubin can be detected by tests previously described for bile pigments.

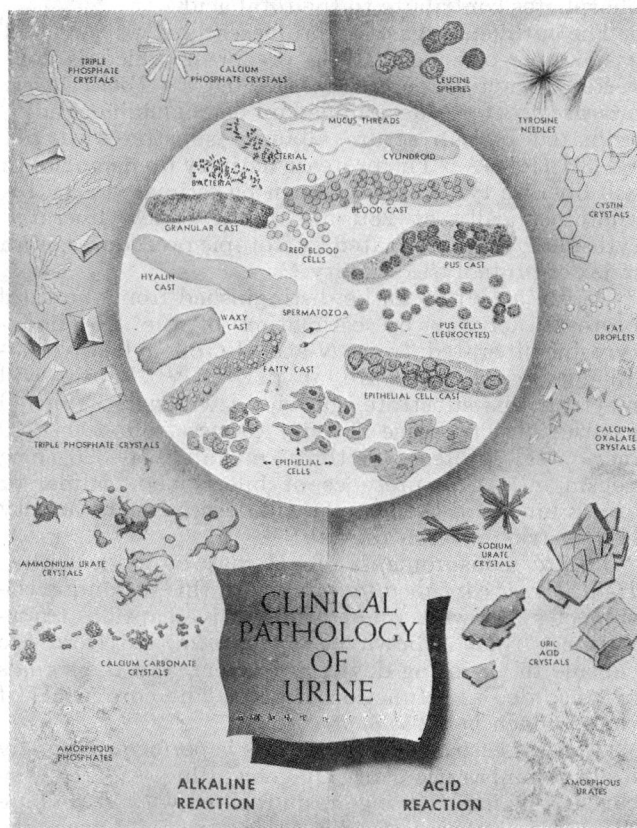

Fig. 426. **Microscopic analysis of urinary sediments (courtesy, MSD).**

Fecal urobilinogen can be determined colorimetrically by reduction of urobilin to urobilinogen with alkaline ferrous sulfate, and then reaction with acidified *p*-dimethylaminobenzaldehyde (Ehrlich's reaction). Fecal urobilinogen is increased from a normal range of 40–280 mg daily to 400–1400 mg in hemolytic jaundice, and is decreased in obstructive jaundice. The presence of intact red cells or digested blood will impart a red to black or tarry appearance to the specimen.

Blood is readily detected by the benzidine or guaiac tests; this is valid only if the patient has been on a meat-free diet for 3 days. The use of ^{51}Cr-tagged erythrocytes has been used to quantitate and locate the source of gastrointestinal bleeding. The subject's red cells are mixed with an isotonic ^{51}Cr solution and then reinjected intravenously. If bleeding occurs, the ^{51}Cr-isotope content of the feces will be increased.

Location of the hemorrhagic area can be determined by an isotopic scan of the abdominal area.

The presence of excessive quantities of mucus is usually indicative of dysentery, colitis, or other inflammatory processes in the intestinal mucosa. Strongly alkaline or acidic reaction in the feces is indicative of excessive quantities of protein or carbohydrate in the diet, respectively.

Quantitative determination of fecal fat and nitrogen are useful in analysis of pancreatic function. In pancreatic disease increases in fecal nitrogen will occur as a result of decreased secretion of pancreatic proteolytic enzymes. The normal individual will excrete 4–13% of ingested nitrogen in the feces; in chronic pancreatitis, 9–30%. Fecal nitrogen can be determined by the Kjedahl digestion procedure. Fecal fat is present in the forms of triglycerides of fatty acids (neutral fat), free fatty acids (FFA), and combined fatty acids (soaps). Fat determinations are based on the solubility of neutral fat and FFA in ether; the soaps are insoluble in ether and have to be acid hydrolyzed to their respective FFA prior to extraction. Neutral fat will liberate FFA only on alkaline hydrolysis. The FFA, isolated from the above fractionations, are then determined by titrimetric, colorimetric, or gaschromatographic procedures.

Determinations of blood, urine, and fecal ^{131}I after oral administration of an iodinated glyceryl trioleate preparation is an index of both liver and pancreatic function and correlates with fecal fat excretion. The bile must emulsify the preparation prior to enzymatic hydrolysis by pancreatic lipase to yield FFA–^{131}I which are subsequently absorbed and metabolized. An increased amount of fat in the feces (steatorrhea) is associated with pancreatic diseases (cystic fibrosis with achylia), obstructive jaundice, malabsorption disease (sprue, celiac disease), and idiopathic steatorrhea.[85]

A microscopic examination[86] of emulsified feces includes analysis for the presence of crystals, food residues, body cells, bacteria, and parasites. Crystals of triple phosphate, calcium oxalate, fat and cholesterol, starch granules, vegetable fibers, and neutral fat globules are normally present. Octahedral needleshaped crystals (Charcot Leyden crystals) are present in parasitic infestation and mucus colitis. Excessive quantities of fat or starch are seen in malabsorption disease.

Adult, larval, or oval phases of parasites may be encountered in the feces. The most common parasitic infestations are caused by *cestodes* (tapeworms), *trematodes* (flukes), *nematodes* (roundworms), and *protozoa* (amoeba).

The characterization of tapeworm segments (*proglottids*) or head (*scolex*) in the feces will differentiate *Taenia saginata* (beef tapeworm) from *T. solium*, which is derived from infested pork. The roundworms are differentiated by the morphology of the ova, larvae, and adult forms; *Necator americanus* (hookworm), *Trichuris trichuria* (whipworm), and *Enterobius vermicularis* (pinworm) are commonly encountered nematodes.

Vegetative or cystic stages of *Schistosoma sp.* or *Fasciola sp.* are seen in blood and liver fluke infestations. The presence of vegetative and cystic stages of *Endamoeba histolytica* is associated with ulcerative colitis and amoebic dysentery. Feces are usually concentrated by sedimentation, centrifugation, or flotation techniques prior to microscopic examination for parasites.

Toxicological Examinations[87,88]

Determination of blood, urine, fecal, or tissue concentrations of various compounds is an important aspect in toxicologic evaluation and treatment. Agents involved in acute and chronic toxicologic syndromes are barbiturates, ethanol, methanol, lead, halogenated hydrocarbons, phenothiazines, strychnine, morphine analogs, amphetamines, bromides, mercury, thallium, beryllium, nitrites, and phenols. Spectrophotometric, fluorometric, chromatographic (gas, paper, and thin-layer), and enzymatic techniques are used in the analysis of such substances.

Blood-alcohol levels may be determined by aeration, distillation, gas-chromatography, or specific enzymatic analysis with alcohol dehydrogenase.

In the chemical techniques the blood sample is either oxidized or distilled into a dichromate–sulfuric acid mixture; the excess dichromate is then determined by titration with potassium iodide or methyl orange–ferrous sulfate solutions. The gas-chromatographic and enzyme procedures are specific for ethanol, whereas the chemical techniques are influenced by other volatile or oxidizable substances in the blood. The enzymatic method is based on the reaction of ethanol and DPN in the presence of alcohol dehydrogenase to form acetaldehyde and DPNH; the acetaldehyde is removed with semicarbazide and the DPNH, formed in the reaction, is estimated spectrophotometrically at 340 mμ.

Ethanol levels of >0.15% are indicative of intoxication and apparent psychomotor disturbance. Levels of 0.40–0.50% are associated with medullary and diencephalic disturbances such as tremors, coma, respiratory depression, peripheral collapse, and death.

The barbiturates—eg, phenobarbital, amobarbital, secobarbital, and pentobarbital—are determined in blood or urine after solvent extraction at an acid pH and subsequent chromatographic or spectrophotometric analysis of the extract. In ultraviolet spectrophotometry the spectrum of an alkaline blood extract is determined at pH 10 and 13.4. Colorimetric methods are based on the reaction of barbiturates with cobalt acetate in methanol–isopropylamine.

In acute poisoning, blood-barbiturate levels are as follows: long-acting (phenobarbital), more than 10 mg/100 ml; intermediate-acting (amobarbital), 7 mg/100 ml; and short-acting (pentobarbital), 3 mg/100 ml. The rate of excretion of these drugs is inversely related to the length of action—eg, phenobarbital, 21%; amobarbital, 48%; pentobarbital, 57% daily decrease in blood levels.

Specific analysis of heavy metals is performed by atomic-absorption spectroscopy. Lead also may be estimated colorimetrically after oxidation of organic matter, extraction with sodium diethyldithiocarbamate, and complex formation with dithizone. Halogenated hydrocarbons are determined by gas-chromatographic procedures.

Analysis of blood for drugs (phenothiazines, amphetamines, alkaloids, and narcotics) is based on solvent extraction, chromatographic and spectrophotometric techniques. Isolation of the substance and confirmation of structure by mass or infrared spectrophotometry, neutron-activation analysis or nuclear magnetic resonance has been introduced recently in forensic medicine.

Gastric Secretions

The chief constituents of gastric juice are hydrochloric acid, gastric proteases (pepsin and gastricsin), hemopoietic factor (intrinsic factor and Vitamin B_{12} binders), and mucus.[89] Tests for gastric function are usually performed on gastric juice samples collected by direct intubation into the stomach. The fasting content (normal, <100 ml) of the stomach is removed and gastric secretion is stimulated by the oral administration of caffeine-benzoate or alcohol, or parenteral administration of histamine, insulin, or the hormone gastrin. Samples are removed at periodic time intervals and analyzed for acidity and gastric protease activity.

Acidity is determined by electrometric titration of a sample of centrifuged gastric juice to pH 3.5, 4.5, and 7.4; the end-points for free acid (HCl), protease activity, and physiological neutrality, respectively. The normal free acidity is 15–45 mEq/liter and total acidity is 25–55 mEq/liter.[90] In addition to free HCl, protein hydrochlorides, organic acids, and acid phosphates contribute to the total acid.

The principle gastric proteases are pepsin and gastricsin; pepsinogen is a precursor which is converted to active pepsin by free HCl. *Total gastric protease activity* is determined on hemoglobin or radioiodinated human serum albumin substrates at pH 1.8–3.1 (RISA-^{131}I); protease activity on hemoglobin will liberate tyrosine which can be estimated spectrophotometrically at 280 mμ; with RISA, liberated tyrosine-^{131}I, as estimated by isotopic procedures, is an index of proteolytic activity.

Pepsin activity can be distinguished from the total protease activity by estimation of the 3,5-diiodotyrosine liberated from *N*-acetyl-L-phenylalanyl-3,5-diiodotyrosine substrate at pH 2.1.[91] Pepsin will react on this substrate, gastricsin will not. Normal gastric juice protease activity ranges from 200–1200 mcg total protease activity/ml and 50–300 mcg pepsin/ml. The presence of bile, blood, saline, or excess mucus in the sample will decrease both acidity and gastric protease activity.

In situ measurements of pH may be made with a *Heidelberger capsule apparatus*. In this technique the subject swallows a small pH-sensitive capsule (transmitter); then radiowaves are transmitted from the capsule to a sensing device (receiver), and the signals are recorded as a function of pH. The normal pH of the stomach is 1.2–1.8.

Tubeless gastric acidity analysis is performed also by oral administration of Diagnex Blue (*Squibb*),[1] a carbacrylic ion-exchange resin reacted with azure blue dye. The hydrogen ions in the gastric juice exchange with the dye on the resin; the dye is absorbed and then excreted in the urine. The dye concentration in the urine is a function of gastric acidity. The normal value is >0.6 mg dye in the urine 2 hr after administration.

The mucosubstances of gastric juice are aminopolysaccharides, mucopolyuronides, mucoids, and mucoproteins. Decreases (hypochlorhydria) in gastric acidity are seen in chronic gastritis; complete absence of acid (achlorhydria) occurs in gastric carcinoma and pernicious anemia. Decreases in acidity are usually accompanied by a decline in gastric protease activity.

Other Body Fluids

Physical, chemical, and microscopic examination of cerebrospinal fluid, synovial fluid, human milk, transudates, and exudates are performed also by the clinical laboratory. The principles of the various determinations are similar to those described for blood and urine.

Microbiology

Medical microbiology[92] is concerned with the isolation and identification of infectious fungi, yeast, bacteria, or virus. The techniques usually involve propagation of the organism on a primary culture medium, selective isolation on special growth media, determination of morphologic and staining characteristics of the organism, biochemical or immunochemical analysis for differentiation and identification, and animal innoculation to determine pathogenicity. Aseptic technique is used in obtaining samples of blood, urine, feces, cerebrospinal fluid, nasopharyngeal secretions, and effusions from infected tissue.

Micrococcus pyogenes var *aureus* (staphylococcus) and *Streptococcus hemolyticus* are Gram-positive cocci (Gram staining reaction) associated with blood, nasopharyngeal, or tissue infections. The specimen is plated on blood agar containing phenylethyl alcohol as an inhibitor of the growth of Gram-negative organisms and then incubated at 37°C; pathogenic staphylococci and streptococci produce zones of hemolysis around the bacterial colonies due to the action of a staphylo- or streptolysin enzyme on the blood cells. The presence of desoxyribonuclease activity and an enzyme—staphylocoagulase—which will clot plasma can be correlated with the virulency of the staphylococci.

Neisseria gonorrheae is a Gram-negative coccus which causes the venereal disease gonorrhea. Identification is based on isolation of the gonococcus from urethral exudates on a hemoglobin agar and confirmation of the oxidase activity of the colonies by reaction with *p*-dimethylaminoaniline which turns oxidase-positive colonies black.

N. intracellularis is the causative agent in bacterial meningitis. Identification is based on isolation of the meningococcus from spinal fluid or nasopharyngeal secretions on a hemoglobin agar containing selective inhibitors of bacteria and fungi growth (vancomycin, colistin, and nystatin), and subsequent identification by biochemical or serologic agglutination techniques with polyvalent antiserum.

The enteric bacilli are Gram-negative, nonsporulating rods which are associated with dysentery (*Shigella sp.*), typhoid fever (*Salmonella sp.*), urinary tract and tissue infections (*Escherichia coli, Proteus sp.*, or *Pseudomonas sp.*), and pulmonary infections (*Klebsiella sp.*). Clinical samples are initially plated on a selective media for the growth of enteric bacilli; MacConkey agar—containing lactose, bile salts, neutral red indicator, and crystal violet—will inhibit the growth of Gram-positive organisms and permit growth of the enteric bacilli. These organisms may be differentiated by biochemical or immunochemical reactions.

The presence or absence of the enzymes cytochrome oxidase, phenylalanine deaminase, urease, and lysine decarboxylase will readily differentiate *Pseudomonas, Salmonella,* and *Proteus.* Tests used in the differentiation of enteric bacilli also include: fermentation of lactose, sucrose, or dextrose; production of hydrogen sulfide, indol, and acetylmethylcarbinol; and utilization of citrate as the sole source of carbon.

Serologic identification of *Salmonella* and *Shigella* species is based on the agglutination of specific thermostable somatic "O," or thermolabile somatic "K" and flagellar "H" antigens by specific antisera.[93] Other Gram-negative rods of medical importance are the hemophilic (*Bordetella pertussis*, whooping cough) and hemorrhagic (*Pasteurella pestis*, bubonic plague)

bacilli. Spore-forming bacilli are the infectious agents in tetanus and gas gangrene. This group of organisms—*Clostridium*—must be cultivated under anaerobic conditions.

The morphology, biochemistry, and virulency of the isolated organisms or their toxins are the basis of selective differentiation. The mammalian tubercle bacilli—*Mycobacterium tuberculosis* var *hominis, bovis,* or *ovium*—is isolated from sputum samples on a special glycerol–egg media or oleic acid–albumin agar. The presence of an acid-fast organism (Ziehl–Neelsen staining), together with a positive skin tuberculin test and x-ray diagnosis, is confirmatory evidence of active tuberculosis.

Bacteriophages are viruses that infest and lyse bacteria. Bacteria may be classified by "phage-typing." In this procedure the bacteria under examination are mixed with a culture of specific bacteriophages; after incubation the cultures are examined for complete lysis of the bacteria. *Staphylococcus, E. coli,* and *Sal. typhosa* have been classified into various subgroups by this procedure.

Medically important fungi[94] include *Tricophyton sp.* (ringworm), *Actinomyces bovis* and *Blastomyces dermatiditis* (pulmonary infections), *Coccidioides immitus* (granuloma), *Histoplasma capsulatum* (systemic febrile disease), and *Candida albicans* (superficial pulmonary moniliasis). The following are used in the analysis of the infective agent: isolation of the organism on selective media; morphologic, biochemical, and immunologic techniques; and skin antigen tests.

Pathogenic fungi may be isolated on peptone–dextrose or brain–heart infusion agar containing bacteriostatic agents such as cycloheximide or chloramphenicol. Demonstration of serum antibodies in active fungal disease is used also in the differentiation of the causative agent; eg, *Histoplasmin* latex agglutination test.

The use of *antibiotic sensitivity tests* is helpful in the determination of the therapeutic agent. A culture of the sample or infectious organism is streaked on a suitable growth media; small filter paper disks impregnated with various antibiotics are placed on the media. After incubation at 37°C for 24 hr, the absence or growth of the organism around the disks is an index of sensitivity to the specific chemotherapeutic.

The laboratory identification of viruses[95,96] is based on growth of an ultrafilterable agent in a tissue culture media or on embryonated eggs, and subsequent determination of the pathogenicity of the isolated organism in animals. The morphology of the virus can be studied with an electron microscope.

Some examples of human viral infections are: respiratory infections (adenovirus), enteric disease (coxsackie or ECHO—enteric cytopathogenic human origin virus), smallpox (variola), measles (rubeola), German measles (rubella), chicken pox (varicella), shingles (herpes zoster), psittacosis and lymphogranuloma venereum (LVG), group polio, and rabies.

Pleuropneumonialike organisms (*PPLO* or Mycoplasmatales) are filterable agents which appear to be between the bacteria and larger viruses. They are filterable agents with no definite cell wall; they can be cultivated on cell-free culture media enriched with serum or ascitic fluid. The L-forms of PPLO reproductive unit have been isolated from the oral cavity and urinary tract of humans.

The technique of immunofluorescence[97,98] has become a powerful tool in immunologic research, experimental pathology, and diagnostic microbiology. Smears or tissue sections containing the antigen (bacteria, fungi, parasite, or virus) are treated with appropriate solutions of an antibody labeled with fluorescein isothiocyanate. The preparations are then washed to remove unreacted antibody and examined under a fluorescence microscope. The appearance of a fluorescent particle indicates a reaction of the specific labeled antibody with its antigen to form a fluorescent antigen–antibody complex. The technique is extremely sensitive and easy to perform. Purified fluorescein-labeled globulin antibody fractions are prepared by fractionation of the serum globulins and purification by adsorption and ion-exchange methods.

Serology

Immunology, serology, and immunochemistry[93] include the study of resistance to disease and the properties and behavior of antigens and antibodies. Although the majority of antigens are proteins, certain complex polysaccharides will induce an antigenic response. An antibody is a modified blood globulin formed in response to an antigenic stimulus. The combination of antigen and antibody can be demonstrated by techniques involving agglutination, precipitation, toxin neutralization, phagocytosis, lysis, and complement fixation. The identification and quantitation of specific antigens and antibodies in blood serum constitute the methods of serology.

Heterophile antibodies are agglutinins which are capable of reacting with antigens that are entirely unrelated to those which stimulate their production. These antibodies, which occur in the serum of patients with infectious mononucleosis[99] or serum sickness, will agglutinate formalized horse erythrocytes. In order to distinguish the specific heterophile agglutinins of infectious mononucleosis, the serum sample is mixed with guinea-pig kidney tissue or beef erythrocyte stromata; the infectious mononucleosis antibody will be absorbed and inactivated by the beef cells but not by the kidney tissue, and subsequent agglutination of horse erythrocytes will occur only in the kidney-tissue system.

C-reactive protein (CRP)[100] is a protein present in the serum of patients in the acute stages of bacterial and viral infections, collagen diseases, and other inflammatory processes. The presence of this antigen in serum is detected by agglutination of polystyrene latex particles sensitized with specific CRP antibody globulin. In the management of rheumatic fever, decreases in CRP blood levels are used to measure the effectiveness of therapy.

Rheumatoid arthritis is characterized by the presence of a reactive group of macroglobulins known as the *rheumatoid factors* (RF)[101] in blood and synovial fluid. Analysis of RF is based on agglutination procedures employing polystyrene latex particles coated with a layer of adsorbed human gamma globulin. The RF–antibody reaction causes a visible agglutination of the inert latex particles.

The laboratory diagnosis of *syphilis*[102] (treponemal disease) is based on the demonstration of an antibody-like substance, reagin, in the blood serum of infected individuals. This can be accomplished with *complement fixation* or agglutination techniques. Complement is a plasma substance which combines with antigen–antibody complexes. In the first phase of complement fixation tests (Wasserman or Reiter Test), the syphilitic serum reagin reacts with a complex phos-phatidic acid antigen (cardiolipin) and complement; the complement is bound and will not lyse hemolysin-sensitized red cells which were added in the second phase of the test. In normal serum the reagin–cardiolipin complex is not formed and the complement is free to react with hemolysin and lyse the erythrocytes.

Flocculation tests for determination of syphilis use a cardiolipin–lecithin–cholesterol antigen which clumps in the presence of serum antilipid reagin occurring in nontreponemal diseases and syphilis (*Venereal Disease Research Laboratory—VDRL Test*).

Increased reagin titers also occur in malaria, leprosy, and infectious mononucleosis. Treponemal antibody can be detected also by reaction of the patient's serum with treponemal antigen and subsequent confirmation with fluorescein-labeled antihuman globulin as an indicator of primary antigen–antibody reaction (*Fluorescent Treponemal Antibody—FTA—Test*).

Febrile antibodies[1] are present in the serum of patients with certain bacterial or rickettsial infections (spotted, typhus, or Q fever). In typhus disease the patient's serum contains a febrile antibody which will agglutinate a suspension of *Proteus OX-19* bacteria (Weil–Felix Reaction). *Salmonella* O–H, *Pasteurella tularensis*, and *Brucella abortus* antigens are used in febrile antibody tests for diagnosis of typhoid or paratyphoid fever, tularemia, and brucellosis, respectively.

Cold agglutinins are antibodies which clump Group O human erythrocytes only at 5°C or lower. The reaction is reversible and agglutinated cells will resuspend if the preparation is warmed to room temperature. Increases in cold agglutinin serum titer are of diagnostic value in severe cases of primary atypical pneumonia.

References

1. Wintrobe, M. M., *Clinical Hematology*, 5th ed., Lea & Febiger, Philadelphia, 1961, p. 214.
2. Damm, H. C., and King, J. W., *Practical Manual for Clinical Laboratory Procedures*, Chemical Rubber Co., Cleveland, 1965.
3. Ingersoll, L. O., *Am. J. Med. Technol.*, **28**, 318 (1962).
4. Mattern, C. F. T., et al, *J. Appl. Physiol.*, **10**, 56 (1957).
5. Seligson, D., *Std. Methods Clin. Chem.*, **2**, 49 (1958).
6. MacFarlane, R. G., and Poole, J. C. F., *Am. J. Clin. Pathol.*, **24**, 67 (1954).
7. Damm, H. C., and King, J. W., *Handbook of Clinical Laboratory Data*, Chemical Rubber Co., Cleveland, 1965, p. 153.
8. Danon, D., et al, *Transfusion*, **4**, 339 (1964).
9. Beutler, E., *Blood*, **28**, 533 (1966).
10. Zinkham, W. H., and Conley, C. L., *Bull. Johns Hopkins Hosp.*, **98**, 102 (1956).
11. Dameshek, W., *Arch. Internal Med.*, **50**, 579 (1932).
12. Brecher, G., and Cronkite, E. P., *J. Appl. Physiol.*, **3**, 365 (1950).
13. Nettis, S., *Am. J. Med. Sci.*, **196**, 177 (1938).
14. Brecher, G., *Am. J. Clin. Pathol.*, **19**, 805 (1949).
15. Campbell, T. J., et al, *J. Lab. Clin. Med.*, **52**, 768 (1958).
16. Szirmai, E., ed., *Nuclear Hematology*, Academic, New York, 1965, pp. 11–36.
17. Schilling, R. F., et al, *J. Lab. Clin. Med.*, **45**, 926 (1955).
18. Quick, A. J., *Ann. Internal Med.*, **55**, 201 (1961).
19. Gaston, L. W., *New Engl. J. Med.*, **260**, 236 (1964).
20. Frankel, S., and Reitman, S., eds., Clinical Laboratory Methods and Diagnosis, 6th ed., Mosby, St. Louis, 1963, p. 1193.
21. Wintrobe, M. M., *Laboratory Medicine—Hematology*, 2nd ed., Mosby, St. Louis, 1962, p. 299.
22. Quick, A. J., *Hemorrhagic Diseases*, Lea & Febiger, Philadelphia, 1957, p. 305.
23. Ware, A. G., and Stragnell, R., *Am. J. Clin. Pathol.*, **22**, 791 (1952).
24. Owren, P. A., *Lancet*, **II**, 754 (1959).
25. Biggs, R., and Douglas, A. S., *Am. J. Clin. Pathol.*, **6**, 23 (1953).
26. Struver, G. P., and Bittner, D. L., *Am. J. Clin. Pathol.*, **38**, 473 (1962).
27. *Manual of Blood Coagulation Technics*, 2nd ed., Warner-Chilcott, Morris Plains, N.J., 1966, p. 12.
28. Harrower, H. W., and Brook, D. L., *Am. J. Clin. Pathol.*, **47**, 2 (1967).
29. *A Manual of Methods for the Coagulation Laboratory*, BD&Co., Rutherford, N.J., 1965, p. 9.
30. Routine procedures in blood banks are compiled in both *Technical Methods and Procedures of the American Association of Blood Banks*, 1962, and *Standards for Blood Transfusion Service*, 4th ed., Am. Assoc. Blood Banks, Chicago, 1963.
31. Griffiths, J. J., and Elliott, J., *Blood Bank Procedures*, Dade Reagents, Miami, Mar., 1967, p. 1.

32. Mollison, P. L., *Blood Transfusion in Clinical Medicine*, 3rd ed., Thomas, Springfield, Ill., 1961, p. 1.
33. A registry of rare blood donors is also available: *Central File for Rare Donors*, Am. Assoc. Blood Banks, Milwaukee.
34. Winsten, S., *Std. Methods Clin. Chem.*, **5,** 1 (1965).
35. *"Vacutainer" Specimen Tubes for Blood Tests*, BD&Co., Rutherford, N.J.
36. Searcy, R. L., *et al, J. Am. Med. Technol.*, **28,** 33 (1966).
37. Berkman, S., *et al, J. Biol. Chem.*, **206,** 937 (1954).
38. Sunderman, F. W., *et al, Am. J. Clin. Pathol.*, **21,** 901 (1951).
39. Young, N. F., *Std. Methods Clin. Chem.*, **1,** 60 (1953).
40. Reinhold, J. G., *Std. Methods Clin. Chem.*, **1,** 65 (1953).
41. Sexton, J. S., and Aull, J. C., *Am. J. Clin. Pathol.*, **42,** 320 (1964).
42. Free, A. H., *Advan. Clin. Chem.*, **6,** 67 (1963).
43. Frankel, S., and Reitman, S., eds., Clinical Laboratory Methods and Diagnosis, 6th ed., Mosby, St. Louis, 1963, p. 89.
44. Donnell, G. N., *Biochem. Med.*, **1,** 29 (1967).
45. Fawcett, J., and Scott, J., *J. Clin. Pathol.*, **13,** 156 (1960).
46. Reardon, J., *et al, Clin. Chim. Acta*, **14,** 403 (1966).
47. Varley, H., *Practical Clinical Chemistry*, 2nd ed., Interscience, New York, 1958.
48. Bittner, D., *et al, Am. J. Clin. Pathol.*, **40,** 423 (1963).
49. *Chromatography in Mass Screening for Disorders of Amino Acid Metabolism*, Hyland Labs., Los Angeles, Calif., Dec., 1966, p. 1.
50. Berlow, S., *Advan. Clin. Chem.*, **9,** 165 (1967).
51. Woolf, L., *Advan. Clin. Chem.*, **7,** 98 (1963).
52. Musago, L., and Benassi, C., *Advan. Clin. Chem.*, **7,** 63 (1964).
53. Peeters, H., *Advan. Clin. Chem.*, **2,** 2 (1959).
54. Rosalki, S., and Wilkinson, J., *Diagnostic Enzymology*, Dade Reagents, Miami, 1966, p. 1.
55. Wilkinson, J., *Introduction to Diagnostic Enzymology*, Edward Arnold, Ltd., London, 1962, p. 1.
56. Vesell, E., *Ann. NY Acad. Sci.*, **151,** 1 (1968).
57. Kontinen, A., *Clin. Chim. Acta*, **18,** 147 (1967).
58. Martin, G. J., *Clinical Enzymology*, Little, Brown, Boston, 1958, p. 1.
59. Paoletti, R., *Lipid Pharmacology (Med. Chem. Ser.*, vol. 2), Academic, New York, 1964, p. 1.
60. Szymanski, H., *Biomedical Applications of Gas Chromatography*, Plenum, New York, 1964, p. 1.
61. Marinetti, G., *J. Lipid Res.*, **3,** 1 (1962).
62. Schwarz, H., *Advan. Clin. Chem.*, **3,** 1 (1960).
63. Searcy, R. L., and Bergquist, L., *Biochemistry of Serum Lipoproteins in Health and Disease*, Thomas, Springfield, Ill., 1969.
64. Sunderman, F. W., *Lipids and Steroid Hormones in Clinical Medicine*, Lippincott, Philadelphia, 1960, p. 158.
65. Davajan, V., *et al, Obstet. Gynecol.*, **29,** 515 (1967).
66. Zettner, A., *Advan. Clin. Chem.*, **7,** 1 (1964).
67. Schales, O., and Schales, S. S., *J. Biol. Chem.*, **140,** 879 (1941).
68. Whitehead, T. P., *Advan. Clin. Chem.*, **9,** 195 (1967).
69. Winters, R. W., *et al, Acid Base Physiology in Medicine*, London Co., New York, 1967, p. 1.
70. Rudolph, G., *et al, Clin. Chim. Acta*, **18,** 187 (1967).
71. Tengstrom, B., *et al, Am. J. Digest. Diseases*, **12,** 853 (1967).
72. Josephson, B., and Ek, J., *Advan. Clin. Chem.*, **1,** 41 (1958).
73. Nordyke, R., *et al, Clin. Res.*, **8,** 116 (1960).
74. Stevens, C., and Levandoski, N., *Clin. Chem.*, **9,** 400 (1963).
75. Nova, M., and De Groot, L., *New Engl. J. Med.*, **266,** 1307 (1962).
76. Nordin, B., *Advan. Clin. Chem.*, **4,** 275 (1961).
77. Reinouts van Hago, P. R., and de Wael, J., *Advan. Clin. Chem.*, **4,** 321 (1961).
78. Dybkaer, R., and Jorgensen, K., *Quantities and Units in Clinical Chemistry*, Williams & Wilkins, Baltimore, 1967, p. 1.
79. Gershenfeld, L., *Urine and Urinalysis*, 2nd ed., Romaine-Pierson, New York, 1948, p. 1.
80. Johnson, R. B., ed., *Std. Methods Clin. Chem.*, **5,** 159 (1965).
81. *"Labstix" and Other Urinalysis Reagents*, Ames, Elkhart, Ind.
82. Belmonte, M., *Diabetes*, **16,** 557 (1967).
83. Sternheimer, R., and Malbon, B., *Am. J. Med.*, **11,** 312 (1951).
84. Fletcher, T., and Pan, S., *Tech. Bull. 1R-8074-M*, Beckman, Fullerton, Calif., 1962, p. 1.
85. Frazer, A. C., *Advan. Clin. Chem.*, **5,** 69 (1962).
86. Faust, E., and Russell, P., *Clinical Parasitology*, 7th ed., Lea & Febiger, Philadelphia, 1964, p. 1.
87. Lindquist, F., and Curry, A., *Methods of Forensic Science*, vols. I–IV, Wiley, New York, 1962–1965.
88. National Clearinghouse for Poison Control Centers, US Dept. HEW, Washington, D.C.
89. Jerzy Glass, G., *Advan. Clin. Chem.*, **7,** 236 (1964).
90. Sun, D., ed., *Ann. NY Acad. Sci.*, **140,** 687 (1967).
91. Chiang, L., *et al, Proc. Soc. Exptl. Biol. Med.*, **122,** 700 (1966).
92. Bailey, R. W., *Diagnostic Microbiology*, 2nd ed., Mosby, St. Louis, 1966, p. 1.
93. Kabat, E., and Mayer, M., *Experimental Immunochemistry*, 2nd ed., Thomas, Springfield, Ill., 1961, p. 1.
94. Emmons, C., *et al, Medical Mycology*, Lea & Febiger, Philadelphia, 1963, p. 1.
95. Burnet, F., and Stanley, W., *The Viruses*, vols. I–III, Academic, New York, 1959.
96. Fenner, F., *Biology of the Animal Viruses*, vols. I–II, Academic, New York, 1968.
97. Cherry, W., and Moody, M., *Bacteriol. Rev.*, **29,** 222 (1965).
98. Schiller, E., *Advan. Clin. Chem.*, **9,** 43 (1967).
99. Lee, C. L., and Davidsohn, I., Am. Soc. Clin. Pathol. Coll. Am. Pathol. Mtg., Chicago, 1967, p. 1.
100. Singer, J., *et al, Am. J. Clin. Pathol.*, **28,** 611 (1957).
101. Golden, M., and Black, A., *Ann. Rheumatic Diseases*, **23,** 485 (1964).
102. *Serological Tests for Syphilis*, No. 411, US Dept. HEW, Washington, D.C., 1964, p. 1.

40 | Chromatography

Development of chromatographic techniques—theory of
chromatography—techniques of chromatography—applications of
chromatography

This chapter was prepared by

John C. Drach, PhD, *Research Biochemist, Research Laboratories, Parke, Davis
and Company, Ann Arbor, Mich.* 48106

Purification and separation procedures are needed
for the preparation of many pharmaceutical products.
They are used from the initial detection and isolation
of trace quantities of synthetic and naturally occurring compounds and for the final large-scale preparation of medicinal agents.

The term "chromatography" refers to a number of
highly efficient techniques for the separation of a wide
variety of substances ranging from inorganic ions to
complex biopolymers. Because chromatography is so
intimately involved in pharmaceutical research and
development, the pharmacist should possess a working
knowledge of its principles and techniques.

*Chromatography is a separation process based upon
the differential distribution of a mixture between two
phases, one of which is percolated through the other.*
This distribution must be reversible, and the substances in the mixture must be of molecular dimensions, the latter requirement usually being met by
putting them into solution or by vaporizing the mixture.

One of these phases is termed the *stationary phase,*
and the other the *mobile phase.* The stationary phase
may be a porous solid, a finely divided solid, or a
liquid that has been bound to some inert supporting
material. The mobile phase may be a solution, gas, or
liquid. By some definitions, this might include such
separation techniques as ultracentrifugation, foam
fractionation and liquid-liquid countercurrent distribution. However these techniques will not be considered in the present discussion.

If the stationary phase is a solid, the process is
termed *adsorption chromatography,* while if the stationary phase is liquid the process is termed *partition
chromatography.* The difference between partition
chromatography and adsorption chromatography lies
in the nature of the forces that determine distribution
of the solute between the two phases.

In adsorption chromatography the mobile phase
passes over the solid stationary phase carrying the
dissolved compounds with it. The rate at which the
solutes move or separate depends on the various degrees of affinity that the solutes have for the stationary
phase.

In partition chromatography a porous matrix, such
as cellulose or silica gel, immobilizes a layer of solvent
which thereby becomes the stationary phase. The
mobile phase is passed over this matrix and the relative
solubility of the compounds in the two liquid phases
is the controlling factor in the separation process.

Ion-exchange chromatography is usually classified
separately. Although it employs a solid phase, adsorption at the liquid–solid interface is not the primary
phenomenon. In this instance ion or electron exchange is the most important single factor. Both
partition and adsorption effects are operative in many
instances, and no single factor governs the entire
chromatographic process.

When a gas is the mobile phase, the method is called
vapor-phase or *gas chromatography* and is further classified as *gas-adsorption* chromatography or as *gas-partition* chromatography, depending on whether the stationary phase is a solid or a liquid. Rather than using a
gas or liquid as the mobile phase, an electrical field may
be applied to produce migration of charged molecules.

Thus, *zone electrophoresis* or *electrochromatography*
utilizes a solid supporting medium which is moistened
by a buffer to permit electrical conduction. This supports the differential migration of molecules having
different net electrical charges.

These techniques and some of their practical applications are described briefly in the following sections.

Development of Chromatography

In the introductory paragraphs chromatographic
principles were generally divided into adsorption
chromatography, where the stationary phase is a solid,
and partition chromatography, where the stationary
phase is a liquid. Each of these methods may be further subdivided depending on the nature of the mobile
phase.

Adsorption chromatography which uses a liquid for
elution, or development, may be called liquid–solid or
liquid-adsorption chromatography (LSC). Likewise,
development with a gas gives gas–solid or gas-adsorption chromatography (GSC). Similarly, partition

techniques result in liquid–liquid or liquid-partition
chromatography (LLC) and gas–liquid or gas-partition
chromatography (GLC). Most chromatographic techniques may be additionally defined based on the
method of mobile phase development.

Elution development, displacement development, and
frontal analysis are the ways in which chromatograms
may be developed. These methods will be introduced
in the following historical overview to aid in the subsequent development of the techniques and applications
of chromatography.

Liquid-Adsorption Chromatography

Frontal analysis of chromatograms was first performed by Day and his associates. In 1897 Day[1] first recognized adsorption chromatography in his work on the origin of Pennsylvania petroleum. He observed that oil samples ranged in color from black, through reddish hues, to some that were nearly white.

To Day this suggested that the oil underwent a fractional filtration process in the ground. Later, he and his associates found that crude petroleum could be percolated through large columns filled with limestone and fuller's earth to give light aliphatic hydrocarbons, followed in turn by aromatic and unsaturated hydrocarbons, and finally by nitrogen and sulfur compounds of increasing complexity. In these instances where the only solution which is passed through the column is the mixture of interest, each succeeding fraction contains one new component in addition to all the preceding ones.

This method of development is referred to as frontal analysis (Fig. 427). Although the technique is of limited value for the isolation of pure compounds from a mixture, it has been used extensively by Claesson[2] and Nobel-laureate Tiselius[3] for determining the number of components in a mixture.

Elution development was first used in the early 1900's by the Russian botanist Tswett[4] for the separation of green leaf pigments. Instead of percolating the solution through a column, he applied a relatively small amount of a petroleum ether extract to the top of a calcium carbonate column. After the pigments had been adsorbed onto the column, pure solvent was applied and like "light rays in the spectrum" the different components of the mixture separated.

For the first time Tswett referred to this technique as the "chromatographic process" or color writing. When the leading component reached the end of the column, the solvent flow was stopped and the adsorbent extruded and sectioned. More conveniently, the development process is continued and the effluent collected in fractions, permitting the qualitative and quantitative evaluation of the individual components (see Fig. 428).

Tswett's achievement was superior to that of Day in that he correctly interpreted the process and also introduced elution development using pure solvent. In spite of this, Tswett's chromatographic methods were little noted until Kuhn, *et al*,[5] revived interest in chromatography by resolving carotenoid isomers on calcium carbonate columns.

Displacement development was introduced by Tiselius.[6] It may be used to elute a column by displacing the solutes on the adsorbent with a more strongly adsorbed compound. The displacing agent "pushes out" the solute which is least firmly adsorbed, followed by other solutes which are more firmly bound. The process continues until the added displacing agent leaves the column.

The elution pattern is very similar to that obtained with frontal analysis except the trailing edge of the solute zone is well defined and does not extend back through the length of the column (Fig. 429). The technique will succeed where tailing would otherwise make separations impossible. While permitting separation, solutes leave the column immediately behind one another thereby causing some overlap of peaks.

Tiselius and Hagdahl[7] improved this technique and used it for the separation of small quantities of amino acids and peptides by interposing a number of alcohols (having intermediate adsorption characteristics) as carriers between the solutes. This *carrier-displacement development* causes the solutes to collect in narrow zones at the boundaries of the much broader carrier zones. Given the proper ratio of carrier to solute, the components of the mixture will elute in narrow, well-defined zones. The contaminating carrier may be removed by evaporation or extraction.

Liquid-Partition Chromatography

A variation in *column applications* of chromatography was introduced by Martin and Synge.[8] Subsequent developments led to applications of such importance that these men jointly received the Nobel

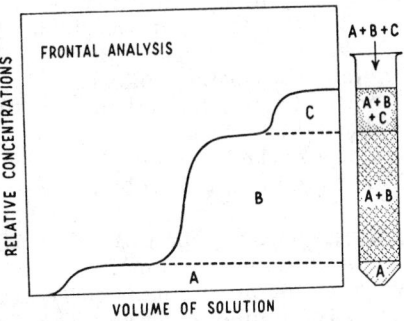

Fig. 427. Frontal analysis for determining the number of components in a mixture. A solution containing a mixture of the Solutes *A*, *B*, and *C* is percolated through the adsorption column at the right. *A* is least strongly adsorbed and appears first in the effluent solution. This is followed by a mixture of *A* + *B* and finally *A* + *B* + *C*. The elution diagram illustrates the increasing concentration of solutes in the effluent.

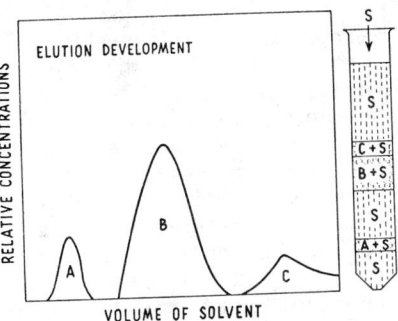

Fig. 428. Elution development for separating components of a mixture. A sample containing Solutes *A* + *B* + *C* is applied to the top of an adsorption column, and the chromatogram developed by percolating pure solvent (*S*) through the column. The components separate as they pass down the column and are collected separately in the effluent.

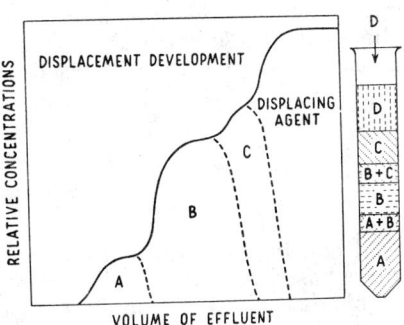

Fig. 429. Displacement development for determining number, nature, and concentration of solutes. A sample containing Solutes *A* + *B* + *C* is applied to the top of an adsorption column. The chromatogram is developed with a solvent containing a displacing agent (*D*) which is more strongly adsorbed on the column than either *A*, *B*, or *C*.

Prize in chemistry for 1953. They found that mixtures of acetylated amino acids could be partially resolved by a process of serially partitioning the components between two immiscible liquids.

This technique of discontinuous countercurrent distribution has been greatly extended by Craig[9] and now finds wide use for both analytical and preparative purposes. However, Martin and Synge succeeded in applying the partition concept to column operation, thereby providing a continuous extraction method which was simpler and more efficient than the discontinuous one.

In their original method silica gel was moistened with an aqueous solution of methyl orange dye and then suspended in water-saturated chloroform containing 1% n-butyl alcohol. This changed the dye color from pink to yellow. The slurry was placed into a tube, permitted to settle, and rinsed with the chloroform-containing mobile phase. Little water-soluble dye was eluted by the rinsing, indicating that the water was indeed bound to the silica gel and would act as the stationary phase.

A solution of acetylated amino acids was applied to the top of the column and eluted with the chloroform solution. The position of the acids was revealed by the dye, which turned from yellow to pink. The single pink band separated into its constituent bands, which moved down the column at rates characteristic of the partitioning of the amino acids between the aqueous and organic solvent phases.

Paper-partition chromatography was introduced by Consden, *et al.*[10] They found that better resolution of amino acids could be obtained by using strips of filter paper as the stationary phase support rather than silica gel. The technique of using filter paper as a stationary support was originally used by Schoenbein[11] and Goeppelsroeder.[12] Their system of "capillary analysis" simply consisted of dipping one end of a paper strip into a solution containing a mixture of solutes. The solutes rose to different heights along the length of the paper because of adsorption phenomena.

In contrast, Consden, *et al*, first placed the filter paper in a sealed tank and permitted the cellulose to equilibrate with a water-saturated organic solvent. The cellulose-bound water then became the stationary phase and amino acids were separated by partition between the bound water and the water-saturated organic solvent which was used to irrigate the paper strip.

Gas-Adsorption Chromatography

In order to analyze the components of gas mixtures, Schuftan[13] devised a system of adsorption chromatography in the early 1930's using the gas as the mobile phase. In the early stages GSC was limited to the analysis of gases or highly volatile solutes. More recently, less volatile and polar compounds have been separated by using specially prepared adsorbents and highly sensitive detectors. The adsorbents which have been used include charcoal, silica gel, alumina, organic polymers, etc.

Techniques of development have included frontal analysis, elution development, and displacement development, although elution development is by far the most widely used. GSC is important due to the unique selectivity of some adsorbents and to the lack of "bleeding" of the stationary phase which occurs in GLC. However, the present use of GSC is rather limited, especially in pharmaceutical applications, and will not be detailed in this chapter.

Gas-Partition Chromatography

When Martin and Synge introduced the concept of partition chromatography in 1941 they clearly stated, "The mobile phase need not be a liquid but may be a vapor."[8] Subsequent developments in chromatography centered upon the use of liquid solvent systems, and the concept of vapor-phase chromatography remained at a standstill for about 10 years.

In the early 1950's James,[14] working in Martin's laboratory, reminded him of his earlier suggestions concerning gas–liquid chromatography (GLC), and they proceeded to experiment with the separation of short-chained fatty acids on columns of Celite coated with mineral oil. The detection device was merely a test tube filled with an aqueous indicator which was titrated dropwise, each drop being timed with a stopwatch. The separations were disappointing, and other packings were tried with equally poor results. Finally, in desperation, a mixture of methylamines was chromatographed and clean separations were obtained on the very first run.

The problem of fatty acid separation was then studied more intensively, and a practical solution to the problem eventually resulted from James and Martin.[15] During much of this period, titration was still used as a rudimentary means of detection. It is worth noting that the basic principles of gas chromatography were evolved with the simplest possible laboratory equipment, and that the more elegant refinements in technique were left to others who perhaps were not as much concerned with the fundamental aspects of gas chromatography.

While the first applications of GLC by James and Martin were in the field of biochemistry, the petroleum industry shortly began to use the method to solve many analytical problems. The combination of extreme sensitivity in detection and efficiency in fractionation assured the adoption of the technique by all branches of chemistry.

Theory of Chromatography

Theoretical considerations of chromatographic processes may be based on either equilibrium or kinetic concepts. This discussion will be limited primarily to equilibrium considerations because the basic ideas are readily developed. For detailed discussion of both concepts the reader is referred to the books by Giddings and Heftmann in the *Bibliography* (page 693).

The *partition coefficient* (α) is used to define the distribution of a solute between two phases, whether gas, liquid or solid. It was defined by Martin and Synge[8] as follows

$$\alpha = \frac{\text{Gm solute per ml of stationary phase}}{\text{Gm solute per ml of mobile phase}} = \frac{c_{st}}{c_m} \quad (1)$$

In partition chromatography α is governed by the relative solute solubility in the two phases, whereas in adsorption chromatography the relative affinity for the stationary phase is the controlling factor. The partition coefficient also depends on temperature and to a much lesser extent on pressure. It is assumed to be independent of concentration. Thus, variation of the temperature or the composition of the mobile phase during chromatography will influence the migration of solutes.

To effectively define the total amount of solute partitioned between the entire stationary and mobile phases a modified expression of the partition coefficient (β) may be calculated by multiplying α by the quotient of the volume (or the surface area, if adsorption chromatography is involved) of the stationary and mobile phases:

$$\beta = \alpha \left(\frac{V_{st}}{V_m} \right) = \frac{c_{st}V_{st}}{c_m V_m} \qquad (2)$$

From the equilibrium, or theoretical plate concept, chromatography may be viewed as a series of discontinuous equilibrations of a solute between the stationary and mobile phases as the mobile phase passes up a paper strip, down a column, etc. In fact, this discontinuous process is exactly the technique of countercurrent distribution where a series of extractions is performed using separatory funnels or a completely automated apparatus.

To illustrate, consider a hypothetical paper strip onto which 80 mcg of a solute with $\beta = 1$ has been placed. The cellulose matrix of the paper (supporting the stationary aqueous phase) is placed into a trough of organic mobile phase which develops the chromatogram by capillary action. As the mobile phase reaches the solute, 40 mcg of it will diffuse into the organic solvent and 40 mcg will remain in the aqueous phase.

This single equilibration between phases is termed a theoretical plate, the term arising from similar considerations in fractional distillation techniques. The height of a column or paper section required for one equilibration is called the height equivalent to one theoretical plate or HETP. This is a theoretical term and is assumed to be constant throughout the length of the stationary phase. It is governed by the rate at which the solute molecules equilibrate between phases within a given plate and is related to the number of theoretical plates by:

$$\text{HETP} = \frac{L}{n} \qquad (3)$$

where L = the total length of the chromatogram and n = the total number of theoretical plates in the chromatogram. Plate height also increases in a chromatogram of given length because of nonequilibrium conditions and diffusion. The usual HETP for a good chromatogram is on the order of 1 mm or less, so that hundreds or even thousands of equilibration steps occur during the development of the chromatogram. Also, it may be said that the chromatogram contained hundreds or thousands of theoretical plates.

Returning to the hypothetical paper chromatogram, let us simplify by assuming there are only five theoretical plates in the chromatogram.

As fresh mobile phase migrates up the paper, 40 mcg of solute will be carried along to the first theoretical plate. Of this, 20 mcg will diffuse into the stationary phase and 20 mcg will remain in the mobile phase. The 40 mcg which remained in the stationary phase from Plate #0 simultaneously partitions with the newly ascended mobile phase. After equilibration the ascending mobile phase will carry 20 mcg of solute

from Plate #1 to Plate #2, and the process continues as depicted in Fig. 430.

This model assumes a discontinuous process where equilibrium is achieved in each plate. In actuality, chromatography is a continuous process where true equilibrium does not exist. However, for purposes of this discussion the equilibrium concept is adequate. Also, in this hypothetical paper chromatogram the solvent flow stops after the leading edge of solvent has passed through the fifth HEPT. The resulting developed paper is considered a *complete chromatogram*.

While it is not possible to continue development of the paper by the ascending solvent flow, *continuous chromatograms* are possible by using descending solvent flow or column techniques.

Aspects of Complete Chromatography

Techniques of complete chromatography include ascending paper chromatography, thin-layer chromatography, and some forms of column chromatography and electrophoresis where the supporting medium is physically sectioned to separate component fractions. This contrasts with continuous chromatography where mobile phase flow continues until solutes are eluted from the end of the stationary phase support. In both complete and flowing chromatograms the fractional distance traveled by a given solute relative to the total distance traveled by the solvent front is termed the R_f value:

$$R_f = \frac{\text{distance traveled by solute}}{\text{distance traveled by solvent front}}$$

In complete chromatograms the distances of movement of solute and solvent are most conveniently expressed as length in cm. from the point where the solute was applied to the stationary phase (origin). Consden, et al,[10] related the R_f value to the partition coefficient (α) by the following expression:

$$R_f = \frac{A_L}{A_L + \alpha A_s} \qquad (4)$$

where A_L = the cross-sectional area or volume (V_m) occupied by the mobile phase and A_s = the cross-sectional area or volume (V_{st}) occupied by the stationary phase. A simplified expression can be calcu-

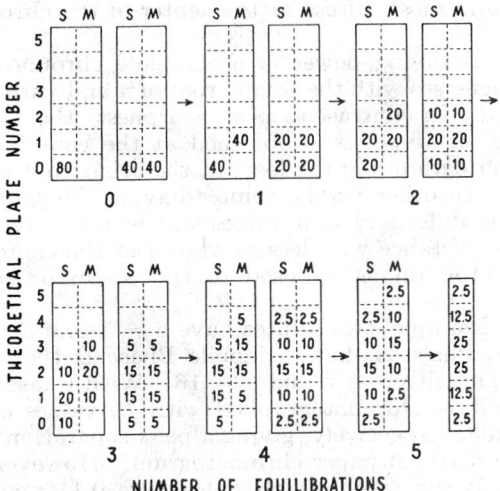

Fig. 430. **Chromatography depicted as a discontinuous equilibrium process.** For purposes of illustration the stationary (S) and mobile (M) phases are shown separately. The mobile phase migrates up the paper strip causing a solute with a partition coefficient of 1 to successively equilibrate between the two phases.

lated by using the volume notations in Eq. 4, solving Eq. 2 for V_m and making the appropriate substitutions:

$$R_f = \frac{1}{1 + \beta} \qquad (5)$$

It is immediately obvious that as the partition coefficient increases (or as more solute is retained in the stationary phase) the R_f value decreases. The R_f value of the solute of Fig. 430 is 0.5 with the peak concentration in the middle of the chromatogram. A closer examination of Fig. 430 reveals that the highest concentration of solute is contained in the center of the part of the paper strip *in use* regardless of the plate number.

As the number of equilibrations increases, the sample spreads over a greater area of the paper but not over a greater percentage of the paper *in use*. In fact, after equilibration number 2, 40 mcg (or 50%) of the total solute is present in the center third of the paper strip. But, after five equilibrations, 50 mcg (or 62.5%) of the solute is concentrated in the center third of the strip. *Therefore, as the number of theoretical plates in a chromatogram increases, the sharpness of the solute peak increases but the R_f value remains unchanged.*

A measure of the sharpness of a chromatographic band is the fraction of solute contained per unit length of the chromatogram at the point of maximum solute concentration. Or, for the same amount of solute, the higher the maximum concentration per length (C_L), the sharper the peak. For complete chromatograms Johnson[16] derived a relationship between C_L and the partition coefficient, chromatogram length, and number of theoretical plates. It may be expressed in relation to the R_f value of a particular solute by:

$$C_L = \frac{1}{L} \sqrt{\frac{n}{2\pi R_f (1 - R_f)}} \qquad (6)$$

where L = the length of the complete chromatogram and n = the number of theoretical plates in the complete chromatogram.

For chromatograms of constant length, the sharpness of solute peaks will increase in proportion to increases in the square root of n. Within the same chromatogram the sharpness of solute peaks varies with the relative position of the peak; ie, depends on β. Peaks are most well defined near the origin and solvent front and most diffuse at the center of the chromatogram.

The resolving power of a complete chromatogram also increases with the square root of n and varies with R_f or β. In contrast to peak sharpness, the greatest resolution of peaks is obtained at the center of the chromatogram and the least at the origin and solvent front. In other words, solutes having the same percentage difference in β values will be separated by a greater distance with less overlap near the center of a chromatogram as opposed to the origin or solvent front.

For example, two solutes have $\beta = 1$ and $\beta = 2$ in mobile Phase A, but in mobile Phase B the solutes partition with $\beta = 8$ and $\beta = 16$. With Phase A the two solutes chromatographed with R_f values of 0.50 and 0.33, respectively, giving a peak separation of 1.7 cm on a 10-cm paper chromatogram. However with Phase B the resultant R_f values are 0.11 and 0.06, respectively, yielding a peak separation of 0.5 cm. It is desirable, therefore, to choose conditions so that solutes of interest migrate with R_f values near 0.5 in the techniques of complete chromatography.

Aspects of Continuous Chromatography

Continuous chromatograms result when the mobile phase development is permitted to continue and elute solutes from the stationary phase. Column applications of this technique include gel filtration, ion-exchange chromatography, gas chromatography, and liquid chromatography. While the ensuing discussion applies to all these techniques, the simplified mathematical relationships must be expanded to include variables which may be involved in one technique but not in another.

In continuous chromatography the relative positions of solutes are expressed in terms of ml of solvent necessary for elution rather than R_f values. The volume of mobile phase present on a column at any one time is equal to the internal volume of the column minus the support and stationary phase volumes. This volume is generally termed the holdup volume (V_H).

If a column were developed with only one V_H, it would be a complete chromatogram as no solutes would be eluted. Continuing the mobile phase flow elutes the solutes in increasing order of partition coefficient (Fig. 431). The volume of mobile phase needed for this elution (V_S) is related to R_f, and by Eq. 5, to β in the following manner:

$$\frac{V_S}{V_H} = \frac{1}{R_f} = \beta + 1 \qquad (7)$$

From Eq. 7 it can be seen that a solute with $\beta = 1.0$ would require two holdup volumes to be eluted from the column. Therefore this solute will undergo two times as many equilibrations as it would if the column were operated as a complete chromatogram *where the number of equilibrations is the same for all solutes.* Thus, a series of solutes with increasing partition coefficients will require increasing volumes of mobile phase to be eluted, resulting in a greater number of theoretical plates for each successively eluted solute.

Where V_S is much larger than V_H (as with gas chromatography and many liquid chromatographic techniques), this may be expressed as:

$$n = \frac{16 (V_S)^{2*}}{w^2} \qquad (8)$$

where w = the baseline width of the solute peak. The baseline width of a solute peak equals 4σ where σ is the standard deviation of the Gaussian concentration profile. The width increases during chromatography due to ordinary molecular diffusion, rate of partition or sorption–desorption of solutes between the two phases, and flow diffusion.

In continuous chromatograms the sharpness of peaks increases with an increasing number of theoretical plates and decreases with increasing values of β. Mayer and Tompkins[17] first derived this relationship and equated these parameters to the fraction of solute in the mobile phase in contact with the plate having maximum solute concentration. This may be converted to the fraction of solute per unit volume by multiplying Mayer and Tompkin's equation by the number of plates per unit volume to give:

$$C_V = \frac{1}{V_H} \sqrt{\frac{n}{2\pi\beta (1 + \beta)}} \qquad (9)$$

where C_V = the maximum concentration per unit vol-

---

* For the derivation, see the book by Gudzinowicz in the *Bibliography* (page 693).

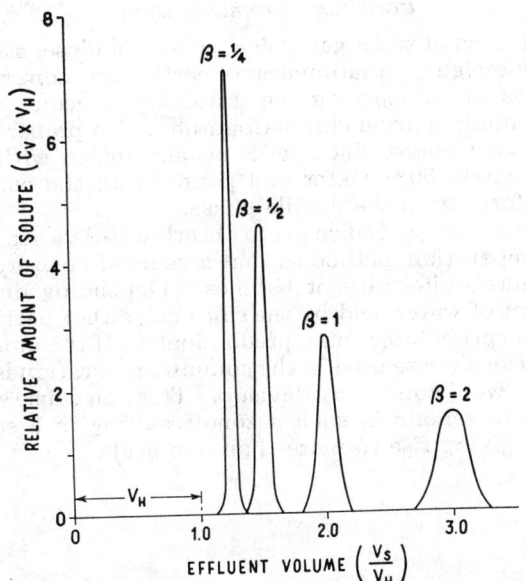

Fig. 431. Elution pattern of solutes from a hypothetical continuous chromatogram. The increases in peak spreading and elution volume are illustrated for solutes having different effective partition coefficients (β). The amount of each solute is taken as unity so that the areas under each curve are equal.

ume expressed as a fraction of the total solute in the eluted mobile phase and n = number of theoretical plates if the column were operated as a complete chromatogram. The term C_V for continuous chromatography is analogous to C_L in complete chromatography. Figure 431 illustrates the principles given by the above equations. For ease of illustration it was constructed using $n = 100$, $V_H = 100$, and Eq. 8 for baseline peak width even though V_S is not greatly

larger than V_H. From this figure it is evident that solute peaks broaden with increasing holdup volumes of solvent needed for elution; ie with increasing β values. This spreading of a solute zone occurs as it migrates down a continuous chromatogram, becoming more diffuse as the length of travel increases.

As mobile phase is percolated through a column to elute a solute, the C_V for that solute *decreases* inversely proportional to the increasing number of holdup volumes needed for elution and *increases* by the square root of the resulting increases in n. Because solute elution will require x-times the holdup volume of solvent, the number of theoretical plates also increases x-fold. This results in a net decrease in C_V by a factor of $1/\sqrt{x}$ or the peak is $\sqrt{x}$ times more diffuse.

In spite of zone spreading being increased by a factor of $\sqrt{x}$, the separation between two solute peaks increases directly with x thereby outdistancing the spreading influences. Thus, slowly eluting solute peaks will be diffuse, but will be proportionately well separated.

From all the foregoing discussion it is apparent that good chromatographic separations depend on maximum values of n or, from Eq. 3, minimum values of HETP. Optimization of the following will yield the minimum HETP values:

1. The *initial sample size* should be small so that the initial solute band will occupy the fewest HETP.
2. *Dead volume* should be minimized. Any volume without stationary phase increases length without increasing n.
3. *Flow velocity* must be optimum to give a minimum HETP. Too rapid a flow will not permit a complete partition of solute molecules, too slow will cause excess molecular diffusion.
4. *Particle diameter* of the stationary phase must be sufficiently small to permit rapid partition of the solute; thus small HETP.
5. *Temperature* must be constant or adequately programed to control the partition coefficient.

Techniques of Chromatography

The basic separation principles of chromatography such as adsorption, partition, and ion exchange can be applied by the use of various techniques. The following discussion will include the application of these different principles involved in chromatographic separations.

Liquid-Column Chromatography

Fundamental Procedures

The essential steps involved in the classic types of column chromatography are:

1. Preparation of the column.
2. Addition of the sample to the top of the column.
3. Development of the chromatogram by percolating a solvent through the column.
4. Recovery of the fractions.

The column is usually a piece of glass tubing which may be anywhere from a few millimeters to 30 cm or more in diameter. The packing material is supported by a sintered glass disc or a plug of glass wool at the bottom of the tube. In larger columns a piece of stainless steel gauze is often used. The column may be filled with dry, powdered adsorbent, or with a slurry of the adsorbing agent suspended in the solvent. Great care must be taken to pack the column evenly.

With slurries, suction or pressure may be applied to produce uniform packing, and the solvent level is always kept above the packing. A small amount of the sample dissolved in the mobile phase is applied to the top of the column where it is adsorbed by the topmost layer of packing material. The developing solvent is percolated slowly through the column, and various constituents of the sample are carried along at different rates of movement.

Adsorption Chromatography

Many different combinations of solvent and adsorbent are possible. Some of the more common agents are listed in Table I. In order to obtain good movement of the components, the adsorbent and solvent should be selected from as close to the top of this list as possible.

A good deal of experimentation may be required before optimum conditions are found, and the success of the operation may depend to a great extent on the skill and ingenuity of the chemist in arriving at the best possible set of conditions. For example, certain compounds will wash rapidly through the column leaving others adsorbed at the top requiring many volumes of solvent for elution. This drawback may be overcome by switching to a more polar solvent at this point.

Another possibility is to change the composition of the mobile phase gradually and continuously during development (*gradient elution*). This involves the use of siphons and mixing devices to produce linear, logarithmic, concave, etc changes in the solvent composition reaching the column (see Bock and Ling[18]). This results in sharp solute peaks even though a great many holdup volumes may be required for elution. Since this may be a time-consuming process, automatic fraction-collecting devices are often used, as shown in Fig. 432.

The factors influencing adsorption are not well understood. The compound being adsorbed may interact with the solvent in which it is dissolved as well as with the adsorbent, and a consideration of all three components is therefore involved.

The electrical dissymmetry or *polarity* of these components is an important factor in determining the degree of adsorption. Polar compounds are more readily adsorbed from nonpolar solvents, while nonpolar compounds are usually adsorbed more readily with increasing molecular size and degree of unsaturation. Saturated hydrocarbons are poorly adsorbed as a rule, with adsorption increasing with the number of double bonds and degree of conjugation, but decreasing with hydrogen bonding. The addition of functional groups to the molecule appears to influence adsorption in the

Table I—Adsorbents and Solvents Used in Column Chromatography

Adsorbents	Eluents
Sucrose ————————(Weakest)—	Petroleum ether
Starch	Carbon tetrachloride
Inulin	Cyclohexane
Talc	Carbon disulfide
Sodium carbonate	Diethyl ether
Calcium carbonate	Acetone
Calcium phosphate	Benzene
Magnesium carbonate	Toluene
Magnesia	Esters
Lime	Chloroform
Silicic acid	Alcohols
Alumina	Water
Charcoal	Pyridine
Fuller's earth ————(Strongest)—	Organic acids

following order: acids and bases > alcohols > primary amines > aldehydes and ketones > esters and halogens > nitro > O-alkyl > alkyl.

In certain cases, the configuration of the molecule may affect its adsorption properties, and even stereoisomers can be separated sometimes by the proper choice of solvent and adsorbent.

In recent years a number of different and highly specific adsorbents have been devised for the separation of nucleic acids. These utilize hydrogen bonding or salt linkages as the adsorptive forces.

Mandell and Hershey[19] first demonstrated that DNA and RNA could be resolved from each other and also subfractionated on columns where methylated serum albumin was adsorbed onto kieselguhr. About the same time others prepared modified celluloses to which purines, pyrimidines, and synthetic and naturally occurring nucleic acids were either adsorbed or covalently bound (eg, see Adler and Rich[20]).

Nucleic acids are adsorbed onto the column by the formation of hydrogen bonds with the base or nucleic acid attached to the column packing. Development is achieved by gradient elution utilizing a changing salt concentration. This technique can result in highly specific fractionations based on bonding between complementary sequences in nucleic acids.

Partition Chromatography

Columns of silica gel (silicic acid), cellulose, starch, and kieselguhr (diatomaceous earth) are commonly used as the support for the stationary aqueous phase in column partition chromatography. To prepare the stationary phase, silica gel is usually mixed with approximately 50% water and poured into the column as a slurry with the mobile phase.

The capacity of silica gel to absorb water varies with the preparation method so that care must be exercised to insure uniformity of batches. Depending on the amount of water held by the silica gel, either partition or adsorption forces may predominate. If the amount of aqueous phase used in the column preparation is too large, "wet" zones may develop. This can cause some solute to remain in such a zone resulting in a single solute giving rise to more than one peak.

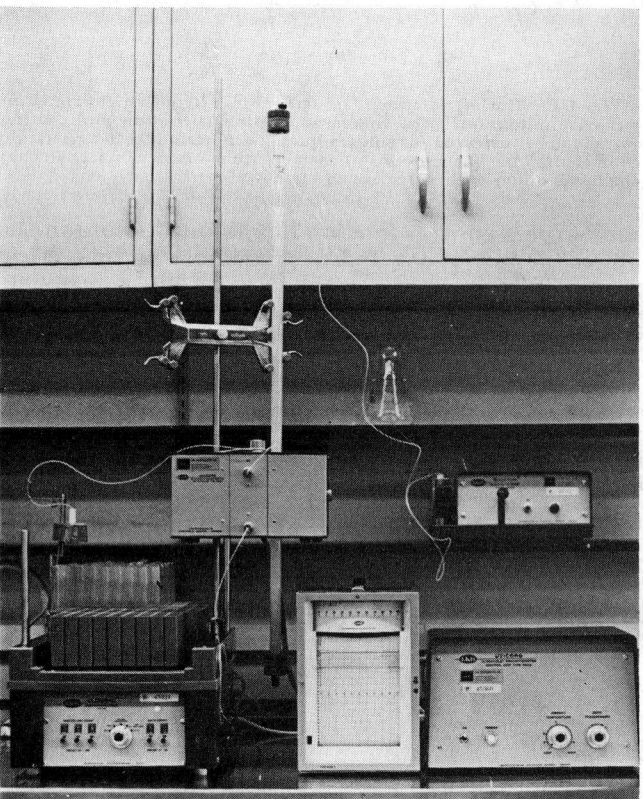

Fig. 432. An LKB type 7000 fraction collector with an ultraviolet flow-through detector. Solvent is pumped from the reservoir in the background to a gel-filtration column. The effluent is continuously monitored for ultraviolet-absorbing materials and the concentration recorded. Effluent then flows to the fraction collector where fraction volume is controlled by a preset photoelectric drop counter.

The use of starch and cellulose as the stationary support also is common. The separation of small amounts of solutes by paper partition chromatography often can be scaled up to preparative separations by using cellulose or starch as the support for column partition chromatography.

Reversed-phase partition chromatography involves the use of packing materials which absorb an organic solvent so that the chromatogram may be developed with an aqueous phase. Columns consisting of benzene or butanol absorbed onto rubber latex or silicone-treated cellulose have been used for the separation of fatty acids and steroids. Elution is performed with aqueous buffers or water:methanol mixtures.

Ion-Exchange Chromatography

A major advance in chromatography was introduced by the development of synthetic ion-exchange resins. A series of publications released by the Atomic Energy Commission in 1947 first described the use of these resins for the separation of rare earth metals from fission products by a modified type of column chromatography. This technique has since been applied to a large number of organic compounds and has proved especially useful for separating acidic and basic substances from mixtures. The advantage of ion-exchange resins over the older types of adsorbents lies in their greater degree of selectivity arising from simultaneous operation of ion-exchange and molecular adsorption mechanisms.

Many types of synthetic ion-exchange resins, possessing widely different physical and chemical properties, are now available. These resins are insoluble in water and most organic solvents and carry polar groups in definite and regularly recurring positions in the molecule. Strong cation exchangers are usually sulfonated resins of the polystyrene type; weaker cation exchangers are usually carboxylic acid resins; most anion-exchange resins are aliphatic amines (weak bases) or quaternary ammonium salts (strong bases). The ion-exchange capacity of cellulose filter papers has also been increased by chemical modification. Diethylaminoethyl cellulose (DEAE-cellulose) and triethylaminoethyl cellulose (TEAE-cellulose) are good anion-exchange materials, and carboxymethyl cellulose (CM-cellulose) has cation-exchange properties. These have been used extensively for the purification of protein and enzyme preparations. In addition, papers loaded with different ion-exchange resins are available commercially, combining the advantages of partition and ion-exchange mechanisms for special applications.

Mechanism—The mechanism of ion exchange depends primarily on the replacement of the dissociable groups of the resin by the ionic species being separated. For example, sodium chloride may be removed from water by a mixture of anion- and cation-exchange resins:

$$(1) \quad Resin\text{-}SO_3H + Na^+ \rightleftharpoons Resin\text{-}SO_3Na + \boxed{H^+}$$
$$(2) \quad Resin^+OH^- + Cl^- \rightleftharpoons Resin^+Cl^- + \boxed{OH^-}$$

At the present time a number of resin mixtures are available commercially which incorporate strong cation and anion exchangers, together with a dye which changes color when the resins are exhausted [Amberlite MB-1, MB-3 (*Rohm & Haas*)]. By passing water slowly through a column of this material, ionizable salts are completely removed and water of exceptional chemical purity is obtained. This resin mixture is used in certain deionizing devices that may be attached to faucets, the water coming through the unit being suitable for use in steam irons and storage batteries and for photographic work. A polystyrene wash bottle fitted to a container of mixed ion-exchange resins is also available, the water being purified as it is forced out of the nozzle. Nonionizable organic compounds are not removed by this procedure, and water containing such contaminants must be pretreated with oxidizing agents or with charcoal. At any rate high-purity water free of objectionable odor may now be obtained without recourse to distillation.

Applications—Ion-exchange resins have found extensive application in the control of the water balance of the body. Certain cation-exchange resins incorporated into the diet will remove sodium ions from the intestinal tract and minimize their absorption. This appears to be a practical form of sodium-reduction therapy in cases of congestive heart failure, nephrosis, and cirrhosis of the liver. The acid resin picks up sodium ions from the intestinal tract and is eliminated in the feces. To prevent depletion of potassium in serum, part of the resin is in the form of its potassium salt. An anion-exchange resin is generally included in the preparation to reduce the hazard of acidosis and to decrease the load on the kidneys by removal of sulfates and phosphates. Resins also have been used in peptic ulcer therapy to reduce the acidity in the stomach without producing the undesirable side effects of some types of antacid therapy, such as gastric irritation, eructation, alkalosis, or constipation.

A novel application of ion-exchange resins is in the so-called "tubeless" gastric acidity tests. Cationic-exchange resins are combined with organic bases such as quinine or Azure A. The complex is administered orally, and the release of base in the stomach is roughly proportional to the gastric acidity. The liberated base is then adsorbed from the intestinal tract and excreted into the urine, where its through-put can be measured by colorimetric means. Combinations of drugs with ion-exchange resins also have been used to retard the rate of intestinal absorption, producing a sustained release of drug over a longer period of time.

Amino acids have been separated on the ion-exchange resin Dowex 50, which is a crosslinked aromatic hydrocarbon chain containing nuclear sulfonic acid groups. They have also been separated on Dowex 2, which is a quaternary ammonium salt of a substituted polystyrene, crosslinked with divinylbenzene. Each can be used successfully, depending on the properties of the amino acids. In the operation of an anion-exchange column the anions of amino acids are first adsorbed on the resin at the top of the column. However, the ionization of the weak acids will be depressed by the stronger acids and they will be displaced by the stronger acids. The weaker acids will thus move down the column ahead of the stronger acids. The order of displacement has been found to correspond roughly with the dissociation constants of the amino acids, modified to some extent by other properties.

Column temperatures should be well controlled to obtain good resolution of the amino acids. The operation of a typical large-scale ion-exchange column is shown in Fig. 433. Columns of ion-exchange resins also have been used to separate various nucleic acids, nucleotides, and peptides, as well as higher-molecular-weight proteins including different hemoglobins, serum proteins, ribonuclease, hyaluronidase, lysozyme, and chymotrypsinogen. When the separation of a large number of solutes is desired, such as the tryptic digest of a protein, gradient elution is especially useful.

Ligand-exchange chromatography is a relatively new technique in which an ion-exchange resin is used to immobilize a metal ion (for a brief review, see Helfferich[21]). The ion-exchange resin is used exclusively to hold the metal ion and does not enter into the sorptive process. Complex formation occurs between the metal ion (or its counter ion) and the complexing substances (ligands) to be separated. High selectivity is possible because the complex formation is much more specific than adsorptive or ion-exchange reactions.

Development of such chromatograms may be by elution using an agent which is less strongly complexed than the substances to be separated, or by displacement development using an agent which complexes more strongly than these substances.

Separation of ammonia, monoamines and diamines,

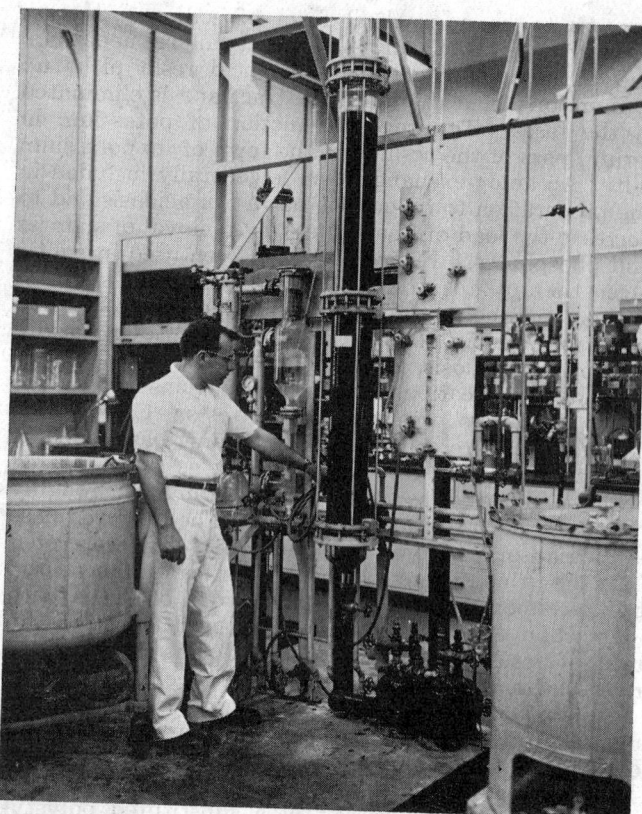

Fig. 433. Pilot-plant operation of an ion-exchange column. The column is made of 6-in. Pyrex pipe, with flanged ends. Dowex 50 is used in this apparatus for the isolation of pure amino acids. The effluent is run into a vacuum concentrator shown behind the operator (courtesy, Parke-Davis).

polyhydric alcohols, organic acids, and olefins have been achieved using cation exchangers in forms as Ag^+, Cu^{2+} and Ni^{2+}.

Gel Filtration

This is a relatively new form of chromatography where separations are based primarily on molecular size and shape. The discovery of the technique was one of those accidental happenings in science. As Tiselius related the story,[22] "Research workers . . . tried to use dextran particles as a filling material in electrophoresis columns. They forgot to turn on the current but observed nevertheless a beautiful separation when buffer solution ran through the column."

The technique was first described by Porath and Flodkin[23] in Sweden, using a crosslinked dextran gel, available commercially as Sephadex (Pharmacia). The dry granules are first allowed to swell in a hydrophilic solvent, following which they are poured into a glass column to serve as the stationary phase and washed. A solution containing the components to be fractionated is applied to the top of the column, and the development process is started by the addition of more solvent. Each component migrates at a different rate, with the largest molecules appearing in the eluate first and the smaller molecules appearing later.

Apparently, the molecules penetrate the gel network to different degrees, depending largely on the steric relationship between the molecular structure of the gel itself and that of the solute, reaching an equilibrium between the solvent within the gel and the solvent outside.

Charged molecules would obviously behave in a more complicated manner. These are usually separated with solvents of high ionic strength to swamp the charge effects, leaving the "molecular sieve" effect as the predominant separation mechanism. Aromatic compounds also behave in a more complicated manner due to adsorption of the molecules onto gel particles.

Another type of gel is available as a molecular sieve. Hjerten and Mosbach[24] introduced the use of polyacrylamide gels which later were marketed under the tradename Bio-Gel (Bio-Rad). Both Sephadex and Bio-gel are available in forms with different degrees of crosslinking to control the size of molecules which will be excluded from the gel particles.

Any molecule exceeding the approximate molecular weight exclusion limit will pass through the column in the holdup volume as it is too large to partition into the gel particle. The various degrees of crosslinking give fractionation ranges for molecules under 700 in molecular weight to those in the range from 500 to 800 thousand. While these fractionation ranges afford excellent separations of many small molecules, proteins, nucleic acids, and polysaccharides, large particles such as viruses or complex nucleic acids will be excluded from the above-mentioned gels.

These limits on fractionation ranges have been extended to molecules (particles) with apparent molecular weights as high as 20 to 30 million by the use of agarose gels. These gels provide a looser network containing no covalent crosslinkages.

Gel filtration has proved to be an extremely useful tool for desalting protein solutions. Hemoglobin, for example, passes readily through a Sephadex column, with inorganic salts trailing behind. By proper choice of conditions it is possible to use the gel-filtration technique for the estimation of molecular size.

It is also finding a useful place in drug–plasma binding studies, since protein-bound drug can be separated easily from unbound drug with this technique. This provides a distinct advance over the time-honored but archaic ultrafiltration techniques using cellophane membranes since errors were often introduced through binding on the membrane itself.

Gel filtration also has been applied to the separation of low-molecular-weight organic compounds, where the adsorption forces and the effects of pH and ionic strength are of greater importance than in the case of high-molecular-weight substances.

More recently dextran has been modified to provide ion-exchange properties. Three different Sephadex ion exchangers are currently available: one anion exchanger (DEAE-Sephadex) and two cation exchangers (CM-Sephadex and sulfoethyl- (SE-) Sephadex). They are weakly basic, weakly acidic, and strongly acidic, respectively. Finer separations are possible when ion exchange is combined with gelfiltration.

The limitation of gel filtration to water-soluble substances has been eliminated by the introduction of a crosslinked dextran in which most hydroxyl groups have been alkylated (Sephadex LH-20). This modification permits the dextran to swell in organic solvents, thereby permitting the fractionation of lipophilic substances.

Electrochromatography

Paper electrophoresis involves the migration of ionized compounds along a paper strip in an electrical field.

The simplest procedure is to spot the mixture of solutes in the middle of a paper strip, moisten the

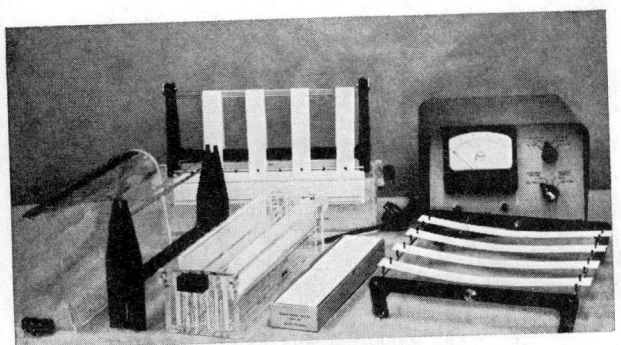

Fig. 434. Typical apparatus for paper electrophoresis. Equipment shown is Beckman/Spinco Model R. Power supply is regulated for constant voltage (0–500 v) or constant current operation (2–50 ma). Electrophoresis cell made of Plexiglas is based on the hanging-strip, inverted-V design originally described by Durrum. The sample is applied as a narrow band at the top of the inverted V. With the rack in position within the cell, the ends of the paper strips are in contact with the electrolyte solution in the lower part of the cell (courtesy, Parke-Davis).

paper with some electrolyte, and place it between two sheets of glass. The ends of the paper strip extending beyond the glass plates are immersed in beakers of the electrolyte. A potential of approximately 5 v/cm of paper length is placed on this system, using a direct current source such as a small radio power supply. Electrophoresis is allowed to continue for a period of several hours. Usually, sufficient movement occurs in that time to obtain good separations, but longer periods are sometimes required.

A weak solution (0.01 M) of acetic acid or of ammonia is commonly used as the conducting electrolyte. For protein separations, the use of buffers such as pyridine–acetic acid mixtures permits the control of the ionic charge on the molecule, thereby controlling the electrical migration.

Many modifications of this apparatus have been described. The paper strips are sometimes placed horizontally in closed chambers with a number of supports to keep them from sagging. Another type of apparatus has the paper strip supported in the middle, hanging like a tent with the ends dipping into the electrolyte compartments (Fig. 434). In this case the sample is applied to the top of the inverted V.

This technique has been used extensively in clinical laboratories for the separation of serum proteins, giving patterns very similar to those obtained by the Tiselius electrophoresis apparatus. The paper strips are generally stained with bromophenol blue, and consecutive sections can be cut out, leached in alcoholic sodium carbonate solutions, and the intensity of color determined directly in a colorimeter. The strips also can be scanned with a photometer and recorded. Analytical values obtained with this technique for normal human serum are shown in Table II.

Table II—Normal Values for Human Serum Proteins Obtained by Paper Electrophoresis[a]

Protein fraction	Concentration (Gm per 100 ml)	
	Mean ± standard deviation	95% Range (± 2 SD)
Total protein	8.14 ± 0.57	7.00 – 9.29
Albumin	5.08 ± 0.51	4.06 – 6.10
α_1-Globulin	0.22 ± 0.07	0.08 – 0.36
α_2-Globulin	0.61 ± 0.17	0.27 – 0.95
β-Globulin	0.92 ± 0.19	0.54 – 1.30
γ-Globulin	1.30 ± 0.30	0.70 – 1.90

[a] Dunn, W. L., and Pearce, R. H., *Can. Med. Assoc. J.*, **84**, 272 (1961).

Many other supporting media have been used for electrophoretic separations. *Cellulose acetate* strips are being used widely in clinical laboratories, producing excellent separations of 7 to 9 protein fractions in a few hours time. This material is exceedingly fine and homogeneous, and little "tailing" is encountered due to negligible adsorption. It is especially useful for separating α_1-globulins from albumin and provides a good background for staining glycoproteins (see Chapter 39, *Clinical Analysis*).

High-voltage paper electrophoresis provides a greatly increased migration rate by using potential gradients up to 100 v/cm. This greatly decreases the amount of diffusion resulting in better separations. Although migration rate increases linearly with increases in potential, the heat generated increases quadratically. This necessitates efficient heat removal to prevent paper charring or distortion of zones by localized overheating. This can be accomplished by using apparatus equipped with either liquid or solid heat exchangers. In the former the paper is immersed in an immiscible liquid, as a light petroleum fraction, from which heat is removed by a series of cooling coils. The latter functions by transferring heat to cooled plates which overlay the paper. The technique has been well applied to the separation of amino acids, peptides, sugars, nucleotides, aldehydes, and ketones.

Peptides resulting from the enzymic degradation of proteins have been investigated by a two-dimensional combination of high-voltage electrophoresis and descending paper chromatography called "fingerprinting." Fine separations result from the combination of the two techniques. Figure 435 illustrates the separation of hemoglobin tryptic peptides in this manner.

Electrophoresis in compact gels also has been used for the separation of protein fractions, depending at least in part on molecular sieving effects to achieve fractionation. *Starch gels* have been particularly valuable in this respect (see Smithies[25]). *Agar gels* and *polyacrylamide gels* also are being used. The latter has been applied to "disc electrophoresis," where the protein fractions in columns of the gel are so sharply defined that they appear as thin discs after staining. (For a recent review, see Poulik.[26])

Polyacrylamide gels also have been used successfully for the fractionation of DNA and RNA.[27] The technique yields separations which are superior to those obtained by zone centrifugation through sucrose den-

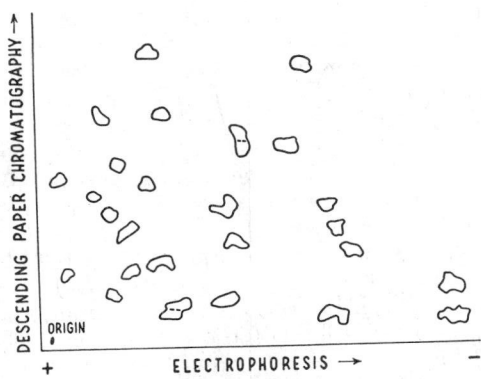

Fig. 435. Fingerprint of rabbit hemoglobin tryptic peptides. The peptide mixture was spotted along a 1-cm strip and the 50 × 110-cm paper moistened with 2.5% pyridine acetate buffer (pH 4.7) containing 5% *n*-butyl alcohol. Electrophoresis of 35 v/cm was applied for 110 min. The paper was dried, cut and developed by descending chromatography for 30 hr at a 90° angle to the direction of electrophoresis. The developing solvent was 27.5% pyridine, 42.5% *n*-butyl alcohol, and 30% water. Peptides were visualized by reaction with ninhydrin.

sity gradients, requiring a greatly reduced period of time.   Larger columns of starch, cellulose, and silica gel are suitable for preparative work, yielding highly purified fractions in sufficient quantity for chemical analysis.

Paper-Partition Chromatography

Partition is the primary principle of separation involved in paper chromatography, but it is likely that adsorption and ion-exchange phenomena also are operative.

The mechanics of operation for paper chromatography are quite simple.   Since no enclosing column is used, the paper must be kept in a closed chamber where the atmosphere is saturated with vapor of the solvent system.   If the developing solvent is to be water-saturated n-butanol, equal volumes of water and butanol are shaken together until they are mutually saturated.   The butanol layer is separated and placed in a reservoir which will be used as the mobile phase to irrigate the paper strips.   The aqueous layer is transferred to a second container.   Both the aqueous and organic phases are placed in a large, covered aquarium jar or other enclosure and allowed to stand until the atmosphere is saturated with the vapor of the solvents. It is obvious that isothermal distillation will not change the composition of the solvents since the two immiscible solvents were mutually saturated with each other before they were separated.

The water which is adsorbed by the filter paper is regarded as the stationary or immobile phase.   Paper in equilibrium with a water-saturated atmosphere at room temperature will take up approximately 22% moisture. A drop of solution containing the unknown mixture is applied a few inches from one end of a strip of filter paper and allowed to dry.   The paper is placed in the chromatography chamber and equilibrated with the vapor for about an hour, this being done to obtain reproducible R_f values.   However, if a standard of known composition is run at the same time for comparative purposes, the waiting period can usually be eliminated.

Much information can be derived by analysis of various parameters of chromatographic migration such as the R_f value.   Martin[28] predicted that the differences between the logarithms of the partition coefficients for adjacent members of a homologous series would be constant, provided the degree of ionization was the same.   This was based on assumptions that (1) the free energy required to transport a given group (eg, —CH$_2$—) from one solvent to another was independent of the rest of the molecule in an ideal system and (2) the total free energy of the molecule was the sum of the free energies of its component groups.

He went on to conclude that the addition of a new group should change the partition coefficient in a predictable manner, based on the nature of the group and the solvents employed but independent of the rest of the molecule.   From the Eq. 4 relating R_f to the partition coefficient, if the ratio of A_L/A_S remains constant over the entire length of the column or paper strip, $R_M = \log (1/R_f - 1)$ should decrease by equal amounts for each added substituent in a homologous series.   This has been confirmed experimentally for many carboxylic acids and phenolic compounds.

By comparing the R_M values obtained in alkaline solvents where the acids are fully ionized, and in acidic solvents where ionization is suppressed, it is possible to predict the number of carboxyl groups in an un-

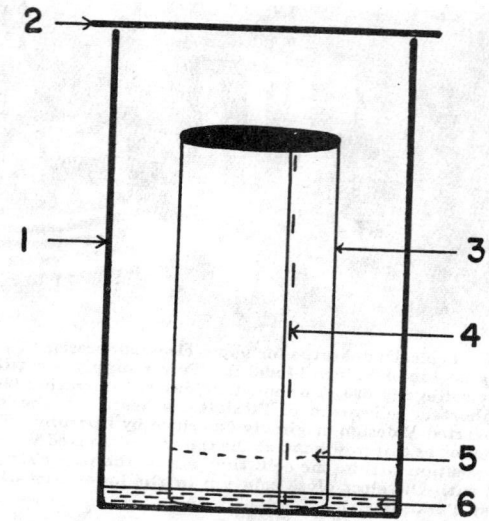

Fig. 436.   Diagram of paper chromatography apparatus employing ascending method.   (1) 9½-gal cylindrical jar;   (2) lid;   (3) sheet of filter paper formed into a cylinder;   (4) staples or pins;   (5) starting line where samples are applied for one- or two-dimensional chromatography;   (6) developing solvent.   A beaker containing the aqueous phase can be placed in the chamber to insure equilibrium conditions.

known acid and to obtain some information concerning the presence and location of aryl, alkyl, amino, hydroxy, and halogen groups in a molecule.   The recent review by Bush[29] is recommended for those desiring additional information.

The development, ie, passage of the mobile solvent over the paper, can be carried out by the *ascending method* or the *descending method*, depending on the direction of solvent flow.   In the ascending method the end of the paper strip nearest the applied sample is dipped into a reservoir of the solvent, which rises upward by capillary forces.   The movement of solvent is somewhat slower than in the descending method, where the strip is hung from a solvent reservoir at the top of the chamber.   The ascending technique has an advantage in that the solvent cannot drip off the end of the strip, but the descending technique is somewhat more convenient. Examples of typical chromatography apparatus are shown in Figs. 436 and 437.

A great many modifications of these basic techniques have been developed.   One of the simplest is known as *circular chromatography*.   A wick is cut from a round sheet of filter paper along one radius, and about 2 mm wide.   A drop of the solute mixture is applied to the center of the sheet close to the attached wick.   The paper is placed over a Petri dish which is partly filled with solvent;   the edges of the filter paper rest on the rim of the dish, and a cover is placed on top.   The solvent rises through the wick and spreads out from the center of the disc, carrying with it the solutes which were applied at that point.   This produces a series of concentric circles, each representing a different solute. An interesting demonstration of this technique is to place a drop of fountain-pen ink at the center of the circle and to chromatograph with water.   A typical, jet-black ink resolves itself into a series of colored bands, each representing different dyes used in the manufacture of the ink.

For complex mixtures of solutes such as amino acids in a protein hydrolysate, a process of *two-dimensional paper chromatography* has been widely used.   A drop of the unknown mixture is applied an inch or two from one corner of a sheet of filter paper.   The sheet is formed into a cylinder by fastening opposite edges together with pins or staples, and the cylinder is placed upright in a glass jar with a pool of solvent at the bottom (Fig. 436). As the solvent rises in the paper, the constituents of the unknown mixture are chromatographed in one direction, resulting in a series of spots along one line. The paper is removed and dried. The fastenings are removed, and the other two edges are brought together to form a cylinder with the line of spots along the lower edge. This cylinder is placed in a second jar containing a different solvent system and chromatographed again, with the second solvent moving at right angles to the direction of the first. This results in a series of spots which are spread out over the sheet of filter paper. (As explained in detail under *Methods of Detection*, if the substances being separated are colorless, their positions on the paper may be determined by spraying the paper with a suitable reagent that produces a color with them.) The use of two solvent systems results in a high degree of resolution, and the R_F values in the two solvents can be used to characterize the unknown compounds. This is analogous to the fingerprinting technique shown in Fig. 435. Their identity can be established by comparing the locations on the sheet with those of known compounds.

Thin-Layer Chromatography

In 1951 Kirchner, *et al*[30] (US Dept. of Agriculture), coated glass strips with a slurry of silicic acid mixed with starch as a binding agent and succeeded in separating a number of terpenes by ascending chromatography. Little attention was paid to this development because of the great interest in paper chromatography at the time. It was generally recognized that lipophilic compounds were better separated by adsorption techniques, and attempts were made to adapt paper strips to adsorption processes by using acetylated cellulose and by impregnating the paper with alumina. These modifications were not too successful, and packed columns generally provided a better solution to these problems.

About 5 years later Stahl[31] in West Germany revived the technique of thin-layer chromatography (TLC) and demonstrated its usefulness in many different applications. He prepared 250-μ layers of silica gel on glass plates using plaster of Paris as a binder and standardized his equipment and coatings to the point where they were made available commercially (*Desaga*, Heidelberg; and *E. Merck*, Darmstadt).

The TLC technique offers considerable advantages over both column and paper chromatography. In column chromatography tailing and poor resolution occur unless the flow rate is well controlled. Among other reasons, this can occur because fluids flowing through a tube have a greater flow velocity at the center, due to frictional resistance at the sides. Additional problems arise from flow resistance and irregularities in the packing of the stationary phase itself.

In TLC these problems are minimized because the solvent flow occurs on a planar surface. Although many features of TLC are similar to paper chromatography, TLC is extremely more versatile because of the

Table III—Sorbents and Solvents Used in Various TLC Techniques

Technique	Sorbents	Solvents
Adsorption TLC	Silica gel Aluminum oxide Calcium phosphate Kieselguhr	Organic solvents usually as mixtures
Partition TLC	Cellulose Kieselguhr Silica gel Superfine Sephadex	Mixtures of organic and aqueous solvents
Reversed-phase partition TLC	Paraffin and silicone oils impregnated on silica gel or kieselguhr Acetylated-cellulose Polyamides	Mixtures of organic and aqueous solvents
Ion-exchange TLC	Modified ion-exchange resins DEAE-cellulose Acetylated-cellulose	Dilute acids, bases, and buffers
Ligand-exchange TLC	Silica gel or kieselguhr impregnated with AgNO$_3$, tungstates, bisulfite	Organic or organic–aqueous mixtures
Gel-filtration TLC	Superfine Sephadex, G-25 to G-200	Dilute acids, bases, salts, buffers
Thin-layer Electrophoresis	Silica gel Cellulose Superfine Sephadex Agar	Aqueous buffers

large number of materials available as stationary phase sorbents. Nor is spreading of solutes as severe because of the quantitative differences between the fibrous structure of paper and the particulate nature of TLC coatings. This permits lower solute detection thresholds in TLC and considerably shortened development time.

Sorbents and Solvents—The availability of many sorbents in particle sizes suitable for thin-layer preparation makes many chromatographic principles adaptable to TLC. Adsorption, partition, ion-exchange, ligand-exchange, gel filtration, and electrophoresis may all be performed on thin-layer plates. These techniques are listed in Table III along with some commonly used sorbents and developing solvents.

Adsorption TLC is highly versatile and useful in the separation of a great many classes of compounds. It is the most commonly used form of TLC. The polarity of the substances to be separated dictates the combination of sorbent and solvent to be used.

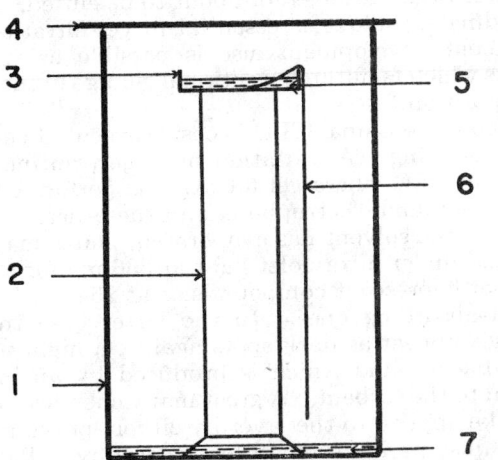

Fig. 437. Diagram of paper chromatography apparatus employing descending method. (1) 9½-gal cylindrical jar, 24-in. high by 12-in. diameter; (2) 2-L cylinder; (3) 6-in. Petri dish or evaporating dish; (4) lid; (5) developing solvent–organic phase; (6) paper strip; (7) aqueous phase saturated with the developing solvent. **Twenty strips can be run easily at one time in this apparatus. The supporting cylinder can be wrapped with a sheet of filter paper with the lower end dipping into the aqueous phase in the bottom of the chamber to facilitate saturation of the atmosphere with the solvent vapor.**

Silica gel (silicic acid) is slightly acidic and therefore is best applied to the separation of neutral and acidic substances. Alumina (aluminum oxide), on the other hand, is basic and should be used for the separation of basic compounds. Alternatively, silica gel can be used for the separation of basic compounds if a dilute base (as ammonia) is added to the developing solvent. Silica gel and alumina are the most active (powerful) adsorbents; less active are calcium phosphate, calcium carbonate, and kieselguhr. The activity of silica gel or alumina can be reduced by mixing with kieselguhr. The most active sorbents are used with the most non-polar compounds and the more inactive ones with polar molecules.

A third variable in selecting chromatographic conditions—the solvent system—gives a great flexibility to the method. An excellent and rapid manner for the selection of a solvent system is to place spots of the sample on several locations on TLC plates prepared with various sorbents. A capillary filled with pure solvent is applied to the gel in the middle of the sample spot. The solvent develops a small, circular chromatogram with the migrating solutes arranged in concentric circles about the origin.

Using a series of polar to nonpolar solvents or solvent mixtures produces at least one sorbent–solvent combination where the solute of interest migrates about halfway between the origin and solvent front. This combination should yield good TLC separations.

Cellulose is the most commonly employed sorbent for *partition TLC*. The same sorbents and procedures which are used in paper chromatography may be successfully applied to TLC. The low adsorptive power of kieselguhr also makes it easily adapted to this method. In addition, silica gel layers have been used for partition where the aqueous solvents decrease its adsorptive power. However, both adsorption and partition forces probably are involved.

The selection of gel-filtration and ion-exchange sorbents is made on the basis of considerations analogous to those required for column applications. The choice of thin-layer electrophoresis sorbents is usually made on the basis of the substances to be separated. For example, silica gel layers have been used to separate amino acids, amines, phenols, and inorganic ions. Sephadex and agar gels have been applied to the separation of proteins, mucopolysaccharides, nucleic acids, and viruses.

Preparation of Plates—To insure a physically stable layer which does not flake, binders may be added to the sorbents. Calcium sulfate, starch, and carboxymethylcellulose are commonly applied for this purpose. Acids or buffers also may be added to the sorbents, and fluorescent indicators may be incorporated to permit detection of ultraviolet-absorbing compounds. Commercially available sorbents are supplied either with or without binders and indicators.

A slurry of the sorbent mixture is made by the addition of water or in some cases an organic solvent. This is poured into a spreading device which is drawn across a series of 5 × 20 or 20 × 20-cm glass plates, depositing a uniform coating on them. Alternatively, reasonably good TLC plates may be made by placing two or three layers of adhesive tape along the edges of the glass plates, placing some slurry on each, and drawing a glass rod across them, supported by the tape. Gradient-making applicators also are available.

Rather than coating a plate with one sorbent, two different sorbents may be applied simultaneously so that the layer is made of a gradient mixture of both.

For example, silica gel and alumina may be used to prepare a pH gradient across the width of the plates. This may yield separations which otherwise would not be possible.

The binder usually sets within a few minutes of being poured and the plates are allowed to air dry in a level position for about an hour. Plates for adsorption TLC are activated by drying in an oven around 100° for an hour. Additional heating is required for alumina plates. They are then stored over a desiccant until used.

Plates for reversed-phase TLC also must be thoroughly dried before impregnation with the stationary phase. This is best done by placing the plate into a shallow trough containing an organic solution of the stationary phase, and permitting the solution to migrate up the plate. Plates for normal-partition TLC may be used while still moist from preparation or moistened at a later time over boiling water. Gel-filtration and electrophoresis plates also must be moistened before use; better, they are used while still moist from preparation. Commercially prepared plates containing binder are available with glass, plastic, or aluminum backing.

Development and Detection Techniques—Samples, which may range from a few micrograms to milligrams, are applied at points about 1.5 cm from one edge of the plate. For ascending development, the plate is placed into a rectangular-shaped tank with the developing solvent covering the bottom to a depth of about 0.5 cm. The inside of the jar is lined with filter paper to insure that the solvent will completely saturate the atmosphere. The cover is replaced and the solvent rises through the layer producing the chromatogram by elution development. The run is usually stopped when the solvent front traverses about $\frac{3}{4}$ of the plate. Rather than using a filter paper-lined jar, "sandwich-type" tanks may be used where the jar edges are very nearly in contact with the plate.

Descending techniques are less commonly used but may be of particular value in separating slowly moving compounds. Solvent is delivered to the plate by filter paper strips which saturate the layer. Solvent is permitted to drip from the end of the plate until solutes of interest are resolved or about to be eluted. The descending technique is essential in gel-filtration TLC. Gradient development also is possible using special tanks which facilitate a continual change in the solvent composition.

Two-dimensional TLC is easily executed as is TLC fingerprinting. A variation of fingerprinting is possible on TLC where gel filtration is performed in one dimension and electrophoresis in the other.

After the solvent has evaporated, plates may be examined under ultraviolet light at 366 mμ for the presence of fluorescent compounds or at 254 mμ for ultraviolet-absorbing ones. In the latter case the compounds appear as dark spots against a highly fluorescent background which is produced by an indicator added to the sorbent. A great many chemical reagents may be applied to the layer by either spraying or dipping, just as in paper chromatography. Thin-layer plates are especially valuable where corrosive reagents are required, such as iodine vapors or sulfuric acid, which detect most organic compounds.

Radioactive compounds may be detected either directly by a scanning device which moves the plate under a G–M tube and records the resulting increase in counting rate or by physically removing sections

nd determining the radioactivity present by liquid-
cintillation counting. The latter method gives great
uantitative accuracy and permits the simultaneous
etection of two or three isotopes.

A combination of this method with ultraviolet detec-
on is used to characterize unknown drug metabolites.
solution of trace amounts of radioactive metabolites
mixed with reference compounds of known structure
nd chromatographed. The reference compounds are
etected by ultraviolet absorption, the radioactive
etabolites by liquid-scintillation spectrometry. Cor-
espondence between radioactive and ultraviolet-
bsorbing peaks indicates identity.

Recent advances in technology also make it possible
obtain infrared, NMR, and mass spectral data on
ery small samples. These may be eluted directly
om TLC plates.

Preparative TLC—Thick layers of sorbents may
e prepared to separate several hundred milligrams on
single 20 × 20-cm plate. However, if the layer is
uch thicker than 2 mm, solvent flow becomes more
olumn-like and the advantages of TLC are lost.
amples are uniformly streaked across the entire width
f the plate and development produces a series of
olute bands which may be eluted for additional char-
cterization. Separations which are achieved on TLC
ay be scaled up to column work when large quanti-
ies of material are needed.

Gas Chromatography

Techniques of gas chromatography are in wide-
pread use because highly selective separations can be
ombined with very sensitive detection procedures.
'his is rather remarkable when you consider that in
955 gas chromatography was almost unknown to re-
earchers in fields that now extensively utilize the
echnique.

Basic Design—Many units now are commercially
vailable such as the one shown in Fig. 438. The gas
asses from a pressurized tank through various regu-
ators into the instrument. It initially passes the
ample injection port which simply may be a sidearm
t the beginning of the column, closed by a self-sealing
ubber septum. A microliter syringe is used to inject
he sample directly into the gas flow at the top of the
olumn.

For liquid samples or solids dissolved in liquids the
njection port is ordinarily heated to a temperature
bove that of the column to insure vaporization of the
ample but not so high as to decompose the sample.
Gaseous samples may be injected directly or a more
laborate system may be required. The vaporized
ample is moved by the carrier gas through the oven-
nclosed column onto the stationary phase. The oven
emperature must be high enough to maintain all the
omponents in the vapor state. The column may be
traight, U-shaped, or coiled and 1–4 M in length and
2–4 mm in diameter. It may be made of glass or stain-
ess steel.

When the solute molecules reach the stationary
phase, distribution occurs between the two phases
based on the partition coefficient. The molecules not
adsorbed or dissolved in the stationary phase are swept
down the column by the carrier gas, thereby causing
he molecules in the stationary phase to diffuse back
nto the gas flow. As with all forms of chromatography, it is this constant movement of solute molecules
between phases that is the basic mechanism of gas
chromatography.

At the column exit there is a continuous flow of carrier gas. When a solute is eluted, a binary mixture of
solute and gas emerge and pass into the detection unit.
The unit may be of several types which in essence
transfers a physical characteristic of the compound
(eg, thermal conductivity, ionizability, radioactivity,
etc) into an electrical signal. This gives a tracing of
peak heights (differential plot) as a function of time.
Recorded peaks most often will be symmetrical because in GLC, and usually in GSC, the amount of
sample is quite small compared to column capacity.

In the theory section (page 672) it was assumed that
α is independent of concentration. This is not always
true; in certain cases the distribution of a solute between the two phases will vary with solute concentration. For example, if a solute is more soluble in the
mobile phase at higher concentrations due to saturation of the stationary phase, the resultant peak will
"tail" from the lagging edge. This occurs because
molecules in the center of the band (most concentrated) will be swept along at a faster rate than those
at the trailing edge of the band where the concentration is lower.

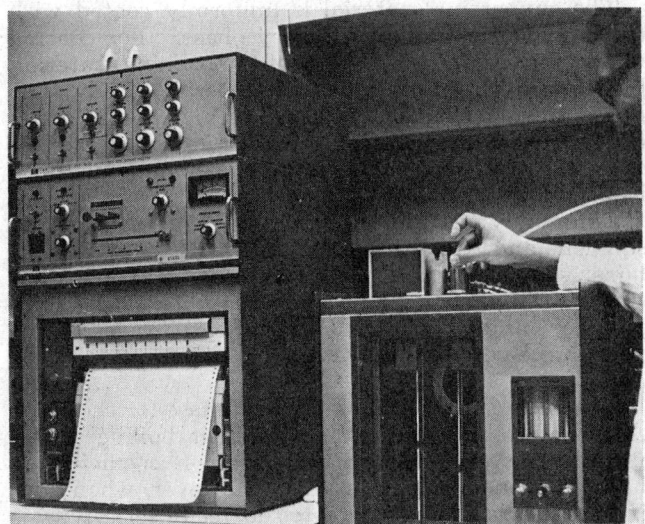

**Fig. 438. Typical gas-chromatography equipment consisting of a
programmed-temperature, dual-column Hewlett-Packard 402 High
Efficiency Gas Chromatograph. The unit at the right of the photograph consists of two packed 4-ft U-shaped columns contained in a
heating oven (opened only for illustration). Two fans located in the
oven recirculate air over the columns and heaters. Flowmeters and
pressure regulators are located to the right of the oven while the injection ports are located near the top of the columns. A hydrogen-
flame detector is connected to each column in back of the injection
port and an electron-capture detector is located just to the left of
one of the hydrogen-flame detectors. The electrometer is located in
the main unit at the left, along with the recorder, temperature regulating devices, and programming controls.**

Another factor affecting the shape of the peak is time
the solute was retained on the column. As this time
(or V_S) increases, the peak height decreases and the
width increases; ie, the concentration decreases. This
was explained previously utilizing plate theory. Or
it may be thought that as the stationary phase solubility of a series of compounds increases, the volume
of gas required to remove the molecules also increases
resulting in a lower solute concentration.

Mobile and Stationary Phases—The carrier gas
may be, in theory, any gas, but in practice the choice
is usually limited to hydrogen, helium, nitrogen, or
argon. One of the most important considerations is
the purity of the gas. An impure gas will result in not
only an unsteady or elevated baseline but may cause

negative (inverted) peaks. These occur when the clean, vaporized sample partitions with the contaminated gas resulting in noncontaminated bands. The negative peaks can introduce both qualitative and quantitative errors.

Carrier gas also must be inert. This is especially important in GSC where a reactive gas would compete with the solute for binding sites on the column. Gases with low viscosity such as hydrogen or helium are desirable in applications requiring high flow rates through long columns. Safety considerations may dictate the use of helium. On the other hand, heavier gases which reduce solute diffusion are favored when more efficient separations are desired.

In GLC the column packing consists of a granular, inert material (around 60–100 mesh) which supports the nonvolatile liquid stationary phase. The most common porous supporting material is kieselguhr, which may have been treated by calcining, heating, or mixing with binder. Nonporous supports such as glass microbeads are occasionally used especially for analysis of high-boiling liquids. In some applications the column itself serves as the support with the liquid coating the inside.

The supporting material is uniformly coated with the nonvolatile, liquid stationary phase. The coating may comprise up to 40% w/w of the packing material, but concentrations of 1–5% are generally used. The liquid must be chemically stable and high boiling, have low viscosity at operating temperatures, and exhibit specific solvent properties toward the components to be separated.

Commonly used liquids include hydrocarbons as squalene and Apiezon grease for separating hydrocarbons; silicone oils and gums which partition on a volatility basis; polyesters which separate polar compounds; and polyalcohols as the carbowaxes which permit the resolution of alcohols, amines, aldehydes, and esters.

The choice of a liquid stationary phase for the separation of compounds having different boiling points presents no problems as the partition coefficient is highly dependent on volatility. However, when boiling points are similar, a greater degree of selectivity is needed. For example, if two slightly polar compounds are not resolved by a given liquid a somewhat more polar phase may give the desired separation.

To facilitate the choice of the stationary phase, it is essential to know the relative polarities of the liquids in question. The Kovats index[32] was developed to permit such comparisons. The index measures where a compound will appear on a chromatogram with respect to a series of n-alkanes. It is determined on both a polar and nonpolar column and the difference (ΔI) is proportional to the column polarity. However, the relative polarity of a stationary phase may depend on the substances being analyzed.

Rohrschneider[33] determined ΔI values for several different compounds representing various polarities. The determinations were made for benzene, ethanol, methyl ethyl ketone, nitromethane, and pyridine on a number of different stationary phase liquids. For example, if a series of polar compounds is not resolved by a particular column and a more polar stationary phase is desired, one of the above five compounds is selected on the basis of similar polarity.

For instance, if ethanol were chosen, a table of Rohrschneider constants would be consulted and the ethanol value determined for the column in use. All that remains is to search the table and find a liquid phase having a constant for ethanol which is numerically higher and use the liquid phase corresponding to that value.

Column Operating Conditions—The majority of available gas chromatographs may be used in either isothermal or programmed-temperature operation modes. In the latter, temperature is automatically raised at a predetermined rate varying from 0.5° to 50°/min. This is analogous to gradient elution in liquid columns. The proper column temperature should be near the boiling points of the two components. However, the components of a complex mixture, such as fatty acid esters, often have widely differing boiling points.

If the column is operated at a high temperature, the low-boiling solutes are rapidly eluted but not resolved. Contrariwise, if the temperature is low, low-boiling solutes will be resolved but the high boilers will require great volumes for elution resulting in peaks which are so diluted that they may be difficult to detect.

By temperature programing, the peaks can be evenly spaced with good peak heights in a drastically reduced period of time. The initial temperature is selected on the basis of the desired retention time for the lowest boiling solute and the final temperature on the basis of the highest—in accord with the maximum allowable temperature of the stationary phase.

On some instruments gas flow rate also may be programed. This has some of the advantages of temperature programing without the necessity of exposing solutes and stationary phases to high temperatures.

Requirements of the mobile and stationary phases are similar whether temperature is programed or not. However, some stationary phase is always being eluted (bleeding) and detected, thereby adding to the baseline. In isothermal operation this is easily cancelled. However, bleeding increases with temperature thus causing an increasing baseline during temperature programing. This can be eliminated by a dual-column system with a differential recording system where the sample is injected onto one column with the other serving as a baseline monitor.

High-pressure gas chromatography recently has been introduced (for a review, see Giddings[34]). Pressures of up to 2000 atmos. are used so that the density of the supercritical carrier gas approaches that of a liquid. This system, unlike the usual GLC, can handle macromolecules and other high-molecular-weight species. Polymers have been separated in this manner as well as carotenoids, sterols, nucleosides, amino acids, and carbohydrates.

Detectors—A great deal of the progress in GLC has evolved because of the development of highly sensitive, rapid, and specific detectors. One of those in common use is the *thermal-conductivity cell*. It consists of a heated metal filament having a large temperature coefficient of resistance, or a thermistor can be used to detect temperature changes.

These devices are used in matched pairs in a Wheatstone-bridge network, with one element being exposed to carrier gas before it enters the column, and the other being exposed to the column effluent. Thermistors are most useful for low-temperature applications, while the hot-wire detectors (katharometers) are excellent for higher temperatures. However, much of the work with biological samples requires a higher degree of sensitivity.

In contrast, the *hydrogen-flame ionization detector* is more sensitive but destroys the sample. Hydrogen gas and air are mixed with the carrier gas from the

olumn and the flame is ignited. The conduction of
an electrical current through the flame is altered when
organic compounds are present and the output is recorded. The hydrogen-flame ionization detector is
relatively insensitive to the presence of water vapor
in the sample, and it has proved to be one of the better
detection devices for biological work.

The *argon-ionization detector* is one of the most
sensitive detection devices available for gas chromatography, capable of detecting 10^{-12} parts by volume.
Argon is used as the carrier gas, and is exposed to a
radioactive source such as ^{90}Sr in the detector cell.
The electron bombardment produces an energized
state in the argon atoms without producing ionization.
The metastable argon atoms then collide with the
organic molecules in the column effluent, transferring
their excitation energy to them and producing ionization. This results in increased conductivity between
two electrodes, producing a current rise or a drop in
potential which can be amplified and recorded.

The *electron-capture detector* also is highly sensitive
and depends on ionization induced by a radioactive
source. In this case, however, specific compounds
which react with, or capture, free electrons are detected through the direct formation of negative ions.
The source of electrons is usually tritium adsorbed
onto a metal surface or ^{63}Ni for high-temperature work
where the tritium might be desorbed. By applying a
low potential across the detection chamber, ions
formed by irradiation cause a decrease in current flow.
Compounds for which electron-capture detectors are
specific include carbonyl-containing compounds and
halogenated compounds such as the organic insecticides.

Specially constructed *ionization chambers* can be
used to detect radioactive compounds in GLC efflu-
ents. The effluent passes into the chamber inducing
the ionization of a suitable gas. This is detected by a
G–M or proportional counter.[35] Much added information may be gathered by splitting the effluent stream
and simultaneously using two detectors. For example,
mass and radioactivity may be detected separately
and the correspondence between the two sets of peaks
used as identity criteria.

Qualitative and Quantitative Aspects—It is
possible to identify chemically the solutes eluted from
GLC by collecting individual fractions as they emerge
from the detector. This can be automated so that the
response from the detector actuates a fraction collector, placing a new receiving flask in position for each
individual fraction. The hydrogen-flame detector is
obviously destructive, and thermal-conductivity detectors are usually used for this purpose. Parallel
columns having identical characteristics also may be
used, with a detector on one and a collector on the
other. Automatic recycling operations also are possible, with a fresh sample being injected into the column on the completion of each run. In this way overnight operation may yield sufficient material for characterization by ultraviolet- and infrared-absorption
techniques.

Alternatively, ultraviolet and infrared spectrometers may be used as detectors by employing flow-
through cells. These may be operated at a single frequency or make scans while the solute of interest is
being eluted.

Probably the most sensitive and versatile GLC techniques are now being performed with a mass spectrometer acting as the detector. The carrier gas is automatically removed from the GLC effluent and the
solute introduced directly into the mass spectrometer.
This combination is highly advantageous because
compounds separated by GLC have sufficient vapor
pressure for direct mass spectral analysis. Much
structural information can be gained from a mass
spectrum obtained from only submicrogram quantities
of GLC-purified solutes.

Highly polar compounds such as carboxylic acids
and phenols plus other compounds such as amino
acids, amines, aldehydes, and ketones may not have
a sufficient volatility to be chromatographed by GLC
or they may decompose under the conditions used.
Derivatives of these compounds must be prepared to
overcome these problems.

N-Trifluoroacetyl methyl esters of amino acids are
satisfactory for GLC, and trimethylsilyl ethers or
esters have been widely used to permit GLC separations of alcohols, phenols, acids, and polyhydroxy
compounds including carbohydrates. In addition,
methyl esters and *N*-acetyl, *N*-butyl, and trifluoroacetyl derivatives are commonly employed to increase
the volatility of compounds.

In *reaction-gas chromatography* injected solutes are
adsorbed or changed during the chromatographic
process. This method has become a field in itself
within the last few years. Reactions may occur in a
specially designed precolumn, on the column itself or
in a short column preceding the detector. Hydrogenation reactions, pyrolysis degradations, subtractive
degradations, and elemental analyses are all possible
with this technique.

Precise quantitative evaluations may be obtained
from GLC data. If the operating conditions are properly selected, the area under each peak will be directly
proportional to concentration. The area can be determined with electronic or mechanical integrators
attached to the recorder or measured with a planim-
eter. Adequate estimates also can be made by relating the area under the curve to the width of the
curve at half-peak height.

One of the real problems in quantitation is to know
the precise volume of sample taken for analysis, which
may be in the 1–10-μl range. To eliminate volume
considerations, we prefer to use the "internal standard" method. The internal standard is a compound
with a structure similar to that of the compound to be
quantitated. It also must be resolvable from the
other compound, but with a similar retention time.

A set of standards containing a constant amount of
the internal standard and a varying amount of the
solute of interest are prepared and chromatographed.
A calibration curve is constructed plotting the ratio of
internal standard peak heights to solute peak heights
against solute concentrations. The same amount of
internal standard is added to samples containing the
solute of interest; they are extracted, concentrated,
and any convenient volume injected into the GLC
unit. The peak-heights ratio is determined and concentration interpolated from the calibration curve.
Using this method it has been possible to determine
drug blood levels in a number of instances with a sensitivity of under 1 mcg/ml of original sample.

Applications of Chromatography

A brief summary of chromatographic procedures applied to compounds of pharmaceutical interest will serve to illustrate the versatility of these techniques. Examples are chosen to show how chromatography has been applied to various types of investigations. The use of TLC, GLC, and paper chromatography is particularly emphasized because of the general usefulness of these techniques. A number of references are listed at the end of this chapter which will serve as a guide to further reading. Official analytical methods involving chromatographic separation are discussed in Chapter 37, *Analysis of Medicinals*.

General Methods of Detection

When highly colored compounds are separated by chromatography, there is no problem in locating the bands on columns, plates, or paper strips. In most biological work, however, the compounds are colorless and so must be located by special means. Furthermore, the methods used for detection must be sufficiently sensitive to detect microgram quantities of material. In column work, of course, larger quantities of sample can be used, and analyses performed in pure solvents. With paper strips and TLC plates, however, extremely sensitive methods of detection must be employed.

One method used routinely is examination under ultraviolet light. If a compound is fluorescent, it can be detected very readily. In some cases compounds will fluoresce on paper strips even though the solid crystalline compound or solutions show little or no fluorescence. On the other hand it is often possible to detect compounds such as purines and pyrimidines by their absorption of ultraviolet light on paper strips. Ultraviolet light sources are available with maximum emission at 365 or 254 mμ. The longer wavelength is especially useful for producing fluorescence, while the shorter wavelength can be used to detect compounds absorbing in this region. Another test of general utility is to expose the plates or paper strips to iodine vapor in a chamber. Bands on the chromatogram will often retain iodine a little longer than the background and stand out with a deeper brown color. Failing all other tests, the paper strip can be cut into sections, leached out with alcohol or water, and the solutions analyzed by standard physical or chemical procedures.

One of the commonest and most widely used methods for detection of bands is to spray the surface with chemical reagents which produce colored derivatives. It has been said that practically any chemical reaction which can be performed in test tubes can also be applied to paper strips. Such a wide variety of tests has been utilized that the statement is essentially correct. For example, aromatic nitro compounds such as chloramphenicol may be detected by successive applications of four separate reagents:

1. A reducing agent (TiCl$_3$) to convert the nitro group to a primary amino group.
2. An oxidizing agent (Br$_2$) to destroy the excess reducing agent.
3. A diazotizing agent (nitrous acid).
4. A coupling reagent (*N*-1-naphthylethylenediamine) to produce a final colored derivative (an azo dye).

In many cases a single color-producing reagent will suffice. Amino acids are detected by spraying with a solution of ninhydrin and then heating the paper in an oven. Carbohydrates may be detected by spraying with ammoniacal silver nitrate solutions; on heating dark spots appear where reducing agents are present. In general, a knowledge of the reactive groups in a given compound will indicate the type of reagent that may be used to give a good color test. The spraying procedure is quite simple. Strips of filter paper are mounted on a clean sheet of paper with adhesive tape or TLC plates are merely leaned against a support and placed in a hood having forced ventilation. Atomizers of various types may be used for spraying.

The quantitative measurement of the visualized spots may be performed in several manners. The area of a spot is roughly proportional to the logarithm of concentration and this can be used to estimate concentration. A direct comparison of spot intensities with a series of known concentrations run at the same time and under identical conditions is probably easiest but no better than ±10%.

Another possibility is to elute each spot from the paper or sorbent and run a chemical assay on the resulting solution. This method suffers from the fact that complete elution of microgram quantities is difficult.

A third choice is direct scanning of the chromatographic surface by a densitometer or fluorometer and recording peak areas. Bush[36] reviewed the techniques involved in this area.

Other methods of detection can be used in special instances. Antibiotics and growth factors can be detected by laying the paper strips upon agar plates seeded with bacterial cultures. Bands of antibiotic will show clear zones of inhibited growth following incubation of the plates, while bands of growth factor will enhance growth in media which are deficient in these factors.

Compounds labeled with radioactive isotopes are readily detected by placing the paper strips in contact with photographic film, allowing adequate time for exposure, and developing the film. This produces a *radioautograph* in the spots where labeled compounds were present. Geiger counters and gas-flow counters also are used for scanning paper strips for radioactivity. These are usually used with rate meters and chart recorders so that a permanent record can be kept for each strip.

An alternative is to section the paper strip or TLC layer, determine radioactivity in a liquid-scintillation spectrometer, convert to solute concentration, and plot the results. This procedure can be automated by using a TLC zonal plate scraper to prepare the liquid scintillation counting vials and inputting the counting data to a computer equipped with an electroplotter (see Snyder and Smith[37]).

Aromatic Amines

Aromatic amines are of considerable importance in the pharmaceutical field because a large number of drugs fall into this category. The Bratton-Marshall test is often used to detect primary aromatic amines on paper strips. Diazotization can be accomplished by spraying with a 2.5% solution of sodium nitrite in 0.5 N sulfuric acid. The coupling reaction is carried out by spraying with a 0.1% solution of *N*-1-naphthyl ethylenediamine dihydrochloride in water. This test has been applied to the detection of aromatic nitro compounds derived from chloramphenicol, in which the nitro group is first reduced to an amine with titanous chloride. Chromatography of urine clearly demonstrated the presence of a water-soluble metabolite, which was isolated and identified as the glucuronic acid conjugate of chloramphenicol.

A second useful test for amines is to spray the surface with a 0.5% solution of Ehrlich's reagent (dimethylaminobenzaldehyde) dissolved in butanol with glacial acetic acid added. In applying this reagent to sulfones (such as diaminodiphenylsulfone), it was found that sulfone metabolites excreted in the urine gave a good color reaction only after prior exposure of the paper strip to hydrochloric acid vapor. This treatment hydrolyzed the N-acetyl metabolites, and good color reactions were obtained from the liberated primary amines.

Still another reagent of value for the detection of primary and secondary aromatic amines is an alkaline solution of sodium β-naphthoquinone sulfonate. The colors appear slowly on standing, but closely related amines may produce different colors. For example, nor-epinephrine may be separated from epinephrine by paper chromatography with acid phenol. The naphthoquinone reagent gives a blue color with nor-epinephrine, while epinephrine produces a pink or red color. This procedure has been used for the estimation of nor-epinephrine in epinephrine preparations isolated from natural sources.

The application of paper chromatography to the identification of sulfonamide mixtures has been studied in a number of laboratories. Spots are identified by spraying with Ehrlich's reagent directly onto the paper after the completion of the run. TLC also has been employed by a great number of investigators for the separation of amines with medical interest.

Literally hundreds of these compounds have been separated by TLC including antihistamines, phenothiazines, and sympathomimetic amines. In addition to the above, Dragendorff's reagent, Mandelin's reagent, acidic ferric chloride, and other compounds have been used as locating agents.

GLC also is used extensively for the determination of amines. Forensic chemists have applied the technique to the identification of many classes of drugs, including the antihistamines.[38] Table IV presents GLC retention times of a number of clinically useful antihistamines. The amount used to elicit a good response from the hydrogen-flame ionization detector was from 1 to 10 mcg of each compound.

Amino Acids, Peptides, and Proteins

Until the advent of paper chromatography, work in this field was severely handicapped by a lack of specific analytical methods for detecting individual amino acids. Microbiological assay techniques provided a tremendous impetus for research in this field, but they were laborious and time consuming. The introduction of two-dimensional paper chromatography provided a means for rapidly establishing the number, identity, and approximate concentration of individual amino acids in highly complex mixtures. Most of the early work involved the use of water-saturated phenol and collidine as solvents.

One of the most useful tests for amino acids and simple aliphatic amines is the color reaction with ninhydrin (1,2,3-triketohydrindene). This reagent is generally applied to paper strips as a 0.2% solution in water-saturated butanol. After spraying, the paper is heated for a few minutes in an oven at 90°C, resulting in the appearance of blue or purple spots corresponding with the location of amino acids. This procedure is extremely sensitive, but it is not limited to amino acids. Interference may also be expected from high concentrations of salts and acids. Mention should also be made of the fluorescence of certain amino acids on paper strips. Most amino acids are not fluorescent in the crystalline state, but when dried with heat on paper, they apparently react with the free aldehyde groups of cellulose to form fluorescent derivatives. This appears to be analogous to the "browning" reaction of amines with carbohydrates.

A number of new amino acids have been discovered with the aid of paper chromatography. These include α-aminobutyric acid in bacteria, γ-aminobutyric acid in potato extracts, bacteria, plants, and brain tissue; β-aminoisobutyric acid, α-aminoadipic acid, and methylhistidine in human urine; 3-hydroxyproline in collagen; and α,ε-diaminopimelic acid in hydrolysates of diphtheria and tuberculosis organisms. Iodinated tyrosine derivatives have been separated from the thyroid gland and blood plasma. The distribution of radioactive I^{131} has been studied extensively with this technique. After chromatographic separation the paper may be dried and radioautograms produced. The location of the spots on the chromatogram thus permits immediate identification of inorganic iodide, mono- and di-iodotyrosine, di- and tri-iodothyronine, and thyroxine.

Peptides have been studied extensively using paper chromatography, ninhydrin reagent being employed for detection. On further hydrolysis the individual amino acid constituents of the peptides can be determined. A preliminary separation of peptides into acidic, basic, and neutral groups is usually desirable, following which paper chromatography is carried out on a two-dimensional scale. The solvents employed are similar to those used for amino acids. Applying this method, the antibiotic polymyxin was found to consist of a mixture of individual polypeptides. Extensive work has also been done on the nature of the hydrolysis products of proteins after partial chemical or enzymatic attack. The amino acid sequence for most of the structure of insulin has been established, and much has been learned about ACTH, polymyxin, and other proteins and polypeptides of biological interest.

The use of *silica gel columns* by Martin and Synge for the separation of acetylated amino acids already has

Table IV—GLC Retention Times for Some Antihistamines[38,a]

Antihistamine	Retention time min
Diphenhydramine HCl	2.9
Doxylamine succinate	3.6
Antazoline HCl	3.8
Tripelennamine base	5.4
Chlorpheniramine maleate	6.2
Methapyrilene HCl	6.3
Carbinoxamine maleate	9.6
Brompheniramine maleate	9.8
Bromdiphenhydramine HCl	11.1
Chlorothen citrate	11.6
Pyrilamine maleate	24.0
Triprolidine HCl	32.6
Methdilazine HCl	50.4

[a] A 5-ft stainless steel column with a 0.093-in. i.d. was employed using a carbowax as the liquid stationary phase. Operating conditions included: injection port temperature, 230°; oven temperature, 190°; nitrogen flow rate, 79 ml/min.

been described. This technique has been applied also in studies on the amino acid composition of gelatin, wool, gramicidin, and tyrocidin. *Starch columns* were later used by Synge,[39] and Moore and Stein at the Rockefeller Institute perfected this technique for routine analyses. Using hydrolysates of lactalbumin and serum albumin, they obtained recoveries of 100 ± 3%. Similar techniques have been used by others for the analysis of oxytocin, vasopressin, bacitracin, and other proteins.

The order of appearance of various amino acids in a typical run is shown in Table V. Moore and Stein[40] have pointed out that these columns probably involve adsorption of the aromatic amino acids as well as partition. Some form of *automatic fraction collector* is generally used so that the column operation can be continued over a period of several days, if necessary, without interruption.

The use of *ion-exchange columns* for the separation of amino acids has become quite popular in recent years. Larger samples can be used than in paper chromatography, and pure amino acids can be obtained on a preparative scale (Fig. 433).

Strongly basic resins (eg, Dowex 2) can be used with dilute acids to obtain separations not possible on the cation exchangers. Leucine thus can be separated from methionine, alanine from glycine, and proline from valine. Moore and Stein[41] developed a complete analytical procedure for amino acids using columns of sulfonated polystyrene (Dowex 50), and eluting with a series of buffers of increasing alkalinity. Each amino acid constituent appears as a distinct peak, permitting a complete analysis to be performed on a 5-mg sample.

This procedure has been completely automated with the equipment commercially available. Ninhydrin color and radioactivity determinations can be made simultaneously on the effluent and peak areas determined by electronic integration.

In recent years GLC has become an important technique for the determination of amino acids (for a review, see Weinstein[42]). Although amino acids possess a low vapor pressure, it is not sufficient for GLC work. To permit GLC determinations, either the α-amino or -carboxyl group, or both, must be removed or converted into a derivative. There are many ways to accomplish this including oxidation, pyrolysis, decarboxylation, esterification, and esterification plus acylation.

Diastereoisomers also have been resolved by GLC using the butyl esters of the N-trifluoroacetyl amino acids. Table VI presents some separations which have been achieved for 21 of the most common amino acids using the trifluoroacetyl methyl ester derivatives. Preparation of N-diethyl phosphate amino acid methyl esters coupled with the use of an alkali-flame detector has permitted the detection of picogram quantities of 11 amino acids.[43]

The most promising separation techniques for proteins appears to be *electrochromatography* and *gel filtration*. Clear-cut separations of plasma proteins are readily obtained by paper electrophoresis (see Fig. 434) and numerous applications to clinical chemistry are being made. Detection of sickle cell anemia is now a relatively simple matter, since the sickle hemoglobin migrates less rapidly than normal hemoglobin in an electrical field. Electrochromatography in starch and polyacrylamide gels has proved to be a valuable tool for the separation of proteins and is finding extensive application in research laboratories.

Alkaloids

A very simple system has been described for the rapid identification of alkaloids in medicolegal investigations. This is based on paper chromatography by the ascending method. Strips of Whatman No. 1 paper are dipped in a 5% solution of sodium dihydrogen citrate, blotted, and dried at 60°C for 25 minutes. After spotting the unknown mixture near one end of the strip, development proceeds in a solvent made up by shaking 50 ml of n-butanol with 50 ml of water and 1 Gm of citric acid. After development with the butanol

Table V—Order of Emergence of Amino Acids and Related Compounds[40,a]

Compound	Position of peak, ml	Compound	Position of peak, ml
Leucine-isoleucine	13.5	Di-iodotyrosine	12.5
Phenylalanine	16.5	Tryptophan	18
Valine	24	α-Amino-n-butyric Acid	38
Methionine	26	α-Amino-adipic Acid	41
Tyrosine	28	Cysteic Acid	64
Proline	52	Taurine	74
Glutamic Acid	59	Hydroxyproline	80
Alanine	59	Sarcosine	84
Threonine	75	Citrulline	98.5
Aspartic Acid	82	Ethanolamine	102
Serine	100	Asparagine	121
Glycine	106	Glucosamine	126
Ammonia	117	Histamine	160
Arginine	136	Ornithine	176
Lysine	149	Hydroxyproline	180
Histidine	163		
Cystine	179		

[a] Determined on columns 0.9 × 30 cm prepared from 13.4 Gm of starch (anhydrous), developed with (1:2:1) n-butanol: n-propanol: 0.1 N HCl and shifted to (2:1) n-propanol: 0.5 N HCl at 83 ml.

Table VI—GLC Retention Times of Trifluoroacetyl Methyl Esters of the Amino Acids[a,b]

Amino acid	Retention time, min Neutral Group I	Neutral + acidic Group II	Neutral + basic Group III
Alanine	9.6		
Valine	10.6		
Isoleucine	14.4		
Threonine (diacyl)	16.5		
Glycine	17.6		
Leucine	18.4	2.6	
Serine (diacyl)		6.7	
Proline		7.4	
Aspartic acid		11.8	
Cysteine (diacyl)		13.0	
Hydroxyproline		15.1	
Methionine		23.2	
Glutamic acid		26.9	
Phenylalanine		30.0	
Histidine (diacyl)			1.0
Tyrosine (diacyl)			1.4
Ornithine (diacyl)			2.9
Lysine (diacyl)			3.9
Tryptophan (diacyl)			5.1
Arginine (diacyl)			6.3
Cystine			21.2

[a] Conditions for chromatography: All groups run on 3/32-in. i.d. stainless steel columns with neopentyl glycol succinate as the liquid stationary phase and nitrogen as the carrier gas. *Group I*: column length, 15 ft; flow rate, 11.4 ml/min; temperature, 137°. *Group II*: column length, 15 ft; flow rate, 29.8 ml/min; temperature, 161°. *Group III*: column length, 19 in; flow rate, 13.3 ml/min; temperature, 204°.
[b] Makisumi, S., and Saroff, H. A., *J. Gas Chromatog.*, **3**, 21 (1965).

phase, the strips are dried and dipped into Dragendorff's reagent (Soln. A = 0.85 Gm bismuth subnitrate + 40 ml water + 10 ml acetic acid; Soln. B = 8 Gm potassium iodide + 20 ml water. For use, take 5 ml A + 5 ml B + 20 ml glacial acetic acid + water to 100 ml). The alkaloids appear as red spots on a pale orange background.

TLC is widely used for alkaloid separations. Practically the same locating reagents are used for TLC as for paper chromatography. All the conventional sorbents may be used but most work has been done on silica gel. The alkaloids are usually chromatographed in the form of the nondissociated bases, and, as previously discussed, alkali must be added to the silica gel or to the developing solvent.

Table VII presents R_f values obtained for several alkaloids chromatographed in two solvent systems on silica gel layers which were made basic by preparation in 0.1N potassium hydroxide. Better resolution of the compounds which were not well separated could be achieved under other conditions.

Alkaloids also have been separated on a preparative scale by column chromatography using activated alumina, ion-exchange resins, and partition columns.

Organic Acids

Organic acids can be separated on adsorption and ion-exchange columns and by partition chromatography on silica gel or on cellulose. Anion-exchange resins are generally useful for removing nonpolar impurities, the acid anions being retained on the column, while carbohydrates, etc, are washed through. The anion exchange appears to depend more on the structure, size, and valence of the anion than on the degree of ionization. Elution can be achieved by gradually increasing the concentration of a displacing agent such as formic acid. Weaker acids will be displaced progressively and travel down the length of the column faster, resulting in separation of the acids.

Fatty acids of low molecular weight have been separated on columns of silica gel. Bromocresol green incorporated in the gel forms yellow zones in the presence of acids. The column is developed with chloroform containing 5% butanol. The various acids appear as yellow bands along the length of the column and are distributed in the order of their partition coefficients, with acetic acid at the top, and propionic, butyric, and valeric acids following in that order. On increasing the concentration of butanol, the bands move more rapidly and can be collected separately in the effluent leaving the column. Good separation of C_5—C_{10} acids has been obtained with iso-octane as the developing solvent, and the use of other solvents has extended the range to C_{11}—C_{19} acids.

The distribution of a carboxylic acid between the stationary and mobile phases in a partition chromatogram depends on the partition coefficient of the undissociated acid and the degree of dissociation of the acid. Using unbuffered solvents, the degree of ionization will vary with the concentration of carboxylic acid, which may produce streaking of the acid band. This can be prevented by incorporating a strong acid in the solvent to suppress the ionization of the acids in the sample. A buffer can also be incorporated in the solvent to maintain a constant salt to acid ratio. The R_f value will depend principally on the partition coefficient of the free acids in the first case or on the partition coefficient plus the dissociation constants when buffered solvents are used.

Using a butanol solvent equilibrated against an equal volume of 1.5 N NH$_4$OH, Reid and Lederer[44] found the following R_f values for lower fatty acids: C_1 = 0.1; C_2 = 0.11; C_3 = 0.19; C_4 = 0.29; C_5 = 0.41; C_6 = 0.53; C_7 = 0.62; C_8 = 0.65; C_9 = 0.67.

In general this procedure is adequate for the lower fatty acids, but poor separations are obtained with fatty acids having chain length greater than C_9. Various derivatives of organic acids also have been chromatographed. The keto acids can be converted to the 2,4-dinitrophenyl hydrazones, and fatty acids to their hydroxamates before chromatography.

After chromatography, the solvents are removed by evaporation at room temperature for several hours, and the acids located by spraying the paper with various indicators such as bromophenol blue or bromocresol green.

A more sensitive method which will detect <5 mcg of many organic acids has been introduced by Schmidt, et al.[45] Paper chromatograms are sprayed with a mixture of 2% sulfanilamide and 0.5% betanaphthol in 95% ethanol, dried, and sprayed with a 1% aqueous sodium nitrite solution. Nitrous acid forms only in those spots occupied by the free acids and consequently diazotization and coupling occurs. The acids appear immediately as deep-orange spots on a pale-pink background.

Phenols

In recent years many chromatographic techniques have been applied to phenol separations. TLC has proved especially valuable for the separation of phenolic acids and hydroxyquinones which are not well resolved on paper. However, paper chromatography is the most important technique for separating this class of compounds.

The butanol–acetic acid–water (40:10:50) solvent used for the paper chromatography of carbohydrates is also suitable for the separation of phenols. A second solvent useful for two-dimensional work is m-cresol-acetic acid-water (50:2:48). R_f values obtained with these two solvents are given in Table VIII. The samples were applied to Whatman No. 1 paper in acid butanol solution, and run by the descending technique.

Table VII—TLC of Alkaloids[a,b]

Compound	R_f value System I	R_f value System II
Atropine	0.09	0.11
Caffeine	0.04	0.55
Cinchonine	0.10	0.37
Cocaine	0.58	0.57
Codeine	0.07	0.28
Diacetylmorphine	0.22	0.39
Dihydrocodeinone	0.06	0.17
Dihydromorphinone	0.05	0.15
Ephedrine	0.08	0.18
Meperidine	0.55	0.48
Morphine	0.02	0.28
Nicotine	0.53	0.52
Papaverine	0.11	0.62
Quinine	0.05	0.47
Scopolamine	0.09	0.54
Strychnine	0.13	0.17

[a] Conditions of chromatography—*Adsorbent:* silica gel G; *Solvent System I:* cyclohexane:benzene:diethylamine (75:15:10); *Solvent System II:* methanol.
[b] Fike, W. W., *Anal. Chem.*, **38**, 1697 (1966).

Table VIII—Paper Chromatography of Phenols[46]

Compound	Butanol acetic acid water (R_f)	m-Cresol acetic acid water (R_f)
Benzoic acid	0.92	0.93
Catechol	0.91	0.74
Cinnamic acid	0.94	0.92
o-Coumaric acid	0.94	0.82
Gallic acid	0.68	0.08
m-Hydroxybenzoic acid	0.91	0.72
p-Hydroxybenzoic acid	0.90	0.72
Orcinol	0.91	0.75
Phloroglucinol	0.76	0.16
Phloroglucinol carboxylic acid	0.55	0.06
Protocatechuic acid	0.85	0.35
Pyrogallol	0.77	0.38
Quinol	0.88	0.69
Resorcinol	0.91	0.63
β-Resorcylic acid	0.93	0.54
Salicylic acid	0.95	0.84
Vanillic acid	0.92	0.81

To insure reproducible R_f values, the following precautions were taken:

1. Temperature was held constant at 20° ± 0.5°C.
2. The solvent mixtures were thoroughly shaken and allowed to stand for 3 days before use.
3. The paper strips were allowed to equilibrate with the solvent vapors for 24 hr before irrigation was started.
4. A control substance was run with every sample to make certain that conditions were constant.
5. Development with the solvent was carried out until the solvent front had traveled a distance of 30–35 cm from the origin.

Such closely controlled conditions are not required for routine work, but it is possible to obtain R_f values reproducible to ±0.02 unit with this procedure.

Phenols can be detected readily on paper chromatograms with an alcoholic solution of diazotized sulfanilic acid (Pauly's Reagent), followed by exposure to ammonia. Ferric chloride or ammoniacal silver nitrate can also be used, but Pauly's Reagent is more sensitive. Exposure to iodine vapor is also a useful technique, and the polyphenols often show fluorescence under ultraviolet light.

The degree of hydroxylation appears to have a marked effect on the R_f value of phenols, with greater number of hydroxyl groups producing lower R_f values. Bate-Smith and Westall[46] found that the addition of one — OH group to the molecule produced almost exactly the same effect on R_f, regardless of the nature of the rest of the molecule. From a critical analysis of these effects, a linear relationship was established between the number of — OH groups and the R_f value.

Lipids

In many instances the complete qualitative and quantitative analysis of a lipid mixture now may be performed by chromatographic techniques alone. Liquid solid chromatography, especially with ion-exchange celluloses, TLC, GLC, and paper chromatography usually permit the desired analysis when used in combination. Preliminary lipid fractionations are required and may be accomplished best by adsorption chromatography. Phospholipids and glycolipids will be retained when a chloroform solution is applied to a silica gel column, the remaining components passing through.

Cholesterol, cholesterol esters, and various triglycerides are weakly adsorbed on alumina columns, while fatty acids and phosphatides are strongly adsorbed. The monoglycerides generally show stronger adsorption than the di- or triglycerides. Natural oils have been fractionated by a single passage through alumina columns into mono-, di-, and triglycerides, sterol esters, and waxes.

Neutral lipids may be separated on TLC layers of silica gel. One-dimensional TLC is usually employed, either by single or multiple development. In the latter, development is achieved in one solvent system, the plate removed, dried, and placed into a second system.

By double-development techniques, hydrocarbons, cholesterol esters, fatty acid methyl esters, triglycerides, free fatty acids, 1,3-diglycerides, 1-2-diglycerides, cholesterol, and polar lipids were resolved in that order. Polar lipids also may be separated on silica gel layers, frequently employing acetic acid or ammonia in the solvent systems to take advantage of the amphoteric nature of various lipid classes. Lysolecithin, sphingomylein, lecithin, phosphatidyl ethanolamine and neutral lipids have been separated in this manner.

GLC probably has been the most significant analytical technique in the area of lipid research. Separations of fatty acid esters have been particularly well developed.

Elution characteristics of solutes are frequently expressed in terms of retention times or volumes. However, because these terms are highly dependent on many chromatographic conditions, slight variations in any one of several conditions produces different retention times. This renders difficult the comparison of data obtained by different investigators. To some extent this may be corrected by relating the retention time of a particular unknown or fatty acid ester to another solute as palmitate or stearate.

Miwa, et al,[47] introduced the concept of "equivalent chain length" (ECL) values to further standardize the description of elution characteristics. These values are derived by establishing a reference curve where the logarithm of retention time is plotted against chain length (number of carbon atoms) of a series of known, straight-chain, saturated, monocarboxylic methyl esters which occur frequently in lipid extracts.

Values for other solutes chromatographed at the same time are interpolated from the curve using the observed retention times. The slope of the curve will vary with temperature but the ECL values remain constant. Saturated, straight-chain compounds, of course, have integral values on any liquid phase whereas unsaturated, branched-chain, or substituted fatty acid methyl esters do not (Table IX).

Identity may be established by the equivalence of ECL values for known compounds and the unknown solutes on several stationary phases. Homologous series are readily apparent and can be characterized with some degree of accuracy as unsaturated, branched-chain, or substituted fatty acid esters or aldehydes on the basis of ECL value shifts between properly selected stationary phases.

In addition to fatty acid determinations, GLC is used for analysis of long-chain aldehydes, long-chain sphingolipid bases, coenzyme A esters, steroids, and bile acids. Chromatographic techniques in lipid analysis are well documented in the book edited by Marinetti.[48]

Paper chromatography has been a valuable adjunct to the study of steroids. An interesting modification is the use of *alumina-impregnated paper strips*. The

Table IX—Equivalent Chain Lengths of Fatty Acid Methyl Esters[47]

Parent acid		ECL value	
		Apiezon L Grease	Resoflex 446
Saturated, straight-chain			
Stearic	(C$_{18}$)	18.0	18.0
Unsaturated, straight-chain			
Monoenoic			
Palmitoleic	(C$_{16}$)	15.7	16.4
Oleic	(C$_{18}$)	17.7	18.4
Petroselinic	(C$_{18}$)	17.7	18.4
Erucic	(C$_{22}$)	21.7	22.4
Dienoic			
Linoleic	(C$_{18}$)	17.6	19.0
Trienoic			
Linolenic	(C$_{18}$)	17.6	19.8
Tetraenoic			
Arachidonic	(C$_{20}$)	19.2	21.6

paper is soaked in a solution of ammonium alum, drained, and left to hang overnight in a chamber containing ammonia gas. The paper is then washed in running water for 6 hours and dried. Progesterone, estrone, estradiol, and the acetates of various corticosteroids can be separated on these strips using benzene as a developing agent. Estrone, testosterone, and androsterone are chromatographed with tetralin as a solvent.

Carbohydrates

Free carbohydrates have been chromatographed on columns of activated earths using alcohols, ketones, acids, water, and pyridine as the developing solvents. Displacement chromatography has also been accomplished on charcoal columns using phenol or ephedrine as the displacing agents. Most column separations involve the preparation of various carbohydrate derivatives, which are more readily separated than the free carbohydrates. For example, carbohydrates have been esterified with p-phenylazobenzoyl chloride to give colored derivatives which can be separated on silica or alumina columns. Partition chromatography appears to be a more useful technique for carbohydrates. Columns of silica gel and powdered cellulose have been used successfully for the separation of carbohydrates, using water-saturated butanol containing ammonia for development.

Paper chromatography, especially as a two-dimensional procedure, is very useful for the separation and identification of carbohydrates. The initial work in this field was carried out by Partridge,[49] at Cambridge. The solvent systems were similar to those used by Consden for amino acids, and the carbohydrates were detected by spraying the sheets with an ammoniacal solution of silver nitrate (equal volumes of 0.3 N AgNO$_3$ and N NH$_4$OH are mixed immediately before use). On standing or heating, brown or black spots appear in the presence of reducing agents. The reagent is sufficiently sensitive to detect less than a microgram of glucose.

Reducing agents other than carbohydrates, such as uric acid, will also produce dark spots. Typical results obtained by Partridge are shown in Table X. Rather than using R_f values to express the mobility of sugars, R_g values may be used. This defines the distance moved by a spot relative to the distance moved by glucose or 2,3,4,6-tetra-O-methylglucose. The term is similar to GLC relative retention time.

While the silver nitrate reagent is effective for the detection of reducing sugars, it will not give a color reaction with nonreducing polysaccharides. A 0.2% solution of naphthoresorcinol in dilute hydrochloric or trichloroacetic acid solution will give intense red colors with ketoses when heated to 100°C. Aniline acid phthalate in water-saturated butanol gives brown colors with aldohexoses, aldopentoses, and hexuronic acids, and red colors with pentoses. A number of other reagents have also been described which assist in the identification of different carbohydrates. Hexosamines can be detected with ninhydrin; glucosamine has been identified in tuberculin preparations with the aid of this reagent.

The structures of a number of naturally occurring polysaccharides have been investigated with paper chromatography, other chemical methods having failed. Reducing substances in urine can be detected readily, and distinctions can be made between glucose, fructose, lactose, and pentoses. The time required is minimal. Strips can be set up in the evening, allowed to develop overnight, and sprayed the following morning. Although the development procedure is time-consuming, no attention is required from the operator during the run.

Extensive studies have been carried out on the metabolism of carbohydrates labeled with radioactive carbon-14 and using paper chromatography combined with radioautography. The intermediates are often phosphorylated derivatives which can also be detected

Table X—R_f Values of Carbohydrates and Related Substances[49]

Whatman No. 1 Paper—Descending Chromatography

	Phenol-H$_2$O + 1% NH$_3$, HCN (R_f)	s-Collidine (H$_2$O satd.) (R_f)	n-Butanol 40%, water 50%, acetic acid 10% (R_f)	Isobutyric acid (R_f)
D-Glucose	0.39	0.39	0.18	0.13
D-Galactose	0.44	0.34	0.16	0.14
D-Mannose	0.45	0.46	0.20	0.15
L-Sorbose	0.42	0.40	0.20	0.16
D-Fructose	0.51	0.42	0.23	0.18
D-Xylose	0.44	0.50	0.28	0.19
D-Arabinose	0.54	0.43	0.21	0.21
D-Ribose	0.59	0.56	0.31	0.22
L-Rhamnose	0.59	0.59	0.37	0.30
D-Oxyribose	0.73	0.60	..	0.32
L-Fucose	0.63	0.44	0.27	..
Lactose	0.38	0.24	0.09	0.07
Maltose	0.36	0.32	0.11	0.09
Raffinose	0.27	0.20	0.05	..
D-Galacturonic acid	0.13	0.14	0.14	0.09
D-Glucuronic acid[a]	0.12	0.16	0.12	0.08
D-Glucurone	0.12	0.72	0.33	0.22
D-Glucosamine·HCl[a]	0.62	0.32	0.13	0.05
Chondrosamine·HCl[a]	0.65	0.28	0.12	..
N-Acetylglucosamine	0.69	0.50	0.26	0.25
L-Ascorbic acid	0.24	0.42	0.38	0.19
Dehydroascorbic acid	0.28	0.47	0.48	0.16
I-Inositol	0.23	0.10	0.09	..

[a] The lactone forms of these compounds have different R_f values.

by spraying the paper strips with an acid molybdate solution and heating. The free phosphoric acid resulting from this treatment interacts with the molybdate to form a complex which is reduced to an intensely blue compound on exposure to hydrogen sulfide gas. Quantitative analyses are even possible by cutting out the blue areas, wet-ashing, and determining the phosphorus content by chemical procedures. Quantities of 1–10 mcg of phosphorus in 4–8 cm² of paper have been determined by this technique with an error of less than 3%.

Antibiotics

Chromatography has proved to be highly useful in isolating new antibiotics and studying their chemical structure through the identification of degradation products. In screening "beers" (fermented broths) for antibiotics, a drop of the Seitz-filtered broth is placed on a small disc of filter paper and transferred to a seeded agar plate. After incubation, bacterial growth occurs everywhere except in the vicinity of antibiotics. The antibacterial spectrum obtained by using different test organisms may give some clue to the nature of the antibiotic. In many instances more than one antibiotic may be present in a single fermentation "beer." For this reason positive cultures are often subjected to paper chromatography at this point to determine whether more than one antibiotic is present. After development of the chromatogram the paper strip is laid down on a seeded agar plate and zones of antibiotic substances are detected by their inhibitory effect on bacterial growth.

The first penicillin isolated by Sir Howard Florey was a crude extract from mold cultures which produced undesirable side reactions in human subjects. Early purification procedures involved adsorption on charcoal, followed by elution with 80% acetone. Repeated chromatography on columns of alumina gave preparations which were free of color and pyrogenic activity. Goodall and Levi[50] found that a number of different penicillins could be separated from crude preparations by paper chromatography. They used paper strips impregnated with a phosphate buffer, and developed the chromatograms with water-saturated ether. At least eight different penicillins have been recognized, using modifications of this basic technique. Columns of buffered silica gel have also been used to isolate a number of different penicillins in preparative quantities. Although chromatographic techniques give clean-cut separations, it is usually desirable whenever possible to use continuous solvent extraction procedures for large-scale operations.

Streptomycin is adsorbed readily from basic solution onto activated charcoal, which can be washed to remove some of the impurities and extracted with acid–methanol to elute the antibiotic. Salts of streptomycin such as the picrate can be prepared from this concentrate and subjected to further chromatography. Alumina columns have been used to separate the picrates of streptomycin and streptothricin, which may occur in the same fermentation broths. Streptomycin B (mannosido-streptomycin) has been separated from streptomycin on alumina columns. Paper chromatography also has been used for the recognition of streptomycin, dihydrostreptomycin, mannosido-streptomycin, streptothricin, lincomycin, kanamycins, and neomycins. A good solvent system for this purpose consists of water-saturated butanol containing 2% p-toluenesulfonic acid.

Antibiotics having a macrocyclic lactone structure include the erythromycins, oleandomycin, spiramycins, and leucomycin. Separations in this class of antibiotics have been accomplished by paper chromatography and TLC on silica gel employing many solvent systems. TLC and paper chromatography also have been used extensively for fractionation of polypeptide antibiotics including the gramicidins and tyrothricins which are composed only of amino acids. Others having heterocyclic, fatty acid or hydroxy acid moieties—such as bacitracins, actinomycins, and polymyxins—have been separated on CM-cellulose and CM-Sephadex columns as well.

Inorganic Chromatography

The applications of paper chromatography to the identification of inorganic constituents of mixtures are varied and useful. The technique is so simple that it may replace older schemes for qualitative analysis. The reagents used to detect heavy metals are usually sensitive enough to detect microgram quantities of materials, and the color reactions themselves, as well as the R_f values, are of considerable assistance in establishing the identity of unknown elements. This technique has been applied to the determination of the metals in the ashed residues of various drugs and fermentation products in the pharmaceutical industry.

A wide range of solvents has been used for inorganic chromatography, including alcohols, ethers, ketones, acids, and esters. The presence of a certain amount of water and acid is required for the chromatography of cations, and complexing agents are sometimes added to increase the solubility of the metals. The heavy metals can be detected readily on paper strips by exposure to hydrogen sulfide gas, preferably after exposure to ammonia. More sensitive reactions can be obtained by spraying the strips with organic compounds such as 8-hydroxyquinoline or diphenylcarbazide to produce different colored derivatives, some of which may fluoresce under ultraviolet light. Typical results obtained with various solvents are shown in Table XI. Special solvents also have been developed for separating various groups of metals and the use of specific reagents further assists in the identification of unknown cations.

Elbeih, et al,[53] described a procedure of particular interest to forensic chemists in which arsenic is separated from other metals by paper chromatography. Water-saturated butanol containing 1% ammonium borate, 1% ammonium tartrate, and 0.5% mannitol is used as the developing solvent. The paper is then sprayed with an alcoholic solution of 1% nitric acid and 5% glycerin, following which it is sprayed with ammoniacal silver nitrate solution. The arsenic band slowly turns brown, with an R_f of 0.45. The other common heavy metals have an R_f of less than 0.2. The sensitivity of this test is great enough to detect less than 1 microgram of arsenic, and the R_f value is presumptive evidence of its identity.

Anions also can be separated and identified by paper chromatography. Neutral or alkaline alcohol solutions are commonly used as the developing solvent. The anions are usually chromatographed in the form of their sodium or ammonium salts, but the movement of the anions appears to be independent of the particular cation present unless metal complexes are formed. Using a solvent consisting of 40 parts butanol, 40 parts pyridine, and 20 parts 1.5 N NH₄OH, Pollard, et al,[54] found the following R_f values for different anions: phosphate 0.04, arsenate 0.05, carbonate 0.06, sulfate

Table XI—Separation of Inorganic Cations

Cation	Solvent 1[a] (R_f)[51]	Solvent 2[b] (R_f)[51]	Solvent 3[c] (R_f)[52]
Ag^+	0.02	0.02	0.15
Hg^+	0.08	. . .	0.43
Pb^{2+}	0.16	0.03	0.09
Hg^{2+}	1.0	0.82	0.43
Bi^{3+}	0.94	0.67	0.23
Cu^{2+}	0.47	0.26	0.12
Cd^{2+}	1.0	0.75	0.12
As^{3+}	0.50	0.43	0.43
Sb^{3+}	0.85	0.77	0.02
Sn^{2+}	0.97	0.83	0.82
Al^{3+}	0.37	0.25	0.09
Cr^{3+}	0.47	0.18	0.09
Fe^{3+}	0.56	0.42	0.43
Zn^{2+}	0.93	0.90	0.10
Mn^{2+}	0.36	0.21	0.11
Co^{2+}	0.32	0.15	0.10
Ni^{2+}	0.34	0.15	0.09

[a] Solvent 1: ethyl alcohol + 10% 5 N HCl.
[b] Solvent 2: 45 parts isopropyl alcohol + 45 parts ethyl alcohol + 10 parts 5 N HCl.
[c] Solvent 3: butanol satd. with 2 N HNO$_3$ containing 1% acetylacetone.

0.07, iodate 0.09, arsenite 0.19, chloride 0.24, bromate and nitrite 0.25, bromide 0.36, nitrate 0.40, chlorate 0.42, iodide 0.47, and thiocyanate 0.56. Use of different color-forming reagents serves to distinguish between compounds having similar R_f values.

References

1. Day, D. T., *Proc. Am. Phil. Soc.*, **36**, 112 (1897).
2. Claesson, S., *Ann. NY Acad. Sci.*, **49**, 183 (1949).
3. Tiselius, A., *Lex Prix Nobel en 1948*, Stockholm, 1949.
4. Tswett, M., *Ber. Deut. Botan. Ges.*, **24**, 316 (1906).
5. Kuhn, R., *et al*, *Z. Physiol. Chem.*, **197**, 141 (1931).
6. Tiselius, A., *Arkiv. Kemi*, **16A** (18) (1943).
7. Tiselius, A., and Hagdahl, L., *Acta Chem. Scand.*, **4**, 394 (1950).
8. Martin, A. J. P., and Synge, R. L. M., *Biochem. J.*, **35**, 1358 (1941).
9. Craig, L. C., *J. Biol. Chem.*, **155**, 519 (1944).
10. Consden, R., *et al*, *Biochem. J.*, **38**, 224 (1944).
11. Schoenbein, C. F., *Verhandl. Naturforsch. Ges. Basel*, **III**, 249 (1861).
12. Goeppelsroeder, F., *Verhandl. Naturforsch. Ges. Basel*, **III**, 268 (1861).
13. Schuftan, P., *Die Technische Gasanalyse*, S. Hirzel, Leipzig, 1931.
14. James, A. T., *Gas Chromatog. Proc. Symp. 2nd Amsterdam*, Academic, New York, 1961, p. 247.
15. James, A. T., and Martin, A. J. P., *Biochem. J.*, **50**, 679 (1952).
16. Johnson, M. J., in Umbreit, W. W., *et al*, eds., *Manometric Techniques*, 4th ed., Burgess, Minneapolis, 1964, p. 233.
17. Mayer, S. W., and Tompkins, E. R., *J. Am. Chem. Soc.*, **69**, 2866 (1947).

18. Bock, R. M., and Ling, N., *Anal. Chem.*, **26**, 1548 (1954).
19. Mandell, J. D., and Hershey, A. D., *Anal. Biochem.*, **1**, 66 (1960).
20. Adler, A. J., and Rich, A., *J. Am. Chem. Soc.*, **84**, 3977 (1962).
21. Helfferich, F., in Giddings, J. C., and Keller, R. A., eds., *Advances in Chromatography*, vol. 1, Marcel De ker, New York, 1965, p. 39.
22. Tiselius, A., *Ann. Rev. Biochem.*, **37**, 1 (1968).
23. Porath, J., and Flodkin, P., *Nature*, **183**, 1657 (1959).
24. Hjerten, S., and Mosbach, R., *Anal. Biochem.*, **3**, 109 (1962).
25. Smithies, O., *Arch. Biochem. Biophys. Suppl.*, **1**, 125 (1962).
26. Poulik, M. D., *Methods Biochem. Analy.*, **14**, 455 (1966).
27. Bishop, D. H. L., *et al*, *J. Mol. Biol.*, **26**, 373 (1967).
28. Martin. A. J. P. *Biochem. Soc. Symp. Cambridge Engl.*, **3**, 4 (1950).
29. Bush, I. E., *Methods Biochem. Analy.*, **13**, 357 (1965).
30. Kirchner, J. G., *et al*, *Anal. Chem.*, **23**, 420 (1951).
31. Stahl, E., *Pharmazie*, **11**, 633 (1956).
32. Wehrli, A., and Kovats, E., *Helv. Chim. Acta*, **42**, 2709 (1959).
33. Rohrschneider, L., *J. Chromatog.*, **22**, 6 (1966).
34. Giddings, J. C., *et al*, *Science*, **162**, 67 (1968).
35. James, A. T., in James, A. T., and Morris, L. J., eds., *New Biochemical Separations*, Van Nostrand, London, 1964, p. 1.
36. Bush, I. E., *Methods Biochem. Analy.*, **11**, 149 (1963).
37. Snyder, F., and Smith, D., *Separation Sci.*, **1**, 709 (1966).
38. Fontan, C. R., *et al*, *Anal. Chem.*, **35**, 591 (1963).
39. Synge, R. L. M., *Biochem. J.*, **38**, 285 (1944).
40. Moore, S., and Stein, W. H., *J. Biol. Chem.*, **178**, 53 (1949).
41. Moore, S., and Stein, W. H., *J. Biol. Chem.*, **192**, 663 (1951).
42. Weinstein, B., *Methods Biochem. Analy.*, **14**, 203 (1966).
43. Ertingshausen, G., *et al*, *Separation Sci.*, **2**, 681 (1967).
44. Reid, R. L., and Lederer, M., *Biochem. J.*, **50**, 60 (1951).
45. Schmidt, G. C., *et al*, *J. Pharm. Sci.*, **52**, 468 (1963).
46. Bate-Smith, E. C., and Westall, R. G., *Biochim. Biophys. Acta*, **4**, 427 (1950).
47. Miwa, T. K., *et al*, *Anal. Chem.*, **32**, 1739 (1960).
48. Marinetti, G. V., ed., *Lipid Chromatographic Analysis*, vol. 1, Marcel Dekker, New York, 1967.
49. Partridge, S. M., *Biochem. J.*, **42**, 238 (1948).
50. Goodall, R. R., and Levi, A. A., *Nature*, **158**, 675 (1946).
51. Lederer, M., *Anal. Chim. Acta*, **5**, 185, 191 (1951).
52. Pollard, F. H., *et al*, *J. Chem. Soc.*, **1951**, 466 (1951).
53. Elbeih, I. I. M., *et al*, *Discussions Faraday Soc.*, **7**, 183 (1949).
54. Pollard, F. H., *et al*, *J. Chem. Soc.*, **1951**, 470 (1951).

Bibliography

Ettre, L. S., and Zlatkis, A., eds., *The Practice of Gas Chromatography*, Interscience, New York, 1967.
Giddings, J. C., in Giddings, J. C., and Keller, R. A., eds., *Dynamics of Chromatography*, Part 1: *Principles and Theory*, vol. 1 of *Chromatographic Science Series*, Marcel Dekker, New York, 1965.
Gudzinowicz, B. J., in Giddings, J. C., and Keller, R. A., eds., *Gas Chromatographic Analysis of Drugs and Pesticides*, vol. 2 of *Chromatographic Science Series*, Marcel Dekker, New York, 1967.
Heftmann, E., *Chromatography*, 2nd ed., Reinhold, New York, 1967.
Kirchner, J. G., in Perry, E. S., and Weissberger, A., eds., *Thin-Layer Chromatography*, vol. XII of *Technique of Organic Chemistry*, Interscience, New York, 1967.
Kunin, R., *Ion Exchange Resins*, 2nd ed., Wiley, New York, 1958.
Lederer, E., and Lederer, M., *Chromatography*, 2nd ed., Elsevier, Amsterdam, 1957.
Schupp, O. E., in Perry, E. S., and Weissberger, A., eds., *Gas Chromatography*, vol. XIII of *Technique of Organic Chemistry*, Interscience, New York, 1968.
Smith, I., *Chromatographic and Electrophoretic Techniques*, vol. 1: *Chromatography*, vol. 2: *Zone Electrophoresis*, Interscience, New York, 1960.
Stahl, E., ed., *Thin-Layer Chromatography*, Academic, New York, 1965.

41 | Instrumental Methods of Analysis

X-ray methods—ultraviolet and visible absorption spectrometry—
infrared spectrometry—nuclear magnetic resonance spectrometry—
emission spectrometry—flame photometry—atomic absorption
spectrometry—fluorescence and phosphorescence spectrometry—
nonabsorptive interaction of matter with EM radiation—light-scattering
spectrometry—refractometry and interferometry—polarimetry—mass
spectrometry—potentiometry—voltametry—high-frequency methods

This chapter was prepared by

Jay Nematollahi, PhD, *Assistant Professor of Pharmaceutical Chemistry, College of
Pharmacy, The University of Texas, Austin, Texas 78712*

In the past two decades man has witnessed many scientific achievements both in space and on the ground. Although laymen have taken great pride and joy in many well-publicized aerospace achievements, it has by no means been obscure to scientists that any spectacular feat owes much of its accomplishment to many sophisticatedly designed and theoretically sound laboratory instruments.

At present many of the conventional physicochemical methods which were used a few years ago are gradually becoming obsolete or playing a minor role in research and development; the so-called "wet" methods of analysis familiar to the classical pharmaceutical educators and researchers are being replaced by more modern instrumental methods.

This chapter includes two major sections: (1) opticometric methods of analysis and (2) electrometric methods of analysis.

Under opticometric methods, the instruments whose principles are based on absorptive or nonabsorptive interaction of matter with electromagnetic (EM) radiation are described and their applications are explored. The instruments utilizing infrared (IR) and ultraviolet (UV) radiation, designed on the absorptive principle, are discussed in the first part of this section and those such as the refractometer and the polarimeter, designed on the nonabsorptive principle, in the latter part.

Under electrometric methods, the electrochemical behavior of matter characterized by measuring different electrical quantities, such as voltage, current, resistance, etc, is discussed.

Opticometric Methods

A study of the theory and application of instrumentation, with a primary objective of employing methods which involve absorption or emission of EM radiation, necessitates a broad understanding of the interaction of matter with radiation.

The concept of the electromagnetic field was first expressed in the latter part of the 19th century by Maxwell. His equations theorized the existence of waves that travel through electromagnetic fields and whose properties are identical to those of light. Hertz succeeded in generating radio waves, the velocity of which was found to be equal to that of light—2.998×10^{10} cm/sec.

The oscillation of an electron gives rise to EM radiation. As is illustrated in Fig. 439, at each point in the direction of the beam, the electric field and magnetic field, represented by two vectors, are perpendicular to each other. The wavelength, λ, is defined as the distance between successive maxima or minima, and is expressed in Angstroms (Å), millimicrons (mμ), or microns (μ). The frequency in cycles per second (cps or Hz) is denoted by ν. The frequency is related to λ by $\nu = c/\lambda$, where c is the velocity of light in vacuum. The time required for the completion of 1 cycle is designated by τ, which is related to ν by $\tau = 1/\nu$. The reciprocal of wavelength, $1/\lambda$, is referred to as wavenumber, $\bar{\nu}$, expressed in reciprocal centimeters, cm^{-1}. The wavenumber is employed particularly in describing the peak maxima of IR spectra.

Electromagnetic Radiation—Initially, the assignment of wave properties to EM radiation for the description of many physicochemical phenomena did not encounter difficulty. Both light and waves share identical properties such as energy, intensity (amplitude), wavelength, frequency, and velocity.

As the field of physics advanced, the wave property of light was found to be unsatisfactory for the explanation of certain effects of light; eg, the photoelectric effect, which is the emission of electrons from the surface of a specific metal upon illumination with light of a relatively low wavelength, such as blue light. Red light, irrespective of its intensity, fails to eject an electron from a similar metal.

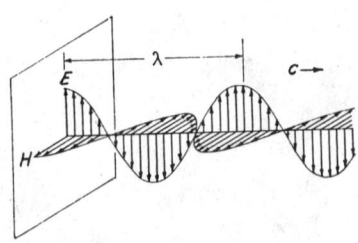

Fig. 439. A plane-polarized electromagnetic radiation. *E:* electric vector; *H:* magnetic vector.

Accordingly, ascribing particle nature to light seemed to be more reasonable. This, however, failed to explain other phenomena such as diffraction of light, wherein EM radiation must function as a wave. Considering these facts, a reliance on the dual nature of the light, behaving both like a wave and a particle, seemed to be indispensable for resolving many phenomena.

Max Planck presented the idea that energy in matter occurs in the form of bundles, referred to as quanta. Light, like any other matter, also consists of bundles of energy called photons. Likewise, electrons, photons, and elementary particles, which behave like particles, were found to manifest properties of wave motion. The mathematical expression of the nature of waves and particles is discussed extensively in texts on quantum mechanics.

The energy in a photon of light is related to wave frequency by the expression

$$E = h\nu = hc/\lambda \qquad (1)$$

where h is Planck's constant, 6.6256×10^{-27} erg-sec.

In 1900 Planck formulated his concept of quantum restriction. He stated that oscillating atoms of a hot body can have only energies that are integral multiples of $h\nu$. In other words, the energy of an oscillator is discontinuous and any change in the energy can occur only by a jump between two energy states.

Interaction between Molecules and EM Radiation—The presence of radiation of a particular frequency is necessary, but is not always sufficient, for inducing a change in the energy level of a molecule. Quantum restriction requires conditions for the interaction of radiation with a molecule. On many occasions energy is absorbed only if the radiation frequency corresponds to the components of the molecular frequency. This is referred to as resonance absorption.

The probability of the occurrence of an energy change is associated with an EM radiation-induced dipole moment, which is the result of transducing the EM oscillation energy into energy associated with a dipole. The magnitude of this dipole, known as the transition dipole, determines the probability of EM radiation—molecule interaction. The higher the probability of interaction and the larger the electrical moment of the excited state, the more intense the absorption.

The position of maximum absorption, λ_{max}, for a molecule in a region of spectrum is a function of the total structure of the molecule with a transition energy corresponding to a given wavelength. The intensity of the absorption maximum, ϵ_{max}, is a function of the probability of EM radiation—molecule interaction and

polarity of the excited state. At room temperature a molecule is normally in its lowest energy state; ie, the ground state. The transition between E_1 and E_2 (two quantum numbers for absorption or emission of radiation) occurs by the interaction of EM radiation with a molecule. The difference between E_1 and E_2 is designated by ΔE, whose frequency of radiation is expressed as $\Delta E = h\nu$ ergs, where $h = 6.62 \times 10^{-27}$ erg-sec/molecule. For a Gm-atom or Gm-molecule this number should be multiplied by the Avogadro number, 6.02×10^{23}.

Often, frequency or wavelength values are used as energy unit equivalents. Thus, the expression, "an energy of 1000 cm^{-1}," means that a separation between two energy levels is associated with a wave number value of 1000 cm^{-1}.

Regions of the Spectrum—The whole range of the EM radiation is divided arbitrarily into a number of regions. Interaction between a molecule and various parts of EM radiation gives rise to a change in the electronic energy and/or kinetic energy of the molecule. Fig. 440 depicts a wavelength and frequency scale of EM radiation.

A particular change in the energy of a molecule due to interaction with various ranges of EM radiation has been utilized by chemists for structural elucidation. Interaction with a particular range of the x-ray, UV, visible, IR, microwave, or radio-frequency spectrum with a molecule gives rise to an absorption of a particular type of molecular energy, thus resulting in the generation of a characteristic spectrum. These spectra serve to elucidate the atomic or molecular structure of unknown substances.

A theoretical and practical description of various types of spectroscopy of primary interest in the pharmaceutical sciences is given in the following sections. An arbitrary order has been adopted in organizing this chapter, beginning with the instrumental methods using the highest frequency EM radiation and proceeding toward the lowest frequency. The length of discussion of each topic is based on the extent of the applicability of the method in pharmacochemical analysis.

X-Ray Methods

The EM radiation section with wavelengths of approximately 0.1 − 10Å is known as the x-ray region. These are the shortest wavelength radiations wherein the energy change of the involved atoms is reversible. X-rays are employed in the structural elucidation of organic and inorganic substances. There are three x-ray methods of analysis: powder diffraction, emission (including fluorescence), and absorption.

X-rays are produced by the bombardment of a heavy metal target with high-speed (high-energy) electrons. The radiation originates from electronic transition between the deepest shells of atoms. The frequency of the emitted radiation is given by

$$\nu = Z^2 \frac{2\pi^2 m e^4}{h^3} \left(\frac{1}{N_1^2} - \frac{1}{N_2^2} \right) \qquad (2)$$

where Z is the atomic number of the atom, m and e are the mass and charge of the electron, h is Planck's constant, and N_1 and N_2 are 1 and 2 for K and L shell, respectively.

An x-ray tube consists of an evacuated tube containing a heated cathode and an anode (target). The emitted electrons are accelerated to the target by

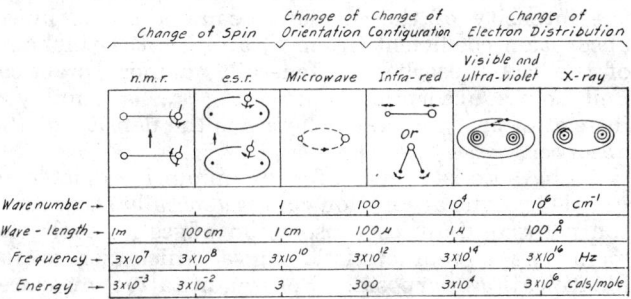

	Change of Spin		Change of Orientation	Change of Configuration		Change of Electron Distribution	
	n.m.r.	e.s.r.	Microwave	Infra-red		Visible and ultra-violet	X-ray
Wavenumber →			1	100	10⁴	10⁶	cm⁻¹
Wave-length →	1m	100cm	1 cm	100μ	1μ	100 Å	
Frequency →	3×10⁷	3×10⁸	3×10¹⁰	3×10¹²	3×10¹⁴	3×10¹⁶	Hz
Energy →	3×10⁻³	3×10⁻²	3	300	3×10⁴	3×10⁶	cals/mole

Fig. 440. A simplified illustration of the interaction of matter with various regions of EM radiation.

imposing a high voltage across the electrodes. Impact of the electrons with the target results in the emission of two types of x-radiation:

1. A continuous spectrum results from the transfer of the kinetic energy of the impinging electrons to the atoms of the target. Since not all electrons lose all their energy and some are less decelerated, a distribution of energy or spectrum occurs.

2. The characteristic x-ray emmision lines occur due to discrete transitions of electrons in the target atoms. These sharp lines are superimposed on the continuous distribution. Fig. 441 depicts the peaks for molybdenum.

The generation of the x-ray spectrum is caused by the expulsion of an electron from the lower quantum levels of the atom. This vacancy is filled by an electron from one of the upper shells, which results in the emission of a photon possessing energy identical to that which was lost by the original electron; ie, $\Delta E = E_1 - E_2$, where E_1 and E_2 are the initial and final energy of the electron, respectively. If the vacancy produced in the K shell is filled with an electron from the L shell, the radiation is called $K\alpha$; if it is filled with an electron from the M shell, $K\beta$. Usual x-ray methods for obtaining a characteristic spectrum of a substance are made by using the sample as an anode or affixing the specimen on the target.

X-Ray Diffraction

X-ray diffraction analysis is employed for characterization of crystalline substances. A crystal diffracts x-rays similar to a diffraction grating, whose plane diffracts ordinary light. The three-dimensional crystal functions like a series of plane gratings stacked one above the other. The wavelength of the x-rays, λ, is related to the angle of incidence, θ, and the interatomic distance, d, by Bragg's equation:

$$n\lambda = 2d \sin \theta \qquad (3)$$

where n is the order of the diffraction, 1, 2, 3, . . .

For a single crystal the diffracted x-rays consist of a few lines; with powder, due to a random distribution of crystals, the diffraction pattern (Fig. 442) consists of a series of concentric cones with a common apex on the sample.

The atoms in a crystal possess the power of diffracting the x-ray beam. Each substance scatters the beam in a particular diffracting pattern, producing a "fingerprint" for each atomic crystal or molecule.

If an unknown powder sample is to be identified, either its diffraction pattern is compared with those of known substances or its d values are calculated from the diffraction diagram and compared with the d values of known compounds. For reference materials the three most intense reflections are listed on the upper left corner of each pattern card. The cards

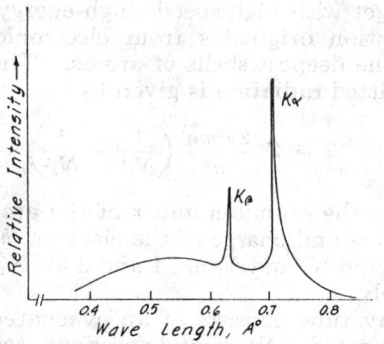

Fig. 441. The x-ray emission spectrum of molybdenum.

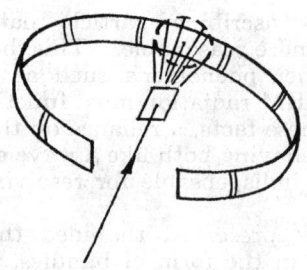

Fig. 442. An x-ray powder diffraction pattern.

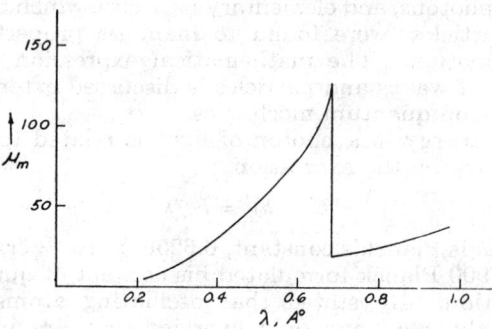

Fig. 443. The x-ray absorption curve of zirconium.

are then arranged in decreasing order of d values of the most intense reflections to facilitate location and comparison of the unknown.

If the diffraction pattern of a single crystal is to be determined, the crystal is mounted on a thin glass capillary and the capillary is fastened to a brass pin. Metal samples are machined into an appropriate shape and plastics are prepared into a desirable shape by extrusion. A substance in powder form can be ground to a fine powder and transformed into a small rod using collodion as a binder.

X-ray diffraction has been employed to determine the existence of polymorphic forms of a substance; eg, carbon in graphite or in diamond. The method also is used to distinguish between various oxides such as FeO and Fe_2O_3. The x-ray diffraction method is applied also in polymer chemistry to determine the degree of orientation of the fibers.

X-Ray Absorption

The wavelength at which a substance absorbs radiation is characteristic of a particular element. The intensity of the absorption is a function of the concentration. The absorption of a monochromatic x-ray beam is given by

$$I = I_0 e^{-\mu l} \quad \text{or} \quad \log \frac{I_0}{I} = \frac{\mu l}{2.303} \qquad (4)$$

where I is the intensity of the transmitted beam, I_0 is the intensity of the incident beam, μ is the linear absorption coefficient in cm^{-1}, and l is the thickness of the cell (absorber). Generally, a more practical unit, mass absorption coefficient, μ_m, is employed instead of μ; $\mu_m = \mu/\rho$, where ρ is the density of the absorber.

A characteristic curve for zirconium is depicted in Fig. 443. The absorption curves generally show some sharp discontinuities (absorption edges). Each element has a characteristic curve which serves for identification purposes. For quantitative measurement, a calibration curve is plotted for known weights of a sample. The method is somewhat similar in principle to absorption photometry used in UV and visible spectroscopy (see below).

The x-ray absorption method is utilized in analyses such as the determination of sulfur in oil, the halogen content of halogenated hydrocarbon polymers, and the measurement of sample thickness.

X-Ray Fluorescence

X-ray fluorescence analysis gives qualitative and quantitative data about the elements in a sample. As a K electron is expelled, either by bombardment with high-energy electrons or by absorption of x-ray, it is replaced by an L or M electron. Emission of energy of a wavelength longer than the excited wavelength is known as fluorescence radiation.

In x-ray fluorescence, the sample is a secondary target and is irradiated by a beam produced by bombarding a primary target with high-energy electrons. The sample is rotated to insure uniformity of exposure. The emitted fluorescence lines, which are characteristic of a given substance, are collimated and directed onto the surface of the analyzing crystal. The analyzing crystal consists of a flat, single crystal plate. The reflected radiation is directed through an exit slit to the detector, where x-ray energy is transformed into electrical impulses.

X-ray fluorescence is applicable to the quantitative determination of elements, such as niobium and the rare earths, for which no reliable analytical methods exist. The method is also complementary for emission spectrometry.

Instrumentation—This consists of an x-ray tube, a monochromator, and a detector.

The x-ray source was discussed briefly in conjunction with the theoretical and practical aspects of x-ray methods, in the previous paragraphs. The monochromator employed in diffraction analysis is a metal foil; in fluorescence analysis, however, a crystal of mica, quartz, or lithium fluoride is employed as the monochromator. A photographic emulsion, a Geiger counter, or a photoelectric x-ray detector tube is used as a detector; the latter type consists of dynodes containing a phosphor to convert x-rays to visible radiation.

Ultraviolet and Visible Absorption Spectrometry

A region of EM radiation, whose interaction with a molecule gives rise to electronic transition, exists at 100–8000Å (10–800 mμ as generally employed units).

The total energy of a diatomic molecule, according to the Born-Oppenheimer approximation, is the sum of electronic energy (E_e), vibrational energy (E_v), and rotational energy (E_r). If a range of radiation in the region of 10–800 mμ interacts with a molecule, a change in the energy of the molecule from the ground

state to a higher level occurs. This transition of energy is due to a displacement of a valence electron.

Accompanying the electronic excitation is a change in vibrational energy and rotational energy of the molecule. The energy requirements for the excitation of the latter two modes is of lesser magnitude than that for the electronic excitation. It should be emphasized, however, that the UV or visible spectrum of a molecule is the result of a change in energy of a molecule as a whole rather than of a particular bond. As mentioned previously, this energy, according to quantum theory, is absorbed or emitted in a discrete manner, expressed as $\Delta E = h\nu$. The excitation of a diatomic molecule is illustrated in Fig. 444.

Laws of Spectrophotometry—If a substance under investigation is placed in the path of an EM beam, a number of events may take place:

1. The intensity of the incident beam (I_0) is identical to the intensity of the emergent beam (I). This indicates that no absorption of radiation has occurred.
2. The intensity of the emergent beam is less than that of the incident beam. This indicates that some absorption has taken place.
3. Reflection, refraction, and scattering may occur.

A given substance will show a constant absorption intensity irrespective of the length of time of irradiation unless, of course, the radiation produces structural changes in the molecule. In other words, a finite number of molecules appear to absorb an infinite quantity of EM radiation. This paradox can be clarified by considering the modes of energy transfer among molecules:

1. The loss of kinetic energy due to the collision of a molecule with neighboring molecules. This results in an increase in the temperature of the medium.
2. The emission of the absorbed radiation is in random directions. The net effect, however, results in an absorption of energy from the impinging beam since re-emitted radiation has as much chance of entering the detector as the source.

If incident light with wavelength λ and intensity I_0 impinges on a solution with concentration, c, and pathlength, l, of 1 cm, the radiant energy of the light is diminished in an exponential fashion. Thus, if a given concentration of a substance absorbs 50% of the incident light, doubling the concentration will not absorb 100% but rather 75% of the light. The thickness of the sample or pathlength has a similar effect on the absorption.

Mathematically, the radiation-concentration and radiation-pathlength relation can be expressed by the following equations:

$$\frac{dI}{dc} = -k_1 I \quad \text{and} \quad \frac{dI}{dl} = -k_2 I \tag{5}$$

Integration of the equations in Eq. 5 give

$$\int_I^{I_0} \frac{dI}{I} = -k_1 \int_0^C dc \quad \text{and} \quad \int_I^{I_0} \frac{dI}{I} = -k_2 \int_0^C dc \tag{6}$$

Evaluation of the integrals between limits, combining the two formulas, and incorporating the value 2.303 (for transforming the natural log into a log of base 10) in the constant provides the more familiar equation used in spectrophotometry:

$$\log (I_0/I) = \epsilon c l \tag{7}$$

where I_0 is the intensity of the incident light, I is the intensity of the emergent light, c is the concentration, l is the thickness of the absorber, and ϵ is the molar absorptivity (formerly expressed as molar extinction coefficient) for concentration in moles/liter.

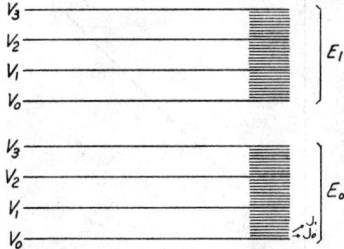

Fig. 444. The excitation of a diatomic molecule. E_0 and E_1: electronic ground and excited states; V_0, V_1, etc: vibrational ground and excited states; J_0, J_1, etc: rotational ground and excited states.

If the concentration is expressed in Gm/liter, absorptivity is designated by a instead of ϵ. The term $\log I_0/I$ or $\log (1/T)$ is referred to as absorbance, A (formerly expressed as optical density, OD). $E_{1cm}^{1\%}$, which is encountered less frequently in the literature, represents a concentration of 1% w/v and a 1-cm cell thickness.

A typical UV absorption curve, shown in Fig. 445, is the result of plotting wavelength vs absorptivity. The wavelength corresponding to maximum absorptivity, ϵ_{max} is denoted by λ_{max}.

UV Terminology—A few of the most generally employed terms in absorption spectrometry follow:

Chromophore—A moiety of a molecule responsible for selective absorption of radiation in a given range.

Auxochrome—A chemical group which does not give rise to an absorption band by itself, but upon being attached to a chromophore alters both the position and intensity of the peak.

Bathochromic Shift—A shift of the peak position (λ_{max}) to a higher wavelength due to the effect of a substituent or solvent (red shift).

Hypsochromic Shift—A shift of λ_{max} to lower wavelength (blue shift).

Hyperchromic and Hypochromic Effect—These terms refer to an increase and decrease in absorptivity, respectively.

Electronic transitions of organic molecules, which give rise to absorption bands, could be ascribed to the σ electron transition, π electron transition, or an n electron transition from the ground state to an excited state. These are designated by σ^* and π^*. Since the σ electron is involved in the construction of a single bond, its transition requires much more energy (usually in far UV) than the n electron (nonbonding electrons) or less tightly bonded π electrons.

Types of Absorption Bands—Four types of absorption bands are known to occur due to the electronic transition of a molecule.

R-Bands—These are observed in compounds containing such groups as C=O or NO₂. They involve $n \rightarrow \pi^*$ transition, which is a forbidden transition. The ϵ_{max} value is less than 100. The band at 279 mμ observed in the UV spectrum of acetone is an example of an R-band.

K-Bands—These arise from $\pi \rightarrow \pi^*$ transition in π-π conjugated systems and show $\epsilon_{max} > 10,000$. 1,3,5-Hexatriene is an example of such a conjugated system.

B-Bands—These are due to aromatic and heteroaromatic systems. The λ_{max} values are between 230 and 270 mμ and $\epsilon_{max} < 2,000$. These bands are also called benzenoid bands. In the presence of K-bands, the position of the B-bands is shifted to a longer wavelength. The UV spectrum of benzaldehyde contains K-bands, R-bands, and B-bands.

E-Bands—These, also known as ethylenic bands, are characteristic of the aromatic system as are the B-bands, except that they occur at lower wavelengths. The presence of an auxochromic group shifts an E-band to a higher wavelength. The ϵ_{max} values for these bands vary

Table I—Type of Transition, λ_{max} and ϵ_{max}, of a Few Commonly Known Compounds[a]

Electronic structure	Example	Transition	λ_{max} (mμ)	ϵ_{max}	Type of band
σ	Ethane	$\sigma \rightarrow \sigma^*$	135	—	—
n	Methanol	$n \rightarrow \sigma^*$	183	500	—
π	Ethylene	$\pi \rightarrow \pi^*$	165	10,000	—
π and n	Acetone	$\pi \rightarrow \pi^*$	188	900	—
		$n \rightarrow \pi^*$	279	15	R
π-π	1,3,5-Hexatriene	$\pi \rightarrow \pi^*$	278	35,000	K
Aromatic π	Benzene	$\pi \rightarrow \pi^*$	200	8,000	E
		$\pi \rightarrow \pi^*$	255	215	B
Aromatic π-π	Styrene	$\pi \rightarrow \pi^*$	244	12,000	K
		$\pi \rightarrow \pi^*$	282	450	B
Aromatic π-π and n	Acetophenone	$\pi \rightarrow \pi^*$	240	13,000	K
		$\pi \rightarrow \pi^*$	278	1,110	B
		$n \rightarrow \pi^*$	319	50	R

[a] Courtesy, Silverstein and Bassler.

from 2,000 to 14,000. The UV band at 210 mμ with ϵ_{max} of 6200 for phenol is an example of an E-band.

The absorption bands and various types of transitions of a few compounds are listed in Table I. Information thus attained serves in the structural elucidation of unknown molecules.

UV spectroscopy is also employed for quantitative measurements. An unknown concentration of a known compound, if it conforms to Beer's law, can be determined by using Eq. 7. A representative calibration curve, shown in Fig. 446, is constructed by plotting absorbance (A) vs concentration (c).

Factors Affecting Electronic Absorption Spectra—*Solvents*—Solvent–solute interaction affects the electronic spectra of a molecule because of an unequal perturbation of the ground and excited electronic states. The fine structure is retained in nonpolar solvents such as saturated hydrocarbons more than in polar solvents such as ethanol.

Solvent effects have the value of differentiating whether an electronic transition is $n \rightarrow \pi^*$ or $\pi \rightarrow \pi^*$. The n electrons interact strongly with polar solvents resulting in a shift to shorter wavelength, referred to as a "blue shift." Usually, but not always, if the $\pi \rightarrow \pi^*$ transition occurs, the shift will be toward the higher wavelength, referred to as a "red shift."

Intermolecular Hydrogen Bonding—Hydrogen bonding between solute–solute or solvent–solute is a factor which affects the absorption spectra, of which benzoic acid is a classic example. It was found that the ϵ_{max} at 230 mμ increases with an increase in the benzoic acid concentration in cyclohexane or in cyclohexane

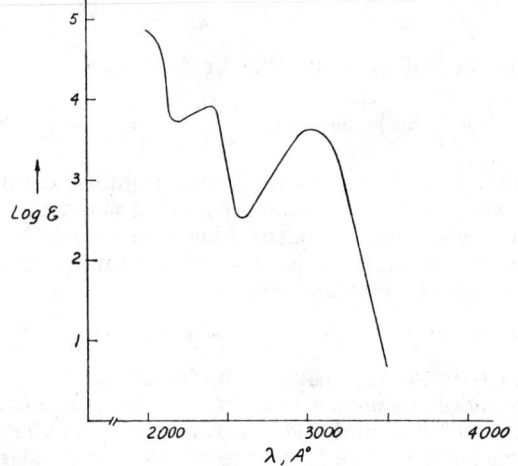

Fig. 445. The UV absorption curve of salicylic acid.

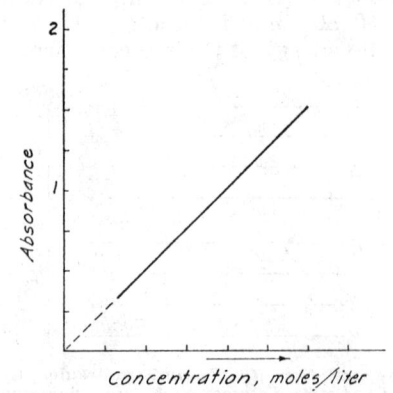

Fig. 446. A representative Beer's law plot.

mixed with a small quantity of ether. Upon increasing the concentration of ether, the concentration dependency of the absorption intensity decreases so that in 100% ether ϵ_{max} becomes concentration independent. This can be interpreted as the predominancy of the monomeric form of benzoic acid when solvent–solute H bonding occurs.

pH—The effect of pH on the spectrum is observed if a functional group such as COOH, OH, NH_2, etc is present in the molecule. The gain or loss of a proton causes a change in the electronic structure of the molecule, thus a chromophoric change. Consequently, the position and intensity of the absorption band becomes altered. Fig. 447 depicts the UV absorption spectrum of 1-methylbarbituric acid at pH values ranging from 1 to 14. The point at which the molar absorptivities of all the ionic species is identical is referred to as the *isobestic point*.

Temperature—A small change in the temperature of the solution under observation usually does not cause a change in the over-all appearance of an absorption spectrum. In general, a lowering of the temperature results in a greater resolution and the appearance of fine structure. The absorptivity is somewhat affected by temperature since increasing the temperature causes a decrease in absorptivity.

Instrumentation—A simplified diagram of a UV-visible spectrophotometer is presented in Fig. 448 and its major components are described below.

Radiation Source—The source for the UV range is usually a high-pressure hydrogen (or deuterium) discharge lamp, which covers a range of 200 to 375 mμ. A xenon arc or a mercury vapor lamp provides a more intense radiation. The source employed for the visible range is a 6- or 12-v tungsten automobile headlamp bulb.

Monochromator—The primary function of a monochromator is the dispersion of polychromatic light by means of a prism or grating. The desired monochromatic ray, whose position is determined by the angular position of the prism or grating, is directed toward the sample compartment.

Sample Compartment—This is the section where monochromatic light encounters the sample. In a double-beam instrument, this compartment contains a light-chopping device or a beam-switching assembly which allows the beam to pass alternatively through the sample and reference cells (about 35 times/sec). This allows the sample-reference relationship to remain unaffected when a change occurs in the source or optics of the instrument.

Detector—The detector is usually a photomultiplier tube. As depicted in Fig. 449, the cathode consists of a surface coated with a light-sensitive layer. It emits electrons upon being impinged with light. A series of electrodes called dynodes, which are also coated with a light-sensitive layer, are connected by a voltage-dividing network of resistors. The electrons are attracted from the cathode to Dynode 1, from Dynode 1 to 2, etc, each impinging quantum thus producing an avalanche of about 10^6 electrons. The collection of electrons on the anode creates a few milliamperes of current which can be measured as voltage across a resistor.

The output from the detector is amplified and observed on a meter or a recorder. The description of the amplifier or the recorder is beyond the scope of this chapter. Interested readers may refer to texts on electronics and instrumentation.

Analytical Procedure—Samples for UV absorption analysis can be utilized in the form of a vapor or a solution. Both polar and nonpolar solvents can be employed for preparing an analytical sample. The cutoff point of a solvent, however, should be recognized. A cutoff point is the wavelength at which the absorbance of a solvent approaches unity, using water as a reference. The cutoff points for many solvents can be found in the literature and in solvent charts supplied by several manufacturers.

Infrared Spectrometry

The range of EM radiation between 0.8μ to 500μ is referred to as infrared (IR) radiation. This radiation was first observed by Herschel in 1800, who detected an increase in the temperature of a thermometer upon placing it in an IR spectrum of the sun obtained with a glass prism. The development of a commercial IR instrument, however, did not begin until the end of World War II. At present the IR spectrophotometer is one of the instruments most frequently employed in the characterization of organic molecules.

The most commonly used region of the IR spectrum in organic chemistry is the region between 2.5μ to 16μ or 25μ, corresponding to 4000 to 625 cm^{-1} or 400 cm^{-1}. Both wavelength units and wave number

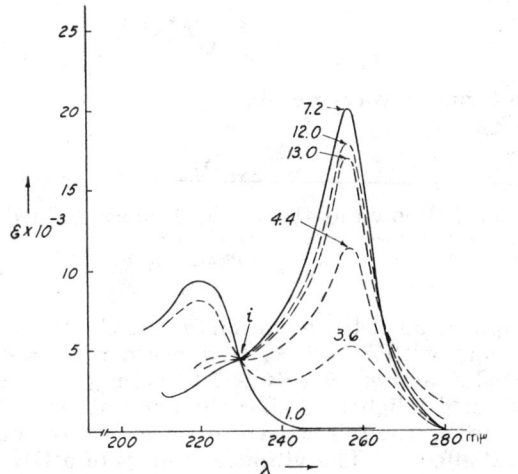

Fig. 447. The UV absorption spectrum of 1-methylbarbituric acid at various pH values; *i*: **isobestic paint.**

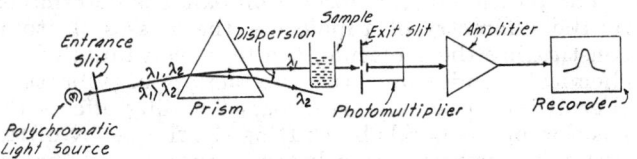

Fig. 448. A UV visible spectrophotometer.

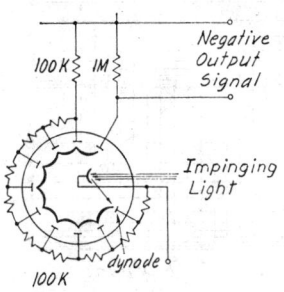

Fig. 449. The circuit of a photomultiplier system.

units are used in the literature to locate the position of the bands. The latter unit will be used throughout this chapter.

The near IR, or overtone region, refers to that part of the spectrum extending from 12,500 to 5,000 cm^{-1}; the far IR, or rotational region, 400 to 20 cm^{-1}.

Theory—The requirements for absorption of EM radiation by a molecule have been discussed previously. In order for IR radiation to be absorbed by a molecule, at least two criteria must be met: (1) the molecule should possess a vibrational or rotational frequency identical to that of the impinging EM radiation and (2) a change in the magnitude or direction of the dipole moment should occur as a result of radiation molecule interaction.

When the IR radiation impinges upon a molecule at the proper frequency, the vibration and/or rotation of the molecule is altered. The change in the vibrational energy creates a greater amplitude of vibration; the change in rotational energy causes a higher frequency of rotation.

The longest wavelength (lowest energy) of IR radiation that induces a change in the vibratory motion of a molecule gives rise to an absorption band known as the *fundamental band*. There is only one fundamental band in a diatomic molecule, although multiples of the band frequency (ν), known as overtones, can occur as 2ν, 3ν, etc.

Since upon absorption of IR radiation both vibrational and rotational modes of a molecule change, a band of absorption frequencies centered upon one frequency is observed. The magnitude of rotational energy changes in a molecule is less than the vibrational energy changes. These changes in the quantum number can be written as $\Delta\nu$ and ΔJ. If the vibrational quantum number denoted by ν'' and ν' is in the order of increasing quantum number, the change from the energy level $\nu' = 0$ to $\nu'' = 1$ is expressed as

$$\Delta\nu = \nu' - \nu'' = 1 - 0 = 1$$

The change in rotational quantum numbers, denoted by J'' and J' in the order of increasing quantum number, is expressed as

$$\Delta J = J' - J'' = 0, \pm 1$$

This concept is illustrated in Fig. 450. The transition at $\Delta J = 0$ is known as the Q-branch. It is a forbidden transition for hydrogen chloride and most of the diatomic molecules. The transition where $\Delta J = +1$ is known as the R-branch and those of $\Delta J = -1$, as the P-branch.

Since the total kinetic energy is a combination of translational, rotational, and vibrational energies of a molecule (ie, $E_t = E_{tr} + E_r + E_v$), a polyatomic molecule consisting of n atoms will have 3n degrees of

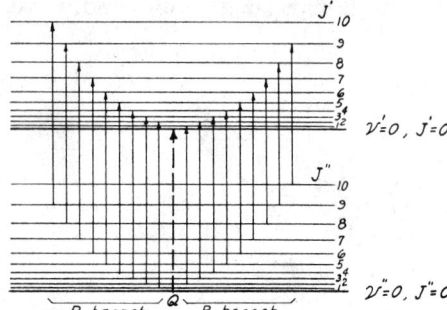

Fig. 450. The vibrational–rotational energy levels of a diatomic molecule.

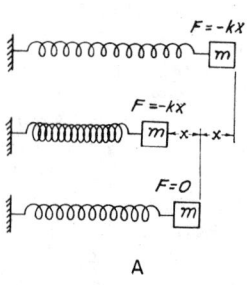

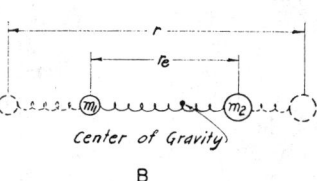

Fig. 451. A: A simple harmonic oscillator (presentation of Hooke's law); B: the vibration of a diatomic molecule.

freedom of motion. The possible fundamental vibrational modes of a molecule can be calculated by subtracting 3 for translational energy and 3 for rotational energy (2, if the molecule is linear). This gives a total of 3n-6 possible vibrational modes. The theoretical number of absorption bands, however, is not observed due to such factors as weak absorptivity, coalescence of several closely located bands, and lack of required change in dipole moment. Application of the laws of mechanical motion to the vibration of atoms in a molecule can be expressed according to Hooke's law, $F = -kx$, illustrated in Fig. 451A. The equation states that the restoring force (F) of a spring is directly proportional to the displacement (x) from its equilibrium position. The proportionality constant (k) is referred to as a force constant (dyne/cm). For a diatomic molecule (Fig. 451B) m_1 and m_2, the frequency of fundamental vibration is expressed by

$$\nu = \frac{1}{2\pi}\sqrt{\frac{k}{\mu}} \tag{8}$$

or in terms of wave number by

$$\bar{\nu} = \frac{1}{2\pi c}\sqrt{\frac{k}{\mu}} \tag{9}$$

where μ is known as the reduced mass, defined by

$$\mu = \frac{m_1 m_2}{m_1 + m_2} \tag{10}$$

Application of the equation for the C—H stretching frequency with $k = 5 \times 10^5$ dynes/cm, $m_1 = 19.8 \times 10^{-24}$ Gm, and $m_2 = 1.64 \times 10^{-24}$ Gm gives the value 3040 cm^{-1} (slightly higher than the observed value, 2950 cm^{-1}, which is caused by neglect of the environmental effect). The vibration modes of a CH_2 group are depicted in Fig. 452. It should be observed that more energy is required for the stretching vibration than for the bending vibration.

The position of the absorption bands is determined by the symmetry of a molecule, the masses of atoms constituting the molecule, the force constants of the chemical bonds, and the interaction of vibrations (Fermi interactions). Hydrogen bonding affects the position of the bands by shifting the frequency of the stretching vibration to a lower frequency and that of the bending vibration to a higher frequency.

Characterization of Molecules—There are two major applications of IR spectrometry in the characterization of various molecules: (1) determination of the identity of a compound by means of spectral comparison with that of an authentic sample and (2) verification for the presence of functional groups in an unknown molecule. The latter aspect is quite important in the structural elucidation of the synthetic organic compounds or substances isolated from natural sources.

A typical IR spectrum is depicted in Fig. 410A. The position of the absorption bands due to stretching and in-plane bending vibrations of the functional groups such as C=O, C—H, N—H, O—H, etc are somewhat independent of the influence of the neighboring groups in the molecule. These bands usually occur at 4000–1300 cm^{-1}. The position of the bands below 1300 cm^{-1} is markedly influenced by neighboring groups in the molecule. The portion of the spectrum from 1300–400 cm^{-1} is referred to as the "fingerprint" region.

Extensive charts and tables of the characteristic group absorption frequencies for common organic functional groups can be found in many of the texts listed in the Bibliography (eg, Colthup charts). Several catalogs of reference spectra have been published, the most voluminous of which is that of the Sadtler Research Laboratories, currently in excess of 33,000 spectra. Only a brief treatment of structure–absorption frequency correlation can be given here.

C—H Stretching and Bending Vibrations—The absorption bands for C—H stretching vibrations occur at 3300–2800 cm^{-1}. Each particular type of hydrocarbon has its own characteristic band position.

Saturated Acyclic Hydrocarbons—The C—H stretching $\bar{\nu}$ occurs at 2960–2850 cm^{-1} and in-plane bending $\bar{\nu}$ at 1470–1360 cm^{-1}. Vibrations at higher frequencies are ascribed to asymmetric stretching or bending and those in lower frequencies to a symmetric mode.

The bands due to CH$_2$ in- and out-of-plane bending (ie, rocking, wagging, and twisting) occur at 1350–1150 cm^{-1} for twisting and at 750–720 cm^{-1} for rocking. Branching in general does not greatly affect the position of the C—H bands. A doublet-like band with peaks at about 1380 and 1365 cm^{-1} is characteristic of a gem-dimethyl group.

Saturated Cyclic Hydrocarbons—Except for small-size (strained) rings such as cyclopropane and cyclobutane, all other alicyclic hydrocarbon bands occur in the same positions as the aliphatic hydrocarbons. The C—H stretching frequency for cyclopropane is about 3100 cm^{-1}, which is probably due to the strained ring altering the normal character of the C—H bond in cyclopropane as compared with the acyclic C—H, of medium-size cyclic, compounds.

Unsaturated Hydrocarbons—
1. The olefinic C—H stretching frequency bands occur at 3090–3000 cm^{-1}. Substituents have some influence on the position of the bands; eg, for 1,2-dialkylethylene the C—H stretching band is observed at 3030–3010 cm^{-1} and at 3090–3070 cm^{-1} for 1,1,2-trialkylethylene. For *trans*-disubstituted olefins the in-plane bending vibration occurs at 1310–1290 cm^{-1}; the out-of-plane bending vibration occurs at 970 cm^{-1}. For *cis* compounds the out-of-plane bending vibration occurs at about 700 cm^{-1}.

2. The acetylenic C—H stretching frequency occurs at 3300–3270 cm^{-1}. This could be ascribed to the similarity in character between the strained rings and the C—H bond of acetylenic hydrocarbon as compared with the saturated hydrocarbons. The out-of-plane bending vibration of acetylene usually occurs at about 650 cm^{-1}.

3. The aromatic C—H stretching vibration band occurs at 3100–3000 cm^{-1}; the C—H out-of-plane bending vibration occurs at 900–650 cm^{-1}. A more characteristic band for the aromatic system is a band at 1610–1590 cm^{-1}, which is due to aromatic skeletal vibration.

In general, the intensity of C—C, C=C, and C≡C stretching modes is quite weak, probably due to a weak dipole moment. The positions of the bands for these three bonds are at 1200–800 cm^{-1}, 1650–1630 cm^{-1}, and 2250–2100 cm^{-1}, respectively.

O—H Vibration—The stretching vibration band for O—H occurs at 3700–3350 cm^{-1}, depending on the extent of hydrogen bonding. Dilution of the O—H-containing molecules with nonpolar solvents, which causes a reduction of intermolecular hydrogen bonding, shifts the O—H stretching vibration to a higher frequency but the bending vibration to a lower frequency. The latter frequency occurs at 1420–1320 cm^{-1}.

C—O Vibration—The bands for C—O stretching vibration occur at 1280–1000 cm^{-1}, depending on the type of molecule. For alcohols and phenols (C—OH) the bands occur at about 1000 cm^{-1} and 1250 cm^{-1}, respectively.

For molecules such as ethers, esters, and anhydrides (which contain the C—O—C system) the absorption bands are at 1250–1050 cm^{-1}, with esters (C—O) at a higher frequency than ethers. The peroxide absorption band occurs at about 850 cm^{-1}.

C=O Vibration—Depending on the type of C=O bond (eg, ketone, acid, ester, anhydride), the position of the C=O stretching bands occur at 1950–1640 cm^{-1}. The C=O bands are quite intense, very conspicuous, and provide a great deal of information about an unknown molecule containing a carbonyl function.

Hydrogen bonding, field effect, and conjugation are some factors which should be considered in the evaluation of the position of the C=O absorption bands. For example, the C=O band position for ethyl benzoate should be expected to occur at a lower frequency than for ethyl hexanoate because the C=O bond of the former compound conjugates with the phenyl ring, rendering less double-bond character to C=O than to the aliphatic ester. Hydrogen bonding has a similar effect on carbonyl absorption.

Halogen substitution at a position α to the C=O, or halogen attached directly to the C=O, results in a high-frequency shift of the carbonyl group of ketones or of acyl halides. Apparently, this shift is due both to the inductive effect and the field effect. The latter effect is more influential since substitution of two halogens on the α carbon does not shift the C=O frequency band beyond that of the monosubstituted derivative. The field effect operates across space, wherein rotation around C—C bond results in the formation of two carbonyl peaks for the two rotational conformers shown below:

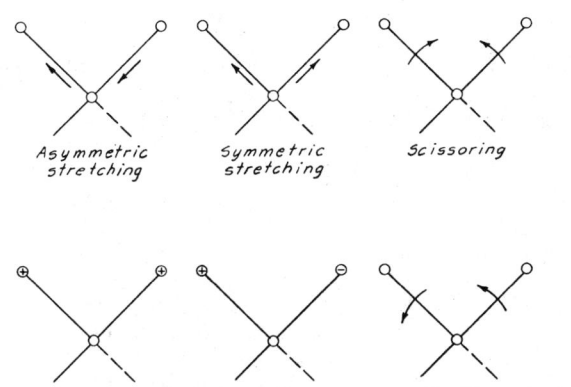

Fig. 452. Vibrational modes of CH$_2$ group. The signs + and − indicate relative movement in and out of the plane of the page, respectively.

A shift of the C=O peak to a higher frequency is

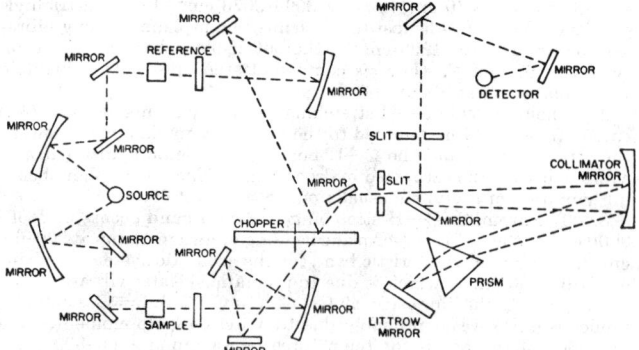

Fig. 453. The optical system of the Beckman IR 5 (courtesy, Beckman).

observed also when C=O is a part of a strained-ring system. Acyclic anhydrides show sharp C=O bands at about 1820 cm^{-1} and 1750 cm^{-1}.

The amide C=O absorption occurs at a lower frequency than esters and ketones. The C=O absorption band at about 1650 cm^{-1} observed for the primary amides (amides of ammonia) is known as the Amide I band. The secondary amide (amides of primary amines) absorbs at about 1640 cm^{-1}. For both primary and secondary amides, peaks are shifted to about 1700 cm^{-1} if the spectra are determined in solution form. The C=O peak of tertiary amides (amides of secondary amines) occurs at about 1650 cm^{-1}, and the position of this peak is independent of the physical state of the substance. The C=O absorption bands for cyclic amides vary according to the size of the ring. The peak frequency shifts from a lower frequency to a higher frequency as the ring becomes smaller (ie, more strained). For example, the δ lactam C=O absorption peak occurs at about 1680 cm^{-1} and the γ lactam at about 1750 cm^{-1}.

The two absorption bands for amides at about 1650 cm^{-1} and 1560 cm^{-1} are ascribed to the Amide I and Amide II bands, respectively. The second band is absent in the spectra of lactams and tertiary amides. The origin of the amide II band is thought to be due to the in-plane NH vibration. However, because of the absence of such peaks in lactams, the correctness of the assignment has become subject to some doubt. An alternative explanation for the origin of the amide II band is the partial double-bond character of C—N. This explanation, likewise, was found to be unsatisfactory because of the absence of such bands for tertiary amides.

N—H Vibration—The N—H stretching vibration frequency occurs at 3500–3300 cm^{-1}, with free N—H at higher frequencies and hydrogen bonded N—H at lower frequencies. The bands for $\overset{+}{N}H_3$, $\overset{+}{N}H_2$, and $\overset{+}{N}H$ occur at about 3200, 2700, and 2000 cm^{-1}, respectively. The band due to in-plane N—H bending is known to occur at 1650–1550 cm^{-1}; out-of-plane deformation occurs at 900–600 cm^{-1}.

C—N Vibration—C—N stretching frequency bands for aliphatic compounds occur at about 1210 cm^{-1} and for aromatic compounds, at 1250–1350 cm^{-1}. The band for C=N occurs at 1680–1640 cm^{-1} and for C≡N, at about 2250 cm^{-1}.

It should be mentioned that IR spectroscopy is generally employed for qualitative identification, rather than quantitative measurement, of unknown molecules. The laws of spectrometry, mentioned under *Ultraviolet and Visible Absorption Spectrometry*, are also applicable to IR spectrometry.

Instrumentation—A brief description of the major components of an IR spectrophotometer is given below, and an IR instrument is illustrated in Fig. 453.

Radiation Source—Generally, IR radiation is obtained by electrically heating a Nernst glower (a mixture of oxides of zirconium, yttrium, and thorium) or a globar unit (a small rod of silicon carbide).

Monochromator—The most commonly used prism materials for dispersion of IR radiation are:
1. NaCl with a refractive index of 1.5442. This provides good dispersion at 2000–650 cm^{-1}, but poor dispersion beyond 2000 cm^{-1}.
2. KBr, with a refractive index of 1.53, disperses at 1600–370 cm^{-1}.
3. CsBr, with a refractive index of 1.69, disperses at 1000–250 cm^{-1}.

In recent years grating systems have been employed more widely than the prism, primarily because of their high resolving power.

Detector—The thermocouple and bolometer are two types of detectors which are used in IR spectrometry, the former being employed to a greater extent. A bolometer is comprised of a resistance in a bridge circuit. A change in the resistance upon heating causes an unbalance signal which can be amplified and recorded.

As depicted in Fig. 453, the source beam is reflected by mirrors to form the sample and reference beam. After passing through the sample and reference, the beams are chopped by a mirror which serves to focus each beam alternately onto the entrance slit of the monochromator. If the sample absorbs part of the radiation, the intensity of the two beams will be unequal. This inequality results in the development of an unbalance signal in the detector. After amplifying and rectifying, the signal is relayed to a comb or wedge to drive the reference beam attenuator to reduce the intensity of the reference beam. As the difference between the two beams becomes zero, the unbalance signal also becomes zero. The pen of a recorder, which is connected to the attenuator, will perform the function of plotting the absorption coordinates on a paper chart. The speed of the chart is a function of wavelength (or frequency), and the resulting tracing of absorbance (or % transmission) vs frequency is known as an IR spectrogram.

Preparation of the Sample—Samples for IR spectra determination can be prepared in the form of a gas, liquid, or solid. Liquid samples are prepared "neat" (pure form) or in solution using a liquid cell. Carbon tetrachloride and carbon disulfide are the two commonly used solvents. With solutions, the solvent should be placed in the path of the reference beam in order to cancel absorption due to the solvent. This method is particularly useful in the study of various types of hydrogen bonding.

Solid samples are prepared either as a KBr disc or in the form of a suspension in mineral oil. A KBr disc of a sample is prepared by grinding the sample with KBr powder, placing the mixture between a punch and die, and applying a pressure of about 50,000 psi. This is the most extensively used method of sample preparation for IR spectrophotometry.

A mineral oil suspension of a sample is usually placed between two sodium chloride windows. This method possesses an inherent disadvantage in that the C—H absorption bands in the sample will be masked by those of the oil.

Attenuated Total Reflectance (ATR)—This IR method has been developed recently for determining the IR spectra of insoluble, opaque materials. The IR spectrum of a substance is developed as a result of the reflection of radiation from the surface of a material rather than transmission through it. The IR radiation from the source enters a trapezoidal prism composed of material with a refractive index greater than 2 through the IR range. The sample is fastened to the base of the prism. The beam of the IR radiation is adjusted to enter the face of the prism at an angle that will contact the sample and penetrate into it about 5μ and reflect back through the other side of the prism. Since this angle is less than the critical angle, total reflectance occurs and the energy of the reflected beam is attenuated in the wavelengths where the sample absorbs the IR radiation. This provides an IR spectrum similar but not identical to the IR spectrum obtained as a result of beam transmission through a compound.

Frustrated multiple internal reflection (FMIR) is a modified version of ATR. The source beam undergoes internal multiple reflections 35 to 50 times, providing an intense absorption spectrum of the substance under investigation.

Nuclear Magnetic Resonance Spectrometry

Since its very recent development, nuclear magnetic resonance (NMR) spectrometry has found its place among the most useful of analytical tools. At present it is one of the most frequently employed techniques in the structural elucidation of organic molecules.

Theory—The association of an electrical charge with the spinning nucleus gives rise to a nuclear dipole, whose magnitude is expressed as a nuclear magnetic moment, μ. In order to simplify certain nuclear behavior, nuclei can be assumed to exist as spinning bar magnets. The angular momentum of the spinning charge is expressed by a spin quantum number, I (in units of $h/2\pi$, where h is Planck's constant). The I value for isotopes may vary by integral values 1, 2, 3, ..., or half-integral values $\frac{1}{2}$, $\frac{3}{2}$, ... $\frac{9}{2}$. An I value equal to zero indicates no spin. The spin number of isotopes can be determined by observing the following rules:

1. Nuclei with an even number of protons and neutrons have a spin number of zero, or no spin (eg, ^{4}He, ^{12}C, ^{16}O).
2. Nuclei with an odd number of protons and neutrons have an integral spin of 1, 2, 3, ... (eg, ^{2}H, ^{14}N, ^{10}B).
3. Nuclei with an odd mass number have a half-integral spin of $\frac{1}{2}$, $\frac{3}{2}$, ... $\frac{9}{2}$ (eg, ^{1}H, ^{19}F, ^{13}C).

The nuclei of an isotope ($I > 0$) placed in a magnetic field will assume a number of orientations equal to $(2I + 1)$. Since I for the proton is $\frac{1}{2}$, there will exist 2 orientations or spin states: (1) a low-energy state, wherein the nuclei are in alignment with the external magnetic field (parallel orientation, N pole near S pole) and (2) a high-energy state, wherein the nuclei are in alignment against the external magnetic field (antiparallel orientation, S pole near S pole) (see Fig. 454). The separation of the energy levels is a function of the nuclear magnetic moment, μ, and the external magnetic field strength, H_0, and inversely proportional to the spin quantum number, I, according to the formula

$$E = \frac{\mu H_0}{I} \tag{11}$$

As shown in Fig. 455, the spin axis of the nucleus precesses about the axis parallel to the field direction. If H_0 is increased, the precessional frequency of the nucleus increases proportionally. The angular velocity of the precessing nucleus, ω_0, is expressed as

$$\omega_0 = \gamma H_0 \tag{12}$$

where γ is the magnetogyric ratio (a nuclear constant). The flipping from one energy state to another

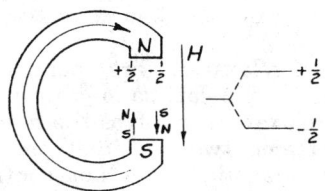

Fig. 454. Orientation of nuclear magnets in an external magnetic field.

can occur by absorption or transmission of radiation according to the formula

$$\nu = \frac{\gamma H_0}{2\pi} \tag{13}$$

where ν is the radio frequency (rf), corresponding to the precessional frequency of the nucleus, which causes nuclear transition from a low-energy to a high-energy state. Restated, if the rotating magnetic vector of rf equal to ω_0 is introduced perpendicular to H_0, the system will be attuned; ie, the frequency of the precessing nucleus and inserted frequency will be in resonance.

Combining Eqs. 12 and 13 gives

$$\omega_0 = 2\pi\nu \tag{14}$$

If H_0 is 14,092 gauss, an external frequency of 60 mHz (a weak magnetic field H_1) is required to induce "flipping" of protons. The direction of the rotating magnetic field, H_1, is perpendicular to the direction of H_0. When resonance occurs, the nuclei flip over (revert to alternate energy states). This results in an induced voltage in a receiving coil placed at a right angle to both H_0 and H_1.

In practice the rf oscillator is maintained at a constant frequency and H_0 is swept over a narrow range (usually of the order of a few milligauss).

Population of nuclei in each energy level is given by

$$N_{\text{upper}}/N_{\text{lower}} = e^{-\Delta E/kT} \tag{15}$$

where k is the Boltzmann constant (1.38×10^{-16} erg degree^{-1}). In the case of proton nuclear spin, $\Delta E = 5 \times 10^{-19}$ erg in a 15,000 gauss field at a temperature of $T = 300°$K, $N_{\text{upper}}/N_{\text{lower}} \approx e^{-5\times10^{-19}/4.2\times10^{-14}}$ or $1-1.2 \times 10^{-5}$ for such nuclei.

Considering such a small number of excess population in the lower energy level, there should be a mechanism to maintain this excess number; otherwise, a preliminary absorption of rf equates the population of the two states and no net absorption of radiation is detected. Therefore, the required condition for nuclear resonance is the maintenance of excess nuclei in the lower energy level. This is accomplished by a process known as relaxation, through which a

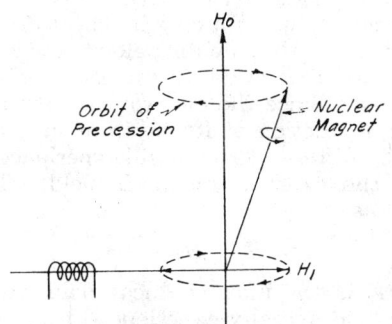

Fig. 455. The spinning and precessing of a nuclear magnet in an external magnetic field.

nucleus returns from the higher to the lower energy state.

Two types of relaxations are operative: spin–spin relaxation and spin–lattice relaxation. Spin–spin (transverse) relaxation involves the mutual exchange of energy between two proximal precessing nuclei. This type of relaxation does not contribute to the maintenance of an excess lower state spin population, but it decreases the lifetime of the excited state nucleus, which affects spectral linewidth.

Spin–lattice (longitudinal) relaxation involves a transfer of the nuclear energy, as a result of transition to a lower state, to the energy of the lattice components. The term lattice refers to the framework of molecules in a system in any physical state. Translational, rotational, and vibrational energies of the molecules are the components of a lattice. Owing to the magnetic properties of these various types of energies, the lattice contains a variety of magnetic fields whose proper alignment with a precessing nucleus can cause transition to a lower state. The energy thus released increases the translational, vibrational, and rotational energies. There is no net change of energy in the system. This process is responsible for maintaining the small excess nuclei in the lower energy level.

Both spin–spin and spin–lattice relaxations are responsible for spectral linewidth. The linewidth is inversely proportional to the lifetime of nuclei in the excited state. In solids or viscous liquids, restriction of molecular motion does not allow frequent occurrence of proper magnetic orientation, resulting in a long spin–lattice relaxation time. This condition, however, creates a proper orientation of nuclei so that the mutual exchange of energy becomes quite facile, thus shortening spin–spin relaxation time which in turn results in the broadening of the spectral line.

Measurement and Interpretation of Spectra— Most of the discussion of this portion of the chapter will relate to *proton* magnetic resonance, since this is the commonly used version of NMR.

Chemical Shift—As discussed previously, when the frequency of the rotating magnetic field, H_1, whose plane is perpendicular to H_0, becomes equal to the precessional frequency of the nucleus, energy will be absorbed and nuclear transition will occur.

An NMR spectrum, which is a display of peaks for various protons in different magnetic environments, would not have existed if the precessional frequencies of all the nuclei in a given magnetic field were identical. This, however, is not the case. The frequency of resonance depends on the magnetic environment of the protons in a molecule. This concept can be elaborated by considering the phenomenon that, when placed in an external magnetic field, electrons in a molecule will circulate. The circulating electrons create a new magnetic field which opposes the external magnetic field, thus reducing its effect on the nucleus. This is known as the shielding effect, and its magnitude is determined by the density of the electrons around the nucleus. Since the electron density around each proton is a function of its environment, protons surrounded by different groups will experience an unequal effect of the external magnetic field. This can be expressed as

$$H = H_0 - \sigma H_0$$

where σH_0 is the induced local field and H is the magnetic field actually experienced by the nuclei.

Environmental variation among the many kinds of protons found in organic compounds seldom produces resonances whose frequencies are spread more than 1000 Hz. An NMR spectrum is a plot of resonant frequencies vs an arbitrary intensity scale. The area under each peak (when properly evaluated, as will be discussed later) is proportional to the number of protons in the environment producing such a peak or combination of peaks. Tetramethylsilane (TMS) is used as a reference standard since all of the protons are equivalent; thus, only one resonant peak is observed and it occurs at a point farther "up field" from most other proton resonances. All other proton resonances are referred to TMS (arbitrarily assigned a value of zero) and are measured from the TMS value using a concept known as a *chemical shift* (distance from the TMS value, measured in ppm—see below). Since the chemical shift is a function of the magnetic field strength, its value will vary if instruments with different rf magnetic fields are employed for measurement (40, 60, 100 mHz). To make the chemical-shift expression independent of field strength, a chemical-

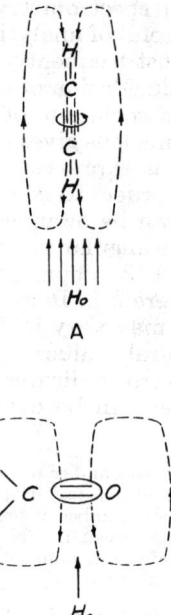

Fig. 456. The electron-induced magnetic lines of force. *A:* Shielded acetylenic proton; *B:* deshielded aldehyde proton.

shift symbol, δ, in dimensionless units of parts per million (ppm) is used.

$$\delta = H_8 - H_{TMS}/H_1 \times 10^6 \qquad (16)$$

where H_8 and H_{TMS} are the field strengths (in Hz) corresponding to resonance for the sample and reference, respectively. H_1 is the frequency of the rf signal used. τ (where $\tau = 10 - \delta$) is also used to designate chemical shift.

It should be emphasized at this point that although the electronegativities of atoms proximal to protons is a contributory factor in determining chemical-shift values, the position of the resonance peak is influenced also by several structural features. A classic example is the peak for acetylenic protons at δ 2.35 which is more shielded than the olefinic proton at δ 4.60.

This apparent anomaly can be explained by considering the diamagnetic anisotropy effect; ie, the orientation of the chemical bond in a magnetic field. In Fig. 456A, the lines of force, induced by circulating π electrons of the acetylenic C≡C bond, shield the

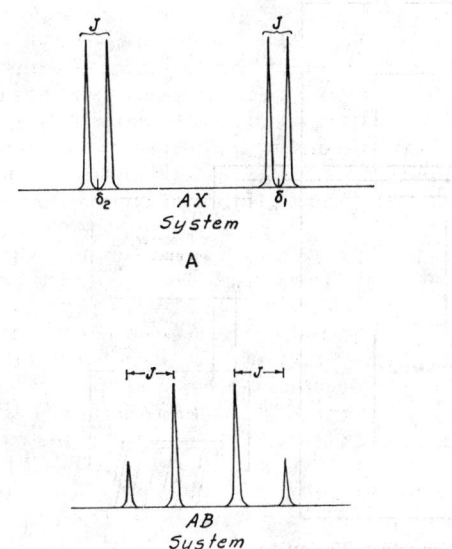

Fig. 457. A typical AX system (*A*) and AB system (*B*).

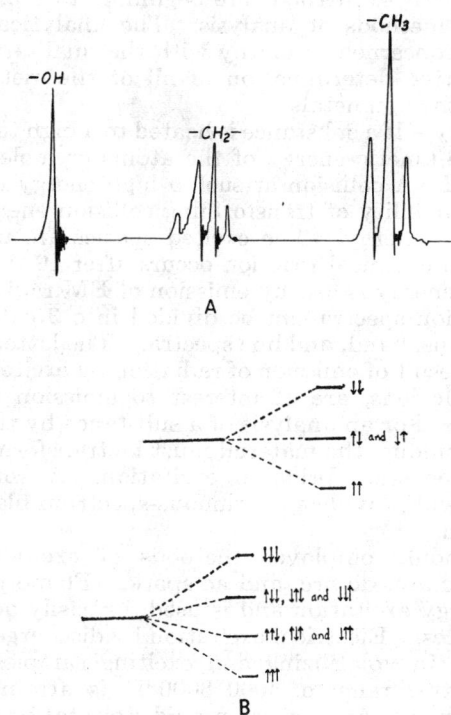

Fig. 458. *A:* A high-resolution NMR spectrum of ethanol; *B:* spin–spin splitting presentation of proximal CH_3 and CH_2.

proton. In contrast, the induced magnetic field deshields an aldehyde proton (Fig. 456*B*).

Spin–Spin Coupling—Fig. 457 depicts the NMR spectrum of ethanol as determined by a high resolution instrument. Instead of observing three distinct peaks indicative of the methyl (CH_3—), methylene (—CH_2—), and hydroxyl (—OH) protons, with peak areas in the relation 3:2:1, several peaks are noted in each area. Each peak representative of certain types of protons has been *split* by coupling with adjacent protons, as is discussed in the following.

The concept of spin–spin coupling can be visualized by considering the effect of one proton on a neighboring proton connected by not more than three bonds

(conjugated systems excepted). The splitting occurs because of the tendency of the electron to pair its spin with that of the nearest proton.

For a simple explanation of spin–spin splitting, assume a molecule with nonequivalent protons, H_1 and H_2, in a magnetic field. If the nucleus H_1 is in an antiparallel position, the field experienced by H_2 becomes augmented, corresponding to a higher precessional frequency. The resonance line for H_2 occurs at a lower field if H_1 is absent. An opposite effect is observed if the nucleus H_1 has the parallel position. A similar effect is exerted on H_1 by H_2. The combination of these effects thus gives rise to two doublets.

Fig. 458*B* illustrates the probable nuclear arrangement of the —CH_2— and —CH_3 groups of ethanol. The multiplicity caused by the effect of one group on a neighboring group is given by the formula $2nI + 1$, where n is the number of equivalent nuclei of spin I. In the case of protons with $I = \frac{1}{2}$, the formula can simply be written as $n + 1$.

In Fig. 458*A* the CH_2 group in ethanol consists of four peaks with intensities of 1:3:3:1; the CH_3 group has three peaks with intensities of 1:2:1. The ratio of the total area of CH_2 to that of CH_3 is 2:3.

The distance between multiplets is referred to as the coupling constant, J, expressed in Hz. For protons, the J value rarely exceeds 20 Hz. The separation of two resonance lines, $\Delta\nu$, is expressed in Hz. Unlike chemical shift, the J value is independent of the strength of the applied magnetic field, H_0, and its magnitude is a function of the extent of coupling between two nuclei. Chemically equivalent protons also undergo spin–spin coupling but the transitions are forbidden.

Recently, the use of the letters A, B, C, ... (in order of decreasing value) for labeling nonequivalent protons has been proposed if their chemical-shift values are similar. The letters M, N, ... and/or X, Y, ... are used for those whose chemical shifts are far apart. Equivalent nuclei are assigned the same number. Ethyl bromide, CH_3—CH_2—Br, eg, is an A_2B_3 system.

The symmetry of multiplets is related to $\Delta\nu$. The CH_3 triplet of *n*-propyl iodide (CH_3—CH_2 = 50 Hz) is less symmetrical than the triplet of ethanol ($\Delta\nu$ of CH_3—CH_2=147 Hz). For an AX system, J and $\Delta\nu$ can be determined directly from the spectra (Fig. 458*A*).

In AB cases, direct determination is not possible. As $J_{AB}/\Delta\nu_{AB}$ increases, the intensity of the inner peaks increases and of the outer peaks decreases (Fig. 457*B*). The J value can be read directly from the spectrum. If the peaks are numbered 1, 2, 3, ..., from left to right, $\Delta\nu_{AB}$ is calculated by

$$|1 - 3| = |2 - 4| = \sqrt{\Delta\nu_{AB}^2 + J_{AB}^2} \qquad (17)$$

and $\pm\frac{1}{2}\Delta\nu$ from the midpoint of the spectrum gives values for the absorption position of unperturbed A and B.

In summary, the structural elucidation of many complex molecules would not have been possible without NMR. Determination of dihedral angles in many molecules, detection of partial C=N character, and barrier to internal rotation in compounds such as dimethylformamide or hydrazones are but a few examples of the complex problems which can be unraveled by NMR.

Instrumentation—Fig. 459 depicts a 60-mHz NMR instrument, consisting of the following major parts:

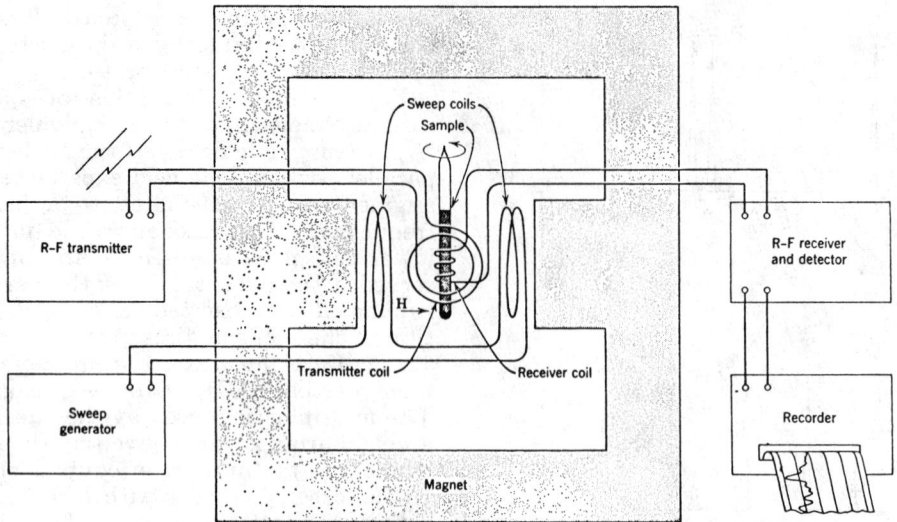

Fig. 459.   A basic NMR instrument (courtesy, Varian).

Magnet—Either a permanent magnet or electromagnet can be employed in NMR to supply H_0. Since chemical shift is a function of magnetic field strength, greater dispersion is achieved at a higher magnetic field strength. In practice, the field is varied over a very small range (about a few milligauss) with the aid of a sweep coil. If a sawtooth voltage is employed to change the field of the large magnet and the same sawtooth is used as an x axis driving voltage, the signal can be observed on a recorder or an oscilloscope.

Radiofrequency Oscillator (Transmitter)—This rf field is provided by a transmitter coil whose magnetic vector component moves in a plane perpendicular to the direction of H_0. The field induces nuclear transitions when its frequency equals ω_0.

Radiofrequency Receiver (Detector)—The flipping of nuclei as a result of rf insertion induces a voltage in the receiving coil, whose axis is at a right angle to the axis of the transmitter coil and H_0.

Oscilloscope and Recorder (Display Device)—The voltage from the receiving coil is amplified and observed in an oscilloscope or a recorder. The peaks of an NMR spectrum are the result of plotting intensity vs frequency of resonance.

Preparation of the Sample—A sample for NMR spectral determination should be dissolved in one of the following solvents: CCl_4, $CDCl_3$, D_2O, $SO(CD_3)_2$, $CO(CD_3)_2$, CF_3COOH, etc. The choice of solvent depends on the nature of the substance and obviously the solute and solvent must not interact.

Usually, 30–70 mg of the compound under investigation is dissolved in about 0.2 ml of the solvent in an NMR tube. A small amount of TMS is added for reference. Due to the insolubility of TMS in some solvents, such as water, an external TMS standard is often used. This is done either by placing a sealed TMS-containing capillary tube inside the NMR tube or by marking the reference point, just prior to determining the spectrum of a sample, with a TMS solution in CCl_4 or $CDCl_3$.

Emission Spectroscopy, Flame Photometry, and Atomic Absorption

Because of common principles shared by emission spectroscopy, flame photometry, and atomic absorption, all three are discussed under one category.

Emission Spectroscopy

If alkali metal solutions are introduced into a flame, by spraying a solution of the metal salt, radiation is emitted. The yellow light visualized by introducing a sodium salt in a flame is an example.

The "wet" analysis of metals is not adequate to satisfy the needs and the enormous demands of ana-

lytical chemistry. The rapidity and accuracy of emission and atomic absorption spectroscopy are reasons why these methods are beginning to replace the classical methods of analysis. The analytical technique is concerned primarily with the qualitative and quantitative determination of all of the metals and most of the nonmetals.

Theory—If a substance is heated to a high temperature, the kinetic energy of the atoms or molecules is increased. A collision at such a high energy incurs a high probability of transforming collision energy into excitation energy. The excited species are unstable and if no chemical reaction occurs after 10^{-4} to 10^{-7} sec, the energy is lost by emission of EM radiation.

Emission spectra can be divided into 3 categories: continuous, band, and line spectra. The latter, which are the result of emission of radiation by excited atoms or atomic ions, are of interest to emission spectroscopists. For an analysis of a substance by the emission technique, the material must be transformed into the vapor state prior to excitation. A condensed system will provide a continuous-spectrum blackbody radiation.

Commonly employed methods of excitation are flame, ac arc, dc arc, and ac spark. Flame provides low-energy excitation and is used for easily activated substances. Electrical excitation by discharge is very effective in volatilizing and exciting samples and a temperature range of 4000–8000°K is attainable by this method. An ac spark provides excitation energies greater than the arc and is produced by application of a high voltage (10–50 kv) across the electrodes. Excitation also can be achieved with an optical ruby laser.

Instrumentation—The optical system of a typical emission spectrograph is shown in Fig. 460. A diffraction grating can be used in place of a prism for radiation dispersion.

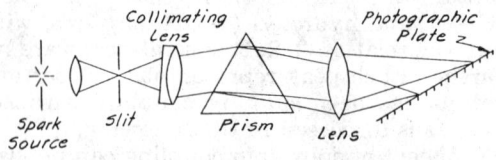

Fig. 460.   A simplified optical diagram of an emission spectrophotometer.

Analytical Procedure—For the qualitative analysis of metallic samples, the metal usually is fabricated into the electrodes. If a quantitative analysis is desired, the sample is prepared in the form of a powder or solution and introduced onto pure graphite or copper electrodes mounted vertically. The lower electrode contains a small depression in the tip for powder samples. A solution may be placed on the electrode and evaporated; the residue then yields an emission spectrum. Unknowns are identified using a densitometer by comparing the lines at various wavelengths with the lines in the previously photographed spectra of known metals. Iron is a valuable internal standard.

Flame Photometry

Flame photometry employs an emission-measuring device and utilizes a gas–air flame (1100–1300°C) for excitation. The detection is limited to group IA and IIA metals of the periodic table which have a low-lying electronic level. Sodium is the most active in the series with a detection limit of 0.0002 ppm and beryllium is the least active with a detection limit of 25 ppm. The detection limit of a few elements is listed in Table II.

Table II—The Detection Limits of Some Elements Using Flame Photometry[a]

Element	Wavelength, mμ	Detection limit, ppm
Barium	553.6	1.3
Calcium	422.7	0.003
Cesium	852.1	0.1
Lithium	670.8	0.002
Magnesium	285.2	0.2
Potassium	766.5	0.001
Sodium	589.3	0.0002

[a] Courtesy, Beckman.

Instrumentation—A flame photometer is composed of the following parts:

The Flame Source—This part consists of pressure regulators and flow meters for the fuel, atomizer, and burner. The burner has inlets for fuel and oxygen or air. In order to insure constant emission, a major requirement of the flame is the maintenance of a steady state. The quality of the burner is important in attaining a proper spectrum.

The Optical System—The optical system is identical to that of the atomic absorption spectrometer. In recent years instruments have been designed to combine both flame photometry and atomic absorption spectrometry. In flame photometric measurement, a chopping device, located between the flame and the monochromator, is employed to provide an ac signal at the detector. The chopping of the flame is stopped when the instrument is being used for absorption purposes. Other parts of the instrument are identical to those required for atomic absorption spectrometry.

Analytical Procedure—Samples are dissolved in a solvent and introduced into the burner via an atomizer. Calibrating solutions for analysis should be similar to the sample since variables such as viscosity and temperature affect the nature of atomization, thus the degree of excitation. In clinical laboratories the quantitative measurement of sodium, potassium, and calcium in biological samples is made by means of flame photometers.

Atomic Absorption Spectrometry

As early as 1860 Kirchhoff described the basic principles of atomic absorption spectra. It was not until 1955, however, that Walsh gave a theoretical background and demonstrated the analytical applications of atomic absorption spectrometry.

Atomic absorption spectrometry can be envisaged as the inverse of emission spectrometry. The simplicity of this technique makes it an attractive tool for the analysis of many elements. At present, many chemical and clinical laboratories use this method for measuring Mg, Na, and Ca in blood, urine, feces, etc.

Theory—The intensity of the emission line, S, arising as a result of the electronic transition from an excited state E_j to the ground state E_0, is proportional to the number of atoms in an excited state, N_j, by the equation

$$S = N_j E_j / \tau \qquad (18)$$

where τ is the lifetime of an atom in an excited state.

N_j is related to N_0, the number of atoms in the ground state, by the equation

$$N_j = N_0 (P_j / P_0) e^{-E_j/kT} \qquad (19)$$

where P_j/P_0 is the ratio of probability of atoms existing in the excited and ground states, k is the Boltzmann constant, and T is the absolute temperature.

Below 3000°K the value of N_j/N_0 is very small and, therefore, N_0 is equal to the total number of atoms, N. This is a satisfactory condition where the object is the production of an atomic vapor. An air–acetylene or nitrous oxide–acetylene flame promotes only 1% of the atoms to an excited state.

If radiation, with intensity I_0, originating in a hollow cathode tube, is directed to the flame with thickness l, and the flame contains vapor of the elements identical to that in the hollow cathode tube, absorption will occur according to the equation

$$I_0/I = e^{K_\nu l} \qquad (20)$$

where K_ν is absorptivity (absorption coefficient) whose value varies with ν. Since the absorption line has a finite width,

$$\int K_\nu d\nu = (\pi e^2/mc) N_\nu f \qquad (21)$$

where e is the electron charge, m is the electron mass, c is the velocity of light, N_ν is the number of atoms/ml capable of absorbing radiation of frequency ν, and f is the oscillator strength (ie, the average number of electrons/atom capable of being excited by the incident radiation).

The width of an absorption line is about 0.02Å. This is affected by the following factors:

1. The Doppler Broadening Effect: due to the movement of the atoms relative to the observer.
2. The Pressure Broadening Effect: due to collisions between neighboring atoms; ie, the absorbing atoms or otherwise.
3. The Stark Broadening Effect: developed as the result of an external electric field effect or by charged particles.

The atomic absorption of any element can be determined if the element can be reduced to the atomic state and if its resonance line can be detected by the instrument. An element under investigation generally absorbs only at the resonance line; ie, a narrow range of wavelengths which correspond to the transition between the lowest excited state and the ground state. Most of the available instruments operate in the visible and the near UV portions of the spectrum.

Elements are transformed into the atomic vapor form by means of an open flame. Both oxyacetylene and nitrous oxide—acetylene flames are employed in the burner. The latter mixture has the advantage of providing a temperature as high, but with a burning velocity as slow as that of the oxyacetylene flame. This feature provides for easy handling of the flame.

The quantity of O_2 in the flame determines the degree of metal oxide formation (MO). The ease of oxide formation varies from one metal to another

$$2M + O_2 \underset{}{\overset{K_{eq}}{\rightleftharpoons}} 2MO$$

where K_{eq} (equilibrium constant) for Ag is $10^{-2.7}$ and for Mg, $10^{-1.9}$.

In an oxidizing flame (ie, excess O_2 present) the formation of MO will be promoted. In a flame in which there is more fuel than O_2, the atomic form of the element $M°$ will be produced from MO.

The flame provides two types of energy: thermal and spectral energy. Both the droplets of liquid and residue formed on evaporation absorb spectral energy emitted by the flame; this absorption speeds their disintegration.

Factors Affecting Atomic Absorption Spectra—
Solvents—In general, an organic solvent enhances the absorption signal. For example, the relative absorption intensity of Ni is 4 in water and 144 in acetone. A solvent may affect the spectrum by one or a combination of the following effects:

1. It may produce spectral emission as a result of combustion.
2. Variation in the viscosity of various solvents may cause a change in the sample feed rate.
3. The size of droplets, which is a function of surface tension, will vary from one solvent to another.

Spectral absorption by the solvent or its combustion products may alter the absorption intensity. Many of the effects can be minimized by measuring the absorption of the solvent alone, then the solution, and computing the difference as the net absorption for the sample.

The enhancement effect of organic solvents is ascribed to an increase in the feed rate. However, the following explanation seems to be more convincing.

Combustion of a water solution:

Ions in H_2O $\xrightarrow{\text{Step 1}}$ hydrated residue $\xrightarrow{\text{Step 2}}$

dehydrated residue $\nearrow$ excited atom (emission)

$\searrow$ neutral atom (absorption)

Combustion of an organic solvent:

Metals in solvent $\xrightarrow{\text{Step 1}}$ solvent burns $\xrightarrow{\text{Step 2}}$ organic addend burns →

Step 3 $\nearrow$ excited atom (emission)

$\searrow$ unexcited atoms (absorption)

In aqueous solvents Steps 1 and 2 are endothermic; in organic solvents they are exothermic. As a result, free atoms are produced more efficiently in an organic solvent.

Cations and Anions—Cations have little or no effect on the signal. Anions, on the other hand, bond strongly with metals and tend to reduce the signal intensity. This effect can be eliminated by using chelating agents such as EDTA (see Chapter 16, *Complexation*).

Metal Binding—Sometimes, the presence of one metal interferes with the signal of another. For ex-

ample, either Si or Al interferes with a proper absorption signal of Sr if both are present in a solution. The signal can be improved by the addition of La which preferentially binds the interferants.

Ionization—If a large quantity of the test element is ionized, a very weak absorption is observed. This is due to the ionic absorption occurring at wavelengths different from that of the atomic one. The condition can be improved by adding a large excess of easily ionized elements; eg, in the measurement of Ca, a large amount of sodium ion is usually added.

Emission from the flame itself is minimized by using a chopper between the lamp and the flame. Since the amplifier is designed to amplify only an ac signal, that of the chopping frequency, the intensity of light from the hollow cathode tube can be observed and recorded. A reduction of intensity due to the presence of the sample in the flame then will be detected. The magnitude of the decrease in intensity is a function of the quantity of the sample in the flame. Fig. 461 shows a list of elements which can be determined by atomic absorption.

The sensitivity of atomic absorption is defined as the concentration of the element which gives an absorption of 1%. The sensitivity thus can be used for comparing the relative efficiency of various burners, fuels, and performances of various instruments.

Instrumentation—An atomic absorption spectrophotometer consists of the following elements:

Source—Single-element or multielement hollow cathode tubes are generally employed as sources in atomic absorption. Less frequently, the bright continuum of a xenon arc has been used as a source. The cathode of the hollow cathode tube is comprised of an element identical to that under investigation in the flame. Upon excitation by an electric current, metal atoms are sputtered off. Collision of these atoms with an inert gas such as argon induces excitation of the metal atoms and subsequent emission of characteristic radiation.

Burner—The quality of the burner, the type of fuel, and the ratio of fuel to oxidant are the most important factors which affect the result of analysis by an atomic absorption instrument. The burner can be compared to a sampling cell in a spectrophotometer. The following characteristics are desirable in a burner: stability, sensitivity, freedom from memory, freedom from background, linearity, and lack of self-emission.

There are two main types of burners: the "total consumption" ("diffusion") type and the "premix" type. In the total consumption type, the fuel, oxidant, and sample all enter separately into an opening where the flame emerges. In the premix type the sample, fuel, and oxidant are mixed prior to entering the flame. Each type has some inherent advantages and disadvantages, a discussion of which is beyond the scope of this chapter. Oxyacetylene, nitrous oxide-acetylene, and oxygen-cyanogen are oxidant-fuel mixtures employed in the burner.

Monochromator, Phototube, and Amplifier—These parts are identical to those employed in UV spectrophotometry. The monochrom-

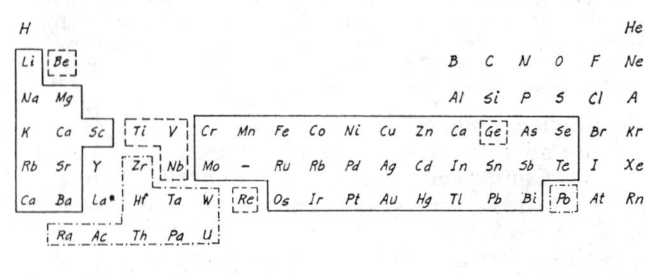

Fig. 461. **Elements which can be detected by atomic absorption spectrometry.**

ator, however, should be able to pass the resonance line and filter out others. A large bandpass causes the absorbance curve to bend. Most of the elements are determined at slitwidths corresponding to bandpasses of 7–40Å; in atomic absorption a 10Å wavelength accuracy is sufficient. This is compared to a good UV instrument which has an accuracy of 1Å.

Analytical Procedure—It is desirable to dissolve the sample in an organic solvent and for higher sensitivity the strongest absorption line must be chosen. In general, the resonance line resulting from the lowest excited state is usually the line exhibiting the strongest absorption. However, light passing through the flame should be scanned over all the emission wavelengths of the source. The instruction manual of each instrument suggests the choice of the line and the sampling technique.

Fluorescence and Phosphorescence Spectrometry

Fluorescence and phosphorescence are two spectrophotometric methods whose basic principle depends on the emission of radiation from excited molecules.

Theory—Fig. 462 depicts an energy-level diagram for a diatomic molecule. Upon absorption of visible or UV radiation by a molecule, the electron from S_0 (singlet ground state) is promoted to S_1 or S_2 (singlet excited states). The excited species, whose lifetime varies from 10^{-8} to 10^{-4} sec, may return to the ground state by dissipation of energy through collision or by vibrational relaxation of the excited state. The vibrationally relaxed species can return to the ground state with the emission of radiation with a wavelength longer than that which originally was absorbed. This radiation is referred to as fluorescence.

There is also a nonradiative process in which the excited state gives off energy and proceeds to a lower energy (triplet) state, T, by a decay process. A return from T to S_0 gives off a long-lived radiation, 10^{-4} to 10 sec. This radiation is called phosphorescence. The absorption and emission of radiation is specific for a particular molecule.

In order for a molecule to fluoresce, an absorbing molecular structure is required. Fluorescence may be expected generally in molecules containing a highly conjugated system. At least one electron-donating group such as NH_2 or OH should be a part of the conjugated system. Electron-withdrawing groups such as $COOH$ or NO_2 diminish, and in some cases prevent, fluorescence. Fluorescence is enhanced as the rigidity of the molecule increases; ie, a reduction in the internal vibration of the molecule.

Table III—Fluorescence Indicators

Compound	pH range	Color change
3,6-Dihydroxyphthalimide	0.0–2.5	colorless–yellow
Chromotropic acid	3.0–4.5	colorless–blue
Fluorescein	4.0–6.0	colorless–green
β-naphthoquinoline	4.4–6.3	blue–colorless
o-Coumaric acid	7.2–90	colorless–green
Naphthol AS	8.2–10.3	colorless–green

The position and intensity of the fluorescence bands are affected by pH. Table III shows a few examples of the effect of pH on fluorescence. The quantum yield, ϕ, of fluorescence is lower than unity due to a "quenching" process; ie, not all of the excited molecules return to the ground state by emitting fluorescence radiation. Energy may be lost by bond dissociation and deactivation.

Beer's law gives the relationship between I and I_0 to indicate the fraction of light energy transmitted through a solution. The fraction of light absorbed is expressed as

$$1 - I/I_0 = (1 - e^{-dC}) \qquad (22)$$

Rearrangement of Eq. 22 to express the amount of light absorbed, is

$$I_0 - I = I_0(1 - e^{-dC}) \qquad (23)$$

The fluorescence intensity, F, is given as

$$F = \phi(I_0 - I) \qquad (24)$$

where ϕ is the quantum efficiency of fluorescence. Thus Eq. 23 can be written as

$$F = \phi I_0(1 - e^{-dC}) \qquad (25)$$

and for dilute solutions where very little light is absorbed, Eq. 25 becomes

$$F = k\phi I_0(2.303 \; dc) \qquad (26)$$

where k is a constant to account for variation among instruments.

Fluorescence spectrometry offers detection limits lower than absorption spectrometry. A quantity of 1.1 mcg/liter can be measured and linearity can be maintained up to 10,000 mcg/liter. The method is applicable in the quantitative determination of fluorescing substances.

Instrumentation—The source of irradiation of the sample is a mercury-discharge lamp or xenon lamp. Selection of the exciting wavelength can be done by means of a filter; this type is called a filter fluorometer. In a true fluorescence spectrophotometer two monochromators usually are employed, one for the excitation source and the other for analyzing fluorescence emission. If the fluorescence spectrum is strong, the excitation spectrum can be determined by placing the desired solution in the instrument and evaluating the fluorescence while varying the wavelength of the exciting light. The detector is a photomultiplier tube whose output is connected to a meter or a recorder. The preparation of the sample is similar to that for UV.

Nonabsorptive Interaction of Matter with EM Radiation

The phenomenon of nonabsorptive interaction of the matter with EM radiation is applied in such analytical procedures as light-scattering photometry, refractive

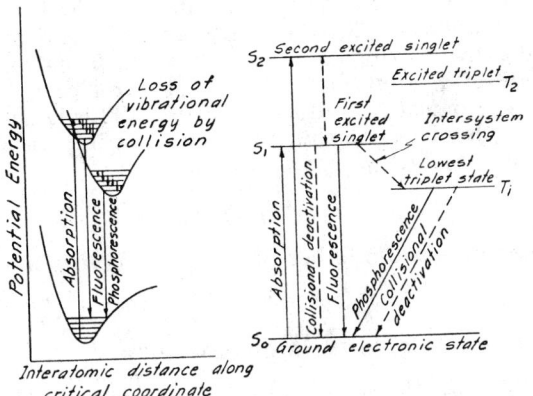

Fig. 462. The energy-level diagram of a diatomic molecule.

index, and polarimetry. These interactions are not quantized and therefore are considered to be non-specific. However, each compound possesses its own characteristic interaction. The differentiation of stereoisomers with a polarimeter, quantitative analysis of various substances with a refractometer, and determination of the molecular weight of macromolecules by light-scattering are examples of this type of instrumentation.

Light-Scattering Spectrometry

Theory—Scattering of EM radiation is analogous to the phenomena of reflection and refraction. Scattering of radiation results from induced secondary emission by particles during exposure to radiation. In order for EM radiation to be scattered by particles, two criteria should be met: (1) the dimensions of particles should be equal to or smaller than the incident wavelengths and (2) the dispersing medium should have a refractive index different from that of the particles.

Particles of 1–10,000 Å scatter EM in the UV and visible regions. If a beam of light is allowed to illuminate a colloidal suspension in a test tube, a pencil of light will be observed in the tube, due to the light-scattering phenomenon. This is known as the *Tyndall effect* and is an indication of the presence of suspended particles.

The simplest kind of scattering is that observed by small, spherical, and optically isotropic particles and is known as *Rayleigh scattering*. The particles should not have a dimension more than 10% of the wavelength of the incident radiation. The scattering intensity, I_s, is given by

$$I_s = \frac{8\pi^4\alpha^2}{\lambda^4 r^2}(1 + \cos^2\theta)I_0 \qquad (27)$$

where α is the polarizability of the particles, λ is the wavelength of the incident radiation, I_0 is the intensity of the incident radiation, θ is the angle between the incident and the scattered ray, and r is the distance between the detector and the scattering site. As is indicated by Eq. 27 the scattering intensity increases as either the particle size becomes larger or the wavelength becomes shorter.

If a beam of light illuminates a nonabsorbing but light-scattering dispersion, the intensity of the transmitted light, I, is given by

$$I = I_0 e^{-\tau l} \qquad (28)$$

where τ is the turbidity and l is the path length of the medium.

The scattering phenomenon has been applied in determining the concentration of macromolecules in a suspension and the molecular weight (particle weight) of proteins and polymers.

Turbidimetry and Nephelometry—These techniques have been employed in determining the properties of macromolecules. Turbidimetry refers to the measurement of transmitted-light intensity at a 0° angle. This gives poor sensitivity when the turbidity is low. Nephelometry refers to the measurement of the scattered-light intensity at an angle of 75°–135°. Such measurements have a high sensitivity at low turbidity. At high turbidity, interparticle interference makes nephelometry somewhat unreliable.

The components of a nephelometer are somewhat similar to a UV-visible spectrophotometer. Both the monochromatic radiation source (eg, the mercury arc) and the polychromatic source (eg, the tungsten lamp) have been used. By employing appropriate filters, light with the desirable wavelength can be provided. The most widely used detector is the photomultiplier tube. The detector is either fixed at a 90° angle to the transmitted light or mounted on a movable disc to allow the measurement of the scattered light at any desirable angle.

Light Scattering in Molecular-Weight Determinations—Macromolecules such as polymers and proteins possess the light-scattering property when dissolved in solvents. Two features need to be considered when molecular-weight determination of high-molecular-weight substances is desired: the size and the concentration of the macromolecules in the solution. As the size of the molecules become larger than $\frac{1}{20}$ of the incident wavelength, a complex asymmetric scattering pattern will be created which in turn will cause an intensity attenuation at angle θ larger than 90° (backward direction). A high concentration causes an intermolecular interference. Observing both variables, the molecular weight of isotropic macromolecules can be obtained by

$$\lim_{\substack{c \to 0 \\ \theta \to 0}} \frac{I_v}{c} = \left[\frac{4\pi^2\eta_0^2(\partial\eta/\partial c)^2}{\lambda^4 N}\right]M \qquad (29)$$

where I_v is the reduced scattered intensity of the vertically polarized light (the value of I_v at 90° is known as Rayleigh's ratio), c is the concentration in Gm/ml, η_0 is the refractive index of the solvent, N is Avogadro's number, λ is the wavelength of incident light, and M is the weight-average molecular weight of the substance. The value $(\partial\eta/\partial c)^2$ can be replaced by $[(\eta - \eta_0)/c]^2$, where η is the refractive index of the solution. These refractive indices usually are determined by means of a differential refractometer (described in the next section).

The value of I_v can be calculated by

$$I_v = i\theta r^2/I_v^0 \qquad (30)$$

where I_v^0 is the intensity of the vertically polarized incident light, $i\theta$ is the excess intensity measured at angle θ (relative to the incident light), and r is the distance from the detector to the center of the solution.

Incorporation of a thermodynamic constant, A_2, and a probability distribution function, $P(\theta)$, in Eq. 29 gives

$$Kc/I_v = 1/MP(\theta) + 2A_2 c \qquad (31)$$

from which the molecular weight of macromolecules can be calculated.

In practice, light-scattering data should be acquired at four or five different concentrations and at one or more angles. Plotting concentration against Kc/I_v and extrapolating to and $c = 0$ to $\theta = 0$ (at which the value of $P(\theta)$ becomes unity), the reciprocal of the molecular weight will be obtained. This is one of the methods of calculating the weight-average molecular weight, $\bar{M}_w$, which is defined as

$$\bar{M}_w = \Sigma n_i M_i^2 / \Sigma n_i M_i \qquad (32)$$

where n_i is the number of particles having molecular weight M_i.

Refractometry and Interferometry

Theory—When electromagnetic radiation impinges obliquely upon the interface of two substances of different densities, an abrupt change in the direction of the beam in the new medium is observed. This phenomenon is known as refraction and is illustrated in Fig. 463. The angle of incidence, θ_1, is equal to the angle of reflection, θ_2. The angle θ_3 is called the angle of refraction and differs from θ_1. The relationship between θ_1 and θ_3 depends on the velocity of light in each medium and is expressed by

$$\sin \theta_1/\sin \theta_3 = v_1/v_2 = \eta \qquad (33)$$

where $\sin \theta_1$ and $\sin \theta_3$ are the sines of the angle of incidence and refraction, respectively, and v_1 and v_2 are the velocities of EM radiation in vacuum and the medium, respectively. The ratio $\sin \theta_1/\sin \theta_3$ is called the *refractive index* of the material and is designated by η. The refractive index is characteristic of the substance and varies with the wavelength of light. It should be observed that the frequency, ν, of the impinging EM radiation is identical in both media, and it is the velocity and the wavelength which vary in each medium.

If the incident light originates in a dense medium and passes into a rarer medium, η is less than 1; in the opposite case, η is greater than 1. Conventionally, the refractive index is expressed relative to air, whose refractive index is assumed to be approximately 1. Absolute refractive indices are found by

$$\eta_{abs} = \eta_{rel} \cdot \eta_{air} = 1.00027 \, \eta_{rel} \qquad (34)$$

The refractive index is calculated by

$$\frac{\eta}{\eta_1} = \frac{\sin \theta_1}{\sin \theta_3} \text{ or } \frac{\sin i}{\sin r} \qquad (35)$$

where i and r are the angles of incidence and refraction, respectively, η_1 is the refractive index of the medium at which the light is incident, and η_D^{20} is the refractive index measured at 20°C using a sodium-D line.

If the EM ray passes from a dense into a rare medium, r is greater than i. If i is increased to a limit where r is 90°, the light does not pass into the second medium, but rather it passes along the surface of the boundary of the two media. This incident angle is referred to as the *critical angle*, which provides a reference line in refractometry. If the angle of incidence is increased beyond its critical value, the ray will be reflected back from the surface. This is referred to as *total reflection*.

Since the refractive index varies with the temperature and pressure, a term has been devised to make the index independent of these variables. This term is known as *specific refraction*, r, and is expressed by

$$r = (\eta^2 - 1)/(\eta^2 + 2)d \qquad (36)$$

where d is the density of the liquid under investigation.

It is known that a given number of atoms in various molecules always contribute the same definite quantity to the molar refraction, which is defined as the product of the specific refraction and the molecular weight. The sum of atomic or group refractions is, therefore, equal to the experimentally determined molar refraction. The atomic refractions of a few

Table IV—Atomic Refractions

Group	M_{rD}
H	1.100
C	2.418
C=C	1.733
C≡C	2.398
O (with C=O)	2.211
O (O—H)	1.525
O (R—O—R)	1.643
N (1° amine)	2.322
N (2° amine)	2.499
N (3° amine)	2.840
C≡N	5.459
Cl	5.967
Br	8.865
I	13.900

elements are listed in Table IV. It is possible to determine the molecular structure of an unknown molecule by this method of computation.

Instrumentation—There are two major types of refractometers: (1) critical-angle and (2) image-displacement refractometers. The former is the most widely used in research and development.

Source—The source of illumination is either white light or monochromatic radiation. The sodium doublet line (sodium-D line) at 589.0 and 589.6 mμ is the most widely used source, as no filter is required. When white light (eg, a tungsten lamp or daylight) is used in the critical-angle instrument, the dispersion causes the critical boundary to be seen as a wide gray band. The necessary compensation for the dispersion is achieved by the use and proper adjustment of *Amici* prisms.

Critical-Angle Refractometers—The three commonly employed refractometers whose function is based on the critical-angle principles are the Abbe, the Pulfrich, and the immersion refractometer. These instruments provide satisfactory precision for the measurement of refractive indices of liquid and solid compounds.

The Abbe Refractometer—The prism system of an Abbe refractometer is depicted in Fig. 464A. The rays from the source, reflected by a mirror, are directed into the lower prism, P_1 (illuminating prism). The upper surface of this prism is rough ground to function as a source for an infinite number of rays. These rays pass through the liquid sample at 90° and enter the upper prism, P_2 (refracting prism). The surface of P_2 is polished and the rays striking it are refracted. Since the refractive index varies with temperature, the prisms are partially hollowed and jacketed to allow for circulation of water which is maintained at a constant temperature.

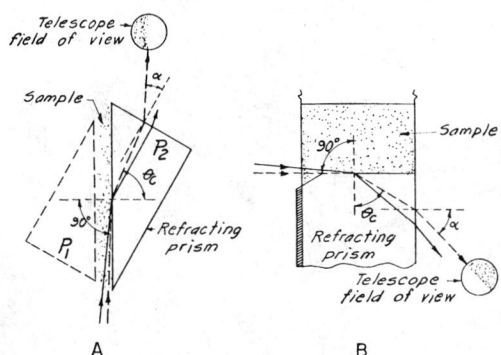

Fig. 463. The reflection and refraction of light; θ_C: critical angle.   Fig. 464. The prisms of the Abbe (A) and Pulfrich (B) refractometers.

The radiation impinges on a thin layer of a sample, held between prisms P_1 and P_2, grazing at or near 90°. The relation between the critical angle, the refractive index η_2 of prism P_2 (Medium 2), and the refractive index η_1 of the sample (Medium 1) is given by

$$\eta_2/\eta_1 = 1/\sin \theta_c \qquad (37)$$

As is noted in Fig. 464A, all incident rays of an angle less than 90° will be refracted at angles smaller than θ_c and a dark–light boundary is formed with the rays incident at 90°. There are two facts which require emphasis at this point: (1) the refractive index of a substance is measurable only if η_2 is greater than η_1 and (2) it is the emergence angle, α, of the critical ray rather than the critical ray itself that is measured by the refractometer. This angle is detected by moving a telescope, connected to P_2, to and fro until the dark–light boundary becomes centered. The scale is calibrated to read the refractive index directly.

If a tungsten lamp is employed as the energy source, a pair of Amici prisms is used to compensate for dispersion. Accuracy with the Abbe refractometer is about 0.0001 and the range of η is from 1.30–1.70.

The Pulfrich Refractometer—As depicted in Fig. 464B, the refracting prism P_2 is located under the sample. As with the Abbe refractometer, the angle α, which is the refracted angle from P_2, is observed by a telescope connected to a graduated arc. The accuracy of the instrument is about 0.0001 unit in η and the range of measurement is 1.33–1.60.

The Immersion Refractometer—This instrument is commonly employed for analyzing solutions. A single prism is mounted rigidly in the telescope and the samples under investigation are placed in small beakers and partly immersed in a constant-temperature water bath. The prism is immersed in the beaker containing the sample, which is illuminated with a mirror which reflects light from the source. As with the Abbe refractometer, an Amici compensator is used also with the immersion instrument. The transparent scale, graduated from −5 to +105 arbitrary units, is located at the focal plane of the eyepiece. Light hitting the face of the prism at all angles up to the grazing angle is refracted to give a light field observed in the scale. Conversion tables are designed to convert the readings of the immersion refractometer into refractive index values or directly into concentrations of sugar, alcohol, etc.

Image-Displacement Refractometers—These instruments are constructed in accordance with the principle that any prism spectrometer is also a refractometer. If the prism of a spectroscope is replaced by a prism-shaped vessel containing the sample, the image of the slit will be displaced proportional to the refractive index of the sample prism. The refractive index value is read from the graduated arc attached to a movable telescope arm, by whose manipulation the refracted slit image can be centered in the field. The accuracy of the instrument is about $\pm 10^{-6}$ in units of η. A large range of wavelengths, UV to IR, can be employed as a source of radiation. In contrast to critical-angle refractometers, these instruments are capable of measuring any value of refractive index.

Differential Refractometers—These refractometers are designed to detect any difference between the refractive index of the sample compared to a reference, when placed separately into two hollow prisms. Any difference between the values of η will cause an angular deviation of the slit image, which is measured by using a stationary telescope. This method is used in gel-permeation chromatography.

A method involving *schlieren* techniques, using the principle of the refractive index phenomenon, has been employed for determining the concentration gradients of protein solutions in an electrophoresis cell and ultracentrifuge. The separated homogeneous layers of protein will show a detectable refractive index change at the interface.

The Interferometer—This instrument is a differential refractometer whose function is based on the interference phenomenon of light; this principle is depicted in Fig. 465A. The analytical results are reliable to the 7th decimal place for liquids and the 8th for gases. As shown, the sample and the reference are placed individually into two matched cells, C_1 and C_2, of equal path length. The velocities of light in the two cells are proportional to their indexes of refraction. The difference between the sample and the reference will appear on the screen; ie, a deviation of the point from its original position. The optical length can be varied by rotating the glass plate P_1 (a plate located at a 45° angle to the beam). The magnitude of rotation, measured by a micrometer, is read as refractive index on a scale.

Application—The refractive index, η, is an intrinsic property of a substance, as are melting point and boiling point. It is complementary to the results from IR, UV, and NMR in determining the identity and purity of a chemical.

Numerous reference books and handbooks list the refractive indexes of various compounds. If, however, the refractive index of a compound is not available, the value can be estimated by adding the atomic refractions of the compound. The refractive index is calculated by using the formula

$$R = [(\eta - 1)/(\eta + 2)]^2 M/d \qquad (38)$$

where R is the molecular refractive index, M is the molecular weight, and d is the density.

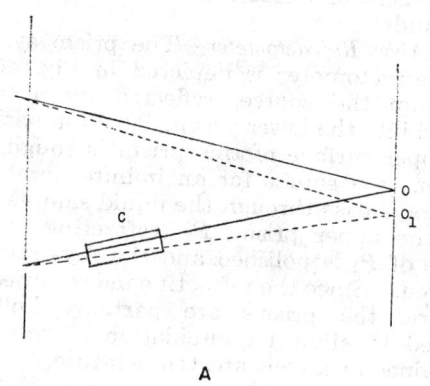

A

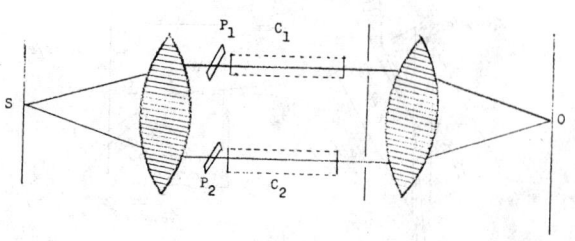

B

Fig. 465. A simplified optical system of two different types of interferometers.

In general, the measurement of refractive index is simple enough to allow laboratory personnel with little training to carry out the procedure with extreme precision and accuracy.

Polarimetry

The fundamental principle of polarimetric analysis is based on the existence of optical activity in a substance; ie, the ability of a material to rotate plane-polarized light. Biot, Fresnel, and Pasteur were the pioneers in the investigation of optical rotation and demonstration of change in rotatory power as a function of wavelength. This latter concept, which was neglected for about a century, is now the basis of optical rotatory dispersion techniques.

Polarimetry is applicable in the determination of the molecular structure of substances which do not have a rotation–reflection symmetry axis (*vide infra*). Determination of the sugar content of foodstuffs is an example of the quantitative application of polarimetry.

Theory—EM radiation consists of perpendicular electric and magnetic vectors vibrating in all orientations mutually perpendicular to the direction of propagation. Plane-polarized light is obtained by passing a beam of light through an anisotropic crystal. By this process, the components of the electric fields and magnetic fields in all directions but two perpendicular planes are excluded. Since the interacting vector with matter is the electric vector, the term plane is appropriate.

The polarization of EM radiation and its interaction with matter requires some description. Light can be polarized by various devices of which Polaroid discs and Nicol prisms are the most widely used. These two polarizers function in the visible and IR EM radiation range. The emergent radiation from a Nicol prism, made of calcite crystals, possesses 50% of the intensity of the incident radiation. As is true in the case of many other crystalline substances, calcite exhibits optical anisotropy; ie, impinging radiation is not affected identically in all directions but, except in the direction of the optical axis, a monochromatic radiation travels through the crystal with varying speeds. This is due to the difference in the spacing of units in the crystal lattice or variation in the quantities of each kind of constituting atoms in various sections of the crystal. A crystal may have one or two optical axes which are uniaxial or biaxial, respectively. The former type, which is of interest in polarimetry, resolves an incident beam into two rays with perpendicular planes, one of which is in the principal plane. A principal plane is constructed between an optical axis and the perpendicular to one of the main faces of the crystal. The ray traveling along the optical axis is known as the *ordinary ray*, and that along the principal plane is known as the *extraordinary ray*. The index of refraction of the latter ray varies with the direction of the beam. This resolution of a beam by an anisotropic crystal into two plane-polarized rays is known as *double refraction* or *optical birefringence*.

Polarization by a Nicol prism is depicted in Fig. 466. In calcite the refractive index of the ordinary ray is 1.66 and that of the extraordinary ray is 1.49. The value of η for Canada balsam is 1.55. Due to the higher value of η for the ordinary ray than that of the balsam, at an angle greater than the critical angle, the ray will be totally reflected. The extraordinary ray, however, will be transmitted because its η value is lower than

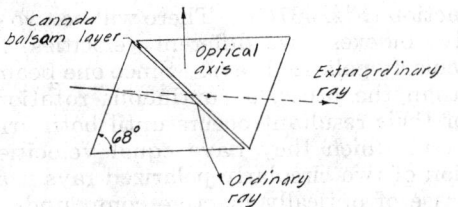

Fig. 466.   The Nicol prism.

that of the balsam. This transmitted ray is the polarized ray.

Since Canada balsam absorbs UV radiation, a Nicol prism is restricted to the visible region only. The Foucault prism, in which the balsam is replaced by air, functions in the UV range. There are also other UV prisms wherein glycerin is used instead of the balsam.

If the polarized light emerging from the Nicol prism is directed into an optically active substance, its plane of polarization will be rotated. In order to have optical activity, a molecule should be devoid of a center of symmetry, a plane of symmetry, and an alternating rotation–reflection axis of symmetry. Since a one-fold alternating axis of symmetry is equivalent to one plane and a two-fold alternating axis is equivalent to a center of inversion, the absence of an alternating rotation–reflection axis of symmetry in a molecule is required for optical activity. The interaction of the electric field of the radiation with the electronic configuration of the molecule causes the electric field of the radiation to change its direction of oscillation. In symmetric molecules no optical rotation is observed because equal rotations in the opposite direction are cancelled. In asymmetric molecules these rotations do not average to zero and the net result is the rotation of plane-polarized light. Another way of expressing this concept is to envisage that the incident plane-polarized light, impinging upon an optically active substance, is resolved into two circularly polarized beams oscillating in opposite directions, clockwise and counterclockwise. In reality, this is *circular double refraction* (Fig. 467A). The magnitude of the resultant of the two vectors varies as a

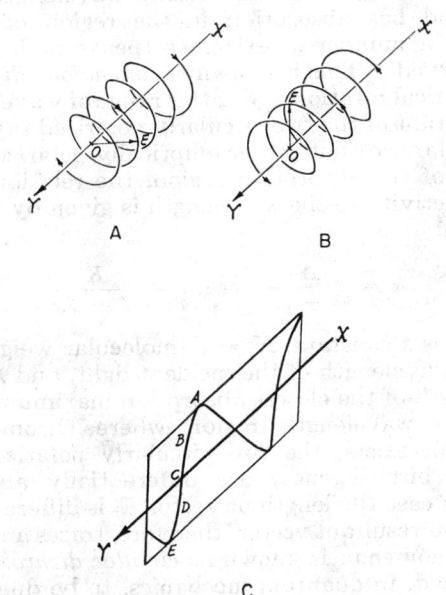

Fig. 467.   *A* and *B*: Right and left circularly polarized light; *C*: the vector sum of *A* and *B*.

sine function (Fig. 467C). There will be two different refractive indexes (two different velocities) for these two circularly polarized rays. Since one beam travels faster than the other, a continuous rotation of the plane of their resultant occurs until both arrive in a medium in which they have equal velocities. The formation of two circularly polarized rays is also true in the case of optically inactive compounds, but the velocities or refractive indexes of the left-hand and right-hand circularly polarized rays are equal.

The relationship between the angle of rotation and the difference in refractive indexes is given by Fresnel's formula:

$$\alpha = 2\pi l \, (\eta_l - \eta_r)/\lambda \tag{39}$$

where λ is the wavelength of EM radiation in a vacuum, l is the pathlength, and η_l and η_r are the refractive indexes of the left-hand and right-hand circularly polarized rays.

The specific rotation α is obtained by

$$[\alpha] = \alpha 1800/c\pi \tag{40}$$

which is derived from Eq. 39, wherein α is in degrees/dm (obtained by using the conversion factor $1800/\pi$) and c is the concentration in Gm/ml of solution.

The molar rotation $[\Phi]$ is given by

$$\Phi = [\alpha]M/100 \tag{41}$$

where M is the molecular weight of the substance.

Optical Rotatory Dispersion—To exhibit optical activity, the medium should be *circularly birefringent;* ie, η_l and η_r for the two circularly polarized beams must be different. The values of η_l and η_r, however, vary with wavelength and, therefore, $[\alpha]$ and $[\Phi]$ vary as a function of wavelength. This is the principle of optical rotatory dispersion.

A plot of $[\alpha]$ vs λ provides the curve shown in Fig. 468A. For compounds which do not have absorption in the wavelength region where optical activity is being examined, the increase in magnitude of optical activity is inversely proportional to the increase in wavelength.

A plain dispersion curve is designated as positive or negative according to the rise or fall of the rotation curve as a function of decreasing wavelength. If a compound has absorption in the region of optical activity, a number of extremes (peaks and troughs) are observed. This is known as *anomalous dispersion* of the optical rotation. For this range of wavelengths, the resultant of the two circularly polarized rays is not plane-polarized, but rather elliptically polarized light. Outside of the absorption region, the relationship of optical activity to the wavelength is given by Drude's equation:

$$\alpha = \frac{A}{\lambda^2 - \lambda_0^2} \quad \text{or} \quad \Phi = \frac{K}{\lambda^2 - \lambda_0^2} \tag{42}$$

where A is a constant, $K = A \cdot$ molecular weight$/100$, λ is the wavelength of the incident light, and λ_0 is the wavelength of the closest absorption maximum.

In the wavelength region where chromophoric absorption exists, the two circularly polarized rays (circular birefringence) are differentially absorbed. In such a case the length of vector E_r is different from E_l. Their resultant vector, therefore, traces an ellipse. This phenomenon is known as *circular dichroism* and is theorized, in quantum mechanics, to be due to the difference in transition probability between right-hand and left-hand circularly polarized light. The angle of

ellipticity, ψ, measured in radians/unit length, is

$$\psi = \pi \, (K_l - K_r)/\lambda \tag{43}$$

where λ is the wavelength of incident light and K_l and K_r are the absorption coefficients for right-hand and left-hand circularly polarized light, respectively. The value of $k = 2.3 \, \epsilon \, c;$ where ϵ is absorptivity and c is the molar concentration.

The term ψ is analogous to α; therefore,

$$[\psi] = \psi/lc \tag{44}$$

where $[\psi]$ is the specific ellipticity, l is the pathlength in dm, and c is the concentration in Gm/ml.

Cotton Effect—Fig. 468B depicts typical optical rotatory dispersion curves for *trans*-8-methylhydrindan-5-one and its *cis* isomer. The compounds are said to exhibit the Cotton effect. A positive Cotton effect is assigned to a curve if the rotation rises to a maximum toward the short wavelength prior to changing sign, as is exhibited by the *trans* isomer. The opposite is a negative Cotton effect. Optical rotatory dispersion is useful in conformational and configurational analysis of organic compounds, particularly the steroids.

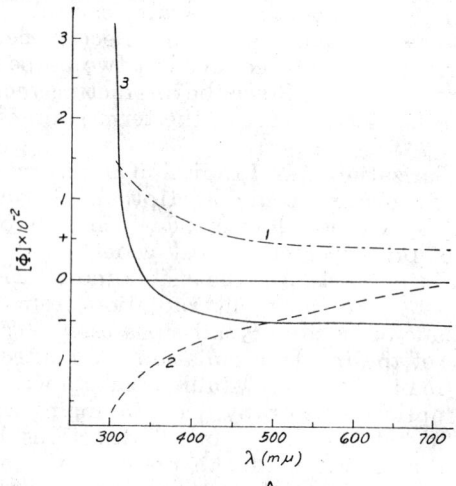

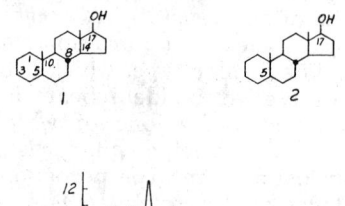

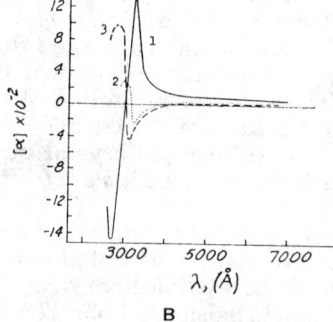

Fig. 468. *A:* **The plain dispersion curve of (+)-17β-hydroxy-5α-androstane (1), (−)-17α-hydroxy-5α-androstane (2), (+) and (−)-α-(o-iodophenoxy)propionic acid.** *B:* **The ORD dispersion curves of (1)** *trans*-8-methylhydrinandan-5-one; **(2)** *cis*-8-methylhydrindan-5-one; **(3)** β-norcoprostan-3-one.

Instrumentation

Instrumentation—A polarimeter consists of the following components:

Source—Monochromatic light source should be employed if determination of the optical rotation of various asymmetric substances is desired. Emission from either a sodium lamp with lines at 5890 and 5896Å or a mercury lamp with lines at 4358, 5461, 5770, and 5791Å can be used. White light can be employed if the polarimeter is to be used for measuring only single substances, or if the dispersion of the optical rotation for each sample can be compensated. A hydrogen lamp or a xenon lamp with a monochromator is employed in the UV region.

Polarizer and Analyzer—The Nicol prism is the most widely used polarizing and analyzing device for use in the visible region. Another method of polarizing radiation is with a Polaroid filter. This consists of a film of dichroic crystals which absorb one of the polarized beams to a greater extent than the other. The Polaroid wavelength range is limited to 5000–6800Å and pure linearly polarized light is not produced by this means. In a polarimeter the intensity of light emerging from an analyzer is given by Malus' law:

$$I = KI_0 \cos^2 \theta \qquad (45)$$

where I is the intensity of light emerging from the analyzer, I_0 is the intensity of light incident on the analyzer, θ is the angle between the direction of transmission of the analyzer and the polarizer, and K is a constant approximately equal to 1; it accounts for reflection and absorption of light by the analyzer.

Sample Tube—This tube should contain parallel glass discs at the ends. These discs should be devoid of strain, otherwise a partial circular polarization occurs. Prior to use, each tube should be tested by filling it with water, placing it in the instrument, and observing the constancy of the zero rotation point (uniform dark field).

Detector—Generally, visual matching of light intensities of a half-shaded device or a dark field is employed for detection. The double-field polarimeter has one auxiliary Nicol prism which covers half the field of the polarizing prism. This gives a field with two parts. An optical rotation for a substance is recorded when the rotation of the analyzer, attached to a graduated disc for direct reading, renders a uniform field.

Application and Analytical Procedure—Quantitative determination of a number of optically active substances is one of the paramount applications of polarimetry. Conventionally, the optical rotation of a substance is expressed in terms of a specific rotation, $[\alpha]_\lambda^t$. The temperature and wavelength at which measurement has been determined is designated as a superscript and subscript, respectively, following α.

To determine the optical rotation of a substance, the pure liquid, or a solution of a liquid or solid, is placed in a sample tube and inserted between the analyzer and polarizer Nicol prisms. The prisms have been previously oriented, without the sample, to give a uniform intensity field when viewed axially. An optically active substance in the sample cell will rotate the plane of polarized light and unbalance the split field. If the analyzer prism must be turned clockwise to restore the original uniform field, the sample substance is said to be dextrorotatory; if counterclockwise, the sample is levorotatory.

Mass Spectrometry

The phenomenon of deflection of ions in electric or magnetic fields was first proposed by Wien in 1898. Using this principle, Thompson in 1912 and Aston in 1919 performed some experimental work on the identification and quantification of isotopes. A mass spectrometer for general use, however, did not become available until the mid-1930's.

Theory and Instrumentation—The theoretical and instrumental aspects of mass spectrometry are somewhat intermingled and it is appropriate, therefore, to discuss them together.

The principle of mass spectrometry consists of the (1) generation of positive ions (primarily from organic molecules), (2) separation of ions according to their mass, and (3) collection of ions and recording the quantity of each species. Molecules up to a mass of 500 can be analyzed by single-focusing (magnetic-focusing) instruments. The double-focusing instruments, in which a combination of electrostatic and magnetic fields has been employed, provide a higher resolution. An accurate molecular weight (to four decimal places) can be obtained by the latter instrument. A mass spectrometer is shown in Fig. 469. The following sequence provides the analytical procedure common to most mass spectrometric measurements.

Introduction of Sample and Ion Production—A gas sample is introduced from a gas bulb into a small glass manifold. A known volume is passed into a reservoir where the pressure is 50–100μ. Liquids are introduced by a micropipet or by injection through a silicone rubber dam using a hypodermic syringe and needle. Due to the vacuum in the reservoir, the liquid is drawn in as a vapor.

Solid samples are ordinarily volatilized by heating and a vapor pressure of 10^{-2} torr is necessary, while a sample is still below its decomposition temperature, in order to introduce sufficient sample into the ionization chamber. In recently developed instruments, the sample can be heated in high vacuum in the proximity of the electron beam. A compound must be stable at a temperature at which its vapor pressure is about 10^{-7} torr. Special handling techniques are required for compounds exhibiting thermal instability. The sample in the vapor form enters the ion-producing chamber via a small orifice, known as *molecular leak*.

The sample vapor can be transformed into ions by various means; the electron bombardment of the vapor is the most widely used. In the case of inorganic substances, ions can be obtained by surface ionization (heating a metal surface) or by the vacuum spark, where a spark is induced between two electrodes of a metal or semiconductor. A rf spark (1 mHz/sec) is used for high-melting solids. The ionization chamber, where the neutral molecules from the molecular leak enter, is maintained at a pressure of 10^{-6} torr.

A hot, carbonized, tungsten filament provides electrons which are drawn off by a pair of positively charged slits and directed on the vaporized sample molecules. The collision of electrons with molecules produces both negative and positive ions. Currently, mass spectrometers only make use of the positive species. The electric field can be varied from 6 to 100 v and *parent ions* and fragments with various mass numbers are produced in this potential range.

The positive parent ions and fragment ions are accelerated toward the analyzing tube by one positively charged repeller slit, placed after the molecular leak, and two negatively charged slits located between the electron beam and the entrance to the analyzer tube. The ions can be accelerated up to 150,000 miles/sec by applying voltages ranging from 400 to 4000 v across the two accelerating slits. The potential energy, eV, of an accelerated ion will be equal to its kinetic energy; ie, $eV = \frac{1}{2}mv^2$, where m is the mass of the ion of charge e and velocity v in terms of the accelerating voltage V.

The Analyzer Tube—This tube which guides the ions to the collector is located between two magnetic poles and maintained at a pressure of 10^{-7} to 10^{-8} torr. The path of the ions is shown in Fig. 469. Varying the current in the electromagnet increases or decreases the force imposed upon the ions; thereby, each ion beam is brought into focus at the exit slit.

Ion Collector—The ion beam, upon passing through the exit slit of the analyzer tube, carries a current of 10^{-18} to 10^{-10} amp. This current is amplified by an electrometer prior to recording.

Recorder—Five separate galvanometers are used to record simultaneously the peaks for fragment ions and the parent ion. The relative sensitivity ratios are 1:3:10:30:100. Also, electrical data from the ion collector may be fed into a computer which assesses the data and prints out the mass and relative abundance of each molecular fragment generated in the ionization chamber.

Resolution in mass spectrometry is defined as the mass divided by the difference between closely related mass numbers; ie, $M/\Delta M$. For example, to differentiate between O_2 of mass 31.9898 and S of mass 31.9721, a resolution of 1800 is necessary.

Mass Spectra and Molecular Structure—With the low-energy electron beams in the order of 8–14 eV it is possible to observe the molecular ion (parent ion). Unlike other analytical methods, mass spectrometry gives an exact molecular weight. The mass spectrograph of toluene shows a peak at $m/e = 92$ (m/e is the mass to charge ratio; for the parent ion this value

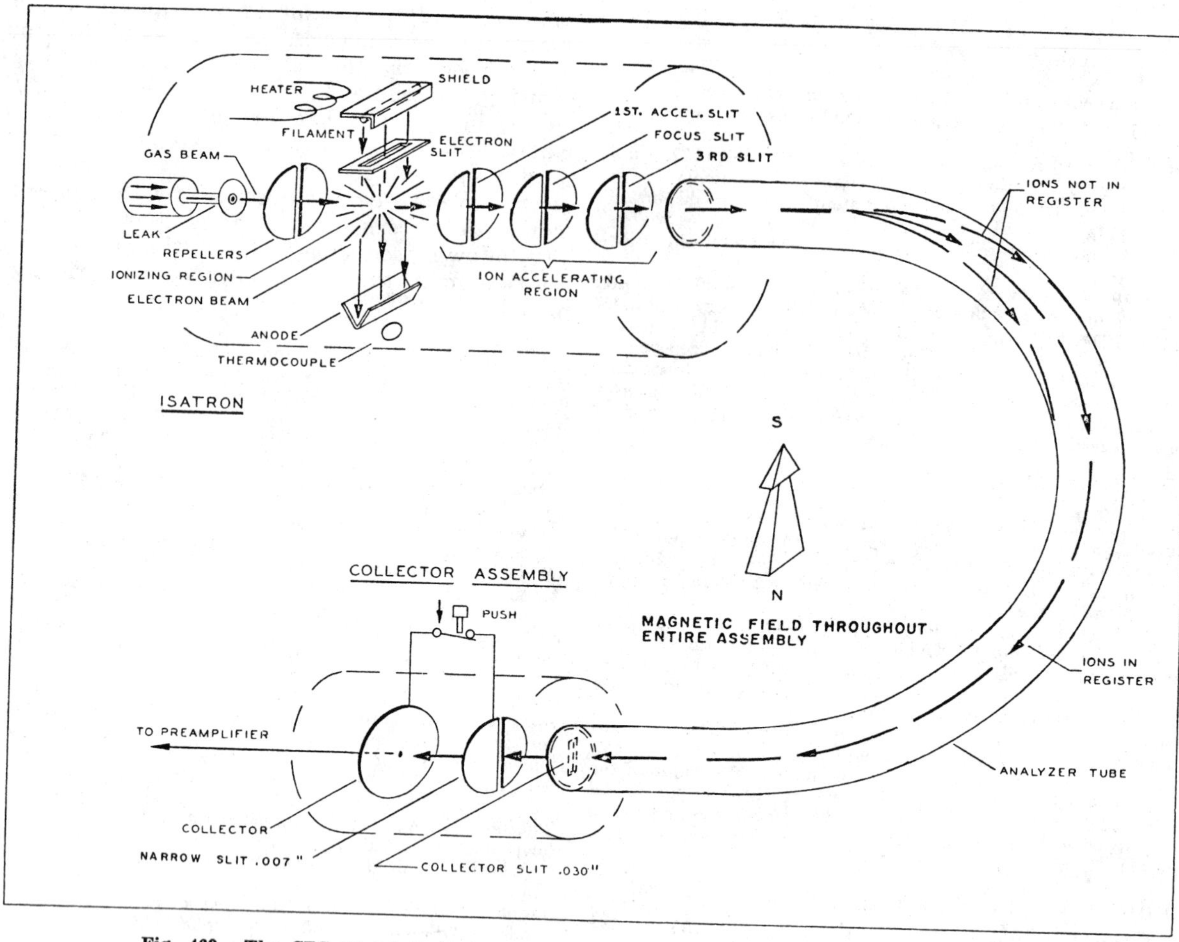

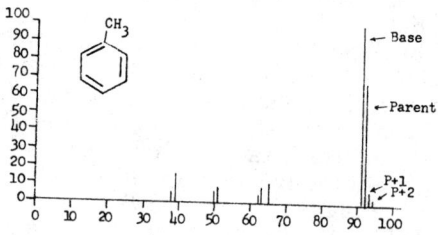

Fig. 469.   The CEC Model 21-103C mass spectrometer (Courtesy, Consol. Electrodynamics).

is also the molecular weight), which is developed according to

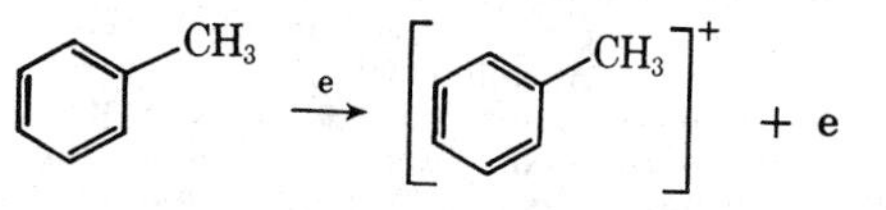

$$\text{(}\bigcirc\text{)}\!-\!CH_3 \xrightarrow{\ e\ } \left[\text{(}\bigcirc\text{)}\!-\!CH_3\right]^+ + e \qquad (46)$$

With a high-energy electron beam, in the order of 70 eV, the parent ion disintegrates, due to the removal of several electrons, giving positively charged and uncharged fragments. Adopting the symbolism for the transfer of a single electron by a single-headed arrow, two typical examples for fragmentation can be given by

$$R\!-\!\overset{\frown}{CH_2}\!-\!NH_2 \longrightarrow R \cdot + CH_2\!\!=\!\!\overset{+}{NH_2}$$

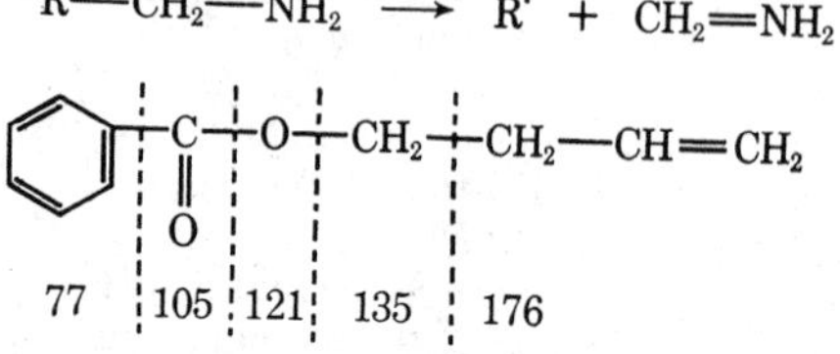

$$\text{(}\bigcirc\text{)}\!-\!\overset{C}{\underset{O}{\parallel}}\!-\!O\!-\!CH_2\!-\!CH_2\!-\!CH\!\!=\!\!CH_2 \qquad (47)$$

77 ¦ 105 ¦ 121 ¦ 135 ¦ 176

The mass spectrum of a compound, therefore, is a display of masses of molecular fragments together with the mass of the parent ion vs the relative abundance of each species as depicted by the peak heights.

The graphic form of the mass spectrum of toluene and its tabular presentation is depicted in Fig. 470.

m/e	o/o OF BASE PEAK	m/e	o/o of P
38	4.4	92 (P)	100
39	16	93 (P+1)	7.37
45	3.9	94 (P+2)	0.29
50	6.3		
51	9.1		
62	4.1		
63	8.6		
65	11		
91	100 (Base)		
92	68 (Parent)		
93	5.3 (P+1)		
94	0.21 (P+2)		

Fig. 470.   Relative abundance of various fragments shown in the mass spectrogram of toluene (courtesy, Silverstein and Bassler[2]).

The most intense mass peak is referred to as the *base peak* and is assigned an arbitrary value of 100; the other peaks are measured relative to this. Since the ratios of fragment abundance for a given compound remains constant, a mass spectrum (like an IR spectrum) becomes a "fingerprint" for each molecule.

Several empirical rules of molecular fragmentation are listed below:

1. Cyclic compounds show an intense parent peak and a peak at the mass number of the ring.
2. Saturated cyclic compounds lose side-chains at the α-carbon. The peaks resulting from the loss of two atoms from the ring is more intense than the peaks from the loss of one atom.
3. In cyclic compounds containing a double bond next to the side-chain, cleavage occurs at the bond β to the ring.
4. In olefins, cleavage occurs β to the double bond.
5. In compounds with heteroatoms, cleavage occurs at the bond β to the heteroatom.
6. In hydrocarbon molecules, the ease of cleavage is in the following order: tertiary > secondary > primary. The positive charge remains on the branched fragment.
7. In carbonyl-containing compounds, cleavage occurs at this group, the positive charge remaining on the $\diagup C{=}O$-containing fragment.

The isotope abundance of atoms such as Cl, Br, S, and Si leads to the detection of these elements by mass spectrometry. For example, the ratio of ^{35}Cl to ^{37}Cl is 100 to 32.5.

For compounds of the general formula $C_wH_xN_yO_z$, contribution from the heavy isotopes can be calculated by

$$100\frac{P+1}{P} = 1.11w + 0.015x + 0.37y + 0.037z \quad (48)$$

and

$$100\frac{P+2}{P} =$$
$$0.0002wx + 0.004wy + 0.006w(w-1) + 0.20z \quad (49)$$

where P is the monoisotopic peak (parent peak; equivalent to the nominal molecular weight value) and $P+1$ and $P+2$ are the monoisotopic mass number plus one and two mass numbers, respectively. The relative isotope abundance of the heavy isotopes of each element determines the height of the $P+1$ and $P+2$ peaks. By consulting special tables of abundance factors for the $P+1$ and $P+2$ peaks, it is possible to determine an exact molecular formula from mass spectral data.

The following example represents the use of isotopic contribution in structural elucidation.

A compound with a mass spectrogram of $P=110$ (100%), $P+1=111$ (5.5%), and $P+2=112$ (0.3%) could be sorted out of the following molecular formulas with the molecular weight of 110:

Formula	$P+1$	$P+2$
$C_3H_2N_4O$	4.84	0.30
$C_4H_2N_2O_2$	5.20	0.51
$C_4H_4N_3O$	5.57	0.33
$C_4H_6N_4$	5.94	0.15
$C_5H_2O_3$	5.55	0.73
$C_5H_4NO_2$	5.93	0.55

The data reveal that the molecular formula of the compound is $C_4H_4N_3O$.

The fragmentation patterns of a few representative chemical classes are illustrated below. More detailed information can be obtained by consulting reference books on mass spectrometry.

Molecular fragmentation may occur by one or a combination of the following processes: simple fission, simple rearrangement, complex fission, and complex rearrangement.

Simple Fission and Simple Rearrangement—

Saturated Hydrocarbons—Peaks varying from one another by a multiple of 14 (CH_2) are observed in the spectrum of the saturated hydrocarbons. If branching is present, fission occurs at the tertiary or quaternary center. This is due to the order of stability of carbonium ion (tertiary > secondary > primary) generated during the ionization stage. By this technique, the position of branching can be recognized:

$$[R_3C - CR_3]^{\cdot+} \rightarrow R_3C^+ + R_3C\cdot \quad (50)$$

Olefins—Usually, allylic cleavage occurs. Migration of the double bond is not unusual. Cyclic olefins depict a distinct parent peak.

Aromatic Hydrocarbons—These molecules, because of high stability, show a large parent peak. The $m/e = 65, 77, 78, 79, 91,$ and 92 in alkyl-substituted benzenes are ascribed to the following rearrangements:

Molecules with Heteroatom C—X—If a heteroatom such as N, O, S, or F is present on the hydrocarbon skeleton, fission occurs at the α carbon–carbon bond. The onium ion is stabilized due to pairing of an odd n electron with the odd electron originating from C—C fission.

The fragmentation of a secondary alcohol will proceed as follows:

Molecules with Heteroatom C=X—The cleavage is similar to the single-bonded heteroatom.

Fragmentation of an aldehyde, ketone, and ester are shown in the following equations:

(56)

(57)

(58)

A rearrangement process may accompany simple fissions. A ketone and a nitrile undergo rearrange-

ments as follows:

(59)

(60)

Further description and discussion in mass spectrometry is beyond the scope of this chapter. The books listed in the *Bibliography* cover the subject extensively.

Electrometric Methods

Chemical analyses in which electrical current, voltage, or resistance is involved are known as electrochemical reactions. To facilitate discussion of this topic, some fundamental concepts of electrical and electrochemical phenomena should be reviewed.

Although the electrical waves associated with the generation of power and lighting equipment are classified under EM radiation, their interaction with matter differs from the relatively high-frequency optical waves such as UV and visible. The signals from the former travel in metal but those from the latter travel in space.

The following are a few commonly employed units in electricity:

Coulomb (Q)—The coulomb is a quantity of electricity. One electron has a charge of 1.602×10^{-19} Q. One Q can deposit 0.0011180 Gm of silver.

Faraday (F)—The Faraday is 96,489 Q, the charge carried by an equivalent weight.

Ampere (I)—The ampere is the unit of electric current. A rate of flow of 1 Q/sec is designated as 1 amp.

Ohm (Ω)—The ohm is the electrical resistance of a uniform column of mercury at 0°C with a mass of 14.4521 Gm, a length of 106.300 cm, and uniform cross section.

Volt (v)—The volt is the potential difference required to produce a current of 1 amp through a resistance of 1 ohm. The symbol for potential is E. Volt is equal to the product of current and resistance (v = IR).

Watt (w)—The watt is the unit of power; work performed at a rate of 1 joule/sec. It is equal to the product of current and voltage (P = EI).

For a proper understanding of electrochemical methods, it is appropriate to describe a few pertinent components and terms.

Electrodes—Gases and liquids which are capable of conducting current, depositing materials at the electrodes, or dissolving the electrodes are known as electrolytes. Metallic conductors immersed in electrolytes are known as electrodes. A negative electrode (cathode) is the supplier of electrons in a chemical cell. An electron emitter in a vacuum tube is called a cathode. A collector of positive ions in a gas-filled tube is also known as an electrode (anode). Electrodes are also discussed under *Potentiometry*.

The standard electrode potential ($E°$) is the potential of the electrode immersed in a solution of its ions at unit activity ($a = 1$). All the electrode potentials are referred to the hydrogen electrode set at $E°_{\text{Pt, H}_2, \text{H}^+} = 0$.

When a cell is operating reversibly, the electrical work (ΔF) obtained per Gm-atom is the maximum work given by

$$\Delta F = -nFE \qquad (61)$$

where n is the valence change, F is a Faraday (96,489 coulombs), and E is the voltage or electromotive force (emf) of the cell.

Electrical Cell—An electrical cell is an electrical circuit which consists of two electrodes and a solution of electrolytes. One electrode functions as an electron acceptor and the other as an electron donor. There are two general types of electrochemical cells:

1. A galvanic cell, in which the chemical energy is converted into electrical energy by spontaneous chemical reaction. The current, which occurs as a result of an oxidation–reduction reaction, continues so long as all the components are available.

2. An electrolytic cell, in which chemical reactions occur as a result of an applied potential.

Electrochemical methods of analysis are divided into two major categories:

1. Potentiometry, which involves determination of the emf of chemical cells. This method is applicable to quantitative chemical measurements.

2. Voltametry, which involves electrolysis. This method provides information on the composition of a solution.

Potentiometry

Potentiometric methods of analysis consist of the measurement of the emf of chemical cells. Two types of electrochemical analyses are performed by potentiometry:

1. A direct determination of electrode potential.
2. The measurement of changes in the emf of a cell vs the quantity of a titrant.

The emf of a cell is the sum of three potentials:

$$E_{\text{cell}} = E_{\text{ref}} + E_{\text{ind}} + E_{\text{jcn}} \qquad (62)$$

where the subscripts denote reference, indicator, and junction potentials, respectively. E_{jcn} is the potential at the liquid junction which is constant. Since the E_{ref} is known, the indicator electrode then can provide information about the concentration of a species involved in electron exchange. An inert electrode, such as platinum, immersed in a solution of an oxidation-reduction system, provides or accepts electrons and indicates the ratio of oxidized to reduced species. A general expression of this phenomenon is given by the Nernst equation:

$$E = E_0 + 0.0591 \log (A_{\text{oxid}}/A_{\text{red}}) \qquad (63)$$

where A is the activity of oxidized or reduced species.

A chemical cell consists of a reference electrode half-cell and an indicator electrode half-cell.

Reference Electrodes—The most widely used reference electrodes are the so-called *electrodes-of-the-second-kind*, which consist of either a mercury-calomel electrode or a silver-silver chloride electrode:

$$Hg \,|\, Hg_2Cl_2(s), \ KCl \ soln$$

or

$$Ag \,|\, AgCl(s), \ HCl \ soln$$

in which a calomel electrode connection to the test solution is made through a saturated solution of KCl and electric connection by a platinum wire in contact with the mercury, for the former. The half-cell reaction is given by

$$2Hg + 2Cl^- = Hg_2Cl_2 + 2e \qquad (64)$$

Indicator Electrodes—Noble metals are widely used as indicator electrodes. For example, platinum is used for the Fe^{2+}, Fe^{3+}, or H_2, H^+ potentiometric system.

There are also indicator *electrodes-of-the-second-kind*, such as Sb-Sb_2O_3 and Hg-Hg_2O (oxide electrodes), that are sensitive to H^+ and are employed in nonaqueous acid–base titrations.

The glass electrode is a membrane-type electrode, whose primary use is for the determination of H^+ concentration in aqueous solutions. The silicate network of the membrane absorbs water and alkali metal ions and becomes hydrated. An exchange of ions from solution to surface and *vice versa* occurs on a limited scale. The inner and outer glass surfaces assume potentials which depend on the solution with which they are in contact. The glass-electrode potential varies only with the pH of the external solution. The membrane of the electrode has a high resistance; ie, 5–1000 megohms at 25°. Considering this, the current drawn from this cell must be kept smaller than 10^{-11} amp if an error greater than 1 mv is to be avoided (10^{-11} amp × 100 megohms = 1 mv).

Metal-ion-sensitive glass electrodes have been constructed by replacing part of the silica in the glass structure with oxides of aluminum or boron. This type of glass electrode responds to univalent cations other than H^+, but not to polyvalent cations. Some of these electrodes are particularly sensitive to Na^+, Ag^+, and other ions.

Measurement of the Cell emf—This measurement is done potentiometrically by the null-balance method. An unknown-cell emf is determined by comparing it with a known-cell emf source. The circuit diagram of a simple potentiometer is depicted in Fig. 471.

Classes of Potentiometric Analyses

Measurement of pH—Determination of the activity of H^+ is done either (1) potentiometrically or (2) by direct reading with a pH meter. For the potentiometric measurement the apparatus consists of a potentiometer whose sensitivity has been increased by electronic amplification of the unbalance current. The second type is a circuit designed to give meter-needle deflection as a function of pH. This is essentially an electronic vacuum tube voltmeter (VTVM) with a high-input resistance.

Acid–Base Titration—An acid–base titration curve can be obtained by using a pH meter with a recorder (or manually plotting points). In an aqueous system, in order to obtain proper curves with well-resolved end-points, the acid or base to be titrated should be stronger than water and the concentration prepared for titration should be higher than the hydrogen or hydroxyl concentration of water. If the emf (E) obtained during the titration is plotted against volume (v) of the titrant, the end-point is the inflection point, or the steepest slope.

Precipitation and Complexation—An ion may be determined by a potentiometric precipitation or complexation titration. This method requires an indicator electrode that can detect one of the ions precisely or that the reaction be accompanied by a change in pH or redox potential. To arrive at an exact equivalence point, the salt formed during the titration should have a low solubility or the complex should demonstrate high stability. Examples of precipitation titrations are the formation of insoluble or undissociated salts of Ag^+ and Hg^+ with Cl^-, Br^-, I^-, CN^-, and CNS^-.

Complexation titration by potentiometry has been employed for quantification of ions such as Cu^{2+}. Ethylenediaminetetraacetic acid (EDTA) in the form of its disodium salt is the most widely used complexing agent. An indicator electrode that is sensitive either to the pH or to the metal ion is employed for detection of the end-point.

$$M^{2+} + H_2(EDTA)^{2-} = M(EDTA)^{2-} + 2H^+ \qquad (65)$$

Titrations in Nonaqueous Systems—Many organic acids and bases are too weak to be titrated in aqueous solvents. As is discussed in Chapter 20, *Ionic Solutions and Electrolytic Equilibria* and Chapter 37, *Analysis of Medicinals* (see analyses utilizing nonaqueous solvents), water is a leveling solvent, hydroxide ion being the strongest base and hydrogen ion the strongest acid which can be titrated. Any substance which is a weaker base or acid than water cannot be effectively titrated in an aqueous medium.

There are three general types of solvents:

1. Amphiprotic solvents, which have both acidic and basic properties. Examples: water, the lower alcohols, and acetic acid.
2. Aprotic solvents, which possess no acidic or basic properties. Due to their low dielectric constant, they have a low ionizing potential. Examples: hydrocarbons and carbon tetrachloride.
3. Basic solvents, which have no acidic properties. Examples: amines, ketones, and ethers.

The acidic strengths of various solute molecules vary as a function of the dielectric constant of the solvent. Generally, a nonaqueous potentiometric titration is unsuitable in solvents with a dielectric constant less than 5. A decrease in the dielectric constant of a solvent increases the acidic strength of a positively charged acid, such as NH_4^+, but lowers that of a negatively charged acid, such as the hydrogen succinate ion. For the titration of weak bases, a solvent with a low basic strength such as acetic acid is suitable; likewise, for weak acids, solvents with moderate basic strength are desirable. In the former case the titrant is usually perchloric acid in dioxane or acetic acid;

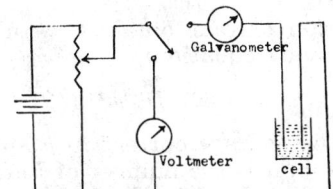

Fig. 471.   **A simplified potentiometer circuit.**

in the latter case, sodium ethoxide in benzene–methanol.

Oxidation–Reduction Reactions—An inert electrode, such as platinum, which is unaffected by oxidizing agents, is used in redox titrations. A calomel electrode can be used as a reference electrode. The electrode generates a potential proportional to the logarithm of the concentration ratio of the two oxidation states of the reactant or titrant. Titration of iron II with cerium IV is an example. The electrode potential changes gradually during the major portion of the titration. As the equivalence point approaches, the concentration ratio changes rapidly.

Voltametry

Voltametry is a method in which an external potential is imposed on a system in order to carry out various electrochemical analyses. The application of an external potential and the use of an appreciable amount of current differentiates voltametric from potentiometric methods of analysis. Two major types of electrochemical analysis based on voltametric principles are:

1. Polarography and amperometry, in which a very small fraction of the test solution is involved in the analysis. These methods can be used both for quantitative and qualitative analysis.
2. Coulometry and electrogravimetry, in which a complete electrolysis of a test solution is required. These methods are used primarily for quantitative analysis.

Both aqueous and nonaqueous solvents are employed in voltametry. The analysis is primarily for inorganic substances, but a number of organic compounds have been analyzed.

Polarography—This method was originated by Heyrovsky in 1922. The analysis is based on the current–voltage curves arising in a cell consisting of a dropping mercury electrode (DME) or a microelectrode and a nonpolarizable current-carrying electrode. Substances in a concentration range of 10^{-5} to $10^{-2}M$ can be analyzed, both qualitatively and quantitatively, provided it can undergo cathodic reduction or anodic oxidation.

Polarography provides (1) a limiting electrolysis current that is proportional to the concentration of a given compound and (2) a half-wave potential, which is characteristic of an individual species.

Fig. 416 (page 615) shows the simple circuit of a polarograph. The voltage applied across the electrodes may be increased gradually and the resulting electrolysis current measured with a galvanometer. The plot of emf (voltage) vs current (μ amp) provides the curve shown in Fig. 472. Until the decomposition potential is reached, there will be only a minor increase in current. The decomposition potential is a function of E° of the reaction and the concentration of the ions

involved. At this point there will be a sharp rise in the current. A further voltage increase will cause the curve to level off. The sharp increase in current, called the diffusion current (i_d), which is due to the diffusion of the ions to the electrodes wherein the ions are plated out. This plating causes the concentration at the solution–mercury interface to be lowered and results in a concentration gradient being established which causes ions to diffuse from the body of the solution into the interface at a rate proportional to the concentration difference. The current-voltage curve levels off when complete concentration–polarization occurs; ie, the diffusion rate becomes constant and proportional to the ion concentration in the body of the solution.

A mixture of two ions, Cd^{2+} and Zn^{2+}, with standard oxidation potentials of $+0.4$ and $+0.76$, respectively, gives the polarogram shown in Fig. 472. The diffusion current for Zn^{2+} is the difference between the total current and that for Cd^{2+}.

In addition to the diffusion current, ions attracted to the DME by electric forces also create some current, referred to as *migration current*. The limiting current is therefore the sum of a migration current and the diffusion current. Current in an electrolytic cell is carried by all the ions present, irrespective of their participation in electrode reaction; therefore, if an inert electrolyte such as KCl (which at the low potentials employed in the polarography of Zn^{2+} or Cd^{2+} is neither oxidized nor reduced) is added in excess to the solution, the migration current will be carried almost entirely by the KCl ions. The limiting current observed then will be the diffusion current for the ions under investigation.

Another type of current that occurs in polarography is residual current. Even with inert ions, it is observed that an increase in voltage gives rise to a small but observable current. This is due to charges acquired by the DME on application of higher voltages. In polarography, compensation is allowed for this residual current.

Mathematically, the rate of diffusion of an ion is expressed by Fick's law:

$$dx/dt = AD(C - C_0)/b \qquad (66)$$

where C_0 is the concentration of ions at the electrode surface, C is the concentration of ions in the bulk of the solution, A is the exposed area of the electrode surface, D is the diffusion coefficient of the ion, and b is the thickness of the hypothetical diffusion layer about the microelectrode.

When equilibrium is established, the rate of discharge of the ion by the current will be equal to the rate of diffusion to the electrode. If i is the current and A is unity, the rate of discharge of ions is

$$i/nF = D(C - C_0)/b \qquad (67)$$

where i is the current, n is the number of electrons involved in the discharge process, and F is a Faraday (ie, the quantity of electricity carried by one equivalent).

The diffusion current obtained with the DME is given by Ilkovic's equation:

$$i_d = 607nD^{1/2}m^{2/3}t^{1/6}C \qquad (68)$$

where i_d is the average current in μ amp during the life of the drop, n is the number of Faradays of electricity required/mole of the electrode reaction, D is the diffusion coefficient of the reducible or oxidizable

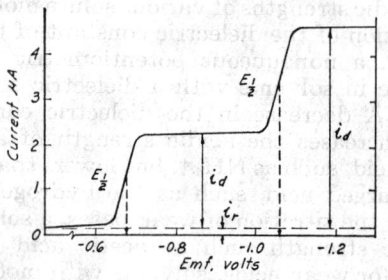

Fig. 472. The polarogram of a solution containing Cd^{2+} and Zn^{2+}. The diffusion current and residual current are denoted by i_d and i_r, respectively.

substance in $cm^2 sec^{-1}$, m is the rate of flow of Hg from the DME capillary in $mg sec^{-1}$, C is the concentration in moles/liter, and t is the drop time in sec (an optimum drop time is 2–5 sec). The equation is simplified by keeping all the factors except C constant:

$$i_d = k_c C \qquad (69)$$

Plotting i_d vs C will give a straight line.

Half-Wave Potential—As shown in Fig. 472, the half-wave potential ($E_{1/2}$) is an oxidation or reduction potential at the current mid-point of a polarographic curve. A half-wave potential is characteristic of an electrolyzable species, is independent of concentration, and is related to the standard electrode potentials (E° values). The half-wave potential of a compound, however, is related to the form in which an oxidizable or reducible molecule exists. For example, it can be shifted by varying the pH of a solution. Two compounds, whose half-wave potentials overlap at a given pH, can possibly be resolved by varying the pH or adding a complexing agent. For example, in acid solutions the half-wave potential of tin and antimony are −0.47 v and 0.20 v, respectively, but in alkaline solutions they are −1.1 v and 1.8 v. Therefore, the latter condition is preferred in determining these ions in a mixture.

Electrodes—In polarography the indicator or polarizable electrode is either a DME for reduction reactions or a platinum electrode (stationary or rotating) for oxidation reactions. The curves provided by these reactions are known as cathodic and anodic waves, respectively. By convention, diffusion currents are designated as follows: reduction, positive; oxidation, negative. The advantages of the DME are that it provides a smooth surface and the diffusion currents obtained are reproducible. However, it has the disadvantage in that at a small positive potential anodic dissociation occurs. Therefore, platinum is preferred. Precision obtainable with a platinum electrode is about ±5%. For a reference electrode either a mercury pool or a saturated calomel electrode is used.

Both manual and recording polarographs are available, of which the recording type is the most widely used.

Amperometry—This method is based on the principle of polarography, with the exception that the voltage is maintained constant during a titration procedure. Substances which cannot be analyzed polarographically, due to the absence of a diffusion current, can be determined amperometrically by using a titrant which yields a diffusion current. Fig. 473A, B, and C illustrate typical amperometric titration curves. The equivalence point is the intersection of the two extrapolated straight lines, whose slopes are a function of the diffusion current. In contrast to a polarographic measurement, in which several ions in a mixture can be determined, the amperometric titration involves determinations of a single substance only. A substance and its half-wave potential must be known prior to titration. A change in volume during the titration is usually minimized by selecting a titrant five to ten times more concentrated than the material to be analyzed. The best potential for the microelectrode is chosen by referring to the half-wave potentials of the sample and titrant. The applied voltage is located on the plateau of the electrolysis wave.

As shown in Fig. 473A, the titration of SO_4^{2-} with Pb^{2+} is carried out at a potential more negative than −0.46 v ($Pb^{2+} + 2e \rightarrow Pb$, −0.46 v half-wave

potential). As sulfate ions are removed and Pb^{2+} concentration is increased, the diffusion current increases. The opposite is true if Pb^{2+} is to be titrated with SO_4^{2-}. In the titration of Pb^{2+} with sodium or potassium dichromate at −1.2 v, when the equivalence point is passed, the excess $Cr_2O_7^{2-}$ gives an increase in the diffusion current.

In amperometric titrations (as in polarography) an inert electrolyte must be added to eliminate the effect of migration current and nitrogen is bubbled through the solution to remove dissolved oxygen. The titrations are performed in an H-shaped cell. Either a DME or a rotating platinum electrode can be used with a saturated calomel electrode (SCE) as the reference electrode.

The amperometric procedure is applied in the measurement of ions which cannot be evaluated potentiometrically. For example, no suitable electrode is available to determine sulfate anion potentiometrically. Amperometrically, however, excellent results are obtained. A similar application is utilized in the determination of fluoride ion with thorium or lanthanum nitrate.

Coulometry and Electrogravimetry—These methods can be included under one heading because fundamentally they both operate on the same principle; ie, exhaustive electrolysis. Both procedures require currents larger than those employed in polarography, plus an unpolarized working electrode. Either constant current or constant voltage techniques can be employed and elaborate electronic regulating devices are commercially available.

In coulometry it is possible to generate a reactant *in situ*; therefore, unstable reagents may be employed in the analytical procedure.

With the electrogravimetric method, the quantity of the metal deposited on the working electrode is determined by weighing, or if a gas is generated, it is collected in a gas buret. The potential necessary for quantitative electrolysis can be determined by the Nernst equation:

$$E' = E^\circ + (0.0591/n) \log C_0 \times 10^{-4} \qquad (70)$$

where E' is the final potential of the working electrode and C_0 is the initial concentration of the substance to be analyzed.

In coulometry, the quantity of the reactant formed

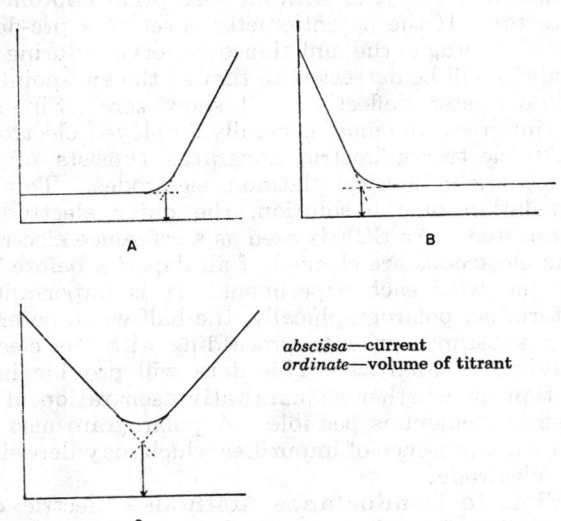

abscissa—current
ordinate—volume of titrant

Fig. 473. Titration of *A:* SO_4^{2-} **with** Pb^{2+}; *B:* Pb^{2+} **with** SO^{2-}; *C:* Pb^{2+} **with** $Cr_2O_7^{2-}$.

is proportional to Q, which can be calculated from Faraday's law:

$$Q = it \qquad (71)$$

where i is the current and t is the time of electrolysis. One Faraday of electricity is 96,487 Q, which causes chemical changes in $1/n$ Gm-ions, where n is the number of electrons. If the current is maintained constant, the weight of the reactant can be calculated by

$$\frac{it}{96{,}487} = \frac{\text{weight of } x}{\text{equivalent weight of } x} \qquad (72)$$

There are two important factors to be considered in coulometric analysis: (1) the substance of interest must be electrolyzed completely and (2) the exact time at which the reaction is completed should be determined.

In the electrical generation of the analytical reagent, three points must be observed: (1) the working electrode must remain inert during analysis—eg, due to the tendency of halide to react with platinum giving PtX_6^{2-}, platinum cannot be employed as an anode when a halide is present, (2) oxygen should be removed, and (3) interference occurring as a result of participation of electrons in the electrolysis of another substance, such as a solvent, must be eliminated. In order to avoid the involvement of the solvent or impurities during an analysis, a constant-current procedure is used for the electrical generation of the reactant. The use of an excess quantity of the inactive form of a reagent (titrant) provides a proper control of the electrode voltage. For example, in the titration of Fe^{2+}, a large excess of Ce^{3+} is added. Upon the passage of current, Ce^{4+} is easily generated at the working electrode (anode) and Fe^{2+} is oxidized.

$$Ce^{4+} + Fe^{2+} \rightarrow Fe^{3+} + Ce^{3+} \qquad (73)$$

Generation of Ce^{4+} ceases at the end-point.

Analytical Procedure and Instrumentation—A constant-current coulometer is the most widely used instrument. A power supply provides a constant current for the cell. Usually a current of less than 250 ma is employed and the time of electrolysis varies from about 10 to 200 sec. An accurate electric timer starts or stops the electrolysis by controlling a switch. The end-point can be detected potentiometrically, amperometrically, or with an absorption photometric detector. If the potentiometer is set at a pre-determined voltage, the unbalance observed during the analysis will be decreased so that at the end-point the galvanometer deflection will show zero. Silver or platinum are the most generally employed electrodes.

An electrogravimetric apparatus consists of two concentric cylindrical platinum electrodes. To allow circulation of the solution, the outer electrode is perforated. An SCE is used as a reference electrode. The electrodes are cleaned of all deposits before proceeding with each experiment. It is important to determine, polarographically, the half-wave potential of a substance prior to proceeding with the electrogravimetric analysis. This data will provide information on whether a quantitative separation of the desired element is possible. A polarogram also will show the presence of impurities which may deposit on the electrode.

Electric Conductance Methods—Electric conductivity of a solution under a given potential is a function of the nature of the solute and its concentration. The current is conducted by the migration of

ions under the influence of an electric field. Conductance, *mho*, is $1/R$, where R is the resistance in ohms. Specific conductance, κ, is the reciprocal of the resistance of a 1-cm cube of liquid and is

$$1/R = \kappa(A/d) \qquad (74)$$

where A is the area of the electrodes and d is the distance between the electrodes. In a cell with electrodes of 1-cm^2 area and 1 cm apart, equivalent conductance, Λ, is

$$\Lambda = (1000/C_s)\kappa \qquad (75)$$

where C_s is the concentration of the solution in moles per liter.

The equivalent conductance of a solution increases upon further dilution due to an increase in ionic mobility. The degree of dissociation of an electrolyte, α, is given by

$$\alpha = \Lambda/\Lambda_0 \qquad (76)$$

where Λ_0 is the equivalent conductance at infinite dilution. Λ_0, which is also denoted by Λ_∞, is the summation of the conductances of the cations and anions in the solution.

$$\Lambda_\infty \equiv \Lambda_0 = \Sigma(\lambda_+) + \Sigma(\lambda_-) \qquad (77)$$

where λ_+ and λ_- are the ionic conductance of cations and anions, respectively, at infinite dilution. The dissociation constant of weak electrolytes can be calculated by

$$K_\alpha = \alpha^2 C_s/(1 - \alpha) \qquad (78)$$

If Λ_0 of a weak electrolyte cannot be obtained directly by extrapolation of the plot Λ vs $\sqrt{C}$, the concept of additivity of ionic conductance known as Kohlrausch's law can be applied for calculation. For example, Λ_0 of a weak acid, HR, can be calculated by

$$\Lambda_0 HR = \Lambda_0 HCl + \Lambda_0 NaR - \Lambda_0 NaCl \qquad (79)$$

Conductance Cells—A conductance cell consists of two platinum plates placed parallel to each other. The electrodes are plated with platinum black to reduce the polarizing effect of the current passed between the electrodes.

Analytical Procedure—In conductance measurements, a solution with a known specific conductance is placed in a cell and the cell constant, $\theta = d/A$, is calculated by measuring the resistance and applying the formula

$$\kappa = \frac{1}{R}\left(\frac{d}{A}\right) = \frac{\theta}{R} \qquad (80)$$

Potassium chloride is a commonly employed solution for the calibration. The κ value at 18° and 25°C for three different KCl concentrations is given below:

Gm of KCl/Kg of solution	κ in ohm^{-1} cm^{-1} 18°C	25°C
71.1352	0.09784	0.11134
7.4191	0.01117	0.01286
0.7453 (0.01M)	0.001221	0.001409

Because a direct current induces some changes in an electrolyte solution, it is necessary to use a rapidly alternating (60-Hz) current of a low-intensity source or an oscillator of about 1000 Hz. The cell is placed in one arm of a wheatstone bridge as shown in Fig. 474. A balanced bridge can be expressed by

$$R_x = R_1 R_3/R_2 \qquad (81)$$

The variable capacitance is used for balancing the capacitance of the cell. The detector can be an ac galvanometer, earphone, or oscilloscope.

High-Frequency Methods

Some substances absorb a broad band of EM radiation in the frequency range from 0.1 to 100 mHz. This absorption is not a specific property of a substance, as with UV or IR. The degree of absorption, however, is characteristic for organic compounds. The method may be used in quantitative analysis for determination of the end-point in a titration or in the measurement of the dielectric constant of organic compounds.

The analysis is performed by placing the vessel containing the sample between plates of a capacitor or in the field of an inductance coil. Since the sample becomes a part of the high-frequency circuit, any variation in its property can be detected. Because there are no electrodes in contact with the solution to cause electrolysis, the use of high-frequency methods of analysis are superior to their low-frequency or direct-current counterparts.

Any change in the sample is detected as a change in the current or voltage of the plate or grid of a vacuum tube oscillator (Fig. 475). The measurement also can be made by using two identical oscillator circuits: one contains the sample (f); the other is used as a reference (f_0). The outputs from the two are fed into a mixer. The difference $(f - f_0)$ can be measured either directly or by a compensatory alteration of a variable capacitor in the circuit to offset the capacitance change in the cell. The beat-frequency shift, measured by a heterodyne-beat method, has been used successfully in high-frequency methods of analysis. The magnitude of the beat-frequency changes for various organic compounds are listed in the literature.

The measurement of dielectric constant is performed by placing the liquid in a glass container and the container between two metal plates. The two types of capacitors—C_g for the glass of the cell and C_s for the sample—are in series. The value of C_s is designated as C_0 when the cell contains air and the dielectric

Table V

Compound	Dielectric constant
Formamide	109.5
Water	81
Acetonitrile	37.5
Methanol	32.6
Ethanol	24.3
Acetone	20.7
Acetic anhydride	20.7
Acetic acid	6.15
Ethyl acetate	6.02
Chloroform	4.8
Benzene	2.4
Carbon tetrachloride	2.23
1,4-Dioxane	2.20

constant of a substance is defined as

$$D = C_s/C_0 \qquad (82)$$

The dielectric constants (D) of water and a few organic compounds are listed in Table V. The D values of many organic substances fall between water and air.

References

1. Silverstein, R. M., and Bassler, G. C., *Spectrophotometric Identification of Organic Compounds*, 2nd ed., Wiley, New York, 1967, p. 151.
2. Silverstein, R. M., and Bassler, G. C., *Spectrophotometric Identification of Organic Compounds*, 2nd ed., Wiley, New York, 1967, p. 8.

Bibliography

Instrumental Methods of Analysis

Bair, E. J., *Introduction to Chemical Instrumentation*, McGraw-Hill, New York, 1962.
Connors, K. A., *A Textbook of Pharmaceutical Analysis*, Wiley, New York, 1967.
Ewing, G. W., *Instrumental Methods of Chemical Analysis*, McGraw-Hill, New York, 1960.
Pecsok, R. L., and Shields, L. D., *Modern Methods of Chemical Analysis*, Wiley, New York, 1968.
Strobel, H. A., *Chemical Instrumentation*, Addison-Wesley, Reading, Mass., 1960.
Willard, H. H., *et al*, *Instrumental Methods of Analysis*, Van Nostrand, New York, 1965.

X-Ray Spectrometry

Birks, L., *X-Ray Spectrochemical Analysis*, Interscience, New York, 1959.
Liebhafsky, H., *X-Ray Absorption and Emission in Analytical Chemistry*, Wiley, New York, 1960.
Nuffield, E., *X-Ray Diffraction Methods*, Wiley, New York, 1966.
Nyburg, S., *X-Ray Analysis of Organic Structures*, Academic, New York, 1961.
Alphabetical and Grouped Numerical Index of X-Ray Diffraction Data (Spec. Tech. Publ. 48E), Am. Soc. Testing Mater., Philadelphia, 1955.

Ultraviolet and Visible Spectrometry

Braude, E. A., in *Determination of Organic Structures by Physical Methods*, Academic, New York, 1955, Chap. 4, pp. 131–194.
Duncan, A. B. F., and Matsen, F. A., in Weissberger, A., ed., *Technique of Organic Chemistry*, vol. IX, Interscience, New York, 1956, pp. 581–706.
Jaffe, H. H., and Orchin, M., *Theory and Application of Ultraviolet Spectroscopy*, Wiley, New York, 1962.
Lang, L., *Absorption Spectra in the Ultraviolet and Visible Region*, vols. 1–5, Academic, New York, 1961–1965.
Rao, C. N. R., *Ultra-Violet and Visible Spectroscopy*, Chemical Applications, Butterworths, London 1961.
Scott, A. I., *Interpretation of the Ultraviolet Spectra of Natural Products*, Pergamon, New York, 1964.
Organic Electronic Spectral Data, vols. I–IV, Interscience, New York, 1960–1963 (covers literature from 1946 to 1959).
ASTM Index to Ultraviolet and Visible Spectra (ASTM Tech. Publ. 357), Am. Soc. for Testing Mater., Philadelphia, 1963.

Infrared Spectrometry

Bellamy, L. J., *The Infra-red Spectra of Complex Organic Molecules*, 2nd ed., Wiley, New York, 1958.
Colthup, N. B., *et al*, *Introduction to Infrared and Raman Spectroscopy*, Academic, New York, 1964.
Davies, M., ed., *Infrared Spectroscopy and Molecular Structure—An Outline of Principles*, Elsevier, Amsterdam and London, 1963.
Dyer, J. R., *Applications of Absorption Spectroscopy of Organic Compounds*, Prentice-Hall, Englewood Cliffs, N.J., 1965.
Kendall, D. N., ed., *Applied Infrared Spectroscopy*, Reinhold, New York, 1966.
Rao, C. N. R., *Chemical Applications of Infrared Spectroscopy*, Academic, New York and London, 1963.
Szymanski, H. A., *IR Theory and Practice of Infrared Spectroscopy*, Plenum, New York, 1964.

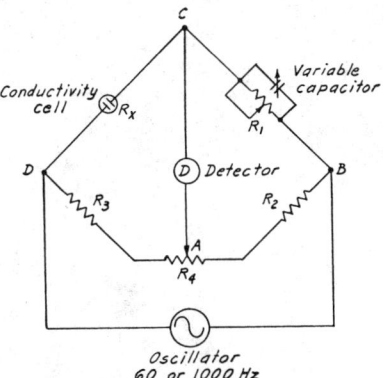

Fig. 474.   A conductivity bridge.

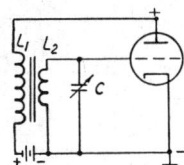

Fig. 475.   The circuit of a high-frequency oscillator.

Szymanski, H. A., *Interpreted Infrared Spectra*, vol. I, Plenum, New York, 1964.

Szymanski, H. A., *Infrared Band Handbook*, Plenum, New York, 1962 (Suppl. 1 and 2 cover the 200–600 cm $^{-1}$ region).

Catalog of Infrared Spectra, Sadtler Res. Labs., Philadelphia.

Silverstein, R. M., and Bassler, G. C., *Spectrometric Identification of Organic Compounds*, 2nd ed., Wiley, New York, 1967.

Nuclear Magnetic Resonance

Bible, R. H., Jr., *Interpretation of NMR Spectra*, Plenum, New York, 1965.

Bible, R. H., Jr., *Guide to the Empirical Method: A Workbook*, Plenum, New York, 1967.

Dyer, J. R., *Applications of Absorption Spectroscopy of Organic Compounds*, Prentice-Hall, Englewood Cliffs, N.J., 1965, Chap. 4.

Jackman, L. M., *Applications of Nuclear Magnetic Resonance Spectroscopy in Organic Chemistry*, Pergamon, New York, 1959.

Nakanishi, K., *et al*, *A Guidebook to the Interpretation of NMR Spectra*, Holden-Day, San Francisco, 1967.

Pople, J. A., *et al*, *High-Resolution Nuclear Magnetic Resonance*, McGraw-Hill, New York, 1959.

Silverstein, R. M., and Bassler, G. C., *Spectrometric Identification of Organic Compounds*, 2nd ed., Wiley, New York, 1967.

Wiberg, K. B., and Nist, B. J., *The Interpretation of NMR Spectra*, W. A. Benjamin, New York, 1962.

Nuclear Magnetic Resonance Spectra, Sadtler Res. Labs., Philadelphia.

High Resolution NMR Spectra Catalogue, vols. 1 and 2, Varian Associates, Palo Alto, Calif., 1962–1963.

Emission Spectrometry, Flame Photometry, and Atomic Absorption Spectrometry

Ahrens, L. H., and Taylor, S. R., *Spectrochemical Analysis*, 2nd ed., Addison-Wesley, Reading, Mass., 1961.

Brode, W. R., *Chemical Spectroscopy*, 2nd ed., Wiley, New York, 1943.

Elwell, W. T., and Gidley, J. A. F., *Atomic Absorption Spectrophotometry*, Pergamon, New York, 1966.

Meggers, W. F., *et al*, "Tables of Spectral-line Intensities," Parts I and II, *Natl. Bur. Std. (US) Monograph*, **32** (1961, 1962).

Mavrodineanu, R., and Boiteux, H., *Flame Spectroscopy*, Wiley, New York, 1965.

Atomic Absorption Newsletter, Perkin-Elmer Corp., Norwalk, Conn.

Fluorescence and Phosphorescence Spectrometry

Guilbault, G. C., *Fluorescence: Theory, Instrumentation and Practice*, Dekker, New York, 1967.

Hercules, D. M., ed., *Fluorescence and Phosphorescence Analysis*, Interscience, New York, 1966.

Udenfriend, S., *Fluorescence Assay in Biology and Medicine*, Academic, New York, 1962.

Light-Scattering, Refractometry, and Polarimetry

Batsanov, S. S., *Refractometry and Chemical Structure. II.*, Consultant Bureau Enterprises, New York, 1961.

Crabbe, P., *Optical Rotatory Dispersion and Circular Dichroism in Organic Chemistry*, Holden-Day, San Francisco, 1965.

Djerassi, C., *Optical Rotatory Dispersion*, McGraw-Hill, New York, 1960.

Stacey, K., *Light-Scattering in Physical Chemistry*, Butterworths, London, 1956.

Weissberger, A., ed., *Physical Methods in Organic Chemistry*, vol. 1, Interscience, New York, 1960, Part II.

Mass Spectrometry

Beynon, J. H., *Mass Spectrometry and Its Application to Organic Chemistry*, Elsevier, Amsterdam, 1960.

Budzikiewicz, H., *et al*, *Interpretation of Mass Spectra of Organic Compounds*, Holden-Day, San Francisco, 1964.

Budzikiewicz, H., *et al*, *Structure Elucidation of Natural Products by Mass Spectrometry*, vols. I and II, Holden-Day, San Francisco, 1964.

Hill, H. C., *Introduction to Mass Spectrometry*, Sadtler Res. Labs., Philadelphia, 1966.

Lederberg, J., *Computation of Molecular Formulas for Mass Spectrometry*, Holden-Day, San Francisco, 1964.

Reed, R. I., *Application of Mass Spectrometry to Organic Chemistry*, Academic, New York, 1966.

Silverstein, R. M., and Bassler, G. C., *Spectrometric Identification of Organic Compounds*, 2nd ed., Wiley, New York, 1967.

Catalog of Mass Spectra Data (Am. Petrol. Inst. Res. Pro. 44), Carnegie Inst. of Technol., Pittsburgh.

Index of Mass Spectral Data (ASTM Spec. Tech. Publ. 356), Am. Soc. for Testing Mater., Philadelphia, 1963.

Electrochemistry

Brezina, M., and Zuman, P., *Polarography in Medicine, Biochemistry, and Pharmacy*, Interscience, Wiley, New York, 1958.

Delakey, P., and Tobias, C., *Advances in Electrochemistry and Electrochemical Engineering*, vols. 1–6, Interscience, New York, 1961–1967.

Hills, G. J., *Polarography*, vols. 1 and 2, Interscience, New York, 1966.

Kolthoff, I. M., and Lingane, J. J., *Polarography*, vols. I and II, Interscience, New York, 1952.

Latimer, W. M., *Oxidation Potential*, Prentice-Hall, Englewood Cliffs, N.J., 1956.

Meites, L., *Polarographic Techniques*, Interscience, New York, 1965.

Mueller, O., *Polarographic Method of Analysis*, Chem. Educ. Publ. Co., Easton, Pa., 1956.

Milner, G. W., and Phillips, G., *Coulometry in Analytical Chemistry*, Pergamon, New York, 1968.

Stock, J. T., *Amperometric Titration*, Wiley, New York, 1965.

Part VI

PHARMACEUTICAL and MEDICINAL AGENTS

PHARMACOLOGY EDITORS

Ewart A. Swinyard, PhD, *Professor of Pharmacology, College of Pharmacy and College of Medicine, University of Utah, Salt Lake City, Utah 84112*

Stewart C. Harvey, PhD, *Associate Professor of Pharmacology, College of Medicine, University of Utah, Salt Lake City, Utah 84112*

CHEMISTRY EDITOR

Clarence T. Van Meter, PhD, *Project Director, Office of Engineering Research, University of Pennsylvania, Philadelphia, Pa. 19104*

PHARMACY EDITORS

Linwood F. Tice, DSc, *Dean, Philadelphia College of Pharmacy and Science, Philadelphia, Pa. 19104*

Allen M. Kratz, PharmD, *Assistant Professor of Clinical Pharmacy, Philadelphia College of Pharmacy and Science, Philadelphia, Pa. 19104*

VETERINARY EDITOR

Richard A. Huebner, VMD, *Director, Veterinary Service, Wyeth Laboratories, Philadelphia, Pa. 19101*

42 | Drug Absorption, Action, and Disposition

**Drug action and effect—drug receptors and receptor theory—
mechanism of drug action—absorption, distribution, and excretion—
drug interaction and combination**

This chapter was prepared by

Stewart C. Harvey, PhD, *Associate Professor of Pharmacology, College of
Medicine, University of Utah, Salt Lake City, Utah 84112*

Although drugs differ widely in their pharmacodynamic effects and clinical application, in penetrance,
absorption, and usual route of administration, in
distribution among the body tissues, and in disposition
and mode of termination of action, there are certain
general principles which help explain these differences.
These principles have both pharmaceutic and therapeutic implications. They facilitate an understanding
of both the features that are common to a class of
drugs and the differentia among the members of that
class.

In order for a drug to act it must be absorbed,
transported to the appropriate tissue or organ, penetrate to the responding subcellular structure, and
elicit a response or alter ongoing processes. The drug
may be simultaneously or sequentially distributed to a
number of tissues, bound or stored, metabolized to
inactive or active products, or excreted. The history
of a drug in the body is summarized in Fig. 476. Each
of the processes or events depicted relates importantly
to therapeutic and toxic effects of a drug, and to the
mode of administration, and drug design must take
each into account. Since the effect elicited by a drug
is its *raison d'etre*, *drug action* and *effect* will be discussed first in the text that follows, even though they
are preceded by other events.

Drug Action and Effect

The word *drug* imposes an action–effect context
within which the properties of a substance are described. The description must of necessity include
the pertinent properties of the recipient of the drug.
Thus, when a drug is defined as an analgesic, it is
implied that the recipient reacts in a certain way,
called pain,* to a noxious stimulus. Both because
the pertinent properties are locked into the complex
and somewhat imprecise biological context and because
the types of possible response are many, descriptions
of the properties of drugs tend to emphasize the qualitative features of the effects they elicit. Thus a drug
may be described as having analgesic, vasodepressor,
convulsant, antibacterial, etc., properties. The specific effect (or use) categories into which the many
drugs may be placed are the subject of Chapters 43
through 70 and will not be elaborated upon in this
chapter. However, the description of a drug does
not end with the enumeration of the responses it may
elicit. There are certain intrinsic properties of the
drug–recipient system that can be described in quantitative terms and which are essential to the full
description of the drug and to the validation of the
drug for specific uses. Under *Definitions and Concepts*, below, certain general terms are defined in
qualitative language; under *Dose–Effect Relationships*
the foundation is laid for an appreciation of some of
the quantitative aspects of pharmacodynamics.

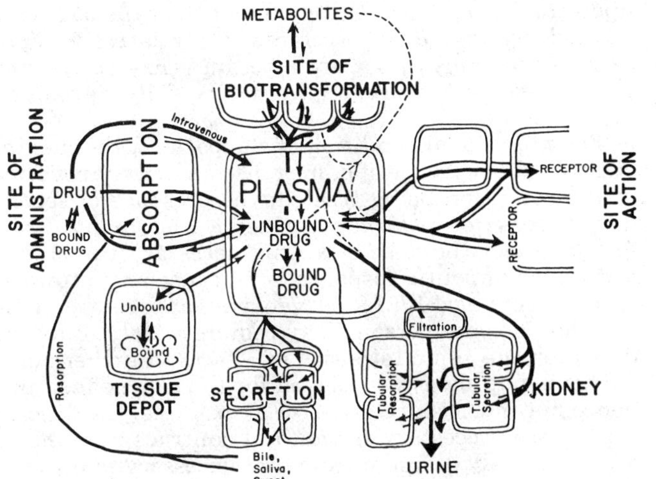

Definitions and Concepts

In the field of pharmacology, the vocabulary that is
unique to the discipline is relatively small, and the
general vocabulary is that of the biological sciences
and chemistry. Nevertheless, there are a few definitions that are important to the proper understanding
of pharmacology. It is necessary to differentiate
among action, effect, selectivity, dose, potency, and
efficacy.

Action vs Effect—The *effect* of a drug is an *alteration of function* of the structure or process upon which
the drug acts. It is common to use the term action as
a synonym for effect. However, action precedes
effect. *Action* is the alteration of condition that
brings about the effect.

The final effect of a drug may be far removed from
its site of action. For example, the diuresis subse-

Fig. 476. The absorption, distribution, action, and elimination of
a drug (arrows represent drug movement). Intravenous administration is the only process whereby a drug may enter a compartment
without passing through a biological membrane. Note that drugs
excreted in bile and saliva may be resorbed.

** Sophisticated studies indicate that pain is not simply the *perception* of a
certain kind of stimulus but rather a *reaction* to the perception of a variety of
kinds of stimuli or stimulus patterns.*

quent to the ingestion of ethanol does not result from an action on the kidney but instead from a depression of activity in the supraopticohypophyseal region of the hypothalamus, which regulates the release of antidiuretic hormone from the posterior pituitary gland. The alteration of supraopticohypophyseal function is, of course, also an effect of the drug, as is each subsequent change in the chain of events leading to diuresis. The action of ethanol was exerted only at the initial step, each subsequent effect being then the action to a following step.

Multiple Effects—No known drug is capable of exerting a single effect, although a number are known which appear to have a single mechanism of action. Multiple effects may derive from a single mechanism of action. For example, the inhibition of acetylcholinesterase by physostigmine will elicit an effect at every site where acetylcholine is produced, is potentially active, and is hydrolyzed by cholinesterase. Thus physostigmine elicits a constellation of effects.

A drug can also cause multiple effects at several different sites by a single action at only one site, providing that the function initially altered at the site of action ramifies to control other functions at distant sites. Thus a drug that suppresses steroid synthesis in the liver may not only lower serum cholesterol, impair nerve myelination and function, and alter the condition of the skin (as a consequence of cholesterol deposition) but also may affect digestive functions (because of a deficiency in bile acids) and alter adrenocortical and sexual hormonal balance.

Although a single action can give rise to multiple effects, most drugs exert multiple actions. The various actions may be related, as, for example, the sympathomimetic effects of metaraminol that accrue to its structural similarity to norepinephrine and its ability partially to suppress sympathetic responses because it occupies the catecholamine storage pools in lieu of norepinephrine; or the actions may be unrelated, as with the actions of morphine to interfere with the release of acetylcholine from certain autonomic nerves, to block some actions of 5-hydroxytryptamine (serotonin), and to release histamine. Many drugs bring about immunologic (allergic or hypersensitivity) responses that bear no relation to the other pharmacodynamic actions of the drug.

Selectivity—Despite the potential most drugs have for eliciting multiple effects, one effect is generally more readily elicitable than another. This differential responsiveness is called *selectivity*. It is usually considered to be a property of the drug, but it is also a property of the constitution and biodynamics of the recipient subject or patient.

Selectivity may come about in several ways. The subcellular structure (receptor) with which a drug combines to initiate one response may have a higher affinity for the drug than that for some other action; atropine, for example, has a much higher affinity for the muscarinic receptors (page 899) that subserve the function of sweating than it does for the nicotinic receptors (page 899) that subserve voluntary neuromuscular transmission, so that suppression of sweating can be achieved with only a tiny fraction of the dose necessary to cause paralysis of the skeletal muscles. A drug may be distributed unevenly, so that it reaches a higher concentration at one site than generally throughout the tissues; chloroquine is much more effective against hepatic than intestinal (colonic) amebiasis because it reaches a many times higher concentration in the liver than in the wall of the colon.

An affected function may be much more critical to or have less reserve in one organ than in another, so that a drug will be predisposed to elicit an effect at the more critical site; some inhibitors of dopa decarboxylase (which is also 5-hydroxytryptophane decarboxylase) depress the synthesis of histamine more than that of either norepinephrine or 5-hydroxytryptamine (serotonin), even though histidine decarboxylase is less sensitive to the drug, simply because histidine decarboxylase is the only step and hence is rate-limiting in the biosynthesis of histamine. Dopa decarboxylase is not rate-limiting in the synthesis of either norepinephrine or 5-hydroxytryptamine until the enzyme is nearly completely inhibited. Another example of the determination of selectivity by the critical balance of the affected function is that of the mercurial diuretic drugs. An inhibition of only 1% in the tubular resorption of glomerular filtrate will usually double urine flow, since 99% of the glomerular filtrate is normally resorbed; aside from the question of the possible concentration of diuretics in the urine, a drug-induced reduction of 1% in sulphydryl enzyme activity in tissues other than the kidney is not usually accompanied by an observable change in function. Selectivity also can be determined by the pattern of distribution of destructive or activating enzymes among the tissues and by other factors.

Dose—Even the uninitiated person knows that the *dose* of a drug is the amount administered. However, the appropriate dose of a drug is not some unvarying quantity, a fact sometimes overlooked by pharmacists, official committees, and physicians, and the practice of pharmacy is entrapped in a system of fixed-dose formulations, so that fine adjustments in dosage are often difficult to achieve. Fortunately, there is usually a rather wide latitude allowable in dosages. It is obvious that the size of the recipient individual should have a bearing upon the dose, and the physician may elect to administer the drug on a body-weight basis rather than as a fixed dose. Usually, however, a fixed dose is given to all adults, unless the adult is exceptionally large or small. The dose for infants and children is often determined by one of several formulas which take into account age or weight, depending upon the age group of the child and the type of action exerted by the drug. Infants are relatively more sensitive to many drugs, often because enzyme systems which destroy the drugs may not be fully developed in the infant.

The nutritional condition of the patient, the mental outlook, the presence of pain or discomfort, the severity of the condition being treated, the presence of secondary disease or pathology, genetic, and many other factors affect the dose of a drug necessary to achieve a given therapeutic response or to cause an untoward effect (see page 1381). Even two apparently well-matched normal persons may require widely different doses for the same intensity of effect. Furthermore, a drug is not always employed for the same effect and hence not in the same dose. For example, the dose of a progestin necessary for an oral contraceptive effect is considerably different from that necessary to prevent spontaneous abortion, and a dose of an estrogen for the treatment of the menopause is much too small for the treatment of prostatic carcinoma.

From the above it is evident that the wise physician knows that *the dose of a drug is "enough"* (ie, no rigid quantity but rather that which is necessary and can be tolerated) and individualizes his regimen accordingly. The wise pharmacist will also appreciate this dictum and recognize that official or manufacturer's recommended doses are sometimes quite narrowly defined and may be very wide of the mark. They should serve only as a useful guide rather than as an imperative. For these reasons throughout the monographs in Part VI, doses other than the official dose are sometimes stated under the heading of *Other Dose Information.*

Potency and Efficacy—The *potency* of a drug is the reciprocal of dose. Thus it will have the units of persons/unit weight of drug or body weight/unit weight of drug, etc. Potency generally has little utility other than to provide a means of comparing the relative activities of drugs in a series, in which case *relative potency*, relative to some prototype member of the series, is commonly used among pharmacologists and in the pharmaceutical industry.

Whether a given drug is more potent than another has little bearing on its clinical usefulness, provided that the potency is not so low that the size of the dose is physically unmanageable or the cost of treatment is higher than with an equivalent drug. If a drug is less potent but more selective, then it is the one to be preferred. Promotional arguments in favor of a more potent drug are thus irrelevant to the important considerations that should govern the choice of a drug. However, it sometimes occurs that drugs of the same class differ in the maximum intensity of effect; that is, some drugs of the class may be less efficacious than others, irrespective of how large a dose is used.

Efficacy connotes the property of a drug to achieve the desired response, and *maximum efficacy* denotes the maximum achievable effect. Even huge doses of codeine often cannot achieve the relief from severe pain that relatively small doses of morphine can; thus codeine is said to have a lower maximum efficacy than morphine. Efficacy is one of the primary determinants of the choice of a drug.

Dose–Effect Relationships

The importance of knowing how changes in the intensity of response to a drug vary with the dose is virtually self evident. Both the physician, who prescribes or administers a drug, and the manufacturer, who must package the drug in appropriate dose sizes, must translate such knowledge into everyday practice. Theoretical or molecular pharmacologists also study such relationships in inquiries into mechanism of action and receptor theory (see page 733). It is necessary to define two types of relationship: (1) the dose–intensity relationship—ie, the manner in which the intensity of effect in the individual recipient relates to dose—and (2) dose–frequency relationship—ie, the manner in which the number of responders among a population of recipients relates to dose.

Dose–Intensity of Effect Relationships—Whether the intensity of effect is determined *in vivo* (eg, the blood-pressure response to epinephrine in the human patient) or *in vitro* (eg, the response of the isolated guinea pig ileum to histamine) the dose–intensity of effect (often called dose-effect) curve usually has a characteristic shape, namely a curve that closely resembles one quadrant of a rectangular hyperbola.

In the dose–intensity curve depicted in Fig. 477, the curve appears to intercept the x axis at 0 only because the lower doses are quite small on the scale of the abscissa, the smallest dose being 1.5×10^{-3} mcg. Actually, the x intercept has a positive value, since a finite dose of drug is required to bring about a

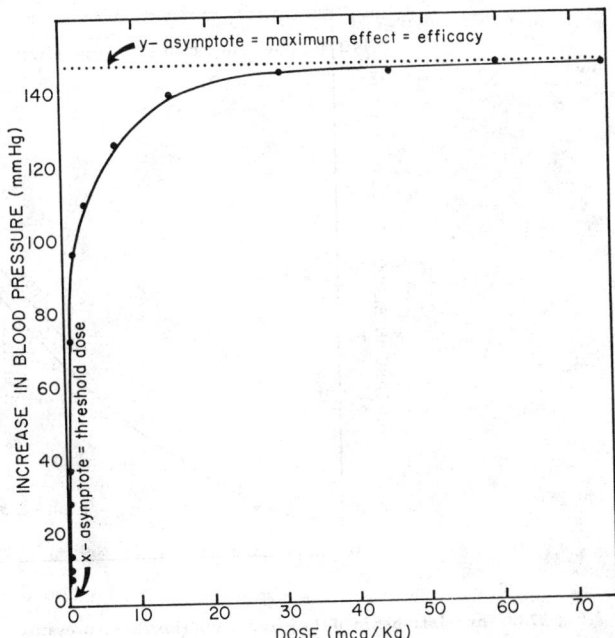

Fig. 477. The relationship of the intensity of the blood-pressure response of the cat to the intravenous dose of levarterenol.

response, this lowest effective dose being known as the threshold dose. Statistics and chemical kinetics predict that the curve should approach the y axis asymptotically. However, if the intensity of the measured variable does not start from zero, the curve may possibly have a positive y intercept (or negative x intercept), especially if the ongoing basal activity before the drug is given is closely related to that induced by the drug.

In practice, instead of an asymptote to the y axis, dose–intensity curves nearly always show an upward concave foot at the origin of the curve, so that the curve has a lopsided sigmoid shape. At high doses the curve approaches an asymptote which is parallel to the x axis, and the value of the asymptote establishes the maximum possible response to the drug, or maximum efficacy. However, experimental data in the regions of the asymptotes are generally too erratic to permit an exact definition of the curve at the very low and very high doses. The example shown represents an unusually good set of data.

Because the dose range may be 100- or 1000-fold from the lowest to the highest dose, it has become the practice to plot dose–intensity curves on a logarithmic scale of abscissa; ie, to plot the log of dose vs the intensity of effect. Fig. 478 is such a semilogarithmic plot of the same data as in Fig. 477. In the figure the intensity of effect is plotted both in absolute units (at the left) or in relative units, as percent (at the right).

Although no new information is created by a semilogarithmic representation, the curve is stretched out in such a way as to facilitate the inspection of the data; the comparison of results from multiple observations and the testing of different drugs is also rendered easier. In the example shown, the curve is essentially what is called a *sigmoid curve* and is nearly symmetrical about the point which represents an intensity equal to 50% of the maximal effect, ie, about the mid-point. The symmetry follows from the rectangular hyperbolic character of the previous Cartesian plot (Fig. 477). The semilogarithmic plot reveals better the dose–effect relationships in the low dose range, which are lost in

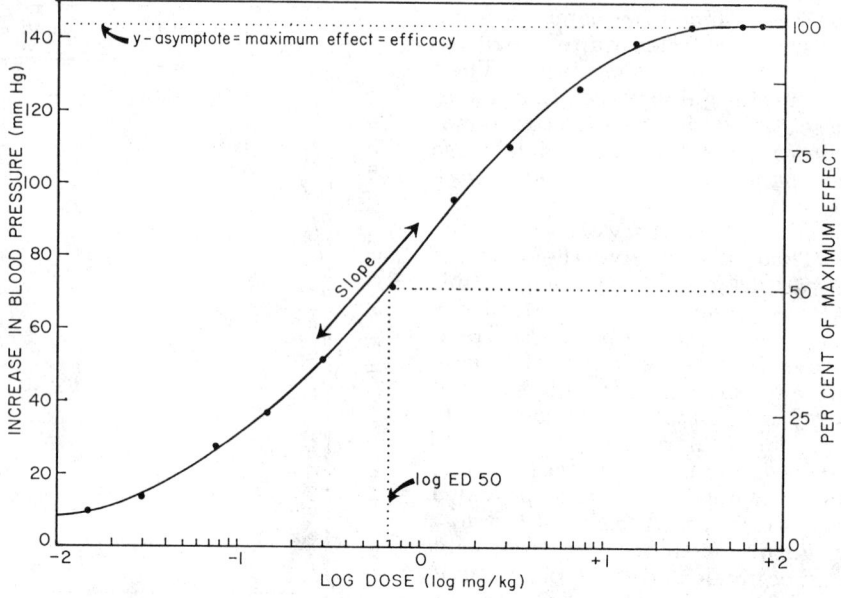

Fig. 478. The relationship of the intensity of the blood-pressure response of the cat to the log of the intravenous dose of levarterenol.

the steep slope of the Cartesian plot. Furthermore, the data about the mid-point are almost a straight line; the nearly linear portion covers approximately 50% of the curve. The slope of the "linear" portion of the curve, or, more correctly, the slope at the point of inflection, has theoretical significance (see *Drug Receptors and Receptor Theory*, page 733).

The upper portion of the curve approaches an asymptote, which is the same as that in the Cartesian plot. If the response system is completely at rest before the drug is administered, the lower portion of the curve should be asymptotic to the *x* axis. Both asymptotes and the symmetry derive from the law of mass action (see page 734).

Dose–intensity curves often deviate from the ideal configuration illustrated and discussed above. Usually, the deviate curve remains sigmoid but not extended symmetrically about the mid-point of the "linear" segment. Occasionally other shapes occur, sometimes quite bizarre ones. Deviations may derive from multiple actions that converge upon the same final effector system, from varying degrees of metabolic alteration of the drug at different doses, from modulation of the response by feedback systems, from non-linearity in the relationship between action and effect, or from other causes.

It is frequently necessary to identify the dose which elicits a given intensity of effect. The intensity of effect that is generally designated is the 50% of maximum intensity. The corresponding dose is called the *50% effective dose*, or *individual ED50* (see Fig. 478). The use of the adjective *individual* distinguishes the ED50 based upon the intensity of effect from the median effective dose, also abbreviated ED50, determined from frequency of response data in a population (see *Dose–Frequency Relationships*, page 731).

Drugs that elicit the same quality of effect may be graphically compared. In Fig. 479, five hypothetical drugs are compared. Drugs *A*, *B*, *C*, and *E* can all achieve the same maximum effect, which suggests that the same effector system may be common to all. *D* may possibly be working through the same effector system, but there are no *a priori* reasons to think this is so. Only *A* and *B* have parallel curves and common slopes. Common slopes suggest, but do not prove,

that *A* and *B* not only act through the same effector system but also by the same mechanism. Although drug–receptor theory (see *Drug Receptors and Receptor Theory*, page 733) requires that the curves of identical mechanism have equal slopes, examples of exceptions are known.

The relative potency of any drug may be obtained by dividing the ED50 of the standard or prototype drug by that of the drug in question. Any level of effect other than 50% may be used, but it should be recognized that when the slopes are not parallel, the relative potency depends upon the intensity of effect chosen. Thus the potency of *A* relative to *C* (in Fig. 479) calculated from the ED50 will be smaller than that calculated from the ED25.

The low maximum intensity inducible by *D* poses even more complications in the determination of relative potency than do the unequal slopes of the other drugs. If its dose–intensity curve is plotted in terms of per cent of its own maximum effect, its relative inefficacy is obscured, and the limitations of relative potency at the ED50 level will not be evident. This dilemma simply underscores the fact that drugs can better be compared from their entire dose–intensity curves than from a single derived figure like ED50 or relative potency.

Drugs that elicit multiple effects will generate a dose–intensity curve for each effect. Even though the various effects may be qualitatively different, the several curves may be plotted together on a common

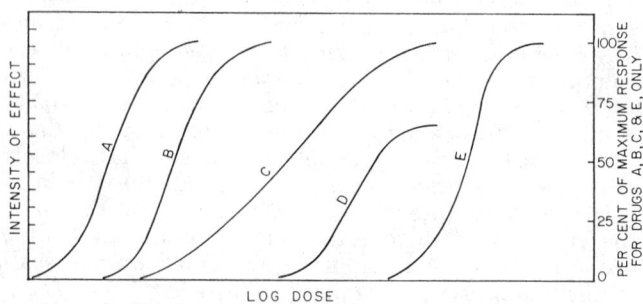

Fig. 479. Log dose–intensity of effect curves of five different hypothetical drugs (see text for explanation).

scale of abscissa, and the intensity may be expressed in terms of percent of maximum effect; thus all curves can share a common scale of ordinates in addition to common abscissa. Separate scales of ordinates could be employed, but would make it harder to compare data.

The selectivity of a drug can be determined by noting what percent of maximum of one effect can be achieved before a second effect occurs. As with relative potency, selectivity may be expressed in terms of the ratio between the ED50 for one effect to that for another effect, or a ratio at some other intensity of effect. Similarly to relative potency, difficulties follow from nonparallelism. In such instances, selectivity expressed in dose ratios varies from one intensity level to another.

When the dose–intensity curves for a number of subjects are compared, it is found that they vary considerably from individual to individual in many respects: threshold dose, mid-point, maximum intensity, etc, and sometimes even slope. By averaging the intensities of the effect at each dose, an average dose–intensity curve can be constructed.

Average dose–intensity curves enjoy a limited application in comparing drugs. A single line expressing an average response has little value in predicting individual responses unless it is accompanied by some expression of the range of the effect at the various doses. This may be done by indicating the standard error of the response at each dose. Occasionally, a simple scatter diagram is plotted in lieu of an average curve and statistical parameters (see Fig. 61, page 124). An average dose–intensity curve may also be constructed from a population in which different individuals receive different doses; if sufficiently large populations are employed, the average curves determined by the two methods will approximate each other.

It is obvious that the determination of such average curves from a population sufficiently large to be statistically meaningful requires a great deal of work. Retrospective clinical data is occasionally treated in this way, but prospective studies are infrequently designed in advance to yield average curves. The usual practice in comparing drugs is to employ a quantal (all-or-none) end-point and to plot the frequency or cumulative frequency of response over the dose range, as discussed below.

Dose–Frequency of Response Relationships— When an end-point is truly all-or-none, such as death, it is an easy matter to plot the number of responding individuals (eg, dead subjects) at each dose of drug or intoxicant. Many other responses that vary in intensity can be treated as all-or-none if simply the presence or absence of a response (eg, cough or no cough, convulsion or no convulsion, etc) is recorded, without regard to the intensity of the response when it occurs.

When the response grades from the basal or control state in a less abrupt manner (eg, tachycardia, miosis, rate of gastric secretion, etc) it may be necessary to designate arbitrarily some particular intensity of effect as the end-point. If the end-point is taken as an increase in heart rate of 20 beats/min, then all individuals whose tachycardia is less than 20/min would be recorded as non-responders, while all those with 20 or above would be recorded as responders. When the percent of responders in the population is plotted against the dose, a characteristic dose-response curve, more properly called a *dose–cumulative frequency* or *dose–percent* curve, is generated. Such a curve is,

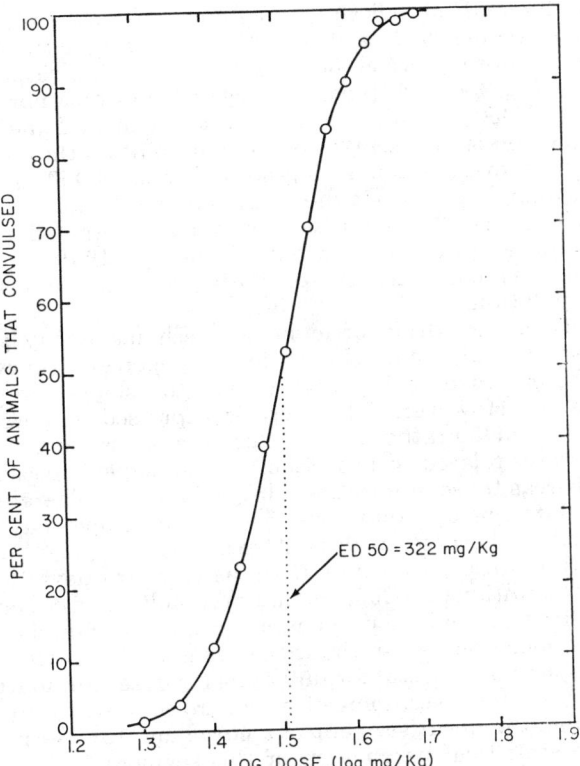

Fig. 480. The relationship of the number of responders in a population of mice to the dose of pentylenetetrazol (courtesy, Dr. D. G. Mc-Quarry and Dr. E. G. Fingl, University of Utah).

in fact, a cumulative frequency–distribution curve, the percent of responders at a given dose being the frequency of response.

Dose–cumulative frequency curves are generally of the same geometric shape as dose–intensity curves (namely, sigmoid) when frequency is plotted against log dose (see Fig. 480). The tendency of the cumulated frequency of response (ie, percent) to be linearly proportional to the log of the dose in the middle of the dose range is called the Weber–Fechner law, although it is not invariable, as a true natural law should be. In many instances, the cumulative frequency is simply proportional to dose rather than log dose. The Weber–Fechner law applies to either dose–intensity or dose–cumulative frequency data. The similarity between dose–frequency and dose–intensity curves may be more than fortuitous, since the intensity of response will usually have an approximately linear relationship to the percent of responding *units* (smooth muscle cells, nerve fibers, etc) and hence is also a type of cumulative frequency of response.

If only the increase in the number of responders with each new dose is plotted, instead of the cumulative percent of responders, a bell-shaped curve is obtained. This curve is the first derivative of the dose–cumulative frequency curve and is a *frequency-distribution* curve (see Chapter 11, *Statistics*). The distribution will be symmetrical—ie, *normal* or Gaussian (see Fig. 65, page 127)—only if the dose–cumulative frequency curve is symmetrically hyperbolic. Because most dose–cumulative frequency curves are more nearly symmetrical when plotted semilogarithmically (ie, as log dose), dose–cumulative frequency curves are usually *log-normal*.

Since the dose–intensity and dose–cumulative frequency curves are basically similar in shape, it follows that the curves have similar defining characteristics, such as ED50, efficacy, and slope.   In dose–cumulative frequency data, the ED50 (*median effective dose*) is the dose to which 50% of the population responds (see Fig. 480).   If the frequency distribution is normal, the ED50 is both the arithmetic mean and median dose and is represented by the mid-point on the curve; if the distribution is log-normal, the ED50 is the median dose but not the arithmetic mean dose.   The efficacy is the cumulative frequency summed over all doses; it is usually but not always 100%.   The slope is characteristic of both the drug and test population.

Even two drugs of identical mechanism may give rise to different slopes in dose–percent curves, whereas in dose–intensity curves the slopes are the same.   However, if the dose is expressed as percent of the ED50 rather than in absolute terms, curves for closely related drugs tend to be superimposable, whereas those of unrelated drugs do not.[1]   Therefore, if data are appropriately plotted, the slope may be used to characterize drug classes.

Statistical parameters (such as standard deviation) —in addition to ED50, maximum cumulative frequency (efficacy), and slope—characterize dose-cumulative frequency relationships (see Chapter 11, *Statistics*).

There are several formulations for dose–cumulative frequency curves, some of which are employed only to define the linear segment of a curve and to determine the statistical parameters of this segment.   For the statistical treatment of dose–frequency data, see Chapter 11, *Statistics*.   One simple mathematical expression of the entire log-symmetrical sigmoid curve is

$$\text{Dose} = K + f \log \left(\frac{\% \text{ response}}{100\% - \text{response}} \right) \quad (1)$$

where percent response may be either the percent of maximum intensity or the percent of a population responding.[1]   The equation is thus basically the same for both log normal dose–intensity and log normal dose–percent relationships. K is a constant that is characteristic of the mid-point of the curve, or ED50, and $1/f$ is characteristically related to the slope of the linear segment, which, in turn is closely related to the standard deviation of the derivative log normal frequency distribution curve.

The comparison of dose–percent relationships among drugs is subject to the same pitfalls indicated for dose–intensity comparisons (see page 730), namely, that when the slopes of the curves are not the same (ie, the dose–percent curves are not parallel), it is necessary to state at which level of response a potency ratio is calculated.   As with dose–intensity data, potencies are generally calculated from the ED50, but potency ratios may be calculated for any arbitrary percent response.   The expression of selectivity is likewise subject to similar qualifications, inasmuch as the dose–percent curves for the several effects are usually nonparallel.

The term *therapeutic index* is used to designate a quantitative statement of the selectivity of a drug when a therapeutic and an untoward effect are being compared.   If the untoward effect is designated as T (for toxic) and the therapeutic effect as E, the therapeutic index may be defined as TD50/ED50 or a similar ratio at some other arbitrary levels of response.   The TD and the ED are not required to express the same percent of response; some clinicians use the ratio TD1/ED99 or TD5/ED95, based on the rationale that if the untoward effect is serious, it is important

to use a most severe therapeutic index in passing judgment upon the drug.

There will be a different therapeutic index for each untoward effect that a drug may elicit, and, if there is more than one therapeutic effect, a family of therapeutic indices for each therapeutic effect.   However, in clinical practice, especially, and often in the laboratory, all untoward effects are lumped together and treated as one effect, namely toxicity, thereby obviating the need for the designation of a spectrum of therapeutic indices.

Variations in Response and Responsiveness— From the above discussion of dose–frequency relationships and the chapter on *Statistics*, it is obvious that in a normal population of persons there may be quite a large difference in the dose required to elicit a given response in the least-responsive member of the population and that to elicit the response in the most-responsive member.   The difference will ordinarily be a function of the slope of the dose–percent curve, or, in statistical terms, of the standard deviation.   If the standard deviation is large, the extremes of responsiveness of responders is likewise large.

In a normal population 95.46% of the population responds to doses within two standard deviations from the ED50 and 99.73% within three standard deviations.   In log normal populations the same distribution applies when standard deviation is expressed as log dose.

In the population represented in Fig. 480, 2.25% of the population (two standard deviations from the median) would require a dose more than 1.4 times the ED50; an equally small percent would respond to 0.7 the ED50.   The physician who is unfamiliar with statistics is apt to consider the 2.25% at either extreme as abnormal reactors.   The statistician will argue that these 4.5% are within the normal population and that only those who respond well outside of the normal population, at least three standard deviations from the median, deserve to be called abnormal.

Irrespective of whether the physician's or the statistician's criteria of abnormality obtain, the term *hyporeactive* applies to those individuals who require abnormally high doses and *hyperreactive* to those who require abnormally low doses.   The terms *hyporesponsive* and *hyperresponsive* may also be used.   It is incorrect to use the terms hyposensitive and hypersensitive in this context; *hypersensitivity* denotes an allergic response to a drug and should not be used to refer to hyperreactivity.   The term *supersensitivity* correctly applies to hyperreactivity that results from denervation of the effector organ; it is often more definitively called denervation supersensitivity.   Sometimes hyporeactivity is the result of an immunochemical deactivation of the drug, or *immunity*.   Hyporeactivity should be distinguished from an increased dose requirement that results from a severe pathological condition.   Severe pain requires large doses of analgesics, but the patient is not a hyporeactor; what has changed is the baseline from which the end-point quantum is measured.   The responsiveness of a patient to certain drugs sometimes may be determined by the history of previous exposure to appropriate drugs.

Tolerance is a diminution in responsiveness as use of the drug continues.   The consequence of tolerance is an increase in the dose requirement.   It may be due to an increase in the rate of elimination of drug, as discussed elsewhere in this chapter, to reflex or other compensatory homeostatic adjustments, to exhaustion of the effector system or depletion of mediators, to the development of immunity, or to other mechanisms. Tolerance may be gradual, requiring many doses and days to months to develop, or acute, requiring only the first or a few doses and only minutes to hours to develop. Acute tolerance is called *tachyphylaxis*.

Drug resistance is the decrease in responsiveness of microorganisms, neoplasms, or pests to chemotherapeutic agents, antineoplastics, or pesticides, respectively. It is not tolerance in the sense that the sensitivity of the individual microorganism or cancer cell decreases; rather it is the survival of normally unresponsive cells which then pass the genetic factors of resistance on to their progeny.

Patients who fail to respond to a drug are called *refractory*. Refractoriness may result from tolerance or resistance, but it may also result from the progression of pathological states that negate the response or render the response incapable of surmounting an overwhelming pathology. Rarely, it may result from a poorly developed receptor or response system.

Sometimes a drug evokes an unusual response that is *qualitatively* different from the expected response. Such an unexpected response is called a *meta-reaction*. A not uncommon meta-reaction is a central nervous stimulant rather than depressant effect of phenobarbital, especially in women. Certain pathological states and pain sometimes favor meta-reactivity. Responses that are different in infants or the aged than in young and middle-aged people are not meta-reactions if the response is usual in the age group. The term *idiosyncracy* also denotes meta-reactivity, but the word has been so abused that it is recommended that it be dropped. Although hypersensitivity may cause unusual effects, it is not included in meta-reactivity.

Drug Receptors and Receptor Theory

Most drugs act by combining with some key substance in the biological milieu that has an important regulatory function in the target organ or tissue. This biological partner of the drug goes by the name of *receptive substance* or *drug receptor*. The receptive substance is mostly considered to be a cellular constituent, although in a few instances it may be extracellular, as the cholinesterases are, in part. The receptive substance is thought of as having a special chemical affinity and structural requirements for the drug. Drugs such as emollients, which have a physical rather than chemical basis for their action, obviously do not act upon receptors. Drugs, such as demulcents and astringents, which act in a nonselective or nonspecific chemical way are also not considered to act upon receptors, since the candidate receptors have neither sharp chemical nor biological definition. Even antacids, which react with the extremely well-defined hydronium ion, cannot be said to have a receptor, since the reactive proton has no permanent biological residence.

Because of early preoccupation with physical theories of action and the classical and illogical dichotomy of chemical and physical molecular interaction, there is a reluctance to admit receptors for drugs such as local anesthetics, general anesthetics, certain electrolytes, etc, which are now generally accepted to combine with cellular or organelle membrane constituents. The word receptor is used often inconsistently and intuitively, and some critics have moved for its abandonment. However, the term is a legitimate symbol for that biological structure with which a drug interacts to initiate a response. The fact that we are ignorant of the identities of most receptors does not detract from but rather increases the importance of the term and general concept.

Once a receptor is identified it is frequently no longer thought of as a receptor, although such identification may afford the basis of profound advances in receptor theory. Since the effects of anticholinesterases are only indirectly derived from inhibition of cholinesterase and no drugs are known which stimulate the enzyme, it may be argued that it is not a receptor. Nevertheless, it is probable that a large number of drugs ultimately will be revealed to act indirectly through the inhibition of such modulator enzymes, and it is important for the theoretician to develop models based upon such indirect interrelations.

Enzymes, of course, readily suggest themselves as candidates for receptors. However, there is more to cellular function than enzymes. Receptors may be intracellular constituents that govern the spatial orientation of enzymes, compartmentalization of the cytoplasm, contractile or compliant properties of subcellular structures, or permeability and electrical properties of membranes. For nearly every cellular constituent there can be imagined a possible way for a drug to affect its function; therefore, few cellular constituents can be dismissed *a priori* as possible receptors.

Occupation and Rate Theories

Two major theories deal with the role of drug–receptor interaction in initiating a response. The first of these, the *occupation theory*,[2] states that a drug continues to act as long as it remains combined with its receptor and that the intensity of effect is directly proportional to the *proportion of receptors occupied*. The second, the *rate theory*,[3] states that a stimulating drug (agonist: see below) continues to act only as long as fresh drug and receptor molecules come into collision and that the intensity of effect is a linear function of the *rate* of drug-receptor reaction.

Probably each theory correctly applies in a particular context and appropriate situation, and the two theories are not necessarily mutually exclusive. However, the occupation theory, the older, dominates the receptor theory.

In both theories the terms agonist, partial agonist, and antagonist are employed. An *agonist* is a drug that combines with a receptor to initiate a response.

In the occupation theory two attributes of the drug are required: (1) *affinity*, a measure of the equilibrium constant of the drug-receptor interaction and (2) *intrinsic activity*, or *efficacy* (not to be confused with efficacy as maximum effect), a measure of the ability of the drug to induce a positive change in the function of the receptor.

In the rate theory two different attributes are required: (1) a large *association constant* (ie, forward rate), so that a high initial rate of reaction is favored and (2) a large *dissociation constant* (ie, backward rate), which enables the free drug and receptor to be readily regenerated and to reassociate again and thus to sustain the reaction rate and the action.

In both theories a *competitive antagonist* is a drug which occupies a significant proportion of the receptors and thereby preempts them from reacting maximally with an agonist. In the occupation theory the prerequisite property is affinity without intrinsic activity. In the rate theory it is a small dissociation constant.

A *partial agonist* is a drug that can elicit some but not a maximal effect and which antagonizes an agonist. In the occupation theory it would be a drug with a favorable affinity but a low intrinsic activity. In the rate theory it would show an intermediate to high association constant but a low dissociation constant. Thus a sufficient amount would remain complexed to slow the association rate.

A *noncompetitive* antagonist may react with the receptor in such a way as not to prevent agonist–receptor combination but to prevent the combination from initiating a response, or it may act to inhibit some subsequent event in the chain of action–effect–action–effect that leads to the final overt response.

The mathematical formulation of the receptor theories derive directly from the law of mass action and chemical kinetics. Certain assumptions are required to simplify calculations. The key assumption is that the intensity of effect is a direct linear function of either the proportion of receptors occupied or the rate of occupation, according to the appropriate theory. The correctness of this assumption is most improbable on the basis of theoretical considerations, but empirically it appears to be a close enough approximation to be useful. A second assumption, in the occupation theory only, is that the drug–receptor interaction is at equilibrium. Another common assumption is that the number of molecules of receptor is negligibly small compared to that of the drug. This assumption is undoubtedly true in most instances and is the reason why drug–receptor kinetics appear to be first-order processes, when they are, in fact pesudomonomolecular.

The first clearly stated mathematical formulation drug–receptor kinetics was that of Clark.[2] In his equation,

$$Kx^n = \frac{y}{100 - y} \qquad (2)$$

where K is the affinity constant, x is the concentration of drug, n is the molecularity of the reaction, and y is the percent of maximum response. Clark assumed that y was a linear function of the percent of receptors occupied by the drug, so that y could also symbolize the percent of receptors occupied. When the equation is rearranged to solve for y,

$$y = \frac{100Kx^n}{1 + Kx^n} \qquad (3)$$

A Cartesian plot of this equation is identical in form to that shown in Fig. 477. When y is plotted against $\log x$ instead of x, the usual sigmoid curve is obtained. Thus it may be seen that the dose–intensity curve derives from mass action equilibrium kinetics, which in turn derive from the statistical nature of molecular interaction. The fact that dose–intensity and dose–percent curves have the same shape shows that they both involve the same kind of statistics.

If Eq. 2 is put into log form,

$$\log K + n \log x = \log \frac{y}{100 - y} \qquad (4)$$

a plot of $\log y/100 - y$ against $\log x$ will then yield a straight line with a slope of n; n is theoretically the number of molecules of drug which react with each molecule of receptor. However, the wide range of empirical values of n suggests unseen factors in this variable.

The probability that a molecule of drug will react with a receptor is a function of the concentration of both drug and receptor. The concentration of receptor molecules cannot be manipulated like the concentration of a drug. But as each molecule of drug combines with a receptor, the population of free receptors is diminished accordingly. If the drug is a competitive antagonist, it will diminish the probability of an agonist–receptor combination in direct proportion to the percent of receptor molecules preempted by the antagonist. Consequently, the intensity of effect will be diminished. However, the probability of agonist–receptor interaction can be increased by increasing the concentration of agonist, and the intensity of effect can be restored by appropriately larger doses of agonist. Addition of more antagonist will again diminish the response, which can, again, be overcome or *surmounted* by more agonist.

Clark[4] showed empirically and by theory that as long as the ratio of antagonist to agonist was constant, the concentration of the competitive drugs could be varied over an enormous range without changing the magnitude of the response (see Fig. 481). Since the presence of competitive antagonist only diminishes the probability of agonist–receptor combination at a given concentration of agonist and does not alter the molecularity of the reaction, it also follows that the effect of the competitive antagonist is to shift the dose–intensity curve to the right in proportion to the amount of antagonist present; neither shape nor slope of the curve is changed (see Fig. 482). Both Figs. 481 and 482 are from Clark's original paper on competitive antagonism.

Many refinements of the Clark formula have been made, but they will not be treated here; details and references[5–8] are available. Most refinements were introduced to facilitate studies of competitive inhibition. The introduction of the concept of intrinsic activity (see Ref. 5), or efficacy,[6] required appropriate changes in mathematical treatment.

Another important concept has been added to the occupation theory, namely the concept of *spare receptors*. Clark assumed the maximal response to occur only when the receptors were completely occupied, which does not account for the possibility that the

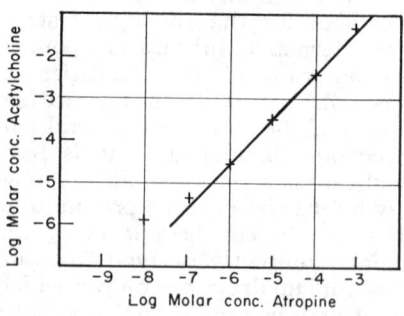

Fig. 481. Direct proportionality of the dose of agonist (acetylcholine) to the dose of antagonist (atropine) necessary to cause a constant degree of inhibition (50%) of the response of the frog heart (courtesy, adaptation, Clark[4]).

maximum response might be limited by some step in the action–effect sequence subsequent to receptor occupation. More recent work with isotopically labelled agonists and antagonists and with dose–effect kinetics has shown that the maximal effect is often achieved when only a small fraction of the receptors are yet occupied. The mathematical treatment of this phenomenon has enabled theorists to explain several puzzling observations that appeared to contradict drug–receptor theory.

The rate theory of receptor action[3] is a marked departure from the original Clark concept, but, strangely, its mathematical formulations are such that the kinetic consequences at equilibrium or steady state are almost the same as those of the occupation theory.

The Nature of Receptor Groups and Models of Receptors

A *receptor group* is that portion of the receptor molecule with which an agonist acts and which is vital to the function of the receptor. Studies of receptor group composition and configuration are too complex for the purposes of this text; consequently, only a brief sketch will be made here to orient casually the reader to the nature of the approach.

From the chemical configuration and reactivity of agonists and antagonists, certain deductions can be made about the structure of a receptor group. For example, all highly active agonists of cholinergic receptors are cations at physiological pH. This suggests that the receptor group contains an anionic group and that the force of attraction is electrostatic, at least in part, which agrees with thermodynamic data. That van der Waals forces may also make an important contribution to binding is suggested by the requirement for *N*-methyl groups and by the low but definite activity of the nonionizable quaternary carbon analog of acetylcholine, 3,3-dimethylbutyl acetate. This establishes a requirement for an auxiliary structure close to the anionic site. Studies of the contribution to activity of ester and carbonyl oxygen among

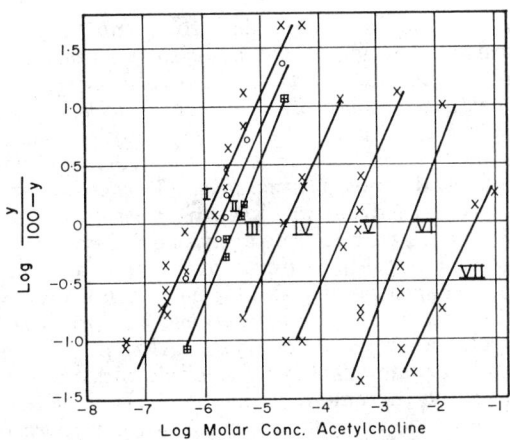

Fig. 482. Effect of an antagonist to shift the log dose–intensity curve to the right without altering the slope. The effector is the isolated heart. *I*: no atropine; *II*: atropine, $10^{-8}M$; *III*: 10^{-7}; *IV*: 10^{-6}; *V*: 10^{-5}; *VI*: 10^{-4}; *VII*: 10^{-3}. Y: % of maximum intensity of response; the function $\log \frac{y}{100-y}$ converts the log dose–intensity relationship to a straight line (courtesy, adaptation, Clark[4]).

analogs of acetylcholine, of intramolecular distances, and of the stereospecificity of various isomers and conformers have indicated a cationic site between 2.5 and 4Å and a region of low electronic density between 5 and 7 Å from the anionic site. Mucopolysaccharides and phosphoproteins have been proposed as models for such a receptor.

The structure–activity relationships among competitive inhibitors must also be consistent with any model of a receptor. However, binding sites additional to the receptor group can be involved, and results are frequently more difficult to interpret than those with agonists. Nevertheless, studies with antagonists have made a substantial contribution to receptor group analysis. There is considerable interest in antagonists that combine irreversibly with the receptor, since such drugs offer a way of marking the receptor for isolation and for identification of the receptor group.

Mechanism of Drug Action

Any metabolic or physiological function provides a potential mechanism of action of a drug. The term *mechanism of action* has been employed in a number of ways. In the past it was often the habit to confuse the site or locus of action with the mechanism of action. For example, the mechanism of the hypotensive action of tetraethylammonium ion was originally described as that of ganglionic blockade, which did nothing more than identify the anatomical structure upon which the drug acted. In a general sense, this was a partial elucidation of the mechanism of action, if mechanism is used in the mechanical sense of the entire linkage between the input and output of a machine. However, there has been a gradual narrowing of the definition of mechanism of action to be restricted to only the first event in the action–effect sequence, that is, only to the alteration of receptor function by the drug. In this sense the mechanism of action of tetraethylammonium is more appropriately defined as that of competition with acetylcholine for nicotinic cholinergic receptors on the postsynaptic ganglion cell membrane, even though the alteration in

receptor function is not defined. The ultimate mechanism of action is known for only a few drugs.

It is customary to speak of a drug as a stimulant or a depressant, of the action as being excitatory or inhibitory, etc. Such terms describe only the effect and not the action, and they have no bearing upon whether the drug augments receptor function or diminishes it. In biological systems positive and negative modulation and feedback occurs at every level, the organ as well as the subcellular. Thus an agonist to a negative modulator may be able to bring about the same effect as an antagonist to a positive modulator. It is possible for an antagonist or inhibitor to elicit an excitatory effect. An example is the convulsant action of strychnine, which results from its antagonism of a mediator of postsynaptic inhibition in the central nervous system. Conversely, it is possible for an agonist to elicit an inhibitory effect. An example is the reflex bradycardia that results from the stimulant action of veratrum alkaloids on chemoreceptors in the left ventricle.

Because of the central role *enzymes play* in cellular

function, it is not surprising that thinking on the mechanism of action of drugs has focused largely upon enzymes. Agonist drugs conceivably could serve as substrates, cofactors, or activators. At the present time, no drug is definitely known to exert its action as a substrate or as a cofactor, exclusive of vitamins and known nutrients. However, at least three classes of drugs are known and several are suspected to work through the activation of enzymes.

The most notable example of enzyme activation is that of epinephrine and similar catecholamines, which activate adenyl cyclase to increase the production of 3′,5′-cyclic adenylic acid (cyclic AMP). The metabolic and cardiac effects of catecholamines are attributable to the increment in cyclic AMP. With very little doubt, adenyl cyclase is the β-adrenergic receptor. Glucagon also owes its hyperglycemic action to activation of hepatic adenyl cyclase. There is thus the interesting phenomenon of one receptor, adenyl cyclase, mediating the action of two chemically unrelated drugs. Since β-adrenergic blocking agents do not antagonize glucagon, it is obvious that glucagon works upon a different reactive group (ie, receptor group) in the enzyme (receptor) than does epinephrine. Epinephrine is thought to act at the active center of the cyclase, where ATP is bound and converted to cyclic AMP, whereas glucagon is thought to act not immediately at the active center but elsewhere, perhaps by inducing a more favorable conformation of the enzyme protein.

Many drugs are inhibitors of enzymes. When the drug is a *competitive inhibitor* of a natural endogenous substrate of the enzyme, it is called an *antimetabolite*. Examples of antimetabolites are sulfonamides, which compete with para-aminobenzoic acid and thus interfere with its incorporation into folic acid, and methotrexate, which competes with folic acid for folic reductase and thus interferes with the formation of folinic acid. It might seem that anticholinesterases are also antimetabolites, although they are never placed into that classification. The reason is that the products of cholinesterase–acetylcholine interaction do not subserve important metabolic functions, as do folic and folinic acids, so that the organism is not deprived of an important metabolite by the action of the cholinesterase inhibitors.

Some drugs are competitive inhibitors of enzyme systems whose natural function appears not to produce useful metabolites but to rid the body of foreign substances. Inhibitors of the hepatic microsomes and probenecid fall into this category; the hepatic microsomes do perform a few biotransformations on endogenous substrates, but the renal tubular anion transport system does not appear to be required to eliminate any important endogenous substances.

Since neither the hepatic microsomes nor the tubular anion transport system seems to be involved in response systems, inhibitors of these enzyme systems are antagonists without corresponding agonists. Indeed, even natural endogenous substrates of enzymes are rarely considered to be agonists.

Noncompetitive enzyme inhibitors among drugs are also known. Examples are cyanide, fluoride, disulfiram, and probably cardiac glycosides. When enzyme inhibition brings about a positive response—eg, the cholinergic effects of the anticholinesterases or the effects of theophylline consequent to inhibition of phosphodiesterase—the drug appears to be an agonist. Yet there can be no competitive antagonist to such an inhibitor, since the competitor to the drug is more

substrate, to which the effect of the drug is actually attributable.

Acetylcholine increases the permeability of the synapse to cations and the heart to potassium, but the mechanism of this effect remains undefined. The mechanism has been generally thought to involve some conformation or other change in a membrane constituent so that pore size or permeability constant is affected, instead of an enzyme. Even though there may now be cogent reasons to reconsider an enzymatic mechanism for acetylcholine, there still remains a high probability that many drugs and toxins, among them local anesthetics, sedative–hypnotics, general anesthetics, and tetrodotoxin, act through *alterations in the structural and physical properties of membranes*. To the extent that some of such substances may disperse themselves generally throughout the lipoid phase of the membrane rather than to combine with special chemical entities, no definite receptors for such drugs can be said to exist.

The mechanism of action of certain drugs, especially autonomic drugs, is often stated to be *mimicry* of a natural neurohumor or hormone. Thus methacholine mimics acetylcholine as an agonist. This does not define the mechanism of action, unless the mechanism of action of the natural substance is known.

Mimicry usually occurs because of a structural similarity between the natural substance and the mimetic drug. Mimicry in agonist functions is easy to demonstrate, but the site of action may not be mimicry of the natural agonist at its receptor but rather at its storage site to *release* the natural agonist.

Examples of mimetics that act by release of the natural mediator are sympathomimetics such as *d*-amphetamine, mephentermine, ephedrine (in part), tyramine, and others, which are now known to act by displacing norepinephrine from storage sites within the adrenergic neurone. Many of such indirectly acting sympathomimetics lack a direct action on the adrenergic receptor, although some, like ephedrine, act both upon the receptor and the storage complex. Another mimetic by a release mechanism is carbachol, which promotes the presynaptic discharge of acetylcholine.

In these examples there is a close structural similarity between the mimetic and the released mediator. In the case of many releasers of histamine (such as tubocurarine, polymyxin, or morphine) no close chemical relationship exists between the releaser and the released. In such instances release probably occur because of activation of an enzyme, lysolecithinase, which attacks the membrane of the storage cell or organelle.

Structural similarity may also aid mimicry by promoting chemical combination with an enzyme of destruction or some other means of disposition. For example, metaraminol, amphetamine, etc *inhibit membrane transport* into the neurone and hence inhibit the neuronal recapture of released norepinephrine. Consequently, the extraneuronal concentration of norepinephrine in the nearby region of the receptors does not drop as rapidly as in the absence of the mimetic, and the action of the mediator is sustained.

Some inhibitors of the enzymes of the destruction of mediators are structurally similar enough to the mediator to have some agonist action. This is true of neostigmine, which has a direct stimulant action on nicotinic receptors in addition to its anticholinesterase action. In contrast, the anticholinesterase physostigmine has some antagonist actions on cholinergic receptors and an effect to interfere with acetylcholine synthesis.

The above multiple actions come about because all the structures that interact with a small molecule mediator (the receptor, synthesizing enzyme, destructive enzyme, storage molecule, membrane transport carrier) must have some common structural features and affinities. A drug that reacts with one of these molecules has a distinct probability of interacting with another.

The recognition of the critical role of *ions* in the function of membranes, the excitability of cells, and the activity of many enzymes has generated a renewed interest in ions in the mechanism of action of certain drugs. The inorganic ions, some of which are used as drugs, lend themselves automatically to a discussion of ionic mechanisms. The repair of electrolyte deficiencies by replacement therapy warrants no further comment here, except to say that the mechanisms of action of these ions are yet poorly understood. Some nonphysiological ions act as imperfect impersonators of physiological ions; lithium partially substitutes for sodium, bromide for chloride and thiocyanate for iodide, and each may owe its pharmacological action, in part, to a sluggish mobility through membrane channels, through which their sister ions normally pass readily when traffic is not impeded by "slowly moving vehicles." Iodide has an effect to increase the penetrance of drugs into caseous and necrotic areas, to aid in the resolution of gummatous lesions, to reduce the viscosity of mucous secretions, and other odd effects; it is thought to do so by increasing the hydration of collagen and mucoproteins by a poorly understood mechanism. The transition and heavy metals have in common the ability to form complexes with a variety of physiologically active substances, particularly the active centers of many enzymes. *Chelation* and other *complexation* are the mechanism of action of several drugs used to treat heavy metal intoxication, diseases that involve abnormal body burdens or plasma levels of heavy metals and hypercalcemia (see pages 1255 and 843).

More recent interest has centered upon the effects of drugs upon ion movements. Cardiac glycosides are known to inhibit an ATPase involved in the membrane transport of sodium and several other substances, but their effects on the heart seem more probably linked with the movements of calcium. The mechanisms of action of local anesthetics, quinidine, and various other drugs are also speculated to involve calcium movements.

Concomitant with the development of molecular biology was the appreciation that drugs act through *nuclear* and *extranuclear genetic mechanisms.* Nitrogen mustards have long been known to interfere with the replication of DNA. Streptomycin, kanamycin, neomycin, and gentamicin cause misreading by the ribosomes of the code incorporated into messenger RNA; tetracyclines, erythromycin, and chloramphenicol inhibit the synthesis of protein at the ribosomes; and chloroquine, novobiocin, and colchicine inhibit DNA polymerase. Other drugs induce the production of enzymes; aldosterone appears to act by inducing the synthesis of the enzyme, membrane ATPase, necessary to sodium transport. The proliferation of work on microsomal enzyme induction will undoubtedly multiply the examples of drugs that affect the genetic apparatus.

A number of drugs have simple mechanisms that do not involve an action at the cellular level. Examples are bulk and saline cathartics, osmotic diuretics, and cholestyramine. Although such drugs usually do not generate much excitement among pharmacologists, they do serve to remind us of the many avenues through which mechanism of action may be expressed. Throughout the various chapters of Part VI specific mechanisms of action may be mentioned.

Absorption, Distribution, and Excretion

No matter by which route a drug is administered it must pass through several to many biological membranes during the processes of absorption, distribution, biotransformation, and elimination. Since membranes are traversed in all of these events, the subject of this section will begin with a brief description of biological membranes and membrane processes and the relationship of the physicochemical properties of a drug molecule to penetrance and transport.

Structure and Properties of Membranes

The concept that a membrane surrounds each cell arose shortly after the cellular nature of tissue was discovered. The biological and physicochemical properties of cells seemed in accord with this view. Nevertheless, from time-to-time the actual existence of the membrane has been questioned by brilliant men, and ingenious explanations have been advanced to explain cellular integrity and the osmotic and electrophysiological properties of cells. Few authorities have taken such challenges seriously, since microchemical, x-ray diffraction, electron microscopic, and other investigations leave virtually no room for doubt. The exact structure of the cell membrane, however, continues to be debated. The description of the membrane that follows is somewhat oversimplified, but it is essentially in accord with the current predominant view and with the general properties of the membrane.

Structure and Composition—The cell membrane has been described as a "mayonnaise sandwich," in which a bimolecular layer of lipid material is entrained between two parallel monomolecular layers of protein. In Fig. 483 the lipid layers are represented as an orderly, closely packed array of lipid molecules associated tail-to-tail, each "tail" being an alkyl chain or steroid group and the "head" being a polar group, such as carboxyl or phosphate. In reality a membrane is probably not so orderly, since its composition is quite complex. Chains of fatty acids of different degrees of saturation and steroid groups cannot array themselves in simple parallel arrangements. Furthermore, the polar heads will assume a number of orientations depending upon the substances and groups involved.

The plasma membrane appears to be asymmetrical. The lipid composition varies from cell type to cell type and perhaps from site to site on the same membrane. There are, for example, differences between the membrane of the endoplasmic reticulum and the plasma

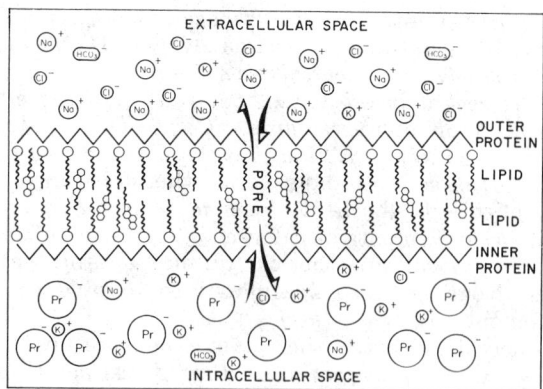

Fig. 483. Simplified cross section of a cell membrane (components are not to scale). The lipid interior of the membrane consists of various phospholipids, fatty acids, cholesterol, and other steroids. Ions are indicated in order to illustrate differences in size relative to the pore. Pr: protein.

membrane, even though the membranes are coextensive. Where membranes are double, the inner and outer layers may differ considerably; the inner and outer membranes of mitochondria have been shown to have strikingly different compositions and properties. Some authorities have expressed doubt as to the existence of the protein layers in biological membranes, although the evidence is preponderantly in favor of at least an outer protein coat.

The cell membrane appears to be perforated by water-filled pores of various sizes, varying from about 4–10 Å, being predominantly around 7Å. Through these pores pass inorganic ions and small organic molecules. Since sodium ions are more hydrated than potassium and chloride ions, they are larger and do not pass as freely through the pores as potassium and chloride. The vascular endothelium appears to have pores at least as large as 40Å, but these may be interstitial passages rather than transmembrane pores. Lipid molecules small enough to pass through the pores may do so, but they have a higher probability of entering into the lipid layer, from where they will equilibrate chemically with the interior of the cell. From work on monolayers, some workers contend that it is not necessary to postulate pores to explain the permeability to water and small water-soluble molecules.

Stratum Corneum—Although the stratum corneum is not a membrane in the same sense as a cell membrane, it offers a barrier to diffusion, which is of significance in the topical application of drugs. The stratum corneum consists of several layers of dead keratinized cutaneous epithelial cells enmeshed in a matrix of keratin fibers and bound together with cementing desmosomes and penetrating tonofibrils of keratin. Varying amounts of lipids and fatty acids from dying cells, sebum, and sweat are contained among the dead squamous cells. Immediately beneath the layer of dead cells and above the viable epidermal epithelial cells is a layer of keratohyaline granules and various water-soluble substances, such as alpha amino acids, purines, monosaccharides, and urea.

The precise location of the cutaneous barrier to penetration of chemical substances is in dispute, both the upper and lower layers of the stratum corneum having been implicated. It is probable that the barrier to penetration from the surface is in the upper layers and the barrier to the outward movement of water is in the lowest layer of the stratum corneum.

Membrane Potentials—Across the cell membrane there exists an electrical potential, always negative on the inside and positive on the outside. If a cell did not have special membrane electrolyte transport processes, its membrane potential would be mainly the result of the Donnan equilibrium (see Chapter 16, *Complexation*) consequent to the semipermeability of the membrane. Such potentials generally lie between 2 and 5 mv.

A cell with a membrane across which diffusible electrolyte distribution is purely passive would be expected to have a high internal concentration of sodium, such as is true for the erythrocytes of some species. However, the interior of most cells is high in potassium and low in sodium, as depicted in Fig. 483. This unequal distribution of cations attests to special electrolyte transport processes and to differential permeabilities of diffusible ions, so that the membrane potential is higher than that which would result from a purely passive Donnan distribution. In nerve and skeletal or cardiac muscle the membrane potential ranges upwards to about 90 mv. The electrical gradient is on the order of 50,000 v/cm, because of the extreme thinness of the membrane. Obviously, such an intense potential gradient will strongly influence the transmembrane passages of charged drug molecules.

Diffusion and Transport

Transport is the movement of a drug from one place to another within the body. The drug may diffuse freely in uncombined form with a kinetic energy, appropriate to its thermal environment, or it may move in combination with extracellular or cellular constituents, sometimes in connection with energy-yielding processes that allow the molecule or complex to overcome barriers to simple diffusion.

Simple Nonionic Diffusion and Passive Transport—Molecules in solution move in a purely random fashion, providing they are not charged and moving in an electrical gradient. Such random movement is called *diffusion*, and if the molecule is uncharged it is called *nonionic diffusion*.

In a population of drug molecules, the probability that during unit time any drug molecule will move across a boundary is directly proportional to the number of molecules adjoining that boundary and therefore to the drug concentration. Except at dilutions so extreme that only a few molecules are present, the actual rate of movement (molecules/unit time) is directly proportional to the probability and therefore to the concentration. Once molecules have passed through the boundary to the opposite side, their random motion may cause some to return and others to continue to move further away from the boundary. The rate of return is likewise proportional to the concentration on the opposite side of the boundary. It follows that, although molecules are moving in both directions, there will be a net movement from the region of higher to that of lower concentration and that the net transfer will be proportional to the concentration differential or gradient. If the boundary is a membrane, which has both substance and dimension, the rate of movement is also directly proportional to the permeability and inversely proportional to the thickness. These factors combine into Fick's Law of Diffusion,

$$\frac{dQ}{dt} = \frac{\bar{D}A(C_1 - C_2)}{x} \tag{5}$$

where Q is the net quantity of drug transferred across the membrane, t is time, C_1 is the concentration on one side and C_2 on the other, x is the thickness of the membrane, A is the area, and $\bar{D}$ is the diffusion coefficient, related to permeability. The equation is more correct if chemical activities are used instead of concentrations. Since a biological membrane is patchy, with pores of different sizes and probably with varying thickness and composition, both $\bar{D}$ and x probably vary from spot to spot. Nevertheless, some mean values can be assumed.

It is customary to combine the membrane factors into a single constant, called a permeability constant or coefficient, P, so that $P = \bar{D}/x$, A in Eq. 5 having unit value. The rate of net transport (diffusion) across the membrane then becomes

$$\frac{dQ}{dt} = P(C_1 - C_2) \tag{6}$$

As diffusion continues, C_1 approaches C_2, and the net rate, dQ/dt, approaches zero in exponential fashion characteristic of a first-order process. Equilibrium is defined as that state in which $C_1 = C_2$. The equilibrium is, of course, dynamic, with equal numbers of molecules being transported in each direction during unit time. If water is also moving through the membrane, it may either facilitate the movement of drug or impede it, according to the relative directions of movement of water and drug; this effect of water movement is called *solvent drag*.

Ionic or Electrochemical Diffusion—If a drug is ionized, the transport properties are modified. The probability of penetrating the membrane is still a function of concentration, but it is also a function of the potential difference or electrical gradient across the membrane. A cationic drug molecule will be repelled from the positive charge on the outside of the membrane, and only those molecules with a high kinetic energy will pass through the ion barrier. If the cation is polyvalent, it may not penetrate at all.

Once inside the membrane, a cation will be simultaneously attracted to the negative charge on the intracellular surface of the membrane and repelled by the outer surface; it is said to be moving along the *electrical gradient*. If it is also moving from a higher towards a lower concentration, it is said to be moving along its *electrochemical gradient*, the electrochemical gradient being the sum of the influences of the electrical field and the concentration differential across the membrane.

Once inside the cell, cations will tend to be kept inside by the attractive negative charge on the interior of the cell, and the intracellular concentration of drug will increase until, by sheer numbers of accumulated drug particles, the outward diffusion or mass escape rate equals the inward transport rate, and electrochemical equilibrium is said to have occurred. At electrochemical equilibrium at body temperature (37°C), ionized drug molecules will be distributed according to the Nernst equation,

$$\pm \log \frac{C_o}{C_i} = \frac{ZE}{61} \tag{7}$$

where C_o is the molar extracellular and C_i the intracellular concentration, Z is the number of charges per molecule, and E is the membrane potential in millivolts. Log C_o/C_i is positive when the molecule is negatively charged and negative when the molecule is positively charged.

Facilitated Diffusion—Sometimes a substance moves more rapidly through a biological membrane than can be accounted for by the process of simple diffusion. This accelerated movement is termed *facilitated diffusion*. It is thought to be due to the presence of a special molecule, called a *carrier*, within the membrane, with which carrier the transported substance combines. There is considered to be a greater permeability to the carrier–drug complex than to the drug alone, so that the transport rate is enhanced. After the complex traverses the membrane it dissociates. The carrier must either return to the original side of the membrane to be reused or be constantly produced on one side and eliminated on the other in order for the carrier process to be continuous. Although facilitated diffusion resembles active transport, below, in its dependence upon a continuous source of energy, it differs in that facilitated diffusion will only transport a molecule along its electrochemical gradient.

Active Transport—Active transport may be defined as energy-dependent movement of a substance through a biological membrane against an electrochemical gradient. It is characterized by the following:

1. The substance is transported from a region of lower to one of higher electrochemical activity.
2. Metabolic poisons interfere with transport.
3. The transport rate approaches an asymptote (ie, saturates) as concentration increases.
4. The transport system usually shows a requirement for specific chemical structures.
5. Closely related chemicals are competitive for the transport system.

Many drugs are secreted from the renal tubules or into the bile by active transport, but the role of active transport of drugs in the distribution into the body compartments and tissues is less well known. Active transport is required for the penetrance of a number of sympathomimetics into neural tissue.

Pinocytosis—Many, perhaps all, cells are capable of a type of phagocytosis called *pinocytosis*. The cell membrane has been observed to invaginate into a saccular structure containing extracellular materials and then pinch off the saccule at the membrane, so that the saccule remains as a vesicle or vacuole within the interior of the cell. Since metabolic activity is required and since an extracellular substance may be transported against an electrochemical gradient, pinocytosis shows some of the same characteristics as active transport. However, pinocytosis is relatively slow and inefficient compared to most active transport, except in gastrointestinal absorption, in which pinocytosis is of considerable importance.

It is not known to what extent pinocytosis contributes to the transport of most drugs, but many macromolecules and even larger particles can be absorbed by the gut. Pinocytosis probably explains the oral efficacy of the Sabin polio vaccine. Some drugs themselves affect pinocytosis; for example, adrenal glucocorticoids markedly inhibit the process in macrophages and other cells involved in inflammation.

Physicochemical Factors in Penetrance

Drugs and other substances may traverse the membrane primarily either through the pores or by dissolution into the membrane lipids and subsequent diffusion from the membrane into the cell sap or other fluid on the far side of the membrane. The physicochemical prerequisites are different according to which route is taken. To pass through the pores the "diameter" of the molecule must be smaller than the pore, but the molecule can be longer than the pore diameter. The probability that a long, thin molecule will be oriented properly is low, unless there is also bulk flow, and the transmembrane passage of large molecules is slow.

Water-soluble molecules with low lipid solubility are usually thought to pass through the membrane mainly via the pores and to a small extent by pinocytosis, but recent work with lipid monolayers suggests that small water-soluble molecules may also be able to pass readily through the lipid, and the necessity of postulating the existence of pores has been questioned. Nevertheless, experimental data on penetrance overwhelmingly favor the concept of passage of water-soluble lipid-insoluble substances through pores. If there is a membrane carrier or active transport system, a low solubility of the drug in membrane lipids is no impediment to penetration, since the drug-carrier complex is assumed to have an appropriate solubility, and energy from an active transport system enables the drug to penetrate the energy barrier "imposed by the lipids." Actually, the lipids are not an important energy barrier; rather the barrier is the force of attraction of the solvent water for its dipolar or polar solute, so that it is difficult for the solute to leave the water and enter the lipid.

Drugs with a high solubility in the membrane lipids, of course, pass easily through the membrane. Even when their dimensions are small enough to permit passage through pores, lipid-soluble drugs primarily pass through the membrane lipids, not only because chemical partition favors the lipid phase but because the surface area occupied by pores is only a small fraction of the total membrane area.

Lipid Solubility and Partition Coefficients—As early as 1902 Overton[9] investigated the importance of lipid solubility to the penetrance and absorption of drugs. Eventually it was recognized that more important than lipid solubility was the lipid–water distribution coefficient; that is to say, a high lipid solubility does not favor penetrance unless the water solubility is low enough that the drug is not entrained in the aqueous phase.

In Fig. 484 is illustrated the relationship between the chloroform–water partition coefficient and the colonic absorption of barbiturates. Chloroform is probably not the optimal lipid solvent for such a study, and natural lipids from nerve or other tissues have been shown to be superior in the few instances in which they have been employed. Nevertheless, the correlation shown in the figure is a convincing one.

When the water solubility of a substance is so low that a significant concentration in water or extracellular fluid cannot be achieved, absorption may be negligible in spite of a favorable partition coefficient. Hence mineral oil, petrolatum, etc are virtually unabsorbed. The optimal partition coefficient for permeation of the skin appears to be lower than that for the permeation of the cell membrane, being perhaps as low as one.

Dipolarity, Polarity, and Nonionic Diffusion— The partition coefficient of a drug depends upon the polarity and the size of the molecule. Drugs with a high dipole moment, even though unionized, have a low lipid solubility and hence poor penetrance. An example of a highly dipolar substance with a low partition coefficient and which does not penetrate into cells

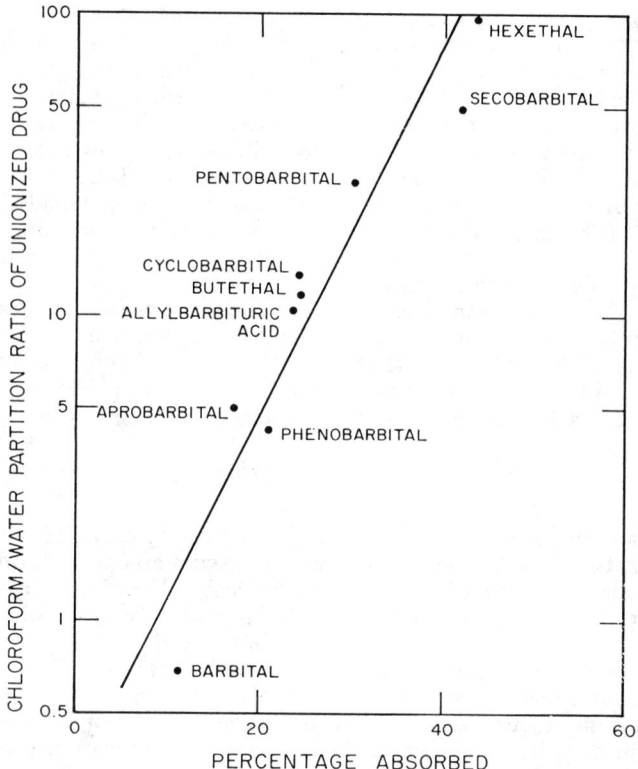

Fig. 484. The relationship of absorption of the unionized forms of drugs from the colon of the rat to the chloroform:water partition coefficient (courtesy, Schanker[10]).

is sulfisoxazole. Sulfadiazine is somewhat less dipolar, has a chloroform–water partition coefficient ten times that of sulfisoxazole, and readily penetrates cells. Ionization not only greatly diminishes lipid solubility but may also impede passage through charged membranes (see *Ionic Diffusion*, page 739).

It is often stated that ionized molecules do not penetrate membranes, except for ions of small diameter. This is not necessarily true, because of the presence of membrane carriers for some ions, which carriers may effectively shield or neutralize the charge (ion-pair formation). The renal tubular transport systems, which transport such obligate ions as tetraethylammonium, probably form ion-pairs. Furthermore, if an ionized molecule has a large nonpolar moiety such that an appreciable lipid solubility is imparted to the molecule in spite of the charge, the drug may penetrate, although usually at a slow rate. For example, various morphinan derivatives are passively absorbed from the stomach even though they are completely ionized at the pH of gastric fluid. Nevertheless, when a drug is a weak acid or base, the unionized form with a favorable partition coefficient passes through a biological membrane so much more readily than the ionized form that, for all practical purposes, only the unionized form is said to pass through the membrane. This has become known as the *principle of nonionic diffusion.*

This principle was appreciated early by Jacobs[11] and applied by Davson and Danelli[12] and by Eagle.[13] This principle is the reason that only the concentrations of the unionized form of the barbiturates are plotted in Fig. 484.

For the purpose of further illustrating the principle, Table I is provided. In the table the permeability constants for penetrance into the cerebral spinal fluid of rats are higher for unionized drugs than for ionized

Table I—Rates of Entry of Drugs in CSF and the Degrees of Ionization of Drugs at pH 7.4[14]

Drug	% binding to plasma protein	pK$_a$[a]	% unionized at pH 7.4	Permeability constant (P min^{-1}) ± S.E.
Drugs mainly ionized at pH 7.4				
5-Sulfosalicylic acid	22	(strong)	0	<0.0001
N′-Methylnicotinamide	<10	(strong)	0	0.0005 ± 0.00006
5-Nitrosalicylic acid	42	2.3	0.001	0.001 ± 0.0001
Salicylic acid	40	3.0	0.004	0.006 ± 0.0004
Mecamylamine	20	11.2	0.016	0.021 ± 0.0016
Quinine	76	8.4	9.09	0.078 ± 0.0061
Drugs mainly unionized at pH 7.4				
Barbital	<2	7.5	55.7	0.026 ± 0.0022
Thiopental	75	7.6	61.3	0.50 ± 0.051
Pentobarbital	40	8.1	83.4	0.17 ± 0.014
Aminopyrine	20	5.0	99.6	0.25 ± 0.020
Aniline	15	4.6	99.8	0.40 ± 0.042
Sulfaguanidine	6	>10.0[b]	>99.8	0.003 ± 0.0002
Antipyrine	8	1.4	>99.9	0.12 ± 0.013
N-Acetyl-4-aminoantipyrine	<3	0.5	>99.9	0.012 ± 0.0010

[a] The dissociation constant of both acids and bases is expressed as a pK$_a$—the negative logarithm of the acidic dissociation constant.
[b] Sulfaguanidine has a very weakly acidic group (pK$_a$ > 10) and two very weakly basic groups (pK$_a$ 2.75 and 0.5). Consequently, the compound is almost completely undissociated at pH 7.4.

ones. The apparent exceptions—barbital, sulfaguanidine, and acetylaminoantipyrine—may be explained by the dipolarity of the unionized molecules. With barbital, the two lipophilic ethyl groups are too small to compensate for the considerable dipolarity of the unionized barbituric acid ring; it may be also seen that barbital is appreciably ionized, which contributes to the relatively small permeability constant. Sulfaguanidine and acetylaminoantipyrine are both very polar molecules. Mecamylamine might also be considered an exception, since it shows a modest permeability even though strongly ionized; there is no dipolarity in mecamylamine elsewhere than the amino group.

Absorption of Drugs

Absorption is the process of movement of a drug from the site of application into the extracellular compartment of the body. Inasmuch as there is a great similarity among the various membranes that a drug may pass through in order to gain access to the extracellular fluid, it might be expected that the particular site of application (or *route*) would make little difference to the successful absorption of the drug. In actual fact, it makes a great deal of difference; many factors other than the structure and composition of the membrane determine the ease with which a drug is absorbed. These factors are discussed in the following sections, along with an account of the ways that drug formulations may be manipulated to alter the ability of a drug to be readily absorbed.

Routes of Administration

Drugs may be administered by many different routes. The various routes include oral, rectal, sublingual or buccal, parenteral, inhalation, topical, etc. The choice of a route depends upon both convenience and necessity.

Oral Route—This is obviously the most convenient route for access to the systemic circulation, providing that various factors do not militate against this route. Oral administration does not always give rise to sufficiently high plasma concentrations to be effective; some drugs are absorbed unpredictably or erratically; patients occasionally have an absorption malfunction. Drugs may not be given by mouth to patients with gastrointestinal intolerance, or who are in preparation for anesthesia, or who have had gastrointestinal surgery. Oral administration is also precluded in coma.

Rectal Route—Drugs that are ordinarily administered by the oral route, usually can be administered by injection or by the alternative *lower enteral* route, through the anal portal into the rectum or lower intestine. With regard to the latter, *rectal suppositories* or *retention enemas* were formerly used quite frequently, but their popularity has abated somewhat, owing to improvements in parenteral preparations. Nevertheless, they continue to be valid and sometimes very important ways of administering a drug, especially in pediatrics and geriatrics. In Fig. 485 the availability of a drug by retention enema may be compared with that by the intravenous route and by oral and rectal suppository administration. It is apparent that the retention enema may be a very satisfactory means of administration but that rectal suppositories may be inadequate where rapid absorption and high plasma levels are required. The illustration is not intended to lead the reader to the conclusion that a retention enema will always give more prompt and higher blood levels than the oral route, for converse findings for the same drug have been reported,[16] but rather to show that the retention enema may offer a useful substitute for the oral route.

Sublingual or Buccal Route—Even though an adequate plasma concentration eventually may be achievable by the oral route, it may rise much too slowly for use in some situations where a rapid response is desired. In such situations parenteral therapy is usually indicated. However, the patients with angina pectoris may get quite prompt relief from an acute

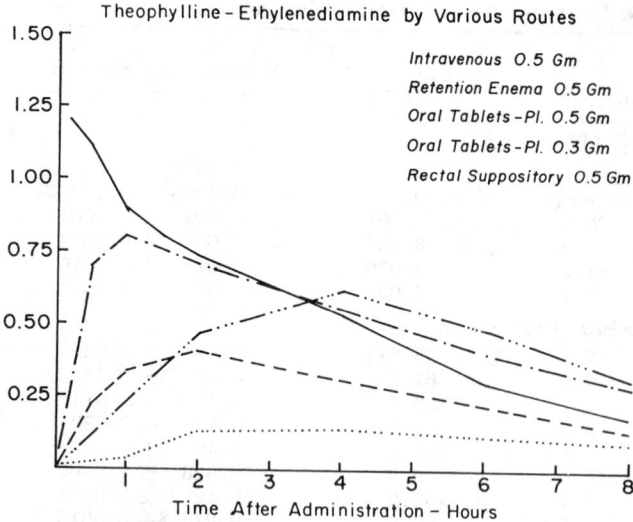

Fig. 485. Blood concentration in mg/100 ml of theophylline (ordinates) following administration to humans of aminophylline in the amounts and by the routes indicated. Doses: per 70 Kg (courtesy, Truitt, et al[15]).

attack by the *sublingual* or *buccal* administration of nitroglycerin, so that parenteral administration may be avoided. When only small amounts of drugs are required to gain access to the blood, the buccal route may be very satisfactory, providing the physico-chemical prerequisites for absorption by this route are present in the drug and dosage form. Only a few drugs may be given successfully by this route.

Parenteral Routes—These routes by definition include any route other than the oral–gastrointestinal (enteral) tract, but in common medical usage the term excludes topical administration and includes only various hypodermic routes. Parenteral administration includes the intravenous, intramuscular, and sub-cutaneous routes. Parenteral routes may be employed whenever enteral routes are contraindicated (see above) or inadequate.

The *intravenous* route may be preferred on occasions even when a drug may be well absorbed by the oral route. There is no delay imposed by absorption before the administered drug reaches the circulation, and blood levels rise virtually as rapidly as the time necessary to empty the syringe or infusion bottle. Consequently, the intravenous route is the preferred route when an emergency calls for an immediate response.

In addition to the rapid rise in plasma concentration of drug, another advantage of intravenous administration is the greater predictability of the peak plasma concentration, which with some drugs can be calculated with a fair degree of precision. Smaller doses are generally required by the intravenous than by other routes, but this usually affords no advantage, inasmuch the sterile injectable dose form costs more than enteric preparations, and the requirement for medical or paramedical supervision of administration may also add to the cost and inconvenience.

Because of the rapidity with which drug enters the circulation, dangerous side effects to the drug may occur which are often not extant by other routes. The principal untoward effect is a depression of cardio-vascular function, which is often called *drug shock*. Consequently, some drugs must be given quite slowly to avoid vasculotoxic concentrations of drug in the plasma. Acute serious allergic responses are also

more likely to occur by the intravenous route than by other routes.

Many drugs are too irritant to be given by the oral, intramuscular, or subcutaneous route, and must of necessity be given intravenously. However, such drugs may also cause damage to the veins (phlebitis) or, if extravasated, cause necrosis (slough) around the injection site. Consequently, such irritant drugs may be greatly diluted in isotonic solutions of saline, dextrose, or other media and given by slow infusion, providing that the slower rate of delivery does not negate the purpose of the administration in emergency situations.

Absorption by the *intramuscular* route is relatively fast, and this parenteral route may be used where an immediate effect is not required but a prompt effect is desirable. Intramuscular deposition may also be made of certain repository preparations, rapid absorption not being desired. Absorption from an intra-muscular depot is often more predictable and uniform than from a subcutaneous site.

Irritation around the injection site is a frequent accompaniment of intramuscular injection, depending upon the drug and other ingredients. Because of the dangers of accidental intravenous injection, medical supervision is generally required. Sterilization is necessary.

In *subcutaneous* administration the drug is injected into the alveolar connective tissue just below the skin. Absorption is slower than by the intramuscular route but nevertheless may be prompt with many drugs. Oftentimes, however, absorption by this route may be no faster than by the oral route. Therefore, when a fairly prompt response is desired, with some drugs the subcutaneous route may not offer much advantage over the oral route, unless for some reason the drug cannot be given orally.

The slower rate of absorption by the subcutaneous route is usually the reason why the route is chosen, and the drugs given by this route are usually those in which it is desired to spread the action out over a number of hours, in order to avoid either too intense a response, too short a response, or frequent injections. Examples of drugs given by this route are insulin and sodium heparin, neither of which is absorbed orally and both of which should be absorbed slowly over many hours. In the treatment of asthma, epinephrine is usually given subcutaneously to avoid the dangers of rapid absorption and consequent dangerous cardio-vascular effects. Many repository preparations, including tablets or pellets, are given subcutaneously. As with other parenteral routes, irritation may occur. Sterile preparations are also required. However, medical supervision is not always required, and self-administration by this route is customary with certain drugs, such as insulin.

Intradermal injections, in which the drug is injected into rather than below the dermis is rarely employed, except in certain diagnostic and test procedures, such as screening for allergic or local irritant responses.

Occasionally, even by the intravenous route it is not possible, practical, or safe to achieve plasma concentrations high enough so that an adequate amount of drug penetrates into special compartments, such as the cerebrospinal fluid, or various cavities, such as the pleural cavity. The brain is especially difficult to penetrate with water-soluble drugs. The name *blood-brain barrier* is applied to the impediment to penetration. When drugs do penetrate, they are often secreted back into the blood very rapidly, so that adequate levels of drugs in the cerebrospinal fluid may be difficult to achieve. Consequently *intrathecal** or *intraventricular* administration may be indicated.

Body cavities such as the pleural cavity are normally wetted by a small amount of effusate which is in diffusion equilibrium with the blood and hence is accessible to drugs. However, infections and inflammations may cause the cavity to fill with serofibrinous exudate which is too large to be in rapid diffusion equilibrium with the blood. *Intracavitary* administration may thus be required. It is extremely important that sterile and nonirritating preparations be used for intrathecal or intracavitary administration.

Inhalation Route—Inhalation may be employed for delivering gaseous or volatile substances into the systemic circulation, as with most general anesthetics. Absorption is virtually as rapid as the drug can be delivered into the alveoli of the lungs, since the alveolar and vascular epithelial membranes are quite permeable, blood flow is abundant, and there is a very large surface for absorption.

Aerosols of nonvolatile substances may also be administered by inhalation, but the route is infrequently used for delivery into the systemic circulation, because of various factors that contribute to erratic or difficult-to-achieve blood levels. Whether or not an aerosol reaches and is retained in pulmonary alveoli depends critically upon particle size: particles greater than 1μ in diameter tend to settle in the bronchioles and bronchi, whereas particles less than 0.5μ fail to settle and are mainly exhaled. Aerosols are mostly employed when the purpose of administration is an action of the drug upon the respiratory tract itself. An example of a drug commonly given as an aerosol is isoproterenol, which is employed to relax the bronchioles in asthma.

Topical Route—Topical administration is employed to deliver a drug at or immediately beneath the point of application. Although occasionally enough drug is absorbed into the systemic circulation to cause systemic effects, absorption is too erratic for the topical route to be used for systemic therapy. Recent work with aprotic solvent vehicles has, however, renewed interest in topical administration for systemic effects. A large number of topical medicaments are applied to the skin, although topical drugs are also applied to the eye, nose and throat, ear, vagina, etc.

In man, percutaneous absorption probably occurs mainly from the surface. Absorption through the hair follicles occurs, but the follicles in man occupy too small a portion of the total integument to be of primary importance. Absorption through sweat and sebaceous glands generally appears to be minor. When the medicament is rubbed on vigorously, the amount of the preparation that is forced into the hair follicles and glands is increased. Rubbing also forces some material through the stratum corneum without molecular dispersion and diffusion through the barrier. Rather large particles of substances such as sulfur have been demonstrated to pass intact through the stratum corneum. When the skin is diseased or abraded, the cutaneous barrier may be disrupted or defective, so that percutaneous absorption may be increased. Since much of a drug that is absorbed through the epidermis diffuses into the circulation without reaching a high concentration in some portions

of the dermis, systemic administration may be preferred in lieu of or in addition to topical administration.

Factors That Affect Absorption

In addition to the physicochemical properties of drug molecules and biological membranes, various factors affect the rate of absorption and determine, in part, the choice of route of administration.

Concentration—It is self-evident that the concentration, or, more exactly, the thermodynamic activity, of a drug in a drug preparation will have an important bearing upon the rate of absorption, since the rate of diffusion of a drug away from the site of administration is directly proportional to the concentration. Thus a 2% solution of lidocaine will induce local anesthesia more rapidly than a 0.2% solution. However, drugs administered in solid form are not necessarily absorbed at the maximal rate (see *Physical State of Formulation and Dissolution Rate* below).

After oral administration the concentration of drugs in the gut is a function of the dose, but the relationship is not necessarily linear. Drugs with a low aqueous solubility quickly saturate the gastrointestinal fluids, so that the rate of absorption tends to reach a limit as the dose is increased. The peptizing and solubilizing effects of bile and other constituents of the gastrointestinal contents assist in increasing the rate of absorption but are in themselves somewhat erratic. Furthermore, many drugs affect the rates of gastric, biliary, and small intestinal secretion, which causes further deviations from a linear relationship between concentration and dose.

Drugs that are administered subcutaneously or intramuscularly also may not always show a direct linear relationship between the rate of absorption and the concentration of drug in the applied solution, because osmotic effects may cause dilution or concentration of the drug, if the movement of water or electrolytes is different from that of the drug. Whenever possible, drugs for hypodermic injection are prepared as isotonic solutions. Some drugs affect the local blood flow and capillary permeability, so that at the site of injection there may be a complex relationship of concentration achieved to the concentration administered.

Physical State of Formulation and Dissolution Rate—When drugs are administered in solid dosage forms (capsules, tablets, powders, suspensions, etc), the rate at which the drug is released into solution may often be slower than other processes involved in absorption, so that dissolution becomes the rate-limiting factor on absorption.

The rate of dissolution depends upon the surface area of the solid, which, in turn, depends upon how finely the drug is subdivided (or comminuted). It also depends upon energy and energy states within the crystals of drug. The Noyes–Whitney equation incorporates the major factors involved in the rate of dissolution, dc/dt:

$$dc/dt = KS(C_s - C_t) \tag{8}$$

where S is the surface area of the particles, K is a constant unique to the chemical substance and incorporates energy and entropy factors, C_s is the concentration at saturation, and C_t is concentration at time t.

K varies widely from drug to drug, and some drugs may have a slow rate of dissolution even despite a fine

---

* Intrathecal administration includes administration into the cerebrospinal fluid at any level of the cerebrospinal axis, including injection into the cerebral ventricles, which is the most common mode of intrathecal administration.

state of subdivision. Some drugs may exist in more than one crystal form, so that there may be more than one K. For example, some preparations of aluminum hydroxide completely dissolve in gastric juice within 30 min, while others show no appreciable dissolution within 1 hr. During storage some drugs change crystal form.

Considerable attention is directed to the dissolution rates of the various salts of drugs that can form salts and to the various crystal forms, in an effort to develop preparations with optimal dissolution rates. Furthermore various substances are often included in tablets, especially, to favor their dispersion (see Chapter 87, *Tablets, Capsules, and Pills*); care must be taken that the drug does not bind with excipients, etc in a way that precludes easy dissolution.

In oil solutions, or in oil-in-water (O/W) emulsions, the rate of absorption may depend on O/W partition coefficients. The rate of absorption of a drug from a viscous solution may be determined by the slow rate of diffusion of drug molecules through the solution, except in the gastrointestinal tract, where the motility tends to break down the drug mass sufficiently that the mean path of diffusion through the viscous material is small enough that the diffusion time is no longer a rate-limiting factor in absorption.

Area of Absorbing Surface—The area of absorbing surface is an important determinant of the rate of absorption. To the extent that the therapist must work with the absorbing surfaces available in the body, the absorbing surface is not subject to manipulation. However, the extent to which the existing surfaces may be utilized is subject to variation. In those rare instances in which percutaneous absorption is intended for systemic administration, the entire skin is available.

Subsequent to subcutaneous or intramuscular injections, the site of application may be massaged in order to spread the injected fluid from a compact mass to a well-dispersed deposit. Alternatively, the dose may be divided into multiple small injections, although this recourse is generally undesirable.

The different areas for absorption afforded by the various routes account, in part, for differences in the rates of absorption by those routes. The large alveolar surface of the lungs allows for extremely rapid absorption of gases, vapors, and properly aerosolized solutions; with some drugs the rate of absorption may be nearly as fast as intravenous injection. In the gut the small intestine is the site of the fastest, and hence most, absorption because of the small lumen and highly developed villi; the stomach has a relatively small surface area, so that even most weak acids are predominately absorbed in the small intestine despite a pH partition factor that should favor absorption from the stomach (see *The pH Partition Principle*, page 746).

Vascularity and Blood Flow—Although the thermal velocity of a freely diffusible average drug molecule is on the order of meters per second, in solution the rate at which it will diffuse away from a reference point will be much slower; collisions with water and/or other molecules, which causes a random motion, and the forces of attraction between the drug and water or other molecules slow the net mean velocity.

The time taken to traverse a given distance is a function of the square of the distance; on the average it would take about $\frac{1}{100}$ sec for a net outward movement of 1μ, 1 sec for 10μ, 100 sec for 100μ, etc.

In a highly vascular tissue, such as skeletal muscle, in which there may be more than 1000 capillaries/sq mm of cross section, a drug molecule would not have to travel more than a few microns, hence less than a second on the average, to reach a capillary from a point of injection.

Once the drug reaches the blood, diffusion is not important to transport, and the rate of blood flow determines the movement. The velocity of blood flow in a capillary is about 1 mm/sec, which is 100 times faster than the mean net velocity of drug molecules 1 mm away from their injection site. The velocity of blood flow is even faster in the larger vessels. Less than a minute is required to distribute drug molecules from the capillaries at the injection site to the rest of the body.

From the above discussion it follows that absorption is most rapid in the vascular tissues. Drugs are absorbed more rapidly from intramuscular sites than from less vascular subcutaneous sites, etc. Despite the small absorbing surface for buccal or sublingual absorption, the high vascularity of the buccal, gingival, and sublingual surfaces favors an unexpectedly high rate of absorption. Because of hyperemia, absorption will be faster from inflamed than from normal areas, unless the presence of edema lengthens the mean distance between capillaries and thus negates the effects of hypermia on absorption.

Vasoconstriction may have a profound effect upon the rate of absorption. When a local effect of a drug is desired, as in local anesthesia, absorption away from the infiltered site may be greatly impeded by vasoconstrictors included in the preparation. Unwanted vasoconstriction sometimes may cause serious problems. For example, in World War II many wounded soldiers were given subcutaneous morphine without evident effect. As a result, injections were sometimes repeated more than once. When the patient was removed to the field hospital, toxic effects would suddenly occur. The explanation is that cold-induced vasoconstriction occurred in the field; when the patient was warmed in the hospital, vasodilation would result and the victim would be flooded with drug. Shock also contributes to the effect, since during shock the blood flow is diminished and there may also be a superimposed vasoconstriction; repair of the shock condition then facilitates absorption.

Molecules too large to pass through the capillary endothelium will of necessity enter the systemic circulation through the lymph. Thus the lymph flow may be important to the absorption of a few drugs.

Movement—A number of factors combine so that movement at the site of injection increases the rate of absorption. In the intestine, segmental movements and peristalsis aid in dividing and dispersing the drug mass. The continual mixing of the chyme helps keep the concentration maximal at the mucosal surface. The pressures developed during segmentation and peristalsis may also favor a small amount of filtration. Movement at the site of hypodermic injection also favors absorption, since it tends to force the injected material through the tissue, increasing the surface area of drug mass and decreasing the mean distance to the capillaries. Movement also increases the flow of blood and lymph. The selection of a site for intramuscular injection may be determined by the amount of expected movement, according to whether the preparation is intended as a fast-acting or a repository preparation.

Gastric Motility and Emptying—The motility of

the stomach is more important to the rate at which an orally administered drug is passed on to the small intestine than it is to the rate of absorption from the stomach itself, since for various reasons, noted above, absorption from the stomach is usually of minor importance.

The average emptying time of the stomach is about 40 min, though it varies according to its contents, reflex and psychological factors, the action of certain autonomic drugs, or disease. The effect of food to delay absorption is due in part to its action to prolong emptying time. The emptying time causes a delay in the absorption of drug, which may be unfavorable or favorable according to what is desired. In the case of therapy with antacids, gastric emptying is a nuisance, since it removes the antacid from the stomach where it is needed.

Solubility and Binding—The dissolution of drugs of low solubility is generally a slow process. Indeed, low solubility is the result of a low rate of departure of drug molecules from the undispersed phase. Furthermore, since the concentration around the drug mass is low, the concentration gradient from the site of deposition to the plasma is small, and the rate of diffusion is low, accordingly.

When it is desired that a drug have a prolonged action but not a high plasma concentration, a derivative of low solubility is often sought. The "insoluble" estolates and other esters of several steroids have durations of action of weeks because of the slow rates of absorption from the sites of injection. Insoluble salts or complexes of acidic or basic drugs are also employed as repository preparations; for example, the procaine salt of penicillin G has a low solubility and is used in a slow release form of the antibiotic.

The solubility of certain macromolecules is critically dependent upon the ionization of substituent groups. When they are amphiprotic, they are least soluble at their isoelectric pH. Insulin is normally soluble at the pH of the extracellular fluid; but by combining insulin with the right proportion of a basic protein, such as protamine, the isoelectric pH can be made to be approximately 7.4, and the complex can be used as a low-solubility prolonged-action drug. For more details, see Chapter 89, *Prolonged-Action Pharmaceuticals*.

Some drugs may bind with natural substances at or near the site of application. The strongly ionized mucopolysaccharides in connective tissue, ground substance, and mucous secretions of the gut are retardants to the absorption of a number of drugs, especially large cationic or polycationic molecules. In the gut, the binding is the least at low pH, which should favor absorption of large cations from the stomach; however, absorption from the stomach is slow (see above), so that the absorption of large cations mainly occurs in the upper duodenum where the pH is still relatively low. Pharmacologically inactive quaternary ammonium compounds are sometimes included in an oral preparation of a quaternary ammonium drug for the purpose of saturating the binding sites of mucin and other mucopolysaccharides and thereby enhancing the absorption of drug.

In addition to mucopolysaccharides in mucous secretions, food in the gastrointestinal tract binds many drugs and slows absorption. Antacids, especially aluminum hydroxide plus other basic aluminum compounds and magnesium trisilicate, bind amine and ammonium drugs and interfere with absorption.

Donnan Effect—The presence of a charged macromolecule on one side of a semipermeable membrane (impermeable to the macromolecule) will alter the concentration of permeant ionized particles according to the Donnan equilibrium (page 747). Accordingly, drug molecules of the same charge as the macromolecule will be constrained to the opposite side of the membrane. The presence of appropriately charged macromolecules not only will influence the distribution of drug ions in accordance with the Donnan equation but will increase the rate of transfer of the drug across the membrane, because of mutual ionic repulsion. This effect is sometimes used to facilitate the absorption of ionizable drugs from the gastrointestinal tract. The Donnan effect also operates to retard the absorption of drug ions of opposite charge; however, the mutual electrostatic attraction of a macromolecule and drug ion generally results in actual binding, which is more important than the Donnan effect.

Vehicles and Absorption Adjuvants—Drugs that are to be applied topically to the skin and mucous membranes are often dissolved in vehicles that are thought to enhance the penetrance. For a long time it was thought that oleaginous vehicles promoted the absorption of lipid-soluble drugs. However, the role and effect of the vehicle has proven to be quite complex and neither yet well understood nor easily predictable. In the skin at least five factors are involved:

1. The effect of the vehicle to alter the hydration of the keratin in the barrier layer.
2. The effect of the vehicle to promote or prevent the collection of sweat at the surface of the skin.
3. The partition coefficient of the drug in a vehicle–water system.
4. The permeability of the skin to the undissolved drug.
5. The permeability of the skin to the vehicle.

The effect of the vehicle to aid in the access of the drug to the hair follicles and sebaceous glands may also be involved, although in man the follicles and glands are probably ordinarily of minor importance to absorption.

A layer of oleaginous material over the skin prevents the evaporation of water, so that the stratum corneum may become macerated and more permeable to drugs. In dermatology it is even sometimes the practice to wrap the site of application with saran wrap or some other waterproof material for the purpose of increasing the maceration of the stratum corneum. However, the layer of perspiration that forms under an occlusive vehicle may itself become a barrier to the movement of lipid-soluble drugs from the vehicle to the skin, but it may facilitate the movement of water-soluble drugs. Conversely, polyethylene glycol vehicles remove the perspiration and dehydrate the barrier, which decreases the permeability to drugs; such vehicles remove the aqueous medium through which water-soluble drugs may pass down into the stratum corneum but at the same time facilitate the transfer of lipid-soluble drugs from the vehicle to the skin.

Even in the absence of a vehicle it is not clear what physicochemical properties of a drug favor cutaneous penetration, high lipid solubility being a prerequisite according to some authorities and an ether–water partition coefficient of approximately 1 according to others. Yet the penetrances of ethanol and dibromomethane are nearly equal,[17] and other such enigmas exist. It is not surprising, then, that the effects of vehicles are not altogether predictable.

A general statement might be made that if a drug

is quite soluble in a poorly absorbed vehicle, the vehicle will retard the movement of the drug into the skin. For example, salicylic acid is 100 times as permeant when absorbed from water than from polyethylene glycol, and pentanol is 5 times as permeant from water as from olive oil.[17] Yet ethanol penetrates 5 times faster from olive oil than from either water or straight ethanol, all of which denies the trustworthiness of generalizations about vehicles.

In recent years there has been much interest in certain highly dielectric aprotic solvents, especially dimethylsulfoxide (DMSO). Such substances generally prove to be excellent solvents for both water- and lipid-soluble compounds and for some compounds not soluble in either water or lipid solvents. The extraordinary solvent properties are probably due to a high polarizability and van der Waals bonding capacity, a high degree of polarization (dipole moment), and a lack of association through hydrogen bonding. As a vehicle, DMSO greatly facilitates the permeation of the skin and other biological membranes by numerous drugs, even including such large molecules as insulin. The mechanism is not understood. Such vehicles have a potential for many important uses, but they are at present only experimental, pending investigations on toxicity.

From time to time a claim is made that a new ingredient of a tablet or elixir enhances the absorption of a drug, and a comparison of plasma levels of the old and new preparations seems to support the claim. Upon further investigation, however, it may be revealed that the new so-called absorption adjuvant is replacing an ingredient that previously bound the drug or delayed its absorption; thus the new "adjuvant" is not an adjuvant but rather it is only a non-deterrent.

Other Factors—A number of other less-well-defined factors affect the absorption of drugs, some of which may operate, in part, through factors already cited above. Disease or injury has a considerable effect upon absorption. For example, debridement of the stratum corneum increases the permeability to topical agents, meningitis increases the permeability of the blood–brain barrier, biliary insufficiency decreases the absorption of lipid-soluble substances from the intestine, acid–base disturbances can affect the absorption of weak acids or bases, etc. Certain drugs, such as ouabain, that affect active transport processes may interfere with the absorption of certain other drugs. The condition of the ground substance, or "intracellular cement" probably bears on the absorption of certain types of molecules. Hyaluronidase, which depolymerizes the mucopolysaccharide ground substance, can be demonstrated to facilitate the absorption of some, but not all, drugs from subcutaneous sites.

Drug Disposition

The term *drug disposition* is used here to include all processes which tend to lower the plasma concentration of drug, as opposed to drug absorption, which elevates the plasma level. Consequently, the distribution of drugs to the various tissues will be considered under Disposition. Some authors use the term disposition synonymously with elimination, that is, to include only those processes which decrease the amount of drug in the body. In the present context, disposition comprises three categories of processes: distribution, biotransformation, and excretion.

Distribution, Biotransformation, and Excretion

The term *distribution* is self-explanatory. It denotes the partitioning of a drug among the numerous locations where a drug may be contained within the body. *Biotransformations* are the alterations in the chemical structure of a drug that are imposed upon it by the life processes. *Excretion* is, in a sense, the converse of absorption, namely, the transportation of the drug or its products out of the body. The term applies whether or not special organs of excretion are involved.

Distribution

The body may be considered to comprise a number of compartments: enteric (gastrointestinal), plasma, interstitial, cerebrospinal fluid, bile, glandular secretions, urine, storage vesicles, cytoplasm or intracellular space, etc. Some of these "compartments," such as urine and secretions, are open ended, but since their contents relate to those in the closed compartments, they must also be included.

At first thought it may seem that if a drug were passively distributed (ie, by simple diffusion) and the plasma concentration could be maintained at a steady level, the concentration of a drug in the water in all compartments ought to become equal. It is true that some substances, such as ethanol and antipyrine, are distributed nearly equally throughout the body water, but they are more the exception than the rule. Such substances are mainly small, uncharged, nondissociable, highly water-soluble molecules.

The condition of small size and high water solubility allows for passage through the pores without the necessity of carrier or active transport. Small size also places a limit on van der Waals binding energy and configurational complementariness, so that binding to proteins in plasma or cells is slight. The presence of a charge on a drug molecule makes for unequal distribution across charged membranes, in accordance with the Donnan distribution (page 747). Dissociability causes unequal distribution when there is a pH differential between compartments, as discussed under *The pH Partition Principle* (see below). Thus, even if a drug is distributed passively, its distribution may be uneven throughout the body. When active transport into or a rapid metabolic destruction occurs within some compartments, uneven distribution is also inevitable.

The pH Partition Principle—An important consequence of nonionic diffusion is that a difference in pH between two compartments will have an important influence upon the partitioning of a weakly acidic or basic drug between those compartments. The partition is such that the unionized form of the drug has the same concentration in both compartments, since it is the form that is freely diffusible; the ionized form in each compartment will have the concentration that is determined by the pH in that compartment, the pK, and the concentration of the unionized form. The governing effect of pH and pK on the partition is known as the *pH partition principle.*

To illustrate the principle, consider the partition of salicylic acid between the gastric juice and the interior of a gastric mucosal cell. Assume the pH of the gastric juice to be 1.0, which it occasionally becomes. The pK_a of salicylic acid is 3.0 (Martin[18] provides one source of pK values of drugs). With the Henderson–Hasselbalch equation (see page 285) it may be calculated that the drug is only 1% ionized at pH 1.0.* The intracellular pH of most cells is about 7.0. Assuming the pH of the mucosal cell to be the same, it may be calculated that salicylic acid will be 99.99% ionized within the cells. Since the concentration of the unionized form is theoretically the same in both gastric juice and mucosal cells, it follows that the total concentration of the drug (ionized + unionized) within the mucosal cell will be 10,000 times that in gastric juice. This is illustrated in Fig. 486. Such a relatively high intracellular concentration can have important osmotic and toxicologic consequences.

Had the drug been a weak base instead of an acid, the high concentration would have been in the gastric juice. In the small intestine, where the pH may range from 7.5 to 8.1, the partition of a weak acid or base will be the reverse of that in the stomach, but the concentration differential will be less, because the pH differential from lumen to mucosal cells, etc, will be less. The reversal of partition as the drug moves from the stomach to the small intestine accounts for the phenomenon that some drugs may be absorbed from one gastrointestinal segment and returned to another. The weak base, atropine, is absorbed from the small intestine, but because of pH partition it is "secreted" into the gastric juice.

The pH partition of drugs has never been demonstrated to be as marked as that illustrated in Fig. 486 and in the text. Not only do many drug ions probably pass through the pores of the membrane to a significant extent, but some may also pass through the lipid phase, as explained above for the morphinans and mecamylamine. Furthermore, ion-pair formation in carrier transport also bypasses nonionic diffusion. All processes which tend toward an equal distribution of drugs across membranes and among compartments will cause further deviations from theoretical predictions of pH partition.

Electrochemical and Donnan Distribution—A drug ion may be passively distributed across a membrane in accordance with the membrane potential, the charge on the drug ion, and the Donnan effect. The relationship of the membrane potential to the passive distribution of ions is quantitatively expressed by the Nernst equation (Eq. 7, page 739) and has already been discussed. Barring active transport, pH partition, and binding, the drug will be said to be distributed according to the electrical gradient or to its "equilibrium" potential. If the membrane potential is 90 mv, the concentration of a univalent cation will be 30 times as high within the cell as without; if the drug cation is divalent, the ratio will be 890. The distribution of anions would be just the reverse. If the membrane potential is but 9 mv, the ratio for a univalent cation will be only 1.4 and for a divalent

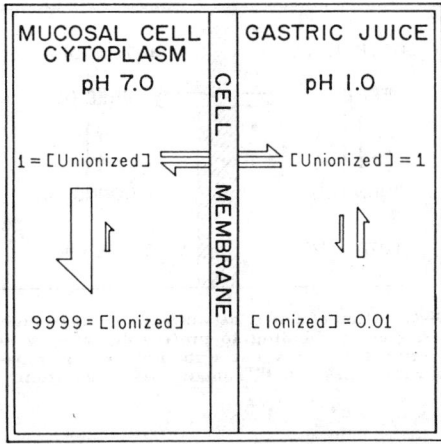

Fig. 486. Hypothetical partition of salicylic acid between gastric juice and the cytoplasm of a gastric mucosal cell. It is assumed that the ionized form cannot pass through the cell membrane. The intragastric concentration of salicylic acid is arbitrarily arranged to provide unit concentration of the unionized form. *Bracketed values:* **concentration;** *arrows:* **relative size depicts the direction in which dissociation–association is favored at equilibrium.**

cation only 2.0. It can thus be seen how important membrane potential may be to the distribution of ionized drugs.

It was pointed out under *Membrane Potentials,* page 738, that large potentials derive from active transport of ions but that small potentials may result from Donnan distribution. Donnan membrane theory is discussed in Chapter 16, *Complexation.* According to the theory, the ratio of the intracellular/extracellular concentration of a permeant univalent anion is equal to the ratio of extracellular/intracellular concentration of a permeant univalent cation. A more general mathematical expression that includes ions of any valence is

$$\left(\frac{A_i}{A_e}\right)^{1/Z_a} = \left(\frac{C_e}{C_i}\right)^{1/Z_c} = r \qquad (9)$$

where A_i is the intracellular and A_e the extracellular concentration of anion, Z_a is the valence of anion, C_i is the intracellular and C_e the extracellular concentration of cation, and r is the Donnan factor. The value of r depends upon the average molecular weight and valence of the macromolecules (mostly protein) within the cell, and the intracellular and extracellular volumes. Since the macromolecules within the cell are negatively charged, the cation concentration will be higher within the cell, that is, $C_i > C_e$. Since a Donnan distribution results in a membrane potential, the distribution of drug ion will also be in keeping with the membrane potential.

The Donnan distribution also applies to the distribution of a charged drug between the plasma and interstitial compartment, because of the presence of anionic proteins in the plasma. Eq. 9 applies by changing the subscript i to p, for plasma, and e to i, for interstitial. The Donnan factor, r, for plasma-interstitial space partition is about 1.05:1.

Binding and Storage—Drugs are frequently bound to plasma proteins (especially albumin), interstitial substances, intracellular constituents, and bone and cartilage. If binding is extensive and firm, it will have a considerable impact upon the distribution, excretion, and sojourn of the drug in the body. Obviously, a drug that is bound to a protein or any other macromolecule will not pass through the mem-

---

* The relationship of ionization and partition to pH and pK has been formulated in several different ways, but the student may calculate the concentrations from simple mass law equations. More sophisticated calculations and reviews of this subject are available.[10,11,19-23]

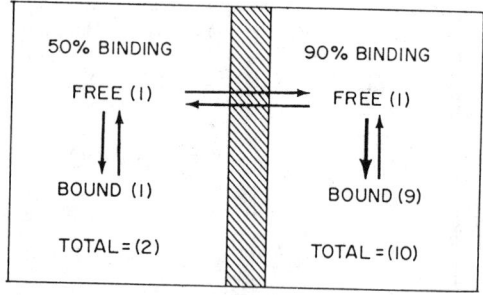

Fig. 487. Distribution of a drug between two compartments between which the degrees of binding to protein differ. The per cent of binding is indicated. Only the unbound drug can pass through the membrane. *Bracketed values:* concentration (courtesy, Schanker[12]).

brane in the bound form; only the unbound form can negotiate among the various compartments.

The partition among compartments is determined by the binding capacity and binding constant in each compartment. As long as the binding capacity exceeds the quantity of drug in the compartment, the following equation generally applies:

$$\log D_b = \log K + a \log D_f \qquad (10)$$

where D_b is the concentration of bound drug, D_f is the concentration of free drug, and a and K are constants characteristic of the drug and binding macromolecule. The equation is that of a Freundlich isotherm. As the binding capacity is approached, the relationship no longer holds. For a nondissociable drug at equilibrium, D_f will be the same in all communicating compartments, so that it would be possible to calculate the partition if K and a are known for each compartment. Except for plasma, the values of a and K are generally unknown, but the percent bound is often known. From the percent bound the partition can also be calculated, as in Fig. 487. However, the logarithmic relationships shown in Eq. 10 serve as a reminder that the percent bound changes with the concentration, so that the partition will vary with the dose. If the drug is a weak acid or base, the unionized free form negotiates among the compartments, but the ionized form is often the more firmly bound, and calculations must take into account the dissociation constant and the different a's and K's of the ionized and unionized forms.

It is commonly misbelieved that binding in the plasma interferes with the activity of a drug and the intracellular binding in a responsive cell increases activity or toxicity. Both binding in plasma and in the tissues decreases the concentration of free drug; but this is easily remedied by adjusting the dose to give a sufficient concentration for pharmacological activity. The distribution and activity of the free form is not affected by binding. The principal effect of binding is to increase the initial dose requirement for drug and to create a reservoir of drug from which the drug may be withdrawn as the free form is excreted or metabolized. However, if the binding is extremely firm and release is slow, the rate of release may not be enough to sustain the free form at a sufficient level for pharmacological activity; in such instances the bound drug cannot be considered a reserve.

The effect of binding upon the sojourn of a drug may be considerable. For example, quinacrine, which may be concentrated in the liver to as much as 15,000 times the concentration in plasma, may remain in the body for months. Some iodine-containing radiopaque diagnostic agents are strongly bound to plasma protein and may remain in the plasma for as long as 2 yr. In pathological conditions, such as nephrosis, diabetes, and cirrhosis, in which plasma protein levels may be decreased, the plasma protein binding, dose, and duration of action may all be decreased.

If a drug is bound to a functional macromolecule, binding may relate to pharmacological activity and toxicity, provided that the binding is at a critical center of the macromolecule. The binding by nucleic acids of certain antimalarials, such as quinacrine, undoubtedly contributes to the parasiticidal actions as well as to toxicity.

Most drugs are bound to proteins by relatively weak forces, such as van der Waals (London, Keesom, or Debye) forces, or hydrogen or ionic bonds. Consequently, binding constants are generally small and binding is usually readily reversible. The larger the molecule, the greater the van der Waals bonding, so that large drug molecules are more likely to be strongly bound than are small ones.

Just as shape and the nature of functional groups is important to drug–receptor combination, so they also are to binding. Drugs of similar shape and/or chemical affinities may bind at the same sites on a binding protein and hence compete with one another. For example, phenylbutazone displaces warfarin from human plasma albumin, which may cause an increase in the anticoagulant effect of warfarin. Some drugs may also displace protein-bound endogenous constituents. For example, sulfisoxazole displaces bilirubin from plasma proteins; in infants with kernicterus the freed bilirubin floods the central nervous system and causes sometimes fatal toxicity.

According to the lipid–water coefficient, a drug may be taken up into fat. The ratio of concentration in fat to that in plasma will not be the same as the partition coefficient because of the content of water and of non-lipids in adipose tissue and because electrolytes and other solutes alter the dielectric constant and hence solubilities from those of pure water. Lipoproteins and even nonpolar substituents on plasma proteins also take up lipid-soluble molecules, so that solubility in plasma can be considerably higher than that in water. The relatively high solubility of ether in plasma makes plasma a pool for ether, the filling of which delays the onset of anesthesia. However, ether and other volatile anesthetics are gradually taken up into the adipose tissue, which acts as a store of the anesthetic. The longer the anesthetic is administered, the greater the store and the longer it takes for anesthesia to terminate when inhalation has been discontinued.

Another notable substance that is readily taken up into fat is thiopental. Even though there is a high solubility of this barbiturate in fat, the low rate of blood flow in fat limits the rate of uptake. Gradually, however, the fat accumulates the drug at the expense of other compartments, including the brain, and the central action is thus terminated. The gradual entry of thiopental into fat at the expense of plasma, muscle, and liver is illustrated in Fig. 488.

Nonequilibrium and Redistribution—Thus far the distribution of drugs have been mainly discussed as though equilibrium or steady state conditions exist after a drug is absorbed and distributed. However, since most drugs are administered at intervals and the body content of drug rises and falls with absorption and destruction—excretion, neither a true equilibrium

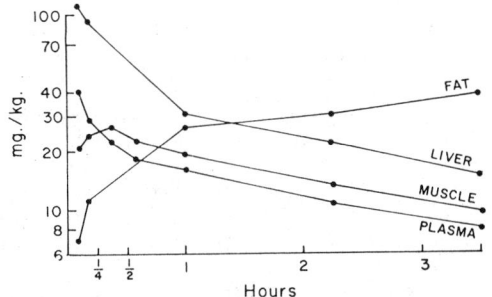

Fig. 488. Predisposition of thiopental for fat.   25 mg/Kg were given to a dog.   After a brief sojourn of thiopental in the more vascular tissues, it gradually transfers to fat, where the lipid-soluble drug dissolves in fat droplets (courtesy, Brodie and Hogben[20]).

among the body compartments nor a steady state exists.

The term equilibrium is misleadingly used to describe the conditions that exist when the plasma concentration and the concentration in a tissue are equal, as exemplified at the point of intersection of the curves for plasma and muscle or plasma and fat in Fig. 488. But such "equilibrium" with fat occurs much later than "equilibrium" with muscle, so that no true equilibrium really exists among all the compartments. Furthermore, the cross-over point for plasma and any one tissue is not necessarily an equilibrium point, because the rates of ingress and egress from the tissue are not necessarily equal when the internal and external concentrations are equal, since there are numerous factors that make for unequal distribution (pH partition, Donnan effect, electrochemical distribution, active transport, binding, etc).

A study of Fig. 488 shows that the distribution of thiopental continually changed during the 3½ hr of observation. At the end of the period, the content in fat was still increasing while that in each of the other compartments was decreasing. This time-dependent shift in partition is called *redistribution*. Eventually, the content in fat would have reached a peak, which peak would represent as nearly a true equilibrium point as could be achieved in the dynamic situation where metabolic destruction and a slight amount of excretion of the drug was taking place. Once the concentration in the fat had reached its peak, its content would have declined in parallel with that in the other tissues, and the partition among the compartments would have remained essentially constant. Redistribution, then, takes place only until the concentration in the slowest filling compartment reaches its peak, so long as the kinetics of elimination are constant.

Volume of Distribution—The *volume of distribution* of a drug is an abstract volume or space which is calculated from the ratio of the amount of drug in the body to the concentration in plasma once partition is stabilized.   Thus

$$V_D = \frac{Q}{C_p} \qquad (11)$$

where V_D is volume of distribution, Q is quantity of drug, and C_p is concentration of the drug in the plasma. V_D is the volume that Q would occupy if it were everywhere distributed at the same concentration, C_p, as in the plasma.

Substances that are concentrated in the tissues may have apparent volumes of distribution greater than that of total body water, so that the volume is not necessarily real in the physical sense.   A drug such as

quinacrine, which is greatly concentrated in the liver and other tissues, may have a volume of distribution of several thousand liters.   If a drug is mainly confined to the plasma, its volume of distribution will be equal to or only slightly greater than *1*.

The word *space* is often used synonymously with volume of distribution.   It is especially employed when the distributed substance has a volume of distribution that is essentially identical to a physical real space or body compartment.   N-acetyl-4-aminoantipyrine is distributed evenly throughout the total body water and is not bound to proteins or other tissue constituents.   Thus the acetylaminoantipyrine space or volume of distribution coincides with that of total body water.   Inulin, sucrose, sulfate, and a number of other substances are essentially confined to extracellular water, so that an inulin space, for example, measures the extracellular fluid volume.   Evans blue is confined to the plasma, so that the Evans blue space is the plasma volume.   Such space measurements with standard space indicators are a necessary part of studies on the distribution of drugs, since it is desirable to compare the volume of distribution of a drug to the standard spaces.

Biotransformations

Most drugs are acted upon by enzymes in the body and converted to metabolic derivatives called metabolites.   The process of conversion is called biotransformation.   Metabolites are usually more polar and less lipid soluble than the parent drug because of the introduction of oxygen into the molecule, hydrolysis to yield more highly polar groups, or conjugation with a highly polar substance.   As a consequence, metabolites often show less penetrance into tissues and less renal tubular resorption than the parent drug, in accordance with the principle of the low penetrance of polar and high penetrance of lipid soluble substances.   For similar reasons metabolites are usually less active than the parent drug, often inactive; even if they are appreciably active, they are generally more rapidly excreted.   Therefore, the usual net effect of biotransformation may be said to be one of *inactivation* or *detoxication*.

There are, however, numerous examples in which biotransformation does not result in inactivation. For example, codeine is metabolized in part to morphine, chloral hydrate to trichloroethanol, mephobarbital and primidone to phenobarbital, aspirin to salicylic acid, thiopental to pentobarbital, phenacetin or acetanilid to acetaminophen, ephedrine to methamphetamine, etc.

There are also examples in which the parent drug has no activity of its own but is converted to an active metabolite.   Parathion, malathion, and certain other anticholinesterases require metabolic activation, inactive chloroguanide is converted to an active triazine derivative, phenylbutazone is hydroxylated to the antirheumatic hydroxyphenylbutazone, inactive pentavalent arsenicals are reduced to their active trivalent metabolites, and there are other examples of an activating biotransformation.

When a delayed or prolonged response to a drug is desired or an unpleasant taste or local reaction is to be avoided, it is a common pharmaceutical practice to prepare an inactive or nonoffending precursor, such that the active form may be generated in the body. This practice has been termed *drug latentiation*.[24] Chloramphenicol palmitate, dichloralphenazone, and the estolates of various steroid hormones are examples of deliberately latentiated drugs. Because inactive metabolites do not always result from biotransformation, the term detoxication[25] should not be used as a synonym for biotransformation.

Biotransformations take place principally in the liver, although the kidney, skeletal muscle, intestine, or even plasma may be important sites of the enzymatic attack of some drugs. Since plasma lacks the enzymes and structures required for electron transport, biotransformations in plasma are mostly hydrolytic.

Endoplasmic Reticulum and Microsomal System—Biotransformations in the liver mainly occur in *smooth endoplasmic reticulum*. The endoplasmic reticulum is a tubular system which courses through the interior of the cell but also appears to communicate with the interstitial space, and its membrane is continuous with the cell membrane. Some of the reticulum is lined with ribonucleoprotein particles, called ribosomes, which are engaged in protein synthesis; this is the *rough* endoplasmic reticulum. Although the smooth endoplasmic reticulum lacks such a granular appearance, it is heavily invested with numerous enzymes which biotransform many drugs and some endogenous substances.

When a broken cell homogenate of the liver is prepared, the reticulum becomes fragmented, and the fragments form vesicular structures called *microsomes*. Although the microsomes are artifacts, it is the practice to refer to the *microsomal drug metabolizing system* rather than to the smooth endoplasmic reticulum.

The microsomal system is peculiar in that both oxidations and reductions usually require the reducing cofactor NADPH (TPNH). This is because microsomal oxidations proceed by way of the introduction of oxygen rather than by dehydrogenation, and NADPH is essential to reduce one of the atoms of O_2.

Some of the enzymes of the microsomal system are quite easily *induced;* that is, a substrate of the enzyme may considerably increase the activity of that enzyme, probably by increasing the biosynthesis of that enzyme. An increase in the amount of smooth reticulum is also sometimes demonstrable concomitantly with enzyme induction.

Treatment of an experimental subject with phenobarbital will greatly increase the rate of metabolism of phenobarbital, which necessitates larger and more frequent doses of the drug in order to maintain a constant sedative effect. Moreover, phenobarbital may induce an increased metabolism of some other but not all barbiturates as well as some unrelated drugs, such as strychnine and warfarin. Oddly, warfarin does not readily induce its own biotransformation. At the present time, both self-induction and cross-induction appear capricious and unpredictable.

Induction may create therapeutic problems. For example, the use of phenobarbital during treatment with warfarin increases the dose requirement for warfarin. If the physician is unaware of this interaction and fails to increase the dose, the patient may suffer a thrombotic episode. If the dose of warfarin has been increased and the phenobarbital is then discontinued, the rate of metabolism of warfarin may drop to its previous level, so that the patient is overdosed, with hemorrhagic consequences. Some drugs inhibit rather than induce the microsomal system, which reduces the dose requirement and may lead to toxicity.

The activity of the microsomal system is affected by many factors other than the presence of drugs. Age, sex, nutritional states, pathological conditions, body temperature, and genetic factors are among the influences that have been identified. Age, particularly, has received considerable attention. Infants have a poorly developed microsomal system, which accounts for the low dose requirement for morphine and explains the high toxicity of chloramphenicol in infants.

The activity and selectivity of the microsomal system varies greatly from species to species, so that care must be exercised in extrapolating experimental findings in laboratory animals to man.

Types of Biotransformations—Biotransformations may be *degradative*, wherein the drug molecule is diminished to a smaller structure, or *synthetic*, wherein one or more atoms or groups may be added to the molecule. Very few drugs are degraded completely. Usually degradation is slight to moderate, the metabolite being then acted upon by the synthetic processes of oxidation or conjugation.

Biotransformations may be placed into five categories: (1) oxidation, (2) reduction, (3) hydrolysis, (4) conjugation, and (5) miscellaneous.

Oxidation—Oxidation is more common than any other type of biotransformation. Oxidations that occur primarily in the liver microsomal system include side-chain hydroxylation, aromatic hydroxylation, deamination (which is oxidative and results in the intermediate formation of RCHO), *N*-, *O*-, and *S*-dealkylation (which probably involves hydroxylation of the alkyl group followed by oxidation to the aldehyde), and sulfoxide formation. *N*-Demethylation involves a different system from *N*-dealkylation of higher radicals.

Oxidations that occur elsewhere than the microsomes are generally dehydrogenations followed by the addition of oxygen or water. Examples are the oxidation of alcohols by alcohol dehydrogenase, the oxidation of aldehyde by aldehyde dehydrogenase, and the deamination of monoamines by monoamine oxidase and diamines by diamine oxidase. The oxidation of purines like caffeine and theophylline is also extramicrosomal.

Reductions—Reductions are relatively uncommon. They mainly occur in liver microsomes, but they occasionally take place in other tissues. Examples are the reduction of nitro and nitroso groups (as in chloramphenicol, nitroglycerin, and organic nitrites), of the azo group (as in prontosil), and of certain aldehydes to the corresponding alcohols (as with the deaminated serotonin metabolite, 5-hydroxytryptophal, to 5-hydroxytryptophol).

Hydrolysis—Hydrolysis is a common biotransformation among esters and amides. Esterases are located in many structures besides the microsomes. For example, cholinesterases are found in plasma, erythrocytes, liver, nerve terminals, junctional interstices, and postjunctional structures, and procaine esterases are found in plasma. Various phosphatases and sulfatases are also widely distributed in tissues and plasma, although few drugs are appropriate substrates. The hydrolytic deamidation of meperidine occurs primarily in the hepatic microsomes.

Conjugation—A large number of drugs or their metabolites are conjugated. Conjugation is the biosynthetic process of combining a chemical compound with a highly polar and water-soluble natural substance to yield a water-soluble, usually inactive product. Conjugations generally involve either esterification, amidation, mixed anhydride formation, hemiacetal formation, or etherization.

Glucuronic acid is the most frequent partner to the drug in conjugation. Actually, the drug reacts with uridine diphosphoglucuronic acid rather than with simple glucuronic acid. The drug or drug metabolite combines at the number 1 carbon (aldehyde end) and not at the carboxyl end of glycuronic acid. The hydroxyl group of an alcohol or a phenol attacks the number 1 carbon of the pyran ring to replace uridine diphosphate. The product is a hemiacetyl-like derivative. Since the product is not an ester, the term *glucuronide* is appropriate. Rarely, thiols and amines may form analogous glucuronides.

Carboxyl compounds form esters, appropriately called *glucuronates*, in replacing the uridine diphosphate. *Sulfuric acid* is also a frequent conjugant, especially with phenols and to a lesser extent with simple alcohols. The sulfurated product is called an *ethereal sulfate*. Occasionally sulfuric acid conjugates with aromatic amines to form *sulfamates*. *Phosphoric acid* also conjugates with phenols and aromatic amines. The conjugation of benzoic acid with glycine to yield hippuric acid is a classical example of an *amidation* conjugative process. Cysteine may take the place of glycine, through the intermediation of glutathione, to yield mercapturic acids with certain aromatic acids.

Amidations with amino acids are less frequent than *acetylation*, partly because few drugs are carboxylic compounds. Aromatic amines and occasionally aliphatic amines or heterocyclic nitrogen are frequently acetylated. Acetyl-CoA is the biological reagent rather than acetic acid itself. Unlike most other conjugates, the acetylate (amide) is usually less soluble than the parent compound. The acetylation of the para-amino group of the sulfonamides is a prime example of this type of conjugation.

Although most conjugations occur in the liver, the microsomal system is not involved. Some conjugations occur in the kidney or in other tissues.

Miscellaneous Biotransformations—Many amines, especially derivatives of β-phenylethylamine and heterocyclic compounds, are methylated in the body. The products are usually biologically active, sometimes more so than the parent compound. *N-methylation* may occur in the cell sap of the liver and elsewhere, especially in chromaffin tissue in the case of phenylethylamines.

Phenolic compounds may be *O*-methylated. *O-methylation* is the principal route of biotransformation of catecholamines such as epinephrine and norepinephrine, the methyl group being introduced on the meta hydroxyl substituent. Both *N*- and *O*-methylation require *S*-methyladenosyl cysteine.

Desulfuration, in which oxygen may replace sulfur, takes place in the liver. Thiopental is in part converted to pentobarbital by desulfuration, and parathion is transformed to paraoxon.

Dehalogenation of certain insecticides and various halogenated hydrocarbons may take place, principally in the liver but not in the microsomes.

Excretion

Some drugs are not biotransformed in the body. Others may be biotransformed, but their products still remain to be eliminated. It follows that excretion is involved in the elimination of all drugs and/or their

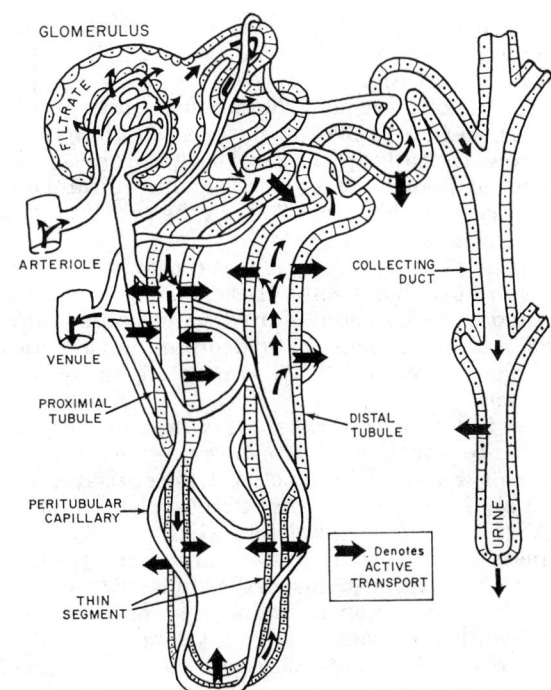

Fig. 489. A mammalian nephron. Note how the lower loops of the postglomerular capillaries course downward and double back along with the tubule. This allows countercurrent distribution to maintain hyperosmolar urine within the thin segment.

metabolites. Although the kidney is the most important organ of excretion, some substances are excreted in bile, sweat, saliva, gastric juice, or from the lungs.

Renal Excretion—The excretory unit of the kidney is called the *nephron* (Fig. 489). There are several million nephrons in the human kidney. The nephron is essentially a filter funnel, called *Bowman's capsule*, with a long stem, called a *renal tubule*. It is also now recognized that the collecting duct is functionally a part of the nephron. The *blood vessels* that invest the capsule and the tubule are also an essential part of the nephron.

Bowman's capsule is packed with a tuft of branching interconnected capillaries (*glomerular tuft*), which provide a large surface area of capillary endothelium ("filter paper") through which fluid and small molecules may filter into the capsule and begin passage down the tubule. The glomerular tuft together with Bowman's capsule constitute the *glomerulus*. The glomerular capillary endothelium and the supporting layer of Bowman's capsule have pores ranging upwards to 40 Å. Consequently, all crystalloid solutes in plasma and even a little albumin pass into the glomerular filtrate.

The postglomerular vessels which lie close to the tubules are critically important to renal function in that substances resorbed from the filtrate by the tubule are returned to the blood along these vessels. The tubule is not straight but rather first makes a number of convolutions (called a *proximal convoluted tubule*), then courses down and back up a long loop (called the *loop of Henle*), makes more convolutions (the *distal convoluted tubule*), and finally joins the collecting duct. The loop of Henle is divided into a *proximal (descending) tubule*, a thin segment, and a *distal (ascending) tubule*.

As the glomerular filtrate passes through the proximal tubule some solute may be resorbed (*tubular resorption*) through the tubular epithelium and returned to the blood. Resorption occurs in part by passive diffusion and in part by active transport, especially with sodium and glucose. Chloride follows sodium obligatorily.

In the proximal region, the tubule is quite permeable to water, so that resorbed solutes are accompanied by enough water to keep the resorbate isotonic. Consequently, although the filtrate becomes diminished in volume by approximately 80% in the proximal tubule, it is not concentrated.

Some *acidification* occurs in the proximal tubule as the result of carbonic anhydrase activity in the tubule cells and the diffusion of hydronium ions into the lumen. In the lumen the hydronium ion reacts with bicarbonate ion, which is converted to resorbable nonionic CO_2.

There is also active transport of organic cations and anions into the lumen (*tubular secretion*), each by a separate system. These active transport systems are extremely important in the excretion of a number of drugs; for example, penicillin G is rapidly secreted by the anion transport system and tetraethylammonium by the cation transport system. Probenecid is an inhibitor of anion secretion and hence decreases the rate of loss of penicillin from the body.

As the filtrate travels through the thin segment it becomes concentrated, especially at the bottom, as a result of active resorption and a countercurrent distribution effect enabled by the recurrent and parallel arrangement of the ascending segment, the parallel orientation of the collecting duct, and the similar recurrent geometry of the associated capillaries.

In the distal tubule sodium resorption occurs partly in *exchange* for potassium (*potassium secretion*) and for hydronium ions. Adrenal mineralcorticoids promote distal tubular sodium resorption and potassium and hydronium secretion. *Ammonia secretion* also occurs, so that the urine may be either acidified or alkalinized, according to acid–base and electrolyte requirements.

Drugs may also be resorbed in the distal tubule; the pH of the urine there is extremely important in determining the rate of resorption,[26] in accordance with the principle of nonionic diffusion and pH partition. The pH of the tubular fluid also affects the tubular secretion of drugs.

As an example of the importance of urine pH, in humans the secondary amine, mecamylamine, is excreted more than four times faster when the urine pH is less than 5.5 than when it is above 7.5;[27] Fig. 490 illustrates the effect of urine pH on the

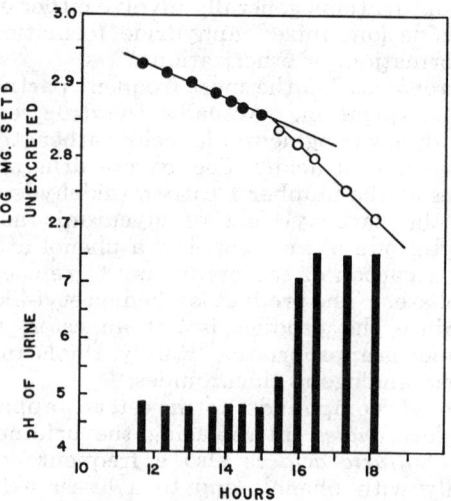

Fig. 491. The effect of urinary pH on the excretion of sulfaethidole in a human subject after oral administration of 2 Gm. *Bars* (lower half): urinary pH; *circles* (open and closed, top): log of the amount of drug remaining in the body; *negative slopes* (of lines defined by the circles): a function of the rate constant of excretion. Note the abrupt increase in rate when the urinary pH is changed from acidic to neutral or slightly alkaline (courtesy, Kostenbauder, *et al*[28]).

excretion of this amine. The effect of urine pH on the excretion of a weak acid,[28] sulfaethidole (for structure, see page 1201), is shown in Fig. 491.

The urine pH and hence drug excretion may fluctuate widely according to the diet, exercise, drugs, time of day, and other factors Obviously, the excretion of weak acids and bases can be partly controlled with acidifying or alkalinizing salts, such as NH_4Cl or $NaHCO_3$, respectively. Beckett has emphasized the importance of controlling urine pH in comparative studies on potency and efficacy in man.[29]

The collecting duct also resorbs sodium and water, secretes potassium, acidifies, and concentrates the urine. Antidiuretic hormone (ADH) controls the permeability to water of both the collecting duct and the distal tubule.

Renal clearance and the kinetics of renal elimination are discussed under *Pharmacokinetics* (page 755).

Biliary Excretion and Fecal Elimination— Many drugs are secreted into the bile and thence pass into the intestine. A drug that is passed into the intestine via the bile may be reabsorbed and not lost from the body. This cycle of biliary secretion and intestinal resorption is called *enterohepatic circulation.* Examples of drugs enterohepatically circulated are morphine and the penicillins. The biliary secretory systems greatly resemble those of the kidney tubules. The enterohepatic system may provide a considerable reservoir for a drug.

If a drug is not completely absorbed from the intestine, the unabsorbed fraction will be eliminated in the feces. An unabsorbable drug that is secreted into the bile will likewise be eliminated in the feces. Such fecal elimination is also called *fecal excretion.* Only rarely are drugs secreted into the intestine through the succus entericus (intestinal secretions), although a number of amines are secreted into gastric juice.

Alveolar Excretion—The large alveolar area and high blood flow make the lungs ideal for the excretion of appropriate substances. Only volatile liquids or gases are eliminated from the lungs. Gaseous and volatile anesthetics are essentially completely eliminated by this route. Only a small amount of ethanol

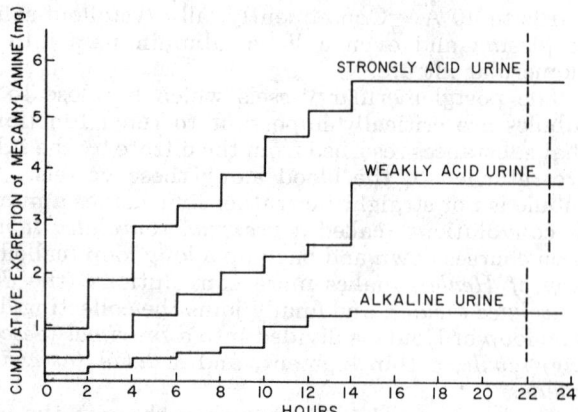

Fig. 490. The effect of urinary pH on the mean cumulative excretion in man of mecamylamine during the first day after oral administration of 10 mg. *Vertical dotted lines:* standard deviation (courtesy, Milne, *et al*[27]).

is eliminated by the lungs, but the concentration in the alveolar air is so constantly related to the blood alcohol concentration that the analysis of expired air is acceptable for legal purposes. The high aqueous solubility and relatively low vapor pressure of ethanol at body temperature account for the retention of most of the substance in the blood. Carbon dioxide from those drugs that are partly degraded to CO_2 also is excreted in the lungs.

Pharmacokinetics

Pharmacokinetics is the discipline that treats of the rates of movement of a drug or its metabolites into the body, among its many compartments, and out of the body and also which treats of the rates of biotransformations of the drug and its metabolites. As in chemistry, it primarily involves following the rate of change in concentration in the appropriate compartment(s), most often in the extracellular fluid (plasma) and/or urine. However, pharmacokinetics is by no means limited to observations on concentration; rates of movement of a drug can be followed by isotopes or other means. The application of pharmacokinetics to drug formulation and treatment regimens is also within the scope of this title.

Kinetics of Absorption

The absorption of a drug by diffusion has the kinetics of a *first-order process;* that is, the rate of absorption is directly proportional to the concentration, in accordance with Fick's Law and Eqs. 5 and 6 (pages 738 and 739); see also *Kinetics of Disposition* (this page). Thus the concentration of drug at the site of administration should fall exponentially with time. Bimolecular absorption processes, such as facilitated diffusion or active transport also usually show first-order kinetics, especially at drug concentrations well below those at which the carrier system will become saturated. At saturation the kinetics become zero order. Even the rate of dissolution of a drug is theoretically a first-order process, provided that the drug is readily soluble. If the solubility is low, it will be a zero-order process as long as there is saturation around the drug.

If the concentration or quantity of drug at the site of administration falls exponentially, the concentration in the plasma ought to rise logarithmically. However, absorption rarely conforms to a simple first-order process, because absorption may take place from more than one site and involve more than one process. After oral administration, a drug is absorbed at different rates from the stomach and different segments of the small intestine, partly simultaneously and partly sequentially. Biliary excretion may also complicate the kinetics.

The curve of plasma concentration is the algebraic sum of all the processes involved in absorption. Furthermore, the processes of distribution, redistribution, biotransformation, and excretion are taking place essentially all during the time of absorption, so that even prior to the time of peak concentration the plasma level reflects much more than absorption alone.

The peak concentration occurs when the rate of absorption equals the rate of disposition; it does not mean that absorption is complete. The time at which the blood concentration is at its peak is the *equilibrium time* for absorption. The time at which absorption is essentially complete is the *absorption*

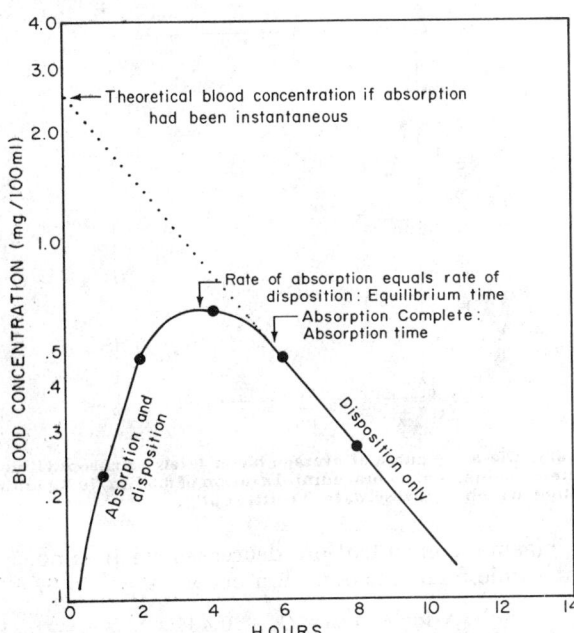

Fig. 492. Kinetics of absorption and disposition of theophylline in a human subject after oral administration of 0.5 Gm of aminophylline. Blood concentration is plotted on a log scale (courtesy, data, Truitt, *et al*[15]).

time. Equilibrium time and absorption time are indicated in Fig. 492. The time of peak plasma concentration must not be confused with the *time of peak effect* (peak time).

Effect often lags behind plasma concentration, sometimes because the tissue concentration at the point of action has not yet reached its peak and sometimes because a response may have a considerable latency. The latency of reserpine or diphenylhydantoin (in its anticonvulsant effect) is measured in hours to days. Occasionally, the time of peak effect may precede the time of peak concentration because of a reflex or other compensatory process which limits effect before the concentration becomes maximal. This is often true with oral ethanol or ephedrine.

Kinetics of Disposition

Unless the rate of disposition of a drug is less than the rate of absorption, the plasma concentration will not usually reach effective levels. If the rate of disposition is sufficiently less, not only will the plasma concentration rise to substantial levels, but the sojourn of the drug in the body will be considerably longer than the time for complete absorption. Consequently, for most useful drugs, the kinetics of disposition largely determine the useful life of a drug within the body. For this reason, the kinetics of disposition evoke more detailed study than do those of absorption.

First-Order Die-Away—Once a drug is absorbed, it is transported in the blood to the tissues, among which it is distributed, metabolized and/or excreted, all of which processes lower the plasma concentration of drug. Each separate process has first-order kinetics. If only a single process were involved, the plasma level would fall according to the equation

$$C = C_o e^{-kt} \tag{12}$$

where t is the time elapsed, C is the concentration at time t, C_o is the concentration at zero time, e is the natural or Naperian logarithmic base, and k is a velocity constant. The minus sign indicates that

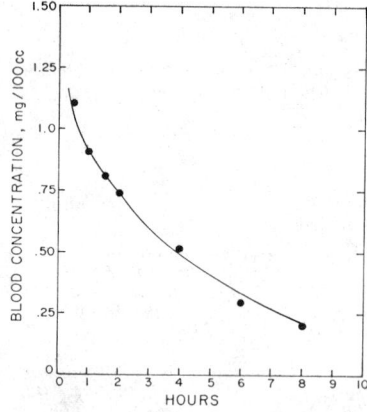

Fig. 493. Die-away curve of average blood levels of theophylline in 11 human subjects after oral administration of 0.5 Gm/70 Kg aminophylline to each (courtesy, data, Truitt, et al[15]).

the plasma concentration decreases with time. In logarithmic form the equation becomes

$$\log C = \log C_o - 0.434kt \qquad (13)$$

Plotted in Cartesian coordinates the so-called *die-away curve* has the typical shape of an exponential decrement. A die-away curve for theophylline in human subjects is shown in Fig. 493. If the data are plotted semilogarithmically or as log dose the die-away curve will become a straight line. Fig. 494 is a semilogarithmic plot of the data of Fig. 493. The extrapolation to zero time (that is, the x intercept) might be thought to be the concentration that obtained immediately upon injection. However, it is likely that the actual zero time concentration was higher than the intercept, because the plotted data was obtained after the drug had been distributed among the tissues; the intercept, then, is an abstraction that represents the plasma concentration at zero time if distribution had been instantaneous. Thus the intercept allows a calculation of the volume of distribution. The intercept of 1.15 mg/100 ml corresponds to a volume of distribution of 34 liters, which is about 68% of the volume of total body water.

Occasionally an elimination process may not exhibit first-order kinetics. This is true of ethanol, the elimination of which shows zero-order kinetics at blood concentrations above 0.040%. This is because the biotransforming enzyme, alcohol dehydrogenase, is saturated above 0.040%. Furthermore, with some

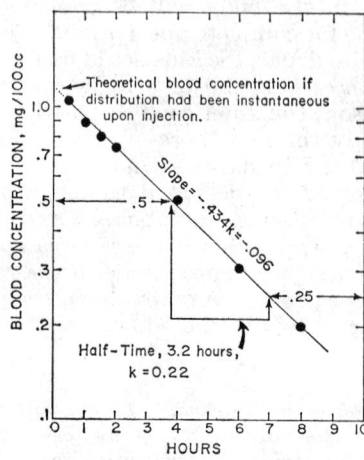

Fig. 494. Semilog plot of the die-away curve in Fig. 493. Note the log scale of the ordinates.

drugs the rate constant is not the same for all doses. With phenylbutazone the rate constant diminishes as the dose increases, presumably by self-inhibition of the enzyme by the substrate or its metabolite.[30]

Biological Half-Life—It is characteristic of exponential decay or die-away that the time required for a given fraction of a substance to disappear is always the same, regardless of the time or concentration at which one begins measurements. The fraction that is usually used as a standard is ½, so that it is customary to speak of the biological half-life, or half-time, of drugs.

The half-life can be determined graphically. A semilogarithmic plot such as that of Fig. 494 offers a slightly more accurate estimation than a Cartesian plot. A Cartesian plot can also be used, but the straight line of a semilogarithmic plot is advantageous. The half-life can then be substituted in Eqs. 14 or 15 in order to calculate the rate constant, k. The half-life from Fig. 494 yields a value of k of 0.22 reciprocal hours; ie, during each hour the plasma concentration drops by 22% of the level at the beginning of the hour. In a semilogarithmic plot the rate constant also closely relates to the slope of the line, as is evident from an analytic geometric comparison of Eq. 13 with the equation for a straight line. The slope will always be $-0.434k$. It must be kept in mind that the log of the concentration must be used, rather than the antilog that is plotted on the log-scaled ordinate in the figure.

Even within a group of closely related drugs, such as the sulfonamides shown in the Table II, there may be wide differences in the rates of elimination among the members. The half-life also may vary widely from species to species; for example, in man the half-life of sulfaethidole is about 8 hr, whereas in cattle it is in less than 2 hr.

Table II—The Approximate Biologic Half-Life in Man of Several Sulfonamides[31]

	$t_{1/2}$, hr
Sulfamethylthiadiazole	2
Sulfaethidole	8
Sulfisoxazole	8
Sulfamethoxypyridazine	34

The biological half-life must not be confused with the time for the response to decline by 50%, since the requirement for a threshold concentration, latency of response, and other factors cause a non-parallelism between blood concentration and intensity of response.

Multiple Processes—When two or more processes are involved in disposition, the over-all or total rate constant, K_t, is the sum of the constants of the individual processes, so that $K_t = k_1 + k_2 + k_3 \ldots + k_n$. The die-away plot in Cartesian coordinates will show more curvature than when only one process is involved. This may be seen in Fig. 495, which illustrates die-away of thiopental and pentobarbital in a human subject.[20] With pentobarbital two processes are especially evident to the eye. However, it is not always evident to the eye how many rate processes are involved.

When the data are plotted semilogarithmically, the separate processes will be evident as distinct rectilinear segments, providing that the rate constants of the processes and hence slopes of the segments are sufficiently different to be discernible.

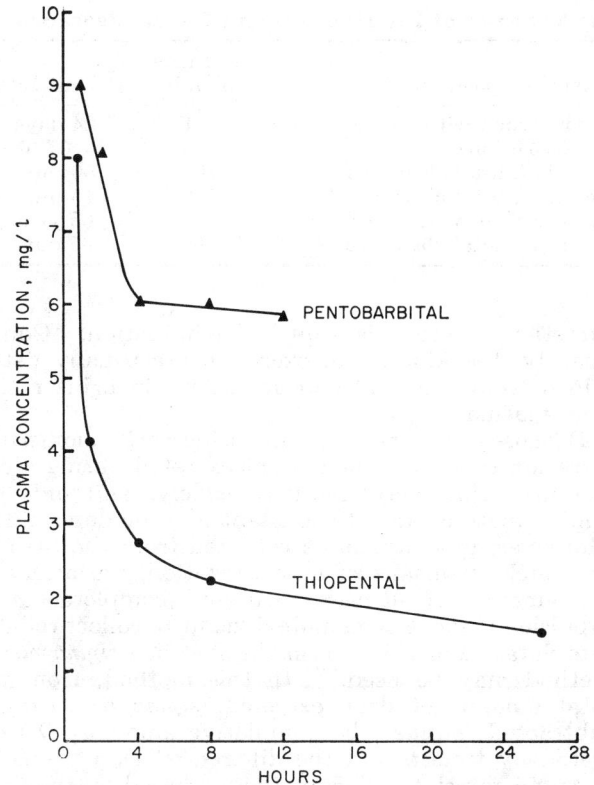

Fig. 495. Plasma concentrations in man of thiopental and pentobarbital after intravenous administration of 750 mg of each drug (courtesy, data, Brodie and Hogben[20]).

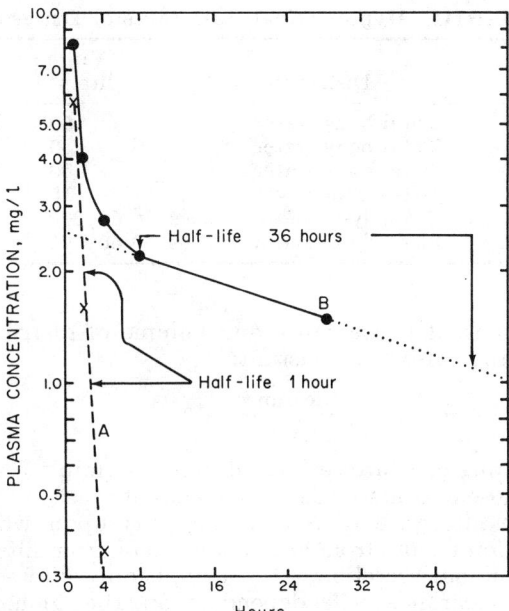

Fig. 496. Semilog plot of the data in Fig. 495. Note the log scale of the ordinates. Dotted lines: extrapolations of the B segment of the solid curve; *dashed line* (A): the result of the dotted line subtracted from the solid curve.

The thiopental data from Fig. 495 are replotted semilogarithmically in Fig. 496. At least two processes are now evident, but it is not clear whether a third process may be shaping the curve from 2 to 8 hr. Therefore, the separate processes were resolved by assuming that the line from 8 to 28 hr (*B*) correctly represents the slowest process, the fastest process (represented by Line *A*) having essentially run its course prior to 8 hr. *B* was then extrapolated to zero time. The value of the extrapolate was then subtracted from each experimental point and a new line, *A*, was plotted from the differences. Since *A* is essentially linear, it may be assumed that only two processes significantly affected the plasma concentration during the 28 hr of observation.

If *A* is extrapolated to zero time, a value of about 20 mg/liter is obtained, from which a volume of distribution of 37.5 liters may be calculated. This is approximately 70% of the volume of total body water. From the intercept of the *B* segment a hypothetical volume of distribution of 294 liters was calculated. This volume of distribution has meaning only if Process *A* is not one of removal of drug from the body.

All experimental data on the excretion and biotransformation of thiopental indicate that *A* was not one of elimination. Therefore, it follows that *A* represents redistribution. The redistribution of thiopental to fat was pointed out on page 748, and kinetics in the dog were illustrated in Fig. 488. It is probable, then, that Process *A* is uptake into fat from the blood.

Distribution to the brain, muscle, liver, and other tissues was probably essentially complete before the first plasma sample was removed at 1 hr. Otherwise, there would have been a third process showing in the plot and a corresponding volume of distribution considerably less than the body water. Process *B* is probably the biotransformation of the drug, which appears to be rate-limiting in the late stages of disposition. The tissue concentrations, including that in fat, during the 8–28-hr interval probably fell in parallel with the plasma concentrations, since the slowness of *B* allowed for the various compartments to come nearly into equilibrium and to a constant partition.

In the above example one of the die-away processes was considered to be redistribution. Usually, however, a relatively constant partition among compartments (approximate equilibrium) is reached more rapidly, often before the first blood sample is removed, so that most die-away curves represent only elimination.

Kinetics of Renal Excretion—The concept of *renal clearance* is helpful to an appreciation of the kinetics of renal excretion. Renal clearance is an abstraction and may be thought of as the hypothetical volume of plasma that the kidney can completely rid, or clear, of an excretable substance in unit time. It is determined as follows:

$$\text{Clearance} = \frac{C_u V_u}{t C_p} \tag{14}$$

where *t* is the time span of urine collection, C_u is the mean concentration of substance in the urine during time *t*, C_p is the mean concentration in the plasma, and V_u is the volume of urine produced during time *t*. The units of clearance are ml/min.

Unless the plasma level is held constant by continuous infusion, both C_w and C_p will fall continuously. However, they fall in a constant ratio, because C_u is directly related to C_p, as a result of both glomerular filtration and the fact that the processes of diffusion, resorption, and secretion obey first-order kinetics. Hence the clearance is independent of time and the plasma concentration at any one moment, and, consequently, clearance is a constant. The volume of distribution, V_D, is also usually constant. Therefore,

Table III—Hypothetical Half-Lives of Drugs of Differing Volumes of Distribution and Renal Clearances

Drug no.	Distribution	V_D, liters	Renal disposition	Clearance, ml/min	Half-Life
1	Total body water	50	Filtered and resorbed with water	1	24 days
2	Total body water	50	Filtered, no resorption	125	4.67 hr
3	Total body water	50	Tubular secretion, total clearance	700	50 min
4	Extracellular water	15	Tubular secretion, total clearance	700	15 min
5	Strongly bound in tissues	50,000	Filtered and resorbed with water	1	66 years
6	Strongly bound in tissues	50,000	Tubular secretion, total clearance	700	35 days

the quotient of clearance and volume of distribution must then also be a constant:

$$\frac{\text{Clearance}}{V_D} = k_e \qquad (15)$$

The units of k_e are reciprocal minutes (min^{-1}), which are those of a first-order rate constant.

The clearance of a drug depends upon whether excretion results from only filtration or from filtration plus tubular secretion. If a drug is only filtered, the renal clearance will depend upon the glomerular filtration rate and the extent of tubular resorption.

In the unusual instance in which there is no tubular resorption, the clearance will be equal to the glomerular filtration rate (GFR), which, in turn, depends upon renal plasma flow (RPF) and the extent of constriction of the afferent arterioles across the nephron. In the average 70-Kg man the effective RPF is about 700 ml/min, and the GFR is about 125 ml/min. Thus a drug which is only filtered and is not resorbed will have a clearance of about 125 ml/min. If the drug is resorbed to the same extent as is salt and water, namely, about 99%, the clearance will be just slightly greater than 1 ml/min. A more complete resorption will reduce the clearance to less than 1 ml/min.

The tubular secretion of some drugs, such as penicillin G, is so rapid that virtually all the drug is removed from the blood to the urine as fast as the blood flows through the kidney; that is, the drug is totally cleared. In such instances the clearance is equal to the renal plasma flow and approaches 700 ml/min. If the tubular secretion does not totally clear the plasma, the clearance will be less than 700 but more than 125 ml/min.

The half-time of a first-order process is $0.693/k$. From Eq. 15 a relationship between biological half-life of an excreted substance, its renal clearance, and volume of distribution may be expressed, as follows:

$$t_{1/2} = 0.693 \frac{V_D}{\text{Clearance}} \qquad (16)$$

Hypothetical half-lives of drugs of different volumes of distribution and renal clearances are shown in Table III. A volume of distribution of 50 liters is that of total body water, 15 liters is that of extracellular water, and 70,000 liters is that of a drug strongly bound in the tissues. Because of biotransformations, few drugs have half-lives longer than a year. However, a few radiopaque iodine-containing diagnostic agents are so tightly bound that their half-lives exceed a year. At the other extreme, a half-life of 15 min by renal elimination is uncommon, because few drugs that are totally cleared have volumes of distribution no larger than that of extracellular water. However, the half-live of penicillin G is about 15 min.

The kinetics of the renal elimination of a drug may be determined from plasma concentrations only if excretion is the sole route of elimination. Consequently, the kinetics of excretion are usually determined from chemical determinations in urine rather than plasma.

Because of variations in urine pH, glomerular filtration rate, etc, the amount excreted during a collection period may fluctuate widely, and only an approximate mean rate constant may be determined. Moreover, unless urine is collected from the bladder or ureter by means of catheterization, variations in the amount of urine voided and completeness of expulsion make it even more difficult to collect reliable rate data. For this reason the so-called *sigma-minus* method may be used.[32] In this method, from the total amount of drug excreted (*sigma* or $D_u\infty$) is subtracted (*minus*) the cumulative amount (D_u) excreted by time t, and the difference, $D_u\infty - D_u$ is plotted against t. This method is based on the first-order equation

$$\ln (D_u\infty - D_u) = \ln D'_o \frac{k_e}{K} - Kt \qquad (17)$$

where k_e is the rate constant of excretion, K the overall rate constant for elimination by all routes, and D'_o is the amount of drug which would have yielded the pattern of drug disappearance had it been present in the body at zero time.

D'_o is real if the drug is given intravenously but is a theoretical abstraction if the drug is given by any other route because of the latency of the appearance of the drug into the blood stream. The equation applies only if the processes of disposition are all first-order processes. A variation of the method is known as the U_{max} method, U_{max} being equal to D'_o.[31] Martin[32] has discussed the advantages of the rate and sigma-minus methods.

Swintosky[33] introduced a sequential dose method which makes it both unnecessary to collect urine until the drug is entirely excreted and to estimate D'_o. When fixed doses of drug are administered at fixed intervals by any route, after an initial lag required to prime the body burden of drug, the amount excreted per dose interval becomes constant (see Fig. 497). The amount excreted per dose is always a constant fraction of the dose and is thus equal to D_u/D'_o of the sigma-minus method. From Eq. 17 it may be determined that D_u/D'_o is equal to k_e/K, so that the method is, in effect, a variation of the sigma-minus method.

Kinetics of Latentiation and Disposition of Drug Metabolites—The amount of a metabolite of a drug in the body at any one time depends upon both the rate of transformation of the drug to metabolite and the rate of disposition of the metabolite. The body content of metabolite will continue to rise as long as the content of precursor is high enough that the rate of biotransformation to metabolite exceeds the rate of elimination of the metabolite. When the concentration of drug or precursor falls to a level

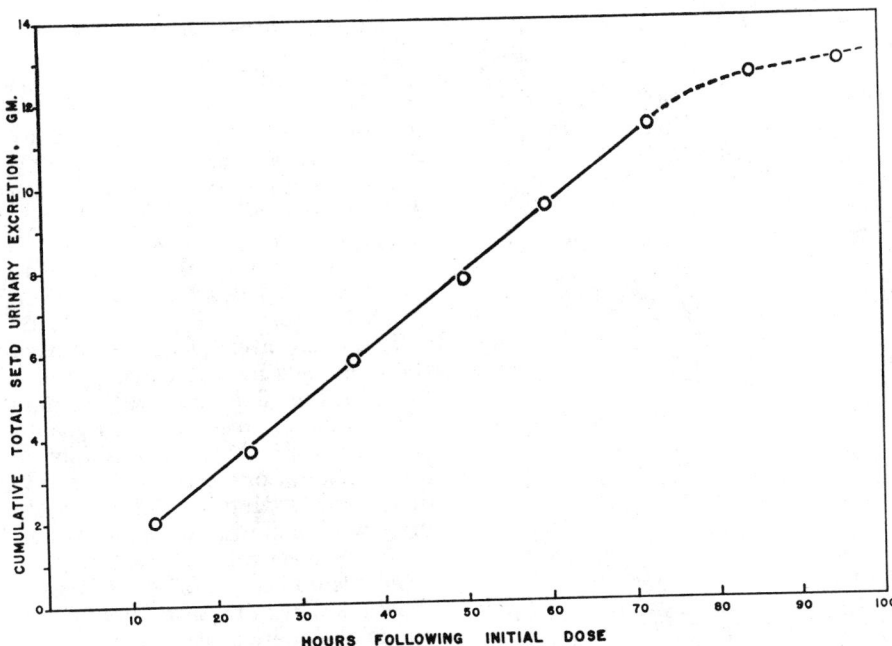

Fig. 497. Average cumulative excretion of sulfaethidole (SETD) in four human subjects after oral administration of 1 Gm every 6 hr to each. *Solid line:* excretion during the time drug was administered; *dashed line:* excretion following discontinuation of the drug (courtesy, data, Swintosky, *et al*[22]).

below which there is no longer a net gain in content of metabolite, the metabolite concentration will fall.

The kinetics of the fall in concentration depends upon which rate is faster, the elimination of drug precursor or the elimination of metabolite. If that of the drug is faster, the content of metabolite will rise above that of the drug, and the drug will soon disappear. This eventually leaves the content of cumulated metabolite to decline according to the kinetics of its own disposition.

In Fig. 498 Drug *B* illustrates the rate-limiting effect of the disposition of a metabolite. When the rate constant for the elimination of the drug or precursor is slower than that of the metabolite, as with Drug *A* in Fig. 498, the content of metabolite never reaches that of the drug and it eventually declines according to the kinetics of biotransformation of the drug. That is, the content of metabolite is mainly that which is being produced moment-to-moment. The figure is adapted from a plot of data from a computer analysis of a multivariable model.[34]

Cummings, *et al*,[35] have also made computer studies of situations in which more than one metabolite is involved. The kinetics of the generation and elimination of a metabolite relative to those of its drug precursor are important when the metabolite is either toxic or therapeutically active. In the latter instance the kinetics are the kinetics of latentiation. Where the metabolite is toxic, a pattern such as in *A* would be less likely to generate toxic concentrations as in *B*.

When the disposition of the drug precursor involves more than one process or when there is more than one metabolite, the kinetics are necessarily more complex than in the illustrations presented above.

Multiple-Dose Administration and Dose Interval—Some drugs may be administered only in a single dose—for example, aspirin for a simple headache, benzathine penicillin for a mild acute infection, nitroglycerin for aborting an attack of angina pectoris, or an anticholinergic to control only nocturnal gastric secretion. More often, however, it is necessary to continue treatment for several to many doses. That

is, the duration of therapy exceeds the effective sojourn of the drug in the body.

The dose intervals are usually prescribed as fixed intervals; ie, every *x* hours, etc, although in practice the interval may be somewhat irregular. From the kinetics of absorption, distribution, and elimination of a single dose of a drug, a dosage regimen may be calculated to provide as nearly as possible the optimal plasma concentration or body content.

The physician is rarely able to make the necessary kinetic determinations and calculations himself, although he may employ clinical criteria and limited laboratory study to adjust the dosage and interval to a suitable regimen. The kinetics of multiple doses are usually made in the laboratories of the drug manufacturer or various specialists in the field of pharmacokinetics. On the basis of kinetic data the manufacturer may recommend a dose schedule, although not all regimens are as yet based upon exacting studies. Furthermore, it must be kept in mind that the variation in drug kinetics among individuals is considerable, and the clinician ultimately has to make the final judgement as to the adequacy of a schedule for any given patient.

If both the dose and interval are fixed, the maximal and minimal plasma concentrations, C_{max} and C_{min}, respectively, are described by

$$C_{max} = \frac{C_o r_1}{1 - r} \qquad (18)$$

and

$$C_{min} = \frac{C_o r}{1 - r} \qquad (19)$$

where C_o is the concentration that would have been achieved if instantaneous absorption had occurred, r_1 and r are the respective functions $10^{-0.434 k_a t_1}$ and $10^{-0.434 kt}$ (t_1 being the time for absorption and t the fixed interval, k_a being the rate constant of absorption and k that for disposition). If administration is intravenous, r_1 drops out of Eq. 18. If the initial

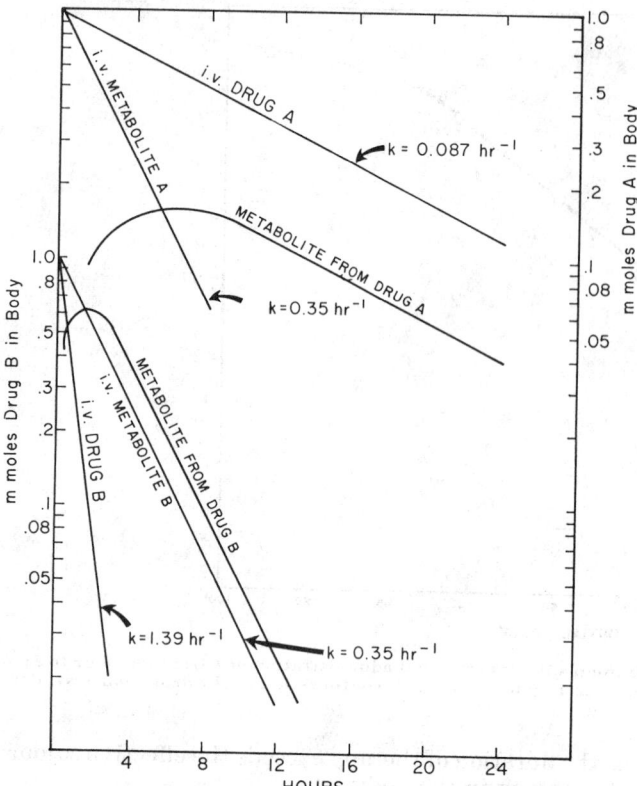

Fig. 498. Computer plot of the relationship of the amount of drug metabolite in the body to the amount of drug in the body at different relative rates of disposition of drug and metabolite. With Drug *A* the metabolite is eliminated at a much faster rate than the parent drug. Curve, "i.v. Metabolite A": the blood concentration when the metabolite is given intravenously; curve, "Metabolite from Drug A": the concentration of metabolite actually biotransformed from Drug *A*. With Drug *B* the metabolite is eliminated at a much faster rate than the parent drug (courtesy, combined replot of two figures, Martin[34]).

(or priming) dose is not the same as the maintenance (ie, subsequent fixed) dose, the equations are more complex.

In Fig. 499, taken from Krüger-Thiemer,[36] the kinetics of fixed-interval fixed-oral maintenance dose administration are illustrated. The importance of the size of the initial dose, D^*, relative to that of the maintenance dose, D, is shown. The desired thera-

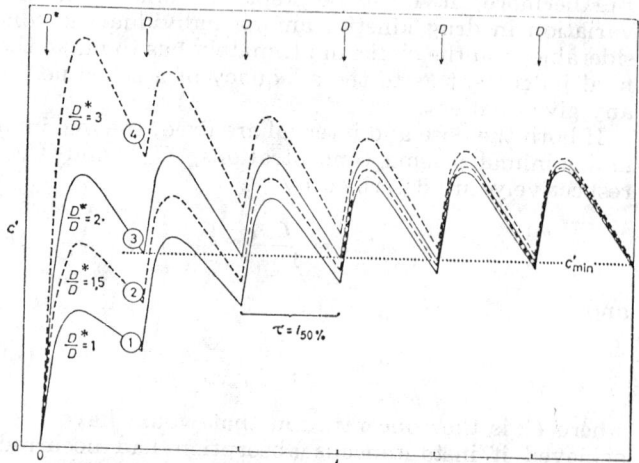

Fig. 499. Variation in the plasma concentration of a drug with time according to different initial and maintenance doses. *C* (ordinate): concentration; *t* (abscissa): time; D^*: initial dose; *D*: maintenance dose (the size of D^* relative to *D* is shown by the ratio for each curve); τ (the dose interval): biological half-life, $t^{1/2}$; C'_{min}: same as C_{min} in Eq. 21 (courtesy, Krüger-Thiemer[36]).

peutic concentration should be just slightly less than C'_{min}.

If the initial dose is too small, the desired therapeutic concentration may not be reached until several doses are given. It is customary to administer digitalis this way, because it avoids overdosing, and heart failure rarely demands an immediate therapeutic effect. If the initial dose is too large, the optimal concentration is greatly exceeded, which is not only wasteful of drug but is potentially toxic with many drugs. The optimal initial dose is about twice that of the maintenance dose.

The dose interval in the illustration of Fig. 499 is the biological half-life, $t_{1/2}$. This is usually considered to be the best fixed interval for maintenance, especially if the rate of absorption is greater than the rate of elimination.[36] With the aid of a few sketches and imagination, or Ref. 36, the interested reader can demonstrate that at intervals shorter than $t_{1/2}$ the drug will accumulate until C'_{min} is too high and that at longer intervals C'_{min} will be too low. With longer intervals and appropriately larger maintenance doses, the peak concentration may be too high and may soar out of the therapeutic range into the toxic range.

Since the plasma concentration will rise after the administration of each dose then subsequently decline, it is not possible to keep the plasma concentration steady, but the fluctuations may be minimized by frequent administration of small doses, limited only by cost and inconvenience to the patient. With oral preparations the effect of repetition at ultrashort intervals can be approximated by the use of capsules containing mixed-release-rate granules, multilayered tablets, etc which effect sustained release.

Kinetics in the Evaluation of Drugs and Drug Products—The utility of pharmacokinetics to the devising of appropriate dosage regimes is obvious. Kinetic studies are also important to the study of the influence of inhibitors of elimination, such as that of probenecid on the excretion of penicillin, and the effect of one drug on the disposition of another.

Plasma or tissue concentrations and their kinetics are not only valid but essential in comparing the availability of a drug from various dosage forms or from preparations of various sources, in which the excipients, adjuvants, etc may vary but the active ingredients are the same. Such data are critical to a proper appraisal of the practice of prescribing drugs by proprietary names.

Kinetics are also employed to compare different drugs, but the meaning of such comparisons is often obscure, and claims of therapeutic superiority based upon kinetics must be accepted cautiously. The kinetics of disposition are important to a comparison of drugs in a class in which toxic effects are frequent; it is often desirable to use a drug with a short biological life, so that a toxic episode may be quickly terminated upon discontinuation of medication. Furthermore, it is valid to compare among drugs the fluctuations in plasma concentration consequent to multiple-dose administration, provided, of course, that for the class of drugs in question the extent of fluctuation has an important bearing on efficacy or toxicity. In the case of penicillin, fluctuations in blood level have very little effect on either efficacy or toxicity.

A comparison of peak or mean blood levels achieved by equal doses of different drugs is not entirely meaningless. It is true that the dose of a drug may be adjusted to compensate for a difference in potency from some reference drug, but it is often difficult for the physician to alter the dose except in multiples of the unit dose provided by the manufacturer. Partly because of the inertia of precedence and habit and partly because it is easier for the physician to memorize doses as a group, closely related drugs whose potencies differ only moderately may all be available in the same dose. Thus tetracyclines are available as "250's" or "500's," even though they are not equipotent, sulfonamides as 1 Gm, etc. It is therefore valid for the physician to choose the drug whose unit dose yields a blood level closest to the optimum. Unfortunately, many physicians do not have the prerequisite knowledge for such a choice and hence may be susceptible to misleading promotional arguments about the superiority of one product over another.

Drug Interaction and Combination

It is frequent that a patient may receive more than one drug concurrently. Case records show that surgical patients commonly receive more than 10 and sometimes as many as 30 drugs and that the patient is often under the influence of several drugs at once, sometimes unnecessarily. Multiple-drug administration is also common to patients hospitalized for infections and for many other disorders. Furthermore, a patient may be suffering from more than one unrelated disorder which demands simultaneous treatment with two or more drugs. In such instances interactions are unsolicited and often unexpected.

In addition to the administration of drugs concurrently for their independent and unrelated effects, drugs are sometimes administered concurrently deliberately to make use of expected interactions.

Types of Interaction and Reasons for Combination Therapy

A drug may effect the response to another drug in a quantitative way. On the one hand, the intensity of either the therapeutic effect or side effect may be augmented or suppressed. On the other hand, a qualitatively different effect may be brought out. The mechanisms of such interactions are many and are not always understood. A drug may not necessarily affect either the quality or initial intensity of effect of another drug but may cause significant to profound changes in the duration of action. The nature of this type of interaction is generally fairly well understood, although it may not yet have been ascertained for any particular drug combination. The deliberate use of combined interacting drugs is most valid when the mechanism of the interaction is understood and the combined effects are both quantifiable and predictable. The rationales of drug combination and the principles involved are discussed below.

Combinations to Increase Intensity of Response or Efficacy—Sometimes the basis for the action of one drug to increase the intensity of response to another is well understood, but often the reason for a positive interaction is obscure. A terminology has grown up[37] that is frequently not enlightening as to mechanisms and principles but also which is somewhat confusing.

Drugs that elicit the same quality of effect and are mutually interactive are called *homergic*, regardless of whether there is anything in common between the separate response systems. Thus the looseness of the term admits a pressor response consequent to an increase in cardiac output to be homergic with one resulting from arteriolar constriction, even though there is not one common responsive element, the blood pressure itself being but a passive indicator. However, homergic drugs usually have in common at least part of a response system. Thus both norepinephrine and pitressin stimulate some of the same vascular smooth muscle, even though they do not excite the same receptors.

Two homergic drugs can be agonists of the same receptor, so that the entire response system is common to both. Such drugs are called *homodynamic*. As discussed under *Drug Receptors and Receptor Theory* (page 733), homodynamic drugs will generate dose–intensity of effect curves with parallel slopes but not necessarily with identical maxima or efficacies, if one of the drugs is a partial agonist.

From mass law kinetics and dose–effect data of the separate drugs it is possible to predict the combined effects of two agonists to the same receptor. If both drugs are full agonists, theory predicts that an EDx of Drug A added to an EDy of Drug B should elicit the same effect as that of an EDy of Drug A added to an EDx of Drug B. An example is shown in Fig. 500.[38] Dose–percent data with homodynamic drugs can be treated in the same way.[39]

Drugs whose combined effects fit the above conditions are called *additive*. If the response to the combination exceeds the expected value for additivity, the drugs are considered to be *supra-additive*. Purely homodynamic drugs do not show supra-additivity; however, if one drug in the pair has an additional action to affect the concentration or penetrance of the other or to prime the response system in some way, two agonists to the same receptor may exhibit supra-additivity. Two homergic drugs are *infra-additive* if their combined effect is less than expected from additivity. As with supra-additivity, infra-additivity

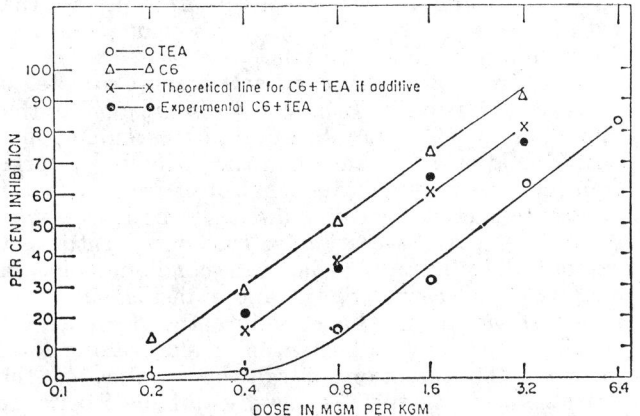

Fig. 500. Additive inhibitory effects of tetraethylammonium (TEA) and hexamethonium (C6) on the superior cervical ganglion of the cat. The theoretical line for additivity was calculated on the basis that an increment of TEA added to an EDx of C6 should have the same effect as if it were added to an EDx of TEA. When TEA and C6 were administered together, an equal amount of each was given. The dose is the sum of the doses of the two components (courtesy, Harvey[38]).

must involve an action elsewhere than on a common receptor.

Two drugs are said to be *summative* if a dose of drug that elicits response x is added to a dose of another drug that elicits response y give the combined response $x + y$. Very little significance can usually be attached to summation. Unless the dose–intensity curve of each drug is linear rather than log-linear, summation cannot be predicted from the two curves. When summation does occur with the usual clinical doses of two drugs, it almost never occurs over the entire dose range; indeed, if the dose of each of the two drugs is greater than an ED50, summation is theoretically impossible unless it is possible to increase the maximal response. At best, summation is an infrequent clinical finding limited to one or two doses.

Two drugs are said to be *heterergic* if the drugs do not cause responses of the same quality. When heterergy is positive, ie, the response to one drug is enhanced by the other, *synergism* is said to occur. The word has often been used to describe any positive interaction, but it should be used only to describe a positive interaction between heterergic drugs. The term *potentiation* has been used synonymously with synergism, but misuse of the term has led to the recommendation that the term be dropped. Synergism is often the result of an effect to interfere with the elimination of a drug and thus to increase the concentration; synergism may also result from an effect on penetrance or upon the responsivity of the effector system. Examples of a synergistic effect in which responsivity is enhanced are the action of adrenalcorticoids to enhance the vasoconstrictor response to epinephrine and the increase of epinephrine-induced hyperglycemia consequent to impairment by theophylline of the enzymatic destruction of the cyclic-AMP which mediates the response.

In clinical practice two homodynamic drugs are rarely coadministered for the purpose of increasing the response, since a sufficient dose of either drug should be able to achieve the same effect as a combination of the two. Most clinical combinations with positively interacting drugs are with heterergic drugs.

Combinations to Decrease Individual Doses and Toxicity—When homodynamic drugs are co-administered, it is usually for the purpose of decreasing toxicity. If the toxicities of two homodynamic drugs are infra-additive, the toxicity of combined partial doses of the two drugs will often be less than with full doses of either drug. This principle is valid for trisulfapyrimidines mixture (see page 1204).

Combinations to Attack a Disease Complex at Different Points—With many diseases more than one organ or tissue may be affected or events at more than one locus may bear upon the ultimate perturbation. For example, in duodenal ulcer psychic factors appear to increase activity in the vagus nerve which modulates gastric secretion, so that it was rational to explore the effects of sedatives, ganglionic blocking drugs, antimuscarinic drugs, and antacids, singly and in combination. In heart failure the decrement in renal plasma flow and changes in aldosterone levels promote the retention of salt and water, so that diuretics and digitalis are usually employed concomitantly. Pain, anxiety, and agitation or depression are frequent accompaniments of various pathological processes, so that it is to be expected that analgesics, tranquilizers, sedatives or antidepressives will frequently be given at the same time, along with other drugs intended to correct the specific pathology.

Combinations to Antagonize Untoward Actions —The side effects of a number of drugs can be prevented or suppressed by other drugs. An antagonist may compete with the drug at the receptor that initiates the side effect, depress the side-effector system at a point other than the receptor, or stimulate an opposing system.

Antagonism at the receptor is *competitive antagonism* if the antagonist attaches at the same receptor group as the agonist (see page 734). Antagonism at a different receptor group or inhibition elsewhere in the response system is *noncompetitive antagonism*. Both competitive and noncompetitive antagonism are classified as *pharmacological antagonism*. The stimulation of an opposing system is *physiological antagonism*.

Clinical examples of pharmacological antagonism are the use of atropine to suppress the muscarinic effects of excess acetylcholine consequent to the use of neostigmine and the use of antihistaminics to prevent the effects of histamine liberated by tubocurarine. Examples of physiological antagonism are the use of amphetamine to correct partially the sedation caused by anticonvulsant doses of phenobarbital and the administration of ephedrine to correct hypotension resulting from spinal anesthesia.

Combinations Which Affect Elimination— Only a few drugs are presently used purposefully to elevate or to prolong plasma levels by interfering with elimination, although continued interest in such drugs will probably increase the number.

Probenecid, which has already been mentioned to antagonize the renal secretion of penicillin, was originally introduced for this purpose. However, the inexpensiveness of penicillin G, repository preparations of penicillin G, and oral preparations (which obviate the need for injection) make it less imperative to retard the excretion of penicillin. The low nonallergenic toxicity of penicillin permits very large doses to be given without concern for the high plasma concentrations that result, which also means that there is little necessity for increasing the biological half-life of the drug. Consequently, probenecid is not used much today in combination with penicillin.

The use of vasoconstrictors to increase the sojourn of local anesthetics at the site of infiltration continues, but few other clinical examples of the deliberate use of one drug to interfere with either the distribution or elimination of another can be cited. Nevertheless, the subject of the effect of one drug on the elimination of another has become immensely active. Innumerable drugs affect the fate of others, and the therapist must be aware of such interactions.

Many drugs enhance the elimination of drugs that are metabolized by the liver microsomes. There would be very little point ordinarily to solicit combinations that would shorten the duration of action unless it were to reduce an overdosage. However, since such combinations are unwittingly or unavoidably used, this type of interaction is of great clinical importance.

Combinations to Alter Absorption—In the section on *Vehicles and Absorption Adjuvants* (page 745) it was mentioned that certain substances facilitate the absorption of others. The use of such absorption adjuvants is generally included under the subject of formulation rather than under drug combination. Although drugs which increase blood flow, motility, etc have an effect to increase the rate of absorption, the use of such drugs has so far not proven to be very practical. When it is desired to slow the absorption of drugs, various physical or physicochemical means prove to be more effective and less troublesome than drug combinations.

Fixed Combinations of Drugs

Concomitant treatment with two or more drugs is frequently unnecessary, and it generally immeasurably complicates therapy and the evaluation of response and toxicity. Nevertheless, it is often warranted, even essential, and cannot be condemned categorically. However, fixed-dose or fixed-ratio combinations, in which the drugs are together in the same preparation, must be condemned, except for a few rare instances like trisulfapyrimidines.

The basis for this condemnation is as follows: patients differ in their responsivity or sensitivity to drugs, and adjustments in dosage or dose-interval may be necessary. If adjustment of only one component of the mixture is required, it is undesirable that the schedule of the second component be obligatorily adjusted, as it is in a fixed combination. According to which way the dose is adjusted, either toxicity or loss of the therapeutic effect may result. Furthermore, when adverse effects to either component occur, both drugs must be discontinued. The fixed combination denies the physician flexible control of therapy. Especially when one component in a mixture is superfluous, as is often the case, the promotion of fixed combinations is reprehensible.

Dangers in Multiple-Drug Therapy

The objections to fixed-dose combinations were stated above. Also the unanticipated effects of drug combinations have been touched upon, particularly with respect to effects upon elimination. But it should be made clear that more is at stake than simply the biological half-life of a drug. On page 750 was given an example of the grave clinical consequences of the effect of phenobarbital to enhance the biotransformation of warfarin. Other examples of dangerous interactions, such as the effect of several antidepressants greatly to synergize catecholamines, may be cited. Even some antibiotics antagonize each other and increase mortality.

In addition to the obvious pitfalls posed by the interactions themselves, the use of multiple-drug therapy fosters careless diagnosis and a false sense of security in the number of drugs employed. Finally, the expense to the patient warrants consideration. Multiple-drug therapy should never be employed without a convincing indication that each drug is beneficial beyond the possible detriments or without proof that a therapeutically equivocal combination is definitely harmless.

References

1. Westerfield, W. W., *Science*, **123**, 1017 (1956).
2. Clark, A. J., *J. Physiol. (London)*, **61**, 530 (1926).
3. Paton, W. D. M., *Proc. Roy. Soc. (London) Ser. B*, **154**, 21 (1961).
4. Clark, A. J., *J. Physiol. (London)*, **61**, 547 (1926).
5. Ariens, E. J., ed., *Molecular Pharmacology*, vol. 1, Academic, New York, 1964, pp. 176–193.
6. Stephenson, R. P., *Brit. J. Pharmacol.*, **11**, 379 (1956).
7. McKay, D. J., *J. Pharm. Pharmacol.*, **18**, 201 (1966).
8. Furchgott, R. F., *Ann. Rev. Pharmacol.*, **4**, 21 (1964).
9. Overton, E., *Arch. Ges. Physiol.*, **92**, 115 (1902).
10. Schanker, L. S., *Advan. Drug Res.*, **1**, 71 (1964).
11. Jacobs, M. H., *Cold Spring Harbor Symp. Quant. Biol.*, **8**, 30 (1940).
12. Davson, H., and Danielli, J. F., *The Permeability of Natural Membranes*, Cambridge, London, 1943, pp. 60–84.
13. Eagle, H., *J. Pharmacol. Exptl. Therap.*, **85**, 222 (1945).
14. Brodie, B. B., *et al*, *J. Pharmacol. Exptl. Therap.*, **130**, 20 (1960).
15. Truitt, E. B., Jr., *et al*, *J. Pharmacol. Exptl. Therap.*, **100**, 309 (1950).
16. Lillehei, J. P., *J. Am. Med. Assoc.*, **205**, 531 (1968).
17. Treager, R. T., *Physical Functions of Skin*, Academic, London, 1966, pp. 9, 17.
18. Martin, A. N., *Physical Pharmacy*, Lea & Febiger, Philadelphia, 1960, pp. 247, 253.
19. Schanker, L. S., *Pharmacol. Rev.*, **14**, 501 (1961).
20. Brodie, B. B., and Hogben, C. A., *J. Pharm. Pharmacol.*, **9**, 345 (1957).
21. Hogben, C. A., *Proc. Federation Am. Soc. Exptl. Biol.*, **19**, 864 (1960).
22. Albert, A., *Pharmacol. Rev.*, **4**, 136 (1952).
23. Ariens, E. J., *et al*, in Ariens, E. J., ed., *Molecular Pharmacology*, vol. 1, Academic, New York, 1964, pp. 7–52.
24. Harper, N. J., *Med. Pharm. Chem.*, **1**, 467 (1959).
25. Williams, R. T., *Clin. Pharmacol. Therap.*, **4**, 234 (1963).
26. Orloff, J., and Berliner, R. W., *Federation Am. Soc. Exptl. Biol.*, **13**, 107 (1954).
27. Milne, M. D., *et al*, *Clin. Sci.*, **16**, 599 (1957).
28. Kostenbauder, H. B., *et al*, *J. Pharm. Sci.*, **51**, 1084 (1962).
29. Beckett, A. H., and Tucker, T. G., *J. Pharm. Pharmacol.*, **18**, 725 (1966).
30. Dayton, P. G., *et al*, *J. Pharmacol. Exptl. Therap.*, **158**, 305 (1967).
31. Swintosky, J. V., *Proc. Am. Pharmacol. Assoc. Coll. Pharm. Teachers Seminar*, **13**, 140 (1961).
32. Martin, B. K., *Brit. J. Pharmacol. Chemotherap.*, **29**, 181 (1967).
33. Swintosky, J. V., *et al*, *J. APhA, Sci. Ed.*, **47**, 753 (1958).
34. Martin, B. K., *Brit. J. Pharmacol. Chemotherap.*, **31**, 420 (1967).
35. Cummings, A. J., *et al*, *Brit. J. Pharmacol. Chemotherap.*, **29**, 136 (1967).
36. Krüger-Thiemer, E., in Ariens, E. J., ed., *Physico-chemical Aspects of Drug Action*, vol. 7, Pergamon, London, 1968, pp. 63–113.
37. Loewe, S., *Pharmacol. Rev.*, **9**, 237 (1957).
38. Harvey, S. C., *Arch. Intern. Pharmacodyn.*, **114**, 232 (1958).
39. Weaver, L. C., *et al*, *J. Pharmacol. Exptl. Therap.*, **113**, 359 (1955).

Bibliography

Albert, A., "Ionization, pH and Biological Activity," *Pharmacol. Rev.*, **4**, 136 (1952).

Albert, A., *Selective Toxicity*, Methuen, London, 1965.

Ariens, E. J., ed., *Molecular Pharmacology*, vol. 1, Academic, New York, 1964.

Ariens, E. J., ed., *Physico-Chemical Aspects of Drug Action*, Pergamon, London, 1968.

Ballard, B., "Biopharmaceutical Considerations in Subcutaneous and Intramuscular Drug Administration," *J. Pharm. Sci.*, **57**, 357 (1968).

Belleau, B., "Conformational Perturbation in Relation to Enzyme and Receptor Behavior," *Advan. Drug Res.*, **2**, 89 (1965).

Binns, T. B., ed., *Absorption and Distribution of Drugs*, Livingston, London, 1964.

Brodie, B. B., and Hogben, C. A., "Some Physico-chemical Factors in Drug Action," *J. Pharm. Pharmacol.*, **9**, 345 (1957).

Brown, A. C., "Passive and Active Transport," in Ruch, T. C., and Patton, H. D., eds., *Physiology and Biophysics*, Saunders, Philadelphia, 1965, Chap. 43.

Conney, A. H., "Pharmacological Implications of Microsomal Enzyme Induction," *Pharmacol. Rev.*, **19**, 317 (1967).

Conney, A. H., and Burns, J. J., "Factors Influencing Drug Metabolism," *Advan. Pharmacol.*, **1**, 31 (1962).

Davson, H., and Danielli, J. F., *The Permeability of Natural Membranes*, 2nd ed., Cambridge, London, 1952.

Furchgott, R. F., "Receptor Mechanisms," *Ann. Rev. Pharmacol.*, **4**, 21 (1964).

Gill, E. W., "Drug Receptor Interactions," *Progr. Med. Chem.*, **4**, 39 (1965).

Gillette, J. R., "Biochemistry of Drug Oxidation and Reduction by Enzymes in Hepatic Endoplastic Reticulum," *Advan. Pharmacol.*, **4**, 219 (1966).

Goldstein, A., "The Interactions of Drugs and Plasma Proteins," *Pharmacol. Rev.*, **1**, 102 (1949).

Goldstein, A., *et al*, *Principles of Drug Action*, Hoeber, New York, 1968.

Goldstein, A., *et al*, *Advan. Drug Res.*, **3**, (1966).

Harper, N. J., and Simmonds, A. B., eds., *Advan. Drug Res.*, **3**, (1966).

Hogben, C. A. M., and Lindgren, P., eds., *Drugs and Membranes*, Macmillan, New York, 1963.

Hogben, C. A. M., "The First Common Pathway," *Proc. Federation Am. Soc. Exptl. Biol.*, **19**, 864 (1960).

Kalow, W., *Pharmacogenetics: Heredity and the Response to Drugs*, Saunders, Philadelphia, 1962.

Kruhoffer, P., "The Pharmacology of Membranes," *J. Pharm. Pharmacol.*, **13**, 193 (1961).

Levine, R. R., and Pelikan, E. W., "Mechanisms of Drug Absorption and Excretion. Passage of Drugs Out and Into the Gastrointestinal Tract," *Ann. Rev. Pharmacol.*, **4**, 69 (1964).

Levy, G., "Biopharmaceutical Considerations in Dosage Form Design and Evaluation," in Sprowls, J. B., Jr., ed., *Prescription Pharmacy*, Lippincott, Philadelphia, 1963, chap. 2.

Martin, B. K., "Potential Effect of the Plasma Proteins on Drug Distribution," *Nature*, **207**, 274 (1965).

McKay, D. J., "The Mathematics of Drug–Receptor Interactions," *J. Pharm. Pharmacol.*, **18**, 201 (1966).

Milne, M. D., "Non-ionic Diffusion and Excretion of Weak Acids and Bases," *Am. J. Med.*, **24**, 709 (1958).

Nelson, E., "Kinetics of Drug Absorption, Distribution, Metabolism, and Excretion," *J. Pharm. Sci.*, **50**, 181 (1961).

Peters, J. H., "Genetic Factors in Relation to Drugs," *Ann. Rev. Pharmacol.*, **8**, 427 (1968).

Porter, C. C., and Stone, C. A., "Biochemical Mechanisms of Drug Action," *Ann. Rev. Pharmacol.*, **7**, 15 (1967).

Ravin, L. J., and Bernardo, P. D., "Pharmaceutical Sciences—1967. A Literature Review of Pharmaceutics," *J. Pharm. Sci.*, **57**, 1075 (1968).

Schanker, L. S., "Passage of Drugs Across Body Membranes," *Pharmacol. Rev.*, **14**, 501 (1961).

Schanker, L. S., "Physiological Transport of Drugs," *Advan. Drug Res.*, **1**, 71 (1964).

Stein, W. D., *The Movement of Molecules Across Cell Membranes*, Academic, New York, 1968.

Stowe, C. M., and Plaa, G. L., "Extrarenal Excretion of Drugs and Chemicals," *Ann. Rev. Pharmacol.*, **8,** 337 (1968).

Swintosky, J. V., "Illustrations and Pharmaceutical Interpretations of First Order Drug Elimination Rate from the Bloodstream," *J. APhA, Sci. Ed.*, **45,** 395 (1956).

Swintosky, J. V., "Biologic Half-Life and Tissue Concentrations," *Proc. Am. Assoc. Coll. Teachers Seminar*, **13,** 140 (1961).

Tedeschi, D. H., and Tedeschi, R. E., *Importance of Fundamental Principles in Drug Evaluation*, Raven Press, New York, 1968.

Wagner, J. G., "Biopharmaceutics: Absorption Aspects," *J. Pharm. Sci.*, **50,** 359 (1961).

Wagner, J. G., "Pharmacokinetics," *Ann. Rev. Pharmacol.*, **8,** 67 (1968).

Wagner, J. G., "Pharmacokinetics 3. Half-Life and Volume of Distribution," *Drug Intelligence*, **2,** 126 (1968).

Weiner, I. M., "Mechanisms of Drug Absorption and Excretion," *Ann. Rev. Pharmacol.*, **7,** 39 (1967).

Wilbrandt, W., "Permeability and Transport Systems in Living Cells," *J. Pharm. Pharmacol.*, **11,** 65 (1959).

Williams, R. T., "Detoxification Mechanisms in Man," *Clin. Pharmacol. Therap.*, **4,** 234 (1963).

Wilson, T. H., *Intestinal Absorption*, Saunders, Philadelphia, 1962.

Woodbury, J. W., "The Cell Membrane: Ionic and Potential Gradients and Active Transport," in Ruch, T. C., and Patton, H. D., eds., *Physiology and Biophysics*, Saunders, Philadelphia, 1965, chap. 1.

43 | Topical Drugs

Protectives—absorbents—demulcents—emollients—astringents—
irritants—rubifacients—vesicants—sclerosing agents—caustics—
escharotics—keratolytics—cleansing agents—miscellaneous topical drugs

This chapter was prepared by

Ewart A. Swinyard, PhD, *Professor of Pharmacology, College of Pharmacy and College of Medicine, University of Utah, Salt Lake City, Utah 84112, and*
Stewart C. Harvey, PhD, *Associate Professor of Pharmacology, College of Medicine, University of Utah, Salt Lake City, Utah 84112*

A large number of chemical agents may be applied to the skin and mucous membranes for their local effects. Many of these, such as antibiotics, antiseptics, and local anesthetics, belong to distinct pharmacological classes treated elsewhere in this text, and will not be discussed in this chapter. The remainder comprise a heterogeneous group of agents which, by exclusion, are mostly nonselective in action.

Those locally acting agents that have limited chemical and pharmacologic activity generally have a *physical* basis of action. Included in this group are protectives, adsorbents, demulcents, emollients, and cleansing agents. The relative inertness of many of these substances renders them of value as vehicles and excipients. Consequently, many in this group are also pharmaceutical necessities and may be treated in Chapter 71 (page 1316).

Those locally acting agents having general *chemical* reactivity include most astringents, irritants, rubefacients, vesicants, sclerosing agents, caustics, escharotics, many keratolytic (desquamating) agents, and a miscellaneous group of dermatologics including hypopigmenting and antipruritic agents.

Although the skin and mucous membranes differ considerably in structure and function, they are similar in penetrability (to chemical agents) and in their response to certain physical and pharmacological stimuli. Thus, many of the agents found in this chapter may be applied to both types of surfaces. On the other hand, it is obvious that many agents, for which there is either contraindication or no rationale for their application to the mucous membranes, may be applied only to the skin.

In its broadest pharmacologic sense a protective is any agent that isolates the exposed surface (skin or mucous membrane) from harmful or annoying stimuli. In common practice only those substances that protect by mechanical or other physical means are considered to be protectives, although the surface action of adsorbents and demulcents cannot be divorced from their chemical properties. Protectives such as demulcents and emollients are customarily placed in separate categories; that practice is followed here.

The abridged category of protectives mainly comprise the dusting powders, adsorbents, mechanical protective agents, and plasters.

Protectives and Adsorbents

Dusting Powders

Certain relatively indifferent (inert and insoluble) substances are used to cover and protect epithelial surfaces, ulcers, and wounds. Usually these substances are very finely subdivided. They generally absorb moisture and therefore also act as cutaneous desiccants. The absorption of skin moisture decreases friction and also discourages certain bacterial growth.

The water absorbent powders should not be administered to wet, raw surfaces because of the formation of cakes and adherent crusts. Starch and other carbohydrate powders may not only become doughy but they may also ferment. Consequently, such powders often contain an antiseptic. Most impalpable powders are to some extent absorptive. Whether absorption of substances other than water contributes to the protection of the skin is uncertain; however, absorption of fatty acids and other constituents of perspiration, along with cutaneous drying, contributes to a deodorant action of the powders. It is generally held that the adsorptive capacity is important to the gastrointestinal protective action of indifferent powders taken internally.

The indifferent dusting powders are not entirely biologically inert, despite the name. When entrained in pores or wounds or left upon parietal surfaces, certain of the dusting powders, eg, talc, may cause irritation, granulomas, fibrosis, or adhesions. Even without direct irritation or obstruction of the perspiration, dust can be troublesome.

Several of the dusting powders are incorporated into ointments, creams, and lotions.

Barium Sulfate—see page 1302.

Boric Acid—see page 1363.

Calcium Carbonate, Precipitated—see page 789.

Chalk, Prepared—see page 793.

Dusting Powder, Absorbable—see page 1876.

Magnesium Stearate USP

Magnesium Stearate is a compound of magnesium with a mixture of solid organic acids obtained from fats, and consists chiefly of variable proportions of magnesium stearate and magnesium palmitate. It contains the equivalent of 6.8–8.0% of MgO (40.31).

Description—A fine, white, bulky powder, having a faint, characteristic odor. Is unctuous, adheres readily to the skin, and is free from grittiness.

Solubility—Insoluble in water, in alcohol, and in ether.

Uses—This salt is used as a *pharmaceutical necessity* (*lubricant*) in the manufacture of compressed tablets and in *baby dusting powders*. When sold for use as a dusting powder for babies, the container should have an automatic closure.

Talc—see page 1375.

Titanium Dioxide—see page 1376.

Zinc Oxide—see page 771.

Zinc Stearate USP

Zinc Stearate is a compound of zinc with a mixture of solid organic acids obtained from fats, and consists chiefly of variable proportions of zinc stearate and zinc palmitate. It contains the equivalent of 12.5–14.0% of ZnO(81.37).

Preparation—Stearic Acid is heated with water until melted, then a slight excess of sodium carbonate over that required for complete neutralization is added, in small portions, and with continuous stirring. A solution of zinc sulfate equivalent to the sodium carbonate is then added to the sodium stearate solution. The precipitate is washed with water until free of sulfate and dried at about 60°.

Description—A fine, white, bulky powder, free from grittiness with a faint, characteristic odor. It is neutral to moistened litmus paper.

Solubility—Insoluble in water, alcohol, or ether but is soluble in benzene.

Identification—It is decomposed by heating with diluted hydrochloric or sulfuric acid, the stearic acid separating on the surface as an oily layer which congeals on cooling, and when the stearic acid is washed well with hot water and dried, then cooled, it solidifies at a temperature not below 54°. The filtrate responds to the identification reactions for zinc.

Uses—Zinc Stearate is used in *water-repellent* ointments and as a *dusting powder* in dermatologic practice for its desiccating and *protective* effect. Poisoning has been reported in infants when the powder has been carelessly and freely applied or when the container has been left within reach of the baby, so that inhalation of the substance has resulted. A form of container having a self-closing aperture has, therefore, been adopted by most manufacturers.

Zinc Stearate is an ingredient in Compound Iodochlorhydroxyquin Powder.

Mechanical Protectives

Several materials may be administered to the skin to form an adherent, continuous coat which may be either flexible or semi-rigid, depending upon the substances and the manner in which they are applied. Such materials may serve three purposes: (1) to provide occlusive protection from the external environment, (2) to provide mechanical support, and (3) to serve as vehicles for various medicaments.

The two principal classes of mechanical protectives are the collodions and plasters. Both are diminishing in use. This is because there is increasing recognition of the beneficial effects of air in maintaining a normally balanced cutaneous bacterial flora of low pathogenicity, and because there is concern over the possibility of plumbism resulting from the lead compounds found in several plasters. Also, the mechanical protectives may of themselves be somewhat irritating because of interference with normal water transport through the skin caused by certain oleaginous and resinous ingredients, especially in plasters. It is also recognized that rubber in adhesive plaster may induce eczema. The cerates may be employed similarly to the plasters. Bandages, dressing, and casts also afford mechanical protection and support, but are considered under *Surgical Supplies* (page 1868). The plasters are considered in greater detail on page 1616.

A number of insoluble and relatively inert powders remain essentially unchanged chemically in the gastrointestinal tract. If the particles possess surface properties that favor their clinging to the gastrointestinal mucosa, and especially if they split up into tabular shapes, they offer mechanical protection against abrasion and may even offer slight protection against toxins and chemical irritants. Many such protectives also are adsorbents (charcoal, bismuth compounds, kaolin), antacids (bismuth compounds), or astringents (bismuth compounds). They are discussed under those categories.

Collodion USP

Collodion contains not less than 5.0%, by weight, of pyroxylin.

Pyroxylin	40 Gm
Ether	750 ml
Alcohol	250 ml
To make about	1000 ml

Add the alcohol and the ether to the pyroxylin contained in a suitable container, and stopper the container well. Shake the mixture occasionally until the pyroxylin is dissolved.

Description—A clear, or slightly opalescent, viscous liquid. It is colorless, or slightly yellowish, and has the odor of ether. Its specific gravity is between 0.765 and 0.775.

Alcohol Content—From 22 to 26% of C_2H_5OH.

Uses—Chiefly employed to seal small wounds or for the preparation of medicated collodions.

Caution—Collodion is highly flammable.

Flexible Collodion USP [Collodium Flexile]—*Preparation*: Weigh the ingredients [Camphor (20 Gm), Castor Oil (30 Gm), and Collodion (qs to make 1000 Gm)], successively, into a dry, tared bottle, insert the stopper in the bottle, and shake the mixture until the camphor is dissolved. *Alcohol Content*: From 21 to 25% of C_2H_5OH. *Uses*: Applied externally to cuts and small burns as a protective. Its application is accompanied by considerable pain, but it is effective as an antiseptic and for excluding air from open wounds. See also *Salicylic Acid Collodion* (page 782).

Absorbable Gelatin Film

[Gelfilm (*Upjohn*)]

Absorbable Gelatin Film is a sterile, nonantigenic, water-insoluble, gelatin film obtained from a specially prepared gelatin-formaldehyde solution by drying on plates at constant temperature and humidity with subsequent sterilization by dry heat at 146° to 149°C for 12 hours.

Description—A light yellow, transparent, brittle sheet with a very slight, bouillon-like odor and taste.

Solubility—Practically insoluble in water; it assumes a rubbery consistency after being in water for a few minutes.

Uses—Absorbable Gelatin Film is used both as a *mechanical protective* and as a *temporary supportive structure* and *replacement matrix* in *surgical repair of defects in membranes*, such as the dura mater and the pleura. When emplaced between damaged or operated structures, it prevents adhesions. When moistened, the film becomes pliable and plastic, so that it can be fitted to the appropriate surface. Absorption requires 1 to 6 months.

Dose—Applied in the form of sheets, previously soaked in isotonic sodium chloride solution and cut to the desired shape. The film blanks are 100 × 125 × 0.16 mm in size.

Petrolatum Gauze USP

[Petrolated Gauze]

Petrolatum Gauze is absorbent gauze saturated with white petrolatum. The weight of the petrolatum in Petrolatum Gauze is 70.0–80.0% of the weight of the gauze. Petrolatum Gauze is sterile. It may be prepared by adding, under aseptic conditions, molten, sterile, white petrolatum to dry, sterile, absorbent gauze, previously cut to size, in the ratio of 60 Gm of petrolatum to each 20 Gm of gauze.

Uses—Petrolatum Gauze is used as a *protective* dressing; also as packing material for postoperative plugs, packs, rolls, and tampons, and as a wick or drain or wrap-around for tubing. It is claimed that there is no danger of tissue maceration and that no growth of granulation tissue through the Gauze occurs.

Zinc Gelatin USP

[Zinc Gelatin Boot; Unna's Boot; Unna's Paste]

Zinc Oxide	100 Gm
Gelatin	150 Gm
Glycerin	400 Gm
Purified Water	350 Gm
To make about	1000 Gm

Gradually add the gelatin to the cold purified water, with constant stirring, allow the mixture to stand for 10 minutes, and then heat on a steam bath until the gelatin dissolves. Add the zinc oxide, which previously has been rubbed to a smooth paste with the glycerin, and stir carefully until a smooth jelly results.

Uses—This preparation is melted and applied in the molten state between layers of bandage to act as a *protective* and to support varicosities and similar lesions of the lower limbs. After a period of about 2 weeks the dressing is removed by soaking with warm water.

Dose—*External use, topically,* as a boot.

Other Mechanical Protectives

Vibesate [Aeroplast Dressing (*Parke-Davis*)]—An ethyl acetate–acetone solution of a polymeric substance composed of hydroxyvinyl chloride acetate, modified rosin ester, and sebacic acid, provided in aerosol form. The liquid solution is clear and colorless, having the odor of the solvents. The dried film is clear, colorless, and odorless. The dried film is soluble in ketone solvents and insoluble in water. *Uses:* Vibesate is used as a film for occlusive dressings, especially when the use of gauze or other materials is undesirable. Thus, it is used to cover burns, or other injured areas, and skin ulcers and eruptions. It prevents the weeping of fluids and electrolytes from the surface; however, it is permeable to water vapor and thus permits drying of the affected area. It also protects the surface from external contaminants and, to some degree, from air. The exclusion of air carries a certain danger of infection from anaerobic organisms. In the open reduction of fractures, it allows the plaster cast to be fitted skin-tight to the limb. The film usually remains intact until healing has occurred. The solvent for the material causes transient smarting of sensitive surfaces; therefore, contact with the eyes should be avoided. The gaseous propellant is flammable, and appropriate precautions are necessary. *Dose:* As an aerosol sprayed on the surface, to generate a film usually 0.05 to 0.08 mm thick.

Demulcents

Demulcents are protective agents which are employed primarily to alleviate irritation (*demulcere*—to smooth down), particularly of mucous membranes or abraded tissues. They are also often applied to the skin. They are generally applied to the surface in viscid sticky preparations which cover the area readily. The local action of chemical, mechanical, or bacterial irritants is thereby diminished, and pain, reflexes, spasm, or catarrh are attenuated. They also prevent drying of the affected surface. The demulcents may be applied to the skin in the form of lotions, cataplasms or wet dressing, to the gastrointestinal tract in the form of demulcent liquors or enemas, and to the throat in the form of pastilles, lozenges, or gargles. When demulcents are applied as solid material (as in lozenges or powders) the liquid is provided by secreted or exuded fluids. Demulcents are frequently medicated. In such instances the demulcent may be an adjuvant, a corrective, or a pharmaceutical necessity. Many of the demulcents are also cathartics (page 796) and are used as such, or they are used with cathartics or antacids for their demulcent and lubricating action.

A variety of chemical substances possess demulcent properties. Among these are mucilages, gums, dextrins, starches, certain sugars, and polymeric polyhydric glycols. Mucus in itself is a natural demulcent. Certain silicates that form silicic acid upon exposure to air or to gastric juice, and glycerol, although it is of low molecular weight and has relatively low binding power, are frequently placed among the demulcents. Also the colloidal hydrous oxides, hydroxides, and subsalts of several metals are widely believed to be demulcent. Many such preparations are listed among the antacids (page 787).

The hydrophilic colloidal properties of most of the demulcents make them valuable emulsifiers and suspending agents in water-soluble ointments and suspensions. They also retard the absorption of many injections and thus may be employed in sundry depot preparations. Many of the demulcents mask the flavor of medicaments by means of at least three physical phenomena: (1) They apparently coat the taste receptors and render them less sensitive; (2) they incorporate many organic solutes into micelles and thereby diminish the free concentration of such solutes; and (3) they coat the surfaces of many particles in suspension. Because of the adhesiveness of the demulcents, they are widely employed as binding agents in tablets, lozenges, and similar dosage forms. Consequently, certain demulcents will be discussed under *Pharmaceutical Necessities* (page 1316).

Acacia—see page 1344.

Acacia Mucilage—see page 1347.

Acacia Syrup—see page 1339.

Benzoin USP

[Gum Benjamin; Benzoe]

Benzoin is the balsamic resin obtained from *Styrax benzoin* Dryander or *Styrax paralleloneurus* Perkins, known in commerce as Sumatra Benzoin, or from *Styrax tonkinensis* (Pièrre) Craib ex Hartwich, or other species of the Section *Anthostyrax* of the genus *Styrax*, known in commerce as Siam Benzoin (Fam. *Styraceæ*).

Sumatra Benzoin yields not less than 75.0% of alcohol-soluble extractive, and Siam Benzoin yields not less than 90.0% of alcohol-soluble extractive.

Constituents—Siam Benzoin contains about 68% of the crystalline ester *coniferyl benzoate* [$C_{17}H_{16}O_4$]; up to 10% of an amorphous form of this compound is also present. Some authorities believe that *coniferyl alcohol* (*m-methoxy-p-hydroxycinnamyl alcohol*, mp 73–74°) occurs in the free state as well. Other compounds which have been isolated are free *benzoic acid* 11.7%, *d-siaresinolic acid* 6%, *cinnamyl benzoate* 2.3%, and *vanillin* 0.3%.

Sumatra Benzoin has been reported to contain the benzoic and cinnamic acid esters of the alcohol *benzoresinol* and probably also of coniferyl alcohol, free *benzoic* and *cinnamic acids*, *styrene*, 2 to 3% of *cinnamyl cinnamate* (also called *styracin*), 1% of *phenylpropyl cinnamate*, 1% of *vanillin*, a trace of *benzaldehyde*, a little *benzyl cinnamate*, and the alcohol *d-sumaresinol* [$C_{30}H_{48}O_4$].

Description—An alcoholic solution of Benzoin is acid to litmus paper and becomes milky upon the addition of water.

Uses—Benzoin is used as a *protective* application for irritations of the skin. When mixed with glycerin and water, the tincture may be applied locally for *cutaneous ulcers, bedsores, cracked nipples*, and *fissures* of the lips and anus. For throat and bronchial inflammation the tincture may be administered on sugar. The tincture and compound tincture are sometimes used in boiling water as steam inhalants for their *expectorant* and *soothing action* in acute laryngitis and croup.

Compound Benzoin Tincture USP [Balsamum Equitis Sancti Victoris, Balsamum Commendatoris Balsamum Catholicum, Balsamum Traumaticum, Balsamum Vulnerarium, Balsamum Persicum, Balsamum Suecium, Balsamum Friari, Balsamum Vervaini, Guttæ Nader, Guttæ Jesuitarium, Tinctura Balsamica, Balsam of the Holy Victorius Knight, Commander's Balsam, Friar's Balsam, Turlington's Drops, Persian Balsam, Swedish Balsam, Vervain Balsam, Turlington's Balsam of Life, Balsam de Maltha, Ward's Balsam, Jerusalem Balsam, Saint Victor's Balsam, Wade's Drops, Wound Elixir, and Balsamic Tincture]—*Preparation:* With Benzoin (in moderately coarse powder, 100 Gm), Aloe (in moderately coarse powder, 20 Gm), Storax (80 Gm), and Tolu Balsam (40 Gm), prepare a tincture (1000 ml) by Process M (page 1590), using alcohol as the menstruum. *History:* This popular preparation has had more different Latin titles and synonyms since its origin in the 15th or 16th century than any other official preparation. Many of these are significant of its uses or its originators, introducers, or patrons, for it has figured as a nostrum as well as in the pharmacopeias of the past 300 years. *Alcohol Content:* From 74 to 80% of C_2H_5OH. *Uses:* Especially valuable in acute *laryngitis*, also in croup, when added to hot water and the vapor inhaled. By adding a teaspoonful of the Tincture to boiling water in an inhaler, and inhaling the vapor, very effective results may be obtained. See page 1908. Also administered, on sugar, for throat and bronchial inflammation and as a local application, when mixed with glycerin and water, for *ulcers, bedsores, cracked nipples*, and *fissures* of the lips and anus. *Dose:* External use, *topically*, as required.

Gelatin—see page 1345.

Glycerin—see page 1359.

Glycerin Suppositories—see page 799.

Glycyrrhiza—see page 1327.

Glycyrrhiza Elixir—see page 1341.

Glycyrrhiza Extract, Pure—see page 1328.

Glycyrrhiza Fluidextract—see page 1328.

Glycyrrhiza Syrup—see page 1340.

Pectin—see page 811.

Plantago Seed—see page 803.

Starch—see page 1374.

Tragacanth—see page 1347.

Tragacanth Mucilage—see page 1348.

Emollients

Emollients are bland, fatty or oleaginous substances which may be applied locally, particularly to the skin, but also to mucous membranes or abraded tissues. Water-soluble irritants, air, and air-borne bacteria are excluded by an emollient layer. The skin is also rendered softer (*emollier*—to soften) and more pliable through penetration of the emollient into the surface layers, through the slight congestion induced by rubbing and massage upon application, and especially through mechanical interference with both sensible and insensible water loss.

Emollients have certain disadvantages. It is now recognized that the retention of perspiration below the emollient and the exclusion of air render conditions favorable to the growth of anaerobic bacteria. Furthermore, the rubbing during application aids in the spreading of cutaneous bacteria. Consequently, the use of emollients to cover burns and abrasions is diminishing.

The liquid emollients may be used for mild catharsis (page 796) and for protection against gastrointestinal corrosives; however, castor oil, because of hydrolysis in the gut to the irritating ricinoleic acid, is employed as an emollient only externally. Orally administered liquid emollients may be aspirated into the trachea and lungs, especially in infants and in the debilitated, and thus induce "oil aspiration pneumonia." This condition may also be induced by emollient nose drops.

The chief use of emollient substances is to provide vehicles for lipid-soluble drugs (as in ointments and liniments). It is widely but incorrectly held that such vehicles facilitate the transport through the skin of their active ingredients. On the contrary, when the oil:water partition coefficient is greater than 1.0, the penetration is retarded, and the emollient vehicle prolongs the action of the active ingredient. Emollient substances also are commonly employed in both cleansing and antiphlogistic creams and lotions. Compound ointment bases, creams, and other medicated applications are treated elsewhere in this book (page 1594). Only the simple emollients and important compounded ointments that are used frequently for their emollient actions are listed below.

Almond Oil NF

[Oleum Amygdalæ Expressum; Sweet Almond Oil; Almond Oil]

Almond Oil is the fixed oil obtained by expression from the kernels of varieties of *Prunus amygdalus* Batsch (Fam. *Rosaceæ*).

Preparation—This oil is obtained equally pure from sweet or bitter almonds. The almonds, having been deprived of a reddish brown powder adhering to their surface, by being rubbed together in a piece of coarse linen, are ground in a mill, and then pressed. The oil, which is at first turbid, is clarified by sedimentation and filtration. Sweet almond yields about 40% and bitter almond 35% of fixed oil. It is not a drying oil and it does not easily turn rancid.

A colorless oil may be obtained by expressing almonds which have been *blanched*—ie, deprived of their testæ by soaking them in hot water and slightly pressing, and afterward drying them to evaporate the water. The fixed oil from peach or apricot kernels is frequently sold for Expressed Almond Oil; it is commercially known as *Oleum Persica* or *Oleum Amygdalarum Gallicum*. While a useful product, it is not intended by the NF that it should be substituted for sweet almond oil.

Description—A clear, pale straw-colored or colorless, almost odorless, oily liquid, with a bland taste. It remains clear at $-10°$, and does not congeal until cooled to nearly $-20°$. Its specific gravity is between 0.910 and 0.915. Iodine value (95 to 105). Saponification value (190 to 200).

Solubility—Slightly soluble in alcohol, but is miscible with ether, chloroform, benzene, and solvent hexane.

Uses—Expressed Almond Oil is used as an *emollient*. It is also a *pharmaceutical necessity*, eg, as an ingredient in *Rose Water Ointment*, page 1353. It must never be confused with the essential (bitter) almond oil. Many customers desiring this oil, simply ask for "almond oil," and if the pharmacist dispenses the poisonous oil without asking any questions, an error is made which might have serious results!

The press cake obtained as a byproduct in the manufacture of Expressed Almond Oil is sometimes recommended as a food product for use by diabetics on account of its high protein and low carbohydrate content. The pharmacist must exercise care in selling almond meal for this purpose so that bitter almond meal which is poisonous is not supplied. Under the name of "*almond meal*" a spurious article consisting of corn meal, soap, etc, is marketed for detergent and cosmetic purposes.

Castor Oil—see page 798.

Cold Cream—see page 1352.

Corn Oil—see page 1342.

Cottonseed Oil—see page 1343.

Dimethicone

$$CH_3-\underset{\underset{CH_3}{|}}{\overset{\overset{CH_3}{|}}{Si}}-O-\left[\underset{\underset{CH_3}{|}}{\overset{\overset{CH_3}{|}}{Si}}-O\right]_n-\underset{\underset{CH_3}{|}}{\overset{\overset{CH_3}{|}}{Si}}-CH_3$$

Dimethicone is a water-repellent silicone oil consisting essentially of dimethyl siloxane polymers of the 200 series of fluids. Since petrolatum lowers the barrier effect of silicones, it is usually formulated in a vanishing cream base. For a discussion of silicones in general, see page 768 under *Other Emollients*.

Description—A water-white, viscous, oil-like liquid.
Solubility—Miscible with chloroform and ether; immiscible with alcohol and water.

Uses—Dimethicone has skin-adherent and water-repellent properties. Applied topically to the skin, it forms a *protective* film which provides a barrier to ordinary soap and water and water-soluble irritants. The film may last for several hours if the skin is exposed mainly to aqueous media. The film provides a less effective barrier to synthetic detergents and lipid-soluble materials, such as organic solvents. Dimethicone should not be applied except in contact dermatoses or dermatoses aggravated by substances that can be repelled by the silicone. It is useful in preventing irritation from ammonia produced by the urine of infants, but it may exacerbate pre-existing irritation. The occlusive protection by the silicone is detrimental to inflamed, traumatized, abraded, or excoriated skin and to lesions that require free drainage. However, applied adjacent to such lesions, it offers protection against irritating discharges and maceration.

Dimethicone is in itself nearly harmless, and does not sensitize skin. However, it does cause a temporary irritation to the eyes.

Dimethicone may be incorporated into a number of ointment bases, according to the need.

Dose—Apply uniformly with rubbing 3 or 4 times for the first 1 or 2 days, then twice daily.
Dosage Form—Ointment: 20 and 30%.

Lanolin—see page 1353.

Lanolin, Anhydrous—see page 1351.

Mineral Oil—see page 804.

Mineral Oil Emulsion—see page 804.

Mineral Oil, Light—see page 1369.

Olive Oil—see page 1349.

Peanut Oil—see page 1343.

Persic Oil—see page 1370.

Petrolatum—see page 1350.

Petrolatum, Hydrophilic—see page 1352.

Petrolatum, White—see page 1350.

Rose Water Ointment—see page 1353.

Sesame Oil—see page 1343.

Theobroma Oil—see page 1376.

White Ointment—see page 1349.

Yellow Ointment—see page 1349.

Other Emollients

Myristyl Alcohol [Tetradecyl Alcohol] [$CH_3(CH_2)_{12}$-CH_2OH]—A white crystalline alcohol. Specific gravity 0.824. Melts at 30°. Insoluble in water; soluble in ether; slightly soluble in alcohol. *Uses:* emollient in cold creams.

Silicones (*polyorganosiloxanes*)—These compounds are organosilicon polymers containing chains of alternating oxygen and silicon atoms with substituent organic groups, frequently methyl or phenyl, on each silicon atom.

Preparation: These polymers may be prepared synthetically by condensing alkylated or arylated *silanols*. Disubstituted *silanediols* [$R_2Si(OH)_2$] form linear polymers having the general formula:

$$HO-\underset{R}{\overset{R}{Si}}-O-\left[\underset{R}{\overset{R}{Si}}-O\right]_n\underset{R}{\overset{R}{Si}}-OH$$

Crosslinked polymers result from condensation of mixtures of substituted silanediols and monosubstituted *silanetriols* [$RSi(OH)_3$]; these may be represented by the following partial formula where R is a hydrocarbon radical:

$$\left[\begin{array}{c} R\quad\quad R\quad\quad R \\ -O-Si-O-Si-O-Si-O- \\ R\quad\quad |\quad\quad R \\ O \\ R\quad\quad\quad\quad R \\ --O-Si-O-Si-O-Si-O- \\ R\quad\quad R\quad\quad R \end{array}\right]_n$$

One method of preparation involves interaction of silicon tetrachloride with appropriate Grignard reagents to yield alkylated or arylated dichlorosilanes. After hydrolysis to produce the corresponding substituted silanols, dehydration procedures are employed to effect condensation polymerization. The over-all reaction, as it involves a disubstituted silanediol, may be represented as follows

$$SiCl_4 \xrightarrow{RMgX} R_2SiCl_2 \xrightarrow{HOH} R_2Si(OH)_2 \xrightarrow{-HOH} HO[Si(R)_2O]_nH$$

| Silicon Tetrachloride | Disubstituted Dichlorosilane | Disubstituted Silanediol | Silicone (Linear Polymer) |

Properties: Silicones with a wide range of properties may be produced by varying the substituent R and by varying the degree of crosslinking. Physically, silicones vary from mobile liquids through viscous liquids and semisolids to solids. Viscosities range from 0.65 to 1,000,000 centistokes. In general, they display high and low temperature stability. They are odorless, tasteless, relatively inert chemically and physiologically, water repellent, and possess anti-foam characteristics. Unmodified silicones are generally insoluble in water; because of this the liquids are often termed *silicone oils;* however, a water-soluble sodium salt of a simple silicone, chemically *sodium methyl siliconate* [$CH_3Si(OH)_2ONa$] has been marketed.

Uses: Preparations containing silicones have various dermatological uses (see *Dimethicone,* page 767), and are used as ingredients of bases for ointments and liniments. In the form of inhalation sprays, silicone preparations have been employed in the treatment of pulmonary edema involving frothing of fluid in the upper respiratory tract. They are also used orally as an antiflatulent. A silicone *bouncing putty* has found acceptance for use as a physical agent in treatment conditions requiring finger exercise. The water-repellent properties of the silicones have found considerable use in a great variety of applications where complete drainage of aqueous fluids from surfaces is desirable.

Silicones are virtually nonirritating; consequently, silicone rubbers are used in various indwelling catheters, tubes, etc, and in some types of prostheses. Liquid silicones are used also to fill in hypoplastic body areas for cosmetic purposes, although they tend to relocate because of flow under gravity and motion.

In addition to uses involving antifoaming, water-repellent, and nonirritating characteristics, silicones are employed also to prevent sticking of one object to another and are then commonly referred to as release agents. Examples of such employment include release of rubber and plastics from molds, food from metal, ice from the wings of aircraft, and capsules and tablets from molds and dyes in which they are fabricated. The use of silicones as a coating for capsules and tablets has been studied.

Astringents

Astringents are locally applied protein precipitants which have such a low cell penetrability that the action is essentially limited to the cell surface and the interstitial spaces. The permeability of the cell membrane is reduced but the cells remain viable. The astringent action is accompanied by contraction and wrinkling of the tissue and by blanching. The cement substance of the capillary endothelium is hardened so that pathological transcapillary movement of plasma protein is inhibited and local edema, inflammation and exudation is thereby reduced. Mucus or other secretions may also be reduced so that the affected area becomes drier.

Many *antiperspirants* act through an astringent mechanism. Astringents are used therapeutically to arrest hemorrhage by coagulating the blood (*styptic action;* page 837) and to check diarrhea, reduce inflammation of mucous membranes, promote healing, toughen the skin, or decrease sweating.

Many astringents are irritants or caustics in moderate to high concentrations. Consequently, strict attention must be paid to the appropriate concentration. Most astringents are also antiseptics.

The principal astringents are (1) the salts of aluminum, zinc, manganese, iron, and bismuth, (2) certain other salts that contain these metals such as permanganates, and (3) tannins, or related polyphenolic compounds. Acids, alcohols, phenols, and other substances that precipitate proteins may be astringent in the appropriate amount or concentration; however, such substances generally are not employed for their astringent effects, because they readily penetrate cells and promote tissue damage. Strongly hypertonic solutions dry the affected tissues and are thus often but wrongly called astringents, unless protein precipitation also occurs.

Alcohol—see page 1357.

Alum NF

[Alumen; Alumen Purificatum; Purified Alum]

Alum, previously dried at 250° to constant weight, contains 99.0–100.5% of $AlNH_4(SO_4)_2$, or 99.0–100.5% of $AlK(SO_4)_2$.

The label of the container must indicate whether the salt is Ammonium Alum [$AlNH_4(SO_4)_2.12H_2O$ = 453.33] or Potassium Alum [$AlK(SO_4)_2.12H_2O$ = 474.39].

History—Potassium Alum was known to the ancients. They were also familiar with its styptic property and hence it was named *stypteria* by Dioscorides. Pliny called it *alumen*. It has also been known as *Cube Alum*. The crude lump alum as it occurs with earth attached has been known as *Rock Alum* (*Alumen Rupeum*) and as *Roman Alum*. It was used in early times, as it is now, as a mordant in dyeing.

Preparation—Alum is prepared from the mineral *bauxite* (a hydrated aluminum oxide) and sulfuric acid, with the addition of ammonium or potassium sulfate for the respective Alums. Ammonium Alum is prevalent on the market because of its lower cost.

Description—Large, colorless crystals, crystalline fragments, or a white powder. It is odorless and has a sweetish, strongly astringent taste. Its solutions are acid to litmus.

Solubility—1 Gm of Ammonium Alum is soluble in 7 ml of water, and 1 Gm of Potassium Alum is soluble in 7.5 ml of water. Both are soluble in about 0.3 ml of boiling water but they are insoluble in alcohol. Alum is freely but slowly soluble in glycerin.

Incompatibilities—When Alum is dispensed in powders with *phenol*, *salicylates*, or *tannic acid*, gray or green colors may be developed due to traces of iron in the Alum. A partial liberation of its water of crystallization permits it to act as an acid toward *sodium bicarbonate*, thus liberating carbon dioxide. Ammonia is liberated simultaneously from Ammonium Alum. *Alkali hydroxides and carbonates, borax,* and *lime water* precipitate aluminum hydroxide from solutions of Alum. It possesses the incompatibilities of the sulfates as described under *Sodium Sulfate* (page 803).

Uses—Alum is a powerful *astringent* in acidic solutions. It is slightly antiseptic, probably due to bacteriostasis through liberation of acid on hydrolysis. It is sometimes used as a local *styptic*, and is frequently employed in making astringent lotions and douches. It is employed especially by athletes to toughen the skin. The dose as an astringent is 0.5 to 5%.

Alum enjoys extensive use in industry and the arts. It is employed in the purification of water, in the tanning of leather, in baking powders, as a mordant in dyeing textiles and calico printing, and in many other processes.

For most purposes the *Ammonium Alum* or the *Potassium Alum* may be used interchangeably.

Soda Alum, known also as *porous alum* [$AlNa(SO_4)_2.12H_2O$], has been used as the acidic element in the so-called *alum baking powders*. It is known in the trade as *S.A.S.* (*sodium aluminum sulfate*). *Concentrated alum* is aluminum sulfate.

Styptic pencils are made by fusing Potassium Alum, usually with the addition of some potassium nitrate, and pouring into suitable molds.

Caution—Do not confuse *styptic* pencils with *caustic* pencils (page 780); the latter contain *silver nitrate*.

Dose—*External use, topically*, as a **0.5** to **5**% solution.

Alum, Dried—see page 781.

Aluminum Acetate Solution USP

[Liquor Burowü; Burow's Solution]

Aluminum Acetate Solution yields, from each 100 ml, 1.20–1.45 Gm of aluminum oxide [Al_2O_3 = 101.96], and 4.24–5.12 Gm of acetic acid [$C_2H_4O_2$ = 60.05], corresponding to 4.8–5.8 Gm of aluminum acetate [$C_6H_9AlO_6$ = 204.12]. Aluminum Acetate Solution may be stabilized by the addition of not more than 0.6% of boric acid.

Caution—This solution should not be confused with Aluminum Subacetate Solution which is a stronger preparation.

Aluminum Subacetate Solution....	545 ml
Glacial Acetic Acid................	15 ml
Water, a sufficient quantity,	
To make.......................	1000 ml

Add the glacial acetic acid to the aluminum subacetate solution and sufficient water to make 1000 ml. Mix, and filter, if necessary.

Note—Dispense only clear Aluminum Acetate Solution.

*Note—*In preparing Aluminum Acetate Solution other methods for producing aluminum acetate may be used. When other methods are used the finished product must meet the requirements of this monograph for strength, quality, and purity.

Aluminum Acetate Solution also may be prepared as follows:

Dissolve lead acetate (150 Gm) and aluminum sulfate (87 Gm) separately in water (525 ml), and mix the cold solutions by pouring the lead acetate solution in a thin stream, with constant stirring, into the aluminum sulfate solution. Set the mixture aside in a cold place (about 10°) for 24 hours. Siphon off 1000 ml of the clear liquid; or, if necessary, transfer the magma to a filter and add sufficient water through the magma to make the product measure 1000 ml.

History—The name Burow's Solution is derived from Dr. August Burow of Königsberg who prescribed a similar solution in 1857. In his original solution alum replaced aluminum sulfate, but the latter is preferable, as no foreign salts, such as potassium acetate or sulfate, remain in solution.

Description—Clear, colorless liquid having a faint acetous odor, and a sweetish, astringent taste. Specific gravity: about 1.022; pH: 3.6–4.4.

Uses—Aluminum Acetate Solution is usually diluted with about 10 to 40 parts of water for use as an antiseptic dressing, also as an astringent and antiseptic mouth wash and gargle. The use of aluminum acetate solution prepared from lead acetate should be condemned.

Veterinary Uses—Burow's Solution is used as an astringent and antiseptic in *burns* and various forms of *dermatitis*, usually diluted with 5 to 10 parts of water.

Dose—*External use, topically*, diluted with 10 to 40 parts of water as a wet dressing.

Aluminum Chloride NF

Aluminum Chloride [$AlCl_3.6H_2O$ = 241.43], contains 95.0–102.0% of $AlCl_3$, calculated on the anhydrous basis.

Preparation—Aluminum Chloride may be prepared by heating aluminum in a current of chlorine and then dissolving the product in water and crystallizing, or by dissolving freshly precipitated aluminum hydroxide in hydrochloric acid and concentrating and crystallizing.

Description—A white or yellowish white, deliquescent, crystalline powder. It is nearly odorless, and has a sweet, very astringent taste. Its solutions are acid to litmus.

Solubility—1 Gm is soluble in about 0.9 ml of water and in about 4 ml of alcohol. It is also soluble in glycerin.

Incompatibilities—*Alkali hydroxides* and *carbonates*, *borax*, and *lime water* precipitate aluminum hydroxide from solutions of Aluminum Chloride. It possesses the incompatibilities of the chlorides. See *Potassium Chloride* (page 839).

Uses—Aluminum Chloride solution is extensively employed on the skin as an *astringent* and *anhydrotic* and forms the basis for many proprietary preparations designed for this purpose. The basic salt [Al(OH)Cl$_2$] is preferable as an astringent and deodorant since it is less acid and therefore less harmful to the clothing and less irritating.

A 50% solution of Aluminum Chloride is used for the "carbonization" of wool.

Dose—*External use, topically,* as a **10 to 25%** solution.

Aluminum Subacetate Solution USP

Aluminum Subacetate Solution yields, from each 100 ml, 2.30–2.60 Gm of aluminum oxide [Al$_2$O$_3$ = 101.96], and 5.43–6.13 Gm of acetic acid [C$_2$H$_4$O$_2$ = 60.05]. It may be stabilized by the addition of not more than 0.9% of boric acid.

Aluminum Sulfate	**145 Gm**
Acetic Acid	**160 ml**
Precipitated Calcium Carbonate	**70 Gm**
Water, a sufficient quantity,	
To make	**1000 ml**

Note—The Aluminum Sulfate official in this Pharmacopeia contains less water of hydration than the corresponding USP XVII article; hence, only 145 Gm of it is required for a Solution of the same strength as that obtained with 160 Gm of the Aluminum Sulfate recognized in USP XVII.

Dissolve the aluminum sulfate in 600 ml of cold water, filter the solution, and add the precipitated calcium carbonate gradually, in several portions, with constant stirring. Then slowly add the acetic acid, mix, and set the mixture aside for 24 hours. Filter the product on a Buchner funnel with the aid of a vacuum if necessary, returning the first portion of the filtrate to the funnel. Wash the magma on the filter with small portions of cold water, until the total filtrate measures 1000 ml.

Note—Other methods and ingredients for producing Aluminum Subacetate Solution may be used. When other methods are used the finished product must meet the official requirements for strength, quality, and purity.

Description—A clear, colorless, or faintly yellow liquid, having an acetous odor. It gradually becomes turbid on standing, due to separation of a more basic salt. Heat accelerates precipitation. It is acid to litmus.

Uses—For external use as an *antiseptic* and *astringent*. It is also used to make Aluminum Acetate Solution.

Dose—*External use, topically,* diluted with 20 to 40 parts of water as a wet dressing.

Aluminum Sulfate USP

[Aluminum Sulfate; Cake Alum; Patent Alum; Concentrated Alum; Pearl Alum; Pickle Alum; "Papermaker's Alum"]

Aluminum Sulfate contains an amount of Al$_2$(SO$_4$)$_3$

(342.15) equivalent to 99.5–101.5% of Al$_2$(SO$_4$)$_3$.14H$_2$O (594.36).

Preparation—Aluminum Sulfate may be prepared by reacting freshly precipitated aluminum hydroxide with an appropriate quantity of sulfuric acid. The resulting solution is evaporated and allowed to crystallize.

Description—A white crystalline powder, shining plates, or crystalline fragments. It is stable in air. It is odorless and has a sweet, mildly astringent taste. The aqueous solution (1 in 20) is acid and has a pH not less than 2.9.

Solubility—1 Gm is soluble in about 1 ml of water; insoluble in alcohol.

Uses—Aluminum Sulfate is a powerful *astringent*, acting much like alum. It is widely used as a *local antiperspirant* and is the effective ingredient in many commercial antiperspiration products. It is used in large quantities for sizing paper, for purifying water, and as a mordant in dyeing textiles. This is the salt used for water purification by means of the "alum flocculation" process. Aluminum Sulfate is a *pharmaceutical necessity* for *Aluminum Subacetate Solution*.

Bismuth Subcarbonate—see page 788.

Bismuth Subnitrate—see page 789.

Calamine USP

[Prepared Calamine; Lapis Calaminaris; Aerosus Lapis; Artificial Calamine]

Calamine is zinc oxide with a small proportion of ferric oxide, and contains, after ignition, 98.0–100.5% of ZnO (81.37).

Preparation—Calamine is made by thoroughly mixing zinc oxide with sufficient ferric oxide (usually 0.5 to 1%) to obtain a product of the desired color.

Calamine was originally obtained by roasting a native zinc carbonate, then known as *calamine;* hence the name. This name is also applied by mineralogists to a native form of zinc silicate, which is not suitable for making medicinal Calamine.

Description—A pink powder, all of which passes through a No. 100 standard mesh sieve. It is odorless and almost tasteless.

Solubility—Insoluble in water, but dissolves almost completely in mineral acids.

Incompatibilities—See *Zinc Oxide* (page 771).

Uses—Its uses are similar to those for zinc oxide, being employed chiefly as an *astringent* and in *protective* and soothing ointments and lotions for *sunburn, ivy poisoning,* etc. It is often prescribed by dermatologists to give opacity and a flesh-like color to lotions or ointments.

Dose—*External use, topically,* in lotions and ointments.

Calamine Lotion USP [Lotio Calaminae]—*Preparation:* Dilute the bentonite magma (250 ml) with an equal volume of calcium hydroxide solution. Mix calamine (80 Gm) and zinc oxide (80 Gm) intimately with the glycerin (20 ml) and about 100 ml of the diluted magma, triturating until a smooth, uniform paste is formed. Gradually incorporate the remainder of the diluted magma. Finally add calcium hydroxide solution (qs) to make 1000 ml, and shake well. If a more viscous consistency in the Lotion is desired, the quantity of bentonite magma may be increased to not more than 400 ml. *Note: Shake the Lotion thoroughly before dispensing.*

Phenolated Calamine Lotion USP [Lotio Calaminae Composita; Compound Calamine Lotion]—*Preparation:* Mix liquefied phenol (10 ml) and calamine lotion (990 ml) to make 1000 ml. See *Calamine*. *Note: Shake the Lotion thoroughly before dispensing.*

Cupric Sulfate—see page 806.

Ferric Chloride Solution—see RPS-13, page 439.

Ferric Chloride Tincture—see RPS-13, page 491.

Ferric Subsulfate Solution—see RPS-13, page 439.

Formaldehyde Solution—see page 1177.

Milk of Bismuth—see page 788.

Potassium Permanganate—see page 1186.

Resorcinol—see page 1187.

Silver Nitrate—see page 779.

White Lotion NF

[Lotio Alba; Lotio Sulfurata]

Zinc Sulfate.....................	**40 Gm**
Sulfurated Potash...............	**40 Gm**
Purified Water, a sufficient quantity,	
To make......................	**1000 ml**

Dissolve the zinc sulfate and the sulfurated potash separately, each in 450 ml purified water, and filter each solution. Add slowly the sulfurated potash solution to the zinc sulfate solution with constant stirring. Then add the required amount of purified water, and mix.

Note—Prepare the Lotion freshly and shake thoroughly before dispensing. For further discussion see *Sulfurated Potash* (page 1375).

Uses—An *astringent* and *protective*. The astringency is attributable to the zinc ion.

Dose—*External use, topically*, as required.

Zinc Chloride USP

Zinc Chloride contains 97.0–100.5% of $ZnCl_2$ (136.28).

Preparation—Zinc chloride is easily prepared by reacting metallic zinc with hydrochloric acid and evaporating the solution to dryness. It may also be prepared by treating zinc oxide with the appropriate amount of hydrochloric acid.

Description—A white, or nearly white, odorless, crystalline powder, or as porcelain-like masses, or in moulded pencils. It is very deliquescent. The aqueous solution (1 in 10) is acid to litmus.

Solubility—1 Gm dissolves in 0.5 ml of water, about 1.5 ml of alcohol, and about 2 ml of glycerin. Its solution in water or in alcohol is usually slightly turbid, but the turbidity disappears upon the addition of a small quantity of hydrochloric acid.

Incompatibilities—Soluble zinc salts are precipitated as zinc hydroxide by alkali hydroxides, including ammonium hydroxide; the precipitate is soluble in an excess of either the fixed or the ammonium hydroxide. *Carbonates, phosphates, oxalates, arsenates,* and *tannin* cause a precipitation. The precipitation with sodium borate can be prevented by addition of an amount of glycerin equal in weight to the sodium borate. In weak aqueous solutions, zinc chloride has a tendency to form the insoluble basic salt by hydrolysis and about one-half its weight of ammonium chloride has been used for the purpose of stabilization. Zinc chloride is very *deliquescent*. It has the incompatibilities of the chlorides, being precipitated by *silver* and *lead salts*.

Uses—An *astringent*. See *Zinc Sulfate* (page 1191). It also is used to desensitize teeth.

Dose—*External use, topically*, to the teeth, as a **10%** solution; to skin and mucous membranes, as a **0.5** to **2%** solution.

Zinc Oxide USP

[Flowers of Zinc; Zinc White; Pompholyx; Nihil Album; Lana Philosophica; Flores Zinci]

Zinc Oxide, freshly ignited, contains 99.0–100.5% of ZnO (81.37).

Preparation—Zinc Oxide can be prepared by exposing zinc carbonate in a shallow dish to a low red heat until all the carbon dioxide and water are expelled.

On a large scale it is made by the "dry process." In this process a ground mixture of coal and a zinc mineral,

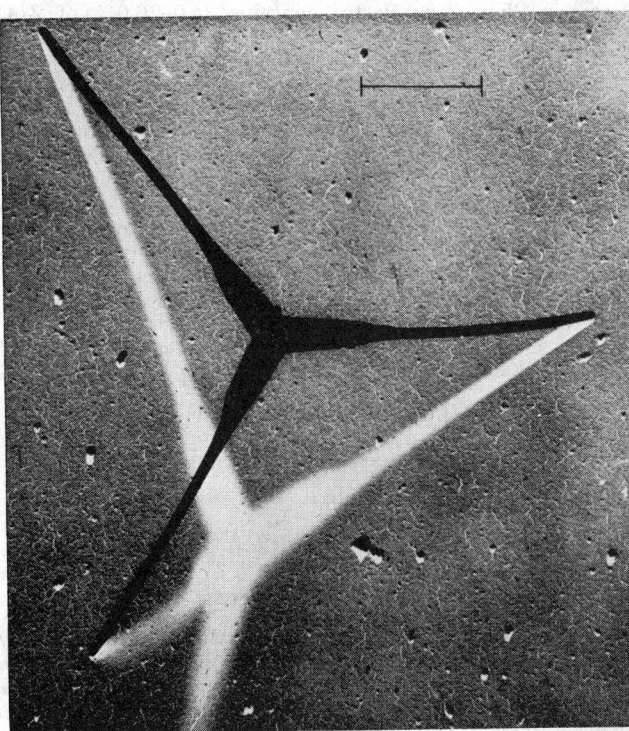

Fig. 101. Zinc oxide smoke crystal micrograph (19,000×) showing how shadowing reveals fourth spike on crystal (courtesy, J. G. Sayre, Argonne National Laboratories and Radio Corporation of America).

such as *calamine, franklinite, willemite,* or *zincite* (red oxide of zinc) is heated in a furnace at a high temperature. The zinc is thereby liberated from its combinations and the hot vaporized metal passes up a tower where it meets a powerful current of air and is thus burned to the oxide.

Description—A very fine, odorless, amorphous, white or yellowish white powder, free from gritty particles. It gradually absorbs carbon dioxide from the air. When strongly heated it assumes a yellow color which disappears on cooling. Its suspension in water is practically neutral.

Solubility—Insoluble in water and in alcohol but is soluble in dilute acids, in solutions of the alkali hydroxides, and in ammonium carbonate solution.

Incompatibilities—Zinc Oxide reacts slowly with the fatty acids in *oils* and *fats* to produce lumpy masses of zinc oleate, stearate, etc. *Vanishing creams* tend to dry out and crumble. Whenever permissible, it is advisable to levigate Zinc Oxide to a smooth paste with a little liquid petrolatum before incorporation into an ointment.

Uses—Zinc Oxide has a mild *astringent, protective,* and *antiseptic* action. In the form of its various official ointments and pastes it is widely employed in the treatment of such skin diseases and infections as *eczema, impetigo, ringworm, pruritus, psoriasis,* and *varicose ulcers.*

Industrially, Zinc Oxide has many applications, eg, as a white pigment in paints, in automobile tires, in the manufacture of glass, in dental cements, and in white glue, etc.

Dose—*External use, topically,* as a **15** to **25**% lotion or ointment.

Zinc Oxide Ointment USP [Zinc Ointment] contains 18.5–21.5% of ZnO. *Preparation:* Levigate zinc oxide (200 Gm) with mineral oil (150 Gm) to a smooth paste, and then incorporate white ointment (650 Gm) to make 1000 Gm.

Zinc Oxide Paste USP [Compound Paste of Zinc Oxide; Lassar's Plain Zinc Paste] contains 24.0–26.0% of ZnO. *Preparation:* Mix zinc oxide (250 Gm), starch (250 Gm), and white petrolatum (500 Gm) to make 1000 Gm.

Zinc Oxide Paste with Salicylic Acid NF [Lassar's Paste; Pasta Zinci; Lassar's Zinc Paste with Salicylic Acid; Zinc and Salicylic Acid Paste] contains 23.5–25.5%, by weight, of ZnO (zinc oxide). *Preparation:* Thoroughly triturate salicylic acid (in fine powder, 20 Gm) with a portion of the paste; then add the remaining paste, and triturate until a smooth mixture is obtained to make 1000 Gm. *Uses:* Frequently used in the treatment of athletes foot and other dermatomycoses. The presence of zinc oxide imparts an *astringent* and *protective* property to this paste. The astringent action is desired to reduce inflammation and to close fissures. The salicylic acid adds keratolytic properties.

Zinc Peroxide, Medicinal—see page 1195.

Zinc Phenolsulfonate—see RPS-13, page 1252.

Zinc Sulfate—see page 1191.

Zinc Undecylenate—see page 1261.

Other Astringents

Aluminum Chlorhydroxide [Aluminum Chlorohydrate; Chlorhydrol]—An aluminum chlorohydroxide complex [Al(OH)$_2$Cl]. *Uses:* Antiperspirant.

Aluminum Paste USP XVII—It contains 9.5–10.5% of Al. *Preparation:* Levigate aluminum (100 Gm), in very fine powder, with mineral oil (50 Gm) to a smooth paste, and then incorporate the mixture with zinc oxide ointment (850 Gm) to make 1000 Gm. *Uses:* A protective dressing applied topically as required. It combines the emollient action of petrolatum with the astringent action of zinc oxide. It is doubtful whether or not the aluminum contributes to the efficacy of the preparation.

Aluminum Citrate [AlC$_6$H$_5$O$_7$]—White powder or scales. Very slowly soluble in cold water, soluble in hot water, readily soluble in ammonia water, with the formation of a complex similar to ferric ammonium citrate. *Uses:* Anhidrotic.

Calamine Ointment NF XII [Turner's Cerate]—*Preparation:* Melt yellow wax (40 Gm) with anhydrous lanolin (40 Gm) and petrolatum (750 Gm). Mix calamine (170 Gm) thoroughly with the melted mixture to produce a smooth, homogeneous ointment.

Ferric Chloride, Iron Perchloride [FeCl$_3$.6H$_2$O]—An oxidizing agent in chemical analysis. Used medicinally as an astringent and styptic.

Lead Acetate NF X [Sugar of Lead]—Purity: not less than 99.5% Pb(C$_2$H$_3$O$_2$)$_2$.3H$_2$O. It occurs as efflorescent, colorless, transparent prisms or plates, or as white crystalline masses having 3 molecules of water. It absorbs carbon dioxide on exposure to air, becoming incompletely soluble in water. Its solutions are slightly alkaline to litmus. It is soluble 1 Gm in 1.6 ml of water. *Uses:* Its use as a local astringent *should be completely abandoned* because of the danger of lead intoxication; for the preparation of lead subacetate solution; as an astringent in veterinary medicine.

Neocalamine, Prepared NF IX—Prepared Neocalamine is a mixture of zinc oxide and ferric oxide which more nearly matches the color of the human skin than does calamine. It contains 93% zinc oxide, 4% yellow ferric oxide, and 3% red ferric oxide. *Uses:* As for calamine. See *Calamine* (page 770).

Tannic Acid USP XVII [Gallotannic Acid; Tannin; Digallic Acid]—A tannin usually obtained from nutgalls, the excrescences produced on the young twigs of *Quercus infectoria* Olivier, and allied species of *Quercus* Linné (Fam. *Fagaceæ*). *Description:* It occurs as yellowish-white to light-brown amorphous powder, glistening scales, and spongy masses; usually odorless with a strong astringent taste; gradually darkens on exposure to air and light. *Solubility:* 1 Gm dissolves in about 0.35 ml water or 1 ml warm glycerin; very soluble in alcohol and acetone, but practically insoluble in chloroform, ether, or carbon tetrachloride. *Incompatibilities:* Solutions of tannic acid gradually darken on exposure to air and light through oxidation of phenolic groups to quinoid structures.

Types of Derivatives: (1) organic esters of tannic acid, represented by *acetyltannic acid* (*tannigen*); (2) coagulated tannin proteinate, represented by exsiccated *tannin albuminate;* (3) *tannin caseinate* (*protan*); and (4) a heterogeneous group of other compounds, such as bismuth salts of tannic acid. The chief criteria for evaluating the tannic acid compounds are their solubilities and speed of hydrolysis during various reaction periods in acid and alkaline solution, with or without the addition of enzymes.

Uses: The therapeutic usefulness of tannic acid is due to its property of precipitating protein. Internally, tannic acid has been used in diarrhea; but if it is given as such, it is rapidly dissolved in the stomach and may then produce excessive gastric irritation, nausea, and even vomiting. The desire to avoid these effects has prompted the introduction of relatively insoluble compounds of tannin, such as acetyltannic acid or albumin tannate, which would act but little, if at all, in the stomach, and whose action would extend further down the intestines. Tannic acid preparations should not be employed as the principal curative agent but as an occasional adjunct to the proper physical and dietetic remedies, when the discharges are unduly profuse.

Tannic acid was once extensively employed in the treatment of burns. A 10% solution was sprayed over the burned area following careful debridement. This resulted in the formation of a firm eschar which helped protect the burned tissue from infection, preserved body fluids, and added greatly to the comfort of the patient. A disadvantage of tannic acid is that it is not an active germicide. It is also absorbed from denuded surfaces and may cause serious systemic toxicity, particularly liver damage. Furthermore, it causes necrosis of viable tissue in the burned area. It has lost favor as an astringent in the treatment of burns and is now rarely used except in very minor cases.

An ointment or spray of tannic acid is also effective in the treatment of bed sores, weeping ulcers, etc. Tannic Acid Glycerite NF XII was formerly used locally for sore throat and stomatitis and to harden the nipples during nursing.

The tannic acid in tea accounts for the use of strong tea in the universal antidote, presumably for the dual purpose of precipitating toxic alkaloids and of hardening the surface of the gastrointestinal mucosa and its mucous layer.

Zinc Oleate [approx. (C$_{17}$H$_{33}$COO)$_2$Zn]—White powder, unctuous to the touch. Insoluble in water; soluble in alcohol, ether, benzene, and carbon disulfide. *Uses:* An antiseptic and astringent. Usually employed in the form of an ointment for the treatment of indolent ulcers, eczema, pruritus, and excoriated surfaces. Also contained in some antiperspirants.

Zinc Phosphate [Zn$_3$(PO$_4$)$_2$.4H$_2$O]—White, odorless, fine powder. Insoluble in water or alcohol; dissolved by dilute mineral acids; also soluble in ammonia and in alkali hydroxide solutions. *Uses:* An antiseptic and astringent in dental cements.

Zirconium Carbonate [approx. 3ZrO$_2$.CO$_2$.H$_2$O]—A basic salt occurring as a white amorphous powder, insoluble in water. The freshly precipitated salt is readily soluble in mineral acids with effervescence. *Uses:* Ingredient of specialties for the treatment of rhus dermatitis (poison ivy, poison sumac) and other dermatoses.

Irritants, Rubefacients, and Vesicants

The *irritants* are drugs which act locally on the skin and mucous membranes to induce hyperemia, inflammation and, when the action is severe, vesication. Agents which induce only hyperemia are known as *rubefacients.* Rubefaction is accompanied by a feeling of comfort, warmth, and sometimes itching and hyperesthesia. Appropriately low concentrations of directly applied or inhaled vapors of volatile aromatic irritants such as camphor or menthol induce a sensation of coolness rather than of warmth. When the irritation is more severe, plasma escapes from the damaged capillaries and forms blisters (vesicles). Agents that induce blisters are known as *vesicants.* Most rubefacients also may be vesicants in higher concentrations. Certain irritants may be relatively selective for various tissues or cell types, so that hypersecretion of the surface, seborrheic abscesses, paresthesia or other effects may be noted in the absence of appreciable hyperemia.

Irritants have been used empirically for many centuries, probably even prehistorically. They may be employed for counterirritation, the mechanism of which is poorly understood. A moderate to severe pain may be obscured by a milder pain arising from areas of irritation appropriately placed to induce reflex stimulation of certain organs or systems, especially respiratory. Sensory and visible effects of irritation sometimes give the patient assurance that he is receiving effective medication. Taken internally, many irritants exert either an emetic or cathartic action. Irritant cathartics are listed on page 796. A few irritants, especially cantharides, upon absorption into the blood stream irritate the urogenital tract and are consequently often dangerously employed as *aphrodisiacs.* Certain irritants also possess a healing action on wounds, possibly the result of local stimulation. Many condiments are irritants.

Alcohol—see page 1357.

Alcohol, Rubbing—see page 1174.

Ammonia Spirit, Aromatic—see page 868.

Anthralin NF

[1,8,9-Anthracenetriol; 1,8-Dihydroxyanthranol; Dithranol; Dioxyanthranol; Cignolin; 1,8,9-Trihydroxyanthracene]

Anthralin contains 95.0–100.5% of $C_{14}H_{10}O_3$ (226.23) calculated on the dried basis.

Preparation—Anthralin is produced from the readily available anthraquinone (made by oxidizing anthracene with bichromate-sulfuric acid). The anthraquinone is first sulfonated. Oleum is used for the sulfonation reaction and 1% mercuric oxide is necessary as a catalyst. On partial dilution of the sulfonation mixture with water, the unwanted 1,5-disulfonic acid is separated and discarded. Further dilution with water precipitates the desired 1,8-disulfonic acid.

The replacement of the sulfonic acid groups by hydroxyl is carried out at 195° to 200° with a mixture of calcium hydroxide and calcium chloride. The resulting 1,8-dihydroxy-9,10-anthraquinone is then reduced with tin and hydrochloric acid to Anthralin.

Description—An odorless, tasteless, yellowish brown, crystalline powder. An aqueous extract is neutral to litmus. Melting point 175° to 181°.

Solubility—Soluble in chloroform, acetone, benzene, and solutions of alkali hydroxides; slightly soluble in alcohol, ether, and glacial acetic acid; insoluble in water.

Uses—A *local irritant,* (*anti-eczematic*) used as a substitute for *Chrysarobin* in *psoriasis* and *chronic dermatoses;* it is less irritating and causes less discoloration of the skin than chrysarobin.

Dose—*External use, topically,* as a **0.1** to **1**% ointment.

Dosage Form—Ointment NF: 0.1, 0.25, 0.5, and 1%.

Anthralin Ointment NF [Strong Dithranol Ointment] is anthralin in a petrolatum or other suitable base. Anthralin Ointment labeled to contain more than 0.1% of anthralin [$C_{14}H_{10}O_3$] contains 90.0–115.0% of the labeled amount of $C_{14}H_{10}O_3$, and that labeled to contain 0.1% or less of anthralin contains 90.0–130.0% of the labeled amount of $C_{14}H_{10}O_3$. *Preparation:* Reduce anthralin (10 Gm) to a very fine powder and mix well with white petrolatum (a small portion of the 990 Gm) until a smooth and homogeneous mixture is obtained. Add the remainder of the white petrolatum and mix thoroughly to make 1000 Gm. *Note*—Due to the slow oxidation of anthralin to 1,8-dihydroxyanthraquinone upon standing, Anthralin Ointments intended not to be used for a reasonable period of time should be prepared with about 5% excess of anthralin for ointments of strengths greater than 0.1%, and a 20% excess of anthralin for ointments of strengths of 0.1% or less.

Benzoin Tincture, Compound—see page 766.

Camphor USP

[2-Bornanone; 2-Camphanone; Gum Camphor; Laurel Camphor]

Camphor [$C_{10}H_{16}O$ = 152.24] is a ketone obtained from *Cinnamomum camphora* (Linné) Nees et Ebermaier (Fam. *Lauraceæ*) (Natural Camphor) or produced synthetically (Synthetic Camphor).

Preparation—Natural crude camphor is obtained by steam distilling chips of the camphor tree. In some places the leaves are also used. Upon cooling, the camphor and any volatile oils separate. After removal of the water, the mixture of the camphor and volatile oil is pressed to remove the liquid volatile oil, and the crude camphor so obtained is purified, usually by sublimation. In one of the processes the crude camphor is mixed with lime before submitting it to sublimation, the object of the lime being to bind any water that may be present in the crude product.

One method of producing synthetic camphor starts with *pinene* [$C_{10}H_{16}$], a hydrocarbon obtained from turpentine oil. The pinene is saturated with hydrogen chloride at 0° thus forming bornyl chloride [$C_{10}H_{17}Cl$]. Upon heating the bornyl chloride with sodium acetate and glacial acetic acid it is converted into isobornyl acetate, which is subsequently hydrolyzed to form isobornyl alcohol [$C_{10}H_{17}OH$]. The latter upon oxidation with chromic acid is converted into camphor.

Synthetic camphor resembles natural camphor in most of its properties except that it is a racemic mixture and therefore lacks optical activity.

When camphor is treated in approximately molecular proportions with chloral hydrate, menthol, phenol, or thymol, liquefaction ensues; such mixtures are known as *eutectic mixtures* (see page 176).

Description—Camphor occurs as colorless or white crystals, granules, or crystalline masses; or as colorless to white, translucent, tough masses. It has a penetrating, characteristic odor, a pungent, aromatic taste, and is readily pulverizable in the presence of a little alcohol, ether, or chloroform. Its specific gravity is about 0.99. It melts between 174° and 179° and slowly volatilizes at ordinary temperature and in steam. The specific rotation of natural camphor determined in an alcohol solution is +41° to +43°.

Solubility—1 Gm dissolves in about 800 ml of water, 1 ml of alcohol, about 0.5 ml of chloroform, and 1 ml of ether; freely soluble in carbon disulfide, in solvent hexane, and in fixed and volatile oils.

Incompatibilities—Camphor forms a liquid or a soft mass when rubbed with *chloral hydrate, hydroquinone, menthol, phenol, phenyl salicylate, resorcinol, salicylic acid, thymol,* and other substances.

It is precipitated from its alcoholic solution by the addition of water. It is precipitated from camphor water by the addition of soluble salts.

Uses—Locally, Camphor is weakly *antiseptic*, mildly *anesthetic* (*antipruritic*), and *rubefacient* when rubbed on the skin. The spirit is applied locally to allay the itching caused by insect stings. The liniment is used in veterinary practice as a counterirritant in pneumonia in dogs and other animals. It is also used as a counterirritant in humans for *inflamed joints, sprains,* and *rheumatic* and other *inflammatory* conditions such as colds in the throat and chest. Although the patient may feel improved, the inflammation is not affected.

When taken internally in small amounts it produces a feeling of warmth and comfort in the gastrointestinal tract, and was therefore formerly much used as a *carminative*. Camphor is a reflexly-active *circulatory* and *respiratory stimulant* by injecting a 20% solution in oil intramuscularly. However, its use as a stimulant is obsolete. It also possesses a slight *expectorant* action.

Camphor is a pharmaceutical necessity for *Flexible Collodion* and *Camphorated Opium Tincture*.

Dose—*External use, topically,* as a **1** to **3%** lotion or ointment.

Camphor Spirit NF [Tinctura Camphoræ; Camphor Tincture] is an alcohol solution containing, in each 100 ml, 9.0–11.0 Gm of $C_{10}H_{16}O$. *Preparation:* Dissolve camphor (100 Gm) in alcohol (about 800 ml), then add alcohol to make the product measure 1000 ml. Filter if necessary. *Alcohol Content:* 80 to 87% (*v/v*) of C_2H_5OH. *Uses:* Formerly used as a *sedative* in hysteria and other forms of nervous excitement, and as an *antispasmodic* in diarrhea. It is applied locally as a *counterirritant* to relieve *headache* and to allay the itching caused by *insect stings*. *Dose: Usual, 1 ml* (unofficial). *Veterinary Dose:* Carminative, *Horses, 30 to 60 ml; Dogs, 0.6 to 2 ml.*

Coal Tar USP

[Pix Carbonis; Prepared Coal Tar BP; Pix Lithanthracis; Gas Tar]

Coal Tar is the tar obtained as a by-product during the destructive distillation of bituminous coal.

Description—A nearly black, viscous liquid, heavier than water, with a characteristic naphthalene-like odor and a sharp burning taste. On ignition it burns with a reddish, luminous, and very sooty flame, leaving not more than 2% of residue.

Solubility—Only slightly soluble in water, to which it imparts its characteristic odor and taste and a faintly alkaline reaction; partially dissolved by alcohol, acetone, methanol, solvent hexane, carbon disulfide, chloroform, or ether; to the extent of about 95% by benzene, and entirely by nitrobenzene with the exception of a small amount of suspended matter.

Uses—Coal Tar is a *local irritant* which is used in the treatment of *chronic skin diseases*. The mechanism of its action is unknown, but it probably is not simply one of irritation.

Dose—*External use, topically,* in ointments and solutions in **1** to **20%** concentration 2 or 3 times a day.

Coal Tar Ointment USP [Unguentum Picis Carbonis]—*Preparation:* Blend coal tar (10 Gm) and incorporate the mixture with polysorbate 80 (5 Gm) to make 1000 Gm. If desired by the physician, the Ointment may be made with washed coal tar. To wash the coal tar, stir or agitate it with about 5 times its volume of purified water, then pour off the separated water. The process may be repeated a number of times. The coal tar may then be dried by heating on a water bath. *Note*—The USP XVIII Ointment differs in strength from that which was official in USP XV, which specified 3% Coal Tar.

Coal Tar Solution USP [Liquor Picis Carbonis; Liquor Carbonis Detergens]—*Preparation:*

Mix coal tar (200 Gm) with washed sand* (500 Gm) and add polysorbate 80 (50 Gm) and alcohol (700 ml). Macerate the mixture for 7 days in a closed vessel with frequent agitation. Filter, and rinse the vessel and the filter with sufficient alcohol to make the product measure 1000 ml. *Alcohol content:* From 81 to 86% of C_2H_5OH. *Uses:* This solution is used *externally*, diluted with 9 volumes of water, in the treatment of *chronic skin diseases*. See *Coal Tar*.

Creosote—see page 1192.

Eucalyptol—see page 1337.

Eucalyptus Oil—see page 1327.

Green Soap—see page 785.

Green Soap Tincture—see page 786.

Ichthammol NF

[Ammonium Ichthosulfonate; Sulfonated Bitumen; Ictiol; Ictiosulfonato Amonico; Ichthyol (*Stiefel*)]

Ichthammol is obtained by the destructive distillation of certain bituminous schists, sulfonating the distillate, and neutralizing the product with ammonia.

Ichthammol yields not less than 2.5% of NH_3 (ammonia) and not less than 10% of total S (sulfur).

History—The prototype of Ichthammol is *Ichthyol*, literally meaning "fish oil" which was first produced from the hydrocarbons of a shale found in Seefeld Tyrol. This shale frequently bears impressions of fish, hence "ichthy" which is derived from the Greek word for fish.

---

* Washed sand may be prepared in the following manner: Digest clean hard sand at room temperature with a mixture of 1 part of hydrochloric acid, and 2 parts of water (about 13% of HCl) for several days, or at an elevated temperature for several hours. Collect the sand on a filter, wash with water until the washings are neutral and show only a slight reaction for chloride, and finally dry. Washed sand meets the following USP tests and limits: *Substances soluble in hydrochloric acid* (0.16%) and *Chloride* (0.003%).

Constituents—Ichthammol belongs to a class of preparations containing as their essential constituents salts or compounds of a mixture of acids containing sulfur and designated by the group name *sulfoichthyolic acid* which are formed by the sulfonation of the oil obtained in the destructive distillation of certain bituminous shales. Sulfoichthyolic acid is characterized by a high sulfur content, the sulfur existing largely in the form of sulfonates, sulfones, and sulfides.

Description and Properties—A reddish brown to brownish black, viscous fluid, with a strong, characteristic, empyreumatic odor.

Solubility—Ichthammol is miscible with water, glycerin, and fixed oils or fats, but is partially soluble in alcohol or ether.

Identification—Upon the addition of hydrochloric acid to a 1 in 10 solution, a dark, resinous precipitate is produced which is insoluble in ether. Addition of sodium hydroxide TS to a similar solution and heating to the boiling point causes evolution of ammonia gas.

Incompatibilities—Ichthammol becomes granular in the presence of *acids* or under the influence of *heat*. In solution, it is precipitated by acids and *acid salts* as a dark, sticky mass. *Alkalies* liberate ammonia. Many *metallic salts* cause precipitation. With *alkaloids* or their salts, less soluble derivatives are formed. An insoluble compound is formed with *potassium iodide*.

Uses—Ichthammol is an *irritant* and *local antibacterial* agent. It is used alone, or in combination with other antiseptics, for the treatment of skin disorders such as *erysipelas, psoriasis,* and *lupus erythematosus,* and to promote healing in chronic inflammations.

The current estimate of the effects of sulfoichthyolic acid preparations is based largely on the use of ichthyol. The sulfoichthyolate preparations were formerly used locally under the supposition that they secure the absorption of swellings and effusions in contusions, burns, etc, and especially in gynecologic practice. They have been tried internally in a great variety of conditions, but evidence that they are of any therapeutic value when used in this way is lacking.

Dose—*Topically* as a **10%** ointment.

Ichthammol Ointment NF—*Preparation:* Thoroughly incorporate ichthammol (100 Gm) with anhydrous lanolin (100 Gm) and then combine this mixture with petrolatum (800 Gm) to make 1000 Gm.

Juniper Tar NF

[Pix Juniperi; Cade Oil; Oleum Juniperi Empyreumaticum]

Juniper Tar is the empyreumatic volatile oil obtained from the woody portions of *Juniperus oxycedrus* Linné (Fam. *Pinaceæ*).

Description—A dark brown, clear, thick liquid, having a tarry odor and a faintly aromatic, bitter taste.

Solubility—Very slightly soluble in water; 1 volume dissolves in 9 volumes of alcohol; it dissolves in 3 volumes of ether, leaving only a slight, flocculent residue; only partially soluble in solvent hexane; miscible with amyl alcohol, chloroform, and glacial acetic acid.

Uses—Juniper Tar is a mildly irritant oil that is employed as a topical antipruritic in several chronic dermatologic disorders, such as *psoriasis, atopic dermatitis, pruritus, eczema,* and *seborrhea.* Since it is irritant to the conjunctiva and also may cause chemosis of the cornea, care should be taken to keep the tar out of the eyes.

Dose—*External use, topically,* as **1** to **5%** ointment. *Other Dose Information*—Juniper Tar is applied once a day; it is also used as a 4% shampoo or 34% bath.

Menthol USP

[*p*-Menthan-3-ol; Peppermint Camphor, Headache Crystals]

Menthol [$C_{10}H_{20}O = 156.27$] is an alcohol obtained from diverse mint oils or prepared synthetically. Menthol may be levorotatory (*l*-Menthol) from natural or synthetic sources, or racemic (*dl*-Menthol).

Preparation—Peppermint oil owes its odor chiefly to Menthol which is obtained from it by fractional distillation and allowing the proper fraction to crystallize, or by chromatographic processes.

In recent years various synthetic menthols have appeared on the market. Among the numerous methods of synthesis of an optically inactive product are the following: (1) the catalytic hydrogenation of thymol (which may be obtained from natural sources or synthesized from *m*-cresol or cresylic acid); (2) the conversion of piperitone (found in certain eucalyptus oils) to menthone, followed by the reduction of this ketone to racemic menthol; (3) the reduction of pulegone (found in oil of pennyroyal) to menthone or menthol by treatment with sodium and alcohol; and (4) from either *p*-menthanol-8 or α-terpineol (both of which are present in American pine oil). The former compound is first dehydrated to Δ³-menthene, which is then oxidized to menthene oxide; this rearranges to menthone, which is then reduced to menthol. The preparation from α-terpineol involves catalytic hydrogenation.

The main process capable of producing a synthetic *l*-menthol of USP grade is one which employs *d*-citronellal, obtained from Java citronella oil, as the starting material. This optically active aldehyde is converted to a mixture of isopulegols by cyclization; upon catalytic hydrogenation an optically active mixture of menthols results, from which by suitable esterification and further treatment pure *l*-menthol can be obtained.

The difficulty involved in the synthesis arises from the fact that menthol contains three asymmetric carbon atoms, and there are thus eight stereoisomers which are designated as *l*- and *d*-menthol, *l*- and *d*-isomenthol, *l*- and *d*-neomenthol, and *l*- and *d*-neoisomenthol. In order to obtain a product meeting USP requirements, it is necessary to separate the *l*-menthol from its stereoisomers, for which purpose fractional crystallization, distillation under reduced pressure, or esterification may be used. The other stereoisomers differ from the official *l*-menthol in physical properties and possibly to some extent in pharmacological action.

Description—Colorless, hexagonal, usually needle-like crystals, or fused masses, or a crystalline powder, with a pleasant, peppermint-like odor. *l*-Menthol melts between 41° and 43°, and *dl*-Menthol congeals at 27° to 28°. The specific rotation [α]$_D^{25}$ of *l*-Menthol, determined in an alcohol solution containing 10 Gm in 100 ml and using a 200-mm tube, is between −45° and −51°, and that of *dl*-Menthol is between −2° and +2°.

Solubility—Very soluble in alcohol, chloroform, ether, and solvent hexane. Freely soluble in glacial acetic acid, mineral oil, and in fixed and volatile oils. Slightly soluble in water.

Identification—When mixed with about an equal weight of camphor, chloral hydrate, phenol, or thymol, Menthol forms a "eutectic" mixture liquefying at room temperature.

Incompatibilities—Menthol produces a liquid or soft mass when triturated with *camphor, phenol, chloral hydrate, resorcinol, thymol,* and numerous other substances. *Chromic acid, potassium permanganate,* and other *oxidizing agents* decompose it. It is thrown out of an alcoholic solution as an oily liquid by the addition of water.

Labeling—The label on the container indicates whether the Menthol is levorotatory or racemic.

Uses—Menthol is extensively used as an ingredient in preparations for the nose and throat, in ointments to relieve local irritations or for *counterirritant* purposes, and in throat lozenges. It is also a satisfactory *antipruritic* in the appropriate concentration. Inhalers containing menthol compressed into blocks or cones are commonly used for the relief of *nasal congestion, headache,* and *neuralgia.* Small amounts of the drug are contained in the so-called "mentholated cigarettes." It is now rarely administered internally.

Dose—*External use, topically,* as a **0.1** to **2%** lotion or ointment.

Peruvian Balsam NF

[Peru Balsam; Balsam of Peru; Indian Balsam; Black Balsam]

Peruvian Balsam is obtained from *Myroxylon pereiræ* (Royle) Klotzsch (Fam. *Leguminosæ*).

Constituents—This Balsam contains from 60 to 64% of a volatile oil termed *cinnamein* and from 20 to 28% of *resin.* The higher the content of volatile oil, the greater is the market price of the drug. Cinnamein is a mixture of numerous compounds, among which the following have been identified: the esters *benzyl benzoate, benzyl cinnamate, cinnamyl cinnamate (styracin),* and the alcohol *peruviol* (considered by some authorities to be identical with the sesquiterpene alcohol *nerolidol,* ($C_{15}H_{26}O$) as ester; free *cinnamic acid;* about 0.05% of *vanillin;* and a trace of *coumarin.* The presence of the following compounds has also been claimed: *dihydrobenzoic acid, farnesol* (a sesquiterpene alcohol), *styrol (phenylethylene),* and a *phytosterol.* The resin consists of the benzoic and cinnamic acid esters of the alcohol *peruresinotannol,* together with some free cinnamic acid.

Description—Peruvian Balsam is a dark brown, viscid liquid. It is transparent and appears reddish brown in thin layers. It has an agreeable odor resembling vanilla, a bitter, acrid taste, with a persistent after-taste, and is free from stringiness or stickiness. It does not harden on exposure to air. Specific gravity 1.150 to 1.170.

Solubility—The Balsam is nearly insoluble in water, but is soluble in alcohol, in chloroform, and in glacial acetic acid, with not more than an opalescence. It is only partly soluble in ether and in solvent hexane.

Uses—Peruvian Balsam is a *local irritant.* It is a valuable dressing to promote the growth of epithelial cells in the treatment of *indolent ulcers, wounds,* and certain *skin diseases,* eg, scabies. Ointments containing both Peruvian Balsam and sulfur present a problem in compounding, since the resinous part of the Balsam tends to separate. This difficulty may be overcome by mixing the Balsam with an equal amount of castor oil, prior to incorporating it into the base; or alternatively, by mixing it with solid petroxolin.

Dose—*External use, topically,* to skin as required, usually in ointment or in alcohol solution.

Pine Needle Oil—see page 1332.

Pine Tar NF

[Pix Pini; Pix Liquida; Tar]

Pine Tar is the product obtained by the destructive distillation of the wood of *Pinus palustris* Miller, or of other species of *Pinus* Linné (Fam. *Pinaceæ*).

History—An aqueous extract of tar was claimed by George Berkeley, Bishop of Cloyne, in the early part of the eighteenth century, to be a panacea for all human ills and he wrote a book on *Tar Water* which makes very interesting reading as an example of misbelief and credulity.

Preparation—Tar is usually obtained as a by-product in the manufacture of charcoal or acetic acid from wood. It is a complex mixture of phenolic bodies for the most part insoluble in water. Among these are *creosol, phlorol, guaiacol, pyrocatechol, cærulignol,* and *pyrogallol* ethers. Traces of *phenol* and *cresols* are also present as well as hydrocarbons of the paraffin and benzene series.

Description—A very viscid, blackish brown liquid. It is translucent in thin layers, but becomes granular and opaque with age. It has an empyreumatic, terebinthinate odor, a sharp, empyreumatic taste, and is more dense than water. Its solution is acid to litmus.

Solubility—Pine Tar is miscible with alcohol, ether, chloroform, glacial acetic acid, and with fixed and volatile oils. It is slightly soluble in water, the solution being pale yellowish to yellowish brown.

Uses—Pine Tar is used externally as a mild *irritant* and *local antibacterial* agent in chronic *skin diseases.* The volatile products of tar are *expectorant;* tar inhalations were formerly used for this purpose. It is also used in veterinary medicine.

Resorcinol—see page 1187.

Resorcinol Ointment, Compound—see page 1188.

Resorcinol Monoacetate—see page 1188.

Storax—see page 1374.

Tolu Balsam—see page 1335.

Turpentine Oil, Rectified—see page 875.

Other Irritants, Rubefacients, and Vesicants

Camphor Liniment NF XII [Camphorated Oil] contains 19–21% of $C_{10}H_{16}O$. *Caution—This preparation is not intended for parenteral use. Preparation:* pour cottonseed oil (800 Gm) into a suitable dry flask or bottle, heat it on a steam bath, add camphor (200 Gm) to make 1000 Gm and stopper the container securely. Dissolve the camphor by agitation without the further application of heat. This liniment should never be made in an open dish, as much of the camphor will be volatilized. Although the synonym "camphorated oil" is often applied to this liniment, this term is also frequently used by physicians to indicate a sterile, 10% solution of camphor in olive or other fixed oil. The two products must not be confused.

Camphor and Soap Liniment NF XII [Soap Liniment; Liquid Opodeldoc; Camphorated Tincture of Soap]—*Preparation:* Dissolve camphor (in small pieces, 45 Gm) and rosemary oil (10 ml) in alcohol (700 ml), add the green soap (120 Gm) and stir or agitate until the mixture is clear. Add purified water (qs) to make the product measure 1000 ml, mix, set it aside in a cool place for 24 hours, and filter. Only the official hard soap should be used; soaps made from animal oils will cause gelatinization. If soap shavings from bar soap are used, dry thoroughly and then run through a mill or grater. *History:* The term opodeldoc sometimes applied to this preparation was first used by Paracelsus in connection with a plaster which had no connection with soap whatever. In the Edinburgh Pharmacopœia of 1722 a formula was provided for an *Unguentum Opodeldoch* which contained soap in addition to a large number of other ingredients. This was undoubtedly the basis for *Steer's Opodeldoc*, which was a solid preparation of soap, and the *Solid Soap Liniment* of NF VIII. *Alcohol Content:* From 62 to 66% of C_2H_5OH. *Uses:* A local *irritant*, mild *rubefacient*, and weak local *anesthetic*, for *sprains*, *bruises*, and *rheumatism*. It also forms the basis for other liniments.

Cantharides NF X [Spanish Flies; Russian Flies]—It consists of the ground, dried insect, *Cantharis vesicatoria* (Linné) De Geer (Fam. *Meloideæ*). It yields not less than 0.6% of cantharidin [$C_{10}H_{12}O_4$]. Also present are fat, resinous substances, acetic acid, and uric acid. *Uses:* As an *obsolete* gastrointestinal and urinary tract irritant for which reason it has an unwarranted reputation as an aphrodisiac. Cantharides is highly toxic when taken orally, hence its therapeutic application is limited to the skin for use as a counter-irritant. Due to percutaneous absorption, it is even dangerous to use in this manner. Used as an ingredient of rubefacient and vesicant preparations in veterinary equine practice. *Caution:* Cantharides having an ammoniacal odor must not be used.

Capsicum NF XI [Cayenne Pepper]—The dried ripe fruit of *Capsicum frutescens* Linné and other species of Capsicum (Fam. *Solanaceæ*). *Uses:* Externally, it is widely used as a rubefacient and is the basis of numerous ointments and liniments. It does not cause blistering even in concentrated solutions. It formerly enjoyed wide use as a carminative. *Dose:* 60 mg. *Veterinary Dose: Horses and Cattle, 1 to 4 Gm; Dogs, 60 to 500 mg.*

Chloroform Liniment NF XII contains, in each 100 ml, 27–30.5 ml of $CHCl_3$. *Preparation:* Mix chloroform (300 ml) and camphor and soap liniment (700 ml) by agitation to make 1000 ml. *Alcohol Content:* 43–47%. *Uses:* A stimulant, *rubefacient* liniment for application to the skin for the production of counterirritation in the treatment and relief of *myalgias*, *neuralgias*, and certain forms of involvement of joints and periarticular structures.

Mustard, Black NF XI [Sinapis Nigra]—The dried ripe seed of *Brassica nigra* (Linné) Koch or of *Brassica juncea* (Linné) Czerniaew, or of varieties of these species (Fam. *Cruciferae*). Black Mustard yields not less than 0.6% of allyl isothiocyanate (CH_2=$CHCH_2$—N=C=S). *Uses:* As a *condiment*, *stimulant*, and *emetic*; externally, it is *rubefacient*. When Black Mustard is prepared as a condiment by the addition of vinegar, salt, and water, the product is known as *German Prepared Mustard*. Both white and black mustard are used in making homemade poultices. It is sometimes used archaically as a counter-irritant in the form of "mustard plasters," made by mixing it with varying amounts of wheat flour and adding sufficient tepid water to make a paste. It is occasionally used as a gastric and intestinal stimulant. It is an active, although unpleasant emetic, in a usual dose of 10 Gm. *Veterinary Dose:* Carminative in horses, 8 to 16 Gm; emetic in dogs, 4 to 8 Gm in cup of warm water.

Myrrh NF XI—The oleo-gum-resin obtained from *Commiphora molmol* Engler, *Commiphora abyssinica* (Berg) Engler, or from other species of *Commiphora* Jacquin (Fam. *Burseraceae*). *Uses:* Sometimes used as a local *stimulant* in diseases of the mouth and as an application for sore gums. It was formerly administered internally as a *carminative* and externally as a *protective*. The volatile oil is used in perfumes of the oriental type and as a fixative.

Pine Tar Ointment NF XII [Unguentum Picis Pini; Unguentum Picis Liquidæ]—*Preparation:* Melt yellow wax (150 Gm) and yellow ointment (350 Gm) together on a water bath, mix well, remove from the heat, and stir until the mixture congeals. Then incorporate pine tar (500 Gm) and mix, to make 1000 Gm.

Thyme Oil NF XII [Common Thyme Oil; Garden Thyme Oil] is a volatile oil distilled from the flowering plant of *Thymus vulgaris* Linné or of *Thymus zygis* Linné and its var. *gracilis* Boissier (Fam. *Labiatæ*). Thyme Oil yields not less than 40%, by volume, of phenols. The most valuable constituent is *Thymol* (page 1190); other constituents include γ-terpinene, cymene, carvacrol, linalool, and bornyl acetate. *Description and Solubility:* A colorless, yellow, or red liquid with a characteristic, pleasant odor, and a pungent, persistent taste. It is affected by light. It dissolves in 2 volumes of 80% alcohol. Uses: Chiefly used in liniments as a *stimulant*. It is also classed as a *flavor*.

Sclerosing Agents

A number of irritant drugs are sufficiently active to damage cells but are not sufficiently active to destroy large numbers of cells at the site of application. Such agents promote fibrosis and are used to strengthen supporting structures and to close inguinal rings, etc. The intimal surface of blood vessels may break down under attack by such agents and thus initiate thrombosis. This action is the basis of the use of sclerosing agents in the reduction of varicose veins and hemorrhoids.

Morrhuic Acid

Cod Liver Oil (page 1020), the fixed oil obtained from the fresh livers of *Gadus morrhua* Linné, consists largely of the glyceryl esters of the unsaturated fatty acids *arachidonic, asellic, clupanodonic, gadoleic, gadinic, jecoleic, jecoric, linolenic, linoleic, oleic, selacholeic, stearidonic, therapic,* and *zoomaric.* Approximately 15% of the oil consists of the glycerides of the saturated fatty acids, *palmitic* and *stearic*. The mixture of free fatty acids obtained from the oil is known as *morrhuic acid*. It is not official, but its sodium salt, in the form of an Injection, appears in the USP.

Sodium Morrhuate Injection USP

Sodium Morrhuate Injection is a sterile solution of the sodium salts of the fatty acids of cod liver oil. It contains, in each ml, 46.5–53.5 mg of sodium morrhuate. A suitable antimicrobial agent, not to exceed 0.5%, and ethyl or benzyl alcohol, not to exceed 3.0%, may be added.

Note—Sodium Morrhuate Injection may show a separation of solid matter on standing. Do not use the material if such solid does not dissolve completely upon warming.

Preparation—This Injection may be prepared by heating cod liver oil with alcoholic sodium hydroxide until completely saponified. After dilution with water the alcohol is removed by distillation. Dilute sulfuric acid is then added to the aqueous solution, and the liberated organic acids are separated or preferably extracted with a suitable immiscible solvent such as ether. Just sufficient aqueous sodium hydroxide is then added to neutralize the acids. About 20 mg of benzyl alcohol per ml of the Injection is usually added to lessen the pain of injection.

Uses—This Injection is used as a *sclerosing* and *fibrosing agent* for obliterating *varicose veins*. Irritants of this type have also been employed for closure of hernial rings, fibrosing of uncomplicated hemorrhoids, the removal of condylomata acuminata, and in other conditions where the ultimate objective is production of fibrous tissue.

Dose—*Intravenous*, by special injection, **0.5 to 5** ml to a localized area; *usual*, **1 ml**.

Dosage Forms—Injection USP: 2, 5, 10, and 30 ml.

Other Sclerosing Agents

Quinine and Urea Hydrochloride USP XVII is a double salt of quinine and urea hydrochlorides. It contains an amount of anhydrous quinine equivalent to 98–110% of $C_{20}H_{24}N_2O_2 \cdot HCl \cdot CH_4N_2O \cdot HCl \cdot 5H_2O$ (547.48). *Preparation:* This double salt may be prepared by dissolving 40 parts of quinine hydrochloride in 30 parts of 10% hydrochloric acid, adding 6 to 6.1 parts of urea, warming to form a solution, filtering if necessary, and allowing the salt to crystallize from solution. *Description and Solubility:* Colorless, translucent prisms, white granules, or a white powder. It is odorless, has a very bitter taste, and is affected by light. A 1 in 20 aqueous solution is acid to litmus. 1 Gm dissolves in 1 ml of water and 3 ml of alcohol. *Uses:* It is used as a *sclerosing agent.* Solutions over 1.0% may cause necrosis. The solution is not to be used for systemic effects. *Dose:* 0.5 to 5 ml; usual, intravenous, by special injection, 1 ml of a 5% solution to localized area.

Sodium Ricinoleate [Soricin; Colidosan]—Sodium ricinoleate consists of the sodium salts of mixed fatty acids from castor oil. It is a white or yellowish, nearly odorless powder. Soluble in water or alcohol. A 5% solution (0.5 to 5 ml) of sodium ricinoleate in water (pH 8.2–8.5) exerts a sclerosing action for the obliteration of varicose veins. Before starting actual treatment, all patients should be tested for possible sensitivity by injection of 0.5 ml of a 2% solution into a small varicosity. *Contraindications*—in obstruction of the deep circulation, phlebitis, infected varicose ulceration, uncontrolled diabetes, arteriosclerosis, and hypertension.

Sodium Tetradecyl Sulfate [STS; Sotradecol Sodium (*Elkins-Sinn*)] is sodium 7-ethyl-2-methyl-4-undecyl sulfate. *Description and Solubility:* A white, waxy, odorless solid. Soluble in water, alcohol, and ether. *Uses:* A *sclerosing agent* similar in action to sodium morrhuate. It is used as a buffered solution in the *obliteration of varicose veins and internal hemorrhoids.* For such purposes, the solution is injected directly into the vein. Injection outside of the vein may cause sloughing. For this reason, the substance is not used to close inguinal rings. The principal untoward effect is pain immediately upon injection, although brief, mild anaphylactoid and idiosyncratic responses rarely occur. Because the substance is an anionic surface-active agent, it is also used as a wetting agent to promote the spreading of certain topical antiseptics.

Dose: By injection directly into the target vein, as a 1, 3, or 5% solution, depending upon the size of the vein. The volume then to be injected at any one site varies from 0.2 to 2.0 ml, depending upon the concentration and the number of previous injections at the site, the larger volumes being given only after several previous injections. No more than 10 ml of the 3% solution or 6 ml of the 5% solution should be given at any one sitting. The interval between injections varies from 5 to 7 days. *Dosage Form:* Injection: 1, 3, and 5% (30 ml).

Caustics and Escharotics

Any topical agent that causes destruction of tissues at the site of application is a *caustic* (or corrosive).

Caustics may be used to induce desquamation of cornified epithelium ("keratolytic" action) and are therefore used to destroy warts, condylomata, keratoses, certain moles, and hyperplastic tissues.

If the agent also precipitates the proteins of the cell and the inflammation exudate, there is formed a scab (or eschar), which is later organized into a scar; such an agent is an *escharotic* (or cauterizant). Most, but not all, caustics are also escharotic. Furthermore, certain caustics, especially the alkalies, redissolve precipitated proteins, partly by hydrolysis, so that no scab or only a soft scab forms; such agents penetrate deeply and are generally unsuitable for therapeutic use. Escharotics are sometimes employed to seal cutaneous and aphthous ulcers, wounds, etc. Since most escharotics are bactericidal, it was formerly thought that chemical cauterization effected sterilization; however, sterilization is not always achieved, especially by those agents which remain bound to the protein precipitate. The growth of certain bacteria may even be favored by the chemically-induced necrosis and by the protection of the scab.

Acetic Acid, Glacial—see page 1362.

Alum—see page 769.

Gentian Violet—see page 1178.

Phenol—see page 1370.

Podophyllum USP

[Mandrake; May Apple]

Podophyllum yields not less than 5.0% of podophyllum resin.

Podophyllum consists of the dried rhizome and roots of *Podophyllum peltatum* Linné (Fam. *Berberidaceæ*).

Constituents—Podophyllum contains from 3 to 6% of resin along with up to 1% of quercetin and podophyllotoxin and peltatin glucosides. All told, some 16 different compounds have been isolated and characterized. The aglycone, *podophyllotoxin* [$C_{22}H_{22}O_8$], is the lactone of 1-hydroxy-2-(hydroxymethyl)-6,7 - methylenedioxy - 4 - (3′,4′,5′ - trimethoxyphenyl)-1,2,3,4-tetrahydronaphthalene-3-carboxylic acid. Hydrolytic rupture of the lactone ring yields *podophyllic acid* [$C_{22}H_{24}O_9$], the 2,3-*trans* form of which is *podophyllinic acid* while the 2,3-*cis* form is *picropodophyllinic acid.* The closely related aglycone, *peltatin* [$C_{21}H_{20}O_8$], is 1-deoxy-4′-demethoxy-4′,8-dihydroxypodophyllotoxin and exists in both α and β forms.

Although podophyllotoxin has been demonstrated to possess marked caustic, cathartic, and toxic properties, it is believed that not it, but an amorphous *resin,* called *podophylloresin,* is the chief cathartic principle of the drug.

Uses—The chief therapeutic use of Podophyllum in humans is as a *caustic* for the removal of *warts* and *papillomas* or as a source of the more effective resin. It was formerly used as a *cathartic* and as a *veterinary purgative.* Its actions differ from those of most caustics in that action is neither direct nor immediate; rather, cell division is arrested and other cellular processes are impaired, which leads eventually to the disruption of the cells and erosion of the tissue. In appropriate concentration, normal tissue is spared.

Dose—See *Podophyllum Resin* below.

Podophyllum Resin USP [Podophyllin] is the powdered mixture of resins removed from podophyllum by percolation with alcohol and subsequent precipitation from the concentrated percolate upon addition to acidified water. *Preparation:* Place podophyllum (in fine powder, 1000 Gm), in a suitable percolator, and percolate alcohol through it slowly. Concentrate the percolate to the consistency of a thin syrup, and pour the residue into a mixture, previously cooled to a temperature between 5° and 10°, of 10 ml of hydrochloric acid in 1000 ml of water. Allow the resin to settle, decant the supernatant liquid, and wash the resin with two 1000-ml portions of cold water. Dry the resin, and powder it.

Description: It occurs as an amorphous powder, varying in color from light brown to greenish yellow, turning darker when subjected to a temperature exceeding 25° or when exposed to light. It has a slight, peculiar, faintly bitter taste. *Solubility:* It dissolves in alcohol with only a slight opalescence; its alcohol solution is acid to litmus paper; only partially soluble in ether and in chloroform. *Caution—Podophyllum Resin is highly irritating to the eye and to mucous membranes in general.*

Uses: Podophyllum resin is the superior form of podophyllum for the topical treatment of *hyperplasms* and *growths*. It has been used frequently as a *caustic* to remove various *papillomas, warts, fibroids,* etc. The resin is also an unpredictable and frequently toxic irritant cathartic; consequently, its cathartic use is mainly restricted to animals. *Dose: External use, topically* to certain papillomas, as a 25% dispersion in compound benzoin tincture or as a solution in alcohol once a week. *Other Dose Information:* It is commonly suspended in mineral oil, 25% for warts, and 1–12% for papillomata of the bladder. Solutions in ethanol (20%) have also been employed in the treatment of warts. *Veterinary Dose: Cattle, 8 to 15 Gm; Dogs, 15 to 30 mg.*

Potassium Hydroxide USP

[Kalii Hydroxidum; Caustic Potash; Lye; Potash Lye; Potassa]

Potassium Hydroxide contains not less than 85.0% of total alkali, calculated as KOH (56.11), including not more than 3.5% of K_2CO_3 (138.21).

Caution—Exercise great care in handling Potassium Hydroxide, as it rapidly destroys tissues. Do not handle it with bare hands.

Preparation—Potassium Hydroxide is prepared on a large scale by electrolysis of a solution of potassium chloride. The electrolysis is carried out in the presence of a porous diaphragm which permits the passage of the current but does not allow the liberated chlorine to react with the newly formed Potassium Hydroxide. The over-all reaction may be represented as follows:

$$2KCl + 2H_2O \rightarrow 2KOH + H_2 + Cl_2$$

An older method of preparation consists of adding a suspension of calcium hydroxide to a hot solution of potassium carbonate. When metathesis is complete and the calcium carbonate has settled, the supernatant KOH solution is decanted and concentrated to form the solid product as described below.

Potassium Hydroxide, known commercially as *caustic potash*, is prepared in the form of sticks, pellets, flakes, or fused masses. Sticks or pellets are made by evaporating a solution of Potassium Hydroxide rapidly in a silver or clean iron vessel until a fluid of oily consistency remains, a drop of which, when removed on a warm glass rod, solidifies on cooling. The hot caustic is poured into suitable molds and while still warm the product is packaged quickly to prevent deliquescence.

Potassa by alcohol and *potassa by baryta* are terms formerly used to designate pure caustic Potassium Hydroxide which was purified with alcohol or barium hydroxide. In the alcohol process the alcohol dissolves only the Potassium Hydroxide. In the baryta process the sulfate and carbonate are separated by treatment of the potassium hydroxide solution with baryta water, which is a solution of barium hydroxide, forming the insoluble barium salts of these respective acids.

Description—White, or nearly white, fused masses, small pellets, flakes, sticks, and other forms. It is hard and brittle and shows a crystalline fracture. Exposed to air it rapidly absorbs carbon dioxide and moisture, and deliquesces. It melts at about 360–380°. When dissolved in water or alcohol, or when its solution is treated with an acid much heat is generated. Solutions of potassium hydroxide, even when highly diluted, exhibit a strong alkaline reaction to litmus paper.

Solubility—One Gm dissolves in 1 ml of water, in about 3 ml of alcohol, and in about 2.5 ml of glycerin at 25°. It is very soluble in boiling alcohol.

Incompatibilities—Bases react with *acids* to form salts, liberate alkaloids from aqueous solutions of *alkaloidal salts,* and promote various hydrolysis reactions such as the decomposition of *chloral hydrate* into chloroform and a formate or the breakdown of *salol* into phenol and a salicylate.

Since the alkalinity of any substance in aqueous solution is considered to be due to the presence of hydroxyl ions, these reactions can be considered applicable to all alkaline substances.

Only the alkali hydroxides are appreciably soluble in water. Nearly all common *metals* will be precipitated as hydroxides when solutions of their salts are added to solutions of the alkali hydroxides. Certain hydroxides, however, notably those of aluminum, zinc, arsenic, and lead, will dissolve in excess of sodium or potassium hydroxide.

Ammonia is liberated from *ammonium compounds* by alkalies and many alkaline salts. Some pharmaceutical preparations are alkaline in reaction and possess this characteristic incompatibility. See *Sodium Hydroxide* (page 1373).

Uses—Potassium Hydroxide is used as a *caustic,* principally in veterinary practice. The end of the stick may be inserted into a section of rubber tubing, or wrapped several times with tin foil, to avoid cauterizing the fingers of the operator. It is used also as a *pharmaceutical necessity* in several pharmacopeial preparations. In industry it is used in the manufacture of soft soap, in electroplating, in paint and varnish removers, and in many other processes.

Silver Nitrate USP

[Argenti Nitras]

Silver Nitrate, powdered and then dried in the dark over silica gel for 4 hours, contains 99.8–100.5% of $AgNO_3$ (169.87).

History—This salt was described by Geber in the seventh century AD. It was first used in medicine in the eighteenth century in Pilulæ Lunares. Christopher Glaser, the apothecary to Louis XIV of France, first prepared it in sticks for use as a caustic.

Preparation—Silver Nitrate is prepared by the action of nitric acid on silver metal, as indicated by the equation:

$$3Ag + 4HNO_3 \rightarrow 3AgNO_3 + NO + 2H_2O$$

The nitric acid is diluted to about 30% with distilled water.

It is most economical to use in this process the purest silver commercially available. Silver metal of 99.9% purity is now readily obtainable from silver smelters. With impure silver the cost of purification of the silver nitrate is considerable. The nitric acid should also be pure, and free from halogens, sulfate, and iron; otherwise the product may not be sufficiently pure to meet the official standards and even more so the very stringent purity required for the manufacture of photographic films and silver mirrors.

By using insufficient nitric acid to dissolve all the silver, the nitric acid is more completely utilized, and most of the iron present in the silver remains with the undissolved silver. The solution, after heating to expel nitrous fumes, is filtered while hot and allowed to crystallize. The crystals are thoroughly dried on a filter and dried on trays at about 40° to 50°. If not sufficiently pure they are recrystallized from hot distilled water.

Description—Colorless or white crystals. On exposure to light in the presence of organic matter it becomes gray or grayish black due to its reduction to metallic silver. Its specific gravity is about 4.3. It melts at 212°. The aqueous solution (1 in 10) is neutral to litmus paper and must be clear and colorless.

Solubility—One Gm is soluble in 0.4 ml of water, in 30 ml of alcohol, in about 250 ml of acetone, in slightly more than 0.1 ml of boiling water, and in about 6.5 ml of boiling alcohol. It is slightly soluble in ether.

Incompatibilities—Silver Nitrate is easily reduced to metallic silver by most *reducing agents*, including *ferrous salts, arsenites, hypophosphites, tartrates, sugars, tannins, volatile oils,* and most other *organic substances*. It darkens readily under the influence of *light*. In neutral or alkaline solutions, it is precipitated by *chlorides, bromides, iodides, borax, hydroxides, carbonates, phosphates, sulfates, chromates, arsenites,* and *arsenates*. *Potassium permanganate, tannic acid,* and the *soluble citrates and sulfates* may cause a precipitate if sufficiently concentrated. In acid solution, only the *chloride, bromide,* and *iodide* are insoluble. *Ammonia water* dissolves many of the insoluble silver salts through formation of the silver diammine complex, $Ag(NH_3)_2{}^+$.

Uses—Silver Nitrate is used as a *caustic, antiseptic, germicide,* and *astringent*. In the form of toughened silver nitrate, it is valuable for the cauterization of wounds and the removal of granulation tissue, warts, etc.

Silver Nitrate is particularly active against gonococci. Most state laws require that a few drops of 1 to 2% Silver Nitrate be dropped in the conjunctival sac of newborn infants for the prophylaxis of ophthalmia neonatorum. The solution is immediately washed out with isotonic saline solution. See *Silver Nitrate Ophthalmic Solution,* page 1188.

Caustic pencils consist of Silver Nitrate mixed with some silver chloride or potassium nitrate to render them less brittle. See *Toughened Silver Nitrate.*

Silver Nitrate serves for the preparation of all other silver salts, including *protein silver*. Silver Nitrate is largely consumed in the manufacture of photographic films and silver mirrors.

Dose—*External use, topically,* as a **0.5**% solution to burned areas of the skin; **0.1** ml of a **1**% solution to the conjunctiva. For *Toughened Silver Nitrate,* see below.

Other Dose Information—A 1:10,000 solution is mildly antiseptic and astringent. It is employed for irrigation of the bladder and urethra. Solutions as strong as 10% are used for local treatment of infected ulcers of the mouth. In conjunction with tannic acid, Silver Nitrate has been employed in the treatment of burns.

Toughened Silver Nitrate USP [Argenti Nitras Induratus; Molded Silver Nitrate; Fused Silver Nitrate; Silver Nitrate Pencils; Caustic Stick or Pencil; Lunar Caustic] contains not less than 94.5% of AgNO₃, the remainder consisting of silver chloride (AgCl). *Preparation:* The official process for making this preparation has been deleted. It was formerly made by fusing silver nitrate with the addition of hydrochloric acid, added in small proportions to produce a small amount of silver chloride, which had the effect of toughening the fused mass and making the sticks less brittle. E. J. Hughes found that when a small proportion of sodium chloride was used instead of the hydrochloric acid, the process was very much improved, and the preparation was equally efficient.

In order to keep the sticks from becoming discolored during the molding process, it is advisable to add a little diluted nitric acid (1 in 5) occasionally to the melted nitrate, and carefully prevent the mass from becoming overheated.

Silver molds are preferably employed in molding the cones. Potassium nitrate is frequently used instead of silver chloride. The pencils made with it do not discolor so readily. Silver nitrate pencils made with 25 or 33% potassium nitrate are "milder" and they are preferred for some applications. *Description:* White, crystalline masses, generally molded as pencils or cones. It breaks with a fibrous fracture. It becomes gray or grayish black on exposure to light, due to the silver chloride. Its solution is neutral to litmus. *Solubility:* Soluble in water to the extent of its nitrate content (there is always a residue of silver chloride); partially soluble in alcohol and slightly soluble in ether. *Uses:* See *Silver Nitrate.* Silver nitrate is toughened to lessen the danger of breakage when applied inside the oral cavity, and to provide pencil-shaped applicators which may be sharpened. A good caustic holder may be made from a glass stirring rod of the same diameter as the cone by joining it to the cone with a short length of rubber tubing. The cone may be protected from the action of the air by slipping over it another short length of rubber tubing, having a very short piece of glass rod in the other end as a stopper. *Dose:* *External use, topically,* after being dipped in water.

Death has resulted more than once through the careless use of silver nitrate in cauterizing the throat, the cone having slipped out of the fingers and then been swallowed by the patient.

Small wooden sticks, dipped in toughened silver nitrate, sufficient for one application, have also been offered.

Silver Nitrate Applicators, consisting of 3- or 6-inch wooden sticks on which is fused a mixture of 75% silver nitrate and 25% potassium nitrate are sometimes used. See *Medicated Pencils* (RPP XII, page 428).

Trichloroacetic Acid USP

CCl₃COOH

Trichloroacetic Acid contains 99.0–100.5% of C_2-HCl_3O_2 (163.39), calculated on the dried basis.

Preparation—This acid, discovered by Dumas in 1838, is usually made by oxidizing chloral hydrate with fuming nitric acid. To the chloral hydrate, previously fused at about 58°, a little over one-third its weight of fuming nitric acid is added and the mixture set aside until the red fumes have disappeared; the liquid is then distilled, and the portion coming over above 190°, which is trichloroacetic acid, is then crystallized.

Description—Colorless, deliquescent crystals having a slight, characteristic odor. The Acid melts at about 58° and boils at 196°–197°.

Solubility—One Gm dissolves in about 0.1 ml of water; it is soluble in alcohol and in ether.

Identification—It is decomposed by alkali hydroxide solution forming chloroform and the carbonate of the alkali used. The chloroform gives the phenyl isocyanide reaction described under *Chloral Hydrate.*

Uses—Trichloroacetic Acid is *keratolytic* and is used as a *caustic* on the skin or mucous membranes, in solution or in crystals. It is extensively employed as a precipitant of protein in the chemical analysis of body fluids and tissue extracts, also as a decalcifier and fixative in microscopy.

Caution—*Trichloroacetic Acid is highly corrosive to the skin.*

Dose—*External use, topically,* as a **15** to **50**% solution.

Other Caustics and Escharotics

Alum, Dried NF XII [Alumen Exsiccatum; Exsiccated Alum; Burnt Alum; Alumen Ustum], dried at 200° for 16 hours, contains not less than 96.5% of $AlNH_4(SO_4)_2$ (237.14) or 96.5–105% of $AlK(SO_4)_2$ (258.21). The label of the container must indicate whether the salt is *Exsiccated Ammonium Alum* or *Exsiccated Potassium Alum*.

Preparation: By placing a thin layer of alum in a tared, shallow, porcelain dish, and heating it cautiously on a sand bath until liquefied. The heat is then continued at a temperature not exceeding 220°, with constant stirring, until aqueous vapors cease to evolve and a dry, white, porous mass is obtained. When cold, reduce the product to a fine powder. Care must be observed in the regulation of the heat during exsiccation as temperatures appreciably above 220° produce insoluble basic aluminum sulfate. The final product should show a weight loss of 47.5% (ammonium alum) or 45.5% (potassium alum).

Description and Solubility: A white, odorless powder with a sweetish, astringent taste which absorbs moisture on exposure to air. 1 Gm is very slowly soluble in 20 ml of water and in about 2 ml of boiling water; insoluble in alcohol.

Uses: An escharotic; it is more powerful than alum, not only because it is more concentrated but, being hygroscopic, it also removes water from the tissues.

Nitric Acid NF X—It contains 67–71 % HNO_3. It is a fuming liquid, very caustic, and has a characteristic, highly irritating odor. It boils at 120°C and has a specific gravity of about 1.41. It is miscible with water. *Uses:* As a cauterizing agent for the immediate sterilization of dangerously infected wounds, such as the bite from a rabid animal. It does not penetrate too deeply and forms a firm-eschar; in the Heller Test to detect albumin in the urine; industrially, in the production of nitrates and numerous synthetic organic medicinal products.

Keratolytics (Desquamating Agents)

The epidermis consists of layers of flat cells, called *stratified squamous epithelial cells.* They are bound together by desmosomes and penetrating tonofibrils, both of which largely consist of keratin. The outer layer of the epidermis, the cornified epithelium or stratum corneum, is made up of the collapsed ghosts of the squamous cells and, as such, is principally a tight network of keratin and lipoprotein. Certain fungi, especially the dermatophytes, utilize keratin and therefore reside in the stratum corneum in those places where the degree of hydration and the pH are sufficiently high. One way such mycoses may be suppressed is that of removal of the stratum corneum, a process that is called *desquamation.* Certain chemical substances, especially among phenols and sulfhydryl compounds, loosen the keratin and thus facilitate desquamation. These substances are called *keratolytics.* Aqueous maceration of the stratum corneum also favors desquamation. In addition to the treatment of epidermophytosis, keratolytics are used to thin hyperkeratotic areas. Most keratolytics are irritant. Irritants also can cause desquamation by causing damage to and swelling of the basal cells.

Resorcinol—see page 1187.

Resorcinol Ointment, Compound—see page 1188.

Silver Nitrate—see page 779.

Salicylic Acid USP

[o-Hydroxybenzoic Acid]

COOH
OH

Salicylic Acid contains 99.5–101.0% of $C_7H_6O_3$ (138.12) calculated on the dried basis.

Preparation—Salicylic Acid may be obtained from several natural sources such as birch or gaultheria oil, but nearly all of the salicylic acid of commerce is obtained according to Kolbe's process by treating *sodium phenolate* with carbon dioxide. For this purpose, the most concentrated caustic soda solution is evaporated with the corresponding amount of phenol to a dry powder. This is then heated to 100° while a stream of dry carbon dioxide is passed over it. The temperature is gradually raised to 180° and then to 220° as soon as phenol distils over, and finally raised to 250° until no more phenol distils. Half of the phenol distils over unchanged and the residue left in the retort is essentially composed of sodium sodio-salicylate $[C_6H_4(ONa)-COONa]$. The disodium salt thus obtained is dissolved in water and decomposed by hydrochloric acid. The salicylic acid is then filtered off, washed, and crystallized from a hot aqueous solution, or more commonly purified by sublimation in a current of superheated steam.

In the Schmitt modification of the Kolbe synthesis, carbon dioxide is reacted with sodium phenolate in closed vessels at a temperature of 130° forming sodium phenyl carbonate which passes into sodium salicylate. By this modification no separation of phenol occurs and the extent of phenol conversion is enhanced.

Salicylic Acid is also made from gaultheria oil by refluxing an alcoholic hydroxide whereby saponification takes place and sodium salicylate is formed; the refluxed mixture is then poured into diluted hydrochloric acid and the separated salicylic acid purified if necessary by recrystallization.

Description—Salicylic Acid occurs as white, fine, needle-like crystals or as a fluffy, white, crystalline powder. Synthetic Salicylic Acid is white and odorless. The Acid prepared from natural salicylate may have a slightly yellow or pink tint and a faint wintergreen-like odor. The Acid has a sweetish, afterward acrid, taste. It is stable in the air. Salicylic Acid melts between 158° and 161°.

Solubility—One Gm of Salicylic Acid dissolves in 460 ml of water, in 3 ml of alcohol, in 45 ml of chloroform, in 3 ml of ether, and in 135 ml of benzene. One Gm of the Acid dissolves in about 15 ml of boiling water.

Identification—Ferric chloride produces a violet color even in dilute solutions of salicylic acid or soluble salicylates. The addition of dilute mineral acids to moderately concentrated solutions of salicylates produces a white crystalline precipitate of the salicylic acid which, when washed with cold water and dried, has the melting point of salicylic acid.

Incompatibilities—See *Sodium Salicylate* (page 1139). Salicylic Acid is incompatible with the usual *vanishing cream* due to the fact that creams of this type are based on the formation of an emulsion with the aid of a soap. The soap is decomposed by reaction with an acid.

Uses—Salicylic Acid is not employed internally as an *analgesic* due to its local irritating effect on the gastrointestinal tract. It is employed *externally* on the skin, where it exerts a slight *antiseptic* action and a marked *keratolytic* action. The latter property makes Salicylic

Acid a beneficial agent in the local treatment of *warts, corns, fungous infections*, and certain forms of *eczematoid dermatitis*. Tissue cells swell, soften, and ultimately desquamate. Salicylic Acid Plaster is often used for this purpose.

Dose—*External use, topically,* as a **2** to **20%** collodion, lotion, or ointment, and as **10** to **40%** plaster.

Salicylic Acid Collodion USP [Corn Collodion; Salicylic Collodion] contains 9.5–11.5% of $C_7H_6O_3$ (138.12).

Preparation: Dissolve salicylic acid (100 Gm) in flexible collodion (about 750 ml), add sufficient flexible collodion to make the product measure 1000 ml, and mix.

Salicylic Acid Plaster USP is a uniform mixture of salicylic acid in a suitable base, spread on paper, cotton cloth, or other suitable backing material. The plaster mass contains 90.0–110.0% of the labeled amount of $C_7H_6O_3$.

Sulfur, Sublimed—see page 1273.

Trichloroacetic Acid—see page 780.

Miscellaneous Dermatologics

Gargles, nasal washes, douches, enemata, etc, generally contain as basic ingredients substances described under other categories in this chapter. These preparations are described elsewhere in this book under *Aqueous Solutions,* page 1478. *Antiphlogistics* include alcohol and several creams and lotions that cool by evaporation. Many antiphlogistic preparations also contain an astringent and a local anesthetic. Commonly employed *antipruritics* also depend largely upon local anesthetics and the soothing effect of cooling, although emollients or demulcents may be included, especially depending upon the etiology of the pruritis. The antipruritic properties of phenol preparations largely derive from superficial local anesthesia. *Vulnerary* and *epithelizing* properties are attributed to numerous irritants and to several dyes; however, few reliable data exist to support most claims to vulnerary action. *Sun screens* contain aromatic compounds, like para-aminobenzoic acid, which efficiently absorb the harmful ultraviolet rays from the incident sunlight and transmit mainly the less harmful wavelengths, or titanium dioxide, which reflects sunlight from the surface of application. *Melanizers* are substances that promote the pigmentation of the skin. Most melanizers produce their effect by sensitizing the skin to ultraviolet light,* so that the effect is principally the same as if the subject had been exposed for a long time to the sun. Skin bleaches, or demelanizers, mostly contain either ammoniated mercury or hydroquinone derivatives. *Hair bleaches* generally contain peroxides. There are no official *depilatories*, although there are a large variety on the market. Many of them are sulfhydryl compounds, especially thioglycollates, which reduce the disulfide bonds of keratin, thus softening the hair to the point where it can be separated easily from the epidermis. *Antiperspirants* have been included among the astringents.

Cetyl Alcohol—see page 1352.

Hydroquinone NF

[*p*-Dihydroxybenzene; Hydroquinol; Quinol; Tecquinol]

OH

OH

Hydroquinone, dried at 105° for 3 hours, contains 99.0–100.5% of $C_6H_6O_2$ (110.11).

Preparation—Various processes are employed. One involves reacting a sulfuric acid solution of aniline with manganese dioxide and reducing the resulting *p*-benzoquinone with sodium bisulfite.

Uses—Hydroquinone is a *hypopigmenting* agent employed percutaneously to lighten localized areas of hyperpigmented skin, such as skin blemishes, freckles, etc. Its action is only temporary, so that it is necessary to repeat the application at frequent intervals. It is a mild irritant, and erythema or rash may develop, which requires discontinuation of the drug. It should not be used near the eyes or in open cuts. It is contraindicated in the presence of sunburn, miliaria, or irritated skin. Hydroquinone is not to be used on children.

Dose—*External use, topically,* as a **2%** ointment to the affected area once or twice daily at 12-hour intervals.

Dosage Forms—Ointment NF: 2%.

Hydrogen Peroxide Solution—see page 1180.

Mercury, Ammoniated—see page 1182.

Methoxsalen

[Ammoidin;   9-Methoxypsoralen;   Xanthotoxin;   Meloxine (*Upjohn*); Oxsoralen (*Elder*)]

OCH$_3$

Methoxsalen is 9-methoxy-7*H*-furo[3,2-*g*][1]benzopyran-7-one. It is frequently literature-indexed as the δ-lactone of 6-hydroxy-7-methoxy-5-benzofuranacrylic acid. On the basis of an alternative ring numbering, this compound is commonly known as 8-methoxypsoralen.

Preparation—Methoxsalen occurs naturally in *Psorales coryfolia, Ammi majus, Ruta chalepensis,* and various other plants. It may be synthesized by methods described in *J. Am. Chem. Soc.,* **79,** 3491 (1957) and US Pat. 2,889,337.

Description—A white to cream-colored, odorless, crystalline solid.

Solubility—Practically insoluble in cold water, sparingly soluble in boiling water, and freely soluble in chloroform. Soluble in boiling alcohol, acetone, and acetic acid. Soluble in aqueous alkalies with ring cleavage; reconstitution occurs upon neutralization. A yellow solution results when it is mixed with concentrated H_2SO_4.

---

* This action is termed a *photodynamic action*. The term has been used loosely to include all instances of enhanced sensitivity to light, but in strict definition it is confined to photosensitization in which the participation of oxygen is required. In the photodynamic process light of wavelengths too long to be ordinarily effective may be utilized, so that the activating spectrum may be shifted toward longer wavelengths.

Uses—Methoxsalen increases the photodynamic pigmentation of skin; it does not induce pigmentation in the absence of ultraviolet light. It is used in the treatment of vitiligo. Severe sunburning can occur. After oral administration gastrointestinal upset and central nervous toxicities, such as vertigo and excitement, also occur. Consequently, the drug should be used only under medical supervision.

Dose—**20 mg** orally once daily. Lotions are **1%**.

Dosage Forms—Lotion: 1% (30 ml); Tablets: 10 mg.

Monobenzone NF

[*p*-(Benzyloxy)phenol; Monobenzyl Ether of Hydroquinone; Benoquin (*Elder*)]

Monobenzone, dried at 105° for 3 hours, contains 98.0–102.0% of $C_{13}H_{12}O_2$ (200.24).

Preparation—Monobenzone may be prepared in various ways. One method involves condensing sodium *p*-nitrophenolate with benzyl chloride to produce benzyl *p*-nitrophenyl ether followed by (1) reduction of nitro to amino, (2) diazotization of amino, and (3) hydrolytic decomposition of the diazonium compound to the corresponding phenol.

Description—It occurs as a white, odorless, crystalline powder possessing very little taste. Melting range 115° to 118°.

Solubility—Freely soluble in alcohol and in acetone. Insoluble in water.

Uses—Monobenzone is a *hypopigmenting agent* or *demelanizer*. It acts by interfering with the formation of melanin, which is the principal cutaneous pigment. It is used in the treatment of lentigo, severe freckling, and other types of hyperpigmentation. Its pigment-decreasing action is somewhat erratic. Irritation of varying degrees occurs in a considerable number of patients.

Dose—*External use, topically*, as a **20%** ointment or **5%** lotion 1 or 2 times daily.

Dosage Forms—Lotion NF: 5%; Ointment NF: 20%.

Sodium Bicarbonate—see page 793.

Sodium Borate USP

[Borax; Sodium Tetraborate; Sodium Pyroborate; Sodium Biborate]

Sodium Borate contains an amount of $Na_2B_4O_7$ (201.22) equivalent to 99.0–105.0% of $Na_2B_4O_7 \cdot 10H_2O$ (381.37).

Preparation—This salt is found in immense quantities in California as a crystalline deposit, at Clear Lake, and near Death Valley. It is probable that this will continue to be the principal source of borax for many years to come. The process of purification consists simply of selecting the large and perfect crystals and washing them. The earth, which is strongly impregnated with borax, is lixiviated; the solution is evaporated and crystallized.

Calcium borate, or *cotton balls*, also occurs in the borax deposits of California, and sodium borate is obtained from it by double decomposition with a solution of sodium carbonate. Borax is also found native in Tibet, Persia, and other localities. It is sometimes called *tincal*.

Description—Colorless, transparent crystals, or a white, crystalline powder. It is odorless. The crystals are often coated with white powder due to efflorescence. Its solution is alkaline to litmus and to phenolphthalein; pH about 9.5. Borax dissolves many metallic oxides when fused with them.

Solubility—One Gm dissolves in 16 ml of water, in about 1 ml of glycerin, and in about 1 ml of boiling water; it is insoluble in alcohol.

Incompatibilities—Sodium Borate precipitates many *metals* as insoluble borates. In aqueous solution it is alkaline in reaction and precipitates *aluminum salts* as aluminum hydroxide, *iron salts* as a basic borate and ferric hydroxide, and *zinc sulfate* as zinc borate and a basic salt. *Alkaloids* are precipitated from solutions of their salts. Approximately equal weights of *glycerin* and boric acid react to produce a decidedly acid derivative generally called glyceroboric acid. Thus the addition of glycerin to a mixture containing sodium borate overcomes those incompatibilities arising from an alkaline reaction.

Uses—Saturated solutions of Sodium Borate have limited usefulness as an *antipruritic* for the skin. Solutions are also sometimes used as a mouth wash in the treatment of *stomatitis* and *gingivitis*. Sodium Borate should not be administered internally. See *Boric Acid* (page 1363).

Pharmaceutically, it is frequently used in small quantities in ointments, in hand lotions, and in other cosmetics. It forms a soap which serves as an emulsifying agent in the preparation of the ointment. It is a frequent ingredient in eye lotions, but is incompatible with zinc sulfate, as insoluble zinc borate is formed.

Industrially, borax is used as flux in soldering, in the manufacture of enamels and glass, in fireproofing of fabrics and wood, in soaps, and in various cleaning compounds.

Titanium Dioxide—see page 1376.

Sodium Fluoride USP

Sodium Fluoride contains 98.0–101.0% of NaF (41.99), calculated on the dried basis.

Description—Sodium Fluoride is a white, odorless powder.

Solubility—1 Gm dissolves in about 25 ml of water; insoluble in alcohol.

Uses—Sodium Fluoride is a *dental prophylactic*. It has now been definitely established that fluoridation of city water supplies is a safe and practical public health measure. A concentration of about 1 ppm of Sodium Fluoride in the water supply results in a 50 to 66% reduction in the incidence of *dental caries* in permanent teeth, and repeated topical application of a 2% solution of Sodium Fluoride to cleaned teeth of children has resulted in a 40% reduction of dental caries.

Sodium Fluoride is widely used in *roach powders* (see page 1281). This salt, as well as sodium and magnesium silicofluorides, are used for *mothproofing* textile fabrics.

Caution—*Sodium Fluoride is very poisonous. When acidified, Sodium Fluoride yields hydrofluoric acid which also is a very poisonous substance.*

Dose—*Usual*, 2.2 mg (the equivalent of **1 mg** of fluoride ion) once a day; *application*, **1.5 to 3 ppm** (equivalent to **0.7 to 1.3 ppm** of fluoride ion) in drinking water; *topically*, as a 2% solution to the teeth.

Veterinary Dose—Despite its poisonous character, the drug may be used as an anthelmintic for swine (against Ascaris lumbricoides) by mixing 1 part by weight with 99 parts of dry, ground feed. The mixture is fed for 1 day only. Extreme caution must be exerted.

Stannous Fluoride NF

[Tin Difluoride; Fluoristan]

Stannous Fluoride [$SnF_2 = 156.69$], dried at 105° for 4 hours, contains not less than 71.2% of Sn^{2+} (stannous tin), and 22.3–25.5% of F (fluoride).

Description—A white, crystalline powder with a bitter, salty taste. It melts at about 213°.

Solubility—Freely soluble in water; practically insoluble in alcohol, ether, and chloroform.

Uses—Stannous Fluoride alters the composition and crystalline structure of the hydroxyapatite-like salts that make up the bulk of enamel, especially, and dentin, so that the tooth material is more resistant to acidic erosion and dental caries (decay). The substance is applied only topically, so that the tooth substance is only affected in the superficial layers, and Stannous Fluoride must be applied periodically. It is most effective when applied to the tooth surface after the teeth have been cleaned thoroughly by a dentist. However, there is good evidence that even when incorporated into tooth pastes the drug has a retardant effect on the development of dental caries.

Dose—*Topically*, to the teeth.

Other Dose Information—Stannous Fluoride is generally used as a 2% solution.

Trioxsalen NF

[2,5,9-Trimethyl-7*H*-furo[3,2-*g*][1]benzopyran-7-one; 6-Hydroxy-β,2,7-trimethyl-5-benzofuranacrylic Acid δ-Lactone; Trisoralen (*Elder*)]

Trioxsalen contains 97.0–103.0% of $C_{14}H_{12}O_3$ (228.25), calculated on the dried basis.

Caution: Avoid contact with the skin.

Preparation—2-Methylresorcinol is cyclized with ethyl acetoacetate with the aid of sulfuric acid to 7-hydroxy-4,8-dimethylcoumarin (I). Treatment with allyl bromide in the presence of potassium carbonate transforms (I) into the 7-allyloxy compound which, on reacting with acetic anhydride in the presence of *N*,*N*-diethylaniline and anhydrous sodium acetate, rearranges and esterifies to give the 7-acetoxy-6-allyl compound (II). Bromination of (II) followed by reaction with sodium methoxide yields Trioxsalen. US Pat. 3,201,421.

(I)   (II)

Description—White to off-white, odorless, tasteless crystalline solid. It is stable in light, air, and heat. It melts between 232° and 234°.

Solubility—Soluble in alcohol; sparingly soluble in chloroform; slightly soluble in alcohol and methylene chloride; practically insoluble in water.

Uses—Trioxsalen facilitates the action of near ultraviolet light to induce melanin (skin pigment) formation. It does not *promote pigmentation* in the absence of light. It is used to cause repigmentation in idiopathic *vitiligo* and to enhance pigmentation to *increase tolerance to sunlight* or for *cosmetic purposes*. The increased tolerance to sunlight does not occur until enhanced pigmentation has occurred, and the user must be cautioned that severe sunburning to a less than normal exposure can occur early during the course of treatment. The increase in dermal pigment occurs gradually over a period of several days of repeated exposure. The manufacturer's recommended schedule of exposure should be used except at high altitudes where exposure times should be appropriately reduced.

Trioxsalen is contraindicated in persons with photosensitizing diseases, such as infectious leukoderma, porphyria, or lupus erythematosus and when photosensitizing drugs are being given. The drug may sometimes cause gastric irritation and emesis. Children under 12 should not take the drug.

Dose—5 to 10 mg; *usual*, 10 mg 2 hours before exposure to sunlight.

Other Dose Information—For the treatment of vitiligo the exposure should be repeated once daily for 4 days, and subsequent exposures should be determined according to the results of the initial 4 days. For the enhancement of pigmentation, treatment should not exceed 2 weeks. Persons who show side effects of the drug should take only 5 mg; the duration of use will be necessarily prolonged.

Dosage Forms—Tablets NF: 5 mg.

Other Miscellaneous Topical Drugs

Chlorophyll Derivatives, Water-Soluble—Consists chiefly of the copper complex of the sodium and/or potassium salts of saponified chlorophyll. These salts occur as a blue-black powder having a fishy odor and are often referred to as chlorophyllins. They are slightly soluble in alcohol and freely soluble in water. A 1% solution has a pH range of 9.5–10.7. *Uses:* For deodorization. A deodorant action has never been objectively demonstrated and is unlikely on physicochemical grounds. Its presumed effect to stimulate granulation and repair is also poorly supported by acceptable studies. Applied topically as an ointment (0.5%) or solution (0.2%).

Red Veterinary Petrolatum [RVP (*Elder*)] contains diacetylamino-azotoluol (2%) in a hydrocarbon oil ointment base. *Uses:* Devoid of antiseptic action and thus unsuitable for the treatment of purulent wounds (until free of infection), it is used to promote epithelialization of damaged or denuded body surfaces. A thin film is applied topically twice daily. It is also used as a sunscreen preparation [RVPlus (*Elder*)] which contains microcrystalline titanium-coated platelets dispersed in a 30% Red Veterinary Petrolatum emulsion base. A thin film is applied to exposed skin areas before going into sunlight.

Sulfur, Colloidal—This form of sulfur is usually marketed in aqueous suspension, stabilized with various colloids such as albumin, casein, or gelatin. Several processes for its preparation have been patented. It may be prepared by adding hydrochloric acid to an aqueous solution of 2 moles of sodium sulfide and 1 mole of sodium sulfite. The sulfur is formed by the interaction of the hydrogen sulfide formed from the sulfide and the sulfur dioxide formed from the sulfite. The mixture is then dialyzed to remove the sodium chloride and free acid. A superior preparation may be made at the site of application by first washing the affected site with vinegar and applying concentrated (25–50%) sodium thiosulfate solution immediately. *Uses:* Colloidal sulfur is the most active form of sulfur. It consists of elemental sulfur in such a minute state of subdivision that it can be placed in aqueous colloidal solution. Solutions of colloidal sulfur have been administered by the intramuscular and intravenous routes in the treatment of a number of diseases. However, no objective evidence indicates that

systemic colloidal sulfur is useful in the treatment of any disease. For topical uses see page 1273. Colloidal sulfur is especially useful in the treatment of *tinea versicolor* and *tinea cruris*.

Cleansing Preparations

The skin may be cleansed with detergents, solvents, or abrasives, singly or in combination. Among the detergents, the soaps have enjoyed the greatest official status, more through custom than through especial merit. The non-soap detergents became important not only as household hand cleansers but also in dermatologic and surgical practice as well. However, because many non-soap detergents do not decompose in sewage disposal plants, there has been a return to real soap. Some of the antiseptic "soaps" still contain synthetic detergents. Soap interferes with the action of many antiseptics, which is the reason synthetic detergents are often used in antiseptic cleansing preparations. Non-soap skin detergents rarely sensitize and thus are prescribed when the user is allergic to soap.

It is commonly but erroneously believed that soap has an antiseptic action. The promotion of either soap or synthetic detergents alone for the control of acne is unwarranted; antiseptic substances must be added to the cleansing material or be used separately. Quantitative studies of the cutaneous flora before and after cleansing with soap or with other anionic detergents show a negligible antiseptic effect. However, the removal of loose epidermis lessens the likelihood that cutaneous bacteria will be transferred from the skin to other structures. Certain cationic detergents employed in dermatology are antiseptic. Detergents are treated under *Surface-Active Agents* (page 315).

The choice of organic solvents to cleanse the skin depends largely upon the nature of the material to be removed. In medical practice ethanol is the most frequently employed organic solvent. Cleansing creams act both as solvents and as detergents.

Alcohol—see page 1357.

Alcohol, Rubbing—see page 1174.

Benzalkonium Chloride—see page 1175.

Green Soap NF

[Sapo Mollis Medicinalis; Soft Soap; Medicinal Soft Soap USP XVI]

Green Soap is a potassium soap made by the saponification of suitable vegetable oils, excluding coconut oil and palm kernel oil, without the removal of glycerin. Green Soap may be prepared as follows:

The Vegetable Oil	380	Gm
Oleic Acid	20	Gm
Potassium Hydroxide (total alkali 85%)	91.7	Gm
Glycerin	50	ml
Purified Water, a sufficient quantity,		
To make about	1000	Gm

Mix the oil and oleic acid, and heat the mixture to about 80°. Dissolve the potassium hydroxide in a mixture of the glycerin and 100 ml of purified water, and add the solution, while it is still hot, to the hot oil. Stir the mixture vigorously until emulsified, then heat while continuing the stirring,

until the mixture is homogeneous and a test portion will dissolve to give a clear solution in hot water. Add sufficient hot purified water to make the product weigh 1000 Gm, continuing the stirring until the Soap is homogeneous.

Note—The vegetable oil to be used in the formula given above may be corn, cottonseed, linseed, olive, soybean, or a similar oil which has a saponification value not greater than 205 and an iodine value not less than 80. These specifications limit the degree of saturation (iodine value) and the average molecular weight of the fatty acids present in the oil (saponification value). Iodine values less than 80 indicate that the oils are not sufficiently unsaturated and are likely to produce a soap which is too hard. Saponification values above 205 indicate molecular weights which are too low. The lower fatty acids produce soaps which are too irritating for this product. For these reasons *coconut* and *palm kernel oils* are excluded. Since glycerin is added only to accelerate the saponification, it may be omitted if desired.

The quantity of potassium hydroxide given in the formula is based on an alkalinity equivalent to 85% KOH. If the potassium hydroxide is of any other strength, a proportionately larger or smaller quantity should be taken. The oleic acid is added to form an emulsion nucleus which aids in dispersion of the fixed oil, thus aiding in its saponification. A slight excess of alkali is desirable to promote detergency.

A variety of soft soap prepared from green colored oils, such as green olive oil, or artificially colored, is known as "Green Soap." The official soap is not green in color. It has been demonstrated that the green color adds nothing to the therapeutic value and linseed oil soap has long been used with satisfaction. On a large scale the soap may be prepared without the addition of alcohol or glycerin, heat and concentrated alkali producing saponification. It should contain a little free alkali, but too much must be avoided. The amount is regulated by NF tests.

Description—A soft, unctuous, yellowish white to brownish or greenish yellow, transparent to translucent mass, with a slight, characteristic odor, often suggesting the oil from which it was prepared, and an alkaline taste. Its solution (1 in 20) is alkaline to bromothymol blue TS.

Incompatibilities—Medicinal Soft Soap is incompatible with *acids*, which liberate the free fatty acids, and with many *metallic salts*, which form insoluble soaps.

Uses—Green Soap has three major uses as a *detergent* to be used *topically* on the skin:

1. The preoperative preparation of operative sites—For this purpose there is required a soap that is a good fat emulsifier which contains just enough reserve alkalinity to make it quickly effective in the removal of sebaceous secretions from the skin. The soap must contain such proportions of unsaturated fatty acids that it is soluble in and lathers with water and is not too easily affected by hard water. The fatty acids must not be of such low molecular weight that they are irritating to the skin, yet the amount of free alkali must be enough to give prompt detergent activity without at the same time having the powerful caustic effect of free alkali upon the skin. The germicidal efficacy of Green Soap is at best only slight. In *Green Soap Tincture* it is the ethanol that is antiseptic.

2. *The cleansing of the skin and hair in dermatological conditions*—Green soap is used when it is necessary to remove greasy substances or greasy preparations that have been added for therapeutic reasons, to produce a clean area where other medicinal agents may be used, or to remove irritating discharges.

3. *The cleansing of the surgical operator and assistants*— The soap for this use likewise must have excellent detergent power, must be fairly resistant to hard water, and must be equally free from irritating effects of fatty acids or alkalies upon the surgeon's hands. Germicidal detergents, generally containing hexachlorophene, have considerably replaced Green Soap in the surgical scrub.

Coconut and *palm oil soaps* are excellent detergents and they are much less easily affected by hard water than are those soaps that are employed in the NF monograph, but they are irritating to the skin and therefore excluded.

Green Soap Tincture is locally irritating.

Dose—*Topically*, to the skin, generally in the form of *Green Soap Tincture*.

Green Soap Tincture NF [Linimentum Saponis Moolis Medicinalis; Soft Soap Liniment; Medicinal Soft Soap Liniment USP XVI; Tinctura Saponis Viridis]—*Preparation:* mix lavender oil (20 ml) with alcohol (300 ml), dissolve in this the green soap (650 Gm) by stirring or by agitation, set the solution aside for 24 hours, filter through paper, and add alcohol (qs) to make 1000 ml. *Alcohol Content:* From 28 to 32% (v/v) of C_2H_5OH. *Dose: External use, topically,* to skin.

Hexachlorophene Liquid Soap—see page 1180.

Isopropyl Rubbing Alcohol—see page 1182.

Soap, Hard—see page 1379.

Sodium Lauryl Sulfate—see page 1347.

44 | Gastrointestinal Drugs

Gastric antacids—digestants—cathartics (irritant, bulk, and emollient)—emetics—antiemetics—adsorbents—miscellaneous gastrointestinal drugs

This chapter was prepared by

Ewart A. Swinyard, PhD, *Professor of Pharmacology, College of Pharmacy and College of Medicine, University of Utah, Salt Lake City, Utah 84112, and*
Stewart C. Harvey, PhD, *Associate Professor of Pharmacology, College of Medicine, University of Utah, Salt Lake City, Utah 84112*

Drugs appropriate for this chapter include gastric antacids, digestants, cathartics, emetics, antiemetics, adsorbents, and some miscellaneous agents which act on the gastrointestinal tract. A number of other drugs not included in this chapter are often administered for their effect on the gastrointestinal tract. Opium and morphine are frequently used to treat diarrhea and to relieve severe abdominal pain; antispasmodics such as papaverine and the parasympatholytic agents are used to suppress gastric acid secretion and to treat gastrointestinal spasm; cholinergics and posterior pituitary are occasionally used to increase the peristaltic activity of the gastrointestinal tract and to allay distention; and the anthelmintics, amebacides, and certain sulfonamides are used in the treatment of infections of the gastrointestinal tract.

Gastric Antacids

Gastric antacids are drugs which on ingestion react with the hydrochloric acid of the gastric contents to lower the acidity. They are prescribed by physicians chiefly for the treatment of hyperchlorhydria and peptic ulcer, and used by the laity for a large variety of symptoms. Indiscriminate use of these agents, as encouraged by the widely advertised nostrums, is to be condemned since such use may lead to severe *uncompensated alkalosis*, a condition which is frequently unrecognized despite its high incidence.

Antacids act to neutralize the continuously secreted acid gastric juice. The ultimate goal of therapy is to bring the gastric contents to a pH between 4 and 5, but it is difficult to maintain the desired pH because antacids do not decrease the activity of secreting gastric cells, and their effects are temporary and disappear when medication is discontinued. Furthermore, acid is usually secreted in greater amounts in the duodenal ulcer patient than in the normal individual.

These agents may be classified as *systemic* or *nonsystemic antacids*; this classification is synonymous with absorbable and nonabsorbable antacids. A systemic antacid is soluble and readily absorbed, produces systemic electrolyte disturbances and symptoms of alkalosis, and imposes on the kidney the burden of electrolyte readjustment. The nonsystemic antacids are either poorly absorbed or not absorbed and, hence, have no systemic effect. It is generally agreed that only nonsystemic antacids should be used when intensive and prolonged antacid therapy is contemplated.

Alumina and Magnesia Oral Suspension USP

[Aludrox (*Wyeth*)]

Alumina and Magnesia Oral Suspension is a mixture containing variable amounts of aluminum oxide (Al_2O_3), in the form of aluminum hydroxide and hydrated aluminum oxide, and magnesium hydroxide [$Mg(OH)_2$]. It contains the equivalent of 3.6–4.0% of aluminum oxide [Al_2O_3], and 1.7–2.2% of magnesium hydroxide [$Mg(OH)_2$]. It contains 5.3–6.2% of combined aluminum oxide (Al_2O_3) and magnesium hydroxide [$Mg(OH)_2$]. It may contain a flavoring agent, and may contain suitable antimicrobial agents in a total amount not exceeding 0.6%.

Preparation—An aqueous solution containing aluminum and magnesium salts in the desired proportion is treated with sodium hydroxide. The co-precipitated aluminum and magnesium hydroxides are collected by filtration, washed free of soluble salts, and stabilized by the addition of a suitable hexitol such as sorbitol.

Description—A white, opaque, viscous suspension, from which small amounts of clear liquid may separate on standing. Its pH is between 7.3 and 7.9.

Uses—Alumina and Magnesia Oral Suspension is used as an *antacid*. The alumina, in the form of the hydroxide, is an antacid, but it is quite constipating. The latter effect is counteracted by the magnesium hydroxide.

This product contains approximately twice as much aluminum oxide and hydroxide as magnesium hydroxide, but the combined aluminum oxide and magnesium hydroxide content is the same (5.3 to 6.6%) as that in *Magnesia and Alumina Oral Suspension* (page 791). Thus, the theoretical neutralizing capacity of the two preparations is essentially the same.

Dose—5 to 120 ml daily; *usual*, 15 ml 4 to 6 times a day.

Dosage Forms—Oral Suspension USP; Tablets USP: 230 mg (aluminum oxide) and 85 mg (magnesium hydroxide).

Aluminum Hydroxide Gel USP

[Colloidal Aluminum Hydroxide]; Amphojel (*Wyeth*)

Aluminum Hydroxide Gel is a suspension each 100 Gm of which contains the equivalent of 3.6–4.4 Gm of aluminum oxide [Al_2O_3 = 101.96], in the form of aluminum hydroxide and hydrated oxide.

It may contain peppermint oil, glycerin, sorbitol, sucrose, saccharin, or other suitable flavors, and it may contain suitable antimicrobial agents in a total amount not exceeding 0.5%.

Preparation—One process for the preparation of this type of aluminum hydroxide is as follows:

Dissolve 1000 Gm of $Na_2CO_3.10H_2O$ in 4000 ml of hot water and filter. Dissolve 800 Gm of ammonium alum in 2000 ml of hot water and filter into the carbonate solution with constant stirring. Then add 4000 ml of hot water and remove all gas. Dilute to 80,000 ml with cold water. Collect and wash the precipitate and suspend it in 2000 ml of purified water flavored with 0.01% peppermint oil and preserve with 0.1% of sodium benzoate. Homogenize the resulting gel.

The principal property desired is a very fine particle size to achieve large surface and thus maximum adsorption capacity.

Description—A white, viscous suspension, from which small amounts of water may separate on standing; translucent in thin layers. It affects both red and blue litmus paper slightly but is not reddened by phenolphthalein.

Incompatibilities—The use of Aluminum Hydroxide Gel and similar materials to reduce the gastrointestinal problems accompanying the use of the tetracycline antibiotics has resulted in complexation and decreased absorption of the antibiotic.

Uses—Aluminum hydroxide is used primarily as an antacid in the treatment of *peptic ulcer*. Contrary to popular views, the compound is not an adsorbent, but reacts chemically to neutralize the gastric contents. Although suspensions of aluminum hydroxide have some demulcent properties, this is of little clinical significance. Aluminum hydroxide has been used for *intestinal toxemia*, but more effective agents are available. The major advantage of aluminum hydroxide is that no systemic alkalosis is produced.

Dose—**5** to **30 ml** up to 12 times daily; *usual*, **15 ml** 4 to 6 times a day.

Dosage Forms—Dried USP; Oral Suspension; Dried, Tablets USP: 300, 500, and 600 mg.

Veterinary Dose—*Dogs*, **2** to **8 ml** diluted with water or milk at 2-hour intervals.

Dried Aluminum Hydroxide Gel USP yields not less than 50.0% of aluminum oxide [Al_2O_3 = 101.96]. *Preparation:* Aluminum hydroxide, prepared as described under *Aluminum Hydroxide Gel*, is dried at a low temperature until it has the required amount of Al_2O_3. *Description:* A white, odorless, tasteless, amorphous powder. The filtrate from the aqueous suspension (1 in 25) is neutral to litmus. *Solubility:* Insoluble in water and in alcohol; soluble in diluted mineral acids and in solutions of fixed alkali hydroxides. *Dose:* The equivalent of 300 mg to 5 Gm of aluminum hydroxide daily; *usual*, the equivalent of 300 mg of aluminum hydroxide, 4 to 6 times a day. *Veterinary Dose: Dogs, 0.2 to 0.6 Gm.*

Aluminum Phosphate Gel NF

[Phosphaljel (*Wyeth*)]

Aluminum Phosphate Gel is a water suspension containing 4.0–5.0% (*w/w*) of $AlPO_4$ [aluminum phosphate = 121.95].

It may contain sodium benzoate, benzoic acid, or other suitable agents, in an amount not exceeding 0.5%, as a preservative.

Preparation—The Gel may be prepared by precipitation from a solution of aluminum chloride with a solution of sodium phosphate. The particle size of the precipitate, which is an important factor in its acid adsorption, is governed by several factors, eg, the concentration of the reactants, the temperature and pH maintained during the process, as well as the manner of addition of the reactants—whether the sodium phosphate is added to the aluminum solution or the reverse. The soluble salts formed in the reaction are removed by washing by decantation with water, or by dialysis.

Description—A white viscous suspension. A small amount of water will usually separate on standing. Its pH at 25° is between 6.0 and 7.2.

Uses—Aluminum Phosphate Gel is used as an *antacid* and functions in much the same manner as *Aluminum Hydroxide Gel* (page 787). It has approximately half the neutralizing capacity of Aluminum Hydroxide Gel but has the advantage over the latter of not interfering with the absorption of phosphate from the intestinal tract.

Dose—**15** to **45 ml**; *usual*, **15 ml** to **30 ml** every 2 hours.

Bismuth Subcarbonate USP

[Bismuth Carbonate; Basic Bismuth Carbonate; Bismuth Oxycarbonate; Bismuthyl Carbonate]

Bismuth Subcarbonate [approximately $(BiO)_2CO_3.$½H_2O = 518.98] is a basic salt, which yields on ignition not less than 90.0% of Bi_2O_3 (465.96), calculated on the dried basis.

Preparation—A nitric acid solution of the washed subnitrate, obtained as described under *Bismuth Subnitrate*, is added, with constant stirring, to an excess of an approximately 20% solution of sodium carbonate (about 2 parts of monohydrated sodium carbonate for each part of bismuth), and allowed to stand for some time:

$$4Bi(NO_3)_3 + 6Na_2CO_3 + H_2O \rightarrow [(BiO)_2CO_3]_2.H_2O \downarrow +$$
$$12NaNO_3 + 4CO_2$$

After filtering and washing until the washings are neutral, the subcarbonate is dried at about 50°.

Description—A white, or pale yellowish white, odorless and tasteless powder. It is stable in air, but is slowly affected by light.

Solubility—Bismuth Subcarbonate is practically insoluble in water and in alcohol, but is dissolved by excess of nitric and hydrochloric acids with copious effervescence, forming the corresponding salts.

Uses—Bismuth Subcarbonate is used topically as a *protective* in lotions and ointments. It is used internally as an *astringent, protective,* and *adsorbent*. In ulcerative lesions of the bowel, the insoluble salt is believed to coat the crater of an ulcer and thus afford mechanical protection. Bismuth Subcarbonate is given in the dose of 1 to 4 Gm every 2 to 4 hours in the treatment of *enteritis, diarrhea, dysentery,* and *ulcerative colitis*.

Dose—*Topically*, in lotions and ointments.

Other Dose Information—The oral range is 1 to 4 Gm; *usual*, 1 Gm 4 times a day.

Veterinary Dose—*Horses* and *Cattle*, **10** to **20 Gm**; *Sheep* and *Swine*, **2** to **4 Gm**; *Dogs*, **0.3** to **2 Gm**.

Milk of Bismuth NF

[Bismuth Magma NF XII; Bismuth Cream]

Milk of Bismuth contains bismuth hydroxide and bismuth subcarbonate in suspension in water, and yields 5.2–5.8% (*w/w*) of Bi_2O_3 (bismuth trioxide = 465.96).

Bismuth Subnitrate	**80 Gm**
Nitric Acid	**120 ml**
Ammonium Carbonate	**10 Gm**
Strong Ammonia Solution, Purified Water, each, a sufficient quantity,	
To make	**1000 ml**

Mix the bismuth subnitrate with 60 ml of purified water and 60 ml of nitric acid in a suitable container, and agitate, warming gently until solution is effected. Pour this solution, with constant stirring, into 5000 ml of purified water containing 60 ml of nitric acid. Dilute 160 ml of strong ammonia solution with 4300 ml of purified water in a glazed or glass vessel of at least 12,000-ml capacity. Dissolve the ammonium carbonate in this solution, and then pour the bismuth solution quickly into it with constant stirring. If the mixture is not distinctly alkaline, add sufficient diluted ammonia solution to make it so, and allow it to stand until the precipitate has settled; then pour or siphon off the supernatant liquid, and wash the precipitate twice with purified water, by decantation. Afterward transfer the magma to a strainer of close texture, so as to provide continuous washing with purified water, the outlet tube being elevated to prevent the surface of the magma from becoming dry, and allow the operation to proceed until the washings cease to yield a pink color with phenolphthalein TS. Then drain the moist preparation, transfer it to a graduated vessel, add sufficient purified water to make the product measure 1000 ml, and mix it thoroughly.

NOTE—The method of preparation as given above may be varied provided the product meets the requirements given in the NF.

Description—A thick, white, opaque suspension which separates upon standing. It is odorless and almost tasteless.
Solubility—Miscible with water and alcohol.

Uses—See *Bismuth Subnitrate.*
Dose—*Usual,* **5 ml.**

Bismuth Subnitrate NF

[Basic Bismuth Nitrate; Bismuth Oxynitrate; Spanish White; Bismuth Paint; Bismuthyl Nitrate]

Bismuth Subnitrate, [approximately $4Bi(OH)_2NO_3 \cdot BiO(OH) = 1461.99$], is a basic salt which, dried at 105° for 2 hours, yields upon ignition not less than 79.0% of Bi_2O_3 (465.96).

Preparation—Bismuth metal of a high degree of purity is dissolved by adding to it twice its weight of nitric acid, the acid having been previously diluted with an equal volume of water; a solution of bismuth nitrate is thus obtained:

$$2Bi + 8HNO_3 \rightarrow 2Bi(NO_3)_3 + 4H_2O + 2NO$$

Air is now bubbled through the solution to expel the nitric oxide, then the solution is diluted with about an equal volume of distilled water, and filtered if necessary. The solution is cooled to about 15°, and a filtered solution of sodium carbonate is slowly added, with continuous stirring, to produce a pH of about 5. The stirring is continued for an additional hour, then the bismuth subnitrate thus formed is collected by filtration, washed with cold water, and dried at about 50° (120°F).

Description—A white, slightly hygroscopic powder. Its suspension in distilled water is faintly acid to litmus paper (pH about 5).
Solubility—It is practically insoluble in water and organic solvents, but dissolves readily in an excess of hydrochloric or nitric acid.
Incompatibilities—Bismuth Subnitrate is slowly hydrolyzed in *water* with the liberation of nitric acid; thus it possesses the incompatibilities of the acid. It decomposes *carbonates,* liberates iodine from *iodides,* and reacts with *salts of organic acids.* The use of the subcarbonate instead of the Subnitrate obviates these difficulties. *Hypophosphites* and other *reducing agents* darken it with the production of metallic bismuth. *Tannic acid* produces a yellow or gray color.

Uses—Bismuth Subnitrate is employed as an *astringent, adsorbent,* and *protective.* In the treatment of *diarrheas,* and intestinal inflammation and ulcerations, the subcarbonate is preferred to the subnitrate because, with the latter drug, there is the distinct danger of the formation of nitrite ion in the lumen of the bowel and the absorption of toxic amounts of this ion with resulting hypotension and cyanosis due to methemoglobinemia. Fatalities have been reported from the oral use of Bismuth Subnitrate, especially in infants suffering from severe infectious diarrheas. This agent, like other insoluble bismuth salts, is used topically in lotions and ointments.
Dose—See *Milk of Bismuth,* above.
Veterinary Dose—Same as for *Bismuth Subcarbonate.*

Precipitated Calcium Carbonate USP

[Calcium Carbonate; Creta Præcipitata; Precipitated Chalk; Precipitated Carbonate of Lime]

Precipitated Calcium Carbonate, dried at 200° for 4 hours, contains calcium equivalent to 98.0–100.5% of $CaCO_3$ (100.09).

Preparation—This carbonate is conveniently made by the double decomposition of calcium chloride and sodium carbonate in aqueous solution. The density and fineness of the Precipitated Calcium Carbonate are governed by the concentration of the solutions, and heavy and light forms are available on the market.

Description—A fine, white, microcrystalline powder, without odor or taste, and is stable in air. Its aqueous suspension is practically neutral to litmus.
Solubility—Practically insoluble in water; its solubility in water is increased by the presence of any ammonium salt and by the presence of carbon dioxide; the presence of any alkali hydroxide reduces its solubility; it is insoluble in alcohol; it dissolves with effervescence in diluted acetic, hydrochloric, and nitric acids.

Uses—Precipitated Calcium Carbonate is a *gastric antacid.* Calcium carbonate is classified as a "nonsystemic" *antacid* in that it does not tend to cause a systemic alkalosis. The salt reacts with hydrochloric acid in the stomach to form calcium chloride, and the latter reacts with sodium bicarbonate in the intestinal tract to form calcium carbonate. The carbonates precipitate, and for this reason calcium salts by mouth are apt to be constipating. For this reason calcium and magnesium antacids are often alternated in therapy.

Precipitated Calcium Carbonate is also employed in dentifrices and is a pharmaceutical necessity for *Aluminum Subacetate Solution.*
Dose—**1** to **10 Gm** daily; *usual,* **1 Gm** 4 to 6 times a day.
Dosage Forms—Tablets NF: 600 mg and 1 Gm.
Veterinary Dose—*Horses,* 30 to **120 Gm;** *Cattle,* **120** to **360 Gm;** *Sheep* and *Swine,* **7.5** to **15 Gm;** *Dogs,* **650 mg** to **4 Gm.**

Calcium Hydroxide Solution—see page 1364.

Calcium Phosphate, Dibasic—see page 839.

Calcium Phosphate, Tribasic—see page 839.

Cholestyramine Resin USP

[Cuemid (*MSD*); Questran (*Mead-Johnson*)]

Cholestyramine Resin is a strongly basic anion-exchange resin in the chloride form, consisting of styrene–divinylbenzene copolymer with quaternary ammonium functional groups. Each Gm exchanges 1.8–2.2 Gm of sodium glycocholate, calculated on the dried basis.

Preparation—Polystyrene trimethylbenzylammonium chloride is copolymerized through cross-linkage with divinylbenzene.

Description—A white to buff-colored, hygroscopic, fine powder. It is odorless or has not more than a slight amine-like odor. Its pH is between 4 and 5, in a slurry (1 in 100).

Solubility—Slightly soluble in water and alcohol; insoluble in benzene, chloroform, and ether.

Uses—Cholestyramine Resin, an ion-exchange resin with an affinity for bile salts, is used for the relief of pruritis associated with bile stasis which occurs in biliary cirrhosis and with various forms of partial obstructive jaundice. The safe use of Cholestyramine Resin during pregnancy has not been established. Chronic use may be associated with a tendency to increased bleeding; hyperchloremic acidosis may also occur.

Dose—10 to **16 Gm** daily; *usual*, **4 Gm** 3 times a day.

Dosage Forms—USP: 4 Gm.

Dihydroxyaluminum Aminoacetate NF

[Basic Aluminum Glycinate; (Glycinato)dihydroxyaluminum; Alglyn (*Brayten*); Alzinox (*Patch*); Robalate (*Robins*)]

Dihydroxyaluminum Aminoacetate yields 35.5–38.5% of Al_2O_3 [Aluminum oxide = 101.96], calculated on the dried basis. Dihydroxyaluminum Aminoacetate ($H_2NCH_2COOAl(OH)_2.xH_2O$) may contain small amounts of aluminum oxide and of aminoacetic acid. The mol wt of the anhydrous salt ($C_2H_6AlNO_4$) is 135.05.

Preparation—The compound precipitates on adding a solution of aluminum isopropoxide in propanol to an aqueous solution of glycine.

Description—A white, odorless powder having a faintly sweet taste. The pH of a 1 in 25 aqueous suspension is between 6.5 and 7.5.

Solubility—Insoluble in water and inorganic solvents; dissolves in dilute mineral acids and in solutions of fixed alkalies.

Uses—Dihydroxyaluminum Aminoacetate is administered orally as an *antacid* in the medical management of *peptic ulcer*. Its actions are almost identical with those of the aluminum hydroxide gel preparations and it has the same advantages and disadvantages. Although Dihydroxyaluminum Aminoacetate is claimed to act somewhat more rapidly than the dried aluminum hydroxide gel, and to be less constipating because of its lower aluminum content, these differences do not appear to be great.

The drug may be employed as a constituent of almost any regimen to control *gastric hyperacidity*. Substitution of another form of antacid therapy may occasionally be necessary to alleviate the constipation which may occur after prolonged use of any of the aluminum preparations.

Dose—**500 mg** to **2 Gm**; *usual*, **500 mg** to **1 Gm** 4 times a day.

Other Dose Information—The dose is 500 mg to 1.0 Gm, in tablet form, usually taken between meals and at bedtime, or alternated with small feedings of milk or similar food.

Dosage Forms—Magma NF: 500 mg/5 ml; Tablets NF: 500 mg.

Dihydroxyaluminum Sodium Carbonate NF

[Aluminum Sodium Carbonate Hydroxide; Rolaids (*Am. Chicle*)]

$$(HO)_2AlOCO_2Na$$

Dihydroxyaluminum Sodium Carbonate [$CH_2AlNaO_5.xH_2O$ = 144.00 (anhydrous)], dried to constant weight at 130°, contains the equivalent of 34.8–38.2% of Al_2O_3 (aluminum oxide), and the equivalent of 28.5–31.5% of CO_2 (carbon dioxide).

Preparation—Aluminum isopropoxide is reacted with a basic solution of sodium bicarbonate. US Pat. 2,783,179.

Description—A fine, white powder that is odorless and tasteless. It is stable in light, slightly hygroscopic at room temperature, and dehydrates and loses CO_2 above 100°.

Solubility—Practically insoluble in water, alcohol, and other organic solvents unless a reaction occurs with an acidic group.

Uses—Dihydroxyaluminum Sodium Carbonate is a single molecule which combines the antacid properties of aluminum hydroxide and sodium bicarbonate. It has a rapid onset of action as gastric acid reacts with the sodium carbonate portion of the molecule; this is followed by a sustained, but less intense, antacid action due to the generated aluminum hydroxide.

Dose—*Usual*, **300** to **600 mg** as required.

Dosage Forms—Tablets NF: 300 mg (anhydrous).

Magaldrate NF

[Tetrakis(hydroxymagnesium)decahydroxydialuminate dihydrate; Riopan (*Ayerst*)]

$$[Mg(OH)_4] [(HO)_4 Al(OH) (HO)Al(OH)_4] . 2HO$$

Magaldrate is a chemical combination of aluminum hydroxide and magnesium hydroxide, corresponding to the approximate formula of $Al_2H_{14}Mg_4O_{14}.2H_2O$ (425.32). It contains the equivalent of 28.0–39.0% of MgO (magnesium oxide), and the equivalent of 17.0–25.0% of Al_2O (aluminum oxide).

Preparation—Magaldrate is prepared by precipitation using aqueous solutions of sodium or potassium aluminate and a magnesium salt under controlled conditions of concentration and temperature. The precipitated product is collected by filtration, washed to remove soluble byproducts, and dried. US Pat. 2,923,660. The formulas shown above have been suggested although the substance is also described as an indefinite mixture of magnesium and aluminum hydroxides.

Description—A white, odorless, crystalline powder.

Solubility—Insoluble in water and alcohol; soluble in dilute solutions of mineral acids.

Uses—Magaldrate, a chemical combination of magnesium and aluminum hydroxides, is used as an *antacid*. It is employed in gastric or duodenal ulcer, gastritis, heartburn, gastrointestinal disorders resulting from dietary indiscretions, food intolerance, excessive smoking, or alcoholic stimulation. It is also useful for the management of hyperacidity associated with corticosteroid therapy or administration of ulcerogenic drugs. It neutralizes gastric acidity within 15 minutes after oral administration; gastric acidity usually returns to pretreatment levels within 45 minutes. Magaldrate disturbs neither electrolyte balance nor bowel function.

Dose—*Usual,* **400** to **800 mg** of magaldrate as required, preferably taken between meals and at bedtime.

Dosage Forms—Oral Suspension NF: 400 mg/5 ml; Tablets NF: 400 mg.

Magnesia and Alumina Oral Suspension USP

[Maalox (*Rorer*)]

Magnesia and Alumina Oral Suspension is a mixture containing magnesium hydroxide [Mg(OH$_2$)], and variable amounts of aluminum oxide [Al$_2$O$_3$] in the form of aluminum hydroxide and hydrated aluminum oxide. It contains 3.4–4.2% of magnesium hydroxide [Mg(OH)$_2$], and the equivalent of 2.0–2.4% of aluminum oxide [Al$_2$O$_3$]. It contains 5.4–6.6% of combined magnesium hydroxide [Mg(OH)$_2$] and aluminum oxide [Al$_2$O$_3$]. It may contain a flavoring agent, and may contain suitable antimicrobial agents in a total amount not exceeding 0.5%.

Preparation—See *Alumina and Magnesia Oral Suspension,* page 787.

Description—Its pH is between 7.3 and 8.3.

Uses—Magnesia and Alumina Oral Suspension is used as an *antacid.* The magnesia, in addition to its antacid properties, is intended to counteract the constipating effect of the aluminum hydroxide.

This product contains approximately ½ as much aluminum oxide and hydroxide as magnesium hydroxide, but the combined aluminum oxide and magnesium hydroxide content is the same (5.3 to 6.6%) as that in *Alumina and Magnesia Oral Suspension USP* (page 787). Thus, the neutralizing capacityo f the two preparations is essentially the same.

Dose—**5** to **120 ml** daily; *usual,* **15 ml** 4 to 6 times a day.

Dosage Forms—Oral Suspension USP; Tablets USP: *of each ingredient*—200 and 200 mg, 400 and 400 mg.

Magnesium Carbonate NF

[Light Magnesium Carbonate; Heavy Magnesium Carbonate; Magnesium Carbonate Hydroxde; Magnesii Carbonas Ponderosus; Magnesii Carbonas Levis; Carbonate of Magnewia]

Magnesium Carbonate is a basic hydrated magnesium carbonate [approximately 4MgCO$_3$.Mg(OH)$_2$.5H$_2$O = 485.65] or a normal hydrated magnesium carbonate [MgCO$_3$.H$_2$O = 102.33]. It contains the equivalent of 40.0–43.5% of MgO (magnesium oxide).

Medicinal Magnesium Carbonate is available in *light* and *heavy* forms; the light, which is 2 to 2½ times as bulky as the heavy, is the most commonly used. The NF recognizes both under the one title.

Preparation—Magnesium Carbonate is largely prepared from *dolomite* [MgCO$_3$.CaCO$_3$] by first calcining it, suspending the calcined product in water and saturating with CO$_2$ under pressure. Some lime also dissolves as calcium bicarbonate, but when the temperature, after the treatment with carbon dioxide, is raised, nearly all of the dissolved lime precipitates as the insoluble carbonate. The filtered solution is then heated to the boiling temperature whereupon the magnesium

bicarbonate loses CO$_2$ and H$_2$O and magnesium carbonate precipitates. This process generally yields the light carbonate.

The heavy carbonate is generally produced by precipitating a hot, concentrated solution of magnesium chloride or sulfate with a solution of sodium carbonate.

Description—Light, white, friable masses, or as a bulky, white powder. It is odorless, but it readily absorbs odors. It is stable in air.

Solubility—Practically insoluble in water, to which however, it imparts an alkaline reaction, but it is appreciably soluble in water containing carbon dioxide; insoluble in alcohol; dissolved by dilute acids with effervescence.

Incompatibilities—*Acids* dissolve Magnesium Carbonate with the liberation of carbon dioxide. A slight alkalinity is imparted to water and suspensions of it will cause precipitation of free *alkaloids* from solutions of alkaloidal salts.

Uses—Magnesium Carbonate is an effective *antacid* and *cathartic* with pharmacologic properties similar to magnesium oxide. It differs from the latter, however, in that carbon dioxide is liberated during neutralization. As an antacid, it is usually alternated with calcium carbonate to overcome the constipating action of the latter salt.

Dose—*Usual,* **500 mg** to **2 Gm** 4 times a day.

Veterinary Dose—*Foals, Calves,* and *Pigs,* **4** to **15 Gm**; *Dogs,* **300 mg** to **4 Gm.**

Magnesium Hydroxide NF

Magnesium Hydroxide, dried at 105° for 2 hours, contains 95.0–100.5% of Mg(OH)$_2$ (58.32).

Preparation—Magnesium Hydroxide is prepared by precipitation using aqueous solutions of magnesium chloride or sulfate and sodium hydroxide. US Pat. 3,127,241. A method for preparing it in various particle sizes is described in US Pat. 3,232,708.

Description—A white, very fine, bulky powder. It slowly absorbs carbon dioxide on exposure to air.

Solubility—Practically insoluble in water and in alcohol, but it dissolves in dilute acids.

Uses—Magnesium Hydroxide has the same uses as *Magnesium Oxide.*

Dose—*Usual,* antacid, **300** to **600 mg**; *cathartic,* **2** to **4 Gm.**

Dosage Forms—Magnesia Tablets USP: 300 mg.

Veterinary Dose—*Foals, Calves,* and *Pigs,* **12** to **20 Gm**; *Dogs,* **1** to **6 Gm.**

Milk of Magnesia USP [Magnesium Hydroxide Mixture; Cream of Magnesia; Magnesia Magma USP XVI] is a suspension of magnesium hydroxide, each 100 Gm of which contains 7.0–8.5% of Mg(OH)$_2$ (58.32). It may contain 0.1% of citric acid, and may contain not more than 0.05% of a volatile oil or a blend of volatile oils, suitable for flavoring purposes. *Note*—The citric acid is allowed to minimize the interaction of glass containers and this preparation. No formula is now included in the USP as there are various satisfactory methods of preparation and any one of these may be used if the finished product conforms to the official specifications. *Description:* A white, opaque, more or less viscous suspension from which varying proportions of water usually separate on standing. It has a pH of about 10. It absorbs carbon dioxide from the air. It is alkaline to litmus and to phenolphthalein. *Incompatibilities:* The fact is occasionally overlooked that milk of magnesia has an alkaline reaction and possesses the incompatibilities typical of such a reaction. Thus, *alkaloids* are liberated from solutions of their salts. *Uses:* Milk of Magnesia is a nonsystemic gastric *antacid* and mild *cathartic.* When used routinely as an antacid, the cathartic effect may be minimized by the occasional use of calcium carbonate. *Dose: 5 to 50 ml daily; usual antacid, 5 ml 4 times a day; usual, cathartic, 15 to 30 ml; Veterinary Dose: Dogs: antacid, 2 to 5 ml; laxative, 8 to 15 ml.*

Magnesium Oxide USP

[Magnesia; Light Magnesia; Calcined Magnesia; Magnesii Oxidum Leve; Magnesii Oxidum Ponderosum; Heavy Magnesium Oxide; Heavy Magnesia; Heavy Calcined Magnesia; Magnesia Usta]

Magnesium Oxide, after ignition, contains 96.0–100.5% of MgO (40.30).

Preparation—Light or Heavy Magnesium Carbonate is exposed to a red heat whereupon carbon dioxide and water are expelled, and Light or Heavy Magnesium Oxide is left. The density of the oxide is also influenced by the calcining temperature, higher temperatures yielding more compact forms.

Description—A very bulky, white powder known as Light Magnesium Oxide or as a relatively dense, white powder known as Heavy Magnesium Oxide. See the USP for relative densities. It readily absorbs moisture and carbon dioxide when exposed to air.

Solubility—Practically insoluble in water to which, however, it imparts an alkaline reaction; insoluble in alcohol, but soluble in dilute acids.

Incompatibilities—Magnesium Oxide hydrates slowly in contact with moisture and, in the presence of a limited amount of *water*, sets to a mass of cement-like hardness. In liquid mixtures, glycerin is frequently used to overcome this tendency. Although Magnesium Oxide has been recommended as a diluent for liquefying ingredients in capsules, it may be objectionable due to the formation of a concrete mass. Magnesium carbonate is generally more satisfactory for the purpose.

Uses—Magnesium Oxide is a popular nonsystemic gastric *antacid* and possesses several desirable features.

It does not neutralize gastric contents excessively and does not liberate carbon dioxide, besides being fairly long acting. It is sometimes employed as a *cathartic*. Either the light or heavy form may be employed.

Light magnesia is preferable to the heavy for administration in liquids because, being a finer powder, it suspends more readily.

Dose—250 mg to 4 Gm daily; *usual*, **250 mg** 4 times a day.

Veterinary Dose—*Foals, Calves,* and *Pigs,* 8 to 15 Gm; *Dogs,* 600 mg to 4 Gm.

Magnesium Phosphate NF

[Tribasic Magnesium Phosphate NF XII]

Magnesium Phosphate [Mg$_3$(PO$_4$)$_2$.5H$_2$O = 352.93], ignited to constant weight, contains 98.0–101.5% of Mg$_3$(PO$_4$)$_2$ (262.86).

Preparation—It is made by precipitation using aqueous solutions of tribasic sodium phosphate and magnesium sulfate or chloride. The precipitate of Magnesium Phosphate is washed with water until practically free of sulfate and then dried at a low temperature.

Description—A white, odorless, and tasteless powder.

Solubility—Almost insoluble in water but is readily soluble in diluted mineral acids.

Uses—Magnesium Phosphate is an *antacid* used like *Tribasic Calcium Phosphate* (page 839). It neutralizes the excess acid of the stomach but produces no excess alkalinization of the system. It has a mild laxative action.

Dose—*Usual,* 1 Gm.

Magnesium Trisilicate USP

[Hydrated Magnesium Silicate; Trisomin (*Lilly*)]

Magnesium Trisilicate [2MgO.3SiO$_2$.xH$_2$O] [molecular weight (anhydrous) = 260.86] is a compound of magnesium oxide and silicon dioxide with varying proportions of water. It contains not less than 20.0% of magnesium oxide [MgO = 40.30] and not less than 45.0% of silicon dioxide [SiO$_2$ = 60.08].

Preparation—Magnesium Trisilicate is produced by precipitating a solution of sodium silicate of the proper composition [Na$_4$Si$_3$O$_8$, or having a ratio of Na$_2$O to SiO$_2$ = 1:1.5] with a solution of magnesium chloride or sulfate. The precipitate of the Magnesium Trisilicate is filtered, washed, and dried at a low temperature.

Description—A fine, white, odorless, tasteless powder, free from grittiness. Its suspension is neutral or only slightly alkaline to litmus.

Solubility—Insoluble in water and in alcohol; readily decomposed by mineral acids with the liberation of silicic acid.

Uses—Magnesium Trisilicate is an effective nonsystemic antacid and adsorbent. The drug is considered to be completely innocuous when taken by mouth. However, a case of siliceous nephrolith has been reported following chronic use. Large doses may cause diarrhea due to the action of the soluble magnesium salts on the enteric tract.

Dose—1 to **16 Gm** daily; *usual*, **1 Gm** 4 times a day.

Dosage Forms—Tablets USP: 500 mg.

Potassium Bicarbonate USP

[Bicarbonate of Potash; Potassium Acid Carbonate]

Potassium Bicarbonate contains 99.0–101.0% of KHCO$_3$ (100.12), calculated on the dried basis.

Preparation—This salt is made by passing carbon dioxide through a solution of potassium carbonate, preferably under pressure, until it is fully saturated, and concentrating the solution by evaporation to the crystallization point at a temperature below 71° (160°F) to prevent decomposition.

Salæratus is a crude potassium bicarbonate obtained by suspending a dish containing a concentrated solution of potassium carbonate within the fermenting tuns of a brewery; the carbon dioxide produced during fermentation is thus utilized.

Description—Colorless, transparent, monoclinic prisms, or as a white, granular powder. It is odorless, and has a saline and slightly alkaline taste. It is stable in air. Its aqueous solutions are neutral or alkaline to phenolphthalein TS. It is readily decomposed even by diluted acids.

Solubility—1 Gm dissolves in 2.8 ml of water; practically insoluble in alcohol.

Incompatibilities—See *Sodium Bicarbonate* (below).

Uses—Potassium Bicarbonate is occasionally employed as a *gastric antacid*. However, it is more expensive than sodium bicarbonate and moreover the potassium ion is more toxic than the sodium ion. The salt is therefore seldom prescribed. Potassium Bicarbonate also has been used occasionally as a *diuretic*. Potassium Bicarbonate is an acceptable product for the administration of potassium in states of potassium depletion only if a source of chloride is also provided.

Dose—**500 mg to 8 Gm** daily; *usual,* **1 Gm** 4 times a day.

Sodium Bicarbonate USP

[Baking Soda;   Sodium Acid Carbonate;   Natrium Bicarbonicum]

Sodium Bicarbonate contains 99.0–100.5% of Na-HCO₃ (84.01), calculated on the dried basis.

Preparation—Sodium Bicarbonate is largely produced by the ammonia-soda process, or *Solvay Process*, as it is usually called. In this process carbon dioxide is passed into a solution of common salt in ammonia water, Sodium Bicarbonate is precipitated, and ammonium chloride, being much more soluble, remains in solution. The ammonium chloride solution is heated with lime whereby the ammonia is regenerated and returned to the process.

Description—A white, crystalline powder. It is odorless and has a saline and slightly alkaline taste. Its solutions, when freshly prepared with cold water without shaking, are alkaline to litmus paper. Its alkalinity increases as the solutions stand, are agitated, or heated. It is stable in dry air, but slowly decomposes in moist air.

Solubility—1 Gm dissolves in 10 ml of water; with hot water it is converted into carbonate; insoluble in alcohol.

Incompatibilities—Sodium Bicarbonate is decomposed by *acids* and *salts having an acid reaction* with the liberation of carbon dioxide. Acid-reacting vehicles are troublesome in this respect, as are some tinctures, fluidextracts, and solutions. *Heating* or *agitating* the aqueous solution partially converts it to the normal carbonate with evolution of carbon dioxide. Sodium Bicarbonate intensifies the darkening which occurs in solutions of *salicylates*. Some *alkaloids* are precipitated from solutions of their salts.

In powder mixtures, atmospheric moisture or water of crystallization from another ingredient sometimes permits Sodium Bicarbonate to react with *boric acid* or a salt such as *alum*. In liquid mixtures containing *bismuth subnitrate*, Sodium Bicarbonate reacts with the acid formed by hydrolysis of the bismuth salt.

Uses—Sodium Bicarbonate is widely employed as a gastric *antacid* and in combating systemic acidosis. The salt is also of great value when it is desirable to render the urine alkaline. As a gastric antacid, Sodium Bicarbonate possesses several outstanding disadvantages. Its reaction with hydrochloric acid results in the production of carbon dioxide, thus giving rise to epigastric distress. Although the onset of action is rapid, the duration of action is short. Sodium Bicarbonate is readily absorbed and thus will produce systemic alkalosis. For these reasons, other gastric antacids are preferred.

In the treatment of *systemic acidosis*, Sodium Bicarbonate is specific in that the salt is composed of the two ions essential to correct this condition.

Sodium Bicarbonate is used locally on the skin in the form of a moist paste or a solution. In this form, it is an effective *antipruritic*. The salt is also an ingredient of many effervescent mixtures, alkaline solutions, douches, etc.

Dose—**300 mg to 16 Gm** daily; *usual*, **300 mg** to **2 Gm** 1 to 4 times a day.

Dosage Forms—Injection USP: 1%/20 ml, 1.4 and 5%/500 ml, 7.5%/50 ml, 8.4%/30 ml; Tablets USP: 300 and 600 mg.

Veterinary Dose—*Horses*, 25 to 50 Gm; *Cattle*, 50 to 100 Gm; *Sheep, Goats,* and *Swine,* 2 to 5 Gm; *Dogs*, 200 mg to 1 Gm.

Other Gastric Antacids

Aluminum Carbonate, Basic [Basaljel (*Wyeth*)] is an aqueous suspension of an aluminum hydroxide carbonate prepared by the interaction of soluble aluminum salts and soluble carbonates. It contains the equivalent of 5.1% of Al₂O₃ and not less than 2.4% of CO₂. *Description:* A white, creamy, thixotropic gel having a pH of 6.6 to 7.0. The preparation, if not kept in tightly closed containers, gradually loses CO₂. *Uses:* To control gastric hyperacidity and as an adjunct in the treatment of peptic ulcer. On a weight basis, its neutralizing power exceeds that of aluminum hydroxide. It is about ⅓ more effective than aluminum hydroxide in binding phosphate and is the agent of choice in the management of nephrolithiasis when the stones are composed of phosphate salts. It combines with the phosphate ion in the intestinal tract to form insoluble aluminum phosphate which is excreted in the stool. When combined with a low phosphorus diet, it keeps the urine relatively free of phosphate; it is thereby of value in individuals who suffer from recurrent stone formation. The drug is relatively nontoxic. It has a tendency to produce constipation which can easily be controlled with a mild laxative. There are no reported contraindications to its use. *Dose:* As an antacid, the average adult oral dose of the drug is 8 ml, repeated every 2 to 4 hours as necessary to control gastric hyperacidity. In the management of phosphatic urinary calculi, larger doses (30 ml 4 times daily) are used to combine with phosphate in the intestine and decrease phosphate absorption.

Ammonium Bicarbonate BP [NH₄HCO₃]—White crystals or crystalline powder, easily decomposed by heat. Soluble in water; insoluble in alcohol. *Uses:* Antacid and stimulant. *Dose:* 0.3 to 1 Gm.

Chalk, Prepared NF XI [Chalk; Drop Chalk]—A native form of calcium carbonate freed from most of its impurities by elutriation, and contains, after drying, not less than 97% CaCO₃. *Uses:* An Antacid, and employed in the treatment of diarrhea. *Dose:* Usual, 1 Gm. *Veterinary Dose:* horses and cattle, 30 to 60 Gm; dogs, 300 mg to 2 Gm.

Gastric Mucin—The fraction precipitated by approximately 60% alcohol from the supernatant liquid after pepsin–hydrochloric acid digestion of hog stomach linings. Gastric mucin is a white to yellow powder or brownish yellow granules. It has a slightly salty taste and characteristic odor indicative of peptones. Both forms yield a viscous gray, opalescent solution when triturated with water. *Uses:* Used in the treatment of peptic ulcer. Currently available preparations of gastric mucin do not effectively neutralize gastric acidity in man. *Dose:* Average dose 2.5 Gm, which can be given at 2-hour intervals.

Polyamine-Methylene Resin [Resinat (*National Drug*)] is an anion-exchange resin described commercially as a polyethylene polyamine methylene substituted resin of diphenylol dimethylmethane (4,4′-isopropylidenediphenol) and formaldehyde in basic form. *Description and Solubility:* A light-amber, granular, freely flowing powder without appreciable odor. Insoluble in water, alcohol, ether, and aqueous solutions of acids and alkalies. *Uses:* For control of symptoms in simple hyperchlorhydria and peptic ulcer. The antacid effect results from temporary binding in the stomach of gastric hydrochloric acid and pepsin which are later released in the intestine. The resin is eliminated unchanged from the gastrointestinal tract without permanent ionic disturbance of the body fluids. *Dose:* For the relief of symptoms in acute or chronic peptic ulcer, 0.5 to 1 Gm in milk or other liquid orally every 2 hours.

Digestants

Digestants are drugs which promote the process of digestion in the gastrointestinal tract. They have limited usefulness in the treatment of conditions characterized by a deficiency of one or more of the specific substances essential for the digestion of foodstuffs in the alimentary canal. Thus, in a general way, they may be classified as drugs used for replacement therapy in deficiency states. The digestants commonly employed are the *choleretics* (bile, bile acids, bile salts) and hydrochloric acid.

Although bile is composed of a variety of substances, only the bile salts (salts of the native bile acids, see this page) are therapeutically important. When given by mouth the bile salts are absorbed from the intestine and re-excreted by the liver in the bile, thus entering the same cyclic process as endogenous bile salts. They are of value in promoting the absorption of fats and fat-soluble vitamins (see Chapter 56, page 1011) from the intestinal tract when the normal biliary output is either reduced or absent.

Hydrochloric acid exerts several physiological functions in the gastrointestinal tract. It converts pepsinogen to active pepsin, renders gastric contents relatively sterile, plays a role in the normal emptying of the stomach, aids in the secretion of intestinal and pancreatic juices, and, finally, is essential for the absorption of certain inorganic salts. Gastric hydrochloric acid secretion is deficient in 10 to 15% of the general population. This condition is commonly called *hypochlorhydria*. *Achlorhydria* is frequently associated with gastritis, gastric carcinoma, pernicious anemia, etc. It may also be present in individuals with no demonstrable gastric lesion. Symptoms usually attributed to achlorhydria include vague epigastric distress, belching, abdominal distention, coated tongue, nausea, vomiting, and diarrhea. Hydrochloric acid or its substitutes are effective in relieving such deficiency symptoms in a significant number of individuals.

Bile, Bile Acids, and Bile Salts

The bile, a viscid, bitter, alkaline (pH 7.8), fluid, isotonic with the blood and yellowish brown to a golden yellow in color, is excreted by adults at the rate of 500 to 1100 ml in 24 hours. The principal organic constituents are bile acids (as salts), bile pigments, cholesterol, lecithin, mucin, neutral fats, nucleoproteins, and phosphatides. The principal inorganic constituents are sodium, calcium, copper, iron, magnesium, potassium, bicarbonate, phosphate, and sulfate.

The bile acids, present as the sodium salts of a mixture of acids, are divided into two groups: (1) the *glycocholic acids* and (2) the *taurocholic acids*. The first group consists of the various cholic acids combined through peptide linkages at their COOH groups with the amino acid *glycine* [H_2NCH_2COOH] and the second group consists of the cholic acids combined in a similar manner with *taurine* [$H_2NCH_2CH_2SO_3H$].

The predominant cholic acids represented in bile are cholic, desoxycholic, and lithocholic. The structural relationships among these and their parent molecule, 5β-cholanic acid, are shown below. The essentially synthetic dehydrocholic acid is included for comparison.

5β-Cholanic Acid

[5β-cholan-24-oic acid]

Cholic Acid—3α,7α,12α-Trihydroxy-5β-cholanic Acid
Deoxycholic Acid—3α,12α-Dihydroxy-5β-cholanic Acid
Lithocholic Acid—3α-Hydroxy-5β-cholanic Acid
Dehydrocholic Acid—3,7,12-Trioxo-5β-cholanic Acid

The composition of bile varies considerably with the species of animal; the glycocholates predominate in human bile whereas the reverse is true of the bile of carnivora. The bile salts can be isolated as stable crystals soluble in water. The free bile acids can be obtained; they are only slightly soluble in water. These acids combine with the fatty acids in varying proportions, depending on the size of the aliphatic acid molecule, by means of secondary valence forces to form *choleic acids*. The latter are responsible for emulsifying, dispersing, and thus promoting the absorption of fats, cholesterol, and the oil-soluble vitamins.

Dehydrocholic Acid NF

[3,7,12-Trioxo-5β-cholan-24-oic Acid; Cholan-DH (*Strasenburgh*); Decholin (*Dome*)]

Dehydrocholic Acid contains 98.5–101.0% of $C_{24}H_{34}O_5$ (402.54), calculated on the dried basis. Dehydrocholic Acid for parenteral use melts between 237° and 242°.

Preparation—Dehydrocholic Acid has been isolated in minute quantities from cow's bile. It is readily prepared from cholic acid, the main steroid constituent of ox bile, by oxidation with chromic acid in acetic and sulfuric acid solution. The use of a large excess chromic acid assures complete oxidation of all the hydroxyl groups to keto groups.

Description—A white, fluffy, odorless, bitter powder. Melting range 231° to 242°, with a range of not more than 3° for a given sample. The higher the melting temperature, the greater is the purity.

Solubility—Practically insoluble in water; slightly soluble in ether and methanol; 1 Gm dissolves in about 100 ml of alcohol and in about 35 ml of chloroform; soluble in glacial acetic acid and in solutions of alkali hydroxides and carbonates.

Uses—Dehydrocholic Acid is the most potent *hydrocholeretic* known.

Dose—250 to **750 mg**; *usual*, **500 mg** 3 times a day.

Dosage Forms—Injection NF (as the sodium salt; see below): 500 mg/10 ml, 600 mg/3 ml, 1 Gm/5 ml, 2 Gm/10 ml; Tablets NF: 250 mg.

Sodium Dehydrocholate Injection NF [Decholin Sodium Injection (*Dome*)] is a sterile solution of $C_{24}H_{33}NaO_5$ (sodium dehydrocholate) in water for injection, usually prepared by neutralizing dehydrocholic acid for parenteral use. It contains 94.0–106.0% of the labeled amount of $C_{24}H_{33}NaO_5$. *Description:* Its pH is between 8.5 and 9.5. *Uses:* See *Dehydrocholic Acid* (above) and *Sodium Dehydrocholate* (page 795). *Dose: Usual, intravenous,* 3 to 5 ml of a 20% solution.

Glutamic Acid Hydrochloride NF

[Acidoride (*Abbott*); Acidulin (*Lilly*); Glutan HCl (*Lederle*)]

Glutamic Acid Hydrochloride, dried at 80° for 4 hours, contains 99.0–101.0% of $C_5H_9NO_4 \cdot HCl$ (183.59).

Description—A white crystalline powder. Its solution is acid to litmus. The *specific rotation* determined in 3.0 *N* hydrochloric acid solution (125 mg per ml) is not less than +23.5° and not more than +25.5°.

Solubility—1 Gm dissolves in about 3 ml of water; almost insoluble in alcohol and in ether.

Uses—Glutamic Acid Hydrochloride is administered orally as a source of hydrochloric acid in *achlorhydria* due to pernicious anemia or other causes, and in *hypochlorhydria*. Since it is administered in capsules, dental enamel is not exposed to the acid. It is less effective than free hydrochloric acid in lowering gastric pH. One 300-mg capsule contains approximately 1.7 mEq of hydrochloric acid.

Dose—*Usual*, **600 mg** to **1.8 Gm** during meals.

Dosage Forms—Capsules NF: 300 mg.

Veterinary Dose—In achlorhydria and hypochlorhydria of all species, ⅕ of the dose of Diluted Hydrochloric Acid.

Diluted Hydrochloric Acid NF

[Dilute Hydrochloric Acid]

Diluted Hydrochloric Acid contains, in each 100 ml, 9.5–10.5 Gm of HCl (36.46).

Diluted Hydrochloric Acid may be prepared as follows:

Hydrochloric Acid................	**234 ml**
Purified Water, a sufficient quantity,	
To make.......................	**1000 ml**

Mix the ingredients.

Description—A colorless, odorless liquid, strongly acid to litmus. Its specific gravity is about 1.05 at 25°.

Uses—Diluted Hydrochloric Acid is used in the treatment of *gastric achlorhydria* and *hypochlorhydria*.

Hydrochloric acid is often given in conjunction with iron therapy in the treatment of *hypochromic anemia*. In the treatment of pernicious anemia, it is also prescribed, if the accompanying achlorhydria gives rise to intestinal symptoms. See also *Glutamic Acid Hydrochloride* (above).

Dose—*Usual*, **5 ml**, well diluted in water.

Other Dose Information—The recommended dose may vary from 1 to 10 ml since there is no unanimity of opinion among physicians as to what constitutes an adequate dose. The acid should be diluted with water and sipped through a glass tube to prevent a solvent reaction upon the dental enamel. It is usually taken during or after meals.

Veterinary Dose—*Horses*, 4 to **10 ml**; *Cattle*, 10 to **20 ml**; *Dogs*, **0.3** to **0.6 ml**.

Malt Extract—see page 1348.

Pancreatin—see page 1051.

Pepsin—see page 1052.

Pepsin Elixir, Lactated—see page 1054.

Resorcinol—see page 1187.

Other Digestants

Betaine Hydrochloride [Lycine Hydrochloride, Oxyneurine Hydrochloride, Trimethylglycocoll Hydrochloride] [$C_5H_{11}NO_2.HCl$]—Crystals melting at about 227–228° with decomposition. Soluble 1:1.7 water and 1:20 alcohol. *Uses:* In water, slowly liberates its acid radical. Used as a substitute for hydrochloric acid in hypochlorhydria. A dose of 0.5 Gm corresponds to 1.1 ml diluted hydrochloric acid.

Deoxycholic Acid [Choleic Acid; Desoxycholic Acid; $3\alpha,12\alpha$-dihydroxy-5β-cholanic acid] $HC_{24}H_{39}O_4$—A steroid lacking the C-7 hydroxyl group of cholic acid. It occurs in the bile of man and of the herbivora. It is soluble to the extent of about 1:4000 in water and 1:5.5 in alcohol; soluble in solutions of alkali hydroxides or carbonates. It forms molecular coordination compounds (choleic acids) with many substances. *Uses:* Choleretic. *Dose:* 0.1 to 0.2 Gm.

Florantyrone [Zanchol (*Searle*)] is γ-oxo-8-fluoranthenebutyric acid [$C_{20}H_{14}O_3$]. *Description and Solubility:* Fine platelets which melt at 195°. Soluble in alcohol, methanol, and aqueous sodium carbonate solutions. *Uses:* A hydrocholeretic agent which has been proposed for the management of chronic inflammation of the gallbladder and bile ducts and in the prevention of biliary calculi. *Dose:* 750 mg to 1 Gm daily.

Sodium Dehydrocholate [Decholin Sodium (*Dome*)] [$C_{24}H_{33}NaO_5$]—Sodium salt of 3,7,12-trioxo-5β-cholanic acid. Colorless, crystalline powder having a very bitter taste, soluble in water and alcohol. *Uses:* Same as those for dehydrocholic acid; also useful diagnostic aid in the determination of arm-to-tongue circulation time. *Dose: intravenously*, 5 to 10 ml of a 20% solution followed by 10 ml on the second and third day; as diagnostic aid, 3 to 5 ml injected rapidly into cubital vein, time noted to bitter taste perception.

Sodium Glycocholate [$C_{26}H_{42}NNaO_6$]—A constituent of ox bile. White to yellowish, hygroscopic, and deliquescent powder with an unpleasant odor and bitter taste. Soluble in water and alcohol. *Uses:* A cholagogue. *Dose:* 0.2 to 0.3 Gm.

Sodium Succinate [$C_4H_4Na_2O_4.6H_2O$]—White, odorless, granules or crystalline powder. Soluble in about 5 parts water; insoluble in alcohol. *Uses:* Formerly used in catarrhal jaundice, gall stones, infection of gall bladder, and biliary passages. *Dose:* 0.3 Gm.

Sodium Taurocholate [$C_{26}H_{44}NNaO_7S$]—A constituent of ox bile. Yellowish gray powder, very soluble in water or alcohol. *Uses:* Choleretic. *Dose:* 120 to 400 mg.

Tocamphyl [$C_{23}H_{37}NO_6$ = 423.53] [Gallogen (*Massengill*); Syncuma (*Philips-Roxane*)] is *p*,α-dimethylbenzyl hydrogen camphorate, diethanolamine salt. *Preparation:* Camphoric anhydride is monoesterified with α,*p*-dimethylbenzyl alcohol and the resulting ester–acid is reacted with an equimolar quantity of diethanolamine. *Description and Solubility:* A pale-yellow to amber, unctuous mass with a faint, aromatic odor and a very bitter taste; it may be clear, or opaque, if crystallized; it is stable in light and air, and is nonhygroscopic; since it is a semiliquid, it has no definite melting point. Soluble in alcohol, acetone, ether, and chloroform; slowly soluble in water becoming turbid on dilution. *Uses:* To increase flow of bile, encourage activity of the gallbladder, and promote functional activity of the biliary system. It acts directly on the hepatic lobule and stimulates the liver to secrete bile. Consequently, it is useful whenever it is desirable to increase the flow of bile. It is a useful adjunct in the management of cholecystectomized patients and in colitis characterized by incomplete digestion of fats and carbohydrates. It is also useful in x-ray visualization to facilitate cholecystography by increasing the output of bile. Tocamphyl is contraindicated in patients with common bile duct obstructions, cholangitis, acute hepatitis, obstructive jaundice, and gallstones. *Dose:* 75 to 100 mg 3 times daily for 3 or 4 weeks; maintenance (adjust to patient's requirements), usually 75 to 100 mg daily.

Cathartics

Cathartics are drugs that facilitate the passage and elimination of feces from the colon and rectum. These agents have been exploited by the patent medicine industry probably more than any other group of drugs. As a result, many cases of both chronic constipation and bowel irritation have been induced by their indiscriminate use. There are only a few conditions in which the use of a *rectal evacuant* is indicated. Legitimate uses include the elimination of drug and food poisons, the medical induction of labor, the presence of painfully hard stools, the presence of certain anorectal lesions during late pregnancy and early puerperium, and the prevention of straining at stool in extreme hypertension, aneurysm, abdominal hernia, or recent coronary occlusion.

The cathartics are so numerous that they require classification. This has been done in a variety of ways. The drugs vary considerably in their intensity of action, and thus, have been classified as *laxatives*, *purgatives*, and *drastics*, in the order of increasing potency. They have also been grouped according to their site of action or the interval of time before they are effective. The most useful classification, however, is based on their mechanism of action. Hence, they are usually divided into four groups: *irritant (stimulant) cathartics*, *bulk cathartics*, *emollient cathartics*, and *fecal softeners*.

Irritant (Stimulant) Cathartics

The irritant (stimulant) cathartics act on the intestinal tract to increase its motor activity. For convenience the irritant cathartics may be divided into four groups: glycoside, resinous, irritant oil, and miscellaneous cathartics. The more commonly employed agents are the anthraquinone cathartics, *cascara sagrada* and *senna;* the diphenylmethane derivatives, *phenolphthalein* and *bisacodyl;* and *castor oil.* These agents have many characteristics in common; they increase peristalsis, cause griping and intestinal cramps, increase mucous secretion, and increase fluidity of the stool. Intensity of effect is related to dosage, but effective doses vary markedly from one individual to another.

The anthraquinone cathartics all contain characteristic derivatives which are present in the free state (aglycones) or in glycosidic combination with glucose, arabinose, or rhamnose. The major active constituents are anthraquinone or anthranol derivatives related to emodin (see below).

Emodin (Frangula Emodin)   **Chrysophanic Acid**

Aloe-Emodin   *iso*-**Emodin**

Their laxative action is generally attributed to the anthraquinone principles. The action of the drugs is also probably associated with the content of resinous principles, but it is possible that the resins contain the anthraquinones in combination.

Since the anthraquinone cathartics act only in the large intestine and since they reach this area through the circulation, the rate and intensity of the cathartic action of the individual drugs containing anthraquinone glycosides vary with a number of factors. Some of these are the rate at which the phenolic anthraquinones are liberated from glycosidic combination and the rate at which absorption occurs in the small intestine. These factors in turn may be influenced by other principles present in the drugs.

The anthraquinone principles may be transferred in sufficient amounts to exert a cathartic action in infants feeding naturally during lactation. Some of these principles are also excreted in the urine, eg, chrysophanic acid, which may color it yellow to violet hues depending on pH, and alarm the patient unless he is forewarned. Long continued use of these cathartics also blackens the rectal mucosa.

The *resinous cathartics* include colocynth, gamboge, ipomea, and jalap, and are generally considered too irritant for human use. These agents are quite irritant, produce profuse watery stools, and are toxic in high dosage. Their locus of action is the small intestine.

Castor oil is the only *irritant oil cathartic* important to modern therapeutics. In the small intestine this oil is hydrolyzed to liberate ricinoleic acid, a markedly irritant substance which is responsible for the cathartic action of castor oil.

The miscellaneous irritant cathartics covered in this section include glycerin suppositories, mild mercurous chloride, and phenolphthalein. Glycerin acts merely as a local irritant.

The precise mechanism of the cathartic action of mercurous chloride and phenolphthalein has not been elucidated but may be due to some selective chemical reaction with cellular enzymes. Phenolphthalein acts primarily on the colon.

Note—The use of cathartics to relieve gastrointestinal symptoms of unknown cause cannot be too emphatically condemned.

Irritant Glycoside Cathartics

Aloe USP

[Aloes]

Aloe is the dried juice of the leaves of *Aloe Perryi* Baker, known in commerce as Socotrine Aloe, or of *Aloe barbadensis* Miller (*Aloe vera* "Linné"), known in commerce as Curaçao Aloe, or of *Aloe ferox* Miller and hybrids of this species with *Aloe africana* Miller and *Aloe spicata* Baker, known in commerce as Cape Aloe (Fam. *Liliaceæ*).

Aloe yields not less than 50% of water-soluble extractive.

Constituents—The active principles of Aloe are the pentosides (glycosides in which the sugar fragment is a pentose): *aloin* (barbaloin, socaloin, or capaloin) [$C_{20}H_{18}O_9$], *beta-barbaloin*, and *iso-barbaloin*. According to Viehoever the resin content of aloe is also an active constituent of the drug.

History—This drug was mentioned by Dioscorides in the first century of the Christian Era. He advised its use in doses of from 1 to 3 drams, especially for *urbani et literatim cupidi* (city men and men of letters) ie, those of sedentary habits. It was an ingredient in the ancient *hieras* (see *Powder of Aloes and Canella*) and in many compound pills and other laxative preparations.

Uses—Aloe is an ingredient in *Compound Benzoin Tincture USP*. Hence, it is categorized officially as a pharmaceutic aid. Nevertheless, Aloe is still widely employed as a cathartic, either alone or in a number of irrational mixtures. The active principle is aloin, a mixture of glycosides which upon hydrolysis in the intestine yields an anthraquinone derivative which is responsible for the cathartic action. The action of Aloe is accompanied by intestinal griping and pelvic vascular congestion. The latter property has given to Aloe the undeserved classification of an emmenagogue. The cathartic action of Aloe occurs 8 to 12 hours after ingestion.

Aloin is often combined with strychnine and belladonna as a cathartic mixture. *Mixtures of this type are irrational.* The purpose of the strychnine is to add tone to the smooth muscle of the bowel, an action which it does not possess. Belladonna is present to prevent griping, but this action would be manifest and over before the cathartic action of aloin is exerted. In the form of candy-covered pills such mixtures have often been the cause of fatal strychnine poisoning in children. The dose is 120 to 250 mg.

The use of Aloe as a cathartic is irritational and should be abandoned.

Veterinary Dose—*Cathartic, Horses*, **15 to 50 Gm** as a single dose.

Cascara Sagrada USP

[Rhamnus Purshiana; Sacred Bark; Chittem; Dogwood; Coffeeberry; Bear-berry; Bitter Bark; Bear-wood]

Cascara Sagrada is the dried bark of *Rhamnus purshiana* De Candolle (Fam. *Rhamnaceæ*).

Note—*Cascara Sagrada should be collected at least one year prior to use.*

Constituents—The identity of the active principles of cascara has engaged the attention of several investigators, and the following substances isolated from the drug have been reported: *Aloe-emodin* (1,8-dihydroxy-3-hydroxymethylanthraquinone), *chrysophanic acid* (1,8-dihydroxy-3-methylanthraquinone), *iso-emodin* (3,5,8-trihydroxy-2-methylanthraquinone), *methylhydrocotoin* (2,4,6-trimethoxybenzophenone), and *purshianin*, a glycoside forming red-brown crystals, melting at 237°. Cascara also contains several *resins*, one of which is very bitter and gives a bright-red color with potassium hydroxide solution.

Uses—Cascara Sagrada is a widely used *cathartic*. Of its several official preparations, the fluidextract or aromatic fluidextract is perhaps the most effective. The action of cascara is mild and is unaccompanied by discomfort or griping. Indeed, it is the least griping of the emodin cathartics. A therapeutic dose causes a single evacuation of the bowel in approximately 8 hours. The stool may be solid or semifluid. Prolonged ingestion of cascara frequently results in characteristic melanotic pigmentation of the rectal mucosa.

Note—When ground Cascara Sagrada is moistened and mixed with magnesium or calcium hydroxide the drug loses its intensely bitter taste, the acid constituents being neutralized and apparently rendered insoluble. Such treatment seems to lessen its activity.

Veterinary Dose—*Dogs*, **300 mg to 2 Gm.**

Cascara Sagrada Extract NF [Cascara Dry Extract; Powdered Cascara Sagrada Extract; Rhamnus Purshiana Extract]—One Gm of Cascara Sagrada Extract represents 3 Gm of cascara sagrada. *Preparation:* Mix cascara sagrada in coarse powder (900 Gm), with boiling water (4000 ml), and macerate the mixture during 3 hours. Then transfer it to a percolator, allow it to drain, and exhaust it by percolation, using boiling water as the menstruum and collecting about 5000 ml of percolate. Evaporate the percolate to dryness, reduce the extract to a fine powder, and add sufficient starch, dried at 100°, to make the product weigh 300 Gm. Mix the powders thoroughly and pass the Extract through a fine sieve. *Dose: Usual, 300 mg. Veterinary Dose: Dogs, 120 to 500 mg; Cats, 15 to 250 mg.*

Cascara Sagrada Fluidextract NF [Cascara Liquid Extract; Rhamnus Purshiana Fluidextract]—*Preparation:* with cascara sagrada (in very coarse powder, 1000 Gm), prepare a fluidextract by Process D (page 1591). Evaporate the percolate until it measures 800 ml, and when it is cold, gradually add 200 ml of alcohol and, if necessary, sufficient water to make the product measure 1000 ml. Mix thoroughly. *Alcohol Content:* From 17 to 19% of C_2H_5OH. *Uses:* A mild and effective *cathartic*, especially valuable because it does not produce habitual or after constipation. Its usefulness is limited because of its intensely bitter taste. See *Cascara Sagrada. Dose: Usual, 1 ml. Veterinary Dose: Dogs, 0.3 to 2 ml.*

Cascara Tablets NF are prepared from cascara sagrada extract. *Dose: Usual, 300 mg of Cascara Sagrada Extract.*

Aromatic Cascara Fluidextract USP [Aromatic Rhamnus Purshiana Fluidextract; Elixir of Cascara Sagrada]—*Preparation:* Mix cascara sagrada (in very coarse powder, 1000 Gm) with magnesium oxide (120 Gm), moisten it uniformly with boiling water (2000 ml), and set it aside in a shallow container for 48 hours, stirring it occasionally. Pack it in a percolator, and percolate with boiling water until the drug is exhausted. Evaporate the percolate, at a temperature not exceeding 100°, to 750 ml, and at once dissolve in it the pure glycyrrhiza extract (40 Gm). When the liquid has cooled, add alcohol (200 ml), in which saccharin (2 Gm), methyl salicylate (0.1 ml), anise oil (0.65 ml), and coriander oil (0.15 ml) have been dissolved, and finally add water (qs) to make 1000 ml, mix. *Alcohol Content:* From 17 to 19% of C_2H_5OH. *Uses:* This mild and effective cathartic is the most frequently employed form of cascara sagrada. The treatment with magnesium oxide (hydroxide in the presence of water) precipitates the acidic constituents and makes the preparation more palatable, particularly in the presence of the aromatic flavoring agents employed. The cathartic activity is also lessened. *Dose: 5 to 15 ml daily; usual, 5 ml. Veterinary Dose: Dogs, 0.3 to 4 ml.*

Danthron NF

[1,8-Dihydroxyanthraquinone; Chrysazin; Dorbane (*Riker*)]

Danthron contains 95.0–105.0% of $C_{14}H_8O_4$ (240.22).

Preparation—It may be prepared from anthraquinone as described in the synthesis of anthralin, page 773. Its chemical structure closely resembles the anthraquinone derivatives which exist in glycosidic combination in cascara sagrada and the other irritant glycoside cathartics.

Description—An orange colored crystalline powder. Melts between 190° and 195°. The ultraviolet absorbance, E (1%, 1 cm), determined in benzene solution at 432 mμ, is between 420 and 465.

Solubility—Practically insoluble in water; soluble in alcohol, in ether, in benzene, in chloroform, and in solutions of sodium hydroxide.

Uses—Danthron is a *cathartic* which produces a soft or semisolid stool in 6 to 8 hours. The drug is eliminated in the urine as a red dye. It has not gained wide acceptance in clinical medicine, but is used mainly in veterinary medicine. It also is an important intermediate in the manufacture of dyes and it forms lakes with calcium, barium, and lead.

Dose—*Usual*, **75 to 150 mg.**

Dosage Forms—Tablets NF: 75 mg.

Veterinary Dose—(As a bolus or electuary mixed with food or fluid) *Horses*, **14 to 38 Gm**; *Cattle*, **20 to 45 Gm**; *Goats* and *Sheep*, **4 to 6 Gm**; *Swine*, **10 to 20 Gm**; *Dogs*, **300 mg to 3 Gm**; *Cats*, **400 mg to 1 Gm.**

Senna NF

[Senna Leaf; Senna Leaves; Glysennid (*Sandoz*); Senokot (*Purdue-Frederick*)]

Senna consists of the dried leaflet of *Cassia acutifolia* Delile, known in commerce as Alexandria Senna, or of *Cassia angustifolia* Vahl, known in commerce as Tinnevelly Senna (Fam. *Leguminosæ*).

Constituents—The principal cathartic constituents of Senna are reported to be: *aloe-emodin* and *rhein* and their glycoside derivatives; *sennaemodin* and an emodin glycoside; *chrysophanic acid* (*chrysophanol*); *cathartic acid* (formerly believed to be the chief purgative principle; *cathartomannite*, and *sennanigrin*. Also present are *sennacrol, sennarhamnetin, kaempferol* [C₁₅H₁₀O₆], its glycoside *kaempferin*, and a small amount of an essential oil. When senna leaves are macerated in strong alcohol, the principles which produce griping and give odor and taste are said to be dissolved while the purgative properties are unaffected. Water and diluted alcohol are good solvents for its active principles.

Uses—Senna is an active *cathartic* causing a single thorough evacuation of the bowels within 6 hours after administration. Its action is usually accompanied by considerable griping.

Dose—*Usual*, **2 Gm.**

Veterinary Dose—*Horses* and *Cattle*, **120 to 150 Gm**; *Sheep* and *Swine*, **30 to 60 Gm**; *Dogs*, **2 to 8 Gm**; *Cats*, **1 to 6 Gm.** Rarely used in veterinary practice.

Senna Fluidextract NF [Fluidextractum Sennæ]—*Preparation:* With senna (in coarse powder, 1000 Gm), prepare a fluidextract by Process A (page 1591) using a mixture of 1 volume of alcohol and 2 volumes of water as the menstruum. Macerate the drug for 24 hours, then percolate at a moderate rate, and reserve the first 800 ml of percolate. *Alcohol Content:* From 23 to 27% of C₂H₅OH. *Uses:* A *cathartic*, frequently producing griping when used alone. It is chiefly used to make other preparations. *Dose: Usual*, 2 ml. *Veterinary Dose: Horses* and *Cattle*, 120 to 150 ml; *Sheep* and *Swine*, 30 to 60 ml; *Dogs*, 2 to 8 ml; *Cats*, 1 to 6 ml.

Senna Syrup NF [Syrupus Sennæ]—*Preparation:* Mix coriander oil (5 ml) with senna fluidextract (250 ml), and gradually add purified water (330 ml). Allow the mixture to stand for 24 hours in a cool place, with occasional agitation, then filter, and pass enough purified water through the filter to obtain 580 ml of filtrate. Dissolve the sucrose (635 Gm) in this liquid, and add sufficient purified water to make the product measure 1000 ml. Mix well and strain. *Alcohol Content:* From 5 to 7% of C₂H₅OH. *Uses:* Senna Syrup is used as a *cathartic*, frequently in combination with other drugs. *Dose: Usual*, 8 ml.

Other Irritant Glycoside Cathartics

Aloin NF XI—A mixture of active principles obtained from aloe. It varies in chemical composition and in physical and chemical properties according to the variety of aloe from which it is obtained. *Uses:* Obsolete cathartic, see *Aloe* (page 796). *Dose: Usual*, 15 mg.

Rhubarb NF XI [Rheum; Chinese Rhubarb; Rhubarb Root]—Consists of the dried rhizome and root of *Rheum officinale* Baillon, or *Rheum palmatum* Linné (Fam. *Polygonaceæ*), grown in China. It contains the active principles, emodin, aloe-emodin, rhein, and chrysophanic acid. *Uses:* A *cathartic*, unique in that its various preparations contain tannin and thus have an *astringent* as well as cathartic action. Consequently, its evacuant action may be followed by a period of constipation. The action is mild, accompanied by little discomfort or griping, and occurs from 4 to 8 hours after the administration of a cathartic dose. Rhubarb and its several preparations are no longer official. *Dose: Usual adult*, 1 Gm. *Veterinary Dose:* Laxative, *Foals* and *Calves*, 5 to 10 Gm; *Pigs*, 2 to 5 Gm; *Dogs*, 0.5 to 1 Gm.

Indian Rhubarb NF XI—Consists of the dried rhizome and root of *Rheum emodi* Wallich, of *Rheum Webbianum* Royle or of some other related species of *Rheum* native to India, Pakistan or Nepal. *Uses:* Introduced into the American market in large quantities during World War II when the varieties official at that time became unobtainable. *Dose: Usual*, 1 Gm.

Irritant Resinous Cathartics

Colocynth NF XI [Bitter Apple]—The dried pulp of the unripe but full-grown fruit of *Citrullus Colocynthis* (Linné) Schrader (Fam. *Cucurbitaceæ*). *Uses:* An intensely irritating resinous cathartic. It has no place in modern medicine either alone or in combination with other agents. *Dose:* 120 mg. *Veterinary Dose* (of Extract): *Swine*, 30 to 130 mg; *Dogs*, 8 to 16 mg.

Gamboge NF XI—The gum resin obtained from *Garcinia Hanburyi* Hooker filius (Fam. *Guttiferae*). *Uses:* An obsolete drastic hydragogue cathartic, usually given in combination with other cathartics. It may produce nausea and vomiting or griping when administered in the full dose. *Dose:* 125 mg. *Veterinary Dose* (with magnesium sulfate): *Cattle*, 15 to 30 Gm (the drug is too drastic for use in horses and dogs).

Ipomea NF XI [Orizaba Jalap; Mexican Scammony]—The dried root of *Ipomaea orizabensis* Ledenois (Fam. *Convolvulaceae*). *Uses:* Obsolete cathartic. It is usually administered in the form of its resin. *Dose:* 1 Gm.

Jalap NF XI [Jalap Root]—The dried tuberous root of *Exogonium purga* (Wenderoth) Bentham (Fam. *Convolvulaceæ*). *Uses:* An obsolete cathartic. Jalap is the least drastic of the resinous cathartics. It causes a fluid stool 3 to 4 hours after administration, with little gastrointestinal irritation. *Dose:* 1 Gm. *Veterinary Dose: Swine*, 4 to 15 Gm; *Dogs*, 300 mg to 4 Gm. (Seldom used; of minimal action in horses and cattle.)

Irritant Oil Cathartics

Only two official monographs fall in this category.

Castor Oil USP

[Oleum Ricini]

Castor Oil is the fixed oil obtained from the seed of *Ricinus communis* Linné (Fam. *Euphorbiaceæ*).

History—The *Palma Christi* tree, as the castor oil plant was called, has been identified as Jonah's Gourd. It is certain that the seeds of this plant and the oil pressed therefrom were used by the ancient Egyptians and are referred to in the Ebers Papyrus.

The name *Ricinus* was the Latin name of the dog-tick and was applied to these seeds on account of their resemblance in appearance to the insect. In Greek the same insect was known as *Kroton*. The name Castor Oil was derived through an erroneous belief during the 16th and 17th centuries that the plant which yielded the seeds was *Agnus Castus*.

Preparation—Castor Oil is prepared by cold expression and subsequent clarification of the oil by heat. It consists chiefly of the glycerides of ricinoleic and iso-ricinoleic acids. The purgative action is supposed to be due to the hydrolysis of ricinolein in the intestine, ricinoleic acid being produced. The seeds contain two principles, *ricin*, a very poisonous albumin (150 mg toxic per os), and *ricinine*, a poisonous base (1,2-dihydro-4-methoxy-1-methyl-2-oxonicotinonitrile). Because of the presence of these toxic substances, the seeds are definitely poisonous.

Description—A pale yellowish or almost colorless, transparent, viscid liquid with a faint, mild odor, and a bland followed by a slightly acrid and usually nauseating taste. Its specific gravity is between 0.945 and 0.965.

Solubility—It is soluble in alcohol and is miscible with dehydrated alcohol and with glacial acetic acid, chloroform, and ether.

Identification—Distinguished from most other fixed oils by its partial solubility in solvent hexane and its solubility in an equal volume of alcohol.

Uses—Castor Oil is used externally as an emollient, internally as a *cathartic*. The oil is bland and soothing to the skin. When ingested it is hydrolyzed in the intestinal tract to ricinoleic acid, which is an irritant. The local irritant action is responsible for the catharsis.

Castor Oil is sometimes employed to initiate labor at term. Hyperemia of the intestinal tract causes reflex stimulation of the uterus.

Dose—**15 to 60 ml** daily; *usual*, **15 ml.**

Other Dose Information—No harm results if this dose is exceeded inasmuch as the cathartic action of the first portion of the oil sweeps the remaining oil through the intestinal tract.

Veterinary Dose—*Horses*, **250 to 750 ml**; *Foals* and *Calves*, **60 to 90 ml**; *Sheep* and *Swine*, **60 to 120 ml**; *Dogs*, **8 to 30 ml**; *Cats*, **4 to 15 ml.**

Aromatic Castor Oil NF [Oleum Ricini Aromaticum]— *Preparation:* Dissolve cinnamon oil (3 ml), clove oil (1 ml), saccharin (0.5 Gm), and vanillin (1 Gm) in alcohol (30 ml), add castor oil (qs), and mix thoroughly to make 1000 ml. *Alcohol Content:* From 2 to 3% of C_2H_5OH. *Uses:* A *cathartic*. The aromatics assist in its administration by masking the disagreeable taste of the castor oil. *Dose: Usual, 15 ml.*

Miscellaneous Irritant Cathartics

Arecoline Hydrobromide—see page 902.

Bisacodyl NF

[4,4'-(2-Pyridylmethylene)diphenol Diacetate (ester); Dulcolax [*Geigy*]]

Bisacodyl contains 98.0–101.0% of $C_{22}H_{19}NO_4$ (361.40), calculated on the dried basis.

Caution—Avoid inhalation and contact with the eyes, skin, and mucous membranes.

Preparation—2-Pyridinecarboxyaldehyde is condensed with phenol with the aid of a suitable dehydrant such as sulfuric acid and the resulting 4,4'-(2-pyridyl)diphenol is esterified by treatment with acetic anhydride and anhydrous sodium acetate. Crystallization is from aqueous ethanol. US Pat. 2,764,590.

Description—A white to off-white, crystalline powder in which particles of the order of 50μ in diameter predominate.

Solubility—Very slightly soluble in water; freely soluble in chloroform and alcohol; soluble in methanol and benzene; slightly soluble in ether.

Uses—Bisacodyl is a contact laxative which acts directly on the colonic mucosa to increase peristalsis throughout the large intestine. It is administered either orally or rectally for constipation and for evacuation of the bowel prior to surgery, proctoscopy, or radiologic examination. Bisacodyl provides satisfactory cleansing of the bowel, obviating the need for an enema. Side effects are usually limited to abdominal cramps. There are no contraindications to the use of Bisacodyl, except for an acute surgical abdomen.

Dose—*Oral*, **10 to 30 mg**; *usual, oral* and *rectal*, **10 mg.**

Dosage Forms—Suppositories NF: 10 mg; Tablets NF: 5 mg.

Glycerin Suppositories NF

Glycerin	**91 Gm**
Sodium Stearate	**9 Gm**
Purified Water	**5 Gm**
To make about	**100 Gm**

Heat the glycerin in a suitable container to about 120°. Dissolve the sodium stearate, with gentle stirring, in the heated glycerin. Then add the purified water, mix, and immediately pour the hot mixture into a suitable mold, which, if made of metal, previously has been heated and is used while hot. Cool the suppositories completely before removal.

Note—If preferred, the sodium stearate for Glycerin Suppositories may be prepared during the making of the Suppositories by the direct reaction between stearic acid and sodium bicarbonate, sodium carbonate, or sodium hydroxide, these being taken in correct proportion. A typical formula is that of the USP X which is as follows:

Glycerin	**80 Gm**
Monohydrated Sodium Carbonate	**2 Gm**
Stearic Acid	**8 Gm**
Water	**10 ml**
To make about	**100 Gm**

Dissolve the monohydrated sodium carbonate in the water and add it to the glycerin contained in a suitable vessel placed in a water bath in such a way that the vessel is well immersed in the boiling water and its contents protected as much as possible from the steam of the bath. Add the stearic acid and heat the mixture for 15 minutes or until the carbon dioxide ceases to be evolved and the liquid is clear. Then pour the melted mass into suitable molds, remove the suppositories when they are completely cold, and preserve them in tightly stoppered glass vessels in a cool place.

Uses—Glycerin Suppositories are occasionally used in *constipation*, especially in children, puppies and kittens to promote peristalsis through local irritation of the mucous membrane of the rectum. This irritation may become excessive through habitual use of the suppositories.

Phenolphthalein NF

[3,3-Bis(*p*-hydroxyphenyl)phthalide]

Phenolphthalein contains 97.0–101.0% of $C_{20}H_{14}O_4$ (318.33), calculated on the dried basis.

Preparation—Phenolphthalein results from the condensation of phthalic anhydride with phenol.

A mixture of 10 parts of phenol, 5 parts of phthalic anhydride, and 4 parts of sulfuric acid is heated at 120° for 10 or 12 hours. The product is extracted with boiling water, then the residue dissolved in dilute sodium hydroxide solution, filtered, and precipitated with acid.

Description—A white or faintly yellowish white, crystalline powder. It is odorless, and is stable in air. It melts not lower than 258°.

Identification—Phenolphthalein dissolves in solutions of alkali hydroxides or carbonates with a red color which is discharged by an excess of acid or by high concentration of alkali hydroxides.

Solubility—Practically insoluble in water; 1 Gm dissolves in about 15 ml of alcohol, and in about 100 ml of ether.

Uses—Phenolphthalein is one of the most widely used of the *cathartic* drugs, being the basis of many proprietary laxatives. When taken orally, it is dissolved by the intestinal juices and bile and stimulates the intestinal musculature, chiefly that of the colon. It acts within 4 to 8 hours after ingestion. In susceptible individuals, Phenolphthalein may cause a skin rash. It should also be remembered that Phenolphthalein colors an alkaline urine red, and small portions may appear in the urine after oral ingestion. It is also used as an indicator in volumetric analysis.

Saline Bulk Cathartics

The *bulk cathartics* (saline salts and hydrophilic colloids and indigestible fibers) increase the contents of the tract and are more physiological in action than the irritant cathartics.

The *saline cathartics* are salts which are not absorbed, or at most only slightly absorbed, from the gastrointestinal tract. Consequently, when given orally in hypertonic solutions, they draw water from the tissues into the intestine, increase peristalsis, and induce a profuse, watery stool.

Magnesium Carbonate—see page 791.

Magnesium Citrate Solution NF

[Citrate of Magnesia, "Citrate"]

Magnesium Citrate Solution contains, in each 100 ml, an amount of magnesium citrate corresponding to 1.55–1.9 Gm of MgO (magnesium oxide).

Dose—*Usual*, 60 mg.
Dosage Forms—Tablets NF: 60 and 120 mg.
Veterinary Dose—*Dogs* and *Cats*, 5 to 250 mg.

Other Miscellaneous Irritant Cathartics

Calomel NF XII [Hydrargyri Chloridum Mite; Hydrargyri Subchloridum; Mercurous Chloride; Mild Mercurous Chloride; Protochloride of Mercury; Subchloride of Mercury], dried over phosphorus pentoxide for 5 hours, contains not less than 99.6% of HgCl (236.04). *Preparation:* Calomel is made by the direct union of hot mercury vapors with chlorine gas, the amount of chlorine being regulated to be between 5 and 10% in excess and thus avoid the possible presence of metallic mercury in the final product. The bichloride formed from the excess chloride is removed by thorough washing with water. A very finely divided Calomel may be obtained by precipitating a solution of mercurous nitrate with diluted hydrochloric acid or a solution of sodium chloride. *Description and Solubility:* A white, heavy, odorless, impalpable powder, becoming yellowish white when triturated with strong pressure; specific gravity, 7.1; stable in air, but gradually darkens when exposed to light. Insoluble in water, alcohol, ether, and cold dilute acids.

Uses: Calomel, once a popular cathartic, has no valid use. It is of interest only because of its mechanism of action. In the intestine, a portion of the Calomel is converted to more soluble mercuric ions that inhibit the active absorption of sodium and other ions from the intestinal lumen. Thus, electrolyte and, consequently, water are retained in the bowel. Liberation of mercuric ions from Calomel is also responsible for the toxic action of the drug. For this reason, the administration of Calomel is usually followed by a saline cathartic to facilitate the excretion of the toxic ions.

The stools following the administration of Calomel are green due to the presence of large amounts of the bile pigment biliverdin. This led to the erroneous impression that Calomel stimulated the secretion of bile. It is now known that the increased biliverdin content of the stools results from the antiseptic action of the mercuric ions, which prevents the normal bacterial conversion of the bile pigment in the bowel, and from the fact that catharsis propels the intestinal contents through the tract before biliverdin has been converted to bilirubin.

Calomel has some action as a diuretic but the organic mercurial diuretics are to be preferred.

Veterinary Uses: Once popular as a cathartic and as an anthelmintic (combined with santonin) in swine and small animals, and as a cathartic (combined with aloe or aloin) in horses, its toxic properties have reduced its use. Doses adequate for catharsis may be toxic.

Magnesium Carbonate	15	Gm
Citric Acid	27.4	Gm
Syrup	60	ml
Talc	5	Gm
Lemon Oil	0.1	ml
Potassium Bicarbonate	2.5	Gm
Purified Water, a sufficient quantity,		
To make	350	ml

Note—An amount of citric acid containing 1 molecule of water of hydration, equivalent to 27.4 Gm of anhydrous citric acid, may be used in the above formula.

Dissolve the anhydrous citric acid in 150 ml of hot purified water in a suitable dish, add slowly the magnesium carbonate, previously mixed with 100 ml of purified water, and stir until it is dissolved. Then add the syrup, heat the mixed liquids to the boiling point, immediately add the lemon oil, previously triturated with the talc, and filter the mixture, while hot, into a strong bottle (previously rinsed with boiling purified water) of suitable capacity. Add enough boiled purified water to make the product measure 350 ml. Stopper the bottle with purified cotton, allow to cool, add the potassium bicarbonate, and immediately stopper the bottle securely. Lastly, shake the solution occasionally until the potassium bicarbonate is dissolved. Keep the bottle on its side in a cool place, preferably in a refrigerator.

Note—In this process the 2.5 Gm of potassium bicarbonate may be replaced by 2.1 Gm of sodium bicarbonate, preferably in tablet form. The Solution may be further carbonated by the use of CO_2, under pressure. Carbon dioxide alone, instead of the potassium or sodium bicarbonates, should not be used, as the citrates formed from the latter have a desired therapeutic effect.

The stability of Magnesium Citrate Solution may be improved by pasteurizing or sterilizing the Solution. For Solutions which are not intended to be pasteurized or sterilized, the stability may be improved by employing 30 Gm of citric acid and a quantity of magnesium carbonate equivalent to 6.0 Gm of MgO for each 350 ml of Solution. The excess is necessary in order to form carbon dioxide when the bicarbonate is added, thus adding to the flavor due to carbonation and to the therapeutic effectiveness through the formation of alkali citrates.

In this connection it should be noted that official Magnesium Carbonate contains the equivalent of 40.0 to 43.5% of MgO, corresponding to from 6.00 to 6.47 Gm of MgO from the 15 Gm of the carbonate.

It was shown[1] that solutions containing amounts of magnesium oxide approaching the lower official limit were more stable than those containing higher percentages. Precipitation on standing is increased by the presence of sucrose and carbon dioxide and decreased by sterilization of the finished product.

If the pharmacist does not have the facilities for sterilization he should at least sterilize the stoppers by boiling them in water for 20–30 minutes.

If the official Solution is too acid for the patient, an additional amount of sugar or syrup will render it more palatable. The use of purified water has been found necessary, as precipitation has frequently been traced to the use of ordinary water.

Description—A colorless to slightly yellow, clear effervescent liquid having a sweet, acidulous taste and a lemon flavor.

Uses—A pleasant *saline cathartic*.

Dose—*Usual*, **200 ml.**

Magnesium Oxide—see page 792.

Magnesium Sulfate USP

[Bitter Salts; Epsom Salts]

Magnesium Sulfate [$MgSO_4.7H_2O$ = 246.47], rendered anhydrous by ignition, contains 99.0–100.5% of $MgSO_4$ (120.37).

History—This salt, which at one time sold for a shilling an ounce, was first obtained from the celebrated spring at Epsom, the English Spa, hence the common name. In continental Europe it is frequently called *Seidlitz Salt*, because it is the principal active constituent in the Seidlitz Spring of Germany. In America it has been called *Crab Orchard Salt*, because it was obtained from the waters of a spring by that name in Kentucky.

Preparation—This well-known and widely used salt can be prepared by neutralizing sulfuric acid with magnesium carbonate or oxide, but it is usually obtained directly from natural sources. Magnesium sulfate in the form of double salt with alkali metals occurs abundantly in several mines, and these form the largest source of the salt. It is also produced in large quantities from the magnesium salts occurring in the brines used for extraction of bromine. The "liquors" after the removal of bromine are treated with calcium hydroxide, thus precipitating magnesium as the hydroxide. Sulfur dioxide and air are passed into an aqueous suspension of the magnesium hydroxide, yielding Magnesium Sulfate:

$$Mg(OH)_2 \ + \ SO_2 \ + \ \tfrac{1}{2}O_2 \ \rightarrow \ MgSO_4 \ + \ H_2O$$

Description—Small, colorless crystals, usually needle-like, and has a cooling, saline, and bitter taste. It effloresces in warm, dry air. At 100° it loses 5 molecules of its water. The aqueous solution is neutral to litmus.

Solubility—1 Gm is soluble in 1 ml of water and is slowly soluble in about 1 ml of glycerin; 1 Gm is soluble in 0.2 ml of boiling water and is sparingly soluble in alcohol.

Incompatibilities—Addition of *alcohol* may cause a precipitation of Magnesium Sulfate from an aqueous solution. *Alkali hydroxides* form insoluble magnesium hydroxide, *alkali carbonates* form a basic carbonate, and the *salicylates* form a basic salicylate. *Arsenates, phosphates,* and *tartrates* may cause precipitation of the corresponding magnesium salts. *Sulfates* are precipitated by lead, barium, strontium, and calcium.

Uses—Magnesium Sulfate is an effective and widely employed *saline cathartic*. The cathartic action results from the fact that Magnesium Sulfate is not absorbed from the intestinal tract, and thus retains sufficient water within the lumen of the bowel to make an isotonic solution. In the event that the salt is given in hypertonic solution, the source of water would be the body fluids, and thus a dehydrating action is exerted. The average oral dose of 15 Gm retains approximately 400 ml of water. It is the increased bulk which promotes the motor activity of the bowel. If dissolved in iced water, its nauseous taste is not so perceptible as when water of ordinary temperature is used; it may be still further disguised by the use of orange juice.

A cold, wet compress of saturated Magnesium Sulfate solution in water has been employed in the treatment of such skin disorders as erysipelas. Hot concentrated, aqueous solutions of Magnesium Sulfate (about 1 pound per pint of water) are sometimes used in the treatment of deep-seated infections, cloths being saturated and applied while hot. The action is much like that of a poultice.

For parenteral use see *Magnesium Sulfate Injection*, page 1099.

Dose—**10 to 30 Gm** daily; *usual*, **15 Gm.**

Veterinary Dose—*Cattle*, 500 to 1000 Gm; *Sheep, Swine,* and *Goats,* 60 to 120 Gm; *Dogs,* 8 to 25 Gm; *Cats,* 2 to 4 Gm. A single dose is unreliable in horses.

Milk of Magnesia—see page 791.

Potassium Sodium Tartrate NF

[Rochelle Salt; Seignette Salt; Sodium Potassium Tartrate]

Potassium Sodium Tartrate [KOOC.CH(OH).CH(OH).COONa.4H$_2$O = 282.23] contains 99.0–100.5% of $C_4H_4KNaO_6$ (210.26), calculated on the dried basis.

History—Rochelle Salt was named for the city in which it was first discovered and manufactured by Peter Seignette, an apothecary of the latter half of the seventeenth century. The secret of its composition was kept undivulged by him and his descendants for nearly a century and it was sold as a proprietary remedy or nostrum. He put it up in individual envelopes and called it *Sal Polychrestum*, or the Salt of Many Virtues. It has also been called Seignette's Salt in honor of its discoverer. The secret of its composition was divulged in 1731 in a paper by Boulduc, a noted Parisian pharmacist, which was deemed of sufficient importance to be published by the French Academy of Sciences and the Transactions of the Philosophical Society of Great Britain. The name Sal Polychestrum has previously been applied to potassium sulfate by Christopher Glaser, apothecary to Louis XIV of France. The first official name of Rochelle Salt in the London Pharmacopœia of 1788 was *Natron Tartarizatum*, which in the edition of 1809 was changed to *Soda Tartarizata*.

Preparation—This salt is made by reacting a double molar portion of potassium bitartrate with a hot solution of sodium carbonate.

Description—Colorless crystals, or a white, crystalline powder, having a cooling, saline taste. It effloresces slightly in warm, dry air. The crystals are often coated with a white powder. The aqueous solution is alkaline to litmus paper, but is not reddened by phenolphthalein.

Solubility—1 Gm dissolves in 1 ml of water; practically insoluble in alcohol.

Incompatibilities—*Acids* cause a precipitation of potassium bitartrate. *Magnesium sulfate* and *calcium* salts produce a precipitate. The tartrates are weak reducing agents.

Uses—Potassium Sodium Tartrate is employed as a *saline cathartic*. Compound Effervescent Powders (Seidlitz Powders) also owe their cathartic properties to the presence of Rochelle Salt. The mechanism of action of the saline cathartics is discussed under *Magnesium Sulfate* (page 801).

Dose—*Usual*, 10 Gm.

Sodium Phosphate NF

[Dibasic Sodium Phosphate; Disodium Orthophosphate; Disodium Hydrogen Phosphate; Secondary Sodium Phosphate]

Sodium Phosphate [$Na_2HPO_4.7H_2O = 268.07$], dried at 105° for 12 hours, contains 98.0–100.5% of Na_2HPO_4 (141.96).

Preparation—The incombustible part of bones called *bone phosphate* or *bone ash*, obtained by heating bones to whiteness, consists chiefly of tribasic calcium phosphate which is used in the manufacture of Sodium Phosphate. The mineral *phosphorite*, which is a tribasic calcium phosphate is also used. The finely ground phosphatic material is mixed with a quantity of sulfuric acid, a little in excess over the amount required to transform the phosphate into monobasic calcium phosphate. The mixture is then leached with hot water, and a concentrated solution of sodium carbonate sufficient to convert half of the phosphate into the dibasic sodium salt is added. The solution is then boiled.

$$CaH_4(PO_4)_2 + Na_2CO_3 \rightarrow CaHPO_4 + Na_2HPO_4 +$$
$$H_2O + CO_2$$

After filtering, the solution is concentrated and the Sodium Phosphate is allowed to crystallize.

Description—Colorless, or white, granular salt. It effloresces in warm, dry air. The solutions are alkaline to litmus and phenolphthalein (pH about 9.5).

Solubility—1 Gm dissolves in 4 ml of water; very slightly soluble in alcohol.

Incompatibilities—Practically all phosphates, except those of ammonium, potassium and sodium, are insoluble in water but are made soluble by acids or alkali citrates. The tribasic alkali phosphates are very alkaline in reaction and

precipitate alkaloids and *metallic salts* from solution. Most *heavy metals* are precipitated as insoluble phosphates, redissolved by acids or alkali citrates.

Uses—Sodium Phosphate is one of the most palatable of the *saline cathartics*.

Caution—This phosphate should not be confused with tribasic sodium phosphate which is very alkaline and has a caustic action.

Dose—4 to 8 Gm; *usual*, 4 Gm.

Veterinary Dose—*Horses*, **500 Gm**; *Cattle*, **500 to 750 Gm**; *Foals* and *Calves*, **25 to 50 Gm**; *Sheep* and *Swine*, **15 to 45 Gm**; *Dogs*, **4 to 8 Gm**; *Cats*, **2 to 4 Gm**.

Dried Sodium Phosphate NF [Exsiccated Sodium Phosphate NF XII] [$Na_2HPO_4.xH_2O$], dried at 105° for 4 hours, contains 98.0–100.5% of Na_2HPO_4 (141.96). *Description:* A white powder which readily absorbs moisture. *Solubility:* 1 Gm dissolves in about 8 ml of water; insoluble in alcohol. *Uses:* Exsiccated Sodium Phosphate is a *saline cathartic*. It is used chiefly in the form of Effervescent Sodium Phosphate for which purpose it should be freshly dried, otherwise it will be variable in its water content. It rapidly absorbs as much as 15 to 20% of water if exposed to a moist atmosphere. *Dose: 2 to 4 Gm.*

Effervescent Sodium Phosphate NF—*Preparation:* Powder citric acid (uneffloresced crystals 162 Gm), mix it intimately with dried sodium phosphate (dried and powdered, 200 Gm) and tartaric acid (in dry powder, 252 Gm), and thoroughly incorporate sodium bicarbonate (in dry powder, 477 Gm) to make about 1000 Gm. Place the mixed powders on a plate of glass or in a suitable dish in an oven previously heated to between 93° and 104°. Manipulate the mixture carefully, with a spatula which is acid-resistant, and when it has become moist rub it through a No. 6 tinned-iron sieve. Dry the granules at a temperature not exceeding 54°, and immediately transfer the salt to suitable containers and seal them tightly. *Note:* The proportions of tartaric acid and citric acid may be varied if desired, but their combined acidity must be equivalent to the acidity indicated in the official formula. *Uses:* This is one of the most pleasant of the *saline cathartics*, being an effervescent mixture which combines the cathartic action of the phosphate and tartrate ions. *Dose: 10 to 20 Gm.*

Sodium Phosphate Solution NF contains, in each 100 ml, the equivalent of 71.0–79.0 Gm of $Na_2HPO_4.7H_2O$. *Preparation:* Add sodium phosphate (755 Gm), citric acid (130 Gm), and glycerin (150 ml) to purified water (150 ml), and digest on a steam bath until solution is effected. Filter, and pass sufficient purified water through the filter to make the product measure 1000 ml. *Note:* 400 Gm of dried sodium phosphate may be used in place of the 755 Gm of sodium phosphate specified in the formula. If this alternative is followed, the 150 ml of purified water specified in the directions should be increased to 500 ml. *Description:* A clear, colorless liquid, of a thick, syrupy consistency, practically odorless, and with a cooling, saline taste. Its specific gravity is about 1.385 at 25°. It is acid to litmus and produces effervescence with sodium carbonate. *Uses:* This Solution, which corresponds to 0.8 Gm of the official hydrated salt in each ml, furnishes a convenient form for the administration of a *saline cathartic*. The citric acid is added to prevent the salt from crystallizing, and the glycerin assists in its preparation, especially in preventing the development of microorganisms. *Dose: Usual, 10 ml* (one usual dose contains about 8 Gm).

Other Saline Bulk Cathartics

Potassium Bitartrate NF XII [Cream of Tartar; Acid Potassium Tartrate; $C_4H_5KO_6$ (188.18)]—*Preparation:* This salt is made by purifying *argol* or *tartar*—a substance deposited in wine casks during the fermentation of grape juice which substance consists of about 80% potassium bitartrate. *Description and Solubility:* Colorless or slightly opaque crystals, or as a white, crystalline powder having a pleasant, acid taste; its saturated solution is acid to litmus.

1 Gm dissolves in 165 ml of water, 8820 ml of alcohol, or 16 ml of boiling water. *Incompatibilities:* Because it contains an acidic hydrogen, it can react with alkaline substances. Its slight solubility sometimes causes difficulty in liquid mixtures. *Uses:* Occasionally employed as a *cathartic.* This salt is one of the ingredients in Compound Jalap Powder, formerly in the NF. It is largely used in baking powders and in the manufacture of hard candies. *Dose: Usual,* 2 Gm. *Veterinary Dose: Diuretic, Horses* and *Cattle,* 15 to 45 Gm; *Dogs,* 600 mg to 2 Gm; *Laxative, Dogs,* 4 to 15 Gm.

Potassium Phosphate NF XII [Dibasic Potassium Phosphate; Dipotassium Hydrogen Phosphate; K_2HPO_4 (174.18)]—*Preparation:* By reacting potassium carbonate or potassium hydroxide with phosphoric acid. *Description and Solubility:* Colorless or white granules or powder; deliquescent when exposed to moist air; its solutions are alkaline to phenolphthalein TS. 1 Gm dissolves in 3 ml of water; very slightly soluble in alcohol. *Uses:* Same as *Sodium Phosphate* (page 802) and is also an official reagent. *Dose: Usual,* 4 Gm.

Seidlitz Powders NF XII [Compound Effervescent Powders]—The mixture in a blue paper weighs 9.5–10.5 Gm, and contains 23–27% of sodium bicarbonate and 73–78% of potassium sodium tartrate (Rochelle Salt). The white paper contains 2–2.4 Gm of tartaric acid. *History:* The name of this preparation is incorrect; it was applied by the originator, Thomas Savory, in 1815, because he thought that the powders owed their value to the mineral properties (magnesium sulfate) of the Seidlitz Spring in Germany. *Preparation:* Mix sodium bicarbonate (30 Gm) intimately with potassium sodium tartrate (90 Gm), divide into 12 equal parts, and wrap each part in a blue paper; then divide tartaric acid (26 Gm) into 12 equal parts and wrap each part in a white paper. *Uses:* See *Potassium Sodium Tartrate* (page 801). *Dose: Usual,* the contents of a white and blue paper, each dissolved in about 60 ml of water, the solutions mixed, and administered after the effervescence begins to subside.

Sodium Sulfate NF XII [Glauber's Salt]—*History:* This compound was first described by Johann Rudolph Glauber in 1651, who had such a high opinion of its virtues that he called it *sal mirabile* (wonderful salt). *Preparation:* It is largely obtained as a byproduct in the manufacture of hydrochloric acid, ammonium chloride, etc; it is also produced by reacting sodium chloride and sulfuric acid. *Description and Solubility:* Large, colorless, odorless, transparent crystals or a granular powder; effloresces rapidly in air; liquefies in its water of hydration at about 33°; at 100° it loses all of its water of hydration; solutions are neutral to litmus. 1 Gm dissolves in 1.5 ml of water; insoluble in alcohol but soluble in glycerin. *Incompatibilities:* Sulfates give precipitates with salts of *lead, barium, strontium, and calcium. Silver* and *mercury* form slightly soluble salts. *Alcohol* throws most sulfates out of solution. Sodium Sulfate is troublesome in powders due to its water of crystallization. *Uses:* An effective *saline cathartic. Dose: Usual,* 15 Gm. *Veterinary Dose: Purgative, Horses,* 250 to 1000 Gm; *Cattle,* 500 to 1000 Gm; *Sheep, Goats,* and *Swine,* 60 to 120 Gm; *Dogs,* 10 to 25 Gm; *Cats,* 2 to 4 Gm. (Laxative doses approximate ⅕ of purgative doses.)

Hydrophilic Colloid Bulk Cathartics

The *hydrophilic colloids* and *indigestible fibers* supplement a diet that is deficient in indigestible residue. Hence, they promote defecation without subjecting the bowel to the undesirable action of irritating drugs.

Agar—see page 1344.

Methylcellulose—see page 1345.

Plantago Seed NF

[Psyllium Seed; Plantain Seed]

Plantago Seed is the cleaned, dried, ripe seed of *Plantago psyllium* Linné, or of *Plantago indica* Linné (*Plantago arenaria* Waldstein et Kitaibel), known in commerce as Spanish or French Psyllium Seed; or of *Plantago ovata* Forskal, known in commerce as Blond Psyllium or Indian Plantago Seed (Fam. *Plantaginaceæ*).

Uses—Plantago Seed, by virtue of its indigestibility and mucilaginous character, acts as a mild *cathartic.*

Dose—4 to 15 Gm; *usual,* 7.5 Gm.

Sodium Carboxymethylcellulose USP

[Carmethose (*Ciba*); C.M.C. (*Stuart*)]

Sodium Carboxymethylcellulose is the sodium salt of a polycarboxymethyl ether of cellulose. It contains 6.5–9.5% of sodium (Na), calculated on the dried basis.

The apparent viscosity of a solution containing 2 Gm of Sodium Carboxymethylcellulose in each 100 Gm is 80–120% of that stated on the label for viscosity types of 100 centipoises or less; and 75–140% of that stated on the label for viscosity types of higher than 100 centipoises.

Description—Occurs as a white powder or granules. The powder is hygroscopic. Its 1 in 100 aqueous suspension has a pH between 6.5 and 8.0.

Solubility—Easily dispersed in water to form colloidal solutions; insoluble in alcohol, in ether, and in most other organic solvents.

Uses—Sodium Carboxymethylcellulose is a synthetic hydrophilic colloid used to treat *chronic constipation.* It forms a bland, demulcent gel which increases stool bulk and softness. Its bulk-forming properties are not as great as methylcellulose, but its lubricating properties are superior, with little tendency to produce intestinal obstruction. Sodium Carboxymethylcellulose is categorized officially as a *thickening agent.* It is used as an *emulsifier* and *suspending agent* for various pharmaceutical preparations.

Dose (unofficial)—*Usual,* **1.5 Gm** 3 times a day with meals.

Dosage Forms—Tablets NF: 500 mg.

Veterinary Dose—*Dogs,* **0.5 to 2 Gm;** *Cats,* **0.25 to 1 Gm.** The dose is given 3 times a day in both species, preferably mixed in small quantities of food or water.

Other Hydrophilic Colloid Bulk Cathartics

Sterculia Gum NF XI [Gum Karaya]—The dried gummy exudation from *Sterculia urens* Roxburgh or other species of *Sterculia* Linné (Fam. *Sterculiaceæ*) or from species of *Cochlospermum* Kunth (Fam. *Bixaceæ*). *Uses:* An indigestible bulk cathartic or mechanical laxative which swells when moistened.

Emollient Cathartics

The *emollient cathartics* (mineral oil and vegetable oils) lubricate the intestinal tract, soften the fecal contents, and facilitate the passage of feces. The many untoward effects induced by mineral oil, such as *aspiration oil pneumonitis* and *lipoid avitaminosis A*, suggest that habitual use be avoided.

Cottonseed Oil—see page 1343.

Mineral Oil USP

[Petrolatum Liquidum; Liquid Paraffin; Liquid Petrolatum; White Mineral Oil; Heavy Liquid Petrolatum]

Mineral Oil is a mixture of liquid hydrocarbons obtained from petroleum. It may contain a suitable stabilizer.

Preparation—After removing the lighter hydrocarbons from petroleum by distillation the residue is again subjected to distillation at a temperature between 330° and 390° and the distillate treated first with sulfuric acid, then with sodium hydroxide, and afterward decolorized by filtering through bone black, animal charcoal, or fuller's earth. The purified product is again chilled, to remove paraffin, and redistilled at a temperature above 330°. In some instances the sulfuric acid treatment is omitted.

Description—A colorless, transparent, oily liquid, free or nearly free from fluorescence. It is tasteless and odorless when cold and develops not more than a faint odor of petroleum when heated. Its specific gravity is between 0.860 and 0.905, and its kinematic viscosity is not less than 38.1 centistokes at 37.8°.

Solubility—Insoluble in water or alcohol; miscible with most fixed oils, but not with castor oil; also soluble in volatile oils.

Uses—Mineral Oil is used as a vehicle, especially for drugs to be applied to the nasal mucous membranes, and internally as a *laxative*. It is now recognized that neither of these procedures is as benign as once supposed.

A small portion of mineral oil may be aspirated into the lungs after topical application to nasal mucous membranes and may cause "lipid" pneumonia.

When taken internally, mineral oil, by its mechanical action, is a mild laxative. It is probably harmless in occasional laxative doses, but if taken continuously in large amounts it may impair appetite, reduce somewhat the absorption of fat-soluble vitamins, and possibly be absorbed to an extent sufficient to cause recognizable changes in the liver and mesenteric lymph nodes.

Dose (unofficial—**15 to 30 ml**; *usual*, **15 ml** 1 or 2 times daily.

Veterinary Dose—*Horses* and *Cattle*, **500 to 1000 ml**; *Goats*, *Sheep*, and *Swine*, **150 to 300 ml**; *Dogs* **5 to 60 ml**; *Cats*, **2 to 10 ml**.

Mineral Oil Emulsion NF [Liquid Petrolatum Emulsion NF XII; Mineral Oil Emulsion; Liquid Paraffin Emulsion]—*Preparation*: Mix mineral oil (500 ml) with acacia in very fine powder (125 Gm) in a dry mortar, add purified water (250 ml) all at once, and emulsify the mixture. Then add, in divided portions, triturating after each addition, a mixture of syrup (100 ml), purified water (50 ml), and vanillin (40 mg), dissolved in alcohol (60 ml). Finally add sufficient purified water to make the product measure 1000 ml, and mix well. *Note*: In preparing Mineral Oil Emulsion, other methods of emulsification may be used and the quantity of acacia may be reduced or it may be replaced by agar, gelatin, tragacanth, or mixtures of any of these emulsifying agents, provided the resulting emulsion is similar in viscosity and appearance to the emulsion made by the formula given. The vanillin may be replaced by not more than 1% of any other official flavoring substance or mixture of official flavoring substances. Sixty ml of sweet orange peel tincture, or 2 Gm of benzoic acid may be used as a preservative in place of the alcohol. Heavy Liquid Petrolatum should be used in preparing this emulsion as that variety is preferable for internal administration and is less likely to cause "leakage." *Alcohol Content:* When present, 4 to 6% of C_2H_5OH. *Uses:* A palatable form of Liquid Petrolatum for administration as an intestinal lubricant and *cathartic. Dose:* Usual, 30 ml. *Veterinary Dose: Dogs*, 10 to 30 ml; *Cats*, 4 to 20 ml.

Light Mineral Oil—see page 1369.

Olive Oil—see page 1349.

Fecal Softeners

The fecal softeners represent the most recent approach to the management of constipation and fecal impaction. Substances included in this category are "surface-acting" or "wetting" agents which are claimed to be nonabsorbable, nontoxic, and pharmacologically inert. Their action is attributed to their surface acting property; by lowering surface tension they permit the intestinal fluids to penetrate the fecal mass more readily, and thus produce soft, easily passed stools. The superiority of this group of agents over the more reliable emollient cathartics, such as mineral oil, remains to be established.

Dioctyl Calcium Sulfosuccinate NF

[Bis(2-ethylhexyl) S-Calcium Sulfosuccinate; Surfak (Hoescht)]

Dioctyl Calcium Sulfosuccinate contains 91.0–100.5% of $C_{40}H_{74}CaO_{14}S_2$ (879.20), calculated on the dried basis.

Preparation—Dioctyl Sodium Sulfosuccinate (page 805) is dissolved in isopropanol and reacted with a methanolic solution of calcium chloride. US Pat. 3,035,973.

Description—A white, gelatinous solid having the characteristic odor of octyl alcohol. It is free of the odor of other solvents.

Solubility—Slightly soluble in water; freely soluble in alcohol and glycerin; very soluble in polyethylene glycol 00 and corn oil.

Uses—Dioctyl Calcium Sulfosuccinate is a *fecal-softening* agent useful in *preventing constipation* or in patients where laxative therapy is undesirable or contraindicated. It does not cause peristaltic stimulation and, therefore, may be used in patients in whom cathartic medication is contraindicated. Except for occasional mild, transitory cramping pains, Dioctyl Calcium Sulfosuccinate is free from side effects and contraindications.

Dose—*Usual*, 240 mg.
Dosage Forms—Capsules NF: 50 and 240 mg.

Dioctyl Sodium Sulfosuccinate USP

[Bis(2-ethylhexyl) S-Sodium Sulfosuccinate; Aerosol OT Dry (*Am. Cyanamid*); Colace (*Mead-Johnson*); DioMedicone (*Medicone*); Doxinate (*Hoescht*)]

$$C_2H_5$$
$$|$$
$$COOCH_2CH(CH_2)_3CH_3$$
$$|$$
$$CH_2$$
$$|$$
$$CH-SO_3Na$$
$$|$$
$$COOCH_2CH(CH_2)_3CH_3$$
$$|$$
$$C_2H_5$$

Dioctyl Sodium Sulfosuccinate, dried at 105° for 2 hours, it contains 98.5–100.5% of $C_{20}H_{37}NaO_7S$ (444.57).

Preparation—Several patents have been issued covering the preparation of this compound. In general, maleic anhydride is treated with 2-ethylhexanol to produce the so-called dioctyl maleate which is then reacted with sodium bisulfite under conditions conducive to saturation of the olefinic bond with simultaneous rearrangement of the bisulfite to the sulfonate structure.

Description—A white, wax-like, plastic solid with a characteristic odor suggestive of octyl alcohol. It usually is available in the form of pellets.

Solubility—1 Gm slowly dissolves in about 70 ml of water; freely soluble in alcohol and glycerin; very soluble in solvent hexane.

Incompatibilities—*Strong alkalies* decompose this substance.

Uses—Dioctyl Sodium Sulfosuccinate is a surface-active agent which is used internally in the management of constipation and fecal impaction. It is used to soften the stools in impaction associated with megacolon, anal fissures, and postoperative anal atresia. It is also useful for constipation in geriatric, pediatric, and obstetric patients.

Dose—50 to **500 mg** daily; *usual*, **100 mg** 2 or 3 times a day.

Other Dose Information—For infants and children the dose is 10 to 20 mg daily.

Dosage Forms—Capsules USP: 50, 60, 100, and 240 mg; Solution NF: 10 mg/ml; Syrup NF: 20 mg/5 ml; Tablets USP: 50, 60, 100, and 125 mg.

Poloxalkol

[Ethylene Oxide-Propylene Oxide Polymer; Magcyl (*Elder*); Polykol (*Upjohn*)]

$$HO(CH_2CH_2O)_a(CHCH_2O)_b(CH_2CH_2O)_cH$$
$$|$$
$$CH_3$$

Poloxalkol is a relatively tasteless, nonionic, surface-active ethylene oxide–propylene oxide polymer having the type structure shown above.

Preparation—Poloxalkol is an oxyalkylene polymer of approximate molecular weight 8000 prepared by reacting ethylene oxide with polypropylene glycol. US Pat. 2,674,619.

Description—White granules or flakes, having a slight soapy taste with a faint bitter after-taste.

Solubility—Freely soluble in water, alcohol, chloroform, in addition to dilute solutions of hydrochloric acid, sodium hydroxide, and ammonium hydroxide; sparingly soluble in ether.

Uses—Poloxalkol is used for the treatment and prevention of constipation associated with dry, hard stools in children. It acts as a fecal softener by lowering the surface tension of intestinal fluids.

Dose—*Oral*, for children under 3 years of age, **100 to 200 mg** once or twice daily; for children 3 to 12 years of age, **200 mg** up to 3 times daily.

Dosage Forms—Capsules: 250 mg; Drops: 200 mg/ml.

Other Cathartics

Croton Oil [Oleum Tiglii]—A pale yellow or brownish yellow, somewhat viscid and slightly fluorescent fixed oil with a faint, characteristic odor, obtained by expression or by percolating the ground seeds of *Croton Tiglium* Linné (Fam. *Euphorbiaceæ*; habitat, Southeastern Asia) with carbon disulfide and distilling the percolate. *Uses:* Powerful purgative, rubefacient, and vesicant.

Magnesium Sulfate, Dried BP [Dried Epsom Salts; Exsiccated Magnesium Sulfate] [approx. $MgSO_4 \cdot 3H_2O$]—Purity: 62–70% $MgSO_4$. A white, odorless powder having a saline bitter taste. At 20° it is soluble in 2 parts of water and more soluble in hot water. A 7.5% aqueous solution is neutral to phenol red solution. *Uses:* In the preparation of effervescent and noneffervescent, aperient powders or granules; in the preparation of Morison's paste, which is employed as an application to carbuncles and boils. *Dose:* orally, 2 to 12 Gm.

Plantago Ovata Coating—A cream colored to brown, granular powder which is practically odorless and tasteless. This preparation consists principally of the separated outer mucilaginous layers of plantago ovata seeds (blond psyllium). *Uses:* Correction of simple constipation of functional or nervous origin due to lack of sufficient bulk in the stool. *Dose:* orally, 5 to 10 Gm 3 times daily in a glass of water or milk.

Psyllium Hydrophilic Mucilloid [Metamucil (*Searle*)] —A white to cream colored, slightly granular powder with little or no odor and a slightly acid taste. It consists of the mucilaginous portion (outer epidermis) of blond psyllium seeds. *Uses:* Adjunctive treatment of constipation. It acts as a fecal softener and also as a demulcent in the presence of inflamed mucosa. It has been mixed with barium sulfate to obtain more uniform dispersion of the barium for x-ray visualization. *Dose:* orally, 4 to 7 Gm 1 to 3 times daily in a glass of liquid followed by an additional glass of liquid.

Senna Fruit BP [Senna Pod]—Consists of the dried ripe

fruits of *Cassia acutifolia* Delile, known in commerce as Alexandrian senna pods, or of *Cassia angustifolia* Vahl, known in commerce as Tinnevelly senna pods. It possesses a slight odor and taste. It contains aloe-emodin, rhein, sennaemodin, chrysophanic acid, cathartic acid, cathartmannite and sennanigrin. *Uses:* As a cathartic causing single, thorough evacuation of the bowels. *Dose: Orally,* Gm.

Emetics

An *emetic* is a drug which induces vomiting. Although vomiting is primarily a respiratory function, the final result of this act is to evacuate the stomach. Therefore, the *emetics* are considered here with the gastrointestinal drugs. Such drugs may act directly by stimulation of the *chemoreceptor trigger zone* located in the area postrema of the medulla oblongata (eg, apomorphine, morphine, Hydergine, and digitalis glycosides) or they may act reflexly by irritant action on the gastrointestinal tract (eg, copper sulfate, mustard, sodium chloride, and zinc sulfate). They may also produce stimulation of the nodose ganglion of the vagus (eg, veratrum) or excitation of receptors in the heart, in the central nervous system rostral to the brain stem, and in other organs. The clinical value of emetics has been lessened by the stomach tube, a safer and more efficient tool for emptying the stomach. Emetics should not be used in patients with severe heart disease, tuberculosis, hernia, or advanced pregnancy. They are also contraindicated in debilitated patients and in poisoning caused by corrosive or petroleum products.

Apomorphine Hydrochloride NF

[Aporphine-10,11-diol Hydrochloride]

Apomorphine Hydrochloride [$C_{17}H_{17}NO_2 . HCl .$ $\frac{1}{2}H_2O = 312.80$] contains 98.5–100.5% of $C_{17}H_{17}NO_2 .$-HCl. For the structure, see page 493.

Preparation—It may be made by heating morphine in a closed tube with a great excess of hydrochloric acid for 2 or 3 hours at a temperature of 140° to 150°. The elements of one mole of H_2O are abstracted from the morphine, resulting in a change in the molecular structure. Upon cooling, crude Apomorphine Hydrochloride crystallizes out, being less soluble in hydrochloric acid than in water. The alkaloid is purified by recrystallization from water in the presence of HCl.

Description—Minute, white or grayish white, glistening crystals or white powder. It gradually acquires a green color on exposure to light and air. It is odorless. Its solutions are neutral to litmus. It is levorotatory in dilute acid; $[\alpha]_D^{25} -49°$ to $-51°$.

Solubility—1 Gm dissolves in about 50 ml of water and about 50 ml of alcohol; 1 Gm dissolves in about 20 ml of water at 80°; very slightly soluble in chloroform and in ether.

Incompatibilities—A green color is rapidly developed in *alkaline solution*. It is precipitated by *tannic acid* and other *alkaloidal precipitants* and decomposed by *oxidizing agents*. See also page 491.

Uses—Apomorphine is an *expectorant* in doses of 1 mg and a powerful *emetic* in doses of 5 mg. It should be employed with caution because in certain conditions (depression of the nervous system from poisons or overdoses of hypnotics) apomorphine may fail to cause emesis and will then cause further depression of the central nervous system. Collapse, coma, and even death have occurred from the injudicious use of this powerful alkaloid. If vomiting does not occur from the first dose, a second should not be given. It is better to administer a gastric tube and lavage the stomach than to employ emetic drugs.

Dose—*Usual, subcutaneous,* **5 mg.**

Dosage Forms—Tablets NF: **6 mg.**

Veterinary Dose—*Dogs* only, **1 to 2 mg** subcutaneously as an emetic.

Cupric Sulfate NF

[Copper Sulfate; Bluestone; Blue Vitriol; Blue Copperas; Cuprum Sulfuricum; Cuprum Vitriolatum]

Cupric Sulfate [$CuSO_4 . 5H_2O = 249.68$], dried at 250° to constant weight, contains 98.5–100.5% of $CuSO_4$ (159.60).

Preparation—This salt is generally made by heating scrap copper with sulfuric acid, the oxygen of the air assisting the reaction:

$$2Cu + 2H_2SO_4 + O_2 \rightarrow 2CuSO_4 + 2H_2O$$

In another largely used process the scrap copper is heated in a reverberatory furnace with sulfur, the reaction being controlled in order to obtain a maximum yield of Sulfate. The mass is then thrown into diluted sulfuric acid and any unchanged oxide or sulfide is converted into Cupric Sulfate.

Description—Deep blue, triclinic crystals, or blue, crystalline granules or powder. It has a nauseous, metallic taste, and effloresces slowly in dry air. Its solution is acid to litmus.

Solubility—1 Gm dissolves in 3 ml of water, in about 500 ml of alcohol, very slowly in 3 ml of glycerin, and in about 0.5 ml of boiling water.

Incompatibilities—The copper ion is precipitated as copper hydroxide by the *alkali hydroxides*. Precipitation is retarded by many organic substances such as citrates, tartrates, salicylates, glycerin, and sugar. *Ammonium hydroxide* gives a precipitate which is soluble in an excess of the reagent due to formation of the copper ammine ion, $[Cu(NH_3)_4]^{++}$. *Alkali carbonates, phosphates, borax,* and *tannic acid* cause a precipitation. *Soluble iodides* reduce the cupric ion to cuprous which precipitates as cuprous iodide with simultaneous liberation of iodine. *Lead, barium, strontium,* and *calcium* form insoluble sulfates.

Uses—Cupric Sulfate, known commercially as *bluestone* or *blue vitriol*, is employed as an *emetic*. It may rarely be used as a *hematinic* in certain forms of nutritional anemias, especially in children. Cupric Sulfate is also employed as an *antidote for phosphorus* and as an *astringent*.

Cupric Sulfate also enjoys many industrial applications. It is used to the extent of about 20 to 30 parts per million in swimming pools for destroying algæ, in *Bordeaux Mixture* (page 1292) for treating fungus diseases of fruit trees, in dyeing cotton and silk, and in electric batteries. It is also used for preserving wood, for preparing Fehling's and Benedict's solutions (extensively used in testing for and the assaying of sugars), and for the manufacture of many other copper salts.

Note—Blue Copperas [$CuSO_4.5H_2O$] *must not be confused with Copperas* [$FeSO_4.7H_2O$].

Dose (unofficial)—*Emetic,* **300 mg;** *hematinic,* for infants, given in milk or fruit juice, **3 mg** daily; for adults, **5** to **10 mg** 3 times daily, in capsules.

Emetine Hydrochloride—see page 1251.

Ipecac—see page 871.

Mustard, Black—see page 777.

Sodium Chloride—see page 842.

Zinc Sulfate—see page 1191.

Antiemetics

The *nausea–vomiting complex* is one of the most frequent symptoms of disease. It is often induced by certain drugs and occurs after operations and radiation therapy, during pregnancy, in gastrointestinal carcinoma, and as the result of certain types of motion in hypersensitive persons. Often it is mild and self-limiting; at times, it is very disturbing. A number of drugs which block this action, the *antiemetics* (*antinauseants*), are therapeutically effective. Useful agents are found among the sedatives, antihistamines, and ataraxics. Of these, the phenothiazine derivatives appear to be the most potent and the only drugs known to depress directly the *chemoreceptor trigger zone* (see page 806). Persistent vomiting results in loss of hydrochloric acid, alkalosis, and dehydration which, in turn, may precipitate further vomiting. Hence, electrolyte therapy may be necessary after vomiting has been present for some time (see page 837).

Chlorpromazine—see page 1106.

Cyclizine Hydrochloride USP

[1-(Diphenylmethyl)-4-methylpiperazine Monohydrochloride; Marezine Hydrochloride (*Burroughs-Wellcome*)]

Cyclizine Hydrochloride contains 98.0–100.5% of $C_{18}H_{22}N_2.HCl$ (302.85), calculated on the dried basis.

Preparation—Benzhydryl chloride is condensed with *N*-carbethoxypiperazine and the carbethoxy group is then split off by heating with potassium hydroxide. The *N*-benzhydrylpiperazine thus formed is isolated from the reaction product and then methylated at the N^4-position by treatment with formic acid and formaldehyde to give cyclizine base. The purified base may be converted conveniently into the hydrochloride by passing hydrogen chloride into a solution of the base in an appropriate organic solvent.

Description—White, crystalline powder or as small colorless crystals. It is odorless or nearly so and has a bitter taste. It melts indistinctly and with decomposition at about 285°. The pH, potentiometrically determined, of a 1 in 50 solution of Cyclizine Hydrochloride in a mixture of 2 volumes of alcohol and 3 volumes of water is between 4.5 and 5.5.

Solubility—1 Gm dissolves in about 115 ml of water, 115 ml of alcohol, and 75 ml of chloroform; insoluble in ether.

Uses—Cyclizine Hydrochloride is an antihistaminic agent which is effective in the prevention and relief of the vertigo, nausea, and vomiting associated with seasickness and airsickness. It also reduces the sensitivity of the labyrinth in the symptomatic relief of vertigo and concomitant symptoms caused by vestibular disorders. Cyclizine Hydrochloride is relatively free from side effects, but high doses may cause drowsiness and dryness of the mouth. Animal studies suggest this drug may possess teratogenic properties. Therefore, it should not be used during pregnancy.

Dose—**50** to **200 mg** daily; *usual,* **50 mg** 3 times a day.

Dosage Forms—Tablets USP: 50 mg.

Dimenhydrinate USP

[8-Chlorotheophylline 2-(Benzhydryloxy)-*N,N*-dimethylethylamine Compound (1:1); Dramamine (*Searle*)]

Dimenhydrinate [$C_{17}H_{21}NO.C_7H_7ClN_4O_2 = 469.98$] contains 53.0–55.5% of diphenhydramine ($C_{17}H_{21}NO$), and 44.0–47.0% of 8-chlorotheophylline ($C_7H_7ClN_4O_2$), calculated on the dried basis.

Preparation—It is prepared by causing dimethylaminoethyl benzhydryl ether to combine with 8-chlorotheophylline by refluxing an isopropyl alcohol solution. The crystalline precipitate of Dimenhydrinate which forms on cooling is collected by filtration, washed with cold ethyl acetate and dried.

Description—A white, crystalline, odorless powder' which melts between 102° and 107°.

Solubility—Slightly soluble in water; freely soluble in alcohol and in chloroform; sparingly soluble in ether.

Uses—An *antihistaminic* compound which is a combination of diphenhydramine (Benadryl, *Parke-Davis*) and 8-chlorotheophylline. The latter contributes little, if anything, to its action as an antiemetic or an antihistaminic agent. It is chiefly employed as an *antinauseant* in *motion sickness* (air-, trans-, sea-sickness, etc). It has also been used with success in the management of the vertigo associated with Ménière's syndrome, radiation sickness, and vestibular dysfunction resulting from streptomycin therapy. See page 1233.

Dose—**25** to **600 mg** daily; *usual,* **50 mg** 4 times a day.

Dosage Forms—Syrup USP; Tablets USP: 50 mg.

Veterinary Dose—To control *motion sickness* in dogs, **2 mg** per **pound** of body weight *orally* 30 minutes before travel.

Diphenhydramine Hydrochloride—see page 1147.

Diphenidol

[Vontrol (SK&F)]

Diphenidol is α,α-diphenyl-1-piperidinebutanol [$C_{21}H_{27}NO = 309.43$].

Preparation—Piperidine is reacted with 1-bromo-3-chloropropane in benzene with the aid of trimethylamine and the resulting 1-(3-chloropropyl)piperidine is converted to a Grignard reagent and reacted with benzophenone in tetrahydrofuran. Hydrolysis of the Grignard reaction complex yields crude Diphenidol which may be purified by recrystallization from isopropanol. US Pat. 2,898,340.

Description—A white, crystalline powder that is odorless and has a slightly bitter taste. It is stable in light and in air. It melts between 103° and 107°.

Solubility—Freely soluble in chloroform, ether, and cyclohexane; sparingly soluble in alcohol; insoluble in water.

Uses—Diphenidol, an antiemetic agent for oral, rectal, intramuscular, or intravenous administration, is useful in the management of nausea and vomiting associated with infectious diseases, malignancies, radiation sickness, general anesthesia, and treatment with antineoplastic agents. It is also useful in the treatment of vertigo of vestibular origin. Experimentally, it has been shown to exhibit weak parasympatholytic actions, but to lack significant sedative, tranquilizing, or antihistaminic properties. Its use should be restricted to patients under close medical supervision, since auditory and visual hallucinations, disorientation, and confusion have been reported. Other untoward effects such as drowsiness, dry mouth, dizziness, skin rash, heartburn, headache, nausea, blurred vision, malaise, etc have been infrequent and minor in nature. Since Diphenidol does possess parasympatholytic properties, it should be used cautiously in patients with glaucoma, prostatic hypertrophy, peptic ulcer, pyloric or duodenal obstruction, or cardiospasm. Animal experiments have revealed no evidence of teratogenic effects.

Dose—*Usual oral* or *rectal*, **25** to **50 mg** 4 times daily; for control of acute symptoms, **20** to **40 mg** by deep IM injection 4 times daily, or an initial dose of **20 mg** intravenously and repeated in 1 hour.

Dosage Forms—Injection (as the hydrochloride): 20 mg/ml; Suppositories: 25 or 50 mg; Oral Suspension (as the pamoate): 20 mg/5 ml; Tablets (as the hydrochloride): 25 mg.

Meclizine Hydrochloride USP

[1-(p-Chloro-α-phenylbenzyl)-4-(m-methylbenzyl)piperazine Dihydrochloride; Bonine Hydrochloride (Pfizer)]

Meclizine Hydrochloride [$C_{25}H_{27}ClN_2.2HCl.H_2O = 481.90$] contains 97.0–100.5% of $C_{25}H_{27}ClN_2.2HCl$ (463.88), calculated on the anhydrous basis.

Preparation—Meclizine (base) is formed by condensing N-(m-methylbenzyl)piperazine with p-chlorobenzyhydryl chloride in the presence of triethylamine. The purified base may then be dissolved in a suitable solvent and converted to the dihydrochloride by a stream of hydrogen chloride.

Description—White or slightly yellowish, crystalline powder. It has a slight odor and is tasteless.

Solubility—Practically insoluble in water and ether; freely soluble in chloroform, pyridine, methylacetamide, and acid–alcohol–water mixtures; slightly soluble in dilute acids and alcohol.

Uses—Meclizine Hydrochloride is a long-acting antihistaminic agent which is effective in the prevention or treatment of *motion sickness*, and in the treatment of *vertigo, labyrinthitis, Ménière's syndrome*, and *radiation sickness*. Like other antihistamines, it may cause drowsiness and other side actions, such as blurred vision, dryness of the mouth and fatigue. The action of a single dose persists for 9 to 24 hours. There is a lack of agreement with respect to the teratogenic effects of this agent. The dose and duration of treatment should be minimal when used during pregnancy. See general statement (page 807).

Dose—**25** to **100 mg** daily; *usual*, **25** to **50 mg** once a day.

Dosage Forms—Tablets USP: 25 mg.

Pheniramine Maleate—see page 1152.

Prochlorperazine NF

[2-Chloro-10-[3-(4-methyl-1-piperazinyl)propyl]phenothiazine;   Compazine (SK & F)]

Prochlorperazine contains 98.0–101.0% of $C_{20}H_{24}ClN_3S$ (373.95).

Preparation—A toluene solution of 1-(3-chloropropyl)-4-methylpiperazine and 2-chlorophenothiazine is refluxed with sodamide for several hours. After filtering and distilling off the toluene, the Prochlorperazine is obtained by short-path distillation under high vacuum.

Description—A clear, pale yellow, viscous liquid. It is sensitive to light.

Solubility—Very slightly soluble in water; freely soluble in alcohol, chloroform, and ether.

Uses—Prochlorperazine is a phenothiazine derivative with actions, uses, and limitations similar to those of *Prochlorperazine Maleate* (see page 809). However, Prochlorperazine, as the base, is administered rectally.

Dose—*Usual, rectal*, **2.5** to **25 mg**.

Other Dose Information—The *child's rectal* dose should not exceed 7.5, 10, and 15 mg for a 20 to 29-pound, 30 to 39-pound, and 40 to 58-pound child, respectively. It is not recommended for children weighing less than 20 pounds.

Dosage Forms—Suppositories NF: 2.5, 5, and 25 mg.

Prochlorperazine Edisylate USP

[2-Chloro-10-[3-(4-methyl-1-piperazinyl)propyl] phenothiazine 1,2-Ethane-disulfonate (1:1); Prochlorperazine Ethanedisulfonate USP XVI; Compa-zine Ethanedisulfonate (*SK & F*)]

Prochlorperazine Edisylate contains 98.0–101.5% of $C_{20}H_{24}ClN_3S.C_2H_6O_6S_2$ (564.15), calculated on the dried basis.

The structure of prochlorperazine is given above.

Preparation—Prochlorperazine (page 808) is dissolved in a suitable solvent and treated with an equimolar portion of 1,2-ethanedisulfonic acid. The official salt precipitates.

Description—A white to very light yellow, odorless, crystalline powder. Its solutions are acid to litmus.

Solubility—1 Gm dissolves in about 2 ml of water and about 1500 ml of alcohol; insoluble in ether and chloroform.

Uses—Prochlorperazine Edisylate has the same actions and uses as prochlorperazine maleate except that it may be administered intramuscularly as well as orally. Parenteral therapy is usually reserved for the treatment of severe nausea and vomiting, for the immediate control of acutely disturbed psychotics or for patients who cannot or will not take oral medication. See *Prochlorperazine Maleate.*

Dose—*Oral*, the equivalent of **5** to **100 mg** of prochlorperazine daily; *usual, oral*, **5 mg** 3 or 4 times a day; *intramuscular* or *intravenous*, **10** to **40 mg** daily; *usual*, **intramuscular, 5** to **10 mg**, repeated after 3 to 4 hours if necessary.

Other Dose Information—No more than 60 mg (40 mg of base) should be injected in any 24-hour period unless the patient is hospitalized and under adequate observation. For acutely disturbed patients, the usual dose is 20 to 40 mg intramuscularly at intervals ranging from 1 to 6 hours. Oral dosage for adults and children is the same as that outlined for *Prochlorperazine Maleate.*

Dosage Forms—Injection USP: 2 and 10 ml; Syrup USP.

Prochlorperazine Maleate USP

[2-Chloro-10-[3-(4-methyl-1-piperazinyl)propyl]phenothiazine Maleate (1:2); Compazine Dimaleate (*SK & F*)]

Prochlorperazine Maleate contains 98.0–101.5% of $C_{20}H_{24}ClN_3S.2C_4H_4O_4$ (606.10), calculated on the dried basis.

Preparation—Prochlorperazine Maleate is synthesized by the method described above for Prochlorperazine Edisylate except that maleic acid is employed instead of ethanedisulfonic acid and it is employed in double equimolar quantity in relation to the prochlorperazine base. The official salt is actually the bisbimaleate.

Description—A white or pale yellow, practically odorless, crystalline powder. Its saturated solution is acid to litmus.

Solubility—Practically insoluble in water and alcohol; slightly soluble in warm chloroform.

Uses—Prochlorperazine Maleate is used as an *antiemetic* and *tranquilizing agent*. It has an antiemetic potency 4 to 5 times that of chlorpromazine and is used to control mild or severe nausea and vomiting due to a variety of causes, such as early pregnancy, anesthesia and surgery, and radiation therapy. As a tranquilizing agent, it is used in mild mental disorders in which anxiety, tension, and agitation predominate. The drug has also been employed in severe psychiatric

disorders such as schizophrenia, mania, involutional psychoses, degenerative conditions and senile and toxic psychoses. Beneficial results ascribed to its action include, among others, reduction in psychomotor agitation and excitement, diminished aggressiveness and destructiveness, loss of hallucinations and delusions and a general calming effect.

When administered in the usual therapeutic dose range, side effects are generally infrequent, mild, transitory, and somewhat less intense than those observed after the administration of chlorpromazine. These include sedation, dizziness, hypotension, tachycardia and xerostomia. Rarely, a skin reaction, tinnitus, vertigo, nasal congestion, miosis or gastric hyperacidity may occur. Although no jaundice or blood dyscrasias have been reported, extrapyramidal involvement characterized by Parkinsonian-like symptoms may be troublesome at the higher dosages. If extrapyramidal symptoms appear, they may be controlled by the downward adjustment of dosage, the concomitant administration of an anti-Parkinson drug or the temporary withdrawal of prochlorperazine.

Dose—The equivalent of **5** to **150 mg** of prochlorperazine daily; *usual*, **5 mg** 3 or 4 times a day.

Other Dose Information—The usual dose is increased gradually until the desired response has been obtained. The usual effective dose in psychoses is 75 to 125 mg (of base) daily.

Dosage Forms—Tablets USP: 5, 10, and 25 mg.

Scopolamine Hydrobromide—see page 918.

Thiethylperazine Maleate NF

[2-(Ethylthio)-10-[3-(4-methyl-1-piperazinyl)propyl]phenothiazine Maleate (1:2); Torecan (*Sandoz*)]

Thiethylperazine Maleate contains 98.0–101.5% of $C_{22}H_{29}N_3S_2.2C_4H_4O_4$ (631.77), calculated on the dried basis.

Preparation—Thiethylperazine (base) is prepared by reacting 2-(ethylthio)-phenothiazine with 1-(3-chloropropyl)-4-methylpiperazine in the presence of sodamide or another appropriate dehydrochlorinating agent. The base is then dissolved in a suitable solvent and reacted with a double molar quantity of maleic acid to produce the official salt. The starting phenothiazine compound may be prepared by condensing phenothiazine with ethanethiol, and the piperazine compound similarly from methylpiperazine and trimethylene chloride. US Pat. 3,336,197.

Description—Faintly yellowish, fine, crystalline, voluminous powder. It is odorless or has a very slight odor and is bitter to the taste. It shows a decomposition point at approximately 183°C, but the exact temperature varies with the conditions of the test.

Solubility—Poorly soluble in water, methanol, and absolute ethanol; very poorly soluble in benzene, ether, and chloroform.

Uses—Thiethylperazine Maleate is a phenothiazine with antiemetic and weak tranquilizing properties. Laboratory studies indicate it acts on both the chemoreceptor trigger zone (CTZ) and the vomiting center in the medulla. It is useful in the control of post-anesthetic nausea and vomiting and in some cases of vertigo. Its usefulness in the management of the nausea and vomiting resulting from ionizing radiation and nitrogen mustard therapy remains to be established. The drug is not particularly effective in the control of the nausea and vomiting which frequently follows the use of morphine or meperidine. The contraindications and side effects are the same as those for other phenothiazines.

Dose—*Usual, oral* and *intramuscular*, **10** to **30 mg** daily.

Other Dose Information—The usual rectal dose is 10 to 30 mg per day.

Dosage Forms—Tablets NF: 10 mg.

Trimethobenzamide Hydrochloride NF

[*N* - [*p* - [2 - (Dimethylamino)ethoxy]benzyl] - 3,4,5 - trimethoxybenzamide Monohydrochloride; Tigan (*Roche*)]

Trimethobenzamide Hydrochloride, dried at 105° for 4 hours, contains 98.5–100.5% of $C_{21}H_{28}N_2O_5 \cdot HCl$ (424.93).

Preparation—4-[2-(Dimethylamino)ethoxy]benzyl-amine is condensed with 3,4,5-trimethoxybenzoyl chloride by refluxing in an inert solvent. The resulting trimethoxy benzamide may be converted to the hydrochloride by dissolving it in a suitable solvent and treating with HCl. The starting amine may be prepared in various ways, eg, by condensing sodium *p*-aminomethylphenoxide with 2-chloro-*N,N*-dimethylethylamine.

Description—Occurs as a white crystalline powder. It has a slight phenolic odor.

Solubility—Soluble in water and in warm alcohol; insoluble in ether and in benzene.

Uses—Trimethobenzamide Hydrochloride is a dimethylaminoethanol derivative which has been reported helpful in alleviating nausea and reducing vomiting in the immediate postoperative period; in pregnancy; in motion sickness; in drug-induced emesis; and in such pathological conditions as malignancy, hepatitis, cholecystitis, radiation sickness, and labyrinthine disease. Its antiemetic potency is about one-tenth that of chlorpromazine when given subcutaneously and one-fourth that of the latter when given orally. Minor side effects which have been reported include drowsiness, vertigo, diarrhea, and local irritation. During the courses of acute febrile illness, encephalitides, gastroenteritis, dehydration, and electrolyte imbalance, especially in children and the elderly and debilitated, CNS reactions such as opisthotonos, convulsions, coma, and extrapyramidal symptoms have been reported with and without the use of the drug. Therefore, caution should be exercised when Trimethobenzamide Hydrochloride is used in these conditions.

Dose—*Usual, oral* and *intramuscular*, **100** to **250 mg** 4 times a day; *rectal*, **200 mg** 3 or 4 times a day.

Dosage Forms—Capsules NF: 100 and 250 mg; Injection NF: 200 mg/2 ml, 2 Gm/20 ml; and Benzocaine Suppositories NF: 200 mg (trimethobenzamide hydrochloride) and 2% (benzocaine).

Adsorbents

Adsorbents are chemically inert powders which have the ability to adsorb gases, toxins, and bacteria. The fine state of subdivision of these inert powders confers high adsorptive capacity upon them. However, in the complex milieu of the gastrointestinal secretions, physical (Van der Waals) adsorbents are more likely to be selective for surface-active substances such as bile salts than for bacterial toxins and other noxious substances. Consequently, only certain materials that possess chemical adsorptive and persorptive properties lend themselves effectively to gastrointestinal detoxification and to the adsorption of gases resulting from abnormal intestinal fermentation. Such substances are kaolin, which is employed supposedly to adsorb bacterial toxins in diarrhea, dysentery, and chronic ulcerative colitis, and activated charcoal, which is employed to adsorb organic intoxicants especially, and gastrointestinal gases. It is doubtful that either are effective adsorbents in the lower gastrointestinal tract since passage through the upper tract saturates and deactivates the agent; however, the effectiveness of these agents in bulk entraining and dispersing bacterial aggregates may contribute to beneficial effects in the lower bowel.

Many of the nonsystemic antacids may serve as internal protectives and adsorbents, especially after regeneration in the alkaline small intestine. Magnesium trisilicate is claimed to exert a protective action also in the stomach by virtue of released silicic acid, which acts more as a demulcent than as a solid protective. *Antacids* are commonly combined with kaolin or other adsorbents. For a description of such preparations see page 811.

Bismuth Subcarbonate—see page 788.

Bismuth Subnitrate—see page 789.

Activated Charcoal USP

[Carbo Activatus; Medicinal Charcoal]

Activated Charcoal is the residue from the destructive distillation of various organic materials, treated to increase its adsorptive power.

Preparation—Under the name *Carbo Ligni* or *Wood Charcoal*, USP X recognized a product made by burning wood out of contact with air, the residue obtained consisting of nearly pure carbon. Charcoal made by this process is variable in its adsorptive powers, frequently being entirely devoid of such properties. It was found that the adsorptive powers of charcoal could be tremendously increased by treating it with various substances such as steam, air, carbon dioxide, oxygen, zinc chloride, sulfuric acid, or phosphoric acid, or a combination of some of these substances, at temperatures ranging from 500° to 900°. This treatment is referred to as activation, the activating agent presumably removing substances previously adsorbed on the charcoal and, in some instances at least, breaking down the granules of carbon into smaller ones having a greater total surface area. It has been estimated that 1 ml of charcoal, finely divided, possesses a total surface of approximately 1000 square meters.

In addition to wood many other substances are used as sources of charcoal, such substances including sucrose, lactose, rice starch, coconut pericarp, bone, blood, various industrial wastes, etc. As many different activated charcoals are available for various purposes, one should be certain to use only the medicinal variety for medicinal purposes.

Description—A fine, black, odorless, and tasteless powder, free from gritty matter.

Solubility—Insoluble in water or the other known solvents.

Uses—Activated Charcoal is used in medicine as an *adsorbent* for the purpose of reducing flatulence. Unfortunately, adsorption is not a specific action, thus nutrients and enzymes, as well as noxious substances, are adsorbed. Therefore, it has little therapeutic value in dyspepsia, diarrhea, and dysentery. Activated Charcoal is the most valuable single agent as an emergency *antidote* in many forms of poisoning because of its adsorptive powers.

Industrially it is used in large quantities in chemical and pharmaceutical manufacturing as a decolorizer.

Activated charcoal is marketed under the names of *Nuchar*, *Darco*, and *Norit*, less pure forms used for decoloration of solutions during manufacturing processes. See *Clarification* (page 387) and *Decoloration* (page 389).

Dose—5 to 50 Gm; *usual*, 10 Gm.

Veterinary Dose—*Horses*, 30 to 60 Gm; *Dogs*, 2 to 8 Gm.

Kaolin NF

[Light Kaolin; White Bole; China Clay]

Kaolin is a native hydrated aluminum silicate, powdered, and freed from gritty particles by elutriation.

History and Occurrence—The name *Kaolin* is derived from the Chinese word *kaoling*, meaning "high ridge"; it is sometimes called *China clay*, or *porcelain clay*, because of its use in pottery, and it is a valuable commercial product. The clays were highly esteemed as remedial agents, given internally, since the time of Hippocrates. *Terra sigillata* or "the earth imprinted with a seal" was a form of clay collected, purified, and authenticated under official supervision. Dr. Herman Schelenz, the eminent historian of pharmacy, says that the use of the seal or imprint upon these clay tablets several thousand years ago was the origin of the trademark. Galen and other early authors wrote voluminously upon their properties. They were considered as alexipharmics or alexiterics which are terms used in ancient medicine and pharmacy to denote antidotes for certain purposes.

That there was some basis for this belief is shown by the modern theories of the adsorptive properties of hydrated siliceous earths.

Preparation—Kaolin is widely distributed in nature. Most Kaolin deposits, however, are frequently contaminated with ferric oxide (hence the red color of ordinary clay) and some other impurities, such as calcium carbonate, magnesium carbonate, etc. To render such Kaolin suitable for pharmaceutical use it has to be purified by treatment with hydrochloric acid or sulfuric acid, or both, then washed well with water.

Kaolin of a high degree of purity, directly suitable for

pharmaceutical use without acid purification, is now mined in the state of Georgia. England has large deposits of a fine grade of Kaolin. The Kaolin from these deposits is freed of coarse particles by elutriation or by screening. Kaolin is essentially a colloid, and the *colloidal kaolin* on the market differs only from ordinary Kaolin in that it contains a larger percentage of fine particles and it is prepared by special screening.

The BP also recognizes a native *Heavy Kaolin* (*Kaolinum Ponderosum*) for use in poultices. The Light Kaolin BP (Kaolin NF) is prepared from the heavy variety by elutriation.

Description—A soft, white, or yellowish white powder, or lumps. It has a characteristic earthy or clay-like taste and, when moistened with water, it becomes darker and develops a pronounced clay-like odor.

Solubility—Insoluble in water, in cold diluted acids, and in solutions of the alkali hydroxides.

Uses—Kaolin, either alone or as *Kaolin Mixture with Pectin*, is used medicinally as an *adsorbent*. It is of value chiefly in the treatment of *diarrhea* caused by agents capable of being adsorbed, as, for example, the diarrhea of food poisoning or dysentery. Kaolin has also been used in the treatment of chronic ulcerative colitis, but it is doubtful whether any adsorptive capacity is retained by the time the preparation reaches the colon.

It has been used as a clarifying and decolorizing medium and as a filtering medium, but it must never be used as a filtering agent for liquids containing alkaloids, as it has been shown that it adsorbs alkaloids, often separating them completely from the liquids filtered.

Dose (unofficial)—It is usually given suspended in water in the dose of from 50 to 100 Gm, at 3-hour intervals.

Veterinary Dose—*Horses*, 50 to **200 Gm**; *Cattle*, 50 to **250 Gm**; *Sheep*, 30 to **60 Gm**; *Swine*, 15 to 30 Gm; *Dogs*, 0.5 to 5 Gm; also used to bind water to form a viscous gel for the suspension of insoluble anthelmintics.

Kaolin Mixture with Pectin NF [Ka-Pek (*APC*)]— *Preparation:* Mix kaolin (200 Gm) with purified water (500 ml). Triturate pectin (10 Gm), powdered tragacanth (5 Gm), and sodium saccharin (1 Gm) with glycerin (20 ml) and add to this, with constant stirring, benzoic acid (2 Gm) dissolved in boiling purified water (300 ml). Allow the mixture to stand until it cools to room temperature and all the pectin is dissolved. Add peppermint oil (0.75 ml) and the kaolin–water mixture, mix thoroughly, and finally add sufficient purified water to make 1000 ml. In order to obtain a product with suitable consistency when larger amounts are prepared, the quantity of tragacanth and, if necessary, the quantity of pectin may be altered. However, if the proportion of pectin in the formula is altered by more than 10%, the pectin content of the preparation must be clearly stated on the label. *Uses:* An *adsorbent demulcent.* See *Kaolin*. *Dose: Usual, 30 ml as needed.*

Magnesium Trisilicate—see page 792.

Pectin NF

Pectin is a purified carbohydrate product obtained from the dilute acid extract of the inner portion of the rind of citrus fruits or from apple pomace. It consists chiefly of partially methoxylated polygalacturonic acids.

Pectin yields not less than 6.7% of methoxy groups and not less than 74.0% of $C_6H_{10}O_7$ (galacturonic acid), calculated on the dried basis.

Pectin may be standardized to the convenient "150 jelly grade" by addition of dextrose or other sugars, and it may contain sodium citrate or other buffer salts. Such pectin is not suitable for medicinal use.

Description—A coarse or fine powder, yellowish white in color, almost odorless, and with a mucilaginous taste.

Solubility—Almost completely soluble in 20 parts of water at 25°, forming a viscous, opalescent, colloidal solution which flows readily and is acid to litmus; insoluble in alcohol or in diluted alcohol, and in other organic solvents; dissolves in water more readily if first moistened with alcohol, glycerin, or simple syrup, or if first mixed with 3 or more parts of sucrose.

Incompatibilities—Pectin is precipitated from solution by an excess of *alcohol*. *Metals*, particularly the heavy metals, form insoluble derivatives. In the presence of *alkalies*, Pectin undergoes progressive hydrolysis resulting in a demethylation followed by a splitting of the glycosidic linkages of the galacturonic acid units. *In cold acid solution* it is more stable; prolonged heating of such a solution causes hydrolysis. Liquefaction of pectin pastes may be due to a hydrolysis which accompanies growth of certain types of *mold*.

Uses—Pectin is a *protective* of value in the treatment of *diarrhea* in infants and children. The unchanged molecules of the polygalacturonic acids may have an *adsorbent* action in the intestine.

Other Adsorbents

Aluminum Hydroxide USP IX [Al(OH)₃]—White, bulky amorphous powder; insoluble in water. *Uses:* A mordant for dyeing, a constituent of colors and lakes, a filtering medium, a desiccant powder, an adsorbent, and an antacid. *Dose:* 0.13 to 0.3 Gm.

Kaolin, Heavy BP [China Clay]—A native, hydrated aluminum silicate, freed from most of its impurities by elutriation and then dried. It occurs as a soft, whitish, odorless, and tasteless powder, free from gritty particles. It is insoluble in water and in mineral acids. When kaolin is prescribed, light kaolin should be dispensed. *Uses:* In the preparation of kaolin poultice.

Kaolin, Light BP—A hydrated aluminum silicate freed from most of its impurities by elutriation and then dried. It occurs as an odorless, tasteless, light, white powder, free from gritty particles. It is insoluble in water and mineral acids. When given orally, it adsorbs substances from the gastrointestinal tract and increases the bulk of feces. *Uses:* In the symptomatic treatment of enteritis, colitis, cholera, dysentery and diarrhea; in the treatment of food and alkaloidal poisoning; as a dusting powder and as an ingredient of toilet powders; as a pill excipient; for clarification purposes. *Dose: orally,* 15 to 60 Gm.

Polycarbophil NF

[Acrylic Acid–Divinyl Glycol Copolymer; ingredient of Sorboquel (*White*)]

Polycarbophil is polyacrylic acid cross-linked with divinyl glycol.

Preparation—Acrylic acid and divinyl glycol (1,5-hexadiene-3,4-diol) are copolymerized in a hot salt slurry using azobis[methylpropionitrile] as the initiator. US Pat. 3,202,577.

Description—White to creamy white granules, having a slight, characteristic, esterlike odor. It contains a maximum of 1.5% water.

Solubility—Swells but is insoluble in water; insoluble in most organic solvents.

Uses—Polycarbophil is a pharmacologically inert substance which has the capacity to bind free fecal water. Hence, it is used in diarrheal disorders to decrease the fluidity or looseness of stools. Orally administered, Polycarbophil exerts its most marked hydrosorptive action only on reaching the slightly acid or alkaline medium of the small intestine and colon. Polycarbophil should not be used in nursing mothers or in patients with glaucoma, prostatic hypertrophy, peptic ulcer, gastrointestinal obstructions, or cardiospasm.

Dose—*Usual,* **500 mg** 4 times a day.

Miscellaneous Gastrointestinal Drugs

A number of miscellaneous gastrointestinal drugs whose therapeutic value has not been fully established are presented in this section. Some of these may be classified arbitrarily either as *bitters* or *carminatives*. In addition, the drug Dexpanthenol is included since its action is confined to the gastrointestinal tract and it is used in the treatment of gastrointestinal atony and distention.

Bitters are substances used empirically to increase salivary and gastric secretions and to improve the appetite. Their action is probably psychic, although they may act reflexly to stimulate the taste buds. They are rarely prescribed in modern medicine.

Carminatives are substances which relieve gaseous distension of the stomach or intestines. Many carminative volatile oils are also used as flavoring agents (see Chapter 71 page 1321).

Anise Oil—see page 1324.

Camphor—see page 773.

Camphor Spirit—see page 774.

Camphor Water—see RPS-13, page 436.

Capsicum—see page 777.

Capsicum Oleoresin—see RPS-13, page 497.

Capsicum Tincture—see RPS-13, page 491.

Caraway—see page 1325.

Caraway Oil—see page 1325.

Cardamom Oil—see page 1336.

Cardamom Seed—see page 1325.

Cardamom Spirit, Compound—see page 1336.

Cardamom Tincture, Compound—see page 1342.

Chlorobutanol—see page 1317.

Chloroform—see page 1056.

Cinnamon—see page 1325.

Cinnamon, Ceylon—see page 1337.

Cinnamon Oil—see page 1326.

Coriander Oil—see page 1326.

Dexpanthenol

[d-Pantothenyl Alcohol;   Cozyme (*Travenol*);   Ilopan (*Warren-Teed*);
Motilyn (*Abbott*)]

$$HOCH_2-\overset{\overset{\displaystyle CH_3}{|}}{\underset{\underset{\displaystyle CH_3}{|}}{C}}-\overset{\overset{\displaystyle OH}{|}}{\underset{\underset{\displaystyle H}{|}}{C}}-CONHCH_2CH_2CH_2OH$$

Dexpanthenol is D(+)-2,4-dihydroxy-N-(3-hydroxy-propyl)-3,3-dimethylbutyramide.

Preparation—Propanolamine is caused to undergo chemical addition to the lactone of D-2.4-dihydroxy-3,3-dimethylbutyric acid through ring rupture. US Pat. 2,413,077.

Description—A viscous, somewhat hygroscopic liquid with a slightly bitter taste.

Solubility—Freely soluble in water and alcohol; slightly soluble in ether.

Uses—Dexpanthenol, the alcohol analogue of D-pantothenic acid, is said to increase the amount of coenzyme A available for the synthesis of acetylcholine. The increased formation of acetylcholine is thought to increase peristalsis and intestinal tone. Hence, Dexpanthol has been proposed for the prevention and treatment of gastrointestinal atony and distention. Side effects are minimal and the drug has no pharmacologic effect on the intestine, cardiovascular, or respiratory systems. Dexpanthenol prolongs bleeding time and, hence, is contraindicated in hemophilia. It should not be used in combination with parasympathomimetic drugs. Since the clinical value of this agent has not been fully established, its use should be considered experimental.

Dose—Usual, adult, 250 or 500 mg intramuscularly repeated in 2 hours and then every 6 hours for the prevention of gastrointestinal atony and distention.

Dosage Forms—Injection: 250 and 500 mg/ml.

Ether—see page 1057.

Fennel Oil—see page 1327.

Peppermint Spirit NF

[Essence of Peppermint]

Peppermint Spirit contains, in each 100 ml, 9.0–11.0 ml of peppermint oil.

Peppermint Oil...................	**100 ml**
Peppermint, in coarse powder.......	**10 Gm**
Alcohol, a sufficient quantity,	
To make......................	**1000 ml**

Macerate the peppermint leaves, freed as much as possible from stems and coarsely powdered, for 1 hour in 500 ml of purified water, and then strongly express them. Add the moist, macerated leaves to 900 ml of alcohol, and allow the mixture to stand for 6 hours with frequent agitation. Filter, and to the filtrate add the oil and sufficient alcohol to make the product measure 1000 ml.

The maceration of the peppermint leaves with water is for the purpose of removing brownish colored pigments. If this processing were not performed, the finished product would not possess a brilliant green color, since the undesirable pigments are also soluble in alcohol. On the other hand, the maceration with water does not remove chlorophyll. For the same reason, maceration with water is performed with spearmint leaves in preparing *Spearmint Spirit* (RPS-13, page 452).

Alcohol Content—From 79 to 85% of C_2H_5OH.

Uses—A *carminative* in *flatulence* and *nausea*.
Dose—*Usual*, 1 ml 3 times a day.
Veterinary Dose—*Horses* and *Cattle*, **8 to 15 ml;** *Dogs*, **0.6 to 2 ml.**

Peppermint Water—see page 1338.

Pimenta Oil—see page 1337.

Spearmint Oil—see page 1334.

Diphenoxylate Hydrochloride NF

[Ethyl 1-(3-Cyano-3,3-diphenylpropyl)-4-phenylisonipecotate Monohydrochloride; ingredient of Lomotil (*Searle*)]

Diphenoxylate Hydrochloride contains 98.0–102.0% of $C_{30}H_{32}N_2O_2 \cdot HCl$ (489.06) calculated on the dried basis.

Preparation—Ethyl 4-phenylisonipecotate (prepared as described under *Meperidine Hydrochloride* (page 1130) except omitting the final step of N-methylation), is condensed with 2,2-diphenyl-4-bromobutyronitrile by refluxing in toluene using either an excess of the ester or another suitable dehydrobrominating agent. Extraction of the filtered reaction product with hydrochloric acid followed by alkalinization of the extract precipitates diphenoxylate (base) which may be converted to the hydrochloride by extracting with ether and treating the extract with hydrogen chloride. US Pat. 2,898,340.

Description—A white, odorless, crystalline powder. A saturated solution has a pH of about 3.3.

Solubility—Soluble in methanol; sparingly soluble in alcohol and acetone; slightly soluble in water and isopropyl alcohol; freely soluble in chloroform; practically insoluble in ether and solvent hexane.

Uses—See *Diphenoxylate Hydrochloride and Atropine Sulfate Solution*.

Dose—5 to 40 mg per day; *usual*, **5 mg** 4 times a day.

Dosage Forms—and Atropine Sulfate Solution NF (see below): 2.5 mg (diphenoxylate hydrochloride) and 25 mcg (atropine sulfate)/5 ml; and Atropine Sulfate Tablets NF: 2.5 mg (diphenoxylate hydrochloride) and 25 mcg (atropine sulfate).

Diphenoxylate Hydrochloride and Atropine Sulfate Solution NF contains 93.0–107.0% of the labeled amount of $C_{30}H_{32}N_2O_2 \cdot HCl$ (diphenoxylate hydrochloride), and 80.0–120.0% of the labeled amount of $(C_{17}H_{23}NO_3)_2 \cdot H_2SO_4 \cdot H_2O$ (atropine sulfate). *Uses:* Diphenoxylate Hydrochloride and Atropine Sulfate Solution contains 2.5 mg of Diphenoxylate Hydrochloride and 0.025 mg of Atropine Sulfate in each 5 ml of solution. This preparation inhibits excessive gastrointestinal propulsion and is indicated in the treatment of *diarrhea* associated with *gastroenteritis, irritable bowel, functional hypermotility, regional enteritis, drugs, acute infections, ulcerative colitis,* and *food poisoning.* It is also useful in the control of *intestinal transit time* in patients with *ileostomies* and *colostomies.* Diphenoxylate Hydrochloride and Atropine Sulfate Solution exerts essentially no analgesia and no evidence for addiction liability has been reported. This preparation is contraindicated in patients with cirrhosis or advanced liver disease. It should be used with caution in patients on barbiturates since the drug may potentiate the activity of the latter agent. Side effects are usually minor and include nausea, sedation, dizziness, vomiting, pruritus, skin eruption, insomnia, and abdominal cramps. Numbness of the extremities, headache, blurring of the vision, swelling of the gums, and general malaise have also been reported. *Dose: Usual,* adult, 10 ml 3 or 4 times daily (unofficial).

Other Miscellaneous Gastrointestinal Drugs

Asafetida NF X, [Gum Asafetida, Devil's Dung]—The oleoresin obtained by incising the living rhizome and roots of *Ferula Assafaetida* Linné, *Ferula rubricaulis* Boissier, and of *Ferula faetida* (Bunge) Regel, and probably of other species of *Ferula* (Fam. *Umbelliferæ*). It occurs as a soft mass or as pliable masses composed of agglutinated tears imbedded in a weak brown to moderately yellowish brown matrix. It hardens on drying. The surface of the freshly fractured tears is white, changing gradually to a moderately yellowish brown. When moistened with water, the tears become orange. The odor is persistent and alliaceous, and the taste is bitter. It contains 60 per cent of resin, which consists chiefly of the ferulic acid ester of the alcohol asaresinotannol, 25 per cent gum, and from 3 to 9 per cent of volatile oil. Vanillin is present in traces. *Uses:* As a carminative, placebo, and formerly as an antispasmodic. *Dose: Orally,* 0.4 Gm.

Gentian NF XI [Gentian Root; Bitter Root]—Dried rhizomes and roots of *Gentiana lutea* Linné (Fam. *Gentianaceæ*). *Uses:* Obsolete bitter tonic. *Dose:* 1 Gm. *Veterinary Dose:* Horses and Cattle, 15 to 30 Gm; Sheep and Swine, 4 to 8 Gm; Dogs, 300 mg to 1 Gm.

Sodium Phytate ($C_6H_9Na_9O_{24}P_6$) [Rencal (*Squibb*)]—A sodium salt of inositol hexaphosphoric acid (phytic acid) derived from corn. *Uses:* Blocks the absorption of calcium from the gastrointestinal tract and is used in the treatment of hypercalciuria. *Dose:* 3 Gm 3 times a day.

References

1. Tice, L. F., and Osol, A., *J. APhA,* **25,** 1108 (1936).

45 | Blood, Fluids, and Electrolytes

Whole blood, blood fractions, and blood substitutes—hematopoietics and hematinics—agents affecting coagulation of the blood—anticoagulants—electrolytes—miscellaneous parenteral fluids and systemic buffers—miscellaneous drugs that affect blood

This chapter was prepared by

Douglas M. Surgenor, PhD, *Provost, Faculty of Health Sciences, State University of New York at Buffalo, Buffalo, N.Y.   14214*

Blood is composed of two major parts, which may be recognized if clotting is prevented while a specimen of blood is observed. One part, which settles to the bottom, consists of the so-called *formed elements*, composed of red blood cells and other particulate components of the blood. These form from 40 to 50% of the bulk of normal human blood. The overlying, straw-colored, translucent liquid, in which the formed elements are suspended, is known as *plasma*. The components of these two major parts of blood may be described in greater detail as follows.

Formed Elements

1.   Red Blood Cells (*erythrocytes*)—of which normally 4.5 to 5 million are present in each cubic millimeter of whole blood. They serve to transport oxygen to tissues and aid in returning carbon dioxide to the lungs. Their major component is the protein hemoglobin, which has a specific affinity for oxygen.

2.   White Blood Cells (*leukocytes*)—in normal blood numbering 5 to 10,000 per cu mm, rising to 20 to 50,000 in the presence of infection and certain other conditions, and to much larger numbers in leukemia. They act as scavengers, taking up foreign matter and attacking invading microorganisms, and may play a role in the formation of antibodies.

3.   Platelets (*thrombocytes*)—small particles which play a vital role in the initiation of blood clotting wherever a blood vessel is cut or injured.

Plasma

1.   Water—in which the other constituents are dissolved.

2.   Inorganic Substances—Sodium, 142 mEq/L*; potassium, 4.3 mEq/L; calcium, 5.0 mEq/L; magnesium, 3.4 mEq/L; chloride, 104 mEq/L; bicarbonate, 27 mEq/L; phosphate, 2.3 mEq/L; sulfate, 0.6 mEq/L. The electrolytes represent about 0.85% of the plasma.

3.   Organic Substances—*lactic acid, urea, amino acids, creatinine, glucose,* etc.—the raw materials of tissue metabolism, in transport to the tissue cells as nutrients, or to the kidney or liver for disposal. Under this heading belong the *hormones* and *proteins*. Normally about 7% of the plasma by weight consists of proteins, classified in general as *albumins* and *globulins*.

4.   Dissolved Gases—aside from the large amounts of *oxygen* and *carbon dioxide* which the red cells are especially equipped to transport, these gases and the others of the atmosphere are dissolved in the plasma as well; so are inhaled gaseous drugs or poisons such as nitrous oxide and hydrogen cyanide.

5.   Miscellaneous Foreign Substances—Any drugs or poisons which are absorbed through the skin or viscera may be present in the plasma—eg, sulfadiazine, alcohol, benzene, and some toxins. Likewise bacteria or other microorganisms may be liberated into the blood stream during the course of infections.

Whole Blood, Blood Fractions, and Blood Substitutes

The blood is both an important regulator and a mirror of the proper functioning of body cells. Although it does not come into direct contact with cells other than the vascular endothelium, the interstitial fluid and lymph so resemble plasma, except that they are nearly devoid of protein, that plasma may be thought of as the culture medium of the tissue cells. Consequently, its electrolyte and organic composition is of the utmost importance. Plasma is, of course, also the vehicle for the transport of most nutrients to, and many wastes from, the tissues. The proteins in plasma are importantly involved in the regulation of the hydration of the tissues by virtue of osmosis resulting from the impermeability of the vascular endothelium to most of the protein. Some of the plasma proteins are intimately involved in the clotting of blood and therefore in its conservation. The erythrocytes are especially involved with oxygen and carbon dioxide transport.

Whole Blood

The National Institutes of Health regulations, which are also widely followed by blood banks not actually under NIH control, provide that blood may be collected for human use only from persons who are certified by a physician as being free of transmissible disease, as far as can be determined from the donor's personal history and physical examination, etc. The usual amount drawn is 500 ml. The blood is collected into acid–citrate–dextrose ("ACD") solution, containing sodium citrate, citric acid, and dextrose in concentrations sufficient to provide the optimum pH and dextrose content for long-term preservation of red cells (see *Anticoagulant Acid Citrate Dextrose Solution*, page 833). A sample of blood is collected at the time of bleeding and submitted to serologic tests to exclude syphilis in the donor.

The introduction of ACD (see page 833) extended the useful life of the red cells with the result that, following storage under proper conditions, the blood can be used with safety for a period of three weeks after collection. The drawing of blood into $\frac{1}{6}$ to $\frac{1}{4}$ of its volume of ACD solution is now universally recommended for blood to be kept on hand for emergencies, and the use of this solution has greatly extended the flexibility of hospital or community blood banks. Particular care must be exercised in collecting blood for this purpose, not only in the maintenance of scrupulously sterile technique, but in drawing the blood into prechilled bottles which are then kept at 4° to 10°, preferably near the lower temperature.

If used as whole blood, it is carefully handled and

---

* mEq = milliequivalents.

stored in the cold without further processing or testing, except for occasional observation to detect evidence of hemolysis or contamination.

Uses for Blood and Blood Derivatives—The many physiological functions of blood derive from the specific roles of its many parts; in addition to the formed elements there are more than 70 discrete proteins in the plasma. When whole blood has been lost, as by hemorrhage, then whole blood is required for replacement. However, the use of whole blood to overcome a deficiency of a single part constitutes a dissipation of the other useful parts. In the majority of instances, the administration of a single component in concentrated form elicits a far better response than the administration of a single component in whole blood. Furthermore, by using the specific parts of the blood, the supply of blood can be used more economically; the net result is utilization of the components of a single donation for several purposes.

The program to make available certain parts of the blood (blood derivatives) as well as whole blood is well under way, although the number of products now available is still far short of the number of known parts of the blood. Thus, for example, the red cells can be made available for treatment of anemia, the albumins for treatment of shock, and the gamma globulins for the prophylaxis of certain infectious diseases. These and other important available blood derivatives are discussed in the following sections.

In the United States the processing of blood into blood derivatives is carried on under both public and private auspices. The blood which is freely given by the American public to the Red Cross, state and other public agencies is processed and made available by the agencies concerned to qualified physicians through designated channels. In addition, several pharmaceutical houses process blood obtained from paid donors or placental sources; the blood derivatives so obtained are marketed in the usual way. Although several products are available through both channels, others are available through one or the other.

The use of blood and blood derivatives is accompanied by the risk of transmission of the virus of homologous serum jaundice. Unfortunately, there is no known method of demonstrating the presence or absence of hepatitis-producing viruses. With single units of blood, the risk depends primarily upon the incidence of the virus in the donor population. When multiple transfusions are employed, the risk mounts accordingly. Similarly, if plasma is pooled, a single infected sample may contaminate the whole pool. On the other hand, the risk may be diminished or indeed eliminated by suitable processing treatments. Thus, gamma globulin prepared by the ethanol-water fractionation procedure is free of virus even without specific viricidal treatment. Carefully documented evidence based on almost 20 years of experience, indicates that *Normal Human Serum Albumin USP* carries no risk of virus transmission, as a result of heating the solution to 60°C for 10 hours. From this experience it is not unlikely that any product which can be heated at 60°C for 10 hours will have a greatly diminished, if not zero, risk of viral transmission, but no absolute statement can be made about such products. Unfortunately, very few products can withstand such rigorous treatment, and other means have been sought to inactivate viruses, but with less than complete success. These include irradiation with ultraviolet light, or with cathode rays, and chemical treatment with various substances such as β-propiolactone. None of these methods, as presently used,

can be relied on to inactivate completely all viruses that might be present, although it is likely that they may diminish the risk associated with use of the material. In short, except for certain products such as albumin and gamma globulin which are known to be free of virus, most blood derivatives must be assumed to involve a risk of virus transmission, and this risk must be weighed against the medical consequences to the patient of withholding the use of the product.

Whole Blood USP

[Citrated Whole Blood (Human); Citrated Whole Human Blood USP XVII]

Whole Blood is blood that has been drawn from a selected donor under rigid aseptic precautions. It contains citrate ion or heparin as an anticoagulant. Its production and distribution are subject to federal regulations (see *Biologics*, page 1425).

Description—A deep red, opaque liquid from which the corpuscles readily settle upon standing for 24 to 48 hours, leaving a clear, yellowish or pinkish supernatant layer. If the blood has been drawn soon after the donor has eaten, it may, on standing, acquire a layer of fatlike material near its surface.

A deep pink or red color in the plasma, or a purplish tint at the surface of the cell portion, usually indicates that the blood is unsatisfactory for use.

Uses—See the general statement (page 815).

Dose—*Intravenous, infusion,* as needed to replenish blood volume; *usual,* **1 unit** (500 ml) repeated as necessary.

Dosage Forms—Between 440 and 500 ml.

Formed Elements

Packed Red Blood Cells, and *concentrated red blood cells* are derivatives of whole blood which frequently can be used in its place, when the primary need is replacement of red cells. "Packed red cells" consist of the red cells and most of the white cells left at the bottom of the container after the plasma has been drawn off. They must be handled with the same extreme care, as regards sterility and uniform chilling, as is required for whole blood. They are kept in the original container, but a small amount of saline diluent may be added to them to render them less viscous just before they are administered to a patient. "Concentrated red cells" are similarly derived from the residue remaining after drawing off the plasma; the buffy layer is discarded. Packed red cells and concentrated red cells must be grouped and typed as for whole blood. The recommended dating period (providing proper refrigeration has been maintained) is not exceeding 10 days from the date of bleeding.

Frozen Packed Red Blood Cells is a preparation in which the red cells are suspended in a glycerol solution and frozen at temperatures ranging from −80°C to −120°C. Such cells can be kept frozen for periods of two years or more without deterioration. Before use, the suspension is thawed and the glycerol medium is replaced with a more physiological solution.

White Cells and Platelets—Although the classical methods for blood collection and processing preserve many of the useful qualities, they do not prevent the rapid deterioration of many of the fragile parts of the blood, such as the white cells, platelets, and certain plasma proteins. In modern processing of blood, procedures are used which preserve many more of the components of blood than when classical methods are used.

Preserved platelets have been successfully re-infused into recipients suffering from platelet deficiency. It now appears that it may be possible to stockpile platelets for use in emergency situations. Studies on the utilization of white cells are not as advanced, primarily because of the complexity of the cells, and also the existence of complex white cell types.

Packed Human Blood Cells USP

[Packed Red Blood Cells (Human)]

Packed Human Blood Cells is whole blood from which plasma has been removed. Packed Human Blood Cells may be prepared at any time during the dating period of the whole blood from which it is derived, except that if centrifuging is used for the separation of plasma and cells, the preparation is made not later than 6 days after the blood has been drawn. Its production and distribution are subject to federal regulations (see *Biologics*, page 1425).

Description—Dark red when packed and may show a slight creamy layer on the surface and a small supernatant layer of yellow or opalescent plasma. Resuspended Human Blood Cells is a dark red fluid.

Uses—Human blood cells may be used as a *blood replenisher* in any condition in which the primary deficiency in the blood is that of the erythrocytes. Thus they are used in the emergency treatment of a number of the anemias which formerly were treated with whole blood transfusions. Human blood cells are not suitable alone as a replacement fluid in hemorrhage, but they may be employed in cases where chronic blood loss is not too great to decrease appreciably the plasma volume and plasma protein content.

Dose—*Usual, intravenous infusion*, the equivalent of 1 unit (500 ml) of whole blood, repeated as necessary.

Dosage Forms—Equivalent to red cells from 1 unit (about 500 ml) of human blood.

Plasma, Plasma Fractions, and Plasma Expanders

Hemorrhage and shock result in loss of blood volume, which, if carried beyond a certain critical point, leads to circulatory failure. Replacement of the plasma proteins, or injection of a substance having similar osmotic properties, will restore the blood volume at least temporarily, so that circulation of oxygen to the tissues may be maintained. Many substances have been employed for this purpose: *whole blood*, which in certain situations is ideal but which is not always immediately available; *human plasma*, which is extremely effective but is unstable in the liquid form, relatively cumbersome in the dry form, involves injection of salt and water, which are in some cases undesirable, and finally, cannot readily be rendered free of pathogenic viruses without rather expensive types of processing; and *normal human serum albumin*, the protein in the plasma which functions to control blood volume (see below).

Plasma Extenders—Much effort has been expended in the search for nontoxic substances, not of human origin, which might be used in an emergency to restore blood volume. It should be emphasized that these substances are in no sense substitutes for plasma; following their emergency use, plasma or blood must be replaced as rapidly as feasible.

Plasma Proteins—Many of the important physiological actions of blood result from the properties of the plasma proteins. Proteins are the most complex chemical entities known. Each is composed of varying numbers of the twenty or more known amino acids, the total number of amino-acid units in each protein molecule ranging from a few hundred to many thousands. Many protein molecules in addition possess various attached phospholipids, carbohydrates, or other organic complexes. A minor shift in the arrangement of any of these components may result in a major change in the properties of the molecule. Physically, proteins may vary greatly, from the egg-shaped albumin molecule with a molecular weight of 70,000 to the needle-like fibrinogen molecule with a molecular weight near 500,-000. By their nature, amino acids contribute both basic and acid properties to protein molecules; this amphoteric property has a fundamental bearing on the behavior of proteins in solution. The numerous free acid or basic groups on the surface bear negative or positive charges, respectively, resulting in a total charge which under given conditions is characteristic for each protein, both in its net algebraic sum and in the evenness or unevenness of its distribution over the surface of the molecule.

Though it is easy to determine the types and numbers of amino acids and other components present in a given protein, the sequence of the individual amino acid residues in the polypeptide chain can be determined only with difficulty. The amino acid sequence in insulin and a few other small proteins is known, but only limited information is available concerning larger proteins. The classification and definition of proteins must therefore be based primarily upon their physicochemical properties: solubility in water, in salt solutions and in organic solvents; molecular weight (determined chiefly by rate of sedimentation in an ultracentrifuge); shape (determined by viscosity measurements and other properties; rate of movement in an electrical field (usually determined by means of the electrophoresis apparatus); net electrical charge; electrical "moment;" and certain other physical properties similar in principle to those mentioned. In addition, certain proteins possess biological properties which aid greatly in characterizing them: eg, ability to form a clot (fibrinogen); catalysis of specific chemical reactions (enzymes); precipitation with bacteria or their products (antibodies), etc. It is upon a knowledge of these various properties that any successful separation and characterization of a pure protein species must be based.

Physiologically, the most clearly established role of albumin appears to be its water-retaining (osmotic) capacity. It is due chiefly to plasma albumin that the water of the plasma, instead of diffusing into the tissues, is retained in the blood stream, maintaining the volume of blood which is necessary for effective heart action and circulation. Albumin, although it comprises less than 60% of the plasma proteins, contributes 80% of the osmotic effect. Another highly important property of albumin is its capacity to bind various chemical substances, including numerous ions and drugs, such as the sulfonamide drugs.

Globulins are extremely varied both in physicochemical and in biological properties. They include *fibrinogen*, from which blood clots are formed; *antibodies* (chiefly gamma globulin), which furnish immunity against infections; *prothrombin*, which under appropriate circumstances is converted to the enzyme *thrombin* which causes fibrinogen to clot; *isoagglutinins*, a group of antibodies which react with specific blood group substances; various enzymes (eg, amylase, lipase, peptidase, phosphatase, serum esterase); a metal-binding beta globulin which serves in the transport of iron

Properties and Interactions of Protein Components of Human Plasma[a]

Protein components	Estimated % plasma proteins	Sedimentation constant $S_{20, w}$	Approximate isoelectric point	Specific chemical interactions
Major protein components				
Serum albumin	52	4.6	4.9	Fatty acids, dyes, bile salts, drugs, and mercury
Mercaptalbumin	(34)	...	...	
α_2-Glycoproteins	1.2	9	4.9	Carbohydrates and barium
α_2-Mucoproteins	0.5	9	4.9	
Fibrinogen	4	9	<5.3	Thrombin
Cold insoluble globulin	0.15	...	<5.3	
α_1-Lipoproteins	3	5	5.2	Steroids and carotenoids
β_1-Lipoproteins	5	7	5.4	
β_1-Lipid-poor euglobulins	{2 {1	7} 20}	5.5	
β_1-Metal-combining protein	3	5.0	5.8	Iron and copper
β_2-Globulins	3	7	6.3	
γ-Globulins	11	{ 7 {10	6.3} 7.3}	Antigens
	86			
Other protein components				
Prothrombin	0.1	...	...	Calcium and thromboplastin
Plasminogen	...	...	...	Streptokinase
Angiotensinogen	...	...	...	Renin
Iodoproteins	...	...	...	
Isoagglutinins	(0.03)	...	6.3	Incompatible red cells
Complement components {C'$_1$ {C'$_2$	0.4	...	...	Antigen-antibody complex
Amylase	...	...	...	Starch
Choline esterase	0.005	...	4.5	Choline esters
Alkaline phosphatase	...	...	...	Phosphate esters
Peptidase	...	...	...	L-Leucylglycylglycine
β-Glucuronidase	...	...	...	β-Glucuronides
Caeruloplasmin	...	...	4.4	Copper
α_1-Small acid protein	0.5	2.9	3.0	
α_1-Bilirubin globulin	0.05	...	4.7	Bilirubin
α_2-Protein	0.1	2.9	...	Barium
β_1-Protein	0.05	5	...	

[a] Courtesy, Cohn, et al.[1]

in the plasma; alpha and beta lipoproteins which probably serve to transport cholesterol, phospholipids, and other fats in the blood; a sizable remainder of alpha and beta globulins to which no specific function has yet been assigned; a variety of other special components, as noted in the table, such as heparin complement, plasminogen, and hypertensinogen, for which definite physiological functions are known; and finally others such as the cold insoluble globulin, for which a function cannot yet be clearly discerned.

Plasma Fractions—The first fractionation of blood consisted in the separation of the plasma from the red cells by centrifugation, or by allowing blood to clot and drawing off the serum which separated from the clot. This laboratory procedure was put to practical use when it was found possible to preserve blood plasma or serum in suitable form (and quantity) for intravenous injection to restore blood volume after hemorrhage, or to correct plasma protein deficiencies. The onset of World War II created a need for a blood substitute more compact and stable than plasma. It was seen that a purified concentrate of albumin in liquid form would provide such a substitute, and the difficult task of preparing such a pure concentrate was undertaken by the late Professor Cohn of Harvard Medical School and his colleagues, working with a diversified team of physicists, immunologists, chemists, and clinicians, and utilizing a part of the large quantity of blood procured through the volunteer blood donor program of the American Red Cross. Despite the inherent difficulties of the problem—notably the tremendous complexity of the mixture of components in plasma, and the great instability of many of these proteins—methods were devised for preparation of human plasma albumin which was over 99% pure. Unlike most plasma proteins, it proved to be extraordinarily stable, so that it did not require desiccation or continuous refrigeration, and therefore could be kept on hand as a 25% solution, ready for instant use. Separation of the albumin left the remaining plasma oteins as by-products. One by one many of these mponents were in turn fractionated, providing highly rified antibody solutions, isoagglutinins in large quan-y, and clotting agents so processed that they could rve previously unmet needs in surgery and medi-e. Subsequent studies have broadened the uses albumin and pointed to new ways in which the her products can be employed. Thus it is now pos-le to derive many specific pharmaceutical agents m one blood donation, enabling more efficient use of given quantity of blood. What started as a wartime udy has therefore developed into a valuable procedure r civilian needs.

Investigations continue to center primarily on im-oving the methods of fractionation so as to obtain portant labile proteins which were damaged under e conditions encountered in the older methods of ocessing.

Normal Human Serum Albumin USP

ormal Serum Albumin (Human); Albumisol (*MSD*); Albuspan (*Parke-Davis*); Proserum (*Pitman-Moore*)]

Normal Human Serum Albumin is a sterile prepara-on of serum albumin obtained by fractionating blood om healthy, human donors. Not less than 96.0% of s total protein is albumin. It is a solution containing, each 100 ml, 25 Gm of the serum albumin osmot-ally equivalent to 500 ml, or 5 Gm equivalent to 100 l, of normal human plasma. It contains no added ntimicrobial agent, but may contain stabilizing gents. Its production and distribution are subject federal regulations (see *Biologics*, page 1425).

Description—A moderately viscous, clear, brownish uid. It is substantially odorless, and, when dried, has a ght yellow to deep cream color.

Preparation—For clinical use Normal Human erum Albumin is made up into a solution. For certain urposes (eg, treatment of edema in kidney diseases and ther conditions) it is essential that the albumin solu-on have a very low salt content. "Salt-poor" prepara-ons contain sodium acetyltryptophanate or sodium cetyltryptophanate and sodium caprylate as stabi-zers; the 25% solution may contain no more than .33% sodium, and no preservative. The 5% solution made up in isotonic sodium chloride solution. They re sterilized in the final container by heating at 60° for 0 hours, in order to kill any pathogenic viruses which ay be present. The presence of the organic stabilizer akes it possible to submit albumin to this intense reatment without denaturing the protein.

Because of its remarkable stability to heat, normal erum albumin may be kept without refrigeration in he liquid state, ready for immediate use in the field. 100-ml package of the 25% solution occupies only ne-sixth the space of a 500-ml package of dried plasma ut has an equal osmotic effect. The viscosity of a 5% albumin solution is relatively low, so that it flows s readily as whole blood.

Uses—In the treatment of *shock* or *hemorrhage*, lbumin serves as an emergency agent for restoration f blood volume, by drawing water from the tissues. ach Gm of albumin holds about 18 ml of water in he blood stream. Because its action depends on avail-bility of tissue water, albumin should not be used in everely dehydrated patients without simultaneous dministration of saline or glucose solutions. It has een used in protein replacement therapy where serum rotein levels are low due to excessive loss as in *nephro-*

sis, certain skin diseases, and other conditions; or due to inadequate formation of proteins resulting from *nutritional disturbances, cirrhosis*, or other causes. However, the value of albumin in the therapy of chronic nephritis or cirrhosis is less impressive than in acute hypo-albuminemia. The "salt-poor" form should be used by preference in protein replacement therapy, since the edema which is associated with protein deficiencies is aggravated by administration of salt.

Low salt content and the high stability of the single protein component present render "salt-poor" albumin the agent of choice in certain types of protein replacement therapy, bearing in mind the following limitations: Albumin does not in any sense replace red cells and therefore should not be used in hemorrhagic shock except as an emergency remedy. It lacks the other proteins contained in plasma, and hence is not an adequate agent for treatment of plasma loss as in burns, or of deficiencies of specific plasma proteins (eg, fibrinogen, prothrombin) such as occur in acute hepatitis. It does not replace lost fluids, and therefore must be given with ample quantities of crystalloid solution when used in dehydrated patients, as noted above.

Dose—*Intravenous*, volumes equivalent to **25 to 125 Gm** of albumin daily; *usual*, a volume equivalent to **25 Gm** of albumin.

Dosage Forms—25 Gm/100 ml (25%): 20, 50, and 100 ml (osmotically equivalent to 100, 250, and 500 ml of plasma); 5 Gm/100 ml (5%): 250 and 500 ml (equivalent to 250 and 500 ml of plasma).

Dextran 40

[LMD (*Abbott*); Rheomacrodex (*Pharmacia*)]

Dextran 40 is a polymer of glucose, with an average molecular weight of about 40,000, in which the glucosidic linkages are predominantly of the $\alpha(1 \rightarrow 6)$ type.

Preparation—Sucrose is subjected to the action of the bacterium, *Leuconostoc mesenteroides* B 512, and the crude, high-molecular-weight dextran thus formed is hydrolyzed and fractionated to an average molecular weight of about 40,000 as measured by light-scattering techniques. US Pat. 2,644,815.

Description—A white, amorphous powder that is odorless and tasteless. Its 10% solution of 5% dextrose in water darkens slightly over a long storage period as with other dextrose-containing solutions; darkening is accelerated by increased ambient temperatures.

Solubility—Freely soluble in water; soluble in dimethyl sulfoxide and formamide; insoluble in acetone, alcohol, and ether.

Uses—Dextran 40 is marketed in the US only for use as an isotonic solution to prime pumps or to improve flow in surgery requiring *cardiopulmonary bypass*. It has the property of preventing the aggregation of erythrocytes, which aggregation has been claimed to occur in such surgery and to increase viscosity, so that capillary flow is impaired. However, the improvement in flow has been shown to be the result of hemodilution. For this reason, 10% Dextran 40 in isotonic saline solution or 5% dextrose is superior to Dextran 40 in whole blood.

The size of the molecule is such that the polysaccharide is excreted more rapidly than larger macromolecules, such as Dextran 70. Consequently, the substance is inferior as a plasma expander for the treatment of shock.

Dextran 40 may cause allergic reactions. Also, cases of renal shutdown following use of the drug have been reported. For this reason, many surgeons prefer to prime their bypass with other solutions. Renal failure and severe dehydration contraindicate the use of this substance.

Dose—*Usual, intravenous, or added to the pump circuit,* as a 10% solution in isotonic saline or 5% dextrose, **10 to 20 mg** per **Kg** of body weight. The total daily dose should not exceed 1000 ml per day.

Dosage Forms—Sterile Solution: 10%/500 ml (in normal saline), 10%/500 ml (in 5% dextrose in water).

Dextran 70

[Gentran (*Travenol*); Macrodex (*Pharmacia*)]

Dextran 70 is a polymer of glucose, with an average molecular weight of about 70,000, in which the glucosidic linkages are predominantly of the α $(1 \rightarrow 6)$ type.

Preparation—The procedure is that described for *Dextran 40* (page 819) except that the hydrolysis and fractionation are adjusted to yield a product of average molecular weight of about 70,000.

Description—A fine, white, amorphous powder that is odorless and tasteless. It is stable in light and is very hygroscopic. Commercial grades usually contain about 5% water.

Solubility—Freely soluble in hot water, dimethyl sulfoxide, and formamide; insoluble in acetone, alcohol, ether, and methanol.

Uses—Dextran 70 is employed as a plasma expander in the prevention or treatment of *hypovolemic shock*. The macromolecule is contained within the plasma and hence contains fluid in the vascular bed by osmosis. Hypertonic solutions cause the dehydration of tissues, the abstracted water being added to the plasma. For this reason it is useful in the treatment of toxemia of pregnancy and nephrosis. Although Dextran 70 is inferior to plasma, it has the advantage that refrigeration is not required or that the solution does not have to be prepared immediately before use. Thus, it may be kept ready for use in emergency vehicles, field kits, etc. It is also less expensive than plasma. Like plasma, it is inferior to whole blood as replacement when hypovolemia is due to hemorrhage. When hypoproteinemia exists, it should not be used in place of plasma.

A small part of Dextran 70, corresponding to the low-molecular-weight molecules, is excreted during the first 1 or 2 days. The remainder is taken up by the reticuloendothelial system and is later metabolized, which requires approximately 10 days.

Dextran 70 may increase clotting time in a few patients, the defect appearing several hours after administration. Allergic reactions (hives, angioedema, bronchospasm, and anaphylaxis) have been observed. The substance may interfere with cross-matching of blood if unsuitable dilutions of erythrocytes and serum are used.

Dose—*Intravenous*, **250 to 4500 ml** in the first day; *usual*, **500 to 1000 ml** of a **6%** solution in isotonic saline or 5% dextrose or invert sugar solution.

Other Dose Information—The rate of infusion is usually 20 to 40 ml per minute but may be accelerated if hypovolemia is severe. For nephrosis or toxemia of pregnancy, 500 ml a 10% solution in 5% dextrose or invert sugar may be given at a rate of about 60 ml per hour.

Veterinary Dose—*Intravenous*, varies widely depending upon requirements, but calculable at **2 to 20 ml** of a **6% solution** per **pound** of body weight;

usual, Horses and *Cattle*, **1000 ml**; *Sheep* and *Swin* **500 ml**. Dogs and cats tolerate the drug well.

Dosage Forms—Sterile Solution: 6%/500 ml (in normal saline).

Normal Human Plasma

[Citrated Normal Human Plasma]

Normal Human Plasma is the sterile plasma obtained by pooling approximately equal amounts of the liquid portion of whole blood from eight or more adult humans who, at the time the blood is drawn, are in condition physically to give blood and are free from evidence of those diseases transmissible by transfusion of plasma, insofar as can be determined from personal history, by physical examination, and by appropriate tests.

The blood is drawn under aseptic conditions into individual, sterile receptacles containing a suitable anticoagulant. The cell-free plasma is separated by centrifugation or by sedimentation in the individual receptacles and is pooled and distributed into final containers through a closed system.

Normal Human Plasma is dispensed as liquid, frozen, or dried plasma. Liquid plasma contains 5% of dextrose as a stabilizer. Liquid and dried plasma may be subjected to ultraviolet radiation during processing.

Because of the high incidence of homologous serum hepatitis in recipients of Normal Human Plasma, the product is no longer marketed in the United States.

Description—*Liquid Normal Human Plasma*, when freshly collected, is a slightly opalescent liquid of a faint yellowish or amber color and is practically odorless. It contains no visible particles and is free from blood cells. Increased opalescence or a precipitate may develop on standing.

Uses—The principal use of normal human plasma is as a *blood volume replenisher*. Because certain of the labile factors involved in blood clotting are inactivated during storage and processing of plasma, stored normal human plasma is ordinarily of little use in treating hemorrhagic states. The risk of transmitting homologous serum hepatitis through Normal Human Plasma is so great that its use is no longer warranted.

Dose—*Intravenous*, **500 to 1500 ml**; *usual*, **500 ml**, repeated as necessary.

Plasma Protein Fraction USP

[Plasma Protein Fraction (Human); (*Hyland*)]

Plasma Protein Fraction is a sterile solution of selected proteins derived from the blood plasma of adult human donors. It contains 4.5–5.5 Gm of protein per 100 ml, of which about 83–90% is albumin, and the remainder is alpha and beta globulins. It contains no microbistatic but may contain suitable stabilizers. Its production and distribution are subject to federal regulations (see *Biologics*, page 1425).

Preparation—Human Plasma Protein Fraction 5% is prepared by a process similar to that by which albumin is made. The product resembles plasma from which certain unstable globulins have been removed, including gamma globulin and certain lipoproteins. The solution is sterilized by heating at 60°C for 10 hours to reduce the risk of virus transmission. The solution is isotonic with normal plasma and is isotonic with respect to diffusible ions, the major ions being sodium and chloride.

Description—Transparent, nearly colorless or slightly brownish liquid. Is nearly odorless. May develop a slight, granular or flaky deposit during storage.

Uses—Like albumin, Plasma Protein Fraction is indicated as a substitute for plasma in treating shock. It is also a convenient source of protein for intravenous nutrition. Because it does not contain any clotting factors, it is not a substitute for fresh plasma in treating hemorrhagic states.

Dose—*Intravenous infusion*, **250 ml** to **1.5 liters** at a rate not exceeding 8 ml per minute; *usual*, **500 ml**.

Dosage Forms—250 and 500 ml.

Antibodies

Human plasma contains antibodies of various types, which are almost entirely concentrated in Fractions II + III. Some of these occur naturally, others arise as a result of infection or artificial immunization.

Isoagglutinins—The serum of all human beings contains antibodies (agglutinins or isoagglutinins) which react with those principal blood group factors (agglutinogens) which the individual does *not* possess.

Thus, for example, 45% of the population in the United States possesses the blood group O factor in its red cells, and agglutinins against the A and B factors in the plasma. Should the whole blood or cells of a Group A individual be injected into a Group O patient, the anti-A agglutinins of the patient will clump the cells received, and will usually destroy (lyse) them, causing a serious reaction in many cases, even if the volume of cells injected is as little as 50 ml. The importance of establishing the blood group of anyone either giving or receiving whole blood is therefore obvious. This is done by mixing a specimen of the cells of the subject with the serum of a selected individual whose group is known; for example, if the cells of an untyped donor are clumped by the serum of a known Group B subject, but not by the serum of a known Group A subject, the donor evidently belongs to Group A. In practice, anti-A isoagglutinins obtained from selected group B subjects, and anti-B isoagglutinins from similarly selected Group A subjects, have for years provided highly effective reagents for identification of the blood groups. It has been demonstrated that administration of small quantities of the specific blood group substances A or B (which can be obtained from red blood cells or, in larger quantities, from other animal tissues) to individuals having the corresponding isoagglutinins will induce a tremendous rise in titer of the agglutinin. In this fashion extremely potent blood grouping sera have been prepared in ample quantities. It is also possible to produce blood grouping sera as a by-product of ethanol fractionation of plasma, since the blood grouping isoagglutinins are greatly concentrated in this process. The rather limited supply of anti-A serum (normally obtained from the small percentage of Group B subjects) can be augmented by using the serum from Group O donors, by mixing it with a small quantity of Group B blood, which absorbs out the anti-B antibodies, leaving a pure anti-A isoagglutinin.

In practice, it is customary not only to determine the blood group of a donor and recipient of a blood transfusion, but to "cross match" the cells of the donor with the serum of the patient and *vice versa*, so as to detect any otherwise unpredictable incompatibility in the

Blood Group Factors

Blood groups (cells) Factors present	Frequency in population	Isoagglutinins (plasma)
O	45%	Anti-A and Anti-B
A	41%	Anti-B
B	10%	Anti-A
AB	4%	None

bloods of the two individuals. This extra precaution is invaluable, not only for the purpose indicated but also as a final check against mistaken identity of the specimens. There are numerous other precautions involved in correct blood grouping, so that it has become a highly specialized technique, which should only be performed by a qualified technician.

The Rh Factor—A much rarer antibody occurs in a small proportion of individuals as a result of injection of so-called "Rh positive blood," or absorption of such blood across the placenta during pregnancy in gravid females. This "Rh factor" actually consists of at least eight different factors, any one or several of which may be present in the red cells of a given individual. Isoagglutinins reacting with these factors do not occur normally in humans, but appear only as a result of accidental "immunization" of an individual with a type of Rh factor which he or she does not possess. At least nine such antibodies have been described. Actually, the blood of about 85% of Western Europeans or Americans contains one or two of the commonest of these factors, which also are the most potent as antigens. Therefore in general practice it is customary and quite permissible to classify individuals simply as either "Rh positive" or "Rh negative." The technique of Rh typing is essentially like that of blood grouping, except that the readings are more delicate, and require somewhat more skill in accurate interpretation. Rh antibodies are peculiar in that they occur in at least three forms, two of which are common and important. One of these forms will cause agglutination of red cells in saline solution, whereas the other ("incomplete") antibody requires the presence of protein in the solution to bring about agglutination. Both may be used in Rh typing, provided the special requirements for use of the latter type are clearly understood. Similarly, the presence of dangerously high titers of such antibodies, in an individual who has been sensitized to one of the Rh factors, may be determined by testing his serum as though it were an Rh isoagglutinin, allowing, of course, for the possibility that the serum may contain only the protein-requiring type of antibody.

Like anti-A and anti-B blood grouping serum, the principal source for Rh typing serum is the blood of human donors who, by chance or intention, have become hyperimmunized to one of the Rh factors. One of the commonest sources is the blood of Rh negative women who have borne several Rh positive infants, absorbed their Rh factor, and thereby have become sensitized. Another source is Rh negative individuals who have been transfused with Rh positive blood. Injection of small amounts of Rh substance in the latter individuals will induce very high antibody titers, rendering them suitable donors of hyperimmune serum for typing purposes. The danger of mismatched transfusion in such individuals is actually decreased, since they become extremely easy to identify.

Several reports have indicated the possibility of isolating a so-called "Rh hapten" from Rh positive red cells, and have suggested the use of this hapten to absorb antibodies in the blood of individuals with dangerously high titers, particularly in pregnant women who are likely to give birth to infants suffering from "erythroblastosis," because of an Rh incompatibility. More recent studies, however, indicate that the Rh hapten may not be specific, and that further work is required to define its properties and functions, before its usefulness can be fully understood.

Gamma Globulins—Adult blood contains antibodies specific for various infectious agents to which the individual has built up a resistance. In pooled plasma some of these are in high enough concentration to have a protective action. This is especially true of measles antibodies. Antibodies from adult plasma will protect against the disease if given after exposure. In certain other conditions, it is possible to select individuals with already detectable antibody levels, and by injection of an appropriate vaccine to raise their antibody level to very high titers, much as was described for blood grouping and Rh typing sera above. This practice has been most widely employed in the production of pertussis hyperimmune serum for the treatment or prophylaxis of whooping cough.

During the fractionation of plasma, most of the antibodies are concentrated into a single fraction (Fraction II); electrophoretically the proteins in this fraction are characterized as gamma globulins. Isolated gamma globulins, dispensed as a 16% solution, represent a concentration of most antibodies approximately 25 times greater than in plasma. As a result, they have been found useful in the prophylaxis of certain infectious diseases, including measles, infectious hepatitis (not to be confused with serum hepatitis), and poliomyelitis. The usefulness derives from the immunity conferred by the *added* antibody. Since, however, the added antibody is slowly metabolized and therefore disappears, the immunity is passive, and lasts only as long as the concentration of antibody is above an effective level, usually from one to two months. Thereafter, the recipient once again becomes susceptible to infection. Alternatively, and particularly when exposure to infection can be ascertained with reasonable accuracy, as in measles, a modifying dose of antibodies may be administered. While failing to prevent active infection, the added antibody lessens the severity of the disease and the patient responds to the infection by producing antibodies of his own. This production of antibodies persists for long periods thereafter, thus conferring long lasting immunity. In measles, the dosage can be adjusted with sufficient accuracy to produce modification of the infection and allow for active immunity with a high degree of success.

At present, gamma globulin is distributed by several commercial firms and by the American Red Cross, through various public health agencies. Gamma globulin is administered intramuscularly; it cannot be used intravenously. Reactions are uncommon and when they do occur are chiefly local and usually mild. Another source of gamma globulin is the blood from normal human placentas. The "placental extract" made from this source some years ago was not wholly satisfactory and caused a number of untoward reactions. Application of the newer methods of processing gamma globulin from human blood, however, has made possible the preparation of a similar globulin from placentas, which also runs 95% gamma globulin or better, is essentially free of reactions, and is almost indistinguishable from the preparation derived from blood. The practically inexhaustible supply of placentas makes it possible to produce gamma globulin of this origin in large quantities at a reasonable cost.

Immune Serum Globulin USP

[Immune Serum Globulin (Human) USP XIV; Gammagee (*MSD*); Gamostan (*Cutter*); Gamulin (*Pitman-Moore*); Immu-G (*Parke-Davis*)

Immune Serum Globulin is a sterile solution of globulins that contains many antibodies normally present in adult human blood. It contains 15–18 Gm of protein per 100 ml, not less than 90.0% of which is globulin. It contains glycine and a suitable antimicrobial agent. Each lot of Immune Serum Globulin is derived from an original plasma or serum pool representing venous or placental blood from at least 1000 individuals. Its production and distribution are subject to federal regulations (see *Biologics*, page 1425).

Description—Immune Serum Globulin is a transparent or slightly opalescent liquid, either colorless or of a brownish color due to denatured hemoglobin. It is nearly odorless; it may develop a slight, granular deposit on aging.

Uses—This Serum Globulin is a *prophylactic* in the prevention and modification of *measles*. It is equal in usefulness to convalescent serum but has the advantage of universal availability. Prevention is, of course, less desirable than modification except where younger children ill with other diseases are apt to contract measles by exposure to a modified case. Otherwise it is more desirable to permit a child to have mild measles so that immunization occurs rather than to prevent the disease and leave the child nonimmune to subsequent attacks of the disease. Protection should not be attempted until definite exposure has taken place.

Gamma globulin contains other antibodies. It appears to be capable of preventing or modifying *infectious hepatitis* in a large proportion of exposed individuals. It has been shown to be effective in the prophylaxis of poliomyelitis as well. Normal gamma globulin does not appear to have value, however, in the *treatment* of serum hepatitis. It has also been found effective in the management of certain rather rare conditions characterized by a deficiency of antibodies or failure to produce antibodies (hyper- or agammaglobulinemia). Gamma globulin from convalescent plasma has been used in the treatment of mumps. It has also proved to be of benefit to persons suffering from certain types of allergies.

Dose—*Usual, intramuscular, prophylactic* (measles) **0.25 ml per Kg**; *prophylactic* (infectious hepatitis) **0.02 ml per Kg**; *modification* (measles) **0.05 ml per Kg**.

Dosage Forms—2 and 10 ml.

Anti-Rh₀(D) Immune Globulin [Rhogam (*Ortho*)] is a sterile concentrated solution of specific gamma globulin (IgG) in which the active ingredient is the anti-Rh₀(D) antibody contained in 15% plus or minus 1.5% serum globulin. *Uses:* Anti-Rh₀(D) Immune Globulin is administered to Rh-negative mothers who deliver Rh-positive (D- or Dᵘ-positive) ABO-compatible infants. The immune globulin must be given within 72 hours after delivery in order for the immune globulin antibodies to neutralize the Rh-positive antigen and hence to prevent Rh-sensitization or isoimmunization (formation of endogenous Rh-positive antibodies within the mother). Thus, if her next infant is Rh-positive, the infant will be protected. Adverse effects include occasional local reactions and occasional fever lasting for about a day. The immunoglobulin is contraindicated prior to delivery, since if transplacental hemorrhage exists, it is also possible that the antibody will enter the fetal circulation and cause hemolysis. *Dose: Intramuscular*, 1.5 ml 72 hours or less after delivery.

Blood Grouping and Typing Serums

The only official representative item of this section that has been given monograph status in the NF follows immediately.

Blood-Group Specific Substances A and B NF

Blood group Specific Substances A and B is a sterile, isotonic solution of the polysaccharide-containing complexes that are capable of reducing the titer of the anti-A and the anti-B isoagglutinins of group O blood. The blood-group specific substance A is usually isolated from hog gastric mucin and the blood-group specific substance B is usually isolated from the glandular portion of horse gastric mucosa. Blood-group Specific Substances A and B contains a suitable preservative.

Its production and distribution are subject to federal regulations (see *Biologics*, page 1425).

Description—It is a clear solution, which may have a slight odor due to the preservative. Its pH is between 6.0 and 6.8.

Uses—Blood group specific substances A and B is added to group O blood as a *neutralizer of isoagglutinins* and hence it makes the blood reasonably safe for transfusions into patients whose blood is of another group. It may also be used to condition plasma. However, conditioned plasma which contains immune anti-A and anti-B agglutinins may cause reactions. Furthermore, it must not be forgotten that blood from group O donors that have previously received conditioned group O blood may contain A and B isohemagglutinins. Such blood is dangerous to use in universal donation unless it is conditioned with blood group specific substances A and B.

Dose—*Intravenous*, one transfusion unit (**10 ml**) in approximately **500 ml** of group O blood.

Dosage Forms—10 ml (to be added to 500 ml of group O blood).

Diagnostic Reagents

The following diagnostic reagents are described in the appendix of the USP, which makes a distinction between items used in clinical tests on the patient's tissues or fluids separated from his body and those items employed in clinical tests which require application directly upon or administration to the patient. Use monographs are provided only for the latter category.

The usefulness of these serums is described on page 821 under *Isoagglutinins*.

Anti-A Blood Grouping Serum USP

Anti-A Blood Grouping Serum is derived from high-titered serums of humans, with or without stimulation by the injection of group-specific red cells or substances. It agglutinates human red cells containing A agglutinogens; ie, blood groups A and AB (including subgroups A_1, A_2, A_3, A_1B, and A_2B). It may contain a suitable antibacterial preservative. Its production and distribution are subject to federal regulations (see *Biologics*, page 1425).

Description—Liquid Anti-A Blood Grouping Serum is a clear or slightly opalescent fluid unless artificially colored, when it has a blue or blue-green color. The dried product is light yellow to deep cream color, unless artificially colored as indicated for liquid serum, and is microscopically of a honeycomb-like structure. It may contain a preservative.

Anti-B Blood Grouping Serum USP

Anti-B Blood Grouping Serum is derived from high-titered serums of humans, with or without stimulation by the injection of group-specific red cells or substances. It agglutinates human red cells containing B agglutinogens; i.e., blood groups B and AB (including subgroups A_1B and A_2B). It may contain a suitable antibacterial preservative. Its production and distribution are subject to federal regulations (see *Biologics*, page 1425).

Description—Liquid Anti-B Blood Grouping Serum is a clear or slightly opalescent fluid unless artificially colored, when it has a yellow to red-orange color. The dried product is light yellow to deep cream color, unless artificially colored as indicated for liquid serum, and is microscopically of a honeycomb-like structure. It may contain a preservative.

Anti-Rh Typing Serums USP

Anti-Rh Typing Serums are derived from the blood of humans who have developed specific Rh antibodies. Anti-Rh Typing Serums are free from agglutinins for A- or B-agglutinogen and from agglutinins other than those for which claims are made in the labeling. They may contain suitable antibacterial agents.

Two varieties of Anti-Rh Typing Serums are recognized: i.e., (1) complete ("saline-agglutinating") serums, which specifically agglutinate human red blood cells in saline TS, and (2) incomplete ("blocking") serums, which agglutinate human red blood cells only in a medium containing protein or other macromolecular substances, which may be furnished in an accompanying diluent. Complete serums commonly are designated "For saline tube test," and the incomplete serums are designated "For slide or modified (rapid) tube test." In liquid form, the latter contain, as additives, the required macromolecular substances.

The left-hand column of the accompanying table lists the designations under which the US Public Health Service licenses the production of the most commonly used anti-Rh typing serums, and the right-hand column lists the blood factor(s) with which each serum specifically reacts. The designations in a second system of nomenclature are given parenthetically.

The production and distribution of each Serum are subject to federal regulations (see *Biologics*, page 1425).

Anti-Rh serum	Rh factor(s) reacting
Anti-Rh_0(Anti-D)	Rh_0(D)
Anti-rh' (Anti-C)	rh'(C)
Anti-rh" (Anti-E)	rh"(E)
Anti-Rh_0'(Anti-CD)	Rh_0(D), rh'(C)
Anti-Rh_0"(Anti-DE)	Rh_0 (D), rh" (E)
Anti-Rh_0rh'rh"	Rh_0 (D), rh' (C),
(Anti-CDE)	rh" (E)
Anti-hr' (Anti-c)	hr'(c)
Anti-hr" (Anti-e)	hr" (e)

Immune Sera

Various biological products obtained from the blood of humans or animals and used for their prophylactic or therapeutic effects, eg, antitoxins, immune sera, and immune globulin, are discussed in the chapter on *Immunizing Agents* (page 1426).

Hematopoietics

Hematopoietics are *antianemics* that aid in production of red and white blood cells; *hematinics* are *antianemics* that increase the hemoglobin content of blood through erythropoiesis or through an increase in hemoglobin content of erythrocytes. The hematinic to be employed is critically dependent upon the nature of the anemia. The hypochromic anemias are nearly all iron deficiency anemias in character and are treated with iron preparations. Occasionally, other accessory factors are indicated in the treatment of the hypochromic anemias. For example, the anemia of nurslings may require copper to facilitate the mobilization of iron from the gut and tissues. Ascorbic acid occasionally helps promote the antianemic action of iron. When given with iron salts, it promotes the absorption of iron, probably by promoting the reduction of ferric ion, which is less well absorbed than the ferrous form. Ferrous salts are easily oxidized so that ascorbate aids in their stabilization. However, ascorbic acid appears to have an additional but obscure role in hematopoiesis. Cobalt and molybdenum probably also play a role in hematopoiesis, but deficiency syndromes in man are unknown, and the inclusion of these metals in hematinic preparations is irrational. The use of cobalt may even be dangerous. Although copper is known to have a hematopoietic function, a deficiency in man severe enough to impair erythropoiesis has never been demonstrated (see page 1047). The macrocytic anemias all respond to cyanocobalamin, but the route of administration and accessory factors are critically dependent upon the particular anemia. In tropical sprue, the absorption of folic acid is impaired to a greater extent than that of vitamin B_{12}, so that folic acid usually elicits the greater hematopoietic response. For reasons stated elsewhere (below and on page 1038), the promiscuous use of folic and folinic acids should be condemned.

Iron and Iron Compounds

Iron has been used in medicine in the following forms: (1) metallic or elementary iron (reduced iron); (2) ferrous compounds (ferrous sulfate, etc); (3) ferric compounds (ferric chloride tincture); and (4) complex compounds of iron (ferric citrochloride tincture).

Complex (nonionic) iron compounds are those compounds of iron whose solutions do not respond to the ordinary tests for ferrous or ferric ions because the iron in them is part of a complex radical. Complex compounds of iron do not have the astringent taste of simple iron solutions. The permanence of these complex radicals differs widely. Some, such as soluble ferric phosphate, are converted to simple ionic iron by action of dilute acids, while others resist treatment with strong acids or with alkalies. The complex iron compounds occurring naturally in animal and vegetable tissues (termed food irons) belong generally to the more resistant class, while the complex iron compounds produced artificially are as a rule decomposed rather readily. There is, however, no sharp line of distinction between the natural complex iron compounds and those products artificially produced, nor is there any good evidence that they differ in therapeutic action.

Uses—The principal use of iron is in the treatment of *hypochromic, iron-deficiency anemias,* that is, in anemias characterized by a deficiency of hemoglobin. The two most common causes of such anemias are nutritional (deficient intake, especially in infancy, in childhood, at puberty, during pregnancy, and late in menstrual life or at the menopause), and chronic blood loss (especially bleeding peptic ulcer, carcinoma of the colon or stomach, bleeding from the urinary tract, or excessive loss of blood during menstruation). Iron therapy is of no particular value in other forms of anemia, such as pernicious anemia, unless the patient has entered an iron-deficiency stage of his disease. Formerly, the most common forms of iron therapy employed in the United States include *Reduced Iron, Ferrous Sulfate, Ferrous Carbonate,* and *Iron and Ammonium Citrates.* However, since 1957 a number of iron organic complexes or salts have been used with increasing frequency.

Reduced iron, which yields ferrous chloride when dissolved in the stomach, acts as a ferrous compound, provided the hydrochloric acid in the gastric fluid is sufficient to permit solution. Complex iron compounds (eg, iron and ammonium citrate) are generally less prone to produce gastric distress than the simple ferrous and ferric compounds; they are also less efficiently utilized physiologically. Indeed, in some complexes the iron may be so effectively chelated as to escape absorption altogether.

Bunge supposed that only "organic iron" could be absorbed and assimilated by the body, the reputed action of inorganic iron being altogether indirect and due to its local effect on the alimentary canal. This theory was modified by Abderhalden to the effect that inorganic iron, while it could not be converted into hemoglobin, nevertheless stimulated the conversion of "organic iron." Later work (Tartakowski), however, proved that inorganic iron is assimilated and converted into hemoglobin and it is in fact therapeutically more effective than natural complex iron compounds. Whipple and his co-workers showed that ferrous carbonate aids recovery from the anemia of repeated hemorrhages. Reiman showed that ferrous salts are effective in bringing about a reticulocyte response, hemoglobin and red blood cell increase in much smaller amounts than ferric salts; 100 mg of iron as ferrous salts daily was shown to be effective.

A difference exists between the different iron preparations in their local irritant and astringent action, which is absent in most of the complex iron compounds; for this reason the less astringent and less irritant ferrous salts are preferred to the ferric salts. These local actions may be desirable in some cases and undesirable in others. This should mainly determine the selection of the particular iron preparation most suitable for each patient. The irritation occurs mostly in the stomach and upper duodenum, where the pH is low. Enteric coatings allow the preparation to pass into the more alkaline portions of the gut before release occurs. However, the absorption of iron from enteric-coated preparations is less than in uncoated ones, especially in persons with bowel hypermotility. Antacids also diminish absorption. Constipation consequent to local actions of iron may be countered by cathartics, properly individualized. Suitable diet (especially liver, kidney, and meat) is sometimes more effective than the iron preparations, presumably by the co-operation of other factors.

Ascorbic Acid—see page 1036.

Dextriferron Injection NF

[Astrafer (*Astra*)]

Dextriferron Injection is a sterile, colloidal solution prepared from a complex of ferric hydroxide with partially hydrolyzed dextrin in water for injection. It contains 95.0–105.0% of the labeled amount of Fe (iron).

Uses—Dextriferron is used in the treatment of *iron-deficiency anemias*. When administered intravenously, the iron of dextriferron is almost quantitatively incorporated into hemoglobin. Within 3 to 7 days the hemoglobin content in blood increases, depending upon the initial level of hemoglobin and the extent of depletion of the iron pool. However, the intravenous administration of iron in this or any other form is rarely necessary. Untoward effects include flushing, nausea, headache, and abdominal pain, immediately upon injection, and stiffness, in the extremities and face, chills and fever, after a latent period.

Dose—*Usual, intravenous, initial trial dose* of **1.5 ml** (equivalent to 30 mg of iron), then increase dose in increments of **1 to 1.5 ml** (equivalent to 20 to 30 mg of iron) per day until a daily dose of **5 ml** (equivalent to 100 mg of iron) is reached.

Other Dose Information—If stored iron is considered to be depleted, 250 mg to 1 Gm of iron may be given.

Dosage Forms—Injection NF: Equivalent of 20 mg iron/ml in 5-ml containers.

Ferrous Fumarate USP

[Iron (2+) Fumarate; *Various Mfgs.*]

$$\begin{array}{c} HC-C\!=\!O \\ O\!=\!C-CH \ \ O \\ O\!-\!\!-\!\!-\!\!Fe \end{array}$$

Ferrous Fumarate contains 96.5–101.0% of $C_4H_2FeO_4$ (169.91).

Preparation—Ferrous sulfate and sodium fumarate are metathesized in hot aqueous solution whereupon the sparingly soluble, anhydrous ferrous fumarate precipitates.

Description—Reddish orange to red-brown, odorless powder. May contain soft lumps that produce a yellow streak when crushed.

Solubility—Slightly soluble in water; very slightly soluble in alcohol; its solubility in dilute hydrochloric acid is limited by the separation of insoluble free fumaric acid.

Uses—Ferrous Fumarate is used in the clinical management of *iron-deficiency anemias*. Its efficacy is about the same as that of Ferrous Sulfate, but the untoward effects are somewhat less severe. The drug may sometimes be employed without difficulty in patients who cannot tolerate other preparations of iron. When side effects occur, they include anorexia, nausea, vomiting, cramping, and constipation or diarrhea; the effects generally subside as therapy is continued.

Dose—**200** to **600 mg** daily; *usual*, **200 mg**, the equivalent of 66 mg of elemental iron, 2 or 3 times a day.

Dosage Forms—Tablets USP: 200 mg.

Ferrous Gluconate NF

[Iron (2+) Gluconate; *Various Mfgs.*]

$$\left[HOCH_2-CH-CH-CH-CH-COO- \atop \quad \overset{|}{OH} \ \overset{|}{OH} \quad \ \overset{|}{OH} \right]_2 Fe \ .2H_2O$$

Ferrous Gluconate [$C_{12}H_{22}FeO_{14}.2H_2O = 428.18$], dried at 105° for 4 hours, contains 95.0–100.5% of $C_{12}H_{22}FeO_{14}$.

Preparation—Ferrous Gluconate may be prepared by metathesis between hot solutions of calcium gluconate and ferrous sulfate whereby ferrous gluconate and insoluble calcium sulfate are formed. The mixture is filtered while hot to minimize the solubility of calcium sulfate and the filtrate is evaporated to crystallization.

It may also be produced by heating freshly prepared ferrous carbonate with the proper quantity of gluconic acid in aqueous solution.

Description—Fine, yellowish gray or pale greenish yellow powder, or granules, with a slight burnt-sugar-like odor. It is affected by light and the ferrous iron slowly oxidizes to ferric on exposure to air. Its aqueous solution is acid to litmus. The color of the solutions depends on pH; they are light yellow at pH 2, brown at pH 4.5, and green at pH 7. The iron rapidly oxidizes at higher pH.

Solubility—1 Gm dissolves in about 10 ml of water with slight heating and in 1.3 ml of water at 100°; practically insoluble in alcohol; it forms supersaturated solutions which are stable for a period of time; its solubility is increased by addition of citric acid or the citrate ion.

Incompatibilities—Approximately neutral solutions undergo rapid oxidation; oxidation is retarded and stability improved by buffering to a pH of 3.5 to 4.5 with citrate buffer. Glycerin also retards oxidation. Solubility is increased by the citrate ion. *Ascorbic acid* and *aminoacetic acid* can cause a dark coloration; with *pyridoxine* a green color is produced. Other members of the B-complex are compatible.

Uses—Ferrous Gluconate is used as a *hematinic*, similar to other ferrous salts. It causes fewer side effects than ferrous sulfate. See general statement under *Iron and Iron Compounds* (page 824).

Dose—**200** to **600 mg**; *usual*, **300 mg** 3 times a day.

Dosage Forms—Tablets NF: 300 mg.

Ferrous Sulfate USP

[Ferri Sulfas; Ferrosi Sulfas; Iron Protosulfate; ±s Aeratum; Iron (2+) Sulfate; Green Vitriol; Copperas*; Feosol (*SK&F*)]

Ferrous Sulfate contains an amount of $FeSO_4$ (151.91), equivalent to 99.5–104.5% of $FeSO_4.7H_2O$ (278.02).

Note—Do not use Ferrous Sulfate that is coated with brownish yellow basic ferric sulfate.

Preparation—The salt may be prepared by dissolving iron in diluted sulfuric acid. The resulting solution is filtered and concentrated, if necessary, to the point of crystallization of ferrous sulfate. Commercially, scrap iron is used in the process.

Description—Pale, bluish green crystals or granules. It is odorless, has a saline, styptic taste, and effloresces in dry air, becoming white. The solution (1 in 10) is acid to litmus having a pH of about 3.7.

Solubility—1 Gm dissolves in 1.5 ml of water and 0.5 ml of boiling water; insoluble in alcohol.

---

* This unfortunate synonym, *copperas*, has led to a great many errors through the impression that this salt must contain copper. It is often confounded with the poisonous copper sulfate, or blue vitriol, and they have been substituted for each other in error.

Incompatibilities—Ferrous salts are oxidized by exposure to *air*, by *mercuric salts* in alkaline solution, and by *oxidizing agents*. Inorganic acids generally favor oxidation; light hinders it, as do alcohol, citric acid, glycerin, sugar, and soluble citrates. A darkening in the color of ferrous salts is evidence of oxidation. Ferrous salts are precipitated by *alkalies* as white ferrous hydroxide which quickly oxidizes to ferroferric hydroxide, then to the reddish brown ferric hydroxide. Sugar, glycerin, and many organic hydroxy acids hinder precipitation. In neutral solutions, the soluble *carbonates*, *phosphates*, and *oxalates* produce precipitates. *Tannic acid* precipitates ferrous tannate which is quickly oxidized to the blue-black ferric salt. *Borax* gives a white precipitate. Acids and the alkali citrates and tartrates favor solution of the precipitates. Aqueous solutions of Ferrous Sulfate are acid in reaction. See also *Sodium Sulfate* (page 803).

Uses—This salt is one of the most commonly employed *hematinic* preparations used in iron-deficiency anemias, as outlined in the general statement under *Iron and Iron Compounds* (page 824). The drug is most commonly dispensed as tablets, coated for protection from air and moisture. The salt is sometimes mixed with glucose or lactose to protect it against oxidation.

Impure ferrous sulfate, called *copperas*, is used as a disinfectant.

Dose—**300 mg** to **1 Gm** daily; *usual*, **300 mg,** the equivalent of 60 mg of elemental iron, 2 or 3 times a day.

Other Dose Information—The usual dose of Ferrous Sulfate Syrup NF is 10 ml (containing about 400 mg of ferrous sulfate).

Dosage Forms—Dried USP (see below); Syrup NF; Tablets USP: 300 mg.

Veterinary Dose—*Horses*, **2** to **8 Gm;** *Cattle*, **8** to **15 Gm;** *Sheep* and *Swine*, **600 mg** to **2 Gm;** *Dogs*, **60** to **300 mg;** *Cats*, **30** to **250 mg.**

Dried Ferrous Sulfate USP [Dried Iron Sulfate] [approximately $FeSO_4.2H_2O$] contains 86.0–89.0% of anhydrous ferrous sulfate [$FeSO_4 = 151.91$]. *Preparation:* It is made by exposing well-crushed crystals of ferrous sulfate to a temperature of 70° to 80°, stirring frequently, and then powdering. *Description:* A grayish white powder. *Solubility:* Slowly soluble in water; insoluble in alcohol. *Uses:* This salt is more stable in air than the fully hydrated Ferrous Sulfate, and is more adaptable for making capsules, pills, and tablets. It may be substituted for Ferrous Sulfate in *Ferrous Sulfate Tablets. Dose:* See *Ferrous Sulfate. Veterinary Dose: Horses, 1 to 5 Gm; Cattle, 5 to 10 Gm; Sheep* and *Swine, 500 mg to 1 Gm; Dogs, 30 to 200 mg; Cats, 20 to 150 mg.*

Ferrous Sulfate Syrup NF [Feosol Syrup (*SK & F*)] contains, in each 100 ml, 3.75–4.25 Gm of $FeSO_4.7H_2O$. *Preparation:* Dissolve the ferrous sulfate (40 Gm), the citric acid (hydrous: 2.1 Gm), the peppermint spirit (2 ml), and sucrose (200 Gm) in purified water (450 ml), and filter the solution until clear. Then dissolve sucrose (625 Gm) in the clear filtrate, and add purified water (qs) to make 1000 ml. Mix well, and filter, if necessary, through a pledget of cotton. *Uses:* See *Ferrous Sulfate. Dose: Usual*, 10 ml (1 usual dose contains about 400 mg of ferrous sulfate).

Iron Dextran Injection USP

[Imferon (*Lakeside*)]

Iron Dextran Injection is a sterile, colloidal solution of ferric hydroxide in complex with partially hydrolyzed dextran of low molecular weight, in water for injection. It contains 95.0–105.0% of the labeled amount of iron. It may contain not more than 0.5% of phenol as a preservative.

Preparation—To an aqueous solution of partially depolymerized dextran (intrinsic viscosity 0.04 to 0.07) is added a solution of alkali and a solution of a ferric salt. The mixture is heated, then cooled to room temperature and clarified by centrifugation, and the solution is dialyzed against running water. After concentrating to the required iron content, the solution is filtered, ampuled, and sterilized by autoclaving.

Description—Dark brown, slightly viscous liquid; pH, 5.2 to 6.0.

Uses—Iron provides a source of iron for treatment of the *iron-deficiency anemias*. Because the iron is strongly chelated by the dextran, it is not locally irritating upon intramuscular injection. Absorption is rapid from an intramuscular site. Thus the drug is used for intramuscular injection in those patients in whom oral therapy can not be tolerated or does not evoke a therapeutic response. If the drug is administered to persons not in an iron-deficiency state, hemosiderosis may occur. Absorption is very slow from a subcutaneous site and a brown stain occurs that may remain for 1 to 2 years. Consequently, in injecting the drug, care must be taken to prevent leakage under the skin. Injections are given deeply into the upper-outer quadrant of the buttock by a special technique called a Z-track injection, which diminishes leakage to subcutaneous sites.

In 1960 Iron-Dextran Complex was withdrawn from the market because of the finding that massive doses of the drug can produce sarcomata in certain experimental animals. Apparently, local accumulation of iron and lymphatic obstruction is necessary. In the human the lymphatic system is well developed and the dose of the complex is relatively low, so that the danger of malignancy is very slight. Consequently, the complex has again been licensed for human use.

Dose—*Intramuscular*, the equivalent of **50** to **250 mg** of iron daily to every other day; *usual*, **100 mg** once a day.

Veterinary Dose—*Horses and Cattle*, **1 ml** (100 mg of elemental iron) per **100 pounds** of body weight; *Dogs and Cats*, **1 ml** per **10 pounds**; *Lambs*, **1** to **2 ml**; *Baby Pigs*, **1** to **2 ml** at 3 days of age *intramuscularly* for the prevention or treatment of iron-deficiency anemia.

Iron Sorbitex Injection USP

[Jectofer (*Astra*)]

Iron Sorbitex Injection is a sterile solution of a complex of iron, sorbitol, and citric acid that is stabilized with the aid of dextrin and an excess of sorbitol. It contains 94.0–104.0% of the labeled amount of iron.

Preparation—Ferric chloride is caused to undergo complexation with sorbitol and citric acid, and the complex is stabilized with a specially purified dextrin.

Description—A dark-brown, clear liquid; pH, 7.2 to 7.9; specific gravity, 1.17 to 1.19 at 20°.

Uses—Iron Sorbitex Injection is used as a source of iron in patients with established *iron deficiency* that are unable to absorb adequate amounts of iron from the gastrointestinal tract or when oral preparations cannot be tolerated. Thus it may be used in chronic hemorrhage, in which the loss outstrips gastrointestinal absorption, or in nontropical sprue or idiopathic steatorrhea, in which iron absorption is impaired, or when oral preparation aggravate ulcerative colitis or peptic ulcers.

Iron Sorbitex may cause flushing, malaise, muscle and joint aches, and weakness. Pain sometimes occurs in the site of injection. As with iron dextran injection (above), subcutaneous deposition may give rise to long-lasting discoloration of the skin; consequently, deep intramuscular administration with the Z-tract technique is used. Hives, a sensation of pressure in the chest, palpitations, sweating, nausea and vomiting, vertigo, hypotension, and collapse also are known to occur. Serious reactions are more probable when the patient is simultaneously taking oral iron, since the serum binding protein, transferrin, may be close to saturation. In hemolytic and certain other anemias in which transferrin is overloaded, the use of Iron Sorbitex is contraindicated. Other conditions in which it is contraindicated are hypersensitivity to iron, hepatitis, renal dysfunction, folic acid deficiency, hypoplastic anemia, hemosiderosis, hemochromatosis, thalassemia, and infections of the urinary tract.

The renal excretion of a considerable fraction of the iron may result in a darkening of the urine as it stands because of the gradual formation of ferrous sulfide. The patient should be advised of this harmless phenomenon.

Dose—*Intramuscular*, the equivalent of **100 to 200 mg** of iron daily; *usual*, **100 mg** once a day.

Other Dose Information—The daily dose should not exceed 200 mg. The total dose should not exceed the calculated iron deficit. It is advisable that the first dose be ½ of the usual dose in order to test the sensitivity of the individual to the drug.

Dosage Forms—Injection USP: The equivalent of 100 mg of iron/2 ml.

Other Hematopoietics and Hematinics

Ferric Ammonium Citrate NF XI [Soluble Ferric Citrate; Iron and Ammonium Citrate]—Contains *ca* 17.5% Fe. *Uses:* A readily soluble complex of ferric citrate used as a source of iron in the treatment of *iron-deficiency anemias*. It is less constipating than inorganic forms of iron. It is free from astringent and irritant properties, and is practically tasteless. However, ferric ion is less well absorbed than ferrous ion, so that its supposed advantages are outweighed by its lesser efficacy. Being very soluble in water, the salt can be dispensed as a solution, a drinking tube being used to prevent staining of the teeth. *Veterinary Uses:* A hematinic, employed especially in canine practice. *Dose: Usual,* 1 Gm. In severe anemias 2 Gm, 2 to 3 times daily, may be given. *Horses* and *Cattle,* 4 to 8 Gm; *Dogs,* 300 to 600 mg; *Cats,* 100 to 300 mg.

Ferric Pyrophosphate, Soluble, is a complex salt of sodium ferricitropyrophosphate containing about 12.0% of iron. *Description and Solubility:* Apple-green, transparent scales, green granules, or a yellowish-green powder that has an acidulous, saline taste; it darkens in light. Freely soluble in water; insoluble in alcohol. *Uses:* Ferric pyrophosphate is used as a source of iron in the treatment of *iron deficiency anemias* and as a prophylactic when iron demands are increased as in pregnancy, or when the dietary source is suspected to be inadequate. *Dose: Oral,* the equivalent of 30 to 90 mg of iron per day.

Ferrocholinate [Chel-Iron (*Kinney*); Ferrolip (*Flint*)] is an iron choline citrate chelate. *Preparation:* By reacting equimolar quantities of freshly precipitated ferric hydroxide with choline dihydrogen citrate. However, in commercial preparations a product which meets specifications is usually prepared by reacting 1.25 moles choline dihydrogen citrate in solution with 1 mole freshly precipitated ferric hydroxide. The compound contains 12.0–13.0% ferric iron, 35.0–37.0% choline base, and as much as 6.0% water. *Description and Solubility:* Varicolored, amorphous, odorless, coarse granules, having a taste resembling citric acid; it is photosensitive, slightly hygroscopic, and decomposes without melting at 300°. Freely soluble in water; soluble in acids and alkalies; practically insoluble in alcohol. *Uses:* A source of iron for treatment of the *iron-deficiency anemias.* Because the iron is sequestered in chelate form by the citrate moiety of the molecule, it is less astringent and hence less toxic to the gastrointestinal tract than dissociable salts of iron, and hence is better tolerated. Nevertheless, mild nausea and diarrhea or constipation may occur, especially in the early course of medication. There is no clinical evidence that Ferrocholinate is superior to other iron preparations with respect to the therapeutic response. *Dose: Oral,* for persons over 6 years of age, 330 to 660 mg 3 times a day, and, for persons under 6 years of age, 104 mg once daily.

Ferroglycine Sulfate Complex [Glycamine Iron; Glyferro; Ferronord; Ferronord (*Cooper*)]—*Uses:* The complexation of ferrous iron in Ferroglycine Sulfate Complex stabilizes the iron against oxidation to ferric ion. The iron is thus claimed to be less irritating and better absorbed than that in noncomplexed forms. The drug is used for the treatment of *iron-deficiency anemia* and to provide iron in pregnancy or postgastrectomy. *Dose: Oral,* 400 mg (equivalent to 75 mg of iron) once or twice a day.

Ferrous Carbonate, Saccharated NFX—*Uses:* Ferrous Carbonate is marketed as a source of iron in the treatment of *iron-deficiency anemias* and in pregnancy or following gastrectomy. There is no evidence that it is superior to other forms of iron. Indeed, insoluble divalent metal carbonates, in general, are slow to dissolve in gastric juice and may be emptied from the stomach before the major portion has been reacted. The claim that the incidence of gastric upset is low is consistent with this generalization. Unreacted ferrous carbonate is probably poorly absorbed in the intestine. For this reason the rationale of choosing this drug in preference to other ferrous compounds is dubious, especially after gastrectomy. *Dose: Oral,* the equivalent of 100 mg of iron twice a day.

Iron, Reduced NF X [Iron by Hydrogen]—Elemental iron obtained by chemical process in powdered form, containing not less than 90% Fe. It may be produced electrolytically, by the decomposition of iron pentacarbonyl, and by the action of hydrogen upon ferric oxide. It occurs as a noncrystalline, odorless, grayish black powder, all of which must pass through a No. 100 sieve. It is stable in dry air, but in moist air it cakes and oxidizes forming ferric hydroxide. It is soluble in diluted mineral acids with the evolution of hydrogen. *Uses:* in the therapy of hypochromic, iron-deficiency anemias. It offers no advantages over ferrous sulfate. *Dose: orally,* 0.5 Gm. In severe iron-deficiency anemias, the adult dose is 1 to 1.5 Gm, 2 or 3 times daily.

Molybdenum Oxide [Molybdenum Sesquioxide] [Mo_2O_3]—*Uses:* Experimentally it has been shown that complete molybdenum deprivation results in anemia and that traces of molybdenum aid the hematinic action of iron compounds. However, no such action of molybdenum has been shown in human beings; furthermore, the human diet contains a superabundance of the metal, which, if required, is needed only in microtrace amounts. Molybdenum Oxide has been incorporated into various shotgun hematinic preparations, but only sales promotion has been thus benefited.

Agents for Macrocytic Anemias

The macrocytic anemias are characterized by the presence of large erythrocytes. They include *pernicious anemia,* the *anemia* of *sprue, macrocytic tropical anemia, fish tapeworm anemia, achrestic anemia,* and anemias resulting from gastric carcinoma and resection or disease of the intestinal tract. In all of these, insufficient intake or absorption of *cyanocobalamin* (vitamin B_{12}) is the cause of the disorder, the vitamin being essential to normal hematopoiesis and to the integrity of the central nervous system. Early work on pernicious anemia had established the need for a dietary factor, called the *extrinsic factor*, and a gastric and upper duodenal secretory factor, called the *intrinsic factor*. It is now well established that cyanocobalamin is the extrinsic factor; the vitamin is also the *antianemia principle* of liver. The intrinsic factor is essential to the proper absorption of vitamin B_{12}. The intrinsic factor is absent in pernicious anemia; in this disease the secretion of hydrochloric acid and pepsin is also diminished or absent. Before the advent of cyanocobalamin, various liver preparations were employed as sources of extrinsic factor and stomach preparations as sources of the intrinsic factor. Since orally administered liver was not reliable because it did not provide the intrinsic factor, it was necessary to administer a stomach preparation at the same time or to administer the liver parenterally. Today, the preparation of choice is cyanocobalamin, which is cheaper and which causes less discomfort at the site of injection than liver. Oral cyanocobalamin, of course, like liver, optimally requires a source of intrinsic factor.

For the patient with uncomplicated pernicious anemia in relapse, the initial dose of cyanocobalamin is 30 mcg daily, parenterally, or every other day for 5 to 10 doses, followed by 15 to 30 mcg once or twice weekly until the blood picture is normal. For maintenance; 40 to 60 mcg every 2 weeks or 80 to 100 mcg once a month is usually adequate. If there is demonstrable neurological damage, it may be necessary to administer 1000 mcg weekly for several months before switching to the maintenance schedule. Therapy must be maintained for life, since the basic deficiency in gastrointestinal physiology remains. Nevertheless, the patient may be kept in good health and may lead a fairly normal life.

Despite the superiority of cyanocobalamin, liver and stomach preparations are still available. The ingestion of 200 to 400 Gm of whole liver may be irregularly effective in inducing a remission in pernicious anemia. Concentrates for oral administration are made from such amounts of liver, but concentration results in some loss of activity. Extracts suitable for parenteral administration may be prepared from 10 to 15 Gm of liver. Similar effects may be produced by the ingestion of 30 to 40 Gm of desiccated stomach; however, the combinations of stomach and liver are required for optimal oral therapy. Liver preparations for injection may be assayed microbiologically, employing *Lactobacillus leichmannii* ATCC 7830, the assay being expressed in terms of vitamin B_{12}. However, since oral preparations are rarely effective, owing to the absence of the intrinsic factor, assay must be made in the human pernicious anemia patient in relapse, and the assay is expressed in terms of NF oral units (see NF XI). No liver preparations are included in the current NF. This absence of an official liver preparation reflects the ridiculousness of using archaic and irregularly effective preparations when the active ingredient, vitamin B_{12} or cyanocobalamin, or derivatives, is readily available and is more easily and safely administered.

Megaloblastic anemia of infancy, megaloblastic anemia of pregnancy, achrestic anemia, and nutritional macrocytic anemia generally respond better to liver preparations than they do to cyanocobalamin, and deficiencies in *folic* and *folinic acid* intake or metabolism are implicated; thus, either of these two acids may evoke a dramatic response in such anemias. Ascorbic acid also may occasionally confer additional benefits. The metabolic functions of folic or folinic acid and vitamin B_{12} converge in certain respects. Thus, folic or folinic acid may induce a remission in the blood pathology in pernicious anemia, but it will not revert or delay the progression of the epithelial and neurological pathology, which may develop insidiously and emerge explosively and irreversibly. Therefore, folic or folinic acid therapy of pernicious anemia is to be condemned. *Equally offensive and irresponsible is the inclusion of these acids in liver or multivitamin-hematinic preparations* because, in allaying the blood pathology of undiagnosed pernicious anemia, they prevent detection of the disease until the neurological pathology has advanced to a dangerous state. Unfortified liver preparations also may contain enough folic acid to constitute the same danger. *In general, a hematinic should be employed only upon accurate diagnosis of the anemia and upon specific indication.* Multiple preparations are to be avoided.

Cobalamin Concentrate—see page 1038.

Cyanocobalamin—see page 1037.

Folic Acid—see page 1038.

Hydroxocobalamin—see page 1038.

Liver Injection NF XII [Injectio Hepatis; Liver Extract for Parenteral Use; Pernaemon (*Organon*)] is a sterile solution in water for injection of that soluble thermostable fraction of mammalian livers which increases the number of red corpuscles in the blood of persons affected with pernicious anemia. Each ml of Liver Injection has vitamin B_{12} activity equivalent to that of either 10 or 20 mcg of cycnocobalamin. The potency is 100–150% of that stated on the label. *Uses:* See the general statement. *Dose: Usual, intramuscular,* in terms of the equivalent weight of cyanocobalamin, 1 mcg daily, preferably administered in amounts of 10 or 15 mcg at appropriate intervals.

Antihematopoietic Drugs

Polycythemia and erythrocytosis are conditions in which there is an increase in the number of circulating erythrocytes. The cause is usually the result of a deficient oxygenation of the arterial blood, and either condition may be corrected by management of the underlying primary disorder. However, in *polycythemia rubra vera* the condition is primary, and therapy is thus directed at the erythrocytes, either by their removal by venesection, their destruction by phenylhydrazines, or the suppression of their formation by antihematopoietic drugs or by x-irradiation. Several of the antineoplastic drugs such as the nitrogen mustards, the antifolic acids, arsenicals, and radiophosphate may be employed. The *leukemias* result from excessive leukocytic hematopoietic activity of a neoplastic nature; either the bone marrow (myelogenous or granulocytic leukemia) or lymphatic tissue (lymphocytic leukemia) may be involved. In myelogenous leukemia there may be anemia because the erythropoietic cells are crowded out by leukopoietic cells. Drugs used in the treatment of the leukemias are treated in the chapter on *Antineoplastic and Immunosuppressive Drugs*, page 1163.

Busulfan—see page 1164.

Chlorambucil—see page 1165.

Mechlorethamine Hydrochloride—see page 1167.

Mercaptopurine—see page 1168.

Methotrexate—see page 1169.

Pipobroman—see page 1169.

Pyrimethamine—see page 1247.

Sodium Phosphate P 32—see page 567.

Thiotepa—see page 1170.

Triethylenemelamine—see page 1171.

Uracil Mustard—see page 1171.

Urethan—see page 1171.

Vincristine Sulfate—see page 1172.

Agents Affecting Coagulation of the Blood

Blood-Clotting Proteins

The clotting of blood depends upon a sequence of reactions involving *thromboplastin* from blood platelets or damaged tissues, several trace proteins of plasma, and calcium. The terminal event in this sequence is the conversion of the soluble plasma protein, fibrinogen, into the insoluble substance *fibrin*, which forms the matrix of the clot. This conversion is brought about by the enzyme *thrombin*, which in turn is generated from a precursor, *prothrombin*. The clotting process may be outlined in a much oversimplified fashion, as follows:

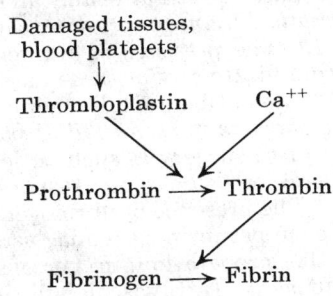

The other factors enter early in the sequence; for example, antihemophilic factor, the factor present in normal plasma which is deficient in hemophilia, participates at one of the first stages.

The synthesis of prothrombin and three other clotting factors in the liver depends on vitamin K. The prothrombopenic anticoagulants such as warfarin act as inhibitors of vitamin K, thus retarding the rate of synthesis of these factors. Not infrequently, deficiencies of single clotting factors are encountered which may result in severe hemorrhagic tendencies. Such deficiencies may be congenital or acquired. Congenital deficiency states, of which hemophilia is an example, have been described for almost every known clotting factor. Because several of the plasma factors are very unstable, it has heretofore been necessary to use fresh plasma or whole blood as a source of clotting factors for therapy. Meanwhile, much effort is presently being expended in attempts to make available concentrates of certain factors in safe, stable form. To date, however, only a few clotting factors can be obtained in a satisfactory state for use.

Aminocaproic Acid NF

[6-Aminohexanoic Acid; Amicar (*Lederle*)]

$$CH_2CH_2CH_2CH_2CH_2COOH$$
$$NH_2$$

Aminocaproic Acid contains 98.5–100.5% of $C_6H_{13}NO_2$ (131.18), calculated on the anhydrous basis.

Preparation—The lactam group of the commercially available caprolactam (hexahydro-2*H*-azepin-2-one) is cleaved at the C-N linkage by heating an aqueous solution with calcium hydroxide. The calcium aminocaproate thus formed is reacted with sulfuric acid to free the official acid and precipitate the calcium. Various other methods of preparation are also available.

Description—A fine, white, crystalline powder that is odorless, or nearly so, and tasteless. It is stable in light and air. It melts at about 205°.

Solubility—Freely soluble in water, acids, and alkalies; slightly soluble in methanol and alcohol; practically insoluble in chloroform and ether.

Uses—Aminocaproic Acid is a competitive inhibitor of plasminogen activators and, to a lesser extent, of fibrinolysin. As a consequence, it suppresses the formation of plasmin, an enzyme which destroys fibrinogen, fibrin, and other clotting components. For vascular integrity a normal low rate of fibrin deposition is essential, and excessive fibrinolysis leads to hemorrhage. Aminocaproic Acid is used in the treatment of *procedures or disorders in which fibrinolysis is enhanced*, such as cardiac bypass, postcaval shunt, major thoracic surgery, prostatic postoperative hematuria, leukemia, metastatic prostatic carcinoma, cirrhosis and other hepatic diseases, eclampsia, intrauterine fetal death, amniotic fluid embolism, and abruptio placentae. The drug is of no value in hemorrhage due to thrombocytopenia, hyperheparinemia, or other coagulation defects, or to vascular disruption.

Aminocaproic Acid may cause itching, erythema, skin rash, diuresis, heart burn, nausea, and diarrhea. It also has an antiadrenergic effect similar to guanethidine, so that nasal stuffiness, conjunctival suffusion, and hypotension may occur. The drug may enhance thrombotic processes by suppression of reactive fibrinolysis, which tends to limit clot formation and to favor clot resolution. The drug is teratogenic in animals and hence should not be used in humans in the first two trimesters of pregnancy and in the third trimester only if its use is imperative.

Aminocaproic Acid is excreted by the kidney; in the presence of renal disease the dose should be reduced.

Dose—*Usual, oral* or *intravenous, initial,* **5 Gm,** followed by **1** to **1.25 Gm** per hour to maintain a plasma concentration of 13 mg per 100 ml. No more than **30 Gm** per 24-hour period is recommended.

Other Dose Information—For intravenous administration the drug should be diluted in isotonic or dextrose solution and injected *slowly*. After 8 hours of treatment, the patient's condition should be re-evaluated.

Dosage Forms—Injection NF: 5 Gm/20 ml; Tablets NF: 500 mg.

Human Antihemophilic Factor

[Antihemophilic Factor (Human) (Method 4); (*Hyland*)]

Human Antihemophilic Factor is a stable dried preparation of human antihemophilic factor (Factor VIII, AHF, AHG) in concentrated form with minimal quantities of other proteins.

Preparation—Antihemophilic factor (AHF) activity is precipitated by glycine from a solution of an AHF-rich first precipitate from pooled normal human plasma following principles of the Wagner, *et al*, method.[2] After treatment to lower the content of glycine and inactive proteins, a solution of the active fraction is sterilized by filtration, aseptically filled into final containers, dried aseptically from the frozen state, stoppered under vacuum, and assayed for AHF content.

Description—A dry powder or coke-like solid that is colorless or opalescent when reconstituted with the diluent provided.

Uses—The coagulation defect in hemophilia is predominately a deficit of the coagulation factor VIII (sometimes factor IX or XI), called antihemophilic factor (AHF). In severe hemorrhage *in the hemophilic* (hemophilia A) *person only*, Human Antihemophilic Factor as a concentrate or in fresh plasma or whole blood, is required to *terminate hemorrhage* or to prevent hemorrhage in surgery or consequent to various procedures in which bleeding may occur. The concentrate is generally preferred, since the AHF titres of blood and plasma are quite variable. For other types of hemophilia (B or C), blood or plasma is indicated.

Dose—*Usual, intravenous, initial,* **1 unit** (equivalent to 1 pint of blood) per **7 Kg** of body weight followed by ½ unit every 12 hours as long as necessary.

Dosage Forms—for Injection: 30 ml.

Fibrinogen USP

[Fibrinogen (Human) (*Hyland; MSD*); Parenogen (*Cutter*)]

Fibrinogen is a sterile fraction of normal human plasma, dried from the frozen state, which in solution has the property of being converted into insoluble fibrin when thrombin is added. It contains no preservative. Its production and distribution are subject to federal regulations (see *Biologics*, page 1425).

Preparation—Human plasma conforming to the requirements of the National Institutes of Health is fractionated with ethanol. The dried residue from the sterile, fibrinogen-containing fraction constitutes the official Fibrinogen.

Description—White or grayish, amorphous substance.

Uses—Fibrinogen (Human) is employed in certain surgical procedures in which it is desirable to create a clot or adhesion *in situ*, in which case it is applied locally, generally along with a solution of thrombin, and for restoring plasma fibrinogen levels to normal in hemorrhagic conditions resulting from *hypofibrino-genemia*, such as may accompany premature separation of the placenta or following drastic thoracic surgery. It is also used in certain procedures for the *assay of plasma prothrombin* content. Its use in the human is not without danger because of the risk of transmitting serum hepatitis to the recipient, and its use should only be undertaken after clear indication based upon laboratory studies (plasma fibrinogen below 100 mg per 100 ml) and urgency of need.

Dose—*Intravenous infusion,* **2 to 8 Gm;** *usual,* **2 Gm.**

Dosage Forms—1 and 8 Gm.

Fibrinogen with Antihemophilic Factor

[Fibro-AHF (*MSD*)]

Fibrinogen with Antihemophilic Factor is obtained from normal human plasma by the Cohn cold ethanol procedure of plasma fractionation.

Uses—The separation of fibrinogen from antihemophilic factor is difficult and adds considerably to the expense of the separate components. Consequently, many physicians prefer to use the more economical complex, Fibrinogen with Antihemophilic Factor, when either fibrinogen or antihemophilic factor is indicated.

The effect of fibrinogen is employed in *abruptio placentae, intrauterine fetal death, amniotic fluid embolism, acute leukemia, terminal cancer, burns, cirrhosis of the liver, cardiac bypass, postcaval shunt,* and after *major thoracic, pancreatic, uterine, or prostatic surgery* or after serious trauma. The presence of antihemophilic factor does not complicate any of these uses.

The effect of the antihemophilic factor is sought to *terminate hemorrhage in the hemophiliac* patient or as a *prophylactic* prior to surgery in such patients. Hemophilia of types B or C does not respond as well as hemophilia A. The presence of fibrinogen complicates therapy, since hyperfibrinogenemia usually results from use of the preparation in persons without a deficit in fibrinogen. Intravascular fibrin deposition and visceral infarction sometimes results. Furthermore, hyperfibrinogenemia may cause erythrocyte agglutination and mild hemolysis and also interfere with blood typing.

Allergic reactions, such as itching, urticaria, facial edemia, chills, fever, and dyspnea occur rarely. As with all blood products, serum hepatitis may occur.

Dose—*Intravenous,* up to **8 Gm** or more according to plasma fibrinogen or AHF level required.

Dosage Forms—1 and 2 Gm.

Antihemophilic Human Plasma USP

[Antihemophilic Plasma (Human); Single-Donor Plasma (Human)]

Antihemophilic Human Plasma is normal human plasma, from a single donor, that has been processed promptly to preserve the antihemophilic factor of the original blood. It is in either the frozen form or the form of a dried solid obtained by cryodesiccation. The production and distribution of Antihemophilic Human Plasma are subject to federal regulations (see *Biologics*, page 1425).

Note—Plasma that is labeled as *Single-Donor Plasma (Human)* is a suitable source of antihemophilic factor only if used within 1 year.

Description—Light yellow to deep cream in color. When viewed microscopically it exhibits a honeycomb-like structure and shows no evidence of fusion.

Uses—The antihemophilic plasma is used for a *temporary* correction of the coagulation defect of *hemophilia*, which correction may be desired for surgery, or in anticipation of other situations in which bleeding may occur, or as may be needed in emergency, to terminate already progressing hemorrhage. It has also been employed for routine administration in the chronic management of hemophilia.

Dose—*Intravenous infusion*, **250 to 500 ml**; *usual*, **250 ml** daily.

Dosage Forms—100 and 250 ml.

Thrombin NF

(*Upjohn*); Thrombin Topical (*Parke, Davis*)]

Thrombin is a sterile protein substance prepared from prothrombin of bovine origin through interaction with added thromboplastin in the presence of calcium. It is capable, without the addition of other substances, of causing the clotting of whole blood, plasma, or a solution of fibrinogen. It may contain a suitable antibacterial agent.

Thrombin complies with the requirements of the United States Public Health Service (see *Biologics*, page 1425).

Note: Solutions of thrombin should be used within a few hours after preparation, and are not to be injected.

Description—Thrombin is a white or grayish, amorphous substance dried from the frozen state.

Uses—Concentrated Thrombin has an extraordinarily potent hemostatic or clotting effect on blood. Its powerful coagulant action is employed in coagulating fibrinogen solution. It is also useful for local application to *cuts* or *injuries*, in the control of minor oozing where the blood flow is not great enough to wash away the clot as it forms. For more extensive or inaccessible *hemorrhage*, a matrix must be applied to hold the thrombin in place and provide a structure for clot formation. Such a matrix is provided by various products, including fibrin foam, gelatin sponge, etc.

Dose—*Topically*, as a powder or as a solution containing **100 units** per ml.

Other Agents Affecting Coagulation of the Blood

Urokinase [(*Abbott*); Win-Kinase (*Winthrop*)] is a clot-dissolving enzyme extracted from human urine. *Description:* An off-white, odorless, lyophilized powder. It should be protected from light and stored in a sealed container at refrigerated temperature. The bulk drug, when frozen at $-20°$, is stable for years.

Uses: Urokinase is an activator of plasminogen. Consequently, when given intravenously, it increases the fibrinolytic activity in the plasma. It has an even greater effect to activate plasminogen in thrombi. Not only does the enhanced fibrinolytic activity limit the extension of intravascular clots in various thromboembolic disorders, but it may also cause clot dissolution in some patients if given within 72 hours of thrombogenesis. Urokinase is advantageous over other fibrinolytic agents in that it is nonpyrogenic and nonantigenic. Furthermore, its fibrinolytic effects are more predictable than with other agents. No toxic effects of the substance have been observed to date, but a slight decline in hematocrit and blood factor 7 sometimes occurs. The drug must not be given to patients who are actively bleeding, patients with recent major surgery (within 7 to 10 days), or persons with coagulation defects. *Dose:* Urokinase is still an experimental drug, and optimal doses have not yet been worked out. The usual intravenous dose is initially 1600 to 2000 CTA units per pound of body weight, to be given slowly over a 10-minute period; thereafter, 1600 to 2000 CTA units per pound per hour are given by continuous slow infusion for 48 hours.

Anticoagulants

Anticoagulants are substances or drugs which delay coagulation of blood. They are of three general types.

1. *Calcium sequestering agents*—Calcium is essential to several steps in the clotting process; hence, its removal prevents clotting. The calcium sequestering agents are employed only in withdrawn blood; systemically they induce the dangerous hypocalcemia syndrome long before the calcium concentration is low enough to prolong clotting time. However, certain complexing agents are used systemically in the treatment of heavy metal poisoning or to reduce the levels of plasma calcium for reasons other than anticoagulation.

2. *Heparin and Heparin Substitutes*—These agents interfere with clotting by inhibiting the conversion of prothrombin to thrombin, the action of thrombin on fibrinogen, and the rupture of blood platelets.

3. *Prothrombopenic Anticoagulants*—In this group bishydroxycoumarin provides the prototype of action but not necessarily of structure. Prothrombopenic anticoagulants competitively inhibit vitamin K in the hepatic production of prothrombinogen, the immediate precursor of plasma prothrombin; the plasma content of prothrombin is thus reduced and coagulation of the blood impaired.

The heparin and prothrombopenic anticoagulants are generally not employed for the same purpose since chronic medication with heparin is expensive and entails the nuisance of parenteral administration. Rather, they may be complementary, heparin being employed acutely or initially, and prothrombopenic anticoagulants being employed for longer term therapy.

Disodium Edetate—see page 843.

Anisindione NF

[2-(*p*-Methoxyphenyl)-1,3-indandione; Miradon (*Schering*)]

Anisindione contains 97.0–103.0% of $C_{16}H_{12}O_3$ (252.27), calculated on the dried basis.

Preparation—3-(*p*-Methoxybenzylidene)phthalide is caused to undergo rearrangement under the influence of sodium methoxide. US Pat. 2,899,359.

Description—A fine, white to cream-white, crystalline powder that is odorless or has a slightly sweet odor. It is stable in light and air. It melts between 152° and 158°.

Solubility—Practically insoluble in water; soluble in methylene chloride; sparingly soluble in sodium hydroxide TS; slightly soluble in ether, methanol, and hydrochloric acid.

Uses—Anisindione is a prothrombopenic anticoagulent with actions and uses similar to those of *Bishydroxycoumarin* (page 832). Its onset of action is 24 to 72 hours, and its duration of action is ordinarily 3 to 5 days. Like other drugs in the class, the effective dose and duration of action is affected by a number of factors, including dietary intake and enteric bacterial synthesis of vitamin K, and concurrent drugs which affect the hepatic "microsomal" drug-metabolizing system.

Untoward effects include hemorrhagic diathesis resulting from an overdose and dermatitis. Overdoses can be antagonized with phytonadione (vitamin K_1), but there is a long delay before prothrombin levels return to a safe range. If fever or dermatitis appears, the drug should be discontinued, because of the possible danger of blood dyscrasias. The drug may cause some orange discoloration of the urine, which may obscure the onset of hematuria, the important sign of impending hemorrhage; it may be distinguished from hematuria by its disappearance upon acidification. The patient should be advised of the possibility of discoloration.

Dose—*Maintenance*, **25** to **250 mg** per day, as determined by prothrombin time determinations; *usual, initial*, **300 mg** the first day, **200 mg** the second day, and **100 mg** the third day; *maintenance*, **75** to **100 mg** per day, as determined by prothrombin time determinations; *usual, maintenance*, **75** to **100 mg** per day.

Dosage Forms—Tablets NF: 50 mg.

Bishydroxycoumarin USP

[Dicoumarol; Dicumarol; Dicoumarin; Biscumarol; Melitoxin; 3,3'-Methylenebis[4-hydroxycoumarin]]

Bishydroxycoumarin contains 98.0–100.5% of $C_{19}H_{12}O_6$ (336.30), calculated on the dried basis.

Preparation—Methyl acetylsalicylate is stirred with sodium at 165°–175° for 1 hour, thus effecting ring closure through demethanolation to form the sodium derivative of 4-hydroxycoumarin. Treatment with hydrochloric acid liberates the 4-hydroxycoumarin which readily forms Bishydroxycoumarin on heating with formaldehyde and water.

Description—White or creamy white, crystalline powder, with a faint, pleasant odor and a slightly bitter taste. Melting range 287° to 293°.

Solubility—Practically insoluble in water, alcohol, and ether; slightly soluble in chloroform; readily soluble in solutions of fixed alkali hydroxides.

Uses—Bishydroxycoumarin is employed as a *prothrombopenic anticoagulant*. It depresses hepatic production of prothrombin, probably by competing with vitamin K; the resultant lowering of the blood level of prothrombin renders the blood less coagulable. The plasma levels of certain other coagulation factors are also depressed; indeed, there is evidence that in some persons the major effect of bishydroxycoumarin is upon these other factors.

Bishydroxycoumarin has advantages over heparin (see page 834) for ambulatory and prolonged anticoagulant therapy in that it is *orally effective*, has a longer duration of action (2 to 7 days) and is considerably less expensive; it is unsuitable for short term or emergency therapy in that the maximal effect of a full initial dose does not occur for 48 to 96 hours after administration. During the period of onset of action, heparin may be given. Bishydroxycoumarin or one of its congeners is employed for long-term therapy to a much greater extent than heparin; however, the neces-

sity for frequent prothrombin tests, which are more difficult to determine than clotting time, restricts the use of Bishydroxycoumarin to physicians having access to properly equipped laboratories and trained personnel. Bishydroxycoumarin may be used in the treatment of the following: *pulmonary embolism*, to prevent further embolism; primary acute and postoperative *thrombophlebitis* and *traumatic injuries to blood vessels*, to forestall *venous thrombosis* and to prevent *thromboemboli*; sudden *arterial occlusion from thrombosis or embolism*; prophylaxis of *postoperative venous thrombosis or embolism; vascular surgery*. In the absence of specific contraindications, it is frequently used routinely in acute *coronary thrombosis* with myocardial infarction. It is also advocated in the treatment of chronic diseases that predispose to thrombi or emboli such as congestive heart failure, persistent phlebitis migrans, recurrent thrombophlebitis, recurrent coronary thrombosis and atrial fibrillation; however, the exact status of such long-term therapy is undetermined.

The aim of treatment is to maintain the blood prothrombin activity at a level of 15 to 25% of normal.

Overdosage, which predisposes to massive hemorrhage, can be antagonized by natural or synthetic vitamin K preparations, or by transfusions of fresh blood. Nausea, vomiting, and diarrhea sometimes occur during the treatment.

Dose—*Usual, initial* **200 mg** to **300 mg** daily, then **50** to **100 mg** daily, according to prothrombin times.

Other Dose Information—Maintenance doses may be given at daily to weekly intervals, according to the prothrombin activity and the dosage schedule employed.

Dosage Forms—Capsules NF: 25, 50, and 100 mg; Tablets USP: 25, 50, and 100 mg.

Diphenadione NF

[2-(Diphenylacetyl)-1,3-indandione; Diphenylacetylindandione; Dipaxin *(Upjohn)*]

Diphenadione 98.0–100.5% of $C_{23}H_{16}O_3$ (340.38) calculated on the dried basis.

Preparation—Dimethyl phthalate is condensed with diphenylacetone using sodium methoxide in dry benzene. After completion of the reaction, a five per cent sodium hydroxide solution is added, and the solid sodium derivative which separates is collected, suspended in water, and acidified with dilute hydrochloric acid. The crude, gummy diphenadione thus formed soon solidifies and is purified by crystallization from ethanol.

Description—Yellow crystals or as yellow crystalline powder which is odorless. Melting range: 144° to 150°.

Solubility—Practically insoluble in water; soluble in benzene, ether, and glacial acetic acid; slightly soluble in acetone and alcohol.

Uses—A *prothrombopenic anticoagulant* (see *Bishydroxycoumarin*). It has an unusually long duration of action, which may be as much as 20 days. It is orally effective. Diphenadione may cause nausea and vomiting.

Dose—**2.5** to **30 mg**; *usual, initial*, **20** to **30 mg** the first day, **10** to **15 mg** the second day; *usual, maintenance*, **2.5** to **5 mg** daily.

Other Dose Information—The initial dose is 20 to 30 mg orally followed by 10 to 15 mg the second day. Thereafter the dose is adjusted according to the plasma prothrombin levels achieved.

Dosage Forms—Tablets NF: 5 mg.

Ethyl Biscoumacetate NF

[Ethyl Bis(4-hydroxy-2-oxo-2*H*-1-benzopyran-3-yl)acetate; 3,3′-(carboxy-methylene)bis[4-hydroxycoumarin] Ethyl Ester]

Ethyl Biscoumacetate, dried at 105° for 2 hours, contains 97.0–101.0% of $C_{22}H_{16}O_8$ (408.37).

Preparation—Two molecules of 4-hydroxycoumarin are condensed with one molecule of glyoxylic acid (OCH.COOH) to yield 3,3′-(carboxymethylene)bis(4-hydroxycoumarin) which is then esterified by lengthy heating with ethanolic HCl. The ester crystallizes out on cooling. US Pat. 2,482,512.

Description—Occurs as a white to yellowish white, crystalline powder.

Solubility—1 Gm dissolves in about 20 ml of acetone; soluble in benzene; slightly soluble in alcohol and in ether; insoluble in water.

Uses—A *prothrombopenic anticoagulant* (see *Bishydroxycoumarin*). Its onset and duration of action are shorter than that of its prototype.

Dose—*Usual, initial*, **1.2** to **1.8 Gm**, then **300** to **900 mg** daily in accordance with prothrombin time determinations.

Dosage Forms—Tablets NF: 150 and 300 mg.

Sodium Citrate—see page 873.

Anticoagulant Sodium Citrate Solution NF

Anticoagulant Sodium Citrate Solution is a sterile solution of sodium citrate in water for injection and contains, in each 100 ml, 3.80–4.20 Gm of $C_6H_5Na_3O_7.$-$2H_2O$ (294.10). It contains no antimicrobial agents.

Sodium Citrate (dihydrate)	**40 Gm**
Water for Injection, a sufficient quantity,	
To make.	**1000 ml**

Note—Anhydrous sodium citrate (35.1 Gm) may be used instead of the dihydrate.

Dissolve the sodium citrate in sufficient water for injection to make 1000 ml, and filter until clear. Place the solution in suitable containers, and sterilize.

Description—A clear, colorless solution possessing a slightly saline taste. The pH of the Solution is not less than 6.4 and not more than 7.5.

Uses—Anticoagulant Sodium Citrate Solution prevents the clotting of blood by forming an undissociated calcium citrate complex; calcium ions are essential for the coagulation of blood. The solution when added to blood both prevents the clotting of blood and prevents either crenation or swelling of the cells. The sterile solution is employed for the preparation of blood for fractionation, for banked blood for transfusion, and for the preparation of citrated human plasma. It is used as an *additive* (50 ml in 500 ml of normal human plasma or blood).

Anticoagulant Citrate Dextrose Solution USP

[Anticoagulant Acid Citrate Dextrose Solution USP XVII; ACD Solution]

Anticoagulant Acid Citrate Dextrose Solution is a sterile solution of citric acid, sodium citrate, and dextrose in water for injection. It contains 95.0–105.0% of the labeled amounts of citric acid [$C_6H_8O_7$ = 192.13], sodium citrate [$C_6H_5Na_3O_2.2H_2O$ = 294.10], and dextrose [$C_6H_{12}O_6.H_2O$ = 198.17]. It contains no antimicrobial agents.

	Solution A	Solution B
Citric Acid (anhydrous)	7.3 Gm	4.4 Gm
Sodium Citrate (dihydrate).	22.0 Gm	13.2 Gm
Dextrose (monohydrate).	24.5 Gm	14.7 Gm
Water for Injection, a sufficient quantity,		
To make.	**1000 ml**	**1000 ml**

Dissolve the ingredients, and mix. Filter the solution until clear, place immediately in suitable containers, and sterilize.

If desired, 8 Gm and 4.8 Gm of monohydrated citric acid may be used instead of the indicated, respective amounts of anhydrous citric acid; 22.4 Gm and 13.4 Gm of anhydrous dextrose may be used instead of the indicated, respective amounts of monohydrated dextrose; and 19.3 Gm and 11.6 Gm of anhydrous sodium citrate may be used instead of the indicated, respective amounts of dihydrated sodium citrate.

Note—Either 15 ml of Solution A or 25 ml of Solution B, providing the several ingredients in approximately the same ratio, is required for each 100 ml of whole blood.

Description—A clear, colorless, and odorless liquid having a pH of between 4.5 and 5.5. It is dextrorotatory. It meets the requirements under *Injections*, page 1519.

Uses—See *Anticoagulant Sodium Citrate Solution*. ACD Solution will preserve whole blood for 21 days. The addition of citric acid to the sodium citrate buffers the blood at a pH at which the blood cells are more stable; both potassium and lipid loss are decreased. Dextrose provides a substrate for glycolysis, so that high-energy phosphates in the blood cells do not disappear as rapidly as with sodium citrate solution alone. Not only is the storage life of the cells improved but also the post-transfusion life.

Anticoagulant Citrate Phosphate Dextrose Solution USP

Anticoagulant Citrate Phosphate Dextrose Solution is a sterile solution of citric acid, sodium citrate, sodium biphosphate, and dextrose in water for injection. It contains 95.0–105.0% of the labeled amounts of citric acid ($C_6H_8O_7$), sodium citrate ($C_6H_5Na_3O_7.$-$2H_2O$), sodium biphosphate ($NaH_2PO_4.H_2O$), and dextrose ($C_6H_{12}O_6.H_2O$). It contains no antimicrobial agents.

Citric Acid (anhydrous).	**3.0 Gm**
Sodium Citrate (dihydrate).	**26.3 Gm**
Sodium Biphosphate (monohydrate; $NaH_2PO_4.H_2O$).	**2.22 Gm**
Dextrose (monohydrate).	**25.5 Gm**
Water for Injection, a sufficient quantity,	
To make.	**1000 ml**

Dissolve the ingredients, and mix. Filter the solution until clear, place immediately in suitable containers, and sterilize.

If desired, 3.27 Gm of monohydrated citric acid may be used instead of the indicated amount of anhydrous citric acid; 23.1 Gm of anhydrous sodium citrate may be used instead of the indicated amount of dihydrated sodium citrate; 1.93 Gm of anhydrous sodium biphosphate may be used instead of the indicated amount of monohydrated sodium biphosphate; and 23.2 Gm of anhydrous dextrose may be used instead of the indicated amount of monohydrated dextrose.

Description—A clear, colorless, odorless liquid. It is dextrorotatory. Its pH is between 5.0 and 6.0.

Uses—See *Anticoagulant Sodium Citrate Dextrose Solution*.

Application—For use in the proportion of 14 ml of Solution for each 100 ml of whole blood.

Sodium Heparin USP

[Heparin; Lipo-Hepin (*Riker*); Liquaemin Sodium (*Organon*); Panheprin (*Abbott*)]

Sodium Heparin is a mixture of active principles, having the property of prolonging the clotting time of blood. It is usually obtained from the lungs, intestinal mucosa, or other suitable tissues of domestic mammals used for food by man. The potency of Sodium Heparin, calculated on the dried basis, is not less than 140 USP Heparin Units* in each mg, and 90.0–110.0% of the potency stated on the label.

Preparation—Heparin is the body's natural anticoagulant, taking part in the physiological function of maintaining the fluidity of the blood. It is produced by the mast cells of Ehrlich, which are clustered in the perivascular connective tissue of the walls of major blood vessels and capillaries. Heparin is a polysulfuric ester of mucoitin.[3,4] The molecular skeleton is constructed from acetylated glucosamine and glucuronic acid. The disaccharide unit is similar to that in *mucoitin sulfuric acid* and *hyaluronic acid*. Protein-free samples of heparin contain about 10% of sulfur present as ester sulfates. Original preparations of heparin contain mixtures consisting of mucoitin disulfuric and trisulfuric acids. The anticoagulant action is greater in preparations with the highest sulfuric content. Heparin in the final, therapeutic form is supplied in a solution made from the sodium salt, but in the steps of its purification the barium salts of heparin are prepared. Heparin, being a mixture of the several sulfuric esters, is not entirely homogeneous, and there is debate as to whether a truly crystalline or homogeneous preparation has been or ever can be prepared.

Heparin is prepared commercially from lung tissue of slaughtered animals. Thus, the name heparin, although given because the anticoagulant was first extracted by Howell from liver, is obviously undesirable. Now it is neither obtained in quantity from the liver nor does it have any of the actions of the well-known liver extracts. Its production by the mast cells is actually a nonhepatic source.

Description—White or pale-colored amorphous powder. Odorless, or nearly so. Hygroscopic. A 1% solution has a pH of 5 to 7.5. It will not dialyze through a parchment membrane, and only slightly through a collodion membrane. Heparin is resistant to all kinds of chemical agents; it gives an insoluble precipitate with protamine and with toluidine blue; and interference with the sulfuric groups reduces its anticoagulant activity. Heparin has a very low osmotic pressure in respect to its high degree of ionization. In contrast to the effect of oxalate, heparin has no osmotic influence on red blood cells. Heparin may be stored for long periods without loss of activity.

Solubility—1 Gm dissolves in 20 ml of water; soluble in methanol, alcohol, acetone, and glacial acetic acid.

Uses—Heparin exerts its *anticoagulant* effects at several stages in the complex process of blood coagulation. It prevents the conversion of prothrombin to thrombin, it antagonizes thromboplastin, it prevents the formation of fibrin from fibrinogen and thrombin, and, lastly, it prevents the agglutination of platelets. The mechanism of these actions is not known; the density of the electrical charge of the Heparin anion, which may affect enzymes involved in blood coagulation, and the ability of Heparin to split certain lipoproteins, such as various thromboplastics, probably are partly responsible for its actions. Its effects on lipoproteins may also relate to its ability to diminish plasma turbidity in alimentary lipemia and to its interference with complement fixation.

Heparin is employed clinically in acute conditions in which a rapid reduction in the coagulability of the blood is desired. Its high cost and oral inefficacy discourage prolonged use, although it is often employed to initiate prolonged anticoagulant therapy in order to cover the latent period of the onset of action of the bishydroxycoumarin-type anticoagulants. Heparin is also used in lieu of the bishydroxycoumarin type of drugs in prolonged therapy when laboratory facilities are unavailable for the determination of prothrombin time. Some of its primary clinical applications are nonfatal *pulmonary embolism*, primary and postoperative *thrombophlebitis*, sudden *arterial occlusion* from thrombosis or embolism, prophylaxis of postoperative *venous thrombosis* or embolism, and *vascular surgery*. It is advocated by some for the immediate therapy of *coronary occlusion*, but its status in that condition is still controversial. The indications for prolonged therapy with heparin are essentially the same as with prothrombopenic anticoagulants (see *Bishydroxycoumarin*, page 832), except for cost and inconvenience. Heparin also has special uses, such as prevention of clotting of blood samples, to *prevent clotting* during blood transfusions, and for the Heparin tolerance test. It is also used to prevent pleural and peritoneal *adhesions*. Hemorrhage is the principal toxic effect, usually the result of overdosage; Tolonium Chloride (Toluidine Blue O) or Protamine, with both of which Heparin combines, may be employed for the immediate control of hyperheparinemia.

Heparin must be administered by the intravenous, intramuscular, or subcutaneous route; it is *inactive orally*. Intravenously it may be given intermittently or by continuous drip. For continuous drip, 10,000 to 20,000 IU (1 mg equals approximately 100 IU) is added to 1 liter of isotonic dextrose or sodium chloride solution, and the flow is usually started at 1 ml per minute. More concentrated solutions may be employed if edema is impending. The rate is finally adjusted to maintain the clotting time (Lee-White) at 15 to 20 minutes.

Dose—*Intravenous*, **5000** to **10,000 USP Units** every 4 to 6 hours; *infusion*, **5000** to **40,000 Units** per **liter** at a rate of **1 ml** per **minute**; *subcutaneous*, **10,000** to **20,000 Units** 2 times daily; *usual, intravenous* or *subcutaneous*, as indicated by prothrombin-time determinations.

Other Dose Information—For intermittent intravenous dosage, 5000 IU is given at 4-hour intervals, but a total daily dose of 25,000 IU is generally not exceeded. The intramuscular dose schedule depends upon the

---

* *Note*—One USP Heparin Unit is the specific activity of that quantity of USP Sodium Heparin Reference Standard which is equivalent to one International Heparin Unit. This Unit is equivalent in activity to 10 mg of the barium salt of the purest ox heparin.

concentration of the Heparin solution; the action of a single ml containing 12,000 IU will endure approximately 8 hours. By the subcutaneous route the duration of action can be further prolonged. Repository preparations containing vasoconstrictors and/or other ingredients to retard absorption are available.

Dosage Forms—Anticoagulant Heparin Solution USP (see below): 2025, 2125, and 2250 Units/container. Injection USP: 1000, 5000, 7500, 10,000, 15,000, 20,000, and 40,000 Units/ml; 22,000 Units/1.1 ml; 2000, 40,000, and 80,000 Units/2 ml; 44,000 and 88,000 Units/2.2 ml; 40,000, 80,000, and 160,000 Units/4 ml; 5000, 50,000, 100,000, and 200,000 Units/5 ml; 10,000, 50,000, 100,000, 200,000, and 400,000 Units/10 ml; 20,000 Units/20 ml; 30,000 Units/30 ml.

Anticoagulant Heparin Solution USP [*Various Mfgs.*] is a sterile solution of sodium heparin in *Sodium Chloride Injection* (see page 843). It exhibits a potency of 90.0–110.0% of the potency stated on the label in terms of USP Heparin Units, and contains 0.85–0.95% of sodium chloride. It contains no antimicrobial agents.

Preparation: Add the sodium heparin (75,000 Units), in solid form or in solution, to the Sodium Chloride Injection (qs) to make 1000 ml, mix, filter if necessary, and sterilize. Its pH is between 5.0 and 7.5. *Uses:* See *Sodium Heparin.* *Application:* For use in the proportion of 6 ml of Solution for each 100 ml of whole blood.

Phenprocoumon NF

[3-(α-Ethylbenzyl)-4-hydroxycoumarin; Liquamar (*Organon*)]

Phenprocoumon contains 99.0–101.0% of $C_{18}H_{16}O_3$ (280.33), calculated on the dried basis.

Preparation—Diethyl (α-ethylbenzyl)malonate is reacted with acetylsalicylic acid chloride by heating with a suspension of powdered sodium in dry benzene. The resulting diethyl (o-acetoxybenzoyl)(α-ethylbenzyl)malonate is dissolved in absolute ether and treated with sodium methylate whereby ethyl acetate is split off with concomitant cyclization to the coumarin derivative, 3-carbethoxy-3-(α-ethylbenzyl)-4-oxodihydrocoumarin. This is saponified and decarboxylated by heating with aqueous sodium hydroxide, following which acidification with sulfuric acid liberates Phenprocoumon. Recrystallization is from 80% ethanol. US Pat. 2,701,804.

Description—A fine, white, crystalline powder that is odorless or has a slight odor. It melts between 177° and 181°.

Solubility—Practically insoluble in water; soluble in chloroform, methanol, and solutions of alkali hydroxides.

Uses—Phenprocoumon is a prothrombopenic anticoagulant with actions and uses similar to those of *Bishydroxycoumarin* (page 832). Its onset of action is 48 to 72 hours, and its duration of action may be as long as 7 days. Like other drugs of this class, the effective dose and duration of action is affected by a number of factors, including dietary intake and enteric bacterial synthesis of vitamin K, and concurrent drugs which affect the hepatic "microsomal" drug metabolizing system.

Overdose of the drug may cause hemorrhagic diathesis; phytonadione (vitamin K₁) can be used to antagonize the overdose, but there is a long delay before prothrombin levels return to a safe range. The drug may cause diarrhea, or other mild gastrointestinal disturbances, and dermatitis. Leukopenia, urticaria, or alopecia, seen with other coumarins, has not yet been reported.

Dose—*Usual, initial,* **21 mg** the first day, **9 mg** the second day, and **3 mg** the third day; *maintenance,* **1 to 4 mg** daily, according to prothrombin level.

Dosage Forms—Tablets NF: 3 mg.

Potassium Warfarin NF

[3-(α-Acetonylbenzyl)-4-hydroxycoumarin Potassium]

Potassium Warfarin contains 98.0–102.0% of $C_{19}H_{15}KO_4$ (346.43), calculated on the dried basis.

Preparation—Warfarin (see under *Sodium Warfarin*) is reacted with an equimolar portion of potassium hydroxide.

Description—Occurs as a white, odorless, crystalline powder, having a slightly bitter taste. It is discolored by light.

Solubility—Very soluble in water; freely soluble in alcohol; very slightly soluble in chloroform and ether.

Uses—See *Sodium Warfarin*. The potassium salt has the same uses as the sodium salt.

Dose—*Usual, initial,* **25 to 50 mg**, then **2.5 to 10 mg** daily in accordance with prothrombin time determinations.

Dosage Forms—Tablets NF: 5 and 25 mg.

Sodium Warfarin USP

[3-(α-Acetonylbenzyl)-4-hydroxycoumarin Sodium; Coumadin Sodium (*Endo*); Panwarfin (Abbott)]

Sodium Warfarin is an amorphous solid or a crystalline clathrate. The clathrate form consists principally of sodium warfarin, isopropyl alcohol, and water, the molecular proportions of which vary between 8:4:0 and 8:2:2. Sodium Warfarin contains 97.0–102.0% of $C_{19}H_{15}NaO_4$ (330.32), calculated on the anhydrous and isopropyl alcohol-free basis.

Preparation—Warfarin may be prepared by causing 4-hydroxycoumarin to undergo addition to benzalacetone under the catalytic influence of a mildly basic substance such as ammonia or piperidine. The reaction is a typical Michael "condensation." Conversion to the official sodium salt is readily effected by reacting the purified warfarin with an equimolar portion of dilute sodium hydroxide solution at room temperature.

Description—It is a white, odorless, crystalline powder, having a slightly bitter taste. It is discolored by light. The pH of a 1 in 100 solution is between 7.2 and 8.3.

Solubility—Very soluble in water, freely soluble in alcohol, and very slightly soluble in chloroform and ether.

Uses—A *prothrombopenic anticoagulant* (See *Bishydroxycoumarin*). Although it is usually administered orally, its chief distinction from other prothrombopenic drugs is the fact that it is water-soluble and may be administered intravenously. By the intravenous route its onset of action is 12 to 18 hours and its duration is 5 to 6 days.

Dose—*Oral, intramuscular,* or *intravenous, initial,* **25 to 75 mg;** *usual, initial,* **50 mg,** then **5 to 10 mg** once a day, in accordance with prothrombin time determinations; *maintenance,* **2 to 10 mg** daily.

Other Dose Information—Maintenance doses for both the oral and intravenous routes are about ⅔ of the initial dose, given at intervals indicated by the plasma prothrombin level.

Dosage Forms—for Injection USP: 50 and 75 mg; Tablets USP: 2, 2.5, 5, 7.5, 10, and 25 mg.

Other Anticoagulants

Acenocoumarol [Sintrom (*Geigy*)] is 3-(α-acetonyl-*p*-nitrobenzyl)-4-hydroxycoumarin [$C_{19}H_{15}NO_6$]. *Description and Solubility:* Crystals which melt between 196° and 199°. Almost insoluble in water or in organic solvents; forms water-soluble salts with alkalies. *Uses:* The most potent of the bishydroxycoumarin-like (prothrombopenic) anticoagulants. After oral administration its peak effect is reached within 3 to 4 days and its effect disappears within 3 to 4 days. Its uses and limitations are those of *Bishydroxycoumarin* (page 832). *Dose: Oral, initial,* 16 to 28 mg with subsequent adjustment according to the response. Maintenance doses are generally 2 to 10 mg daily.

Phenindione [Danilone (*Schieffelin*); Hedulin (*National Drug*)] is 2-phenyl-1,3-indandione [$C_{15}H_{10}O_2$]. *Description and Solubility:* A pale-yellow, crystalline material. Very soluble in alcohol; slightly soluble in water. *Uses:* A prothrombopenic anticoagulant that has a more rapid onset of action than *Bishydroxycoumarin* (page 832). Its therapeutic effect is obtained within 18 to 24 hours and lasts 24 to 48 hours after medication is discontinued. As with all short-acting prothrombopenic drugs, its actions are erratic, and its short duration of action is of no real therapeutic advantage. Untoward effects include liver and renal damage, leukopenia, and rarely, agranulocytosis. The drug frequently imparts a red or orange color to the urine which the patient may confuse with hematuria; therefore, he should be forewarned. The obscuring of hematuria masks an important early sign of impending hemorrhagic diathesis. For this reason more serious hemorrhagic episodes occur with this drug than with other prothrombopenic drugs. *Dose: Oral, initial,* 200 to 300 mg in 2 divided doses at 12-hour intervals, and 25 to 50 mg twice daily for maintenance.

Potassium Oxalate [$K_2C_2O_4 \cdot H_2O$]—The oxalate anion of potassium oxalate combines with calcium ions to form the very insoluble calcium oxalate. Thus when it is added to withdrawn (shed) blood it acts as an anticoagulant, for which purpose it may be employed in clinical laboratory procedures. It may also be used as a reagent in the determination of serum or other calcium by the permanganate method, the washed precipitated calcium oxalate being redissolved in acid and the oxalate titrated with permanganate. The reducing properties of the oxalate anion make this substance useful as a cleaning and bleaching agent, especially for straw. Care must be exercised in its storage and use because it is highly toxic.

Sodium Oxalate [$Na_2C_2O_4$]—The actions and uses of sodium oxalate are virtually identical to those of *Potassium Oxalate,* above.

Anticoagulant Antagonists

Anticoagulant therapy carries the risk of serious hemorrhage, so that there may be need to arrest the anticoagulant action. Bishydroxycoumarin-type anticoagulants, as expected from their mode of action, are antagonized by vitamin K or its synthetic substitutes. Not all vitamin K preparations are equally effective, vitamin K_1 (phytonadione) being superior and menadione inferior. The efficacy of vitamin K preparations also varies according to the anticoagulant, but all agents of the bishydroxycoumarin group may be antagonized by an appropriate dose of vitamin K_1. The antagonism is not manifested immediately, since normal coagulation is obtained only after the liver has had time to replenish the prothrombin and prothrombinogen. Heparin is antagonized by various amines, ammonium compounds, and basic proteins, which precipitate the polysulfate. Circulating heparinoid substances in the blood can also be assayed with such substances.

Menadiol Sodium Diphosphate—see page 1021.

Menadione—see page 1022.

Menadione Sodium Bisulfite—see page 1022.

Phytonadione—see page 1022.

Protamine Sulfate USP

Protamine Sulfate is a purified mixture of simple protein principles obtained from the sperm or testes of suitable species of fish, which has the property of neutralizing heparin. Each mg of Protamine Sulfate,

calculated on the dried basis, neutralizes not less than 85 USP Units of heparin activity derived from lung tissue and not less than 120 USP Units of heparin activity derived from intestinal mucosa.

Preparation—Frozen ripe salmon testes are ground, water-washed, centrifuged, and dehydrated by means of solvents and vacuum drying. The dried material is then extracted with 10% sulfuric acid and, after filtering, a protamine sulfate-rich fraction is precipitated from the filtrate with cold alcohol. After collecting, this fraction is dissolved in hot water, and the protamine sulfate separates as an oil upon cooling. This protamine-rich oil is dissolved in hot water and fractionated again with cold alcohol. After collecting, this fraction is dehydrated by means of solvents and vacuum drying.

Description—A fine, white or faintly colored, amorphous or crystalline powder.

Solubility—Sparingly soluble in water.

Uses—Protamine Sulfate is a *heparin antagonist.* Because it is a strongly basic macromolecule, it combines strongly with heparin, which is a polyanionic macromolecule. It is injected slowly intravenously after suitably diluting with physiological salt solution, to counteract the effect of *overmedication with heparin.*

Dose—*Usual, intravenous,* **50 mg,** repeated as necessary.

Other Dose Information—Not more than 50 mg is administered at one time. It is also injected in the treatment of certain *hemorrhagic conditions.* The total daily dose is 5 to 6 mg per Kg, injected in two equal portions 6 hours apart. The dose is diluted to 300 ml with physiological salt solution and slowly administered intravenously.

Dosage Forms—Injection USP: 50 mg/5 ml, 250 mg/25 ml; for Injection USP: 50 mg.

Other Anticoagulant Antagonists

Tolonium Chloride [Toluidine Blue; Blutene (*Abbott*)] is 3-amino-7-(dimethylamino)-2-methylphenazathionium chloride [$C_{15}H_{16}ClN_3S$]. *Description and Solubility:* A dark-green powder. 1 Gm dissolves in about 26 ml of water, yielding a blue to violet solution, and in about 175 ml of alcohol, yielding a blue solution. *Uses:* It precipitates heparin. It is used for the treatment of overdosage of heparin and for the treatment of certain hemorrhagic states, some of which, but not all, are associated with elevated blood heparinoid levels. The organs are stained blue and the urine becomes pale blue-green. Nausea, vomiting, burning sensation upon urination, and tenesmus may occur, but they may be avoided by adequate fluid intake. *Dose: Oral,* 200 to 300 mg daily for menorrhagia; *intramuscular* or *slow intravenous,* for heparin overdosage, 100 mg. *Veterinary Dose: Oral, Dogs and Cats, 200 to 300 mg daily.*

Hemostatics and Styptics

Many substances not especially related to the clotting mechanism are capable of promoting clotting. Upon contact with most surfaces, platelets disintegrate, thereby liberating a thromboplastin. Spongy and gauzy materials, which provide a large surface area, are thus used to arrest bleeding; absorbable sponges may be left permanently at the site of bleeding. Fibrin, fibrinogen, and thrombin are also potent hemostatics (see page 829). Astringents (see Chapter 43, page 768) also initiate clotting by precipitating proteins and by labilizing platelets; ferric salts are mostly employed as styptics.

Alum—see page 769.

Cellulose, Oxidized—see page 1876.

Estrogens, Conjugated—see page 991.

Ferric Chloride—see page 772.

Fibrinogen—see page 830.

Fibrinogen with Antihemophilic Factor—see page 830.

Absorbable Gelatin Sponge USP

[Gelfoam (*Upjohn*)]

Absorbable Gelatin Sponge is gelatin in the form of a sterile, absorbable, water-insoluble sponge.

Description—A light, nearly white, nonelastic, tough, porous, hydrophilic solid. A 10-mm cube weighing approximately 9 mg will take up approximately 45 times its weight of well-agitated oxalated whole blood. It is stable in dry heat at 150° for 4 hours.

Solubility—Insoluble in water, but absorbable in body fluids; completely digested by a solution of pepsin.

Uses—Absorbable Gelatin Sponge is a *hemostatic* and *coagulant* used to control bleeding. It is moistened with thrombin solution or sterile normal saline and may then be left in place following the closure of a surgical incision. It is absorbed in from 4 to 6 weeks.

Human Antihemophilic Factor—see page 830.

Antihemophilic Human Plasma—see page 830.

Protamine Sulfate—see page 836.

Thrombin—see page 831.

Thromboplastin—see page 1376.

Tolonium Chloride—see this page.

Other Hemostatics and Styptics

Carbazochrome Salicylate [Adrenosem (*Massengill*); Adrestat (*Organon*)]—An adrenochrome monosemicarbazone [3-hydroxy-1-methyl-5,6-indolinedione-5-semicarbazone] sodium salicylate complex [$C_{10}H_{12}N_4O_3 \cdot C_7H_5NaO_3$] occurring as a fine, orange-red, odorless powder with a sweetish saline taste. It is soluble in both alcohol and water. A 13% aqueous solution has a pH range of 6.7–7.3. *Uses:* Proposed for the systemic control of capillary bleeding of various types. Its clinical usefulness for this purpose is scientifically unjustified. *Dose: Oral,* 1 to 5 mg 4 times daily; *intramuscular,* 5 mg every 2 to 4 hours.

Ferric Subsulfate [approx. $Fe_4O(SO_4)_5 \cdot H_2O$]—Used and prepared only as a solution. Ferric Subsulfate Solution was official in NF XI. It is prepared by oxidizing ferrous sulfate with nitric acid. The solution contains 20–22 Gm Fe per 100 ml. It is reddish brown and has an astringent, sour taste. It is miscible with alcohol. *Uses:* An important styptic solution. The solution is less irritating than ferric sulfate because of the lesser amount of sulfuric acid present. It is occasionally used to control surface bleeding and as an astringent in a variety of skin disorders. It should not be used in vesicular, bulbous, or exudative dermatoses, because it may then cause permanent pigmentation of the skin.

Fibrin Foam Human—A dry artificial sponge of human fibrin, prepared by clotting with thrombin a foam of a solution of human fibrinogen. The clotted foam is dried from the frozen state and heated at 130° for 3 hours to sterilize. It appears as a fine, white sponge of firm texture. It is insoluble in water. *Uses:* A mechanical coagulant of blood in case of hemorrhage, especially in surgery of the brain, liver, kidneys, and other organs where ordinary methods of hemostasis are ineffective or inadvisable. This preparation is used by impregnating it with a freshly prepared solution of thrombin in normal saline solution and then applying the foam to the bleeding area. In time, the foam is absorbed.

Electrolytes

The concentration of several of the electrolytes in the plasma is critical for the proper functioning of the cells, especially those of the excitable tissues. For the normal plasma concentration of the principal electrolytes, see page 815. The proper balance of the several ions is complex; it depends not alone upon the concentration in the extracellular fluid (of which plasma is one compartment) but also upon the intracellular concentration, the ratio across the cell membrane being an essential factor, and upon the ratio of one ion type to another. Thus, the plasma electrolyte concentrations provide only a crude clue to the electrolyte status of the patient.

and balance or other ancillary studies are often necessary to determine the true electrolyte needs. Certain of the electrolytes, for example calcium and phosphate, serve also as structural elements in the hard tissues (bone, teeth, etc) and may be employed for that purpose. Others, for example the chlorides of sodium, potassium, or calcium, may be occasionally employed as diuretics (see Chapter 53, page 936).

Calcium Chloride USP

[Muriate of Lime; Calcaria Muriatica]

Calcium Chloride contains an amount of $CaCl_2$ (110.99) equivalent to 99.0–107.0% of $CaCl_2.2H_2O$ (147.02).

Preparation—Calcium Chloride may be prepared by saturating hydrochloric acid with chalk or marble, then making the solution alkaline with calcium hydroxide and boiling. The treatment with calcium hydroxide precipitates magnesium, iron, and other metals. After filtering, the filtrate is neutralized with hydrochloric acid and evaporated to dryness at a temperature not exceeding 200° until it contains about 24% of water.

Description—White, hard, odorless fragments or granules. It is deliquescent.

Solubility—1 Gm is soluble in 1.2 ml water, about 10 ml of alcohol at 25°, 0.7 ml of boiling water, and about 2 ml of boiling alcohol.

Incompatibilities—Soluble calcium salts are precipitated by *borates, carbonates, citrates, oxalates, phosphates, sulfates, and tartrates*. For chloride ion incompatibilities, see *Potassium Chloride*, page 839.

Uses—Calcium Chloride is an acid-forming *diuretic* by virtue of the fact that the calcium ion is excreted by the bowel or deposited in bone leaving the chloride ion free to combine with fixed base. As a diuretic, it is used for the same purposes and in the same dosage as ammonium chloride.

Calcium Chloride provides an immediate source of calcium ions in the treatment of *tetany* arising from a low concentration of calcium in the blood regardless of etiology. For this purpose, 5 to 20 ml of a 5% solution is given by slow intravenous injection. Calcium Chloride is also *antispasmodic* to smooth muscle and is of special value in the treatment of colic arising from *lead poisoning*. It is administered intravenously in the same dosage as above. Calcium salts are also effective in relieving the abdominal pain and diarrhea of *intestinal tuberculosis*. For this purpose, they are given orally. A neutral salt is to be preferred.

Calcium Chloride has been used as an *antiallergic* to prevent serum sickness after the injection of antitoxins and antisera and also in the treatment of hay fever, urticaria, asthma, and other conditions resulting from allergy. The salt is the specific antidote in cases of *magnesium poisoning*.

A saturated solution of the salt mixed with finely powdered bentonite forms an *electrode paste* for attaching electrodes to the skin so that good contact is achieved during the tracing of electroencephalograms.

Anhydrous calcium chloride is used as a dryer for gases and many liquids and as a desiccant in desiccators for abstracting water from moist substances.

As an *electrolyte replenisher* Calcium Chloride is a pharmaceutical necessity for *Ringer's Injection, Lactated Ringer's Injection,* and *Ringer's Solution.*

Unofficial Dose Information—The usual oral and intravenous dose is 1 Gm 4 times a day.

Dosage Forms—Injection: 1 Gm/10 ml.
Veterinary Dose—*Intravenous, Horses* and *Cattle*, 15 to 50 Gm; *Sheep* and *Swine*, 2 to 3 Gm; *Dogs*, 500 mg to 1 Gm.

Calcium Gluconate USP

[Calcinol; Calglucon (*Sandoz*)]

$$\left[\underset{\text{HO } \text{OH } \text{OH}}{\text{HOCH}_2\text{CHCHCHCHCHCOO}-} \underset{}{\overset{\text{OH}}{|}} \right]_2 \text{Ca}$$

Calcium Gluconate contains 98.0–102.0% of $C_{12}H_{22}CaO_{14}$ (430.38), calculated on the dried basis.

Preparation—D-Glucose is oxidized to gluconic acid in the presence of calcium carbonate. The oxidation may be effected by certain molds, eg, *Aspergillus niger*, or by bromine.

Description—White, crystalline granules or powder, without odor or taste. It is stable in air and does not lose its water on drying without undergoing decomposition. Its solution is neutral to litmus paper. It is decomposed by dilute mineral acids into gluconic acid and the calcium salt of the mineral acid used.

Solubility—1 Gm dissolves slowly in about 30 ml of water and about 5 ml of boiling water; insoluble in alcohol and many other organic solvents.

Identification—It responds to the identification tests for *Calcium* and to the following *Test for Gluconic Acid:* To 5 ml of a warm aqueous solution of Calcium Gluconate (1 in 10) 0.7 ml of glacial acetic acid and 1 ml of freshly distilled phenylhydrazine are added, and the mixture is heated on a water bath for 30 minutes. After allowing it to cool, the inner surface of the tube is scratched with a glass stirring rod. Crystals of gluconic acid phenylhydrazide form.

Incompatibilities—The incompatibilities of the soluble calcium salts are discussed under *Calcium Chloride* (this page). Calcium Gluconate is precipitated from its aqueous solution by the addition of *alcohol*. Due to its limited solubility, this salt must frequently be suspended in liquid mixtures and tragacanth is useful as a suspending agent.

Uses—Calcium Gluconate is an *electrolyte replenisher*. It is used as a source of calcium ion in the treatment of *low-calcium tetany*. It is less irritating than calcium chloride and may be given orally or by intramuscular or intravenous injection.

Dose—*Oral* or *intravenous*, 1 to 15 Gm daily; *usual, oral*, 1 Gm 3 or more times a day; *usual, intravenous*, 1 Gm 1 or more times a day.

Other Dose Information—For injection purposes a 10% solution is employed.

Dosage Forms—Injection USP: 1 Gm/10 ml; Tablets USP: 500 mg and 1 Gm.

Veterinary Uses—This salt is widely used as a source of calcium in the treatment of various acute and chronic hypocalcemic conditions. Calcium gluconate is preferred to lactate or chloride because it is less irritating to the tissues and may be administered intramuscularly and subcutaneously. It is indicated in *milk fever* (parturient paresis) of cattle and hypocalcemic conditions of cows, ewes, does, mares, *parturient eclampsia* of the bitch, and *transport tetany* of cows and ewes, given parenterally. It is also used as a source of calcium given orally when indicated.

Veterinary Dose—*Horses* and *Cattle*, 25 to 100 Gm, intravenously, subcutaneously, or intramuscularly; *Sheep, Goats,* and *Swine*, 4 to 5 Gm, intramuscularly or intravenously; *Dogs*, 1 to 2 Gm, intramuscularly or intravenously. The same or larger doses are used for oral administration.

Calcium Lactate NF

Calcium Lactate [$C_6H_{10}CaO_6 \cdot xH_2O$] contain 98.0–101.0% of [$CH_3CH(OH)COO]_2Ca$ (218.22), calculated on the dried basis.

Preparation—Calcium Lactate is made by fermenting hydrolyzed starch with a suitable mold in the presence of calcium carbonate, and purifying until the product meets NF purity requirements. It is also obtained, now in decreasing quantities, by fermentation of the mother liquors resulting from the production of milk sugar.

Description—A white, almost odorless powder or granules. It is somewhat efflorescent. Becomes anhydrous at 120°. Aqueous solutions of calcium lactate are prone to become moldy.

Solubility—1 Gm dissolves in about 20 ml of water; practically insoluble in alcohol.

Incompatibilities—Calcium Lactate has the incompatibilities of the soluble calcium salts as described under *Calcium Chloride* (page 915).

Uses—Calcium Lactate is an excellent source of calcium ion in the treatment of *calcium deficiency*. It is given, usually in association with lactose.

Dose—*Usual*, 1 to 5 Gm 3 times a day.

Dosage Forms—Tablets NF: 300 and 600 mg (pentahydrate).

Veterinary Uses—A source of calcium when this element is deficient. It is seldom used intravenously, however, because calcium gluconate is considered to be the drug of choice for parenteral injection. Given *per os*, it is less likely to irritate the gastric mucosa than calcium chloride.

Veterinary Dose—*Horses* and *Cattle*, 50 to 100 Gm; *Sheep* and *Swine*, 4 to 5 Gm; *Dogs*, 1 to 2 Gm.

Dibasic Calcium Phosphate NF

[Dicalcium Orthophosphate; Calphate (*Merrell*); D. C. P. (*Parke, Davis*)]

Dibasic Calcium Phosphate is anhydrous or contains two molecules of water of hydration. After ignition at 800° to 825° to constant weight, it contains an amount of calcium pyrophosphate ($Ca_2P_2O_7$) equivalent to 98.0–100.5% of $CaHPO_4$ (136.06).

Preparation—A phosphate mineral, eg, *apatite*, or preferably ignited animal bone, is decomposed with sulfuric acid, resulting in the production of phosphoric acid and calcium sulfate. After filtering off the calcium sulfate, the proper quantity of calcium hydroxide is added to form dibasic calcium phosphate.

It may also be prepared from animal bones as described under the preparation of *Tribasic Calcium Phosphate*, using only sufficient calcium hydroxide to form the dibasic salt.

Description—A white, odorless, tasteless powder. It is stable in the air and its aqueous suspension is neutral to litmus.

Solubility—Almost insoluble in water; readily soluble in diluted hydrochloric and nitric acids; insoluble in alcohol.

Uses—See *Tribasic Calcium Phosphate*, below. Dibasic Calcium Phosphate is an excellent *source of calcium* and *phosphorus* during pregnancy, lactation, or calcium deficiency diseases in a mild form, eg, *low-calcium tetany*. If the tetany is severe, intravenous cal-

cium medication is administered. See *Calcium Gluconate Injection* (page 838).

Dose—1 to 5 Gm; *usual*, 1 Gm 3 times a day.

Tribasic Calcium Phosphate NF

[Calcium Phosphate; Calcium Orthophosphate; Tricalcic Phosphate; Precipitated Calcium Phosphate]

Tribasic Calcium Phosphate consists of a variable mixture of calcium phosphates having the approximate composition $10CaO \cdot 3P_2O_5 \cdot H_2O$ (1004.64). It contains an amount of phosphate (PO_4) equivalent to not less than 90.0% of tribasic calcium phosphate [$Ca_3(PO_4)_2$ = 310.18], calculated on the ignited basis.

Preparation—This phosphate is usually obtained from animal bones which contain about 80% of Tribasic Calcium Phosphate. The bones are calcined until white, then ground and digested with hydrochloric acid (sulfuric acid is frequently employed instead of hydrochloric). After filtration, the solution is treated either with ammonia or more generally with calcium hydroxide whereby calcium phosphate is precipitated.

It may also be prepared from calcium chloride and sodium phosphate in the presence of ammonia water at boiling temperature.

Tribasic Calcium Phosphate of commerce is a somewhat basic salt, hence the low percentage of $Ca_3(PO_4)_2$ stated in the purity rubric.

Description—A white, odorless, and tasteless powder which is stable in air.

Solubility—Almost insoluble in water; dissolves readily in diluted hydrochloric and nitric acids; insoluble in alcohol.

Uses—This salt is an excellent *source of both calcium and phosphorus* useful in supplementing calcium intake, as, for example, during pregnancy and lactation, or as a source of calcium in diseases of calcium deficiency. The dose is 1 to 2 Gm with meals, taken as a suspension in water or milk, or sprinkled on food. It is ineffective as an *antacid*.

Tribasic Calcium Phosphate is also used to the extent of about 1 per cent in table salt and other products to prevent caking and to render them free-flowing. It functions in this application by converting traces of deliquescent impurities into nonhygroscopic phosphates.

Dose—*Usual*, 1 to 5 Gm 3 times a day.

Veterinary Dose—*Horses*, 30 to 60 Gm; *Dogs*, 2 to 10 Gm.

Potassium Acetate—see page 871.

Potassium Bicarbonate—see page 792.

Potassium Chloride USP

[Kalii Chloridum; Kaochlor (*Warren-Teed*)]

Potassium Chloride contains 99.0–100.5% of KCl (74.56), calculated on the dried basis.

Preparation—This salt occurs in sea water and in many mineral springs. Formerly the salt was largely imported from Germany where it is mined at Stassfurt, occurring there as *carnallite* [$KCl \cdot MgCl_2 \cdot 6H_2O$] and as *sylvite* [KCl]. The demand for Potassium Chloride is now met by the Searles Lake deposit in the Mojäve Desert of southern California and from recently found deposits of carnallite and sylvite in New Mexico and Texas. Another source of Potassium Chloride which has been worked during the past few years is the Dead Sea, where considerable quantities are found as dissolved carnallite. This double salt, in aqueous solution, is treated with live steam, the two separate salts form, and the less soluble salt, potassium chloride, crystallizes out as the solution cools. In the laboratory it may be prepared from potassium carbonate or bicarbonate and hydrochloric acid.

Description—Colorless, elongated, prismatic, or cubical crystals, or as a white granular powder. It is odorless, has a saline taste, and is stable in air. The aqueous solution is neutral to litmus paper (pH about 7).

Solubility—1 Gm dissolves in 2.8 ml of water at 25° and about 2 ml of boiling water; insoluble in alcohol.

Incompatibilities—Chlorides form precipitates by reaction with *lead* and *silver salts*. Strong *oxidizing agents* such as *potassium chlorate* liberate chlorine from hydrochloric acid and acidic solutions of chlorides.

Uses—Potassium Chloride is the salt most frequently employed when the action of the potassium cation is desired. It is used when *hypokalemia* exists, as after prolonged diarrhea or vomiting or consequent to adrenal steroid therapy or treatment with certain diuretics, especially the thiazides. It is also used when it is desired to elevate normal plasma potassium levels, as in the treatment of digitalis intoxication. It may be used as a diuretic. Potassium Chloride is also of value for the relief of the symptoms of *familial periodic paralysis*, a rare disease characterized by recurrent attacks of muscular weakness. Potassium salts have also been found to relieve the symptoms of *Ménière's disease*. Potassium Chloride is an ingredient of *Lactated Potassic Saline Injection, Ringer's Solution, Lactated Ringer's Injection, and Ringer's Injection*.

Potassium Chloride is irritant to the gastrointestinal tract; oral preparations may cause nausea, vomiting, epigastric distress, abdominal discomfort, and diarrhea. Enteric coating lessens the incidence of such side effects but favors the development of small bowel lesions when thiazides are concurrently used. Noncoated tablets are less irritating if taken with a full glass of water.

Overdoses may cause paresthesias, generalized weakness, flaccid paralysis, listlessness, vertigo, mental confusion, hypotension, cardiac arrhythmias, and heart block. Death may ensue. Signs of toxicity may even occur with apparently normal blood levels; consequently, the signs must be frequently monitored, and the ambulatory patient must be apprised of premonitory symptoms. Most patients can be managed adequately and more safely with foods high in potassium and low in sodium (fruits, especially dried, and cereals).

Potassium Chloride must be administered cautiously in the presence of heart disease.

Dose—*Oral*, **1** to **10 Gm** daily; *usual, oral*, **1 Gm** 2 to 6 times a day; *intravenous infusion*, **1** to **3 Gm** daily; *usual, intravenous infusion*, **1000 ml** of a **0.3%** solution over a period of 4 hours.

Other Dose Information—Clinicians think in terms of milliequivalents (mEq) in repairing potassium deficiency. 3 Gm of KCl provides 40 mEq. Potassium chloride for injection is marketed in units of 20 ml containing 40 mEq, the so-called "15%" solution. For infusion, this solution must be diluted to 1000 ml with isotonic saline or dextrose solution.

Dosage Forms—Injection USP: 1.5 Gm/10 ml, 3 Gm/12.5 and 20 ml, 4.5 and 6 Gm/30 ml; Tablets USP: 300 mg and 1 Gm.

Potassium Citrate—see page 872.

Potassium Gluconate NF

[Kaon (*Warren-Teed*)]

$$\underset{\underset{\text{OH}}{|}}{\text{HOCH}_2}\overset{\overset{\text{H}}{|}}{\text{C}}\overset{\overset{\text{H}}{|}}{\underset{\underset{\text{OH}}{|}}{\text{C}}}\overset{\overset{\text{OH}}{|}}{\underset{\underset{\text{H}}{|}}{\text{C}}}\overset{\overset{\text{H}}{|}}{\underset{\underset{\text{OH}}{|}}{\text{C}}}\text{COOK}$$

Potassium Gluconate contains 97.0–103.0% of $C_6H_{11}KO_7$ (234.25), calculated on the dried basis.

Preparation—Glucose may be oxidized to gluconic acid by various processes, eg, electrolytic oxidation of an alkaline solution, reaction with hypobromites, or by fermentation using *Aspergillus niger* or various other microorganisms. Neutralization with potassium hydroxide provides the official salt.

Description—A white to yellowish white, crystalline powder or as granules. It is odorless and has a slightly bitter taste. It is stable in air, and its solutions are slightly alkaline to litmus.

Solubility—Freely soluble in water; practically insoluble in dehydrated alcohol, ether, benzene, and chloroform.

Uses—Potassium Gluconate is used as a source of potassium for the management of hypokalemic states, such as occur consequent to adrenocorticosteroid therapy or the use of thiazide diuretics, or for the deliberate production of hyperkalemia, as for the treatment of digitalis intoxication. The gluconate anion supposedly makes the compound better tolerated in the gastrointestinal tract than is potassium chloride. It is also claimed that the potassium of the gluconate is absorbed high in the gastrointestinal tract, above the location where mucosal lesions sometimes occur in combined thiazide–potassium therapy, whereas other salts are not so quickly absorbed. Such faulty suppositions and claims ignore the unavoidable chemical fact that irrespective of the salt used, potassium is completely dissociable and hence is unaffected in its irritant actions and absorption by the anion in the compound. Sugar-coated Potassium Gluconate tablets dissolve at a higher level than do enteric-coated tablets of potassium chloride but, by this very fact, are free to cause the irritation for which the chloride tablet was coated. The fact that Potassium Gluconate may cause nausea, vomiting, diarrhea, and abdominal discomfort shows that the gluconate has no advantage over non-enteric-coated potassium chloride tablets. A full glass of water taken with either greatly reduces the irritant effects of either salt. Hypochloremia is a frequent accompaniment of hypokalemia; in such instances the chloride is definitely preferred. Furthermore, since gluconate metabolizes to bicarbonate, it contributes to alkalosis, which may also be present in hypokalemia. Thus it is difficult to find situations in which the gluconate would be superior.

The use and toxicity of and contraindications to Potassium Gluconate are the same as those for *Potassium Chloride* (this page).

Dose—*Usual*, the equivalent of 10 mEq of potassium 4 times daily.

Dosage Forms—Elixir NF: 4.68 Gm/15 ml, equivalent to 20 mEq (782 mg) of K; Tablets NF: 1.17 Gm, equivalent to 5 mEq (195.5 mg) of K.

Lactated Potassic Saline Injection NF

[Darrow's Solution]

Lactated Potassic Saline Injection is a sterile solution of KCl (potassium chloride), NaCl (sodium chloride), and $C_3H_5NaO_3$ (sodium lactate) in water for injection. It contains, in each 100 ml, 126–147 mg of potassium (K, equivalent to 240–280 mg of KCl), 262–294 mg of sodium (Na, equivalent to 380–420 mg of NaCl, and 550–630 mg of $C_3H_5NaO_3$), 344–388 mg of chloride ion (Cl, as KCl and NaCl), and 437–501 mg of lactate ion ($C_3H_5O_3$, as $C_3H_5NaO_3$). It contains no bacteriostatic agents.

Note—The potassium and sodium contents of Lactated Potassic Saline Injection are approximately 3.5 and 12 milliequivalents per 100 ml, respectively.

Uses—Lactated Potassic Saline Injection is employed parenterally to correct *potassium deficiencies*, especially those arising in conjunction with *dehydration* and *acidosis*. Severe diarrheas, such as infantile diarrhea, cause loss of both potassium and bicarbonate, and such disorders are the principal indication for Darrow's solution. Diabetic acidosis is also sometimes treated with the solution. It should not be employed routinely for the treatment of electrolyte disturbances that can be corrected by other repair solutions. It is particularly contraindicated in alkalosis. The potassium chloride in the solution serves to replenish potassium. The sodium lactate is metabolized to sodium bicarbonate, and thus tends to correct acidosis and to prevent further electrolyte distortions caused by the chloride in the solution. Cardiac changes from potassium overdosage can result; slow administration, electrocardiograms and blood potassium determinations should be made. (For details of the toxicity, see *Potassium Chloride*, page 840.)

Hypodermoclysis is the preferred route of administration, although intravenous infusion may be employed in emergencies.

Dose—*Usual, intravenous* and *subcutaneous*, **40 to 80 ml** per **Kg** of body weight per day, given slowly over a period of 4 to 12 hours.

Other Dose Information—The total daily dose is usually given at intervals throughout a period of 8 to 12 hours at such a rate that the total time of actual administration is greater than 4 hours. For infants, it should be diluted with two parts of 5% dextrose solution.

Dosage Forms—Injection NF: 150, 250, 500, and 1000 ml.

Ringer's Injection USP

[Ringer's Solution No. 3 USP XIV; Isotonic Solution of Three Chlorides]

Ringer's Injection is a sterile solution of sodium chloride, potassium chloride, and calcium chloride in water for injection. It contains, in each 100 ml, 820–900 mg of sodium chloride (NaCl), 25–35 mg of potassium chloride (KCl), and 30–36 mg of calcium chloride ($CaCl_2.$-$2H_2O$). Ringer's Injection contains no antimicrobial agents.

Sodium Chloride............	8.6 Gm
Potassium Chloride..........	0.3 Gm
Calcium Chloride...........	0.33 Gm
Water for Injection, a sufficient quantity,	
To make.....................	1000 ml

Dissolve the three salts in the water for injection, filter until clear, place in suitable containers, and sterilize.

Description—A colorless, odorless solution having a salty taste. The pH is between 5.0 and 7.5.

Uses—Ringer's Injection is theoretically superior to Sodium Chloride Injection as a *fluid and electrolyte replenisher* in that it supplies the three important cations of the extracellular fluid. However, in actual practice, the addition of potassium and calcium increases only slightly the therapeutic value of an isotonic sodium chloride solution. Neither potassium nor calcium is present in sufficient concentration to render Ringer's Injection useful for the repair of deficits of these ions. Further, while administration of large volumes of Ringer's Injection would result in minimal distortion of the cation composition of the extracellular fluid, like *Sodium Chloride Injection*, it would alter acid–base balance. Ringer's Injection is frequently used to prime pumps for cardiopulmonary bypass in heart surgery.

Dose—*Usual, intravenous infusion*, **1000 ml.**

Other Dose Information—The usual intravenous range is 500 to 1000 ml and the usual intravenous dose is 500 ml.

Dosage Forms—Injection USP: 500 and 1000 ml.

Lactated Ringer's Injection USP

[Lactated Ringer's Solution USP XIV; Hartmann's Solution]

Lactated Ringer's Injection is a sterile solution of calcium chloride, potassium chloride, sodium chloride, and sodium lactate in water for injection. It contains, in each 100 ml, 18–22 mg of calcium chloride ($CaCl_2.$-$2H_2O$), 27–33 mg of potassium chloride (KCl), 570–630 mg of sodium chloride (NaCl), 290–330 mg of sodium lactate ($C_3H_5NaO_3$). Lactated Ringer's Injection contains no antimicrobial agents.

Sodium Chloride............	8.6 Gm
Potassium Chloride..........	0.3 Gm
Calcium Chloride...........	0.33 Gm
Water for Injection, a sufficient quantity,	
To make.....................	1000 ml

Dissolve the three salts in the water for injection, filter until clear, place in suitable containers, and sterilize.

Note—The calcium, potassium, and sodium contents of Lactated Ringer's Injection are approximately 2.7, 4, and 130 milliequivalents per liter, respectively.

Description—It has a pH between 6.0 and 7.5.

Uses and Dose—See *Ringer's Injection*. Except for the concentration of lactate and absence of bicarbonate, the composition of Lactated Ringer's Injection closely approximates that of the extracellular fluids. It is employed as a *fluid and electrolyte replenisher*. The lactate ultimately metabolizes to bicarbonate and thus has an alkalinizing effect in the body. The absence of bicarbonate from the solution stabilizes the calcium; which sometimes tends to precipitate as calcium carbonate from heated solutions which contain bicarbonate.

Dose—*Usual, intravenous* infusion, **1000 ml.**

Other Dose Information—The usual intravenous range is 500 to 1000 ml and the usual intravenous dose is 500 ml.

Dosage Forms—Injection USP: 150, 250, 500, and 1000 ml.

Locke-Ringer's Solution

Reagent Sodium Chloride......	9	Gm
Reagent Potassium Chloride...	0.42	Gm
Reagent Calcium Chloride......	0.24	Gm
Reagent Magnesium Chloride..	0.2	Gm
Sodium Bicarbonate...........	0.5	Gm
Dextrose....................	.5	Gm
Water recently distilled from a hard glass flask, a sufficient quantity,		
To make....................	1000	ml

The solution must be freshly made each day. The constituents (except the dextrose and the sodium bicarbonate) may be made up in a more concentrated stock solution and diluted as needed.

Uses—Locke-Ringer's Solution is not a therapeutic solution; rather, it is a medium in which test organs are bathed in bioassay procedures.

Ringer's Solution NF

[Ringer's Solution No. 1 USP XIV; Compound Injection of Sodium Chloride]

Ringer's Solution is a solution of NaCl (sodium chloride), KCl (potassium chloride), and CaCl$_2$.2H$_2$O (calcium chloride) in purified water. It contains, in each 100 ml, 323.0–354.0 mg of sodium (Na, equivalent to 820.0–900.0 mg of NaCl); 13.0–18.0 mg of potassium (K, equivalent to 25.0–35.0 mg of KCl); 8.20–9.80 mg of calcium (Ca, equivalent to 30.0–36.0 mg of CaCl$_2$.2H$_2$O); and 523.0–580.0 mg of chloride (Cl, as NaCl, KCl, and CaCl$_2$.2H$_2$O).

Caution—Do not use Ringer's Solution for parenteral administration or in preparations to be used parenterally. For such purposes use Ringer's Injection (page 841).

Sodium Chloride...................	8.6 Gm
Potassium Chloride...............	0.30 Gm
Calcium Chloride................	0.33 Gm
Purified Water, recently boiled, a sufficient quantity,	
To make......................	1000 ml

Dissolve the three salts in a sufficient quantity of recently boiled purified water to make 1000 ml, and filter until clear.

Uses—A *physiological salt solution for topical application.*

Dose—*Topically,* as required.

Sodium Acetate NF

Sodium Acetate [CH$_3$COONa.3H$_2$O = 136.08], dried at 80° overnight and followed by drying at 120° for 4 hours, contains 99.0–101.0% of C$_2$H$_3$NaO$_2$ (82.03).

Preparation—This salt is now largely obtained as a by-product from the manufacture of acetanilid, acetylsalicylic acid, and similar acetylated compounds. It is most easily prepared by neutralizing acetic acid with sodium carbonate and evaporating the solution to crystallization.

Description—Colorless, transparent crystals or granular, crystalline powder. It is odorless or has a faint, acetous odor. It effloresces in warm, dry air. It melts at about 60°.

Solubility—1 Gm is soluble in about 0.8 ml of water and about 19 ml of alcohol.

Identification—It responds to the tests for *Sodium* and for *Acetate,* and it yields an alkaline residue on ignition which effervesces with acids (Na$_2$CO$_3$).

Incompatibilities—see *Potassium Acetate.*

Uses—The acetate ion is rapidly and completely metabolized by the body, and consequently the administration of sodium acetate is an effective method of increasing the body reserve of fixed base. It is metabolized to sodium bicarbonate, so that it is eventually equivalent to giving sodium bicarbonate. Solutions of sodium acetate are stable and readily sterilized, and this salt is popular for the parenteral therapy of *acidotic conditions.* It is both a *systemic* and a *urinary alkalizer.*

Dose—*Usual,* 1.5 Gm.

Sodium Bicarbonate—see page 793.

Sodium Chloride USP

[Natrii Chloridum; Salt; Table Salt; Rock Salt; Sea Salt]

Sodium Chloride contains 99.5–100.5% of NaCl (58.44), calculated on the dried basis. It contains no added substance.

Preparation—Common salt is widely distributed over the world, and may be obtained by mining, as rock salt, by evaporating a purified solution of saline deposits, or by evaporating sea water, and purifying afterward. If perfectly free from contaminating salts, it is not hygroscopic.

Description—Colorless, hexahedral crystals, or a white crystalline powder. It is odorless and has a saline taste. The solution is practically neutral. A 23% solution of sodium chloride in water freezes at −20°.

Solubility—1 Gm dissolves in 2.8 ml of water, about 10 ml of glycerin, and 2.7 ml of boiling water; slightly soluble in alcohol.

Incompatibilities—Precipitates are formed by reaction with *lead,* and *silver salts.* Strong *oxidizing agents* liberate chlorine from acidified solutions of sodium chloride.

Uses—Solutions of Sodium Chloride more closely approximate the composition of the extracellular fluid of the body than solutions of any other single salt. For example, more than 90% of the cation of the extracellular fluid is sodium, more than 60% of the anion is chloride. Furthermore, a 0.9% solution of Sodium Chloride has approximately the same osmotic pressure as body fluids, ie, is isotonic with body fluids. Thus, an isotonic Sodium Chloride solution (injection) can be injected without affecting the osmotic pressure of the body fluids and without causing any appreciable distortion in chemical composition. An isotonic solution of Sodium Chloride is therefore the choice as a vehicle for many drugs which have to be administered parenterally. The solution has the added advantage of being nonirritating to tissue. Isotonic solutions of Sodium Chloride may be applied topically to intact or exposed tissues for purposes of irrigation, to keep tissues moist, or as a vehicle for other agents. Sodium Chloride Solution is also isotonic and sterile but is not pyrogen free and should not be injected parenterally.

Sodium Chloride Injection is also used as an *electrolyte replenisher* for maintenance or replacement of deficits of extracellular fluid. Since the solution is potentially capable of producing metabolic acidosis and does not supply all major cations or the extracellular fluid, other solutions, such as Lactated Ringer's Injection, may be preferred if large volumes of fluids are to be administered. Other solutions of appropriate composition must also be employed if the composition of the extracellular fluid is markedly distorted. Sterile solutions are administered, usually by the intravenous route.

Sodium Chloride is administered orally for the prevention of *heat cramps* (Miner's Cramps, Low Sodium Syndrome) caused by the depletion of sodium salts through copious perspiration. A beverage containing only 0.5% of Sodium Chloride will prevent development of the symptoms. This salt is also given in adrenal cortical insufficiency (*Addison's Disease*) where it decreases the requirement for adrenal cortical extract.

Sodium Chloride is largely used as a condiment. Most commercial varieties of table salt are unfit for use in pharmacy, as they contain foreign substances added to diminish their hygroscopic quality. It is largely used in medicine as Sodium Chloride Injection, commonly known as Isotonic Sodium Chloride Solution. Common salt is used as a preservative; 6% or more prevents the growth of *Cl. botulinum* and other pathogens.

Dose—*Oral,* 3 to 6 Gm daily; *usual, oral,* **1 Gm** 3 times a day; *usual, intravenous infusion,* **1 liter** of a **0.9%** solution; *topically,* as a **0.9%** solution.

Other Dose Information—Intravenous, 500 ml to 5 liters; usual, intravenous, 500 ml of a 0.9% solution; usual, topical, as necessary.

Dosage Forms—Injection USP: 100, 150, 250, 500, and 1000 ml; Bacteriostatic Injection USP: 2, 5, 10, 20, and 30 ml; Solution USP (see below); Tablets USP: 600 mg, and 1 and 2.25 Gm; Sodium Chloride and Dextrose Tablets NF: 200 mg (sodium chloride) and 450 mg (dextrose).

Veterinary Dose—*Horses,* 25 to 50 Gm; *Cattle,* 50 to 100 Gm; *Sheep* and *Swine,* 2 to 5 Gm; *Dogs,* **200 mg** to **1 Gm.**

Sodium Chloride Solution USP is a solution of sodium chloride in purified water. It contains 0.85–0.95% of NaCl. Caution: *Do not use Sodium Chloride Solution for parenteral administration or for irrigations that may result in absorption of the Solution into the blood. For such purposes use Sodium Chloride Injection. Preparation:* Dissolve sodium chloride (9 Gm) in purified water (qs) to make 1000 ml. Filter the prepared solution until clear. *Description:* A clear, colorless solution.

Sodium Lactate Injection USP

Sodium Lactate Injection is a sterile solution of lactic acid ($C_3H_6O_3$) in water for injection prepared with the aid of sodium hydroxide. It contains 95.0–110.0% of the labeled amount of $C_3H_5NaO_3$ (112.06).

Note—Sterilize Sodium Lactate Injection preferably by steam under pressure. See Chapter 81, *Sterilization* (page 1501).

Preparation—A weighed quantity of lactic acid assayed by the USP method, sufficient to yield the desired amount of sodium lactate, is diluted with several times its weight of water for injection. A volume of an assayed concentrated sodium hydroxide solution, equivalent to the quantity of lactic acid as calculated from the assay, is then added and the mixture gently boiled until all the lactic anhydride also has been converted into sodium lactate. After quickly cooling, the solution is diluted with water for injection to the proper volume, promptly filtered if necessary, ampuled, and sterilized. One part of absolute lactic acid yields 1.24 parts of sodium lactate.

Description—Its pH, diluted, if necessary, to about ⅕ molar (25 mg per ml), is between 6.0 and 7.3.

Uses—Sodium Lactate, like sodium acetate, may be employed as a substitute for sodium bicarbonate in solutions for *parenteral fluid* and *electrolyte therapy.* Since the lactate ion is rapidly metabolized in the body, Sodium Lactate is a potential source of fixed cation for correction of meta bolic *acidosis.* Sodium Lactate is preferred to sodium bicarbonate because its solutions may be sterilized by boiling. Sodium Lactate is also used to accelerate the heart in hypopotassemia.

Dose—*Usual, intravenous,* **1 liter** of a ⅙ *M* solution.

Other Dose Information—For antagonizing the cardiac effects of hypopotassemia, 100 ml of a 1 molar solution are given in 2–5 minutes, after which infusion is continued at a rate of 30 to 60 drops per minute until the desired effect is achieved.

Dosage Forms—Injection USP: ⅙ *M* solution in 150-, 250-, 500-, and 1000-ml containers.

Cation Complexing Agents

The monovalent cations do not form strong complexes with sequestering agents; thus, hyperkalemia and hypernatremia cannot be treated by simple chemical means. However, the divalent and polyvalent cations do form complexes easily and can be removed from the plasma; thus, hypercalcemia is a frequent target for complexing agents. It is generally difficult to complex magnesium in the presence of calcium; however, disorders of magnesium metabolism are rare. The complexing agents may also be employed for removing certain foreign toxic cations from the body.

N-Acetylpenicillamine—see page 1256.

Dimercaprol—see page 1225.

Penicillamine—see page 1256.

Disodium Edetate USP

[Disodium Ethylenediaminetetraacetate; Disodium(Ethylenedinitrilo)tetraacetate]

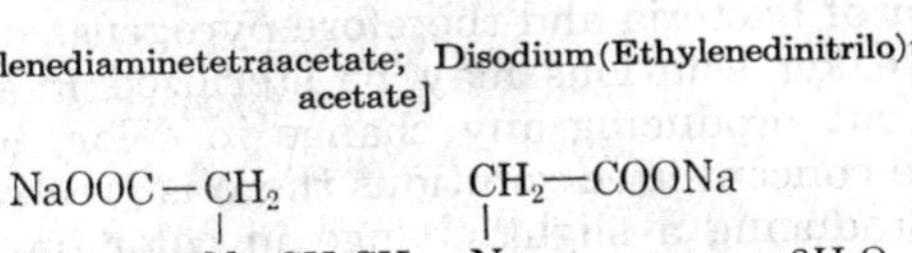

$$
\begin{array}{ccc}
NaOOC-CH_2 & & CH_2-COONa \\
| & & | \\
& N-CH_2CH_2-N & \cdot 2H_2O \\
| & & | \\
HOOC-CH_2 & & CH_2-COOH
\end{array}
$$

Disodium Edetate contains 99.0–100.5% of $C_{10}H_{14}N_2Na_2O_8 \cdot 2H_2O$ (372.24).

Preparation—(Ethylenedinitrilo)tetraacetic acid is dissolved in a hot solution containing two equivalents of sodium hydroxide and the disodium salt is allowed to crystallize. The starting acid is prepared by condensing ethylenediamine with sodium monochloroacetate with the aid of sodium carbonate. An aqueous solution of the reactants is heated to about 90°C for 10 hours, then cooled and acidified with HCl whereupon the acid precipitates. US Pat. 2,130,505.

Description—White, crystalline powder.
Solubility—Freely soluble in water.

Uses—Disodium Edetate readily chelates calcium, so that it may be employed to remove free calcium ions from solution. Thus it may be employed as an *anticoagulant* in the same manner as sodium citrate. Intravenously, it temporarily *lowers plasma calcium* concentration, but the effect is too brief to be of value. Constant infusion can yield a more sustained effect. It is employed occasionally to *terminate* abruptly *the effects of injected calcium* in the digitalis tolerance and other tests. Disodium Edetate can also dissolve precipitated calcium salts. It has been given by retrograde injection to dissolve *urinary calculi;* irritation of the mucous membrane results. Intravenous Disodium Edetate sometimes has a nephrotoxic action.

Dose—*Usual, intravenous infusion,* **50 mg** per **Kg** of body weight in 3 to 4 hours, once a day.

Other Dose Information—The dose depends upon the use and the amount of calcium to be sequestered; 1 Gm chelates 0.12 Gm of calcium. The drug is usually employed as a 3% solution in isotonic saline or glucose. It is given by slow intravenous drip.

Dosage Forms—Injection USP: 3 Gm/20 ml.

Sodium Polystyrene Sulfonate USP

[Kayexalate (*Winthrop*)]

Sodium Polystyrene Sulfonate is a cation-exchange resin prepared in the sodium form. Each Gm exchanges 110–135 mg of potassium, calculated on the anhydrous basis.

Description—A golden brown, fine powder that is odorless and tasteless.

Solubility—Insoluble in water.

Uses—Sodium Polystyrene Sulfonate is an ion-exchange resin used for the treatment of hyperkalemia resulting from acute renal failure. The resin is given orally by a stomach tube or as a high retention enema. The sodium moiety of the resin is in part replaced by potassium which is subsequently eliminated from the body when the resin is excreted in the feces or in the enema. The potassium-removing capacity of the resin is approximately ⅓ of that possible when measured under conditions in which potassium is the only cation present. The resin should be an adjunct to other therapeutic measures, such as restriction of electrolyte intake, control of acidosis, and high caloric diet. Untoward effects include anorexia, nausea, vomiting, and constipation. Constipation and fecal impaction can be minimized by the administration of 70% sorbitol solution every 2 hours as needed to produce watery stools. Serum potassium levels should be determined daily in order to avoid hypokalemia. The drug should be used with caution in patients with actual or impending cardiac failure; the release of sodium in the intestine may be hazardous in such patients and the drug may also exaggerate the effect of digitalis.

Dose—15 Gm 1 to 4 times a day.

Other Dose Information—Each dose should be suspended in a small quantity of water or syrup. By enema, 30 Gm in 150 to 200 ml of water as retention enema once or twice daily.

Dosage Forms—454 Gm.

Other Cation Complexing Agents

Deferoxamine Mesylate [Desferrioxamine; $C_{25}H_{48}$-$N_6O_8.CH_4SO_3$; Desferal Mesylate (*Ciba*)] is *N*-{5-[3-[(5-Aminopentyl)hydroxycarbamoyl]propionamido]pentyl] - 3-[[5 - (*N* - hydroxyacetamido)pentyl]carbamoyl]propionohydroxamic Acid Methanesulfonate (656.81). *Preparation:* Deferoxamine may be isolated from cultures of *Streptomyces pilosus* by the method of Bickel, *et al*,[5] or it may be synthesized by the method of Prelog and Walser.[6] *Description and Solubility:* White crystals; reconstituted solutions of the drug are stable for 2 weeks at room temperature. Freely soluble in water. *Uses:* Deferoxamine Mesylate is a chelating agent that is specific for iron. It is used for the *treatment of iron intoxication* or *iron storage disease*. Stoichiometrically, 100 mg of Deferoxamine sequesters 8.5 mg of ferric iron. Although it does not appreciably bind ferrous ion, it has nevertheless proven useful in the treatment of intoxication by ferrous as well as by ferric salts, probably partly because some of the toxicity of ferrous salts is due to ferric ion resulting from oxidation of the divalent ion and partly because complexation of the ferric ion favors further oxidation of ferrous ion and so promotes a diminution in the content of the divalent form. The iron chelate (ferrioxamine) is excreted by the kidney and imparts a reddish color to the urine; in severe renal disease the drug is contraindicated. The drug is not absorbed orally and must be given parenterally. Pain and induration may occur at the site of an intramuscular injection. Other untoward effects include diarrhea, blurring of vision, abdominal discomfort, muscular spasms in the legs, itching, tachycardia, and fever. In long-term therapy, various allergic reactions, including anaphylaxis, have been reported.

Dose: Intramuscular, 1 Gm initially, 500 mg twice at 4-hour intervals, then 500 mg every 4 to 12 hours, not to exceed 6 Gm per day; *intravenous*, 1 Gm initially, to be given at a rate no more than 15 mg per Kg of body weight per hour, then 500 mg at two successive 4-hour intervals and 500 mg every 4 to 12 hours, thereafter, not to exceed 6 Gm per day.

Miscellaneous Parenteral Fluids and Systemic Buffers

Various non-electrolytes have a considerable effect on the volume and composition of the extracellular fluid (which includes plasma). Some of these, such as dextrose, may be used for several different purposes and hence appear arbitrarily in this chapter. Some organic compounds affect the acid–base status of the extracellular fluid, even though they are not classical inorganic fixed acids or bases. Tromethamine is an example.

Dextrose Injection USP

[Injection of Glucose]

Dextrose Injection is a sterile solution of dextrose in water for injection. It contains 95.0–105.0% of the labeled amount of $C_6H_{12}O_6.H_2O$. Dextrose Injection contains no antimicrobial agents.

Preparation—Dextrose Injection undoubtedly represents one of the most extensively used injections, especially in hospital practice. The strength of the solution may vary from 5%, which is generally considered satisfactory as an isotonic solution, to 10, 20, 25, and 50%. Usually the 5% solution is used in hospitals.

Quantities which are administered may vary from 100 ml to 1000 ml or more. With such large amounts being administered, a hospital will require considerable quantities of this solution daily, and many short-cuts have been developed for its manufacture. It is general practice to prepare concentrated solutions and then to dilute these with water for injection, thus saving an immense amount of labor and time, particularly in the filtration operation.

Care should be exercised in the selection of dextrose, since the sugar itself may be a source of pyrogens, and extreme care must be observed throughout the preparation of the dextrose injections to prevent contamination, for the conditions are practically ideal for the development of bacteria and therefore pyrogens.

Weaker solutions may be sterilized in an autoclave without producing any change in color, but with the more concentrated solutions there is greater possibility of producing a slight change in color on sterilization with high temperatures. Consequently, sterilization by filtration is often resorted to in these cases.

The pH of dextrose solutions is lowered upon heating and in the past buffers were frequently used in an attempt to maintain stability. At present, however, buffers are seldom added directly to the solution during its preparation since this was often the cause of discoloration and the buffer capacity was frequently overwhelmed after the solution had stood for a period of time. Where buffers are desired, they should be dispensed separately so that the physician may add the buffer extemporaneously when the preparation is to be administered. Dextrose solutions should be tested for mold.

Note—Bacteriostatic agents are prohibited since such large quantities of dextrose are administered at one time that excessive doses of the bacteriostatic agent would thus be given.

Description—A clear, colorless solution having a pH between 3.5 and 6.5.

Uses—Dextrose provides a readily metabolized nutrient. It is a carbohydrate which can be given parenterally. During periods of inanition, intravenous injection of isotonic solutions of dextrose *provides both fluid and carbohydrate.* Body protein is spared and starvation ketosis and acidosis are prevented. Dextrose injection is also employed for parenteral fluid therapy when it is desired to supply water unaccompanied by electrolyte. The injection also provides a suitable vehicle for the slow intravenous infusion of numerous drugs.

Dextrose is usually administered intravenously as a 5.5% solution which is isosmotic with body fluids. Subcutaneous injection of dextrose solution is less desirable since such solutions are irritating. In addition, such solutions cause temporary sequestration of extracellular electrolyte in the subcutaneous depot. If the subcutaneous route is to be employed, *Dextrose* and *Sodium Chloride Injection* should be used.

When administered intravenously, hypertonic solutions of dextrose cause cellular dehydration which may be of benefit in the treatment of *cerebral edema, shock,* and *circulatory collapse.* Hypertonic solutions of dextrose are also administered intravenously to initiate *osmotic diuresis.* Dextrose in the glomerular filtrate in excess of that which can be reabsorbed by the renal tubule causes excretion of an osmotic equivalent of water. Additional quantities of extracellular electrolyte also escape renal tubular reabsorption during the osmotic diuresis.

Dose—*Usual, intravenous,* **1 liter.**

Other Dose Information—The usual diuretic dose is 50 ml of a 50% solution.

Dosage Forms—Injection USP: 2.5, 5, 10, 20, 25, and 50% in various sizes. See USP.

Veterinary Dose—Varies with concentration of solution and its therapeutic purpose. *Usual, intravenous* (50% solution), *Horses* and *Cattle,* **100 to 500 ml;** *Sheep* and *Swine,* **50 to 100 ml;** *Dogs,* **10 to 50 ml;** *Pigs,* showing hypoglycemia, *subcutaneous* or *intraperitoneal,* **4 to 8 ml.**

Dextrose and Sodium Chloride Injection USP

[Sodium Chloride and Dextrose Injection]

Dextrose and Sodium Chloride Injection is a sterile solution of dextrose and sodium chloride in water for injection. It contains 95.0–105.0% of the labeled amount of $C_6H_{12}O_6 \cdot H_2O$ and of NaCl. It contains no antimicrobial agents.

Preparation—This preparation may represent a highly concentrated solution for use as a sclerosing agent, or may represent much weaker solutions to be used in a manner similar to the use of 5 or 10% dextrose solution. This may be a mixture of equal parts of isotonic sodium chloride solution and isotonic dextrose solution, or it may represent 5% of dextrose in isotonic sodium chloride solution. Both of these should be prepared according to the suggestions given for the preparation of *Dextrose Injection.*

Description—A clear, colorless solution having a pH between 3.5 and 6.0.

Uses—Dextrose and Sodium Chloride Injection may be employed to provide dextrose as a nutrient (see above) in a medium that does not hydrate the tissues, or it may be employed as a source of isotonic sodium chloride, or both. Since dextrose, alone, cannot safely be given by the subcutaneous route (see *Dextrose Injection,* above), Dextrose and Sodium Chloride Injection is the preferred preparation.

Dose—*Usual, intravenous* **1 liter.**

Dosage Forms—Various percentages of each ingredient, in various sizes. See USP.

Fructose Injection—see page 1046.

Fructose and Sodium Chloride Injection—see page 1046.

Protein Hydrolysate Injection—see page 1044.

Tromethamine NF

[2-Amino-2-(hydroxymethyl)-1,3-propanediol; Tham-E (*Abbott*)]

$$\begin{array}{c} CH_2OH \\ | \\ HOCH_2CCH_2OH \\ | \\ NH_2 \end{array}$$

Tromethamine contains 99.0–101.0% of $C_4H_{11}NO_3$ (121.14), calculated on the dried basis.

Preparation—Nitromethane is caused to additively react with formaldehyde to yield tris(hydroxymethyl)nitromethane, and the nitro compound is then hydrogenated with the aid of Raney nickel. US Pat. 2,174,242.

Description—A white, crystalline powder with a slight, characteristic odor and a faint, sweet, soapy taste. It is stable in light and air. It melts between 168° and 172°.

Solubility—Freely soluble in water and the lower aliphatic alcohols; practically insoluble in chloroform, benzene, and carbon tetrachloride.

Uses—Tromethamine is a weak amine base with a pK_b of 7.8 at body temperature. This is close to the plasma pH (7.4), so that the compound is well suited to the preparation of a buffer mixture for controlling the extracellular pH. Furthermore, at pH 7.4 it is 30% unionized and hence easily penetrates cells, where it may also buffer the intracellular contents. Tromethamine can react with any proton donor, and the notion that it reacts primarily with carbonic acid or carbon dioxide is erroneous. By removing protons from hydronium ions, the ionization of carbonic acid is shifted so as to decrease pCO_2 and to increase bicarbonate. The excess bicarbonate is then gradually excreted in the kidney. This is an especially useful way to manage excessively high pCO_2 in *respiratory acidosis* (respiratory distress syndrome, asphyxia neonatorum, status asthmaticus, chronic respiratory insufficiency, drug intoxication, etc), in which pulmonary ventilation is inadequate. However, Tromethamine is equally useful in the management of *metabolic acidosis* (drug intoxications, cardiac surgery, diabetic acidosis, etc), especially when the intracellular pH is low, since it readily penetrates cells. Ionized Tromethamine is excreted by the kidney, so that the effect is that of excretion of hydrogen ions. The elimination of the drug from the body is entirely by renal excretion. The excretion of Tromethamonium ion is accompanied by osmotic diuresis, since the clinical doses of the drug considerably add to the osmolarity of the glomerular filtrate. Tromethamine is also used to buffer blood for transfusions.

The principal untoward effects are related to its buffering action, namely that overdoses may cause alkalosis. Also, it is locally irritant because of its alkalinity, and a slough may develop at a site of extravasation, and venospasm and thrombosis may also occur. The fact that about 70% remains in extracellular space means that a sufficient amount of water must be given to prevent hyperosmolarity and hence to avoid tissue dehydration and the hemodynamic consequences of an increased blood volume. Plasma hyperosmolarity, in general, causes hepatic and renal damage, and Tromethamine is no exception. The hemorrhagic liver necrosis seen frequently in newborn infants treated with the drug may possibly have another origin, perhaps related to the route of administration (umbilical vein). The drug also causes hyperkalemia, hypoglycemia, and may depress the respiratory center.

Dose—*Usual, intravenous,* **300 mg** per **Kg** of body weight as a single dose with the average total dose being about **25 Gm** given over a period of not less than 1 hour. Doses of up to 500 mg per Kg may be required depending upon the severity and progression of the acidosis.

Other Dose Information—Tromethamine may be given orally, but it must first be neutralized with citric or lactic acid to lessen the irritant effects; the acids are metabolized and have no lasting effect on the buffering properties of Tromethamine.

Dosage Forms—for Injection: 36 Gm (tromethamine), 370 mg (potassium chloride), and 1.75 Gm (sodium chloride).

Miscellaneous Drugs That Affect Blood

Methylene Blue USP

[3,7-Bis(dimethylamino)phenazathionium Chloride; Cœruleum Methylenum; Methylthionine Chloride; Aniline Violet]

$$\left[(CH_3)_2N-\underset{S}{\overset{N}{\bigcirc}}-N(CH_3)_2\right] Cl^- \cdot 3H_2O$$

Methylene Blue [$C_{16}H_{18}ClN_3S.3H_2O = 373.90$] contains 98.0–103.0% of ($C_{16}H_{18}ClN_3S$) (319.86), calculated on the dried basis.

Preparation—This thiazine dye is made by treating a hydrochloric acid solution of *N,N*-dimethyl-*p*-phenylenediamine with hydrogen sulfide, and ferric chloride as the oxidizing agent.

Description—Dark green crystals or a crystalline powder, having a bronze-like luster; odorless or having a slight odor. It is stable in air. Solutions of Methylene Blue have a deep blue color.

Solubility—1 Gm dissolves in about 25 ml of water and about 65 ml of alcohol; soluble in chloroform.

Incompatibilities—Methylene Blue is easily salted out of solution and is therefore unsuitable for coloring solutions of *salts*. *Mercuric chloride, potassium iodide, potassium permanganate,* and *potassium dichromate* cause a precipitation. Strong solutions of *potassium* or *sodium hydroxide* behave similarly. *Reducing agents* destroy the color.

Uses—Methylene Blue is readily reduced to leukomethylene blue, which, in turn, is readily re-oxidized to Methylene Blue. Thus, it is useful as a reversible *oxidation–reduction* indicator. Its principal therapeutic use stems from this use; namely, that it is employed in the *treatment of methemoglobinemia*. Methylene Blue acts as an electron-acceptor in the transfer of electrons from reduced pyridine nucleotides (NADPH and NATPH) to methemoglobin, thus facilitating the reduction of ferric to ferrous iron. However, if the dose of Methylene Blue is high, the oxidation potential favors the formation of methemoglobin from hemoglobin. This effect is used in the *treatment of cyanide poisoning*. The methemoglobin so formed complexes cyanide, which tends to spare the cytochrome system. However, other drugs are superior.

Methylene Blue was formerly employed as a urinary *antibacterial* agent, but this use is now obsolete. Likewise, its use as an *analgetic, antipyretic,* and *parasiticide* has been abandoned. This dye is also used as a *bacteriological stain*.

Dose—*Usual, intravenous,* **50 ml** of a **1%** solution.

Other Dose Information—The usual oral dose in chronic cases of idiopathic methemoglobinemia is 300 mg daily. In acute drug-induced methemoglobinemia the intravenous dose is 1 to 2 mg per Kg. The official dose is much too high for this use, but may be used in cyanide poisoning.

Dosage Forms—Injection USP: 1, 10, and 50 ml.

Veterinary Use—Formerly employed in the treatment of infectious diseases and as a urinary and/or mammary disinfectant. Antidote in cyanide and nitrate poisoning.

Veterinary dose—*Intravenous,* in **1%** solution. *Horses* and *Cattle,* **2 Gm**; *Swine,* **100 to 500 mg.**

Sodium Nitrite USP

[Natrii Nitris]

Sodium Nitrite contains 97.0–101.0% of $NaNO_2$ (69.00), calculated on the dried basis.

Preparation—Sodium Nitrite is made by heating sodium nitrate until it fuses, then adding sufficient metallic lead to completely reduce the nitrate to nitrite. The heating is continued until the reaction is complete. The mixture is lixiviated with water, filtered, partially evaporated, and allowed to crystallize.

Description—A white to slightly yellow, granular powder, or white or nearly white, opaque, fused masses or sticks. It has a mild, saline taste and is deliquescent in air. Its solution is alkaline to litmus.

Solubility—One Gm dissolves in 1.5 ml of water. It is sparingly soluble in alcohol.

Incompatibilities—Nitrites react with most *acids* to produce nitrous acid which is capable of acting either as an oxidizing or as a reducing agent. It liberates iodine from *iodides* and bromine from *ammonium bromide;* other bromides are not readily affected. *Hypophosphites* are oxidized to phosphates and *sulfites* to sulfates. *Potassium chlorate, potassium permanganate* and some *metallic salts* are reduced. *Tannic acid* or preparations containing this substance decompose it with the liberation of gaseous oxides of nitrogen. A number of organic compounds produce colored derivatives; thus, *acetanilid or acetophenetidin* gives a yellow color, *antipyrine* gives a green, *phenol* a yellow which changes to red-brown, *salicylates* a red-brown *thymol* a green or a brown, and *morphine* a yellow.

Nitrous acid is an unstable substance and continually undergoes decomposition resulting in the liberation of gaseous oxides of nitrogen. Hence, nitrites cannot be dispensed in acidic vehicles.

Sodium Nitrite reacts with acid substances such as *citrated caffeine* and *acetylsalicylic acid* in capsules and powder mixtures, particularly in the presence of (atmospheric) moisture or water of crystallization. It may also cause trouble due to its hygroscopicity. Sticky masses are usually produced, accompanied by the evolution of gases.

Uses—Sodium Nitrite causes relaxation of smooth muscles, especially those of small blood vessels. However, it is no longer used for these actions. Its major use is for the treatment of *cyanide poisoning*. Use is made of the fact that the nitrite ion causes methemoglobinemia. In cyanide poisoning, Sodium Nitrite is injected intravenously in very large doses to produce methemoglobin which combines with the highly lethal cyanide ion and renders it temporarily inactive in the form of cyanmethemoglobin. *Sodium Thiosulfate* (page 1260) is then injected intravenously to form the nontoxic thiocyanate. Solutions of Sodium Nitrite are unstable and should be prepared directly before use.

Dose—*Usual, intravenous,* **10** to **15 ml** of a **3%** solution.

Veterinary Dose—*Horses* and *Cattle, intravenous* or, if necessary, *intraperitoneal,* **5** to **10 Gm** (in 10 to 20% solution; maximum volume, 50 ml); may be repeated after 10 minutes.

References

1. Cohn, E. J. *et al*, *J. Am. Chem. Soc.*, **72**, 465 (1950).
2. Wagner, R. H., *et al*, *Thromb. Diath. Haemorrh.*, **11**, 64 (1964).
3. Wolfrom, M. L., and Rice, F. A. H., *J. Am. Chem. Soc.*, **68**, 532 (1946).
4. Wolfrom, M. L., *et al*, *J. Am. Chem. Soc.*, **72**, 5796 (1950).
5. Bickel, H., *et al*, *Helv. Chim. Acta*, **43**, 2118 (1960).
6. Prelog, V., and Walser, A., *Helv. Chim. Acta*, **45**, 631 (1962).

46 | Cardiovascular Drugs

Hypotensive (antihypertensive) drugs—peripheral vasodilators—
coronary drugs—digitaloid drugs—antiarrhythmic drugs—drugs
affecting blood lipids—miscellaneous cardiovascular drugs

This chapter was prepared by

Ewart A. Swinyard, PhD, *Professor of Pharmacology, College of Pharmacy and
College of Medicine, University of Utah, Salt Lake City, Utah 84112, and*
Stewart C. Harvey, PhD, *Associate Professor of Pharmacology, College of
Medicine, University of Utah, Salt Lake City, Utah 84112*

Any drug that affects the heart or blood vessels, directly or indirectly, is a cardiovascular drug, although the term generally connotes only those drugs which are used for their cardiovascular actions. A large number of such drugs exists. Nearly every autonomic drug has clinically applicable cardiovascular actions. *Sympathomimetics* (see Chapter 48, page 880) may be used to elevate blood pressure, stimulate the heart, slow the heart reflexly, etc, depending on the particular agents and the clinical conditions. *Adrenergic blocking drugs* (see Chapter 50, page 908) may be used in vasospastic conditions, in the diagnosis and management of pheochromocytoma, and rarely in malignant and toxemic hypertensive crises. *Cholinergic Drugs* (see Chapter 49, page 899) may be used as vasodilators, and under unusual conditions as cardio-decelerators in atrial

tachycardia, although their usual action is to speed the heart reflexly. Atropine and other *cholinergic blocking agents* (see Chapter 51, page 914) may be used to block the cardiac vagus nerve in Adams-Stokes syndrome and certain other bradycardias. The *ganglionic blocking agents* are treated in this chapter. Most of the *antihypertensive agents* can be considered autonomic drugs. A large number of drugs other than the autonomic agents have useful cardiovascular actions. *Digitalis* and its allies, the coronary and peripheral dilators, and the *antiarrhythmic agents* are included below. *Parenteral fluids* (see Chapter 45, page 815), which may be used in the treatment of shock, *diuretics* (see Chapter 53, page 936), which are adjuvants in the treatment of heart failure and hypertension, are discussed elsewhere, as are numerous miscellaneous drugs.

Hypotensive (Antihypertensive) Drugs

Hypotensive (antihypertensive) drugs are used mainly in the treatment of hypertension, although certain ones enjoy scattered uses in other therapeutic, diagnostic, and surgical procedures. The predominant types of hypertension are essential and malignant hypertension, the latter generally considered to be a severe, progressive phase of the former. Unfortunately, there is no specific therapy for these diseases, and individual cases vary widely in response to various drugs.

At present, the drug therapy of hypertension is in flux because of the large number of agents introduced since 1958. The finding that the diuretic, chlorothiazide (see page 945), not only is mildly antihypertensive but also greatly potentiates the antihypertensive effects of other drugs initiated a revolution in the medical management of hypertension. Closely following chlorothiazide came guanethidine, syrosingopine (see page 913), and later alphamethyldopa, certain monoamine oxidase inhibitors (see Chapter 62), mebutamate (see the index) and various experimental drugs that necessitated revisions in concepts and approach. At the present time in the United States the tendency is not to treat mild hypertension. The treatment of moderate hypertension is begun with either chlorothiazide of other antihypertensive diuretics or a rauwolfia alkaloid. If neither type of drug is effective alone, then the two are used in combination. More severe hypertension is popularly treated with guanethidine or alphamethyldopa, generally in combination with a diuretic. The ganglionic blocking agents have largely been pushed aside by the newer drugs. Hydralazine

still finds application in combination with other drugs, especially rauwolfia alkaloids, when other drugs do not appear to lower the blood pressure. Diuretics and guanethidine or hydralazine, and to a lesser extent veratrum alkaloids and ganglionic blocking agents, are employed in the treatment of hypertensive crises, such as eclampsia. It is difficult to anticipate how and when the treatment of hypertension will stabilize, but it seems likely that diuretics, rauwolfia alkaloids, guanethidine, and alphamethyldopa, or drugs having similar mechanisms of action, will continue to dominate the field.

Ganglionic Blocking Agents

All of the currently used ganglionic blocking agents are presumed to act by competing with acetylcholine for the cholinergic receptors of the autonomic postganglionic neurones. However, mecamylamine appears to have ganglionic depressant actions in addition to competition with acetylcholine. Like acetylcholine, most of these agents are quaternary ammonium agents, although a few outstanding amines also possess ganglionic blocking properties. Since the ganglia of both the sympathetic and parasympathetic nervous systems are cholinergic, these drugs interrupt the outflow through both systems; thus, it is not possible to achieve a therapeutic block of autonomic outflow to a given locus without a number of undesirable but unavoidable side effects resulting from the blockage of other autonomic nerves.

The ganglionic blocking agents are used mostly for

their interruption of the sympathetic outflow in *hypertension*, *vasospastic disorders*, and *peripheral vascular disease*, thus lowering the blood pressure and increasing the peripheral blood flow. This is not to imply, however, that increased sympathetic activity occurs in all disorders for which these agents are used; rather, a reduction in even normal sympathetic tone is conducive to symptomatic improvement. In *arterial embolism*, *herpes zoster*, *acute thrombophlebitis*, *acrocyanoses*, *trench foot*, *immersion foot*, *reflex dystrophy*, and *Raynaud's disease* sympathetic hyperactivity may occur at some point in the disease; in essential and malignant hypertensions, diabetic gangrene, thromboangiitis obliterans, and arteriosclerosis obliterans there is no evidence of significant sympathetic hyperactivity. The ganglionic blocking agents are also sometimes used for their interruption of parasympathetic nervous outflow, as in *intestinal hypermotility* and *peptic ulcer*, but more specific anticholinergic agents are superior.

Mecamylamine Hydrochloride USP

[*N*,2,2,3-Tetramethyl-2-norbornanamine Hydrochloride; Inversine Hydrochloride (*MSD*)]

Mecamylamine Hydrochloride contains 95.0–100.5% of $C_{11}H_{21}N \cdot HCl$ (203.76), calculated on the dried basis.

Preparation—*dl*-Camphene (I) is treated with an excess of hydrogen cyanide under strongly acidic conditions at about 5°C to yield 2-formamido-2,3,3-trimethylnorcamphane (II). The reaction may be viewed as involving addition of the hydrogen cyanide to the 2,8-double bond of camphene to yield the 2-isocyanate followed by hydration of the isocyano group to form-amido. Reduction of the formyl group in (II) with lithium aluminum hydride yields mecamylamine base which may be converted into the hydrochloride by dissolving it in a suitable organic solvent and introducing a stream of hydrogen chloride.

I   **II**

Description—White, odorless or practically odorless, crystalline powder which melts at about 245° with some decomposition.

Solubility—Freely soluble in water and in chloroform, slightly soluble in benzene, practically insoluble in ether. One Gm dissolves in about 28 ml of isopropyl alcohol.

Uses—Mecamylamine is employed primarily for the treatment of *hypertension*. To a lesser extent it is used in the treatment of *peripheral vascular diseases* in which vasospasm is a component of the disease. It differs from most other ganglionic blocking agents in that it is not a quaternary ammonium compound; it is poorly ionized in the small intestine and thus is readily and completely absorbed. Consequently its actions are more predictable than those of most other ganglionic blocking agents, and it is also more potent by the oral route. Its nonionic form permits it to pass into the central nervous system, so that occasional bizarre cen-

tral disturbances may result. It has a low renal clearance and hence a longer duration of action than most ganglionic agents.

Like the ganglionic blocking agents in general, Mecamylamine may produce a variety of unpleasant unavoidable side effects that result from the interruption of both sympathetic and parasympathetic outflow. Orthostatic hypotension, blurring of vision, dry mouth, diarrhea followed by constipation, occasional paralytic ileus, nausea and vomiting, urinary retention, fatigue, sedation and impotence are among these general side effects. Tremor and delusions or hallucinations may occur; these actions are not shared by the quaternary ammonium ganglionic blocking agents.

Dose—2.5 to 60 mg daily; *usual, initial,* **2.5 mg** 2 times a day, increased by **2.5-mg** increments at intervals of not less than 2 days as required; *maintenance,* **7.5 mg** 3 times a day.

Dosage Forms—Tablets USP; 2.5 and 10 mg.

Trimethaphan Camsylate USP

[(+)-1,3-Dibenzyldecahydro-2-oxoimidazo[4,5-c]thieno[1,2-*a*]thiolium 2-Oxo-10-bornanesulfonate; Arfonad Camphorsulfonate (*Roche*)]

Trimethaphan Camsylate contains 99.0–101.5% of $C_{32}H_{40}N_2O_5S_2$ (596.81) calculated on the dried basis.

Preparation—Silver *d*-camphor-10-sulfonate is metathesized with an equimolar portion of the trimethaphan bromide in aqueous medium. After filtering off the silver bromide, the filtrate is evaporated to dryness, and the residue of crude product is purified by crystallization from a suitable solvent. The required trimethaphan bromide is readily prepared from an intermediate produced in the synthesis of biotin.

Description—It occurs as white crystals or crystalline powder, which may have a slight odor. Its 1 in 10 solution is clear and has a pH between 5.5 and 6.5. Melting range 230° to 235°. Specific rotation +20° to +23°.

Solubility—Freely soluble in water, alcohol, and chloroform; insoluble in ether.

Uses—Trimethaphan is a ganglionic blocking agent with an extremely brief duration of action. Thus the hypotension induced is subject to moment-to-moment control simply by varying the rate of intravenous infusion. Its only use is for the *induction of brief hypotension*, as for surgical procedures in an otherwise bloody field or for certain diagnostic procedures.

Dose—*Intravenous infusion,* **0.2** to **5 mg** per **minute** in **500 ml** of isotonic solution at a rate adjusted to maintain blood pressure; *usual,* **500 mg.**

Dosage Forms—Injection USP: 500 mg/10 ml (to be diluted before use).

Trimethidinium Methosulfate NF

[1,3,8,8 - Tetramethyl - 3 - [3 - (trimethylammonio)propyl] - 3 - azonia-bicyclo[3.2.1]octane Bis(methyl sulfate); Ostensin (*Wyeth*)]

Trimethidinium Methosulfate contains 97.0–102.0% of $C_{19}H_{42}N_2O_8S_2$ (490.68), calculated on the anhydrous basis.

Preparation—Camphoric anhydride is condensed with *N,N*-dimethyl-1,3-propanediamine under reflux in xylene followed by removal of the solvent under vacuum. The residual liquid, which consists of *N*-[3-(dimethylamino)propyl]camphorimide, is dissolved in a suitable ether and reacted with lithium aluminum hydride whereupon both carbonyl groups are reduced to methylene, thus producing the di-tertiary amine. After purification by fractional vacuum distillation, the amine is doubly quaternized with methyl sulfate to form the official article. US Pat. 2,786,834.

Description—White, crystalline, hygroscopic powder. It is practically odorless or has a slight camphoraceous odor.

Solubility—Soluble in water and alcohol; very slightly soluble in acetone; insoluble in ether.

Uses—Trimethidinium Methosulfate is a quaternary ammonium ganglionic blocking agent with the same actions and uses as other ganglionic blocking agents. Since it is quaternary, absorption may be incomplete and erratic. It should be given on an empty stomach. Its duration of action is 7 to 12 hours. It has all the side effects of other ganglionic blocking agents.

Dose—**40** to **300 mg** daily in divided doses; *usual, initial,* **20 mg** 2 times a day, with 20-mg increments every third day until the desired response is obtained.

Other Dose Information—The usual maintenance dose range is 40 to 300 mg daily in divided doses.

Dosage Forms—Tablets NF: 20 mg.

Other Ganglionic Blocking Agents

Hexamethonium Chloride is hexamethylenebis [trimethylammonium chloride] [$C_{12}H_{30}Cl_2N_2$]. *Description and Solubility:* A white, crystalline, hygroscopic powder which decomposes between 289° and 292°; pH (10% aqueous solution), 5.5 to 6.5. Freely soluble in water; soluble in alcohol; practically insoluble in chloroform and ether. *Uses:* For nearly a decade hexamethonium chloride, bromide, and tartrate dominated the field of ganglionic blocking agents. However, the more reliably absorbed and longer acting agents displaced the hexamethonium drugs. It is of limited usefulness as a therapeutic and diagnostic agent in the management of *peripheral vascular diseases,* especially those in which a vasospastic component exists. It has also been used in the treatment of various *causalgias.* Its greater use has been in the treatment of *hypertension,* especially for episodes of severely elevated blood pressure. Tolerance develops. By the oral route hexamethonium is sometimes absorbed erratically; consequently, parenteral routes are preferred. *Dose: Oral, initial,* 125 mg 4 times daily, to be gradually increased as needed up to 3 Gm daily; *parenteral,* 50 to 100 mg every 6 hours; however, debilitated or severely ill patients should receive an initial trial dose of 1.3 to 6.5 mg. *Veterinary Dose:* (*Experimental*) *parenteral, Horses, Goats,* and *Dogs,* 0.2 to 1.6 mg per pound of body weight.

Pentolinium Tartrate [Ansolysen (*Wyeth*)] is 1,1′-pentamethylenebis[1-methylpyrrolidinium hydrogen tartrate] [$C_{23}H_{42}N_2O_{12}$]. *Description and Solubility:* A white to light-cream-colored, crystalline powder with an acid taste; decomposes at 203°; pH (10% aqueous solution), 3.0 to 4.0. 1 Gm dissolves in 0.4 ml of water and 810 ml of alcohol; insoluble in ether and chloroform. *Uses:* A ganglionic blocking agent whose actions closely resemble those of *Hexamethonium* (this page); like hexamethonium, its use has diminished sharply. *Dose: Oral, initial,* 20 mg every 8 hours, with 20-mg increments every 2 to 7 days until the maximum effect is achieved, generally between 60 and 600 mg; *parenteral, initial,* 2.5 to 3.5 mg, with 0.5- to 1-mg increments at 4- to 6-hour intervals, up to a *maintenance* dose of 30 to 60 mg daily, in divided doses at 6- to 8-hour intervals.

Tetraethylammonium Bromide [TEAB {[$(C_2H_5)_4$-N$^+$]Br$^-$}]—Deliquescent crystals. Freely soluble in water, alcohol, chloroform, acetone; slightly soluble in benzene. *Uses:* diagnostic and therapeutic agent in peripheral vascular disorders. Diagnostic in hypertension. See *Tetraethylammonium Chloride* (below). *Dose: intravenously,* 0.2 to 0.5 Gm; *intramuscularly,* 1 to 2 Gm.

Tetraethylammonium Chloride [$(C_2H_5)_4$N$^+$]Cl$^-$; [TEA Chloride; Etamon Chloride (*Parke-Davis*)] is the quaternary ammonium compound formed by the chemical addition of ethyl chloride to triethylamine. *Description and Solubility:* Deliquescent crystals; pH (10% aqueous solution), 6.48; the pH is not changed by heating for 28 hours at 95°. Freely soluble in water, alcohol, chloroform, and acetone; slightly soluble in benzene.

Uses: Tetraethylammonium (TEA) Chloride was the first known ganglionic blocking drug, and hence it is of historical interest. It produces a blockade of both sympathetic and parasympathetic ganglia and most of its effects on the intact organism can be explained on this basis. It produces a marked peripheral vasodilation and orthostatic hypotension. Vasodilation is particularly prominent in areas where a considerable element of vascular spasm exists. This agent also relaxes the gastrointestinal musculature, markedly decreases neurogenic gastric secretion, and delays gastric emptying.

TEA Chloride has largely been replaced by superior ganglionic blocking drugs, both as a therapeutic and as a diagnostic agent, partly because of the shorter duration and lesser selectivity of action of TEA and because it is not effective orally. Formerly, TEA was employed in a variety of clinical disorders, particularly those of the cardiovascular system in which it is desirable to improve peripheral blood flow and in which interruption of the sympathetic pathways would be expected to be of benefit.

By an unknown mechanism TEA can sometimes relieve visceral and cardiac pain, paresthesias, the pain of causalgia and related post-traumatic states, herpes zoster, and certain chest pains, and it is occasionally used for these purposes. It has also been used in the treatment of certain gastrointestinal disorders temporarily to relieve spasm and pain. It can evoke typical hypertensive crises in pheochromocytoma, and it has occasionally been so employed as a diagnostic agent.

Dose: Intravenous, 200 to 500 mg in a 10% solution may be given over a period of 30 to 60 seconds; the duration of action is 15 minutes to 1 hour. *Intramuscular,* should not exceed 20 mg per Kg and should be divided between two injection sites; the duration of action is about 4 to 6 hours.

Veratrum Alkaloids

The description and chemistry of the Veratrum Alkaloids may be found in Chapter 30 on *Natural Products* (page 500).

Uses—The pharmacology of the veratrum alkaloids is complex; not only does each alkaloid manifest a variety of actions, but the alkaloids differ from one another both quantitatively and qualitatively. Fur-thermore, their actions vary from species to species and with the dose and route of administration. The *veratrine* alkaloids (from *V. Sabadilla*) exert complex actions on nerve fibers and skeletal muscles; at present they find no clinical application and need not be discussed. The veratrum alkaloids (principally from *V. viride* and *V. album*) primarily affect the cardiovascular system and respiration; only the ester veratrum alkaloids, and not the alkamine or glycoside alkaloids, are of clinical significance.

In clinical doses, the veratrum alkaloids lower the blood pressure by *vasodilation* and slow the heart; these effects result from inhibition of sympathetic tone and from vagal stimulation, reflexly initiated by stimulation of sensory receptors in the left ventricle and in the lung. There may also be minor contributions to the cardiovascular effects by reflexes arising elsewhere and by central actions. Somewhat higher doses, occasionally reached in man, depress respiration, also by a combination of reflex stimulation and central inhibition.

The principal use of the veratrum alkaloids is in the treatment of *essential and malignant hypertension* and of *toxemias of pregnancy;* however, the veratrum alkaloids are used infrequently. In essential hypertension their efficacy is unpredictable, especially when the oral route is used. Toxic effects frequently require discontinuation of therapy. Parenteral administration is inconvenient for ambulant patients and is not without danger. In toxemias of pregnancy, parenterally administered veratrum alkaloids frequently are beneficial and occasionally spectacular in their salutary effects. Veratrum alkaloids are also sometimes employed in the therapy of hypertension resulting from certain kidney diseases.

The range between the therapeutic and the toxic dose is quite narrow; in patients, the veratrum alkaloids frequently cause epigastric and substernal burning, unpleasant taste, salivation, sweating, hiccough, nausea and vomiting, and other lesser side effects. Overdosage can cause severe hypotension and cardiovascular collapse. Atropine and ephedrine can counteract the bradycardia and hypotension, respectively. The physician must select his therapeutic regimen carefully and adjust the dosage to the patient's needs and response. Dosage schedules are complex and must continually be readjusted; tolerance may also develop. For each individual preparation it is advisable to consult the manufacturer's recommendations.

With a carefully adjusted dosage schedule of cryptenamine acetates, blood pressure can be reduced for 3 to 6 hours daily without producing nausea, vomiting, or tolerance to the medication. Restoration of vision in malignant hypertension and relief of hypertensive headaches and encephalopathy are occasional beneficial effects. It is emphasized that management of the hypertensive patient with veratrum alkaloids is palliative rather than curative, and that its field of particular usefulness is in alleviating symptoms and lowering blood pressure in patients in whom ganglionic blocking agents, rauwolfia preparations or other measures are unsuccessful and inapplicable. The veratrum alkaloids are usually given in combination with a rauwolfia alkaloid or a thiazide diuretic. However, fixed drug combinations of veratrum alkaloids and other drugs are an abuse of optimal therapy.

Alkavervir [Veriloid *(Riker)*] is a mixture of alkaloids obtained by the selective extraction of *Veratrum viride* with various organic solvents and selective precipitation from acidic and basic solutions. *Description and Solubility:* A light-yellow powder, strongly sternutatory. Freely soluble in alcohol; practically insoluble in water. *Uses:* See the general statement on *Veratrum Alkaloids* (above). Alkavervir causes a higher incidence of side effects than cryptenamine and the protoveratrines. The oral route is preferred in the absence of a hypertensive crisis. Oral Alkavervir exerts a maximal hypotensive effect in about 2 hours and the effect lasts 4 to 6 hours. Parenteral administration is re-

served for selected cases of hypertensive encephalopathy, pre-eclampsia and eclampsia; the onset of action is nearly immediate but the effect lasts only 1½ to 3 hours. *Dose: Oral,* 3 to 5 mg every 6 to 8 hours; *intramuscular,* 0.25 mg per 50 pounds of body weight at 2- or 3-hour intervals; *intravenous,* 0.06 mg per 10 pounds of body weight, diluted to 10 ml with isotonic sodium chloride or dextrose solution, given very slowly, at 1½- to 3-hour intervals.

Cryptenamine Acetates [Unitensen Aqueous *(Neisler)*] is the acetate salts of a mixture of alkaloids derived from an extract of *Veratrum viride. Description and Solubility:* A white to tan, amorphous powder that is odorless, stable in aqueous solution, and melts over a wide range. Very soluble in water and alcohol. *Uses:* See the general statement on *Veratrum Alkaloids* (page 850). Cryptenamine is better tolerated than other veratrum alkaloids; nevertheless, its use is frequently accompanied by untoward effects. Cryptenamine Acetates are employed only in selected cases of hypertensive encephalopathy, pre-eclampsia, and eclampsia. They are given only by the intravenous or intramuscular routes; the hypotensive effect is prompt and lasts 3 to 6 hours. *Dose: Intravenous,* 1 mg. diluted with 20 ml of isotonic dextrose solution, to be infused at the rate of 1 ml per minute and to be repeated as needed; *intramuscular, initial,* 1 mg at hourly intervals until the hypertension is controlled, then at 3- to 6-hour intervals; 0.2-mg increments may be necessary.

Cryptenamine Tannates [Unitensen *(Neisler)*] is the tannate salts of a mixture of alkaloids derived from an extract of *Veratrum viride. Description and Solubility:* A tan, amorphous powder that is odorless, stable in light and air, and melts over a wide range. Soluble in alcohol; very slightly soluble in water. *Uses:* See the general statement on *Veratrum Alkaloids* (page 850) and *Cryptenamine Acetates* (above). The tannates are given only by the oral route and are preferred only in the absence of a hypertensive crisis. *Dose, Oral, initial,* 2 mg twice daily. Increments may be made at weekly intervals, if necessary, by increasing the number of daily doses rather than the size of the individual dose.

Protoveratrine A [$C_{41}H_{63}NO_{14}$] [Protalba *(Pitman-Moore)*] is one of the several ester–alkaloids isolated from *Veratrum alba* and *Veratrum viride.* For its structure, see page 501. *Description and Solubility:* Cubic leaflets, melting between 259° and 262° (copper block) or 302° and 304° (Kofler block, with effervescence and decomposition). Soluble in chloroform, pyridine, and hot alcohol. *Uses:* See the general statement on *Veratrum Alkaloids* (page 850). Protoveratrine A is the more potent of the two alkaloids, *Protoveratrines A and B* (below). However, in hypotensive doses it produces the same incidence of side effects as the mixture and hence offers no particular advantage over the mixture. After oral administration, the duration of action is about 8 hours. *Dose: Oral, initial,* 0.2 mg 4 times daily, with upper or lower adjustments as necessary.

Protoveratrines A and B [Veralba *(Pitman-Moore)*] is a mixture of protoveratrine A [$C_{41}H_{63}NO_{14}$] and protoveratrine B [$C_{41}H_{63}NO_{15}$], two of the ester–alkaloids isolated from *Veratrum album* and from *Veratrum viride.* For the structures, see page 501. *Description and Solubility:* A white, odorless, slightly bitter, crystalline powder with a strongly sternutatory action; decomposes between 256° and 262°; a saturated solution in water is nearly neutral; stable to light and air; solutions with a pH between 4.0 and 6.0 are stable for several months, but the substance is rapidly destroyed in alkaline and in alcoholic solutions. Freely soluble in chloroform; very slightly soluble in ether; practically insoluble in water; soluble in dilute aqueous acid solutions. *Uses:* See the general statement on *Veratrum Alkaloids* (page 850). Protoveratrines A and B may be given either parenterally or orally. Their action is erratic by the oral route, so that either the blood pressure or untoward effects may be hard to control. Oral administration is to be used only in the absence of a hypertensive crisis. During a crisis, a parenteral route is employed, generally initially intravenous then intramuscular for maintenance. The duration of action of an oral dose is about 8 hours; an intramuscular dose, 3 to 8 hours; and an intravenous dose, 1½ to 3 hours. *Dose: Oral,* 0.4 to

1.5 mg 4 times daily; *intramuscular*, 0.12 to 4 mg every 4 to 8 hours; *intravenous, initial*, 0.06 to 0.1 mg at 4-hour intervals, with adjustments by steps of 0.01 mg, as needed. Various schedules of interrupted intravenous infusion are also used, such that usually 0.08 to 0.16 mg are accumulated before an adequate blood pressure response is obtained.

Protoveratrines A and B Maleates [Provell Maleate (*Lilly*)] is a mixture of the maleate salts of the two alkaloids, protoveratrine A and protoveratrine B. *Description and Solubility:* A white to buff-colored powder with a faint, characteristic odor and a strongly sternutatory action; de-composes between 210° and 222°; pH (0.2% aqueous solution), 4.1 to 4.7. Freely soluble in alcohol, water, and chloroform; practically insoluble in ether. *Uses:* The actions are the same as those of *Protoveratrines A and B* (above), except that the maleates are not given parenterally and hence are limited to use in moderate to severe essential malignant hypertension in which no hypertensive crisis exists. *Dose: Oral, initial,* 0.5 mg 3 times daily, with gradual increments of 0.125 mg until the desirable effect is obtained. As total daily dose is increased, the number of dose divisions may be increased to 5.

Miscellaneous Hypotensives (Antihypertensives)

A large number of substances are capable of lowering the blood pressure, at least briefly. Few of these, however, are employed for their hypotensive action. Examples of drugs with prominent hypotensive actions that are rarely used for such actions are the nitrites, histamine, parasympathomimetics, azapetine, and tolazoline; however, they may be used to increase peripheral blood flow. The dihydrogenated ergot alkaloids (see Chapter 30, page 498) were used briefly as antihypertensives. Adrenergic blocking agents (page 908) may also be hypotensive.

Diuretics are antihypertensive by their effect to reduce body sodium content and to decrease plasma volume. Thiazide diuretics also have an antihypertensive action beyond that of diuresis alone.

Bendroflumethiazide—see page 944.

Benzthiazide—see page 944.

Chlorothiazide—see page 945.

Chlorthalidone—see page 948.

Cyclothiazide—see page 945.

Deserpidine—see page 913.

Ethacrynic Acid—see page 948.

Furosemide—see page 949.

Guanethidine Sulfate—see page 910.

Hydralazine Hydrochloride NF

[1-Hydrazinophthalazine Monohydrochloride; Apresoline (*Ciba*)]

Hydralazine Hydrochloride contains 98.0–100.5% of $C_8H_8N_4 \cdot HCl$ (196.64), calculated on the dried basis.

Preparation—Phthalazone (lactim form shown in I) is converted to 1-chlorophthalazine (II) by treatment with phosphorus oxychloride. (II) is isolated by precipitation with water and is then condensed with hydrazine hydrate in an organic solvent to form 1-hydrazinophthalazine. After drying, the base is converted to the hydrochloride by treatment with hydrochloric acid. The salt is purified by recrystallization from hydrochloric acid.

Description—A white, odorless, crystalline powder. Melting range 270° to 280°.

Solubility—1 Gm dissolves in about 25 ml of water and in about 500 ml of alcohol; very slightly soluble in ether.

Uses—Hydralazine is a hypotensive agent, the actions of which are complex. It depresses the vasomotor center, but there are indications its antihypertensive action may not be wholly attributable to its central action; both its action to increase renal blood flow and to induce a relative adrenal insufficiency may possibly contribute to the clinical response. Although in high doses it antagonizes adrenergic neurohumors (epinephrine and norepinephrine) and certain other endogenous pressor agents, it is unlikely that the hypotension can be attributed to such actions. Hydralazine may be used in the treatment of *essential* and *early malignant hypertension*, virtually always in conjunction with rauwolfia alkaloids or ganglionic blocking agents; however, mainly because of its side effects, it is generally not used until other safer therapy has failed.

The principal serious toxic effects of Hydralazine Hydrochloride are syndromes resembling rheumatoid arthritis or lupus erythematosus, the appearance of which necessitates withdrawal of the drug. Frequent side effects include tachycardia and palpitation, dizziness, headache and cardiomegaly. It tends to exacerbate angina pectoris.

Dose—*Usual, oral, initial,* **10 mg** 4 times a day; *maintenance,* up to **100 mg** 4 times a day; *usual, intramuscular* or *intravenous,* **20** to **40 mg** repeated as necessary.

Dosage Forms—Injection NF: 20 mg/ml; Tablets NF: 10, 25, 50, and 100 mg.

Hydrochlorothiazide—see page 946.

Hydroflumethiazide—see page 946.

Isocarboxazid—see page 1115.

Mebutamate—see page 1094.

Methychlothiazide—see page 946.

Methyldopa—see page 911.

Methyldopate Hydrochloride—see page 911.

Nialamide—see page 1116.

Phenelzine—see page 1117.

Phentolamine Hydrochloride—see page 909.

Pargyline Hydrochloride NF

[*N*-Methyl-*N*-2-propynylbenzylamine Hydrochloride; Eutonyl (*Abbott*)]

$$\left[\bigcirc\!\!-CH_2-\overset{+}{\underset{\underset{CH_3}{|}}{N}H}-CH_2C\equiv CH \right] Cl^- $$

Pargyline Hydrochloride contains 98.0–101.0% of $C_{11}H_{13}N \cdot HCl$ (195.69), calculated on the anhydrous basis.

Preparation—2-Propynyl bromide is reacted with *N*-methylbenzylamine by refluxing in ethanol for several hours in the presence of anhydrous sodium carbonate. The reaction mixture is filtered, the ethanol is removed by distillation, and the pargyline (base) is extracted from the residue with ether. A stream of hydrogen chloride precipitates the hydrochloride from the ether solution. US Pat. 3,155,584.

Description—A fine, white or practically white, crystalline powder, having a slight, characteristic odor. It sublimes slowly at elevated temperatures. It is stable in light and air and has a melting range of 158° to 162°.

Solubility—Very soluble in water; freely soluble in alcohol and chloroform; very slightly soluble in acetone, benzene, and isooctane.

Uses—Pargyline Hydrochloride is an inhibitor of monoamine oxidase. It has a weak *antihypertensive* action. It does not appreciably lower the blood pressure of hypertensive patients when they are recumbent, but only when they are standing. Thus it effects only an orthostatic hypotension and has little demonstrable peripheral action or influence on the disease process. The mechanism of its action is unknown; it appears to promote the exchange of the weak sympathomimetic, octopamine, for norepinephrine in the adrenergic terminals. Pargyline has been claimed to have a euphoriant or antidepressant action, but controlled clinical observation has not shown the effect to be significant. Untoward effects of the drug are vertigo, weakness, and syncope (the result of orthostatic hypotension), nausea and vomiting, constipation, dry mouth, sweating, headache, nervousness, insomnia, nightmares, impotence, and difficulty in ejaculation. It potentiates dangerously the effects of narcotics, sedatives (including alcohol), psychomotor stimulants, sympathomimetics, antihistaminics, and hypotensives. Because it inhibits monoamine oxidase, which normally destroys tyramine and other pressor amines in cheese, hypertensive crises sometimes occur upon the eating of certain cheeses. It may cause the emergence of concealed psychoses. Thus both physician and patient are required to be on continuous alert. It also promotes increased appetite and fluid retention, which may lead to serious weight gain.

Dose—*Usual, initial,* **10** to **25 mg** once daily, then increase daily dose in increments of **10 mg** once a week until the desired response is obtained.

Other Dose Information—If used in combination with other antihypertensives, or in elderly or sympathectomized patients, the initial dose should be 10 to 25 mg.

Dosage Forms—Tablets NF: 10, 25, and 50 mg.

Other Miscellaneous Hypotensives

Diazoxide [Hyperstat (*Schering*)] is 7-chloro-3-methyl-2*H*-1,2,4-benzothiadiazine 1,1-dioxide ($C_8H_7ClN_2O_2S$). *Description* and *Solubility:* White to creamy white crystals or a crystalline powder; it is odorless; it is stable in light, air, and heat; it melts at about 325°. Insoluble in water. *Uses:* Diazoxide is chemically related to the benzothiadiazine diuretics but is devoid of diuretic action. Indeed, in contrast to the thiazide diuretics, it causes salt and water retention and expands the extracellular fluid volume. Nevertheless, Diazoxide has a hypotensive action that is prompt in onset. The fall in blood pressure results from arteriolar dilatation. Hypotension is not accompanied by postural hypotension, which is an advantage over that produced by certain other prominent antihypertensives. However, because of several disadvantageous side effects, Diazoxide is not used in the chronic treatment of *essential hypertension*, but it may be used in the short term management of *hypertensive crises*. In addition to salt and water retention, which may be corrected by simultaneous administration of a thiazide diuretic, hiruitism, gastrointestinal upsets, and dermatoses occur with chronic use. The drug may cause hyperglycemia acutely, which is useful in the treatment of *hypoglycemia*, especially in children. The mechanism of hyperglycemic action appears to be both an inhibition of hepatic phosphodiesterase, an enzyme that hydrolyzes 3′,5′-cyclic AMP, and an inhibition of insulin release. *Dose:* For *hypertension, intravenous,* 200 to 400 mg; for *hypoglycemia, oral,* 6 to 18 mg per Kg of body weight per day in 3 to 4 divided doses.

Dioxyline Phosphate [Paveril Phosphate (*Lilly*)] is 1-(4-ethoxy-3-methoxybenzyl)-6,7-dimethoxy-3-methylisoquinoline sesquiphosphate ($C_{22}H_{25}NO_4 \cdot 1\frac{1}{2}H_3PO_4$). *Description* and *Solubility:* White to off-white crystals or a white crystalline powder; it is practically odorless and has a slightly bitter taste; it melts between 196.5° and 201.5°; light may cause a slight discoloration; it is not hygroscopic, but may absorb some water if the humidity is high. 1 Gm dissolves in about 25 ml of water and about 320 ml of alcohol. *Incompatibilities:* See *Alkaloids* (page 491). *Uses:* Dioxyline has actions and uses similar to those of papaverine (see *Papaverine Hydrochloride*, page 854). *Dose:* Oral, 90 to 360 mg 3 to 4 times daily.

Peripheral Vasodilators

Peripheral vasodilators are substances which dilate the arterioles and increase blood flow in the numerous systemic vascular beds, especially in the extremities. To the pharmacologist, the word *peripheral* may indicate that the action is directly on the arterioles, but to the clinician the word merely indicates the site of the final effect. Thus, centrally acting, reflexly acting, or ganglionic blocking drugs that reduce sympathetic tone to the periphery are peripheral vasodilators, clinically speaking; consequently, all of the hypotensives listed in the previous section may be considered to be peripheral dilators, but only the ganglionic blocking agents and the veratrum alkaloids are employed for the purpose of increasing blood flow to any specific peripheral area. Some sympathomimetics with prominent beta receptor stimulant actions are employed for their peripheral vasodilator effects. The adrenergic blocking drugs are also used to improve flow through specific peripheral vascular beds.

Peripheral vasodilators are employed in the treatment of vasospastic disorders such as *Raynaud's disease*, *causalgias* and *reflex dystrophy*, vasospasm associated with *arterial embolism* and *thrombophlebitis*, *immersion foot*, *trench foot*, *herpes zoster*, *decubitous ulcers*, and degenerative arterial diseases such as *thromboangiitis obliterans*, *arteriosclerosis obliterans*, *acrocyanosis*, and *diabetic gangrene*.

Aminophylline—see page 1154.

Carbachol—see page 900.

Histamine Phosphate—see page 1142.

Isoxsuprine Hydrochloride—see page 888.

Methacholine Chloride—see page 900.

Niacin—see page 1039.

Nitrates and Nitrites (see Coronary Drugs)—see pages 855 to 858.

Nylidrin Hydrochloride—see page 892.

Papaverine Hydrochloride NF

[6,7-Dimethoxy-1-vertarylisoquinoline Hydrochloride; *Various Mfgs.*]

Papaverine Hydrochloride contains 98.0–100.5% of $C_{20}H_{21}NO_4 \cdot HCl$ (375.86), calculated on the dried basis.

Papaverine Hydrochloride is the hydrochloride of an alkaloid obtained from opium or prepared synthetically.

Preparation—Papaverine, along with narcotine, thebaine, and some other opium alkaloids, is found in the mother liquors remaining after the precipitation of morphine with ammonia from the aqueous opium extract in the presence of dilute alcohol, or in the precipitate obtained by treating the opium extract with sodium acetate. It may be roughly separated from the accompanying alkaloids in alcohol solution as the acid oxalate and the base obtained from it purified by crystallization from alcohol.

The great demand for papaverine is now largely satisfied through synthetic preparation using vanillin as the starting material, and involving 10 to 12 major steps. Homoveratryl–homoveratroylamine is the final intermediate from which Papaverine is produced by ring closure and dehydrogenation.

Papaverine was synthesized from o-dimethoxybenzene (veratrol) by Pictet and Gams in 1909.[1]

Description and Properties—White crystals or a white, crystalline powder. It is odorless, and has a slightly bitter taste. It is optically inactive. Its solutions are acid to litmus.

Solubility—1 Gm is soluble in about 30 ml of water, about 120 ml of alcohol; soluble in chloroform; practically insoluble in ether.

Incompatibilities—See *Alkaloids* (page 491).

Uses—Papaverine Hydrochloride is a *smooth muscle relaxant* in general, although different organs are affected in a varying degree.

It is most effective in hypertonic conditions; it does not interfere materially with the normal movements, for instance, of the intestines. It is also a rather feeble central analgetic and a local anesthetic. Its toxicity is low, and neither tolerance nor habituation has been reported. These actions have prompted its use, with reported success, in various spasmodic conditions of the smooth muscles, especially in all kinds of gastric and *intestinal spasms*, in *biliary colic*, and in *bronchial spasm*. Perhaps the chief use of Papaverine is in peripheral arterial or pulmonary *embolism*, where it may be life-saving. *Its action is to dilate the arteries* and allow collateral blood supply to reach the obstructed region. For this purpose, it is given intravenously. Papaverine also dilates the coronary arteries, and it may be used in *angina pectoris;* however, its effect to stimulate the heart tends to negate the benefits of coronary vasodilation. In normal subjects, Papaverine dilates the cerebral vessels. Consequently, it is used to treat cerebral ischemia, although its vasodilator effect on diseased cerebral vessels is less marked. The alkaloid also affects the refractory period of cardiac muscle, and is useful in the treatment of *extrasystoles*, particularly of ventricular origin.

In general, the more successful therapeutic applications of the actions of Papaverine are those listed above for the heart and blood vessels, rather than for relief of spasm of smooth muscle of the bronchi, ureter, or gastrointestinal tract. More effective antispasmodics are available for these last-named structures. The content of Papaverine in opium or in "concentrated opium" is not sufficient to impart to these drugs the actions of papaverine.

Caution—Although it is not a narcotic, Papaverine requires a physician's narcotic prescription before it can be dispensed, and inasmuch as it is an alkaloid of opium, its sale and use come under the *Harrison Narcotic Law*.

Dose—*Oral*, 60 to 200 mg; *usual*, *oral*, 100 mg; *intramuscular*, 30 to 60 mg; *usual*, *intramuscular*, 30 mg.

Other Dose Information—In urgent situations the drug may be given intravenously, slowly over a period of 2 minutes. In the oral treatment of angina pectoris, intestinal spasm, biliary colic, or bronchial spasm, the drug may be given 3 to 4 times daily.

Dosage Forms—Injection NF: 30 mg/ml, 60 mg/2 ml, 300 mg/10 ml; Tablets NF: 30, 60, 100, and 200 mg.

Veterinary Uses and Dose—A reduction in size of myocardial infarcts in dogs has followed 8 weeks' therapy with twice-daily doses as follows: *intramuscular*, 30 mg; *oral*, 60 to 200 mg.

Phentolamine Hydrochloride—see page 909.

Phentolamine Mesylate—see page 909.

Other Peripheral Vasodilators

Aluminum Nicotinate [Tris(nicotinato)aluminum; Nicalex (*National Drug*)]—A white, practically odorless, amorphous powder with a slight, acidulous taste. Insoluble in water and alcohol; soluble in dilute mineral acids. *Uses:* For peripheral vasodilation in certain peripheral vascular disorders. The active moiety of the drug is the nicotinate, which is *niacin* (see page 1028). Like niacin, the nicotinate has a potential for lowering blood lipids, but the recommended dose is much too small for this purpose. *Dose:* 125 to 625 mg daily in divided doses.

Azapetine Phosphate [Ilidar Phosphate (*Roche*)] is 6-allyl-6,7-dihydro-5H-dibenz[*c,e*]azepine phosphate [$C_{17}H_{17}$-N.H_3PO_4]. *Description and Solubility:* A white, crystalline powder that is odorless or has a faint odor and is stable in air; melts between 210° and 213°. 1 Gm dissolves in about 25 ml of water and 500 ml of absolute alcohol; practically insoluble in ether and chloroform. *Uses:* Generally classified as an adrenergic blocking agent. However, like tolazoline, which it closely resembles, its prominent actions are those of direct vasodilation. Adrenergic blockade with the usual clinical doses is lacking; however, vasodilation with improved peripheral blood flow is the important action, whatever the mechanism. Azapetine is employed in the therapy of *vasospastic states* and *acute arterial occlusion;* its efficacy in the organic occlusive vascular diseases is doubtful. *Dose: Intravenous,* 50 to 75 mg 3 times a day. A preliminary 7-day test period with ⅓ the above dose should be made.

Cyclandelate [Cyclospasmol (*Ives*)] is 3,3,5-trimethylcyclohexyl mandelate [$C_{17}H_{24}O_3$]. *Description and Solubility:* Crystals which melt at 50° to 53°. Insoluble in water; soluble in lipoids and their solvents. *Uses:* An antispasmodic drug with actions similar to those of papaverine. It relaxes vascular smooth muscle and erratically increases blood flow. It is used in the treatment of *thrombophlebitis, Raynaud's disease, thromboangiitis obliterans, diabetic angioses, intermittent claudication, arteriosclerosis, erythrocyanosis, frostbite,* and *refractory skin ulcers.* Side effects include flushing and tingling, vertigo, nausea, headache, and sweating. *Dose: Oral,* 100 to 200 mg 4 times daily.

Ethaverine [$C_{24}H_{29}NO_4$] [Neopaverine (*Savage*)] is a synthetic analog of papaverine in which ethoxy groups replace the four methoxy groups. Its uses are the same as those of papaverine. Despite claims to the contrary, it is not a useful antihypertensive. See *Papaverine Hydrochloride* (page 854). *Dose: Oral, initial,* 60 to 180 mg; *maintenance,* 30 to 90 mg every 4 to 6 hours; *intramuscular,* 15 to 60 mg. *Veterinary Uses* and *Dose: Oral, spasmolytic* and *antitussive, Dogs* and *Cats,* 15 mg.

Nicotinyl Alcohol [3-Pyridine Methanol; $C_5H_4NCH_2$-OH; Roniacol (*Roche*)]—A colorless, hygroscopic liquid. Slightly soluble in water and diethyl ether; readily soluble in petroleum ether. *Uses:* See *Nicotinyl Tartrate* (below), which is the form of the alcohol used in all solid dosage forms. Nicotinyl Alcohol as the free base is dispensed as an elixir containing 50 mg of the alcohol per 5 ml. *Dose:* 50 to 100 mg 3 times daily.

Nicotinyl Tartrate [Roniacol Tartrate (*Roche*)] is 3-pyridinemethanol tartrate (1:1)[$C_6H_7NO.C_4H_6O_6$]. *Description and Solubility:* Crystals having a sour taste; that melt between 147° and 148°. Freely soluble in water and alcohol; soluble in ether. *Uses:* Its actions are due to its component of nicotinyl alcohol. The function of the tartaric acid is purely pharmaceutical, namely, to convert the hygroscopic liquid alcohol to a solid salt that lends itself to a tablet form. In the body, nicotinyl alcohol is converted to nicotinic acid, and it is believed that the pharmacologic properties of the alcohol are mediated through the acid. Given in very large oral doses, it is a peripheral vasodilator and causes flushing of the skin in the blush area and a feeling of warmth and tingling. Consequently, the drug is employed in the treatment of *vasospastic disorders,* such as *Raynaud's disease, acrocyanosis,* and *chillblains.* However, no sound clinical studies have established that the usual doses effect any beneficial action in these diseases. Even more dubious are scattered claims to effectiveness in the treatment of obliterative vascular diseases. The duration of action is brief except when given in sustained-release form. Side effects include flushing on the face and neck, tingling, mild swelling of the extremeties, nausea, vomiting, and rarely, syncope. *Dose: Oral,* 50 to 100 mg 3 times daily, except 150 to 300 mg twice daily in sustained-release form.

Tolazoline Hydrochloride [$C_{10}H_{12}N_2$.HCl] [Benzazoline Hydrochloride; 2-Benzyl-2-imidazoline Hydrochloride; Priscoline Hydrochloride (*Ciba*)]—*Preparation:* Benzyl cyanide and ethylene diamine are heated together in the presence of carbon disulfide, whereby hydrogen sulfide and ammonia are liberated, and tolazoline base is formed. After purification by distillation, the base is converted to the hydrochloride by passing dry hydrogen chloride gas into a solution of the base in a suitable organic solvent. *Description and Solubility:* A white or creamy white, crystalline powder; its solutions are slightly acid to litmus; melting range, 172° to 176°. Very soluble in water; freely soluble in alcohol. *Uses:* A smooth muscle relaxant and *vasodilator.* In sufficient doses in man the drug can effect an adrenergic blockade of short duration; however, its clinical usefulness does not depend upon adrenergic blockade but rather upon a direct peripheral vasodilation. Tolazoline stimulates the heart, so that the blood pressure may actually be elevated; it also stimulates the gastrointestinal tract; and it induces mydriasis. It promotes the gastric secretion of acid; consequently, it has found limited application as a substitute for histamine in tests for gastric secretion. Tolazoline is employed in a variety of peripheral vascular disorders such as *Raynaud's disease, Buerger's disease, arteriosclerotic peripheral vascular disease, acute arterial occlusion* and *cerebral vascular accidents, phlebothrombosis,* and *thrombophlebitis.* Side effects which may be encountered include palpitation, increased gastrointestinal motility, chills, apprehension, and occasionally, anginal pain. *Dose: Oral* and *parenteral,* 25 to 75 mg *usual,* 50 mg 4 times a day.

Coronary Drugs

Most vasoactive substances dilate the coronary vessels, even though their peripheral effects may be that of constriction. Thus, sympathomimetics, which are peripheral vasoconstrictors, dilate the coronary beds. But, a useful coronary *vasodilator* should have minimal effects on the blood pressure and should not increase cardiac work. Thus, most autonomic agents, hypotensives and peripheral vasodilators do not fall in this class. The principal coronary dilators are smooth muscle relaxants in general and may be employed as spasmolytics in certain instances. However, coronary dilatation makes a minimal contribution to the antianginal effects. Rather, arteriolar dilation, which reduces peripheral resistance, and venous dilation, which reduces venous return and hence stroke volume, combine to reduce cardiac work and thus give relief.

At present much attention is being given to the prevention or eradication of coronary atherosclerosis. Many claims of the efficacy of polyunsaturated fats and certain dietary factors in the reduction of atherosclerosis have been made, but no claim has yet been widely accepted by authorities in the field.

A few drugs, such as posterior pituitary and the ergot alkaloids, constrict the coronary vessels. Dihydroergotamine (see page 953) is occasionally used as a coronary constrictor in the tests of coronary competence.

Aminophylline—see page 1154.

Amyl Nitrite NF

[Isoamyl Nitrite; Isopentyl Nitrite]

$$CH_3$$
$$|$$
$$CH_3—CH—CH_2—CH_2—O—N=O$$

Amyl Nitrite contains 95.0–105.0% of $C_5H_{11}NO_2$ (117.15). It consists chiefly of isoamyl nitrite [(CH_3)$_2$-

CHCH$_2$CH$_2$ONO] but other isomers are also present.

Preparation—A good grade of commercial amyl alcohol (isoamyl alcohol) boiling above 125° is mixed with an aqueous solution of sodium nitrite sufficient to furnish 15 to 20% excess nitrous acid. While stirring, diluted sulfuric acid (1 in 3) is slowly added to the mixture. The odor of amyl alcohol should completely disappear; if it does not, more sodium nitrite and acid should be added. After allowing the liquids to separate, the upper layer of Amyl Nitrite is washed with a cold solution of sodium carbonate to remove free sulfuric acid, then with cold water, and finally shaken with anhydrous potassium carbonate to absorb the water held by the ester.

Description—A clear, yellowish liquid with a peculiar, ethereal, fruity odor and a pungent, aromatic taste. It boils at about 97° but is volatile even at low temperatures and it is flammable. It slowly decomposes on exposure to air and light. Moisture accelerates decomposition. The specific gravity of Amyl Nitrite is between 0.871 and 0.875. The specific gravity of pure Amyl Nitrite is 0.875.

Solubility—It is practically insoluble in water; miscible with alcohol, chloroform, and ether.

Uses—Amyl Nitrite, being exceedingly volatile, can be inhaled in order to obtain the therapeutic effects of the nitrite ion in the body rapidly. In actual practice however, Amyl Nitrite is employed but rarely, except as a *vasodilator* in the treatment of attacks of *angina pectoris*. An unusual but at times life-saving use for Amyl Nitrite is in the emergency treatment of *cyanide poisoning*, where nitrites are given to produce methemoglobin, which temporarily inactivates the toxic cyanide ion by combining with it to form cyanmethemoglobin. For this purpose, sodium nitrite is employed intravenously, but Amyl Nitrite may be inhaled while the solution of sodium nitrite is being prepared. In angina pectoris, pain is eased by the vasodilatation of the coronary arteries produced by Amyl Nitrite. It is administered by crushing a glass *pearl of amyl nitrite* in a handkerchief and inhaling the liquid which volatilizes, or by dropping a small quantity on a handkerchief and inhaling the vapor.

Caution—Amyl Nitrite is very flammable. Do not use where it may be ignited.

Dose—*Usual, inhalation*, **0.3 ml** as required.

Veterinary Dose—*Inhalation, Horses* and *Cattle*, **2 to 4 ml**; *Dogs*, **0.1 to 0.3 ml**.

Dioxyline Phosphate—see page 853.

Ethaverine—see page 855.

Isocarboxazid—see page 1115.

Diluted Erythrityl Tetranitrate NF

[Erythritol Tetranitrate; Cardilate (*Burroughs-Wellcome*)]

CH$_2$ONO$_2$

HCONO$_2$

HCONO$_2$

CH$_2$ONO$_2$

Diluted Erythrityl Tetranitrate is a dry mixture of erythrityl tetranitrate [C$_4$H$_6$N$_4$O$_{12}$ = 302.11] with lactose or other suitable inert excipients, to permit safe handling and compliance with federal Interstate Commerce Commission regulations pertaining to interstate shipment. It contains 90.0–110.0% of the labeled amount of C$_4$H$_6$N$_4$O$_{12}$.

Caution: Undiluted erythrityl tetranitrate is a powerful explosive, and proper precautions must be taken in handling. It can be exploded by percussion or by excessive heat. Only extremely small quantities should be isolated.

Preparation—Erythritol is reacted with nitric acid in the presence of sulfuric acid under controlled temperature.

Description—A white powder having a slight odor of nitric oxides and a bitter taste. It is unstable in light and heat. It melts at 61°.

Solubility—Soluble in acetone, acetonitrile, ether, and alcohol; slightly soluble in alcohol and chloroform; practically insoluble in water.

Uses—Erythrityl Tetranitrate is a *vasodilator* similar in action to the other organic nitrates. It has a relatively long duration of action within its class. Its principal use is in the prophylaxis of *angina pectoris*. Prominent authorities consider it the drug of choice for prophylaxis. As with nitroglycerin and other organic nitrates, its peripheral effects undoubtedly contribute more to relief than does coronary vasodilation (see general statement, page 855). Tolerance can occur, but a week or two of discontinuation restores sensitivity.

Dose—*Usual, oral, initial*, **10 mg** of erithrityl tetranitrate 3 times a day; *sublingual, initial*, **5 mg** of erithrityl tetranitrate 3 times a day. These doses may be increased in 2 or 3 days if needed.

Dosage Forms—Tablets NF: 5, 10, and 15 mg.

Mannitol Hexanitrate

[Maxitate (*Strasenburgh*); Nitranitol (*Merrell*)]

O$_2$NO ONO$_2$

O$_2$NOCH$_2$CHCHCHCHCH$_2$ONO$_2$

O$_2$NO ONO$_2$

Mannitol Hexanitrate is C$_6$H$_8$N$_6$O$_{18}$ (452.17).

Description—It occurs as long needles in regular clusters, melting between 106° and 108°. It reduces Fehling's solution. It will explode on percussion. Because of its stability at ordinary temperatures, it may be used commercially, but is distinctly less stable than nitroglycerin at 75°. It is used in pharmaceutical preparations only in admixture with carbohydrate substances in dilutions corresponding to 1 part of the drug to 9 parts of carbohydrate; in this dilution it is considered nonexplosive.

Solubility—Soluble in alcohol and in ether; insoluble in water.

Uses—Mannitol Hexanitrate is a vasodilator with the same qualitative actions and toxicity as nitroglycerin; however, its onset of action is slower and its duration much longer than that of nitroglycerin. Its principal use is in the prophylaxis of attacks of *angina pectoris*.

Dose—*Oral* or *sublingual*, **15 to 60 mg** every 4 to 6 hours.

Dosage Forms—Tablets: 15 and 30 mg.

Veterinary Dose—*Dogs*, **15 to 30 mg**.

Nialamide—see page 1116.

Nitroglycerin Tablets USP

[Glyceryl Trinitrate Tablets USP XVI; Trinitrin Tablets; Nitrobid (*Marion*); Nitroglyn (*Key*); Nitrospan (*USV*)]

Nitroglycerin Tablets contain 80.0–112.0% of the labeled amount of glyceryl trinitrate [C$_3$H$_5$N$_3$O$_9$ = 227.09].

Preparation—Nitroglycerin (glyceryl trinitrate) is a practically colorless, odorless liquid with a sweet taste. It is made by nitrating glycerin with a mixture of nitric and sulfuric acids called "nitration acid." This acid usually consists of 3 parts of concentrated nitric acid and 5 parts of sulfuric acid, the latter acid acting as a dehydrating agent thus making the nitration more complete.

Uses—Like amyl nitrite, Nitroglycerin is a general relaxant of, but does not paralyze, smooth muscle. Its actions are directly on the smooth muscle and are independent of the type of innervation; its actions cannot be prevented by any known agent. It acts as a *vasodilator* on the finer blood vessels and therefore causes a fall in blood pressure. The hypotensive action is only occasionally sought clinically; however, the peripheral vasodilation and venous pooling find extensive clinical application in the prophylaxis and of attacks of *angina pectoris* (see the general statement, page 855). It does not have a direct effect on the myocardium. It does occasionally induce coronary dilatation. The drug is poorly absorbed from the stomach and intestines but is effectively absorbed from the buccal or sublingual mucosae. By the sublingual route, the vasodilator effects of the drug appear in 2 to 3 minutes and last for about 20 minutes. Nitroglycerin is also sometimes employed for the relief of *biliary* and *ureteral spasm;* it is rarely efficacious in the treatment of bronchial asthma or gastrointestinal spasm. Hypotension consequent to the administration of Nitroglycerin may decrease coronary blood flow; consequently, it is contraindicated in patients with recent myocardial infarction. Cerebral vasodilatation may cause transient headaches.

Veterinary Use—Nitroglycerin has been used for *pulmonary edema, pulmonary congestion,* and *spasmodic bronchial asthma* of the dog.

Dose—*Sublingual,* **300 mcg** to **10 mg** daily; *usual,* **400 mcg,** repeated as necessary.

Dosage Forms—Tablets USP: 150, 300, 400, and 600 mcg.

Veterinary Dose—*Horses* and *Cattle,* **10 to 30 mg;** *Dogs,* **0.4 to 1 mg.**

Papaverine Hydrochloride—see page 854.

Diluted Pentaerythritol Tetranitrate NF

[2,2-Bis(hydroxymethyl)-1,3-propanediol Tetranitrate; Niperyt; Penthrit; Pentaerythrityl Tetranitrate; PETN; Pentritol (*Armour*); Peritrate (*Warner-Chilcott*); Vasodiatol (*Rowell*)]

$$O_2NOCH_2 \quad CH_2ONO_2$$
$$C$$
$$O_2NOCH_2 \quad CH_2ONO_2$$

Diluted Pentaerythritol Tetranitrate is a dry mixture of pentaerythritol tetranitrate [$C_5H_8N_4O_{12}$ = 316.14] with lactose or mannitol or other suitable inert excipients, to permit safe handling and compliance with federal Interstate Commerce Commission regulations pertaining to interstate shipment. It contains 90.0–110.0% of the labeled amount of $C_5H_8N_4O_{12}$.

Caution—Undiluted pentaerythritol tetranitrate is a powerful explosive, and proper precautions must be taken in handling. It can be exploded by percussion or by excessive heat. Only extremely small amounts should be isolated.

Preparation—Pentaerythritol is added to 98% nitric acid while maintaining the temperature by agitation and cooling so that it does not exceed 20°.

After washing with water and sodium carbonate solution, the initial product is crystallized from aqueous acetone. The pentaerythritol is usually made by reacting acetaldehyde with formaldehyde in the presence of calcium or sodium hydroxide.

Description—A white to ivory colored powder having a faint, mild odor.

Solubility—Soluble in acetone; slightly soluble in alcohol and ether; practically insoluble in water.

Uses—Pentaerythritol Tetranitrate slowly releases nitrite ions in the body. The nitrite ion induces vasodilation and reduced cardiac work (see the general statement, page 855). The Tetranitrate is much longer acting than nitroglycerin but slower in onset. Hence it is useful in the prophylaxis of attacks of *angina pectoris* but not in the management of the acute attack. It is of no value in the management of hypertension. Transient headache and nausea may accompany its use; thus far, methemoglobinemia has not been observed, but there is every reason to expect that this action, common to all other organic nitrates and nitrites, is possible. It is not absorbed sublingually. Tolerance may develop; it can be remitted by withholding the drug for 1 to 2 weeks.

Dose (pentaerythritol tetranitrate)—**10 to 20 mg;** *usual,* **10 mg** 3 or 4 times a day.

Dosage Forms—Diluted NF: 7 to 35% concentrations; Extended-Release Oral Solid: 30 and 80 mg; Tablets NF: 10 and 20 mg.

Propranolol Hydrochloride—see page 910.

Trolnitrate Phosphate

[Aminotrate Phosphate; Triethanolamine Trinitrate Diphosphate; Metamine (*Pfizer*); Nitretamine (*Squibb*)]

$$\left[HN \begin{array}{c} CH_2CH_2ONO_2 \\ CH_2CH_2ONO_2 \\ CH_2CH_2ONO_2 \end{array} \right] H_2PO_4^-\cdot H_3PO_4$$

Trolnitrate Phosphate [$C_6H_{12}N_4O_9.2H_3PO_4$] is 2,2′,2″-nitrilotriethanol trinitrate (ester) phosphate (1:2) (salt).

Description—A colorless, crystalline powder. It undergoes hydrolytic decomposition if exposed to moist air. Explosions have been experienced while handling and storing the undiluted compound. Under anhydrous conditions the purified compound appears to be quite stable. It melts with decomposition between 101° and 103°.

Solubility—Soluble in alcohol; insoluble in ether and chloroform; dissociates in water with the liberation of phosphoric acid and the formation of an insoluble oil, trinitrotriethanolamine, which is soluble in chloroform, ether, and alcohol.

Uses—Trolnitrate Phosphate produces a mild prolonged relaxation of smooth muscle, especially of the coronary vessels and certain other vascular beds. It does not lower blood pressure or induce reflex tachycardia. Its toxicity is the same as that of the other organic nitrates and nitrites which are used as coronary dilators, but is much less frequent. The main use of trolnitrate is the prophylaxis of attacks of *angina pectoris.* Trolnitrate is irritating and hence is not administered sublingually. Like other nitrates, tolerance can develop.

Dose—*Oral,* 8 to **16 mg** in 4 divided doses; 3 to 7 days may be required for its maximal effect.

Dosage Forms—Extended-Release Oral Solid: 10 mg; Tablets: 2 and 10 mg.

Other Coronary Drugs

Dipyridamole [2,2′,2″,2‴-(4,8-Dipiperidinopyrimidino-[5,4-*d*]pyrimidine-2,6-diyldinitrilo)tetraethanol; $C_{24}H_{40}N_8$-O_4; Persantin (*Geigy*)]—*Uses:* marketed as a coronary dilator. Although it can induce coronary dilatation after intravenous administration, it does not do so after oral administration, which is the route for which the commercial item is prepared. In carefully conducted clinical studies, the drug has been shown to be no better than a placebo. *Dose:* orally, 25 to 50 mg 2 or 3 times daily.

Isosorbide Dinitrate [1,4:3,6-dianhydrosorbitol 2,5-dinitrate; $C_6H_8N_2O_8$; Isordil (*Ives*); Sorbitrate (*Stuart*)]—*Uses:* an organonitrate coronary vasodilator and is thus used in the management of *coronary insufficiency* and *angina pectoris*. It has a latency of 30 to 45 minutes after oral ingestion; its effects last 4 to 5 hours. It is thus intended for prophylaxis rather than for relief of the acute anginal attack. Initial reports on the efficacy of isosorbide dinitrate were favorable, but later clinical studies have raised doubts about initial findings. It must be kept in mind that the psychological effects of the trial of a new drug in patients with angina invariably bring about improvement. The status of isosorbide has yet to be determined. *Dose: oral,* 10 to 40 mg 4 times a day; *sublingual,* 5 to 40 mg 4 times a day.

Prenylamine [*N*-(3,3-Diphenylpropyl)-α-methylphenethylamine; $C_{24}H_{27}N$]—*Uses:* used in the treatment of *angina pectoris.* Its action is relatively long, and the drug appears from preliminary studies to be roughly equivalent to pentaerythritol tetranitrate. When used in conjunction with nitroglycerin, the consumption of nitroglycerin tablets is diminished. The mechanism of action of prenylamine is not clear. In dogs, coronary flow is increased. However, the drug also diminishes the content of tissue catecholamines, which may result in an adrenergic neuronal block of cardiac sympathetics. The resulting decrease in cardiac work could also give relief of anginal pain. *Dose: oral,* 90 mg initially 3 times a day, then 2 times a day for maintenance.

Digitaloid Drugs

The digitaloid drugs are frequently referred to as cardiac glycosides or simply as digitalis. However, not all are glycosides, nor are they all derived from species of digitalis. But the aglycones, which are the noncarbohydrate portions of glycoside molecules (see page 474), are all chemically similar, and the actions of the various digitaloid agents are nearly identical except for onset and duration. These *cardiotonics* increase the strength of contraction of the heart muscle. These drugs are used mainly in the treatment of *congestive heart failure* and they are unexcelled in this use. In higher doses they may induce heart block. They may be used in the treatment of *atrial flutter* and *fibrillation* to prevent the majority of too frequent atrial impulses from reaching the ventricle. They may also induce nausea and vomiting, various neuralgic pains, headache, fatigue, drowsiness and rarely hallucinations or convulsions. They may occasionally induce ominous ventricular arrhythmias. Because of the clinical and historical importance of digitalis and its service as a prototype, it is considered in detail on page 858.

Acetyldigitoxin NF

[α-Digitoxin Monoacetate; Acylanid (*Sandoz*)]

$C_{18}H_{30}O_9$—$COCH_3$
(acetyltridigitoxose)

Acetyldigitoxin contains 95.0–100.5% of $C_{43}H_{66}O_{14}$ (807.00), calculated on the dried basis.

Caution—Acetyldigitoxin is extremely poisonous.

Acetyldigitoxin is the α-form of a glycoside known as β-acetyldigitoxin. The latter occurs naturally in *Digitalis ferruginea* and can also be derived from lanatoside A, a glycoside present in *Digitalis lanata*, by enzymatic cleavage of the terminal (glucose) component of its carbohydrate moiety. In their structure, both acetyldigitoxins differ from digitoxin (page 861) only in that the terminal digitoxose residue is monoacetylated. The α and β forms differ in the locus of the acetyl on the digitoxose residue, and the β form can be caused to rearrange to the α form by heating suitably prepared solutions. US Pat. 2,776,963.

Description—A white, odorless, microcrystalline powder which melts between 217° and 221° and is hygroscopic. It displays a specific rotation $[\alpha]_D^{20}$ of +5.0° when measured using a solution containing 0.7 Gm/100 ml pyridine.

Solubility—Soluble in methanol; sparingly soluble in chloroform; slightly soluble in alcohol; practically insoluble in water.

Uses—Acetyldigitoxin is a digitaloid drug and as such has the same general actions and uses as *Digitoxin* (page 861). See also the uses under *Digitalis* (page 859). However, its onset and duration of action are much shorter than those of digitoxin. The drug is administered orally. About ⅔ of an oral dose is absorbed.

Dose—*Rapid digitalization,* **1.6** to **2.2 mg;** *usual, initial,* **1.8 mg** in 1 dose or several divided doses given within 24 hours; *slow digitalization,* **1.8** to **3.2 mg;** *usual, initial,* **2.4 mg** in divided doses given over a period of 2 to 6 days; *maintenance,* **100** to **200 mcg;** *usual,* **150 mcg** per day.

Dosage Forms—Tablets NF: 100 and 200 mcg.

Deslanoside USP

[Desacetyl-lanatoside C; Cedilanid D (*Sandoz*)]

$C_{18}H_{30}O_9$—$C_6H_{11}O_5$
(tridigitoxose)   (glucose)

Deslanoside is desacetyl lanatoside C. It contains 95.0–100.5% of $C_{47}H_{74}O_{19}$; (943.10), calculated on the dried basis.

Deslanoside's side chain consists of 3 molecules of digitoxose and 1 molecule of glucose in glycosidic linkage. Hydrolysis yields the aglycone, digoxigenin ($C_{23}H_{34}O_5$).

Preparation—It may be prepared by deacetylating Lanatoside C, *qv*, by treatment with alkali.

Description—Colorless or white crystals or a white, crystalline, odorless powder. It is hygroscopic, absorbing about 7% of moisture when exposed to air. Melts indistinctly between 220° and 235°. The specific rotation of a 2% solution in anhydrous pyridine, calculated on the dried basis, is between +7.0° and +8.5°.

Solubility—Very slightly soluble in water; 1 Gm dissolves in about 300 ml of alcohol and in about 200 ml of methanol; very slightly soluble in chloroform.

Uses—The *cardiotonic* actions and uses of Deslanoside are essentially the same as those of lanatoside C; even the dose and duration of action are the same; its latency by the intravenous route is about ten minutes. For intravenous administration its greater stability and solubility give it advantages over lanatoside C injection.

Dose—*Usual, intramuscular* or *intravenous*, for *digitalization*, **1** to **1.6 mg** in ½ day; *usual*, **1.6 mg**, in 1 or 2 doses.

Other Dose Information—The above dose corresponds to the initial dose. The usual maintenance dose is 400 mcg.

Caution—*Handle Deslanoside with exceptional care, since it is highly potent.*

Dosage Forms—Injection USP: 400 mcg/2 ml, 800 mcg/4 ml.

Digitalis USP

[Foxglove; Digitalis folium; Digitalis Leaf; Fairy Cap; Lady's Glove, Fingers, Thimbles, or Bells; Digifortis (*Parke-Davis*); Digitora (*Upjohn*)]

Digitalis is the dried leaf of *Digitalis purpurea* Linné (Fam. *Scrophulariaceæ*).

The potency of Digitalis is such that, when assayed as directed, 100 mg is equivalent to not less than 1 USP Digitalis Unit. One *United States Pharmacopeial Digitalis Unit* represents the potency of 100 mg of the USP Digitalis Reference Standard.

Note—*When Digitalis is prescribed, Powdered Digitalis is to be dispensed.*

History—The common name Foxglove is a corruption of an old vernacular name "foxes glew" which meant "foxes music." The Norwegian name means "fox bells." The German name "fingerhut" means thimble, and Füches, a German botanist of the sixteenth century, Latinized this name as Digitalis. It was first official in the London Pharmacopœia of 1650. Its later extensive use in medicine arose from the publicity given it by Dr. William Withering, Birmingham, England, in 1785. It was used as a diuretic for the treatment of dropsy, the importance of a cardiotonic action for this use not having been recognized.

Constituents—Digitalis has been the subject of long and exhaustive investigation. The constituents which are now recognized as being of the greatest importance as cardiovascular agents are *digitoxin* [$C_{41}H_{64}O_{13}$], *gitoxin* [$C_{41}H_{64}O_{14}$], *digoxin* [also $C_{41}H_{64}O_{14}$], and *lanatoside C* [$C_{49}H_{76}O_{20}$]. The latter two are obtained from *Digitalis lanata*. Digitoxin (the most active principle), Digoxin, and Lanatoside C are official. The *French Digitaline* of Nativelle (*Homolle's digitalin*) consists chiefly of digitoxin and is very active.

Digitonin, or *digitin* [$C_{56}H_{92}O_{29}$], a saponin-like glycoside of digitalis, is practically devoid of digitalis action but is widely used as a reagent for the determination of cholesterol. It is a specific precipitant for steroids having a 3-hydroxyl group with the β configuration as long as they do not contain a methyl group with an epi configuration at C_{10}.

Other constituents of digitalis are *digitoflavin*, *digitophyllin*, fat etc. *German digitalin* is a purified mixture of the glycosides of digitalis seed. It is soluble in water but is much less active than French digitaline or Nativelle. *Digitalin True (Schmiedeberg's Digitaline* or *Digitalinum Verum Kiliani*) originally assumed to be a pure, individual principle, was probably also somewhat of a mixture of the glycosides from the seed of *Digitalis purpurea*.

Uses—The chief therapeutic use for Digitalis is in the treatment of *congestive heart failure*. It is of value regardless of whether the failure is predominantly of the right or left side of the heart. Arrhythmias and valvular defects may modify the response to Digitalis, but their presence neither indicates nor contraindicates the use of the drug. However, it is generally true that the most dramatic responses are seen in patients with *both auricular fibrillation and congestive heart failure*. Badly damaged hearts do not respond well. When the failure is due to an acute toxic or infectious process, like typhoid fever or diphtheritic myocarditis, rather than to a chronic degenerative process like arteriosclerosis or failure secondary to hypertensive heart disease, Digitalis may give poor results and may even be contraindicated. Congestive failure in patients with myxedema, hyperthyroidism, and thiamine deficiency is likewise not much benefited. Also, heart failure secondary to cardiovascular syphilis yields poorly to Digitalis therapy. Digitalis may be indicated in peripheral circulatory collapse, shock, etc.

The mechanism by which Digitalis and all allied cardiac glycosides exert beneficial effects on the failing heart is identical, namely, a direct *cardiotonic action* on the myocardium to increase the force of contraction and to increase cardiac tone. Concomitantly the refractory period of cardiac muscle is prolonged, the muscle is less excitable to abnormally frequent impulses transmitted over the conduction system, and the improved coronary blood supply which comes in the wake of a compensated circulation improves the nutrition and strength of the heart. Slowing of the cardiac rate occurs only when the rate was originally rapid due to the failure. When the failure is abolished, there is no longer any need for the compensatory tachycardia and consequently the heart rate slows to normal. This slowing has mistakenly been attributed to a "vagal action" of Digitalis. The toxic dose of Digitalis may slow the heart by a direct action on auriculoventricular conduction or on the sino-auricular node. Toxic doses also give rise to serious ventricular arrhythmias.

The signs and symptoms of heart failure are in large measure abolished by Digitalis, but bed rest, sedatives, and often diuretics and restriction of salt intake may be required to obtain best results. Exertional and paroxysmal nocturnal dyspnea disappears; cough, cyanosis, ascites, edema, and chronic passive congestion of the lungs and abdominal viscera are relieved; the enlarged diastolic size of the heart is decreased; engorged veins due to increased venous pressure are returned to normal; cardiac output, stroke volume, and circulatory velocity are enhanced; and the diastolic rest period in each cardiac cycle is prolonged. All this is accomplished by the direct action of Digitalis or its allied cardiac glycosides on the heart muscle, an action which tends to make the heart a more efficient pump. Digitalis is not a true diuretic, even though it increases urine flow and abolishes edema. It acts to improve the circulation so that the mechanism of edema formation no longer operates. It also relieves chronic passive congestion of the kidneys and permits more normal renal function.

Once Digitalis is required to alleviate congestive heart failure, it must usually be taken for the remainder of one's life. There is some evidence that elderly people with arteriosclerosis or hypertension who sooner or later develop heart failure may be benefited by the prophylactic use of Digitalis. In patients with atrial fibrillation, the indication for the use of Digitalis rests not on the arrhythmia but on the presence or absence of congestive failure. Digitalis glycosides do not cure the arrhythmia, but they improve the heart and abolish the failure. The atrial fibrillation usually persists. Even if atrial fibrillation is not abolished, heart block may decrease the ventricular rate toward a more optimal value. In an occasional case of auricular flutter, the proper use of fairly large doses of Digitalis may abolish the arrhythmia. Digitalis also occasionally stops attacks of paroxysmal tachycardia. In the presence of acute coronary thrombosis, Digitalis must be used with caution and then in reduced amounts. The presence of angina pectoris is not a deciding factor in itself as to whether Digitalis is indicated in any particular patient.

The choice of preparation in the administration of digitalis offers considerable difficulty to many practitioners. Both the official purified glycosides and the USP Powdered Digitalis will produce excellent results in the majority of cases. The major instances in which the galenical preparations are not adequate are the rare cases in which intravenous therapy is essential. Both the crude digitalis preparations and purified digitoxin are adequately absorbed after oral administration, and the latter is now only slightly more expensive. When other purified digitalis glycosides are substituted for galenical preparations, their incomplete absorption after oral administration must be taken into consideration. When absorbed in adequate amounts, all the active digitalis principles produce identical effects on the myocardium, and their toxic effects are essentially the same. They differ from each other largely in speed of onset of action and duration of cardiac effects.

Although the purified principles make acceptable digitalis preparations, their action on the heart is no different from that obtainable by the use of digitalis powder itself. The active principles are no less toxic.

The *lanatosides*, native glycosides derived from *Digitalis lanata*, do not differ in any essential respect from similar glycosides of *Digitalis purpurea*, and in fact both groups share two glycosides in common, namely, digitoxin and gitoxin. In addition, each group yields one distinctive glycoside as follows: gitalin, in the case of *D. purpurea;* digoxin, in the case of *D. lanata*. It is digilanid C, called lanatoside C, which yields digoxin, and the claim that lanatoside C is a unique, more effective, and safer cardiac principle is entirely unfounded. While it is true that the mixture of digilanids A, B, and C is an acceptable Digitalis preparation for oral use, the claims for lanatoside C itself are exaggerated. Being soluble, it can be employed parenterally and in this respect deserves to be placed in the same category as ouabain and strophanthin. It is also true that, being a pure crystalline principle, it can be assayed gravimetrically. This is no great advantage over bio-assay, however, due to the fact that the dose of Digitalis varies considerably from patient to patient and therefore clinical assay must be performed in each patient.

Digitalis leaf is used for making the various digitalis preparations; also for the production of digitoxin. Ordinary powdered digitalis leaf should not be dispensed on prescriptions; instead only the official standardized *Powdered Digitalis* should be used.

Dose—*Initial*, 1 to 2 **Gm** in 1 or 2 days; *usual*, **1.5 Gm** divided over 24 to 48 hours; *maintenance*, **100** to **200 mg** daily; *usual*, **100 mg** once a day.

Other Dose Information—Two types of Digitalis dosage are recognized, initial dose for digitalization, and maintenance dose for chronic therapy. Initial digitalization may be accomplished rapidly or slowly, depending on the urgency of the case. The vast majority of patients with congestive heart failure are not *in extremis* and can be digitalized over a period of several days to a week. Digitalization is usually complete when the patient has ingested the equivalent of a total of 1.2 Gm (12 USP Units) of powdered Digitalis in a period of 48 to 96 hours. This amount can be divided into several equal daily doses, and the total daily dose is usually divided into two or three equal amounts. For example, one USP unit may be taken three times daily with meals for four days, at the end of which time full digitalis effects will usually be evident. A larger increment of the digitalizing dose may have to be given at one time if the case requires, and it is not unusual to digitalize a patient in 12 or 24 hours by giving half the calculated dose at once, and the remainder in two or three divided doses at intervals of 6 hours. No fixed formula or rule of thumb can be employed. Each case is a law in itself, and the physician must constantly watch his patient to observe the developing effects of the drug, and to prevent unpleasant or serious toxic effects from overdosage. Usually the patient should be seen immediately before an additional dose is given, when the rapid method of digitalization is employed.

In rare cases it may be necessary to inject intravenously ouabain, strophanthin, deslanoside, or some other purified parenteral preparation in order to save life. Such patients are usually *in extremis* and may die before Digitalis given by mouth can exert its effect (within 2 hours). Small doses are employed as a rule and digitalization with an orally efficacious preparation is then completed by the oral route.

By maintenance dose is meant that daily dose which will give optimal digitalis effects and replace the glycoside which is constantly being destroyed or excreted. Optimal effects can be obtained without toxic effects, and the optimal dose is not necessarily the largest tolerated dose. It can be found only by careful observation of the patient.

Dosage Forms—Powdered Digitalis USP (see below); Capsules NF: 60 and 100 mg; Tablets USP: 30, 50, 55, 60, 83, and 100 mg.

Powdered Digitalis USP [Prepared Digitalis] is digitalis dried at a temperature not exceeding 60°, reduced to a fine or a very fine powder, and adjusted, if necessary, to conform to the official potency by admixture with sufficient lactose, starch, or exhausted marc of digitalis, or with a powdered digitalis having either a lower or a higher potency. The potency of Powdered Digitalis is such that, when assayed as directed, 100 mg is equivalent to 1 USP Digitalis Unit. *Note—When Digitalis is prescribed, Powdered Digitalis is to be dispensed. Dose: See Digitalis. Veterinary Dose: Horses, 1 to 15 Gm; Dogs, 15 to 200 mg.* Orally, it is emetic in cats but valueless in ruminants.

Digitoxin USP

[Crystodigin (*Lilly*); Digitaline Nativelle (*Fougera*); Myodigin (*Davies-Rose*); Purodigin (*Wyeth*)]

(tridigitoxose)

Digitoxin is a cardiotonic glycoside obtained from *Digitalis purpurea* Linné, *Digitalis lanata* Ehrh, and other suitable species of *Digitalis*. Digitoxin contains 90.0–101.0% of $C_{41}H_{64}O_{13}$ (764.96), calculated on the dried basis.

The side chain of Digitoxin consists of 3 molecules of digitoxose in glycosidic linkage. Removal of the side chain by hydrolysis yields the aglycone, digitoxigenin ($C_{23}H_{34}O_4$).

Description—A white or pale buff, odorless, micro-crystalline powder. Pure digitoxin has a specific rotation of $+18°$ to $+19°$ in chloroform solution.

Solubility—Insoluble in water; 1 Gm dissolves in about 150 ml of alcohol or 40 ml of chloroform; very slightly soluble in ether.

Uses—Digitoxin is the primary active glycosidal constituent of USP digitalis and consequently its absorption, cumulative properties, duration of action, and therapeutic effects are essentially the same as for digitalis itself. It is by far the most commonly employed purified glycoside of digitalis and is now only slightly more expensive, dose for dose, than the powdered leaf. It has the theoretical advantage of greater accuracy of dosage because it is a pure substance, but the wide variations in the responses of different patients to any of the digitalis glycosides or galenical preparations make it necessary to adapt the dose of Digitoxin to each individual patient treated, by a process of trial and error. The reduced gastrointestinal irritant property of Digitoxin as compared to crude digitalis is not an important factor except when a single, full digitalizing dose is administered orally. Digitoxin is almost completely absorbed after oral administration.

Dose—*Initial*, 1 to 1.5 mg divided over 24 to 48 hours; *usual, initial*, **1.5 mg**; *maintenance*, **100 to 200 mcg** daily; *usual, maintenance*, **100 mcg** once a day.

Other Dose Information—The practice of giving a single fixed digitalizing dose of 1.2 mg of Digitoxin is not recommended. Few patients require such rapid digitalization; although this is approximately the average dose required, it is inadequate for some cases and causes overdigitalization in other patients.

Dosage Forms—Injection NF: 100 and 200 mcg/ml; Tablets USP: 50, 100, 150, and 200 mcg.

Caution—Handle Digitoxin with exceptional care, since it is highly potent.

Veterinary Dose—*Oral, total digitalization, Dogs,* **0.14 mg** per **10 pounds** of body weight; *maintenance,* may vary from $\frac{1}{10}$ to $\frac{1}{5}$ of the digitalization dose; *intravenous*, **0.14 mg** per **10 pounds** of body weight; $\frac{1}{2}$ the calculated digitalization dose may be given at once and injections of $\frac{1}{10}$ to $\frac{1}{8}$ the digitalization dose may be continued at 2-hour intervals, if necessary.

Digoxin USP

[Davoxin (*Davies-Rose*); Lanoxin (*Burroughs-Wellcome*)]

(tridigitoxose)

Digoxin is a cardiotonic glycoside obtained from the leaves of *Digitalis lanata* Ehrh. (Fam. *Scrophulariaceae*). Digoxin contains 96.0–101.0% of $C_{41}H_{64}O_{14}$ (780.96), calculated on the dried basis.

The side chain of Digoxin consists of 3 molecules of digitoxose in glycosidic linkage. Hydrolytic cleavage yields the aglycone, digoxigenin ($C_{23}H_{34}O_5$).

Description—Clear to white crystals or a white crystalline powder. It is odorless. Its specific rotation at 546.1 mμ, $[\alpha]^{25}$, in anhydrous pyridine solution is between $+13.6°$ and $+14.2°$. It melts with decomposition above 235°.

Solubility—Digoxin is insoluble in water, chloroform, or ether, but is freely soluble in pyridine and also soluble in dilute alcohol.

Uses—The *cardiotonic* actions and uses of Digoxin are similar to those of USP digitalis. Because it is a purified preparation, it is frequently used intravenously for very rapid digitalization. Intravenously its action becomes manifest in 5 to 30 minutes. Orally its action is manifest within a few hours. Its duration of action is one-seventh to one-third as long as that of digitoxin. Consequently, with Digoxin, merely by interrupting therapy, it is easier to correct over-digitalization than with digitalis or digitoxin; but, by the same token, it is easier to lose control of digitalization if a dose is missed. Considerable attention to appropriate spacing of maintenance doses is required for smooth digitalization.

Dose—*Oral: initial*, **750 mcg to 3 mg** in 1 day; *usual*, **2 to 3 mg**, divided over 24 hours; *maintenance*, **250 mcg to 1 mg** daily; *usual*, **250 mcg** 1 to 3 times a day. *Intramuscular, or intravenous: initial*, **500 mcg to 2 mg** in $\frac{1}{2}$ day; *usual*, **500 mcg to 1.5 mg**, divided over 12 hours; *maintenance*, **250 to 500 mcg** daily; *usual*, **250 mcg** 1 or 2 times a day.

Dosage Forms—Elixir USP; Injection USP: 500 mcg/2 ml.

Veterinary Dose (*total digitalization*)—Oral, Horses, **3 mg** per **100 pounds** of body weight; Dogs, **0.03 to 0.1 mg** per **pound** of body weight. *Intravenous*, Cattle, **0.4 mg** per **100 pounds** of body weight; Dogs, **0.02 to 0.03 mg** per **pound** of body weight.

Gitalin NF

[Gitalgin (*Schering*)]

Gitalin is a cardiotonic glycosidal constituent obtained from *Digitalis purpurea* Linné (Fam. *Scrophulariaceæ*). It contains 13.0–19.0% of gitoxin, 13.0–19.0% of gitaloxin, and 14.0–20.0% of digitoxin, calculated on the dried basis.

Preparation—A cold-water extract of *Digitalis purpurea* is purified and evaporated to dryness. The residue (Gitalin) consists of the cardioactive glycosides gitaloxin (16-formylgitoxin), gitoxin, and digitoxin, with smaller amounts of strospeside, formylstrospeside, odoroside H, and aglycones, together with other natural solubilizing substances. A review of the preparation and composition of Gitalin is available in the literature.[2]

Description—A white or pale buff, amorphous powder. It decomposes with liquefaction between 120° and 150°.

Solubility—Slightly soluble in water; freely soluble in acetone, alcohol, chloroform, and ether.

Uses—The actions and uses are essentially identical to those of *Digitalis* (page 859). It differs from digitalis and digitoxin in that its onset of action is more prompt and its duration of action is shorter. The short duration of action is an advantage when toxicity occurs. The drug is only administered by the oral route; it is well absorbed.

Dose—*Usual, initial, rapid digitalization*, **2.5 mg.** followed by **750 mcg** every 6 hours until therapeutic effect or toxicity develops, with a total dose of about 6 mg being given in 24 hours; *slow digitalization*, **1.5 mg** daily for 4 to 6 days; *maintenance*, **250 mcg** to **1.25 mg** daily; *usual*, **0.5 mg** daily.

Dosage Forms—Tablets NF: 500 mcg.

Lanatoside C NF

[Digilanide C; Cedilanid (*Sandoz*)]

$(C_6H_{10}O_3)_2 - C_8H_{12}O_4 - C_6H_{11}O_5$

(digitoxose)₂ (acetyl- (glucose)
digitoxose)

Lanatoside C contains 98.0–102.0% of $C_{49}H_{76}O_{20}$ (985.14), calculated on the dried basis.

Caution—Lanatoside C is extremely poisonous.

Lanatoside C is a glycoside obtained from the leaves of *Digitalis lanata* Ehrhart (Fam. *Scrophulariaceæ*). Its aglycone is identical with that of digoxin.

Description—Colorless or white crystals or a white crystalline powder. It is odorless. Lanatoside C is hygroscopic and will absorb about 7% of water on exposure to air. Its $[\alpha]_D^{20}$ in methanol solution is between +32.0° and +34.5°. It melts indistinctly, and with decomposition at about 240°.

Solubility—Insoluble in water; 1 Gm dissolves in about 45 ml of alcohol, 20 ml of methanol, and about 2000 ml of chloroform; soluble in pyridine and dioxane; practically insoluble in ether and solvent hexane.

Uses—Lanatoside C has the same *cardiotonic* uses as official galenical preparations of *Digitalis purpurea* but is usually employed orally, inasmuch as it is water-insoluble. A specially compounded injection is available, however, which is administered in certain rare cardiac emergencies by intravenous injection, in a manner similar to ouabain and strophanthin, over which it has no compelling advantages. For a complete discussion of the actions and uses of digitaloids, and the principles governing the choice of preparations, see *Digitalis*.

Dose—*Usual, initial,* **7.5** to **10 mg;** *maintenance,* **0.5** to **1.5 mg.**

Dosage Forms—Tablets NF: 500 mcg.

Ouabain USP

[G-Strophanthin]

Ouabain contains 95.0–100.5% of $C_{29}H_{44}O_{12} \cdot 8H_2O$ (728.79).

Caution—Ouabain is extremely poisonous.

It is a glycoside obtained from the seeds of *Strophanthus gratus* (Wall. et Hook.) Baillon and from the wood of *Acokanthera Schimperi* (A. DC.) Schwf. (Fam. *Apocynaceæ*). The side chain of Ouabain consists of a molecule of rhamnose in glycosidic linkage. Hydrolytic cleavage yields the aglycone, oubagenin ($C_{23}H_{34}O_8$).

Description—White, odorless crystals, or a crystalline powder. It is stable in air, but is affected by light. Its solutions are neutral to litmus paper. It melts indistinctly and with decomposition at about 190°. The specific rotation, $[\alpha]_D^{25}$, of anhydrous Ouabain in aqueous solution is between −31° and −32.5°.

Solubility—1 Gm dissolves slowly in about 75 ml of water, and in about 100 ml of alcohol; more soluble in hot water and in hot alcohol.

Uses—This *cardiotonic* glycoside has actions on the heart identical to those exhibited by digitalis (page 859). Its oral use is unsafe because of its slow and irregular absorption from the gastrointestinal tract. Being water soluble, its chief use is for parenteral administration when rapid digitalis-like effects are desired with *congestive heart failure in extremis*. The actions and uses of the cardiotonic glycosides and the choice of preparations are discussed under Digitalis.

Dose—*Usual, intravenous,* for digitalization, **500 mcg** to **1 mg,** divided over 24 hours.

Other Dose Information—The dose of Ouabain varies from 0.1 to 1 mg, repeated if necessary, depending on the urgency of the case, and digitalization is usually completed by the oral route. The precautions to be observed are outlined under *Digitalis*, page 859.

Dosage Forms—Injection USP: 1 and 2 ml.

Veterinary Dose (*total digitalization*)—*Intravenous, Horses,* **0.6** to **1 mg** per **100 pounds** of body weight in fractional doses at 2-hour intervals with total dose maximum of 10 mg; *Cattle,* **0.6** to **1 mg** per **100 pounds** of body weight repeated after 24 to 36 hours; *Dogs,* **0.01** to **0.015 mg** per **pound** of body weight repeated at 24- to 36-hour intervals for 3 to 5 days followed by *oral maintenance* with digoxin. Careful supervision for evidence of toxicity during both initial and maintenance therapy is required.

Other Digitaloid Drugs

Digilanid (*Sandoz*)—A mixture of the isomorphous crystallized cardioactive glycosides, lanatoside-A (47%), lanatoside-B (16%), and lanatoside-C (37%), obtained by extraction of the wet leaves of *Digitalis lanata*. *Uses:* for increasing myocardial contractility in patients with congestive heart failure; in the treatment of auricular fibrillation to slow the ventricular rate by inducing heart block. *Dose:*

nitial *oral* dose 0.67 to 1.33 mg daily until the desired effect s obtained, then a maintenance dose of 0.33 to 0.67 mg daily. *Intravenously*, 0.8 mg given slowly, or intramuscu-larly, 0.8 mg, in 1 or 2 divided doses at least 12 hours apart; maintenance should be oral. The same precautions should be observed as when giving any digitalis preparations.

Antiarrhythmic Drugs

Cardiac arrhythmias may result from disturbances in pacemaker function of the *sinoatrial node,* from altera-tions in conduction path and velocity, so that heart block or a self-perpetuating "circus rhythm" occurs, or from activation of dormant pacemakers outside of the sinus node. Arrhythmias originating at the sinoatrial node may be tachycardia, bradycardia, and even cardiac arrest. Autonomic drugs are usually sufficient to manage such arrhythmias. For example, sinus tachycardia may be slowed by reflex action resulting from the pressor effects of certain vasoconstrictors, usually sympathomimetics which lack significant direct actions on the heart (see Chapter 48, page 881), or they may be slowed directly by cholinergic drugs. Sym-pathomimetics are also used to revive an arrested heart and to relieve certain types of heart block. Circus rhythms include certain tachycardias, some atrial flutters and some atrial fibrillations. Circus rhythm may be terminated by drugs that increase atrial con-duction velocity (digitalis) so that the circular-moving wave of excitation catches up with itself and thus dies in its own refractory zone, or by *cardiac depressants* that increase the refractory period of the heart muscle (procainamide, etc). Aberrant pacemakers, or ectopic foci, give rise to certain atrial tachycardias, some atrial flutters, some atrial fibrillations, nodal rhythms, ventricular tachycardias, ventricular extrasystoles, and ventricular fibrillation. They may be suppressed by drugs (quinidine, procainamide, etc) that decrease the myocardial excitability and increase the refractory period. Digitalis is also used to invoke heart block in unmanageable cases of atrial tachycardia, flutter, and fibrillation, so that the ventricle is not overwhelmed with impulses of atrial origin.

Digitalis and Digitaloid Drugs—see pages 858–863.

Diphenylhydantoin—see page 1099.

Ephedrine Sulfate—see page 855.

Epinephrine—see pages 886 and 887.

Ethaverine—see page 855.

Hydroxyamphetamine Hydrobromide—see page 887.

Hydroxyzine Hydrochloride—see page 1093.

Hydroxyzine Pamoate—see page 1093.

Isoproterenol—see page 888.

Lidocaine—see page 1071.

Methacholine Chloride—see page 901.

Methoxamine Hydrochloride—see page 891.

Papaverine Hydrochloride—see page 854.

Phenylephrine Hydrochloride—see page 893.

Procainamide Hydrochloride USP

[*p*-Amino-*N*-[2-(diethylamino)ethyl]benzamide Monohydrochloride; Pron-estyl Hydrochloride (*Squibb*)]

$$\left[NH_2-\!\!\!\bigcirc\!\!\!-CONH-CH_2CH_2-\overset{H}{\underset{}{N}}{}^{+}(C_2H_5)_2 \right] Cl^{-}$$

Procainamide Hydrochloride contains 98.0–100.5% of $C_{13}H_{21}N_3O \cdot HCl$ (271.79), calculated on the dried basis.

Preparation—Among other ways, procainamide (base) may be prepared by condensing *p*-nitrobenzoyl chloride with β-diethylaminoethylamine and then re-ducing the nitro group to amino by any of the usual methods. The hydrochloride forms readily when a stream of hydrogen chloride is passed into a solution of the base in an appropriate organic solvent.

Description—A white to tan, crystalline powder. It is odorless. Its 1 in 10 solution has a pH between 5 and 6.5. Melting range between 165° and 169°. Chemically it dif-fers from procaine only in having an amide linkage (—CO-NH—) instead of the ester structure (—COOR).

Solubility—Very soluble in water; soluble in alcohol; slightly soluble in chloroform; very slightly soluble in ben-zene and in ether.

Uses—Procainamide is an antiarrhythmic and anti-fibrillatory agent. Its *cardiac depressant* effects are essentially identical to those of *Quinidine* (page 864). Myocardial excitability is depressed, conduction is slowed, and the refractory period, particularly that of the atrium, is increased. Procainamide is useful in *arrhythmias* of ventricular origin, including ventricular extrasystoles, paroxysmal ventricular tachycardia, and ventricular fibrillation. Although less satisfactory re-sults have been obtained in cases of atrial arrhythmias, the drug is also effective in paroxysmal atrial tachy-cardia, atrial flutter, and atrial fibrillation. In cases of paroxysmal atrial tachycardia, other measures and agents of choice should be employed before Procain-amide is tried. Many cardiologists employ Procain-amide and quinidine interchangeably. However, either drug may be effective in an individual patient who has failed to respond to maximally tolerated doses of the other agent.

Procainamide is usually well tolerated. Gastro-intestinal distress may be noted when the drug is given orally, and hypotension almost invariably occurs when the intravenous route is employed. Hypersensitivity to the drug has been reported and fatal agranulocytosis has occurred. Cross sensitivity to procaine and related drugs should be anticipated. In addition, untoward responses may result from actions of the drug on an abnormal myocardium, such as ventricular asystole or fibrillation in patients with marked disturbances of atrioventricular conduction.

Dose—*Oral* or *intramuscular,* **500 mg** to **6 Gm** daily; *usual,* **500 mg** to **1 Gm** 4 to 6 times a day *intravenous,* **50 mg** to **1 Gm** daily; *usual,* **50 to 100 mg** per minute up to a total dose of 1 Gm.

Other Dose Information—The usual oral dose in cases of ventricular arrhythmias is 500 mg to 1.0 Gm at intervals of 3 to 6 hours. Larger doses are required in cases of atrial arrhythmias, and 500 mg to 1.0 Gm may be administered every 2 hours to the limit of tolerance or until the arrhythmia is interrupted. Parenteral medication may be employed if necessary. The intramuscular dose is 500 mg to 1.0 Gm, repeated every 6 hours. It should not be administered intravenously faster than 25 to 50 mg per minute.

Dosage Forms—Capsules USP: 250 and 500 mg; Injection USP: 10 ml.

Propranolol Hydrochloride—see page 910.

Quinidine Gluconate USP

[Quinidine Monogluconate (Salt); Quinaglute (*Cooper*)]

Quinidine Gluconate is the gluconate of an alkaloid that may be obtained from various species of *Cinchona* and their hybrids, or from *Remijia pedunculata* Flückiger (Fam. *Rubiaceæ*), or prepared from quinine. Quinidine Gluconate contains 99.0–100.5% of $C_{20}H_{24}$-$N_2O_2 \cdot C_6H_{12}O_7$ (520.58), calculated on the dried basis. For the structure of quinidine, see page 494.

Description—A white powder. It is odorless and has a very bitter taste.

Solubility—Freely soluble in water; only slightly soluble in alcohol.

Uses—Quinidine Gluconate is an antiarrhythmic drug with the same uses as *Quinidine Sulfate*, but is preferred for *intramuscular* use, since it is nonirritating and stable in solution. The *intravenous* administration of quinidine is only occasionally warranted, but sometimes is a lifesaving measure in certain desperate conditions such as *ventricular tachycardia* with acute pulmonary edema or severe congestive failure. The cardiac effect may be observed in 15 to 20 minutes after intramuscular injection. Hypotension is frequent.

Dose—*Intramuscular* or *intravenous*, **300 mg to 2.4 Gm** daily; *usual*, **400 mg** repeated every 2 hours if necessary.

Dosage Forms—Injection USP: 10 ml; Extended-Release Oral Solid: 330 mg.

Quinidine Sulfate USP

[Quinidine Sulfate (2:1) (Salt); Quinidex (*Robins*); Quinora (*Davies-Rose*)]

Quinidine Sulfate $(C_{20}H_{24}N_2O_2)_2 \cdot H_2SO_4 \cdot 2H_2O$ = 782.96] is the sulfate of an alkaloid obtained from various species of *Cinchona* and their hybrids and from *Remija pedunculata* Flückiger (Fam. *Rubiaceae*), or prepared from quinine. It contains 99.0–101.0% of $(C_{20}H_{24}N_2O_2)_2 \cdot H_2SO_4$, calculated on the anhydrous basis.

Quinidine is a stereoisomer of quinine (page 494) and occurs in cinchona bark in amounts ranging from 0.3 to over 1%, although in some barks it may be practically absent. Quinidine of commerce is usually accompanied

by about 25% of *hydroquinidine* (which is quinidine with an ethyl group replacing the vinyl) which, however, is therapeutically as potent as quinidine and no more toxic.

Preparation—Quinidine may be made by treating quinine with a metallic alkoxide[3] or by oxidizing quinine to quininone and then reducing the latter with sodium isopropoxide.[4]

Although the USP admitted the alkaloid made from quinine because of the war emergency, actually no significant quantities have ever been produced by this process and none is made now because of the expensiveness of the process, and the availability of the natural product.

Quinidine is obtained from the mother liquors remaining after removal of the quinine sulfate and is separated from cinchonine and the other alkaloids by special processes.

Description—Fine, needle-like, white crystals, frequently cohering in masses. It is odorless, has a very bitter taste, and darkens on exposure to light. Its solutions are neutral or alkaline to litmus. Its specific rotation is $+223°$ to $+231°$.

Solubility—One Gm dissolves in about 100 ml of water, and 10 ml of alcohol, in 5 ml of boiling water, and in 15 ml of chloroform, but is insoluble in ether.

Uses—Quinidine depresses myocardial excitability. It also prolongs conduction time and the effective refractory period. The decreased excitability and prolonged refractory period tend to abolish premature systoles of the atrium and ventricle and to prevent *atrial fibrillation* and *ventricular tachycardia*. However, the slowed conduction tends to favor certain types of fibrillation, and its clinical usefulness as an antifibrillatory agent depends upon the predominance of its actions on excitability and refractory period over its action on conduction. Quinidine decreases myocardial contractility and also tends to lower the blood pressure, particularly in large doses. Combined with digitalis, quinidine may induce bizarre abnormalities of rhythm. Occasionally it may cause ventricular tachycardia, fibrillation, or standstill. It may also induce cinchonism and hypersensitivity. Its principal use is in the treatment of atrial tachycardia, flutter, and fibrillation. The gluconate is employed for intramuscular and intravenous administration. See also *Quinidine Gluconate*.

Dose—**100 mg** to **4 Gm** daily; *usual*, **100 to 200 mg** 1 to 4 times a day.

Dosage Forms—Capsules USP: 100, 200, and 300 mg; Tablets USP: 100, 125, 200, and 300 mg.

Veterinary Dose (*atrial fibrillation*)—Oral, Horses, 1st day: **5 Gm**, 2nd day: **10 Gm** 2 times a day, 3rd and 4th days: **10 Gm** 3 times a day, 5th and 6th days, **10 Gm** 4 times a day, 7th and 8th days, **10 Gm** 5 times a day (minimum dose interval: 4 hours); *Dogs*, 1st day: **50 to 100 mg**, next 3 days: **3 to 6 mg** per **pound** of body weight every 2 hours 4 or 5 times a day. Qualified supervision is imperative to recognize impending toxic effects.

Other Antiarrhythmic Drug

Quinidine Polygalacturonate $[(C_{20}H_{24}N_2O_2 \cdot C_6H_{10}O_7 \cdot H_2O)_x]$ [Cardioquin (*Purdue-Frederick*)]—*Uses:* Those of *Quinidine Sulfate* (this page). It is claimed that the polygalacturonate causes a lesser incidence of gastrointestinal side effects; however, gastrointestinal side effects do not number among the serious reactions to quinidine. Well-controlled clinical studies of the drug have yet to be made. *Dose:* Oral, 275 mg up to 6 times a day as necessary.

Drugs Affecting Blood Lipids

Drugs that affect blood lipids may be classified as cardiovascular drugs because of the probable relation of blood lipids to atherosclerosis. Atherosclerosis is regarded by many as a disorder in lipid metabolism or as a normal effect of a diet high in certain lipids. Since one of the major lipids in the atheroma is cholesterol, much attention has been centered upon cholesterol in the diet and blood. There is a correlation between blood cholesterol content and the incidence of coronary occlusion, although it is far from a perfect one. Experimentally, a diet high in cholesterol can promote or exacerbate atherosclerosis in certain species. Consequently, there has been interest in drugs that affect the absorption of cholesterol from the intestine. However, in clinical studies the blood cholesterol level is affected more by other lipids than cholesterol itself. Saturated fats induce higher blood cholesterol levels than do unsaturated fats. Polyunsaturated fats are not only the least offensive in elevating blood cholesterol but may also actually suppress the elevation by saturated fats. The blood β-lipoprotein and serum triglyceride levels also correlate somewhat with the incidence of coronary occlusion and with the type of fat in the diet. It is evident that the blood lipids are only one of a number of factors that cause atherosclerosis and coronary occlusion. Thus it should not be expected that manipulation of the blood lipids will necessarily bring about improvement in the disease.

Cholestyramine Resin—see page 790.

Clofibrate NF

[Ethyl 2-(p-Chlorophenoxy)-2-methylpropionate; Atromid S (Ayerst)]

Cl—⟨benzene ring⟩—O—C(CH₃)(CH₃)—COOCH₂CH₃

Clofibrate contains 97.0–103.0% of $C_{12}H_{15}ClO_3$ (242.70), calculated on the anhydrous basis.

Preparation—Clofibrate may be prepared by condensing phenol with ethyl 2-chloro-2-methylpropionate in the presence of a suitable dehydrochlorinating agent and then chlorinating.

Description—Stable, colorless to pale-yellow liquid with a faint, characteristic odor and a characteristic taste. Its boiling point is 158° to 160°.

Solubility—Insoluble in water; soluble in acetone, alcohol, benzene, and chloroform.

Uses—Clofibrate *lowers the total serum lipids*, the principal reduction occurring in the triglyceride and cholesterol fractions. The reduction in cholesterol levels is moderate to pronounced in women and only slight to moderate in men. The effect on blood lipids is more consistent and attended with fewer side effects than with other hypocholesteremic drugs. The mechanism of action is unknown, and reports on the effect of cholesterol biosynthesis are somewhat contradictory. There is some evidence that fecal excretion of cholesterol is increased. Clofibrate increases the anticoagulant effects of prothrombopenic drugs, especially warfarin, so that appropriate adjustments in dose of anticoagulant are mandatory. Urticaria, pruritus, and stomatitis occasionally occur, and alopecia areata rarely occurs. Nausea and dyspepsia occur in about 10% of patients.

Dose—*Usual,* **500 mg** 4 times daily.

Other Dose Information—In hyperlipemia, if no response occurs within 3 months, the drug should be discontinued. Administration may be continued longer for resorption of xanthomas.

Dosage Forms—Capsules NF: 250 and 500 mg.

Safflower Oil

Safflower Oil is an oily liquid extracted from the seeds of the safflower, *Carthamus tinctorius*, containing 74.5% linoleic acid ($C_{17}H_{31}COOH$) and 6.6% saturated fatty acids, the former being an essential fatty acid.

Description—An edible drying oil with an acid value of 1.0 to 9.7, a saponification value of 188 to 194, and an iodine value of 140 to 150. Its specific gravity at 25° is 0.9211 to 0.9215. It thickens and becomes rancid on prolonged exposure to air.

Solubility—Soluble in the usual fat and oil solvents.

Uses—Safflower Oil is a polyunsaturated oil (see the general statement, this page). Consequently, when used in the diet in lieu of more saturated fats and oils, the blood cholesterol is not elevated to the extent as with the more saturated lipids. There is some evidence that it may also partially suppress the hypercholesteremic effect of saturated fats. To do so, approximately three times as much Safflower Oil as dietary saturated fat must be ingested. Thus, unless the saturated fat intake is greatly reduced, the addition of safflower oil markedly increases the caloric intake. It is probably better simply to reduce the fat intake in the diet as much as possible and to use polyunsaturated oils in cooking where fat or oil cannot be eliminated. There is no good evidence that Safflower Oil is superior to other polyunsaturated oils marketed as ordinary food items.

Dose—*Oral,* supposedly **75 ml** of a 65% emulsion in divided doses. However, see above with respect to the required ratio of Safflower Oil to dietary saturated fat.

Sitosterols NF

[Cytellin (Lilly)]

CH₂CHCH₂CH₂CH(C₂H₅)CH(CH₃)₂

β-Sitosterol

Sitosterols is a mixture of β-sitosterol (stigmast-5-en-3β-ol) ($C_{29}H_{50}O$) (414.72) and related sterols of plant origin. It contains not less than 95.0% of total sterols and not less than 85.0% of unsaturated sterols, calculated on the dried basis as β-sitosterol.

Literally translated, the term *sitosterols* means *grain-sterols;* it is used broadly to refer to sterols (see page 479) present in the lipoidal extractive from higher order plants such as wheat, corn, rye, cotton, soy and rice. Several varieties of sitosterols are recognized, eg, α_1, α_2, α_3, β, and γ, which, although closely related, differ slightly from each other in molecular weight, degree of saturation, and/or stereoconfiguration. The complete structures of some are still uncertain, but β-sitosterol has been shown to be stigmast-5-en-3β-ol, ie, 24-ethyl-5-cholesten-3β-ol or 24-ethylcholesterol, *cf* page 811.

Preparation—Sterol fractions rich in β-sitosterol are isolated from the still-bottoms (about 2 to 4% by weight of sterols) remaining after distillation of the commercially usable oils from tall oil (results from Kraft paper processing of pine shavings), corn seed oil, cottonseed oil, or soya bean oil. Enrichment to between 40 and 60% sterols is accomplished, after a saponification step, by means of countercurrent liquid-liquid extractions using immiscible solvent pairs. By means of carbon decolorization and fractional crystallization in organic solvents, the sterols are then brought to a final purity of 85 to 100% β-sitosterol. Soya β-sitosterol must undergo further counter-current purification to separate it from stigmasterol prior to the final crystallizations.

Description—Occurs as a white, essentially odorless tasteless powder. Specific rotation $-25°$ to $-38°$ (when previously dried at 100° for 3 hours and determined in a solution in chloroform containing 200 mg in each 10 ml).

Solubility—Freely soluble in chloroform and in carbon disulfide; practically insoluble in water; slightly soluble in alcohol.

Uses—Because of their close structural relationship to cholesterol, the sitosterols have been studied as possible competitive inhibitors of cholesterol absorption, but there is no clear evidence that they lower serum cholesterol levels (*antihypercholesterolemics*). It is not established that in man the dietary intake of cholesterol has any relationship to the development of atherosclerosis. Moreover, there is some evidence that the sitosterols may themselves be deposited in the vessels. It is surprising that this drug has maintained official status.

Dose—**9** to **30 Gm** daily; *usual*, **3 Gm** 3 times a day before meals.

Dosage Forms—Suspension NF: 3 Gm/15 ml.

Sodium Heparin—see page 834.

Sodium Dextrothyroxine NF

[Sodium D-3-[4-(4-Hydroxy-3,5-diiodophenoxy)-3,5-diiodophenyl]alanine; Choloxin (*Flint*)]

Sodium Dextrothyroxine contains 97.0–103.0% of $C_{15}H_{10}I_4NNaO_4$ (798.86), calculated on the dried basis.

Preparation—Using D-thyroxin, the process is analogous to that described for *Sodium Levothyroxine*, page 985.

Description—A light-yellow to buff-colored, odorless, tasteless powder. It is stable in dry air but may assume a slight pink color upon exposure to light. The pH of a saturated solution is about 8.9.

Solubility—1 Gm dissolves in about 700 ml of water and about 300 ml of alcohol; insoluble in acetone, chloroform, and ether; soluble in solutions of alkali hydroxides and in hot solutions of alkali carbonates.

Uses—Sodium Dextrothyroxine is employed to *lower serum cholesterol* and other lipids. All thyroid hormones have this effect on the blood lipids, but they cannot ordinarily be used because of the increased metabolism and attendant cardiovascular dangers. However, the general metabolic actions of Dextrothyroxine are proportionately less than with levothyroxine, so that it is possible to lower blood lipids with lesser increases in basal metabolic effect and other indices of thyrotoxicity. When used in combination with estrogenic substances, such as stilbestrol, the lipid-lowering effect is enhanced and the dose of Dextrothyroxine may be reduced, but side effects of the estrogen may make use of the combination undesirable, especially in men.

Untoward effects of Dextrothyroxine include increased metabolic rate, tachycardia, and increased frequency of anginal attacks in persons with coronary insufficiency.

Dose—**1.0** to **8.0 mg** daily; *usual, initial,* **1.0** to **2.0 mg** daily; *maintenance,* **4.0** to **8.0 mg** daily.

Other Dose Information—When used in combination with estrogens or other hypolipemic drugs, 2 mg. The usual dose of stilbestrol used in combination with Dextrothyroxine is 0.25 mg.

Dosage Forms—Tablets NF: 2 and 4 mg.

Other Drugs Affecting Blood Lipids

Potassium Heparin is the potassium salt of heparin standardized in terms of the International Unit, each IU representing the activity of 0.0077 mg of sodium heparin (page 834). *Uses:* Although Potassium Heparin has the same anticoagulant actions as *Sodium Heparin* (page 834), it is not employed as an anticoagulant. Rather, it is used for its effects on the physicochemical state of the plasma lipids. Heparin, whether as the sodium or potassium salt, converts the larger chylomicrons (fat droplets) to smaller ones and converts lipoproteins of low density to high density. Since some workers believe that the low-density lipoproteins contain cholesterol and also that they are the source of the lipid in the arterial lesion in atherosclerosis, heparin has been advocated in the prevention and treatment of *atherosclerosis*. However, a beneficial effect of heparin in the disease or its prevention has not been demonstrated. The potassium salt has no particular advantage over the sodium salt; neither is absorbed well or consistently sublingually, but an effect on blood lipids can sometimes be shown after large doses of the drug. No effect on blood coagulability occurs after sublingual administration. *Dose: Sublingual,* 1500 units 3 times a day after meals.

Miscellaneous Cardiovascular Drugs

Angiotensin Amide NF

[*N*-[1-[*N*-[*N*-[*N*-(*N*²-L-asparaginyl-L-arginyl)-L-valyl]-L-tyrosyl]-L-valyl]-L-histidyl]-L-prolyl]-3-phenylalanine; 1-L-Asparagine-5-L-valineangiotensin II; Hypertensin (*Ciba*)]

Angiotensin Amide contains not less than 77.0% of $C_{49}H_{70}N_{14}O_{11}$ (1031.19).

It is a synthetic octapeptide which is identical with natural angiotensin II, except that the terminal aspartic acid unit has been replaced by asparagine.

Description—White to slightly off-white amorphous powder. It is odorless and is stable in dry air. It is supplied in sealed vials and ampuls as a sterile white cake or powder in combination with lactose or mannitol.

Solubility—Soluble in water; slightly soluble in methanol; insoluble in ether, chloroform, and benzene. It gradually decomposes in aqueous solution into ammonia and α-L-Angiotensin II.

Uses—Angiotensin Amide is the amide of angiotensin II. Its actions are those of angiotensin II.

Angiotensin II is an octapeptide formed in the blood by the action of a converting enzyme on the decapeptide precursor, angiotensin I. Angiotensin I is formed from angiotensinogen through the action of renin, an enzyme produced by the juxtaglomerular apparatus of the kidney. Angiotensin II stimulates the adrenal secretion of aldosterone. The renal renin–angiotensin–aldosterone system is considered to play a role in electrolyte and body fluid homeostasis and to be involved in edematous states, such as congestive heart failure, and hypertension.

Angiotensin Amide raises blood pressure by an action on systemic arterioles, especially of the viscera. It does not greatly affect systemic veins and hence does not impair venous return to the right heart; it also does not greatly affect pulmonary arteries and veins and hence does not impair venous return to the left heart. For this reason it has been employed in hypovolemic shock and also in other types of *shock*. In hypovolemic shock a better effect is obtained if levarterenol is given simultaneously to constrict veins. Since Angiotensin Amide is rapidly destroyed by angiotensinase and other numerous peptidases in blood and tissues, extravascular angiotensin does not remain long enough to cause damage to tissues. Angiotensin has an oxytocic action, the clinical implications of which have not been fully determined.

Dose—*Intravenous, infusion, usual,* **3** to **10 mcg** per minute as determined by the blood pressure response.

Other Dose Information—Each 0.5 mg is diluted with 1 ml of sterile water. Appropriate volumes of this solution are then added to 500 ml of isotonic saline solution, isotonic glucose solution, or 5% dextran solution and infused at a rate which elicits the desired pressor reponse. Because of tachyphylaxis, it may be necessary to increase the rate to 100 mcg per minute. Sometimes the dose needs to be adjusted downward as the cardiovascular system improves.

Dosage Forms—for Injection NF: 500 mcg and 2.5 mg.

References

1. A review of the synthetic methods for preparing papaverine has appeared in the *United Nations Bulletin on Narcotics*, Vol. IV, No. 3, p. 27 (July–Sept., 1952).
2. Mitchell, H. I., *Am. J. Pharm.*, **136**, 71 (1964).
3. Doering, W. E., *et al*, *J. Am. Chem. Soc.*, **69**, 1700 (1947).
4. Woodward, R. B., *et al*, *J. Am. Chem. Soc.*, **67**, 1428 (1945).

47 | Respiratory Drugs

Respiratory stimulants—expectorant and antitussive drugs—
therapeutic gases

This chapter was prepared by

Ewart A. Swinyard, PhD, *Professor of Pharmacology, College of Pharmacy and College of Medicine, University of Utah, Salt Lake City, Utah 84112, and* **Stewart C. Harvey, PhD,** *Associate Professor of Pharmacology, College of Medicine, University of Utah, Salt Lake City, Utah 84112*

A number of pharmacologic agents have in common the property of acting on the respiratory system. Alcohol, anesthetic agents, barbiturates and other hypnotic drugs, morphine and other narcotic drugs, in addition to acetanilid and related antipyretic and analgesic drugs exert undesirable side actions which depress the respiratory system. Although vomiting is a respiratory act, emetic drugs are discussed with the gastrointestinal drugs (see page 806) because they are used to evacuate the stomach in case of food and drug poisoning. The nitrites, belladonna, stramonium, ephedrine, epinephrine, and aminophylline are powerful bronchodilators and are employed to relieve or prevent the paroxysms of asthma; these agents also have other valuable therapeutic actions and are described elsewhere. Included in this chapter are the respiratory stimulants, the expectorant and antitussive agents, and the therapeutic gases.

Respiratory Stimulants

Respiration is controlled by a respiratory center in the medulla oblongata. This center is stimulated by the presence of carbon dioxide in the blood. An increase in the carbon dioxide content of blood, as in exercise, stimulates the respiratory center and increases the respiratory rate. Other drugs which act directly on the center to increase respiratory rate include atropine, caffeine, pentylenetetrazol, and picrotoxin. Respiration is partly controlled by both chemical and sensory stimuli from the carotid body and carotid sinus, and drugs such as nikethamide exert at least part of their respiratory effect through this mechanism. The rate of respiration is also modified by numerous forms of sensory stimuli reaching the brain from the skin, nose, mouth, throat, etc, and drugs such as ammonia act through this mechanism. Finally, respiration may be modified voluntarily through the higher brain centers, and drugs which restore the functional activity of depressed higher centers, such as pentylenetetrazol and picrotoxin, act to increase respiration.

Aromatic Ammonia Spirit NF

[Spirit of Sal Volatile]

Aromatic Ammonia Spirit contains, in each 100 ml, 1.7–2.1 Gm of total NH₃ (17.03), and ammonium carbonate corresponding to 3.5–4.5 Gm of (NH₄)₂CO₃ (96.09).

History—This Spirit first found an official place in the London Pharmacopœia of 1721 under the name *Spiritus Salis Volatilis Oleosus.* The present name was first adopted in the London Pharmacopœia of 1809. The formula and process have changed repeatedly during the several centuries in which the preparation has been used.

Ammonium Carbonate, in translucent pieces	**34 Gm**
Strong Ammonia Solution	**36 ml**
Lemon Oil	**10 ml**
Lavender Oil	**1 ml**
Myristica Oil	**1 ml**
Alcohol	**700 ml**
Purified Water, a sufficient quantity, To make	**1000 ml**

Dissolve the ammonium carbonate in the strong ammonia solution and 195 ml of purified water by gentle agitation, and allow the solution to stand for 12 hours. Dissolve the oils in the alcohol, contained in a graduated bottle or cylinder, and gradually add the ammonium carbonate solution and enough purified water to make the product measure 1000 ml. Set the mixture aside in a cool place for 24 hours, occasionally agitating it, and then filter, using a covered funnel.

The ammonium carbonate in this preparation must be in translucent pieces. The soft, chalky variety is chiefly ammonium bicarbonate, a deteriorated product. See *Ammonium Carbonate* (page 869) for a discussion of the chemistry involved in this preparation.

Description—A nearly colorless liquid when recently prepared, but gradually acquires a yellow color on standing. It has the taste of ammonia, has an aromatic and pungent odor, and is affected by light. Its specific gravity is about 0.90.

Alcohol Content—From 62 to 68% of C₂H₅OH.

Incompatibilities—*Water* causes separation of the oils contained in this preparation. *Alkaloids* are liberated from solutions of their salts but are frequently soluble in the alcohol of the Spirit.

Uses—This preparation is given orally as a *reflex* respiratory *stimulant.* It should be well diluted with water.

Dose—By inhalation of vapor as required. *Other Dose Information*—Usual, oral, **2 ml.**

Veterinary Dose—*Horses*, **15 to 90 ml**; *Dogs*, **0.3 to 4 ml.**

Ammonium Carbonate NF

[Ammonia Crystal; Sal Volatile; Ammonium Sesquicarbonate]

Ammonium Carbonate consists of ammonium bicarbonate [$NH_4HCO_3 = 79.06$] and ammonium carbamate [$NH_2.COONH_4 = 78.07$] in varying proportions. It yields 30.0–34.0% of NH_3.

The purity rubric given above corresponds to an equimolar mixture of the two compound salts.

Preparation—Ammonium Carbonate is prepared by sublimation from an intimate mixture of ammonium sulfate and calcium carbonate.

$$2(NH_4)_2SO_4 + 2CaCO_3 \rightarrow NH_4HCO_3.NH_4NH_2CO_2 + NH_3 + 2CaSO_4 + H_2O$$

If ammonium carbamate is dissolved in water, it is soon changed to normal ammonium carbonate.

$$NH_4NH_2CO_2 + H_2O \rightarrow (NH_4)_2CO_3$$

Hence an aqueous solution of commercial ammonium carbonate contains both the normal and acid carbonates.

If, however, the ammonium carbonate is dissolved in diluted ammonia solution, not only is the carbamate converted by the water to the normal carbonate according to the equation given above, but the bicarbonate which is present is also converted by the ammonia to the normal salt. The following equation summarizes the complete reaction.

$$NH_4HCO_3.NH_4NH_2CO_2 + NH_4OH \rightarrow 2(NH_4)_2CO_3$$

The above reactions are involved in the use of diluted ammonia solution for the preparation of *Aromatic Ammonia Spirit* (page 868). The normal carbonate is soluble in the alcohol used as part of the vehicle.

If the official Ammonium Carbonate is exposed to dry air, the carbamate portion gradually changes into gaseous NH_3 and CO_2 ultimately leaving a white, powdery residue of ammonium bicarbonate:

$$NH_4NH_2CO_2 \rightarrow 2NH_3 + CO_2$$

In the presence of atmospheric moisture the ammonium carbamate loses ammonia and is converted to ammonium bicarbonate:

$$O=C\underset{NH_2}{\overset{ONH_4}{<}} + H_2O \rightarrow O=C\underset{OH}{\overset{ONH_4}{<}} + NH_3$$

Through the absorption of carbon dioxide and moisture from the air conversion to ammonium bicarbonate proceeds as follows:

$$O=C\underset{NH_2}{\overset{ONH_4}{<}} + CO_2 + 2H_2O \rightarrow 2O=C\underset{OH}{\overset{ONH_4}{<}}$$

Description—A white powder or hard, white or translucent masses, having a strong odor of ammonia, without empyreuma, and with a sharp, ammoniacal taste. It is affected by light. On exposure to air, it loses ammonia and carbon dioxide, becoming opaque, and is finally converted into friable, porous lumps or a white powder of ammonium bicarbonate. It is decomposed by hot water and by weak acids.

Solubility—1 Gm is very slowly soluble in about 4 ml of water and is partly (the carbamate portion) soluble in alcohol. It is decomposed by hot water. Its solution has the odor of ammonia and is alkaline to litmus.

Incompatibilities—*Acids* and *acid salts* decompose Ammonium Carbonate as do liquid preparations having an acid reaction. Many *metals* form insoluble carbonates or basic salts. *Alkaloids* are generally precipitated although atropine, hyoscyamine, codeine, and caffeine are among the exceptions. *Resorcinol* gives a brown color which changes to blue; *calomel* is converted partly to a dark mixture of ammoniated mercury and metallic mercury.

Uses—Ammonium Carbonate is employed as an *expectorant* in the dose of 300 to 500 mg every hour or two. It is more apt to cause gastric irritation than is ammonium chloride. Ammonium Carbonate is the basis of *smelling salts*, valuable as a restorative in hysterical syncope. For this purpose, ¼- to 1-inch cubes of the salt are generally used. Ammonium Carbonate is occasionally used as a leavening agent and in consequence is sometimes called *baker's ammonia*. It is used as a *pharmaceutical necessity* in the preparation of *Aromatic Ammonia Spirit* (page 868).

Dose (unofficial)—Up to **300 mg** in dilute solutions.

Veterinary Dose—*Horses*, 4 to **15 Gm**; *Cattle*, 15 to **30 Gm**; *Sheep* and *Swine*, 1 to 2 Gm; *Dogs*, 200 to **500 mg.**

Atropine Sulfate—see page 915.

Caffeine—see page 1155.

Caffeine and Sodium Benzoate—see page 1156.

Camphor—see page 773.

Carbon Dioxide USP

[After-damp; Aer Fixus; Carbonic Acid Gas]

Carbon Dioxide contains not less than 99.0%, by volume, of CO_2 (44.01).

Preparation—See *Carbon Dioxide* (page 869).

Description—An odorless, colorless gas. One liter of it at 760 mm and 0° weighs 1.977 Gm.

Solubility—One volume dissolves in about 1 volume of water at 25°; it is more soluble at lower than at higher temperatures, also less soluble in alcohol and other solvents. Its solutions are slightly acid to litmus and have a slightly acid taste.

Identification—Carbon Dioxide extinguishes a flame and produces a white precipitate, soluble in acetic acid with effervescence, when passed into barium hydroxide TS.

Uses—The principal therapeutic use of Carbon Dioxide is as a *respiratory stimulant*. When breathed into the lungs, it elevates the carbon dioxide content of the blood. At low to moderate concentrations, the carbon dioxide in the blood stimulates the respiratory, vasomotor, and cardioaccelerator centers. For these effects, the optimal concentration in inhaled air or gas mixtures is 10%. Above this concentration it is less effective, and higher concentrations may induce respiratory depression, dyspnea, and disorientation, either immediately or following a transient period of stimulation; stimulation of the vasomotor center may continue with concentrations as high as 20%, but cardiac function may be impaired at this concentration. Concentrations of 20 to 30% and above are *rapidly fatal*, convulsions and respiratory depression occurring in devastating combination.

Carbon Dioxide has very little indication as a stimulant of a depressed respiratory center, although it is still occasionally and unwisely used in asphyxia neonatorum and resuscitation. In respiratory depression, the carbon dioxide content of the blood is already high and further increases cannot be expected to be of value; indeed, further elevations may exacerbate respiratory depression. Only when coma or respiratory depression is accompanied by a low carbon dioxide tension in the blood is administration of Carbon Dioxide rational and safe. However, the gas finds applications as a respiratory stimulant in patients with nondepressed respiratory centers in whom it is desirable to increase respiratory minute volume. Carbon Dioxide is therefore used to hasten the excretion of toxic gases and vapors from the blood via the lungs or to cause the lungs to expand to a maximum, for example, to prevent or treat *postoperative atelectasis* or atelectatic complications of pneumonia and oxygen therapy. It is also occasionally employed as a depressant in the treatment of *hiccough* and as an *expectorant*.

Carbon Dioxide is administered by inhalation, most conveniently through a tight-fitting mask. The gas is employed in conjunction with oxygen. Concentrations of 5 to 7.5% are employed; 5% is the usual concentration.

Dose—By *inhalation*, up to 7% in oxygen.

Doxapram Hydrochloride NF

[1-Ethyl-4-(2-morpholinoethyl)-3,3-diphenyl-2-pyrrolidinone   Monohydrochloride; Dopram (*Robins*)]

Doxapram Hydrochloride [$C_{24}H_{30}N_2O_2 \cdot HCl \cdot H_2O = 433.00$], dried at 105° for 2 hours contains 98.0–100.5% of $C_{24}H_{30}N_2O_2 \cdot HCl$ (414.98).

Preparation—1-Ethyl-3-pyrrolidinol is reacted with thionyl chloride to form the corresponding 3-chloro compound which is then condensed with diphenylacetonitrile in toluene solution with the aid of sodamide. The resulting α-(1-ethyl-3-pyrrolidinyl)-diphenylacetonitrile is hydrolyzed with 70% sulfuric acid to the corresponding acid. On treatment with thionyl chloride, the acid is converted into the acid chloride which immediately isomerizes to 4-(2-chloroethyl)-3,3-diphenyl-1-ethyl-2-pyrrolidinone. Condensation of this with morpholine in a suitable dehydrohalogenating environment yields doxapram (base) which, on reacting with an equimolar quantity of hydrochloric acid, gives the official salt.

Description—A white to off-white, odorless, crystalline powder that is stable in light and air. It melts between 217° and 221°.

Solubility—Soluble in chloroform; sparingly soluble in water and alcohol; practically insoluble in ether.

Uses—Doxapram Hydrochloride is a respiratory stimulant for intravenous administration. It acts mainly to increase tidal volume, but it also moderately increases respiratory rate. The respiratory stimulation is usually accompanied by a slight increase in blood pressure and heart rate. Doxapram Hydrochloride is contraindicated in epilepsy and other convulsive states, incompetence of the respiratory mechanism due to muscle paresis, flail chest, pneumothorax, airway obstruction, and extreme dyspnea; severe hypertension and cerebrovascular accidents; and drug hypersensitivity. More clinical research is necessary before it can be concluded that Doxapram Hydrochloride is more effective and less toxic than other agents such as aminophylline.

Dose—*Usual, intravenous,* **500 mcg** to **1.0 mg/Kg** of body weight given as a single injection or **1.5 to 2.0 mg/Kg** of body weight given as injections of **500 mcg** to **1.0 mg/Kg** of body weight at 5-minute intervals.

Dosage Forms—Injection NF: 400 mg/20 ml.

Veterinary Uses—This drug is used to stimulate respiration during and after general anesthesia with barbiturates and to speed awakening and return of reflexes after anesthesia in dogs and cats.

Veterinary Dose—*Intravenous, Dogs* and *Cats,* **2.5** to **5 mg** per **pound** of body weight; if necessary, the dose may be repeated after 15 to 20 minutes.

Nikethamide—see page 1159.

Pentylenetetrazol—see page 1160.

Picrotoxin—see page 1160.

Expectorant and Antitussive Drugs

Expectorants are drugs used to assist in the removal of secretion or exudate from the trachea, bronchi, or lungs and, hence, they are useful in the treatment of cough. Expectorants may also have anesthetic, antiseptic, diuretic, or other activity. For convenience, these drugs may be classified as sedative expectorants, stimulant (irritant) expectorants, and centrally acting expectorants and antitussive agents.

Sedative Expectorants

Drugs in this classification act to soothe acute inflammation by aiding the secretion of protective mucus. This group includes the saline expectorants, which increase bronchial secretion and "loosen" the cough; the nauseant expectorants, which are expectorant in small doses and nauseant and emetic in large doses; and the demulcent expectorants, which are mucilaginous or syrupy and coat and protect the mucous membranes of the upper respiratory tract.

Acacia—see page 1344.

Acetylcysteine

[Mucomyst (*Mead-Johnson*)]

$$CH_2(SH)CHCOOH$$
$$|$$
$$NHCOCH_3$$

Acetylcysteine [$C_5H_9NO_3S = 163.20$] is *N*-acetyl-L-cysteine.

Preparation—Acetylcysteine may be prepared by direct acetylation of naturally occurring L-cysteine.

Description—A white, crystalline powder which has a very slight odor and a characteristic sour taste. It is stable in ordinary light, nonhygroscopic (oxidizes in moist air), and stable at temperatures up to 120°. It melts between 104° and 110°.

Solubility—Soluble in water, alcohol, hot isopropyl alcohol, methyl acetate, and ethyl acetate.

Uses—Acetylcysteine is used to reduce the viscosity of pulmonary secretions and facilitate their removal. Hence, it is used as an adjuvant therapy in bronchopulmonary disorders when mucolysis is desirable. It is thought the sulfhydryl group in the molecule "opens" the disulfide bonds in mucus and lowers the viscosity. Side effects are rare. However, stomatitis, nausea, and rhinorrhea have been observed and bronchospasm has been reported in highly sensitive asthmatic patients using the drug. Acetylcysteine is a relatively new drug and final evaluation must await more definitive clinical study.

Dose—*Aerosol*, for most patients, **3 to 5 ml** every 3 or 4 hours; *direct instillation*, **1 to 2 ml** (full or half strength) every 1 to 4 hours.

Ammonium Carbonate—see page 869.

Ammonium Chloride—see page 936.

Antimony Potassium Tartrate—see page 1265.

Glycerin—see page 1359.

Glycyrrhiza— see page 1327.

Hydriodic Acid Syrup—see page 1340.

Ipecac and Opium Powder—see RPS-13, page 561.

Ipecac USP

[Ipecacuanha; Ipecacuanhae Radix]

Ipecac consists of the dried rhizome and roots of *Cephaëlis Ipecacuanha* (Brotero) A. Richard, known in commerce as *Rio* or *Brazilian Ipecac*, or of *Cephaëlis acuminata* Karsten, known in commerce as Cartagena, Nicaragua, or Panama Ipecac (Fam. *Rubiaceæ*). Ipecac yields not less than 2.0% of the ether-soluble alkaloids of ipecac.

History—The first mention of this Brazilian drug is by *Purchas*, a famous traveler, in 1625. Its first introduction into European medicine was in 1686 when Louis XIV purchased from a quack named *Helvetius* the secret of a nostrum used successfully in the treatment of diarrhea and dysentery, and Ipecac was found to be the essential ingredient.

Constituents—Ipecac contains *emetine* (*methylcephaëline*) [$C_{29}H_{40}N_2O_4$], *cephaëline*, [$C_{28}H_{38}N_2O_4$], *psychotrine* [$C_{28}H_{36}N_2O_4$], *emetamine* [$C_{29}H_{36}N_2O_4$], *ipecamine*, also *ipecacuanhic acid*, pectin, starch, resin, sugar, etc. All of the alkaloids are interrelated and may be synthesized from each other. Brazilian roots yield as much as 2.5% of total alkaloids and Cartagena root 2.0%. The apothegmatic matter, which is dissolved by hydroalcoholic liquids when percolating it, is slowly precipitated when added to water or syrup. It may be separated by allowing the aqueous liquid to stand until the separation is completed and then filtering.

Uses—Ipecac has *expectorant*, *emetic*, and *amebicidal properties*. The syrup is preferred for use as an expectorant and emetic. Emetic doses of Ipecac may be used in patients with *paroxysmal auricular tachycardia*, the vagal impulses arising from the excitation of the medullary vagal vomiting mechanism acting to bring about the cessation of the arrhythmia. Ipecac has amebicidal potency by virtue of its content of emetine, but is almost never used in the therapy of amebiasis.

Veterinary Uses—Ipecac may be used as an *emetic* for dogs, cats, and pigs and as an *expectorant*.

Veterinary Dose—*Emetic in Swine*, 2 to 3 Gm; *Dogs*, 0.3 to 2 Gm, and *Cats*, 0.25 to 0.75 Gm; *Expectorant in Horses*, 4 to 8 Gm, *Swine*, 0.1 to 0.3 Gm and *Dogs*, 10 to 50 mg.

Powdered Ipecac USP is ipecac reduced to a fine or a very fine powder and adjusted to a potency of 1.9–2.1% of the ether-soluble alkaloids of ipecac, by the addition of exhausted marc of ipecac or of other suitable inert diluent or by the addition of powdered ipecac of either a lower or a higher potency. *Description:* Pale brown, weak yellow, or light olive-gray powder.

Ipecac Syrup USP yields, from each 100 ml, 123–157 mg of ether-soluble alkaloids of ipecac. *Preparation:* Exhaust powdered ipecac (70 Gm) by percolation, using a mixture of 3 volumes of alcohol and 1 volume of water as the menstruum, macerating for 72 hours, and percolating slowly. Reduce the entire percolate to a volume of 70 ml by evaporation at a temperature not exceeding 60° and preferably in vacuum, and add water (140 ml). Allow the mixture to stand overnight, filter, and wash the residue on the filter with water. Evaporate the filtrate and washings to 40 ml, and to this add hydrochloric acid (2.5 ml) and alcohol (20 ml), mix, and filter. Wash the filter with a mixture of 30 volumes of alcohol, 3.5 volumes of hydrochloric acid and 66.5 volumes of water, using a volume sufficient to produce 70 ml of filtrate. Add glycerin (100 ml) and syrup (qs) to make the product measure 1000 ml, and mix. *Alcohol Content:* From 1 to 2.5% of C_2H_5OH. *Uses:* Emetic and nauseant expectorant. Ipecac Syrup is the emetic of choice in the management of poisonings in children, wherein evacuation of the stomach contents is desirable and not specifically contraindicated. The syrup is especially valuable for croupous *bronchitis* in children. *Dose—Emetic:* 10 to 30 ml; *usual*, 15 ml. *Other Dose Information*—Expectorant, 1 to 2 ml; croupous bronchitis, 5 "drops" for the first year of age, and 1 additional drop for each additional year. *Veterinary Dose:* Emetic in Dogs, 4 to 15 ml; expectorant in Dogs, 1 to 2 ml.

Potassium Acetate NF

CH₃COOK

Potassium Acetate, dried at 150° for 2 hours, contains 99.0–100.5% of $C_2H_3KO_2$ (98.15).

Preparation—This salt may be made by adding potassium bicarbonate or potassium carbonate to glacial acetic acid, previously diluted with water, until effervescence ceases. After the addition of a slight excess of the acid the solution is cautiously evaporated to dryness in a porcelain or aluminum evaporating dish. Great care is necessary to avoid contamination with iron.

Description—Colorless, monoclinic crystals or a white, crystalline powder, rapidly deliquescing in moist air. It has a saline and slightly alkaline taste. Its aqueous solution is alkaline to litmus paper, but does not affect phenolphthalein TS.

Solubility—1 Gm dissolves in about 0.5 ml water, about 3 ml alcohol, and about 0.2 ml of boiling water.

Incompatibilities—See *Acetic Acid* (page 1433). *Mineral acids* liberate acetic acid and because of the feeble ionization of this acid, acetates act as buffers toward mineral acids, decreasing to some extent the hydrogen ion concentration.

Uses—Potassium Acetate is sometimes used as an *expectorant*, in the dose of from 1 to 2 Gm, every 1 or

2 hours. The salt should be liberally diluted with water or fruit juice, to avoid gastric distress. Potassium Acetate also has a limited usefulness as a *diuretic* and systemic *alkalizer*. It tends to cause alkalosis and an alkaline urine.

Veterinary Uses—An *expectorant* and *diuretic*.

Dose—*Usual*, 1 Gm.

Veterinary Dose—*Horses*, 25 to 50 Gm; *Cattle*, 50 to 100 Gm; *Dogs*, 500 mg to 2 Gm.

Potassium Citrate NF

[Tripotassium Citrate; Citrate of Potash]
CH₂(COOK)C(OH)(COOK)CH₂COOK.H₂O

Potassium Citrate [$K_3C_6H_5O_7.H_2O$ = 324.42], dried at 180° for 4 hours, contains 99.0–100.5% of $C_6H_5K_3O_7$ (306.41).

Preparation—This salt is made by adding potassium bicarbonate or carbonate to a solution of citric acid until effervescence ceases, filtering the solution and evaporating to granulation.

Description—Transparent crystals, or a white, granular powder. It is odorless, has a cooling, saline taste, and is deliquescent in moist air. Its aqueous solution is alkaline to litmus, but is not reddened by phenolphthalein TS.

Solubility—1 Gm dissolves in about 1 ml of water at 25°; almost insoluble in alcohol.

Incompatibilities—Aqueous solutions of potassium citrate are slightly alkaline and will react with *acidic substances*. *Alkaloidal salts* may be precipitated from their aqueous or hydroalcoholic solutions. Acidification or addition of alcohol will restore the solution. *Calcium* and *strontium salts* cause a precipitation of the corresponding citrates.

Hydroalcoholic solutions may be caused to separate into layers by the addition of fairly large quantities of potassium citrate. The upper layer is alcoholic and contains whatever alcohol-soluble ingredients were present; the lower is aqueous and contains most of the citrate. Dilution with water promotes the miscibility.

Uses—Potassium Citrate is employed as an *expectorant*, systemic *alkalizer*, and *diuretic*.

Veterinary Use—An *expectorant*.

Dose—*Usual*, 1 Gm.

Other Dose Information—It is used in the dose of 1 to 2 Gm every few hours, diluted with at least ½ glassful of water or fruit juice.

Veterinary Dose—*Horses*, 25 to 50 Gm; *Cattle*, 50 to 100 Gm; *Dogs*, 500 mg to 2 Gm.

Potassium Iodide USP

[Kalii Iodidum]

Potassium Iodide contains 99.0–101.5% of KI (166.01), calculated on the dried basis.

Preparation—A hot aqueous solution of potassium hydroxide is treated with iodine in slight excess to form a mixture of potassium iodide and potassium iodate.

$$6KOH + 3I_2 \rightarrow 5KI + KIO_3 + 3H_2O$$

The solution is concentrated by heating over a free flame in an iron kettle, then an excess of powdered charcoal is added and well incorporated. The mixture is evaporated to dryness, then ignited. The charcoal (carbon) reduces the iodate to iodide and all of the iodine is thus obtained as Potassium Iodide. The mass is lixiviated with water, filtered, evaporated to a suitable concentration, and set aside to crystallize, or it is granulated from the hot solution.

Potassium Iodide is also prepared by first forming ferroso–ferric iodide through the reaction between iron wire and iodine in the presence of water. A solution of pure potassium carbonate is then added until the solution is faintly alkaline, boiled for a few moments, and filtered; the filtrate is concentrated and set aside to crystallize.

$$Fe_3I_8 + 4K_2CO_3 \rightarrow 8KI + Fe_3O_4 + 4CO_2$$

Potassium Iodide is always crystallized from an alkaline solution and to prevent discoloration due to formation of free iodine, a small amount of free alkali is permitted. See also the equations under *Potassium Bromide*, page 1090.

Description—Hexahedral crystals, either transparent and colorless or somewhat opaque and white, or a white, granular powder. It is stable in dry air, but slightly hygroscopic in moist air. On prolonged keeping it may become yellowish through the formation of free iodine by oxidation. The aqueous solution is neutral or slightly alkaline to litmus, and gradually becomes yellow because of the formation of free iodine. The addition of small amounts of sodium thiosulfate removes the yellow color.

Solubility—1 Gm dissolves in 0.7 ml of water, 22 ml of alcohol, 2 ml of glycerin, 75 ml of acetone at 25°, and 0.5 ml of boiling water. When dissolved in water heat is absorbed. 100 ml of its aqueous solution saturated at 25° contains 100 Gm of KI.

Incompatibilities—Iodides are water-soluble except the *lead, silver, mercury*, and *cuprous salts*. These are soluble in the presence of alkali iodides, the lead and silver iodides least readily.

In the presence of *acid*, iodides are decomposed rapidly with the liberation of iodine. Sugar retards the reaction. *Oxidizing agents* liberate iodine with simultaneous reduction of the agent. Thus, by reaction with *cupric sulfate*, iodine is liberated and cuprous iodide is precipitated; with *ethyl nitrite spirit*, iodine and nitric oxide (which forms brown NO_2 on contact with air) are evolved. Ammonium iodide, calcium iodide, and zinc iodide decompose spontaneously under the influence of *light*.

The alkali iodides precipitate most *alkaloids*. Addition of alcohol will frequently preserve the solubility. *Mercurous chloride* in the presence of an excess of potassium iodide produces metallic mercury and mercuric iodide, the latter forming the soluble double salt, potassium mercuric iodide.

Difficulties may be encountered in preparing capsules and powders containing iodides due to their deliquescence. Use may be made of dried ingredients and suitable diluents in order to obtain satisfactory products.

Uses—Potassium Iodide is the salt usually employed when the action of the iodide ion is desired. Iodides have been used so extensively in therapy that only the more important therapeutic uses can be discussed here.

In regions where little iodine is obtained in the diet, iodides are completely effective in the *prevention of goiter*. Only minute doses are required and these small amounts can best be administered in the form of iodized salt (1 part of Potassium Iodide to 100,000 parts of salt). Saturated solution of Potassium Iodide may also be used in the place of Lugol's Solution for the treatment of *toxic goiter*, in the dose of 0.3 ml, 3 times daily. See *Strong Iodine Solution* (page 1181).

Iodides were formerly extensively employed in the treatment of syphilis.

Potassium Iodide is one of the most valuable of the saline expectorants and is widely employed in the treatment of *bronchitis* and *asthma* where it affords relief by liquefying tenacious sputum.

Mild untoward reactions frequently occur with iodide medication. The syndrome is known as iodism. The symptoms include salivation, lacrimation, coryza soreness of the teeth and gums, swelling of the salivary glands and eruption of the skin. The symptoms disappear when the drug is discontinued. Serious reactions occur only very rarely.

Dose—**300 mg to 2 Gm** daily; *usual,* **300 mg 4** times a day.

Other Dose Information—An expectorant dose is 0.3 Gm taken with a glassful of water.

Veterinary Uses—Potassium Iodide has been used for over 100 years in the treatment of *actinomycosis* and *actinobacillosis* in cattle; it is also employed in the treatment of *sporotrichosis* and *botryomycosis*. In regions where there is an iodine deficiency, Potassium Iodide is administered to prevent *hypothyroidism*. For the prevention of hypothyroidism, Potassium Iodide is frequently made available to animals in the form of iodized salt containing 0.02% potassium iodide.

Veterinary Dose—*Horses* and *Cattle,* **4 to 10 Gm;** *Sheep* and *Swine,* **1 to 3 Gm;** *Dogs,* **100 to 600 mg.**

Potassium Iodide Solution NF [Saturated Potassium Iodide Solution; S.S.K.I.] contains, in each 100 ml, 97.0–103.0 Gm of KI. *Preparation:* Dissolve potassium iodide (1000 Gm) in hot purified water (680 ml), cool to about 25°, and add sufficient purified water to make 1000 ml; filter, if necessary. *Note:* If the solution is not to be used within a short time, 500 mg of sodium thiosulfate should be added to each liter. *Description:* A clear, colorless, and odorless solution having a characteristic, strongly salty taste. It is neutral or slightly alkaline to litmus paper. Its specific gravity is about 1.700. *Incompatibilities:* See *Potassium Iodide. Uses:* Antigoitrogenic and expectorant; see *Potassium Iodide. Dose:* Usual, 0.3 ml, equivalent to 300 mg of Potassium Iodide.

Sodium Citrate USP

[Trisodium Citrate: Natrii Citras]

CH₂(COONa)C(OH)(COONa)CH₂COONa . 2H₂O

Sodium Citrate $[C_6H_5Na_3O_7.2H_2O = 294.10]$ is anhydrous or contains two molecules of water of hydration. It contains 99.0–100.5% of $C_6H_5Na_3O_7$ (258.07), calculated on the anhydrous basis.

Preparation—This salt is usually prepared by adding sodium carbonate to a solution of citric acid until effervescence ceases, evaporating, and granulating the product.

Description—Colorless crystals, or a white, crystalline powder. It has a cooling, saline taste. It is stable in the air. The aqueous solution is slightly alkaline to litmus but should not be reddened by phenolphthalein.

Solubility—1 Gm dissolves in 1.5 ml of water at 25° and in 0.6 ml of boiling water; insoluble in alcohol.

Incompatibilities—See *Potassium Citrate* (page 872).

Uses—Sodium Citrate is used as an *expectorant, systemic antacid, anticoagulant,* and *pharmaceutic aid.* As a pharmaceutic aid, Sodium Citrate is used to prevent darkening when iron is added to preparations containing tannin.

Dose (unofficial)—*Usual,* expectorant, **1 to 2 Gm,** well diluted with water, taken every 2 hours; *systemic antacid,* **1 to 4 Gm** 4 times a day.

Anticoagulant Sodium Citrate Solution—see page 833.

Anticoagulant Citrate Dextrose Solution—see page 833.

Sodium Iodide USP

[Natrii Iodidum]

Sodium Iodide contains 99.0–101.5% of NaI (149.89), calculated on the anhydrous basis.

Preparation—Sodium Iodide may be prepared from iodine and sodium hydroxide, but metathesis between ferrosoferric iodide and sodium carbonate is preferred. See *Potassium Iodide* (page 872).

Description—Colorless, odorless crystals, or a white, crystalline powder. In moist air Sodium Iodide cakes and then deliquesces, and frequently undergoes decomposition, developing a brown tint. Its solution in water is neutral or slightly alkaline to litmus and gradually becomes yellow because of the formation of free iodine. In contrast to potassium iodide, when Sodium Iodide is dissolved in water heat is liberated due to the formation of the dihydrate [NaI.2H₂O].

Solubility—1 Gm dissolves in 0.6 ml of water, about 2 ml of alcohol, and about 1 ml of glycerin.

Incompatibilities—See under *Potassium Iodide* (page 872). Sodium Iodide is *deliquescent* and in the damp state is easily oxidized by *air,* taking on a brown color.

Uses—Sodium Iodide can be used interchangeably with potassium iodide, as a therapeutic agent, except where sodium ion is contraindicated. See *Potassium Iodide* (page 872).

Dose—*Oral,* **300 mg to 2 Gm** daily; *usual,* **300 mg** 2 to 4 times a day; *intravenous infusion,* **1 to 3 Gm** daily; *usual,* **1 Gm.**

Veterinary Dose—*Horses* and *Cattle,* **4 to 10 Gm;** *Sheep* and *Swine,* **1 to 3 Gm;** *Dogs,* **100 to 600 mg.**

Sodium Iodide I 125 Capsules—see page 570.

Sodium Iodide I 125 Solution—see page 566.

Sodium Iodide I 131 Capsules—see page 566.

Sodium Iodide I 131 Solution—see page 566.

Other Sedative Expectorants

Ammonium Iodide NF X—Purity: not less than 98% NH₄I. It may contain not more than 1% of ammonium hypophosphite as a stabilizing agent. It occurs as minute, colorless, cubic crystals, or a white, hygroscopic, granular powder. It is odorless and has a sharp, salty taste. It becomes yellow or yellowish brown on exposure to air and light, due to the loss of ammonia and the liberation of iodine, if no stabilizing agent is added. Its aqueous solution is neutral or acid to litmus. 1 Gm is soluble in 0.6 ml of water, 0.5 ml of boiling water, about 3.7 ml of alcohol, and about 1.5 ml of glycerin. *Uses:* Expectorant. *Dose:* Orally, 0.3 Gm.

Calcium Iodide [CaI₂.6H₂O]—A yellowish white, deliquescent powder; becomes yellow in the air due to liberation of iodine. Very soluble in water, soluble in alcohol. *Uses:* A source of calcium and iodide. *Dose:* 0.3 to 0.6 Gm.

Ipecacuanha, Prepared BP [Prepared Ipecac]—Finely powdered ipecac adjusted, if necessary, by admixture in suitable proportion of powdered exhausted ipecac, or of powdered lactose, to contain 2% of the total alkaloids of ipecac, calculated as emetine (limits, 1.9 to 2.1%). It occurs as a light gray to yellowish brown powder having a slight odor and bitter taste. *Uses:* As an expectorant and emetic; as a diaphoretic when combined with opium in the treatment of the common cold. *Dose:* Orally, expectorant, 25 to 125 mg; emetic, 1 to 2 Gm (unofficial).

Levopropoxyphene [Novrad (*Lilly*)] is the alpha form of (−) - 4 - (dimethylamino) - 3 - methyl - 1,2 - diphenyl - 2-butanol propionate (ester). It is a slightly bitter, white crystalline solid which is very slightly soluble in water. *Uses:* Antitussive, indicated for the symptomatic treatment of cough. When taken orally, it decreases the frequency and intensity of cough associated with acute and chronic respiratory diseases. See also *Levopropoxyphene Napsylate,* page 877. *Dose:* 50 to 100 mg every 4 hours.

Lobelia NF X [Indian Tobacco; Emetic Weed; Asthma Weed]—It consists of the dried leaf and top of *Lobelia inflata* Linné (Fam. *Lobeliaceæ*). Its principal constituent is the alkaloid lobeline. *Uses:* Formerly as an expectorant and emetic; however, it is now obsolete. *Dose: Orally,* 0.1 Gm.

Lobeline [*l*-Lobeline; sometimes designated as α-lobeline to differentiate from the mixture of the total alkaloids of the plant] [$C_{22}H_{27}NO_2$]—From herb and seeds of *Lobelia inflata* L., *Lobeliaceæ.* Colorless crystals. Melts 130° to 131°. $[\alpha]_D^{15}$ is −42.8° in alcohol. Very slightly soluble in water or in petroleum benzin; soluble in hot alcohol, or in chloroform, benzene, ether. *Uses:* It has been employed as a respiratory stimulant, especially for resuscitation of the newborn. It acts by stimulation of the chemoreceptors of the carotid body in a manner analogous to nicotine. Its action is brief in duration and better respiratory stimulants are available. The adult dose is 3 to 10 mg, given hypo-dermically. Lobeline has also been used to control symptoms in patients undergoing withdrawal treatment for the tobacco habit. For this purpose, it is taken orally (8-mg capsules) as necessary.

Lobeline Hydrochloride [Lobelini Hydrochloridum PhI] [$C_{22}H_{27}NO_2$.HCl]—White, granular, bitter powder. Melts at about 180°. $[\alpha]_D^{20}$ is − 42.5°. 1 Gm dissolves in 40 ml water, 12 ml alcohol; very soluble in chloroform. The aqueous solution is slightly acid to litmus. *Uses:* As a respiratory stimulant in respiratory failure from diseases, drowning or other accidents, and from narcotic or CO_2 poisoning. Has also been suggested for tobacco addiction. *Dose: Subcutaneously* or *intramuscularly,* 15 mg, *intravenously,* 5 to 10 mg.

Stimulant (Irritant) Expectorants

Drugs in this classification act to stimulate repair in chronic inflammatory processes of the mucous membranes of the respiratory tract. The principal agents employed are terpin hydrate and the balsams; they are used primarily in chronic bronchitis.

Creosote—see page 1192.

Eucalyptol—see page 1337.

Eucalyptus Oil—see page 1327.

Glyceryl Guaiacolate NF

[3-(*o*-Methoxyphenoxy)-1,2-propanediol; ingredient of Robitussin (*Robins*) and of 2/G (*Pitman-Moore*)]

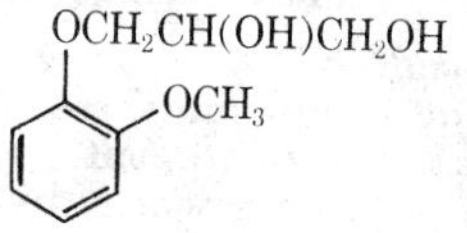

OCH₂CH(OH)CH₂OH
OCH₃

Glyceryl Guaiacolate contains 98.0–102.0% of $C_{10}H_{14}O_4$ (198.22), calculated on the dried basis.

Preparation—Guaiacol and 3-chloro-1,2-propanediol are condensed via dehydrochlorination by warming a mixture of the reactants with a base.

Description—A white to slightly gray, crystalline powder having a bitter taste. It may have a slight charcteristic odor. It is stable in light and heat and is nonhygroscopic. It melts between 81° and 82°.

Solubility—1 Gm dissolves in 15 ml of water; soluble in alcohol, chloroform, glycerin, and propylene glycol; insoluble in petroleum ether.

Uses—Glyceryl Guaiacolate is extensively used as an *expectorant.* It acts to increase respiratory tract fluid, thereby reducing viscosity of tenacious secretions. It is an ingredient in a number of proprietary expectorant formulations.

Dose—*Usual,* **100 mg** every 3 or 4 hours.

Dosage Forms—Syrup NF: 100 mg/5 ml.

Veterinary Uses—Experimentally, this drug has been used as a preanesthetic agent and, alone, for anesthesia of short duration in horses.

Veterinary Dose — *Experimental, intravenous, Horses,* **1 ml** (of 5% solution) per **pound** of body weight.

Pine Needle Oil—see page 1332.

Potassium Guaiacolsulfonate NF

[Potassium Hydroxymethoxybenzenesulfonate]

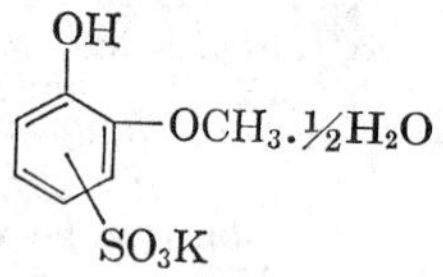

OH
OCH₃.½H₂O
SO₃K

Potassium Guaiacolsulfonate [$C_7H_7KO_5S.\frac{1}{2}H_2O$ = 251.30] contains 98.0–102.0% of $C_7H_7KO_5S$ (242.30), calculated on the anhydrous basis.

It is reported to be a mixture of the 3- and 5-sulfonate isomers.

Preparation—Guaiacol is treated with sulfuric acid at a temperature of 70° to 80° to form guaiacolsulfonic acid. After dilution with water the excess of sulfuric acid is removed by adding barium carbonate which converts the sulfuric acid to the insoluble barium sulfate. After removing the barium sulfate by filtration, sufficient potassium carbonate is added to neutralize the guaiacolsulfonic acid and to precipitate any excess barium. After a second filtration, the solution of potassium guaiacolsulfonate is concentrated to crystallization.

Description—White crystals, or a white crystalline powder. It has a slightly aromatic odor, and a slightly bitter taste. It is affected by light. Its aqueous solution is neutral or slightly alkaline to litmus.

Solubility—1 Gm dissolves in about 7.5 ml of water; insoluble in alcohol and in ether.

Uses—Potassium Guaiacolsulfonate is a stimulant *expectorant.* It does not disturb digestion, is comparatively tasteless, and is not toxic.

Dose—*Usual,* **500 mg.**

Veterinary Dose—*Dogs,* **300 mg to 1 Gm.**

Storax—see page 1374.

Terpin Hydrate NF

[*cis-p*-Menthane-1,8-diol Hydrate; Terpinum; Terpinol]

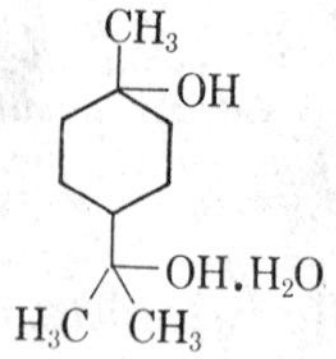

CH₃
OH
OH.H₂O
H₃C CH₃

Terpin Hydrate [$C_{10}H_{20}O_2.H_2O$ = 190.29] contains 98.0–100.5% of $C_{10}H_{20}O_2$, calculated on the anhydrous basis.

Preparation—The manufacture of terpin hydrate is based on the hydration of the pinenes in turpentine oil (or pine oil). The oil, which should contain a high proportion of *pinene* hydrocarbons, is stirred with 2 to 3 times its volume of about 30% sulfuric acid at a temperature of between 20° and 30°. After continuous stirring for 4–6 days, at the same time blowing air through the mixture to assure intimate contact, crystals of Terpin Hydrate separate. The yield depends on the quality of the oil, as well as on the temperature. Higher temperatures than 30° decrease the yield. It is generally preferable to work at a temperature of about 20°, but at this temperature the reaction is slower and the stirring has to be continued for a day or two longer. The crude terpin hydrate is purified by crystallization from alcohol.

The initial reaction involves a rupture of the 1,6-methano bridge of the pinene with simultaneous rearrangement and addition of H_2SO_4 at the double bond. Upon hydrolysis of the latter, two molecules of H_2SO_4 are regenerated, and the glycol *terpin* (*cis-p*-menthane-1,8-diol) is formed. On standing terpin forms the hydrate $[C_{10}H_{18}(OH)_2 . H_2O]$ which crystallizes out. The official identification test is dependent upon the dehydration of terpin to α-, β-, and γ-*terpineol*, an aromatic mixture of cyclic alcohols.

Description—Occurs as colorless, lustrous crystals, or as a white powder. It has a slight odor, and is efflorescent in dry air. A hot 1:100 aqueous solution is neutral to litmus. When dried over sulfuric acid in a vacuum, it melts between 102° and 105°.

Solubility—1 Gm dissolves in about 200 ml of water, 13 ml of alcohol, 140 ml of chloroform, and about 140 ml of ether, at 25°; 1 Gm dissolves in about 35 ml of boiling water and about 3 ml of boiling alcohol.

Identification—A hot solution of Terpin Hydrate becomes turbid and developes a strongly aromatic odor on the addition of a few drops of sulfuric acid.

Incompatibilities—The slight solubility of terpin hydrate in water and vehicles of low alcohol content leads to dispensing difficulties. In some instances alcohol may be added, in others the terpin hydrate may be suspended.

Uses—Terpin Hydrate is used in *bronchitis* as an *expectorant*. Note that Terpin Hydrate Elixir contains too little of the compound to be effective and is employed mainly as a vehicle for cough mixtures.

Dose—*Usual,* **125** to **300 mg** every 6 hours.

Terpin Hydrate Elixir NF contains, in each 100 ml, 1.53–1.87 Gm of $C_{10}H_{20}O_2 . H_2O$. *Preparation:* Dissolve terpin hydrate (17 Gm) in the alcohol (430 ml); add successively sweet orange peel tincture (20 ml), benzaldehyde (0.05 ml), glycerin (400 ml), syrup (100 ml), and purified water (qs) to make the product measure 1000 ml; mix well and filter, if necessary, until the product is clear. *Note*—The sweet orange peel tincture may be replaced by 1 ml of orange oil dissolved in 15 ml of alcohol. *Alcohol Content:* From 39 to 44% of C_2H_5OH. The high alcoholic content in this Elixir is required for the solution of the Terpin Hydrate. *Incompatibilities:* Dilution of this elixir with water or liquids of low alcohol content causes precipitation of the terpin hydrate. *Dose: Usual,* 5 ml equivalent to 85 mg of Terpin Hydrate. *Veterinary Dose: Dogs,* 2 to 4 ml.

Terpin Hydrate and Codeine Elixir NF contains, in each 100 ml, 1.53–1.87 Gm of $C_{10}H_{20}O_2 . H_2O$ (terpin hydrate), and 180–220 mg of $C_{18}H_{21}NO_3 . H_2O$ (codeine). *Preparation:* Dissolve codeine (2 Gm) in terpin hydrate elixir (qs) to make the product measure 1000 ml. *Alcohol Content:* From 39 to 44% of C_2H_5OH. *Uses:* This elixir is an *expectorant* and *sedative* used to allay excessive coughing. Its value resides primarily in its content of codeine. *Caution*—This elixir is sometimes used by addicts, by whom it is known as *GI Gin,* for its alcohol and codeine content. In some states pharmacists are required to register and limit its sale. Its repeated sale to an individual should be noted and stopped. *Dose: Usual,* 5 ml, equivalent to 10 mg of codeine and 85 mg of Terpin Hydrate. *Veterinary Dose: Dogs,* 2 to 4 ml.

Terpin Hydrate and Dextromethorphan Hydrobromide Elixir NF contains, in each 100 ml, 1.53–1.87 Gm of $C_{10}H_{20}O_2 . H_2O$ (terpin hydrate), and 180–220 mg of $C_{18}H_{25}NO.$-$HBr.H_2O$ (dextromethorphan hydrobromide). *Preparation:* Dissolve dextromethorphan hydrobromide (2 Gm) in a sufficient quantity of terpin hydrate elixir to make the product measure 1000 ml. *Uses:* The same indications as Terpin Hydrate and Codeine Elixir. It is used in the control of coughs associated with the common cold, laryngitis, tracheitis, and bronchitis. Dextromethorphan acts to elevate the threshold for coughing. Unlike codeine, it rarely produces drowsiness or gastrointestinal disturbances. *Dose: Usual,* 5 ml, equivalent to 10 mg dextromethorphan hydrobromide and 85 mg of terpin hydrate. *Other Dose Information:* The usual adult dose is 5 to 10 ml 1 to 4 times daily; total daily dose should not exceed 40 ml. Children, 4 to 12 years, 2.5 to 5 ml 4 times a day; total dose should not exceed 20 ml. Children, 2 to 4 years, 1 to 2.5 ml 1 to 4 times daily; total daily dose should not exceed 10 ml.

Tolu Balsam—see page 1335.

Tolu Balsam Syrup—see page 1335.

Tolu Balsam Tincture—see page 1335.

Other Stimulant Expectorants

Creosote Carbonate NF IX—A mixture of the carbonates of various constituents of creosote. A clear, colorless or yellowish, viscid liquid. It is odorless and tasteless, or has a slight odor and taste of creosote. Its specific gravity is not less than 1.145. It is insoluble in water but is miscible with alcohol, petroleum benzin, fixed oils, chloroform, and benzene. *Uses:* Stimulant expectorant. *Dose:* 1 Gm.

Guaiacol NF X—A liquid consisting principally of $C_6H_4(OH)(OCH_3)$-1,2, usually obtained from wood creosote, or a solid, usually prepared synthetically. It occurs as a colorless or yellowish liquid. The solid drug is crystalline and is colorless or yellowish. It becomes darker on exposure to light. It has an agreeable aromatic odor. The specific gravity of the liquid is not less than 1.112 and that of the solid is about 1.132. The solid melts at about 28°C. 1 Gm dissolves in about 65 ml of water and about 1 ml of glycerin, but it separates from the latter when water is added. It is miscible with alcohol, chloroform, ether, and glacial acetic acid. Poisoning from this drug resembles and is treated similarly to phenol intoxication. *Uses:* Stimulant expectorant and local anesthetic. *Dose: Orally,* 0.5 ml.

Guaiacol Carbonate [Guaiacolis Carbonas] $[C_{15}H_{14}O_5]$ —Small, colorless crystals or white, crystalline powder. It is odorless and tasteless, or is but slightly aromatic in odor and taste. It is insoluble in water; 1 Gm is soluble in 60 ml of alcohol, 1 ml of chloroform, 18 ml of ether. Freely soluble in boiling alcohol or benzene, and slightly soluble in glycerin or fixed oils. Melts between 86° and 88°C. *Uses:* Expectorant. *Dose:* 1 Gm.

Turpentine Oil, Rectified NF XI—A colorless liquid prepared by treating turpentine oil with sodium hydroxide and water. *Uses:* As a stimulant *diuretic, anthelmintic, carminative,* and *expectorant.* The Rectified Oil provides a purer form of the Oil for internal administration; its odor is much more fragrant and less objectionable than that of the crude Oil. The alkali with which the crude Oil is treated in the distillation process holds back the resinous oxidation or polymerization products which form on aging. As this Oil deteriorates upon keeping, by ozonizing and finally resinifying, it should not be kept on hand for a long time before using. *Note: Rectified Turpentine Oil is to be dispensed when Turpentine Oil is required for internal use. Oil that has become turbid must not be dispensed. Dose: Usual,* 0.3 ml. *Veterinary Doses: Carminative: Horses* and *Cattle,* 30 to 60 ml; *Sheep* and *Swine,* 4 to 15 ml; *Dogs,* 0.6 to 2 ml. *Expectorant: Horses* and *Cattle,* 10 to 25 ml. *Ruminatoric: Cattle,* 25 to 50 ml; *Sheep* and *Goats,* 2 to 4 ml.

Centrally Acting Expectorants and Antitussive Agents

The centrally acting expectorants consist primarily of the phenanthrene alkaloids of opium; their actions and uses are discussed elsewhere (see Chapter 63, page 1120). Synthetic agents not derived from the opium derivatives, but which exhibit antitussive action, are included in this section. These agents, like the opium alkaloids, are thought to act selectively on the medullary centers to suppress the cough reflex. They differ from the opium alkaloids, however, in that they have little, if any, analgesic action or effect on respiration.

Apomorphine Hydrochloride—see page 806.

Benzonatate NF

[2,5,8,11,14,17,20,23,26-Nonaoxaoctacosan-28-yl *p*-(Butylamino)benzoate; Tessalon (*Ciba*); Ventussin (*Warren-teed*)]

$$CH_3(CH_2)_3 \overset{H}{\underset{}{N}} - C_6H_4 - \overset{O}{\underset{}{C}} - OCH_2CH_2(OCH_2CH_2)_nOCH_3$$

Average: *n* = 8

Benzonatate contains 95.0–105.0% of $C_{30}H_{53}NO_{11}$ (average: 603).

Benzonatate is a mixture of the *p*-butylaminobenzoate esters of the monomethyl ethers derived from a mixture of polyethylene glycols having the average composition of a nonaethylene glycol. The NF subtitle is specific for the average compound. A generic chemical name often used to denote the mixture is ω-methoxypoly(ethyleneoxy)ethyl *p*-(butylamino)benzoate.

Preparation—Ethyl *p*-(butylamino)benzoate is caused to undergo transesterification with a polyethyleneglycol monomethyl ether fraction of boiling range 180°–220° at 1 mm Hg. A mixture of the two components is heated *in vacuo* under conditions whereby a stream of xylene passes up through it. When the last traces of moisture and volatile materials have been removed, a solution of sodium methoxide in methanol is introduced, xylene is again added *in vacuo*, and the mixture is heated for about 2 to 3 hours at 100°. The crude ester is purified by extracting its benzene solution with sodium carbonate solution whereby the ester remains in the benzene layer. US Pat. 2,714,606.

Description—Pale yellow, clear, viscous liquid with a faint characteristic odor and a bitter taste followed by a sense of numbness.

Solubility—Freely soluble in chloroform, alcohol, and benzene; miscible with water in all proportions.

Uses—Benzonatate is an *antitussive*. It exerts an inhibitory effect on the respiratory mucosa similar to that induced by the topical application of a local anesthetic. In addition, it inhibits transmission of impulses of the cough reflex in the vagal nuclei of the medulla and strongly depresses polysynaptic spinal reflexes. Although its antitussive potency is essentially the same as codeine when evaluated against experimentally induced cough in animals and man, it is somewhat less effective than codeine against cough associated with clinical illness.

Benzonatate is well tolerated in therapeutic doses. Untoward effects reported to date include drowsiness, nausea, skin eruption, nasal congestion, a sensation of burning of the eyes, and numbness or tightness in the chest. If the capsules are allowed to dissolve in the mouth, they exert a local anesthetic effect which is disagreeable to a few patients. Habituation, euphoria, respiratory depression, or constipation have not been reported.

Dose—**100** to **200 mg**; *usual*, **100 mg** 3 times a day.

Other Dose Information—The capsules should not be chewed.

Dosage Forms—Capsules NF: 50 and 100 mg; Injection: 5 mg/ml.

Carbetapentane Citrate NF

[2-[2-(Diethylamino)ethoxy]ethyl 1-Phenylcyclopentane-1-carboxylate Citrate (1:1)]

$$[-\overset{O}{\underset{}{C}}OCH_2CH_2OCH_2CH_2\overset{+}{N}H(C_2H_5)_2] \cdot H_2C_6H_5O_7^-$$

Carbetapentane Citrate contains 98.0–100.5% of $C_{20}H_{31}NO_3 \cdot C_6H_8O_7$ (525.60), calculated on the anhydrous basis.

Preparation—1-Phenylcyclopentanecarbonyl chloride (I) is esterified with 2-[2-(diethylamino)ethoxy]ethanol (II). The carbetapentane (base) thus formed may be converted readily into the citrate by dissolving it in alcohol or another suitable solvent and reacting it with an equimolar portion of citric acid.

(I) may be synthesized by the following sequence of reactions: (a) Grignardizing cyclopentanone with phenylmagnesium bromide to produce 1-phenylcyclopentanol (III); (b) converting (III) to the bromide with PBr_3; (c) refluxing the bromide with alcoholic NaCN to produce the nitrile; (d) hydrating the nitrile to the acid; and (e) converting the acid to (I) with PCl_5.

(II) is synthesized readily from diethylamine and a double molar portion of ethylene oxide.

Description—Occurs as a white, or practically white, odorless, crystalline powder. Melting range 90° to 95°.

Solubility—Freely soluble in water; slightly soluble in alcohol; practically insoluble in ether.

Uses—Carbetapentane Citrate is an *antitussive* agent which exhibits atropine-like and local anesthetic properties. The drug is reported to suppress the cough reflex by selectively depressing the medullary centers. It is effective in *acute coughs* associated with common upper respiratory infections.

Dose—*Usual*, **15** to **30 mg** 3 to 4 times a day.

Codeine—see page 1124.

Codeine Phosphate—see page 1124.

Codeine Sulfate—see page 1125.

Dextromethorphan Hydrobromide NF

[(+)-3-Methoxy-17-methyl-9α,13α,14α-morphinan Hydrobromide; *d*-1,3,4,9,10,10a-Hexahydro-6-methoxy-11-methyl-2H-10,4a-iminoethanophenanthrene Hydrobromide; Dormethan (*Dorsey*); Romilar (*Roche*)]

Dextromethorphan Hydrobromide contains 98.0–100.5% of $C_{18}H_{25}NO \cdot HBr \cdot H_2O$ (370.33), calculated on the anhydrous basis.

Preparation—Dextromethorphan (base) [d-3-methoxy-N-methylmorphinan] is prepared from the corresponding d-3-hydroxy compound by methylation with phenyltrimethylammonium hydroxide. The procedure is analogous to that employed for the methylation of morphine to produce codeine (page 1124). Treatment of the base with hydrogen bromide yields the official hydrobromide which may be purified by recrystallization.

The starting d-3-hydroxy compound is synthesized as described under Levorphanol Tartrate (page 1127) except that the d-enantiomorph of compound (IV) is employed in the final step.

Description—Practically white crystals, or crystalline powder, having a faint odor. Melting range: 125° to 128°. Specific rotation: +26° to +28°. pH: 5.2 to 6.5.

Solubility—1 Gm dissolves in about 65 ml of water; freely soluble in alcohol and chloroform; insoluble in ether.

Uses—Dextromethorphan Hydrobromide, a synthetic morphine derivative, is employed exclusively as an *antitussive* agent. It is devoid of analgesic properties and produces little or no depression of the central nervous system. Addiction has not been observed after the administration of rather large doses for prolonged periods. The side effects reported to date have been slight, and there is some doubt that those which have been reported are due to the drug.

Dose—*Usual*, **15 to 30 mg** 1 to 4 times a day.

Dosage Forms—Syrup NF: 15 mg/5 ml.

Ethylmorphine Hydrochloride—see page 1125.

Hydrocodone Bitartrate—see page 1126.

Levopropoxyphene Napsylate NF

[(−)-α-4-(Diethylamino)-3-methyl-1,2-diphenyl-2-butanol Propionate (ester)
2-Naphthalenesulfonate (salt); Novrad Napsylate (*Lilly*)]

Levopropoxyphene Napsylate $[C_{22}H_{29}NO_2 \cdot C_{10}H_8O_3S \cdot H_2O = 565.73]$ contains 97.0–101.0% of $C_{22}H_{29}NO_2 \cdot C_{10}H_8O_3S$ (547.72), calculated on the anhydrous basis.

Preparation—The racemate of the α-diastereoisomer of the substituted butanol corresponding to Propoxyphene is prepared as described on page 1139 and resolved with (+)-camphorsulfonic acid. The (−)-alcohol thus obtained is esterified with propionic anhydride to form (−)-propoxyphene (base) which is then caused to combine with an equimolar quantity of 2-naphthalenesulfonic acid to form the official salt.

Description—A white powder that is essentially odorless and has a bitter taste. It melts between 158° and 165° (previously dried at 105°).

Solubility—Soluble in methanol, alcohol, chloroform, and acetone; very slightly soluble in water.

Uses—Levopropoxyphene Napsylate is used as an antitussive agent. In contrast to *Propoxyphene* (page 1139), this isomer is devoid of analgesic activity. It is

somewhat less potent than codeine in the treatment of cough; 50 to 100 mg appears to be as effective as 15 mg of codeine in experimental cough. Untoward effects are usually mild; headache, lightheadedness, skin rash, dryness of the mouth, nausea and vomiting, urinary urgency, and tremors have been reported. Since the drug does not induce physical dependence, it is particularly valuable when long-term antitussive therapy is necessary.

Dose—*Usual*, **50 to 100 mg** every 4 hours.

Dosage Forms—Capsules NF: 50 and 100 mg.

Methadone Hydrochloride—see page 1131.

Morphine Hydrochloride—see page 1125.

Morphine Sulfate—see page 1123.

Noscapine NF

[(−)-Narcotine; Nectadon (*MSD*)]

Noscapine contains 99.0–100.5% of $C_{22}H_{23}NO_7$ (413.43), calculated on the anhydrous basis.

It is the naturally occurring (l-form) of the alkaloid, narcotine. For the structural formula, see page 493.

Preparation—Noscapine is isolated from opium in which it is present in amounts ranging from 3 to 10%.

Description—A fine, white, or practically white, crystalline powder. It is odorless. Because of its very bitter taste, it is unacceptable in solutions for oral use. It is stable in the presence of light and air. Its solution in chloroform is levorotatory, but aqueous solutions of its salts with mineral acids are dextrorotatory. Melting range 174° to 176°.

Solubility—Practically insoluble in water; freely soluble in chloroform; soluble in acetone and in benzene; slightly soluble in alcohol and ether.

Uses—Noscapine, an isoquinoline alkaloid of opium also known commonly as narcotine, is an *antitussive* agent which depresses the medullary centers and suppresses the cough reflex. The drug reduces the frequency and intensity of coughing paroxysms. Its antitussive potency, onset, and duration of action is approximately equal, milligram for milligram, to those of codeine.

Therapeutically effective doses of Noscapine are essentially devoid of the unpleasant side effects of codeine, and, except for occasional nausea, its side effects are negligible. The drug has no morphine-like effects and has no effect on the morphine abstinence syndrome. Tolerance to the antitussive effect has not been observed. Hence, Noscapine is classified as an especially exempted preparation under the federal narcotic law.

Dose—**15 to 30 mg**; *usual*, **15 mg** up to 4 times a day.

Noscapine Hydrochloride NF XII

[Noscapinium Chloride; l-Narcotine Hydrochloride; Nectadon Hydrochloride (*MSD*)]

Noscapine Hydrochloride contains not less than 99.0% of $C_{22}H_{23}NO_7 \cdot HCl$ (449.89), calculated on the dried basis. For the structure, see page 493.

Description—It occurs as a fine, white, or practically white, crystalline powder. It is odorless or has a slight odor of ethyl alcohol. Its solution in water is dextrorotatory. The pH of a solution (1 in 20) is between 2.5 and 3.5.

Solubility—Freely soluble in water, chloroform, and methanol; soluble in ethanol; sparingly soluble in acetone; practically insoluble in ether.

Uses—See *Noscapine*.
Dose—*Usual*, **15 to 30 mg**, 3 to 4 times a day.

Other Centrally Acting Expectorants and Antitussive Agents

Brown Mixture NF XII [Mistura Opii et Glycyrrhizæ Composita; Compound Opium and Glycyrrhiza Mixture NF XI: Mistura Glycyrrhizæ Composita; Compound Mixture of Glycyrrhiza]—*Preparation:* Dilute glycyrrhiza fluidextract (120 ml) with glycerin (120 ml) and purified water (500 ml), add antimony potassium tartrate (0.24 Gm), dissolved in hot purified water (12 ml), then add paregoric (120 ml) and alcohol (30 ml), and purified water (qs) to make the product measure 1000 ml. This formula in which glycyrrhiza extract is replaced by the fluidextract will contain a precipitate, but it is intended to be dispensed without filtering to retain its universally known classification as a mixture. *Alcohol Content:* 9–11%. *Uses:* A needlessly complex therapeutic survival of another day, although occasionally employed by certain physicians. It is prescribed for coughs, often combined with ammonium chloride. *Dose: Usual,* 5 ml, equivalent to 1.2 mg of antimony potassium tartrate and 0.6 ml of paregoric. *Veterinary Dose: Horses* and *Cattle,* 40 ml; Dogs, 3 to 6 ml.

Chlophedianol Hydrochloride [2-chloro-α-[2-(dimethylamino)ethyl]benzhydrol hydrochloride; $C_{17}H_{20}ClNO.HCl$; ULO (*Riker*)]—*Uses:* A non-narcotic cough suppressant with some local anesthetic and anticholinergic properties. It is used to control the cough associated with upper respiratory infections, common cold, influenza, pneumonia, bronchitis, tracheitis, laryngitis, croup, pertussis, pleurisy, etc. It has a slower onset of action and a more prolonged action than the narcotic expectorants. Side effects include excitation, hyperirritability and nightmares. Tolerance or addiction have not been reported. *Dose: Usual adult,* 25 mg (one teaspoonful of the syrup) 4 times daily as required for cough.

Dimethoxanate Hydrochloride [Cothera (*Ayerst*)] is 2-[2-(dimethylamino)ethoxy]ethyl phenothiazine-10-carboxylate hydrochloride [$C_{19}H_{22}N_2O_3S.HCl$]. *Description and Solubility:* White, odorless, crystalline powder which discolors on exposure to daylight; melts at 156°. Very soluble in water, lower alcohols, and chloroform. *Uses:* An *antitussive, local anesthetic,* and *mild antispasmodic.* This phenothiazine derivative acts centrally to depress the cough reflex. It is somewhat less effective and has a shorter duration of action than codeine. Untoward effects are generally mild and include drowsiness, nausea, dizziness, and occasionally, lip numbness caused by its local anesthetic action. *Dose: Usual,* 25 to 50 mg 3 or 4 times daily; the dose for children has not been established.

Pholcodine BP—The 3-[2-(4-morpholinyl)ethyl] ether of morphine [$C_{23}H_{30}N_2O_4$]. Occurs as a white or almost white, crystalline powder; odorless; very bitter taste; Soluble, at 20°, in 50 parts of water and in 3 parts of absolute alcohol; very soluble in chloroform and acetone; soluble in dilute hydrochloric acid. *Uses:* Cough suppressant. *Dose:* 5 to 15 mg.

Pipazethate [2-(2-piperidinoethoxy)ethyl 10*H*-pyrido-[3,2-*b*] [1,4]benzothiazine-10-carboxylate; $C_{21}H_{25}N_3O_3S$; Theratuss (*Squibb*)]—*Uses:* Depresses the cough center in the medulla. Hence, it is useful in the control of cough arising from a variety of conditions including bronchitis, asthmatic states, chronic pleurisy, sarcoidosis, influenza, pneumonia, acute respiratory infections, etc. The drug is usually effective within 10 to 30 minutes and provides relief for 4 to 6 hours. Although side effects are minimal, nausea, vomiting, and gastric upset have been reported in some patients. Moderate tachycardia has also been observed. The drug should not be used in children under 7 years of age. *Dose: Usual adult oral,* 20 to 40 mg 3 or 4 times daily according to the severity of the cough.

Therapeutic Gases

A number of pharmacologic agents are gaseous at normal temperatures and pressures, whereas others are liquids or even solids with such high vapor pressures that they yield vapors in sufficiently high concentration to exhibit pharmacological properties. Since these gases and vapors are absorbed by way of the respiratory tract, they could be included in this section. However, only those gases which have therapeutic application are presented here. Aside from the anesthetic gases and vapors, which are discussed elsewhere (see Chapter 58, page 1055), the most important therapeutic gases are carbon dioxide, oxygen, and helium. Although helium is not a pharmacologically active agent, it does possess valuable therapeutic properties attributable to its unique physical properties; hence, it is included in this section.

Carbon Dioxide—see page 869.

Helium USP

Helium [He = 4.0026; At. No. 2] contains not less than 99.0% by volume of He. The remainder consists mainly of nitrogen.

History, Occurrence and Preparation—See page 403.

Description—A colorless, odorless, tasteless, chemically inert gas. A liter of the gas at 760 mm and 0° weighs not less than 174.5 mg and not more than 232.5 mg.

Solubility—Very slightly soluble in water.

Identification—A burning splinter of wood is extinguished when plunged into Helium. It does not react with hydrogen.

Uses—Helium is used as a diluent for medicinal gases. It owes its pharmacological actions exclusively to its physical properties. A mixture of 80 parts Helium and 20 parts oxygen is only one-third as heavy as air. Such mixtures are used in the treatment of *respiratory obstruction* and are of great value in relieving *status asthmaticus* and the symptoms arising from inflammatory obstructions. When administered in *asphyxia*, the light mixture penetrates the air passages more readily than mixtures of nitrogen and oxygen.

Dose—By *inhalation*, **60** to **80%**, with oxygen 20 to 40%.

Oxygen USP

Oxygen contains not less than 99.0% by volume of O_2 (32.00).

Preparation—See page 418.

Description—A colorless, odorless, tasteless gas. It supports combustion more energetically than air. A liter of Oxygen at a pressure of 760 mm (1 atm) and at 0°C weighs 1.429 Gm.

Solubility—One volume of Oxygen dissolves in about 32 volumes of water or in about 7 volumes of alcohol at 20°C and 760 mm pressure.

Identification—A glowing splinter of wood held in Oxygen bursts into flame.

Uses—Oxygen is widely employed in the treatment of *anoxia*. It is usually administered by means of an oxygen tent, or a special face mask in concentrations ranging from 40 to 100%. Pure Oxygen should be given only for limited periods of time, inasmuch as it is apt to injure the epithelial lining of the lung.

Oxygen exerts its greatest benefit in the treatment of conditions of anoxia which arise from inadequate oxygenation of the blood passing through the lungs. Chief among these are *pneumonia* and *pulmonary edema*. The gas also offers relief in the treatment of severe *asthma*. The symptoms of *acute coronary occlusion* are also somewhat mitigated by high concentrations of Oxygen. Patients in *shock* are greatly benefited by the gas.

A special indication for Oxygen is in the treatment of *carbon monoxide poisoning*. The inhalation of a high concentration of Oxygen, especially when combined with carbon dioxide, speeds the conversion of carboxyhemoglobin formed by the carbon monoxide to oxyhemoglobin.

Oxygen is routinely employed during the administration of anesthetic gases or vapors by the "closed" method. Anesthetic agents which are sufficiently potent so as to permit the simultaneous administration of a high concentration of oxygen possess advantages (see *Cyclopropane*, page 1060) over those which are less active (see *Nitrous Oxide*, page 1060).

Dose—By *inhalation*, as required.

48 | Sympathomimetic Drugs

This chapter was prepared by

Ewart A. Swinyard, PhD, *Professor of Pharmacology, College of Pharmacy and College of Medicine, University of Utah, Salt Lake City, Utah 84112, and*
Stewart C. Harvey, PhD, *Associate Professor of Pharmacology, College of Medicine, University of Utah, Salt Lake City, Utah 84112*

The next five chapters treat specifically of autonomic drugs, and several other chapters (eg, Chapters 44, 46, 62, and 65) include references to a number of autonomic drugs. Consequently, it will be helpful to review briefly the autonomic nervous system and the classification of drugs which act upon or simulate components of that system.

Autonomic Nervous System and Autonomic Drugs

The *autonomic (involuntary) nervous system* is generally defined as that system of motor (efferent) nerves which contains cell bodies and corresponding synapses (ie, ganglia) outside of the cerebrospinal axis. The definition includes the sensory (efferent) nerves that subserve functions mediated by the autonomic motor nerves, although a given sensory nerve may also subserve somatic motor functions. This system modulates or controls the activities of smooth (involuntary) muscles of the body, including those that control the caliber of blood vessels, the heart muscle, and the digestive, salivary, sweat, and some endocrine glands. Unconsciously (without conscious control) it tends to maintain a constant state (homeostasis) of the vital functions of the body, constantly adjusting one factor to attempt to restore an equilibrium upset by external or internal influences; cerebral blood flow, body temperature, visual accommodation, blood sugar, and body fluid composition, for example, are kept remarkably constant by means of servoadjustments mediated through the autonomic nerves. However, it should be noted that the *somatic (voluntary) nervous system* also unconsciously subserves vital functions such as respiration, swallowing, defecation, motor reflexes, body temperature, and many less vital but important unconscious modulations of muscle tone; however, the degree of conscious modulation of this control is much greater than in the autonomic nervous system. These involuntary somatic motor functions are coordinated with autonomic functions.

There are two main motor divisions to the autonomic nervous systems—the *sympathetic* (thoracolumbar) and the *parasympathetic* (craniosacral) divisions. Most organs or systems (effectors) receive innervation from both these divisions; generally, but not invariably, the two divisions are qualitatively opposed in their action on a given effector. An abridged list of responses is presented in Table I.

The opposition of the two divisions of the autonomic nervous system reflects the fact that the chemical substances (mediator, transmitter, or neurohumor) liberated by the postganglionic nerve terminals are not the same for the two divisions. Parasympathetic postganglionic nerves liberate acetylcholine, and hence are

Table I—Response of Human Effector Organs to Autonomic Nerve Impulses

Effector system	Sympathetic nerve impulses	Parasympathetic nerve impulses
Systemic blood vessels	Constrict Dilate[a]	Innervate few systemic vessels, but dilate
Pulmonary blood vessels	Constrict	Dilate
Coronary blood vessels	Dilate	Dilate
Bronchioles	Dilate	Constrict
Stomach motility and tone	Decrease	Increase
Gastric secretion	Little Effect	Increase
Intestinal motility and tone	Decrease	Increase
Urinary bladder sphincter	Constrict	Dilate
Heart	Increase rate and strength	Decrease rate and strength; block
Pupil of eye	Dilate	Constrict
Salivary glands	Stimulate to viscid saliva	Stimulate to watery saliva
Sweat glands	Stimulate[a]	Not innervated
Lacrimal glands	Not innervated	Stimulate

[a] *Cholinergic* sympathetic postganglionics mediate response.

called *cholinergic* nerves. Most sympathetic postganglionic nerves liberate norepinephine(levarterenol); however, sympathetics to the sweat glands and certain blood vessels, especially those of the skeletal muscles, liberate acetylcholine (ie, are cholinergic). Some sympathetic nerves also appear to liberate histamine. The normal adrenal medulla, which is innervated by sympathetic preganglionics, liberates mostly epinephrine, originally known as adrenaline; since adrenaline was early thought to be the sympathetic transmitter, norepinephrine-releasing nerves are termed *adrenergic.*

At the ganglia, preganglionic nerves of either division liberate acetylcholine (ie, are cholinergic), but the character of the acetylcholine ganglionic receptors is different from those in the neuroeffectors, so that the two types of receptors are not blocked by the same drugs. Somatic motor nerves also liberate acetylcholine (ie, are cholinergic) and are similar to autonomic preganglionics in this regard.

Autonomic drugs are classified according to their relation to the chemical mediator that they either mimic or block. Thus, a drug is cholinergic if it either mimics or blocks stimulation by adrenergic nerves. The terms *cholinomimetic* and *adrenomimetic* have been advanced for the appropriate mimetic agents. There prevails, however, an older terminology based on the erroneous belief that all sympathetic postganglionic nerves yielded the same transmitter. Hence, adrenomimetics are usually called *sympathomimetics* (this chapter) and cholinomimetics are often called *parasympathomimetics* (Chapter 49, page 899); but it should be recalled that two types of cholinergic receptor exist, and the use of the term parasympathomimetic best fits those drugs that act upon the cholinergic neuroeffectors (ie, are muscarinic), not the ganglionic synapses. Agents which block the receptors are called *blocking agents*, according to the nature of the chemical transmitter with which they compete. Thus, there are *adrenergic blocking agents* (Chapter 50, page 908) and *antimuscarinic agents* (Chapter 51, page 914), the latter term again restricted to those drugs that block acetylcholine at the neuroeffector receptors. Those agents that block acetylcholine at the ganglionic synapse are simply called *ganglionic blocking agents* (Chapter 46, page 848); their somatic motor counterpart (generally loosely included among the autonomic drugs) are called *neuromuscular blocking agents* (*curarimimetics*) (Chapter 52, page 928). The suffix lytic sometimes is used in lieu of the word *blocking;* thus a sympatholytic agent is an adrenergic blocking agent. No terminology has been developed for those agents that act at afferent (sensory or reflex) or central autonomic loci. Also, agents, such as the anticholinesterases, which enhance autonomic transmission by preserving the transmitter from enzymatic destruction are endowed with no definitive designation; the *anticholinesterases* (Chapter 49, page 902) are awkwardly classified as cholinomimetics or parasympathomimetics.

An autonomic mediator not only is liberated at different sites and exerts different effects, but it may also act upon different receptors. The actions of acetylcholine upon the exocrine glands, smooth muscle and heart differ from those on autonomic ganglia and the voluntary neuromuscular junction. The former (and not the latter) effects are blocked by atropine, whereas the latter (and not the former) are blocked by tubocurarine. Since muscarine exerts the former actions (and not the latter), the corresponding receptors are called *muscarinic;* since nicotine exerts the latter actions (and not the former), the corresponding receptors are called *nicotinic.* In the adrenergic system there are also two main types of receptors. The *alpha* adrenergic receptors subserve smooth muscular stimulant and some intestinal relaxant functions, adrenergic sweating, adrenergic salivating, and lipolysis. The *beta* adrenergic receptors subserve smooth muscle relaxant functions everywhere, except possibly in some veins, and also cause stimulation of the heart and glycolysis. As in the cholinergic system, the different receptors are inhibited by different blocking agents, the alpha receptors being selectively blocked by phenozybenzamine and the beta receptors by propranolol. Dopamine excites a receptor that is blocked by haloperidols; this receptor does not appear to be activated by other adrenergic stimulants. There are also at least two receptors for histamine.

Sympathomimetics

Both levarterenol (norepinephrine) and epinephrine are natural to the body. Although levarterenol is the principal transmitter of the adrenergic nerves, epinephrine was first isolated (from the adrenal medulla) and serves as the historical prototype. Neither drug is simple in its actions. Epinephrine differs from the adrenergic transmitter in having prominent vasodilator actions in low concentrations; especially in the skeletal muscle vascular bed, dilation may occur even in relatively high concentrations. Vasoconstrictor actions at physiological concentrations are prominent only in the cutaneous and renal vascular beds, although at higher concentrations constriction may be general. Epinephrine also has prominent metabolic actions to elevate the blood glucose and lactate concentrations and other effects. By utilizing the appropriate portion of the epinephrine molecule, it is possible to design sympathomimetic molecules that accentuate one action and minimize another so that there are pressor agents without prominent cardiac effects, general depressor agents, vasodilators for certain vascular beds only, etc. Epinephrine also is a central stimulant, and it is possible to mimic this action with a minimal amount of the cardiovascular actions. Absorption and duration can also be altered by the appropriate molecular substituents. Aliphatic amines longer than *n*-butylamine are sufficient for pressor activity, but the aromatic rings markedly enhance potency. However, the unsubstituted aromatic ring also increases central stimulant activity. Single hydroxyl groups in the 3 or 4 position of the ring increase vasoconstrictor potency. Two hydroxyl groups (3,4) increase the tendency to induce vasodilation when other optimal molecular substituents are present. Cardiac and metabolic actions are also enhanced by the 3,4-dihydroxy substitution. N-substituents favor vasodilation, the optimal substituent being an isopropyl group, and metabolic effects, the optimal substituent being a methyl group. Substitution on the side chain immediately adjacent to the amino group prevents enzymatic destruction, which confers oral efficacy and prolonged duration of action. Topical efficacy and central stimulant activity are favored by a minimum of polar groups in the molecule or by increasing the size of nonpolar substituents. Levo forms (of the β-hydroxyl) are the more active in any of the actions except the central actions; this fact makes selective *central stimulants* possible.

Many sympathomimetics do not actually mimic the actions of levarterenol or epinephrine at the effector receptor. Rather, they induce the release of levarterenol from the sympathetic postganglionic adrenergic nerves. The structural prerequisite for a prominent direct action on the adrenergic receptor is two hydroxyl groups in the molecule, either both on the ring (in the 3,4 positions) or one on the ring and one at the 2 position of the side chain. Those sympathomimetics which do not meet this prerequisite mainly act indirectly by the release of the true adrenergic mediator. Indirectly acting sympathomimetics are less effective in patients treated with norepinephrine-depleting drugs, such as the rauwolfia alkaloids, or other adrenergic neurone blockers.

Catecholamines such as norepinephrine and epinephrine are attacked by both monoamine oxidase (MAO) and catechol-O-methyl transferase (COMT); COMT seems to be the more important enzyme in the periphery, but MAO is more important in the CNS. Consequently, sympathomimetics with central stimulant properties are contraindicated when MAO inhibitors are being used. Furthermore, several noncatecholic sympathomimetics are mainly biotransformed by MAO even in the periphery, so that dangerous pressor responses may occur with usual doses when MAO inhibitors are being used. Consequently, it is a wise precaution to avoid the concomitant use of sympathomimetics of any kind and MAO inhibitors.

Amphetamine

[Amphetamine USP XIV; Benzedrine (*SK&F*);   *dl*-α-Methyl-β-phenyl-
ethylamine; (±)-α-Methylphenethylamine]

Amphetamine [$C_9H_{13}N$ = 135.21] is now official only
in the form of certain salts. The unqualified term,
Amphetamine, signifies the racemic mixture.

Preparation—Amphetamine may be prepared by
several methods, the most important of which utilize
phenylacetone as the intermediate. In one method,
the phenylacetone is converted into its oxime which is
then reduced with hydrogen to amphetamine. In
another method the phenylacetone is directly converted into amphetamine by heating it with formamide
at about 190°.

Description—Colorless, mobile liquid with a characteristic odor and acrid taste. Volatilizes at ordinary temperatures. Readily absorbs carbon dioxide from the air and its
solutions are alkaline to litmus. Specific gravity 0.930 to
0.936. Distilling range 200° to 203°, with slight decomposition.

Solubility—Slightly soluble in water; soluble in alcohol,
in ether, and diluted mineral acids.

Uses—Amphetamine has *sympathomimetic* properties related to those of epinephrine and ephedrine. It
does not stimulate adrenergic effectors directly but acts
indirectly through the release of levarterenol from the
adrenergic nerves. It thus stimulates smooth muscles
and gland cells innervated by sympathetic (adrenergic)
nerves. In addition it has a potent excitatory effect on
the central nervous system. Amphetamine does not
share all the actions of ephedrine and related compounds
and thus is not useful in asthma, or, with a few exceptions, for cardiovascular or gastrointestinal purposes.
It does constrict small vessels when applied locally and
thus, in the form of an inhaler or a solution in oil, was
formerly widely employed to shrink mucosa in *hay
fever, acute coryza, vasomotor rhinitis, acute sinusitis*, etc;
however, because of an upsurge of amphetamine addiction, less addicting sympathomimetics have completely
replaced amphetamine in over-the-counter preparations.
It can also be employed in *orthostatic hypotension* and in
syncope due to abnormal carotid sinus reflexes. In
ophthalmological work, the drug is occasionally used as
a *mydriatic*. It is also helpful in *myasthenia gravis*.
Its use in *epilepsy* along with phenobarbital has definite
therapeutic value. It is also fairly specific for the
oculogyric crises of *postencephalitic parkinsonism*, and
is often prescribed in this disorder in combination with
belladonna alkaloids. Other uses of the central actions
of amphetamine include the acute poisoning by central
nervous system depressant drugs, such as morphine
and barbiturates;   the symptomatic treatment of
narcolepsy; psychogenic disorders including acute and
chronic *alcoholism*, and *migraine*. Amphetamine also
has an effect to suppress appetite (anorexic effect),
and it is often used in the treatment of obesity.
However, dextroamphetamine and certain other
related amines are more selective in this action and
are thus more rational to use. Moreover, the effect
is not lasting, and the patient reverts to previous
eating habits quickly after discontinuation of treatment. Because of this and of the danger of drug
abuse, Amphetamine (and probably all anorexic
amines) should not be used in the treatment of obesity.

Reserpine does not abolish the central effects o:
Amphetamine.
Dose—See under the monographs of the salts below

Amphetamine Sulfate NF

[(±)-α-Methylphenethylamine Sulfate (2:1); Racemic Amphetamine Sul
fate; *dl*-1-phenyl-2-aminopropane sulfate; Benzedrine Sulfate *SK&F*)

Amphetamine Sulfate, dried at 105° for 2 hours, con
tains 98.0–100.5% of $(C_9H_{13}N)_2 \cdot H_2SO_4$ (368.50).
For the structure of the base, see *Amphetamine*
this page.

Description—A white, odorless, slightly bitter, crystal
line powder. Its solutions are acid to litmus, having a pH
of 5 to 6.
Solubility—1 Gm dissolves in about 9 ml of water an
about 500 ml of alcohol; insoluble in ether.

Uses—See *Amphetamine*.
Dose—*Oral*, 5 to 30 mg daily; *usual, oral*, 5 mg
times a day; *intravenous*, 10 to 50 mg; *usual, intra
muscular* and *slow intravenous*, for barbiturate poison
ing, 10 mg.
Dosage Forms—Injection NF: 20 mg/ml, 60
mg/30 ml; Tablets NF: 5 and 10 mg.
Veterinary Dose—*Horses* and *Cattle, subcutaneously
100 to 300 mg; Dogs, *parenterally*, 0.5 to 2.0 m;
per **pound** of body weight; *Cats*, 0.5 to 1 mg pe
pound of body weight to combat depression asso
ciated with encephalomyelitis and CNS depressants.

Benzphetamine Hydrochloride NF

[(+)-*N*-Benzyl-*N*,α-dimethylphenethylamine Hydrochloride;   Didr
(*Upjohn*)]

Benzphetamine   Hydrochloride   contains   98.0
101.0% of $C_{17}H_{21}N \cdot HCl$ (275.82), calculated on th
dried basis.
Preparation—(+)-Desoxyephedrine is benzylate
by reaction with benzyl chloride in the presence c
sodium carbonate. The benzphetamine (base) thu
formed is distilled from the product under reduce
pressure, dissolved in a suitable solvent, and precip
tated as the hydrochloride by means of hydroge
chloride.

Description—Odorless, white to off-white, crystallin
powder. It is polymorphic with one form melting at abou
130° and another at about 150° and higher with decompos
tion.
Solubility—1 Gm dissolves in about 1.5 ml of wate
1.5 ml of alcohol, and in 1.5 ml of chloroform; slightly so
uble in ether.

Uses—Benzphetamine is an indirectly acting sym
pathomimetic drug and central nervous system stimu
lant derived from Amphetamine. Its principal clinica
use is as an *appetite suppressant*. It is not intended fo
use as a peripheral sympathomimetic or as a genera
central nervous system stimulant. It has a euphori
action. As an anorexigenic agent it is about as effica
cious as Dextroamphetamine. See *Amphetamin
(above) regarding limitations to anorexic therapy.
Untoward effects include nervousness, dizzines
insomnia, tachycardia, palpitation, dry mouth, loss o

taste, nausea, vomiting, constipation, tachycardia, palpitation, polyuria, and dermatitis. Its addicting potentialities have not been determined.

Dose—*Usual*, **25** to **50 mg**, 1 to 3 times a day.

Dosage Forms—Tablets NF: 25 and 50 mg.

Cyclopentamine Hydrochloride NF

[*N*,α-Dimethylcyclopentaneëthylamine Hydrochloride;   Clopane (*Lilly*)]

$$\left[\begin{array}{c} CH_2CHNH_2CH_3 \\ | \\ CH_3 \end{array} \right] Cl^-$$

Cyclopentamine Hydrochloride, dried at 80° for 3 hours, contains 98.0–100.5% of $C_9H_{19}N \cdot HCl$ (177.72).

Preparation—Acetoacetic ester is reacted in alcohol solution with sodium ethoxide to produce the sodio derivative (I). Cyclopentyl bromide (II) is added and the mixture is refluxed whereupon sodium bromide precipitates with the formation of (III). After filtering to remove the sodium bromide and evaporating in vacuo to remove the alcohol, (III) is hydrolyzed by heating with sodium hydroxide solution to yield cyclopentylacetone (IV). Simultaneous treatment of (IV) with hydrogen and anhydrous methylamine under the catalytic influence of Raney nickel causes reduction to the corresponding carbinol followed by condensation with the amine to yield cyclopentamine (base). After purification by distillation under reduced pressure, the base is dissolved in ether and treated with anhydrous hydrogen chloride whereupon the official salt precipitates in crystalline form.

C_2H_5OCO CHCOCH_3
|
Na
I

Br
II

C_2H_5OCO CHCOCH_3
III

CH_2COCH_3
IV

Description—White, crystalline powder, possessing a mild characteristic odor and a bitter taste. It melts between 113° and 116°, and has a pH of about 6.2.

Solubility—1 Gm dissolves in about 1 ml of water, 2 ml of alcohol, 25 ml of benzene, and about 1 ml of chloroform; slightly soluble in ether.

Uses—Cyclopentamine is an indirectly acting sympathomimetic which has vasoconstrictor and pressor actions accompanied by only slight cardiac or central actions. It relaxes the bronchioles and the bowel and induces mydriasis. It does not act directly on adrenergic receptors but rather indirectly through the release of levarterenol from adrenergic nerves. It is used to *maintain blood pressure* in operative procedures, especially by spinal anesthesia, and in cardiovascular collapse and for *nasal decongestion*.

Dose—*Usual, intramuscular*, **25 mg**; *intravenous*, **5** to **10 mg**; *intranasal*, **1** or **2 drops** of a **0.5** or **1%** solution every 3 or 4 hours.

Dosage Forms—Injection NF: 25 mg/ml; Solution NF: 0.5 and 1%.

Dextroamphetamine Phosphate NF

[Monobasic Dextro-amphetamine Phosphate;   Monobasic   (+)-α-Methylphenethylamine Phosphate (1:1)]

Dextroamphetamine Phosphate, dried at 105° for 2 hours, contains 98.5–100.5% $C_9H_{13}N \cdot H_3PO_4$ (233.21).

For the structure of the base, see *Amphetamine*, page 882.

Preparation—It may be prepared by resolving *dl*-amphetamine bitartrate, liberating and extracting the *d*-amphetamine content, followed by neutralizing the *d*-amphetamine with an equimolar portion of phosphoric acid. By using suitable solvents, the neutralization reaction may be conducted in such fashion as to cause precipitation of the crystalline salt as it is formed.

Description—A white, odorless, crystalline powder having a bitter taste. The pH of a 1 in 20 solution is between 4 and 5. The specific rotation of a 4% aqueous solution of a dried sample is between +15° and +19°.

Solubility—1 Gm dissolves in 20 ml of water; slightly soluble in alcohol; practically insoluble in benzene, chloroform, and ether.

Uses—The actions and uses of Dextroamphetamine are very similar to those of racemic amphetamine (see *Amphetamine*), but the peripheral actions are considerably weaker. As a central stimulant, the dextrorotatory isomer is approximately twice as potent (on a weight basis) as the racemic mixture and three to four times as potent as the levorotatory isomer. Because of its *central stimulant* effects, Dextroamphetamine is of value in *narcolepsy*, and, in combination with belladonna alkaloids, it is useful in *postencephalitic parkinsonism*. The drug is also employed as an adjuvant to psychotherapy in the treatment of *chronic alcoholism*, and for its anorexigenic action in the treatment of *obesity*. It is a valuable adjuvant to phenobarbital in the therapy of *grand mal epilepsy;* it counteracts the ataxia and drowsiness produced by phenobarbital and allows sufficient amounts of the latter drug to be employed to control seizures. It serves a similar purpose when combined with trimethadione in the treatment of *petit mal epilepsy.*

Dextroamphetamine has been used in the treatment of a variety of psychogenic disorders, but its efficacy in these states is controversial. Although this agent has been widely used to *alleviate sleepiness and fatigue* in individuals not under medical supervision, its indiscriminate use for this purpose is to be condemned. The cardiovascular action of Dextroamphetamine is of value in the treatment of certain cases of *orthostatic hypotension;* the results obtained appear to be as good as those obtained with ephedrine. Dextroamphetamine has also been employed to control *nausea and vomiting of pregnancy*, but more specific drugs have eclipsed a full investigation for this use.

Dose—**5** to **10 mg**; *usual*, **5 mg** every 4 to 6 hours.

Dosage Forms—Tablets NF: 5 mg.

Dextroamphetamine Sulfate USP

[(+)-α-Methylphenethylamine Sulfate (2:1);   Dexamphetamine Sulphate; *d*-1-Phenyl-2-aminopropane Sulfate; *d*-Amfetasul (*Pitman–Moore*); Dexedrine Sulfate (*SK&F*)]

Dextroamphetamine Sulfate, the dextrorotatory isomer of amphetamine sulfate, contains 98.0–101.0% of $(C_9H_{13}N)_2 \cdot H_2SO_4$ (368.50), calculated on the dried basis.

For the structure of the base, see *Amphetamine*, page 882.

Description—A white, odorless, crystalline powder. Its 1 in 20 solution has a pH between 5 and 6. The specific rotation of a 4% aqueous solution of a dried sample is between +20° and +23.5°.

Solubility—1 Gm dissolves in about 10 ml of water and about 800 ml of alcohol; insoluble in ether.

Uses—See *Dextroamphetamine Phosphate*.

Dose—5 to **50 mg** daily; *usual*, **2.5 to 5 mg** 1 to 3 times a day.

Dosage Forms—Elixir USP; Extended-release Oral Solid: 5, 10, and 15 mg; Tablets USP: 5 and 10 mg.

Diethylpropion Hydrochloride NF

[2-(Diethylamino)propiophenone Hydrochloride; Tenuate (*Merrell*); Tepanil (*National Drug*)]

$$
\left[\underset{\underset{\overset{+}{N}H(C_2H_5)_2}{|}}{\underset{}{C_6H_5-\overset{\overset{O}{\|}}{C}-CH-CH_3}} \right] Cl^-
$$

Diethylpropion hydrochloride contains 97.0–103.0% of $C_{13}H_{19}NO \cdot HCl$ (241.76), calculated on the anhydrous basis.

Preparation—Propiophenone is brominated with bromine to form 2-bromopropiophenone which is then condensed with diethylamine to yield diethylpropion (base). The purified base is dissolved in a suitable solvent and treated with hydrogen chloride to form the official salt. US Pat. 3,001,910.

Description—White or creamy white, small crystals or crystalline powder. It has a characteristic, mildly aromatic odor, and is stable in dry air. It melts between 171° and 173° with decomposition.

Solubility—1 Gm dissolves in approximately 0.6 ml of water, 1.6 ml of chloroform, 1 ml of absolute methanol, and 1 ml of 95% alcohol; insoluble in ether.

Uses—Its cardiovascular actions are minimal, but its central actions, particularly anorexigenesis, are prominent. Thus it is used to suppress appetite in the management of obesity. As with other central stimulant appetite suppressants, it may interfere with sleep and thus not be used at night when obese persons often overeat most; successful management requires concomitant diet therapy and retraining in eating habits. The drug may be abused for its central stimulant effects. It should not be used if the patient is under treatment with monoamine oxidase inhibitors.

Dose—*Usual*, **25 mg** 3 times a day.

Other Dose Information—25 mg may be taken midevening if insomnia is not a problem.

Dosage Forms—Extended-release Oral Solid: 75 mg; Tablets NF: 25 mg.

Ephedrine NF

[(−)-Erythro-α-[1-(methylamino)ethyl]benzyl Alcohol]

$$
C_6H_5-\underset{\underset{OH}{|}}{CH}-\underset{\underset{NHCH_3}{|}}{CHCH_3}
$$

Ephedrine is anhydrous, or contains not more than one-half molecule of water of hydration. Anhydrous Ephedrine contains 98.5–100.5% of $C_{10}H_{15}NO$ (165.24). Hydrated Ephedrine [ephedrine hemihydrate, $C_{10}H_{15}NO \cdot \frac{1}{2}H_2O = 174.24$] contains 98.5–100.5% of $C_{10}H_{15}NO$, calculated on the anhydrous basis.

It is an alkaloid which may be obtained from *Ephedra equisetina* Bunge, and other species of *Ephedra* (Family *Gnetaceæ*), but is usually produced synthetically.

Preparation—Ephedrine was first obtained by Nagai in 1887 from a Chinese herb, *ma huang*. Structurally, it is closely related to epinephrine, but it is more stable. Ephedrine may be obtained by alkalinizing powdered *ma huang* with milk of lime or sodium carbonate solution, and extracting the base with alcohol or benzene. It is now, however, almost exclusively produced by synthetic methods. The most economic process (Neuberg) for synthetic production commences with fermenting a mixture of benzaldehyde and molasses to form the ketoalcohol, $C_6H_5CH(OH)\text{-}COCH_3$. This is mixed with a solution of methylamine [CH_3NH_2] and treated with hydrogen. The keto group is thereby reduced to—CHOH—which condenses with the methylamine.

Description—An unctuous, almost colorless solid, or white crystals or granules. It gradually decomposes on exposure to light. It melts between 33° and 40°, the variability in the melting point being due to differences in the moisture content, anhydrous Ephedrine having a lower melting point than the hemihydrate of Ephedrine. Its solution is alkaline to litmus. The specific rotation of an aqueous solution of the hydrochloride is between −33° and −35.5°.

Solubility—Soluble in water, alcohol, chloroform, and ether, and is moderately and slowly soluble in liquid petrolatum, the solution in the latter becoming turbid if the Ephedrine contains more than about 1% of water.

Incompatibilities—Ephedrine differs from most alkaloids in being soluble in water, producing a solution which has a strongly alkaline reaction. Incompatibilities may occur because of this alkalinity. Rosin, Eger, and Mack, *J. APhA, Sci. Ed.*, **31**, 71 (1942), have recorded the solubility of the anhydrous alkaloid in light liquid petrolatum at 20° as 2.2 Gm in 100 ml of solution. The hemihydrate which contains about 5% of water was soluble only to the extent of 0.84 Gm in 100 ml of solution at the same temperature. Both substances were more soluble at 25°. This striking difference in solubility indicates the importance of using the anhydrous variety in the preparation of oil solutions.

After frequent and prolonged exposure to a moist atmosphere, Ephedrine may absorb sufficient moisture to prevent the preparation of a clear solution in oil due to the separation of droplets of water. Anhydrous calcium chloride has been suggested as a means of clarifying such a solution. The alkaloid is rendered more soluble in liquid petrolatum by trituration with an equal weight of oleic acid. Camphor, menthol, thymol, cinnamon oil, and thyme oil also increase its solubility.

A compound insoluble in either water or oil is formed with *iodine*. *Tannic acid* precipitates the alkaloid but not its salts. Ephedrine reduces *silver salts* in aqueous solution to metallic silver. (See also *Ephedrine Hydrochloride*.) Because of its alkalinity, ephedrine is incompatible with *chlorobutanol* causing that substance to decompose with the liberation of hydrochloric acid. In an oil solution the ephedrine hydrochloride thus formed is insoluble.

Uses—Ephedrine is a *sympathomimetic* amine which shares some of the actions and uses of epinephrine, but which differs from the latter drug in several important ways. In ordinary doses ephedrine acts indirectly through the release of levarterenol from adrenergic nerves. Thus its actions more nearly resemble those of levarterenol. In higher doses it has a direct sympathomimetic action. It penetrates membranes and the brain better than levarterenol or epinephrine. Ephedrine, due to its stability, can be given by mouth, a distinct advantage when chronic therapy is required. The duration of action of Ephedrine is longer than that ordinarily obtained with epinephrine. The constrictor effect of Ephedrine on arterioles is less prominent than that of epinephrine; but Ephedrine does not have a biphasic action on small blood vessels, such as has epinephrine which, for example, results in late vascular congestion ("after-congestion") of mucosa after initial shrinkage. Ephedrine exerts a mydriatic action of value in ophthalmology, an effect elicitable with epinephrine only under special circumstances. Ephedrine also possesses a powerful *central nervous system stimulant* action, and thus has uses not enjoyed by epinephrine, such as in the treatment of *narcolepsy* and in the therapy of poisoning by central nervous system depressants. Finally, Ephedrine differs from epinephrine in that it is of value in the treatment of *myasthenia gravis*.

The therapeutic uses made of the actions of Ephedrine on the cardiovascular system are numerous. Ephedrine is employed to support the blood pressure in patients undergoing spinal anesthesia. It is also employed in *postural hypotension*. When wisely employed, it may be of benefit in certain forms and certain stages of *shock*. It is also used in patients with complete *heart block*. The bronchodilator actions of Ephedrine are made use of in the treatment of *bronchial asthma*. The constrictor action of Ephedrine on the small blood vessels is applied therapeutically in *hay fever, acute coryza, acute rhinitis, acute sinusitis*, etc. In such conditions, sprays, solutions, and jellies are of value to relieve the troublesome mucosal congestion. Ephedrine is applied in ophthalmology as a *mydriatic*, frequently in combination with homatropine.

Ephedrine is a cortical and respiratory stimulant occasionally useful in treating morphine and barbiturate overdosage and similar types of drug poisoning. In *narcolepsy*, Ephedrine counteracts the irrepressible desire to sleep, relieves the inversion of the sleep cycle, and abolishes the cataleptic seizures. In *myasthenia gravis*, Ephedrine may give moderate to dramatic symptomatic relief in selected cases, but is not as generally useful as neostigmine. It is often combined with neostigmine therapy. Finally, Ephedrine is an important agent used to prevent or treat a variety of allergic syndromes, including *angioneurotic edema, drug reactions, chronic urticaria*, etc.

As a rule, the salts of Ephedrine are employed instead of the free base.

Ephedrine Hydrochloride NF

[(−)-α-[1-(Methylamino)ethyl]benzyl Alcohol Hydrochloride]

Ephedrine Hydrochloride, dried at 105° for 3 hours, contains 98.0–100.5% of $C_{10}H_{15}NO \cdot HCl$ (201.70).

For the structure of the base, see *Ephedrine*, page 884.

Description—Fine, white, odorless crystals or powder. It is affected by light. Melting range 217° to 220°. Specific rotation −33° to −35.5°.

Solubility—1 Gm dissolves in about 3 ml of water and about 14 ml of alcohol; insoluble in ether.

Incompatibilities—Ephedrine salts differ from the base in being insoluble in liquid petrolatum and in the fact that their aqueous solutions are slightly acid in reaction. Ephedrine sulfate appears to be compatible with silver salts whereas the base has a reducing action upon them and the hydrochloride gives a precipitate. Colloidal silver chloride or iodide is compatible with ephedrine sulfate.

Iodine and other *Alkaloidal precipitants* cause a precipitation.

Uses—See *Ephedrine.*
Dose—*Usual,* **25** to **50 mg** every 3 or 4 hours.
Veterinary Dose—*Dogs,* 8 to **25 mg.**

Ephedrine Sulfate USP

[(−)-α-[1-(Methylamino)ethyl]benzyl Alcohol Sulfate (2:1)]

Ephedrine Sulfate contains 98.0–101.0% of $(C_{10}H_{15}NO)_2 \cdot H_2SO_4$ (428.55), calculated on the dried basis.

For the structure of the base, see *Ephedrine*, page 884.

Description—Fine, white, odorless crystals or a powder. It is affected by light, and its aqueous solution is practically neutral to litmus. Ephedrine Sulfate has a specific rotation of −30.0° to −32.0°.

Solubility—1 Gm dissolves in about 1.3 ml of water and about 90 ml of alcohol; insoluble in ether.

Incompatibilities—See *Ephedrine Hydrochloride.*

Uses—See *Ephedrine.* Additional information regarding the uses of specific dosage forms of Ephedrine Sulfate follows. *Ephedrine Sulfate Injection USP:* See *Ephedrine;* the sulfate contains less actual ephedrine than the hydrochloride, but it is used in preference to the hydrochloride since it produces less reaction in the form of a stinging sensation when injected. The preparation is used in the treatment of asthma and hay fever, and it is sometimes used for raising the blood pressure during spinal anesthesia. *Ephedrine Sulfate Solution USP:* For use on mucous membranes this solution is diluted with an equal volume of isotonic sodium chloride solution. *Ephedrine Sulfate and Phenobarbital Capsules NF:* See *Ephedrine;* the phenobarbital is incorporated into this preparation as a corrective for the central stimulant actions of ephedrine. The preparation is thus employed for the peripheral actions of ephedrine.

Dose—*Oral* or *parenteral,* **100** to **200 mg** daily; *usual,* **25 mg** 4 to 6 times a day; *topically, intranasal,* **0.2** to **0.6 ml** of a 1 to 3% solution 4 to 6 times a day.

Other Dose Information—20 mg (as 5 ml of Ephedrine Sulfate Syrup) to 25 mg; the usual dose of Ephedrine Sulfate and Phenobarbital Capsules is 25 mg of ephedrine sulfate and 30 mg of phenobarbital.

Dosage Forms—Capsules USP: 25 and 50 mg; Injection USP: 25 and 50 mg/ml, 500 mg/10 ml, 750 mg/30 ml; Solution USP: 3%; Syrup USP (see below); Tablets NF: 25 and 50 mg; and Phenobarbital Capsules NF (see below): 25 and 50 mg (ephedrine sulfate) and 15 and 30 mg (phenobarbital).

Veterinary Dose—*Dogs,* 8 to 25 mg.

Ephedrine Sulfate Syrup USP—*Preparation:* Dissolve ephedrine sulfate (4 Gm), citric acid (1 Gm), and caramel (0.4 Gm) in purified water (450 ml) and add lemon oil (0.125 ml), orange oil (0.25 ml), benzaldehyde (0.06 ml), and vanillin (0.016 Gm) previously dissolved in alcohol (25 ml). To this add amaranth solution (4 ml) and sucrose (800 Gm), and dissolve the latter by agitation. Finally add sufficient purified water to make the product measure 1000 ml. *Alcohol Content:* 2–4%.

Ephedrine Sulfate and Phenobarbital Capsules NF contain 91.0–109.0% of the labeled amounts of $(C_{10}H_{15}NO)_2 \cdot H_2SO_4$ (ephedrine sulfate) and of $C_{12}H_{12}N_2O_3$ (phenobarbital). *Dose:* Ephedrine Sulfate, 25 mg; Phenobarbital, 30 mg. *Dosage Forms:* Capsules NF: 25 and 50 mg (ephedrine sulfate) and 15 and 30 mg (phenobarbital).

Epinephrine USP

[Adrenaline; Suprarenalin; Nephridine; (−)-3,4-Dihydroxy-α-[(methylamino)methyl]benzyl Alcohol; Adrenalin (*Parke-Davis*); Suprarenin (*Winthrop*)]

Epinephrine contains 97.0–100.5% of $C_9H_{13}NO_3$ (183.21), calculated on the dried basis.

History—Epinephrine, the blood-pressure-raising constituent of the suprarenal glands, originally trade-marked as adrenalin, was discovered by Dr. John J. Abel. Fuerth also claimed the discovery of an active principle which he called *suprarenin* (*suprarenalin*) and Takamine obtained and introduced it as a crystalline substance and named it *adrenalin*, a name which became official in Britain. These substances proved to be identical and the official name is that given to it originally by Abel.

Preparation—Epinephrine may be prepared by digesting finely cut adrenal glands with acidulated water. The acid combines with the epinephrine which is a base to form a water-soluble salt. The mixture is then heated to coagulate albuminoid material and filter-pressed. The digestion with acidified water is repeated to effect a more complete extraction. The liquid, freed from fats, is concentrated in a vacuum, mixed with alcohol to precipitate inert ingredients, filtered, and made alkaline with ammonia to precipitate the epinephrine. The crude product so obtained is purified by dissolving in acidified alcohol and reprecipitating with ammonia.

Epinephrine may also be prepared by several synthetic processes. A common one proceeds as follows:

Catechol → **(Chloroacetyl)catechol** → **(Methylaminoacetyl)catechol** → **dl-Epinephrine**

The racemic form is resolved with *d*-tartaric acid.

Description—A white or light brownish, microcrystalline, odorless powder, gradually darkening on exposure to light and air. It combines with acids, forming salts which are readily soluble in water, and from these solutions the base may be precipitated by ammonia water or by alkali carbonates. Its solutions are alkaline to litmus. The specific rotation of Epinephrine, determined in a solution of 1 Gm of the sulfuric acid-dried material in 20 ml of $0.5N$ hydrochloric acid, is between $-50°$ and $-53.5°$.

Solubility—Very slightly soluble in water and in alcohol; insoluble in ether, chloroform, and fixed and volatile oils.

Incompatibilities—Solutions of epinephrine are usually prepared with the aid of hydrochloric acid and an acid reaction is essential to the stability of such solutions not only because of possible precipitation but also because of the possibility of rapid oxidation to inert products. Oxidation is generally evidenced by development of a pink to brown color. Air, light, heat, and alkalies promote deterioration. Solutions buffered to a pH of 4.2 and containing a suitable antioxidant such as 0.1% sodium metabisulfite are stable for prolonged periods of time if protected from light, heat, and undue exposure to air.

Metals, notably *copper, iron*, and *zinc*, destroy its activity.

Uses—Epinephrine, the *sympathomimetic* adrenal hormone, in its actions mimics many of the effects of sympathetic nerve impulses in the body. It acts on smooth muscle cells, gland cells, and the heart to produce responses similar to those evoked by stimulation of the corresponding sympathetic (adrenergic) nerves. Thus Epinephrine stimulates the heart, increases the heart rate, raises the blood pressure, relaxes the musculature of the bronchi and intestine, etc, in high concentrations it constricts the arterioles of all vascular beds, but in physiological concentrations it dilates the arterioles of the splanchnic and skeletal muscle beds, especially. Its therapeutic applications are thus manifold, but like other drugs which act on many organs, not much selectivity of response is possible. Thus, in order to obtain the effects on the heart, it is necessary to tolerate the many other actions of Epinephrine in the body. To some extent this disadvantage can be overcome by local application of Epinephrine, eg, to the nasal or bronchial mucosa. Epinephrine has very little mydriatic action by either parenteral or topical routes, because of poor penetration into the eye.

The actions of Epinephrine on the cardiovascular system have numerous therapeutic applications. The drug is employed topically in the control of *superficial hemorrhages*, as, for example, to obtain a clear field in operative procedures on the nose or throat. In acute *coryza, sinusitis, hay fever, allergic rhinitis*, etc, a solution of Epinephrine topically applied gives considerable symptomatic but brief relief, and may be followed by more mucosal congestion than before the Epinephrine (after-congestion). Ephedrine or phenylephrine is to be preferred. Epinephrine is used in combination with local anesthetic solutions. By causing local vasoconstriction, Epinephrine keeps the local anesthetic in the desired area thus prolonging its action and preventing it from being absorbed and exerting toxic systemic effects. In shock and circulatory collapse, Epinephrine is not of much value and its injudicious use may be harmful. In complete *heart block*, Epinephrine is very valuable. It is of less service in resuscitation after cardiac arrest, and of very little value in acute heart failure, although it is frequently employed in these two syndromes. In those cases of *cardiac asthma* in which an element of bronchial spasm may be operative, small doses of Epinephrine may be used as an adjuvant to more primary therapy, such as morphine, theophylline, and digitalis.

The use of Epinephrine in *bronchial asthma* is quite extensive, and the drug not only gives dramatic relief in most acute cases, but also may be life saving in status asthmaticus. The drug can be injected subcutaneously or intramuscularly (preferred) as an aqueous solution or suspension in oil; or it may be inhaled from an all-glass nebulizer as an aqueous solution.

Epinephrine is of benefit in a variety of *allergic disorders*, giving symptomatic relief in many cases of *giant urticaria, serum reactions, serum sickness, angioneurotic edema*, etc. It has a number of miscellaneous uses including the hastening of the onset of inoculation malaria (by contraction of the splenic capsule and extrusion of plasmodia into the blood stream), the temporary relief of hypoglycemic reacions (by mobilization of liver glycogen), etc.

Note: Do not use any Epinephrine dosage form if it is brown in color or contains a precipitate.

Dose—*Intramuscular* or *subcutaneous*, **200 mcg** to **1 mg** (0.2 to 1 ml) in a **0.1%** solution, or **1** to **3 mg** (0.5 to 1.5 ml) in a **0.2%** oil suspension, repeated as necessary; *usual, intramuscular*, **300** to **500 mcg** (0.3 to 0.5 ml) in a **0.1%** solution, or **1 mg** (0.5 ml) in a **0.2%** oil suspension, repeated as necessary; *usual, subcutaneous*, **300** to **500 mcg** (0.3 to 0.5 ml) in a **0.1%** solution, repeated as necessary; *oral inhalation*, a **0.1** to **1%**

solution applied as a fine mist as required; *topically*, *intranasal*, a **0.1**% solution as required.

Other Dose Information—Epinephrine may be injected subcutaneously, intramuscularly, or intravenously as the 1:1000 solution; injected subcutaneously or intramuscularly (preferred) as the 1:500 suspension in oil; inhaled as the 1:100 aqueous solution; applied topically, usually in solution in water; or used in ointment, suppository, jelly, or emulsion form. For topical application in operative procedures on the nose and throat, solutions of 0.002 to 0.05%, freshly prepared from the official 0.01% solution, may be used.

Dosage Forms—Inhalation USP; Injection USP: 1 and 30 ml; Solution USP: 30 ml; Sterile Suspension USP: 1 ml.

Additional information regarding the dosage forms of Epinephrine follows.

Epinephrine Injection USP—This solution is extremely sensitive to air, light, and alkali and its decomposition is activated by heat. At a pH of about 4 to 4.5 the solution will be amply protected against the possible alkalinity of the glass even when sterilized by heat. The addition of 0.1% of sodium bisulfite preserves the solution almost indefinitely, maintaining a colorless solution. At times it has been filled under CO_2 or N_2, but this procedure is probably not necessary if the sodium bisulfite is used. It is a 1:1000 solution intended for parenteral administration.

Epinephrine Solution USP—*Note:* This preparation is nonsterile and cannot be employed for injection, its use being reserved for *topical* application.

Sterile Epinephrine Suspension USP [Sus-Phrine (*Brewer*)]—Epinephrine is more slowly absorbed and hence has a longer duration of action when injected intramuscularly in oily suspension than in aqueous solution.

Veterinary Dose—1:1000 solution: *subcutaneously* or *intramuscularly*, *Horses* and *Cattle*, **4** to **8 ml**; *Sheep* and *Swine*, **1** to **3 ml**; *Dogs* and *Cats* **0.2** to **0.6 ml**; *intravenously* or *intracardially*, *Horses* and *Cattle*, **0.5** to **4 ml**; *Dogs*, **0.03** to **0.5 ml**.

Epinephrine Bitartrate USP

[Epinephrine Tartrate (1:1); Adrenaline Bitartrate BP; Adrenaline Acid Tartrate Adrenatrate (*Crookes-Barnes*); Epitrate (*Ayerst*); Lyophrin (*Alcon*)]

Epinephrine Bitartrate contains 97.0–102.0% of $C_9H_{13}NO_3 \cdot C_4H_6O_6$ (333.30), calculated on the dried basis.

For the structure of the base, see *Epinephrine*, page 885.

Preparation—It may be prepared by reacting epinephrine with an equimolar portion of tartaric acid and precipitating by the addition of alcohol.

Description—A white, grayish white, or light brownish gray crystalline powder. Odorless. Slowly darkens on exposure to air and light. Melting range 147° to 152°. The pH of a 1% solution is 3.5. Its specific rotation, determined by dissolving an accurately weighed 200 mg sample in sufficient 0.5 N hydrochloric acid to make 10 ml, is between −50° and −53.5°.

Solubility—1 Gm dissolves in about 3 ml of water and about 550 ml of alcohol; almost insoluble in chloroform and in ether.

Uses—Epinephrine Bitartrate is applied *topically* to the eye, in an ointment or as a solution (see below); the ophthalmic preparations are used to decrease conjunctival and scleral *inflammation* and *edema*. It is much more stable and less irritating than the hydrochloride.

Dose—*Topically*, **0.1 ml** of a **2**% solution to the conjunctiva 2 times a day to once every other day.

Dosage Forms—Ophthalmic Solution USP: 1 and 2%.

Hydroxyamphetamine Hydrobromide USP

[(±)-*p*-(2-Aminopropyl)phenol Hydrobromide;   Paredrine Hydrobromide (*SKF*)]

$$\left[HO\!-\!\!\left\langle \right\rangle\!\!-\!CH_2\overset{\displaystyle |}{\underset{\displaystyle CH_3}{C}}H\overset{+}{N}H_3 \right] Br^-$$

Hydroxyamphetamine Hydrobromide contains 98.0–101.5% of $C_9H_{13}NO \cdot HBr$ (232.12), calculated on the dried basis.

Preparation—Among other methods, this compound may be synthesized by reducing *p*-methoxybenzyl methyl ketoxime followed by hydrolysis of the methoxy group with mineral acids. The free base may then be liberated with alkali, and, after extraction, may be converted into the salt by treatment with hydrobromic acid.

Description—A white, crystalline powder. Its solutions are slightly acid to litmus, having a pH of about 5. Melting range 189° to 192°.

Solubility—1 Gm dissolves in about 1 ml of water and about 2.5 ml of alcohol; slightly soluble in chloroform; almost insoluble in ether.

Uses—Hydroxyamphetamine, the chemical structure of which resembles that of both tyramine and amphetamine, is a more stable sympathomimetic amine than epinephrine and is practically devoid of ephedrine-like actions on the central nervous system. Its action is mainly indirect. Its principal therapeutic usefulness is therefore dependent on its peripheral effects. The drug is employed to *shrink nasal mucosa;* at equal dosage levels, it is about twice as effective as ephedrine for this purpose. Instilled into the eye it produces adequate *mydriasis* for ophthalmic examination. As an adjuvant to atropine and homatropine, it permits the use of lower concentrations of the alkaloids and hence diminishes the duration of cycloplegia. By injection or oral administration the drug produces *pressor effects* which are of value in supporting blood pressure during spinal anesthesia, in preventing syncopal attacks in *Stokes-Adams disease*, in relief of *heart block*, in aborting attacks of *paroxysmal tachycardia*, and in the treatment of *orthostatic hypotension*.

Although Hydroxyamphetamine shares the general properties of other sympathomimetic amines, it also presents some interesting anomalies. The drug does not cause vasoconstriction when injected intradermally; consequently, it does not prolong the duration of action of local anesthetics. In addition, its actions on the bronchi and gastrointestinal tract are not of sufficient intensity to be useful clinically.

Hydroxyamphetamine should not be employed if the patient is under treatment with monoamine oxidase inhibitors.

Dose—*Topically*, **0.1 ml** of a **0.25** to **1**% solution, to the conjunctiva, repeated as necessary.

Other Dose Information—Topically, to nasal mucosa, as a 0.5 to 1% solution; oral, 60 mg or more for postural hypotension, 20 to 60 mg repeated as necessary for carotid sinus syndrome, and 20 to 60 mg every 3 to 4 hours for heart block.

Dosage Forms—Ophthalmic Solution USP: 15 ml.

Isoproterenol Hydrochloride USP

[Isopropylarterenol Hydrochloride; 3,4-Dihydroxy-α-[(isopropylamino)-methyl]benzyl Alcohol Hydrochloride; Isuprel Hydrochloride (*Winthrop*)]

$$\left[\text{HO} \underset{\text{HO}}{\overset{}{\bigcirc}} \text{CHCH}_2\overset{+}{\text{NH}}_2\text{CH(CH}_3)_2 \atop \text{OH} \right] \text{Cl}^-$$

Isoproterenol Hydrochloride contains 97.0–101.5% of $C_{11}H_{17}NO_3 \cdot HCl$ (247.72), calculated on the dried basis.

Preparation—Isoproterenol base may be prepared by the synthetic procedure given for *Epinephrine* (page 886), using isopropylamine in place of methylamine. The base is then converted to the hydrochloride without resolution.

Description—A white to nearly white, odorless, crystalline powder, having a slightly bitter taste. Gradually darkens on exposure to air and light. Solutions become pink to brownish pink on standing exposed to air, and almost immediately so when rendered alkaline. Its 1% aqueous solution has a pH of about 5. Melting range between 167° and 172°.

Solubility—1 Gm dissolves in 3 ml of water and 50 ml of alcohol; less soluble in dehydrated alcohol; insoluble in chloroform and ether.

Uses—Isoproterenol is a close congener of epinephrine which elicits primarily beta adrenergic stimulant effects. Thus it exerts inhibitory effects on smooth muscle, causes a decrease in blood pressure, relaxes the smooth muscle of the gastrointestinal tract and bronchial tree, and is a potent *cardiac stimulant*. It has a greater positive effect on the heart rate and the contractile force of the myocardium than has epinephrine.

Isoproterenol is a valuable *bronchodilator* and is useful clinically in the treatment of *asthma*. The drug affords almost complete relief in mild and moderately severe asthma and is of value in *status asthmaticus*. The most effective method of administration is by the oral inhalation of a suitable aerosol at the onset of an attack (systemic administration should be avoided because of the marked action on the myocardium). Following oral inhalation the drug tends to liquefy tenacious mucus, thus exerting a mild expectorant action. Isoproterenol is somewhat more active than epinephrine and is often effective in the patient who is no longer responsive to epinephrine. The sublingual administration of 10 mg of isoproterenol also affords relief in mild asthma, but the incidence of side reactions is high. In fact, the sublingual route is sometimes used in the isoproterenol treatment of *ventricular bradycardia* in patients with heart block and to *prevent cardiac standstill* caused by carotid sinus stimulation. Parenteral administration is also employed for this purpose. Common side effects include palpitation, precordial pain, headache, nausea, nervousness, tremor, dizziness, weakness, and sweating. The incidence of side actions is low following oral inhalation of an aerosol, somewhat higher following inhalation of the powder, and is highest (about 30%) in patients treated with sublingual tablets, syrup, or injection.

Note—Do not use any dosage forms of Isoproterenol Hydrochloride if they are brown in color or contain a precipitate.

Dose—*Sublingual*, **10** to **60 mg** daily; *usual*, **10** to **15 mg** 3 to 4 times a day; by *oral inhalation*, **125** to **750 mcg** in 2 hours; *usual*, **125** to **250 mcg** of a **0.25%** solution, repeated at 1-, 5-, and 10-minute intervals as necessary; *parenteral*, **10** to **200 mcg**; *usual*, *intramuscular* or *subcutaneous*, **200 mcg**, repeated as necessary; *usual*, *intravenous*, **10** to **20 mcg**, repeated as necessary; *infusion*, **2 mg** in **500 ml** of **5%** Dextrose Injection at a rate adjusted to maintain blood pressure.

Other Dose Information—The usual inhalation dose is 0.1 to 0.3 ml of a 1:100 solution or 0.5 ml of a 1:200 solution. Inhalant powders are also effective. The usual sublingual dose is 10 mg.

Dosage Forms—Inhalation USP: 0.5 and 1%, 0.25% in metered aerosols; Injection USP: 1 and 5 ml; Tablets USP: 10 and 15 mg.

Isoproterenol Sulfate USP

[Isopropylarterenol Sulfate; 3,4-Dihydroxy-α-[(isopropylamino)methyl]-benzyl Alcohol Sulfate (2:1); Norisodrine (*Abbott*)]

Isoproterenol Sulfate contains 98.0–100.5% of $(C_{11}H_{17}NO_3)_2 \cdot H_2SO_4 \cdot 2H_2O$ (556.63).

For the structure of the base, see Isoproterenol Hydrochloride, this page.

Preparation—An alcoholic solution of 2-chloro-3',4'-dihydroxyacetophenone is condensed with isopropylamine. The resulting, 3',4'-dihydroxy 2-(isopropylamino)acetophenone is isolated as the sulfate and the carbonyl group is then reduced to carbinol by catalytic hydrogenation.

Description—A white to nearly white, odorless, crystalline powder, having a slightly bitter taste. It gradually darkens on exposure to air and light. Its solutions become pink to brownish pink on standing exposed to air, and almost immediately so when rendered alkaline. Its 1 in 100 solution has a pH of about 5. Melting range 125° to 129°.

Solubility—Freely soluble in water; slightly soluble in alcohol; very slightly soluble in benzene and ether.

Uses—See *Isoproterenol Hydrochloride*.

Dose—*Oral inhalation*, **0.5 ml** of a **0.5%** solution.

Dosage Forms—Aerosol NF: 2 mg/ml (delivers 80 mcg/inhalation); Inhalation USP: 0.2% in metered aerosols.

Isoxsuprine Hydrochloride NF

[*p*-Hydroxy-α-[1-[(1-methyl-2-phenoxyethyl)amino]ethyl]benzyl Alcohol Hydrochloride; Vasodilan (*Mead-Johnson*)]

$$\left[\text{HO} \underset{\text{HO}}{\overset{}{\bigcirc}} \underset{\text{NH}_2\text{CHCH}_2\text{O}}{\overset{\text{CHCHCH}_3}{}} \underset{\text{CH}_3}{\overset{+}{\bigcirc}} \right] \text{Cl}^-$$

Isoxsuprine Hydrochloride contains 97.0–103.0% of $C_{18}H_{23}NO_3 \cdot HCl$ (337.85), calculated on the dried basis.

Preparation—*p*-Hydroxypropiophenone is benzoylated at the hydroxy position and then brominated to give the 2-bromo compound. The bromo compound is then condensed with 1-methyl-2-phenoxyethylamine to yield the *O*-benzoylated phenone corresponding to Isoxsuprine. In the form of its hydrochloride, this phenone is simultaneously debenzoylated and reduced by hydrogenation with the aid of palladium on charcoal to give a mixture of the *erythro* and *allo* forms of the corresponding carbinol. The *erythro* form (Isoxsuprine) is extracted with acetone and converted to the hydrochloride. US Pat. 3,056,836.

Description—A white, crystalline powder which is odorless and has a bitter taste. It melts between 201° and 208°.

Solubility—Slightly soluble in water; sparingly soluble in alcohol.

Uses—Isoxsuprine Hydrochloride is a *sympathomimetic* with actions that resemble *Isoproterenol* (see above), except that it has less pronounced effects on the heart. It is used clinically mainly for its vasodilator actions, in order to increase circulation in certain *peripheral vascular diseases*, to *increase cerebral blood flow*, and to *increase flow in the skeletal muscle* vascular bed. It does not increase cutaneous blood flow. Because the drug relaxes the uterus, it also has been used in the treatment of *dysmenorrhea* and *threatened abortion;* however, its use in these conditions has not gained acceptance. Side effects include nausea, vomiting, dizziness, weakness, palpitation, and occasional cardioacceleration.

Dose—*Usual,* **10** to **20 mg**, 3 or 4 times a day.

Dosage Forms—Injection: 5 mg/ml; Tablets NF: 10 mg.

Other Dose Information—Intramuscular, 5 to 10 mg 2 to 3 times a day.

Levarterenol Bitartrate USP

[(−)-α-(Aminomethyl)-3,4-dihydroxybenzyl Alcohol Tartrate (1:1); *l*-Norepinephrine Bitartrate; Noradrenaline Acid Tartrate; Levophed Bitartrate (*Winthrop*)]

$$\left[HO-\underset{HO}{\bigcirc}-\underset{OH}{\overset{\overset{+}{\underset{|}{CHCH_2NH_3}}}{}} \right] HC_4H_4O_6^- \cdot H_2O$$

Levarterenol Bitartrate [$C_8H_{11}NO_3 \cdot C_4H_6O_6 \cdot H_2O$ = 337.29] contains 97.0–102.0% of $C_8H_{11}NO_3 \cdot C_4H_6O_6$ (319.27), calculated on the anhydrous basis.

Preparation—Levarterenol base may be prepared by the synthetic procedure given for *Epinephrine* (page 886), using ammonia in place of methylamine. The base is then converted to the bitartrate and resolved.

Description—A white or faintly gray, crystalline powder. Odorless. Slowly darkens on exposure to air and light. Solutions are acid to litmus, having a pH of about 3.5. Melts, without previous drying, between 100° and 106° to form a turbid melt. Specific rotation between −10° and −12°.

Solubility—1 Gm dissolves in about 2.5 ml of water and about 300 ml of alcohol; practically insoluble in chloroform and in ether.

Uses—Levarterenol is the major pressor amine found in postganglionic adrenergic nerves, and all available evidence indicates that it is the predominant adrenergic mediator liberated by their stimulation. In addition, it constitutes 10 to 18% of the catecholamine content of the adrenal medulla and as much as 97% of that of some pheochromocytomas.

The pharmacological actions of Levarterenol are similar to those of epinephrine, but important quantitative differences exist. When Levarterenol is administered by slow intravenous infusion, peripheral vasoconstriction is more marked than vasodilatation, so total peripheral resistance is increased rather than decreased as in the case of infusion of epinephrine. The positive chronotropic action of the drug on the myocardium is less prominent than that of epinephrine because it is masked by compensatory vagal bradycardia. Peripheral blood flow except in the kidney and skin is maintained by the increase in mean arterial pressure. Large doses of Levarterenol are required to produce hyperglycemia and other metabolic effects. It does not share the bronchodilatory actions and uses of epinephrine in

allergic disorders such as bronchial asthma. Actions upon the central nervous system are usually somewhat less prominent than those following administration of epinephrine. Like epinephrine, Levarterenol has a very short duration of action and is ineffective when administered orally.

The most important use of Levarterenol is for the *support of blood pressure* as an adjunct to fluid replacement therapy in certain types of *shock*. However, despite adequate restoration of blood pressure, failures occur in approximately 50% of cases. The drug is also included in local anesthetic preparations; the local vasoconstrictor effect slows the flow of blood and lymph and thus prolongs the sojourn of local anesthetic at that site.

Levarterenol is usually administered by continuous intravenous infusion. Normally, infusion of a solution containing 4 mcg of Levarterenol base (8 mcg of the bitartrate) per ml, at the rate of 2 to 4 mcg per minute, is adequate. The infusion must never be left unattended and blood pressure must be determined at least every 15 minutes and more frequently during the initial adjustment of the rate of infusion.

Untoward effects are usually minimal. Subjective symptoms of anxiety, respiratory difficulty, awareness of the slow, forceful heart beat, and transient headache are noted most often. Severe hypertension with violent headache, photophobia, stabbing retrosternal pain, pallor, intense sweating, and vomiting may occur in some patients. Extravasation of the drug during infusion has caused necrosis and sloughing at the site of injection. Like epinephrine, Levarterenol can induce cardiac arrhythmias and its use during cyclopropane anesthesia is contraindicated.

Note—*Do not use any dosage forms of Levarterenol Bitartrate if they are brown in color or contain a precipitate.*

Dose—*Usual,* intravenous infusion, **8 mg**, the equivalent of 4 mg of levarterenol, in **500 ml** of 5% **Dextrose Injection,** at a rate adjusted to maintain blood pressure (usually 1 to 10 mcg/minute).

Dosage Forms—Injection USP: 400 mcg/2 ml, 8 mg/4 ml.

Veterinary Uses—Levonordefrin is used to combat vascular shock or disastrous hypotension, particularly in animals pretreated with phenothiazine-derived ataraxics or with antibiotics.

Veterinary Dose—*All animals, intravenous infusion,* **2 mcg** per ml (in 5% dextrose solution) at the rate of 5 to 15 drops per minute (to provide approximately 0.005 to 0.01 mcg per pound of body weight per minute), depending on blood-pressure response which must be continuously, or at least frequently, monitored.

Levonordefrin NF

[(−)-α-(1-Aminoethyl)-3,4-dihydroxybenzyl Alcohol; *l*-3,4-Dihydroxynorephedrine]

$$HO-\underset{HO}{\bigcirc}-\underset{OH\ \ NH_2}{\overset{CH-CHCH_3}{}}$$

Levonordefrin, dried in vacuum at 60° for 15 hours, contains 98.0–102.0% $C_9H_{13}NO_3$ (183.21).

Preparation—*dl*-Nordefrin may be resolved by dissolving it in an alcoholic solution of *d*-tartaric acid and separating the enantiomorphs as the *d*-tartrates by fractional crystallization. The *l*-nordefrin *d*-tartrate is then treated with alkali to liberate levonordefrin (base) which is extracted with a suitable organic solvent and purified. For the preparation of *dl*-nordefrin, see *Nordefrin Hydrochloride*, page 897.

Description—It occurs as a white to buff-colored, odorless, crystalline solid. Melting range 205° to 215°. Specific rotation −28° to −31°.

Solubility—Practically insoluble in water; slightly soluble in acetone, chloroform, alcohol, and ether; freely soluble in aqueous solutions of mineral acids.

Uses—Levonordefrin is a directly acting sympathomimetic vasoconstrictor with negligible central effects as ordinarily used. Since dextronordefrin, which makes up ½ of the base of nordefrin, is negligibly active as a vasoconstrictor, Levonordefrin is twice as potent as the racemic nordefrin base. On the other hand, dextronordefrin has weak central stimulant actions, and removal of the dextro isomer to yield Levonordefrin results in a lesser central stimulant potency. However, as a *vasoconstrictor in local anesthetic solutions*, which is the primary use of this drug, or as a *nasal decongestant*, the central actions are of no significance, so that Levonordefrin has no advantage over Nordefrin Hydrochloride. There is no reason why Levonordefrin cannot be employed for its systemic vasopressor actions, although it is not marketed in a suitable form.

Dose—No official dose.

Other Dose Information—In local anesthetic solutions, as a 0.005% solution.

Mephentermine Sulfate USP

[*N*,α,α-Trimethylphenethylamine Sulfate (2:1); Mephenterminium Sulfate; Mephine; Wyamine Sulfate (*Wyeth*)]

$$\left[\text{CH}_2\text{—}\overset{\overset{\text{CH}_3}{|}}{\underset{\underset{\text{CH}_3\ \text{CH}_3}{|}}{\text{C}}}\text{—}\overset{+}{\text{NH}}_2 \right]_2 \text{SO}_4^= \cdot 2\text{H}_2\text{O}$$

Mephentermine Sulfate [($C_{11}H_{17}N$)$_2$.H_2SO_4.$2H_2O$ = 460.64] contains 99.0–101.0% of ($C_{11}H_{17}N$)$_2$.H_2SO_4 (424.61), calculated on the dried basis.

Preparation—As described in US Pat. 2,590,079, Mephentermine may be made by the following process. Isobutyrophenone is reacted with benzyl bromide in the presence of an alkali metal amide or alcoholate to form 1,3-diphenyl-2,2-dimethylpropanone-1. This compound is isolated and cleaved with sodamide to form 3-phenyl-1-amino-2,2-dimethylpropanone-1. This latter compound is then reacted with an alkali metal hypohalite (such as KOBr) to form di-(β-phenyl-α-α-dimethylethyl)urea. This derivative is then decomposed in the presence of calcium hydroxide and water to yield ω-phenyl-tertiary-butylamine. The *N*-methyl substituted compound is obtained by the condensation of ω-phenyl-tertiary-butylamine with an aromatic aldehyde in the presence of ethanol to form a Schiff base which is then reacted with an alkylating agent such as methyl iodide or methyl bromide. By hydrolysis the reaction product is *N*-methyl-ω-phenyl-tertiary-butylamine (Mephentermine). Salts of this amine, such as the sulfate, are prepared in the usual manner by treatment with the corresponding acid.

Description—White, odorless crystals or a crystalline powder. Its solutions are acid to litmus, having a pH of about 6.

Solubility—1 Gm dissolves in 20 ml of water and about 150 ml of alcohol; practically insoluble in chloroform.

Uses—Mephentermine, an indirectly acting *sympathomimetic* amine (see general statement under *Sympathomimetics*, page 881), is employed parenterally to support blood pressure in hypotensive states or topically as the sulfate in aqueous solution as a *nasal decongestant* and *vasoconstrictor*. Parenteral injections of the drug produce a very prompt and prolonged increase in blood pressure. The pressor response is primarily from peripheral vasoconstriction. It may also be used as a *mydriatic*, but the free base is much more effective. The drug does not possess other prominent sympathomimetic actions. The central stimulant actions are weak relative to the cardiovascular actions. The use of Mephentermine as a corrective for the central depressant effects of certain drugs, such as promethazine, thus appears to be irrational. The drug is absorbed orally.

Dose—*Oral*, *intramuscular*, or *intravenous*, the equivalent of **12.5** to **80 mg** of mephentermine or mephentermine sulfate, repeated as necessary; *usual oral*, **12.5** to **25 mg** 1 or 2 times a day; *usual*, *intramuscular* or *intravenous*, **15** to **30 mg**; by *infusion*, **150 mg** in **500 ml** of an isotonic solution at a rate adjusted to maintain the blood pressure.

Other Dose Information—In various oral preparations, the dose varies between 3 and 7.5 mg, which is too small to be effective for the purposes marketed.

Dosage Forms—Injection USP (in terms of mephentermine base; parenthetic expressions denote equivalent amounts of mephentermine sulfate): 15 mg (20 mg)/ml, 30 mg (40 mg)/l and 2 ml, 60 mg (80 mg)/2 ml, 150 mg (200 mg)/10 ml; 300 mg (400 mg)/10 ml; Tablets USP: 12.5 and 25 mg.

Veterinary Dose—For systemic pressor effect, *Dogs*, *intravenous*, **10** to **25 mg** slowly; for less rapid but more prolonged effect, *intramuscular*, **10** to **40 mg**.

Metaraminol Bitartrate USP

[(−)-α-(1-Aminoethyl)-*m*-hydroxylbenzyl Alcohol Tartrate (1:1); *l*-*m*-Hydroxy-norephedrine Bitartrate; Aramine (*MSD*)]

$$\left[\text{HO}\text{—}\bigcirc\text{—}\overset{\overset{}{|}}{\underset{\underset{\text{OH}}{|}}{\text{CH}}}\text{—}\overset{\overset{}{|}}{\underset{\underset{\overset{+}{\text{NH}}_3}{|}}{\text{CH}}}\text{CH}_3 \right] \text{HC}_4\text{H}_4\text{O}_6^-$$

Metaraminol Bitartrate contains 98.0–101.0% of $C_9H_{13}NO_2$.$C_4H_6O_6$ (317.30), calculated on the dried basis.

Preparation—*m*-Hydroxybenzaldehyde is fermented with yeast in the presence of additives to yield *m*-(hydroxyphenyl) acetylcarbinol (I). An ethanolic solution containing (I) and also an equimolar quantity of benzylamine (II) is then subjected to hydrogenation in the presence of palladium or some other suitable catalyst. The probable course of the reaction is condensation of (I) and (II) to yield the Schiff base type compound (III) followed by hydrogenation of the C≡N

I

II

III

linkage and reductive cleavage at the resulting NH—CH_2 linkage. The metaraminol (base) thus produced is purified and may be converted to the official bitartrate by dissolving it in ethanol and reacting it with an equimolar quantity of tartaric acid.

Description—A white, practically odorless, crystalline powder which has a melting range between 170° and 176° and a pH between 3.2 and 3.5.

Solubility—1 Gm dissolves in about 100 ml of alcohol; freely soluble in water; practically insoluble in chloroform and ether.

Uses—Metaraminol is a directly acting *sympathomimetic* with prominent vasoconstrictor and moderate cardiac actions. Consequently it elevates both diastolic and systolic pressures. The alpha methyl group prolongs its action to four or five times that of norepinephrine. The meta hydroxyl group diminishes central stimulant activity; otherwise, the drug is similar to ephedrine.

Metaraminol is used systemically to elevate or to maintain blood pressure in such acute hypotensive conditions as *spinal anesthesia* and *shock* or locally in *nasal congestion* of various etiology.

Dose—*Intravenous*, the equivalent of **500 mcg** to **5 mg** of metaraminol; by *infusion*, **15** to **100 mg** per **500 ml**; *usual*, *intravenous*, **500 mcg**; *usual*, by *infusion*, **50 mg** in **500 ml** of an isotonic solution at a rate adjusted to maintain blood pressure. *Intramuscular* or *subcutaneous*, **2** to **12 mg**; *usual*, **2** to **5 mg**.

Dosage Forms—Injection USP: 1 and 10 ml.

Methamphetamine Hydrochloride USP

[(+)-N,α-Dimethylphenethylamine Hydrochloride; Deoxyephedrine Hydrochloride; Methylamphetamine Hydrochloride; *d*-1-Phenyl-2-methylaminopropane Hydrochloride; (*Various Mfgs.*)]

Methamphetamine Hydrochloride contains 98.5–100.5% of $C_{10}H_{15}N \cdot HCl$ (185.70), calculated on the dried basis.

Preparation—Methamphetamine may be prepared by the catalytic hydrogenation of ephedrine in acetic acid containing a small quantity of perchloric acid as an activator. The hydrogenation is carried out at 80° to 90° using palladium black as the catalyst.

The product is isolated by first removing the perchloric acid as the insoluble potassium salt and distilling under reduced pressure to remove the acetic acid. The residue is dissolved in water made alkaline and extracted into ether. The addition of an ether solution of hydrogen chloride precipitates Methamphetamine Hydrochloride.

Description—White crystals or a white, crystalline powder. It is odorless. Its solutions are acid to litmus. Melting range 171° to 175°. Specific rotation +16° to +19°.

Solubility—1 Gm dissolves in 2 ml of water, 3 ml of alcohol, and 5 ml of chloroform; very slightly soluble in absolute ether.

Uses—The actions of Methamphetamine Hydrochloride are very similar to those of amphetamine. It is more frequently employed for its *central nervous system stimulant* actions in depressing appetite in the therapy of *obesity*, in *narcolepsy*, in *postencephalitic parkinsonism* and in the therapy of *depressant states*. It may be administered with agents such as antihistaminics and phenobarbital and may eliminate the sedative effects of these agents without antagonizing the antihistaminic or antiepileptic actions. Methamphetamine has also been used to support the blood pressure during spinal anesthesia, although it is difficult to see the advantage of a substance with prominent central nervous system stimulant actions and relatively weak vasoconstrictor action in this application. Hypertension and cardiovascular disease are usually considered to be contraindications, as in the case of amphetamine. Methamphetamine should not be administered late in the day because it frequently causes insomnia. It should not be used when the patient is under treatment with monoamine oxidase inhibitors.

Methylamphetamine is widely abused for its central stimulant actions. It is the drug usually called "speed" in drug abuse circles, although other centrally acting sympathomimetics are often given the same name.

Dose—**2.5** to **50 mg** daily; *usual*, **2.5** to **5 mg** 1 to 3 times a day.

Other Dose Information—In most cases a dose of 2.5 mg should be employed first and then increased if necessary. Doses larger than 10 mg are required only in special cases.

Dosage Forms—Tablets USP: 2.5, 5, 7.5, 8, and 10 mg.

Methoxamine Hydrochloride USP

[α-(1-Aminoethyl)-2,5-dimethoxybenzyl Alcohol Hydrochloride; Vasoxyl Hydrochloride (*Burroughs-Wellcome*)]

Methoxamine Hydrochloride contains 98.0–100.5% of $C_{11}H_{17}NO_3 \cdot HCl$ (247.72), calculated on the dried basis.

Preparation—Among other ways, Methoxamine Hydrochloride may be prepared from 2',5'-dimethoxypropiophenone through reaction with nitrous acid to form the 2-isonitroso derivative followed by catalytic hydrogenation which reduces both the carbonyl function to carbinol and the isonitroso function to amino. The methoxamine (base), dissolved in a suitable organic solvent, is readily converted to the hydrochloride by a stream of hydrogen chloride.

Description—Colorless or white, plate-like crystals, or a white, crystalline powder. Odorless or has only a slight odor. Its solutions are acid to litmus, having a pH of about 5. Melts between 212° and 216°.

Solubility—1 Gm dissolves in about 2.5 ml of water and 12 ml of alcohol; almost insoluble in chloroform and in ether.

Uses—Methoxamine is a *sympathomimetic* amine which is employed solely for its pressor action and for consequent reflex bradycardia. The prompt and prolonged pressor response produced by methoxamine results almost exclusively from increased peripheral resistance. The drug is useful for the treatment of *hypotensive states* when it is desired to raise blood pressure without cardiac stimulation. The reflex bradycardia is employed in the management of *paroxysmal* *atrial tachycardia*. Methoxamine also possesses direct antiarrhythmic properties. The drug is also applied topically as a *nasal decongestant*. Methoxamine has little inhibitory effect on bronchial muscles, causes little or no central stimulation, and does not increase the irritability of the cyclopropane-sensitized heart. Contraindications to the use of this drug are similar to those for epinephrine and other pressor amines. More extensive clinical experience is needed before the value of Methoxamine can be ascertained in relation to well-established sympathomimetic amines.

Methoxamine is usually administered intramuscularly. The intravenous route can be employed in an emergency.

Dose—*Usual, intramuscular,* **10** to **20 mg**; *intravenous,* **5** to **10 mg**; *infusion,* **60 mg** in **500 ml** of an isotonic solution at a rate adjusted to maintain blood pressure.

Dosage Forms—Injection USP: 20 mg/ml, 100 mg/10 ml.

Methylphenidate Hydrochloride—see page 1116.

Naphazoline Hydrochloride NF

[2-(1-Naphthylmethyl)-2-imidazoline Monohydrochloride; Privine Hydrochloride (*Ciba*)]

Naphazoline Hydrochloride, dried at 105° for 2 hours, contains 98.0–100.5% of $C_{14}H_{14}N_2 . HCl$ (246.74).

Preparation—Naphazoline Hydrochloride is prepared in almost quantitative yields by heating 1-naphthylacetonitrile with ethylenediamine monohydrochloride at 175° to 200°C for 1 hour. Ammonia is formed as a by-product. The 1-naphthylacetonitrile, is made from naphthalene by chloromethylation with formaldehyde and hydrochloric acid followed by treatment of the resulting 1-naphthylmethyl chloride with potassium cyanide.

Description—A white, crystalline, odorless, bitter powder. Melting range 253° to 258°.

Solubility—Freely soluble in water and alcohol; very slightly soluble in chloroform; practically insoluble in ether.

Uses—Although its structure differs markedly from that of most *sympathomimetic* agents, Naphazoline has vasoconstrictor properties very similar to those of epinephrine and other phenylethylamines. It is employed as a *local vasoconstrictor* for the relief of *nasal congestion* of infectious or allergic origin. It also may be used to relieve nasal congestion consequent to treatment with reserpine, etc, since its actions are mainly direct. Care should be exercised in its prolonged use because Naphazoline, in common with most locally applied vasoconstrictors, may cause a rebound congestion which simulates the condition for which it was originally employed; it also induces chemical rhinitis. Mere discontinuation of ill-advised vasoconstrictor therapy has been noted to produce dramatic relief of chronic nasal congestion in some cases. Although only small amounts of Naphazoline are absorbed from the nasal mucosa, it may produce some sedation in children. Naphazoline is also used as an ophthalmic solution for the relief of *ocular congestion* and *blepharospasm*.

Dose—*Topically*, to the nasal mucosa, **2 drops** of a **0.05%** no more frequently than every 3 hours.

Other Dose Information—A few drops of a 0.1 or 0.05% aqueous solution of Naphazoline may be instilled into each nostril every 3 hours. The more dilute solution is specifically prepared for children, but it is frequently adequate for adults and should be tried before the more concentrated solution is prescribed. This agent is also available as a 0.05% nasal jelly and as a 0.05% ophthalmic solution.

Dosage Forms—Solution NF: 0.05%.

Nylidrin Hydrochloride NF

[p-Hydroxy-α-[1-[(1-methyl-3-phenylpropyl)amino]ethyl]-benzyl Alcohol Hydrochloride; Arlidin· (*USV*)]

Nylidrin Hydrochloride, dried at 60° in vacuum for 3 hours, contains 98.0–102.0% of $C_{19}H_{25}NO_2 . HCl$ (335.88).

Preparation—Among other ways, nylidrin (base) may be prepared by dissolving p-hydroxynorephedrine (I) and benzylacetone (II) in alcohol and then hydrogenating in the presence of Raney nickel or another suitable catalyst. The reaction may be looked upon as involving initially an addition of (I) to the carbonyl group of (II) to form the aminoalcohol derivative (III), followed by reduction of the newly formed carbinol group. After isolation and purification, the base may be dissolved in ethanol or another suitable solvent and precipitated as the hydrochloride by means of a stream of hydrogen chloride.

Description—A white, odorless, practically tasteless crystalline powder. The pH of a 1 in 100 solution is between 4.5 and 6.5.

Solubility—1 Gm dissolves in about 65 ml of water and about 40 ml of alcohol; very slightly soluble in chloroform and ether.

Uses—Nylidrin is a sympathomimetic amine which dilates the blood vessels, especially those which supply the skeletal musculature. There is little effect on the cutaneous vasculature. It exerts a mild stimulatory effect on the heart. The drug is used in the treatment of vascular disorders of the extremities that may involve the skeletal muscle vessels, such as *intermittent claudication, thrombophlebitis,* and, to a lesser extent, *diabetic vascular disease*. It has been advocated for use in thromboangiitis obliterans, endarteritis obliterans, Raynaud's disease and ischemic ulcers; inasmuch as the drug fails to increase significantly cutaneous blood flow, such use cannot be expected to be of benefit.

Side effects consist of nervousness and palpitation.

Dose—*Oral,* **3** to **12 mg;** *usual, oral,* **6 mg** 3 times a day; *parenteral,* **2.5** to **5 mg;** *usual, parenteral,* **5 mg** 1 or more times a day.

Dosage Forms—Injection NF: 5 mg/ml, 50 mg/10 ml; Tablets NF: 6 mg.

Oxymetazoline Hydrochloride NF

[6-*tert*-Butyl-3-(2-imidazolin-2-ylmethyl)-2,4-dimethylphenol Monohydrochloride; Afrin (*Schering*)]

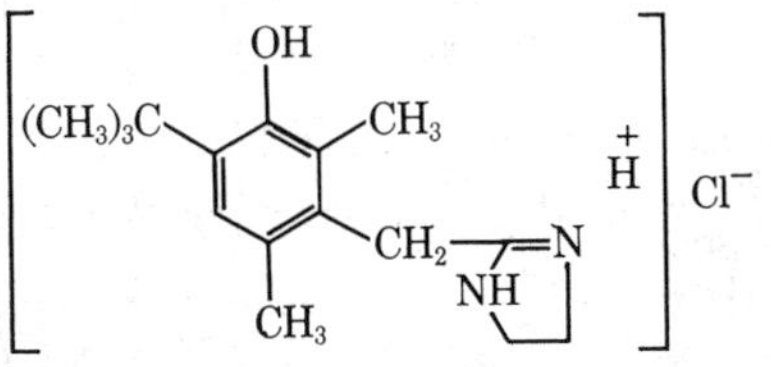

Oxymetazoline Hydrochloride, dried at 105° for 3 hours, contains 98.5–101.5% of $C_{16}H_{24}N_2O \cdot HCl$ (296.84).

Preparation—2,4-Dimethyl-6-*tert*-butylphenol is converted into the benzyl cyanide intermediate (I). This is then reacted with ethylenediamine *p*-toluenesulfonate whereupon, through addition and deammoniation, the imidazoline ring is formed. The oxymetazoline (base) is then isolated and converted to the official salt through interaction with an equimolar quantity of hydrogen chloride. US Pat. 3,147,275.

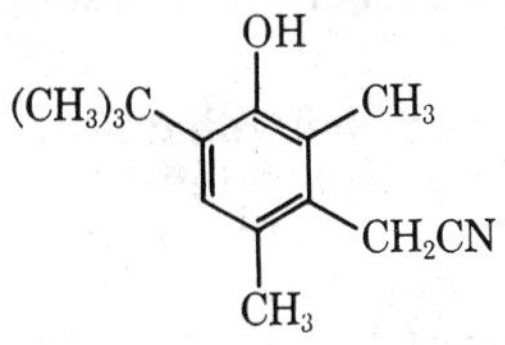

I

Description—A white to nearly white, fine, crystalline powder that is odorless. It is stable in light and heat, and is nonhygroscopic. It melts at 300° with decomposition.

Solubility—Soluble in water and alcohol; practically insoluble in benzene, chloroform, and ether.

Uses—Oxymetazoline is a sympathomimetic with prominent vasoconstrictor actions. It is only used topically to decongest the nasopharyngeal membranes in *acute rhinitis, nasopharyngitis, sinusitis, vasomotor rhinitis, hay fever, otitis media,* and *aerotitis media.* After-congestion is less prominent than with naphazoline.

Dose—*Nasally,* **2** to **4 drops** of a **0.05%** solution instilled into each nostril twice a day.

Dosage Forms—Solution NF: 0.05%.

Phenmetrazine Hydrochloride NF

[3-Methyl-2-phenylmorpholine Hydrochloride; A66; Psychamine A66; Preludin (*Geigy*)]

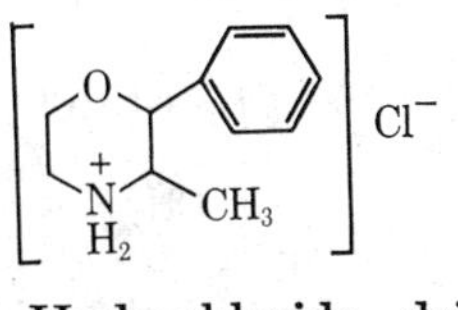

Phenmetrazine Hydrochloride, dried at 105° for 2 hours, contains 98.0–102.0% of $C_{11}H_{15}NO \cdot HCl$ (213.71).

Preparation—Phenmetrazine base may be prepared by cyclizing α-[1-[(2-hydroxyethyl)amino]ethyl]benzyl alcohol with the aid of strong sulfuric acid or other suitable dehydrants. The alcohol may be synthesized through the addition reaction involving ethylene oxide and α-(1-aminoethyl)benzyl alcohol [norephedrine]. The base reacts readily with an equimolar quantity of HCl to form the official salt.

Description—Occurs as a white to off-white, crystalline powder.

Solubility—1 Gm dissolves in about 0.4 ml of water, in 2 ml of alcohol, and about 2 ml of chloroform.

Uses—Phenmetrazine is a *sympathomimetic* with actions similar to dextroamphetamine (see *Dextroamphetamine Phosphate*). It depresses appetite and therefore is employed in the management of obesity. As an anorexigenic agent it is about equal to dextroamphetamine, but the side effects of euphoria, insomnia, nervousness and hyperexcitability are less frequent.

Dose—*Usual,* **25** to **75 mg** per day, in divided doses, administered 1 hour before meals.

Dosage Forms—Extended-release Oral Solid: 75 mg; Tablets NF: 25 mg.

Phentermine

[Phenyl-*tert*-butylamine]

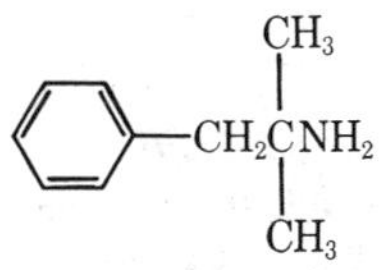

Phentermine is α,α-dimethylphenethylamine [$C_{10}H_{15}$-N = 149.23].

Preparation—According to one method, benzyl chloride is Grignardized with acetone, the resulting α,α-dimethylphenethyl alcohol is reacted with sodium cyanide in an acetic acid-sulfuric acid environment to form the corresponding 2-formamido compound, and this is then hydrolyzed to liberate the Phentermine.

Description—Colorless, mobile, oily liquid with an odor characteristic of amines. It boils at about 200° and yields a benzoyl derivative which melts at approximately 111°.

Solubility—Soluble in chloroform, ether, alcohol, and dilute acids; slightly soluble in water.

Uses—Phentermine is said to have an *anorectic* drug (ie, appetite suppressant) action. It is chemically related to sympathomimetic drugs such as amphetamine. However, its cardiovascular actions are extremely weak. The central stimulant actions are also less prominent than with the amphetamines. Consequently, use of the drug is accompanied by a low incidence of side effects. However, its anorectic effects are also weaker. Clinical trials do not show an unequivocal efficacy. It is marketed as a complex with an ionic resin [phenyl-*tert*-butylamine resin—Ionamin (Strasenburgh)], the purpose of which is to provide a more sustained release after oral ingestion.

Dose—**15** to **30 mg** in terms of the amine base, to be taken upon rising.

Dosage Forms—Capsules: 15 and 30 mg.

Phenylephrine Hydrochloride USP

[(−)-*m*-Hydroxy-α-[(methylamino)methyl]benzyl Alcohol Hydrochloride; Neo-Synephrine Hydrochloride (*Winthrop*)]

Phenylephrine Hydrochloride contains 97.5–102.5% of $C_9H_{13}NO_2 \cdot HCl$ (203.67), calculated on the dried basis.

Preparation—Phenylephrine is prepared from *m*-hydroxyphenacyl bromide by reaction with methylamine followed by catalytic hydrogenation of the resulting compound, the two reactions taking place readily at room temperature:

Phenylephrine

The phenylephrine base so formed, dissolved in ether or other suitable solvent, is treated with hydrochloric acid to form the hydrochloride.

Description—White or nearly white, odorless, bitter crystals. Its solutions are acid to litmus. Melting range 140° to 145°. Specific rotation −42° to −47.5°.

Solubility—Freely soluble in water and in alcohol.

Uses—The *sympathomimetic* actions and the uses of Phenylephrine Hydrochloride are similar to those of levarterenol, but the drug has very weak cardiac, vasodilator, and metabolic actions; it has essentially no central actions and is effective after oral administration. It has a direct action. The topical application is useful for reducing *nasal congestion* accompanying sinusitis, vasomotor rhinitis, and hay fever. Phenylephrine has several uses in ophthalmology; it is employed as a *decongestant* for minor irritations of the conjunctiva, as a temporary *vasoconstrictor*, and as a *mydriatic*. Preparations of Phenylephrine are incompatible with butacaine.

Phenylephrine is superior to ephedrine for sustaining blood pressure during spinal anesthesia because it causes neither central neural effects nor loses its efficacy as a *pressor agent* upon repeated administration. The drug is also employed to retard the systemic absorption and to prolong the duration of action of local anesthetics.

Oral administration has proved effective in the treatment of *orthostatic hypotension*. Pressor doses injected intravenously cause reflex bradycardia which can abort attacks of *paroxysmal tachycardia*. Phenylephrine Hydrochloride, in a nebula, is effective in the treatment of *asthma*.

Dose—*Subcutaneous* or *intramuscular*, 1 to 20 mg; *usual*, 5 mg, repeated in 10 minutes if necessary; *usual*, intravenous infusion, 10 to 20 mg in 500 ml of an isotonic infusion solution at a rate adjusted to maintain blood pressure; *topically*, 0.1 ml of a 0.125 to 10% solution to the conjunctiva, repeated as necessary; 0.2 to 0.6 ml of a 0.125 to 1% solution 4 to 6 times a day.

Other Dose Information—The oral dose is 10 to 25 mg, repeated as indicated. The drug is marketed in solutions of several strengths (see below) for topical application; a 0.125% ophthalmic solution is used for conjunctival decongestion, a 10% ophthalmic solution or emulsion for conjunctival vasoconstriction, or a 1.0% emulsion or a 2.5% ophthalmic solution for mydriatic effects. In local anesthetic solutions it is used in a concentration of 0.05%.

Dosage Forms—Injection USP: 4 mg/2 ml, 10 mg/ml, 50 mg/5 ml; Ophthalmic Solution USP: 0.125, 0.2, 2.5, and 10%; Solution USP: 0.125, 0.167, 0.25, 0.5, and 1%.

Phenylpropanolamine Hydrochloride NF

[(±)-Norephedrine Hydrochloride; (±)-α-(1-Aminoethyl)benzyl Alcohol Hydrochloride; Propadrine Hydrochloride (*MSD*)]

Phenylpropanolamine Hydrochloride contains 98.0–101.0% of $C_9H_{13}NO \cdot HCl$ (187.67), calculated on the dried basis.

Preparation—Phenylpropanolamine (base) may be prepared by reacting benzaldehyde with nitroethane in 95% ethanol in the presence of sodium hydroxide to form α-(1-nitroethyl)benzyl alcohol and then reducing this nitroalcohol to the corresponding amino compound. A stream of hydrogen chloride passed into a suitable solution of the base gives the hydrochloride. US Pat. 2,151,517. For an improved industrial process, see US Pat. 3,028,429.

Description—A white, crystalline powder having a slight aromatic odor. It is affected by light. It melts between 191° and 196°. The pH of a solution (3 in 100) is between 4.2 and 5.5.

Solubility—Freely soluble in water and alcohol; insoluble in ether.

Uses—Phenylpropanolamine is an indirectly acting sympathomimetic with prominent peripheral adrenergic effects and weak central stimulant actions. Its pattern of peripheral actions is similar to that of *Ephedrine* (page 884), and it is used similarly. Its actions are more prolonged than those of ephedrine. It produces less anxiety and other manifestations of central stimulation. The principal use of Phenylpropanolamine is as a nasal decongestant in hay fever, for which it may be given orally or topically. It is also used as a *bronchodilator* and *bronchial decongestant* in *asthma*. It is peculiar that most commercial preparations of phenylpropanolamine hydrochloride contain a mixture of drugs. Under such circumstances, the assessment of the true contribution of phenylpropanolamine to any therapeutic response is difficult. Phenylpropanolamine should not be used in hyperthyroid or hypertensive patients.

Dose—*Usual*, 25 to 50 mg every 3 or 4 hours.

Other Dose Information—Topically, as a 0.1 to 0.3% aqueous solution.

Dosage Forms—Capsules: 25 and 50 mg; Powder: 15 Gm; Elixir: 20 mg/5 ml.

Propylhexedrine NF

[*N*,α-Dimethyl-cyclohexaneethylamine; Benzedrex (*SK&F*)]

Propylhexedrine contains 98.0–101.0% of $C_{10}H_{21}N$ (155.29).

Preparation—As described in US Pat. 2,454,746, it may be synthesized as follows. A solution of commercially available cyclohexylacetone in formic acid is caused to react with *N*-methylformamide by heating for 4 hours at 160° to 180°C. The resulting formyl derivative of propylhexedrine is then hydrolyzed by refluxing with 50% sulfuric acid for about 4 hours, after which the hydrolysate is extracted with ether to remove acid-insoluble material. The aqueous solution is then rendered strongly alkaline with sodium hydroxide and the liberated amine is extracted with ether and purified by distillation under reduced pressure.

Cyclohexylacetone   ***N*-Formyl-propylhexedrine**

Description—A clear, colorless liquid, having a characteristic, aminelike odor. Volatilizes slowly at room temperature. Its solutions are alkaline to litmus, and it absorbs carbon dioxide from the air. Specific gravity between 0.848 and 0.852. Boils at about 205°.

Solubility—Very slightly soluble in water; miscible with alcohol, chloroform, and ether.

Uses—Propylhexedrine is a volatile *sympathomimetic* amine which, because of its lack of central excitatory effects and addiction liability, was introduced as a substitute for amphetamine for use in inhaler cartridges. One or two inhalations through each nostril produce *vasoconstriction* and a *decongestant* effect on nasal mucous membranes. Because of its wide margin of safety and relative freedom from toxic side effects, the use of Propylhexedrine by inhalation is not contraindicated in patients in whom an ephedrine-like action would be undesirable. It is considered safe for self-medication by adults, but children should not have unsupervised access to an inhaler. The drug is an indirectly acting sympathomimetic, so that it will have limited efficacy in the treatment of nasal stuffiness consequent to treatment with reserpine, guanethidine, and other adrenergic neurone blockers and catecholamine depletors.

Dose—By *inhalation* as required.

Other Dose Information—Propylhexedrine is marketed in inhalers which contain 250 mg of the drug. The usual dose is 2 inhalations through each nostril, repeated as required to obtain relief.

Dosage Forms—Inhalant NF.

Pseudoephedrine Hydrochloride NF

[(+)-[α-(1-Methylamino)ethyl]benzyl Alcohol Hydrochloride;   Ro-Fedrin (*Robinson*); Sudafed (*Burroughs-Wellcome*)]

Pseudoephedrine Hydrochloride contains 98.0–100.5% of $C_{10}H_{15}NO \cdot HCl$ (201.70), calculated on the dried basis.

Preparation—(−)-Ephedrine hydrochloride is acetylated to produce (+)-*N*-acetylpseudoephedrine hydrochloride which is then deacetylated to yield the official article. Ephedrine and pseudoephedrine are diastereoisomers, the former having the *erythro* and the latter the *threo* configuration.

Description—Fine, white to off-white crystals or a powder having a faint, characteristic odor. Its solutions are neutral to litmus.

Solubility—Soluble in water, alcohol, and chloroform.

Uses—Pseudoephedrine differs from *Ephedrine*

(page 884) in that it is relatively weaker in its pressor, cardiac, mydriatic, and central stimulant actions. Its nasopharyngeal vasoconstrictor and bronchodilator actions are about the same. Consequently, it is used in the treatment of *nasal congestion, sinusitis, vasomotor rhinitis, eustachian salpingitis, acute aerotitis media, bronchospasm,* and *bronchial asthma*. Pseudoephedrine may cause mild central stimulation. It should not be used in hypertensive or hyperthyroid patients.

Dose—**30** to **60 mg** 3 or 4 times a day; *usual,* **30 mg** 3 times a day.

Other Dose Information—Children of age 7 to 12 years should take ½ the adult dose; children 4 months to 6 years of age should be given only ¼ the adult dose.

Dosage Forms—Syrup NF: 30 mg/5 ml; Tablets NF: 30 and 60 mg.

Tetrahydrozoline Hydrochloride NF

[2-(1,2,3,4-Tetrahydro-1-naphthyl)-2-imidazoline Monohydrochloride;   Tyzine (*Pfizer*);   Visine (*Lemming*)]

Tetrahydrozoline Hydrochloride contains 98.0–100.5% of $C_{13}H_{16}N_2 \cdot HCl$ (236.75), calculated on the dried basis.

Preparation—Ethyl phenylacetate (I) is caused to undergo a typical Michael condensation and cyclization with methyl acrylate (II) in the presence of a suitable catalyst such as sodium ethoxide, followed by treatment with acid to liberate 4-keto-1,2,3,4-tetrahydro-1-naphthoic acid (III). The keto group is then reduced to methylene by hydrogenation with the aid of Raney nickel, and the resulting 1,2,3,4-tetrahydro-1-naphthoic acid is condensed with ethylenediamine in the presence of concentrated hydrochloric acid.

Description—It occurs as a white, odorless solid. Melting range 253° to 259°.

Solubility—Freely soluble in water and in alcohol; very slightly soluble in chloroform; practically insoluble in ether.

Uses—The actions and uses of Tetrahydrozoline Hydrochloride are substantially the same as those of Naphazoline, which is a close chemical congener. See *Naphazoline Hydrochloride* (page 892). However, it is somewhat like epinephrine in having a prominent vasodilator component in its action in man. Prolonged use as a *nasal decongestant* may induce chemical rhinitis. Excessive doses may cause drowsiness and profuse sweating, and severe respiratory depression, coma and shock in young children after overdosage have been reported.

Dose—*Usual,* applied as a **0.05** or **0.1%** solution as nasal drops or spray at 4-hour intervals; to the eye as a **0.05%** solution.

Other Dose Information—Intranasally, 2 or 3 drops of a 0.1% solution every 3 hours or longer. For children 6 years of age or younger, 1 to 3 drops of a 0.05%

solution should be used at intervals no less than 4 hours. For ophthalmic use, 1 to 2 drops of a 0.05% solution into the conjunctival sac, as needed.

Dosage Forms—Solution NF: 0.05 and 0.1%; Ophthalmic Solution NF: 0.05%.

Tuaminoheptane Sulfate NF

[1-Methylhexylamine Sulfate (2:1); Tuamine Sulfate (*Lilly*)]

$$\left[\begin{array}{c} CH_3(CH_2)_4CH\overset{+}{N}H_3 \\ | \\ CH_3 \end{array} \right]_2 SO_4^=$$

Tuaminoheptane Sulfate yields 96.5–100.5% of $(C_7H_{17}N)_2.H_2SO_4$ (328.52), calculated on the dried basis.

Preparation—Tuaminoheptane may be prepared by several methods. A common one involves reduction of commercially available 2-nitroheptane with tin and HCl followed by liberation of the amine by treatment with alkali and extraction of the amine with ether. Salts such as the sulfate are conveniently prepared by treating the purified ether solution with sulfuric acid whereupon the salt is precipitated.

Description—A white, odorless powder.
Solubility—Freely soluble in water; soluble in alcohol; sparingly soluble in ether.

Uses—Tuaminoheptane Sulfate is an indirectly acting *sympathomimetic* aliphatic amine salt which is a potent *vasoconstrictor*, applied locally for prompt relief of *nasal congestion* in the form of a spray, or tampons, or as drops.

Dose—*Topically*, to the nasal mucosa as a **0.5 to 2%** solution.

Dosage Forms—Solution NF (see below): 1%.

Tuaminoheptane Sulfate Solution NF is a solution of tuaminoheptane sulfate in water adjusted to a suitable pH and tonicity. It contains a preservative. It contains 90.0–110.0% of the labeled amount of $(C_7H_{17}N)_2.H_2SO_4$. —*Preparation:* Dissolve sodium hydroxide (227 mg) in purified water (900 ml), then dissolve phenylmercuric nitrate (20 mg), monobasic potassium phosphate (6.9 Gm), sodium chloride (900 mg), and tuaminoheptane sulfate (10 Gm) in this solution, and adjust the pH, if necessary, to between 5.8 and 6.2. Add purified water (qs) to make 1000 ml, mix thoroughly, and filter.

Xylometazoline Hydrochloride NF

[2-(4-tert-Butyl-2,6-dimethylbenzyl)-2-imidazoline Monohydrochloride; Otrivin Hydrochloride (*Ciba*)]

Xylometazoline Hydrochloride contains 99.0–100.5% of $C_{16}H_{24}N_2.HCl$ (280.84), calculated on the dried basis.

Preparation—Utilizing (4-*tert*-butyl-2,6-dimethylphenyl)acetonitrile as the participating nitrile, Xylometazoline Hydrochloride may be prepared by the method described for *Naphazoline Hydrochloride*, page 892.

Description—A white, odorless, crystalline powder. It melts above 300° with decomposition.
Solubility—1 Gm dissolves in about 30 ml of water; freely soluble in alcohol; sparingly soluble in chloroform; practically insoluble in benzene and ether.

Uses—Xylometazoline Hydrochloride is a sympathomimetic chemically related to *Naphazoline Hydrochloride* (page 892) and *Tetrahydrozoline Hydrochloride* (page 895). It is used as a local vasoconstrictor for nasal decongestion. Its effects are prompt in onset and last for several hours but do not seem to be followed by as much reactive hyperemia (rebound congestion) as does naphazoline. Side effects are infrequent and mild but include local stinging or burning, dry nose, rebound congestion, chemical rhinitis, palpitation, headache, and drowsiness.

Dose—*Nasally*, **2 or 3 drops** of a **0.05 or 0.1%** solution every 4 to 6 hours.

Other Dose Information—For children, 1 or 2 squeezes of a plastic spray tube containing a 0.05% solution. A 0.1% solution is also available for adults.

Dosage Forms—Solution NF: 0.05 and 0.1%.

Other Sympathomimetic Drugs

Amphetamine Phosphate NF XII [Monobasic Racemic Amphetamine Phosphate; Monobasic *dl*-Amphetamine Phosphate; (±)-α-Methylphenethylamine Phosphate (1:1); Raphetamine Phosphate (*Strasenburgh*)], dried at 105° for 2 hours, contains not less than 98.0% of $C_9H_{13}N.H_3PO_4$ (233.21). *Preparation:* A solution of amphetamine in alcohol or other suitable solvent is treated with an equimolar portion of phosphoric acid. *Description and Solubility:* A white, odorless, crystalline powder having a bitter taste; pH (1 in 20 solution): 4–5. Freely soluble in water (more soluble than the sulfate); slightly soluble in alcohol; practically insoluble in benzene, chloroform, and ether. *Uses:* See *Amphetamine*, page 882. *Dose:* Usual, oral, 5 mg.

Amphetamine Phosphate Dibasic NF XI [$(C_9H_{13}N)_2.H_3PO_4$ = 368.42][Dibasic Racemic Amphetamine Phosphate]—A white, odorless crystalline powder having a slightly bitter taste. One Gm dissolves in about 20 ml of water and about 650 ml of alcohol; insoluble in ether. *Uses:* see *Amphetamine* (page 882).

Amphetamine Tannate [Tanphetamin]—A tan amorphous powder, freely soluble in alcohol, slightly soluble in water. It is a complex salt of amphetamine with tannic acid. One Gm is equivalent to 0.388 Gm dibasic amphetamine phosphate. *Uses:* See *Amphetamine* (page 882).

Chlorphentermine Hydrochloride [$C_{10}H_{14}ClN.HCl$ (220.14); Pre-Sate (*Warner-Chilcott*)] is 4-chloro-α,α-dimethylphenethylamine. *Preparation:* p-Chlorobenzyl chloride is Grignardized with acetone, the resulting 1-(p-chlorophenyl)-2-methyl-2-propanol is reacted with sodium cyanide in an acetic acid–sulfuric acid environment to form the corresponding 2-formamido compound, and this is then hydrolyzed with alkali to form chlorphentermine (base). Treatment with hydrogen chloride in a suitable solvent yields the hydrochloride. *Description and Solubility:* A white to off-white powder that is odorless and has a bitter taste; stable in light and air; melts between 232° and 235°. Freely soluble in water and alcohol; sparingly soluble in chloroform; practically insoluble in ether. *Uses:* An anorexigenic *sympathomimetic* with very little central stimulant activity. Its cardiovascular effects are also weak, so that the drug has been recommended especially for use in the treatment of obesity complicated by cardiovascular disorders. As an anorexigenic the drug appears to be as good as but not superior to other prominent anorexigenic drugs. Chlorphentermine is contraindicated in glaucoma and in patients under treatment with monoamine oxidase inhibitors. *Dose:* Oral, 65 mg of the base once a day, usually after breakfast.

Dextroamphetamine Phosphate Dibasic NF XI [$(C_9H_{13}N)_2.H_3PO_4$ = 368.42][(+)-α-Methylphenethylamine Phosphate (2:1)]—A white, odorless, crystalline powder having a slightly bitter taste. The specific rotation of a 4% aqueous solution is between +20° and +23°. One Gm dissolves in about 20 ml of water and about 650 ml of alcohol; insoluble in ether. *Uses:* see *Dextroamphetamine Phosphate* (page 883).

Ethylnorepinephrine Hydrochloride [α-(1-Aminopropyl)-3,4-dihydroxybenzyl alcohol hydrochloride] [C_6H_3-$(OH)_2$CH(OH)CH(NH_2)CH_2CH_3.HCl; Bronkephrine (*Breon*)]—It is a sympathomimetic with actions and uses similar to *Isoproterenol* (see page 888). However, in man its vasodilator, cardiostimulatory, and central stimulant actions are weak, while the bronchodilator actions are prominent. It is used as a bronchodilator. *Dose: subcutaneously, intramuscularly, or intravenously,* 0.5 to 2 mg; by *inhalation* as a mist, 2% solution.

Isometheptene Hydrochloride [Methylisooctenylamine Hydrochloride; Octanil Hydrochloride; Octon Hydrochloride; $C_9H_{19}N$.HCl; Octin Hydrochloride (*Knoll*)] is N,1,5-trimethyl-4-hexenylamine hydrochloride. *Description and Solubility:* Extremely hygroscopic crystals, melting at about 68°. Soluble in water and alcohol. *Uses:* An indirectly acting vasoconstrictor *sympathomimetic* that also exerts antispasmodic actions on those structures that are normally inhibited by sympathetic stimulation. It also mildly stimulates the heart. It has been used for the treatment of *urinary tract and gastrointestinal tract spastic conditions* and for the relief of *migraine* attacks. *Dose: Oral,* 4 doses of 15 to 20 drops of a 10% solution at half-hour intervals; *intramuscular,* 50 to 100 mg for acute control of pain, to be later replaced by oral therapy. *It should never be administered intravenously.*

Isometheptene Mucate [Methylisooctenylamine Mucate; Octanil Mucate; Octon Mucate; Octin Mucate (*Knoll*)] is N,1,5-trimethyl-4-hexenylamine mucate [(C_9-$H_{19}N$)$_2$.$C_6H_{10}O_8$]. *Description and Solubility:* A white, crystalline powder with a bitter taste. 1 Gm dissolves in about 20 ml of alcohol; freely soluble in water; almost insoluble in ether and chloroform. *Uses:* It has the same actions and uses as *Isometheptene Hydrochloride* (see above). However, it is never administered parenterally. *Dose: Oral,* 120 mg every half hour for 4 doses; *rectal,* by suppository, 250 mg, which may be repeated after 1 hour if necessary.

Levamphetamine Succinate [$C_9H_{13}N$·$C_4H_6O_4$; Amodril (*N. Am. Pharm.*); Cydril (*Tutag*); Maigret (*Ferndale*)] is (−)-α-methylphenethylamine succinate (1:1). *Description and Solubility:* A white, crystalline powder. Slightly soluble in water; sparingly soluble in alcohol. *Uses:* Its uses are the same as those of *Levoamphetamine Sulfate* (see below). *Dose: Oral,* 7 mg 3 times a day or 21 mg daily as a sustained-release preparation.

Levoamphetamine Sulfate [($C_9H_{13}N$)$_2$·H_2SO_4; Ad-Nil (*Medics*)] is (−)-α-methylphenethylamine sulfate (2:1). *Description and Solubility:* A white, crystalline powder. Slightly soluble in water; sparingly soluble in alcohol. *Uses:* The central stimulant potency of Levoamphetamine is considerably less than that of dextroamphetamine. Euphoria is less frequent. Consequently, the drug is promoted as an anorexigenic agent which will not be abused. However, it has not been clearly established that the anorexigenic is not also less. If a dose is employed with which the central stimulant actions are equal to those of dextroamphetamine, the cardiovascular effects are more apparent than with the dextro isomer. *Dose:* The only marketed form is a sustained-release capsule containing 15 mg, to be taken daily.

Mephentermine [Mephine; Vialin; Wyamine (*Wyeth*)] is N,α,α-trimethylphenethylamine [$C_{11}H_{17}N$]. For the structure, see *Mephentermine Sulfate,* page 890. *Description and Solubility:* A clear, colorless to pale-yellow liquid with a fishy, amine odor. Freely soluble in alcohol; soluble in ether; practically insoluble in water. *Uses:* An indirectly acting *sympathomimetic.* Because it is a free amine base, rather than a salt, and lacks strongly polar groups, it is volatile. Consequently, it can be administered as an inhalant vasoconstrictor for *nasal decongestion.* It readily penetrates the cornea, and hence may be used as a *mydriatic,* although it is little used as such. Its systemic actions are the same as those of *Mephentermine Sulfate. Dose: 1 or 2 inhalations* in each nostril is generally sufficient to provide relief.

Methoxyphenamine Hydrochloride [Ortodrinex Hydrochloride; Orthoxine Hydrochloride (*Upjohn*)] is o-methoxy-N,α-dimethylphenethylamine hydrochloride ($C_{11}H_{17}NO$.HCl]. *Description and Solubility:* A bitter, odorless, white, crystalline powder, melting between 124° and 128°; pH (5% aqueous solution), 5.3.–5.7. Freely soluble in water, alcohol, and chloroform; slightly soluble in ether and benzene. *Uses: A sympathomimetic* with weak vasopressor activity but with relatively prominent bronchodilator and smooth muscle relaxant actions on adrenergically inhibited organs. It is used in the treatment of *bronchial asthma, allergic rhinitis, acute urticaria,* and *gastrointestinal allergy.* It may cause drowsiness, nausea, faintness, and dry mouth. *Dose: Oral,* 50 to 100 mg every 3 or 4 hours.

Methylhexaneamine [Forthane (*Lilly*)] is 4-methyl-2-hexylamine [$C_7H_{17}N$]. *Description and Solubility:* A colorless to pale-yellow liquid with an ammonialike odor. Freely soluble in alcohol, chloroform, ether, and dilute acids; very slightly soluble in water. *Uses:* An indirectly acting *sympathomimetic.* The free base is volatile; consequently, the highly dissociable carbonate salt is used as an inhalant vasoconstrictor for *nasal decongestion.* Its systemic actions include vasoconstriction and mydriasis. It also produces mydriasis by topical application. Side effects include nervousness, tremors, excitement, and headache and require discontinuation of the drug. *Dose: 1* or *2 inhalations* in each nostril is generally sufficient to provide relief; the interval between doses should be no shorter than ½ hour. The presently marketed inhaler contains 250 mg of the base.

Naphazoline Nitrate BP—Purity: 98.5% of $C_{14}H_{14}$-N_2.HNO$_3$. A white, odorless, crystalline powder having a bitter taste. It is soluble in 36 parts of water and in 16 parts of alcohol, very slightly soluble in chloroform, and almost insoluble in ether. A 1% aqueous solution has a pH of 5.0 to 6.5. *Uses* and *Dose:* see *Naphazoline Hydrochloride* (page 892).

Nordefrin Hydrochloride NF XII [(±)-α-(1-Aminoethyl)-3,4-dihydroxybenzyl Alcohol Hydrochloride; dl-3,4-Dihydroxynorephedrine Hydrochloride], dried in a vacuum desiccator over phosphorus pentoxide for 24 hours, contains 98.0–102.0% of $C_9H_{13}NO_3$·HCl (219.67). *Preparation:* 3′,4′-Dihydroxypropiophenone is first converted into its dibenzyl ether to protect the ring against nitrosation and oxidation, and is then converted into its isonitroso derivative. Pressure treatment with hydrogen in the presence of platinized or palladinized charcoal results in (1) reduction of isonitroso to amino and of carbonyl to carbinol and (2) hydrogenolytic cleavage of the benzyl-oxy linkages to regenerate the phenolic hydroxyls. The nordefrin (base) thus obtained may be dissolved in a suitable organic solvent and converted into the salt by means of a stream of hydrogen chloride. *Description and Solubility:* A white, crystalline solid; melting range, 175°–180°. Soluble in water and alcohol; practically insoluble in ether. *Uses:* A directly acting *sympathomimetic* which differs from levarterenol in that the side chain has an alpha methyl group. Its pharmacology is essentially that of *Levarterenol* (page 889), except that Nordefrin is only about ⅒ to ½ as potent in most actions. Also its duration of action is prolonged. It is employed as a *vasoconstrictor* in local anesthetic solutions, as a local *nasal decongestant,* and rarely as a pressor agent in various hypotensive states. However, it has no advantages over either epinephrine or levarterenol or over levonordephrine. *Dose: Locally,* as a 1:10,000 solution.

Phendimetrazine Tartrate [Plegine (*Ayerst*)] is (+)-3,4-dimethyl-2-phenylmorpholine tartrate (1:1). *Description and Solubility:* A white, odorless, crystalline powder, having a bitter taste; melts at 186° with decomposition. Soluble in water, methanol, and alcohol. *Uses:* Closely related to *Phenmetrazine* (page 893) both chemically and pharmacologically. It is an indirectly acting *sympathomimetic* with predominantly central nervous stimulant actions. It is used as an *appetite suppressant* and not as a general central stimulant or sympathomimetic. Common untoward effects include insomnia, nervousness, dizziness, headache, tachycardia, palpitation, hypertension, abdominal cramps, nausea, constipation, glossitis, dry mouth, urinary inertia, and cystitis. It is contraindicated when monoamine oxidase inhibitors are being used. *Dose: Oral,* 17.5 to 70 mg 2 or 3 times daily 1 hour before meals.

Phentermine Hydrochloride [Wilpo (*Dorsey*)] is $C_{10}H_{15}N \cdot HCl$. For the structure of the base, see *Phentermine* (page 893). *Description and Solubility:* A white, crystalline powder that is odorless or has a faint characteristic odor and melts at about 203°. Very soluble in water, chloroform, and alcohol; insoluble in ether; very slightly soluble in acetone and benzene. *Uses:* See *Phentermine.* *Dose: Oral, 8 mg* to be taken 30 minutes before mealtime; *24 mg* daily with sustained-release preparations.

Protokylol Hydrochloride [Caytine (*Lakeside*)] is α-[(α-Methyl-3,4-methylenedioxyphenethylamino)methyl]-protocatechuyl alcohol hydrochloride [$C_{18}H_{21}NO_5 \cdot HCl$]. *Description and Solubility:* A white to light-cream powder that melts between 170° and 176°. 1 Gm dissolves in approximately 18.5 ml of water, 39.4 ml of absolute alcohol, and 4.9 ml of methanol. *Uses:* A *sympathomimetic* which resembles *Isoproterenol* (page 888) in its actions and uses; its bronchodilator actions are somewhat stronger in proportion to its cardiac actions. It is used in the treatment of *bronchial asthma;* in long-term treatment it is about as effective as ephedrine. It is frequently effective after refractoriness has developed to other bronchodilators. It also is used in the treatment of *chronic pulmonary emphysema, pulmonary fibrosis, chronic bronchitis, and bronchiectasis.* Side effects include tachycardia, palpitation, tremulousness, tension, insomnia, vertigo, and nausea. *Dose: Oral, 2 to 4 mg 4* times daily; *intramuscular* or *subcutaneous, 0.1 to 0.5 mg,* for subacute or acute episodes; *inhalation,* by nebulization of a *1:100* solution 4 to 6 times a day. *Veterinary Dose: Dogs* and *Cats, intramuscular* or *subcutaneous,* 0.1 to 0.5 mg; *oral,* 1 to 4 mg (*Puppies* and *Kittens,* 0.25 to 1 mg).

Racephedrine Hydrochloride NF XII [*dl*-Ephedrine Hydrochloride; (±)-α[1-(Methylamino)ethyl]benzyl Alcohol Hydrochloride], dried at 105° for 3 hours, contains 98.2–100.7% of racemic $C_{10}H_{15}NO \cdot HCl$ (201.70). *Preparation:* It may be synthesized by a number of methods, generally the same as those for synthesizing ephedrine, except that the step involving resolution of the racemic mixture is omitted. One patented method consists of reacting 2-bromopropiophenone with methylamine and reducing the resulting 2-(methylamino)propiophenone catalytically with hydrogen. *Description and Solubility:* Fine, white, odorless crystals or powder; affected by light; its solutions are optically inactive. 1 Gm dissolves in about 4 ml of water and about 25 ml of alcohol; insoluble in ether. *Uses:* Similar to those of *Ephedrine* (page 884). *Dose: Usual, oral, 25 mg.*

Tuaminoheptane [2-Aminoheptane; Heptamine; Heptedrine; Tuamine (*Lilly*)] is 1-methylhexylamine [$C_7H_{17}N$]. *Preparation:* See *Tuaminoheptane Sulfate,* page 896. *Description and Solubility:* A colorless to pale-yellow liquid, boiling between 142° and 144°; pH (1% aqueous solution), about 11.5. Freely soluble in alcohol, chloroform, and ether; slightly soluble in water. *Uses:* An indirectly acting *sympathomimetic.* Because the free base is volatile, it is given by inhalation as a vasoconstrictor for *nasal decongestion.* Systemic effects include hypertension, tachycardia, mydriasis, and intestinal spasm, but no use is made of these effects. *Dose: 1* or *2 inhalations* in each nostril, no more frequently than once per hour. The present marketed inhaler contains 325 mg.

49 | Cholinomimetic (Parasympathomimetic) Drugs

Cholinomimetics—anticholinesterases

This chapter was prepared by

Ewart A. Swinyard, PhD, *Professor of Pharmacology, College of Pharmacy and College of Medicine, University of Utah, Salt Lake City, Utah 84112, and*
Stewart C. Harvey, PhD, *Associate Professor of Pharmacology, College of Medicine, University of Utah, Salt Lake City, Utah 84112*

The terms *cholinomimetic* (*cholinergic*) and *parasympathomimetic* are not equivalent, but they are popularly treated as synonyms. It will be recalled (see General Statement on *Autonomic Nervous System and Autonomic Drugs*, page 880) that acetylcholine is liberated not only at parasympathetic *post*ganglionic nerve endings but also at all autonomic *pre*ganglionic nerve endings, at somatic motor nerve endings, and probably at certain central synapses. Thus, a cholinomimetic can be a ganglionic or neuromuscular stimulant (ie, can be nicotinic—see *Nicotine*, page 902), possibly even a centrally acting drug, with or without also being a parasympathomimetic. A parasympathomimetic drug is literally an agent whose cholinomimetic action is limited to the parasympathetic neuroeffectors (ie, it is muscarinic—see *Muscarine*, page 902). Most muscarinic substances also possess varying degrees of action on autonomic ganglia and neuromuscular junctions (ie, nicotinic actions). Even methacholine, which is generally held to be strictly muscarinic, exerts nicotinic actions on the neuromuscular junction in myasthenia gravis or on the

adrenal medulla in pheochromocytoma. There are muscarinic receptors in autonomic ganglia. Their normal function is elusive and complex. There are sympathetic cholinergic neuroeffectors that are indistinguishable in receptor type from those of the parasympathetic system, so that every parasympathomimetic also is a mimetic of sympathetic cholinergic activity.

Acetylcholine is hydrolyzed to choline and acetic acid by the enzyme *acetylcholinesterase* at or near the site of liberation of the neurohumor. Similar specific and nonspecific esterases are also present in plasma, erythrocytes, and other tissues. Drugs that inhibit these enzymes prolong the life of acetylcholine at the cholinergic neuroeffectors and synapses and thereby facilitate the normal transmission of cholinergic nervous impulses. Although this action of anticholinesterases is one of support rather than mimicry of acetylcholine, the anticholinesterases are generally loosely classified as cholinomimetics. They are therefore included in this chapter also. The section on *Anticholinesterases* can be found on page 902.

Cholinomimetics

Acetylcholine, the natural cholinomimetic, is too rapidly destroyed by cholinesterases in the blood to be of much clinical value. Clinically useful parasympathomimetics are only slowly or not at all hydrolyzed by these enzymes. Changes in chemical structure may alter the proportion of truly parasympathomimetic (muscarinic) actions to ganglionic or neuromuscular (nicotinic) actions. Most of the cholinomimetics are quaternary ammonium compounds structurally related to acetylcholine salts, shown below:

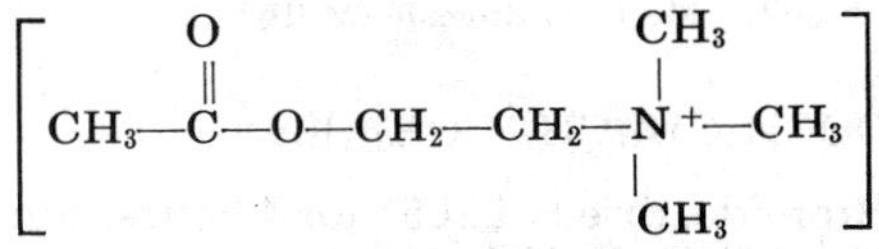

$$\left[CH_3-\overset{\overset{O}{\|}}{C}-O-CH_2-CH_2-\overset{\overset{CH_3}{|}}{\underset{\underset{CH_3}{|}}{N^+}}-CH_3 \right] A^- \quad (A^- = anion)$$

The muscarinic (parasympathomimetic) actions can be blocked by atropine and its congeners, which serve as antidotes to overdosage, and the ganglionic and neuromuscular (nicotinic) stimulant actions can be respectively antagonized by ganglionic blocking and neuromuscular blocking agents.

Bethanechol Chloride USP

[Carbamylmethylcholine Chloride; (2-Hydroxypropyl)trimethylammonium Chloride Carbamate; Myocholine (*Glenwood*); Urecholine Chloride (*MSD*)]

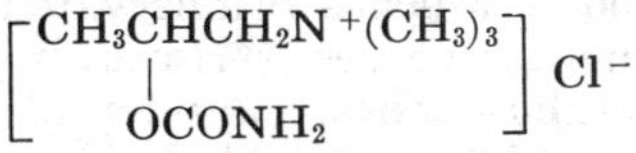

$$\left[\begin{matrix} CH_3CHCH_2N^+(CH_3)_3 \\ | \\ OCONH_2 \end{matrix} \right] Cl^-$$

Bethanechol Chloride contains 98.0–101.5% of $C_7H_{17}ClN_2O_2$ (196.68), calculated on the dried basis.

Preparation—It may be prepared by treating propylene chlorohydrin with phosgene, reacting the condensation product (2-chloro-1-methylethyl chloroformate) with ammonia in ether solution, and heating the resulting urethan with trimethylamine.

Description—Colorless or white crystals or a white crystalline powder, usually having a slight, amine-like odor. It is slightly hygroscopic. Its 1% solution has a pH between 5.5 and 6.5. Exhibits polymorphism; one form melts at about 211° and the other at about 219°.

Solubility—1 Gm dissolves in 1 ml of water, and in 10 ml of alcohol; less soluble in dehydrated alcohol; insoluble in chloroform and in ether.

Uses—The pharmacological properties of Bethanechol Chloride are similar to those of acetylcholine. Since it is not hydrolyzed by the enzyme cholinesterase, it has a relatively prolonged *parasympathomimetic* effect. Its actions are primarily muscarinic (on smooth muscle and exocrine glands) rather than nicotinic (on skeletal muscle and autonomic ganglia). The effects of the drug are readily blocked by atropine. The gastrointestinal tract and urinary bladder are stimulated by doses which produce few cardiovascular effects. Thus it does not share the usefulness of methacholine in paroxysmal atrial tachycardia. However, it is of particular value in *functional urinary retention*, postoperative and postpartum *intestinal ileus*, and in the treatment of *postvagotomy gastric atony*. Limited clinical trial also indicates that topical therapy with bethanechol is of value as a *miotic* and is serviceable in chronic noncongestive *glaucoma*.

Bethanechol is supplied for subcutaneous administration and also for oral administration. The drug should not be administered by the intravenous or intramuscular route. It is applied topically to the conjunctival sac in 1% solution.

Dose—*Oral*, **30** to **120 mg** daily; *usual, oral*, **10** to **30 mg** 3 times a day; *subcutaneous*, **2.5** to **30 mg** daily; *usual, subcutaneous*, **2.5 mg** 3 times a day.

Dosage Forms—Injection USP: 5 mg/ml; Tablets USP: 5, 10, and 25 mg.

Carbachol USP

[Carbamoylcholine Chloride; Choline Chloride Carbamate; Lentin; Carbamiotin (*Crookes-Barnes*); Carcholin (*MSD*); Isopto-Carbachol (*Alcon*)];

$$[NH_2COO.CH_2CH_2.N^+(CH_3)_3]Cl^-$$

Carbachol contains 99.0–101.0% of $C_6H_{15}ClN_2O_2$ (182.65), calculated on the dried basis.

Preparation—Ethylene chlorohydrin is treated with phosgene. The resulting chloroethyl chloroformate upon treatment with ammonia is converted into chloroethyl urethan, which yields Carbachol when reacted with aqueous trimethylamine.

Description—White or faintly yellow crystals or a crystalline powder. Odorless or has a slight, amine-like odor and is hygroscopic. Its solutions are neutral to litmus. It melts between 201° and 205°.

Solubility—1 Gm dissolves in about 1 ml of water and 50 ml of alcohol; practically insoluble in chloroform and ether.

Uses—Carbachol shares with acetylcholine the property of stimulating those smooth muscle and gland cells of the body which are innervated by *cholinergic* (parasympathetic) nerves. However, Carbachol is much more stable, shows considerable selectivity of action, and stimulates particularly the urinary bladder and intestinal tract. It has been employed in *urinary retention, intestinal paresis,* and *peripheral vascular disease,* and topically in *ozena* and *glaucoma*. See *Methacholine Chloride*. It is applied topically to the eye or nasal mucosa.

Dose—*External use, topically,* **0.1 ml** of a **0.75** to 3% solution instilled into the conjunctival sac, 2 or 3 times a day.

Other Dose Information—*Oral*, 0.2 to 0.8 mg 3 times a day; *subcutaneous*, 0.2 to 0.4 mg.

Caution!—Carbachol must not be dispensed in more than ¼ mg dose for glaucoma.

Dosage Forms—Ophthalmic Solution USP: 0.75, 1.5, 2.25, and 3%.

Veterinary Dose—*Horses, Cattle,* and *Swine,* **2** to **4 mg**; *Sheep* and *Goats* (Caution) **0.1** to **0.2 mg**; *Colts,* **0.5** to **1 mg**; *Foals,* **0.25** to **0.5 mg**; *Calves,* **0.5** to **2 mg**; *Dogs,* **0.05** to **0.4 mg**; *Cats,* **0.05** to **0.1 mg.** Administered *subcutaneously*.

Edrophonium Chloride USP

[Ethyl(*m*-hydroxyphenyl)dimethylammonium Chloride; Tensilon Chloride (*Roche*)]

Edrophonium Chloride contains 98.0–100.5% of $C_{10}H_{16}ClNO$ (201.70), calculated on the dried basis.

Preparation—The commercially available *m*-dimethylaminophenol is dissolved in a suitable organic solvent and quaternized with ethyl iodide. The dimethylethyl(3-hydroxyphenyl)ammonium iodide precipitates and is collected and washed. It may then be converted to the chloride in various ways, one of which involves treatment with moist silver oxide to form the quaternary base followed by neutralization with hydrochloric acid.

Description—White, odorless crystalline powder. Its 1 in 10 solution is practically colorless and has a pH of 4.0–5.0. It melts between 167° and 170°.

Solubility—1 Gm dissolves in about 0.5 ml of water and about 5 ml of alcohol; insoluble in chloroform and ether.

Uses—Edrophonium Chloride is a cholinomimetic drug with prominent neuromuscular actions and weak ganglionic and cholinergic neuroeffector stimulant actions. It also moderately inhibits cholinesterase at the neuromuscular junction, so that its neuromuscular actions are both direct and indirect. It is used to *abolish neuromuscular paralysis due to d-tubocurarine* or similarly acting motor endplate stabilizing drugs, with which edrophonium apparently competes for the receptor, or as a *diagnostic agent for myasthenia gravis,* and occasionally as an agent to treat *myasthenic crises.* Transient blurring of vision, lacrimation, perspiration and dizziness may accompany its use. It causes muscle fasciculations in the normal human.

Dose—*Intravenous*, **5** to **40 mg** in one episode; *usual*, **10 mg**, repeated in 5 to 10 minutes if necessary.

Other Dose Information—The above official dose is used to antagonize curare overdosage or as a diagnostic agent; 5 mg to terminate mild curarization. It is administered by continuous intravenous drip in myasthenic crises.

Dosage Forms—Injection USP: 10 mg/ml, 100 mg/10 ml.

Methacholine Bromide NF

[Acetyl-β-methylcholine Bromide; (2-Hydroxypropyl)trimethylammonium Bromide Acetate; Mecholyl Bromide (*MSD*)]

$$[CH_3COOCH(CH_3)CH_2\overset{+}{N}(CH_3)_3]Br^-$$

Methacholine Bromide, dried at 105° for 4 hours, contains 98.0–102.0% of $C_8H_{18}BrNO_2$ (240.14).

Preparation—Aqueous trimethylamine is reacted with propylene oxide [$CH_3—CH—O—CH_2$] to yield 2-(hydroxypropyl)trimethylammonium hydroxide. After neutralization with hydrobromic acid, the reaction mixture is dried and the residue of 2-(hydroxypropyl)-

trimethylammonium bromide is esterified by treatment with acetic anhydride.

Description—It occurs as a white, crystalline powder, possessing a slight amine-like odor. It is very hygroscopic. The pH of a freshly prepared solution (1 in 20) is about 5. Melting range 147° to 150°.

Solubility—Freely soluble in water and alcohol; practically insoluble in benzene and ether.

Uses—Methacholine Bromide has the same actions and uses as the chloride (see *Methacholine Chloride*, below). Because the bromide is the less hygroscopic, it is the more suitable for oral preparations.

Dose—**200** to **600 mg;** *usual*, **200 mg** 2 or 3 times a day.

Other Dose Information—If a total daily dose of more than 2 Gm is required, the chloride should be used to avoid bromism.

Dosage Forms—Tablets NF: 200 mg.

Methacholine Chloride NF

[(2-Hydroxypropyl)trimethylammonium chloride Acetate; Mecholyl Chloride (*MSD*)]

$$[CH_3COOCH(CH_3)CH_2\overset{+}{N}(CH_3)_3]Cl^-$$

Methacholine Chloride, dried at 105° for 4 hours, contains 98.0–102.0% of $C_8H_{18}ClNO_2$ (195.69).

Preparation—This choline derivative may be prepared from propylene chlorohydrin (or propylene oxide + HCl), trimethylamine and acetic anhydride by the steps shown in the following scheme:

$$CH_2ClCHOHCH_3 \xrightarrow{\ N(CH_3)_3\ }$$

$$[HOCH(CH_3)CH_2\overset{+}{N}(CH_3)_3]Cl^- \xrightarrow{\ (CH_3CO)_2O\ }$$

$$[CH_3COOCH(CH_3)CH_2\overset{+}{N}(CH_3)_3]Cl^-$$

Description—Colorless or white crystals, or a white, crystalline powder. It is odorless or has a slight odor, and is very deliquescent. Its solutions are neutral to litmus. It melts between 170° and 173°. It is hydrolyzed by alkali hydroxide solutions with the splitting off of the acetyl group and chloride; it is similarly but slowly affected by water.

Solubility—Very soluble in water; freely soluble in alcohol and chloroform.

Uses—Methacholine Chloride resembles acetylcholine in its actions in the body in that it stimulates those organs innervated by parasympathetic (cholinergic) nerves. It is much more stable than acetylcholine and hence lends itself better to therapeutic application. It is more muscarinic than nicotinic in its actions. Its actions on the cardiovascular system are more prominent than those on the gastrointestinal and genitourinary systems. It is employed in certain disorders of cardiac rhythm (especially *paroxysmal tachycardia*), in peripheral vascular diseases (*Raynaud's disease, thromboangiitis obliterans*), in *intestinal ileus*, in *atonic constipation*, in *megacolon*, in *urinary retention*, etc. It is also used locally by iontophoresis in certain *arthritides*. It may also be used in the treatment of *myasthenia gravis* and as a diagnostic agent in *pheochromocytoma*. Atropine is a complete pharmacological antagonist to methacholine.

Dose—*Subcutaneous*, **10** to **40 mg;** *usual, initial*, **10 mg;** then may give **25 mg** 10 to 30 minutes later.

Other Dose Information—*Usual, oral*, 50 to 100 mg; for *iontophoresis*, 0.25 to 1% aqueous solution.

Dosage Forms—Sterile NF: 25 mg.

Pilocarpine Hydrochloride USP

[Pilocarpine Monohydrochloride; Almocarpine (*Ayerst*); Isopto-Carpine (*Alcon*); Pilocar (*Smith, Miller & Patch*)]

Pilocarpine Hydrochloride contains 98.5–100.5% of $C_{11}H_{16}N_2O_2.HCl$ (244.72), calculated on the dried basis.

Preparation—It is prepared as described under *Pilocarpine Nitrate*, except that hydrochloric acid is used in place of the nitric acid.

Description—Colorless, translucent, odorless, faintly bitter crystals. It is hygroscopic and is affected by light. Its solutions are acid to litmus. It melts between 200° and 203°, and has a specific rotation of +88.5° to +91.0°.

Solubility—1 Gm dissolves in 0.3 ml of water, about 3 ml of alcohol, or about 360 ml of chloroform; also in 1.5 ml of alcohol at 60°; insoluble in ether.

Incompatibilities—See *Alkaloids* (page 491). Since the free alkaloid is quite soluble in water, *alkalies* do not readily cause a precipitation when added to solutions of its salts. It reduces *silver nitrate*. *Permanganate* destroys it.

Uses—Pilocarpine acts in the body to stimulate all smooth muscles and gland cells innervated by parasympathetic (cholinergic) nerves, and thus shares many of the properties of acetylcholine and muscarine. Clinically, however, its uses are largely limited to its actions *on the eye to cause miosis, on the salivary glands to cause secretion,* and *on the sweat glands to cause profuse diaphoresis.* It is also occasionally employed to overcome some of the antimuscarinic side effects of other drugs, especially those used in the treatment of Parkinsonism. The applications of pilocarpine in therapy are thus few, and the drug is not indispensable.

It is employed as an ophthalmic solution or ointment or in lamellæ. Atropine is a complete antagonist. The uses are the same for the nitrate, which because of a lesser hygroscopicity it is more convenient to handle.

Dose—*External use, topically,* **0.1 ml** of a **0.5** to **6%** solution to the conjunctiva 1 to 6 times a day.

Other Dose Information—*Oral*, 5 to 20 mg.

Dosage Forms—Ophthalmic Solution USP: 0.25, 0.5, 1, 2, 3, 4, 5, 6, 7, 8, and 10%.

Veterinary Uses—This drug is applied topically to the conjunctiva and administered parenterally for its cholinomimetic effects on the gastrointestinal tract and salivary glands.

Veterinary Dose—*Subcutaneous, Horses,* **100** to **200 mg;** *Cattle,* **200 to 400 mg** (*ruminatoric,* **50 to 60 mg**); *Swine,* **2 to 50 mg;** *Dogs,* **5 to 20 mg;** *Cats,* **1 to 3 mg.**

Pilocarpine Nitrate USP

[Pilocarpine Mononitrate; P.V. Carpine (*Allergan*)]

Pilocarpine Nitrate contains 98.5–100.5% of $C_{11}H_{16}N_2O_2.HNO_3$ (271.28), calculated on the dried basis.

Preparation—The total alkaloids are extracted from the dried crushed leaves of *Pilocarpus microphyllus*, or other suitable *Pilocarpus* species, with alcohol containing a small amount of hydrochloric acid. The solvent is distilled off, the aqueous residue neutralized with ammonia, and allowed to stand until the resins are all deposited. It is then filtered, and the filtrate evaporated to a small bulk. Ammonia is added in excess and the free alkaloids extracted with chloroform. After removing the solvent by distillation, the residue is dissolved in a small quantity of dilute nitric acid and allowed to crystallize.

Description—Shining, white crystals. It is stable in air but is affected by light. Its solutions are acid to litmus. Melts between 170° and 175° and has a specific rotation of +79.5° to +82.0°.

Solubility—1 Gm dissolves in 4 ml of water and 75 ml of alcohol; insoluble in chloroform and ether.

Incompatibilities—See *Pilocarpine Hydrochloride.*

Uses and Dose—See *Pilocarpine Hydrochloride.*

Dosage Forms—Ophthalmic Solution USP: 0.5, 1, 2, 3, 4, and 6%.

Other Cholinomimetics

Acetylcholine (ion)—The chemical transmitter at parasympathetic postganglionic, some sympathetic postganglionic, all autonomic preganglionic and somatic motor nerve endings. Acetylcholine is the natural prototype with which cholinomimetics are compared. It dilates nearly all blood vessels, but may constrict certain veins. It lowers the blood pressure and slows and decreases the strength of the heart and may induce heart block. However, the direct cardiac actions are manifested only at relatively high doses, and the usual cardiac effect is reflex acceleration consequent to the hypotension. Gastrointestinal smooth muscle is stimulated, but genitourinary smooth muscle is stimulated or depressed, depending upon its location. It is only weakly miotic, owing to poor absorption. It stimulates gastric secretion, salivation, sweating, and other exocrine discharges as well as those of the pancreatic islets. In addition to the above-listed muscarinic actions (see *Muscarine*), acetylcholine possesses stimulant actions on postganglionic neurons and the neuromuscular junction (Nicotinic Actions) (see *Nicotine*). Owing to rapid destruction by blood and tissue cholinesterases, its duration of action is too brief to be of clinical use.

Areca NF XII [Areca Nut; Betel Nut; Areca Seed] is the dried ripe seed of *Areca catechu* Linné (Fam. *Palmae*). It contains not less than 0.35% of ether-soluble alkaloids calculated as arecoline. *History:* Areca, a tall palm tree of southeast Asia, bears fruits which contain the seeds or betel nuts of commerce. These "nuts" are chewed by the natives and impart a red color to the saliva, teeth, and feces. *Uses:* Not employed on man. See *Arecoline Hydrobromide* (below) for its actions. *Veterinary Uses:* A *vermifuge;* expulsion is accomplished by the drug's marked stimulation of peristalsis. *Veterinary Doses:* Proportional to the weight of the animals. *Horses* and *Cattle,* 100 to 250 Gm; *Foals,* 10 to 63 Gm; *Sheep,* 4 to 8 Gm; *Swine* and *Calves,* 4 to 15 Gm; *Dogs,* 2 to 4 Gm; *Cats,* 0.5 to 1 Gm.

Arecoline Hydrobromide NF XII [Methyl 1,2,5,6-Tetrahydro-1-methylnicotinate Hydrobromide; $C_8H_{13}NO_2.HBr$ (236.12)] is the hydrobromide of an alkaloid obtained from the dried ripe seed of *Areca catechu* Linné (Fam. *Palmae*), or produced synthetically. *Preparation:* Although it may be prepared from finely ground areca (13th ed., page 977), a simple synthesis involves the reduction of the methiodide of methyl nicotinate with potassium borohydride; the arecoline is then treated with alcoholic hydro-

gen bromide and crystallized. *Description and Solubility:* White, crystalline powder, or white crystals; odorless and bitter-tasting; affected by light; melts between 170° and 175°. 1 Gm dissolves in about 1 ml of water and about 10 ml of alcohol; slightly soluble in ether or chloroform. *Uses:* Not employed in human therapy. It exerts a direct cholinomimetic action on smooth muscle and exocrine glands. It also stimulates autonomic ganglia and skeletal muscle. *Veterinary Uses:* A *cathartic* for horses, injected hypodermically, when rapid action is essential. It may be used as a *ruminatoric* in cattle, but the dose must be very carefully regulated. *Veterinary Dose: Cathartic, subcutaneous,* in *Horses,* 4 to 30 mg; *ruminatoric, subcutaneous,* in *Cattle,* 4 to 8 mg; *teniafuge, oral, Dogs,* 1 to 15 mg; *Cats,* 1 to 2 mg.

Muscarine—This contains the quaternary ammonium ion, trimethyl(tetrahydro-4-hydroxy-5-methylfurfuryl)ammonium $[(CH_3)_3\overset{+}{N}CH_2CHCH_2CH(OH)CH(CH_3)O]$. It exists as salts, eg, muscarine chloride, $[C_9H_{20}\overset{+}{N}O_2]\overset{-}{C}l$. *Uses:* Muscarine was studied long before acetylcholine and other parasympathomimetics were discovered. Like acetylcholine it acts on smooth muscle, heart and exocrine glands, but it does not ordinarily stimulate postganglionic neurons of the neuromuscular junction. Hence upon systemic administration it somewhat more faithfully simulates parasympathetic stimulation than does the real parasympathetic neurohumor, acetylcholine. Because of this and because of its temporal priority, muscarine has been a time-honored prototype of parasympathomimetics, and the neuroeffector actions of parasympathomimetics are designated as *muscarinic* actions. These actions are readily blocked by atropine. Muscarine has no clinical uses, but it has clinical significance in that, in the form of a quaternary salt, it is the toxic agent in the red variety of the deadly mushroom *Amanita muscaris.*

Nicotine, 1-Methyl-2-(3-pyridyl)pyrrolidine [CH₃NCH-(C₅H₄N)CH₂CH₂CH₂]—From *Nicotiana Tabacum.* A poisonous, oily liquid. It has an unpleasant tobacco-like odor, a burning taste, and a strongly alkaline reaction.

Nicotine is the prototype of cholinomimetics of the so-called nicotinic type. The action of nicotine in the body is characterized by a primary transient stimulation followed by a persistent depression of all sympathetic and parasympathetic ganglia. The actions are explained by a common mechanism, namely, that of depolarization of the postsynaptic membrane. During the onset of depolarization, nerve action potentials are generated. Once the postsynaptic membrane becomes fully depolarized, further action potentials cannot be initiated, since they require a polarized postsynaptic membrane at their outset. Thus a block of synaptic transmission results from the persisting depolarization induced by nicotine. Even after the membrane is restored, the block may persist. The synaptic stimulatory and depressant effects of nicotine cannot be overcome by atropine.

Nicotine likewise stimulates then paralyzes skeletal muscles and thus induces a curariform action, which is the major reason for the toxic effect of the alkaloid on respiration. However, nicotine is more active on ganglia than on skeletal muscles, whereas the reverse is true of curare. In addition to the above well established actions, nicotine also first stimulates then paralyzes the central nervous system. There is also evidence that the alkaloid possesses activity as a vasoconstrictor and that it increases intestinal motility.

Anticholinesterases

The anticholinesterases increase activity at cholinergic loci. Both parasympathetic and sympathetic postganglionic nervous activity is increased by facilitation at the ganglia, and some sympathetic components of action may be apparent with certain anticholinesterases; but, since the anticholinesterases also increase

cholinergic neuroeffector transmission, thus allowing for facilitation twice in the parasympathetic pathway, the predominant autonomic effects are heightened parasympathetic and sympathetic cholinergic activity. Thus, miosis, sweating, salivation, increased bowel activity, urination, and bradycardia may occur, although the several agents vary widely in their actions on the numerous structures. The blood pressure may rise or fall. Since neuromuscular facilitation also occurs, heightened muscular tone results, and with excessive doses muscular fasciculations and fibrillation occur. Certain anticholinesterases, particularly the organophosphates* and physostigmine, may exert central actions with components of both stimulation and depression; the quaternary ammonium agents do not readily penetrate the blood–brain barrier and hence do not exert prominent central actions. The quaternary ammonium agents also have varying degrees of direct cholinomimetic actions, especially at the neuromuscular junctions.

The amine and quaternary ammonium anticholinesterases combine reversibly with the enzymes and consequently have a limited duration of action which may last from a few minutes to a few hours. Because of the possible central actions, lability, and cost of physostigmine, only the quaternaries are in regular use, except for the ophthalmological use of physostigmine. The organophosphate anticholinesterases combine quite firmly with the enzymes; the dialkyl moiety combines with the esteratic site with the formation of a stable coordinate covalent bond. Consequently, the organophosphate anticholinesterases have durations of action from days to months. Some are extremely potent, and since they are absorbed even through the skin, they are dangerous. They are mainly employed as insecticides and some have been studied for possible use as war gases; the only clinical use of any of these agents is the topical ophthalmological use of isoflurophate or echothiophate, except for the sporadic use of certain of these agents in the therapy of myasthenia gravis. But the pharmacist should be alert to the several organophosphate insecticides that are sold in pharmacies. (See page 1287). Although the pharmacist may not dispense any, or only a few, of the organophosphate insecticides, he may receive emergency queries from physicians about the content and actions of insecticides; consequently, a number of nontherapeutic anticholinesterases are listed on pages 1287 and 1288) in Chapter 69 on *Pesticides*.

Formerly, the only antidote was heavy medication with atropine (6 to 40 mg, *initially*, and 1 to 2 mg every 1 to 2 hours), but now several oximes are in use as antagonists of the organophosphates.

Ambenonium Chloride NF

[Oxalylbis(iminoethylene)]-bis(o-chlorobenzyl)diethylammonium Dichloride]; Mysuran; Mytelase (*Winthrop*)]

Ambenonium Chloride is anhydrous or may occur as the tetrahydrate. It contains 97.0–103.0% of $C_{28}H_{42}Cl_4N_4O_2$ (608.48), calculated on the dried basis.

* The term *organophosphate* is commonly used with no specific structural connotation to refer to any organic compound which contains phosphorus and which displays anticholinesterase activity.

Preparation—N,N-Diethylethylenediamine is reacted with ethyl oxalate to give N,N'-bis[2-(diethylamino)ethyl]oxamide which is then doubly quaternized with 2-chlorobenzyl chloride. US Pat. 3,096,373.

Description—Crystals, melting at 184°.
Solubility—Freely soluble in water.

Uses—Ambenonium Chloride is a quaternary ammonium *anticholinesterase* drug with actions similar to those of *Neostigmine* (see page 904), but Ambenonium is 2 to 4 times more potent and its duration of action is somewhat longer. It is also claimed to have a lower incidence of side effects than Neostigmine, particularly of the gastrointestinal tract. It is used in the treatment of *myasthenia gravis*. Side effects include excessive salivation, miosis, urinary urgency, sweating, diarrhea, vomiting and abdominal cramps. Atropine will antagonize the side effects without affecting the neuromuscular actions.

Dose—5 to **50 mg**; *usual, initial,* **5 mg,** gradually increased as required up to **5 to 25 mg** 3 or 4 times a day.
Dosage Forms—Tablets NF: 10 and 25 mg.

Demecarium Bromide USP

[(m-Hydroxyphenyl)trimethylammonium Bromide Decamethylenebis-[methylcarbamate]; Tosmilen; Humorsol (*MSD*)]

Demecarium Bromide contains 95.0–102.0% of $C_{32}H_{52}Br_2N_4O_4$ (716.61), calculated on the dried basis.

Preparation—N,N' - Dimethyl - 1,10 - decamethylenediamine is added to molten 3-(dimethylamino)-phenyl carbonate to produce 1,10-decamethylenebis[3-(dimethylamino)phenyl N-methylcarbamate]. After purification this ester, which is a viscous oil, is dissolved in ethanol and doubly quaternized with the aid of an acetone solution of methyl bromide. US Pat. 2,789,981.

Description—A white, slightly hygroscopic powder which decomposes between 162° and 167°. Aqueous solutions are neutral.

Solubility—Freely soluble in water and in alcohol; sparingly soluble in acetone; insoluble in ether.

Uses—Demecarium Bromide is a quaternary ammonium *anticholinesterase* drug which has a high topical penetrability into the eye. In the eye it induces contraction of the ciliary body and miosis. Its ocular actions may last for a week. It is used in the treatment of *wide angle glaucoma* and *accommodative convergent strabismus*. Untoward effects include myopia, photophobia, blurred vision, browache, blepharospasm, conjunctival and intraocular injection, iridocyclitis, pigment cysts of the iris, rarely retinal detachment, and occasional contact dermatitis. A transient but dangerous rise in intraocular pressure may occur shortly after administration. Systemically absorbed drug can be cumulative and give rise to salivation, nausea, vomiting, diarrhea, abdominal cramps, and dyspnea; convulsions are possible. Atropine will successfully antagonize these effects, but it will also suppress the ocular actions.

Dose—*Topically,* **0.03** to **0.06** ml of a **0.125** to **0.25**% solution twice a week to 1 or 2 times a day, to the conjunctiva.

Dosage Forms—Ophthalmic Solution USP: 0.125 and 0.25%.

Echothiophate Iodide USP

[(2-Mercaptoethyl)trimethylammonium Iodide *S*-Ester with *O,O*-Diethyl Phosphorothioate;   Phospholine Iodide (*Ayerst*)]

$$\left[(CH_3)_3\overset{+}{N} - CH_2CH_2 - S - \overset{\displaystyle O}{\underset{\displaystyle OC_2H_5}{\overset{\uparrow}{P}}} \begin{array}{c} OC_2H_5 \\ \end{array} \right] I^-$$

Echothiophate Iodide contains 88.0–100.5% of $C_9H_{23}INO_3PS$ (383.23).

Preparation—β-(Dimethylamino)ethanol, in benzene solution, is reacted with sodium and the resulting sodium alkoxide is condensed with *O,O*-diethyl phosphorochloridothioate [ClP(S)(OC₂H₅)₂] to yield crude *S*-[2-(dimethylamino)ethyl] *O,O*-diethyl phosphorothioate. This ester, after purification by vacuum distillation, is dissolved in an inert solvent and quaternized with methyl iodide.   US Pat. 2,911,430.

Description—White, crystalline, hygroscopic solid having a slight mercaptan-like odor. Its solutions have a pH of about 4.

Solubility—1 Gm dissolves in about 1 ml of water, about 3 ml of methanol, and about 25 ml of dehydrated alcohol; practically insoluble in other organic solvents.

Uses—Echothiophate is an *anticholinesterase* drug that is both a quaternary ammonium and organosphosphate compound.   Like *Isoflurophate* (see below), it has a long duration of action.   Applied topically to the eye it cau~~ses~~ intense miosis and contraction of the ciliary ~~muscle. T~~he effects begin in 10 to 45 minutes and last for ~~several~~ weeks.   It is used for the treatment of *wide-angle* ~~gl~~aucoma.   Side effects include ocular pain from ciliary spasm, browache, blepharospasm, conjunctival and intraocular injection, fibrinous iritis, iridocyclitis, and pigment cysts of the iris.   Systemic absorption may give rise to an accumulative action resulting in salivation, nausea, vomiting, diarrhea, and abdominal cramps; atropine will control these effects, but it will also suppress the ocular actions.   Echothiophate does not penetrate into the central nervous system.

Dose—*External use, topically,* **0.1** ml of a **0.06** to **0.125**% solution to the conjunctiva, 1 or 2 times a day.

Other Dose Information—Solutions are not marketed and must be made from commercial powder by dissolution into isotonic sodium chloride solution containing 0.5% chlorobutanol; solutions are stable for over a year at 4°C and for over a month at room temperature.

Dosage Forms—for Ophthalmic Solution USP: 3, 6.25, 12.5, and 125 mg.

Edrophonium Chloride—see page 900.

Isoflurophate

[Isopropyl Phosphorofluoridate;   Isopropyl Fluophosphate;   Diisopropyl Fluorophosphate;   DFP;   Floropryl (*MSD*)]

$$(CH_3)_2CHO - \overset{\displaystyle F}{\underset{\displaystyle O}{\overset{|}{\underset{\|}{P}}}} - OCH(CH_3)_2$$

Isoflurophate is $C_6H_{14}FO_3P$ (184.15).

Preparation—Isoflurophate may be prepared by various processes.   A well known one involves the following steps:

1.   Interaction of isopropyl alcohol and phosphorus trichloride to produce diisopropyl phosphite:

$$3(CH_3)_2CHOH + PCl_3 \rightarrow [(CH_3)_2CHO]_2POH + \\ KCl + HCl;$$

2.   Oxidation of the phosphite by means of chlorine to produce diisopropyl phosphorochloridate:

$$[(CH_3)_2CHO]_2POH + Cl_2 \rightarrow [(CH_3)_2CHO]_2PO(Cl) + HCl;$$

3.   Metathesis of the phosphorochloridate with sodium fluoride:

$$[(CH_3)_2CHO]_2PO(Cl) + NaF \rightarrow \\ [(CH_3)_2CHO]_2PO(F) + NaCl.$$

Description—A clear, colorless or faintly yellow liquid. It boils at 183°, and has a specific gravity of about 1.05. Its vapor is extremely irritating to the eye and mucous membranes.   In the presence of moisture, it decomposes with formation of hydrogen fluoride and loss of its anticholinergic activity.

Solubility—Sparingly soluble in water;   soluble in alcohol and vegetable oils.

Uses—Isoflurophate is an *organic phosphate* ("*organophosphate*") *anticholinesterase* (see page 902) for ophthalmic use.   It is applied topically as a 0.01 to 0.1% solution or as a 0.025% ophthalmic ointment 1 to 3 times a day.

Isoflurophate is the most potent and the most persistent *miotic* known.   It is of value in the symptomatic treatment of *glaucoma*.   One drop of Isoflurophate Ophthalmic Solution instilled in the conjunctival sac at intervals of one day to one week usually produces satisfactory reduction in intraocular tension.

Caution—When handling Isoflurophate in open containers, protect the eyes, nose, and mouth with a suitable mask, and avoid contact with the skin.

Dose—*External use, topically,* to *conjunctiva, ointment,* apply once every 3 days 3 times a day; *solution,* **1** to **3 drops** 3 times a day to once every 3 days.

Dosage Forms—Ophthalmic Ointment NF: 0.025%;   Ophthalmic Solution USP: 0.1%.

Neostigmine Bromide USP

[(*m*-Hydroxyphenyl)trimethylammonium Bromide Dimethylcarbamate;   Prostigmin Bromide (*Roche*)]

$$\left[\begin{array}{c} \overset{\displaystyle N^+(CH_3)_3}{\bigcirc} \\ O - C - N(CH_3)_2 \\ \| \\ O \end{array} \right] Br^-$$

Neostigmine Bromide contains 98.0–102.0% of $C_{12}H_{19}BrN_2O_2$ (303.21), calculated on the dried basis.

Preparation—It may be prepared by reacting dimethylcarbamoylchloride [(CH₃)₂NCOCl] with potassium *m*-(dimethylamino)phenolate, then quaternizing with methyl bromide.

Description—A white, crystalline powder.   It is odorless, and has a bitter taste.   Its solutions are neutral to litmus.   It melts with decomposition at about 167°.

Solubility—1 Gm dissolves in about 0.5 ml of water; soluble in alcohol;   practically insoluble in ether.

Uses—Neostigmine is a quaternary ammonium anticholinesterase (see *Anticholinesterases,* page 902). It acts at the esteratic site of the enzyme to form the inactive dimethylcarbamoyl enzyme. Neostigmine has widespread actions, but fortunately its effects are more prominent on certain structures than on others, being particularly useful on the bowel, urinary bladder, and skeletal muscle, and not affecting to any significant degree the pupil, the heart, blood pressure, secretions, etc., in doses that are ordinarily effective on the structures listed above.

Neostigmine is used in conditions of *urinary bladder atony* due to postanesthetic depression or to neurological disorders; in the prevention and treatment of post-anesthetic *intestinal paresis;* and in the symptomatic therapy of *myasthenia gravis.* In the latter disorder Neostigmine is almost specific, and can be employed as a diagnostic test, especially after symptoms have been purposely accentuated by the administration of quinine. Neostigmine has also been used in *atrophic rhinitis,* in *ozena,* as a diagnostic test of early pregnancy, in *peripheral vascular diseases,* as an *antagonist to curare* and certain other curariform drugs, and as a *diagnostic test agent in myotonia congenita,* in which condition Neostigmine aggravates the symptoms.

Neostigmine is administered subcutaneously or intramuscularly as the methylsulfate salt and orally as the bromide salt. *It is not to be injected intravenously,* and should not be employed along with acetyl-β-methylcholine (Methacholine) or other choline esters. Solutions of the methylsulfate have also been used topically as a nasal spray.

Caution—Neostigmine is a very potent drug and must be administered with care. Atropine will antagonize completely the muscarine-like actions of Neostigmine.

Dose—15 to **375 mg** daily; *usual,* **15** to **30 mg** 3 to 6 times a day.

Dosage Forms—Tablets USP: 15 mg.

Neostigmine Methylsulfate USP

[(*m*-Hydroxyphenyl)trimethylammonium Methyl Sulfate Dimethylcarbamate; Prostigmin Methylsulfate (*Roche*)]

Neostigmine Methylsulfate contains 98.0–102.0% of $C_{13}H_{22}N_2O_6S$ (334.39), calculated on the dried basis.

Preparation—It is made by the method outlined under *Neostigmine Bromide,* using dimethyl sulfate in place of methyl bromide.

Description—A white, crystalline powder. It is odorless, and has a bitter taste. Its solutions are neutral to litmus. It melts between 142° and 145°.

Solubility—Very soluble in water; soluble in alcohol.

Uses—See *Neostigmine Bromide.*

Dose—*Intramuscular or subcutaneous,* **1** to **5 mg** daily; *usual,* **500 mcg** 4 to 8 times a day.

Dosage Forms—Injection USP: 250 and 500 mcg/ml, 5 and 10 mg/10 ml.

Physostigmine USP

[1,2,3,3a,8,8a-Hexahydro-1,3a,8-trimethylpyrrolo[2,3-*b*]indol-5-ol Methylcarbamate (Ester)]

Physostigmine is an alkaloid usually obtained from the dried ripe seed of *Physostigma venenosum* Balfour (Fam. *Leguminosæ*). It contains 97.0–102.0% of $C_{15}H_{21}N_3O_2$ (275.35), calculated on the dried basis.

Description—White, odorless, microcrystalline powder. Acquires a red tint when exposed to heat, light, air, or contact with traces of metals.

Solubility—Slightly soluble in water; very soluble in chloroform and dichloromethane; freely soluble in alcohol; soluble in benzene and fixed oils.

Uses—Physostigmine is the oldest of the anticholinesterases. It combines with the enzyme at the esteratic site to yield the inactive methylcarbamoyl enzyme. It shares with neostigmine marked stimulatory actions on the bowel, but causes more secretion of glands, more effect on blood pressure, more constriction of the pupil, and less action on skeletal muscle. Since it is a tertiary amine, it penetrates into the central nervous system and can exert central actions when given in overdoses. Its main use in medicine is locally in the eye, to reduce intraocular pressure in *glaucoma.* Lamellae may also be employed. In alternation with atropine, physostigmine is used to *break adhesions between the iris and lens.* The alkaloid is occasionally employed to bring a drug-dilated pupil back to normal size. It is also prescribed for *marginal corneal ulcers.* Occasionally, physostigmine is employed for *intestinal distention of paresis,* but prostigmine is preferred because of its fewer side effects. The same important precautions as outlined for neostigmine should be observed in the use of physostigmine.

Physostigmine is generally used as the salicylate or sulfate salt; the salicylate has the advantage of being less deliquescent than the sulfate. The addition of a few grains of boric acid to a solution of the salt is said to inhibit the formation of the red decomposition product which is produced by alkalies and which frequently occurs in solutions of physostigmine salts which have been dispensed upon prescriptions. A red or discolored solution should not be used.

Caution—The dose for internal administration (oral or by hypodermic injection) should not exceed 3.0 mg. Atropine is an effective antagonist to all the muscarine-like actions of physostigmine.

Dose—*External use, topically,* as a **0.25%** ointment to the conjunctiva 1 to 4 times a day.

Veterinary Uses—It is used as a miotic and to stimulate motility of the gastrointestinal tract. Its cathartic action in cattle often is painful. It is contraindicated in advanced pregnancy, immovable intestinal obstruction, cardiac or pulmonary diseases, and in aged or debilitated animals.

Veterinary Dose—*Subcutaneous,* with caution, *Horses,* **50** to **100 mg;** *Cattle,* **30** to **50 mg** (as ruminatoric) with maximum dose 200 mg; *Sheep* and *Swine,* **5** to **20 mg;** *Dogs,* **0.5** to **3 mg;** *Cats,* **0.25** to **0.5 mg.**

Physostigmine Salicylate USP

[Eserine Salicylate; Isopto-Eserine (*Alcon*)]

Physostigmine Salicylate contains 97.0–102.0% of $C_{15}H_{21}N_3O_2 \cdot C_7H_6O_3$ (413.48), calculated on the dried basis.

Preparation—Physostigmine is prepared by extracting powdered *Physostigma* seeds with hot alcohol. After distilling off the alcohol, the residue is mixed with sodium carbonate and extracted with ether, from which solution the physostigmine is removed by means of dilute sulfuric acid. The free alkaloid may be obtained by alkalinizing the acid solution. The salicylate may be made by adding 2 parts of physostigmine to a solution of 1 part of salicylic acid in 35 parts of boiling distilled water, and allowing the salt to crystallize on cooling.

Description—White or faintly yellow odorless powder or shining crystals. It acquires a red tint when exposed to light and air. Its specific rotation in aqueous solution is between −91° and −94°. A cold, saturated solution is neutral or acid to litmus.

Solubility—1 Gm dissolves in 75 ml of water, 16 ml of alcohol, 6 ml of chloroform, and about 250 ml of ether.

Incompatibilities—Aqueous solutions of Physostigmine Salicylate tend to develop a red color on standing; a pink solution does not necessarily indicate complete ineffectiveness but as the color deepens to red, the product rapidly loses its value. Boric acid retards the change but alkalies hasten decomposition. Alkali-free glass should be used. It is precipitated by the usual alkaloidal precipitants. See also page 491.

Uses—See *Physostigmine.*

Dose—*External use, topically,* **0.1 ml** of a **0.25** to **0.5%** solution instilled into the conjunctival sac 1 to 4 times a day.

Veterinary Dose—See *Physostigmine.*

Dosage Forms—Ophthalmic Solution: 0.25 and 0.5%.

Physostigmine Sulfate USP

[Physostigmine Sulfate (2:1)]

Physostigmine Sulfate contains 97.0–102.0% of $(C_{15}H_{21}N_3O_2)_2 \cdot H_2SO_4$ (648.78), calculated on the dried basis.

Description—White, odorless, microcrystalline powder. Is deliquescent in moist air and acquires a red tint when long exposed to heat, light, air, or contact with traces of metals.

Solubility—1 Gm dissolves in 4 ml of water, 0.4 ml of alcohol, and about 1200 ml of ether.

Uses—See *Physostigmine.*

Dose—*External use, topically,* **0.1 ml** of a **0.25** to **0.5%** solution instilled into the conjunctival sac 1 to 4 times a day.

Veterinary Dose—See *Physostigmine.*

Pyridostigmine Bromide USP

[3-Hydroxy-1-methylpyridinium Bromide Dimethylcarbamate; Mestinon *(Roche)*]

Pyridostigmine Bromide contains 98.5–100.5% of $C_9H_{13}BrN_2O_2$ (261.13), calculated on the dried basis.

Preparation—3-Pyridinol is condensed with dimethylcarbamoyl chloride in the presence of a suitable basic catalyst such as dimethylaniline, magnesium oxide, etc. The resulting ester, 3-pyridyl dimethyl-

carbamate, is isolated, dissolved in a suitable organic solvent, and quaternized with methyl bromide.

Description—White or practically white, crystalline powder, having an agreeable, characteristic odor. It is hygroscopic. It melts between 154° and 157°.

Solubility—Freely soluble in water, alcohol, and chloroform; slightly soluble in solvent hexane; practically insoluble in ether.

Uses—Pyridostigmine is a quaternary ammonium anticholinesterase which is approximately ¼ as potent as neostigmine at the neuromuscular junction and about ⅛ as potent on the bowel, genitourinary tract, and exocrine glands. Its onset of action by the oral route is about 30 minutes, which is more than twice that of neostigmine and is a disadvantage, but its duration of action is 2 to 6 times that of neostigmine and is an advantage. Because of its relative affinity for the neuromuscular junction, its principal use is in the treatment of *myasthenia gravis*, in which use it causes fewer side effects than neostigmine. It is also superior to neostigmine in that the patient may be carried through the night without the necessity of interrupting sleep for medication. However, in some patients it provides less control of muscular weakness than neostigmine.

Dose—**60 mg** to **1.5 Gm** daily; *usual*, **60** to **120 mg** 3 to 6 times a day.

Other Dose Information—Orally, 60 mg will serve as an initial trial dose, every 2 to 6 hours; however, the average daily dose is about 780 mg and daily doses as high as 6 Gm have been reported.

Dosage Forms—Syrup USP: 60 mg/5 ml; Tablets USP: 60 mg.

Other Anticholinesterases

Benzpyrinium Bromide NF XII [1-Benzyl-3-hydroxypyridinium Bromide Dimethylcarbamate], dried at 80° for 4 hours, contains not less than 98.5% of $C_{15}H_{17}BrN_2O_2$ (337.22). *Preparation:* Sodium 3-pyridinesulfonate is fused with potassium hydroxide and then treated with hydrochloric acid to yield 3-pyridinol. Condensation with dimethylcarbamoyl chloride in the presence of triethylamine produces pyridine 3-dimethylcarbamate, which is dissolved in benzene and quaternized with benzyl bromide. *Description and Solubility:* White to slightly yellow, crystalline powder; melts between 114° and 123°; pH (1 in 100 solution): 4.5–5.5. Very soluble in water and alcohol; practically insoluble in ether. *Uses:* Same actions and uses as neostigmine (see *Neostigmine Bromide* and also the *General Statement*). It is administered by the intramuscular route only. *Dose:* Usual, *intramuscular*, 2 mg every 2 to 3 hours, except for simple delayed menstruation, in which case it is administered only once daily for 2 to 3 days.

Malathion [The *S*-(1,2-dicarbethoxyethyl) ester of *O,O*-dimethyl phosphorodithioate; $(CH_3O)_2P(:S)[SCH(COO-C_2H_5)CH_2COOC_2H_5]$]—An organophosphate anticholinesterase employed as an insecticide. It was the first organophosphate approved for household use and is consequently the major organophosphate insecticide with which community pharmacists will have contact. Its toxicity to man is the lowest of the agents in this group, 60 Gm being the estimated fatal oral dose.

Cholinesterase Reactivators

Several substances are capable of displacing dialkylphosphate groups (from organophosphate anticholinesterases) and methyl- or dimethylcarbamoyl groups (from physostigmine or neostigmine) from the esteratic sites of cholinesterases poisoned by the anticholinesterases. At present all such substances of promise contain oxime groups, which

engage in a nucleophilic attack on the attached phosphate or carbamoyl group and rupture the bond between the inhibiting group and the esteratic site. This action is especially important in the treatment of intoxication by organophosphate anticholinesterases, since the organophosphates have such a long duration of action. The reactivation of carbamoylated enzyme is less prominent. Unfortunately, within a period of minutes to hours after poisoning with an organophosphate, there is a change in the phosphorylated enzyme ("aging"), so that the alkylphosphate–enzyme bond becomes too stable to be displaced by reactivators. The efficacy of any one reactivator varies according to which anticholinesterase is involved because of differences in electrophilicity of the phosphorus in the various phosphate radicals; one anticholinesterase, octamethylphosphoramide, is refractory to displacement by anticholinesterase reactivators. Atropine also must be used concomitantly with reactivators for optimal therapy. The reactivators may be used prophylactically.

Pralidoxime Chloride USP

[2-Formyl-1-methylpyridinium Chloride Oxime; 2-PAM Chloride;
Protopam Chloride (*Ayerst*)]

Pralidoxime Chloride contains 97.0–103.0% of $C_7H_9ClN_2O$ (172.62), calculated on the dried basis.

Preparation—Picolinal is converted to its oxime which is then quaternized with dimethyl sulfate. Metathesis of the resulting pralidoxime methosulfate with hydrochloric acid yields the official chloride. US Pat. 3,123,613.

Description—A white to pale-yellow, crystalline powder free from odor. It is stable in air, light, and heat. It melts between 215° and 228° with decomposition.

Solubility—Freely soluble in water; slightly soluble in absolute alcohol; moderately soluble in methanol; insoluble in acetone.

Uses—Pralidoxime is an anticholinesterase reactivator. The quaternary portion of the molecule attaches to the anionic site of the cholinesterase molecule and brings the oxime into close proximity to the poisoned esteratic site. The drug is used in the treatment of poisoning by organophosphate anticholinesterases, especially, but also in poisoning by neostigmine or physostigmine. The therapeutic effect (remission) usually occurs within an hour. When Pralidoxime is injected more rapidly than the recommended rate, dizziness, nausea, headache, mild weakness, blurred vision, diplopia, or tachycardia may result.

Dose—*Usual, intravenous,* **1 Gm** injected in a period of not less than 2 minutes; *infusion,* **1 Gm in 250 ml** of Sodium Chloride Injection over a period of 30 minutes. Repeat in 1 hour if necessary. *Usual, oral,* **1 Gm,** repeated in 3 hours if necessary.

Other Dose Information—The oral dose ranges from 1 to 3 Gm initially. If signs and symptoms of cholinesterase poisoning already exist, more than two doses will probably be of little extra value. If the drug is given prophylactically after exposure before signs of poisoning ensue, up to 5 oral doses of 3 Gm each may be given, to protect against slowly absorbing anticholinesterase. Intravenously, for a cholinergic crisis due to echothiophate it is often the practice to start with 50 mg and increase the dose every 5 minutes until a remission occurs. For cholinergic crisis due to neostigmine, ambenonium, or pyridostigmine, an initial dose of 1 to 2 Gm may be given, followed by 250 mg every 5 minutes until a remission occurs.

Dosage Forms—Sterile USP: 1 Gm; Tablets USP: 500 mg.

Veterinary Uses—This drug is used for the treatment of organophosphate insecticide poisoning in dogs, usually in combination with atropine.

Veterinary Dose—*Dogs, intravenous,* **3 to 5 mg** per **pound** of body weight.

50 | Adrenergic Blocking Drugs

Adrenergic blocking agents—adrenergic neurone blocking (antiadrenergic) agents

This chapter was prepared by

Ewart A. Swinyard, PhD, *Professor of Pharmacology, College of Pharmacy and College of Medicine, University of Utah, Salt Lake City, Utah 84112, and* Stewart C. Harvey, PhD, *Associate Professor of Pharmacology, College of Medicine, University of Utah, Salt Lake City, Utah 84112*

The term *blockade* is rather loosely used to indicate interference with a response system such that the final effect is prevented. A *blocking drug* is the agent to that interference. *Adrenergic* blockade indicates that the particular response system affected is that which normally involves the catecholamine neurohumoral transmitters, epinephrine (*adren*aline) and norepinephrine (nor*adren*aline, levarterenol). The term adrenergic refers to any of the cellular apparatus concerned with the elaboration, storage, release, transmission, reception or action of these catecholamines or to their mimetics. Thus the locus of action of an adrenergic blocking agent might be any of these adrenergic sites. Until the discovery of the catecholamine-depleting effects of reserpine, the only adrenergic blocking agents were those that blocked at the adrenergic neuroeffector receptor as competitive antagonists to the catecholamines or their mimetics. At present, drugs are known which can block the adrenergic response system by inhibiting the synthesis, storage or release of catecholamines. Such drugs prevent the response to stimulation of the sympathetic adrenergic nerves by preventing delivery of catecholamines to the neuroeffector receptor; they do not prevent the actions of catecholamines or sympathomimetics on the neuroeffector receptor as do the "classical" adrenergic blocking agents. Thus far, no universal terminology has been adopted to distinguish those drugs that block the catecholamines and sympathomimetics from those that prevent the delivery of catecholamines to the receptor. The term *adrenergic blocking agent* might better be applied to the former class, in accordance with previous custom, and the term *adrenergic neurone blocking agent*, or antiadrenergic drug, be applied to the latter class. The adrenergic blocking agents are also sometimes called *sympatholytics*, because they abolish the response to stimulation of the sympathetic nerves, or *adrenolytics*, because the classical adrenergic blocking drugs abolished certain responses to epinephrine (*adren*aline). Adrenergic neurone blocking agents are sympatholytic but not adrenolytic.

Adrenergic Blocking Agents

Two principal types of adrenergic effector receptors exist. Those that initiate salivation, adrenergic sweating, and contraction of smooth muscle (except in the gut) are classified as alpha receptors. Those that increase the frequency and strength of the heart beat and that initiate relaxation of smooth muscle (except in the gut) and metabolic effects are classified as beta receptors. Alpha receptor blocking agents have been known since 1906, when Dale demonstrated the reversal by ergotoxine of the vasopressor effects of epinephrine. The reversal results because the alpha receptors, which initiate vasoconstriction, are blocked but the beta receptors, which initiate vasodilation, normally masked by the overriding vasoconstriction, are not. Since the stimulant effects on the heart are subserved by beta receptors, alpha receptor blocking drugs do not block the classical cardiac effects of adrenergic stimuli. Drugs whose clinical usefulness derives from blockade of alpha receptors include phenoxybenzamine, phentolamine and piperoxan. Although the ergot alkaloids can effect adrenergic blockade under experimental conditions, they do not do so in clinically tolerated doses; lowering of sympathetic activity and interference with sympathetically mediated reflexes derives from a depressant action on the vasomotor centers. The ergot alkaloids are described under *Uterine Drugs*, page 951.

Several other drugs, such as tolazoline and azapetine are frequently classified as alpha adrenergic blocking drugs, but their clinical usefulness derives from direct peripheral vasodilator properties. Similarly, adrenergic blocking properties are often ascribed to hydralazine, but such properties are never manifested in clinical doses. Piperoxan is too weak a blocking agent in clinical doses to prevent the alpha effects of sympathetic nerve impulses, which release high local concentrations of norepinephrine, but is strong enough to block the alpha effects of circulating neurohumors, as from the adrenal medulla or pheochromocytoma; consequently, piperoxan will lower the blood pressure of the patient with hypertension because of a pheochromocytoma but not that of a patient with any other type of hypertension or that of a normal person.

Several drugs that can block beta receptors are now known. At present, only one drug of this class, Propranolol, has been cleared for clinical use. The prototype of this class, dichloroisoproterenol, has too many side effects to be clinically useful.

Azapetine Phosphate—see page 855.

Hydralazine Hydrochloride—see page 852.

Phenoxybenzamine Hydrochloride

[Dibenzyline Hydrochloride (*SKF*)]

Phenoxybenzamine Hydrochloride is *N*-(2-chloroethyl) - *N* - (1 - methyl - 2 - phenoxyethyl)benzylamine hydrochloride.

Description—Crystals, melting between 137.5° and 140°.

Solubility—Soluble in alcohol and in propylene glycol; sparingly soluble in water.

Uses—Phenoxybenzamine is the most nearly specific of the commercial adrenergic blocking drugs in that once it is absorbed and distributed there is but one side effect, namely drowsiness, that cannot definitely be attributed to adrenergic blockade; postural hypotension, drooping eyelids, and nasal stuffiness are consequent to adrenergic blockade. It combines irreversibly with the smooth muscle adrenergic excitatory receptors, through alkylation, so that a complete blockage, once induced, may last for several days. Adrenergic cardiac and inhibitory actions are not affected by the drug. It is effective orally, which is an advantage over many other β-haloalkylamine agents in this category. However, while the drug is in the gastrointestinal tract it may cause irritation; therefore, it is given in several divided doses, generally with milk. Immediately during moderately fast intravenous administration there may be central excitation with possible nausea, vomiting, and even convulsions and vascular collapse unless barbiturate prophylaxis has been rendered. Extravasation may result in local necrosis. Phenoxybenzamine is useful in the treatment of *Raynaud's disease*, *acute arterial occlusion*, and other conditions in which there is a component of vasospasm, and in *phlebitis*, *phlebothrombosis*, and *chronic skin ulcers*. It is occasionally effective in the treatment of essential and malignant hypertensions, but it is tried only when more common measures have failed. It is sometimes dramatic in the relief of *hypertensive encephalopathy*, *retinopathy*, and *oliguria*. It is used in the chronic and preoperative management of the patient with *pheochromocytoma*, as well as in the diagnosis. It has also been found to be useful in the treatment of *shock*, especially to protect the kidney from irreparable damage from reflex ischemia. Preliminary reports indicate that it may have prophylactic value as a presurgical medicament to prevent ischemic tissue damage and shock, especially in poor-risk candidates for heart surgery. It may be useful in the treatment of *acute angle glaucoma*.

Dose—*Orally*, **20 to 200 mg** per day in 2 to 6 divided doses, generally with milk. *Intravenously*, **0.5 to 2.0 mg per Kg** in 250–500 ml of isotonic dextrose or sodium chloride, generally given over a period of an hour.

Dosage Forms—Capsules: 10 mg.

Phentolamine Hydrochloride NF

m-[*N*-(2-Imidazolin-2-ylmethyl)-*p*-toluidino] phenol Monohydrochloride;
Regitine Hydrochloride (*Ciba*)

Phentolamine Hydrochloride, dried at 60° in vacuum for 2 hours, contains 98.0–100.5% of $C_{17}H_{19}N_3O \cdot HCl$ (317.82).

Preparation—*m*-(*p*-Toluidino)phenol is refluxed in xylol solution with 2-chloromethylimidazoline hydrochloride and the crude compound is purified by recrystallization.

m-(*p*-Toluidino)phenol   2-Chloromethylimidazoline

Description—A white or slightly grayish, crystalline, odorless powder. Its solutions are acid to litmus, having a pH of about 5, and foam on shaking. Melting range 238° to 242°.

Solubility—1 Gm dissolves in about 50 ml of water and about 120 ml of alcohol; very slightly soluble in chloroform and ether.

Uses—The actions of Phentolamine Hydrochloride are the same as those given for *Phentolamine Mesylate;* however, its use is limited to oral medication.

Dose—**50** to **100 mg;** *usual,* **50 mg** 4 to 6 times a day.

Dosage Forms: Tablets NF: 50 mg.

Phentolamine Mesylate USP

[*m*-[*N*-(2-Imidazolin-2-ylmethyl)-*p*-toluidino]phenol Monomethanesulfonate (Salt); Phentolamine Methanesulfonate USP XVI; Regitine Methanesulfonate (*Ciba*)]

Phentolamine Mesylate contains 98.0–102.0% of $C_{17}H_{19}N_3O \cdot CH_4SO_3$ (377.47), calculated on the dried basis. For the structure and chemical name of phentolamine, see *Phentolamine Hydrochloride*.

Preparation—It may be prepared by treating phentolamine base with an equimolar portion of methanesulfonic acid.

Description—A white, odorless, crystalline powder. Its solutions are acid to litmus, having a pH of about 5, and slowly deteriorate. Melting range between 175° and 180°.

Solubility—1 Gm dissolves in about 1 ml of water, 4 ml of alcohol, and about 700 ml of chloroform.

Uses—Phentolamine Mesylate is an alpha adrenergic blocking agent related to tolazoline both chemically and pharmacologically. It is more potent that tolazoline as an adrenergic blocking agent and is somewhat weaker as a vasodilator and cardiac stimulant, but the vasodilator actions nevertheless make important contributions to its therapeutic efficacy in certain conditions. The drug finds considerable application as a *diagnostic agent for pheochromocytoma;* it is sometimes employed to control the hypertension of pheochromocytoma, especially during surgery. It is also employed in the treatment of *Raynaud's disease,* acute arterial occlusion, and other conditions characterized by *arteriolar spasm.* It is occasionally effective in the treatment of *hypertensive emergencies,* but it is not useful in the chronic treatment of essential hypertension. Patients may experience tachycardia, orthostatic hypotension, nasal stuffiness, and gastrointestinal disturbances, especially after repeated doses.

Dose—*Intramuscular* or *intravenous,* usual, **5 mg.**

Other Dose Information—As a diagnostic agent for pheochromocytoma, 5 mg are given intravenously.

This dose is sufficient to block the hypertensive effects of circulating adrenal medullary hormones and sometimes to block the adrenergic sympathetic ouflow. For other purposes the usual intravenous or intramuscular dose is 0.05 to 0.1 mg per Kg, 4 to 6 times a day.

Dosage Forms: for Injection USP: 5 mg.

Tolazoline Hydrochloride—see page 855.

Propranolol Hydrochloride

[Inderal (*Ayerst*)]

$$\left[\underset{OH}{OCH_2CHCH_2\overset{+}{N}H_2CH(CH_3)_2} \right] Cl^-$$

Propranolol Hydrochloride [$C_{16}H_{21}NO_2 \cdot HCl$ = 295.80] is 1-(isopropylamino)-3-(1-naphthyloxy)-2-propanol hydrochloride.

Preparation—α-Naphthol is reacted with epichlorhydrin in aqueous alkali to form 2,3-epoxypropyl α-naphthyl ether and the epoxy ring is then ruptured by reaction with isopropylamine. The base is converted to the hydrochloride with hydrochloric acid.

Description—A white or almost white powder that is odorless and has a bitter taste. It is stable in heat, unstable in light, and nonhygroscopic. It melts between 163° and 164°.

Solubility—1 Gm dissolves in 20 ml of water and 20 ml of alcohol; slightly soluble in chloroform.

Uses—Propranolol Hydrochloride is a β-adrenergic blocking agent. As such, it is capable of suppressing the heart rate and contractility and bronchodilation to the extent that these functions are supported by adrenergic acvitity, and to increase vasoconstriction in those vascular beds where there may be some degree of masked β-adrenergic vasodilator activity. The effect to reduce heart rate and contractility reduces cardiac work and hence is of benefit in *angina pectoris;* however, it has not yet been released for this use in the US. Coronary dilation is not involved; indeed,

propranolol may even induce a mild degree of coronary constriction by blocking coronary β-adrenergic receptors and by reducing myocardial oxygen consumption. It is also employed to suppress tachycardia and increased myocardial work in *hyperthyroidism, pheochromocytoma,* and *idiopathic hypertrophic subaortic stenosis.* Propranolol is also useful as an *antiarrhythmic,* especially for *ventricular tachycardias* of any origin and *digitalis-induced tachyarrhythmias,* including *atrial tachycardia, premature ventricular contractions,* and *ventricular tachycardia.* It is less useful in the management of atrial flutter and fibrillation. If atrioventricular conduction is impaired, however, the drug may cause complete heart block by removing facilitatory β-adrenergic function. Likewise, it may precipitate frank congestive heart failure in a weakened heart; but if an existing failure is the result of a tacharrhythmia, failure may sometimes be relieved by the drug. The antiarrhythmic effects are independent of β-adrenergic blockade; indeed, the *d*-isomer is the better antiarrhythmic yet is nearly devoid of β-adrenergic blocking activity.

Propranolol may cause nausea, vomiting, mild diarrhea, light-headedness, and mental depression. Side effects consequent to diminished cardiac output and hence to β-adrenergic blockade are hypotension, with attendant orthostatic hypotension, weakness, dizziness, or syncope. When pre-existing heart disease exists, it is wise to digitalize the patient to prevent heart failure. β-Adrenergic blockade may also occasionally precipitate bronchospasm, laryngospasm, or other respiratory distress. The drug is relatively contraindicated in bronchial asthma, cardiogenic shock, congestive heart failure, hay fever, sinus bradycardia, and advanced heart block.

Dose—*Intravenous,* for *arrhythmias,* **1** to **3 mg** at a rate not to exceed 1 mg/min. The dose may be repeated in a few minutes, if necessary. *Oral,* for *arrhythmias,* **10** to **30 mg** 3 to 4 times a day; for *angina pectoris* (not in US), **40** to **60 mg** 3 to 4 times a day; for *hypertrophic subaortic stenosis,* **20** to **40 mg** 3 to 4 times a day.

Dosage Forms—Injection: 1 mg/ml; Tablets: 10 and 40 mg.

Adrenergic Neurone Blocking Agents

(Antiadrenergic Drugs)

The biosynthesis of the adrenergic neurohumor, norepinephrine (levarterenol), takes place in the postganglionic sympathetic adrenergic neurone. The substrate is 3,4-dihydroxyphenylalanine (DOPA), which is formed in the adrenergic neurone by the hydroxylation of tyrosine. DOPA is acted upon by the enzyme, dopadecarboxylase. The product of the decarboxylation is the catecholamine, dopamine (3,4-dihydroxy-β-phenylethylamine). Within the adrenergic neurone in the region of the nerve endings are granular organelles which contain the enzyme, dopamine β-oxidase, which introduces the side chain hydroxyl group into dopamine to make norepinephrine. The norepinephrine is stored in the same granular organelle. By an unknown mechanism the norepinephrine can be released from the granule by a nerve impulse. It can also be released by indirectly acting sympathomimetics (see Chapter 48) and drugs such as reserpine, guanethidine and alphamethyldopa (methyldopa). After the

norepinephrine is initially released from the granules by reserpine or guanethidine, newly formed or transported norepinephrine cannot be reincorporated into the depleted granules; furthermore, residual norepinephrine in the granules, of which there is considerable after guanethidine, cannot be released. The total effect is that no norepinephrine is available for delivery to the effector in response to nerve stimulation. With methyldopa, a metabolite (methylnorepinephrine) replaces norepinephrine in the granules.

Guanethidine Sulfate USP

[2-(Hexahydro-1(2H)-azocinyl)ethyl]guanidine Sulfate (2:1); Ismelin Sulfate (*Ciba*)]

$$\left[\underset{H_2C \quad CH_2}{N-CH_2CH_2NH-\underset{NH_2}{C}=\overset{+}{N}H_2} \right]_2 SO_4^{=}$$

Guanethidine Sulfate contains 95.0–105.0% of $(C_{10}H_{22}N_4)_2 \cdot H_2SO_4$ (494.70).

Preparation—Cycloheptanone oxime is caused to undergo Beckmann rearrangement to form hexahydro-2(1H)azocinone $[\overline{CH_2(CH_2)_5CONH}]$ which is then reduced to heptamethyleneimine $[\overline{CH_2(CH_2)_6NH}]$. This is then condensed with chloroacetonitrile and the resulting nitrile is hydrogenated to 1-(2-aminoethyl)heptamethyleneimine. Condensation with 2-methyl-2-thiopseudourea $[HN:C(SCH_3).NH_2]$ sulfate eliminates CH_3-SH to produce crude Guanethidine Sulfate which is purified by recrystallization.

Description—White, crystalline powder, having a strong, characteristic odor.

Solubility—Very soluble in water; slightly soluble in alcohol; practically insoluble in chloroform.

Uses—Guanethidine Sulfate is an adrenergic neurone blocking agent that partially depletes the adrenergic nerve of its norepinephrine (levarterenol) and prevents the release of that which remains. Its onset of action is slow, requiring several hours to 2 or 3 days for its full effect, and its duration of action may be 4 or more days. As an antihypertensive it appears to be superior to any other drug, especially when used in conjunction with thiazide diuretics. Tolerance is rare and is of a low degree. The most common untoward effects are those that obligatorily accrue to the effects of sympathetic blockade. They include orthostatic hypotension with its attendant vertigo, weakness, lassitude, nausea, and occasional syncope, bradycardia, nasal stuffiness, diarrhea and failure of ejaculation. Fatigue and dyspnea from exertion also occur frequently. Like reserpine the drug may cause edema and azotemia as a result of a deficient renal blood flow consequent to decreased cardiac output.

Dose—10 to **100 mg** daily; *usual, initial,* **25 to 50** once a day.

Other Dose Information—The average dose is 50 to 75 mg daily, but it may range upward to several hundred mg. In combination with other antihypertensive drugs the dose may be lower.

Dosage Forms—Tablets USP: 10 and 25 mg.

Methyldopa USP

[(−)-3-(3,4-Dihydroxyphenyl)-2-methylalanine; Alphamethyldopa; Aldomet (*MSD*)]

Methyldopa contains 98.0–101.0% of $C_{10}H_{13}NO_4$ (211.22), calculated on the anhydrous basis.

Preparation—The product of the reaction of 3,4-dimethoxyphenylacetonitrile with sodium ethoxide is hydrolyzed with acid to give 3,4-dimethoxyphenylacetone. This is then reacted with ammonium carbonate and potassium cyanide to form a substituted hydantoin intermediate which, on alkaline hydrolysis, yields the racemic methyldopa. The acetylated form of this racemate is resolved using (−)-α-methylbenzylamine. The isolated acetylated (−)-methyldopate salt is then deacetylated with base and treated with mineral acid to liberate the (−)-Methyldopa. US Pat. 2,868,818.

Description—White to yellowish white, odorless, fine powder, which may contain friable lumps. It is almost tasteless and relatively stable in both light and air. It melts above 290° with decomposition.

Solubility—Sparingly soluble in water; very soluble in diluted hydrochloric acid; slightly soluble in alcohol; practically insoluble in ether.

Uses—Methyldopa is the alphamethyl congener of the catecholamine precursor, 3,4-dihydroxyphenylalanine (Dopa). Methyldopa appears to induce release of norepinephrine from storage sites and to interfere with release in response to stimuli, probably through the action of the decarboxylated metabolites of methyldopa, methyldopamine, and methylnorepinephrine. The effects accumulatively result in adrenergic neuronal block. Methyldopa also has a hypotensive action independent of its antiadrenergic actions. Its action begins in about 2 hours, becomes maximal in 6 to 8 hours, and lasts from 18 to 24 hours. Methyldopa also depletes tissue 5-hydroxytryptamine by interference with tryptophandecarboxylase. The drug is employed as an *antihypertensive* in the treatment of moderate to severe essential hypertension; it appears to be at least equal to reserpine but somewhat inferior to guanethidine. However, the degree of orthostatic hypotension with Methyldopa is considerably less than with guanethidine. Its action is erratic, and a third of treated patients may not respond to the drug. Tolerance sometimes develops in up to a third of initially responsive patients. The drug also has some usefulness in the treatment of *pheochromocytoma* and *carcinoid tumor*. It acts to inhibit dopa decarboxylase (which is also 5-hydroxytryptophan decarboxylase) and thus to suppress the biosynthesis of norepinephrine, epinephrine, and 5-hydroxytryptamine (serotonin). Side effects consequent to its blockade of sympathetic nerves include occasional orthostatic hypotension with vertigo, nausea, weakness and headache, bradycardia, nasal stuffiness, diarrhea, and impotence. Other side effects include frequent drowsiness, dry mouth, and skin rashes. Like reserpine, it may cause edema and rarely psychic depression and nightmares, parkinsonism, arthralgia, and myalgia. Lactation and breast enlargement occur rarely. Depression of liver function characterized by fever and malaise and occasionally jaundice may occur.

Dose—**500 mg** to **2 Gm** daily; *usual,* **250 mg** 3 times a day.

Other Dose Information—The usual maintenance dose is 1 to 1.5 Gm, in divided doses, daily.

Dosage Forms—Tablets USP: 250 mg.

Methyldopate Hydrochloride USP

[(−)-3-(3,4-Dihydroxyphenyl)-2-methylalanine Ethyl Ester Hydrochloride; Aldomet Ester Hydrochloride (*MSD*)]

Methyldopate Hydrochloride contains 98.0–101.0% of $C_{12}H_{17}NO_4 \cdot HCl$ (275.73), calculated on the dried basis.

Preparation—Methyldopate Hydrochloride may be prepared by converting Methyldopa (this page) to its ethyl ester and passing hydrogen chloride into a solution of the ester in a suitable organic solvent.

Description—A white or practically white crystalline powder which is odorless or practically odorless and has a bitter taste. It is relatively stable both in light and air. It melts at about 160°.

Solubility—Freely soluble in water, alcohol, and methanol; slightly soluble in chloroform; practically insoluble in ether.

Uses—The actions and uses of methyldopate hydrochloride are the same as those of *Methyldopa*. The ester is employed for intravenous use in hypertensive crises. In the body the ethyl group is removed by hydrolysis to yield methyldopa. Since the onset of action by the oral route is relatively rapid and only slightly longer than that by the intravenous route, intravenous administration is not indicated, unless the patient is unable to take substances by mouth.

Dose—*Intravenous infusion*, **100 mg** to **4 Gm** daily; *usual*, **250** to **500 mg** in **100 ml** of **5%** Dextrose Injection over a period of 30 to 60 minutes 4 times a day.

Dosage Forms—Injection USP: 5 ml.

Rauwolfia Serpentina NF

[(*Various Mfgs.*)]

Rauwolfia Serpentina is the dried root of *Rauwolfia serpentina* (Linné) Bentham ex Kurz (Fam. *Apocynaceæ*), sometimes with fragments of rhizome and aerial stem bases attached. It contains not less than 0.15% of reserpine–rescinnamine group alkaloids, calculated as reserpine.

Uses—Rauwolfia Serpentina produces the sum of the actions of the total alkaloids contained in the whole root. The component alkaloids exhibit the sedative–antihypertensive–bradycrotic action characteristic of reserpine, the latter of which accounts for approximately 50% of the total activity. The actions, uses, and limitations are the same as those for reserpine. See *Reserpine*.

Dose—*Usual*, *initial*, **200 mg** daily for 1 to 3 weeks; *maintenance*, **50** to **300 mg** daily.

Dosage Forms—Powdered NF (see below); Tablets NF, 50 and 100 mg.

Powdered Rauwolfia Serpentina NF is rauwolfia serpentina reduced to a fine or very fine powder, and adjusted if necessary to conform to the official requirements for reserpine–rescinnamine group alkaloids by admixture with lactose or starch or with a powdered rauwolfia serpentina containing a higher or lower content of these alkaloids. It contains 0.15–0.20% of reserpine–rescinnamine group alkaloids, calculated as reserpine.

Rescinnamine NF

[Methyl Reserpate Ester with 3,4,5-Trimethoxycinnamic Acid; Methyl 18β-Hydroxy-11,17α-dimethoxy-3β,20α-yohimban-16β-carboxylate 3,4,5-Trimethoxycinnamate (Ester); Moderil (*Pfizer*)]

Rescinnamine, dried at 60° for 3 hours, contains 95.0–100.5% of $C_{35}H_{42}N_2O_9$ (634.73).

For the structural formula, see page 500.

Preparation—Rescinnamine is extracted from *Rauwolfia vomitora* and other species of *Rauwolfia* by adaptation of the usual procedures for isolating alkaloids.

It may also be produced synthetically starting with the more plentiful alkaloid, reserpine, by the following steps: (*a*) saponification with alcoholic potassium hydroxide and subsequent acidification to form reserpic acid (I); (*b*) reacting (I) with diazomethane to produce methyl reserpate [—COOCH₃ at the 16β-position] and (*c*) esterifying the hydroxyl at the 18β-position with trimethoxycinnamoyl chloride.

I (Reserpic Acid)

Description—It occurs as a white, or pale buff to cream-colored, odorless, crystalline powder. It darkens slowly on exposure to light, but more rapidly when in solution. Melting range 220° to 232° (when previously dried at 60° for 3 hours). Specific rotation −87° to −97° (when previously dried at 60° for 3 hours and determined in a solution in chloroform containing 100 mg in each 10 ml). The NF provides tests for *Identification*.

Solubility—Soluble in chloroform and in acetic acid. Slightly soluble in alcohol, and practically insoluble in water.

Uses—Rescinnamine, a purified ester alkaloid of the alseroxylon fraction of rauwolfia, has the same order of effectiveness and the same uses as reserpine. Thus, rescinnamine is useful for the management of mild, labile hypertension and as a tranquilizing agent in agitated patients with simple neuroses and frank psychoses. Except that sedation and bradycardia occur less frequently and in milder form with rescinnamine, the incidence of other side effects such as weakness and fatigue, nasal congestion, dizziness, confusion, increased appetite and weight gain is about the same as with reserpine. Both drugs, however, are subject to the same precautions and contraindications. See *Reserpine*.

Dose—**250 mcg** to **2 mg** daily; *usual*, *initial*, **500 mcg** 1 or 2 times a day for up to 2 weeks; *maintenance*, **250 mcg** daily.

Other Dose Information—The daily dose is increased or decreased by increments of 0.25 mg, to achieve the desired therapeutic response. The daily oral dose for institutionalized psychotic patients ranges from 3 to 12 mg.

Dosage Forms—Tablets NF: 250 and 500 mcg.

Reserpine USP

[Methyl Reserpate Ester with 3,4,5-Trimethoxybenzoic Acid; Methyl 18β-Hydroxy-11,17α-dimethoxy-3β,20α-yohimban-16β-carboxylate 3,4,5-Trimethoxybenzoate (Ester); (*Various Mfgs.*)]

Reserpine contains 97.0–101.0% of $C_{33}H_{40}N_2O_9$ (608.69) calculated on the dried basis.

Reserpine is a purified alkaloid isolated from several species of *Rauwolfia*. The structure of reserpic acid is shown above. For the structural formula of *Reserpine*, see page 500.

History—This alkaloid was isolated and described in 1952.[1] Since then intensive chemical and pharmacological investigations of its properties have been conducted in several countries.

Description—White or pale buff to slightly yellowish, odorless, crystalline powder. It darkens slowly on exposure to light, but more rapidly when in solution. It melts between 255° and 265° with decomposition.

Solubility—Insoluble in water; very slightly soluble in ether; 1 Gm dissolves in about 1800 ml of alcohol and about 6 ml of chloroform; slightly soluble in benzene; freely soluble in acetic acid.

Uses—Reserpine, the first rauwolfia alkaloid to be officially recognized, was first used for the symptomatic management of patients with anxiety or tension psychoneuroses or chronic psychoses involving anxiety, psychomotor hyperactivity, or compulsive aggressive behavior. Higher doses of the drug are required in the management of grossly disturbed psychoses than in anxiety-tension states. However, in both types of patients the drug must be administered for 1 or 2 weeks before the optimal level of dosage can be determined. The tranquilizing effect of the drug makes the patient more cooperative, less destructive, and more amenable to psychotherapy. Unless the dosage is carefully adjusted, the drug may induce a paradoxical form of anxiety and adverse reactive depression. In chronic psychoses, the drug does not appear to alter the basic psychopathological state. Because of the seriousness of side effects, reserpine is no longer used much as a tranquilizer.

Reserpine has a firmly established position in modern antihypertensive therapy. Because the doses used are generally considerably smaller than those for its tranquilizing effects, the drug may be used for its hypotensive effects with more safety than as a psychopharmacologic drug. The drug is chiefly used for the management of mild, labile hypertension, in conjunction with potent hypotensive agents, for the management of *essential hypertension* and hypertension associated with *toxemia of pregnancy*. The use of oral reserpine alone is considered to be of little value for severe hypertension, but it is useful to augment or to prolong the action of potent hypotensive agents, to reduce dosage and side effects. The value of reserpine for routine use as a prophylactic against progressive vascular changes in patients with early hypertension is unwarranted. Intravenous reserpine is quite useful in the management of severe hypertension and hypertensive crises. The antihypertensive action of reserpine derives from adrenergic neuronal blockade consequent to depletion of the catecholamine-containing granules of the postganglionic sympathetic neurone. The mechanism of the central effects is unknown. It depletes both brain serotonin and catecholamines.

Reserpine is claimed to be adequately absorbed from the gastrointestinal tract, but the difference in efficacy of oral and intravenous doses raises doubts about the adequacy of absorption. It characteristically has a long latency of onset and a prolonged duration of action. For example, with daily oral administration the effects of the drug usually are not fully manifest for several days to 2 weeks and may persist for as long as 4 weeks after oral medication is discontinued. Tolerance to the drug does not develop with continued administration. Nasal congestion, weight gain, and diarrhea are the most frequently noted side effects. Suicidal depression is the most serious untoward effect. The drug may reactivate old peptic ulcers because it increases hydrochloric acid secretion by the stomach. Other serious reactions are excessive drowsiness, orthostatic hypotension, fatigue, weakness, insomnia, nightmares, excitement, irrational behavior, and incipient parkinsonism.

Dose—*Oral*, **100 mcg** to **1 mg** daily; *usual*, **250 mcg** 1 or 2 times a day; *intramuscular*, **250 mcg** to **10 mg** daily; *usual*, **2.5 mg** 1 to 3 times a day.

Other Dose Information—In anxiety or tension psychoneuroses, 0.5 to 2 mg daily. In disturbed psychotics, 3 to 5 mg orally in conjunction with 5 to 10 mg daily by intramuscular injection.

Dosage Forms—Injection USP: 5 mg/2 ml, 25 and 50 mg/10 ml; Tablets USP: 0.1, 0.25, 0.5, 1, 2, and 5 mg.

Veterinary Use—Tranquilizer and sedative.

Veterinary Dose—*Horses*, **1 mg** per **1000 pound** body weight *parenterally; Cattle*, **7.0** to **7.5 mg** per **1000 pound** body weight *parenterally; Dogs* and *Cats*, **0.01** to **0.03 mg** per **pound** body weight *orally* or *parenterally.*

Syrosingopine NF

[Methyl Reserpate Ester with Syringic Acid Ethyl Carbonate; Methyl 18β-Hydroxy-11,17α-dimethoxy-3β,20α-yohimban-16β-carboxylate 4-Hydroxy-3,5-dimethoxybenzoate Ethyl Carbonate (Ester); Singoserp (*Ciba*)]

Syrosingopine, dried at 60° in vacuum for 3 hours, contains 97.0–101.0% of $C_{35}H_{42}N_2O_{11}$ (666.73).

For the structural formula, see page 500.

Preparation—Gallic acid is exhaustively methoxylated with dimethyl sulfate and the 4-methoxy group is then selectively cleaved with sulfuric acid to form syringic acid [3,5-dimethoxy-4-hydroxybenzoic acid]. This acid is then carbethoxylated with ethyl chloroformate and the resulting syringic acid ethyl carbonate is converted to the acid chloride with thionyl chloride. Condensation of the acid chloride with methyl reserpate (produced by selective saponification of reserpine) yields Syrosingopine.

Description—Occurs as a white or slightly yellowish, crystalline, odorless powder. It is stable in air, but is affected by light.

Solubility—Practically insoluble in water; slightly soluble in ether; 1 Gm dissolves in about 200 ml of methanol and about 4 ml of chloroform; freely soluble in acetic acid.

Uses—Syrosingopine is an adrenergic neurone blocking agent which is closely related chemically and pharmacologically to reserpine. Although Syrosingopine is less potent and less toxic than reserpine, the two drugs have approximately the same margin of safety. Syrosingopine alone may be effective in some cases of mild or moderate labile essential *hypertension*, but it is ineffective in severe hypertension, unless used in conjunction with more potent antihypertensive drugs. Syrosingopine has relatively little central action; otherwise, its advantages, limitations, and untoward effects are similar to those of reserpine. See *Reserpine.*

Dose—*Usual, initial*, **1** to **2 mg** daily; *maintenance*, **500 mcg** to **3 mg** daily.

Dosage Forms—Tablets NF: 1 mg.

Other Adrenergic Neurone Blocking Agents

Deserpidine [11-desmethoxyreserpine; Harmonyl (*Abbott*)] is an alkaloid derived from *Rauwolfia canescens* which differs structurally from reserpine in the absence of its 11-methoxy group. It occurs as a white to light-yellow, crystalline powder. Insoluble in water; very slightly soluble in alcohol. *Uses:* Deserpidine is an adrenergic neurone blocking drug of the rauwolfia class (see *Reserpine*, page 912). Like reserpine, it is used mainly for the treatment of mild essential hypertension in conjunction with thiazide diuretics. Ten to 14 days are generally required before an effect becomes evident. It is also occasionally used as a tranquilizer in the treatment of mild anxiety states. Like the other rauwolfia alkaloids, for the management of psychoses, higher doses are required, which often cause serious side effects, so that this use is no longer common. The side effects and contraindications are the same as for Reserpine. *Dose: Usual, oral, initial*, for hypertension, *0.25 mg* 3 or 4 times a day, tapering off to a *maintenance* dose of *0.25 mg* 1 or 2 times a day; for mild anxiety states, *initially, 0.1 mg* per day with graded increments, if necessary.

References

1. Mueller, J. M., *et al*, *Experientia*, **8**, 338 (1952).

51 | Antimuscarinic Drugs

Solanaceous antimuscarinic drugs—synthetic antimuscarinic drugs

This chapter was prepared by

Ewart A. Swinyard, PhD, *Professor of Pharmacology, College of Pharmacy and College of Medicine, University of Utah, Salt Lake City, Utah 84112, and*
Stewart C. Harvey, PhD, *Associate Professor of Pharmacology, College of Medicine, University of Utah, Salt Lake City, Utah 84112.*

Cholinergic transmission occurs not only at the neuroeffectors innervated by the parasympathetic and certain sympathetic postganglionic nerves but also at all autonomic ganglia, the somatic neuromuscular junction, and certain central synapses (see introductory statement, Chapter 48, page 880). The term *cholinergic blocking drug,* loosely used by some as synonymous with antimuscarinic drug, denotes any drug that can antagonize cholinergic stimuli at any of these sites. Thus, cholinergic blocking drugs properly include drugs, such as ganglionic and neuromuscular blocking agents, that block nicotinic cholinergic effects, as well as antimuscarinic drugs. Synonyms for the term antimuscarinic are *anticholinergic, cholinolytic, parasympatholytic, and parasympathetic blocking drugs.* Since "cholinergic," ganglionic, and neuromuscular blocking drugs have in common the antagonism of acetylcholine, it is to be expected certain of these drugs may block at more than one cholinergic locus and that structural requirements for one type of blocking activity have some relationship to those for activity at other cholinergic sitse.

The effects of antimuscarinic drugs on the whole are readily predicted by considering the consequences of interruption of parasympathetic (and sympathetic cholinergic) nerve stimulation. Thus, the effects are decreased gastrointestinal motility, decreased gastric secretion, dry mouth, drying of the mucous membranes in general, mydriasis and loss of accommodation (and a *para passu* tendency to increased intraocular pressure), urinary retention, decreased sweating and compensatory cutaneous flush, bronchial and biliary dilatation, tachycardia (although effective block of the cardiac inhibitory nerves is difficult to achieve), etc.

In addition to the more common effects, the tertiary amine agents penetrate the central nervous system where they may increase the level of excitability, as with atropine, or decrease the level, as with scopolamine. In high doses they antagonize the central effects of anticholinesterases. They also aid in the control of tremors and rigidity of Parkinson's disease and related states (see Chapter 52, page 928).

The quaternary ammonium agents essentially lack central actions, but they exert moderate blocking actions at the autonomic ganglia, which lessen the intensity of neuroeffector activity to be overcome at the periphery. Some of the quaternaries are slightly more selective for gastrointestinal receptors than they are for other neuroeffector sites. Consequently, they are the primary parasympathetic blocking agents employed in antiulcer therapy and in the treatment of intestinal hypermotility. However, some of the early quaternaries proved to cause serious intolerance in patients who often covertly or overtly discontinued medication. Moreover, gastric secretion proved to be difficult to suppress except by parenteral administration. Consequently, synthetic antimuscarinics fell into disrepute for the management of peptic ulcer and bowel disorders. Medical acceptance of the superior newer antimuscarinic drugs has been slow and grudging. Certain prominent authorities express doubt that they are superior to conventional parasympathetic blocking agents, under normal conditions of use, but the superiority of certain of the synthetic antimuscarinic drugs now seems almost incontrovertible.

The therapeutic uses of parasympathetic blocking drugs derive logically from their actions. They are largely outlined under the two prototypes. These are: (1) *Atropine* (below), which is one of the solanaceous alkaloids found in belladonna, hyoscyamus, etc, and (2) *Methantheline* (page 921), which was the first important synthetic quaternary ammonium antimuscarinic drug to be introduced.

Solanaceous Antimuscarinic Drugs

Atropine NF

[1αH,5αH-Tropan-3α-ol: (±)-Tropate Ester]

Atropine contains 99.0–100.5% of $C_{17}H_{23}NO_3$ (289.38).

Atropine is an alkaloid usually obtained from botanical sources, or produced synthetically.

Caution—Atropine is extremely poisonous.

*Note—*Actually, Atropine has not been shown to occur in natural sources as an alkaloid; it is a racemic mixture of *d-* and *l-*hyoscyamine (see *Preparation,* below).

For the structural formula, see page 496.

Preparation—Atropine was isolated by Vaquelin in 1809 and its alkaloidal nature recognized by Brandes in 1819. It is claimed that the alkaloid does not occur as such in any of the solanaceous plants, but is the product of the racemization of *l-*hyoscyamine present in these plants. *Hyoscyamus muticus* from Egypt is the preferred source for the manufacture of atropine because of its high alkaloid content, with stramonium next in order. The powdered drug is thoroughly moistened with an aqueous solution of sodium carbonate and extracted with ether or benzene. The alkaloidal bases are extracted from the solvent with acetic acid, the acid solution is shaken with ether as long as the latter takes up coloring matter, then precipitated with sodium carbonate. The precipitate of the bases, after washing and drying, is dissolved in ether or acetone, the solution dehydrated with anhydrous sodium sulfate, and filtered. After concentration and cooling of the solution, the bases consisting of atropine and hyoscyamine crystallize from solution. The crude crystalline mass is filtered off and dissolved in alcohol, sodium hydroxide solution is added, and the solution is allowed to stand until racemization is complete (as indicated by absence of optical activity). The crude atropine is purified by crystallization from acetone.

Description—White crystals, usually needle-like, or a white, crystalline powder. Its saturated solution is alkaline to phenolphthalein TS. It is optically inactive, but usually contains some levorotatory hyoscyamine. It melts between 114° and 118°.

Solubility—1 Gm dissolves in about 460 ml of water, about 2 ml of alcohol, about 27 ml of glycerin, about 1 ml of chloroform, and about 25 ml of ether; 1 Gm dissolves in 90 ml of water at 80°; soluble in hot benzene.

Incompatibilities—The difficulty which is sometimes experienced in preparing solutions in *liquid petrolatum* is overcome by the use of oleic acid. The alkaloid is dissolved in a drop or two of alcohol and warmed with a little oleic acid until the alcohol has evaporated. Additional oleic acid is then added to make the product 25 times the weight of the Atropine, and this solution is dissolved in the liquid petrolatum.

Uses—Galenical preparations of belladonna are active chiefly by virtue of their content of Atropine, a potent and useful alkaloid; atropine owes its activity to the *l*-hyoscyamine isomer. Atropine typifies in its actions the entire group of belladonna alkaloids. It has two main types of actions, one on the central nervous system to cause respiratory stimulation and selective sedation (in certain diseases), and the other to depress smooth muscles and secretory glands innervated by parasympathetic (cholinergic) nerves. Having such widespread effects in the body, Atropine enjoys many therapeutic uses but does not exert much selectivity of action. Thus, if it is employed for its effects on the bowel, the unwanted actions on the eye, the salivary glands, heart, etc, must be tolerated.

The central actions of Atropine are employed to *stimulate respiration*, to give symptomatic relief in *paralysis agitans* and *postencephalitic parkinsonism*, and in certain types of *spastic* and *rigid states* due to central nervous system injury or disease. They are also used in the antagonism of the central actions of anticholinesterases. A few practitioners use deliberately toxic doses of atropine in the treatment of *schizophrenia*.

The peripheral actions of atropine are concerned with the eye, the bronchial muscles, the secretions of the bronchio-respiratory glands, the heart, the gastrointestinal tract, the urinary tract, the sweating mechanism, and the uterus. In ophthalmology, Atropine is used to *dilate the pupil* and to *paralyze the accommodation*. It is usually administered topically for this purpose as the sulfate salt, but occasionally the free alkaloidal base in oil solution, in an ointment, or in gelatin disks (lamellæ) is placed in the conjunctival sac. Atropine is sometimes combined with cocaine, amphetamine, or hydroxyamphetamine for ophthalmic use. In *bronchial asthma*, Atropine causes relaxation of the bronchial muscles and drying up of bronchial secretions. It is not as effective as epinephrine but is used in mild or chronic cases, or in the intervals between attacks. In acute *coyrza, hay fever*, and *rhinitis*, Atropine is sometimes employed to dry up the annoying excessive secretions. Proprietary "cold" tablets

often contain Atropine for this purpose. Atropine is almost routinely employed prior to inhalation anesthesia to *inhibit excessive salivation or bronchial secretions*.

With respect to the heart, Atropine is sometimes employed to abolish extrasystoles and partial or complete heart block, or syncope due to hyperactive carotid sinus reflexes. Abnormal cardiac slowing due to drugs or to poisoning by certain species of mushrooms may also yield to Atropine therapy.

In spastic conditions of the bowel, Atropine may be employed, particularly for *spastic colitis, pylorospasm, cardiospasm*, etc; the extract and tincture of belladonna are common forms of atropine used for these purposes. It is of limited value in the therapy of *ulcer of the stomach or duodenum*. Atropine counteracts to some extent the intestinal spasm of lead colic, morphine constipation, and similar states. Atropine is often used to relieve *ureteral colic*, frequently in combination with morphine. It is also employed to control *enuresis* in children, and to relieve urinary frequency and urgency. It is a frequent constituent of drug mixtures for the relief of *dysmenorrhea*. Finally Atropine is given to *suppress sweating*, and also to control excessive salivation.

The cycloplegia induced by atropine may result in an increase in intraocular pressure in some persons, especially the elderly. For this reason, the drug is contraindicated in persons whose intraocular pressure is already elevated (ie, in glaucoma). It is also contraindicated in the presence of prostatic hypertrophy. In the larger therapeutic doses atropine may cause dizziness, restlessness, tremor, fatigue, and locomotor difficulties. It is also sometimes sensitizing. Dry mouth, blurred vision, photophobia, anhidrosis, and constipation are unavoidable side effects of the drug. Large doses may cause extreme thirst, hyperpyrexia, disorientation, hallucinations, delerium, convulsions, and circulatory or respiratory collapse.

Atropine is usually employed in the form of its sulfate salt. It can be given orally, hypodermically, or intravenously, and in the case of the eye it is applied topically.

Dose—*Usual*, **250 mcg** 3 times a day.

Other Dose Information—The dose is usually taken ½ hour before meals.

Veterinary Dose—See *Atropine Sulfate*.

Atropine Sulfate USP

[1αH,5αH-Tropan-3α-ol (±)-Tropate (Ester) Sulfate (1:1)]

Atropine Sulfate [$(C_{17}H_{23}NO_3)_2.H_2SO_4.H_2O$ = 694.85] contains 98.5–101.0% of $(C_{17}H_{23}NO_3)_2.H_2SO_4$, calculated on the anhydrous basis.

Caution—*Atropine Sulfate is very poisonous*.

For the structural formula of atropine, see page 496.

Preparation—Atropine Sulfate is prepared by dissolving atropine base in warm acetone and adding just sufficient dilute sulfuric acid to furnish the necessary amount of H_2SO_4. The salt is then allowed to crystallize from solution.

Description—Colorless and odorless crystals or a white crystalline powder. It effloresces in dry air and is slowly affected by light. When previously dried at 120° for 3 hours it melts at a temperature not below 188°. The aqueous solution of Atropine Sulfate is practically neutral or only faintly acid to litmus.

Solubility—1 Gm dissolves in 0.5 ml of water, 5 ml of alcohol, and about 2.5 ml of glycerin; 1 Gm dissolves in 2.5 ml of boiling alcohol.

Uses—See *Atropine*.

Dose—*Oral* or *parenteral*, **300 mcg** to **4 mg** daily; *usual*, **500 mcg** 3 or 4 times a day; *topically*, as a **1%** ointment or **0.1 ml** of a **0.5** to **3%** solution to the conjunctiva 3 to 5 times a day.

Dosage Forms—Injection USP: 400 mcg/0.5 ml; 300, 400, 500, and 600 mcg, land 1.2 mg/ml; 4 and 10 mg/10 ml; 8, 10, and 24 mg/20 ml; 50 mg/25 ml; 9, 12, 15, 18, and 36 ml/30 ml. Ophthalmic Solution USP: 0.5, 1, 2, 3, and 4%. Tablets: 300, 400, and 600 mcg.

Veterinary Dose—*Subcutaneous, Horses* and *Cattle*, **15** to **60 mg;** *Sheep* and *Goats*, **5** to **30 mg;** *Swine*, **2** to **8 mg;** *Dogs*, **0.3** to **5 mg;** *Cats*, **0.1** to **0.3 mg.** Doses in high range are administered intravenously or intramuscularly and repeated if necessary as an antidote in organophosphate poisoning.

Diphenoxylate Hydrochloride and Atropine Sulfate Tablets—see page 813.

Belladonna Leaf USP

[Belladonnæ Folium; Deadly Nightshade Leaf; Belladonna Herb; Black Cherry Leaf; Dwale; Dwayberry Leaf]

Belladonna Leaf consists of the dried leaf and flowering or fruiting top of *Atropa belladonna* Linné or of its variety *acuminata* Royle ex Lindley (Fam. *Solanaceæ*).

Belladonna Leaf yields not less than 0.35% of the alkaloids of belladonna leaf.

Uses—Same as those for *Belladonna Tincture, Belladonna Extract*, and *Atropine*. See *Atropine* for discussion of actions and uses. Belladonna Leaf itself is rarely employed in humans. Belladonna Leaf Fluidextract is only rarely employed and is not preferred to the tincture or extract of belladonna, or to the purified alkaloids such as atropine or scopolamine. Belladonna Tincture, which is made from the leaf, is one of the few galenical preparations of belladonna which is widely employed in medicine. It is used especially for its antispasmodic effect on the gastrointestinal tract, which it exerts chiefly by virtue of its atropine content.

Veterinary Dose—*Horses* and *Cattle*, **1** to **4 Gm;** *Sheep*, **0.2** to **0.6 Gm;** *Swine*, **0.1** to **0.5 Gm;** *Dogs*, **60** to **300 mg;** *Cats*, **15** to **30 mg.**

Belladonna Extract NF [Belladonna Dry Extract] contains, in each 100 Gm, 1.15–1.35 Gm of the alkaloids of belladonna leaf. *Pilular Belladonna Extract:* Prepare an extract by percolating 1000 Gm of belladonna leaf, using a mixture of 3 volumes of alcohol and 1 volume of water as the menstruum. Macerate the drug during 16 hours and then percolate it at a moderate rate. Evaporate the percolate to a pilular consistence under reduced pressure and at a temperature not exceeding 60°, and adjust the remaining extract, after assaying, by dilution with liquid glucose so that the finished Extract will contain, in each 100 Gm, 1.25 Gm of the alkaloids of belladonna leaf. *Powdered Belladonna Extract:* Prepare an extract by percolating 1000 Gm of belladonna leaf, using alcohol has the menstruum. Macerate the drug during 16 hours and then percolate it slowly. Evaporate the percolate to a soft extract under reduced pressure and at a temperature not exceeding 60°, add 50 Gm of dry starch, and continue the evaporation, at the same temperature, until the product is dry. Powder the residue. The extract may be deprived of its fat by treating either the soft extract first obtained, or the dry and powdered extract, as directed under *Extracts* (page 1591). Assay the powdered residue and add sufficient starch, dried at 100°, to make the finished Extract contain, in each 100 Gm, 1.25 Gm of the alkaloids of belladonna leaf. Mix the powders thoroughly and pass the Extract through a fine sieve. *Uses:* The NF has introduced both Pilular and Powdered Extracts of Belladonna Leaves under the one title. This provides the powdered form for pills and capsules should the pharmacist prefer to use it and the Pilular Extract, which contains no insoluble diluent, and consequently is much better adapted for the making of ointments or suppositories. *Dose: Usual, 15 mg 3 times daily. Veterinary Dose: Horses, 0.3 to 1 Gm; Cattle, 0.3 to 1.5 Gm; Sheep, 60 to 200 mg; Swine, 30 to 120 mg; Dogs, 20 to 60 mg; Cats, 5 to 10 mg.*

Belladonna Leaf Fluidextract NF contains, in each 100 ml, 270–330 mg of the alkaloids of belladonna leaf. *Preparation:* The Fluidextract is prepared from belladonna leaf (in moderately coarse powder, 1000 Gm) by Process A, as modified for assayed fluidextracts (page 1591), or by Process E (page 1591). By Process A, use a mixture of 3 volumes of alcohol and 1 volume of water as the menstruum, macerate the drug during 48 hours, and percolate at a moderate rate. By Process E, use a mixture of 2 volumes of alcohol and 1 volume of water as the menstruum and proceed as follows: Mix 1000 Gm of ground drug with 400 ml of the menstruum, so that it is evenly and distinctly damp. Allow the dampened drug to stand for about 1 hour, then pack into a cylindrical percolator, or a series of such percolators joined together, with a length equal to about 30 times the diameter. Saturate the drug at a slow rate by forcing the menstruum under 6 to 15 pounds of air pressure through the packed drug. Allow to macerate during 48 hours, and proceed with percolation by forcing the menstruum through under pressure at a rate of about 1.5 ml per minute until 950 ml has been collected. Adjust the concentrated fluid to contain, in each 100 ml, 300 mg of the alkaloids of belladonna, and 60% of C_2H_5OH. *Alcohol Content:* From 57 to 63% of C_2H_5OH. *Dose: Usual, 0.06 ml 3 times a day. Veterinary Dose: Horses* and *Cattle, 2 to 6 ml; Dogs, 0.06 to 0.2 ml.*

Belladonna Tincture USP [Belladonna Leaf Tincture] yields, from each 100 ml, 27–33 mg of the alkaloids of belladonna leaf. *Preparation:* With belladonna leaf (in moderately coarse powder, 100 Gm) prepare a tincture by Process P as modified for assayed tinctures (page 1590) using a mixture of 3 volumes of alcohol and 1 volume of water as the menstruum. Finally adjust the Tincture to contain, in each 100 ml, 30 mg of the alkaloids of belladonna leaf. *Alcohol Content:* From 65 to 70% of C_2H_5OH. *Dose: 0.3 to 4 ml daily; usual, 0.6 to 1 ml 3 or 4 times a day. Veterinary Dose: Horses* and *Cattle, 15 to 40 ml; Dogs, 0.3 to 2 ml.*

Homatropine Hydrobromide USP

[1αH,5αH-Tropan-3α-ol Mandelate (Ester) Hydrobromide]

Homatropine Hydrobromide contains 98.5–100.5% of $C_{16}H_{21}NO_3 \cdot HBr$ (356.26), calculated on the dried basis.

It is the hydrobromide of tropine mandelate. For the structural formula, see page 496.

Preparation—It is made by heating *tropine* [$C_8H_{15}NO$] with *mandelic acid* in the presence of hydrochloric acid; ammonia is added, and the homatropine which is liberated is dissolved out by chloroform; the solution is evaporated, hydrobromic acid added, and the crystals of Homatropine Hydrobromide purified by recrystallization.

Description—White crystals, or a white crystalline powder. It is affected by light. It melts between 214° and 217° with slight decomposition. Its aqueous solution is practically neutral or only faintly acid to litmus.

Solubility—1 Gm dissolves in 6 ml of water, 40 ml of alcohol, and about 420 ml of chloroform; insoluble in ether.

Uses—Homatropine may be viewed as a weakened atropine in its *cholinergic blocking* actions. The drug is used solely for its *mydriatic* effects. It is sometimes preferred to atropine because its effects are shorter in duration, and there is no protracted cycloplegia. It is often combined with ephedrine or hydroxyamphetamine in ophthalmic practice.

Caution—*Homatropine Hydrobromide is extremely poisonous.*

Dose—*External use, topically,* **0.1 ml** of a **2** to **5%** solution to the conjunctiva, repeated in 5 minutes.

Dosage Forms—Ophthalmic Solution USP: 2 and 5%.

Homatropine Methylbromide NF

[3α-Hydroxy-8-methyl-1αH,5αH-tropanium Bromide Mandelate; 8-Methylhomatropinium Bromide; Novatropine; Mesopin (*Endo*)]

Homatropine Methylbromide contains 98.5–100.5% of $C_{17}H_{24}BrNO_3$ (370.29), calculated on the dried basis. For the structural formula, see page 496.

Preparation—This synthetic antispasmodic may be prepared by adding a moderate excess of methyl bromide to an alcohol or ether solution of homatropine base.

Description—An odorless, white powder. It slowly darkens on exposure to light. Its solutions are practically neutral to litmus. It melts between 190° and 198°.

Solubility—Very soluble in water; freely soluble in alcohol; almost insoluble in ether and acetone; freely soluble in acetone containing 20% of water.

Uses—Homatropine Methylbromide is a quaternary ammonium *cholinergic blocking* agent and is consequently much less active than atropine on the central nervous system. Like homatropine, it is a weaker and less toxic autonomic blocking agent than atropine. It is used mainly for *gastrointestinal disorders,* for which it can be employed in the same manner as atropine.

Dose—*Usual,* **2.5** to **5 mg** 4 times a day.

Dosage Forms—Tablets NF: 2.5 and 5 mg.

Hyoscyamine Hydrobromide NF

[1αH,5αH-Tropan-3α-ol (−)-Tropate (Ester) Hydrobromide]

Hyoscyamine Hydrobromide contains 98.5–100.5% of $C_{17}H_{23}NO_3 \cdot HBr$ (370.29), calculated on the dried basis.

Caution—Hyoscyamine Hydrobromide is extremely poisonous.

For the structure of hyoscyamine, see page 496.

Preparation—Hyoscyamine Hydrobromide may be prepared by passing hydrogen bromide into a concentrated solution of hyoscyamine in ethanol and then diluting with ether.

Description—White, odorless, crystals or as a crystalline powder. Its solutions, freshly prepared, are neutral to litmus. It is affected by light.

Solubility—Freely soluble in water, alcohol, and chloroform; very slightly soluble in ether.

Uses—The uses of Hyoscyamine Hydrobromide are the same as those of the sulfate (see below).

Dose—*Usual,* **250 mcg** to **1 mg.**

Hyoscyamine Sulfate NF

1αH,5αH-Tropan-3α-ol (−)-Tropate (Ester) Sulfate (2:1); Daturine Sulfate]

Hyoscyamine Sulfate $(C_{17}H_{23}NO_3)_2 \cdot H_2SO_4 \cdot 2H_2O =$ 712.86) contains 98.5–100.5% of $(C_{17}H_{23}NO_3)_2 \cdot H_2SO_4$, calculated on the anhydrous basis.

Caution: Hyoscyamine Sulfate is extremely poisonous.

Hyoscyamine Sulfate is the sulfate of an alkaloid usually obtained from species of *Hyoscyamus* Linné or other genera of Fam. *Solanaceæ.*

For the structural formula of hyoscyamine, see page 496.

Description—White, odorless crystals or a crystalline powder. It is deliquescent. It is affected by light. Its solutions are acid to litmus. When previously dried at 105° for 4 hours, does not melt below 200°. Specific rotation not less than −24° (water solution containing 500 mg in each 10 ml).

Solubility—1 Gm dissolves in about 0.5 ml of water and about 5 ml of alcohol; practically insoluble in ether.

Uses—Hyoscyamine is a *cholinergic blocking* agent. The base, hyoscyamine, is the levo isomer comprising ½ of the racemic mixture known as atropine (page 914), and it is the primary active component of the mixture.

Dose—*Usual,* **125** to **250 mcg** 3 or 4 times a day.

Dosage Forms—Tablets NF: 125 and 250 mcg.

Methscopolamine Bromide NF

[6β,7β-Epoxy-3α-hydroxy-8-methyl-1αH,5αH-tropanium Bromide (−)-Tropate; N-methylscopolammonium Bromide; Scopolamine Methylbromide; Pamine Bromide (*Upjohn*)]

Methscopolamine Bromide contains 98.0–101.0% of $C_{18}H_{24}BrNO_4$ (398.30), calculated on the dried basis.

For the structural formula, see page 496.

Preparation—Benzene solutions of scopolamine and methyl bromide are mixed and allowed to stand. Quaternization occurs and the crystalline compound precipitates.

Description—Occurs as white crystals, or as a white, odorless, crystalline powder.

Solubility—Freely soluble in water; slightly soluble in alcohol; insoluble in acetone and in chloroform.

Uses—Methscopolamine Bromide is a quaternary ammonium derivative of scopolamine. It has greater selectivity than scopolamine or atropine in blocking vagal impulses to the gastrointestinal tract, but it is not free of such side effects as dry mouth, mydriasis, blurred vision, and urinary retention. Constipation is the inevitable result of its gastrointestinal actions. It is used in the treatment of *peptic ulcer,* since it decreases gastric emptying and sometimes decreases gastric motility, *bowel hypermotility,* and *functional diarrhea.* In some persons it decreases the output of gastric acid secretion. It may be used against *hyperhidrosis* and *sialorrhea.*

Dose—*Oral,* **2.5** to **5 mg;** *usual, oral,* **2.5 mg** 4 times a day; *parenteral,* **250 mcg** to **1 mg;** *usual,* **500 mcg** up to 4 times a day.

Dosage Forms—Injection NF: 1 mg/ml; Tablets NF: 2.5 mg.

Methscopolamine Nitrate

[6β,7β-Epoxy-3α-hydroxy-8-methyl-1αH,5αH-tropanium Nitrate (−)-Tropate; Skopyl (*Pharmacia*)]

Methscopolamine Nitrate $(C_{18}H_{24}N_2O_7)$ is *N*-methylscopolammonium nitrate. It is commonly known as scopolamine methylnitrate. For the structure of the cation, see *Methscopolamine Bromide*, page 496.

Description—A white, odorless, tasteless, crystalline powder. A 0.05% solution in water is acidic (pH 5.0–5.4).

Solubility—Freely soluble in alcohol and water.

Uses—The actions and uses of Methscopolamine Nitrate and *Methscopolamine Bromide* (see above) are identical, the active quaternary ammonium moiety being the same in both compounds.

Dose—*Orally,* **2.5** to **5 mg** 4 times daily; *subcutaneously* or *intramuscularly,* **0.25** to **0.5 mg** 3 or 4 times daily.

Dosage Forms—Capsules: 5 mg; Drops: 2.5 mg/ml.

Scopolamine Hydrobromide USP

[6β,7β-Epoxy-1αH,5αH-tropan-3α-ol (−)-Tropate (Ester) Hydrobromide; Hyoscine Hydrobromide]

Scopolamine Hydrobromide [$C_{17}H_{21}NO_4 \cdot HBr \cdot 3H_2O$ = 438.32] contains 98.5–102.0% of $C_{17}N_{21}NO_4 \cdot HBr$ (384.28), calculated on the anhydrous basis.

For the structural formula of scopolamine, see page 496.

Preparation—This alkaloid is recovered from the mother liquors remaining after crystallization of hyoscyamine. It is, however, most economically prepared from the leaves of *Datura Metel*, India, or from *D. meteloides* (Mexico) as the alkaloid content of these plants is predominantly scopolamine (hyoscine).

Description—Colorless or white crystals or a white, granular powder. It is odorless, and is slightly efflorescent in dry air. The anhydrous salt melts between 195° and 199°, previously dried at 105° for 3 hours, and the $[\alpha]_D^{25}$, determined in an aqueous solution and calculated to the anhydrous salt, is −24° to −26°.

Solubility—1 Gm dissolves in 1.5 ml of water and 20 ml of alcohol; slightly soluble in chloroform; insoluble in ether.

Uses—Scopolamine Hydrobromide (hyoscine hydrobromide) is an *antimuscarinic* drug similar to atropine in many ways but differs in the following important respects, which represent the basis for its selective therapeutic uses: scopolamine differs from atropine in that it is a sedative and tranquilizing depressant to the central nervous system. In its peripheral actions, Scopolamine depresses smooth muscles and secretory glands innervated by parasympathetic (cholinergic) nerves, but differs from atropine in that it is a stronger blocking agent for the iris, ciliary body, and salivary, bronchial, and sweat glands. On the other hand, Scopolamine is weaker than atropine in its action on the heart, the intestinal tract, and bronchial musculature.

Scopolamine is employed for its central depressant actions as a *sedative*. Frequently it is given for this purpose to prevent *motion sickness* and prior to anesthesia, under which circumstances it also inhibits secretions. It is used in *maniacal states*, in *delirium tremens*, and in obstetrics (combined with morphine as "twilight sleep"). It is also employed in *paralysis agitans*, in *postencephalitic parkinsonism*, and in certain *spastic states* due to nervous system injury. It is used for its peripheral actions on the eye in ophthalmology, as a *mydriatic* and *cycloplegic*. Mydriasis is somewhat shorter in duration, and intraocular pressure is affected less markedly than is the case after atropine.

Caution—*Scopolamine Hydrobromide is extremely poisonous.*

Dose—*Oral* or *parenteral*, **300 mcg** to **4 mg** daily; *usual*, **600 mcg** 3 or 4 times a day; *topically*, **0.1 ml** of a **0.2** to **0.5**% solution to the conjunctiva, 3 to 5 times a day.

Dosage Forms—Injection USP: 400 mcg/0.5 ml, 300, 400, 500, and 600 mcg and 1 mg/ml; Tablets USP: 300, 400, and 600 mcg.

Veterinary Use—Occasionally administered in combination with morphine as a preanesthetic narcotic in dogs; not reliable.

Veterinary Dose—*Dogs*, **0.3** to **0.6 mg.**

Other Solanaceous Antimuscarinic Drugs

Atropine Methonitrate [Metropine (*Strasenburgh*); Atropine Methylnitrate; 8-Methylatropinium Nitrate; $C_{17}H_{23}NO_3 \cdot CH_3NO_3$]—The methylnitrate quaternary salt of the alkaloid, atropine. It occurs as colorless, odorless crystals that are soluble, at 20°, in less than 1 part of water and in 13 parts of alcohol, but insoluble in ether and in chloroform. It melts between 166° and 168°C. Aqueous solutions are unstable and must not be kept for more than 1 week; they should be freshly prepared. Alcoholic solutions are stable for about 1 year. It has antispasmodic and mydriatic properties similar to those of atropine but is much less toxic. *Uses*: in the treatment of congenital hypertrophic pyloric stenosis of infants; for the relief of pylorospasm and cardiospasm in adults, to inhibit the action of the salivary glands in dentistry; as an ingredient of spray solutions for the relief of asthma and hay fever. *Dose*: orally, 1 to 2 mg; in the treatment of congenital hypertrophic pyloric stenosis of infants, 2 to 6 ml of a 0.01% aqueous solution, ½ hour before feeding.

Atropine Methylbromide [Methylatropine Bromide; 8-Methylatropinium Bromide] [$C_{17}H_{23}NO_3 \cdot CH_3Br$]—White crystals. Very poisonous! Melts at 222° to 223°. Soluble in 1 part water; slightly soluble in alcohol; almost insoluble in chloroform, ether. *Uses*: mydriatic, anhidrotic, antispasmodic. Externally instead of sulfate in ophthalmology. *Dose*: orally, 1 to 2 mg., *subcutaneously*, 0.1 to 0.3 mg.

Homatropine Hydrochloride [$C_{16}H_{21}NO_2 \cdot HCl$]—Small white crystals, soluble in water and alcohol. *Uses*: to cause paralysis of accommodation in ophthalmological procedures; recovery from cycloplegic effect is complete in one day. Must be used with care in persons disposed to glaucoma. Its actions are identical to those of *Homatropine Hydrobromide*, page 916. *Dose*: topically, to the eye in 1% solution.

Scopolamine Butylbromide [Buscopan; Hyoscine Butylbromide; *N*-Butylscopolammonium Bromide] [$C_{21}H_{30}BrNO_4$]—*Uses*: exhibits mild anticholinergic and spasmolytic atropine-like actions, but possesses rather marked ganglionic blocking and curariform properties. It is devoid of the central stimulant action of atropine. Reduces peristalsis without loss of tone in peptic ulcer therapy; reduces spasm in gastrointestinal, biliary, and renal conditions. *Dose*: 10 to 20 mg up to 5 times a day.

Synthetic Antimuscarinic Drugs

Benztropine Mesylate—see page 931.

Clidinium Bromide NF

[3-Hydroxy-1-methylquinuclidinium Bromide Benzilate; Quarzan, an ingredient of Librax (*Roche*)]

Clidinium Bromide contains 99.0–100.5% of $C_{22}H_{26}BrNO_3$ (432.36), calculated on the dried basis.

Preparation—3-Quinuclidinol is esterified to the benzilate either by transesterification with methyl benzilate or by reaction with benzilic acid chloride, and the resulting 3-quinuclidinyl benzilate is quaternized with methyl bromide. US Pat. 2,648,667.

Description—A white or nearly white, crystalline powder that is almost odorless. It is optically inactive. It should not be exposed to excessive light and heat. It melts between 240° and 244°.

Solubility—Soluble in water and alcohol; very slightly soluble in ether and benzene.

Uses—Clidinium Bromide is a quaternary ammonium *antimuscarinic* drug. Like most other quaternary antimuscarinic agents, it also possesses ganglionic blocking activity. It has a somewhat selective action on the gastrointestinal tract, so that it is employed in the treatment of the *irritable bowel syndrome, spastic colitis, ulcerative colitis, duodenitis, gastritis,* and *peptic ulcer.* Clidinium is a new drug with which there has been too little experience to establish its true efficacy and toxicity in the above conditions. Furthermore, it is marketed only in combination with chlordiazepoxide, so that it is difficult to ascertain the contribution of Clidinium alone. For this reason, it seems strange that Clidinium Bromide would be so prematurely accepted into the NF.

Clidinium may cause dry mouth, mydriasis, cycloplegia, and difficulty in urination. It is contraindicated in the presence of prostatic hypertrophy, benign bladder neck obstruction, or glaucoma.

Dose—2.5 to 5 mg 3 or 4 times a day; *usual,* 2.5 mg 3 times a day.

Cyclopentolate Hydrochloride USP

[2-(Dimethylamino)ethyl 1-Hydroxy-α-phenylcyclopentaneacetate Hydrochloride; Cyclogyl (*Schieffelin*)]

Cyclopentolate Hydrochloride contains 98.0–100.5% of $C_{17}H_{25}NO_3 \cdot HCl$ (327.85), calculated on the dried basis.

Preparation—The acid moiety of the ester, 1-hydroxy-α-phenylcyclopentaneacetic acid (III), may be prepared as follows. Sodium phenylacetate is added to an ethereal solution of isopropyl magnesium bromide whereupon propane is evolved and sodium phenylacetate magnesium bromide (I) is formed. Treatment with an ethereal solution of cyclopentanone results in Grignard addition with the formation of (II) which is then hydrolyzed by treatment with hydrochloric acid to give (III).

The ester is produced by metathesis between the sodium salt of (III) and 2-dimethylaminoethyl chloride using isopropyl alcohol as the reaction medium. After purification by crystallization from acetone, the ester may be converted into the official hydrochloride by dissolving it in an appropriate organic solvent and introducing a stream of hydrogen chloride.

Description—A white, crystalline powder, which upon standing develops a characteristic odor. Its solutions are acid to litmus. It melts between 137° and 141°. The pH (1 in 100) is between 5.0 and 5.4.

Solubility—Freely soluble in alcohol; very soluble in water; insoluble in ether.

Uses—Cyclopentolate hydrochloride is an *antimuscarinic* drug which is used primarily for its *ophthalmologic* actions. After local installation in the eye there is a rapid, intense cycloplegia and mydriasis of moderate duration. It is used as mydriatic in *refraction* studies, in the management of *iritis, iridocyclitis,* and in *keratitis* and *choroiditis,* and in *hyperpigmented irides.* It is also used to *prevent* or *break lenticular adhesions* during and after ocular infections and to *prevent spasms* of the sphincter in inflammation. It is about one-half as active as atropine.

Dose—*Topically,* 0.1 ml of a 0.5 to 2% solution to the conjunctiva, 3 to 5 times a day.

Other Dose Information—Deeply pigmented irides may require the higher concentration. For refraction, a second application may be given after ten minutes. In ocular inflammation it may be repeated every 6 to 8 hours. For lenticular adhesions it is repeated at 24-hour intervals, with interspersed courses of pilocarpine nitrate.

Dosage Forms—Ophthalmic Solution: 0.5, 1, and 2%.

Cycrimine Hydrochloride—see page 932.

Dicyclomine Hydrochloride NF

[2-(Diethylamino)ethyl [Bicyclohexyl]-1-carboxylate Hydrochloride; Bentyl Hydrochloride (*Merrell*)]

Dicyclomine Hydrochloride contains 99.0–102.0% of $C_{19}H_{35}NO_2 \cdot HCl$ (345.96), calculated on the dried basis.

Preparation—Cyclohexanol is reacted with hydrogen chloride to form cyclohexyl chloride which is then Grignardized with ethyl formate to yield dicyclohexyl carbinol (α-cyclohexylcyclohexanemethanol). Oxidation of the carbinol with sodium dichromate yields the corresponding ketone which is then chlorinated with sulfuryl chloride to give 1-chlorocyclohexyl cyclohexyl ketone. Reaction of the ketone with the sodium derivative of 2-(diethylamino)ethanol furnishes an intermediate which rearranges to dicyclomine (base). The purified base is dissolved in an appropriate solvent and treated with hydrogen chloride to form the official hydrochloride. US Pat. 2,474,796.

Description—A fine, white, crystalline powder that is practically odorless and has a very bitter taste. It is stable in air and to moderate heat. It melts between 169° and 174°.

Solubility—1 Gm dissolves in 15 ml of water, 5 ml of alcohol, 2.5 ml of chloroform, and 6000 ml of ether; insoluble in an alkaline aqueous medium.

Uses—Dicyclomine is an *antimuscarinic* drug used for its atropine-like effects on the gastrointestinal tract. Some authorities deny that it has significant antimuscarinic properties and contend that its effects result from a nonspecific antispasmodic action. It decreases the motility but does not suppress gastric secretion. It is used in the treatment of irritable colon, spastic constipation, mucous colitis, spastic colitis, pylorospasm, and biliary dyskinesia. In the treatment of peptic ulcer it is used to delay gastric emptying. Side effects include dizziness and a feeling of abdominal fullness.

Dose—*Usual,* **10** to **20 mg** 3 or 4 times a day.

Other Dose Information—Oral or intramuscular, 5 mg for infants, 10 mg for children, and 20 mg for adults, 3 or 4 times a day. Occasionally doses may need to be higher.

Dosage Forms—Capsules NF: 10 mg; Injection: 10 mg/ml; Syrup NF: 10 mg/5 ml; Tablets: 20 mg.

Diphemanil Methylsulfate NF

[4-(Diphenylmethylene)-1,1-dimethylpiperidinium Methyl Sulfate; Prantal (*Schering*)]

Diphemanil Methylsulfate contains 97.0–103.0% of $C_{21}H_{27}NO_4S$ (389.52), calculated on the dried basis.

Preparation—Methyl N-methylisonipecotate (I) is subjected to the typical Grignard reaction for esters using an excess of phenylmagnesium bromide. The resulting α,α-diphenyl-N-methyl-4-piperidinemethanol (II) is dehydrated with sulfuric acid to yield diphemanil (base) (III). Quaternization of the purified base is accomplished by dissolving it in benzene and adding dimethyl sulfate. The quaternary compound precipitates.

Description—White or nearly white crystalline solid, having a bitter taste and a faint characteristic odor. Melting range: 189° to 196°. pH: 4.0 to 6.0 (1 in 100 solution). Stable to heat and light and is somewhat hygroscopic.

Solubility—1 Gm dissolves in about 33 ml of water, alcohol, and chloroform.

Uses—Diphemanil Methylsulfate is a quaternary ammonium *antimuscarinic* agent; consequently it also exerts a moderate ganglionic blocking action. Its most prominent action is the relief of *pylorospasm.* It may reduce gastric secretion moderately by the oral route and considerably by the parenteral route; large but poorly tolerated parenteral doses may markedly suppress gastric secretion for a brief time. The drug also effectively suppresses sweating and exerts bronchodilator actions at relatively low doses. Thus it is also used in the management of *peptic ulcer, gastric hyperacidity,* and *hypermotility,* as in chronic hypertrophic gastritis, and *hyperhidrosis.* Its side effects are other effects of cholinergic blockade and include dry mouth, mydriasis and blurred vision, tachycardia, urinary retention, and constipation or diarrhea. It is poorly absorbed by the oral route and should be given between meals.

Dose—*Oral,* **50** to **200 mg;** *usual, oral,* **100 mg** every 4 to 6 hours; *usual, intramuscular* and *subcutaneous,* **25 mg** 4 times a day.

Dosage Forms—Injection NF: 25 mg/ml, 250 mg/10 ml; Tablets NF: 100 mg.

Veterinary Dose—*Intramuscular, Horses,* **25 mg** per **100 pounds** of body weight; *Dogs* and *Cats,* **0.75** to **1 mg** per **pound** of body weight twice daily.

Eucatropine Hydrochloride USP

[1,2,2,6-Tetramethyl-4-piperidyl Mandelate Hydrochloride]

Eucatropine Hydrochloride contains 99.0–100.5% of $C_{17}H_{25}NO_3 \cdot HCl$ (327.85), calculated on the dried basis.

Preparation—This synthetic mydriatic is the hydrochloride of the mandelic acid ester of 1,2,2,6-tetramethyl-4-piperidinol, which ester may be obtained by heating the two components in alcohol solution.

Description—A white, granular, odorless powder. Its melting range is between 183° and 186°. It is stable in air but is affected by light. Its aqueous solution is neutral to litmus.

Solubility—Very soluble in water; freely soluble in alcohol and chloroform; insoluble in ether.

Uses—Eucatropine produces prompt mydriasis free from anesthetic action, pain, corneal irritation, or increase in intraocular tension. It has little or no effect on accommodation, and such effect as it has disappears more rapidly than with atropine, cocaine, homatropine, etc. It is useful as an aid in *ophthalmoscopic examinations* in place of atropine, homatropine, etc. Its lack of a prominent cycloplegic action is advantageous in the elderly and patients with glaucoma, but it precludes a refractive examination.

Dose—*Topically,* **0.1 ml** of a **2** to **5%** solution to the conjunctiva, repeated in 5 minutes.

Glycopyrrolate NF

[3-Hydroxy-1,1-dimethylpyrrolidinium Bromide α-Cyclopentylmandelate; Robinul (*Robins*)]

Glycopyrrolate, dried at 105° for 3 hours, contains 98.0–100.5% of $C_{19}H_{28}BrNO_3$ (398.34).

Preparation—α-Phenylcyclopentaneglycolic acid is esterified by refluxing with methanol in the presence of hydrochloric acid and the resulting ester is transesterified with 1-methyl-3-pyrrolidinol using sodium as a catalyst. The transester is then reacted with methyl bromide and recrystallization of the quaternary to constant melting point gives the racemate which is Glycopyrrolate.

Description—A white, crystalline powder that is odorless and has a bitter taste. It is stable in light and heat and is nonhygroscopic. It melts between 193° and 198°.

Solubility—1 Gm dissolves in 20 ml of water; soluble in alcohol; practically insoluble in chloroform, benzene, and ether.

Uses—Glycopyrrolate is a quaternary ammonium *antimuscarinic* drug which has a moderate degree of selectivity for the gastrointestinal tract. The drug not only prolongs gastric emptying time, which favors the retention of antacids, but decreases gastric acid production in many patients. Consequently, Glycopyrrolate is used especially in the treatment of *peptic ulcer*. It is also used for *spastic colon, spastic duodenum, colitis, biliary spasm*, and other gastrointestinal disorders associated with spasm. Although the incidence of side effects is low with the recommended doses, they do occur. They include dry mouth, mydriasis with attendant photophobia, cycloplegia with blurred vision, urinary hesitancy or retention, constipation, tachycardia, nausea, weakness, dizziness, headache, drowsiness, and rash. It may elevate intraocular tension in susceptible persons; it is contraindicated in glaucoma. It is also contraindicated in pyloric obstruction, intestinal obstruction, urinary bladder neck obstruction, prostatic hypertrophy, cardiospasm, and achalasia of the esophagus.

Dose—1 to **2 mg**; *usual*, **1 mg** 3 times a day.

Other Dose Information—The dose must be individualized. In acute severe conditions the total daily dose may exceed 8 mg. Once symptoms subside the dose should be reduced to the minimum necessary for relief.

Dosage Forms—Tablets NF: 1 and 2 mg.

Isopropamide Iodide NF

[(3-Carbamoyl-3,3-diphenylpropyl)diisopropylmethylammonium   Iodide;
Darbid (*SK&F*)]

Isopropamide Iodide, dried in vacuum at 60° for 2 hours, contains 98.0–101.0% of $C_{23}H_{33}IN_2O$ (480.44).

Preparation—4 - (Diisopropylamino) - 2,2 - diphenylbutyronitrile is hydrated to the corresponding butyramide by heating with moderately concentrated sulfuric acid. The amide is then isolated and quaternized with methyl iodide to form crude Isopropamide Iodide which is recrystallized by dissolving in a hot isopropanol/methanol mixture and precipitating with hexane. The starting nitrile may be produced by condensing (3-chloro-2,2-dimethylpropyl)diethylamine with diphenylacetonitrile under the influence of lithium amide. US Pat. 2,823,233.

Description—White or nearly white powder, which is practically odorless and has a bitter taste. It melts at about 183°. The dry powder is stable at room temperature for 2 years, stored in glass bottles.

Solubility—Freely soluble in water (at 100°) and in chloroform; soluble in 95% ethanol; sparingly soluble water (at room temperature) and 0.1N HCl; slightly soluble in acetone.

Uses—Isopropamide Iodide is a quaternary ammonium *antimuscarinic* drug with very little ganglionic blocking action at regular doses. It is advocated for use in the therapy of peptic ulcer and other conditions of gastrointestinal hyperactivity, but it has no special selectivity for this system. However, its long duration

of action (12 hours) makes it especially useful for managing the troublesome nocturnal secretion of the peptic ulcer patient. Side effects are dry mouth, mydriasis, blurred vision, and urinary retention.

Dose—10 to **20 mg** daily; *usual*, **5 mg** 2 times a day.

Dosage Forms—Tablets NF: 5 mg.

Veterinary Dose—To control gastrointestinal hyperactivity, *Dogs* and *Cats, oral* or *subcutaneous*, **0.1** to **0.2 mg** per **pound** of body weight twice daily.

Mepenzolate Bromide NF

[3-Hydroxy-1,1-dimethylpiperidinium Bromide Benzilate; Cantil (*Lakeside*)

Mepenzolate Bromide contains 98.0–102.0% of $C_{21}H_{26}BrNO_3$ (420.35), calculated on the dried basis.

Preparation—3-Pyridinol is quaternized with methyl bromide and the resulting 3-hydroxy-1-methylpyridinium bromide is catalytically reduced to 1-methyl-3-piperidinol. Transesterification of methyl benzilate with this alcohol in the presence of sodium methoxide affords 1-methyl-3-piperidyl benzilate which, on quaternization with methyl bromide, yields the official article. US Pat. 2,918,408.

Description—White or light-cream powder, which melts with decomposition between 230° and 237°.

Solubility—1 Gm dissolves in 112 ml of water, 7.6 ml of methanol, 121 ml of absolute ethanol at room temperature.

Uses—Mepenzolate Bromide is an *antimuscarinic* drug that has the same qualitative actions as *Atropine* (see page 914). However, the actions of Mepenzolate on the gastrointestinal tract are proportionately greater than those on other cholinergic structures, as is generally the case with other quaternary ammonium cholinergic blocking drugs. The agent reduces motility in the colon, small intestine, and stomach, the effect on the colon supposedly being greatest. Given parenterally or in large oral doses, it can reduce gastric acid secretion of hydrochloric acid, but the effect does not occur during ordinary clinical use. Mepenzolate also relaxes the sphincter of Oddi. It is used in the treatment of *spastic colon, irritable bowel, regional ileitis, infectious diarrhea, ulcerative colitis, gaseous distention of the colon*, and *duodenal ulcer*. Side effects include dry mouth, blurred vision, constipation, vertigo, headache, and difficulty in urination.

Dose—25 to **50 mg**; *usual*, **25 mg** 4 times a day.

Dosage Forms—Tablets NF: 25 mg.

Methantheline Bromide NF

Diethyl(2-hydroxyethyl)methylammonium Bromide Xanthene-9-carboxylate; Banthine Bromide (*Searle*)]

Methantheline Bromide contains 98.0–102.0% of $C_{21}H_{26}BrNO_3$ (420.35), calculated on the dried basis.

Preparation—Xanthene-9-carboxylic acid is reacted with β-diethylaminoethyl chloride in boiling isopropyl alcohol yielding the corresponding ester hydrochloride, β-diethylaminoethyl xanthene-9-carboxylate hydrochloride. The ester hydrochloride is treated with an aqueous solution of sodium carbonate, and the resulting ester-free base, β-diethylaminoethyl xanthene-9-carboxylate, is extracted with benzene. After the benzene is removed by evaporation, the ester-free base is dissolved in butanone and converted by addition of methyl bromide to the ester quaternary salt, β-diethylaminoethyl xanthene-9-carboxylate methobromide, which is filtered and dried.

Description—A white or nearly white, practically odorless powder, having a bitter taste. Its solutions are acid, having a pH of about 5. Melting range between 171° and 177°.

Solubility—Very soluble in water; freely soluble in alcohol and chloroform; practically insoluble in ether; aqueous solutions decompose on standing.

Uses—Methantheline Bromide is a synthetic quaternary ammonium *antimuscarinic* drug which effectively blocks the response of smooth muscle, cardiac muscle, and secretory cells to injected as well as endogenously released acetylcholine. In larger amounts it also exerts anticholinergic actions on autonomic ganglia and skeletal muscles. In man, therapeutic doses of the drug produce pupillary dilation, diminished ocular accommodation, dryness of the mouth, and decreased sweating. Moderate tachycardia appears in some patients. The major effects are on the gastrointestinal tract and resemble those produced by atropine; gastric contractions are diminished, emptying time of the stomach delayed, gastric secretory volume variably reduced, and the amount of total and free acid erratically decreased. In tolerated doses, the gastrointestinal effects of Methantheline Bromide are greater and more prolonged than those of atropine.

Side effects observed after Methantheline Bromide include dry mouth, blurred vision, mydriasis, a feeling of epigastric fullness, heart burn, difficulty in urination, decreased libido, and constipation. These effects are usually mild and can sometimes be minimized by adjustment of the dose. Central nervous system symptoms such as restlessness, euphoria, and fatigue occur in some patients, and rare instances of psychotic episodes have been reported. Skin rashes, including exfoliative dermatitis, have been observed. The drug should be used with caution in individuals with prostatic hypertrophy, in order to avoid acute urinary retention. It is contraindicated in patients with glaucoma, cicatricial duodenal stenosis, achalasia, cardiospasm, organic pyloric obstruction, coronary insufficiency, and cardiac failure.

Methantheline Bromide has been used primarily for the *adjunct treatment of duodenal ulcer*. It may relieve both the pain and the symptoms which accompany this condition. The mechanism whereby it relieves the pain of duodenal ulcer is probably mostly the reduction in gastrointestinal motility. However, objective roentgenological improvement is not always apparent. Patients with gastric ulcer are not appreciably benefited by the drug. Instances of duodenal ulcer recurrence as well as the development of gastric ulcer have been reported in individuals receiving prophylactic doses of the drug for healed duodenal ulcer. Furthermore, a large percentage of patients discontinue the drug because they refuse to tolerate the side effects.

Of the numerous drugs used in the treatment of peptic ulcer, methantheline appears to cause the highest incidence of intolerance. Its continuing official status is mostly from deference to its historical precedence rather than from its therapeutic efficacy. Other conditions in which the methantheline has been used successfully include the following: *"hyperacidity" syndrome, chronic hypertrophic gastritis, biliary, dyskinesia, pylorospasm, acute and chronic pancreatitis, diverticulitis, "irritable colon" syndrome, regional ileitis, ulcerative colitis, hyperhidrosis,* and *sialorrhea*. It has also been employed in urological patients to relieve *renal colic, ureteral colic, neurogenic enuresis,* and *urinary bladder pain.*

Dose—**50 to 100 mg;** *usual,* **50 mg** 4 times a day.

Other Dose Information—The usual oral adult dose in active peptic ulcer is 50 to 100 mg, every 6 hours day and night. The night dose is particularly important in order to control the high free acidity of nocturnal gastric secretion. The maintenance dose in cases of peptic ulcer is usually ½ of the therapeutic dose.

Dosage Forms—Tablets NF: 50 mg.

Veterinary Dose—In general, *oral* or *intramuscular,* **0.5 mg** per **pound** of body weight at 6-hour intervals.

Oxyphencyclimine Hydrochloride NF

[(1,4,5,6-Tetrahydro-1-methyl-2-pyrimidinyl)methyl α-Phenylcyclohexaneglycolate Monohydrochloride; Daricon (*Pfizer*); Vio-Thene (*Rowell*)]

Oxyphencyclimine Hydrochloride, dried in vacuum at 60° for 2.5 hours, contains 98.0–101.0% of $C_{20}H_{28}$-N_2O_3.HCl (380.92).

Preparation—Glycolonitrile is heated with ethanol and hydrogen chloride in chloroform solution to form ethyl glycolimidate hydrochloride which is then condensed with *N*-methyltrimethylenediamine in ethanol solution to give 1,4,5,6-tetrahydro-1-methyl-2-pyrimidinemethanol. Reaction with thionyl chloride converts the methanol group to chloromethyl and the chloromethyl compound is refluxed with α-phenylcyclohexaneglycolic acid in isopropanol solution to yield Oxyphencyclimine Hydrochloride. The α-phenylglycolic acid required for the last step may be prepared through Grignardization of benzoylformic acid with cyclohexyl bromide.[1]

Description—A white, odorless, crystalline powder having a characteristic bitter taste. It melts between 231° and 233° with decomposition.

Solubility—Soluble in water; slightly soluble in absolute alcohol and methylene chloride; insoluble in ether.

Uses—Oxyphencyclimine Hydrochloride is an *antimuscarinic* drug with the same qualitative actions as *Atropine* (see page 914). Its actions on the gastrointestinal and genitourinary systems are prominent. In large doses, it can decrease the secretion of gastric acid, but with the usual daytime dose its gastric effects are usually limited to decreased motility.

After oral administration its effects are manifested in 1 to 2 hours and the peak effect is reached in 6 to 8 hours. The effects last longer than 12 hours. Its principal use is in the treatment of *peptic ulcer*. Many gastroenterologists consider oxyphencyclimine to be the best antimuscarinic available for the treatment of peptic ulcer. Side effects include dry mouth, blurred vision, constipation, difficulty in urination, palpitation, elevated intraocular tension and drowsiness.

Dose—10 to **50 mg** daily, in divided doses; *usual*, **10 mg** 2 times a day.

Dosage Forms—Tablets NF: 10 mg.

Penthienate Bromide NF

[Diethyl(2-hydroxyethyl)methylammonium Bromide α-Cyclopentyl-2-thiopheneglycolate; Monodral (*Winthrop*)]

Penthienate Bromide, dried at 60° in vacuum to constant weight, contains 98.0–100.5% of $C_{18}H_{30}BrNO_3S$ (420.41).

Preparation—Sodium α-cyclopentyl-2-thiopheneglycolate is metathesized with 2-diethylaminoethyl chloride using a suitable nonpolar organic solvent as the reaction medium. After filtering and removing the solvent by evaporation, the residue of ester may be dissolved in an appropriate organic solvent and precipitated as the official quaternary salt by the addition of methyl bromide.

Description—It occurs as a white, odorless, crystalline powder. Melting range 122° to 128°.

Solubility—Soluble in water and alcohol; freely soluble in chloroform; practically insoluble in acetone and ether.

Uses—Penthienate Bromide is a quaternary ammonium *antimuscarinic* agent. It has been claimed to have characteristically greater actions on the gastrointestinal tract, especially the upper portions, than on the other neuroeffectors. Consequently it is used in the treatment of *pylorospasm, peptic ulcer, spastic colon* and to a lesser extent, *hyperhidrosis*. However, careful clinical studies show it to be *less selective for the gastrointestinal tract than even atropine*. Consequently, it is difficult to rationalize the official status of this drug. Side effects result from generalized parasympathetic blockade and include dry mouth, mydriasis, often with headache, blurred vision, constipation, urinary retention, and less commonly tachycardia and vertigo.

Dose—2.5 to **10 mg**; *usual*, **5 mg** 3 or 4 times a day.

Dosage Forms—Tablets NF: 5 mg.

Propantheline Bromide USP

[(2-Hydroxyethyl)diisopropylmethylammonium Bromide Xanthene-9-carboxylate; Pro-Banthine (*Searle*)]

Propantheline Bromide contains 98.0–102.0% of $C_{23}H_{30}BrNO_3$ (448.41), calculated on the dried basis.

Preparation—Sodium xanthene-9-carboxylate is caused to undergo metathesis with β-diisopropylaminoethyl chloride. The ester is extracted from the reaction product by means of chloroform and quaternized with methyl bromide. The crude product remaining after removal of the chloroform is purified by crystallization.

Description—White or nearly white crystals. It is odorless and has a bitter taste. It melts between 155° and 160°, with decomposition.

Solubility—Very soluble in water, alcohol, and chloroform; practically insoluble in ether and benzene.

Uses—Propantheline bromide is a quaternary ammonium *antimuscarinic* agent closely related to methantheline, which it greatly resembles in action and use (see *Methantheline Bromide*, page 921). It is somewhat more potent and induces a lesser severity of side effects. Beneficial effects in *peptic ulcer* mostly derive from decreased gastric motility, although some suppression of gastric secretion occurs after parenteral administration. Although it is superior to methantheline, it is inferior to several more recently introduced antimuscarinic drugs.

Dose—*Oral*, 30 to **75 mg** daily; *usual*, **15 mg** 4 times a day. *Parenteral*, 30 to **240 mg** daily; *usual*, **15 to 30 mg** 4 times a day.

Dosage Forms—Sterile USP: 30 mg; Tablets USP: 7.5 and 15 mg.

Veterinary Dose—Gastrointestinal sedative, *Dogs*, oral, **5 mg** 3 times daily for animal of average size (ie, approx. 30 pounds).

Thihexinol Methylbromide NF

[4-(Hydroxydi-2-thienylmethyl)cyclohexyl]trimethylammonium Bromide; Ingredient of Sorboquel (*White*)]

Thihexinol Methylbromide, dried at 105° for 3 hours, contains 98.0–102.0% of $C_{18}H_{26}BrNOS_2$ (416.45).

Preparation—Hydrolysis of the product of the reaction between two moles of thienyllithium and one mole of *trans* ethyl 4-(dimethylamino)-cyclohexylcarboxylate yields the tertiary alcohol (thixinol) which is then quaternized with methyl bromide. US Pat. 2,764,519.

Description—It occurs as a white to creamy white, crystalline powder. It melts at about 235° with decomposition.

Solubility—Sparingly soluble in water and chloroform; soluble in alcohol; very slightly soluble in acetone and ether.

Uses—Thihexinol Methylbromide is a quaternary antimuscarinic drug which is employed to *depress intestinal motility*, especially in diarrhea. Unlike other quaternary antimuscarinics, the drug is essentially devoid of ganglionic blocking actions in experimental animals; a clinical assessment of ganglionic function has not been made. Thihexinol Methylbromide appears to be devoid of an action on gastric secretion in the highest doses tested. At present, the drug is marketed only in combination with a bulk cathartic, for use in diarrheal conditions. Only two limited studies of the use of Thihexinol Methylbromide alone have been reported. Consequently, its true range of usefulness, efficacy, and limitations remains to be defined. It is surprising that a drug with so little published background has acceded to official status. Definitive studies on the rate of onset, duration of action, and fate of the drug given in official doses, are lacking. When doses of 25 to 50 mg are administered, the duration of action is longer than 2 hours.

As with other antimuscarinics, Thihexinol Methylbromide may cause side effects. With the low official dose, dry mouth and throat are the principal untoward effects that have been reported. However, a potential for other effects at other loci exists, and mydriasis, tachycardia and palpitation, blurred vision, increased intraocular pressure, vertigo, weakness, drowsiness, headache, nausea and vomiting, constipation, and urinary hesitancy and retention may occur. The drug is thus contraindicated in glaucoma, bladder neck hypertrophy, and in nursing mothers. Known or suspected obstructions in the gastrointestinal tract also contraindicate the use of the drug; it is to be avoided in duodenal obstruction, other suspected intestinal obstruction, pyloric obstruction, stenosing peptic ulcer, and cardiospasm.

Dose—*Usual*, **15 mg** 4 times a day.

Other Dose Information—The above dose is for use in combination with a bulk cathartic. It is a suboptimal dose, so that the incidence of side effects is reduced. It is questionable whether this dose actually exerts an appreciable action. 50 mg 6 times a day has been published as an effective dose. However, the cathartic employed in the marketed combination limits the dose that may be taken.

Tridihexethyl Chloride NF

[(3-Cyclohexyl-3-hydroxy-3-phenylpropyl)-triethylammonium Chloride; 3-Diethylamino-1-phenyl-1-cyclohexylpropanol Ethochloride; Pathilon (*Lederle*)]

$$\left[\underset{\underset{\bigcirc}{|}}{\overset{\overset{OH}{|}}{\underset{\bigcirc}{C}}} - CH_2 - CH_2 - \overset{+}{N}(C_2H_5)_3 \right] Cl^-$$

Tridihexethyl Chloride, dried at 105° for 2 hours, contains 98.0–100.5% of $C_{21}H_{36}ClNO$ (353.98).

Preparation—Acetophenone, formaldehyde, and diethylamine are caused to undergo the Mannich condensation by refluxing a solution of the reactants in 60 per cent ethanol. The resulting β-diethylaminopropiophenone is then subjected to a Grignard reaction with cyclohexylmagnesium bromide to yield the tridihexethyl (base). Conversion to the official quaternary compound may be effected by dissolving the purified base in a suitable organic solvent and treating with ethyl chloride.

Description—It occurs as a white, odorless, crystalline powder. Melting range 198° to 202°.

Solubility—Freely soluble in water, methanol, and chloroform; practically insoluble in ether and in acetone.

Uses—Tridihexethyl Chloride is a quaternary ammonium *antimuscarinic* agent similar to other agents in this class. (See the general statement, page 914, and

Methantheline Bromide, page 921.) It is used in the treatment of *peptic ulcer*, *gastric hyperacidity* and *hypermotility*, *spastic colon*, *functional diarrhea* and *pylorospasm*. Given orally, it does not decrease gastric secretion. Side effects are low in incidence but may include dry mouth, mydriasis, blurred vision, constipation, urinary retention and tachycardia.

Dose—**25** to **75 mg** up to 4 times a day; *usual*, **25 mg** 3 times a day and **50 mg** at bedtime.

Other Dose Information—Parenteral, 10 to 20 mg every 6 hours; oral therapy should be substituted as soon as it can be tolerated by the patient.

Dosage Forms—Tablets NF: 25 mg.

Trihexyphenidyl Hydrochloride—see page 934.

Tropicamide USP

[*N*-Ethyl-2-phenyl-*N*-(4-pyridylmethyl)hydracrylamide; Mydriacyl (*Alcon*)]

$$\underset{\underset{C_2H_5}{|}}{\underset{|}{\overset{\overset{CH_2OH}{|}}{\underset{\bigcirc}{CH}}}} - CON - CH_2 - \bigcirc N$$

Tropicamide contains 99.0–101.0% of $C_{17}H_{20}N_2O_2$ (284.36), calculated on the dried basis.

Preparation—Tropic acid is esterified with acetyl chloride and the resulting tropic acid acetate is converted to the corresponding acid chloride by reaction with thionyl chloride. Condensation of the acid chloride with 4-[(ethylamino)methyl]pyridine in the presence of an appropriate dehydrochlorinating agent yields the tropicamide acetate ester which saponifies readily to Tropicamide. US Pat. 2,726,245.

Description—A fine, white or practically white, crystalline powder that is odorless, or has not more than a slight odor, and has a bitter taste. It is stable in air, is nonhygroscopic, and is not overly light sensitive; in solution, it is highly heat stable. It melts between 96 and 100.

Solubility—1 Gm dissolves in 3 ml of chloroform, 3 ml of 2N hydrochloric acid, and 500 ml of water; freely soluble in alcohol, chloroform, and solutions of strong acids.

Uses—Tropicamide is an *antimuscarinic* drug that is used to induce *mydriasis* and *cycloplegia* in ophthalmologic practice. Applied topically to the eye it has short duration of action. The time to a maximal effect is usually 20 to 25 minutes. The duration of maximal effect is only about 15 to 20 minutes, but full recovery requires 5 to 6 hours. However, photophobia and other subjective indices of an effect may disappear as early as 2 hours after application. The drug thus has an obvious advantage over belladonna alkaloids in its shorter duration of action and over homatropine in its ability to induce cycloplegia. It is disadvantageous in that the ophthalmologist must time his examination to coincide with the time of maximal effect and that he has a brief time for examination or else that it is necessary to repeat administration at 30-minute intervals in order to obviate the timing problem.

Although Tropicamide does not increase intraocular pressure in normal persons it may do so in patients with glaucoma or those who have certain structural deformities of the anterior chamber of the eye. It should thus be used cautiously in such patients. If an antimuscarinic must be employed in such patients, Tropicamide is indicated because of its brief duration of action. Irritation or local allergic reactions have not been reported thus far nor have systemic effects.

Dose—*Topically*, **0.1 ml** of a **0.5** to **1**% solution to the conjunctiva, repeated in 5 minutes.

Other Dose Information—Topical, for mydriasis, 1 or 2 drops of a 0.5% solution instilled only once into the conjunctive sac; for refraction, 1 or 2 drops of a 1% solution instilled twice at 5-minute intervals.

Dosage Forms—Ophthalmic Solution USP: 0.5 and 1%.

Valethamate Bromide NF

[Diethyl(2-hydroxyethyl)methylammonium Bromide 3-Methyl-2-phenyl-valerate; Murel (*Ayerst*)]

$$\left[\begin{array}{c} C_2H_5 \\ | + \\ CH_3NCH_2CH_2-O-C-CHCHCH_2CH_3 \\ | \qquad\qquad\quad | \\ C_2H_5 \qquad\qquad CH_3 \end{array} \right] Br^-$$

Valethamate Bromide contains 97.0–100.5% of $C_{19}H_{32}BrNO_2$ (386.38), calculated on the dried basis.

Preparation—Benzyl cyanide is reacted in ether with 2-bromobutane in the presence of sodamide to form α-(1-methylpropyl)phenylacetonitrile and the nitrile is converted to the corresponding acid and thence to the acid chloride by the usual processes. Condensation of the acid chloride with *N,N*-diethylethanolamine in the presence of pyridine gives the 2-(diethylamino)ethyl ester of α-(1-methylpropyl)-phenylacetic acid and quaternization of the ester in ether with methyl bromide yields Valethamate Bromide. US Pat. 2,948,746.

Description—White, odorless, crystalline powder, which melts at 122°.

Solubility—Very soluble in water; soluble in ethanol and chloroform; slightly soluble in acetone, ether, and ethyl acetate.

Uses—Valethamate Bromide is a quaternary ammonium *antimuscarinic* drug with actions characteristic of *Atropine* (see page 914), except that its actions are more prominent on the gastrointestinal tract. It also has mild direct antispasmodic actions. It does not decrease gastric acid secretion; consequently, its use in *peptic ulcer* rests on its effect to decrease gastric motility. It is also used to treat *intestinal hypermotility* and *intestinal, biliary*, and *genitourinary spasm*. In acute, severe spasm the drug may be administered parenterally. Side effects include dry mouth, blurred vision, constipation, difficulty in urination, and tachycardia, although such side effects are infrequent.

Dose—*Usual, intramuscular* and *intravenous*, **10** to **20 mg** every 4 to 6 hours up to a maximum dosage of **60 mg** in a 24-hour period.

Other Dose Information—Oral, 10 to 20 mg 3 to 4 times a day.

Dosage Forms—Injection NF: 50 mg/5 ml; Extended-Release Oral Solid: 40 mg; Tablets: 10 mg.

Other Antimuscarinic Drugs

Aminopentamide Sulfate [4-(Dimethylamino)-2,2-diphenyl-valeramide sulfate] [$C_{19}H_{24}N_2O.H_2SO_4$]—A tertiary amine with parasympathetic blocking action having predominantly atropine-like pharmacologic actions. It is a white, odorless, crystalline powder, freely soluble in alcohol

and in water. A 2.5% solution has a pH range of 1.3 to 2.2. *Uses:* in the adjunctive management of peptic ulcer, pylorospasm, and chronic hypertrophic gastritis when associated with gastric hyperacidity and hypermotility; for the postoperative care of ileostomy patients. Clinical results accord the drug no special status. Side effects are those of atropine. *Dose:* orally, 0.5 mg 3 or 4 times daily.

Amprotropine Phosphate [$C_{18}H_{29}NO_3.H_3PO_4$]—The phosphate of *dl*-tropic acid ester of 3-(diethylamino)-2,2-dimethyl-1-propanol. White, crystalline powder, soluble in water. *Uses:* the main pharmacological effect of Amprotropine, one of the older synthetic substitutes for atropine, is to relax, by direct spasmolytic action, the musculature of the gastrointestinal and genitourinary tracts. It has little effect on the bronchi, uterus, and gastric secretion. Conventional therapeutic doses are practically devoid of pupillary, salivary, secretory, or cardiovascular effect. Amprotropine has topical anesthetic potency; the direct local anesthetic action following oral administration may interrupt local gastrointestinal reflexes and thus be a factor in reducing smooth muscle spasm. Although the drug has been recommended for the symptomatic relief of gastrointestinal, vesical, and urethral spasm and for dysmenorrhea, recent reports deny that it has clinically useful spasmolytic action. *Dose:* orally, 50 to 100 mg, repeated 3 or 4 times daily.

Anisotropine Methylbromide [Valpin (*Endo*)] is 8-methyltropinium bromide 2-propylvalerate [$C_{17}H_{32}BrNO_2 = 362.33$]. *Preparation:* Tropine (base) is esterified with 2-propylvaleryl chloride and the ester is then quaternized with methyl bromide. US Pat. 2,962,499. *Description and Solubility:* A white, glistening powder or plates that are probably odorless; when inhaled, one is immediately aware of an extremely bitter taste with a choking sensation; it is stable in light, heat, and air; its melting range varies; ie, if the capillary tube is set into the bath at 272° (heating rate: 2°/minute), it will sublime quite suddenly at about 305°; between 305° and 339° (heating rate (2°/minute), melting will be observed between 315° and 318°. Soluble in water and chloroform; sparingly soluble in alcohol; slightly soluble in acetone; insoluble in ether.

Uses: Anisotropine Methylbromide is a quaternary ammonium antimuscarinic drug. It appears to be relatively selective for the gastrointestinal tract and to cause a low incidence of side effects at recommended doses. However, it probably has very little effect on gastric secretion. It is used in the treatment of *mucous colitis* and *irritable colon, spastic colitis, biliary dyskinesia, cholelithiasis, pylorospam, gastritis duodenitis*, and *peptic ulcer*. Its effect in ulcer is mainly to lessen gastric motility in order that antacids be better retained in the stomach. *Dose:* 10 mg 3 or 4 times a day, before meals and at bedtime.

Dibutoline Sulfate [Dibuline Sulfate (*MSD*)] is bis-[ethyl-2(hydroxyethyl)dimethylammonium] sulfate bis-(dibutylcarbamate) [$C_{30}H_{66}N_4O_8S$]. *Description and Solubility:* An extremely hygroscopic powder which decomposes at 166°; pH (5% aqueous solution), 6.75 to 7.50; aqueous solutions are stable at room temperature for 1 year, but decompose when heated at 100°; therefore, sterilization by filtration is recommended. Soluble in water and benzene. *Uses:* Structurally closely related to carbachol, but the *N*-substituents are larger. The drug combines with the cholinergic (muscarinic) receptor but is incapable of exciting it; hence the drug is an *antimuscarinic*. It is advocated for the therapy of peptic ulcer and other gastrointestinal hyperactivity, but it has no special selectivity for the gastrointestinal tract and hence is inferior to many other agents. In general its actions and usefulness are very similar to those of *Atropine* (page 914). However, as a mydriatic and cycloplegic it has the advantage of rapid onset and short duration of action. It is not absorbed by the oral route, so that systemic use requires parenteral administration. *Dose:* Subcutaneous or intramuscular, 5 to 40 mg every 4 to 6 hours; topically, to eye, 7.5% aqueous solution.

Hexocyclium Methylsulfate [Tral (*Abbott*)] is 4-(β-cyclohexyl - β - hydroxyphenethyl) - 1,1 - dimethylpiperazinium dimethylsulfate [$C_{21}H_{36}N_2O_5S$]. *Description and Solubility:* Crystals which melt between 200° and 210°. 1 Gm dissolves in about 2 ml of water; slightly soluble in chloroform; insoluble in ether. *Uses:* A quaternary ammonium *antimuscarinic* agent with mild ganglionic blocking properties. However, it has no special selectivity for the gastrointestinal tract, and its variable effect on gastric secretion makes it inferior to several other more selective agents. Its actions, side effects and uses are those of *Atropine* (page 914). *Dose: Oral,* 25 mg 4 times a day, with dosage adjustments as needed.

Methixene Hydrochloride [Trest (*Dorsey*)] is 1-methyl-3-(thioxanthen-9-ylmethyl)piperidine hydrochloride [$C_{20}H_{23}$-NS.HCl = 345.94]. *Preparation:* 3-Pyridinemethanol is reacted with methyl iodide and the resulting quaternary is hydrogenated to form *N*-methyl-3-piperidinemethanol. This alcohol is then reacted with thionyl chloride and the 3-(chloromethyl)-1-methylpiperidine thus formed is coupled with thioxanthene sodium. US Pat. 2,905,590. *Description and Solubility:* A white powder which is practically odorless and has a bitter taste; stable in air; darkens slowly in light; melts between 213° and 217°. Soluble in water, alcohol, and chloroform; insoluble in ether.

Uses: Methixene is an *antimuscarinic* drug. Although it is a tertiary rather than quaternary amine, it has a relatively high selectivity for the gastrointestinal tract. It is used in the management of conditions in which there is hypermotility, as in *pylorospasm, biliary dyskinesia, spastic colon, duodenitis* and *gastritis,* and in other disorders in which it is desirable to diminish even normal motility, as in *duodenal ulcer.* It does not diminish gastric secretion. Although it is recommended for use in gastric ulcer, a decrease in motility can result in retention of acid and hence sometimes exacerbate the erosive process. The incidence of side effects is low with the usual doses. Side effects include dry mouth, blurred vision, and urinary retention. The drug is contraindicated in pyloric obstruction, intestinal obstruction, cardiospasm, prostatic hypertrophy, urinary bladder neck obstruction, duodenal stenosis, and stenosing peptic ulcer. *Dose: Oral,* 1 to 2 mg 3 times a day.

Oxyphenonium Bromide [Antrenyl Bromide (*Ciba*)] is diethyl(2-hydroxyethyl)methylammonium bromide α-phenylcyclohexaneglycolate [$C_{21}H_{34}BrNO_3$]. *Description and Solubility:* A white, crystalline powder that melts between 193° and 196°; its aqueous solutions are neutral. Freely soluble in water and alcohol; insoluble in ether and acetone. *Uses:* A quaternary ammonium *antimuscarinic* agent with a moderate selectivity for the gastrointestinal tract. It decreases gastric motility and in large doses transiently decreases gastric secretion; the effects on secretion are not elicited under ordinary conditions of use. It also reduces intestinal motility. It is used in the treatment of *peptic ulcer,* in *intestinal hypermotility,* and *spastic colon.* It may cause dry mouth, mydriasis and blurring of vision, constipation, difficulty in urination, and, less commonly, weakness, dizziness, drowsiness, nausea, vomiting, headache, and tachycardia. *Dose: Oral,* 10 mg 4 times daily, with adjustments; *subcutaneous* or *intramuscular,* 1 to 2 mg every 6 hours.

Pentapiperide Methylsulfate [Quilene (*Warner-Chilcott*)] is 4-hydroxy-1,1-dimethylpiperidinium methyl sulfate 3-methyl-2-phenylvalerate ($C_{20}H_{23}NO_6S$). *Uses:* An antimuscarinic drug promoted especially for its effect to suppress gastric secretion. Thus its principal use is in the management of peptic ulcer. However, it may also be used to decrease gastrointestinal motility. Pentapiperide is the most recent of the antimuscarinic drugs. Consequently, several years of clinical experience will be required to ascertain the true therapeutic value of this drug. Side effects include dry mouth, cycloplegia with blurring of vision, mydriasis and photosensitivity, difficulty in urination, constipation, nausea, headache, and hypersensitivity. The drug is contraindicated in the presence of gastric retention, stenosing peptic ulcer, pyloric obstruction or stenosis, prostatic hypertrophy and urinary bladder neck obstruction, any other known or suspected obstruction in the gastrointestinal or genitourinary tracts, megaesophagus, organic cardiospasm, glaucoma, and hypersensitivity to the drug. *Dose:* 10 to 20 mg 3 to 4 times a day; an extra 10 mg may be taken at bedtime. The dose should be individualized on the basis of gastric function tests and individual tolerance.

Pipenzolate Bromide [Piptal (*Lakeside*)] is 3-hydroxy-1-ethyl-1-methylpiperidinium bromide benzilate [$C_{22}H_{28}$-BrNO$_3$]. *Description and Solubility:* A white to light-cream powder that melts with decomposition between 176° and 182°. 1 Gm dissolves in 1.5 ml of water, 5.1 ml of chloroform, 0.69 ml of methanol, and 10.2 ml of absolute alcohol. *Uses:* A quaternary ammonium derivative of *Piperidolate Hydrochloride* (below). It has *antimuscarinic* actions with moderate selectivity for the gastrointestinal tract. It relaxes gastrointestinal smooth muscle and hence finds use in the treatment of *irritable colon, ileitis, diarrhea,* etc, and also *biliary spasm.* In large doses, but not under ordinary conditions of use, it briefly decreases the secretion of gastric acid. Its efficacy in the treatment of peptic ulcer is mainly due to decreased gastric motility. Its side effects are those of *Atropine* (page 914), but they are generally much more mild. *Dose: Oral,* 4 mg 3 times daily before meals and 5 to 10 mg at bedtime, subject to individual adjustments.

Piperidolate Hydrochloride [Dactil (*Lakeside*)] is 1-ethyl-3-piperidyl diphenylacetate hydrochloride [$C_{21}H_{25}$-NO$_2$.HCl]. *Description and Solubility:* A white powder that melts with decomposition between 194° and 198°. 1 Gm dissolves in 18.3 ml of water, 3.6 ml of chloroform, 4.7 ml of methanol, and 52.5 ml of absolute alcohol. *Uses:* An *antimuscarinic* agent with spasmolytic actions mainly on the upper gastrointestinal tract, but it does not relax biliary smooth muscle. It also does not decrease gastric secretion. It is mainly used in the treatment of cardiospasm, pylorospasm, gastroduodenal spasm, and biliary dyskinesia. It is relatively free of atropine-like side effects (see *Atropine,* page 914) but such may occur occasionally. *Dose: Oral,* 50 mg 4 times daily.

Poldine Methylsulfate [Nacton (*McNeil*)] is 2-(hydroxymethyl)-1,1-dimethylpyrrolidinium methyl sulfate benzilate ($C_{22}H_{29}NO_7S$). *Description and Solubility:* A creamy white, crystalline compound; soluble in water. *Uses:* An antimuscarinic drug claimed to have a selective effect on gastrointestinal functions. Thus, it is promoted for use in the treatment of "hyperacidity," peptic ulcer, gastritis, ulcerative colitis, duodenitis, enteritis, dumping syndrome, and pancreatitis. Although early reports were that the drug may suppress gastric secretion by more than 50%, very little effect on gastric secretion occurs with tolerated oral doses, and authoritative gastroenterologists do not recommend the drug for the management of peptic ulcer. However, the drug does somewhat suppress gastrointestinal hypermotility. Side effects include dry mouth, mydriasis, cycloplegia with blurring of vision, constipation, tachycardia, and difficulty in urination. The drug is contraindicated in urinary bladder neck obstruction, prostatic hypertrophy, glaucoma, gastric retention, pyloric obstruction or stenosis, stenosing peptic ulcer, other known or suspected obstructions of the gastrointestinal tract, megaesophagus, and organic cardiospasm. *Dose:* 4 mg 3 to 4 times a day.

Thiphenamil Hydrochloride [2-diethylaminoethyl diphenylthioacetate hydrochloride; $C_{20}H_{25}NOS$.HCl; Trocinate (*Poythress*)]—White powder, with a bitter taste and a potent local anesthetic effect. Melting point at 129°. Soluble 1:25 in water; soluble in alcohol. *Uses:* antispasmodic for gastrointestinal and genitourinary spasms. *Dose: 200 mg,* 4 times a day.

Tricyclamol Chloride [Elorine (*Lilly*)] is 1-(3-cyclohexyl - 3 - hydroxy - 3 - phenylpropyl) - 1 - methylpyrrolidinium chloride [$C_{20}H_{32}ClNO$]. *Description and Solubility:* A white, extremely bitter-tasting, crystalline powder that has a faint odor; stable in light, air, and heat. Soluble in alcohol and water. *Uses:* A quaternary ammonium derivative of procyclidine and possesses the general properties of quaternary ammonium antimuscarinic agents. It thus is moderately selective for the gastrointestinal tract, suppressing hypermotility but not gastric secretion. It is used in the treatment of *peptic ulcer, chronic hypertrophic gastritis, pylorospasm,* and *irritable colon.* It lacks the central actions and uses of the parent tertiary compound. Side effects include dry mouth, occasional mydriasis, and blurring of vision and occasional urinary retention. *Dose: Oral,* 50 to 500 mg (average, 100 to 150 mg) 4 to 6 times daily.

Miscellaneous Antispasmodics

Several antispasmodics are not antimuscarinic drugs, although they may nonselectively suppress a cholinergically induced spasm. A few, such as adiphenine (see below) were synthesized in quest of antimuscarinic drugs but did not prove to have significant anticholinergic activity. Others, such as alverine, were offshoots of efforts to create new adrenergic drugs. Such miscellaneous antispasmodics are included in this chapter only for convenience, since the nonselective antispasmodics do not comprise a large enough group to warrant a separate chapter.

Alverine Citrate NF

[N-Ethyl-3,3',-diphenyldipropylamine Citrate (1:1); Profenil (*Smith, Miller & Patch*); Spacolin (*Philips-Roxane*)]

Alverine Citrate contains 99.0–102.0% of $C_{20}H_{27}N \cdot C_6H_8O_7$ (473.57), calculated on the dried basis.

Preparation—3-Phenylpropyl bromide is condensed with ethylamine in an alkaline medium. The alverine (base) thus formed is dissolved in a suitable solvent and reacted with an equimolar portion of citric acid to form the official salt.

Description—A white to off-white powder having a sweet odor and a slightly bitter taste. It melts between 100° and 102°.

Solubility—Slightly soluble in water and chloroform; sparingly soluble in alcohol; very slightly soluble in ether; soluble in dilute acids.

Uses—Alverine Citrate is a nonselective *antispasmodic*. It is used in the management of gastrointestinal disorders in which hypermotility or spasm is involved, such as *spastic colon, diarrhea, duodenitis, gastritis* or *achalasia*, in *biliary dyskinesia* and *cholelithiasis*, and in *genitourinary spasm*, such as may accompany the passage of a stone, urinary tract infection, or prostatic hypertrophy. Since antimuscarinics are contraindicated in prostatic hypertrophy, alverine enjoys a special status in the management of this disorder. Although alverine has been once claimed to decrease gastric secretion, there is no evidence that it does so under ordinary conditions of use. Any benefits in peptic ulcer derive from a lessening of gastrointestinal motility and a prolongation of the retention of antacids in the stomach. It may also be used in certain *primary dysmenorrheas* and to aid in various *endoscopic examinations*. Hypotension, drowsiness, and dizziness are the most frequent side effects.

Dose—*Usual*, **120 mg** 1 to 3 times a day.
Dosage Forms—Tablets NF: 120 mg.

Ethaverine Hydrochloride—See page 855.

Isometheptene—See page 897.

Papaverine Hydrochloride—see page 854.

Other Miscellaneous Antispasmodics

Adiphenine Hydrochloride [Trasentine (*Ciba*)]—The hydrochloride of 2-(diethylamino)ethyl diphenylacetate [$C_{20}H_{25}NO_2 \cdot HCl$]. Crystals. Melting point 113° to 114°. Freely soluble in water. *Uses:* a synthetic antispasmodic. The compound exerts a direct spasmolytic action on the musculature of the gastrointestinal and genitourinary tracts, but effects on the pupil, secretions, and cardiovascular system are insignificant. Adiphenine is structurally related to the local anesthetics; it is more potent and less toxic than cocaine. It has been suggested that a directly local anesthetic effect on gastric mucosa may be a factor in the rapid relief from pain that it affords in certain cases of peptic ulcer and that this effect may, by interrupting local reflex pathways necessary for local gastrointestinal tone and motility, account for part of the drug's spasmolytic action. Adiphenine has been employed for the symptomatic relief of gastrointestinal disorders characterized by spasm; for spastic conditions of the gall bladder and biliary ducts; for dysmenorrhea; for ureteral colic; and for neurogenic bladder and certain other types of dysuria. Although the drug is relatively nontoxic, it should not be used in close sequence with morphine; the combination appears to cause apprehension and tachycardia. *Dose:* 75 to 150 mg, 2 or 3 times daily.

Carbofluorene Aminoester [Pavatrine Hydrochloride (*Searle*); Robitrin (*Robins*)] is 2-(diethylamino)ethyl 9-fluorenecarboxylate hydrochloride [$C_{20}H_{23}NO_2 \cdot HCl$]. Crystals. Melting point 143° to 144°. Soluble in water.

Uses: A synthetic antispasmodic; the smooth muscle relaxant properties are due in part, but not completely, to antimuscarinic actions. It is promoted for use in the treatment of spastic colon and spasms of the duodenum and stomach. It may provide relief in cholecystitis by relaxing the sphincter of Oddi. It is also claimed to be of benefit in urinary tenesmus and in dysmenorrhea, when uterine hypertension is present. Side effects attributable to antimuscarinic actions occur; they include, especially, dry mouth and constipation, but a potential for other antimuscarinic untoward effects, such as cycloplegia and difficulty in micturition, exists. Dizziness also occurs. Carbofluorene Aminoester should not be administered in patients with glaucoma or with known or suspected stenoses or obstructions in the gastrointestinal or genitourinary tracts. *Dose:* 125 mg 2 or 3 times a day.

References

1. Faust, J. A., *et al, J. Am. Chem. Soc.*, **81**, 2214 (1959).

This chapter was prepared by

Ewart A. Swinyard, PhD, *Professor of Pharmacology, College of Pharmacy and College of Medicine, University of Utah, Salt Lake City, Utah 84112, and* Stewart C. Harvey, PhD, *Associate Professor of Pharmacology, College of Medicine, University of Utah, Salt Lake City, Utah 84112*

Skeletal muscle may be relaxed by blocking the effect of somatic motor nerve impulses or by depressing the appropriate neurones within the central nervous system so that somatic motor nerve impulses fail to be generated. Interruption of certain afferent reflex pathways, as by local anesthesia, may also effect relaxation of circumscribed muscle groups; local anesthetic block of efferent somatic motor outflow is also sometimes employed to relieve localized skeletal muscle spasm. In this chapter only those drugs that act at the myoneural junction, the *neuromuscular blocking drugs*, and those drugs that act upon central neurones, the *centrally acting muscle relaxants*, will be treated. The *antiparkinson drugs* are covered in the latter section.

Neuromuscular Blocking Drugs

Neuromuscular blocking drugs act by rendering the motor end plate membrane of the myoneural junction incapable of responding to acetylcholine, the normal transmitter. Drugs of the curare type, which generally contain two, but at least one, quaternary ammonium groups and a bulky structure, appear to compete with acetylcholine and, hence, prevent access of the transmitter to the receptors. Such drugs are called *stabilizing* neuromuscular blocking drugs. On the other hand, certain of the simple skeleton-like bisquaternary synthetics, such as decamethonium or succinylcholine, have an initial phase of action in which they mimic acetylcholine and depolarize the motor end-plate membrane; initial blockade is the result of persisting depolarization, so that the membrane cannot repolarize to accept new stimuli. Such agents are called *depolarizing* neuromuscular blocking agents. However, there develops a later phase of action during which the membrane repolarizes, and yet the block persists. In this phase, the drugs resemble the stabilizing agents. Different muscle fibers may vary with respect to the predominant phase at any one time. Stabilizing blocking agents can be antagonized with anticholinesterases, such as neostigmine (see Chapter 49, page 902), which also compete with the blocking drug. Edrophonium and neostigmine both combine anticholinesterase and cholinomimetic actions. The "depolarizing" agents are difficult to antagonize because anticholinesterases or cholinomimetics may either potentiate or antagonize, depending upon the phase of action of the blocking drug.

The neuromuscular blocking agents are mainly used to promote muscular relaxation during surgery, during orthopedic manipulations, and to relax the laryngeal muscles for bronchoscopy.

Several of these agents, prepared in specially constructed cartridge-needle units and propelled by compressed air from a rifle, have been used in the capture of wild and/or unruly animals. Mortality among the targets is comparatively high; the advantage, of course, is that the risk of physical injury to the captor is minimized.

Dimethyl Tubocurarine Iodide NF

[(+)-*O,O'*-Dimethyltubocurarine Diiodide; Metubine Iodide (*Lilly*)]

Dimethyl Tubocurarine Iodide, dried in vacuum at 75° for 8 hours, contains 95.0–105.0% of $C_{40}H_{48}I_2N_2O_6$ (906.65).

Dimethyl Tubocurarine Iodide is the dimethyl ether of *d*-tubocurarine iodide.

For the structure of tubocurarine, see *Tubocurarine Chloride*, page 929.

Preparation—It may be prepared by methylation of the naturally occurring *d*-tubocurarine, with methyl iodide or dimethyl sulfate, and then forming the diiodide.

Description—An odorless, white or pale yellow crystalline powder.

Solubility—Slightly soluble in water, diluted hydrochloric acid, and diluted solutions of sodium hydroxide; very slightly soluble in alcohol; practically insoluble in benzene, chloroform, and ether.

Uses—Dimethyl Tubocurarine Iodide has essentially the same actions and uses as *Tubocurarine Chloride* (page 929). In man, Dimethyl Tubocurarine Iodide is approximately three times more potent than *d*-tubocurarine chloride.

Dose—*Usual, intravenous, initial,* **1.5** to **8 mg** given over a 60-second period; *maintenance,* **500 mcg** to **1 mg** every 25 to 90 minutes.

Other Dose Information—The initial dose depends on the anesthetic employed; with ether: 1.5 to 3 mg; with cyclopropane: 2 to 4 mg; with nitrous oxide–thiopental: 3 to 8 mg. Supplementary doses, which may be required after 25 to 90 minutes, should be 0.5 to 1 mg. All doses are given *intravenously*.

Dosage Forms—Injection NF: 5 mg/10 ml, 10 mg/10 ml, 40 mg/20 ml, 50 mg/50 ml.

Gallamine Triethiodide USP

[v-Phenenyltris(oxyethylene)]tris[triethylammonium] Triiodide; [1,2,3-Tris-(β-diethylaminoethoxy)benzene Triethiodide; Flaxedil (*Lederle*)]

$$\left[\begin{array}{c} OCH_2CH_2\overset{+}{N}(C_2H_5)_3 \\ OCH_2CH_2\overset{+}{N}(C_2H_5)_3 \\ OCH_2CH_2\overset{+}{N}(C_2H_5)_3 \end{array}\right] 3\,I^-$$

Gallamine Triethiodide contains 98.0–101.0% of $C_{30}H_{60}I_3N_3O_3$ (891.54), calculated on the dried basis.

Preparation—Pyrogallol is condensed with 2-chloro-triethylamine and the resulting triamine [2,2''',2'''''''-(v-phenenyltrioxy)tris(triethylamine)] is quaternized with ethyl iodide in boiling acetone. The crude product which precipitates is purified by repeated crystallization from hot ethanol.

Description—Occurs as a white, odorless, amorphous powder. It is hygroscopic.
Solubility—Very soluble in water; sparingly soluble in alcohol; very slightly soluble in chloroform.
Note—Gallamine Triethiodide exhibits a pharmaceutical incompatibility with meperidine hydrochloride (solutions must not be mixed).

Uses—Gallamine triethiodide is a neuromuscular blocking drug similar in its actions and uses to *d*-tubocurarine (see *Tubocurarine Chloride*, this page. However, it has very little action on autonomic ganglia. It also does not release histamine.
Dose—*Usual, intravenous, initial,* **1 mg** per **Kg** of body weight, then **500 mcg to 1 mg** at 30- to 60-minute intervals if necessary.
Dosage Forms—Injection USP: 100 mg/ml, 200 mg/10 ml.

Succinylcholine Chloride USP

[Suxamethonium Chloride; Choline Chloride Succinate (2:1); Anectine Chloride (*Burroughs-Wellcome*); Quelicin Chloride (*Abbott*); Sucostrin Chloride (*Squibb*); Sux-Cert (*Travenol*)]

$$\left[\begin{array}{c} COOCH_2CH_2\overset{+}{N}(CH_3)_3 \\ (CH_2)_2 \\ COOCH_2CH_2\overset{+}{N}(CH_3)_3 \end{array}\right] 2Cl^-$$

Succinylcholine Chloride usually contains approximately two molecules of water of hydration. It contains 98.0–101.0% of $C_{14}H_{30}Cl_2N_2O_4$ (361.31), calculated on the anhydrous basis.
Preparation—It may be prepared by condensing succinyl chloride with β-dimethylaminoethanol and quaternizing the resulting ester with methyl chloride.

Description—A white, odorless, crystalline powder. Its solutions are acid to litmus, having a pH of about 4. Melting range between 158° and 164°, without previous drying.
Solubility—1 Gm dissolves in about 1 ml of water and about 350 ml of alcohol; slightly soluble in chloroform; practically insoluble in ether.

Uses—Succinylcholine Chloride is a neuromuscular blocking agent of the so-called depolarizing type (see the *General Statement*, page 928). It usually has very transient duration of action because of rapid hydrolysis of the drug by cholinesterases. The effects of a single injection usually last only a few minutes. Prolonged muscular relaxation is achieved by continuous intravenous infusion, and the intensity of muscle paralysis is readily controlled by adjustment of the infusion rate.

Succinylcholine Chloride does not cause liberation of histamine and the drug is well tolerated. Muscle aching resulting from its transient stimulatory action is minimized by slow initial administration. Premedication with atropine or scopolamine is necessary to prevent salivation. No specific pharmacological antagonist of the skeletal muscle effects is available. Its actions may be prolonged in individuals with reduced plasma cholinesterase activity.

Single doses of Succinylcholine Chloride are employed *to facilitate endotracheal intubation, to relax laryngospasm,* and *to reduce the severity of convulsions* in psychiatric patients undergoing *electroconvulsive therapy.* Administered by continuous intravenous infusion, the drug is also serviceable for production of skeletal muscle relaxation during longer surgical procedures such as open heart surgery. Succinylcholine Chloride appears to be a valuable addition to the list of adjuncts available to the anesthesiologist.
Dose—*Intravenous,* **10 to 40 mg;** *usual,* **30 mg;** *infusion,* **2.5 mg** of a **0.1 to 0.2%** solution per minute.
Other Dose Information—Dosage is highly individualized and varies from 0.6 to 7.5 mg per minute for maintenance of adequate relaxation. The average adult dose is 2 to 3 mg per minute.
Dosage Forms—Injection USP: 200 and 500 mg and 1 Gm/10 ml; Sterile USP: 500 mg and 1 Gm.
Veterinary Dose—In restraint of horses for procedures such as castration, dentistry, therapeusis, bandaging, ligations or during surgical procedures where a muscle relaxant is desirable. To produce muscular relaxation and recumbency, single intravenous injection of **4 mg** per **100 pounds** of body weight given rapidly (10 to 30 seconds). If initial dose is inadequate, allow 5 minutes for effect to dissipate then repeat injection, adding 4 to 8 mg per animal to previously calculated dose. Horses, who have high pseudo-cholinesterase levels, metabolize the drug very rapidly by hydrolysis; species with low plasma cholinesterase levels (cattle, sheep and goats) exhibit prolonged respiratory paralysis requiring artificial respiration. Paralytic effect of the drug is not antagonized by cholinesterase inhibitors such as neostigmine, physostigmine and edrophonium but it is generally intensified and prolonged.

Tubocurarine Chloride USP

[(+)-Tubocurarine Dichloride; *d*-Tubocurarine Chloride]

Tubocurarine Chloride [$C_{38}H_{44}Cl_2N_2O_6.5H_2O$ = 785.77] contains 98.0–102.0% of $C_{38}H_{44}Cl_2N_2O_6$, calculated on the anhydrous basis.

Tubocurarine Chloride is the hydrated chloride of a quaternary base obtained from the bark and stems of *Chondodendron tomentosum* and related species.
Preparation—Tubocurarine Chloride is isolated from the stems and bark of the freshly gathered plant *Chondodendron tomentosum* which is extracted with small portions of water. The aqueous extracts are concentrated to a brownish black syrupy paste which

is autoclaved and then evaporated to dryness. The residue is extracted with an aqueous solution of tartaric acid and the extracts are treated with excess lead subacetate. The precipitated lead salts are separated and the filtrate, after removal of the soluble lead as its sulfide, is made slightly alkaline and extracted with chloroform to remove other alkaloids. The chloroform-extracted water solution is acidulated with sulfuric acid to pH 3 and treated with picric acid. The insoluble picrate is separated, purified by recrystallization from a mixture of acetone and ethanol, and converted to tubocurarine chloride by treatment with dilute hydrochloric acid in the presence of toluene. The product distributes in the aqueous acid layer and picric acid distributes in the toluene layer. Tubocurarine crystallizes from the aqueous acid layer on chilling. Further purification is achieved by recrystallization from 6% hydrochloric acid.

Description—A white or yellowish white to grayish white, odorless, crystalline powder. It melts with slight decomposition at about 270°.

Solubility—1 Gm dissolves in about 20 ml of water and about 45 ml of alcohol; insoluble in acetone, chloroform, and ether.

Uses—Tubocurarine Chloride is a neuromuscular blocking agent which possesses the actions typical of curare. Its primary effect is inhibition of the transmission of nervous impulses to skeletal muscle by a competitive blockade of acetylcholine. Consequently, its effects can be antagonized by cholinesterase inhibitors, such as neostigmine and edrophonium. The neuromuscular effects of tubocurarine are potentiated by ether, so that only one-third of the usual dose of the blocking agent may be required. It produces muscular relaxation without significant nervous system depression. It may cause a fall in blood pressure and bronchospasm by releasing histamine from the tissues. The principal use of this agent is to supplement gas or thiopental anesthesia and thus to provide adequate skeletal muscular relaxation with small amounts of the primary agent. The paralyzant effects usually last from 30 to 60 minutes. The muscles of respiration are usually the most resistant, but the drug is a powerful relaxing agent and should be employed only by adequately trained personnel under conditions which allow for artificial respiration and, if necessary, for the intratracheal administration of oxygen in case of mishap. Tubocurarine chloride is also employed to decrease the severity of muscle contraction during pentamethylenetetrazol and electroshock therapy. It has received trial to decrease muscle tone in various spastic conditions, but the results have usually been disappointing. Small doses may be employed with care in the diagnosis of myasthenia gravis, the myasthenic patient being extremely sensitive to the paralytic effects of curare.

In cases of overdosage, in addition to artificial positive-pressure respiration with oxygen, parenteral neostigmine or edrophonium may be cautiously employed as an antidote to the paralyzing effect on neuromuscular junctions.

Dose—*Usual, intravenous,* **6 to 9 mg** in 30 to 90 seconds, followed in 5 minutes by **3 to 6 mg** more if necessary.

Other Dose Information—Tubocurarine Chloride is given *intravenously,* occasionally intramuscularly. Except when ether anesthesia is employed, the *usual* initial dose for *surgery* is 6 to 9 mg (40–60 units) *slowly,* if necessary, in 3 to 5 minutes an additional 3 to 4.5 mg may be given; this dose may be repeated at appropriate intervals. If ether anesthesia is employed, the above doses should be cut to one-third. In *shock therapy,* 3 mg per 18 Kg of body weight may be given. In the *diagnosis of myasthenia gravis,* 0.3 mg per 18 Kg are given.

Dosage Forms—Injection USP: 15 mg/ml, 30 mg/10 and 20 ml.

Other Neuromuscular Blockings Drugs

Curare—A name applied to extracts principally of the bark and of other parts of plants of certain species of *Chondodendron* or *Strychnos,* especially *Chondodendron tomentosum* and *Strychnos toxiferin,* prepared by South American Indians of the Upper Amazon and Orinoco basins for use as arrow poisons. The extracts contain neuromuscular paralyzant alkaloids and numerous other contaminants. The chondodendron alkaloids contain tertiary and quaternary benzylisoquinoline derivatives such as *d*-tubocurarine (see *Tubocurarine Chloride*), *curine,* and related compounds. The strychnos alkaloids contain β-carboline alkaloids such as the toxiferins and calabash *curarines.* None of the crude preparations is currently used in therapeutics. Only purified preparations or alkaloids from *Chondodendron tomentosum* are commercially available.

Decamethonium Bromide [Syncurine (*Burroughs-Wellcome*)] is decamethylenebis[trimethylammonium bromide]. *Description and Solubility:* Crystals which decompose at 255° and 267°. Aqueous solutions are stable and therefore may be autoclaved. Freely soluble in water and alcohol; very slightly soluble in chloroform; insoluble in ether. *Uses:* A neuromuscular blocking agent of the so-called depolarizing type (see the *General Statement,* page 928). After intravenous injection, skeletal muscle paralysis is maximal within 3 to 4 minutes and has passed by 20 to 30 minutes, the drug thus having shorter duration of action than *d*-tubocurarine but longer than that of succinylcholine. It is employed for muscle relaxation during short surgical procedures, manipulations such as bronchoscopy and the setting of fractures, and to prevent injury during electroshock therapy. *Dose: Intravenously,* 0.5 to 3 mg.

Dimethyl Tubocurarine Chloride [Mecostrin Chloride (*Squibb*)] is the dimethyl ether of *d*-tubocurarine chloride, page 929. *Description and Solubility:* Crystals which decompose at about 236° with effervescence. Soluble in water and dilute sodium hydroxide; sparingly soluble in alcohol, dilute hydrochloric acid, and chloroform; practically insoluble in benzene and ether. *Uses:* Essentially those of *Tubocurarine Chloride* (page 929); the dimethyl derivative is about 3 times as potent. *Dose: Intravenously,* 2 to 3 mg over a period of ½ to 1 minute, with a 1- to 15-mg supplement in 3 to 5 minutes, if needed. After the effect of the primary dose has begun to wane (about 45 minutes) an additional dose of 1.5 to 2 mg may be given. When the general anesthetic is an ether, the above doses should be cut to 33%. For *shock therapy* and *manipulative procedures,* 0.05 to 0.08 mg per Kg of body weight.

Hexafluorenium Bromide [Mylaxen (*Neisler*)] [hexamethylenebis[fluorene-9-yldimethyl ammonium bromide]]— *Uses:* A neuromuscular paralyzant with an unknown mechanism of action. Although it stabilizes the motor end-plate it potentiates rather than antagonizes succinylcholine, a depolarizer. The neuromuscular block caused by Hexafluorenium is not antagonized by anticholinesterases or acetylcholine. The drug has anticholinesterase properties of its own. It is used mainly in combination with succinylcholine; the effective dose of succinylcholine is thereby reduced, the paralysis is more complete, and muscular fasciculations and consequent postoperative muscle soreness is virtually eliminated. On the one hand, because of the anticholinesterase properties of Hexafluorenium, the hydrolysis of succinylcholine is impaired; thus, the action of succinylcholine may be prolonged unless the dose is small. On the other hand, the build-up of succinylmonocholine and choline is prevented, so that apnea from these products is avoided. *Dose:* To be determined by the anesthesiologist; the range is *40 to 200 mg.*

Centrally Acting Muscle Relaxants and Antiparkinson Drugs

The cell bodies of the somatic motor nerves lie within the spinal cord and, hence, within the central nervous system. They have very little spontaneous activity, and motor activity is initiated by afferent impulses directly or indirectly from the sensory nerves and by nerves descending from voluntary and involuntary motor areas in the brain. The motor neurones may also be inhibited by appropriate afferent impulses directly and indirectly from the sensory nerves and by inhibitory nerves descending from various regions of the brain. Thus, the control of motor nerve activity is complex, and pharmacological agents may influence a given motor neurone from a number of possible loci in the brain and in the spinal cord. At the present, all practical centrally acting relaxants appear to depress neuronal activity rather than to stimulate inhibitory nerves. On the other hand, in the usual therapeutic doses none of them acts directly on the motor neurone, but rather upon impinging exciting neurones. The *interneurone depressants* such as mephenesin, meprobamate, phenaglycodol, etc. depress the internuncial neurones that mediate between sensory or descending nerve fibers and the motor neurone. The selectivity for the interneurone does not result from qualitative differences between interneurone and motor neurone; rather, it results from the fact that impulse generation in the interneurone is more critically balanced than in the motor neurone. In higher dosage, interneurone depressants will depress the motor neurone directly. Interneurone depressants are especially indicated to induce muscle relaxation in spasticity or rigidity in which spinal reflex activity contributes considerably to the excited state of the motor neurone, provided there are interneurones in the reflex arc. In paralysis agitans (Parkinsonism) and similar drug-induced states (eg, by major tranquilizers; see Chapter 62), where the neurological deficit is in a much more removed, subtle, and intricate portion of the central nervous system (ie, in basal ganglia and thalamus), the interneurone depressants are less effective. Instead, a separate group of agents, the *antiparkinsonism drugs*, which for unknown reasons are also anticholinergic agents or close derivatives (see Chapter 51, page 914), are generally more effective. The antiparkinsonism drugs do not have appreciable interneurone depressant activity. Since general anesthetics may depress all neurones, it follows that they may induce skeletal muscle relaxation at several loci, including the motor neurone itself, within the central nervous system. This effect is sought for surgical anesthesia, but, of course, the effect does not lend itself to the therapy of the spastic and related states, where ambulation and nearly normal voluntary motor control is desirable.

The basal ganglia contain a high content of L-dopamine, the immediate biological precursor of norepinephrine. L-Dopamine resides within neurones in the basal ganglia, as well as in other central nervous structures, and it undoubtedly plays a transmitter role in some central synaptic transmission. In Parkinson's disease, the L-dopamine content of the basal ganglia is considerably lower than normal; it is the basal ganglia which are also dysfunctional in Parkinson's disease. Consequently, a trial of L-dihydroxyphenylalanine (L-dopa), which enters the brain more readily than L-dopamine and is rapidly decarboxylated to the amine once inside the nerve cell, was logical, especially since L-dopamine has prominent cardiovascular actions and is not orally efficacious. Clinical trials of the amino acid have produced dramatic results, and it is possible that the therapy of Parkinsonism will be drastically revised in the near future.

Certain antidepressants are efficacious in relieving apathy and depression, which afflict patients with Parkinsonism.

Amphetamine Salts—see page 882.

Atropine—see page 914.

Benztropine Mesylate USP

[Benztropinium Methanesulfonate; Benztropine Methanesulfonate USP XVI; 3-(Diphenylmethoxy)-1αH,5αH-tropane Methanesulfonate; Cogentin Mesylate (*MSD*)]

Benztropine Mesylate, dried in vacuum over phosphorus pentoxide for 12 hours, contains 98.0–110.0% of $C_{21}H_{25}NO \cdot CH_4O_3S$ (403.54).

Preparation—Bromodiphenylmethane, formed by direct bromination of diphenylmethane, is condensed with tropine. This may be accomplished by the Williamson ether synthesis using the sodium alkoxide derivative of tropine. After purification, the benztropine base thus obtained is dissolved in a suitable organic solvent and precipitated by reacting it with an equimolar quantity of methanesulfonic acid.

Description—A white, colorless, slightly hygroscopic, crystalline powder. Melting range 142° to 144°.

Solubility—Very soluble in water; freely soluble in alcohol; very slightly soluble in ether.

Uses—Benztropine Mesylate combines chemical features of both atropine and antihistaminics of the diphenhydramine type. It is thus an *antimuscarinic* drug of potency ¼ that of atropine sulfate and an antihistaminic of potency equal to that of pyrilamine maleate. It also possesses local anesthetic properties. However, only its central actions to suppress tremor and rigidity are employed therapeutically. These actions are similar to those of atropine; but unlike atropine, it possesses sedative and other effects similar to those of diphenhydramine. Since some patients, particularly the elderly, are often excited by other antiparkinson drugs, the sedative property is of special value. Benztropine Mesylate is used mainly in the treatment of *paralysis agitans* to control tremor and rigidity and also to relieve sialorrhea, oculogyric crises, mask-like facies and pain secondary to muscle spasm. It may be used alone or in combination with other drugs. Side effects include dry mouth, blurred vision, nausea, and nervousness, and less frequently they may include vomiting, mental confusion, sedation or excitement and difficulty in urination.

Dose—*Oral, intramuscular,* or *intravenous,* **500 mcg** to **8 mg** daily; *usual,* **1** to **2 mg,** 1 or 2 times a day.

Dosage Forms—Injection USP: 1 mg/ml; Tablets USP: 500 mcg and 1 and 2 mg.

Biperiden NF

[α-5-Norbornen-2-yl-α-phenyl-1-piperidinepropanol;   Akineton (*Knoll*)]

Biperiden contains 98.0–101.0% of $C_{21}H_{29}NO$ (311.47), calculated on the dried basis.

Preparation—Acetophenone is caused to undergo a Mannich condensation with formaldehyde and piperidine hydrochloride. The resulting 3-piperidino-propiophenone is Grignardized in benzene with 5-chloro-2-norbornene to yield the tertiary carbinol, Biperiden, which is extracted with methanol. US Pat. 2,789,110.

Description—A white, practically odorless, crystalline powder that is stable in light and nonhygroscopic. It melts between 112° and 116°.

Solubility—Freely soluble in chloroform; sparingly soluble in alcohol; practically insoluble in water.

Uses—Biperiden is an *antimuscarinic* drug with *antiparkinson* actions similar to those of trihexyphenidyl. In the treatment of *paralysis agitans* it reduces tremor, akinesia, muscle rigidity, drooling, and sweating. It also may decrease the incidence and severity of oculogyric crises. Biperiden sometimes appears to be of value in lessening spasticity in certain disorders of the pyramidal tract. Untoward effects result from the antimuscarinic properties and include dry mouth, blurring of vision, and urinary retention. The patient should be carefully monitored if glaucoma or urinary bladder neck obstruction exist.

Biperiden is not used as the free base but rather in salt form. The hydrochloride is used in oral medicaments and the lactate for parenteral administration (rarely necessary). Once a sufficient measure of control is obtained by parenteral administration, a switch to oral administration should be attempted.

Dose—*Usual, intramuscular*, **2 mg** (as the lactate) which may be repeated every half-hour until relief is obtained, but no more than four consecutive doses should be given in a 24-hour period; *intravenous*, **5 mg** (as the lactate) given slowly, this dose may be repeated once in a 24-hour period.

Dosage Forms—Lactate Injection NF: 5 mg/ml.

Biperiden Hydrochloride NF

[α-5-Norbornen-2-yl-α-phenyl-1-piperidinepropanol Monohydrochloride; Akineton Hydrochloride (*Knoll*)]

Biperiden Hydrochloride contains 98.0–101.0% of $C_{21}H_{29}NO\cdot HCl$ (347.93), calculated on the dried basis.

For the structure of the base, see *Biperiden*, this page.

Preparation—A methanolic solution of *Biperiden* (this page) is treated with a stream of hydrogen chloride.

Description—A white, crystalline powder that is practically odorless and has a slightly bitter taste. It is stable in light, nonhygroscopic, and stable at ambient temperatures. It melts at about 270° with decomposition. It is optically inactive.

Solubility—Sparingly soluble in methanol; slightly soluble in alcohol and chloroform; very slightly soluble in water and ether.

Uses—See *Biperiden*.

Dose—*Usual*, **2 mg** 3 to 4 times a day.

Other Dose Information—An initial oral dose of 0.5 mg is given 3 or 4 times daily, then a gradual increase in dosage until the individual dose is 2 mg.

Dosage Forms—Tablets NF: 2 mg.

Chlorphenoxamine Hydrochloride

[Systral;   Phenoxene (*Pitman-Moore*)]

Chlorphenoxamine Hydrochloride [$C_{18}H_{22}ClNO\cdot HCl$ = 340.30] is 2-[(*p*-chloro-α-methyl-α-phenyl-benzyl)oxy]-*N,N*-dimethylethylamine hydrochloride.

Preparation—*p*-Chlorobenzoquinone is Grignardized with methyl chloride to yield *p*-chloro-α-methyl-α-phenylbenzyl alcohol which is then etherified by treatment with 2-(dimethylamino)ethyl chloride in the presence of a strong base. The chlorphenoxamine (base) thus obtained is dissolved in a suitable solvent and converted to the hydrochloride by a stream of hydrogen chloride. US Pat. 2,785,202.

Description—Needle-like crystals which melt at 128°.

Solubility—Soluble in water.

Uses—Chlorphenoxamine is a close chemical congener of diphenhydramine. However, it is not used for its antihistaminic actions but rather for its central effects to reduce muscle rigidity and akinesia in certain patients with *Parkinson's disease*. Speech, gait, and posture are frequently markedly improved, but it has little effect on tremor. The drug has *antimuscarinic* properties. It causes sedation, vertigo, dry mouth, nausea, indigestion, or anorexia in one-fifth of cases. Other side effects include vomiting, burning sensation in the mouth, numbness and swelling of the extremities, epigastric pressure, nervousness, excessive sweating, blurred vision, confusion, apathy, asthenia, and urinary retention. It should not be used in patients with glaucoma, prostatic hypertrophy, gastrointestinal obstruction, cardiospasm, or stenosing peptic ulcer.

Dose—**50** to **100 mg** 3 to 4 times a day; *usual*, **50 mg** 3 times a day.

Dosage Forms—Tablets: 50 mg.

Cycrimine Hydrochloride NF

[α-Cyclopentyl-α-phenyl-1-piperidinepropanol Hydrochloride; Pagitane (*Lilly*)]

Cycrimine Hydrochloride, dried at 105° for 5 hours, contains 97.0–100.5% of $C_{19}H_{29}NO\cdot HCl$ (323.91).

Preparation—An ethanolic solution containing piperidine hydrochloride, acetophenone, paraformaldehyde, and hydrochloric acid is refluxed for several hours whereupon a typical Mannich reaction (condensation) occurs with formation of 3-piperidinopropiophenone which crystallizes after partial removal of the alcohol followed by cooling. This is then subjected to a typical Grignard reaction with cyclopentylmagnesium bromide which yields cycrimine (base). Treatment of a solution of the base in a suitable solvent with hydrogen chloride forms the official salt which is purified by recrystallization from alcohol.

Description—White, odorless solid, possessing a bitter taste. It melts with decomposition between 241° and 244°, and has a pH between 5.2 and 5.8.

Solubility—1 Gm dissolves in about 175 ml of water, 35 ml of chloroform, and 50 ml of alcohol.

Uses—Cycrimine Hydrochloride has actions very close to those of *Trihexyphenidyl* (see page 934), from which it differs only in having a cyclopentyl instead of a cyclohexyl ring. It is thus an *antimuscarinic* agent (see Chapter 51), half as potent as atropine as an antispasmodic and mydriatic and one-tenth as potent against the cardiac vagus and sialorrhea. It also has local anesthetic activity. It is slightly less potent than atropine in its central actions. It is used in the treatment of all forms of *paralysis agitans*. Side effects include dry mouth, soreness of the mouth and tongue, blurred vision, epigastric distress, anorexia and nausea, weakness, and occasionally vertigo or disorientation. Caution should be observed in elderly patients with arteriosclerosis, glaucoma, or any tendency toward urinary retention.

Dose—1.25 to **5** mg; *usual, initial*, **1.25** mg 3 times a day; *maintenance*, to be determined by the ohysician.

Dosage Forms—Tablets NF: 1.25 and 2.5 mg.

Dextroamphetamine Salts—see page 883.

Diazepam—see page 1092.

Diphenhydramine—see page 1147.

Isocarboxazid—see page 1115.

Mephenoxalone—see page 1094.

Meprobamate—see page 1094.

Methocarbamol NF

[3-(o-Methoxyphenoxy)-1,2-propanediol 1-Carbamate; Neuraxin; Robaxin (*Robins*)]

O—CH$_2$CHCH$_2$—OCONH$_2$
OCH$_3$ OH

Methocarbamol contains 98.0–102.0% of C$_{11}$H$_{15}$NO$_5$ (241.25).

Preparation—3-(o-Methoxyphenoxy)-1,2-propanediol participates in a transesterification reaction with ethyl carbonate in the presence of an alkaline catalyst to eliminate ethanol and produce the cyclic carbonate of the starting diol. Subsequent treatment with ammonia ruptures the cyclic carbonate ring at the locus required to form the primary carbamate of the starting compound. US Pat. 2,770,649.

Description—A fine, white powder; odorless or has a slight characteristic odor; melts between 93° and 97°.

Solubility—Freely soluble in alcohol; sparingly soluble in water and chloroform; insoluble in benzene and *n*-hexane.

Uses—Methocarbamol is a *centrally acting muscle relaxant*. Because it is less soluble than Mephenesin, it is absorbed more slowly from the gastrointestinal tract, which confers both a longer onset and duration of action. After parenteral administration, its action is prompt and intense enough to *facilitate orthopedic procedures*. Methocarbamol is used in the *treatment of muscle spasm* resulting from injury, musculoskeletal disorders, tetanus and other disorders. It is also used in the treatment of *paralysis agitans*, *cerebral palsy*, *multiple sclerosis*, and *cerebrovascular accidents* (with spastic manifestations). Side effects include drowsiness, vertigo, gastrointestinal upsets and rarely syncope. After parenteral administration there may be also muscular incoordination, nystagmus, diplopia, hypotension, bradycardia and metallic taste. Extravasated injections are locally irritating. The vehicle for commercial solutions, polyethylene glycol, causes uremia in persons with renal dysfunction, and parenteral administration is contraindicated in the presence of renal disease.

Dose—*Usual, oral*, **1.5** to **2 Gm** 4 times a day for the first 2 or 3 days, then **1 Gm** 4 times daily; *intramuscular*, **1 Gm** every 8 hours; *intravenous*, **1** to **3 Gm** per day given at a rate not exceeding 3 ml (0.30 Gm) per minute.

Other Dose Information—For children, the daily oral dose should not exceed 30 mg per pound.

Dosage Forms—Injection NF: 1 Gm/10 ml; Tablets NF: 500 and 750 mg

Methylphenidate—see page 1116.

Nialamide—see page 1116.

Orphenadrine Citrate NF

[*N,N*-Dimethyl-2-[(o-methyl-α-phenylbenzyl)oxy]ethylamine Citrate (1:1); Norflex (*Riker*)]

CHO—CH$_2$CH$_2$NH(CH$_3$)$_2$
CH$_3$ H$_2$C$_6$H$_5$O$_7^-$

Orphenadrine Citrate contains 98.0–101.5% of C$_{18}$H$_{23}$NO·C$_6$H$_8$O$_7$ (461.52), calculated on the dried basis.

Preparation—2-Methylbenzhydrol is etherified through reaction with the sodium derivative of 2-(dimethylamino)ethanol and the resulting orphenadrine (base) is caused to react, in a suitable solvent, with an equimolar quantity of citric acid. US Pats. 2,567,351 and 2,991,225.

Description—White, crystalline powder with a bitter taste and practically no odor. It melts between 134° and 138°.

Solubility—1 Gm dissolves in about 70 ml of water and 400 ml of alcohol; insoluble in chloroform, benzene, and ether; very slightly soluble in acetone; soluble in acid solutions; orphenadrine base precipitates from aqueous alkaline solutions.

Uses—Orphenadrine Citrate reduces voluntary muscle spasm by a central action and resembles atropine in this respect. It is used in the symptomatic management of *Parkinson's disease*. In addition to the decrease in spasticity, oculogyra, and blepharospasm, it also may reduce sialorrhea and diaphoresis. However, tremor may be exacerbated. Consequently, the drug is useful only as an adjunct to other therapy. Orphenadrine also is used in the management of *acute spastic disorders* of the skeletal muscles, especially those resulting from trauma, vertebral disk dislocation, or tension, but a clearcut efficacy has not been shown. Orphenadrine sometimes induces a mild euphoria in fatigued or depressed patients. Mild excitement sometimes occurs. Peripheral atropine-like actions are mild, but dry mouth may occur. Other side effects include nausea, vertigo, and occasional hallucinations.

By the oral route the citrate and the hydrochloride (page 935) are equally efficacious, if allowance in dose is made for the difference in molecular weight. The manufacturer's recommendations of a longer interval between doses of the citrate than of the hydrochloride is based upon the retarding effect of the plasticized matrix in which the oral citrate is compounded. The citrate may be given parenterally.

Dose—*Usual, oral,* **100 mg** 2 times a day; *parenteral,* **60 mg** every 12 hours.

Dosage Forms—Injection: 60 mg/2 ml; Tablets: 100 mg.

Phenaglycodol—see page 1096.

Phenelzine—see page 1117.

Phenindamine Tartrate—see page 1148.

Phenyramidol—see page 1138.

Scopolamine Hydrobromide—see page 918.

Trihexyphenidyl Hydrochloride USP

[α-Cyclohexyl-α-phenyl-1-piperidinepropanol Hydrochloride; Artane (*Lederle*); Pipanol (*Winthrop*); Tremin (*Schering*)]

Trihexyphenidyl Hydrochloride contains 98.0–100.5% of $C_{20}H_{31}NO.HCl$ (337.94), calculated on the dried basis.

Preparation—Acetophenone and piperidine are caused to undergo a Mannich condensation with formaldehyde by refluxing a solution of the reactants in 60% ethanol. The 3-piperidinopropiophenone thus produced is isolated and subjected to a typical Grignard reaction with cyclohexylmagnesium chloride to yield after hydrolysis, trihexyphenidyl base. The hydrochloride is conveniently prepared by dissolving the base in a suitable solvent and precipitating with a stream of hydrogen chloride.

Description—It occurs as a white or slightly off-white, crystalline powder, having no more than a very faint odor.

Solubility—Slightly soluble in water; soluble in alcohol and chloroform.

Use—Trihexyphenidyl Hydrochloride is an antiparkinsonism drug with weak *antimuscarinic* and *antispasmodic* actions. It reduces the muscular rigidity and mental inertia of *paralysis agitans* and

also decreases *tremors* and *sialorrhea*. Its anticholinergic side effects, such as blurred vision, mydriasis, dry mouth are minimal, and it does not tend to precipitate glaucoma in elderly patients. Dizziness and mild nausea occur occasionally but tend to disappear upon continued use of the drug.

Dose—1 to **15 mg** daily; *usual,* **2 mg** 3 or 4 times a day.

Other Dose Information—Orally, **1 mg** the first day, with 1- to 2-mg daily increments until 6 to 10 mg is reached. The daily dose is divided into 3 or 4 doses.

Dosage Forms—Elixir USP: 2 mg/5 ml; Tablets USP: 2 and 5 mg.

Other Centrally Acting Muscle Relaxants

Carisoprodol [Rela (*Schering*); Soma (*Wallace*)] is *N*-isopropyl-2-methyl-2-propyl-1,3-propanediol dicarbamate. *Description and Solubility:* Crystals which melt between 92° and 93°. Very slightly soluble in water; soluble in most common organic solvents; insoluble in vegetable oils. *Uses:* Like *Meprobamate*, which it closely resembles, Carisoprodol is a sedative drug with skeletal muscle relaxant properties. The relaxant effect is the result of a depressant action on reticulospinal facilitation. Carisoprodol also possesses analgesic activity. Early reports that the drug is useful in the control of cerebral palsy are subject to challenge. However, it appears to be useful in the alleviation of *muscle spasm* of local origin, such as that resulting from sprains, strains, and the low-back syndrome. Part of its action may result from analgesia, sedation, and the alleviation of anxiety. Side effects include urticaria, weakness, lassitude, and sedation. *Dose:* Orally, usually 350 mg 4 times daily for adults and 250 mg 2 or 3 times daily for children over 5 years old.

Chlormezanone [Trancopal (*Winthrop*)] is 2-(*p*-chlorophenyl)tetrahydro-3-methyl-4*H*-1,3-thiazin-4-one 1,1-dioxide. *Description and Solubility:* Crystals which melt between 116.2° and 118.2°. Soluble less than 0.25% w/v in water (at 25°); soluble less than 1.0% w/v in alcohol (at 25°). *Uses:* A metathiazanone derivative with somewhat greater skeletal muscle relaxant properties and slightly less sedative-tranquilizing activity than meprobamate. It is used in the management of various conditions characterized by muscle spasm and tension. The incidence of untoward reactions is about 3% and minor in nature; nausea, drowsiness, dizziness, and weakness are most frequently observed. *Dose:* Usual, oral, 100 to 200 mg 3 or 4 times daily.

Chlorphenesin Carbamate [$C_{10}H_{12}ClNO_4$ = 245.68; Maolate (*Upjohn*)] is 3-(*p*-chlorophenoxy)-1,2-propanediol 1-carbamate. *Preparation:* *p*-Chlorophenol is caused to undergo addition to glycidol (2,3-epoxy-1-propanol) by the catalytic influence of a tertiary amine to form 3-(*p*-chlorophenoxy)-1,2-propanediol and the 1-hydroxy group is then esterified by reaction with carbamoyl chloride. US Pats. 3,214,336 and 3,161,567. *Description and Solubility:* White to off-white powder that is odorless and practically tasteless; stable in light, air, and at ordinary temperatures; melts between 86° and 92°. Freely soluble in alcohol; sparingly soluble in chloroform; very slightly soluble in water.

Uses: A centrally acting skeletal muscle relaxant similar in its actions to *Mephenesin* (page 935). It is employed to diminish *skeletal muscle spasms* resulting from trauma, inflammation, vertebral disk syndrome, osteoarthritis, and rheumatoid arthritis. Side effects include drowsiness, dizziness, epigastric distress, nausea, skin rash, headache, insomnia, nervousness, and agitation. The incidence of side effects is low. *Dose:* Oral, 400 to 800 mg 2 to 4 times a day.

Chlorzoxazone [Paraflex (*McNeil*)] is 5-chloro-2-benzoxazolol. *Description and Solubility:* White or creamy white, odorless, glistening, crystalline powder; melts between 189° and 194°. Moderately soluble in acetone and methanol; very slightly soluble in water; when an excess of HCl is added to a solution of it in 3.1*N* NaOH, a precipitate is obtained. *Uses:* A centrally acting muscle relaxant for the treatment of painful muscle spasm associated with musculoskeletal disorders, such as fibrositis, bursitis, myositis, spondylitis, sprains, and muscle strains. It may be of some benefit in vertebral disk disorders and cervical root syndrome. It is of little use in spasticity resulting from lesions of the central nervous system. Untoward effects, infrequent and generally mild, include rash or petechiae, nausea and vomiting, vertigo, malaise, headache, and drowsiness. Gastrointestinal bleeding and jaundice have occurred, but the causal role of the drug has not been firmly established. The drug causes occasional hypersensitivity. *Dose: Orally*, for adults, 250 to 753 mg 3 or 4 times daily.

Ethopropazine Hydrochloride [Profenamine Hydrochloride; Parsidol (*Warner-Chilcott*)] is 10-[2-(diethylamino)-propyl]phenothiazine hydrochloride. *Description and Solubility:* White or slightly off-white, odorless, crystalline solid, melting at about 225° with decomposition. Sparingly soluble in alcohol; slightly soluble in water. *Uses:* In the treatment of *paralysis agitans*, especially for the control of rigidity, but also for the spasm tremor, sialorrhea, and oculogyric crises. It has weak *antimuscarinic* and *antihistaminic* actions, the former providing most of the side effects, which are dry mouth, mydriasis, and blurred vision. Lassitude, sense of limb heaviness, and epigastric discomfort also occur. *Dose: Initial*, 50 mg, increasing gradually to 500 mg daily in accordance with the needs of that patient. Therapy usually begins with 10 mg per dose with 10-mg increments until the desired effect is achieved.

Levodihydroxyphenylalanine [L-Dopa] is 3-(3,4-dihydroxyphenyl)-L-alanine ($C_9H_{11}NO_4$). *Description and Solubility:* Needles which melt with decomposition between 276° and 278°. 1 Gm dissolves in about 600 ml of water. *Uses:* Levodihydroxyphenylalanine is an experimental antiparkinson drug of such extraordinary potential that a paragraph is warranted here, even though the use of the drug has not yet been approved by the FDA. The rationale for its use is discussed in the general statement (page 931). The drug is currently being tested in the treatment of idiopathic and postencephalopathic parkinsonism. The drug relieves most symptoms, to some degree; however, there is usually more improvement in the akinesia and rigidity than in the tremor. Clinical improvement, varying from modest to dramatic, occurs in approximately 75% of patients. Whether clinical improvement can be maintained over long periods of time remains to be determined. Untoward effects of the drug include transient nausea and vomiting, orthostatic hypotension, arrhythmias, granulocytopenia, and a reversible abnormal movement of the head. The toxic effects of long-term use are not yet known. *Dose: Oral, usual*, 4 to 8 Gm daily. The maintenance dose is achieved by starting with a small daily dose (usually 0.3 Gm) and building up to the large dose in daily increments (usually 0.3 Gm).

Mephenesin NF XII [3-o-Tolyloxy-1,2-propanediol; (*Various Mfgs.*)] contains not less than 97.0% of $C_{10}N_{14}O_3$ (182.22), calculated on the anhydrous basis. *Preparation:* By reacting 3-chloropropane-1,2-diol (α-chlorohydrin) with sodium o-cresolate. *Description and Solubility:* White, crystalline powder with a faint characteristic odor and a bitter taste producing tongue numbness; melts between 70° and 73.5°. 1 Gm dissolves in about 100 ml of water; freely soluble in alcohol, chloroform, and ether; sparingly soluble in benzene.

Uses: A *centrally acting skeletal muscle relaxant* which produces reversible muscular relaxation without loss of consciousness. It is used in the treatment of *cerebral palsy* and *parkinsonism*. Unfortunately, its value is markedly restricted because of its brief duration of action and the unpredictability of benefit following oral medication. It may be of value as a diagnostic aid and adjunct to physiotherapy in *acute muscle spasm*, and it may afford relief in certain cases of *intractable "thalamic"* pain. Phlebothrombosis and intravascular hemolysis may result if solutions more concentrated than 2% are administered intravenously.

Other untoward effects noted frequently are the result of excessive central depression and of gastrointestinal distress when the drug is administered by mouth. *Dose: Oral*, 2 to 3 Gm 3 to 5 times a day; *intravenous*, 30 to 150 ml of a 2% solution at a rate of 6 or 7 ml per minute.

Mephenesin Carbamate [Tolseram (*Squibb*)] is 3-o-toloxy-1,2-propanediol 1-carbamic acid ester ($C_{11}H_{15}NO_4$). *Preparation:* By interacting mephenesin with phosgene and treating the reaction product with ammonia (US Pat. 2,609,386). *Description and Solubility:* Crystals which melt at 93°. 1 Gm is soluble in about 333 ml of water and about 50 ml of chloroform; freely soluble in alcohol. *Uses:* Mephenesin Carbamate, the carbamate ester of mephenesin, is absorbed and excreted more slowly than the parent compound. Except for a longer duration of action, its actions and uses are the same as mephenesin. *Dose: Usual*, 400 mg 3 or 4 times a day. *Dosage Forms:* Oral Suspension: 1 Gm/5 ml; Tablets: 500 mg.

Metaxalone [Skelaxin [(*Robins*)] 5-(3,5-Dimethylphenoxymethyl)-2-oxazolidinone]—*Uses:* Metaxalone is reputed to have muscle relaxant properties with a central nervous locus of action. It is marketed as a drug for the relief of acute muscle spasm resulting from various injuries or strains. However, its efficacy is in serious question, and there seems to be no reason to use the drug in lieu of drugs that are obviously more effective. Furthermore, the toxicity of Metaxalone is greater than that of more efficacious drugs; toxic effects include anorexia, nausea, vomiting, vertigo, drowsiness, nervousness, mental confusion, dry mouth, urinary retention, pruritus, dermatitis, rarely leucopenia, anemia and jaundice, and possible pyuria, albuminuria and nephrolithiasis. It may also exacerbate grand mal epilepsy. *Dose: Orally*, for adults 2.4 to 3.2 Gm daily for no more than 10 consecutive days.

Orphenadrine Hydrochloride [Disipal (*Riker*)] is N,N-dimethyl - 2 - [(o - methyl - α - phenylbenzyl)oxy]ethylamine hydrochloride. *Description and Solubility:* Crystals which melt between 156° and 157°; pH of an aqueous solution: about 5.5. Soluble in water, alcohol, and chloroform; sparingly soluble in acetone and benzene; insoluble in ether. *Uses:* The actions, uses, and side effects of Orphenadrine Hydrochloride are exactly the same as those of *Orphenadrine Citrate* (page 933). *Dose: Oral*, 50 mg 3 times a day with adjustments.

Procyclidine Hydrochloride [α-Cyclohexyl-α-phenyl-1-pyrrolidinepropanol Hydrochloride; Kemadrin (*Burroughs-Wellcome*)] is the pyrrolidine analog of Trihexyphenidyl Hydrochloride. *Description and Solubility:* Crystals which decompose between 226° and 227°. Moderately soluble in water (about 3 Gm/100 ml); more soluble in alcohol and chloroform; very slightly soluble in ether. *Uses:* An *antimuscarinic* agent similar to atropine in its actions. However, its pronounced antispasmodic effects on smooth muscle have not been much employed clinically. Rather, its central actions to relieve spasticity in voluntary muscle in *paralysis agitans* are mainly sought. Tremor may be relieved or exacerbated by the drug. Dry mouth, mydriasis and blurring of vision, lightheadedness, and disorientation are the principal side effects. *Dose: Orally, initially*, 7.5 mg per day increasing gradually to as high as 60 mg (usual, 15 to 30 mg) per day, in 3 divided doses.

Styramate [Sinaxar (*Armour*)] is β-hydroxyphenethyl carbamate. *Description and Solubility:* Fine, pearly white, crystalline powder which is odorless and tasteless; stable in both light and air; melts between 110° and 113°. Soluble in alcohol; sparingly soluble in ethyl acetate; slightly soluble in water and chloroform. *Uses:* A *centrally acting skeletal muscle relaxant* with actions and uses similar to those of *Mephenesin* (this page). However, its true clinical efficacy has not been proven. Its duration is 2 to 3 times that of mephenesin. Toxic effects include drowsiness, headache, vertigo, and possibly skin eruptions. *Dose: Orally*, 200 mg 4 times daily; the total daily dose may be revised upward to 1.6 Gm.

53 | Diuretic Drugs

Osmotic diuretics—inhibitors of renal tubular transport—miscellaneous renal agents

This chapter was prepared by

Ewart A. Swinyard, PhD, *Professor of Pharmacology, College of Pharmacy and College of Medicine, University of Utah, Salt Lake City, Utah 84112, and*
Stewart C. Harvey, PhD, *Associate Professor of Pharmacology, College of Medicine, University of Utah, Salt Lake City, Utah 84112*

Diuretics are drugs used to increase the volume of urine excreted by the kidneys. They are employed principally for the relief of edema and ascites. These conditions occur in diseases of the heart, kidneys, and liver. Diuretics are most effective in the treatment of cardiac edema, particularly that associated with congestive heart failure. They are also used in the ascites of cirrhosis, the nephrotic syndrome, and the edema of pregnancy. Some diuretics have highly specialized uses in glaucoma, hyperpotassemia, bromide intoxication, anginal syndrome, epilepsy, migraine, hypertension, and in premenstrual depression, these being conditions in which edema is not present or at least not definitely established.

The formation of urine from the blood, in simplest terms, consists of glomerular filtration and selective tubular reabsorption and secretion. As the glomerular filtrate passes through the tubules, substances essential to the blood and tissues—water, glucose, salts, and amino acids—are reabsorbed. Other substances in the glomerular filtrate, such as urea, are not as readily absorbed by the tubules. Thus, it is thought that in the renal tubule there is a specific mechanism for the transport of each ionic species, the capacities of which are quite different. For example, the capacity of the renal tubule to reabsorb sulfate ion is limited. The tubular capacity for the reabsorption of phosphate is such that sufficient is reabsorbed to maintain the normal extracellular level and any excess is excreted. On the other hand, much larger amounts of bicarbonate ion and chloride ion can be reabsorbed.

Under normal circumstances the glomerular filtration rate is about 100 ml per minute. About 99 ml of the fluid is returned to the blood and only 1 ml is excreted as urine. It follows, therefore, that drugs may increase the rate of urine formation in two ways: (1) by increasing glomerular filtration and (2) by depressing tubular reabsorption. Increasing glomerular filtration is not an efficient mechanism and usually causes only a moderate increase in urine formation. If, for example, the per cent of fluid reabsorbed by the renal tubules is assumed to remain constant, glomerular filtration rate would have to be increased two-fold in order to double the urinary output. On the other hand, a 1% decrease in the tubular reabsorption of water, induced either by the administration of excessive quantities of electrolytes or nonelectrolytes (osmotic diuretics) or by agents which alter selective reabsorption of substances in the renal tubules, would evoke a two-fold increase in urinary output. Most powerful diuretics act to depress tubular reabsorption.

Agents employed clinically as diuretics may be divided into two groups: (1) osmotic diuretics and (2) agents which inhibit renal tubular transport. In this presentation a third category, miscellaneous renal agents, is provided for obsolete diuretic substances and for agents such as ion-exchange resins and probenecid which are not true diuretics.

Osmotic Diuretics

The capacity of the renal tubule to reabsorb various electrolytes and nonelectrolytes is limited and, as previously mentioned, varies for each ionic species. If large amounts of these substances are administered to an individual, their concentration in the body fluids and, subsequently, in the glomerular filtrate exceeds the reabsorption capacity of the tubule, and the excess appears in the urine accompanied by an increased volume of water. Substances which increase urine formation in this manner are called osmotic diuretics.

This group of diuretics includes osmotic electrolytes (potassium and sodium salts), osmotic nonelectrolytes (urea, glucose, sucrose, and mannitol), and acid-forming salts (ammonium and calcium salts). The basic mechanism for all of these agents is essentially the same. The acid-forming salts have only limited use as a primary diuretic; their chief value is for the potentiation of mercurial diuretics.

Acacia—see page 1344.

Ammonium Chloride USP

[Muriate of Ammonia; Sal Ammoniac]

Ammonium Chloride contains 99.5–100.5% of NH_4Cl (53.49) calculated on the dried basis.

Preparation—Ammonium Chloride is made by the following processes:

1. The ammoniacal liquid obtained from gas works during the destructive distillation of coal is neutralized with hydrochloric acid, and the crude product is subsequently purified.
2. The vapors of ammonia from synthetic processes are absorbed in hydrochloric acid.
3. It is also obtained as a byproduct in the Solvay process for sodium bicarbonate (page 793).

Description—Colorless crystals, or a white, fine or coarse, crystalline powder. It has a cool, saline taste, and is somewhat hygroscopic. When it is dissolved in water the temperature of the solution is lowered. The aqueous solution is slightly acid to litmus.

Solubility—1 Gm is soluble in about 3 ml of water, about 100 ml of alcohol, about 8 ml of glycerin, and about 1.4 ml of boiling water.

Incompatibilities—Ammonium Chloride has the reactions of the ammonium salts described under *Ammonium Bromide* (page 1089) and of the chlorides described under *Sodium Chloride* (page 842).

Uses—Ammonium Chloride is widely employed as a *diuretic* and *expectorant*. It is also used as a *systemic acidifier*. Ammonium Chloride is a combination of a labile cation and a fixed anion. When the ammonium ion is converted to urea, the liberated hydrogen ion reacts with bicarbonate and other body buffers. The end result is that chloride ion displaces bicarbonate ion, the latter is converted to CO_2. Thus, the chloride load to the kidneys is increased and an appreciable amount escapes reabsorption along with an equivalent amount of cation (predominantly sodium) and an iso-osmotic quantity of water. This is the basic mechanism by which Ammonium Chloride brings about a net loss of extracellular fluid and promotes the mobilization of edema fluid.

Ammonium Chloride is sometimes employed alone for its diuretic action but usually it is given in conjunction with mercurial diuretics, the action of which it potentiates.

The fact that Ammonium Chloride causes systemic acidosis makes the salt of some value in the treatment of alkalosis. It also renders the urine acid and is prescribed for this purpose in conjunction with methenamine. In the rare instances when it is desired to produce an acidosis, Ammonium Chloride may be used. An example is in the treatment of lead poisoning where an acidosis is desired to hasten the excretion of lead.

It should never be combined with potassium chlorate, a mixture that in the dry state may explode, especially at elevated temperatures.

Dose—*Oral*, 4 to **12 Gm** daily; *usual, oral*, 1 to 2 **Gm** 4 times a day; *intravenous*, **100** to **1000 ml** of 2% solution; *usual, intravenous*, **500 ml** of a 2% solution infused over a 3-hour period.

Other Dose Information—The oral dose may vary from 8 to 12 Gm daily in divided doses. The drug is usually taken with or after meals to avoid gastric irritation.

Veterinary Dose—*Horses*, 4 to **15 Gm**; *Cattle*, **15** to **30 Gm**; *Sheep* and *Swine*, 1 to 2 **Gm**; *Dogs*, 200 to **500 mg.**

Dosage Forms—Injection USP: 160 mg/30 ml, 600 mg/100 ml, 10.7 Gm/500 ml, 21.4 Gm/1000 ml; Tablets USP: 500 mg and 1 Gm.

Glucose, Liquid—see page 1367.

Mannitol USP

[D-Mannitol; Mannite; Manna Sugar; Osmitrol (*Travenol*)]

$$HO-CH_2-\overset{\displaystyle |}{C}H-\overset{\displaystyle OH}{\underset{\displaystyle |}{C}H}-\overset{\displaystyle OH}{\underset{\displaystyle |}{C}H}-\overset{\displaystyle |}{\underset{\displaystyle OH}{C}}H-CH_2-OH$$

Mannitol contains 98.0–102.0% of $C_6H_{14}O_6$ (182.17), calculated on the dried basis.

History—Mannitol is a hexahydric alcohol which occurs rather widely distributed in the tissue fluids of various plants. It is the major constituent of *Manna*, which was official in NF VII and described therein as "the dried exudation of *Fraxinus Ornus* Linné (Fam.

Oleaceae)." It is recorded in biblical history that manna was an extremely important foodstuff available to the Israelites as they made their memorable exodus from Egypt following generations of oppression.

Preparation—Mannitol may be extracted from manna and other natural sources by means of hot alcohol or other selective solvents. Commercially it is produced by the catalytic or electrolytic reduction of certain monosaccharides such as mannose and glucose. Manufacture is somewhat complicated due primarily to the need for separation of stereoisomers. For example, a prime producer has reported that the following seven steps are involved in preparing mannitol from a monosaccharide (sugar) catalytically: (1) preparing the reaction slurry by dissolving the refined sugar in water and mixing with nickel catalyst; (2) continuous catalytic reduction of the sugar to a mixture of sorbitol and mannitol with hydrogen in a specially designed high-pressure reaction system; (3) filtering off the spent catalyst and reprocessing it for return to the system; (4) purifying the solution by ion exchange and decolorizing it by activated carbon; (5) separation of the mannitol by crystallizing it from the solution; (6) purifying the mannitol by recrystallization from water solution and drying; and (7) grinding the dry mannitol to a uniform powder.

Description—A white, crystalline powder, odorless and having a sweetish taste. Density about 1.52 at 20°. Melting range between 165° and 168°.

Solubility—1 Gm dissolves in about 5.5 ml of water; slightly soluble in pyridine; very slightly soluble in alcohol; soluble in aniline and alkaline solutions; insoluble in ether.

Identification—Mannitol is identified officially by its ability to prevent precipitation of ferric hydroxide and by the melting point of its acetyl derivative.

Uses—Mannitol is used as a *diuretic* and a *diagnostic agent for kidney function*. The intravenous administration of hypertonic solutions of Mannitol, as of dextrose, causes cellular dehydration and initiates *osmotic diuresis*. Mannitol is superior to dextrose in that it is only slightly metabolized in the body and is only slightly reabsorbed by the renal tubule.

Since only a negligible amount of Mannitol which appears in the glomerular filtrate is reabsorbed by the renal tubule, Mannitol has been employed for the measurement of *glomerular filtration rate*.

Dose—*Usual, intravenous infusion*, **50** to **200 Gm** daily.

Other Dose Information—The usual *diuretic* dose is 50 to 100 Gm, administered as a 25% solution.

Dosage Forms—Injection USP: 5 and 10% (in 500 and 1000 ml), 15% (in 150 and 500 ml), 20% (in 250 and 500 ml), 25% (in 50 ml); and Sodium Chloride Injection (see below): *of each ingredient*—5 and 0.3% (in 500 and 1000 ml), 10 and 0.3% (in 500 and 1000 ml), 15 and 0.45% (in 150 and 500 ml), 20 and 0.45% (in 250 and 500 ml).

Veterinary Uses—Mannitol is used in dogs as an osmotic diuretic causing cellular dehydration, to reduce intraocular pressure in glaucoma, and to reduce cerebral edema following surgery or injury.

Veterinary Dose—*Dogs, intravenous*, in hypertonic (20–25%) solution, **0.5 Gm** per **pound** of body weight twice daily, usually for 3 days.

Mannitol and Sodium Chloride Injection USP [Various Mfgs.] is a sterile solution of mannitol and sodium chloride in water for injection. It contains 95.0–105.0% of the labeled amounts of $C_6H_{14}O_6$ and NaCl. It contains no bacteriostatic agents. *Description*: Its pH is between 4.5 and 7.0. *Uses* and *Dose*: See *Mannitol*.

Potassium Acetate—see page 871.

Potassium Bicarbonate—see page 792.

Potassium Chloride—see page 839.

Potassium Citrate—see page 872.

Sodium Bicarbonate—see page 793.

Sodium Biphosphate NF

[Sodium Acid Phosphate; Sodium Dihydrogen Phosphate; Monosodium Orthophosphate; Monobasic Sodium Phosphate]

Sodium Biphosphate [$NaH_2PO_4 \cdot H_2O$ = 137.99] contains 98.0–100.5% of NaH_2PO_4 (119.98), calculated on the anhydrous basis.

Preparation—Sodium Biphosphate is prepared by adding phosphoric acid to a hot concentrated solution of disodium phosphate until the liquid ceases to give a precipitate with barium chloride. The solution is then concentrated to the crystallization point by evaporation.

Description—Colorless crystals or a white, crystalline powder. It is odorless and is slightly deliquescent. The solution is acid to litmus and to phenolphthalein TS but is neutral, or practically neutral, to methyl orange TS. Its solution produces effervescence with sodium carbonate.

Solubility—Freely soluble in water; practically insoluble in alcohol.

Incompatibilities—Since Sodium Biphosphate is an acid salt, it is incompatible with *carbonates* and *alkalies* in general. In solution with *methenamine* it causes a slow evolution of formaldehyde.

Uses—Sodium Biphosphate is most frequently employed as a *urinary acidifier*, as, for example, during therapy with methenamine. In large doses it is laxative.

Dose—**500 mg** to **1 Gm** 1 to 6 times a day; *usual*, **600 mg** 4 times a day.

Veterinary Dose—*Horses* and *Cattle*, **250** to **1000 Gm** (large doses may cause marked gastrointestinal distress); *Dogs*, **300 mg** to **1 Gm.**

Sodium Chloride—see page 842.

Sodium Sulfate—see page 803.

Sucrose—see page 1334.

Urea USP

[Carbamide; Carbonyldiamide; Ureaphil (*Abbott*); Urevert (*Travenol*)]

$$H_2N - \overset{\overset{\displaystyle O}{\|}}{C} - NH_2$$

Urea contains 99.0–100.5% of CH_4N_2O (60.06).

History—Rouelle in 1773 discovered the presence of urea in urine. It occurs chiefly in the urine of carnivora. Human urine contains about 2.5%, and results from decomposition of proteins. In 1828 Wöhler obtained it by evaporating a solution of potassium cyanate with ammonium sulfate. This was purported to be the first synthesis of an organic compound from inorganic materials.

Preparation—Urea is now prepared on a large scale by heating calcium cyanamide with water under pressure:

$$CaNCN + 3H_2O \rightarrow CO(NH_2)_2 + Ca(OH)_2$$

Description—Colorless to white, prismatic crystals or a white, crystalline powder. It is almost odorless and has a cooling, saline taste. It may gradually develop a slight odor of ammonia, especially in the presence of moisture. It melts between 132° and 134°. Its aqueous solution is neutral to litmus, but on standing or on heating, it decomposes into NH_3 and CO_2.

Solubility—1 Gm dissolves in 1.5 ml of water, about 10 ml of alcohol, and about 1 ml of boiling alcohol; practically insoluble in chloroform or ether.

Identification—Urea and certain compounds similar to Urea are characterized by giving what is known as the *biuret reaction* which is carried out as follows:

The urea is cautiously heated in a test tube until it liquefies and the odor of ammonia is evolved. The heating is continued until the liquid becomes turbid. After cooling, the fused mass is dissolved in a few ml of water to which 1 ml of 10% sodium hydroxide has been added, then 1 drop of cupric sulfate TS is added. The solution acquires a reddish violet color. Urea is also characterized by yielding with a moderate excess of nitric acid a white precipitate of urea nitrate.

Uses—Urea is used orally as a *diuretic*. It is largely rejected by the renal tubules and in the course of its excretion carries fluid with it. It does not enjoy widespread use, however, because of the large dose required, its disagreeable taste, and its relative ineffectiveness. Urea is used intravenously in hypertonic solutions to reduce intracranial and intraocular pressure. It has also been shown to be effective in status epilepticus. It is devoid of toxicity and thus can be given in high dosage. Industrially it is employed in fertilizers, in the manufacture of barbiturates and plastics, as a stabilizer in explosives, and in celluloid products.

It has been used in *otitis media, infected wounds*, and *indolent ulcers*. It appears to potentiate the antibacterial activity of the sulfonamides.

Dose—*Usual, intravenous infusion*, **100 mg** to **1 Gm** per **Kg** of body weight daily, as a **30%** solution in Dextrose Injection at a rate not exceeding 6 ml per minute.

Other Dose Information—It is usually administered in fruit juices or syrups to mask its taste in the single dose of 20 Gm taken 2 to 5 times daily.

Dosage Forms—Sterile USP: 40 and 90 Gm.

Veterinary Dose—*Horses*, 50 to 250 Gm; *Dogs*, 1 to 15 Gm.

Other Osmotic Diuretics

Potassium Nitrate NF XI [Niter; Nitre; Nitrate of Potash; Saltpeter; KNO_3 = 101.11]—Colorless, transparent prisms, or a white, crystalline powder. It is odorless, has a salty taste, and produces a cooling sensation in the mouth. It is slightly hygroscopic in moist air. 1 Gm dissolves in 3 ml of water, about 620 ml of alcohol, and 0.5 ml of boiling water. Nitrates are oxidizing agents and if triturated with oxidizable material, particularly organic matter such as sugar, or glycerin, it may cause an explosion due to the vigor of the reaction. In acidic solution, potassium nitrate will readily oxidize organic substances, hypophosphites, arsenites, ferrous salts, *etc.* Iodides and bromides are gradually decomposed with the liberation of the free halogens; in solution in the presence of free acid, the decomposition is accelerated. *Uses:* Potassium Nitrate is used chiefly as a *diuretic*. It is also used as an explosive. *Black Gunpowder* consists of sulfur 10 parts, charcoal 15 parts, and potassium nitrate 75 parts. *Caution—Many amateur chemists have been seriously injured attempting to make this substance for fireworks displays. The inexperienced should not attempt its preparation. Dose: Usual*, 1 Gm. As a diuretic, the dose is 5 to 10 Gm daily, given orally in divided portions at mealtime. It is conveniently administered in the form of enteric capsules. *Veterinary Dose: Horses*, 8 to 15 Gm; *Dogs* 300 mg to 1 Gm, administered twice daily.

Inhibitors of Renal Tubular Transport

The most powerful and consistently effective diuretics are those which depress tubular mechanisms responsible for the active reabsorptive transport of certain ions. Drugs which induce diuresis in this way may be divided into five groups: xanthines, mercurials, carbonic anhydrase inhibitors, aldosterone antagonists and benzothiadiazine and related derivatives.

The xanthines—notably caffeine, theobromine, and theophylline—in addition to their pharmacological properties described elsewhere, exert an appreciable diuretic action. This activity and their relative freedom from toxicity have led to the clinical use of these agents as diuretics. These agents are among the most extensively studied and least understood of the diuretic drugs. Although the xanthines increase glomerular filtration rate, this is not the primary mechanism by which they induce diuresis. Their effect appears to be primarily one of inhibiting renal tubular reabsorption of sodium and chloride; the diuretic effect is secondary to their saluretic action.

The inherent potency of the xanthine diuretic agents is neither sufficiently great nor sufficiently long to make them uniformly useful in edematous states attending cardiac decompensation. Therefore, diuresis induced by administration of the xanthine derivatives in combination with more effective mercurial diuretics has superseded the use of xanthines alone. The xanthine derivatives used as diuretics are discussed in the chapter on *Central Nervous System Stimulants* (see page 1154).

Aminophylline—see page 1154.

Caffeine—see page 1155.

Theobromine—see page 1156.

Theobromine Calcium (also **Sodium**) **Salicylate**—see page 1158.

Theophylline—see page 1157.

Theophylline Sodium Acetate—see page 1157.

Mercurial Diuretics

Although the diuretic action of mercury compounds has been known for centuries, the introduction of merbaphen in 1920 marked the beginning of the modern use of these agents. The organic mercurial diuretics now have the justified reputation of being among the most effective of all diuretic drugs. Their potency is increased and their irritant properties are decreased by admixture with an equimolecular amount of a xanthine derivative, usually theophylline. The efficiency of mercury-xanthine diuretics can be increased still further by the simultaneous administration of acidosis-producing salts such as ammonium chloride.

There is a lack of agreement as to the mechanism by which mercurials produce diuresis. Plasma-protein dilution, increased glomerular filtration rate, and decreased tubular reabsorption have been implicated. Available evidence indicates that these agents produce a temporary and partial inhibition of SH-activated enzyme systems which are essential for the reabsorption of certain ions. Precisely which ionic species is involved is not clear; both sodium and chloride have been implicated, but most investigators favor chloride. Two observations favor this view. First, chloride is the major urinary anion during diuresis and second, there is some degree of correlation between plasma chloride level and the diuretic response. In metabolic alkalosis induced by sodium bicarbonate, plasma chloride is low and mercurial diuretics are ineffective; in metabolic acidosis induced by ammonium chloride, on the other hand, the chloride level is high and mercurial diuresis is enhanced. These observations suggest that fixed cation is lost secondarily to the anionic excretion. As a result of a proportionally greater loss of chloride than bicarbonate from extracellular fluid, a mercurial diuresis tends to produce a hypochloremic alkalosis.

Mercurial diuretics are used for the treatment of cardiac edema, nephrotic edema, ascites of liver disease, and for carefully selected cases of subacute and chronic nephritis complicated by cardiac edema. Mercurials are contraindicated in acute nephritis and should be used with caution in chronic kidney disease. Hypersensitivity reactions characterized by stomatitis, gastric disturbances, vertigo, febrile reactions, and cutaneous eruptions have been observed; hence, initial sensitivity tests and careful regulation of dosage are prerequisites to the safe, effective use of these agents. Patients on prolonged mercurial therapy should be examined periodically for the presence of albumin, casts and blood cells in their urine.

Chlormerodrin NF

[Chloro(2-methoxy-3-ureidopropyl)mercury; [3-(Chloromercuri)-2-methoxypropyl]urea; Neohydrin (*Lakeside*)]

$$ClHg-CH_2-CH-CH_2-NH-C-NH_2$$
$$| \qquad \qquad ||$$
$$OCH_3 \qquad \quad O$$

Chlormerodrin contains 98.8–100.7% of $C_5H_{11}Cl-HgN_2O_2$ (367.20), calculated on the dried basis.

Preparation—Allylurea is acetoxymercurated by refluxing with mercuric acetate in methanol. Saturation occurs simultaneously resulting in the introduction of the 2-methoxy. Aqueous NaCl is then added whereupon metathesis ensues and the Chlormerodrin, which precipitates, is filtered, washed, and dried.

Description—Occurs as a white, odorless, bitter powder.

Solubility—1 Gm dissolves in about 60 ml of water, about 100 ml of methanol, and about 300 ml of absolute alcohol; practically insoluble in acetone and ether.

Uses—Chlormerodrin, an orally effective mercurial *diuretic*, is useful in the management of cardiac and nephrotic *edema*, *ascites* of liver disease, and in selected cases of subacute and chronic *nephritis*. In some patients, a parenteral mercurial may be required to replace or supplement oral medication.

Dose—*Usual*, 55 to 110 mg (equivalent to 30 to 60 mg of mercury) daily.

Other Dose Information—The dose depends on the severity of edema or circulatory failure.

Dosage Forms—Tablets NF: 18.3 mg.

Meralluride USP

[3 - [3 - (3 - Carboxypropionyl)ureido] - 2 - methoxypropyl](theophyllinato)-mercury;   N-[[2-Methoxy-3-[(1,2,3,6-tetrahydro-1,3-dimethyl-2,6-dioxo-purin-7-yl)mercuri]propyl]carbamoyl]succinamic Acid;   Mercuhydrin (Lakeside)]

$$CH_2CHCH_2NHCONHCOCH_2CH_2COOH$$

Meralluride contains 94.0–102.0% of $C_{16}H_{22}HgN_6O_7$ (610.98), calculated on the dried basis.

Preparation—By one method, allylurea is heated with succinic anhydride to form the corresponding ureide which is then boiled in methanol with mercuric acetate to give the socalled mercuri component of Meralluride, viz, [3-[3-(3-carboxypropionyl)ureido]-2-methoxypropyl]hydroxymercury. Condensation with an equimolar portion of theophylline yields Meralluride. US Pat. 2,208,941.

Description—White to slightly yellow powder. Slowly affected by light. Its saturated solution is acid to litmus.

Solubility—Slightly soluble in water; soluble in hot water; soluble in glacial acetic acid and solutions of alkali hydroxides.

Uses—Meralluride is a mercurial *diuretic* proposed for use in the *edema* of cardiorenal disease and of nephrosis, *ascites* of liver disease, and other conditions in which a mercurial diuretic may be indicated. It is well tolerated systemically and seldom causes pain at the site of injection when given intramuscularly. It is rapidly absorbed following intramuscular injection. It is also administered by intravenous injection. Contraindications and side effects are similar to those for other mercurial diuretics. See the general statement, page 939.

Dose—*Parenteral*, **1** to **2 ml**; *usual*, **1 ml** [equivalent to 39 mg of mercury and 43.6 mg of anhydrous theophylline (48 mg of hydrous theophylline)] 1 or 2 times a week.

Dosage Forms—Injection USP: the equivalent of 39 mg of mercury and 43.6 mg of anhydrous theophylline (48 mg of hydrous theophylline)/ml (in 1, 2, and 10 ml).

Mercurous Chloride, Mild—see page 800.

Sodium Mercaptomerin USP

[Sterile Mercaptomerin Sodium (USP XV); [3-(3-Carboxy-2,2,3-trimethyl-cyclopentanecarboxamido)-2-methoxypropyl](hydrogen mercaptoacetato)-mercury Disodium Salt; Sodium [[[3-(3-Carboxy-2,2,3-trimethylcyclopentanecarboxamido)-2-methoxypropyl]thio]mercuri]acetate; Thiomerin Sodium (Wyeth)]

$$NaOOC \quad CONHCH_2CHCH_2HgSCH_2COONa$$
$$OCH_3$$

Sodium Mercaptomerin contains 95.0–105.0% of $C_{16}H_{25}HgNNa_2O_6S$ (606.01), calculated on the dried basis.

Preparation—As described in US Pat. 2,576,349, Sodium Mercaptomerin may be prepared by reacting 3-[[3-(hydroxymercuri)-2-methoxypropyl]carbamoyl]-1,2,2-trimethylcyclopentanecarboxylic acid with sodium thioglycollate in aqueous NaOH solution, and

obtaining the product either by evaporation or by precipitation with suitable solvents. See below under *Mercurophylline* for preparation of the acid moiety.

Description—A white, hygroscopic powder or amorphous solid having a characteristic honeycomb structure. Its 1 in 50 solution is neutral or slightly alkaline to litmus.

Solubility—Freely soluble in water; soluble in alcohol; slightly soluble in chloroform and ether.

Uses—Mercaptomerin is a mercurial *diuretic* with actions and clinical uses similar to those of other agents in this class. See the general statement, page 939. It causes less local tissue reaction at the site of injection than do most other mercurial diuretics and hence may be administered subcutaneously. When administered frequently, the incidence of sensitization is higher than that from other agents of this class. Injected intravenously, Mercaptomerin is much less toxic to the myocardium than are the other organic mercurials.

Dose—*Parenteral*, **25** to **250 mg** daily to weekly; *usual*, **125 mg** once a day.

Dosage Forms—Injection USP: 1, 2, 10, and 30 ml; Sterile USP: 1.4 and 4.2 Gm.

Mercurophylline NF XII

[Mercupurin; Novurit]

Mercurophylline consists of the sodium salt of 3-[[3-(hydroxymercuri) - 2 - methoxypropyl]carbamoyl]-1,2,2-trimethylcyclopentanecarboxylic acid (the mercuri compound, $C_{14}H_{24}HgNNaO_5$, mol wt 509.93), and theophylline, in approximately molecular proportions. Dried at 105° for 4 hours, it contains 94–106% of the labeled amount of the mercuri compound and of anhydrous theophylline [$C_7H_8N_4O_2$].

The structural formula shown above represents the condensation product of these two components.

Preparation—Mercurophylline is prepared by a series of reactions starting with camphor. The first step is oxidation of camphor to camphoric acid with nitric acid.

The conversion of camphoric acid to its anhydride is next accomplished by heating for a short while at 100° with acetic anhydride in the presence of zinc chloride. The opening of the anhydride with allylamine is then accomplished. This occurs almost exclusively in the direction desired because of steric hindrance about one side of the anhydride system. The last step consisting of mercuration of the double bond, with simultaneous addition of the methoxy group, takes place readily by heating a mixture of the amine, mercuric acetate, and methanol. It is finally converted into the sodium salt and thus made soluble by the addition of the required amount of sodium hydroxide.

Description—A white or slightly yellow, odorless powder. Moderately hygroscopic and slowly darkens on exposure to light. Its solutions are alkaline to litmus.

Solubility—1 Gm dissolves in about 5 ml of water; soluble in alcohol; insoluble in ether and mineral oils.

Uses—This combination of an organic mercury compound and theophylline is a *diuretic*. It is used in the same manner and dosage as *Mersalyl and Theophylline Injection*. Also see the general statement, page 939.

Dose—*Usual intramuscular*, **135 mg** (in 1 ml) once or twice a week; *usual*, *oral*, **200 mg** daily.

Dosage Forms—Injection: 100 mg/ml; Tablets.

Merethoxylline Procaine

[Dicurin Procaine (*Lilly*)]

Merethoxylline Procaine is a mixture of procaine merethoxylline and theophylline is the ratio of 1 mole of the former to 1.4 moles of the latter. The procaine merethoxylline is an equimolar combination of procaine and merethoxylline. Merethoxylline is the inner salt of [*o*-[[3-(hydroxymercuri)-2-(2-methoxyethoxy)propyl]-carbamoyl]phenoxy] acetic acid; its structure is shown below.

Description—Merethoxylline is a white or practically white powder. It is stable in light and air. It melts between 138° and 141°.

Solubility—Merethoxylline is soluble in alkaline solutions; practically insoluble in water.

Uses—Merethoxylline Procaine has the same actions, uses, and limitations as other mercurial diuretics. See the general statement on mercury compounds (page 939). The procaine component minimizes the discomfort of local irritation that may be produced by the mercurial compound when injected into tissues. Sensitivity to procaine also is a contraindication in susceptible patients.

Dose—*Usual* daily, **0.5 to 2.0 ml** (containing 195 mg of the salt per ml) *intramuscularly* or *subcutaneously*. Intravenous administration is not recommended.

Dosage Forms—Injection: 100 mg/ml.

Other Mercurial Diuretics

Mercumatilin—[Mercumallylic Acid, 8-[3-(Hydroxymercuri)-2-methoxypropyl]-2-oxo-2*H*-1-benzopyran-3-carboxylic acid [$C_{14}H_{14}HgO_6$], and theophylline in approximately equimolar proportions. *Uses:* Mercurial diuretic, given orally to supplement parenteral injection of sodium mercumatilin. *Dose:* 67 to 134 mg daily.

Mersalyl NF XI [Sodium *o*-{[3-(hydroxymercuri)-2-methoxypropyl]carbamoyl}phenoxyacetate] [$C_{13}H_{16}HgN-NaO_6$]—*Uses:* Mersalyl is an organic mercurial diuretic which is employed to promote the excretion of *edema* fluid in such conditions as heart failure, renal disease, etc. Diuretic activity may be enhanced by giving Mersalyl with an acid-forming salt. Mersalyl is given in 10% solution by intravenous or intramuscular injection. A test dose of 0.5 ml is usually given the day before the full therapeutic dose of 1 to 2 ml is administered.

Mersalyl Acid BP—A mixture of *o*-{[3-(hydroxymercuri)-2-methoxypropyl]carbamoyl}phenoxyacetic acid and its anhydrides. Purity: it contains the equivalent of 97–103% of $C_{13}H_{17}HgNO_6$, calculated on the dried basis. An odorless, slightly hygroscopic, white powder that is sparingly soluble in water and in dilute mineral acids but readily soluble in sodium hydroxide solution. *Uses:* In the preparation of *Mersalyl Injection BP*, which is employed as a mercurial diuretic.

Sodium Mercumatilin [Cumertilin Sodium (*Endo*)]—a sterile aqueous solution of approximately equimolar quantities of sodium mercumallylate [$C_{14}H_{13}HgNaO_6$] and theophylline. *Uses:* Sodium Mercumatilin produces the same diuretic effect as other mercury-theophylline compounds. Its injection causes local irritation similar to that produced by other organic mercurial diuretics which are suitable only for intramuscular or intravenous injection. *Dose*—*Usual*, 0.5 to 2 ml (containing 132 mg in 1 ml) *intramuscularly* or *intravenously*, at biweekly intervals.

Carbonic Anhydrase Inhibitors

Carbonic anhydrase is an ubiquitous enzyme which is responsible for the catalytic reversible hydration of carbon dioxide and dehydration of carbonic acid, a process critical to the transport of carbon dioxide in the erythrocyte and its exchange in the parenchyma of the lungs. This enzyme is also found in the renal cortex, gastric mucosa, pancreas, eye, and central nervous system. The renal tubular cells also contain substantial amounts of carbonic anhydrase, and the CO_2 produced metabolically in the cells of the renal tubule is immediately converted to carbonic acid by the enzyme. Urine is acidified by the secretion of hydrogen ions derived from carbonic acid formed in the tubular cells in exchange for sodium ions in the lumen of the tubule. When carbonic anhydrase is inhibited, the amount of hydrogen ions available for exchange with sodium is decreased; the excess sodium ions retained in the tubule combine with bicarbonate and are excreted by the kidney with an increased volume of water. The diuretic effect is self-limited, however, since the subsequent metabolic acidosis prevents further diuretic action by the carbonic anhydrase inhibitor.

Although the carbonic anhydrase inhibitors were originally developed as diuretics, their major usefulness is in glaucoma. Inhibition of carbonic anhydrase in the ciliary body of the eye markedly reduces the secretion of aqueous humor; the oral or parenteral administration of carbonic anhydrase inhibitors decreases intraocular pressure in most patients with this ocular defect. These agents have also been used in some cases of petit mal and grand mal epilepsy refractory to other anticonvulsants.

Acetazolamide USP

N-(5-Sulfamoyl-1,3,4-thiadiazol-2-yl)acetamide; Diamox (*Lederle*)]

Acetazolamide contains 98.0–102.0% of $C_4H_6N_4O_3S_2$ (222.25), calculated on the anhydrous basis.

Preparation—Hydrazine hydrate is reacted with a double equimolar quantity of ammonium thiocyanate to produce 1,2-bis(thiocarbamoyl)hydrazine which is then caused, through loss of ammonia and rearrangement, to yield 5-amino-2-mercapto-1,3,4-thiadiazole. This is then acetylated and the acetyl compound, in aqueous medium, is oxidized to the 2-sulfonyl chloride with chlorine. The final step consists of amidation by treatment with ammonia.

Description—Occurs as a white to faintly yellowish white, crystalline, odorless powder.

Solubility—Very slightly soluble in water; sparingly soluble in hot water (90° to 100°); slightly soluble in alcohol.

Uses—Acetazolamide is a sulfonamide-type organic compound which inhibits the activity of the enzyme carbonic anhydrase (see introductory statement, page 941). It is rapidly absorbed from the stomach, reaches a peak plasma level within 2 hours, and is eliminated unchanged in the urine within 8 to 12 hours.

Acetazolamide has been used as a *diuretic* in the treatment of edema associated with congestive heart failure. It is most effective in the treatment of mild or moderate cases of congestive heart failure; however, it has largely been replaced in these conditions by the thiazide diuretics. Acetazolamide is also used in the treatment of *petit mal* and *grand mal epilepsy*, in obstetric and gynecologic conditions associated with edema, and in the treatment of *glaucoma*. In glaucoma, the drug is used as an adjunct to the usual miotic therapy.

The drug is also used in premenstrual tension, in obesity where water retention is a problem, in drug-induced edema, and as adjunctive therapy to eliminate excess fluid in the pregnant patient.

Acetazolamide is sometimes the diuretic of choice where careful following of blood electrolytes is not possible, as in outpatients. It has low toxicity.

Dose—**250 mg** to **1 Gm** daily; *usual*, **250 mg** 2 to 4 times a day.

Other Dose Information—In *glaucoma*, 250 mg every 4 hours.

Dosage Forms—Tablets USP: 125 and 250 mg.

Dichlorphenamide USP

[4,5-Dichloro-*m*-benzenedisulfonamide; Daranide (*MSD*); Oratrol (*Alcon*)]

Dichlorphenamide contains 97.0–100.5% of C_6H_6-$Cl_2N_2O_4S_2$ (305.16), calculated on the dried basis.

Preparation—*o*-Chlorophenol is reacted with chlorosulfonic acid to produce 5-chloro-4-hydroxy-1,3-benzenedisulfonyl chloride which is then treated with PCl_5 to replace the 4-hydroxy with chlorine. Ammonolysis of the sulfonyl chloride yields the disulfonamide.

Description—White or nearly white, crystalline powder having not more than a slight characteristic odor. It melts between 235° and 240°.

Solubility—Very slightly soluble in water; freely soluble in pyridine and in 1*N* sodium hydroxide; soluble in alcohol and in 2*N* sodium carbonate; slightly soluble in ether.

Uses—Dichlorphenamide, a carbonic anhydrase inhibitor, is used in the treatment of *primary glaucoma*, the acute phase of *secondary glaucoma*, and in the preoperative control of intraocular tension. The drug lowers intraocular pressure by reducing the rate of secretion of aqueous humor. Although it has diuretic properties, it is not promoted for this purpose. Side effects are the same as those induced by other carbonic anhydrase inhibitors and include anorexia, nausea and

vomiting, confusion, ataxia, tremor, dizziness, paresthesias, depression, and lassitude. Hypersensitivity reactions have been observed. Prolonged therapy may induce electrolyte abnormalities, such as hypokalemia. The drug is contraindicated in patients with hyperchloremic acidosis, adrenocortical insufficiency, and renal failure.

Dose—**50** to **300 mg** daily; *usual*, **25** to **50 mg** 1 to 3 times a day.

Dosage Forms—Tablets USP: 50 mg.

Ethoxzolamide USP

[6-Ethoxy-2-benzothiazolesulfonamide; Cardrase (*Upjohn*); Ethamide (*Allergan*)]

Ethoxzolamide contains 97.0–103.0% of C_9H_{10}-$N_2O_3S_2$ (258.32), calculated on the dried basis.

Preparation—6-Ethoxy-2-benzothiazolethiol, prepared as described by Sebrell and Boord,[1] is converted to the sulfenamide by reaction with sodium hypochlorite and ammonia. Oxidation with potassium permanganate yields the sulfonamide. US Pat. 2,868,800.

Description—White or slightly yellow, odorless, crystalline powder.

Solubility—Very soluble in alcohol; slightly soluble in acetone, chloroform, and ether; practically insoluble in water.

Uses—Ethoxzolamide is a diuretic agent with actions and uses similar to those of the chemically related sulfonamide compound, acetazolamide. Both drugs are potent inhibitors of carbonic anhydrase and are believed to influence fluid mobilization by the same basic mechanism of action (see introductory statement). Although on a weight basis Ethoxzolamide appears to be approximately twice as active as acetazolamide, both compounds have approximately the same duration of action, 8 to 12 hours after a single oral dose.

Ethoxzolamide is used to produce *diuresis* in patients with mild to moderate congestive heart failure. Like acetazolamide, Ethoxzolamide has largely been replaced in these conditions by the thiazide diuretics. Other reported uses of Ethoxzolamide include *petit mal* and *grand mal* epilepsy, glaucoma, and obstetric conditions associated with edema.

Commonly reported side effects include nausea, dizziness, and paresthesia of the fingers and toes. Other less frequently reported reactions include drowsiness, fatigue, headache, and dryness of the mouth. The drug should be used cautiously in patients with hepatic cirrhosis and is contraindicated in patients with renal failure, hyperchloremic acidosis, and Addison's disease.

Dose—**62.5 mg** to **1 Gm** daily; *usual*, **125 mg** 2 to 4 times a day.

Dosage Forms—Tablets USP: 125 mg.

Methazolamide USP

[*N*-(4-Methyl-2-sulfamoyl-Δ²-1,3,4-thiadiazolin-5-ylidene)acetamide; Neptazane (*Lederle*)]

Methazolamide contains 96.0–100.5% of $C_5H_8N_4$-O_3S_2 (236.27).

Preparation—2 - Acetamido - 5 - mercapto - 1,3,4-thiadiazole, prepared as described under *Acetazolamide* (page 941), is treated with *p*-chlorobenzyl chloride to produce the *p*-chlorobenzylmercapto derivative (I) which, upon treatment with methyl bromide in the presence of sodium methylate, undergoes methylation and rearrangement to yield the acetylimino thiadiazoline derivative (II). Oxidation of (II) with chlorine water produces the sulfonyl chloride (III) which yields Methazolamide on amidation with ammonia. For structure proof, see J. Am. Chem. Soc., **78**, 4649 (1956).

Description—White or faintly yellow, crystalline powder having a slight odor. Melts at about 213°.

Solubility—Very slightly soluble in water and in ethanol; soluble in dimethylformamide; slightly soluble in acetone.

Uses—Methazolamide, a *carbonic anhydrase inhibitor* chemically related to acetazolamide, is used either alone or in combination with acetazolamide in the treatment of glaucoma. Significant reduction in intraocular pressure occurs in 6 to 8 hours and persists for 8 to 10 hours. It is indicated in patients who do not respond to acetazolamide or in those who are intolerant to it. The incidence and nature of side effects are similar to those induced by acetazolamide, except for a lesser incidence of skin rashes and gastrointestinal complaints.

Dose—**100** to **600 mg** daily; *usual*, **50** to **100** mg 2 to 3 times a day.

Dosage Forms—Tablets USP: 50 mg.

Sterile Sodium Acetazolamide USP

[Diamox Sodium (*Lederle*)]

Sterile Sodium Acetazolamide is prepared from acetazolamide with the aid of sodium hydroxide. It is suitable for parenteral use. It contains 98.0–100.5% of $C_4H_5N_4NaO_3S_2$ (244.23).

For the structure of acetazolamide, see page 941.

Preparation—Acetazolamide is dissolved in aqueous sodium hydroxide solution containing an equimolar quantity of NaOH whereupon the acidic H of the —SO_2NH_2 group is replaced by Na. The solid sodium compound may then be produced by various drying or crystallization techniques.

Description—The pH of a freshly prepared solution (1 in 10) is between 9.0 and 10.0.

Uses—See *Acetazolamide*.

Dose—*Intravenous*, the equivalent of **250 mg** to **1 Gm** of acetazolamide daily; *usual*, **250 mg** 2 to 4 times a day.

Dosage Forms—Sterile USP: 500 mg.

Veterinary Uses—This drug is used in all species as a diuretic in edematous conditions resulting from metabolic dysfunction, local infections, heart failure, and glaucoma.

Veterinary Dose—The *initial intramuscular* or *intraperitoneal* dose is followed by *oral maintenance* therapy. Daily doses per pound of body weight follow. *Horses, parenteral,* **0.5** to **1 mg**; *oral,* **1** to **2 mg**. *Cattle, parenteral,* **0.5** to **1 mg**; *oral* **3** to **4 mg**. *Swine, parenteral* or *oral,* **2** to **4 mg**. *Dogs, parenteral* or *oral,* **5** to **15 mg**. The daily total should be administered in 2 or more divided doses.

Aldosterone Antagonists

The aldosterone antagonists represent a new approach to diuretic therapy. They differ from other inhibitors of renal tubular transport in their mechanism of action and in their profile of electrolyte effects. These agents block the renal tubular actions of aldosterone, the natural sodium-retaining factor of the body. Hence, they are ineffective when endogenous aldosterone secretion is low and their diuretic action may be overcome by increasing the concentration of aldosterone. The aldosterone antagonists increase the excretion of sodium and chloride, reduce the excretion of potassium and ammonium, and decrease the titratable acidity of the urine. They are effective in the management of edema associated with *congestive heart failure, hepatic cirrhosis with ascites, the nephrotic syndrome,* and *idiopathic edema*. The aldosterone antagonists should not be used in patients with severe renal insufficiency; patients on the drug should be watched for the development of hyponatremia and hyperkalemia. No other contraindications have been established.

Spironolactone USP

[17-Hydroxy-7α-mercapto-3-oxo-17α-pregn-4-ene-21-carboxylic Acid γ-Lactone Acetate; Aldactone (*Searle*)]

Spironolactone contains 97.0–101.5% of $C_{24}H_{32}O_4S$ (416.58).

Preparation—Spironolactone is synthesized by treating dehydroepiandrosterone (prepared from cholesterol or sitosterol) with acetylene to form the 17α-ethynyl-17β-hydroxy derivative which is carbonated to the 17α-propiolic acid. Reduction of the unsaturated acid in alkaline solution affords the saturated acid which spontaneously cyclizes to the lactone on acidification. Bromination to the 5,6-dibromo compound, followed by oxidation of the 3-hydroxyl group to the ketone, then dehydrobromination yields the 7α-hydroxyl derivative, which is esterified with thioloacetic acid to form Spironolactone.

Description—Light cream-colored to light tan, crystalline powder; has a faint to mild mercaptan-like odor; is stable in air.

Solubility—Practically insoluble in water; freely soluble in benzene and chloroform; soluble in ethyl acetate and alcohol; slightly soluble in methanol and fixed oils.

Uses—Spironolactone is a *diuretic* effective in the management of *edema* associated with *congestive heart failure, hepatic cirrhosis* with ascites, the *nephrotic syndrome,* and *idiopathic edema.* It has also been reported to exert an antihypertensive effect; this requires further clinical study. Spironolactone, by blocking the sodium-retaining effects of aldosterone on the distal convoluted tubule, corrects one of the most important mechanisms responsible for the production of edema. Its onset of diuretic action is gradual and it requires 4 or 5 days to achieve full diuretic effect. It is most useful when employed as an adjunct to other diuretics, such as the mercurials and thiazides. When used in this combined manner, it enhances the excretion of sodium and decreases the excretion of potassium. Further increase in diuresis may be obtained by the use of a glucocorticoid with spironolactone in combination with another diuretic. Side effects include hyponatremia, hyperkalemia, and drowsiness. Some patients on spironolactone develop a skin rash; however, this disappears when the drug is stopped. Spironolactone should not be used in patients with severe renal insufficiency.

Dose—*Usual,* **25 mg** 2 to 4 times a day.

Other Dose Information—If satisfactory diuretic effect is not achieved in 5 days, a mercurial or thiazide diuretic should be added to the regime.

Dosage Forms—Tablets USP: 25 mg.

Benzothiadiazine Diuretics

A number of nonmercurial diuretics inhibit renal tubular transport, but have either chemical structures or mechanisms of action which differ from those of the xanthines and the carbonic anhydrase inhibitors. These agents are classified as benzothiadiazine, phthalimidine, quinazoline, and pyrimidinedione derivatives. The benzothiadiazine derivatives (chlorothiazide and related compounds) have chemical structures which resemble, at least in some respect, those of the carbonic anhydrase inhibitors, but their effect on the kidney differs markedly from that of acetazolamide. Indeed, the pharmacodynamic characteristics of these agents appear to be intermediate to those of acetazolamide and the organic mercurial diuretics. Thus, these agents are potent inhibitors of the renal tubular reabsorption of sodium. In appropriate doses they cause only a slight increase in excretion of bicarbonate and a considerable increase in the excretion of chloride. In low doses, bicarbonate excretion is increased as a result of mild carbonic anhydrase inhibitory action, but this effect is not responsible for the major excretion of sodium and chloride. All of the benzothiadiazine diuretics are similar in diuretic and hypotensive effectiveness, in extent of potassium loss, and in untoward effects. The difference in milligram potency among the different drugs has no clinical significance. Benzothiadiazines, in combination with potassium salts or potassium salts administered alone, have been shown to cause ulcerative lesions of the small intestines. These small lesions have caused obstruction, hemorrhage, and perforation. Surgery is frequently required and deaths have occurred. Therefore, the NAS/NRC drug efficacy panel has recommended that potassium-containing formulations be withdrawn from the market. Two agents included in this section, chlorthalidone and quinethazone, are phthalimidine and quinazoline derivatives, respectively; their mechanisms of action and therapeutic indications are similar to the benzothiodiazines. The pyrimidinedione derivatives (amisometradine and aminometradine) also inhibit the renal tubular reabsorption of sodium, but have much less effect on the excretion of chloride. These agents have no effect on carbonic anhydrase, renal blood flow, or glomerular filtration rate in the dosage usually employed. The exact mode of action of the benzothiadiazine, phthalimidine, quinazoline, and pyrimidinedione derivatives on the renal tubular reabsorption of sodium has not been fully defined.

Bendroflumethiazide NF

[3-Benzyl-3,4-dihydro-6-(trifluoromethyl)-2*H*-1,2,4-benzothiadiazine-7-sulfonamide 1,1-Dioxide; Bristuron (*Bristol*); Naturetin (*Squibb*)]

Bendroflumethiazide contains 98.0–102.0% of $C_{15}H_{14}F_3N_3O_4S_2$ (421.42), calculated on the anhydrous basis.

Preparation—One method consists of cyclization of 4-amino-6-trifluoromethyl-*m*-benzenedisulfonamide through condensation with phenylacetaldehyde.[2]

Description—A white to cream colored, finely divided, crystalline powder which is odorless or has a slight, characteristic floral odor. It melts at about 220°.

Solubility—Freely soluble in alcohol and acetone; practically insoluble in water.

Uses—Bendroflumethiazide is a potent orally effective *diuretic* and antihypertensive agent. It is indicated in the control of *edema, congestive heart failure, nephrosis* and *nephritis, cirrhosis* and *ascites,* and other *edematous states.* It is also of value in *hypertension* alone or when combined with other antihypertensives. Side effects and contraindications are similar to those reported for chlorothiazide. See *Chlorothiazide* (page 945) and the general statement (this page).

Dose—*Diuretic, initial,* **5 to 20 mg** daily; *maintenance,* **2.5 to 5 mg** daily; *antihypertensive, initial,* **5 to 20 mg** daily; *maintenance,* **2.5 to 15 mg** daily.

Dosage Forms—Tablets NF: 2.5 and 5 mg.

Benzthiazide NF

[3-[(Benzylthio)methyl]-6-chloro-2*H*-1,2,4-benzothiadiazine-7-sulfonamide 1,1-Dioxide; Aquatag (*Tutag*); Exna (*Robins*)]

Benzthiazide contains 98.0–101.5% of $C_{15}H_{14}ClN_3O_4S_3$ (431.94), calculated on the dried basis.

Preparation—4-Amino-6-chloro-*m*-benzenedisulfonamide is reacted with chloroacetic anhydride to give 2,3'-dichloro-4',6'-disulfamoylacetanilide which is then caused to condense and cyclize by treatment with benzyl mercaptan in the presence of sodium hydroxide. US Pat. 3,111,517.

Description—A fine, white, crystalline powder having both a characteristic odor and taste. It is stable in both light and air. It melts at about 242°.

Solubility—Freely soluble in dimethylformamide and solutions of fixed alkali hydroxides; slightly soluble in acetone; practically insoluble in water, ether, and chloroform.

Uses—Benzthiazide is a *diuretic* and *antihypertensive* agent with pharmacological characteristics similar to the thiazides. It is about 10 times as potent on a milligram basis as chlorothiazide. Side effects and contraindications are also similar to other benzothiodiazines. See *Chlorothiazide*, this page.

Dose—*Usual, diuretic, initial*, **50** to **200 mg** daily; *maintenance*, **50** to **150 mg** daily; *usual, antihypertensive, initial*, **25** to **50 mg** twice daily; *maintenance*, adjust to the response of the patient with a maximal dose of **50 mg** 3 times a day.

Dosage Forms—Tablets NF: 50 mg.

Chlorothiazide NF

[6-Chloro-2*H*-1,2,4-benzothiadiazine-7-sulfonamide 1,1-Dioxide; Diuril (*MSD*)]

Chlorothiazide contains 98.0–100.5% of $C_7H_6ClN_3O_4S_2$ (295.72), calculated on the dried basis.

Preparation—3-Chloroaniline is acylated with chlorosulfonic acid to produce the 4,6-disulfonyl chloride which is then amidated with ammonia to give the 4,6-disulfonamide. Heating the latter with formic acid results in cyclization through double condensation.

Description—White or practically white, odorless, crystalline powder which melts at about 355°.

Solubility—Very slightly soluble in water; freely soluble in dimethylformamide and dimethylsulfoxide; slightly soluble in methanol and pyridine; practically insoluble in ether, benzene, and chloroform.

Uses—Chlorothiazide, a potent inhibitor of the renal tubular reabsorption of sodium (see introductory statement), is a potent, orally effective *diuretic* agent. Its diuretic effectiveness is greater than that of other oral diuretics and it almost equals that of the parenteral mercurials. Diuretic effects are apparent within 2 hours after oral administration and persist for about 6 to 12 hours. Refractoriness to the drug is relatively uncommon even after prolonged periods of continuous administration.

Chlorothiazide is a valuable adjunct in the management of edema associated with *congestive heart failure*. The drug may be used alone or to supplement mercurials and is effective in severe as well as mild congestive failure. Chlorothiazide has been used with good results in the treatment of *edema* associated with *adrenocorticosteroid medication*, certain types of *nephrosis* and *nephritis*, *cirrhosis*, *toxemia* of pregnancy, and *premenstrual fluid retention*. The drug may be effective in some patients who have become refractory to other saluretic agents. Like all diuretics, it can be expected to be ineffective in patients with severe renal disease and impaired glomerular filtration.

Chlorothiazide also is useful as an adjunct in the management of *hypertension*. The drug exerts a potentiating effect on other antihypertensive drugs such as rauwolfia and veratrum alkaloids, hydralazine, and ganglionic blocking agents; indeed with ganglionic blocking drugs, it may produce an excessive fall in blood pressure. When given alone, the drug generally has minimal lowering effects on blood pressure.

Chlorothiazide decreases arterial responsiveness to norepinephrine. Hence, thiazide therapy should be discontinued 48 hours prior to elective surgery. Since the drug may precipitate acute gout, it should be used with caution in patients with hyperuricemia or a history of gout. The drug may cause hypercalcemia and glycosuria in patients with latent diabetes; it also modifies the insulin requirements in diabetic patients.

Chlorothiazide is apparently well tolerated and few serious immediate side effects have been reported. Nausea, vomiting, dizziness, and diarrhea have been observed. Moderate muscular weakness and fatigue may appear initially, but these symptoms usually disappear with continued treatment. The most important side effect is excessive loss of potassium, causing general muscular weakness and heart irritability. Marked potassium loss is more likely to occur when the drug is given at relatively high dosage levels (2 Gm or more daily) or when it is used with adrenocortical steroids, which also induce potassium loss. Potassium loss potentiates the action of digitalis drugs and may aggravate disturbances in heart rhythm associated with coronary-artery insufficiency. Accordingly, the dosage of the drug should be reduced in patients with coronary artery disease or those taking digitalis. A drug rash has been observed in an occasional patient. The possibility of allergic hypersensitivity reactions should be kept in mind.

Dose—*Antihypertensive*, **250** to **500 mg**; *usual, antihypertensive*, **250 mg** 3 times a day; *diuretic*, **500 mg** to **1 Gm**; *usual, diuretic*, **500 mg** 1 or 2 times a day.

Other Dose Information—Dosage must be highly individualized according to the response of the individual patient and the severity of the condition under treatment.

Dosage Forms—Oral Suspension NF: 250 mg/5 ml; Tablets NF: 250 and 500 mg; Sodium Chlorothiazide for Injection NF: 500 mg.

Veterinary Uses—Chlorothiazide is used as an oral diuretic in the treatment of congestive heart failure, renal edema, ascites, and other edematous conditions.

Veterinary Dose—*Oral, Cattle*, **2 Gm** once or twice daily; *Dogs*, **5** to **10 mg** per **pound** of body weight daily in divided doses.

Cyclothiazide NF

[6-Chloro-3,4-dihydro-3-(5-norbornen-2-yl)-2*H*-1,2,4-benzothiadiazine-7-sulfonamide 1,1-Dioxide; Anhydron (*Lilly*)]

Cyclothiazide contains 97.0–101.5% of $C_{14}H_{16}ClN_3O_4S_2$ (389.88), calculated on the anhydrous basis.

Preparation—The process is analogous to that for *Chlorothiazide* (this page), except that 5-norbornene-2-carboxaldehyde is employed in the cyclization step instead of formic acid. US Pat. 3,275,625.

Description—A white to nearly white, practically odorless powder.

Solubility—Freely soluble in acetone, ethyl acetate, and methanol; sparingly soluble in alcohol; practically insoluble in water, chloroform, and ether.

Uses—Cyclothiazide is an orally effective *diuretic* and *antihypertensive* agent. Its site and mechanism of action, pattern of electrolyte excretion, untoward effects, and clinical applications are similar to those of other thiazides. See *Chlorothiazide*, page 945. Like other agents of this type, it may be used as an adjunct to other antihypertensive agents, such as reserpine and the ganglionic blocking agents. See the general statement, page 944.

Dose—*Usual, diuretic, initial*, **1** to **2 mg** daily; *maintenance*, **1** to **2 mg** every other day or 2 or 3 times a week; *usual, antihypertensive*, **2 mg** 1 to 3 times a day.

Dosage Forms—Tablets NF: 2 mg.

Hydrochlorothiazide USP

[6-Chloro-3,4-dihydro-2*H*-1,2,4-benzothiadiazine-7-sulfonamide 1,1-Dioxide; Esidrix (*Ciba*); HydroDiuril (*MSD*); Oretic (*Abbott*)]

Hydrochlorothiazide contains 97.0–101.5% of $C_7H_8ClN_3O_4S_2$ (297.74), calculated on the dried basis.

Preparation—The process is identical with that for *Chlorothiazide* (page 945) except that formaldehyde is employed in the final cyclization step instead of formic acid.

Description—White, or practically white, odorless, crystalline powder. Melts with decomposition at about 268°.

Solubility—Slightly soluble in water; freely soluble in sodium hydroxide solution, *n*-butylamine, and dimethylformamide; sparingly soluble in methanol; insoluble in ether, chloroform, benzene, and dilute mineral acids.

Uses—Effective diuresis, comparable to that produced by 500 mg of chlorothiazide twice daily, is induced with 50 mg of Hydrochlorothiazide twice daily. Otherwise, the pharmacological actions, clinical uses, and untoward effects are the same as for chlorothiazide. *Chlorothiazide* (page 945). See also the general statement (page 944).

Dose—**25** to **200 mg** daily; *usual*, **50 mg** 1 or 2 times a day.

Dosage Forms—Tablets USP: 25 and 50 mg.

Veterinary Dose—*Intravenous* or *intramuscular*, once or twice daily, *Horses* and *Cattle*, **125** to **250 mg**; *Swine*, **25** to **75 mg**. *Initial parenteral* therapy may be sustained with *oral* treatment. The total *oral* daily dose for *all species* is calculated at **1 mg** per **pound** of body weight.

Hydroflumethiazide NF

[3,4-Dihydro-6-(trifluoromethyl)-2*H*-1,2,4-benzothiadiazine-7-sulfonamide 1,1-Dioxide; Saluron (*Bristol*)]

Hydroflumethiazide contains 98.0–102.0% of $C_8H_8F_3N_3O_4S_2$ (331.29), calculated on the anhydrous basis.

Preparation—4 - Amino - 6 - (trifluoromethyl) - *m*-benzenedisulfonamide is heated with formaldehyde in a sulfuric acid environment thus effecting concomitant condensation and cyclization to Hydroflumethiazide. US Pat. 3,254,076.

Description—A white to cream colored, finely divided, crystalline powder. It is odorless. It melts between 270° and 275°. The pH of a 1 in 100 dispersion in water is between 4.5 to 7.5.

Solubility—Very slightly soluble in water; soluble in alcohol; freely soluble in acetone.

Uses—Hydroflumethiazide is a potent orally administered *diuretic* useful in the management of edema associated with cardiac failure, hepatic cirrhosis, premenstrual tension, and steroid administration. It is also recommended for the treatment of mild to moderate hypertension either alone or in combination with other antihypertensive agents. Since Hydroflumethiazide potentiates the actions of other antihypertensive agents, the dose of other agents may need to be reduced when this drug is added to the regimen. Except for the fact that a smaller dosage is required for Hydroflumethiazide, there is no convincing evidence of significant differences in therapeutic, metabolic, or toxic or sensitization in edemic or hypertensive patients over that of the parent compound, flumethiazide, or the prototype chlorothiazide. See *Chlorothiazide* (page 945) and the general statement (page 944).

Dose—**25** to **200 mg**; *usual*, **50** to **100 mg** per day.

Other Dose Information—Refractory cases may require as much as 200 mg per day in divided doses. Dosage should be adjusted to provide the minimum effective dose for the individual patient.

Dosage Forms—Tablets NF: 50 mg.

Methyclothiazide NF

[6-Chloro-3-(chloromethyl)-3,4-dihydro-2-methyl-2*H*-1,2,4-benzothiadizine-7-sulfonamide 1,1-Dioxide; Enduron (*Abbott*)]

Methyclothiazide contains 97.0–102.0% of $C_9H_{11}Cl_2N_3O_4S_2$ (360.24), calculated on the dried basis.

Preparation—By a process analogous to that for *Chlorothiazide* (page 945), 4-amino-6-chloro-*N*³-methyl-*m*-benzenedisulfonamide is cyclized through condensation with monochloroacetaldehyde or an acetyl thereof. US Pat. 3,163,644.

Description—A white or practically white, crystalline compound. It is odorless or has a slight odor and is tasteless. It chars slightly below 220° and decomposes at 220°.

Solubility—Freely soluble in acetone and pyridine; sparingly soluble in methanol; slightly soluble in alcohol; very slightly soluble in water, benzene, chloroform, and isopropyl alcohol.

Uses—An orally effective diuretic and antihypertensive agent of the thiazide group. Except for its enhanced potency and longer duration of action, its pharmacological actions, therapeutic uses, side effects, and contraindications are similar to chlorothiazide and related agents. See *Chlorothiazide* (page 945). Diuresis comparable to that produced by 500 mg of chlorothiazide twice a day is induced with 2.5 mg once a day. See the general statement (page 944).

Dose—*Usual*, **2.5** to **10 mg** once daily, 10 mg being the maximum single effective dose.

Other Dose Information—*Usual, maintenance* and *antihypertensive*, 2.5 to 5 mg once daily.

Dosage Forms—Tablets NF: 2.5 and 5 mg.

Polythiazide NF

[6-Chloro-3,4-dihydro-2-methyl-3-[[(2,2,2-trifluoroethyl)thio]methyl]-2H-1,2,4-benzothiadiazine-7-sulfonamide 1,1-Dioxide; Renese (*Pfizer*)]

Polythiazide, dried in vacuum at 60° for 2 hours, contains 97.0–101.0% of $C_{11}H_{13}ClF_3N_3O_4S_3$ (439.88).

Preparation—6 - Amino - 4 - chloro - N^1 - methyl-*m*-benzenedisulfonamide is condensed with the dimethyl acetal of 2,2,2-trifluoroethylmercaptoacetaldehyde by refluxing a solution of the components in the dimethyl ether of ethylene glycol. A small amount of ethyl acetate saturated with hydrogen chloride is also present to catalyze the condensation. The crude Polythiazide, which precipitates when the reaction mixture is added to cold water, is recrystallized from isopropanol. US Pat. 3,009,911.

Description—White, crystalline powder.
Solubility—Soluble in methanol, acetone, and dimethylformamide; practically insoluble in water and chloroform.

Uses—Polythiazide is an orally effective long-acting diuretic and antihypertensive agent of the thiazide class. Its clinical effectiveness, untoward reactions, and contraindications are similar to those of other benzothiadiazine diuretics. When compared on a milligram basis, 2 mg has approximately the same diuretic activity as 500 mg of chlorothiazide. See *Chlorothiazide* (page 945) and the general statement (page 944).

Dose—*Usual*, **1** to **4 mg** daily.
Other Dose Information—Antihypertensive, 2 to 4 mg adjusted to achieve desired results.

Dosage Forms—Tablets NF: 1, 2, and 4 mg.

Quinethazone USP

[7-Chloro-2-ethyl-1,2,3,4-tetrahydro-4-oxo-6-quinazolinesulfonamide; Hydromox (*Lederle*)]

Quinethazone contains 98.0–102.0% of $C_{10}H_{12}ClN_3O_3S$ (289.74), calculated on the dried basis.

Preparation—4′-Chloro-*o*-acetotoluidide is subjected to chlorosulfonation and subsequent amination to form 2-amino-4-chloro-5-sulfamoylbenzamide. Refluxing with an acidulated alcoholic solution of the diethylacetal of propionaldehyde effects the required condensation cyclization to yield Quinethazone. US Pat. 2,976,289.

Description—A white to yellowish white, odorless, crystalline powder that has a bitter taste. It discolors in the presence of strong light and alkaline materials. It melts between 250° and 252°.

Solubility—1 Gm dissolves in 20 ml of polyethylene glycol 300, 125 ml of propylene glycol, and 500 ml of alcohol; freely soluble in solutions of alkali hydroxides and carbonates; sparingly soluble in pyridine; very slightly soluble in water.

Uses—This is a quinazoline derivative with *diuretic* and *antihypertensive* actions similar to the thiazides. It differs chemically from the benzothiazide type only in the replacement of a sulfur atom by a carbon. Available clinical evidence indicates that its site, mechanism, duration of action, electrolyte excretion pattern, therapeutic actions, and untoward effects are similar to those of chlorothiazide and related agents. See *Chlorothiazide* (page 945) and the general statement (page 944).

Dose—**50** to **200 mg** daily; *usual*, **50** to **100 mg** once a day.

Dosage Forms—Tablets USP: 50 mg.

Trichlormethiazide NF

[6-Chloro-3-(dichloromethyl)-3,4-dihydro-2H-1,2,4-benzothiadiazine-7-sulfonamide 1,1-Dioxide; Metahydrin (*Lakeside*); Naqua (*Schering*)]

Trichlormethiazide, dried at 105° for 3 hours, contains 97.5–102.5% of $C_8H_8Cl_3N_3O_4S_2$ (380.66).

Preparation—Trichlormethiazide may be prepared by reacting 4-amino-6-chloro-*m*-benzenedisulfonamide with dichloroacetaldehyde, or an acetal thereof, in a suitable condensation environment. US Pats. 3,163,645 and 3,264,292.

Description—A white, crystalline powder that is odorless and tasteless. It is light sensitive, but is stable in air and heat. It melts at about 274° with decomposition.

Solubility—1 Gm dissolves in about 10 ml of acetone, 50 ml of alcohol, 1200 ml of water, and 5000 ml of chloroform.

Uses—Trichlormethiazide is an orally effective and long-acting *diuretic* and *antihypertensive* of the thiazide class. Pharmacological actions, therapeutic uses, untoward effects, and contraindications are also similar to the parent substance, chlorothiazide. See *Chlorothiazide* (page 945) and the general statement (page 944). On a milligram basis, it is approximately 250 times more active than chlorothiazide.

Dose—*Usual*, **2** to **4 mg** twice daily, then **2** to **4 mg** once daily.

Dosage Forms—Tablets NF: 2 and 4 mg.

Miscellaneous Inhibitors of Renal Tubular Transport

A number of diuretics with diverse chemical structure are potent inhibitors of renal tubular transport. Some of these agents, such as chlorthalidone and furosemide, are chemically related to the sulfonamides. Other agents, such as ethacrynic acid and triamterene, are chemically unrelated to other diuretics. Despite their unrelated chemical structures, all these substances act by inhibiting renal tubular transport of various ions. Hence, they are described under this section.

Chlorthalidone USP

[2-Chloro-5-(1-hydroxy-3-oxo-1-isoindolinyl)benzenesulfonamide;   Hygroton (*Geigy*)]

Chlorthalidone contains 98.0–102.0% of $C_{14}H_{11}Cl$-N_2O_4S (338.77).

Preparation—3 - Amino - 4 - chlorobenzophenone-2-carboxylic acid is diazotized and the resulting diazonium chloride is reacted in the cold with sulfur dioxide in glacial acetic acid in the presence of cupric chloride to form 4-chloro-2'-carboxybenzophenone-3-sulfonyl chloride (I).   Heating (I) with thionyl chloride yields 3-chloro-3-(3'-chlorosulfonyl-4'-chlorophenyl)phthalide which is isolated, dissolved in chloroform, and reacted with ammonia in the cold in the presence of ethanol.   Removal of the solvent and treatment of the residue with hydrochloric acid yields crude Chlorthalidone which is recrystallized from aqueous ethanol.   US Pat. 3,055,904.

Description—A white to yellowish white, crystalline powder.   It melts with decomposition between 215° and 222°.

Solubility—Soluble in methanol; slightly soluble in alcohol;   practically insoluble in water, ether, and chloroform; forms easily soluble salts with Na_2CO_3 and NaOH.

Uses—This phthalimide derivative is an orally effective *diuretic* useful in the treatment of edema associated with *congestive heart failure, renal disease, hepatic cirrhosis, pregnancy, obesity,* and the *premenstrual syndrome.*   The diuretic effects start within 2 hours after administration, reach a peak in 6 hours, and persist for 48 to 72 hours.   Therefore, the drug usually is given only every other day.   Biochemical studies suggest that the prolonged duration of action is due to slow gastrointestinal absorption and enterohepatic recirculation.   The drug is excreted unchanged by the kidney.   Chlorthalidone also exerts an antihypertensive effect and may be administered with other agents, such as reserpine, ganglionic blocking agents, hydralazine, and guanethidine.   Since Chlorthalidone contains a sulfonamide group, its pharmacological actions and many of its untoward effects are similar to those of other orally administered diuretics.   Chlorthalidone is contraindicated in patients with severe renal or hepatic disease.   Patients on this drug should be watched closely for symptoms of renal damage or of electrolyte disturbance.

Dose—**50** to **200 mg** daily or every other day; *usual,* **100 mg** once a day.

Other Dose Information—Usual, antihypertensive, 100 mg every other day or 50 mg daily.

Dosage Forms—Tablets USP: 50 and 100 mg.

Ethacrynic Acid USP

[2,3-Dichloro-4-(2-methylenebutyryl)phenoxy]acetic Acid;   Edecrin (*MSD*)

Ethacrynic Acid contains 97.0–102.0% of $C_{13}H_{12}$-Cl_2O_4 (303.14), calculated on the dried basis.

Caution—Use care in handling Ethacrynic Acid, since it irritates the skin, eyes, and mucous membranes.

Preparation—2,3-Dichlorophenoxyacetic acid is subjected to a Friedel–Crafts reaction with butyryl chloride to form the 4-butyryl derivative.   This is then caused to undergo a Mannich reaction with formaldehyde and dimethylamine, the product of which is readily decomposed thermally to introduce the methylene group.

Description—A white or practically white, crystalline powder that is odorless or practically odorless and has a bitter taste.   It is relatively stable in light and at room temperature and is nonhygroscopic.   It melts between 121° and 125°.

Solubility—1 Gm dissolves in about 1.6 ml of alcohol, about 3.5 ml of ether, and about 6 ml of chloroform;   very slightly soluble in water.

Uses—Ethacrynic Acid is a *diuretic agent* chemically unrelated to other oral or parenteral diuretics.   Maximum water and sodium diuresis is similar to that with furosemide, but greatly exceeds that with thiazides or organomercurial diuretics.   Ethacrynic Acid is used in the treatment of *fluid retentive states* caused by *congestive heart failure, cirrhosis of the liver,* and *renal disease.*   Its usefulness in essential hypertension has not been fully established.   It exerts its action largely on the ascending loop of Henle, where it affects both the concentrating and diluting mechanisms of the kidney.   Ethacrynic Acid causes the excretion of virtually an iso-osmotic urine by preventing sodium reabsorption from the loop of Henle; chloride excretion is even greater than sodium.   After oral administration, diuresis begins within 1 hour, reaches a peak in 2 or 3 hours and persists for 6 to 8 hours.   After intravenous administration, diuresis begins immediately and reaches a maximum within 30 minutes.   Ethacrynic Acid can be used with additive effect with diuretics having different sites of action.   Side effects include hypotension, low blood volume, hypokalemia, hyponatremia, and hypochloremic alkalosis.   Nausea, vomiting, and severe diarrhea may occur after either oral or intravenous administration of the drug.   Transient deafness, tinnitus, and vertigo have been observed.   Both hypoglycemia and hyperglycemia have been reported.   Reversible agranulocytosis, rashes, blurred vision, and uric acid retention have also occurred in some patients.   Patients on Ethacrynic Acid should have their blood urea nitrogen, serum carbon dioxide and electrolytes, and white blood cell counts checked frequently.

Dose—**50** to **200 mg** daily;   *usual,* **50 mg** 2 times a day or 2 times every other day.

Other Dose Information—Dosage must be carefully regulated to prevent excessive fluid and electrolyte loss.

Dosage Forms—Tablets USP: 25 and 50 mg.

Sodium Ethacrynate for Injection USP

[Sodium   [2,3-Dichloro-4-(2-methylenebutyryl)phenoxy]acetate;   Lyovac Sodium Edecrin (*MSD*)]

Sodium Ethacrynate for Injection is a sterile, cryodesiccated powder prepared by the neutralization of ethacrynic acid with the aid of sodium hydroxide. It contains an amount of sodium ethacrynate equivalent to 90.0–110.0% of the labeled amount of $C_{13}H_{12}Cl_2O_4$ (303.14).

Preparation—Ethacrynic acid (page 948) is dissolved in an equimolar portion of aqueous sodium hydroxide and the resulting salt is either crystallized through concentration or precipitated by the addition of a suitable organic liquid.

Uses—See *Ethacrynic Acid*.

Dose—*Intravenous*, the equivalent of **50 to 100 mg** of ethacrynic acid; *usual*, the equivalent of **50 mg** of ethacrynic acid.

Dosage Forms—USP: 50 mg.

Furosemide USP

[4-Chloro-*N*-furfuryl-5-sulfamoylanthranilic Acid; Lasix (*Hoechst*)]

Furosemide contains 98.0–101.0% of $C_{12}H_{11}ClN_2O_5S$ (330.75), calculated on the dried basis.

Preparation—2,4-Dichlorobenzoic acid is heated with chlorosulfonic acid and the resulting 5-chlorosulfonyl derivative is reacted with concentrated ammonia to convert it to the 5-sulfamoyl analog (I). Refluxing (I) with furfurylamine in large excess or in the presence of sodium bicarbonate yields crude Furosemide which is recrystallized from aqueous ethanol. Protection of the chlorine atom adjacent to the sulfamoyl group is achieved by controlling the temperature of the furfurylamination. US Pat. 3,058,882.

Description—A fine, white to slightly yellow, crystalline powder that is odorless and practically tasteless. It is unstable in light but stable in air. It melts between 203° and 205° with decomposition.

Solubility—Freely soluble in acetone, dimethylformamide, and solutions of alkali hydroxides; soluble in methanol; sparingly soluble in alcohol; slightly soluble in ether; very slightly soluble in chloroform; practically insoluble in water.

Uses—Furosemide is a *diuretic* chemically related to the sulfonamide diuretics, but with much greater maximum diuretic effect. Furosemide produces a good diuretic response in patients with *edema due to congestive heart failure, hepatic cirrhosis,* or *renal disease.* It is also useful in the management of *hypertension.* Like ethacrynic acid, Furosemide acts primarily on the ascending limit of the loop of Henle to inhibit sodium and water reabsorption. Administered orally, the diuretic effect begins within 1 hour, reaches a peak in 1 or 2 hours, and persists for 4 to 6 hours. Adverse effects which may result from therapy with Furosemide include reduction of renal, cerebral, and cardiac blood flow, potassium loss with resultant cardiac and neuromuscular abnormalities, elevation of blood uric acid and blood sugar levels, allergic reactions, and blood dyscrasias (thrombcytopenia and leukopenia). Paresthesia, blurring of vision, postural hypotension, nausea, vomiting, or diarrhea may occur. Diuresis induced by Furosemide has also been accompanied by weakness, fatigue, lightheadedness or dizziness, muscle cramps, thirst, and urinary frequency. Excessive Furosemide therapy can lead to profound diuresis with water and electrolyte depletion. Patients on this drug should be tested at frequent intervals for blood urea nitrogen, sodium, potassium, chloride, and carbon dioxide concentrations. The drug should not be used in cirrhotic patients, unless they do not respond to other therapy. The safety of Furosemide in children and pregnant women has not been fully established.

Dose—**40 to 200 mg** daily; *usual,* **40 to 80 mg** once a day.

Dosage Forms—Injection: 10 mg/ml; Tablets USP: 40 mg.

Veterinary Dose—*Horses, parenteral,* **250 to 500 mg** (5 to 10 ml of a 5% solution) daily or intermittently; *Dogs* and *Cats, oral, intramuscular,* or *intravenous,* **2 mg** per **pound** of body weight once or twice daily.

Triamterene USP

[2,4,7-Triamino-6-phenylpteridine; Dyrenium (*SKF*)]

Triamterene contains 98.0–102.0% of $C_{12}H_{11}N_7$ (253.27), calculated on the dried basis.

Preparation—5 - Nitroso - 2,4,6 - triaminopyrimidine is refluxed with phenylacetonitrile in the presence of sodium methoxide. The solid which separates on cooling is collected, decolorized with charcoal, suspended in deionized water, and warmed for 15 minutes. US Pat. 3,081,230.

Description—A yellow, odorless, crystalline powder. It is stable to temperature and light.

Solubility—Soluble in formic acid; sparingly soluble in 2-methoxyethanol; very slightly soluble in acetic acid, alcohol, and dilute mineral acids; practically insoluble in water, benzene, chloroform, ether, and dilute alkaline hydroxides.

Uses—This pteridine diuretic is used in the treatment of edema associated with *congestive heart failure, cirrhosis,* the *nephrotic syndrome,* and late pregnancy. It is also employed for the management of *idiopathic edema* and edematous patients unresponsive to other therapy. It was originally thought to be a nonsteroidal antagonist of aldosterone; however, subsequent work demonstrated it to be effective in both adrenalectomized and normal animals. This indicates that Triamterene directly inhibits the reabsorption of sodium and chloride independent of aldosterone. Although it promotes the excretion of sodium and chloride, it is believed to conserve potassium by reducing the transport of this ion from the tubular cell to the tubular lumen. Hence, it should not be used with potassium supplements and should be used with caution in patients with pre-existing elevated serum potassium. It is also contraindicated in patients with severe kidney and liver disease. Side effects are usually mild and consist of nausea, vomiting, gastrointestinal disturbances, weakness, headache, dry mouth, and rash.

Dose—**100 mg** every other day to **300 mg** daily; *usual,* **100 mg** once a day.

Other Dose Information—The usual dose should be taken after meals. For *maintenance,* 100 mg daily or every other day. The total dose should not exceed 300 mg daily.

Dosage Forms—Capsules USP: 100 mg.

Other Miscellaneous Inhibitors of Renal Tubular Transport

Amisometradine NF XI [Rolicton (*Searle*)] is 6-amino-methyl-1-(2-methylallyl)uracil [$C_9H_{13}N_3O_2$]. *Description and Solubility:* A white, crystalline powder; it is odorless and has a mild, slightly unpleasant taste; it melts between 170° and 176°. Slightly soluble in water; freely soluble in alcohol; insoluble in ether. *Uses:* An orally effective non-mercurial *diuretic* which has been successfully employed in patients with mild to moderate congestive heart failure, hepatic cirrhosis, and the nephrotic syndrome. It has also been used for the management of water and salt retention during pregnancy and in the premenstrual period. Nausea and vomiting occur in 10 to 15% of patients when it is employed. *Dose:* Usual, *400 mg* 4 times daily.

Miscellaneous Renal Agents

Probenecid USP

[*p*-(Dipropylsulfamoyl)benzoic Acid; Benemid (*MSD*)]

$$(CH_3CH_2CH_2)_2NSO_2\!-\!\!\bigcirc\!\!-\!COOH$$

Probenecid contains 98.0–100.5% of $C_{13}H_{19}NO_4S$ (285.36), calculated on the dried basis.

Preparation—Toluene is reacted with chlorosulfonic acid, and the resulting *p*-toluenesulfonyl chloride is hydrolyzed to *p*-toluenesulfonic acid. Oxidation of the methyl group with potassium permanganate produces *p*-carboxybenzenesulfonic acid. This acid is then converted into the corresponding sulfonyl chloride by treatment with chlorosulfonic acid, and the final step consists of condensing the sulfonyl chloride with di-*n*-propylamine. Crude Probenecid is precipitated by pouring the reaction mixture into cold water. The precipitate is collected, washed, and purified by recrystallization from a suitable solvent such as alcohol.

Description—White or nearly white, fine, crystalline powder. It is practically odorless. It melts between 198° and 200°.

Solubility—Soluble in dilute alkali, alcohol, and acetone; practically insoluble in water and dilute acids.

Uses—Probenecid is an effective *uricosuric* agent for the treatment of gout and gouty arthritis. It inhibits the tubular reabsorption of urate, thus increasing urinary excretion of uric acid and decreasing serum uric acid levels. The drug also inhibits the renal tubular excretion of certain organic compounds such as penicillin, cephalothin, aminosalicylic acid, and phenolsulfonphthalein. It therefore, is useful as an adjunct to intensive therapy with penicillin, cephalothin, or aminosalicylic acid to increase and prolong the plasma concentrations of these anti-infective agents. However, it is rarely necessary to resort to Probenecid to increase blood and tissue levels of these agents or to lengthen the interval between doses. The drug also inhibits tubular reabsorption of erythromycin, but this effect is of little importance since the liver and biliary tract are the major excretory pathways for these agents. Probenecid has no effect on the excretion of streptomycin, chloramphenicol, chlortetracycline, or oxytetracycline. Its suppression of the renal clearance of phenolsulfonphthalein (phenol red) is of significance in the application of that kidney excretion test as a clinical guide to the effectiveness of Probenecid.

Probenecid is well tolerated, but occasional patients may experience nausea. Rarely, sensitivity may be manifested by the appearance of a skin rash, in which case therapy should be discontinued.

Dose—500 mg to 2 Gm daily; *usual*, **500 mg** 2 to 4 times a day.

Dosage Forms—Tablets USP: 500 mg.

Sulfinpyrazone—see page 1140.

Other Miscellaneous Renal Agents

Carbacrylamine Resins [Carbo-Resin (*Lilly*)]—A mixture of 87.5% of cation exchangers (⅔ polyacrylic carboxylic acid resin and ⅓ potassium salt of this resin) and 12.5% anion exchanger (polyaminemethylene resin). A light buff, free-flowing powder, practically odorless, and practically insoluble in acids, alkalies, alcohol, ether, and water. *Uses:* When ingested in their hydrogen or ammonium cycle, cation exchange resins interfere with the intestinal absorption of dietary sodium and promote fecal excretion of sodium, potassium and, to a lesser extent, calcium. The high affinity of these resins for potassium provides an effective means of reducing dangerously high potassium levels in anuric patients with hyperkalemia.

However, when Carbacrylamine Resins, which contain a portion of the cation exchange resin in the potassium cycle, are administered, a negative potassium balance is only rarely produced. Thus, Carbacrylamine Resins are employed as adjuncts to mercurial diuretic therapy and dietary electrolyte restriction for mobilization of edema fluid and maintenance of the edema-free state, particularly in patients with congestive heart failure. They are also useful in other conditions, such as hypertension, in which dietary sodium restriction may be of value.

Anorexia, nausea, and vomiting may occur in some patients and many patients refuse resin therapy because of the large bulk required and the unpleasant taste. The major untoward effects are disturbances in electrolyte metabolism. If renal function is inadequate, severe uncompensated hyperchloremic acidosis may occur. Vigorous resin therapy, especially when combined with diuretic agents and with dietary salt restriction, has led to excessive negative sodium balance and the signs and symptoms of "low-salt syndrome." If the resins are to be employed for a long period, supplementary calcium intake is advisable to prevent disturbances in calcium metabolism. *Dose:* Dosage is highly individualized. The usual initial dose is 16 Gm, 3 times daily, taken between meals. The maximum single dose recommended is 24 Gm; when it is necessary to prescribe more than 72 Gm daily, the number of doses should be increased. Each Gm will remove approximately 1 mEq of sodium from the intestinal tract.

References

1. Sebrell and Boord, *J. Am. Chem. Soc.*, **45**, 2390 (1923).
2. *J. Am. Chem. Soc.*, **81**, 4807 (1959).

This chapter was prepared by

Ewart A. Swinyard, PhD, *Professor of Pharmacology, College of Pharmacy and College of Medicine, University of Utah, Salt Lake City, Utah 84112, and*
Stewart C. Harvey, PhD, *Associate Professor of Pharmacology, College of Medicine, University of Utah, Salt Lake City, Utah 84112*

Drugs that stimulate the smooth muscle of the uterus are known as *oxytocics*. Only two chemical types of oxytocics are clinically used: (1) the oxytocic fraction (oxytocin) of the posterior pituitary extract and (2) certain ergot alkaloids. However, a number of other agents possess mild to intense oxytocic actions. Some of these, eg, hydrastis, have been used formerly but are now archaic. Others, eg, quinine, are used by the lay public without medical approval. The lay public, and sometimes also the physician, employ cathartics and abdominal congestants such as castor oil reflexly to induce uterine movement, but it is doubtful whether such agents are effective until the uterus is prepared to present the fetus normally.

The response of the uterus to oxytocics depends upon estrogenic and progestational hormonal influences, the progestational influences being the more conducive to responsiveness. Consequently, and fortunately, during the first two terms of pregnancy, oxytocics are generally incapable of inducing labor. During the third term, uterine responsiveness rises sharply in advance of pelvic relaxation, cervical dilatation, and the coordination of uterine contractions necessary to proper delivery of the fetus. Consequently, the premature induction of labor by oxytocics can result in harm to both mother and infant and may result in stillbirth if premature separation of the placenta, placental vasoconstriction, or umbilical strangulation occur consequent to the actions of the oxytocic. Therefore, only under rare circumstances should oxytocics be used to induce labor; indeed, they are generally withheld *during* labor until the cervix is dilated and presentation of the fetus has occurred (ie, until the third stage of labor). The oxytocic is then given to hasten the delivery of the placenta and to diminish uterine bleeding, which diminution is the result of contractile compression of the blood sinuses and of vasoconstriction. Oxytocics may also be employed during the puerperium to aid in the involution of the uterus to normal.

Nonoxytocic ergot alkaloids are listed in this section because of their relationship to the oxytocic prototypes.

The so-called uterine sedatives comprise an ill defined class of drugs which diminish or supposedly diminish uterine activity. They are employed to interrupt premature labor, to diminish pain in dysmenorrhea, and to diminish premenstrual discomfort. Some of these agents, such as central nervous system sedatives, have a central locus, and it is questionable whether uterine activity is affected at all. Uterine activity and premature labor may be decreased after opiates have been administered. Ammonium chloride and other diuretics may give relief in dysmenorrhea, not by their effects on uterine activity, but by the relief of pelvic congestion and edema. Both estrogens and progestational hormones (see Chapter 55, page 988) have been employed in the treatment of dysmenorrhea. Though the estrogens may suppress uterine motility under certain circumstances, the prophylactic action in this instance is through the prevention of ovulation. Progestational hormones may decrease uterine motility in appropriate circumstances, but the mechanism of their action in dysmenorrhea is undetermined, except that it is not a proliferative effect. The balance between estrogens and progestational hormones may be more important to uterine activity than either type of hormone alone. The hormone relaxin is claimed to decrease uterine motility. Miscellaneous "uterine sedatives," may be no more than placebos.

Ergonovine Maleate USP

[(+)-9,10-Didehydro-*N*-[(*S*)-2-hydroxy-1-methylethyl-6-methylergoline-8β-carboxamide Maleate (1:1) (Salt); Ergometrine Maleate; Ergotrate Maleate (*Lilly*)

Ergonovine Maleate contains 98.0–101.0% of $C_{19}H_{23}N_3O_2 \cdot C_4H_4O_4$ (441.49), calculated on the dried basis.

For the structural formula of ergonovine, see page 499.

Preparation—Ergonovine maleate may be prepared from the natural alkaloid ergonovine by dissolving the latter in a suitable solvent and reacting it with an equimolar portion of maleic acid.

Ergonovine alkaloid is also prepared synthetically from isolysergic acid which is obtained by the alkaline hydrolysis of ergot alkaloids. One of the methods of synthesis involves the following steps: (1) conversion of the acid to its methyl ester by reaction with diazomethane; (2) hydrazinolysis of the ester to lysergic acid hydrazide; (3) condensation of the hydrazide with nitrous acid to form the azide; (4) metathesis of the azide with D-2-amino-1-propanol to form the amide; and (5) isomerization of the amide to the normal form by treatment with acetic or phosphoric acid. Schematically:

$$R-\overset{\overset{\displaystyle O}{\|}}{C}-OH \xrightarrow{CH_2N_2} R-\overset{\overset{\displaystyle O}{\|}}{C}-OCH_3 \xrightarrow{N_2H_4} R-\overset{\overset{\displaystyle O}{\|}}{C}-NH\cdot NH_2$$

$$\downarrow HNO_2$$

$$\text{Ergonovine} \xleftarrow[\text{then isomerization}]{CH_3\cdot CH(NH_2)\cdot CH_2OH;} R-\overset{\overset{\displaystyle O}{\|}}{C}-N\cdot N:N$$

where R represents lysergic acid (see page 499) minus its carboxyl group.

Description—A white, or faintly yellow, odorless, micro-crystalline powder. It is affected by light. It has a specific rotation of +51° to +56° in aqueous solution.

Solubility—1 Gm dissolves in about 36 ml of water and about 120 ml of alcohol; insoluble in ether and chloroform.

Uses—Ergonovine is the most valued of the ergot alkaloids for obstetrical use. It is a powerful *uterine stimulant* and is active after both oral or parenteral administration. It is less toxic than the other active alkaloids of ergot and is much less prone to cause gangrene (see *Ergot*, page 953). Ergonovine Maleate is given after the delivery of the placenta for the purpose of contracting the uterus in order to *reduce postpartum bleeding*. It may also be administered during the puerperium to *promote involution of the uterus*.

Dose—*Oral, intravenous,* or *intramuscular,* **400 mcg** to **1.6 mg** daily; *usual, oral* **200 mcg** 3 or 4 times a day; *usual, intravenous,* or *intramuscular,* **200 mcg**, repeated after 2 to 4 hours if necessary.

Dosage Forms—Injection USP: **1** ml; Tablets USP: 200 mcg.

Veterinary Dose—*Intramuscular, Mares* and *Cows,* **10** to **20 mg**; *Ewes, Goats,* and *Sows,* **0.4** to **1 mg**; *Bitches,* **0.2** to **0.5 mg**; *Queens,* **0.07** to **0.125 mg**. In severe bleeding a repeat injection may be required after 2 to 4 hours.

Ergotamine Tartrate USP

[Ergotamine Tartrate (2:1); Gynergen (*Sandoz*)]

Ergotamine Tartrate contains 97.0–100.5% of $(C_{33}H_{35}N_5O_5)_2 \cdot C_4H_6O_6$ (1313.44), calculated on the dried basis.

For the structural formula of ergotamine, see page 499.

Description—Colorless crystals or a white to yellowish white, crystalline powder, usually containing solvent of crystallization. These crystals lose the solvent of crystallization in a high vacuum. It melts at about 180° with decomposition. The $[\alpha]_D^{20}$ of ergotamine base in chloroform solution, obtained by suspending Ergotamine Tartrate in sodium bicarbonate solution (1 in 20) and extracting the liberated alkaloid with chloroform, is −150° to −160°.

Solubility—1 Gm dissolves in about 500 ml of water and about 500 ml of alcohol; slightly more soluble in the presence of a slight excess of tartaric acid.

Uses—Ergotamine Tartrate possesses the characteristic actions of the ergot alkaloids (see *Ergot*, page 953). At one time it was extensively employed in obstetrics, but ergonovine has proved to be a more valued preparation, chiefly because of more rapid onset of action, better absorption after oral administration, and lessened toxicity.

Ergotamine Tartrate is an effective drug in the treatment of *migraine*, for which purpose ergonovine cannot be substituted. It contracts the painfully dilated cerebral vessels in this disease. The drug is most effective if given early in the course of the attack. It is best administered by subcutaneous or intramuscular injection. The toxic potentialities of this drug are discussed under Ergot, page 953.

Dose—*Oral* or *rectal,* **2** to **10 mg** weekly; *usual, oral, initial,* **2 mg**, followed by **1 mg** every 30 minutes, if necessary, to a maximum of **6 mg** per attack; *intramuscular* or *subcutaneous,* **250 mcg** to **1 mg** weekly; *usual,* **250** to **500 mcg**, repeated in 1 hour is necessary; *usual, rectal,* **2 mg**, repeated in 1 hour if necessary.

Other Dose Information—No more than 1 mg should be given parenterally during a 24-hour period. The usual suppository dose is 2 mg.

Dosage Forms—Injection USP: 0.5 and 1 ml; Tablets USP: 1 mg.

Ergotamine Tartrate and Caffeine Suppositories NF

[Cafergot Suppositories (*Sandoz*)]

Ergotamine Tartrate and Caffeine Suppositories contain 90.0–110.0% of the labeled amounts of $(C_{33}H_{35}N_5O_5)_2 \cdot C_4H_6O_6$ (Ergotamine tartrate) and of $C_8H_{10}N_4O_2$ (caffeine).

Uses—See *Ergotamine Tartrate and Caffeine Tablets,* below.

Dose—*Usual, rectal,* **2 mg** of ergotamine tartrate with **100 mg** of caffeine; this dose may be repeated once only in 1 hour if necessary.

Dosage Forms—NF: 2 mg (ergotamine tartrate) and 100 mg (caffeine).

Ergotamine Tartrate and Caffeine Tablets NF

[Cafergot Tablets (*Sandoz*)]

Ergotamine Tartrate and Caffeine Tablets contain 90.0–110.0% of the labeled amounts of $(C_{33}H_{35}N_5O_5)_2 \cdot C_4H_6O_6$ (ergotamine tartrate) and of $C_8H_{10}N_4O_2$ (caffeine).

Uses—Ergotamine Tartrate and Caffeine are used in combination for the treatment of *migraine headache.* This use and the side effects and contraindications of Ergotamine Tartrate were discussed under *Ergotamine Tartrate,* above. Caffeine synergizes the action of ergotamine, probably because caffeine also constricts the cerebral blood vessels, distention of which is believed to be the cause of the pain.

Dose—*Usual, initial,* **2 mg** of ergotamine tartrate and **200 mg** of caffeine, followed by 1/2 this dose every 30 minutes until relief is obtained, but not to exceed a total dose of **6 mg** of ergotamine tartrate.

Dosage Forms—NF: 1 mg (ergotamine tartrate) and 100 mg (caffeine).

Methylergonovine Maleate USP

[(+)-9,10-Didehydro-*N*-[(*S*)-1-(hydroxymethyl)propyl]-6-methylergoline-8β-carboxamide Maleate (1:1) (Salt); Methergine (*Sandoz*)]

Methylergonovine Maleate contains 97.0–103.0% of $C_{20}H_{25}N_3O_2 \cdot C_4H_4O_4$ (455.52), calculated on the dried basis.

For the structural formula of methylergonovine, see page 499.

Preparation—Methylergonovine (base) is prepared by the synthetic method described above for ergonovine alkaloid except that in step (4), D-2-amino-1-butanol is employed. The base, dissolved in a suitable solvent, readily yields the official maleate by reaction with an equimolar quantity of maleic acid.

Description—A white to pinkish tan, microcrystalline powder, which is odorless and possesses a bitter taste. It must be protected from light and heat. Specific rotation +44° to +50°. The pH of a 1 in 5000 solution is between 4.4 and 5.2.

Solubility—Slightly soluble in water; sparingly soluble in alcohol; very slightly soluble in chloroform and ether.

Uses—Methylergonovine maleate is similar in its actions to ergonovine, and it shares the same uses (see *Ergonovine Maleate*). It may induce uterine contractions upon either oral or parenteral administration.

The intensity and duration of its action is greater than that of ergonovine but less than that of ergotamine. It is weaker than ergonovine and ergotamine in elevating the blood pressure and consequently may be used despite the presence of eclampsia or pre-eclampsia.

Dose—*Oral, intramuscular,* or *intravenous,* **200** to **800 mcg** daily; *usual, oral,* **200 mcg** 3 or 4 times a day; *usual, intramuscular* or *intravenous,* **200 mcg,** repeated after 2 to 4 hours if necessary.

Other Dose Information—This drug may be administered intramuscularly or intravenously at intervals of 3 or 4 times daily during subinvolution or postpartum convalescence. The tablets are not used during the third stage of labor, inasmuch as the onset of action is too slow.

Dosage Forms—Injection USP: 1 ml; Tablets USP: 200 mcg.

Methysergide Maleate NF

[(+)-9,10-Didehydro-*N*-[1-(hydroxymethyl)propyl]-1,6-dimethylergoline-8β-carboxamide Maleate (1:1) (Salt) (Sansert (*Sandoz*)]

Methylsergide Maleate contains 97.0–103.0% of $C_{21}H_{27}N_3O_2 . C_4H_4O_4$ (469.54), calculated on the dried basis.

For the structural formula of methysergide, see page 499.

Preparation—Methylergonovine (base) is methylated at the indole nitrogen with methyl iodide and the resulting methysergide (base) is dissolved in a suitable solvent and reacted with an equimolar portion of maleic acid. For the preparation of methylergonovine (base), see page 952. US Pat. 3,113,133.

Description—White to yellowish white, crystalline powder. The melting point is uncharacteristic showing decomposition above approx. 165°. It is odorless or has not more than a slight odor.

Solubility—1 Gm dissolves in 250 ml of water, in approx. 120 ml of methanol, and in approx. 9000 ml of chloroform (all at 20°); slightly soluble in alcohol; practically insoluble in ether.

Uses—Methysergide is the N-methyl derivative of methylergonovine. However, its oxytocic activity is much weaker, and it is not employed as an oxytocic. Its principal therapeutic use is in the treatment and prophylaxis of *migraine headache,* for which the drug is quite effective. Since methysergide has only weak vasoconstrictor activity, cerebral vasoconstriction has been discounted as the mechanism of action against migraine; thus its action would differ from that of Ergotamine (see *Ergotamine Tartrate,* page 952). However, direct proof in man that cerebral vasoconstriction does not occur has not been offered; the fact that Methysergide induces anginal pain and intermittent claudication in some persons strongly suggests a significant degree of vasoconstrictor activity. It has been suggested that it may induce vasoconstriction indirectly through central vasomotor stimulation or through sensitization to other endogenous vasoconstrictors, but this hypothesis is unsatisfactory on both pharmacological and physiological grounds. Methysergide is a potent serotonin antagonist, and it has been suggested that its usefulness against migraine is based in this action; nevertheless, various facts render this mechanism unlikely. The drug is not effective in tension and other types of headache. Side effects occur in more than a third of patients. They include especially nausea, abdominal pain, excitement and insomnia or drowsiness, paresthesias of limbs, epigastric pain (with increased secretion of gastric acid), and psychic disturbances.

Less frequent effects include vomiting, diarrhea, constipation, myalgia and arthralgia, vertigo, ataxia, skin rash, edema, weakness, coronary and peripheral arterial insufficiency, and induction of premature labor. Prolonged therapy has been known to cause retroperitoneal fibrosis. It has also been suspected to cause pleuropulmonary, myocardial, and aortic fibrosis, the last-named to the point of obstruction. Many of the side effects diminish after continued administration of the drug. Methysergide should be taken with meals.

Dose—*Usual,* **4 mg** to **8 mg** daily in divided doses, preferably with meals.

Dosage Forms—Tablets NF: 2 mg.

Oxytocin Injection USP

[Injectio Oxytocini; Alpha-Hypophamine; Pitocin (*Parke-Davis*); Syntocinon (*Sandoz*)]

Oxytocin Injection is a sterile solution in water for injection of an oxytocic principle prepared by synthesis or obtained from the posterior lobe of the pituitary of healthy, domestic animals used for food by man. Each ml of Oxytocin Injection possesses an oxytocic activity equivalent to 10 USP Posterior Pituitary Units.

For the structural formula of oxytocin, see page 959.

Preparation—The synthesis of this polypeptide hormone constitutes a milestone in biochemistry. It was accomplished by du Vigneaud and his colleagues at the Cornell University Medical College. Detailed description is beyond the scope of this text other than to relate that it involves the separate synthesis of *N*-carbobenzoxy-*S*-benzyl-L-cysteinyl-L-tyrosine and the heptapeptide amide L-isoleucyl-L-glutaminyl-L-asparaginyl-*S* - benzyl - L - cysteinyl - L - prolyl - L - leucylglycinamide which are then caused to undergo condensation, and the resulting substituted peptide amide is then subjected to appropriate reduction and oxidation operations. For the detailed description, see *J. Am. Chem. Soc.,* 76, 3107, 3110, 3113, 3115 (1954).

Uses—Oxytocin Injection is used to stimulate uterine contraction in obstetrical practice, chiefly to *prevent postpartum bleeding.*

Dose—*Intramuscular,* **0.3** to **1 ml**; *usual, intramuscular,* **1 ml,** repeated in 30 minutes if necessary; *usual, intravenous infusion,* **1 ml** in 1000 ml of isotonic solution at a rate of 0.5 to 2 ml per minute.

Veterinary Dose—*Subcutaneous, intramuscular,* or *intravenous Mares and Cows,* **40** to **100 units;** *Sows* and *Ewes,* **30** to **50 units;** *Bitches,* **5** to **30 units;** *Queens,* **5** to **10 units.**

Other Uterine Drugs

Dihydroergotamine [$C_{33}H_{37}N_5O_5$; D.H.E. 45 (*Sandoz*)] —The smooth muscle stimulant effects of dihydroergotamine are somewhat weaker than those of ergotamine (see page 952). Nevertheless, they are significant enough that the drug may be used in the treatment of migraine headache and that ergotism may occasionally accrue to its chronic use or to overdose. It is also oxytocic and has been employed in the third stage of labor, although it is inferior to the official ergot alkaloids. Dihydroergotamine induces a greater depression of the vasomotor center than does ergotamine and causes vasodepression by virtue of reduced sympathetic activity. However, the alkaloid has proven to be of no value as an antihypertensive. Its adrenergic blocking effects cannot be achieved in man in nontoxic doses. Toxicity mainly consists of nausea and vomiting, but gangrene may rarely occur. *Dose: Orally,* 1 to 1.5 mg.

Ergot NF XI [Ergota; Rye Ergot; Secale Cornutum PhI; Rye Mother; Rye Smut; Spurred Rye; Horn-seed] is the dried sclerotium of *Claviceps purpurea* (Fries) Tulasne (Fam. *Hypocreaceæ*) developed on plants of rye, *Secale* *cereale* Linné (Fam. *Gramineæ*). *History:* The malady (gangrene) that "devoured by an invisible fire" and known to the ancients as St. Anthony's fire was the result of milling into flour, for breadmaking, rye contaminated with the fungus, ergot, which is now successfully cultivated for use as a drug. *Constituents:* Ergot yields not less than 0.15% of the total alkaloids of Ergot calculated as ergotoxine, and water-soluble alkaloids equivalent to not less than 0.01% of ergonovine. *Uses:* Ergot contains a number of pharmacologically active ingredients. The most important of these are the ergot alkaloids. The other substances present contribute little to the pharmacological actions of Ergot, in spite of the fact that several are physiologically active. All ergot alkaloids are similar in action, but each possesses outstanding features. Only two are used in therapy—ergotamine and ergonovine. However, several derivatives and semisynthetic ergot alkaloids are used. The ergot alkaloids are classified as *oxytocics* in that they are capable of causing the uterus to contract. Even an immature uterus is stimulated by the active natural alkaloids. After small doses, uterine contractions are strong, but quite normal in character, relaxation occurring after each. After large doses, the contractions are more powerful and spasm may occur. Spastic contractions of the pregnant uterus can be very dangerous. Therefore, the therapeutic use of the ergot alkaloids is reserved until after delivery of the fetus and placenta. At this time they are used to *reduce postpartum bleeding* and to *hasten involution of the uterus.*   The semisynthetic ergot alkaloid, methylergonovine, is also a uterine stimulant. The semisynthetic lysergic acid diethylamide (LSD), page 1119, is essentially devoid of uterine actions but has bizarre hallucinogenic actions. The dihydrogenated ergot alkaloids have weaker uterine actions than the parent compounds, but dihydroergotamine nevertheless has appreciable uterine

stimulation actions. The relative advantages of the various preparations are discussed under the individual drugs. The ergot alkaloids stimulate smooth muscle in general, especially that of the vascular tree. Indeed, the reduction of postpartum bleeding is in part due to vasoconstriction. These drugs also have an action on small peripheral blood vessels, causing them to contract and actually causing pathological changes in the intima of the vessels. As a result, if they are used in too large doses, or over too long a period of time, gangrene of the hands or feet may occur (see under *History* above). Ergonovine is the only active natural alkaloid of ergot which does not possess this action on blood vessels to a marked degree. The natural alkaloids induce hypertension; the dehydrogenated alkaloids may induce hypotension by a central depression of the vasomotor center, but a direct peripheral vasoconstrictor action is demonstrable, and ergotistic gangrene is possible. The vasoconstrictor action of ergotamine and dihydroergotamine on the cerebral vessels is employed in the treatment of migraine, to reduce the pain consequent to vascular dilatation. The ergot alkaloids, except ergonovine and methylergonovine, are adrenergic blocking agents, but adrenergic blockade in man cannot be achieved because of contravention of serious toxic effects. Central suppression of vascular reflexes has been misconstrued as evidence of adrenergic blockade. However, the dihydroergot alkaloids, especially those of the ergotoxine group, are more potent adrenergic blocking agents. Adrenergic blockade in man has probably been achieved with dihydrogenated ergot alkaloids mixture. No therapeutic uses accrue to these actions. Ergot poisoning, especially of cattle, occurs occasionally from the ingestion of ergotized forage crops and may cause serious losses. *Veterinary Dose: Horses,* 15 to 25 Gm; *Cattle,* 25 to 30 Gm; *Sheep and Swine,* 4 to 8 Gm; *Dogs,* 0.5 to 2 Gm; *Cats,* 0.1 to 1 Gm.

55 | Hormones

The pituitary hormones—the adrenal hormones—the pancreatic
hormones—the parathyroid hormone—the thyroid hormones—the sex
hormones

This chapter was prepared by

Ewart A. Swinyard, PhD, *Professor of Pharmacology, College of Pharmacy and
College of Medicine, University of Utah, Salt Lake City, Utah   84112, and*
Stewart C. Harvey, PhD, *Associate Professor of Pharmacology, College of
Medicine, University of Utah, Salt Lake City, Utah   84112*

Hormones are substances secreted by the endocrine, or ductless, glands which serve to integrate metabolic processes. The regulatory function of the hormones differs from other regulatory mechanisms (such as the nervous system and other glandular secretions) in that the hormones are transported to the affected tissues by the blood. Some of the hormones affect nearly all the tissues of the body; the action of others is restricted to but a few tissues or organs.

Chemically, the hormones represent a very diverse group of compounds. Some, like epinephrine and thyroxine, are relatively simple amino acid derivatives. Several groups of hormones, including those produced by the adrenal cortex and the gonads, are steroids, while the pituitary, parathyroid, and pancreatic hormones are polypeptides or proteins; the molecular weights of the latter range from about 1000 to 30,000 or more.

In the majority of instances, the existence of a physiologically important hormone was usually first recognized when degeneration or destruction of a gland by disease or accident in humans or its experimental removal from animals was found to result in unfavorable physiological consequences. Attempts were then made to reverse such untoward effects by implanting tissues from healthy animals (frequently at other sites) or by supplying extracts prepared from them. Once the type of physiological activity attributable to any one gland has been recognized and a biologically effective extract has been produced, the way is opened for the development of an assay method by means of which the hormone content of various preparations can be compared. The ultimate goal with each extract is to obtain a demonstrably pure active substance, to establish its chemical structure, and to develop either a method of synthesis or a convenient method of preparation from natural sources so as to make it available for therapeutic or experimental use. Frequently, the successful conclusion of attempts to isolate, purify, and identify a hormone has also permitted the development of chemical methods for its determination—for example, in body fluids. However, for some of the hormones, available chemical methods for identification and quantitative determination are still inferior to biological methods as regards specificity and sensitivity.

Standardization—Many of the hormones, or substances which possess nearly identical biological properties, have been prepared in chemically pure (usually crystalline) form, either from natural sources, or by synthesis. For such materials, the standard practice is prescription in terms of weight. With others, especially some of the polypeptide or protein hormones, potency is expressed in terms of biological activity. In such instances, a unit of biological activity is established as the amount necessary to produce a predetermined response in a test animal, or by comparison with an arbitrarily accepted standard preparation. For some preparations, eg, insulin and the posterior lobe hormones, the custom of designating dosage in terms of biological "units" has persisted even after the substance has become available in chemically pure form. In any event, no hormone preparation should be used therapeutically unless it is a pure substance or its activity can be assayed biologically.

Administration—A few of the hormones can be administered *orally* with full effect, as, for example, thyroid and certain steroid hormones. There is usually some loss due to destruction of the hormone in the digestive tract, to its elimination from the circulation, or inactivation while it is in transit through the liver immediately after absorption. Some hormones must be administered by injection, either *hypodermically* or *intramuscularly*, because they are inactivated in the digestive tract. The intramuscular injection is usually chosen, and it gives rapid absorption if the hormone is in aqueous solution, or slower absorption if the hormone is in oil. This use of oil is not ideal, for oil is not readily removed from the site of injection, and oils are difficult to free from allergens. Therefore, another technique is the *implantation* of compressed pellets of those hormones which are only slightly soluble in tissue fluid; these pellets are placed in the subcutaneous tissues and are absorbed during a period of a few months. This technique has the disadvantage of requiring a careful surgical procedure, and, even with good technique, certain pellets may be extruded due to infection, or they may be of no value because of fibrous tissue barriers which develop about the pellets in some cases. Efforts have been made to perfect a method to inject the hormone hypodermically in the form of microscopic crystals suspended in water, and thus aqueous microcrystalline suspensions of various steroid hormones are actually preferred by some in place of oil solutions. Still another form is the buccal tablet of very highly compressed steroid hormone. These tablets are held in the mouth for periods up to 45 minutes, and during this time there is absorption through the buccal mucous membrane, providing direct access of the steroid to the systemic circulation. This is said to avoid the disadvantage of the oral route, by which steroids must pass through the liver where they are largely inactivated. Some of the synthetic or semisynthetic hormones are so structured as to greatly diminish enzymatic destruction in the liver and hence are effective orally. Notable among these are the oral contraceptives.

The Pituitary Hormones

The pituitary body (hypophysis) comprises anterior, intermediate, and posterior portions or lobes, which have distinguishing structures and functions. Active principles have been discovered in extracts prepared in various ways from all three portions of the pituitary, and these will be listed and discussed separately.

The Anterior Pituitary

The pituitary body is known as the "master gland" because it has so many important actions in the body and it regulates the function of several of the other glands. Without the anterior portion of the pituitary gland, the sex functions and growth cease, and the functions of the adrenal cortex, the thyroid, and the parathyroids decrease markedly. Through studies in experimental animals, chiefly with the use of the hypophysectomized rat, we now know that the anterior lobe of the pituitary has at least *six* different important actions, apparently due to separate hormones.

1. **Growth Hormone** (*Somatotropin, STH*)—This hormone causes an increase in weight and length of the body. The increase in length is especially prominent, due to bone growth, but its effect is manifested in nearly all the tissues of the body. Human growth hormone also possesses most of the activities of lactogenic hormone. For maximum action of growth hormone, all the essential and quasi-essential amino acids must be present in abundance.

The growth hormone from human pituitaries has been isolated as a crystalline, apparently homogeneous protein of molecular weight 29,000. Its biological properties can be assayed by observing the growth of hypophysectomized young rats in response to injections of the hormone, or by measuring the extent of bone growth (tibia) adjacent to the epiphyseal line. The daily injection of as little as 0.010 mg of purified growth hormone will cause a measurable increase in the weight of young hypophysectomized rats.

In humans, the protein anabolic action of growth hormone is most readily measured by its nitrogen-retaining effect.

In addition to its effects upon protein metabolism, growth hormone also affects the metabolism of carbohydrates and fats. These effects include (a) maintenance of a normal amount of muscle glycogen in hypophysectomized animals, (b) decreased responsiveness to insulin, and (c) increasing the concentration of nonesterified fatty acids in plasma. Human growth hormone also exerts prominent effects on the kidney and electrolyte metabolism.

Unlike corticotropin, insulin, and some of the other protein hormones, a considerable species difference has been observed in response to growth hormone administration. Thus, growth hormone active in fishes can be isolated from fish pituitaries, but this substance is inactive in mammals (eg, rats). Bovine growth hormone is active in fishes, rats, dogs (and presumably in cattle) but is inactive in monkeys and men, whereas growth hormone prepared from simian or human pituitaries is active in both primate species, as well as in nearly all lower orders of animals in which it has been tested. These differences appear to be reflections of significant differences in the chemical composition of the hormones from various sources. For example, the molecular weight of primate growth hormone is much smaller than that of the bovine variety (29,000 vs 46,000).

These facts explain why attempts to demonstrate beneficial effects when growth hormone preparations from domestic animals are used clinically have been disappointing. Human growth hormone has been isolated from human pituitaries and has been used successfully in stimulating growth (height and weight increase) in hypopituitary dwarfs for long periods. The usual dose is 2 to 4 mg 3 times weekly, given intramuscularly. An interesting diagnostic application of human growth hormone is based upon its ability to increase the concentration of free fatty acids in the blood. Patients suffering from acromegaly (a disease caused by excessive secretion of growth hormone) are sometimes treated by radiation therapy. In order to assess the effects of the treatment, growth hormone is administered and its effects upon plasma free fatty acid is determined. The administration of growth hormone to an untreated acromegalic causes no change in plasma free fatty acid, since the concentration of growth hormone in the circulation is already very high. If the treatment is successful, production of endogenous growth hormone diminishes or ceases; subsequent injection of growth hormone will cause an increase in free fatty acids in the plasma.

2. **The Gonadotropic Hormones**—Three separate gonadotropins are secreted by the anterior pituitary. These three hormones, acting both in concert and sequentially, control the sexual (estrus) cycle in lower animals and the menstrual cycle in primates.

a. Follicle-stimulating Hormone (FSH)—This substance promotes maturation of the primordial follicle and in combination with small amounts of LH (see below), stimulates secretion of estrogen by the developing follicle. Human FSH has a molecular weight of 17,000. The carbohydrate content is 8 to 9%.

b. Luteinizing Hormone (LH)—The secretion of LH increases near the middle of the cycle. As noted above, small amounts of LH, acting with FSH, stimulate the secretion of estrogen by the ovarian follicle. As the amount of LH increases, ovulation occurs, and the corpus luteum begins to form. Human LH has a molecular weight of 26,000. The carbohydrate content is 3.5%.

LH also acts upon the male gonads, specifically upon the interstitial cells of the testis, to produce testosterone. Because of this property, LS is also sometimes referred to as interstitial cell-stimulating hormone (ICSH).

c. Luteotropic Hormones (LtH)—The luteotropic hormone maintains the corpus luteum in a functioning state; in combination with LH, it causes the corpus luteum to secrete progesterone. LtH also stimulates milk secretion by the mammary gland: synonyms for LtH are *prolactin, mammotropin,* and *lactogenic hormone.* The molecular weight of LtH is 23,500.

Other Gonadotropic Preparations—In addition to the anterior pituitary glands, three other sources of gonadotropic activity are known. Two are produced by the chorionic cells of the placentae of women and mares, respectively. The third is a gonadotropin (menotropins) present in the serum of postmenopausal women and is, undoubtedly, actually a true adenohypophyseal gonadotropin (FSH) or a mixture of FSH and a small amount of LH. Human chorionic gonadotropin (HCG) is secreted into the maternal blood and is excreted in the urine, where it may be detected within 48 hours after the ovum is implanted. The biological properties of HCG approximate most closely those of LH and LtH in combination, although it differs substantially from either in chemical properties. Thus, like LtH, HCG maintains the secretion of the corpus luteum, enabling pregnancy to continue. Like LH, it will act upon gonadal interstitial cells. Unlike FSH, it will not act upon the ovary of the hypophysectomized rat, although it will exert a marked synergism with FSH in this respect.

Human chorionic gonadotropin has been isolated in a form which is chromatographically and electrophoretically homogeneous. It appears to be a glycoprotein of molecular weight 30,000; the carbohydrate content is about 28%.

Unlike HCG, the gonadotropin of pregnant mare serum (PMS) is not excreted in the urine. Its biological effects are similar to those of both FSH and LH; thus, it will stimulate both follicular and luteal development of the rat ovary. The molecular weight of purified PMS is about 23,000; its carbohydrate content is 45%.

Uses of Gonadotropic Hormones—Although many attempts have been made to demonstrate in humans an effect of pituitary gonadotropins from domestic animals, the evidence obtained so far has been equivocal or frankly negative. This may be due to a species specificity of the kind already noted in connection with growth hormone preparations. Preparations of FSH from human pituitaries or menotropins from the serum of postmenopausal women have been found to induce ovulation in women suffering from diminished pituitary function. However, evidence of superovulation (production of more than one ovum) is sometimes obtained following administration of FSH or menotropins of human origin. Human chorionic gonadotropin has been used for stimulation of androgen secretion by testicular interstitial cells, and for expediting the descent of the tests in boys and young men with cryptorchidism. It has also been found to be effective in prolonging luteal function and in inducing ovulatory cycles in anovulatory women with metropathia hemorrhagica. However, human chorionic gonadotropin appears to induce ovulation only when a mature ovarian follicle is present. Unfortunately, a mature follicle is not common in anovulatory women. Pregnant mare serum gonadotropin, as a source of both FSH- and LH-like activity, has found some efficacy in the treatment of hypogonadotropic hypogonadism, although its use must be attended with care because of the possibility of sensitivity to horse serum. Because of the foreign proteins present, immunity to its effects may develop.

The international unit of HCG is defined as the activity of 0.1 mg of the international standard. Purified HCG contains approximately 12,000 IU per mg. Purified PMS, standardized by methods similar to those used for HCG, contains about 16,000 IU per mg.

3. **Thyrotropic Hormone** (*Thyrotropin, TSH*)—This substance sustains the activity of the thyroid gland, promoting increased uptake of inorganic iodine and release of organically bound iodine. In the absence of TSH, the thyroid gland atrophies, producing only small amounts of thyroid hormone. An excess of TSH causes hypertrophy and hyperplasia of the thyroid, and a clinical picture resembling Graves' disease.

The most potent TSH preparations which have been obtained thus far are still impure. TSH obtained from beef pituitaries is a glycoprotein of molecular weight of about 25,000. TSH assays depend upon the measurement of the weight, acinar cell height, or iodine content of thyroids of chicks or guinea pigs. Methods based upon the discharge of thyroid iodine, which decreases when TSH is administered, are to be preferred. The use of radioactive iodine as a tracer in the latter procedure represents an elegant refinement of this technique.

In Graves' disease an abnormal thyrotropic substance is present in the blood. Because of its long duration of action it is called long-acting thyroid stimulator (LATS). Its physiological and chemical relationship to TSH remains to be determined.

4. Adrenal Corticotropic Hormone (*Corticotropin, ACTH*)—This hormone maintains and controls the function of the adrenal cortex, and thus indirectly affects carbohydrate, protein, and mineral metabolism (see section on *Adrenal Hormones*). Adrenocorticotropin is a polypeptide containing 39 amino acid residues with a molecular weight of about 4500.

The hormones from pituitaries of various species of animals differ with respect to the sequence of amino acids 25–32, but these differences do not affect their biological actions. When corticotropin is treated briefly with pepsin, 11 amino acid residues at the C-terminal end are removed. The product (β-corticotropin) retains full biological activity. In contrast, even slight alteration of the N-terminal end of the molecule results in substantial inactivation.

A synthetic polypeptide containing the first 23 amino acid residues of naturally occurring corticotropin has been found to possess essentially all of the biological and clinical properties of corticotropin. Several peptides have been synthesized which are more potent than natural ACTH.

Physiological Effects—Since the known physiological actions of corticotropin are mediated through the adrenal cortex, its effects are similar to those of the adrenal cortical hormones, especially the glucocorticoids (see section on *Adrenal Hormones*). ACTH also enhances the adrenal cortical output of aldosterone and hence has an action on mineral metabolism. However, aldosterone secretion is also under the control of the rennin–angiotensin system.

The first 13 amino acids of ACTH are identical in sequence to those of α-MSH (melanocyte-stimulating hormone); consequently, ACTH causes some hyperpigmentation of the skin. ACTH also causes ketosis, adipokinesis, hypoglycemia, and insulin resistance in high doses; these effects are not necessarily mediated through adrenal corticoids.

5. Other Pituitary Principles—From time to time the existence of anterior pituitary hormones other than those listed above have been postulated. Generally, the effects attributed to them have been shown to be referable to one or more of the known pituitary hormones. Thus, for example, the diabetogenic effect of anterior pituitary extracts has been shown to be due to the action of somatotropin under conditions of limited insulin supply. Several of the anterior lobe hormones possess fat-mobilizing (adipokinetic) properties. In addition, a unique peptide with adipokinetic activity has been isolated from pituitary residues remaining after corticotropin extraction. This substance is of molecular weight about 5000. Although it is very active in laboratory animals, as little as 1 mg causing persistent lipemia in rabbits, it has no demonstrable effect in human beings.

The release of the anterior pituitary tropic hormones is under the control of the hypothalamus, which secretes a different releasing factor for each tropic hormone. The releasing factor, in turn, is released according to the plasma levels of the ultimate hormone. For example, when the plasma levels of thyroid hormone fall below a critical level, the hypothalamus releases the thyrotropin-releasing factor (TRF), which stimulates the adenohypophysis to release more thyrotropic hormone, which, in turn, stimulates the thyroid to produce more thyroid hormone. Thus, there is a negative feedback mechanism which regulates the plasma concentration of each hormone and which is vital to endocrine homeostasis.

Chorionic Gonadotropin USP

[*Various Mfgs.*]

Chorionic Gonadotropin is a gonad-stimulating principle obtained from the urine of pregnant women. Its potency is not less than 1500 USP Chorionic Gonadotropin Units in each mg, and 80.0–125.0% of the potency stated on the label.

Description—White or practically white, amorphous powder.

Solubility—Freely soluble in water.

Uses—*See Uses of Gonadotropic Hormones* in the *General Statement* (page 956). Although Chorionic Gonadotropin alone rarely induces ovulation in anovulatory women, in sequence with Menotropins (page 959), which favors the maturation of ovarian follicles, ovulation may be effected. There have been claims that Chorionic Gonadotropin may be effective in the treatment of fertility in women who have a luteal hypofunction and hence do not produce enough progesterone to develop a normal secretory endometrium, but acceptable evidence of a sufficient luteinizing effect is lacking. Likewise, there is a paucity of evidence of a usefulness of Chorionic Gonadotropin in the treatment of male sterility. Some authorities consider Chorionic Gonadotropin to be superior to either oral or parenteral androgens for replacement therapy in androgenic insufficiency, but the necessity for the injection of Chorionic Gonadotropin is disadvantageous. Chorionic Gonadotropin may cause virilization; some evidence exists that it may favor thromboembolism and rupture of ovarian cysts.

Dose—*Intramuscular*, **500** to **5000 USP Units** weekly; *usual*, **500** to **1000 Units** 2 or 3 times a week.

Other Dose Information—If the hormone is going to have an effect in cryptorchidism, 4000 IU a day for 3 successive days will effect descent of the testicles in 2 to 3 weeks without the risk of virilization and premature arrest of normal bone growth.

Dosage Forms—For Injection USP: 5000, 10,000, and 20,000 Units.

Corticotropin Injection USP

[ACTH Injection; Adrenocorticotropin Injection; (*Various Mfgs.*)]

Corticotropin Injection is a sterile preparation of the principle or principles derived from the anterior lobe of the pituitary of mammals used for food by man, which exert a tropic influence on the adrenal cortex. It possesses a potency of 80.0–125.0% of that stated on the label in USP Corticotropin Units. It may contain a suitable antimicrobial agent.

Note—Corticotropin Injection labeled for intramuscular or subcutaneous administration is assayed by subcutaneous injection. Corticotropin Injection labeled for intravenous administration only is assayed by intravenous injection. Corticotropin Injection may be labeled for administration either subcutaneously or intramuscularly or intravenously provided the ratio of the observed potency by subcutaneous assay and that by intravenous assay is 0.80–1.25.

Preparation—Most commercial preparations of *corticotropin* are obtained from either hog or sheep pituitary glands, although beef and whale glands have also been used. Two types of preparations are available: short- and long-acting. The short-acting preparations consist of a lyophilized powder or a stable aqueous solution containing 1% phenol. The powder is dissolved in physiological saline or other suitable medium before injection. Short-acting preparations are administered either intramuscularly or by intravenous infusion.

Long-acting preparations (repository corticotropin, corticotropin gel) contain *corticotropin* incorporated in a gelatin menstruum designed to delay the rate of absorption and increase the period of effectiveness. Combination of corticotropin with zinc hydroxide suspension also delays the rate of absorption. These are injected intramuscularly.

Corticotropin is standardized by the Sayers assay. The clinical effectiveness, however, varies with the mode of administration. The difference is particularly evident in comparisons of short-acting preparations injected intramuscularly with long-acting preparations similarly administered. For this reason, gel preparations are labeled in terms of "clinical units" to conform more nearly to their expected physiological potency. Fourteen USP Units in gelatin medium possess the approximate clinical efficacy of 40 USP Units of aqueous corticotropin solution by intermittent intramuscular injection.

Description—A colorless or light straw-colored liquid, or a soluble amorphous solid obtained by drying such liquid from the frozen state. It is odorless or has the odor of an antibacterial agent. The pH of the liquid form or after reconstitution from the solid state is between 3.0 and 7.0.

Uses—*Diagnostically*, the fall in circulating eosinophils and increase of urinary steroid excretion following the injection of a standard dose of corticotropin affords a means of assessing the functional capacity of the adrenal. This is at present the most important clinical use of this agent.

Therapeutically, Corticotropin has been found to be valuable as a nonspecific therapeutic agent in a wide variety of disorders. These include various forms of *rheumatic or articular disease, collagen diseases, skin disorders*, and a number of *inflammatory conditions*. It may also provide benefits in *Hodgkin's disease, lymphosarcoma, multiple myeloma*, and especially *acute leukemia*, but its usefulness is only temporary. In general, with the exception of primary adrenal insufficiency, corticotropin is effective in all of the conditions for which adrenal cortical steroids (cortisone, hydrocortisone) are found useful. Unlike the latter, however, corticotropin is ineffective when applied locally. There is no evidence that ACTH can achieve any therapeutic effect that cannot be achieved by appropriate doses of adrenal corticoids.

The diversity of the metabolic derangements for which corticotropin is employed therapeutically, as well as the variation in individual response, precludes the establishment of a definitive therapeutic use. This is especially true since the margin between optimum clinical effectiveness and undesirable side effects is frequently narrow.

The continued administration of large amounts of corticotropin may result in one or more of the manifestations of Cushing's syndrome, may exacerbate the symptoms of latent or frank diabetes, and, because of its anti-inflammatory action, may mask symptoms of infection. The need for adequate medical supervision durings its use, therefore, cannot be overemphasized.

Abrupt cessation of corticotropin injections may be followed by withdrawal effects which take the form of symptoms of adrenal insufficiency. These result from pituitary inhibition which occurs during treatment with corticotropin and may be minimized or eliminated by gradually reducing the amount injected.

Dose—*Intramuscular,* **40** to **160 USP Units** daily; *usual, intramuscular,* **20 USP Units** 4 times a day.

Other Dose Information—For an initial clinical response, 50–100 USP Units per day injected intramuscularly in divided doses every 6–8 hours, or 40–100 USP Units of repository corticotropin, or 20–25 USP Units by intravenous infusion during eight hours is frequently effective. After the establishment of a

satisfactory response, if therapy is to be continued, the dose may be lowered to a suitable maintenance level.

Dosage Forms—Injection USP: (liquid form) 40 Units/2 ml, 200 Units/5 and 10 ml; (dry form) 25 and 40 Units; Repository Injection USP: 40 and 80 Units/ml, 200 and 400 Units/5 ml; Sterile Zinc Hydroxide Suspension USP: 200 Units/5 ml.

Veterinary Dose—*Parenteral, Horses* and *Cattle,* **100** to **600 USP Units;** *Sheep,* **10** to **25 Units;** *Dogs,* **1 Unit** per **pound** of body weight

---

Repository Corticotropin Injection USP [*Various Mfgs.*] is corticotropin in a solution of partially hydrolyzed gelatin. It possesses a potency of 80–125% of that stated on the label in USP Corticotropin Units. It may contain a suitable antibacterial agent. *Description:* A colorless or light straw-colored liquid which may be quite viscid at room temperature. It is odorless or has an odor of an antibacterial agent. *Uses:* See *Corticotropin Injection. Dose: Intramuscular,* 10 to 160 *USP Units daily; usual, intramuscular,* 40 *USP Units* 1 or 2 times a day. *Veterinary Dose:* See *Corticotropin Injection.*

Sterile Corticotropin Zinc Hydroxide Suspension USP [Cortrophin-Zinc (*Organon*)] is a sterile suspension of corticotropin adsorbed on zinc hydroxide. It possesses a potency of 80–125% of that stated in USP Corticotropin Units. It contains 0.45–0.55 mg of zinc for each 20 USP Corticotropin Units. *Description:* A flocculent, white, aqueous suspension, free from large particles following moderate shaking. The pH, determined electrometrically, is between 7.0 and 8.0. *Uses:* The complex of corticotropin with zinc hydroxide results in a product whose absorption is delayed in comparison to corticotropin. Therefore, therapy may be maintained with less frequent administration. *Dose: Intramuscular,* 10 to 160 *USP Units daily; usual, intramuscular,* 40 *USP Units* 1 or 2 times a day. *Veterinary Dose:* See *Corticotropin Injection.*

Thyrotropin

[Thytropar (*Armour*)]

Thyrotropin is the thyrotropic hormone secreted by the basophilic cells of the bovine anterior pituitary.

Preparation—This glycoprotein may be prepared from extracts of the anterior lobe of the pituitary gland of domesticated animals by adjusting the pH to the isoelectric point and then either precipitating the product with a suitable buffer salt or extracting it with appropriate solvents. For a detailed discussion of Thyrotropin, see the monograph entitled *Thyrotropin*.[1]

Uses—Thyrotropin (TSH) is the anterior pituitary hormone which stimulates the thyroid gland. Exogenous Thyrotropin increases the uptake of iodide into and the release of thyroid hormone from a functional thyroid gland. If the gland is incapable of proper function (primary thyroid failure), TSH will not induce as much of an effect on iodine metabolism. Thus the hormone is used diagnostically *to distinguish hypothyroidism secondary to anterior pituitary failure* to produce endogenous TSH *from primary thyroid failure.* In the former, various indices of thyroid function and iodine metabolism, such as thyroid uptake of ^{131}I, renal excretion of ^{131}I, protein bound iodine content, etc, will show an appropriate response to Thyrotropin, whereas in the latter they will not. Thyrotropin is not used for replacement therapy in anterior pituitary failure.

Dose—*Intramuscular* or *subcutaneous,* **10 USP Units.**

Dosage Forms—for Injection: 10 USP Units/3 ml.

Other Hormones of the Anterior Pituitary

Corticotropin, Purified, is prepared by the absorption of corticotropin from a dilute acetic acid solution on oxycellulose and the subsequent elution of the adsorbed material with dilute hydrochloric acid. *Uses:* The same as *Corticotropin Injection* (page 957). On a weight basis, the purified hormone is 10 to 40 times more potent than the USP material. Expression of the dose in terms of USP Units does not adjust entirely for the difference in purity; for some inexplicable reason, by the subcutaneous or intramuscular route, but not by the intravenous route, Purified Corticotropin is clinically 3 to 4 times more potent, unit for unit, than is Corticotropin USP. Thus it is customary to express dosage in terms of clinical equivalents to USP Units; so expressed, the dose is the same as that of Corticotropin USP, when the intramuscular or subcutaneous route is employed. When the intravenous route is employed, the dose in clinical units of Purified Corticotropin is ¼ to ⅓ that of Corticotropin USP. Purified Corticotropin is incorporated into a depot form with gelatin; in this form the duration of action is 18 to 24 hours. *Dose:* See the statement above. *Subcutaneous* or *intramuscular*, usually 40 to 50 USP Units equivalent daily in 4 divided doses; if the gel form is used, the entire daily dose may be given in one injection. *Intravenous*, 1.7 to 7 USP Units equivalent infused over an 8-hour period; the powder or commercial solution is diluted with 500 ml of isotonic dextrose or saline solution to provide the solution for infusion.

Gonadotrophin, Serum PhI [Pregnant Mares' Serum Gonadotrophin; P. M. S. G.; Equinex (*Ayerst*)]—A sterile preparation containing the follicle-stimulating substance from the serum of pregnant mares. See *Other Gonadotropic Preparations* under the *General Statement*, page 956. It occurs as a white powder containing not less than 100 units per mg. It is a glycoprotein with an isoelectric point at pH 2.6 and is soluble in water. It is produced in the placenta and endometrium of the pregnant mare, and is found in the serum after the 37th day of pregnancy. It has actions similar to a mixture of pituitary follicle-stimulating hormone and luteinizing hormone, with the former more predominant. Its clinical value is doubtful. Unlike other gonadotropins, it is not excreted by the kidneys and has a prolonged action. *Uses:* to supplement the action of estrogens in the treatment of delayed puberty, amenorrhea and hypomenorrhea; in the treatment of functional uterine bleeding, habitual and threatened abortion, and cryptorchidism in the male. *Dose: intramuscularly*, 200 to 1000 units twice weekly.

Menotropins [Human Follicle Stimulating Hormone; Humegon (*Organon*); Pergonal (*Cutter*)] is an extract of postmenopausal urine containing primarily the follicle-stimulating hormone (FSH).

Uses: Menotropins is a gonadotropin, the actions of which are probably mostly due to follicle stimulating hormone from the anterior pituitary. The preparation also has some luteinizing hormonal activity, which also probably aids in maturation of the follicle and the secretion of estrogen. It is employed in the treatment of *infertility* in women when infertility is the result of anovulation. Side effects primarily result from overstimulation of the ovary. They include ovarian enlargement with pain, discomfort, and mild abdominal distention or even ascites. There also tends to be a high incidence of multiple pregnancy. At present, menotropins is only an experimental drug, but it is highly likely to be released in the near future. *Dose: Intramuscular*, 150 to 225 IU a day until evidence of adequate follicular stimulation (by changes in cervical mucus). Generally 7 to 10 days are required. Chorionic gonadotropin in a dose of 5000 IU per day is either added to menotropins or in a dose of 12,000 IU divided over 1 to 3 days substituted for menotropins until ovulation occurs. Chorionic gonadotropin may also be given for a few days in advance of menotropins.

The Intermediate Lobe

The intermediate lobe of the pituitary produces a substance, *intermedin,* or *melanocyte-stimulating hormone* (MSH) which disperses the pigment granules in the melanophores and other chromatophores in some amphibians and fishes. The biological assay of MSH depends upon its capacity for darkening the skin of frogs either *in vivo* or *in vitro*.

Extracts of mammalian pituitaries contain two substances with MSH activity: α- and β-MSH. These are polypeptides containing 13 and 18 amino acids, respectively; the amino acid sequences in both are known. Although MSH has no known physiological role in mammals, alkali-treated MSH (which has a more prolonged action than the native material) will cause some darkening of the skin in man. Purified ACTH possesses intrinsic MSH activity, probably due to similarity of structure between ACTH and α-MSH. It has been suggested that the hyperpigmentation of Addison's disease is due to excessive ACTH secretion.

The Posterior Pituitary

Extracts of the posterior lobe of the pituitary gland exert four typical effects: (1) an antidiuretic action (through increased renal tubular reabsorption of water), (2) a pressor action (through peripheral vasoconstriction), (3) an oxytocic action (through direct stimulation of uterine smooth muscle), and (4) a milk-ejecting action (through contraction of the myoepithelial cells of the mammary gland). From such extracts two purified octapeptides have been isolated. One, *oxytocin* (*pitocin*), page 953, possesses the oxytocic and milk-ejecting actions; the other, *vasopressin* (*pitressin*), page 960, exerts the pressor and antidiuretic actions. In addition, the latter fraction also stimulates smooth muscle of the intestinal tract. Commercially available extracts representing these two fractions contain a maximum of 5% of the other fraction.

Each of the octapeptides has been synthesized. Oxytocin has the structure:

Oxytocin

The structure of vasopressin from human, monkey, dog, cat, ox, camel, rabbit, and rat pituitaries is identical with that of oxytocin, except that the isoleucine and leucine residues are replaced by residues of phenylalanine and arginine, respectively. Vasopressin prepared from pig pituitaries contains lysine instead of arginine.

The synthesis of oxytocin by du Vigneaud and his students in 1953 represented the first synthesis of a peptide hormone. The synthetic product is qualitatively and quantitatively identical in biological properties with the purified natural hormone. Purified oxytocin contains 500 to 600 USP Units per mg.

Purified oxytocin, whether natural or synthetic, is nearly devoid of pressor activity. However, purified vasopressin possesses some oxytocic activity, which appears to be an intrinsic property of the vasopressin molecule, rather than to contamination by oxytocin.

By the use of mild extraction procedures, it has been possible to isolate, from posterior lobes, a protein of molecular weight 20,000 to 30,000, which contains both pressor and oxytocic activity in constant ratio, and which appears to be a homogeneous protein by all available criteria. It is likely that this substance represents the form in which the two hormones are secreted by the gland, and is perhaps the form which circulates in the blood.

The successful synthesis of the naturally occurring posterior lobe hormones has provided the impetus for the synthesis of a number of analogues of both oxytocin and vasopressin. Thus, substances in which one or more of the amino acids of the native hormones have been replaced by others, or containing fewer or additional amino acid residues, have been prepared and their pharmacological properties explored. One of these was the compound vasotocin, containing the pentapeptide ring of oxytocin and the tripeptide side chain of vasopressin. This substance possesses the biological properties of both neurohypophyseal hormones, although in lesser degree. Subsequently, it was shown that vasotocin is in fact the naturally occuring neurohypophyseal hormone of birds and amphibians.

It has become rather common practice to name those synthetic analogs of oxytocin and the two vasopressins in which one or more of the amino acids of the native hormones have been replaced by others by the simple expedient of assigning consecutive numbers to the amino acid residues in the native hormone and using these numbers to denote the alterations represented in the synthetic. Exemplifying with oxytocin, for which the numbering scheme is

$$
\begin{array}{ccc}
1 & 2 & 3 \\
\text{cysteine} - \text{tyrosine} - \text{isoleucine} \\
| \quad 6 & 5 & 4 \\
\text{cysteine} - \text{asparagine} - \text{glutamine} \\
7 & 8 & 9 \\
\text{proline} - \text{leucine} - \text{glycinamide,}
\end{array}
$$

a synthetic in which the leucine moiety is replaced by arginine is named simply 8-arginineoxytocin. Altered vasopressins are handled similarly; thus the name 2-(phenylalanine)-8-lysinevasopressin signifies a vasopressin which differs from native 8-lysinevasopressin in that the No. 2 amino acid residue (tyrosine) of the natural hormone has been replaced by phenylalanine.

Uses—The three actions of pharmacological importance in posterior pituitary (oxytocic, pressor, and antidiuretic) all have therapeutic applications. The oxytocic principle causes contraction of the uterus. The action is shorter in duration than that caused by the ergot alkaloids. Posterior pituitary is used after delivery of the fetus and placenta to promote contraction of the uterus and *reduce postpartum bleeding*. Also if used cautiously it may be employed to *initiate labor at term* (see Chapter 54). The usual dose for the former purpose is 10 units given by injection in the form of oxytocin injection. For the induction of labor very small doses are employed by intravenous infusion. Use of the milk-ejecting activity has been made clinically in the treatment of breast engorgement.

Vasopressin is specific replacement therapy in the treatment of *diabetes insipidus* (*not diabetes mellitus*). The large urine volume can be reduced toward normal by the intramuscular injection of 10 Units twice daily. Its action to stimulate the smooth muscle of the intestinal tract has been employed in the treatment of *postoperative intestinal ileus*. However, for these purposes, it is probably inferior to the choline esters and anticholinesterases. The pressor actions were formerly sought to support blood pressure during surgery, but vasopressin is no longer recommended for this purpose. Safer and more effective agents, such as certain of the sympathomimetic amines, are available.

The active principles of the posterior pituitary are destroyed by the digestive enzymes of the gastrointestinal tract. For this reason they are not effective when given orally. The common route of administration is by intramuscular or subcutaneous injection of active extracts. However, posterior pituitary powder or solution can be applied to the nasal mucous membrane and significant absorption occurs. This method of administration has been employed for the induction of labor and for the control of the polyuria of diabetes insipidus.

Posterior Pituitary NF

[Pituitary; Hypophysis Sicca]

Posterior Pituitary is a powder prepared from the clean, dried, posterior lobe of the pituitary of domestic animals used for food by man. Each mg of Posterior Pituitary possesses an oxytocic activity equivalent to not less than 1 USP Posterior Pituitary Unit.*

Description—A yellowish or grayish, amorphous powder having a characteristic odor.

Solubility—It is only partially soluble in water.

Uses—Since relatively purified extracts of vasopressin and oxytocin are available commercially, there is little need to employ extracts such as Posterior Pituitary Injection which possesses all the pharmacologic activities of the gland. However, Posterior Pituitary Injection may be substituted for either of the purified fractions. The chief use of posterior pituitary powder is for the control of *diabetes insipidus*, either through (1) the nasal insufflation of the fine powder, or probably a better alternative method is (2) the subcutaneous injection of long-acting insoluble vasopressin tannate in oil suspension, in doses of 0.25 ml intramuscularly at intervals of from 24 to 48 hours.

Dose—By *insufflation*, 5 to 20 mg; *usual*, 10 mg as snuff 3 or more times a day as needed; *subcutaneous*, up to 10 USP Units; *usual*, 10 USP Units.

Dosage Forms—Injection NF: 10 USP Units/ ml, 100 USP Units/10 ml.

Veterinary Dose—*Cows* and *Mares*, 5 to 10 ml; *Sows* and *Ewes*, 3 to 5 ml; *Bitches*, 0.5 to 3 ml; *Queens*, 0.5 to 1 ml.

Vasopressin Injection USP

[Beta-Hypophamine; Pitressin (*Parke-Davis*)]

Vasopressin Injection is a sterile solution in water for injection of the water-soluble, pressor principle prepared by synthesis or obtained from the posterior lobe of the pituitary of healthy domestic animals used for food by man. Each ml of Vasopressin Injection possesses a pressor activity equivalent to 20 USP Posterior Pituitary Units.

Description—A clear, colorless or practically colorless liquid, with a faint, characteristic odor.

---

* One USP Posterior Pituitary Unit represents the potency of 0.5 mg of USP Posterior Pituitary Reference Standard.

Uses—See the general discussion (page 960). Vasopressin Injection is employed for its *antidiuretic* effect and for its action upon the smooth muscle of the intestinal tract. It should *not* be used as a pressor agent.

Dose—*Intramuscular*, **0.25** to **2 ml** daily; *usual*, **0.5 ml.**

Veterinary Dose—*Intramuscular, Dogs,* **5 to 10 USP Units.**

Vasopressin Tannate

[β-Hypophamine; Pitressin Tannate (*Parke-Davis*)]

Vasopressin Tannate is the water-insoluble tannate of the pressor principle of the posterior lobe of the pituitary of healthy domesticated animals used as food by man.

Preparation—An aqueous solution containing the pressor and antidiuretic principles of the posterior lobe of pituitary glands is made alkaline with sodium hydroxide. Tannic acid is added to combine with the protein fraction. The excess tannic acid is removed and the Vasopressin Tannate is dried and powdered.

Glass or stainless steel vessels should be used throughout. Contact with iron or copper must be avoided.

Description—A dark-brown amorphous solid with a faint, characteristic odor. It is stable at room temperature.

Solubility—At least 1 Gm dissolves in 100 ml of acetic acid; insoluble in water and alcohol.

Uses—The uses of Vasopressin Tannate are the same as those of *Vasopressin Injection* (above). See also the general statement under *The Posterior Pituitary* (page 960). Vasopressin Tannate has a longer duration of action than Vasopressin. Furthermore, it is more suitable for suspension in oil, so that depot preparations can be made conveniently from the tannate. Because of embolism, Vasopressin Tannate and Vasopressin Tannate in Oil should *never be given intravenously*.

Dose—*Intramuscularly*, **1.5** to **5 units** every 36 to 48 hours. *Do not give intravenously!*

Dosage Forms—Injection (in oil): 5 units/ml.

Veterinary Dose—*Intramuscular, Dogs*, **1 to 5 Units** every 36 to 48 hours.

The Adrenal Hormones

The adrenal hormones include both the adrenocorticoids from the adrenal cortex and epinephrine and norepinephrine from the adrenal medulla. The discussion below will deal only with the adrenocorticoids. Epinephrine and norepinephrine are treated in Chapter 48, *Sympathomimetic Drugs.*

The cortex, or outer portion of the adrenal gland is one of the endocrine structures most vitally necessary for normal metabolic function. While it is possible for life to continue in the complete absence of adrenal cortical function, serious metabolic derangements ensue, and the capacity of the organism to respond to physiological or environmental stress is completely lost. The vital role of the adrenal cortex is due to its production of a group of hormones, all *steroid* in nature.

Physiology—Three general patterns of adrenal cortical hormone action have been described: (1) retention of sodium ions in extracellular fluid and potassium ions within cells, thus maintaining the normal distribution of water and chloride ion and resulting maintenance of blood volume and blood pressure; (2) maintenance of normal blood glucose levels and facilitation of liver glycogen deposition; and (3) enhanced mobilization of tissue protein and gluconeogenesis from protein. In addition, cortical hormones exert a regulatory influence upon lymphocytes, erythrocytes, and eosinophils of the blood, and upon the structure and function of lymphoid tissue. The relative or complete absence of adrenocortical function, known as *Addison's disease*, is accompanied by loss of sodium chloride and water, retention of potassium, lowering of blood glucose and liver glycogen levels, increased sensitivity to insulin, nitrogen retention, and lymphocytosis. The disturbances in electrolyte metabolism are the cause of morbidity and mortality in most cases of severe adrenal insufficiency. All of these disorders may be corrected by administration of adrenal cortical extract or the pure adrenal cortical steroids now available.

Structures—Over 44 steroids have been shown to be present in the adrenal cortex. Only seven of these, however, have been shown to exert a significant biological effect related to adrenal cortical function. However, the adrenal cortex also produces androgenic steroids. All of the adrenal cortical steroids contain 21

carbon atoms, an α,β-unsaturated ketone in ring A, and an α-ketol side chain (—COCH$_2$OH) attached to ring D. They differ in the extent of oxygenation or hydroxylation at carbons 11, 17, or 19. Depending upon whether the predominant biological effect is related to electrolyte and water metabolism, or to carbohydrate and protein metabolism, the cortical steroids are classified as either *mineralocorticoid* or *glucocorticoid*, respectively. The presence of oxygen at position 11 is necessary for significant glucocorticoid activity but not for mineralocorticoid activity; the 11β-hydroxy group is more potent than the 11-keto group; the 11-keto group is converted to the active β-hydroxy group in the body. The 17α-hydroxy group is also important to glucocorticoid activity. The 21-hydroxy group is essential to mineralocorticoid activity; it favors but is not required for glucocorticoid activity. Fluorination in the 9α position enhances both glucocorticoid and mineralocorticoid activity. All adrenal corticoids require the 3-keto group and 4–5 unsaturation.

Biological Activity—For biological testing of adrenal cortical hormones, a number of different types of assay have been used. All of the above compounds will prolong the lives of adrenalectomized animals, although their relative effectiveness varies widely, the mineralocorticoids being 10–30 times as potent as the glucocorticoids. Desoxycorticosterone and aldosterone are likewise considerably more effective in maintaining normal kidney function in adrenalectomized animals. One method of assaying effects on electrolyte metabolism involves the determination of the relative amounts of radioactive sodium (^{24}Na) and potassium (^{42}K) excreted during one hour after their injection. In adrenalectomized animals the ratio (^{24}Na:^{42}K) is high, but is restored to normal upon the injection of microgram amounts of mineralocorticoids. Glucocorticoid activity is most conveniently measured by determining the capacity to restore normal liver glycogen levels in adrenalectomized mice or rats. 17-Hydroxycorticosterone (hydrocortisone) and 11-dehydro-17-hydroxycorticosterone (cortisone) are two to five times as active as corticosterone and 11-dehydrocorticosterone in this test; the 11-desoxycorticoids are essentially inactive. Topical glucocorticoids may also be assayed by their vasoconstrictor effect in the skin of the human.

In its biosynthesis of the steroid hormones, the adrenal cortex uses cholesterol which is present in large amounts in the gland; during periods of secretory activity it also consumes large quantities of ascorbic acid, which is likewise present in high concentration. Control of adrenal gland secretion appears to be of two kinds. The production of mineralocorticoids, chiefly aldosterone, appears to be controlled in part by sodium intake and consequent changes in intravascular fluid volume and in part by the anterior pituitary. For normal development and normal capacity to meet the routine homeostatic requirements, adrenal cortical function must be stimulated by adrenocorticotropin (see *Pituitary Hormones*, page 957); adrenal cortical activity is enhanced through release of corticotropin from the anterior pituitary. In emergency states or during stress, adrenal cortical activity is increased, which prepares for a prolonged duration of the state of stress.

As indicated above, adrenal cortical activity is shared by a number of steroids. However, only three of these have found general therapeutic applications, *viz.,* desoxycorticosterone, cortisone, and hydrocortisone. In addition, extracts of adrenal glands containing corticoids are occasionally employed. The latter must be standardized biologically.

In general, clinical experience has indicated that the anti-inflammatory activity of adrenal cortical steroids in man correlates well with their glucocorticoid activity. The undesirable side effects (sodium retention, edema) are associated with mineralocorticoid activity. Synthetic steroids possessing higher glucocorticoid and lower mineralocorticoid activity than cortisone or cortisol have been prepared and marketed. Additional unsaturation in ring A enhances the anti-inflammatory and antirheumatic properties while at the same time reducing the sodium-retaining effect. Thus, prednisolone has 4 times the anti-inflammatory activity of cortisol and yet has only 0.8 of the mineralocorticoid activity. Introduction of either methyl or hydroxyl groups at position 16 markedly reduces mineralocorticoid activity but only slightly alters glucocorticoid and anti-inflammatory activity. Thus, none of paramethasone (16α-methyl), betamethasone (16β-methyl), dexamethasone (16α-methyl), and triamcinolone (16α-hydroxy) have significant mineralocorticoid activity. 6α-Methylation has unpredictable effects: it enhances the mineralocorticoid activity of cortisol but virtually abolishes that of prednisolone. The 9-fluoro group enhances both glucocorticoid and mineralocorticoid activities, but the effects of substituents at the 6 and 16 positions override this effect. Further examples will become apparent from the discussions provided in the following individual monographs.

Betamethasone NF

[9-Fluoro-11β,17,21-trihydroxy-16β-methylpregna-1,4-diene-3,20-dione; Celestone (*Schering*)]

Betamethasone contains 96.0–104.0% of $C_{22}H_{29}FO_5$ (392.47), calculated on the dried basis.

Preparation—Betamethasone is prepared from 16-dehydropregnenolone (see under *Progesterone*, page 1002) by treatment with methyl magnesium iodide to insert the 16β-methyl group, catalytic reduction of the remaining double bond, enol acylation at position-20, and reaction with peracetic acid followed by hydrolysis to the 16β-methyl-17α-hydroxy compound. Bromination and acetoxylation gives the 3β-hydroxy-21-acetoxy derivative which is oxidized to the 3-oxo compound with chromic acid. Dibromination at positions 1 and 4 followed by dehydrobromination with dimethylformamide to the 1,4-diene then incubation with *Pestalotia foedans* (or a similar organism) results in the 11α-hydroxy derivative. Esterification at the 11-position with ethyl chloroformate, elimination of the ester function with acetic acid to form the 1,4,9(11)-triene, treatment with *N*-bromoacetamide and perchloric acid gives the 9α-bromo-11β-hydroxy compound. Abstraction of HBr with potassium acetate affords the 9β,11β-epoxy derivative which by treatment with HF in a halogenated hydrocarbon yields the 9α-fluoro-11β-hydroxy analog, Betamethasone.

Description—Occurs as a white to practically white, odorless, crystalline powder. When tested by the method for *Class Ia*, page 594, it melts at about 240° with some decomposition.

Solubility—Sparingly soluble in acetone, alcohol, dioxane, and methanol; very slightly soluble in chloroform and ether; insoluble in water.

Uses—Betamethasone is an extremely potent adrenal corticoid with all of the anti-inflammatory actions and clinical uses of cortisone (see *Cortisone Acetate*, below). However, it only rarely induces sodium and water retention and potassium loss such as accompanies treatment with cortisone and many other adrenal corticoids; on occasion, Betamethasone may even increase sodium excretion and induce diuresis. In the usual doses, the incidence of characteristic adrenal corticoid untoward effects such as anorexia, protracted weight loss, vertigo, headache, and muscle weakness is quite low.

Dose—**600 mcg to 8.4 mg** daily; *usual, initial,* **2.4 to 4.8 mg** daily in divided doses; *maintenance,* **600 mcg to 1.2 mg** daily; *topically,* as a **0.2% cream** applied to the skin 2 or 3 times a day.

Dosage Forms—Cream NF: 0.2%; Tablets NF: 600 mcg.

Veterinary Dose—*Horses* and *Cattle, intramuscular,* **10 to 30 mg**; *intra-articular or periarticular,* **5 to 40 mg**. *Dogs* and *Cats, oral,* **6 mcg** per **pound** of body weight daily in divided doses; *intra-articular or periarticular,* **5 to 10 mg**.

Betamethasone Acetate NF

[Betamethasone 21-Acetate]

Betamethasone Acetate contains 97.0–103.0% of $C_{24}H_{31}FO_6$ (434.51), calculated on the anhydrous basis.

For the structure of the base, see *Betamethasone*.

Preparation—*Betamethasone* (this page) is acetylated with acetic anhydride in the presence of pyridine. US Pat. 3,164,618.

Description—A white to creamy white, odorless powder. It sinters and resolidifies at about 165° and remelts with decomposition between 200° and 220°.

Solubility—Practically insoluble in water; freely soluble in acetone; soluble in alcohol and chloroform.

Uses—The actions of Betamethasone Acetate are the same as those of the parent compound, *Betamethasone*. However, the acetate is less soluble, so that intramuscular or intra-articular injections of Betamethasone Acetate have a more sustained action than betamethasone. At present, the acetate is marketed only in combination with the sodium phosphate.

Dose—See *Sterile Betamethasone Sodium Phosphate and Betamethasone Acetate Suspension* (below).

Betamethasone Sodium Phosphate NF

[Betamethasone 21-(Disodium Phosphate)]

Betamethasone Sodium Phosphate contains 97.0–103.0% of $C_{22}H_{28}FNa_2O_8P$ (516.42), calculated on the anhydrous basis.

For the structure of the base, see *Betamethasone*.

Preparation—Starting with *Betamethasone* (page 962), this disodium phosphate ester may be prepared by the method described for *Dexamethasone Sodium Phosphate* (page 965). US Pat. 3,164,618.

Description—A white to practically white, odorless powder. It is hygroscopic.

Solubility—1 Gm dissolves in 1.6 ml of water and 6.25 ml of methanol; practically insoluble in acetone and chloroform.

Uses—The actions of Betamethasone Sodium Phosphate are those of betamethasone, to which the disodium phosphate is converted in the body. However, the disodium phosphate ester is much more soluble. Consequently, following injection the plasma or synovial fluid levels rise at a rapid rate to high levels, which effects a prompt response. At present, the sodium phosphate is marketed only in combination with the acetate.

Dose—See *Sterile Betamethasone Sodium Phosphate and Betamethasone Acetate Suspension* (below).

Sterile Betamethasone Sodium Phosphate and Betamethasone Acetate Suspension NF

[Celestone Soluspan (*Schering*)]

Sterile Betamethasone Sodium Phosphate and Betamethasone Acetate Suspension is a sterile preparation of betamethasone sodium phosphate in solution and betamethasone acetate in suspension in water for injection. It contains an amount of $C_{22}H_{28}FNa_2O_8P$ (betamethasone sodium phosphate) equivalent to 90.0–115.0% of the labeled amount of $C_{22}H_{29}FO_5$ (betamethasone), and 90.0–115.0% of the labeled amount of $C_{24}H_{31}FO_6$ (betamethasone acetate).

Uses—See *Betamethasone Acetate* and *Betamethasone Sodium Phosphate*. The combination is intended for use in glucocorticoid-responsive disease (see *Cortisone Acetate*) in patients in whom oral medication cannot be achieved, in acute self-limiting disease in which a single dose is sufficient, and to initiate treatment in severe diseases where a prompt response is desired prior to switching to a drug with a slower onset and longer duration of action. Although the injection may be given intra-articularly, there is evidence that repeated intra-articular glucocorticoids sometimes effect a painless destruction of the joint.

Dose—*Usual, intramuscular,* **1 ml** (equivalent to **3 mg** of betamethasone acetate and **3 mg** of betamethasone) repeated at intervals of 3 days to 1 week; *intra-articular,* **0.25 to 2 ml** depending on the size of the joint.

Dosage Forms—Sterile Suspension NF: Betamethasone sodium phosphate (equivalent to 15 mg of betamethasone) and 15 mg (betamethasone acetate)/5 ml.

Betamethasone Valerate NF

[Betamethasone 17-Valerate; Valisone (*Schering*)]

Betamethasone Valerate contains 97.0–103.0% of $C_{27}H_{37}FO_6$ (476.59), calculated on the dried basis.

For the structure of the base, see *Betamethasone*.

Preparation—A solution of *Betamethasone* (page 962) in an organic solvent is treated with a lower alkyl orthovalerate such as trimethyl orthovalerate [$C_4H_9C(OCH_3)_3$] to produce betamethasone-17,21-ylene alkyl orthovalerate. This is then hydrolyzed with dilute acid and the resulting crude betamethasone 17-valerate is extracted and crystallized from a suitable organic solvent. US Pat. 3,312,590.

Description—A white to practically white, odorless, crystalline powder. It melts at about 190° with decomposition.

Solubility—Practically insoluble in water; freely soluble in acetone and chloroform; soluble in alcohol; slightly soluble in benzene and ether.

Uses—The actions of Betamethasone Valerate are the same as those of the parent compound, *Betamethasone*. However, the physicochemical properties of the compound favor penetration into the skin. It is thus employed for the treatment of the inflammatory and allergic dematoses and dermatitides, such as *psoriasis, eczema, seborrheic dermatitis, contact dermatitis, atopic dermatitis, lichen planus, intertrigo, anogenital pruritus, milaria,* and *stasis dermatitis.*

Unless extensive areas of the skin are dressed with Betamethasone Valerate cream under occlusion, systemic effects are unlikely to occur. However, prolonged topical use may cause cutaneous and subcutaneous atrophy and consequent striae. Irritation, folliculitis, or sensitization is rare.

Dose—*Topically,* as a cream containing the equivalent of **0.1%** of betamethasone to the affected area 1 to 3 times a day.

Dosage Forms—Cream NF: 0.1% (of the equivalent of betamethasone); Ointment: same strength as Cream).

Cortisone Acetate USP

[Kendall's Compound E Acetate; 17,21-Dihydroxypregn-4-ene-3,11,20-trione 21-Acetate; KE Acetate; Wintersteiner's Compound F Acetate; Reichstein's Substance Fa Acetate; Cortogen Acetate (*Schering*); Cortone Acetate (*MSD*)]

Cortisone Acetate contains 97.0–102.0% of $C_{23}H_{30}O_6$ (402.49), calculated on the dried basis.

Preparation—Cortisone is prepared by a variety of methods using easily obtainable starting materials such as ergosterol, diosgenin or hecogenin from plant materials and cholesterol or desoxycholic acid from animal sources. The cortisone is esterified with acetic anhydride to give the acetate.

Description—A white or practically white, odorless, crystalline powder. It is stable in air and melts at about 240° with some decomposition when tested by the method for *Class Ia*.

Solubility—Insoluble in water; 1 Gm dissolves in about 350 ml of alcohol, 4 ml of chloroform, 30 ml of dioxane, and 75 ml of acetone.

Uses—Cortisone Acetate is a natural glucocorticoid with a slight degree of mineralocorticoid activity. It is used specifically, in combination with desoxycorticosterone acetate, in *adrenal cortical insufficiency*. Cortisone Acetate may also be used to suppress oversecretion of the adrenal cortex in *bilateral adrenal hyperplasia*.

Cortisone Acetate is also used nonspecifically in the treatment of a wide variety of disorders, including *rheumatic* and *articular disease, lupus erythematosus, ulcerative colitis, inflammatory* and *allergic conditions, bronchial asthma, nephrosis,* and some *chronic infections.* The physiological basis for the successful application of the cortical steroids in so many different afflictions is unknown. However, the hormone is known to stabilize membranes, including those of lysosomes, and to diminish the activity of macrophages and other phagocytes. Cortisone and its cogeners may favorably affect the course of *acute leukemia,* complete remissions occasionally occurring. However, the effect is temporary, and the patient eventually becomes refractory to steroid therapy. *Hodgkin's disease, lymphosarcoma,* and *multiple myeloma* may also be temporarily suppressed by cortisone and its cogeners, especially with respect to pain.

Like corticotropin, cortisone may lead to exacerbation of diabetic symptoms, and may suppress some of the symptoms of acute infection. Its use, therefore, must be accompanied by careful medical supervision. Suppression of the inflammatory response favors bacteria and viral invasion; is especially contraindicated in tuberculosis and herpes simplex. Other side effects, mainly of chronic use, include fluid and electrolyte disturbances, "moon face," "buffalo hump," subclavicular fat pads, obesity, cutaneous striae, ecchymoses, acne, hirsutism, osteoporosis, myopathy, negative potassium balance, activation of peptic ulcers, hyperglycemia, glycosuria, convulsions, and psychoses. Also, when treatment is discontinued, adrenal cortical hypofunction ensues. Withdrawal symptoms, due to anterior pituitary inhibition, can be controlled by gradual reduction in dosage.

Dose—*Oral* or *intramuscular,* **10** to **400 mg** daily; *usual oral,* **25 mg** 4 times a day; *usual, intramuscular,* **100 mg** daily; *topically,* **0.1 ml** of a 0.5 to 2.5% suspension to the conjunctiva 6 to 12 times a day.

Other Dose Information—A satisfactory initial response to Cortisone Acetate can usually be obtained with 150–300 mg daily, either intramuscularly in a single dose, or orally in divided doses. Subsequently, the dose is gradually lowered to the minimum which provides satisfactory maintenance.

Dosage Forms—Ophthalmic Suspension USP: 0.5 and 2.5%; Sterile Suspension USP: 250 mg/10 ml, 500 mg/10 and 20 ml; Tablets USP: 5, 10, and 25 mg.

Veterinary Uses—Cortisone is recommended for use in the treatment of *bovine ketosis, canine rheumatoid arthritis,* certain skin conditions, and inflammation of the external eye.

Veterinary Dose—*Horses* and *Cattle, intramuscular,* **1** to **1.5 Gm** daily; *intra-articular,* **50** to **250 mg**. *Dogs* and *Cats, intramuscular,* **1** to **2 mg** per **pound** of body weight daily; *oral,* same as *intramuscular,* but divided in 3 or 4 doses.

Desoxycorticosterone Acetate USP

[21-Hydroxypregn-4-ene-3,20-dione Acetate; 11-Deoxycorticosterone Acetate; Desoxycorticosteroni Acetas; Desoxycortone Acetate; Deoxycortone Acetate; Cortate (*Schering*); D.O.C.A. (*Organon*); Percorten (*Ciba*)]

Desoxycorticosterone Acetate contains 97.0–103.0% of $C_{23}H_{32}O_4$ (372.51), calculated on the dried basis.

History—This steroid was first isolated from the adrenal cortex in 1938. It has also been synthesized from *stigmasterol,* a phytosterol obtained from soya bean. See *Sterols* (page 479).

Preparation—Desoxycorticosterone is condensed with acetyl chloride in pyridine solution. Dilution of the reaction product with water precipitates the ester which is collected, washed with acid and then with water, dried, and recrystallized from a suitable organic solvent.

Description—A white, or creamy white, crystalline powder. It is odorless and is stable in air. It melts between 155° and 161°, and has a specific rotation $[\alpha]_D^{20}$ of +168° to +176° when determined in dioxane solution.

Solubility—Practically insoluble in water; sparingly soluble in alcohol, acetone, and dioxane; slightly soluble in vegetable oils.

Uses—Desoxycorticosterone is a natural mineralocorticoid (see the general statement, page 961). Physiologically it is of much less importance than aldosterone, but the cost of the latter is too prohibitive for clinical use. Treatment of *Addison's disease* has been greatly advanced by the use of desoxycorticosterone. Although the defects in carbohydrate and protein metabolism are not corrected by this particular compound, life can be maintained by its intelligent administration.

Since Addison's disease is a permanent disorder, treatment is for life, and a long duration of action is therefore desirable. Consequently, desoxycorticosterone is administered in the form of intramuscular oil solutions or as subcutaneous pellets. With pellet implantation the hormone is slowly absorbed (0.5 mg per day), and a single implantation of an adequate number of pellets may be effective for as long as 6 months or more.

Patients receiving desoxycorticosterone should be careful to maintain an adequate intake of salt and carbohydrate and, during periods of acute adrenal insufficiency, carbohydrate must be specially administered. In crisis, extracts containing the glycogenic corticoids should be administered.

The principal side effects are due to the renal action to promote sodium and water retention and potassium loss. Weight gain, "moon face," and hypokalemic alkalosis may result.

Dose—*Intramuscular,* **1** to **10 mg** daily; *usual,* **1** to **5 mg** once a day.

Other Dose Information—Buccal, 2 to 10 mg.

Dosage Forms—Injection USP: 50 mg/10 ml; Pellets NF: 75 and 125 mg; Tablets: 2 mg.

Veterinary Dose—*Cattle, intramuscularly*, **20 mg**; *Dogs*, **2.5 to 5 mg.**

Desoxycorticosterone Pivalate NF

[21-Hydroxypregn-4-ene-3,20-dione Pivalate; 11-Deoxycorticosterone Pivalate; Percorten Trimethylacetate (*Ciba*)]

Desoxycorticosterone Pivalate contains 97.0–103.0% of $C_{26}H_{38}O_4$ (414.59), calculated on the dried basis.

For the structure of desoxycorticosterone, see *Desoxycorticosterone Acetate* (page 964).

Preparation—This ester is prepared as described above for the acetate except that trimethylacetyl chloride is employed.

Description—Occurs as a white, or creamy white, crystalline powder. It is odorless and is stable in air. It melts between 198° and 204°. Specific rotation +153°–+161° in a solution in dioxane containing 100 mg in each 10 ml.

Solubility—Practically insoluble in water; slightly soluble in alcohol, methanol, ether, and vegetable oils; sparingly soluble in acetone; soluble in dioxane.

Uses—The actions of Desoxycorticosterone Pivalate are the same as those of *Desoxycorticosterone Acetate* (above), except that intramuscular microcrystalline suspensions of the trimethylacetate (pivalate) have a very long duration of action. Consequently, it is used only for the treatment of chronic primary and secondary adrenal cortical insufficiency.

Dose—*Usual, intramuscular*, **50 to 100 mg**, repeated in not less than 30 days.

Dosage Forms—Sterile Suspension NF: 100 mg/4 ml.

Dexamethasone USP

[9-Fluoro-11β,17,21-trihydroxy-16α-methylpregna-1,4-diene-3,20-dione; (*Various Mfgs.*)]

Dexamethasone contains 97.0–102.0% of $C_{22}H_{29}FO_5$ (392.47), calculated on the dried basis.

Preparation—This material is prepared in a manner quite similar to that for *Betamethasone* (page 962), the difference being that the 16-methyl group is inserted in the α-configuration.

Description—Occurs as a white to practically white, odorless, crystalline powder. It is stable in air, and when tested by the method for *Class Ia*, page 1548, melts at about 250° with some decomposition.

Solubility—Sparingly soluble in acetone, alcohol, dioxane, and methanol; slightly soluble in chloroform; very slightly soluble in ether; practically insoluble in water.

Uses—Dexamethasone is a synthetic adrenal steroid derived from prednisolone. It possesses glucocorticoid activity and has the appropriate clinical uses (see the general statement, page 961, and *Cortisone Acetate*, page 963). It is especially used as an antiinflammatory and antiallergic agent. Topically it is employed in the treatment of glucocorticoid-responsive dermatoses. In ophthalmology it is used in the treatment of ocular and periocular inflammations; for these purposes, it is used only as the sodium phosphate. Its potency is about 35 times that of cortisone. It is capable of inducing all the usual side effects of the adrenal corticoids. It has the same side effects as cortisone, except that they are less pronounced. After systemic administration weight gain, edema, dyspnea, nausea, weakness, increased appetite, peptic ulceration, and central nervous stimulation may occur.

Dose—**500 mcg to 5 mg** daily; *usual*, **750 mcg** 2 to 4 times a day; as an *aerosol*, spray affected area for 1 to 2 seconds 2 or 3 times a day.

Dosage Forms—Aerosol NF: 3.3 mg/30 Gm, 10 mg/90 Gm; Elixir NF: 500 mcg/5 ml; Tablets USP: 250, 500, and 750 mcg, and 1.5 mg.

Veterinary Dose—*Intravenous* or *intramuscular, Horses*, **2.5 to 5 mg**; *Cattle*, **5 to 20 mg**; *Dogs*, **0.25 to 1 mg**; *Cats*, **0.125 to 0.5 mg.** *Oral*, total daily doses approximately the same.

Dexamethasone Sodium Phosphate USP

[Dexamethasone 21-(Disodium Phosphate); Decadron Phosphate (*MSD*); Hexadrol Phosphate (*Organon*)]

Dexamethasone Sodium Phosphate contains 95.0–100.5% of $C_{22}H_{28}FNa_2O_8P$ (516.42), calculated on the water-free and alcohol-free basis.

For the structure of the base, see *Dexamethasone*.

Preparation—Dexamethasone is esterified with methanesulfonyl chloride at the 21-position, and the ester is refluxed with sodium iodide in ethanol to form the 21-iodo derivative. This is treated with silver dihydrogen phosphate and the resulting 21-(dihydrogen phosphate) is neutralized with sodium hydroxide.

Description—A white or slightly yellow, crystalline powder. It is odorless or has a slight odor of alcohol. It is very hygroscopic.

Solubility—1 Gm dissolves in about 2 ml of water; insoluble in dioxane; slightly soluble in alcohol; insoluble in ether and chloroform.

Uses—Dexamethasone Sodium Phosphate has the same actions as *Dexamethasone*. It is one of the most soluble adrenalcorticoid compounds. Thus it lends itself well to intravenous administration, local injection, inhalation, and to solutions and water based ointments for topical application, especially for ophthalmalogic use. The aerosol is used in the management of bronchial asthma. Although it may be given intraarticularly, it is usually not recommended by this route because of the danger of painless joint destruction. The contraindications are those of the other glucocorticoids; however, the products for ophthalmic use are especially dangerous in the presence of herpes simplex, and the inhalant is particularly proscribed in tuberculosis.

Dose—*USP: Intravenous* or *intramuscular*, **2 to 50 mg** daily; *usual*, the equivalent of **2 to 4 mg** of dexamethasone phosphate 6 to 8 times a day; by inhalation, **3 inhalations** of an aerosol containing 18 mg of dexamethasone sodium phosphate per 12.6 Gm of suspension (approximately 0.1 mg of dexamethasone sodium phosphate per inhalation) 3 or 4 times a day.

NF: Topically as 0.05% ointment or 0.1% solution 1 to 3 times a day to the eye or 3 or 4 drops 1 to 3 times a day to the ear; as 0.1% cream to affected area 2 or 3 times a day.

Dosage Forms—Cream NF: 0.1%; Injection: 4 mg/ml; Ophthalmic Ointment NF: 0.05%; Ophthalmic Solution NF: 0.1%.

Neomycin Sulfate and Dexamethasone Sodium Phosphate Cream NF

[Neo-Decadron Phosphate Cream (MSD)]

Neomycin Sulfate and Dexamethasone Sodium Phosphate Cream contains an amount of $C_{22}H_{28}$-FNa_2O_8P (dexamethasone sodium phosphate) equivalent to 90.0–115.0% of the labeled amount of $C_{22}H_{30}$-FO_8P (dexamethasone phosphate), and an amount of neomycin sulfate equivalent to 90.0–135.0% of the labeled amount of neomycin base. Neomycin Sulfate and Dexamethasone Sodium Phosphate Cream conforms to the regulations of the federal Food and Drug Administration concerning certification of antibiotic drugs.

Uses—Neomycin Sulfate and Dexamethasone Sodium Phosphate Cream combines the glucocorticoid properties of Dexamethasone (see *Dexamethasone* and *Dexamethasone Sodium Phosphate*, above) with the antibacterial properties of *Neomycin Sulfate* (see page 1219). The uses are the same as those of *Dexamethasone Sodium Phosphate*, except the mixture is not used in the treatment of exfoliative dermatitis. The purpose of the neomycin is to prevent infections that may occur as the result of suppression of the inflammatory response or to control infections which are secondary to the dermatological disorder. The cream is contraindicated in tuberculosis, chicken pox, and herpes simplex.

Dose—*Topically*, to the affected area 2 or 3 times a day.

Other Dose Information—Marketed preparations contain 0.1% Dexamethasone Sodium Phosphate and 0.35 or 0.5% Neomycin Sulfate.

Fluocinolone Acetonide NF

[6α,9-Difluoro-11β,16α,17,21-tetrahydroxypregna-1,4-diene-3,20-dione Cyclic 16,17-Acetal with Acetone; Fluonid (*Marion*); Synalar (*Syntex*)]

Fluocinolone Acetonide contains 97.0–103.0% of $C_{24}H_{30}F_2O_6$ (452.50), calculated on the dried basis.

Preparation—Fluocinolone acetonide is prepared from the 21-acetate of 16α,17α-epoxy-3β,21-dihydroxy-pregn-5-en-20-one (available by synthesis from naturally occurring sapogenins such as diosgenin). Treatment of this pregnene with HF and *N*-bromoacetamide, followed by chromic acid oxidation and then treatment with HBr in acetic acid gives the Δ⁴-16β-bromo-6α-fluoro derivative. This latter compound on refluxing with potassium acetate in acetic acid and then saponifying with sodium carbonate affords the 6α-fluoro-16α,17α-dihydroxy compound which when incubated with minced, defatted bovine adrenals adds an 11β-hydroxyl group. From the 16,21-diacetate, with dimethylformamide and methanesulfonyl chloride, the 4,9-diene is synthesized, which is converted to the 9β,11β-epoxide and then to the 9α-fluoro-11β-hydroxy compound in a manner similar to that for *Betamethasone* (page 962). Oxidation of this product with selenium dioxide yields the 1,4-diene (fluocinoline)

which on reaction with acetone and perchloric acid yields the acetonide.

Description—A white, crystalline powder that is odorless. It is stable in light, nonhygroscopic, and decomposes in heat. It melts between 272° and 278°.

Solubility—Soluble in alcohol, acetone, and methanol; slightly soluble in chloroform; insoluble in water.

Uses—Fluocinolone Acetonide is a glucocorticoid with potent anti-inflammatory and metabolic actions and negligible mineralocorticoid actions. It is employed topically in the treatment of various *dermatoses*, such as atopic dermatitis, contact dermatitis, chronic lichen simplex, lichen planus, chronic familial benign pemphigus, seborrheic dermatitis and psoriasis. Even in instances in which nearly the whole body has been covered by a cream containing the corticoid, evidences of systemic side effects are rare. However, folliculitis or striae is a frequent complication, especially if occlusive dressings are used. Topical Fluocinolone is contraindicated in the presence of tuberculosis, fungal infections, and most viral lesions of the skin (vaccinia, varicella, herpes simplex, etc). Neomycin is often included in topical preparations of Fluocinolone Acetonide to suppress infections secondary to the inflammatory process or which result from the use of the glucocorticoid.

Dose—*Topically*, as a **0.01** to **0.2%** cream, ointment, or solution.

Dosage Forms—Cream: 0.01 and 0.025%; Ointment: 0.025%; Solution: 0.01%.

Fluorometholone NF

[9-Fluoro-11β,17-dihydroxy-6α-methylpregna-1,4-diene-3,20-dione; Oxylone (*Upjohn*)]

Fluorometholone contains 97.0–103.0% of $C_{22}H_{29}$-FO_4 (376.47), calculated on the dried basis.

Preparation—6α-Methyl-9α-fluoroprednisolone is esterified with *p*-toluenesulfonyl chloride to give the 21-*p*-toluenesulfonate. This is treated with sodium iodide in acetone solution to give the corresponding 21-iodo compound which is then reduced with sodium bisulfite to Fluorometholone. US Pats. 2,852,511 and 2,867,637.

Description—White to yellowish-white, odorless, crystalline solid. It melts at about 290° with decomposition.

Solubility—Slightly soluble in alcohol and acetone; very slightly soluble in water and ether.

Uses—Fluorometholone is a glucocorticoid with the actions and uses of *Hydrocortisone* (see page 968). By the oral route it is equipotent to hydrocortisone, but by topical administration it is 40 times as potent. Consequently, it is used for the topical treatment of *chronic dermatoses* such as contact dermatitis, atopic dermatitis, seborrheic dermatitis, pruritus with lichenfication, and nonspecific anogenital pruritus.

Dose—*Topically*, as a **0.025%** cream, 1 to 3 times a day.

Dosage Forms—Cream NF: 0.025%.

Fluprednisolone NF

[6α-Fluoro-11β,17,21-trihydroxypregna-1,4-diene-3,20-dione; Alphadrol (*Upjohn*)]

Fluprednisolone contains 97.0–103.0% of $C_{21}H_{27}FO_5$ (378.44), calculated on the dried basis.

Preparation—The 3-ethylene glycol ketal of methyl 3,11-dioxopregna-4,17(20)-dien-21-oate is reacted with peracetic acid to form the 5,6-epoxide (I). Reaction of (I) with HF in methylene chloride produces methyl 3,11-dioxo-6β-fluoro-5α-hydroxypregn-17(20)-en-21-oate (II). The 3-ketal of (II) is prepared with ethylene glycol in the presence of *p*-toluenesulfonic acid, and this is reduced with lithium aluminum hydride in anhydrous ether to the 3-ethylene ketal of 6β-fluoro-5α,11β,21-trihydroxypregn-17(20)-en-3-one. Conversion to the 21-acetate is effected with acetic anhydride and pyridine and this ester is then oxidized in *tert*-butanol solution with α-methylmorpholine oxide peroxide and osmium tetroxide to 5α,11β,17α-trihydroxy-6β-fluoro-21-acetoxy-pregnane-3,20-dione 3-ethylene ketal. The 3-ketal is hydrolyzed and dehydration at position 5 is carried out in dimethylformamide solution with hydrochloric acid. Introduction of the Δ¹ double bond is accomplished with *Septomyxa affinis* under conditions which also effect 21-deacetylation. Isomerization to the 6α-fluoro compound (Fluprednisolone) may be effected by streaming dry HCl into a cold chloroform/ethanol solution of the 6β epimer. US Pat. 2,841,600.

Description—A white to off-white, odorless, crystalline powder. It melts at about 210°.

Solubility—Sparingly soluble in alcohol, methanol, and ethyl acetate; slightly soluble in chloroform, ether, and ethylene dichloride; very slightly soluble in benzene; practically insoluble in water.

Uses—Fluprednisolone is a glucocorticoid that is approximately 2½ times as potent as prednisolone and 40 times as potent as cortisone. However, occasionally it does not always appear to be able to control allergic or inflammatory conditions that can be controlled with other glucocorticoids. Whether this occasional erratic behavior is the result of an intrinsic defect in the drug or to inexperience with dosage remains to be determined. Fluprednisolone is used for the same purposes as *Cortisone Acetate* (page 963), and it has the same side effects, except that steroid myopathy has not been reported. Fluprednisolone also has erratic mineralocorticoid activity.

Dose—*Usual,* 750 mcg to **5.25 mg** 1 to 4 times daily.

Other Dose Information—Once a therapeutic response has been achieved with an initial dose regimen, the dose should be reduced to the lowest that will provide adequate control but not necessarily complete relief.

Dosage Forms—Tablets NF: 750 mcg and 1.5 mg.

Flurandrenolone

Flurandrenolone [$C_{21}H_{29}FO_6$ = 396.46] is 6α-fluoro-11β,16α,17,21 - tetrahydroxypregn - 4 - ene - 3,20-dione.

Preparation—6α - Fluoro - 11β,16α,17,21 - tetrahydroxypregn-4-ene-3,20-dione is caused to undergo condensation with acetone under the influence of a dehydrating agent such as hydrogen chloride, anhydrous copper sulfate, or perchloric acid. US Pat. 3,126,375. The starting steroid may be prepared by the methods described in US Pat. 2,997,489.

Description—Fine, white, crystals that are odorless and tasteless. It is stable to light and nonhygroscopic. It melts between 240° and 245°.

Solubility—Readily soluble in alcohol; soluble in methanol, acetone, ethyl acetate, chloroform, and acetic acid; practically insoluble in water.

Uses—Flurandrenolone is a potent glucocorticoid intended for topical use which is effective in alleviating and controlling pruritus and in inflammation associated with various *dermatoses*. The addition of a 6α-fluoro substitute to hydrocortisone has resulted in a compound which is more effective than the parent drug in reducing inflammation of the skin. However, there are superior topical glucocorticoids. Local side effects include irritation or burning in some instances and striae after prolonged use. Hypertrichosis and hypopigmentation are seen occasionally. Systemic side effects do not occur with topical administration unless a large area is chronically treated under an occlusive dressing.

Dose—*Topically,* as a **0.05**% cream or ointment, 2 or 3 times a day.

Flurandrenolide NF

[6α-Fluoro-11β,16α,17,21-tetrahydroxypregn-4-ene-3,20-dione Cyclic 16,17-Acetal with Acetone; Flurandrenolone Acetonide; Cordran Acetonide (*Lilly*)]

Flurandrenolide contains 95.0–100.5% of $C_{24}H_{33}FO_6$ (436.53), calculated on the dried basis.

For the structure of the base, see *Flurandrenolone*.

Preparation—Flurandrenolone (6α-fluoro-16α-hydroxycortisol) is condensed with acetone by treating its solution in acetone with 70% perchloric acid. US Pat. 3,126,375.

Description—A white to off-white, fluffy, odorless, crystalline powder.

Solubility—Freely soluble in chloroform; soluble in methanol; sparingly soluble in alcohol; practically insoluble in water and ether.

Uses—Flurandrenolone Acetonide is a glucocorticoid which has a high potency topically but low potency systemically, owing to rapid destruction in the liver. Consequently, its use is limited to the management of the appropriate dermatologic disorders; systemic side effects are rare. It is used in the treatment of *sunburn, diaper rash, milaria, anogenital pruritus, dyshidrosis, eczemas, intertrigo, lichen planus, lichen simplex, neurodermatitis, psoriasis, seborrheic dermatitis, stasis dermatitis,* and *otitis externa.* Local side effects are uncommon but include irritation and burning, hypertrichosis, hypopigmentation, and striae. Neomycin is often included in topical preparations of flurandrenolide to suppress infections secondary to the inflammatory process or to the use of the glucocorticoid.

Dose—*Topically,* as a **0.025 to 0.05**% cream or ointment to the affected area 2 or 3 times a day.

Dosage Forms—Cream NF: 0.025 and 0.05%; Lotion: 0.05%; Ointment NF: 0.025 and 0.05%; Tape.

Hydrocortisone USP

[11β,17,21-Trihydroxypregn-4-ene-3,20-dione; Cortisol; Compound F; Reichstein's "Substance M"; Cortef (*Upjohn*); Cortril (*Pfizer*); Hydrocortone (*MSD*)]

Hydrocortisone contains 97.0–102.0% of $C_{21}H_{30}O_5$ (362.47), calculated on the dried basis.

Preparation—The most attractive commercial synthesis of Hydrocortisone involves the oxidation of 17α,21-dihydroxypregn-4-ene-3,20-dione, which is readily obtainable from diosgenin. Microbiological hydroxylation at the 11β-position is effected on the diacetate of the above compound employing organisms of the *Rhizopus, Aspergillus* or *Streptomyces* species. Saponification then yields Hydrocortisone.

Description—A white to practically white, odorless, crystalline powder. Melting range 212° to 220° except that when in the form of a fine powder, such that at least 95% passes through a No. 325 standard sieve, it may begin to melt at 209°. Absorptivity of a solution in methanol (1 in 100,000) at 242 mμ does not differ by more than 2.5% from a similarly prepared standard. The specific rotation $[\alpha]_D^{25}$ (calculated on the dried basis and measured in dioxane solution) is between +150° and +156°.

Solubility—Very slightly soluble in water and in ether; 1 Gm dissolves in 40 ml of alcohol and about 80 ml of acetone; slightly soluble in chloroform.

Uses—See *Cortisone Acetate* (page 963). Except for the greater potency of hydrocortisone, cortisone and hydrocortisone are to be considered identical.

Dose—10 to **300 mg** daily; *usual, oral,* **10 to 20 mg** 3 to 4 times a day; *topically,* as a **0.5 to 2.5**% cream or ointment, or as a **0.125, 0.25, 0.5,** or **1**% lotion 3 or 4 times a day.

Other Dose Information—For intravaginal use, the dose is 10 mg.

Dosage Forms—Cream USP (see below): 0.125, 0.25, 0.5, 1, 2, and 2.5%; Lotion NF: 0.125, 0.25, 0.5, and 1%; Ointment USP: 0.125, 0.25, 0.5, 1, 2, and 2.5%; Tablets USP: 5, 10, and 20 mg.

Hydrocortisone Cream USP is hydrocortisone in a suitable cream base. It contains 90.0–110.0% of the labeled amount of $C_{21}H_{30}O_5$. *Preparation:* Levigate hydrocortisone (the labeled quantity) with mineral oil (10 Gm) to make a smooth paste, and incorporate into hydrophilic ointment (qs) to make 1000 Gm. *Uses* and *Dose:* See *Hydrocortisone.*

Hydrocortisone Acetate USP

[Hydrocortisone 21-Acetate; Cortef Acetate (*Upjohn*); Cortril Acetate (*Pfizer*); Hydrocortone Acetate (*MSD*)]

Hydrocortisone Acetate contains 97.0–102.0% of $C_{23}H_{32}O_6$ (404.51), calculated on the dried basis.

Preparation—Hydrocortisone (this page) is esterified with acetic anhydride in pyridine to give the 21-acetate.

Description—A white, to practically white, odorless, crystalline powder. Melting range 216° to 222°. Specific rotation +158° to +165° (calculated on the dried basis, in dioxane solution containing 100 mg per 10 ml). Absorptivity of a solution in methanol (1 in 100,000) at 242 mμ does not differ by more than 2.5% from a similarly prepared standard.

Solubility—Insoluble in water; 1 Gm dissolves in 230 ml of alcohol and 200 ml of chloroform.

Uses—Hydrocortisone Acetate has the same actions and side effects as *Hydrocortisone* and is similar in many ways to *Cortisone Acetate.* However, cortisone appears not to be reduced in the skin to the active form, cortisol, so that cortisone has a low topical efficacy. The use of Hydrocortisone Acetate is limited principally to topical therapy of dermatoses, such as *contact dermatitis, atopic dermatitis, seborrheic dermatitis, anogenital pruritus, lichenified pruritus, dyshidrosis, intertrigo, lichen planus, neurodermatitis, psoriasis, seborrheic dermatitis, stasis dermatitis, eczemas, milaria, diaper rash,* and *sunburn,* to local injection into synovial fluid or tendon cysts, and local ophthalmologic therapy of *ocular and periocular inflammations.* It may cause local irritation and burning, folliculitis, or striae. Systemic effects can result from local application.

The inclusion of neomycin in lotions and creams containing hydrocortisone acetate is for the purpose of protecting against bacterial infections that might be favored by the suppression of the inflammatory response and of clearing up infections secondary to the inflammatory condition.

Dose—*Intra-articular,* **10 to 50 mg** at each site 1 to 4 times a month; *usual,* **25 mg** at each site every 2 weeks; *topically,* as a **0.5 to 2.5**% ointment or suspension.

Dosage Forms—Ointment USP: 1 and 2.5%; Ophthalmic Ointment USP: 0.5, 1.5, and 2.5%; Ophthalmic Suspension USP: 0.5, 2.0, and 2.5%; Sterile Suspension USP: 25 and 50 mg/ml, 125 and 250 mg/5 ml, 250 and 500 mg/10 ml.

Neomycin Sulfate and Hydrocortisone Acetate Lotion NF

Neomycin Sulfate and Hydrocortisone Acetate Lotion is neomycin sulfate and hydrocortisone acetate suspended in a suitable aqueous vehicle. It contains an amount of neomycin sulfate equivalent to 90.0–135.0% of the labeled amount of neomycin base, and 90.0–110.0% of the labeled amount of hydrocortisone acetate ($C_{23}H_{32}O_6$). Neomycin Sulfate and Hydrocortisone Acetate Lotion conforms to the regulations of the federal Food and Drug Administration concerning certification of antibiotic drugs (see page 1206).

Uses—See *Neomycin Sulfate* (page 1219) and *Hydrocortisone Acetate* (above).

Dose—*Topically,* to the affected area 1 to 3 times a day.

Dosage Forms—NF: 0.35% (neomycin base) with 0.5 or 1% (hydrocortisone acetate).

Veterinary Dose—*Horses* and *Cattle*, *intramuscular*, **0.5** to **1.5 Gm**, repeated if necessary. *Dogs* and *Cats*, *oral* or *intramuscular*, **1** to **5 mg** per pound of body weight 2 to 4 times daily. Dose must be adjusted to the response of the patient.

Hydrocortisone Tebutate

[Hydrocortone T.B.A. (*MSD*)]

Hydrocortisone Tebutate [$C_{27}H_{40}O_6$ = 460.62] is hydrocortisone 21-(3,3-dimethylbutyrate).

For the structure of the base, see *Hydrocortisone*.

Preparation—Hydrocortisone (page 968) is esterified by treatment with 3,3-dimethylbutyryl chloride in the presence of pyridine.

Description—Dimorphic crystals that melt between 168° and 169° and between 229° and 230°.

Solubility—1 Gm dissolves in about 12.5 ml of boiling alcohol.

Uses—Hydrocortisone Tebutate is intended only for local use by intra-articular injection or injection into soft tissue. Its slight solubility promotes a relatively prompt onset of action after injection, yet favors a duration of action longer than that of more soluble preparations. By the intra-articular route it is used in the management of various *arthritides*. It is injected into soft tissues in the treatment of *bursitis, tendonitis, myositis, bunions, helomata, ganglia fibrositis, sprains, strains, whiplash* and other *acute rheumatic conditions*, and many other rheumatic and inflammatory disorders. As with other glucocorticoids, chronic intra-articular administration may occasionally result in painless joint destruction.

Dose—To be determined by the physician according to the need.

Other Dose Information—*Intra-articular*, large joints, 25 to 37.5 mg; small joints, 10 to 12.5 mg; *by local injection*, bursae, 25 to 37.5 mg; tendon sheaths, 5 to 12.5 mg; helomata, 10 to 25 mg; ganglia, 12.5 to 25 mg; soft tissue infiltration, 25 to 75 mg.

Dosage Forms—Suspension: 25 mg/ml.

Hydrocortisone Sodium Phosphate USP

[Hydrocortisone 21-(Disodium Phosphate); Hydrocortone Phosphate (*MSD*)]

Hydrocortisone Sodium Phosphate contains 96.0–102.0% of $C_{21}H_{29}Na_2O_8P$ (486.41), calculated on the dried basis.

For the structure of the base, see *Hydrocortisone*.

Preparation—Hydrocortisone Sodium Phosphate may be prepared from hydrocortisone by a method similar to that used for *Dexamethasone Sodium Phosphate* (page 965). US Pat. 2,870,177.

Description—A white to light-yellow, odorless or practically odorless, bitter-tasting powder. It is relatively stable in light and heat and is very hygroscopic. The pH of a 1% solution is 7.5 to 8.5.

Solubility—1 Gm dissolves in about 1.5 ml of water; slightly soluble in alcohol; practically insoluble in chloroform, dioxane, and ether.

Uses—Hydrocortisone Sodium Phosphate has the same actions and uses as *Hydrocortisone* (page 968). However, the phosphate is quite soluble and hence has a special usefulness as a parenteral form of hydrocortisone in emergency situations in which a rapid response is essential or when oral medication cannot be tolerated. Emergency states in which it is indicated are severe, *life-threatening allergic reactions, status asth-*maticus, acute *life-threatening infections* (only when appropriate antibiotic therapy is also undertaken!), *thyroid crisis* and *acute thyroiditis, lupoid crisis, severe croup, pre-* and *post-operative* management of patients undergoing *bilateral adrenalectomy* or *hypophysectomy*, and so-called *irreversible shock*.

Dose—*Intravenous* or *intramuscular*, the equivalent of **100** to **1000 mg** of hydrocortisone daily; *usual*, the equivalent of **100** to **250 mg** of hydrocortisone.

Other Dose Information—The total daily dose should not exceed 1 Gm. In children, the dose is 25 to 75 mg.

Dosage Forms—Injection USP: 100 mg/2 ml.

Hydrocortisone Sodium Succinate USP

[Hydrocortisone 21-(Sodium Succinate); Solu-Cortef (*Upjohn*)]

Hydrocortisone Sodium Succinate contains 97.0–102.0% of $C_{25}H_{33}NaO_8$ (484.53), calculated on the dried basis.

Preparation—Hydroxycortisone 21-(hydrogen succinate) is first prepared by reacting hydrocortisone with succinic anhydride dissolved in pyridine. When the reaction is complete, the mixture is added to cold, dilute HCl whereupon the acid ester precipitates. It is collected, washed with water, dried, and purified by recrystallizing from acetone. The sodium salt is then prepared by neutralizing the acid with dilute sodium hydroxide solution followed by drying the solution from the frozen state.

Description—White or nearly white, odorless, hygroscopic, amorphous solid.

Solubility—Very soluble in water and alcohol; insoluble in chloroform; very slightly soluble in acetone.

Uses—The actions and uses of Hydrocortisone Sodium Succinate are the same as those of hydrocortisone (see *Hydrocortisone*), into which it is converted in the body. However the sodium succinate derivative is highly soluble and hence is the preferred form for infusion concentrates and for intravenous or intramuscular administration when intense rapid action is desired, as in *shock-like syndromes* resulting from *acute adrenal cortical insufficiency, acute hypersensitivity, status asthmaticus, disseminated lupus erythematosus* and *overwhelming infections*. It is intended only for short-term emergency therapy or for *local application to mucous membranes*.

Dose—*Intravenous* or *intramuscular*, the equivalent of **100** to **1000 mg** of hydrocortisone daily; *usual*, the equivalent of **100** to **250 mg** of hydrocortisone.

Dosage Forms—for Injection USP: 100 and 250 mg.

Veterinary Use—Emergencies where immediate high levels of circulating hydrocortisone are required.

Veterinary Dose—*Dogs* and *Cats*, **5** to **20 mg** *intravenously, initially*, followed by **2** to **10 mg** at 1, 3, 6, and 10 hours as required.

Methylprednisolone NF

[11β,17,21-Trihydroxy-6α-methylpregna-1,4-diene-3,20-dione;   6α-Methylprednisolone; Medrol (*Upjohn*)]

Methylprednisolone contains 97.0–103.0% of $C_{22}H_{30}O_5$ (374.48), calculated on the dried basis.

Preparation—For the preparation of Methylprednisolone, *Progesterone* (page 1002) is converted to the 6α-methyl derivative in the same manner as indicated in the synthesis of *Medroxyprogesterone Acetate* (page 999). Incubation of the 6α-methyl compound with an Ascomycete, such as *Pestalotia*, forms the 11α-hydroxy derivative which is oxidized to the 3,11-diketo compound with chromic acid. Further treatment with ethyl oxalate followed by bromination, rearrangement with sodium methoxide and debromination with zinc dust gives the methyl ester of the 4,17(20)-diene-21-carboxylate. With pyrrolidine, lithium aluminum hydride reduction and treatment with alkali, the 11β,21-dihydroxy-4,17(20)-diene is formed which is converted to the 21-acetate and then oxidatively hydroxylated to 6α-methylhydrocortisone acetate. Saponification, followed by dehydrogenation with *Septomyxa affinis* gives the 1,4,17(20)-triene, which is again converted to the 21-acetate, oxidatively hydroxylated to yield the 17α-hydroxy derivative and saponified to give Methylprednisolone.

Description—Occurs as a white to practically white, odorless, crystalline powder. When tested by the method for *Class Ia*, page 594, it melts at about 240° with some decomposition.

Solubility—Sparingly soluble in alcohol, dioxane, and methanol; slightly soluble in acetone and in chloroform; very slightly soluble in ether; insoluble in water.

Uses—Methylprednisolone is a glucocorticoid that has the same uses as *Prednisolone* (page 971). However, it induces considerably less retention of sodium and water than the parent prednisolone. It is employed for its anti-inflammatory actions in the treatment of *rheumatic*, *allergic*, and *ocular disorders*, and it is efficacious in all conditions for which glucocorticoids are indicated; it also causes side effects characteristic of glucocorticoids (see *Cortisone Acetate*, page 963). It may be given as a retention enema for ulcerative colitis. Because methylprednisolone possesses only weak mineralocorticoid activity, it is not employed in the management of acute adrenal insufficiency.

Dose—2 to **60 mg** daily; *usual*, **4 mg** 4 times a day.
Dosage Forms—Tablets NF: 2, 4, and 16 mg.

Methylprednisolone Acetate NF

[Methylprednisolone 21-Acetate; Depo-Medrol and Medrol Acetate Veriderm (*Upjohn*)]

Methylprednisolone Acetate contains 97.0–103.0% of $C_{24}H_{32}O_6$ (416.52), calculated on the dried basis.
For the structure of the base, see *Methylprednisolone*.
Preparation—Methylprednisolone Acetate is the 21-acetate compound obtained in the synthesis of *Methylprednisolone* (this page), just prior to the final saponification.

Description—Occurs as a white or practically white, odorless, crystalline powder. When tested by the method for *Class Ia*, page 594, it melts at about 215° with some decomposition.
Solubility—Soluble in dioxane; sparingly soluble in acetone, alcohol, chloroform, and methanol; slightly soluble in ether; insoluble in water.

Uses—The actions of Methylprednisolone Acetate are the same as those of *Methylprednisolone* (this page), into which it is converted in the body. It has no advantage over Methylprednisolone in systemic ther-

apy; thus the acetate is employed principally for local therapy. As a suspension it may be given intra-articularly for rheumatoid arthritis and osteoarthritis and by local injection for bursitis and tendinitis. However, it should be kept in mind that chronic intra-articular glucocorticoids appear to cause occasional destruction of the joint. Methylprednisolone Acetate is applied topically in the treatment of pruritus, allergic dermatoses, atopic dermatitis, contact dermatitis, and seborrheic dermatitis. Methylprednisolone Acetate is employed topically, with or without neomycin; the function of neomycin is to prevent activation of infections as well as to suppress infections secondary to the inflammatory disorder. Systemic effects sometimes result from local administration.

Dose—*Intra-articular* or *intramuscular*, **10** to **80 mg**; *usual*, **40 mg**.
Other Dose Information—Topically, as a 0.25 to 1% cream. For maintenance therapy in chronic conditions, initial doses should be reduced gradually until smallest effective individual dose is established. When treatment is withdrawn after prolonged therapy, dose should be reduced gradually.
Dosage Forms—Cream: 0.25 and 1%; Sterile Suspension NF: 40 mg/ml; 100 and 200 mg/5 ml.
Veterinary Dose—Varies with size of animal patient, severity of condition under treatment, and response to therapy. Intramuscular injection results in prolonged systemic effects: *Horses, usual, intramuscular,* **200 mg**, repeated as necessary; *Dogs, average, weekly,* **20 mg** (2 mg weekly in miniature breeds, 40 mg in medium breeds, 120 mg in extremely large breeds or dogs with severe involvement); *Cats, average, weekly,* **10 mg to 20 mg** weekly.

Methylprednisolone Sodium Succinate NF

[Methylprednisolone 21-(Sodium Succinate); Solu-Medrol (*Upjohn*)]

Methylprednisolone Sodium Succinate contains 97.0–103.0% of $C_{26}H_{33}NaO_8$ (496.54), calculated on the dried basis.
For the structure of the base, see *Methylprednisolone*.

Preparation—*Methylprednisolone* (page 969) is treated with succinic anhydride in pyridine and added to dilute hydrochloric acid to precipitate the hemisuccinate which is neutralized with sodium hydroxide in aqueous acetone solution and the solvent removed by lyophilization.

Description—Occurs as a white, or nearly white, odorless, hygroscopic, amorphous solid.
Solubility—Very soluble in water and alcohol; insoluble in chloroform; very slightly soluble in acetone.

Uses—The actions of Methylprednisolone Sodium Succinate are the same as those of *Methylprednisolone* (this page), into which it is converted in the body. The solubility of the sodium succinate makes the drug advantageous for parenteral administration when a rapid and intense action is desired. It is used only for short-term treatment. Its side effects are those of Methylprednisolone. It has been employed successfully as a retention enema in the local treatment of mild ulcerative colitis; no side effects have been observed.

Dose—*Intravenous* or *intramuscular*, the equivalent of **10** to **125 mg** of methylprednisolone; *usual*, the equivalent of **40 mg** of methylprednisolone every 6 to 24 hours.
Dosage Forms—for Injection NF: 40 and 125 mg.

Paramethasone Acetate NF

[6α-Fluoro-11β,17,21-trihydroxy-16α-methylpregna-1,4-diene-3,20-dione
21-Acetate; Haldrone (*Lilly*)]

Paramethasone Acetate contains 95.0–101.0% of $C_{24}H_{31}FO_6$ (434.51).

Preparation—Paramethasone Acetate may be prepared from the well-known 3-hydroxy-16α-methyl-pregn-5-en-20-one acetate (16α-methylpregnenolone acetate). This starting compound is first subjected to a series of standard steroid reactions to form 6α-fluoro-17,21 - dihydroxy - 16α - methylpregn - 4 - ene - 3,20-dione. This is then hydroxylated at the 11β position by incubation with bovine adrenal glands and then converted to the 21-acetate ester. Dehydrogenation with selenium dioxide in the presence of pyridine completes the synthesis with creation of the 1,2 double bond.

Description—A fluffy, practically white, odorless, crystalline powder. Exposure to light should be avoided. It melts at about 240° with decomposition.

Solubility—Very soluble in alcohol; soluble in acetone, chloroform, and methanol; practically insoluble in water.

Uses—Paramethasone Acetate is a glucocorticoid which is used for its antiallergic and anti-inflammatory drug properties in the treatment of *rheumatoid arthritis* and other *collagen disorders, certain hematologic conditions,* and other conditions in which glucocorticoids are indicated (see *Cortisone Acetate,* page 963). It is 12 times as potent as cortisone, but potency does not confer any particular advantages. The drug lacks mineral corticoid activity; indeed, it promotes the excretion of sodium, chloride and, to a slight extent, potassium.

Paramethasone Acetate causes adverse effects similar to those of other glucocorticoids (see Cortisone Acetate). However, increased appetite and weight gain occur in only about ⅓ of patients. The catabolic effects, such as protein depletion and osteoporosis, are only moderate with low to moderate doses of the drug.

Dose—*Usual, initial,* 4 to **12 mg** daily in 3 or 4 divided doses; *maintenance,* **1** to **8 mg** daily in divided doses.

Dosage Forms—Tablets NF: 1 and 2 mg.

Prednisolone USP

[11β,17,21-Trihydroxypregna-1,4-diene-3,20-dione; Delta-Cortef (*Upjohn*); Hydeltra (*MSD*); Meticortelone (*Schering*); Paracortrol (*Parke-Davis*); Predne-Dome (*Dome*); Prednis (*USV*); Sterane (*Pfizer*); Sterolone (*Rowell*)]

Prednisolone is anhydrous or contains one and one-half molecules of water of hydration. It contains 97.0–102.0% of $C_{21}H_{28}O_5$ (360.45), calculated on the dried basis.

Preparation—Prednisolone may be prepared from hydrocortisone by a microbiologic process utilizing *Corynebacterium simplex* which selectively dehydrogenates hydrocortisone at the 1 and 2 positions.

In practice, a nutrient medium of yeast extract is prepared in a fermentation tank, sterilized, and inoculated with a pure culture of *C. simplex.* The culture is allowed to grow under continuous aeration and agitation. Upon completion of the growth period, hydrocortisone is added directly to the culture mixture. When the reaction is complete, the fermentation broth is extracted with chloroform, and the extract is concentrated to a slurry, chilled, and filtered. The crude solid Prednisolone thus obtained is purified by recrystallizing from acetone.

Description—White to practically white, odorless, crystalline powder. When tested by the method for *Class Ia* (page 594), it melts at about 235° with some decomposition. The specific rotation is +97° to +103°.

Solubility—Very slightly soluble in water; 1 Gm dissolves in about 30 ml of alcohol, 180 ml of chloroform, and about 50 ml of acetone; soluble in methanol and dioxane.

Uses—Prednisolone is similar to Cortisone and Hydrocortisone in its actions and uses (see *Cortisone Acetate*), especially as regards its glucocorticoid properties. It is relatively somewhat weaker as a mineralocorticoid, but sodium retention and potassium depletion can occur. It has a relatively high solubility and hence is suitable for intra-articular injection. Except for its higher solubility, it may be considered exactly equivalent to Prednisone (see *Prednisone*).

Dose—5 to 80 mg daily; *usual, oral, initial,* **5 mg** 2 to 4 times a day; *maintenance,* **5 mg** 1 or more times a day.

Other Dose Information—Topically, as a 0.5% ointment applied 3 or 4 times a day. It is also used as an 0.33% aerosol.

Dosage Forms—Tablets USP: 1, 2.5, and 5 mg.

Veterinary Use—*Parenterally,* for its anti-inflammatory effects in joint disease, dermatitides, burns, allergic manifestations, ocular diseases, and nephritis.

Veterinary Dose—*Intra-articularly, Horses* and *Cattle,* 50 to 100 mg; *Dogs,* 5 to 25 mg; *Cats,* 5 to 25 mg; *intramuscularly, Horses* and *Cattle,* 50 to 100 mg; *Dogs,* 20 to 50 mg; *Cats,* 10 mg; *orally, Dogs,* 20 to 25 mg; *Cats,* 10 mg.

Prednisolone Acetate USP

[Prednisolone 21-Acetate; Meticortelone (*Schering*); Nisolone (*Ascher*); Sterane (*Pfizer*)]

Prednisolone Acetate contains 97.0–102.0% of $C_{23}H_{30}O_6$ (402.49), calculated on the dried basis.

Preparation—This ester may be conveniently prepared from *Prednisolone,* qv, by reaction with acetic anhydride. The crude ester is precipitated upon the addition of water and is then purified by recrystallization from a suitable organic solvent.

Description—White to practically white, odorless, crystalline powder. When tested by the method for Class Ia, it melts at about 235° with some decomposition. The specific rotation is +112° to +119°.

Solubility—Practically insoluble in water; 1 Gm dissolves in about 120 ml of alcohol; slightly soluble in chloroform and acetone.

Uses—The actions and uses of Prednisolone Acetate are the same as those of Prednisolone (see *Prednisolone*), into which it is converted in the body. The acetate is relatively nonirritating to the tissues and hence is preferred for intramuscular or local injection. It may be used particularly in those situations in which oral Prednisolone is not feasible, but there are no contraindications to substitution of the parenteral Prednisolone Acetate for oral prednisolone for any purpose. The side effects and therapeutic limitations of the acetate ester are the same as those of the parent Prednisolone.

Dose—*Intra-articular*, **5** to **50 mg** 1 to 4 times a month; *usual*, **10** to **25 mg** at each site every 2 weeks; *intramuscular*, **5** to **80 mg** daily; *usual*, **5 mg** 4 times a day.

Dosage Forms—Sterile Suspension USP: 125 mg/5 ml.

Prednisolone Sodium Phosphate USP

[Prednisolone 21-(Disodium Phosphate); Hydeltrasol (*MSD*)]

Prednisolone Sodium Phosphate contains 96.0–102.0% of $C_{21}H_{27}Na_2O_8P$ (484.40), calculated on the dried basis.

Preparation—Prednisolone Sodium Phosphate is prepared from *Prednisolone* (page 971) by a method similar to that used for *Dexamethasone Sodium Phosphate* (page 965).

Description—White or slightly yellow, friable granules or powder. Is odorless or has a slight odor. Is slightly hygroscopic.

Solubility—1 Gm dissolves in 4 ml of water and 13 ml of methanol; slightly soluble in alcohol and chloroform; very slightly soluble in acetone and dioxane.

Uses—Prednisolone Sodium Phosphate has the same actions as *Prednisolone* (page 971), into which it is converted in the body. However, because of its high solubility, it has a more rapid onset and shorter duration of action when administered parenterally. It is employed parenterally in emergency situations in which an intense glucocorticoid action is required. Since absorption by the intramuscular route is quite rapid, the intravenous route is essentially never employed, although it may be used. The high solubility of the drug also lends itself well to intrasynovial injection in the treatment of arthritides and bursitides and to local injection for inflammatory cysts and soft tissue inflammations. It is also employed in the local treatment of a number of inflammatory eye diseases and for inflammatory and pruritic dermatoses, bites and burns.

Dose—*Intramuscular* or *intravenous*, **10** to **200 mg** daily; *usual*, *intramuscular* or *intravenous*, **20 mg**. *Topically*, **0.1 ml** of a **0.5**% solution to the conjunctiva 6 to 12 times a day.

Other Dose Information—In addition to the doses given above, it is also used as follows: intrasynovial and infiltration, 5 to 30 mg.

Dosage Forms—Injection USP: 40 mg/2 ml, 100 mg/5 ml; Ophthalmic Solution USP: 0.5%.

Prednisolone Succinate NF

[Prednisolone 21-(Hydrogen Succinate)]

Prednisolone Succinate contains 98.0–102.0% of $C_{25}H_{32}O_8$ (460.53), calculated on the dried basis.

For the structure of the base, see *Prednisolone*.

Preparation—Prednisolone is reacted with succinic anhydride in the presence of pyridine.

Description—A fine, creamy white, practically odorless powder with friable lumps. It melts at about 205° with decomposition.

Solubility—Very slightly soluble in water; freely soluble in alcohol; soluble in acetone.

Uses—Prednisolone Sodium Succinate has all the actions of *Prednisolone* (page 971), to which the sodium succinate is converted in the body. It is a highly soluble compound and hence is used for parenteral administration, especially intravenous, in emergency situations in which a rapid response is important. Such situations include so-called *irreversible shock*, *severe allergic reactions*, *status asthmaticus*, *prevention of transfusion reactions*, and pre- and postoperative management of candidates for bilateral adrenalectomy or hypophysectomy.

Dose—*Usual*, *intravenous*, the equivalent of **25** to **50 mg** of prednisolone given over a 1-minute period, repeated every 3 or 4 hours for 4 doses.

Dosage Forms—for Injection NF (sodium salt): 50 mg.

Prednisone USP

[17,21-Dihydroxypregna-1,4-diene-3,11,20-trione; (*Various Mfgs.*)]

Prednisone contains 97.0–102.0% of $C_{21}H_{26}O_5$ (358.44), calculated on the dried basis.

Preparation—Prednisone may be prepared as described above for *Prednisolone* except that cortisone is used instead of hydrocortisone.

Description—White to practically white, odorless, crystalline powder. When tested by the method for Class 1a, it melts at about 225° with some decomposition. The specific rotation is +167° to +175°.

Solubility—Very slightly soluble in water; 1 Gm dissolves in about 150 ml of alcohol and about 200 ml of chloroform; slightly soluble in methanol and dioxane.

Uses—Prednisone is a simple dehydrogenated derivative of Cortisone and shares its actions, uses and most of its limitations. It has relatively somewhat less of mineralocorticoid activity, but sodium retention and potassium depletion may occur. Its use has been primarily in the therapy of the collagen diseases, such as *rheumatoid arthritis*, *lupus erythematosus*, *periarteritis nodosa*, *dermatomyositis* and *scleroderma* and in the symptomatic management of the allergic states, especially *bronchial asthma*. It is of value in every condition in which systemic cortisone is of value (see *Cortisone Acetate*, page 963), except, perhaps, acute adrenal insufficiency, in which considerable mineralocorticoid activity is desired.

Dose—**5** to **80 mg** daily; *usual*, *initial*, **5 mg** 2 to 4 times a day; *maintenance*, up to **5 mg** 1 or more times a day.

Dosage Forms—Tablets USP: 1, 2.5, and 5 mg.

Veterinary Use—Parenterally for the treatment of ketosis in cattle; for the treatment of arthritides and dermatitides.

Veterinary Dose—*Horses* and *Cattle*, **100** to **400 mg** *intramuscularly*; *Dogs*, **20** to **25 mg** *intramuscularly* for 3 to 5 days followed by **2.5** to **10 mg** *orally* daily.

Triamcinolone USP

[9-Fluoro-11β,16α,17,21-tetrahydroxypregna-1,4-diene-3,20-dione;   Aristocort (*Lederle*); Kenacort (*Squibb*)]

Triamcinolone contains 97.0–102.0% of $C_{21}H_{27}FO_6$ (394.44), calculated on the dried basis.

Preparation—Triamcinolone can be synthesized from *Hydrocortisone Acetate* (page 968) via the 3,20-bisketal by treatment with thionyl chloride, refluxing with potassium hydroxide and acetylation to give 21-acetoxy-4,9,11(16)-pregnatriene-3,20-dione. Oxidation with osmium tetroxide to the 16α,17α-dihydroxy derivative and subsequent insertion of the 9α-fluoro and 11β-hydroxy groups as indicated for *Betamethasone* (page 962), gives a product lacking only a double bond at the 1-position. This latter step is accomplished by incubation with *Nocardia corallina*, followed by saponification of the acetate to yield Triamcinolone. Alternatively, the compound can be made from *Fludrocortisone* by enzymatically inserting the 16α-hydroxyl group and dehydrogenation as above at the 1,2-position.

Description—A fine, white or practically white, crystalline powder having not more than a slight odor. Its polymorphic forms and/or solvates melt between 248° and 250°, 260° and 263°, and 269° and 271°.

Solubility—1 Gm dissolves in about 5000 ml of water, 70 ml of propylene glycol, and less than 20 ml of dimethyl sulfoxide; slightly soluble in alcohol and chloroform.

Uses—Triamcinolone is structurally related to hydrocortisone and shares most of its actions and uses, except usefulness in the treatment of adrenal insufficiency (see *Hydrocortisone*). As a glucocorticoid and antirheumatic it is 7 to 13 times more potent than hydrocortisone. It has been claimed that therapeutic doses of Triamcinolone are nearly devoid of mineralocorticoid and other side effects of hydrocortisone, but the mineralocorticoid actions vary from patient to patient. It appears that the drug may induce naturesis, negative sodium balance with weight loss in most patients (along with headache, dizziness, and fatigue), and sodium retention with weight gain, moon face, etc, in others. Nearly every side effect seen with hydrocortisone has been seen with Triamcinolone, but the relative frequencies are less. It does not increase appetite and thus differs from other glucocorticoids. Glucocorticoid side effects, such as impairment of carbohydrate utilization and negative protein and calcium balance, osteoporosis, peptic ulcer, "buffalo hump," etc, are undesirable results of long-term therapy.

Dose—1 to 32 mg daily; *usual, initial*, **4 mg** 1 to 4 times a day; *maintenance*, **1** to **4 mg** 1 to 2 times a day.

Other Dose Information—For acute bursitis, initially 2 to 16 mg daily with later downward adjustments; for rheumatoid arthritis or various dermatoses, initially 8 to 16 mg daily and 1 to 2 mg daily maintenance; for hemolytic diseases, 12 to 24 mg daily; for nephrotic syndrome, initially 16 to 20 mg daily, with downward adjustments after massive diuresis ensues; for rheumatic fever, initially 16 to 20 mg and 6 to 20 mg maintenance; for disseminated lupus erythematosus, initially 20 to 30 mg daily and 3 to 30 mg daily maintenance; in leukemia and lymphomatous diseases, 16 to 40 mg daily or 1 to 2 mg per Kg of body weight in children with acute leukemia.

Dosage Forms—Tablets USP: 1, 2, 4, 8, and 16 mg.

Veterinary Dose—*Dogs*, **0.25 to 2 mg** daily; *Cats*, **0.25 to 0.5 mg** daily in 2 or more divided doses. For short-term therapy (2 days) of acute conditions, treat at twice the highest recommended dose. Overdosage may cause polyuria, polydipsia, and anorexia; discontinue treatment until these symptoms disappear, then reconstitute dosage at lower level.

Triamcinolone Acetonide USP

[Triamcinolone 16,17-Cyclic Acetal with Acetone;   Aristocort Acetonide (*Lederle*); Aristoderm (*Lederle*); Kenalog (*Squibb*)]

Triamcinolone Acetonide contains 97.0–102.0% of $C_{24}H_{31}FO_6$ (434.51), calculated on the dried basis.

Preparation—*Triamcinolone* (above) is treated with acetone and perchloric acid followed by neutralization and vacuum concentration.

Description—A white to cream-colored, crystalline powder having not more than a slight odor. It melts between 290° and 294°.

Solubility—Practically insoluble in water; very soluble in dehydrated alcohol, chloroform, and methanol; sparingly soluble in acetone and ethyl acetate; slightly soluble in alcohol.

Uses—Triamcinolone acetonide is a simple derivative of *Triamcinolone* (above) and shares its *glucocorticoid* activity. It is intended only for local application, in which circumstances it is as efficacious as *Hydrocortisone* (see page 968) and is more potent. It is used in the treatment of allergic and inflammatory dermatoses, pruritus, arthritis, bursitis, tendonitis, and synovitis. It should not be applied to infected areas of the skin unless antibiotics are concomitantly applied.

Dose—*Usual, intra-articular*, **2.5 to 15 mg**; *intramuscular*, **40 to 80 mg** once a week; *topically*, as a **0.1%** ointment, cream, or lotion, or as an aerosol applied to the affected area 1 to 3 times a day.

Other Dose Information—Intra-articular, 2.5 to 15 mg at intervals of 1 to several weeks.

Dosage Forms—Aerosol NF: 66 mcg/Gm in 50- and 150-Gm containers; Cream USP: 0.025, 0.1, and 0.5%; Ointment USP: 0.025 and 0.1%; Sterile Suspension USP: 50 and 200 mg/5 ml.

Veterinary Dose—In *bovine ketosis, intramuscular,* **2.5 to 10 mg**, repeated after 48 hours if necessary. Concomitant use of dextrose is recommended.

Triamcinolone Diacetate NF

[Triamcinolone 16,21-Diacetate; Aristocort Diacetate (*Lederle*)]

Triamcinolone Diacetate contains 97.0–103.0% of $C_{25}H_{31}FO_8$ (478.52), calculated on the dried basis.

For the structure of the base, see *Triamcinolone*.

Preparation—Triamcinolone Diacetate may be prepared by direct acetylation of triamcinolone.

Among other ways, it has also been prepared from $11\beta,16\alpha,17,21$ - tetrahydroxypregn - 4 - en - 3,20-dione (16α-hydroxyhydrocortisone) through the following sequence of reactions: (a) microbiological oxidation with *Nocardia corallina* or *Corynebacterium simplex* to the pregna-1,4-diene analog, (b) acetylation yielding the $16\alpha,21$-diacetate, (c) selective dehydration involving the 11-hydroxy with thionyl chloride to form the 1,4,9(11)-pregnatriene compound, (d) addition of hypobromous acid to the 9,11 double bond followed by treatment with potassium acetate in ethanol to form the 9,11-epoxy compound, and (e) rupturing the epoxy ring with hydrogen fluoride to introduce the 9α-fluorine.

Description—Fine, white or slightly off-white crystals that have not more than a slight odor and a slight, bitter taste. Prolonged heating above 100° will convert the hydrate to the anhydrous form; otherwise, the compound is reasonably stable to heat, light, and moisture. The hydrated form melts between 145° and 158°; the anhydrous form melts between 170° and 185°.

Solubility—Soluble in alcohol and chloroform; practically insoluble in water.

Uses—Triamcinolone Diacetate has actions and uses identical with those of *Triamcinolone* (see page 973). However, its slight solubility is such that by injection it has a reasonably prompt onset of action yet a duration of action longer than that of more soluble preparations. It is used both for local (intralesional) and systemic treatment for all disorders in which glucocorticoids are indicated (see *Cortisone Acetate*, page 963).

Dose—*Oral* or *intramuscular*, 4 to **30 mg** daily; *usual,* **4 mg** daily.

Dosage Forms—Sterile Suspension NF: 40 mg/ml, 125 and 200 mg/5 ml; Syrup NF: 2 and 5 mg/5 ml.

Other Adrenal Hormones

Adrenal Cortex Extract—An extract of adrenal glands, from domesticated animals used as food for man, containing the cortical steroids essential for the maintenance of life in adrenalectomized animals. Only traces of epinephrine are present. *Uses:* Although active by mouth the results are not dependable; usually administered subcutaneously, intramuscularly, or intravenously. The extract is of value in the treatment of Addison's disease or adrenal insufficiency of other types. *Dose:* Governed by clinical response of the patient; may vary from 500 to 5000 dog units per day (50 dog units = 2.5 rat units = 0.1 mg hydrocortisone), supplemented by sodium chloride.

Adrenal Cortex Injection NF XII [Adrenal Cortex Extract (Injectable) (*Armour; Upjohn*); Eschatin (*Parke-Davis*)] is a sterile solution in alcohol and water for injection containing a mixture of the endocrine principles derived from the cortex of adrenal glands of healthy domestic animals used for food by man. Each ml of Adrenal Cortex Injection exhibits a biological activity equivalent to that of 100 mcg of USP Hydrocortisone Reference Standard. It contains a suitable antibacterial agent. *Description:* A clear, colorless, or faintly colored solution with a pH between 4.0 and 6.0. *Uses:* Aqueous adrenal extract has been used in maintenance therapy of patients with Addison's disease, although it has largely been replaced by combinations of natural, semisynthetic, or synthetic adrenal corticoids. Aqueous adrenal extract is still useful in the therapeutic management of acute adrenal crisis, especially in the absence of preparations of cortisone and hydrocortisone for intravenous use. *Dose:* Usual, *intramuscular* and *intravenous,* 10 ml, repeated as necessary.

Fludrocortisone Acetate [Florinef Acetate (*Squibb*)] is 9α - fluoro - $11\beta,17,21$ - trihydroxypregn - 4 - ene - 3,20 - dione

21-acetate. *Preparation:* One method starts with *Hydrocortisone Acetate* (page 968) which is first dehydrated to the 4,9-diene. The 9α-fluoro and 11β-hydroxy groups are inserted by a method similar to that used for *Betamethasone* (page 962). *Description and Solubility:* A fine, white to pale yellow powder that is odorless and has a slightly bitter taste. It is stable in both light and air. It melts at about 225° with some decomposition. Soluble in alcohol, acetone, and chloroform; slightly soluble in water. *Uses:* The same actions and uses as *Hydrocortisone Acetate* (page 968. It may be effective in slightly lesser doses than hydrocortisone, but untoward effects also appear at slightly lesser doses, so that its therapeutic index is about the same as that of hydrocortisone. Although it may be given orally for maintenance in Addison's disease, it is usually used topically for the treatment of glucocorticoid-responsive dermatoses and ocular inflammations. *Dose:* Topically, as a 0.05 to 0.25% lotion or ointment 2 to 4 times daily; as an ophthalmic solution, 0.1%; oral, 0.1 to 0.3 mg daily.

Fludrocortisone Hemisuccinate [Florinef Hemisuccinate (*Squibb*)] is 9α-fluoro-$11\beta,17,21$-trihydroxypregn-4-ene-3,20-dione 21-(hydrogen succinate). *Preparation:* From *Fludrocortisone Acetate* by hydrolysis of the acetate with a weak base to the alcohol which is then treated with succinic anhydride. *Description and Solubility:* White or nearly white, nearly odorless, crystalline powder. It melts at about 205°. Avoid heat and light. Soluble in water (pH 7) and the lower alcohols. *Uses:* The same actions as *Fludrocortisone Acetate* and other glucocorticoids. However, its uses are generally confined to ophthalmology for the treatment of allergic and inflammatory ocular and periocular disorders. The greater solubility of the hemisuccinate is an advantage over the acetate in the preparations of solutions for topical application to wet surfaces. *Dose:* As the equivalent of fludrocortisone acetate, 0.1% solution; 1 or 2 drops are placed into the conjunctival sac 2 to 4 times a day.

Flumethasone Pivalate [Locorten (*Ciba*)] is $6\alpha,9\alpha$-difluoro-$11\beta,17,21$-trihydroxy-16α-methylpregna-1,4-diene-3,-20-dione 21-pivalate. *Preparation:* The method described for *Betamethasone* (page 962) may be adapted to Flumethasone by incorporating a step employing one of the several known methods for introducing the 6-fluorine. Esterification to the pivalate may be accomplished by treatment with trimethylacetic acid anhydride in the presence of pyridine. *Description and Solubility:* A fine, white, crystalline powder that is odorless. It is stable at 40° and at 50° for 12 weeks. It melts between 263° and 272°. Slightly soluble in alcohol and methanol; very slightly soluble in water, chloroform, and methylene dichloride; insoluble in carbon tetrachloride and isooctane. *Uses:* A glucocorticoid which, is about 800 times more potent than cortisone acetate in local anti-inflammatory activity. When applied locally, there are only weak systemic side effects, owing to metabolic destruction of absorbed circulating drug. It is used primarily as an anti-inflammatory agent for the treatment of chronic dermatologic disorders in dogs. It is marketed (in a veterinary form) in a mixture which also contains the antimicrobial agent, *Iodochlorhydroxyquin* (page 1252). *Dose:* Locally, as a 0.02% cream, 2 to 4 times a day. No more than 10% of the body surface of a pregnant dog should be medicated. The commercial preparation also contains 3% iodochlorhydroxyquin.

Hydrocortamate Hydrochloride [Ulcort (*Ulmer*)] is hydrocortisone 21-(diethylamino)acetate hydrochloride ($C_{27}H_{41}NO_6 \cdot HCl$). *Description and Solubility:* A white or creamy white, crystalline powder; it melts between 213° and 214°. Very soluble in water, but gradually hydrolyzes on standing. *Uses:* Hydrocortamate Hydrochloride is similar to the hormone *Hydrocortisone Acetate* (page 968) in its glucocorticoid actions and uses. However, the aminoacetate moiety affects its absorption and distribution, and it appears to be especially suited to topical application. Topically, it is about twice as potent as hydrocortisone but no more efficacious. However, systemic effects from topical application are uncommon. It is used in the treatment of acute or chronic dermatoses which have an inflammatory or allergic basis. *Dose:* Topically, as a 0.5% ointment.

Hydrocortisone Cypionate [Cortef Fluid (*Upjohn*)] is

the 21-cyclopentanepropionate ester of hydrocortisone. *Description and Solubility:* A white, tasteless, odorless solid which melts between 177° and 183°. Insoluble in water; soluble in ether, glycols, and vegetable oils; freely soluble in chloroform; sparingly soluble in alcohol. *Uses:* The same actions, molecular potency, and uses as *Hydrocortisone* (page 968). However, it is absorbed more slowly from the gastrointestinal tract and also has a more pleasant taste. *Dose:* As an equivalent of hydrocortisone, oral, 20 to 300 mg daily in 2 or 3 divided doses; usual, 40 to 60 mg.

Prednisolone Tebutate [Prednisolone *tert*-Butylacetate; Hydeltra T.B.A. (*MSD*)] is prednisolone 21-(3,3-dimethylbutyrate). *Preparation:* From *Prednisolone* (page 971) by esterification of the 21-hydroxyl group with 3,3-dimethylbutyryl chloride. *Description and Solubility:* A white to slightly yellow powder that is odorless or has not more than a moderate, characteristic odor, and is almost tasteless. It is relatively stable in light; the monohydrate is relatively stable in air, but the dried material is hygroscopic and absorbs moisture until it equilibrates at the monohydrate. It melts between 240° and 250°. Freely soluble in dioxane; soluble in chloroform; sparingly soluble in alcohol and methanol; slightly soluble in ether; insoluble in water. *Uses:* The same actions and potential uses as *Prednisolone* or *Prednisolone Acetate.* However, its use is mostly confined to local injection or infiltration therapy of inflammatory disorders of the joints, tendons, and bursae. Its very slight solubility results in a slow onset of action (24 to 48 hours) and long duration of action (2 to 3 weeks) after intra-articular and soft tissue injection. It is slightly more potent than hydrocortisone acetate. Temporary local discomfort may follow the injection. It must be kept in mind that chronic intra-articular glucocorticoids probably cause joint destruction in some instances. *Dose: Intra-articular* or *soft tissue injection* only, 4 to 30 mg, depending on the site and the seriousness of the disorder.

Nonsteroid Antirheumatic and Anti-Inflammatory Drugs

Several drugs not obviously related to the adrenocortical steroid suppress certain features of the rheumatic and inflammatory processes. Chief among these drugs is aspirin, which is frequently the agent of choice for the initial treatment of rheumatic fever. Certain other analgesics, such as aminopyrine and phenylbutazone also possess antirheumatic and anti-inflammatory properties, but their use involves more risk than does that of acetylsalicylic acid or adrenal steroids. Gold compounds are still employed in the treatment of arthritis, but, used improperly, their toxicity makes their use hazardous; nevertheless some authorities place the gold compounds ahead of adrenal steroids in efficacy. Colloidal gold is of no value in the treatment of rheumatoid arthritis, and the use of such suspensions should be discouraged. Because certain prominent authorities have considered that the inflammatory diseases were immune or autoimmune disorders, certain antineoplastics, which are also immunosuppressives, have been tried as antirheumatic drugs. Antimalarial immunosuppressives are also being used in the management of rheumatic disorders. The mechanism of antirheumatic action of most of the non-steroid drugs is unknown, and the extent of adrenocortical involvement remains to be determined. Although none of the several drugs listed below is a steroid hormone analog, they are listed in this section because the rheumatic diseases and their treatment are so closely allied to adrenocortical function.

Amodiaquine—see page 1245.

Aspirin—see page 1134.

Aurothioglucose USP

[(1-Thio-D-glucopyranosato)gold; Gold Thioglucose; Solganal (*Schering*)]

Aurothioglucose contains 95.0–105.0% of C₆H₁₁AuO₅S (392.18), calculated on the dried basis. It is stabilized by the addition of not more than 5.0% of sodium acetate.

Preparation—It may be prepared by refluxing an aqueous solution of thioglucose with gold tribromide in the presence of sulfur dioxide. The compound is thus precipitated, and is purified by dissolving in water after which it is reprecipitated by the addition of alcohol.

Description—A yellow powder, odorless or nearly so, and stable in air. The pH of a 1 in 100 solution is about 6.3. Aqueous solutions are unstable on long standing.

Solubility—Freely soluble in water; practically insoluble in acetone, alcohol, chloroform, and ether.

Uses—Aurothioglucose is an *antirheumatic* used for the treatment of active *rheumatoid arthritis* and non-disseminated *lupus erythematosus.* The adrenal steroids once largely displaced gold compounds from the therapeutic armamentarium, but recognition of the dangers of steroid therapy has renewed interest in gold. Some authorities consider gold compounds the more efficacious if used properly. The best therapy is based upon the daily excretion rate of gold in the individual patient. The aim is to build up slowly the body burden of gold to the point of obvious improvement of the condition or of minimal toxicity then maintain with doses that just balance the amount of gold excreted. In the absence of determinations of urinary gold to guide maintenance therapy, it is best to increase the weekly dosage in small steps so that more than twelve weeks are required to reach a maximum dose. Maintenance is then achieved by lengthening the interval between doses to three or four weeks. Pruritus is generally the first sign of toxicity and calls for a slight reduction in dose. Other toxic manifestations are dermatitis, stomatitis, gastritis, colitis, rarely blood dyscrasias, hepatitis and neuritis.

Dose—*Intramuscular,* 10 to 50 mg per week; *usual, initial,* 10 mg, increased to 25 mg and then to 50 mg per week to a total dose of 750 mg, then in decreasing amounts.

Other Dose Information—The dose is given until signs of improvement or toxicity appear (see above). Maintenance doses vary from 5 to 50 mg every 2 to 4 weeks.

Dosage Forms—Injection USP: 50 and 100 mg/ml.

Azathioprine—see page 1164.

Bismuth Sodium Triglycollamate—see page 1254.

Chloroquine Phosphate—see page 1245.

Corticotropin—see page 957.

Cyclophosphamide—see page 1165.

Gold Sodium Thiomalate USP

[(Disodium Mercaptosuccinato)gold; (1,2-Dicarboxyethyl)thio] gold Disodium Salt; Auri Sodii Thiomalas; Sodium Aurothiomalate; Myochrysine (*MSD*)]

$$\text{AuS—CHCH}_2\text{COONa} \quad \cdot \text{H}_2\text{O}$$
$$\text{|}$$
$$\text{COONa}$$

Gold Sodium Thiomalate contains 96.0–101.5% of $C_4H_3AuNa_2O_4S.H_2O$ (408.09).

Preparation—Sodium thiomalate is reacted with gold chloride. Details are provided in US Pat. 1,994,-213.

Description—A white to yellowish white, odorless, fine powder. It is affected by light. The pH of a 1 in 10 solution is between 5.8 and 6.5.

Solubility—Very soluble in water; insoluble in alcohol, ether, and most organic solvents.

Uses—Gold Sodium Thiomalate is an *antirheumatic* with the same uses and toxicity as *Aurothioglucose* (page 975). It is given intramuscularly only.

Dose—*Intramuscular*, **10** to **50 mg** per week; *usual*, *initial*, **10 mg**, increasing to **25 mg** and then to **50 mg** per week to a total dose of **750 mg**, then in decreasing amounts.

Other Dose Information—Note: The official dose differs slightly from that of *Aurothioglucose* (*qv*), but it should be the same. It is given until signs of improvement or toxicity appear. Maintenance doses vary from 5 to 50 mg every 2 to 4 weeks.

Dosage Forms—Injection USP: 10, 25, 50, and 100 mg/ml, 500 mg/10 ml.

Gold Sodium Thiosulfate NF XII

[Auri Sodii Thiosulfas; Aurocidin; Aurous Sodium Thiosulfate; Crisalbine; Sanocrysin; Sodium Aurothiosulfate]

Gold Sodium Thiosulfate contains 97.9–100.6% of $Na_3Au(S_2O_3)_2.2H_2O$ (526.22).

Preparation—It may be prepared by treating aurous iodide [AuI], obtained by adding potassium iodide solution to a solution of auric chloride, with an aqueous solution of sodium thiosulfate in the proportion of two moles of the latter to one mole of the former, then adding alcohol. Gold Sodium Thiosulfate, being only slightly soluble in alcohol, slowly precipitates in brilliant white crystals.

Description—White, needle-like or prismatic, small, glistening crystals. It slowly darkens on exposure to light. Its solution (1 in 20) is neutral or alkaline to litmus.

Solubility—1 Gm of the salt dissolves in about 2 ml of water; insoluble in alcohol and most other organic solvents.

Uses—Gold Sodium Thiosulfate has the same actions, uses, and toxicity as *Aurothioglucose* (page 975). The thiosulfate has the reputation of being more toxic than Aurothioglucose or Gold Sodium Thiomalate; in experimental animals it is more toxic, but no statistically acceptable clinical proof has been achieved. The drug is often given by the intravenous route, which may elicit immediate toxic responses not observed after intramuscular injection. It is best given intramuscularly, although it may be given intravenously.

Note—See the dosage schedule given for *Aurothioglucose*, page 975.

Hydroxychloroquine Sulfate—see page 1246.

Indomethacin—see page 1136.

Mefenamic Acid—see page 1136.

Oxyphenbutazone—see page 1137.

Phenylbutazone—see page 1138.

Quinacrine—see page 1247.

Salicylamide—see page 1139.

Sodium Salicylate—see page 1139.

Sodium Suramin—see page 1254.

Other Nonsteroid Antirheumatic and Anti-Inflammatory Drugs

Aurothioglycanide [Aurothioglycolanilide; Aurothioglycolic Acid Anilide; Lauron (*Endo*)] is 2-(auromercapto)-acetanilide. *Description and Solubility:* A grayish yellow powder which melts between 238° and 241°. Insoluble in water, acids, bases, ether, and chloroform. *Uses:* In the same manner as other aurothio compounds in the treatment of *rheumatoid arthritis* and *nondisseminated lupus erythematosus* (see *Aurothioglucose*, page 975). Because of its insolubility, it is absorbed more slowly from the site of injection than the official gold compounds. Claims that it is less toxic have not been validated by clinical experience; it is the body burden of gold and not the rate of absorption that relates to toxicity. Aurothioglycanide should be employed with the same precautions attendant upon gold therapy of any kind. *Dose: Intramuscular.* The gold content of the drug is nearly the same as that of aurothioglucose; for a dosage schedule see *Aurothioglucose*.

The Pancreatic Hormones

The larger portion of the pancreas consists of glandular tissue which secretes digestive enzymes, but there are also isolated groups of cells, called *Islets of Langerhans*, the beta cells of which produce an internal secretion known as *insulin* and the alpha cells a factor known as *glucagon*.

Insulin—Insulin is the catalyst which facilitates the processes by which the various tissues in all parts of the body may use glucose, either as a fuel for the liberation of energy, or as a store, converted to the less soluble form known as glycogen or to the more permanent deposit in the form of fat. When the supply of insulin is inadequate glucose accumulates rapidly in the body fluids, and as the blood glucose concentration increases beyond a certain point it is excreted by the kidneys. This causes a continual waste of this essential nutrient,

and at the same time even more serious consequences related to the reduced ability to use glucose, producing a depression of the functions of the brain, muscle, and many other tissues. In extreme cases due to the faulty metabolism of fats and carbohydrates a condition of acidosis occurs, and if this extreme condition is not treated promptly and adequately, death will ensue after the individual has become comatose.

This disease condition is known as *diabetes mellitus*, the familiar "sugar diabetes." It is probable that the disease may be produced by conditions other than a simple lack of insulin; but, even so, administration of adequate doses of insulin will save life, improving health as long as suitable insulin treatment is maintained. Conversely, with too much insulin, serious or dangerous symptoms from hypoglycemia may result, causing sweating, hunger, incoherence, convulsions, coma, and death. Glucose administration relieves the symptoms of overdosage.

Insulin is obtained by extraction of beef, sheep, swine, or whale pancreas and was one of the first proteins obtained in crystalline form. Insulin (monomer) is a polypeptide of molecular weight 6000; it consists of two peptide chains containing 21 and 30 amino acids, respectively, the two chains being held together by disulfide (—S—S—) bonds of cystine. In aqueous solution, the insulin monomer polymerizes to form macromolecules of molecular weight 12,000 or 36,000, depending on pH and concentration. The isoelectric point of insulin is 5.3. Preparations of crystalline insulin invariably contain about 0.5% zinc, the function of which is unknown.

The arrangement of the amino acids in each of the two chains of insulin has been determined for insulins from several species of animals, including man.* Although the species differences are relatively small, involving mainly substitutions among amino acids 8–10 of the shorter (A) chain, antibodies to insulin can be prepared in some animals.

Successful syntheses of both chains of bovine insulin have been achieved. When synthetic A chain was combined with synthetic B chain, a product possessing some insulin activity was obtained.

As indicated below, several types of insulin preparations are currently in use. The differences between them are principally differences in solubility, and consequently in speed of onset and duration of action.

Crystalline Zinc Insulin—By the addition of appropriate amounts of zinc salts, insulin may be crystallized. This achieves a superior degree of purification, which is of advantage when treating diabetics who demonstrate an allergic sensitivity to Insulin Injection, the earlier and more commonly used, but less highly purified type. The speed and duration of action of these two types of insulin are so nearly identical that they may be used interchangeably. The Reference Standard of the USP is made up of dried Zinc-Insulin Crystals, and is defined as containing 22 USP Units per milligram. Either form will meet USP specifications. The materials prepared from crystals may be labeled as USP Insulin Injection.

Distinguishing Characteristics—Federal Food and Drug regulations require that the labels of various insulin preparations shall have distinctive colors.

Glucagon (*Hyperglycemic Factor*)—In addition to insulin, the pancreas also produces a substance which exerts an effect upon blood sugar opposite to that of insulin. This *hyperglycemic factor*, or glucagon is produced by the alpha cells of the Islets of Langerhans. Contamination of insulin preparations by glucagon is manifested by a transitory *increase* in blood glucose following insulin injection. Some insulins, for example the Danish *Novo* insulins, do not contain this *hyperglycemic factor* (HGF).

Glucagon is a peptide of molecular weight 3464 and consists of a single chain of 29 amino acid residues in the following sequence:

NH₂
|
His-Ser-Glu-Gly-Thr-Phe-Thr-Ser-Asp-Tyr-
  NH₂
  |
Ser-Lys-Tyr-Leu-Asp-Ser-Arg-Arg-Ala-Glu-
  NH₂   NH₂
  | |
Asp-Phe-Val-Glu-Tyr-Leu-Met-Asp-Thr

Glucagon exerts its hyperglycemic effect by stimulating the conversion of liver glycogen to glucose. It also increases the rate of degradation of liver protein. Although its true physiological significance is in dispute, it has found some utility as a diagnostic aid in glycogen storage disease and in the treatment of insulin-induced hypoglycemia.

Glucagon USP

[*Lilly*]

Glucagon is a polypeptide occurring in the pancreas glands of domestic mammals used for food by man, which has the property of increasing the blood glucose concentration.

It is employed as the hydrochloride.

Description—Fine, white to off-white, crystalline powder. Is practically odorless and tasteless.

Solubility—Soluble in dilute alkali and acid solutions; insoluble in most organic solvents.

Uses—Glucagon converts liver phosphorylase B to the active phosphorylase A, thereby promoting the breakdown of liver glycogen. The end result is the release of glucose and an elevation of blood glucose. After parenteral injection the response is quite prompt. The action lasts but 45 to 90 minutes. Glucagon is used primarily to terminate hypoglycemic coma, such as may occur from an overdose of insulin. It is dubious that it offers any compelling advantage over intravenous dextrose for this purpose. Its value in idiopathic hypoglycemia, islet cell carcinoma, and glycogen storage disease has not yet been fully determined. Side effects include nausea and vomiting and hypotension.

Dose—*Parenteral*, 0.5 to 1 USP Glucagon Unit, repeated as necessary; *usual*, 0.5 Unit, repeated in 20 minutes if necessary.

Dosage Forms—for Injection USP: 1 and 10 USP Glucagon Units.

Insulin Injection USP

[Insulin; Insulin Hydrochloride; Iletin (*Lilly*)]

Insulin Injection is a sterile, acidified solution of the active principle of the pancreas which affects the metabolism of glucose. It has a potency of 95.0–105.0% of the potency stated on the label, expressed in USP Insulin Units, the potency being 40, 80, 100, or 500 USP Insulin Units in each ml.

Description—When containing in each ml not more than 100 USP Units it is a colorless or almost colorless liquid. That containing 500 Units may be straw-colored. It is substantially free from turbidity and from insoluble matter. It contains from 0.1 to 0.25% (*w/v*) of either phenol or cresol and 1.4 to 1.8% (*w/v*) of glycerin. The pH of Insulin Injection is between 2.5 and 3.5 when determined potentiometrically.

Uses—The specific therapeutic use of insulin is in the treatment of *diabetes mellitus*. Dosage varies with the individual case. Insulin must be given by hypodermic injection, the hormone being destroyed in the gastrointestinal tract. Diabetic individuals are trained to inject themselves. For this purpose a special syringe measuring the dosage of insulin directly in units is employed. The number of injections required daily and the strength of solution employed is determined by the

---

* The determination of the structure of beef insulin by F. Sanger in 1954 was the first example of the elucidation of the complete structure of a protein.

severity of the diabetes. The amount of sugar in the urine is a rough index of the severity of the diabetes and may be used to approximate the amount of insulin necessary for treatment.

The limited ability of the cells of the diabetic individual to metabolize glucose and the consequent increase in fat utilization leads to the accumulation in the blood of many of the end products of the oxidation of fatty acids. These are organic acids which can combine with fixed base. As a result, if diabetes remains untreated, severe acidosis leading to *diabetic coma* develops, which demands heroic treatment with insulin.

Insulin is rapidly absorbed and exerts its maximum action within three hours. Therefore in severe diabetes, injections must be spaced throughout the day, usually being given before meals. During the night, when no insulin is available, the blood sugar rises and is usually at its highest point before the morning dose. This erratic behavior on the level of blood sugar can be more adequately controlled by the use of preparations of insulin which are absorbed more slowly and thus can exert a continuous even action over a period as long as 24 hours. Globin zinc insulin, isophane insulin, protamine zinc insulin and crystalline zinc insulin are such preparations. The isoelectric point of globin zinc insulin, isophane insulin, or protamine zinc insulin is near pH 7.3. This means that at the pH of body fluids they are very insoluble. Crystalline zinc insulin has a higher solubility than the protein complexes but goes into solution at a very slow rate. Protamine zinc insulin is injected as a suspension. It only goes into solution slowly and this limits the rate of absorption. By the use of protamine zinc insulin the number of injections required to control the level of blood sugar can often be reduced to one daily. What is more important, wide fluctuations in the level of blood sugar are less likely to occur. In certain cases combinations of protamine zinc insulin and regular insulin may be employed.

The time interval from a hypodermic injection of insulin until its action can be demonstrated is about one hour, but it is longer with the protein–insulin complexes. The duration of action is relatively short and is not linearly proportional to the size of the dose, but is a simple function of the logarithm of the dose; ie, insulin is inactivated in the body at a rate proportional to the amount in the body at the time; if 1 unit will last four hours, 10 units will last 8 hours. Since the usual duration is from 4 to 8 hours, the insulin injection usually is planned in 2 to 4 daily doses for proper control of severe diabetes. This is ordinarily timed a few minutes before the ingestion of food, in order to avoid an unpleasant reduction of the blood glucose level.

In the event that too much insulin is given to a diabetic patient, symptoms of hypoglycemia ensue. These chiefly affect the nervous system and, if severe, a hypoglycemic convulsion may occur. Specific treatment of this condition is a soluble carbohydrate or fruit juice, or glucagon. The diabetic patient often carries some source of sugar to prevent the occurrence of hypoglycemic reactions.

Insulin is occasionally employed in nondiabetic cases. For example, it has been used to produce convulsive shock seizures for the treatment of certain psychiatric cases. It is also used in the treatment of underweight individuals, the purpose being to stimulate the appetite by lowering the level of blood sugar. Such uses of insulin are rare, however. More recently, there have been claims that topical insulin is efficacious in the treatment of decubitous ulcers, but the true value of such therapy remains to be determined.

Dose— 5 to 20 USP Units daily; *intravenous*, 30 to 60 Units, followed by 20 Units at 30-minute intervals as necessary; *subcutaneous*, 5 to 40 USP Units 1 to 3 times daily.

Other Dose Information—There is no standard dosage for insulin; each case must be studied individually. The hormone is administered by injection into the loose subcutaneous tissue of the body; the short-acting insulins are injected 30 minutes before meals. In practice, the amount of insulin given is based upon the amount of dextrose the patient utilizes from his diet.

In cases of coma or severe acidosis an initial dose of 30 to 60 units may be given (in coma one-half the amount intravenously and one-half subcutaneously) followed at ½-hour intervals by doses of 20 units or more subcutaneously. Some physicians administer 1 Gm of dextrose for each unit of insulin used. The patient should never become hypoglycemic. The urine should be examined hourly for dextrose. If it becomes sugar-free, more dextrose must be given. More than 150 units of insulin in 12 hours occasionally is needed. Young children with diabetes of recent onset usually require smaller doses and seldom more than 80 units in the first 12 hours.

Dosage of insulin always should be expressed in units rather than in cubic centimeters or minims. The volume of a dose of insulin containing a certain number of units will vary with the strength of the solution employed. It is advisable to keep the volume per injection at 0.25 to 0.75 cc, choosing the strength of insulin which will give the required number of units within this range.

Veterinary Dose—*Horses* and *Cattle*, **100 to 250 Units**; *Dogs*, **1 to 3 Units** per **Kg** of body weight daily in divided doses. These dosages are usually modified according to need.

Globin Zinc Insulin Injection USP

[Injectio Zinco Insulini Globini; Globin Insulin with Zinc; Globin Zinc Insulin (*Burroughs-Wellcome; Squibb*)]

Globin Zinc Insulin Injection is a sterile solution of insulin modified by the addition of zinc chloride and globin. The globin used is obtained from globin hydrochloride prepared from beef blood. The globin used and the Globin Zinc Insulin Injection conform to the regulations of the federal Food and Drug Administration concerning certification of drugs composed wholly or partly of insulin.

In the preparation of Globin Zinc Insulin Injection, the amount of insulin used is sufficient to provide either 40 or 80 USP Insulin Units for each ml of the Injection.

Description—An almost colorless liquid, substantially free from turbidity and insoluble matter. It contains from 1.3 to 1.7% (w/v) of glycerin and either from 0.15 to 0.20% (w/v) of cresol or from 0.20 to 0.26% (w/v) of phenol. It contains from 0.25 to 0.35 mg of zinc and from 3.6 to 4.0 mg of globin (calculated as 6.0 times the nitrogen content of the globin) for each 100 USP Insulin Units. The pH is 3.4 to 3.8, determined potentiometrically.

Uses—See *Insulin Injection*, page 977. Globin Zinc Insulin Injection is administered by injection usually into the loose subcutaneous tissue. *It is never administered intravenously.* Globin Zinc Insulin is intermediate in its action both with respect to onset time and duration; its action begins in 1 to 2 hours, reaches a peak in 8 to 16 hours, and lasts 18 to 24 hours.

Dose—*Subcutaneous*, 10 to 80 USP Units daily; *usual*, according to the needs of the patient.

Veterinary Dose—The dose is to be determined by the veterinarian in accordance with the needs of the patient.

Note—*Globin Zinc Insulin Injection differs in its action from that of other insulin injections in the USP in both time of onset and duration.*

Isophane Insulin Suspension USP

[Isophane Insulin; Isophane Insulin Injection; NPH Insulin (*Squibb*); NPH Iletin (*Lilly*)]

Isophane Insulin Suspension is a sterile suspension of zinc-insulin crystals and protamine in buffered water for injection, combined in a manner such that the solid phase of the suspension consists of crystals composed of insulin, protamine, and zinc. The protamine is prepared from the sperm or from the mature testes of fish belonging to the genus *Oncorhynchus* Suckley, or *Salmo* Linné (Fam. *Salmonidæ*), and conforms to the regulations of the federal Food and Drug Administration concerning certification of drugs composed wholly or partly of insulin.

Each ml of Isophane Insulin Suspension is prepared from sufficient insulin to provide either 40 or 80 USP Insulin Units of insulin activity.

Description—A white suspension of rod-shaped crystals approximately 30μ in length and free from large aggregates of crystals following moderate agitation. Isophane Insulin Suspension contains either (1) 1.4 to 1.8% (w/v) of glycerin, 0.15 to 0.17% (w/v) of metacresol, and 0.06 to 0.07% (w/v) of phenol, or (2) 0.42 to 0.45% (w/v) of sodium chloride, 0.7 to 0.9% (w/v) of glycerin, and 0.18 to 0.22% (w/v) of metacresol.

Isophane Insulin Suspension contains 0.15 to 0.25% (w/v) of dibasic sodium phosphate. It contains also 0.016 to 0.04 mg of zinc and 0.3 to 0.6 mg of protamine for each 100 USP Insulin Units. When examined microscopically, the insoluble matter in the Suspension is crystalline, and contains not more than traces of amorphous material. The pH is between 7.1 and 7.4, determined potentiometrically.

Uses—See *Insulin Injection*. The action of Isophane Insulin Suspension begins in 1 to 2 hours, reaches a peak in 10 to 20 hours, and lasts 28 to 30 hours. *It is never given intravenously.*

Dose—*Subcutaneous*, 10 to 80 USP Units daily; *usual*, according to the needs of the patient.

Note—*Isophane Insulin Suspension differs in it actions from that of other insulin injections in the USP in both time of onset and duration. To secure accuracy of dosage, the preparation must be brought into uniform suspension by careful shaking before use.*

Insulin Zinc Suspension USP

[Lente Insulin; Lente Iletin (*Lilly*)]

Insulin Zinc Suspension is a sterile suspension of insulin in buffered water for injection, modified by the addition of zinc chloride in a manner such that the solid phase of the suspension consists of a mixture of crystalline and amorphous insulin in a ratio of approximately 7 parts of crystals to 3 parts of amorphous material.

Each ml of Insulin Zinc suspension is prepared from sufficient insulin to provide either 40 or 80 USP Insulin Units of insulin activity.

Description—An almost colorless suspension of a mixture of characteristic crystals predominantly 10 to 40 microns in maximum dimension and many particles which have no uniform shape and do not exceed 2 microns in maximum dimension. It contains 0.15 to 0.17% (w/v) of sodium acetate, 0.65 to 0.75% (w/v) of sodium chloride, and 0.09 to 0.11% (w/v) of methylparaben. It contains also, for each 100 USP Insulin Units, 0.20 to 0.25 mg of zinc of which 40 to 65% is in the supernatant liquid. The pH range is between 7.1 and 7.5.

Uses—"Amorphous" zinc insulin has a duration of action of 12 to 16 hours and crystalline zinc insulin a duration of longer than 36 hours, owing to the slowness with which the larger crystals dissolve. An appropriate dose of the 3 : 7 mixture used in Insulin Zinc Suspension has an intermediate duration of action which is very close to that of Isophane Insulin Suspension (28 to 30 hours), with which preparation it may be used interchangeably. The advantage of Zinc Insulin Suspension is its freedom from foreign proteins, such as globin or protamine, to which certain patients are sensitive.

Dose—*Subcutaneous*, 10 to 80 USP Units daily; *usual*, according to the needs of the patient.

Other Dose Information—10 units daily with adjustments for newly developed moderate cases or 80% of an established dose of unmodified insulin (eg, *Insulin Injection*) or protamine zinc insulin for cases of longer standing.

Veterinary Dose—For treatment of *diabetes mellitus* in *dogs*, *initially* 4 units, increased daily by 2 units until laboratory findings and clinical response indicate satisfactory dose has been reached (usual daily effective dose 10 to 25 units).

Extended Insulin Zinc Suspension USP

[Ultra-Lente Iletin (*Lilly*)]

Extended Insulin Zinc Suspension is a sterile suspension of insulin in buffered water for injection, modified by the addition of zinc chloride in a manner such that the solid phase of the suspension is crystalline.

In its preparation, sufficient insulin is used to provide either 40 or 80 USP Insulin Units for each ml of the suspension.

Description—Almost colorless suspension of a mixture of characteristic crystals the maximum dimension of which is predominantly 10–40 μ. The preparation contains, for each 100 USP Units of Insulin, 0.20–0.25 mg of zinc (of which 40–65% is in the supernatant liquid), and not more than 0.70 mg of nitrogen. The preparation contains also 0.15–0.17% (w/v) of sodium acetate, 0.65–0.75% (w/v) of sodium chloride, and 0.09–0.11% (w/v) of methylparaben.

Uses—The crystals in Extended Insulin Zinc Suspension are of sufficient size to have a slow rate of dissolution. Consequently, the duration of action is usually in excess of 36 hours, which is slightly longer than that of *Protamine Zinc Insulin*. Since Extended Insulin Zinc Suspension is free of protamine and other foreign proteins, the incidence of allergic reactions is minimized. The dose needs to be individualized to the patient on the basis of a study of responses of blood and urine glucose to trial doses of the drug. This suspension is administered by deep subcutaneous injection.

Dose—*Subcutaneous*, 10 to 80 USP Units daily; *usual*, according to the needs of the patient.

Prompt Insulin Zinc Suspension USP

[Semi-Lente Iletin (*Lilly*)]

Prompt Insulin Zinc Suspension is a sterile suspension of insulin in buffered water for injection, modified by the addition of zinc chloride in a manner such that the solid phase of the suspension is amorphous.

In its preparation, sufficient insulin is used to provide either 40 or 80 USP Insulin Units for each ml of the Suspension.

Description—Almost colorless suspension of particles that have no uniform shape and the maximum dimension of of which does not exceed 2μ. The preparation contains, for each 100 USP Units of Insulin, 0.20–0.25 mg of zinc (of which 40–65% is in the supernatant liquid), and not more than 0.70 mg of nitrogen. The preparation contains also 0.15–0.17% (w/v) of sodium acetate, 0.65–0.75% (w/v) of sodium chloride, and 0.09–0.11% (w/v) of methylparaben.

Uses—The zinc insulin in Prompt Insulin Zinc Suspension is a mixture of amorphous and extremely fine crystalline materials. Consequently, the rate of dissolution is nearly maximal for the substance. Even so, the rate is slow enough that the suspension has a duration of action (12 to 16 hours) comparable to that of *Globin Zinc Insulin*. Because Prompt Zinc Insulin Suspension is essentially free of foreign proteins, the incidence of allergic reactions is extremely low. The suspension is administered by deep subcutaneous injection.

Dose—*Subcutaneous*, **10 to 80 USP Units** daily; *usual*, according to the needs of the patient.

Protamine Zinc Insulin Suspension USP

[Injectio Zinco Insulini Protaminati; Protamine Zinc Insulin; Protamine Zinc Insulin Injection (*Squibb*); Protamine Zinc and Iletin (*Lilly*)]

Protamine Zinc Insulin Suspension is a sterile suspension of insulin in buffered water for injection, modified by the addition of zinc chloride and protamine. The protamine is prepared from the sperm or from the mature testes of fish belonging to the genus *Oncorhynchus* Suckley, or *Salmo* Linné (Fam. *Salmonidæ*), and conforms to the regulations of the federal Food and Drug Administration concerning certification of drugs composed wholly or partly of insulin.

In the preparation of Protamine Zinc Insulin Suspension, the amount of insulin used is sufficient to provide either 40 or 80 USP Insulin Units for each ml of the Suspension.

Description—A white, or almost white, suspension, free from large particles following moderate agitation. It must contain from 1.4 to 1.8% (w/v) of glycerin, and either from 0.18 to 0.22% (w/v) of cresol or from 0.22 to 0.28% (w/v) of phenol. It contains from 0.15 to 0.25% (w/v) of Na_2HPO_4. It must contain from 0.20 to 0.25 mg of zinc and from 1.0 to 1.5 mg of protamine for each 100 USP Insulin Units. The pH, determined potentiometrically, is between 7.1 and 7.4.

Uses—Because of its slower onset of action (4 to 6 hours) this insulin need not be given with any definite time relation to food intake, and it must not be depended upon when very prompt action is needed, as in diabetic acidosis and coma. Also, due to the prolonged action (24 to 36 hours), the protamine zinc insulin need not be given more often than once daily, but this should be done at a fairly uniform, scheduled time. Since each dose continues to demonstrate activity for three of four days, the dose should be adjusted at intervals of not less than 3 days.

Protamine zinc-insulin and the more rapidly acting insulin have been mixed in various proportions and in different ways. Such variations produce mixtures that give intermediate patterns of speed and duration of physiological activity. This method, however, makes it possible through the long-acting insulin to take care of the sugar requirements during the night, while short-acting insulin causes full utilization of food taken during the day. It thus permits one to avoid large doses of the long-acting insulin such as might cause hypoglycemia in the early morning hours. However, the need to individualize the insulin schedule makes commercial fixed mixtures impractical and places the responsibility for the preparation in the hands of the physician. Except for the inconvenience of an extra injection, the short-acting insulin can just as well be administered by separate injection.

Protamine Zinc Insulin Suspension is administered by injection usually into the loose subcutaneous tissue. It is never administered intravenously.

Dose—*Subcutaneous*, **10 to 80 USP Units** daily; *usual*, according to the needs of the patient.

Veterinary Dose—Should be determined by the veterinarian depending on the need of the individual patient.

Note—Protamine Zinc Insulin Suspension differs in its action from that of other insulin injections in the USP in both time of onset and duration. To secure accuracy of dosage, the preparation must be brought into uniform suspension by careful shaking before use.

Oral Hypoglycemic and Hyperglycemic Drugs

For several decades it has been known that certain substances could effect hypoglycemia, ie, reduce blood sugar concentrations. A few of these received clinical trial but were abandoned as insulin became more popular and manageable. In 1954 Franke and Fuchs discovered that carbutamide (1-butyl-3-sulfanilylurea) had hypoglycemic actions, and they initiated clinical trials in diabetic patients. Although carbutamide proved to be dangerously toxic, its ability to control hyperglycemia stimulated activity in the field of oral hypoglycemics, and several useful sulfonylureas were evolved. The best known of these compounds are derivatives of benzenesulfonylurea:

$$R_1-\underset{\displaystyle\underset{O}{\|}}{\overset{\displaystyle\overset{O}{\|}}{S}}-NH-\underset{\displaystyle\underset{}{}}{\overset{\displaystyle\overset{O}{\|}}{C}}-NH-R_2$$

Analogues of earlier hypoglycemics, especially of Synthalin, were also studied, and several promising biguanides (formamidyliminoureas) were discovered, of which phenformin is outstanding.

The oral hypoglycemics were received enthusiastically by the medical profession. However, the new agents, especially the sulfonylureas, have proved to be efficacious only in certain types of diabetes, primarily in mild early adult diabetes mellitus. The limitations to the usefulness of the oral hypoglycemics are most certainly connected with the mechanism of their hypoglycemic action and with the nature of the metabolic deficiency in each of the various types of diabetes. The principal action of the sulfonylureas seems to be to increase secretion of insulin, and some pancreatic beta cell function must be present for sulfonylureas to lower blood sugar; in addition, hepatic glucogenesis is decreased. The biguanides apparently lower blood sugar indirectly by inhibiting gluconeogenesis and increasing insulin sensitivity. They are effective in a wider variety of patients than are the sulfonylureas. Oddly, phenformin will not lower blood sugar in nondiabetic individuals.

A few drugs increase the blood sugar and hence have received attention as possible agents for treating hypoglycemia. Epinephrine and related catecholamines are not used for this purpose because of their strong cardiovascular effects and because they are poorly effective orally. Diazoxide, which has received considerable attention as an antihypertensive, also elevates the blood sugar, especially in hypoglycemic patients, mostly infants and young children, who are responsive to leucine. The prognosis of leucine-sensitive hypoglycemic children is poor, so that despite serious side effects, Diazoxide is used. Further information on Diazoxide may be found on page 853.

Acetohexamide NF

[1-[(*p*-Acetylphenyl)sulfonyl]-3-cyclohexylurea; Dymelor (*Lilly*)]

Acetohexamide contains 97.0–101.0% of $C_{15}H_{20}N_2O_4S$ (324.40), calculated on the dried basis.

$$CH_3CO-\underset{}{\bigcirc}-SO_2NHCONH-\bigcirc$$

Preparation—*p*-Acetylbenzenesulfonamide is treated with anhydrous potassium carbonate and the resulting potassium salt of the sulfonamide is then reacted with cyclohexyl isocyanate. After removal of the acetone, the residue (potassium salt of acetohexamide) is dissolved in water and acidified with hydrochloric acid to precipitate the Acetohexamide. Purification is by recrystallization from aqueous ethanol. US Pat. 3,320,312.

Description—A white, practically odorless, crystalline powder. It melts between 184° and 189°.
Solubility—Practically insoluble in water and ether; slightly soluble in alcohol and chloroform; soluble in pyridine and dilute solutions of alkali hydroxides.

Uses—Acetohexamide is a sulfonylurea oral hypoglycemic drug with actions and uses similar to those of *Tolbutamide* (page 982). Thus it is used in the treatment of mild to moderately severe *diabetes mellitus* of the maturity-onset, nonketotic type in patients in whom diet alone cannot control glycosuria. It is ineffective in juvenile-onset, unstable, or brittle diabetes and is contraindicated in diabetes complicated by acidosis ketosis, severe infections, coma, severe trauma, or major surgery.

The side effects of Acetohexamide are similar to those of other sulfonylureas. They include gastrointestinal irritation, which causes nausea, gastritis, and rarely hemorrhage; photosensitivity; skin eruptions; and occasional headache, nervousness and tingling, which may be the result of hypoglycemia.
Dose—**250 mg to 1.5 Gm** daily; *usual*, **250 mg to 1 Gm** daily.
Dosage Forms—Tablets NF: 250 and 500 mg.

Chlorpropamide USP

[1-[(*p*-Chlorophenyl)sulfonyl]-3-propylurea; Diabinese (*Pfizer*)]

$$Cl-\underset{}{\bigcirc}-SO_2-NH-\overset{\overset{\displaystyle O}{\|}}{C}-NH-CH_2CH_2CH_3$$

Chlorpropamide contains 97.0–103.0% of $C_{10}H_{13}ClN_2O_3S$ (276.74), calculated on the dried basis.
Preparation—*p*-Chlorobenzenesulfonamide is caused to undergo addition to propyl isocyanate by warming a solution consisting of equimolar quantities of the two reactants in a suitable inert solvent.

Description—White, crystalline powder, having a slight odor.
Solubility—Practically insoluble in water; soluble in alcohol; sparingly soluble in chloroform.

Uses—Chlorpropamide is an oral hypoglycemic agent with actions and uses essentially the same as those of *Tolbutamide* (page 982). As with Tolbutamide its use is limited to patients with stable, mild to moderately severe diabetes mellitus who still have some residual pancreatic beta cell function. If the patient requires more than 40 units of insulin per day, he usually will not respond to chlorpropamide. Refractoriness sometimes develops. The duration of action (half-life 30 to 36 hours) is much longer than that of Tolbutamide. The side-effects are of the same type as with Tolbutamide but have a somewhat higher incidence. They include cholestatic jaundice, diarrhea, allergic reactions and dermatoses, leukopnea, agranulocytosis and thrombocytopenia.
Dose—**100 to 750 mg** daily; *usual*, **100 to 250 mg** 1 or 2 times a day.
Other Dose Information—The oral, initial dose is 100 to 250 mg daily, with later adjustments at 3 to 5 day intervals. The maintenance dose is usually 100 to 500 mg daily; doses above 500 mg are generally no more effective than lower doses and greatly increase the danger of untoward effects.
Dosage Forms—Tablets USP: 100 and 250 mg.

Phenformin Hydrochloride USP

[1-Phenethylbiguanide Monohydrochloride; PEDG; DBI (*USV*)]

$$\left[\bigcirc-CH_2CH_2-\underset{\underset{NH_2}{|+}}{N}H\overset{}{C}N\overset{\|}{H}\overset{\|}{C}NH_2\right]Cl^-$$

Phenformin Hydrochloride contains 99.0–100.5% of $C_{10}H_{15}N_5 \cdot HCl$ (241.73), calculated on the dried basis.
Preparation—Equimolar quantities of phenethylamine and dicyanodiamide (cyanoguanidine) are mixed and neutralized with aqueous hydrochloric acid. Water is distilled off until the mixture boils (at about 129°) after reflux is allowed to continue for three hours. The crude product may be recrystallized from isopropanol. US Pat. 2,961,377.

Description—A white or practically white, odorless, crystalline powder, having a bitter taste.
Solubility—Freely soluble in water; slightly soluble in alcohol; practically insoluble in chloroform, ether, and solvent hexane.

Uses—Phenformin is an oral hypoglycemic drug of the biguanide (or formamidinyliminourea) group. It increases the clearance of insulin into muscle, thereby promoting muscle uptake of glucose and lowering blood glucose levels. It is of interest that it will not lower blood sugar in normal humans. It is used in the management of *diabetes mellitus*. Unlike the sulfonylureas (see *Tolbutamide*), phenformin may be efficacious even in severe cases of diabetes, although severe cases require high doses. However, it is a much less effective hypoglycemic agent than insulin, so that its use is generally restricted to the same kind of patients who respond to the sulfonylureas. If the patient requires more than 40 units of insulin per day, he is unlikely to respond to Phenformin. Phenformin also lowers plasma cholesterol concentration, by interfering with cholesterol synthesis, and reduces serum triglyceride levels. It is not clear how these effects relate to the hypoglycemic action. The drug reduces body weight in obese persons with hyperinsulinism and abnormal glucose tolerance. Serum fibrinolytic activity is elevated by Phenformin, probably secondarily to its effects on lipid metabolism. There is a high incidence of gastrointestinal upset during the first week of therapy and weight loss, fatigue, and malaise after 4 to 16 weeks of therapy.

Dose—**25 to 300 mg** daily; *usual*, **25 to 50 mg** 1 to 3 times a day.

Other Dose Information—Maintenance doses may require up to 150 mg daily. Doses above that amount generally induce gastrointestinal upsets.

Dosage Forms—Capsules: 50 mg; Tablets USP: 25 mg.

Tolazamide USP

[1-(Hexahydro-1*H*-azepin-1-yl)-3-(*p*-tolylsulfonyl)urea; Tolinase (*Upjohn*)]

$$CH_3 \text{—} SO_2\text{—NHCONH—N}$$

Tolazamide contains 98.0–101.0% of $C_{14}H_{21}N_3O_3S$ (311.41), calculated on the dried basis.

Preparation—Methyl *p*-tolylsulfonylcarbamate is caused to undergo an ammonolysis type of reaction with 1-aminohexamethyleneimine. US Pat. 3,063,903.

Description—A white to off-white, crystalline powder that is odorless or has a slight odor.

Solubility—Very slightly soluble in water; freely soluble in chloroform; soluble in acetone; slightly soluble in alcohol.

Uses—Tolazamide is a sulfonylurea oral hypoglycemic drug with actions and uses similar to *Tolbutamide* (see below). Thus it is used in the treatment of mild to moderately severe *diabetes mellitus* of the maturity-onset, nonketotic type in patients in whom glycosuria cannot be controlled by diet alone. It is ineffective in juvenile-onset, unstable or brittle diabetes and is contraindicated in diabetes complicated by acidosis, ketosis, severe infections, coma, severe trauma, or major surgery. After oral administration the peak plasma levels reach a peak in 4 to 8 hours. The duration of maximal action is about 10 hours, and blood sugar levels begin to rise after 14 to 16 hours.

The total incidence of side effects is about 5%; about 2% of patients find it necessary to discontinue the drug. Side effects include gastrointestinal irritation characterized by nausea, vomiting, and gastritis, skin rashes, pruritus, and hypoglycemic symptoms such as vertigo, malaise, and headache.

Dose—**100 mg to 1 Gm** daily; *usual*, **250 mg** 1 or 2 times a day.

Dosage Forms—Tablets USP: 100 and 250 mg.

Tolbutamide USP

[1-Butyl-3-(*p*-tolylsulfonyl)urea; Orinase (*Upjohn*)]

$$\begin{matrix} & & O \\ & & \| \\ H_3C \text{—} & SO_2\text{—NH—C—NH—}(CH_2)_3CH_3 \end{matrix}$$

Tolbutamide contains 98.0–101.0% of $C_{12}H_{18}N_2O_3S$ (270.35), calculated on the dried basis.

Preparation—Tolbutamide may be prepared by the following sequence of reactions. Toluene is treated with chlorosulfonic acid and the resulting *p*-toluenesulfonyl chloride is converted into *p*-toluenesulfonamide by interaction with ammonia. Condensation of the sulfonamide with ethyl chloroformate in the presence of pyridine or another suitable basic catalyst yields the ester, ethyl *N*-*p*-toluenesulfonylcarbamate. Aminolysis with butylamine in ethylene glycol monomethyl ether solution yields Tolbutamide. The solvent is removed by distillation and water is added to the residue. The crude solid tolbutamide thus obtained is dissolved in dilute ammonia solution, decolorized with charcoal, precipitated with hydrochloric acid, and crystallized from 50% ethanol.

Description—It occurs as a white, or practically white, crystalline powder. It is slightly bitter and practically odorless. Melting range 126° to 132°.

Solubility—Insoluble in water; soluble in alcohol and chloroform.

Uses—Tolbutamide is a sulfonylurea that is orally active as a hypoglycemic drug. The drug stimulates the pancreatic islet beta cells to release extra insulin. It is useful in the treatment of selected cases of *diabetes mellitus*, namely mild uncomplicated, stable diabetes of adult onset and which cannot be controlled by diet alone. These persons have some remaining functional islet beta cells which can be stimulated by the drug. If the patient requires more than 40 units of insulin per day, he generally will not respond to Tolbutamide. In diabetic patients the peak effect is reached in 5 to 8 hours. The duration of action is usually less than 24 hours, so that two daily doses are required in most patients. The hypoglycemia induced by even high doses of Tolbutamide is generally not as severe as can be induced by insulin, hence the incidence of acute hypoglycemic reactions is lower with Tolbutamide. Refractoriness to Tolbutamide sometimes develops. Toxic effects of Tolbutamide include gastrointestinal upset, weakness, headache, tinnitus, paresthesias, and alcohol intolerance. Impaired liver function may occur, and the drug is contraindicated in the presence of liver damage. Furthermore, because the hypoglycemic action of Tolbutamide is mild, the patient is more susceptible to loss of control of the blood sugar through dietary indulgence or infections.

Dose—**500 mg to 2 Gm** daily; *usual*, **500 mg** 2 times a day.

Other Dose Information—Doses greater than 3 Gm are usually no more effective than smaller doses and greatly increase the likelihood of toxicity.

Dosage Forms—Tablets USP: 500 mg.

Sodium Tolbutamide USP

[1-Butyl-3-(*p*-tolylsulfonyl)urea Monosodium Salt; [*N*-(Butylcarbamoyl)-*p*-toluenesulfonamido] sodium; Orinase Diagnostic (*Upjohn*)]

$$\begin{matrix} & & Na \\ & & | \\ CH_3 \text{—} & SO_2NCONH(CH_2)_3CH_3 \end{matrix}$$

Sodium Tolbutamide contains 97.0–101.0% of $C_{12}H_{17}N_2NaO_3S$ (292.33), calculated on the dried basis.

Preparation—*Tolbutamide* (this page) dissolves readily in aqueous sodium hydroxide to form the sodium derivative.

Description—A white to off-white, practically odorless, crystalline powder, having a slightly bitter taste.

Solubility—Freely soluble in water; soluble in alcohol and chloroform; very slightly soluble in ether.

Uses—For the actions of Sodium Tolbutamide, see *Tolbutamide* (above). Because of its water solubility, Sodium Tolbutamide may be given intravenously. By this route, its rapid onset of action lends itself to the *diagnosis of diabetes mellitus* in persons in whom the usual indices are equivocal. Since normal persons have better pancreatic islet function than diabetic ones, the normal person responds with a more rapid and intense drop in blood glucose content than does the diabetic, especially during the first hour after injection. Persons with *pancreatic insulinoma* respond with a prolonged hypoglycemia, so that the drug may also be used diagnostically when that condition is suspected.

Dose—*Usual, intravenous*, the equivalent of **1 Gm** of tolbutamide.

Dosage Forms—Sterile USP: 1 Gm.

The Parathyroid Hormone

Spontaneous atrophy, or injury (as at thyroidectomy) of the parathyroid glands is followed by a decrease in the concentration of serum calcium and an increase in serum phosphorus. These changes can be reversed by the parenteral administration of suitably prepared extracts of the parathyroids of domestic animals. The active principle of the parathyroid gland appears to be a protein of molecular weight 8500. Depending on the procedures used, active substances of lower molecular weight (3800 and 6900) can also be isolated from para-thyroid tissue. These products possess ¼ to ½ the specific calcium-mobilizing activity of the larger molecular-weight preparation, and probably represent partially degraded molecules.

Secretion of parathyroid hormone is stimulated by a fall in the Ca^{++} concentration of the plasma. The hormone then acts to restore Ca^{++} concentration by: (1) increasing reabsorption of calcium and increasing the excretion of phosphate by the kidney, (2) increasing resorption of bone, with release of Ca^{++}, and (3) increasing absorption of calcium from the gastrointestinal tract. Vitamin D_2 (calciferol) and dihydrotachysterol can simulate the hypercalcemic effect of parathyroid hormone; these compounds, moreover, are active orally. Overdosage with any of these compounds can lead to dangerously high calcium concentrations in the blood with attendant complications such as calcification of kidneys and blood vessels. Their use, therefore, should have careful medical supervision and be controlled by frequent determinations of blood calcium.

The thyroid gland produces a hormone, thyrocalcitonin (see page 984), that reduces serum calcium concentration. Its biological function seems to be to prevent excessive hypercalcemia from parathyroid hormone activity.

Dihydrotachysterol USP

[Dihydrotachysterol₂; Hytakerol (*Winthrop*)]

Dihydrotachysterol is $C_{28}H_{46}O$ (398.68).

Preparation—Calciferol (activated ergosterol) is dissolved in a suitable organic solvent and subjected to catalytic hydrogenation until the proper amount of hydrogen has reacted.

Description—Occurs as colorless or white crystals, or as a white, crystalline powder. It is odorless. It melts between 123.5° and 129°. Specific rotation—+100° to +103°.

Solubility—Practically insoluble in water; soluble in alcohol; freely soluble in ether and chloroform; sparingly soluble in vegetable oils.

Uses—Dihydrotachysterol is chemically closely related to vitamin D_2 (Calciferol) and is consequently frequently classified as a D vitamin. However, it possesses very weak antirachitic activity, being only about ¼₀₀ as potent as calciferol in this respect. But it has potent calcemic activity (ie, raises plasma calcium concentration) and is similar to parathyroid hormone in this action. Consequently, it has long been used in lieu of parathyroid hormone in the treatment of *hypocalcemia* and *hypoparathyroidism*. Its calcemic action may be of value in the treatment of vitamin D-resistant rickets. Other uses of Dihydrotachysterol, such as in scleroderma and the tetany of pregnancy are not well established by objective clinical studies. The drug should not be used in the presence of renal insufficiency or hyperphosphatemia. Extreme care must be used to prevent overdosage.

Dose—*Usual, initial*, **750 mcg** to **2.5 mg** once a day; *maintenance*, **250 mcg** to **1.75 mg** once a week.

Dosage Forms—Capsules: 125 mcg; Solution (in oil): 250 mcg/ml.

Parathyroid Injection USP

[Parathyroid Solution; Parathyroid Extract; Paroidin (*Parke, Davis*)]

Parathyroid Injection is a sterile solution in water for injection of the water-soluble principle or principles of the parathyroid glands that have the property of increasing the calcium content of the blood. Each ml of Parathyroid Injection possesses a potency of not less than 100 USP Parathyroid Units.

Note—*One USP Parathyroid Unit represents one one-hundredth of the amount of Parathyroid Injection required to raise the calcium content of 100 ml of the blood serum of normal dogs 1 mg within 16 to 18 hours after administration.*

Preparation—It is obtained from the fresh parathyroid glands of healthy domesticated animals used for food by man; the animal source of each preparation should be stated. The parathyroid glands are removed from the animals immediately after slaughtering, and then extracted at once or kept frozen until extracted. The glands are freed from gross fat and connective tissue, ground, extracted, and the extract purified to make it suitable for parenteral administration. The Injection is then adjusted to the proper potency.

Description—The pH is between 2.5 and 3.0.

Uses—The parathyroid hormone is one of the factors which regulates the concentration of calcium in the blood. A deficiency in the secretion of the hormone results in a hypocalcemia, which in turn causes tetany. See the general statement (page 983). The specific indication for the parathyroid hormone is in the treatment of *hypoparathyroidism*. The hormone is inactive by mouth and must be given by subcutaneous or intramuscular injection.

The onset of action of the parathyroid hormone is relatively slow, maximal effects on the level of blood calcium not being obtained for 18 hours. Therefore, for the immediate control of symptoms the intravenous injection of a soluble calcium salt may be necessary. The effects of a single dose of hormone are evident for 36 hours. For this reason, injections are made at 24- to 48-hour intervals.

Treatment with parathyroid hormone is inconvenient due to the necessity of injections. Also the action of the hormone is difficult to control. Therefore dihydrotachysterol, a drug which affects the level of blood calcium in much the same way as the parathyroid hormone

and which can be taken orally, is a more favored preparation in the treatment of hypoparathyroidism.

Parathyroid hormone is occasionally employed for the treatment of conditions other than parathyroid deficiency. The hormone promotes the excretion of urine and in rare instances is used for its *diuretic* action. It also promotes the excretion of lead, and it was formerly employed in the treatment of *lead poisoning*. It is also of limited value in the treatment of certain types of *hemorrhage*, the calcium ion being one of the essentials for the normal clotting of blood.

Dose—*Intramuscular*, **20** to **100 USP Units** daily; *usual*, **40 USP Units** every 12 hours.

Other Dose Information—In severe cases as much as 100 Units may be given without the danger of producing hypercalcemia. In less drastic cases, a dose of 10 to 20 Units suffices. Therapy should be regulated by frequent reference to the actual serum calcium and phosphate concentrations of the patient, and high values should be avoided.

Dosage Forms—Injection USP: 500 USP Units/5 ml.

Veterinary Dose—*Dogs*, **2 to 25 Units.**

The Thyroid Hormones

The thyroid gland modulates the energy metabolism and certain nonenergetic metabolic functions of the body. In the absence of the thyroid gland the basal metabolic rate is less than 55% of normal, and growth and development are impaired. In the presence of a hyperactive gland the metabolic rate may be up to 160% of normal; the excitability of irritable tissues is increased, and tachycardia, nervousness, etc, result. Thyroid "hormone" is mainly used clinically to replenish the corporal hormone supply in conditions of thyroid insufficiency (hypothyroidism), such as may result from a natural thyroid or pituitary pathology or from thyroid surgery. The "hormone" is rarely administered to increase the metabolic rate and organic activity above normal, and such iatrogenic hyperthyroidism may indeed be dangerous.

The mediator by which the thyroid gland stimulates the tissues to a higher activity and rate of metabolism is called the *thyroid hormone*, but it is clear that not one but four active substances, all iodinated thyronines, are released by the gland. Thyroxine (L-3,5,3',5'-tetraiodothyronine) is found in the greatest amount in blood (about 75% of the thyroid hormone content of the plasma), and the moderately less active L-3,3'-*diiodothyronine* is present in the next greatest amount (25%). L-3,5,3'-*triiodothyronine* (Liothyronine), which is 3 to 10 times as active as thyroxine, and L-3,3',5'-*triiodothyronine* comprise less than 3% of the plasma thyroid hormone content. But since the triiodothyronines disappear more rapidly from blood than thyroxine, they probably comprise a somewhat larger proportion of the glandular secretion; in the thyroid gland they account for about ⅕ of the hormone content and as much as 40% of its hormone activity. Furthermore, there is evidence to suggest that in the tissues, thyroxine may be converted to Liothyronine, possibly the true active form of thyroxine. In the colloid of the thyroid gland these thyronine derivatives are bound to a globulin, *thyroglobulin*, which was formerly thought to be the thyroid hormone. The reaction *in vitro* between iodine and certain tyrosine-containing proteins, such as

casein, also results in the formation of bound iodothyronines; such iodinated proteins have been used in lieu of natural thyroid hormones.

The mechanism by which the thyroid hormones increase the metabolic rate and organic function of the body is not known. Certain *in vitro* actions, such as uncoupling of oxidative phosphorylation, cannot yet be related to the physiological actions, inasmuch as many other uncouplers lack thyroid hormone activity.

The thyroid gland concentrates iodide ion from the plasma and converts it to free iodine, which then reacts with tyrosine moieties within the substance of the gland eventually to produce the thyroid hormones. The glandular accumulation of iodide and the conversion to the intermediate, 3,5-diiodotyrosine are under the control of the thyrotropic hormone (see page 956). Iodine deficiency results in a compensatory increase in the size of the thyroid gland in a usually fruitless homeostatic attempt to manufacture more hormone. Iodine administration corrects this type of goiter and permits the normal production of the thyroid hormones. The incorporation of sodium iodide into table salt helps protect against iodine deficiency thyroid disorders.

Thyroid hormones lower plasma lipid concentrations. However, because of their effect to increase the metabolic rate, they are not used clinically to lower blood lipids. The lipid-lowering action is also possessed by the dextro isomers of thyroid hormones, but the dextro forms have only a very weak effect on the metabolic rate. Consequently, dextrothyroxine is employed to lower blood lipids.

Thyrocalcitonin is also a thyroid hormone, but its effects are to decrease plasma calcium concentration rather than to affect energy and lipid metabolism. It plays a role in the homeostasis of blood calcium. When plasma calcium levels are elevated, thyrocalcitonin is released in increased quantities. Thus it tends to oppose parathyroid hormone. The molecular weight of thyrocalcitonin is about 4500. It is a polypeptide of 32 amino acid units.

Potassium Iodide—see page 872.

Sodium Dextrothyroxine—see page 866.

Sodium Iodide—see page 873.

Sodium Levothyroxine USP

[Sodium L-3-[4-(4-Hydroxy-3,5-diiodophenoxy)-3,5-diiodophenyl] alanine; Sodium L-3,3′,5,5′-tetraiodothyronine; Letter (*Armour*); Synthroid (*Flint*); Titroid (*Century*)]

Sodium Levothyroxine is the sodium salt of the levo isomer of thyroxine, an active physiological principle obtained from the thyroid gland of domesticated animals used for food by man, or prepared synthetically. It contains 61.6–65.5% of iodine, corresponding to 97.0–103.0% of $C_{15}H_{10}I_4NNaO_4$ (798.86), calculated on the anhydrous basis.

Preparation—L-Thyroxine is dissolved in dilute sodium hydroxide solution and the resulting sodium salt is precipitated by saturating the solution with sodium chloride.

Thyroxine may be prepared from thyroid glands and by synthesis. Preparation from the glands (fresh or desiccated) involves extraction with dilute sodium hydroxide followed by acidification with hydrochloric acid whereupon a very crude form of thyroxine is precipitated. Purification involves repeated solubilization by means of sodium hydroxide and reprecipitation with acid, these operations being conducted under increasingly refined conditions and with the aid of auxiliary operations designed to enhance the purity of the final precipitate of thyroxine.

The key compound in the synthesis of thyroxine is 3,5-diiodo-4-(*p*-methoxyphenoxy)nitrobenzene (I) which is readily formed by condensing *p*-methoxyphenol with 3,4,5-triiodonitrobenzene under the influence of anhydrous potassium carbonate. Initial subsequent operations involve (*a*) reduction of nitro to amino; (*b*) replacement of amino by cyano by treatment with cuprous cyanide and butyl nitrite; (*c*) hydration of cyano to carboxyl; and (*d*) reduction of carboxyl to formyl. The resulting aldehyde may be converted into thyroxine in various ways. One involves condensation with 2-phenyl-2-oxazolin-5-one to produce (II) which is then simultaneously hydrogenated, demethylated, and reductively cleaved by hydrogen iodide in the presence of phosphorus and acetic anhydride to give the DL-form of 3-[4-(4-hydroxyphenoxy)-3,5-diiodophenyl]alanine (III). (III) is then resolved and the isolated L-enantiomorph is iodinated with ammoniacal potassium triiodide solution at the 3,5-positions on the phenoxy ring to give levothyroxine (IV). Neutralization of this acid with sodium hydroxide yields the official salt.

Description—A light yellow to buff-colored, odorless, tasteless, hygroscopic powder. It is stable in dry air but may assume a slight pink color upon exposure to light. The pH of a saturated solution is about 8.9. The specific rotation (determined in a mixture of 1 part of $1N$ sodium hydroxide and 2 parts of alcohol containing 300 mg in each 10 ml) is between $-5°$ and $-6°$.

Solubility—1 Gm dissolves in about 700 ml of water and about 300 ml of alcohol; insoluble in acetone, chloroform, and ether; soluble in solutions of alkali hydroxides and hot solutions of alkali carbonates.

Uses—Sodium Levothyroxine is the sodium salt of L-thyroxine, the most abundant of the thyroid hormonal substances. Its actions, uses, side effects, and limitations are those of *Thyroid* (see page 986). It is claimed that the sodium salt is better absorbed orally than is the free amino acid, but since the salt is converted in the stomach to the same acid hydrochloride as the free amino acid, this claim is hardly credible. Approximately 50% of an oral dose is absorbed. The time for the intensity of its effect to fall to one-half of its initial value is 9 to 12 days, and some residual effects may be apparent for several weeks after the last dose. Although the L-form is twice as active as the racemic mixture, it offers no particular therapeutic advantage over the DL-form.

Dose—**25 mcg to 1 mg** daily; *usual*, **100 to 400 mcg** once a day.

Dosage Forms—Tablets USP: 25, 50, 100, 150, 200, 300, and 500 mcg.

Sodium Liothyronine USP

[Sodium L-3-[4-(4-Hydroxy-3-iodophenoxy)-3,5-diiodophenyl]alanine; Cytomel (*SK&F*)]

Sodium Liothyronine is the sodium salt of L-3,3′,5-triiodothyronine. It contains 53.7–57.1% of iodine, corresponding to 95.0–101.0% of $C_{15}H_{11}I_3NNaO_4$ (672.96), calculated on the dried basis.

Preparation—3,5-Diiodo-L-thyronine [the L-enantiomorph of compound (III) in the thyroxine synthesis described under Sodium Levothyroxine above] is dissolved in methanol and iodinated only at the 3-position by treatment with ammonia and iodine at room temperature. The liothyronine (acid) is then liberated by acidifying the reaction mixture. It is collected, purified, and neutralized with sodium hydroxide to give the official salt.

Description—It occurs as a light tan, odorless, crystalline powder. Specific rotation is not less than $+18°$ and not more than $+21°$, calculated on the dried basis.

Solubility—Very slightly soluble in water; slightly soluble in alcohol; practically insoluble in most other organic solvents.

Uses—Sodium Liothyronine is the sodium salt of one of the thyroid hormones (see the general statement, page 984). It is 3 to 10 times more potent than Sodium Levothyroxine (see *Sodium Levothyroxine*). Certain evidence suggests that Liothyronine may be the active form into which thyroxine is converted in the tissues. The actions and uses of Liothyronine are those of thyroid and sodium levothyroxine, except that it is considered to be more suitable for the treatment of a vague syndrome known as *metabolic insufficiency*, which perhaps is due to a deficiency in the tissue utilization of thyroxine, and experimentally for the treatment of *male infertility* and certain *menstrual disorders* associated with hypothyroidism. Liothyronine has also been used to *reduce goiter*, since the drug effectively reduces the anterior pituitary release of thyrotropic hormone. Liothyronine has a rapid onset (one to two days) and a short duration of action compared to thyroxine. The prompt onset and rapid offset are considered to be an advantage over thyroid or levothyroxine. The time for the intensity of its effect to fall to one-half of its initial value is 4 to 10 days. Liothyronine is erratically absorbed from the gastrointestinal tract, and 30 to 40% may be recovered from the stools. Liothyronine is only loosely bound to plasma proteins and hence does not elevate the plasma protein bound iodine (PBI) significantly like levothyroxine; indeed, PBI may actually be lowered, because of a homeostatic decrease in thyroxine release from the thyroid gland.

Dose—The equivalent of **5 to 100 mcg** of liothyronine daily; *usual*, the equivalent of **25 to 75 mcg** of liothyronine once a day.

Dosage Forms—Tablets USP: 5, 25, and 50 mcg.

Veterinary Dose—*Dogs*, **0.5 to 1 mcg** per **pound** of body weight daily in single or divided doses. Dose must be adjusted to the response of the patient.

Thyroglobulin

[Proloid (*Warner-Chilcott*)]

Thyroglobulin is the form in which thyroid hormone is stored in the colloid of the thyroid gland.

Preparation—Hog thyroid glands are ground and extracted with dilute aqueous sodium chloride solution. Adjusting the pH to the isoelectric point with acetic acid and heating precipitates the crude product which is then defatted with an appropriate solvent, dried, milled, and blended.

Description—A cream to tan, free-flowing powder that has a characteristic odor and taste. It is stable in air, heat, and light, although it may deteriorate on prolonged exposure to strong light.

Solubility—Insoluble in water, alcohol, and other common organic solvents.

Uses—The actions and uses of Thyroglobulin are the same as Thyroid (this page). However, it is less likely to cause hypersensitivity, although it is not completely free of contaminating proteins; to this extent it may have some advantage over thyroid, but it is difficult to see any advantage over sodium levothyroxine or sodium liothyronine.

Dose—**30 to 300 mg** a day; *usual, maintenance,* **180 mg** a day.

Dosage Forms—Tablets: ¼, ½, 1, 1½, 3, and 5 gr.

Thyroid USP

[Thyroideum; Thyroidea; Desiccated Thyroid; Thyroid Extract; Thyroid Gland]

Thyroid is the cleaned, dried, and powdered thyroid gland previously deprived of connective tissue and fat. It is obtained from domesticated animals that are used for food by man.

Thyroid contains 0.17–0.23% of iodine (I) in thyroid combination, and is free from iodine in inorganic or any form of combination other than that peculiar to the thyroid gland. A desiccated thyroid of a higher iodine content may be brought to this standard by admixture with a desiccated thyroid of a lower iodine content or with lactose, sodium chloride, starch, or sucrose.

Description—A yellowish to buff-colored, amorphous powder, having a slight characteristic, meat-like odor and a saline taste.

Uses—The thyroid hormone is essential for normal metabolism and development. The congenital absence of thyroid hormone results in a condition known as *cretinism*. In childhood or adult life, absence of thyroid hormone causes *myxedema*. These conditions are characterized by an abnormally low basal metabolic rate. The primary therapeutic use of thyroid is in their treatment.

Thyroid is often given to individuals with *low metabolic rates* unassociated with myxedema. For example, patients with chronic constipation, menstrual disorders, sterility, arthritis, etc., associated with a low metabolic rate are often benefited by thyroid hormone.

Employment of thyroid as an aid to reduce *excessive weight* is a frequent practice, often futile, and sometimes fraught with danger. It should never be attempted without medical supervision.

Thyroid has a very slow onset of action. A given dose does not exert its maximum effect for several days and will continue to have some degree of action for 2 to 3 months. Therefore caution must be exercised in judging the dose of thyroid in that cumulative effects must be anticipated.

Dose—**15 to 300 mg** daily; *usual,* **60 to 180 mg** once a day.

Other Dose Information—In the treatment of adult myxedema, the average patient requires at least 100 mg daily. In the treatment of cretinism much lower doses are employed, depending upon the age.

Dosage Forms—Tablets USP: 15, 30, 60, 125, 200, 250, and 300 mg.

Veterinary Uses—Thyroid therapy has been used in small animal practice for the treatmeat of various conditions including rickets, osteomalacia, chronic eczema, delayed union of fractures, and obesity from over feeding.

Veterinary Dose—*Dogs*, 15 to 300 mg.

Other Thyroid Hormones

Thyroxin USP XIII [Thyroxine; Thyroxin Fraction

$$HO-\text{⟨ring⟩}-O-\text{⟨ring⟩}-CH_2CHCOOH$$
with I substituents and NH_2

(Squibb)][$C_{15}H_{11}I_4NO_4$]—An active physiological principle obtained from the thyroid gland or prepared synthetically. It contains not less than 64% of iodine as an integral part of the thyroxin molecule. *Uses:* Same as for Thyroid. It has no advantages over the latter except that suitably prepared solutions of the sodium salt may be administered intravenously. *Dose:* 0.5 mg a day.

Antithyroid Compounds

Several investigators, while using sulfaguanidine in an attempt to prevent the synthesis of certain vitamins by the intestinal flora of test animals, noticed a hypertrophy of the thyroid gland with concurrent lowering of the basal metabolism. When administration of thyroxine subsequently reversed these effects, further research with numerous compounds revealed the fact that a number of linear and heterocyclic derivatives of thiourea inhibit the production of thyroid hormone by the thyroid gland. The mechanism of action is that of an interference with the incorporation of inorganic iodine into the organic form. The decline in thyroid hormone output and the resultant lowering of plasma levels of the thyroid hormones is sensed in the hypothalamus, which through the intermediation of the thyrotropin-releasing factor stimulates the adreno-hypophysis to produce more thyrotropic hormone. Consequently, the thyroid gland is stimulated to enlarge, even though the enlarged gland cannot produce more thyroid hormone. Because of the thyroid enlargement consequent to the use of the thiourea class of antithyroid compounds, such compounds are called goitrogens. The goitrogens are employed in the control of hyperthyroidism. Glandular enlargement, with the concomitant friability and vascularity of the gland, makes surgery difficult. Therefore, iodine (or a thyroid hormone), which reduces the size of the gland, is added to the regimen preparatory to thyroid surgery.

Several other classes of compounds are also antithyroid agents. Compounds such as thiocyanates and perchlorates competitively inhibit the iodine uptake mechanism. Large doses of iodine inhibit the enzyme tyrosine iodinase and thus interfere with the production of thyroid hormone. Therefore, iodine also may be used in the treatment of hyperthyroidism. Curiously, this action of iodine is not goitrogenic; in fact, iodine opposes the goitrogenic effects of certain antithyroid drugs. Radioiodine (I 131) is antithyroid by virtue of tissue destruction caused by radiation. Thyroid hormones are antigoitrogenic by a homeostatic mechanism to reduce the hypothalamic release of thyrotropin-releasing factor.

Methimazole USP

[1-Methylimidazole-2-thiol; Tapazole (*Lilly*)]

Methimazole contains 98.0–101.0% of $C_4H_6N_2S$ (114.17), calculated on the dried basis.

Preparation—One method consists of cyclizing (methylamino)acetaldehyde diethyl acetal with thiocyanic acid via de-ethanolation. Details are provided in *J. Am. Chem. Soc.*, **71**, 4000 (1949).

Description—A white to pale buff, crystalline powder, having a faint, characteristic odor. Its solutions are practically neutral to litmus. Melting range 144° to 147°.

Solubility—1 Gm dissolves in about 5 ml of water, about 5 ml of alcohol, about 4.5 ml of chloroform, and about 125 ml of ether.

Uses—Methimazole is an antithyroid drug that is employed for the preparation of the hyperthyroid patient for surgery and for the total treatment of *hyperthyroidism*. Methimazole is approximately 10 times as potent as *Propylthiouracil* and is more prompt in eliciting an antithyroid response. The drug also exhibits a more prolonged action than propylthiouracil; a single dose of 5 mg may inhibit the synthesis of thyroid hormone for 24 hours.

The toxic side effects are similar to those of propylthiouracil and include skin rashes, urticaria, joint pains, and agranulocytosis. Approximately 6% of patients taking the drug experience some untoward effect. Thus, the incidence of untoward reactions is somewhat higher than with propylthiouracil, but considerably lower than with other antithyroid drugs.

Dose—**5** to **60 mg** daily; *usual*, **10 mg** 3 times a day.

Other Dose Information—Methimazole is given initially in the above dose until hyperthyroidism is controlled (up to two months!), after which the dose is generally adjusted downward for maintenance.

Dosage Forms—Tablets USP: 5 and 10 mg.

Methylthiouracil NF

[Antibason; 6-Methyl-2-thiouracil]

Methylthiouracil contains 97.0–100.5% of $C_5H_6N_2OS$ (142.18), calculated on the dried basis.

Preparation—Acetoacetic ester is condensed via dehydration and de-ethanolation with thiourea. Details are provided in *J. Am. Chem. Soc.*, **67**, 2197 (1945).

Description—A white, odorless, crystalline powder. It melts with decomposition at about 330°.

Solubility—Very slightly soluble in water; sparingly soluble in alcohol; slightly soluble in chloroform and ether; freely soluble in ammonia and solutions of alkali hydroxides.

Uses—Methylthiouracil, the methyl analog of *Propylthiouracil*, has actions and uses essentially like those of the latter agent; it is employed in the preparation of the hyperthyroid patient for surgery and for the treatment of hyperthyroidism. The side effects of the drug are also similar to those of propylthiouracil and include skin rashes, urticaria, joint pains, and agranulocytosis. Unfortunately, the incidence of side effects from Methylthiouracil is approximately six times higher than that for propylthiouracil. Therefore, its use should be restricted to those patients who are unable to tolerate or are refractory to other antithyroid drugs. Patients receiving the drug should be kept under the same close observation as those under propylthiouracil therapy.

Dose—*Usual*, 50 mg 4 times a day.

Other Dose Information—The daily dose should not exceed 300 mg.

Veterinary Dose—Daily: *Cattle*, **0.5** to **4 Gm**; *Sheep* and *Swine*, **100** to **500 mg**; *Dogs*, **20** to **100 mg**.

Potassium Iodide—see page 872.

Propylthiouracil USP

[6-Propyl-2-thiouracil; Propacil; (*Various Mfgs.*)]

$$CH_3CH_2CH_2 \quad \underset{\underset{NH}{\overset{HN}{|}}}{\overset{S}{\diagdown}}$$

Propylthiouracil contains 98.0–100.5% of $C_7H_{10}N_2$-OS (170.23), calculated on the dried basis.

Preparation—As described for *Methylthiouracil* (above), except using ethyl 3-oxocaproate instead of acetoacetic ester.

Description—A white, powdery, crystalline substance. It is starch-like in appearance and to the touch, and has a bitter taste. Melting range 218° to 221°.

Solubility—Slightly soluble in water; sparingly soluble in alcohol; slightly soluble in chloroform and ether; soluble in ammonia and alkali hydroxides.

Uses—Propylthiouracil interferes with the synthesis of thyroid hormone by the thyroid gland, an action which has been applied in the management of *hyperthyroidism*. Since the drug does not interfere with the release or utilization of stored thyroid hormone, the period which elapses between the beginning of medication and the manifestations of its antithyroid action is dependent upon the quantity of thyroid hormone stored in the gland. The marked hyperplasia of the thyroid gland which follows Propylthiouracil administration is a result of a compensatory increase in adenohypophyseal thyrotrophic activity consequent to a reduction in the thyroid hormone titer of the blood.

Propylthiouracil is employed in the preparation of the hyperthyroid patient for surgery. When treatment with the drug has brought the basal metabolic rate to normal (euthyroidism) or nearly so, iodine is administered to reduce the marked vascularity and friability of the gland. Propylthiouracil is also used in the total (medical) treatment of hyperthyroidism. However, at least half the patients so treated may be expected to have a remission 6 to 12 months after cessation of medication.

Propylthiouracil exerts toxic actions in a small but significant number of patients. The most serious of these toxic actions are granulocytopenia, leucopenia, drug fever, and dermatitis. The over-all incidence of untoward reactions to Propylthiouracil is approximately 2%; the incidence of agranulocytosis approaches 0.5%. Therefore, the patient who receives chronic medication with this drug should be kept under close surveillance.

Dose—**50** to **500 mg** daily; *usual*, **100 mg** 3 times a day.

Dosage Forms—Tablets USP: 50 mg.

Veterinary Dose—Daily: *Cattle*, **0.25** to **1 Gm**; *Sheep* and *Swine*, **50** to **125 mg**; *Dogs*, **15** to **20 mg**.

Sodium Iodide—see page 873.

Sodium Iodide I 131—see page 566.

Sodium Liothyronine—see page 985.

Other Antithyroid Compounds

Iothiouracil Sodium [Itrumil Sodium (*Ciba*)] is sodium 5-iodo-2-thiouracil. *Description and Solubility:* An odorless, white to light-yellow, crystalline powder. It melts between 242° and 244° with decomposition; pH (2% aqueous solution), 8.5 to 9.5. In the usual form (the dihydrate) it is reasonably stable to moisture and sunlight at room temperature. Soluble in water; slightly soluble in alcohol. *Uses:* Combines the thyroid involuting cations of iodide and the antithyroid action of thiouracil, the former suppressing the vascularization of the thyroid gland and goitrogenic effects of the latter action. However, the drug is not superior to the combination of iodide with other antithyroid agents. It is used in the treatment and preoperative management of hyperthyroidism. Its toxic effects are those of the other thiouracils (see *Methylthiouracil* and *Propylthiouracil*, page 987 and this page, respectively. *Dose:* Oral, 150 to 300 mg daily in divided doses. For preoperative management, 4 to 8 weeks may be required.

The Sex Hormones

The sex hormones, like the hormones of the adrenal cortex, are steroids. They may be classified into the following groups, according to chemical structure and physiological activity:

(1) estrogenic hormones (female);
(2) progestational hormone (female);
(3) androgenic hormones (male).

Groups (1) and (2) are collectively known as the *ovarian hormones*. They include synthetic as well as natural products.

Structure—The natural estrogens are all steroids (see Chapter 30, page 479) containing 18 carbon atoms, oxygenated at carbons 3 and 17. Ring A of all the estrogens is aromatic; some estrogenic hormones found in the urine of the *equidae* possess further unsaturation in ring B.

Progesterone, the hormone of the corpus luteum, is a 21-carbon atom steroid, possessing, like the adrenal cortical steroids, an α,β-unsaturated ketone component in ring A. It differs from the latter in that its C_{17} does not carry hydroxyl.

The natural androgenic steroids are 19-carbon atom compounds. They are characterized by a partly or completely saturated ring A, and by either a hydroxyl or a keto group at C_3 and C_{17}.

As with all other classes of steroids, stereoisomerism is of fundamental importance with the sex hormones; and the α and β configuration conventions are applied in drawing the structural formulas.

The Ovarian Hormones

The ovaries serve the dual purpose of secreting the female hormones and producing the ova which, after the woman's maturity, are liberated normally at the rate of one every four weeks. The ovaries secrete two principal types of hormones which are intimately related to the entire process of sex development and function. The first category of these hormones to be recognized chemically is the group of steroids named *estrogens*. The second category of hormone secreted by the ovaries, also steroidal, is the *luteal* or *progestational hor-*

mone named *progesterone*. The ovaries also secrete small amounts of androgens, adrenal steroids, and the nonsteroidal hormone, relaxin (page 1004).

The ovarian production of hormones is regulated by the gonadotropic hormones of the anterior pituitary (see page 956). However, the hypothalamic control of pituitary gonadotropin production is, in turn, modulated by the estrogens and progesterone, which in low plasma concentrations appear to stimulate and at high concentrations inhibit the production of FSH, LH, and LTH. Thus a complex positive and negative feedback system subserves the cyclic phenomena of ovulation and menstruation. The exact details in this concert are not completely known for woman. It is known that in women ovulation can be prevented by estrogens as the result of suppression of FSH production. Estrogen alone is not satisfactory for oral contraception, owing to what is termed "break through" bleeding, except when dangerously high doses of estrogen are used. In impractically large doses, progesterone also inhibits ovulation, presumably because of suppression of luteinizing hormone production; furthermore, it can favor infertility by a second mechanism, namely, that of maintaining the endometrium in a hypoproliferative and hyposecretory state which is unfavorable to implantation of the fertilized ovum. It is now known that some progestogens have an antifertility effect at doses well below those necessary to suppress endometrial proliferation and secretion. Interest in oral contraceptives originally started with progestogens. However, intermenstrual bleeding occurs during continuous treatment with many progestogens, and it was found desirable to add estrogens, which, although they favor endometrial proliferation, have a hemostatic effect on uterine bleeding. Furthermore, the 19-norprogestogens were originally synthesized by a route that contaminated the intended product with an estrogen. It was gradually accepted that the estrogen not only helped normalize cyclic bleeding but also contributed to the contraceptive effect. In fact, some authorities argued that the estrogen was alone responsible for the antifertility effect and that the progestogen was only promoting a normal mense. Now it is appreciated that progestogens alone can be contraceptive in low doses which do not disturb the menses of many users. However, the antifertility use of progestogens alone is still under investigation. Progestogens alone would avoid the drawbacks of estrogens, namely nausea, vomiting, headache, and a tendency to venous thrombosis. In the meantime, sequential therapy, in which anovulatory doses of estrogen are followed later by a progestogen, has come in vogue.

Natural Estrogenic Hormones and Derivatives

Natural estrogenic hormones are secreted by the ovarian follicles. They stimulate or regulate the growth and development of the uterus, the vaginal mucous membrane, and also other structures such as the mammary glands, subcutaneous fat, axillary and pubic hair, and certain elements in the skin. These latter comprise the secondary sex characteristics. Therefore the estrogens are also called *female sex hormones*. Of the estrogens the most potent occurring naturally is *β-estradiol*, and its two principal metabolic products which are also estrogenic are *estrone* and *estriol*. Several other products of metabolic change occur in smaller amounts, but these are not offered as single substances for therapy. Estrogens are secreted throughout the period of activity of the ovaries, but at varying rates at different times of the menstrual cycle.

The naturally occurring estrogens can be prepared synthetically, but at greater cost than by extraction from natural materials or by simple chemical processing of natural estrogens as they occur in urine. An interesting improvement of the natural estrogen has been the synthetic modification of β-estradiol, the most potent of natural estrogens, by the addition of a side chain, producing *ethinyl estradiol*. This has a very high activity when administered orally. The potencies of these estrogens were originally measured entirely in terms of biologically determined units, but in the cases of purified, crystalline products, weights may now be used. Biological units are still commonly mentioned and depend upon the reaction of spayed rats to injections of the hormones, which induce rapid development of cornified cells in the vaginal mucosa, detectable by the vaginal smear technique.

Uses—Estrogens are used as substitution therapy when *menopausal symptoms* occur after cessation of ovarian function, following castration or x-ray or radium therapy; or in the natural menopause (also called the climacteric). The purpose of the treatment is to afford relief from any of a long list of subjective complaints which are widely recognized as characteristic of the menopause. The doses needed for such relief vary from patient to patient, and from time to time, in any one woman. The duration of the disturbance which is susceptible to such treatment is from a few days to several years. It represents a transition period during which the body is becoming adjusted to the absence of estrogen stimulation. Use of minimal doses which will provide comfort during this transition does not prolong the adjustment, and under medical supervision may be used with confidence. Furthermore, there is good evidence that estrogens retard postmenopausal atherosclerosis, angina pectoris, and osteoporosis, and possibly even retards the onset of senility.

Other uses of estrogens include *stimulation of development of the uterus*, or of *secondary sex characteristics* in women with delayed or inadequate development, and in the treatment of a variety of conditions, including dysmenorrhea, amenorrhea, premenstrual distress, functional uterine bleeding, etc. Estrogens are also used to inhibit the growth of *prostatic cancer* of men and *carcinoma of the breast* or carcinoma elsewhere in the reproductive tract of women who are more than 4 years beyond the menopause (see Chapter 66, page 1163). Another important use of estrogenic substances is in *oral contraception* (see *Ovarian Hormones*, above). Large doses of estrogens given within a few days after coitus have an effect to prevent pregnancy. This application is especially helpful in managing cases of rape.

There is a choice of compounds for estrogenic therapy. Estrone is commonly employed by intramuscular injection. Considerable activity is lost if the oral route is used. Ethinyl estradiol is the most active of all oral estrogens, and its oral activity is nearly equal to its injection activity. Per milligram, estradiol benzoate is more powerful in action than estrone. Its action is also more sustained. It is commonly given by intramuscular injection. Estriol is considerably less active than estrone when given hypodermically, and its activity following oral administration is probably too low to make it important. Conjugated estrogens (see page 991) retain much of their activity on oral administration and are used extensively by this route. Estrogens can also be given by inunction. In addition various concentrates of estrogenic hormones are available.

Synthetic compounds, of which the best known is

Diethylstilbestrol, possess most of the actions of the natural estrogenic hormones and are often cheaper. Since they lose little activity after oral administration they have replaced the natural estrogens in many fields of treatment.

Estradiol NF

[Estra-1,3,5(10)-triene-3,17β-diol;   17-*Beta*-estradiol;   Dihydrotheelin; Aquadiol (*National Drug*); Progynon (*Schering*)]

Estradiol contains 97.0–103.0% of $C_{18}H_{24}O_2$ (272.39), calculated on the dried basis.

Preparation—Estradiol has been isolated from ovarian follicular fluid and from placental tissue, and is the most potent of the natural estrogens. It is usually prepared through reduction of the 17-keto group of *Estrone* (page 991).

It is curious that the urine of stallions and of the males of other *Equidæ* contains 3 to 5 times as much estradiol as that of the female of the species.

Description—White or creamy white, small crystals or a crystalline powder. It is odorless and stable in air. It melts between 173° and 179°. Its specific rotation is not less than +76° and not more than +83° in dioxane solution.

Solubility—Almost insoluble in water; soluble in alcohol, acetone, dioxane, and solutions of fixed alkali hydroxides; sparingly soluble in vegetable oils.

Uses—See the general use statement under *Natural Estrogenic Hormones and Derivatives* (page 989). Estradiol is mainly employed to supplement parenteral therapy with esters of estradiol. Parenteral estradiol may be used, but the hormone is rapidly destroyed, and the esters are superior.

Dose—*Usual, implantation,* **25 mg,** repeated when necessary; *intramuscular,* **220 mcg** to **1.5 mg** 2 or 3 times a week; *oral,* **200** to **500 mcg** 1 to 3 times a day.

Other Dose Information—Maintenance doses usually are as follows: oral, 0.2 mg 3 times daily; intramuscular, 0.5 to 1.5 mg 2 or 3 times weekly; locally, by vaginal suppository, 0.4 mg at bedtime. Implants are repeated about every 3 months.

Dosage Forms—Pellets NF: 25 mg; Sterile Suspension NF: 250 mcg and 1 mg/ml, 2.2, 2.5, 4.4, and 11 mg/10 ml, 5.5 mg/25 ml; Tablets NF: 200 and 500 mcg.

Veterinary Dose—Administered *hypodermically,* *Mares* and *Cows,* 1 to **5 mg;** *Ewes,* **0.3** to **2.5 mg;** *Bitches,* **0.1** to **1 mg** (doses not well established).

Estradiol Benzoate NF

[Estradiol 3-Benzoate;   Beta-estradiol Benzoate;   Progynon Benzoate (*Schering*)]

Estradiol Benzoate contains 97.0–103.0% of $C_{25}H_{28}$-O_3 (376.50), calculated on the dried basis.

For the structure of the base, see *Estradiol.*

Preparation—This compound is prepared by benzoylation of the 3-hydroxyl of *Estradiol.*

Description—A white or creamy white crystalline powder, odorless, and stable in air. It melts between 190° and 196°. Its specific rotation, $[\alpha]_D^{25}$, is not less than +58° and not more than +63° in dioxane solution.

Solubility—Almost insoluble in water; soluble in alcohol, acetone, benzene, and dioxane; slightly soluble in ether; sparingly soluble in vegetable oils.

Uses—This compound is an oil-soluble ester from which *beta*-estradiol is slowly released at the site of intramuscular injection. This provides a depot-action which is prolonged for several days. The sustained low levels of estrogen thus provided are more effective than larger doses of the more rapidly destroyed estrogens, such as estradiol itself. The benzoate is used in the treatment of the same conditions described under estrone but is several times more active.

Estradiol Benzoate has intrinsic biological activity about half that of estradiol, but owing to its sustained action, it is more efficacious.

Dose—*Usual, intramuscular, initial,* **1.0** to **1.66 mg** 2 or 3 times a week for 2 or 3 weeks; *maintenance,* **330 mcg** to **1.0 mg** twice weekly.

Other Dose Information—Estradiol Benzoate is most often administered intramuscularly in doses of from 1 to 1.66 mg 2 or 3 times a week for 2 to 3 injections, gradually adjusting thereafter to a maintenance dose of 0.33 to 1.66 mg 2 or 3 times a week, depending upon the condition.

Dosage Forms—Injection NF: 10 and 33.3 mg/10 ml.

Estradiol Cypionate NF

[Estradiol 17-Cyclopentanepropionate;   Estradiol Cyclopentylpropionate NF XI; Depo-Estradiol (*Upjohn*)]

Estradiol Cypionate contains 97.0–103.0% of C_{26}-$H_{36}O_3$ (396.58), calculated on the dried basis.

For the structure of the base, see *Estradiol.*

Preparation—Estradiol is esterified at both the 3- and 17-positions by treatment with cyclopentylpropionyl chloride in pyridine, the diester being recovered in the usual way by pouring the reaction mixture into an excess of cold, dilute hydrochloric acid. The solid 3,17-diester is collected and treated with potassium carbonate in aqueous methanol whereby saponification is effected only at the 3-position. Water is then added, and the crude 17-ester which precipitates is collected and crystallized from 80% methanol.

Description—It is a white to practically white, odorless, crystalline powder. Melting range 149° to 153°. Specific rotation +39° to +44°.

Solubility—Insoluble in water; soluble in alcohol, acetone, chloroform, and dioxane; sparingly soluble in vegetable oils.

Uses—Estradiol Cypionate has the same actions and uses as Estradiol (see *Estradiol*) and its other official esters (see *Estradiol Benzoate, Valerate,* and *Estradiol Dipropionate*). However, intramuscularly injected vegetable oil solutions of the cyclopentylpropionate (cypionate) have a more prolonged action than do those of the benzoate, valerate, or dipropionate. The average duration of action is 3 to 8 weeks.

Dose—*Usual, intramuscular, initial,* **1** to **5 mg** weekly for 2 to 3 weeks; *maintenance,* **2** to **5 mg** every 3 to 4 weeks.

Dosage Forms—Injection NF: 10 and 50 mg/10 ml, 25 mg/5 ml.

Veterinary Use—Treatment of various reproductive disorders and for the chronologic regulation of estrus in ewes.

Veterinary Dose—*Mares* and *Cows,* 5 to **10 mg;** *Ewes,* 1 to **2 mg;** *Sows,* **1.0 mg;** *Dogs,* 1 to **2 mg;** *Cats,* **0.25** to **0.50 mg.**

Estradiol Dipropionate NF

[1,3,5(10)-Estratriene-3,17β-diol Dipropionate;   Ovocylin Dipropionate
(*Ciba*)]

Estradiol Dipropionate contains 97.0–103.0% of $C_{24}H_{32}O_4$ (384.52), calculated on the dried basis.

For the structure of the base, see *Estradiol*.

Preparation—Estradiol is esterified at both the 3- and 17-positions by treatment with propionyl chloride in pyridine. The diester is recovered in the usual way by pouring the reaction mixture into an excess of cold, dilute HCl.

Description—Small, white or slightly off-white crystals or crystalline powder. It melts between 104° and 109°. Its specific rotation, in dioxane solution, is not less than +37° and not more than +41°.

Solubility—Practically insoluble in water; soluble in acetone and in alcohol; sparingly soluble in vegetable oils.

Uses—Estradiol Dipropionate is half as potent as *Estradiol Benzoate*, but because of a more sustained depot-action the dipropionate is more potent with respect to cumulative maintenance dosage.

Dose—*Usual, intramuscular, initial,* **1** to **5 mg** every 1 to 2 weeks; *maintenance,* **1** to **2.5 mg** every 10 days to 2 weeks.

Dosage Forms—Injection NF: 2.5 mg/ml, 10 and 50 mg/10 ml.

Estradiol Valerate USP

[Estra-1,3,5(10)-triene-3,17β-diol 17-Valerate;   Delestrogen (*Squibb*);   Dura-
trad (*Ascher*)]

Estradiol Valerate is $C_{23}H_{32}O_3$ (356.51).

Preparation—This ester may be prepared by the method described above for the cypionate, using valeryl chloride as the esterificant.

Description—White, crystalline powder. Is usually odorless but may have a faint, fatty odor.

Solubility—Practically insoluble in water; soluble in castor oil, methanol, benzyl benzoate, and dioxane; sparingly soluble in sesame oil and peanut oil.

Uses—Estradiol Valerate is very slowly absorbed from an oil suspension injected intramuscularly; the duration of action of suspensions in oil is about 3 weeks. Its actions, uses and contraindications are those of other estrogens (see the general statement under *Natural Estrogenic Hormones and Derivatives*, page 989, and *Estrone*, this page). In the management of primary or secondary amenorrhea and junctional uterine bleeding, Estradiol Valerate may be administered along with the progestational agent employed.

Dose—*Intramuscular,* **5** to **40 mg** every 1 to 3 weeks; *usual,* **5** to **30 mg** every 2 weeks.

Other Dose Information—Its intramuscular dose, for menstrual disorders or uterine or ovarian dysfunction, is 5 to 20 mg once per menstrual period, and for postpartum breast engorgement, 10 to 25 mg; topical dose, for senile vaginitis, kraurosis vulvae, or pruritus vulvae, 10 to 20 mg every 2 or 3 weeks.

Dosage Forms—Injection USP: 10 and 20 mg/ml, 50, 100, and 200 mg/5 ml.

Conjugated Estrogens USP

[Amnestrogen (*Squibb*); Conestron (*Wyeth*); Menest (*Massengill*); Premarin
(*Ayerst*)]

Conjugated Estrogens is a mixture of the sodium salts of the sulfate esters of the estrogenic substances, principally estrone and equilin, that are of the type excreted by pregnant mares. The content of total estrogens is 90.0–110.0% of the labeled amount. Conjugated Estrogens contains 50.0–65.0% of sodium estrone sulfate, and 20.0–35.0% of sodium equilin sulfate, calculated on the basis of the total estrogens content.

Preparation—The urine of pregnant mares is subjected to a solvent extraction process. US Pats. 2,565,115 and 2,720,483.

Description—A fine, light-brown powder. Since this is a biological, heat and exposure to air and moisture should be avoided. Any exposure will cause the equilin content to lose potency. The odor is pungent, characteristic, and unpleasant.

Solubility—Soluble in water.

Uses—See *Estrone*, this page. Estrone sulfate, the principal constituent of Conjugated Estrogenic Substances, retains a greater potency by the oral route than does Estrone, so that it is superior for oral administration.

Conjugated Estrogens have been advocated for rapid control of spontaneous "capillary bleeding" and to reduce "capillary bleeding" in surgery. However, in controlled studies no hemostatic effect of the conjugated estrogens has been found, and expert medical opinion holds that there is no acceptable evidence for a hemostatic effect.

Dose—*Oral,* **1.25** to **30 mg** daily; *usual, oral,* **1.25** to **2.5 mg** 1 to 3 times a day; *intramuscular or intravenous,* **20** to **40 mg** daily; *usual, intramuscular or intravenous,* **20 mg.**

Other Dose Information—Oral, in the menopause, 1.25 mg daily, and in mammary cancer, 30 mg daily; topical, in senile vaginitis, kraurosis vulvae, and pruritus vulvae, 1.25 to 3.75 mg daily.

Dosage Forms—for Injection USP: 20 mg; Tablets USP: 300 and 625 mcg, 1.25 and 2.5 mg.

Esterified Estrogens USP

Esterified Estrogens is a mixture of the sodium salts of the sulfate esters of the estrogenic substances, principally estrone, that are of the type excreted by pregnant mares. The content of total estrogens is 90.0–110.0% of the labeled amount. Esterified Estrogens contains 70.0–85.0% of sodium estrone sulfate, and 7.5–12.0% of sodium equilin sulfate, calculated on the basis of the total estrogens content.

Description—A buff-colored, amorphous powder. It is odorless or has a slight characteristic odor.

Uses and **Dose**—See *Conjugated Estrogens.*

Dosage Forms—Tablets USP: 300 and 625 mcg, 1.25 and 2.50 mg.

Estrone NF

[3-Hydroxyestra-1,3,5(10)-trien-17-one;   Folliculin;   Menformin (*Organon*);
Theelin (*Parke-Davis*);   Wynestron (*Wyeth*)]

Estrone contains 97.0–103.0% of $C_{18}H_{22}O_2$ (270.37).

Preparation—Estrone was the first sex hormone isolated in pure form (Doisy and Allen in 1929). It is present, along with traces of other estrogens, in the urine of pregnant mares to the extent of about 10 mg per liter and was formerly obtained exclusively from this source. It has also been prepared "synthetically" from stigmasterol, a phytosterol found in soya bean oil. Urinary estrone is regarded as resulting from the metabolic oxidation of the 17-hydroxy group of estradiol to a ketone group.

Estrone is currently prepared from the Mexican yam (*Dioscorea*) via 16-dehydropregnenolone acetate as outlined in the synthesis of *Progesterone* (page 1002). The side chain at position-17 is degraded by first forming the 20-oxime and then effecting Beckmann rearrangement with *p*-acetamidobenzenesulfonyl chloride to the 17-acetamido derivative which on treatment with dilute sulfuric acid forms the enamine acetate and is hydrolyzed to the 17-keto compound, Estrone.

Note—The estrogenic activity of 0.1 mcg of crystalline Estrone constitutes the International Unit of estrogenic activity.

Description—Small, white crystals, or a white to creamy white, crystalline powder. It is odorless and is stable in air. It melts between 256° and 262°. Its specific rotation, $[\alpha]_D^{25}$, is not less than +158° and not more than +165° in dioxane solution.

Solubility—Practically insoluble in water; soluble in alcohol, acetone, dioxane, vegetable oils, and solutions of fixed alkali hydroxides.

Uses—See the general use statement under *Natural Estrogenic Hormones and Derivatives* (page 989).

Dose—*Intramuscular*, **200 mcg** to **5 mg** per week; *usual*, **1 mg** 1 or more times a week as required; reduce to *maintenance* dose as soon as response is obtained.

Dosage Forms—Injection NF: 200 and 500 mcg and 1 mg/ml, 10 mg/10 ml.

Ethinyl Estradiol USP

[17-Ethynylestradiol;   19-Nor-17α-pregna-1,3,5(10)-trien-20-yne-3,17-diol;   Ethynylestradiol;   Estinyl (*Schering*);   Lynoral (*Organon*)]

Ethinyl Estradiol contains 97.0–102.0% of $C_{20}H_{24}O_2$ (296.41), calculated on the dried basis.

Preparation—Ethinyl Estradiol may be prepared by the Nef reaction, or a modification thereof, whereby estrone is caused to react with sodium acetylide in liquid ammonia. Hydrolysis of the sodoxy addition complex yields the desired carbinol. It may also be prepared by a typical Grignard reaction from estrone and ethynyl magnesium bromide.

Description—A white to creamy white, odorless, crystalline powder. In dioxane solution it exhibits a slight dextrorotation. Melting range 142° to 146°; also exists in a polymorphic modification melting between 180° and 186°. Absorptivity 69 to 73 (1%, 1 cm, 281 mμ, 0.05 mg per ml of alcohol solution). The benzoate melts between 200° and 202°.

Solubility—Insoluble in water; soluble in alcohol, chloroform, ether, vegetable oils, and solutions of the fixed alkali hydroxides.

Uses—The actions, uses, and limitations of Ethinyl Estradiol are those of the other estrogens (see the general use statement under *Natural Estrogenic Hormones and Derivatives*, page 989). It has an anovulatory effect at relatively low doses. However, for oral contraceptive action it is usually combined or given sequentially with a progestogen. The ethinyl radical delays the decomposition of the estradiol molecule that occurs during absorption by the oral route. It is one of the most potent oral estrogens known. Ethinyl Estradiol may sometimes cause nausea and vomiting, diarrhea, cramping, headache, skin rashes, and breast engorgement.

Dose—**20 mcg** to **3 mg** daily; *usual*, **50 mcg** 1 to 3 times a day.

Other Dose Information—In the treatment of the menopausal syndrome, a minimal controlling dose should be sought; this may be as low as 20 mcg every other day. For functional uterine bleeding the initial dose is 500 mcg 1 or 2 times a day until bleeding stops, then 50 mcg 1 to 3 times a day during the first 2 weeks of the cycle, after which a progestogen is substituted. For postpartum breast enlargement, 500 mcg are given daily for 3 days, followed by a gradual reduction to 50 mcg over a 7-day period, after which therapy is discontinued. For carcinoma of the breast, 500 mcg 3 times daily. For prostatic carcinoma, 50 to 500 mcg 3 to 6 times a day. As an oral contraceptive, 100 mcg daily in a sequential regimen (this dose is not yet firmly established).

Dosage Forms—Tablets USP: 10, 20, 50, and 500 mcg.

Veterinary Dose—See *Estradiol*.

Ethinyl Estradiol and Dimethisterone Tablets—see page 997.

Ethinyl Estradiol and Medroxyprogesterone Acetate Tablets—see page 1000.

Ethinyl Estradiol and Norethindrone Acetate Tablets—see page 1001.

Other Natural Estrogenic Hormones and Derivatives

Estriol [Theelol (*Parke-Davis*)] [Estra-1,3,5(10)-triene-3,16α,17β-triol ($C_{18}H_{24}O_3$)]—White crystalline powder insoluble in water but soluble in ethanol and oils. A natural estrogenic steroid isolated from the urine of pregnant women; much less estrogenic activity than estrone when injected. *Uses*: Same as for other orally effective estrogenic substances. *Dose*: *Orally*, 0.06 to 0.12 mg 1 to 4 times a day.

Piperazine Estrone Sulfate [Ogen (*Abbott*)]—A white or yellowish-white, crystalline powder. It melts at about 190° forming a light brown syrup, which solidifies on further heating, and finally melts with decomposition at about 245°. It is slightly soluble in alcohol; soluble in water. *Uses*: It has the same actions and uses as *Estrone* (above). It is the piperazine salt of the same sulfate conjugate of estrone that is found in *Conjugated Estrogenic Substances* and, as such, is more effectively absorbed than the other estrogens. *Dose*: *Orally*, 1.5 to 4.5 mg daily; 4.5 mg 6 times daily for postpartum breast engorgement.

Synthetic Estrogens

The exciting discovery by Dodds and co-workers in 1938 that diethylstilbestrol and other relatively simple nonsteroidal organic compounds possessed estrogenic activity gave considerable impetus to research in this field during the next decade. This research was designed to discover compounds which had more favorable therapeutic indexes because of either greater potency or lesser toxicity. Hundreds of compounds were synthesized and tested and numerous methods for the synthesis of these compounds starting with readily available materials have been devised.

Attempts to explain why such non-steroidal compounds are estrogenically potent have been intriguing. Dodds pointed out that when the formulas are written appropriately there is a spatial resemblance between them and the true hormone estradiol. Others have focused attention on the closeness of the dimensions of the synthetics (especially length, width, and distance between OH groups) with those of estradiol. It has been proposed that such spatial considerations suggest a steric fitting of the hormone (or of the synthetics) with some enzyme system. However, the configuration of methallenestril does not conform to the hypothetical dimensions prerequisite to activity.

These synthetic materials cost less to manufacture than do the natural materials, and also there is less loss of potency when therapy by the oral route is compared with the parenteral. Regarding the latter comparison it must be recalled that the oral doses of natural estrogens, with the possible exception of ethinyl estradiol (a derivative of a natural estrogen), may have to be five or more times that of the parenteral doses to secure similar results. This appears due to metabolic changes in the liver and also loss due to excretion into the bile, as well as to destruction in the digestive tract. One disadvantage of some synthetic estrogenic compounds is that nausea follows use of even the minimum effective dose in some women, but probably not over 20% of those who use the materials carefully. In such women the synthetic materials must be replaced by natural products. One other slight difference which is possibly debatable is the general impression that the natural estrogens give the patient a greater feeling of well-being than do the synthetics.

Benzestrol NF

[4,4'-(1,2-Diethyl-3-methyltrimethylene)diphenol; (*Various Mfgs.*)]

Benzestrol, dried at 105° for 1 hour, contains 98.5–100.5% of $C_{20}H_{26}O_2$ (298.43).

Preparation—Benzestrol may be prepared by the following series of reactions. *p,p'*-Dimethoxy-2-ethyl-3-methylchalcone (I) is subjected to a Grignard reaction with ethylmagnesium bromide. The resulting unsaturated alcohol is hydrogenated in alcohol solution with the aid of Raney-nickel catalyst to form benzestrol dimethylether. This is then demethylated by heating with alcoholic potassium hydroxide under pressure. The crude product is purified by vacuum distillation. The starting chalcone (I) may be prepared

I

by condensing 1-*p*-methoxypropiophenone with 1-*p*-methoxybutyrophenone with the aid of dry hydrogen chloride or other suitable dehydrating agents.

Description—White, crystalline powder. A 1 in 50 solution in ether is clear and colorless. A 1 in 50 solution in previously neutralized 80% alcohol is neutral. It melts between 161° and 163°.

Solubility—Practically insoluble in water and in dilute mineral acids; readily soluble in acetone, ethanol, ether, methanol, and sodium hydroxide TS; soluble in vegetable oils; moderately soluble in glacial acetic acid; slightly soluble in dilute alcohol, benzene, chloroform, and solvent hexane.

Uses—Benzestrol has the uses, actions and limitations of the other estrogens (see the general use statement under *Natural Estrogenic Hormones and Derivatives* (page 989). One mg of Benzestrol is equivalent to 2.5 mg of estrone. The incidence of toxicity with Benzestrol is low. Intramuscular doses are generally the same as oral doses.

Dose—500 mcg to 5 mg; *usual,* 1 to 2 mg daily.

Dosage Forms—Tablets NF: 1, 2, and 5 mg.

Chlorotrianisene NF

[Chlorotris(*p*-methoxyphenyl)ethylene; Tri-*p*-anisylchloroethylene; Tace (*Merrell*)]

Chlorotrianisene, dried at 80° for 18 hours, contains 97.0–103.0% of $C_{23}H_{21}ClO_3$ (380.88).

Preparation—An alcoholic solution of anisaldehyde is refluxed with potassium cyanide to yield anisoin which may be converted to deoxyanisoin (I) by reduction with zinc and hydrochloric acid. Performing a Grignard reaction on (I) with *p*-methoxyphenylmagnesium bromide yields 1,1,2-tri-*p*-anisylethanol (II). Dehydration of (II) by treatment with phosphoric acid produces 1,1,2-tri-*p*-anisylethene which is chlorinated directly in carbon tetrachloride solution. The resulting crude chlorotrianisene is purified by recrystallization from an acetone-alcohol mixture.

Description—Small white crystals, or as a crystalline powder. It is odorless and stable in air. It melts between 115° and 117°, and has a pH between 5 and 7.

Solubility—1 Gm dissolves in about 4200 ml of water, 360 ml of ethanol or methanol, 28 ml of ether, 7 ml of acetone, 2.5 ml of benzene, and about 1.5 ml of chloroform; practically insoluble in 2,2,4-trimethylpentane.

Uses—Chlorotrianisene is an estrogen with most of the actions, uses and limitations of the other estrogens. See the general use statement under *Natural Estrogenic Hormones and Derivatives* (page 989). However, it is unique in that its potency is greater by the oral than by any other route, a fact that suggests that the drug is converted in the liver to a more active form. Also, it apparently induces less anterior pituitary and adrenal hyperplasia than other estrogens. In fact, it appears to be *anti*estrogenic at the hypothalamic locus that regulates adenohypophyseal gonadotropin release. Furthermore, it causes a lesser incidence of withdrawal bleeding. It is stored in the fat, from which it is slowly released to give a sustained action.

Dose—12 to 50 mg; *usual,* 24 mg daily.

Dosage Forms—Capsules NF: 12, 25, and 72 mg.

Dienestrol NF

[4,4'-(Diethylidineethylene)diphenol; Dienœstrol; Restro (*Central*); Synestrol (*White*)]

Dienestrol contains 98.0–100.5% of $C_{18}H_{18}O_2$ (266.34), calculated on the dried basis.

Preparation—Among other methods, Dienestrol may be prepared from diethylstilbestrol diacetate. Saturation of the olefinic bond with bromine yields the dibromo derivative which is then dehydrobrominated by refluxing with pyridine to yield dienestrol diacetate. Saponification then yields Dienestrol.

Description—Dienestrol occurs as colorless or white, or practically white, odorless needle-like crystals or as a white, crystalline powder. It melts between 227° and 231°.

Solubility—Practically insoluble in water; soluble in alcohol, acetone, ether, methanol, propylene glycol, and solutions of fixed alkali hydroxides; slightly soluble in chloroform and fatty oils.

Uses—Same as for *Diethylstilbestrol* (below). However, it gives rise to fewer untoward effects than does Diethylstilbestrol.

Dose—*Oral*, **100 mcg** to **1.5 mg**; *usual, oral*, **500 mcg** daily; *vaginal*, **5 Gm** of a **0.01**% cream once or twice a day for 7 to 14 days, then once every 48 hours for 7 to 14 days.

Dosage Forms—Cream NF: 0.01%; Tablets NF: 100 and 500 mcg.

Diethylstilbestrol USP

[(E) α,α'-Diethyl-4,4'-stilbenediol; Stilbœstrol; Stilbetin (*Squibb*)]

Diethylstilbestrol contains 97.0–100.5% of $C_{18}H_{20}O_2$ (268.36), calculated on the dried basis.

Preparation—Diethylstilbestrol is a synthetic estrogen first synthesized by Dodds, *et al*, in 1938. As to be expected, the compound exists in 2 geometric isomeric forms. The *cis*-isomer, which has less than one-tenth the activity of the *trans* and does not form readily, is unstable and tends to revert to the *trans*-isomer; hence the official product is *trans*-diethylstilbestrol.

Several methods of synthesis have been devised. That of Kharasch and Kleiman[2] uses anethole hydrobromide as the starting material and is most convenient.

Description—A white, odorless, crystalline powder. It melts between 169° and 172°.

Solubility—Almost insoluble in water; soluble in alcohol, ether, chloroform, fatty oils, and dilute alkali hydroxides.

Uses—Diethylstilbestrol is used for the same conditions for which natural estrogens are employed and the contraindications are also the same. See the general use statement under *Natural Estrogenic Hormones and*

Derivatives (page 989) and *Synthetic Estrogens* (page 992). It is advantageous because it is well absorbed orally. The ratio of single oral to parenteral dose varies from 2 to 5. However, because the interval between oral doses is usually the shorter, the maintenance oral dose is nearly the same as the parenteral dose.

Nausea, vomiting, and headache may frequently accompany its use. Nausea and vomiting appear to be caused, in part, by local actions of the drug. Enteric coatings on tablets slow the rate of release and lessen the incidence and intensity of such local effects. It is advised to start with the smaller doses for patients who tend to develop disagreeable symptoms such as nausea.

The dipropionate ester provides a longer action when administered in oil solution intramuscularly.

Dose—*Oral*, **100 mcg** to **15 mg** daily; *intramuscular*, **100 mcg** 2 times a week to **5 mg** 3 times a day; *usual, oral, intramuscular*, or *vaginal*, **100 mcg** to **1 mg** once a day.

Dosage Forms—Injection USP: 1 and 5 mg/ml, 50 and 250 mg/10 ml, 30, 60, 150, and 750 mg, and 1.5 Gm/30 ml; Suppositories USP: 100 and 500 mcg and 1 mg; Tablets USP: 50, 100, 250, and 500 mcg and 1, 2, 5, 10, 25, 50, and 100 mg.

Veterinary Use—Replacement therapy for under-developed females; incontinence, vaginitis of spayed bitches. To induce heat in anestrus. In uterine inertia, pyometra. To check milk secretion in pseudopregnancy; prevent conception in mismated bitches. In hypertrophy of prostate in dogs. Chemical caponization of poultry.

Veterinary Dose—*Intramuscularly, Horses*, **10 to 25 mg**; *Cows, Heifers*, and *Small Breeds*, **10 to 20 mg**; *Large breeds*, **20 to 25 mg**; *Sheep*, **2 to 3 mg**; *Swine*, **3 to 10 mg**; *Dogs*, **0.2 to 1.0 mg** intramuscularly or orally. *Pyometra, Cows*, **30 to 50 mg** intramuscularly. *Caponization of poultry*, **15 to 30 mg** subcutaneously. *Caution:* Lactation, pregnancy.

Diethylstilbestrol Dipropionate NF

[(E) α,α'-Diethyl-4,4'-stilbenediol Dipropionate]

Diethylstilbestrol Dipropionate contains 98.0–100.5% of $C_{24}H_{28}O_4$ (380.49), calculated on the dried basis.

For the structure of the diol, see *Diethylstilbestrol;* both hydroxyl groups are esterified.

Preparation—Diethylstilbestrol may be propionylated by dissolving it in a mixture of propionic anhydride and propionic acid and refluxing. The crude ester precipitates upon dilution of the reaction mixture with water and is purified by recrystallization from ethanol or another suitable solvent.

Description—White, odorless, tasteless, crystalline powder. A 1 in 100 suspension in diluted alcohol is neutral to litmus. Melting range: 105° to 107°.

Solubility—Very slightly soluble in water and dilute mineral acids; insoluble in solutions of alkali hydroxides; soluble in vegetable oils; readily soluble in acetone, benzene, chloroform, ether, hot ethanol, and hot methanol.

Uses—The actions and uses of Diethylstilbestrol Dipropionate are those of the estrogens in general (see the general use statement under *Natural Estrogenic Hormones and Derivatives*, page 989). However, the dipropionate is more soluble in oil than is Diethylstilbestrol, and oil solutions are often given intramuscularly for their depot action. Nausea and vomiting are less frequent with the dipropionate than with the parent Diethylstilbestrol.

Dose—*Usual*, **100 mcg** to **1 mg** per day.

Other Dose Information—Usual doses are as follows: oral, 0.1 to 1 mg 3 times a day; intramuscular, 0.5 to 2 mg 2 or 3 times a week except 3 mg daily for prostatic cancer or 5 mg 1 or 2 times a day for breast engorgement.

Dosage Forms—Injection: 0.5, 1, and 5 mg/ml; Tablets NF: 500 mcg, 1 and 5 mg.

Veterinary Dose—See *Diethylstilbestrol*.

Mestranol USP

[3-Methoxy-19-nor-17α-pregna-1,3,5(10)-trien-20-yn-17-ol; (*Lilly*)]

Mestranol contains 97.0–100.5% of $C_{21}H_{26}O_2$ (310.44).

Preparation—Estrone is converted to its 3-methoxy analogue by reaction with methyl sulfate. The ethynyl group may then be introduced at position 17 either through reaction with sodium acetylide in liquid ammonia followed by hydrolysis of the sodoxy compound, or through Grignardization with ethynyl bromide. US Pat. 2,666,769.

Description—White to off-white, odorless powder, occasionally in the form of small plates. It melts between 148° and 154°.

Solubility—Freely soluble in chloroform; sparingly soluble in ether; slightly soluble in alcohol; insoluble in water.

Uses—Mestranol possesses estrogenic activity. It is readily absorbed by the oral route and hence has advantages over several of the natural estrogens. In high doses the drug inhibits the release of pituitary gonadotropins and is thus useful for suppressing ovulation in the treatment of endometriosis and as an oral contraceptive. It was a contaminant in early preparations of norethynodrel. Such impure preparations were superior to pure norethynodrel for oral contraception. Therefore, Mestranol is incorporated with Norethynodrel in the now famous oral contraceptive, *Norethynodrel and Mestranol* (page 1002) and with Norethindrone in *Norethindrone and Mestranol* (page 1000). When it occurs, it is likely that inhibition of pituitary gonadotropin production is more attributable to the estrogenic ether than to the norethynodrel or norethindrone. However, oral contraceptive preparations containing Mestranol do not suppress ovulation in a large fraction of users, and the oral contraceptive effect cannot thus be correctly attributed to an anovulatory effect of the estrogen.

Dose—**USP**: **50** to **150 mcg** daily in combination with a progestin; *usual*, **50** to **80 mcg** once a day in combination with a progestin. **NF**: **80** to **100 mcg** daily for 20 days of each menstrual cycle.

Dosage Forms—Tablets NF: 80 to 100 mcg. See also combinations referred to, below.

Chlormadinone Acetate and Mestranol Tablets—see page 997.

Ethynodiol Diacetate and Mestranol Tablets—see page 999.

Norethindrone and Mestranol Tablets—see page 1000.

Norethynodrel and Mestranol Tablets—see page 1002.

Other Synthetic Estrogenic Hormones

Diethylstilbestrol Diphosphate [Stilphostrol (*Dome*)] is α,α′-diethyl-4,4′-stilbenediol diphosphoric acid ester ($C_{18}H_{22}O_8P_2$). *Preparation:* By esterifying *Diethylstilbestrol* (page 994) through reaction with phosphorus oxychloride in the presence of pyridine. *Description* and *Solubility:* A voluminous, white, crystalline powder that melts with decomposition between 204° and 206°. Sparingly soluble in water.

Uses: The actions of Diethylstilbestrol Diphosphate are the same as those of Diethylstilbestrol (page 994). It is claimed that it is better tolerated than Diethylstilbestrol, but the basis for the claim is tenuous. However, it can be given intravenously, which is advantageous in those rare circumstances in which intravenous administration is indicated. Although the drug may be used in all situations in which other estrogens are used, however, it is promoted principally for the treatment of *prostatic carcinoma*, a disorder which demands very large doses of estrogen. The manufacturer contends that it is often effective when other estrogens fail to exert an effect, although it is difficult to explain why this should be so. *Dose: Intravenous, initial*, 500 mg, dispersed in 250 to 300 ml of isotonic saline or dextrose; *maintenance*, 1 Gm; *oral, initial*, 50 mg 3 times a day; *maintenance*, up to 200 mg 3 times a day.

Hexestrol NF XI [Dihydrodiethylstilbestrol; 4,4′-(1,2-Diethylethylene)diphenol]—A white, odorless crystalline powder with a melting range of 185° to 188°. It is freely soluble in ether; soluble in acetone, alcohol, and methanol; slightly soluble in benzene and chloroform; practically insoluble in water and dilute mineral acids. It dissolves in vegetable oils and in solutions of fixed alkali hydroxides. *Uses:* A synthetic estrogen. See *Estrone* (page 991). *Dose:* 200 mcg to 3 mg; *orally*, 2 to 3 mg daily until symptoms are controlled and then 0.2 to 1 mg daily; *intramuscular*, in oil, 1 mg 3 times weekly.

Methallenestril [Vallestril (*Searle*)] is β-ethyl-6-methoxy-α,α-dimethyl-2-naphthalenepropionic acid. *Description and Solubility:* A white, microcrystalline powder which has a slight characteristic odor. It melts between 135° and 141°. Freely soluble in chloroform; soluble in ether and alcohol; insoluble in water. *Uses:* A synthetic estrogen the actions and uses of which are those of the estrogens in general (see the general use statement under *Natural Estrogenic Hormones and Derivatives*, page 989). Its potency is about that of estrone and $\frac{1}{10}$ that of diethylstilbestrol. The incidence of nausea and vomiting is less than that of diethylstilbestrol and about the same as that of other synthetic estrogens. The incidence of withdrawal bleeding may be less than with other estrogens. *Dose: Oral, initial*, 6 to 9 mg daily, except 20 mg daily for breast engorgement or prostatic carcinoma, with gradual adjustments to a *maintenance* dose of 3 mg daily.

Promethestrol Dipropionate [o,o′-Dimethylhexestrol Dipropionate; Meprane Dipropionate (*Reed & Carnrick*)] is 4,4′-(1,2-diethylene)di-o-cresol dipropionate. *Description and Solubility:* Crystals which melt at 115°. A solution in alcohol (90%) is neutral to litmus. Freely soluble in ether, ethyl acetate, and benzene; slightly soluble in alcohol; practically insoluble in water, dilute acids, and dilute alkalies. *Uses:* Its actions and uses are those of the other estrogens, especially *Diethylstilbestrol* (page 994). See also the general use statement under *Natural Estrogenic Hormones and Derivatives* (page 989). *Dose: Oral, initial*, 1 mg 3 times daily with gradual reduction to once daily.

Antiestrogens

In a broad sense, antiestrogens are substances which suppress the effects of estrogens, regardless of mechanism. Androgens and progestogens would thus qualify as incomplete antiestrogens, since they are antagonists to estrogens in some of their effects. With the advent of competitive antagonists of estrogens the term antiestrogen has become restricted in use to apply only to such drugs. A number of estrogens have been found which reduce the intensity of response to other estrogens, behavior as partial agonists, as it were. Some substances appear to exert antiestrogenic effects only on some but not all target organs; for example, chlorotrianisene is estrogenic in the periphery but antiestrogenic in the hypothalamus, so that it interrupts the normal negative feedback system that modulates anterior pituitary gonadotropin release. A closely related compound, clomiphene, has even a stronger antiestrogenic action in the hypothalamus but is sufficiently weak in the periphery so as not to interfere with the peripheral effects of endogenously released estrogens. By blocking the effects of endogenous estrogen to suppress adenohypophyseal release of gonadotropins, antiestrogens allow the anterior pituitary to produce more gonadotropins than normally. The ovaries are thus stimulated to a greater extent and follicular development and maturation are enhanced. In cases of infertility resulting from failure to ovulate this effect may result in ovulation and the development of fertility.

Clomiphene Citrate [$C_{26}H_{28}ClNO.C_6H_8O_7$ (598.10); Clomid (*Merrell*)] is 2-[p-(2-chloro-1,2-diphenylvinyl)phenoxy]triethylamine citrate (1:1). *Preparation:* 4-Hydroxy-benzophenone is condensed with 2-(diethylamino)ethyl chloride in toluene in the presence of alkali. The 4-[2-(diethylamino)ethoxy]benzophenone thus formed is Grignardized with benzyl chloride and the tertiary carbinol thus produced is dehydrated to give 2-[p-(1,2-diphenylvinyl)phenoxy]triethylamine. This compound is chlorinated to yield clomiphene (base) which is permitted to react with an equimolar quantity of citric acid. *Description and Solubility:* A white, crystalline powder that is odorless and tasteless. It is not appreciably hygroscopic. It melts with decomposition between 117° and 119°. Sparingly soluble in alcohol; slightly soluble in water and chloroform; insoluble in ether. *Uses:* Clomiphene Citrate is an antiestrogen (see the General Statement above) that is employed to induce ovulation and hence to *promote fertility* in anovulatory women who have functional adenohypophysis and ovaries. In patients who have reached the menopause or who have gonadal dysgenesis, panhypopituitarrism, or Sheehan's syndrome the drug is of no benefit. Some of the untoward effects of the drug are attributable to the increase in gonadotropin levels caused by the drug. Enlarged ovaries and ovarian cysts are the principal disorders. Also, a disproportionate number of multiple births occur among treated women. Hot flashes and vasomotor reactions may occur, but it is not clear whether they are consequent to ovarian stimulation or are a direct effect. Blurred vision, scintillation, and scotomata sometimes occur but disappear after cessation of treatment. A reversible thinning of hair also occurs. The drug should be used cautiously in the presence of ovarian cysts or in persons who have a history of cysts or in any condition of abnormal uterine function. The drug is contraindicated in patients with liver disease. *Dose:* 50 mg daily for 5 days, starting at anytime if there have been no recent menses or on the 5th day of the extrapolated menstrual cycle. If ovulation does not occur, additional courses with 100-mg doses may be tried, but it is imperative that the dose not exceed 100 mg.

Progestational Substances and Oral Contraceptives

The second type of hormone produced in the ovaries is *progesterone*, which is excreted in the form of pregnanediol glucuronide. Although it originates in cells which also may produce estrogen and although it has a molecular structure very similar to that of the estrogens, progesterone has a unique physiological action. Under its influence the numerous minute glands which line the uterine cavity are transformed into secreting glands. This alteration is a part of the change which is essential to provide for the implantation of a fertilized ovum and for the continuing development of the placenta. This endometrial alteration requires the cooperation of an estrogen; in the absence of an estrogen, a progestogen that is devoid of estrogenic activity will exert an atrophic effect on the endometrium. Progestins also cause a change in the cervical secretions to suppress "ferning," a dendritic crystallization of cervical mucopolysaccharides. When the cervical mucus is not dendritic, it forms a tight net of fibers, through which it is believed sperm cannot pass. The antifertility effect of some progestogens may possibly be due to the suppression of ferning. Progesterone has the ability to stimulate development of the glandular portions of the mammæ, and also exerts some effects upon the capacity of tissues to retain water in the intercellular spaces.

Most oral contraceptives contain both an estrogen and a progestogen or estrogens and progestogens are used sequentially. The use of certain progestogens alone is still exploratory. Oral contraceptive mixtures are included here, rather than under *Estrogens*, simply because historically interest in contraception began with progestogens.

Chlormadinone Acetate NF

[6-Chloro-17-hydroxypregna-4,6-diene-3,20-dione Acetate; Lormin (*Lilly*)]

Chlormadinone Acetate contains 97.0–102.0% of $C_{23}H_{29}ClO_4$ (404.94), calculated on the dried basis.

Preparation—Chlormadinone Acetate may be prepared from 17-hydroxypregna-4,6-diene-3,20-dione acetate. Reaction with peroxyphthalic acid attacks the 6-double bond forming the corresponding 6α,7α-oxidopregn-4-ene compound. Subsequent treatment with hydrogen chloride ruptures the oxido bridge forming the 6-chloro-7-hydroxy compound which readily dehydrates to recreate the 6-double bond.[3]

Description—An off-white to pale yellow, fluffy, crystalline powder that is odorless. It is stable in light and is nonhygroscopic. It melts between 206° and 214°.

Solubility—Freely soluble in chloroform; slightly soluble in acetone, alcohol, ether, and chloroform; practically insoluble in water.

Uses—Chlormadinone Acetate is a progestogen that is used primarily as an oral contraceptive. In high doses (2 to 4 mg per day) it inhibits ovulation, suppresses the endometrium, and reduces the fluidity and ferning of the cervical mucus. At low doses (0.5 mg per day) its effects are only on the cervical mucus. Nevertheless, in low doses it still exerts a strong contraceptive effect and Chlormadinone is one of the progestogens that is under investigation as an oral contraceptive that does not require the inclusion of an estrogen. It appears that it may be used successfully in low doses continuously in most instances without interfering with a normal estrous cycle and menses or with nursing. However, menstrual irregularities, such as breakthrough bleeding or amenorrhea, occur in up to 12% of continuous users of this drug. In the US the contraceptive use of Chlormadinone alone is not officially approved, and the drug is marketed in a sequential combination with mestranol. Chlormadinone may be used for other progestational uses (see *Progesterone*, page 1002).

In addition to menstrual irregularities when used alone, in 1 to 5% of patients Chlormadinone may cause pelvic fullness, abdominal and pelvic cramping, mastalgia, chloasma, irritability, or acne.

Dose—See *Chlormadinone Acetate and Mestranol Tablets*.

Other Dose Information—Oral, 2 mg or as determined by the physician according to the needs of the patient.

Chlormadinone Acetate and Mestranol Tablets NF

[C-Quens (*Lilly*)]

Chlormadinone Acetate and Mestranol Tablets contain 90.0–110.0% of the labeled amount of $C_{23}H_{29}ClO_4$ (chlormadinone acetate), and of $C_{21}H_{26}O_2$ (mestranol).

Uses—Chlormadinone Acetate and Mestranol are used in a sequential regimen for oral contraception. For the actions of the separate components, see *Chlormadinone Acetate* (above) and *Mestranol* (page 995). The estrogen is given first, and it promotes a proliferative endometrium; the progestogen converts the endometrium to the secretory type. Within a few days after medication is interrupted, menstruation begins. Thus a normal menstrual cycle is simulated. The antifertility effect is due to mestranol, which is used in a higher dose than in the oral contraceptive mixtures. The effect is mainly an anovulatory one. The most frequent side effects are mostly those of Mestranol. They are nausea, abdominal cramps, breakthrough bleeding and other menstrual irregularities (including amenorrhea), malaise, anorexia, and vomiting. Breast tenderness, diarrhea, drowsiness, nervousness, premenstrual tension, edema and weight gain, and headache also occur.

Dose—Beginning on day 5 of menstrual cycle, **80 mcg** of mestranol daily for 15 days, then **80 mcg** of mestranol and **2 mg** of chlormadinone acetate daily for 5 days.

Dosage Forms—Tablets NF: 2 mg (chlormadi-

none acetate) and 80 mcg (mestranol) in separate tablets.

Dimethisterone NF

[17β-Hydroxy-6α-methyl-17-(1-propynyl)androst-4-en-3-one]

Dimethisterone contains 97.0–103.0% of $C_{23}H_{32}O_2 \cdot H_2O$ (358.52).

Preparation—Epoxidation of 17α-(1-propynyl)-androst-5-ene-3β-17β-diol with perphthalic acid gives 5α,6α - epoxy - 17α - (1 - propynyl)androstane - 3β,17β-diol. After protecting the 3β-hydroxyl by propylation, treatment with methylmagnesium bromide yields 6β - methyl - 17α - (1 - propynyl)androstane - 3β,5α,-17β-triol. Oppenauer oxidation of this triol followed by dehydration of the 5α-hydroxyl and an acid catalyzed epimerization gives Dimethisterone.

Description—A white, crystalline powder. It is odorless and tasteless. It is stable in light and is nonhygroscopic. It melts at about 110° with decomposition.

Solubility—1 Gm dissolves in 0.7 ml of chloroform; 1 ml of pyridine, and 3 ml of alcohol; slightly soluble in acetone; practically insoluble in water.

Uses—Dimethisterone is a progestogen with actions and uses similar to *Norethindrone* (page 1000), of which it is a dimethyl derivative. However, its estrogenic and androgenic actions are both weaker. Although it probably is as efficacious as other progestogens in the various types of progestational therapy, it is presently promoted only for use in sequence with a suitable estrogen (marketed with Ethinyl Estradiol) for oral contraception (see the general statement under *Ovarian Hormones*). Side effects include edema and weight gain and breast engorgement and tenderness.

Dose—See *Ethinyl Estradiol and Dimethisterone Tablets* (below).

Other Dose Information—An estrogen is given alone on the 5th through the 16th day of the cycle. Dimethisterone plus estrogen are given on the 21st through the 25th days.

Ethinyl Estradiol and Dimethisterone Tablets NF

[Oracon (*Mead-Johnson*)]

Ethinyl Estradiol and Dimethisterone Tablets contain 90.0–115.0% of the labeled amount of $C_{20}H_{24}O_2$ (ethinyl estradiol), and 90.0–110.0% of the labeled amount of $C_{23}H_{32}O_2 \cdot H_2O$ (dimethisterone).

Uses—Ethinyl Estradiol and Dimethisterone are primarily intended for use in a sequential regimen for oral contraception. For the actions of the separate components, see *Ethinyl Estradiol* (page 992) and *Dimethisterone* (above). The estrogen is given first, and it promotes a proliferative endometrium. When the progestogen is administered, the endometrium is converted to the secretory phase. Menstruation follows within a few days after the pause in treatment. Thus a normal menstrual cycle is simulated. The antifertility effect is the result of interference with pituitary release of gonadotropin (especially FSH) and is due to the estrogen. The adverse effects are mainly those of Ethinyl Estradiol; they result in discontinuation of medication in 4 to 5% of users. Nausea is the most frequent side effect. Vomiting, abdominal cramps, anorexia, malaise, bloating, breakthrough bleeding, changes in the amount and duration of menstrual flow (including amenorrhea), and mucorrhea are also common. It is not definite whether rare venous thrombosis is caused by the estrogen component. Headache, changes in libido, nervousness, weight gain, breast tenderness, dizziness, diarrhea, drowsiness, and premenstrual tension also occur; several of these effects are due to Dimethisterone.

Dose—*Usual, ethinyl estradiol*, **100 mcg** daily for 20 days of each menstrual cycle; *dimethisterone*, **25 mg** daily for 5 days of each cycle.

Other Dose Information—What the above ambiguously stated official dose really means is, ethinyl estradiol is given alone for the first 15 days, *then* ethinyl estradiol plus dimethisterone are given for the next 5 days; however, according to the manufacturer and clinical experience, ethinyl estradiol should be taken for *16*, not 15, days.

Dosage Forms—Tablets NF: 100 mcg (ethinyl estradiol) and 25 mg (dimethisterone).

Dydrogesterone NF

[9β,10α-Pregna-4,6-diene-3,20-dione; Isopregnenone; Duphaston (*Philips-Roxane*); Gynorest (*Mead-Johnson*)]

Dydrogesterone contains 98.0–102.0% of $C_{21}H_{28}O_2$ (312.46), calculated on the dried basis.

Preparation—This compound will be recognized as a dehydrogenated stereoisomer of progesterone; ie, 6,7-didehydro-9β,10α-progesterone. It has been referred to as 6-dehydro*retro*progesterone, the *retro* implying that the C_9-C_{10} stereoconfiguration is opposite to that observed in the natural hormone.

Dydrogesterone may be prepared from lumista-4,6,22-trien-3-one which is the ketone related to a lumisterol produced by ultraviolet irradiation of ergosterol and in which the C_9-C_{10} stereoconfiguration is of the *retro* variety. The over-all process consists of changing the C_9H_{19} group at C_{17} in the starting ketone to the required $COCH_3$ group. The process is lengthy and is described in detail in US Pat. 3,198,792 along with procedures for preparing various other *retro*-steroids. Descriptions are also given in *Rec. Trav. Chim.*[4,5]

Description—A white to pale yellow, odorless and tasteless, crystalline powder. It melts between 167.5° and 170.5°.

Solubility—Freely soluble in alcohol, chloroform, and methanol; slightly soluble in water.

Uses—Dydrogesterone is a *progestogen*. Its actions and uses are similar to those of *Progesterone* (page 1002). Unlike progesterone, it is orally effective. It also differs in that it is not thermogenic. In doses several times the usual dose it does not appear to inhibit pituitary output of gonadotropin or interfere with the normal development of the corpus luteum. However, when estrogens are concomitantly administered, the combination can inhibit ovulation and delay menstruation. It has neither estrogenic nor androgenic activity.

Dose—**10** to **30 mg**; *usual*, **10** to **20 mg** daily in divided doses.

Other Dose Information—For threatened abortion, initial, 20 to 40 mg and usually 5 to 10 mg daily until symptoms cease; for habitual abortion, 10 mg daily following the first missed period; for primary and secondary amenorrhea, 10 to 20 mg daily on the 15th through the 25th days after menstruation begins; for primary dysmenorrhea, 10 to 20 mg daily for 21 days beginning on the 5th day after menstruation begins, for 2 or 3 cycles; for endometriosis, 20 mg daily; for pregnancy test, 10 mg daily for 5 days.

Dosage Forms—Tablets NF: 5, 10, and 20 mg.

Ethisterone NF

[17-Hydroxy-17α-pregn-4-en-20-yn-3-one; Pregneninolone; 17-Ethinyltestosterone; Anhydrohydroxyprogesterone; Pranone (*Schering*); Progestoral (*Organon*)]

Ethisterone contains 98.0–102.0% of $C_{21}H_{28}O_2$ (312.46), calculated on the dried basis.

Preparation—Among various other methods, it may be prepared by causing acetylene to react with dehydroepiandrosterone in the presence of potassium *tert*-butoxide followed by Oppenauer oxidation. The over-all effects are addition of acetylene to the 17-carbonyl group forming the ethynyl carbinol group, oxidation of the carbinol group at the 3-position to carbonyl, and rearrangement of the 5,6 double bond in the starting compound to the 4,5 position.

Description—White or slightly yellow crystals or a crystalline powder. It is odorless and is stable in air, but is affected by light. It melts between 267° and 275°. The specific rotation, $[\alpha]_D^{25}$, determined in pyridine solution is between +29° and +33°.

Solubility—Practically insoluble in water; slightly soluble in alcohol, ether, chloroform, or vegetable oils; moderately soluble in dioxane, methanol, and pyridine.

Uses—Ethisterone is a *progestogen* with the same uses as *Progesterone*, but this steroid hormone has approximately ⅕ the progesterone action when taken orally as has progesterone itself given intramuscularly. In many progestational uses, such as the treatment of threatened abortion, Ethisterone has not proved to be very satisfactory, and many authorities decline to use it, although the supposed oral efficacy obviously should be attractive. As with progesterone, it is likely that the usual doses are too small. It is mainly used in conjunction with an estrogen for the treatment of *functional amenorrhea, dysfunctional uterine bleeding*, and *dysmenorrhea*. Such combinations are also used as a test for pregnancy; if uterine bleeding occurs within 2 to 10 days following a 3-day course, started in the first week after the menses is missed, the patient is *not* pregnant.

Dose—*Usual*, **25 mg** up to 4 times a day.

Dosage Forms—Tablets NF: 5, 10, and 25 mg.

Ethynodiol Diacetate USP

[19-Nor-17α-pregn-4-en-20-yne-3β,17-diol Diacetate]

Ethynodiol Diacetate contains 97.0–102.0% of $C_{24}H_{32}O_4$ (384.52).

Preparation—Ethynodiol Diacetate may be prepared from *Norethindrone* (page 1000) by reducing the keto group to the carbinol state and then esterifying the 3- and 17-hydroxyls with acetyl chloride in the presence of pyridine.

Description—A white, odorless, crystalline powder. It is stable in air. It melts between 126° and 132°.

Solubility—Insoluble in water; very soluble in chloroform; freely soluble in ether; soluble in alcohol; sparingly soluble in fixed oils.

Uses—Ethynodiol Diacetate is a *progestogen* with actions and uses similar to *Norethindrone* (page 1000), to which it is closely related chemically. However, because of the hydroxyl rather than keto character of the 3 position of the A ring, Ethynodiol has stronger estrogenic activity and is essentially devoid of androgenic activity. It is useful in the treatment of all conditions in which progestogens are indicated (see the General Statement, page 996, and *Progesterone*, page 1002). Ethynodiol Diacetate is promoted as an *oral contraceptive*, for which purpose it is combined with an estrogen (marketed with Mestranol); however, because of its inherent estrogenic activity, Ethynodiol Diacetate could probably be used alone. It suppresses the midcycle elevation of luteotropin that is the immediate stimulus to ovulation. Side effects include breast engorgement and tenderness, edema and weight gain, and thermogenesis.

Dose—*Usual*, **1 mg** once a day as component of combination with estrogen.

Ethynodiol Diacetate and Mestranol Tablets

[Ovulen (*Searle*)]

Uses—Ethynodiol Diacetate and Mestranol is an *oral contraceptive mixture* that differs little from other mixtures of this type. For the actions of the separate components, see *Ethynodiol Diacetate* (above) and *Mestranol* (page 995). The mixture prevents ovulation, more by a suppression of the release of LH than of FSH. The mixture also moderately suppresses the proliferative development of the endometrium. The mixture may also be used in other conditions in which progestogens are indicated, particularly in those situations in which anovulation is desired (see *Progesterone*, page 1002). In large doses it may also be used to arrest dysfunctional uterine bleeding. Adverse effects in decreasing order of incidence are nausea, spotting, breakthrough bleeding, headache, dizziness, depression, edema, amenorrhea, breast tenderness, vomiting, and several miscellaneous effects of uncommon occurrence. Like all such mixtures, it is probable but uncertain that the mixture favors rare venous thrombosis.

Dose—*For contraception*, **1 mg** of Ethynodiol Acetate and **100 mcg** of Mestranol daily for 21 days, starting on the 5th day after menstruation begins.

Dosage Forms—Tablets: Ethynodiol Diacetate (1 mg) and Mestranol (100 mcg).

Hydroxyprogesterone Caproate USP

[17-Hydroxypregn-4-ene-3,20-dione Hexanoate; Delalutin (*Squibb*)]

Hydroxyprogesterone Caproate is $C_{27}H_{40}O_4$ (428.62).

Preparation—Hydroxyprogesterone is esterified by heating with caproic anhydride in the presence of *p*-toluenesulfonic acid under an atmosphere of nitrogen. US Pat. 2,753,360.

Description—White or creamy white, crystalline powder which is odorless or has a slight odor. It melts at about 122°. The crystals should not be exposed to heat and light.

Solubility—Insoluble in water; 1 Gm is soluble in about 20 ml of ether and 800 ml of benzene.

Uses—Hydroxyprogesterone caproate is a *progestogen* with actions and uses like *Progesterone* (page 1002). It is several times more potent, and its duration of action is longer, but its onset of action is also slower. A single injection of a solution of Hydroxyprogesterone Caproate in oil will exert progestational effects for 1 to 2 weeks. It does not prevent ovulation. It is not converted to progesterone or hydroxyprogesterone in the body. When used to regulate an irregular estrus cycle, it is usually combined with an estrogen.

Hydroxyprogesterone Caproate occasionally causes hypersensitivity, coughing, or dyspnea. In rare instances it may cause virilization of the female fetus.

Dose—*Intramuscular*, **125** to **1000 mg** once a month; *usual, cyclic therapy*, **250 mg** every 4 weeks; *continuous therapy*, **250 mg** once a week.

Dosage Forms—Injection USP: 250 mg/2 ml, 1.25 Gm/5 and 10 ml.

Medroxyprogesterone Acetate USP

[17-Hydroxy-6α-methylpregn-4-ene-3,20-dione Acetate; Provera (*Upjohn*)]

Medroxyprogesterone Acetate contains 97.0–103.0% of $C_{24}H_{34}O_4$ (386.54), calculated on the dried basis.

Preparation—This compound is prepared from 17α-hydroxyprogesterone by first forming the 3,21-bis-ethylene acetal with ethylene glycol, then treatment with peracetic acid to give a mixture of the 5α,6α- and 5β,6β-epoxides. With methyl magnesium iodide the α-epoxide isomer yields the 5α-hydroxy-6β-methyl derivative which dehydrates and epimerizes with hydrogen chloride in chloroform to the Δ⁴-6α-methyl compound, Medroxyprogesterone. Acylation with acetic anhydride and p-toluenesulfonic acid in acetic acid gives Medroxyprogesterone Acetate.

Description—White to off-white, odorless, crystalline powder. Is stable in air.

Solubility—Insoluble in water; freely soluble in chloroform; soluble in acetone and dioxane; sparingly soluble in alcohol and methanol; slightly soluble in ether.

Uses—Medroxyprogesterone acetate is a *progestogen* with actions and uses similar to those of *Progesterone* (page 1002). Its oral efficacy is an advantage over progesterone. For this reason, in combination with an estrogen, Medroxyprogesterone is used in oral contraceptives. Aqueous suspensions administered intramuscularly have a duration of action of 2 to 4 weeks.

Dose—*Cyclic therapy*, oral, **2.5** to **10 mg** daily for 5 to 10 days, during second half of menstrual cycle; *continuous therapy*, oral, **10** to **40 mg** daily; *intramuscular*, **50** to **100 mg** weekly or every 2 weeks. *Usual*, oral, **10 mg** once daily; *intramuscular*, **50 mg** once weekly.

Dosage Forms—Sterile Suspension USP: 50 mg/ml, 250 mg/5 ml; Tablets USP: 2.5 and 10 mg.

Veterinary Dose—*Mares*, follicular ovarian cysts with persistent estrus, **125** to **250 mg**; early habitual abortion, **250 mg** at 40 to 60 days of pregnancy; impending abortion, **250** to **500 mg,** repeated if signs recur; prevention of estrus, **125** to **250 mg** during anestrus, repeated at 30-day intervals. *Bitches*, prevention of estrus, **50** to **150 mg** during anestrus, repeated at 6-month intervals; abbreviation of estrus, **250 mg**; pseudopregnancy, **250 mg.** *Cats*, prevention of estrus, **50** to **150 mg** during anestrus, repeated at 6-month intervals; abbreviation of estrus, **50** to **150 mg.** In *Mares*, dose is given as a single *intramuscular* or *subcutaneous* injection in the cervical region. In *Bitches* and *Cats*, dose is given as a single *subcutaneous* injection; because a semipermanent bleb may result, administration should be made in an unobservable site. Because 250 mg of the drug has produced mammary swelling and lactation in *Greyhound* bitches, it should not be administered to this breed. (*Note*—Recent reports of undesirable uterine side effects have brought the drug ill repute.)

Ethinyl Estradiol and Medroxyprogesterone Acetate Tablets

[Provest (*Upjohn*)]

Uses—Ethinyl Estradiol and Medroxyprogesterone is an *oral contraceptive mixture* that differs little from other mixtures of this type. However, the marketed product is lower in estrogenic activity than most oral contraceptive mixtures. For the actions of the separate components, see *Ethinyl Estradiol* (page 992) and *Medroxyprogesterone* (above). The antifertility effect appears to be due more to the progestogen than to the estrogen. The mixture may also be used in other conditions in which progestogens are indicated, particularly in those situations in which anovulation is desired (see *Progesterone*, page 1002). In large doses it may also be used to arrest dysfunctional uterine bleeding. The adverse effects are essentially those of *Ethynodiol Diacetate and Mestranol Tablets* (page 999), but they are of lesser incidence because of the low estrogen content.

Dose—*For contraception*, **10 mg** of Medroxyprogesterone and **50 mcg** of Ethinyl Estradiol daily for 20 days, starting on the 5th day after menstruation begins.

Dosage Forms—Ethinyl Estradiol (50 mcg) and Medroxyprogesterone Acetate (10 mg).

Norethindrone USP

[17-Hydroxy-19-nor-17α-pregn-4-en-20-yn-3-one; Norethisterone; Norlutin (*Parke-Davis*)]

Norethindrone contains 97.0–102.0% of $C_{20}H_{26}O_2$ (298.43), calculated on the dried basis.

Preparation—The methyl ether of estrone is reacted with lithium metal in liquid ammonia to reduce Ring A to the 4-ene state and the reduced compound is then oxidized with chromic acid in aqueous acetic acid to form estr-4-ene-3,17-dione (I). In order to prevent the 3-keto group from participating in the ensuing ethynylation reaction, (I) is now reacted with ethyl orthoformate in the presence of pyridine hydrochloride to form the 3-ethoxy-3,5-diene compound (II). Acetylene is then passed into a solution of (II) in toluene, previously admixed with a solution of sodium in *tert*-amyl alcohol, to form the 17-ethynyl-17-hydroxy compound. Hydrolysis at the 3-ethoxy linkage by heating with dilute HCl is accompanied by a rearrangement of the 3-hydroxy-3,5-diene compound to the 3-oxo-4-ene state. US Pat. 2,744,122.

Description—White to creamy white, crystalline powder. It is odorless and stable in air.

Solubility—Practically insoluble in water; sparingly soluble in alcohol; soluble in chloroform and dioxane; slightly soluble in ether.

Uses—Norethindrone is a *progestogen* very closely related to *Ethisterone* in structure and action (see page 998), and like ethisterone it is orally effective. For the actions and uses of the progestogens see the general statement, page 996, and *Progesterone*, page 1002. In addition to its progestational actions, Norethindrone has weak estrogenic actions, owing to biotransformation to an estrogenic metabolite. Among the progestational drugs, Norethindrone ranks high in ability to postpone menstruation, and it is used for this purpose for both medical and social reasons. In high doses it prevents ovulation by suppressing pituitary gonadotropin output. In lower doses it suppresses the endometrium and decreases the fluidity of the cervical mucus. Consequently, the steroid is one of the important oral contraceptives. As an oral contraceptive it is combined with an estrogen, especially *Mestranol* (page 995); see also *Norethindrone and Mestranol Tablets* (below). Norethindrone has weak androgenic properties and may cause deepening of the voice, hirsutism and acne, and it may cause masculinization of the fetus.

Dose—USP: **1** to **40 mg** daily; *usual*, **1** to **10 mg** once a day. NF: **5** to **30 mg** daily.

Dosage Forms—Tablets NF: 5 mg.

Norethindrone and Mestranol Tablets

[Various Mfgs.]

Uses—Norethindrone and Mestranol has become well known as an *oral contraceptive* mixture. The two components act in a concerted manner to suppress pituitary release of gonadotropins and hence to prevent ovulation, which is the basis of the contraceptive effect in the higher dose forms. In addition to its role in the anovulatory effect, Mestranol antagonizes some of the androgenic actions of Norethindrone. The mixture may be used in nearly all conditions in which progestogens are indicated (see *Progesterone*, page 1002), particularly in those situations where anovulation is desirable. It is especially used to regularize erratic estrous cycles and to arrest dysfunctional uterine bleeding.

Norethisterone and mestranol are also used in a sequential oral contraceptive regimen in which the estrogen is given first and the progestogen is given after a proliferative endometrium is established. In this regimen a higher dose of mestranol is used, and it is the mestranol to which the antifertility effect must be attributed.

Dose—1 to **10 mg** of norethindrone and **80 to 100 mcg** of mestranol daily from the 5th through the 24th day of the menstrual cycle, except through the 25th day when the 1-mg dose is used.

Other Dose Information—Oral, in a sequential regimen, 80 mcg of mestranol daily for 16 days starting on the 5th day after menstruation begins, and 2 mg of norethindrone daily for 5 days, starting on the 21st day after menstruation begins.

For cyclic therapy in dysmenorrhea, functional uterine bleeding, premenstrual tension, amenorrhea, or idiopathic infertility, 1 2- or 10-mg tablet daily for 20 days of the cycle, beginning on the 5th; for emergency control of functional or dysfunctional uterine bleeding, 1 10-mg tablet 2 or 3 times daily until bleeding is arrested, then once daily; to delay menstruation, 1 to 2 10-mg tablets daily, beginning at least 1 week before the expected menstruation.

Dosage Forms—Tablets: Norethindrone (1,2, and 10 mg) and Mestranol (50 and 80 mcg).

Norethindrone Acetate NF

[17-Hydroxy-19-nor-17a-pregn-4-en-20-yn-3-one Acetate;   Norlutate (*Parke-Davis*)]

Norethindrone Acetate contains 97.0–103.0% of $C_{22}H_{28}O_3$ (340.47), calculated on the dried basis.

Preparation—*Norethindrone* (page 1000) is acetylated by treatment with acetic anhydride in the presence of pyridine.

Description—White to creamy white crystals or crystalline powder.

Solubility—Practically insoluble in water; soluble in alcohol; very soluble in chloroform; freely soluble in dioxane; soluble in ether.

Uses—The actions, uses, and side effects of Norethindrone Acetate are identical to those of *Norethindrone* (page 1000). However, it is 2 to 3 times as potent as the parent steroid. Although Norethindrone Acetate may be employed alone as a progestogen, it is most commonly employed in combination with an estrogen (marketed with Ethinyl Estradiol; see below) for oral contraceptive or cyclic therapy.

Dose—5 to **15 mg**; *usual*, **10 mg** daily.

Other Dose Information—Oral, for cyclic therapy, 2.5 to 10 mg daily from the 5th through the 25th day of the menstrual cycle; for continuous therapy, 2.5 to 10 mg twice daily, except 5 to 15 mg daily in the treatment of endometriosis.

Dosage Forms—Tablets NF: 5 mg.

Ethinyl Estradiol and Norethindrone Acetate Tablets

[Gestest (*Squibb*); Norlestrin (*Parke-Davis*)]

Uses—Ethinyl Estradiol and Norethindrone is an *oral contraceptive mixture* that differs little from other mixtures of this type. However, the marketed product is lower in estrogenic activity than most oral contraceptive mixtures. For the actions of the separate components, see *Ethinyl Estradiol* (page 992) and *Norethindrone Acetate* (above). The antifertility effect appears to be due more to the progestogen than the estrogen. The mixture may also be used in other conditions in which progestogens are indicated, particularly in those situations in which anovulation is desired (see *Progesterone*, page 1002). Adverse effects are essentially the same as those of *Norethindrone and Mestranol Tablets* (page 1000).

Dose—*For contraception*, **1** to **2.5 mg** of norethindrone and **50 mcg** of ethinyl estradiol daily for 21 days, starting on the 5th day after menstruation begins.

Dosage Forms—Tablets: Ethinyl Estradiol (50 mcg) and Norethindrone Acetate (2.5 mg).

Norethynodrel USP

[17-Hydroxy-19-nor-17α-pregn-5(10)-en-20-yn-3-one]

Norethynodrel contains 97.0–101.0% of $C_{20}H_{26}O_2$ (298.43).

Preparation—Dehydroepiandrosterone acetate is simultaneously saponified and oxidized by a series of reactions to 19-hydroxyandrost-5(6)-ene-3,17-dione. The hydroxymethyl group at the 10 position is then oxidized to carboxyl. The resulting acid is decarboxylated with simultaneous shifting of the double bond to give estr-5(10)-ene-3,17-dione. Selective addition of acetylene at the expense of the 17-one group yields Norethynodrel. US Pat. 2,725,389.

Description—A white or nearly white, odorless, crystalline powder. It is stable in air. It melts between 174° and 184°, but the range between beginning and ending of melting does not exceed 3°.

Solubility—Freely soluble in chloroform; sparingly soluble in alcohol and ether; very slightly soluble in water and solvent hexane.

Uses—Norethynodrel is a *progestogen* which is isomeric with *Norethindrone* (page 1000). However, the shift of the double bond in the A ring abolishes the weak androgenic properties found in Norethindrone. In fact, Norethynodrel exerts weak estrogenic actions, because it is biotransformed to an estrogenic metabolite. Nevertheless, for progestational therapy or for oral contraception it is usual to supplement Norethynodrel with an estrogen, both to prevent withdrawal bleeding and to favor an anovulatory effect. The prevention of ovulation is the result of suppression of pituitary gonadotropin release. However, contraception occurs also by other mechanisms. The drug is the primary ingredient of an important oral contraceptive (see *Norethynodrel and Mestranol*, below). It is not advocated for infertility and maintenance of pregnancy, since it appears not to promote an endometrium which is favorable to nidation and support of the fetus. Furthermore, it causes some masculinization of the fetus, even though it otherwise lacks androgenic properties. This androgenic activity is somewhat antagonized by the estrogenic actions of mestranol and other estrogens. Norethynodrel is not used separately from its estrogenic adjuvant even in general progestational therapy.

Dose—**2.5** to **30 mg** daily; *usual,* **2.5** to **10 mg** once a day.

Norethynodrel and Mestranol Tablets

[Enovid (*Searle*); Enovid E (*Searle*)]

For the structures, see pages 1001 and 995.

Uses—Norethynodrel and Mestranol became famous the world over as an oral contraceptive and has been dubbed "The Pill." However, it is also used in other progestational therapy. The oral contraceptive activity is attributable to both ingredients. Although Norethynodrel alone in large doses can prevent ovulation, the presence of *Mestranol* (see page 995) greatly increases the potency to suppress pituitary production of gonadotropins. The contraceptive action is not entirely the result of prevention of ovulation; the endometrium is rendered inhospitable to the fertilized ovum, so that nidation cannot take place. Nevertheless, the mixture may be used in the treatment of infertility if it is the result of endometrial hypoplasia; the mixture is administered cyclically for 3 cycles, then discontinued, and conception may be successful in the next few cycles. Also, if infertility is due to luteal insufficiency, administration of the drug from 3 days after ovulation through the 5th month of pregnancy is used. Nevertheless, the mixture does not support pregnancy experimentally and does not appear to do so in humans; furthermore, it causes some virilization of the fetus. In addition to oral contraception, it is used to postpone menstruation and in the treatment of dysfunctional uterine bleeding, endometriosis, premenstrual tension and dysmenorrhea.

Side effects of the mixture include bleeding irregularities, nausea, and vomiting in about $\frac{1}{4}$ of all users, breast fullness, chloasma, headache, weakness, dizziness, and diarrhea. The effects diminish with continual use. Sometimes fluid retention and acne occur. Cholestatic jaundice occurs rarely. It is uncertain whether the mixture increases the incidence of thrombophlebitis.

Dose—Norethynodrel (**2.5, 5,** or **9.85 mg**) plus Mestranol (**100, 75,** or **150 mcg**), respectively, daily for 20 days, starting on the 5th day after menstruation begins.

Dosage Forms—Tablets: Norethynodrel (2.5 mg) and Mestranol (100 mcg).

Other Dose Information—The so-called 5-mg tablet contains 5 mg of norethynodrel with 0.075 mg of mestranol and the 10-mg tablet contains 9.85 mg of norethynodrel and 0.15 mg of mestranol. For cyclic therapy in dysmenorrhea, functional uterine bleeding (once it is controlled), premenstrual tension, amenorrhea (once a menses has been accomplished), or idiopathic infertility, one 5- or 10-mg tablet daily for 20 days of each cycle, beginning on the 5th day after menstruation begins; for emergency control of functional or dysfunctional uterine bleeding, one 10-mg tablet 2 or 3 times a day until bleeding is arrested, then once daily through the 24th day after menstruation began; for endometriosis, one 5- or 10-mg tablet daily for 2 weeks, beginning on the 5th day after menstruation begins, increasing in dosage every 2 weeks until 20 mg a day is being given, to be continued for 6 to 9 months; to delay menstruation, one to two 10-mg tablets daily, beginning at least 1 week in advance of the expected menstruation; to advance menstruation, one 5- or 10-mg tablet for 10 days, beginning on the 5th day after the start of menstruation.

Progesterone NF

[Pregn-4-ene-3,20-dione; Proluton (*Schering*)]

Progesterone contains 98.0–102.0% of $C_{21}H_{30}O_2$ (314.47), calculated on the dried basis.

Preparation—Progesterone is obtained from animal ovaries, synthesized from stigmasterol, or better from diosgenin (extracted from *Dioscorea mexicana,* a Mexican yam). The latter synthesis involves acetolysis, chromic acid oxidation, cleavage of the ketoester diacetate with boiling acetic acid to 16-dehydropregnenolone acetate, which on catalytic reduction yields pregnenolone acetate. Saponification of the acetate ester to the 3β-alcohol followed by Oppenauer oxidation affords Progesterone. Progesterone in pure form was first isolated in 1934 by Butenandt.

Description—A white or creamy white, crystalline powder. It is odorless and stable in air. It melts between 128° and 133°; a polymorphic modification melts at about 121°. Its specific rotation, in dioxane solution $[\alpha]_D^{25}$, is not less than +175° and not more than +183°.

Solubility—Practically insoluble in water; soluble in alcohol, acetone, and dioxane; sparingly soluble in vegetable oils.

Uses—Therapy with Progesterone is chiefly to sustain the secretory type of endometrium (uterine glands) during the third and fourth weeks of the menstrual cycle, with the hope that this will allow successful implantation and retention of a fertilized ovum, or by extending this same type of action *to sustain the conditions favorable for pregnancy* during the first three or four months of a pregnancy. This is especially indicated in women who have previously had a history of several abortions which may be attributable to a deficient secretion of progesterone by the ovaries. Such secretion by the ovaries normally becomes supplanted after about the third month of pregnancy by a placental supply of progesterone.

Progesterone may be useful if administered early to women who show signs of *impending abortion.* Doses may have to be as much as 50 mg or more daily. Early failures with progesterone might have been the result of insufficient dosage. However, leading gynecologists state that progesterone cannot prevent threatened or habitual abortion. Similar doubts exist about the efficacy of newer progestational hormones in the maintenance of pregnancy.

Progesterone is also used in so-called *cyclic therapy,* especially in sequence after estrogen or in combination with estrogen, in order to secure more regular rhythm of menstrual intervals and less prolonged flowing. This applies to those women who have decidedly irregular and unpredictable menses, and who tend to flow very profusely for periods longer than five days (*functional uterine bleeding*). However, authorities are still dubious about the efficacy of progesterone for this purpose; it is likely that the usual doses are too small. The hormone is used to lessen premenstrual tension; the mechanism is not clear. Extremely high doses may prevent ovulation. This effect of Progesterone is not used for contraception but it is sometimes used to circumvent *dysmenorrhea* and discomfort resulting from *endometriosis*. Very high doses may be required to arrest *dysfunctional uterine bleeding;* ordinarily, an estrogen–progestogen combination is used for this purpose.

Progesterone is ineffective orally except by buccal or sublingual administration, in which case it is questionably effective, possibly because the usual doses are too small. In view of this fact and the fact that several other progestational hormones are quite effective by the oral route, the use of oral preparations of Progesterone should be discouraged. In fact, tablets have virtually disappeared among commercial preparations of Progesterone.

Progesterone causes some salt and water retention, so that continuous therapy may be accompanied by edema and weight gain. Breast engorgement and painful breasts, resulting from a concerted action of Progesterone and endogenous estrogens, may occur. Progesterone also has a thermogenic action, which, however, is of minor consequence.

Dose—*Usual, buccal,* **10 mg** up to 4 times a day; *intramuscular,* **2 to 25 mg.**

Dosage Forms—Injection NF: 5, 10, 25, 50, and 100 mg/ml, 50 and 125 mg/5 ml, 100, 250, and 500 mg/ 10 ml; Sterile Suspension NF: 10, 25, and 50 mg/ml, 250 and 500 mg/10 ml; Tablets NF: 10 and 25 mg.

Veterinary Use—For the control of habitual abortion and to delay estrus and ovulation in cattle, swine, and dogs.

Veterinary Dose—*Cattle,* **50 mg** daily; *Swine,* **50 to 100 mg** daily; *Dogs,* **50 to 75 mg** of repository form.

Other Progestogens and Oral Contraceptives

Flurogestone Acetate [Synchro-Mate (*Searle*)] is 9-fluoro-11β-17-dihydroxypregn-4-ene-3,20-dione 17-acetate [$C_{23}H_{31}FO_5$ = 406.50]. *Preparation:* 16,17-Epoxypregna-4,9(11)-diene-3,20-dione is reacted with hydrogen iodide in acetic acid to form the corresponding 17-hydroxy-16β-iodo compound. The 16-iodine is then removed by hydrogenation with Raney nickel and the resulting 17-hydroxypregna-4,9(11)-diene-3,20-dione is acetylated with acetic anhydride and *p*-toluenesulfonic acid to give the 17-acetate ester. Treatment with hypobromous acid attacks the 9(11) double bond and the resulting 9-bromo-11β-hydroxy compound is converted to the 9,11β-epoxy analog by reaction with sodium carbonate in aqueous tetrahydrofuran. Rupture of the epoxy ring with hydrogen fluoride in tetrahydrofuran yields Flurogestone Acetate [*J. Am. Chem. Soc.,* **81**, 4432 (1959)]. *Uses:* Flurogestone Acetate is a progestogen which in sheep and cattle is about 25 times as potent as progesterone. It is employed in animal husbandry, principally for the purpose of controlling the time at which female stock come into heat and hence to regulate the time of breeding. Flurogestone Acetate suppresses ovulation during the time of exposure to

the drug; upon withdrawal, the female comes into estrus in a few days. A large percentage of such females mates and is impregnated during the first or second estrus after withdrawal. Pregnant mare's serum may be given to enhance ovulation and conception. In this way, lambing and calving can be synchronized among all the stock so as to occur at the most advantageous time and also to favor more than one crop of young a year. *Veterinary Dose: Intravaginal,* as an impregnated polyurethane sponge pessary, *Ewes* and *Goats,* 20 to 30 mg; *Cows,* 100 mg. The pessary is usually left in place for 10 to 20 days.

Hydroxyprogesterone Acetate [Prodox (*Upjohn*)] [17-Hydroxyprogesterone Acetate]—A white, crystalline solid which is slightly soluble in water; soluble in alcohol. *Uses:* A progestational steroid with actions and uses like *Progesterone* (page 1002). However, hydroxyprogesterone acetate is quite active by the oral route and is considerably more potent than ethisterone by this route. The acetate is presently only administered orally, but it is also active by parenteral routes. The acetate has been replaced largely by the caproate (see *Hydroxyprogesterone Caproate,* page 999). *Dose: Orally,* 25 to *50 mg* daily except 200 to 400 mg daily for habitual abortion.

Megestrol Acetate [17-Hydroxy-6-methylpregna-4,6-diene-3,20-dione Acetate ($C_{24}H_{32}O_4$)]—A white or slightly off-white, crystalline powder that is stable in air and unaffected by moisture. It melts between 216° and 219°. Insoluble in water; soluble in alcohol, methanol, benzene, and ethyl acetate; very soluble in chloroform; sparingly soluble in petroleum ether. *Uses:* A progestational agent chemically related to *Dydrogesterone* (page 998). It is very potent in inhibiting ovulation; consequently, it is employed as an oral contraceptive. For such purposes, it is supplemented with an estrogen, generally ethinylestradiol. The compound has no estrogenic or androgenic properties of its own. Side effects include nausea and vomiting, headache, tiredness, breast discomfort and weight gain. *Dose: Orally,* as tablets also containing 1.25 mg ethinylestradiol, *2 to 4 mg* daily from the 5th through the 24th day of the menstrual cycle.

Norgestrel [$C_{21}H_{28}O_2$ = 312.46] is (±)-13-ethyl-17-hydroxy-18,19-dinor-17α-pregn-4-en-20-yn-3-one. *Preparation:* Norgestrel is a product of total, stereoselective chemical synthesis based on the concept of condensing 1,2,3,4-tetrahydro-6-methoxy-1-vinyl-1-naphthol with 2-ethyl-1,3-cyclopentanedione to obtain initially a tricyclic intermediate (secosteroid) containing all of the carbon atoms of the gonane skeleton. Cyclization of the secosteroid via dehydration yields a 13-ethylgona-1,3,5(10),8,14-pentane structure which is then successively reduced and ethynylated in a series of reactions to the end product. *Description and Solubility:* A white to nearly white powder that is odorless and tasteless. It is stable in light and heat and is nonhygroscopic. It melts between 205° and 212° within a 4° range. Soluble in chloroform and acetone; sparingly soluble in alcohol; insoluble in water. *Uses:* Norgestrel is a *progestogen* that is similar to the other orally effective progestogens. It may be used in any of those conditions for which progestogens are employed (see *Progesterone,* page 1002) and it promotes the same adverse effects. It is marketed in combination with Ethinyl Estradiol for oral contraceptive use (below).

Norgestrel and Ethinyl Estradiol Tablets [Ovral (*Wyeth*)]. *Uses:* An oral contraceptive mixture similar in action and side effects to *Ethynodiol Diacetate and Mestranol Tablets* (page 999). *Dose: For contraception,* 0.5 mg in combination with 50 mcg of ethinyl estradiol daily for 21 days, beginning on the 5th day after menstruation begins.

Polypeptide Ovarian Hormones

In addition to the steroid hormones mentioned above, the ovary also produces one or more nonsteroid substances which are concerned in the reproductive physiology of various species of animals. A polypeptide compound present in aqueous extracts of the ovaries of pregnant sows and the blood of pregnant humans, to which the name *relaxin* has been given, causes relaxation of the symphysis pubis in estrogen-treated guinea pigs and mice. Other characteristic physiological properties of relaxin-containing extracts include effects upon uterine endometrium and myometrium and upon cervical musculature although much of this activity is attributable to a contaminant, the "*uterine relaxing factor*" (Lututrin). Very active relaxin preparations which are substantially homogeneous electrophoretically have been isolated. Relaxin is a protein of molecular weight 10,000–12,000 which appears to be free of nonamino acid constituents. Relaxin preparations are standardized in terms of their ability to cause pelvic relaxation in estrogen-primed guinea pigs or mice. Another water-soluble ovarian preparation, lututrin, is assayed in terms of its ability to inhibit spontaneous contractions of the guinea pig uterus.

Much of the human physiology of Relaxin and Lututrin remains to be elucidated. There is considerable doubt that a deficiency of these hormones exists in the human and hence that there are rational indications for their use.

These preparations have been used in the treatment of dysmenorrhea, premature labor, cervical dystocia, and scleroderma, but evidence for their therapeutic effectiveness is still equivocal.

Other Polypeptide Ovarian Hormones

Lututrin [Lutrexin (*Hynson*)]—A water-soluble, polypeptide, uterine-relaxing factor obtained from the corpus luteum of sow ovaries by a process of salting out followed by dialysis. *Uses:* Lututrin ("uterine relaxing factor") can induce relaxation of the uterus, and the clinical uses are based on this effect. Good results are sometimes obtained in the treatment of functional dysmenorrhea; if anatomical abnormalities or psychosomatic factors are present, it is not indicated. It is probably of little value in the remission of premature labor or threatened abortion. As many as 75,000 units have been given in a day without untoward effects.

Dose: Orally, for dysmenorrhea *6000* to *12,000 units* every 3 or 4 hours as needed; for premature labor or threatened abortion, initially *12,000 units*, *9000 units* at 1 hour, *6000 units* hourly until contractions cease, and *3000* to *6000* 2 to 4 times daily thereafter.

Relaxin—A naturally occurring protein or polypeptide of relatively low molecular weight produced by the corpus luteum during pregnancy and extracted from the ovaries of pregnant sows. It is capable of relaxing the symphysis pubis and the uterine smooth muscle in experimental animals. There is some evidence that it can also relax the uterus and soften the cervix in pregnant humans, but more evidence is needed. *Uses:* The actions of Relaxin are listed in the *General Statement*, above. Although Relaxin has been used for the same purposes as Lututrin (see above), namely, in the treatment of dysmenorrhea, premature labor, and threatened abortion, clinical interest centers mainly on its effects on the uterine cervix. It is claimed to soften and facilitate the cervix and hence to shorten labor; clinical opinion is divided, with the majority holding that it is of little value. It might be expected to be detrimental because of the uterine relaxing effect; since most prolonged labor is the result of uterine inertia rather than the failure of the cervix to dilate, the use of Relaxin would appear to be irrational. When uterine contractions are vigorous, normally or after oxytocin, Relaxin may shorten the course of labor. It may possibly aid in the delivery of retained dead fetuses. The effect of the substance to soften the skin has found use in the treatment of scleroderma, apparently with variable success. Allergic reactions, including anaphylaxis, have occurred after injection. *Dose: Intravenously*, for cervical softening, *40* to *120 mg* in 250 to 500 ml of sterile diluent, given at a rate of 4 to 8 ml per minute; for premature labor *40* to *80 mg* in 1 L of isotonic dextrose, given at the rate of 4 ml per minute. *Intramuscularly*, for cervical softening, *40 mg* every 2 hours for 3 doses; for premature labor, *40 mg*, followed by *20 mg* every 2 hours; for dysmenorrhea, *20 mg* every 4 hours; for scleroderma, *20 mg* per day initially, to be reduced when improvement is apparent; for delivery of retained dead fetus, *60 mg* every 2 hours for 6 doses.

The Testicular Hormone

The testis has a dual function, to produce the germ cell (the *sperm*) and to supply the male hormone (*testosterone*). Two clearly defined groups of cells are found in the testes; the one group in the tubules produces the sperm, while the other, clustered in between the tubules, consists of interstitial cells. The first or spermatogenic tissue is thought by some investigators to produce an internal secretion, but if this is true, the hormone involved has not yet been identified, nor is there agreement about its existence.

The interstitial cells are the seat of production of a steroid hormone, testosterone, which stimulates and maintains the secondary sex organs; these are the penis, the prostate, seminal vesicles, vas deferens, and scrotum. It also exerts sustaining effects upon the spermatogenic cells, and it stimulates the development of bone, muscle, skin, and hair growth, and emotional responses to produce the characteristic adult masculine traits. This group of combined actions of this hormone is termed *androgenic actions*. Testosterone also antagonizes a number of the effects of estrogens, and is sometimes employed clinically for this purpose. This is especially important in the suppression of metastatic carcinoma of the breast. Since it promotes the development of the clitoris, which is an anatomic homolog of the penis, androgens may increase the libido of women.

The naturally occurring androgens are derivatives of androstane (androsterone, testosterone). Testosterone and its esters (testosterone propionate) and derivatives (methyltestosterone) are the most commonly used androgenic steroids. In addition to their androgenic properties, however, these compounds exert widespread anabolic effects; in attempts to dissociate the virilizing and anabolic properties (for use in women) a number of compounds with high anabolic: androgenic ratios have been prepared. However, it has not yet been possible to abolish completely the androgenic effects.

Dromostanolone Propionate NF

[17β-Hydroxy-2α-methyl-5α-androstan-3-one Propionate; Drolban (*Lilly*)]

Dromostanolone Propionate contains 95.0–102.0% of $C_{23}H_{36}O_3$ (360.54), calculated on the dried basis.

Preparation—Testosterone is reacted with ethyl formate and alkali metal hydride to form 2-(hydroxymethylene)testosterone (I).[6] Refluxing a benzene suspension of (I), methyl iodide, and sodium hydride under nitrogen produces 2-formyl-2-methyltestosterone which is then decarbonylated by passage through a column of alkalinized alumina to yield 2α-methyltestosterone (II). Esterification of (II) with propionic anhydride in pyridine solution forms (II) propionate which yields Dromostanolone Propionate on hydrogenation in the presence of palladium on barium sulfate or various other catalysts. US Pat. 3,118,915.

Description—A white to creamy white, crystalline powder. It is odorless or has a faint odor.
Solubility—Practically insoluble in water; soluble in chloroform, ether, and methanol.

Uses—Dromostanolone Propionate is an *androgen* similar in its actions to *Testosterone Propionate* (page 1009), but it appears to be somewhat less virilizing. Its use has been restricted to the treatment of metastatic carcinoma of the breast. With respect to efficacy in the regression of the carcinoma, it is about equivalent to testosterone propionate, but its lesser virilizing activity makes Dromostanolone advantageous. The drug may improve anemia and the patient's sense of well being, but these effects are unrelated to regression of the disease.

The untoward effects of Dromostanolone are mainly those which result from virilization and include facial hair growth, deepening of the voice, acne, and enlargement of the clitoris, which occasionally may give rise to an increase in libido. The virilizing effects develop slowly and may not reach their peak for several months. Fluid retention with edema may occur. Effects on serum calcium are not untoward but rather reflect the success of the drug on osteolytic metastases; if regression occurs, serum calcium falls. Jaundice has not been reported, but the potential exists. Dromostanolone should be used with caution in the presence of liver disease, heart failure, kidney disease, and pregnancy.

Dose—*Usual, intramuscular,* **100 mg** 3 times a week.
Dosage Forms—Injection NF: 50 mg/ml, 500 mg/10 ml.

Fluoxymesterone USP

[9-Fluoro-11β,17β-dihydroxy-17-methylandrost-4-en-3-one; Halotestin (*Upjohn*); Ora-Testryl (*Squibb*); Ultandren (*Ciba*)]

Fluoxymesterone contains 97.0–102.0% of $C_{20}H_{29}FO_3$ (336.45), calculated on the dried basis.
Preparation—This material is synthesized from 17-methyltestosterone first by introduction of a hydroxyl group at position 11 through oxidation with a microorganism (such as *Pestalotia* or *Aspergillus*), followed by dehydration, epoxidation and treatment with HF, as for *Betamethasone* (page 962).

Description—White, odorless, tasteless solid. It melts at about 240° with decomposition.
Solubility—Soluble in alcohol; slightly soluble in chloroform; practically insoluble in water.

Uses—Fluoxymesterone has the same actions, uses, and limitations as *Testosterone* (see page 1008) and its

congeners, except that it is approximately 5 times more potent and is orally effective.
Dose—**2** to **30 mg** daily; *usual*, **2** to **4 mg** 1 to 3 times a day.
Other Dose Information—For breast cancer, 30 mg daily.
Dosage Forms—Tablets USP: 2, 5, and 10 mg.

Methandrostenolone NF

[17β-Hydroxy-17-methylandrosta-1,4-dien-3-one; Methandienon; Dianabol (*Ciba*)]

Methandrostenolone contains 97.0–103.0% of $C_{20}H_{28}O_2$ (300.44), calculated on the dried basis.
Preparation—*Methyltestosterone* (this page) is dehydrogenated, either by microbial methods or by reaction with selenium dioxide, to create the Δ^1 double bond. US Pat. 2,900,398.

Description—White crystals or as a white, crystalline powder. It is odorless. It melts between 160° and 166° with decomposition.
Solubility—Soluble in alcohol, chloroform, and glacial acetic acid; slightly soluble in ether; insoluble in water.

Uses—Methandrostenolone is an androgenic steroid with relatively strong anabolic and weak androgenic activity. Consequently, it is employed mainly to *promote nitrogen anabolism* and weight gain in cachexia and debilitating diseases and after serious infections, burns, trauma, or surgery. It may relieve pain in certain types of *osteoporosis*, and it favors the retention of calcium, which assists in arresting the disease. It also helps to relieve pain and to promote a sense of well being in the arthritides. Side effects include virilization and acne, especially in women and children, sodium retention and edema, and cholestatic jaundice. Methandrostenolone potentiates prothrombopenic anticoagulants and hence may favor hemorrhagic diatheses in persons taking such drugs.
Dose—*Usual,* **2.5** to **5 mg** daily.
Other Dose Information—Continuous therapy should consist in repeated courses of no longer than 6 weeks, separated by intervals of 2 to 4 weeks.
Dosage Forms—Tablets NF: 2.5 and 5 mg.

Methyltestosterone NF

[17β-Hydroxy-17-methylandrost-4-en-3-one; Metandren (*Ciba*); Neo-Hombreol M (*Organon*); Oreton (*Schering*)]

Methyltestosterone contains 98.0–102.0% of $C_{20}H_{30}O_2$ (302.46), calculated on the dried basis.
Preparation—Methyltestosterone can be readily synthesized from dehydroepiandrosterone (prepared from cholesterol) by subjecting it to a Grignard reaction with CH_3MgI followed by an Oppenauer oxidation. The first reaction creates the tertiary carbinol structure at C_{17}, while the second oxidizes the secondary carbinol

group at position 3 to carbonyl and causes a rearrangement of the double bond from the 5,6 to the 4,5 position.

Description—White or creamy white crystals or a crystalline powder. It is odorless and is stable in air but slightly hygroscopic. It is affected by light. It melts between 163° and 168°. If specific rotation, determined in benzene solution, is between +84° and +87°.

Solubility—Insoluble in water; soluble in alcohol, methanol, ether, and other organic solvents; sparingly soluble in vegetable oils.

Uses—The actions, uses, and limitations of Methyltestosterone are the same as those of *Testosterone* (page 1008), except that Methyltestosterone is effective orally. It is also combined with various estrogens for use in the treatment of menorrhagia, menopausal symptoms, dysmenorrhea, osteoporosis, malnutrition, and to suppress postpartum lactation. It may cause a rare type of cholestatic jaundice.

Dose—*Oral,* **10** to **50 mg** per day; *usual, oral,* **10 mg** 3 times a day; *buccal,* **5** to **25 mg** per day; *usual, buccal,* **5 mg** up to 4 times a day.

Dosage Forms—Tablets NF: 5, 10, and 25 mg.

Nandrolone Decanoate NF

[17β-Hydroxyestr-4-en-3-one Decanoate; Deca-Durabolin (*Organon*)]

Nandrolone Decanoate contains 96.0–104.0% of $C_{28}H_{44}O_3$ (428.66), calculated on the dried basis.

Preparation—A dry benzene solution of 17β-hydroxyestr-4-en-3-one (19-nortestosterone) and pyridine is mixed with a dry benzene solution of decanoyl chloride and the esterification is allowed to proceed overnight in an atmosphere of nitrogen. After washing successively with acid, alkali, and water, the solvent is evaporated and the crude ester is recrystallized from petroleum ether or some other suitable solvent. US Pat. 2,998,423.

Description—A fine, white to creamy white, crystalline powder. It is odorless or may have a slight odor. It melts between 33° and 37°.

Solubility—Soluble in chloroform, alcohol, acetone, and vegetable oils; practically insoluble in water.

Uses—The actions and uses of Nandrolone Decanoate are the same as those of *Nandrolone Phenpropionate* (see below). Oil solutions of the Decanoate have a duration of action 3 to 4 times longer than that of the phenpropionate.

Dose—*Usual, intramuscular,* **50** to **100 mg** every 3 to 4 weeks.

Dosage Forms—Injection NF: 50 mg/ml, 100 mg/2 ml.

Nandrolone Phenpropionate NF

[17β-Hydroxyestr-4-en-3-one Hydrocinnamate; Durabolin *Organon*)]

Nandrolone Phenpropionate contains 97.0–103.0% of $C_{27}H_{34}O_3$ (406.57), calculated on the dried basis.

For the structure of the steroid moiety, see *Nandrolone Decanoate.*

Preparation—19-Nortestosterone is esterified with hydrocinnamoyl chloride by the method described for *Nandrolone Decanoate.*

Description—A fine, white to creamy white, crystalline powder having a slight characteristic odor.

Solubility—Soluble in alcohol, chloroform, dioxane, ether, and vegetable oils; practically insoluble in water.

Uses—Nandrolone phenpropionate is a synthetic androgen with actions intermediate to those of *Testosterone* (page 1008) and *Norethandrolone* (below). Although Nandrolone Phenpropionate is less androgenic than testosterone in doses which exert anabolic actions, virilization may occur after high doses or during chronic administration. Indeed, the androgenic virilizing actions are sought in the treatment with this agent of *inoperable breast cancer* in women. Used in the treatment of *chronic wasting diseases* and *conditions in which negative nitrogen balance exists.* Low doses may *accelerate growth of children* with retarded growth without excessively accelerating bone age; higher doses accelerate bone maturation more than body growth. The phenylpropionate ester moiety confers a long duration of action to suspensions in oil injected intramuscularly. Nandrolone Phenpropionate does not appear to cause cholestatic jaundice, probably because it lacks an alkyl group on carbon 17.

Dose—*Usual, intramuscular,* **25** to **50 mg** each week.

Other Dose Information—For children of ages 2 to 13 years, 25 mg every 2 to 4 weeks; for infants, 12.5 mg or 1 mg per Kg of body weight every 2 to 4 weeks.

Dosage Forms—Injection NF: 25 mg/ml, 100 mg/2 ml, 125 mg/5 ml.

Norethandrolone NF

[17-Hydroxy-19-nor-17α-pregn-4-en-3-one; 7α-Ethyl-19-nortestosterone; Nilevar (*Searle*)]

Norethandrolone contains 96.0–102.0% of $C_{20}H_{30}O_2$ (302.46), calculated on the dried basis.

Preparation—*Mestranol* (page 995) is subjected to a two-step hydrogenation which converts (a) the 17-ethynyl group to ethyl and (b) the benzenoid ring A to the 1,4-dihydro state, thus producing 3-methoxy-19-nor-17α-pregna-2,5(10)-dien-17-ol. Demethylation of the methoxy group under acidic conditions is accompanied by a rearrangement of Ring A from the 3-hydroxy-2,5(10)-diene state to the 3-oxo-4-ene state. US Pat. 2,721,871.

Description—A white, odorless, crystalline powder. It is stable in air but darkens slightly under prolonged exposure to light. It melts between 130° and 136°.

Solubility—Practically insoluble in water; sparingly soluble in ether; freely soluble in alcohol and acetone; very soluble in chloroform.

Uses—Norethandrolone is a synthetic androgen with actions closely related to *Testosterone* (page 1008). However, its anabolic potency is proportionately stronger than its androgenic potency, so that it is employed for the treatment of conditions and *wasting diseases in which negative protein balance exists.* However, unless a proper diet accompanies treatment, positive nitrogen balance is only transient. It decreases body loss of calcium in certain conditions. Therefore, it is employed *when retention of calcium* is *desirable*. The steroid does cause virilizing effects. It also has progestational activity which may cause menstrual irregularities in women. Nausea and vomiting, edema, fluid retention, and cholestatic jaundice also occur occasionally.

Dose—*Usual*, **10 mg** 2 or 3 times a day.

Other Dose Information—As much as 100 mg per day may be given, but androgenic effects will usually result. For children, oral, 0.5 mg per Kg of body weight per day.

Dosage Forms—Injection: 25 mg/ml; Oral Solution: 8.3 mg/ml (approx. 250 mcg/drop); Tablets NF: 10 mg.

Oxandrolone NF

[17β-Hydroxy-17-methyl-2-oxa-5α-androstan-3-one; Anavar (*Searle*)]

Oxandrolone contains 97.0–100.5% of $C_{19}H_{30}O_3$ (306.45), calculated on the dried basis.

Preparation—Methyldihydrotestosterone is converted into the corresponding 1,2-dehydro compound by bromination followed by dehydrobromination. Ring A is then ruptured through ozonization and subsequent hydrolysis to yield the aldehyde-acid (I). Reduction of the formyl group in (I) yields the expected hydroxy acid implied in the partial structure (II) which is lactonized to Oxandrolone.

(I)   (II)

Description—A white, odorless, crystalline powder. It is stable in air but darkens when exposed to light. It melts between 225° and 233°.

Solubility—Practically insoluble in water; sparingly soluble in alcohol and acetone; freely soluble in chloroform.

Uses—Although Oxandrolone is not strictly speaking a steroid, its configuration is that of a 17-methyl androgenic steroid. Its anabolic actions are strong relative to its androgenic actions. Consequently, it is used in the treatment of *chronic wasting diseases* and conditions in which *negative nitrogen balance* exists. In children with *retarded growth*, low doses of Oxandrolone may increase height and weight without increasing bone age to a comparable degree, but large doses may advance bone age and cause closure of the epiphyses. The drug favors calcium retention and bone reconstruction and hence may be used to treat *osteoporosis*; however, in females it is probably usually better to use estrogens for that purpose. The drug may cause virilization, especially in children or in adults if the recommended doses are exceeded. Oxandrolone can cause sodium and fluid retention. It may adversely affect liver function tests, and the possibility of cholestatic jaundice must be kept in mind. Leucopenia has also been reported. It is contraindi-cated in prostatic cancer and also in breast cancer in some women.

Dose—*Usual, initial,* **5** to **10 mg** daily; *maintenance,* **2.5** to **5 mg** daily.

Other Dose Information—The usual dose should not be taken any longer than 3 months in one course.

Dosage Forms—Tablets NF: 2.5 mg.

Oxymetholone NF

[17β-Hydroxy-2-(hydroxymethylene)-17-methyl-5α-androstan-3-one; Adroyd (*Parke-Davis*); Anadrol (*Syntex*)]

Oxymetholone contains 97.0–103.0% of $C_{21}H_{32}O_3$ (332.49), calculated on the dried basis.

Preparation—17β-Hydroxy-17-methylandrostan-3-one (17-methyldihydrotestosterone) is reacted with ethyl formate and sodium hydride by stirring the mixture under nitrogen for several hours thus forming the 2-(sodoxymethylene) derivative. Treatment of the washed sodium compound with cold dilute hydrochloric acid liberates the Oxymetholone which may be purified by recrystallization from ethyl acetate.[7]

Description—White to creamy white crystals or crystalline powder. It is odorless and stable in air. It is tautomeric in nature and can exist as either tautomer or as a mixture of both, the exact composition depending on solvent and rate of crystallization. It melts between 174° and 182°.

Solubility—Practically insoluble in water; sparingly soluble in alcohol; freely soluble in chloroform; soluble in dioxane; slightly soluble in ether.

Uses—Oxymetholone is an androgenic steroid with relatively greater anabolic activity than androgenic activity. Consequently, it is mainly employed to *promote nitrogen anabolism* and weight gain in cachexia and debilitating diseases and after serious infections, burns, trauma or surgery. It may relieve pain in certain types of *osteoporosis*, and it promotes calcium retention, so that the condition of the bone may improve. Side effects include virilization, especially in women and children, sodium retention and edema, and hepatic dysfunction.

Dose—**5 to 30 mg**; *usual,* **5** to **10 mg** daily.

Other Dose Information—Continuous therapy should consist in repeated courses of no longer than 6 weeks, separated by intervals of 2 to 4 weeks. For prepubertal children the daily dose is 2.5 to 5 mg daily; a pediatric course should not exceed 30 days.

Dosage Forms—Tablets NF: 2.5, 5, and 10 mg.

Stanozolol NF

[17-Methyl-2'H-5α-androst-2-eno[3,2-c]pyrazol-17β-ol; Winstrol (*Winthrop*)]

Stanozolol contains 98.0–100.5% of $C_{21}H_{32}N_2O$ (328.50), calculated on the dried basis.

Preparation—17 - Methyl - 5α - androstan - 17β-ol-3-one is reacted with ethyl formate and sodium methoxide, then acidified with acetic acid to form the 2-hydroxymethylene derivative. This is then condensed with hydrazine hydrate. US Pat. 3,030,358.

Description—Nearly colorless, odorless, crystalline powder. It exists in two forms: one melts between 153° and 156°, the other between 230° and 242°.

Solubility—Soluble in dimethylformamide; sparingly soluble in chloroform and alcohol; slightly soluble in ether, ethyl acetate, and acetone; very slightly soluble in benzene; insoluble in water.

Uses—Stanozolol is an androgenic steroid with relatively strong anabolic and weak androgenic activity. Consequently, it is employed mainly to *promote nitrogen anabolism* and weight gain in cachexia and debilitating diseases and after serious infections, burns, trauma, or surgery. Although it may relieve pain in certain types of *osteoporosis*, it appearly does not affect bone density. Side effects include virilization, especially in women and children, sodium retention and edema, and hepatic dysfunction.

Dose—*Usual*, **2 mg** 3 times a day.

Other Dose Information—For children, 2 to 6 mg daily.

Dosage Forms—Tablets NF: 2 mg.

Veterinary Dose—*Oral*, small *Dogs* and *Cats*, **1** to **2 mg** twice daily; large *Dogs*, **2** to **4 mg** twice daily, depending on body weight.

Testosterone NF

[17β-Hydroxyandrost-4-en-3-one; Androlin (*Lincoln*); Neo-Hombreol-F (*Organon*); Oreton-F (*Schering*); Synandrets (*Pfizer*)]

Testosterone contains 97.0–103.0% of $C_{19}H_{28}O_2$ (288.43), calculated on the dried basis.

It is commonly considered to be the natural male hormone of the human testes.

The term *androgen* applies to this and to other steroids and various chemical derivatives having similar but usually less activity. Many steroids have some androgen activity and several derivatives of testosterone are known. Only one, other than testosterone and its propionate ester, is used for therapy; this is methyltestosterone, a synthetic compound, which is more effective for oral administration. Testosterone for injection is usually supplied as the propionate ester, which is oil soluble and slowly yields the free hormone with a depot-type action.

Preparation—Testosterone was first isolated in crystalline form by Laquer in 1935 who obtained it from animal testes. Although small amounts of testosterone may be extracted from testicular material, the synthetic commercial supply is derived from cholesterol. The key intermediate in the synthesis is dehydroepiandrosterone which can be treated further, by either chemical or microbiological processes, to yield testosterone.

Description—White or slightly creamy white crystals or crystalline powder. It is odorless and stable in air. Melting range: 153° to 157°. Its specific rotation, $[\alpha]_D^{25}$ is +101° to +105° in dioxane.

Solubility—Insoluble in water; 1 Gm dissolves in about 6 ml of dehydrated alcohol, 2 ml of chloroform, and 100 ml of ether; soluble in dioxane and vegetable oils.

Uses—Testosterone is employed in substitutional therapy in men who have climacteric symptoms, or in men or youths with *impaired* or *destroyed testicular function*. It has been employed to facilitate development of adult masculine characteristics when the adolescent process has been delayed. It is also very useful in therapy of patients with *hypopituitarism* and with *Addison's disease*. Use of testosterone for relief of impotence not associated with other evidence of testicular underactivity (psychic causes) is known to be futile in most cases. Testosterone has been used to accelerate growth when stature is subnormal.

Testosterone therapy may be efficacious in the treatment of the *menopausal syndrome*, and, especially in combination with estrogens, in functional *dysmenorrhea*. It may also be used in the treatment of postpartum *breast engorgement* and for the *suppression of lactation*.

Testosterone and related compounds find widespread application in the palliative treatment of *cancer of the breast* in women who are premenopausal or early post-menopausal. Its use in men with prostatic cancer is, however, contraindicated.

Side effects of testosterone and other androgens are hirsutism, deepening or hoarseness of the voice, increased libido (in both male and female!), enlargement of the clitoris in the female, flushing, acne, weight gain, edema, and hypercalcemia. Hypercalcemia requires discontinuation of therapy, and edema requires diuretic therapy. Except in the treatment of breast cancer, a reduction in dosage is indicated upon virilization in women. Testosterone is not effective orally because it is destroyed in the liver upon absorption.

Dose—*Usual, buccal*, **10 mg** daily; *usual, implantation* **300 mg**; *usual, intramuscular*, **25 mg** twice a week to once daily, depending on condition being treated.

Dosage Forms—Pellets NF: 75 mg; Sterile Suspension NF: 250 and 500 mg/10 ml.

Veterinary Dose—*Intramuscular*, *Dogs*, 10 to 25 mg; *Horses*, 50 to 125 mg.

Testosterone Cypionate USP

[Testosterone Cyclopentylpropionate USP XVI; 17β-Hydroxyandrost-4-en-3-one Cyclopentanepropionate; Depo-Testosterone Cypionate (*Upjohn*)]

Testosterone Cypionate contains 97.0–103.0% of $C_{27}H_{40}O_3$ (412.62), calculated on the dried basis.

Preparation—Testosterone is esterified by interaction with 3-cyclopentylpropionyl chloride [C_5H_{11}-CH_2CH_2COCl] in the presence of pyridine. The solid ester is recovered by pouring the reaction mixture into cold 6N sulfuric acid, extracting the crude ester with isopropyl ether, washing the extract with water, drying the solution, removing the solvent, and crystallizing from hexane.

Description—It occurs as a white or creamy white, crystalline powder which is odorless and is stable in air. It melts between 98° and 104°. Its specific rotation is not less than +85° and not more than +92°.

Solubility—Insoluble in water; freely soluble in alcohol, chloroform, dioxane, and ether; soluble in vegetable oils.

Uses—The actions, uses, and limitations of Testosterone Cypionate are the same as those of *Testosterone* (see above), except that the cypionate has a much longer duration of action when administered intramuscularly in oil.

Dose—*Usual, intramuscular,* **100** to **400 mg** 1 or 2 times monthly.

Other Dose Information—For eunuchism the dose is 100 to 150 mg weekly. In women the dose in menstrual disorders is 25 mg 1 week in advance of the mense menorrhagia and once weekly for metrorrhagia and 100 mg once only for the suppression of lactation and postpartum breast engorgement. For the palliation of breast cancer, virilizing doses of at least 100 to 250 mg weekly are in the right range.

Dosage Forms—Injection USP: 100 and 200 mg/ml, 500 mg and 1 and 2 Gm/10 ml.

Testosterone Enanthate USP

[Testosterone Heptanoate; Delatestryl (*Squibb*)]

Testosterone Enanthate contains 97.0–103.0% of $C_{26}H_{40}O_3$ (400.61).

Preparation—A solution of enanthic acid in benzene is refluxed for about one hour after which it is allowed to cool, testosterone is added, and the mixture is refluxed for about 21 hours. The resulting light brown solution is cooled, extracted with a sodium hydroxide to remove surplus enanthic acid, washed with water, and dried over magnesium sulfate. After removal of solvent, the crude ester is distilled in a molecular still at 280°C under 0.8 micron Hg pressure.

Description—It occurs as a white or creamy white, crystalline powder or as a viscous, amber-colored liquid. It is odorless or has a faint odor characteristic of enanthic acid. It melts between 34° and 39°, the initial temperature of the bath not exceeding 20°. Its specific rotation is not less than +77° and not more than +82°.

Solubility—Insoluble in water; 1 Gm dissolves in about 0.3 ml of ether; soluble in vegetable oils.

Uses—The actions, uses, and limitations of Testosterone Enanthate are the same as those of *Testosterone* (page 1008), except that when administered intramuscularly in oil it has a much longer duration of action. The effects of a single intramuscular injection may last 3 to 4 weeks.

Dose—*Intramuscular,* **100** to **400 mg** 1 or 2 times a month.

Other Dose Information—There is not much difference in the recommended dose for various uses in either sex. Only one dose is given for the suppression of lactation and postoperative breast engorgement or once one week in advance of the menses in menorrhagia.

Dosage Forms—Injection USP: 200 mg/ml, 500 mg and 1 Gm/5 ml, 1 and 2 Gm/10 ml.

Testosterone Propionate USP

[17β-Hydroxyandrost-4-en-3-one Propionate; Andronaq (*Central*); Neo-Hombreol (*Organon*); Oreton (*Schering*); Perandren (*Ciba*)]

Testosterone Propionate contains 97.0–103.0% of $C_{22}H_{32}O_3$ (344.50), calculated on the dried basis.

Preparation—It is readily prepared from testosterone by refluxing with propionic anhydride.

Description—White or creamy white crystals or crystalline powder. It is odorless and is stable in air. It melts between 118° and 123°. The specific rotation, $[\alpha]_D^{25}$, determined in a solution in dioxane, is between +83° and +90°.

Solubility—Insoluble in water; freely soluble in alcohol, dioxane, ether, and other organic solvents; soluble in vegetable oils.

Uses—The actions, uses, and limitations of Testosterone Propionate are the same as those of *Testosterone*

(page 1008). Intramuscular injection of the propionate provides a somewhat more intense action than with testosterone, but the duration of action is somewhat shorter. The other esters of testosterone and synthetic congeners have considerably diminished the importance of the propionate.

Dose—*Intramuscular,* **25** to **150 mg** weekly; *usual,* **25 mg** 3 times a week.

Other Dose Information—In males, the usual dose is 10 to 50 mg 2 to 6 times a week; in females, 10 to 25 mg triweekly, not to exceed a total monthly dosage of 150 mg, except when 150 to 300 mg is administered weekly for breast cancer or when 50 to 75 mg is administered in 2 or 3 days for suppression of lactation and breast engorgement; the buccal dose, in males is 5 to 10 mg daily.

Dosage Forms—Injection USP: 10, 25, 50, and 100 mg/ml, 100, 250, and 500 mg and 1 Gm/10 ml.

Veterinary Uses—Deficiency of androgenic hormone in all species, impotence, testicular deficiency, cryptorchidism due to androgenic deficiency (not anatomic anomalies).

Veterinary Dose—*Horses* and *Cattle,* **100** to **300 mg**; *Sheep,* **100 mg**; *Dogs,* **20** to **50 mg**, injected *intramuscularly* or *subcutaneously* only.

Other Androgenic Hormones

Ethylestrenol [$C_{20}H_{32}O$ (288.46); Maxibolin (*Organon*)] is 17α-ethylestr-4-en-17-ol. *Preparation:* A solution of 3-ethoxy-17α-ethylestradiol in ether is reacted in the cold with dry ethylamine to which lithium has been added in small pieces. Following a suitable solvent extraction process, the crude dry product is distributed between equal parts of petroleum ether and 70% methanol. The petroleum ether layer is separated and evaporated to yield the Ethylestrenol. US Pat. 3,112,328. *Description and Solubility:* A white to creamy white, crystalline powder that is odorless and tasteless. It is unstable in heat and light and is nonhygroscopic. It melts between 83° and 95°. Freely soluble in alcohol; soluble in chloroform, acetone, and methanol; practically insoluble in water.

Uses: Ethylestrenol is an anabolic steroid related to the androgens. It promotes tissue building, a renewal of vigor, a feeling of well being, and bone matrix reconstruction. Consequently, there is an increase in appetite and body weight. It is used in treating the wasting diseases to facilitate convalescence from prolonged illness, and to arrest osteoporosis. It is also used to antagonize certain catabolic effects of corticosteroid therapy. Its most serious side effect is cholestatic jaundice in common with other anabolic steroids. Although its androgenic actions are weak, the drug may induce withdrawal bleeding and amenorrhea in women, and it is contraindicated in prostatic carcinoma. *Dose: Oral,* 4 to 8 mg once a day for up to 6 weeks; after a 4-week pause, an additional course may be administered if indicated.

Methandriol [Methylandrostenediol; Stenediol (*Organon*)] [17-methylandrost-5-en-3β,17β-diol]—Methandriol is one of several well-known anabolic androgens possessing low androgenic activity with less virilizing effect than testosterone. It occurs as an odorless, white crystalline powder that melts at 198°–206°. It is insoluble in water, readily soluble in methyl alcohol and ethyl alcohol, soluble in ethyl acetate and sparingly soluble in ether. *Uses:* In the treatment of nervous anorexia, retarded growth, convalescence, and dysmenorrhea; for the prophylaxis and treatment of negative nitrogen balance in senile osteoporosis; spinal paraplegia, and decubitus ulcer; in the treatment of inoperable breast cancer. *Dose: Orally* and *sublingually,* 0.03 to 0.3 Gm daily, depending on use.

Testolactone [Teslac (*Squibb*)] is 1,2,3,4,4a,4b,7,9,10-,10a-decahydro-2-hydroxy-2,4b-dimethyl-7-oxo-1-phenanthrenepropionic acid δ-lactone ($C_{19}H_{24}O_3$). *Description:* Crystals which melt between 218° and 219°. *Uses:* An androgenic steroid employed for palliative treatment of advance or metastatic carcinoma of the breast in postmenopausal women who would otherwise be candidates for androgen treatment. In premenopausal women the drug is not recommended until after surgical or radiation castration. It appears that the drug is devoid of androgenic or any other steroid hormonal activity and that its effect is a cytotoxic one of unknown mechanism. However, Testolactone is new, and claims must be corroborated by additional objective studies. Side effects include irritation and inflammation at the site of injection, with slight pain, macupapular erythema, and hypertension. In instances in which large doses of the drug follow adrenal corticoids, alopecia has been reported. Nausea and vomiting, paresthesias, myalgia, and arthralgia, which are also symptoms of the disease, have been reported. *Dose: Intramuscular,* 100 mg 3 times a week. Although responses often appear to be prompt, as long as 3 months may be required before evidence of remission occurs.

Testosterone Phenylacetate [Perandren Phenylacetate (*Ciba*)] [$C_{27}H_{34}O_3$]—White, crystalline powder, insoluble in water, soluble in chloroform and vegetable oils. Melting range is 125° to 131°. *Uses:* Testosterone Phenyl-

acetate has the same actions, uses and limitations as *Testosterone* (page 1008). However, injected intramuscularly as a crystalline suspension, it has a very long duration of action, approached only by the enanthate. A single intramuscular injection may exert an action for as long as a month. *Dose: Intramuscularly,* for male climacteric or prepubertal hypogonadism, 50 mg every 3 to 4 weeks; for eunuchoidism, 50 to 200 mg every 3 to 5 weeks; for osteoporosis, 100 mg in the male and 25 mg in the female every 3 to 4 weeks; for nitrogen anabolism, 25 to 40 mg every 4 weeks; in breast cancer, 150 to 300 mg monthly; in menorrhagia, 25 mg 1 week before the mense; in metrorrhagia, 25 mg every 2 to 3 weeks.

References

1. *Thyrotropin* (monograph), Thomas, Springfield, Ill., 1963.
2. *Medicinal Chemistry,* Vol. II, Wiley, New York, 1956.
3. Brückner, K., et al, *Chem. Ber.,* **94,** 1225 (1961).
4. *Rec. Trav. Chim.,* **79,** 771 (1960).
5. *Rec. Trav. Chim.,* **80,** 43 (1961).
6. *J. Am. Chem. Soc.,* **76,** 552 (1954).
7. *J. Am. Chem. Soc.,* **81,** 427 (1959).

56 | Vitamins and Other Nutrients

Fat-soluble vitamins—water-soluble vitamins—multivitamin
preparations—proteins and amino acids—sugars—fats—trace minerals

This chapter was prepared by

O. L. Kline, PhD, *American Institute of Nutrition, Bethesda, Md.   20014, and*
J. W. Boehne, BS, *Division of Nutrition, Food and Drug Administration,*
Washington, D. C.   20204

The principal purpose of food consumed by man is to provide energy for growth, maintenance of body functions, and work. This energy is furnished by carbohydrates, fats, and proteins. The proportion of each of these constituents of the diet varies widely according to the local economy, culture, and personal taste of the individual. However, normal physiological and metabolic function, growth, and repair require adequate ingestion of other nutriments which serve structural, osmotic, and catalytic functions, but do not necessarily provide energy. The chief structural substances of the body are proteins, lipoproteins, ground substance (a complex mucopolysaccharide), and "bone salts." Dietary requirements for this purpose are calcium, phosphate, and an adequate level of protein with its appropriate pattern of essential amino acids. The trace minerals of importance in nutrition are treated separately from minerals which function as electrolytes. These electrolytes are principally sodium, potassium, chloride, and magnesium, which are presented in Chapter 45, page 815. An understanding of the place of vitamins and other nutrients in human physiology has evolved largely from research studies on lower forms of life, mainly bacteria and animals such as the chick, rat, guinea pig, and dog. Added to this are the illuminating studies on clinical evaluation of malnutrition that is found in underdeveloped countries.

Vitamins

Vitamins are organic compounds which are required for the normal growth and maintenance of life of animals, including man, who as a rule, are unable to synthesize these compounds by anabolic processes that are independent of environment other than air, and which compounds are effective in small amounts, do not furnish energy, and are not utilized as building units for the structure of the organism, but are essential for the transformation of energy and for the regulation of the metabolism of structural units. They or their precursors are found in plants and, so far as is known, have specific metabolic functions to perform in plant cells. Plant tissues are the sources to the animal kingdom of these protective nutritional factors. In addition to carbohydrates, fats, proteins, mineral salts, and water, it is essential that the food of man and animals contain small amounts of these organic substances called *vitamins*. If any one of at least 13 of these compounds is lacking in the diet, there occurs eventually a breakdown of the normal metabolic processes that results in a reduced rate or complete lack of growth in children, and in symptoms of malnutrition that are classed as the *deficiency diseases*.

The vitamins are unlike each other in their chemical composition and their function in nature. They are alike only in that they cannot be synthesized at all or at least at an adequate rate in the tissues of animals. The functions they serve fall into two categories, the maintenance of normal structure and of normal metabolic functions. For example, vitamin A is essential for the maintenance of normal epithelial tissue; vitamin D functions in the absorption of normal bone salts for the formation and growth of a sound bony structure. Certain vitamins of the water-soluble group, among them thiamine, riboflavin, pantothenic acid, and niacin, are known to be essential constituents of the respiratory enzymes that are required in the utilization of energy from oxidative catabolism of sugars and fats.

It is convenient in a discussion of this subject to divide these nutritional substances into two groups, the *fat-soluble* and the *water-soluble factors*. Vitamins A, D, E, and K fall into the fat-soluble group, since they can be extracted with fat solvents and are found in the fat fractions of animal tissues. The water-soluble vitamins include ascorbic acid and the B group of vitamins, which consists of some 10 or more well-defined compounds. The characterization of vitamins as essential metabolic factors with discrete chemical structures included their isolation in pure form from natural sources and subsequent laboratory synthesis. Commercial chemical or microbiological syntheses, some from relatively simple compounds, are the source of most of the vitamins now used in pharmaceutical preparations, dietary supplements, and fortified foods.

Standardization—Vitamin activity or potency is measured by three different types of methods. (1) *Biological procedures* in which rats, mice, guinea pigs, and chickens serve as the assay animals, have been extensively used, and for some of the vitamins are the most reliable means of assay. (2) *Microbiological assay methods* which employ bacteria that require certain of the water-soluble vitamins, are rapid, specific, and precise. Such methods are used for manufacturing and laboratory control of the production of some vitamins. (3) *Chemical methods*, utilizing a sensitive reac-

Table I—Minimum Daily Requirements for Vitamins and Minerals Established by the Food and Drug Administration[a]

	Vitamin A, USP Units	Vitamin D, USP Units	Vitamin C, mg	Thia-min, mg	Ribo-flavin, mg	Nia-cin, mg	Cal-cium, Gm	Phos-phorus, Gm	Iron, mg	Iodine, mg
Infants	1500	400	10	0.25	0.6	[b]	[b]	[b]	[b]	[b]
1–6 years	3000	400	20	0.50	0.9	5.0	0.75	0.75	7.5	0.1
6–12 years	3000	400	20	0.75	0.9	7.5	0.75	0.75	10.0	0.1
12 years or more	4000	400	30	1.0	1.2	10.0	0.75	0.75	10.0	0.1
Pregnant or lactating women[c]	4000	400	30	1.0	1.2	10.0	1.5	1.5	15.0	0.1

[a] Taken from regulations under Section 403(j), Federal Food, Drug and Cosmetic Act. Values vary somewhat from Recommended Dietary Allowances of the Food and Nutrition Board, National Academy of Sciences–National Research Council.
[b] No value established.
[c] Minimum daily requirements for calcium and iron are established specifically for pregnant or lactating women. Other values represent requirements for all persons 12 years of age or older, except for vitamin D, which applies to the entire population (infants, children, and adults).

tion specific for the compounds, are available for most vitamins in uncomplicated mixtures. The status of vitamin methods of assay is now such that manufacturers of vitamin preparations find it possible to state with precision the potency of their products, and tables of vitamin content of foods are quite complete. Methods of assay are described briefly in the individual vitamin sections.

In the interest of improvement and uniformity of expressing the results of such assays, the World Health Organization of the United Nations has sponsored the preparation and distribution of Standards. As a rule, an International Standard is no longer provided once the substance responsible for its characteristic activity has been isolated, identified, and made readily available. The USP has set up comparable Reference Standards in this country with biological potency of vitamins A and D expressed in USP Units that are equal to International Units. International Units are still in common use for vitamin A (1 IU = 0.344 mcg all-*trans*-retinyl acetate), carotene (1 IU = 1 IU vitamin A [rat] = 0.5 IU vitamin A [man] = 0.6 mcg all-*trans*-β-carotene), vitamin D (1 IU = 0.025 mcg cholecalciferol or ergocalciferol, as measured by rat assay) and vitamin E (1 IU = 1 mg dl-α-tocopheryl acetate). However, availability of all the vitamins in pure form encourages a transition from use of units to use of weight in expressing amounts present in vitamin products. There are official *USP Reference Standards* for ascorbic acid, calcium pantothenate, cholecalciferol (vitamin D_3), choline chloride, cyanocobalamin, ergocalciferol (vitamin D_2), folic acid, niacinamide, pyridoxine hydrochloride, riboflavin, thiamine hydrochloride, vitamin A, vitamin D capsules, and vitamin D oil.

Requirements—Requirements of man and animals for each of the vitamins have been the subject of extensive study. Our knowledge is not complete, but it has been possible to construct tables of requirement values that have been useful in surveying the nutritional status of population groups in this country and in many other parts of the world. A table of Recommended Dietary Allowances for certain nutrients (vitamins, minerals, protein, and calories) has been formulated by the Food and Nutrition Board of the National Academy of Sciences–National Research Council. These values shown in Table II are the amounts estimated to meet the need for maintaining good nutrition of practically all healthy people in this country.

Both the Food and Drug Administration and National Research Council engage actively in reviewing the minimal daily requirements, requirements in deficiency, therapeutic claims, and vitamin combinations

and multivitamin use. Both new guidelines and regulations are expected in the near future.

Under the Food, Drug and Cosmetic Act, regulations pertaining to foods for special dietary use have been promulgated, which include a statement of minimum daily requirements for certain of the vitamins and minerals. These values are for the purpose of labeling foods and pharmaceutical preparations which come under the purview of this Act and are listed in Table I.

In addition to the vitamins listed in Table I, it is recognized that vitamin E, vitamin K, pantothenic acid, pyridoxine, folic acid, biotin, and vitamin B_{12} are essential in human nutrition, but for purposes of these regulations minimum daily requirement values for them have not been established.

Widespread use of vitamins has served to control and eradicate to a large extent the important deficiency diseases which have occurred in both the animal and the human population of this country. Since 1930 the deficiency disease, rickets, has become exceedingly rare. This has resulted from an extensive use of foods and pharmaceutical preparations that contain added vitamin D. Pellagra, prevalent during the 1930's in the southern part of the United States, is now rarely seen and is controlled in part by means of the addition of niacin to the diet in the form of enriched foods, and by the use of a variety of foods that go to make up a well-balanced diet.

Nutrition Misinformation

There is a vast amount of confusion in the public mind about the influence which various foods or specially prepared products, such as vitamin supplements, have on the preservation or promotion of good health and even the prevention or cure of a variety of diseases. It is indeed difficult to impress the impressionable with the simple fact about nutrition—that if appetizing meals include a wide variety of foods individually chosen with reasonable judgement, adequate if not abundant amounts of all essential nutrients can be obtained. Instead, many people are prey to the misrepresentations and outright false claims made for "health foods," including dietary supplements, by self-styled doctors and pseudo-nutritionists. Such charlatans, through lectures, advertising, or even door-to-door canvassing, often convincingly use technical language that persuades the uninformed and frequently physically suffering individual to purchase the nostrums offered for sale. A simple test of the truthfulness of an "expert" is usually this: If claims are made that particular foods or combinations of foods

Table II—Food and Nutrition Board, National Academy of Sciences–National Research Council Recommended Daily Dietary Allowances,[a] Revised 1968[b]
Designed for the Maintenance of Good Nutrition of Practically All Healthy People in the USA

	Age[c] (years) From	Age[c] (years) To	Weight (Kg)	Weight (lb)	Height (cm)	Height (in.)	Kcal	Protein (Gm)	Vitamin A Activity (IU)	Vitamin D (IU)	Vitamin E Activity (IU)	Ascorbic Acid (mg)	Folacin[d] (mg)	Niacin (mg equiv)[e]	Riboflavin (mg)	Thiamin (mg)	Vitamin B6 (mg)	Vitamin B12 (mcg)	Calcium (Gm)	Phosphorus (Gm)	Iodine (mcg)	Iron (mg)	Magnesium (mg)
Infants	0	1/6	4	9	55	22	kg × 120	kg × 2.2[f]	1,500	400	5	35	0.05	5	0.4	0.2	0.2	1.0	0.4	0.2	25	6	40
	1/6	1/2	7	15	63	25	kg × 110	kg × 2.0[f]	1,500	400	5	35	0.05	7	0.5	0.4	0.3	1.5	0.5	0.4	40	10	60
	1/2	1	9	20	72	28	kg × 100	kg × 1.8[f]	1,500	400	5	35	0.1	8	0.6	0.5	0.4	2.0	0.6	0.5	45	15	70
Children	1	2	12	26	81	32	1,100	25	2,000	400	10	40	0.1	8	0.6	0.6	0.5	2.0	0.7	0.7	55	15	100
	2	3	14	31	91	36	1,250	25	2,000	400	10	40	0.2	8	0.7	0.6	0.6	2.5	0.8	0.8	60	15	150
	3	4	16	35	100	39	1,400	30	2,500	400	10	40	0.2	9	0.8	0.7	0.7	3	0.8	0.8	70	10	200
	4	6	19	42	110	43	1,600	30	2,500	400	10	40	0.2	11	0.9	0.8	0.9	4	0.8	0.8	80	10	200
	6	8	23	51	121	48	2,000	35	3,500	400	15	40	0.2	13	1.1	1.0	1.0	4	0.9	0.9	100	10	250
	8	10	28	62	131	52	2,200	40	3,500	400	15	40	0.3	15	1.2	1.1	1.2	5	1.0	1.0	110	10	250
Males	10	12	35	77	140	55	2,500	45	4,500	400	20	40	0.4	17	1.3	1.3	1.4	5	1.2	1.2	125	10	300
	12	14	43	95	151	59	2,700	50	5,000	400	20	45	0.4	18	1.4	1.4	1.6	5	1.4	1.4	135	18	350
	14	18	59	130	170	67	3,000	60	5,000	400	25	55	0.4	20	1.5	1.5	1.8	5	1.4	1.4	150	18	400
	18	22	67	147	175	69	2,800	60	5,000	400	30	60	0.4	18	1.6	1.4	2.0	5	0.8	0.8	140	10	400
	22	35	70	154	175	69	2,800	65	5,000	—	30	60	0.4	18	1.7	1.4	2.0	5	0.8	0.8	140	10	350
	35	55	70	154	173	68	2,600	65	5,000	—	30	60	0.4	17	1.7	1.3	2.0	5	0.8	0.8	125	10	350
	55	75+	70	154	171	67	2,400	65	5,000	—	30	60	0.4	14	1.7	1.2	2.0	6	0.8	0.8	110	10	350
Females	10	12	35	77	142	56	2,250	50	4,500	400	20	40	0.4	15	1.3	1.1	1.4	5	1.2	1.2	110	18	300
	12	14	44	97	154	61	2,300	50	5,000	400	20	45	0.4	15	1.4	1.2	1.6	5	1.3	1.3	115	18	350
	14	16	52	114	157	62	2,400	55	5,000	400	25	50	0.4	16	1.4	1.2	1.8	5	1.3	1.3	120	18	350
	16	18	54	119	160	63	2,300	55	5,000	400	25	50	0.4	15	1.5	1.2	2.0	5	1.3	1.3	115	18	350
	18	22	58	128	163	64	2,000	55	5,000	400	25	55	0.4	13	1.5	1.0	2.0	5	0.8	0.8	100	18	350
	22	35	58	128	163	64	2,000	55	5,000	—	25	55	0.4	13	1.5	1.0	2.0	5	0.8	0.8	100	18	300
	35	55	58	128	160	63	1,850	55	5,000	—	25	55	0.4	13	1.5	1.0	2.0	5	0.8	0.8	90	18	300
	55	75+	58	128	157	62	1,700	55	5,000	—	25	55	0.4	13	1.5	1.0	2.0	6	0.8	0.8	80	10	300
Pregnancy							+200	65	6,000	400	30	60	0.8	15	1.8	+0.1	2.5	8	+0.4	+0.4	125	18	450
Lactation							+1,000	75	8,000	400	30	60	0.5	20	2.0	+0.5	2.5	6	+0.5	+0.5	150	18	450

[a] The allowance levels are intended to cover individual variations among most normal persons as they live in the United States under usual environmental stresses. The recommended allowances can be attained with a variety of common foods, providing other nutrients for which human requirements have been less well defined. See text for more detailed discussion of allowances and of nutrients not tabulated.

[b] Courtesy, *Recommended Dietary Allowances* (NAS-NRC Publ. 1694), 7th rev. ed., Food and Nutrition Board, NAS-NRC, Washington, D.C., 1968.

[c] Entries on lines for age range 22–35 years represent the reference man and woman at age 22. All other entries represent allowances for the midpoint of the specified age range.

[d] The folacin allowances refer to dietary sources as determined by *Lactobacillus casei* assay. Pure forms of folacin may be effective in doses less than ¼ of the RDA.

[e] Niacin equivalents include dietary sources of the vitamin itself plus 1 mg equivalent for each 60 mg of dietary tryptophan.

[f] Assumes protein equivalent to human milk. For proteins not 100 percent utilized factors should be increased proportionately.

Table III—Vitamin Nomenclature

Vitamin	Synonym or descriptive terms
A group	antixerophthalmic vitamin
A₁	retinol, axerophthol
A₂	dehydroretinol
Provitamins A	carotene (alpha, beta, & gamma), cryptoxanthin (hydroxy beta-carotene). Plant carotenoid pigments converted to vitamin A in animal body
B group	water-soluble B, formerly vitamin B complex
Thiamine	vitamin B₁, aneurin, antiberiberi vitamin
Riboflavin	vitamin B₂, lactoflavin
Niacin and niacinamide	nicotinic acid and nicotinamide, pellagra-preventive factor
Pantothenic acid	formerly vitamin B₃
Pyridoxine	vitamin B₆ group: three naturally occurring compounds with interchangeable potential vitamin activity—pyridoxine, pyridoxal, pyridoxamine
Biotin	anti-egg white injury factor
Folic acid	pteroyl (mono) glutamic acid, PGA, folacin. Folic acid also generic term for pteroylglutamates containing several glutamic acid residues (tri-, hepta-, etc.) formerly known as Norite eluate factor, L. casei factor. Folinic acid, formyltetrahydro PGA, formerly known as citrovorum factor
B₁₂	cyanocobalamin, anti-pernicious anemia vitamin, extrinsic factor, erythrocyte maturation factor, vitamin B₁₂ᵦ (aquocobalamine or hydroxocobalamin), vitamin B₁₂ᶜ (nitritocobalamin)
C	L-ascorbic acid, antiscorbutic vitamin
D group	antirachitic vitamin
D₂	ergocalciferol (formerly calciferol), activated ergosterol
D₃	cholecalciferol, activated 7-dehydrocholesterol
E group	tocopherols
α-tocopherol β-tocopherol γ-tocopherol	Possess vitamin E activity in varying degrees. Occur as fatty acid esters
K group	antihemorrhagic vitamin
K₁ K₂	phytonadione, phylloquinone / farnoquinone — naturally occurring
K₃ K₄₋₇	menadione / biologically active analogs of menadione — synthetic

are related to either the production or prevention of cancer, arthritis, heart disease, or several other diseases, or that particular foods will give a superior level of health, one can assume at once that the experts or writers are unreliable and should be received skeptically. Serious consequences may result when the purchaser accepts the advice of the purveyor of a falsely labeled product in place of proper and needed treatment of diseases such as cancer.

The Food and Drug Administration has an important responsibility to control interstate traffic in products falsely promoted through food faddism and nutritional quackery. Food faddism thrives on myths that our crops are produced on impoverished and depleted soils and are therefore "devitalized"; that our foods are inadequate sources of vitamins because of losses during shipping, storage, and cooking; that vitamin deficiency disease is widespread in this country; and that the only salvation for the prospective buyer is the purchase of the vitamin product offered. If the labeling includes false or misleading statements, the Food and Drug Administration can institute legal action. By its countrywide activity of monitoring the labeling as well as the composition of the myriad of packaged foods on the market, some degree of compliance with regulations that ensure fair and honest practices is accomplished.

The suspicion of fraudulent practices in dissemination of nutrition misinformation, especially through labeling, should be reported by pharmacists to the nearest Food and Drug Administration office.

Since their dramatic discovery during the first half of this century, vitamins and trace elements have had special appeal for the enthusiastically health-minded but inadequately informed public. The Council on Foods and Nutrition of the American Medical Association summarizes the value of vitamin preparations in a report entitled "Vitamin Preparations as Dietary Supplements and as Therapeutic Agents."[1] This is an authoritative evaluation of the conditions in which vitamin preparations may be useful, and sets forth the combinations of ingredients and amounts of vitamins that are used rationally for diet supplementation or for therapy.

It must be recognized that, particularly in the field of nutrition where misinformation may endanger the public health, the consumer must be helped by a continuous and effective program of nutrition education. The pharmacist, because of his day-to-day contact with the public most directly concerned, has an important responsibility to be well informed, to allay the fears that are created in the pseudo-scientific writings of the unscrupulous, and to protect the purse as well as the health of his patron.

The Fat-Soluble Vitamins

Vitamin A and Carotene

Vitamin A was the first fat-soluble vitamin discovered. Animal nutritionists observed growth failures in calves born of cows maintained on wheat or oats alone, whereas whole cornplant supported growth and development of the animals. The vitamin was found to be related to chlorophyll and carotenoid-containing plants. Later study revealed that the vitamin is essential for the maintenance of normal tissue structure and for other important physiologic functions such as vision and reproduction.

Chemistry and Assay—Vitamin A is represented primarily by the cyclic polyene alcohol vitamin A₁ (retinol) with an empirical formula of $C_{20}H_{30}O$ and whose four conjugated double bonds in the side chain are in the *trans* arrangement.

$$CH_3 \quad CH_3 \qquad CH_3 \qquad\qquad CH_3$$
$$-CH=CHC=CHCH=CHC=CHCH_2OH$$
$$CH_3$$

Vitamin A (Retinol) (Vitamin A₁)

Another representative of vitamin A occurring in nature is vitamin A_2, which has an additional double bond in the ring at the 3-4 position. It has only about ¼ to ½ the biological activity of vitamin A_1 for the rat and has no commercial significance. A third such representative is neovitamin A-a in which the terminal double bond in the side chain of vitamin A_1 is *cis*. It has low biological activity.

Vitamin A_1 is a pale yellow crystalline compound, is soluble in fat solvents, and has an ultraviolet absorption maximum at 328 mμ wavelength. The vitamin is not readily destroyed by heat but is easily oxidized and is less stable in acid than in alkaline solution. The esters of vitamin A_1 with the fatty acids, acetic and palmitic, are commercially important since they are considerably more stable than the alcohol.

The source of most of the vitamin A in animals, birds, and fish is the carotenoid pigments, the yellow-colored compounds in all chlorophyll-containing plants. At least 10 different carotenoids exhibit provitamin A activity, but only alpha- and beta-carotene and cryptoxanthin (found in yellow corn) are important in animal nutrition, beta-carotene being the most important.

β-Carotene

Stoichiometrically, one molecule of beta-carotene can yield two molecules of vitamin A_1, whereas alpha-carotene and cryptoxanthin can yield only one molecule. The conversion of the provitamin to vitamin A occurs primarily in the walls of the small intestine and perhaps to a lesser degree in the liver. Like vitamin A_1, the carotenes are soluble in fat solvents, in crystalline form appear deep orange or copper-colored, and have characteristic absorption spectra.

Total synthesis of vitamin A_1 and beta-carotene is achieved commercially, vitamin A usually being prepared as the acetate. Concentration of vitamin A from animal fats and fish liver oil is still important. The principal steps in the process are molecular distillation, saponification, and crystallization of the distillate and conversion to the desired ester.

The USP Unit for vitamin A is identical to the International Unit. The USP Reference Standard for vitamin A is a solution of crystalline vitamin A acetate in cottonseed oil such that there is contained 1 USP Unit (0.344 mcg) per 0.1 mg of solution. Although there is no USP Unit for carotene, there is an International Unit; the relation between carotene and vitamin A is 6 to 3.44 by weight of the respective pure compounds.

Vitamin A can be assayed by direct measurement of its ultraviolet absorption, by photometric evaluation of the color reaction with antimony trichloride in chloroform (the Carr–Price reaction), or by a biologic method based on the resumption of growth of rats when the vitamin activity is added to a vitamin A-deficient diet. The Carr–Price method is the most widely used. The chemical or physicochemical determination of beta-carotene depends upon measurement of the yellow color of its solutions in organic solvents. Chromatographic separation of associated carotenoids is usually necessary before an accurate analysis of the biologically active compounds can be made.

Metabolic Functions—Of the known functions of vitamin A in the body, its role in the visual process is established best. The retina of man contains two distinct photoreceptor systems. The rods, which are the structural components of one system, are especially sensitive to light of low intensity. A specific vitamin A aldehyde is essential for the formation of rhodopsin (the high molecular weight glycoprotein part of the visual pigment within the rods) and the normal functioning of the retina. By virtue of this relation to the visual process, vitamin A alcohol has been named retinol and the aldehyde form named retinal. A vitamin A-deficient person has an impaired dark adaptation ("night-blindness").

Vitamin A also participates in the maintenance of the integrity of the epithelial membranes such that normal structures may be substituted by stratified keratinizing epithelium in the eyes and paraocular glands, respiratory, alimentary and genitourinary tracts under the stresses of a deficiency. The basal cells do not lose their function under such conditions, however, and are able to be restored to normal when sufficient vitamin A is absorbed. Abnormalities of nerve and connective tissue and of bones are further consequences of a dietary deficiency of the vitamin. In severe deficiency the affected epithelial and connective tissue may become the site of infections due to the cells' reduced resistance to bacterial invasion. This gave rise to the notion that administration of vitamin A was useful in the treatment of skin infections. However, several decades of expert medical opinion hold this application to be an abuse and that the vitamin has no anti-infective value in the absence of a specific deficiency. Nevertheless, there has been a flurry of recent reports that both topical and oral vitamin A, and especially vitamin A acid, improve the condition of the skin in acne vulgaris; further well-controlled clinical trials are required to establish the validity of these claims.

The common severe deficiency symptoms are increased susceptibility to microbial infections, xerophthalmia and other eye disorders, loss of appetite and weight, and sterility, conditions which require a long time for their development. Although the recommended daily allowance is no more than 8000 Units per day, in a deficiency much greater amounts are indicated. For example, the usual therapeutic oral dose range is from 10,000 to 20,000 Units daily for 7 to 10 days for infants and growing children and 25,000 to 100,000 Units daily for older children and adults.

If large doses of vitamin A or of carotene are ingested for long periods of time, manifestations of toxicity develop. In the absence of a deficiency, chronic administration of vitamin A of 50,000 to 75,000 Units daily induce pathologic changes in bone and periosteal tissues, skin and mucous membranes, liver, and changes in behavior. Doses as low as 18,500 Units of a water-dispersed vitamin A preparation daily for 1 to 3 months are reported to be toxic for infants 3 to 6 months of age.

Dietary Requirement and Food Sources—According to the National Research Council's "Recommended Dietary Allowances," the requirement for vitamin A appears to be proportional to body weight. The recommended allowance for the maintenance of good nutrition of healthy adults in the US is 5,000 Units of vitamin A activity daily, although the adult requirement for maintenance of normalcy in important vitamin A functions is about ½ this value. Somewhat more vitamin A than the allowance should be provided during the latter two-thirds of pregnancy and even more during lactation. These increments would assure the nutritional well being of the rapidly growing fetus and nursing infant, who are dependent on the mother's vitamin A intake.

About ½ of the vitamin A activity in the average American diet comes from carotene and related compounds. The other half is provided by the vitamin itself present in foods of animal origin. Not all of the carotene present in the food eaten is converted into vitamin A. Some passes through the digestive tract and is excreted as such. The richest sources of carotene are yellow and green (leafy) vegetables and yellow fruits. Preformed vitamin A_1 is supplied primarily from the fat of dairy products and egg-yolk, but other important sources in some diets are liver, kidney, and fish. Federal regulations provide for the optional addition of 15,000 USP Units of vitamin A per pound of margarine. Almost all margarine is so fortified. There are also provisions for marketing vitamins A & D fortified nonfat dry milk containing 500 Units vitamin A and 100 Units vitamin D per reconstituted 8 fluid ounces.

Vitamin D

Vitamin D is the antirachitic vitamin effective in promoting calcification of the bony structures of man and animals. It is sometimes popularly known as the "sunshine" vitamin because it is formed by the action of the sun's ultraviolet rays on precursor sterols in the skin. Exposure to sunlight, therefore, has a powerful antirachitic effect. The term rachitic denotes the condition of a person or animal affected with the deficiency disease rickets.

Chemistry and Assay—The two immediate biological precursors (provitamins) to the vitamins D are the steroid alcohols ergosterol (ergosta-5,7,22-trien-3β-ol) and 7-dehydrocholesterol (cholesta-5,7-dien-3β-ol). Under the influence of ultraviolet light, each undergoes scission of the 9(10) bond of the steroid nucleus with the simultaneous creation of a 10(19) double bond yielding, respectively, vitamin D_2 (ergocalciferol) and vitamin D_3 (cholecalciferol).

Vitamin D_2 (Ergocalciferol)
Vitamin D_3 (Cholecalciferol):
same except C_{17} side chain is

Pure vitamins D_2 and D_3 are white, odorless crystals that are soluble in fat solvents such as ether, alcohol or chloroform, but insoluble in water. The compounds have characteristic absorption spectra, which property is useful in their identification. Both forms of the vitamin are stable to oxidation by air and to moderate heat in neutral and alkaline solutions. Upon alkaline saponification of fats, the vitamin appears in the nonsaponifiable fraction. It withstands autoclaving temperatures of 120° in the absence of air, but at this temperature is subject to oxidation, and it is completely destroyed by heating at 170°. Vitamin D is

stable over long periods of storage in oil solution but is quite unstable in the presence of mineral salts, such as tricalcium phosphate, when compounded in tablet form. It may be stabilized by dispersion in gelatin or a similar protective coating.

The international standard for vitamin D is a crystalline preparation of pure vitamin D_3 assigned a potency of 40 million units per Gm. The USP adopted an equivalent standard of vitamin D_3 with the same assigned potency, distributed in the form of a cottonseed oil solution.

The provitamins D are found in both plant and animal tissue; 7-dehydrocholesterol is principally found in animal skin and ergosterol in relatively large amounts in yeasts, although it was first isolated from ergot. The vitamin D which is absorbed through the intestinal wall from dietary sources or which is formed in the skin from 7-dehydrocholesterol enters the circulatory system, and excesses are stored. Like vitamin A, vitamin D is stored in animal body fats, principally in the liver. The liver oils, particularly of fish, are the most potent natural sources of the vitamin. The vitamin D of commerce is now principally synthesized from readily available structurally related compounds, such as cholesterol, which are often obtained as packinghouse byproducts.

There are two methods available for quantitative physicochemical assay of vitamin D; however, the biological assay based on the curative effects of the vitamin on experimental rickets in young rats is the method of choice for accurately measuring the total biological activity of the vitamin in complex materials of low potency. Minimal amounts of the vitamin are needed by the rat; therefore, the rachitic condition is produced by using an abnormal high-calcium, low-phosphorus diet. For relatively concentrated solutions of vitamin D in alcohol (but not in oil), ultraviolet spectrophotometric determination is made at the wavelength of maximum absorption. Antimony trichloride reacts with various vitamins D in a Carr–Price reaction yielding a yellow color whose intensity is proportional to the vitamin D present. The reaction is satisfactory only for concentrated preparations; cholesterol and vitamin A interfere only when present in amounts in excess of certain limits.

Metabolic Functions—Vitamin D aids in the absorption of calcium from the intestinal tract and the resorption of phosphate in the renal tubule. It induces the formation or elaboration of a calcium-binding factor by intestinal mucosa, the factor being a protein. The vitamin acts, therefore, as an initiator of the synthesis of enzymes in the mucosa which, in turn, are involved in the active transport of ingested available calcium. Vitamin D is necessary for normal growth in children, but whether this is a general metabolic effect or whether it is related specifically to calcification and growth of the long bones is not clear.

A deficiency of vitamin D leads to inadequate absorption of calcium from the intestinal tract and retention of phosphorus in the kidney and thence to faulty mineralization of bone structures. The inability of the soft bones to withstand the stress of weight results in skeletal malformations. Early rickets is difficult to diagnose, but fully developed cases in infants and children present characteristic signs. These include delayed closure of the fontanelles and softening of the skull, soft fragile bones with bowing of the legs and spinal curvature, enlargement of wrist, knee, and ankle joints, poorly developed muscles, restlessness, and nervous irritability. A form of "adult rickets" called osteomalacia similarly may occur. It, too, represents a failure of the process of calcification caused by simple vitamin D lack and calcium inadequacy.

With adequate calcium–phosphorus intake, adult osteomalacia and uncomplicated rickets can be cured by ordinary daily allowances of 400 Units of vitamin D. Larger doses (about 1600 Units or more daily) are more rapidly effective, the first evidence of improvement—a rise in serum phosphorus—occurring in about 10 days.

Vitamin D has a serious toxic potential. Amounts of the order of 1000 to 3000 Units per Kg of body weight per day, which are only about 80 to 100 times the recommended dietary intake, may lead to hypercalcemia and attendant complications, such as metastatic calcification and renal calculi. In advanced stages, demineralization of bones occurs, and multiple fractures may result from very slight trauma.

Dietary Requirement and Food Sources—The requirement for vitamin D can be met entirely by skin irradiation, so that the need for ingested vitamin D is influenced by the amount of exposure to ultraviolet light. There are few reliable data concerning minimum vitamin D requirements, except for infants. Long experience has shown that 400 Units per day are sufficient to meet the requirements of practically all healthy individuals, assuming no exposure to ultraviolet light. In normal full-term infants, intakes of as little as 100 Units per day have prevented rickets. There is no evidence that diets need supply more than 400 Units per day for normal growth of infants and children.

Vitamin D is the one vitamin of which our foods supply very little. Egg yolks, which are the best food source, vary in content from winter to summer depending most upon the content of the vitamin in the hen's diet. Dairy products contain some vitamin D, but again the potency varies with the season. Varieties of fish, whose muscle tissues contain substantial quantities of oil and fat, may supply an appreciable part of the dietary requirement. The livers of a number of fish, or the oils extracted from the livers, are extremely rich in vitamin D. Addition of vitamin D to appropriate foods has been an important factor in the prevention of any significant incidence of rickets in this country. Vitamin D-fortified whole milk and evaporated milk containing 400 Units per quart (or reconstituted quart in the case of evaporated milk) are particularly effective because of their use in infant feeding during the stage of growth most susceptible to rachitic changes. Fortification is accomplished by addition of vitamin D concentrates, mainly in the form of vitamin D_3. Fortification of other foods, such as processed cereals, nonfat dry milk, and margarine, is practiced to a limited degree.

Vitamin E

Vitamin E designates the group of compounds with biological activity called tocopherols. Studies which led to its discovery as an essential factor in animal metabolism showed that it was, among other things, necessary for reproduction in rats. It is erroneously termed the antisterility vitamin, since it is not known to specifically function in this capacity in humans.

Chemistry and Assay—As with several of the other vitamins, there are a series of closely related compounds, tocopherols, known to occur in nature. Biological activity associated with the vitamin nature of the group is exhibited by four major compounds: alpha-, beta-, gamma- and delta-tocopherol, each of which can exist in various stereoisomeric forms. These are all methyl-substituted tocols; alpha-tocopherol, the most important member of the series because of its activity and occurrence, is 5,7,8-trimethyltocol, ie, 2,5,7,8-tetramethyl-2-(4,8,12-trimethyltridecyl)-6-chromanol.

The tocopherols are oily liquids at room temperature. High temperatures and acids do not affect the stability of vitamin E, but oxidation does take place readily in the presence of iron salts or in rancid fats. The tocopherols themselves act as antioxidants, the delta-tocopherol having the greatest antioxidant power. Decomposition also occurs in ultraviolet light. Tocopherols are isolated on a commercial scale from vegetable oils, usually by molecular distillation, extraction with organic solvents, or absorption chromatography. Alpha-tocopherol is usually the most important homolog isolated from these sources; it also can be prepared synthetically and made available as the acetate and acid succinate esters.

The international standard for vitamin E used as a reference in all assays for this vitamin is a solution of *dl*-alpha tocopheryl acetate in coconut oil. Each 0.1 Gm of this solution contains 1 mg of the acetate. Results of an assay are expressed in terms of mg of the vitamin. The following relationship exists between International Units (there are no USP Units) of the

alpha-tocopherol

vitamin and the respective weights of the common forms:

> 1 IU = 1 mg *dl*-alpha tocopheryl acetate = 0.91 mg *dl*-alpha tocopherol = 0.735 mg *d*-alpha tocopheryl acetate (the ester of the natural form) = 0.671 mg *d*-alpha tocopherol (the natural form)

The Unit represents biological activity as determined by the rat antisterility test.

The usual methods for quantitative assay of vitamin E depend either directly or indirectly upon the ease with which free alpha-tocopherol is oxidized. The esters, which are almost exclusively used in pharmaceuticals, must first be hydrolyzed. The free alcohol then, because of its instability, must be handled with care in all other analytical operations. The physicochemical methods generally applied employ either of two oxidation–reduction reactions: (1) the formation of a red orthoquinone by treatment of the tocopherol with concentrated nitric acid and (2) the reduction of ferric chloride in the presence of α,α'-dipyridyl which forms a red-colored complex with ferrous ions. Both methods are relatively nonspecific and are suitable only when combined with adequate separation procedures.

The classical biological method is the rat assay in which female rats are depleted of vitamin E and mated with normal males. The dose of the material to be tested and of the standard is distributed over a period of several days after conception. On the 20th day of pregnancy the female rats are killed and the numbers of living and dead fetuses, and resorption sites are recorded. Another more simple bioassay is based on the dialuric acid hemolysis test in which the red blood cell fragility is measured as a criterion of vitamin E status in the rat.

Metabolic Functions, Dietary Requirement, and Food Sources—The exact biochemical mechanism whereby vitamin E functions in the body is still unknown. Since these compounds are antioxidants they may participate in an oxidation–reduction system vital to life. They are probably cellular antioxidants connected with the stabilization of certain fats and sulfur-containing amino acids and of vitamin A. Interestingly enough, however, the order of antioxidant power among the tocopherols, as measured by their effect on the rate of peroxide formation in fats, is the reverse of the order of biological potencies. Other physiological functions probably include participation in nucleic acid metabolism, and it also appears that the tocopherols may be a component of the cytochrome reductase segment of the terminal respiratory chain in intermediary metabolism. In general, it appears that vitamin E plays an important role in insuring the stability and integrity of cellular membranes; thus far in man, the only such demonstrated effect is on the red blood cell. The effect is also modified by the level of polyunsaturated fatty acids in the diet. The therapeutic effectiveness of vitamin E in the prevention of abortion, in certain menstrual disorders, in the improvement of lactation, in muscular dystrophy, or in cardiovascular diseases has not been substantiated, and the promotion of vitamin E for such purposes is fraudulent.

A clearly defined uncomplicated vitamin E deficiency disease has not been recognized as a public health problem. A deficiency state with respect to vitamin E has been demonstrated in human subjects, especially in premature and newborn infants and in infants with steatorrhea. The evidence rests mainly on determinations of *in vitro* hemolysis and blood tocopherol level. Vitamin E requirement apparently is not related to body weight directly or to caloric intake, but seems to be related to body weight in kilograms to the three-quarter power, sometimes designated as physiologic or metabolic size. According to the National Research Council's Recommended Dietary Allowances, the daily vitamin E activity allowances are as follows: infants, 3 to 6 IU; children, 10 to 15 IU; adults, 20 to 30 IU.

Vitamin E is ubiquitous in its distribution and is found particularly in cereals, nuts, and leafy green and yellow vegetables. Some of the vegetable oils are good sources of the vitamin. It is found stored to some extent in animal tissues, particularly in the fat fractions; hence significant sources also include eggs and meat.

Vitamin E is so widely distributed in nature that it is difficult to prepare a diet deficient in it and hard to see how a vitamin E deficiency in diets for humans might occur. Indeed, in adults the plasma concentration does not fall until the subject has been on a very stringent experimental diet for several months; even after the plasma level falls, no clinical signs and symptoms are currently demonstrable.

Vitamin K

Vitamin K refers to a group of substances, widespread in nature, having similar biologic activity; one form was isolated first from alfalfa and the other from putrefied fish meal. The primary activity which makes the vitamin essential in human metabolism is its involvement in the blood-clotting system through synthesis of prothrombin and other clotting factors.

Chemistry and Assay—The parent structure of the K family of vitamins is 2-methyl-1,4-naphthoquinone or menadione. This fat-soluble compound and several water-soluble derivatives such as the sodium bisulfite and diphosphoric acid ester are the common commercial forms used in medical practice. Vitamin K_1 (isolated from alfalfa) is 2-methyl-3-phytyl-1,4-naphthoquinone.

vitamin K_1—phylloquinone; phytonadione

Vitamin K_2 exists as a chemical series which, instead of the phytyl side-chain in the 3-position, have side-chains of varying number of unhydrogenated isoprene units depending on the bacterial source. The vitamin K_2 having a 35-carbon side-chain and originally isolated from the putrefied fish meal is 2-methyl-3-*all-trans*-farnesylgeranylgeranyl-1,4-naphoquinone.

vitamin K₂(₃₅) (farnoquinone)

The naturally occurring substances in pure form are light-yellow solids or oils, insoluble in water, but soluble in fat solvents. Transparent colloidal solutions of vitamin K_1 can be prepared by means of nonionic surfactants. Although menadione, too, is fat soluble, it is easily soluble in boiling water and it is also slightly volatile at room temperature. Vitamins K_1 and K_2 as well as menadione are redox substances stable in the quinone form. In this respect there is a structural analogy between the vitamins K and E and a recently isolated series of naturally occurring quinones called ubiquinones. The latter do not possess any vitamin activity. Vitamins K have characteristic absorption spectra in the ultraviolet and are sensitive to alkali, light, and ionizing radiation.

There is neither an International nor USP Standard (or Unit) for vitamin K. There is, however, an NF Reference Standard of menadione. The activity of test materials is generally measured in terms of biological equivalency to milligrams or micrograms of menadione in a chick feeding test.

After extraction and separation from interfering substances, the vitamins K can be determined by their ultraviolet spectra or by color reactions. They react with sodium ethylate to give a blue color, which changes to brown. A more sensitive reaction occurs with sodium diethyldithiocarbamate to give a transient blue color. The method prescribed in the NF for assay of menadione is the photometric assay of Menotti, in which 2,4-dinitrophenylhydrazine in ethanol is heated with menadione in the presence of HCl. The vitamin is thus converted to the hydrazone, which when treated with ammonia yields a blue-green color.

The chick is particularly suited for the biological assay of vitamin K because of the ease in producing a dietary vitamin deficiency and the high requirement, and the criterion of activity (blood "prothrombin time") is readily measurable.

Metabolic Functions, Dietary Requirement, and Food Sources—Vitamin K is necessary for the formation of prothrombinogen and other blood clotting factors in the liver. During clotting, circulating prothrombin is required for the production of thrombin; in turn, the thrombin converts fibrinogen to fibrin, the network of which constitutes the clot. It is obvious from this description that interference with formation of prothrombin will reduce the clotting tendency of the blood. In a deficiency of the vitamin, a condition of hypoprothrombinemia occurs, and blood-clotting time may be greatly, or even indefinitely, prolonged. Internal or external hemorrhages may ensue either spontaneously or following injury or surgery.

A group of substances termed vitamin K antagonists are characterized by their property to decrease plasma prothrombin levels and their usefulness in medicine as anticoagulants (see page 831). Representative of this group is dicoumarol, originally isolated from spoiled sweet clover hay, in which it is formed by bacterial action on coumarin. An important use of vitamin K is in the treatment of hypoprothrombinemia consequent to prothrombopenic anticoagulant therapy.

Vitamin K_1 is the preferred form. Large doses of salicylates also antagonize vitamin K.

Dicoumarol

A few chemically related derivatives of dicoumarol are commercially used as rodenticides. Another compound with similar antagonist activity is sulfaquinoxaline, a sulfonamide drug used in veterinary medicine for treatment of various infectious intestinal diseases. It increases the animal's requirement for vitamin K in some undetermined manner probably by eliminating vitamin K-synthesizing enteric bacteria, upon which the animal depends, in part, for a source of the vitamin. Extended treatment with antibacterial drugs that alter the enteric flora also increases the dietary vitamin K requirement in man.

Optimal absorption of the vitamins K requires the presence of bile or bile salts in the intestine. Menadione, however, is easily absorbed in the absence of bile. The average diet apparently contains adequate amounts of vitamin K, since few if any malnourished humans have presented findings of dietary lack of vitamin K uncomplicated by intestinal disease, which prevents absorption. Because of the lack of reliable information concerning human intakes of vitamin K and because of other factors shown to be operative in experimental animals, but not yet evaluated in man, an absolute daily allowance for this vitamin has not been established. The daily requirement is probably below the equivalent of 2 mg of menadione administered intravenously.

The premature infant appears to be particularly sensitive to a lack of the vitamin, and also to an excess, particularly in the case of menadione. Because of this potential toxicity, the inclusion of menadione in over-the-counter supplements for the gravid female is prohibited. Vitamin K_1 does not exhibit this toxicity and is the preferred form. For newborn infants and especially those born prematurely (and anoxic), a single dose of 1 mg of vitamin K_1, immediately after birth, is often a routine measure to prevent hemorrhagic disease. Vitamin K_1 may be administered to the mother 12 to 24 hours prior to the expected delivery, or at the first sign of labor, especially if the mother has been receiving prothrombopenic anticoagulants.

Although extensive measurements of dietary intakes and food content of the vitamins K have not been made, primarily because suitable analytical methods have not been developed, enough information is known to say that the vitamin is widely distributed in a variety of foods. The green, leafy vegetables, tomatoes, cauliflower, egg yolk, soybean oil, and liver of all kinds are good sources. Since it is insoluble in water, there is no loss in ordinary cooking. The human also utilizes vitamin K synthesized by certain enteric bacteria.

Cholecalciferol USP

[Vitamin D₃; Activated 7-Dehydrocholesterol USP XVI]

Cholecalciferol[$C_{27}H_{44}O = 384.65$] is activated 5,7-cholestadien-3β-ol. It is an antirachitic vitamin obtained from natural sources or prepared synthetically.

For the structure, see page 1016.

Preparation—Vitamin D₃, a very potent antirachitic substance, was first prepared by irradiating 7-dehydrocholesterol in Windaus' laboratory, in 1935. Almost simultaneously, Brockmann, working with Windaus, isolated the vitamin from tunny-liver oil. The sources and chemistry of this substance are discussed on pages 1016 and 1017.

Description—White, odorless crystals. Is affected by air and by light.

Solubility—Insoluble in water; soluble in alcohol, chloroform, and fatty oils.

Uses—The only valid nutritional uses of Cholecalciferol are in the treatment of vitamin D *deficiency* or in the *prophylaxis* of deficiency in persons with a known deficiency, a high requirement, or an absorption defect. However, the substance may be employed to treat *hypocalcemic tetany* and *hypoparathyroidism*. A description of the pathology and metabolic disorders that accrue to deficiency and of the toxicity is found under *Metabolic Functions* (page 1017). Cholecalciferol should not be employed in the presence of renal insufficiency or hyperphosphatemia.

Dose—See the general statement, page 1017.

Cod Liver Oil NF

[Oleum Morrhuæ; Oleum Jecoris Aselli; Oleum Gadi]

Cod Liver Oil is the partially destearinated fixed oil obtained from fresh livers of *Gadus morrhua* Linné and other species of the Family *Gadidæ*. Cod Liver Oil contains, in each Gm, not less than 255 mcg (850 USP Units)* of vitamin A and not less than 2.125 mcg (85 USP Units) of vitamin D.

Cod Liver Oil may be flavored by the addition of not more than 1% of a suitable flavoring substance or a mixture of such substances.

Preparation—The highest grade of medicinal Cod Liver Oil is manufactured from strictly fresh cod livers. These should be from healthy fish, and they should be removed from the fish within a few hours after they are caught. The oil is separated from the livers by steam cooking. For this purpose, low-pressure steam is conducted directly into the cooking kettles containing the livers, and ordinarily it requires only a short time to cook livers sufficiently so that the oil is released from the weakened tissues surrounding the oil cells. The oil is then quickly separated from all water and liver tissue.

When livers of high quality are used and the manufacturing procedure is carried out under carefully controlled, sanitary conditions the resulting crude oil is of a light yellow color, and of good flavor and odor. Such an oil requires no purification or chemical refining.

Due, however, to long-established trade demands, it is necessary to remove the cod liver stearin so that the oil will remain clear at all temperatures above freezing. To accomplish this, the cod liver oil manufacturer chills the crude medicinal oil. After the cod liver stearin has crystallized out, it is a simple matter to separate the stearin and nonfreezing oil by filter pressing. In order to preserve the natural vitamin content of Cod Liver Oil, it should be stored out of contact with air or light and preferably in a cool place.

Constituents—Cod Liver Oil consists chiefly of unsaturated glycerides but contains *palmitin* and *stearin*, as well as traces of *chlorine, bromine, phosphorus*, and *sulfur*. American cod liver oils may contain as much as 3 parts per million of arsenic, but there is little evidence as to how completely it may be assimilated. American cod liver oils are rich in *iodine*—one sample was found to contain nearly 15,000 parts of iodine per billion parts of oil, and it is reported that the iodine content of the blood is increased to about the same degree by the use of Cod Liver Oil and iodized salt. Hence the iodine content of 10 ml of cod liver oil per day, if assimilated, would contribute materially to the physiological needs of the average human adult.

It has been shown that the vitamin value of Cod Liver Oil resides in the unsaponifiable fraction. Since some persons object to taking oils, much attention has been given to preparing tablets and capsules which contain the unsaponifiable fraction of cod liver oil. Several patents have been granted for such processes. In general the procedure consists of saponifying the cod liver oil, separating the unsaponifiable portion, and extracting it with suitable solvents. The extract is diluted with corn oil and packed in capsules or mixed with solid materials and manufactured into tablets. The vitamin potency of these preparations can be adjusted to the patient's requirements but obviously they do not supply the constituents present in the saponifiable portion of the cod liver oil from which they were prepared.

Description—A thin, oily liquid, with a characteristic, slightly fishy, but not rancid, odor and a fishy taste. Its specific gravity: 0.918 to 0.927.

Solubility—Slightly soluble in alcohol; freely soluble in ether, chloroform, carbon disulfide, and ethyl acetate.

Uses—Cod Liver Oil is a valued source of vitamins A and D. The vitamins are present in such proportion that the oral dose of 5 ml provides the daily requirements for children or adults of both of these dietary essentials. Cod Liver Oil is extensively employed in the prophylaxis of rickets in infants. It offers the advantages of being relatively inexpensive, the disadvantage of the large volume dosage in comparison with concentrates.

Dose—5 ml containing **1170 mcg** (3900 USP Units) of vitamin A and **9.7 mcg** (386 USP Units) of vitamin D.

Veterinary Dose—*Horses* and *Cattle*, **60 to 120 ml**; *Swine*, **20 to 40 ml**; *Dogs*, 4 to 8 ml; *Chickens* and *Turkeys*, **300** to **900 ml** per **100 pounds** of feed.

Note—Cod Liver Oil containing more than the minimum NF requirements for both vitamin A and vitamin D may be administered in proportionally smaller doses.

Nondestearinated Cod Liver Oil NF [Oleum Morrhuæ Non-Destearinatum] is the entire fixed oil obtained from fresh livers of *Gadus morrhua* Linné and other species of the Family *Gadidæ*, containing not more than 0.5% by volume

---

* In 1931, "Units" were adopted to express the biological activity of vitamin A and vitamin D. The biological activity of the USP Unit and the International Unit in the case of each vitamin is identical; however, the base of reference has changed from time to time. Present-day physical and chemical assay methods have practically eliminated the need for a biological assay of vitamin A. On this basis, the weight of vitamin A is to be preferred to "Units," as evidenced in the USP. A biological assay for vitamin D is still used in the NF.

of water and liver tissue. Nondestearinated Cod Liver Oil contains, in each Gm, not less than 255 mcg (850 USP Units) of vitamin A and not less than 2.125 mcg (85 USP Units) of vitamin D. *Description:* A thin, oily liquid at room temperature, with a characteristic, slightly fishy, but not rancid, odor, and a fishy taste. It congeals or deposits stearin upon chilling. *Solubility:* Slightly soluble in alcohol; freely soluble in ether and chloroform. *Uses:* Nondestearinated Cod Liver Oil is the high-grade medicinal oil as separated from the livers but before the excess of stearins has been removed. It was not expected that it would be used directly as a medicinal oil, but by giving it official recognition its importation was established. This oil should, therefore, be destearinated before being sold.

Dihydrotachysterol—see page 983.

Ergocalciferol USP

[Calciferol USP XVI; Vitamin D_2; Viosterol]

Ergocalciferol [$C_{28}H_{44}O$ = 396.66] is irradiated ergosta-5,7,22-trien-3β-ol.

For the structure, see page 1016.

Preparation—Ergocalciferol is obtained by exposing ergosterol to ultraviolet light for the proper length of time. See page 1016. Insufficient irradiation results in the production of products with little or no antirachitic activity and prolonged exposure causes the production of toxic products.

Description—White, odorless crystals. Affected by light and by air. Melting range: 115°–118°.

Solubility—Insoluble in water; soluble in alcohol, chloroform, ether, and fatty oils.

Uses—Ergocalciferol is known as Vitamin D_2, and, like other forms of Vitamin D, it exhibits both antirachitic and calcemic effects (see the general statement under *Vitamin D, Metabolic Functions*, page 1017). It has a relatively high potency and is thus especially useful for the treatment of severe or refractory *rickets*. It may also be used in the management of *hypocalcemia* and *hypoparathyroidism*. Care must be exercised to prevent overdosage (see page 1017). It should not be employed when renal insufficiency or hyperphosphatemia prevails.

Dose—*Usual*, daily, **10 mcg** (400 USP Vitamin D Units); in *rickets*, *prophylactic*, **10 mcg** (400 Units), and *therapeutic*, **30 mcg** (1200 Units); in *hypocalcemic tetany*, up to **5 mg** (200,000 Units).

Dosage Forms—Capsules USP: 1.25 mg (50,000 Units); Solution USP.

Veterinary Dose—*Therapeutic: Horses*, up to **25 mcg** (1000 Units) per **100 pounds** of body weight; *Oxen*, **37.5** to **75 mcg** (1 500 to 3000 Units) per **100 pounds** of body weight; *Swine*, **50 mcg** (2000 Units) per **100 pounds** of body weight.

Oleovitamin A and D NF

[Concentrated Vitamins A and D Solution]

Oleovitamin A and D is a solution of vitamin A and vitamin D in fish liver oil or in an edible vegetable oil. The vitamin D is from natural sources or is present as ergocalciferol or cholecalciferol or the products obtained by the activation of either ergosterol or 7-dehydrocholesterol. Oleovitamin A and D contains not less than 90.0% of the labeled amounts of vitamins A and D.

Description—A yellow to red oily liquid. It is a clear liquid at temperatures above 65°, and it may crystallize on cooling. It may be nearly odorless or may have a fish-like odor. It does not have a rancid odor or taste. It is unstable in air, and in light.

Solubility—Insoluble in water and glycerin; very soluble in ether and chloroform; soluble in dehydrated alcohol and vegetable oils.

Uses—Since the vitamins A and D content of Oleovitamin A and D may be varied, the uses also vary according to the composition. Thus it may be used to supply primarily either vitamin A or vitamin D. However, it is generally used as a source of both vitamins for use when the vitamin requirement is high or when there is a diminished absorption from the gastrointestinal tract.

Dose—*Usual*, to be determined by the physician according to the needs of the patient.

Dosage Forms—Capsules NF.

Menadiol Sodium Diphosphate USP

[Tetrasodium 2-Methyl-1,4-naphthalenediol Bis(dihydrogen phosphate); Vitamin K_4; Kappadione (*Lilly*); Synkayvite Sodium Diphosphate (*Roche*)]

Menadiol Sodium Diphosphate [$C_{11}H_8Na_4O_8P_2 \cdot 6H_2O$ = 530.18] contains 97.5–102.0% of $C_{11}H_8Na_4O_8P_2$ (422.09), calculated on the anhydrous basis.

Preparation—One method involves reduction of menadione to the diol compound by treatment with zinc in the presence of acid followed by double esterification with HI, metathesizing the resulting 1,4-diodo compound with AgH_2PO_4, and neutralizing the bis(dihydrogen phosphate) ester thus formed with NaOH.

Description—A white to pink powder, having a characteristic odor. It is hygroscopic. Its solutions are neutral or slightly alkaline to litmus, having a pH between 7 and 9.

Solubility—Very soluble in water; insoluble in alcohol.

Uses—See *Menadione* (below) and *Phytonadione* (page 1022). Menadiol Sodium Diphosphate in the body is converted to menadione, and consequently it has the same uses and limitations, except that it is water soluble and does not require the presence of bile salts for its absorption; therefore, it is especially useful in the presence of bile obstruction.

Other Dose Information—The dose for oral, subcutaneous, intramuscular, or intravenous administration is the same. The usual doses are as follows: for hypoprothrombinemia, usually 3 to 6 mg daily; to antagonize prothrombopenic anticoagulants, 75 mg intramuscularly, to be repeated as needed; to antagonize the prothrombopenic actions of salicylates, 10 to 25 mg daily, in 3 divided doses; to prevent hypoprothrombinemia of the newborn, either 6 to 12 mg parenterally to the mother during labor or 3 mg to the infant shortly after birth.

Dose—*Parenteral*, **5** to **75 mg** daily; *usual*, **5 mg** once a day.

Dosage Forms—Injection USP: 5 and 10 mg/ml, 75 mg/2 ml; Tablets NF: 5 mg.

Menadione NF

[2-Methyl-1,4-naphthoquinone; Menaphthone; Menaphthene]

Menadione contains 98.5–101.0% of $C_{11}H_8O_2$ (172.19), calculated on the dried basis.

Caution—Menadione powder is irritating to the respiratory tract and to the skin, and a solution of it in alcohol is a vesicant.

Preparation—Menadione is usually made by the action of chromic acid on 2-methylnaphthalene in the presence of H_2SO_4.

Description—Bright yellow, crystalline powder which is nearly odorless. It is affected by sunlight. It melts between 105° and 107°.

Solubility—Practically insoluble in water; 1 Gm dissolves in 60 ml of alcohol and 10 ml of benzene; sparingly soluble in chloroform and carbon tetrachloride; soluble in vegetable oils.

Incompatibilities—Menadione is incompatible with alkalies. Reducing agents convert it to a hydroquinone. It is affected by light.

Uses—See *Phytonadione* (this page). In some of its actions menadione appears to be more potent than phytonadione. However, menadione is inferior to natural vitamin K_1 in the antagonism of anticoagulants of the bishydroxycoumarin type. Because of the insolubility of menadione, bile salts should be coadministered when bile obstruction exists.

Dose—*Oral* and *parenteral*, 2 to 5 mg; *usual*, 2 mg daily.

Dosage Forms—Injection NF: 2 and 5 mg/ml; Tablets NF: 2, 5, and 10 mg.

Veterinary Dose—*Dogs, oral*, 3 to 10 mg; *intramuscular*, 0.5 to 5 mg.

Menadione Sodium Bisulfite NF

[2-Methyl-1,4-naphthoquinone Sodium Bisulfite; Menadione Bisulfite; Menaphthone Sodium Bisulfite; Hykinone (*Abbott*)]

Menadione Sodium Bisulfite [$C_{11}H_9NaO_5S \cdot 3H_2O$ = 330.29], dried in vacuum for 3 hours, contains 94.0–100.5% of $C_{11}H_9NaO_5S$.

Preparation—It may be prepared by reacting menadione with sodium bisulfite. The reaction may be visualized as consisting of the typical addition of $NaHSO_3$ to a ketone forming the $R(OH)(SO_3Na)$ compound which then rearranges at the expense of one degree of unsaturation of the quinonoid nucleus. The compound readily regenerates menadione on treatment with mild alkali and thus behaves as a typical ketone-$NaHSO_3$ addition compound.

Description—A white, crystalline, odorless, hygroscopic powder.

Solubility—1 Gm dissolves in 2 ml of water; slightly soluble in alcohol; practically insoluble in ether and benzene.

Uses—Menadione Sodium Bisulfite is an addition product of menadione and sodium bisulfite, and it is converted in the body to menadione. Consequently,

its actions and uses are those of menadione (see *Menadione*, above, and *Phytonadione*, below). Because of its aqueous solubility, the presence of bile salts is not needed for its absorption from the small intestine.

Dose—*Usual, intravenous* and *subcutaneous*, 2 mg daily.

Other Dose Information—*Parenterally*, for hypoprothrombinemia, 0.5 to 2 mg daily; to prevent hypoprothrombinemia of the newborn, 1 mg shortly after birth; to antagonize prothrombopenic anticoagulants, 50 to 100 mg by slow intravenous injection.

Dosage Forms—Injection NF: 2.5 mg/0.5 ml, 5 and 10 mg/ml, 72 mg/10 ml.

Veterinary Dose—*Parenteral, Swine*, 0.5 to 10 mg; *Dogs*, 0.5 to 2 mg. In emergencies of bleeding, larger doses may be given at intervals of 4, 6, or 8 hours.

Phytonadione USP

[Vitamin K_1; Phylloquinone; Mephyton and Aqua-Mephyton (*MSD*); Konakion (*Roche*)]

Phytonadione [$C_{31}H_{46}O_2$ = 450.71] is 2-methyl-3-phytyl-1,4-naphthoquinone.

For the structure, see page 1018.

Description—A clear, yellow, very viscous, odorless or nearly odorless liquid. Specific gravity about 0.967. It is stable in air, but decomposes on exposure to sunlight. A solution (1 in 20) in alcohol is neutral to litmus. Refractive index 1.5230 to 1.5252 at 25°.

Solubility—Insoluble in water; soluble in dehydrated alcohol, benzene, chloroform, ether, and vegetable oils.

Uses—Phytonadione is the natural product, vitamin K_1. For the metabolic functions of vitamin K, see page 1019.

Vitamin K_1 has a more prompt and prolonged action than menadione and other synthetic analogs of vitamin K, and it is the more reliable in restoring prothrombin to the blood in conditions of *hypoprothrombinemia*. *Hypoprothrombinemia in the newborn* may be prevented or treated by the administration of Phytonadione to the mother shortly before parturition or by giving the infant a single dose shortly after birth. In *hypoprothrombinemia consequent to prothrombopenic anticoagulant therapy*, an adequate intravenous injection will usually stop hemorrhage within 3 to 4 hours and restore the plasma prothrombin level to normal in 12 to 24 hours. In hypoprothrombinemia resulting from liver disease it may have limited value, especially if the disease is hepatocellular; in *biliary obstruction or fistula*, in which only the absorption of vitamin K is impaired, hypoprothrombinemia responds promptly to parenteral Phytonadione. In other enteric diseases in which absorption is defective—as in *sprue, regional enteritis, enterocolitis, ulcerative colitis, dysentery*, and in *extensive bowel resection*—Phytonadione will correct hypoprothrombinemia if given parenterally.

It must be emphasized that Phytonadione cannot be used to check bleeding irrespective of its origin. It is of no benefit in diseases of the blood-forming organs, thrombocytopenic purpura, hemophilia, etc.

Excessive doses of Phytonadione may occasionally cause hyperprothrombinemia and a tendency toward thrombosis.

Dose—*Oral* or *intramuscular*, 1 to 50 mg daily; *usual, oral*, 10 mg; *usual, intramuscular*, 5 mg, repeated as necessary.

Other Dose Information—Dosage schedules: *Oral*, for hypoprothrombinemia, 1 to 25 mg. *Intravenous*, in emergency treatment, 10 to 25 mg, preferably in a somewhat dilute emulsion. It may be diluted with sterile water or 5% dextrose; 5 to 7 ml of diluent is added to each ml of emulsion. It should not be given at a rate faster than 10 mg per minute; *intravenous* or *intramuscular*, to prevent hypoprothrombinemia of the newborn, 0.5 to 2 mg to the mother 12 to 24 hours prior to delivery or to the infant immediately after delivery.

Dosage Forms—Injection USP: 1 mg/0.5 ml, 10 mg/ml, 25 mg/2.5 ml, 50 mg/5 ml; Tablets USP: 5 mg.

Veterinary Dose—*Intravenous, Horses,* **250** to **500 mg**; *Dogs,* **1** to **2 mg** (50 mg as antidote for warfarin poisoning).

Vitamin A USP

Vitamin A contains a suitable form of retinol ($C_{20}H_{30}O$; vitamin A alcohol) and possesses vitamin A activity equivalent to not less than 95.0% of that declared on the label. It may consist of retinol or esters of retinol formed from edible fatty acids, principally acetic and palmitic acids. It may be diluted with edible oils, or it may be incorporated in solid, edible carriers or excipients, and it may contain suitable antimicrobial agents, dispersants, and antioxidants. For the structure of retinol, see page 1015.

Description—Yellow to red, oily liquid that may solidify upon refrigeration. In solid form, it has the appearance of any diluent that has been added. May be nearly odorless or may have a fishy odor, but has no rancid odor or taste. Is unstable to air and light.

Solubility—In liquid form, it is insoluble in water and glycerin; soluble in absolute alcohol and vegetable oils; very soluble in ether and chloroform. In solid form, it may be dispersible in water.

Uses—The only valid uses of Vitamin A are in the treatment of vitamin A *deficiency* or in the *prophylaxis* of deficiency in persons with a known dietary deficiency, a high requirement, or an absorption defect. A description of the pathology and metabolic disorders that accrue to deficiency and of the toxicity is found under *Metabolic Functions* (page 1018). In persons without deficiency the vitamin does not improve the skin, prevent infections, or improve the eyes.

Dose—*Prophylactic,* **1.2** to **2.4 mg** (4000 to 8000 USP Vitamin A Units) daily; *usual, prophylactic,* **1.5 mg** (5000 Units) once a day; *therapeutic,* **7.5** to **60 mg** (25,000 to 200,000 Units) daily; *usual, therapeutic,* **7.5 mg** (25,000 Units) once a day.

Dosage Forms—Capsules USP: 1.5, 7.5, 15, and 30 mg (5,000, 25,000, 50,000, and 100,000 Units).

Vitamin E NF

Vitamin E is a suitable form of alpha tocopherol [$C_{29}H_{50}O_2$ = 430.72]. It may consist of *d-* or *dl-*alpha tocopherol ($C_{29}H_{50}O_2$), *d-* or *dl*-alpha tocopheryl acetate [$C_{31}H_{52}O_3$ = 472.76], *d-* or *dl*-alpha tocopheryl acid succinate [$C_{33}H_{54}O_5$ = 530.80], mixed tocopherols concentrate, or *d*-alpha tocopheryl acetate concentrate. The concentrates are obtained from edible vegetable oils or from the by-products of their refining.

d- or *dl-*Alpha tocopherol, *d-* or *dl*-alpha tocopheryl acetate, and *d-* or *dl*-alpha tocopheryl acid succinate contain 97.0–100.5% of $C_{29}H_{50}O_2$, $C_{31}H_{52}O_3$, or $C_{33}H_{54}O_5$, respectively.

Mixed tocopherols concentrate contains not less than 34.0% of total tocopherols and may be so adjusted by the addition of an edible vegetable oil. Of the total tocopherols present, not less than 50.0% consists of *d*-alpha tocopherol, the content of which may be adjusted by physical or chemical means.

d-Alpha tocopheryl acetate concentrate contains not less than 25.0% of *d*-alpha tocopheryl acetate and may be so adjusted by the addition of an edible vegetable oil. Of the total tocopheryl acetates present, not less than 64.0% consists of *d*-alpha tocopheryl acetate, the content of which may be adjusted by physical or chemical means.

Alpha tocopherol (also written α-tocopherol) is a trivial generic name (which embraces all eight stereoisomeric forms of 2,5,7,8-tetramethyl-2-(4,8,12-trimethyltridecyl)-6-chromanol. The term *d*-alpha tocopherol is employed in the pharmaceutical field in the sense adopted by the American Institute of Nutrition and by the Food and Drug Administration, ie, to designate that form of the compound which (a) occurs naturally and (b) is dextrorotatory. The term *dl*-alpha tocopherol designates the mixture of stereoisomers prepared synthetically, commonly from racemic isophytol.

The structural formula of alpha tocopherol is shown on page 1017. The phenolic hydroxyl is readily susceptible to acylation and the resulting esters, eg, the acetate and acid succinate, are much more resistant to oxidation and discoloration on exposure to air and light than the phenolic form.

Description—Vitamin E has little or no odor or taste. *The alpha tocopherols and alpha tocopheryl acetates:* clear, yellow, viscous oils. *d-Alpha tocopheryl acetate:* may solidify in the cold. *Alpha tocopheryl acid succinate:* a white powder; the *d*-isomer melts within the range of about 73° to 78°, and the *dl*-isomer melts within the range of about 68° to 74°. *The concentrates:* clear, yellow to brownish-red, viscous oils. *The esters:* stable to air and to light but are unstable to alkali; *the acid succinate:* also unstable when held molten. *The alpha tocopherols:* unstable to air and to light, particularly when in alkaline media.

Solubility—*Alpha tocopheryl acid succinate:* insoluble in water; slightly soluble in alkaline solutions; soluble in alcohol, ether, acetone, and vegetable oils; very soluble in chloroform. *Other forms of Vitamin E:* insoluble in water; soluble in alcohol; miscible with ether, acetone, vegetable oils, and chloroform.

Uses—The only valid use of Vitamin E is as a supplement to the diet of the newborn infant, especially if premature, or in the treatment of the infant with steatorrhea, in which the gastrointestinal absorption of vitamin E is impaired. No need for administration to children or adults has been demonstrated. For a discussion of the functions and daily allowance, see *Metabolic Functions, Dietary Requirements, and Food Sources* (page 1018).

Dose—*Usual, prophylactic,* from **5** to **30 IU** of Vitamin E; *therapeutic,* to be determined by the physician according to the needs of the patient.

Other Fat-Soluble Vitamins

Vitamin K₅ [Synkamin (*Parke-Davis*)] is 4-amino-2-methyl-1-naphthol ($C_{11}H_{11}NO$). *Description* and *Solubility* (of the hydrochloride): Needles that darken at 262° and melt with decomposition between 280° and 282°; turn pink to dark violet on exposure to air and light. Freely soluble in water; slightly soluble in alcohol; insoluble in ether. *Uses:* Vitamin K₅ is used as the hydrochloride, the solubility of which lends itself to intravenous administration. The free amine is also relatively soluble and does not require bile salts for absorption. Its uses are those of *Menadione* (page 1022) and *Menadione Sodium Bisulfite* (page 1022). *Dose:* Usual, oral, 4 mg; *intravenous,* 1 to 5 mg.

The Water-Soluble Vitamins

Except for ascorbic acid, all the vitamins in this water-soluble category belong to the B-group of vitamins. Some still retain their original individual designations, such as B_1, B_6, and B_{12}, whereas comparable names for other vitamins have become obsolete.

In 1930, when it was clear that vitamin B was of multiple nature, the term vitamin B complex was coined to refer to the group of water-soluble animal growth factors found in relatively high concentrations in such products as liver, yeast, and rice bran. This was a convenient term to use in the early scientific literature, but it was not intended to be a specific name for pharmaceutical preparations that contain skin varying proportions of the B vitamins. The term was intended to apply to a group of vitamins whose identity was being sought, rather than to a group of compounds whose identity had been established. Since the nature of the "complex" has been characterized, the term vitamin B complex is no longer appropriate.

Ascorbic Acid (Vitamin C)

Vitamin C, or ascorbic acid, is necessary for the prevention and cure of the deficiency disease scurvy (antiscorbutic vitamin).

Scurvy has been recognized since the Middle Ages and was found widespread in northern Europe and among the crews of sailing ships. During the 18th century it was learned that when fresh fruit was made available aboard sailing vessels, scurvy was avoided. In 1907 Holst and Frolich observed a scurvy-like syndrome in guinea pigs that was similar to human scurvy and cured it by feeding citrus juices. This gave an experimental means for the rapid development of our knowledge of vitamin C, to which many workers contributed.

Chemistry and Assay—Ascorbic acid is a white, crystalline compound structurally related to the monosaccharides. It exists in nature in both a reduced, and the oxidized form, dehydroascorbic acid. These substances are in a state of reversible equilibrium in biological systems, and both have the same biological activity.

L-Ascorbic Acid   Dehydroascorbic Acid

Ascorbic acid is stable in the dry state but is easily oxidized in aqueous solution in the presence of air. Oxidation is accelerated by heat, light, alkalies, oxidative enzymes, and traces of copper and iron. Because of its relative instability, ascorbic acid is readily lost during cooking if simple precautions to avoid aeration are not taken. Also, because of its high aqueous solubility, the vitamin is lost to a considerable extent when large amounts of cooking water are discarded. Progressive loss of vitamin C in fresh fruits and vegetables occurs during storage.

Solutions of ascorbic acid are strongly reducing, and the vitamin is easily oxidized. In animal tissues the greater part of the vitamin is in the reduced form, but, as scurvy develops, the ratio of oxidized to reduced form rises. This property of reversible oxidation–reduction is the most likely basis for the role of the vitamin in biochemical reactions.

The article of commerce is produced exclusively by synthesis. Sorbitol, a hexose occurring in several fruits but commercially obtained by hydrogenating dextrose, is the raw material for production of ascorbic acid. Amounts of ascorbic are expressed in terms of weight, as milligrams. The USP provides a Reference Standard of L-ascorbic acid for assay purposes. The practical methods of ascorbic acid assay are based on its powerful reducing properties which enable determination by oxidimetric titration. The three most-used reagents for this titration are chloroamine-T, 2,6-dichlorophenolindophenol, and iodine. Another practical assay is based on the conversion of ascorbic acid to oxalic acid 2-nitrophenylhydrazide by treatment with diazotized 2-nitroaniline. This yields a colored compound which is measured photometrically. Still another is the photometric assay of total ascorbic acid (ascorbic acid plus dehydroascorbic acid) by conversion of the vitamin to its 2,4-dinitrophenylhydrazone.

Metabolic Function, Dietary Requirement, and Food Sources—Vitamin C is known to be essential for the formation of intercellular collagen. In scorbutic tissues the amorphous ground substance, and the fibroblasts in the area between the cells appear normal but without the matrix of collagen fibers. These bundles of collagenous material appear within a few hours after the administration of ascorbic acid. This points to the relationship of the vitamin in maintenance of tooth structures, matrix of bone, and the walls of capillaries. In scurvy, these are the tissues found to be faulty.

The picture of clinical scurvy in humans is one that can be related to the general breakdown of intercellular collagen substance. Bleeding is common, particularly at sites of pressure. The occurrence of petechiae, pinpoint hemorrhages that occur in the skin under reduced pressure, has been used as a diagnosis of scurvy. This is an indication of weakness or fragility of the walls of capillaries. Bones become brittle and cease to grow, and normal structures are replaced by connective tissue that contains calcified cartilage. Anemia is a common occurrence in scurvy, indicating a breakdown in the blood-forming organs. Tooth enamel, cementum, and particularly dentin change in structure, and the gums about the teeth become spongy and bleed easily.

Vitamin C is essential for the healing of bone fractures. Such fractures heal slowly in a patient deficient in vitamin C. This is true also of wound healing.

There is evidence to indicate that the vitamin functions in the metabolism of tyrosine. There is an abnormal excretion of homogentisic, p-hydroxyphenylpyruvic, and p-hydroxyphenyllactic acids in scorbutic guinea pigs following administration of tyrosine, which, of course, is corrected with ascorbic acid. The excretion of "tyrosyl" derivatives in humans on a vitamin

C-low diet given 20 Gm of tyrosine daily is also affected by ascorbic acid administration. In some newborn, the occurrence of tyrosinemia possibly accruing to high protein intakes suggests that this relationship be taken into consideration in evaluating the ascorbic acid requirement for the infant.

An intake of 10 to 20 mg of ascorbic acid is sufficient to protect an adult from classical scurvy. However, this represents only a fraction of that needed to maintain desirable plasma ascorbic levels, about 1 mg per 100 ml plasma. The recommended allowance (Food and Nutrition Board, National Research Council) for persons beyond 12 years old has been calculated as 2.5 mg per Kg of body weight to the three-fourths power, representing metabolic body size. This gives a figure of 60 mg daily for a 70-Kg man. For infants, the allowance of 35 mg of ascorbic acid provides about the same amount as supplied daily by 850 ml of milk from mothers living in the US. The vitamin C requirements are increased following trauma, during infections, and during periods of vigorous physical activity; in such circumstances the requirement may be 100 to 200 mg daily.

For therapeutic purposes in treatment of adult scurvy, 1000 mg of ascorbic acid daily in divided doses for 1 week is recommended, then 500 mg until all signs disappear. It is also used in the treatment of idiopathic methemoglobinemia to reduce the ferric iron in heme to the ferrous state. Ascorbic acid is essentially nontoxic, and large doses may be given without harm to the individual.

Vitamin C is found in all living plant cells, is synthesized during the germination of seeds, and is relatively concentrated in the rapidly growing parts of the plant. It is present in all animal tissues as well, but only guinea pigs, the primates, and man are unable to meet body needs by synthesis, and must rely upon a dietary source.

Although Vitamin C appears to be present in all living tissues, our best sources of supply are fresh fruits such as citrus fruits, strawberries and currants, and green vegetables such as lettuce and cabbage. Potatoes do not contain large amounts of ascorbic acid, but, nevertheless, because of the great quantities consumed, they constitute one of our major sources. It is a common practice, and a sound one, to rely to a large extent upon citrus fruits and juices as important vitamin C carriers, particularly in infant feeding. An ounce of orange or lemon juice per day is sufficient to prevent scurvy in humans on an otherwise vitamin C-low diet.

It is fairly common practice to add ascorbic acid to foods for technical purposes; eg, as an antioxidant to protect natural flavors and colors.

The B Vitamins

The "water-soluble B" of McCollum, or the "anti-beriberi vitamine" of Funk, has now been differentiated into at least eleven separate and distinct chemical entities. It has been established that eight of these are required in human nutrition. They are *thiamine, riboflavin, niacin, folic acid, pyridoxine, biotin, pantothenic acid, and vitamin B₁₂.* Para-aminobenzoic acid, choline, and inositol have an essential part in cellular metabolism in plants and animals, but this does not constitute presumptive evidence of their importance in human nutrition. When the dietary intake of methionine is adequate, choline can be synthesized endogenously; therefore, the human requirement is relative to the methionine intake, similarly to the relationship between niacin and tryptophan. It can be stated categorically that the human does not require either an exogenous or endogenous source of para-aminobenzoic acid. A human need for inositol has not been established.

There is no one natural source of the B vitamins as a group that is necessarily superior to another source. No natural source contains all the water-soluble factors in the proportions that are needed in human nutrition, and the therapeutic value of any vitamin-containing material depends upon the needs of the individual to whom it is being administered. Nevertheless, multiple deficiencies to B-vitamins often coexist, especially to thiamine and niacin. Furthermore, the repair of one B-vitamin deficiency may increase the need for another; thus, the administration of thiamine in clinical or subclinical beriberi increases the need for riboflavin. Consequently, there is some justification for multivitamin therapy with those five B vitamins for which *clinical* deficiencies occur (thiamine, niacin, riboflavin, folic acid, and vitamin B₁₂) human deficiencies in biotin and pantothenic acid have only been produced experimentally, and pyridoxine deficiency is only a rare occurrence in infants fed on an unfortified formula.

It should be emphasized that *synthetic B vitamins are equal to the naturally occurring ones* in their biological and therapeutic effects.

Biotin

[*cis*-Hexahydro-2-oxothieno[3,4-*d*]imidazole-4-valeric acid]

Before this nutritional factor was identified as a discrete chemical substance, it was variously called vitamin H, anti-egg white injury factor, coenzyme R, Bios II, and others. Its discovery was an outgrowth of studies on the "toxicity" of large amounts of unheated egg white as the sole source of protein for rats.

Chemistry and Assay—Biotin is a colorless, crystalline monocarboxylic acid, only slightly soluble in water and alcohol (its salts are quite soluble). Water solutions are stable at 100°, and the dry substance is both thermostable and photostable. Biotin is unstable, however, in strong acids and alkaline solutions and in oxidizing agents. The vitamin is optically active and the natural isomer, which alone possesses biological activity, is the *d*-form (rings are *cis*-fused and the isomer is designated (+)-biotin).

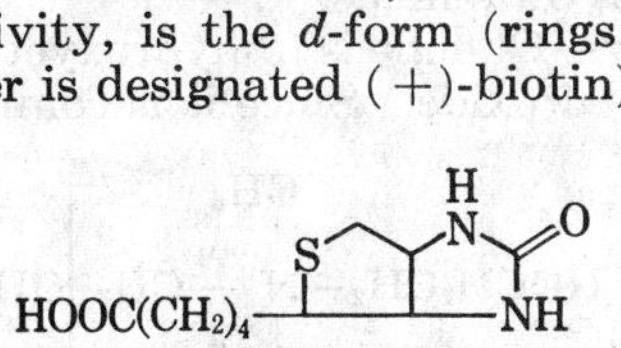

Biotin

Although biotin with the above structure is the compound present in food sources, the sulfur atom can be replaced with an oxygen atom without reduction of its metabolic activity. Biotin occurs in animal and plant tissues primarily in combined forms which are liberated by enzymatic hydrolysis during digestion. One of the simplest such complexes is biocytin, ε-*N*-biotinyl-L-lysine. The amount of the vitamin in a product is expressed solely in terms of the weight of the chemically pure substance, the free monocarboxylic acid.

Only microbiological methods are feasible for the quantitative assay of biotin because of their sensitivity to the low concentrations usually encountered. After simple aqueous or acid extraction combined with heating, a microbiological assay using growth of the test organisms *Allescheria boydii* or *Lactobacillus arabinosus* as the criterion is carried out.

Metabolic Functions, Dietary Requirement, and Food Sources—Attempts to induce biotin deficiency in man by inclusion of large amounts (200 Gm) of dried unheated egg white for several days in the diet have resulted in the appearance of vague symptoms such as change in skin color and dermatoses, slight change in lingual papillae of the tongue, muscle pains, loss of appetite, sleeplessness, and extreme lassitude. Raw egg white contains a protein, avidin, which combines with biotin and prevents absorption of the vitamin from the intestine. Rapid relief from such symptoms was observed with administration of biotin. This condition is difficult to produce in human subjects and, since a frank and specific deficiency disease is not discernible, there is uncertainty as to the exact nature of the deficiency syndrome as well as the need for a dietary source of biotin in human nutrition. Intestinal synthesis is undoubtedly the important factor in the supply of biotin to the body.

Biotin functions in carbon dioxide fixation reactions in intermediary metabolism, transferring the carboxyl group to acceptor molecules. It similarly acts also in decarboxylation reactions. For its part in these vital enzymatic steps, in catalyzing deamination of amino acids, and in oleic acid synthesis, biotin is essential in human metabolism and presumed to be a dietary essential in the absence of microbial synthesis in the intestine.

Diets providing a daily intake of 150 to 300 mcg of biotin are considered adequate. And these amounts are readily met and exceeded when milk, meat, and eggs are frequent items of the diet.

Choline

The propriety of classifying choline as a vitamin and a member of the B group is questionable because it is synthesized in the human body, and there is no evidence that a lack of choline has a disturbing effect on human metabolism. Nevertheless, choline plays an important role both as a structural component of tissues and in biological methylation reactions. Dietary deficiency of it leads to gross pathology in several species of animals.

Chemistry—Choline is (β-hydroxyethyl)trimethylammonium hydroxide. Since it is completely dissociated, it is comparable to alkali hydroxides as a base.

$$\left[\begin{array}{c} CH_3 \\ | \\ HOCH_2CH_2-N^+-CH_3 \\ | \\ CH_3 \end{array} \right] OH^-$$

choline

ated, it is comparable to alkali hydroxides as a base. Consequently, it does not exist as such at body pH but rather as a salt, the anion of which is that in its immediate biological environment. The β-(hydroxyethyl)trimethylammonium cation is the biologically important moiety. The cation is incorporated into phospholipids, such as lecithin and sphingomyelin, and acetylcholine, a substance released at cholinergic nerve junctions during transmission of nerve impulses. Acid hydrolysis of phospholipids yields the free choline salt which is very soluble in water, and to a lesser extent in ethanol.

Metabolic Functions, Dietary Requirement, and Food Sources—Besides its vital function as a precursor of acetylcholine, which is important in the sequence of nerve-muscle stimulations, choline is an important contributor of methyl groups needed for the *in vivo* synthesis of metabolites and perhaps some hormones. The biogenesis of choline appears to be universal in nature, and is the result of the three-step transfer of methyl groups to an acceptor, which may be either free aminoethanol or phosphatidyl aminoethanol. Such transfers require methionine as a methyl donor (actually, S-adenosylmethionine). Choline is indirectly a source of methyl groups; it is first oxidized to betaine, which then may transfer a methyl group to homocysteine to form methionine. By thus regenerating methionine lost in transmethylation reactions, exogenous choline can spare the amino acid for use in protein synthesis. Methionine is an essential amino acid.

Choline has the property of preventing the deposition of excess fat, or of causing the removal of excess fat from the liver of experimental animals fed high-fat diets and, because of this, is often classified as a "lipotropic agent." The lipotropic action probably relates to the incorporation of choline into phosphatidyl choline (lecithin), which, in turn, is incorporated into phospholipids and lipoproteins. The lipotropic action is independent of the function of choline as a reservoir of methyl groups.

Choline has never been associated in man with a specific deficiency syndrome, even though it has been experimentally induced in several animal species. A dietary requirement for choline, therefore, cannot be given. An average mixed diet consumed by man in the US has been estimated to contain 500 to 900 mg choline per day, an amount known to be adequate when compared with animal requirements. Foods that supply large amounts of choline are liver, kidney, brain, muscle meats, fish, nuts, beans, peas, and eggs. Moderate amounts exist in cereals, milk, and a number of vegetables.

Folic Acid (Folacin)

The vitamin derives its name from the Latin word *folium*, leaf. It was first isolated from spinach leaves where it is now known to occur in relatively minute amounts, compared to other food sources. Several apparently unrelated factors had been isolated in various laboratories before realization that they had in common the same parent compound, pteroyl-L-glutamic acid: Factor U (a chick growth factor), vitamin M (a factor for monkeys), vitamin B$_c$ (a chick anti-anemia factor), liver and yeast *L. casei* factors (bacterial growth factors), and others. In 1960 the International Union of Pure and Applied Chemistry decided that the name *folic acid* be applied generically to all pteroylglutamic acids possessing vitamin activity and that pteroylglutamic acid itself, which had hitherto been given the name folic acid (or folacin), be designated simply as *pteroylglutamic acid*. However, the USP continues to call pteroylglutamic acid folic acid, and common practice usually does the same.

Chemistry and Assay—Pteroylglutamic acid crystallizes from cold water, in which it is only slightly soluble, as yellow spear-shaped platelets. It is readily destroyed by boiling in acid solution and its solutions will deteriorate in sunlight. It is insoluble in alcohol and the usual organic solvents but readily dissolves in dilute solutions of alkali hydroxides and carbonates. The characteristic ultraviolet absorption spectrum of pteroylglutamic acid in dilute NaOH is used to aid in identification and measurement of the compound.

A series of folic acids with several molecules of glutamic acid attached to the first glutamic acid radical in peptide linkage have been synthesized. Compounds with one, two, three and seven glutamic acid groups have been isolated. The latter three are known as conjugates. Some animals and man can utilize them as a source of pteroylglutamic acid presumably, because appropriate digestive enzymes can hydrolyze them. Microorganisms can use them to only a variable and limited extent, unless they are first hydrolyzed to the free form with liver, kidney, or pancreatic enzymes, called conjugases.

Pteroyl(mono)glutamic acid (PGA; formerly called folic acid or folacin)

The functional form of this vitamin group called folic acid is basically the 5,6,7,8-tetrahydro PGA in which a formyl group (—CHO), when present, is attached at either or both the N^5 or N^{10} positions. The hydrogenated N^5-formyl compound is named *folinic acid*, or leucovorin, which is available, as is the monosodium salt of PGA, as a discrete pharmaceutical preparation. These compounds similarly serve as standards during assay of the vitamin. A USP Reference Standard Folic Acid is available. Separately, the three moieties which make up the PGA molecule (pteroic acid, *p*-aminobenzoic acid, and glutamic acid) have no vitamin activity.

The quantitative assay of folic acid in natural products is mainly by biological or microbiological methods. In the chick assay, the birds are placed on a folic acid-free diet until they become anemic, after which folic acid supplements and the test material are administered. The degree of recovery is related to the quantity of reference folic acid fed. The two organisms most used in the microbiological method are *Lactobacillus casei* and *Streptococcus faecalis*. The method is based on the fact that pteroylglutamic acid is a required growth factor for each; however, the assay is complicated when biological material is analyzed, because naturally occurring folic acid derivatives do not all have the same biological activity for the two organisms.

Folic acid can be determined by either of two physicochemical methods, provided the compound is present in relatively pure form. One method is the spectrophotometric measurement of the extinction maxima of the ultraviolet absorption curve; the other is the photometric measurement after oxidative fission of folic acid to 4-aminobenzoylglutamic acid followed by diazotization and coupling to give an azo dye.

Metabolic Functions—Folic acid is one of the important hematopoietic agents necessary for proper regeneration of the blood-forming elements and their functioning. Although the mechanism whereby PGA performs this vital role is not understood, much is known about the involvement of folic acid as a coenzyme in intermediary metabolic reactions in which one-carbon units are transferred. These reactions are important in interconversions of various amino acids and in purine and pyrimidine synthesis. This role is in contrast to that of choline in furnishing and transferring so-called labile methyl groups in transmethylation reactions. The biosynthesis of purines and pyrimidines is ultimately linked with that of nucleotides and ribo- and deoxyribo-nucleic acids, functional elements of all cells.

The concept of antivitamins or vitamin antagonists is exemplified in a particular aspect of folic acid metabolism. By virtue of its structural similarity, sulfanilamide competes with *p*-aminobenzoic acid in the biological synthesis of folic acid. The organism is thus deprived of needed folic acid. Sulfonamides act, therefore, as growth inhibitors of certain pathogenic organisms, a competitive antagonism which is responsible for the antibacterial action of sulfa drugs. Since mammals use preformed folic acid, sulfonamides do not disrupt the host metabolism.

Numerous analogs of pteroylglutamic acid have been prepared which exhibit potent anti-folic acid activity. Several compounds, notably aminopterin (4-aminopteroylglutamic acid) and methotrexate (4-amino-N^{10}-methylpteroylglutamic acid), compete with PGA in nucleic acid synthesis and have been used in the treatment of leukemia and other cancers.

Dietary Requirement and Food Sources—Folic acid deficiency results in megaloblastic anemia, glossitis, diarrhea, and weight loss. A deficiency is best diagnosed by the demonstration of low levels of the vitamin in serum or blood by microbiological assay or by the hematological response to a physiological dose of folic acid, 50 to 200 mcg intramuscularly per day for 10 days. The condition of megaloblastic anemia arising as a result of dietary deficiency of folic acid occurs most frequently after the age of 65 years, in persons suffering from malabsorption syndromes, in women during the last trimester of pregnancy, and in infants receiving unfortified proprietary formulas or goats' milk. In the treatment of megaloblastic or macrocytic anemia in the elderly, folic acid should be administered as the sole therapeusis only when the possibility of pernicious anemia and other primary diseases of the small bowel have been absolutely excluded because of the vitamin's ability to mask other diagnostic signs of these conditions.

The minimum amount of folic acid required by the normal adult is about 0.05 mg per day, though pregnancy and other stressful situations, including various disease states and the consumption of alcohol, increase the requirement. Since the vitamin exists in nature predominantly in the combined form which has limited availability, the daily dietary allowances recommended by the Food and Nutrition Board, National Research Council take this into account. Their recommendations are 0.4 mg for adolescents and adults, 0.8 mg during pregnancy, 0.5 mg during lactation, and from 0.05 to 0.2 mg for infants and children.

A balanced American diet for adults contains approximately 0.2 to 0.6 mg of total folic acid activity, and the intestinal microflora also provide some absorbable amounts of the vitamin. The best food sources of folic acid are liver, kidney, dry beans, asparagus, mushrooms, broccoli, and collards. Other good sources include spinach, peanuts, lima beans, cabbage, sweet corn, chard, turnip greens, lettuce, milk, and whole wheat products.

Niacin (Nicotinic Acid) and Nicotinamide

Nicotinic acid (niacin) and nicotinamide (niacinamide) have identical properties as vitamins. Both compounds had been known for sometime before their biological significance was realized. In 1867 nicotinic acid was synthesized by the oxidation of nicotine with nitric acid. But it was not until 1937 that it was isolated from biological sources and found to be effective in the cure of black tongue in dogs and, later, pellagra in humans. The vitamin has none of the pharmacological properties of nicotine, however. In the 1940's the term "niacin' was adopted as a synonym for food labeling purposes to avoid association with the nicotine of tobacco. The term "niacin" is sometimes used generically to include both nicotinic acid and nicotinamide.

Chemistry and Assay—Nicotinic acid is 3-pyridine carboxylic acid. The structures of nicotinic acid and nicotinamide are shown below.

Niacin, the most stable of the vitamins, is not destroyed by heating in acid or alkaline solution. It withstands mild oxidation, and retains its biological activity during the processing of food and the preparation and storage of pharmaceuticals. It is readily soluble in water and alcohol but insoluble in ether and chloroform. Niacinamide, on the other hand, may be extracted from water solution with ether. The amide is readily hydrolyzed to the free acid by heating in acid or alkaline solution.

The usual commercial synthesis of nicotinic acid used in foods and drugs is by the oxidation of quinoline with potassium permanganate or manganous dioxide, and mono-decarboxylation of the purified quinolinic acid with controlled heating. Nicotinamide is usually prepared by esterifying nicotinic acid with methanol followed by ammonolysis.

The activity of both forms of the vitamin is expressed in milligrams of the chemically pure substance. Because they have identical biological activity and their molecular weights are nearly identical, they are equivalent on a weight basis. An NF Reference Standard Niacin is available from the American Pharmaceutical Association and a Niacinamide Reference Standard is available from the USP.

Niacin may be determined in food, drugs, and biological materials by microbiological assay or by chemical methods. No animal biological method exists. The chemical determination involves reaction of the pyridine ring with cyanogen bromide and coupling of the fission product with an aromatic amine. The yellow polymethine dye which is formed is measured in a photometer at 436 mμ. In natural products niacin occurs mainly in combined form as a coenzyme and must be liberated by acid hydrolysis before assay.

The microbiological assay employs *Lactobacillus arabinosus* as the test organism. A quantitative discrimination between nicotinic acid and nicotinamide in a sample is possible by assaying with both the latter organism which utilizes both forms and *Leuconostoc mesenteroides* which can utilize only nicotinic acid.

Metabolic Functions—In the body niacin is converted to niacinamide, which is an essential constituent of coenzymes I and II that occur in a wide variety of enzyme systems involved in the anaerobic oxidation of carbohydrates. The coenzyme serves as a hydrogen acceptor in the oxidation of the substrate. These enzymes are present in all living cells and take part in many reactions of biological oxidation.

Coenzyme I—known also as nicotinamide-adenine dinucleotide (NAD)—is the inner salt of the 5'-ester of 3-carbamoyl-1-β-D-ribofuranosylpyridinium hydroxide with adenosine 5'-pyrophosphate, and has the structure shown below. Coenzyme II—known also as nicotinamide-adenine dinucleotide phosphate (NADP) —differs only in that the adenosine moiety is esterified at its 2'-position with phosphoric acid.

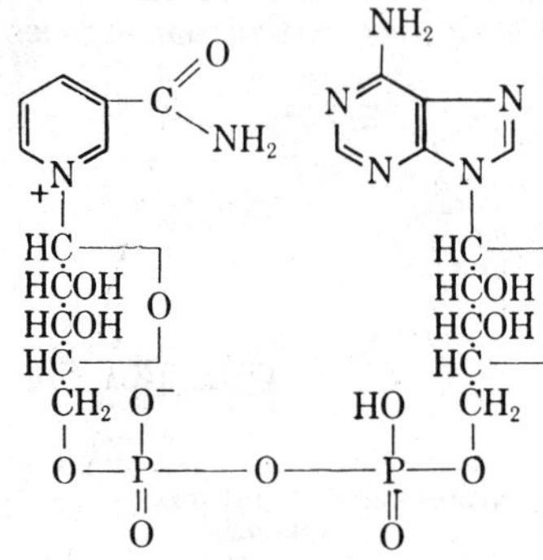

Coenzyme I (NAD)

These coenzymes are synthesized in the body and have a part in the metabolism of all living cells. Since they are of such widespread and vital importance, it is not difficult to see why serious disturbance of metabolic processes occurs when the supply of niacin to the cell is interfered with.

The observations of numerous nutritionists that the daily requirement for niacin is influenced by the amount and kind of dietary protein led to the discovery that the amino acid tryptophan functions as a potential precursor of niacin. The efficiency of the conversion indicates that 60 mg of dietary tryptophan is equivalent to 1 mg of niacin. This relationship has given rise to the use of the term "niacin equivalent," which is defined for the purpose of estimating the adequacy of diets in this vitamin as 1 mg of niacin or 60 mg of dietary tryptophan.

Niacin is readily absorbed from the intestinal tract, and large doses may be given orally or parenterally, with equal effect.

The principal excretory product of niacin in the urine is *N*-methylnicotinamide, a fluorescent compound formed in the liver. On a normal diet approximately one-fourth of the niacinamide ingested is excreted as *N*-methylnicotinamide. With increased levels of niacin intake the percent of ingested niacin excreted as the fluorescent substance is decreased.

Dietary Requirement and Food Sources—Pellagra, which means rough skin, is the primary deficiency disease due to lack of sufficient niacin in the diet, and it appears only after months of dietary deprivation. The condition involves the gastrointestinal tract, the skin, and the nervous system. Loss of weight, anorexia, weakness, insomnia, headache, and diarrhea are common and appear without obvious cause. Other early symptoms may include abdominal pain, nervousness, and mental confusion.

Typical manifestations of pellagra in a well-advanced stage are diarrhea, dermatitis, and dementia. Gastrointestinal difficulties vary in severity, and absence of gastric secretion is a common finding. In the more advanced state, diarrhea is severe. Dermatitis has a characteristic appearance and occurs at those sites subject to exposure or irritation. The skin lesions are usually bilaterally symmetrical and appear first as erythematous patches, changing to brown pigmented areas, followed by desquamation and thickening. Glossitis is common; it is characterized by swelling and redness at the margins and tip of the tongue. Because of inflammation and superficial desquamation, the tongue, gums, and lips appear scarlet and smooth. Mental symptoms vary in occurrence and intensity; they include irritability, mental depression, and emotional instability. A confused mental state with hallucinations, mania, and delirium are seen in advanced stages of the disease. Pellagra is a complex deficiency, and symptoms of riboflavin, thiamine, and folic acid deficiency frequently complicate the clinical picture.

Treatment of the disease requires immediate change to a well-balanced diet and the administration of niacin or niacinamide. Where neurological symptoms are present, use of thiamine and riboflavin may be necessary as well. Recovery from the acute condition is dramatic in most instances, and occurs within 24 to 48 hours. Small doses given frequently during the day have been found to be more effective than a single large daily dose. Niacinamide is of advantage to niacin in that it does not produce vasodilation in the skin with sensations of itching, burning, or tingling. With severe nausea and diarrhea, intravenous injection of niacinamide is of additional advantage.

In considering dietary requirement and the foods which contribute to it, one must consider the content of preformed niacin and the niacin available by conversion from tryptophan, an essential amino acid present in all good-quality proteins. The minimum requirement for niacin milligram equivalents to prevent pellagra is about 4.4 per 1000 Kcal per day. The recommended daily allowance of the Food and Nutrition Board is 6.6 per 1000 Kcal and not less than 13 at caloric intakes of less than 2000 Kcal. Most diets consumed in the US supply from 500 to 1000 mg or more of tryptophan daily and 8 to 17 mg of preformed niacin, equalling a range of 16- to 33-mg equivalents of niacin.

Poultry, meats, and fish constitute the most important single food group insofar as niacin is concerned. Organ meats are somewhat superior to muscle tissue. Potatoes, legumes, and some green leafy vegetables contain moderate amounts of preformed niacin, as do whole grains. An important public health nutrition practice, begun in the 1940's, is the nutrient enrichment of cereal products: wheat flour, farina, corn products, rice, macaroni and noodle products, and bread. Niacin, thiamine, riboflavin, and iron are mandatory ingredients in those products which are labeled "enriched." The level of enrichment for niacin is such that a significant proportion of the daily requirement is obtainable from a generous serving of these foods.

Inositol

Inositol is hexahydroxycyclohexane (1,2,3,5/4,6-cyclohexanol; *i*-inositol; *meso*-inositol). Actually, there are nine stereoisomeric cyclohexanols, which all are

Inositol

now commonly referred to as inositols. Several occur in nature; the isomer described above is by far the most prevalent and is the only one that is biologically active.

Inositol occurs normally in nearly all plant and animal cells, either free or combined, suggesting that it is an essential cell constituent. There is no direct evidence of its possible function except that it has been found as a constituent of an amylase enzyme system. On low inositol diets, mice are stunted, and they develop alopecia. There has as yet been no demonstration of need for inositol in human nutrition. Since the substance is so widely distributed, it is possible that the failure to show a deficiency syndrome is the result of the difficulty in obtaining a truly deficient diet; furthermore, intestinal flora also synthesize the compound.

Although inositol possesses weak lipotropic activity, it is not as effective as methionine or choline. There is no valid nutritional or therapeutic use of the compound, and the promotion of inositol must be considered a commercial abuse.

Pantothenic Acid

Knowledge of the identity and importance of pantothenic acid grew principally from experimental studies on microorganisms and chicks. Because of its wide distribution in nature it was named "pantothenic" from the Greek word *pantothen*, from all sides. The terms vitamin B_3 and chick antidermatitis factor were once applied to variously purified concentrates of the factor, but they are now obsolete. No known therapeutic value exists for pantothenic acid, except perhaps in the treatment of frank or suspected cases of combined nutritional deficiencies.

Chemistry and Assay—Pantothenic acid is optically active. Maximum vitamin activity resides only in the D-form, and it is readily available as either the sodium or calcium salts which are crystalline substances. Another commercially available form used in liquid preparations is D-pantothenyl alcohol (panthenol). Chemically, pantothenic acid is a composite structure of β-alanine and 2,4-dihydroxy-3,3-dimethylbutyric acid γ-lactone, connected in peptide linkage.

Pantothenic Acid

The free acid is fairly stable in neutral solution but sensitive to acids, bases, and heat. The salts are somewhat more stable, but even these are destroyed by autoclaving.

Pantothenic acid, its salts and alcohol, can be assayed by both chemical and microbiological methods. A chick growth method has been used but it is time-consuming and has been replaced since suitable methods are available for releasing the bound vitamin (a protein enzyme) from its firm combination in plant and animal tissue. The first step in chemical assay is acid or alkaline hydrolysis. This cleaves the molecule at the peptide linkage into an alanine part and a pantoic acid part. These fission products can then be determined photometrically by suitable color reactions. *Saccharomyces carlsbergensis* and *Lactobacillus plantarum* are used for the microbiological assay of pantothenic acid and its salts. There is available a USP Reference Standard Calcium Pantothenate.

Metabolic Functions, Dietary Requirement, and Food Sources—Pantothenic acid is of the highest biological importance because of its incorporation into Coenzyme A (CoA), which is involved in many vital enzymatic reactions transferring a two-carbon compound (the acetyl group) in intermediary metabolism. It is involved in the release of energy from carbohydrate, in the degradation and metabolism of fatty acids, and in the synthesis of such compounds as sterols and steroid hormones, porphyrins, and acetylcholine. CoA is composed of one mole each of adenine, ribose, and β-mercaptoethylamine and three moles of phosphate for each mole of pantothenate.

Many microorganisms depend on the same metabolic pathways for their growth and reproduction as do animal species and humans and in this respect require pantothenic acid. Some have the ability to synthesize pantothenic acid at a life sustaining rate from proper precursors. Synthesis by the bacterial flora of the intestine in man appears to be an important source of the vitamin and is the probable explanation, in part, that pantothenic acid deficiency in man is seldom encountered. A deficiency syndrome has been experimentally induced in human volunteers by the oral administration of a pantothenic acid antagonist, ω-methyl-pantothenic acid, imposed on a pantothenic acid-deficient diet. It has been impossible so far to induce an isolated deficiency of the vitamin in less than at least 9 months on anything resembling a natural diet alone because of the occurrence of significant amounts of pantothenic acid in such a wide variety of foods.

The symptoms which appear to be specific for a lack of available pantothenic acid from the studies using the antivitamin are neuromuscular disorders (paresthesias of the hands and feet and cramping of the legs and impairment of motor coordination), loss of normal eosinopenic response to adrenal corticotrophic hormone (ACTH), heightened sensitivity to a test dose of insulin, and, in concert with pyridoxine, a loss of antibody production. Fatigue, malaise, headache, sleep disturbances, nausea, abdominal cramps, epigastric distress, occasional vomiting and an increase in flatus were subjective observations of the pantothenic acid-deficient human volunteers.

Usual diets of adult Americans furnish about 10 to 15 mg of pantothenic acid daily, with a probable range of 6 to 20 mg. A daily intake of 5 to 10 mg is probably adequate for children and adults, and there is no evidence for or against a greater requirement during pregnancy or lactation. Human milk contains about 2 mg per liter; cow's milk, about 3.5 mg per liter. Liver and other organ meats and eggs are particularly good sources. Broccoli, cauliflower, white and sweet potatoes, tomatoes, and molasses are quite high in pantothenic acid. Muscle tissue of beef, pork, lamb, and chicken are also good sources.

Pyridoxine (Vitamin B₆)

Vitamin B₆ does not denote a single substance but is rather a collective term for a group of naturally occurring pyridines that are metabolically and functionally interrelated; namely, pyridoxine, pyridoxal, and pyridoxamine. They are interconvertible *in vivo* in their phosphorylated form. There is no information on the relative biologic activity of the three compounds in humans, and since pyridoxine is the most stable, it probably contributes the most vitamin activity to the diet.

Chemistry and Assay—Pyridoxine as the free base has a bitter taste and is readily soluble in water, alcohol, and acetone. It crystallizes as the hydrochloride and is prepared in this form for commercial use. Pyridoxine is one of the more stable vitamins and in the alcohol form withstands heating in acid or alkaline solution. Pyridoxal and pyridoxamine are less stable, however, and are known to undergo destruction in the more severe heat treatments sometimes used in food processing. Under most conditions of processing and storage of foods and pharmaceutical preparations the vitamin is well retained.

The structures of the three active forms of the vitamin and the phosphorylated form of one of them, pyridoxal phosphate, are shown below.

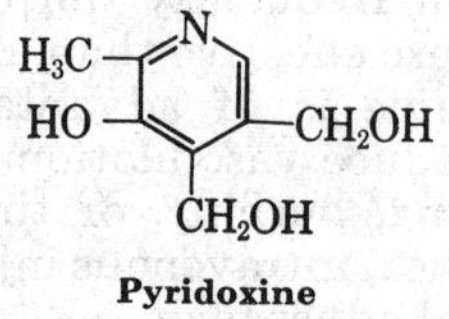

Pyridoxine

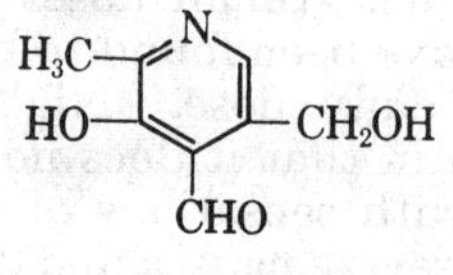

Pyridoxal

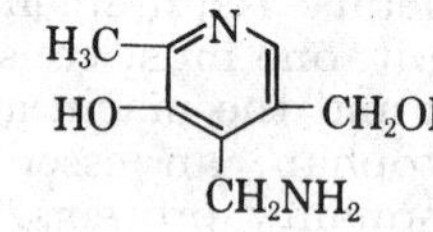

Pyridoxamine

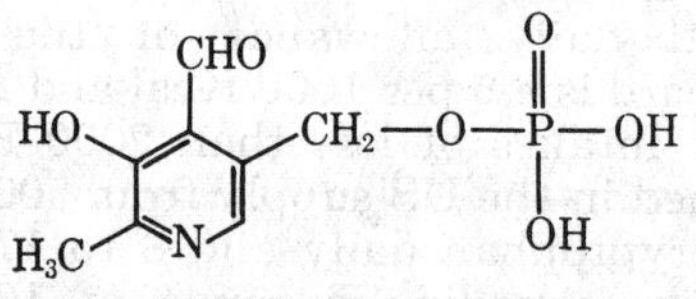

Pyridoxal Phosphate

The biological activity of the vitamin is expressed in milligrams of the chemically pure substance, usually pyridoxine hydrochloride, for which a USP Reference Standard is available. Chicks and rats have been used for the biologic assay of vitamin B₆ by placing the animals on a deficient basal diet which, when supplemented with known amounts of the test vitamin, supports a degree of growth related to the amount present. Physicochemical methods can be used only to a limited extent for assaying vitamin B₆ quantitatively in natural products, because they are nonspecific for the three forms. Microbiological assays, however, will discriminate between the individual vitamin B₆ components and thus yield a more accurate estimate of total biologic activity. A very useful technique employed in this type of assay is the preliminary separation of the different vitamin forms by a column chromatographic procedure using an ion exchanger. The column eluates are then analyzed by procedures suited to the vitamin form present in the eluates. The organisms most commonly used are

Saccharomyces carlsbergensis, Lactobacillus casei, and *Streptococcus faecalis.*

Metabolic Functions, Dietary Requirement, and Food Sources—Vitamin B_6 in the form of pyridoxal phosphate or pyridoxamine phosphate functions in carbohydrate, fat, and protein metabolism; its major functions are most closely related to protein and amino acid metabolism. The vitamin is a part of the molecular configuration of many enzymes (a coenzyme), notably glycogen phosphorylase, various transaminases, decarboxylases and deaminases. The latter three are essential for the anabolism and catabolism of proteins.

The biologic activity of vitamin B_6 seems to be a function of the molecule as a whole, since small changes in structure render it inactive. Deoxypyridoxine, a derivative of the vitamin in which one of the methanol groups is reduced to a methyl group, has potent antivitamin activity, but it is of limited experimental use in man because of its toxicity. The antivitamin isonicotinic acid hydrazide (isoniazid) has been widely used in the treatment of tuberculosis. It is chemically related to pyridoxine and acts also as an antagonist, thus requiring the physician to be alert to the pyridoxine nutriture of his patients so treated. A similar antagonism is possible during treatment of hypertension with the drug hydralazine.

No classic syndrome of pyridoxine deficiency exists, probably because it is widely distributed in nature and unique or unusual dietary habits have not so far produced an uncomplicated deficiency. That it is essential for the growth of animals and human infants is well established. Other manifestations of deficiency in humans are probably an acrodynia-like syndrome characterized by edema and loss of hair, nerve degeneration resulting in behavioral changes and, in infants, convulsive seizures. The latter symptom was shown to result when infants were fed a proprietary milk-based formula, unsupplemented with pyridoxine, in which the natural vitamin content was destroyed inadvertently during sterilization. Clearly, in this instance, marked changes in electroencephalogram patterns of the infants were produced; and they returned to normal minutes after pyridoxine administration.

In infants, although daily requirements of the vitamin are met by consumption of adequate quantities of normal breast milk, the protein-vitamin B_6 relationship is critical. General experience with proprietary formulas suggests that metabolic requirements are satisfied if the vitamin is present in amounts of 0.015 mg per Gm of protein, or 0.04 mg per 100 Kcal. The recommended daily allowances of the Food and Nutrition Board for adolescents and adults, including conditions of pregnancy and lactation, range from 1.4 to 2.5 mg.

The best food sources of vitamin B_6 are muscle meats, liver, green vegetables and whole-grain cereals. The bran from the cereal grains has especially large amounts. Nuts, corn, eggs, and milk are also good sources.

Riboflavin

Riboflavin was formerly known as vitamin B_2 or G and lactoflavin. It owes its discovery as one of the components of the B vitamin group to its characteristic fluorescence and pigmenting quality in such common foods as milk and egg yolk. Isolation and characterization of the yellow protein enzyme originally from yeast led to studies on the essential nature of the flavin pigment part of the enzyme in human metabolism, growth, and health.

Chemistry and Assay—Riboflavin is a yellow to orange-yellow, crystalline powder having a slight odor. When dry, it is not appreciably affected by diffused light, but in solution, especially in the presence of alkalies, it deteriorates quite rapidly, the deterioration being accelerated by light.

In alkaline solution it is readily soluble, but quite unstable to heat and to light, forming lumiflavin, a fluorescent degradation product that is without biological activity. Riboflavin is more stable to heat in acid solution, particularly from pH 1.0 to 6.5 but upon irradiation forms lumichrome, also biologically inactive. Riboflavin is readily adsorbed from acid or neutral solution on such agents as frankonite, fuller's earth, and certain zeolites, and eluted with acetone or pyridine solutions. Adsorbates have been used in pharmaceutical preparations, but from some of these the vitamin has been found to be unavailable to the human because of difficulty of elution in the intestinal tract.

Solutions of riboflavin have a characteristic yellow-green fluorescence that has a maximum absorption at 565 mμ in the acid pH range. This property is made use of in the chemical determination of riboflavin. It is rapidly reduced by hydrosulfite, or by hydrogen in the presence of zinc in acid solution, to the leuco form which is colorless and nonfluorescent. The leucoriboflavin is easily reoxidized by shaking in air. This oxidation–reduction property (see below) is the probable basis for the biological importance of riboflavin in the respiratory enzyme systems.

One gm dissolves in from 3000 to about 20,000 ml of water, the variations in the solubility being due to differences in the internal crystalline structure of the riboflavin; it is more soluble in isotonic sodium chloride or alkaline solution than in water, and less soluble in alcohol. It is insoluble in most lipid solvents. Derivatives such as the phosphate or acetate have been prepared for use in pharmaceutical preparations when higher concentrations are desired.

Riboflavin

Leucoriboflavin

The bulk of the product of commerce is produced synthetically. The basic materials for this synthesis are 3,4-xylidine (4-amino-o-xylene), the sugar ribose, and barbituric acid or alloxan.

The activity of riboflavin is expressed in milligrams of the chemically pure substance, and a USP Reference Standard Riboflavin is available for assay purposes. In early work, the riboflavin content of substances was measured by a rat growth bioassay method, but this has been replaced by both physicochemical and microbiological methods.

Chemical determinations are based on colorimetric and fluorimetric procedures. Straightforward measurement of the intrinsic yellow color of riboflavin is often sufficient for assaying pharmaceutical preparations. The fluorometric method is more sensitive and free of interferences and is therefore more suited to the assay of the vitamin in foods. It depends upon the extraction of the vitamin with dilute acid, filtration, treatment of the filtrate with permanganate and hydrogen peroxide to destroy interfering pigments, and measurement of the fluorescence.

Lactobacillus casei is used as the test organism for microbiological assay of riboflavin. It is determined by measurement of the growth stimulation of the organism or by alkaline titration of the acid produced during incubation.

Metabolic Functions—Riboflavin plays its physiological role as the prosthetic group of a number of enzyme systems that are involved in the oxidation of carbohydrates and amino acids. It functions in combination with a specific protein either as a mononucleotide, containing phosphoric acid, or as a dinucleotide combined through phosphoric acid with adenine.

Flavin-adenine dinucleotide (FAD)

The specificity of each of the enzymes is determined by the protein in the complex. By a process of oxidation–reduction, riboflavin in the system either gains or loses hydrogen. The substrate, either carbohydrate or amino-acid, may be oxidized by a removal of hydrogen. The first hydrogen acceptor in the chain of events is coenzyme I or coenzyme II, the di- or tri-nucleotide containing nicotinic acid and adenine. The oxidized riboflavin system then serves as hydrogen acceptor for the coenzyme system and in turn is oxidized by the cytochrome system. The hydrogen is finally passed on to the oxygen to complete the oxidative cycle. A number of flavoprotein enzymes have been identified, each of which is specific for a given substrate.

There is evidence now that some of the flavin enzymes contain metallic constituents. These metallo-flavoproteins may contain iron, copper, or molybdenum. Succinic dehydrogenase, for example, contains iron, and xanthine oxidase contains molybdenum, as well as iron.

Riboflavin is absorbed after phosphorylation from the intestinal tract, and excreted in the urine. A human adult on an ordinary diet excretes from 0.5 to 1.5 mg in 24 hours, depending on the content of the diet. Of a 10-mg dose taken by mouth, 50 to 70% is excreted within 24 hours. In riboflavin deficiency there is little or none found in the urine. Measure of excretion has been used as a diagnostic sign of deficiency. Riboflavin, like thiamine, is stored to a limited extent, and constant dietary supply is needed to maintain normal body levels. Liver, kidney, and heart tissues contain relatively large amounts of riboflavin because of their high enzyme content.

Dietary Requirement and Food Sources—Symptoms of human ariboflavinosis include cheilosis (reddening of the lips and the appearance of fissures at the corners of the mouth), characteristic changes in color of the mucous membranes, inflammation of the tongue, and denuding of the lips. Lesions of a seborrheic nature have also been observed as a result of riboflavin deficiency. Ocular manifestations that appear in man and animals are characterized chiefly by corneal vascularization, in which the cornea is extensively invaded by small capillaries. This is usually accompanied by sensations of itching, burning, and roughness of the eyelid, lacrimation, photophobia, and visual fatigue. Some of these conditions may, of course, arise from other causes and are not necessarily indicative of riboflavin deficiency.

Riboflavin deficiency in humans has not been found to be widespread in any part of the world, but is undoubtedly a complicating factor in other deficiency diseases such as pellagra. For therapeutic purposes, doses of 1 to 10 mg daily have been given. Rapid disappearance of symptoms of ariboflavinosis occurs with 10-mg doses, and there is some question of the need for administering amounts larger than this.

Studies dealing with the quantitative riboflavin requirement of the human indicate that it is related to body size, metabolic rate, and rate of growth. And the parameter used to express these most closely is metabolic body size, represented as Kg of body weight taken to the 0.75 power. The recommended daily allowance of the Food and Nutrition Board for riboflavin is 0.4 to 0.6 mg for infants, 0.6 to 1.2 mg for children up to 10 years, 1.3 to 1.7 mg for adolescents and adults and slightly higher for women during pregnancy and lactation. In general, the minimum requirement for riboflavin is about 0.3 mg for adults and 0.8 mg for infants on a 1000-Kcal intake basis. From a physiological point of view, an intake of more than 0.5 to 0.6 mg per 1000 Kcal may be of little extra value in normal adult persons.

Riboflavin is widely distributed in nature, in both plants and animals, as an essential constituent of all living cells, and is therefore found widely distributed in small amounts in foods. It is quite stable during the processing of food, except where there is excessive exposure to light. Because of its water solubility, there is moderate loss of riboflavin in cooking when the cooking water is discarded. This loss, however, is generally smaller than that of thiamine, niacin, or ascorbic acid.

Foods that make important contributions of riboflavin to the diet are liver and other organ tissues, milk, and eggs. Vegetables and fruits furnish a small but constant supply.

Many species of microorganisms are capable of synthesizing riboflavin, and because of the extensive bacterial growth in the human intestinal tract, this may form an important and constant source of supply of riboflavin and may account for the limited occurrence of deficiency in humans.

When it was recognized that cereal products would be a good vehicle to use to improve the content of riboflavin in many diets, its mandatory addition as an enriching ingredient was adopted. In concert with thiamine, niacin and iron, riboflavin is present in nutritionally significant amounts in enriched wheat flour, farina, corn products, bread and macaroni and noodle products. Because of certain cooking habits and the unacceptability of the unnatural yellow color, the enrichment of rice with riboflavin has been resisted.

Thiamine

Concentrates of thiamine, often termed vitamin B_1, were given the latter name by early workers in this country who recognized that at least two accessory dietary factors were needed for normal growth of laboratory rats, one in butter fat and the other in "milk sugar." The names they suggested for these factors were fat-soluble vitamin A and water-soluble vitamin B. It was shown subsequently by a number of investigators that the latter consisted of a group of substances rather than a single compound, but vitamin B_1 was finally the first pure compound of the group to be laboriously isolated from rice polishings. In the pioneer studies on this substance it was found that a thiamine concentrate prevented polyneuritis in chickens, which later was found to be caused by the absence of thiamine in their diet. Deriving from this observation, an early name for the factor is aneurin (from antineuritic), which has persisted in some quarters.

Chemistry and Assay—Thiamine is a generic term applied to all substances possessing vitamin B_1 activity, regardless of the anion attached to the molecule. The cationic portion of the molecule, which is the part that may properly be called "thiamin," is made up of a substituted pyrimidine ring connected by a methylene bridge to the nitrogen of a substituted thiazole ring. A general structural formula is

where A is any appropriate anion. In addition, ammonium salts may be formed with the amine substituent on the pyrimidine ring. The common nomenclature is confusing, but, in general, the term mono, as in thiamine mononitrate or thiamine monophosphate, designates the thiazolium type salt. Thiamine hydrochloride is the ammonium salt formed by reacting thiamine chloride with hydrochloric acid (see page 1040).

Thiamine compounds are usually readily soluble in water and in alcohol but insoluble in fat solvents. They are stable in acid solution, and may be heated without decomposition, but unstable in neutral or alkaline solution. At neutral or alkaline pH splitting occurs at the methylene bridge upon heating in the presence of moisture. Splitting of the molecule takes place quantitatively in the presence of bisulfite ions, a reaction that is made use of in preparing dietary constituents free of thiamine for bioassay purposes.

Thiamine is oxidized in alkaline solution to thiochrome, a biologically inactive, highly fluorescent substance. This reaction is the basis for the chemical method of estimating thiamine. The pure vitamin is not readily oxidized in air.

An alternate commercial form of vitamin B_1 widely used because of its greater stability than the hydrochloride is the mononitrate.

The activity of the vitamin is expressed in milligrams of the chemically pure substance and a USP Reference Standard Thiamine Hydrochloride is available.

The determination of thiamine in food, biological materials, and pharmaceutical products is almost exclusively done by the thiochrome fluorometric method. On oxidation with ferricyanide in alkaline solution, thiamine is transformed into thiochrome which has a strong blue fluorescence. It is a very sensitive method and correlates well with bioassay results. The sequence in the determination involves extraction of the vitamin, enzyme hydrolysis, adsorption, elution and oxidation to thiochrome which is extracted with isobutanol and determined fluorometrically.

Before the development of suitable physicochemical methods, thiamine was determined in a typical rat-growth assay which is based on the growth response of young thiamine-depleted rats to supplemental doses of a reference standard and to the test material either fed in or separate from the diet or injected parenterally.

Metabolic Functions—In a phosphorylated form, thiamine (thiamine pyrophosphate; cocarboxylase) serves as the prosthetic group of enzyme systems that are concerned with the decarboxylation of α-keto-acids. For example, pyruvic acid is formed which is decarboxylated to form a two-carbon residue. This process of decarboxylation is catalyzed by the pyruvic acid decarboxylase enzyme system which consists of a specific protein, manganese ions, and diphospho-thiamine. An α-hydroxyethyl group (the "acetaldehyde" residue of the decarboxylated pyruvic acid) attaches to the 2-carbon of the thiazole ring. The hydroxyethyl group (active "acetate," active "acetaldehyde," or two-carbon fragment) attaches to one of the sulfur atoms of lipoamide, from which it is removed by coenzyme A. Pyrophosphorylated thiamine is effective in the decarboxylation of other α-keto-acids as well. Some decarboxylation processes are reversible, so that synthesis (condensation) may be achieved; thus thiamine is also important to the biosynthesis of keto-acids. It is involved in trans-ketolase reactions.

Thiamine is readily absorbed in aqueous solution from both the small and large intestine, and is then carried to the liver by the portal circulation. In the liver, as well as in all living cells, it normally combines with phosphate to form cocarboxylase. It may be stored in the liver in this form or it may combine further with manganese and specific proteins to become active enzymes known as carboxylases.

Thiamine is excreted in the urine in amounts that reflect the amount taken in and the amounts stored in the tissues. Measurement of the urinary excretion of thiamine after giving a small dose of thiamine is useful in determining whether body stores are adequate or deficient.

Dietary Requirement and Food Sources—Polyneuritis (disfunctioning of the nervous system) or beriberi is the frank disease associated with thiamine deficiency in man. Peripheral neuritis is a pathological condition of the nerves of the extremities; usually both legs are affected and sometimes the arms as well. The symptoms include loss of sensation, muscle weakness, and paralysis. In beriberi this condition is also associated with edema and abnormal electrocardiogram patterns.

Severe cases of beriberi are commonly found in the Orient among people whose diets consist principally of milled or polished rice, from which the vitamin, contained in the bran and germ of the cereal, is largely removed during the milling process. American dietaries generally furnish sufficient thiamine to meet requirements, and with the use of a varied diet, including whole grain cereals or enriched bread or flour, adequacy of thiamine in most instances is beyond question. Symptoms of thiamine deficiency have been observed among chronic alcoholics, who use alcohol in place of food as a source of energy. Deficiency also occurs in cases of chronic diarrhea, in which absorption is interfered with over a period of time and during pregnancy complicated with anorexia and nausea.

In the diagnosis of thiamine deficiency, symptoms to be noted in particular are anorexia, fatigue, loss of weight, sensation of burning in the soles of the feet, tenderness in calf muscles, muscle cramps, and general muscular weakness. Such signs are not in themselves specific, however, without supplementary laboratory findings that indicate a reduced thiamine content of blood and urine.

For treatment of beriberi or thiamine deficiency in humans, the first requisite is a nutritionally complete, well-balanced diet. Good diet is essential, because beriberi in most instances results from a complex or multiple deficiency, and administration of thiamine alone may precipitate a condition resulting from a lack of other water-soluble factors. Doses of 10 to 100 mg of thiamine has been used in severe cases to bring about a cure, but evidence of superiority of the larger doses is lacking. As size of the dose is increased, the proportion of thiamine retained rapidly decreases, the excess being excreted rapidly in the urine. Frequent small doses are to be preferred to a single large daily dose. Only in the most severe cases, or in patients with impaired intestinal absorption, does parenteral administration appear advantageous. Pharmaceutical preparations of many types and potencies are available commercially.

It is generally assumed that thiamine need is related to calorie need, particularly to those calories derived from carbohydrate. The Food and Nutrition Board considers that 0.5 mg per 1000 Kcal will maintain satisfactory thiamine nutriture under normal conditions in the US. As the caloric allowance varies with age, so does the recommended daily dietary allowance for thiamine; for infants, 0.2 to 0.5 mg; for children up to 12 years, 0.6 to 1.3 mg; for adolescents and adults, 1.0 to 1.5 mg, the highest allowance being for boys and men 12 to 35 years. The literature on thiamine needs in maternal and child nutrition suggests an increased need for thiamine during pregnancy, and an additional 0.2 mg per day is recommended, in accordance with the increased calorie recommendation.

Thiamine is found widely distributed in foods. Thiamine is found in all plants, and is synthesized by some microorganisms, particularly yeasts. No one food can be considered of particular importance above all others, although the cereal grains, milk, legumes, nuts, eggs, and pork probably furnish the larger proportion of thiamine in diets used in this country. Sophistication and processing of foods generally tend to reduce the thiamine supply. For example, in the preparation of wheat flour, separation of the bran coat and germ removes three-fourths or more of the thiamine present in the whole wheat. This is true for other cereal grains as well. Much of the white flour, corn grits, and rice used in this country is enriched to approximately the whole grain level. Because of the lability of thiamine to heat, cooking and baking processes reduce the raw food content of the vitamin.

The loss of thiamine in home cooking is not considered excessive, except with foods cooked in large amounts of water that is then discarded. Because of its solubility, the thiamine content of the cooking water is always appreciable.

Vitamin B$_{12}$

Vitamin B$_{12}$, the most recently discovered of the B group, was isolated from liver fractions in crystalline form in 1948 and was soon after shown to be specific for the treatment of Addisonian pernicious anemia. It has been established that extracts of liver, employed for more than 30 years in the control of pernicious anemia, contain vitamin B$_{12}$ as their active principle. Liver continues to be an important dietary source of the vitamin, but liver injection is no longer used in the treatment of pernicious anemia, because of the ready availability of crystalline forms of the vitamin.

Chemistry and Assay—Vitamin B$_{12}$ is a complex water-soluble compound which crystallizes as small red needles that have a specific rotation in dilute aqueous solution of $-59°$. Characteristic absorption spectrum maxima occur at 278 mμ, 361 mμ, and 550 mμ. The crystalline substance blackens without melting at 300°C. The compound is a cobalt coordination complex, in which the cobalt is trivalent and has a coordination number of six. The complex is neutral. Vitamin B$_{12}$ is composed of two heterocyclic systems, a benzimidazole and a modified porphyrin nucleus, with the following structure:

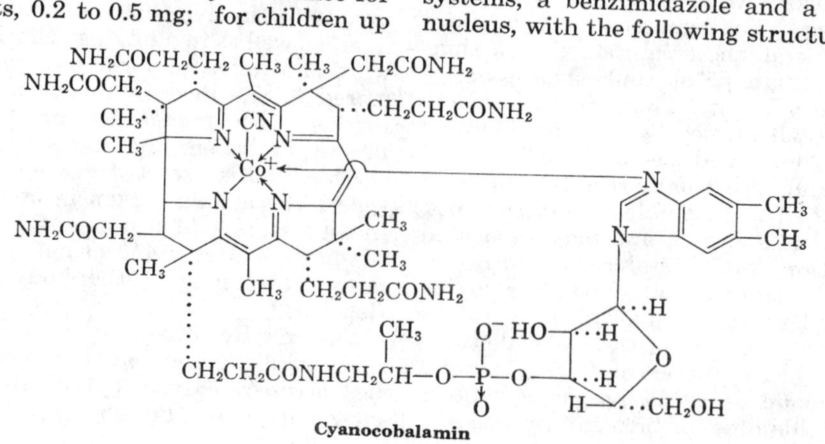

Cyanocobalamin

Actually, the cyanide group coordinated to the cobalt is not a part of the true vitamin but rather is an artifact caused by isolation of the vitamin on charcoal; in the liver the ligand is 5'-deoxyadenosyl anion. Nevertheless, by strict organic chemical definition, by virtue of the fact that the cyanide was the first form of the vitamin to be isolated, cyanocobalamin *is* vitamin B_{12}. When the ligand is hydroxide instead of cyanide, the compound is *vitamin B_{12a}* (hydroxocobalamin); when it is water, the substance is *vitamin B_{12b}* (aquocobalamin); when it is nitro, the compound is *vitamin B_{12c};* the 5'-deoxyadenosyl form is *coenzyme B_{12};* if the ligand is methyl, the compound is *methyl B_{12}.* Sulfito- and thio-cyanatocobalamins also are known. In practice, all of these compounds are vitamin B_{12}. A similar situation obtains with respect to the name *cobalamin*, which strictly is synonymous with cyanocobalamin but in loose practice applies to any active compound containing the α-(5,6-dimethylbenzimidazoyl)cobamide structure. *Cobamides* is a more appropriate generic term for these compounds.

Vitamin B_{12} (cyanocobalamin) in an atmosphere of hydrogen with a platinum catalyst is reduced to a red crystalline compound with slightly changed ultraviolet absorption maxima, and a reduced stability to heat. Vitamin B_{12a} results from such reduction; Vitamin B_{12b}, another reduced form, occurs in natural sources.

Commercially vitamin B_{12} is obtained from the fermentation of *Streptomyces griseus*. The vitamin is precipitated from aqueous solutions saturated with ammonium sulfate by *n*-butanol. Purification is achieved by chromatography, using bentonite or aluminum silicate as the adsorbent. Sharply defined red bands are formed during the development of the chromatograms indicating the location of the vitamin. The red band is separated mechanically and eluted with water. The concentrated water solution on addition of acetone gives the crystalline vitamin which can be further purified by recrystallization from aqueous acetone.

The USP provides a Reference Standard Cyanocobalamin for use in assay of the vitamin. The most important physicochemical method for determining vitamin B_{12} involves measurement of light absorbance at certain specific wavelengths characteristic for cyanocobalamin. This method is only applicable to relatively concentrated solutions of the compound, such as in pharmaceutical preparations.

Vitamin B_{12} is one of the most active biological factors known, its activity for bacteria is measured in terms of millimicrograms. Because of this sensitivity of some bacteria to such low levels of the vitamin and the fact that foods contain exceptionally low concentrations of the vitamin, microbiological methods are widely used. The following three organisms, which require vitamin B_{12} for growth, are used: *Lactobacillus leichmannii, Ochramonas malhamensis,* and *Euglena gracilis.*

Metabolic Functions, Dietary Requirement, and Food Sources—The vitamin is essential for the normal functioning of all cells, but particularly for cells of the bone marrow, the nervous system, and the gastrointestinal tract. It appears to facilitate reduction reactions and participate in the transfer of methyl groups. Evidence exists that vitamin B_{12} is involved in protein, carbohydrate, and fat metabolism, but its chief importance in mammalian tissues seems to be, together with folic acid, in the anabolism of deoxyribo-

nucleic acid in all cells. Coenzyme forms of vitamin B_{12}, in which the vitamin is linked to adenine and a sugar, which catalyze specific reactions in intermediary metabolism have been isolated from bacterial cultures and probably have similar vitamin roles in mammalian cells.

The biochemical fault in pernicious anemia, a condition caused by a prolonged deficiency of vitamin B_{12}, is a failure of elaboration of the intrinsic factor, normally present in the secretions of the stomach mucosa. This intrinsic factor, which is essential for the absorption of the vitamin through the intestinal wall, is known to form a complex with vitamin B_{12}. Intrinsic factor, now available in a purified form, is reported to be a mixture of mucoproteins.

Vitamin B_{12} is a requisite for normal blood formation, and certain macrocytic anemias respond to its administration. In pernicious anemia, unless accompanied by intrinsic factor, the vitamin is not orally absorbed in effective amounts and must be administered parenterally in microgram quantities. Preparations containing vitamin B_{12} and intrinsic factor concentrate are now available for oral use, and have been shown for short-term use at least, to be equivalent in value to the injections. Clinical studies indicate that if milligram amounts of the vitamin are administered orally, in the absence of intrinsic factor, enough of the vitamin passes through the intestinal wall to be effective in maintaining the pernicious anemia patient. However, the injectable form of vitamin B_{12} continues to be the drug of choice because of the desirability of occasional but regular attention of a physician to the condition of the patient.

The evidence indicating that vitamin B_{12} is the anti-pernicious anemia factor, and fully as effective in the treatment of macrocytic anemias as liver extract, appears to be complete. In treating pernicious anemia, vitamin B_{12}, administered intramuscularly, produces a maximal reticulocyte response in 4 to 9 days, and a restoration of red and white cell count in 4 to 6 weeks. The change in bone marrow, from a megaloblastic to a normoblastic state is dramatic, and occurs within a few hours after the injection of as little as 1 mcg of the vitamin. Vitamin B_{12} is considered to be the extrinsic factor of Castle, the absorption of which from the intestinal tract is facilitated by the intrinsic factor present in normal gastric juice. The biochemical defect in pernicious anemia then, is a failure of elaboration of the intrinsic factor. Because of this relationship, vitamin B_{12} given orally is much less effective in the pernicious anemia patient, and entirely ineffective if there is complete absence of intrinsic factor.

The vitamin is effective in preventing the occurrence of neurological changes common to pernicious anemia. Acute symptoms of combined system disease have been found to disappear rather promptly after B_{12} administration, but recovery appears to depend more on the chronicity of the disease than on the extent of neurological involvement, and conditions of long standing are less apt to show recovery.

A simple nutritional concept of pernicious anemia which seems valid is that of essentially an uncomplicated deficiency of vitamin B_{12} conditioned by the lack of intrinsic factor and, hence, the inability to absorb the vitamin from ingested food. This validation rests on several types of evidence, of which particularly convincing is the comparison of the clinical development of vitamin B_{12} deficiency in vegans, in patients following total gastrectomy (resulting in removal of intrinsic factor and interference with absorption of the vitamin) and the relapse following withholding of therapy from previously adequately treated patients with pernicious anemia. Simple experimental dietary deficiency of vitamin B_{12} has not yet been produced in the adult human under conditions of careful continuous observation. It seems probable that the requirements of parenterally administered (or absorbed) vitamin B_{12} by the patient with pernicious anemia or gastrectomy is similar to the requirements of the normal subject.

The recommended daily dietary allowance of the Food and Nutrition Board for vitamin B_{12} ranges from 1 to 8 mcg; the lowest value is for infants up to 2 months, and the highest value (3 mcg higher than the average adult allowance) is for women during pregnancy.

Vitamin B_{12} occurs in meat and dairy products but is not present to any measurable extent in plants or cereal grains. It is probable that indigenous bacteria in plant foods synthesize sufficient vitamin B_{12} to meet the requirement of those individuals whose dietary habits preclude the use of animal foods.

Official Water-Soluble Vitamins

Ascorbic Acid USP

[Vitamin C; Cevitamic Acid; Hexuronic Acid; Cecon (*Abbott*); Cevalin (*Lilly*); Ce-Vi-Sol (*Mead-Johnson*)]

Ascorbic Acid contains 99.0–100.5% of $C_6H_8O_6$ (176.13). For the structure, see page 1024.

Preparation—The article in commerce is produced exclusively by synthesis. Sorbitol, a hexose sugar, occurring in several fruits but commercially obtained by hydrogenating dextrose in the presence of a Cu–Cr catalyst, is the raw material for the production of Ascorbic Acid. The D-sorbitol in aqueous solution is converted by the action of the organism *Acetobacter suboxydans* to L-sorbose, which is a ketose. The L-

sorbose is then condensed with acetone by means of sulfuric acid to form diacetone sorbose. The object of the acetonation is to protect the hydroxyl groups from oxidation in the subsequent steps. The diacetone sorbose, after suitable purification, is oxidized by potassium permanganate and then hydrolyzed forming 2-keto-L-gulonic acid. This acid is esterified with methanol and an intermediate sodio compound is formed with sodium methoxide. Hydrolysis with aqueous HCl removes the methyl group and sodium and lactonizes it yielding ascorbic acid. The process is illustrated on this page.

Description—White or slightly yellow crystals or powder. It is odorless and on exposure to light it gradually darkens. In the dry state it is reasonably stable in air, but in solution it rapidly deteriorates in the presence of air. It melts at about 190°. Its specific rotation in aqueous solution is between +20.5° and +21.5°. Its solution is acid to litmus paper. Its solutions have an acid taste. Its aqueous solution has the acidic properties of a monobasic acid and it forms salts with metallic ions. It is easily oxidized particularly in the presence of copper.

Solubility—1 Gm dissolves in about 3 ml of water and 30 ml of alcohol; insoluble in chloroform, ether, and benzene.

Incompatibilities—Ascorbic Acid is stable in the dry state but in solution oxidizes rapidly in the presence of air. The reaction is accelerated by *alkalies* and certain *metals*, especially *copper*; it is retarded by acids. Aqueous solutions are strongly acidic, having a pH of 2 to 3.

Uses—In addition to the uses described in the general statement (page 1035), vitamin C is sometimes given with iron salts in the treatment of iron-deficiency anemia; it functions to keep the iron in the ferrous state and hence to improve absorption. Apart from coadministration of vitamin C and iron preparations, a few cases of hypochromic anemia improve upon increasing the intake of the vitamin.

No more than the recommended daily allowance should be given to the pregnant woman; the metabolism of the fetus adapts to high levels of the vitamin, and scurvy may develop after birth when the intake drops to normal levels.

Dose—*Daily, oral* or *parenteral*, **40 mg to 1 Gm;** *usual, requirement,* **60 mg** once a day; *therapeutic,* **250 mg** 2 times a day.

Other Dose Information—The USP daily requirement, given above, does not conform to the Food and Nutrition Board, National Academy of Sciences–National Research Council recommended daily allowances (see page 1013).

Dosage Forms—Injection USP: 100 and 500 mg/ml, 100, 200, and 500 mg/2 ml, 500 mg and 1 Gm/5 ml, 1 Gm/10 ml; Tablets USP: 25, 50, 100, 250, and 500 mg.

D-Glucose → D-Sorbitol → L-Sorbose → Diacetone L-Sorbose → 2-Keto-L-gulonic Acid → L-Ascorbic Acid

Sodium Ascorbate USP

[Cenolate (*Abbott*)]

Sodium Ascorbate contains 99.0–101.0% of $C_6H_7NaO_6$ (198.11), calculated on the dried basis.

Description—White or very faintly yellow crystals, or crystalline powder. Odorless or practically odorless. Relatively stable in air. On exposure to light it gradually darkens. The pH of a 1 in 10 solution is about 7.5.

Solubility—1 Gm dissolves in 1.3 ml of water; insoluble in alcohol.

Uses—Sodium Ascorbate is a pharmaceutical necessity for *Ascorbic Acid Injection* (page 1036). It is also used as an antioxidant and in the processing of meat.

Dose—See *Ascorbic Acid* (page 1036).

Ascorbyl Palmitate—see page 1316.

Calcium Pantothenate USP

[Calcium D(+)-Pantothenate; Dextro Calcium Pantothenate; Pantholin (*Lilly*)]

[HO.CH₂.C(CH₃)₂.CH(OH).CO.NH.(CH₂)₂COO]₂Ca

Calcium Pantothenate [$C_{18}H_{32}CaN_2O_{10}$ = 476.54] is the calcium salt of the dextrorotatory isomer of pantothenic acid. It contains the equivalent of 90.0–100.5% of dextrorotatory calcium pantothenate, calculated on the dried basis.

Description—A slightly hygroscopic, white powder. It is odorless, has a bitter taste, and is stable in air. It is unstable to heat both in the dry state and in acid or alkaline solution. It is most stable at pH 5.5 to 6.5 and its solutions may be autoclaved at this pH for a short time without appreciable loss. Its solutions are neutral or slightly alkaline to litmus, having a pH of 7 to 9. Specific rotation (calculated on the dried basis and in a 5% solution) +25° to +27.5°.

Solubility—1 Gm dissolves in about 3 ml of water; soluble in glycerin; practically insoluble in alcohol, chloroform and ether.

Uses—See the general statement on *Pantothenic Acid* (page 1029). Since a deficiency to pantothenic acid, alone, is virtually unknown, the primary indication for use is a general nutritional deficiency. Clinical cases have been too few to supply creditable data on dosage; consequently, the dose that follows is more customary than meaningful. Pantothenic acid is so ubiquitous that there is no need to supplement any eucaloric diet, regardless of balance, with Calcium Pantothenate.

Dose—10 to **50 mg** daily; *usual,* **10 mg** once a day.
Dosage Forms—Tablets USP: 10 mg.

Racemic Calcium Pantothenate USP

[Calcium (±)-Pantothenate]

Racemic Calcium Pantothenate [$C_{18}H_{32}CaN_2O_{10}$ = 476.54] is a mixture of the calcium salts of the dextrorotatory and levorotatory isomers of pantothenic acid. It contains the equivalent of not less than 45.0% of dextrorotatory calcium pantothenate, calculated on the dried basis.

Note—The physiological activity of Racemic Calcium Pantothenate is approximately one-half that of Calcium Pantothenate.

Description—A white, slightly hygroscopic powder. It is odorless, has a bitter taste, and is stable in air. Its solutions are neutral or alkaline to litmus, having a pH of 7 to 9. It is optically inactive.

Solubility—Freely soluble in water; soluble in glycerin; practically insoluble in alcohol, chloroform, and ether.

Uses—See *Calcium Pantothenate* (above) and the general statement on *Pantothenic Acid* (page 1030). Since biological activity resides only in the dextro isomer, the racemic compound is only ½ as potent as calcium pantothenate.

Dose—**20** to **100 mg** daily; *usual,* **20 mg** (equivalent to approximately 10 mg of dextrorotatory calcium pantothenate) once a day.

Cyanocobalamin USP

[α-5,6-Dimethylbenzimidazolylcobamide Cyanide; Vitamin B₁₂ USP XIV; Cycobemin; (*Various Mfgs.*)]

Cyanocobalamin contains 96.0–100.5% of $C_{63}H_{88}CoN_{14}O_{14}P$ (1355.40), calculated on the dried basis.

For the structure, see page 1034.

Preparation—Vitamin B₁₂ can be isolated from aqueous liver extracts and from *Streptomyces griseus* fermentation. Commercially, it is obtained from the latter source. The vitamin is precipitated from aqueous solutions saturated with ammonium sulfate by *n*-butanol. Purification is achieved by chromatography, using bentonite or aluminum silicate as the adsorbent. Sharply defined red bands are formed during the development of the chromatograms indicating the location of the vitamin. The red band is separated mechanically and eluted with water. The concentrated water solution on addition of acetone gives the crystalline vitamin which can be further purified by recrystallization from aqueous acetone.

Description—Dark red, hygroscopic crystals or amorphous or crystalline powder. When the anhydrous compound is exposed to air it may absorb about 12% of water.

Solubility—1 Gm dissolves in 80 ml of water; soluble in alcohol; insoluble in acetone, chloroform, and ether.

Uses—The metabolic functions, dietary requirement, and food sources of vitamin B₁₂ are described on pages 1035 and 1036. Cyanocobalamin and other forms of vitamin B₁₂ are used to treat various megaloblastic anemias, especially *pernicious anemia* and other anemias in which the secretion of the intrinsic factor is impaired, as in *gastric cancer, gastric atrophy, total* or even *subtotal gastrectomy*. It may also be used to treat the megaloblastic anemias of *tropical sprue, idiopathic steatorrhea, gluten-induced enteropathy, regional ileitis, ileal resection, malignancies, granulomas, strictures, or other structural disorders of the ileum* in which vitamin B₁₂ absorption is impaired; in most of these, folate deficiency is even more severe, and combined therapy is indicated. The megaloblastic anemia associated with *fish tapeworm infestation* also responds to vitamin B₁₂. The megaloblastic anemias of pregnancy, infancy, alcoholism, and poverty are usually due to folic acid deficiency and only infrequently respond to vitamin. B₁₂. The vitamin is *not useful* in the treatment of infectious hepatitis, multiple sclerosis, trigeminal neuralgia, anorexia, miscellaneous neuropathies, thyrotoxicosis, retarded growth, aging, or various psychiatric disorders, and claims to the contrary and promotion therefore represent an abuse.

In addition to intrinsic factor, gastrointestinal absorption requires an alkaline pH. In the presence of pancreatic disease it may be necessary to administer oral vitamin B_{12} with bicarbonate or give the vitamin parenterally.

Dose—*Intramuscular*, **30 mcg** to **1 mg** per dose; *maintenance*, **100 mg** once a month; *therapeutic*, **100 mcg** once a week.

Other Dose Information—The dose of Cyanocobalamin varies with the severity of the *anemia*, its response to therapy and with other signs and symptoms of the disease. For the patient with uncomplicated pernicious anemia in relapse, the initial intramuscular dose of cyanocobalamin is 30 mcg injected daily or every other day for 5 to 10 doses; then 15 to 30 mcg injected once or twice weekly until the blood picture is normal. Maintenance dosage of 40 to 60 mcg every 2 weeks or 80 to 100 mcg every month usually suffices. Critically ill patients and those with intercurrent infection or with neurological complications require vigorous parenteral treatment, and larger doses for both initial and maintenance therapy must be employed. However, there is no acceptable evidence that doses in excess of 30 mcg per day achieve more than does 30 mcg per day.

Dosage Forms—Cobalamin Concentrate NF; Injection USP: 100 mcg and 1 mg/ml, 5 mg/5 ml, 300, 500, and 600 mcg, and 1 and 10 mg/10 ml, 3 and 30 mg/30 ml.

Veterinary Dose—In general, *intramuscular*, **1 mcg** per **pound**.

Folic Acid USP

[PGA; *N*-{*p*-{ [(2-Amino-4-hydroxy-6-pteridinyl)methyl]amino}benzoyl}-glutamic Acid; Folacin; Pteroylglutamic Acid; Liver *L. casei* Factor; Folvite (*Lederle*)

Folic Acid contains 98.0–102.0% of $C_{19}H_{19}N_7O_6$ (441.41), calculated on the anhydrous basis.

For the structure, see page 1027.

Preparation—Commercially the production of pteroylglutamic acid is effected by synthetic methods by any of several different processes. In one of the better known methods the synthesis is accomplished as follows:

2,3-Dibromopropionaldehyde, dissolved in a water-miscible organic solvent (alcohol, dioxan), is added to a solution of equal molecular quantities of 2,4,5-tri-amino-6-hydroxypyrimidine and *p*-aminobenzoyl-glutamic acid, maintaining a pH of about 4 by the controlled addition of alkali as the reaction progresses. The scheme of the reaction is analogous to that described for *Methotrexate* (page 1169), the only difference being in the starting pyrimidine compound.

Description and Properties—A yellow or yellowish orange, odorless, crystalline powder. Its specific rotation is +18° to +23°. It is readily destroyed by boiling in acid solution, but is relatively stable to processing and storage in pharmaceutical preparations. The compound has a characteristic absorption in the ultraviolet range of the spectrum, with maxima at wave lengths 256, 283, and 365 mμ, and the ratio A_{256}/A_{365} is between 2.80 and 3.00. It is easily oxidized to a degradation product that exhibits a bright blue-green fluorescence when exposed to ultraviolet light.

Solubility—Very slightly soluble in water; insoluble in alcohol and the usual organic solvents; readily dissolves in dilute solutions of alkali hydroxides and carbonates, and is soluble in hot diluted hydrochloric or sulfuric acid, forming very pale yellow solutions.

Uses—The only valid therapeutic use of Folic Acid is in the treatment of a deficiency of the vitamin or prophylactically in instances in which the folic acid

requirement is increased, as in the third trimester of pregnancy. *Megaloblastic anemias* in which folic acid deficiency occurs may result from malabsorption syndromes, such as *sprue, idiopathic steatorrhea, celiac disease, intestinal reticulosis, regional jejunitis, jejunal diverticulosis, blind loop syndrome, and gastroenterostomy*. Megaloblastic anemia of infancy is generally the result of generalized malnutrition, as is nutritional megaloblastic anemia. In all of the above-named megaloblastic anemias vitamin B_{12} deficiency often coexists, and Folic Acid, alone, may be inadequate. Pernicious anemia should be ruled out, lest the Folic Acid mask the disease (see below). In the megaloblastic anemias of deficiency, a low serum folic acid level will obtain. However, in megaloblastic anemias consequent to treatment with pyrimethamine, diphenylhydantoin and related substances, or methotrexate, the serum folic acid levels may be normal; the signs of deficiency result from the antimetabolite effects of the drugs, and they may be overcome competitively by increasing the intake of folic acid. Folic Acid is not effective in the treatment of aplastic anemia, leukemia, anemias of infection and nephritis, and general reduction in bone marrow activity of unknown origin.

The vitamin is readily absorbed from the gastrointestinal tract and from parenteral sites of administration. The portion of administered folic acid which is excreted in the urine varies directly with the dose; only a small fraction appears in the urine following the oral ingestion of 0.1 mg, but up to 90% may be excreted by the kidney when a single dose of 15 mg is ingested. The fate of the unrecovered folic acid is unknown. The indications for parenteral folic acid are rare. Sodium Folate (page 1042) is the preferred form for injection.

Folic Acid is capable of bringing about an incomplete and temporary hematopoietic response in pernicious anemia, which may cause the physician to overlook the basic disorder. But folic acid does not affect the progressive neurological lesions of the disease, which may appear explosively and in an irreversible stage. Doses of Folic Acid which will correct a folic acid deficiency but which will not generally cause a remission in pernicious anemia are on the order of 0.1 mg; consequently, doses of more than 0.1 mg per day require a prescription.

Folic Acid is practically nontoxic, and doses greatly in excess of those necessary to prevent nutritional deficiency are devoid of pharmacodynamic action.

Dose—*Usual maintenance, oral*, **100 mcg** once a day; *therapeutic, oral* or *intramuscular*, **250 mcg** to **1 mg** once a day.

Other Dose Information—The USP estimated requirement, above, does not conform to the Food and Nutrition Board, National Academy of Sciences–National Research Council daily recommended allowances (see page 1013).

Dosage Forms—Injection USP: 15 mg/ml, 150 mg/10 ml; Tablets USP: 100 and 400 mcg and 5, 10, and 20 mg.

Hydroxocobalamin

[Vitamin B_{12a}; (*Various Mfgs.*)]

Hydroxocobalamin [$C_{62}H_{89}CoN_{13}O_{15}P$ = 1346.41] is cobinamide hydroxide phosphate, 3'-ester with 5,6-dimethyl-1-α-D-ribofuranosylbenzimidazole, inner salt.

Hydroxocobalamin is an analog of *Cyanocobalamin* (page 1034) in which a hydroxyl function has replaced the cyano function.

Preparation—Cyanocobalamin in solution is hydrogenated at room temperature with the aid of Raney nickel. The solution is then exposed to air and diluted with acetone. Oxidation takes place and, upon standing, the hydroxocobalamin crystallizes.

Description—Dark red crystals that are odorless or practically odorless and tasteless. For stability purposes, it is stored, under nitrogen, in tightly sealed light-resistant containers below 15°.

Solubility—1 Gm dissolves in about 100 ml of water; it is preferable to make solutions in acetate buffer at pH 3.5–4.5 in which 1 Gm dissolves in about 100 ml.

Uses and **Dose**—See *Cyanocobalamin* (page 1037).

Dosage Forms—Injection: 100 and 1000 mcg/ml.

Niacin NF

[Nicotinic Acid USP XVI; 3-Pyridinecarboxylic Acid]

Niacin contains 99.5–101.0% of $C_6H_5NO_2$ (123.11), calculated on the dried basis.

For the structure, see page 1028.

Description—Occurs as white crystals or crystalline powder. It is odorless or has a slight odor.

Solubility—1 Gm dissolves in about 60 ml of water; freely soluble in boiling water, boiling alcohol, and also solutions of alkali hydroxides and carbonates; practically insoluble in ether.

Uses—The vitaminergic actions, metabolic functions, and daily requirements of Niacin are discussed in the general statement (pages 1028 and 1029). Niacin is chiefly used in the treatment of pellagra, a disease common among the poor in sub-tropical countries due to diet deficiency. It has also been found useful in conjunction with vitamin B_1 and riboflavin in the treatment of nutritional deficiency in chronic alcoholism.

In doses of 20 mg or more in humans, Niacin elicits a vasodilator effect that occurs a few minutes after oral ingestion, or immediately after intravenous injection, and lasts for a few minutes to an hour. Symptoms of flushing, itching, burning, or tingling occur, along with an increased skin temperature and increased motility and gastric secretion. Nicotinyl alcohol also shares this vasodilator property, and at one time both nicotinic acid and the alcohol were popularly used in the treatment of peripheral vascular disease and senility (as a cerebral vasodilator). These uses of nicotinic acid are now obsolete and now are but an annoying side effect of large doses. The vasodilator effect of oral Niacin is less if the Niacin is given with a meal.

Large doses of Niacin lower blood cholesterol, phospholipids, triglycerides, and free fatty acids, and the drug has been used in the treatment of hypercholesterolemia and atherosclerosis. Nicotinamide does not possess the hypolipemic or the vasodilator property.

Large doses of nicotinic acid, comparable to those used to lower blood lipids, cause abnormalities in liver function, including jaundice.

Niacin is well absorbed orally, and the oral and parenteral doses are the same. With large doses, a considerable amount is excreted into the urine, so that it is advisable to give several small doses during the day rather than one large one.

Dose—*Usual, oral, requirement,* **20 mg** daily; *oral and parenteral, therapeutic,* **50 mg** 3 to 10 times a day.

Other Dose Information—To meet daily requirement, 10 mg; to meet recommended daily allowance, 5 to 20 mg; for treatment of deficiency, 50 to 500 mg daily, in 3 to 10 divided doses; as a peripheral vaso-

dilator, 50 to 200 mg orally or 10 to 50 mg parenterally 3 to 6 times daily; for hypercholesteremia, 3 to 6 Gm daily, in 10 divided doses.

Dosage Forms—Injection NF: 50 and 100 mg/ml; Tablets NF: 25, 50, and 100 mg.

Niacinamide USP

[Nicotinamide USP XVI: Nicotinic Acid Amide]

Niacinamide contains 98.5–101.0% of $C_6H_6N_2O$ (122.13), calculated on the dried basis.

For the structure, see page 1028.

Description—A white, crystalline powder. It is odorless or nearly so, and has a bitter taste. Its solutions are neutral to litmus paper. It melts between 128° and 131°C.

Solubility—1 Gm dissolves in 1 ml of water, 5.5 ml of alcohol, and 10 ml of glycerin.

Uses—See the general statement under *Metabolic Functions* (page 1028) and *Niacin* (above). Niacinamide lacks the vasodilator, gastrointestinal, hepatic, and hypolipemic actions of niacin. Consequently, it is preferred to niacin in the treatment of deficiency. The essential absence of untoward effects explains the USP status of Niacinamide in preference to niacin.

Dose—*Oral or parenteral,* 20 to **500 mg** daily; *usual, prophylactic,* **20 mg** once a day; *therapeutic,* **50 mg** 3 to 10 times a day.

Other Dose Information—The USP "prophylactic" dose, above, corresponds to the highest recommended daily allowance of the Food and Nutrition Board, National Academy of Sciences–National Research Council for niacin (see page 1013), which nutritionally is equivalent to Niacinamide.

Dosage Forms—Injection USP: 100 mg/2 ml, 500 mg/5 ml, 1 Gm/10 ml, 3 and 6 Gm/30 ml; Tablets USP: 25, 50, and 100 mg.

Pyridoxine Hydrochloride USP

[5-Hydroxy-6-methyl-3,4-pyridinedimethanol Hydrochloride; Vitamin B_6; Vitamin B_6 Hydrochloride; Hexabetalin (*Lilly*)]

Pyridoxine Hydrochloride contains 98.0–100.5% of $C_8H_{11}NO_3 \cdot HCl$ (205.64), calculated on the dried basis.

Description—Colorless or white crystals or a white, crystalline powder. It is stable in air, and is slowly affected by sunlight. Its solutions are acid to litmus, having a pH of about 3. Melting range 204° to 208° with some decomposition.

Solubility—1 Gm dissolves in 5 ml of water and 100 ml of alcohol; insoluble in chloroform and ether.

Uses—For the metabolic functions and characteristics of deficiency, see *Pyridoxine* (page 1031). Since pyridoxine deficiency in adults is extremely difficult to induce, it is doubtful that there is ever a therapeutic need for pyridoxine, alone, in the adult. However, it is justified to give pyridoxine along with other B-vitamins when there is evidence of a *multiple B-vitamin deficiency*. Occasionally a deficiency occurs in infants on a proprietary formula in which sterilization has destroyed the pyridoxine and which had not been supplemented; pyridoxine alone is indicated in such instances. Pyridoxine may be used prophylactically to prevent peripheral neuritis in *patients treated with* *isoniazid*. It has been claimed that pyridoxine controls the *nausea and vomiting of pregnancy* or of *radiation sickness*, but unequivocal proof has never been marshalled. The vitamin also appears to aid in the dissolution of renal stones of calcium oxalate, possibly because of increased excretion of calcium-chelating citric acid. Pyridoxine is of *no value* in the treatment of various neurological, neuromuscular, or dermatological disorders, and promotion for such uses is an abuse.

Dose—*Usual, oral* or *parenteral, prophylactic,* **2 mg** once a day; *therapeutic,* **5** to **150 mg** daily.

Other Dose Information—The USP "prophylactic" dose, above, is less than the highest recommended daily allowance (2.5 mg) of the Food and Nutrition Board, National Academy of Sciences–National Research Council (see page 1013).

The dose for malnutrition is 5 to 10 mg daily; for hyperemesis gravidum and emesis of radiation sickness is 10 to 100 mg daily. Oral and parenteral doses are the same for comparable therapy, but the parenteral doses are usually higher owing to the generally more serious condition of the patient who cannot tolerate oral alimentation.

Dosage Forms—Injection USP: 50 and 100 mg/ml, 500 mg and 1 Gm/10 ml, 3 Gm/30 ml; Tablets USP: 10, 25, 50, and 100 mg.

Riboflavin USP

[Lactoflavin; Riboflavine; Vitamin B₂; Vitamin G]

Riboflavin contains 98.0–102.0% of $C_{17}H_{20}N_4O_6$ (376.37), calculated on the dried basis.

For the structure, see page 1031.

Description—A yellow to orange-yellow, crystalline powder having a slight odor. It melts at about 280°. Its saturated solution is neutral to litmus. When dry, it is not appreciably affected by diffused light, but when in solution, light induces quite rapid deterioration, especially in the presence of alkalies.

Solubility—Very slightly soluble in water, alcohol, and isotonic sodium chloride solution; very soluble in dilute solutions of alkalies; insoluble in ether and chloroform.

Uses—For the metabolic functions, human requirements, and characteristics of deficiency, see the general statement on *Riboflavin* (page 1032). Riboflavin is used to treat ariboflavinosis (riboflavin deficiency) and also to supplement other B vitamins in the treatment of pellagra and beriberi.

Dose—*Oral* or *parenteral,* **2** to **15 mg** daily; *usual, oral* or *parenteral, prophylactic,* **2 mg** once a day; *therapeutic,* **10 mg** once a day.

Other Dose Information—The USP "prophylactic" dose, above, corresponds to the highest recommended daily allowance of the Food and Nutrition Board, National Academy of Sciences–National Research Council.

Dosage Forms—Injection USP: 5 mg/ml, 350 mg/10 ml; Tablets USP: 1, 2, 5, 10, and 25 mg.

Thiamine Hydrochloride USP

[Thiamin Chloride; Vitamin B₁; Vitamin B₁ Hydrochloride; Aneurine Hydrochloride; Betalin-S (*Lilly*)]

Thiamine Hydrochloride contains 98.0–102.0% of $C_{12}H_{17}ClN_4OS \cdot HCl$ (337.27), calculated on the dried basis.

Preparation—This vitamin consists of two ring systems, a pyrimidine portion and a thiazole portion joined by a methylene bridge.

The *pyrimidine* may be prepared by several processes, one of which is as follows: Ethyl acrylate [$CH_2 = CHCOOC_2H_5$] is heated with ethyl alcohol forming β-ethoxypropionic ester [$C_2H_5OCH_2CH_2COOC_2H_5$] which is condensed in the presence of sodium metal with formic acid to form ethyl sodioformyl-β-ethoxypropionate [$C_2H_5OCH_2CNa(CHO)COOC_2H_5$]. This is then condensed with acetamidine yielding 2-methyl 5-ethoxymethyl-6-hydroxypyrimidine. This compound is treated with phosphorus oxychloride thereby replacing the OH on carbon 6 with Cl, and by reacting the resulting chloro derivative with ammonia, the Cl is replaced by NH_2. Finally on treating the latter product with HBr, 2-methyl-5-bromomethyl-6-aminopyrimidine hydrobromide is produced.

The *thiazole* portion of the thiamine molecule may be built up in the following manner: Ethyl acetoacetate [$CH_3COCH_2COOC_2H_5$] is treated with ethylene oxide [C_2H_4O] and the resulting acetyl-butyryl lactone, when reacted with sulfuryl chloride, yields chloroacetyl butyro-lactone. This compound is decarboxylated when heated with HCl, splitting off CO_2 and chloroacetopropanol. The latter, when condensed with thioformamide yields the thiazole, 4-methyl-5-hydroxy-ethylthiazole.

The final step of this process is the combination of the pyrimidine and the thiazole to form a thiazolium halide. Since this is a simple addition of an alkyl halide (the bromo pyrimidine) to a tertiary amine (the thiazole) it is readily effected by bringing the two components together in a suitable solvent. The vitamin-bromohydrobromide so obtained is transformed into the corresponding chlorine compound, thiamine with freshly precipitated silver chloride. The silver combines with the bromine to form the less soluble silver bromide and the chloride from the silver chloride replaces the bromine.

Acetamidine   Enol form of Ethyl Sodioformyl-β-ethoxypropionate

2-Methyl-5-bromoethyl-6-aminopyrimidine Hydrobromide

Acetoacetic Ester

γ-Chloro-γ-acetyl Propanol

4-Methyl-5-(β-hydroxyethyl)-thiazole

Thiamine Chloride Hydrochloride (the official vitamin)

Description—Small white crystals or a crystalline powder usually having a slight, characteristic odor. When exposed to air, the anhydrous product rapidly absorbs about 4% of water. Its solutions are acid to litmus paper. The pH of a solution (1 in 100) is between 2.7 and 3.4. It melts, with some decomposition, at about 248°.

Solubility—1 Gm dissolves in about 1 ml of water and about 100 ml of alcohol; soluble in glycerin; insoluble in ether or benzene.

Incompatibilities—Thiamine Hydrochloride in the dry state is stable. Acidic solutions having a pH below 5.5, preferably from 5.0 to 3.5, are also relatively stable. *Alkalies* destroy it. It is precipitated from solution by several of the *alkaloidal reagents* such as *mercuric chloride, iodine, picric acid, tannin,* and *Mayer's reagent.* It is sensitive to both *oxidizing* and *reducing agents.*

Elixirs of thiamine hydrochloride are necessarily acid in reaction and are, therefore, incompatible with any acid-neutralizing substance. *Phenobarbital sodium* has been an occasional offender in this respect, the result frequently being such as to cause precipitation of the phenobarbital as well as a partial lowering of the acidity of the mixture with consequent deterioration of the vitamin. Phenobarbital, not the sodium derivative, may be dispensed in such an instance provided that sufficient alcohol is present to keep it in solution. If a part of the elixir is replaced with alcohol for this purpose, an amount of thiamine hydrochloride equivalent to that contained in the volume so replaced must be added to the product.

Uses—For a description of the metabolic functions and of a deficiency, see *Thiamine* (page 1033). Thiamine is used to treat *beriberi* and also *general B vitamin deficiency.* The fact that thiamine cures the neuropathologies of beriberi has given rise to a widespread use of thiamine in nearly any type of neuropathology. Although such indescriminatory use can do no organic harm to the patient, it constitutes an unnecessary expense; the promotion of the vitamin for such promiscuous use constitutes an abuse.

Dose—*Oral* or *parenteral, daily,* **2 to 100 mg;** *usual, prophylactic,* **2 mg** once a day; *therapeutic,* **10 to 15 mg** 2 or 3 times a day.

Dosage Forms—Injection USP: 100 mg/ml, 200 mg/2 ml, 500 mg and 1 Gm/10 ml, 2 Gm/20 ml, 2.5 Gm/5, 10, and 25 ml, 3 and 6 Gm/30 ml; Tablets USP: 5, 10, 25, 50, 100, and 250 mg.

Veterinary Dose (not well established)—*Prophylactic, Horses,* **2.5 mg** per **100 pounds** of body weight; *Dogs,* **0.3 to 0.6 mcg** per **pound** of body weight; *therapeutic, Dogs,* **0.6 to 2 mg** daily.

Thiamine Mononitrate USP

[Thiamine Nitrate; Vitamin B₁ Mononitrate]

Thiamine Mononitrate contains 98.0–102.0% of $C_{12}H_{17}N_5O_4S$ (327.36), calculated on the dried basis.

Description—White crystals or crystalline powder, usually having a slight, characteristic odor.

Solubility—1 Gm dissolves in about 35 ml of water; slightly soluble in alcohol and chloroform.

Uses—Thiamine Mononitrate is more stable than thiamine hydrochloride. Its vitaminergic actions and uses are identical to those of the hydrochloride. See *Thiamine Hydrochloride* (this page) and the general statement on *Thiamine* (page 1033).

Other Water-Soluble Vitamins

Aminobenzoic Acid NF XII [*p*-Aminobenzoic Acid; PABA], dried at 105° for 2 hours, contains not less than 98.5% of $C_7H_7NO_2$ (137.14). The aminobenzoic acid of biological significance is para-aminobenzoic acid (PABA). *Preparation:* From *p*-nitrobenzoic acid by reduction with iron and hydrochloric acid. The required *p*-nitrobenzoic acid is obtained by oxidation of the readily available *p*-nitrotoluene with potassium permanganate or potassium dichromate in the presence of sulfuric acid. *Description and Solubility:* White or slightly yellow, odorless crystals or a crystalline powder. It discolors on exposure to air or light. It melts between 186° and 189°.

Uses: PABA is an essential nutrient for a number of microorganisms, especially those that synthesize folic acid. The failure of growth of rats, chicks and mice, and achromotrichia in black rats has been observed in the absence of PABA. Consequently, PABA has long been included among the vitamins. However, it now appears that the nutrient action is indirect, mediated through folic acid and other vitamins synthesized by enteric bacteria. Since mammals utilize preformed folic acid, PABA is not required in the diet to support the biosynthesis of folic acid, and no other biological loci for the compound have been shown. Consequently, there is no need for PABA in human nutrition, and continued promotion of the compound represents an abuse. For this reason Aminobenzoic Acid has been dropped from the NF. Aminobenzoic Acid acts as a sun screen and is incorporated into some sunscreen ointments.

Calcium Leucovorin USP XVI [(*Lederle*); Calcium Folinate-SF; Calcium 5-Formyl-5,6,7,8-tetrahydrofolate; Calcium *N*-[*p*-[[2-Amino-5-formyl-5,6,7,8-tetrahydro-4-hydroxy-6-pteridinyl)methyl]amino]benzoyl]glutamate; Citrovorum Factor]—*Purity:* 90–110% of $C_{20}H_{21}CaN_7O_7 \cdot 5H_2O$. A yellowish white or yellow, odorless, microcrystalline powder. Very soluble in water; practically insoluble in alcohol. *Uses:* Leucovorin (folinic acid) is the biological formyl derivative and the active form of folic acid (see *Folic Acid*), and the calcium salt is simply a convenient pharmaceutical form that is preferred for intramuscular injection. Consequently its uses and limitations in the *treatment of the megaloblastic anemias* are the same as for folic acid. However, it is superior to folic acid in *counteracting the excessive effects of the folic acid antagonists* (methotrexate, etc; see page 1169), since the antagonists competitively antagonize the conversion of folic acid to leucovorin and not the leucovorin itself. *Dose: Intramuscularly,* for the counteraction of folic acid antagonists, 3 to 6 mg daily; for the treatment of megaloblastic anemias, 10 mg daily for 10 to 15 days; as an adjunct to cyanocobalamin therapy, 0.2 to 15 mg daily.

Choline Bitartrate NF XI [(2-Hydroxyethyl)trimethylammonium Bitartrate]*—A white, crystalline powder. It is hygroscopic when exposed to air. It is freely soluble in water and slightly soluble in alcohol; insoluble in ether, chloroform, and benzene. *Uses:* See *Choline Chloride* (this page). The bitartrate anion does not affect the physiological actions of choline. *Dose:* 2 Gm. [*$C_9H_{19}NO_7$.]

Choline Chloride is (2-hydroxyethyl)trimethylammonium chloride.† *Preparation:* For the preparation of choline, see *Choline Dihydrogen Citrate* (below). *Description and Solubility:* White, deliquescent crystals. A 10% aqueous solution has a pH of about 4.7. Very soluble in water or alcohol. *Uses:* For the metabolic effects of *Choline,* see the general statement (page 1026). Choline Chloride is used to reduce fatty infiltration of the liver and thus supposedly to prevent degeneration and cirrhosis. Such infiltration may occur after exposure to certain chemical intoxicants, such as carbon tetrachloride, chloroform, various other halogenated hydrocarbons (including several general anesthetics), divinyl ether, etc. Moderate to severe ethanol intoxication and habitual ingestion of ethanol also predispose to fatty infiltration of the liver. Patients who are acutely ill and cannot eat or persons on a high-fat diet frequently develop fatty livers, for which choline may be given. In none of these conditions has there been a clearly demonstrable efficacy. Furthermore, a high-protein diet, especially one that includes eggs, meat, liver, and milk, not only provides some choline but also methionine, which promotes the endogenous synthesis of *Choline* (see the general statement, page 1026). Once cirrhosis occurs, it is probably too late for any possible benefits. There is no evidence that choline is helpful in infectious hepatitis. For the above reasons, there is no longer any official preparation of choline. Since the anion is irrelevant to the metabolic effects, the chloride is neither superior nor inferior to other salts. [†C$_5$H$_{14}$ClNO.]

Choline Dihydrogen Citrate NF XII [(2-Hydroxyethyl)trimethylammonium Dihydrogen Citrate] contains not less than 98.0% of C$_{11}$H$_{21}$NO$_8$ (295.29), calculated on the anhydrous basis. *Preparation:* Choline may be prepared by treating aqueous trimethylamine with ethylene oxide. Conversion to the dihydrogen citrate is conveniently effected by dissolving the base in a suitable solvent such as ethanol and treating with an equimolar portion of citric acid. *Description and Solubility:* Colorless, translucent crystals, or a white, granular to fine, crystalline powder. It is odorless or may have a faint trimethylamine odor and has an acidic taste. It is hygroscopic when exposed to air; melts between 103° and 107.5°. 1 Gm dissolves in 1 ml of water and 42 ml of alcohol; very slightly soluble in ether, chloroform, and benzene. *Uses:* See *Choline Chloride* (above) and the general statement on *Choline* (page 1026).

Rutin NF XI [Eldrin; Melin; Myrticolorin; Phytomelin; Rutoside]$\ddagger$—The 3-rhamnoglucoside of 5,7,3′,4′-tetrahydroxyflavonol obtained from buckwheat, *Fagopyrum esculentum* Moench (Fam. *Polygonaceae*), or from other sources. Enzymatic hydrolysis yields the sugar *rutinose* and the aglycone *quercetin*. It is a tasteless, greenish yellow powder or microscopic, needle-shaped crystals. It becomes plastic at 190° and decomposes at about 215°. It is insoluble in water; slightly soluble in alcohol; soluble in isopropyl alcohol and methyl alcohol; insoluble in chloroform, ether and benzene. *Uses:* It is alleged to decrease capillary fragility, but evidence of any physiologic effect in humans is lacking. Its fall from official status reflects the fact that sound medical opinion holds the substance to be of no therapeutic value. *Dose:* Its continued promotion represents an abuse. [$\ddagger$C$_{27}$H$_{30}$O$_{16}$.]

Sodium Folate [Folvite Sodium (*Lederle*)] is the monosodium salt of folic acid.§ For the structure of the acid, see page 1027. *Description and Solubility:* A clear, mobile liquid having a yellow to orange-yellow color; pH, 8.5 to 11.0; *Uses:* Sodium Folate has the actions of *Folic Acid* (page 1038). However, the salt is preferred for parenteral use. *Dose:* 5 to 15 mg daily. [§C$_{19}$H$_{18}$N$_7$NaO$_6$.]

Vitamin B$_{12}$ with Intrinsic Factor Concentrate NF XI—A dry, slightly yellow, amorphous powder. It possesses vitamin B$_{12}$ activity made more readily absorbable from the gastrointestinal tract of patients suffering from pernicious anemias by combination with suitable preparations of the mucosa of the stomach or intestine of domestic animals used for food by man. It has a vitamin B$_{12}$ activity equivalent to that of not more than 15 mcg of cyanocobalamin and contains not more than 300 mg of the preparation constituting the intrinsic factor concentrate, per dose. *Uses:* hematopoietic preparation of vitamin B$_{12}$ intended for oral administration. It is employed chiefly in those patients who refuse parenteral administration. Oral cyanocobalamin therapy is usually not adequate for critically ill patients, or those with intercurrent infection or with neurological impairment. *Dose:* 1 NF unit (oral) daily in two divided doses.

Multivitamin Preparations

In the preceding text and in various monographs, in several instances attention has been called to the fact that it is desirable at times to administer more than one vitamin for what appears to be the symptoms of a single deficiency. The quotation "In the shadow of pellagra walks beriberi" has considerable substance in fact. Diets deficient in niacin are frequently also deficient in thiamine and also in other B vitamins of similar dietary source. The same relationship holds frequently for folic acid and vitamin B$_{12}$. Malabsorption syndromes affect the assimilation of several vitamins. Furthermore, the repair of a deficiency of one vitamin may increase the requirement of another; for example, repletion of thiamine increases the need for riboflavin. Diseases in which there is increased metabolism, such as thyrotoxicosis, increase the need for most of the vitamins, as do periods of hard physical work, stress, pregnancy, and lactation. Therefore, multivitamin therapy is often rational. However, most non-deprived persons other than the aged and debilitated, consume a well enough balanced diet that routine multivitamin consumption is not indicated in the US, and advertising that suggests otherwise should be condemned.

The Food and Drug Administration is revising its regulations regarding labeling and content of *Multivitamin Supplement* and *Multivitamin and Mineral Supplement*, and such regulations will be published probably in the near future.

Official Multivitamin Preparations

Decavitamin Capsules USP

Decavitamin Capsules contain, in each Capsule, not less than 1.2 mg (4000 USP Units) of retinol in the form of vitamin A, 10 mcg (400 USP Units) of vitamin D from natural sources or as ergocalciferol or cholecalciferol or the products obtained by the activation of either ergosterol or 7-dehydrocholesterol, 70 mg of ascorbic acid (C$_6$H$_8$O$_6$), 10 mg of calcium pantothenate (C$_{18}$H$_{32}$CaN$_2$O$_{10}$) or its equivalent as racemic calcium pantothenate, 5 mcg of cyanocobalamin (C$_{63}$H$_{88}$CoN$_{14}$O$_{14}$P), 100 mcg of folic acid (C$_{19}$H$_{19}$N$_7$O$_6$), 20 mg of niacinamide (C$_6$H$_6$N$_2$O), 2 mg of pyroxidine hydrochloride (C$_8$H$_{11}$NO$_3$.HCl), 2 mg of riboflavin (C$_{17}$H$_{20}$N$_4$O$_6$), 2 mg of thiamine hydrochloride (C$_{12}$H$_{17}$ClN$_4$OS.HCl) or its equivalent as thiamine mononitrate, and a suitable form of alpha tocopherol in an amount equivalent to 11 mg of *d*-α-tocopheryl acetate or 15 mg of *d,l*-α-tocopheryl acetate, all amounts corresponding to not less than 100% of the molecular formula where stated.

Uses—A *multivitamin* preparation which supplies in each capsule no less than the adult recommended daily allowance of the vitamins contained therein.

Dose—*Usual,* **1 capsule** daily.

Decavitamin Tablets USP

Decavitamin Tablets contain in each Tablet, not less than 1.2 mg (4000 USP Units) of retinol in the form of vitamin A, 10 mcg (400 USP Units) of vitamin D from natural sources or as ergocalciferol or cholecalciferol or the products obtained by the activation of either ergosterol or 7-dehydrocholesterol, 70 mg of ascorbic acid ($C_6H_8O_6$), 10 mg of calcium pantothenate ($C_{18}H_{32}CaN_2O_{10}$) or its equivalent as racemic calcium pantothenate, 5 mcg of cyanocobalamin ($C_{63}H_{88}CoN_{14}$-$O_{14}P$), 100 mcg of folic acid ($C_{19}H_{19}N_7O_6$), 20 mg of niacinamide ($C_6H_6N_2O$), 2 mg of pyridoxine hydrochloride ($C_8H_{11}NO_3$.HCl), 2 mg of riboflavin ($C_{17}H_{20}N_4O_6$), 2 mg of thiamine hydrochloride ($C_{12}H_{17}ClN_4OS$.HCl) or its equivalent as thiamine mononitrate, and a suitable form of alpha tocopherol in an amount equivalent to 11 mg of d-α-tocopheryl acetate or 15 mg of d,l-α-tocopheryl acetate, all amounts corresponding to not less than 100% of the molecular formula where stated.

Uses—See *Decavitamin Capsules* (page 1042).

Dose—*Usual*, **1 tablet** daily.

Hexavitamin Capsules NF

Hexavitamin Capsules contain, in each capsule, not less than 1.5 mg (5000 USP Units) of retinol in the form of vitamin A; not less than 10 mcg (400 USP Units) of vitamin D from natural sources or as ergocalciferol or cholecalciferol or the products obtained by the activation of either ergosterol or 7-dehydrocholesterol; not less than 75 mg of ascorbic acid; not less than 2 mg of thiamine hydrochloride or an equivalent amount of thiamine mononitrate; not less than 3 mg of riboflavin; and not less than 20 mg of niacinamide.

Uses—Hexavitamin Capsules is a multivitamin preparation which supplies in one capsule no less than the adult recommended daily allowance of the vitamins contained therein.

Dose—*Usual*, to be determined by the physician according to the needs of the patient.

Hexavitamin Tablets NF

Hexavitamin Tablets contain, in each tablet, not less than 1.5 mg (5000 USP Units) of retinol in the form of vitamin A; not less than 10 mcg (400 USP Units) of vitamin D from natural sources or as ergocalciferol of cholecalciferol or the products obtained by the activation of either ergosterol or 7-dehydro-

cholesterol; not less than 75 mg of ascorbic acid; not less than 2 mg of thiamine hydrochloride, or an equivalent amount of thiamine mononitrate; not less than 3 mg of riboflavin; not less than 20 mg of niacinamide.

Uses—See *Hexavitamin Capsules*.

Dose—*Usual*, to be determined by the physician according to the needs of the patient.

Dried Yeast NF

[Brewer's Yeast; Dry Yeast; Saccharomyces Siccum]

Dried Yeast consists of the dried cells of any suitable strain of *Saccharomyces cerevisiæ* Meyan (Fam. *Saccharomycetaceæ*) or *Candida utilis* (Hanneberg) Lodder and Kreger-Van Rij (Fam. *Cryptococcaceæ*), commonly called Torula Yeast. Dried Yeast may be obtained by growing suitable strains of the above species in media other than those required for beer production using appropriate environmental conditions. Such yeasts, properly designated as to species, are commonly known as "Primary Dried Yeasts." Dried Yeast may also be obtained as a by-product from the brewing of beer. Such yeasts are washed free of beer residues prior to drying. The washing step may include one or more alkaline washes for the purpose of removing the insoluble acetic bitter resins deposited on the yeast cells from the hops. These yeasts are commonly known, respectively, as "Brewer's Dried Yeast" and "Debittered Brewer's Dried Yeast."

Dried Yeast contains not less than 45.0% of protein and, in each Gm, the equivalent of not less than 300 mcg of niacin, 40 mcg of riboflavin, and 120 mcg of thiamine hydrochloride.

Description—Yellowish white to weak yellowish orange flakes, granules, or powder, with an odor and taste characteristic of the type. Dried Yeast is inactive in fermenting power.

Uses—As a source of B vitamins and protein. At one time it was less expensive to administer yeast for its vitamins than to administer the pure vitamins. However, today, with astute purchasing, the pure vitamins can be bought considerably less expensively. Thus the only recommendation for the use of yeast is as a source of high-quality protein.

Dose—*Usual*, **10 Gm** 4 times a day.

Other Dose Information—The usual total daily dose comes close to providing the recommended daily dietary allowance of niacin and exceeds that of thiamin.

Dosage Forms—Tablets NF: 500 mg.

Amino Acids and Proteins

This section includes monographs only for naturally occurring amino acids and proteins. With the exception of the hydrochlorides of glutamic acid, aminoacetic acid, arginine, and the salts of aspartic acid, all are employed primarily as nutrients.

For information relevant to the classification and structure of proteins and the uses for amino acids and proteins, see pages 482*ff*. Naturally occurring amino acids and proteins that have specific non-nutritional uses (eg, as for immunization, enzymes, blood, etc) are treated elsewhere.

Aminoacetic Acid NF

[Glycocoll; Glycine]

Aminoacetic Acid [$H_2N.CH_2.COOH = 75.07$], dried at 105° for 2 hours, contains 98.5–101.5% of $C_2H_5NO_2$.

Description—A white, odorless, crystalline powder, having a sweetish taste. Its solution is acid to litmus.

Solubility—1 Gm dissolves in about 4 ml of water; very slightly soluble in alcohol and ether.

Uses—Unmixed Aminoacetic Acid is occasionally

in the therapy of *myasthenia gravis*. It is much less effective than ephedrine or neostigmine, but is sometimes used in combination with one of these two agents. The mechanism of action of glycine in myasthenia gravis is unknown, and some investigators doubt whether the compound is of any value in this disorder. Aminoacetic acid is also sometimes used as a bladder irrigant. The acid is also used in various antacid preparations, sometimes as a complex salt. However, its limited buffering capacity does not warrant the expense of most of such preparations.

Dose—*Usual*, **30 Gm** daily, in divided doses; *application*, irrigating solution as a **1.5%** solution.

Dosage Forms—Sterile Solution NF: 1.5%/1500, 2000 and 3000 ml, 15% (concentrate)/1000 ml.

Glutamic Acid Hydrochloride—see page 794.

Methionine NF

[DL-Methionine; DL-2-Amino-4-(methylthio)butyric Acid; Meonine (*Ives*)]

Methionine contains 99.0–100.5% of $C_5H_{11}NO_2S$ (149.21), calculated on the dried basis.

Description—White, crystalline platelets or powder. It has a characteristic odor.

Solubility—1 Gm dissolves in about 30 ml of water; soluble in dilute acids and solutions of alkali hydroxides; very slightly soluble in alcohol; practically insoluble in ether.

Uses—Methionine is a sulfur-containing amino acid which is considered an indispensable dietary component. It is available in synthetically prepared racemic form that may be administered in sufficient quantity to provide amounts equivalent to the biologically active levo form. Methionine shares the lipotropic actions and uses of choline (see *Choline*, page 1026) and likewise is considered useful as an adjunct in the treatment of liver disease for those patients who cannot take an adequate diet. There is some evidence to suggest that overdosage may be harmful.

Dose—3 to **20 Gm** per day; *usual*, **3 Gm** 1 to 3 times a day.

Other Dose Information—As a supplement to a high protein diet, 3 to 6 Gm is usually administered daily in tablet form. In severe cases 10 to 20 Gm have been used. When oral administration is not feasible, crystalline methionine 5 to 10 Gm may be given daily by slow intravenous drip as a 3% solution in *Dextrose Injection USP* or *Water for Injection USP* that has been further sterilized by autoclaving.

Dosage Forms—Capsules NF: 200 and 500 mg; Tablets NF: 250 and 500 mg.

Protein Hydrolysate Injection USP

[C.P.H. (*Cutter*); Solution Amigen (*Baxter*); Solution Aminosol (*Abbott*)]

Protein Hydrolysate Injection is a sterile solution of amino acids and short-chain peptides which represent the approximate nutritive equivalent of the casein, lactalbumin, plasma, fibrin, or other suitable protein from which it is derived by acid, enzymatic, or other method of hydrolysis. It may be modified by partial removal and restoration or addition of one or more amino acids. It may contain alcohol, dextrose, or other carbohydrate suitable for intravenous infusion. Not less than 50.0% of the total nitrogen present is in the form of α-amino nitrogen.

Description—A yellowish to reddish amber, transparent liquid.

Uses—Protein hydrolysates, as artificial hydrolytic digests of suitable proteins, supply, in the form of constituent amino acids and short-chain peptides, the approximate nutritive equivalent of the source protein. More than half of their total nitrogen is in the form of α-amino nitrogen. They are used for parenteral alimentation to maintain positive nitrogen balance in conditions in which there is interference with the ingestion, digestion, or absorption of food. Such conditions most frequently occur during severe illness, after surgical operations upon the gastrointestinal tract, or in cases of severe peptic ulcer. The protein hydrolysates are intended for repair and must be spared for such by adequate intake of other caloric foods; consequently, dextrose is frequently included in the preparations. Intravenous injection may induce nausea, vomiting, fever (especially after repeated administration), flushing and hypotension, abdominal pain, convulsions, phlebitis and thrombosis, and edema at the injection site. Protein hydrolysates may be given orally in conditions where absorption is adequate, but they are distasteful and frequently rejected by the patient. They are also used in nonallergenic diets for infants. Insufficient information exists to enable an exact statement of dose. Forty-five to 70 Gm of protein is sufficient to maintain positive nitrogen balance in the normal adult, but the needs may be greater in pathological conditions.

Dose—*Intravenous*, **250** to **1500 ml**; *usual*, **500 ml** of a **5%** solution.

Dosage Forms—See USP.

Other Amino Acids and Proteins

Arginine Hydrochloride [The hydrochloride of L-2-amino-5-guanidinovaleric acid; Modumate (*Abbott*); R-Gene (*Cutter*)] [$H_2NC(:NH)NHCH_2CH_2CH_2CH(NH_2)$-$COOH.HCl$]—Crystalline plates or prisms that are soluble in water and slightly soluble in hot alcohol. An amino acid with pharmacological actions and clinical uses similar to those of sodium glutamate. Intravenous administration causes a lowering of blood ammonia levels. Since it is sodium free it is better tolerated than equivalent amounts of sodium glutamate. *Uses:* symptomatic management of gravely ill patients with encephalopathies associated with ammoniacal azotemia, usually the result of severe liver dysfunction. The amino acid combines with ammonia with the consequent formation of asparagine. Lowering of the blood ammonia level may occasionally bring about a reversion of the neurological status from stupor to consciousness. Expert medical opinion holds that arginine is of very little efficacy. Therapy with this amino acid should be considered to be only adjunctive to other measures designed to reduce blood ammonia levels. *Dose: intravenously*, 20 Gm in 1000 ml of dextrose injection, given over a period of 4 hours.

Casein—A phosphoprotein which comprises 80% of the total protein content of milk. It is white, amorphous, nearly odorless and tasteless powder, insoluble in water, but soluble in aqueous alkalies or dilute mineral acid. Its isoelectric point is about pH 4.7. *Uses:* dietary supplement; as a source of protein in hypoproteinemia, burns, infections, gastric and duodenal ulcers, pregnancy, geriatrics and pre- and postoperative care. *Dose:* 20 to 30 Gm 4 times daily, as required.

Glutamic Acid [α-Aminoglutaric Acid] [$HOOCCH_2CH_2$-$CH(NH_2)COOH$]—White, crystalline powder with a mild acid taste and peculiar aftertaste. Melting range: 224° to 225°. 1 Gm dissolves in 100 ml of water, 1500 ml of alcohol. Soluble in alkalies and dilute acids. Prepared by acid hydrolysis of vegetable and animal proteins, such as gelatin and wheat kernels. *Uses:* The only legitimate systemic use of glutamic acid is in the treatment of encephalopathies associated with azotemia, usually as the result of severe liver dysfunction. Even in this condition, its value is questionable. For this purpose, the sodium salt is generally used (see below). The substance combines with ammonia to form glutamine, thereby lowering the blood ammonia and urea. The hydrochloride is used as a source of hydrochloric acid for digestion (see page 794). Few substances have been promoted for so many nonsense and unethical purposes. It is of no value in the correction of any sexual or psychosexual disorders, such as impotence, frigidity, gonadal hypofunction, amenorrhea, functional uterine bleeding, etc, is worthless in all types of mental and neurological aberrations, including grand mal, mental retardation, poor memory, psychiatric disorders, anorexia, etc, and it has no effect on atherosclerosis. *Dose:* 8 to 20 Gm daily.

Potassium and Magnesium Aspartates [Spartase (*Wyeth*)]—A mixture of equal amounts by weight of potassium hydrogen and magnesium hydrogen L-aminosuccinates. *Uses:* It has been claimed that this preparation of aspartates relieves the fatigue syndrome. The syndrome itself is so vague, subjective, and erratic that it is easy for the physician to fool himself and the patient, so that a degree of placebo effect is possible. Biochemical and critical clinical evidence show these aspartates to be of no essential value. Side effects include nausea, gastrointestinal discomfort and diarrhea; these reactions are less severe if the aspartates are taken after meals. *Dose: Orally,* 1 Gm twice a day.

Protein Hydrolysates, Oral is an oral powder of amino acids and short-chain peptides prepared from the same sources and in the same manner as are the parenteral preparations, and they conform to the same nutritional standards. It may be prepared from the same protein sources and are digested in the same manner and to the same extent as those for intravenous use (see *Protein Hydrolysate Injection,* page 1044). *Uses:* For *alimentation* of patients who need a high-protein intake but who, for various reasons, cannot ingest or digest ordinary proteinacious foods. They are especially indicated in the diet of infants who are allergic to milk; however, other dietary ingredients must also be incorporated into the diet, generally as a formula including protein hydrolysates. It is a common misconception that protein hydrolysates are effective gastric antacids in the management of peptic ulcer; not only is their buffer capacity low and the duration of buffer action evanescent, but also they stimulate a high rate of secretion of gastric acid. Thus they must not be used in lieu of effective mineral gastric antacids. *Dose:* The dose must be adjusted to the need and the intake of protein in other forms. The average daily protein requirement is about 1 Gm per Kg of body weight per day. Approximately 2 Gm of hydrolysate is nutritionally equivalent to 1 Gm of protein.

Sodium Glutamate [NaOOC.CH₂.CH₂.CH(NH₂).COOH; Glutavene (*Crookes-Barnes*)]—The monosodium salt of L-α-aminoglutaric acid that decreases blood and tissue ammonia levels by combining with ammonia to form sodium glutamine. *Uses:* To reduce blood ammonia levels in ammoniacal azotemia, such as may accompany hepatic insufficiency or intensive chlorothiazide therapy. Control of the azotemia occasionally prevents coma and encephalopathy. However, the substance infrequently lowers the plasma ammonia levels, and expert medical opinion holds glutamate to be of little value. This agent is contraindicated in renal impairment or in other conditions in which sodium intake is critical. Also alkalosis and hypokalemia may result, and the acid-base balance of the patient should be monitored. This drug is also used as a condiment, supposedly to accent the natural flavor in foods. The substance is also promoted for most of the illegitimate and unethical uses described under *Glutamic Acid* (above). *Dose: Intravenously,* initial dose of 29 Gm diluted to 1000 ml with 5% sterile dextrose solution, to be given over a 4 hour period. No more than 58 Gm should be given per day.

Sugars

Sugars are carbohydrates that are sweet to the taste and highly soluble in water. They may be either monosaccharides or disaccharides. The chemistry of the sugars is discussed in Chapter 30, page 469. In the section below are listed only those sugars that are used in medicine as aliments. Some of the sugars also have important uses as pharmaceutical necessities, in parenteral fluids, as diuretics, as osmotic "stuffing" for injection of other drugs, etc; consequently, the monographs of certain nutrient sugars may be found elsewhere in this volume.

Dextrose—see page 1366.

Dextrose Injection—see page 844.

Dextrose and Sodium Chloride Injection—see page 845.

Liquid Glucose—see page 1367.

Sucrose—see page 1334.

Syrup—see page 1340.

Fructose NF

[D(−)-Fructose; Levulose; β-D(−)Fructopyranose; Levugen (*Baxter*)]

Fructose, dried in vacuum at 70° for 4 hours, contains 98.0–102.0% of C₆H₁₂O₆ (180.16).

Fructose is a sugar usually obtained by the inversion of aqueous solutions of sucrose and subsequent separation of fructose from glucose.

Preparation—Sucrose is inverted by treatment with dilute acid at moderate temperature, and the fructose is separated by precipitation of the lime-fructose complex. Fructose is released from the complex by means of carbon dioxide which precipitates the calcium as carbonate. After filtering, the fructose solution is purified with the aid of activated carbon and ion exchange resins and evaporated to dryness.

Description—Colorless crystals or as a white, crystalline or granular powder, which is odorless and has a sweet taste. Specific rotation: −89° to −91°.

Solubility—1 Gm dissolves in about 15 ml of alcohol and about 14 ml of methanol; freely soluble in water.

Uses—Fructose is used as a *parenteral aliment.* It is converted to liver glycogen and metabolized more rapidly than dextrose. Consequently, it can be infused intravenously in higher (twice) concentration than dextrose without as much temporary plasma hypertonicity; also, because of the smaller volume of water infused, when the fructose is converted from the blood there is less residual hydremia. Thus, when alimentation rather than hydration or osmotic diuresis is the aim of sugar infusion, fructose is advantageous. It is especially indicated for the alimentation or hydration of diabetics, since the diabetic has a nearly normal tolerance for fructose. The subcutaneous route is not recommended, because sugars given subcutaneously may cause electrolyte distortions, which occasionally may be severe.

Dose—*Intravenous* and *subcutaneous*, as required.

Dosage Forms—Injection NF: 100 Gm/1000 ml; Fructose and Sodium Chloride Injection NF: 100 Gm (fructose) and 9 Gm (sodium chloride)/1000 ml.

Other Sugars

Invert Sugar—An equimolar mixture of glucose and fructose (dextrose and levulose) obtained by the hydrolysis of sugar. Invert sugar forms clear, colorless solutions having a pH of 3.5 to 6.0. *Uses:* instead of dextrose, for parenteral administration of carbohydrate. While it has the same caloric value as dextrose (4 Kcal. per Gm), invert sugar is more rapidly utilized and may be administered intravenously twice as fast as dextrose. *Dose:* 1 liter of a 5 or 10% solution in either water or isotonic sodium chloride solution. Invert sugar may be administered intravenously, or subcutaneously, observing the same precautions as with other forms of parenteral feeding.

Maltose [Malt Sugar] [$C_{12}H_{22}O_{11}.H_2O$]—Obtained by the action of diastase on starch. White crystalline powder. $[\alpha]_D^{20}$ is $+128.6°$. Very soluble in water; slightly soluble in alcohol; insoluble in ether. *Uses:* nutrient; sweetener; in culture media.

Fats and Fixed Oils

Fats and oils yield more than twice as many calories per gram as carbohydrates and proteins. This is the basis of the well-known use by mountaineers and others of chocolate for an energy source. However, clinically, fats and oils have not enjoyed much use as aliments, partly because their parenteral administration carries the danger of fat embolism and numerous other untoward effects. If fat or oil is the only aliment given the patient, acidosis also is a possible complication. The use of high-fat diets for reducing body weight has not been found satisfactory. Much attention has been given to possible essential fatty acids, and it seems clear that linoleic acid is required for normal metabolism. The need is met when the diet contains linoleic acid to the extent of 1 to 2% of the dietary fat. The polyunsaturated fats of the *cis-cis* methylene interrupted type have also received much attention in connection with a protective effect against the onset as well as the crisis of atherosclerosis (see Chapter 46, page 865). It is evident that a diet in which polyenic fats have been substituted for unsaturated fats effects a lowering of serum cholesterol in the hypercholesterolemic patient.

Corn Oil—see page 1342.

Olive Oil—see page 1349.

Peanut Oil—see page 1343.

Safflower Oil—see page 865.

Fixed Oils

Arachidonic Acid [5,8,11,14-Eicosatetraenoic Acid] [$C_{20}H_{32}O_2$]—An *essential fatty acid*. Occurs in liver, brain, glandular organs, and depot fats of animals, small amounts in human depot fats. It melts at $-49.5°$. *Uses:* recommended with other unsaturated fatty acids in infant eczema and dermatitis.

Cottonseed Oil Emulsion—A 15% oil-in-water emulsion of the refined fixed oil (see *Cottonseed Oil*, page 1343) obtained from the seeds of cultivated plants of various varieties of *Gossypium hirsutum* Linné or of other species of *Gossypium*. *Uses:* as a parenteral aliment for severely malnourished patients who are unable to take food orally. Approximately 750 Kcal are provided by 500 ml of the emulsion. Immediately upon administration certain side effects may occur, such as, back and chest pain, dyspnea, flushing, urticaria, fever, nausea, vomiting, headache, vertigo, tachycardia, and hypertension. Also, delayed reactions may occur, such as abdominal pain, hepatomegaly, mild anemia, hemorrhage, and fat embolism. *Dose: intravenous drip,* 250 to 500 ml daily, extremely slow infusion.

Linoleic Acid [Linolic acid; *cis*-9, *cis*-12-Octadecadienoic acid] [$CH_3(CH_2)_4CH:CHCH_2CH:CH(CH_2)_7COOH$] and **Linolenic Acid** [9,12,15-Octadecatrienoic acid] [$CH_3-(CH_2CH:CH)_3(CH_2)_7.COOH$)] are unsaturated acids occurring as the glycerides in linseed, cottonseed, poppy seed, and most drying oils. They are colorless or practically colorless liquids. Specific gravity of linolenic acid is about 0.91. Both acids are insoluble in water, but are soluble in organic solvents. *Uses:* recommended in infantile eczema and dermatitis.

Trace Mineral Nutrients

Trace elements of interest in nutrition are those inorganic constituents of foods and biological fluids (other than electrolytes discussed in Chapter 45, page 815), present in minute quantities, usually less than 50 ppm, which play a specific role as nutrients. In the ash constituents of the human body, as many as $\frac{4}{5}$ of the elements listed in the periodic table have been identified. The absence from the diet of only a few of these has been shown to produce specific deficiency symptoms. A few additional elements are known to be involved in essential metabolic functions and are therefore probably dietary essentials. On this basis it is appropriate to discuss the nutrient relationships of iron, iodine, zinc, copper, and manganese.

The function of these trace elements has been identified as a result either of their relationship to specific disease in man or animals, or of observations of animals given highly purified diets devoid of one or another of the trace elements. Also of importance are the biochemical studies of enzyme systems involved in intermediary metabolism of living cells, which have demonstrated that trace elements act as cofactors for certain enzymatic reactions. Trace elements may appear as reactive components of complex nitrogenous structures called metalloenzymes in which they are strongly bound. Metal–enzyme complexes, in which there is a loose binding of the metal to the protein, are active in intermediary metabolism as the transfer enzymes in the citric acid cycle. A third class of compounds contain trace elements as integral parts of nonprotein molecules. Examples are such compounds as vitamin B_{12}, in which cobalt is a firmly fixed component, and thyroxine, in which iodine is firmly bound.

Except for iron and iodine, the significance of trace elements in practical human nutrition is of little everyday concern. With a diet made up of a variety of foods, the trace elements essential to nutrition occur in an ubiquitous fashion. Iodine is readily supplied in the ordinary diet in the form of iodized salt for cooking and table use. Only in the case of iron is there any well-defined need for food supplementation.

Imbalance in the intake of trace minerals may lead to inhibited absorption. For example, excess molybdenum in the rations of cattle causes an anemia, effectively treated by the addition of copper to the ration. Here molybdenum antagonizes the intestinal absorption of copper. Similar imbalances have been observed with other trace mineral combinations. Therefore it is unwise to modify the diet with supplements of trace minerals which may be irrational.

Fluoride

Although fluoride has not been established as an essential nutrient, there is no doubt but that it is essential to the optimal well being of the individual. It is incorporated into bone salts and tooth enamel as a fluoroapatite, which increases the strength of bone and increases the resistance of the tooth enamel to acid and hence to *caries*. Consequently, it is not only a dental medicament but also may be used in the treatment of *osteoporosis*. There is also some evidence that it retards the development of arteriosclerosis. The optimal daily intake is not well established, but it is probably about 1 mg of a soluble form (calcium fluoride is poorly absorbed). A concentration of 1 ppm in drinking water, recommended to lessen the incidence of dental caries, provides approximately this amount. When the intake exceeds this amount, there is an increased tendency to mottling of the tooth enamel; with high intake, osteosclerosis and exostoses occur. In the treatment of osteoporosis, the dose is 50 mg 3 times a day, for a period to be determined by the physician and radiological evidence of bone consolidation.

Iron

Iron is a component of hemoglobin, myoglobin, the cytochromes, catalase, peroxidase and certain other enzyme systems which serve important functions in oxygen transport and cellular respiration. Dietary deficiency of iron leads to development of hypochromic microcytic anemia. The dietary allowances recommended by the Food and Nutrition Board are adequate for all ordinary needs. Those recommendations show that the dietary intake of children from under one year to over 12 years should increase from 6 to 18 mg during this period. The recommended daily dietary allowances for men and women are 10 and 18 mg, respectively, including the conditions of pregnancy and lactation for the latter. A diet which includes one egg and one serving of meat per day, assures at least a 15-mg intake. Iron is administered orally preferably in the form of ferrous salts because they are more efficiently absorbed. Iron and iron compounds are discussed and listed in the section on *Hematopoietics and Hematinics* in Chapter 45, page 824.

Iodine

Iodine is an essential component of the thyroid hormone, thyroxine and the related active thyronine derivatives. The hormone is a master regulator of the rates of the many metabolic reactions involved in cellular oxidation. Unless the body has a functional thyroid gland into which dietary ionic iodine is absorbed from the blood stream and iodination and condensation of tyrosine molecules accomplished to synthesize thyroxine, growth and cell differentiation and reproductive activity of the organism fail. Similarly, if iodine intake or absorption from the gastrointestinal tract or into the gland is depressed to the point below which sufficient iodine enters the thyroid gland for maintaining adequate thyroxine levels, the gland attempts to compensate by enlarging and thereby enhancing its capacity for synthesis. This condition is known as goiter. When the deficiency is more severe or occurs in the young and remains untreated, various health problems associated with cretinism, feeble-mindedness, deaf mutism and general physical and mental degeneration may occur. Although the exact requirement for iodine is not known, estimates indicate that it is about 100 μg daily for adults and 30 μg daily for infants. The adult daily dietary allowances of the Food and Nutrition Board are about 50 mcg per 1000 Kcal intake. Iodized salt for cooking and table use fully meets these needs. Pharmaceutical iodide salt preparations for use as antigoitrogens are described in Chapter 47, page 868.

Zinc

Zinc is normally distributed more widely and in higher concentration in the organs and tissues of the body than any other trace element except iron. It is an essential component of the enzyme, carbonic anhydrase, which catalyzes the liberation of carbon dioxide into alveolar air and is, therefore, important to carbon dioxide transport, as hemoglobin is to oxygen transport. Zinc is also an essential component of the proteolytic metalloenzyme, carboxypeptidase, which splits terminal amino acids from certain peptides in the intestinal tract. The occurrence of high concentrations of zinc in the prostate gland, sperm and testis and the effects of low zinc intakes on survival of germinal epithelium, appearance of testicular atrophy and reduced spermatogenosis, suggest a vital role for zinc in the metabolism of the reproductive organs. Primary dietary zinc deficiency has been postulated as responsible for syndromes of dwarfism and hypogonadism in young male humans whose diets were high in cereal content, whose drinking water was low in zinc and who habitually practiced geophagia (clay-eating). The average daily intake of zinc by adults consuming normal, well-balanced diets is about 10 to 15 mg. Even though zinc is poorly absorbed from the gastrointestinal tract, the body has a great capacity for conserving plasma and tissue stores in the form of protein-bound zinc and little is excreted in the urine. Recent interest has centered on studies which indicate that relatively large doses of zinc promote wound healing. The current practice is to give $ZnSO_4$ in a dose of 220 mg. More carefully controlled clinical trials are needed to establish the true value of this agent.

Copper

Copper is essential primarily for the formation of hemoglobin. It is tightly bound to heme, a coenzyme of the cytochrome oxidase system in terminal oxidation, in which form it undergoes oxidation-reduction as an electron carrier in the vital electron transport process. Copper is also found in a number of other enzymes, mostly oxidative, which catalyze a variety of metabolic reactions. Tyrosinase, lactase, ascorbic acid oxidase, and butyryl coenzyme A dehydrogenase are all copper-containing enzymes dependent for activity on the presence of a copper–protein bond. Nutritional deficiency of copper in man has not been recorded even though a range of experimental conditions develop in different animal species and even within the same species, depending on the age, as a result of dietary deficiency of copper. Estimates of copper requirements for man from balance experiments reveal that dietary intakes of 1 to 2 mg daily may be sufficient. The American diet furnishes 2 to 5 mg on the average per day.

Manganese

Manganese is an activator of liver arginase and several other enzymes such as mitochondrial respiratory enzyme systems, cholinesterase and enolase, the latter an enzyme of importance in the anaerobic metabolism of carbohydrates which catalyzes the reversible removal or addition of a molecule of water from its substrate. Activation of these enzymes shows a more or less broad metal-ion specificity. Manganese, magnesium, zinc or iron can activate enolase, for example, in an isolated *in vitro* system. It is not yet known whether manganese is a component of a specific metalloenzyme required in human metabolism thus essentiality of manganese for man has not been established. Primary manganese deficiency has been produced experimentally in laboratory and domestic animals, in which growth, bone formation and reproduction are all adversely affected. Lack of manganese has not been linked with any disability or disease in humans. The usual American diets provide about 3 to 9 mg manganese per day.

Reference

1. *J. Am. Med. Assoc.*, **169**, 41 (Jan. 3, 1959).

Bibliography

History

Beeuwkes, A. M., *et al*, *Essays on History of Nutrition and Dietetics*, American Dietetic Association, Chicago, 1967.
Darby, W. J., *J. Am. Med. Assoc.*, **180**, 816 (1962).
Elvehjem, C. A., *J. Am. Dietetic Assoc.*, **38**, 236 (1961).
McCollum, E. V., *A History of Nutrition*, Houghton-Mifflin, Boston, 1957.

Assay

The United States Pharmacopeia, 18th rev., Mack Publ. Co., Easton, Pa., 1970.
The National Formulary, 13th ed., Mack Publ. Co., Easton, Pa., 1970.
Official Methods of Analysis, 10th ed., Association of Official Agricultural Chemists, Washington, D.C., 1965.
Strohecker, R., and Henning, H. M., *Vitamin Assay—Tested Methods*, Verlag Chemie., Weinheim/Bergstr., Germany, 1965.

Freed, M., ed., *Methods of Vitamin Assay*, 3rd ed., Interscience, New York, 1966.

Clinical

Davidson, S., and Passmore, R., *Human Nutrition and Dietetics*, 3rd ed., Williams & Wilkins, Baltimore, 1966.
Mitchell, H. S., *et al*, *Cooper's Nutrition in Health and Disease*, 15th ed., Lippincott, Philadelphia, 1968.
Fomon, S. J., *Infant Nutrition*, Saunders, Philadelphia, 1967.
Pareira, M. D., *Therapeutic Nutrition with Tube Feeding*, Thomas, Springfield, Ill., 1959.
Robinson, C. H., *Proudfit-Robinson's Normal and Therapeutic Nutrition*, 13th ed., Macmillan, New York, 1967.
West, E. S., *et al*, *Textbook of Biochemistry*, 4th ed., Macmillan, New York, 1966.
Wohl, M. G., and Goodhart, R. S., *Modern Nutrition in Health and Disease*, 3rd ed., Lea & Febiger, Philadelphia, 1964.

General

Beaton, G. H., and McHenry, E. W., eds., *Nutrition—A Comprehensive Treatise*, Academic, New York, 1964.
Dyke, S. F., *The Chemistry of the Vitamins*, Interscience, New York, 1965.
Burton, B. T., *Heinz Handbook of Nutrition*, 2nd ed., McGraw-Hill, New York, 1965.
Gyorgy, P., and Pearson, W. N., *The Vitamins*, vols. VI and VII, 2nd ed., Academic, New York, 1967.
Lowenberg, M., *et al*, *Food and Man*, Wiley, New York, 1968.
Nutrient Requirements of Domestic Animals (Poultry, Swine, Dairy and Beef Cattle, Sheep, Horses, Mink and Foxes, Dogs, Rabbits, Laboratory Animals), National Academy of Sciences–National Research Council, Washington, D. C., 1962 and later.
Pike, R. L., and Brown, M. L., *Nutrition: An Integrated Approach*, Wiley, New York, 1967.
Sebrell, W. H., Jr., and Harris, R. S., eds., *The Vitamins*, vols. I–V, 2nd ed., Academic, New York, 1967.
Underwood, E. J., *Trace Elements in Human and Animal Nutrition*, 2nd ed., Academic, New York, 1962.
Chaney, M. S., and Ross, M. L., *Nutrition*, 7th ed., Houghton-Mifflin, Boston, 1966.

Books for Lay Readers

Leverton, R. M., *Food Becomes You*, Iowa State Univ. Press, Ames, Iowa, 1965; also available as a paperback from Doubleday, Garden City, New York.
McHenry, E. W., *Food without Fads*, Lippincott, Philadelphia, 1960.
McWilliams, M., *Nutrition for the Growing Years*, Wiley, New York, 1967.
Mickelson, O., *Nutrition Science and You*, Scholastic Books, Englewood Cliffs, N.J., 1964.
White, P. L., *Let's Talk about Food*, American Medical Association, Chicago, 1967.
Yearbook of Agriculture, 1959 (Food), US Dept. of Agriculture, Washington, D.C., 1959; available from USGPO, Washington, D.C.
Yearbook of Agriculture (Protecting Our Food), US Dept. of Agriculture, Washington, D.C., 1966; available from USGPO, Washington, D.C.

Food and Composition

Church, C. F., and Church, H. N., *Bowes and Church's Food Values of Portions Commonly Used*, 10th ed., Lippincott, Philadelphia, 1966.
Orr, M. L., and Watt, B. K., *Amino Acid Content of Foods* (Home Econ. Res. Rept. No. 4), US Dept. of Agriculture, Washington, D.C., 1957; available from USGPO, Washington, D.C.
Fatty Acids in Food Fats (Home Econ. Res. Rept. No. 7), US Dept. of Agriculture, Washington, D.C., 1959; available from USGPO, Washington, D.C.
Nutritive Value of Foods (Home and Garden Bull. No. 72), US Dept. of Agriculture, Washington, D.C., 1963; available from USGPO, Washington, D.C.
Watt, B., and Merrill, A. L., *Composition of Foods—Raw, Processed, Prepared* (Handbook No. 8), US Dept. of Agriculture, Washington, D.C., 1963; available from USGPO, Washington, D.C.

57 | Enzymes

Properties, nomenclature, and types of enzymes

This chapter was prepared by

James W. Gibb, PhD, Assistant Professor of Pharmacology, College of Pharmacy and College of Medicine, University of Utah, Salt Lake City, Utah 84112

The functions of all living organisms depend on chemical reactions. For example, the conversion of sugar to carbon dioxide and water proceeds through a series of chemical reactions each of which requires a biologic catalyst for the reaction to occur. Enzymes are proteins which serve as biologic catalysts. Without these enzymes conditions for reaction would be required which would be incompatible with the life of the cell. Thus, enzymes play a vital role in the function of the normal cell.

The importance of enzymes in normal body function is dramatically illustrated in conditions where one enzyme is nonfunctional as a result of a disease state or a congenital abnormality. Patients with these "inborn errors of metabolism" are strikingly abnormal. Phenylketonuric infants who are born without the enzyme phenylalanine hydroxylase (which is responsible for the conversion of phenylalanine to tyrosine) develop motor disturbances, light coloration of the skin, hair, and eyes, and in early childhood (if not in infancy) remain mentally retarded to the point of idiocy.

Since most chemical reactions in the body require the action of an enzyme, these biologic catalysts often serve as the focal point for regulation of body function. Increased enzyme activity accelerates the production of a given product which may be essential for a particular function. The synthesis of norepinephrine illustrates this principle well. Heart rate will increase when norepinephrine is released from the sympathetic nerves. Norepinephrine is synthesized through a series of enzymatic reactions of which the rate-limiting, and therefore the most important, regulating enzyme is tyrosine hydroxylase. Increased tyrosine hydroxylase activity brings about the conversion of more tyrosine to dihydroxyphenylalanine (DOPA), which is converted by dopa decarboxylase to dopamine. Dopamine is converted to norepinephrine by the enzymatic activity of dopamine-β-hydroxylase. The formation of norepinephrine can be regulated by a feedback mechanism. Increased levels of norepinephrine inhibit the enzyme tyrosine hydroxylase so that less norepinephrine is synthesized. Thus, levels of norepinephrine can control the amount of norepinephrine synthesized.

The pharmacologic actions of an increasing number of drugs depend on an enzyme–drug interaction. Good examples of enzyme–drug interactions are (1) monoamine oxidase inhibitors, which prevent the breakdown of biogenic amines by the enzyme monoamine oxidase and (2) allopurinol, a relatively new drug used in the treatment of gout. The actions of this drug depend on its ability to inhibit xanthine oxidase, an enzyme responsible for conversion of xanthine to uric acid.

These examples illustrate the importance of drug–enzyme interactions in the pharmacologic actions of therapeutic agents. The actions of drugs of the future will undoubtedly depend on drug–enzyme interaction. Indeed, the pharmacologic action of many drugs currently being prescribed by the physician probably will eventually be found to involve such interplay. Since enzymes are so intricately involved in regulation of function, it is only logical to suppose that drugs may increase or decrease function by stimulating or depressing enzyme activity, respectively. A knowledge of enzymes and their properties, therefore, becomes increasingly important to the pharmacist in order to understand the action of drugs.

Properties—Four properties of enzymes make them exceptional catalysts.

1. Most enzymes will catalyze only a specific range of reactions and in many cases only one reaction will be catalyzed by a given enzyme. Some enzymes have a low degree of specificity; eg, pepsin hydrolyzes almost all soluble native proteins but the hydrolysis is limited to certain very specific peptide linkages. On the other hand, urease is a highly specific enzyme; its only known substrate is urea. Almost all enzymes show a high degree of spatial specificity. Arginase acts only on L-arginine; it does not attack D-arginine. The specificity of enzymes is one of their most fundamental and important properties.

2. Enzymes are exceedingly efficient. Most enzymatic reactions, under optimal conditions, proceed 10^8 to 10^{11} times more rapidly than the corresponding nonenzymatic reactions.

3. Enzymes as a group are exceptionally versatile catalysts. For example, enzymes effectively catalyze hydrolytic reactions, dehydrations, acyl transfer reactions, oxidation–reduction reactions, polymerizations, aldol condensations, and free radical reactions.

4. Enzymes are subject to a variety of cellular controls. Their final concentration and rate of synthesis are under genetic control. In addition, enzymes are present in the cell in both inactive as well as active forms. The rate of conversion from inactive to active form is influenced by environmental changes; eg, phosphorylase b is converted to phosphorylase a very rapidly through a series of reactions which are triggered by release of catecholamines.

Nomenclature—Enzymes are usually named in terms of the reactions that are catalyzed. Usually the suffix "-ase" is added to the name of the substrate upon which the enzyme acts; ie, the enzyme which attacks urea is urease, and arginine is acted upon by arginase. Enzymes are also classified according to the reaction they catalyze; eg, reductases and dehydrogenases. Some older names, which are unrelated to the function of the enzyme, remain in usage; eg, rennin, trypsin, and pepsin.

The Commission on Enzymes of the International Union of Biochemistry has established a complete but rather complex system of classification and nomenclature. According to this classification enzymes are divided into six general groups:

1. *Oxidoreductases*—catalyzing oxidation–reduction reactions.
2. *Transferases*—catalyzing a chemical group from one molecule to another.
3. *Hydrolases*—catalyzing hydrolytic enzymes.
4. *Lyases*—catalyzing the addition of groups to double bonds or vice versa.

5. *Isomerases*—catalyzing intramolecular rearrangements.

6. *Ligases* (also known as synthetases)—catalyzing the condensation of two molecules coupled with the cleavage of a pyrophosphate bond of ATP or similar triphosphate.

In this system every enzyme is coded in a four-number system according to the type of reaction catalyzed, type of isomerization, type of bond hydrolyzed, etc.

A more comprehensive description of this system is described in the literature.[1]

Many enzymes possess nonprotein chemical groups. Thus, an enzyme can often be dissociated into a protein component, apoenzyme, and a nonprotein component, prosthetic group. Prosthetic groups are also referred to as coenzymes or cofactors. Vitamins and certain metals are examples of these prosthetic groups.

Preparations of enzymes are of limited use in the following conditions: (1) debridement, ie, as aids in resolving and removing blood clots or fibrinous or purulent accumulations; (2) replacement therapy to correct certain gastrointestinal deficiencies; and (3) locally in certain inflammatory conditions after either topical application or hypodermic injection.

Chymotrypsin NF

[Avazyme (*Wampole*); Chymar (*Armour*); Chymotest (*Testagar*); Enzeon (*Breon*)]

Chymotrypsin is a proteolytic enzyme crystallized from an extract of the pancreas gland of the ox, *Bos taurus* Linné (Fam. *Bovidæ*). When assayed as directed in the NF, it contains not less than 1000 NF Chymotrypsin Units in each mg, calculated on the dry basis, and 90.0–110.0% of the labeled potency.

Note: Determine the suitability of the substrate and check the adjustment of the spectrophotometer by performing the assay using NF Chymotrypsin Reference Standard. Determine the suitability of the substrate in the limit test for Trypsin by using the appropriate amount of NF Trypsin Crystallized Reference Standard.

Description—Occurs as a white to yellowish white, odorless, crystalline or amorphous powder.

Solubility—An amount equivalent to 100,000 NF Chymotrypsin Units is soluble in 10 ml of water or in 10 ml of saline TS.

Uses—Chymotrypsin topically is used alone or in combination with trypsin for the debridement of necrotic wounds, ulcers, abscesses, empyemas, and fistulas. It is used also for the liquefaction of blood and exudates that have not become organized by fibrous tissue. Chymotrypsin is inactivated rapidly when injected into closed cavities. The effectiveness of orally, buccally or intramuscularly administered chymotrypsin and other proteolytic enzymes for the treatment of inflammation and edema in traumatized tissue and other disease processes has not been adequately demonstrated clinically.

Chymotrypsin causes local irritation and occasional ulceration. Its use has resulted in a variety of histamine-like allergic reactions including anaphylaxis which has been treated with antihistamine.

Dose—*Usual, intramuscular,* **2500** to **5000 NF Units** 1 to 3 times a day; *application, for zonule lysis,* **150** to **500 NF Units** as a **1:5000** solution.

Other Dose Information—*Ophthalmic,* about 2 ml of a solution of 150 units per ml into the posterior chamber; *orally,* 50,000 to 100,000 units 4 times daily; *buccally,* 10,000 units 4 times daily; *intramuscularly,* as an

aqueous solution or suspension in oil, 2500 to 5000 units in 0.5 to 1 ml once or twice daily.

Dosage Forms—Injection NF: 5000 NF units/ ml, 25,000 NF units/5 ml; Sterile NF: 750 NF units.

Hyaluronidase for Injection NF

[Alidase (*Searle*); Hyazyme (*Abbott*); Wydase (*Wyeth*)]

Hyaluronidase for Injection is a sterile, dry, soluble, enzyme product prepared from mammalian testes and capable of hydrolyzing mucopolysaccharides of the type of hyaluronic acid. Its potency, in NF Hyaluronidase Units, is not less than the labeled potency. Hyaluronidase for Injection contains not more than 0.25 mcg of tyrosine for each NF Hyaluronidase Unit. It may contain a suitable stabilizer.

Description—A white, amorphous solid. It is destroyed by heat. Its solutions are colorless and odorless.

Uses—Intercellular cement, which binds together the parenchymal cells of organs, appears to be a gel of highly polymerized hyaluronic acid. The latter is present in all organs but is most abundant in tissues of mesenchymal origin (eg, connective tissue and blood vessels); the testis is the richest source in mammals. Hyaluronidase hydrolyzes hyaluronic acid by splitting the glucosaminidic bond between carbon-1 of the glucosamine moiety and carbon-4 of glucuronic acid. Hyaluronidase accelerates the subcutaneous spread of both particulate matter and solutions by depolymerizing the hyaluronic acid. This results in a larger area of distribution of drugs in the tissue spaces and facilitates their absorption.

The chief clinical use of hyaluronidase is to facilitate the administration of fluids by hypodermoclysis. The enzyme also can be injected directly into local accumulations of transudate or blood to facilitate their spread and absorption. It has been used to facilitate absorption of penicillin and diagnostic agents. Its use with local anesthetics is not recommended. The use of hyaluronidase in obstetrics requires further study.[2,3] Hyaluronidase should not be used in infected areas because of the danger of spreading the infection. Additional information about hyaluronidase may be found in the literature.[4-6]

Dose—*Usual, hypodermoclysis,* **150 NF Units.**

Other Dose Information—A dose of 150 NF units is dissolved in 1 ml of isotonic sodium chloride solution and either added to 1000 ml of hypodermoclysis fluid or injected at the proposed site of infusion. In order to avoid overhydration the rate of administration should not exceed that employed for intravenous infusion.

Dosage Forms—NF: 150 and 1500 NF Units.

Veterinary Dose—See *Dose* above.

Malt Extract—see page 1348.

Pancreatic Dornase

[Dornavac (*MSD*)]

Pancreatic Dornase is a stabilized preparation of the enzyme, deoxyribonuclease, prepared by fractional precipitation of aqueous acid extracts of beef pancreas followed by dialysis, sterilization by filtration, and lyophilization. The activity of pancreatic dornase is determined by measuring the rate at which it reduces the viscosity of thymus deoxyribonucleic acid, potency being expressed in terms of units. One unit is an amount of enzyme which causes a drop of one viscosity unit in 10 minutes at 30°C, where the flow-time of water is taken as one viscosity unit.

Description—White, fluffy powder having a slight characteristic protein odor. It is thermally unstable.

Solubility—Soluble in water; insoluble in nonaqueous systems.

Uses—The name "dornase" derives from an elision of deoxyribonuclease. Derived from beef pancreas, pancreatic dornase depolymerizes deoxyribonucleoprotein of extracellular accumulations and disintegrated cells. Like streptodornase, it does not act on living matter. Clinical experience with pancreatic dornase has been disappointing in allergic asthma except in special instances in which infection with grossly purulent sputum has dominated the picture. The Committee on Therapy of the American Thoracic Society[7] states that proteolytic enzymes used to reduce the viscosity of sputum "have many side effects and are of questionable value." Irritation of the nose, throat, eyes, and respiratory tract and allergic reactions have been reported with proteolytic agents. Occasionally, anaphylactic shock has occurred.

Dose—*Inhalation*, **50,000** to **100,000 units** 1 to 4 times daily. The freeze-dried powder of purified enzyme is reconstituted with 2 ml of isotonic sodium chloride solution immediately prior to use. It is most often used as an aerosol.

Dosage Forms—for Solution: 100,000 units.

Pancreatin NF

[Panteric (*Parke-Davis*)]

Pancreatin is a substance containing enzymes, principally amylase, protease, and lipase, obtained from the pancreas of the hog, *Sus scrofa* Linné var. *domesticus* Gray (Fam. *Suidæ*) or of the ox, *Bos taurus* Linné (Fam. *Bovidæ*). Pancreatin converts not less than 25 times its weight of NF Potato Starch Reference Standard into soluble carbohydrates, and not less than 25 times its weight of casein into proteoses. Pancreatin of a higher digestive power may be labeled as a whole-number multiple of the two minimum activities or may be diluted by admixture with lactose, or with sucrose containing not more than 3.25% of starch, or with pancreatin of lower digestive power.

Preparation—Pancreatin is made by cutting the fresh pancreas into small pieces, kneading thoroughly with water, straining the liquid, and then filtering; an equal volume of alcohol is added to the filtrate and the precipitate is dried and powdered. The constituent *amylopsin* converts starch into maltose and forms small amounts of dextrose. Slight acidity checks this reaction and destroys the enzyme. *Trypsin* acts upon proteins and nucleoproteins, changing them into peptones and polypeptides. An excess of mineral acid soon decomposes it, although it keeps fairly well in 25 to 50% alcohol and best in 50% glycerin. Both ferments are most active at 40° in a slightly alkaline medium.

Description—A cream-colored, amorphous powder, having a faint, characteristic, but not offensive odor. It changes protein into proteoses and derived substances, and converts starch into dextrins and sugars. Its greatest activities are in neutral or faintly alkaline media; more than traces of mineral acids or large amounts of alkali hydroxides render it inert. An excess of alkali carbonate also inhibits its action.

Solubility—Slowly and incompletely soluble in water; insoluble in alcohol.

Incompatibilities—*Mineral acids* or excess *alkali hydroxides* or carbonates render pancreatin inert. It is precipitated by *strong alcoholic solutions* and by many *metallic salts*.

Uses—Pancreatin is indicated in the treatment of patients with cystic fibrosis (mucoviscidosis), chronic pancreatitis, partial or complete surgical pancreatectomy, and other conditions associated with exocrine pancreatic insufficiency. The administration of pancreatin decreases the nitrogen and fat content of the stool. The use of pancreatin except in pancreatic insufficiency is of no known value. The efficacy of pancreatin in the treatment of gaseous distention has not been demonstrated. When treating pancreatic insufficiency, a high-caloric diet which is high in protein and low in fat is recommended. Multivitamin supplements in water-soluble form are also desirable. Dietary and enzyme regimens are best based on repeated clinical evaluation and, in hospitalized patients, periodic measurements of fecal fat and nitrogen loss. Since the underlying pancreatic deficiency is unchanged, replacement pancreatin therapy is permanent.

Dose—*Usual*, **500 mg** to **1 Gm.**

Other Dose Information—Pancreatin and similar preparations are more effective when the dose is given at frequent intervals throughout the day.

Dosage Forms—Capsules: 5 gr; Granules: 12 and 20 gr; Tablets: 5 gr.

Pancrelipase

[Cotazym (*Organon*)]

Pancrelipase is a preparation of whole hog pancreas containing the enzymes amylase, trypsin, and lipase to which calcium and a buffer are added to activate the lipase.

Description—Creamy white to light-tan, amorphous powder having a characteristic odor.

Solubility—Not completely insoluble in water forming a suspension.

Uses—Pancrelipase essentially has the same actions as *Pancreatin* (this page), of which it is a more concentrated form. However, the lipase activity is increased out of proportion to that of amylase and trypsin. It is employed as replacement therapy in *pancreatic insufficiency* to promote the absorption of fat and diminish steatorrhea.

Dose—*Orally*, as capsules containing approximately 300 mg, **1** to **3 capsules** with each meal and 1 capsule with each piecemeal.

Dosage Forms—Capsules: 2000 units.

Penicillinase

[Neutrapen (*Riker*)]

Penicillinase is a specially purified enzyme preparation obtained by fermentation from cultures of a strain of *Bacillus cereus*.

Description—White, odorless, mixed crystals which are stable in dry form in both air and light.

Solubility—Soluble in water.

Uses—Penicillinase catalyzes the conversion of penicillin to the inactive penicilloic acid. Penicillinase has been used to treat patients who have developed reactions to penicillin since the enzyme has been found to produce rapid disappearance of the circulating drug in man. It should not be depended upon for relief of immediate anaphylactic reactions. After the anaphylactic emergency has been controlled by epinephrine, and other drugs, however, the effects of penicillinase may be used to control such delayed allergic symptoms as urticaria, dermatitis, arthralgias, and fever. Penicillinase, however, also has the potential hazard of precipitating severe allergic reactions to the enzyme itself.

Penicillinase finds a large area of application in the isolation of organisms from the blood and cultures of patients receiving penicillin. It should be included in all media in which material obtained from individuals treated with penicillin is being cultured, in order to remove the suppressive effect of any transferred penicillin that may be present.

Dose—*Usual, intramuscular,* **800,000 units.**
Dosage Forms—Injection: 800,000 units.

Pepsin NF XII

Pepsin is a substance containing a proteolytic enzyme obtained from the glandular layer of the fresh stomach of the hog, *Sus scrofa* Linné *var. domesticus* Gray (Fam. *Suidæ*).

Pepsin, when assayed as directed (see NF XII, page 294), digests not less than 3000 and not more than 3500 times its weight of coagulated egg albumen. A pepsin of higher digestive power may be reduced to the official standard by admixture with a pepsin of lower power or with lactose.

Preparation—Pepsin is made from hogs' stomachs which are macerated in water acidulated with hydrochloric acid, for several days, with frequent stirring. The strained liquid, if not clear, is clarified by allowing it to stand for 24 hours, and decanting. Sodium chloride, or other suitable precipitating medium is then dissolved in the solution to cause the precipitation of the pepsin, which comes to the surface. After several hours the floating pepsin is skimmed from the surface and purified by solution and reprecipitation. *Purified pepsin,* or *scale pepsin,* is made by concentrating an acidulated solution of pepsin in a vacuum apparatus and spreading the thick solution on glass plates to form scales, as is done with the scale salts of iron. It is in the form of yellowish scales. It is sometimes prepared in thicker scales which are broken up to form *granular pepsin.* When in these forms, pepsin is very soluble, and analysis has shown the presence of as much as 10% of free hydrochloric acid. One of the best forms of commercial pepsin is the *spongy* variety said to be produced by drying the pepsin solution in vacuum driers which causes the pepsin to puff and assume a spongy form.

An insoluble pepsin free from acid is also largely used for dispensing in powders and capsules, as it is not hygroscopic, and can be dispensed without becoming moist. This form is said to consist of the dried and pulverized stomach tissue containing the unremoved pepsin.

Description and Properties—Lustrous, transparent or translucent scales; granular or spongy masses, ranging in color from weak yellow to light brown; or a fine, white, to weak yellow amorphous powder, free from offensive odor and having a slightly acid or salty taste. Pepsin is not more than slightly hygroscopic.

Dry pepsin is not injured by heating to 100°. The activity of pepsin in solution is destroyed by alkalies or by temperatures exceeding 70°.

Solubility—Freely soluble in water, the solution being more or less opalescent; practically insoluble in alcohol, chloroform and ether.

Incompatibilities—The activity of pepsin is destroyed by *alkalies, strong acids,* temperatures above 70° or prolonged *agitation.* It is precipitated by strong *alcohol, tannin,* and many *metallic salts. Bismuth subcarbonate* precipitates it but the *subnitrate* does not.

Uses—Pepsin is the *proteolytic enzyme* secreted by the gastric glands. It functions in the initial stages of the digestion of protein. Presumably it should be effective in the treatment of digestive disturbances associated with a decrease in gastric secretory activity. Clinically a deficiency of pepsin in gastric juice is associated with an inadequate secretion of hydrochloric acid. In the treatment of this condition, results are just as favorable if diluted HCl alone is given, although pepsin is sometimes prescribed simultaneously. Apparently the digestion of protein proceeds adequately in the intestine without the action of pepsin in the stomach.

Dose—*Usual,* **500 mg.**
Veterinary Dose—*Horses,* **4 to 10 Gm;** *Dogs,* **100 mg to 1 Gm;** *Swine,* **2 to 4 Gm;** *Calves* and *Sheep,* **2 to 4 Gm.**

Streptokinase–Streptodornase Injection

[Varidase (*Lederle*)]

Streptokinase–streptodornase is a mixture of enzymes produced by a strain of *Streptococcus hemolyticus.* The mixture contains phosphate buffer at pH 7.5.

Description—White, flaky powder.
Solubility—The contents of each vial (20,000 units) is freely soluble in 2 ml of distilled water.

Uses—Streptokinase, which is elaborated by a strain of hemolytic streptococci, activates naturally occurring plasminogen in the fibrin deposits to the fibrinolytic enzyme, plasmin, which facilitates autodigestion of the thrombus. Streptokinase also reduces the levels of coagulation factors such as fibrinogen and Factors V and VIII.[8,9]

Streptodornase elaborated during the growth phase of hemolytic streptococci is a deoxyribonuclease which acts directly on deoxyribonucleic acid (DNA) to yield free purine and pyrimidine bases. Nucleic acids and nucleoproteins derived from degenerated leukocytes and injured tissue cells comprise 30 to 70% of the solids of viscid purulent matter. Streptodornase rapidly hydrolyses the polymer into smaller units and thus decreases the viscosity of the thick, slimy exudates. Unlike streptokinase, the action of streptodornase does not depend on activation of an endogenous substance like plasminogen. Streptodornase does not act on living cells.

Streptokinase-streptodornase is employed to facilitate the liquefaction and drainage of fibrinous and purulent exudates resulting from trauma or inflammation. When streptokinase-streptodornase is used in the treatment of infected areas it should be employed only as an adjunct to surgical debridement and drainage. Its use in nonsuppurative inflammations is not established.

Like some of the other enzymes reported in this chapter, the intramuscular, oral, and buccal administration of streptokinase-streptodornase has been proposed for treatment of edema associated with inflammation as may occur in thrombophlebitis, cellulitis, fractures, sprains, etc. However, favorable results with systematically administered enzymes have been demonstrated in animals only with 10 to 20 times the recommended clinical dose and then only when the enzymes were given before the production of the inflammation.[10] Therefore, these claims require further verification. Streptokinase requires the presence of plasminogen and areas of compromised blood flow may not provide sufficient amounts of the plasminogen. Furthermore, repeated application of the enzymes often elicits specific antibodies which tend to neutralize their effects. Streptokinase has been employed for the treatment of thromboemboli but its use in this condition is still in the experimental stages of investigation.[11,12]

The enzyme mixture is contraindicated in the presence of active hemorrhage since it may interfere with clotting. It should not be used where breakdown of surrounding tissue is contraindicated as for example in active tuberculosis or acute cellulitis.

Dose—Streptokinase and streptodornase must not be administered intravenously. When injected into cavities provision must be made for release of the increased fluid resulting from the liquefying action of the enzymes. The enzyme combination is used topically as a freshly prepared solution in phosphate buffer of pH 7.5. Depending on the amount of coagulation present, a solution containing from 1000 to 200,000 units of streptokinase with 250 to 50,000 units of streptodornase is applied once daily as a wet soak for a 4- to 6-hour period. The preparation may be used in conjunction with antibiotic agents.

Dosage Forms—Injection: 20,000/5,000 units; Jelly: 100,000/25,000 units; for Sterile Solution: 100,000/25,000 units; Tablets (buccal): 10,000/2,500 units; Tablets (oral): 10,000/2,500 units.

Trypsin Crystallized NF

[Parenzyme (*National Drug*); Tryptar (*Armour*)]

Trypsin Crystallized is a proteolytic enzyme crystallized from an extract of the pancreas gland of the ox, *Bos taurus* Linné (Fam. *Bovidæ*). When assayed as directed in the NF, it contains not less than 2500 NF Trypsin Units in each mg, calculated on the dried basis, and 90.0–110.0% of the labeled potency.

Note: Determine the suitability of the substrates and check the adjustment of the spectrophotometer by performing the assay using NF Trypsin Crystallized Reference Standard.

Preparation—One of the better known methods involves repeated fractional precipitation of crude trypsin with ammonium sulfate and crystallizing the partially purified material thus obtained from its concentrated solution in a borate buffer at pH 9.0.

Description—It occurs as a white to yellowish white, odorless, crystalline or amorphous powder.

Solubility—An amount of Trypsin Crystallized, equivalent to 500,000 NF Trypsin Units, is soluble in 10 ml of water or in 10 ml of saline TS.

Uses—Trypsin is a proteolytic enzyme which degrades a large number of proteins. Nevertheless, it does not attack susceptible proteins in viable tissue and plasma; however, it does accomplish some dissolution of fibrin in clots and exudates before it is completely inhibited.

In general, it has the same spectrum of activity and is subject to the same limitations as chymotrypsin; ie, its effectiveness by intramuscular, buccal, or oral administration for systemic effects is not established. It is used either alone or in combination with chymotrypsin for debridement of infected surface areas or in

infected areas with adequate drainage to the exterior.

Trypsin frequently produces local pain, and there may be induration at the site of injection. Occasionally allergic reactions occur, generally of minor but sometimes of serious degree. Antihistaminics diminish the intensity of such reactions.

Dose—*Usual, intramuscular,* **12,500** to **25,000 NF Units** daily. *Buccal,* **12,500 NF Units** 4 times daily. *Topical,* as a wet dressing of a solution containing **10,000 NF Units** per **ml.**

Veterinary Uses—For use in the debridement or removal of necrotic tissues. Effective in: osteomyelitis, surface ulcers, soft tissue abscesses, bovine foot rot, paranasal sinusitis, suppurative bursitis (fistulous withers), suppurative arthritis, equine foot canker, purulent and gangrenous mastitis, pyometra, metritis, suppurative otitis, infected compound fractures, infected amputation stumps.

Veterinary Dose—*Topically,* dry powder may be sprinkled on surface lesions, ie, ulcers, gangrene, and open infected wounds. When necessary the solution may be instilled by means of a hypodermic syringe into infected areas. The amount necessary varies from **200,000** to **800,000 NF Units** depending on the area treated.

Dosage Forms—for Injection, Aqueous: 5 mg/ml, 25 mg/5 ml; for Topical Solution: 125,000 units/20 ml, 250,000 units/30 ml.

Other Enzymes

Alpha Amylase [Buclamase (*Rystan*); Fortizyme (*Breon*)]—A starch-splitting enzyme derived from a nonpathogenic bacterium in the *Bacillus subtilis* class. *Description and Solubility:* Off-white, practically odorless powder. The presence of oxidizing agents, moisture, and heat should be avoided. Soluble in water; denatured by alcohol. *Uses:* Starch digestion occurs primarily in the small intestine by the action of pancreatic α-amylase. The amylases have, therefore, been used as digestants. Taken sublingually, alpha amylase is claimed to have an anti-inflammatory effect. It has been particularly recommended for the treatment of pain, edema, and hematomas in sports injuries. The effectiveness of this therapy has not been established.

Alpha-Chymotrypsin [Alpha Chymar (*Armour*); Quimotrase (*Smith, Miller & Patch*); Zolyse (*Alcon*)]—α-Chymotrypsin is obtained by a chymotrypsin-catalyzed cleavage of the dipeptide bonds of chymotrypsin. *Uses:* α-Chymotrypsin is the most stable member of the chymotrypsin family and has been used in cataract surgery. Following incision of the cornea, application of the enzyme for 2 to 4 minutes causes lysis of the zonules holding the lens, thus facilitating removal of the lens. Complications, however, include delay of healing and loss of vitreous humor. *Dose: Topically,* a few drops of a solution containing 150 units per ml.

Bromelains [Ananase (*Rorer*)]—A mixture of proteolytic enzymes derived from the stem of the pineapple plant, *Ananas comosus* (L.) Merr. *Description and Solubility:* Buff-colored, amorphous powder with a faint, characteristic odor. Partially soluble in water; insoluble in acetone, alcohol, ether, and chloroform. *Uses:* Bromelains have been suggested for decreasing the inflammation and edema resulting from surgery and injury. The proposed rationale for their use is similar to agents already discussed. Swelling that accompanies inflammation is theorized to be caused by occlusion of the tissue spaces with fibrin. It is claimed that Bromelains resolves the fibrin deposits blocking the vessels, reduces the inflammatory process, and thus enhances the healing of tissue. The evidence for the oral effectiveness of the Bromelains in reducing inflammation and edema is at present controversial[13,14] so that evaluation of these enzymes must await further investigation.

Collagenase [Collagenase ABC (*Agr. Biol.*)]—A product

of *Clostridium histolyticum*, which breaks down native collagen at physiological pH and temperature. It is a fermentation-produced enzyme complex. *Description and Solubility:* Amorphous and heat-labile. Soluble in water and alcohol. *Uses:* It has been recommended for debridement of wounds, second and third degree burns, and dermal ulcers. No clinical studies have been reported comparing the effectiveness of Collagenase to other agents already in use for similar purposes. It is compounded in white petrolatum or cholesterolized lanolin. The enzyme is compatible with antibiotics such as Polymyxin B sulfate or Neomycin. Collagenase is adversely affected by heavy metal antiseptics, detergents, and hexachlorophene so that these agents must be removed before using the enzyme. *Dose:* The ointment (0.5% w/w) is applied daily or every other day to the lesions and covered with sterile dressings.

Fibrinolysin [Thrombolysin (*MSD*)]—Fibrinolysin is a proteolytic enzyme also known as *plasmin* which is prepared by activating one of the normal components of human plasma, profibrinolysin (plasminogen). The normal *in vivo* activator is fibrinokinase but other activators are urokinase (see page 831) and streptokinase. Fibrinolysin has the property of lysing fibrin clots such as occur in a number of thromboembolic diseases. The commercial preparation named above contains both fibrinolysin and also some purified streptokinase which latter substance assists in the action of the former by acting on endogenous profibrinolysin. It is supplied in the form of a lyophilized powder which is restored with water for injection or 4% dextrose for further dilution in isotonic dextrose followed by slow intravenous injection. While there is some question regarding its clinical usefulness, it does seem to be of value in phlebothrombosis, thrombophlebitis, and pulmonary embolism. It is not recommended in cerebral or coronary thromboembolism.

Fibrinolysin and Desoxyribonuclease [Elase (*Parke-Davis*)]—This is a mixture of fibrinolysin of bovine origin and desoxyribonuclease obtained from beef pancreas. These two enzymes function together when used topically to lyse fibrin and liquefy pus (see *Pancreatic Dornase*, page 1050), thus aiding in the removal of necrotic material both from the skin and certain body cavities. It is not suitable for parenteral use and is not to be used in thromboembolic diseases. The commercial product named above is supplied as a lyophilized powder, from which a solution for topical use may be prepared, and in ointment form.

Papain [Papase (*Warner-Chilcott*)]—A proteolytic enzyme from the fruit of the tropical melon tree, *Carica papaya*. The enzyme exhibits broad spectrum specificity. Peptides, amides, esters, and thioesters are all susceptible to papain-catalyzed hydrolysis. *Uses:* Papain has long been employed to tenderize meat. It has been used, without evidence of effectiveness, as an aid to digestion. Large parenteral doses soften the cartilage in the ears of rabbits

and also cause severe damage to the aortas in this species. The oral use of papain for the prevention of adhesions and for the reduction of inflammation and edema remains to be clearly substantiated. Applied locally, it may aid in debridement of necrotic tissue. The possibility of allergic reactions must be considered when using this agent.

Lactated Pepsin Elixir NF XII [Compound Pepsin Elixir; Compound Digestive Elixir] possesses in each 100 ml, a proteolytic activity equal to not less than 1.75 Gm of NF Reference Pepsin. *Preparation:* Add pepsin (35 Gm) to cold purified water (500 ml) containing lactic acid (1 ml), and allow the mixture to stand in a cool place until the pepsin is thoroughly softened; then stir very gently until dissolved and add glycerin (250 ml). Dissolve orange oil (2 ml) in alcohol (200 ml), add amaranth solution (14 ml), and gradually add this solution to the pepsin solution with gentle stirring. Then add sufficient purified water to make the product measure 1000 ml, and filter, if necessary, until the product is clear. *Note:* Pepsin solutions are reduced in proteolytic activity by agitation and storage, particularly at or above normal room temperature. In order to compensate for this, an excess of pepsin has been used in the formula. *Alcohol Content:* From 16 to 19% of C_2H_5OH. *Incompatibilities:* Although this elixir finds frequent use as a vehicle for a great variety of substances it is doubtful if it is actually the vehicle of choice in most instances. Even when the pepsin is not thrown out of solution by the added ingredient it has a fair chance of being inactivated. It is generally "salted out" of solution by moderate concentrations of *bromides, acetates, etc. Phenobarbital* is liberated from the sodium derivative by the slight acidity of the elixir. *Sodium bicarbonate* effervesces and *sodium nitrite* is decomposed with the liberation of gaseous oxides of nitrogen. As a vehicle for *tinctures* it causes a separation of extractive matter due to its relatively low alcohol content. *Alkalies* inactivate the pepsin. *Uses:* A vehicle for nauseating medicines. *Dose: Usual, 10 ml.*

References

1. Florkin, M., and Stolz, E. H., eds., *Comprehensive Biochemistry*, vol. 13, Elsevier, New York, 1964.
2. Green, P. S., *Am. J. Obstet. Gynecol.*, **99**, 337 (1967).
3. O'Leary, J. A., and Erez S., *Obstet. Gynecol.*, **26**, 66 (1965).
4. Fishman, W. H., in Sumner, J. B., and Myrback, K., eds., *The Enzymes: Chemistry and Mechanism of Action*, vol. 1, part 2, Academic, New York, 1951, p. 769.
5. *Ann. NY Acad. Sci.*, **52**, 945 (1950).
6. Brimacombe, J. S., and Webber, J. M., Mucopolysaccharides: Chemical Structure, Distribution, and Isolation, Elsevier, Amsterdam and New York, 1964.
7. *Am. J. Respirat. Diseases*, **92**, 513 (1965).
8. Hiemeyer, V., *Ger. Med. Monthly*, **12**, 461 (1967).
9. Verstraete, M., *Scand. J. Clin. Lab. Invest.* Suppl., **93**, 190 (1967).
10. Sherry, S., and Fletcher, A. P., *Clin. Pharmacol. Therap.*, **1**, 202 (1960).
11. Hirsh, J., *et al*, *Lancet*, II, 593 (1967).
12. Dahlstrom, H., *Scand. J. Clin. Lab. Invest. Suppl.*, **93**, 187 (1967).
13. Gylling, U., *et al*, *Acta Chir. Scand.*, **131**, 193 (1966).
14. Seltzer, A. P., *Eye, Ear, Nose and Throat Monthly*, **46**, 1281 (1967).

Inhalation anesthetics—intravenous anesthetics—basal anesthetics

This chapter was prepared by

Ewart A. Swinyard, PhD, *Professor of Pharmacology, College of Pharmacy and College of Medicine, University of Utah, Salt Lake City, Utah 84112, and*
Stewart C. Harvey, PhD, *Associate Professor of Pharmacology, College of Medicine, University of Utah, Salt Lake City, Utah 84112*

Anesthetics are drugs which produce anesthesia, a condition of inability to appreciate sensation. Two types of anesthesia are usually recognized: (1) local anesthesia, in which the anesthesia is confined to a portion of the body and under which the patient is conscious and (2) general anesthesia, in which the anesthesia extends to the entire body and under which the patient is unconscious, in a state of muscular relaxation and insensibility to pain. The latter type is employed for most surgical operations.

Two classes of anesthetic drugs are described in this book: (1) local anesthetics, presented in Chapter 59, are agents which anesthetize only that part of the body to which they are applied and (2) general anesthetics, to be discussed in this chapter, are agents which anesthetize the entire organism. The general anesthetics may, for convenience in presentation, be divided into three groups: inhalation anesthetics, intravenous anesthetics, and those which are used only to induce basal anesthesia. The first group includes the volatile liquids and gases; the second group, the ultra short-acting barbiturates; and the third group, tribromethanol and certain barbiturates.

The safety, effectiveness, and general usefulness of general anesthesia have been greatly extended by the use of preanesthetic medications which are used to prepare the patient for anesthesia. The barbiturates and also narcotics are given prior to anesthesia to produce serenity and amnesia for the events preceding the operation and to act as a base for the anesthetic to be given. The phenothiazine-type tranquilizers are used for their sedative actions, to increase effects of central nervous system depressants, and to reduce the incidence of post-operative nausea and vomiting. Atropine or scopolamine is used to lessen the secretion of saliva and to reduce undesirable reflex action through the vagus nerve. Scopolamine has the added effect of producing amnesia. Curare and related compounds are used to increase muscle relaxation. These preanesthetic medications are mentioned elsewhere under the monograph for the particular agent (eg, see *Skeletal Muscle Relaxants*, page 928).

Inhalation Anesthetics

Volatile liquids and gases are commonly used to induce anesthesia by progressively increasing the amount of volatile anesthetic in the inspired air and thus in the blood and brain. The administration of an anesthetic results in progressive depression of the central nervous system, which may be preceded by varying degrees of excitation. These drugs first depress the cerebral cortex and then the basal ganglia and cerebellum. This is followed first by sensory and then motor paralysis of the functions of the spinal cord from below, upward. If the administration of the anesthetic is continued, the medullary centers are involved, and death may result from paralysis of the respiratory and vasomotor centers.

Four more or less definite stages of anesthesia may be recognized. These stages vary considerably in character and duration, depending upon the nature of the anesthetic as well as the speed of induction and the manner in which it is administered. They are most clearly seen with ether. When induction is rapid, as with cyclopropane, the early stages are less clearly defined. When anesthesia is induced by intravenous administration, as with the thiobarbiturates, unconsciousness occurs so promptly that the preliminary stages of anesthesia are not observed. The four stages of anesthesia, as originally described by Dr. A. E. Guedel, are presented below.

Stage I: Analgesia—This stage starts with the first inhalation of anesthetic gas and ends with the onset of unconsciousness. The patient is conscious and experiences sensations of warmth, remoteness, drifting, falling, and giddiness. There is a marked reduction in the perception of painful stimuli. This stage is often useful in obstetrics and minor surgery.

Stage II: Delirium or Excitement—This stage begins with the loss of consciousness. The inhibitory control of the higher centers is removed, and the subconscious emotions take over. The responses in this stage vary with different individuals; some patients pass through this stage peacefully and quietly, others become very excited and may exhibit excessive and even violent, struggling movements. Blood pressure, heart rate, and respiratory rate are all increased. All reflexes are present. It is desirable to pass through this stage as quickly as possible.

Stage III: Surgical Anesthesia—This is the stage of unconsciousness and paralysis of reflexes. In this stage the patient reflects complete tranquillity. Respiration is full and regular; the pulse is slow, full, and strong; the face is calm and expressionless; the body's musculature becomes soft and pliable; and the pupils become constricted. This stage is divided into four planes on the basis of the disappearance of various reflexes and the degree of respiratory depression. All surgical procedures are carried out in this stage.

Stage IV: Medullary Paralysis—This stage begins with central respiratory paralysis and ends with cardiac failure and death unless restorative measures are instituted. This stage should be avoided, except under unusual circumstances controlled by a skilled anesthetist.

Recovery—If the anesthetic is removed and the respiration is re-established and sustained before the heart stops, the symptoms may be reversed, and the body regains its normal physiological faculties. As recovery proceeds, the signs of the various stages occur in the reverse order, Stage I being the last stage to reappear.

The inhalation anesthetics are usually administered by one of two methods.

1. *Open Method*—The liquid anesthetic is dropped on a cotton or gauze mask held over the patient's nose or mouth. Air is the diluent and no anesthetic machine is required.

2. *Closed Method*—The gaseous or liquid anesthetic is contained in a special apparatus which, when attached to the patient's nose and mouth, constitutes a closed system. The patient is continually rebreathing the contents of the system. Provision is made for the removal of carbon dioxide with soda lime and the addition of oxygen as needed.

Sometimes, a semiclosed method, a modification of the second method, is used. This method employs a closed method type of apparatus, but a valve on the mask permits ready respiration outside the system, under which circumstances rebreathing is not excessive and no provision is made for removal of CO_2 or water.

Liquid Inhalation Anesthetics

The principal liquid anesthetics are ether, chloroform, vinyl ether, ethyl chloride, and trichloroethylene. Except for ethyl chloride, which boils at 12°C, the anesthetics in this group are liquids at room temperature and have a boiling point above 20°C. All of these agents are capable of producing surgical anesthesia when administered in appropriate concentrations and, unassisted by preanesthetic medication, can carry anesthesia to the stage of medullary paralysis. Hence, they are sometimes referred to as 100% anesthetic agents.

Halothane is probably the most frequently employed liquid inhalation anesthetic. Ether continues to be used, however, and serves as a standard by which all general anesthetics are measured. Chloroform is still employed in the tropics, but, because of the greater toxicity, it has largely been abandoned in this country. Vinyl ether induces anesthesia smoother and more rapidly than ether or chloroform; it is approximately 7 times as potent as ether. Although ethyl chloride is not frequently employed as a general anesthetic, it is a very potent and rapidly acting anesthetic agent. Trichloroethylene exhibits the typical actions of the inhalation anesthetics, but induction is long and laborious, and recovery is slow.

The ideal liquid anesthetic has yet to be discovered. All available agents exhibit toxic properties which tend to limit their usefulness. Chloroform and trichloroethylene sensitize the myocardium to sympathoadrenal discharges and to epinephrine. Consequently, serious and sometimes fatal cardiac arrhythmias may occur while patients are under the influence of these agents. Except for ether, which is not a hepatotoxic agent, all halogenated liquid anesthetics are capable of producing liver damage.

Chloroform NF

[Chloroformum Anæsthesicum; Trichloromethane]

Chloroform [$CHCl_3$ = 119.38] contains 99.0–99.5% of $CHCl_3$, the remainder consisting of alcohol.

Caution—*Care should be taken not to vaporize Chloroform in the presence of a flame, because of the production of harmful gases* (hydrogen chloride and phosgene).

Preparation—Chloroform was formerly made by the action of chlorinated lime (calcium chloride hypochlorite) on alcohol at a temperature of about 40°. In the past few decades, however, acetone and calcium hypochlorite have been advantageously used instead of alcohol and chlorinated lime. The reaction is more rapid and the yield is nearly quantitative. The reactions taking place in the acetone process are complicated, but the over-all effect is frequently represented by the following simplified equation:

$$2CH_3COCH_3 + 3Ca(OCl)_2 \rightarrow$$
$$2CHCl_3 + Ca(C_2H_3O_2)_2 + 2Ca(OH)_2$$

Chloroform is also being made by the reduction of carbon tetrachloride with water and iron and by the controlled chlorination of methane.

Absolutely pure chloroform readily decomposes on keeping, particularly if exposed to moisture and sunlight, giving rise to the formation of phosgene (carbonyl chloride [$COCl_2$]) and other products. The presence of a small amount of alcohol greatly retards or prevents this decomposition; hence the NF requires that chloroform contain 0.5% to 1% of alcohol. The alcohol combines with any phosgene forming ethyl carbonate which is nontoxic.

Description—A clear, colorless, mobile liquid of a characteristic, ethereal odor and a burning, sweet taste. It is not flammable but its heated vapors burn with a green flame. It is affected by light and by moisture. Its specific gravity is 1.474 to 1.478, indicating not less than 99 per cent and not more than 99.5% of $CHCl_3$. It boils at about 61°. Chloroform is not affected by acids, but is decomposed by alkali hydroxide into alkali chloride and sodium formate:

$$CHCl_3 + 4NaOH \rightarrow 3NaCl + HCOONa + 2H_2O$$

Solubility—Soluble in 210 volumes of water; miscible with alcohol, ether, benzene, solvent hexane, acetone, and with fixed and volatile oils.

Incompatibilities—Chloroform is occasionally prescribed in aqueous mixtures in which it is insoluble. The difficulty is sometimes overcome by the use of a quantity of the spirit equivalent to the required amount of chloroform. At times it is necessary to use an alcoholic solution of chloroform of greater strength than the official spirit in order to avoid too large a volume. One must be sure, in such a case, that the chloroform remains in solution in the completed product.

Uses—Chloroform is used as an *anesthetic* by inhalation. Although it possesses advantages of non-flammability and great potency, it is rarely used due to the serious toxic effects it produces on the heart and liver. Taken internally, in small doses, it is a *carminative*. Externally it is *irritant* and when used in liniments it may produce blisters.

Chloroform is used as a *preservative* during the aqueous percolation of vegetable drugs to prevent bacterial decomposition in the process of manufacture. In most instances it is evaporated before the product is finished. Chloroform is an excellent solvent for alkaloids and many other organic chemicals, and is therefore used in the manufacture of these products and in chemical analyses. Chloroform is also used in the manufacture of organic chemicals such as chlorobutanol.

Dose (unofficial)—By *inhalation* as required.

Other Dose Information—As a carminative, 0.3 to 1 ml.

Ether USP

[Æther Anæsthesicus; Ethyl Ether; Diethyl Ether; Sulfuric Ether]

$$CH_3CH_2—O—CH_2CH_3$$

Ether contains from 96.0–98.0% of $C_4H_{10}O$ (74.12), the remainder consisting of alcohol and water.

Caution—Ether is highly volatile and flammable. Its vapor, when mixed with air and ignited, may explode.

History—Valerius Cordus in 1517 described ether or a very similar product under the name *Oleum Vitriolo Dulce*. Later it was called *Spiritus Vini Æthereius* and still later *Ether Sulphuricus*.

In 1842 Dr. Crawford Long of Athens, Ga., first used ether as a general anesthetic. In 1844 Dr. Horace Wells, of Hartford, Conn., used it independently for the same purpose. Drs. C. T. Jackson and William Morton of Boston, Mass., had also used it earlier. The first hospital operation under ether anesthesia was performed in Boston, in 1846 by Dr. Warren.

Preparation—Ether may be made by reacting alcohol with sulfuric acid between the temperatures of 130° and 137°, which is known as the etherifying temperature. The sulfuric acid is regenerated in the process as shown below.

$$C_2H_5OH + H_2SO_4 \rightarrow C_2H_5HSO_4 + H_2O$$

$$C_2H_5HSO_4 + C_2H_5OH \rightarrow (C_2H_5)_2O + H_2SO_4$$

A large portion of the Ether produced in the United States is made starting with ethylene. It is treated with sulfuric acid to form ethylsulfuric acid, and the synthesis then proceeds as above.

Description—Ether is a transparent, colorless, mobile liquid, having a characteristic odor, and a burning sweetish taste. It is highly volatile and flammable, and its vapor, when mixed with air and ignited, may explode violently. It is slowly oxidized by the action of air, moisture, and light, with the formation of peroxides. The specific gravity of Ether is between 0.713 and 0.716 at 25°, corresponding to a $C_4H_{10}O$ content of 96 to 98%, the lower the specific gravity of the Ether the higher the absolute ether content. The specific gravity of absolute Ether is 0.7097 at 25°. Ether boils at about 35°.

Solubility—Dissolves in about 12 times its volume of water at 25°C with slight contraction of volume; miscible with alcohol, benzene, chloroform, solvent hexane, and with fixed and volatile oils.

Uses—Ether is used principally as an *anesthetic*, and, notwithstanding the many efforts made to supplant it, continues to be used for producing insensibility to pain in surgical operations. It is occasionally given by mouth as a *carminative*. It is a *solvent* for volatile and fixed oils, many resins and balsams, tannic acid, and most of the alkaloids. It dissolves iodine and bromine freely, and sulfur and phosphorus sparingly. Its power to dissolve corrosive sublimate makes it a useful agent in the manipulations for detecting that poison.

Official "Ether" to be used for anesthesia is directed to be specially packaged to avoid oxidation and the de-velopment of aldehydes or peroxides which are believed by many to render it unsuited for anesthetic use.

Caution—Ether to be used for anesthesia must be preserved in tight containers of not more than 3-Kg capacity, and is not to be used for anesthesia if it has been removed from the original container longer than 24 hours. Ether to be used for anesthesia may, however, be shipped in larger containers for repackaging in containers as directed above, provided the ether at the time of repackaging meets the requirements of the tests of the USP.

While anesthetic Ether may be used as a solvent or reagent, "*solvent ether*" or *Ethyl Oxide NF XII*, with less rigid tests for aldehydes and peroxides, is more suitable for this purpose.

Special care should be observed in pouring ether from one vessel to another in the presence of a flame, as the vapor is heavy—two and a half times as heavy as air—and it readily ignites with explosive violence, when mixed with air.

Ether, although not the most frequently employed inhalation anesthetic, is the standard against which all other general anesthetic agents are measured. It has a wide field of usefulness, is sufficiently potent for the most painful surgical procedures, and is relatively benign so far as the metabolic processes of the body are concerned. Its chief disadvantages are its flammability and explosibility, and a tendency to cause bronchopulmonary irritation. It can be administered by the ordinary drip method or by use of a gas machine allowing ether to be mixed with oxygen. It can also be given rectally in oil to produce anesthesia.

Ether is also employed as a surface antiseptic and cleansing agent. It is sometimes incorporated in rubefacient liniments. Finally, Ether is occasionally employed in expectorant cough mixtures.

Dose—By *inhalation* as required.

Veterinary Uses—Ether is sometimes employed as a carminative in *flatulent colic* of the horse and ox. Its most important use, however, is in *general anesthesia*; it is suitable for use on dogs, cats, and small pigs, but not for sheep, horses, cattle, or large swine.

Veterinary Dose—*Horses* and *Cattle*, 25 to 50 ml; *Dogs*, 2 to 4 ml.

Ethyl Chloride NF

[Chloroethane; Monochloroethane; Kelene]

Ethyl Chloride contains 99.5–100.5% of C_2H_5Cl (64.52).

Caution—Ethyl Chloride is highly flammable. Do not use where it may be ignited.

Preparation—Ethyl Chloride is generally prepared by distilling a mixture of alcohol, sodium chloride, and sulfuric acid, the reaction taking place as shown by the following equation:

$$C_2H_5OH + NaCl + H_2SO_4 \rightarrow C_2H_5Cl + NaHSO_4 + H_2O$$

Description—A gas at temperatures above 12°. At temperatures below 12° or under sufficient pressure, it is a colorless, mobile, and very volatile liquid, boiling between 12° and 13° at ordinary pressure. Its specific gravity is about 0.921 at 0°. Ethyl Chloride has a characteristic ethereal odor and a burning taste. When it is liberated at ordinary room temperature from its sealed container it rapidly vaporizes and produces a lowering of the temperature. It burns with a smoky greenish flame and formation of hydrogen chloride.

Solubility—Slightly soluble in water; freely soluble in alcohol or ether.

Uses—Ethyl Chloride is used as a *local anesthetic* by "freezing"; its great volatility requires special methods for dispensing; hermetically sealed tubes are used, so made that when the end is broken off, or the metallic orifice opened, and the tube held in the hand, the heat causes expansion and expels the liquid in a fine stream which is directed against the part to be anesthetized. It can also be employed as a *general anesthetic* by inhalation, especially for minor operations.

However, neither as a local nor general anesthetic is Ethyl Chloride indispensable. When employed locally, Ethyl Chloride actually freezes the tissues, thawing is painful, healing is delayed, and tissues may be damaged. As a general anesthetic, Ethyl Chloride has potentialities similar to chloroform for causing serious disturbances of the cardiac rhythm and damage to the liver. It is rarely employed as a general anesthetic.

Dose—*External use, topically,* as spray on intact skin.

Fluroxene NF

[2,2,2-Trifluoroethyl Vinyl Ether; Fluoromar (*Ohio Medical*)]

$$CF_3CH_2—O—CH=CH_2$$

Fluroxene contains 99.0–100.0% of $C_4H_5F_3O$ (126.08). It contains a suitable stabilizer.

Caution—Fluroxene is highly volatile and flammable. Its vapor, when mixed with air and ignited, may explode.

Preparation—Under moderate pressure in the presence of a basic catalyst, 2,2,2-trifluoroethanol is caused to undergo addition to acetylene. The crude ether is removed from the reaction mixture as an azeotrope and purified. US Pats. 2,830,007 and 2,870,218.

Description—Clear, colorless, volatile liquid having a mild ethereal odor. It boils at 43.2°.
Solubility—1 ml dissolves in 250 ml of water (at 30°).

Uses—Fluroxene is a highly volatile, pleasant smelling liquid which is used as a *general inhalation anesthetic.* Muscular relaxation is difficult to obtain and concomitant use of relaxant drugs is usually necessary. When administered in combination with oxygen or nitrous oxide, induction is generally smooth and rapid; excessive salivation is not encountered. This is a potent anesthetic agent and the depth of anesthesia may change quickly; therefore, the blood pressure and respiratory volume must be carefully monitored. It is used most frequently for procedures which require only the first or upper second plane of anesthesia, such as *cardiac, dental, orthopedic, obstetric,* and certain types of *gynecologic* and *urologic surgery.* Recovery is rapid and postoperative nausea and vomiting is infrequent. Fluroxene is an excellent analgesic. Althought hepatic toxicity has not been reported, the possibility can not be excluded without more extensive clinical study.

Dose—*By inhalation* as required.
Other Dose Information—For surgical anesthesia, concentrations of 3 to 8% are required.
Dosage Forms—Liquid: 125 ml.

Halothane USP

[2-Bromo-2-chloro-1,1,1-trifluoroethane; Fluothane (*Ayerst*)]

$$
\begin{array}{ccc}
 & Br & F \\
 & | & | \\
H— & C—C & —F \\
 & | & | \\
 & Cl & F
\end{array}
$$

Halothane [$C_2HBrClF_3$ = 197.39] contains 0.008–0.012% of thymol, by weight, as a preservative.

Preparation—Commercially available 2-chloro-1,1,1-trifluoroethane is subjected to direct bromination and Halothane is isolated from the reaction product by fractional distillation.

Description—Colorless, mobile, nonflammable, heavy liquid, having a characteristic odor resembling that of chloroform. Its taste is sweet and produces a burning sensation.
Solubility—Slightly soluble in water; miscible with alcohol, chloroform, ether, and fixed oils.

Uses—Halothane, a volatile, nonflammable liquid, is the most frequently employed *general inhalation anesthetic.* Induction with halothane is smooth and fairly rapid. The signs of anesthesia resemble those of chloroform anesthesia, and any depth of anesthesia can be obtained without hypoxia. The vapors are not unpleasant and are not irritating to mucous membranes. Like cyclopropane and chloroform, halothane sensitizes the myocardium to the action of epinephrine and levarterenol and injection of these amines during halothane anesthesia may induce ventricular tachycardia or fibrillation. Although serious hepatic damage is rare, the drug should be held suspect because of its chemical structure. Halothane should not be used in patients in whom previous exposure was accompanied by fever and/or jaundice. It is seldom used alone. Halothane is usually employed in conjunction with nitrous oxide and muscle relaxants to provide general anesthesia for operations of all types. It should be used with caution as an obstetrical anesthetic since it is not a potent analgesic and it depresses uterine tone.

Dose—*By inhalation* as required.

Methoxyflurane NF

[2,2-Dichloro-1,1-difluoroethyl Methyl Ether; Penthrane (*Abbott*)]

$$CHCl_2CF_2—O—CH_3$$

Methoxyflurane contains 99.9–100.0% of $C_3H_4Cl_2F_2O$ (164.97). It may contain a suitable stabilizer.

Preparation—1,1-Dichloro-2,2-difluoroethane is reacted with methanol in the presence of strong alkali or a basic ion-exchange resin to produce a mixture consisting largely of Methoxyflurane with small amounts of 2,2-dichloro-1-fluorovinyl methyl ether. Purification consists of removing the latter unsaturated component and may be accomplished by treatment with ozone, peroxy compounds, or other oxidizing agents to form readily removable oxidation products, and subsequent distillation. US Pat. 3,264,356.

Description—Clear, mobile liquid having a characteristic fruity odor.
Solubility—Very slightly soluble in water (at 37°); miscible with olive oil (in all proportions), chloroform, 95% ethyl alcohol, acetone, and benzene.

Uses—For inhalation as general anesthetic and inhalation analgesic in obstetrics. Induction of anesthesia is relatively slow and recovery is prolonged. The drug causes constriction of the pupil; hence, the depth of anesthesia must be judged by the blood pressure, respiratory volume, and degree of muscle relaxation. Postoperative nausea and vomiting are infrequent. Since methoxyflurane is a halogenated hydrocarbon the concurrent use with epinephrine should be avoided because of the potential danger of cardiac arrhythmias. The anesthetic agent is contraindicated in patients with cirrhosis or other liver disease.

At room temperature this volatile liquid is nonflammable and nonexplosive.

Dose—By *inhalation* as required.

Other Dose Information—Administered by the closed or semiclosed technique in a concentration of 1.5 to 3%.

Dosage Forms—Liquid: 125 ml.

Trichloroethylene USP

[Trilene (*Ayerst*); Trimar (*Ohio Medical*)]

CHCl:CCl₂

Trichloroethylene contains not less than 99.5% of C_2HCl_3 (131.39). It contains 0.008–0.012%, by weight, of thymol as an antimicrobial agent. A dye certified for use in drugs by the federal Food and Drug Administration may be added to impart a blue color to Trichloroethylene.

Preparation—Trichloroethylene may be prepared by the abstraction of the elements of HCl from *sym*-tetrachloroethane by means of lime.

Trichloroethylene is unstable in light and moisture. Its decomposition may, however, be retarded by various additives, hence the presence of thymol.

Description—A clear, colorless, or blue, mobile liquid with a characteristic, chloroform-like odor. It is not flammable, but is slowly decomposed by moisture, light accelerating the decomposition. Its specific gravity is between 1.458 and 1.463 indicating a content of not less than 99.5% and not more than 100.0% of C_2HCl_3. It boils between 86° and 88°, and solidifies at −83°. It has a refractive index of 1.4782 at 20°.

Solubility—Practically insoluble in water; miscible with alcohol, chloroform, ether, and many other organic liquids; dissolves most fixed and volatile oils.

Uses—Trichloroethylene has been sporadically employed as a *general inhalation anesthetic*. It is not a satisfactory anesthetic alone since it does not produce adequate muscle relaxation; hence, it is usually used to supplement nitrous oxide anesthesia. It is serviceable as an *analgetic* in certain cases of *trigeminal neuralgia*. The availability of pure preparations and the development of special inhaler devices have served to popularize the use of the vapor for *obstetrical analgesia*. However, it is slow in onset of analgesia and potentially cardiotoxic.

Industrially, it is used as a solvent for various organic compounds, fats, oils, etc.

Dose—By *inhalation* as required.

Other Dose Information—Trigeminal neuralgia, a frangible glass ampul containing 1.0 ml is broken and the contents inhaled. A second inhalation may be necessary after a few minutes, if relief is not obtained, and further administrations are repeated 3 or 4 times daily for several weeks.

Dosage Forms—USP: 300 ml.

Vinyl Ether NF

[Æther Vinylicus; Divinyl Ether; Divinyl Oxide; Vinethene (*MSD*)]

CH₂:CH—O—CH:CH₂

Vinyl Ether for anesthesia contains 96.0–97.0% of C_4H_6O (70.09), the remainder consisting of dehydrated alcohol. It may contain not more than 0.025% of a suitable preservative.

Caution—*Do not use Vinyl Ether for anesthesia if the original container has been opened longer than 48 hours. It is flammable.*

Preparation—This olefin ether corresponds to its paraffin analogue, ethyl ether (*Ether USP*). It is made from β,β′-dichloroethyl ether by dehydrochlorination with the aid of potassium hydroxide.

Because of its unsaturation this ether is prone to decompose by oxidation and to polymerize into a solid gel-like substance, especially in the presence of traces of acid, but in the presence of a small amount of preservative (antioxidant) and alcohol it is stable for 2 years or longer in the unopened container. The alcohol also reduces the volatility of the ether and thus minimizes the tendency for ice formation on the anesthesia mask and in the gas machines employed in the process. This is the prime reason for the presence of about 4% alcohol in the preparation.

Description—A clear liquid of a characteristic odor. It is colorless or has a slight purple fluorescence from the preservative. It has a specific gravity of 0.767 to 0.771, and boils at about 30°.

Solubility—Slightly soluble in water; miscible with alcohol, acetone, chloroform, and ether.

Uses—Vinyl Ether is employed as a *general inhalation anesthetic*, in a manner similar to ethyl ether. It is more potent than ether and is more rapid in its action. The recovery period is likewise shorter. Vinyl Ether is administered by the open drop method (by the use of a face mask or a few thicknesses of fluffed gauze), or by the closed method with oxygen in a gas machine. When anesthesia over one-half hour's duration is needed Vinyl Ether should be given with oxygen by the closed technique. It should not be employed longer than 1 hour, and should not be used repeatedly in the same patient due to the danger of cumulative hepatic damage. Vinyl Ether finds its main usefulness for short surgical procedures, changing of painful dressings, extraction of teeth, setting of fractures, etc. Its disadvantages are that a trained anesthetist is required for its proper and safe use, and that there is possibility of hepatic damage. Atropine must be employed with this ether because the latter causes salivation. Finally, Vinyl Ether is highly volatile and cannot be employed in the tropics.

Dose—By *inhalation* as required.

Gaseous Inhalation Anesthetics

The gaseous anesthetic agents are vapors at ordinary room temperature and, in general, have boiling points at less than 20°C. Consequently, they are confined under high pressure in cylinders and administered by the closed method with an anesthetic machine. These agents vary greatly in anesthetic potency, and their successful use often depends upon the proper premedication of the patient. For example, even under the most favorable circumstances, nitrous oxide-oxygen and ethylene-oxygen mixtures will carry patients only 15 and 25%, respectively, through the surgical stage of anesthesia. Thus, nitrous oxide and ethylene are referred to as 15 and 25% anesthetic agents, respectively. In marked contrast, cyclopropane, irrespective of previous preparation of the patient, will carry anesthesia through to medullary paralysis; hence, it is a 100% anesthetic agent. Nitrous oxide is nonirritating and causes no untoward side actions if anoxia is avoided.

Ethylene allows a rapid, pleasant, and safe induction, excitement is minimal, recovery is rapid, and post-operative complications infrequent. Cyclopropane allows more oxygen throughout all depths of anesthesia than ethylene or nitrous oxide, produces greater skeletal muscle relaxation than other anesthetic gases, and provides a wide margin of safety between the anesthetic and lethal concentrations. Cyclopropane can cause serious disorders of cardiac rhythm, and certain precautions must be exercised to diminish danger from this action of the gas.

Cyclopropane USP

[Trimethylene]

$$\underset{H_2C \!-\! CH_2}{\overset{\overset{\displaystyle H_2}{C}}{}}$$

Cyclopropane contains not less than 99.0%, by volume, of C_3H_6 (42.08).

Caution—Cyclopropane is highly flammable. Do not use where it may be ignited. Use same precautions as those given under Ethylene.

Preparation—Among other methods, Cyclopropane may be prepared by several patented processes which involve treating 1,3-dichloropropane with zinc in the presence of sodium iodide.

Description—A colorless gas resembling solvent hexane in odor; has a pungent taste. 1 liter at 760 mm Hg pressure and 0° weighs 1.879 Gm.

Solubility—1 volume of Cyclopropane dissolves in about 2.7 volumes of water at 15°; freely soluble in alcohol; soluble in fixed oils.

Note—Maintain cylinders of Cyclopropane at 25 ± 2° for at least 6 hours prior to withdrawing samples for the tests and assay, and correct the results to 25° and 760 mm of mercury.

Uses—Cyclopropane is employed as *general anesthetic*. It is the most potent of the anesthetic gases, being approximately five times as potent as ethylene and seven times as potent as nitrous oxide. This fact gives rise to its chief advantage, namely, that it allows sufficient room in the gas mixture for a plenitude of oxygen. Indeed, with proper preanesthetic medication, 15 to 20 volumes % of Cyclopropane permits anesthesia sufficiently deep for most major surgical procedures. Cyclopropane requires the use of a modern anesthesia machine and an experienced anesthetist. It has the disadvantages that it is highly explosive and also that it produces irregularities of the heart in the deeper planes of anesthesia. Cyclopropane continues to be a popular and useful anesthetic agent. Its outstanding merits include safety, controllability, and versatility.

Dose—By *inhalation* as required.

Ethylene NF

[Ethene; Olefiant Gas]

$$CH_2\!=\!CH_2$$

Ethylene contains not less than 99.0% by volume of C_2H_4 (28.05).

Caution—Ethylene is highly flammable. Do not use where it may be ignited.

Note—A mixture of it with oxygen or air will explode when brought in contact with a flame or other cause of ignition.

Preparation—Ethylene may be prepared by abstracting 1 molecule of water from 1 molecule of ethyl alcohol. This may be accomplished by passing alcohol through a red-hot tube containing aluminum oxide or through a tower of coke impregnated with glacial phosphoric acid (metaphosphoric acid). It is now available cheaply and in almost unlimited quantities from the "cracking process" of petroleum (page 442).

Description—A colorless gas, somewhat lighter than air, and has a slightly sweet odor and taste. A liter of Ethylene at 760 mm Hg pressure and 0° weighs 1.260 Gm.

Solubility—1 volume of Ethylene dissolves in about 4 volumes of water at 0°, and in about 9 volumes of water at 25°; in about 0.5 volume of alcohol at 25° and in about 0.05 volume of ether at 15.5°.

Note—Maintain cylinders of Ethylene at 25 ± 2° for at least 6 hours prior to withdrawing samples for the tests and assay, and correct the results to 25° and 760 mm of mercury.

Uses—Ethylene is employed as a *general inhalation anesthetic*. It is considerably weaker than cyclopropane, but stronger than nitrous oxide. Unless sufficient preanesthetic medication is employed, Ethylene will not produce adequate relaxation for the more painful or extensive surgical procedures. Inasmuch as high concentrations must be used (85 to 90%), the available space in the mixture for adequate amounts of oxygen is encroached upon. Ethylene is probably the most nontoxic of all general anesthetics, and no deaths have been reported from its use. It has the disadvantage of being explosive and fatal accidents have occurred from explosions during Ethylene anesthesia. Consequently, the use of Ethylene has declined markedly in recent years.

Dose—By *inhalation* as required.

Nitrous Oxide USP

[Dinitrogen Monoxide; Laughing Gas]

Nitrous Oxide contains not less than 99.0%, by volume, of N_2O (44.01).

The remainder is chiefly nitrogen.

Preparation—It is usually prepared by heating ammonium nitrate to about 170°.

$$NH_4NO_3 \rightarrow N_2O + 2H_2O$$

It is also produced by heating a mixture of ammonium sulfate and sodium nitrate. The crude gas is purified to free it from acid and alkaline substances (nitrous anhydride and ammonia) by passing it through acidulated dilute potassium permanganate solution to oxidize any nitrogen trioxide, and then through sodium hydroxide solution to free it from acid substances and halogens.

Nitrous Oxide is furnished in compressed form in metallic cylinders.

Description—A colorless gas, without appreciable odor or taste. Its specific gravity is 1.53. 1 liter of it, at a pressure of 760 mm Hg at 0° weighs 1.977 Gm.

Solubility—1 volume dissolves in about 1.5 volumes of water at 20° under normal pressure; freely soluble in alcohol; soluble in ether and oils.

Uses—Nitrous Oxide is the weakest but probably the safest inhalation *general anesthetic*. Therefore, its potency is increased by the use of halothane, trichloroethylene, or ethyl ether, and its muscle relaxant properties are enhanced by the concomitant use of a neuromuscular blocking drug. Thus, an anesthetic regimen is built around nitrous oxide, since it cannot by itself provide sufficient hypnosis, analgesia, and muscle relaxation. During its administration some patients become hysterical and because of this characteristic it is often called *laughing gas*. It causes only the lighter grades of anesthesia unless the patient has had considerable preanesthetic medication (morphine, scopolamine, barbiturate, etc) or unless supplemental anesthesia (ether, cyclopropane, etc) is used. Inasmuch as high concentrations of Nitrous Oxide are required, little room is left in the mixture for oxygen. This may result in serious anoxia and tissue damage, especially to the central nervous system. For this reason, considerable experience is required for the proper use of Nitrous Oxide as an anesthetic, and care must be exercised in the proper selection of cases. Due to the pleasant, rapid induction, Nitrous Oxide is often employed to initiate anesthesia, prior to the use of ether. Nitrous Oxide is also commonly used in dental surgery because of the rapid recovery which it allows. It is also frequently employed in obstetrics to produce analgesia.

Dose—By *inhalation* as required.

Intravenous Anesthetics

Intravenous anesthesia offers the advantages of rapid, pleasant induction, simplicity of administration, and freedom from explosion hazards. Further advantages include lack of pulmonary irritation and a rapid recovery without nausea or vomiting. Although all barbiturates that are used clinically as sedatives and hypnotics will produce anesthesia and are often used for this purpose in laboratory animals, the duration of action is too long to render them safe for routine use as general anesthetics in man. The ultrashort-acting barbiturates, however, are useful as intravenous anesthetics because their very short action allows a control of the depth and safety of anesthesia approaching that obtained by inhalation anesthesia. Since they are poor analgesics, they are seldom used alone, but are usually supplemented with an inhalation anesthetic, such as nitrous oxide in oxygen. The general principles which apply to the use of barbiturates for intravenous anesthesia are the same as those which govern the use of other general anesthetic agents.

Sodium Hexobarbital NF XII

[Sodium 5-(1-Cyclohexen-1-yl)-1,5-dimethylbarbiturate; Hexobarbitone Sodium; Cyclural Sodium; Evipal Sodium (*Winthrop*)]

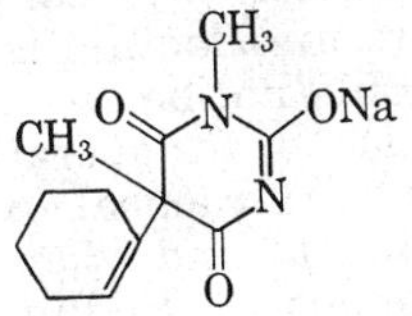

Sodium Hexobarbital contains 98.5–101.0% of $C_{12}H_{15}N_2NaO_3$ (258.25), calculated on the dried basis.

Preparation—The diethyl ester of methyl cyclohexenyl malonic acid is prepared by the general method described under *Barbital* (page 1080), and is then condensed with *N*-methylurea in the presence of sodium ethylate.

Description—A white, crystalline, odorless, hygroscopic powder, with a slightly bitter taste. Becomes discolored on exposure to air. The pH of an aqueous 1 in 10 solution is between 10.5 and 12.

Solubility—Very soluble in water; soluble in alcohol; practically insoluble in ether; solutions decompose on standing.

Uses—Hexobarbital Sodium is one of the "ultrashort-acting" *Barbiturates* (see page 1079) employed as a *general anesthetic* by the *intravenous* route.

Dose—To be determined by the physician according to the needs of the patient.

Sodium Methohexital for Injection NF

[Sodium 5-Allyl-1-methyl-5-(1-methyl-2-pentynyl)barbiturate; Brevita Sodium (*Lilly*)]

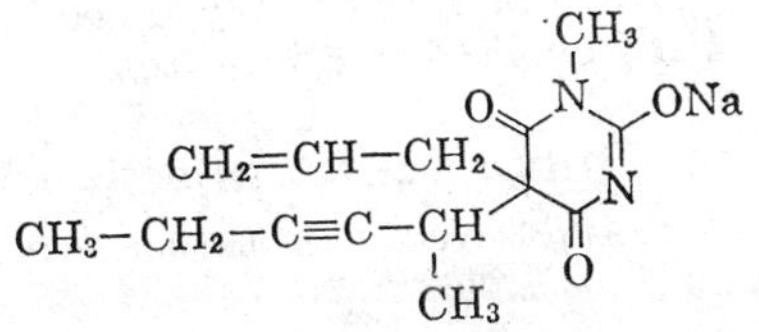

Sodium Methohexital for Injection is a sterile mixture of sodium methohexital and anhydrous sodium carbonate as a buffer. It contains 93.0–107.0% of the labeled amount of $C_{14}H_{17}N_2NaO_3$ (284.29), calculated on the dried basis.

Preparation—1-Butynyl magnesium bromide is Grignardized with acetaldehyde and the resulting alcohol is treated with PCl_5 to produce 2-chloro-3-pentyne. Condensation with ethyl cyanoacetate in the presence of sodium ethylate yields ethyl 1-methyl-2-pentynyl-cyanoacetate which, on similar further condensation with allyl bromide yields ethyl (1-methyl-2-pentynyl)allyl-cyanoacetate (I). Reaction of I with *N*-methylurea yields the iminobarbituric acid (II) which hydrolyzes under the influence of proton to methohexital. Neutralization with NaOH yields the official barbiturate.

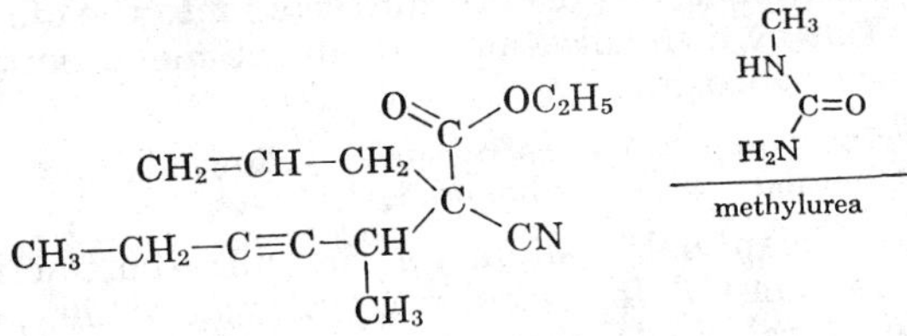

I

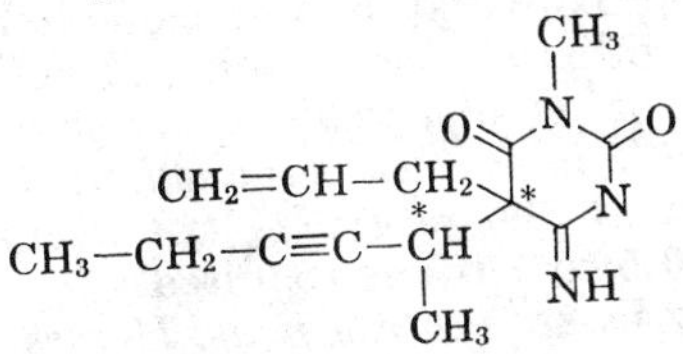

II

Note: As indicated in formula (II), the barbituric acid contains two asymmetric C atoms and hence exists in two diastereoisomeric forms. These have been designated as α and β forms in the literature. The α-form is the one used medicinally (the β-form causes undesirable side effects) and is formed almost exclusively by the above process. The malonic ester synthesis described under *Barbital* on page 1080 is not used because it yields mainly the unwanted β-form.

Description—Occurs as a white to off-white hygroscopic powder. It is essentially odorless. Its solutions are alkaline to litmus.

Uses—An ultrashort-acting barbiturate useful for intravenous *general anesthesia*. Although Sodium Methohexital is similar in action to thiopental sodium, it is more potent and less firmly bound to fatty tissue than the latter agent. Induction of anesthesia is about as rapid as with thiopental sodium, but recovery is more rapid. Hence, it is particularly useful for brief procedures, such as *reduction of fractures, gynecologic examination, electroconvulsive therapy, genitourinary procedures,* and *oral surgery.* Untoward effects include muscle twitching, sneezing, coughing, hiccuping, laryngospasm and respiratory stridor. The drug is contraindicated in patients with severe hepatic dysfunction, respiratory obstruction, asthma, severe hypotension or hypertension, myocardial disease, congestive heart failure, anemia, and extreme obesity.

Dose—*Usual, intravenous, induction,* **7.5 ml** of **1%** solution, at the rate of **1 ml** every 5 seconds; *maintenance,* **2 to 4 ml** every 4 to 6 minutes.

Sodium Thiamylal for Injection NF

[Sodium   5-Allyl-5-(1-methylbutyl)-2-thiobarbiturate;   Surital   Sodium (*Parke-Davis*)]

$$CH_2=CH-CH_2 \quad \underset{CH_3CH_2CH_2CH}{\overset{O\ \ \ H}{\underset{\underset{CH_3}{|}}{}}} SNa$$

Sodium Thiamylal for Injection is a sterile mixture of sodium thiamylal with anhydrous sodium carbonate as a buffer. It contains 93.0–107.0% of the labeled amount of $C_{12}H_{17}N_2NaO_2S$ (276.34), calculated on the dried basis.

Preparation—The thiobarbituric acid, thiamylal, may be prepared by the general process described under *Barbital,* page 1080, except using allyl bromide and 1-methylbutyl bromide as the alkylating agents instead of ethyl bromide, and condensing the resulting allyl 1-methylbutyl malonic ester with thiourea instead of urea. The free acid is readily converted into the official sodium salt by neutralization with an equimolar portion of sodium hydroxide.

Description—Occurs as a pale yellow, hygroscopic powder, having a disagreeable odor.

Uses—Thiamylal sodium is an ultrashort-acting barbiturate useful for *intravenous anesthesia* in procedures of relatively short duration. Its anesthetic potency is approximately one and one-half times that of pentothal, otherwise its profile of action and untoward effects are similar to the other thiobarbiturates.

Dose—*Usual, intravenous, induction,* **3 to 6 ml** of **2.5%** solution at the rate of **1 ml** every 5 seconds; *maintenance,* **0.5 to 1 ml** as required.

Veterinary Dose—*Intravenous,* Horses, **1 Gm** (as a 0.5% solution to animals weighing 500 to 1000 pounds); for *deeper anesthesia,* **1 ml** of a **4%** solution per **12 pounds** of body weight (1 Gm per 300 pounds);

Cattle, **1 ml** of a **2%** solution per **5 pounds** of body weight or **1 ml** of a **4%** solution per **7 pounds**; *Swine,* **1 ml** of a **4%** solution per **5 pounds** of body weight; *Dogs* and *Cats, initial,* approximately **1 ml** of a **4%** solution per **5 pounds** of body weight, followed by fractional supplements if required.

Sodium Thiopental USP

[Sodium 5-Ethyl-5-(1-methylbutyl)-2-thiobarbiturate; Thiopentone Sodium; Thiopentone Soluble; Thiopental Sodium with Sodium Carbonate; Pentothal Sodium (*Abbott*)]

$$\underset{CH_3CH_2CH_2CH}{\overset{CH_3CH_2}{}}\ \underset{\underset{CH_3}{|}}{}\ \overset{O\ \ \overset{H}{N}}{\underset{O}{}}\ SNa$$

Sodium Thiopental contains 97.0–102.0% of $C_{11}H_{17}N_2NaO_2S$ (264.32), calculated on the dried basis.

Sodium Thiopental intended for rectal use may be suitably colored and may be buffered with anhydrous sodium carbonate.

Preparation—Thiopental is made in the same manner as *Barbital,* using 2-bromopentane $[CH_3(CH_2)_2-CHBrCH_3]$ to react with one of the hydrogens in the CH_2 group instead of one C_2H_5Br molecule, and the ethyl 1-methylbutyl malonic ester is condensed with thiourea $[CS(NH_2)_2]$ instead of urea. See page 1080.

Description—A white to off-white, crystalline powder or a yellowish white hygroscopic powder. It may have a disagreeable odor. Its aqueous solution is alkaline to litmus. Its solutions decompose on standing, and on boiling precipitation occurs. Carbon dioxide also causes precipitation in the solution.

Solubility—Soluble in water and alcohol; insoluble in absolute ether, benzene, and solvent hexane.

Incompatibilities—Same as *Sodium Phenobarbital* (page 1083).

Uses—Sodium Thiopental is employed in therapeutics almost exclusively as an *intravenous general anesthetic,* for short operative procedures. It must be administered by an anesthetist thoroughly trained in its use and well acquainted with its contraindications and dangers. The duration of action is quite brief. Sodium Thiopental should not be used as a surgical anesthetic in office practice, or for operations of long duration. Facilities for intratracheal oxygen administration should always be at hand when injecting Sodium Thiopental intravenously. Sodium Thiopental is contraindicated in patients with a complete absence of suitable veins or a history of barbiturate hypersensitivity, status asthmaticus, or porphyria.

Dose—*Usual, intravenous, induction,* **6 to 12 ml** of a **2.5%** solution at intervals of 30 to 60 seconds; *maintenance,* **0.5 to 2 ml** as required; *usual, rectal,* **30 to 50 mg** per **Kg** of body weight, in a 5 to 10% solution, or a 20% suspension in oil, to a total dose of **3 Gm**.

Dosage Forms—for Injection USP: 500 mg, and 1, 5, 6.25, 10, and 12.5 Gm.

Veterinary Dose—*Intravenous* (per pound of body weight), *Horses, Cattle, Sheep,* and *Swine,* **4 to 7 mg**; *Calves,* **7 to 10 mg**; *Dogs* and *Cats,* **8 to 15 mg**.

Basal Anesthetics

Basal anesthesia is a state of unconsciousness produced by the use of certain central nervous system depressants. The unconsciousness produced by these agents is not of sufficient depth to permit surgical procedures. Basal anesthesia provides pleasant induction, freedom from mental distress and respiratory irritation incident to the use of certain inhalation anesthetics, reduction in the amount of inhalation anesthetic required, and a long, post-anesthetic period of sedation. The chief disadvantage of the basal anesthetics, principally that of tribromethanol, is that it is a nonvolatile anesthetic given by a route which prevents adequate control by the anesthetist once it is administered.

Magnesium Sulfate Injection—see page 1099.

Paraldehyde—see page 1088.

Phencyclidine Hydrochloride

[Sernylan (*Parke-Davis*)]

Phencyclidine Hydrochloride [$C_{17}H_{25}N.HCl$ = 279.84] is 1-(1-phenylcyclohexyl)piperidine hydrochloride.

Preparation—An aqueous solution of potassium cyanide and piperidine is added to a cooled slurry of cyclohexanone sodium bisulfite to form 1-piperidinocyclohexanecarbonitrile. The nitrile is reacted with phenylmagnesium bromide after which the mixture is treated with aqueous hydrobromic acid, neutralized with potassium carbonate, and extracted with isooctane to give phencyclidine (base). Hydrogen chloride passed into an isopropanol solution of the base yields the hydrochloride. US Pat. 3,097,136.

Description—A white to creamy white, crystalline powder or granules that are odorless and have a slightly bitter taste. It is stable in light and in air. It melts between 222° and 228°.

Solubility—Freely soluble in water, alcohol, and chloroform; sparingly soluble in dilute hydrochloric acid.

Uses—Phencyclidine Hydrochloride, a piperidine derivative, is used as an *immobilizing agent* for primates. The effects produced are unlike those produced by the classical anesthetics. Even though the animal is completely incapacitated simple reflexes such as patellar, palpebral, corneal, and pupillary are not completely eliminated, the eyes remain open, muscle tone is increased in most cases, and respiration and blood pressure are not usually depressed except after deliberate overdosage. When Phencyclidine Hydrochloride is used prior to an anesthetic agent, such as ether or a barbiturate, a greatly reduced amount of the anesthetic will produce surgical anesthesia. Side effects observed include disorientation, salivation, anxiety, restlessness, convulsions, muscular tremors, hyperpnea, respiratory arrest, cardiac arrest, and emesis. Decreased body temperature, shock, and death have also been observed in the *Macacus irus* monkey and *Anubis* baboon. The shock is *best* prevented by the application of heating pads to the animal. Phencyclidine Hydrochloride should not be used in animals other than primates. *It is especially contraindicated in animals whose meat, milk, or eggs are to be used for food.* Phencyclidine Hydrochloride is a stable chemical which is not degraded at temperatures normally used in cooking or in freezing foods. The persistence

time of drug residues in milk or tissues of animals has not been determined.

Dose—**0.5 to 2 mg per Kg;** *usual, intramuscular,* **0.8 mg per Kg.**

Sodium Hexobarbital—see page 1061.

Sodium Hexobarbital, Sterile—see page 1061.

Sodium Thiamylal for Injection—see page 1062.

Sodium Thiopental—see page 1062.

Tribromoethanol NF

[2,2,2-Tribromoethanol; Tribromoethyl Alcohol; Avertin (*Winthrop*)]

Tribromoethanol contains the equivalent of 99.0–101.8% of $C_2H_3Br_3O$ (282.77), calculated on the dried basis.

Preparation—This anesthetic may be prepared by reacting a solution of bromal with aluminum ethylate (aluminum ethoxide) or preferably aluminum isopropoxide, whereby the bromal is reduced to tribromoethanol and the isopropyl alcohol is oxidized to acetone:

$$3Br_3C.CHO + 3H_2O + \left(\begin{matrix}CH_3\\CH_3\end{matrix}\right)CH.O\Big)_3Al \rightarrow$$

$$3Br_3C.CH_2OH + 3CH_3COCH_3 + Al(OH)_3$$

The aluminum hydroxide is removed by filtration and the acetone by distillation, and the residual solution containing the tribromoethanol is evaporated under reduced pressure to crystallization.

Description—A white, crystalline powder having a slight, aromatic odor and taste. It decomposes on exposure to air and light, becoming discolored and acquiring an acid reaction. It is rapidly and similarly decomposed in solution. It melts between 79° and 82°, and at a pressure of 10 mm Hg it boils at about 93°. Upon heating with aqueous alkali hydroxides, alkali bromide and various organic decomposition products are formed.

Solubility—1 Gm dissolves in about 35 ml of water; very soluble in amylene hydrate; soluble in alcohol, ether, and benzene.

Uses—Tribromoethanol, in the form of Tribromoethanol Solution, is employed as a *basal anesthetic* by rectal instillation. This once popular agent is infrequently used today because of its tendency to produce hypotension, its potential hepatic and renal toxicity, and the relative uncontrollability of drug absorption. The chief advantage of this type of anesthesia is the pleasant induction free from apprehension and irritating vapors. Very rigid technique must be followed for proper preparation and administration of this form of anesthesia, and a careful test of the solution must first be made to insure freedom from irritating decomposition products.

In addition to its use as a basal anesthetic, Tribromoethanol is employed wherever prolonged, light anesthesia is desirable, as in *status asthmaticus*, and in certain convulsive disorders, particularly *tetanus, status epilepticus*, and *eclampsia*. Repeated rectal instillations may be required over a period of days.

Dose—*Usual, rectal,* **60 to 80 mg per Kg** of body weight, not to exceed **8 Gm** for woman, **10 Gm** for man.

Dosage Forms—Solution NF (see below.

Tribromoethanol Solution NF [Liquor Tribromoæthanolis; Tribromoethyl Alcohol Solution; Bromethol] is a solution of tribromoethanol in amylene hydrate. It contains, in each 100 ml, 95.0–105.0 Gm of $C_2H_3Br_3O$. *Preparation:* Dissolve tribromoethanol (100 Gm) in amylene hydrate (50 ml), and add sufficient amylene hydrate to make 100 ml. *Description:* A clear, colorless liquid with a camphor-like odor and a burning taste. A freshly prepared 1:40 aqueous solution is neutral to congo red at 40°. *Note: For administration of the Solution as an anesthetic, dilute the Tribromoethanol Solution just before use with warm purified water in the proportion of 2.5 ml of Solution to 100 ml of the dilution. Mix 5 ml of this dilution with 1 drop of congo red TS: it has the same color as a mixture of 5 ml of purified water and 1 drop of congo red TS.*

Other Basal Anesthetics

Fentanyl Citrate and Droperidol Injection [Innovar Injection (*McNeil*)]—*Uses:* Fentanyl citrate [Sublimaze (*McNeil*), 0.05 mg] and droperidol [Inapsine, 2.5 mg/ml] is employed as premedication for anesthesia and as an adjunct for induction and maintenance of anesthesia. It is also used as the only agent in diagnostic procedures such as arteriograms and pneumoencephalograms in which patient cooperation is desired. Fentanyl citrate is a narcotic analgesic with a profile of action similar to morphine, except it produces the same degree of analgesia with 1/150 the dose and is virtually devoid of emetic properties. Droperidol is a neuroleptic which produces general quiescence and decreased responsiveness to environmental stimuli. Fentanyl Citrate and Droperidol Injection is contraindicated in children under 2 years of age and in patients with bronchial asthma or myasthenia gravis. It should not be used in patients on MAO inhibitors. *Dose: Premedication, intramuscular,* 0.5 to 2 ml 45 to 60 minutes preoperatively; *induction, intravenous,* 1 ml per 20 to 25 pounds of body weight; *maintenance, intravenous,* 0.5 to 1 ml as indicated by changes in vital signs. *Dosage Forms:* 0.05 mg (fentanyl citrate) and 25 mg/ml (droperidol).

Hydroxydione Sodium Succinate [Viadril (*Pfizer*)] is 21-hydroxy-5β-pregnane-3,20-dione 21-sodium succinate. *Description and Solubility:* Fluffy white powder which decomposes between 193° and 203°. pH (2% aqueous solution): 8.5–9.8. Soluble in water, acetone, and chloroform. *Uses:* A steroid compound which produces central nervous system depression leading to *hypnosis* and *general anesthesia.* It is used intravenously as a *basal anesthetic* or for the induction of general anesthesia prior to maintenance with gaseous anesthetic agents. Induction is slow but smooth, and recovery is relatively free from nausea and vomiting. The drug exerts an amnesic effect. It provides little, if any, analgesia, does not effect glandular secretions, and only moderately relaxes skeletal muscle. The usual anesthetic dose produces little respiratory depression, but apnea, tachypnea, and hypotension may occur in some patients. Pain at the site of injection is frequently encountered. *Dose: Usual,* 25 ml of a 1% solution per minute administered into the tubing of a rapidly running intravenous solution (isotonic sodium chloride or 5% dextrose).

59 | Local Anesthetics

This chapter was prepared by

Ewart A. Swinyard, PhD, *Professor of Pharmacology, College of Pharmacy and College of Medicine, University of Utah, Salt Lake City, Utah 84112, and*
Stewart C. Harvey, PhD, *Associate Professor of Pharmacology, College of Medicine, University of Utah, Salt Lake City, Utah 84112*

Local anesthetics are drugs which produce a condition of anesthesia in a limited area around the site of application or injection of the drug. They are used to prevent pain in surgical procedure, injury, and disease. Methods of producing local anesthesia vary with the site of application and the technique of administration. Hence, local anesthetics may be divided into three general groups: (1) those which produce anesthesia through the production of cold, such as ether and ethyl chloride, (2) certain protoplasmic poisons such as phenol, and (3) those which specifically affect the sensory nerves or their endings, such as cocaine and the large number of synthetic anesthetics. Agents included in the first two groups are rarely used for local anesthesia today, but agents in the latter group have numerous local anesthetic applications.

The synthetic local anesthetic agents may be divided into two groups: the soluble compounds and the slightly soluble compounds. Only soluble compounds of relatively low toxicity should be injected.

Local anesthesia induced by injectable agents is designated according to the technique or anatomic site of the injection. *Infiltration anesthesia* refers to injection directly into the area that is painful or to be subjected to surgical trauma. *Nerve block anesthesia,* as the name implies, refers to injection in proximity to specific nerve trunks innervating a particular anatomic site. Particular nerve block injections are named according to the point chosen for interruption of nerve transmission. In *spinal anesthesia* the drug is injected within the dural membrane surrounding the spinal cord and the nerve roots. In *extradural* or *epidural anesthesia* the anesthetic solution is deposited immediately outside the dural membrane and within the bony spinal or caudal canals. Examples of the latter type are caudal or sacral anesthesia. Other nerve blocks such as paravertebral, conduction, and regional anesthesia, are designated according to their location along the course of nerve trunks or their way to peripheral tissues.

The insoluble local anesthetics (as well as many soluble agents) are used for surface (topical) application, since their slow absorption renders them safe for use on ulcers, wounds, and mucous surfaces. The anesthesia which they induce is not as complete as that induced by soluble compounds, but it is more lasting.

The mechanism by which local anesthetics induce their effect is not known for a certainty. It is generally agreed their action is to interfere with the initiation and transmission of the nerve impulse. Present theory holds that local anesthetics prevent the depolarization of the nerve membrane and, hence, the propagation of the impulse. This is thought to be due to interference with the mutual exchange of sodium and potassium ions across the membrane. As a consequence, a negative electric potential necessary for a propagated discharge does not develop. The possibility that certain local anesthetics may interrupt conduction by competitive inhibition of acetylcholine at receptor sites cannot be excluded.

When infiltration, conduction, or regional techniques are employed, both nerve fibers and nerve endings are anesthetized. The ease in which a nerve fiber may be anesthetized is related to its size. Small nerve fibers concerned with vasoconstriction, temperature, and surface pain are most easily anesthetized, whereas large fibers associated with the sensation of touch, pressure, deep pain, and the sensations from joints and tendons are anesthetized with more difficulty. In spinal anesthesia, it is probable that both sensory and motor nerve fibers are anesthetized. In surface (topical) anesthesia, the sensory nerve endings are the chief nerve structures affected.

The comparative potency and effectiveness of topical anesthetics in man have been studied by Adriani and Zepernick.[1] They found the order of decreasing duration of action of the topical agents, at the maximum effective concentration of each, to be: tetracaine, 1%; dibucaine, 0.5%; cocaine, 20%; dyclonine, 1%; lidocaine, 4%; piperocaine, 5%; pramoxine, 2%; and hexylcaine, 5%. Tetracaine, cocaine, and dibucaine were the most effective and longest lasting drugs in the entire series. Exceeding the maximum effective concentrations or mixing two drugs at their optimal dose levels neither enhanced the anesthesia nor prolonged the duration of action.

The speed of onset, the size of area affected, and the duration of local anesthesia may be markedly altered by the judicious use of certain adjuvant drugs. Hyaluronidase in combination with local anesthetic agents facilitates distribution of the anesthetic. Unless a vasoconstrictor agent is also employed, there is a more rapid absorption, shorter duration of anesthesia, and a higher rate of systemic reactions. Because of these disadvantages, hyaluronidase is seldom used today. Since local anesthetics produce paralysis of vasoconstrictor nerves, the injection of a local anesthetic solution is usually followed by vasodilation. For this reason a vasoconstrictor drug such as epinephrine hydrochloride is almost always added to local anesthetic solutions. Epinephrine in a concentration of not less than 1:200,000 and not more than 1:50,000 induces sufficient vasoconstriction to reduce the volume of solution required, prolong the duration of anesthesia, and lessen the danger of toxic reactions. Except for solutions to be used for spinal anesthesia and for solutions to be injected in the fingers and toes, epinephrine may be added to all local anesthetic solutions. Other vasoconstrictor agents less commonly employed include phenylephrine (1:2500 to 1:5000) and cobefrin (1:10,000 to 1:20,000).

All local anesthetics are toxic, and the tolerance of

patients varies. Safe dosage, therefore, is limited for each drug and must be individualized. Choice of drug, concentration, rate and site of injection, age, and emotional and physical status of the patient represent a few factors which must be considered. In general, the smallest amount of the least toxic drug that will serve the purpose should be used, if reactions are to be avoided. Premedication with a barbiturate is advisable to prevent or decrease toxic reactions. Many local anesthetics occasionally give rise to dermatitis. When this is severe, the use of the anesthetic should be discontinued.

Benzocaine NF

[Benzocaine; Anæsthesin; Anesthesin; Ethyl *p*-Aminobenzoate; Ethyl Aminobenzoate NF XI]

$$H_2N-\langle\ \rangle-COOC_2H_5$$

Benzocaine, dried over phosphorus pentoxide for 3 hours, contains 98.0–101.0% of $C_9H_{11}NO_2$ (165.19).

Preparation—*p*-Nitrobenzoic acid, obtained by nitration of toluene and oxidation of the resulting *p*-nitrotoluene, is converted into the ethyl ester by heating with alcohol and sulfuric acid. The resulting ethyl *p*-nitrobenzoate is treated with tin and hydrochloric acid. This reduces the nitro to the amino group. The crude product so obtained is recrystallized from alcohol.

Description—Small, white, odorless crystals or as a white crystalline powder. It melts between 88° and 92°, and it is stable in the air. It is decomposed by alkali hydroxides into the salt of the acid and alcohol. It exhibits local anesthetic properties when placed upon the tongue.

Solubility—1 Gm dissolves in about 2500 ml of water, 5 ml of alcohol, 2 ml of chloroform, 4 ml of ether, 30 to 50 ml of expressed almond oil or olive oil; also soluble in dilute mineral acids.

Incompatibilities—A soft or liquid mass is produced by trituration with *menthol, phenol, camphor,* or *resorcinol*. It is hydrolyzed by *alkalies* into alcohol and para-aminobenzoic acid salt. With a mixture of *acetylsalicylic acid* and *acetophenetidin,* it can produce a hard, black, shrunken mass; with either ingredient alone it appears to be stable. Ethyl aminobenzoate is but poorly soluble in water or glycerin in which it is sometimes prescribed; 30 to 50 parts of olive or almond oil dissolve it with the aid of gentle heat.

Since derivatives of para-aminobenzoic acid have an antisulfonamide action, ethyl aminobenzoate is contra-indicated during therapy with these agents.

Uses—Benzocaine is a *local anesthetic*. Its slight solubility renders it unsuitable for injection, but its slow absorption renders it safer than other anesthetics, especially for *ulcers, wounds,* and *mucous surfaces*. The anesthesia is usually not so complete as with the soluble local anesthetics but is more lasting.

It is employed for painful wounds, ulcers, etc, of the skin and accessible mucous membranes; for instance, after dental operations.

Dose—*Topically,* as a **1** to **20**% ointment to the skin.

Dosage Forms—Ointment NF: 1, 2.5, 5, 10, and 20%.

Benzyl Alcohol NF

[Phenylcarbinol]

$$\langle\ \rangle-CH_2OH$$

Benzyl Alcohol is phenylmethanol [C_7H_8O = 108.14].

Preparation—Benzyl Alcohol occurs in nature as the esters of benzoic and cinnamic acids in storax, Peruvian balsam, and tolu balsam. The product on the market is made synthetically from benzyl chloride [C_6H_5.CH_2Cl] by distilling it from an aqueous solution of potassium carbonate with thorough agitation.

Description—A colorless liquid with a sharp, burning taste and a faint aromatic odor. Its specific gravity is between 1.042 and 1.047 at 25°. It distils between 202.5° and 206.5°, and has a refractive index of 1.5385 to 1.5405. It boils without decomposition at about 206°. It slowly oxidizes in the air. Its aqueous solutions are neutral to litmus.

Solubility—1 Gm dissolves in about 30 ml of water, or 1.5 ml of diluted alcohol; miscible with alcohol, ether, and chloroform.

Identification—When 2 or 3 drops of Benzyl Alcohol are treated with potassium permanganate solution acidified with dilute sulfuric acid, it is quickly oxidized to benzaldehyde, recognizable by its characteristic almond-like odor.

Uses—Benzyl Alcohol is a *local anesthetic* by injection and by application to mucous membranes. By injection it is administered in a 1 to 4% solution. Externally it is applied as an ointment or as a lotion of equal parts of Benzyl Alcohol, ethyl alcohol, and water, to relieve cutaneous itching. It is also used as a *bacteriostatic agent* in various parenteral preparations.

Butethamine Hydrochloride NF

[2-(Isobutylamino)ethanol *p*-Aminobenzoate (Ester) Monohydrochloride; Monocaine Hydrochloride (*Phila. Pharm.*)]

$$\left[H_2N-\langle\ \rangle-COOCH_2CH_2\overset{+}{N}H_2CH_2CH(CH_3)_2\right]\ Cl^-$$

Butethamine Hydrochloride, dried at 105° for 2 hours, yields 98.5–100.5% of $C_{13}H_{20}N_2O_2\cdot HCl$ (272.78).

Preparation—Butethamine Hydrochloride may be prepared by causing *p*-nitrobenzoyl chloride to react with 2-(isobutylamino)ethanol, followed by stannous chloride reduction of the nitro group to amino, and then treatment with hydrochloric acid to form the hydrochloride.

Description—Small, white crystals or a white crystalline powder, odorless, stable in air. Exhibits local anesthetic properties when placed upon the tongue. Melts between 192° and 196°. The pH of a 1 in 100 solution is about 5.

Solubility—Sparingly soluble in water; slightly soluble in alcohol and chloroform; very slightly soluble in benzene; practically insoluble in ether.

Uses—Butethamine Hydrochloride is a *local anesthetic* similar to procaine in its applications but it is about one-third more anesthetic and toxic. For minor surgery *nerve block* a 1% solution, containing 1:75,000 epinephrine, is injected and for major surgery nerve block a 1.5% solution, containing 1:100,000 epinephrine, is used.

Dose—*Usual, local injection,* **1.8** to **2.2 ml** of a **1.5**% solution with epinephrine **1:100,000** or a **2**% solution with epinephrine **1:50,000.**

Dosage Forms—and Epinephrine Injection NF: 1% (butethamine hydrochloride) and 1:75,000 (epinephrine)/5 ml; 1.5% and 1:100,000/5 and 30 ml; 1.5% and 1:30,000/5 ml; 2% and 1:50,000/1.8, 2, 2.2, 2.5, 30, 60, and 125 ml.

Butyl Aminobenzoate NF

[*n*-Butyl *p*-Aminobenzoate; Butesin (*Abbott*)]

$$H_2N- C_6H_4 -\overset{O}{\underset{}{C}}-O-CH_2CH_2CH_2CH_3$$

Butyl aminobenzoate, dried over phosphorus pentoxide for 3 hours, contains 98.0–101.0% of $C_{11}H_{15}NO_2$ (193.25).

Preparation—It may be made by esterifying *p*-nitrobenzoic acid with *n*-butyl alcohol, then reducing the nitro group with stannous chloride or iron filings and hydrochloric acid.

Description—A white, odorless, and tasteless crystalline powder, melting between 57° and 59°. When boiled with water it slowly hydrolyzes into aminobenzoic acid and butyl alcohol: alkali hydroxides accelerate the hydrolysis.

Solubility—1 Gm dissolves in about 7000 ml of water; soluble in dilute acids, alcohol, chloroform, or ether and in fixed oils.

Incompatibilities—See *Benzocaine* (page 1066).

Uses—Butyl Aminobenzoate is a *local anesthetic* of low solubility used in the same manner and for the same purposes as *Benzocaine*. It is claimed to be more effective than the ethyl ester when applied to intact mucous membranes.

Chlorbutanol—see page 1317.

Chloroprocaine Hydrochloride NF

[2-(Diethylamino)ethyl 4-Amino-2-chlorobenzoate Monohydrochloride; Nesacaine Hydrochloride (*Strasenburgh*)]

$$\left[H_2N- C_6H_3(Cl) -COO-CH_2CH_2\overset{+}{N}H(C_2H_5)_2 \right] Cl^-$$

Chloroprocaine Hydrochloride contains 98.0–102.0% of $C_{13}H_{19}ClN_2O_2 \cdot HCl$ (307.22), calculated on the dried basis.

Preparation—2-Chloro-4-nitrobenzoic acid is reacted with thionyl chloride and the resulting acid chloride is condensed with 2-(diethylamino)ethanol. Reduction of the nitro ester with iron and acidulated water yields chloroprocaine base which may be converted into the hydrochloride by dissolving in a suitable solvent and introducing hydrogen chloride.

Description—White, crystalline powder. Is odorless and is stable in air. Its solutions are acid to litmus. Exhibits local anesthetic properties when placed on the tongue.

Solubility—1 Gm dissolves in about 20 ml of water and about 100 ml of alcohol; very slightly soluble in chloroform; practically insoluble in ether.

Uses—Chloroprocaine Hydrochloride is a local anesthetic agent similar in chemical structure and pharmacological action to the parent compound, procaine hydrochloride. It is more rapid in onset and has an anesthetic potency at least twice that of procaine. Its toxicity is low and qualitatively similar to procaine. It is used to produce anesthesia by techniques of infiltration, field block, and regional nerve block, including caudal and epidural block.

Dose—Up to **1 Gm** of **0.5 to 3%** solution; *usual, infiltration,* **100 ml** of **0.5%** solution; *peripheral nerve block,* **50 ml** of **1%** solution.

Other Dose Information—*Epidural,* 25 ml of 3% solution.

Dosage Forms—Injection NF: 300 and 600 mg/30 ml.

Clove Oil USP

[Oleum Caryophylli BP; Oil of Cloves]

Clove Oil is the volatile oil distilled with steam from the dried flower buds of *Eugenia caryophyllus* (Sprengel) Bullock et Harrison (formerly *E. caryophyllata* Thunberg) (Fam. *Myrtaceæ*). It contains not less than 85.0% by volume of total phenolic substances, chiefly eugenol ($C_{10}H_{12}O_2$).

Constituents—The chief constituent is the phenol *Eugenol* (page 1070) which occurs in amounts up to 85%, and is official in the USP. The odor of the Oil is modified by the presence of less than 1% of *methyl pentyl ketone*. Other constituents include about 3% of *aceteugenol*, a mixture of the sesquiterpenes α- and β-*caryophyllene*, and small amounts of *furfural, furfuryl alcohol, methyl heptyl ketone*, the methyl esters of *salicylic* and *benzoic acids*, the benzyl ester of *phenylacetic acid, vanillin*, and *caryophyllin* [$C_{30}H_{48}O_3$]. The percentage of eugenol present is regarded as an index to the Oil's quality.

Description—A colorless or pale yellow liquid, becoming darker and thicker by aging or exposure to the air, and having the characteristic odor and taste of clove. Specific gravity: 1.038 to 1.060 at 25°. Angular rotation: inactive, or does not exceed −1° 30′ in a 100-mm tube at 25°. Refractive index: 1.5270 to 1.5350 at 20°. The Oil is soluble in 2 volumes of 70% alcohol.

Uses—Clove Oil is a powerful *germicide* but is too irritant for most purposes. It is applied topically to alleviate toothache (see *Toothache Drops*, page 1076). It acts as an *obtundant*, relieving pain caused by an exposed dentine.

Dose—*Topically* to dental cavities, as required.

Cocaine NF

[Methyl 3β-Hydroxy-1αH,5αH-tropane-2β-carboxylate Benzoate (Ester); [Cocain; Cocaina; Methylbenzoylecgonine]

Cocaine, dried over phosphorus pentoxide for 3 hours, contains 99.0–101.0% of $C_{17}H_{21}NO_4$ (303.36).

Cocaine is an alkaloid obtained from the leaves of *Erythroxylon coca* Lamarck and other species of *Erythroxylon* Linné (Fam. *Erythroxylaceæ*), or by synthesis from ecgonine or its derivatives.

History—Cocaine was isolated by Gaedken in 1844 from Brazilian coca leaves and until two decades ago the latter was the only source of cocaine. Today the alkaloid is obtained principally from Java coca leaves. Brazilian coca leaves contain from 0.5 to 1% of methyl benzoyl ecgonine or cocaine, whereas the Java leaves contain very little cocaine as such. However, there are present in the latter such derivatives as benzoylecgonine, cinnamoylecgonine, methylecgonine, etc., to the extent of 1.5 to 2%, all of which are converted to cocaine in the manufacturing process. For the structural relationships among the ecgonine derivatives, see page 497.

Preparation—It may be made by moistening ground coca leaves with sodium carbonate solution, percolating with benzene or other solvents such as petroleum benzin, shaking the liquid with diluted sulfuric acid, and adding to the separated acid solution an excess of sodium carbonate. The precipitated alkaloids are removed with ether, and, after drying with sodium carbonate, the solution is filtered and the ether distilled off. The residue is dissolved in methyl alcohol and the solution heated with sulfuric acid or with alcoholic hydrogen chloride. This treatment splits off any acids from the ecgonine and esterifies the carboxyl group. After dilution with water, the organic acids which have been liberated are removed with chloroform. The aqueous solution is then concentrated, neutralized, and cooled with ice, whereupon methylecgonine sulfate crystallizes. This is now benzoylated by heating with benzoyl chloride or benzoic anhydride at about 150°C. Upon adding water and sodium hydroxide, methyl benzoyl ecgonine or cocaine is precipitated. The cocaine is extracted with ether and the solution concentrated to crystallization. For the purification of cocaine, recrystallization from a mixture of acetone and benzene is generally preferred.

The total synthesis has been accomplished.[2]

Description—Colorless to white crystals, or a white, crystalline powder. It is odorless. It melts between 96° and 98° and its solution in diluted hydrochloric acid is levorotatory. Its saturated solution is alkaline to litmus.

Solubility—1 Gm dissolves in about 600 ml of water, 7 ml of alcohol, 1 ml of chloroform, 3.5 ml of ether, about 12 ml of olive oil, and from 80 to 100 ml of liquid petrolatum; very soluble in warm alcohol.

Incompatibilities—Moisture absorbed by cocaine causes cloudiness in liquid petrolatum solutions. The alkaloid can be dried over sulfuric acid in a suitable desiccator or it can be heated carefully on a water bath. Cocaine and its salts have the general incompatibilities of the *alkaloids* (page 491).

Uses—Cocaine was the first local anesthetic to be discovered. At present it is considered too toxic for any anesthetic procedure requiring injection,[3] but it is still employed for anesthesia of the nose and throat. For this purpose a 10% solution of the hydrochloride is employed. It is also used for corneal anesthesia, but many substitutes are superior.

Cocaine is a central stimulant, but is never employed clinically for this purpose. Cortical stimulation from Cocaine is of such a nature as to be indulged in licentiously by certain individuals. Addiction and a certain amount of tolerance result. Because of these properties, the sale of Cocaine and its salts is regulated by the *Harrison Narcotic Act.*

Dose—*Topical,* to mucous membrane as a 1% solution.

Cocaine Hydrochloride USP

[Methyl 3β-Hydroxy-1αH,5αH-tropan-2β-carboxylate Benzoate (Ester) Monohydrochloride; Neurocaine Hydrochloride]

Cocaine Hydrochloride contains 99.0–101.0% of $C_{17}H_{21}NO_4 \cdot HCl$ (339.82), calculated on the dried basis.

For the structure of cocaine, see page 1067.

Preparation—It may be made by adding cocaine to an alcoholic solution of hydrochloric acid and crystallizing.

Description—Colorless crystals or a white crystalline powder; usually it is odorless. It has a specific rotation of −71° to −73° in water (200 mg per 10 ml).

Solubility—1 Gm is soluble in 0.5 ml of water, 3.5 ml of alcohol, and 15 ml of chloroform; soluble in glycerin and insoluble in ether.

Incompatibilities—Cocaine Hydrochloride has the general incompatibilities of the alkaloidal salts (page 491). The free alkaloid is liberated by *sodium borate;* use of boric acid avoids precipitation. With *silver nitrate* a precipitate of silver chloride is formed.

Uses—Cocaine Hydrochloride is used in solution as a *local anesthetic* when applied to the mucous membrane or injected hypodermically; it is also a cerebral stimulant. See *Cocaine.*

Dose—*Topically,* as a 2 to 10% solution to mucous membranes.

Dosage Forms—Solution: 2 to 10%; Tablets NF: 8 and 15 mg.

Cyclomethycaine Sulfate

[Surfacaine (*Lilly*)]

Cyclomethycaine Sulfate is 2-methyl-1-piperidine-propanol *p*-(cyclohexyloxy)benzoate sulfate (2:1).

Description—White, odorless, crystalline powder.

Solubility—Sparingly soluble in water, alcohol, chloroform, and isopropyl alcohol; very slightly soluble in acetone, ether, and dilute acids.

Uses—Cyclomethycaine Sulfate is an effective topical anesthetic for use in thermal and chemical burns; in proctology; dermatological lesions, sunburn and skin abrasions; in urology, obstetrics, gynecology, and anesthetic procedures. As with all topical anesthetic agents, Cyclomethycaine Sulfate carries a slight but predictable sensitizing potential when utilized on patients with allergies or in conditions of prolonged use.

Dose—*Topically,* 0.25 to 1.0% in suitable form.

Dosage Forms—Jelly: 0.75%; Ointment: 0.5 and 1%; Suppositories (rectal or vaginal): 10 mg.

Dibucaine NF

[2-Butoxy-*N*-[2-(diethylamino)ethyl]cinchoninamide]

Dibucaine contains 97.0–100.5% of $C_{20}H_{29}N_3O_2$ (343.47), calculated on the dried basis.

Preparation—Dibucaine is prepared by the following series of reactions which begins with the readily available isatin:

Isatin   *N*-Acetylisatin

2-Hydroxycinchoninic Acid   2-Chlorocinchoninoyl Chloride

$$\underset{asym\text{-Diethylethylenediamine}}{(C_2H_5)_2NCH_2CH_2NH_2} \longrightarrow$$

CONHCH$_2$CH$_2$N(C$_2$H$_5$)$_2$

**2-Chloro-*N*-[2-(diethylamino)ethyl]
cinchoninamide**

CONHCH$_2$CH$_2$N(C$_2$H$_5$)$_2$

$$\underset{\text{Sodium Butoxide}}{NaOCH_2CH_2CH_2CH_3}$$

OCH$_2$CH$_2$CH$_2$CH$_3$

Dibucaine

The rearrangement of *N*-acetylisatin with alkali to the quinoline compound is known as the *Pfitzinger reaction*. The introduction of the diamine grouping is carried out at room temperature in order to avoid reaction with the less reactive 2-chloro-substituent.

Isatin may be readily prepared by oxidizing indigo with sodium dichromate in the presence of sulfuric acid.

Description—A colorless or almost colorless powder. Odorless, somewhat hygroscopic, and darkens on exposure to light. It melts between 62° and 65°.

Solubility—Soluble in 1 *N* hydrochloric acid and ether; slightly soluble in water.

Uses—See *Dibucaine Hydrochloride*.

Dose—*Topically*, as a **0.5**% cream or a **1**% ointment several times a day.

Dosage Forms—Cream NF: 0.5%; Ointment NF: 1%.

Dibucaine Hydrochloride USP

[2-Butoxy-*N*-[2-(diethylamino)ethyl]cinchoninamide Monohydrochloride; Cinchocaine Hydrochloride; Percaine; Nupercaine Hydrochloride (*Ciba*)]

N—OCH$_2$CH$_2$CH$_2$CH$_3$

Cl$^-$

O=C—NH—CH$_2$CH$_2$NH(C$_2$H$_5$)$_2$

Dibucaine Hydrochloride contains 97.0–100.5% of C$_{20}$H$_{29}$N$_3$O$_2$.HCl (379.93), calculated on the dried basis.

Preparation—Dibucaine base is dissolved in an appropriate organic solvent or solvent mixture and precipitated with a stream of hydrogen chloride.

Description—Colorless or white crystals, or a white, crystalline powder. Odorless, somewhat hygroscopic, and darkens on exposure to light. Its solutions are acid to litmus, pH of 5 to 6. Melts between 95° and 100°. It has a bitter, acrid taste and exhibits a prolonged anesthetic action when applied to the tongue.

Solubility—1 Gm dissolves in about 2 ml of water; freely soluble in alcohol, acetone, and chloroform; only slightly soluble in cold benzene, ethyl acetate, and toluene.

Uses—Dibucaine Hydrochloride is the most potent, most toxic, and longest acting of the commonly employed *local anesthetics*. It acts like cocaine when applied to mucous membranes but is several times more active. It acts like procaine or cocaine when injected, but is many times more active than procaine when injected subcutaneously and about 5 times more toxic than cocaine when injected intravenously. For *infiltration anesthesia*, 1:1000 to 1:2000 solutions (not more than 50 ml of a 1:1000 solution) are injected. As a *spinal anesthetic*, not more than 7.5 to 10 mg is administered in a 1:1500 solution. In *sacral anesthesia*, 25 to 35 ml of a 1:1000 solution is given.

Dose—*Subarachnoid*, **5** to **18 ml** of a **0.067**% (1 in 1500) solution, or **0.5** to **2 ml** of a **0.5**% (1 in 200) solution; *usual*, **10 ml** of a **0.067**% (1 in 1500) solution or **1.5 ml** of a **0.5**% (1 in 200) solution.

Dosage Forms—Injection USP: 0.5% (1:200)/2 ml, 0.067% (1:1500)/20 ml.

Dimethisoquin Hydrochloride NF

[3-Butyl-1-[2-(dimethylamino)ethoxy]isoquinoline Monohydrochloride; Quotane (*SK&F*)]

OCH$_2$CH$_2$NH(CH$_3$)$_2$

Cl$^-$

CH$_2$CH$_2$CH$_2$CH$_3$

Dimethisoquin Hydrochloride, dried at 105° for 2 hours, contains 98.0–101.0% of C$_{17}$H$_{24}$N$_2$O.HCl (308.85).

Preparation—A solution of α-*n*-butylphenethylamine (I) in an organic solvent is reacted with phosgene to form α-butylphenethyl isocyanate (II) which, upon heating with anhydrous aluminum chloride, cyclizes through rearrangement to produce 3-*n*-butyl-3,4-dihydro-1(2*H*)-isoquinolone (III). Catalytic dehydrogenation of (III) at the 3,4-positions followed by reaction of phosphorus oxychloride on the lactim form of the dehydrogenated compound (IV) yields 3-*n*-butyl-1-chloroisoquinoline (V). Condensation of V with β-dimethylaminoethanol (VI) is then effected by treating a solution of the two compounds in an inert organic solvent with metallic sodium. The crude dimethisoquin base thus formed is purified by distillation under reduced pressure, dissolved in a suitable organic solvent, and reacted with an equimolar portion of hydrogen chloride to produce the official salt.

NH$_2$

CH$_2$—CH—C$_4$H$_9$

I

O=C=N

CH$_2$—CH—C$_4$H$_9$

II

O

NH

C$_4$H$_9$

III

OH

N

C$_4$H$_9$

IV

Cl

N

C$_4$H$_9$

V

HOCH$_2$CH$_2$N(CH$_3$)$_2$

VI

Description—It occurs as a white to off-white, colorless, crystalline powder. Melting range 144° to 148°. pH 3.5 to 5.0.

Solubility—1 Gm dissolves in about 8 ml of water, 2 ml of chloroform, and 3 ml of alcohol; very slightly soluble in ether.

Uses—Dimethisoquin hydrochloride is a surface anesthetic which is used topically in a 0.5% lotion or ointment for the relief of itching, irritation, burning or pain in dermatoses, including nonspecific pruritus, and mild sunburn. Its lack of systemic toxicity and low index of sensitization permit the drug's unsupervised use as a topical remedy for symptomatic relief of simple irritations which accompany undiagnosed minor skin conditions.

Dose—*Topically*, to the skin as a **0.5**% ointment or lotion 2 to 4 times a day.

Dosage Forms—Lotion NF: 0.5%; Ointment NF: 0.5%.

Dyclonine Hydrochloride USP

[4'-Butoxy-3-piperidinopropiophenone Hydrochloride; Dyclone (*Pitman-Moore*)]

Dyclonine Hydrochloride contains 98.0–102.0% of $C_{18}H_{27}NO_2 \cdot HCl$ (325.88), calculated on the dried basis.

Preparation—*p*-Hydroxyacetophenone is reacted with butyl bromide in a basic environment to produce the corresponding butoxy compound. This is then reacted with piperidine hydrochloride and formaldehyde in an organic solvent under acidic conditions. US Pat. 2,771,391 and 2,868,689.

Description—White crystals or white, crystalline powder, which may have a slight odor. It exhibits local anesthetic effect when placed on the tongue.

Solubility—Soluble in water, acetone, alcohol, and chloroform.

Uses—Dyclonine Hydrochloride is an effective topical anesthetic. The onset, intensity, and duration of action is similar to that of other topical anesthetics. Dyclonine Hydrochloride is used to allay the pain associated with certain examinations and surgical procedures in dermatology, ophthalmology, urology, proctology, otolaryngology, dentistry, and radiology. It is also used for the relief of itching in dermatology, proctology, and gynecology. When instilled into the conjunctival sac, it induces anesthesia without miosis or mydriasis. Dyclonine Hydrochloride also has antimicrobial properties. The clinical significance of this property has not been determined.

Dose—*Topically*, as a **0.5** to **1**% solution, to the mucous membranes.

Dosage Forms—Solution USP: 0.5 and 1%.

Ethyl Chloride—see page 1057.

Eugenol USP

[Synthetic Clove Oil; 4-Allyl-2-methoxyphenol]

Eugenol [$C_{10}H_{12}O_2 = 164.21$] is obtained from clove oil and from other sources.

Preparation—Eugenol is found in the volatile oils from clove, pimenta, bay leaves, Ceylon cinnamon, camphor, sassafras, massoy bark, canella, culilawan, and other oils. It is principally obtained, however, from clove oil. The oil is treated with an excess of sodium hydroxide solution which dissolves the Eugenol and the mixture is then shaken with ether to remove the other constituents. The aqueous solution of sodium

eugenol is treated with hydrochloric acid, and the separated Eugenol is purified by repeated washing.

Description—A colorless or pale yellow liquid, having a strongly aromatic odor of clove and a pungent, spicy taste. Exposure to air causes it to become darker and thicker. Eugenol is optically inactive. Its specific gravity is 1.064 to 1.070. Its refractive index is 1.5400 to 1.5420 at 20°. Eugenol distils between 250° and 255°.

Solubility—Slightly soluble in water; miscible with alcohol, chloroform, ether, and fixed oils; soluble in twice its volume of 70% alcohol.

Uses—Eugenol is a *dental obtundent* and *topical anesthetic* used extensively to replace clove oil, principally by dentists, who also employ it for its disinfectant action in filling root canals (see *Zinc–Eugenol Cement*, page 1377). Eugenol is only rarely administered internally. It is the basic material in one of the processes for the production of vanillin.

Dose—*Topically*, in dental protectives, (eg, *Zinc Oxide Paste*, page 772).

Hexylcaine Hydrochloride NF

[1-(Cyclohexylamino)-2-propanol Benzoate (Ester) Hydrochloride; Cyclaine (*MSD*)]

Hexylcaine Hydrochloride, dried in vacuum over phosphorus pentoxide for 4 hours, contains 98.0–102.0% of $C_{16}H_{23}NO_2 \cdot HCl$ (297.83).

Preparation—A solution of 1-(cyclohexylamino)-2-propanol (I) in a mixed solvent composed of benzene and tetrachloroethane is treated with benzoyl chloride. Esterification and salt formation occur simultaneously. (I) may be prepared by causing cyclohexylamine to undergo either addition to propylene oxide or condensation with α-propylene chlorohydrin.

Description—A white powder, possessing a bitter taste and not more than a slight aromatic odor. Melting range 182° to 184°. The pH of a 1 in 20 solution is between 4.0 and 6.0.

Solubility—1 Gm dissolves in about 17 ml of water; freely soluble in alcohol and chloroform; practically insoluble in ether.

Uses—Hexylcaine Hydrochloride is a soluble all-purpose local anesthetic agent. It is employed for infiltration anesthesia in a concentration of 1%; for nerve block anesthesia in 1 and 2% solution; for single-dose spinal anesthesia in a 2.5% solution containing 10% dextrose; and for topical application to the skin and mucous membranes, in a concentration of 1 to 5%. When used locally, it is as potent as an equal concentration of cocaine; when used for infiltration and nerve block anesthesia, it is faster and longer acting than an equal concentration of procaine. Hexylcaine Hydrochloride shares the toxic potentialities of other local anesthetic agents and should be employed with the same care and in accordance with established techniques of administration.

Dose—*Topically* or by *injection* according to site and condition.

Dosage Forms—Injection NF: 1%/30, 50, and 100 ml, 2%/20 ml, 2.5% (with 10% dextrose)/2 ml; Solution NF: 5%.

Veterinary Use—Topical, infiltration, nerve block and spinal anesthesia of longer duration than that from procaine hydrochloride.

Veterinary Dose—5% solution for *topical* use; 1% for infiltration and nerve block; **2.5**% with **10**% glucose for spinal anesthesia; **1** or **2**% solution for topical anesthesia of cornea.

Isobucaine Hydrochloride NF

[2-(Isobutylamino)-2-methyl-1-propanol Benzoate (Ester) Hydrochloride]

Isobucaine Hydrochloride, dried at 105° for 4 hours, contains 98.0–102.0% of $C_{15}H_{23}NO_2.HCl$ (285.82).

Preparation—2-(Isobutylamino)-2-methyl-1-propanol is condensed with benzoyl chloride in toluene solution with the aid of sodium hydroxide. The toluene layer is separated, washed, dried, and diluted with isopropyl alcohol. Introduction of HCl gas precipitates the final compound.

Description—Occurs as a white, odorless, crystalline solid.

Solubility—Freely soluble in water, alcohol, and chloroform; sparingly soluble in 2-propanol; very slightly soluble in ether.

Uses—Isobucaine, a *local anesthetic* used primarily in *dentistry*, is similar in chemical structure to meprylcaine. Like the latter, Isobucaine is several times more toxic and exhibits a shorter duration of action than procaine. It has a rapid onset of action (1 to 4 minutes) and a duration of 2 to 2½ hours, unaccompanied by side effects.

For infiltration, 1 ml of a 2% solution is used with epinephrine 1:65,000; for nerve block, 1.5 to 1.8 ml is used.

Dosage Forms—and Epinephrine Injection NF: 2% (isobucaine hydrochloride) and 1:65,000 (epinephrine)/1.8 ml.

Lidocaine USP

[2-(Diethylamino)-2′,6′-acetoxylidide; Xylocaine (*Astra*)]

Lidocaine contains 99.0–101.0% of $C_{14}H_{22}N_2O$ (234.34), calculated on the dried basis.

Preparation—Lidocaine may be prepared by chloroacetylation of 2,6-xylidine and condensing the resulting chloroacetoxylidide with diethylamine.

Description—A white or slightly yellow, crystalline powder, with a characteristic odor. Stable in air. Melts between 66° and 69°.

Solubility—Very soluble in alcohol and chloroform; freely soluble in benzene and ether; practically insoluble in water; dissolves in oils.

Uses—Lidocaine is a potent *local anesthetic* with a potency about twice that of an equal concentration of procaine. Lidocaine has approximately the same toxicity as procaine when injected subcutaneously as a 0.5% solution, but as the concentration is increased, its toxicity exceeds that of procaine; at 2%, it is 50% more toxic. Systemic side reactions and local irritant effects are few. Nausea and vomiting, muscular twitching, and chills have been observed.

Lidocaine is employed for *infiltration anesthesia* in a concentration of 0.5%; for *nerve block*, in a concentration of 1.0 and 2.0%; for *peridural anesthesia* in a concentration of 0.6 to 1.5%; and for *saddle block anesthesia* in a concentration of 5% made hyperbaric with 7.5% dextrose. Lidocaine is also used topically on mucous membranes as a 1 to 4% aqueous solution or 2% jelly, and on minor burns, abrasions, and anorectal lesions as a 2.5 or 5.0% ointment. The drug may be combined with epinephrine to delay absorption, prolong its action, and reduce its toxic effects. Because it is also effective without a vasoconstrictor, it appears to be the anesthetic of choice for use in those individuals who are sensitive to epinephrine and its congeners. In addition, it is so dissimilar in chemical structure to procaine and related local anesthetics that it is the agent of choice in individuals sensitive to procaine.

Clinical experience shows Lidocaine also to be an effective and safe antiarrhythmic for use in cardiac surgery. It causes less vasodepression than procainamide. For this purpose it is usually given in a dose of 1 to 2 mg per kg intravenously.

Dose—*Topically*, as a **2.5** to **5**% ointment or a solution to mucous membranes.

Dosage Forms—Ointment USP: 2.5 and 5%.

Lidocaine Hydrochloride USP

[2-(Diethylamino)-2′,6′-acetoxylidide Monohydrochloride; Lignocaine Hydrochloride BP; Xylocaine Hydrochloride (*Astra*)]

Lidocaine Hydrochloride [$C_{14}H_{22}N_2O.HCl.H_2O$ = 288.82] contains 99.0–101.0% of $C_{14}H_{22}N_2O.HCl$ (270.81), calculated on the anhydrous basis.

For the structure and preparation of the base, see *Lidocaine*.

Description—White, odorless, crystalline powder, having a slightly bitter taste.

Solubility—Very soluble in water and alcohol; soluble in chloroform; insoluble in ether.

Uses—See *Lidocaine*.

Dose—*Infiltration, peripheral nerve block,* or *epidural*, up to **60 ml** (100 ml with epinephrine), as a **0.5**% solution; up to **27 ml** (45 ml with epinephrine), as a **1**% solution; up to **20 ml** (33 ml with epinephrine), as a **2**% solution. *Usual, infiltration,* **50 ml** of a **0.5**% solution. *Usual, peripheral nerve block,* **25 ml** of a **1.5**% solution. *Usual, epidural,* **15** to **25 ml** of a **1.5**% solution. *Topically,* up to **250 mg** as a 2 to 4% solution or as a **2**% jelly, to mucous membranes.

Dosage Forms—Injection USP: 0.5%/50 ml, 1%/2, 5, 20, 50, and 100 ml, 1.5%/20 and 30 ml, 2%/2, 10, 20, and 50 ml, 4%/5 ml; Jelly USP; 2%; Ointment: 2.5 and 5%; Suppositories: 0.1 Gm; Viscous: 2%.

Menthol Ointment, Compound—see RPS-13, page 542.

Mepivacaine Hydrochloride NF

[(±)-1-Methyl-2′,6′-pipecoloxylidide Monohydrochloride; Carbocaine Hydrochloride (*Winthrop*)]

Mepivacaine Hydrochloride, dried at 105° for 4 hours, contains 98.0–102.0% of $C_{15}H_{22}N_2O.HCl$ (282.82).

Preparation—Picolinic acid (2-pyridinecarboxylic acid) is condensed with 2,6-xylidine to yield 2',6'-picolinoxylidide which is then reacted with dimethyl sulfate in xylene solution. Platinum catalyzed hydrogenation of the quaternary compound in acetic acid solution followed by alkalinization yields mepivacaine base which is then dissolved in an inert solvent and reacted with an equimolar quantity of HCl.

Description—Occurs as a white, odorless, crystalline solid.

Solubility—Freely soluble in water and methanol; very slightly soluble in chloroform; practically insoluble in ether.

Uses—Mepivacaine Hydrochloride is a local anesthetic employed for infiltration, nerve block, peridural, and caudal anesthesia. Its usefulness as a topical anesthetic has not been established. Mepivacaine Hydrochloride has an action similar to *Lidocaine;* hence, it is approximately twice as potent as procaine. However, its duration of action is considerably longer than lidocaine, even without epinephrine. Thus, Mepivacaine Hydrochloride is particularly indicated in circumstances in which epinephrine is contraindicated.

Dose—[*Infiltration and nerve block,* not to exceed **20 ml of 1 or 2% Mepivacaine** in sterile saline. For *caudal and peridural,* **15 to 30 ml of 1%, 10 to 25 ml of 1.5%,** or **10 to 20 ml of a 2% Mepivacaine** in modified Ringer's solution: unofficial.]

Dosage Forms—Injection NF: 3%/1.8 ml, 1 and 1.5%/30 ml, 2%/20 ml, 1 and 2%/50 ml; and Levonordefrin Injection NF: 2% (mepivacaine hydrochloride) and 1:20,000 (levonordefrin)/1.8 and 20 ml.

Meprylcaine Hydrochloride NF

[2-Methyl-2-(propylamino)-1-propanol Benzoate (Ester) Hydrochloride]

Meprylcaine Hydrochloride, dried in a vacuum desiccator over phosphorus pentoxide for 6 hours, contains 98.5–101.5% of $C_{14}H_{21}NO_2 \cdot HCl$ (271.79).

Preparation—Meprylcaine Hydrochloride may be prepared from 2-methyl-2-(propyalmino)-1-propanol by direct benzoylation as described above for Hexylcaine Hydrochloride. Among other ways, the 2-methyl-2-(propylamino)-1-propanol may be prepared by the interaction of isobutylene oxide [2-methyl-1,2-epoxypropane) and propylamine.

Description—It occurs as a white, odorless, crystalline solid. Melting range 150° to 152°. The pH of a solution (1 to 50) is about 5.7.

Solubility—Freely soluble in water, alcohol, and chloroform; slightly soluble in acetone.

Uses—Meprylcaine hydrochloride, a local anesthetic used primarily in dentistry, has a potency substantially greater than that of procaine. The drug is rapidly destroyed and, hence, the anesthesia induced is of relatively short duration. Acute toxicity is similar to that of procaine.

Dose—[*Infiltration* and *nerve block,* **1 to 2 ml** of a 2% solution with 1:50,000 epinephrine: unofficial.]

Dosage Forms—and Epinephrine Injection NF: 2% (meprylcaine hydrochloride) and 1:50,000 (epinephrine)/2, 2.5, and 20 ml.

Metabutethamine Hydrochloride NF

[2-(Isobutylamino)ethanol *m*-Aminobenzoate (Ester) Monohydrochloride]

Metabutethamine Hydrochloride, dried in a vacuum desiccator over phosphorus pentoxide for 6 hours, contains 98.5–100.5% of $C_{13}H_{20}N_2O_2 \cdot HCl$ (272.78).

Preparation—Metabutethamine Hydrochloride, a position isomer of Butethamine Hydrochloride, is prepared as described previously for the latter using *m*-nitrobenzoyl chloride instead of the *p*-compound.

Description—It occurs as a white, odorless, crystalline solid. Melting range 181° to 184°. The pH of a solution (1 in 50) is about 6.0.

Solubility—Soluble in water; slightly soluble in alcohol, acetone, and chloroform.

Uses—Metabutethamine hydrochloride is a local anesthetic used primarily in dentistry. A 3.8% solution of metabutethamine hydrochloride with epinephrine is somewhat more potent than a 2% solution of procaine, but the anesthesia is of relatively short duration. On a weight basis, the drug is considerably less toxic than procaine when the two drugs are administered by the subcutaneous or intraperitoneal route, but equally toxic when they are administered by intravenous injection.

Dose—[*Infiltration* and *nerve block,* **1 to 2 ml** of a **3.8%** solution with 1:60,000 epinephrine: unofficial.]

Dosage Forms—and Epinephrine Injection NF: 3.8% (metabutethamine hydrochloride) and 1:60,000 (epinephrine)/2 and 30 ml.

Peppermint Oil—see page 1331.

Phenacaine Hydrochloride NF

[*N,N'*-Bis(*p*-ethoxyphenyl)acetamidine Monohydrochloride; Holocaine Hydrochloride]

Phenacaine Hydrochloride [$C_{18}H_{22}N_2O_2 \cdot HCl \cdot H_2O = 352.86$], dried at 105° for 6 hours, yields 98.0–102.0% of $C_{18}H_{22}N_2O_2 \cdot HCl$ (334.85).

Preparation—Among other methods, it may be prepared by condensing phenetidin with acetophenetidin, using phosphorus oxychloride as the condensing agent.

Description—Small, white, odorless crystals or crystalline powder. It has a faintly bitter taste, producing transient numbness of the tongue, and is stable in air. The melting temperature of the dried substance is not below 190°.

Solubility—1 Gm dissolves in 50 ml of water; freely soluble in alcohol or chloroform; insoluble in ether.

Incompatibilities—This substance is precipitated by *alkaloidal precipitants* and by *alkalies.* The alkalinity of a soft glass container may be sufficient to cause precipitation of the base from aqueous solutions of Phenacaine Hydrochloride.

Uses—Phenacaine Hydrochloride is one of the oldest of the synthetic *local anesthetics.* It is used in a 1% solution mainly for producing local *anesthesia of the eye.*

It is slightly irritating. Therefore, anesthesia is preceded by some smarting and discomfort.

Dose—To the conjunctiva as a **1**% solution or as a **1** to **2**% ointment.

Dosage Forms—Ophthalmic Solution: **1**%.

Pramoxine Hydrochloride NF

[4-[3-(*p*-Butoxyphenoxy)propyl]morpholine Hydrochloride;   Tronothane (*Abbott*)]

Pramoxine Hydrochloride, dried at 105° for 1 hour, contains 98.0–100.5% of $C_{17}H_{27}NO_3 \cdot HCl$ (329.87).

Preparation—An aqueous mixture of 4-(3-chloropropyl)morpholine and *p*-butoxyphenol is refluxed until the condensation is complete. The reaction mixture is then cooled and the pramoxine (base) is extracted with benzene. After evaporation of the benzene, the base may be purified by distillation, dissolved in a suitable solvent, and converted to the hydrochloride by means of a stream of hydrogen chloride.

Description—A white to nearly white, crystalline powder, having a numbing taste. It may have a slight aromatic odor. The pH of a 1 in 100 solution is about 4.5. Melting range 169° to 172°.

Solubility—1 Gm is soluble in about 35 ml of chloroform; freely soluble in alcohol and water; very slightly soluble in ether.

Uses—Pramoxine hydrochloride is a surface anesthetic which has low indices of sensitization and toxicity, and is unrelated structurally to the procaine-type drugs. It is applied locally in a **1**% concentration for the relief from discomfort and pain in hemorrhoids and rectal surgery, episiotomies, anogenital pruritus, itching dermatoses, certain intubation procedures, moderate burns and sunburn. It is too irritating to be used in the eye.

Dose—*Topically,* as a **1**% cream or jelly every 3 to 4 hours.

Dosage Forms—Cream NF: **1**%; Jelly NF: **1**%.

Prilocaine Hydrochloride NF

[2-(Propylamino)-*o*-propionotoluidide Monohydrochloride;   Citanest Hydrochloride (*Astra*)]

Prilocaine Hydrochloride contains 99.0–101.0% of $C_{13}H_{20}N_2O \cdot HCl$ (256.78), calculated on the dried basis.

Preparation—*o*-Toluidine is condensed with 2-bromopropionyl bromide and the resulting 2-bromo-*o*-propionotoluidide is in turn condensed with propylamine to yield prilocaine (base). An acetone solution of the base treated with hydrogen chloride yields the official salt. Brit. Pat. 839,943.

Description—White, odorless, crystalline powder having an initially acidic and then bitter taste. It is stable in light and air. It melts between 167° and 168°.

Solubility—Freely soluble in water and alcohol; slightly soluble in chloroform; very slightly soluble in acetone; practically insoluble in ether.

Uses—Prilocaine Hydrochloride, an agent chemically similar to lidocaine and mepivacaine, is used for *local* and *regional-block anesthesia.* In a concentration of 1% to 3% its onset of action and effectiveness are said to be equivalent to lidocaine and mepivacaine in a 1% to 2% concentration. Its duration of action is intermediate to the shorter-acting lidocaine and the longer-acting mepivacaine. Prilocaine Hydrochloride is used in infiltration anesthesia, therapeutic nerve blocks such as intercostal and paravertebral blocks, regional anesthesia such as brachial plexus and sciatic-femoral blocks, and blockade of major nerve trunks via the peridural and caudal routes. Prilocaine Hydrochloride solutions are used without epinephrine. Hence, they are particularly useful for patients who cannot tolerate vasopressor agents; eg, patients with hypertension, diabetes, thyrotoxicosis, or other cardiovascular disorders. Except for methemoglobinemia, side effects are similar to those observed with other local anesthetics. Prilocaine Hydrochloride has been shown capable of inducing methemoglobinemia in laboratory animals and in man. When methemoglobinemia occurs, it can be reversed by the intravenous injection of methylene blue (1 mg/kg). As with other local anesthetics, Prilocaine Hydrochloride is contraindicated in the presence of shock, severe cardiovascular disease, or heart block.

Dose—*Usual, therapeutic nerve block,* **3** to **5 ml** of a **1** or **2**% solution; *infiltration,* **20** to **30 ml** of a **1** or **2**% solution; *regional anesthesia, peridural and caudal,* **15** to **20 ml** of a **3**% solution or **20** to **30 ml** of a **1** or **2**% solution; *infiltration* and *nerve block in dentistry,* **0.5** to **5.0 ml** of a **4**% solution.

Dosage Forms—Injection NF: **1** and **2**%/30 ml, **3**%/20 ml, **4**%/1.8 ml.

Procaine Hydrochloride USP

[Ethocaine; Procaine; Syncaine; 2-(Diethylamino)ethyl *p*-Aminobenzoate Monohydrochloride; Novocaine (*Winthrop*)]

Procaine Hydrochloride contains 99.0–101.0% of $C_{13}H_{20}N_2O_2 \cdot HCl$ (272.78), calculated on the dried basis.

Preparation—This local anesthetic is produced by the following process: 2-(diethylamino)ethanol is made by reacting ethylene chlorohydrin or bromohydrin with diethylamine. The diethylaminoethanol is then heated with *p*-nitrobenzoyl chloride forming diethylaminoethyl-*p*-nitrobenzoate. The NO_2 group is reduced with iron or tin and hydrochloric acid.

Description—Small, white, odorless crystals or a white crystalline powder. It melts between 153° and 156°. It is stable in air and its aqueous solution is acid to litmus. It exhibits local anesthetic properties when placed on the tongue. Procaine is readily differentiated from cocaine by the fact that its solution, acidulated with dilute sulfuric acid, decolorizes permanganate solution while cocaine does not decolorize it.

Solubility—1 Gm dissolves in 1 ml of water or 15 ml of alcohol; slightly soluble in chloroform; practically insoluble in ether.

Incompatibilities—*Alkaloidal reagents* including solutions of iodine and mercuric chloride cause a precipitation and *alkalies* liberate insoluble procaine base. Because of its relationship to *p*-aminobenzoic acid, a known inhibitor of sulfa drug activity, procaine is contraindicated during *sulfa drug* therapy.

Uses—Procaine Hydrochloride is one of the least toxic and most widely employed of the *local anesthetics*. It is not very effective when applied to mucous membranes, but is used extensively for *infiltration, nerve block,* and *spinal anesthesia*. It owes its popularity to several factors: minimal systemic toxicity, lack of local irritation, ease of sterilization, reasonable duration of action, and low cost. It is usually employed in a solution containing epinephrine, 1:50,000; absorption is retarded, the anesthetic solution remains in contact with nerve fibers for a longer period of time, and the duration of action is very much prolonged.

The usual concentrations of solutions of Procaine Hydrochloride employed for infiltration anesthesia are 0.25 to 0.5%; for nerve block 1.0 to 2.0%. A total of 0.5 Gm or more may be conservatively employed during the course of a surgical procedure. For spinal anesthesia, the average dose is 100 to 150 mg.

Procaine has been administered intravenously for a variety of conditions, including the control of medical and surgical pain, the treatment of delayed serum sickness and urticaria, and the treatment of premature aging. However, the degree of analgesia is only slightly better than a placebo, antihistamines are much more effective in serum sickness and urticaria, and the geriatric use of procaine has not been established.

Procaine in combination with butethamine, tetracaine, or propoxycaine and a vasoconstrictor agent such as epinephrine, phenylephrine, levarterenol, or levonordefrin is used as a local anesthetic in dentistry. Such combinations are intended to alter the potency, onset, and/or duration of anesthetic action and to be useful in patients who may be sensitive to one or another of the vasoconstrictor agents. Although such combinations may have a more rapid onset or a longer duration of action than either agent used singly, combinations of local anesthetics in fixed ratio present the same inherent limitations as are common to all fixed-dose mixtures.

Dose—*Infiltration, peripheral nerve block,* or *epidural,* up to **160 ml** of a **0.5%** solution, **70 ml** of a **1%** solution, or **30 ml** of a **2%** solution; *usual, infiltration,* **50 ml** of a **0.5%** solution; *usual, peripheral nerve block,* **25 ml** of a **1** or **2%** solution; *usual, epidural,* **25 ml** of a **1.5%** solution.

Dosage Forms—Injection USP (procaine hydrochloride and epinephrine, respectively): 1% and 1:100,000/30 ml, 1% and 1:50,000/30 ml, 2% and 1:50,000/30 ml; Sterile USP: 50, 100, 125, 150, and 500 mg. Procaine Hydrochloride and Levonordefrin Injection NF: 2%—1:20,000/2 ml; Procaine and Phenylephrine Hydrochlorides Injection NF: 2 or 4%—1:2500; Procaine and Propoxycaine Hydrochlorides and Levarterenol Bitartrate Injection NF: 2%–0.4%—1:30,000/1.8, 2.2, and 30 ml; Procaine and Propoxycaine Hydrochlorides and Levonordefrin Injection NF: 2%–0.4%—1:20,000/2 ml; Procaine and Tetracaine Hydrochlorides and Levarterenol Bitartrate Injection NF: 2%–0.15%—1:30,000/2 ml; Procaine and Tetracaine Hydrochlorides and Levonordefrin Injection NF: 2%–0.15%—1:20,000/2 and 30 ml; Procaine, Tetracaine, and Phenylephrine Hydrochlorides Injection NF: 2%–0.15%—1:2500/2 ml.

Proparacaine Hydrochloride USP

[2-(Diethylamino)ethyl 3-Amino-4-propoxybenzoate Monohydrochloride; Ophthaline (*Squibb*); Ophthetic (*Allergan*)]

$$\left[CH_3CH_2CH_2O - \underset{NH_2}{\underset{|}{\bigcirc}} - COOCH_2CH_2\overset{+}{N}H(C_2H_5)_2 \right] \bar{C}l$$

Proparacaine Hydrochloride contains 97.0–103.0% of $C_{16}H_{26}N_2O_3 \cdot HCl$ (330.86), calculated on the dried basis.

Preparation—*p*-Hydroxybenzoic acid is reacted with *n*-propyl chloride in alkaline solution and the resulting *p*-propoxybenzoic acid is nitrated to the 3-nitro compound. Treatment with thionyl chloride yields the acid chloride which is then coupled with 2-(diethylamino)ethanol. The resulting nitro ester is reduced to form proparacaine base which reacts with an equimolar quantity of HCl to form the hydrochloride.

Description—White to off-white, or faintly buff-colored, odorless, crystalline powder. On heating or exposure to air the compound tends to discolor. Solutions exposed to air slowly discolor and finally become dark, with some loss of potency. The crystals melt within a 2° range, between 178° and 185°. Its solutions are neutral to litmus.

Solubility—1 Gm dissolves in about 30 ml of water, 30 ml of acids, and 30 ml of warm alcohol or methanol; insoluble in ether and benzene; in contact with alkali the free base is liberated.

Uses—Proparacaine Hydrochloride is an effective surface anesthetic with a potency slightly greater than that of an equal amount of tetracaine. It is a useful anesthetic in ophthalmology and induces little or no initial irritation. Its onset of action is rapid; surface anesthesia of sufficient intensity to permit tonometry can generally be obtained within about 20 seconds after the instillation of 1 or 2 drops of a 0.5% solution. The duration of such anesthesia is about 15 minutes. Proparacaine Hydrochloride is useful for most ocular procedures that require topical anesthesia such as tonometry, removal of foreign bodies and sutures, gonioscopy, conjunctival scraping for diagnosis, and short operative procedures involving the cornea and conjunctiva. The drug has also been employed as the sole anesthetic for cataract extractions and glaucoma surgery. Although Proparacaine is too toxic for use as an injection anesthetic, its ophthalmic use has been relatively free from side effects or untoward reactions.

Dose—*Topically,* **0.05 ml** of a **0.5%** solution to the conjunctiva, repeated at 5- to 10-minute intervals if necessary.

Dosage Forms—Ophthalmic Solution USP: 0.5%.

Propoxycaine Hydrochloride NF

[2-(Diethylamino)ethyl 4-Amino-2-propoxybenzoate Monohydrochloride; Blockain (*Breon*)]

$$\left[H_2N - \underset{OC_3H_7}{\underset{|}{\bigcirc}} - COO - (CH_2)_2\overset{+}{N}H(C_2H_5)_2 \right] Cl^-$$

Propoxycaine Hydrochloride, dried at 105° for 3 hours, contains 98.0–102.0% of $C_{16}H_{26}N_2O_3 \cdot HCl$ (330.86).

Preparation—Sodium 2-propoxy-4-nitrobenzoate is metathesized with 2-chlorotriethylamine in isopropyl alcohol and the nitro group is then reduced to amino with tin and hydrochloric acid.

Description—It occurs as a white, odorless, crystalline solid which discolors on prolonged exposure to light and to air. Melting range 146° to 151°. The pH of a solution (0.4 to 2 in 100) is about 5.4.

Solubility—Very soluble in water, slightly soluble in alcohol and in chloroform, and practically insoluble in acetone and in ether.

Uses—Propoxycaine Hydrochloride is a local anesthetic with a potency seven or eight times that of procaine; anesthesia is also more rapid in onset and longer in duration than that obtained with the latter. Propoxycaine hydrochloride is used only for infiltration and nerve block anesthesia.

Dose—[*Usual*, 2 to 5 ml of a 0.5% solution; total dose should not exceed 20 ml: unofficial.]

Dosage Forms—Injection NF: 150 mg/30 ml; Propoxycaine and Procaine Hydrochlorides and Levonordefrin Injection NF: 0.4%–2%—1:20,000/2 ml.

Pyrrocaine Hydrochloride NF

[1-Pyrrolidineaceto-2',6'-xylidide Monohydrochloride; Endocaine (*Endo*)]

Pyrrocaine Hydrochloride contains 98.0–100.5% of $C_{14}H_{20}N_2O \cdot HCl$ (268.79), calculated on the dried basis.

Preparation—A solution of 2,6-xylidine in glacial acetic acid is treated with chloroacetyl chloride and the resulting 2-chloro-2',6'-acetoxylidide is precipitated with sodium acetate, dissolved in benzene containing suspended sodium carbonate, and treated with pyrrolidine to produce pyrrocaine (base). The purified base is dissolved in isopropyl alcohol and converted to the hydrochloride by a stream of hydrogen chloride. US Pat. 2,949,470.

Description—A white, odorless, crystalline powder. It melts between 200° and 204°.

Solubility—Soluble in water, alcohol, and isopropanol; practically insoluble in chloroform and ether.

Uses—Pyrrocaine Hydrochloride, 2% solution with Epinephrine [Dynacaine (*Graham*)] is used in dentistry for *infiltration* and *block anesthesia*. Clinical trials indicate that the intensity of anesthesia is similar to that obtained with the same formulation of lidocaine. Indeed, the two anesthetics appear to be approximately of the same potency and duration of action and to produce similar effects on blood pressure and heart rate. Since Pyrrocaine differs in chemical structure from procaine and related compounds, it may be useful in those rare instances where the dentist or patient may be sensitive to the procaine type of local anesthetic.

Dose—*Usual, infiltration*, 1 ml of a 2% solution; *nerve block*, 1.5 to 2 ml of a 2% solution.

Other Dose Information—*Usual*, 1 ml of a 2% Pyrrocaine Hydrochloride with Epinephrine (1:150,000 or 1:250,000) to be used for infiltration anesthesia and 1.5 to 2 ml to be used for nerve-block anesthesia.

Dosage Forms—Pyrrocaine Hydrochloride and Epinephrine Injection NF: 2%—1:100,000, 1:150,000 or 1:250,000/1.8 ml.

Tetracaine NF

[2-(Dimethylamino)ethyl *p*-(Butylamino)benzoate]

$$CH_3(CH_2)_3NH\!-\!\!\bigcirc\!\!-\!COOCH_2CH_2N(CH_3)_2$$

Tetracaine contains 98.0–101.0% of $C_{15}H_{24}N_2O_2$ (264.37), calculated on the dried basis.

Preparation—Ethyl *p*-aminobenzoate is butylated by refluxing an ethanolic solution of it and *n*-butyl bromide in the presence of sodium carbonate. The resulting ethyl *p*-butylaminobenzoate is then caused to undergo transesterification by heating a solution of it in 2-(dimethylamino)ethanol in the presence of sodium ethoxide under conditions such that the liberated ethanol is continuously distilled from the reaction mixture. The crude product may be purified by crystallization from aqueous ethanol.

Description—It occurs as a white, or light yellow, waxy solid. Melting range: 41° to 46°.

Solubility—Very slightly soluble in water; soluble in alcohol, ether, benzene, and chloroform.

Uses—See *Tetracaine Hydrochloride*.

Dose—*Topically*, as a 0.5% ointment, to the conjunctiva.

Dosage Forms—Ophthalmic Ointment NF.

Veterinary Use—For *topical anesthesia*, particularly in the eye, 0.5 to 1% concentrations.

Tetracaine Hydrochloride USP

[Amethocaine Hydrochloride; 2-(Dimethylamino)ethyl *p*-(Butylamino)-benzoate Monohydrochloride; Pantocain; Anethaine; Decicain; Butethanol; Pontocaine Hydrochloride (*Winthrop*)]

Tetracaine Hydrochloride contains 98.5–101.0% of $C_{15}H_{24}N_2O_2 \cdot HCl$ (300.83), calculated on the anhydrous basis.

For the structure of the base, see *Tetracaine*.

Preparation—Tetracaine Hydrochloride may be prepared by dissolving Tetracaine (base) in a suitable organic solvent such as benzene and passing hydrogen chloride into the solution whereupon the salt precipitates. For the preparation of the base, see Tetracaine above.

Description—Fine, white, crystalline, odorless powder. It has a slightly bitter taste followed by a sense of numbness. Solutions are neutral to litmus. Melts at about 148°; 2 polymorphic modifications melt at about 134° to 139°, respectively. Mixtures of these may melt between 134° and 147°.

Solubility—Very soluble in water; soluble in alcohol; insoluble in ether and benzene.

Uses—Tetracaine Hydrochloride is an all-purpose local anesthetic. The effects are longer lasting than are those of procaine.

Dose—*Subarachnoid*, 1 to 3 ml; *usual*, 2 ml as a 0.5% solution; *topically*, 0.1 ml of a 0.5% solution to the conjunctiva repeated at 5- to 10-minute intervals if necessary; 1 ml of a 2% solution to the nose and throat.

Dosage Forms—Injection USP: 1%/2 ml, 0.15%/100 ml; Sterile USP: 10 and 20 mg.

Other Local Anesthetics

Amolanone Hydrochloride [hydrochloride of 3-(2-Diethylamino)ethyl]-3-phenyl-2-benzofuranone] [$C_{20}H_{23}NO_2 \cdot HCl$]—This is a substituted γ-butyrolactone with both anticholinergic and local anesthetic actions. Crystals, soluble in water. *Uses:* As a topical anesthetic of the lower urinary tract in carrying out certain urological procedures such as catheterization, urethral dilatation, cystoscopy, and pan-endoscopy. Further clinical experience is necessary, however, to determine its usefulness as a topical anesthetic. *Dose:* By *intra-urethral instillation*, the urethra being filled with a 0.33% solution and the meatus closed off with a penile clamp. After 3 to 5 minutes the clamp is removed and the urological procedure begun. This solution should not be injected into the tissue.

Amydricaine Hydrochloride [1-(dimethylamino)-2-[(dimethylamino)methyl]-2-butanol benzoate monohydrochloride] [$C_{16}H_{26}N_2O_2$. HCl]—This anesthetic occurs as a white, crystalline powder, soluble in water, alcohol, and chloroform, but insoluble in ether. Aqueous solutions are stable to boiling for not more than 5 minutes; 2 to 4% aqueous solutions are stable but weaker solutions are likely to become moldy. *Uses:* Local anesthetic equal to cocaine, but not a mydriatic. *Dose:* Ophthalmology, 2 to 4%; rhinolaryngology, 5 to 10%; urology, 1 to 4%; dentistry, 2%; and minor surgery, 0.5 to 2% solutions.

Benoxinate Hydrochloride USP XVI [2-(Diethylamino)ethyl 4-amino-3-butoxybenzoate monohydrochloride; Dorsacaine (*Dorsey*)] [$C_{17}H_{28}N_2O_3$. HCl]—White crystals or crystalline powder. It is odorless and has a salty taste and produces local anesthesia of the tongue. It melts at about 155°. Very soluble in water and chloroform; soluble in alcohol; insoluble in ether. *Uses:* Benoxinate Hydrochloride, a benzoic acid ester related to procaine, is an effective *surface anesthetic* useful in ophthalmology. It also has bacteriostatic properties. Benoxinate Hydrochloride is used in a 0.4% solution for tonometry, gonioscopy, removal of foreign bodies in the cornea, and for short operative procedures involving the cornea and conjunctiva. A single instillation produces significant anesthesia within 60 seconds and 3 drops at 90-second intervals induces sufficient anesthesia for the removal of foreign objects from the cornea; full anesthesia persists for 20 to 30 minutes and the sensitivity of the cornea returns to normal in 1 hour. Although signs of hypersensitivity have followed its prolonged use in the eye, it should be used with the usual precautions for surface anesthesia, and should be used sparingly in patients with allergies, cardiac disease, hyperthyroidism or open lesions. *Dose: Topically,* 0.05 to 0.2 ml of 0.4% solution in the eye.

Butacaine Sulfate NF X [3-(Dibutylamino)-1-propanol *p*-aminobenzoate (ester) sulfate (2:1); Butyn Sulfate (*Abbott*)] [$(C_{18}H_{33}N_2O_2)_2$. H_2SO_4]—A white, odorless, crystalline powder which is affected by light and rapidly produces a numbness when placed on the tongue. It is slowly soluble in its own weight of water producing a solution neutral to litmus, very soluble in warm alcohol and acetone, and insoluble in ether. It is a more active local anesthetic than either cocaine or procaine. Its action is more prolonged and more rapid than that of cocaine. Locally, it is more toxic than procaine, but less toxic than cocaine. Parenterally, it is more toxic than cocaine. It acts through intact mucous membranes. *Uses: Local anesthesia,* particularly of the eye. Several instillations of a 2% solution about 3 minutes apart permit most surgical procedures.

Butamben Picrate [Butesin Picrate (*Abbott*)]—A compound consisting of 1 molecule of trinitrophenol and 2 molecules of butyl aminobenzoate. *Uses:* In burns, ulcers, and other denuded painful lesions of the skin. The drug should be discontinued if a rash develops following its use. *Dose:* as a 1% ointment.

Butethamine Formate [2-(Isobutylamino)ethyl *p*-aminobenzoate monoformate [$C_{13}H_{20}N_2O_2$.HCHO]₂—For the structure of butethamine, see page 1066. White crystals, soluble in water and alcohol. *Uses:* in spinal anesthesia. Its action is qualitatively identical with that of procaine but only ¾ the dose usually employed for procaine need be given.

Diperodon Hydrochloride [3-Piperidino-1,2-propanediol dicarbanilate (ester) monohydrochloride; Diothane (*Merrell*)] [$C_{22}H_{27}N_3O_4$. HCl]—White crystals; soluble in alcohol, slightly soluble in water. *Uses:* similar to cocaine. Intravenous toxicity 3 times that of procaine. Used on skin

and mucous membranes; in hemorrhoids. *Dose:* locally in 1% solution; 0.5% solution for infiltration anesthesia.

Metabutoxycaine Hydrochloride NF XII [2-(Diethylamino)ethyl 3-Amino-2-butoxybenzoate Monohydrochloride], dried in a vacuum desiccator over phosphorus pentoxide for 6 hours, contains 98.5–101.5% of $C_{17}H_{28}H_{28}N_2O_3$. HCl (344.89). *Preparation:* The ester is conveniently prepared by metathesis between sodium 2-butoxy-3-nitrobenzoate and 2-chlorotriethylamine using isopropyl alcohol as the reaction medium, followed by reduction of nitro to amino by means of tin and hydrochloric acid. The base thus formed may be converted into the hydrochloride by dissolving it in a suitable organic solvent and precipitating the salt by introducing a stream of hydrogen chloride. *Description and Solubility:* White, odorless, crystalline solid; pH (1.5 to 2 in 100 solution): about 5.5; melts between 117° and 120°. Very soluble in water and alcohol; sparingly soluble in acetone and chloroform; very slightly soluble in ether.

Uses: A relatively short-acting local anesthetic intended primarily for use in dentistry. Its potency as a conduction anesthetic is somewhat greater than that of an equal concentration of procaine. Laboratory studies indicate the acute toxicity of Metabutoxycaine is approximately the same as that of procaine. *Dose: Infiltration* and *nerve block,* 1 to 2 ml of a 1.5% solution with 1:50,000 epinephrine.

Orthocaine BP [Methyl *m*-amino-*p*-hydroxybenzoate] [$C_8H_9NO_3$]—White, crystalline powder; insoluble in water, soluble in alcohol. *Uses:* Local anesthetic for relief of pruritus and pain in 2 to 5% concentration.

Piperocaine Hydrochloride USP XVI, BP [2-Methyl-1-piperidinepropanol benzoate (ester) hydrochloride; Metycaine Hydrochloride (*Lilly*)] [$C_{16}H_{23}NO_2$. HCl]—Small, white crystals or a white, crystalline powder which is odorless and stable in air. Melting range 172° to 175°. 1 Gm dissolves in 1.5 ml of water and 4.5 ml of alcohol; readily soluble in chloroform; almost insoluble in ether and fixed oils. *Uses:* Piperocaine Hydrochloride is a *local anesthetic* which produces prompt anesthesia either by subcutaneous *injection* or *topical application*. Its subcutaneous toxicity is comparable to that of procaine; its intravenous toxicity is three times that of procaine. It is equivalent in action to procaine for spinal anesthesia.

For ophthalmological use, 2 to 4% solutions or 4% ophthalmic ointments are employed; for nose and throat, 2 to 10% solutions; and for use in the urethra, 1 to 4% solutions. For *infiltration anesthesia,* 0.5 to 1% solutions; for *nerve block,* 1 to 2%; and for *spinal anesthesia,* 1.5 to 5% solutions and with a maximum of 0.75 mg per pound of body weight. *Dose: Usual,* 0.25 to 5% solution as required by route of administration; for *external use, topically* as a 2% solution or 4% ointment to the conjunctiva.

Salicyl Alcohol [Saligenin; Saligenol; Salicain; *o*-Hydroxybenzyl alcohol] [$C_6H_4(CH_2OH)(OH)$-1,2]—Prepared by the action of emulsin on salicin, or by heating phenol with methylene chloride and aqueous NaOH. Crystalline powder. Melts 86°–87°. Soluble in water and benzene; very soluble in alcohol, chloroform, and ether. *Uses:* 2 to 8% solution for infiltration and mucous membrane anesthesia.

Toothache Drops NF XI [Odontalgicum]—A preparation consisting of 25 Gm of chlorobutanol dissolved in a sufficient quantity of clove oil to make 100 ml. *Uses:* A local analgetic, applied on a pledget of cotton to the cavities of aching teeth.

Tutocaine Hydrochloride [Butamin; 3-(Dimethylamino)-1,2-dimethylpropyl *p*-aminobenzoate monohydrochloride] [$C_{14}H_{22}N_2O_2$.HCl]—Faintly bitter crystals producing a sense of numbness on the tongue. Stable in air. It melts between 212° and 215°. 1 Gm dissolves in about 4 ml of water and about 40 ml of alcohol. *Uses:* 0.2 to 5% solution for surface and infiltration anesthesia.

References

1. Adriani, J., and Zepernick, R., *J. Am. Med. Assoc.,* **188,** 711 (1964).
2. Willstäter, R., *et al,* Ann., 434, 111 (1923).
3. See *Procaine* and analogs, page 1073.

60 | Sedatives and Hypnotics

Barbiturates—nonbarbiturates—miscellaneous (mild tranquilizers) sedative hypnotic agents

This chapter was prepared by

Ewart A. Swinyard, PhD, *Professor of Pharmacology, College of Pharmacy and College of Medicine, University of Utah, Salt Lake City, Utah 84112, and*
Stewart C. Harvey, PhD, *Associate Professor of Pharmacology, College of Medicine, University of Utah, Salt Lake City, Utah 84112*

The term *sedative* refers to a quieting effect accompanied by relaxation and rest, but not necessarily sleep. Sedative drugs are used to allay excitement and reduce motor activity without inducing sleep. The term *hypnotic* refers to the production of sleep and is synonymous with somnifacient and soporific. Hence, hypnotic drugs are used to induce sleep when sleeplessness is not due to a definite stimulus, such as pain, dyspnea, or itching which prevents sleep or awakens the patient. Both sedative and hypnotic actions usually reside in the same drug; a small dose of a drug may act as a sedative, whereas a large dose of the same drug may act as a hypnotic.

Agents used as sedatives and hypnotics include a large number of compounds of diverse chemical structure and pharmacological properties which have in common the ability to induce a nonselective, reversible depression of the central nervous system. Thus, inorganic salts (bromide), chloral derivatives (chloral hydrate), acetylenic alcohols (ethchlorvynol), cyclic ethers (paraldehyde), carbamic acid esters of alcohols (ethinamate), carbamic acid esters of glycols (meprobamate), monoureides (ectylurea), diureides (barbiturates), piperidinedione derivatives (glutethimide), disubstituted quinazalones (methaqualone), benzodiazepines (chlordiazepoxide), and some miscellaneous aromatic tertiary alkylamines, such as antihistaminics (diphenhydramine) and parasympatholytics (scopolamine) all exhibit pronounced sedative and hypnotic effects. Some of these agents, such as diphenhydramine and scopolamine, exhibit primary pharmacological actions which dictate they should be classified in other sections of this text. On the other hand, the "minor tranquilizers" such as meprobamate, chlordiazepoxide and related agents, exhibit primary pharmacological actions which characterize them as sedative and hypnotic agents. Therefore, the latter group will be discussed in this chapter. For convenience, the sedatives and hypnotics presented herein will be divided into three groups: barbiturates; nonbarbiturates; and miscellaneous (minor tranquilizers) sedative and hypnotic agents. The latter group could more properly be included with the nonbarbiturate sedatives and hypnotics. They are separated here to emphasize the fact that these newer agents belong in this chapter and that they exhibit pharmacological properties characteristic of other sedative and hypnotic agents.

Agents included in this chapter are extensively used as *sedatives, hypnotics, anticonvulsants, preanesthetic medication,* and *diagnostic* and *therapeutic aids* in psychiatry. As *sedatives,* these drugs are used in the management of neuroses and to allay the anxiety and apprehension which accompanies various disease states, such as hypertension, cardiac failure, and coronary artery disease. There is no convincing evidence that the newer agents afford any distinct advantage over appropriate doses of the well-established barbiturates or minor tranquilizers as daytime sedatives for the relief of anxiety and tension. Therefore, the physician is well advised to prescribe such well understood agents as phenobarbital, meprobamate, or chlordiazepoxide for this purpose.

As *hypnotics,* they are frequently used to induce sleep. The choice of hypnotic agent depends to a large extent on the characteristics of the insomnia. Some patients have difficulty only in falling asleep and, once asleep, need no drug assistance; a rapidly acting hypnotic drug with a short duration of action will suffice for these patients. Other patients fall asleep readily, but experience one or more periods of wakefulness during the night; a hypnotic drug with a long duration of action is usually indicated in such cases. Still other patients have trouble falling and in staying asleep; a rapidly acting hypnotic drug which exerts an effect throughout part or most of the night is required for such patients. In all cases, however, consideration should be given to what the patient does on the day following a night of drug-induced sleep. Persons who must be alert the following day will usually object to drugs which leave residual sedation, whereas hospitalized patients, or individuals with no place to go and nothing to do may actually benefit from such after effects.

A number of these agents have *anticonvulsant* properties. However, only phenobarbital, mephobarbital, and metharbital are sufficiently selective in this regard to be clinically useful as *antiepileptics.* A number of benzodiazepines have excellent anticonvulsant actions and some of these have been used in epilepsy. Final evaluation of their usefulness, however, must await more extensive clinical trial.

Sedative and hypnotic agents are frequently used as *preanesthetic medication* and as *adjunctive therapy* in psychiatry. Short-acting barbiturates are commonly used to allay anxiety and apprehension prior to surgery. In psychiatry, short-acting barbiturates have been used in *narcoanalysis* and *narcotherapy.*

It is generally agreed that prolonged overdosage with most of these drugs can result in habituation and physical dependence liability. Thus, many of these agents qualify as addicting drugs. It should be emphasized that with usual hypnotic doses and close medical supervision, the problem of drug addiction with these agents is seldom encountered.

Barbiturates

The barbiturates are among the most frequently employed hypnotic and sedative drugs. They are all substituted derivatives of barbituric acid, a synthetic condensation product of malonic acid and urea. Several hundred derivatives of barbituric acid have been synthesized and more than 50 of these have been introduced as therapeutic agents. Many of the clinically available barbiturates do not differ significantly in their pharmacological or therapeutic properties. Indeed, major variations occur in the duration of depressant action, the locus of destruction in the body, and the suitability for special therapeutic purposes, such as in epilepsy and surgical anesthesia. Therefore, they will be discussed as a group and only important differences in actions or uses of specific barbiturates will be mentioned in the monographs for each drug.

In pharmaceutical and medical parlance, the class name "barbiturates" is used to refer both to the free barbituric acids and to their salts (usually sodium or calcium).

Chemically, the barbiturates are classified as ureides (see page 460). The parent molecule, barbituric acid, is the cyclic ureide, malonylurea. It may exist as a "keto" form (I) or as an "enol" form (II):

Barbituric acid itself does not possess hypnotic properties. These are conferred when the hydrogens on the carbon in position 5 are replaced by organic groups. Most of the clinically useful barbiturates have two aliphatic radicals substituted for the hydrogen atoms although a few have one alicyclic (eg, hexobarbital) or one aromatic (eg, phenobarbital) radical. Other variations in structure include the substitution of halogen for one of the hydrogens on alkyl side chains, the substitution of an organic radical for the hydrogen attached to either of the nitrogens, and the replacement of the oxygen attached to the carbon in position 2 with sulfur to form a thiobarbiturate. The structural relationships of the official barbiturates are shown in Table I

Barbiturates are classified, rather arbitrarily, by the duration of their clinical effects into "long," "intermediate," "short," and "ultrashort" acting compounds. Comparison of experimental with clinical data on the duration of activity shows considerable variation among different investigators. On the basis of certain general conclusions, the compounds may be classified as indicated in Table I.

The rapidity of onset of their therapeutic effects, for the most part, parallels their duration of action. A long-acting drug, such as phenobarbital, may require 30 to 60 minutes for induction following the oral administration of a somnifacient dose. The "sleep" may last 4 to 6 hours or longer and leave a moderate "hangover." Those drugs of short duration, such as pentobarbital, usually produce their effects in from 15 to 30 minutes and cause sleep of 2 to 4 hours, often without the postsomnial lassitude. By reason of this dissimilarity in therapeutic activity the physician can select the drug which most satisfactorily fits the situation.

The long-acting barbiturates are excreted largely by the kidney; the short-acting barbiturates are destroyed to a large extent in the liver. The ultrashort-acting barbiturates are first deposited in body fat, but are eventually dependent on the liver and kidney for metabolic degradation and elimination. Most of the intermediate-acting barbiturates are first degraded by the liver and then excreted by the kidney.

Uses—The derivatives of barbituric acid are effective sedatives and hypnotics, and as such are widely employed in a variety of diseases and syndromes where sedation or sleep is needed. They are useful in insomnia, hyperthyroidism, acute maniacal states, delirium tremens, and certain psychoneurotic disorders. The barbiturates are useful in anxiety and tension states associated with hypertension, coronary artery disease, and functional gastrointestinal disorders. Although the barbiturates are not analgesic when administered in doses which do not cause unconsciousness, they do potentiate the analgesic effects of the so-called coal-tar analgesic drugs; hence, they are used in combination with these agents for the relief of pain. Barbiturates are very useful in the management of convulsive disorders, and when certain types of acute convulsions are present, the soluble salt of effective compounds may be injected intravenously. Such conditions include tetanus, eclampsia, status epilepticus, poisoning by convulsant drugs, etc. They also protect against the toxic effects of local anesthetics, and should routinely be given by mouth in full sedative doses for the prophylactic purpose whenever local anesthesia is contemplated. Certain barbiturates, ie, phenobarbital, metharbital, and mephobarbital, are useful in the treatment of epilepsy. They also have a number of uses in anesthesia; namely, the preanesthetic medication to insure sleep and rest, basal anesthesia, obstetrical amnesia, and complete surgical anesthesia. For the latter purpose, the long-acting barbiturates such as barbital and phenobarbital are not used, but preference is given to the ultrashort-acting drugs such as hexobarbital, thiamylal, and thiopental, which are widely employed for surgical operations of short duration.

The elixirs of certain barbiturates have proved satisfactory as somnifacients and sedatives for children. Their palatability combined with other desirable therapeutic effects have been found of aid in the relief of colic, excitation, and restlessness due to illness. Sedative doses may be administered as frequently as 3 to 4 times a day in cases of pylorospasm, whooping cough, nausea and vomiting of functional origin, etc. Small doses administered orally or, if necessary, rectally have proved of value in pediatric office procedures in which little or no pain is occasioned.

Inasmuch as barbiturate derivatives can cause acute and chronic poisoning, and also because some patients manifest idiosyncrasy to these agents, their indiscriminate use must be avoided. Accidental and suicidal deaths from acute barbiturate poisoning and barbiturate addiction are encountered frequently. Treatment varies with the degree of intoxication. Unabsorbed barbiturate is removed from the stomach by lavage. In mild degrees of intoxication symptomatic therapy is usually sufficient. In severe intoxication, analeptics such as picrotoxin and Metrazol are employed to

Table I—Relation of Structure and Activity of Barbiturates

Nonproprietary name	Chemical name[a]	Substituents[b]			Duration of action
		R	R'	Other groups	
Barbital	5,5-Diethylbarbituric acid	CH₃CH₂—	CH₃CH₂—		Long
Mephobarbital	5-Ethyl-1-methyl-5-phenyl-barbituric acid	CH₃CH₂—	C₆H₅— CH₃—		"
Phenobarbital[d]	5-Ethyl-5-phenylbarbituric acid	CH₃CH₂—	⬡		"
Amobarbital[d]	5-Ethyl-5-isopentylbarbituric acid	CH₃CH₂—	(CH₃)₂CHCH₂CH₂—		Intermediate
Aprobarbital	5-Allyl-5-isopropylbarbituric acid	CH₂=CHCH₂—	(CH₃)₂CH—		"
Sodium Butabarbital	5-sec-Butyl-5-ethylbarbituric acid	CH₃CH₂—	CH₃CH₂CH(CH₃)—		"
Butalbital	5-Allyl-5-isobutylbarbituric acid	CH₂=CHCH₂—	(CH₃)₂CHCH₂—		"
Butallylonal	5-2-Bromoallyl-5-sec-butyl-barbituric acid	CH₂=CBrCH₂—	CH₃CH₂CH(CH₃)—		"
Butethal	5-n-Butyl-5-ethylbarbituric acid	CH₃CH₂—	CH₃CH₂CH₂CH₂—		"
Diallylbarbituric Acid	5,5-Diallylbarbituric acid	CH₂=CHCH₂—	CH₂C=CHCH₂—		"
Sodium Probarbital	5-Ethyl-5-isopropylbarbituric acid	CH₃CH₂—	(CH₃)₂CH—		"
Talbutal	5-Allyl-5-sec-butylbarbituric acid	CH₂=CHCH₂—	CH₃CH₂CH—|\nCH₃		"
Vinbarbital[d]	5-Ethyl-5-(1-methyl-1-butenyl)barbituric acid	CH₃CH₂—	CH₃CH₂CH=C(CH₃)—		"
Calcium Cyclobarbital	5-(1-Cyclohexen-1-yl)-5-ethylbarbituric acid	CH₃CH₂—	⬡		Short
Sodium Heptabarbital	5-(1-Cyclohepten-1-yl)-5-ethylbarbituric acid	C₂H₅—	⬡		"
Sodium Pentobarbital	5-Ethyl-5-(1-methylbutyl)-barbituric acid	CH₃CH₂—	CH₃CH₂CH₂CH(CH₃)—		"
Secobarbital[d]	5-Allyl-5-(1-methylbutyl)-barbituric acid	CH₂=CHCH₂—	CH₃CH₂CH₂CH(CH₃)—		"
Sodium Hexobarbital	5-(1-Cyclohexen-1-yl)-1,5-dimethylbarbituric acid	CH₃—	⬡	CH₃—	Ultrashort[c]
Sodium Methohexital	dl-5-Allyl-1-methyl-5-(1-methyl-2-pentynyl)barbituric acid	CH₂=CHCH₂—	CH₃CH₂C≡CCH—|\nCH₃	CH₃—	" "
Sodium Thiamylal	5-Allyl-5-(1-methylbutyl)-2-thiobarbituric acid	CH₂=CHCH₂—	CH₃CH₂CH₂CH(CH₃)—	S=	" "
Sodium Thiopental	5-Ethyl-5-(1-methylbutyl)-2-thiobarbituric acid	CH₃CH₂—	CH₃CH₂CH₂CH(CH₃)—	S=	" "

[a] Names are those of the barbituric *acids*. The sodium and calcium barbiturates are salts of the named acids.
[b] The substituents R and R' are at the 5-position. Of the other groups, methyl is at the 1-position and thio is at the 2-position.
[c] Anesthetic doses are given intravenously in the form of sterile aqueous solutions of the sodium salts.
[d] Data applies also to the sodium salt which is also official.

stimulate the vital centers, but peritoneal dialysis or use of the artificial kidney may be lifesaving.

Chronic barbiturate poisoning involves a large number of individuals in this country. Some authorities consider the problem of chronic barbiturate poisoning as serious as morphine addiction and believe the barbiturates should be included in the Narcotic Act. Serious withdrawal symptoms may occur when barbiturate is withheld from patients addicted to it, including convulsions and psychoses. In some chronically intoxicated individuals, even though they have no previous history of epilepsy, major convulsive seizures follow the sudden withdrawal of barbiturate. It is advisable to reduce the dose of barbiturate gradually in both epileptic and nonepileptic patients when cessation of chronic barbiturate medication is contemplated.

Amobarbital USP

[5-Ethyl-5-isopentylbarbituric Acid; Amylobarbitone; Amytal (*Lilly*); Isoamyl Ethyl Barbituric Acid]

Amobarbital contains 98.5–101.0% of $C_{11}H_{18}N_2O_3$ (226.28), calculated on the dried basis.

Preparation—It may be prepared by the general method described under *Barbital* (see below), using ethyl bromide and isopentyl bromide as alkylating agents at the 5-position.

Description—A white, crystalline, odorless, bitter powder. Its solutions are acid to litmus. Melting range: 156° to 161°, but the range between beginning and end of melting does not exceed 3°.

Solubility—1 Gm dissolves in about 1300 ml of water, 5 ml of alcohol, about 17 ml of chloroform, and 6 ml of ether; soluble in solutions of fixed alkali hydroxides and carbonates.

Uses—Amobarbital is a *hypnotic* and *sedative*. It is one of the intermediate-acting *Barbiturates* (see page 1079). It has a wide spectrum of action; central depression ranging from minimal sedation to preanesthetic hypnosis may be achieved with appropriate doses.

Dose—50 to 200 mg daily; *usual*, **100 mg** at bedtime.

Dosage Forms—Elixir NF (below); Tablets USP: 15, 30, 50, and 100 mg.

Veterinary Dose—*Dogs*, 50 to 300 mg; *Cats*, 25 to 50 mg.

Amobarbital Elixir NF contains, in each 100 ml, 418–462 mg of $C_{11}H_{18}N_2O_3$. *Preparation:* Dissolve amobarbital (4.4 Gm), sodium saccharin (1 Gm), orange oil (0.26 ml), lemon oil (0.15 ml), cinnamon oil (0.03 ml), caraway oil (0.006 ml), coriander oil (0.0018 ml), and anise oil (0.02 ml) in alcohol (300 ml). Add propylene glycol (310 ml), methenamine (4.4 Gm), caramel (11.25 ml), and sufficient purified water to make the product measure 1000 ml. Mix well, allow the product to stand 24 hours, and filter until the elixir is clear. The methenamine increases the solubility of the amobarbital. *Alcohol Content:* 26 to 32% of C_2H_5OH. *Dose: Usual, 5 ml*, equivalent to 22 mg of Amobarbital.

Aprobarbital NF

[Allylisopropylmalonylurea; 5-Allyl-5-isopropylbarbituric Acid; Alurate (*Roche*)]

Aprobarbital, dried at 105° for 2 hours, contains 98.5–101.0% of $C_{10}H_{14}N_2O_3$ (210.23).

Preparation—It may be prepared by the general method described under *Barbital* (see below), using allyl bromide and isopropyl bromide as alkylating agents at the 5-position.

Description—A fine, white, odorless, crystalline powder having a slightly bitter taste. Stable in air. A saturated aqueous solution is acid to litmus. Melting range between 141.5° and 143.5°.

Solubility—Very slightly soluble in cold water; soluble in alcohol, in chloroform, and in ether.

Uses—Aprobarbital is one of the intermediate-acting *Barbiturates* (see page 1079).

Dose—*Usual, sedative*, **20 to 40 mg** 3 times daily; *hypnotic*, **40 to 160 mg** at night.

Dosage Forms—Elixir NF: 40 mg/5 ml.

Barbital

[Barbitone; Diethylmalonylurea; ingredient of Neuronidia (*Schieffelin*)]

Barbital $[C_8H_{12}N_2O_3 = 184.20]$ is 5,5-diethylbarbituric acid.

Preparation—Monochloroacetic acid is treated with sodium cyanide; the resulting cyanoacetic acid is treated with hydrochloric acid in the presence of alcohol, yielding the diethyl ester of malonic acid. This ester, in absolute alcohol solution, is treated with the theoretical quantity of metallic sodium to replace one hydrogen of the CH_2 group, and thereupon a slight excess of the theoretical amount of an ethylating agent, such as ethyl bromide, is added. The second hydrogen is then similarly replaced. The diethyl ester of diethylmalonic acid thus obtained is heated in an alcoholic solution and in the presence of sodium with urea. Sodium barbital is formed, from which the barbital is liberated with hydrochloric acid.

The alkylation of the CH_2 group of the malonic ester, whether the alkyls be both the same as in barbital or different as in pentothal, may be done in two stages, introducing one alkyl group at a time.

Description—Colorless or white crystals or as a white crystalline powder. It is odorless, has a slightly bitter taste, and is stable in the air. It melts between 188° and 192°. An aqueous solution of Barbital is acid to litmus.

Solubility—1 Gm dissolves in 130 ml water, about 15 ml alcohol, 75 ml chloroform, 35 ml ether, and about 13 ml boiling water; soluble in acetone and ethyl acetate.

Incompatibilities—Barbital is decomposed by *alkalies* with the liberation of ammonia. See *Phenobarbital* (this page).

Uses—Barbital, the oldest of the barbiturates, is a "long-acting barbiturate." It is seldom used in modern therapeutics. See also the general discussion on *Barbiturates* (page 1078).

Dose—*Usual*, **300 mg**.

Dosage Forms—Elixir: 175 mg/ml; Tablets: 300 mg.

Veterinary Dose—*Horses*, **2 to 8 Gm**; *Swine*, **0.25 to 1.5 Gm**; *Dogs*, **150 mg to 1 Gm**; *Cats*, **100 to 200 mg**.

Butalbital NF

[5-Allyl-5-isobutylbarbituric Acid; Allylbarbituric Acid NFX; Itobarbital; Sandoptal; Ingredient of Fiorinal (*Sandoz*)]

Butalbital, dried at 105° for 2 hours, contains 97.5–101.5% of $C_{11}H_{16}N_2O_3$ (224.26).

Preparation—Butalbital may be prepared by the general method described under *Barbital* (page 1080) using allyl bromide and isobutyl bromide as the alkylating agents at the 5-position.

Description—A white, crystalline powder that is odorless, has a slightly bitter taste, and is stable in air. Its saturated solution is acid to litmus.

Solubility—Freely soluble in alcohol, ether, and chloroform; slightly soluble in cold water and soluble in boiling water; soluble in solutions of fixed alkalies and alkali carbonates.

Uses—Butalbital, a barbiturate with an intermediate duration of action, is used both as a hypnotic and sedative. When administered in hypnotic doses, sleep is induced in 15 to 30 minutes and lasts 6 to 8 hours. In sedative doses, the drug is used in patients with tension and anxiety, neurasthenia, hysteria, delirium tremens, hypertension, coronary disease, gastrointestinal disorders, and hyperthyroidism. See the general statement on *Barbiturates* (page 1078).

Dose—50 to 100 mg; *usual*, **50 mg** every 6 hours.
Dosage Forms—Tablets: 30, 50, and 120 mg.

Calcium Cyclobarbital NF XII

[Calcium 5-(1-Cyclohexen-1-yl)-5-ethylbarbiturate; Phanodorn (*Winthrop*)]

Calcium Cyclobarbital contains 97.5–102.5% of $C_{24}H_{30}CaN_4O_6$ (510.61), calculated on the dried basis.

Preparation—Cyclobarbital may be prepared by the general method described under *Barbital* (page 1080), using ethyl bromide and cyclohexenyl bromide as alkylating agents at the 5-position. Cyclobarbital is also prepared by hydrogenation of phenobarbital in alcoholic solution using colloidal palladium as catalyst. The slightly soluble calcium salt is prepared by dissolving cyclobarbital in a solution containing an equimolar quantity of sodium hydroxide and metathesizing with a solution of calcium chloride. The precipitate is washed with water and dried.

Description—White or almost white powder. A saturated solution is alkaline to litmus.
Solubility—1 Gm dissolves in about 100 ml of water; practically insoluble in alcohol, chloroform, and ether.

Uses—Calcium Cyclobarbital is one of the short-acting *Barbiturates* (see page 1079).
Dose—*Usual*, **200 mg.**
Dosage Forms—Tablets: 200 mg.

Mephobarbital NF

[5-Ethyl-1-methyl-5-phenylbarbituric Acid; Prominal; Phemitone; Mebaral (*Winthrop*)]

Mephobarbital, dried at 105° for 4 hours, contains 98.0–100.5% of $C_{13}H_{14}N_2O_3$ (246.27).

Preparation—The diethyl ester of ethylphenylmalonic acid is prepared by the general method described under *Barbital* (page 1080), and is then condensed with N-methylurea in the presence of sodium ethylate. The resulting sodium mephobarbital is treated with hydrochloric acid, whereupon Mephobarbital crystallizes out; it is purified by recrystallization from alcohol.

The N-methylurea is prepared as follows. Methylamine is gassed into a mixture of sulfuric acid and absolute alcohol until the mixture is alkaline. Potassium cyanate is then added and the mixture is refluxed overnight whereupon the monomethyl ammonium cyanate produced initially by metathesis rearranges (Wöhler) to N-methylurea. The solution on hand is suitable for continuing with the synthesis of mephobarbital without isolating the N-methylurea.

Description—A white crystalline powder. Stable in air. A saturated solution is neutral to litmus. Melts between 176° and 181°.
Solubility—Soluble in chloroform; slightly soluble in alcohol, ether, and water; soluble in solutions of fixed alkali hydroxides or carbonates.

Uses—Mephobarbital is one of the long-acting *Barbiturates* (see page 1079). It is used as a sedative and hypnotic, and also employed in the treatment of *grand mal* and *petit mal epilepsy*. See the general statement, page 1078.
Veterinary Use—Has been employed to control epileptiform convulsions but, in the dog, is poorly absorbed and converted to phenobarbital.
Dose—*Usual*, anticonvulsant, **400 to 600 mg** daily; *usual*, sedative, **32 to 100 mg** 3 or 4 times a day.
Dosage Forms—Tablets NF: 32, 50, 100, and 200 mg.

Metharbital—see page 1100.

Phenobarbital USP

[5-Ethyl-5-phenylbarbituric Acid; Phenylethylmalonylurea; Phenobarbitone; Gardinal; Luminal (*Winthrop*)]

Phenobarbital contains 98.0–101.0% of $C_{12}H_{12}N_2O_3$ (232.24).

Preparation—Benzyl chloride is converted into phenylacetic ester (ethyl phenylacetate) by treating with sodium cyanide and then hydrolyzing with acid in the presence of alcohol.

The ethyl phenylacetate is condensed in the presence of alcohol and metallic sodium with ethyl oxalate, forming diethyl sodium phenyloxaloacetate.

Hydrochloric acid is added to liberate the liquid diethyl phenyloxaloacetate which, on being distilled at about 180°, splits off carbon monoxide, and phenylmalonic ester $[C_6H_5CH(COOC_2H_5)_2]$ is formed. The hydrogen of the CH in the phenylmalonic ester is then ethylated and the resulting ethylphenylmalonic ester condensed with urea as described under *Barbital* (page 1080).

Description—White, odorless, glistening, small crystals, or a white crystalline powder, which may exhibit polymorphism. Stable in air. Its saturated aqueous solution is acid to litmus. Melts between 174° and 178°.

Solubility—1 Gm dissolves in about 1000 ml of water, 10 ml of alcohol, about 40 ml of chloroform, and 15 ml of ether; soluble in solutions of the fixed alkali hydroxides or carbonates.

Incompatibilities—Most of the difficulties encountered in the use of Phenobarbital arise from its limited solubility in vehicles of low alcohol content. The fault may be remedied either by addition of alcohol, by substitution of phenobarbital sodium, or by the use of a suspending agent. The addition of alcohol, provided too large a quantity is not required, is usually the method of choice. Sodium phenobarbital can be used only in neutral or alkaline media since it is converted to Phenobarbital in the presence of acid. See page 1083.

Uses—Phenobarbital has the same field of usefulness as a *sedative* and *hypnotic* as other long-acting barbiturates. In appropriate doses, it is probably the drug of choice for the management of neuroses and related tension states. Phenobarbital may also be used when mild, prolonged sedation is indicated, as in hypertension, coronary artery disease, functional gastrointestinal disorders, and preoperative apprehension. In addition, Phenobarbital has specific usefulness in the symptomatic therapy of *epilepsy*. It is especially helpful in grand mal, less so in petit mal, and may make psychomotor equivalent seizures worse. It differs from diphenylhydantoin in that effective doses usually produce a certain degree of drowsiness or sluggishness. Phenobarbital is often employed in epilepsy in combination with a ketogenic diet, diphenylhydantoin, or other therapeutic measures. If large doses are required to control attacks, the drowsiness they entail can be abolished by the concomitant use of amphetamine. With the exception of Metharbital and Mephobarbital, Phenobarbital is the only barbiturate effective in epilepsy. Like other barbiturates it lacks analgetic potency and should not be given alone in the presence of pain. See the general statement, page 1078.

Dose—*Anticonvulsant, sedative,* and *hypnotic,* **50** to **200 mg** daily; *usual, anticonvulsant* and *sedative,* **15** to **30 mg** 3 or 4 times a day; *usual, hypnotic,* **100 mg** at bedtime.

Dosage Forms—Elixir USP (see below): Tablets USP: 15, 30, 60, and 100 mg.

Veterinary Dose—*Dogs,* 30 to 300 mg; *Cats,* 15 to 60 mg.

Phenobarbital Elixir USP contains, in each 100 ml, 370–430 mg of $C_{12}H_{12}N_2O_3$. *Preparation:* Dissolve phenobarbital (4 Gm) in alcohol (150 ml), and add orange oil (0.75 ml), glycerin (450 ml), syrup (150 ml), and amaranth solution (10 ml), then add sufficient purified water to make the product measure 1000 ml. Mix, and filter, if necessary. *Alcohol Content:* 12 to 15% of C_2H_5OH. *Incompatibilities:* The alcohol content of this preparation is almost the very minimum required to keep the phenobarbital in solution. Consequently, the addition of water or a liquid of lower alcohol content may cause a precipitation.

Secobarbital USP

[5-Allyl-5-(1-methylbutyl)barbituric Acid; Seconal (*Lilly*)]

Secobarbital contains 97.5–100.5% of $C_{12}H_{18}N_2O_3$ (238.29), calculated on the dried basis.

Preparation—Secobarbital may be prepared by the general method described under *Barbital* (page 1080) using allyl bromide and 1-methylbutyl bromide as alkylating agents at the 5-position.

Description—A white, amorphous, odorless powder, having a slightly bitter taste. Its saturated solution is acid to litmus. Melting range 96° to 100°.

Solubility—Slightly soluble in water; very soluble in alcohol and ether; very slightly soluble in solvent hexane; 1 Gm dissolves in approximately 8.5 ml of $0.5N$ sodium hydroxide.

Uses—Secobarbital is one of the short-acting barbiturates. See the general use statement under *Barbiturates*, page 1078.

Dose—**50** to **200 mg** daily; *usual,* **100 mg** at bedtime.

Dosage Forms—Elixir USP.

Veterinary Dose—*Dogs* and *Cats, orally,* **30** to **200 mg,** depending on size of animal.

Sodium Amobarbital USP

[Sodium 5-Ethyl-5-isopentylbarbiturate; Amobarbital Sodium USP XV Sterile Amobarbital Sodium USP XV; Amytal Sodium (*Lilly*)]

Sodium Amobarbital contains 98.5–100.5% of $C_{11}H_{17}N_2NaO_3$ (248.26), calculated on the dried basis.

Preparation—Sodium Amobarbital may be prepared by reacting amobarbital with a solution containing a chemically equivalent quantity of sodium hydroxide or sodium carbonate, evaporating to dryness, and crystallizing the residue from a solution in a suitable solvent such as alcohol.

Description—White, friable, hygroscopic, odorless, granular powder with a bitter taste.

Solubility—Very soluble in water; soluble in alcohol; practically insoluble in ether and chloroform.

Uses—Sodium Amobarbital is used as a hypnotic and sedative. It is one of the intermediate-acting barbiturates. It has a spectrum of action which ranges from minimal sedation to hypnosis.

Dose—**50** to **200 mg** daily; *usual, oral, intramuscular,* or *subcutaneous,* **100 mg** at bedtime.

Dosage Forms—Capsules USP: 60 and 200 mg; Sterile USP: 60, 125, 250, and 500 mg, and 1 Gm.

Sodium Butabarbital NF

[Sodium 5-*sec*-butyl-5-ethylbarbiturate; Butisol (*McNeil*)]

Sodium Butabarbital contains 98.2–100.5% of $C_{10}H_{15}N_2NaO_3$ (234.23), calculated on the dried basis.

Preparation—Sodium Butabarbital may be prepared by treating an alcoholic solution of butabarbital with an equimolar quantity of sodium hydroxide and removing the solvent by evaporation.

Description—White, bitter powder. The pH of a 1 in 100 solution is between 9.0 and 10.2.

Solubility—1 Gm is soluble in about 2 ml of water and about 7 ml of alcohol; practically insoluble in benzene and absolute ether.

Uses—Sodium Butabarbital is an intermediate-acting barbiturate with pharmacologic actions similar to those of other barbiturates. Since initial effect after oral administration is observed within 30 minutes and sedation is sustained for approximately 5 to 6 hours, it exerts a more continuous depression of the central nervous system than the short-acting barbiturates.

Dose—*Sedative*, **7.5 to 60 mg**; *usual, sedative*, **15 to 30 mg** 3 or 4 times a day; *hypnotic*, **100 to 200 mg**; *usual, hypnotic*, **100 mg.**

Dosage Forms—Capsules NF: 15, 30, 50, and 100 mg; Elixir NF (see below): 30 mg/5 ml; Tablets NF: 15, 30, 50, and 100 mg.

Sodium Butabarbital Elixir NF contains, in each 100 ml, 560–630 mg of $C_{10}H_{15}N_2NaO_3$. *Preparation:* Dissolve sodium butabarbital (6 Gm), sodium saccharin (1 Gm), compound orange spirit (1.5 ml), and anethole (0.034 ml) in alcohol (300 ml). Add propylene glycol (350 ml). Add tartrazine (FD&C Yellow No. 5, 0.1 Gm) dissolved in purified water (50 ml), and add sufficient purified water to make the product measure 1000 ml. Mix well, and filter if necessary, to produce a clear elixir. *Alcohol Content:* 25 to 31% of C_2H_5OH. *Dose:* 5 ml, which contains 30 mg of Sodium Butabarbital.

Sodium Hexobarbital—see page 1061.

Sodium Hexobarbital, Sterile—see page 1061.

Sodium Methohexital for Injection—see page 1061.

Sodium Pentobarbital USP

[Pentobarbitone Sodium; Soluble Pentobarbital; Sodium 5-Ethyl-5-(1-methylbutyl)barbiturate; Embutal; Nembutal (*Abbott*); Pental (*Mallinckrodt*); Napental (*Massengill*)]

Sodium Pentobarbital contains 98.5–101.0% of $C_{11}H_{17}N_2NaO_3$ (248.26), calculated on the dried basis.

Preparation—This barbiturate is prepared by the process given for barbital, using 2-bromopentane [$CH_3(CH_2)_2CHBr(CH_3)$] to react with one of the hydrogens in the CH_2 of the malonyl group instead of one of the CH_3CH_2Br molecules. It is then converted into the soluble sodium salt by the addition of the required amount of sodium hydroxide.

Description—White, odorless, crystalline granules or a white powder with a slightly bitter taste. Its solution is alkaline to litmus and to phenolphthalein. Its solutions decompose on standing, heat accelerating the decomposition.

Solubility—Very soluble in water; freely soluble in alcohol; practically insoluble in ether.

Incompatibilities—Same as *Sodium Phenobarbital* (below).

Uses—Sodium Pentobarbital is a short-acting *hypnotic* and *sedative*. It is useful for daytime sedation in mild tension states and neuroses as well as bedtime sedation in insomnia. It is also used as a sedative in a wide variety of ailments, including functional gastro-intestinal disorders, preoperative apprehension, hypertension, and coronary disease. It is given parenterally for the control of *convulsive syndromes* as outlined under the general statement, page 1078. It has neither analgetic potency nor antiepileptic action.

Veterinary Use—The drug is employed in animals as a *surgical anesthetic* in the intraperitoneal or intravenous dose of approximately 29 mg per Kg.

Dose—*Oral*, **50 to 200 mg** daily; *usual*, **100 mg** at bedtime; *intravenous*, **50 to 200 mg** daily; *usual*, **100 mg** at bedtime.

Other Dose Information—It can also be instilled rectally in solution in the dose of 300 mg.

Dosage Forms—Capsules USP: 30, 50, and 100 mg; Elixir USP (see below); Injection USP: 100 mg/2 ml, 250 mg/5 ml, 1 Gm/20 ml.

Veterinary Dose—*Sedative, Dogs,* **100 to 200 mg**; *Cats,* **30 to 50 mg.**

Sodium Pentobarbital Elixir USP [Pentobarbital Elixir] contains, in each 100 ml, 375–425 mg of $C_{11}H_{17}N_2NaO_3$. *Preparation:* Sodium Pentobarbital Elixir may be prepared as follows: Dissolve sodium pentobarbital (4 Gm) in purified water (200 ml), then add glycerin (450 ml), alcohol (150 ml), orange oil (0.75 ml), caramel (2 Gm), and syrup (150 ml). Mix, and add diluted hydrochloric acid (6 ml) and sufficient purified water to make the product measure 1000 ml. Mix, and filter, if necessary. *Alcohol Content:* 12 to 18% of C_2H_5OH.

Sodium Phenobarbital USP

[Sodium 5-Ethyl-5-phenylbarbiturate; Phenobarbital Sodium USP XV; Sterile Phenobarbital Sodium USP XV Soluble Phenobarbital; Phenobarbitone Sodium; Phenobarbitalum Natri cum; Luminal Sodium (*Winthrop*)]

Sodium Phenobarbital contains 98.5–101.0% of $C_{12}H_{11}N_2NaO_3$ (254.22), calculated on the dried basis.

Preparation—Sodium Phenobarbital may be prepared by dissolving phenobarbital in a calculated amount of sodium hydroxide solution in alcohol and evaporating at a low temperature.

Description—White flaky crystals, crystalline granules, or powder. It is odorless, has a bitter taste and is hygroscopic. It decomposes on exposure to air and moisture with the formation of free phenobarbital. Its solution is alkaline to litmus and to phenolphthalein. Its solutions decompose on standing, heat accelerating the decomposition.

Solubility—Very soluble in water and alcohol; practically insoluble in ether or chloroform.

Incompatibilities—Sodium Phenobarbital, like other soluble barbiturates, has an alkaline reaction in aqueous solution and exhibits the incompatibilities of the alkalies, leading usually to the precipitation of phenobarbital. Thus, it reacts with *acids*, *acid salts* including many *alkaloidal salts*, and many of the common *vehicles* which have an acid reaction. All *elixirs* and *syrups of thiamine hydrochloride* liberate phenobarbital from the sodium compound and subsequent solution or precipitation of this substance depends on the alcohol concentration of the product. However, even if precipitation does not occur, the combination is incompatible due to the neutralizing effect of the sodium compound on the acidity of the liquid with resultant destruction of the thiamine. In such a situation, phenobarbital should be used in place of the sodium salt and, if necessary, alcohol added to keep it in solution. It may also be necessary to add thiamine hydrochloride equivalent to that contained in the vehicle being replaced by alcohol.

Sodium Phenobarbital liberates ammonia from *ammonium salts* and decomposes *chloral hydrate* with the formation of chloroform. With *alkaloidal salts*, phenobarbital and the free alkaloid are produced and may be precipitated.

Other soluble barbiturates have the same incompatibilities as Sodium Phenobarbital.

Uses—Because of its solubility, Sodium Phenobarbital may be administered hypodermically. This barbiturate can also be injected intravenously for the control of acute convulsive syndromes. See also *Phenobarbital*, page 1081.

Dose—*Parenteral, anticonvulsant* and *hypnotic*, **50** to **600 mg** daily; *usual, parenteral, anticonvulsant*, **300 mg**; *usual, parenteral, hypnotic*, **100 mg,** repeated if necessary.

Dosage Forms—Injection USP: 50 and 125 mg/ml, 300 mg/2 ml, 125 and 300 mg/5 ml, 1.5 Gm/10 ml; Sterile USP: 60, 125, 200, and 300 mg.

Sodium Secobarbital USP

[5-Allyl-5-(1-methylbutyl)barbrituric Acid Sodium Salt; Soluble Secobarbital; Quinalbarbitone Sodium; Seconal Sodium (*Lilly*)]

Sodium Secobarbital contains 98.5–100.5% of $C_{12}H_{17}N_2NaO_3$ (260.27), calculated on the dried basis.

Preparation—Secobarbital may be prepared by the general method described under *Barbital* (page 1079), using allyl bromide and 2-bromopentane as alkylating agents at the 5-position. It is converted into Sodium Secobarbital by treatment with a chemically equivalent portion of sodium hydroxide as described under *Sodium Phenobarbital* (this page).

Description—A white, odorless, hygroscopic powder, having a bitter taste. Its solutions are alkaline to litmus and to phenolphthalein.

Solubility—Very soluble in water; soluble in alcohol; practically insoluble in ether.

Uses—Sodium Secobarbital is one of the short-acting *Barbiturates* (see page 1079). It is useful in obstetrics, neuropsychiatry, and dental procedures or whenever a rapidly acting sedative or hypnotic effect is desirable. It is used orally and rectally for insomnia, preoperative sedation, and sedation in obstetrics.

Dose—*Oral* or *parenteral*, **50** to **200 mg** daily; *usual*, **100 mg** at bedtime.

Dosage Forms—Capsules USP: 30, 50, and 100 mg; Sterile USP: 100 and 250 mg.

Sodium Secobarbital and Sodium Amobarbital Capsules NF

[Tuinal (*Lilly*)]

Sodium Secobarbital and Sodium Amobarbital Capsules contain 90.0–110.0% of the labeled amounts of $C_{12}H_{17}N_2NaO_2$ (sodium secobarbital) and of $C_{11}H_{17}N_2NaO_3$ (sodium amobarbital).

Uses—Sodium Secobarbital and Sodium Amobarbital, a mixture of equal parts of these two barbiturates, is a rapidly effective, moderately long-acting hyp-

notic. It is used in conditions in which a prompt and moderately sustained hypnosis is required. It is not suitable for continuous daytime sedation. Adverse reactions, contraindications, and addiction liability are the same as for other barbiturates. See the general statement on *Barbiturates*, page 1078.

Dose—*Usual hypnotic dose range of sodium secobarbital,* **50** to **200 mg** at bedtime; *of sodium amobarbital,* **50** to **200 mg** at bedtime.

Dosage Forms—Capsules NF: 25, 50, and 100 mg of each.

Sodium Vinbarbital Injection NF

[Sodium 5-Ethyl-5-(1-methyl-1-butenyl)barbiturate Injection; Delvinal Sodium Injection (*MSD*)]

Sodium Vinbarbital Injection is a sterile solution of sodium vinbarbital in a suitable solvent. It contains 90.0–105.0% of the labeled amount of $C_{11}H_{15}N_2NaO_3$ (sodium vinbarbital) (246.24).

Note—Solutions of sodium vinbarbital in water decompose on standing.

Description—The pH is between 8 and 10.

Uses—See *Vinbarbital*.
Dose—*Usual, parenteral*, **60 mg**.
Dosage Forms—Injection NF: 60 mg/ml.

Talbutal

[Lotusate (*Winthrop*)]

Talbutal is 5-allyl-5-sec-butylbarbituric acid ($C_{11}H_{16}N_2O_3$).

Description—Crystals that melt between 108° and 110°. It has a slightly bitter taste. Its saturated aqueous solution is acid to litmus.

Solubility—Practically insoluble in water and petroleum ether; soluble in alcohol, chloroform, ether, acetone, glacial acetic acid, and solutions of fixed alkali hydroxides.

Uses—Talbutal is a barbiturate with an intermediate duration of action (see general statement, page 1078). It is used as a sedative and hypnotic. In sedative doses, it is used in patients with tension and anxiety states, neurasthenia, hysteria, delirium tremens, hypertension, coronary disease, gastrointestinal disorders, and hyperthyroidism. In full hypnotic doses, it induced sleep in 15 to 30 minutes which lasts 6 to 8 hours. Untoward effects are usually mild and generally include slight "hangover," drowsiness, or headache.

Dose—*Usual, hypnotic*, **120 mg** before bedtime; *sedative*, **30 mg** 2 or 3 times daily.

Dosage Forms—Capsules: 30, 50, and 120 mg.

Vinbarbital NF

[5-Ethyl-5-(1-methyl-1-butenyl)barbituric Acid; Delvinal (*MSD*)]

Vinbarbital, dried at 105° for 2 hours, contains 98.5–100.5% of $C_{11}H_{16}N_2O_3$ (224.26).

Preparation—Vinbarbital may be prepared by condensing methyl *n*-propyl ketone with ethyl cyanoacetate to form 1-methylbutylidenecyanoacetic ester, followed by treatment with diethyl sulfate to produce the ethyl ester of ethyl-1-methyl-1-butenylcyanoacetic acid, and subsequent condensation with urea to form 5-ethyl-5-(1-methyl-1-butenyl) barbituric acid (Vinbarbital).

Description—A white powder with a bitter taste and characteristic odor. Melting range 160° to 163°.

Solubility—Very slightly soluble in water; soluble in alcohol; sparingly soluble in ether.

Uses—Vinbarbital, a *central depressant*, is one of the intermediate-acting *Barbiturates* (page 1079). It is used as a depressant in certain psychoneurotic states, for induction of obstetrical amnesia and anesthesia, and for preoperative sedation.

Dose—*Usual, hypnotic,* **100 to 200 mg** at bedtime. *Other Dose Information*—The usual sedative dose is 30 mg 3 or 4 times a day.

Dosage Forms—Capsules NF: 100 mg.

Other Barbiturates

Barbital Sodium NF XI [Soluble Barbital; Soluble Barbitone; Barbitone Sodium] [$C_8H_{11}N_2NaO_3$]—White, odorless powder having a bitter taste. It is stable in air. 1 Gm dissolves in about 5 ml of water; slightly soluble in alcohol; insoluble in ether. *Uses:* Barbital Sodium has the same uses as *Barbital,* but is more readily absorbed because it is more soluble. In sterile solution, it can be injected subcutaneously, intramuscularly, or intravenously for the production of central nervous system depression, as outlined under the general discussion, page 1078. The intravenous injection of Barbital Sodium is usually reserved for the control of convulsive disorders. *Note:* Solutions of sodium barbiturates are not stable and therefore should be prepared extemporaneously as required for use. A 10% solution (pH about 10) of Barbital Sodium, heated at 100° for 1 hour, loses about 2.5% of its activity. The decomposition increases with increasing pH. *Dose: Usual,* 300 mg. *Veterinary Dose:* Dogs, 150 mg to 1 Gm, Cats, 100 to 300 mg.

Butallylonal NF X [5-(2-Bromoallyl)-5-*sec*-butylbarbituric acid]—Purity: 98.5–101.5% $C_{11}H_{15}BrN_2O_3$. A fine, white, crystalline powder with a slightly bitter taste, melting at 130–133°C. Very slightly soluble in water, freely soluble in alcohol, ether, and alkaline solutions. *Uses:* Hypnotic with intermediate duration of action. *Dose: Orally,* 0.2 Gm.

Butethal NF X [Butobarbitone BP; 5-Butyl-5-ethyl-barbituric acid]—Purity: not less than 98% $C_{10}H_{16}N_2O_3$. A white crystalline powder having a slightly bitter taste and melting at 124–127°C. 1 Gm dissolves in about 5 ml alcohol, 10 ml ether, but is practically insoluble in water. *Uses:* Hypnotic with intermediate duration of action. *Dose: Orally,* 0.1 to 0.2 Gm, maximum in 24 hours is 0.4 Gm.

Cyclobarbital NF X [5-(1-Cyclohexen-1-yl)-5-ethyl-barbituric acid]—Purity: not less than 98.5% $C_{12}H_{16}N_2O_3$. A white, crystalline, odorless powder with a bitter taste, melting at 171–174°C. Very slightly soluble in cold water but soluble in hot water; 1 Gm dissolves in 5 ml alcohol and in 10 ml of ether. *Uses:* A hypnotic and sedative of short duration of action. *Dose: Orally,* 0.1 to 0.4 Gm.

Diallylbarbituric Acid NF X [Allobarbital; 5,5-Diallyl-barbituric acid]—Purity: not less than 98.5% $C_{10}H_{12}N_2O_3$. White, odorless, glistening, small crystals or a white crystalline powder with a bitter taste, melting at 171–173°C. 1 Gm dissolves in about 300 parts cold water, 50 parts boiling water, 20 parts cold alcohol, and 20 parts ether. *Uses:* Sedative and hypnotic of intermediate duration of action. *Dose: Orally,* for *sedation,* 30 mg; for *hypnosis,* 0.1 to 0.3 Gm.

Heptabarbital [Medomin (*Geigy*)] is 5-(1-cyclohepten-1-yl)-5-ethylbarbituric acid ($C_{13}H_{18}N_2O_3$). *Description* and *Solubility:* Crystals with a slightly bitter taste; it melts at 174°. Very sparingly soluble in water, more soluble in alcohol; soluble in alkaline solutions; forms water-soluble calcium, magnesium, and sodium salts. *Uses:* A mild sedative with a medium duration of hypnotic action. The drug should not be used in patients with intermittent porphyria, severe respiratory depression, or severe circulatory depression. It is also contraindicated in patients known to be dependent on or sensitive to barbiturates. *Dose: Usual, sedative,* 50 to 100 mg 2 or 3 times daily; *hypnotic,* 200 to 400 mg. Occasionally larger doses may be required. *Dosage Forms:* Tablets, 200 mg.

Hexobarbital PhI [Hexobarbitone; 5-(1-Cyclohexen-1-yl)-1,5-dimethylbarbituric acid; Sombulex (*Riker*); Somnalert (*Warren-Teed*)] [$C_{12}H_{16}N_2O_3$]—Purity: not less than 98.4%. Colorless, odorless crystals or tasteless, white, crystalline powder, melting at 144–147°C. It is soluble in 3000 parts of water, in 250 parts of boiling water, in about 45 parts of ethyl alcohol and soluble in ether, chloroform, and solutions of alkali hydroxides but not in solutions of alkali carbonates. Sleep is induced within 10 to 20 minutes and lasts for 3 to 6 hours with this drug. *Uses:* Hypnotic with a short duration of action. *Dose: Orally,* 0.25 to 0.5 Gm.

Pentobarbital [5-Ethyl-5-(1-methylbutyl)barbituric acid] [$C_{11}H_{18}N_2O_3$]—White, granular powder, freely soluble in alcohol, slightly soluble in water, soluble in alkali hydroxide solutions. *Uses:* Short-acting barbiturate. *Dose: Orally,* 0.12 Gm.

Pentobarbital Calcium—Fine, white powder; sparingly soluble in water and alcohol. *Uses and Dose:* As of *Sodium Pentobarbital* (see page 1083). The calcium salt is better suited for making compressed tablets.

Probarbital Sodium NF X [Sodium 5-ethyl-5-isopropyl-barbiturate; Ipral (*Squibb*)]—Purity: not less than 98% $C_9H_{13}N_2NaO_3$. A white, odorless, hygroscopic powder. It is freely soluble in water, forming a solution which is alkaline to litmus; slightly soluble in alcohol and insoluble in ether. Its aqueous solutions are unstable. *Uses:* Sedative and hypnotic of intermediate duration of action. *Dose: Orally,* 0.05 to 0.5 Gm.

Nonbarbiturate Sedatives and Hypnotics

In addition to the various derivatives of barbituric acid discussed in the previous section, there are a number of other agents which possess useful sedative and hypnotic properties. Among these are the newer nonbarbiturate amides, the century-old bromides, the occasionally used alcohols, and time-proved chloral hydrate. Disulfiram [Antabuse (*Ayerst*)], an antioxidant agent devoid of sedative and hypnotic properties, is included in this section because of its use as an adjunct in the management of alcoholism. The effective hypnotic dose of nonbarbiturates is usually larger than that for the barbiturates. Although some of the newer agents are said to be less toxic, there is no reason for believing that any of the newer hypnotics differ qualitatively from the barbiturates in their desirable or undesirable effects. Many of these agents will produce physical dependence and habituation when taken chronically in excessive doses. The chief value of the newer agents is their occasional usefulness in patients who fail to benefit from the older, well-established, and cheaper drugs such as the barbiturates and chloral hydrate.

Alcohol—see page 1357.

Amylene Hydrate—see page 1359.

Chloral Betaine NF

[Chloral Hydrate Betaine (1:1) Compound; Beta-Chlor (*Mead-Johnson*)]

$$CCl_3CH(OH)_2 \cdot (CH_3)_3\overset{+}{N}CH_2CO\overset{-}{O}$$

Chloral Betaine [$C_7H_{14}Cl_3NO_4$ = 282.55] is an adduct formed by the reaction of chloral hydrate with betaine. It contains 56.0–59.5% of $C_2H_3Cl_3O_2$ (chloral hydrate), and 40.0–44.0% of $C_5H_{11}NO_2$ (betaine).

Preparation—Chloral Betaine may be prepared by warming an equimolar mixture of betaine hydrate and chloral hydrate.

Description—A white, crystalline powder with a faint, aromatic, penetrating, slightly acrid odor characteristic of chloral hydrate, and a slightly bitter taste. It darkens slightly with long exposure to light and is slightly hygroscopic. It melts with decomposition between 120° and 128°.

Solubility—Very soluble in water; freely soluble in alcohol; very slightly soluble in chloroform.

Uses—Chloral Betaine, an addition compound representing one molecule each of chloral hydrate and betaine, is used as a **sedative** and **hypnotic** agent. This agent is virtually devoid of undesirable gastro-intestinal effects but retains the characteristic effect of chloral hydrate on the central nervous system. Onset and duration of sleep is similar to that for an equivalent amount of chloral hydrate.

Dose—*Usual,* **870 mg** to **1.74 Gm** 15 to 30 minutes before bedtime.

Dosage Forms—Tablets NF: 870 mg (equivalent to 500 mg of chloral hydrate).

Chloral Hydrate USP

[Chloral; Hydrated Chloral; Kessodrate (*McKesson*); Noctec (*Squibb*); Somnos (*MSD*)]

Chloral Hydrate contains 99.5–102.5% of $C_2H_3Cl_3O_2$ (165.40).

The *gem*-diol structure of Chloral Hydrate is indicated by the avidity with which chloral combines not only with water but also with other compounds such as ammonia and hydroxylamine to form *stable* addition compounds. It is also explicable on theoretical grounds in terms of the electron-withdrawal effect of the three chlorine atoms which renders the carbonyl carbon relatively positive and thus more receptive to hydroxyl and other electron-rich reagents.

Preparation—Chloral Hydrate is prepared by the action of chlorine on alcohol. An amount of chlorine gas, closely approximating 4 mols per mol of alcohol used, is slowly passed into alcohol. Heating during chlorination greatly accelerates the process. When all of the chlorine has been absorbed, the oily, crude product is stirred with sulfuric acid which aids in the escape of occluded hydrogen chloride and dissolves some of the side products. The separated crude chloral is then fractionally distilled, and the fraction coming over between about 95° to 98°, and consisting largely of anhydrous chloral, is mixed with the calculated quantity of water

to form the hydrate. It is then allowed to stand undisturbed until no more crystallizes out.

Description—Colorless or white crystals, having an aromatic, penetrating, slightly acrid odor, and a slightly bitter, caustic taste. It melts at about 55°, but liquefies at room temperature when triturated with an equal quantity of camphor, menthol, or thymol. It slowly volatilizes in the air.

Solubility—1 Gm dissolves in 0.25 ml of water, 1.3 ml of alcohol, 2 ml of chloroform, and 1.5 ml of ether; very soluble in olive oil; freely soluble in turpentine oil, petroleum benzin, and carbon tetrachloride.

Identification—Chloral Hydrate is decomposed by alkali and alkaline earth hydroxides into chloroform and a formate of the base. This is the principle involved in the official assay. When Chloral Hydrate is warmed with a few drops each of aniline and sodium hydroxide TS, phenyl isocyanide, which has an intensely disagreeable odor, is formed (phenyl isocyanide is *poisonous*). The phenyl isocyanide is formed by reaction between the aniline and the chloroform formed by the action of the NaOH on the Chloral.

Incompatibilities—A liquid or soft mass is produced on trituration with *acetanilid, acetophenetidin, antipyrine, camphor, menthol, phenol, phenyl salicylate, thymol,* and many other organic compounds, as well as certain hydrated salts such as *quinine sulfate, sodium phosphate,* etc. Up to about 15% of chloral hydrate can be incorporated into theobroma oil without the melting point being lowered sufficiently to require added stiffening agent. Twenty per cent of spermaceti in the theobroma oil permits the inclusion of 30% of chloral hydrate.

In aqueous solution, chloral hydrate slowly decomposes with the formation of acid. *Alkaline substances* cause its decomposition into chloroform and a formate. The *soluble barbiturates* are therefore incompatible, causing not only a breakdown of the chloral hydrate but a precipitation of the barbiturate as well. In solution with *potassium iodide,* chloral hydrate is slowly decomposed with the liberation of chloroform and iodine.

In *hydroalcoholic solutions* in the presence of *salts,* chloral alcoholate is formed and may remain in solution or may separate as an oily liquid depending on the concentration of the alcohol and the amount of salt present. If less than 10% of alcohol is present, separation does not occur regardless of the salt or chloral hydrate concentration. In the presence of more than 50% of alcohol, no separation occurs. Chloral alcoholate is no more toxic than chloral hydrate but there is danger of uneven dosage if it separates. *Sugar* behaves similarly to salt in inducing separation. In most instances, separation may be prevented by increasing or decreasing the alcohol content, the latter as by simple dilution with water.

Uses—Chloral Hydrate is employed as a *sedative* and *soporific.* It has little or no analgesic action, and should not be used alone in the presence of pain. Chloral Hydrate is used as a sedative in hysteria and chorea. It is frequently employed in persons undergoing *withdrawal therapy for barbiturate or alcohol addiction,* and has been rather widely employed in the management of *eclampsia* (Stroganoff treatment). It is not to be preferred to intravenously administered barbiturates in convulsive syndromes when convulsions are actually present. Patients with serious heart, kidney, or liver disease should not be given Chloral Hydrate. If gastritis is present, the drug may be administered by rectum in olive oil as a retention enema.

For oral use, it is usually given in a flavored syrup. Also alkalies and alkaline salts are to be avoided because of the decomposition of Chloral Hydrate which they cause.

Dose—**250 mg** to **2 Gm** daily; *usual,* **500 mg** at bedtime.

Dosage Forms—Capsules USP: 250 and 500 mg, and 1 Gm; Syrup USP: 250, 500, and 800 mg/5ml.

Veterinary Dose—Deep narcosis or light anesthesia: *Light Horses*, **5** to **6 Gm** per **100 pounds** of body weight; *Heavy Horses*, **4.5** to **5 Gm** per **100 pounds** of body weight, given intravenously in dilute solution; *Cattle*, **5** to **6 Gm** per **100 pounds** of body weight, given intravenously in dilute solution; *Sheep*, **4** to **8 Gm** per **100 pounds** of body weight, given by slow intravenous injection to effect; *Swine*, mature, **0.15** to **0.17 Gm** per **Kg** of body weight, given by slow intravenous injection; *Young Pigs*, **0.3 Gm** per **Kg** of body weight, injected intraperitoneally in 5% solution.

Sedative: *Horses* and *Cattle*, **30** to **60 Gm**; *Dogs*, **300** to **400 mg**.

Narcotic: *Horses* and *Cattle*, **75** to **125 Gm**, per os or rectum; *Dogs*, up to **4 Gm** in 30 ml of cold water per rectum for each 25 pounds of body weight.

Diphenhydramine Hydrochloride—see page 1147.

Disulfiram

[Alcophobin (*Consolidated*); Antabuse (*Ayerst*)]

$$(C_2H_5)_2N-\overset{\overset{\displaystyle S}{\|}}{C}-S-S-\overset{\overset{\displaystyle S}{\|}}{C}-N(C_2H_5)_2$$

Disulfiram is bis(diethylthiocarbamoyl)disulfide [$C_{10}H_{20}N_2S_4 = 296.54$].

Preparation—For commercial methods of preparation, consult US Pats. 1,796,977 and 1,782,111.

Description—It occurs as crystals which melt at 70°.

Solubility—Soluble in alcohol, ether, acetone, benzene, chloroform, and carbon disulfide; practically insoluble in water.

Uses—Disulfiram is used as an adjunct in the treatment of alcoholism. It blocks the oxidation of alcohol at the acetaldehyde stage, which then accumulates in the body and produces unpleasant symptoms characterized by flushing, palpitation, dyspnea and hyperventilation, increased pulse rate, nausea and vomiting, cyanosis and decreased blood pressure, and occasionally profound collapse. These symptoms are usually followed by drowsiness and sleep, following which the patient has fully recovered.

The drug should not be used without the patient's full knowledge and consent. Extreme caution is necessary during its use because severe and alarming reactions (and some deaths) have been reported in patients on Disulfiram. These include cardiovascular complications involving unusual fall in blood pressure, cardiac arrhythmia, and electrocardiographic evidence of myocardial ischemia and even myocardial infarction. Some patients complain of mild drowsiness, fatigability, impotence, headache or peripheral neuritis, and occasionally skin rashes.

Patients on Disulfiram should avoid contact with alcohol in a partially disguised form such as cough syrup or other medicinals containing it and alcoholic lotions applied to the skin. In addition to alcohol-induced reactions, physicians should be alert to drug-induced psychotic episodes that may occur during therapy. Disulfiram should not be used in patients recently treated with paraldehyde, and paraldehyde should not be given to patients receiving Disulfiram.

Dose—*Usual, oral, initial*, **500 mg** daily for the first 2 or 3 weeks; *usual, maintenance*, **125** to **500 mg** daily.

Dosage Forms—Tablets: 500 mg.

Ethchlorvynol NF

[1-Chloro-3-ethyl-1-penten-4-yn-3-ol; β-Chlorovinyl Ethyl Ethynyl Carbinol; Placidyl (*Abbott*)]

$$HC\equiv C-\overset{\overset{\displaystyle OH}{|}}{\underset{\underset{\displaystyle CH_2CH_3}{|}}{C}}-CH=\overset{\overset{\displaystyle H}{|}}{C}-Cl$$

Ethchlorvynol contains 95.0–102.0% of C_7H_9ClO (144.60), calculated on the anhydrous basis.

Preparation—Ethchlorvynol may be prepared by reacting ethyl chlorovinyl ketone (I) with lithium acetylide under Grignard reaction conditions. The alkoxide addition complex reacts readily with dilute acid to form crude ethchlorvynol which is extracted with a suitable, water-immiscible organic solvent such as ether and is subsequently purified by distillation. (I) may be prepared in good yield by causing propionyl chloride to undergo addition to acetylene at a temperature of about 40°C in the presence of a small quantity of zinc chloride.

Description—It occurs as a colorless to yellow liquid possessing a characteristic pungent odor. It darkens on exposure to light and to air. Specific gravity 1.068 to 1.071. Refractive index 1.4765 to 1.4800.

Solubility—Immiscible with water; miscible with most organic solvents.

Uses—Ethchlorvynol is a mild hypnotic with a short onset of action and a duration of action of approximately 5 hours. Its effect is less profound and not as predictable as that obtained with barbiturates. The excessive chronic use of large doses of Ethchlorvynol has been reported to cause psychic and physical dependence, tolerance, and withdrawal symptoms, including convulsions, when the drug is discontinued. It should not be used in patients with a history of drug abuse, and the drug should be gradually withdrawn from patients taking excessive quantities. The drug is metabolized primarily by the liver. Side effects, such as nausea, mental confusion, headache, and dermatitis, have been observed in some patients.

Dose—*Sedative*, **100** to **200 mg**; *usual, sedative*, **100 mg** 2 or 3 times a day; *hypnotic*, **500 mg** to **1 Gm**; *usual, hypnotic*, **500 mg**.

Dosage Forms—Capsules NF: 100, 200, and 500 mg.

Ethinamate NF

[1-Ethynylcyclohexanol Carbamate; Valmid (*Lilly*)]

$$\overset{\displaystyle O-\overset{\overset{\displaystyle O}{\|}}{C}-NH_2}{\underset{\displaystyle C\equiv CH}{\bigcirc}}$$

Ethinamate contains 98.0–100.5% of $C_9H_{13}NO_2$ (167.21), calculated on the dried basis.

Preparation—Ethinamate may be prepared by condensing 1-ethynylcyclohexanol with carbamoyl chloride in the presence of pyridine or another suitable basic catalyst. The crude ester is obtained by treating the reaction mixture with dilute hydrochloric acid. It may be purified by crystallization from an ethanol-water mixture. The 1-ethynylcyclohexanol may be synthesized by a typical Grignard reaction using cyclohexanone and ethynylmagnesium bromide.

Description—White, essentially odorless powder. Melting range: 95° to 98°. pH (saturated solution): 6.5 to 7.0.

Solubility—1 Gm dissolves in about 500 ml of water; freely soluble in alcohol, chloroform, and ether.

Uses—Ethinamate is a short-acting mild hypnotic which produces little or no after effect. It is useful for the prompt induction of sleep in simple insomnia. Although Ethinamate is rapidly destroyed in the body, the principal site of destruction is unknown; it is *not* destroyed by the liver. Hence, it is useful in the presence of impaired liver and kidney function. Side effects are minimal. Habituation and physical dependence may result from excessive use of the drug. It should be used with caution in patients with a history of drug abuse.

Dose—500 mg to 1 Gm; *usual*, 500 mg.
Dosage Forms—Tablets NF: 500 mg.

Glutethimide NF

[2-Ethyl-2-phenylglutarimide; Doriden (*Ciba*)]

Glutethimide, dried at 45° over phosphorus pentoxide to constant weight, contains 98.0–101.0% of $C_{13}H_{15}NO_2$ (217.27).

Preparation—Benzyl cyanide in toluene solution is treated with ethyl chloride in the presence of sodamide to yield α-ethylbenzyl cyanide. This is then caused to undergo addition (Michael condensation) to methyl acrylate under the catalytic influence of piperidine or another suitable basic catalyst, thus forming methyl 4-cyano-4-phenylhexanoate (I). After purifying by low pressure distillation, (I) is cyclized in acid medium. The cyclization may be represented as involving hydration of the cyanide group to amide and saponification of the ester, thus yielding (II) which cyclizes through dehydration between the amide and carboxyl groups. The crude product may be purified by recrystallization from an ethanol-water mixture.

Description—White, crystalline powder. The saturated solution is slightly acid. Melting range 86° to 89°.

Solubility—Freely soluble in ethyl acetate, acetone, and chloroform; soluble in alcohol and methanol; practically insoluble in water.

Uses—Glutethimide is a hypnotic and sedative which produces alterations in the electroencephalographic pattern similar to those observed after administration of chloral hydrate or barbiturates. The onset of action begins about one-half hour after the administration of a hypnotic dose and generally lasts from 4 to 8 hours. Hence, it is useful for the induction of sleep in patients with simple and nervous insomnia. In sedative doses, it relieves anxiety usually without impairing psychomotor function. Glutethimide appears to be about as effective as the usually employed short-acting barbiturate hypnotics, but it possesses no particular advantage over the latter except in patients

who cannot tolerate barbituric acid derivatives. Side effects include nausea and, infrequently, skin rash. Habituation and physical dependence may result from the prolonged administration of excessive doses. The drug should be used with caution in patients with a history of drug abuse.

Dose—*Usual*, *sedative*, 125 to 250 mg up to 3 times a day; *hypnotic*, 500 mg to 1 Gm.
Dosage Forms—Tablets NF: 125, 250, and 500 mg.

Magnesium Sulfate Injection—see page 1099.

Methyprylon NF

[3,3-Diethyl-5-methyl-2,4-piperidinedione; Noludar (*Roche*)]

Methyprylon contains 98.0–101.0% of $C_{10}H_{17}NO_2$ (183.25), calculated on the dried basis.

Preparation—3,3 - Diethyl - 2,4(1*H*,3*H*) - pyridinedione (I) is hydroxymethylated at the 5-position by treatment with formaldehyde in the presence of an alkaline catalyst. The resulting methylol derivative (indicated in II) is then subjected to catalytic hydrogenation whereupon the ring is saturated and the hydroxymethyl group is deoxygenated.

Description—It occurs as a white, or nearly white, crystalline powder that has a slight characteristic odor. Melting range 74° to 77°.

Solubility—Soluble in water; very soluble in alcohol, chloroform, ether, and benzene.

Uses—Methyprylon, a piperidine derivative, is a sedative and hypnotic with an onset and duration of action similar to pentobarbital. Hence, it is useful as a hypnotic in patients with simple and nervous insomnia. Side effects, such as vertigo and nausea, are infrequent and mild. Methyprylon is dehydrogenated to a tetrahydropyridine compound that appears in the urine and bile. Since an analogous tetrahydropyridine has been implicated as a causative agent in agranulocytosis, caution should be exercised in administering Methyprylon. Habituation and physical dependence have been reported to occur when excessive doses are taken over an extended period of time.

Dose—*Usual*, 50 to 400 mg at bedtime.
Other Dose Information—Sedative, 50 to 100 mg; usual, 50 mg 3 or 4 times a day; hypnotic, 200 to 400 mg; usual, 200 mg.
Dosage Forms—Capsules NF: 300 mg; Tablets NF: 50 and 200 mg.

Paraldehyde USP

[2,4,6-Trimethyl-*s*-trioxane; Paraldehydum; Paracetaldehyde]

Paraldehyde [$C_6H_{12}O_3$ = 132.16] is a trimer of acetaldehyde.

Caution—Paraldehyde is subject to oxidation to form acetic acid. It may contain a suitable stabilizer.

Preparation—It may be made by treating acetaldehyde with small quantities of sulfur dioxide, hydrochloric acid, carbonyl chloride, or zinc chloride; almost complete conversion occurs, and by freezing the liquid and then distilling the crystallized material, if necessary, pure Paraldehyde is produced.

Description—A colorless, transparent liquid with a disagreeable taste and a strong, characteristic, but not unpleasant or pungent odor. Its specific gravity is about 0.99. It congeals not below 11° and distils between 120° and 126°. In contact with air it slowly oxidizes to acetic acid.

Solubility—1 ml dissolves in about 10 ml of water and about 17 ml of boiling water; miscible with alcohol, chloroform, ether, and volatile oils.

Identification—When it is heated with dilute sulfuric acid it breaks up (depolymerizes) into acetaldehyde [CH_3-CHO]. The latter is a gas at room temperature, having a characteristic odor. When conducted into silver ammonium nitrate TS contained in a clean test tube, a "silver mirror" is produced.

Incompatibilities—*Acids* convert paraldehyde into acetaldehyde, which is prone to oxidation.

Uses—Paraldehyde is one of the oldest and best *hypnotics*. Its chief disadvantage is that, being in part excreted through the lungs, it imparts an odor to the exhaled air. Also, Paraldehyde has an unpleasant taste and may irritate the throat and gastric mucosa unless dispensed in suitable vehicles. It is poorly soluble in water; hence, it is usually prescribed in combination with alcoholic liquors, elixirs, etc. The drug can also be taken in milk, fruit juices, iced tea, or with cracked ice. Finally, it can be administered as a rectal retention enema in olive oil. Paraldehyde is occasionally employed as an *obstetrical analgetic*, in which case large doses are administered, usually by rectum. The drug is also frequently used in *delirium tremens*, and in patients undergoing *withdrawal therapy for alcoholism.*

Dose—*Oral*, **5 to 30 ml** daily; *usual, oral or rectal*, **10 ml,** repeated as necessary; *usual, intramuscular,* **5 ml.**

Dosage Forms—Sterile USP: 2, 5, and 10 ml.

Sodium Bromide NF XII

Sodium Bromide, dried at 105° for 4 hours, contains not less than 99% of NaBr (102.90).

Preparation—A process frequently used in making this salt consists in first making ferroso–ferric bromide by reacting iron with bromine in the presence of water, and then adding it to a solution of sodium carbonate. The reaction proceeds as described under *Potassium Bromide* (page 1090).

Sodium Bromide may also be made by a method similar to that outlined under *Potassium Bromide* (page 1090) in which bromine and sodium hydroxide are combined to form Sodium Bromide and bromate, the latter being afterward converted into bromide by ignition with charcoal.

Description—White, odorless cubic crystals, or a white, granular powder with an intensely saline taste. It absorbs moisture from the air, but does not deliquesce.

Solubility—1 Gm dissolves in 1.2 ml of water and 30 ml of alcohol.

Incompatibilities—In relatively high concentrations soluble bromides are *alkaloidal precipitants*. About 20% of

alcohol prevents the precipitation. *Strong oxidizing agents* liberate bromine. *Mercurous chloride* is partially converted to mercuric salt by the alkali bromides, the mixture becoming dark due to the simultaneous formation of metallic mercury. *Lead, silver, manganese, antimony,* and *mercurous salts* cause a precipitation. *Enzymes* are "salted out" of solution by bromides in fairly high concentration. In contrast to potassium bromide, sodium bromide is hygroscopic and due to this may cause trouble in powder and capsule formulations.

Uses—Sodium Bromide has a variety of uses, as a *sedative* and *mild hypnotic*. It is also used in the symptomatic treatment of *epilepsy*, being fairly effective in grand mal, less so in petit mal, and rather ineffective in most cases of psychomotor equivalent seizures. The bromide ion causes a large number of toxic reactions in the body when its concentration is too high, and some of the symptoms which it causes resemble rather closely many clinical diseases and syndromes. For this reason, the bromides should not be looked upon as innocuous, and should be carefully prescribed. The promiscuous use of bromides in a variety of sedative nostrums can only be deplored. The caution "Non. rep." should be written by the physician on every prescription for bromides. Except where sodium is contraindicated, Sodium Bromide is to be preferred over the many other available bromide salts and preparations, because it is inexpensive and least irritating to the stomach. It may be dispensed as tablets, capsules, or in a variety of liquid forms.

Dose—*Usual*, **900 mg** daily.

Dosage Forms—Elixir.

Veterinary Dose—*Horses* and *Cattle*, **25 to 50 Gm;** *Sheep* and *Swine*, **2 to 5 Gm;** *Dogs*, **300 mg to 2 Gm.**

Other Nonbarbiturate Sedatives and Hypnotics

Acetylcarbromal [1-Acetyl-3-(2-bromo-2-ethylbutyryl)-urea; Sedamyl (*Riker*)] [(C_2H_5)$_2$CBr.CO.NH.CO.NH.-COCH$_3$]—Crystals having a slightly bitter taste and melting at 109°C. Slightly soluble in water, freely soluble in alcohol and ethyl acetate. *Uses*: Sedative in hysteria and nervous irritability. *Dose*: Usual, 0.25 to 0.50 Gm.

Ammonium Bromide NF XII, dried at 105° for 2 hours, contains 99.0–101.0% of NH$_4$Br (97.95). *Preparation*: It may be prepared by any one of the following processes—(1) addition of ammonia water or ammonium carbonate to a solution of ferrosoferric bromide; (2) gradual addition of bromide to a cool aqueous solution containing an excess of ammonia; or (3) neutralizing hydrobromic acid with ammonium hydroxide or ammonium carbonate. *Description and Solubility*: Colorless crystals, or a yellowish-white, crystalline powder having no odor; it is somewhat hygroscopic and its solution is slightly acid to litmus. 1 Gm dissolves in about 1.3 ml of water, 40 ml of alcohol, 1 ml of boiling water, and 1.2 ml of boiling alcohol. *Incompatibilities*: *Alkalies* and *alkaline salts* liberate gaseous ammonia from solutions of the ammonium salts. Some ammonium salts decompose spontaneously with the liberation of ammonia. See also *Sodium Bromide* (this page). *Uses*: For the *sedative* effect of the bromide ion. It is inferior to *Sodium Bromide* (page 1089) and should not be employed because it often causes gastrointestinal distress, is unstable, and is an acid-forming salt tending to produce acidosis; also, it turns yellow on exposure to air and gives off free bromine. *Dose*: Usual, 1 Gm.

Brandy NF XI [Spiritus Vini Vitis; Spiritus Vini Gallici; Eau de Vie; Spiritus Vini; Cognac]—An alcoholic liquid obtained by the distillation of the fermented juice of sound ripe grapes and containing 48–54% by volume of ethyl alcohol. It must have been stored in wood containers for a period of at least 2 years before use. It is a pale, amber liquid with a characteristic odor and taste and an acid reaction to litmus. *Uses*: See *Alcohol* (page 1357).

Bromides, Three, Elixir NF XII contains, in each 100 ml, 23–25 Gm of total bromides. *Preparation:* Dissolve ammonium bromide (80 Gm), potassium bromide (80 Gm), and sodium bromide (80 Gm) in compound benzaldehyde elixir (800 ml), add amaranth solution (3 ml) and compound benzaldehyde elixir (qs) to make the product measure 1000 ml; then filter, if necessary, until the product is clear. *Alcohol Content:* 3–5%. *Incompatibilities:* The ammonium bromide in this elixir appears to be the chief source of difficulty. *Nitrites* are decomposed with evolution of gaseous oxides of nitrogen and *sodium phenobarbital* is converted to phenobarbital which may precipitate. *Alkalies* liberate ammonia, detectable with moist litmus paper if masked by the flavor of the Elixir. *Alkaloids* may be precipitated. *Uses:* For the *sedative* action of the bromide ion. It has no advantages over *Sodium Bromide* (page 1089). *Dose:* Usual, 5 ml.

Bromides, Three, Tablets NF XII (consisting of ammonium bromide, potassium bromide, and sodium bromide in equal proportions) show a content of Br which is 70.0–81.0% of the labeled amount of total bromides, including all tolerances. The tablets show a content of ammonium bromide, which is 30.8–35.8% of the labeled amount of total bromides. *Uses:* For the *sedative* action of the bromide ion with no therapeutic advantage over *Sodium Bromide* (page 1089). *Dose:* Usual, 300 mg of each bromide.

Bromisovalum NF XI—$[C_6H_{11}BrN_2O_2]$—It consists chiefly of 2-bromo-3-methylbutyryl urea with trace amounts of the next higher and lower homologs and their isomers. It occurs as small, white, needle-shaped or scale-like crystals having a faintly bitter taste. It sublimes upon heating; it melts between 147° and 150°. Soluble in alcohol and ether. *Uses:* A *central depressant* employed as a *hypnotic* and *sedative.* It should be used with the same care as other bromide-containing compounds. *Dose: Sedative,* 300 mg; *hypnotic,* 600 mg.

Bromoform PhI [Tribromomethane] $[CHBr_3]$—Prepared by adding bromine to a mixture of acetone and dilute sodium hydroxide and warming. A colorless, heavy liquid with a sweet taste and an odor resembling chloroform. Sp gr 2.902. Boils at 149 to 150°. Soluble in 800 parts of water, miscible with organic solvents. Preserved by the addition of 3 to 4% of alcohol. *Uses:* Formerly in whooping cough and seasickness but unreliable. *Dose: Usual,* 0.03 to 0.12 ml.

Calcium Bromide NF XI—A hydrated salt, containing 84–94% $CaBr_2$. It occurs as a white, odorless, granular salt. It is very deliquescent. It is very soluble in water and freely soluble in alcohol; insoluble in chloroform and ether. *Uses:* Employed for the sedative action of the bromide ion. It has no advantage over sodium and potassium bromide and is not preferred to these. See *Sodium Bromide* (page 1089). *Dose: Usual,* 1 Gm.

Carbromal NF XI [Bromodiethylacetylurea; (2-Bromo-2-ethylbutyryl)urea] $[C_7H_{13}BrN_2O_2]$—A white, odorless, crystalline powder, melting between 116° and 119°; 1 Gm dissolves in about 3000 ml of water, 18 ml alcohol, 3 ml chloroform, and 14 ml ether. *Uses:* A weak *hypnotic* and is but infrequently used in modern therapeutics. It is readily oxidized to urea in the body and is practically nontoxic. Nevertheless, it should be used with the same care as other bromide-containing compounds. Due to its feeble *central depressant* effects, its action is often unreliable and disappointing. *Dose: Usual, oral,* 500 mg.

Dichloralantipyrine—A molecular complex formed by combining 2 moles of chloral hydrate and 1 mole of antipyrine. *Uses:* As a hypnotic in the treatment of insomnia. It also has a mild analgesic action. It is contraindicated in patients with severe renal or hepatic disease and should be discontinued if a skin rash appears during therapy. *Dose: Orally,* 0.6 to 1.2 Gm with full glass of water before retiring.

Ectylurea [*cis*-(2-Ethylcrotonoyl)urea; Levanil (*Upjohn*)] $[C_7H_{12}N_2O_2]$—Needle-like crystals which melt between 191° and 198°. Very slightly soluble in ether, hot alcohol, and other organic solvents; soluble in concentrated aqueous solutions of alkalies and acids. *Uses:* It produces mild depression of the central nervous system and is used as a mild sedative in the treatment of simple anxiety and nervous tension. The site of metabolic breakdown and the precise mechanism of action of this drug are not known. However, two-thirds of an orally administered dose appears in the urine as urea within 12 hours. Side effects in the form of an occasional skin rash appears in less than 1% of patients. Habituation and addiction liabilities are not known. *Dose: Usual, sedative,* 150 to 300 mg *orally* 3 or 4 times a day.

Lithium Bromide NF XI [LiBr]—A white or pinkish white, granular, odorless powder with a sharp, slightly bitter taste. It is very deliquescent. The drug is very soluble in water, freely soluble in alcohol, and soluble in ether. *Uses:* It was employed for the sedative effect of the bromide ion, but, because of the inherent toxicity of the lithium ion, it is a much less desirable therapeutic agent than either sodium or potassium bromide. See *Sodium Bromide* (page 1089). Because of the low atomic weight of lithium its bromide contains a larger percentage of bromine (92%) than any other salt.

Methylparafynol [3-Methyl-1-pentyn-3-ol; Maparfynol; Dormison (*Schering*)] $[C_6H_{10}O]$—It occurs as a liquid having an acrid odor and a burning taste. It is soluble in water to the extent of 12.8 Gm per 100 ml; soluble in ether; miscible with acetone, benzene, and carbon tetrachloride. *Uses:* Methylparafynol, an unsaturated carbinol, was introduced as hypnotic agent. On a weight basis, it is much less potent than the barbiturates, but more potent than paraldehyde. It has been used for insomnia and as a sedative for electroencephalographic examination. It is not particularly effective as a daytime sedative or hypnotic. Furthermore, belching and a bad aftertaste limit patient acceptability of the drug. Untoward effects include exfoliative dermatitis and laboratory evidence of potential hepatotoxicity has been demonstrated. The tendency to produce hepatotoxicity requires careful study. *Dose: Usual adult oral,* 0.25 to 0.75 Gm with water or milk at bedtime.

Petrichloral [Pentaerythritol Chloral; Periclor (*Ives*); $[C[CH_2OCH(OH)CCl_3]_4]$ $[C_{13}H_{16}Cl_{12}O_8]$—A derivative of chloral that is a hypnotic and sedative with pharmacological properties similar to those of chloral hydrate. It is devoid of strong odor and aftertaste; hence, it is better tolerated than chloral hydrate. It has a wide margin of safety and low toxicity. *Uses:* In any situation for which mild sedation or hypnotic action is indicated. *Dose: Orally, hypnotic,* 600 mg at bedtime.

Potassium Bromide NF XII [Kalii Bromidum], dried at 105° for 4 hours, contains 99.0–101.0% of KBr (119.01). *Preparation:* In a formerly official method, ferroso-ferric bromide $[Fe_3Br_8]$ is treated with potassium carbonate; a mixture of ferrous carbonate and ferric hydroxide is precipitated, and potassium bromide is recovered from solution. In another method, bromine is added to a hot solution of potassium hydroxide, producing potassium bromide and bromate; the bromate is then reduced to bromide, with carbon monoxide escaping. *Description and Solubility:* White, odorless, cubical crystals or a granular powder that is stable in air. 1 Gm dissolves in 1.5 ml of water, 400 ml of alcohol, and 20 ml of glycerin. *Incompatibilities:* See *Sodium Bromide* (page 1089). *Uses:* For the *sedative* effect of the bromide ion. For this purpose, *Sodium Bromide* (page 1089), rather than this salt, is indicated. *Dose: Usual,* 1 Gm daily. *Veterinary Dose: Horses* and *Cattle,* 30 to 60 Gm; *Dogs,* 300 mg to 4 Gm.

Strontium Bromide NF X—Purity: not less than 98% $SrBr_2.6H_2O$. Colorless, transparent, hexagonal crystals having no odor but a bitter, salty taste. It deliquesces in moist air but effloresces in dry air. 1 Gm dissolves in 0.35 ml of water to make a solution neutral to litmus. It is soluble in alcohol but insoluble in ether. *Uses:* A sedative having no advantages over the sodium or potassium bromides. *Dose: Orally,* 1 Gm.

Whisky NF XI [Spiritus Frumenti; Whiskey]—An alcoholic liquid obtained by the distillation of the fermented mash of wholly or partly malted cereal grains and containing 47–53%, by volume, of ethyl alcohol. It must have been stored in previously unused charred wood containers for a period of at least two years before use. *Uses:* A central depressant; see *Alcohol* (page 1357).

Miscellaneous Sedatives and Hypnotics

(Mild Tranquilizers)

The miscellaneous sedatives and hypnotics (minor tranquilizers) include a heterogenous group of agents which have in common the ability to produce a mild sedation in doses unlikely to effect adversely the clarity of consciousness and the quality of psychomotor performance. Many of these agents have secondary central and peripheral effects which are sufficiently varied to permit some pharmacological generalizations. Chlordiazepoxide, chlormezanone, emylcamate, hydroxyphenamate, mephenoxalone, meprobamate, and oxanamide are characterized by their central sedative, skeletal muscle relaxant, and anticonvulsant actions. Although the clinical usefulness of the two latter actions has not been unequivocally established, it is interesting to note that muscle tension may contribute to the uneasiness characteristic of neuroses and that diphenylhydantoin, a clinically useful anticonvulsant, is effective in the management of certain behavioral disorders in children. Hydroxyzine and buclizine produce antihistaminic, anticholinergic, antiemetic, and antiarrhythmic effects in addition to their central sedative effects. Consequently, these agents have been employed for the management of allergic conditions, gastrointestinal hypermotility and hypersecretion, cardiac arrhythmias, and nausea and vomiting associated with motion sickness and pregnancy. Although favorable results have been reported in some instances, their value in these conditions remains to be proven. The minor tranquilizers, like other sedatives and hypnotics, are used primarily in the treatment of transient tension states and simple neuroses. Habituation and physical dependence have been observed to follow prolonged administration with high doses of certain of these agents.

Azacyclonol Hydrochloride NF XII

α,α-Diphenyl-4-piperidinemethanol Hydrochloride; Frenquel Hydrochloride (*Merrell*)]

Azacyclonol Hydrochloride, dried at 105° for 2 hours, contains 98–102% of $C_{18}H_{21}NO.HCl$ (303.84).

Preparation—α,α-Diphenyl-4-pyridinemethanol (I) is hydrogenated in acetic acid solution at 75 to 80°C and 100 to 500 psi pressure with the aid of platinum oxide. After filtering to remove the catalyst and removing the acetic acid by distillation under reduced pressure, azacyclonol base is liberated by treatment with aqueous alkali. The base is then dissolved in ethanol and treated with hydrogen chloride, whereupon the hydrochloride precipitates. (I) may be prepared by the usual Grignard procedure using 4-benzoylpyridine and phenylmagnesium bromide.

Description—Small white crystals, or a crystalline powder which is odorless and stable in dry air. It melts between 270° and 281° with decomposition. The pH of a 1 in 200 solution is between 5 and 7.

Solubility—1 Gm dissolves in about 200 ml of water and about 1 L of alcohol. Practically insoluble in chloroform, ether, acetone, and solvent hexane.

Uses—Azacyclonol Hydrochloride is a diphenylmethane derivative of questionable usefulness in reducing the incidence of *hallucinations*, *delusions*, *assaultiveness*, *agitation*, and *seclusiveness*. Clinical results to date have been highly variable; some investigators report decidedly beneficial results in some, but not all, patients, whereas other workers find the drug entirely without value. Untoward reactions and side effects are negligible, even after very large doses.

Dose—*Usual*, 20 mg 3 times a day.

Dosage Forms—Injection: 5 mg/ml; Tablets 20 and 100 mg.

Buclizine Hydrochloride

[Softran (*Stuart*)]

Buclizine Hydrochloride ($C_{28}H_{33}ClN_2.2HCl$) is 1-(*p-tert*-butylbenzyl)-4-(*p*-chloro-α-phenylbenzyl)piperazine dihydrochloride.

Preparation—Methods of manufacture are described in US Pat. 2,709,169.

Description—White to slightly yellow, microcrystalline powder. It is odorless and tasteless.

Solubility—Insoluble in water; slightly soluble in alcohol; soluble in chloroform.

Uses—Buclizine Hydrochloride, an agent similar in chemical structure and pharmacological action to some of the antihistamines, has central nervous system depressant, antiemetic, and antihistaminic properties. Consequently, Buclizine Hydrochloride has been used as a tranquilizing agent in the treatment of insomnia, mild tension states, and senile agitation. It appears to be an effective antihistaminic with actions and uses common to this group. It is also useful for the control of nausea and vomiting of motion sickness. Buclizine Hydrochloride is contraindicated during early pregnancy. Drowsiness is a common untoward effect and patients taking the drug should be cautioned against driving an automobile, piloting a plane, or other activities which demand alertness.

Dose—*Usual*, *oral*, 50 mg 1 to 3 times daily.

Dosage Forms—Tablets: 25 and 50 mg.

Chlordiazepoxide NF

[7-Chloro-2-(methylamino)-5-phenyl-3*H*-1,4-benzodiazepine 4-Oxide; Libritabs (*Roche*)

Chlordiazepoxide contains 99.0–101.0% of $C_{16}H_{14}ClN_3O$ (299.76), calculated on the dried basis.

Preparation—For the preparation of Chlordiazepoxide, see *Chlordiazepoxide Hydrochloride*, this page.

Description—A yellow, practically odorless, crystalline powder. It is sensitive to sunlight.

Solubility—Sparingly soluble in chloroform and alcohol; insoluble in water.

Uses—See *Chlordiazepoxide Hydrochloride*, this page.

Dose—5 to 25 mg; *usual,* 5 or 10 mg 3 or 4 times a day.

Dosage Forms—Tablets: 5, 10, and 25 mg.

Chlordiazepoxide Hydrochloride USP

[7-Chloro-2-(methylamino)-5-phenyl-3H-1,4-benzodiazepine 4-Oxide Mono-hydrochloride; Librium (*Roche*)]

Chlordiazepoxide Hydrochloride contains 99.0–101.0% of $C_{16}H_{14}ClN_3O \cdot HCl$ (336.22), calculated on the dried basis.

For the structure of the base, see page 1091.

Preparation—The final step in the process consists of reacting 6-chloro-2-chloromethyl-4-phenylquinazoline 3-oxide (I) hydrochloride with ice cold 25% methanolic methylamine whereupon condensation and rearrangement, resulting in ring enlargement of the pyrimidine moiety, occur thus producing chlordiazepoxide base.

I

poxide base. The hydrochloride is formed by dissolving the base in methanol containing an equivalent quantity of HCl and then precipitating by dilution with ether and petroleum ether. (I) is synthesized from 2-amino-5-chlorobenzophenone oxime through condensation cyclization by treatment with chloroacetyl chloride. For details, see US Pat. 2,893,992.

Description—Occurs as a white or nearly white, odorless, crystalline powder. It is sensitive to sunlight.

Solubility—Soluble in water and alcohol; insoluble in solvent hexane.

Uses—Chlordiazepoxide Hydrochloride is useful in the symptomatic relief of anxiety associated with various psychoneurotic or psychophysiologic disorders. Its usefulness in psychoses has not been established. Chlordiazepoxide Hydrochloride also has skeletal muscle relaxant and anticonvulsant properties. It is of some value in musculoskeletal disorders associated with emotional disturbances, but has little or no effect on muscle spasm of organic nature. Its usefulness in convulsive disorders remains to be established. Adverse effects reported to date include drowsiness, ataxia, and lethargy. Syncope has occurred following the administration of large doses. Paradoxical reactions of rage, excitement, stimulation, hostility, and depersonalization have sometimes followed administration to severely disturbed patients. Skin rashes, nausea, headache, agranulocytoses, and decreased tolerance to alcohol have also been reported. The chronic administration of large doses of Chlordiazepoxide Hydrochloride may result in the development of tolerance and physical dependence.

Dose—*Oral,* 10 to 300 mg daily; *usual, oral,* 5 to 10 mg 3 or 4 times a day; *intramuscular* or *intravenous,* 25 to 300 mg in 6 hours; *usual, intramuscular* or *intravenous,* 50 to 100 mg, repeated in 4 to 6 hours if necessary.

Other Dose Information—Elderly or debilitated patients should be restricted to 10 to 20 mg daily. Children are usually given 5 mg 2 to 4 times daily or 10 mg 2 to 3 times daily.

Dosage Forms—Capsules USP: 5, 10, and 25 mg; Sterile USP: 100 mg.

Chlormezanone—see page 934.

Diazepam NF

[7-Chloro-1,3-dihydro-1-methyl-5-phenyl-2H-1,4-benzodiazepin-2-one; Valium (*Roche*)]

Diazepam contains 98.5–101.0% of $C_{16}H_{13}ClN_2O$ (284.75), calculated on the dried basis.

Preparation—2-(Methylamino)-5-chlorobenzophenone in ethereal solution is reacted with bromoacetyl bromide to form 2-(2-bromo-N-methylacetamido)-5-chlorobenzophenone. The latter is then reacted with ammonia in methanol solution whereby the bromine is replaced by amino followed by cyclization through a dehydration involving the hydrogens of the amino group and the oxygen of the starting phenone. The crude Diazepam may be purified by recrystallization from ether. US Pat. 3,136,815.

Description—White, odorless, crystalline powder which is stable in the air. It melts between 131° and 135°.

Solubility—1 Gm dissolves in 400 ml of water, 17 ml of alcohol, 2 ml of chloroform, and 40 ml of ether.

Uses—Diazepam is structurally related to chlordiazepoxide and has the same clinical applications. It is used to relieve the symptoms of anxiety and insomnia in patients with emotional disorders and the muscle spasm associated with a number of neuromuscular disorders. It has been used with reported benefit not only in the muscle spasm of arthritis and bursitis, but also in choreo-athetosis, disseminated sclerosis, cerebral palsy and other nervous system diseases associated with muscle spasm or spasticity. It does not have the antipsychotic properties of the phenothiazines and should not be used for this purpose. Side effects with Diazepam generally resemble those with chlordiazepoxide. Drowsiness is most common, but incoordination and ataxia also occur with recommended doses. Skin rashes have also been reported. Abrupt cessation after prolonged therapy with large doses may produce withdrawal symptoms similar to those seen with barbiturates, meprobamate, and chlordiazepoxide. Patients on the drug should be cautioned not to drive an automobile or to operate dangerous machinery until a few days after the drug has been stopped.

Dose—*Usual, oral,* 2 to 10 mg 2 to 4 times a day; *intramuscular* or *intravenous,* 2 to 10 mg, repeated in 3 to 4 hours, if necessary, but no more than 30 mg should be given in an 8-hour period.

Dosage Forms—Injection NF: 10 mg/2 ml; Tablets NF: 2, 5, and 10 mg.

Droperidol—see Fentanyl Citrate and Droperidol Injection, page 1064.

Emylcamate

[Striatran (*MSD*)]

$$CH_3CH_2\overset{\overset{\displaystyle C_2H_5}{|}}{\underset{\underset{\displaystyle CH_3}{|}}{C}}-OCONH_2$$

Emylcamate ($C_7H_{15}NO_2$) is 1-ethyl-1-methylpropyl carbamate.

Preparation—Emylcamate may be prepared by reacting 3-methyl-3-pentanol with carbamoyl chloride in the presence of a suitable dehydrochlorinating agent.

Description—Needles, having a slight odor of camphor, which melt between 56° and 58.5°.

Solubility—Freely soluble in alcohol, ether, and benzene; slightly soluble in water.

Uses—Emylcamate is a mild sedative with actions and uses similar to meprobamate. When compared on a milligram for milligram basis, it is about twice as potent as meprobamate. It is most useful in the suppression of tension and anxiety associated with various disorders. Side effects are usually mild and transitory. Drowsiness, nausea, vomiting, dizziness, headache, xerostomia, and skin rashes have been reported. Patients exhibiting drowsiness or dizziness should be cautioned not to drive an automobile while on the drug. Although tolerance and physical dependence have not been reported, the drug should be held suspect because of its structural and pharmacological similarity to meprobamate.

Dose—*Usual, oral, adult,* **200 mg** 3 or 4 times daily immediately before meals.

Dosage Forms—Tablets: 200 mg.

Hydroxyphenamate

[Listica (*Armour*)]

$$\overset{\overset{\displaystyle C_2H_5}{|}}{\underset{\underset{\displaystyle OH}{|}}{C}}-CH_2OCONH_2$$

Hydroxyphenamate ($C_{11}H_{15}NO_3$) is β-ethyl-β-hydroxyphenethyl carbamate.

Preparation — β - Ethyl - β - hydroxyphenethyl alcohol is condensed with ethyl chloroformate with the aid of an agent such as sodamide and the resulting ester is deethanolated through ammonolysis. US Pat. 3,066,164

Description—A fine, white, crystalline powder which is odorless and has a bitter taste. It is stable in both light and air. It melts between 56° and 58° and decomposes at 150°.

Solubility—Freely soluble in alcohol, chloroform, ether, and ethyl acetate; sparingly soluble in water.

Uses—Hydroxyphenamate is a mild sedative useful in the management of mild tension states. It is ineffective in psychoses. Drowsiness is the most common untoward effect, but urticaria and hypotension have also been observed. Physicians should be alert to the possibility of habituation and tolerance in patients taking large doses of the drug over extended periods of time.

Dose—*Usual, oral, adult,* **200 mg** 3 or 4 times a day.

Dosage Forms—Tablets: 200 mg.

Hydroxyzine Hydrochloride NF

[2-[2-[4-(*p*-Chloro-α-phenylbenzyl)-1-piperazinyl]ethoxy]ethanol Dihydrochloride; Atarax (*Roerig*)]

Hydroxyzine Hydrochloride, dried at 105° for 2 hours, contains 98.0–100.5% of $C_{21}H_{27}ClN_2O_2 \cdot 2HCl$ (447.84).

Preparation—Hydroxyzine (base) may be prepared readily by condensing *p*-chlorobenzhydryl chloride (I) with *N*-[2-(2-hydroxyethoxy)ethyl]piperazine (II). Conversion to the official hydrochloride may be effected by dissolving the base in a double molar quantity of hydrochloric acid and evaporating the solution to dryness.

(I) may be synthesized by treating benzaldehyde with *p*-chlorophenylmagnesium bromide in the usual Grignard fashion and reacting the resulting *p*-chlorobenzhydrol with a suitable halogenating agent such as phosphorus trichloride or thionyl chloride. (II) may be synthesized by causing piperazine to undergo controlled addition with ethylene oxide.

Description—It occurs as a white, odorless powder. Melting range 196° to 204°.

Solubility—1 Gm dissolves in about 11 ml of chloroform; very soluble in water; slightly soluble in acetone; practically insoluble in ether.

Uses—Hydroxyzine Hydrochloride is a mild central nervous system depressant with antispasmodic, antihistaminic, anticholinergic, and antiarrhythmic properties. It is employed clinically for the symptomatic treatment of a wide variety of emotional and mental disorders characterized by anxiety, tension, and agitation. It has also been used for the management of acute and chronic urticaria and other manifestations of allergic dermatoses. Although the drug is used as an antispasmodic and antiarrhythmic agent, its effectiveness has not been fully established. The potentiating action of Hydroxyzine Hydrochloride must be considered when the drug is used in conjunction with central nervous system depressants such as narcotics and barbiturates. The toxicity of Hydroxyzine Hydrochloride is very low and is usually characterized by transient drowsiness.

Dose—**25** to **100 mg**; *usual,* **25 mg** 3 times a day. *Other Dose Information*—The usual intramuscular dose is 50 to 100 mg every 4 to 6 hours.

Dosage Forms—Injection NF: 25 and 50 mg/ml; 100 mg/2 ml, 250 and 500 mg/10 ml; Syrup NF: 10 mg/5 ml; Tablets NF: 10, 25, and 100 mg.

Hydroxyzine Pamoate NF

[Vistaril (*Pfizer*)]

Hydroxyzine Pamoate contains 97.0–100.5% of $C_{21}H_{27}ClN_2O_2 \cdot C_{23}H_{16}O_6$ (763.29), calculated on the anhydrous basis.

It is hydroxyzine 4,4'-methylenebis[-3-hydroxy-2-naphthoate] (1:1). For the structure of the base, see *Hydroxyzine Hydrochloride*.

Preparation—Hydroxyzine (base), prepared as described under *Hydroxyzine Hydrochloride* (above), is reacted with an equimolar portion of 4,4'-methylenebis[3-hydroxy-2-naphthoic acid].

Description—A bright-yellow powder having a slight, bitter taste.

Solubility—Insoluble in water.

Uses and **Dose**—See *Hydroxyzine Hydrochloride*.

Dosage Forms—Capsules NF: 25, 50, and 100 mg; Oral Suspension NF: 25 mg/5 ml.

Mebutamate

[Capla (*Wallace*)]

$$H_2N-\overset{O}{\overset{\|}{C}}-O-CH_2-\overset{CH_3}{\underset{CH_3CHCH_2CH_3}{\overset{|}{\underset{|}{C}}}}-CH_2-O-\overset{O}{\overset{\|}{C}}-NH_2$$

Mebutamate ($C_{10}H_{20}N_2O_4$) is 2-*sec*-butyl-2-methyl-1,3-propanediol dicarbamate, a homolog of *Meprobamate*.

Preparation—Starting with the appropriate diol, it may be prepared by the method described above for *Meprobamate*.

Description—White, essentially odorless, crystalline powder having a characteristic bitter taste.

Solubility—1 Gm dissolves in about 153 ml of water, 2 ml of chloroform, 3 ml of alcohol, 200 ml of benzene, and about 1000 ml of carbon tetrachloride.

Uses—Mebutamate, a congener of meprobamate, is a mild sedative which has been recommended for the management of labile hypertension. Although Mebutamate has been shown to lower blood pressure in laboratory animals, the drug has little antihypertensive action in man when given in nonsedative doses. Thus, any antihypertensive effect observed clinically is probably due to the sedative properties of Mebutamate. The drug is more sedative than meprobamate, but it has no known advantages over the older and well-established sedative agents. Other actions and limitations are similar to those of meprobamate. The development of tolerance and physical dependence after chronic administration of the drug have not been reported; nevertheless, the drug should be held suspect because of its enhanced sedative properties and chemical similarity to meprobamate.

Dose—*Usual*, *oral*, **300** to **1200 mg** daily in 3 or 4 divided doses.

Dosage Forms—Tablets: 300 mg.

Mephenoxalone

[Lenetran (*Lakeside*); Tranpoise (*Whittier*); Trepidone (*Lederle*)]

Mephenoxalone ($C_{11}H_{13}NO_4$) is 5-[(o-methoxyphenoxy)methyl]-2-oxazolidinone.

Preparation—Methods of synthesis are described in US Pat. 2,895,960.

Uses—Mephenoxalone is a mild sedative which may be useful in the suppression of tension and anxiety associated with somatic disorders. It is not effective in the treatment of psychoses. At higher dose levels, Mephenoxalone may exhibit skeletal relaxant properties; this effect is probably due to the sedative action of the drug. Side effects are usually mild and transient. Drowsiness, headache, dizziness, insomnia, nausea, and skin rashes represent the common adverse reactions. Patients who become drowsy or dizzy while taking the drug should be cautioned not to operate a motor vehicle.

Dose—*Usual*, *oral*, *adult*, **400 mg** 4 times a day.

Dosage Forms—Tablets: 400 mg.

Meprobamate USP

[2-Methyl-2-propyl-1,3-propanediol Dicarbamate; 2-Methyl-2-propyltrimethylene Dicarbamate; Equanil (*Wyeth*); Miltown (*Wallace*); Viobamate (*Rowell*)]

$$H_2N-\overset{O}{\overset{\|}{C}}-O-CH_2-\overset{CH_3}{\underset{CH_2CH_2CH_3}{\overset{|}{\underset{|}{C}}}}-CH_2-O-\overset{O}{\overset{\|}{C}}-NH_2$$

Meprobamate contains 97.0–100.5% of $C_9H_{18}N_2O_4$ (218.25), calculated on the dried basis.

Preparation—2-Methyl-2-*n*-propyl-1,3-propanediol, in toluene solution, is condensed at about 0°C with phosgene in the presence of dimethylaniline to yield the chloroformate diester, which is then subjected to ammonolysis to form the dicarbamate ester. The crude product is purified by crystallization from diluted alcohol.

Description—White powder, which has a characteristic odor and a bitter taste. It melts between 103° and 107°.

Solubility—Slightly soluble in water; freely soluble in alcohol and acetone; sparingly soluble in ether.

Uses—Meprobamate is a propanediol derivative chemically related to mephenesin and shares with this compound the ability to depress polysynaptic reflexes and relax skeletal muscle. Hence, it is sometimes useful as an antispastic agent in conditions characterized by muscle spasms. It also has some anticonvulsant effect in experimental animals, but its value in epilepsy is limited to idiopathic petit mal. The drug is useful as a mild hypnotic in simple insomnia or as a psychotherapeutic agent that can be employed in place of potent sedatives and along with psychotherapy in the management of psychoneurotic anxiety and tension states. Meprobamate is useful as premedication in electroshock therapy to allay preshock anxiety and postshock confusion and headache. It may be used in the treatment of alcoholism and as an adjuvant to other therapies in the management of frank psychoses.

The over-all toxicity of Meprobamate is low, but it is capable of producing a variety of side effects and untoward reactions. Most common are those related to hypersensitivity such as skin rashes and pruritus. Drowsiness may be a complication where not desired. Large doses have induced coma, shock and vasomotor and respiratory collapse, and drug-induced attempts at suicide have been recorded. Withdrawal symptoms, including convulsions in some patients, have been observed when the drug is discontinued abruptly after prolonged administration of large doses. This suggests that physical as well as psychic dependence on the drug may develop. Uncommon side effects include gastric discomfort, a paradoxical reaction with extreme excitement, intestinal hyperactivity with abdominal cramping, severe diarrhea with rice-water stools, palsy of extraocular muscles with diplopia, and generalized muscular paralysis. It is evident, therefore, that the drug should be employed with the same discretion as other therapeutic agents and with due cognizance of the possibility of untoward effects.

Dose—*Oral*, 1 to 2.4 Gm daily; *usual*, *oral*, **400 mg** 3 or 4 times a day; *usual*, *intramuscular*, **400 mg** every 3 or 4 hours.

Dosage Forms—Injection USP: 400 mg/5 ml; Oral Suspension NF: 200 mg/5 ml; Tablets USP: 200 and 400 mg.

Veterinary Dose—*Orally* in *dogs* **100 to 400 mg** 2 to 4 times daily depending on body weight and degree of excitation.

Methaqualone

[Parest (*Parke-Davis*); Quaalude (*Rorer*); Sopor (*Arnar-Stone*)]

Methaqualone [$C_{16}H_{14}N_2O = 250.29$] is 2-methyl-3-*o*-tolyl-4(3*H*)-quinazolinone.

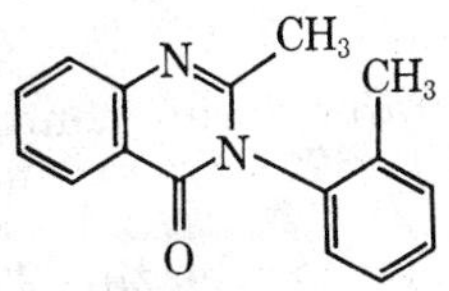

Preparation—*N*-Acetylanthranilic acid is cyclized through condensation with *o*-toluidine in the presence of phosphoryl chloride, and the mixture is then rendered alkaline to precipitate the crude product. Purification is via recrystallization from isopropanol.

Description—A white, crystalline powder with little or no odor and a bitter taste. It is stable in light and air. Its aqueous solution is alkaline to litmus. It melts at about 115°.

Solubility—Freely soluble in alcohol and dilute hydrochloric acid; soluble in ether; very slightly soluble in water.

Uses—Methaqualone is a nonbarbiturate sedative and hypnotic. It induces sleep within 10 to 30 minutes which lasts 6 to 8 hours. The drug also exhibits antispasmodic and antitussive actions which suggest that it may be useful in the management of insomnia complicated by cough or gastrointestinal distress. The drug should be used with caution in patients with depression or suicidal tendencies and those with liver dysfunction. Side effects encountered are usually mild and transient and include headache, drowsiness, nausea, fatigue, epigastric discomfort, dizziness, dry mouth, emesis, restlessness, tachycardia, anorexia, diarrhea, urticaria, and paresthesia. One case of aplastic anemia, possibly related to Methaqualone, has been reported. The drug is contraindicated in women who are or may become pregnant.

Dose—*Hypnotic*, **150 to 300 mg** at bedtime; *sedative*, **75 mg** after each meal and at bedtime.

Oxanamide

[Quiactin (*Merrell*)]

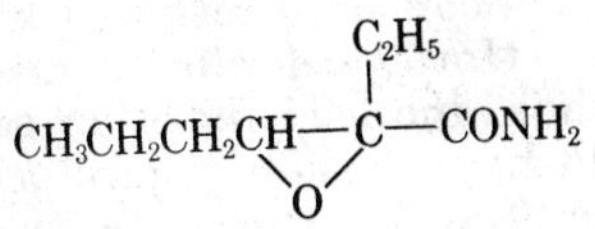

Oxanamide ($C_8H_{15}NO_2$) is 2,3-epoxy-2-ethylhexanamide.

Preparation—A method of preparation is given in *J. Org. Chem.*, **25**, 1021 (1960).

Description—Light, fluffy, white, odorless powder. It melts between 90° and 94°.

Solubility—Soluble in chloroform, methanol, ethanol, ether, and acetone; insoluble in petroleum ether (40° to 60° fraction), hexane, and water.

Uses—Oxanamide is a mild sedative similar in its pharmacologic actions and clinical usefulness to meprobamate. Large doses produce skeletal muscle relaxation as a result of a partial blockade of internuncial neurones and central sedation. Relatively few untoward effects have been reported. Until more clinical experience with the drug has been gained, the usual precautions for drugs of this type should be applied to Oxanamide.

Dose—*Usual*, *oral*, **400 mg** 4 times daily.

Dosage Forms—Tablets: 400 mg.

Oxazepam NF

[7 - Chloro - 1,3 - dihydro - 3 - hydroxy - 5 - phenyl - 2*H* - 1,4 - benzodiazepin-2-one; Serax (*Wyeth*)]

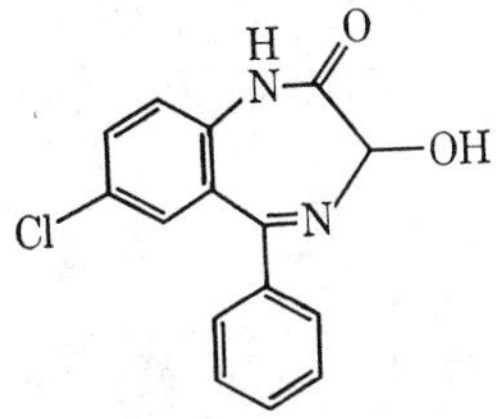

Oxazepam contains 98.0–102.0% of $C_{15}H_{11}ClN_2O_2$ (286.72), calculated on the dried basis.

Preparation—2-Amino-5-chlorobenzophenone is acylated with chloroacetyl chloride and the product is refluxed with sodium iodide to form the iodoacetamido compound (I). Reaction of (I) with hydroxylamine effects dehydration and dehydrochlorination to form the benzodiazepine derivative (II). Treatment of (II) with acetic anhydride causes rearrangement to Oxazepam which is simultaneously esterified to the acetate. Saponification of the ester liberates Oxazepam.

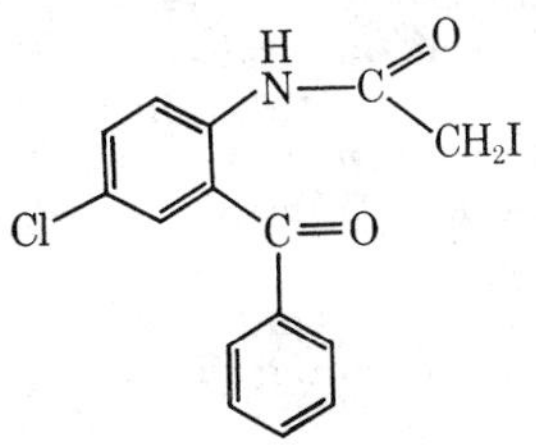

(I) 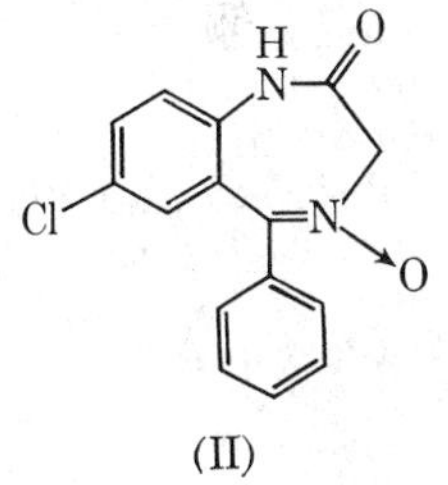   (II)

Description—A creamy white to pale-yellow powder that is odorless and has a bitter taste. It is stable in light and is nonhygroscopic. Its melting point is indefinite.

Solubility—Slightly soluble in alcohol and chloroform; very slightly soluble in water.

Uses—Oxazepam, a benzodiazepine, is a congener of chlordiazepoxide and diazepam. Oxazepam is a mild sedative useful in the management and control of anxiety, tension, agitation, irritability, and related symptoms. This profile of pharmacologic action is similar to that of other benzodiazepines. Excessive and prolonged use may result in the development of physical dependence to the drug. Withdrawal symptoms following abrupt discontinuance of Oxazepam are similar to those seen with barbiturates. As with other sedative agents, patients on this drug should be cautioned against driving automobiles or operating dangerous machinery. Untoward effects include transient mild drowsiness, dizziness, vertigo, headache, and rarely syncope. Mild paradoxical reactions such as excitement and excessive stimulation have also been recorded. Other side effects which have been observed include skin rashes, nausea, lethargy, edema, slurred speech, tremor, and altered libido. More severe reactions include leukopenia and jaundice. Fortunately, the latter reactions are only occasionally observed. The drug should be used with caution in elderly individuals. Patients on the drug should be observed carefully for the appearance of other untoward effects characteristic of benzodiazepine drugs.

Dose—**10** to **30 mg**; *usual*, **10** to **15 mg** 3 or 4 times daily.

Dosage Forms—Capsules NF: 10, 15, and 30 mg; Tablets: 15 mg.

Phenaglycodol

[Ultran (*Lilly*)]

Phenaglycodol ($C_{11}H_{15}ClO_2$) is 2-(*p*-chlorophenyl)-3-methyl-2,3-butanediol.

Preparation—Methods of preparation are described in US Pat. 2,812,363.

Description—White to cream-colored powder having a faint odor.

Solubility—Soluble in alcohol, chloroform, and ether; practically insoluble in water, dilute acids, and bases.

Uses—Phenaglycodol is chemically related to mephenesin and meprobamate and exhibits mild sedative and weak muscle-relaxing properties similar to the latter agent. Phenaglycodol has been used to calm patients with simple *emotional instability, anxiety-tension states*, and functional disorders. However, its action is essentially that of sedation, and the drug cannot properly be classified as a tranquilizer. The toxicity of this agent is low; drowsiness is the only side effect observed and this generally follows the administration of high doses.

Dose—*Usual, oral*, **300 mg** 3 or 4 times a day.

Dosage Forms—Capsules: 300 mg; Tablets: 200 mg.

Pipethanate Hydrochloride

[Piperilate Hydrochloride; Sycotrol; Ingredient of Modutrol (*Reed & Carnrick*)]

Pipethanate Hydrochloride ($C_{21}H_{25}NO_3 \cdot HCl$) is 1-piperidineethanol benzilate (ester) hydrochloride.

Preparation—A method of synthesis is described in *J. Chem. Soc.*, **1947**, 55.

Description—White, finely crystalline substance which is practically odorless.

Solubility—1 Gm dissolves in about 40 ml of water, about 40 ml of alcohol, and about 10 ml of methanol; insoluble in ether.

Uses—Pipethanate Hydrochloride, closely related in chemical structure to benactyzine hydrochloride, is a mild sedative with peripheral anticholinergic actions. It is proposed for use in the management of anxiety and tension associated with peptic ulcer and other somatic disorders. Drowsiness is the only untoward effect reported to date. Nevertheless, patients receiving the drug should be carefully observed for possible adverse effects.

Dose—*Usual, oral*, **3 to 6 mg** 3 times daily.

Dosage Forms—Tablets: 3 mg.

Propiomazine Hydrochloride NF

[1-[10-[2-(Dimethylamino)propyl]phenothiazin-2-yl]-1-propanone Monohydrochloride; Largon (*Wyeth*)]

Propiomazine Hydrochloride contains 98.0–102.0% of $C_{20}H_{24}N_2OS \cdot HCl$ (376.95), calculated on the anhydrous basis.

Preparation—1-(Phenothiazin - 2 - yl) - 1 - propanone is condensed with 2-(dimethylamino)-1-methylethyl chloride with the aid of a dehydrochlorinating agent such as sodamide. The propiomazine (base) thus formed is dissolved in a suitable organic solvent and reacted with an equimolar portion of hydrogen chloride to yield the official salt.

Description—A yellow powder that is practically odorless. It is slowly oxidized when moistened or in aqueous solution on prolonged exposure to air and/or light. It melts between 201° and 206°.

Solubility—1 Gm dissolves in about 4.5 ml of water; soluble in alcohol; insoluble in benzene.

Uses—Propiomazine Hydrochloride is a substituted phenothiazine which is used primarily for its sedative properties. It is closely related chemically to promethazine, and like this agent it has antihistaminic, sedative, and antiemetic actions. Its sedative properties, however, are more prominent than those of promethazine, but its antihistaminic activity is considerably less. Propiomazine Hydrochloride is used to provide nighttime, surgical, or obstetrical sedation. It relieves apprehension and induces light sleep from which the patient may be readily wakened. In combination with meperidine or other analgesics, it may be used for preoperative medication, control of postoperative pain, and for postoperative sedation. It is also employed as a sedative drug during early stages of labor; in combination with meperidine it provides analgesia and sedation, and also controls nausea and vomiting during labor. Like other phenothiazines, Propiomazine Hydrochloride potentiates the action of other central nervous system depressants, and thereby permits the reduction of the dosage of such drugs when they are used conconcomitantly with Propiomazine Hydrochloride. Untoward effects are usually mild and resemble those induced by other sedative phenothiazines. Mild hypotension occurs occasionally and tachycardia has been reported.

Dose—*Intramuscular* or *intravenous*, **10 to 40 mg**; *usual*, **20 mg**.

Other Dose Information—Since severe chemical irritation may occur when perivascular extravasation of the solution occurs, care should be exercised when the intravenous route is employed.

Dosage Forms—Injection NF: 20 mg/ml; 40 mg/2 ml.

Tybamate NF

[2-(Hydroxymethyl)-2-methylpentyl Butylcarbamate Carbamate; Solacen (*Wallace*); Tybatran (*Robins*)]

$$CH_3(CH_2)_3NHCOO{-}CH_2\overset{\overset{\displaystyle CH_3}{|}}{\underset{\underset{\displaystyle CH_2{-}OCONH_2}{|}}{C}}CH_2CH_2CH_3$$

Tybamate contains 98.0–102.0% of $C_{13}H_{26}N_2O_4$ (274.36), calculated on the dried basis.

Preparation—Diethyl methylpropylmalonate is reacted in ether with lithium aluminum hydride and then with diluted sulfuric acid to form 2-methyl-2-propyl-1,3-propanediol (I). Reaction of (I) with phosgene in toluene with the aid of dimethylaniline yields 2-methyl-2-propyl-3-hydroxypropyl chlorocarbonate which is reacted with butylamine to give 2-methyl-2-propyl-3-hydroxypropyl butylcarbamate (II). The hydroxyl function in (II) is converted to carbamate by treatment with ethylurethane in the presence of aluminum isopropoxide. The reaction is conducted in boiling xylene and thus the ethanol liberated during the transesterification is constantly removed from the reaction mixture as an azeotrope with xylene. US Pat. 2,937,119.

Description—A white, crystalline power or clear, viscous liquid which may congeal to a solid on standing. It has a mild, characteristic odor and a bitter taste. It is stable in light and heat. The powder melts between 49° and 54°.

Solubility—Very soluble in alcohol and acetone; freely soluble in ether; very slightly soluble in water.

Uses—Tybamate, a congener of meprobamate, has actions and uses similar to those of the latter agent. Hence, it is useful in a variety of psychoneurotic disorders, especially in the treatment of the anxiety and tension components of psychoneuroses. In general, the pharmacologic properties, contraindications, and untoward effects of Tybamate are similar to those for meprobamate. Tybamate should not be administered to psychotic patients on phenothiazines or other central nervous system depressants; such combinations have been reported to be associated with the occurrence of grand mal or petit mal seizures. The possibility that Tybamate may induce teratogenic effects if taken in early pregnancy or physical dependence if taken chronically in excessive doses has not been excluded.

Dose—**750 mg to 2 Gm** daily in divided doses.

Dosage Forms—Capsules NF: 125, 250, and 350 mg.

Other Miscellaneous Sedatives and Hypnotics

Captodiamine Hydrochloride [2-[[*p*-(Butylthio)-α-phenylbenzyl]thio]-*N,N*-dimethylethylamine Hydrochloride; Suvren (*Ayerst*)][$C_{21}H_{29}NS_2HCl$]—*Description and Solubility:* A white, crystalline powder. Freely soluble in water and alcohol. *Uses:* A mild sedative agent which has been proposed for the management of anxiety and tension states, including psychosomatic diseases such as intestinal hyperirritability and colitis. It has also been reported to be useful in the treatment of hyperactive children with brain damage. It has relatively low toxicity and no serious side effects have been noted. *Dose: Usual,* 100 mg 3 or 4 times a day.

61 | Antiepileptics

Drugs for grand mal, petit mal, psychomotor, and focal epilepsy

This chapter was prepared by

Ewart A. Swinyard, PhD, *Professor of Pharmacology, College of Pharmacy and College of Medicine, University of Utah, Salt Lake City, Utah 84112, and* **Stewart C. Harvey, PhD,** *Associate Professor of Pharmacology, College of Medicine, University of Utah, Salt Lake City, Utah 84112*

Epilepsy may be defined as a paroxysmal, self-sustaining, and self-limiting cerebral dysrhythmia characterized by an abnormal and excessive EEG discharge and by a disturbance of consciousness; it may or may not be associated with body movements or hyperactivity of the autonomic nervous system. The epileptic attack is initiated by an abnormal focus of electrical discharge, originating either in the grey matter or other part of the brain. The discharge spreads to other parts of the central nervous system and results in convulsions and other manifestations of the disorder.

A widely employed clinical classification divides epilepsy into four main types: grand mal, petit mal triad (pyknoepilepsy; myoclonic jerks; akinetic seizures), psychomotor, and focal or Jacksonian epilepsy.

In grand mal epilepsy, the convulsion is often preceded by a premonitory aura which consists of some auditory stimulation, a feeling of strangeness, fear, or epigastric discomfort; this is followed by a loss of consciousness and tonic-clonic convulsions.

Petit mal epilepsy, a type most frequently observed in children, is characterized by brief periods of clouding or loss of consciousness during which the patient stops his activities and after a moment or two resumes them without being aware of the interruption.

Psychomotor epilepsy consists of episodes of abnormal sensations or behavior. Their manifestation may on occasion be bizarre to the point of being considered hysterical or psychotic symptoms. The episodes are usually followed by amnesia.

Focal or Jacksonian epilepsy, normally associated with an organic lesion of the cerebral cortex, is characterized by convulsive twitching of isolated muscle groups; these seizures may remain localized or progress to generalized convulsions with loss of consciousness.

The only effective way of controlling seizures is by the use of antiepileptic drugs. The many medical therapies of antiquity have been replaced by a rational therapeutic approach which had its origin in the beginning of the nineteenth century. It has progressed from the use of bromides in 1857 and phenobarbital in 1912 to the modern era marked by the introduction of diphenylhydantoin in 1938. The clinical efficacy of the latter drug established the fact that chemicals effective in epilepsy need not be hypnotics and stimulated the laboratory search for other effective anticonvulsant agents. As a result, a number of new anticonvulsant barbiturates, hydantoins, oxazolidinediones, acetylureas, succinamides, and acetazolamides have been introduced in the last 25 years. As a result of these advances in drug therapy, 80% of all victims of epileptic disorders can be satisfactorily controlled with available drugs.

Because of the variety of clinical types of epilepsy and their differences in response to drugs, a battery of tests is usually employed for the laboratory study of candidate anticonvulsant drugs in animals. In general, these tests measure the ability of drugs to elevate the threshold for minimal seizures or to modify the pattern of maximal convulsions induced in laboratory animals by electrical or chemical stimulation of the brain. These tests not only reveal the spectrum of activity of candidate drugs with a view to detection of clinically useful properties, but also provide information as to the mechanism of action of drugs employed in the therapy of seizures. With regard to the latter, at least three distinct actions on neuronal processes are thought to underlie the effects of anticonvulsants on electrically induced experimental seizures: stabilization of the neuronal membrane, decrease in tendency to repetitive discharge, and reduction in spread of seizure discharge. Only the first two actions appear to be concerned in altering electrical seizure threshold, whereas all three actions probably underlie alterations in maximal seizure pattern. In addition, chemically induced seizures may be altered by drugs which specifically antagonize the convulsant drug as well as by the above mentioned neuronal processes.

Clinically, it is generally assumed that antiepileptic drugs control seizures by acting (1) on non-neural lesions, (2) on pathologically altered neurons to reduce or prevent their excessive discharge, or (3) on normal neurons to prevent their detonation by excessive discharge from elsewhere. In the first category are drugs which act at some extraneural site, such as an abnormal vascular supply, whereas in the second category are drugs which selectively alter hyperactive neurons without altering the function of normal brain cells. The third category is probably most important and includes drugs which prevent seizure spread; all clinically useful antiepileptics appear to protect normal neurons from invasion by seizure activity of abnormal foci. The exact mechanism for this has yet to be established.

No one anticonvulsant drug is equally effective in all types of epilepsy. Hence, antiepileptic therapy must be individualized and drug therapy selected on the basis of seizure type. In all types of seizures, except petit mal, the initial drugs of choice are diphenylhydantoin and/or phenobarbital. In petit mal, trimethadione, paramethadione, phensuximide, and methsuximide are usually effective. Once the drug or drugs for a particular patient have been selected, administration should be started at a minimum dose and gradually increased until either seizures are controlled or toxic actions to the drug develop. If the latter occurs without seizure control, the dosage of the drug is reduced to a nontoxic level and a second drug is given following the same principle of increasing dosage. This system of pyramiding drug administration allows for the establishment of a reservoir of two or more anticonvulsant drugs, the combined action of which is more effective than any one drug by itself. When new drugs are introduced, previous medication should not be discontinued until an optimum dose level has been established for the new medicament.

Antiepileptic agents have several uses in the nonepileptic patient. They have been used to soften the seizures in patients undergoing electroshock therapy, to control convulsions occurring in dementia paralytica and tetanus, and to lessen muscular rigidity in certain cases of cerebral palsy. Diphenylhydantoin administered intravenously has been reported to be effective in suppressing recurrent cardiac arrhythmias. In addition, diphenylhydantoin, trimethadione, and phenacemide have been employed for the treatment of disturbed nonepileptic psychotic patients, particularly in catatonic excitement states, and in the management of children with behavioral disorders. The latter use is especially intriguing and warrants a careful clinical study.

Acetazolamide—see page 941.

Amphetamine Sulfate—see page 882.

Caffeine, Citrated—see page 1156.

Chlorpromazine Hydrochloride—see page 1106.

Dextroamphetamine Sulfate—see page 883.

Dimenhydrinate—see page 807.

Diphenhydramine Hydrochloride—see page 1147.

Diphenylhydantoin USP

[5,5-Diphenyl-2,4-imidazolidinedione]

Diphenylhydantoin contains 98.5–100.5% of $C_{15}H_{12}N_2O_2$ (252.28), calculated on the dried basis.

Preparation—Acidification of an aqueous solution of Sodium Diphenylhydantoin results in a practically quantitative precipitation of Diphenylhydantoin which is collected by filtration, washed, and dried. The synthesis of Sodium Diphenylhydantoin is described on page 1101.

Description—White, odorless powder. Melts between 292° and 299°.

Solubility—Practically insoluble in water; soluble in hot alcohol; slightly soluble in cold alcohol, chloroform, and ether.

Uses—See *Sodium Diphenylhydantoin.*

Dose—**300** to **600 mg** daily; *usual*, **100 mg** 3 or 4 times a day.

Dosage Forms—Capsules USP: 100 mg; Oral Suspension NF: 6, 20, and 25 mg/ml; Tablets USP: 50 mg.

Veterinary Dose—*Dogs*, 30 to 200 mg every 6 to 8 hours to control epileptiform convulsions.

Ephedrine Sulfate—see page 885.

Ethosuximide USP

[2-Ethyl-2-methylsuccinimide; Zarontin *(Parke-Davis)*]

Ethosuximide contains 98.0–101.0% of $C_7H_{11}NO_2$ (141.17), calculated on the dried basis.

Preparation—Methyl ethyl ketone is condensed with ethyl cyanoacetate to yield ethyl 2-cyano-3-methyl-2-pentenoate which, in ethanolic solution, adds hydrogen cyanide to form ethyl 2,3-dicyano-3-methylpentanoate. Proton-catalyzed saponification of the latter ester is accompanied by decarboxylation to produce 2-methyl-2-ethylsuccinonitrile. This, on heating with aqueous ammonia, forms the corresponding diamide which, through loss of ammonia, cyclizes to yield Ethosuximide. US Pat. 2,993,835.

Description—A white to off-white crystalline powder or waxy solid that has a characteristic odor. It is stable in light, air, and heat at 37°. It melts between 47° and 52°.

Solubility—Very soluble in alcohol and ether; freely soluble in water and chloroform; very slightly soluble in solvent hexane.

Uses—Ethosuximide has been reported by some clinicians to be the most effective succinimide derivative in the treatment of petit mal. The drug is also indicated in patients whose petit mal seizures are resistant to less toxic agents. Anorexia, nausea, vomiting, and drowsiness are troublesome side effects, and leukopenia and agranulocytosis have occurred. Periodic blood and urine tests should be made on patients on the drug.

Dose—**500 mg** to **1 Gm** daily; *usual*, **250 mg** 2 or 3 times a day.

Dosage Forms—Capsules USP: 250 mg.

Magnesium Sulfate—see page 801.

Magnesium Sulfate Injection USP

[Magnesium Sulfate Ampuls]

Magnesium Sulfate Injection is a sterile solution of magnesium sulfate in water for injection. It contains magnesium sulfate equivalent to 93.0–107.0% of the labeled amount of $MgSO_4 \cdot 7H_2O$ (246.47).

Preparation—The magnesium sulfate is dissolved in water for injection, and the solution, suitably filtered until free from suspended matter, is placed in cleansed and sterile ampuls. These are sealed and suitably sterilized.

Since the water of hydration content of magnesium sulfate may vary sufficiently to be troublesome in making solutions of required concentration, some operators have found it advisable to prepare solutions slightly stronger than required and to have these assayed promptly, thereafter making up to final volume of the exact strength desired according to the assay results. The stock solution, in the meantime, is kept under refrigeration to protect it.

Uses—Magnesium Sulfate has been used as a central depressant, especially as an *anticonvulsant* in convulsive syndromes, such as occur in eclampsia and tetanus, but it has been largely replaced with more reliable agents such as the barbiturates. It has also been employed in *obstetrical anesthesia* to augment the action of general anesthetics, but one must constantly guard against respiratory failure when using the salt as a central and neuromuscular depressant.

Dose—*Intramuscular* and *intravenous*, **1 to 10 Gm** daily; *usual, intramuscular,* **1 Gm** in a **25 to 50%** solution; *usual, intravenous,* **4 Gm** in a **10%** solution.

Other Dose Information—In *eclampsia*, the usual dose is 10 ml of a 25% solution given intramuscularly, and repeated in 5-ml amounts every half hour until relief is obtained.

Dosage Forms—Injection USP: 1 Gm/2 and 10 ml, 2 Gm/20 ml, 15 Gm/30 ml.

Mephobarbital—see page 1081.

Meprobamate—see page 1094.

Metharbital NF

[5,5-Diethyl-1-methylbarbituric Acid; Gemonil (*Abbott*)]

Metharbital, dried at 105° for 4 hours, contains 98.0–100.5% of $C_9H_{14}N_2O_3$ (198.22).

Preparation—Metharbital is prepared by the method described on page 1081 for *Mephobarbital* except that the diethyl ester of diethylmalonic acid is used instead of the diethyl ester of ethylphenylmalonic acid.

Description—A white to nearly white, crystalline powder, possessing a faint aromatic odor. Its saturated solution has a pH of about 6.0. Melting range 151° to 155°.

Solubility—1 Gm dissolves in about 830 ml of water, about 23 ml of alcohol, and about 40 ml of ether.

Uses—Metharbital, an *N*-methylated derivative of barbital, has anticonvulsant properties similar to phenobarbital, but is less potent and less toxic. It is rapidly demethylated to barbital by the liver, but its anticonvulsant activity appears to be independent of this degradation product. It is particularly effective in the control of massive spasms in very young children with brain damage, as evidence in part by gross dysrhythmia of the electroencephalogram. Unfavorable side effects, although relatively infrequent, include drowsiness, increased irritability, rash, dizziness, and stomach distress. In some patients, the drug appears to be less hypnotic and depressing than phenobarbital.

Dose—**100 to 800 mg** per day; *usual, initial,* **100 mg,** up to 3 times a day.

Dosage Forms—Tablets NF: 100 mg.

Methsuximide NF

[N,2-Dimethyl-2-phenylsuccinimide; Celontin (*Parke, Davis*)]

Methsuximide contains 97.0–103.0% of $C_{12}H_{13}NO_2$ (203.24), calculated on the dried basis.

Preparation—2-Methyl-2-phenylsuccinic acid is dissolved in excess 40% methylamine. The water and excess amine are distilled off and the residue consisting

of the di(methylamine) salt of the acid is pyrolyzed at about 250°C until no more distillate is formed. The residue of crude Methsuximide may be purified by vacuum distillation or by dissolving in a suitable solvent, charcoaling, and precipitating by the addition of water. US Pat. 2,643,257.

Description—Occurs as a white to grayish white, crystalline powder. It is odorless or has not more than a slight odor.

Solubility—Slightly soluble in hot water; freely soluble in alcohol and ether; very soluble in chloroform.

Uses—Methsuximide is an antiepileptic agent which is more potent and effective than phensuximide in the treatment of petit mal. Although not the agent of choice for minor seizures, it may prove useful in patients refractory to other therapy, especially if added to established treatment regime. The drug may also be used in combination with other therapy for the management of psychomotor seizures. It is rarely of value in patients with grand mal and may even increase the frequency of such seizures. Minor untoward effects, such as gastrointestinal disturbances, central nervous system depression, skin eruptions, fever, and periorbital hyperemia, occur in approximately 30% of patients. Except for the skin and periorbital hyperemia, most untoward effects disappear when the dose of the drug is reduced. Patients with psychomotor seizures should be watched closely for the appearance of behavioral changes, these may progress to an acute psychosis unless the drug is discontinued. Patients on Methsuximide therapy should be examined periodically for evidence of blood dyscrasias and for liver and kidney function.

Dose—*Usual, initial,* **300 mg** daily; *maintenance,* **300 mg to 1.2 Gm** daily.

Dosage Forms—Capsules NF: 150 and 300 mg.

Paramethadione USP

[5-Ethyl-3,5-dimethyl-2,4-oxazolidinedione; Paradione (*Abbott*)]

Paramethadione contains 98.0–100.5% of $C_7H_{11}NO_3$ (157.17).

Preparation—Ethyl α-hydroxy-α-methylbutyrate and urea are refluxed for 24 hours in the presence of sodium methoxide, resulting in condensation cyclization with the formation of the sodium derivative of 5-ethyl-5-methyl-2,4-oxazolidinone. After distilling off the alcohol, dimethyl sulfate is slowly added to effect the desired *N*-methylation.

Description—It occurs as a clear, colorless liquid. It may have an aromatic odor. Its 1 in 40 solution has a pH of about 6. Refractive index 1.4490 to 1.5010.

Solubility—Sparingly soluble in water; freely soluble in alcohol, benzene, chloroform, and ether.

Uses—Paramethadione is used in the treatment of petit mal epilepsy and other conditions in which trimethadione is used. Although it is slightly less potent and induces photophobia and skin rashes in somewhat fewer patients, it has the same limitations and exhibits the same side reactions as the latter drug. See *Trimethadione*, page 1102.

Dose—**300 mg to 2.1 Gm** daily; *usual,* **300 mg** 3 or 4 times a day.

Dosage Forms—Capsules USP: 150 and 300 mg; Solution USP: 50 ml.

Phensuximide NF

[*N*-Methyl-2-phenylsuccinimide; Milontin (*Parke, Davis*)]

Phensuximide contains 97.0–103.0% of $C_{11}H_{11}NO_2$ (189.22), calculated on the anhydrous basis.

Preparation—Phensuximide may be prepared by the method described above for *Methsuximide* using phenylsuccinic acid as the starting compound, or by other methods. US Pat. 2,643,258.

Description—Occurs as a white to off-white, crystalline powder. It is odorless or has not more than a slight odor.

Solubility—Slightly soluble in water; soluble in alcohol; very soluble in chloroform.

Uses—Phensuximide is a succinimide derivative used in the treatment of petit mal epilepsy. It is generally considered to be less effective than trimethadione and paramethadione, but may be effective in some patients who do not respond to the latter drug.

Phensuximide, although relatively free from serious toxic effects, may produce such side reactions as nausea, vomiting, muscular weakness, drowsiness, and occasional skin eruptions. Patients treated with moderate to large doses may exhibit microscopic hematuria and a urinalysis should be performed monthly. Although hematopoietic complications have not been reported, periodic blood studies are advisable in patients taking the drug for prolonged periods.

Dose—*Usual*, **500 mg** to **1 Gm** 2 or 3 times a day, irrespective of age.

Dosage Forms—Capsules NF: 250 and 500 mg; Oral Suspension NF: 62.5 mg/ml.

Primidone USP

[5-Ethyldihydro-5-phenyl-4,6(1*H*,5*H*)-pyrimidinedione; Primaclone; Mysoline (*Ayerst*)]

Primidone contains 98.0–102.0% of $C_{12}H_{14}N_2O_2$ (218.26), calculated on the dried basis.

Preparation—A solution of ethylphenylmalonamide (I) in a large molar excess of formamide (II) is refluxed for two hours. The cyclization may be looked upon as being brought about by a Cannizaro type of disproportionation of (II) followed by a deammoniation and a dehydration between (I) and the highly reactive methanolamine resulting from the disproportionation.

Description—A white, odorless, crystalline powder, which has a slightly bitter taste. Melting range 279° to 284°.

Solubility—1 Gm dissolves in about 2000 ml of water and about 200 ml of alcohol; very slightly soluble in most organic solvents.

Uses—Primidone is useful in the control of grand mal, which is resistant to phenobarbital or a mixture of phenobarbital and diphenylhydantoin, and it is the drug of choice in psychomotor epilepsy. Clinical response in petit mal, minor motor or focal type of seizures is inconsistent and variable. Side effects include drowsiness, ataxia, psychosis, vertigo, anorexia, irrita-

bility, malaise, nausea, vomiting, dermatitis, painful gums, and edema of the legs and eyelids. Most side effects are mild and disappear with continuing therapy.

Dose—**125 mg** to **2 Gm** daily; *usual*, **250** to **500 mg** 3 times a day.

Dosage Forms—Oral Suspension USP: 250 mg/5 ml; Tablets USP: 50 and 250 mg.

Veterinary Use—Reduction of frequency and severity of true idiopathic epileptiform convulsions in the dog.

Veterinary Dose—*Dogs*, **12** to **50 mg** per **pound** of body weight daily.

Quinacrine Hydrochloride—see page 1247.

Sodium Bromide—see page 1089.

Sodium Diphenylhydantoin USP

[Sodium 5,5-Diphenyl-2,4-imidazolidinedione; Phenytoin Sodium; Soluble Phenytoin; Alepsin; Epanutin; Eptoin; Dilantin Sodium (*Parke-Davis*); Diphenetoin (*Massengill*)]

Sodium Diphenylhydantoin contains 98.5–100.5% of $C_{15}H_{11}N_2NaO_2$ (274.26), calculated on the dried basis.

Preparation—The basic components for the production of this chemical are benzaldehyde and urea. By treating benzaldehyde with a solution of sodium cyanide, 2 moles of benzaldehyde are condensed (benzoin condensation) into one mole of benzoin. Upon treating the benzoin with nitric acid or cupric sulfate it is oxidized to benzil. The benzil is then heated with urea in the presence of sodium ethoxide or isopropoxide in an excess of the alcohol, resulting in the formation of diphenylhydantoin. In the latter step two reactions take place: the benzil is first converted into an ester of benzilic acid which then condenses with the urea.

Phenylethylhydantoin (*Nirvanol*), closely related chemically, was one of the first hypnotics synthesized.

Description—A white, odorless powder. It is somewhat hygroscopic and on exposure to air gradually absorbs carbon dioxide with the liberation of diphenylhydantoin.

Solubility—Freely soluble in water, the solution usually being somewhat turbid due to partial hydrolysis and absorption of carbon dioxide; soluble in alcohol; practically insoluble in ether and chloroform.

Incompatibilities—This compound presents little difficulty in this respect since it is almost invariably prescribed alone. Otherwise, its incompatibilities are similar to those of the barbiturates. See *Sodium Phenobarbital*, page 1083.

Uses—Sodium Diphenylhydantoin is employed in the symptomatic therapy of *epilepsy* and other states characterized by involuntary movements such as chorea and Parkinson's syndrome. It also has been employed intravenously for the control of premature ventricular contractions and paroxysmal ventricular and supraventricular tachycardias, and to reduce the rate in patients with atrial flutter or fibrillation. However, the drug is not offered by the manufacturer or approved by FDA for use in cardiac arrhythmias. Furthermore, such intravenous use is hazardous and may induce hypotension, shock, bradycardia, and respiratory or cardiac arrest. Other uses include the treatment of migraine, trigeminal neuralgia, and certain psychoses.

Diphenylhydantoin is the drug of choice for preventing major convulsive seizures (grand mal). It is more effective in controlling *psychomotor equivalent seizures*, a form of epilepsy in which phenobarbital or bromide rarely is of benefit and often makes the patient worse. Diphenylhydantoin is rarely of benefit in petit mal. The drug has the outstanding advantage over bromide or phenobarbital in that it does not cause drowsiness or sedation. It is not effective in convulsions other than those associated with epilepsy. It is often combined with phenobarbital, trimethadione, ketogenic diet, or other measures employed in epilepsy. Many epileptic patients manifest mental improvement as a result of taking the drug. Among the toxic reactions to it may be mentioned hyperplasia of the gums, giddiness, ataxia, diplopia, slurring of speech, tremors, apathy, confusion, acute gastric upsets (due to alkalinity of the drug), dermatitis with fever and leukocytosis, purpura, exfoliative cutaneous lesions, and hirsutism in adolescent girls.

Dose—*Oral*, **200** to **600 mg** daily; *usual, oral,* **100 mg** up to 4 times a day; *usual, intravenous,* **150** to **250 mg,** followed if necessary by **100** to **150 mg** 30 minutes later; *usual, intramuscular,* **100** to **200 mg** every 6 to 8 hours, for a total of 3 or 4 injections.

Dosage Forms—Capsules USP: 30 and 100 mg; Sterile USP: 100 and 250 mg.

Sodium Phenobarbital—see page 1083.

Trimethadione USP

[Troxidone; 3,5,5-Trimethyl-2,4-oxazolidinedione; Tridione (*Abbott*)]

CH₃ O   O
CH₃ —C
   O —— N—CH₃

Trimethadione contains 98.0–102.0% of $C_6H_9NO_3$ (143.14), calculated on the dried basis.

Preparation—Trimethadione is prepared by a series of reactions beginning with acetone and involving the following steps:

$(CH_3)_2CO$ $\xrightarrow{HCN}$ $(CH_3)_2C\text{—CN}$ (with OH) $\xrightarrow{H_2SO_4 + C_2H_5OH}$
Acetone　　　　　　**Acetone**　　　　　Hydrolysis,
　　　　　　　　　　　Cyanohydrin　　Esterification

$(CH_3)_2C\text{—COOC}_2H_5$ (with OH) $\xrightarrow[\text{Urea}]{NaOC_2H_5}$ $(CH_3)_2C\text{...}C=O$ (ring with O, O=C——NH)
Ethyl Dimethylglycolate

5,5-Dimethyloxazolidine-2,4-dione

$\xrightarrow[\substack{\text{Dimethyl}\\ \text{Sulfate}}]{NaOH}$ Trimethadione

The condensation with urea is carried out in ethanol at the boiling point of the mixture.

Description—White, crystalline granules having a slight, camphor-like odor. Melting range: 45° to 47°.

Solubility—Soluble in water; freely soluble in alcohol, ether, and chloroform.

Uses—Trimethadione can prevent or modify electrical and chemical *convulsions* in animals and *epileptic seizures* in man. Trimethadione finds its chief use in the treatment of the *petit mal triad* (pyknoepilepsy, myoclonic epilepsy, akinetic epilepsy). The drug not only prevents clinical seizures but also abolishes the characteristic spike and dome irregularity in the electroencephalogram. Complete remission is obtained in many patients during Trimethadione medication. Following cessation of therapy, the patient may remain symptom-free for weeks or months. When seizures reappear they may be again controlled by the drug.

Trimethadione alone is of no value in the treatment of *grand mal* epilepsy. In some cases, however, the combination of Trimethadione with phenobarbital or diphenylhydantoin is of greater therapeutic value than any of these drugs given alone. When given alone it is of little or no value in the treatment of psychomotor seizures. However, in some cases where diphenylhydantoin does not give satisfactory relief, the combination of primidone and Trimethadione may afford better control of the seizures. It is sometimes used in the treatment of *tetanus, status epilepticus, behavior problems* in children, and *athetoses*. The drug has occasionally been used as an *analgetic*.

Sedation is a common side-action in the therapeutic use of trimethadione. Drowsiness may be overcome by the use of a stimulant such as amphetamine. Hemeralopia occurs frequently in adults, but rarely in young children. Dermatitis may develop in a few patients. Serious blood dyscrasias, such as leukopenia, agranulocytosis, thrombopenic purpura, and aplastic anemia, are rare but unfortunate consequences of Trimethadione medication. Nephrosis and hepatitis have also been observed.

Dose—**900 mg** to **2.4 Gm** daily; *usual,* **300** to **600 mg** 3 or 4 times a day.

Other Dose Information—The adult dose for the treatment of epilepsy is 900 mg to 2.1 Gm daily, in divided amounts. For infants and children the dose ranges from 300 to 900 mg daily.

Dosage Forms—Capsules USP: 300 mg; Solution USP: 40 mg/ml; Tablets NF: 150 mg.

Other Antiepileptics

Albutoin [Co-Ord (*Travenol*)] is 3-allyl-5-isobutyl-2-thiohydantoin ($C_{10}H_{16}N_2OS$). *Description* and *Solubility:* Needle-shaped, white crystals. It has a characteristic odor and a bitter taste. It is stable in light, nonhygroscopic, and stable below 80°. It melts between 108° and 110°. 1 Gm dissolves in about 9000 ml of water and 20 ml of alcohol; very soluble in acetone and chloroform; soluble in benzene and ether; insoluble in petroleum ether and isopropyl ether. *Uses:* Albutoin, an anticonvulsant equal in efficacy to diphenylhydantoin in the treatment of grand mal, psychomotor, and focal (tonic-clonic) seizures, is under clinical investigation. It is particularly effective against grand mal and psychomotor seizures. The drug is ineffective against myoclonic and akinetic epilepsy and may cause exacerbation of these seizure patterns. The incidence of side effects is said to be somewhat lower than that induced by diphenylhydantoin. Mild transient drowsiness and an occasional skin rash have been observed. Clinical tests to date indicate no significant abnormality in blood counts, urinalyses, liver functions, or thyroid attributable to Albutoin therapy.

Since Albutoin is a new anticonvulsant which as yet is not available for general clinical use, its final evaluation must await the results of more definitive clinical studies. *Dose:* 5.0 to 7.5 mg per Kg per day in divided doses.

Carbamazepine [Tegretol (*Geigy*)] is 5*H*-dibenz[*b,f*]-azepine-5-carboxamide [$C_{15}H_{12}N_2O$ = 236.26]. *Preparation:* 5*H*-Dibenz[*b,f*]azepine, which may be prepared by thermal deammoniation of 2-(*o*-aminostyryl)aniline hydrochloride, is condensed with carbamoyl chloride by refluxing in an inert solvent in the presence of sodamide. US Pat. 2,948,-718. *Description* and *Solubility:* A white, crystalline powder; it melts within a range of no more than 3° between 187° and 193°. Insoluble in water; soluble in propylene glycol. *Uses:* Carbamazepine, an iminostilbene derivative originally employed as an anticonvulsant, is used for the relief of pain associated with trigeminal neuralgia. Since effectiveness in other facial neuralgias is equivocal, Carbamazepine is not recommended in these conditions. Furthermore, the drug should not be considered a simple analgesic and administered casually for relief of trivial facial aches or pains. Serious untoward effects including aplastic anemia agranulocytosis, thrombocytopenia, and transient leukopenia have been observed. Therefore, all patients should be subjected to a complete blood test before being placed on the drug; additional blood tests should be done at weekly intervals during the first month of therapy, every 2 weeks during the second and third month, and at monthly intervals as long as the patient is on the drug. If any blood abnormality is observed, the drug should either not be used or stopped if the patient is already on the drug. Other adverse effects include dizziness, drowsiness, unsteadiness, and nausea and vomiting. Carbamazepine should not be used in combination with other drugs; other tricyclic compounds (amitriptyline, desipramine, imipramine, etc.) and MAO inhibitors are particularly contraindicated. *Dose:* 200 to 1200 mg; *usual*, 100 mg twice daily the first day and increased by 100 mg every 12 hours until pain is relieved. *Dosage Forms:* Tablets, 200 mg.

Ethotoin BP [Peganone (*Abbott*); 3-Ethyl-5-phenylhydantoin]—It occurs as a white, crystalline powder, which melts at about 90°. It is insoluble in water; freely soluble in alcohol, benzene, and dilute aqueous solutions of alkali hydroxides; soluble in ether. *Uses:* A hydantoin-type anticonvulsant useful in grand mal epilepsy and of limited usefulness in psychomotor and petit mal epilepsy. When used alone it may not afford complete control, but it does reduce the incidence of such seizures. It is considerably less toxic than many of the commonly used antiepileptics and is less likely to cause ataxia and gingival hyperplasia than other hydantoin derivatives. Occasionally encountered side effects include skin rash, dizziness, anorexia, nausea and vomiting, diplopia, nystagmus, epigastric distress, and depression. The usual precautions for early detection of signs of blood dyscrasias should be taken. It should be noted also that systemic lupus erythematosus and lymphadenopathy have been reported in patients taking hydantoins. *Dose: Usual, oral,* 500 mg 4 to 6 times a day after food.

Mephenytoin [5-Ethyl-3-methyl-5-phenylhydantoin Methoin BP; Mesantoin (*Sandoz*)]—Colorless, odorless, tasteless, lustrous plates melting at 137–138°C. It is soluble in 1500 parts of water, 13 parts of alcohol, 2.3 parts of chloroform, 85 parts of ether, and in aqueous solutions of alkali hydroxides. *Uses:* An anticonvulsant with little or no hypnotic effect. It is particularly indicated in grand mal epilepsy and has given good results in psychomotor and Jacksonian seizures. The major side effects are blood dyscrasias such as pancytopenia, agranulocytosis, and aplastic anemia. Thus, the patient should be instructed to report the occurrence of a sore throat or fever. Severe dermatitis has also been reported. It is not effective in petit mal epilepsy. *Dose: Orally,* 100 mg daily, increasing to 600 mg in accordance with the needs of the patient.

Phenacemide [Phenurone (*Abbott*); (Phenylacetyl)urea] [$C_6H_5CH_2CONHCONH_2$]—A synthetic anticonvulsant possessing minor sedative action. It occurs as a white to creamy white, odorless, tasteless, crystalline solid. It is slightly soluble in alcohol and very slightly soluble in water. *Uses:* In the treatment of psychomotor, grand mal, and petit mal epilepsy. This drug has serious side effects. Personality changes, hepatic damage, and bone marrow depression, as evidenced by leukopenia and aplastic anemia, have followed use of the drug. It should be employed only by physicians experienced in the treatment of epilepsy and only in patients whose seizures are difficult or impossible to control with other recognized anticonvulsants. *Dose: Orally,* 0.5 Gm 3 times a day with meals. The dose should be determined according to the response of the patient and the degree of control already obtained with other anticonvulsant agents.

62 | Psychopharmacologic Agents

Tranquilizing agents for psychoses and for neuroses—antidepressant agents—psychogenic agents

This chapter was prepared by

Ewart A. Swinyard, PhD, *Professor of Pharmacology, College of Pharmacy and College of Medicine, University of Utah, Salt Lake City, Utah 84112, and* **Stewart C. Harvey, PhD,** *Associate Professor of Pharmacology, College of Medicine, University of Utah, Salt Lake City, Utah 84112*

Drugs which alter the mind and behavior have attracted the attention of man since the beginning of recorded history. Without the benefits of science and medicine, mankind has sought emotional comfort or novelty through the use of drugs for a venerable period of time. To cite but two examples, alcohol and opium have been used for this purpose since antiquity. However, it was the inadvertent discovery of the unusual psychotomimetic properties of lysergic acid diethylamide in 1947 and the subsequent demonstration that these effects were similar to those induced by mescaline which marked the start of current interest in psychopharmacology. Additional interest in this new science was created with the introduction of chlorpromazine for the empiric treatment of mental disorders; a host of new drugs quickly followed the successful clinical use of this agent. These developments and the realization that behavior can be objectively studied in laboratory animals have assured psychopharmacology a place among the medical sciences.

Psychopharmacology is the science which deals with facts and theories about drugs used clinically or experimentally to alter the mental state and behavior of human and nonhuman subjects. To qualify as a psychopharmacologic agent, drugs must produce such effects consistently when given in safe ranges of dosage. This qualification distinguishes them from the drugs which alter behavior when given in toxic amounts or to subjects who react idiosyncratically. Moreover, if psychopharmacologic agents are to be used for chronic treatment of mental disorders, their effects upon awareness and mentation must be such that they do not preclude continued, organized effort on the part of the patient to achieve more successful adjustment to his environment. Thus, a primary characteristic of psychopharmacologic drugs, in contrast to the many other drugs which act upon the central nervous system, is that they alter the mental state and behavior in a predictable way.

Human mental disorders can, in general, be divided into two groups: psychoses and neuroses.

The psychoses may be further categorized as either organic or functional. The organic psychoses include drug intoxication (eg, bromide intoxication), withdrawal syndromes (eg, delirium tremens), and mental disturbances secondary to degenerative diseases of the central nervous system. They have in common some form of impairment of the neurophysiological processes which are requisite for normal behavior. The functional psychoses, including schizophrenia and affective disorders such as involutional depression and manic-depressive psychoses, reflect abnormal ways of organizing perceptions and thought processes for the purpose of environmental adjustment. The psychoses are a disturbance of total personality and are expressed in major deviations from normal behavior and thinking.

The neuroses, on the other hand, include a group of mental disorders in which symptom formation affords partial protection to the individual against some overwhelming anxiety. The neuroses are a partial disturbance in personality, centering on a specific conflict which affects a limited area of ones total adjustment. They produce relatively minor deviations from normal behavior.

Since the symptomatology of human mental disorders consists in part of disturbances in thought processes and because man and animals do not have comparable means of communication, it is impossible accurately to produce these disturbances in laboratory animals. On the other hand, some of the overt behavioral features of psychoses, such as states of overwhelming fear, exaggerated overactivity, or abandonment of all purposeful activity, as in catatonia, can be studied in subhuman species. These as well as behavior patterns generated by conditioned learning can serve as models for the laboratory assessment of psychopharmacologic drug activity.

Drugs used in the treatment of behavioral disorders and those which are known to mimic certain of these disorders in man have been classified in various ways. For the purpose of this presentation, the psychopharmacologic drugs (psychochemicals) are divided into tranquilizing agents, antidepressant agents, and psychogenic agents.

Tranquilizing Agents

Tranquilizing agents are drugs used in the treatment of psychoses and neuroses. These drugs, in contrast to the cortical and subcortical actions of sedative agents, act primarily on the lower brain areas to produce emotional calmness and relaxation without significant sedation, hypnosis, motor impairment, or euphoria.

Many of these agents also exhibit clinically useful properties, such as antihypertensive, skeletal muscle relaxant, antiepileptic, and antiemetic properties.

Numerous attempts have been made to classify the tranquilizing agents, most of which are tentative and incomplete. At one time it was suggested that these drugs be divided into major (for psychoses) and minor (for neuroses) tranquilizing agents. Such an arbitrary classification is invalid, since there is no convincing evidence that agents included in the former category are useful in neuroses and those usually listed in the latter category are more properly classified with the sedative drugs (see page 1091). Thus, this section will be restricted to agents used in the treatment of psychoses with only a brief cross-reference to agents used in the treatment of neuroses.

Agents for the Treatment of Psychoses

The tranquilizing agents used in the treatment of psychoses include the phenothiazine derivatives and rauwolfia and its alkaloids. The latter agents are used primarily for their hypotensive action and are described in another chapter (see page 912).

Experimentally, the phenothiazines suppress or abolish conditioned reflexes in trained rats, prevent morphine-induced mania in cats, and reduce the toxicity of amphetamine in aggregated mice. Many of these compounds also suppress vomiting from apomorphine, irradiation, and motion sickness, but, in laboratory animals, do not effect the emesis from morphine, veratrum alkaloids, digitalis, and copper sulfate. The phenothiazines also exhibit weak adrenolytic, hypotensive, antispasmodic, hypothermic, and antihistaminic effects and potentiate the action of many pharmacological agents.

Rauwolfia and its alkaloids, on the other hand, are characterized in the laboratory by actions on the central and peripheral nervous systems which produce a nonhypnotic sedation, ptosis of the eyelids, sinus bradycardia, increased secretory and motor activity of the gastrointestinal tract, and a lowering of arterial blood pressure. These substances act to release norepinephrine and serotonin. It is the effect on norepinephrine which is thought largely to be responsible for the hypotensive effect of these substances. The rauwolfia alkaloids reduce the norepinephrine content of the heart and certain areas of the brain, peripheral tissue, arterial walls, and peripheral nerve endings. There is, therefore, interference with sympathetic nerve impulse transmission and less norepinephrine release, both of which contribute to the hypotensive effect of these agents. The central reduction of sympathetic action as mediated by the hypothalmic centers may also contribute to the hypotensive effect. There are many other aspects of these interesting agents which as yet are not clearly defined. Rauwolfia and its alkaloids have largely been displaced in the pharmacotherapy of mental disorders.

The phenothiazines are of questionable value in relieving anxiety and tension in non-psychotic patients. They are the drugs of choice for relieving agitation and other symptoms characteristic of schizophrenia, such as hallucinations, delusions, and paranoid tension. Notwithstanding claims to the contrary, there is no convincing evidence that there are significant differences in the effectiveness of commonly prescribed phenothiazines, such as chlorpromazine, thioridazine, and fluphenazine, in acute schizophrenia. Some side effects, such as orthostatic hypotension, are common to all phenothiazines. Extrapyramidal symptoms characterized by rigidity, tremors, and excessive salivation are more characteristic of the piperazine phenothiazines. Although extrapyramidal symptoms are usually reversible after short-term therapy, prolonged phenothiazine administration can produce permanent extrapyramidal disorders (persistent dyskinesia). Long-continued treatment with these agents may also cause corneal and lenticular deposits. The phenothiazines have also been reported to cause serious blood dyscrasias. They do not produce habituation or dependency.

Acetophenazine Maleate NF

[10-[3-[4-(2-Hydroxyethyl)-1-piperazinyl]propyl]phenothiazin-2-yl Methyl Ketone Maleate (1:2); Tindal (*Schering*)]

Acetophenazine Maleate, dried at 65° for 4 hours, contains 97.0–103.0% of $C_{23}H_{29}N_3O_2S \cdot 2C_4H_4O_4$ (643.72).

Preparation—Piperazineethanol is condensed with 10-(3-chloropropyl)phenothiazin-2-yl methyl ketone (I) by refluxing the mixture in an inert solvent in the presence of a dehydrochlorinating agent such as sodamide. The resulting acetophenazine (base) is then reacted with a double equimolar portion of maleic acid. (I) is prepared from phenothiazine through the following sequence: (a) acetylation with acetic anhydride and aluminum chloride to the 2,10-diacetyl compound, (b) deacetylation at the 10 position with alkali, and (c) condensing the 2-acetylphenothiazine with 1-bromo-3-chloropropane with the aid of sodamide. US Pat. 2,985,654.

Description—A fine, yellow, powder that is odorless and has a bitter taste. It is sensitive to light and reasonably stable in dry air. It melts with decomposition between 165° and 175°.

Solubility—Soluble in water; slightly soluble in alcohol and acetone.

Uses—Acetophenazine Maleate is a piperazine-substituted phenothiazine suggested for use in chronic brain syndrome and severe neurotic conditions in which tension, anxiety, agitation, and hyperexcitability predominate. It has only limited usefulness in simple neuroses. In doses larger than usual, it is used in the management of psychotic patients. Untoward effects are similar to those for other phenothiazines, except extrapyramidal symptoms occur more frequently after administration of piperazine-substituted phenothiazines.

Dose—40 to 80 mg per day; *usual*, **20 mg** 3 times a day.

Dosage Forms—Tablets NF: 20 mg.

Butaperazine Maleate

[Repoise Maleate (*Robins*)]

Butaperazine Maleate $[C_{24}H_{31}N_3OS.2C_4H_4O_4 = 641.74]$ is 1 - [10 - [3 - (4 - methyl - 1 - piperazinyl)-propyl]phenothiazin-2-yl]-1-butanone maleate (1:2).

Preparation—1-Methylpiperazine is condensed with 10-(3-chloropropyl)phenothiazin-2-yl propyl ketone (I) by refluxing the mixture in an inert solvent in the presence of a dehydrochlorinating agent such as sodamide. The resulting butaperazine (base) is then reacted with a double equimolar portion of meleic acid. (I) may be prepared by appropriate modification of the method described under *Acetophenazine Maleate* (page 1005) for the corresponding methyl ketone. US Pat. 2,985,654.

Description—A bright-yellow powder that is practically odorless and has a moderately bitter taste. It is unstable in light (subject to oxidative degradation) and excessive heat, but not appreciably hygroscopic. Its melting point has not been established as it degrades before it melts.

Solubility—1 Gm dissolves in 400 ml of water; soluble in dimethylformamide; sparingly soluble in alcohol and methanol; insoluble in acetone, chloroform, and ether.

Uses—Butaperazine Maleate, a phenothiazine of the piperazine type, is used in the management of chronic schizophrenia. Available clinical evidence does not demonstrate that this agent has any significant advantages over the older, clinically established phenothiazines. Tremor and other extrapyramidal side effects characteristic of the phenothiazines have also been observed after Butaperazine. Other side effects include drowsiness, postural hypotension, and syncope. Agranulocytosis or jaundice have not been reported, but physicians should be alert for other side effects common to the phenothiazines.

Dose—*Usual,* 5 to 10 mg 3 times a day.

Other Dose Information—This dose may be increased by 5 to 10 mg every few days until maximum response is achieved or untoward effects appear. Total daily dose should not exceed 100 mg.

Dosage Forms—Tablets: 5, 10, and 25 mg (of the base as the maleate).

Carphenazine Maleate NF

[1- [10- [3- [4-(2-Hydroxyethyl)-1-piperazinyl]propyl]phenothiazin-2-yl]-1-propanone Maleate (1:2); Proketazine Maleate (*Wyeth*)]

Carphenazine Maleate contains 98.0–102.0% of $C_{24}H_{31}N_3O_2S \cdot 2C_4H_4O_4$ (657.75), calculated on the anhydrous basis.

Preparation—Phenothiazine is propionylated at the 2 and 10 positions through a Friedel-Crafts reaction with propionyl chloride and then depropionylated at the 10 position by alkaline hydrolysis. The resulting phenothiazin-2-yl-1-propanone is then condensed with trimethylene chlorobromide with the aid of sodium hydride to produce the 10-(3-chloropropyl) derivative, and the latter is further condensed with 1-piperazineethanol in a refluxing solvent to yield carphenazine (base). Treatment of an ethanolic solution of the base with maleic acid yields the maleate. US Pat. 2,985,654.

Description—A yellow, finely divided, odorless powder.

Solubility—Slightly soluble in water and alcohol; practically insoluble in ether.

Uses—Carphenazine Maleate is a phenothiazine-antipsychotic drug structurally related to acetophenazine, fluphenazine, and perphenazine. It is used in the treatment of hospitalized chronic or acute *schizophrenic* patients. It is most effective in *paranoid, catatonic,* and *undifferentiated types of schizophrenia;* the hebephrenic type is least responsive. Untoward effects reported resemble those encountered with other phenothiazines and include extrapyramidal reactions, convulsions, dry mouth, blurred vision, diaphoresis, somnolence, weakness, faintness, dizziness, hypotension, agitation, anxiety, tenseness, edema, puffiness of the eyes, headache, and incontinence. Patients on Carphenazine Maleate should be observed carefully for the appearance of other untoward effects characteristic of phenothiazine derivatives.

Dose—*Usual,* 12.5 to 50 mg 3 times a day; increased by 12.5 to 50 mg daily at intervals of from 4 days to 1 week. The maximal daily dose recommended is 400 mg.

Dosage Forms—Tablets NF: 12.5, 25, and 50 mg.

Chlorpromazine USP

[2-Chloro-10-[3-(dimethylamino)propyl]phenothiazine; Thorazine (*SK&F*)]

Chlorpromazine contains 98.0–101.0% of $C_{17}H_{19}ClN_2S$ (318.87), calculated on the dried basis.

For the structure, see *Chlorpromazine Hydrochloride* (below).

Description—A white or slightly creamy white, crystalline powder. It darkens on prolonged exposure to light.

Solubility—Practically insoluble in water and dilute alkali hydroxides; freely soluble in alcohol, benzene, chloroform, ether, and dilute mineral acids.

Uses—See *Chlorpromazine Hydrochloride* (below).

Dose—*Rectal,* 100 to 400 mg daily; *usual,* 100 mg 3 to 4 times a day, as necessary.

Dosage Forms—Suppositories USP: 25 and 100 mg.

Chlorpromazine Hydrochloride USP

[2-Chloro-10-[3-(dimethylamino)propyl]phenothiazine Monohydrochloride; Thorazine Hydrochloride (*SK&F*)]

Chlorpromazine Hydrochloride contains 98.0–101.5% of $C_{17}H_{19}ClN_2S.HCl$ (355.33), calculated on the dried basis.

Preparation—The free base is prepared by refluxing a toluene solution of 2-chlorophenothiazine and 3-(chloropropyl)dimethylamine in the presence of sodamide for several hours, then filtering and distilling off the toluene under reduced pressure. The pure chlorpromazine base is then obtained by short-path distillation of the residue under high vacuum. Conversion to the hydrochloride is effected by passing hydrogen chloride into a solution of the base in a suitable organic solvent.

Description—White or slightly creamy white, odorless crystalline powder. It darkens on prolonged exposure to light. Its solutions are acid to litmus. Melts between 195° and 198°.

Solubility—1 Gm dissolves in less than 1 ml of water and about 1.5 ml of alcohol and of chloroform; insoluble in ether and benzene.

Uses—Chlorpromazine Hydrochloride, the first *tranquilizer* of the phenothiazine group of compounds, is used in the treatment of *anxiety, tension, agitation,* and in *lessening motor activity* in psychotics. These include selected cases of schizophrenia, mania, and toxic and senile psychoses. Drugs of the phenothiazine type are of questionable value in the treatment of anxiety in the nonpsychotic patient. It is of value also in the treatment of *acute alcoholism.* It is also useful in the control of hiccups refractory to other forms of therapy and in the treatment of *status asthmaticus.*

The *antiemetic* effects of chlorpromazine are valuable in the treatment of the nausea and vomiting associated with carcinomatosis, uremia, acute infections, nitrogen mustard therapy, radiation sickness and vomiting of pregnancy. It is not effective in the control of vomiting from morphine, veratrum and digitalis, nor in motion sickness.

Chlorpromazine also appears to *potentiate* the action of a large number of drugs including sedatives and hypnotics, analgesics and anesthetics; hence, it should be used with caution in the presence of these agents.

Toxic reactions and side effects are fairly frequent. *Orthostatic hypotension* is a common side effect and the drug should be given with extreme caution in patients with cardiovascular disease in whom a sudden drop in blood pressure may be undesirable. Sedation and drowsiness may be desirable in some situations, undesirable in others. Tachycardia, hypothermia, dryness of the mouth, dermatitis and photosensitivity, nausea and vomiting, and a Parkinson-like syndrome may also occur. Recent evidence suggests that prolonged treatment with large doses may result in permanent extrapyramidal disorders (persistent dyskinesia). Long-term treatment with high doses may also result in corneal and lenticular deposits. Jaundice occurs in a significant number of patients, usually in the first two weeks of therapy and requires immediate cessation of therapy. Cases of severe and fatal blood dyscrasias, including agranulocytosis, in some instances associated with hypoplastic anemia and leukopenia, have been reported. These symptoms also require immediate discontinuance of the drug.

Dosage is extremely variable and requires strict individualization. Administration is oral, intramuscular, or intravenous. Parenteral administration should be reserved for bedfast or hospitalized patients. If used in ambulatory patients, the patient must remain in a supine position for at least one hour after the injection. Alarming reactions with failure to respond to pressor agents have been reported from even small intravenous doses. Epinephrine should never be used in treating these cases since the adrenolytic action of the Chlorpromazine may cause epinephrine reversal. Phenylephrine or levarterenol may be used to control the hypotension.

Dose—*Oral,* **10 mg** to **1 Gm** daily; *usual, oral,* **25 mg** 4 times a day; *intramuscular* or *intravenous,* **25 mg** to **1 Gm** daily; *usual, intramuscular* or *intravenous,* **25 mg,** repeated in 2 to 4 hours if necessary.

Dosage Forms—Injection USP: 1, 2, and 10 ml; Syrup USP; Tablets USP: 10, 25, 50, 100, and 200 mg.

Veterinary Dose (per pound of body weight)— *Oral, Sheep* and *Goats,* **1 mg;** *Dogs* and *Cats,* **1.5 mg.** *Intravenous, Horses,* **0.1 mg;** *Cattle,* **0.1 to 0.5 mg;** *Sheep, Goats, Dogs,* and *Cats,* **0.25 to 2 mg.** *Intramuscular, Horses,* **0.5 to 1.8 mg;** *Cattle,* **0.5 to 1 mg;** *Sheep, Goats,* and *Cats,* **1 to 3 mg;** *Dogs,* **0.5 to 3 mg.**

Chlorprothixene NF

[(*E*)-2-Chloro-*N,N*-dimethylthioxanthene-Δ$^{9,\gamma}$-propylamine; Taractan (*Roche*)]

Chlorprothixene contains 99.0–101.0% of $C_{18}H_{18}$-ClNS (315.87), calculated on the dried basis.

Preparation—One of the methods of preparation consists of cyclizing 5-chloro-2-(phenylthio)benzoic acid with the aid of polyphosphoric acid to form 2-chlorothioxanthen-9-one followed by reaction of the latter with [3-(dimethylamino)propylidene]triphenylphosphorane to introduce the 9-substituent. US Pat. 3,115,502 describes a process for converting the *cis* form of the compound to the therapeutically active *trans* form which involves heating in the presence of a strongly basic agent such as an alkali metal hydroxide, alkoxide, or amide.

Description—A yellow, crystalline powder. It has a slight amine-like odor and is unstable when exposed to light and air. It melts between 96.5° and 101.5°.

Solubility—Practically insoluble in water; 1 Gm dissolves in 25 ml of alcohol, 2 ml of chloroform, and 10 ml of ether.

Uses—Chlorprothixene is a thioxanthene derivative which is chemically and pharmacologically related to chlorpromazine. In place of the nitrogen in the phenothiazine ring, Chlorprothixene has a carbon atom with a double bond to the dimethylaminopropyl side chain. This structural difference is not associated with any striking pharmacological difference; Chlorprothixene, like chlorpromazine and other phenothiazines, exhibits sedative, antihistaminic, anticholinergic, hypothermic, adrenolytic, and antiemetic effects. Hence, its spectrum of clinical usefulness is also similar to that of chlorpromazine. Thus, it has been used in the treatment of acute and chronic schizophrenia and in psychotic and severe neurotic conditions in which anxiety, agitation, and tension predominate. It has also been used for the management of nausea and vomiting associated with radiation therapy, surgery, or emotional disturbances. Because of its structural similarity to the phenothiazines, all the known serious side effects associated with phenothiazine therapy should be borne in mind.

Dose—*Usual, moderate anxiety,* **10 mg** 3 or 4 times a day (up to 60 mg daily); *severe neurotic and psychotic states,* **25 to 50 mg** 3 or 4 times daily (up to 600 mg daily).

Dosage Forms—Injection: 12.5 mg/ml; Tablets NF: 10, 25, 50, and 100 mg.

Fluphenazine Enanthate NF

[4-[3-[2-(Trifluoromethyl)phenothiazin-10-yl]propyl]-1-piperazineethanol Heptanoate (ester); Prolixin Enanthate (*Squibb*)]

Fluphenazine Enanthate contains 97.0–103.0% of $C_{29}H_{38}F_3N_3O_2S$ (549.70), calculated on the dried basis.

Preparation—Fluphenazine is esterified through reaction with enanthoyl chloride in the presence of pyridine. For the preparation of fluphenazine (base), see *Fluphenazine Hydrochloride*, this page. US Pat. 3,058,979.

Description—A pale-yellow to yellow-orange, clear to slightly turbid, viscous liquid that has a characteristic odor. It is not recommended to be tasted. It is unstable in strong light, but it is stable in air at room temperature.

Solubility—Freely soluble in alcohol, ether, benzene, and chloroform; insoluble in water.

Uses—Fluphenazine Enanthate, except for duration of action, has actions, uses, contraindications, and untoward effects similar to those of fluphenazine hydrochloride. The esterification of fluphenazine with the enanthate moiety markedly prolongs the drug duration of action without unduly attenuating its beneficial effects. The onset of action generally appears between 24 to 72 hours after injection, and the effects of the drug on psychotic symptoms become significant within 48 to 96 hours. Amelioration of symptoms continues for 1 to 3 weeks or longer, with an average duration of effect of about 2 weeks. See *Fluphenazine Hydrochloride*.

Dose—*Intramuscular* or *subcutaneous*, **12.5 to 100 mg**; *usual*, **25 mg** every 2 weeks.

Dosage Forms—Injection NF: 25 mg/ml, 125 mg/5 ml, 250 mg/10 ml.

Fluphenazine Hydrochloride NF

[4-[3-[2-(Trifluoromethyl)phenothiazin-10-yl]propyl]-1-piperazineethanol Dihydrochloride; Permitil Hydrochloride (*White*); Prolixin Hydrochloride (*Squibb*)]

Fluphenazine Hydrochloride, dried at 65° for 3 hours, contains 97.0–103.0% of $C_{22}H_{26}F_3N_3OS \cdot 2HCl$ (510.45).

Preparation—Fluphenazine (base) may be prepared by condensing 2-(trifluoromethyl)-10-(3-chloropropyl)phenothiazine with 1-piperazineethanol in toluene with the aid of sodamide. Reaction of the purified base with a double molar quantity of hydrogen chloride yields the official salt. The starting phenothiazine compound may be prepared in the usual way by heating 3-(trifluoromethyl)diphenylamine with sulfur and condensing the resulting 2-(trifluoromethyl)phenothiazine with 1-bromo-3-chloropropane. US Pat. 3,058,979.

Description—A white or nearly white, odorless, crystalline powder. It melts within a range of 5° above 225°.

Solubility—Freely soluble in water; slightly soluble in acetone, alcohol, and chloroform; practically insoluble in benzene and ether.

Uses—Fluphenazine Hydrochloride is a trifluoromethyl phenothiazine derivative intended for the management of *anxiety* and *tension* states, *severe mental disorders*, and *behavioral problems* in children. Although the pharmacologic effects of Fluphenazine

Hydrochloride are, in general, similar to those of other phenothiazines, laboratory and clinical studies indicate that this drug exhibits several important differences. The drug is more potent, exhibits a more prolonged duration of action, is less likely to induce hypotension, is less sedative, and does not potentiate central nervous system depressants and anesthetics to the same degree as other phenothiazines. It appears to be particularly effective in modifying psychotic behavior patterns and ameliorating such symptoms as agitation, delusions, and hallucinations. Fluphenazine Hydrochloride is contraindicated in patients with subcortical brain damage since a hyperthermic reaction with temperatures in excess of 104° F may occur. Like other phenothiazines, Fluphenazine Hydrochloride should not be used in patients receiving large doses of hypnotics, and should be used with caution in patients with a history of convulsive disorders. Side effects induced by Fluphenazine Hydrochloride are similar to those encountered with other phenothiazines. Those most frequently encountered include reversible extrapyramidal symptoms including Parkinsonism, dystonia, dyskinesia, akathisia, oculogyric crises, opisthotonos, and hyperreflexia; liver damage manifest by jaundice or biliary stasis; blood dyscrasias, including leukopenia, agranulocytosis, thrombocytopenic purpura, eosinophilia, and pancytopenia; skin disorders such as itching, erythema, urticaria, and even exfoliative dermatitis; peripheral edema, endocrine disturbances, and autonomic reactions. Hypotension has rarely been a problem with Fluphenazine Hydrochloride. Patients given this drug should be under medical supervision and observed carefully for other untoward effects characteristic of phenothiazine agents.

Dose—*Usual*, **0.5 to 2 mg** daily.

Other Dose Information—Initial oral or intramuscular daily dosage, 2.5 to 10 mg in divided doses administered at 6- to 8-hour intervals. Maintenance, 1 to 5 mg orally as a single daily dose. Dosages exceeding 20 mg orally or 10 mg intramuscularly should be used with caution.

Dosage Forms—Injection NF: 25 mg/10 ml; Tablets NF: 250 mcg, and 1, 2.5, 5, and 10 mg.

Haloperidol NF

[4-[4-(*p*-Chlorophenyl)-4-hydroxypiperidino]-4'-fluorobutyrophenone; Haldol (*McNeil*)]

Haloperidol, dried in vacuum at 60° for 3 hours, contains 98.0–102.0% of $C_{21}H_{23}ClFNO_2$ (375.87).

Preparation—4-(*p*-Chlorophenyl)-4-piperidinol condenses readily with 4-chloro-4'-fluorobutyrophenone by heating a toluene solution of the reactants in the presence of a small quantity of potassium iodide. The Haloperidol thus formed is isolated from the reaction mixture and recrystallized from a suitable solvent such as diisopropyl ether. The starting substituted piperidinol may be prepared from *p*-chloro-α-methylstyrene by the method described by Schmidle and Mansfield.[1] The starting substituted butyrophenone may be prepared by a Friedel–Crafts reaction between 4-chlorobutyryl chloride and fluorobenzene.

Description—A white to faintly yellowish, odorless, amorphous or microcrystalline powder. It is light-sensitive and nonhygroscopic. Its saturated solution is neutral to litmus. It melts between 146° and 151°.

Solubility—Practically insoluble in water; soluble in chloroform; sparingly soluble in alcohol; slightly soluble in ether.

Uses—Haloperidol, a butyrophenone derivative, is an antipsychotic agent useful in the management of *acute* and *chronic schizophrenia*. It is also effective in the management of the manic phase of *manic-depressive psychosis, psychosis associated with organic brain damage*, and symptoms associated with organic brain damage. Haloperidol has been reported to be useful in *Gilles de la Tourette's disease* (motor tics, unusual barking, and hissing sounds). Like the phenothiazines, Haloperidol frequently produces extrapyramidal reactions such as Parkinsonism, dystonia, dyskinesia, oculogyric crises, and akathisia. Severe depression has been observed following the use of the drug in some patients. Hence, it is contraindicated in patients with a history of depressive tendencies. Care should be exercised when antihypertensive agents, general anesthetics, hypnotics, alcohol, analgesics, and other central nervous system depressants are used concomitantly with Haloperidol, since it may potentiate their actions. Haloperidol has been reported to decrease the anticoagulant effect of phenindione. The safety of the drug in pregnancy has not been established.

Dose—1 to **5 mg**; daily doses greater than 15 mg are not recommended; *usual*, 1 to **2 mg** 2 or 3 times a day.

Dosage Forms—Concentrate: 2 mg/ml; Solution NF: 2 mg/ml; Tablets NF: 0.5, 1, 2, and 5 mg.

Lithium Carbonate

[Eskalith (*SK & F*)]

Lithium Carbonate is Li$_2$CO$_3$ (73.89).

Description—A white, light, alkaline powder that melts at 618°.

Solubility—1 Gm dissolves in 78 ml of cold water and 140 ml of boiling water; insoluble in alcohol; dissolved by dilute acids.

Uses—Lithium Carbonate has been used for the treatment of the manic phase of manic-depressive psychoses. It has been effective in many patients not responding to the phenothiazines. It is less effective in hyperactive states in schizophrenia and other psychoses. Since the effect of Lithium Carbonate is usually not apparent for 3 to 10 days, initial treatment should be started with a phenothiazine, preferably parenterally. Nausea, vomiting, and diarrhea are presumptive evidence of toxicity and indicate the dose should be reduced. The most common untoward effects are slight tremor and polyuria; these do not ordinarily require a reduction in dosages. Central nervous system effects, such as slurred speech, blurred vision, confusion, and lethargy, require immediate withdrawal of the drug and the administration of sodium chloride (at least 4 Gm extra per day) to facilitate the excretion of lithium. Lithium Carbonate should not be used in patients with cardiovascular or renal disease.

Dose—*Usual*, **0.3** to **0.6 Gm** 3 times a day. When the effect becomes apparent, the dose should be reduced by 0.3 Gm every 5 to 7 days until a maintenance dose is reached.

Dosage Forms—Capsules: 300 mg.

Mepazine Acetate

Mepazine Acetate (C$_{19}$H$_{22}$N$_2$S.C$_2$H$_4$O$_2$) is 10[(1-methyl-3-piperidyl)methyl]phenothiazine monoacetate.

Preparation—3-Chloromethyl-1-methylpiperidine is condensed with phenothiazine with the aid of a suitable dehydrochlorinating agent such as sodium hydride, and the mepazine (base) thus formed is reacted with an equimolar quantity of acetic acid.

Description—A white, slightly caked crystalline powder having a faint acetic acid odor. It is subject to oxidation and develops a pink tint on exposure to light or air. It melts between 70° and 73.5°.

Solubility—Soluble in water; insoluble in isopropanol.

Uses and Dose—See *Mepazine Hydrochloride*.
Dosage Forms—Injection: 25 mg/ml.

Mepazine Hydrochloride

Mepazine Hydrochloride is C$_{19}$H$_{22}$N$_2$S.HCl. For the structure of the base, see *Mepazine Acetate*, this page.

Preparation—Mepazine (base) is reacted with an equimolar portion of hydrogen chloride. For preparation of the base, see *Mepazine Acetate*, above.

Description—Photosensitive, slightly bitter crystals which decompose between 171° and 174° by the capillary tube method and between 185° and 188° by the micro-block method.

Solubility—Freely soluble in absolute alcohol; soluble in chloroform; very slightly soluble in water; practically insoluble in ether and benzene.

Uses—Mepazine Hydrochloride is a phenothiazine derivative with actions and uses similar to, but not identical with, those of chlorpromazine. Pharmacologically it differs from chlorpromazine in that it neither lowers the body temperature in rats nor antagonizes the waltzing syndrome in mice and it augments carotid sinus reflexes in cats. The significance of these differences with respect to clinical usefulness is not clear. Although it is somewhat less potent, the drug has the same clinical uses as chlorpromazine. Hence, it is useful for its calming or tranquilizing action in the management of psychoses in which *anxiety, tension, agitation*, and increased psychomotor activity are present. It also exerts an *antiemetic* effect which is useful in the control of nausea and vomiting from a variety of causes and its tranquilizing action is useful in *narcotic withdrawal* to control restlessness and agitation, in chronic alcoholism to lessen anxiety and tensions, and in advanced *neoplastic states* to reduce the quantity of narcotics needed for control of pain.

The types of side effects induced by Mepazine are about the same as for chlorpromazine, but the former drug induces more agranulocytosis, seizures, and atropine-like actions. The most serious untoward effects attributed to Mepazine are depression of the bone marrow and jaundice. Because it potentiates the action of other central nervous system depressants, Mepazine is contraindicated in patients under the influence of large doses of narcotics, barbiturates, or large quantities of alcohol.

Dose—*Usual, oral*, **25 mg** 3 or 4 times a day increased every week by 25 mg per day until the desired effect has been attained. For *nausea* and *vomiting*, **50 to 100 mg** per day orally.

Dosage Forms—Tablets: 25, 50, and 100 mg.

Perphenazine NF

[4-[3-(2-Chlorophenothiazin-10-yl)propyl]-1-piperazineethanol;   Trilafon *(Schering)*]

$$CH_2CH_2CH_2-NN-CH_2CH_2OH$$

Perphenazine, dried at 65° in vacuum for 3 hours, contains 98.0–102.0% of $C_{21}H_{26}ClN_3OS$ (403.98).

Preparation—A toluene solution of 2-chloro-10-(3-chloropropyl)phenothiazine and 1-piperazineethanol is refluxed with sodamide and the resulting crude Perphenazine is purified by high vacuum distillation. The starting phenothiazine compound may be prepared by condensing 2-chlorophenothiazine with trimethylene chlorobromide with the aid of sodium hydride. US Pat. 2,838,507.

Description—White creamy-white powder which is almost odorless and has a bitter taste. It melts between 96° and 100°.

Solubility—Practically insoluble in water; freely soluble in alcohol and chloroform; soluble in acetone; sparingly soluble in ether; practically insoluble in sesame oil.

Uses—Perphenazine, a phenothiazine compound, differs chemically from prochlorperazine only with respect to the substitution of a hydroxyethyl group for the methyl group of the latter drug. Perphenazine is approximately twice as potent, milligram for milligram, as prochlorperazine and exhibits depressant actions, clinical uses, and side effects similar to those of chlorpromazine. See *Chlorpromazine Hydrochloride*.

Dose—*Usual, oral*, nonhospitalized patients, **2 to 8 mg** 3 times a day; hospitalized patients, **8 to 16 mg** 2 to 4 times a day; *intramuscular*, **5 to 10 mg** initially, followed by **5 mg** in 6 hours.

Dosage Forms—Injection NF: 5 mg/ml, 50 mg/10 ml; Tablets NF: 2, 4, 8, and 16 mg.

Veterinary Dose—*Cattle, intravenously*, **75 to 100 mg**; *intramuscularly*, **100 to 150 mg**; *Swine, parenterally*, **10 mg** per **100 pounds** of body weight; *Dogs, orally*, **4 mg** per **10 pounds** of body weight twice daily; *parenterally*, **5 mg** per **20 pounds** of weight. Do not inject subcutaneously. Contraindicated in horses.

Piperacetazine

[Quide *(Dow)*]

Piperacetazine is 10-{3-[4-(2-hydroxyethyl)piperidino]propyl}phenothiazin-2-yl methyl ketone ($C_{24}H_{30}N_2O_2S$).

Preparation—A method of preparation may be found in Brit. Pat. 861,807 (1961).

Uses—Piperacetazine, a potent phenothiazine with tranquilizing and sedative properties, is proposed for the control of hyperactivity, agitation, and anxiety associated with schizophrenic reactions. Although useful in chronic schizophrenic states of long duration, response to therapy is more prominent in the acute forms of the disease. Side effects and contraindications are the same as those for other phenothiazines (see *Chlorpromazine Hydrochloride* page 1106). Piperacetazine is contraindicated during pregnancy and lactation. It is not recommended in children under 12 years of age because conditions for its safe use have not been established.

Dose—*Initial*, **10 mg** 2 to 4 times daily; *maintenance*, up to **160 mg** daily in divided doses. If side effects appear, dosage should be reduced or discontinued.

Dosage Forms—Tablets: 10 mg.

Prochlorperazine—see page 808.

Prochlorperazine Edisylate—see page 809.

Prochlorperazine Maleate—see page 809.

Promazine Hydrochloride NF

[10-[3-(Dimethylamino)propyl]phenothiazine Monohydrochloride; Sparine Hydrochloride *(Wyeth)*]

$$\left[CH_2CH_2CH_2\overset{+}{N}H(CH_3)_2 \right] Cl^-$$

Promazine Hydrochloride, dried at 105° for 2 hours, contains 98.0–102.0% of $C_{17}H_{20}N_2S.HCl$ (320.89).

Preparation—Phenothiazine is dissolved in a suitable inert solvent and condensed with 3-chloro-*N,N*-dimethylpropylamine in the presence of sodium hydride to yield promazine. After purification, the base is dissolved in an appropriate organic solvent and reacted with an equimolar quantity of hydrogen chloride.

Description—Occurs as a white to slightly yellow, practically odorless, crystalline powder. It oxidizes upon prolonged exposure to air, and acquires a blue or pink color.

Solubility—Freely soluble in water and chloroform.

Uses—Promazine Hydrochloride lacks a chlorine atom on the ring structure, otherwise it is chemically identical to chlorpromazine hydrochloride and has the same general pharmacological properties as the latter; the chief difference is the lower acute toxicity of Promazine after oral and parenteral administration to experimental animals.

Promazine has the same therapeutic applications and limitations as chlorpromazine. Although some of the more serious toxic effects of chlorpromazine have not been encountered with Promazine, it should be used with the same degree of caution. See *Chlorpromazine Hydrochloride*.

Dose—*Usual, oral, intramuscular*, and *intravenous*, **10 to 200 mg**, every 4 to 6 hours.

Other Dose Information—Total daily dose ranges from 25 to 300 mg to a maximum of 1 Gm daily.

Dosage Forms—Injection NF: 25 and 50 mg/ml, 50 and 100 mg/2 ml, 250 and 500 mg/10 ml; Syrup NF: 10 mg/5 ml; Tablets NF: 10, 25, 50, 100, and 200 mg.

Veterinary Dose—*Intravenous* or *intramuscular*, ataraxic or preanesthetic, *Horses, Cattle, Sheep*, and *Swine*, **0.2 to 0.5 mg** per **pound** of body weight; *oral* or *parenteral, Dogs* and *Cats,* **1** to **3 mg** per **pound** of body weight at intervals of 4 to 6 hours.

Rauwolfia Serpentina—see page 912.

Rescinnamine—see page 912.

Reserpine—see page 912.

Syrosingopine—see page 913.

Thiopropazate Hydrochloride NF

[4-[3-(2-Chlorophenothiazin-10-yl)propyl]-1-piperazineethanol Acetate Dihydrochloride; Dartal (*Searle*)]

Thiopropazate Hydrochloride contains 98.0–100.5% of $C_{23}H_{28}ClN_3O_2S.2HCl$ (518.94), calculated on the anhydrous basis.

Preparation—10-(3-Chloropropyl)phenothiazine is condensed with piperazine in butanone solution and the resulting 10-[3-(1-piperazinyl)propyl]phenothiazine is then further condensed with 2-bromoethyl acetate with the aid of a suitable dehydrobrominating agent such as sodamide to form thiopropazate (base). Reaction of the base with a double molar portion of hydrogen chloride yields the official salt.

Description—Light-tan, microcrystalline powder having a slight sharp odor. It melts between 223° and 229° when placed in the bath within 5° of fusion and heated at a rate of 1.5° per minute.

Solubility—Freely soluble in water; slightly soluble in alcohol; insoluble in chloroform and ether.

Uses—Thiopropazate Hydrochloride is a potent phenothiazine which produces comparable pharmacological effects with doses that are considerably less than those of chlorpromazine. Its spectrum of clinical usefulness is similar to that of other phenothiazines and it is subject to similar limitations. The principal clinical application of Thiopropazate Hydrochloride is in the management of *psychoses* in which *agitation, tension, combativeness,* and *aggressiveness* predominate. Some patients with *psychomotor retardation, apathy,* and *lethargy* are said to be benefited by the drug. It also suppresses involuntary muscular activity in *Huntington's chorea.*

Typical phenothiazine side effects, such as sedation and hypotension, have been reported to be less frequent and less severe with Thiopropazate than with other agents of this class. The drug has produced leukopenia, but no cases of granulocytopenia or jaundice were recorded during its clinical trial; nevertheless, physicians should be alert for such untoward reactions. Extrapyramidal involvement characterized by Parkinson-like symptoms are more likely to occur with this agent since the margin between effective doses and those that cause motor system manifestations is rather narrow. See *Chlorpromazine Hydrochloride.*

Dose—**5** to **10 mg;** *usual,* **10 mg** 3 times a day, adjusted upward or downward in daily increments of 10 mg, at intervals of 3 or 4 days, according to response.

Dosage Forms—Tablets NF: 5 and 10 mg.

Thioridazine

[Mellaril (*Sandoz*)]

Thioridazine [$C_{21}H_{26}N_2S_2 = 370.58$] is 10-[2-(methyl-2-piperidyl)ethyl]-2-(methylthio)phenothiazine.

Preparation—2-(Methylthio)phenothiazine, which may be prepared by reacting 2-chlorophenothiazine with (methylthio)sodium, is condensed with 2-(1-methyl-2-piperidyl)ethyl chloride with the aid of a suitable dehydrochlorinating agent such as sodamide. US Pat. 3,239,514.

Description—Crystals that melt between 72° and 74°.

Uses and **Dose**—See *Thioridazine Hydrochloride.*

Thioridazine Hydrochloride USP

[10-[2-(1-Methyl-2-piperidyl)ethyl]-2-(methylthio)phenothiazine Monohydrochloride; Mellaril Hydrochloride (*Sandoz*)]

Thioridazine Hydrochloride contains 99.0–101.0% of $C_{21}H_{26}N_2S_2.HCl$ (407.04), calculated on the dried basis.

For the structure and preparation of the base, see *Thioridazine.*

Description—A white to slightly yellow, granular powder with a faint odor and a very bitter taste. It is stable in moderate heat, is nonhygroscopic, and darkens upon exposure to light. It melts between 159° and 163°.

Solubility—Freely soluble in water and methanol; slightly soluble in benzene; insoluble in ether.

Uses—Thioridazine Hydrochloride is a piperidyl-type phenothiazine tranquilizer with central sedative and behavioral effects similar to those of chlorpromazine. It has minimal antiemetic action and produces minimal extrapyramidal stimulation. Sedation and drowsiness are less intense with Thioridazine than with chlorpromazine and related compounds. Thioridazine is useful in the management of a variety of mental disorders including anxiety and tension states, acute and chronic psychoneuroses, acute and chronic schizophrenia, and manic psychoses. Untoward effects, such as extrapyramidal reactions, sedation, and drowsiness are less intense and occur less frequently with Thioridazine than with any other phenothiazine. Dryness of the mouth, orthostatic hypotension, and other symptoms of autonomic blockade occur occasionally in patients on large doses of the drug. Gastric irritation, skin eruptions, nasal stuffiness, and stimulation of lactation are minor effects. Agranulocytosis and toxic retinitis and inhibition of ejaculation have also been reported. Electrocardiographic changes resembling those caused by quinidine and hypokalemia have been observed. Other precautions and contraindications are similar to those for chlorpromazine.

Dose—**20** to **800 mg** daily; *usual,* **25** to **50 mg** 3 or 4 times a day.

Dosage Forms—Solution USP; Tablets USP: 10, 25, 50, 100, 150, and 200 mg.

Thiothixene

[Navane (*Roerig*)]

Thiothixene [$C_{23}H_{29}N_3O_2S_2$ = 443.63] is *N,N*-dimethyl - 9 - [3 - (4 - methyl - 1 - piperazinyl)propylidene]thioxanthene-2-sulfonamide.

Preparation—2-Chlorobenzoic acid is converted into its 5-dimethylsulfamoyl derivative by successive reaction with chlorosulfonic acid and dimethylamine. The chlorine is then replaced by the phenylthio group through treatment with benzenethiol in the presence of alkali and the resulting 2-phenylthio derivative is cyclized through dehydration with polyphosphoric acid to form *N,N*-dimethyl-9-oxothioxanthene-2-sulfonamide. Reaction of this compound with [3-(4-methyl-1-piperidyl)propylidene]triphenylphosphorane results in the replacement of the oxo oxygen by the appropriately substituted propylidene group to yield Thiothixene. US Pat. 3,310,553.

Description—A white to light-tan, fine, crystalline powder that is odorless and has a very bitter taste. It is unstable in light. It melts between 149° and 150°.

Solubility—Soluble in chloroform; sparingly soluble in acetone; slightly soluble in alcohol and carbon tetrachloride; practically insoluble in water.

Uses—Thiothixene, a thioxanthene derivative, is an antipsychotic agent used in the treatment of schizophrenia. It is also helpful in the management of psychosis and secondary symptoms of schizophrenia, such as, hallucinations, tension, and suspiciousness. Thiothixene is contraindicated in patients with circulatory collapse, comatose states, central nervous system depression, and blood dyscrasias. Potentiation of central nervous system depressants (opiates, analgesics, antihistamines, barbiturates, alcohol) has not been observed. Since Thiothixene resembles the phenothiazines both chemically and pharmacologically, all of the known side effects of the latter class of agents should be kept in mind when it is employed. Thus, extrapyramidal symptoms, such as Parkinson-like syndromes, dystonic reactions, and akathisia have been reported.

Dose—**6 to 60 mg** daily in 3 divided doses; *usual,* **2 to 10 mg** 3 times a day. Exceeding a total daily dose of 60 mg rarely increases the beneficial response.

Dosage Forms—Capsules: 1, 2, 5, and 10 mg.

Trifluoperazine Hydrochloride NF

[10-[3-(4-Methyl-1-piperazinyl)propyl]-2-(trifluoromethyl)phenothiazine Dihydrochloride; Stelazine Hydrochloride (*SK&F*)]

Trifluoperazine Hydrochloride, dried in vacuum at 60° for 4 hours, contains 98.0–101.0% of $C_{21}H_{24}F_3N_3S$ · 2HCl (480.43).

Preparation—Trifluoperazine Hydrochloride may be prepared by the process described for *Trifluprom-*

azine Hydrochloride (this page) except that 1-(3-chloropropyl)-4-methylpiperazine is used as the condensing amine in place of (3-chloropropyl)dimethylamine. US Pat. 2,921,069.

Description—A white to pale-yellow, crystalline powder. It is practically odorless and has a bitter taste.

Solubility—Freely soluble in water; soluble in alcohol; sparingly soluble in chloroform; insoluble in ether and benzene.

Uses—Trifluoperazine Hydrochloride is a piperazine phenothiazine used in the treatment of psychoses. In low doses, Trifluoperazine is said to be effective in agitation and tension in selected psychosomatic patients. In larger doses, the drug is employed in the treatment of psychotic patients; it is effective in acute and chronic schizophrenias, manic-depressive psychoses, and involutional psychoses and in chronic brain syndrome. Trifluoperazine exhibits greater antiemetic properties than either chlorpromazine or prochlorperazine. On the other hand, the hypotensive and sympatholytic effects of Trifluoperazine are substantially less than those of chlorpromazine or prochlorperazine when the comparison is made on the basis of equipotent doses of the drugs. Likewise, the drug is considerably less sedative than is chlorpromazine. Untoward effects are usually infrequent and mild when the drug is employed in small doses for psychosomatic patients. With large doses, untoward effects are more frequent and severe. Extrapyramidal symptoms occur more frequently with Trifluoperazine than with chlorpromazine. Excitement and increased suggestibility are occasionally encountered. Other untoward effects include temporary stimulation, transient drowsiness, dizziness, muscular weakness, anorexia, rash, lactation, and blurred vision. Jaundice, allergic purpura, and agranulocytosis have been reported on occasion. Since Trifluoperazine may potentiate the action of antihypertensive agents, as well as that of general anesthetics, hypnotics, alcohol, and other central nervous system depressants, caution should be observed in the concomitant use of any of these drugs with Trifluoperazine. The antiemetic action of Trifluoperazine may mask signs of overdosage of toxic drugs or may obscure diagnosis of intestinal obstruction or brain tumor. Trifluoperazine is contraindicated in patients with central nervous system depression or in those who are comatose.

Dose—*Usual, oral,* nonhospitalized patients, **1 to 2 mg** twice daily; hospitalized patients, **2 to 5 mg** daily initially, gradually increasing to the optimum level of **15 or 20 mg** daily, although a few patients may require **40 mg** a day or more; *intramuscular,* **1 to 2 mg** every 4 to 6 hours as required.

Dosage Forms—Injection NF: 20 mg/10 ml; Tablets NF: 1, 2, 5, and 10 mg.

Triflupromazine Hydrochloride NF

[10-[3-(Dimethylamino)propyl]-2-(trifluoromethyl)phenothiazine Monohydrochloride; Vesprin (*Squibb*)]

Triflupromazine Hydrochloride contains 97.0–102.0% of $C_{18}H_{19}F_3N_2S$·HCl (388.89), calculated on the dried basis.

Preparation—2-(Trifluoromethyl)phenothiazine is condensed with (3-chloropropyl)dimethylamine by refluxing in dry benzene in the presence of sodamide. The triflupromazine (base) thus formed is extracted and purified by distillation under high vacuum. Conversion to the hydrochloride is effected by passing hydrogen chloride into an ethanolic solution of the base. The starting phenothiazine compound may be prepared by heating 3-(trifluoromethyl)diphenylamine with sulfur.   US Pat. 2,921,069.

Description—A white to pale-tan, crystalline powder with a slight, characteristic odor. It melts between 170° and 178°.

Solubility—Soluble in water, alcohol, and acetone; insoluble in ether.

Uses—Triflupromazine Hydrochloride is the 2-(trifluoromethyl) analog of chlorpromazine hydrochloride. Except that it is somewhat more potent, Triflupromazine has the same actions, uses, and limitations as chlorpromazine. See *Chlorpromazine Hydrochloride*.

Dose—*Usual, oral*, **30** to **150 mg** daily; *intramuscular*, **5** to **10 mg**, repeated in 4 hours, if necessary; *intravenous*, **1** to **3 mg**, repeated in 4 hours, if necessary.

Dosage Forms—Tablets NF: 10, 25, and 50 mg.

Agents for the Treatment of Neuroses

Many different chemical agents which produce mild depression of the central nervous system have been used to reduce the emotional tension characteristic of neuroses. For example, certain antihistaminics (diphenhydramine), acetylenic carbinols (ethchlorvynol), monoureides (carbromal), barbiturates (phenobarbital), piperidinediones (methyprylon), propyl alcohol derivatives (meprobamate), benzodiazepines (chlordiazepoxide), etc can logically be used for this purpose. Although the newer mild sedative agents have gained favor among many physicians for the treatment of neuroses, no one agent has been shown to be selectively effective in neuroses. All agents used for this purpose have in common the ability to produce mild sedation in doses unlikely to effect adversely the clarity of consciousness and the quality of psychomotor performance. Likewise, many of these drugs exhibit other pharmacological properties, such as skeletal muscle relaxant and anticonvulsant actions. Habituation and/or physical dependence may follow prolonged administration with most of these agents. Therefore, arbitrary classification of the newer sedatives based on their use in neuroses is unwarranted. For this reason the agents listed are discussed in Chapter 60 (page 1091) with the conventional sedative and hypnotic agents.

Azacyclonol Hydrochloride

Buclizine Hydrochloride

Captodiamine Hydrochloride

Chlordiazepoxide Hydrochloride

Diazepam

Emylcamate

Hydroxyphenamate

Hydroxyzine Hydrochloride

Hydroxyzine Pamoate

Mephenoxalone

Meprobamate

Mebutamate

Oxanamide

Oxazepam

Phenaglycodol

Pipethanate Hydrochloride

Tybamate

Antidepressant Agents

Antidepressant agents are drugs which enhance alertness and may result in an increased output of behavior. When compared on the basis of their pharmacologic properties, these agents fall into three groups. The first group include the monoamine oxidase inhibitors; these substances increase the concentrations of serotonin and norepinephrine in the brain. Consequently, they should not be administered simultaneously with sympathomimetic drugs (amphetamine, ephedrine, etc) or with foods containing amines (cheese), because of the danger of inducing an acute hypertensive crisis. The monoamine oxidase inhibitors which contain a hydrazine moiety (phenelzine sulfate and nialamide) are slow to evoke a response (2 to 3 weeks), whereas those without a hydrazine group (tranylcypromine sulfate) act more promptly (7 days). A second group (imipramine hydrochloride and amitriptyline hydrochloride) elicit mild atropine-like effects and exhibit actions similar to those of the phenothiazines.

These agents should not be given concomitantly with, or immediately after, monoamine oxidase inhibitors. The combination may produce severe reactions, such as tremors, hyperpyrexia, convulsions, and even death. The third group, represented by deanol acetamidobenzoate, is thought to act by cholinergic reinforcement. In addition, perphenazine (a phenothiazine tranquilizing drug) and amitriptyline (an antidepressant drug) have been combined [Etrafon (*Schering*); Triavil (*MSD*)] for the treatment of patients with neuroses or psychoses characterized by both anxiety and depression. Clinically, these drugs have been used in a variety of emotional and psychiatric disorders when the predominant symptom is depression. They should be used in conjunction with other measures such as psychotherapy, reduction in environmental stresses, and improved social setting. Some agents (nialamide, phenelzine sulfate, and isocarboxazid) have been said to reduce the incidence and severity of attacks of angina pectoris. The results achieved have not been highly predictable. Furthermore, some of these agents have been reported to be quite toxic. Continued research should be directed toward the discovery of more reliable and less toxic agents with psychomotor stimulant properties in depressed subjects. Among the more frequent side effects are dizziness, ataxia, loss of muscular tonus, hypotension, accommodation disturbances, headache, dry mouth, flushing, sweating, euphoria, confusion, restlessness, and depression. Edema, dyspnea, cardiac failure, and neuralgic pain have also been observed. Jaundice is the most serious toxic effect and must be considered as an ominous sign since this may be followed by fulminating hepatitis which can be fatal. It follows, therefore, that these agents are contraindicated in patients with either a history or the presence of jaundice, liver disease, or impaired hepatic function. Likewise, they should not be given to epileptic patients who are overactive, or stimulated, or agitated. Since these substances potentiate the action of alcohol, ether, barbiturates, meperidine, cocaine, procaine, and phenylephrine, they should be used with caution when these drugs are employed.

Amitriptyline Hydrochloride USP

[10,11-Dihydro-*N*,*N*-dimethyl-5*H*-dibenzo(*a*,*d*)cycloheptene-Δ$^{5,\gamma}$-propyl-amine Hydrochloride; Elavil Hydrochloride (*MSD*)]

Amitriptyline Hydrochloride contains 99.0–100.5% of $C_{20}H_{23}N \cdot HCl$ (313.87), calculated on the dried basis.

Preparation—Phthalic anhydride is reacted with phenylacetic acid to form 3-benzylidenephthalide which is then hydrogenated to 2-phenethylbenzoic acid. Conversion to the acid chloride followed by intramolecular dehydrochlorination yields the ketone (5*H*-dibenzo[*a*,*d*]cyclohepten-5-one) which is then caused to undergo Grignardization with 3-(dimethylamino)-propyl chloride. Dehydration of the resulting tertiary carbinol gives amitriptyline (base) which is dissolved in a suitable solvent and converted to the hydrochloride by a stream of hydrogen chloride. US Pat. 3,205,264.

Description—A white or practically white, odorless or practically odorless, crystalline powder or small crystals. It melts between 196° and 197°.

Solubility—Freely soluble in water, alcohol, chloroform, and methanol; insoluble in ether.

Uses—Amitriptyline Hydrochloride, a compound chemically and pharmacologically related to imipramine hydrochloride, is useful in the management of the depressed phases of *anxiety* and *manic-depressive states*, and in the treatment of *involutional melancholia*. It is less useful in *neurotic depressive reactions*. Although the incidence of adverse effects appear to be less with Amitripyline Hydrochloride than with other effective antidepressants, drowsiness, xerostomia, tremor, fatigue, weakness, blurring of vision, constipation, urinary retention, edema, tachycardia, orthostatic hypotension, etc have been observed. Most untoward effects can be controlled by a reduction in dosage. Patients taking large doses over an extended period of time should be watched closely for possible changes in liver

and hematopoietic functions. See also the general statement, page 1113.

Dose—*Oral*, **30** to **300 mg** daily; *usual, oral*, **25 mg** 2 to 4 times a day; *intramuscular*, **80** to **120 mg** daily; *usual, intramuscular*, **20** to **30 mg** 4 times a day.

Dosage Forms—Injection USP: 100 mg/10 ml; Tablets USP: 10, 25, and 50 mg.

Deanol Acetamidobenzoate

[Deaner (*Riker*)]

Deanol Acetamidobenzoate [$C_{14}H_{11}NO \cdot C_9H_9NO_3$ = 268.31] is 2-(dimethylamino)ethanol *p*-acetamidobenzoate (salt).

Preparation—Deanol (base), prepared by reacting equimolar quantities of dimethylamine and ethylene oxide, is dissolved in a suitable solvent and reacted with an equimolar quantity of *p*-acetamidobenzoic acid.

Description—White to off-white, crystalline powder with little or no odor. It melts between 159° and 163°.

Solubility—1 Gm dissolves in about 2 ml of water and 25 ml of alcohol; slightly soluble in ether and chloroform; insoluble in benzene.

Uses—Deanol Acetamidobenzoate is a mild antidepressant with amphetamine-like properties. It is used primarily to relieve shortened attention spans in children with behavior problems and learning difficulties. It is also proposed for the symptomatic relief of a variety of vague complaints, such as chronic fatigue, neurasthenia, and neurotic depression. Final assessment of its therapeutic value must await more extensive, carefully controlled clinical studies than have been reported to date.

Dose—*Orally, initially*, **50 mg** daily with a *maintenance* dose of **25** to **100 mg** a day; for behavior problems in children, *initially*, **75 mg** with a *maintenance* dose of **75** to **150 mg** a day.

Dosage Forms—Tablets: 25 and 100 mg (of the base).

Desipramine Hydrochloride NF

[10,11-Dihydro-5-[3-(methylamino)propyl]-5*H*-dibenz[*b*,*f*]azepine Monohydrochloride; Norpramin (*Lakeside*); Pertofrane (*Geigy*)]

Desipramine Hydrochloride, dried at 105° for 2 hours, contains 98.0–102.0% of $C_{18}H_{22}N_2 \cdot HCl$ (302.85).

Preparation—Oxidative coupling of *o*-nitrotoluene provides 4,4'-dinitrobibenzyl which is catalytically reduced to the corresponding diamine. Pyrolysis of the methanesulfonate of this amine results in cyclization with the formation of 10,11-dihydro-5*H*-dibenz[*b*,*f*]-azepine. This is then condensed with *N*-(3-chloro-propyl)-*N*-methylbenzylamine in the presence of alkali to form the *N*-benzylated desipramine (base) which, following debenzylation through reductive cleavage, is reacted with an equimolar quantity of hydrochloric acid. Brit. Pat. 908,788.

Description—A white to off-white, crystalline powder that is odorless and has a bitter taste. It is unstable after long exposure to light, heat, and air. It melts within a range of 5° between 208° and 218°.

Solubility—1 Gm dissolves in about 4 ml of chloroform, 20 ml of water, and 20 ml of alcohol; freely soluble in methanol; insoluble in ether.

Uses—Desipramine Hydrochloride, a primary metabolite of imipramine, is used in the management of *depressive states*. Desipramine is reported to be of benefit in endogenous *depressions* such as *manic depressive reactions*, and *reactive depressions*. Desipramine Hydrochloride is contraindicated in patients on monoamine oxidase therapy. Since the drug possesses anticholinergic and epinephrine potentiating properties, it should not be given to patients with glaucoma, urethral or ureteral spasm, or those who have had a myocardial infarction within 3 weeks. It is also contraindicated in patients with severe coronary heart diseases or with active epilepsy. Final evaluation of its place in the management of various depressions must await further clinical study.

Dose—50 to **200 mg** per day; *usual*, **150 mg** per day in divided doses.

Other Dose Information—Initial response may be expected within 7 to 10 days and optimal response within 2 to 3 weeks.

Dosage Forms—Capsules NF: 25 mg; Tablets NF: 25 and 50 mg.

Doxepin Hydrochloride

[Sinequan (*Pfizer*)]

Doxepin Hydrochloride is *N,N*-dimethyldibenz[*b,e*]-oxepin-$\Delta^{11(6H),\gamma}$-propylamine hydrochloride ($C_{19}H_{21}$-NO.HCl).

Uses—Doxepin Hydrochloride, a dibenzoxepin derivative, is a psychotherapeutic agent with antianxiety and antidepressant properties. It is recommended for the management of anxiety and/or depressive states associated with psychoneurosis, psychosis, alcoholism, and organic disease. Adverse reactions, such as dry mouth, blurred vision, constipation, tachycardia, hypotension, and drowsiness, are usually mild and tend to subside as therapy is continued. Other side effects infrequently encountered include extrapyramidal symptoms, gastrointestinal disturbances, increased sweating, weakness, dizziness, fatigue, edema, paresthesia, flushing, chills, tinnitus, photophobia, decreased libido, rash, and pruritus. Doxepin Hydrochloride is contraindicated in patients with glaucoma or a tendency to urinary retention. The drug should not be administered to patients either on MAO inhibitors or who have been on such agents within the prior 2 weeks. The drug may also potentiate the depressant effect of alcohol. The use of Doxepin Hydrochloride in the pregnant patient or in children under 12 years of age is not recommended, because safe conditions for its use have not been established.

Dose—*Initial*, **25 to 50 mg** 3 times a day. Dosage may be increased or decreased according to individual response. The optimal daily dose range is usually 75 to 300 mg. Very mild emotional symptoms may be controlled with daily doses of 25 to 50 mg.

Dosage Forms—Capsules: 25 mg.

Imipramine Hydrochloride USP

[5-[3-(Dimethylamino)propyl]-10,11-dihydro-5*H*-dibenz[*b,f*]azepine Monohydrochloride; Tofranil (*Geigy*)]

Imipramine Hydrochloride contains 98.0–102.0% of $C_{19}H_{24}N_2.HCl$ (316.88), calculated on the dried basis.

Preparation—2-(*o*-aminophenethyl)aniline hydrochloride is heated to yield 10,11-dihydro-5*H*-dibenz-[*b,f*]azepine which is then condensed with 3-chloro-*N,N*-dimethylpropylamine by refluxing in benzene solution with the aid of sodamide. The basic constituents are then extracted with aqueous HCl and the extract is rendered alkaline and extracted with ether. After drying, the solvent is evaporated and the residue is vacuum distilled to yield imipramine base. Treatment with alcoholic HCl produces the hydrochloride. US Pat. 2,554,736.

Description—Occurs as a white to off-white, odorless crystalline powder.

Solubility—1 Gm dissolves in about 5 ml of water, about 10 ml of alcohol, and about 15 ml of acetone; insoluble in ether and benzene.

Uses—Imipramine Hydrochloride differs from other antidepressant drugs in that it is neither a stimulant like amphetamine, nor an amine oxidase inhibitor like nialamide. The exact mechanism of action is unknown. Preliminary studies indicate Imipramine Hydrochloride is highly effective in depressive syndromes, particularly those associated with *manic-depressive* and *involutional psychoses*, and to a lesser degree with *reactive depressions*. Side effects are common, especially in patients over 65. Most side effects occur in patients receiving more than 200 mg daily and include hypotension, seizures, tremors, diplopia, involuntary staring, visual hallucinations, and agitation. Because of possible congenital malformations associated with the use of this drug, Imipramine Hydrochloride should not be used during the first trimester of pregnancy. Imipramine should not be used in patients on monoamine oxidase inhibitors. The ultimate place of imipramine hydrochloride in psychiatric therapy must await more clinical investigation and evidence with the drug.

Dose—*Oral* or *intramuscular*, **50 to 200 mg** daily; *usual*, **25 mg** 3 or 4 times a day.

Other Dose Information—The initial dose may be increased cautiously after several weeks until a total daily dosage of 150 to 200 mg per day is attained. At least 7 days should elapse before it is given to patients previously on monoamine oxidase inhibitors.

Dosage Forms—Injection USP: 2 ml; Tablets USP: 10, 25, and 50 mg.

Isocarboxazid NF

[5-Methyl-3-isoxazolecarboxylic Acid 2-Benzylhydrazide; Marplan (*Roche*)]

Isocarboxazid contains 98.5–100.5% of $C_{12}H_{13}N_3O_2$ (231.26), calculated on the dried basis.

Preparation—Acetonylacetone is reacted with nitric acid under controlled conditions of temperature and concentration to form 5-methyl-3-isoxazolecarboxylic acid which is then converted to its ethyl ester by treatment with ethanol and sulfuric acid. The ester is then reacted with hydrazine hydrate to form the corresponding acid hydrazide which is then condensed with benzaldehyde to yield the corresponding 2-benzylidenehydrazide. Reduction of the last-named product in anhydrous ether with lithium aluminum hydride yields crude Isocarboxazid which is purified by recrystallization from methanol. US Pat. 2,908,688.

Description—A white or nearly white, crystalline powder. It has a slight, characteristic odor and is stable in dry air. It melts between 105° and 107° with decomposition.

Solubility—1 Gm dissolves in 1000 ml of water, 20 ml of alcohol, and 3 ml of chloroform.

Uses—Isocarboxazid is a potent monoamine oxidase inhibitor which has been proposed for use in a wide variety of psychiatric disorders with symptoms of depression. It has also been suggested for use as an antianginal and antihypertensive agent; its role in these conditions remains to be established. As with other amine oxidase inhibitors, patients treated with Isocarboxazid should be kept under close medical supervision. Untoward effects are those characteristic of monoamine oxidase inhibitors in general. See general statement (page 1113). The drug should be discontinued at the first sign of jaundice or impaired liver function. It is contraindicated in patients with a history of liver disease or impaired liver function.

Dose—*Usual, initial*, **30 mg** daily as a single dose or in divided doses; *maintenance*, **10 to 20 mg** daily.

Dosage Forms—Tablets NF: 10 mg.

Methylphenidate Hydrochloride USP

[Methyl α-Phenyl-2-piperidineacetate Hydrochloride; Ritalin (*Ciba*)]

Methylphenidate Hydrochloride contains 98.0–100.5% of $C_{14}H_{19}NO_2 \cdot HCl$ (269.77), calculated on the dried basis.

Preparation—2-Chloropyridine is condensed with phenylacetonitrile and the resulting α-phenyl-2-pyridineacetonitrile is hydrated to its corresponding amide. The pyridine ring is then hydrogenated and the amide is converted to its corresponding carboxylic acid. Esterification with methanol with the aid of hydrogen chloride yields the final product.

Description—Occurs as a white, odorless, fine, crystalline powder. Its solutions are acid to litmus.

Solubility—Freely soluble in water and methanol; soluble in ethanol; slightly soluble in chloroform and acetone.

Uses—Methylphenidate Hydrochloride is a mild central nervous system stimulant with a potency intermediate to caffeine and amphetamine. Its sympathomimetic and cardiovascular effects are less than either of the latter two agents and, in ordinary doses, it does not influence blood pressure, heart rate, or circulation time. Methylphenidate Hydrochloride is used to counteract the depression produced by chlorpromazine and reserpine in neurotic or psychotic patients and by

rauwolfia or its alkaloids in hypertensive patients and for improving the mood, behavior, and mental activity in patients with certain neuroses and psychoses characterized by depression; neurotic patients respond better than those with psychoses. The drug is relatively nontoxic, but occasionally patients experience nervousness, insomnia, anorexia, dizziness, palpitation, headache, and nausea. Tolerance may develop on long-term administration of the drug. Methylphenidate Hydrochloride is contraindicated in patients with hyperexcitability and agitation and should be used with caution in those with epilepsy or hypertension.

Dose—*Oral* or *parenteral*, **20** to **60 mg** daily; *usual*, **10 mg** 3 times a day.

Dosage Forms—for Injection USP: 100 mg; Tablets USP: 5, 10, and 20 mg.

Nialamide NF

[Isonicotinic Acid 2-[2-(Benzylcarbamoyl)ethyl]hydrazide; Niamid (*Pfizer*)]

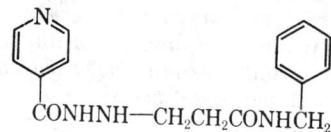

CONHNH—CH₂CH₂CONHCH₂

Nialamide contains 98.0–101.0% of $C_{16}H_{18}N_4O_2$ (298.35), calculated on the dried basis.

Preparation—The methyl ester of 3-[2-(isonicotinyl)hydrazino]propionic acid is condensed with benzylamine by heating a mixture of the components at 130° for three hours. The cooled reaction mass is then recrystallized from ethyl acetate. The starting ester may be prepared in various ways. One convenient method consists of causing isonicotinic acid hydrazide to undergo addition to methyl acrylate by heating an equimolar mixture of the reactants in an inert solvent, such as a tertiary alcohol, in the presence of a catalytic quantity of acetic acid. US Pat. 2,894,972.

Description—A white, practically odorless, crystalline powder having a slight, bitter taste. It melts between 151° and 155°.

Solubility—Soluble in alcohol and acidic solutions; sparingly soluble in water.

Uses—Nialamide is a monoamine oxidase inhibitor useful in the management of various depressive syndromes; it is most effective in endogenous depressions; its value in exogenous or reactive depressions is less clearly defined. It has also been proposed as an antianginal agent; it is of dubious value in this condition. Nialimide is said to produce full effect within 7 to 14 days and to induce few untoward effects; hypotension has been observed. Although no jaundice has been reported in patients receiving Nialamide, the possibility of hepatic reactions should be kept in mind and the drug should be used with caution, if at all, in patients with a history of liver disease. Nialamide should be used with caution in overactive, overstimulated, or agitated persons. Large doses of the drug potentiates barbiturates, meperidine, ether, cocaine, procaine, sympathomimetic amines, opiates, antihypertensive drugs, and similar agents. The drug should be used with caution in the seriously depressed, nonhospitalized patient with suicidal tendencies.

Dose—*Usual, initial*, **75** to **100 mg** daily, which may be decreased or increased in increments of 12.5 to 25 mg at weekly intervals according to response, then reduce gradually to maintenance level.

Dosage Forms—Tablets NF: 25 and 100 mg.

Nortriptyline Hydrochloride NF

[10,11-Dihydro-*N*-methyl-5*H*-dibenzo [*a,d*]cycloheptene-Δ$^{5,\gamma}$-propylamine Hydrochloride; Aventyl Hydrochloride (*Lilly*)]

Nortriptyline Hydrochloride contains 97.0–101.5% of $C_{19}H_{21}N.HCl$ (299.85), calculated on the dried basis.

Preparation—10,11 - Dihydro - 5*H* - dibenzo [*a,d*]-cyclohepten-5-one, which may be prepared as described under *Cyproheptadine Hydrochloride* (page 1152), is reacted with an alkali metal derivative of *N*-methyl-2-propynylamine and the product hydrolyzed to form the carbinol (I). The acetylenic bond in (I) is then saturated by hydrogenation and the resulting carbinol is dehydrated to yield nortriptyline (base). Reaction of the base with hydrogen chloride produces the hydrochloride.

(I)

Description—A white to off-white powder with a slight, characteristic odor. It melts between 215° and 221°.

Solubility—Soluble in water and chloroform; sparingly soluble in methanol; practically insoluble in ether, benzene, and most organic solvents.

Uses—Nortriptyline Hydrochloride, an analog of amitriptyline and imipramine, is an antidepressant agent. Pharmacological studies indicate it inhibits the activity of such diverse agents as histamine, 5-hydroxytryptamine, and acetylcholine. It also increases the pressor effect of norepinephrine but blocks the pressor response of phenethylamine. Studies to date suggest that Nortriptyline Hydrochloride interferes with the transport, release, and storage of catacholamines. Pharmacologic studies further show that Nortriptyline Hydrochloride has a combination of stimulant and depressant properties. In some clinical studies, the drug appeared to cause excitement or increased agitation in some patients and to have sedative effects in others. Similar effects have been observed with other drugs of this general type. Untoward side effects include dryness of the mouth, drowsiness, and a confusional state. Tremulousness and orthostatic hypotension have also been reported. Since drugs of this type can produce a sinus tachycardia and a first-degree heart block, they should be used with great caution in patients with vascular disease. Nortriptyline Hydrochloride should not be used in combination with a monoamine oxidase inhibitor. The potentiation of adverse effects can be serious, even fatal. It is advisable to discontinue the monoamine oxidase inhibitor for at least 10 to 21 days before starting treatment with Nortriptyline. Nortriptyline should be used with caution in patients with glaucoma or urinary retention. Epileptiform seizures may be associated with Nortriptyline. Therefore, patients on this drug should be supervised closely during the initial phase of treatment.

Dose—*Usual*, an amount of Nortriptyline Hydrochloride equivalent to **20** to **100 mg** of nortriptyline base daily in divided doses.

Dosage Forms—Capsules NF: 10 and 25 mg.

Pargyline Hydrochloride—see page 853.

Phenelzine Sulfate USP

[Phenethylhydrazine Sulfate (1:1); Nardil (*Warner-Chilcott*)]

Phenelzine Sulfate contains 97.0–100.5% of $C_8H_{12}N_2.H_2SO_4$ (234.28), calculated on the dried basis.

Preparation—Phenethyl alcohol is reacted with thionyl chloride in the presence of pyridine to give phenethyl chloride which is then added to hydrazine hydrate in isopropanol at controlled temperature to yield phenethylhydrazine hydrochloride. Reaction with sodium hydroxide liberates the phenylhydrazine which is then reacted with an equimolar quantity of sulfuric acid in isopropanol to form the official article. US Pat. 3,314,855.

Description—White to yellowish white powder with a characteristic odor. It is subject to oxidation and must be protected from heat and light. Storage must be in tightly sealed containers protected from light. It melts between 164° and 168°.

Solubility—1 Gm dissolves in about 7 ml of water; very soluble in dimethylformamide; slightly soluble in the alcohols; moderately soluble in acetic acid; practically insoluble in alcohol, ethers, and ketones.

Uses—Phenelzine Sulfate is a monoamine oxidase inhibitor effective in relieving endogenous depression, depressive phase of manic depressive psychosis, exogenous depression, and depression associated with chronic illness. It is useful for mild to severe depression associated with either psychoses or chronic diseases. Maximal effects appear only after 1 to 2 weeks of therapy. Phenelzine Sulfate is contraindicated in elderly, debilitated patients, or to patients with a cerebralvascular defect, cardiovascular disease, hypertension, history of headache, pheochromocytoma, or a history of liver disease. Side effects to date have been minor; hypotension, nausea, ankle edema, delayed micturition, and constipation have been observed. Physicians should be alert to more serious toxic effects characteristic of this class of drugs. See the general statement, page 1113.

Dose—**7.5** to **75 mg** daily; *usual*, the equivalent of **15 mg** of phenelzine once a day or every other day.

Dosage Forms—Tablets USP: 15 mg.

Protriptyline Hydrochloride

[Vivactil Hydrochloride (*MSD*)]

Protriptyline Hydrochloride [$C_{19}H_{21}N.HCl$ = 299.83] is *N*-methyl-5*H*-dibenzo [*a,d*]cycloheptene-5-propylamine hydrochloride.

Preparation—5*H* - Dibenzo[*a,d*]cyclohepten - 5-one, prepared as described under *Cyproheptadine Hydrochloride* (page 1152), is reduced to the corresponding carbinol which is then converted to the 5-chloromethyl compound (I). Reaction with the Grignard reagent of (3-chloropropyl)dimethylamine converts (I) into the 5-[3-(dimethylamino)propyl] compound which, on monodemethylation by treatment with cyanogen bromide and then hydrolysis, yields protriptyline (base). Reaction with an equimolar quantity of hydrogen chloride gives the hydrochloride.

Description—A white to yellowish powder that is odorless or has not more than a slight odor and has a bitter taste. It is reasonably stable in light, stable in air, and stable in heat under the usual prevailing temperature conditions. It melts between 165° and 171°.

Solubility—1 Gm dissolves in about 2 ml of water, about 2 ml of methanol, about 2.3 ml of chloroform, and about 4 ml of alcohol.

Uses—Protriptyline Hydrochloride is a tricyclic (dibenzocycloheptene) antidepressant drug. It induces effects similar to those of amitriptyline except for less sedation. Like other tricyclic antidepressants, it is most useful in depressed patients who are withdrawn, retarded, or apathetic. The drug may aggravate anxiety, and it should not be used in anxious depressed patients unless it is given with a sedative drug, such as a phenothiazine with sedative effects (chlorpromazine), or a more conventional sedative drug such as chlordiazepoxide, meprobamate, or a barbiturate. Protriptyline also possesses anticholinergic properties and, hence, should not be used in patients with pyloric obstruction, glaucoma, or urinary retention. This agent is also contraindicated in patients taking any of the MAO inhibitor antidepressants, such as nialamide, isocarboxazid, tranylcypromine, or phenelzine. Antidepressants of this type reverse the effects of antihypertensive drugs such as guanethidine and should not be used concurrently with them. Untoward effects reported include dryness of the mouth, blurred vision, dizziness and tremors, tachycardia, and postural hypotension. One case of agranulocytosis has also been reported. As with other tricyclic antidepressants, cholostatic jaundice is a possible complication.

Dose—*Usual*, **20 to 60 mg** daily.

Dosage Forms—Tablets: 5 and 10 mg.

Tranylcypromine Sulfate NF

[(±)-*trans*-2-Phenylcyclopropylamine Sulfate (2:1); Parnate (*SK&F*)]

Tranylcypromine Sulfate, dried in vacuum at 60° for 2 hours, contains 98.0–101.0% of $(C_9H_{11}N)_2 \cdot H_2SO_4$ (364.47).

Preparation—Styrene is reacted with ethyl diazoacetate under nitrogen at high temperature to form ethyl 2-phenylcyclopropanecarboxylate. Saponification of this ester with sodium hydroxide and subsequent acidification yields a mixture of the *cis* and *trans* forms of the corresponding acid and the *trans* form is isolated by fractional crystallization from water. The *trans* acid is then subjected to the Curtius reaction whereby carboxyl is transformed successively through the acyl chloride, acyl azide, and isocyanate states to yield finally tranylcypromine (base). Reaction of the base with a ½ equimolar quantity of sulfuric acid gives the official sulfate. US Pat. 2,997,422.

Description—A white, crystalline powder that is either odorless or has a faint, cinnamaldehyde-like odor and a slightly acid taste. It is stable in light, heat, and air. It melts with decomposition at 218°.

Solubility—Soluble in water; very slightly soluble in alcohol and ether; practically insoluble in chloroform.

Uses—Tranylcypromine Sulfate, a nonhydrazine monoamine oxidase inhibitor, is used in the treatment of depression. It is especially useful in severe psychotic depressions in which apathy, immobility, and nonreactiveness, are dominant characteristics. The drug resembles amphetamine in chemical structure and produces an amphetamine-like excitation of the central nervous system. It has a rapid onset of action; antidepressant activity may be apparent within a period of only 2 or 3 days. The incidence and severity of side effects caused by Tranylcypromine are greater with doses above 40 mg daily; effects most commonly experienced are restlessness, insomnia, postural hypotension, headache, vertigo, and loss of appetite. Hypotensive effects are sometimes marked in hypotensive patients, and the drug should be used with caution in such persons. A number of deaths have resulted in patients on Tranylcypromine; death is usually attributed to intracranial hemorrhage. Severe reactions may appear without warning and develop rapidly. This drug, like other antidepressant agents, should only be used under close medical supervision.

Dose—*Usual, initial,* **10 mg** in the morning and afternoon daily for 2 weeks; if no response appears, increase dosage to **20 mg** in the morning and **10 mg** in the afternoon daily for another week; *maintenance,* **10 to 20 mg** per day.

Dosage Forms—Tablets NF: 10 mg.

Other Antidepressant Agents

Pipradrol Hydrochloride NF XII [α,α-Diphenyl-2-piperidinemethanol Hydrochloride; α-(2-Piperidyl)benzhydrol Hydrochloride; Meratran (*Merrell*)], dried at 105° for 2 hours, contains 98.0–102.0% of $C_{18}H_{21}NO \cdot HCl$ (303.84). *Preparation:* By hydrogenating an acetic acid solution of α,α-diphenyl-2-pyridinemethanol (prepared by the Grignard reaction from 2-benzoylpyridine and phenylmagnesium bromide) in the presence of platinum oxide catalyst at 100 to 500 psi hydrogen pressure and 40° to 50°C. After filtering off the catalyst and removing the acetic acid by low-pressure distillation, the residue is dissolved in water and treated with aqueous alkali, and the free base is extracted with ether. The ether is evaporated and the residue of base is dissolved in alcohol and treated with hydrogen chloride, whereupon the hydrochloride precipitates. It is purified by recrystallization from alcohol. *Description and Solubility:* Small, white crystals or a crystalline powder that is odorless and stable in air; melting range (with decomposition), 285° to 295°; pH (1 in 100 solution), 5 to 7. 1 Gm dissolves in about 33 ml of water, 8 ml of methanol, and 50 ml of alcohol; very slightly soluble in chloroform; insoluble in ether.
Uses: A mild central nervous system stimulant, chemically unrelated to the sympathomimetic amines, but exhibiting some of the pharmacologic actions of amphetamine. It produces less anorexia, insomnia, and euphoria than does amphetamine and in therapeutic doses has little effect on heart rate, blood pressure, or respiration. Pipradrol has been used as a supramedullary stimulant in depressive states that are not associated with strong anxiety or compulsive behavior. It has also been used to elevate the mood depres-

sions often encountered in old age and chronic disease. Pipradrol Hydrochloride has a wide margin of safety and reported side effects, such as hyperexcitability, anorexia, and insomnia, can be attributed to its stimulant action. The drug is contraindicated in agitated, prepsychotic patients, paranoia, and in cases in which hyperexcitability, anxiety, chorea, or obsessive-compulsive states are present. *Dose: Usual*, 2.5 mg 2 times a day.

Psychogenic Agents

Psychogenic agents are drugs that consistently induce temporary abnormalities of the mental state of human subjects or the behavior of animals. This definition serves to separate the psychogenic agents from the many drugs which may produce similar effects when taken in excessive amounts or when given to susceptible individuals. Psychogenic drugs produce major disturbances of sensory perception and alter the ability of the subject to organize perceptions and thoughts for the purpose of adaptative behavior. In so doing they produce subjective effects such as hallucinations and alterations in gross behavior which bear some similarity to certain features of the major psychoses. However, there is a serious question as to whether this resemblance is more than superficial. Intensive investigation is directed toward elucidating those features which are common to both "clinical" and "experimental" psychoses. There are no recognized therapeutic applications for these agents and none of them are available for prescription use. These agents are, however, subjected to intensive abuse, a practice which can only be condemned.

Cannabis [Marihuana]—Dried flowering tops of the pistillate plants of *Cannabis sativa* (Fam. *Moraceæ*). *Uses:* no rational or indispensable therapeutic use in modern medicine. Formerly used in migraine, insomnia, neuralgia, and other syndromes, the drug is no longer prescribed. Its sale and use are controlled by federal regulations. The drug is frequently smoked in the form of cigarettes. It produces aggressive tendencies and a stimulation of the senses so that external stimuli are magnified and distorted. There is a relationship between its use and crime. Cannabis causes habituation but, unlike morphine, not true addiction.

Lysergic Acid Diethylamide [*d-N,N*-Diethyllysergamide; LSD-25; LSD] [$C_{20}H_{25}N_3O$]—Closely related structurally (page 499) to ergonovine, one of the principal alkaloids of ergot, but it is distinctly different in its physiological actions. It is an extremely potent agent; as little as 1 mcg per Kg of body weight will induce a hallucinogenic effect. Persons who have taken the drug experience a mental intoxication which has many of the features common with the perceptual disturbances of some cases of schizophrenia. Persons under the influence of lysergic acid diethylamide experience ataxia, tremor, auditory and visual hallucinations, depersonalization and disturbances in space, olfactory, and taste perception, but retain the knowledge that these unusual effects are induced by the drug. Contact with reality is not lost, except after massive doses. Repeated administration of the drug produces serious mental disturbances in some individuals. The drug is also known to induce chromosomal damage and fetal abnormalities if taken during early pregnancy.

The drug has been used in schizophrenic patients to render them more accessible to psychotherapy. Under the influence of the drug, past traumatic experiences which heretofore were kept secret are often communicated.

The first effects from an oral dose of lysergic acid diethylamide appear within $\frac{1}{2}$ hour, reach a peak intensity in $1\frac{1}{2}$ hours, and disappear within 8 hours. Recovery is usually complete, except for some residual depression which may persist for as long as 24 hours after taking the drug. Tolerance to the drug develops within 3 to 7 days after repeated administration. When tolerance has developed a 4-fold dosage increase fails to evoke the hallucinatory syndrome.

Lysergic acid diethylamide should be considered, at least for the present, a tool for the study of "experimental psychoses." Final assessment of its use as an adjunct to psychotherapy must await the results of more clinical experience. The indiscriminate use of the agent cannot be too severely condemned.

Mescaline [3,4,5 - Trimethoxyphenethylamine] [$C_{11}H_{17}NO_3$]—Knowledge of mescaline psychosis dates back to antiquity, since, as the principal alkaloid of peyote, the dried flowering tops of the cactus *Lophophora Williamsii* Coulter, it has been used by various American Indian tribes for religious purposes. Recent interest in mescaline stems from its use as an experimental tool for the investigation of schizophrenia and other psychotic states, and for the study of visual hallucinations. It has also been used as an adjunct to psychotherapy in depth interviews.

Current interest in mescaline centers on the fact that when given orally or intravenously to normal subjects in doses of 5.0 to 7.0 mg per Kg of body weight it causes unusual psychic effects and visual hallucinations. Diffuse anxiety is one of the early symptoms. Other symptoms include sympathomimetic autonomic effects, hyperreflexia of the limbs, static tremors, and vivid hallucinations which are usually visual and consist of brightly colored lights, geometric designs, animals, and, occasionally, human images; color and space perception is often impaired but, otherwise, the sensorium is normal and insight is retained. An extreme anxiety state may develop in some schizophrenic patients given mescaline, and the hallucinations in others may be sexual in character. The effects induced by a single full dose of mescaline appear within one hour and persist for about 12 hours. In some respects, the psychic changes are similar to those caused by lysergic acid diethylamide. Mescaline-induced psychoses are of academic interest only and the drug has no therapeutic application.

References

1. Schmidle, C. J., and Mansfield, R. C., *J. Am. Chem. Soc.*, **78**, 1702 (1956).

63 | Analgesics and Antipyretics

Opiate analgesics—nonopiate addicting analgesics—nonaddicting
analgesics and antipyretics

This chapter was prepared by

Ewart A. Swinyard, PhD, *Professor of Pharmacology, College of Pharmacy and
College of Medicine, University of Utah, Salt Lake City, Utah 84112, and*
Stewart C. Harvey, PhD, *Associate Professor of Pharmacology, College of
Medicine, University of Utah, Salt Lake City, Utah 84112*

Analgesics are agents which relieve pain by acting centrally to elevate pain threshold without disturbing consciousness or altering other sensory modalities. Antipyretics are drugs which reduce elevated body temperature. These two actions are commonly, but not necessarily, found in the same drug. Hence, drugs which exhibit one or both of these actions are considered in this chapter.

Despite the fact that pain is a universal experience of all mankind and everybody knows what is meant by it, attempts to define this term have not proved entirely satisfactory. Pain has been defined in psychologic language as a particular type of sensory experience perceived by nerve tissue distinct from sensations such as touch, pressure, heat, and cold. Since there are several types of pain (bright, dull, aching, pricking, cutting, burning, etc) and it may arise from different causes (injury, body derangements, or disease), it is apparent that this definition is incomplete. Furthermore, it is now generally agreed that pain involves a large psychic component. Thus, it must be concluded that pain cannot be defined, except as one defines it introspectively for himself.

All persons in good health have the ability to perceive pain. The point at which pain is perceived is referred to as the "pain threshold." If this threshold is raised, more stimuli are required before pain is experienced. On the other hand, if this threshold is lowered, less stimuli induce the pain experience. Unfortunately, many factors such as sex, circulatory change, skin temperature, sweating, carbon dioxide tension, anxiety, fear, emotion, etc, alter the pain threshold. Consequently, pain threshold is not constant from individual to individual, or from one time to another in the same individual. Thus, data obtained from laboratory and clinical studies on the effect of drugs on pain threshold are difficult to interpret.

The mechanism by which analgesic drugs raise the pain threshold is not clearly understood. Most studies seem to indicate that these drugs act by interfering with pain impulses carried over sensory nerve tracts at subcortical levels of the brain. Since many analgesics serve also as antipyretics, it has been suggested that this interference takes place in the vicinity of the thalamus, an area of the brain concerned with the relay of sensory impulses to the cerebral cortex. This explanation is based on the fact that the heat regulating center is located in the hypothalamus, which is just ventral to the thalamus. However, the fact that some analgesics are more effective against visceral pain and induce euphoria and narcosis, whereas others are more effective against integumental pain and do not alter mental clarity, precludes the possibility that all presently available analgesics obtund pain by a single mechanism.

Many drugs used to relieve pain are not analgesics. The general anesthetics obtund pain by producing a hiatus in consciousness, the local anesthetics prevent pain by blocking peripheral nerve fibers, the antispasmodics relieve certain kinds of pain by relaxing smooth muscle, and the adrenal corticoids relieve pain associated with rheumatoid arthritis by an anti-inflammatory action. These drugs are considered elsewhere.

Agents which are used principally for the symptomatic relief of pain may for convenience in presentation be divided into three groups: (1) opiate analgesics; (2) nonopiate, addicting analgesics; and (3) nonopiate, nonaddicting analgesics and antipyretics. The drugs considered in this section are classified according to this scheme.

Opiate Analgesics

The opium group of narcotic drugs are among the most powerfully acting and clinically useful drugs producing depression of the central nervous system. Drugs of this group are used principally as analgesics, but possess numerous other useful properties. Morphine, for example, is used to induce sleep in the presence of pain, check diarrhea, suppress cough, ease dyspnea, and facilitate anesthesia.

Unfortunately, morphine also depresses respiration; it increases the activity and tone of the smooth muscles of the gastrointestinal, biliary, and urinary tracts causing constipation, gall bladder spasm, and urinary retention; it causes nausea and vomiting in some individuals; and it may induce cutaneous pruritus. In addition to these actions, morphine and related compounds have other qualities which tend to limit their usefulness. If these agents are given over a long period of time, tolerance to the analgesic effect develops so that the dose must be increased periodically to obtain equivalent pain relief. Tolerance and physical dependence develop, which combined with euphoria result in excessive use and addiction of those patients who have susceptible personalities. For these reasons, it is generally agreed that morphine and its derivatives should not be used for pain when some other analgesic will suffice.

The preparations of opium and its alkaloids are numerous and for convenience are divided into three groups: opium preparations, opium alkaloids, and semisynthetic opium alkaloids.

Opium and its preparations exhibit analgesic and narcotic effects which are directly proportional to their morphine content. Traditionally, these agents are more frequently employed in the form of tinctures for diarrhea and dysenteries. Because of its disagreeable odor and taste, powdered opium is seldom used therapeutically; it is primarily a pharmaceutical necessity used in the preparation of Paregoric USP.

Opium USP

[Gum Opium; Crude Opium; Raw Opium; Thebaicum; Meconium]

Opium is the air-dried milky exudate obtained by incising the unripe capsules of *Papaver somniferum* Linné or its variety *album* De Candolle (Fam. *Papaveraceæ*). It yields not less than 9.5% of anhydrous morphine.

History—Opium as a medicinal drug has been known and cultivated for many centuries, but it was not until the investigations of Sertürner, published in 1817, that it was known that the drug contained certain definite principles now called *alkaloids*.

Dioscorides, in the second century, was the first writer to discuss opium and its uses at length. He gave the recipe for a preparation called *diacodion* which is the prototype of the formerly official syrup of poppies. Paracelsus used opium extensively in the fifteenth century and referred to it as the "stone of immortality." Van Helmont, early in the seventeenth century, used opium so freely that he was referred to as Doctor Opiatus. Sydenham, a little later in the same century, praised opium as the most valuable gift of God to man.

The principal opium exporting countries are: Turkey, Iran (Persia), Yugoslavia, and India. The Turkish and Yugoslav products are nearly alike in their physical properties: color, odor, and consistency. Persian and Indian opiums, while closely resembling each other, differ from the former in physical properties—they are darker, have a somewhat different odor and consistency. There is also a marked difference between the two groups in the amounts of the principal opium alkaloids as shown in Table I.

Table I—Alkaloidal Content of Opiums[a]

Exporting Country	% Morphine	% Narcotine	% Codeine	% Papaverine	% Thebaine
Turkey	11 –12	3–4	0.8–1.4	1–1.5	1.0–1.5
Yugoslavia	13 –15	3	1.1–1.5	1–1.5	0.8–1.2
Iran	9.5–10.5	5–6	2.5–4	2–2.5	3 –4
India	10 –11	...	2.5–3.5	0.8	0.5–1

[a] *Note*—For medicinal preparations only Turkish or Yugoslav opium is used.

The United Nations is conducting a program designed to devise physical and chemical means for identifying the country of origin of opium seized in illicit traffic.[1]

Constituents—Opium owes its value to the narcotic alkaloids present in it. Twenty-five alkaloids have been proved to exist in various kinds of opium, and several more have been announced, but their existence has not been confirmed. Three acids are found combined with the alkaloids in opium—*viz*, meconic, lactic, and sulfuric acids. Also present are three neutral principles *meconin* [$C_{10}H_{10}O_4$], *meconoisin* [$C_8H_{10}O_2$], and *opionin* as well as pectin, glucose, mucilage, caoutchouc, wax,

and odorous, fatty, and coloring matters. *Meconic acid* is colored red by ferric salts, the color not being discharged by solution of mercuric chloride. A solution of potassium thiocyanate is colored in a similar manner by ferric salts, but this color is discharged by solution of mercuric chloride. The known alkaloids are tabulated and classified on page 489.

Description—More or less rounded, oval, brick-shaped, or elongated, somewhat flattened masses, usually about 8 to 15 cm in diameter and weighing about 300 Gm to 2 Kg each; externally, it is pale olive-brown or olive-gray having a coarse surface and covered with a thin coating consisting of fragments of poppy leaves and, at times, with fruits of a species of *Rumex* adhering from the packing; it is more or less plastic when fresh, becoming hard or tough on keeping; internally, it is reddish brown and coarsely granular. It has a very characteristic odor, and a very bitter taste.

Uses—Opium owes its chief pharmacological effects to its content of morphine, other alkaloids not being present in sufficient amount to modify significantly the morphine type of action. Thus, Opium has many of the same uses as morphine, but the latter drug is nearly always preferred, inasmuch as it can be given in a variety of ways. The average adult dose of Opium is 60 mg, taken orally. This is the equivalent of 6 mg of morphine. Opium in the form of the tincture is more commonly employed than the powder itself. Like morphine, Opium has *analgetic* and *narcotic* effects. It acts as an *antiperistaltic* agent by virtue of the fact that it causes spasm of the bowel musculature and prevents propulsive movements. Traditionally, Opium or its tincture is used for *diarrheas* and *dysenteries* rather than morphine. Opium produces *sedation* and *sleep*. It also controls *cough* and *dyspnea*. Opium thus has a variety of therapeutic uses in medicine and surgery.

Caution—Its sale and use, like those of all Opium derivatives and related synthetic compounds, are subject to rigid federal regulations under the *Harrison Narcotic Law* (page 1970) and under laws passed by many states. It should not be dispensed except upon the presentation of a physician's prescription. See *Morphine*.

Powdered Opium USP is opium dried at a temperature not exceeding 70°, and reduced to a very fine powder. Powdered Opium yields 10.0–10.5% of anhydrous morphine. It may contain any of the diluents, with the exception of starch, permitted for powdered extracts under *Extracts* (page 1591). *Description:* Light brown to moderate yellowish brown, consisting chiefly of yellowish brown to yellow, more or less irregular and granular fragments of latex, varying from 15 to 150μ in diameter; a few fragments of strongly lignified, thick-walled, 4- to 5-sided or narrowly elongated, epidermal cells of the poppy capsule; very few fragments of tissues of poppy leaves, poppy capsules, and occasionally *Rumex* fruits. In addition there will be the microscopic characteristics of the diluent if any has been used in the preparation of the powder. *Uses:* A pharmaceutical necessity for *Paregoric*. See *Opium* and *Morphine*. *Veterinary Dose: Horses*, 4 to 20 Gm; *Cattle*, 10 to 25 Gm; *Foals*, *Calves*, and *Sheep*, 1 to 2 Gm; *Dogs*, 30 to 200 mg.

Paregoric USP [Camphorated Opium Tincture USP XVI; Paregoric Elixir; Compound Tincture of Camphor; Tinctura Opii Benzoica; Tinctura Thebaica Benzoica] yields, from each 100 ml, 35–45 mg of anhydrous morphine. *Preparation:* Macerate powdered opium (4.3 Gm), anise oil (3.8 ml), benzoic acid (3.8 Gm), and camphor (3.8 Gm) for 5 days, with occasional agitation, in a mixture of diluted alcohol (900 ml) and glycerin (38 ml). Then filter, and pass enough diluted alcohol through the filter to obtain 950 ml of total filtrate. Assay a portion of this filtrate as directed in the USP, and dilute the remainder with a sufficient quantity of diluted alcohol containing, in each 100 ml, 0.4 ml of anise oil, 400 mg of benzoic acid, 400 mg of camphor, and 4 ml of glycerin, to produce a solution containing, in each 100 ml, 40 mg of anhydrous morphine. It may also be prepared as follows: Dissolve opium tincture (40 ml), anise oil (4 ml), benzoic acid (4 Gm), and camphor (4 Gm) in diluted alcohol (900 ml), and add glycerin (40 ml), and sufficient diluted alcohol to make the product measure 1000 ml. Agitate the mixture and filter. *History:* This preparation was originated by Professor LeMort of the University of Leyden about 1715. It was official in the 1721 edition of the London Pharmacopæia under the name *Elixir Asthmaticum,* which name was changed to *Elixir Paregoricum,* meaning soothing elixir, in 1746. It has also been known as *Tinctura Camphoræ Composita* and *Tinctura Opii Benzoica,* and the formula has changed in minor details many times sunce its introduction into medicine. The word *Paregoric* was used by the ancient writers on pharmacy and medicine in a generic sense to denote an anodyne or soothing preparation. *Alcohol Content:* From 44 to 46% of C_2H_5OH. *Uses:* An *antidiarrheal agent* and mild *anodyne* in *cough, nausea,* and *abdominal pains.* It should never be used to quiet restless infants, as a habit may be induced. It contains 0.4 to 1% of opium. Paregoric is one of the exempted preparations under the *Harrison Narcotic Law,* but its sale is subject to strict regulations under the Act, and the pharmacist is held strictly accountable for its legitimate distribution. In certain states it is nonexempt. *Dose:* 5 to 50 ml daily; *usual,* 5 to 10 ml 1 to 4 times a day. *Veterinary Dose: Foals* and *Calves,* 15 to 40 ml; *Dogs,* 4 to 15 ml.

Other Opiate Analgesics

Granulated Opium USP XVI Opium dried at a temperature not exceeding 70°, and reduced to granules, all of which will pass through a number 10 standard mesh sieve and not more than 10% through a number 60 standard mesh sieve. It yields 10–10.5% anhydrous morphine. It may contain any of the diluents, with the exception of starch, permitted for powdered extracts under *Extracts* (page 1591). *Uses:* A pharmaceutic necessity for *Opium Tincture.* See *Opium* and *Morphine.*

Opium Alkaloids

The pharmaceutically important opium alkaloids are commonly subdivided into two chemical groups: (1) the isoquinoline derivatives which are, as a general rule, antispasmodic drugs, such as papaverine and narcotine (see page 854) and (2) the phenanthrene derivatives described in this section, such as morphine and codeine, which are analgesic and narcotic.* Heroin is many more times addictive than morphine, but it cannot be made or imported into this country legally. Furthermore, the Narcotic Act of 1956 requires that all heroin in the hands of pharmacists, physicians, veterinarians, hospitals, etc, must be surrendered to the federal government. Hence, this agent is no longer available for general therapeutic use and is not included in this section.

Morphine

History—Morphine was the first alkaloid discovered. In the seventeenth and eighteenth centuries many attempts were made to separate from opium the principle to which its activity was due. Preparations claimed to represent these active principles, but which were really extracts, were employed in medicine under the name of *Magisterium Opii.* Bucholz was the first to endeavor to obtain a crystalline product from opium. About 1800 a number of learned apothecaries of the time were devoting their attention to the separation of the suspected active principle. One of these apothecaries, Derosne, succeeded in isolating narcotine in 1803, and the following year Seguin read a paper to the Institute of France describing the isolation of a substance which is now recognized as morphine. He did not publish his paper, however, until 1814 and in 1806, Friedrich William Adam Sertrüner, an apothecary of Einbeck, Germany, announced the separation of a basic crystalline substance which existed in opium in combination with a special acid. He later published, in 1817, the results of further investigation in which he named the substance *morphium* and described it as a *vegetable alkali.* Liebig, in 1831, assigned to it the formula $C_{34}H_{36}N_2O_6$, which was later modified by Laurent to the present formula, $C_{17}H_{19}NO_3$ (285.35).

It was only after almost one hundred years of intensive research by very many able chemists that the cor-rect structural formula (page 493), which adequately explains the multitudinous chemical transformations of morphine, could be proposed.[2] Final confirmation of this structure came with the successful total syntheses of morphine.[3]

Preparation—The isolation of morphine from opium in a quality and purity to meet official standards requires skill and experience. Several processes are in use. In all or nearly all of them the morphine and most of the other opium alkaloids are extracted from the opium with water alone or with slightly acid water. In one of the processes, the extract after concentration is neutralized, excess of a solution of calcium chloride is added, and the mixture is filtered and further concentrated. Crude morphine hydrochloride crystallizes out and is purified by precipitation with ammonia and recrystallized as the sulfate or hydrochloride. In another process the concentrated water extract is mixed with alcohol and made strongly alkaline with ammonia. The morphine, being but slightly soluble in dilute alcohol, separates out while the greater part of the other alkaloids remain in solution. The crude morphine so obtained is purified by repeated crystallization as the sulfate or hydrochloride and reprecipitation if necessary in the presence of alcohol.

Description—Colorless or white shining, rhombic prisms, fine needles, or a crystalline powder, permanent in the air. A saturated aqueous solution of morphine is alkaline to litmus. It melts with decomposition at about 250°. In methanol solution (1%) morphine has a specific rotation of about −132° and in diluted sulfuric acid −116°. It exists as the monohydrate (303.36).

Solubility—1 Gm dissolves in about 5000 ml of water, 210 ml of alcohol (more soluble in methanol), 1220 ml of chloroform, about 6500 ml of ether, 100 ml of lime water, 1075 ml of boiling water, and 98 ml of boiling alcohol; insoluble in benzene; readily soluble in solutions of the fixed alkali and alkaline earth hydroxides from which it is repre-cipitated by ammonium chloride or sulfate.

Identification—In addition to giving precipitates, even in dilute solutions, with most of the alkaloidal precipitants, morphine is particularly characterized by the following color reactions which may be obtained with a few mg or less of morphine: (1) Sulfuric acid, containing 5 mg of selenious acid per ml (*Mecke's reagent*), gives with Morphine Sulfate a blue color, changing to green and then to brown (codeine yields a green color, changing to blue and afterward to grass-green). (2) Sulfuric acid, containing 5 mg of molybdic acid per ml (*Frohde's reagent*), gives with Morphine Sulfate a

---

* For a more detailed classification of the opium alkaloids, see page 493.

purple color, changing to blue. (3) Sulfuric acid, each ml containing one drop of formaldehyde TS (*Marquis' reagent*), yields an intensely purple color with Morphine Sulfate. (4) Add potassium ferricyanide TS, containing 1 drop of ferric chloride TS in each ml, to an aqueous solution of Morphine Sulfate (1 in 100): a deep blue color is produced at once (difference from codeine), due to reduction by morphine of ferricyanide to ferrocyanide which gives Prussian Blue with the ferric chloride. (5) Morphine solutions acidified with sulfuric acid give a yellow to brown color on the addition of 1 to 2 drops of an aqueous solution of potassium iodate or of iodic acid (codeine gives a green color).

Uses—Morphine is one of the most important drugs in the physician's armamentarium, and few would care to practice medicine without it. When wisely used, it can do great good; when unwisely prescribed, it can do untold harm. It is almost indispensable for the relief of pain, *analgesia* being one of its main actions. Unfortunately, Morphine causes euphoria and addiction, and its repeated administration is fraught with the possibility that the patient may become addicted to the alkaloid. No other drug is so generally useful in relieving various categories of severe pain. Morphine is also a *sedative* and *soporific*, and causes tranquil relaxation and in larger doses stupefaction. It also depresses the respiration. Use is made of this last-named property in the treatment of *cough*, and certain forms of *dyspnea*, especially cardiac (but not bronchial!) asthma. Yet the respiratory depression constitutes the chief drawback and hazard in the use of Morphine, and death from acute overdosage is due to depression of breathing.

An important development was the discovery that if the nitrogen-methyl group of morphine is replaced by allyl, propyl, or certain other substituents, products result which antagonize the respiratory depressant effect of Morphine. *Nalorphine*, for example, is a specific antagonist in cases of acute intoxication by Morphine, by its derivatives, or by its synthetic substitutes.

Morphine stimulates smooth muscles of the bronchi, biliary tract, enteric tract, and ureters. For example, it acts on the bowel to cause spastic constipation. This particular side effect of Morphine is put to therapeutic use in the treatment of *diarrheas* and *dysenteries*. Morphine should not be employed in the treatment of convulsant disorders or of acute poisoning by stimulants of the nervous system, such as strychnine. Preference is given to the barbiturates.

Morphine should be given for the least period of time compatible with the needs of the patient's illness. The patient as a rule need not be told that he is being given a narcotic. Under no circumstances should the patient be allowed to inject the drug himself, if injections are required. Morphine is not a specific therapy, and gives only symptomatic relief. Its misuse may obscure symptoms or the progress of the disease. This is especially true if given for abdominal pain before an accurate diagnosis is made. In cases of hopeless diseases such as cancer, where Morphine must be given in ever larger doses, one expects that addiction will occur. This is permissible, and represents the price that must be paid for relief of pain.

The search for effective analgetic substitutes for Morphine without addicting liability is a primary field of endeavor of pharmacologists and synthetic chemists. Numerous synthetic substitutes have been made and subjected to clinical trials. However, the ideal synthetic morphine substitute has yet to be discovered.

The salts of Morphine are used rather than the alkaloidal base. The salt most commonly employed is the sulfate. (See *Morphine Sulfate*). Morphine salts can be given orally, sublingually, hypodermically, and intravenously (in an emergency). The dose varies from 5 to 15 mg, and the usual dose is 10 mg. A large variety of morphine-containing preparations are official, many having little or no advantage over Morphine itself. A large number of derivatives of Morphine is available. The actions of opium are in large measure attributable to its Morphine content.

Caution—The provisions of the *Harrison Narcotic Act* must be scrupulously observed in the sale and use of Morphine. It must not be dispensed except upon presentation of a physician's prescription, properly written.

Morphine Injection USP

Morphine Injection is a sterile solution of a suitable salt of morphine in water for injection. It contains 93.0–107.0% of the labeled amount of the morphine salt, the name of which is stated on the label. Suitable microbistatics, totaling not more than 0.7%, may be added.

Preparation—This injection is usually made with morphine sulfate or less commonly with morphine hydrochloride or tartrate. Solutions of morphine sulfate at a pH above 7 decompose quickly even at room temperature. At a pH of less than 5.5 no change is reported in a 1% solution heated for 1 hour. The pH should not be below 3. Sterilization should be conducted with a minimum of heat.

Uses and Dose—See *Morphine*.

Morphine Sulfate USP

[7,8-Didehydro-4,5α-epoxy-17-methylmorphinan-3,6α-diol Sulfate (2:1)]

Morphine Sulfate [$(C_{17}H_{19}NO_3)_2 \cdot H_2SO_4 \cdot 5H_2O$ = 758.85] contains 98.0–101.0% of $(C_{17}H_{19}NO_3)_2 \cdot H_2SO_4$ (668.77), calculated on the anhydrous basis.

For the structural formula of morphine, see page 493.

Description—White, feathery, silky crystals, as cubical masses of crystals, or as a white crystalline powder. It is odorless and when exposed to air gradually loses water of hydration. It darkens on prolonged exposure to light. Specific rotation: −107° to −109.5°.

Solubility—1 Gm dissolves in 16 ml of water, 570 ml of alcohol, 1 ml of water at 80°, and about 240 ml of alcohol at 60°; insoluble in chloroform and ether.

Incompatibilities—See *Alkaloids* (page 491). Morphine reduces *iodates*, *chlorates*, *alkaline permanganate*, and other oxidizing agents. *Silver nitrate* is reduced and gives a red color. Morphine is precipitated from fairly concentrated solution of its salts by *codeine alkaloid*.

Uses—Morphine Sulfate is much more largely prescribed in the United States than any other salt of morphine. See *Morphine*.

Dose—*Parenteral*, **5** to **75 mg** daily; *usual*, **10 mg** 4 to 6 times a day, as necessary.

Dosage Forms—Tablets USP: 8, 10, 15, and 30 mg; Morphine and Atropine Sulfates Tablets NF (see below): 8, 10, 15 and 30 mg (morphine sulfate) and 400 mcg (atropine sulfate).

Veterinary Dose—*Oral* or *subcutaneous*, Dogs, **10** to **250 mg.**

Morphine and Atropine Sulfates Tablets NF contain 91.0–109.0% of the labeled amounts of $(C_{17}H_{19}NO_3)_2 \cdot H_2SO_4 \cdot 5H_2O$ (morphine sulfate) and of $(C_{17}H_{23}NO_3)_2 \cdot H_2SO_4 \cdot H_2O$ (atropine sulfate). *Uses:* See *Morphine* (this page) and *Atropine* (page 914). This combination of alkaloids invites the same objection that all drug mixtures do, namely, that of fixed dosages. Nevertheless, atropine and morphine are commonly used together, especially for *preanesthetic medication*, and for the relief of *visceral pain*, where atropine relaxes smooth muscles and hence counteracts the spasmodic effect of morphine. Thus, for example, morphine and atropine together give smoother relief of pain in *gall bladder colic* or *ureteral colic* than does morphine alone. *Dose:* Morphine Sulfate, *5 to 20 mg;* Atropine Sulfate, *300 mcg to 1.2 mg.*

Codeine NF

[7,8-Didehydro-4,5α-epoxy-3-methoxy-17-methylmorphinan-6α-ol; Methyl-morphine]

Codeine [$C_{18}H_{21}NO_3 \cdot H_2O$ = 317.39], dried at 80° for 4 hours, contains 98.5–100.5% of $C_{18}H_{21}NO_3$.

Codeine is an alkaloid obtained from opium or prepared from morphine by methylation.

For the structural formula, see page 493.

History—Codeine was isolated from opium by the French chemist Robiquet in 1832, and the name given it by the discoverer is derived from the Greek word meaning poppy capsules.

Preparation—While some Codeine is obtained from opium directly the quantity is not sufficient to meet the extensive use of this alkaloid as a very valuable medicinal agent. Much more codeine is used than morphine. This need is met by making it by partial synthesis from morphine. The process involves methylating the phenolic OH of the latter. The methylating agent generally used is phenyltrimethylammonium hydroxide prepared separately or *in situ* from phenyltrimethylammonium methosulfate or phenyltrimethylammonium chloride. (These salts are prepared in turn, from dimethylaniline and dimethyl sulfate or methyl chloride, respectively.)

Dry morphine is dissolved in the theoretical amount of potassium hydroxide dissolved in absolute alcohol, the required quantity of the methylating agent added, and the solution heated at about 130°. After cooling, water is added, the solution is acidified with sulfuric acid, the dimethylaniline formed is separated, and the alcohol is removed by distillation. Treatment with caustic soda solution precipitates the Codeine, while any unreacted morphine is held in solution by the sodium hydroxide. The crude Codeine is purified by crystallization as the sulfate.

Description—Colorless or white crystals, or a white, crystalline powder. It effloresces slowly in dry air and is affected by light. When rendered anhydrous by drying at 80° it melts between 154° and 158°. Codeine is levorotatory and the specific rotation in acid or alcohol is −137° and in chloroform −112°. A saturated aqueous solution of Codeine is alkaline to litmus. The pH of the saturated aqueous solution is about 9.8.

Solubility—1 Gm dissolves in 120 ml of water, 2 ml of alcohol, about 0.5 ml of chloroform, 50 ml of ether, and about 20 ml of benzene. When heated in an amount of water insufficient for complete solution, Codeine melts to oily drops which crystallize on cooling.

Incompatibilities—Codeine is precipitated from its aqueous solution by most of the *alkaloidal precipitants* but not by sodium, potassium, or ammonium carbonate or sodium bicarbonate. Aqueous solutions are sufficiently alkaline to precipitate other less soluble alkaloids from solutions of their salts. Ammonia may be liberated from *ammonium salts.* See also page 491.

Uses—Codeine may be viewed as a weakened morphine, which fails to produce proportionately greater narcotic effects as the dose is increased. Indeed, large amounts of Codeine may cause excitement. Average doses are *sedative* and *analgetic*, and obtund the cough reflex. Codeine is only one-sixth as analgetic as morphine, on a weight basis, and if 60 mg of the drug fails to relieve pain, larger doses are unlikely to do so. Like morphine, Codeine also produces cortical and respiratory depression, but serious degrees of either are practically unknown. Codeine is less apt than morphine to cause nausea, vomiting, constipation, and miosis. Both tolerance and *addiction* to Codeine occur, however, and the same precautions should be observed in its use as for morphine. *Nalorphine* is a specific antagonist in cases of acute Codeine intoxication.

Codeine, like morphine, is employed as an *analgetic, sedative, hypnotic, antiperistaltic*, and *antitussive* agent. The provisions of the *Harrison Narcotic Law* (page 1970) must be observed when dispensing or prescribing Codeine.

Dose—*Analgesic*, **15** to **60 mg;** *usual, analgesic*, **30 mg** every 4 hours; *usual, antitussive*, **5** to **10 mg** every 4 hours.

Other Dose Information—The dose varies from 15 to 60 mg, and the drug may be taken orally or injected parenterally as a solution of one of its water-soluble salts, such as the phosphate or sulfate. See *Morphine.*

Veterinary Dose—*Dogs*, **4** to **60 mg.**

Codeine Phosphate USP

[7,8-Didehydro-4,5α-epoxy-3-methoxy-17-methylmorphinan-6α-ol   Phosphate (1:1)]

Codeine Phosphate [$C_{18}H_{21}NO_3 \cdot H_3PO_4 \cdot \frac{1}{2}H_2O$ = 406.38] contains 99.0–101.5% of $C_{18}H_{21}NO_3 \cdot H_3PO_4$ (397.37), calculated on the anhydrous basis.

Preparation—It may be prepared by dissolving codeine in an equimolecular quantity of aqueous phosphoric acid, adding alcohol, and allowing the salt to crystallize from solution.

Description—Fine, white, needle-shaped crystals or a white, crystalline powder. It is odorless. It readily loses water of hydration on exposure to air and is affected by light. It solutions are acid to litmus and levorotatory.

Solubility—1 Gm dissolves in 2.5 ml of water, 325 ml of alcohol, 0.5 ml of water at 80°, and 125 ml of boiling alcohol.

Uses—See *Codeine* and *Morphine.* Being more soluble than codeine sulfate, the phosphate is often preferred to the sulfate.

Dose—**5** to **60 mg;** *usual, oral* or *subcutaneous*, **15 mg** every 4 hours.

Dosage Forms—Injection USP: 30 and 60 mg/ml, 600 mg/20 ml, 1.8 Gm/30 ml; Tablets USP: 15, 30, and 60 mg.

Veterinary Dose—*Dogs*, **4** to **60 mg.**

Codeine Phosphate, Aspirin, Phenacetin, and Caffeine Tablets NF

[APC with Codeine; Empirin Compound with Codeine (Burroughs-Wellcome)]

Codeine Phosphate, Aspirin, Phenacetin, and Caffeine Tablets contain 93.0–107.0% of the labeled amount of $C_{18}H_{21}NO_3 \cdot H_3PO_4 \cdot \frac{1}{2}H_2O$ (codeine phosphate), and 90.0–110.0% of $C_9H_8O_4$ (aspirin), of $C_{10}H_{13}NO_2$ (phenacetin), and of $C_8H_{10}N_4O_2$ (caffeine).

Uses—This popular combination, having both analgesic and antitussive actions, is used for the relief of pain of all degrees of severity, up to that which requires morphine.

Dose—*Usual*, **8** to **60 mg** (codeine phosphate), **600 mg** (aspirin), **300 mg** (phenacetin), and **200 mg** (caffeine).

Dosage Forms—Tablets NF: 8, 15, 30, and 60 mg (codeine phosphate), 230 mg (aspirin), 150 mg (phenacetin), and 30 mg (caffeine).

Codeine Sulfate NF

[7,8-Didehydro-4,5α-epoxy-3-methoxy-17-methylmorphinan-6α-ol   Sulfate (2:1)]

Codeine Sulfate [($C_{18}H_{21}NO_3)_2$. H_2SO_4 . $3H_2O$ = 750.87], dried at 105° for 3 hours, contains 98.5–100.5% of ($C_{18}H_{21}NO_3)_2$. H_2SO_4 (696.82).

Preparation—Codeine Sulfate is made by crystallization from a solution of codeine in diluted sulfuric acid.

Description—White crystals, usually needle-like, or a white, crystalline powder. It effloresces in dry air and is affected by light. Its aqueous solution is practically neutral or only slightly acid to litmus. Codeine Sulfate has a specific rotation of −112.5° to −115°.

Solubility—1 Gm dissolves in 30 ml of water, 1280 ml of alcohol, and in about 6.5 ml of water at 80°; insoluble in chloroform and ether.

Incompatibilities—See *Alkaloids* (page 491). Codeine Sulfate reacts with *phenobarbital sodium* to produce the free alkaloid and phenobarbital, both of which may precipitate unless the vehicle contains a moderate proportion of alcohol.

Uses—See *Codeine* and *Morphine*.

Dose—*Analgesic*, 15 to **60 mg**; *usual, analgesic*, **30 mg** every 4 hours; *usual, antitussive*, **5 to 10 mg** every 4 hours.

Dosage Forms—Tablets NF: 15, 30, and 60 mg.

Veterinary Dose—*Dogs*, 4 to **60 mg**.

Other Opium Alkaloids

Codeine Hydrobromide [$C_{18}H_{21}NO_3$.HBr.$2H_2O$]—White crystals. The anhydrous salt melts at 190° to 192°. $[\alpha]_D^{22}$ is −96.6°. 1 Gm dissolves in 60 ml water, 110 ml alcohol. *Uses* and *Dose*: As for the sulfate, especially in cough.

Codeine Hydrochloride [$C_{18}H_{21}NO_3$.HCl.$2H_2O$]—White, fine, small needles. Melts at about 280° with some decomposition. $[\alpha]_D^{22}$ is −108°. 1 Gm dissolves in 20 ml water, 1 ml boiling water, 180 ml alcohol. pH about 5. *Uses* and *Dose*: As for the sulfate.

Codeine Methylbromide, Eucodin [$C_{18}H_{21}NO_3$.CH_3Br] —White crystals or powder. Melts about 260°. Soluble in water (2 to 3 parts), hot methanol; sparingly soluble in alcohol; insoluble in chloroform, ether. *Uses:* Instead of codeine for coughs. *Dose:* 20 to 50 mg.

Diacetylmorphine, Heroin [$C_{21}H_{23}NO_5$]—An alkaloid prepared from morphine by acetylation. When alkaloidal morphine is heated with acetyl chloride, the synthetic alkaloid, diacetylmorphine, is produced. A white crystalline powder without odor. Its saturated alcoholic solution is alkaline to moistened litmus paper. 1 Gm dissolves in about 1700 ml of water, 31 ml of alcohol, 1.4 ml of chloroform, and 100 ml of ether at 25°C. *Uses:* This alkaloid was formerly much used as a sedative in cough mixtures and to relieve moderate pain, but the Narcotic Act of 1956 requires that all heroin must be turned in to the federal government because of its dangerous habit-forming character. Codeine is largely used in its place. *Dose:* Was 0.003 Gm. For the structure, see page 493.

Diacetylmorphine Hydrochloride [Heroin Hydrochloride; Diamorphine Hydrochloride BP] [$C_{21}H_{23}NO_5$.HCl.-H_2O]—White, odorless, bitter, crystalline powder. Melts about 230° with decomposition. $[\alpha]_D^{20}$ is −153° in water. Soluble in 1.6 parts water and chloroform; soluble in alcohol; insoluble in ether. The manufacture or importation of this narcotic is prohibited by federal law. It was official in USP IX and was used like morphine sulfate in doses of 3 to 5 mg.

Morphine Acetate [$C_{17}H_{19}NO_3$.$C_2H_4O_2$.$3H_2O$]—Yellowish white powder; slight acetic odor. Decomposes with age, losing acetic acid and discoloring. $[\alpha]_D^{15}$ is −77° in water. 1 Gm dissolves in 2.25 ml water, 2 ml boiling water, 22 ml alcohol, 2 ml alcohol at 60°, 4.5 ml glycerin, 4.75 ml chloroform; insoluble in ether. *Uses* and *Dose*: As for the sulfate.

Morphine Hydrochloride USP XV, BP, PhI [$C_{17}H_{19}$-NO_3.HCl.$3H_2O$]—An odorless, white, crystalline powder or white, needle-like crystals having a bitter taste. When exposed to air it gradually loses a portion of its 3 molecules of water. It darkens on prolonged exposure to light. 1 Gm is soluble in 18 ml of water to give a solution having a pH of about 5. It is soluble in alcohol and glycerin but insoluble in chloroform and ether. It has the same actions, uses, and dose as morphine sulfate. See *Morphine Sulfate* (page 1123).

Morphine Tartrate [($C_{17}H_{19}NO_3)_2$.$C_4H_6O_6$.$3H_2O$]—White, crystalline powder. Soluble in 11 parts of water; slightly soluble in alcohol; insoluble in chloroform, ether, carbon disulfide. *Uses* and *Dose*: As for the sulfate.

Semisynthetic Opium Alkaloids

In an effort to obtain an agent which would possess the advantages of morphine or codeine without their disadvantages, chemists have modified the structure of these natural alkaloids of opium. Some of these modifications, eg, hydrocodone, hydromorphone, ethylmorphine, nalorphine, etc, result from making minor chemical alterations in the natural alkaloids, the iminoethanophenanthrene nucleus (see page 467) remaining intact. Others, eg, dextromethorphan, levorphanol, levallorphan, etc, are truly synthetic compounds constructed around the nonopiate morphinan nucleus (see page 467) which is readily synthesizable from coal tar derivatives. For pharmacologic convenience, all of these agents are classified here as semisynthetic opium alkaloids. In general, the pharmacological properties exhibited by these agents differ quantitatively from those of the parent substance, but qualitatively they are similar. The several semisynthetic agents which are clinically employed appear below.

Dextromethorphan Hydrobromide—see page 876.

Ethylmorphine Hydrochloride NF

[7,8-Didehydro-4,5α-epoxy-3-ethoxy-17-methylmorphinan-6α-ol Hydrochloride; Dionin (*MSD*)]

Ethylmorphine Hydrochloride [$C_{19}H_{23}NO_3$. HCl . $2H_2O$ = 385.89] contains 99.0–100.5% of $C_{19}H_{23}NO_3$. HCl (349.86), calculated on the anhydrous basis.

Ethylmorphine Hydrochloride is a salt of the synthetic ethoxy analog of codeine. For the structure, see page 493.

Preparation—Among other ways, ethylmorphine may be prepared by ethylation of morphine with diethyl sulfate in the presence of sodium ethylate. Conversion to the hydrochloride is effected conveniently by dissolving the base in an appropriate solvent such as chloroform and introducing a stream of hydrogen chloride. The crude salt is purified by treatment with decolorizing carbon and crystallization.

Description—A white, or faintly yellow, odorless microcrystalline powder. It melts with decomposition at about

123°; when anhydrous it melts at about 170°. Specific rotation: −102° to −105°.

Solubility—1 Gm dissolves in 10 ml of water and 25 ml of alcohol; slightly soluble in ether and chloroform.

Incompatibilities—See page 491.

Uses—Ethylmorphine Hydrochloride, sold under the name *Dionin*, is used as a substitute for morphine, as it is less likely to cause nausea and depression. In its systemic actions, Ethylmorphine Hydrochloride very closely resembles codeine, but does not enjoy the wide use of the latter alkaloid. Administered systemically, it is used to allay cough and relieve pain. Applied locally to mucous membranes or abraded skin, it causes irritation and marked hyperemia. It is this property which makes it useful in chronic inflammatory conditions of the eye (*indolent corneal ulcers, uveal exudates, vitreous opacities*), where the reactive hyperemia produced by Dionin has beneficial effects. A 2 to 10% solution or 10% ointment is employed. See *Codeine*.

Caution—As a derivative of morphine it is subject to the *Harrison Narcotic Act*.

Dose—*Topically*, as a **1** to **5**% solution in the eye.

Dosage Forms—Powder.

Hydrocodone Bitartrate USP

[Dihydrocodeinonium Tartrate (1:1); 4,5α-Epoxy-3-methoxy-17-methyl-morphinan-6-one Tartrate (1:1); Dihydrocodeinone Bitartrate USP XVI; Dicodid (*Knoll*); Hycodan (*Endo*)]

Hydrocodone Bitartrate contains 98.0–102.0% of $C_{18}H_{21}NO_3 . C_4H_6O_6 . 2\frac{1}{2}H_2O$ (494.50).

For the structure of hydrocodone, see page 493.

Preparation—This synthetic alkaloid is 7,8-dihydrocodeinone. It is prepared either by catalytic rearrangement of codeine or by controlled hydrolysis and oxidation of dihydrothebaine.

Description—Fine white crystals or a fine white crystalline powder. It is affected by light.

Solubility—1 Gm dissolves in 16 ml of water; slightly soluble in alcohol; insoluble in ether and chloroform.

Uses—This alkaloid possesses the *antitussive* and *analgetic* activity of *Codeine* (page 1124). It is a narcotic which causes addiction, and is controlled by the *Harrison Narcotic Act*.

Dose—5 to **50 mg** daily; *usual*, **5** to **10 mg** 3 to 4 times a day.

Dosage Forms—Syrup USP (see below): 5 mg/5 ml; Tablets USP: 5 mg.

Hydrocodone Bitartrate Syrup USP contains 90.0–110.0% of the labeled amount of $C_{18}H_{21}NO_3 . C_4H_6O_6 . 2^1/_2H_2O$. *Preparation:* Dissolve hydrocodone bitartrate (1 Gm) in purified water (50 ml) by warming gently, and add cherry syrup (qs) to make the product measure 1000 ml. *Alcohol Content:* 1 to 2%. *Uses* and *Dose:* See *Hydrocodone Bitartrate*.

Hydromorphone Hydrochloride NF

[4,5α-Epoxy-3-hydroxy-17-methylmorphinan-6-one Hydrochloride; Dihydromorphinone Hydrochloride USP XVI; Dilaudid (*Knoll*)]

Hydromorphone Hydrochloride, dried at 105° for 2 hours, contains 98.0–101.0% of $C_{17}H_{19}NO_3 . HCl$ (321.81).

Hydromorphone Hydrochloride is 7,8-dihydromorphinone hydrochloride. For the structure, see page 493.

Preparation—Dihydromorphinone hydrochloride is made by passing hydrogen into a solution of morphine hydrochloride in the presence of palladium or platinum as a catalyst.

Description—A fine, white, odorless, crystalline powder, affected by light. Specific rotation: −136° to −139°. Its aqueous solution is practically neutral or only slightly acid to litmus.

Solubility—1 Gm dissolves in about 3 ml of water; sparingly soluble in alcohol; practically insoluble in ether.

Incompatibilities—Reactions characteristic of alkaloids are generally applicable to this substance. See page 491.

Uses—Hydromorphone Hydrochloride (Dilaudid) is allied both chemically and pharmacologically to morphine and has the same general actions and uses as morphine. However, it differs in certain respects. It is more analgetic and more toxic on a weight basis and hence is given in doses one-fourth as large as for morphine. The duration of analgesia is definitely shorter than for morphine and thus the interval between doses may have to be shorter. Slower absorption and hence longer relief from pain can be obtained from the use of Hydromorphone Hydrochloride in suppository form. Hydromorphone Hydrochloride causes less tendency to sleep than morphine when given in equivalent analgetic doses, and thus relief from pain can be obtained without sleep or stupefaction. It is claimed that Hydromorphone Hydrochloride causes less constipation and vomiting than morphine. Also, it produces less euphoria. However, *tolerance* and *addiction* do occur with Hydromorphone Hydrochloride, and the drug must be used with the same precautions as for morphine. It can be given by mouth, by rectum in suppository form, or injected subcutaneously or intravenously (in emergency).

Caution—This drug, being a morphine derivative, is subject to the *Harrison Narcotic Law*. *Nalorphine* (page 1127) is a specific antagonist in cases of acute Hydromorphone intoxication.

Dose—*Oral* and *subcutaneous*, **1** to **4 mg**; *usual*, **2 mg** every 4 hours as necessary.

Dosage Forms—Injection NF: 1, 2, 3, and 4 mg/ml, 20 mg/10 ml, 40 mg/20 ml; Tablets NF: 1, 2, 3, and 4 mg.

Levallorphan Tartrate USP

[(−)-17-Allylmorphinan-3-ol Tartrate (1:1); *l-N*-Allyl-3-hydroxymorphinan Bitartrate; Lorfan Tartrate (*Roche*)]

Levallorphan Tartrate contains 98.5–100.5% of $C_{19}H_{25}NO . C_4H_6O_6$ (433.51), calculated on the dried basis.

Preparation—The over-all process involves demethylation of levorphanol (base) followed by allylation and conversion to the tartrate. The levorphanol base (synthesized as described under *Levorphanol Tartrate*, page 1127) is reacted with cyanogen bromide (von Braun cleavage) whereby the —N—CH₃ is converted to

—N—CN. On alkaline hydrolysis, this cyano compound behaves as a typical cyanamide giving rise to the corresponding —NH compound (demethylated levor-

phanol). This may then be allylated in various ways such as treating it with an equimolar quantity of allyl bromide in the presence of a suitable basic catalyst. The resulting levallorphan (base) is then reacted with an equimolar portion of tartaric acid and the bitartrate thus formed is purified by recrystallization.

Description—White or practically white, odorless, crystalline powder. It melts between 174° and 177°. Specific rotation is not less than −37.0° and not more than −39.2°.

Solubility—1 Gm dissolves in about 20 ml of water and about 60 ml of alcohol; practically insoluble in ether; insoluble in chloroform.

Uses—Levallorphan Tartrate is a potent narcotic antagonist. It is used in obstetrics for the prevention and treatment of respiratory depression in the mother, fetus, and newborn infant caused by the administration of narcotics. It is also used to counteract respiratory depression when narcotics are employed preoperatively or postoperatively in the relief of pain, and to combat narcotic overdosage. It is ineffective against the respiratory depression caused by barbiturates, anesthetics, other nonnarcotic agents, or diseased conditions. Levallorphan Tartrate relieves respiratory depression of narcotic agents without affecting the analgesia. Since respiratory depression is observed when Levallorphan Tartrate is administered alone, it should only be given before, along with, or after narcotic administration.

Dose—*Parenteral,* **500 mcg** to **2 mg,** repeated if necessary; *usual,* **1 mg,** repeated 2 times at 3-minute intervals if necessary.

Dosage Forms—Injection USP: 1 and 10 ml.

Levorphanol Tartrate NF

[(−)-17-Methylmorphinan-3-ol Tartrate (1:1); Dihydrate; Levo-Dromoran (*Roche*)]

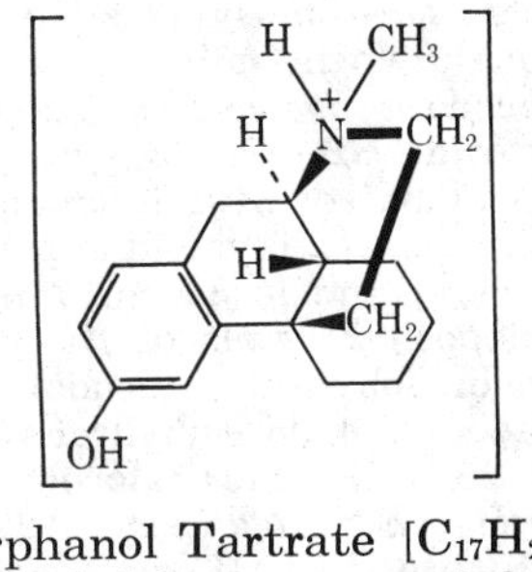

Levorphanol Tartrate [$C_{17}H_{23}NO \cdot C_4H_6O_6 \cdot 2H_2O$ = 443.50], dried in vacuum at 90° to constant weight, contains 99.0–101.0% of $C_{17}H_{23}NO \cdot C_4H_6O_6$ (407.47).

Preparation—Levorphanol (base) is prepared as follows. 5,6,7,8-Tetrahydro-2-methylisoquinolinium bromide (I) is metathesized with *p*-methoxybenzyl magnesium bromide (II), and the product rearranges at the expense of the 1,2-double bond to form 1-(*p*-methoxybenzyl)-2-methyl-1,2,5,6,7,8-hexahydroisoquinoline (III). (III) may be redrawn as shown below to display the ensuing reactions more clearly. A solution of the hydrochloride of (III) is then hydrogenated at the 3,4-positions with the aid of platinized charcoal, and subsequent treatment with ammonia liberates the *dl*-1,2,3,4,5,6,7,8-octahydro compound (IV) which may be resolved into its *d*- and *l*-enantiomorphs by the usual procedures. The final step in the preparation of the base involves heating the *l*-enantiomorph with phosphoric acid at 150°C whereby cyclization between the isoquinoline residue and the benzene ring occurs at the expense of the remaining double bond of the isoquino-

line. During the treatment with phosphoric acid, the methoxy group is simultaneously converted to hydroxy, thus producing levorphanol (V).

The official tartrate may be produced by dissolving the base in aqueous tartaric acid solution and crystallizing.

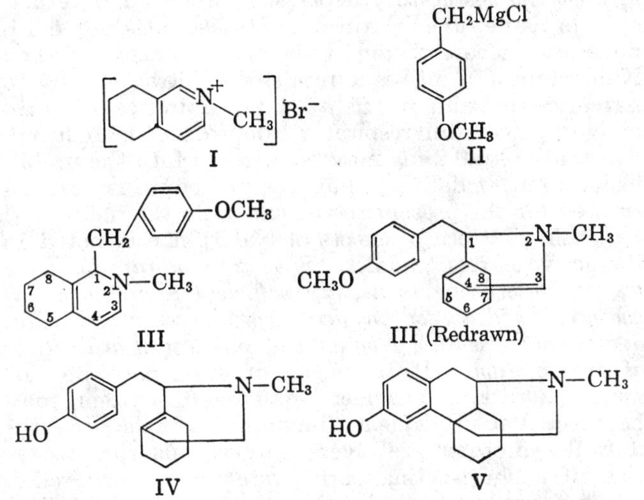

Description—It occurs as a practically white, odorless, crystalline powder. Melting range 114° to 116°. Specific rotation −13.5° to −15.0°.

Solubility—1 Gm dissolves in about 60 ml of water; slightly soluble in alcohol; insoluble in chloroform and ether.

Uses—Levorphanol Tartrate is a potent synthetic analgesic related chemically and pharmacologically to morphine. It produces analgesia in smaller doses than morphine and its action is more prolonged. It may cause addiction.

Dose—*Oral* and *subcutaneous,* **1** to **3 mg;** *usual,* **2 mg.**

Dosage Forms—Injection NF: 2 mg/ml, 20 mg/10 ml; Tablets NF: 2 mg.

Nalorphine Hydrochloride USP

[17-Allyl-7,8-didehydro-4,5α-epoxymorphinan-3,6α-diol Hydrochloride *N*-Allylnormorphine Hydrochloride; Nalline Hydrochloride (*MSD*)]

Nalorphine Hydrochloride contains 97.0–103.0% of $C_{19}H_{21}NO_3 \cdot HCl$ (347.85), calculated on the dried basis. It is the *N*-allyl analog of morphine. For the structure, see page 493.

Preparation—This narcotic is prepared commercially by allylation of normorphine (demethylmorphine). See the papers by McCawley *et al,* and Weijlard *et al.*[4]

Description—A white or practically white, odorless, crystalline powder, slowly darkening on exposure to air and light. Its solutions are acid to litmus, having a pH of about 5. Melting range: 260° to 263°. Specific rotation: −122° to −125°.

Solubility—1 Gm dissolves in about 8 ml of water and about 35 ml of alcohol; insoluble in chloroform and ether; soluble in diluted alkali hydroxide solution.

Uses—The pharmacological effects of Nalorphine Hydrochloride depend upon whether morphine or some related narcotic has previously been administered. In the previously non-medicated individual, its effects resemble those of morphine and it is nearly as effective as morphine in relieving postoperative pain in human patients. Withdrawal following its chronic administration does not induce symptoms of abstinence.

The most useful property of Nalorphine is its ability to antagonize many of the actions of morphine and related analgetics (meperidine, methadone, etc). It is a *specific antidote in acute narcotic intoxication.* Respiratory and circulatory depression is reduced but diminution of narcosis is less prominent. It is not effective against the respiratory depression produced by ether, cyclopropane, or barbiturate. Its use does not minimize the necessity for supportive therapy. When Nalorphine (10 mg) is administered intravenously to narcotic-treated parturients a few minutes prior to delivery, neonatal respiratory depression is reduced. Alternatively, 0.2 mg may be injected into the umbilical vein after delivery, but this procedure is best entrusted for the present to the expert in the field.

A third pattern of effects of Nalorphine is noted in the active narcotic addict. *Subcutaneous injection of 3 mg of Nalorphine is usually sufficient to produce unequivocal evidence of physical dependence in the active addict not presenting symptoms of withdrawal at the time of examination.* If the signs of abstinence do not appear, additional increments of 5 and finally 8 mg may be injected at subsequent 20-minute intervals. If withdrawal symptoms are severe, intravenous administration of a short-acting barbiturate may afford relief. The most valuable application of this action of Nalorphine is its use as an experimental tool for the analysis of the phenomena of physical dependence and tolerance.

The alkaloid is a narcotic controlled by the *Harrison Narcotic Act.*

Dose—*Parenteral,* **2** to **10 mg** per dose; *usual,* **5 mg,** repeated 2 times at 3-minute intervals if necessary.

Other Dose Information—The usual adult dose of 5 to 10 mg intravenously is repeated at intervals of 10 to 15 minutes until pulmonary ventilation is adequately increased. Excessive Nalorphine may cause increased respiratory depression and total dosage should not exceed 40 mg.

Dosage Forms—Injection USP: 200 mcg and 5 mg/ml, 10 mg/2 ml, 50 mg/10 ml.

Veterinary Dose—*Parenteral,* for *narcotic intoxication, Dogs,* **1 mg** per **5 pounds** of body weight, not exceeding 5 mg in a single dose; if respiratory function does not increase, the dose may be repeated at 10- to 15-minute intervals.

Oxymorphone Hydrochloride NF

[(4,5α-Epoxy-3,14-dihydroxy-17-methylmorphinan-6-one   Hydrochloride; Numorphan (*Endo*)]

Oxymorphone Hydrochloride contains 97.0–102.0% of $C_{17}H_{19}NO_4 \cdot HCl$ (337.81), calculated on the dried basis.

For the structure, see page 493.

Preparation—Thebaine is dissolved in aqueous formic acid and treated with 30% hydrogen peroxide, after which neutralization with aqueous ammonia yields 14-hydroxycodeinone. This is then dissolved in acetic acid and hydrogenated with the aid of pal-

ladium-charcoal catalyst to form 14-hydroxy-7,8-dihydrocodeinone (Oxycodone). In the form of its hydrochloride, this compound is demethylated by heating with pyridine hydrochloride to yield crude Oxymorphone Hydrochloride, which is then purified. US Pat. 2,806,033.

Description—White, acicular crystals or as a white or slightly off-white powder. It is odorless. It darkens on prolonged exposure to light. Its aqueous solutions are acid to litmus, having a pH of about 5. The base melts to a black liquid between 246° and 249°.

Solubility—1 Gm dissolves in 4 ml of water; sparingly soluble in alcohol and ether.

Uses—A semisynthetic narcotic analgesic agent with actions, uses, and side effects similar to those of hydromorphone and morphine. It satisfactorily controls postoperative pain, the more severe pain of advanced neoplastic diseases, and other types of pain that can ordinarily be controlled by morphine. It produces an intensity of analgesia comparable to that of morphine in a parenteral dose ⅛ to ¹⁄₁₀ that of morphine. Except that it is somewhat less constipating, the over-all incidence and severity of side effects are similar to those of morphine. Its addiction liability is about the same as morphine.

Dose—*Usual, oral,* **10 mg** every 4 to 6 hours, with a maximum dose of **40 mg** per day; *subcutaneous* and *intramuscular,* **1.0** to **1.5 mg** every 4 to 6 hours as needed; *intravenous,* **0.5 mg** *initially,* repeated in 4 to 6 hours if necessary.

Dosage Forms—Injection NF: 1 mg/ml, 1.5 mg/1.5 ml, 3 mg/2 ml, 15 mg/10 and 15 ml; Suppositories: 2 and 5 mg; Tablets NF: 10 mg.

Other Semisynthetic Opium Alkaloids

Benzylmorphine Hydrochloride [Peronine] [$C_{24}H_{25}NO_3 \cdot HCl$]—White crystalline powder. 1 Gm dissolves in about 100 ml water, 270 ml alcohol or chloroform, 120 ml methanol; slightly soluble in acetone, ether, amyl alcohol. *Uses:* Where contraindications or idiosyncrasy to morphine exist; also to relieve cough when indicated in phthisis, bronchitis, and whooping cough. *Dose: Usual,* 20 to 40 mg.

Nalorphine Hydrobromide BP—Purity: not less than 98% of $C_{19}H_{21}NO_3 \cdot HBr$ calculated with reference to the dried substance. A white, odorless, crystalline powder. It is soluble in 24 parts of water and in 35 parts of alcohol. Aqueous solutions may deposit crystals of the dihydrate which are readily soluble in dehydrated alcohol, but this solution rapidly yields a deposit of the anhydrous salt. Its actions, uses, and dose are the same as for nalorphine hydrochloride. See *Nalorphine Hydrochloride* (page 1127).

Oxycodone Hydrochloride PhI [Dihydrohydroxycodeinone hydrochloride;   Eukodal]—The hydrochloride of 4,5α - epoxy - 14 - hydroxy - 3 - methoxy - 17 - methylmorphinan-6-one [$C_{18}H_{21}NO_4 \cdot HCl$]. For the structure of the latter, see page 493. An odorless, white, crystalline powder having a saline, bitter taste. 1 Gm is soluble in 10 ml water and 60 ml ethyl alcohol. The crystals melt at 274–278°C. *Uses:* Narcotic analgesic and antitussive. *Dose: Orally,* or *subcutaneously,* 5 to 20 mg with a maximum of 60 mg in 24 hours.

Nonopiate Addicting Analgesics

The many undesirable side-actions of morphine and the dependence on the Mediterranean and Near East countries for opium have stimulated the search for synthetic drugs as analgesic as morphine, but with fewer side-actions and less addiction liability. The ideal drug, as yet undiscovered, will eventually make

morphine and other opium derivatives obsolete as analgesics.

It is generally agreed that an ideal analgesic drug should (1) not become ineffective through the development of tolerance, (2) not be habit-forming or addicting, (3) have a high ratio between the toxic dose and the effective analgesic dose, (4) be effective against all types of pain, (5) possess a short latent period and a long duration of action, (6) not alter sensory modalities, (7) not depress respiration or the cardiovascular system, (8) not affect the gastrointestinal tract, (9) be effective both orally and parenterally, and (10) be relatively inexpensive.

Since all the potent synthetic analgesics developed for clinical use are addicting, mimic some of the pharmacological properties of morphine, and are antagonized to some extent by nalorphine, it should be obvious that the ideal analgesic agent has yet to be developed. Nevertheless, currently available synthetic agents have valuable analgesic and pharmacological properties which are described in this section.

Alphaprodine Hydrochloride NF

[(±)-1,3-Dimethyl-4-phenyl-4-piperidinol Propionate Hydrochloride; Nisentil Hydrochloride (*Roche*)]

Alphaprodine Hydrochloride contains 98.0–100.5% of $C_{16}H_{23}NO_2 \cdot HCl$ (297.83), calculated on the dried basis.

Having two different centers of asymmetry, the chemical exists in two diastereoisomeric forms which have come to be referred to commercially as the α and β forms. As the NF title indicates, it is the α form which is official and the melting range provided identifies it as such.

Preparation—Under the influence of sodium ethoxide, the ethyl methyl ester of 2′-methyl-3,3′-(methylimino)dipropionic acid (I) is caused to undergo intramolecular Claissen condensation to yield 1,3-dimethyl-

4-piperidone (II). Reduction with lithium phenyl followed by hydrolysis yields the corresponding phenylated piperidinol which is then esterified using propionic acid anhydride.

Description—Occurs as a white, crystalline powder. It has a slight odor.

Solubility—1 Gm is soluble in about 1 ml of water; freely soluble in alcohol and chloroform; insoluble in ether.

Uses—Alphaprodine Hydrochloride is a synthetic narcotic analgesic chemically similar to meperidine. Its analgesic potency is intermediate to that of morphine and meperidine, but its action is more prompt and of shorter duration. It is suited primarily for temporary analgesia in obstetrics, for urological examinations, for preoperative use in surgery and for minor surgical procedures, especially in orthopedics, ophthalmology, rhinology, and laryngology. The drug may be used in conjunction with nerve block or inhalation anesthesia and with barbiturate sedation when allowance is made

for the added depressant effect. Tolerance and addiction may develop.

Dose—*Subcutaneous*, **20 to 60 mg;** *usual, subcutaneous,* **20 to 40 mg;** *intravenous,* **20 to 30 mg;** *usual, intravenous,* **20 mg.**

Dosage Forms—Injection NF: 40 and 60 mg/ml, 600 mg/10 ml.

Anileridine NF

[Ethyl 1-(*p*-Aminophenethyl)-4-phenylisonipecotate; Leritine (*MSD*)]

Anileridine contains 98.5–101.0% of $C_{22}H_{28}N_2O_2$ (352.48), calculated on the anhydrous basis.

Preparation—Ethyl 4-phenylisonipecotate (I) is heated with *p*-nitrophenethyl bromide and sodium carbonate in ethanol solution and the resulting ethyl 1-(*p*-nitrophenethyl)-4-phenylisonipecotate is hydrogenated to Anileridine over palladium-charcoal. For the synthesis of (I), see *Meperidine Hydrochloride*, page 1130.

Description—A white to yellowish white, odorless to practically odorless, crystalline powder, having a slightly bitter taste. It oxidizes and darkens both in air and on exposure to light. It exhibits polymorphism, and of two crystalline forms observed, one melts at about 80° and the other at about 89°.

Solubility—Freely soluble in alcohol and chloroform; soluble, although it may show turbidity, in ether; very slightly soluble in water.

Uses—See *Anileridine Hydrochloride.*

Dose—*Subcutaneous* or *intramuscular*, **25 to 75 mg;** *usual,* **25 to 50 mg** of Anileridine, present as the phosphate, repeated every 6 hours, if necessary.

Dosage Forms—Injection NF (as the phosphate): 25 mg/ml, 50 mg/2 ml, 750 mg/30 ml.

Anileridine Hydrochloride NF

[Ethyl 1-(*p*-Aminophenethyl)-4-phenylisonipecotate Dihydrochloride; Leritine Hydrochloride (*MSD*)]

Anileridine Hydrochloride contains 96.0–102.0% of $C_{22}H_{28}N_2O_2 \cdot 2HCl$ (425.40), calculated on the dried basis.

For the structure of anileridine, see this page.

Preparation—Anileridine (this page) is dissolved in ethanol containing hydrogen chloride, and the dihydrochloride is allowed to crystallize.

Description—Occurs as a white or nearly white, crystalline, odorless powder. It is stable in air. It melts at about 270° with decomposition. pH of a solution (1 in 20) is between 2.5 and 3.0.

Solubility—Freely soluble in water; sparingly soluble in alcohol; practically insoluble in ether and chloroform.

Uses—Anileridine Hydrochloride is a synthetic analgesic closely related to meperidine in chemical structure and in its pharmacological actions. It appears to be about 2½ times as potent as equal amounts of meperidine and ¼ as potent as the same weight of morphine. In general, Anileridine has the same usefulness and same limitations as meperidine. It is used to relieve moderate to severe pain in many medical, surgical, obstetrical, and dental situations. Its addiction liability is equal to that of morphine.

Dose—**25** to **50 mg**; *usual,* **25 mg** of anileridine, present as the dihydrochloride, repeated every 6 hours if necessary.

Dosage Forms—Tablets NF: 25 mg.

Fentanyl Citrate

[Sublimaze, ingredient of Innovar (*McNeil*)]

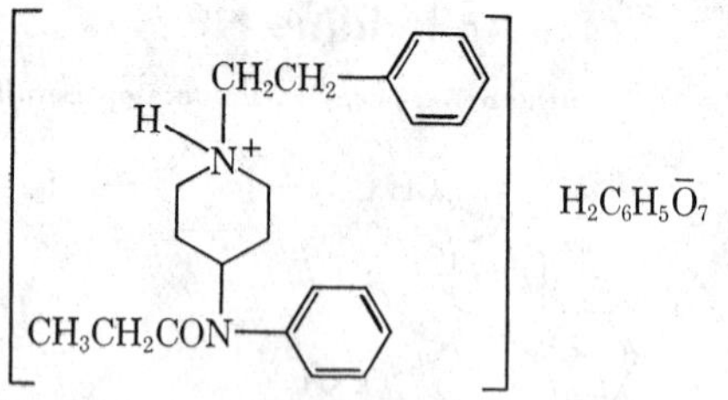

Fentanyl Citrate [$C_{22}H_{28}N_2O \cdot C_6H_8O_7$ = 528.61] is *N*-(1-phenethyl-4-piperidyl)propionanilide Citrate (1:1).

Preparation—One method of preparing fentanyl (base) consists of condensing propionyl chloride with *N*-(4-piperidyl)aniline followed by condensing the resulting *N*-(4-piperidyl)propionanilide with phenethyl chloride, aiding each condensation by the presence of a suitable dehydrochlorinating agent. Reaction of the base with an equimolar portion of citric acid yields the (1:1) citrate. US Pat. 3,164,600.

Description—A white, crystalline powder or glistening crystals that are odorless and tasteless (*Note:* because this compound is extremely potent, no taste test is recommended). It is stable in air. It melts between 147° and 152°.

Solubility—1 Gm dissolves in 40 ml of water, 140 ml of alcohol, and 350 ml of chloroform.

Uses—Fentanyl Citrate, a piperidine derivative, is a potent narcotic analgesic with a rapid onset and a short duration of action. It has a profile of pharmacologic action similar to morphine, except that it does not cause emesis or release histamine. Equianalgesia can be obtained with a dose $\frac{1}{150}$ that of morphine. After intravenous injection, peak analgesia appears within 3 to 5 minutes and lasts 30 to 60 minutes. Fentanyl produces signs and symptoms typical of narcotic analgesics, such as miosis, euphoria, and respiratory depression. Fentanyl is used primarily as an analgesic for the control of pain associated with all types of surgery. It is also an ingredient in *Fentanyl Citrate and Droperidol Injection,* page 1064. Fentanyl is contraindicated in children 2 years of age and younger, in asthmatic patients, in comatose patients, and in patients with a history of myasthenia gravis.

Dose—*Usual, intravenous* or *intramuscular,* **0.05** to **0.10 mg.**

Veterinary Dose—*Analgesic* and *ataraxic* (preceded by a standard dose of atropine sulfate), *Dogs, intramuscular,* **0.02 mg** per **pound** of body weight.

Meperidine Hydrochloride USP

[Ethyl 1-Methyl-4-phenylisonipecotate Hydrochloride; Meperidinium Chloride; Pethidine Hydrochloride; Dolantin, Dolantol, Eudolat, Isonipecaine; Mepadin (*Merrell*); Demerol Hydrochloride (*Winthrop*)]

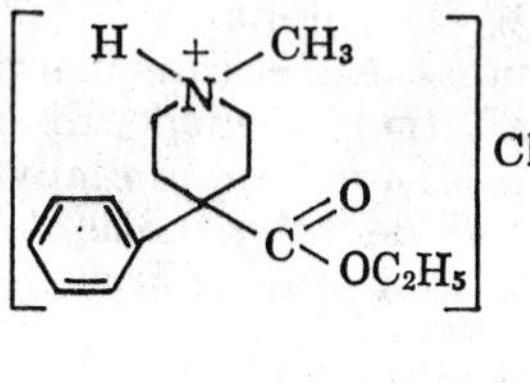

Meperidine Hydrochloride contains 98.0–101.0% of $C_{15}H_{21}NO_2 \cdot HCl$ (283.80), calculated on the dried basis.

Preparation—Meperidine Hydrochloride may be prepared by several methods. One of the better methods utilizes the commercially available benzyl chloride, diethanolamine, and benzyl cyanide in the following principal steps:

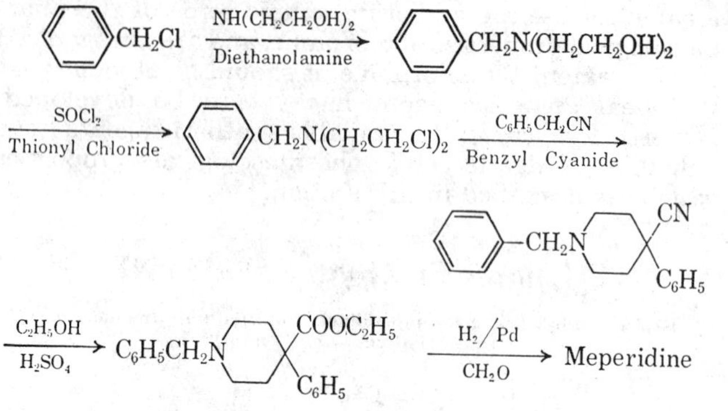

The product of the first step is not isolated but treated directly with the thionyl chloride. The alkylation-ring closure reaction of the chloramine and benzylcyanide is carried out in xylene in the presence of sodamide, resulting in the production of *N*-benzyl-4-phenyl-4-cyanopiperidine. The cyano group is converted to carbethoxy by heating the compound with ethanol and sulfuric acid. Removal of the *N*-benzyl group is accomplished by catalytic hydrogenation in acetic acid solution using a palladium catalyst. The addition of formaldehyde to the reduction mixture followed by further catalytic hydrogenation leads to meperidine. The free base is converted to the hydrochloride by neutralization with hydrochloric acid.

Description—Fine, white, crystalline, odorless powder. It is stable in air at ordinary temperatures. Its solution (1 in 20) is acid to litmus (pH is about 5). Melting range: 186° to 189°.

Solubility—Very soluble in water; soluble in alcohol; sparingly soluble in ether.

Uses—Meperidine Hydrochloride, a synthetic analgetic drug, bears chemical and pharmacological resemblances both to morphine and to atropine. Contrary to earlier claims, Meperidine Hydrochloride does not relax visceral smooth muscles and may even increase spasm in the same manner as morphine. Drowsiness and sleep occur from relatively large doses, but confusion and after-depression do not seem to result. Analgesia is possible with doses which do not cause stupefaction, a decided advantage over morphine. Pain is usually relieved within 20 minutes to 1 hour, analgesia lasting from 2 to 5 hours. The drug is far more analgetic than the salicylates and related compounds, and approaches morphine in its potency. All types of pain are relieved, and the drug has been employed in a manner similar to morphine.

Meperidine Hydrochloride causes less respiratory depression than does morphine, and large doses even cause excitement, tremors, and convulsions. Nausea and vomiting occur in about 5% of patients. Like morphine, it causes euphoria, and has *addicting* liability. Therefore it must be employed with caution. Its ability to cause drug addiction, however, is less than for morphine. Tolerance also develops to the drug but not to a significant extent. It has no untoward renal, metabolic, hepatic, or respiratory effects in the body. In general, it has all the uses of morphine, except that it has no antiperistaltic action and is not useful to stop cough or relieve dyspnea. See *Morphine*.

Nalorphine is a specific antagonist in cases of acute Meperidine intoxication.

Caution—Meperidine is a narcotic governed by the *Harrison Narcotic Act*.

Dose—*Oral* and *parenteral*, **25** to **500 mg** daily; *usual*, **50** to **100 mg** 4 to 6 times a day.

Other Dose Information—The average adult dose is 50 to 100 mg, *orally* or *intramuscularly*.

Dosage Forms—Injection USP: 20, 50, 75, and 100 mg/ml, 100 mg/2 ml, 1.5 Gm/30 ml, 2 Gm/20 ml; Syrup NF: 50 mg/5 ml; Tablets USP: 50 and 100 mg.

Veterinary Dose—*Intramuscularly, Horses* and *Cattle*, **300** to **800 mg**; *Dogs*, 5 to **10 mg** per **pound** of body weight; *Cats*, **2.5** to **5 mg** per **pound** of body weight.

Methadone Hydrochloride USP

[(±)-6-(Dimethylamino)-4,4-diphenyl-3-heptanone Hydrochloride; Amidone Hydrochloride; Dolophine Hydrochloride (*Lilly*)]

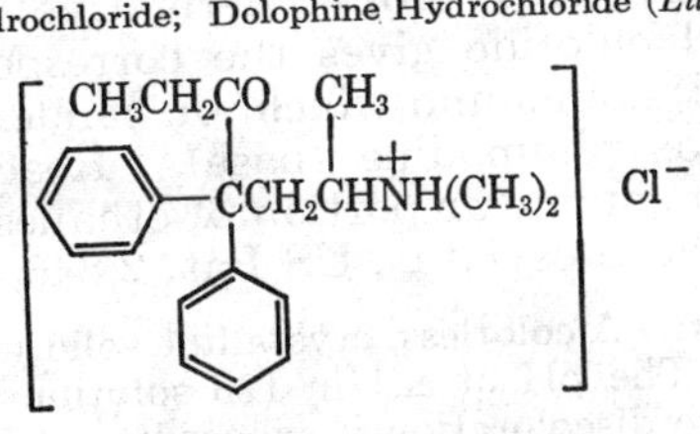

Methadone Hydrochloride contains 98.5–100.5% of $C_{21}H_{27}NO \cdot HCl$ (345.92), calculated on the dried basis.

Preparation—Diphenylacetonitrile is condensed with 2-chloro-1-dimethylaminopropane in the presence of sodamide yielding 4-(dimethylamino)-2,2-diphenyl-valeronitrile and an unwanted isomeric nitrile in approximately equal amounts. The isomers are separated and the above-named one is caused to undergo Grignard addition with ethyl magnesium bromide. Subsequent hydrolysis in the presence of hydrochloric acid yields Methadone Hydrochloride.[5]

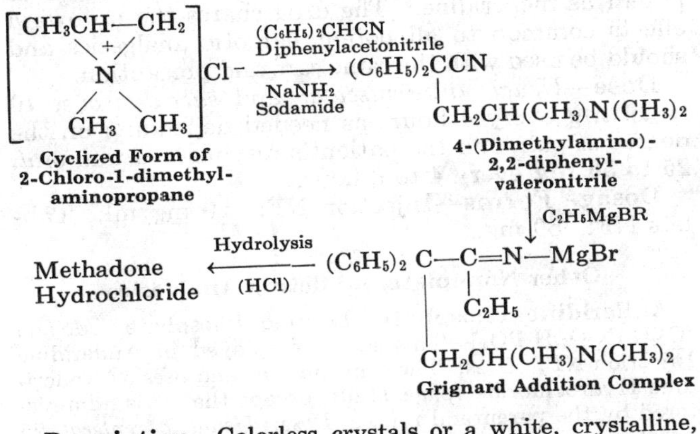

Description—Colorless crystals or a white, crystalline, odorless powder. The pH of an aqueous solution is between 4.5 and 6.5. It is optically inactive (racemic). Only the levo isomer is active analgetically.

Solubility—Soluble in water; freely soluble in alcohol and chloroform; practically insoluble in ether and glycerin.

Uses—The *analgetic* action of Methadone Hydrochloride may be somewhat greater, and its sedative, respiratory depressant and smooth muscle stimulating actions are weaker than those of morphine. Nausea and vomiting after parenteral administration are less common than with morphine, but occur not infrequently after oral administration, particularly in ambulatory pa-

tients. Methadone Hydrochloride may be substituted for morphine in the control of most types of severe pain. Tolerance develops less rapidly to Methadone Hydrochloride than to morphine. It also has useful antitussive properties, but is not desirable as a preanesthetic agent because it is not a sedative. Although dependence to it develops more slowly than to morphine, Methadone Hydrochloride possesses definite addicting properties. Euphoria is not prominent except in morphine addicts. Withdrawal symptoms are less severe and develop more slowly than with morphine, and this agent has been employed successfully as a substitute for morphine prior to morphine withdrawal to ameliorate the withdrawal symptoms.

Nalorphine is an effective antagonist in cases of acute Methadone intoxication. The use of Methadone is subject to the regulations of the *Harrison Narcotic Law*.

Dose—*Oral* or *parenteral*, **2.5** to **50 mg** daily; *usual*, **5** to **10 mg** 3 to 6 times a day.

Other Dose Information—Methadone Hydrochloride is usually employed in doses of 5.0 to 10.0 mg administered orally every 3 to 4 hours, although it may be injected intramuscularly for the rapid relief of severe pain. The usual antitussive dose is 1.0 to 2.5 mg, given orally every 3 hours if necessary.

Dosage Forms—Injection USP: 1 and 20 ml; Tablets USP: 5 mg.

Veterinary Dose—*Preanesthetic, subcutaneously, Dogs*, 1 mg per **Kg** of body weight ½ hour before administration of thiobarbiturate.

Pentazocine NF

[1,2,3,4,5,6-Hexahydro-*cis*-6,11-dimethyl-3-(3-methyl-2-butenyl)-2,6-methano 3-benzozocin-8-ol; Talwin (*Winthrop*)]

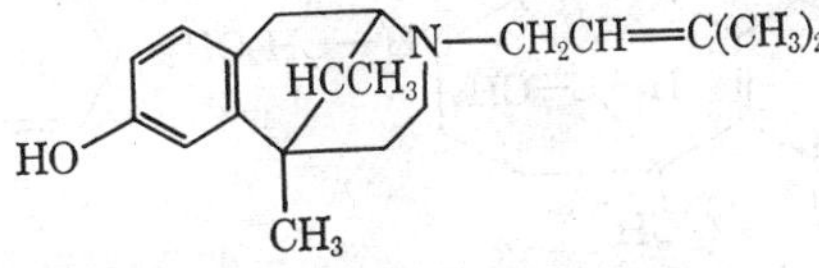

Pentazocine contains 98.0–101.5% of $C_{19}H_{27}NO$ (285.43), calculated on the dried basis.

Preparation—1,2,3,4,5,6 - Hexahydro - 6,11 - dimethyl-2,6-methano-3-benzazocin-8-ol (I) is condensed with 1-bromo-3-methyl-2-butene by refluxing in *N,N*-dimethylformamide in the presence of sodium bicarbonate. The reaction mixture is filtered and the crude Pentazocine is isolated by means of a suitable solvent extraction process and finally crystallized from aqueous methanol. US Pat. 3,250,678. The starting compound (I) may be prepared by the following route:

3,4-dimethylpyridine methiodide

p-methoxybenzylmagnesium chloride

1,3,4-trimethyl-2-(*p*-methoxybenzyl)-1,2-dihydropyridine

sodium borohydride

1,3,4-trimethyl-2-(*p*-methoxybenzyl)-1,2,5,6-tetrahydropyridine

cyclizing agent, e.g., H_3PO_4 or HBr

1,2,3,4,5,6-hexahydro-3,6,11-trimethyl-2,6-methano-3-benzazocin-8-ol

acetic anhydride; then cyanogen bromide

3-cyano-1,2,3,4,5,6-hexahydro-6,11-dimethyl-2,6-methano-3-benzazocin-8-ol acetate (ester)

dilute HCl

Compound (I)

Description—A white to very pale tan, crystalline powder that is odorless and has a slightly bitter taste. It is stable in light, in heat (ambient room temperature), and in air. It melts between 147° and 158°.

Solubility—Freely soluble in chloroform; soluble in alcohol, acetone, ether, and acidic solutions; sparingly soluble in benzene and ethyl acetate; practically insoluble in water.

Uses—Pentazocine, a benzazocine derivative, is a synthetic *analgesic* agent with narcotic antagonist properties. Pentazocine in a dose of 40 to 60 mg is equal in analgesic effectiveness to 10 mg of morphine or 60 to 70 mg of meperidine. Significant analgesia occurs within 15 to 20 minutes after intramuscular injection or 2 to 3 minutes after intravenous administration. When given in equianalgesic doses, Pentazocine produces as much sedation, dizziness, nausea, vomiting, sweating, and other subjective complaints as do morphine and other narcotic analgesics. Likewise, in equianalgesic doses it appears to be as depressant to the respiration as morphine. Pentazocine, like other narcotic antagonists, can precipitate an acute abstinence or withdrawal syndrome in patients physically dependent on narcotics. Repeated administration does not induce drug dependence of the narcotic type. The drug is not subject to federal narcotic control.

Dose—*Parenteral*, **20** to **60 mg** (as the lactate); *usual*, **30 mg** every 3 to 4 hours.

Dosage Forms—Lactate Injection NF: 30 mg (of base)/ml; Tablets: 50 mg.

Phenazocine Hydrobromide

Phenazocine Hydrobromide [$C_{22}H_{27}NO \cdot HBr$ = 402.38] is 1,2,3,4,5,6-hexahydro-6,11-dimethyl-3-phenethyl-2,6-methano-3-benzazocin-8-ol hydrobromide.

Preparation—Using phenethyl bromide instead of 1-bromo-3-methyl-2-butene, phenazocine (base) may be prepared by the method described for Pentazocine (page 1131). Conversion to the hydrobromide may be effected by passing hydrogen bromide into a solution of the base in a suitable organic solvent.

Description—Off-white to white powder. The pH of a 1% solution is 5.9 (at 26°). It melts between 163° and 166° with decomposition; the free base melts between 180° and 181°.

Solubility—Freely soluble in alcohol; sparingly soluble in water and acetone; insoluble in ether and carbon tetrachloride.

Uses—Phenazocine Hydrobromide is a non-opiate analgesic which is used as an adjunct to anesthesia (both before and during surgery), for relief of postoperative and obstetrical pain (labor and delivery, as well as postpartum pain), and for relief of other pain states, both acute and chronic. Although it is effective in smaller doses than morphine, no qualitative differences in type of analgesic activity is apparent, and it has a similar margin of safety. Side effects are usually low and consist of nausea, vomiting, and constipation. Rarely, respiratory depression, hypotension, bradycardia, and tachycardia have occurred. During labor, some patients have experienced dizziness and facial

pruritis. Phenazocine Hydrobromide has an addiction liability equal to that of morphine.

Dose—*Usual*, *intravenous* or *intramuscular*, **0.25** to **2.0 mg**, adjusted to the severity of the pain.

Dosage Forms—Injection: 2 mg/ml.

Piminodine Esylate NF

[(Ethyl 1-(3-Anilinopropyl)-4-phenylisonipecotate Monoethanesulfonate; Alvodine Ethanesulfonate (*Winthrop*)]

Piminodine Esylate contains 97.0–100.5% of $C_{23}H_{30}N_2O_2 \cdot C_2H_6O_3S$ (476.64), calculated on the dried basis.

Preparation—Normeperidine (ethyl 4-phenylisonipecotate) is condensed with 3-chloro-1-propanol to yield the 1-(3-hydroxypropyl) derivative. Treatment with thionyl chloride gives the corresponding 1-(3-chloropropyl) compound which, on condensation with aniline, yields piminodine (base). Reaction of the base with an equimolar portion of ethanesulfonic acid forms the official esylate. US Pat. 2,846,437.

Description—A colorless, crystalline solid with a slightly bitter taste. The pH of a 1 in 125 solution is about 4.8. It will undergo discoloration if exposed to strong light. It melts between 128° and 135°.

Solubility—Freely soluble in alcohol and chloroform; slightly soluble in water and ether.

Uses—A synthetic narcotic agent chemically related to meperidine and with similar properties and therapeutic uses. Its analgesic action is approximately equal to that of morphine, but its hypnotic effect is considerably less than morphine. Contrary to some claims, the drug is not entirely devoid of sedative effects. Piminodine, milligram for milligram, is about equal in analgesic potency to morphine and about 5 times as potent as meperidine. The drug shares the untoward effects common to all potent narcotic analgesics and should be used with the same care and precaution.

Dose—*Usual*, *intramuscular* and *subcutaneous*, **10** to **20 mg** every 4 hours as needed depending on the degree of pain and the patient's response; *usual*, *oral*, **25** to **50 mg** every 4 to 6 hours.

Dosage Forms—Injection NF: 20 mg/ml; Tablets NF: 50 mg.

Other Nonopiate, Addicting Analgesics

Anileridine Phosphate [Leritine Phosphate (*MSD*)] [$C_{22}H_{28}N_2O_2 \cdot H_3PO_4$]—This salt is employed in Anileridine Injection NF. *Uses:* The same actions and uses as Anileridine Hydrochloride (page 1129), except that it is administered by the parenteral route. *Dose: Usual, parenteral*, 25 to 50 mg every 4 to 6 hours.

Dextromoramide [A tartrate salt of *d*-4-[2-methyl-4-oxo-3,3-diphenyl-4-(1-pyrrolidinyl)butyl]morpholine] [$C_{25}H_{32}N_2O_2 \cdot C_4H_6O_6$]—Crystals which melt at 180–184°C, and are soluble in water. It is available as the tartrate. Its actions and uses are similar to those of methadone. Nalorphine is an effective antagonist. Adverse side effects may occur as respiratory depression, nausea, dizziness, headache, ataxia, visual disturbances, and psychic disturbances. It is contraindicated in asthma and depressed respiratory states. *Uses:* Narcotic analgesic, claimed to be more potent than morphine and less addictive. *Dose: Intravenously*, 1 to 2 mg; *orally, rectally,* or *intramuscularly*, 5 to 20 mg.

Dipipanone Hydrochloride BP [*dl*-4,4-diphenyl-6-piperidinoheptan-3-one hydrochloride] [C$_{24}$H$_{31}$NO.HCl]—A white, crystalline powder; almost odorless; bitter taste followed by a sensation of numbness and burning. Soluble in 40 parts of water, 1.5 parts of alcohol, and 6 parts of acetone; insoluble in ether. It melts between 124° and 127°. *Uses:* Narcotic analgesic. *Dose: Subcutaneous or intramuscular,* 25 to 50 mg.

Phenadoxone Hydrochloride [Morphodone Hydrochloride; 6-Morpholino-4,4-diphenyl-3-heptanone hydrochloride] [C$_{23}$H$_{29}$NO$_2$.HCl]—A colorless crystalline powder with a bitter taste. It is soluble in 25 parts water and in 10 parts alcohol. *Uses:* Narcotic analgesic causing true addiction. *Dose: Orally,* 2 to 50 mg; *subcutaneously or intramuscularly,* 5 to 15 mg.

Nonaddicting Analgesics and Antipyretics

The analgesic and antipyretic drugs include a small, heterogeneous group of compounds which, unlike those presented in the two preceding sections, are without addiction liability. Most of these agents affect both pain and fever. Consequently, they are widely used for minor aches and pains, headaches, and the general feeling of malaise that accompanies febrile illnesses, and to alleviate the symptoms of rheumatic fever, arthritis, gout, and other musculoskeletal disturbances. Colchicine is included for its pain-relieving properties in acute gout, but since it is of no value in other types of pain, it cannot be classed as a true analgesic.

Acetaminophen NF

[4'-Hydroxyacetanilide; N-Acetyl-p-aminophenol; p-Acetamidophenol; Tempra (*Mead-Johnson*); Tylenol (*McNeil*)]

HO—⟨⟩—NHCOCH$_3$

Acetaminophen contains 98.0–100.5% of C$_8$H$_9$NO$_2$ (151.17), calculated on the anhydrous basis.

Preparation—p-Nitrophenol is reduced and the resulting p-aminophenol is acetylated by heating with a mixture of acetic anhydride and glacial acetic acid. The crude product may be purified by recrystallization from an ethanol–water mixture or from other suitable solvents.

Description—White, odorless, crystalline powder, possessing a slightly bitter taste. It melts between 169° and 172°. The pH of a saturated solution is between 5.5 and 6.5.

Solubility—1 Gm dissolves in about 20 ml of boiling water, about 10 ml of alcohol, and about 15 ml of sodium hydroxide.

Uses—Acetaminophen, an analgesic compound said to be formed in the decomposition of acetanilid and acetophenetidin, is used to relieve the pain of headaches, myalgias, arthralgic, and other pains arising from muscles and joints, and peripheral nerve affections. Acetaminophen lacks the anti-inflammatory action of aspirin; hence, it is of only limited usefulness in inflammatory rheumatic disorders. It is less toxic than the salicylates and does not produce the methemoglobinemia, agranulocytosis, anemia, and liver damage which sometimes results from the long continued use of acetanilid and acetophenetidin. Although kidney damage has not been reported as due to this agent, it should be remembered that this is a decomposition product of phenacetin. The label on Acetaminophen drugs carries the following statement: *Warning—Do not give to children under 3 years of age or use for more than 10 days unless directed by a physician.*

Dose—**325** to **650 mg,** not to exceed 2.6 Gm per 24-hour period; *usual,* **650 mg** every 4 hours.

Dosage Forms—Elixir NF: 100 mg/ml, 120 mg/5 ml; Tablets NF: 325 mg.

Allopurinol USP

[1*H*-Pyrazolo[3,4-*d*]-pyrimidin-4-ol; Zyloprim (*Burroughs-Wellcome*)]

Allopurinol contains 97.0–102.0% of C$_5$H$_4$N$_4$O (136.11), calculated on the dried basis.

Preparation—(Ethoxymethylene)malononitrile is reacted with hydrazine hydrate via deethanolation and addition thus cyclizing to form 3-aminopyrazole-4-carbonitrile. Controlled hydration of the nitrile forms the corresponding carboxamide which, on condensation with formamide, yields Allopurinol. US Pat. 2,868,803.

Description—A fluffy white to off-white powder which has only a slight odor and is tasteless. It is stable in light and air. It melts above 300° with decomposition.

Solubility—Soluble in solutions of fixed alkali hydroxides and dimethylsulfoxide; very slightly soluble in alcohol; insoluble in water and common organic solvents.

Uses—Allopurinol is used in the long-term treatment of *gout.* It has also been used as adjunctive therapy to the uricosuric drugs. Allopurinol is not uricosuric; it inhibits xanthine oxidase, thus preventing the formation of uric acid from xanthine. It is particularly useful in patients who are resistant to or cannot tolerate uricosuric drugs and in patients with renal function so reduced as to not respond to conventional drugs. Allopurinol precipitates acute gouty arthritis in early therapy more frequently than uricosuric drugs. This can be minimized by starting therapy on a small dose and increasing the dose gradually. Untoward effects include a rash, usually maculopapular; less frequently exfoliative, urticarial, or purpuric; the rash may be accompanied by fever, leukopenia, arthralgias, or other symptoms of hypersensitivity. Diarrhea is frequently observed. Isolated cases of peripheral neuritis, depression of the bone marrow, cataracts, and reversible hepatic damage have been reported. Allopurinol has been observed in experimental studies to increase hepatic iron concentration; therefore, it should not be administered with iron. The drug should not be used during pregnancy or lactation.

Dose—**100** to **600 mg** daily; *usual,* **100 mg** 3 times a day.

Dosage Forms—Tablets USP: 100 mg.

Antipyrine NF

[2,3-Dimethyl-1-phenyl-3-pyrazolin-5-one; Analgesine; Parodyne; Phenazone; Sedatine]

Antipyrine, dried at 60° for 2 hours, contains 99.0–100.5% of $C_{11}H_{12}N_2O$ (188.23).

Preparation—Antipyrine, discovered by Knorr in 1883, is made by condensing equivalent quantities of ethyl acetoacetate and phenylhydrazine, the latter being used in a benzene solution. After heating to evaporate the benzene, 1-phenyl-3-methylpyrazolon is obtained which, upon methylation with a suitable methylating agent (methyl iodide or dimethyl sulfate), yields Antipyrine.

Description—Colorless crystals, or a white crystalline powder. It is odorless, has a slightly bitter taste, and its solutions are neutral to litmus. Melting range 110° to 112.5°.

Solubility—1 Gm dissolves in less than 1 ml of water, 1.3 ml of alcohol, 1 ml of chloroform, and 43 ml of ether.

Incompatibilities—Antipyrine liquefies or forms a soft mass when triturated with *acetanilid, chloral hydrate, phenyl salicylate, resorcinol, sodium salicylate, or thymol*. When triturated with *calomel* in the presence of (atmospheric) moisture, the powder darkens and the calomel is partially decomposed into mercuric chloride and metallic mercury. It is precipitated by *alkaloidal precipitants* such as *tannic acid, iodine, potassium mercuric iodide*, etc.

Ferric salts cause a red color; *acacia* a brown; *nitric acid* a yellow which later turns red.

Uses—Antipyrine is an *analgetic* and *antipyretic*. Its field of usefulness is similar to that for sodium salicylate and aspirin, except that it is not employed in gout or acute rheumatic fever. Antipyrine is traditionally employed more for its antipyretic action than for analgesia, but there is no sound pharmacological basis for this practice. It shares the local antiseptic property of the salicylates, but is too weak in its action to be of medicinal value. Antipyrine is also a weak local anesthetic, but the former practice of using it on the mucosa of the mouth, nose, and throat is obsolete.

Dose—See *Antipyrine and Benzocaine Solution*.

Veterinary Dose—*Horses*, 8 to **15 Gm**; *Cattle*, **12 to 25 Gm**; *Sheep* and *Swine*, 0.5 to 2 **Gm**; *Dogs*, 200 to **600 mg**; *Cats*, 60 to 200 mg.

Antipyrine and Benzocaine Solution NF [Auralgan (*Ayerst*)] is a solution of antipyrine and benzocaine in glycerin. It contains 90.0–110.0% of the labeled amounts of $C_{11}H_{12}N_2O$ (antipyrine) and $C_9H_{11}NO_2$ (benzocaine). *Uses*: Antipyrine and Benzocaine Solution represents an approximately 4 to 1 mixture of these agents in glycerin. It is indicated for the relief of pain and the reduction of inflammation in the congestive and serous stages of acute otitis media; and for the relief of minor discomfort of the ear such as "swimmer's ear." It is also useful for children, and in facilitating the removal of excessive or impacted cerumen. Antipyrine and Benzocaine Solution can also be used as adjuvant therapy when antibiotics or sulfonamides are administered systematically for ear infections. *Application*: Instilled into the ear canal from 3 times a day to every 1 to 2 hours as needed.

Aspirin USP

[Salicylic Acid Acetate; Acetylsalicylic Acid USP XVI; Acetosal; Acetosalin; Empirin; Aspro; Aceticyl; Acetophen; Saletin; Salacetin; Helicon; Salcetogen]

Aspirin contains 99.5–100.5% of $C_9H_8O_4$ (180.16), calculated on the dried basis.

Preparation—Salicylic acid is acetylated directly with acetic anhydride and the crude material is purified by recrystallization from benzene or various other nonaqueous solvents.

A granulated form of Aspirin, either white or colored, is also available commercially for compression into tablets.

Description—White crystals, commonly tabular or needle-like, or a white, crystalline powder. It is odorless or has a faint odor and is stable in dry air, but in moist air it gradually hydrolyzes into salicylic and acetic acids, the odor of the latter becoming noticeable. It melts at about 135°, but the exact melting temperature varies with the conditions of the test. An alcoholic solution of the Acid is not colored violet by ferric chloride (distinction from salicylic acid).

Solubility—1 Gm dissolves in about 300 ml of water, 5 ml of alcohol, 17 ml of chloroform, and from 10 to 15 ml of ether; less soluble in absolute ether; dissolves with decomposition in aqueous solutions of alkali hydroxides and carbonates.

Incompatibilities—Aspirin can form a damp to pasty mass when triturated with *acetanilid, acetophenetidin, antipyrine, aminopyrine, methenamine, phenol*, or *phenyl salicylate*. Powders containing acetylsalicylic acid with an alkali salt such as *sodium bicarbonate* may become gummy on contact with atmospheric moisture due to a partial solution and subsequent hydrolysis of the acetylsalicylic acid. Hydrolysis likewise occurs in admixture with salts containing water of crystallization.

Solutions of the alkaline acetates and citrates, as well as alkalies themselves, dissolve acetylsalicylic acid, but the resulting solutions hydrolyze rapidly to form salts of acetic and salicylic acids. Sugar and glycerin have been shown to hinder the decomposition.

Aspirin very slowly liberates hydriodic acid from *potassium* or *sodium iodide*. Subsequent oxidation by the air produces free iodine.

Uses—Aspirin, as well as the salts of salicylic acid (for example, sodium salicylate), is employed as an *antipyretic* and *analgetic* in a variety of conditions. The popular opinion that aspirin is harmful to the heart has no foundation in fact. Likewise, it is not true that aspirin prevents or relieves colds or acute respiratory infections, although it may afford some symptomatic relief. Many individuals employ Aspirin as a gargle for sore throats, but a warm aqueous moderately hypertonic sodium chloride solution does as much good. In *gout* and in *acute rheumatic fever*, the salicylates, including Aspirin, have a fairly specific action. In gout, large doses must be given fairly often, and the results obtained are somewhat less dramatic than with phenylbutazone or allopurinol. In acute rheumatic fever, full doses are given every hour until salicylism occurs (ringing in ears, dizziness), and then every 4 hours for days or weeks. In neither of the above-mentioned conditions are the salicylates a cure, and other forms of treatment are simultaneously employed.

Aspirin is more potent on a weight basis than the salts of salicylic acid, and also is less irritating to the gastric mucosa. However, the two major gastrointestinal disturbances caused by Aspirin are *dyspepsia* (heart burn) and *bleeding*. The causes of the dyspepsia are not known. Occult gastrointestinal bleeding is observed only after chronic treatment with large doses (3.6 Gm daily).

Salicylates account for approximately 25% of all accidental poisonings, and may result from the promiscuous use of large doses of these agents by the laity. In addition, some few people manifest idiosyncrasy in the form of an allergic sensitivity to salicylates, especially aspirin, and may suffer from serious if not fatal asthma after ingestion of a single 0.3-Gm dose.

Dose—*Oral*, **300 mg** to **8 Gm** daily; *rectal*, **300 mg** to **2 Gm** daily; *usual, oral or rectal*, **600 mg** 4 to 6 times a day as necessary.

Dosage Forms—Capsules NF: 300 mg; Suppositories USP: 60, 125, 200, 300, and 600 mg; Tablets USP: 60, 75, 200, 300, 500, and 600 mg; Aspirin, Phenacetin, and Caffeine Tablets NF (APC Tablets): 230 mg (aspirin), 150 mg (phenacetin), and 15 and 30 mg (caffeine).

Veterinary Dose—*Horses* and *Cattle*, **10** to **50 Gm**; *Sheep* and *Swine*, **1** to **3 Gm**; *Dogs*, **0.25** to **1 Gm**; *Cats*, **100** to **200 mg**. In the last two species, gastric irritation, toxicity, and death have been reported following therapeutic doses.

Aluminum Aspirin NF

[Hydroxybis(salicylato)aluminum Diacetate; Aluminum Acetylsalicylate; Aspirin Dulcet (*Abbott*)]

Aluminum Aspirin contains not less than the equivalent of 80.0% of $C_9H_8O_4$ (aspirin), calculated on the anhydrous basis, corresponding to not less than 90.0% of $C_{18}H_{15}AlO_9$ (402.30). Aluminum Aspirin yields 12.0–17.0% of Al_2O_3 (aluminum oxide = 101.96), calculated on the anhydrous basis.

Preparation—An aqueous solution of sodium acetylsalicylate (prepared by treating a suspension of aspirin with a not greater than 50% stoichiometric excess of sodium carbonate) is treated with an amount of aqueous aluminum chloride solution sufficient to react with both the sodium acetylsalicylate and the surplus sodium carbonate. The gelatinous precipitate which forms consists of a mixture of aluminum aspirin and aluminum hydroxide. It is collected by filtration, washed, and dried.

Description—White to off-white powder or granules. Odorless, or has only a slight odor.

Solubility—Insoluble in water and organic solvents; soluble, with decomposition, in aqueous solutions of alkali hydroxides and carbonates.

Uses—Aluminum Aspirin is used as an analgesic and antipyretic when a salicylate effect is desired. It is reported to be relatively free from acetic odor and taste, to possess greater physical stability than aspirin, and to be absorbed as readily after oral administration as aspirin. Untoward effects are characteristic of the salicylates.

Dose—*Usual*, **670 mg**, equivalent to about 600 mg of aspirin, every 4 hours as necessary; *children's dose*, **75 mg** every 4 hours.

Dosage Forms—Tablets NF: 75 mg.

Carbamazepine—see page 1103.

Colchicine USP

Colchicine [$C_{22}H_{25}NO_6$ = 399.45] is an alkaloid obtained fron various species of *Colchicum*.

Caution—*Colchicine is extremely poisonous.*

Preparation—Colchicine may be obtained by extracting the corm or seed with alcohol. After distilling off the alcohol, the syrupy residue is diluted with water to precipitate fats and resins and filtered. The filtrate is digested with some lead carbonate, refiltered, evaporated to a small volume and extracted with chloroform. Upon concentration of the chloroform solution the colchicine crystallizes out with 2 moles of chloroform of crystallization. When these crystals are heated with water the chloroform is dispelled.

Description—Pale yellow, amorphous scales, or powder. It is odorless or nearly so, and darkens on exposure to light. It melts at about 145°. Colchicine is levorotatory in chloroform and in aqueous solution, showing in the latter solvent an $[\alpha]_D^{25}$ of −410° to −435°.

Solubility—1 Gm dissolves in 25 ml of water and about 220 ml of ether; freely soluble in alcohol and chloroform.

Uses—Colchicine is the agent of choice in the symptomatic treatment of *acute* attacks of *gout*. It is also used in combination with either phenylbutazone, oxyphenbutazone, or allopurinol in the management of acute gout. Its mechanism of action is unknown, and it appears to differ from the salicylates and cinchophen in its metabolic effects in gout. It is practically useless in chronic gout but its routine administration does lessen the frequency and severity of acute attacks. The alkaloid is very toxic, and its use should be discontinued at the first evidence of toxicity, namely, diarrhea, nausea, vomiting, and abdominal pain.

Dose—**1** to **8 mg** daily, *usual, initial*, **1 mg** every 1 or 2 hours for 6 to 8 doses, as tolerated; *maintenance*, **500 mcg** 2 times a day.

Dosage Forms—Tablets USP: 500 and 600 mcg.

Ethoheptazine Citrate NF

[Ethyl Hexahydro-1-methyl-4-phenyl-1*H*-azepine-4-carboxylate Citrate (1:1); Zactane Citrate (*Wyeth*)]

Ethoheptazine Citrate, dried at 60° in vacuum for 3 hours, contains 97.0–102.0% of $C_{16}H_{23}NO_2 \cdot C_6H_8O_7$ (453.49).

Preparation—4 - (Dimethylamino) - 2 - phenylbutyronitrile is cyclized with 1-bromo-3-chloropropane in the presence of sodamide to yield the quaternized nitrile (I). After dequaternization by refluxing in tetralin and conversion of cyano to ethoxycarbonyl by treating with ethanolic HCl, ethoheptazine base is liberated by alkalinization, extracted with ether, and reacted with an equimolar portion of citric acid.

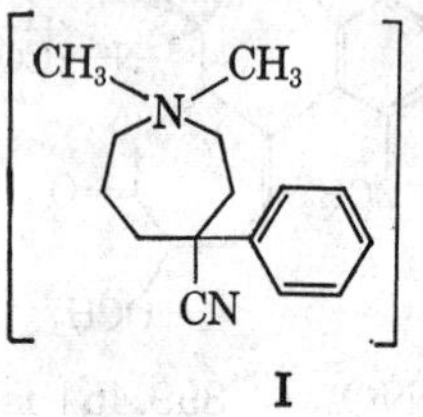

I

Description—Occurs as a white to nearly white, practically odorless powder.

Solubility—Sparingly soluble in water; very slightly soluble in alcohol; insoluble in ether.

Uses—A synthetic, nonnarcotic analgesic of moderate potency, structurally related to meperidine. It is ineffective in relieving severe pain and less effective than aspirin for postpartum pain. A combination of this drug with aspirin appears to be as effective as codeine and aspirin combination for relief of pain in arthritis and other musculoskeletal disorders. Ethoheptazine is apparently devoid of antipyretic, anti-inflammatory, and addicting properties. The incidence of side effects after usual doses of this drug is relatively low. Nausea, vomiting, epigastric distress, dizziness, and pruritus have been observed. Its metabolic fate and routes of excretion are unknown.

Dose—75 to **150 mg**; *usual*, **75 mg** 3 or 4 times a day.

Dosage Forms—Tablets NF: 75 mg.

Veterinary Dose—*Dogs* and *Cats*, **75 to 150 mg** 3 or 4 times a day depending on the severity of pain.

Indomethacin NF

[1-(*p*-Chlorobenzoyl)-5-methoxy-2-methylindole-3-acetic Acid;   Indocin (*MSD*)]

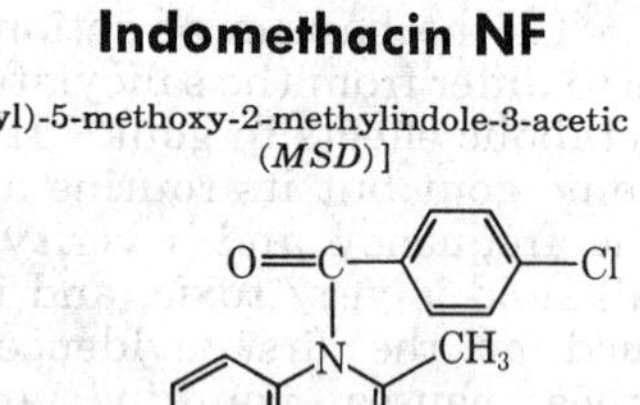

Indomethacin contains 98.0–101.0% of $C_{19}H_{16}$-$ClNO_4$ (357.80), calculated on the dried basis.

Preparation—*p*-Anisidine is diazotized and the diazonium compound reduced with sodium sulfite. The resulting *p*-methoxyphenylhydrazine is caused to undergo the Fisher indole synthesis with methyl levulinate. The steps involved include formation of the hydrazone (I), rearrangement of (I) to the enamine compound (II), and cyclization of (II) through

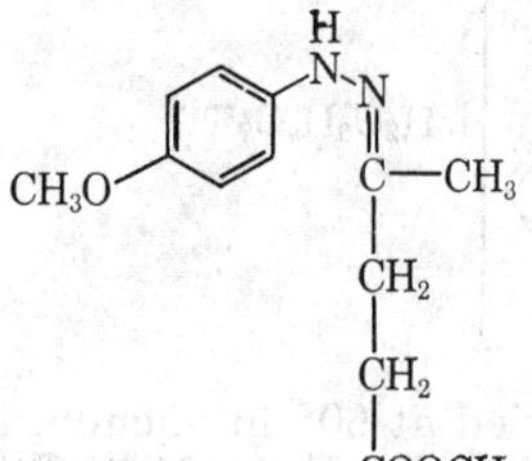

(I) 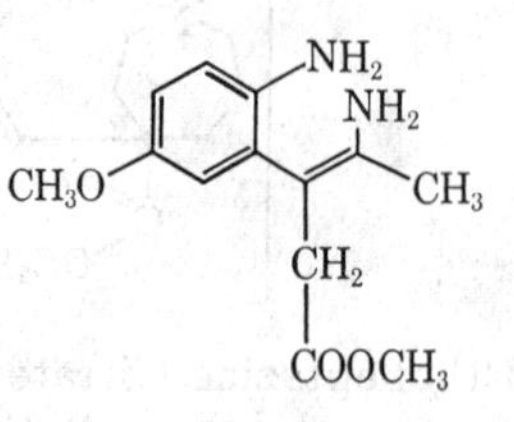   (II)

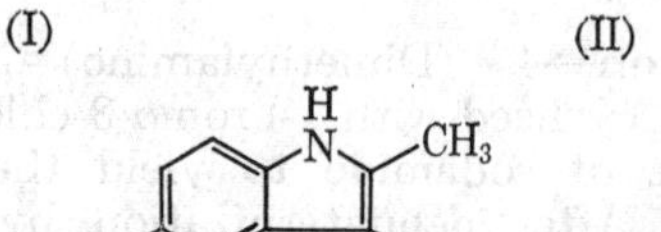

(III)

loss of ammonia to form (III).   (III) is then hydrolyzed to the acid which is re-esterified via the anhydride to give the *tert*-butyl ester.   Acylation with *p*-chloroacetyl chloride followed by debutylation yields Indomethacin.   US Pat. 3,161,654.

Description—A pale-yellow to yellow-tan, crystalline powder that is odorless, or has a slight odor, and has a slightly bitter taste. It is light-sensitive, stable in air, and stable in heat under the usual prevailing temperature conditions. One polymorphic form melts at about 155°, the other at about 162°.

Solubility—1 Gm dissolves in about 30 ml of chloroform, about 45 ml of ether, and about 50 ml of alcohol; practically insoluble in water.

Uses—Indomethacin is a nonsteroid indole derivative used for the treatment of *rheumatoid arthritis, ankylosing (rheumatoid) spondylitis, osteoarthritis,* and *gouty arthritis*. It exhibits both analgesic and anti-inflammatory properties. A mass of conflicting studies on Indomethacin have appeared since it was introduced in 1965. Despite conflicting reports, Indomethacin appears to be a useful drug, but its usefulness is compromised by frequent and sometimes severe side effects. The drug appears to have about the same anti-inflammatory and analgesic effectiveness as aspirin in patients with rheumatoid arthritis and effectiveness similar to phenylbutazone in ankylosing spondylitis. Indomethacin also appears to be effective in the treatment of acute gouty arthritis; some reports indicate that it acts more rapidly than colchicine or phenylbutazone in this condition. The incidence of untoward effects has been reported to vary from a few percent to 75% of patients. Most frequent untoward actions include headaches, vertigo, and gastrointestinal disturbances. Peptic ulceration with bleeding, cholestatic jaundice, and mental depression have been observed. Leukopenia, thrombocytopenia, and agranulocytosis have also been reported. Indomethacin is said to decrease resistance to infection and to activate latent infections. Both the incidence and severity of side effects appear to be dose related.

Dose—*Usual*, **25** or **50 mg** 2 or 3 times a day.

Other Dose Information—The dose is gradually increased until optimum control is achieved. A dose of 150 mg a day should not be exceeded because of the high incidence of adverse effects.

Dosage Forms—Capsules NF: 25 and 50 mg.

Mefenamic Acid

[Ponstel (*Parke-Davis*)]

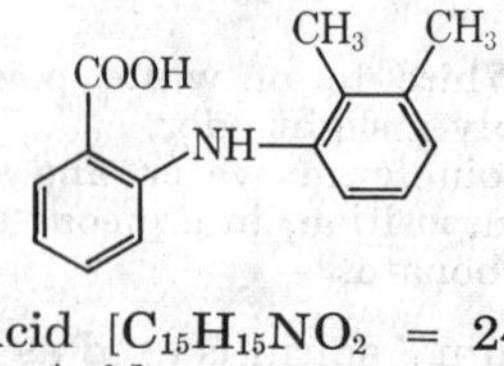

Mefenamic Acid [$C_{15}H_{15}NO_2$ = 241.28] is *N*-(2,3-xylyl)anthranilic Acid.

Preparation—*o*-Benzoyl chloride is condensed with 2,3-xylidine with the aid of potassium carbonate and the resulting potassium salt is treated with mineral acid to liberate the desired acid.   US Pat. 3,138,636.

Description—A white to off-white, crystalline powder that is odorless and has very little initial taste, but it has a bitter aftertaste. It darkens on prolonged exposure to light, is nonhygroscopic, and is stable at 25°, 37°, and 45°; it decarboxylates at temperatures above its melting point (at 300°, 100% is decarboxylated in 3 min). It melts between 227° and 232°.

Solubility—1 Gm dissolves in 26 ml of dimethylformamide and 220 ml of alcohol; insoluble in water.

Uses—Mefenamic Acid is an anthranilic acid drug which is claimed to have *analgesic, antipyretic*, and *anti-inflammatory properties*. It is promoted for the management of *pain* not severe enough to require narcotics. The margin of safety of Mefenamic Acid is reduced at higher doses and after long administration; hence, *it is used only for short term therapy not exceeding one week in duration*. Untoward effects include diarrhea, gastrointestinal ulcerations and bleeding, headache, drowsiness, nausea, and nervousness. Evidence of renal, hepatic, and hematopoietic toxicity has also been reported. Although no direct connection has been established, agranulocytosis, thrombocytopenic purpura, and megaloblastic anemia have occurred in patients on the drug. Until the full range of toxicity has been firmly established, physicians would be well advised to use the more well established analgesic agents.

Dose—*Usual*, **500 mg**, followed by **250 mg** every 6 hours.

Caution: Do not use for more than 7 days.

Dosage Forms—Capsules: 250 mg.

Methotrimeprazine NF

[10-[3-(Dimethylamino)-2-methylpropyl]-2-methoxyphenothiazine; Levoprome (*Lederle*)]

Methotrimeprazine contains 98.0–101.0% of $C_{19}H_{24}N_2OS$ (328.48), calculated on the dried basis.

Preparation—Methotrimeprazine may be prepared by the following route: (1) condensation of *o*-chlorobenzoic acid with *m*-anisidine via dehydrochlorination with potassium carbonate and a copper catalyst to form 2-(*m*-anisidino)benzoic acid; (2) decarboxylation of the acid via pyrolysis to form 3-methoxydiphenylamine; (3) cyclization of the amine by heating with sulfur to form 2-methoxyphenothiazine; and (4) condensation of the 2-methoxyphenothiazine with 2-methyl-3-(dimethylamino)propyl chloride via dehydrochlorination with sodamide.

Description—A fine, white, practically odorless, crystalline powder. It is unstable in light and nonhygroscopic. It melts at about 126°.

Solubility—Practically insoluble in water; sparingly soluble in methanol; freely soluble in chloroform and ether; sparingly soluble in alcohol at 25° but is freely soluble in boiling alcohol.

Uses—Methotrimeprazine, a phenothiazine derivative, is a *nonaddicting analgesic drug*. It is available only in a form for intramuscular administration. It is as effective as morphine or meperidine in relieving severe pain; 20 mg of Methotrimeprazine is approximately as effective as 10 mg of morphine or 75 mg of meperidine in postoperative pain and pain associated with cancer. The drug produces marked sedation and hypotension, which limit its use to nonambulatory patients. Preliminary studies indicate that usual doses of Methotrimeprazine does not depress respiration; thus, it may be particularly useful for obstetrical

analgesia and in patients with pulmonary insufficiency. Methotrimeprazine has also been employed as preanesthetic medication; it provides deeper and longer lasting sedation than morphine or meperidine. Although this drug shares the antiemetic properties of the phenothiazines, the effect of this agent on the incidence of postoperative nausea and vomiting has not been adequately investigated. Untoward effects, other than the previously mentioned sedation and orthostatic hypotension, include disorientation, nasal stuffiness, and urinary retention. Agranulocytosis and cholestatic jaundice have been reported in some patients on long-term, high-dosage therapy with the drug. Since this is a phenothiazine, the physician should be alert for other untoward effects characteristic of these agents.

Dose—*Intramuscular*, **5 to 40 mg**; *usual*, **10 to 30 mg** every 4 to 6 hours.

Other Dose Information—For preanesthetic medication, intramuscularly, 10 to 20 mg.

Dosage Forms—Injection NF: 20 mg/ml.

Oxyphenbutazone NF

[4-Butyl-1-(*p*-hydroxyphenyl)-2-phenyl-3,5-pyrazolidinedione; Tandearil (*Geigy*)]

Oxyphenbutazone [$C_{19}H_{20}N_2O_3 \cdot H_2O$ = 342.40] contains 98.0–100.5% of $C_{19}H_{20}N_2O_3$, calculated on the anhydrous basis.

Preparation—Diethyl butylmalonate is condensed with *p*-benzyloxyhydrazobenzene, with the aid of a solution of sodium ethoxide in anhydrous ethanol, to form 1-(*p*-benzyloxy)-2-phenyl-4-butyl-3,5-pyrazolidinedione (I). Completion of the reaction is effected by adding xylene and heating the mixture to about 140° for several hours, thus removing the alcohol released by the cyclizing condensation. Debenzylation of (I) is effected by Raney nickel hydrogenation at ambient temperature and pressure. Recrystallization of the initial product is via ether/petroleum ether. US Pat. 2,745,783.

Description—White, crystalline compound melting as the monohydrate at approx. 96°.

Solubility—Soluble in ethanol, methanol, chloroform, benzene, and ether; easily soluble in water as the sodium salt.

Uses—A derivative of phenylbutazone which exhibits the same antipyretic and analgesic properties as the parent drug. Except that Oxyphenbutazone causes less gastrointestinal distress, its effectiveness, indications, contraindications, and adverse reactions are the same as those for *Phenylbutazone*, page 1138.

Dose—**100 to 600 mg**; *usual*, **400 mg** daily in divided doses.

Other Dose Information—It should always be taken immediately after meals or with a full glass of milk, to minimize gastric irritation.

Dosage Forms—Tablets NF: 100 mg.

Phenacetin USP

[Acetophenetidin USP XVI; Acetphenetidin; *p*-Acetophenetidide; *p*-Ethoxyacetanilid]

$$C_2H_5O-\langle\bigcirc\rangle-NHCOCH_3$$

Phenacetin contains 98.0–101.0% of $C_{10}H_{13}NO_2$ (179.22), calculated on the dried basis.

Preparation—*o*-Nitrophenol, dissolved in sodium hydroxide solution, is condensed with ethyl bromide or another suitable ethylating agent and the *p*-nitrophenetole so obtained is reduced with sodium sulfide or other suitable reductant. The resulting *p*-phenetidine is acetylated by refluxing with acetic anhydride.

Description—White, glistening crystals, usually in scales, or as a fine, white, crystalline powder. It is odorless, has a slightly bitter taste, and is stable in air. Its saturated solution is neutral to litmus. Melting range 134° to 136°.

Solubility—1 Gm dissolves in about 1300 ml of water, 15 ml of alcohol, 15 ml of chloroform, and about 130 ml of ether; 1 Gm dissolves in 85 ml of boiling water and about 3 ml of boiling alcohol.

Incompatibilities—Phenacetin forms eutectics with *aspirin, aminopyrine, chloral hydrate,* etc. It is decomposed by *alkalies* or *strong acids*. *Oxidizing agents* usually produce a red color. *Ethyl nitrite spirit* slowly gives a yellow color which finally deepens into a reddish brown. With *iodine* an insoluble compound is formed.

Uses—Phenacetin is an *analgetic* and *antipyretic* having the same general field of usefulness as the salicylates. Phenacetin, however, lacks the specific effect on the polyarthritis of acute rheumatic fever, and therefore is not used in this syndrome. Also, it lacks the uricosuric action of the salicylates in gout, and is not employed in this disease. In general, the compound is more toxic than salicylates and cannot be employed so continuously or in such large doses. Methemoglobinemia, sulfhemoglobinemia, and hemolytic anemia are chief toxic effects. Excessive use of Phenacetin may cause severe renal injury. Hence, all preparations containing Phenacetin must carry the following statement: *Warning—This medication may damage the kidneys when used in large amounts or for a long period of time. Do not take more than the recommended dosage, nor take regularly for longer than 10 days without consulting your physician.* However, kidney damage is unlikely if Phenacetin is taken in doses less than 1 Gm daily and for short periods of time.

Phenacetin owes its pharmacological activity to *N*-acetyl-*p*-aminophenol, to which it is largely altered in the body. See *Acetaminophen* (page 1133).

Dose—**300 mg** to **2 Gm** daily; *usual,* **300 mg** 4 to 6 times a day.

Dosage Forms—Tablets USP: 300 mg.

Veterinary Dose—*Horses* and *Cattle,* **6 to 25 Gm;** *Sheep, Swine,* and *Goats,* **2 Gm;** *Dogs,* **100 mg to 1 Gm.**

Phenylbutazone USP

[4-Butyl-1,2-diphenyl-3,5-pyrazolidinedione; Butazolidin (*Geigy*)]

Phenylbutazone contains 98.0–100.5% of $C_{19}H_{20}N_2O_2$ (308.38), calculated on the dried basis.

Preparation—Butylmalonyl chloride is condensed with hydrazobenzene in ether solution at 0°C with the aid of pyridine. After extracting the pyridine with aqueous HCl, the phenylbutazone is extracted with aqueous Na_2CO_3 and then precipitated by addition of HCl. US Pat. 2,562,830.

Description—A white to off-white, odorless, crystalline powder.

Solubility—1 Gm dissolves in about 20 ml of alcohol; very slightly soluble in water; freely soluble in acetone and ether.

Uses—Phenylbutazone, a synthetic pyrazolone derivative chemically related to aminopyrine, exerts similar analgesic and antipyretic properties in animals. It is used chiefly in the treatment of acute gout which has failed to respond to colchicine, and, to a lesser extent, ankylosing spondylitis, rheumatoid arthritis, painful shoulder, and, occasionally, osteoarthritis. Phenylbutazone produces untoward effects in about 40% of patients; approximately 15% have to discontinue the drug because of toxic effect. Consequently, Phenylbutazone should be employed only in those patients who fail adequately to respond to less hazardous substances. The most frequently encountered untoward effects are water retention, nausea, rash, epigastric pain, vertigo, and stomatitis. Other less frequent but more severe effects include hepatitis, hypertension, transient psychosis, moderate leukopenia, agranulocytosis, and thrombocytopenia. Central nervous system stimulation, visual symptoms, anemia, lethargy, constipation, diarrhea, gastrointestinal hemorrhage, fever, and cardiac arrhythmias have also been observed.

Phenylbutazone is contraindicated in the presence of edema, threatened cardiac decompensation, and patients with peptic ulcer and a history of allergy or blood dyscrasia. It should not be used in patients on coumarin drugs, since it displaces the latter from protein binding sites, thus potentiating the anticoagulant action.

This drug should be taken with milk or with meals to minimize gastric irritation.

Dose—**100** to **600 mg** daily; *usual,* **100 mg** 1 to 4 times a day.

Dosage Forms—Tablets USP: 100 mg.

Veterinary Dose—*Horses, oral,* **2 to 4 Gm** per **1000 pounds** of body weight, not to exceed 4 Gm daily; *intravenous,* **1 to 2 Gm** per **1000 pounds** of body weight, by slow and careful injection; limit administration to a maximum of 5 successive days. *Dogs, oral,* **100 mg** per **5 pounds** of body weight in 3 divided doses daily (a maximum of 800 mg per day regardless of weight); *intravenous,* **10 mg** per **pound** of body weight, not to exceed 800 mg daily, by slow injection with a fine-gauge needle; extravascular administration may result in swelling or necrosis at the injection site; if swelling results, discontinue; intravenous dosage should be limited to 2 successive days but may be followed by oral administration.

Phenyramidol Hydrochloride

Phenyramidol Hydrochloride [$C_{13}H_{14}N_2O.HCl$ = 250.72] is α-[(2-pyridylamino)methyl]benzyl alcohol hydrochloride.

Description—A fine, white, crystalline solid that is odorless. It is stable in air in aqueous solutions. It melts between 138° and 140°. Its aqueous solution is colorless and has a pH of 4.

Solubility—1 Gm dissolves in slightly less than 5 ml water.

Uses—Phenyramidol Hydrochloride is a moderately effective analgesic agent which has been used to relieve the pain of musculoskeletal origin and dysmenorrhea. It is said to have approximately the same analgesic effectiveness as the salicylates with no demonstrable advantage over the older drugs. The drug does not possess clinically significant skeletal muscle relaxant, anti-inflammatory, or antipyretic properties. Side effects are relatively minor and include nausea, epigastric distress, drowsiness, and, occasionally, skin rash. Phenyramidol should be used with caution in patients on anticoagulant drugs; it inhibits their metabolic degradation and enhances their effect.

Dose—*Usual,* **200** to **400 mg** 3 or 4 times daily.

Dosage Forms—Capsules: 400 mg; Syrup (as the salicylate): 100 mg/ml; Tablets: 200 mg.

Propoxyphene Hydrochloride USP

[(+)-α-4-(Dimethylamino)-3-methyl-1,2-diphenyl-2-butanol Propionate Hydrochloride; Darvon (*Lilly*)]

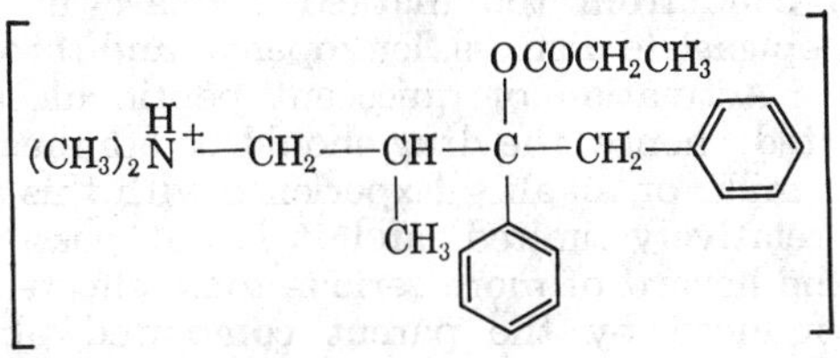

Propoxyphene Hydrochloride contains 98.0–101.0% of $C_{22}H_{29}NO_2.HCl$ (375.94), calculated on the dried basis.

Preparation—The Mannich base (I) formed by condensing propiophenone and dimethylamine with formaldehyde is Grignardized with benzyl magnesium chloride to produce a mixture of the racemates of the two diastereoisomers (designated commercially as α and β) of the alcohol (II). The desired α-*dl* form is isolated by fractional crystallization and resolved by means of *d*-camphorsulfonic acid. The desired α-*d* enantiomorph is propionylated with propionic acid in the presence of trimethylamine to form propoxyphene which adds an equivalent of HCl in forming the hydrochloride.

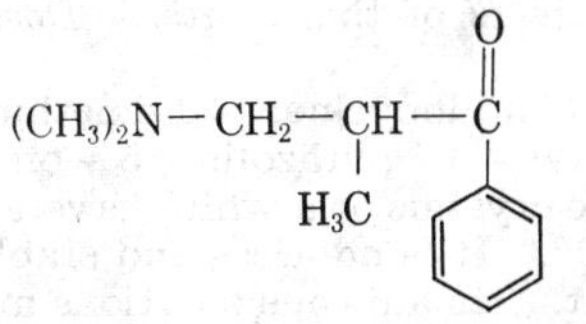

I

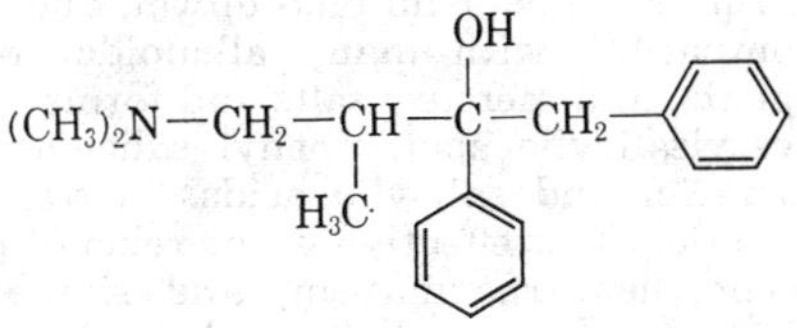

II

Description—White, crystalline powder. Is odorless, and has a bitter taste.

Solubility—Freely soluble in water; soluble in alcohol, chloroform, and acetone; practically insoluble in benzene and ether.

Uses—Propoxyphene Hydrochloride is a synthetic, nonantipyretic, orally effective analgesic which is related pharmacologically to codeine. A dose of 65 mg appears to be approximately equivalent in analgesic effectiveness to 650 mg of aspirin. It produces no respiratory depression, and has little or no antitussive activity. In general, it is useful for the relief of mild pain in patients not controlled by codeine or aspirin. Propoxyphene Hydrochloride has little or no addiction liability.

Dose—**30** to **500 mg** daily; *usual,* **60 mg** 3 or 4 times a day as necessary.

Dosage Forms—Capsules USP: 32 and 65 mg.

Propoxyphene Hydrochloride and Aspirin Capsules NF [Darvon A.S.A. (*Lilly*)] contain 90.0–110.0% of the labeled amounts of $C_{22}H_{29}NO_2.HCl$ (propoxyphene hydrochloride) and of $C_9H_8O_4$ (aspirin). *Uses:* These capsules combine the analgesic properties of these two agents in a single dosage form. Indications, side effects, and contraindications are the same as for *Propoxyphene Hydrochloride. Dose: Usual,* 325 mg (aspirin) every 4 hours and 65 mg (propoxyphene hydrochloride) 3 or 4 times a day.

Salicylamide NF

[Salicim (*Neisler*); Salrin (*Warren-Teed*)]

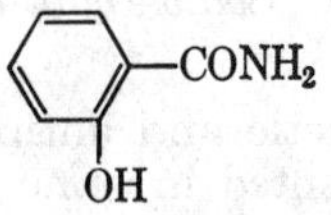

Salicylamide contains 98.0–102.0% of $C_7H_7NO_2$ (137.14), calculated on the anhydrous basis.

Preparation—Among other ways, Salicylamide may be prepared by the ammonolysis of ethyl salicylate. This is usually conducted under pressure in the presence of ammonium sulfite.

Description—A white, almost odorless, crystalline powder. Melting range 139° to 142°. The absorptivity (1%, 1 cm) in alcohol at 236 mμ and 302 mμ is about 548 and 302, respectively.

Solubility—1 Gm dissolves in about 500 ml of water, about 15 ml of alcohol, 100 ml of chloroform, 35 ml of ether, and 20 ml of propylene glycol; freely soluble in solutions of alkalies.

Uses—Salicylamide, the amide of salicylic acid, shares the actions and uses of aspirin. Clinical studies indicate that its analgesic potency, antipyretic, and anti-inflammatory properties are similar, but not superior, to those of aspirin. Patients allergic to aspirin have been reported not to be sensitive to Salicylamide.

Dose—*Usual,* **300** to **600 mg** every 3 or 4 hours.

Other Dose Information—The antirheumatic dose is 1 to 2 Gm every 4 hours.

Dosage Forms—Oral Suspension NF: 65 mg/ml; Tablets NF: 300 and 600 mg.

Sodium Salicylate USP

[Natrii Salicylas]

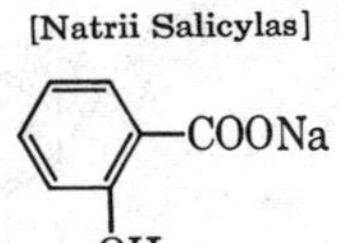

Sodium Salicylate contains 99.5–100.5% of $C_7H_5NaO_3$ (160.11) calculated on the dried basis.

Preparation—Salicylic acid is mixed with sufficient distilled water to form a paste, then sufficient pure sodium carbonate is added in small portions to neutralize all but a small fraction of the salicylic acid. The resulting solution is filtered through a filter free from iron, as even slight contact with iron will discolor the product. The filtered solution is evaporated at a low temperature to dryness, preferably in a vacuum.

Description—An amorphous or a microcrystalline powder or scales. It is colorless or has not more than a faint, pink tinge. It is odorless, or has a faint, characteristic odor, and a sweet, saline taste. It is affected by light. The aqueous solution is neutral or acid to litmus paper.

Solubility—1 Gm dissolves in 1 ml of water, 10 ml of alcohol, or about 4 ml of glycerin; very soluble in boiling water and in boiling alcohol.

Incompatibilities—Solutions of salicylates slowly darken in color due to an *oxidation reaction* influenced by the presence of *alkalies* or *iron* and leading to a quinoid structure. The reaction is retarded by the presence of more easily oxidized substances such as sodium bisulfite, sodium hypophosphite, or sodium thiosulfate. Salicylates give a violet or reddish violet color with *ferric ion*, a green with *copper*, and a brown with *nitric* or *nitrous acids*. *Ethyl nitrite spirit* gives a yellow color which slowly darkens to red-brown. In neutral solutions, *ferric salts* form insoluble basic ferric salicylate. *Lead, bismuth,* and *mercury* behave similarly.

Mineral acids liberate salicylic acid from solutions of the salicylates; this will precipitate except in the presence of sufficient alcohol. The alkali acetates, citrates, and phosphates increase the solubility of salicylic acid by converting it to the salicylate ion. *Soluble quinine salts* are precipitated as quinine salicylate.

Uses—The analgetic and antipyretic actions of the salicylates are presented in some detail under *Aspirin* (page 1134). Like the latter compound, Sodium Salicylate is widely employed for the *relief of pain* and the *reduction of fever*. It is also serviceable in the symptomatic therapy of *gout* and in acute *rheumatic fever*. It is about ⅓ less potent, on a weight basis, than aspirin, and therefore the equivalent analgetic dose is somewhat higher. The sodium salt tends to cause gastric irritation due to the liberation of free salicylic acid by the acid gastric juice. For this reason, an equivalent amount of sodium bicarbonate is usually employed along with Sodium Salicylate. The drug is dispensed in tablets or capsules. Solutions of Sodium Salicylate are generally to be avoided because they have a sweetish, nauseant taste which is difficult to mask completely, and because they become discolored on standing. If bicarbonate is present in the solution, a black precipitate may form. The addition of a very small quantity of sodium bisulfite or sodium sulfite (65 mg to an 8-ounce mixture) retards the development of the black color.

Dose—**300 mg** to **4 Gm** daily; *usual*, **600 mg** 4 to 6 times a day.

Dosage Forms—Tablets USP: 300 and 600 mg.

Veterinary Dose—*Horses* and *Cattle*, **25 to 50 Gm**; *Dogs*, **250 mg to 1 Gm.**

Sulfinpyrazone USP

[1,2-Diphenyl-4-[2-(phenylsulfinyl)ethyl]-3,5-pyrazolidinedione; Anturane *Geigy*)]

Sulfinpyrazone contains 98.5–101.5% of $C_{23}H_{20}N_2O_3S$ (404.49), calculated on the dried basis.

Preparation—[2 - (Phenylsulfinyl)ethyl]malonic acid diethyl ester is condensed with hydrazobenzene with the aid of a solution of sodium ethoxide in absolute ethanol. The reaction is completed by adding xylene and heating at about 130° whereby the residual ethanol and that liberated during the condensation is removed. The Sulfinpyrazone is isolated by a solvent extraction process and recrystallized from ethanol. US Pat. 2,700,671.

Description—A white to off-white powder. It melts between 130.5° and 134.5°.

Solubility—1 Gm dissolves in 10 ml of acetone and in 10 ml of 0.5 N sodium hydroxide; practically insoluble in water and solvent hexane; soluble in alcohol and acetone; sparingly soluble in dilute alkali.

Uses—Sulfinpyrazone, a pyrazolone derivative chemically related to phenylbutazone, is a potent uricosuric agent which is used in the prevention, rather than the treatment, of acute gouty arthritis. In chronic gout, Sulfinpyrazone suppresses formation of new tophi and may reduce the size of old tophaceous deposits and alleviate joint pain and stiffness. Most patients require the concomitant use of colchicine or of other drugs for adequate symptomatic relief, since Sulfinpyrazone has only weak, if any, analgesic or anti-inflammatory action. Salicylates, even in small doses, antagonize the uricosuric action of Sulfinpyrazone. Side effects include marked exacerbation of acute gout, urolithiasis, and renal colic from the marked increase in urate excretion, epigastric distress, leukopenia, and thrombocytopenia. Activation of quiescent peptic ulcer has been reported; hence, the drug should be administered with food, milk, or alkali. Experience with this agent has been relatively limited, and it is not possible to estimate the hazard of more serious toxic effects, such as those induced by the parent compound phenylbutazone.

Dose—**200** to **800 mg** daily; *usual*, **100 mg** 4 times a day.

Dosage Forms—Capsules: 200 mg; Tablets USP: 100 mg.

Other Nonaddicting Analgesics and Antipyretics

Acetanilid NF X [Antifebrin; *N*-Phenylacetamide; $C_6H_5NHCOCH_3$]—White, shiny crystals, usually in scales or a white, crystalline powder melting at 113–115°. 1 Gm dissolves in 190 ml water, 3.5 ml alcohol, 4 ml chloroform, and 5 ml glycerin. It is incompatible with ethyl nitrite, alkalies, alkali bromides and iodides, ferric salts, and it forms a eutectic mixture with phenol, resorcinol, and thymol. *Uses:* Analgesic and antipyretic. It is particularly effective as an analgesic in pain of the neuralgic type, although it will also potentiate the analgesic effects of the opiates. *Dose: Orally,* 0.2 to 0.5 Gm.

Aminopyrine NF X, PhI [Amidopyrine; 4-Dimethylamino - 2,3 - dimethyl - 1 - phenyl - 3 - pyrazolin - 5 - one] [$C_{13}H_{17}N_3O$]—Colorless or white crystals or a white, crystalline powder melting at 107–109°. It is odorless and stable in air, but it is affected by light. Its aqueous solutions are slightly alkaline to litmus. 1 Gm dissolves in 18 ml water, 1.5 ml alcohol, 1 ml chloroform, and 13 ml ether. It is incompatible with many alkaloidal precipitants, oxidizing agents, and mercury salts and forms a eutectic mixture with acetylsalicylic acid, phenyl salicylate, phenol, and citric, tartaric, and salicylic acids. *Uses:* Analgesic and antipyretic. It is effective in the relief of pain in neuralgia, dysmenorrhea, rheumatism, and similar painful conditions. Granulocytopenia, with a high mortality rate, occurs in sensitive individuals. The leukocyte count and differential should be checked during the administration of large doses or continued use of small doses. *Dose: Orally,* 0.13 to 0.3 Gm.

Aspirin, Phenacetin, and Caffeine Capsules NF XII
[APC Capsules] contain 90.0–110.0% of the labeled amounts of aspirin ($C_9H_8O_4$), phenacetin ($C_{10}H_{13}NO_2$), and caffeine ($C_8H_{10}N_4O_2$). *Uses:* An *analgetic.* The widely held assumption that the combination of aspirin, phenacetin, and caffeine has greater analgesic effectiveness than the equivalent doses of aspirin alone has never been supported by carefully controlled clinical studies. All preparations containing phenacetin must bear the warning indicating that kidney damage may result if the recommended dosage is exceeded. See *Phenacetin,* page 1138. *Dose: Usual,* Aspirin, 600 mg; Phenacetin, 300 mg; Caffeine, 200 mg.

Cinchophen NF X [2-phenyl-4-quinolinecarboxylic acid] —Purity: not less than 99.5% $C_9H_5N(C_6H_5)(COOH)$-2,4. Occurs as odorless, small, white, needle-like crystals having a slight bitter taste. They are stable in air but affected by light. 1 Gm dissolves in 120 ml alcohol, 400 ml chloroform, and 100 ml ether; practically insoluble in water. *Uses:* Analgesic in acute gout, acting more promptly than colchicum and without undesirable side effects. However, a serious and often fatal type of toxic hepatitis may develop unpredictably and suddenly in some patients following high doses or long-continued therapy. For this reason, cinchophen is rarely used in modern therapy. *Dose: Orally,* 0.5 Gm.

Ethyl Salicylate [Sal-ethyl; $C_6H_4(OH)COOC_2H_5$]—The salicylic acid ester of ethyl alcohol analogous to methyl salicylate (oil of wintergreen). A transparent, colorless volatile liquid, possessing a pleasant characteristic odor and taste. Its specific gravity is 1.132 at 20° and it boils at from 230° to 232°. It is insoluble in water, but soluble in alcohol. *Uses:* Ethyl salicylate has the same action as methyl salicylate, but is said to be less irritant and less toxic. *Dose:* 0.3 to 0.6 ml.

Gentisic Acid [2,5-dihydroxybenzoic acid; $C_6H_3(OH)_2$-COOH]—Needle-like crystals soluble in water about 1:100, soluble in alcohol and ether, insoluble in benzene. *Uses:* The sodium salt is used as an antirheumatic.

Hydroxyphenylcinchoninic Acid [HPC; Oxycinchophen; 3-hydroxy-2-phenyl-4-quinolinecarboxylic acid; $C_{16}H_{11}NO_3$]—Minute, deep yellow prisms that decompose at 206–207 °C. It is soluble in acetic acid, alkalies, hot alcohol, and benzene but sparingly soluble in water. It has antipyretic, antidiuretic, and uricosuric activity, but probably no greater than that of the salicylates. It is poorly tolerated in patients, particularly during prolonged administration. Anorexia, weight loss, nausea, diarrhea, dermatitis, tinnitus, and drug fever may occur with average doses. *Uses:* In the treatment of rheumatic fever, rheumatoid arthritis, and other collagen diseases as well as gout. *Dose: Orally,* 10 to 20 mg per Kg body weight per day.

Methopholine [dl-1-(4-chlorophenethyl)-1,2,3,4-tetrahydro-6,7-dimethoxy-2-methylisoquinoline] [$C_{20}H_{24}ClNO_2$] —A white crystalline powder with a melting point of 109° to 110 °C. The substance is practically odorless, but has a bitter taste. It is insoluble in water. *Uses:* A synthetic, orally effective, nonnarcotic analgesic of value for the relief of mild to moderately severe degrees of acute, chronic or recurrent pain. Milligram for milligram, Methopholine is equal to codeine in analgesic effectiveness and is equal, or perhaps superior, to propoxyphene; its onset and duration of action are similar to those of codeine. Unlike codeine and other opium derivatives, however, methopholine does not produce sedation and its prolonged use does not lead to physical dependence. In fact, its abuse liability is even less than that of propoxyphene. Moreover, patients do not develop tolerance to the analgesic effect of Methopholine. It does not exhibit the anti-inflammatory or antipyretic properties of the salicylates, though it may be used advantageously in combination with salicylates for additive therapeutic effects. Respiratory depression or changes in pulse rates have not occurred with the oral administration of methopholine. The rare instances of side effects noted with the recommended therapeutic doses of Methopholine— nausea, drowsiness, vomiting and dizziness—were very mild in degree, apparently no more frequent or severe than the "reactions" which might be expected with the administration of placebo. *Dose: Orally,* 60 mg every 4 hours as needed.

Neocinchophen NF XI [Ethyl 6-methyl-2-phenylcinchoninate] [$C_{19}H_{17}NO_2$]—A white to pale yellow, crystalline powder. It is odorless and tasteless, is stable in air, but is affected by light. Melting range 74° to 77°. It is nearly insoluble in water; soluble in hot alcohol; very soluble in ether and chloroform. *Uses:* It resembles cinchophen in all its pharmacological actions and therapeutical uses. The discussion under cinchophen of the danger of liver damage also holds with respect to neocinchophen. Neocinchophen has been employed as an *analgetic* for gout. See *Cinchophen* (above). *Dose:* 300 mg. *Veterinary Dose:* 300 to 500 mg.

Phenetsal [Salophen; $C_6H_4(OH)COOC_6H_4NHCOCH_3$] —The salicylic acid ester of 4′-hydroxyacetanilide. Small plates melting between 187° and 188°. Almost insoluble in cold water, more soluble in warm water. Soluble in alcohol, ether, and benzene. *Uses:* As an analgesic, antipyretic, and intestinal antiseptic.

Sodium Gentisate [sodium 2,5-dihydroxybenzoate; $C_6H_3(OH)_2COONa.5\frac{1}{2}H_2O$]—Crystals which rapidly lose water on exposure to air. Soluble in water. *Uses:* Antirheumatic. A biological oxidation product of salicylates which may be responsible for the antirheumatic activity of the salicylates. *Dose:* Up to 10 Gm a day in divided doses.

References

1. See, for example, *United Nations Bulletin on Narcotics,* 1949 to present.
2. Gulland and Robinson, *Mem. Proc. Manchester Lit. Phil. Soc.,* **69,** 79 (1925).
3. Gates, M., and Tschudi, G., *J. Am. Chem. Soc.,* **74,** 1109 (1952); Elad, D., and Ginsburg, D., *Ibid.,* **76,** 312 (1954).
4. McCawley, Hart, and Marsh, *J. Am. Chem. Soc.,* **63,** 314 (1941); Weijlard and Erickson, *Ibid,* **64,** 869 (1942); Hart and McCawley, n. *Pharmacol.* **82,** 339 (1944).
5. See also *United Nations Bulletin on Narcotics,* **5,** 32–43 (Jan.–Mar., 1953) for a review of methods.

64 | Histamine and Antihistamines

This chapter was prepared by

Ewart A. Swinyard, PhD, *Professor of Pharmacology, College of Pharmacy and College of Medicine, University of Utah, Salt Lake City, Utah 84112, and*
Stewart C. Harvey, PhD, *Associate Professor of Pharmacology, College of Medicine, University of Utah, Salt Lake City, Utah 84112*

Despite the fact that histamine is of relatively little therapeutic importance few agents have commanded more attention from biochemists, pharmacologists, and physiologists. This ubiquitous substance is a natural constituent of many tissues, both animal and plant; it is found in skin, subcutaneous tissues, viscera, peripheral and central nervous systems, nerves, brain, skeletal muscle, blood, blood plasma, gastric juice, saliva, urine, sputum, mast cells, and the fluid found in blisters. It is also found in the common stinging nettle. Histamine evokes a variety of pharmacological effects in concentrations compatible with the possibility that the endogenous release of this substance may be the causative agent in a number of physiologic and pathologic reactions, such as allergy and anaphylactic shock.

The subsequent demonstration that histamine was the factor responsible for allergic and anaphylactic phenomena stimulated the search for histamine antagonists. In 1937, Bovet and Staub demonstrated that certain phenolic ethers were able to block many of the pharmacological actions of histamine. This observation provided the stimulus which resulted in the discovery and development of many useful antihistaminic agents.

Another amine, 5-hydroxytryptamine, is also widely distributed in animals and is present in some plants. This substance, discovered independently by three groups of workers, is also known as *enteramine*, and *serotonin*. It is found in largest amounts in brain, blood, spleen, stomach, intestine, lungs, and skin. It has been suggested that 5-hydroxytryptamine may be involved in the regulation of vascular tone, motor and secretory activity of the gastrointestinal tract, and kidney function. It has been postulated also that 5-hydroxytryptamine serves as a neurotransmitter in the brain and that it may be involved in mental function. These observations and the demonstration that tumors of the argentaffin cells of the intestinal mucosa (argentaffinomas or carcinoids) secrete large amounts of 5-hydroxytryptamine have stimulated the search for 5-hydroxytryptamine antagonists. A number of substances, including ergot alkaloids and derivatives, indole derivatives, adrenergic blocking agents, anticholinergic drugs, morphine-like analgesics, and some phenothiazines have been shown to possess this property. In addition, at least one agent which exhibits both antihistaminic and anti-5-hydroxytryptamine properties is available to clinicians and more selective 5-hydroxytryptamine antagonists are under clinical investigation. Therefore, 5-hydroxytryptamine antagonists also will be included in this chapter.

Histamine Phosphate USP

[4-(2-Aminoethyl)imidazole Phosphate (1:2); Histamine Acid Phosphate]

$$\left[H_2NCH_2CH_2 - \underset{N}{\overset{\overset{H}{N}}{\diagdown}} \quad 2H \right]^{+} 2H_2PO_4^{-}$$

Histamine Phosphate contains 98.0–101.0% of $C_5H_9N_3 \cdot 2H_3PO_4$ (307.14), calculated on the dried basis.

Preparation—Histamine occurs in very small amounts in ergot. It is among the products of the bacterial decomposition of histidine, and this constitutes one of the methods for its production. It is also produced synthetically from imidazolylpropionic acid by the Pyman method,[1] from α-aminobutyrolactone by the Garford and Pyman method,[2] and by other methods.

Description—Colorless, odorless, long prismatic crystals. It is stable in the air but is affected by light. Its aqueous solution is acid to litmus. When dried at 105° for 2 hours, it melts at about 140°.

Solubility—1 Gm dissolves in about 4 ml of water.

Pharmacology—Although many tissues contain a lethal amount of histamine in a bound or inactive form, no effect is produced until it is released in a free form into body fluids as a result of certain stimuli. Since histamine is destroyed in the intestinal tract by the enzyme histaminase, it is ineffective when taken orally. After injection, histamine constricts certain smooth muscles such as the bronchi, uterus, and intestines and dilates the capillary bed. Characteristically, an increased capillary permeability accompanies the dilatation, and there is a seepage of fluid, plasma proteins, and even some cellular elements of the blood into the extracellular spaces. Dilatation of the capillaries and arterioles produces a flushing of the face, a fall in blood pressure, and an increase in skin temperature.

Histamine stimulates all types of glandular secretions—gastric, duodenal, salivary, and lacrimal. An important effect in man is the stimulation of the gastric glands which increases the hydrochloric acid of the stomach. This effect is the basis of a diagnostic test to differentiate between nonspecific hypochlorhydria and that caused by pernicious anemia (see page 1312).

One highly characteristic effect of histamine is the "triple response" induced by the intracutaneous injection of small amounts of this agent. It consists of (1) local reddening at the site of the injection, (2) a wheal or patch of localized edema which obscures the original red spot, and (3) the scarlet flare which surrounds the wheal. The initial red spot is mostly due to local vaso-dilatation, and the wheal develops from an increased capillary permeability. The flare is a local phenomenon produced by an axon reflex involving peripheral sensory nerves. Since the flare does not appear in the presence of atrophy or degeneration of the nerve, this reaction has been used as a diagnostic test to distinguish between real and pseudo anesthesia.

When injected intravenously, histamine provokes an increased output of epinephrine from the adrenal medulla as indicated by a secondary rise in blood pressure. Clinical use is made of this action on the adrenals by employing histamine as a test agent in the diagnosis of pheochromocytoma.

Despite the fact that histamine has yet to become established as a therapeutic agent, the several diagnostic uses justify its official recognition.

Uses—The therapeutic uses of histamine are limited. It is employed chiefly as a *diagnostic aid* in testing for the *functional capacity of the gastric glands.* If no acid is secreted following the injection of 0.25 to 0.5 mg (usually as a 1:1000 solution), a true gastric achylia exists.

Histamine is employed in the *diagnosis of pheo-chromocytoma.* In patients with adrenal medullary tumors, intravenous administration of the compound is followed by a dramatic rise in blood pressure due to the release of excessive quantities of epinephrine and nor-epinephrine from the neoplasm.

Certain allergic conditions are thought to be the result of the liberation of histamine in the body, especially physical allergies as, for example, cold allergy. Histamine has been employed with questionable success to desensitize such individuals.

The drug has been tried in a variety of other conditions, but its true worth is not yet established. Included in this category are rheumatoid arthritis and Ménière's disease.

Upon local application, Histamine Phosphate causes vasodilatation. It has been incorporated in an ointment base for the treatment of indolent ulcers.

Dose—*Subcutaneous,* **800 mcg** to **2 mg** (the equivalent of 300 to 700 mcg of histamine base); *usual,* **800 mcg** (the equivalent of 300 mcg of histamine base).

Dosage Forms—Injection USP: 100 and 364 mcg and 1 mg/ml, 1 and 5 mg/5 ml, 3.64 and 10 mg/10 ml, 2 mg/20 ml, 11 mg/30 ml.

Antihistamines

Following the suggestion by Dale and Laidlaw in 1911 that the symptoms of histamine shock resembled those in anaphylaxis many experimenters added findings tending to substantiate the concept that release of histamine from the tissues is responsible for the anaphylactic reaction. It is true that some of the manifestations of anaphylaxis cannot be explained by histamine effect, but it was argued that histamine is at least the major mechanism. The histamine concept was gradually adopted to explain the allergic reaction in man after Lewis, in 1924, claimed that the histamine effects in man were identical with those of allergy. Many attempts were then made in animals and man to raise the tolerance to histamine by injections of the latter. The preponderance of evidence indicates that a tolerance to histamine only infrequently can be acquired in that manner. Evidence that obtaining such tolerance in man can be obtained by the administration of conjugated histamine (histamine-azo-protein or *Hapamine*) has not been established.

Although many substances had been previously demonstrated to antagonize responses to histamine and certain manifestations of antigen–antibody reactions, it was not until 1942 that sufficiently specific and non-toxic agents became available for this action to be of clinical importance. As a result of intensive research in this field, a very large number of effective agents are now on the market. These differ in antihistaminic potency, length of action, untoward effects, toxicity, and cost. A knowledge of these factors is essential for proper drug selection.

Uses—All presently available *antihistamines (anti-histaminics* or antihistaminic agents) are effective in preventing histamine shock in guinea pigs, bronchospasm induced in guinea pigs by nebulized histamine solutions, whealing on the skin, and many other responses to histamine. The hypotension induced by histamine is more difficult to block and the increased salivation and gastric secretion are not inhibited. The antihistamines also have antianaphylactic properties in large doses and are antipruritic and analgesic. Some have bowel or bladder smooth muscle antispasmodic action; some produce sedation and others central nervous system stimulation.

Clinically, the antihistamines are most effective in *seasonal vasomotor rhinitis* (especially during the earlier part of the season), *acute urticaria* and *acute reactions to sulfonamides, penicillin, and other medicaments.* However, it must be remembered that they produce only symptomatic relief and do not correct the underlying disorder. The relief lasts only as long as medication continues or as the disorder is corrected by other means. These agents are also frequently effective in treating various types of *contact dermatitis,* certain features of *serum reactions, pruritus vulvæ, pruritus ani,* and *insect bites.* Chronic rhinitis, asthma, and erythema nodosa-type of sensitivity reactions are rarely benefited. Pruritus is frequently relieved by the local application of antihistamines, probably to a large extent because of their local anesthetic properties. Certain antihistamines are useful in the prevention and treatment of motion sickness (see page 807). Claims have been made for the efficacy of antihistamine therapy of the common cold, but carefully controlled clinical studies fail to support the claims; however, certain *nasopharyngeal allergic conditions* that simulate the common cold are benefited.

The more severe the affection the larger the dose of antihistamine required and the less the chance of obtaining benefit. These agents may be employed to supplement desensitization procedures, and their administration one hour prior to injection of specific antigens may allow the administration of larger doses of antigen and thus speed the process of desensitization. The response to antihistamines is usually not as rapid or complete as that to epinephrine or intravenous aminophylline, but some workers have found that intravenous administration of antihistamines is of definite value in combating acute allergic episodes. Certain antihistamines cannot be given parenterally because of strong irritating properties.

The sedative antihistamines are sometimes used as

substitutes for barbiturates in the management of insomnia. In addition, they have been used for their antitremor effect in Parkinson's disease and in the treatment of behavioral disorders in children.

Some antihistamines, such as tripelennamine, diphenhydramine, and antazoline, have antiarrhythmic properties and exert effects on the heart similar to those of quinidine. They may terminate ventricular tachycardia, multifocal ventricular premature systoles, and nodal tachycardia. They also may terminate atrial tachycardia and atrial extrasystoles, but not atrial flutter or fibrillation. They are particularly indicated in patients who cannot tolerate quinidine or other antiarrhythmic drugs.

The antihistamines produce a variety of undesirable side effects; these are similar for all of the available agents except phenindamine, although their incidence varies considerably, ranging from less than seven to as high as eighty per cent. The drugs may even produce sensitivity reactions of the type which they usually inhibit. Sensitivity to one antihistamine is ordinarily not an indication that the patient is sensitive to others. Sedation is the most common untoward reaction and is directly related to the dosage employed. In some cases this response may disappear after several days of medication. The reaction is particularly serious when the drug is taken without adequate medical supervision. Sedation may be largely eliminated by the judicious use of small doses of central nervous system stimulants such as amphetamine and methamphetamine. In a few individuals, certain antihistaminics produce signs of central excitation such as insomnia and nervousness. Large doses produce convulsions in experimental animals. Other side effects include anorexia, nausea, vomiting, gastrointestinal pain, diarrhea, and dryness of the mouth and nose.

Dose—The usual oral dose of various agents varies from 2 to 100 mg every 3 to 6 hours. The lower dosage is usually employed first and gradually increased until the limit of tolerance of the particular patient is reached or the desired therapeutic effect is obtained. The dosage should be kept at the minimum necessary to provide relief. Intravenous or intramuscular injection of 25 to 50 mg of certain agents marketed for these parenteral routes of administration may be employed, but the procedure should be limited to exceptional acute cases.

Antazoline Phosphate NF

[2-[(N-benzylanilino)methyl]-2-imidazoline Phosphate (1:1); Antistine Phosphate (Ciba)]

$$\left[\begin{array}{c} HN \\ N \end{array} \right. C - CH_2 - N - CH_2 - C_6H_5 \left. \right]^{2H^+} HPO_4^=$$

Antazoline Phosphate contains 98.0–100.5% of $C_{17}H_{19}N_3 \cdot H_3PO_4$ (363.36), calculated on the dried basis.

Preparation—N-Benzylaniline is converted to N-benzyl-N-phenylaminoacetonitrile by reaction with paraformaldehyde and sodium cyanide in acetic acid solution. Reaction with anhydrous ethylenediamine, catalyzed by carbon disulfide, liberates ammonia with simultaneous closure of the imidazoline ring, thus producing antazoline base. After purification by recrystallization, the base is dissolved in a suitable

solvent and precipitated as the phosphate by reaction with an equimolar portion of phosphoric acid.

Description—A white, crystalline powder, possessing a bitter taste. The pH of a 1 in 50 solution is between 4.0 and 5.0. It melts with decomposition between 194° and 198°.

Solubility—Soluble in water; sparingly soluble in methanol; practically insoluble in benzene and in ether.

Uses—This antihistamine is somewhat weaker than most of the other antihistamines. In addition to the usual clinical indications for antihistaminic drugs, Antazoline is also used as an antiarrhythmic agent. See the general statement on page 1143. It is also used as a 0.5% ophthalmic solution, because it is milder and less irritating to the tissues than other drugs of this group.

Antazoline hydrochloride has over twice the local anesthetic potency of procaine and also exhibits anticholinergic actions.

Dose—*Usual*, 1 or 2 drops of a 0.5% solution in each eye every 3 or 4 hours.

Other Dose Information—The dose as an antiarrhythmic is 400 to 800 mg orally or up to 10 mg per Kg intravenously; for ophthalmic use it is 1 or 2 drops of a 0.5% solution in each eye every 3 or 4 hours.

Dosage Forms—Ophthalmic Solution NF: 0.5%.

Veterinary Use—Antihistaminic. The ophthalmic solution is applied every 4 hours to the eyes in the treatment of canine chronic conjunctivitis.

Veterinary Dose—*Horses* and *Cattle*, 25 mg per 100 pounds of body weight; *Dogs*, 25 to 75 mg 1 to 4 times daily.

Betahistine Hydrochloride

[Serc (Unimed)]

$$\left[\begin{array}{c} H \\ N^+ \\ \end{array} - CH_2CH_2\overset{+}{N}H_2CH_3 \right] 2\bar{Cl}$$

Betahistine Hydrochloride [$C_8H_{12}N_2 \cdot 2HCl$ = 209.12] is 2-[2-(methylamino)ethyl]pyridine dihydrochloride.

Preparation—Methylamine hydrochloride is caused to undergo addition to 2-vinylpyridine by refluxing in isopropanol. The suitably purified product, 2-[2-(methylamino)ethyl]pyridine hydrochloride is reacted with alkali to form betahistidine (base) which is extracted from the reaction mixture with chloroform, purified by vacuum distillation, and reacted with a double molar quantity of hydrogen chloride.

Description—A white or creamy white, crystalline powder that is odorless and has a bitter taste. It is stable in light and hygroscopic. It melts between 151° and 154°.

Solubility—Freely soluble in water and methanol; soluble in alcohol; practically insoluble in chloroform, acetone, ether, and benzene.

Uses—Betahistine Hydrochloride is a histamine-like agent used to reduce the frequency of vertigo in Ménière's syndrome. Clinical evaluation has been concerned primarily with patients having a frequency of vertiginous episodes ranging from one a day to one in two weeks. There is no evidence that the drug is effective in the management of the tinnitus and/or the decreased auditory acuity in Ménière's syndrome. The drug is contraindicated in patients with peptic ulcer and should be used with care in patients with pheochromocytoma. The safety of the drug in pregnancy has not been established. Betahistine should not be used concurrently with antihistamines.

Dose—Usual, **4 mg** 2 to 4 times a day.

Other Dose Information—Total daily dosage should not exceed 32 mg.

Dosage Forms—Tablets: 4 mg.

Bromodiphenhydramine Hydrochloride NF

[2-[(*p*-Bromo-α-phenylbenzyl)oxy]-*N,N*-dimethylethylamine Hydrochloride; Ambodryl Hydrochloride (*Parke-Davis*)]

Bromodiphenhydramine Hydrochloride contains 98.0–101.0% of $C_{17}H_{20}BrNO \cdot HCl$ (370.72), calculated on the dried basis.

Preparation—Benzoyl chloride is subjected to a Friedel–Craft reaction with bromobenzene and the resulting *p*-bromobenzophenone is reduced to its benzhydrol analog with aluminum isopropoxide. Esterification with hydrogen chloride forms the corresponding chloride which, on reacting with the sodium derivative of 2-(dimethylamino)ethanol, yields bromodiphenhydramine (base). The official hydrochloride may be produced by passing a stream of hydrogen chloride into a suitable solution of the base.

Description—A white to pale-buff, crystalline powder having no more than a faint odor and a very bitter taste. Its solutions are unstable in direct sunlight; it is stable in air and stable as a dry powder up to 37°. It melts between 148° and 152°.

Solubility—1 Gm dissolves in 1 ml of water, 2 ml alcohol, and about 25 ml isopropyl alcohol; insoluble in ether and solvent hexane.

Uses—Bromodiphenhydramine Hydrochloride is an antihistaminic agent useful in the treatment of clinical states in which release of histamine or histamine-like substances are involved. Although the incidence of unpleasant side effects is low, Bromodiphenhydramine Hydrochloride induces untoward reactions characteristic of this group of drugs. See general statement (page 1143).

Dose—**25 to 50 mg**, usual, **25 mg** 3 times daily.

Other Dose Information—Some patients may require up to 150 mg daily.

Dosage Forms—Capsules NF: 25 mg; Elixir NF: 12.5 mg/5 ml.

Brompheniramine Maleate NF

[2-[*p*-Bromo-α-[2-(dimethylamino)ethyl]benzyl]pyridine Maleate (1:1); Dimetane (*Robins*)]

Brompheniramine Maleate, dried at 105° for 3 hours, contains 98.0–100.5% of $C_{16}H_{19}BrN_2 \cdot C_4H_4O_4$ (435.32).

Preparation—α-(*p*-Bromophenyl)-2-pyridineacetonitrile is converted to its sodium derivative by reaction with sodium amide and the sodium derivative is then condensed with 2-chloro-*N,N*-dimethylethylamine. The resulting nitrile is then converted to its

corresponding acid which is then decarboxylated by treatment with sulfuric acid. After rendering the mixture alkaline, brompheniramine base is solvent extracted and reacted with an equimolar portion of maleic acid.

Description—Occurs as a white, odorless, crystalline powder.

Solubility—1 Gm dissolves in about 5 ml of water, about 15 ml of alcohol, and about 15 ml of chloroform; slightly soluble in ether and benzene.

Uses—Brompheniramine Maleate, the bromine analog of chlorpheniramine, is an antihistaminic agent with a high order of effectiveness and a low incidence of side effects. It is useful in the treatment of any condition considered amenable to therapy with histamine-antagonizing agents.

Dose—**4 to 8 mg**; usual, **4 mg** 1 to 4 times a day.

Other Dose Information—The parenteral dose, by all routes, is 5 to 20 mg.

Dosage Forms—Elixir NF: 2 mg/5 ml; Tablets NF: 4 mg.

Carbinoxamine Maleate NF

[2-[*p*-Chloro-α-[2-(dimethylamino)ethoxy]benzyl]pyridine Maleate (1:1); Clistin (*McNeil*)]

Carbinoxamine Maleate, dried at 105° for 2 hours, contains 98.0–102.0% of $C_{16}H_{19}ClN_2O \cdot C_4H_4O_4$ (406.87).

Preparation—Picolinaldehyde and *p*-chlorophenylmagnesium bromide are reacted in Grignard fashion to produce *p*-chloro-α-(2-pyridyl)benzyl alcohol. This is converted into its sodium alkoxide derivative by treating it, in xylene solution, with sodamide. Freshly distilled β-dimethylaminoethyl chloride is added and the mixture is refluxed to effect the condensation which yields carbinoxamine (base). After isolation and purification, the base is dissolved in a suitable solvent and converted into the maleate by reaction with an equimolar quantity of maleic acid.

Description—It occurs as a white, odorless, crystalline powder. Melting range 116° to 121° (in a bath preheated to 111°). pH 4.6 to 5.1.

Solubility—Very soluble in water; freely soluble in alcohol and chloroform; very slightly soluble in ether.

Uses—A potent antihistaminic agent with a low incidence of side effects. It also exhibits weak atropine-like anticholinergic activity.

Dose—**4 to 8 mg**; usual, **4 mg** 3 or 4 times a day.

Dosage Forms—Elixir NF: 4 mg/5 ml; Tablets: 4 mg.

Chlorcyclizine Hydrochloride NF

[1-(*p*-Chloro-α-phenylbenzyl)-4-methylpiperazine Monohydrochloride; Perazil (*Burroughs Wellcome*)]

Chlorcyclizine Hydrochloride contains 98.0–100.5% of $C_{18}H_{21}ClN_2 \cdot HCl$ (337.30), calculated on the dried basis.

Preparation—Chlorcyclizine base may be prepared by condensing *p*-chlorobenzhydryl chloride with *N*-methylpiperazine in the presence of sodamide. Treatment of a solution of the base in a suitable organic solvent with hydrogen chloride results in the precipitation of the official hydrochloride.

Description—A white, odorless or almost odorless, crystalline powder. Its solutions are acid to litmus, and the pH of a 1 in 100 solution is between 4.8 and 5.5. Melts between 222° and 227°.

Solubility—1 Gm dissolves in about 2 ml of water, 11 ml of alcohol, and about 4 ml of chloroform; practically insoluble in ether and benzene.

Uses—A mildly sedative antihistaminic agent with a prolonged action and a low incidence of toxic side effects. Chlorcyclizine Hydrochloride has slight anticholinergic and antispasmodic actions and enhances the action of epinephrine. It also has some local anesthetic action. See page 1143.

Dose—25 to **100 mg**; *usual*, **50 mg** up to 4 times a day.

Dosage Forms—Tablets NF: 25 and 50 mg.

Chlorothen Citrate NF

[Chloromethapyrilene Citrate; 2-[(5-Chloro-2-thenyl)[2-(dimethylamino)ethyl]amino]pyridine Citrate (1:1); Tagathen (*Lederle*)]

Chlorothen Citrate, dried in vacuum over phosphorus pentoxide for 5 hours, contains 98.0–100.5% of $C_{14}H_{18}ClN_3S \cdot C_6H_8O_7$ (487.96).

Preparation—Chlorothen base may be prepared by condensing 5-chloro-2-thenylchloride with *N,N*-dimethyl-*N'*-(2-pyridyl)-ethylenediamine in the presence of sodamide. Treatment of the base with an equimolar quantity of citric acid yields the citrate.

Description—A white, crystalline powder, usually having a faint odor. Melts between 112° and 116°; gradually solidifies on further heating, and remelts between 125° and 140° with decomposition. Its solutions are acid to litmus.

Solubility—1 Gm dissolves in about 35 ml of water; slightly soluble in alcohol; practically insoluble in chloroform, ether, and benzene.

Uses—An antihistaminic agent with mild sedative properties. See general statement (page 1143).

Dose—*Usual*, **25 mg** every 3 or 4 hours, should not exceed 150 mg in a 24-hour period.

Dosage Forms—Tablets NF: 25 mg.

Chlorpheniramine Maleate USP

[(±)-2-[*p*-Chloro-α-[2-(dimethylamino)ethyl]benzyl]pyridine Maleate (1:1); Chlorpheniraminium Maleate; Chlorprophenpyridamine Maleate; Chlor-Trimeton Maleate (*Schering*); Drize (*Ascher*); Teldrin (*SK&F*)]

Chlorpheniramine Maleate contains 98.0–100.5% of $C_{16}H_{19}ClN_2 \cdot C_4H_4O_4$ (390.87), calculated on the dried basis.

Preparation—Chlorpheniramine base may be prepared by condensing 2-[*p*-chloro-α-(2-chloroethyl)benzyl]pyridine with dimethylamine in the presence of sodamide. Treatment of the base with an equimolar portion of maleic acid results in the formation of the official maleate.

Description—A white, odorless, crystalline powder. Its solutions are acid to litmus, having a pH between 4 and 5. Melts between 130° and 135°.

Solubility—1 Gm dissolves in about 4 ml of water, 10 ml of alcohol, and about 10 ml of chloroform; slightly soluble in ether and benzene.

Uses—An *antihistaminic* agent with good therapeutic efficacy and low incidence of side effects. See the general statement (page 1143).

Dose—*Oral*, **2** to **24 mg** daily; *usual, oral*, **2** to **4 mg** 3 or 4 times a day; *usual, parenteral*, **10** to **20 mg.**

Other Dose Information—For prophylaxis of blood transfusion reactions, 10 mg to a flask of blood.

Dosage Forms—Elixir USP; Injection NF: 10 mg/ml, 100 mg/10 ml, 200 mg/2 ml. Tablets USP: 4 mg.

Veterinary Dose—*Farm animals, intramuscularly*, doses 2 or 3 times daily. *Dogs and Cats, orally* or *parenterally*, **1 mg** per **6 pounds** of body weight divided in 3 or 4 equal doses.

Clemizole Hydrochloride

[Allercur (*Roerig*); Reactrol (*Purdue-Frederick*)]

Clemizole Hydrochloride [$C_{19}H_{20}ClN_3 \cdot HCl$ = 362.31] is 1-(*p*-chlorobenzyl)-2-(1-pyrrolidinylmethyl)benzimidazole monohydrochloride.

Preparation—*p*-Chlorobenzylamine is condensed with *o*-chloronitrobenzene and the resulting *N*-(*p*-chlorobenzyl)-2-nitroaniline is hydrogenated in the presence of Raney nickel to form the corresponding 2-amino compound (I). Condensation of (I) with chloroacetyl chloride aided by pyridine yields *N*-(*p*-chlorobenzyl) - *N'* - chloroacetyl - *o* - phenylenediamine which, under reflux with pyrrolidine in toluene and subsequent extraction and acidification with hydrochloric acid, produces a mixture of the hydrochlorides of *N*-(*p*-chlorobenzyl)-*N'*-pyrrolidylacetyl-*o*-phenylenediamine (II) and the cyclized (via dehydration) compound, Clemizole (III). Boiling in nitrobenzene converts (II) into (III). The crude Clemizole Hydrochloride may be purified by crystallization from butanol. US Pat. 2,689,853.

Description—White crystals or powder. It is odorless and has a bitter taste. It melts between 245° and 247°.

Solubility—Soluble in ethanol and chloroform; sparingly soluble in water; insoluble in ether.

Uses—An antihistaminic agent with actions, uses, and limitations similar to those of other agents in this pharmacological class. See general statement (page 1143).

Dose—*Usual*, **40 to 80 mg** daily in divided doses.
Dosage Forms—Tablets: 20 and 40 mg.

Cyclizine Hydrochloride—see page 807.

Dexbrompheniramine Maleate NF

[(+)-2-[p-Bromo-α[2-(dimethylamino)ethyl]benzyl] pyridine Maleate (1:1); Disomer (*White*)]

Dexbrompheniramine Maleate, dried at 65° for 4 hours, contains 98.0–102.0% of $C_{16}H_{19}BrN_2 \cdot C_4H_4O_4$ (435.32).

Preparation—The compound may be prepared in a manner analogous to that described for *Dexchlorpheniramine Maleate*, this page.

Description—A white, odorless, crystalline powder. The pH of a 1 in 100 solution is about 5.
Solubility—Freely soluble in water; soluble in alcohol and chloroform.

Uses—Dexbrompheniramine Maleate is the dextro isomer of brompheniramine maleate. The major portion of the antihistaminic activity is said to reside in the dextro isomer; the levo form is relatively inactive. It has actions, untoward effects, and therapeutic applications similar to brompheniramine maleate and other antihistaminics. See general statement (page 1143).
Dose—2 to 12 mg a day; *usual*, **2 mg** 4 times a day.
Dosage Forms—Tablets NF: 2 mg.

Dexchlorpheniramine Maleate NF

[(+)-2-[p-Chloro-α-[2-(dimethylamino)ethyl]benzyl]pyridine Maleate (1:1); Polaramine Maleate (*Schering*)]

Dexchlorpheniramine Maleate, dried at 65° for 4 hours, contains 99.0–100.5% of $C_{16}H_{19}ClN_2 \cdot C_4H_4O_4$ (390.87).
Preparation—Racemic chlorpheniramine (see *Chlorpheniramine Maleate*, page 1146) is resolved with the aid of *d*-phenylsuccinic acid. The *d*-enantiomorph of the base is then liberated from its *d*-phenylsuccinate by treatment with sodium hydroxide and reacted with an equimolar portion of maleic acid.

Description—Occurs as a white, odorless, crystalline powder.
Solubility—1 Gm dissolves in about 4 ml of water; soluble in alcohol and chloroform; slightly soluble in benzene and ether.

Uses—Dexchlorpheniramine Maleate, the dextro isomer of chlorpheniramine, is an antihistaminic agent which has about twice the potency of chlorpheniramine and a wider margin of safety. Its uses and limitations are similar to those for other agents of this type. See general statement (page 1143).
Dose—1 to 2 mg; *usual*, **2 mg** 3 or 4 times a day.
Other Dose Information—The usual dose of 2 mg is

given 3 or 4 times a day; the dose for children under 12 years is ½ the above dose.
Dosage Forms—Syrup NF: 2 mg/5 ml; Tablets NF: 2 mg.

Dimenhydrinate—see page 807.

Dimethindene Maleate NF

[2-[1-[2-[2-(Dimethylamino)ethyl]inden-3-yl]ethyl]pyridine Maleate (1:1); Forhistal (*Ciba*)]

Dimethindene Maleate contains 98.0–102.0% of $C_{20}H_{24}N_2 \cdot C_4H_4O_4$ (408.50), calculated on the dried basis.
Preparation—1-(2-Pyridyl)ethyllithium, generated by the interaction of phenyllithium and 2-ethylpyridine, is caused to undergo addition to 2-[2-(dimethylamino)ethyl]indan-1-one. Hydrolysis with the aid of dilute aqueous acid yields the tertiary carbinol which readily dehydrates on warming to form dimethindene (base). Reaction with an equimolar quantity of maleic acid yields the official salt. The starting indanone compound is readily prepared by appropriate application of the method by Hoffmann, et al.[3]

Description—White crystals or crystalline powder with a faint characteristic odor. It is stable in dry air, but it is sensitive to light. It melts between 159° and 163°.
Solubility—1 Gm dissolves in about 200 ml of water; freely soluble in ethanol and chloroform; practically insoluble in ether; soluble in dilute aqueous acids, but it precipitates as the oily free base in alkaline solution.

Uses—Dimethindene Maleate, an indene compound, is a potent antihistaminic agent with actions, uses, and limitations similar to other drugs of this pharmacological class. Since it is chemically different than other antihistamines, it may be useful in patients not responding to other agents. See general statement (page 1143).
Dose—*Usual*, **1 to 2 mg** 1 to 3 times a day.
Dosage Forms—Extended-release Oral Solid: 2.5 mg; Oral Solution: 500 mcg/0.6 ml; Syrup NF: 1 mg/5 ml; Tablets NF: 1 mg.

Diphenhydramine Hydrochloride USP

[2-(Diphenylmethoxy)-N,N-dimethylethylamine Hydrochloride; β-Dimethylaminoethyl Benzhydryl Ether Hydrochloride; Benadryl Hydrochloride (*Parke-Davis*); Valdrene (*Vale*)]

Diphenhydramine Hydrochloride contains 98.0–100.5% of $C_{17}H_{21}NO \cdot HCl$ (291.82), calculated on the dried basis.
Preparation—Diphenhydramine Hydrochloride is prepared by heating diphenylbromomethane, β-dimethylaminoethanol, and sodium carbonate in toluene at 120° to 125°C for 5 hours. The free base is obtained from the reaction product, after distilling off the tolu-

ene, by distillation under reduced pressure, and is converted to the hydrochloride by treatment with hydrogen chloride in an organic solvent.

Description—White, odorless, crystalline powder. Slowly darkens on exposure to light. Its solutions are practically neutral to litmus. Melting range 167° to 172°.

Solubility—1 Gm dissolves in about 1 ml of water, 2 ml of alcohol, 2 ml of chloroform, and 50 ml of acetone; very slightly soluble in benzene and ether.

Uses—This antihistamine is likely to produce sedation in most patients and is often used before retiring by allergic patients for this purpose. This effect is characteristic of antihistamines which are ethanolamine derivatives. It is also a useful antiemetic (see page 807) and anti-Parkinson agent (see page 931). It is also used in the management of certain cardiac arrhythmias. See general statement (page 1143). The incidence of side effects is about 30 to 60%.

Dose—*Oral* and *parenteral*, **10** to **400 mg** daily; *usual, oral,* **25** to **50 mg** 3 to 4 times a day; *usual, intramuscular* and *intravenous,* **10** to **50 mg**.

Dosage Forms—Capsules USP: 25 and 50 mg; Elixir USP; Injection USP: 50 mg/ml, 100 mg/10 ml, 300 mg/30 ml.

Veterinary Dose—*Usual,* **0.2** to **1 mg** per **pound** of body weight twice daily. *Intravenous, Horses* and *Cattle,* **25** to **50 mg** per **100 pounds** of body weight twice daily or **1 mg** per **pound** of body weight once daily; *Dogs,* **1 mg** per pound of body weight.

Methapyrilene Hydrochloride NF

[2-[[2-(Dimethylamino)ethyl]-2-thenylamino]pyridine Monohydrochloride; Thenylpyramine Hydrochloride; Histadyl (*Lilly*); Lullamin Drops (*Reed & Carrick*); Semikon Hydrochloride (*Massengill*)]

$$\left[\begin{array}{c} \text{CH}_2\text{—N—CH}_2\text{CH}_2\text{N(CH}_3)_2 \\ \end{array} \right] \text{H}^+ \middle| \text{Cl}^-$$

Methapyrilene Hydrochloride, dried at 105° for 3 hours, contains 98.0–100.5% of $C_{14}H_{19}N_3S \cdot HCl$ (297.85).

Preparation—Methapyrilene base may be prepared by condensing 2-(2-thenyl)-aminopyridine with 2-(dimethylamino)ethyl chloride in the presence of sodamide. The base is reacted with an equimolar quantity of hydrogen chloride to produce the hydrochloride.

Description—A white, crystalline powder, usually having a faint odor. Its solutions are slightly acid to litmus, having a pH of about 5 to 6. Melts between 161° and 165°.

Solubility—1 Gm dissolves in about 0.5 ml of water, about 5 ml of alcohol, and about 3 ml of chloroform; practically insoluble in ether and benzene.

Uses—An antihistaminic agent with a mild sedative action and low incidence of side effects. It also has some local anesthetic activity. See general statement (page 1143).

Dose—50 to **100 mg**; *usual,* **50 mg** up to 4 times a day.

Dosage Forms—Capsules NF: 25, 50, and 100 mg; Tablets NF: 50 mg.

Methdilazine NF

[10[(1-Methyl-3-pyrrolidinyl)methyl phenothiazine; Tacaryl (*Mead-Johnson*)]

Methdilazine contains 97.0–103.0% of $C_{18}H_{20}N_2S$ (296.44).

Preparation—Phenothiazine is condensed with 1-methyl-3-pyrrolidinylmethyl chloride (I) in an inert medium using either sodium (or lithium) amide as the condensing agent. (I) is prepared from dimethyl itaconate through the following sequence: (a) condensation with methylamine to form methyl 1-methyl-5-oxo 3-pyrrolidinecarboxylate, (b) reduction of this ester with lithium aluminum hydride to 1-methyl-3-pyrrolidinemethanol, and (c) reacting this carbinol with thionyl chloride. US Pat. 2,945,855.

Description—A light-tan, crystalline powder having a characteristic odor. It melts between 77° and 81°. It is unstable in light or oxidizing agents.

Solubility—Freely soluble in diluted hydrochloric acid; soluble in alcohol and chloroform; practically insoluble in water.

Uses—See *Methdilazine Hydrochloride* (this page).

Dose—*Usual,* **7.2 mg** (equivalent to 8 mg of methdilazine hydrochloride) 2 to 4 times a day.

Dosage Forms—Tablets NF: 3.6 mg.

Methdilazine Hydrochloride NF

[10[(1-Methyl-3-pyrrolidinyl)methyl]phenothiazine Monohydrochloride; Tacaryl Hydrochloride (*Mead-Johnson*)]

Methdilazine Hydrochloride contains 97.0–103.0% of $C_{18}H_{20}N_2S \cdot HCl$ (332.90).

For the structure of the base, see Methdilazine, this page.

Preparation—Methdilazine (base) is reacted with an equimolar quantity of hydrogen chloride in a suitable nonaqueous solvent.

Description—A light-tan, crystalline powder which has a slight characteristic odor and a bitter anesthetic taste. It is nonhygroscopic under normal ambient conditions and is stable to temperatures up to 120°. Its solutions are unstable in light. It melts between 184° and 190°.

Solubility—Freely soluble in water, alcohol, chloroform, and hot isopropyl alcohol.

Uses—Methdilazine Hydrochloride is an effective antihistaminic agent with actions, uses, and limitations similar to those of other members of this group. It is also said to be useful in the management of pruritus of nonallergic origin. See general statement (page 1143).

Dose—*Usual,* **8 mg** 2 to 4 times a day.

Dosage Forms—Syrup NF: 4 mg/5 ml; Tablets NF: 8 mg.

Phenindamine Tartrate NF

[2,3,4,9-Tetrahydro-2-methyl-9-phenyl-1*H*-indeno-[2,1-*c*]pyridine Tartrate (1:1); Thephorin (*Roche*)]

Phenindamine Tartrate contains 98.0–101.5% of $C_{19}H_{19}N.C_4H_6O_6$ (411.46), calculated on the dried basis.

Preparation—An aqueous solution of methylamine hydrochloride is reacted with molar quantities of acetophenone and paraformaldehyde by refluxing in alcohol. The 3,3′-methyliminobis(propiophenone) hydrochloride so obtained is refluxed with hydrobromic acid to form 2,3-dihydro-1-methyl-9-phenyl-1H-indeno[2,1-c]pyridine hydrobromide, which is then hydrogenated catalytically until an equimolar portion of hydrogen is taken up, after which treatment with alkali yields phenindamine base. Treatment of the base with an equimolar portion of tartaric acid produces the official tartrate.

$$C_6H_5COCH_3 \xrightarrow[\text{CH}_3\text{NH}_2\cdot\text{HCl}]{(\text{CH}_2\text{O})_3} (C_6H_5COCH_2CH_2)_2NCH_3\cdot HCl$$

Description—A creamy white powder, usually having a very faint odor. Its solutions are acid to litmus. Melts between 160° and 162°; on continued slow heating, it resolidifies at about 163°, and melts again, with decomposition, at about 168°.

Solubility—1 Gm dissolves in about 40 ml of water and about 350 ml of alcohol; practically insoluble in chloroform, ether, and benzene.

Uses—This antihistamine often produces central nervous stimulation—only rarely sedation. It has also been used in *Parkinson's disease*. See general statement (page 1143).

Dose—25 to **50 mg**; *usual*, **25 mg** up to 4 times a day as necessary.

Dosage Forms—Tablets NF: 25 mg.

Promethazine Hydrochloride USP

[10-[2-(Dimethylamino)propyl]phenothiazine Monohydrochloride: Phenergan (*Wyeth*)]

Promethazine Hydrochloride contains 97.0–101.5% of $C_{17}H_{20}N_2S.HCl$ (320.89), calculated on the dried basis.

Preparation—Promethazine base may be prepared by reacting phenothiazine with 1-chloro-2-(dimethylamino)propane hydrochloride in the presence of sodamide and sodium hydroxide in xylene. The reaction mixture is acidified, and the separated aqueous layer is rendered alkaline. Following ethereal extraction and rectification of the base by distillation under reduced pressure, the base is reacted with an equimolar quantity of hydrogen chloride to form the official hydrochloride.

Description—A white to faint yellow, practically odorless crystalline powder. It is slowly oxidized, particularly when moistened, on prolonged exposure to air, becoming blue in color. The pH of a 1 in 20 solution is between 4.5 and 5.5. A 1 in 10 solution in water and a 1 in 10 solution in chloroform are practically clear and show not more than a light yellow color. Melts within a 3° range between 215° and 225°.

Solubility—Very soluble in water, hot dehydrated alcohol, and chloroform; practically insoluble in ether, acetone, and ethyl acetate.

Uses—Promethazine Hydrochloride is a phenothiazine antihistaminic of marked potency and prolonged duration of action. It is useful in the management of all allergic conditions amenable to antihistaminic therapy, for night-time, surgical, and obstetrical sedation, and for potentiating the action of central nervous system depressants. It is also a useful antitussive and antiemetic agent. See general statement (page 1143).

Dose—*Oral*, or *parenteral*, **5** to **75 mg** daily; *usual*, **25 mg**, repeated after 4 hours if necessary.

Dosage Forms—Injection USP: 25 and 50 mg/ml, 250 and 500 mg/10 ml; Syrup USP: 6.25 and 25 mg/5 ml; Tablets USP: 12.5, 25, and 50 mg.

Veterinary Use—As an antihistaminic to treat allergic reactions, urticaria, pruritus, etc. Useful in azoturia, laminitis and lymphangitis in horses, in bloat and acute metritis in cattle. Used in the control of acute nephritis and motion sickness in dogs.

Veterinary Dose—*Intramuscularly*, in 2.5 to 5% solution. *Horses* and *Cattle*, **0.25** to **1.0 Gm**; *Sheep* and *Swine*, **0.1** to **0.5 Gm**; *Dogs*, **25** to **125 mg**. *Orally*, *Dogs* and *Cats*, **12.5** to **25 mg** 4 times daily.

Pyrilamine Maleate NF

[2-[[2-(Dimethylamino)ethyl](*p*-methoxybenzyl)amino]pyridine Maleate (1:1); Antallergan Maleate; Anthisan Maleate; Pyranisamine Maleate; (*Various Mfgs.*)]

Pyrilamine Maleate, dried in vacuum over phosphorus pentoxide for 5 hours, contains 98.0–100.5% of $C_{17}H_{23}N_3O . C_4H_4O_4$ (401.47).

Preparation—Pyrilamine base may be prepared by condensing 2-[[2-(dimethylamino)ethyl]amino]pyridine with *p*-methoxybenzyl chloride in the presence of sodamide. Treatment of the pure base with an equimolar quantity of maleic acid yields the maleate.

Description—A white, crystalline powder, usually having a faint odor. Its solutions are acid to litmus. Melts between 99° and 103°.

Solubility—1 Gm dissolves in about 0.5 ml of water, 3 ml of alcohol, and about 2 ml of chloroform; slightly soluble in ether and benzene.

Uses—An antihistaminic agent with a low incidence of sedative effects. See general statement (page 1143).

Dose—25 to **50 mg**; *usual*, **25 mg** up to 4 times a day.

Dosage Forms—Tablets NF: 25 and 50 mg.

Veterinary Dose—*Intramuscularly*, in 2.5 to 5% solution, *Horses* and *Cattle*, **0.5** to **1.5 Gm**; *Sheep* and *Swine*, **0.25** to **0.5 Gm**; *Dogs*, **25** to **125 mg**. *Orally*, *Dogs*, **12.5** to **25 mg** 4 times daily.

Pyrrobutamine Phosphate NF

[1-[γ-(p-Chlorobenzyl)cinnamyl]pyrrolidine Phosphate (1:2); Pyronil (Lilly)]

Pyrrobutamine Phosphate contains 98.0–101.0% of $C_{20}H_{22}ClN.2H_3PO_4$ (507.85), calculated on the dried basis.

Preparation—The Mannich base (I) prepared by the condensation of acetophenone and pyrrolidine with formaldehyde is Grignardized with p-chlorobenzyl magnesium chloride and the resulting alcohol (II) is dehydrated with PBr_3 to give the unsaturated pyrrobutamine (base). The base reacts with a bimolar quantity of phosphoric acid to form the official diphosphate.

I   II

Description—Occurs as a white, or almost white, crystalline powder, usually having a faint odor.

Solubility—Soluble in water; slightly soluble in alcohol; practically insoluble in chloroform and ether.

Uses—Pyrrobutamine Phosphate is an antihistaminic which is used in the treatment of conditions amenable to therapy with histamine-antagonizing agents. It has a low incidence of sedation and other side effects. See general statement (page 1143).

Dose—15 to 30 mg: *usual*, **15 mg** 3 times a day.

Dosage Forms—Tablets NF: 15 mg.

Thonzylamine Hydrochloride NF XII

[2-[[2-(Dimethylamino)ethyl](p-methoxybenzyl)amino]pyrimidine Monohydrochloride; Anahist (Anahist Co.); Neohetramine Hydrochloride (Warner-Chilcott)]

Thonzylamine Hydrochloride, dried at 105° for 2 hours, contains not less than 98% of $C_{16}H_{22}N_4O.HCl$ (322.84).

Preparation—2-Aminopyrimidine is condensed with anisaldehyde in the presence of formic acid, and the resulting secondary amine is then condensed with 2-(dimethylamino)ethyl chloride with the aid of sodamide to yield thonzylamine (base). Reacting the purified base with an equimolar quantity of hydrogen chloride produces the official hydrochloride.

Description—A white, crystalline powder, usually having a faint odor. Its solutions are slightly acid to litmus, having a pH of about 5 to 6. Melts between 173° and 176°.

Solubility—1 Gm dissolves in about 1 ml of water, 6 ml of alcohol, and about 4 ml of chloroform; practically insoluble in ether and benzene.

Uses—An antihistaminic agent. Its outstanding advantage is that sedation is less frequent and less severe than with most other antihistamines. See general statement (page 1143).

Dose—*Usual*, **50 mg** up to 4 times a day.

Dosage Forms—Tablets: 25 and 50 mg.

Trimeprazine Tartrate NF

[10-[3-(Dimethylamino)-2-methylpropyl]phenothiazine Tartrate (2:1); Temaril (SKF)]

Trimeprazine Tartrate, dried in vacuum at 60° for 4 hours, contains 98.0–101.0% of $(C_{18}H_{22}N_2S)_2.C_4H_6O_6$ (747.00).

Preparation—A xylene solution of phenothiazine is refluxed with sodamide for 2 hours after which a solution of (3-chloro-2-methylpropyl)dimethylamine in xylene is added and the refluxing continued for 20 hours. The trimeprazine (base) thus formed is extracted with aqueous acid and then liberated with alkali and extracted with ether. After removal of the ether, the base is distilled under reduced pressure and reacted with a ½ equimolar portion of tartaric acid. US Pat. 2,837,518.

Description—A white to off-white, odorless, crystalline powder which darkens on exposure to light. It melts between 160° and 164°.

Solubility—Freely soluble in water and chloroform; soluble in alcohol; very slightly soluble in ether and benzene.

Uses—Trimeprazine Tartrate is a phenothiazine compound which is structurally and pharmacologically related to promazine. Although trimeprazine exerts most of the actions of the phenothiazine derivatives, some of these actions, especially the antiemetic, hypotensive, and potentiating effects, are not so prominent as with other phenothiazine derivatives. On the other hand, the *histamine-antagonizing action* of trimeprazine is from one and one-half to five times that of promethazine, a closely related substance. It also exerts an *antipruritic* action which is more pronounced than any of its other effects. Hence, trimeprazine is recommended exclusively for the symptomatic treatment of *mild and severe pruritus*, whether acute or chronic. Clinical studies indicate the drug relieves pruritus accompanying dermatoses of allergic, inflammatory, metabolic, hemovascular, and psychic origins. It often relieves itching which is not relieved by other therapies, and, in many cases, the administration of trimeprazine permits the reduction or elimination of concomitant topical and systemic medication. The antipruritic effect is not directly related to its antihistaminic, tranquilizing, or sedative actions.

In general, all of the precautions applicable to other phenothiazine compounds should be observed when using trimeprazine. Mild and transient drowsiness is the most frequently observed side effect. Although jaundice has not been observed, patients receiving this drug should be watched for the appearance of this and other side reactions characteristic of the phenothiazines. See *Chlorpromazine Hydrochloride* (page 1146).

Dose—10 to 40 mg daily; *usual*, **2.5 mg** 4 times a day.

Dosage Forms—Syrup NF: 2.5 mg/5 ml; Tablets NF: 2.5 mg.

Veterinary Dose—In general, *all routes, all species,* **0.5** to **2 mg** per **pound** of body weight. *Dogs,* **2.5 mg** per **10 pounds** of body weight up to 40 pounds; patients over 40 pounds, **15 mg** twice daily. After 4 days reduce the dose to ½ the initial dose.

Tripelennamine Citrate USP

[2-[Benzyl[2-(dimethylamino)ethyl]amino]pyridine Citrate (1:1); Pyribenzamine Citrate (*Ciba*)]

Tripelennamine Citrate contains 98.0–100.5% of $C_{16}H_{21}N_3 \cdot C_6H_8O_7$ (447.49), calculated on the dried basis.

Preparation—Tripelennamine (base) is reacted with an equimolar portion of citric acid in a suitable solvent which may then be removed by evaporation. For the preparation of the base, see *Tripelennamine Hydrochloride,* below.

Description—White, crystalline powder. Solutions are acid to litmus. It melts at about 107°.

Solubility—1 Gm dissolves in about 1 ml of water; freely soluble in alcohol; very slightly soluble in ether; practically insoluble in chloroform and benzene.

Uses—An antihistaminic agent which is more palatable than the hydrochloride for oral administration. Otherwise the actions and uses are the same. See *Tripelennamine Hydrochloride.*

Tripelennamine Citrate is administered in a dose ⅓ larger than the hydrochloride, because of the difference in molecular weights of these compounds.

Dose—**37.5** to **900 mg** daily; *usual,* **75 mg** 1 to 3 times a day.

Dosage Forms—Elixir USP: 7.5 mg/ml.

Tripelennamine Hydrochloride USP

[2-[Benzyl[2-(dimethylamino)ethyl]amino]pyridine   Monohydrochloride; Pyribenzamine (*Ciba*)]

Tripelennamine Hydrochloride contains 98.0–100.5% of $C_{16}H_{21}N_3 \cdot HCl$ (291.83), calculated on the dried basis.

For the structure of the base, see *Tripelennamine Citrate,* above.

Preparation—Tripelennamine may be prepared as follows: α-Aminopyridine, prepared by the action of sodamide on pyridine, is reacted with β-dimethylaminoethyl chloride in the presence of sodamide, and the resulting 2-[2-(dimethylamino)ethylamino]pyridine is condensed with benzylbromide in the presence of sodamide. The hydrochloride is formed from the base by treatment with hydrogen chloride in an organic solvent.

Description—A white, crystalline powder which slowly darkens on exposure to light. Its solutions are practically neutral to litmus. Melting range 188° to 192°.

Solubility—1 Gm dissolves in 1 ml of water, 6 ml of alcohol, 6 ml of chloroform, and about 350 ml of acetone; insoluble in benzene, ether, and ethyl acetate.

Uses—An antihistaminic agent with a low incidence of side reactions; gastrointestinal irritation is common, but not severe; sedation is moderate, and central nervous system stimulation occurs occasionally. It has also been employed for the management of certain cardiac arrhythmias. See general statement (page 1143). The incidence of side effects is about 20 to 35%.

Dose—*Oral,* **25** to **600 mg** daily; *usual, oral,* **50 mg** 1 to 3 times a day; *parenteral,* **25** to **100 mg** daily; *usual, parenteral,* **25 mg** 2 times a day.

Dosage Forms—Injection USP: 25 mg/ml, 250 mg/10 ml; Tablets USP: 25 and 50 mg.

Veterinary Use—In the treatment of eczema, asthma, and conjunctivitis in dogs; laminitis, food allergy, bee stings, and pulmonary edema in horses; urticaria, asthma, anaphylactic shock, toxemias associated with bacterial infections, or digestive diseases in cattle.

Veterinary Dose—*Intravenously,* by slow injection, *all species,* **0.5 mg** per **pound** of body weight; *orally,* **0.5** to **1 mg** per **pound.** Doses may be repeated at 2-to 8-hour intervals.

Triprolidine Hydrochloride NF

(*E*)-2-[3-(1-Pyrrolidinyl)-1-*p*-tolylpropenyl]pyridine Monohydrochloride; Actidil (*Burroughs-Wellcome*)]

Triprolidine Hydrochloride [$C_{19}H_{22}N_2 \cdot HCl \cdot H_2O$ = 332.88], dried in vacuum at 50° to constant weight, contains 98.0–101.0% of $C_{19}H_{22}N_2 \cdot HCl$.

Preparation—4′-Methylacetophenone is reacted with formaldehyde and pyrrolidine to form 3-(1-pyrrolidinyl)-4′-methylpropiophenone. Reaction with 2-pyridylsodium and subsequent hydrolysis produces the expected tertiary carbinol, α-[2-(1-pyrrolidinyl)-ethyl]-α-*p*-tolyl-2-pyridinemethanol, which is then dehydrated with sulfuric acid to create the propenyl double bond. Alkalinization liberates the base compound which is purified and reacted with an equimolar portion of hydrochloric acid. US Pats. 2,712,-020 and 2,712,023.

Description—A white, crystalline powder having no more than a slight, but unpleasant, odor and a bitter taste. Its solutions are alkaline to litmus, and it melts at about 115°. It is light-sensitive, nonhygroscopic, and stable to reasonable heat.

Solubility—Soluble in water, alcohol, and chloroform; insoluble in ether.

Uses—Triprolidine Hydrochloride is an unusually potent antihistaminic agent with a rapid onset of action. The maximum effect occurs in about 3½ hours; the duration of effect is about 12 hours. The actions, uses, and incidence of side effects are comparable to those of other antihistaminic agents. See general statement (page 1143).

Dose—*Usual,* **2.5 mg** 2 or 3 times a day.

Dosage Forms—Tablets NF: 2.5 mg.

Other Antihistamines

Antazoline Hydrochloride USP XV [Antazolinium chloride][$C_{17}H_{19}N_3 \cdot HCl$]—White, odorless, crystalline powder having a bitter taste and producing temporary numbness of the tongue. It melts at 237–241°. 1 Gm dissolves in about 40 ml water and about 25 ml alcohol, but it is practically insoluble in chloroform, ether, and benzene. The pH of a 1% solution is 6.3. *Uses:* Antihistaminic agent. *Dose: Orally,* 100 mg up to 4 times a day.

Chlorpheniramine Gluconate is $C_{16}H_{19}ClN_2.C_6H_{12}O_7$ (470.96). For the structure of chlorpheniramine, see *Chlorpheniramine Maleate* (page 1146). *Preparation:* With the substitution of gluconic acid for maleic acid, Chlorpheniramine Gluconate may be prepared by the method described for *Chlorpheniramine Maleate* (page 1146). *Uses:* Chlorpheniramine Gluconate is an antihistamine with actions similar to those for *Chlorpheniramine Maleate* (page 1146). Combined with *Prednisolone Acetone* (page 971), it is available as Metreton Nasal Spray (*Schering*) and Metreton Ophthalmic Suspension (*White*) for the control of acute and chronic inflammatory conditions of the nasal passages and the eyes. Although these preparations are usually well tolerated, their topical application should follow the same precautions as those for the topical application of steroids (see page 961).

Diphenylpyraline Hydrochloride [Diafen (*Riker*); Sumadil (*Summers*)] is 4-(diphenylmethoxy)-1-methyl-piperidine hydrochloride [$C_{19}H_{23}NO.HCl$]. *Description and Solubility:* Crystals which melt at 206°. Soluble in water, alcohol, and isopropyl alcohol; insoluble in ether and benzene. *Uses:* An antihistaminic with a low incidence of side effects. Recommended for various allergic conditions and for the symptomatic relief of upper respiratory infections. See general statement (page 1143). *Dose: Usual,* 2 mg 3 or 4 times daily or one 5-mg capsule (extended-release) every 12 hours.

Doxylamine Succinate NF XII [2-[α-[2-(Dimethyl-amino)ethoxy]-α-methylbenzyl]pyridine Succinate (1:1); Decapryn Succinate (*Merrell*)] contains 97.0–102.0% of $C_{17}H_{22}N_2O.C_4H_6O_4$ (388.47), calculated on the dried basis. *Preparation:* Methyl phenyl 2-pyridyl carbinol is converted into its sodium alcoholate, and this is refluxed in toluene with 2-(dimethylamino)ethyl chloride for about 10 hours. Sodium chloride is precipitated and is removed by filtration. Evaporation of the filtrate under reduced pressure yields doxylamine base, which is reacted with an equimolar quantity of succinic acid in warm acetone, and a precipitate of the crystalline succinate forms on cooling. *Description and Solubility:* A white or creamy white powder with a characteristic odor; its solutions are acid to litmus; it melts between 100° and 104°. 1 Gm dissolves in about 1 ml of water, 2 ml of alcohol, and 2 ml of chloroform; very slightly soluble in ether and benzene. *Uses:* An antihistaminic agent which produces marked sedation when used in full therapeutic doses. See general statement (page 1143). *Dose: Usual,* 25 mg up to 4 times a day as necessary.

Methaphenilene Hydrochloride [*N,N*-Dimethyl-*N'*-phenyl-*N'*-(2-thenyl)ethylenediamine monohydrochloride] [$C_{15}H_{20}N_2S.HCl$]—It occurs as crystals which melt between 186° and 187°. It is freely soluble in water; soluble in alcohol. *Uses:* An antihistaminic agent which is moderately effective in various allergic conditions and in the symptomatic relief of upper respiratory infections. Untoward effects include moderate sedation and gastrointestinal irritation, in a small number of patients. *Dose: Orally,* 50 mg 4 times a day.

Pheniramine Maleate NF XII [Prophenpyridamine Maleate; 2-[α-[2-(Dimethylamino)ethyl]benzyl]pyridine Maleate (1:1); Trimeton (*Schering*)], dried at 65° for 6 hours, contains not less than 99.0% of $C_{16}H_{20}N_2.C_4H_4O_4$ (356.43). *Preparation:* The base may be prepared by condensing 1-phenyl-1-(2-pyridyl)-3-chloropropane with dimethylamine in the presence of sodamide. Treatment of the base with an equimolar portion of maleic acid results in the formation of the maleate. *Description and Solubility:* A white, crystalline powder with a faint, amine-like odor; pH of a 1 in 100 solution, 4.5–5.5; melts between 104° and 108°. 1 Gm dissolves in 5 ml of water; very soluble in alcohol; slightly soluble in benzene and ether. *Uses:* An antihistaminic with moderate sedation and side effects similar to other members of this group of drugs. See general statement (page 1143). *Dose: Usual,* 40 mg.

Rotoxamine [Twiston (*McNeil*)] is (−)-2-[*p*-chloro-α(2-dimethylaminoethoxy)benzyl]pyridine. *Uses:* Rotoxamine, the active isomer of carbinoxamine (page 1145), is used in the *d*-tartrate salt as an antihistamine. It is used for allergic disorders, urticaria, drug reactions, and pruritic skin conditions. It is also used as adjunct therapy in the management of asthma. Limitations, side effects, and contraindications are the same as those for other agents of this class. *Dose:* 2 to 4 mg.

5-Hydroxytryptamine Antagonists

The pharmacologic actions of 5-hydroxytryptamine are varied and complex. Liberation of excessive amounts in man, as in argentaffin cell tumors, produce episodic flushing, tachycardia, and hypertension followed by cyanosis and diarrhea, asthma, and pulmonary stenosis. 5-Hydroxytryptamine antagonists have been employed in the management of this malignancy as well as certain skin diseases and psychoses. The most likely effective clinical application of these antagonists, however, is in the treatment of malignant carcinoid.

In addition to the agents described below, methysergide maleate exhibits 5-hydroxytryptamine antagonist properties. It also has other more prominent actions and uses; consequently, it is described in another chapter (see page 953).

Cyproheptadine Hydrochloride NF

[4-(5*H*-Dibenzo[*a,d*]cyclohepten-5-ylidene)-1-methylpiperidine Hydrochloride; Periactin Hydrochloride (*MSD*)]

Cyproheptadine Hydrochloride [$C_{21}H_{21}N.HCl.1\frac{1}{2}H_2O = 350.89$], dried in vacuum at 100° to constant weight, contains 98.5–100.5% of $C_{21}H_{21}N.HCl$ (323.93).

Preparation—Phthalic anhydride is reacted with phenylacetic acid to form 3-benzylidenephthalide which, on isomerization and hydrogenation, gives 2-phenethylbenzoic acid. This is converted to its acid chloride which then undergoes condensation to close the 7-membered ring and give 10,11-dihydro-5*H*-dibenzo[*a,d*]cyclohepten-5-one. Bromination at the 10 position followed by dehydrobromination introduces the 10,11 double bond. Grignardization of this ketone with 4-chloro-1-methylpiperidine followed by dehydration of the resulting carbinol yields cyproheptadine (base) which, on reacting with an equimolar quantity of hydrogen chloride, forms the official salt. US Pat. 3,014,911.

Description—A white to slightly yellow, crystalline powder that is odorless or practically odorless and has a slightly bitter taste. It is relatively stable in light, stable at room temperature, and nonhygroscopic. The sesquihydrate is stable in air. The anhydrous form melts at about 250° and the sesquihydrate melts at about 162°.

Solubility—1 Gm dissolves in about 1.5 ml of methanol, about 16 ml of chloroform, about 35 ml of alcohol, and about 275 ml of water; practically insoluble in ether.

Uses—Cyproheptadine Hydrochloride, an agent with both antihistaminic and antiserotonin properties, is used as an antipruritic. It is useful in relieving pruritus associated with various dermatoses. The drug has also been reported efficacious in relieving the symptoms of hay fever and asthma of allergic origin in children. Drowsiness, dryness of the mouth, men-tal confusion, ataxia, dizziness, irritability, fatigue, nausea, headache, and anorexia are occasionally en-countered during treatment with Cyproheptadine.

There is evidence that this drug improves the appe-tite in children and results in weight gain.

Dose—4 to **20 mg** a day; *usual*, **4 mg** 3 or 4 times a day.

Dosage Forms—Syrup NF: 2 mg/5 ml; Tablets NF: 4 mg.

References

1. Pyman, *J. Chem. Soc.*, **99**, 668 (1911).
2. Garford and Pyman, *J. Chem. Soc.*, **99**, 489 (1935).
3. Hoffman, *et al*, *Helv, Chim, Acta*, **39**, 607 (1956).

65 | Central Nervous System Stimulants

Xanthine derivatives—analeptics—miscellaneous central nervous system stimulants

This chapter was prepared by

Ewart A. Swinyard, PhD, *Professor of Pharmacology, College of Pharmacy and College of Medicine, University of Utah, Salt Lake City, Utah 84112, and* **Stewart C. Harvey, PhD,** *Associate Professor of Pharmacology, College of Medicine, University of Utah, Salt Lake City, Utah 84112*

Central nervous system stimulants are drugs which increase the activity of some portion of the brain or spinal cord. Drugs which act upon the sensory areas in the brain, (eg, caffeine and its various combinations) increase alertness, brighten spirits, and combat mental fatigue; those which act directly or reflexly on the medulla (eg, nikethamide, pentylenetetrazol, and picrotoxin) stimulate the respiratory center; those which act on the spinal cord (eg, nux vomica and strychnine) facilitate and exaggerate spinal reflexes.

Although the central nervous system stimulants are sometimes dramatic in their pharmacological effects, they are much less important therapeutically than the central nervous system depressants. It is not possible to stimulate the central nervous system over a long period of time because heightened nervous activity is followed by depression, proportional in degree to the intensity and duration of the stimulation. Consequently, therapeutic excitation of the central nervous system is usually of brief duration and reserved for the emergency management of central depression. Those agents which stimulate depressed respiration have special value; those which act on the vasomotor or chemoreceptor vomiting center in the medulla also have some usefulness; and those which possess the ability to lessen narcosis, referred to collectively as analeptics, are of value in the treatment of drug-induced depression. Because the central nervous system stimu-

lants act at various levels of the central nervous system, they are sometimes classified by site of action as cerebral, medullary, and spinal agents. However, any such classification is quite arbitrary since the various stimulants affect tracts and nuclei other than those at the anatomic site of definition. Indeed, a number of central nervous system stimulants have therapeutically useful actions on other parts of the body, and a number of drugs not included in this chapter stimulate the central nervous system when administered in toxic doses. For example, caffeine, a classical central nervous system stimulant, has clinically useful actions on the heart, blood vessels, and kidneys. On the other hand, atropine and ephedrine, drugs with primary actions on the peripheral autonomic nervous system, stimulate the central nervous system.

Only those drugs which have central stimulation as their predominant action are listed in this section. Those agents whose central stimulant properties are secondary (atropine, sympathomimetic amines, cocaine, nicotine, lobeline, carbon dioxide, cyanide, apomorphine, and emetine) and those whose central stimulant properties are induced only with toxic doses (phenol, salicylates, local anesthetics, ergot alkaloids, etc) are listed in other chapters. For convenience, the drugs described are divided into three groups: xanthine derivatives, analeptics, and miscellaneous central nervous system stimulants.

Xanthine Derivatives

Caffeine, theobromine, theophylline, and the newer, related xanthine derivatives are similar in their pharmacological properties but differ markedly in the intensity of their actions on various structures. For example, theobromine and theophylline surpass caffeine in their diuretic, cardiac, and muscular actions, whereas caffeine is a more potent central stimulant and theophylline surpasses theobromine in diuretic efficacy. Therefore, in the therapeutic application of these drugs for a specific effect, side actions can be minimized and the desired effect intensified by the selection of the proper xanthine. The clinically useful therapeutic actions of the xanthines include the ability to stimulate the central nervous system, the action on the kidney to produce diuresis, the stimulating effect on cardiac muscle, and the relaxation of certain smooth muscle structures, particularly the coronary arteries and bronchi. The relative usefulness of the various xanthines in producing these and other clinical effects is indicated in the monographs which follow.

Aminophylline USP

[Theophylline Ethylenediamine Compound(2:1)]

Aminophylline [$C_{16}H_{24}N_{10}O_4 \cdot xH_2O$] is anhydrous or contains not more than two molecules of water of hydration (mol wt, anhydrous form = 420.43). Aminophylline contains 84.0–86.0% of anhydrous theophylline [$C_7H_8N_4O_2$ = 180.17], and 14.0–15.0% of ethylenediamine [$C_2H_8N_2$ = 60.10], both calculated on the anhydrous basis.

Preparation—Aminophylline may be prepared by adding, with vigorous stirring, a weighed quantity of theophylline to a volume of ethylenediamine solution containing the required equivalent quantity of the diamine previously diluted with several volumes of anhydrous alcohol. After standing a few hours, the precipitate of aminophylline is filtered with suction, washed with cold alcohol, and dried at a low temperature.

Description—White or slightly yellowish granules or powder, having a slight ammoniacal odor and a bitter taste. On exposure to air it gradually loses ethylenediamine and absorbs carbon dioxide with liberation of free theophylline. Its solution is alkaline to litmus.

Solubility—1 Gm dissolves in about 5 ml of water, but, owing to hydrolysis, separation of crystals of less aminated theophylline begins in a few minutes, these crystals dissolving on the addition of a small amount of ethylenediamine. When, however, 1 Gm is dissolved in 25 ml of water, the solution remains clear; insoluble in alcohol and ether.

Incompatibilities—Its aqueous solutions are alkaline and display the incompatibilities of the alkalies. *Acids* cause a precipitation of theophylline; even *carbon dioxide* of the air behaves thus. Acid-reacting vehicles cannot therefore be used. When "dry" formulations containing aminophylline are prepared, care should be used in selecting dry ingredients and in preventing the future introduction of atmospheric moisture. Light magnesium carbonate has been used in some capsule formulations to enhance stability.

Uses—A *smooth muscle relaxant* used for the treatment of bronchospasm and coronary disease. Thus, it is used in the treatment of bronchial asthma, cardiac asthma, and pulmonary edema; arteriosclerosis and hypertensive headache; in biliary colic and in various pruritic dermatoses. It also shares other properties of the xanthines (central stimulation, diuresis, etc), but these are insignificant with usual doses. Absorption from the gastrointestinal tract after oral or rectal administration is incomplete, slow, and variable. It is most effective when given intravenously; if given slowly in dilute solution, the drug is relative nontoxic. See *Theophylline.*

Dose—*Oral,* **300** to **800 mg** daily; *usual,* **200 mg** 3 times a day. *Intravenous,* slowly, **250 mg** to **1.5 Gm** daily; *usual,* slowly, **500 mg** 1 to 3 times a day. *Rectal,* **250 mg** to **1 Gm** daily; *usual,* **500 mg** 1 or 2 times a day.

Dosage Forms—Injection USP: 250 mg/10 ml, 500 mg/20 ml (see below); Suppositories USP: 100, 125, 250, and 500 mg; Tablets USP: 100 and 200 mg.

Veterinary Dose—*Dogs,* 30 to **100 mg,** *orally.*

Aminophylline Injection USP [Theophylline Ethylenediamine Injection] is a sterile solution of aminophylline in water for injection, or is a sterile solution of theophylline in water for injection prepared with the aid of ethylenediamine. It contains, in each 100 ml, 2.325–2.675 Gm of $C_{16}H_{24}N_{10}O_4.2H_2O$. Aminophylline Injection may contain an excess of ethylenediamine, but no other substance added for the purpose of pH adjustment, in an amount not exceeding 20 mg of $C_2H_8N_2$ per Gm of $C_{16}H_{24}N_{10}O_4.2H_2O$. *Stabilization:* The aminophylline in this injection absorbs carbon dioxide from the air resulting in the liberation of free theophylline. The USP recognizes the difficulties experienced with the aminophylline injection and, for purposes of stabilization, permits the use of additional *Ethylenediamine* (see page 1317) to the extent of 63 mg for each 1 Gm of aminophylline. However, even this amount may not solve the problem. Since aminophylline absorbs carbon dioxide, thus liberating free theophylline, every precaution should be taken to protect this substance from undue exposure to air and, as far as possible, fresh stock should be used. In this respect it might even be advisable to prepare the solution directly from calculated quantities of theophylline and

of ethylenediamine, thus entirely eliminating the possibility of previous absorption of carbon dioxide. It has been found helpful to ampul the solution while hot, seal it at once, thus producing a slight vacuum in the ampul, and then sterilize the ampul immediately by autoclaving before seed crystals can start to form. Some operators prefer to repeat the sterilization operation, believing that this also helps to prevent subsequent precipitation.

Caffeine USP

[Coffeina; Coffeinum; 1,3,7-Trimethylxanthine; Theine]

Caffeine is anhydrous or contains one molecule of water of hydration. It contains 98.5–101.0% of $C_8H_{10}N_4O_2$ (194.19), calculated on the anhydrous basis.

For the structural formula, see page 497.

History—This alkaloid was discovered by Robiquet in coffee in 1821 while searching for quinine which he believed to be present. In 1827 Oudry found an alkaloid in tea and called in *theine.* In 1838 Jobst and Mülder proved the identical character of the two principles.

Preparation—Caffeine is obtained from tea and coffee, chiefly the former. It also occurs in some other plants, eg, Kola and Guarana. Percentages of caffeine in various substances are as follows: in tea, 1 to 4.8; in kola nuts, 2.7 to 3.6; in coffee, 1 to 1.5; in maté, 1.25 to 2; in guarana, 3 to 5.

Caffeine may be prepared from tea or coffee by boiling with water in the presence of lime or magnesium oxide, which serves to precipitate the tannins and some of the coloring matter. After filtration, the crude caffeine which separates is recrystallized from hot water after treatment with decolorizing charcoal. A source of the commercial supply is tea dust or sweepings; increasing quantities of caffeine are now obtained as a by-product in the manufacture of "decaffeinized coffee." It is also produced by methylation of theobromine (partial synthesis) and by total synthesis from urea or dimethylurea by variations of Traube's classic process.[1] The essential steps of a synthesis of theophylline and caffeine from urea are shown below:

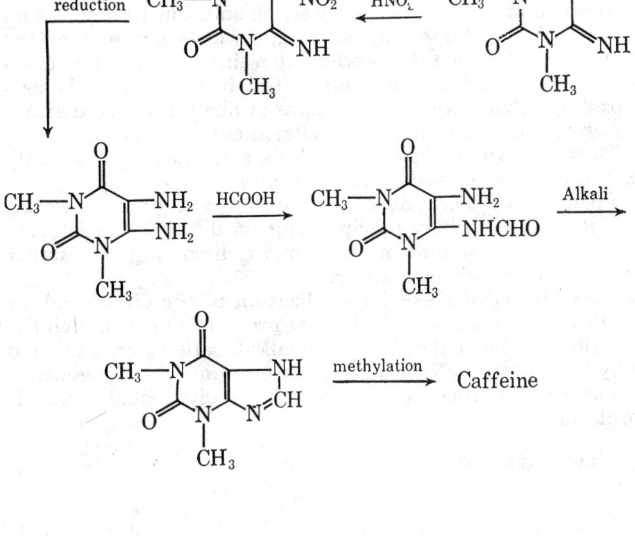

Description—A white powder or white, glistening needles, usually matted. It is odorless and has a bitter taste. Solutions of Caffeine are neutral to litmus. The hydrate is efflorescent in air and loses all its moisture at 80°. Caffeine when rendered anhydrous by drying melts between 235° and 237.5°.

Solubility—1 Gm of hydrous Caffeine dissolves in about 50 ml of water, 6 ml of water at 80°, 75 ml of alcohol, about 25 ml of alcohol at 60°, about 6 ml of chloroform, and 600 ml of ether. Being a weak base, caffeine does not form stable salts, and even its salts of strong acids, such as the hydrochloride or hydrobromide, are readily hydrolyzed by water. The solubility of caffeine in water is increased by the presence of organic acids or their alkali salts, eg, benzoates, salicylates, cinnamates, or citrates and this is the reason for the official recognition of several such preparations.

Uses—Caffeine belongs to a group of drugs known as the xanthines, the other important members being theobromine and theophylline. All possess certain actions in common, but to different degrees. They stimulate the central nervous system, are myocardial stimulants, increase blood flow through the coronary arteries, relax the smooth muscle of bronchi, and are active diuretics. In the case of Caffeine, its action on the central nervous system is the most prominent and the drug is used almost exclusively as a *central stimulant*. For oral administration, Caffeine itself or citrated caffeine is employed. Caffeine and sodium benzoate is the preparation of choice for parenteral injection.

Caffeine is often used in combination with analgetic drugs for the relief of headaches. The clinical superiority of such combinations remains to be proven. In addition, caffeine is sometimes used to stimulate the secretion of hydrochloric acid in the diagnosis of gastric anacidity.

Dose—100 to 500 mg; *usual*, **200 mg** as necessary.

Veterinary Dose—*Horses* and *Cattle*, **5 to 10 Gm**; *Sheep* and *Swine*, **0.5 to 3 Gm**; *Dogs*, **100 to 300 mg**.

Citrated Caffeine NF

Citrated Caffeine is a mixture of caffeine and citric acid containing, when dried at 80° for 4 hours, 48.0–52.0% of $C_8H_{10}N_4O_2$ (anhydrous caffeine) and 48.0–52.0% of $C_6H_8O_7$ (anhydrous citric acid). The sum of the percentages of anhydrous caffeine and anhydrous citric acid is 98.5–101.0.

Preparation—The formula of USP IX was:

Caffeine.........................	**50 Gm**
Citric Acid......................	**50 Gm**
Distilled Water, hot..............	**100 ml**

Dissolve the citric acid in the hot distilled water, add the caffeine, and evaporate the resulting solution to dryness on a water bath, constantly stirring towards the end of the operation. Reduce the product to a fine powder and transfer it to well-closed containers. It is, however, usually prepared by mixing equal proportions of finely powdered anhydrous caffeine and anhydrous citric acid.

Description—White, odorless powder having a slightly bitter, acid taste, and an acid reaction.

Solubility—1 Gm dissolves in about 4 ml of warm water, the caffeine gradually precipitating on diluting the solution with an equal volume of water but redissolving on further dilution with sufficient water.

Incompatibilities—Neutralization of the citric acid by *alkalies* or *alkaline salts* will cause precipitation of caffeine if in sufficient concentration. The alkali salts of organic acid may form either caffeine or the free organic acid. In general, it displays the incompatibilities of the citric acid which it contains.

Uses—See *Caffeine*.

Dose—100 to 500 mg; *usual*, **300 mg** as necessary.
Dosage Forms—Tablets NF: 60 and 150 mg.
Veterinary Dose—*Dogs*, **120 to 500 mg**.

Caffeine and Sodium Benzoate Injection USP

[Injectio Coffeini et Natrii Benzoas]

Caffeine and Sodium Benzoate Injection is a sterile solution of caffeine and sodium benzoate in water for injection. It contains an amount of anhydrous caffeine ($C_8H_{10}N_4O_2$) equivalent to 45.0–52.0%, and an amount of sodium benzoate ($C_7H_5NaO_2$) equivalent to 47.5–55.5%, of the labeled amounts of caffeine and sodium benzoate.

Description—Its pH is between 6.5 and 8.5.

Dose—*Parenteral*, **200 mg** to **1 Gm**; *usual*, **500 mg**, repeated as necessary.

Oxtriphylline NF

[Choline Theophyllinate; Choledyl (*Warner-Chilcott*)]

Oxtriphylline [$C_{12}H_{21}N_5O_3$ = 283.33] contains 41.9–43.6% of $C_5H_{15}NO_2$ (choline), and 61.7–65.5% of $C_7H_8N_4O_2$ (theophylline), calculated on the dried basis.

Preparation—An aqueous solution of choline bicarbonate is reacted with theophylline in isopropanol. After concentration by vacuum distillation, the crude product is crystallized from isopropanol–methanol solution. US Pat. 2,776,287 and 2,776,288.

Description—It occurs as white granules containing about 60% of anhydrous theophylline.
Solubility—1 Gm dissolves in 1 ml of water.

Uses—Oxtriphylline, a theophylline compound, is more soluble, more stable, better absorbed from the gastrointestinal tract, and produces less gastric irritation than aminophylline, but has pharmacological actions similar to other xanthine derivatives. Hence, it is effective orally in the management of bronchial asthma, paroxysmal cardiac dyspnea, Cheyne–Stokes respiration, and chronic edema secondary to congestive heart failure. Its usefulness in premenstrual tension or in dysmenorrhea has not been established.

Dose—200 to 400 mg; *usual*, **200 mg** 4 times a day.
Dosage Forms—Tablets NF: 100 and 200 mg.

Theobromine NF XII

[3,7-Dimethylxanthine]

Theobromine [$C_7H_8N_4O_2$ = 180.17] is an alkaloid prepared from the dried ripe seed of *Theobroma cacao* Linné (Fam. *Sterculiaceæ*), or made synthetically.
For the structural formula, see page 497.

Description—A white, crystalline powder with a bitter taste. It sublimes at about 260°.
Solubility—1 Gm is soluble in about 1800 ml of water, about 2400 ml of alcohol, about 6000 ml of chloroform, and about 150 ml of boiling water; soluble in solutions of fixed

alkali hydroxides, concentrated acids, and is slowly soluble in ammonia solution; insoluble in benzene, carbon tetrachloride, and ether.

Uses—Theobromine possesses actions common to the xanthine derivatives (see *Caffeine*). Its action on the central nervous system is minimal, however, and thus it can be used for its other effects without the attending side-action of central stimulation. Theobromine is employed as a diuretic, its action on the kidney being more lasting than other xanthines. It acts by inhibiting reabsorption in the renal tubules. It is practically devoid of toxicity and thus can be employed on occasions when the more toxic diuretics are contraindicated, as, for example, when renal function is poor. The wide choice of more effective diuretics has limited the use of theobromine for this purpose.

Theobromine salts are also employed to some extent for their action on the coronary arteries. Although their value in angina pectoris is controversial, they are used in this condition on the premise that they increase coronary blood flow. Xanthine preparations are apt to cause gastric irritation and are best given during meals. The salts are less irritating than the alkaloidal bases.

Dose—*Usual*, **500 mg.**

Theophylline USP

[1,3-Dimethylxanthine; Elixophyllin (*Sherman*); Optiphyllin (*Fougera*); Theolix (*Vale*)]

Theophylline [$C_7H_8N_4O_2.H_2O = 198.18$] contains one molecule of water of hydration or is anhydrous. It contains 98.5–101.0% of $C_7H_8N_4O_2$, calculated on the dried basis.

For the structural formula, see page 497.

Preparation—Theophylline is present in tea but in too small an amount to make it an economical source. It has been made from caffeine, but is more successfully produced by total synthesis. See page 1155.

Description—A white, odorless, crystalline powder having a bitter taste. It is stable in air. It melts between 270° and 274°, and its saturated aqueous solution is neutral or slightly acid to litmus. Theophylline is weaker as a base than caffeine or theobromine and scarcely forms salts even with the strong acids, but is more "acidic" than those and readily dissolves in ammonia water.

Solubility—1 Gm dissolves in about 120 ml of water and about 80 ml of alcohol; more soluble in hot water; sparingly soluble in ether and chloroform; freely soluble in solutions of alkali hydroxides and ammonia.

Uses—Theophylline is the most versatile of the xanthine alkaloids and is employed more widely than any other member of the group. It is an effective *diuretic*, having a more powerful but somewhat less sustained action than theobromine. As a diuretic it is used in the treatment of *cardiac* and *nephrotic edema*.

Theophylline is used in the treatment of *angina pectoris*, but the same limitations apply for this drug as for theobromine.

Theophylline is more effective than any other xanthine in relaxing bronchial muscle. It is of special value in cases of *status asthmaticus* that are resistant to epinephrine. The particular preparation employed is theophylline ethylenediamine. Theophylline salts are also effective in the prophylaxis of asthma.

The cardiac actions of Theophylline are of value in the treatment of *paroxysmal nocturnal dyspnea* resulting from left ventricular failure. In this instance stimulation of the myocardium and relaxation of bronchial muscles contribute to the symptomatic relief. The-

ophylline ethylenediamine is used for this purpose. The central actions of Theophylline are of value in the treatment of Cheyne–Stokes respiration, this type of periodic respiration being immediately relieved by the injection of theophylline ethylenediamine.

Theophylline is used in the preparation of *Mersalyl* and of *Mercurophylline*.

Dose—*Usual*, **200 mg** 3 or 4 times a day.

Other Dose Information—The diuretic dose of Theophylline itself is 0.25 Gm 3 to 5 times daily, taken orally. The dose of its various salts is 0.5 Gm 3 to 5 times daily. It is given by slow intravenous injection in the dose of 0.25 to 0.50 Gm.

Dosage Forms—Tablets NF: 100 and 200 mg.

Theophylline, Ephedrine Hydrochloride, and Phenobarbital Tablets NF

[Tedral Tablets (*Warner Chilcott*)]

Theophylline, Ephedrine Hydrochloride, and Phenobarbital Tablets contain 90.0–110.0% of the labeled amounts of $C_7H_8N_4O_2.H_2O$ (theophylline), of $C_{10}H_{15}NO.HCl$ (ephedrine hydrochloride), and of $C_{12}H_{12}N_2O_3$ (phenobarbital).

Uses—Theophylline, Ephedrine Hydrochloride, and Phenobarbital is widely used in the symptomatic relief of bronchial asthma, asthmatic bronchitis, and bronchospastic disorders. It is also used to abort or minimize asthmatic attacks and is of value in the management of seasonal asthma. The theophylline and ephedrine induce bronchodilation, whereas the phenobarbital is intended to counteract possible stimulation by ephedrine and as a mild, long-acting sedative for the apprehensive asthmatic patient. This combination should be used with caution in patients with cardiovascular disease, severe hypertension, prostatic hypertrophy, or glaucoma. Adverse reactions include epigastric distress, palpitation, tremulousness, insomnia, difficult micturition, and CNS stimulation. It should be remembered that phenobarbital may be habit forming.

Dose—*Usual*, Theophylline, **130** to **260 mg** every 4 hours; Ephedrine Hydrochloride, **24** to **48 mg** every 4 hours; Phenobarbital, **8** to **16 mg** every 4 hours.

Dosage Forms—NF: 130 mg (theophylline), 24 mg (ephedrine hydrochloride), and 8 mg (phenobarbital).

Theophylline Sodium Acetate NF

[Theophyllinum Natricum et Natrii Acetas; Theophylline and Sodium Acetate]

Theophylline Sodium Acetate is a hydrated mixture of $C_7H_7N_4NaO_2$ (202.15) (sodium theophylline) and $C_2H_3NaO_2$ (82.03) (sodium acetate) in approximately equimolecular proportions. It yields 55.0–65.0% of $C_7H_8N_4O_2$ (180.17) (anhydrous theophylline).

Preparation—A quantity of sodium hydroxide equivalent in NaOH content to the quantity of theophylline to be used is dissolved in alcohol and the theophylline is then dissolved in this solution. An equivalent amount of sodium acetate is added and the mixture evaporated on a steam bath with frequent stirring. The dry residue is then quickly powdered and put into tight containers.

Description—A white, odorless, crystalline powder having a bitter, salty taste. It gradually absorbs CO_2 from the air and liberates free theophylline. Its solution is alkaline to phenolphthalein TS.

Solubility—1 Gm dissolves in about 25 ml of water; insoluble in alcohol, ether, and chloroform.

Incompatibilities—Aqueous solutions are alkaline and display the incompatibilities of the alkalies. *Acids,* including *carbon dioxide* from the air, liberate theophylline.

Uses—See *Theophylline.*
Dose—*Usual,* **200 mg** to **300 mg** 3 times a day.
Dosage Forms—Tablets NF: 100 and 200 mg.

Theophylline Sodium Glycinate NF

[Glytheonate (*Patch*); Synophylate (*Central*)]

Theophylline Sodium Glycinate is an equilibrium mixture containing $C_7H_7N_4NaO_2$ (sodium theophylline) and $C_2H_5NO_2$ (aminoacetic acid) in approximately equimolecular proportions buffered with an additional mole of aminoacetic acid. Dried at 105° for 4 hours, it yields 49.0–52.0% of $C_7H_8N_4O_2.H_2O$ (theophylline).

Description—A white, crystalline powder. It has a slight ammoniacal odor, and a bitter taste. The pH of a saturated solution is between 8.5 to 9.5.
Solubility—Freely soluble in water; very slightly soluble in alcohol; practically insoluble in chloroform.

Uses—Theophylline Sodium Glycinate is a *smooth muscle relaxant* which is used in the treatment of bronchospasm and coronary artery disease. It should not be used in patients who might be harmed by myocardial stimulation.
Dose—*Usual,* **300 mg** every 4 to 6 hours.
Dosage Forms—Tablets NF: 150, 300, and 330 mg.

Other Xanthine Derivatives

Caffeine and Sodium Salicylate NF X—Purity: 48–52% anhydrous caffeine and 48–52% sodium salicylate. A white odorless, amorphous powder, or granular mass having a bitter, saline taste. One Gm dissolves in 2 ml water and 50 ml alcohol. Its actions and uses are the same as for caffeine, the sodium salicylate being present to increase the solubility of the alkaloid. See *Caffeine* (page 1155). *Dose: Orally,* 0.2 Gm.

Dyphylline [7-(2,3-Dihydroxypropyl)theophylline; Neothylline (*Lemmon*)] [$C_{10}H_{14}N_4O_4$]—A white, extremely bitter, amorphous solid, with a melting point between 155° and 160°. It is freely soluble in water and soluble to the extent of 2 Gm in 100 ml alcohol. The pH of a 1% solution is between 6.5 and 7.0. *Uses:* Peripheral vasodilator and bronchodilator actions characteristic of theophylline derivative.

It is effective orally but has not been shown to be superior to theophylline-sodium glycinate. It also has typical diuretic and myocardial stimulant effects. It is not recommended for use in coronary disease or angina pectoris until it can be shown that increased coronary blood flow precedes rather than follows myocardial stimulation. Its toxicity in mice is considerably less than that of aminophylline. *Dose:* Orally, 0.2 Gm 3 times a day, then individualized dosage.

Theobromine Calcium Salicylate NF XI [Theocalcin (*Knoll*)]—A double salt or complex in equimolar proportions of theobromine calcium and calcium salicylate. It contains 46–50% theobromine. A white, odorless powder having a saline taste. It is slightly soluble in water; insoluble in alcohol. *Uses:* Same uses as for *Theobromine Sodium Salicylate* (below) but is less of a gastric irritant. *Dose:* 500 mg.

Theobromine Sodium Acetate NF XI [Thesodate (*Brewer*)]—A hydrated mixture of theobromine sodium and sodium acetate in approximately equimolecular proportions. It yields 55–65% theobromine. A white, bitter, crystalline powder. It is moderately hygroscopic. On exposure to air, the powder or its solution gradually absorbs CO_2 with liberation of theobromine. 1 Gm dissolves in about 1.5 ml of water. It is slightly soluble in alcohol. *Uses:* Used for the same purposes and in approximately the same dosage as *Theobromine Sodium Salicylate* (below). *Dose:* 500 mg.

Theobromine Sodium Salicylate NF XI—A mixture of theobromine sodium and sodium salicylate in approximately equimolecular proportions. It yields not less than 46.5% of theobromine and not less than 35% of salicylic acid. A white, or essentially white, powder, having a sweetish, salty and somewhat alkaline taste. It is odorless or has a slight peculiar (ozone-like) odor. On exposure to air it absorbs CO_2 and becomes incompletely soluble in water. Its solution (1 in 20) is alkaline. 1 Gm dissolves in about 1 ml of water; slightly soluble in alcohol. *Uses:* A diuretic and smooth muscle relaxant. Its action on the central nervous system is minimal. It is practically devoid of toxicity and can be employed when the more toxic diuretics are contraindicated. Its value in the treatment of angina pectoris is controversial. *Dose:* 1 Gm. *Veterinary Dose: Horses* and *Cattle,* 8 to 15 Gm; *Dogs,* 300 mg to 1 Gm.

Theophylline-Meglumine—An equimolecular mixture of theophylline monohydrate and N-methylglucamine [1-deoxy-1-(methylamino)-D-glucitol]. *Uses:* Identical in action and uses to aminophylline, over which it has no advantage. More soluble than theophylline sodium acetate. *Dose: Orally,* 0.15 to 0.75 Gm; *rectally,* 0.5 Gm.

Theophylline Monoethanolamine [Theophylline Ethanolamine; Monotheamin (*Lilly*)] is $C_7H_8N_4O_2$.-$HOCH_2CH_2NH_2$. It contains anhydrous theophylline (75%) and ethanolamine (25%). *Description* and *Solubility:* A white, crystalline, nonhygroscopic powder. Soluble in water. *Uses:* Has the same actions and uses as *Aminophylline* (page 1154). *Dosage Forms:* Suppositories, 500 mg.

Analeptics

Analeptics are central nervous system stimulants which are employed primarily to counteract drug-induced respiratory depression. This action is largely the result of a direct stimulation of the respiratory center. Excessive quantities of analeptics cause the stimulation to spread to other areas of the brain and may thereby precipitate convulsions. Convulsions may also result when an ordinary dose is used for mild depressions. The most commonly employed analeptics include bemegride, ethamivan, nikethamide, pentylenetetrazol, and picrotoxin. The value of analeptics in the management of acute barbiturate poisoning remains unsettled. Some authorities claim that the use of these agents in selected patients with severe respiratory depression may be lifesaving; others argue that their use is dangerous and never justified. All agree, however, that the use of these agents should not supplant the usual medical measures to support the patients vital functions. Hence, the airway is kept clear by suction or by endotracheal tube, the patient is turned regularly, and oxygen is administered as needed. Shock is overcome by the use of blood or plasma expanders and vasopressors. Where available, dialysis is used to remove the drug. When an analeptic is employed, the dosage is individualized in accordance with the patient's response to the drug.

Bemegride USP XVII

[3-Ethyl-3-methylglutarimide; Megimide (*Abbott*)]

Bemegride contains 98.5%–101.0% of $C_8H_{13}NO_2$ (155.20), calculated on the anhydrous basis.

Preparation—Ethyl methyl ketone is condensed with two molecules of ethyl cyanoacetate by means of saturated alcoholic ammonia to yield the Guareschi-type imide, α,α'-dicyano-β-ethyl-β-methylglutarimide, which is then treated with hot 50% H_2SO_4 to form β-ethyl-β-methylglutaric acid. The acid is converted into its anhydride by heating with acetic anhydride at 175°, and interaction of the anhydride with fused urea at 200° yields Bemegride. The crude product is purified by recrystallization from water.

Description—White or creamy white, almost odorless, flakes or crystalline powder.

Solubility—Slightly soluble in water; soluble in alcohol; freely soluble in chloroform and solutions of alkali hydroxides.

Uses—Bemegride is an analeptic agent with non-specific stimulating effects similar to other members of the class. It is used mainly as an adjunct in the treatment of barbiturate poisoning. Its onset, duration of action, and margin of safety are similar to those of pentylenetetrazol. Hence, overdosage may result in hyperreflexia, muscular twitching, and convulsive episodes. The value of analeptics in the management of poisoning from central nervous system depressants remains controversial. Most physicians recommend the use of mechanical respirators and symptomatic therapy.

Dose—50 to 150 mg; *usual, intravenous*, **50 mg.**

Other Dose Information—The *intravenous* dose for barbiturate intoxication is 50 mg at intervals of 3 to 5 minutes until signs of clinical improvement or toxicity appear. The dose required will depend on the degree of depression as well as other factors, necessitating careful evaluation of the individual patient.

Dosage Forms—Injection: 50 mg/10 ml.

Doxapram—see page 870.

Ethamivan NF

[*N,N*-Diethylvanillamide; Emivan (*USV*)]

Ethamivan contains 98.0–102.0% of $C_{12}H_{17}NO_3$ (223.27), calculated on the dried basis.

Preparation—Vanillin is subjected to the Cannizzaro reaction in a KOH/NaOH melt at about 200°. The vanillic acid thus formed is first acetylated at the phenolic hydroxyl and then reacted with diethylcarbamoyl chloride to form the acetylated ethamivan. Deacetylation with aqueous sodium hydroxide yields the official article. US Pat. 2,641,612.

Description—A white or practically white, crystalline powder having a faint, characteristic odor. It is stable in both light and air. It melts between 94° and 97°.

Solubility—Very soluble in chloroform; freely soluble in alcohol, acetone, and benzene; sparingly soluble in water and ether.

Uses—Ethamivan is a central nervous system stimulant and analeptic which is recommended for the management of severe respiratory depression secondary to barbiturate poisoning and carbon dioxide narcosis. It has also been used to shorten postanesthetic recovery in patients who have received barbiturate as adjuncts to anesthesia. Some reports indicate it may be used orally to relieve the symptoms of mild hypoventilation. Ethamivan, like other analeptics, can cause generalized central nervous system stimulation. Thus, excessive doses may induce hyperexcitability and convulsions.

Dose—*Usual, intravenous*, **0.5 to 5 mg** per **Kg** of body weight, given slowly as a single injection; and then may follow with continuous intravenous infusion at the rate of 10 mg per minute as determined by response of the patient.

Other Dose Information—The oral dose is 20 to 60 mg 2 to 4 times a day.

Dosage Forms—Injection NF: 100 mg/2 ml, 500 mg/10 ml; Tablets: 20 mg.

Nikethamide NF

[*N,N*-Diethylnicotinamide; Nicethamidum; Coramine (*Ciba*)]

Nikethamide contains 99.0–101.0% of $C_{10}H_{14}N_2O$ (178.24), calculated on the anhydrous basis.

Preparation—Nikethamide may be made by the conventional methods for the preparation of *N*-alkylated amides, that is either (1) by treating the ethyl or methyl ester of nicotinic acid with diethylamine, or (2) by reacting nicotinyl chloride with the amine. The nicotinyl chloride required in method (2) may be obtained by the action of phosphoryl chloride [$POCl_2$] or thionyl chloride [$SOCl_2$] on nicotinic acid.

Nikethamide has also been prepared directly from nicotinic acid by heating the latter with diethylamine in the presence of phosphorus pentoxide.

Description—A clear, colorless to pale yellowish, somewhat viscous liquid, which crystallizes on standing in the cold and melts again as the temperature rises. It has a faint, characteristic, aromatic odor, and a peculiar, bitter taste. Its solutions are clear and nearly colorless, and have no more than a faint odor of diethylamine. Specific gravity: 1.058 to 1.066. Congealing range: 22° to 24°. Refractive index: 1.522 to 1.524 at 25°.

Solubility—Miscible with water, alcohol, and ether.

Uses—Nikethamide is used as a *respiratory stimulant* in the event of excessive depression resulting from the use of central depressants. It is not as effective as bemegride, pentylenetetrazol, or picrotoxin. It is of little value as a cardiovascular stimulant. It also has a nicotinic acid-like effect and may be used in the treatment of pellagra. Toxic doses (10 times the minimal effective dose) may cause convulsions and death by respiratory paralysis.

Dose—*Usual, intramuscular* and *intravenous*, **375 mg** to **3.75 Gm** repeated as needed.

Dosage Forms—Injection NF: 375 mg/1.5 ml, 1.25 Gm/5 ml, 5 Gm/20 ml.

Veterinary Dose—*Dogs*, **0.25 Gm** for every **15 pounds** of body weight, *parenterally*. In profound depression, considerably larger doses may be given depending on the response of the subject.

Pentylenetetrazol NF

[6,7,8,9-Tetrahydro-5*H*-tetrazoloazepine; Leptazol; Penetetrazol; Pentamethylenetetrazol: Metrazol (*Knoll*)]

Pentylenetetrazol, previously dried over phosphorus pentoxide for 18 hours, contains 99.0–101.0% of $C_6H_{10}N_4$ (138.17).

Preparation—Pentylenetetrazol can be prepared from hydrazoic acid and cyclohexanone. The reaction proceeds in two steps, the intermediate (not isolated) being the seven-membered cyclic amide (a lactam known as 2-ketohexamethylenimine) formed by ring enlargement of cyclohexanone.

The preparation is carried out by slowly adding concentrated sulfuric acid to a benzene solution of cyclohexanone and hydrazoic acid maintained at 0° to 5°. The product is transferred to water by extraction of the benzene reaction mixture with iced water. The water extract is made alkaline and extracted exhaustively with ether. The product is obtained from ether by concentration and distillation under reduced pressure.

Cyclohexanone is commercially available, being prepared from cyclohexanol by oxidation. The latter, in turn, is prepared by high-pressure catalytic hydrogenation of phenol.

Description—White odorless crystals with a slightly pungent, bitter taste. A solution (1 in 10) is neutral to litmus. Melting range: 58° to 61°.

Solubility—Freely soluble in water and alcohol; soluble in ether, chloroform, and carbon tetrachloride.

Uses—Pentylenetetrazol is used as a *central nervous system stimulant* in the treatment of poisoning by central nervous system depressants and as an analeptic to lessen the degree of anesthesia. It is rapidly detoxified in the body and therefore its action can be well controlled. It is of doubtful value in circulatory collapse other than that due to central vasomotor depression. The drug has been used in the treatment of *schizophrenia* in doses which induce convulsions. Since this can be accomplished more effectively by electroshock, pentylenetetrazol is seldom used for this purpose. It has also been used to activate the EEG in the diagnosis of epilepsy.

Dose—*Intravenous* and *subcutaneous*, **100 mg to 2 Gm**; *usual, initial,* **500 mg,** then adjust dosage and repeat at 30-minute intervals as needed.

Dosage Forms—Injection NF: 100 mg/ml, 300 mg/3 ml, 3 Gm/30 ml, 10 Gm/100 ml.

Veterinary Dose—*Parenterally, Horses* and *Cattle,* **1 to 3 Gm;** *Dogs* and *Cats* of 20 pounds of body weight or less, **3 to 5 mg** per pound of body weight; over 20 pounds of body weight, **100 to 300 mg.**

Picrotoxin NF

[Cocculin]

Picrotoxin [$C_{30}H_{34}O_{13}$ = 602.60] is an active principle obtained from the seed of *Anamirta Cocculus* (Linné) Wight et Arnott (Fam. *Menispermaceæ*).

Preparation—According to Clark, Picrotoxin may be prepared as follows: The ground berries (seeds) are boiled with alcohol and filtered hot. The filtrate is concentrated and two volumes of hot water added. After cooling with ice it is filtered and the filtrate evaporated under reduced pressure. Picrotoxin crystallizes out during evaporation and is purified by solution in hot acetone and precipitation with water. The yield is about 1.4%.

Description—Flexible, shining, prismatic crystals or a micro-crystalline powder. It is odorless, and stable in air, but is affected by light. Its solutions are neutral to litmus. Picrotoxin melts between 198° and 200°.

Solubility—1 Gm dissolves in about 350 ml of water, about 30 ml of boiling water, and about 3 ml of boiling alcohol; more readily soluble in diluted acids and alkalies; sparingly soluble in ether and chloroform.

Uses—Picrotoxin is a powerful *central nervous system stimulant* and *convulsant* that acts chiefly on the higher centers. Thus, when the mid-brain and pons are removed in mammals, the convulsive effect disappears, although signs of medullary stimulation may persist. Its sole valid clinical use is in the *treatment of acute barbiturate intoxication*. It acts on the medulla and brain stem to improve respiration and circulation, hasten the return of swallowing and cough reflexes, and induce restlessness and movement which prevent dangerous circulatory stasis. The duration of picrotoxin action is short; the half-life is approximately 100 minutes. The metabolism of the drug is unknown.

Dose—*Usual, intravenous,* to be determined by the physician according to the needs of the patient.

Other Dose Information—Picrotoxin is injected intravenously in a continuous infusion at a rate of 1 to 2 mg per minute, or intermittently (6 to 12 mg every 10 to 20 minutes) until corneal and swallowing reflexes appear; subsequently, the drug is injected intramuscularly in doses of 3 to 6 mg at intervals of 15 to 30 minutes, as needed.

Dosage Forms—Injection NF: 3 mg/ml.

Veterinary Dose—*Dogs, parenterally,* **1.5 to 6 mg** in dilute solution.

Pipradrol Hydrochloride—see page 1118.

Racephedrine Hydrochloride—see page 898.

Other Stimulants Acting on the Medulla

Camphor, Monobromated NF X [3-Bromo-*d*-2-bornanone [$C_{10}H_{15}BrO$]—Colorless, prismatic needles or scales or a powder having a mild camphoraceous odor and taste, melting at 74–76°C. It is stable in air but is decomposed by prolonged exposure to sunlight. 1 Gm dissolves in 6.5 ml alcohol, 0.5 ml chloroform, and 1.6 ml ether but is practically insoluble in water. *Uses:* Has been used for headache and various neurologic conditions, but its action is largely that of camphor. *Dose: Orally,* 0.12 to 0.3 Gm.

Miscellaneous Central System Stimulants

A number of drugs which stimulate the central nervous system may quite properly be classified as either sympathomimetic or anorexigenic agents. Appropriate cross references to these substances are listed below. Other drugs, such as flurothyl, strychnine, and nux vomica, act primarily on the central nervous system and are described herein. There are no official preparations of either strychnine or nux vomica. Although strychnine has no valid place in modern therapeutics, it is important, not only from a historical point of view but also as a physiological tool for the study of the mechanism of action of other drugs, as a pesticide for destroying agricultural rodents and predatory animals, and as a frequently encountered cause of poisoning in man.

Amphetamine Phosphate—see page 896.

Amphetamine Sulfate—see page 882.

Benzphetamine Hydrochloride—see page 882.

Camphor—see page 773.

Dextroamphetamine—see page 883.

Dextroamphetamine Phosphate—see page 883.

Dextroamphetamine Phosphate, Dibasic—see page 896.

Dextroamphetamine Sulfate—see page 883.

Diethylpropion—see page 884.

Flurothyl NF

[Bis(2,2,2-trifluoroethyl) Ether; Indoklon (*Ohio Medical*)]

$$CF_3CH_2—O—CH_2CF_3$$

Flurothyl contains 99.6–100.0% of $C_4H_4F_6O$ (182.07), calculated on the dried basis.

Preparation—2,2,2-Trifluoroethyl *p*-toluenesulfonate is caused to undergo metathesis with sodium 2,2,2-trifluoroethoxide and the crude ether thus obtained is distilled and purified. US Pat. 3,363,006.

Description—A clear, colorless, volatile liquid having a pleasant, mild, ethereal odor; boils at about 64°.
Solubility—Slightly soluble in water; miscible with alcohol, ether, propylene glycol, and halogenated solvents.

Uses—Flurothyl, an agent known to produce clonic and tonic convulsions in laboratory animals, is used as an alternate for electroconvulsive therapy in the treatment of mental disorders. It has no important advantages over electroconvulsive therapy in most patients. Flurothyl is effective after either inhalation or parenteral administration. Convulsions start within 15 to 20 seconds after administration of the drug; the initial myoclonic jerks are followed by an intense tonic phase which lasts from 30 to 90 seconds. Recovery is prompt and uneventful. Many patients are said to prefer the drug to electroshock. On the other hand, flurothyl convulsions are less predictable and less easily induced than are electroshock seizures. Memory impairment, skeletal fractures, and prolonged apnea are occasional complications of both electroconvulsive therapy and drug-induced convulsions. Arterial spasm and gangrene may follow perivenous administration. Furthermore, the possibility that repeated administration of the halogenated compound might induce liver damage should not be ignored.

Dose—*Usual*, **1 ml** by special inhalation.
Other Dose Information—Intravenous, 6 to 8 ml of a 10% solution.
Dosage Forms—Inhalation: 2 ml.

Methylphenidate—see page 1116.

Phendimetrazine Tartrate—see page 897.

Phenmetrazine Hydrochloride—see page 893.

Phentermine—see page 893.

Strychnine

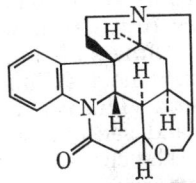

Strychnine [$C_{21}H_{22}N_2O_2 = 334.42$] is an alkaloid obtained chiefly from Nux Vomica. Woodward has effected a total synthesis[2] and has reviewed the work concerning structure.[3]

History—This alkaloid was first discovered in Ignatia bean in 1818 by the French pharmacists, Pelletier and Caventou, who gave it at that time the name which it still bears. They discovered brucine in 1819. It occurs in numerous plants belonging to the *Strychnos* species. In nux vomica seeds (*Strychnos Nux-vomica*) a little less than one-half of the alkaloid is Strychnine, while in Ignatia beans (*Strychnos Ignatia*) and in nux vomica from Saigon about ⅔ is strychnine; each contains from 2 to 3% of total alkaloids. Both brucine and Strychnine are present in other portions of the plants. These species are mainly Asiatic, while the bark of a South American species furnishes the product *Curare* (page 930).

Preparation—Comminuted nux vomica is thoroughly moistened with sodium carbonate and extracted with hot mineral oil or toluene. The alkaloids are removed from these solvents with diluted sulfuric acid and the acid solution is concentrated. The less soluble brucine bisulfate crystallizes from solution first. Upon neutralization and concentration of the mother liquor, strychnine sulfate crystallizes out, and is properly purified. The alkaloid is made from it by precipitation with ammonia. Nearly all Strychnine salts except the sulfate are made from the base by combining it with the desired acid.

Description—Colorless, transparent, prismatic crystals, or a white, crystalline powder. It is odorless, has a very bitter taste, and is stable in the air. Saturated solutions of Strychnine are alkaline to litmus.
Solubility—1 Gm dissolves in about 6420 ml of water, about 136 ml of alcohol, about 5 ml of chloroform, and about 180 ml of benzene; soluble in about 3100 ml of boiling water and about 34 ml of boiling alcohol; very slightly soluble in ether.

Uses—Strychnine is one of the most powerful of the central nervous system stimulants. It acts predominantly to block the inhibitory substance in the spinal cord. Hence, incoming sensory stimuli discharge all motor nerves with the result that all voluntary muscles of the body contract simultaneously. The actions of the stronger muscles predominate and a spinal convulsion results. With subconvulsive doses of strychnine, all spinal reflexes are exaggerated.

Strychnine was once widely employed as a bitter tonic, in combination with cathartic drugs, and as a cardiovascular stimulant. It has no therapeutic use which cannot be obtained with other less toxic and safer agents. Therefore, it has no valid place in modern therapeutics. Strychnine was formerly used in the treatment of poisoning from central nervous system depressants, especially barbiturates; it has been replaced by picrotoxin and other agents. Strychnine is contraindicated in morphine poisoning. The alkaloid is largely used as a pesticide for destroying agricultural rodents and predatory animals and for trapping fur animals.

The symptoms of strychnine poisoning are primarily those of stimulation of the central nervous system. The first symptom begins 10 to 30 minutes following ingestion, and is usually stiffness of the muscles of the neck and face. The patient next exhibits heightened reflex activity or excitability. This progresses to spontaneous muscle twitchings, and sensory stimuli may result in spinal convulsions. The characteristic picture is one of opisthotonos, trismus, and risus sardonicus. The convulsions may involve all voluntary muscles, including the diaphragm, thus interfering with the ability to breathe and resulting in cyanosis. Death is by respiratory failure.

Treatment of strychnine poisoning consists of prevention of asphyxia by maintaining a patent airway and adequate pulmonary ventilation, controlling the convulsions by the administration of a soluble barbiturate, ridding the body of the unabsorbed poison by gastric lavage with 1:10,000 potassium permanganate solution, and general supportive therapy. If the patient can be kept alive for 5 to 6 hours after ingestion of the drug, the prognosis is very good.

Caution—Strychnine is extremely poisonous.

Dose—*Usual*, **1.5 mg.**

Veterinary Dose—*Subcutaneously, Dogs*, **0.3 to 1 mg;** *Horses* and *Cattle*, **16 to 130 mg;** *Cats*, **0.12 to 0.5 mg.**

Other Miscellaneous Central Nervous System Stimulants

Brucine [$C_{23}H_{26}N_2O_4.4H_2O$]—An alkaloid of nux vomica. It differs from strychnine in that it contains 2 methoxy groups. The alkaloid occurs as colorless crystals or as a white, crystalline powder, losing its water of crystallization at 100°. When anhydrous it melts at about 178° and has a specific rotation of −85° in absolute alcohol. Brucine is more soluble in water than strychnine. One part is soluble in 320 parts of water; it is freely soluble in alcohol or chloroform. *Uses:* It has a feeble strychnine-like effect. It is used as a denaturant for alcohol and imported inedible vegetable oils. It is used as a reagent for nitrate and for resolving the optical isomerides of some organic acids.

Brucine Sulfate NF IX [$(C_{23}H_{26}N_2O_4)_2.H_2SO_4.7H_2O$]—The sulfate of an alkaloid obtained from *Strychnos Nux-vomica* Linné (Fam. *Loganiaceæ*). Small white crystals or powder. It is affected by light. 1 Gm dissolves in about 70 ml of water at 25°; more soluble in boiling water; sparingly soluble in alcohol. *Uses:* It exerts a feeble strychnine-like effect and is also used as a bitter. *Dose:* 2 mg.

Caffeine and Sodium Benzoate USP XVII [Caffeine with Sodium Benzoate; Caffeine Sodio-Benzoate] is a mixture of caffeine and sodium benzoate that contains 47.0–50.0% of anhydrous caffeine [$C_8H_{10}N_4O_2$], and 50.0–53.0% of sodium benzoate [$C_7H_5NaO_2$], calculated on the anhydrous basis. The sum of the percentages of anhydrous caffeine and of sodium benzoate found is 98.0–102.0. *Preparation:* It may be prepared by triturating together equal parts of caffeine and sodium benzoate, in a mortar, with enough alcohol to form a smooth paste, drying at a moderate heat, and powdering. *Description and Solubility:* White, odorless powder with a slightly bitter taste. Its solution is practically neutral to litmus. 1 Gm dissolves in 1.2 ml of water with partial precipitation of the caffeine on standing, and in about 30 ml of alcohol; slightly soluble in chloroform (the caffeine). *Incompatibilities:* Addition of acid causes a precipitation of benzoic acid and, usually, caffeine. *Uses:* See *Caffeine. Dose:* 200 to 500 mg usual, intramuscular, and subcutaneous, 500 mg, repeated as necessary. *Veterinary Dose: Parenterally, Horses* and *Cattle*, 1 to 8 Gm; *Dogs*, 30 to 200 mg.

Nux Vomica NF XI [Strychni Semen; Dog Button; Quaker Button; Poison Nut]—The dried ripe seed of *Strychnos Nux-vomica* Linné (Fam. *Loganiaceæ*). It contains not less than 1.15% of strychnine. *Uses:* Has been used in therapy for its strychnine content in the average dose of 100 mg. See *Strychnine* (page 1161). It was formerly official as an extract, administered in a dose of 15 mg; as a fluidextract, with a dose of 0.1 ml; and as a tincture, used in a dose of 1 ml.

Strychnine Nitrate NF X [$C_{21}H_{22}N_2O_2.HNO_3$]—Colorless, odorless needles or white, crystalline powder having a bitter taste. It is stable in air. 1 Gm dissolves in 42 ml water, 50 ml glycerin, about 150 ml alcohol, and about 105 ml chloroform. *Caution: very poisonous. Uses:* See *Strychnine* (page 1161). *Dose: Orally*, 2 mg.

Strychnine Phosphate NF XI—[$C_{21}H_{22}N_2O_2.H_3PO_4.2H_2O$] White crystals or a white powder. It is odorless, has a very bitter taste, and is stable in air. 1 Gm is slowly soluble in about 30 ml of water; slightly soluble in alcohol. *Uses:* See *Strychnine* (page 1161). *Dose:* 2 mg.

Strychnine Sulfate NF XI—[$(C_{21}H_{22}N_2O_2)_2.H_2SO_4.5H_2O$] Colorless or white crystals, or a white, crystalline powder without odor, and efflorescent in dry air. It is levorotatory and slowly affected by light. 1 Gm dissolves in 35 ml water, 85 ml alcohol, and about 220 ml chloroform, 7 ml boiling water, and 25 ml alcohol at 70°; freely soluble in glycerin; insoluble in ether. *Uses:* See *Strychnine* (page 1161).

Thebaine [$C_{19}H_{21}NO_3$]—This alkaloid was obtained originally by Thiboumery, who named it *paramorphine*. It is obtained from opium and contains the iminoethano-phenanthrofuran nucleus typical of morphine and codeine; thus it is not structurally related to strychnine. Crystallized from alcohol in white leaflets of an acrid and styptic rather than bitter taste, [α]D −218.6° in alcohol, melting at about 193°. Slightly soluble in water; very soluble in alcohol, chloroform, and benzene; sparingly soluble in ether when cold and even more insoluble when heated. Alkalies precipitate it from its acid solutions. Unlike morphine, it is not reddened by nitric acid, nor does it become blue with solutions of ferric salts. It is colored blood-red by sulfuric acid which on warming turns orange-yellow and finally olive-green. Unlike opium alkaloids, it is not narcotic; in its effects on the system, it resembles strychnine, producing tetanic spasms in the dose of 60 mg.

References

1. Traube, W., *Ber.*, **33**, 3052 (1900).
2. Woodward, R. B., *et al*, *J. Am. Chem. Soc.*, **76**, 4749 (1954).
3. Woodward, R. B., *Experentia, Suppl. II*, 14th International Congress of Pure and Applied Chemistry, 1955, pp. 213–228.

66 | Antineoplastic and Immunosuppressive Drugs

This chapter was prepared by

Ewart A. Swinyard, PhD, *Professor of Pharmacology, College of Pharmacy and College of Medicine, University of Utah, Salt Lake City, Utah 84112, and*
Stewart C. Harvey, PhD, *Associate Professor of Pharmacology, College of Medicine, University of Utah, Salt Lake City, Utah 84112*

Antineoplastics—Antineoplastic drugs are chemical agents which are employed to suppress the growth and extension of neoplasms. Except for the hormones, they are all generally cytotoxic, and none has a specificity for cancerous tissue. They appear to interfere with nuclear functions concerned with cell division so that the proliferative tissues, including neoplasms, are the most affected. It follows that the major undesirable side effects (except for the hormones) are exerted upon highly proliferative normal tissue such as the bone marrow, lymph tissue, gastrointestinal and buccal mucosae, gonads, hair follicles, etc.

Prior to the 1940's the principal nonsurgical treatment of neoplasms was x-ray and radium therapy, although certain arsenicals and urethane were also in use. During the 1940's there were three main developments: radioisotopes, nitrogen mustards, and antifolic acid agents. The use of sex hormones for the treatment of certain types of neoplasms, and of adrenal corticoids and ACTH for the treatment of leukemia also developed considerably during these years. The nitrogen mustards have been followed by a series of other types of alkylating radiomimetics, whereas the antifolic acids have been followed by other antimetabolites that interfere with the biochemistry of the cell nucleus. The use of radioisotopes has diminished, although there have been important advances in specific techniques with radioisotopes. The antineoplastic drugs have not retired x-irradiation from the scene. Refractoriness to each of the drugs develops so that x-irradiation may ultimately be required; oftentimes x-irradiation is used before or concurrently with antineoplastic drugs. Unfortunately, neither the chemical nor physical agent causes a permanent recession of the neoplasm. Antineoplastic drugs may prolong life in acute leukemia in children, carcinoma of the prostate, and choriocarcinoma in women; they may possibly prolong life in several other neoplastic diseases, but this is often difficult to prove. However, even as mere palliative agents the antineoplastic drugs are valuable. Progress in the elucidation of the pathogenesis and extension of neoplasms will undoubtedly bring more selective and probably even curative drugs.

The nitrogen mustards and other alkylating antineoplastics are called *radiomimetics*, because they mimic the mutagenic and cytotoxic effects of radiation. Their mechanism of action is not proved, but it is thought that they alkylate certain nucleotides in desoxyribonucleic acid (DNA). However, the clinically effective alkylating radiomimetic drugs have two or more alkylating moieties per molecule; it is thought that cross linking of DNA molecules is important to their action. Certain arsenicals and urethane are also radiomimetic, but their mechanism of action is unknown. The mechanism of action of the radioisotopes is self evident. Their specific usefulness depends on selective uptake by certain tissues. Thus, radioiodine is concentrated in the thyroid gland, radiogold colloid in the phagocytosing lymph system, and radiophosphate in proliferating tissues in general, since the phosphorus metabolism in such tissues proceeds at a rapid pace. Radioisotopes employed in needles, pessaries, etc, are not, of course, selected because of any metabolic relation to the neoplastic tissue, but rather because of the characteristics of their radiation. The radioisotopes are discussed in Chapter 34 (page 552).

The activity in the field of antimetabolites, generated by the elucidation of the mechanism of action of sulfanilamide and the discovery of folic acid and its role in nucleotide synthesis, led to the introduction of antimetabolites of folic acid for the treatment of leukemia and other neoplastic disorders. As the metabolism of nuclear constituents was revealed, new antimetabolites were tested, and efficacious drugs were found among purines and pyrimidines.

Adrenocortical steroids stimulate the bone marrow. They are especially useful in the management of chronic lymphocytic leukemia and acute leukemia, especially if secondary auto-immune hemolytic anemia, thrombocytopenia (with hemorrhage), granulocytopenia, or emaciation and debility occurs. They may be used to overcome some of the toxic effects of the antimetabolites. They may also be palliative in certain other types of carcinoma. The adrenal corticoids are discussed in Chapter 55 (page 961).

In cancer of the secondary sex organs, especially, and to a lesser extent of the gonads, androgens or estrogens may be employed, depending upon the type of cancer and age and sex of the patient. Breast cancer is usually treated with androgens (and oophorectomy) in the premenopausal and early postmenopausal woman and with estrogens in the late (more than four years) postmenopausal woman. Androgens may also be used in the treatment of ovarian carcinoma. Prostatic carcinoma may be treated with estrogens. The sex hormones are discussed in Chapter 55 (page 988).

Drugs that induce local inflammation and fibrosis may suppress effusions secondary to various neoplasms. Thus, quinacrine may be given into the pleural and peritoneal cavities to control such effusions. Since the neoplastic process is unaffected, quinacrine is not truly neoplastic.

Immunosuppressives—The immune response involves antigen processing, information transfer, and activation of the thymic and lymph systems to differentiate and proliferate plasma cells and sensitized lymphocytes. The predilection of antineoplastics for proliferating cell systems and genetic information transfer enables such drugs to interrupt the immune response. Consequently, a number of antineoplastics are in use as immunosuppressives. However, not all immunosuppressives are antineoplastics. Antilymphocytic serum is a specific immunosuppressive. Certain antimalarials (eg, pyrimethamine and chloroquine) also possess some immunosuppressive activity. The adrenal steroids, of course, suppress the inflammatory phase of the immune response.

Much current interest in immunosuppressives centers around their use to prevent rejection of organ transplants in man. They are, however, also of interest as agents for the treatment of known autoimmune diseases, probable autoimmune diseases (such as rheumatoid arthritis, lupus erythematosus, and ulcerative colitis), and various sensitivities. These potential uses are far more important than those in organ transplantation.

Immunosuppressive drugs are divided into three classes: *Class I*, in which the agent is effective *only* when given *prior* to the immune stimulus; *Class II*, in which the agent is effective *only* when given *after* the immune stimulus; and *Class III*, in which the agent is effective whether given *before or after* the immune stimulus. For the treatment of autoimmune diseases or prolongation of organ grafts, Class II or III drugs are indicated; for bone marrow grafts, prior treatment with drugs of Classes I or III are indicated, since Class II or III drugs given after the transplantation would kill the transplant.

The cytotoxic (ie, neoplastic) immunosuppressives have adverse effects on the hematopoietic and other proliferative systems, so that their use is not without danger. Usually, such drugs are employed in toxic but tolerable doses. Furthermore, the suppression of the immune response by any immunosuppressive drug may result in various infections, especially those caused by cytomegalic viruses, fungi, or yeasts.

Azathioprine

[Imuran (*Burroughs-Wellcome*)]

Azathioprine [$C_9H_7N_7O_2S$ = 277.29] is 6-[(1-methyl-4-nitroimidazol-5-yl)thio]purine.

Preparation—*N,N'*-Dimethyloxaldiamide is reacted with phosphorus pentachloride to give 5-chloro-1-methylimidazole. This is nitrated and the resulting 5-chloro-1-methyl-4-nitroimidazole is condensed with purine-6-thiol (mercaptopurine) in an appropriate dehydrohalogenating environment. US Pat. 3,056,-785.

Description—A yellow, matted powder that is odorless and has a slightly bitter taste. It is light sensitive, non-hygroscopic, and stable to reasonable temperatures. It decomposes at about 245°.

Solubility—Soluble in dilute alkali solutions (unstable) and dimethylsulfoxide; insoluble in water, most organic solvents, and dilute acids.

Uses—Azathioprine is a derivative of *Mercaptopurine* (page 1168) which it resembles in its actions. However, it is used only as a Class II *immunosuppressive* drug. It probably has been used more than any other immunosuppressive drug in *kidney transplantations*. However, a definitive comparison with other agents has not yet been made. At present, about ½ of kidney transplants survive for longer than 3 years when Azathioprine is used, but other measures also contribute to this rate of success. It is used in other organ transplantations, but since such operations are less frequent, reliable data are not yet available. Azathioprine also appears to bring about a satisfactory response in a high percentage of patients with *ulcerative colitis* or *refractory idiopathic thrombocytopenic purpura*, although to date the studies in various possible autoimmune diseases and chronic allergies have been desultory.

Toxicity or intercurrent infection (see *General Statement*, this page) occurs in about ⅓ of patients under treatment with Azathioprine. Bone marrow depression is the most frequent, occurring in about 11% of patients; leukopenia, thrombocytopenia, and to lesser extent anemia or pancytopenia are manifested. Pancreatitis, alopecia, arthralgia, skin rashes, serum sickness, stomatitis, esophagitis, steatorrhea, retinopathy, peritoneal hemorrhage, and pulmonary edema may also occur in a small percent of cases. Jaundice has been reported, so that in the presence of liver dysfunction the drug should be withheld.

Dose—*Usual*, **3 to 5 mg** per **Kg** of body weight a day; *maintenance*, **2 to 3 mg** per **Kg** a day.

Other Dose Information—In the presence of renal damage or *Allopurinol* (page 1133) the dose should be reduced to ¼ to ⅓ of the above.

Dosage Forms—Tablets: 50 mg.

Busulfan USP

[1,4-Butanediol Dimethanesulfonate; Tetramethylene Dimethanesulfonate; Myleran (*Burroughs-Wellcome*)]

$$CH_3SO_2O(CH_2)_4OSO_2CH_3$$

Busulfan contains 98.0–100.5% of $C_6H_{14}O_6S_2$ (246.30), calculated on the dried basis.

Caution—*Busulfan is very poisonous. Great care should be taken to prevent inhaling particles of Busulfan and exposing the skin to it.*

Preparation—This typical sulfonate ester is readily prepared by esterifying 1,4-butanediol [$HOCH_2CH_2$-CH_2CH_2OH] with methanesulfonyl chloride [CH_3SO_2-Cl] in the presence of pyridine. The crude solid ester may be obtained by pouring the reaction mixture into a large excess of cold dilute hydrochloric acid and filtering. Purification may be accomplished by recrystallization from appropriate solvents.

Description—Occurs as a white, crystalline powder. It has a melting range of 115° to 118°.

Solubility—Very slightly soluble in water; slightly soluble in alcohol; 1 Gm dissolves in about 45 ml of acetone.

Uses—Busulfan is an alkylating radiomimetic which is efficacious in certain cases as a *neoplastic suppressant*. Its principal distinction is that in the usual doses it exerts very little action on rapidly proliferative tissues other than bone marrow. At low doses granulocytopoiesis can be selectively suppressed without affecting erythropoiesis. Thus, it is employed for the treatment of *chronic granulocytic* (myelogenous, myeloid) *leukemia*. It is not to be used in terminal or acute phases of the disease. Since it has little effect on lymphopoiesis, it is of no value in lymphocytic leukemia, Hodgkin's disease, or malignant lymphoma. It is useless against solid tumors. Its chief toxicity is *thrombocytopenia* (with hemorrhagic manifestations) and generalized bone marrow depression. *Lymphocytopenia* is uncommon. A complete differential blood count (including thrombocytes) once a week is mandatory. Nausea, vomiting, diarrhea, impotence, amenorrhea, sterility, and fetal malformation occasionally occur. Granulocyte destruction results in a high rate of excretion of urates, the precipitation of which may cause renal damage; cotreatment with *Allopurinol* (page 1133) may avoid such damage. Busulfan also sometimes causes cheilosis, glossitis, pulmonary fibrosis, anhidrosis, skin pigmentation, and gynecomastia.

Busulfan is not immunosuppressive.

Dose—1 to 4 mg; *usual*, **2 mg** daily.

Other Dose Information—The dose above is given daily until clinical improvement occurs or toxicity supervenes. If maintenance during remission is desired, the usual dose for this purpose is 1 to 3 mg daily.

Dosage Forms—Tablets USP: 2 mg.

Chlorambucil USP

[4-[*p*-[Bis(2-chloroethyl)amino]phenyl]butyric Acid; Leukeran(*Burroughs-Wellcome*)]

$$(ClCH_2CH_2)_2N-\!\!\!\langle\bigcirc\rangle\!\!\!-CH_2CH_2CH_2COOH$$

Chlorambucil contains 98.0–101.0% of $C_{14}H_{19}Cl_2NO_2$ (304.22), calculated on the anhydrous basis.

Caution—*Chlorambucil is very poisonous. Great care should be taken to prevent inhaling particles of Chlorambucil and exposing the skin to it.*

Preparation—4-Phenylbutyric acid is nitrated and the resulting *p*-nitro acid is esterified with isopropyl alcohol. The nitro ester is then hydrogenated to the aminoester. Reaction with ethylene oxide converts the —NH_2 into —$N(CH_2CH_2OH)_2$ which is then converted into —$N(CH_2CH_2Cl)_2$ by treatment with $POCl_3$. Hydrolysis of the ester yields the acid, Chlorambucil.

Description—Off-white, slightly granular powder.

Solubility—Very slightly soluble in water; soluble in dilute alkali; 1 Gm dissolves in 2 ml of acetone.

Uses—Chlorambucil is a nitrogen mustard with actions and uses similar to mechlorethamine hydrochloride. One of its chief advantages is that it is active by the oral route and is more completely and predictably absorbed than is triethylenemelamine. It is more selective for lymphoid tissue than is mechlorethamine and hence it induces less bone marrow depression and nausea and vomiting. It is used in the treatment of *Hodgkin's disease*, *chronic lymphocytic* and *myelocytic leukemias*, *lymphosarcoma*, *testicular tumors*, and *ovarian carcinoma*. Although Chlorambucil is somewhat selective for lymphoid tissue, it has been only cursorily investigated as an immunosuppressive. Chlorambucil is the slowest acting and least toxic of the currently used nitrogen mustards.

Dose—2 to 12 mg daily; *usual*, **6 mg** once a day.

Other Dose Information—The dose for maintenance during remission is 0.03 to 1 mg per Kg of body weight daily.

Dosage Forms—Tablets USP: 2 mg.

Chloroquine—see page 1245.

Chloroquine Phosphate—see page 1245.

Cyclophosphamide USP

[2-[Bis(2-chloroethyl)amino]tetrahydro-2*H*-1,3,2-oxazaphosphorine 2-Oxide; Cytoxan (*Mead-Johnson*)]

$$\begin{array}{c}\text{O}\!\!\nearrow\!\!\text{O}\\ \text{P}\\ \text{NH}\end{array}\!\!N(CH_2CH_2Cl)_2{\cdot}H_2O$$

Cyclophosphamide contains 95.0–105.0% of $C_7H_{15}Cl_2N_2O_2P{\cdot}H_2O$ (279.10).

Caution: Great care should be taken to prevent inhaling particles of Cyclophosphamide and exposing the skin to it.

Preparation—3-Amino-1-propanol is condensed with *N*,*N*-bis(2-chloroethyl)phosphoramidic dichloride [(ClCH₂CH₂)₂N—POCl₂] in dioxane solution under the catalytic influence of triethylamine. The condensation is double, involving both the hydroxyl and the amino groups, thus effecting the cyclization. After filtering to remove the triethylamine hydrochloride and vacuum evaporating to remove the dioxane, the residue is dissolved in ether. Saturation of the ethereal solution with water and subsequent refrigeration yields crystalline Cyclophosphamide.

Description—Occurs as a white, crystalline powder. It liquefies upon loss of its water of crystallization.

Solubility—1 Gm dissolves in about 25 ml of water; soluble in alcohol.

Uses—Cyclophosphamide is an alkylating antineoplastic drug similar in action and usefulness to *Mechlorethamine* (page 1167). However, it does not readily cyclize to the active ethyleneimonium form until tissue phosphamidases remove the phosphamoryl group. Thus the substance is stable in the gastrointestinal tract, is well tolerated and effective by the oral and parenteral routes, and does not cause local vesication, necrosis, phlebitis, or even pain. Furthermore, phosphamidase activity in malignant tissues is somewhat higher than in normal tissue, so that some degree of selective action is possible. Its efficacy is good in the treatment of *lymphosarcoma, Hodgkin's disease, chronic lymphocytic leukemia, giant follicular lymphoma,* and *reticulum cell sarcoma*. It is the drug of choice in the treatment of *Burkitt's lymphoma*. It may be of value in the treatment of multiple myeloma, chronic myelogenous leukemia, acute leukemias, bronchogenic carcinoma, neuroblastoma, and ovarian carcinoma. Cyclophosphamide is a Class III immunosuppressive drug. Preliminary studies of the use of the drug in the treatment of rheumatoid arthritis are promising.

Side effects include anorexia, nausea and vomiting (regardless of the route of administration), mucosal ulcerations, dizziness, leukopenia, occasional thrombocytopenia, alopecia, nail ridging, cutaneous pigmentation, and occasional hepatic dysfunction. Weekly blood counts are required.

Cyclophosphamide may also be given intramuscularly, into body cavities, or by infiltration.

Dose—*Usual*, oral, **2 to 4 mg** per **Kg** of body weight daily; *intravenous infusion*, **5 to 10 mg** per **Kg** of body weight daily for 4 to 10 days.

Other Dose Information—Dose ranges are from 1 to 40 mg per Kg of body weight per day. Usual, oral, maintenance, 1 to 3 mg per Kg; usual, intravenous, maintenance, 3 to 5 mg per Kg.

Dosage Forms—for Injection USP: 100, 200 and 500 mg; Tablets USP: 50 mg.

Dromostanolone Propionate—see page 1004.

Dactinomycin USP

[Actinomycin D; Meractinomycin; Lyovac Cosmegen (*MSD*)]

Dactinomycin contains, in each mg, an amount of $C_{62}H_{86}N_{12}O_{16}$ (1255.45) equivalent to the antibiotic activity of not less than 900 mcg of dactinomycin, calculated on the dried basis. It conforms to the regulations of the federal Food and Drug Administration concerning antibiotic drugs (see page 1206).

Caution—Handle Dactinomycin with exceptional care, to prevent inhaling particles of it and exposing the skin to it.

Preparation—Dactinomycin is elaborated during the culture of *Streptomyces antibioticus*. After extracting from the fermentation broth, it is purified through chromatographic and crystallization processes. US Pat. 2,378,876.

Description—A bright-red crystalline powder. It is light-sensitive and should be protected appropriately; it should also be protected from excessive heat and moisture. It melts between 245° and 248° with decomposition.

Solubility—1 Gm dissolves in about 8 ml of alcohol, 25 ml of water (at 10°), 1000 ml of water (at 37°), and about 1666 ml of ether.

Uses—Dactinomycin is an antineoplastic drug which inhibits RNA polymerase. It is primarily indicated for the treatment of *Wilm's tumor, rhabdomyosarcoma,* and *carcinoma of the testis and uterus.* It also may be of value in the treatment of osteogenic sarcoma, malignant melanoma, Ewing's sarcoma, sarcoma botyroides, neuroblastoma, lymphomas, and breast and lung cancers, but its status in these neoplasms is not well defined. A large percent of patients will not respond to this drug; even with Wilm's tumor, only about 30% respond favorably. Radiation treatment increases the response to Dactinomycin. Tumors that fail to respond to systemic treatment sometimes respond to local perfusion. Dactinomycin is a Class II immunosuppressive.

Nausea and vomiting is usual and occurs within the first few hours after administration of Dactinomycin.

Anorexia, abdominal pain, diarrhea, and gastrointestinal ulceration follow. The patient may also experience malaise, fatigue, lethargy, myalgia, and fever. Cheilitis, ulcerative stomatitis, and pharyngitis are common. Because agranulocytosis, leukopenia, pancytopenia, thrombocytopenia, and anemia frequently occur, the blood picture must be monitored daily. Cutaneous eruptions, alopecia, hyperpigmentation, and erythema also occur. Side effects appear to be reversible. The drug is locally toxic, and extravasation may cause serious local tissue damage. Venous thrombosis may also result from local effects.

Dose—*Usual, intravenous,* **500 mcg** daily for 5 days.

Dosage Forms—for Injection USP: 500 mcg.

Fluorouracil USP

[5 F. U.; 5-Fluorouracil (*Roche*)]

Fluorouracil contains 98.5–101.0% of $C_4H_3FN_2O_2$ (130.08), calculated on the dried basis.

Caution—Great care should be taken to prevent inhaling particles of Fluorouracil and exposing the skin to it.

Preparation—Potassium fluoroacetate is reacted with methyl bromide to form methyl fluoroacetate which is then subjected to a Claisen condensation with methyl formate and sodium ethoxide to produce the potassium enolate of the methyl ester of α-fluoromalonaldehydic acid (I). Cyclization of (I) is effected through condensation under anhydrous conditions with S-benzylisothiourea. The resulting 2-(benzylthio) compound is readily hydrolyzed in the presence of acid to Fluorouracil. US Pat. 2,802,005.

Description—White to practically white, practically odorless, crystalline powder. It is stable when exposed to air. It melts between 281° and 283°.

Solubility—1 Gm dissolves in 80 ml of water, 170 ml of alcohol, and 55 ml of methanol; practically insoluble in chloroform, ether, and benzene; the solubility in aqueous solutions increases with increasing pH of the solution.

Uses—Fluorouracil is a congener of uracil which acts both as a surrogate and an antimetabolite of that nucleotide. It ultimately blocks the synthesis of thymidylic acid and hence of deoxyribonucleic acid; as fluorouridine diphosphate, it also incorporates into ribonucleic acid. Uracil is preferentially utilized by neoplastic tissue; thus the antimetabolite has some degree of selectivity for the neoplasm. It may bring about the regression of a number of neoplasms. It is the antineoplastic of choice in the treatment of *carcinoma of the breast, colon,* or *rectum,* and it may be useful in the treatment of neoplasma of the stomach, gall bladder, ovary and liver, and, to a lesser extent, those of the uterus, cervix, pancreas, esophagus, larynx, thyroid, pharynx and urinary bladder. Fluorouracil is also used topically in the treatment of precancerous dermatoses, especially actinic keratosis. The drug does not affect nonkeratotic lesions. Fluorouracil is a Class II immunosuppressive drug and has been used in *organ transplantation.*

The drug is quite toxic, about $\frac{2}{3}$ of patients showing signs of toxicity; the mortality rate is about 3%. Toxic effects include diarrhea, stomatitis, nausea, vomiting, alopecia, dermatitis, pharyngitis, esophagitis, epistaxis, and leukopenia. Death usually occurs from septicemia, so that concomitant antibiotic therapy is advisable. Topically, Fluorouracil may induce photosensitization, although some persons appear to be resistant to this effect.

Dose—*Intravenous*, **6** to **15 mg** per **Kg**, not exceeding **1 Gm** daily; *usual*, **12 mg** per **Kg** of body weight once a day for 4 or 5 days.

Other Dose Information—The course may be repeathed monthly. It may also be given by regional infusion. For topical administration it is employed as a 1% solution in propylene glycol.

Dosage Forms—Injection USP: 10 ml.

Gold Au 198—see page 565.

Hydroxystilbamidine Isethionate—see page 1258.

Mechlorethamine Hydrochloride USP

[Nitrogen Mustard; 2,2'-Dichloro-*N*-methyldiethylamine Hydrochloride; HN2; Mustargen Hydrochloride (*MSD*)]

$$[CH_3\overset{+}{N}H(CH_2CH_2Cl)_2]Cl^-$$

Mechlorethamine Hydrochloride contains 97.5–100.5% of $C_5H_{11}Cl_2N \cdot HCl$ (192.52), calculated on the anhydrous basis.

Caution—*Mechlorethamine Hydrochloride is a vesicant, and the powder or its solution is irritating to the respiratory tract.*

History—The medical uses for nitrogen mustards were discovered as a result of chemical warfare research on vesicant agents during World War II. After noting that these agents brought about dissolution of lymphoid tissue, Goodman, Gilman, and T. Dougherty were prompted to study the effect of nitrogen mustards on transplanted lymphosarcoma in mice. The first clinical trial with these agents was conducted in collaboration with G. E. Lindskog at Yale University in the fall of 1942.

Preparation—Among other ways, mechlorethamine (base) may be synthesized by reacting methylamine with a double equimolar portion of ethylene oxide to produce *N*-methyldiethanolamine, which is then reacted with thionyl chloride. After purification, the base may then be converted conveniently to the hydrochloride by dissolving it in a suitable organic solvent and passing HCl into the solution.

Description—A white, crystalline, hygroscopic powder. It melts between 108° and 111°, and the pH of a 1:500 aqueous solution is between 3.0 and 5.0.

Solubility—Very soluble in water; soluble in alcohol.

Uses—Mechlorethamine is a *cytotoxic* agent which can be regarded as the prototype and most important member of a series of agents called the nitrogen mustards, which in certain respects simulate radiation in their actions. It *inhibits mitosis and cell division* in all germinal tissues; relatively undifferentiated germinal cells are nonproliferative and hypertrophied during exposure to the drug, but the more differentiated germinal cells disintegrate. Certain neoplastic growths, particularly of the lymph nodes and bone marrow, are somewhat more sensitive to the drug than are the normal more slowly proliferative tissues.

Nitrogen mustard therapy is used as a complement and supplement to radiation therapy, especially when the neoplastic disease is too diffuse for safe radiotherapy or when radiation resistance occurs. It is used in the treatment of diffuse and sometimes localized *Hodgkin's disease*, and regression of the disease may be dramatic; however, life expectancy is not greatly affected, and refractoriness to Mechlorethamine will develop. *Lymphosarcoma* often responds similarly, but the effect of the drug in this disease, especially in small-cell and reticulum-cell types, is less predictable. Mechlorethamine therapy may be palliative in *chronic leukemia*, but it does not alter the eventual outcome of the disease; the temporary remissions are more adequate in myelocytic than in lymphocytic leukemia. Acute leukemia hardly responds to the nitrogen mustard. Certain types of *bronchogenic carcinoma* may temporarily respond to Mechlorethamine. It also may be of value in the treatment of *carcinoma of the nasopharynx, ovary,* and *breast,* and in *seminoma, chorioepithelioma, neuroblastoma,* and *Wilm's tumor.* Satisfactory temporary remissions have also been obtained in a number of cases of *mycosis fungoides* and *lymphoblastomas.* In *polycythemia vera,* remissions of several months to two years have been achieved. All of the above diseases eventually develop resistance to nitrogen mustards. Mechlorethamine is an immunosuppressive drug, but it has been investigated less for this use than have other antineoplastics. In the treatment of *"malignant" rheumatoid arthritis* it effects a good initial response in nearly all patients; maintenance is carried on with cyclophosphamide.

Nausea and vomiting commonly occur following Mechlorethamine therapy, but sedative agents greatly diminish the incidence of such untoward actions originating centrally. Bone marrow depression may result in leukopenia and thrombocytopenia, and also in bleeding tendencies. Hyperheparinemia also may rarely lead to hemorrhagic complications. Skin eruptions are rarely noted, but herpes zoster (shingles) commonly occurs, especially in the nitrogen mustard or radiation treatment of malignant lymphoma. Sometimes temporary menstrual irregularities occur in females. Severe local reactions to Mechlorethamine, as well as rapid chemical breakdown of the drug, require that therapy be limited to the intravenous route; even so, extravasation may cause tender local induration and sloughs, and irritation from within the lumen of the vessel may cause phlebothrombosis or thrombophlebitis, especially if the infusion rate is too rapid or the concentration of solution is too high.

Dose—*Intravenous*, **200** to **600 mcg** per **Kg**, per course of treatment; *usual*, **100 mcg** per **Kg** of body weight daily for 4 days.

Other Dose Information—A course of Mechlorethamine therapy consists of a total dose of 0.4 mg per Kg of body weight; it may be 0.1 mg per Kg intravenously, once daily for 4 days, 0.2 mg per Kg twice in a single day, or given in a single dose. The single dose is preferable, since it spares the patient the unnecessary repitition of bouts of nausea and vomiting. Patients with normal bone marrow function can sometimes tolerate up to twice the usual dose, although serious bone marrow depression will result at the higher doses. Courses may be repeated only when bone marrow function has recovered, as indicated by the cellular composition of the peripheral blood; the required wait is usually not less than 6 weeks. The drug is best injected into intravenous tubing which is rapidly conducting some isotonic fluid; the injection should be made slowly but completed within a few minutes.

Dosage Forms—for Injection USP: 10 mg.

Veterinary Use—As a neoplastic suppressant for the treatment of mass cell sarcoma and lymphosarcoma in dogs and of leukosis in fowl.

Veterinary Dose—*Dogs*, **0.1 mg** per **Kg** of body weight *intravenously* daily for 4 days; *Fowl*, **2 mg** per **Kg** *intravenously*.

Melphalan USP

[L-3-[*p*-[Bis(2-chloroethyl)amino]phenyl]alanine; Alkeran (*Burroughs-Wellcome*)]

$$(ClCH_2CH_2)_2N-\!\!\!\!\bigcirc\!\!\!\!-CH_2CHCOOH$$
$$NH_2$$

Melphalan contains 93.0–100.5% of $C_{13}H_{18}Cl_2N_2O_2$ (305.21), calculated on the dried basis.

Caution—*Do not inhale.*

Preparation—L-3-Phenylalanine is nitrated and the *p*-nitro compound is reduced to L-3-(*p*-aminophenyl)alanine. This is reacted with ethylene oxide to form the corresponding bis(2-hydroxyethyl)amino compound which is then treated with phosphoryl chloride to yield Melphalan.

Description—An off-white to buff powder having a faint odor. It is sensitive to light, heat, and moisture. It melts about 180° with decomposition.

Solubility—Soluble in dilute mineral acids; slightly soluble in alcohol and methanol; practically insoluble in water, chloroform, and ether.

Uses—Melphalan is an *antineoplastic* of the nitrogen mustard type. It has not yet been established to what extent its spectrum differs from that of *Mechlorethamine* (page 1167), but the two drugs differ somewhat. Melphalan is the drug of choice in the treatment of *multiple myeloma;* 70 to 80% of patients show subjective improvement and 33 to 50% show objective improvement for periods from ½ to 2 years, and life expectancy may be increased even when no objective signs of improvement obtain. Melphalan appears to be of some benefit in the treatment of *seminoma, Ewing's tumor, reticulum cell sarcoma, thymoma,* and *ovarian carcinoma.* In osteogenic sarcoma, melanoma, angioendothelioma, cholaniocarcinoma, and mixed tumors of the testes the drug is less effective or quite erratic. It is of no value in the treatment of the acute leukemias.

Melphalan is a Class I immunosuppressive drug.

Adverse effects include mild nausea and vomiting after large doses, bone marrow depression with anemia, neutropenia, thrombocytopenia, and occasional azotemia. Oral ulceration and gastrointestinal hemorrhage also occur occasionally.

Dose—*Usual, initial,* **6 mg** once a day; *maintenance,* **2 mg** once a day.

Other Dose Information—The usual initial oral dose of 6 mg daily is given for 2 or 3 weeks or until the leukocyte or platelet count falls; the usual maintenance dose is 2 mg a day. The drug may be given intermittently, with an initial 7 to 10 day course of 10 mg a day, which causes slowly appearing leukopenia and thrombocytopenia. When the leukocyte count returns to 4,000/cu mm or more, treatment is resumed with 1 to 3 mg a day, to maintain the leukocyte count at 3,000 to 3,500/cu mm.

Dosage Forms—Tablets USP: 2 mg.

Mercaptopurine USP

[Purine-6-thiol; 6 MP; Purinethol (*Burroughs-Wellcome*)]

Mercaptopurine [$C_5H_4N_4S.H_2O$ = 170.19] contains 97.0–102.0% of $C_5H_4N_4S$ (152.18), calculated on the anhydrous basis.

Preparation—Thiourea and ethyl cyanoacetate are reacted in the presence of sodium methylate to give 2-thiol-4-amino-6-hydroxypyrimidine (I) which is then converted to the 5-nitroso derivative (II) by treating with sodium nitrite and acetic acid. Reduction of (II) with sodium hydrosulfite yields the corresponding diamino compound (III) which is then desulfurized by hydrogenolysis in the presence of Raney nickel to yield 4,5-diamino-6-hydroxypyrimidine (IV). The imidazole ring closure is then effected by double condensation of (IV) with formic acid (V), and the resulting hypoxanthine (lactim form shown in VI) is thiolated with P_2S_5.

Description—Yellow, crystalline powder which is odorless or practically odorless. It melts with decomposition above 308°.

Solubility—Insoluble in water, acetone, and ether; soluble in hot alcohol and dilute aqueous alkali; slightly soluble in diluted sulfuric acid.

Uses—Mercaptopurine is an analog and antimetabolite of the nucleotides, adenine and hypoxanthine. Consequently, it interferes in nucleic acid biosynthesis. Mercaptopurine is primarily used in the treatment of *acute leukemia,* in which disease it may induce partial or complete remissions of a few weeks to months in duration. It is not the drug of choice alone for the induction of remissions in children, ranking behind vincristine, folic acid antagonists, and adrenal hormones. Mercaptopurine is inconsistent but sometimes of value in the therapy of *chronic myelogenous leukemia.* However, in combination with prednisone it ranks with vincristine plus prednisone as the agent of choice for initiating treatment. For maintenance, Mercaptopurine or methotrexate is the drug of choice. In *chronic granulocytic leukemia* it may be used for maintenance, but busulfan is ordinarily superior. However, it is important to be aware that no cross-resistance to Mercaptopurine occurs from treatment with other classes of agents, so that it is a back-up drug for the myelogenous and granulocytic anemias. It is not useful in the treatment of lymphocytic leukemia, Hodgkin's disease, lymphosarcoma, and solid tumors. Mercaptopurine is a Class II immunosuppressive drug.

The toxicity of Mercaptopurine consists of hypoplasia of the bone marrow with thrombocytopenia (and hemorrhage), leukopenia, and rarely anemia and ulceration of the gastrointestinal mucosae, although in this respect it is less toxic than the folic acid antagonists. Nausea and vomiting indicate the onset of gastrointestinal toxicity. Frequent blood counts are mandatory.

Dose—2.5 to **5 mg** per **Kg** daily; *usual,* **2.5 mg** per **Kg** of body weight once a day.

Dosage Forms—Tablets USP: 50 mg.

Methotrexate USP

[N-[*p*-[[(2,4-Diamino-6-pteridinyl)methyl]methylamino]benzoyl]glutamic Acid; 4-Amino-10-methylfolic Acid Amethopterin; (*Lederle*)]

Methotrexate is a mixture of 4-amino-10-methylfolic acid and closely related compounds, and it contains not less than 85.0% of $C_{20}H_{22}N_8O_5$ (454.45), calculated on the anhydrous basis.

Caution—Methotrexate is extremely poisonous.

Preparation—2,3-Dibromopropionaldehyde (I) is condensed in aqueous medium with 2,4,5,6-tetraminopyrimidine (II). The condensation is multiple, consisting of: (*a*) dehydrobromination, involving one hydrogen of the 5-amino group and the 2-bromine; (*b*) dehydration, involving the two hydrogens of the 6-amino group and the oxygen in (II); and (*c*) dehydrogenation, involving the remaining hydrogen of the 5-amino group and the 2-hydrogen of (II). The dehydrogenation in step (*c*) is brought about by another molecule of (II) which, by effecting the dehydrogenation, is reduced to 2,3-dibromo-1-propanol. The overall effect of these condensations is the cyclization of (I) with (II) to produce 6-bromomethyl-2,4-diaminopteridine (III).

Further condensation [dehydrobromination, involving the bromine in (III) and the hydrogen of the methylamino group in N-[*p*-(methylamino)benzoyl]glutamic acid (IV)] yields crude Methotrexate which is then purified to meet the official specifications.

Description—Orange-brown, crystalline powder.

Solubility—Practically insoluble in water, alcohol, chloroform, and ether; freely soluble in dilute solutions of alkali hydroxides and carbonates; slightly soluble in dilute hydrochloric acid (1 in 2).

Uses—Methotrexate is the folic acid antimetabolite of choice for the treatment of *acute leukemia* in children, although it is not necessarily the drug of choice, especially for the initiation of therapy. For main-

tenance, it ranks with mercaptopurine as the drug of choice. In acute leukemia in children a temporary complete remission may occur and survival may be prolonged by weeks to two years. Furthermore, Methotrexate is useful in the treatment of *choriocarcinoma,* for which it is the treatment and drug of choice. It is useful in the treatment of *squamous cell carcinomas* of the head and neck. Methotrexate may be given by intra-arterial infusion into the affected region in the treatment of a variety of carcinomata; the local concentrations achieved may be high enough to be effective and yet low enough in the rest of the body not to be toxic. Folinic acid is also often given systemically to prevent generalized toxicity. Methotroxate is a Class II immunosuppressive drug and has been used in organ transplantations. It also has been used with some success in the treatment of psoriasis and psoriatic arthritis.

The toxic effects of Methotrexate are an extension of its antimetabolite effects, and sometimes toxicity occurs first. They include bone marrow hypoplasia with leukopenia, thrombocytopenia (with hemorrhage), and anemia. Depression of cellular proliferation along the gastrointestinal tract results in ulcerative stomatitis, hemorrhagic enteritis and perforation and diarrhea. Alopecia may also occur. Daily blood counts are mandatory. The toxicity and therapeutic effects may be antagonized by leucovorin (page 1041).

Dose—*Oral, intramuscular,* or *intravenous,* 2.5 to **10 mg** daily or every other day; *usual,* **2.5 to 5 mg** once a day or every other day.

Other Dose Information—Orally, for children, 2.5 mg daily, initially; after 7 to 10 days the dose may be increased to 3.75 mg daily, and eventually 5 mg daily may be given if toxicity is absent. It now appears that an intramuscular dose of 30 mg/M^2 of body surface twice weekly is superior to the daily oral schedule. In the treatment of psoriasis and psoriatic arthritis, 2.5 mg daily is given initially, then increased by 2.5 mg at intervals no less than 4 weeks until stomatitis or gastritis develops, upon which treatment is interrupted and folic acid is given. When symptoms subside, treatment is continued with a lower dose. Remissions take 6 to 12 months.

Dosage Forms—for Injection USP (as the sodium salt): 5 and 50 mg; Tablets USP: 2.5 mg.

Oxychlorosene—see page 1194.

Pipobroman NF

[1,4-Bis(3-bromopropionyl)piperazine; Vercyte (*Abbott*)]

Pipobroman contains 98.0–101.5% of $C_{10}H_{16}Br_2N_2O_2$ (356.06), calculated on the dried basis.

Preparation—Piperazine, in dry chloroform solution, is doubly condensed with 3-bromopropionyl chloride using an excess of piperazine to encourage the dehydrochlorination. The crude product is crystallized from isopropyl alcohol.

Description—A white or practically white, crystalline powder, having a sharp, fruity odor and a slight bitter taste. It is stable in light and air. It melts between 102° and 105°.

Solubility—Freely soluble in chloroform; soluble in methanol and acetone; sparingly soluble in alcohol and benzene; slightly soluble in water; very slightly soluble in ether.

Uses—Pipobroman is an antineoplastic drug of the alkylating type. At the present its use is mainly limited to the treatment of *polycythemia vera* and *chronic granulocytic leukemia*. Even in these disorders, however, there is no acceptable evidence that Pipobroman is superior to older modes of treatment. Until there is more experience with the drug, the Council on Drugs of the American Medical Association recommends that Pipobroman be held in reserve for use in patients that have become refractory to x-irradiation and busulfan, and in the case of polycythemia vera, radiophosphorus.

Adverse effects include severe anemia, in part of a hemolytic nature, and reticulocytosis. Leukopenia and thrombocytopenia, of course, are the result of the intended action of the drug, but the leukocyte count should be kept above 3000/cu mm and the platelet count above 100,000/cu mm. Transient nausea, vomiting, abdominal cramps, and diarrhea also sometimes occur.

Dose—*Usual*, **1 to 3 mg** per **Kg** of body weight daily, depending on condition being treated and patient response.

Other Dose Information—For *polycythemia vera*: usual, initial, 1 to 1.5 mg per day; maintenance, 0.1 to 0.2 mg per Kg. For chronic granulocytic leukemia: usual, initial, 1.5 to 2.5 mg per Kg; maintenance, to be determined by the physician according to the leukocyte response and the need of the patient.

Dosage Forms—Tablets NF: 10 and 25 mg.

Podophyllum—see page 778.

Podophyllum Resin—see page 778.

Pyrimethamine—see page 1247.

Quinacrine—see page 1247.

Sodium Iodide I 131—see page 566.

Sodium Phosphate P 32—see page 567.

Testolactone—see page 1009.

Thioguanine NF

[2-Aminopurine-6-thiol (*Burroughs-Wellcome*)]

$$\cdot \tfrac{1}{2} H_2O$$

Thioguanine is anhydrous or contains one-half molecule of water of hydration. After drying in vacuum for 5 hours, it contains 97.0–100.5% of $C_5H_5N_5S$ (167.20).

Preparation—Thioguanine may be prepared, among other ways, by thiation of guanine with phosphorus pentasulfide. US Pat. 2,884,667.

Uses—Thioguanine is an antineoplastic and immunosuppressive drug with a mechanism of action similar to that of mercaptopurine, and its uses are essentially identical (see page 1168). Neither drug may be considered superior to the other. Cross-resistance exists between the two agents. Likewise, the toxicities of the two drugs are essentially the same.

Dose—*Usual, initial,* **2 mg** per **Kg** of body weight per day; *maintenance,* to be determined according to the needs of the patient.

Other Dose Information—The dose is administered as the multiple of 20 mg that is nearest to the calculated 2 mg per kg. If a response does not occur by the 26th day, the treatment should be deemed ineffective, and the drug should be supplanted by one from another class.

Dosage Forms—Tablets NF: 40 mg.

Thiotepa USP

[Tris(1-aziridinyl)phosphine Sulfide; Thio-Tepa (*Lederle*)]

Thiotepa contains 97–102% of $C_6H_{12}N_3PS$ (189.22), calculated on the anhydrous basis.

Caution—*Thiotepa is extremely poisonous.*

Preparation—Ethylenimine is condensed with thiophosphoryl chloride [$SPCl_3$] in the presence of triethylamine as the acid acceptor.

Description—Fine, white crystalline flakes, having a faint odor.

Solubility—Freely soluble in water, ether, and alcohol.

Uses—Thiotepa is an alkylating antineoplastic drug with actions on cell growth similar to *Mechlorethamine* (page 1167). However, it is not locally irritating or caustic and hence may be given safely by any route, although it is not effective orally. It is of value in the treatment of certain carcinomas, especially, metastatic *carcinoma of the breast* and *ovary*. It may be infiltrated directly into the tumor. Since it can be instilled locally into cavities, it is of especial value in controlling serous effusions consequent to such carcinomas. It may bring about brief remissions in *bronchogenic carcinoma*. It is effective in the treatment of *chronic leukemias*, especially chronic myelogenous leukemia, but it does not rank among the top four drugs for this purpose. It is also helpful in the management of *malignant lymphomas*. Thiotepa has been given by local injection to reduce obstructive lesions of the anus and rectum.

Side effects include anorexia, nausea, vomiting, headache, fever, and serious depression of the bone marrow, characterized by neutropenia, thrombocytopenia, and variable anemia. Close attention to the blood cell count and marrow function is mandatory. Unfortunately, the bone marrow effects have a long latency and may not appear until some time after the drug has been discontinued.

Dose—*Parenteral*, **2.5 to 60 mg** every 5 to 20 days; *usual*, **10 to 30 mg** once a week.

Other Dose Information—The intravenous maintenance dose is to be determined by the physician according to the therapeutic and toxicologic response of the patient. Maintenance doses range from 5 to 60 mg, depending on the leukocyte count; treatment is temporarily suspended if the count falls below 3000. *Local injection, intrapleural, intraperitoneal,* or *intracardiac,* 60 mg for patients over 12 years of age, except 40 mg for debilitated persons. When intravenous drug is also being given, the local dose should be reduced by half. In chronic lymphocytic leukemia the intravenous dose is 10 to 60 mg daily for 5 days and a *maximum* of 10 mg every 1 to 3 weeks thereafter.

Dosage Forms—for Injection USP: 15 mg.

Triethylenemelamine NF

[2,4,6-Tris(1-aziridinyl)-*s*-triazine;   2,4,6-Tris-(ethylenimino)-*s*-triazine
Tretamine; TEM; Triethylene Melamine (*Lederle*)]

Triethylenemelamine contains 98.0–100.5% of $C_9H_{12}N_6$ (204.24), calculated on the anhydrous basis.
Caution—Triethylenemelamine is very poisonous.
Preparation—Ethylenimine (I) is condensed with cyanuric acid (II) in a cold aqueous alkaline medium. The reaction mixture is extracted with chloroform, and the crude triethylenemelamine which remains after evaporation of the chloroform is purified by crystallization from an appropriate solvent.

The ethylenimine is conveniently prepared by heating the acid sulfate ester of ethanolamine with sodium hydroxide. The cyanuric acid is readily prepared from carbonyldiurea [$CO(NHCONH_2)_2$] through loss of ammonia by pyrolysis.

Description—It occurs as a white, crystalline powder. It is odorless or has a slight, amine-like odor. It melts to a clear liquid at about 160°, and in this state polymerizes vigorously.
Solubility—Freely soluble in water and chloroform; soluble in alcohol, acetone, benzene, and carbon tetrachloride.

Uses—Triethylenemelamine (TEM) is an alkylating radiomimetic closely related to the nitrogen mustards. Unlike most nitrogen mustards, however, it can be administered orally. Its therapeutic actions and limitations are those of the nitrogen mustards (see *Mechlorethamine* page 1167), except that it lacks the local vesicant activity. Thus it is used for the palliative treatment of certain generalized but not terminal neoplastic disorders of the lymphatic and hematopoietic systems. The best results have been achieved in *Hodgkin's disease*. It is useful but less satisfactory in the treatment of *lymphosarcoma* and *chronic lymphocytic leukemia*. It may be occasionally employed as an adjunctive or desperation agent in chronic granulocytic leukemia. It may be rarely effective in the treatment of mycosis fungoides, polycythemia vera, ovarian carcinoma and bronchogenic carcinoma.

The onset of action of TEM is slower and the duration of action is longer than that of mechlorethamine, and its cumulative toxicity is greater. However, TEM is advantageous in that its oral efficacy permits ambulatory therapy. Also, there is less nausea and vomiting with TEM than with mechlorethamine.
Dose—*Usual, initial,* **2.5 mg** daily for 2 to 3 days; *maintenance,* **0.5 to 1 mg** weekly to **2.5 to 5 mg** every 2 to 5 days.
Other Dose Information—The initial dose is given on each of 2 or 3 successive mornings according to the effect of each successive dose; 7 to 10 days may be required before a therapeutic effect becomes evident. Doses may range from 0.5 to 5 mg every 2 to 14 days,

according to the responsiveness of the condition. When the white cell count falls below 4000, therapy should be discontinued. Each dose must be buffered with 2 Gm of sodium bicarbonate, given simultaneously.
Dosage Forms—Tablets NF: 5 mg.

Uracil Mustard

[(*Upjohn*)]

Uracil Mustard [$C_8H_{11}Cl_2N_3O_2$ = 252.10] is 5-[bis(2-chloroethyl)amino] uracil.
Preparation—5-Aminouracil is reacted with a double molar quantity of ethylene oxide in aqueous acetic acid solution and the dried reaction product, 5-[bis(2-hydroxyethyl)amino]uracil is converted to the corresponding 2-chloroethyl compound by treatment with thionyl chloride. US Pat. 2,969,364.
Uses—The structure of Uracil Mustard combines the features of a nitrogen mustard and a nucleotide antimetabolite. However, its antineoplastic effects are strictly those of its bis-chloroethylamine moiety. Its spectrum of activity and usefulness is the same as that of other nitrogen mustards (see *Mechlorethamine Hydrochloride*, page 1167), and there is no evidence that it is superior to other drugs of this class; indeed, some authorities do not think it is quite as efficacious, especially against chronic granulocytic leukemia. However, it may be more consistent in the management of thrombocytosis. The fact that it is well absorbed orally is advantageous over Mechlorethamine but not over other orally effective alkylating agents.

With the lower dose, Uracil Mustard elicits milder adverse reactions than do other alkylating antineoplastics. The most common effects are nausea, vomiting, and diarrhea. Pruritus, dermatitis, and partial alopecia do occur, but less frequently than with cyclophosphamide. Nervousness, irritability, and depression occur infrequently. Bone marrow depression with leukopenia, thrombocytopenia, and even anemia may occur, and the blood picture must be monitored twice a week during the first month of treatment.
Dose—*Usual, initial,* **3 to 5 mg** per day for 7 days, not to exceed a total dose of 0.5 mg per Kg, or **1 to 2 mg** per day until a remission or bone marrow depression occurs; *maintenance,* **1 mg** per day for 3 weeks out of each 4 week period.
Dosage Forms—Capsules: 1 mg.

Urethan NF

[Ethyl Carbamate; Urethane (*Lilly*)]

$$H_2N-\overset{\overset{\textstyle O}{\|}}{C}-O-CH_2CH_3$$

Urethan contains 99.0–101.0% of $C_3H_7NO_2$ (89.09), calculated on the anhydrous basis.
Preparation—Ethyl chloroformate is prepared by reacting carbonyl chloride (phosgene) with absolute alcohol. This, upon treatment with an excess of ammonia, yields Urethan. Urethan may also be prepared by the interaction of alcohol with carbamyl chlo-

ride, the latter being prepared by treating ammonium chloride with phosgene.

Description—Colorless crystals or a white, granular powder. It is odorless, or nearly so, and has a cool, saline taste. It melts between 48° and 50°, and boils at about 183°. Its aqueous solution is neutral to litmus.

Solubility—1 Gm dissolves in about 0.5 ml of water, about 1 ml alcohol, about 3 ml glycerin, about 1 ml chloroform, about 2 ml ether, and about 35 ml of olive oil.

Incompatibilities—Urethan forms eutectics with *antipyrine, camphor, chloral hydrate, menthol, phenol, phenyl salicylate, resorcinol, thymol*, etc. It is decomposed by *acids* and *alkalies*.

Uses—Urethan is no longer much employed as an *antineoplastic* since it has been replaced by more effective and less toxic drugs. Most effective results are obtained in the treatment of *chronic myeloid leukemia* where the drug has a palliative effect. The leukocytes are markedly reduced in number, the erythrocyte count is increased, the hemoglobin rises, and the spleen is reduced in size. Urethan is less effective in the treatment of chronic lymphatic leukemia. It is possibly of some benefit in multiple myeloma and carcinoma of the prostate, but is of no value in the management of acute leukemia, lymphosarcoma, or Hodgkin's disease. Urethan was the first drug to effect objective improvement in *plasma cell myeloma*, but melphalan and cyclophosphamide have proven to be superior. It is surprising that Urethan has not been deleted from the NF.

Urethan is a hypnotic agent, but its action is so feeble in man that it is not used for this purpose in modern therapeutics. It is combined with quinine hydrochloride as a sclerosing solution for the treatment of varicose veins.

When given orally, Urethan may induce nausea, vomiting, and occasionally diarrhea. Rectal or parenteral administration will obviate in large measure these undesirable side-effects. Drowsiness may occur, particularly after parenteral administration. Severe leukopenia, anemia, and thrombopenia may occur after the prolonged use of Urethan and excessive amounts can cause death. Liver damage has followed its use.

Dose—2 to 6 Gm; *usual*, **3 Gm** daily.

Dosage Forms—Tablets NF: 300 mg.

Veterinary Uses—It is rapid and potent in its action as a *hypnotic*, although infrequently employed, and is often employed as a *laboratory anesthetic* in animals.

Veterinary Dose—*Horses*, **15 to 30 Gm**; *Swine*, **2 to 4 Gm**; *Dogs* and *Cats*, **0.6 to 2.0 Gm**.

Vinblastine Sulfate USP

[Vincaleukoblastine Sulfate (1:1); Velban (*Lilly*)]

Vinbalstine Sulfate contains 96.0–100.5% of $C_{46}H_{58}N_4O_9 \cdot H_2SO_4$ (909.07), calculated on the dried basis.

For the structure of Vinblastine, see page 502.

Preparation—Vinblastine may be obtained by extracting the leaves, bark, or stems of *Vinca rosea* with aqueous or aqueous–alcoholic sulfuric acid, isolating the alkaloid from the extract by the usual precipitation and solvent techniques, and purifying by chromatography on aluminum oxide. Conversion to the (1:1) sulfate may be effected by dissolving the alkaloid in an equimolar quantity of dilute sulfuric acid and either evaporating to dryness or precipitating with a suitable organic solvent. US Pat. 3,097,137.

Uses—Vinblastine Sulfate is an *antineoplastic* drug which is mainly used in the treatment of *Hodgkin's disease*. In the induction of remission it is approxi-mately as efficacious as *Cyclophosphamide* (page 1165) or *Mechlorethamine* (page 1167). However, it is usually reserved for treatment when refractoriness to x-rays and alkylating drugs occurs. There is no cross-resistance between Vinblastine and other classes of antineoplastics. It may be of some value in the treatment of *choriocarcinoma* that has become resistant to methotrexate or dactinomycin. The drug may also be of varying degrees of benefit in lymphosarcoma, reticulum cell sarcoma, Letterer–Siwe's disease, mycosis fungoides, and some solid tumors.

Vinblastine is a Class II immunosuppressive drug.

Nausea, vomiting, headache, and paresthesias occur within 4 to 6 hours in 5 to 20% of patients, according to the dose used. Diarrhea, constipation, anorexia, and stomatitis also occur and are premonitory of neurotoxic effects, such as severe headache, malaise, mental depression, and loss of deep tendon reflexes. Central nervous system damage is occasionally permanent when excessive doses have been used. Blindness and death have been reported. Alopecia occurs in about 10% of users, but it is generally reversible. Bone marrow depression with thrombocytopenia and leukopenia occurs in a high percentage of patients and may require discontinuation of the drug. The blood cell count must be determined each week. The drug is locally toxic, and extravasation should be avoided.

Dose—*Intravenous*, **100** to **500 mcg** per **Kg** of body weight (the latter amount divided into two doses given on successive days) weekly; *usual*, **150 to 200 mcg** per **Kg** of body weight once a week.

Other Dose Information—100 mcg per Kg of body weight per week are usually given, with increments of 50 mcg until a response occurs or the leukocyte count falls to 3000/cu mm or a total of 500 mcg per Kg is reached; maintenance, 50 mcg less than the terminal initial dose, to be given every 1 or 2 weeks.

Dosage Forms—Sterile USP: 10 mg.

Vincristine Sulfate USP

[Leurocristine Sulfate (1:1); Oncovin (*Lilly*)]

Vincristine Sulfate contains 95.0–105.0% of $C_{46}H_{56}N_4O_{10} \cdot H_2SO_4$ (923.06), calculated on the dried basis.

For the structure of Vincristine, see page 502.

Preparation—Using suitable modifications in the chromatographic part of the process, Vincristine Sulfate may be prepared as described above for Vinblastine Sulfate. US Pat. 3,205,220.

Uses—Vincristine Sulfate is an antineoplastic drug that is mainly effective in the treatment of *acute leukemia* in children. The combination of Vincristine plus prednisone shares with mercaptopurine plus prednisone the status of drug of choice in inducing a remission; the remission rate is about 85%. Without prednisone the rate is about 50 to 60%. Vincristine is not used for maintenance, because of its toxic effects. Methotrexate or mercaptopurine is used for maintenance. In children with *Hodgkin's disease, Wilm's tumor, neuroblastoma, rhabdomyocarcoma, lymphosarcoma*, or *retinoblastoma*, Vincristine frequently brings about a favorable response; 30 to 50% of adults with Hodgkin's disease will respond favorably to the drug. It may also be useful in the treatment of *reticulum cell sarcoma* and *lymphoblastic lymphoma* and to a lesser extent *lymphosarcoma*, but remissions are usually of short duration.

The effects of Vincristine on the bone marrow are

less severe than with most other antineoplastics, but leukopenia occurs frequently, and blood counts should be made after each dose. Other frequent untoward reactions include nausea, vomiting, constipation, abdominal cramps and weight loss; these effects are readily reversible. The drug may also cause slowly reversible reactions, such as alopecia and peripheral neuropathy. Serious neuropathic effects may occur; they include loss of deep tendon reflexes, neuritic pain, numbness of the extremities, headache, ataxia, and visual defects; paresis or paralysis and atrophy of certain extensor muscles may occur late; paralysis of cranial nerves 2, 3, 6, and 7 may occur. Neuropathies may persist for several months. Severe hypertension, agitation, or mental depression also may transiently occur. The drug is locally toxic, and extravasation should be avoided.

Dose—*Intravenous*, **50** to **150 mcg** per **Kg** of body weight weekly; *usual*, **50** to **75 mcg** per **Kg** of body weight once a week.

Other Dose Information—Dosage is preferably calculated on the basis of 2 mg per M² of body surface; this corresponds to 50 to 150 mcg per Kg for infants, 30 to 100 mcg for a 10 year old child, and 25 to 75 mcg per Kg for adults. For adults the initial dose is usually 50 mcg per Kg, with weekly increments until a remission occurs or 150 mcg per Kg is reached. For maintenance, 25 mcg per Kg per week is recommended;

neurotoxicity invariably develops if 50 mcg per Kg per week is used for maintenance. Many authorities do not use Vincristine Sulfate for maintenance but prefer to switch to a less toxic drug.

Dosage Forms—for Injection USP: 1 and 5 mg.

Other Antineoplastic and Immunosuppressive Drugs

Cytarabine Hydrochloride—see page 1263.

Hydroxyurea [Hydrea (*Squibb*)][$CH_4N_2O_2$]—*Description* and *Solubility:* A moisture-labile, white, crystalline powder that melts between 133° and 136°. Freely soluble in water; slightly soluble in alcohol. *Uses:* Hydroxyurea inhibits the synthesis of DNA and hence suppresses the division of rapidly proliferating cells, especially those of the bone marrow. Its principal use is in the treatment of myelocytic leukemia, and control of the disorder has been maintained for several months. However, critical authoritative opinion does not hold the drug to be as reliable as busulfan or mercaptopurine. In patients with chronic myelocytic leukemia who have become resistant to busulfan or mercaptopurine, Hydroxyurea has not been shown to be capable of exerting hematological control. Although Hydroxyurea has been claimed to be useful in malignant melanoma, at best only a slight transient regression of tumor nodules occurs in some patients. Untoward effects include nausea, vomiting, diarrhea, abdominal pain, leukopenia, thrombocytopenia and serious hemorrhagic episodes, and anemia. *Dose:* 20 to 30 mg per Kg daily or 80 mg per Kg every 3 days.

67 | Antimicrobial Drugs

Antiseptics—systemic antibacterial drugs (sulfonamides, antibiotics, antibiotic antagonists, and other systemic antibacterial drugs)— antimalarials—amebacides—miscellaneous antiprotozoal drugs— antifungal drugs

This chapter was prepared by

Ewart A. Swinyard, PhD, *Professor of Pharmacology, College of Pharmacy and College of Medicine, University of Utah, Salt Lake City, Utah 84112, and*
Stewart C. Harvey, PhD, *Associate Professor of Pharmacology, College of Medicine, University of Utah, Salt Lake City, Utah 84112*

The antimicrobial drugs occupy a unique niche in the history of medicine. The germ theory of disease was the vehicle of a dramatic revolution in medicine, and aseptic procedures and antiseptic drugs were its agents. During the entire preceding history of medicine, fewer than a handful of drugs had a known locus of action, and even fewer had been submitted to systematic laboratory investigation. The first systemic antimicrobial drugs revolutionized the treatment of certain protozoal infections, especially syphilis, but the second major revolution in medicine in which the anti-microbial drugs played a major role awaited the appearance of sulfanilamide and penicillin; the exponential development in the antibiotic and systemic antibacterial field is the inevitable result of the momentum created by those two agents.

The term *microbe* is sometimes applied only to the unicellular microphytes. However, in its broader sense it includes not only the multicellular microphytes but the microzoa as well. Therefore, this chapter includes the antifungal and antiprotozoal agents as well as the antibacterial agents.

Antiseptics

The words *antiseptic, disinfectant,* and *germicide* all connote an agent which kills microbes upon contact, although certain denotations are more rigid and discriminatory. Drugs in this category are applied locally, although a few may be applied systemically as well. Thousands of chemical compounds have germicidal properties, and hundreds are now available. Unfortunately, many of these are poorly effective in the presence of serum or other organic media, or else they are excessively damaging to the tissues. Tissue damage, of course, is not of concern when such agents are employed for the disinfection of inanimate objects; on the other hand, corrosiveness, stain, and other effects then become important considerations. Many of the official antiseptics listed below do not warrant their exalted status, and many excellent antiseptics are unexploited.

It is commonly believed that antiseptics are non-selective and that they have a continuous spectrum of activity. Although this is approximately true, certain significant absolute exceptions exist, and the relative susceptibilities of the numerous microorganisms must be considered in antiseptic use. For example, hexachlorophene is primarily effective against Gram-positive organisms, cationic antiseptics are not effective against sporulating organisms, etc. Certain bacteria are even capable of growing in 70% ethanol. But bichloride of mercury and iodine have very broad and therapeutically complete spectra of efficacy.

Many antiseptics are also antifungal agents, and certain antiseptics will be treated in the section on antifungal drugs.

No really satisfactory classification of antiseptics exists. The most widely used scheme is the chemical classification. Nevertheless, the drugs listed below are not arranged according to chemical type. However, it will be noted that the major chemical categories represented are oxidizing agents (including the halogens and halogen-releasing compounds), phenols and related compounds, compounds of heavy metals (especially of mercury), surface-active agents (especially the cationic detergents), and a variety of dyes. Scattered representatives from the alcohols and glycols, aldehydes, and acids may also be noted. Locally effective antibiotics are discussed with the antibiotics.

Acetarsone—see page 1254.

Acetic Acid, Diluted—see page 1362.

Acrisorcin—see page 1262.

Alcohol—see page 1357.

Rubbing Alcohol NF

[Alcohol Rubbing Compound NF XI]

Rubbing Alcohol and all preparations coming under the classification of Rubbing Alcohols must be manufactured in accordance with the requirements of the Internal Revenue Service, US Treasury Department, using *Formula 23-H* (8 parts by volume of acetone, 1.5 parts by volume of methyl isobutyl ketone, and 100 parts by volume of ethyl alcohol). It contains 68.5–71.5% by volume of absolute ethyl alcohol, the remainder consisting of water and the denaturants, with or without color additives, and perfume oils. Rubbing Alcohol contains in each 100 ml not less than 355 mg of sucrose octaäcetate or not less than 1.40 mg of denatonium benzoate. The preparation may be colored with one or more color additives, listed by the Food and Drug Administration for use in drugs. A suitable stabilizer may also be added. Rubbing Alcohol complies with the requirements of the Internal Revenue Service of the United States Treasury Department.

Note—Rubbing Alcohol must be packaged, labeled, and sold in accordance with the regulations issued by the Internal Revenue Service, US Treasury Department.

Description—A transparent, colorless or colored as desired, mobile, volatile liquid, with an extremely bitter taste, and in the absence of added odorous substances, a characteristic odor. It is flammable. The specific gravity of *Formula 23-H* is between 0.8691 and 0.8771 at 15.56°.

Uses—Rubbing Alcohol is applied externally as a *cooling, soothing* application for bedridden patients and athletes. It is also widely used for cleansing the surgeon's hands and instruments. As an *antiseptic* it is good against vegetative bacteria and fair against fungi and viruses. It is ineffective against spores. In order to reduce the skin bacterial count to 5% of normal, it must be left on the skin for at least 2 minutes. It is also a feeble *anesthetic*, and a mild *counterirritant*. See *Alcohol* (page 1357). *It is not potable.*

Aluminum Acetate Solution—see page 769.

Aluminum Subacetate Solution—see page 770.

Bacitracin—see page 1209.

Benzalkonium Chloride USP

[Alkylbenzyldimethylammonium Chloride; Benasept (*Blue Line*); Zephiran Chloride (*Winthrop*)]

Benzalkonium Chloride is a mixture of alkylbenzyldimethylammonium chlorides of the general formula, $[C_6H_5CH_2N(CH_3)_2R]Cl$, in which R represents a mixture of alkyls, including all or some of the group beginning with $n\text{-}C_8H_{17}$ and extending through higher homologs, with $n\text{-}C_{12}H_{25}$, $n\text{-}C_{14}H_{29}$ and $n\text{-}C_{16}H_{33}$ comprising the major portion. On the anhydrous basis, the content of $n\text{-}C_{12}H_{25}$ homolog is not less than 40.0%, and the content of the $n\text{-}C_{14}H_{29}$ homolog is not less than 20.0%, of the total alkylbenzyldimethylammonium chloride content. The amounts of the $n\text{-}C_{12}H_{25}$ and $n\text{-}C_{14}H_{29}$ homolog components comprise together not less than 70.0% of the total alkylbenzyldimethylammonium chloride content. The total alkylbenzyldimethylammonium chloride content, calculated on the anhydrous basis, allowance being made for the amount of residue on ignition, is 97.0–103.0% of $[C_6H_5CH_2N(CH_3)_2R]Cl$ of average molecular weight 360.

Preparation—It may be prepared by treating a solution of *N*-alkyl-*N*-methylbenzylamine in a suitable organic solvent with methyl chloride, the solvent being so chosen that the quaternary compound precipitates as it is formed.

Description—A white or yellowish white, amorphous powder. Also occurs in gelatinous pieces. It has an aromatic odor, and a very bitter taste. Its solutions are alkaline to litmus and foam strongly when shaken.

Solubility—Very soluble in water and in alcohol. 1 Gm of the anhydrous form dissolves in about 6 ml of benzene and in about 100 ml of ether.

Incompatibilities—Like other cationic surface-active agents, Benzalkonium Chloride is incompatible with *soap*

and other *anionic agents*. The large organic ions of the two agents, being oppositely charged, are attracted to each other and, in sufficient concentration, precipitate from solution. *Nitric acid* and *nitrates* cause precipitation.

Uses—Benzalkonium Chloride, a rapidly acting nonirritating cationic surface-active agent, is a useful all-purpose *local antibacterial* agent for application to skin, tissues, and mucous membranes. Solutions of Benzalkonium Chloride have low surface tension and possess detergent and emulsifying actions. It has relatively low systemic toxicity, but poisoning from oral ingestion has been reported. Like other cationic surface-active agents, it has certain limitations. It cannot be relied upon to kill clostridial spores, it is inactivated by soap and other anionic surface-active agents, and when applied to the skin it has a tendency to form a film under which bacteria remain viable. It is a good disinfectant for fungi but is ineffective against viruses.

Dose—*Topically,* **0.02** to **0.1**% solution; to the conjunctiva, **0.1** ml of a **0.01**% solution.

Other Dose Information—Benzalkonium Chloride tincture 1:1000 to 1:750 (tinted or stainless) is employed for the preoperative disinfection of unbroken skin or treatment of superficial injuries or fungus infections. Benzalkonium Chloride solutions are used for the *preoperative disinfection* of mucous membranes and denuded skin in 1:10,000 to 1:2000 concentration; for instillation or irrigation of the *eye* or *vagina*, 1:5000 to 1:2000; for irrigation of widely *denuded surfaces,* 1:10,000 or 1:5000; for irrigation of the *urinary bladder* and *urethra*, 1:20,000; for retention lavage of the bladder, 1:40,000; for disinfection of *deep lacerations,* 1:1000; for irrigation of infected *deep wounds*, 1:3000; for treatment of infected denuded areas with wet dressings, 1:5000; for *sterile storage of metallic instruments and rubber articles*, 1:1000 to 1:750. When the drug is used for the sterile storage of metal instruments, sodium nitrite (0.5%) is added to the solution containing Benzalkonium Chloride to prevent corrosion of the metal.

Benzalkonium Chloride is marketed as a colorless or tinted tincture (1:750), as an aqueous solution (1:750), and as a concentrated aqueous solution (17%) which is used to make the tincture or solution.

Dosage Forms—Solution USP: 0.1 (1 in 1000), and 0.133% (1 in 750) topical solution; 10 and 17% concentrate.

Benzethonium Chloride NF

[Benzyldimethyl[2 - [2 - [p - (1,1,3,3 - tetramethylbutyl)phenoxy]-ethoxy] ethyl]ammonium Chloride; Phemerol Chloride (*Parke-Davis*)]

$$\left[(CH_3)_3C-CH_2C(CH_3)_2-\!\!\!\bigcirc\!\!\!-O-CH_2-CH_2-O-CH_2-CH_2-\overset{+}{\underset{\underset{CH_2}{|}}{N}}(CH_3)_2 \right] Cl^-$$

Benzethonium Chloride contains 97.0–103.0% of $C_{27}H_{42}ClNO_2$ (448.09), calculated on the dried basis.

Preparation—4 - (1,1,3,3 - Tetramethylbutyl)phenol, commonly termed *p*-diisobutylphenol, is condensed in the presence of a basic catalyst with β,β'-dichlorodiethyl ether to yield 2{2-[4-(1,1,3,3-tetramethylbutyl)phenoxy]ethoxy}ethyl chloride. Alkaline dimethylamination at the expense of the chlorine gives the corresponding tertiary amine which, after purification by distillation, is dissolved in a suitable organic solvent and treated with benzyl chloride to precipitate the final quaternary compound.

Description—Colorless, odorless crystals, having a bitter taste. Its 1 in 100 solution is slightly alkaline to litmus. Dried at 105° for 4 hours, it melts between 160° and 165°.
Solubility—Soluble in water, alcohol, and chloroform; only slightly soluble in ether.

Uses—Benzethonium Chloride is used as a general all-purpose germicide and antiseptic. It is employed in aqueous solution (1:750) or tincture (1:500) for *disinfection of wounds, lacerations, and infected skin surfaces*. The aqueous solution (1:750), diluted with four parts of water, is preferred for use in the *nose* and *eye*. Like related cationic detergents, its action is opposed by anionic detergents such as ordinary soap, is reduced by organic matter, and is not reliable against clostridial spores. It is of only limited value in the treatment of fungous infections.
Dose—*Topically*, as a **1:750** solution to the skin or **1:5000** solution nasally.
Other Dose Information—Benzethonium Chloride is marketed as an aqueous solution (1:750) and as a tincture (1:500); both preparations are used undiluted, except when applied to the nose or eyes; then the 1:5000 aqueous solution is employed.
Dosage Forms—Solution NF: 1:750 and 3%.

Benzoic Acid—see page 1316.

Benzyl Alcohol—see page 1066.

Butylparaben USP

[Butyl *p*-Hydroxybenzoate]

$$HO\!-\!\!\bigcirc\!\!-\!COOCH_2CH_2CH_2CH_3$$

Butylparaben contains 99.0–100.5% of $C_{11}H_{14}O_3$ (194.23), calculated on the dried basis.
Preparation—Using butanol instead of methanol, Butylparaben is prepared by the method described for *Methylparaben*, page 1184.

Description—Small, colorless crystals or white powder.
Solubility—Very slightly soluble in water and glycerin; very soluble in acetone, alcohol, ether, and propylene glycol.

Uses—The actions and uses of Butylparaben are similar to those of *Methylparaben* (see page 1184), with which it is often used in combination. Butylparaben appears to be the best antifungal agent among the parabens. Butylparaben is also used in antiseptic creams and ointments.

Cadmium Sulfide

[Capsebon (*Pitman-Moore*)]

Cadmium Sulfide is CdS.

Preparation—Hydrogen sulfide is passed into a solution of cadmium sulfate.

Description—Light-yellow or orange-colored powder.
Solubility—Insoluble in water; soluble in hot, moderately diluted mineral acids.

Uses—Cadmium Sulfide is an antibacterial agent useful in the treatment of *seborrheic dermatitis* of the scalp and *seborrheic sicca*. Under ordinary conditions of use, it is nontoxic, and hence it has advantages over selenium sulfide. It also does not cause rebound oili-

ness like selenium sulfide, and it also lacks the offensive odor. However, it is somewhat less effective. Cadmium Sulfide can cause photosensitization if applied to skin that may be subsequently exposed to sunlight. If the substance is not thoroughly rinsed off after treatment, it may discolor light-colored hair.
Dose—*Topically*, as a **1%** detergent suspension. A lather of the suspension is massaged into the wet scalp, whereupon the scalp is rinsed. The application is repeated, and the drug is allowed to remain in contact with the scalp for 5 to 10 minutes before the final rinse. The drug is applied daily to weekly, according to the severity of the condition.

Calomel—see page 800.

Cetylpyridinium Chloride NF

[1-Hexadecylpyridinium Chloride; Ceepryn Chloride (*Merrell*)]

$$\left[\bigcirc\!\!\!\!\!\overset{+}{N}\!\!-\!(CH_2)_{15}CH_3\right]Cl^-.H_2O$$

Cetylpyridinium Chloride [$C_{21}H_{38}ClN.H_2O$ = 358.01] contains 99.0–102.0% of $C_{21}H_{38}ClN$ (340.00), calculated on the anhydrous basis.
Preparation—The anhydrous compound is prepared by heating a mixture of cetyl chloride and a slight excess of pyridine at 140°C for about 60 hours. The crude product is decolorized with charcoal and recrystallized from a mixed solvent composed of methyl ethyl ketone and alcohol. It is then washed with ether and vacuum dried at 50 to 60°C. Recrystallization from water yields the official monohydrate. The cetyl chloride may be prepared by reacting cetyl alcohol with thionyl chloride in the presence of a small amount of zinc chloride.

Description—White powder with a slight, characteristic odor. The melting range is between 80° and 84°, the preliminary drying treatment being omitted.
Solubility—Very soluble in water, alcohol, and chloroform; slightly soluble in benzene and ether.

Uses—Cetylpyridinium Chloride is a *local anti-infective* which possesses surface active as well as antiseptic properties against sensitive nonsporulating bacteria. It is used for preoperative preparation of the skin for the prophylactic antisepsis of minor wounds and for the irrigation of or topical application to the mucous membranes. It is also incorporated into mouthwashes. Its action is inhibited by soap, serum, and tissue fluids.
Dose—*Topically*, as a **1:100** to **1:1000** solution to intact skin; **1:1000** for minor lacerations; **1:2000** to **1:10,000** to mucous membranes.
Dosage Forms—Solution NF: 1:1000.
Veterinary Use—In tincture (**1:500**) or aqueous solution (**1:1000**) for preoperative skin antisepsis. Aqueous concentrations of **1:1000** and **1:5000** as topical treatment for wounds.

Chiniofon—see RPS-13, page 1309.

Cresol NF

[Cresylol; Tricresol]

Cresol [$CH_3C_6H_4OH$ = 108.14] is a mixture of isomeric cresols obtained from coal tar or from petroleum. It contains not more than 5.0% of C_6H_6O (phenol).

History—Soon after the introduction of phenol (carbolic acid) into use as an antiseptic it was discovered that some of the homologous constituents of *crude carbolic acid* were more active than the phenol which it contained. Cresol or *cresylic acid*, as it was then called, was the most important among these, and experience has developed its value. Official Cresol consists of a mixture of three isomers, existing, according to Schulze, in coal tar approximately in the proportion of 40% of *m-cresol*, 35% of *o-cresol*, and 25% of *p-cresol*. Cresol has a higher boiling point than phenol and is separated from it by fractional distillation. NF Cresol usually contains 3 to 4% phenol.

Laws in some states require that preparations of this type shall state upon the label their germicidal activity as compared with phenol. This figure is known as the *Phenol Coefficient* (RPS-13, page 1608).

The official Cresol usually shows a phenol coefficient varying from 2 to 3, but higher boiling fractions, known as "tar acids," are also commercially available and these frequently show a phenol coefficient of from 12 to 25. This modestly increased germicidal activity, while indicated by the test organism, the typhoid bacillus, is not equally manifest with other common organisms and is therefore misleading. The NF has intentionally retained a rather limited boiling-point product, of uniform and dependable activity, so that when the official products are directed by physicians they may depend upon their efficacy.

Description—A colorless, or yellowish to brownish yellow, or a pinkish, highly refractive liquid, becoming darker with age and on exposure to light. It has a phenol-like, sometimes empyreumatic odor. Specific gravity 1.030–1.038. Not less than 90% of it distils between 195° and 205°. A saturated aqueous solution of Cresol is neutral or slightly acid to litmus and gives a bluish violet color with ferric chloride.

Solubility—1 ml dissolves in about 50 ml of water, usually forming a cloudy solution; miscible with alcohol, ether, and glycerin; dissolved by solutions of the fixed alkali hydroxides.

Uses—Cresol is a *disinfectant* and a pharmaceutical necessity as a *preservative* for injections, etc. Compared to modern antiseptics, its potency is low; its continued use rests mainly on force of habit and low cost. It resembles phenol in its medicinal properties, but owing to its greater insolubility in water, it is nearly always employed in combination with alkalies associated with fatty bodies, or soaps which render it very soluble (see *Saponated Cresol Solution*). Cresol is a good disinfectant against vegetative bacteria and fungi, but it is poor against viruses and ineffective against spores. It is used as a disinfectant on dishes, utensils, and other inanimate objects.

Application—1 to 5% solution on dishes, utensils, and other inanimate objects.

Saponated Cresol Solution NF [Compound Cresol Solution; Cresol and Soap Solution] contains, in each 100 ml, 46–52 ml of cresol. It is prepared by the saponification of a mixture of cresol with vegetable oils, or the mixed fatty acids derived therefrom, excluding coconut and palm kernel oils. The vegetable oil may be corn, cottonseed, linseed, or soya bean, or similar oils which have a saponification value not greater than 205, and an iodine value not less than 100. *Preparation:* It may be prepared extemporaneously in the following manner: Mix the vegetable oil (350 ml) and alcohol (55 ml). Dissolve potassium hydroxide (73 Gm) in purified water (100 ml) and immediately add this hot solution to the oil while vigorously stirring the mixture with a mechanical stirrer. Continue the stirring

until a small portion of the soap dissolves in hot purified water to form a clear solution. Add cresol (500 ml) to the soap, stir until a clear solution is obtained, and add sufficient purified water to make the Solution measure 1000 ml. *Note*—If desired, potassium hydroxide (58 Gm) may be replaced by sodium hydroxide (37 Gm). It is also permissible to replace alcohol with oleic acid (20 ml), in which case the oil should be warmed to 85° before the addition of the solution of the alkali hydroxide, and the mixture heated, if necessary, to complete saponification. The quantities of potassium hydroxide and sodium hydroxide here directed have been determined upon the basis of the official minimum percentages of strength, namely, 85% and 95%, respectively. If either or both of the hydroxides used should have a different percentage of strength, corresponding alterations in the quantities should be made. *Alcohol Content:* Not more than 5% of C_2H_5OH. *Uses:* Saponated Cresol Solution is widely used as a *disinfectant* for inanimate objects and excrement. A 1:500 solution is sometimes used as a mildly antiseptic *vaginal douche*. This liquid was introduced into medical practice to supply a need for an antiseptic solution which will mix readily with water. Saponated Cresol Solution must be used with caution as it is about equal to phenol in its poisonous character. Today it has been largely replaced by other germicidal solutions.

Diiodohydroxyquin—see page 1250.

Eucalyptol—see page 1337.

Eucalyptus Oil—see page 1327.

Ethylparaben USP

[Ethyl *p*-Hydroxybenzoate]

$$HO-\!\!\left\langle\right\rangle\!\!-COOC_2H_5$$

Ethylparaben contains 99.0–100.5% of $C_9H_{10}O_3$ (166.18), calculated on the dried basis.

Preparation—Using ethanol instead of methanol, Ethylparaben is prepared by the method described for *Methylparaben*, page 1184.

Description—Small, colorless crystals or white powder.
Solubility—Slightly soluble in water and glycerin; freely soluble in acetone, alcohol, ether, and propylene glycol.

Uses—The actions and uses of Ethylparaben are quite similar to those of *Methylparaben* (page 1184), with which Ethylparaben is often used in combination. Ethylparaben is also used in antiseptic creams and ointments.

Formaldehyde Solution USP

[Formol; Formalin]

Formaldehyde Solution contains not less than 37.0%, by weight, of formaldehyde [$CH_2O = 30.03$], with methanol added to prevent polymerization.

Preparation—This liquid, commonly known as *formaldehyde* or *formalin*, is made by mixing the vapor of boiling methyl alcohol, while under pressure, with air in proper quantity, and allowing the mixed vapors to pass over heated copper tubes, and then condensing the vapors by passing them into a copper tank provided with the means for reducing the temperature to 0°. Sufficient water is added to the product to make it contain 37% by weight of HCHO.

Description—A clear, colorless or nearly colorless liquid, having a pungent, irritating odor. The vapor from Formaldehyde Solution irritates the mucous membrane of the throat and the nose. On long standing, especially in the cold, the Solution sometimes becomes cloudy due to separation of paraformaldehyde (trioxymethylene). Such cloudiness disappears on warming the Solution. It is usually slightly acid. The specific gravity of the Solution is about 1.08 at 25°, and when the Solution is evaporated on a water bath most of the formaldehyde polymerizes to paraformaldehyde which remains as a white residue.

Solubility—Miscible with water and alcohol.

Uses—Formaldehyde Solution or "Formalin" is used as a *disinfectant* and *deodorant*. Its action derives from its ability to condense with amino groups of amino acids and biogenic amines. Its employment for preserving milk, meat, and other articles of food likely to spoil through fermentation is prohibited by both national and state laws. It is, however, used for disinfecting apartments which have been subjected to infection by spraying it on sheets hung in the room or the vapor may be conducted into the room from a generator. Formaldehyde is a good disinfectant not only against vegetative bacteria and fungi but also against spores and viruses. A solution of 20% formaldehyde and 50% ethanol is even superior. Formaldehyde is contained in some dental preparations for reducing the sensitivity of teeth. It is also used to preserve cadavers and zoological specimens.

Veterinary Uses—Formaldehyde has been used for various skin diseases such as *eczema* and *acne* of large animals and combined with 2 to 4 parts of dilute alcohol for the treatment of *demodectic mange* in the dog. Also, it had been used undiluted in the treatment of *canker of the frog* of the horse.

Application—For disinfection of inanimate objects, in **full strength** or as a solution containing **10%** of formaldehyde.

Furazolidone NF

[3-[(5-Nitrofurfurylidene)amino]-2-oxazolidinone; Furoxone (*Eaton*)]

Furazolidone contains 97.0–103.0% of $C_8H_7N_3O_5$ (225.16), calculated on the dried basis.

Preparation—Furazolidone is a typical aldehyde condensation product of 5-nitro-2-furaldehyde (I) and 3-amino-2-oxazolidinone (II). It is prepared by heating the "diacetate" of (I) with an acidified solution of (II). (II) may be prepared by condensing 2-hydroxyethylhydrazine with ethyl carbonate in the presence of sodium methoxide under conditions such that the ethanol of condensation distils off as it is formed.

Description—It occurs as a yellow, odorless, crystalline powder that is tasteless at first, developing a bitter aftertaste.

Solubility—Practically insoluble in water, alcohol, and carbon tetrachloride.

Uses—Furazolidone is an antimicrobial agent used for the peroral treatment of *bacterial enteritis* and *dysentery*. It is bactericidal *in vitro* to many of the usual enteric pathogens, both gram-negative and gram-positive, including many species of Salmonella, Shigella, Escherichia, Proteus, Streptococcus, Staphylococcus and those organisms classed as coliform and enterococci. Clinically it may control some, but not all, diarrheal disorders and enteritis caused by these organisms. It should not be employed to treat the carrier

state. It is also effective against Giardia lamblia enteritis. It is available in tablet and liquid form. The liquid also contains kaolin and pectin, to which some of its efficacy must be attributed. Furazolidone is poorly absorbed from the gut, but breakdown products of absorbed drug may color the urine brown. It is also used for the local treatment of certain vaginal infections, generally in combination with Nifuroxime (see *Furazolidone and Nifuroxime*, below). Untoward effects of oral therapy include nausea and vomiting and occasional headache. Rarely it may cause arthralgia, fever, or rash. Dizziness and partial deafness have also been reported in one patient.

Dose—There is no official dose. Unofficially, the oral daily dose is 5 mg per Kg (2.3 mg per pound) in 4 divided doses over 24 hours.

Veterinary Uses—Fowl typhoid, paratyphoid, pullorum, blackhead, and paracolon in chickens and turkeys. Hexamitiasis in turkeys. Infectious hepatitis, coccidiosis, CRD (air sac), synovitis (arthritis due to a filtrable agent), and nonspecific enteritis in chickens. Bacterial scours, bacterial enteritis and vibrionic dysentery in pigs. Pasteurella-type pneumonia and enteritis in rabbits.

Veterinary Dose—*Prophylaxis*, **0.0055%** in the feed; treatment, **0.011%** in the feed.

Furazolidone and Nifuroxime Powder NF [Tricofuron Powder (*Eaton*)] 0.09–0.11% of $C_8H_7N_3O_5$ (furazolidone), and 0.45–0.55% of $C_5H_4N_2O_4$ (nifuroxime) in a suitable, slightly acidified powder base. *Description:* The pH of a dispersion (1 in 25) is between 3.0 and 4.5. Not less than 99% of the Powder passes through a No. 100 sieve (see page 1638). *Uses:* For the treatment of vaginitis caused by *Trichomonas vaginalis*, *Candida* (*Monilia*) *albicans*, or *Haemophilus vaginalis*—as individual or mixed infections. The actions of the separate active components of this powder are described elsewhere (see *Furazolidone*, above, and *Nifuroxime*, page 1259). *Application: Vaginal insufflation*, 1 or 2 times a week. *Other Dose Information:* The usual amount insufflated is about 5 Gm.

Furazolidone and Nifuroxime Suppositories NF [Tricofuron Suppositories (*Eaton*)] contain 0.225–0.275% of $C_8H_7N_3O_5$ (furazolidone), and 0.337–0.413% of $C_5H_4N_2O_4$ (nifuroxime). *Uses:* See *Furazolidone and Nifuroxime Powder*. *Dose: Usual, vaginal*, 1 suppository 1 or 2 times a day. *Other Dose Information:* After the first week the dose is generally reduced to 1 per day.

Gentian Violet USP

[Methylrosaniline Chloride USP XVI; *N,N,N',N',N'',N''*-Hexamethylpararosaniline Chloride; Methyl Violet; Crystal Violet]

Gentian Violet is hexamethylpararosaniline chloride, usually admixed with pentamethylpararosaniline chloride and tetramethylpararosaniline chloride. It contains not less than 96.0–100.5% of gentian violet, calculated on the anhydrous basis as hexamethylpararosaniline chloride [$C_{25}H_{30}ClN_3 = 407.99$].

Preparation—Several processes are available for the production of the "rosanilines" which represent a large class of dyestuffs. They are generally made by oxidizing a mixture of aniline and *p*-toluidine. The oxidizing agent most commonly used is arsenic acid. Nitrobenzene is also employed. By using methylated anilines, eg, di- or monomethylaniline, methylrosanilines are produced. Pure hexamethylrosaniline may be made by the action of carbonyl chloride (phosgene) on *N,N*-dimethylaniline.

Description—A dark green powder, or greenish glistening pieces having a metallic luster and not more than a faint odor.

Solubility—Soluble in water; 1 Gm dissolves in about 10 ml alcohol and about 15 ml glycerin; soluble in chloroform; insoluble in ether.

Uses—Gentian Violet is an *anthelmintic* and *anti-infective* agent. It is bactericidal to gram-positive organisms in very high dilutions. It also acts against the causative organism of Vincent's angina and against many strains of *Monilia, Torula, Epidermophyton,* and *Trichophyton.* Among the many conditions which have been treated with this dye may be listed *Vincent's angina, cystitis,* and *urethritis, suppurating joint infections, eczematoid dermatitis, furunculosis, recurrent dermatomycosis, monilial paronychia, chronic ulcers, bed sores, impetigo, infectsiosa, pruritus ani,* etc. The drug has been largely outmoded by the antibiotics and systemic antibacterial drugs.

The dye has also been employed in the treatment of *burns.* This forms a pliable eschar and helps to control infection from Gram-positive organisms. However, it is little used today for this purpose.

Gentian Violet is also an effective anthelmintic useful in the treatment of *Strongyloides* and *Oxyuris* infestations.

Dose—*Topically,* in a 1% solution 2 times a day.

Other Dose Information—For direct application to tissues, the dye is employed in a concentration of 1:500 to 1:1000. For instillation in closed cavities a 1:10,000 solution is employed. As an aerosol foam or as a vaginal cream it is used in a concentration of 1.35%. In a tampon 5 mg is used. Vaginal tablets contain 1 mg. For the treatment of burns a 1% solution is sprayed over the burned tissue at 2-hour intervals.

Gentian Violet Solution USP contains, in each 100 ml, 0.95–1.05 Gm of gentian violet, calculated as hexamethylpararosaniline chloride ($C_{25}H_{30}ClN_3$). *Preparation:* Mix alcohol (100 ml) with purified water (800 ml), dissolve the gentian violet (10 Gm), by agitation, in the mixture, add sufficient purified water to make 1000 ml, and mix. *Description:* A purple liquid having a slight odor of alcohol. A 1 in 100 dilution is deep purple in color when viewed through a depth of 1 cm. *Alcohol Content:* From 8 to 10% of C_2H_5OH.

Glycobiarsol—see page 1251.

Gramicidin—see page 1218.

Halazone USP

[*p*-(Dichlorosulfamoyl)benzoic Acid]

Halazone contains 91.5–100.5% of $C_7H_5Cl_2NO_4S$ (270.09).

Preparation—Halazone may be prepared starting with toluene and chlorosulfonic acid. The resulting *p*-toluenesulfonchloride is converted to the amide, which is treated with hypochlorite to form *p*-toluenesulfondichloramide. The methyl group is then oxi-

dized with dichromate or permanganate to form Halazone.

Description—A white, crystalline powder having a chlorine-like odor. It melts with decomposition at about 195°, and is affected by light.

Solubility—Slightly soluble in water or chloroform; soluble in solutions of alkali hydroxides or carbonates, forming the corresponding salts; soluble in glacial acetic acid.

Uses—Halazone is used for the extemporaneous *disinfection of drinking water,* as tablets.

Application—2 to 5 ppm, in drinking water.

Other Dose Information—A concentration of 2 to 5 ppm is produced by adding one 4-mg tablet to 1 quart of water. A 30-minute wait is required before the water may be considered potable. See *Water* (page 1338).

Dosage Forms—Tablets for Solution USP: 4 mg.

Hexachlorophene USP

[2,2'-Methylenebis[3,4,6-trichlorophenol]: G-11; AT-7; Gamophen (*Ethicon*); Hex-O-San (*Retort*); Surgi-Cen (*Central*)]

Hexachlorophene contains 98.0–100.5% of $C_{13}H_6Cl_6O_2$ (406.91), calculated on the dried basis.

Preparation—Hexachlorophene is prepared by the Baeyer condensation reaction involving two molecules of 2,4,5-trichlorophenol, and one molecule of formaldehyde. Sulfuric acid is employed as the dehydrant.

Description—A white to light tan, crystalline powder. Odorless or only a slightly phenolic odor. Melting range between 161° and 167°.

Solubility—Insoluble in water; freely soluble in acetone, alcohol, and ether; soluble in chloroform and dilute solutions of fixed alkali hydroxides.

Uses—Hexachlorophene is an *anti-infective* agent for external use. It is employed primarily in *deodorant* and *germicidal* soaps (see *Hexachlorophene Liquid Soap,* below). When incorporated into soaps only one of the phenolic hydroxy groups is neutralized; therefore this chlorinated bisphenol retains its high germicidal activity. When soaps containing Hexachlorophene are used daily, residual amounts of the phenol are retained on the surface of the skin and the normal bacterial flora is greatly reduced, providing the Hexachlorophene film is not removed by other cleansing agents, including ethanol and water. It is effective mainly against Gram-positive organisms. However, on inanimate objects it is a good disinfectant against fungi.

Preparations containing Hexachlorophene are widely used as antiseptic scrubs by physicians, dentists, food handlers, etc. The incidence and severity of *pyogenic skin infections* is reduced by routine use of a Hexachlorophene soap; however, a thorough surgical scrub is still mandatory. The soap is also of value as a *deodorant,* since it inhibits the bacterial decomposition of organic products in the perspiration responsible for body odor.

Dose (unofficial)—*Topically* to skin.

Other Dose Information—The optimal concentration is 2 to 3% in bar and liquid soaps and 0.5 to 1% in lotions or other preparations that are applied to the skin without dilution. As a disinfectant of inanimate objects, 3 to 4%.

Hexachlorophene Liquid Soap USP is a solution of hexachlorophene in a 10.0 to 13.0% solution of a potassium soap. It contains, in each 100 Gm, 225–260 mg of $C_{13}H_6Cl_6O_2$. It may contain suitable water hardness controls. *Note:* Hexachlorophene Liquid Soap may be prepared also in solutions having higher concentration of hexachlorophene and of potassium soap, where the ratios of these components are consistent with the limits stated in the preceding paragraph, but it must be diluted prior to use. *Note: The inclusion of non-ionic detergents in Hexachlorophene Liquid Soap in amounts greater than 8% on a total weight basis may decrease the bacteriostatic activity of the Soap. Description:* A clear, amber-colored liquid. It has a slight, characteristic odor. Its 1 in 20 solution is clear and has an alkaline reaction. *Dose: Topically* to the skin as the sole detergent.

Hexylresorcinol—see page 1266.

Hydrogen Peroxide Solution USP

[Hydrogen Dioxide Solution; "Peroxide"]

Hydrogen Peroxide Solution contains, in each 100 ml, 2.5–3.5 Gm of H_2O_2 (34.01). Suitable preservatives, totaling not more than 0.05%, may be added.

Preparation—Hydrogen Peroxide Solution is generally prepared by diluting the commercially available concentrated (70 and 90%) solutions. The latter are commonly produced by electrolysis.

Description—A colorless liquid, odorless, or having an odor resembling that of ozone. It is slightly acid to the taste and to litmus paper, and produces a froth in the mouth. It usually deteriorates upon standing or upon protracted agitation, and rapidly decomposes when in contact with many oxidizing, as well as reducing, substances. When rapidly heated, it may decompose suddenly. Light accelerates its decomposition. Its specific gravity is about 1.01.

Incompatibilities—Hydrogen Peroxide Solution is decomposed by practically all *organic matter* and other *reducing agents*. It reacts with many materials to liberate oxygen. *Metals, metallic salts, alkalies, light, agitation,* and *heat* catalyze its decomposition into water and oxygen. Hydrogen Peroxide Solution mixed with *phenol* darkens within a few hours, the phenol being oxidized.

Uses—Hydrogen Peroxide Solution is a *germicide* which is active by virtue of the fact that it releases nascent oxygen. It is a very short acting compound for the reason that this release occurs rapidly.* Thus it is a relatively feeble germicide with poor penetrability. Its chief value is in the cleansing of wounds where the effervescence caused by the release of oxygen affords a mechanical means for the removal of tissue debris from inaccessible regions. It is also an effective mouth wash in the treatment of *Vincent's stomatitis.* Its continued use for this purpose may lead to the condition known as "hairy tongue." It may be employed in the treatment of *Trichomonas vaginalis vaginitis,* and of *balanitis.* It is also popularly employed as a hair bleach. Because of the low germicidal efficacy of hydrogen peroxide, it is surprising that it has been retained in the USP.

Dose—*Topically*, to the skin and mucous membranes as required.

Other Dose Information—For cleansing wounds, 1.5 to 3% solution; as a mouthwash, 3% solution; intravaginal, 2% solution.

---

* *Note*—An interesting experiment demonstrates the availability of oxygen when acted upon by catalase, an enzyme found in nearly all body tissues: a small quantity of hydrogen peroxide solution, poured onto a little liver, ground up and placed in a beaker, produces such copious quantities of froth that it immediately flows over the sides of the container.

Iodine USP

Iodine contains 99.8–100.5% of I (126.90).
Preparation—See page 423.

Description—Iodine occurs in the form of heavy, grayish black plates or granules, having a metallic luster and a characteristic odor. Its specific gravity is about 4.9. It melts at about 114°C but volatilizes even at room temperature.

Solubility—1 Gm dissolves in about 3000 ml of water, 13 ml of alcohol, about 4 ml of carbon disulfide, 10 ml of benzene, and 80 ml of glycerin; freely soluble in chloroform, carbon tetrachloride, ether, and glacial acetic acid; soluble in solutions of iodides or hydriodic acid.

Identification—Solutions of Iodine in chloroform, carbon tetrachloride, and carbon disulfide, of concentrations on the order of 1 in 1000, have a violet color. A saturated aqueous iodine solution is colored blue upon the addition of starch TS.

Incompatibilities—Iodine oxidizes *hypophosphites, sulfites,* the lower valence forms of some *metals,* and *other reducing agents,* the Iodine being reduced to an iodide. *Thiosulfates* (hyposulfites) also react with free iodine. It reacts with *fixed oils* to form addition compounds, and with *volatile oils* to form various derivatives. The reaction with *turpentine oil* is violent. An explosive iodide of nitrogen may be formed with *ammonia water* or *ammoniated mercury.* *Alkali hydroxides* and *carbonates* react with iodine to form iodides or iodates depending on temperature. Many *alkaloids* are precipitated from aqueous solutions of their salts. In *alcoholic solution* Iodine slowly forms hydrogen iodide if alkali iodide is absent.

Uses—Elemental Iodine in the form of aqueous or alcohol solutions is widely used as a *germicide* and *fungicide.* It remains the best all-around antiseptic, provided that appropriate dilutions are used. Unfortunately, aqueous iodine solutions are poorly effective against spores. In isopropyl alcohol it is fairly effective against spores. Its therapeutic index is among the highest of the effective antiseptics; iodine burns are largely the result of the use of concentrations higher than is necessary. Iodine salts also have a variety of therapeutic applications. A 2% solution of iodine in glycerin is the iodine preparation of choice for application to mucous membranes. Iodine may be used as a *disinfectant* of inanimate objects, but both its limited ability to kill spores and its ability to attack metals and other materials must be kept in mind. A more detailed discussion of the therapeutic uses of Iodine and iodides appears under the individual preparations. Iodine is used extensively in operations involving chemical synthesis and analysis.

The radioactive isotopes, iodine-125 and iodine-131, have various diagnostic and therapeutic applications (see page 570).

Iodine Ampuls NF [Iodine Swabs] contain, in each 100 ml, 1.8–2.2 Gm of I and 2.1–2.6 Gm of NaI. *Note: Iodine Ampuls contain Iodine Tincture USP. Alcohol Content:* From 44 to 50% of C_2H_5OH. *Uses:* These ampuls are not used for parenteral administration, but, as the synonym "Iodine Swabs" indicates, they are used for first aid treatments. They usually consist of ampuls covered with gauze or some absorbent material. When the iodine is required for use, the tip of the ampul is broken, the gauze absorbs the iodine and provides a means of applying it directly to the wound. Some Iodine Ampuls are found in the form of fine capillary tubes, which are broken when needed, and the iodine solution is applied directly to the place where it is needed for its *local antibacterial* or *irritant* actions.

Iodine Solution NF contains, in each 100 ml, 1.8–2.2 Gm of I, and 2.1–2.6 Gm of NaI. *Preparation:* Dissolve iodine (20 Gm) and sodium iodide (24 Gm) in purified water (50 ml), then add sufficient purified water to make the product measure 1000 ml. *Description:* A transparent liquid, having a reddish brown color and the odor of iodine. *Incompatibilities:* See *Iodine* (page 1180). *Uses:* Iodine Solution is an effective nonirritating *germicide* and *fungicide* despite its relatively low content of free iodine. Indeed, it may be diluted several fold and still remain one of the most effective antiseptics. Irritation or "iodine burns" are uncommon with this concentration. *Uses:* see *Strong Iodine Solution. Dose:* There is no official statement on dose or application; the solution is applied topically to the skin or to wounds, abrasions, etc.

Strong Iodine Solution USP [Lugol's Solution; Aqueous Solution of Iodine; Solutio Iodi Aquosa; Compound Iodine Solution] contains, in each 100 ml, 4.5–5.5 Gm of iodine (I), and 9.5–10.5 Gm of potassium iodide (KI). *Preparation:* Dissolve iodine (50 Gm) and potassium iodide (100 Gm) in purified water (100 ml), then add sufficient purified water to make the product measure 1000 ml. The potassium iodide is added only to increase the solubility of the iodine. *Description:* A transparent liquid having a deep brown color, and the odor of iodine. *Identification:* A drop of Strong Iodine Solution added to 1 ml of starch TS previously diluted with 10 ml of water, produces a deep blue color. The ignited residue from the Solution responds to the identification tests for potassium and for iodide. *Incompatibilities:* See *Iodine* (page 1180). *Uses:* Strong Iodine Solution is traditionally used in the treatment of many conditions in which the action of the iodide ion is desired. For example, in the treatment of *thyrotoxicosis,* Strong Iodine Solution is employed in order to reduce the metabolic rate prior to operation on the thyroid. For such purposes, however, potassium iodide is equally effective. The presence of free iodine in Strong Iodine Solution makes this preparation of great value as a *germicide* and *fungicide.* Thus, it retains most of the desirable properties of tincture of iodine without the attending irritation which results from the presence of alcohol in the latter preparation. Either Strong Iodine Solution or Iodine Solution can be used for the treatment of those conditions described under the tincture. Aqueous solutions of iodine have the advantage of being less painful than alcoholic solutions when applied to cuts, and they can be made isotonic with the blood (a 2% solution of iodine with alkali iodide is isotonic), but they are subject to freezing and they do not dry rapidly. On the other hand, alcoholic solutions dry rapidly and do not freeze. *Dose: 0.1* to *3 ml* daily; *usual, 0.1* to *0.3 ml* 3 times a day.

Iodine Tincture USP [Mild Tincture of Iodine; Solutio Iodi Spirituosa; Weak Solution of Iodine] contains, in each 100 ml, 1.8–2.2 Gm of iodine (I), and 2.1–2.6 Gm of sodium iodide (NaI). *Preparation:* Dissolve iodine (20 Gm) and sodium iodide (24 Gm) in alcohol (500 ml) and then add sufficient purified water to make the product measure 1000 ml. Sufficient sodium iodide is present to stabilize the tincture and make it miscible with water in all proportions. More than enough iodide is present to combine, theoretically, with all the iodine to form NaI₃, and thus the iodine does not react with the alcohol to form acetaldehyde and hydrogen iodide. If hydriodic acid was formed, the solution would be more painful when applied to wounds. Sodium iodide is used in this Tincture, instead of the potassium salt formerly used, as it is less irritating when applied to open wounds. *Description:* A transparent liquid having a reddish brown color and the odors of iodine and alcohol. *Identification:* One drop of the Tincture added to a mixture of 1 ml of starch TS and 9 ml of water produces a deep blue color. The residue on evaporation from a sample of the Tincture responds to the flame test for *sodium. Alcohol Content:* From 44 to 50% of C₂H₅OH. *Incompatibilities:* See *Iodine* (page 1180). *Uses:* Iodine Tincture is one of the oldest and most effective of the *germicides* and *fungicides.* For disinfection of the skin, the alcoholic vehicle facilitates spreading and penetration. If the stronger tinctures are employed, vesication and desquamation may occur, if the excess iodine is not removed with alcohol. For application to wounds and abrasions, the more dilute tinctures or aqueous solutions of iodine and iodide should be employed. The dilute tincture is also the preparation of choice in the treatment of skin infections due to bacteria and fungi. Elemental

iodine is effective for the *purification of drinking water* in emergencies; 5 to 10 drops of Tincture to a quart of water is both *amebicidal* and *bactericidal,* if allowed to stand for 15 minutes; Iodine Solution in the same dilution is equally effective. Elemental iodine is also an alkaloidal precipitant and the tincture or solution may be employed as a chemical antidote in the treatment of *poisoning by alkaloids* in the dilution of 1 scant teaspoonful to a quart of water. It should be administered by stomach tube and removed by gastric lavage. *Dose: Topically,* to the skin 2 or 3 times a day.

Iodochlorohydroxyquin—see page 1252.

Iodoform NF

[Triiodomethane]

Iodoform, previously dried over phosphorus pentoxide for 4 hours, contains 99.0–100.5% of CHI₃ (393.73).

Preparation—A popular method utilizes the action of iodide and hypochlorite on acetone:

$$CH_3COCH_3 + 3\bar{I} + 3\,Cl\bar{O} \rightarrow$$
$$CHI_3 + 3\bar{Cl} + CH_3CO\bar{O} + 2\bar{OH}$$

The precipitate of Iodoform is filtered from the reaction products, washed with water until free from soluble matter (chlorides), and dried at about 35° to 40°.

Description—A fine, greenish yellow powder or lustrous crystals. It has a peculiar, very penetrating and persistent odor. Iodoform is slightly volatile, even at ordinary temperatures and distils slowly with steam. It melts at about 115° and decomposes at higher temperatures, emitting vapors of iodine. Its specific gravity is about 4.1.

Solubility—Practically insoluble in water to which, however, it imparts its odor and taste; 1 Gm dissolves in about 70 ml of alcohol, 80 ml of glycerin, 10 ml of chloroform, about 6.5 ml of ether, about 34 ml of olive oil, and about 16 ml of boiling alcohol.

Incompatibilities—Iodoform is decomposed by *exposure to air* in direct sunlight. *Peruvian balsam, tannin,* and other *organic substances* slowly decompose it.

Uses—Iodoform has a weak *bactericidal* action as a result of a slow release of elemental iodine. It is so insoluble that it is difficult to achieve effective concentrations. Medicine has had no confidence in the efficacy of Iodoform for several decades. It was formerly widely employed for the dressing of wounds but is now obsolete. It is surprising that it has retained official status.

Dose—There is no official statement on dose or application.

Isopropyl Alcohol NF

[Isopropanol; 2-Propanol]

OH
|
CH₃CHCH₃

Isopropyl Alcohol contains 99.0–100.5%, by weight, of C₃H₈O (60.10).

Preparation—Most of the Isopropyl Alcohol prepared commercially is obtained by treating propylene with sulfuric acid followed by hydrolysis. The olefin is obtained in the cracking of petroleum.

Some of the alcohol is also obtained by the reduction of acetone through high-pressure hydrogenation.

Description—A transparent, colorless, mobile, volatile liquid with a characteristic odor and slightly bitter taste. Specific gravity: 0.783 to 0.787. Distilling range: 81° to 83°. Refractive index: 1.376 to 1.378 at 20°.

Solubility—Miscible with water, alcohol, ether, and chloroform.

Identification—A white or yellowish precipitate, or turbidity, is produced when a mixture of 2 ml of the alcohol, 3 ml of water, and 1 ml of mercuric sulfate TS is warmed gently.

Uses—Isopropyl alcohol is used for the disinfection of hypodermic syringes and needles and, as the rubbing alcohol, it is used as a skin antiseptic. Isopropyl alcohol compares favorably with ethyl alcohol in regard to its *antiseptic* properties. All concentrations greater than 70% are effective skin disinfectants. It does not appear to affect the potency of subcutaneous insulin and hence may be used to prepare the skin for injection. It does promote bleeding at an injection site, which may make reading of allergic tests difficult. Isopropyl Alcohol can not be relied on to destroy the spores of organisms as *Clostridium tetani, Clostridium welchii,* or *Bacillus anthracis.* It is not potable and should not be given by mouth. It is also used in hair and scalp preparations, hand and face lotions, aftershave lotions, liniments, and in the *Isopropyl* Rubbing Alcohol described below. It is also used as a solvent in the extraction of drugs which is the category recognized by the NF. The Isopropyl Rubbing Alcohol is recognized as a rubefacient, although it is more widely used as an antiseptic.

Dose—There is no official statement on dose or application. As an antiseptic it is applied to the skin in concentrations greater than 70% *v/v.* It should be left on the skin for at least 2 minutes.

Isopropyl Rubbing Alcohol NF [Isopropanol Rubbing Compound] contains 68.0–72.0% of isopropyl alcohol, by volume, the remainder consisting of water, with or without color additives certified by the federal Food and Drug Administration for use in drugs, suitable stabilizers, and perfume oils. *Description:* A transparent, mobile, volatile liquid with a slightly bitter taste and, in the absence of odorous constituents, a characteristic odor. Its specific gravity is between 0.869 and 0.879. *It is not potable.*

Yellow Mercuric Oxide NF

[Mercuric Oxide; Yellow Precipitate]

Yellow Mercuric Oxide, dried at 105° for 2 hours, contains 99.5–100.5% of HgO (216.59).

Preparation—To a concentrated aqueous solution of mercury bichloride a moderate excess of a 5% solution of sodium hydroxide is gradually added with continuous stirring. The precipitated Oxide is washed a few times by decantation with purified water, then collected on a filter and washed with purified water until the washings no longer color red litmus paper bluish and cease to give a reaction for chloride with silver nitrate. It is then dried in the dark at about 50°.

The color of the Oxide depends on the concentration of the reactants, the temperature, and the rate of addition of the sodium hydroxide. Lower temperatures during precipitation and higher concentrations produce a lighter colored oxide. In practice higher concentrations of the bichloride are employed, this being attained by the use of sodium chloride which increases the solubility of the mercury bichloride due to the formation of the freely soluble sodium tetrachloromercurate [Na_2HgCl_4].

Description—A yellow to orange-yellow, heavy, impalpable powder. It is odorless and is stable in air, but becomes discolored and decomposes on exposure to light. It is not alkaline when moistened with hot water.

Solubility—Practically insoluble in water; insoluble in alcohol; readily dissolved by diluted hydrochloric or nitric acids forming colorless solutions.

Incompatibilities—By triturating mercuric oxide with *reducing agents* mercurous compounds and metallic mercury may be formed. In the preparation of ointments, contact with *metal* must be avoided. Salts are formed with many *acids.*

Uses—Yellow Mercuric Oxide is used in making mercury oleate and the official ointment, which are employed externally for their *antibacterial* action. The official ointment is used largely for *inflammation of the eyes, pruritus ani,* and *epidermophytosis.* However, it has been replaced largely by newer and safer agents.

Dose—To the conjunctiva as a **1%** ointment.

Yellow Mercuric Oxide Ophthalmic Ointment NF [Unguentum Hydrargyri Oxidi Flavi; Oculentum Hydrargyri Oxidi; Mercuric Oxide Eye Ointment] contains 0.9–1.1% of HgO. *Preparation:* Levigate yellow mercuric oxide (in very fine powder, 10 Gm) with mineral oil (10 Gm) until the mixture is smooth, and then incorporate the white ointment (980 Gm) to make 1000 Gm. *Caution—During its manufacture and storage, Yellow Mercuric Oxide Ophthalmic Ointment must not come in contact with metallic utensils or containers except those made of stainless steel, tin, or tin-coated material [because mercuric oxide is reduced by contact with such metals as copper, iron, zinc, etc].*

Ammoniated Mercury USP

[White Precipitate; Mercury Amide Chloride; Amminomercuric Chloride; Mercurammonium Chloride]

Ammoniated Mercury contains 98.0–100.5% of $HgNH_2Cl$ (252.07).

History—White precipitate was first described by Beguin, a chemist and writer, in 1632. A soluble double chloride of mercury and ammonium was known to the alchemists by the names *sal alembroth* and *sal sapientiæ.*

Preparation—The compound precipitates on pouring an aqueous solution of mercury bichloride, with constant stirring, into a large excess of an aqueous solution of ammonia.

Description—White pulverulent pieces, or a white amorphous powder, sometimes with a pearly sheen. It is odorless, and is stable in air, but darkens on exposure to light.

Solubility—Ammoniated Mercury is insoluble in water and in alcohol, but is readily soluble in warm hydrochloric, nitric, and acetic acids. It also dissolves in a cold saturated solution of sodium thiosulfate with the evolution of ammonia, and when the solution is heated for a short time red mercuric sulfide is precipitated.

Uses—Ammoniated Mercury is used chiefly in the form of the official ointment. It is of value in the treatment of cutaneous infections, *impetigo, ringworm, psoriasis, pruritus ani, pinworm,* and *crab louse infestation.* The compound sensitizes the skin, and patients need to be watched for drug-induced lesions.

Dose—*Topically,* as a **5%** ointment 2 or 3 times a day.

Ammoniated Mercury Ointment USP [White Precipitate Ointment] contains 4.5–5.5% of $HgNH_2Cl$. *Note:* Ammoniated Mercury Ointment BP is 2.5%. *Preparation:* Levigate ammoniated mercury (in very fine powder, 50 Gm) with mineral oil (30 Gm) to a smooth paste, and then incorporate with white ointment (920 Gm) to make 1000 Gm.

Methenamine NF

[Hexamethylenamine; Hexamethylenetetramine; Aminoform; Cystamin; Cystogen; Hexamine; Uritone (*Parke-Davis*); Urotropin (*Warner-Chilcott*)]

Methenamine, dried over phosphorus pentoxide for 4 hours, contains 99.0–100.5% of $C_6H_{12}N_4$ (140.19).

Although a cyclic tetramine, the therapeutic action of this compound depends exclusively on its ability to liberate formaldehyde under suitable environmental conditions.

Preparation—It is made by adding a moderate excess of ammonia water to formaldehyde solution, and evaporating to dryness.

Description—Colorless, lustrous crystals or a white crystalline powder. It is practically odorless. Its aqueous solution is alkaline to litmus. It sublimes at about 260°. When ignited it burns with a smokeless flame.

Solubility—1 Gm dissolves in 1.5 ml of water, 12.5 ml of alcohol, and about 10 ml of chloroform; very slightly soluble in ether.

Incompatibilities—Methenamine is alkaline in reaction and forms salts with weak acids. *Strong acids* and concentrated solutions of organic acids decompose it with the liberation of formaldehyde. With prolonged contact, weak acids also decompose it, as do acidic vehicles. A precipitate is formed with *tannic acid*, most *alkaloids*, and some *metallic salts*. *Ferric, mercuric,* and *silver salts* may be reduced and precipitated.

It liquefies, in some cases with decomposition, when rubbed with *acetylsalicylic acid, antipyrine, benzoic acid, lithium carbonate, menthol, phenol, phenyl salicylate, potassium acetate, sodium benzoate, sodium salicylate* etc. *Ammonium salts* and *alkalies* darken it. In capsules, it may slowly combine with the gelatin, thus rendering it insoluble.

Uses—Methenamine is an effective *urinary tract anti-infective,* provided it is acting in an acid medium. It is rapidly excreted and thus reaches effective antiseptic concentrations in the urine. The drug depends for its action upon the liberation of formaldehyde. This occurs to the extent of 20% of theoretical at pH 5.0 and not at all at pH 7.6. Consequently, precaution must be taken to maintain an acid urine during medication with Methenamine. This is usually accomplished by the administration of sodium biphosphate or mandelic acid.

Methenamine is of particular value in the treatment of *E. coli* infections of the urinary tract. It also is especially useful in patients with renal insufficiency. Because of its low toxicity, failure to excrete the drug causes no harmful consequences.

Approximately 10 to 30% is converted to formalde-

Sodium Biphosphate Tablets are administered, the usual dose is 500 mg.

Dosage Forms—Tablets NF: 300 and 500 mg; and Sodium Biphosphate Tablets NF: 300 mg and 500 mg of each constituent.

Veterinary Uses—Methenamine in conjunction with acid sodium phosphate has been employed as a *urinary antiseptic* in canine practice. It has also been recommended for use in herbivorous animals but evidence is inconclusive.

Veterinary Dose—*Horses,* 4 to 8 Gm; *Dogs,* 200 to 500 mg.

Methenamine Mandelate USP

[Mandelic Acid Hexamethylenetetramine Compound (1:1); Hexamethylene-tetramine Mandelate; Mandelamine (*Warner-Chilcott*)]

Methenamine Mandelate contains not less than 96.0% of $C_6H_{12}N_4 . C_8H_8O_3$ (292.34) and not less than 50.0% of mandelic acid [$C_8H_8O_3 = 152.15$], calculated on the dried basis.

For the structure of the base, see *Methenamine,* above.

Preparation—It may be prepared by reacting equimolar quantities of methenamine and mandelic acid in water or alcohol and concentrating until crystallization occurs.

Description—A white, crystalline powder, practically odorless and having a sour taste. Melting range between 127° and 130°. Its solutions are acid to litmus (pH about 4).

Solubility—Very soluble in water; 1 Gm dissolves in about 10 ml of alcohol, 20 ml of chloroform, and 350 ml of ether.

Uses—Methenamine Mandelate is a *urinary tract anti-infective.* See *Methenamine* (above). Mandelic acid also possesses antiseptic activity at pH's below 5.5, which facilitates the action of the formaldehyde released from methenamine. Furthermore, mandelic acid itself tends to decrease urine pH and aid the action of both components. Because mandelic acid is excreted into the urine, Methenamine Mandelate is contraindicated in renal insufficiency, whereas methenamine alone is not.

Dose—3 to 4 Gm daily; *usual,* **1 Gm** 4 times a day.

Dosage Forms—Oral Suspension USP: 250 and 500 mg/5 ml; Tablets USP: 250 and 500 mg, and 1 Gm.

Methylbenzethonium Chloride NF

[Benzyldimethyl[2-[2-[[4-(1,1,3,3-tetramethylbutyl)tolyl]oxy]ethoxy]ethyl]-ammonium Chloride; Ammorid (*Kinney*); Diaparene Chloride (*Breon*)]

hyde by the acid stomach contents unless enteric capsules are employed. With a 24-hour urine volume of 1200 ml, the dosage of 2 Gm of Methenamine will result in a urinary concentration of approximately 1:5000 of formaldehyde.

Dose—**500 mg** to **1.5 Gm;** *usual,* **1 Gm** 4 times a day.

Other Dose Information—When Methenamine and

Methylbenzethonium Chloride [$C_{28}H_{44}ClNO_2 . H_2O = 480.14$] contains 97.0–103.0% of $C_{28}H_{44}ClNO_2$ (462.12), calculated on the dried basis.

Preparation—It is prepared by the method described on page 1175 for *Benzethonium Chloride* except that cresol is employed instead of phenol. Inasmuch as the starting cresol contains both the *o-* and *m-*isomers, the corresponding isomers of the quaternary are both present in the final product.

Description—Odorless, colorless crystals, having a very bitter taste. Its solutions are neutral or slightly alkaline to litmus. It melts between 161° and 163°.

Solubility—Soluble in water, alcohol, and chloroform; slightly soluble in ether.

Uses—Methylbenzethonium Chloride is a cationic antiseptic with properties similar to the other cationic detergents. It is ineffective against sporulating organisms. To date its only firmly established use is the treatment of *ammonia dermatitis*, by application both to the skin and to diapers, undergarments, and bed linens. It is inactivated by soap and inhibited by organic matter.

Dose—*Topically* as a **0.055%** ointment or powder.

Other Dose Information—It is also used in creams and lotions in a concentration of 0.1%; topical solution. 1:10,000 to 1:100; fabrics, 1:25,000 for 3 minutes, and without rinse.

Dosage Forms—Powder NF: 0.055%.

Methylene Blue—see page 846.

Methylparaben USP

[Methyl *p*-Hydroxybenzoate; Solbrol; Methyl Parasept; Nipagin M]

COOCH$_3$

OH

Methylparaben contains 99.0–100.5% of C$_8$H$_8$O$_3$ (152.15), calculated on the dried basis.

Preparation—Methylparaben is made by esterifying *para*-hydroxybenzoic acid with methanol as described under *Methyl Salicylate* (page 1329). The *para*-hydroxybenzoic acid is obtained by passing carbon dioxide under pressure into dry potassium phenolate heated to about 200°. The resulting potassium salt is decomposed with hydrochloric acid yielding the free *para* acid.

Description—Colorless crystals or a white crystalline powder. It is odorless or has a faint, characteristic odor, and has a slight burning taste. It melts between 125° and 128°.

Solubility—1 Gm is soluble in 400 ml of water, 3 ml of alcohol, 10 ml of ether, and 50 ml of water at 80°; slightly soluble in benzene and carbon tetrachloride; soluble in acetone, glycerin, oils, and fats.

Uses—Methylparaben is used as a *preservative* for galenicals in concentrations ranging from 0.05 to 0.25%. It is also used in cosmetic preparations containing vegetable and animal fats and oils that are susceptible to decomposition. When desired to give a strong *antiseptic* effect, 3 to 5 times the above concentration may be used. Methylparaben and other esters of *para*-hydroxybenzoic acid are odorless, oil-soluble, and harmless to the skin in the proportions usually employed. The esters are usually dissolved in boiling water and then added to the preparation, but when no water is present in the formula they may be dissolved in alcohol, acetone, triethanolamine, glycerin, perfume oils, or melted fats. A combination of two or more esters of *para*-hydroxybenzoic acid has a "synergistic" antiseptic value, ie, the antiseptic effect of the combination is greater than the total effect as calculated from the values of the individual components; thus a preparation containing 0.15% of the propyl ester (propylparaben) and 0.05% of the benzyl ester has a

stronger antiseptic value than 0.2% of either ester alone. The benzyl ester has a high antiseptic value and is suitable for the preparation of antiseptic creams. The ethyl ester and the butyl ester are also used for the same purposes.

All of the parabens are capable of sensitizing the skin and inducing cutaneous allergic responses, although the incidence of such reactions is low. Allergy from oral ingestion or parenteral administration has not been reported. Because parabens are widely used as preservatives in many antibiotic or corticosteroid products, it is possible that sensitivity attributed to the antibiotic or corticosteroid is actually that of a paraben.

Topical antibiotic or corticosteroid preparations usually contain 0.3% parabens; however, ointments of the tetracyclines contain 3% and some surgical powders of tetracyclines contain as much as 20% parabens. A combination of 0.18% Methylparaben and 0.02% Propylparaben has been approved for use as a preservative for certain parenteral solutions, eg, aqueous procaine penicillin suspensions.

Neomycin—see page 1219.

Nitrofurazone NF

[5-Nitro-2-furaldehyde Semicarbazone; Furacin (*Eaton*)]

O$_2$N—furan—CH=N—NH—C(=O)—NH$_2$

Nitrofurazone, dried at 105° for 1 hour, contains 98.0–102.0% of C$_6$H$_6$N$_4$O$_4$ (198.14).

Preparation—It may be prepared by condensing 5-nitro-2-furaldehyde with semicarbazide hydrochloride in the presence of sodium acetate.

Description—An odorless, lemon-yellow, crystalline powder. Nearly tasteless, but develops a bitter aftertaste. Darkens slowly on exposure to light. Turns brownish black on heating to high temperatures and decomposes between 236° and 240°. The pH of a saturated solution is between 5.0 and 7.5.

Solubility—1 Gm dissolves in 4200 ml of water, 590 ml of alcohol, 350 ml of propylene glycol, and polyethylene glycol mixtures up to about 1%; practically insoluble in chloroform and ether.

Uses—Nitrofurazone is a local antibacterial agent with a broad spectrum of activity. Most bacteria of surface infections of the skin or mucosal surfaces are sensitive to the drug. It is applied topically in a powder, or in solutions or ointments in the treatment of mixed infections of superficial wounds and diseases of the eye, ear, nose, skin, and vagina. For best effect it should be applied for at least 24 hours. It is also available as inserts and suppositories for treatment of bacterial infections of the genitourinary tract. Nitrofurazone retains its antibacterial activity in blood, serum, and pus; phagocytosis is not inhibited and it does not interfere with healing. Approximately 0.5 to 2% of patients become sensitized to the drug, sometimes within 5 days of initiation of treatment.

Caution (for all Nitrofurazone dosage forms)—Avoid exposure at all times to direct sunlight, excessive heat, and alkaline materials.

Dose—*Topically* in various dosage forms in strengths ranging from **0.02** to **1%**.

Other Dose Information—Solutions generally contain 0.2% Nitrofurazone, except for ophthalmic or nasal solutions, which are 0.02%. Topical and vaginal creams are 0.2%. Vaginal inserts and suppositories contain 0.3% (6 mg). Urethral inserts contain 0.2% (2.6 mg). Soluble dressings contain 0.2%.

Dosage Forms—Cream NF: 0.2%; Ointment NF: 0.2%; Solution NF: 0.2% (w/w).

(Note: These dosage forms are *not* intended for ophthalmic use.)

Veterinary Uses—For the prevention or treatment of surface bacterial infections; treatment of mastitis, of bacterial ear infections in dogs, of genital tract infections, of gray diarrhea in mink, of necrotic enteritis in swine, of infections and impaired fertility of the female reproductive tract, and for the control of outbreaks of cecal and intestinal coccidiosis in chickens.

Nitromersol NF

[5 - Methyl - 2 - nitro - 7 - oxa - 8 - mercurabicyclo [4.2.0]octa - 1,3,5 - triene; [4-Nitro-3-hydroxymercuri-o-cresol] Anhydride; Metaphen (*Abbott*)

$$\begin{array}{c} NO_2 \\ | \\ Hg-C=C-CH \\ | \qquad \qquad \parallel \\ O-C=C-CH \\ | \\ CH_3 \end{array}$$

Nitromersol, dried at 105° for 2 hours, contains 98.0–100.5% of $C_7H_5HgNO_3$ (351.71).

Preparation—Nitromersol may be prepared by mercuration of *p*-nitro-*o*-cresol as follows: The nitrocresol is dissolved in just sufficient sodium hydroxide to form a solution and the required quantity of mercuric acetate, dissolved in water, is added. The mixture is heated until the supernatant liquid is substantially free of mercuric ions. The precipitate of Nitromersol is filtered, washed, and purified by dissolving in sodium hydroxide, filtering, and reprecipitating from the filtrate with diluted acid.

Description—A yellow to brownish yellow powder or granules. It is odorless, tasteless, and stable in the air.

Solubility—Insoluble in water; almost insoluble in alcohol, acetone, and in ether; soluble in solutions of alkalies and ammonia.

Uses—Nitromersol is a *local antibacterial* agent used only in the form of the sodium salt. It ranks among the best of the organic mercurials; however, against staphylococci it is much inferior to iodine. Nitromersol Tincture is more germicidal than the Solution; however, it is questionable to what extent the mercurial contributes to the efficacy of the Tincture, since the vehicle alone has an equal efficacy against the skin flora. It is relatively nonirritating when applied to mucous membranes or the skin and is without deleterious action on metallic instruments or rubber. It is relatively nontoxic.

Nitromersol is used in the treatment of gonorrhea and other *infections of the eye;* for the *disinfection of skin, surgical instruments* and *rubber* if no sporulating pathogenic organisms are present.

Dose—*Topically,* as a **0.2%** solution or **0.5%** tincture.

Nitromersol Solution NF yields, from each 100 ml 180.0–220.0 mg of $C_7H_5HgNO_3$. *Preparation:* Dissolve sodium hydroxide (0.4 Gm) and monohydrated sodium carbonate (4.25 Gm) in purified water (50 ml), add nitromersol (2 Gm) and stir until dissolved. Gradually add a sufficient quantity of purified water to make 1000 ml. *Caution: Dilutions of Nitromersol Solution should be prepared as needed as they tend to precipitate upon standing.* Description: A clear, reddish orange solution, affected by light. Its specific gravity is between 1.005 and 1.010.

Nitromersol Tincture NF yields, from each 100 ml, 450.0–550.0 mg of $C_7H_5HgNO_3$. *Preparation:* Dissolve nitromersol (5 Gm) in a mixture of acetone (100 ml), alcohol (525 ml), and sodium hydroxide (1 Gm) dissolved in purified water (50 ml) and finally add a sufficient quantity of purified water to make the product measure 1000 ml. *Note:* Nitromersol Tincture may be colored by the addition of any suitable color additive or combination of colors certified by the federal Food and Drug Administration for use in drugs. *Description:* A clear liquid having the odor of acetone and alcohol. It is affected by light. Its specific gravity is between 0.905 and 0.915.

Novobiocin—see page 1221.

Parachlorophenol NF

[*p*-Chlorophenol; 4-Chlorophenol]

$$Cl-\langle\rangle-OH$$

Parachlorophenol contains 99.0–100.5% of C_6H_5ClO (128.56).

Preparation—This germicide is most economically prepared by the chlorination of melted phenol with sulfuryl chloride; little or none of the *ortho* compound is formed.

Parachlorophenol may also be obtained by the direct chlorination of phenol, without a solvent at a temperature above 40°. A mixture of *ortho-* and *para-*phenols is produced in which the latter predominates. Any unreacted phenol is separated from chlorophenol by extraction with an aqueous solution of sodium carbonate. The unreacted phenol is not soluble in the alkali carbonate while the chlorinated products, being more acidic, are dissolved by it. The mixture of the two chlorophenols, obtained after acidifying their solution in the sodium carbonate, is readily separated by fractional distillation since the *ortho-* and *para-*isomers differ in boiling point by 41°.

Description—White or pink crystals, having a characteristic phenolic odor. When undiluted, it whitens and cauterizes the skin and mucous membranes. Melting point about 42°. Congealing temperature 42° to 44°.

Solubility—Very soluble in alcohol, glycerin, chloroform, ether, and fixed and volatile oils; soluble in petrolatum; sparingly soluble in water and liquid petrolatum.

Uses—Parachlorophenol is a *local antibacterial* agent similar in properties and uses to Phenol. The introduction of halogen atoms in phenolic molecules tends to increase the germicidal properties. However, the toxicity and caustic action are also both increased. It is used principally in dental practice for root canal therapy. It is often used in a mixture with metacresyl acetate.

Unofficial Dose Information—It is generally used in concentrations of 25 to 35%.

Camphorated Parachlorophenol NF contains 33.0–37.0% of [parachlorophenol] C_6H_5ClO and 63.0–67.0% of [camphor] $C_{10}H_{16}O$. The sum of the percentages of parachlorophenol and camphor is 97.0–103.0%. *Preparation:* Triturate parachlorophenol (350 Gm) and camphor (650 Gm) together until they liquefy and are thoroughly mixed to make 1000 Gm. *Uses:* Camphorated Parachlorophenol is a *local antibacterial* agent for root canals in dentistry.

Peppermint Oil—see page 1331.

Phenazopyridine Hydrochloride NF

[2,6-Diamine-3-(phenylazo)pyridine Monohydrochloride; Pyridium (*Warner-Chilcott*)]

Phenazopyridine Hydrochloride contains 99.0–101.0% of $C_{11}H_{11}N_5 \cdot HCl$ (249.70), calculated on the dried basis.

Preparation—Aniline is diazotized with sodium nitrite and excess hydrochloric acid, and the resulting benzenediazonium chloride is coupled with 2,6-diaminopyridine.

Description—A light or dark red to dark violet, crystalline powder. It is odorless or has a slight odor. It melts at about 240° with decomposition.

Solubility—Slightly soluble in water, alcohol, and chloroform.

Uses—Phenazopyridine Hydrochloride is an antiseptic drug which is used in the management of *genitourinary tract infections*. When taken systemically it is quickly excreted into the urine, so that a high local concentration is reached. Thus the drug may be administered either orally or instilled locally. However, a considerable proportion of the drug is metabolically converted to an inactive form, so that large oral doses are required to exert a therapeutic effect. Although the drug may often bring about rapid relief of discomfort, such as pain, burning, urgency and frequency, in the urinary tract infections, bacteriological control of the infection is less frequent. The relief of discomfort is mostly attributable to a local anesthetic action. When instilled locally in cystitis, the anesthetic effect may allow other therapeutic measures to be executed with a minimum of pain. Phenazopyridine may occasionally cause gastrointestinal irritation. After oral administration the color of the urine may be orange red to dark red, if the urine is acidic. The drug is contraindicated in renal insufficiency. Phenazopyridine is often combined with sulfonamides.

Dose—*Usual*, **100 mg** 3 or 4 times a day.

Other Dose Information—Topically, as a 1% solution.

Dosage Forms—Tablets NF: 100 and 200 mg.

Phenol—see page 1370.

Phenylethyl Alcohol—see page 1331.

Phenylmercuric Acetate NF

[Acetoxyphenylmercury]

$$CH_3COOHg-\text{(phenyl ring)}$$

Phenylmercuric Acetate contains 98.0–100.5% of $C_8H_8HgO_2$ (336.74).

Preparation—Phenylmercuric Acetate is readily formed by heating benzene with mercuric acetate.

Description—A white to creamy white, crystalline powder or as small white prisms or leaflets. It is odorless. It melts between 149° and 153°.

Solubility—Slightly soluble in water; soluble in alcohol and acetone.

Uses—The actions and uses of Phenylmercuric Acetate are similar to those of *Phenylmercuric Nitrate* (below). However, it is also used in contraceptive gels and foams. It is used as a preservative in various drug preparations. It is also used as a herbicide, especially for crabgrass, and as a garden fungicide.

Dose—There is no official statement on dose. For application to the skin it is used as a 0.2% solution in 50% ethanol; as a preservative it is used in concentrations of 0.002% to 0.125%; in vaginal suppositories and jellies, 0.02%; in vaginal tablets, 3 mg.

Phenylmercuric Nitrate NF

[Merphenyl Nitrate (*Hamilton*)]

Phenylmercuric Nitrate is a mixture of phenylmercuric nitrate [$C_6H_5HgNO_3$ = 339.70] and phenylmercuric hydroxide [C_6H_5HgOH = 294.70] containing 87.0–87.9% of phenylmercuric ions ($C_6H_5Hg^-$), and 62.75–63.50% of Hg (mercury).

This chemical is a basic salt of fairly definite composition, namely, $C_6H_5HgOH \cdot C_6H_5HgNO_3$ containing theoretically 63.3% of Hg. The normal nitrate, $C_6H_5HgNO_3$, has also been prepared, but is unstable, decomposing rapidly into the basic compound on contact with water.

Preparation—Phenylmercuric acetate (see above) is refluxed in benzene with ammonium nitrate and the normal phenylmercuric nitrate thus formed is subjected to hydrolysis to form the official basic salt.

Description—A white, crystalline powder, affected by light. Its saturated aqueous solution is acid to litmus. It melts between 175° and 185°.

Solubility—Very slightly soluble in water; slightly soluble in alcohol and glycerin; more soluble in the presence of either nitric acid or alkali hydroxides.

Uses—Phenylmercuric Nitrate is a *local antibacterial* agent recognized for external use in solution or ointment as an antiseptic for the prophylactic and therapeutic disinfection of the *skin, superficial abrasions, lacerations, wounds,* and *infections*. It is also used in vaginal preparations to reduce odor and to maintain bacterial, trichomonal, and fungal growth at a minimum. Like all the mercurials, it is inferior to iodine against the staphylococci of the skin.

Dose—There is no official statement on dose. For topical application to the skin or mucosae, as a 0.1 to 0.2% solution, generally in 50% ethanol; for disinfection of instruments, 0.001 to 0.1%; as a preservative in pharmaceuticals, 0.0025%.

Phenyl Salicylate—see page 1379.

Pine Tar—see page 776.

Polymyxin B Sulfate—see page 1231.

Potassium Permanganate USP

[Permanganate of Potash; Chameleon Mineral]

Potassium Permanganate contains 99.0–100.5% of $KMnO_4$ (158.04), calculated on the dried basis.

Caution—Observe great care in handling Potassium Permanganate, as dangerous explosions may occur if it is brought into contact with organic or other readily oxidizable substances, either in solution or in the dry state.

Preparation—The manufacturing process consists of two steps. The first step is the production of potassium manganate by heating manganese dioxide with potassium hydroxide and an oxidizing agent such as potassium chlorate or nitrate. In the second step the solution of the potassium manganate is further oxidized to potassium permanganate by passing chlorine or a current of air and carbon dioxide through the hot solution.

Description—Potassium Permanganate occurs in the form of dark purple crystals almost opaque by transmitted light and of a blue metallic luster by reflected light. It is more commonly available as small crystals of a dark bronze-like color. Potassium permanganate is stable in air and light, but is readily decomposed by many reducing substances, such as ferrous salts, iodides, oxalates, citrates, and most other organic substances including alcohol, especially in the presence of an acid. It is also decomposed by hydrochloric or concentrated sulfuric acid with the liberation of chlorine or oxygen, respectively. Solutions are unstable.

Solubility—1 Gm dissolves in 15 ml of water and 3.5 ml of boiling water.

Incompatibilities—Potassium Permanganate is a powerful oxidizing agent and under suitable conditions the vigor of its reaction is sufficient to produce an explosion. It must not be triturated with *organic matter* or such easily oxidizable substances as *charcoal, sulfur, reduced iron,* and *hypophosphites*. In solution it oxidizes *hypophosphites, sulfites, tartrates, mercurous salts, cuprous salts,* and *ferrous salts*. Chlorine, iodine, and bromine are produced from *chlorides, iodides,* and *bromides*, respectively. It liberates oxygen from *hydrogen peroxide*. *Alcohol* is oxidized to acetaldehyde or acetic acid depending on conditions, *phenol* to oxalic acid and carbon dioxide.

Uses—Potassium Permanganate is a valuable *anti-infective*, which is active by virtue of the fact that it is a strong oxidizing agent. Its most common clinical application is in the treatment of *urethritis*. Irrigation of the bladder with a solution of Potassium Permanganate is sometimes effective in the treatment of persistent urinary infections. It is sometimes employed for the vesicular lesions of *epidermophytosis*, in the vesicular stage of *eczema-dermatitis* and in the treatment of *ivy poisoning;* in these uses its astringent properties are employed.

Potassium Permanganate is capable of oxidizing certain drugs and venoms. In the treatment of *poisoning* following the oral ingestion of barbiturates, chloral hydrate, and many of the alkaloids, *gastric lavage* with a solution of Potassium Permanganate helps to destroy the poison and thus prevent absorption. Permanganate solutions should not be left in the stomach. The application of crystals of Potassium Permanganate to snake bites to promote oxidation of the venom not only probably does not destroy the venom sufficiently but is contrary to the present-day principles of snake bite therapy.

Dose—*Topically*, as a **0.004** to **1%** solution 2 or 3 times a day or in a wet dressing.

Other Dose Information—For urethritis, 0.025%; for bladder irrigation, 0.02%; for ivy poisoning or eczema, 0.01%; for epidermophytosis, 1%; for gastric lavage, 0.02%.

Dosage Forms—Tablets for Solution USP: 60, 125, and 300 mg.

Veterinary Use—Potassium Permanganate is frequently employed as an *antiseptic* and in the treatment of foul ulcers, abscesses, fetid stomatitis, nasal catarrh, etc, and as a chemical *antidote* for morphine, strychnine, and other alkaloids.

Veterinary Dose—*Horses*, **1** to **4 Gm;** *Cattle*, **2** to **3 Gm;** *Dogs*, **30** to **200 mg.**

Povidone-Iodine NF

[Poly [1-(2-oxo-1-pyrrolidinyl)ethylene] Iodine Complex; Betadine (*Purdue-Frederick*); Isodine (*Isodine Co.*)]

Povidone-Iodine is a complex of iodine with povidone. Dried at 105° to constant weight, it contains 9.0–12.0% of available I (iodine).

Preparation—*Povidone* (page 1346) having an average molecular weight of 40,000 is heated with elemental iodine in the presence of a little water whereby a small amount of the iodine enters into loose organic union with the polymer to form a complex which contains approximately 10% of available iodine.

Description—Occurs as a yellowish-brown, amorphous powder, having a slight, characteristic odor. Its aqueous solution is acid to litmus.

Solubility—Soluble in water and alcohol; practically insoluble in chloroform, carbon tetrachloride, ether, solvent hexane, and acetone.

Uses—Povidone-Iodine slowly releases its iodine after it has been applied to the surface. The slow release attenuates the antiseptic potency of the iodine, but the prolongation of action is claimed partially to compensate for the decreased concentration of free iodine. However, it cannot be considered equivalent to iodine solutions of equal per cent. Indeed, the concentration of free iodine in Povidone-Iodine solution is too low to be detected by starch, and it is difficult to see how a strong antiseptic action can be attributed to dissociated iodine. The low content of free iodine, the absence of KI, and the demulcent nature of polyvinylpyrrolidone contribute to the fact that this preparation rarely produces smarting or irritation. Povidone-Iodine may be used as a disinfectant of inanimate objects; however, its destructive effects on spores and fungi is poor.

Dose—*Topically*, in various dosage forms which contain available iodine in the range of **0.5** to **3%.**

Other Dose Information—Solutions of 0.05 to 0.15% in iodine may be applied to the oral or vaginal mucosae; for disinfection of inanimate objects, 1%.

Dosage Forms—Aerosol NF: 5.0% of povidone-iodine (equivalent to 0.5% of available iodine); Solution NF: 5, 7.5, 10, and 30% of povidone-iodine (equivalent to 0.5, 0.75, 1, and 3% of available iodine).

Propylparaben USP

[Propyl *p*-Hydroxybenzoate]

$$COOCH_2CH_2CH_3$$

OH

Propylparaben contains 99.0–100.5% of $C_{10}H_{12}O_3$ (180.21), calculated on the dried basis.

Preparation—Same as *Methylparaben* (page 1184) but propyl alcohol is used for esterification.

Description—Colorless crystals or a white powder. It is odorless or has a faint odor. It melts between 95° and 98°.

Solubility—1 Gm dissolves in about 2500 ml of water, in about 1.5 ml of alcohol, in about 3 ml of ether, and in about 400 ml of boiling water.

Uses—As an *antifungal* preservative. See *Methylparaben* (page 1184).

Resorcinol USP

[Resorcin; *m*-Dihydroxybenzene]

OH

OH

Resorcinol contains 99.0–100.5% of $C_6H_6O_2$ (110.11), calculated on the dried basis.

Preparation—Resorcinol is usually prepared by fusing sodium *m*-benzenedisulfonate with sodium hydroxide followed by acidification.

Description—White, or nearly white, needle-shaped crystals, or powder. It has a faint, characteristic odor and a sweetish, followed by a bitter, taste. It acquires a pink tint on exposure to light and air. It melts between 109° and 111°, and its aqueous solution (1 in 20) is neutral or acid to litmus, and does not emit the odor of phenol when warmed.

Solubility—1 Gm dissolves in about 1 ml of water and about 1 ml of alcohol; freely soluble in glycerin and ether; slightly soluble in chloroform.

Incompatibilities—Resorcinol forms a liquid or soft mass when triturated with *acetanilid, antipyrine, camphor, chloral hydrate, menthol, phenol,* and other substances. It becomes pink on exposure to air or on contact with *iron. Alkalies* hasten the color formation. Most *oxidizing agents* produce a red to violet color. A dilute solution of *ferric chloride* colors it violet.

Uses—Resorcinol is an *antifungal, antibacterial,* and *local irritant* agent. It is employed in the treatment of *ringworm, eczema, psoriasis, seborrheic dermatitis, acne rosacae,* etc. Resorcinol possesses mild keratolytic actions and may be used in preparations for the removal of corns, warts, callouses, etc, and in the treatment of athlete's foot. It may cause irritation or sensitization of the skin. It has no legitimate internal uses.

Dose—*Topically* as a **2 to 20%** lotion or ointment.

Compound Resorcinol Ointment NF—*Preparation:* Melt yellow wax (100 Gm) and anhydrous lanolin (280 Gm) in a dish on a steam bath. Triturate zinc oxide (60 Gm) and bismuth subnitrate (60 Gm) with petrolatum (290 Gm) until smooth, and add it to the melted mixture. Dissolve resorcinol (60 Gm) in glycerin (130 Gm); incorporate the solution with the warm mixture just prepared; then add juniper tar (20 Gm), and stir the Ointment until it congeals to make 1000 Gm. *Dose: Topically,* to the skin as required.

Resorcinol Monoacetate NF

[Resorcin Acetate; Euresol (*Knoll*)]

OH

⬡—OCOCH₃

Resorcinol Monoacetate is *m*-hydroxyphenyl acetate [$C_8H_8O_3 = 152.15$].

Preparation—It may be prepared by gently heating resorcinol with an equal weight of acetic anhydride and about 20% of glacial acetic acid, then washing with small quantities of cold water to remove the acetic acid and drying at a low temperature.

Description—A viscous, pale yellow or amber liquid with a faint characteristic odor and a burning taste. Its specific gravity is between 1.203 and 1.207. It boils at about 283° with decomposition. A saturated aqueous solution is acid to litmus.

Solubility—Dissolves in alcohol and most organic solvents; sparingly soluble in water.

Uses—Resorcinol Monoacetate slowly liberates resorcinol, thus yielding a milder but longer lasting effect. Its uses are the same as those of *Resorcinol* (see above).

Dose—In topical preparations for application to the scalp.

Other Dose Information—In creams and ointments, 1.5 to 3%.

Salicylic Acid—see page 781.

Selenium Sulfide NF

[Selenium Disulfide]

Selenium Sulfide [$SeS_2 = 143.09$] contains 52.0–55.5% of Se [selenium = 78.96].

Preparation—Among other ways, selenium sulfide may be prepared by adding an aqueous solution of selenious acid to an aqueous solution containing hydrogen sulfide in stoichiometric excess [$H_2SeO_3 + 2H_2S \rightarrow SeS_2 \downarrow + 3H_2O$]. The precipitate is collected, suitably washed, and dried.

Description—A bright-orange powder, having not more than a faint odor.

Solubility—Practically insoluble in water and organic solvents.

Uses—Selenium Sulfide is an *antibacterial* agent which is used in the local treatment of the nonexudative *seborrheas* of the scalp, eyelids, external ear, and glabrous skin. Selenium Sulfide has mild *antifungal* activity against certain skin pathogens; it is effective in the treatment of *pityriasis versicolor*. It is also useful in the management of *acne vulgaris* and *juvenilis* and *atopic eczema*. Some authorities attribute its efficacy to irritant rather than antibacterial properties. It induces inflammation of the mucous membranes and exposed tissues, so that care should be exercised in the application of the compound. It also causes "rebound" oiliness of the scalp. Furthermore, it is highly toxic by the oral route, and the user must carefully avoid ingestion. The hands and even the fingernails should be carefully cleaned after use. It should not be allowed to get into the eyes. Occasionally it causes loss of hair.

Dose—*Topically* to scalp, **5 or 10 ml** of a **2.5%** suspension for 5 minutes, then wash off thoroughly.

Dosage Forms—Detergent Suspension NF [Selsun (*Abbott*)]: 2.5%.

Veterinary Uses—As a 1% suspension, in treatment of nonspecific dermatoses of dogs and cats such as eczema, fungus infections, etc. (During treatment, protect eyes with ophthalmic ointment and scrotum with petrolatum coating.) **30 to 60 ml** of emulsion is worked through wet hair coat into skin, permitted to remain 5 minutes, then completely rinsed away; treatment may be repeated weekly if necessary. Because of toxic and irritant activity, complete rinsing of both patient and operator is essential.

Silver Nitrate—see page 779.

Silver Nitrate Ophthalmic Solution USP

Silver Nitrate Ophthalmic Solution is a solution of silver nitrate in a water medium. It contains 0.95–1.05% of $AgNO_3$. The solution may be buffered by the addition of sodium acetate.

Description—A clear, colorless solution. The pH is between 4.5 and 6.0.

Uses—Many state laws still require that 1 or 2% Silver Nitrate solution be applied to the conjunctiva of new-born infants for the *prophylaxis of ophthalmia neonatorum*.

Dose—*Topically,* **0.1 ml** of a **1%** solution, to the conjunctiva; to burned skin, **0.5%** solution (wet dressing).

Other Dose Information—The solution is immediately rinsed out with isotonic saline solution.

Mild Silver Protein NF

[Mild Protein Silver; Mild Protargin; Argyrol (*Crookes-Barnes*); Silvol (*Parke, Davis*); Solargentum (*Squibb*)]

Mild Silver Protein is silver rendered colloidal by the presence of, or combination with, protein. It contains 19.0–23.0% of Ag (silver).

Caution: Solutions of Mild Silver Protein should be freshly prepared or contain a suitable stabilizer [and should be dispensed in amber-colored bottles].

The long-continued use of any silver preparation may produce irremediable discoloration of the skin or mucous membrane (argyria).

Various types of colloidal silver preparations were formerly widely used as antiseptics, especially on the eyes and mucous membranes. Their popularity was due primarily to their nonionic character which rendered them relatively noncorrosive and nonirritating yet retaining much of the antiseptic action of silver ion. With the advent of the quaternary ammonium, sulfonamide, and antibiotic antimicrobials, however, the colloidal silvers gradually fell into disuse and are now nearly obsolete. Mild Silver Protein is representative of the most popular type which consisted of a silver protein salt in combination with an excess of the denatured protein. For a detailed discussion of colloidal silver preparations, see the eleventh edition of this text, page 482.

Description—Dark brown or almost black, shining scales or granules. It is odorless, is frequently hygroscopic, and is affected by light.

Solubility—Freely soluble in water, forming a dark-colored solution; practically insoluble in alcohol, chloroform, and in ether.

Incompatibilities—Silver protein solutions slowly form a deposit on prolonged storage. Dilute solutions of the halides give no precipitation; if a silver halide is formed it remains in colloidal form. *Mercuric chloride* causes an immediate precipitation; *ferric chloride* after a time. Other silver precipitants may react on standing if in sufficient concentration. *Alkaloids* are precipitated from solutions of their salts. Solutions are most readily prepared by sprinkling the substance on the surface of water and dissolving by rapid stirring. If triturated in a mortar a mass is formed which dissolves very slowly.

Uses—Although Mild Silver Protein contains more silver than strong silver protein, it is milder in that less of its silver is in the ionic form. The preparation was formerly widely used in the treatment of *conjunctivitis, cystitis, nose and throat infections,* and in the *prophylaxis of gonorrhea.* It is presently employed only sporadically.

Both local and generalized *argyria* can follow its indiscriminate application to the mucous membranes.

Dose—*Topically,* as a **5** to **25**% solution to the skin or mucous membrane several times a day as required.

Sodium Benzoate USP

C₆H₅COONa

Sodium Benzoate contains 99.0–100.5% of $C_7H_5NaO_2$ (144.11), calculated on the dried basis.

Preparation—Benzoic acid is added to a hot concentrated solution of sodium carbonate until effervescence ceases. The solution is evaporated, cooled, and allowed to crystallize, or evaporated to dryness and granulated.

Description—A white, odorless, or nearly odorless, granular or crystalline powder. It is stable in air. The aqueous solution is slightly alkaline to litmus (pH about 8). It is decomposed by dilute mineral acid liberating benzoic acid.

Solubility—1 Gm dissolves in 2 ml of water, 75 ml of alcohol, 50 ml of 90% alcohol, and 1.4 ml of boiling water.

Incompatibilities—*Inorganic acids* precipitate benzoic acid from aqueous solutions of benzoates. *Ferric salts* precipitate ferric benzoate, except in presence of complexing agents such as citrates and tartrates. *Silver, lead,* and *mercury salts* cause precipitation.

Uses—Sodium Benzoate is extensively used as a *food* and *pharmaceutical preservative,* as it is the only legally authorized preservative for many classes of food products. To be effective it must be used in acid media of pH not above 4. It is not bactericidal, but rather it is bacteriostatic.

Sodium Hydroxide—see page 1373.

Sodium Hypochlorite Solution NF

Sodium Hypochlorite Solution contains 4.0–6.0% of NaClO (sodium hypochlorite = 74.44).

Caution—This Solution is not suitable for application to wounds.

Preparation—The solution was formerly made by reacting chlorinated lime with sodium carbonate followed by filtration. It is now largely manufactured by passing the proper quantity of chlorine gas into a cold solution of sodium hydroxide or sodium carbonate.

Sodium Hypochlorite Solution may also be prepared by passing a direct current of electricity through a sodium chloride solution. By the passage of the current, chlorine is given off at the anode and sodium hydroxide is formed at the cathode and if the cell is so constructed that the two are permitted to react with each other at ordinary temperature, sodium hypochlorite and sodium chloride are produced.

Description—A clear, pale greenish yellow liquid, affected by light and having a slight odor of chlorine.

Identification—At first, the Solution colors red litmus blue and then bleaches it. When treated with acid, the odor of chlorine is pronounced. It responds to the flame test for sodium.

Uses—Sodium Hypochlorite Solution is used as a powerful *disinfectant* and *deodorant,* also as a *bleaching agent.* Not only is it very good as a disinfectant against vegetative bacteria, but it is also good against viruses and fair against spores and fungi. It is diluted in the preparation of diluted sodium hypochlorite solution (below) and also extensively used in dairies for disinfecting milk cans and other dairy apparatus. It is not to be given internally. For therapeutic uses, see *Diluted Sodium Hypochlorite Solution.*

Note—If "Labarraque's Solution" is ordered, Sodium Hypochlorite Solution, diluted with an equal volume of water, is to be dispensed.

Diluted Sodium Hypochlorite Solution NF

[Surgical Chlorinated Soda Solution; Modified Dakin's Solution]

Diluted Sodium Hypochlorite Solution is a solution of chlorine compounds of sodium containing, in each 100 ml, 450.0–500.0 mg of NaClO.

These amounts of sodium hypochlorite are equivalent approximately to 430–480 mg of available chlorine.

Preparation—Diluted Sodium Hypochlorite Solution may be prepared as follows:

Sodium Hypochlorite Solution.....	**1000 ml**
Sodium Bicarbonate,	
Purified Water, of each, a sufficient quantity.	

Dilute the Sodium Hypochlorite Solution with 5000 ml of purified water and add 40 ml of a 5% solution of sodium bicarbonate in cold purified water, and mix well. Remove about 20 ml of the mixture, add to it about 20 mg of powdered phenolphthalein, and shake it gently for 2 minutes. If a red color appears, add more of the sodium bicarbonate solution, and test with powdered phenolphthalein as just described, repeating the procedure as often as necessary until no red color is produced. Assay the liquid and dilute it with sufficient purified water to make the final solution contain, in each 100 ml, 480 mg of NaClO.

This solution was developed during World War I to provide an inexpensive but efficient germicide for the treatment of wounds. The alkalinity of Labarraque's solution rendered it unfit for such use, and in the first attempts to develop a neutral solution suitable for wound dressing, boric acid was employed. Sodium bicarbonate was later suggested by Daufresne and others as a more efficient alkalinity reducing agent.

It is of primary importance that the strength of this preparation be accurately adjusted and it should be re-tested if kept for more than a few days.

Description—Colorless or slightly yellow liquid. It has an odor suggesting chlorine, and rapidly deteriorates on exposure to air or to elevated temperatures. Its specific gravity is not more than 1.025.

Uses—Diluted Sodium Hypochlorite Solution is employed in full strength and should be freshly prepared. The solution is used in the treatment of *suppurating wounds*, often by continuous irrigation (Carrel technique). Not only does the solution exert a *germicidal* action but it also *dissolves necrotic tissue*. Disadvantages are that sodium hypochlorite solutions dissolve blood clots, delay clotting, and are irritating to the skin. For the prophylaxis of *epidermophytosis*, Diluted Sodium Hypochlorite Solution is sometimes employed as a foot bath. Hypochlorite solutions are also *deodorant*.

Dose—*Topically*, full strength or diluted with 1 to 3 volumes of water.

Sodium Tetradecyl Sulfate—see page 778.

Sulfur Dioxide—see page 1318.

Sulfur, Sublimed—see page 1272.

Thimerosal NF

[Sodium [(*o*-Carboxyphenyl)thio]ethylmercury; Sodium (Ethylmercurithio)-salicylate; Thiomersal; Merthiolate (*Lilly*)]

Thimerosal, dried to constant weight in a vacuum over phosphorus pentoxide, contains 97.0–101.0% of $C_9H_9HgNaO_2S$ (404.81).

Preparation—An ethanolic solution of thiosalicyclic acid is treated with ethylmercuric chloride (or hydroxide) in the presence of sodium hydroxide.

Description—A light cream-colored, crystalline powder with a slight characteristic odor. The pH of a 1 per cent solution is about 6.7. It is affected by light.

Solubility—1 Gm dissolves in about 1 ml of water and about 12 ml of alcohol; almost insoluble in benzene and ether.

Uses—Thimerosal is a relatively nontoxic *antibacterial* agent with both weak bacteriostatic and mild fungistatic properties. Spore-forming bacteria are particularly resistant. It is inferior to iodine. On the skin, Thimerosal Tincture is less effective than is the solvent alone. However, it is somewhat more effective than the Solution. It is used to *disinfect skin surfaces*. It is also applied to wounds and abrasions, and also the eye, nose, throat, and urethra.

Dose—*Topically*, as a **0.1%** solution or tincture.

Dosage Forms—Aerosol NF (see below); Solution NF (see below); Tincture NF (see below).

Thimerosal Aerosol NF is an alcoholic solution of thimerosal mixed with suitable propellants in a pressurized container. It contains 85.0–115.0% of the labeled amount of $C_9H_9HgNaO_2S$. The preparation may be colored with one of more color additives, certified by the federal Food and Drug Administration for use in drugs. *Preparation:* To alcohol (433 ml) add monoethanolamine (292 mcg) and ethylenedinitrile tetraacetic acid (edetic acid, 21.1 mcg). Dissolve thimerosal (1.0 Gm) in purified water (6.1 ml), and add to the alcohol mixture. Add acetone (100 ml) and alcohol (qs) to make 1000 ml. Mix thoroughly and filter. Add sufficient propellant during filling. *Caution: Manufacture and store Thimerosal Aerosol in glass or suitable resistant metal containers. Alcohol Content:* 18.7 to 25.3%. *Uses* and *Dose:* See *Thimerosal*.

Thimerosal Solution NF contains, in each 100 ml, 95–105 mg of $C_9H_9HgNaO_2S$. The preparation may be colored with one or more color additives certified by the federal Food and Drug Administration for use in drugs. *Caution: Manufacture and store Thimerosal Solution in glass or suitable resistant metal containers. Preparation:* To purified water (250 ml) add ethylenediamine (200 mg) and monoethanolamine (1 Gm). Dissolve sodium chloride (8 Gm), sodium borate (1.4 Gm), and thimerosal (1 Gm) in this solution, and add sufficient purified water to make 1000 ml. Mix thoroughly and filter. *Description:* A clear liquid having a slight characteristic odor. It is affected by light. Specific gravity between 1.004 and 1.010. The pH is between 9.8 and 10.3.

Thimerosal Tincture NF contains, in each 100 ml, 95–105 mg of $C_9H_9HgNaO_2S$. The preparation may be colored with one or more color additives, certified by the federal Food and Drug Administration for use in drugs. *Caution: Manufacture and store Thimerosal Tincture in glass or suitably resistant metal containers. Preparation:* To purified water (250 ml) add ethylenediamine (200 mg) and monoethanolamine (1 Gm), and dissolve thimerosal (1 Gm) in this mixture. Add alcohol (525 ml), acetone (100 ml), and sufficient purified water to make 1000 ml. Mix thoroughly and filter. *Description:* A transparent, mobile liquid with the characteristic odor of alcohol and acetone. It is affected by light. Specific gravity between 0.9070 and 0.9130. *Alcohol Content:* From 47 to 53% of C_2H_5OH.

Thymol USP

[2-Isopropyl-5-methylphenol; Thyme Camphor]

Thymol contains 99.0–101.0% of $C_{10}H_{14}O$ (150.22).

Preparation—Thymol is obtained from the volatile oil of *Thymus vulgaris* Linné (Fam. *Labiatæ*) and some other volatile oils by fractional distillation, which separates the terpenes. The portion distilling above 190° is collected, agitated with sodium hydroxide solution to separate more of the terpenes, and cooled. The compound of Thymol with sodium hydroxide is then reacted with hydrochloric acid, and the Thymol recrystallized from alcohol. Thymol has also been obtained from *Monarda didyma* Linné, *M. punctata* (horsemint), *Ammi copticum*, *Ocymum basilicum*, and *Ptychotis agowan*. A process for the synthesis of Thymol consists of reacting equivalent quantities of *m*-cresol and isopropyl chloride at $-10°$ in the presence of a solvent, using aluminum chloride as the catalyst. Thymol may also be prepared from *p-cymene*.

Description—Thymol occurs as colorless crystals, often large, or as a white, crystalline powder, having an aromatic, thyme-like odor and a pungent taste. It is affected by light. It melts between 48° and 51°, but when melted it remains liquid at a considerably lower temperature. Thymol is heavier than water, but when liquefied by fusion it is lighter than water. Its solution in alcohol is neutral to litmus paper. When Thymol is triturated with an equal weight of camphor, menthol, chloral hydrate, and some other substances, the mixture liquefies.

Solubility—1 Gm dissolves in about 1000 ml of water, 1 ml of alcohol, 1 ml of chloroform, 1.5 ml of ether, and about 2 ml of olive oil; soluble in glacial acetic acid and fixed or volatile oils.

Uses—Thymol is an *antifungal* and *antibacterial* agent. It is useful in the treatment of *epidermophytosis*, in which it may be used alone or as an additive to Whitfield's Ointment. It has been used both locally and orally for the treatment of *actinomycosis*, but there is generally little reason to consider it in lieu of penicillin. Thymol is incorporated into various mouthwashes for its antiseptic action, but such mouthwashes have been shown to be of little germicidal efficacy; for this reason NF Antiseptic Solution (NF XII) has been dropped from official status. Its phenol coefficient is about 50. It was formerly employed internally as an *intestinal antiseptic* and *anthelmintic*, especially against *hookworm*.

Dose—There is no official dose statement. Oral, anthelmintic, 1.5 to 2 Gm daily in 3 to 4 divided doses; topically, antiseptic and antifungal, as a 1% tincture or 2% powder.

Triclobisonium Chloride NF

[Hexamethylenebis[dimethyl[1 - methyl - 3 - (2,2,6 - trimethylcyclohexyl)-propyl]-ammonium] Dichloride; N,N'-*bis*[1-methyl-3-(2,2,6-trimethylcyclohexyl)propyl]-N,N'-dimethyl-1,6-hexanediamine bis(methochloride); Triburon Chloride (*Roche*)]

Triclobisonium Chloride contains 99.0–100.5% of $C_{36}H_{74}Cl_2N_2$ (605.91), calculated on the dried basis.

Preparation—β-Ionone in methanol solution is hydrogenated with Raney nickel in the presence of methylamine to give methyl[1-methyl-3-(2,6,6-trimethyl-1-cyclohexen-1-yl)propyl]amine which is then methylated through reaction with formaldehyde and formic acid to give the correspondingly substituted dimethylamine. This tertiary amine is then subjected to hydrogenation with platinum oxide and the resulting dimethyl[1-methyl-3-(2,2,6-trimethylcyclohexyl)-propyl]amine is quaternized with 1,6-dichlorohexane using a double equimolar portion of the amine. US Pat. 3,064,052.

Description—White, crystalline powder. It is odorless or has a slight irritating odor. It is stable in air, although it readily absorbs moisture. It melts at about 243°.

Solubility—1 Gm dissolves in 2 ml of water, 2 ml of alcohol, and about 4 ml of chloroform; insoluble in ether and benzene.

Uses—Triclobisonium Chloride is topical antiseptic with a spotty efficacy. It is quite effective against some strains of *Staphylococcus aureus* but not others. Strains of *Streptococcus pyrogenes*, *Diplococcus pneumoniæ*, *Listeria monocytogenes*, and *Salmonella typhi* are generally quite susceptible. *Trichomonas Vaginalis* and *Escherichia coli* are susceptible in high concentrations of the drug. In the presence of blood and exudates, it is less potent. It is used in the treatment of *impetigo contagiosa*, *acute folliculitis*, *furunculosis*, *infectious eczematoid dermatitis*, *infected burns*, *postoperative wounds*, *trichomonal vaginitis*, and *monilial vaginitis*. The status of Triclobisonium Chloride in some of the above conditions is not yet firmly established. The drug occasionally causes irritation and also sensitization.

Dose—*Topically*, as a **0.1%** ointment, 3 or 4 times a day; *vaginal*, **5 ml** of a **0.1%** cream every night for 2 weeks.

Dosage Forms—Cream NF: 0.1%; Ointment NF: 0.1%.

Tyrothricin—see page 1235.

Zinc Sulfate USP

[White Vitriol; Zinc Vitriol]

Zinc Sulfate contains 55.6–61.0% of $ZnSO_4$ (161.43), corresponding to 99.0–108.7% of the hydrated salt [$ZnSO_4 . 7H_2O = 287.54$].

Preparation—Zinc Sulfate is made by reacting metallic zinc or zinc oxide with diluted sulfuric acid. The resulting solution is freed from the contamination of iron by first passing chlorine into it to oxidize the iron to the ferric state, then adding a moderate excess of zinc oxide or carbonate and boiling. The iron is thereby precipitated as the insoluble ferric hydroxide which is removed by filtration. The small quantity of zinc chloride formed, being very soluble, remains in the mother liquor after the crystallization of the sulfate. Zinc Sulfate is also prepared by roasting zinc sulfide in a limited supply of oxygen and extracting the sulfate with water.

Description—Colorless, transparent prisms, or small needles, or a granular, crystalline powder. It is odorless and has an astringent metallic taste. It is efflorescent in dry air. Its solutions are acid to litmus.

Solubility—1 Gm dissolves in 0.6 ml of water and about 2.5 ml of glycerin; insoluble in alcohol.

Incompatibilities—See *Zinc Chloride* (page 771). Combinations of Zinc Sulfate and *sodium borate* with or without *boric acid* to be used as collyria are frequently troublesome due to a precipitation of zinc borate. A quantity of glycerin, equal in weight to the borate, suffices to maintain a clear solution. There is also a tendency for solutions of Zinc Sulfate to form a slight cloudiness due to the separation of a basic salt formed through partial hydrolysis.

Insoluble sulfates are formed with *lead, barium, strontium,* and *calcium* salts. *Silver* and *mercury* form slightly soluble salts. Zinc sulfate exercises a dehydrating action on *methylcellulose* suspensions which leads to precipitation of the latter. *Acacia, proteins,* and *tannins* may also be precipitated.

Uses—Zinc Sulfate is *antiseptic, astringent,* and *emetic.* Its antiseptic and astringent properties make it a valuable agent for use as an eyewash (aqueous solution) for the treatment of *conjunctivitis* caused by Morax-Axenfeld bacillus. Antibiotics have largely replaced it in general ophthalmic antiseptics. It may also be applied to the skin as a solution or as *White Lotion* (see page 771) for the treatment of *acne, ivy poisoning, lupus erythematosus,* and *impetigo.* A nasal spray of Zinc Sulfate has been used to shrink the mucous membranes and to promote drainage of infected accessory nasal sinuses; the salutary effect of such treatment is limited because the drug inhibits ciliary activity of the respiratory mucous membrane. It is the principal ingredient in many *deodorant anhydrotics.* Recent interest has centered on claims that large (but subemetic) doses of zinc accelerate the healing of wounds. Further studies are necessary to substantiate these claims.

Dose—*Topically,* **0.1 ml** of a **0.25%** aqueous solution to the conjunctiva 3 or 4 times a day.

Other Dose Information—Zinc Sulfate is a prompt emetic in doses of 0.6 to 2.0 Gm. Oral, for vulnerary effect, 220 mg.

Dosage Forms—Ophthalmic Solution USP: 0.25%.

Veterinary Uses—In addition to its use externally for its *astringent* properties, zinc sulfate is used as a local *emetic* in canine practice. Also used *topically* in ophthalmic solution as for human use.

Veterinary Dose—*Dogs,* emetic, **300 mg to 2 Gm** dissolved in 60 to 100 ml of tepid water.

Other Antiseptics

Aminacrine Hydrochloride [9-Aminoacridine hydrochloride monohydrate; Acramine Yellow] [$C_{13}H_{10}N_2 \cdot HCl \cdot H_2O$]—Pale yellow, odorless, crystalline powder having a bitter taste. 1 Gm is soluble in 300 ml water, 150 ml alcohol, and is soluble in glycerin. The pH of a 0.2% solution is 5.0–6.5. It is highly fluorescent. *Uses:* Aminacrine is a broad spectrum antimicrobial drug which is effective against Gram-negative and Gram-positive bacteria, trichomonads, and various fungi, especially *Monilia.* It retains activity in the presence of body fluids, pus, and secretions. Its principal use in the treatment of infections of the vagina and exocervix, such as moniliasis, trichomonal vaginitis, etc, or as a prophylactic agent in various gynecological procedures. However, it is also used in the treatment of mastitis. *Dose: Intravaginal,* as a 0.1% powder, 0.02% jelly, 140 mg in a suppository, or 3 mg in a tampon.

Benzylparaben [Benzyl *p*-Hydroxybenzoate; Benzyl Parasept] [$C_{14}H_{12}O_3$]—*Uses:* Benzylparaben is an antiseptic agent with actions and uses similar to those of *Methylparaben* (page 1184), with which it is often used in combination. It is also incorporated into antiseptic ointments and creams.

Bithionol NF XII [2,2'-Thiobis(4,6-dichlorophenol); Actamer (*Monsanto*)], dried at 105° for 4 hours, contains not less than 98.0% of $C_{12}H_6Cl_4O_2S$ (356.06). *Preparation:* A solution of 2,4-dichlorophenol in carbon disulfide or carbon tetrachloride is treated with sulfur chloride (S_2Cl_2) in the presence of aluminum chloride as a catalyst. For details, consult Ger. Pat. 583,055. *Description and Solubility:* A white or grayish white, crystalline powder; odorless or has a slight aromatic or phenolic odor; melting range, 186°–189°. Insoluble in water; freely soluble in acetone, alcohol, and ether; soluble in chloroform and dilute solutions of fixed alkali hydroxides. *Uses:* A local *anti-infective* which has

uses similar to those of *Hexachlorophene* (page 1179). *Dose:* Topically as 0.5 to 1% in a soap solution.

Chlorothymol NF XII [6-Chlorothymol; Monochlorothymol] is 4-chloro-2-isopropyl-5-methylphenol [$C_{10}H_{13}ClO$ = 184.67]. *Preparation:* By the action of sulfuhydryl chloride on thymol dissolved in carbon tetrachloride or petroleum benzin. *Description and Solubility:* White crystals, or a crystalline, granular powder, possessing a characteristic odor, and an aromatic, very pungent taste; it usually becomes discolored with age, acquiring a yellowish or brownish color, and is affected by light; melting range, 59°–61°. 1 Gm dissolves in about 0.5 ml of alcohol, 2 ml of benzene, 2 ml of chloroform, 1.5 ml of ether, and 10 ml of solvent hexane; practically insoluble in water. *Uses:* This substance has greater *antibacterial activity* than thymol and is added to Antiseptic Solution NF XII to increase its efficacy. Nevertheless, it is questionable whether or not that solution is effective. The antibacterial activity of Chlorothymol is considerably reduced in the presence of organic matter.

Chlorquinaldol [5,7-Dichloro-2-methyl-8-quinolinol]—[$C_{10}H_7Cl_2NO$]—A yellow, crystalline powder, insoluble in water. A mild antiseptic that may be used in the topical treatment of minor cutaneous infections. It is probably superior to other isoquinolines, especially against resistant staphylococci. In the management of dermatomycoses, the predominating keratoplastic effect of this compound may be more significant than its fungistatic action. *Uses:* A mild antiseptic in the topical treatment of minor cutaneous bacterial and mycotic infections. *Dose: Topically,* as a 3% cream or ointment applied twice daily.

Cloflucarban [Irgasan CF3 (*Geigy*)] is 4,4'-dichloro-3-(trifluoromethyl) carbanilide ($C_{14}H_9Cl_2F_3N_2O$). *Uses:* Cloflucarban is an antibacterial and antifungal agent incorporated into antiseptic and deodorant soaps and other cleansing preparations.

Creosote NF XII [Wood Creosote] is a mixture of phenols obtained from wood tar. *Preparation:* This is a product of the distillation of wood tar, consisting mainly of the following phenols—*guaiacol,* $C_7H_8O_2$, bp *ca* 205°; *cresol,* $C_8H_{10}O_2$, bp *ca* 220°; methylcresol, $C_9H_{12}O_2$, bp *ca* 216°; and *phlorol,* $C_8H_{10}O$, bp *ca* 208°. *Description and Solubility:* An almost colorless or yellowish, highly refractive, oily liquid, having a penetrating, smoky odor, and a burning, caustic taste; it does not readily become brownish on exposure to light; it is combustible, burning with a luminous, smoky flame; specific gravity, not less than 1.076; at least 90% by volume distils between 203° and 220°. Slightly soluble in water; miscible with alcohol, ether, and fixed or volatile oils; soluble in solutions of the fixed alkali hydroxides.

Uses: An expectorant, antiseptic, and *disinfectant.* It is used empirically as an expectorant to lessen the amount of mucus in the chronic stages of *bronchitis* and *bronchiectasis.* It is frequently prescribed for its stimulant expectorant action as a constituent of a steam inhalant. The antiseptic action of Creosote is weak and not clinically useful. The same applies to its antipyretic action. Occasionally, it has been employed as a *local anesthetic* in dentistry, in a manner similar to thymol. It is applied upon cotton to exposed nerve tissue in teeth. It is occasionally employed externally for its *disinfectant* action. Internally, undiluted, and in large doses, it is a powerful poison (see page 1989). Side effects from clinical doses are mainly referable to irritation of the gastrointestinal tract. In large doses, cardiovascular collapse is prominent. *Antidote:* The character and treatment of creosote poisoning are similar to those given for *Phenol* (Chapter 100). The administration of mucilaginous drinks, and the prompt evacuation of the stomach by the stomach pump, is the best treatment, no antidote to poisoning by Creosote being known. *Veterinary Dose: Horses and Cattle,* 4 to 8 ml; *Sheep* and *Swine,* 0.3 to 1 ml; *Dogs,* 0.03 to 0.2 ml.

Dibromsalan is dibromosalicylanilide ($C_{13}H_9Br_2NO_2$). *Description and Solubility:* A white to off-white, free-flowing powder; it has a slight odor (typical of brominated salicylanilides) and is tasteless; it melts between 225° and 227.3°. Insoluble in water; slightly soluble in alcohol.

Uses: Dibromsalan is an antibacterial and antiseptic substance that is incorporated into deodorant and antiseptic soaps and other cleansing preparations. It may cause occasional hypersensitivity, which is increased by strong light.

Furazolium Chloride is 6,7-dihydro-3-(5-nitro-2-furyl)-5H-imidazo[2,1-b]thiazolium chloride [$C_9H_8ClN_3O_3S$ = 273.70]. *Preparation:* Bromomethyl 5-nitrofurfuryl ketone is reacted with 1,3-ethylene-2-thiourea in dimethylformamide to form a thiazolium intermediate which, after treatment with aqueous sodium carbonate, is converted to the chloride. US Pat. 3,169,970. *Description and Solubility:* Yellow to yellowish-orange crystals that are odorless and have a bitter taste; it is light-sensitive, especially to UV light and especially in dilute solution; stable in heat (saturated aqueous solution) as follows: 1 hour at 100° and 24 hours at 37°; nonhygroscopic at 70% RH and 37°; melts at about 250° with decomposition. 1 Gm dissolves in about 24 ml of water, 370 ml of alcohol, and 100,000 ml of ether and chloroform. *Uses:* Furazolium Chloride is an antibacterial with a relatively broad spectrum of activity. At present, its use is limited to veterinary practice, for the treatment of wounds, lacerations, abrasions, pyogenic dermatitis, and following surgery, especially in horses and dogs. *Veterinary Dose:* Topically, as a 0.231% ointment, to be applied to the affected area several times a day.

Glutaraldehyde [Cidex (*Ethicon*)] is $C_5H_8O_2$.
Uses: Glutaraldehyde is a disinfectant that is very good not only against vegetative bacteria but also against spores. Its efficacy against fungi and viruses is good. It is the disinfectant of choice for the cold sterilization of surgical instruments. Glutaraldehyde aerosols are also used to "sterilize" hospital rooms, operating areas, etc. *Application:* as a 2% solution.

Hexetidine [Triocil] is 5-amino-1,3-bis(2-ethylhexyl)-hexahydro-5-methylpyrimidine [$C_{21}H_{45}N_3$ = 339.59]. *Description and Solubility:* A liquid that boils at 160°; it has good thermal stability. Soluble in petroleum ether, methanol, and benzene. *Uses:* Hexethidine is an antimicrobial drug that has activity *in vitro* against a variety of Gram-positive and Gram-negative bacteria, *Trichomonas vagialis,* and *Monilia albicans.* Although it has been promoted for the treatment of vaginitis caused by *Monilia* or *Trichomonas,* its efficacy against these infections is questionable. It is probably that many of the responding infections are not caused by yeasts of trichomonads but by bacteria, especially *Hemophilus,* against which the drug is highly effective. Thus its main use is in the treatment of *nonspecific bacterial vaginitis.* The drug is found at the site of application for as long as 72 hours. It is inactivated by soap, so that soap should not be used if the vagina is to be cleansed prior to application of the drug. It occasionally causes irritation of the vulva. *Dose:* Topically, 7 ml of a 0.1% vaginal gel inserted high into the vaginal vault on each of 6 successive nights.

Lime, Chlorinated BP [Calx Chlorinata; Bleaching Powder; Chloride of Lime]—Purity: not less than 30% w/w of available chlorine. A dull white powder, with an odor of chlorine, obtained by the action of chlorine upon calcium hydroxide. It is partly soluble in water and in alcohol. On exposure to air it becomes moist and decomposes. *Uses:* a disinfectant, deodorant, and bleach; to disinfect feces, urine, and sanitary utensils; for the purification of drinking water (1 oz to 2000 gal); for the disinfection of swimming pool water (0.25 to 1 ppm of free chlorine); for the removal of dyes from the skin. It is a common household bleach.

Merbromin NF XII [Mercuranin; Mercurochrome (*Hynson*); $C_{20}H_8Br_2HgNa_2O_6$ (750.67)] is the disodium salt of 2′,7′-dibromo-4′-(hydroxymercuri)fluorescein. When dried at 105° for 5 hours, Merbromin contains 24.0–26.7% of Hg, and 18.0–21.3% of Br. *Preparation:* Dibromofluorescein is dissolved in just sufficient dilute sodium hydroxide solution to form the sodium salt. Then the required quantity of mercuric acetate, dissolved in water, is added, and the solution is boiled until a sample of the filtered mixture gives no reaction for mercury ions. The precipitate of the acid mercury compound, after filtering and washing well with water, is dissolved in the required amount of sodium hydroxide solution and evaporated to dryness, preferably under reduced pressure.

Description and Solubility: Iridescent, green scales or granules; odorless and stable in air; a dilute aqueous solution (1 in 2000) has a yellow-green fluorescence; since the mercury is not in ionic combination, Merbromin does not give the usual reactions for mercury. Freely soluble in water; practically insoluble in alcohol and acetone; insoluble in chloroform and ether. *Incompatibilities:* With *acids, acid salts, heavy metals, hydrogen peroxide,* and most *alkaloids* and *local anesthetics;* the incompatibility is usually evidenced by a precipitation.

Uses: Merbromin once had a high reputation as an antiseptic. On the skin or in wounds it cannot be relied on to reduce the bacterial population by more than half. The efficacy of tinctures of merbromin can be attributed largely to the alcohol content. The drug is tolerated in a strength of 1% by the bladder, renal pelvis, and urethra; a 2% solution applied to the anterior urethra causes only temporary discomfort. No systemic effects have been observed following its local application in the human. Merbromin has been used in *cystitis* and *urethritis;* also in affections of the eye and ear, such as *otitis media.* Although Merbromin has been injected intravenously, such use may produce toxic symptoms.

Mercury Bichloride NF XII [Corrosive Mercuric Chloride; Corrosive Sublimate; Mercuric Chloride; Perchloride of Mercury], dried over phosphorus pentoxide for 4 hours, contains not less than 99.5% of $HgCl_2$ (271.50). *Caution: Mercury Bichloride is extremely poisonous.* *Preparation:* Now largely made by direct combination of mercury in the vapor state with chlorine. *Description and Solubility:* Heavy, colorless, odorless crystals, crystalline masses, white granules, or powder; the aqueous solution (1 in 20) is acid to litmus, but becomes neutral upon the addition of sodium chloride due to the formation of sodium tetrachloromercurate (Na_2HgCl_4). 1 Gm dissolves in 13.5 ml of water, 3.8 ml of alcohol, 12 ml of glycerin, 25 ml of ether, 2.1 ml of boiling water, and 1.6 ml of boiling alcohol.

Incompatibilities: Its solubility and stability in water are increased by sodium chloride, ammonium chloride, and hydrochloric acid. It is precipitated by *arsenates, borax, carbonates, hydroxides,* and *phosphates,* as well as by *oxalates,* and some other organic salts. Precipitation is retarded by citrates, glycerin, sugar, and acacia. *Albumin, gelatin, tannin,* and some *alkaloids* are also precipitated. *Alkali hydroxides* in excess produce yellow mercuric oxide, lesser quantities the red oxychloride. *Ammonium hydroxide* and *ammonium carbonate* precipitate white ammoniated mercury. *Soluble iodides* precipitate red mercuric iodide which is soluble in excess of the soluble iodide. *Reducing agents* convert mercuric chloride to mercurous chloride and, usually, to metallic mercury, as evidenced by a darkening in color. Light catalyzes the reduction.

Uses: An *antiseptic* formerly used chiefly for the *disinfection of inanimate objects* and the unabraded skin. It is used as a preservative in the tanning of leather, for the disinfection of seed potatoes, and for the production of many mercury compounds. *Application:* 1 in 1000 solution on inanimate objects.

Metacresyl Acetate [$C_9H_{10}O_2$]—The acetic acid ester of metacresol. It is a colorless, oily liquid, which is insoluble in water or glycerin; soluble in animal or vegetable oils and fats, and in alcohol. *Uses:* an antiseptic and analgesic which is used in the treatment of otomycosis; furunculosis of the external auditory canal; various mycotic skin infections; and especially in infected root canals and sockets. *Dose:* applied *topically.*

Methenamine Hippurate [Hiprex (*Riker*)] is hexamethylenamine monohippurate [$C_6H_{12}N_4$; $C_9H_9NO_3$ (319.37)]. *Preparation:* A methanolic solution containing equimolar quantities of methenamine and hippuric acid is refluxed and the salt crystallizes out on cooling. US Pat. 3,004,026. *Description and Solubility:* A fine, white, crystalline powder that is practically odorless and has a sour taste with a mildly bitter aftertaste; stable in light and air, but is hygroscopic in high-humidity conditions; melts at about 115°. Freely soluble in water, alcohol, and chloroform.

Uses: Methenamine Hippurate is a urinary tract antiseptic which depends upon formaldehyde released from the methenamine part of the drug for its antibacterial action (see *Methenamine*, page 1182). The hippuric acid component of the drug aids in lowering urine pH and thus assists the conversion of the methenamine component to the active formaldehyde. Hippuric acid is secreted by the renal tubular anion transport system, so that urine concentrations are initially higher than those of mandelic acid from the mandelate. But, since the plasma is cleared of hippuric acid faster, the concentrations in the urine of the tubules, collecting ducts, calyx, and ureter are lower. The concentration in the urine in the bladder will be intermediate and tend toward a mean which is about the same as that of mandelic acid. It is not yet clear whether the wide fluctuations in urine levels of hippuric acid are beneficial or detrimental to the therapeutic action of the methenamine. Nausea, dysuria, and rash occasionally occur. *Dose:* 1 Gm 2 times a day. The dose for children of ages 6 to 12 is 500 mg to 1 Gm.

Oxychlorosene [Clorpactin XCB (*Guardian*)] is described commercially as a complex hypochlorous acid derivative of a mixture of long-chain alkylbenzenesulfonates. It is thus both an antiseptic and surfactant. *Uses:* A topical *antiseptic* by virtue of its hypochlorite content. It is effective against most bacteria and their spores, viruses, yeasts, and fungi. Perhaps its most significant use is as a *local irrigant during surgery of neoplasms*, to destroy loose viable neoplastic cells and hence to prevent iatrogenic metastasis. *Dose: Topically*, as a 0.5% solution of the calcium salt.

Sodium Oxychlorosene [Clorpactin WCS-90 (*Guardian*)]—*Uses:* The same actions as *Oxychlorosene* (above). However, it has been stabilized so as to prolong its activity. It is used as a topical antiseptic for treating localized infections. It is not used in surgery of neoplasms. *Dose: Topically*, as a 0.4% solution in water or isotonic saline, except 0.1 to 0.2% in ophthalmology and urology.

Oxyquinoline Sulfate [8-hydroxyquinoline sulfate; Chinosol; $(C_9H_7NO)_2.H_2SO_4$]—Yellow, crystalline powder; slight saffron odor; burning taste. Melts between 175° and 178°. Freely soluble in water; soluble in about 100 parts of glycerin; slightly soluble in alcohol; insoluble in ether. *Uses:* A bactericide, fungicide (especially against *monilia*), and trichomonacide; *externally*, in 1:1000 solution; as nasal spray, douche, or eyewash, 1:3000; as gargle, 1:2000; as vaginal douche, 1:1000, increasing if required.

Pine Oil NF XII is a volatile oil composed chiefly of tertiary and secondary terpene alcohols obtained by extraction and fractionation or by steam distillation of the wood of *Pinus palustris* Miller or of other species of *Pinus* Linne (Fam. *Pinaceae*). *Constituents:* The mixture which constitutes the official Pine Oil comprises less than 2% of the total volume of the steam-distilled turpentine oil. It is a high-boiling fraction consisting mainly of the tertiary alcohol *α-terpineol* (bp 221°); the secondary alcohols *borneol* (bp 212°) and *fenchyl alcohol* (bp 201°) are present in smaller amounts. *Description and Solubility:* A colorless to light-amber liquid having a characteristic pinaceous odor. Miscible with alcohol in all proportions.

Uses: A valuable *disinfectant* in veterinary practice, for which purpose an emulsion concentrate (RPS-13, page 455) is used in diluted form. As an *insecticide*, Pine Oil is useful in cattle sprays as a carrier for pyrethrins, rotenone, or derris root. The Oil is also used in flotation processes in mining, in the preparation of wetting and emulsifying agents in textile manufacture, as a source of substances used in the essential oil and perfume industries, and also in the manufacture of certain paints and synthetic resins.

Sodium Perborate NF XII contains not less than 9.0% available oxygen corresponding to about 86.5% of NaBO₃.-4H₂O (153.86). *Preparation:* By mixing 248 parts of boric acid with 78 parts of sodium peroxide, pouring the mixture slowly into 2000 parts of cold water, acidifying with sulfuric acid, and separating and drying the crystals at a temperature not above 50°C.

Description and Solubility: White, crystalline granules or a white powder; odorless and has a saline taste; stable in cool, dry air, but decomposed in warm or in moist air or in solution (see under *Incompatibilities*); decomposition is accelerated by heat; its solution is alkaline to litmus and to phenolphthalein. 1 Gm dissolves in about 40 ml of water;

decomposed by hot water. *Incompatibilities:* With *reducing agents* due to its oxidizing ability; it causes precipitation of some *alkaloids* including *cocaine, morphine, quinine,* and *strychnine*. *Acids* liberate oxygen; *water*, especially if warmed, causes its decomposition into hydrogen peroxide and sodium metaborate.

Uses: Releases nascent oxygen upon contact with organic matter. It was once popular as a mouthwash in a 2% solution, the alkaline residue as well as the germicidal action of the oxygen supposedly exerting benefit. A paste of Sodium Perborate, water, and glycerol was formerly employed in the treatment of *Vincent's angina*, although antibiotics have virtually eclipsed the perborate. Continued use of Sodium Perborate may lead to hypertrophy of the papillae of the tongue, but this condition disappears when the drug is discontinued.

Succinchlorimide NF IX [*N*-Chlorosuccinimide] [$C_4H_4ClNO_2$]—A white, crystalline powder having a chlorine-like odor. It contains 25–27% of active Cl. Melts between 148° and 149°. 1 Gm dissolves in about 70 ml of water, 150 ml of alcohol, 50 ml of benzene; it is sparingly soluble in ether, chloroform, and carbon tetrachloride. *Uses:* a germicide. It has been used for disinfecting drinking water in military camps. 0.12 Gm will sterilize 10 liters of water in 20 minutes at room temperature.

Thiram [Ingredient of Rezifilm (*Squibb*)] is bis(dimethylthiocarbamoyl) disulfide [$C_6H_{12}N_2S_4$ = 240.44]. *Description and Solubility:* A fine, white, crystalline powder; it is odorless (*caution—avoid direct inhalation and contact with skin*) and it is toxic (*caution—do not taste*); it melts between 151° and 159°. Insoluble in water; slightly soluble in alcohol; sparingly soluble in acetone, benzene, and chloroform.

Uses: Thiram has a wide spectrum of antibacterial activity and is also effective against several dermatophytes. Serum does not appear to suppress its activity. At present it is marketed only as a component of a plastic film that is sprayed onto dry surgical wounds for the purpose of preventing postoperative infections. It has not been proven that this Thiram-containing film does, in fact, reduce the incidence of infections. Since it can only be applied to dry wounds, it is not in use during the early period most critical to the prevention of an infection. *Dose:* As a film containing 0.5% Thiram.

Tribromsalan is 3,4′,5-tribromosalicylanilide ($C_{13}H_8$-Br_3NO_2). *Description and Solubility:* A white to off-white, free-flowing powder; it has a slight odor (typical of brominated salicylanilides) and is tasteless; it melts between 225° and 227.3°. Insoluble in water; very soluble in acetone; soluble in alcohol, ether, and benzene; sparingly soluble in chloroform.

Uses: Tribromsalan is a bacteriostatic and antifungal agent that is incorporated into deodorant and antiseptic soaps and other cleansing preparations. It may cause occasional hypersensitivity; sensitization is enhanced by strong light.

Triclocarban [*Monsanto*] is 3,4,4′-trichlorocarbanilide ($C_{13}H_9Cl_3N_2O$). *Description and Solubility:* A fine, white to off-white powder; it has a slight, characteristic odor; tasting is not recommended; it is very stable in light, but decomposes at high temperatures (250° to 255°). 1 Gm solves in 25 ml of acetone and in about 3 ml of dimethyl formamide; practically insoluble in water.

Uses: Triclocarban is an antifungal and antibacterial agent that is incorporated into antiseptic and deodorant soaps and other cleansing preparations.

Undecoylium Chloride-Iodine [Virac (*Ruson*)] is a complex of iodine with mixed cationic, quaternary ammonium surfactants, acyl(s)colaminoformylmethylpyridinium chloride. *Uses:* A topical *antiseptic* which combines the action of a quaternary ammonium detergent and low concentrations of elemental iodine; most of the antibacterial activity is attributable to the iodine, which is slowly released, especially in contact with tissues. The wetting action of the detergent aids in the spread of the drug over surfaces and into crevices. The drug is employed for pre- and postoperative antisepsis of the skin, perineum, and genital tract, for the treatment of dermatologic infections, for disinfection of wounds, as a vaginal douche, and in the treatment of mycoses of scalp and feet. No stinging or irritation of skin or mucous membranes has accured to its application. It does not stain skin or clothing, because of the extremely low concentration of free elemental iodine present; for the same reason, its potency is much lower than that of iodine solutions or tincture. Soap interferes with its actions and should not be used concomitantly. The drug sometimes causes local hypersensitivity reactions. It should not be used in the presence of known sensitivity to iodine. *Dose: Topically,* as a solution containing 0.2, 0.6, 0.8, or 3.2% iodine.

Zinc Peroxide is ZnO_2 (97.37). *Description and Solubility:* A fine, white, or only faintly yellow, odorless powder. Almost insoluble in water and organic solvents; readily soluble in dilute mineral acids. *Incompatibilities:* It is a powerful oxidizing agent. It is gradually decomposed by *water* liberating oxygen, and by *diluted acids* liberating hydrogen peroxide. In the presence of moisture it is decomposed by practically all *organic matter* and other *reducing agents.* It reacts with many materials to liberate oxygen. It must be protected from atmospheric moisture and carbon dioxide. *Uses:* Zinc Peroxide slowly releases nascent oxygen, leaving a residue of zinc oxide. The former exerts a *germicidal,* the latter, an *astringent* action. Medicinal Zinc Peroxide USP XVII, which also contained zinc carbonate and zinc hydroxide, was formerly used widely in the treatment of infections from anaerobic organisms. For oral infections, the powder is suspended in 4 parts of water and used as a wash. For tissues, a 40% suspension is employed. Zinc Peroxide is heated prior to use, heating appearing to increase its activity. *Dose: Topically,* as a 40% suspension in water.

Systemic Antibacterial Drugs

During the early part of this century giant strides were made in the systemic treatment of certain microzoal infections. Nevertheless, these advances did not greatly affect directly the over-all practice of medicine. The advent of sulfanilamide in 1935 marked the beginning of a major revolution in the practice of medicine. The subsequent profusion of antibacterial agents overwhelmed the physician with golden tools. Several leading causes of death have been deposed to a minor status and some to a mere nuisance. The consequent lengthening of the life span turned medicine toward the degenerative diseases and the problems of aging. The social, economic, and political consequences of these effects will reverberate for generations. Meanwhile, certain of the arts of "non-drug" management of infection have nearly been forgotten, and carelessness has been fostered by the glitter and security of the "wonder drugs." The realization that certain microorganisms are successfully resisting our mightiest champions not only will impel a ceaseless search for new systemic antibacterial agents but also will force a sober return to certain ancillary arts of the medical and surgical management of infectious disease.

Although certain of the drugs listed in this section are used only for their local actions, their obvious relationship to parent systemic agents warrants their inclusion.

Sulfonamides

History—The compound *p*-aminobenzenesulfonamide, now known as *sulfanilamide,* was first synthesized in 1908, but it was many years before its therapeutic value was discovered. In 1932, a German firm prepared a red dye, 4-(4′-sulfamylphenylazo)-*m*-phenylenediamine or *p′*-sulfamylchrysoidine, and in 1935 Domagk reported remarkable curative effects of this compound and named it *Prontosil.* In the same year, a group of French investigators (Trefouel, *et al*) found that the bactericidal property of the drug resided in the *p*-aminobenzenesulfonamide portion of the molecule. In 1937 Ewins and Phillips of England synthesized sulfapyridine, which was the first sulfonamide used with great success in combating pneumonia. Then followed sulfathiazole, sulfadiazine, and a large number of other sulfonamides. Over 3300 sulfonamides have since been prepared, but only a few have been accepted for medicinal use.

All the official, and generally all the therapeutically useful, antimicrobial sulfonamides are characterized by the following structure:

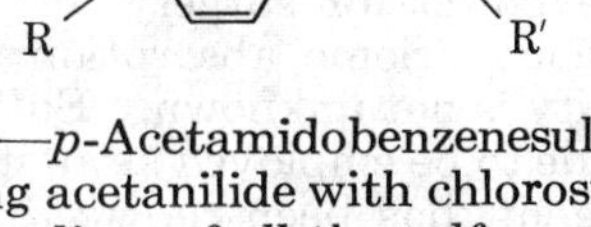

Preparation—*p*-Acetamidobenzenesulfonyl chloride, made by treating acetanilide with chlorosulfonic acid, is the basic intermediate of all the sulfonamides. This is treated with the desired amine in the presence of a weak base such as pyridine, and the resulting acetyl compound is deacetylated via proton or hydroxyl-catalyzed hydrolysis. The reactions taking place in the synthesis of sulfadiazine are illustrated by the following equations.

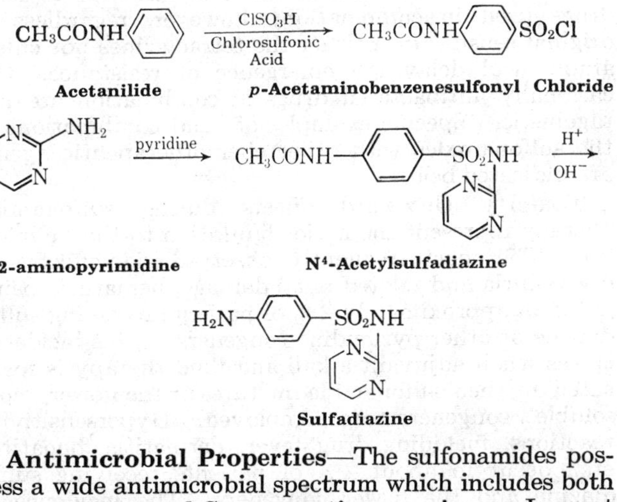

Antimicrobial Properties—The sulfonamides possess a wide antimicrobial spectrum which includes both Gram-positive and Gram-negative organisms. In most circumstances, these agents exert only a bacteriostatic action, and ultimate elimination of the invading microorganisms is dependent upon the cellular and humoral defense mechanisms of the host, which are neither enhanced nor inhibited by the sulfonamides. However, bactericidal concentrations of these agents are sometimes attained in the urinary and intestinal tracts.

The sulfonamides also have a low degree of efficacy against malarial parasites.

The mechanism of the antimicrobial action of the sulfonamides has been analyzed extensively. The sulfonamides compete with p-aminobenzoic acid and prevent its normal cellular utilization, particularly its incorporation into folic acid (pteroylglutamic acid, PGA). Thus, sulfonamide-sensitive organisms are primarily those which must synthesize their own folic acid. Organisms which are able to utilize preformed folic acid or which do not require this metabolite are not generally affected by these agents. This mechanism is of importance as an example of the general concepts of *biological antagonism* and *antimetabolites*. The efficacy of sulfonamides is generally enhanced when the drugs are used in combination with the folic acid antagonist, trimethoprim.

Microorganisms initially sensitive to the sulfonamides may become resistant to these drugs. The clinical importance of such acquired bacterial resistance is attested by the fact that the majority of the strains of *Neisserria gonorrheæ* now isolated from patients with gonococcal urethritis are resistant to these agents, whereas the sulfonamides were once the agents of choice against such organisms. Numerous other examples could be cited, including the occurrence of epidemics among military populations caused by sulfonamide-resistant microorganisms after mass oral prophylactic use of these drugs. While such epidemics have fortunately not yet been of importance in civilian medicine, they do emphasize the necessity for proper precautions to minimize the development of acquired bacterial resistance. The sulfonamides should be employed only when specific indications exist for such medication. Further, when these agents are employed, they should be administered in adequate dosage as early in the course of the infection as possible.

Certain combinations of the sulfonamides with various antibiotics minimize the development of bacterial resistance and achieve chemotherapeutic results not attainable with either agent alone. However, not all combinations of chemotherapeutic agents have a rational basis. The microbe must be sensitive to both drugs used in combination; however, regardless of original sensitivity, neither the tetracyclines nor chloramphenicol delay the emergence of resistance. Occasionally antibacterial drugs in combination are antagonistic. Specific examples of valid combinations of the sulfonamides with other chemotherapeutic agents are indicated below.

Toxicity—Untoward effects during sulfonamide therapy represent the major limitation to their clinical use. The most frequently observed side-effects are crystalluria and related renal damage, hematuria being noted in approximately 2% of patients receiving sulfadiazine or other pyrimidine congeners. This incidence is less when adjuvant alkali and fluid therapy is instituted or when sulfonamide mixtures or the newer, more soluble congeners are employed. Hypersensitivity reactions, including drug fever, dermatitis, hepatitis, etc., occur in about 2% of patients receiving sulfadiazine and the newer congeners. The incidence of hypersensitivity reactions is higher in patients receiving sulfanilamide, sulfathiazole, or sulfapyridine. Agranulocytosis, aplastic anemia, leukopenia, and thrombocytopenia have been noted during sulfonamide therapy, but the incidence is low when sulfadiazine and the other newer congeners are employed. Long-acting sulfonamides, especially, may cause exudative erythema multiforma (Stevens-Johnson syndrome). Central nervous system effects are infrequently observed during sulfadiazine therapy, and cyanosis, acid–base disturbances and other miscellaneous toxic effects formerly common during therapy with sulfanilamide, sulfathiazole, or sulfapyridine are only rarely observed during administration of sulfadiazine.

Because the sulfonamides may cause serious untoward effects, they should be administered only when bacteriological diagnosis indicates that these agents can be expected to be superior to drugs of other classes. Constant medical surveillance, preferably daily, is necessary, and periodic blood counts and urinalyses are mandatory.

Types and Choice of Preparations—The antimicrobial spectrum of all sulfonamides is essentially the same. However, on the basis of solubility and degree of absorption from the gastrointestinal tract, the sulfonamides can be divided into two broad classes, namely, those employed for systemic chemotherapy and those intended only for intestinal chemotherapy. Sulfonamides employed for their systemic actions include sulfachlorpyridazine, sulfadiazine, sulfaethidole, sulfamerazine, sulfameter, sulfamethazine, sulfadimethoxine, sulfamethoxazole, sulfacetamide, sulfisoxazole, sulfisomidine, sulfamethizole, sulfamethoxypyridazine, and the sulfonamide mixtures (see below). These agents are readily absorbed from the gastrointestinal tract and adequate blood concentrations are easily maintained. Since these compounds are excreted almost entirely by the kidney, high urinary concentrations are also attained and these agents are thus employed in certain urinary tract infections. Differences exist among these sulfonamides regarding degree of acetylation, degree of binding by plasma proteins, renal tubular resorption and rapidity of renal excretion, and degree of penetration into the cerebrospinal fluid. Such differences modify their dosage schedules, but choice between them is difficult and frequently merely a matter of personal preference. However, these sulfonamides do differ markedly regarding solubility in urine, and sulfonamide mixtures and particularly certain congeners cause a lower incidence of crystalluria and related renal toxicity than do the other sulfonamides. Sulfanilamide, sulfathiazole, and sulfapyridine are distinctly more toxic than the other sulfonamides employed for systemic chemotherapy and can no longer be recommended for therapeutic use.

Oral administration of the sulfonamides is preferred. However, when medication cannot be taken by mouth, the soluble sodium salts may be given parenterally. They are administered in 0.9% sodium chloride, Ringer's Injection, or $M/6$ sodium lactate solution. The intravenous route is preferred, concentrations up to 5% being injected slowly over a period of at least 10 minutes. Lower concentrations (0.5 to 2.5%) can be given subcutaneously.

On the other hand, certain insoluble sulfonamide congeners, such as succinylsulfathiazole and phthalylsulfathiazole, are poorly absorbed from the gastrointestinal tract. Subsequent hydrolysis of these compounds in the large bowel releases active sulfonamide in high concentration and permits their use for preoperative preparation of the bowel for surgery and for certain intestinal infections. Some absorption does occur and systemic toxicity is not unknown. Sulfaguanidine, the first sulfonamide to be employed as an intestinal chemotherapeutic agent, has been replaced by superior insoluble sulfonamides.

After administration of adequate doses of the insoluble sulfonamides, the intestinal coliform count is markedly reduced. The stool becomes less bulky, semifluid, gelatinous in appearance, and relatively odorless. Further, the abdomen becomes less distended and the bowel free from gas and gross fecal matter. Thus, after several days of medication, the patient is in proper condition for intestinal surgery, and exhausting enemas and dehydrating purgatives can be avoided. These sulfonamides are employed in conjunction with a low-residue diet for 3 to 7 days prior to surgery. Therapy is resumed postoperatively as soon as the patient can take sufficient warm water by mouth. The postoperative course is usually smooth, abdominal distention is absent, gas pains are mild, and peritonitis and deep abscesses do not develop even if the open technique for intestinal anastomoses has been employed. However, the routine use of bowel "sterilization" has been criticized, and most authorities prefer to reserve bowel sterilization for cases in which the bowel is infected.

An enormous number of sulfonamide preparations intended for topical application to cutaneous and mucosal surfaces have been made available and at one time enjoyed much popularity. It is now recognized that topical chemotherapy is rarely effective except in the most superficial infections and indeed may be dangerous. Local application of such agents is one of the major causes of drug sensitization, and the low concentrations of these drugs usually achieved favor the development of acquired bacterial resistance. For these reasons, topical administration of the sulfonamides, with the possible exception of sulfacetamide sodium, is not recommended and strongly discouraged.

Sulfonamide Mixtures—Sulfonamide mixtures are designed to minimize the incidence of crystalluria and related renal injury associated with systemic use of sulfonamides. Since the solubility of a particular sulfonamide is not influenced by the presence of others in the same solution, a higher total concentration of sulfonamide can be attained in the urine without precipitation after administration of a mixture than is possible if a single sulfonamide is given. Employment of mixtures reduces the dose of sodium bicarbonate necessary to maintain the sulfonamides in solution in the urine and may obviate such need completely. Mixtures of equal weights of two or three sulfonamides are commonly employed. Those most frequently used include sulfadiazine, sulfamerazine, sulfamethazine, or sulfacetamide. Sulfonamide mixtures are available only for oral administration, but mixtures of parenteral preparations have been prepared extemporaneously and employed to advantage.

The antimicrobial potency and spectrum and the therapeutic uses of sulfonamide mixtures are the same as those of the individual components. The incidence of renal toxicity is definitely reduced even without concomitant administration of alkalinizing salts and can be reduced further if such adjuvant alkali therapy is employed. The incidence of hypersensitivity reactions is not enhanced and may be reduced. Precautions for use of sulfonamide mixtures are the same as those for use of the individual congeners. Adequate 24-hour urine volume should be assured by fluid therapy if necessary. The dosage for the sulfonamide mixtures is essentially the same as that for the components.

Uses—In spite of the dominance of the antibiotics, the sulfonamides still retain an important place in the chemotherapy of infectious diseases. In some infections, a sulfonamide remains the agent of choice; in others, particularly in serious infections, a sulfonamide is frequently employed in combination with an appropriate antibiotic. In addition, the sulfonamides have certain important prophylactic uses. Major advantages of the sulfonamides are their low cost and ease of administration; the major disadvantage is their untoward effects.

The sulfonamides are still the agent of choice in *chancroid* and *nocardiasis*. They share a first choice status with other agents in *infections of the urinary tract* caused by *E. coli* or *A. Aerogenes* and in *uncomplicated bubonic plague*. In combination with another drug they are first choice in the treatment of various infections caused by *H. influenzae* and in *trachoma*. Most strains of *meningococcus* are more sensitive to sulfonamides than to any other antibiotic, but the occurrence of Type B resistant strains has made penicillin G the drug of first choice. They are also of use in urinary tract infections caused by *Salmonella*, *Shigella*, and *Staphylococcus*. Combined use of sulfonamide with streptomycin has yielded excellent results in *plague*, and combined therapy with streptomycin or a tetracycline is beneficial in *influenzal meningitis* and *brucellosis*. The sulfonamides may be combined with penicillin in *actinomycosis* and may be of value in certain *selected* cases of *subacute bacterial endocarditis* not responsive to antibiotics. In regions in which there is a problem of resistance of malarial parasites to the usual antimalarials, sulfonamides may be given in combination with other antimalarials or with trimethoprim.

Important prophylactic uses of the sulfonamides include their employment to reduce the *meningococcal* carrier rate and thus decrease the spread of meningococcal infections in congested populations and for mass chemoprophylaxis during outbreaks of *bacillary dysentery*. The sulfonamides are inferior to penicillin for the prevention of *streptococcal* infections, especially on a mass scale, but may be employed advantageously for this purpose within a household where proper medical surveillance is possible. The sulfonamides are of benefit in the prevention of bacteremia and subacute bacterial endocarditis consequent to oral surgery, tonsillectomy, child birth, etc., and in the prevention of recrudescences of rheumatic fever.

The sulfonamides have been *replaced by the antibiotics in the treatment of streptococcal, staphylococcal, pneumococcal, and gonococcal infections*. Similarly, they are no longer employed in anthrax infections, psittacosis, ornithosis, lymphogranuloma inguinale, or infections caused by *Klebsiella*. Among the diseases in which the sulfonamides are *ineffective* are syphilis, yaws, malaria, tuberculosis, leprosy, typhoid, tetanus, tularemia, pertussis, diphtheria, and most viral and rickettsial infections.

The insoluble sulfonamides intended for intestinal chemotherapy are employed chiefly for *preoperative* preparation of the bowel prior to surgery. Certain of these agents are also employed alone or combined with systemic sulfonamide therapy in acute and chronic *bacillary dysentery*, in *ulcerative colitis*, and *regional enteritis*. These sulfonamides may also be employed as adjuvant agents in the therapy of *intestinal amebiasis*.

Incompatibilities—The sodium derivatives are soluble in water, invariably imparting to the solution a marked alkalinity. Hence such solutions are incompatible with all acidic substances. In combination with alkaloidal salts such as ephedrine sulfate, both the free alkaloid and the sulfonamide are precipitated in most instances. Aqueous solutions of the sodium derivatives deteriorate rapidly. Solutions of the sulfonamides obtained by the addition of acid or alkali may undergo hydrolytic or other decomposition and are, therefore, unsafe for use.

Local anesthetics related to para-aminobenzoic acid antagonize the action of the sulfonamides. *Ethyl aminobenzoate, propyl aminobenzoate, butyl aminobenzoate, procaine, isocaine, butacaine, tetracaine,* and *monocaine* are so related.

Acetyl Sulfisoxazole NF

[*N* - (3,4 - Dimethyl - 5 - isoxazolyl) - *N* - sulfanilylacetamide; N^1 - Acetyl - N^1 - (3,4 - dimethyl - 5 - isoxazolyl)sulfanilamide; N^1 - Acetylsulfisoxazole; Gantrisin Acetyl (*Roche*)]

Acetyl Sulfisoxazole contains 98.0–100.5% of $C_{13}H_{15}N_3O_4S$ (309.35), calculated on the dried basis.

Preparation—Sulfisoxazole is selectively acetylated at the N^1-position by converting it into its sodium salt which may then be metathesized with an equimolar quantity of acetyl chloride or acetic anhydride.

Description—A white or slightly yellow, crystalline powder. Melting range 192° to 195°.

Solubility—Practically insoluble in water; slightly soluble in alcohol; sparingly soluble in chloroform.

Uses—Acetyl Sulfisoxazole is converted to Sulfisoxazole in the gastrointestinal tract. Thus, its actions and toxicity are identical to those of the parent compound (see *Sulfisoxazole*, page 1203). However, Acetyl Sulfisoxazole is tasteless and hence is the more suitable for liquid oral preparations.

Dose—1.15 to 2.3 Gm every 4 to 6 hours; *usual, initial,* 4.6 Gm, the equivalent of 4 Gm of sulfisoxazole, then 1.15 Gm, the equivalent of 1 Gm of sulfisoxazole, every 4 to 6 hours.

Dosage Forms—Oral Suspension NF: 500 mg/5 ml.

Veterinary Use—In treatment of respiratory and urinary tract infections.

Veterinary Dose—*Oral,* 140 to 220 mg per Kg of body weight daily.

Phthalylsulfacetamide NF

[4′-(Acetylsulfamoyl)phthalanilic Acid; Enterosulfon (*CMC*); Thalamyd (*Schering*)]

Phthalylsulfacetamide, dried at 105° for 4 hours, contains 99.0–100.5% of $C_{16}H_{14}N_2O_6S$ (362.36).

Preparation—Sulfacetamide (*qv,* page 1199) is reacted with phthalic anhydride by refluxing in ethanol.

Description—White or creamy white crystals or a crystalline powder, possessing a slight odor. Decomposes with liquefaction between 186° and 202°.

Solubility—Very slightly soluble in water; soluble in acetone; freely soluble in solutions of alkali hydroxides.

Incompatibilities—See page 1197.

Uses—Phthalylsulfacetamide is a poorly absorbed *intestinal anti-infective* recommended chiefly for acute

bacillary dysentery and for preparation of the bowel prior to surgery. (See general statement, page 1197.) Benefit in *ulcerative colitis* and in *cholera* has also been claimed. Systemic toxicity is low. Its status is inferior to that of succinylsulfathiazole and phthalylsulfathiazole.

Dose—1.5 to 4 Gm; *usual,* 2 Gm 3 times a day.

Other Dose Information—The oral dosage recommended in bacillary dysentery is 3 Gm, 3 times daily for 5 to 10 days. As an adjunct prior to bowel surgery, the daily dose of 0.2 Gm per Kg of body weight, in divided portions, is started 3 to 5 days preoperatively and continued at least 2 days postoperatively.

Dosage Forms—Tablets NF: 500 mg.

Phthalylsulfathiazole NF

[4′-(2-Thiazolylsulfamoyl)phthalanilic Acid; Sulfathalidine (*MSD*)]

Phthalylsulfathiazole contains 98.0–100.5% of $C_{17}H_{13}N_3O_5S_2$ (403.44), calculated on the dried basis.

Preparation—Phthalic anhydride is caused to undergo addition to sulfathiazole by refluxing in a suitable solvent.

Description—A white or faintly yellowish white, crystalline powder. It has a slightly bitter taste and is odorless. It may slowly darken on long exposure to light. Melts with decomposition at about 275°.

Solubility—Practically insoluble in water and chloroform; slightly soluble in alcohol; very slightly soluble in ether; readily soluble in solutions of alkali hydroxides and their carbonates, and in hydrochloric acid.

Incompatibilities—See page 1197.

Uses—Phthalylsulfathiazole is employed solely as an intestinal *antibacterial* agent, chiefly in preparation for *bowel surgery.* (See general statement, pages 1196 and 1197.) For this purpose it is probably the sulfonamide of choice. Advantages over succinylsulfathiazole include its smaller dose, its effectiveness even in the presence of watery diarrhea, and the fact that it produces soft rather than semi-liquid stools.

Like succinylsulfathiazole, Phthalylsulfathiazole is sometimes beneficial in obstinate cases of urinary tract infections caused by *E. coli,* effectiveness usually being attributed to reducing the coliform reservoir in the bowel. Phthalylsulfathiazole lacks the value of succinylsulfathiazole in bacillary dysentery. It is occasionally of benefit in *chronic ulcerative colitis, regional enteritis,* and *intestinal amebiasis.*

Toxicity is low and similar to that of sulfathiazole. It may cause low-grade fever, malaise, headache, and anorexia, which, however, do not require discontinuation of the drug. The occurrence of a skin rash does require cessation of treatment. Precautions to be employed are the same as for other sulfonamides.

Dose—4 to 12 Gm daily; *usual,* 1 Gm every 4 hours.

Other Dose Information—The recommended oral dosage prior to operative procedures on the intestinal tract is 125 mg per Kg of body weight per day, divided in equal portions given at 6- to 8-hour intervals. The diet should be low in residue and mineral oil is to be avoided. Treatment is started 3 to 5 days prior to surgery and continued for 1 to 2 weeks postoperatively. For infections and ulcerative lesions of the colon, the daily dose is 50 to 100 mg per Kg of body weight, administered in equal portions every 6 to 8 hours.

Dosage Forms—Tablets NF: 500 mg.

Veterinary Dose—*Cattle*, 100 to 250 mg per Kg of body weight daily in divided doses; *Swine*, 100 mg per Kg of body weight daily in divided doses; *Dogs*, 150 mg per Kg of body weight daily in divided doses; *Cats*, 140 to 500 mg per Kg of body weight daily in divided doses; *Rabbits*, 500 mg per Kg of body weight daily in divided doses; *Turkeys*, 4 pounds to each ton of mash.

Succinylsulfathiazole USP

[4'-(2-Thiazolylsulfamoyl)succinanilic Acid; Sulfasuxidine (*MSD*)]

Succinylsulfathiazole [$C_{13}H_{13}N_3O_5S_2 . H_2O = 373.41$] contains 99.0–100.5% of $C_{13}H_{13}N_3O_5S_2$ (355.39), calculated on the anhydrous basis.

Preparation—As with phthalylsulfathiazole, this sulfonamide may be made by causing sulfathiazole to undergo addition with succinic anhydride.

Description—A white or yellowish white, crystalline powder, which melts with decomposition between 185° and 195°. It is odorless and is stable in air, but slowly darkens on exposure to light. It is hydrolyzed by hot mineral acids and by solutions of alkali hydroxides into sulfathiazole and succinic acid or alkali succinate.

Solubility—1 Gm dissolves in about 4800 ml of water; soluble in solutions of alkali hydroxides and solutions of sodium bicarbonate with the evolution of carbon dioxide; sparingly soluble in alcohol and acetone; insoluble in chloroform and ether.

Incompatibilities—See introduction to this section (page 1197).

Uses—Succinylsulfathiazole is a poorly absorbed *antibacterial* agent employed for intestinal chemotherapy. (See general statement, pages 1196 and 1197.) Benefit in both acute and chronic *bacillary dysentery* is comparable to that obtained with sulfadiazine. In addition, it sharply reduces the carrier rate and may be of value as a prophylactic agent. However, antibiotics have diminished the importance of this use of the drug. Succinylsulfathiazole is a useful adjunct prior to *bowel surgery*, but phthalylsulfathiazole is probably the sulfonamide of choice. The actions of Succinylsulfathiazole are impeded by diarrhea, hard stools, water, and liquid petrolatum. Both sulfonamides are sometimes beneficial in obstinate cases of *urinary tract infections* caused by *E. coli*, effectiveness usually being attributed to reduction of the coliform reservoir of the colon which serves as the source of reinfection. Succinylsulfathiazole is occasionally of value in *chronic ulcerative colitis*. It is ineffective in typhoid fever.

Toxicity occurs infrequently and results from sulfathiazole which is absorbed to a limited extent from the colon. Low-grade fever, malaise, headache, or anorexia may occasionally occur. Rash is rare, but it requires discontinuation of the drug when it occurs. Precautions to be observed during Succinylsulfathiazole therapy are the same as those for the other sulfonamides.

Dose—6 to 18 Gm daily; *usual*, 3 Gm 6 times a day.

Other Dose Information—The initial oral dosage for bacillary dysentery is 250 mg per Kg of body weight, followed by 250 mg per Kg per day, given in equal portions at 4-hour intervals. Administration is continued until fever and diarrhea are absent for at least 2 days and stool cultures are negative. Similar dosage schedule is recommended when the drug is employed as an adjunct prior to bowel surgery. Therapy is started 5 to 7 days preoperatively and continued for 10 to 14 days postoperatively. The patient should be on a low-residue diet, and mineral oil should be avoided.

Dosage Forms—Tablets USP: 500 mg.

Veterinary Dose—*Calves*, 500 mg to 1 Gm per Kg of body weight daily in divided doses; *Swine*, 200 to 300 mg per Kg of body weight daily in divided doses; *Dogs* and *Cats*, 500 mg per Kg of body weight daily in divided doses.

Sulfacetamide NF

[*N*-Sulfanilylacetamide]

Sulfacetamide, dried at 105° for 2 hours, contains 99.0–100.5% of $C_8H_{10}N_2O_3S$ (214.24).

Preparation—Sulfacetamide may be prepared by reacting sulfanilamide with acetic anhydride, followed by controlled alkaline hydrolysis to remove the N^4-acetyl group and subsequent acidification to a pH of about 4.

Description—A white, crystalline powder. Odorless and has a characteristic, sour taste. Melts between 181° and 184°. Solutions of Sulfacetamide are sensitive to light, and are unstable when strongly acid or strongly alkaline.

Solubility—1 Gm is soluble in about 140 ml of water; soluble in alcohol; slightly soluble in ether; very slightly soluble in chloroform; practically insoluble in benzene; freely soluble in dilute mineral acids and solutions of potassium and sodium hydroxides.

Incompatibilities—See page 1197.

Uses—Since it is rapidly excreted by the kidney, Sulfacetamide is employed chiefly as an *antibacterial* agent in the therapy of *urinary tract infections* caused by sulfonamide-sensitive microorganisms. (See general statement, page 1196.) However, it is now recognized that penetration of tissues is as important as the concentration in the urine in the eradication of urinary tract infections, especially of the prostate, seminal vesicals, and vas deferens; consequently, soluble sulfonamides have fallen somewhat into disfavor, since they do not penetrate tissues as well as does sulfadiazine. The drug is soluble up to 2% in urine and causes a low incidence of crystalluria and related untoward effects on the urinary tract. Alkalinization of the urine is unnecessary for its safe use. Other systemic toxicity is similar to that caused by sulfadiazine.

Dose—*Usual, initial*, 4 Gm; *maintenance*, 1 Gm every 4 hours.

Other Dose Information—For urinary tract infections, the drug is administered in a 10-day course. For adults 1 Gm is administered every 4 hours for 4 days, followed by 1 Gm 3 times daily for 3 days, and finally 0.5 Gm 4 times daily for the last 3 days.

Dosage Forms—Tablets NF: 500 mg.

Sodium Sulfacetamide USP

[Soluble Sulfacetamide; Sulphacetamide Sodium; Sodium *N*-Sulfanilyl-acetamide; (*N*¹-Acetylsulfanilamido)sodium; Bleph (*Allergan*); Sodium Sulamyd (*White*); Sulf-30 (*Smith, Miller & Patch*)]

Sodium Sulfacetamide [C₈H₉N₂NaO₃S.H₂O = 254.24] contains 99.0–100.5% of C₈H₉N₂NaO₃S (236.23), calculated on the anhydrous basis.

For the structure of sulfacetamide, see above.

Description—A white, crystalline, odorless powder with a bitter taste. The pH of a 1 in 20 solution is between 8.0 and 9.5.

Solubility—1 Gm dissolves in 2.5 ml of water; sparingly soluble in alcohol; practically insoluble in benzene, chloroform, and ether.

Incompatibilities—See page 1197.

Uses—The *antibacterial* spectrum of Sodium Sulfacetamide is similar to that of the other sulfonamides. Employed in high concentration by local application, it is of benefit in various *ophthalmologic infections*. Since the drug is nonirritating even in high concentration, it can be employed in sufficient concentration to achieve penetration of the ocular tissues. Although the high local concentrations thus attained obviate certain of the undesirable aspects of local chemotherapy, the usual limitations and dangers of such therapy are not completely eliminated. In many infections, systemic chemotherapy may also be necessary.

Dose—*Topically*, as a **10%** ointment or **0.1 ml** of a **30%** solution to the conjunctiva 2 to 8 times a day.

Dosage Forms—Ophthalmic Ointment USP; Ophthalmic Solution USP.

Sulfacetamide, Sulfadiazine, and Sulfamerazine Oral Suspension NF

[Tricombisul (*Schering*)]

Sulfacetamide, Sulfadiazine, and Sulfamerazine Suspension contains 90.0–110.0% of the labeled amounts of C₈H₁₀N₂O₃S (sulfacetamide), of C₁₀H₁₀N₄O₂S (sulfadiazine), and of C₁₁H₁₂N₄O₂S (sulfamerazine), in a buffered, aqueous suspension.

Description—A buffered, aqueous suspension which may contain suitable flavoring agents, suspending agents, preservatives, and certified color additives.

Uses—The *antibacterial* spectrum and therapeutic uses of sulfonamide mixtures are the same as those of the individual components. An advantage of such mixtures is the lesser incidence of crystalluria and renal injury associated with their use. (See general statement, page 1197.)

Dose—*Usual*, initial, **4 Gm**, then **500 mg to 1 Gm** every 4 hours.

Sulfacetamide, Sulfadiazine, and Sulfamerazine Tablets NF

[Tricombisul (*Schering*)]

Sulfacetamide, Sulfadiazine, and Sulfamerazine Tablets contain 90.0–110.0% of the labeled amounts of C₈H₁₀N₂O₃S (sulfacetamide), of C₁₀H₁₀N₄O₂S (sulfadiazine), and of C₁₁H₁₂N₄O₂S (sulfamerazine).

Uses and **Dose**—See *Sulfacetamide, Sulfadiazine, and Sulfamerazine Oral Suspension.*

Sulfadiazine USP

[*N*¹-2-Pyrimidinylsulfanilamide; Coco Diazine (*Lilly*); Eskadiazine (*SK&F*)]

Sulfadiazine contains 99.0–100.5% of C₁₀H₁₀N₄O₂S (250.28), calculated on the dried basis.

Preparation—Sulfadiazine is prepared by combining *p*-acetamidobenzenesulfonyl chloride (see page 1195) with 2-aminopyrimidine (2-amino-1,3-diazine) in the presence of a mild alkaline agent, then splitting off the acetyl group by hydrolyzing with acid or alkali.

Description—A white or slightly yellow powder. It is odorless or nearly so, and is stable in air, but slowly darkens on exposure to light. It melts between 253° and 257°.

Solubility—1 Gm dissolves in about 13,000 ml of water; sparingly soluble in alcohol and acetone; 1 Gm dissolves in about 620 ml of human serum at 37°; freely soluble in dilute mineral acids, solutions of potassium and sodium hydroxides, and ammonia TS.

Incompatibilities—See page 1197.

Uses—Sulfadiazine is the single sulfonamide most widely employed at the present time when the *systemic antibacterial* actions of these agents are desired. It serves as the prototype for comparison of the other sulfonamides and their mixtures. (See general statement, page 1195.)

Sulfadiazine is bound to the extent of 17 to 56% by the plasma proteins, and hence concentrations of the drug in the cerebrospinal fluid vary from 50 to 80% of those in the plasma. This is a good tissue concentration, as antibacterial agents go. However, higher concentrations in the cerebrospinal fluid are attained when the meninges are inflamed, and intrathecal administration of the drug is usually not necessary. Approximately 15 to 40% of the drug in the urine is acetylated. The tissue-penetrating properties of sulfadiazine have proven to be of importance in combatting urinary tract infections, so that the drug is displacing the more soluble sulfonamides.

Untoward effects occur in approximately 6 to 8% of patients receiving Sulfadiazine therapy. Crystalluria and related renal damage can be minimized by administration of adjuvant alkalinizing salts and by maintenance of an adequate 24-hour urine volume. Urinary volume in the adult should be maintained at more than 1500 ml per 24 hours. If adjuvant alkali therapy is employed, an initial dose of 4 Gm of sodium bicarbonate and subsequent doses of 2 Gm at intervals of 4 hours are necessary to achieve adequate alkalinization of the urine. Hypersensitivity reactions are observed in 1 to 2% of patients, but agranulocytosis and other serious blood dyscrasias have been reported only rarely.

The therapeutic uses of Sulfadiazine have been described in the general statement (page 1197).

Dose—2 to 8 Gm daily; *usual*, initial, **4 Gm**, then **1 Gm** 4 to 6 times a day.

Other Dose Information—In severe infections, the initial oral dose for adults of 100 mg per Kg of body weight is followed by 1.0 to 1.5 Gm every 4 hours day and night until the temperature has been normal for 5 to 7 days. In severe infections in children, the initial dose is 100 to 150 mg per Kg of body weight. Subsequent doses of ¼ the initial dose are administered every 6 hours. In moderate or mild infections in both adults and children, an initial dose of 50 mg per Kg of body weight and maintenance doses ⅓ of the initial dose at intervals of 4 to 6 hours are adequate.

Dosage Forms—Tablets USP: 250, 300, and 500 mg.

Veterinary Dose—*Calves*, **140 mg** per **Kg** of body weight daily in divided doses for 2 or 3 days. The dose may be reduced by 50% and administration continued 2 or 3 days longer if advisable.

Sulfadiazine and Sulfamerazine Tablets NF

[Duozine (*Abbott*)]

Sulfadiazine and Sulfamerazine Tablets contain 90.0–110.0% of the labeled amounts of $C_{10}H_{10}N_4O_2S$ (sulfadiazine) and $C_{11}H_{12}N_4O_2S$ (sulfamerazine).

Uses—See *Sulfadiazine, Sulfamerazine,* and the general statement (page 1197).

Dose—*Usual, initial,* **4 Gm,** then **2 Gm** every 4 hours.

Sodium Sulfadiazine USP

[Sodium N^1-2-Pyrimidinylsulfanilamide; Soluble Sulfadiazine]

Sodium Sulfadiazine contains 99.0–100.5% of $C_{10}H_9$-N_4NaO_2S (272.26), calculated on the dried basis.

For the structure of sulfadiazine, see page 1200.

Preparation—This sulfonamide may be prepared by dissolving sulfadiazine in the required quantity of sodium hydroxide solution and evaporating to dryness or precipitating the compound with alcohol.

Description—A white powder. On prolonged exposure to humid air it absorbs carbon dioxide with the liberation of sulfadiazine and becomes incompletely soluble in water. Its solutions are alkaline to phenolphthalein. It is affected by light.

Solubility—1 Gm dissolves in about 2 ml of water; slightly soluble in alcohol.

Incompatibilities—See introduction to this section (page 1197).

Uses—See *Sulfadiazine.* Because of the solubility of the sodium salt, it is used for parenteral therapy.

Dose—*Intravenous,* **2** to **8 Gm** daily; *usual, initial,* **4 Gm** in a 5% solution, then **2 Gm** 3 times a day.

Other Dose Information—If parenteral medication is indicated, sulfadiazine sodium may be administered intravenously in an initial dose of 100 mg per Kg of body weight to a maximum dose of 5 Gm. Maintenance doses of 30 to 50 mg per Kg of body weight are given every 6 to 8 hours until oral medication can be instituted. Daily blood level determinations and urinalyses are mandatory during intravenous sulfonamide medication. Sulfadiazine sodium may also be administered subcutaneously; dosage by this route is 65 to 100 mg per Kg of body weight every 12 hours.

Dosage Forms—Injection USP: 10 ml.

Sulfadimethoxine NF

[N^1-(2,6-Dimethoxy-4-pyrimidinyl)sulfanilamide; Madribon (*Roche*)]

Sulfadimethoxine, dried at 105° for 3 hours, contains 99.0–100.5% of $C_{12}H_{14}N_4O_4S$ (310.33).

Preparation—Sulfadimethoxine is prepared by the general method for N^1-substituted sulfanilamides (page 1195) using 4-amino-2,6-dimethoxypyrimidine as the amine participating in the condensation with the sulfonyl chloride.

Description—Occurs as a white, odorless, crystalline powder.

Solubility—1 Gm dissolves in about 200 ml of alcohol and about 50 ml of 2 N hydrochloric acid; insoluble in water; slightly soluble in ether, chloroform, and solvent hexane; readily soluble in 2 N sodium hydroxide.

Uses—The actions and uses of sulfadimethoxine are those of the antimicrobial sulfonamides in general (see the general statement, page 1195). However, it is characterized by slow renal excretion, and hence has not only a long duration of action but also a negligible incidence of crystalluria. Other toxicity can be considered to be the same as that of other sulfonamides. However, as with all long-acting sulfonamides, the Stevens-Johnson syndrome is a significant danger. A disadvantage to its long duration of action is that when toxicity occurs, the drug can not be removed quickly from the body.

Dose—**500 mg** to **1 Gm;** *usual, initial,* **2 Gm,** then **1 Gm** daily.

Dosage Forms—Oral Suspension NF: 250 mg/5 ml; Tablets NF: 250 and 500 mg.

Veterinary Dose—*Horses* and *Pigs, parenterally,* **25 mg** per **pound** of body weight; *Dogs* and *Cats, parenterally* or *orally,* **12.5 mg** per **pound** as first dose, followed by **6.25 mg** per **pound** at 24-hour intervals. Increased dosage (to 25 mg per pound 1 to 3 times daily) is indicated in severe infections. Do not administer to pigs over 6 weeks old or to animals intended for use as food.

Sulfaethidole NF

[N^1-(5-Ethyl-1,3,4-thiadiazol-2-yl)sulfanilamide; Sulfaethylthiadiazole; Sul-Spansion and Sul-Spantab (*SK&F*)]

Sulfaethidole, dried at 105° for 2 hours, 98.5–100.5% of $C_{10}H_{12}N_4O_2S_2$ (284.36).

Preparation—Sulfaethidole may be prepared by the general method for N^1-substituted sulfanilamides described on page 1195 using 5-ethyl-2-amino-1,3,4-thiadiazole for the condensation with the sulfonyl chloride.

Description—It occurs as crystals which melt between 185.5° and 186.0°. It is faintly acid to litmus.

Solubility—1 Gm dissolves in 4000 ml of water, 40 Gm of methanol, 30 Gm ethanol, 10 Gm acetone, 1350 Gm ether, 2800 Gm chloroform, and 20,000 Gm of benzene.

Uses—Sulfaethidole shares the antimicrobial actions and uses of *Sulfadiazine* (page 1200), except that it poorly penetrates the blood–brain barrier and hence cannot be employed to treat meningitis. It has a biologic half-life of about 8 hours in man, but with sustained-release preparations a much longer duration of action is achieved. The degree of acetylation of the drug in the body is low; only 5 to 10% of the drug in the urine is in the conjugate form. Since the solubility of the unchanged drug is fairly high, the incidence of crystalluria is considerably lower than that of sulfadiazine.

Dose—**1.3** to **3.9 Gm** daily; *usual, initial,* **2.6 Gm,** then **1.3 Gm** every 12 hours.

Sulfamerazine USP

[N^1-(4-Methyl-2-pyrimidinyl)sulfanilamide; Sulfamethyldiazine]

$$H_2N \text{—} \text{⟨ ⟩} \text{—} SO_2NH$$
(pyrimidine ring with CH$_3$)

Sulfamerazine contains 99.0–100.5% of $C_{11}H_{12}N_4O_2S$ (264.31), calculated on the dried basis.

Preparation—Sulfamerazine may be prepared by the method described for sulfadiazine, using 4-methyl-2-aminopyrimidine instead of 2-aminopyrimidine.

Description—White or faintly yellowish white crystals or powder. It has a slightly bitter taste and is odorless or nearly so. It is stable in air, but slowly darkens on exposure to light. It melts between 234° and 238°.

Solubility—1 Gm dissolves in about 6250 ml of water at 20° and about 3300 ml at 37°; readily soluble in dilute mineral acids and solutions of potassium, ammonium, and sodium hydroxides; sparingly soluble in acetone; slightly soluble in alcohol; very slightly soluble in ether and chloroform.

Incompatibilities—See introduction to this section (page 1197).

Uses—Sulfamerazine closely resembles sulfadiazine in its *antibacterial* properties, toxicity, and therapeutic uses. It is widely employed alone and in sulfonamide mixtures in those infections in which the systemic antimicrobial actions of the sulfonamides are indicated. (See general statement, page 1197, and *Sulfadiazine,* page 1200.)

Sulfamerazine is more completely absorbed from the gut and more slowly excreted by the kidneys than is sulfadiazine. Hence doses of Sulfamerazine required to maintain effective blood levels are smaller and are administered at slightly greater intervals than are those of sulfadiazine. Sulfamerazine is bound to plasma proteins to a greater extent than is sulfadiazine and its concentration in the cerebrospinal fluid is 30 to 70% of that in plasma. Consequently, it is necessary to maintain a higher blood level with Sulfamerazine in order to achieve an efficacy equal to that of sulfadiazine. Approximately 35 to 60% of the drug in the urine is in the inactive acetylated form. Both the free and acetylated forms are less soluble than those of sulfadiazine, so that crystalluria may occur, even despite a lower rate of excretion than with sulfadiazine.

Dose—**2** to **8 Gm** daily; *usual, initial,* **4 Gm,** then **1 Gm** 4 to 6 times a day.

Other Dose Information—In severe infections, the initial oral dose for adults of 3 to 4 Gm is followed by maintenance doses of 1 Gm every 6 hours until temperature has been normal for 5 to 7 days. Doses for children and infants and for moderate or mild infections in both adults and children are appropriately reduced.

Dosage Forms—Tablets NF: 500 mg.

Veterinary Dose—*Average oral dose,* **150 mg** per **Kg** of body weight daily for 2 days, then ½ this amount for 2 days longer.

Sodium Sulfamerazine

[Sulfamerazine Sodium USP XV]

Sodium Sulfamerazine [$C_{11}H_{11}N_4NaO_2S$ = 286.29] is sodium N^1-(4-methyl-2-pyrimidinyl)sulfanilamide.

Uses—See *Sulfamerazine.* Because the sodium salt is soluble, it is employed for parenteral administration.

Dose—*Usual, intravenous,* **2 Gm.**

Dosage Forms—Injection: 5%.

Veterinary Dose—*Cattle,* **200 mg** per **pound** of body weight.

Sulfamethazine USP

[Sulphadimidine; N^1-(4,6-Dimethyl-2-pyrimidinyl)sulfanilamide]

$$H_2N \text{—} \text{⟨ ⟩} \text{—} SO_2NH$$
(pyrimidine ring with two CH$_3$ groups)

Sulfamethazine contains 99.0–100.5% of $C_{12}H_{14}N_4O_2S$ (278.33), calculated on the dried basis.

Preparation—Sulfamethazine may be prepared by the general method for N^1-substituted sulfanilamides described on page 1195 using 2-amino-4,6-dimethylpyrimidine for the condensation with the sulfonyl chloride.

Description—A white or yellowish white, almost odorless powder which may darken on exposure to light. It has a slightly bitter taste. Melts between 197° and 200°.

Solubility—Very slightly soluble in water and ether; slightly soluble in alcohol; soluble in acetone.

Uses—Sulfamethazine closely resembles sulfamerazine in its antimicrobial properties, toxicity, and therapeutic uses. It is employed alone and as a component in sulfonamide mixtures in those infections in which the systemic antimicrobial actions of the sulfonamides are indicated. (See general statement, page 1197 and *Sulfamerazine,* this page.)

Sulfamethazine, like sulfamerazine, is more slowly excreted by the kidney than is sulfadiazine. Hence doses of sulfamethazine required to maintain effective blood levels are smaller and are administered at slightly longer intervals than are those of sulfadiazine.

Sulfamethazine is a pharmaceutical necessity for *Oral Trisulfapyrimidines Suspension* and *Trisulfapyrimidines Tablets.*

Dose—There is no official dose form for Sulfamethazine alone. However, it may be used separately from Trisulfapyrimidines combination.

Other Dose Information—In severe infections, the initial oral dose is 100 mg per Kg of body weight, regardless of age, but it should not exceed a total dose of 5 Gm. Maintenance doses of 1 Gm are administered every 6 hours in adults; in children, ¼ the initial dose is given every 6 hours. Appropriately smaller doses may be employed in mild or moderate infections.

Sulfamethizole NF

[N^1-(5-Methyl-1,3,4-thiadiazol-2-yl)sulfanilamide; Thiosulfil (*Ayerst*)]

$$H_2N \text{—} \text{⟨ ⟩} \text{—} SO_2NH$$
(thiadiazole ring with CH$_3$ and S, N—N)

Sulfamethizole, dried at 105° for 2 hours, contains 99.0–100.5% of $C_9H_{10}N_4O_2S_2$ (270.33).

Preparation—Sulfamethizole may be prepared by the general method for N^1-substituted sulfanilamides described on page 1195 using 5-methyl-2-amino-1,3,4-thiadiazole for the condensation with the sulfonyl chloride.

Description—It occurs as white crystals or powder. It has a slightly bitter taste and is almost odorless; it has no odor of hydrogen sulfide. Melting range 209° to 212°.

Solubility—1 Gm dissolves in about 2000 ml of water; freely soluble in solutions of ammonium, potassium, and sodium hydroxides; soluble in dilute mineral acids; soluble in acetone; sparingly soluble in alcohol; very slightly soluble in chloroform and ether; practically insoluble in benzene.

Uses—The antibacterial actions, uses, and toxicity of Sulfamethizole are those of the other sulfonamides (see general statement, page 1195); however, it has a high solubility, so that it is especially useful in the treatment of urinary tract infections. It only rarely induces crystalluria. There is very little cross-sensitization between sulfamethizole and other sulfonamides, so that it often may be used when sensitivity exists to other sulfonamides.

Dose—**500 mg** to **1 Gm**; *usual*, **500 mg** 4 times daily.

Dosage Forms—Oral Suspension NF: 250 mg/5 ml; Tablets NF: 250 mg.

Sulfamethoxazole NF

[N^1-(5-Methyl-3-isoxazolyl)-sulfanilamide; Gantanol (*Roche*)]

Sulfamethoxazole, dried at 105° for 4 hours, contains 98.5–100.5% of $C_{10}H_{11}N_3O_3S$ (253.28).

Preparation—Sulfamethoxazole may be prepared by the general method for N^1-substituted sulfanilamides (page 1195) using 3-amino-5-methylisoxazole as the coupling amine. The latter may be prepared by heating ethyl 5-methylisoxazole-3-carbamate with aqueous sodium hydroxide. US Pat. 2,888,455.

Description—White, crystalline powder. It is odorless and is stable in air. It melts between 169° and 171°.

Solubility—Practically insoluble in water, ether, and chloroform; 1 Gm dissolves in 50 ml of alcohol and about 4 ml of acetone; it dissolves in HCl or NaOH solutions through salt formation.

Uses—Sulfamethoxazole is closely related chemically to *Sulfisoxazole* (this page), which it resembles in its antibacterial spectrum. It is used in the treatment of infections of the skin and of pyodermata, as well as for urinary tract infections. Its efficacy in gonorrhea, meningitis, and serious respiratory tract infections has not been established. In fact, much of its usefulness remains to be determined. It is slowly and incompletely absorbed and is excreted more slowly than is sulfisoxazole, so that its duration of action is longer. Its toxicity is typical of sulfonamides, including crystalluria.

Dose—*Usual, initial,* **2 Gm**, then **1 Gm** 2 or 3 times daily.

Dosage Forms—Oral Suspension NF: 500 mg/5 ml; Tablets NF: 500 mg.

Sulfapyridine USP

[N^1-2-Pyridylsulfanilamide]

Sulfapyridine contains 99.0–100.5% of $C_{11}H_{11}N_3O_2S$ (249.29), calculated on the dried basis.

Preparation—Sulfapyridine is prepared by the general method for N^1-substituted sulfanilamides (page 1195) using 2-aminopyridine as the coupling amine. The latter may be prepared by slowly adding sodamide to pyridine and hydrolyzing the resulting 2-sodamidopyridine.

Description—White or faintly yellowish white crystals, granules, or powder. It is odorless or nearly so, and is stable in air, but slowly darkens on exposure to light. It melts between 191° and 193°.

Solubility—1 Gm dissolves in about 3500 ml of water, about 440 ml of alcohol, and about 65 ml of acetone; freely soluble in dilute mineral acids and aqueous solutions of potassium and sodium hydroxides.

Incompatibilities—See introduction to this section (page 1197).

Uses—Sulfapyridine has been largely replaced by equally effective and less toxic congeners. It induces a high incidence of leukopenia, agranulocytosis, drug fever, and dermatoses. It is now only of historical interest and cannot be recommended for therapeutic use, except as an *anti-infective* in *dermatitis herpetiformis*, for which use this drug has maintained its official status.

Dose—**2** to **6 Gm** daily; *usual,* **500 mg** to **1 Gm**, 4 times a day.

Dosage Forms—Tablets USP: 500 mg.

Veterinary Dose—*Average dose,* **60** to **90 mg** per **pound** of body weight daily in divided doses.

Sulfisoxazole USP

[N^1-(3,4-Dimethyl-5-isoxazolyl)sulfanilamide; Gantrisin (*Roche*); Entusul (*USV*)]

Sulfisoxazole contains 99.0–101.0% of $C_{11}H_{13}N_3O_3S$ (267.31), calculated on the dried basis.

Preparation—Sulfisoxazole is prepared by the general method for N^1-substituted sulfanilamides described on page 1195 using 3,4-dimethyl-5-amino isoxazole for the condensation with the sulfonyl chloride.

Description—A white to slightly yellowish, odorless, crystalline powder. Melts between 194° and 199°.

Solubility—1 Gm dissolves in about 6700 ml of water and about 10 ml of boiling alcohol; soluble in diluted hydrochloric acid.

Uses—The *antibacterial* properties and therapeutic uses of Sulfisoxazole resemble those of sulfadiazine. However, it is not always effective against infections which are sensitive to other sulfonamides. On the other hand, urinary tract infections caused by *Proteus* group bacteria respond favorably; consequently, the drug finds favor in the treatment of urinary tract infections. However, Sulfisoxazole does not penetrate cells and hence is not able to reach intracellular bacteria. It is secreted into prostatic fluid but it is not known whether it is secreted into other genitourinary fluids. Sulfisoxazole is rapidly excreted by the kidney and reaches high concentrations in the urine. Since both the free and acetylated forms of Sulfisoxazole are highly soluble, even in acidic urine, adjuvant alkali therapy is not necessary and fluids need not be forced. The incidence of renal toxicity is lower than that caused by sulfadiazine or the sulfonamide mixtures. With this exception, untoward effects during Sulfisoxazole therapy are similar to those caused by the other sulfonamides.

Dose 1 to 8 Gm daily; *usual, initial,* **4 Gm,** then **1 Gm** 4 to 6 times a day.

Other Dose Information—In *meningitides,* the total dose during the first day of medication should be 8 to 12 Gm.

Dosage Forms—Tablets USP: 500 mg.

Sulfisoxazole and Phenazopyridine Hydrochloride Tablets NF

[Azo-Gantrisin (*Roche;* Azo-Entusul *USV*]

Sulfisoxazole and Phenazopyridine Hydrochloride Tablets contain 95.0–105.0% of the labeled amount of $C_{11}H_{13}N_3O_3S$ (sulfisoxazole), and 90.0–110.0% of the labeled amount of $C_{11}H_{11}N_5 \cdot HCl$ (phenazopyridine hydrochloride).

Uses—Sulfisoxazole and Phenazopyridine Hydrochloride combination is employed only for treatment of susceptible urinary tract infections. For the actions of the separate components, see *Sulfisoxazole* (page 1203) and *Phenazopyridine Hydrochloride* (page 1186).

The patient should be advised of the effect of the Phenazopyridine to color the urine (see page 1186).

Dose—*Usual,* sulfisoxazole, **1 Gm** 4 times a day; phenazopyridine hydrochloride, **100 mg** 4 times a day.

Dosage Forms—Tablets NF: 500 mg (sulfisoxazole) and 50 mg (phenazopyridine hydrochloride).

Trisulfapyrimidines Oral Suspension USP

[Oral Trisulfapyrimidines Suspension (USP XV); (*Various Mfgs.*)]

Trisulfapyrimidines Oral Suspension contains, in each 100 ml, 9.3–10.7 Gm of total sulfapyrimidines. It contains, in each 100 ml, 3.0–3.7 Gm of $C_{10}H_{10}N_4O_2S$ (sulfadiazine), of $C_{11}H_{12}N_4O_2S$ (sulfamerazine), and of $C_{12}H_{14}N_4O_2S$ (sulfamethazine). Trisulfapyrimidines Oral Suspension may contain either sodium citrate or sodium lactate, and may contain a suitable antimicrobial agent.

Uses—The *antibacterial* spectrum and therapeutic uses of sulfonamide mixtures are the same as those of the individual components. An advantage of such mixtures is the lesser incidence of crystalluria and renal injury associated with their use. (See general statement, page 1197.)

Dose—20 to 80 ml daily; *usual, initial,* **40 ml** (4 Gm of trisulfapyrimidines), then **10 ml** (1 Gm) 4 to 6 times a day.

Trisulfapyrimidines Tablets USP

Trisulfapyrimidines Tablets contain 95.0–105.0% of the labeled amount of total sulfapyrimidines, consisting of $C_{10}H_{10}N_4O_2S$ (sulfadiazine), $C_{11}H_{12}N_4O_2S$ (sulfa-

merazine), and $C_{12}H_{14}N_4O_2S$ (sulfamethazine). The amount of each of the three sulfapyrimidines is 31.5–35.0% of the labeled amount of total sulfapyrimidines.

Uses—See *Trisulfapyrimidines Oral Suspension.*

Dose—2 to 8 Gm daily; *usual, initial,* **4 Gm;** then **1 Gm** 4 to 6 times a day.

Other Sulfonamides

Acetyl Sulfamethoxypyridazine [Kynex Acetyl (*Lederle*); Midicel Acetyl (*Parke-Davis*)] is N^1-acetyl-N^1-(6-methoxy-3-pyridazinyl)sulfanilamide [$C_{13}H_{14}N_4O_4S$]. *Description and Solubility:* A fine, white to yellowish white powder, which is essentially tasteless and odorless; it melts between 186° and 187°. 1 Gm dissolves in about 5000 ml of water, 500 ml of alcohol, 500 ml of propylene glycol, and 5 ml of dimethylacetamide. *Uses:* The same as those of *Sulfamethoxypyridazine* (page 1205), to which it is in a large part converted in the body. Because it is tasteless, it is better suited to liquid medication, especially for pediatric use. *Dose:* Oral, for children, 250 mg per 20 pounds of body weight on the first day and thereafter 125 mg per 20 pounds daily or 250 mg per 20 pounds every other day: for adults, the dose is that of *Sulfamethoxypyridazine* (page 1205).

Mafenide Acetate [Sulfamylon Acetate (*Winthrop*)] is α-amino-*p*-toluenesulfonamide acetate. *Uses:* Mafenide is a sulfonamide developed in Germany during World War II. Although it enjoyed considerable use in Europe, in the US it was never much used. In recent years it has been revived, owing to its moderate efficacy against infections caused by *Staphylococcus aureus* and *Pseudomonas aeruginosa,* which are the two most common offenders in surgical infections and in infections in burns. Although it has been used systemically, its present-day use is topical only. Its mechanism of action is different from the other sulfonamides, so that it has a usefulness in sulfa-resistant infections. Untoward effects include vesicular eruptions, erythematous pruritus, and occasional erythema multiforme. *Dose: Topical,* as an 8.5% (of the base) cream. Clinical reports indicate that higher concentrations are more effective.

Mafenide Hydrochloride [Sulfamylon Hydrochloride (*Winthrop*)] is α-amino-*p*-toluenesulfonamide hydrochloride. *Description:* Crystals that melt at 256°; it is neutral in solution. *Uses:* See *Mafenide Acetate,* above. The hydrochloride in solution leaves the site of application much more rapidly than the acetate in the cream, so that the acetate cream is generally preferred. *Dose: Topical,* as a 5% (of the base) solution.

Para-Nitrosulfathiazole NF XI [*p*-Nitro-*N*-2-thiazolylbenzenesulfonamide; Nisulfazole (*Breon*)] [$C_9H_7N_3O_4S_2$]—A yellow, odorless powder having a slightly bitter taste. Melts between 258° and 266°. It is very slightly soluble in water, chloroform, or ether; slightly soluble in alcohol; freely soluble in solutions of fixed alkali hydroxides. *Uses:* An *antibacterial* agent employed solely by rectal instillation in the local treatment of *proctitis* and *chronic ulcerative colitis.* The drug is effective probably by reduction to sulfathiazole and subsequent alteration of the bacterial flora of the colon and rectum. It is poorly absorbed and systemic toxicity is negligible. The drug is available as a 10% suspension. The usual initial dose is 10 to 60 ml of a 10% suspension instilled rectally 4 times daily. After improvement, 10 to 30 ml are administered once nightly until 2 to 4 weeks after the mucosa has returned to normal. *Dose: Usual, rectally,* 100 mg.

Salicylazosulfapyridine [Azulfidine (*Pharmacia*)] is 5-[*p*-(2-pyridylsulfamoyl)phenylazo]salicylic acid [$C_{18}H_{14}N_4O_5S$]. *Description and Solubility:* Brownish yellow crystals which decompose between 240° and 245°. Practically insoluble in water, chloroform, and ether; slightly soluble in alcohol. *Uses:* Degraded in the body to salicylic acid and sulfapyridine, to which most of its action may be attributed. Consequently, the drug shares the high toxicity of *Sulfapyridine* (page 1203). Careful monitoring of the hematologic status of the patient is essential. Claims that it is selectively retained in connective tissue and hence has a special usefulness in ulcerative colitis are unsubstantiated. It probably has the same efficacy in ulcerative colitis as other sulfonamides, especially sulfapyridine. Relapses occur in about ⅓ of treated cases. To an alkaline urine the drug imparts a yellow color. *Dose: Usual,* 1 Gm 4 to 6 times a day. If a satisfactory response is obtained, the dose should be reduced to 500 mg 3 times daily.

Sodium Sulfabromomethazine NF XII [Sodium N^1-(5-Bromo-4,6-dimethyl)-2-pyrimidinyl)sulfanilamide] contains 97.0–102.0% of $C_{12}H_{12}BrN_4NaO_2S.H_2O$ (397.23), calculated on the dried basis. *Preparation:* By the general method for N^1-substituted sulfanilamides described on page 1195 using 2-amino-5-bromo-4,6-dimethyl pyrimidine for the condensation with the sulfonyl chloride. Reaction of the amide with an equimolar portion of NaOH yields the sodium salt. *Description and Solubility:* A white to light yellow, odorless or practically odorless powder; on prolonged exposure to air it absorbs carbon dioxide with the liberation of sulfabromomethazine and becomes incompletely soluble in water; it may darken on exposure to light. Freely soluble in water; slightly soluble in alcohol; very slightly soluble in ether, chloroform, and acetone. *Uses:* In cattle for infections susceptible to sulfonamide therapy, particularly bacterial infections such as shipping fever, pneumonia, foot rot, septic metritis, and in bovine coccidiosis. By the parenteral route its action lasts approximately 24 hours; by the oral route, 48 hours. *Veterinary Dose: Cattle, usual, oral,* 165 mg per Kg; *intraperitoneal,* 100 mg per Kg; *intravenous,* 50 mg per Kg.

Sulfachlorpyridazine [Sonilyn (*Mallinckrodt*)] is N^1-(6-chloro-3-pyridazinyl)sulfanilamide [$C_{10}H_9ClN_4O_2S$]. *Description and Solubility:* A yellow, crystalline powder having no more than a faint odor. Its loss on drying at 105° for 3 hours does not exceed 0.5%. At 37° in buffered media of pH 5, 6, and 7.5: 70, 200, and 500 mg%, respectively.

Uses: Sulfachlorpyridazine is similar to *Sulfisoxazole* (page 1203) in its actions and uses. It is useful in the treatment of urinary tract infections, especially those caused by *E. coli.* However, sometimes subjective improvement occurs in the absence of a demonstrable decrease in bacteriuria, so that frequent urine cultures should be made. It is absorbed rapidly from the gut and is excreted rapidly. Therefore, the urine concentration is high but the duration of action is brief. Although the drug is quite soluble and less than 50% acetylated, crystalluria does occur, and water intake should be increased. Other side effects are those of sulfonamides in general. If urticaria, rash, fever, sore throat, or hematuria occur, the drug should be discontinued. *Dose: Usual, initial,* 1 to 4 Gm; *usual, maintenance,* 1 Gm 3 to 6 times a day; *for children,* initially 65 mg per kg of body weight and 130 mg per kg per day in divided doses for maintenance.

Sulfaguanidine NF XI [N^1-Amidinosulfanilamide] [$C_7H_{10}N_4O_2S.H_2O$]—A white, needle-like, crystalline powder. It is odorless and stable in air. It melts between 190° and 193°. 1 Gm dissolves in about 1000 ml of water at 25°. It is sparingly soluble in alcohol and acetone. It is freely soluble in dilute mineral acids but insoluble in solutions of sodium hydroxide. *Uses:* Because it is poorly absorbed from the gastrointestinal tract, Sulfaguanidine was formerly employed as an *antibacterial* agent in intestinal chemotherapy. However, it is now *chiefly of historical interest* as the first sulfonamide to be so used, having been largely replaced by newer, more effective, and less toxic congeners. Its continued promotion is reprehensible. *Dose: Usual,* 2 Gm. If employed in bacillary dysentery, conventional oral dosage is 50 to 100 mg per Kg of body weight every 6 or 8 hours.

Sulfameter [Sulla (*Robins*)] is N^1-(5-methoxy-2-pyrimidinyl)sulfanilamide [$C_{11}H_{12}N_4O_3S$]. *Preparation:* By the general method for N^1-substituted sulfanilamides (page 1195) using 5-methoxy-2-aminopyrimidine as the coupling amine. *Description and Solubility:* A fine, white to yellowish white powder that is odorless and has a weak, bitter taste; it is stable in light, air, and heat; it melts between 207° and 211°. 1 Gm dissolves in about 80 ml of acetone; practically insoluble in water, alcohol, ether, carbon tetrachloride, chloroform, and solvent hexane.

Uses: Sulfameter is a long-acting sulfonamide similar to *Sulfadimethoxine* (page 1201) and *Sulfamethoxypyridazine* (this page), over which it has no advantage. Like the other long-acting sulfonamides, the persistence of high concentrations in the plasma appears to contribute to the incidence, seriousness, and slow onset of adverse reactions. Fatalities due to erythema multiforme exudativum (Stevens–Johnson syndrome) have occurred following Sulfameter. For this reason, medical authorities recommend that short-acting sulfonamides be used instead of Sulfameter. The slow rate of excretion of Sulfameter keeps the urine concentration low, which avoids crystalluria but which also renders the drug less effective in the treatment of urinary tract infections than short-acting sulfonamides. The drug should not be used in children under 12, pregnant women near term, or nursing mothers. *Dose: Usual, initial,* 1.5 Gm; *maintenance,* 500 mg a day.

Sulfamethoxypyridazine USP XVII [N^1-(6-Methoxy-3-pyridazinyl)sulfanilamide; Kynex (*Lederle*); Midicel (*Parke-Davis*)] contains not less than 99.0% of $C_{11}H_{12}N_4O_3S$ (280.31), calculated on the dried basis. *Preparation:* Sulfanilamide is fused with 3,6-dichloropyridazine to yield N^1-(6-chloro-3-pyridazinyl) sulfanilamide. Condensation with sodium methoxide replaces the 6-chlorine with methoxy. The compound may also be prepared by the general method for N^1-substituted sulfanilamides described on page 1195 using 3-amino-6-methoxypyridazine for the condensation with the sulfonyl chloride. *Description and Solubility:* A white or yellowish white, crystalline powder that is odorless or nearly so, and stable in air but slowly darkens on exposure to light; it has a bitter aftertaste; melting range, 180° to 183°. Very slightly soluble in water; sparingly soluble in alcohol and acetone; freely soluble in dilute mineral acids and solutions of alkali hydroxides.

Uses: Possesses antibacterial activity approximately equivalent to that of sulfadiazine. However, it is more completely absorbed from the gastrointestinal tract than sulfadiazine. Effective blood levels can be achieved more reliably and with a smaller dose because its rate of excretion is very slow, so that it has an exceptionally long duration of action for a sulfonamide. Consequently, it is quite useful in prophylaxis, as for example, in the prevention of streptococcal infections in rheumatic fever patients. It is also useful in *urinary tract* and *upper respiratory infections, bacillary dysenteries, dermatitis herpetiformis, acne vulgaris,* and many *soft tissue infections.* Because of the low rate of excretion, lower urine levels are achieved than with other sulfonamides. Therefore, crystalluria is rare. Except for less crystalluria, its toxicity is comparable to that of sulfadiazine, except that skin rashes are more likely to occur than with shorter acting sulfonamides. However, when toxicity does occur, the slow dissipation of the drug is a distinct disadvantage. For this reason, shorter acting sulfonamides are preferred. *Dose:* 500 mg to 1 Gm; *usual, initial,* 1 Gm, then 500 mg daily. *Veterinary Uses:* For the treatment of sulfa-susceptible bacterial infections of the urogenital, respiratory, and gastrointestinal tracts of dogs and cats. *Veterinary Dose: Dogs and Cats,* 20 to 30 mg per pound of body weight once or twice daily. Avoid excessive dosage. Continue treatment until patient is symptom-free for 48 hours.

Sulfanilamide NF XI [Sulfamidyl; *p*-Aminobenzene-sulfonamide] [$C_6H_8N_2O_2S$]—White crystals, granules or powder. It melts between 164.5° and 166.5°. 1 Gm dissolves in about 125 ml water, about 37 ml alcohol, and about 5 ml acetone; it is also soluble in glycerin, hydrochloric acid, and solutions of potassium and sodium hydroxide; insoluble in chloroform, ether, and benzene. *Uses:* It has largely, if not entirely, been replaced by its equally effective but less toxic congeners. It is now only of historic interest and cannot be recommended for therapeutic use. Its continued use in topical preparations is a violation of the principles of chemotherapy and should be condemned. *Dose:* 2 Gm.

Sulfaphenazole [N^1-(1-phenylpyrazol-5-yl)sulfanilamide; Sulfabid (*Purdue-Frederick*)] [$C_{15}H_{14}N_4O_2S$]—White to light-yellow, fine, crystalline powder. It melts between 179° and 183°. It is practically insoluble in water; freely soluble in acetone, acetic acid, and methanol; soluble in dilute alkalies and dilute mineral acids. *Uses:* A long-acting sulfonamide with actions, uses, and toxicity comparable to those of other sulfonamides. See the general statement, page 1195. Its long duration of action is advantageous in the convenience of administration but disadvantageous when toxicity occurs. *Dose: orally,* initially, 2 to 3 Gm and 1 Gm every 12 hours thereafter.

Sulfathiazole NF XI [N^1-2-Thiazolylsulfanilamide]— [$C_9H_9N_3O_2S_2$]—White or faintly yellow-white crystals, granules or powder. It melts between 200° and 204°. 1 Gm dissolves in about 1700 ml of water and about 200 ml of alcohols. It is soluble in acetone, diluted mineral acids, and aqueous solutions of alkali hydroxides. *Uses:* It has been largely now only of historical interest and cannot be recommended for therapeutic use. Its continued use in topical preparations for application to the nasopharynx or vagina is a violation of the principles of antibacterial therapy and can only be condemned, especially since Sulfathiazole is one of the two sulfonamides most likely to cause hypersensitivity. *Dose:* 0.5 to 1.0 Gm 4 times daily.

Sulfisomidine [Sulphasomidine BP; Elkosin (*Ciba*)] is N^1 - (2,6 - dimethyl - 4 - pyrimidinyl)sulfanilamide ($C_{12}H_{14}$-N_4O_2S). *Description:* Needles which melt at 243°. Aqueous solutions are neutral to litmus. Compared with sulfanilamide, it is but slightly acetylated in the body. *Note: Do not confuse with sulfamethazine.* Solubility: In water (at 15°), 0.12 Gm per 100 ml; in water (at 30°), 0.30 Gm per 100 ml; more soluble in hot water (about 1 Gm in 60 ml); in urine (at 37°), 360 mg per 100 ml at pH 5.5 as compared to 1100 mg per 100 ml at pH 7.5; slightly soluble in alcohol and acetone; practically insoluble in benzene, ether, and chloroform.

Uses: The drug is used for the same purposes as the rest of the antimicrobial sulfonamides. Since very little of the drug is acetylated in the body and the free form is soluble in acid urine, crystalluria is uncommon, and alkalization of the urine is unnecessary. The drug is especially used in the treatment of urinary tract infections. *Dose: Initial,* oral, 100 mg per Kg of body weight; *maintenance,* ⅙ the initial dose, given every 4 hours until control of the infection is effected, whereupon the dose is given every 6 hours.

Sulfisoxazole Diethanolamine USP XVI [The diethanolamine salt of sulfisoxazole, $C_{11}H_{13}N_3O_3S.C_4H_{11}NO_2$]— A slightly yellowish crystalline powder. Melting range 120° to 123°. It is very soluble in water and soluble in alcohol; very slightly soluble in chloroform; practically insoluble in ether. *Uses:* Salt is more soluble than the parent compound at physiological pH. Consequently, it is employed for the parenteral administration of sulfisoxazole. Its action are those of *Sulfisoxazole* (page 1203). The salt is also employed in ophthalmic preparations. *Dose:* As a 40% solution for *intramuscular* or slow *intravenous* drip. No more than 5 ml should be given into any one intramuscular site. For *subcutaneous* administration, 5%, or less, solutions are used. The total dose should not exceed that of *Sulfisoxazole* (page 1203). 4 Gm every 8 to 12 hours may be used in lieu of the more frequent *oral* administration. *Topically* to the eye, as a 4% solution or ointment, 3 or 4 times daily.

Antibiotics

Antibiotic substances are chemical compounds produced as a result of the metabolic activities of living cells and which inhibit, in very low concentrations, the growth of microorganisms. While antibiotics have been isolated from tissues of higher plants and animals, the term generally has come to refer to inhibitory substances of microbial origin. The antagonistic effect of one microorganism upon the development of others has been recognized since the early days of bacteriology, and the formation of inhibitory substances is but one expression of microbial antagonism.

From the standpoint of chemotherapy and pharmacology, two milestones mark the historical development of the field of antibiotics: (1) discovery by Chain, Florey, and associates at Oxford University of the unusually favorable therapeutic and pharmacological properties of extracts of cultures of the mold *Penicillium notatum,* found to produce *penicillin* by Fleming in 1929; and (2) Dubos' discovery in 1939 of *tyrothricin* and its *in vivo* efficacy against certain virulent bacterial infections. As a result of these studies, and particularly because of the demands due to World War II, a remarkable impetus was imparted to the search for new antibiotics. During the decade 1940–1950 a large number were described, and in the following nine years still more were reported and research in this field continues unabated.

The increased use of antibiotics in man and animals and the extension of uses to areas other than the treatment and prophylaxis of disease has created unsuspected problems that during the past few years have become more acute. More and more strains of organisms have emerged resistant to the available antibiotics and this is particularly true of penicillin, the most widely used. The staphylococci have created the greatest problem and in "closed populations" such as hospitals frequently 90% of the strains isolated are resistant to penicillin G.

The wide use of antibiotics, particularly penicillin, in animal nutrition and in agriculture as well as in disease, has resulted in the sensitization of a relatively large number of the susceptible people, many of whom react violently in contact with these drugs.

In this chapter Penicillin is considered in considerable detail since it is typical. It was the first antibiotic to be produced commercially and still assumes a position of major importance in this field.

Detection and Isolation of Antibiotic-Producing Organisms

The detection of these organisms is based on a distinctive property of antibiotics, namely, the ability to inhibit certain test bacteria under controlled conditions *in vitro.* The nature of the antibiotic found can, to some extent, be influenced by the specific test organism employed. Thus, the use of a certain strain of *S. aureus* as the test organism will detect all antibiotics inhibitory to that organism, but the antibiotic may or may not also be effective against *E. coli,* for example, or even against various other strains of *S. aureus.* To insure securing a valid antibacterial spectrum, a number of species and types of strains must be used in the testing.

Antibiotic-producing organisms can be obtained by: (1) testing pure cultures of organisms available in culture collections or isolated from natural sources, and (2) "screening," or selection through suitable techniques from the vast heterogeneous mixed population of the soil or other natural habitations of microorganisms. In the first case the practice consists simply of adding to broth or agar cultures, seeded with the test organism, suitable quantities or culture filtrates of the cultures being examined, incubating, and inspecting for inhibition of the test organism. The screening method involves plating out in serial dilution an aqueous extract of soil or other natural substrate using agar medium previously seeded with the test organism. During incubation the various organisms of the soil population develop, and those forming antibiotic substances are distinguished by a clear zone or halo around the colony, indicative of inhibition of the test organism which, in the region beyond the clear zone, grows abundantly in the form of a marked turbidity throughout the agar. Innumerable modifications of this principle are possible, depending on the objective of the investigator and upon his ingenuity. Thus, use of different media will expose for screening different types of soil organisms; the same applies to the pH of the medium, temperature of incubation, etc. These must, however, not be incompatible with the growth of the particular test organism employed. Theoretically, the best chance for detecting the largest possible number of antagonists lies in the preincubation for a few days of the agar cultures containing the soil dilutions, but without the test bacteria. This is followed by a secondary incubation after the test organism is applied to the plate by streaking or spraying. In this manner slow-growing soil organisms are given the opportunity to develop and manifest antibiotic-producing ability.

Once detected, the antagonist is isolated in pure culture and identified, and the conditions for maximum production of the antibiotic substance produced by it are investigated. Generally, this involves finding the optimum temperature, pH, and age of the culture. Important also is the composition of the medium. Different organic and inorganic nitrogenous substances are tested, with and without various carbohydrates, minerals, heavy metals, etc. Once a favorable medium is established, other known strains of the antagonist, obtained either from stock culture collections or isolated from nature, are compared for the character and amount of the antibiotic produced, and the highest yielding strain selected for further work. The antibacterial spectrum is obtained, ie, the relative effectiveness of the antibiotic in inhibiting the growth of a large variety of Gram-positive and Gram-negative bacteria, rickettsiæ, viruses, and fungi, especially those which are pathogenic. This identifies those infections in which it may be useful chemotherapeutically. Several concentrates of the antibiotic, not necessarily pure, are then examined for toxicity in mice. Only low toxicity preparations and, in particular, those in which toxicity is inversely proportional to the antibacterial potency are of interest. Toxicity and pharmacological data are obtained in animals and, if favorable, in clinical trials on human beings. If the clinical trials show the antibiotic to be a promising therapeutic agent, attention is turned to large-scale manufacture. Chemical studies of the structure of the pure compound will indicate the feasibility of chemical synthesis. Generally, antibiotics are complex, rather large molecular weight substances whose synthesis may be extremely difficult of at least uneconomical, compared to microbiologic production. This is the case now with most of the successful antibiotics, such as penicillin, streptomycin, chlortetracycline, etc.

The gradual increase in numbers of strains of microorganisms resistant to antibiotics, especially the staphylococci, and the numbers of individuals developing sensitivity to them make it extremely desirable that screening programs for the isolation and development of new agents be continued. A number of the antibiotics have been used in combinations. In certain diseases such as bacterial endocarditis, tuberculosis, and brucellosis such use has been quite successful. The emergence of resistant organisms has been delayed or prevented and markedly superior results in treatment have been obtained. In mixed infections combinations of antibiotics and combinations of an antibiotic with one or more of the sulfonamides have been used with excellent results in selected cases.

Production of Antibiotics

The development and operation of the large-scale commercial production of antibiotic substances may be exemplified by a description of the manufacture of penicillin. In general, the approach and methods employed are typical. Two types of processes for the microbiological production of antibiotics are known: (1) *the surface process*, in which the antibiotic-producing organism grows in the form of a pad on the surface of a liquid medium in trays or bottles, or on the surface of a finely divided moist solid substrate such as wood shavings, wheat bran, etc; (2) *the submerged process*, in which the organism develops in a liquid medium, maintained continuously under mechanical agitation and aeration, so that the organism develops uniformly and homogeneously in the form of a suspension of single cells, or small aggregates or colonies, throughout all portions of the culture liquid. The penicillin is excreted into the culture fluid. The molds used industrially today are derived from *Penicillium chrysogenum*.

The Submerged Process—This process, in which growth is greatly accelerated and the handling of large quantities greatly facilitated, is considerably more efficient than surface processes, and hence is the only feasible method for large-scale commercial production. Stationary, closed, iron, or stainless steel cylindrical-shaped tanks, known as fermenters, of 5000 to 30,000 gallons capacity, are used in penicillin manufacture. Most of these are equipped with vertical single shaft propeller or turbine type agitators and with a mechanical means of comminuting and distributing sterile air, introduced for maximum dispersal effect in the region of the agitator. Some use sterile air only for agitation. The tanks have a detachable manhold on the top, sight glasses, and outlets to valve-closed sampling lines and accessory feed chambers, enabling inoculation by hand if necessary, particularly in small seed tanks, and the addition whenever necessary of other (sterile) materials, such as antifoam agents, during the fermentation. All outlets from the tank are exposed continuously to flowing steam to minimize chances of contamination. The culture medium is sterilized by high-pressure steam and cooled by brine. Temperature control during growth of the mold is maintained automatically at 23–25°. The compressed air, which is introduced into the fermenters, is sterilized by filtration through steam-sterilized cartridges of suitable size and filled, for example, with glass wool.

Inoculum for large tanks is obtained by building up the amount of growth successively through a series of seed tanks, from tank to tank, and transferring under air pressure through sterile pipe lines. Generally this massive inoculum amounts to 5 to 10% of the main batch, and consequently, seed tanks are about $\frac{1}{10}$ the volume of the next larger tank. The first and smallest seed tank is inoculated with a laboratory-prepared culture, consisting either of spores or of a small flask of submerged growth obtained on a laboratory, rotary, or reciprocal-type shaking machine.

The stock or master culture of the penicillin-producing mold is dry and cold-preserved in the form of spores. Continuous vegetative transfer of the mold on artificial media leads to loss of penicillin-producing power (physiological degeneration). Hence, the number of intermediate transfers between master culture and the final batch is kept at a minimum.

A Typical Production Medium

Corn-steep liquor (solids)	2 to 5%
Crude lactose	2 to 3%
Calcium carbonate	0.5 to 1%

The culture medium used for commercial penicillin production almost invariably contains a natural, complex, nitrogenous material, corn-steep liquor, which is a by-product of the corn-milling industry. This has a unique stimulating effect on penicillin formation due in part to its content of certain amino acids, minerals, and precursors which are utilized for direct conversion into the penicillin molecule. The penicillin potency is followed by assay every 3 to 6 hours and, at the time when the potency stops rising, the batch is harvested. Maximum activity generally is reached in 50 to 90 hours. Due to the instability of penicillin at ordinary temperatures, the batch is cooled to 5° and the mycelium filtered off by pressure filtration.

The penicillin is extracted and concentrated by two general processes: (1) charcoal adsorption, and (2) solvent extraction.

In the *charcoal adsorption process*, activated charcoal adsorbs the penicillin, and after filtration, the penicillin is eluted with a solvent such as an 80% solution of acetone in water. The eluate is concentrated by evaporation, cooled to 0°, and acidified with mineral acid to pH 2.0. Penicillin, a rather strong acid, is extractable at this pH into organic solvents; amyl acetate is generally used. The low temperature minimizes losses due to the extreme instability of penicillin at pH 2.0.

In the *solvent extraction process* the penicillin is extracted from the filtrate by a water-immiscible solvent after the solution has been adjusted to pH of 2 to liberate the acid form of penicillin, which is soluble in organic solvents while the sodium salt is insoluble. A number of successive extractions, at carefully adjusted pH values, reduces the volume and separates the large majority of impurities. From the immiscible solvents the penicillin is re-extracted with a dilute solution of sodium bicarbonate, thus forming *penicillin sodium* which is soluble in water but not in the immiscible solvent. This aqueous solution ("rich water") is rendered sterile and pyrogen-free by passage through suitable filters, and a sample taken for the determination of the potency. The liquid is frozen to prevent any decomposition while the analysis is being made. After the analysis is completed, the frozen liquid is melted and again filtered through suitable filters to further insure freedom from bacterial and pyrogenic contaminations. The required volume of the solution, to yield the unitage required, is placed in sterile and pyrogen-free bottles, and the latter are then placed in vacuum chambers capable of being highly refrigerated. After the liquid has frozen the vacuum is turned on, causing the water to sublime leaving a dry amorphous powder.

Freeze-drying is no longer used commercially. All penicillin now available is crystalline and produced by solvent extraction processes.

Improvements in Production—The greatest advancements in the production of penicillin have been (1) the use of the submerged or tank method of production, (2) the use of corn-steep liquor, and (3) progressive improvement in the penicillin-producing capacity of the mold.

The earliest widely used strain in tank production was *Penicillium notatum*, No. 832, which yielded 50 to 60 units per ml. Later, a strain of *Penicillium chrysogenum*, No. 1951B25, with maximum yields of 250 units per ml, was discovered. Spores of this organism, exposed to x-ray irradiation and tested from single spore isolates led to selection of a mutant strain X1612 producing approximately 500 units per ml. Strain X1612 was subjected to ultraviolet irradiation and strain Q176, yielding penicillin potencies of more than double that of X1612, was obtained. This strain has been widely used in commercial production, but industry has even improved on it. Some variant strains produce several thousand units per ml. The improvement in strains suitable for the surface production of penicillin followed a similar path although these were obtained by testing single spore isolates from parent cultures. A strain excellent in submerged culture is not necessarily good for surface culture, and *vice versa*. Surface culture methods are no longer used for commercial production of any of the presently useful antibiotics.

A large number of different fungi are now known to produce penicillin. Up to now some 20 different species of fungi belonging to the genera *Aspergillus* and *Penicillia* have been reported to produce penicillin, and, in addition, the dermatophyte *Trichophyton mentogrophytes* and a thermophilic fungus *Malbranchea pulchella*.

Antibiotic Control

Federal control of antibiotics dates back to an amendment of the 1938 Food and Drug Cosmetic Act (Section 507) under which the Food and Drug Administration was required to pretest all forms of penicillin and its preparations before releasing them for sale. This certification covered potency, demonstration of nontoxicity, and moisture content (the presence of excess moisture makes penicillin less stable). When intended for parenteral use, it was also tested for freedom from pyrogens, for sterility, and for the clarity and pH of its solutions.

This amendment included the provision that when it was found by the Federal Security Administrator (now Secretary of the Department of Health, Education, and Welfare) that the pretesting of penicillin or its preparations was no longer necessary to insure safety and efficacy of such drugs, they could be exempted from the pretesting requirement.

Under this provision of the Act the Federal Security Agency, FDA Division, finding that certain new, highly purified forms of penicillin no longer required pretesting, issued a notice in the Federal Register of April 13, 1949, exempting Crystalline Penicillin G Potassium and Crystalline Penicillin G Sodium from this provision.

In March, 1947, the Congress of the United States placed streptomycin under the certification system and in July of 1949 included chlortetracycline, chloramphenicol, and bacitracin. Since these amendments included all derivatives as well, both dihydrostreptomycin and tetracycline, as well as pyrrolidinomethyl tetracycline and demeclocycline were certifiable drugs.

In May, 1963, the Drug Amendments passed by Congress in 1962 became effective and superseded all previous rulings. These now provide that *all* antibiotics used in humans are subject to certification. Furthermore, those certifiable prior to passage of these latest amendments, ie, chlortetracycline, bacitracin, streptomycin, penicillin, and chloramphenicol, must also be certified for veterinary use.

Amphotericin B—see page 1256.

Bacitracin USP

[Ayfivin; Penitracin; Topitracin; Zutracin]

Bacitracin is a polypeptide produced by the growth of the *licheniformis* group of *Bacillus subtilis* (Fam. *Bacillaceæ*). It has a potency of not less than 40 USP Units* of bacitracin activity per mg, except that when intended for parenteral use its potency is not less than 50 Units per mg. Bacitracin conforms to the regulations of the federal Food and Drug Administration concerning antibiotic drugs (see page 1206).

Bacitracin is a mixture of several polypeptides, mostly Bacitracin A, with a molecular weight of about 1460. The structure of Bacitracin A has been shown to be

in which the detailed structure at the upper right represents a cyclic condensation moiety derived from cysteine and isoleucine.

Preparation—A method for the production of Bacitracin was patented by Commercial Solvents in 1958, although it was prepared in 1945 by shallow culture of *Bacillus subtilis.*[1-3]

Description—A white to pale buff powder, odorless, or has a slight odor. It is hygroscopic. Its solutions rapidly deteriorate at room temperature. Bacitracin is precipitated from its solutions and is inactivated by salts of many of the heavy metals. Bacitracin solutions retain their potency for several weeks if kept in a refrigerator.

Solubility—Freely soluble in water; soluble in alcohol, methanol, and glacial acetic acid, although the solution in the organic solvents usually shows some insoluble residue; insoluble in acetone, chloroform, and ether.

Uses—Bacitracin is largely limited in its use to infections which can be treated by topical application or local infiltration. The high incidence of nephrotoxicity which follows its parenteral administration precludes systemic use except in life-endangering infections in which other antibiotics have proved to be ineffective. However, this drug has proved to be life saving in a large number of cases. At the present time it is available for parenteral use with warnings concerning its possible toxic reactions.

Bacitracin is employed in *surgical infections* caused by pathogens sensitive to the antibiotic; these infections include carbuncles, felons, superficial and deep abscesses, infected traumatic and operative wounds, infected ulcers, and chronic osteomyelitis.

Bacitracin is effective in the treatment of the following *cutaneous bacterial infections* where the pathogen is bacitracin-sensitive: impetigo contagiosa, folliculitis, pyoderma, ecthyma, furunculosis, decubitus ulcer, infectious eczematoid dermatitis, scabies, and dermatophytosis. The drug is used in the treatment of *ophthalmological conditions* including styes, acute and chronic conjunctivitis, corneal ulcer, keratitis, and dacryocystitis. *Infections of the ear, mouth, and nasopharynx* such as Vincent's angina, pharyngitis, chronic suppurative otitis media, and mastoiditis have been successfully treated with bacitracin.

Bacitracin has been effectively used orally for the management of *intestinal amebiasis*, but more potent amebicides are available.

Development of organism resistance is much less frequent and slower for bacitracin than for penicillin, and for most organisms is essentially nil. The drug is not inactivated by the metabolic products of mixed infections.

In addition to renal damage, toxic effects of parenteral bacitracin include pain, induration and petechiæ at the site of injection, skin rash, malaise, anorexia, nausea, and vomiting. In a few instances tinnitus and a peculiar taste in the mouth may be noted. Oral administration of commonly employed doses induces no toxic effects; it is poorly absorbed from the gastrointestinal tract. Topical application is usually not irritating and rarely induces allergic reactions.

Dose—*Intramuscular,* **30,000 to 100,000 Units** daily; *usual, intramuscular,* **10,000 to 20,000 Units** 3 to 4 times a day; *topically,* as ointment containing **500 Units** per **Gm** 2 or 3 times a day.

Other Dose Information—Ointments are applied directly to the involved area one or more times daily. Troches are dissolved slowly in the mouth for superficial infections of the oral mucosa. The dry powder (or soluble tablets if to be used locally) is dissolved in sufficient isotonic sodium chloride solution to yield a final concentration of 500 to 1000 units of bacitracin per ml, which is usually considered optimal for topical use on skin and mucous membranes, for aerosol inhalation, and for local infiltration. Procaine solution, 2% in isotonic sodium chloride solution, may be used as a diluent for solutions injected intramuscularly, using a quantity sufficient to make a concentration of 10,000 units per ml. Procaine should not be used in bacitracin solutions injected into cerebral tissue or into spinal fluid. Bacitracin solutions retain their potency for several weeks if kept in a refrigerator.

Dosage Forms—Ointment USP (see below); Ophthalmic Ointment; Sterile USP: 10,000 and 50,000 Units.

Bacitracin Ointment USP is bacitracin or zinc bacitracin in an anhydrous ointment base. It contains, in each Gm, not less than 500 USP Units of bacitracin activity. *Preparation:* Levigate bacitracin (500,000 Units) with mineral oil (65 Gm), and incorporate it with white petrolatum (925 Gm) to make about 1000 Gm. For a firmer preparation, replace up to 40 Gm of the mineral oil by an equal amount of white petrolatum.

Zinc Bacitracin USP

Zinc Bacitracin is the zinc salt of bacitracin. It has a potency of not less than 40 Units of bacitracin activity per mg. Zinc Bacitracin conforms to the regulations of the federal Food and Drug Administration concerning antibiotic drugs (see page 1206).

Description—White to pale tan powder, odorless or having a slight odor; hygroscopic.

Solubility—Sparingly soluble in water.

---

* The USP Unit of Bacitracin is the bacitracin activity exhibited by the weight of USP Bacitracin Reference Standard indicated on the label of the Standard. The USP unit and that defined by the federal Food and Drug Administration are equivalent.

Uses—Zinc Bacitracin is incorporated into various ointments for topical antibiotic therapy (see *Bacitracin*, page 1209). It is more stable than bacitracin, and the zinc may enhance the activity of the antibiotic.

Dose—*Topically*, as an ointment containing **500 Units** per **Gm** 2 or 3 times a day.

Bacitracin, Zinc, Neomycin Sulfate, and Polymyxin B Sulfate Ointment—see page 1220.

Candicidin—see page 1257.

Chloramphenicol USP

[D-*threo*-(−)-2,2-Dichloro-N-[β-hydroxy-α-(hydroxymethyl)-p-nitrophen-ethyl]acetamide; Amphicol (*McKesson*); Chloromycetin (*Parke-Davis*); Cylphenicol (*Trent*); Tega-Cetin (*Ortega*)]

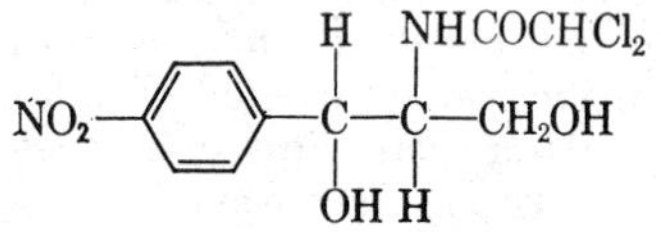

Chloramphenicol contains not less than 90.0% of $C_{11}H_{12}Cl_2N_2O_5$ (323.13). It conforms to the regulations of the federal Food and Drug Administration concerning antibiotic drugs (see page 1206).

Preparation—Chloramphenicol is believed to be the first naturally occurring compound studied thus far which contains a nitro group or which is a derivative of dichloroacetic acid. It is optically active and it is related to *l-norpseudo*ephedrine stereochemically. Using planar formulas, it is represented by the above structure where the secondary hydroxyl group and the acylamido group are on opposite sides. Of the four stereoisomers having the basic structure of Chloramphenicol only the one represented by the natural product has antibiotic activity.

Chloramphenicol can be obtained from the filtrate of a *Streptomyces* culture by extraction with ethyl acetate. If the charcoaled extract is rich in Chloramphenicol the latter can be crystallized from the ethylacetate by diluting with many volumes of kerosene.

Several synthetic methods for the preparation of Chloramphenicol are known. One of the best-known commences with *p*-nitroacetophenone and proceeds as follows:

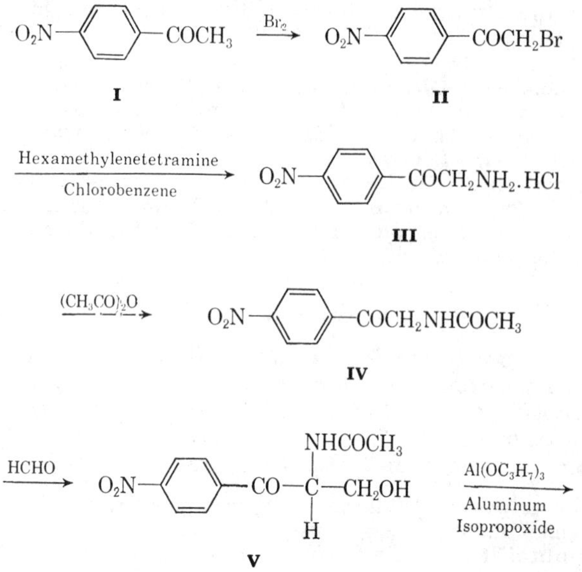

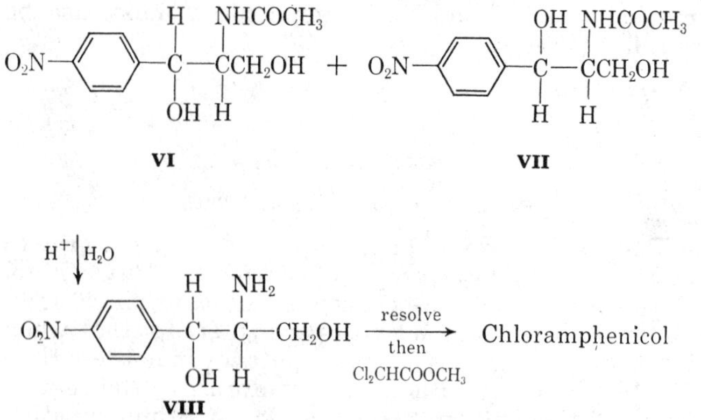

The conversion of *p*-nitro-2-bromoacetophenone, **II**, to the *p*-nitro-2-aminoacetophenone hydrochloride, **III**, is accomplished by mixing the bromo compound with hexamethylenetetramine in chlorobenzene, separation of the complex salt, and hydrolysis of the latter with hydrochloric acid. It should be noted that the reduction of **V** with aluminum isopropoxide in isopropyl alcohol produces two *dl*-mixtures, **VI** and **VII**, and that only **VI** is useful for conversion to Chloramphenicol. The amino-diol **VIII** is resolved using *d*-camphorsulfonic acid. The levo rotating base obtained from the resolution is heated with methyl dichloroacetate to form chloramphenicol.

Description—Fine white to grayish white or yellowish white, needle-like crystals or elongated plates. Odorless. Intensely bitter taste. Its solutions are neutral to litmus. It is reasonably stable in neutral or moderately acid solutions but is rapidly destroyed in alkaline solutions. Melting range: 149° to 153°. Specific rotation in dehydrated alcohol +17° to +20° (C = 5).

Solubility—1 Gm dissolves in about 400 ml of water; freely soluble in alcohol, acetone, butanol, propylene glycol, and ethyl acetate; slightly soluble in ether and chloroform; insoluble in benzene and petroleum ether.

Uses—Chloramphenicol has a wide spectrum of antibacterial activity. The drug is effective in the following: *rickettsial diseases* including epidemic, murine, and scrub typhus, Rocky Mountain spotted fever, rickettsial pox, and Q fever; *virus diseases* including the psittacosis-lymphogranuloma group; and *many bacterial infections* including those caused by *A. aerogenes*, *E. coli*, *K. pneumoniae*, *H. pertussis*, *E. typhosa*, *Brucella*, and *V. cholerae*. Because of serious toxic reactions, the systemic use of the drug has been sharply curtailed. However, it is still used much too promiscuously. It is still the drug of choice for typhoid fever, except in infants. Medical authorities are divided on whether it should be first choice over ampicillin for meningitis or severe respiratory infections caused by *H. influenzae* or with streptomycin in *Klebsiella pneumonia*. It should never be used in mild infections. Chloramphenicol is used topically for conjunctival infections and blepharitis caused by susceptible organisms.

Bone marrow injury is the major toxic effect of Chloramphenicol. Thrombocytopenia, granulocytopenia, and aplastic anemia are the most serious hematopoietic disturbances observed and have resulted in a number of fatalities. The mechanism of the bone marrow injury is unknown. Any patient under treatment with Chloramphenicol must be given a leukocyte and differential count every other day. Minor untoward effects such as transient mild euphoria, skin rash, and gastrointestinal disturbances (occasional nausea and vomiting, gaseous distention, loose stools, and pruritus ani) have been observed. Occasional untoward effects include glossitis, stomatitis, and pharyngitis. Very rarely, optic neuritis may result from Chloramphenicol therapy. The use of Chloramphenicol, as with other antibiotics, may result in an overgrowth of micro-organisms not susceptible to the drug. In neonates Chloramphenicol may cause fatal cyanosis, vomiting, abdominal distention, and loose, green stools, owing to the inability of the infant to metabolize the drug in consequence of glucuronyl transferase deficiency.

Chloramphenicol is rapidly absorbed from the gastro-intestinal tract; significant serum levels are obtained in 30 minutes and peak blood concentrations of 40 to 60 mcg per ml (after 4-Gm dose) are reached in about 2 hours; the drug is no longer detectable in the blood after 12 to 18 hours. Sixty per cent of Chloramphenicol in the blood is bound to serum albumin. The microsomal system of liver is the major site of degradation. The antibiotic is excreted in the urine; 80 to 92% of a single dose is excreted in 24 hours, only 5 to 10% of which is in a biologically active form.

Dose—*Oral* or *intravenous*, **50** to **100 mg** per **Kg**; *usual*, *oral*, **50 mg** per **Kg** of body weight daily, in 4 divided doses; *usual*, *intravenous*, **50 mg** per **Kg** of body weight daily, in 2 or 3 divided doses; *intramuscular*, **1 Gm** every 8 hours; *topically*, as a **0.16** to **1%** ointment or solution 4 to 12 times a day.

Dosage Forms—Capsules USP: 50, 100, and 250 mg; Ophthalmic Ointment USP: 1%; for Ophthalmic Solution USP: 25 mg; Sterile for Suspension NF: 1 Gm.

Note—The Food and Drug Administration no longer permits the marketing of preparations for intramuscular use, even though the NF lists the Sterile Suspension.

Veterinary Dose—The suggested dosage for dogs and cats is **25** to **75 mg** per **pound** of body weight daily in 3 doses. In large animals a daily intramuscular dose of 2 mg per pound has been found effective.

Chloramphenicol Palmitate USP

[Chloramphenicol α-Palmitate; Chloromycetin Palmitate (*Parke-Davis*)]

Chloramphenicol Palmitate ($C_{27}H_{42}Cl_2N_2O_6$ = 561.55) contains 55.5–59.5% of chloramphenicol ($C_{11}H_{12}Cl_2N_2O_5$ = 323.13). Chloramphenicol Palmitate conforms to the regulations of the federal Food and Drug Administration concerning antibiotic drugs (see page 1206).

Preparation—Chloramphenicol is esterified by treatment with palmitoyl chloride [$CH_3(CH_2)_{14}COCl$] in the presence of pyridine. The crude ester is obtained by pouring the reaction product into a large excess of dilute hydrochloric acid and filtering. It is then purified by recrystallization from an appropriate solvent.

Description—A fine, white, unctuous, crystalline powder, having a faint odor and a bland, mild taste. It melts between 86° and 92°.

Solubility—Insoluble in water; very slightly soluble in solvent hexane; soluble in ether; sparingly soluble in alcohol; freely soluble in acetone and chloroform.

Uses—Chloramphenicol Palmitate lacks the bitter flavor of chloramphenicol. It is hydrolyzed in the upper intestinal tract to chloramphenicol. Therefore, its oral uses are those of the parent drug (see *Chloramphenicol*); however, it does not share the topical efficacy of the parent drug. Its toxicity is likewise that of chloramphenicol; thus it should not be used unless certain severe criteria of indication are met. Since the absorption of the chloramphenicol depends upon the hydrolysis of the palmitate ester, the blood levels of chloramphenicol rise more slowly after an oral dose than with the parent chloramphenicol, and its duration of action is somewhat longer.

Dose—The equivalent of **50** to **100 mg** of chloramphenicol per **Kg** daily; *usual*, the equivalent of **12.5 mg** of chloramphenicol per **Kg** of body weight 4 times a day.

Dosage Forms—Oral Suspension USP: the equivalent of 1.875 Gm of chloramphenicol/60 ml.

Chloramphenicol Sodium Succinate USP

Chloramphenicol α-(Sodium Succinate); Chloromycetin Succinate (*Parke-Davis*)]

Chloramphenicol Sodium Succinate contains an amount of chloramphenicol sodium succinate [$C_{15}H_{15}Cl_2N_2NaO_8$ = 445.19] equivalent to not less than 90.0% of the labeled content in terms of chloramphenicol, calculated on the anhydrous basis. It conforms to the regulations of the federal Food and Drug Administration concerning antibiotic drugs (see page 1206).

Preparation—Chloramphenicol is reacted with an equimolar portion of succinic acid anhydride to yield chloramphenicol hydrogen succinate which, after purification by recrystallization, is neutralized with sodium hydroxide to give the official ester-salt.

Description—Light yellow, crystalline powder.
Solubility—Freely soluble in water and alcohol.

Uses—Chloramphenicol Sodium Succinate is useful for parenteral administration by virtue of its high aqueous solubility. Its effectiveness *in vivo* depends on the liberation of the parent compound by hydrolysis, and, therefore, its uses are similar to those of chloramphenicol. Chloramphenicol Sodium Succinate may be preferred when oral therapy is not feasible, or when rapid attainment of a high blood level is desired. The toxicity of Chloramphenicol Sodium Succinate is similar to that of the parent drug; thus it should not be used unless certain severe criteria of indication are met.

Dose—*Intravenous*, the equivalent of **50** to **100 mg** of chloramphenicol per **Kg** daily; *usual*, the equivalent of **12.5 mg** of chloramphenicol per **Kg** of body weight 4 times a day.

Dosage Forms—Sterile USP: 250 mg and 1 Gm.

Chlortetracycline Hydrochloride NF

[7 - Chloro - 4 - (dimethylamino) - 1,4,4a,5,5a,6,11,12a - octahydro - 3,6,10,-12,12a - pentahydroxy - 6 - methyl - 1,11 - dioxo - 2 - naphthacenecarboxamide Monohydrochloride; 7-Chlortetracycline Hydrochloride; Chlortetracyclinium Chloride; Aureomycin Hydrochloride (*Lederle*)]

Chlortetracycline Hydrochloride contains not less than 90.0% of $C_{22}H_{23}ClN_2O_8 \cdot HCl$ (515.35). Chlortetracycline Hydrochloride conforms to the regulations of the federal Food and Drug Administration concerning certification of antibiotic drugs (see page 1206).

Preparation—*Streptomyces aureofaciens*, Duggar, is grown in an appropriate nutrient medium under controlled conditions of temperature, pH, and aeration. The chlortetracycline produced is recrystallized from various solvents at controlled acidity and is converted to the hydrochloride.

Description—A yellow, odorless, bitter, crystalline powder, which is stable in air. It is slowly affected by light.

Solubility—1 Gm dissolves in 75 ml of water and about 560 ml of alcohol; soluble in solutions of alkali carbonates and hydroxides; practically insoluble in acetone, chloroform, dioxane, and ether.

Uses—Chlortetracycline Hydrochloride is a broad spectrum *antibiotic* and *antiprotozoan* which suppresses the growth of most Gram-positive bacteria, many Gram-negative bacteria, spirochetes, amebæ, and certain large viruses. Its clinical spectrum comprises most of the infections amenable to therapy with penicillin and streptomycin, with the important exception of tuberculosis. The drug is effective against certain other diseases in addition; however, even among bacterial genera and species generally susceptible to chlortetracycline, there are found naturally drug-resistant strains and there is an increasing number of strains with acquired resistance. Staphylococci, particularly, have largely become resistant to the drug. Acquired resistance usually develops more slowly and to a lesser degree than with penicillin. Cross-resistance to all other tetracyclines is automatic.

Among the bacterial infections in which Chlortetracycline Hydrochloride may be employed, although not necessarily as the drug of choice in each instance, are *most coccal infections* including those caused by sensitive hemolytic streptococci, staphylococci, pneumococci, meningococci, and gonococci; *subacute bacterial endocarditis;* many urinary tract infections, especially those caused by certain staphylococci, streptococci, *E. coli, A. aerogenes;* bacillary infections such as *brucellosis, tularemia, influenza,* certain *meiningitides, pertussis, peritonitis,* and *E. coli* infections, and some infections caused by *Salmonella* and *Shigella; chancroid; rat bite fever;* clostridial infections; several *ocular infections;* and numerous other diseases. The antibiotic is used orally to "sterilize" the bowel prior to bowel surgery. Rickettsial diseases such as *Rocky Mountain spotted fever, murine and endemic typhus,* and *Q-fever* respond well to Chlortetracycline therapy. *Syphilis* responds to Chlortetracycline treatment, but penicillin remains the drug of choice. In *intestinal amebiasis* the antibiotic has a place, but it is inferior to the related oxytetracycline and to several other agents. Chlortetracycline is also of value in the treatment of certain viral diseases such as *lymphogranuloma venereum* and *psittacosis.*

Untoward effects during therapy with Chlortetracycline are usually mild, but serious effects may occur. After oral administration, as the result of local irritation, epigastric distress, heartburn, anorexia, nausea, and vomiting may develop; antacids, milk, or other food taken with the drug reduce the incidence of such effects. The oropharyngeal and other mucous membranes become irritated, and lesions, some of which are caused by emergent yeast and fungi as the floral balance is upset, may appear. Alterations in intestinal flora, especially upon repeated oral ingestion of the antibiotic, cause diarrhea; occasionally emergent enterococci or other organisms cause serious and sometimes fatal gastroenteritis. Chlortetracycline causes local irritation, especially when unbuffered; rapidly ad-ministered intravenous doses may cause phlebitis, and intramuscular injections frequently produce pain or tenderness at the site of injection. Large intravenous doses may temporarily induce hepatic dysfunction. Drug fever and hypersensitivity reactions are rare but are on the increase.

Chlortetracycline may form a stable calcium complex in any bone-forming tissue. No serious harmful effects have been reported thus far in humans; however, use of this drug during tooth development may cause discoloration of the teeth. This results mostly from long-term use, but it has also occurred during short courses of treatment.

Chlortetracycline is incompletely absorbed from the gastrointestinal tract, especially with total daily doses above 1 Gm. Food in the stomach or upper intestine interferes with absorption. Also, calcium-containing antacids, aluminum hydroxide, or magnesium trisilicate complex or adsorb the drug and diminish absorption. Plasma levels remain in the effective range for longer than 6 hours; the half-life of the drug in the body is about 6 hours. The drug is distributed generally throughout the body; however, it enters the cerebrospinal fluid and certain other body fluids poorly, although meningitis will augment penetration into the cerebrospinal fluid. The drug is concentrated in bile. The antibiotic is partly excreted, and urinary concentrations may be high.

Chlortetracycline is usually orally administered. Large oral priming doses are no longer given because of the ceiling to the amount absorbed by this route. When the patient is unable to take the drug by mouth, a buffered solution may be given intravenously. Absorption from intramuscular sites is erratic. Intrathecal administration is not advised and may be dangerous. A variety of solutions and ointments are used topically, especially for ophthalmic purposes.

Dose—**250** to **500 mg**; *usual,* **250 mg** 4 times a day. *topically,* ophthalmic, **1** or **2 drops** of a **0.5**% solution every 2 hours,

Other Dose Information—Intravenous, 250 to 500 mg; topically, in solution to the lids or conjunctiva as required. In mild infections, 250 mg every 6 hours is the usual regimen; in severe infections, the size of the dose or the frequency of administration may be doubled. In infants and children, 25 to 50 mg per Kg of body weight. Some diseases are treated in courses: amebiasis, 10 days; pinworm, 7 days; acute gonorrhea, 2 doses of 500 mg at 6-hour intervals; bacterial endocarditis, 6 to 8 weeks longer than the termination of symptoms; hemolytic streptococcal infections, 10 days; brucellosis, 1 Gm 2 times a day the first week, then 1 Gm daily for 2 more weeks, to be supplemented with concurrent streptomycin treatment.

Dosage Forms—Capsules NF: 50, 100, and 250 mg; for Injection NF: 500 mg; Ophthalmic NF: 25 mg.

Veterinary Dose—*Orally,* except in herbivorous animals, **10** to **25 mg** per **pound** of body weight followed every 12 hours by 5 to **12.5 mg** per **pound** of body weight; *intravenously,* 2 to **5 mg** per **pound** of body weight followed by ½ this dose at 12-hour intervals (a 2.5% solution is usually employed).

Colistin Sulfate NF

[Coly-Mycin S Pediatric (*Warner-Chilcott*)]

Colistin Sulfate is the sulfate salt of an antibacterial substance produced by the growth of *Bacillus polymyxa* var. *colistinus.* It consists primarily of colistin

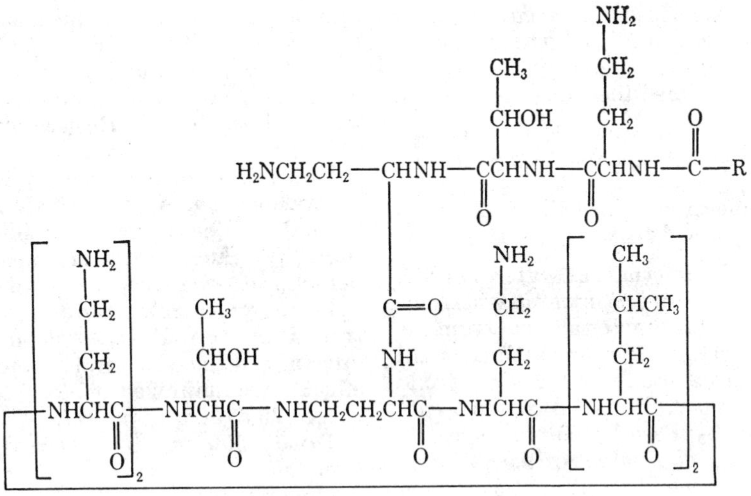

Colistin A R = 5 methylheptyl
Colistin B R = 5 methylhexyl

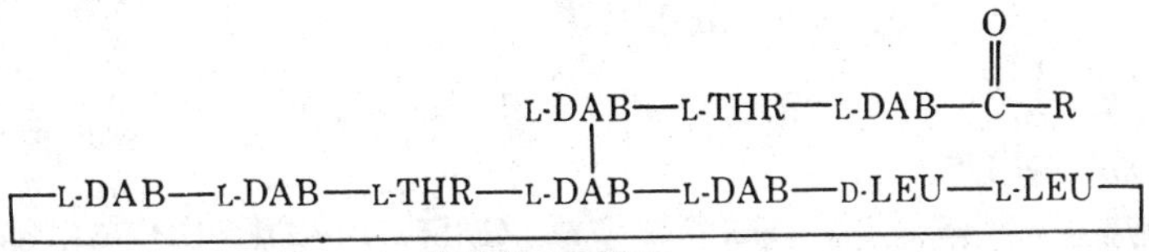

L-DAB—L-THR—L-DAB—C—R

—L-DAB—L-DAB—L-THR—L-DAB—L-DAB—D-LEU—L-LEU—

Colistin Sulfate

A with small amounts of colistin B. It has a potency of not less than 500 mcg of colistin base activity per mg. Colistin Sulfate conforms to the regulations of the federal Food and Drug Administration concerning certification of antibiotic drugs (see page 1206).

The colistins are monoacylated decapeptides with seven of the amino acid residues in cyclic union. Colistin B [$C_{52}H_{98}N_{16}O_{13}$ = 1155.46] is but a deshomologue of Colistin A [$C_{53}H_{100}N_{16}O_{13}$ = 1169.49]. The scheme beneath the structure identifies the individual amino acids; the notation DAB signifies 2,4-diaminobutyric acid.

Description—White to slightly yellow, odorless, fine powder. Its solutions are more stable at an acidic pH than

treatment of children with acute enteritis caused by *Pseudomonas* and *E. coli*. Colistin Sulfate is not absorbed orally except in infants, in whom significant blood levels can be obtained by this route of administration. Infants receiving colistin sulfate should be examined frequently for impairment of renal function.

Dose—*Usual*, 3 to 5 mg of the base per **Kg** of body weight daily in 3 divided doses.

Dosage Forms—for Oral Suspension NF: 300 mg (base activity)/70-ml container.

Sodium Colistimethate USP

[Pentasodium Colistinmethanesulfonate; Sodium Colistinmethanesulfonate; Polymyxin E; Coly-Mycin M Injectable (*Warner Chilcott*)]

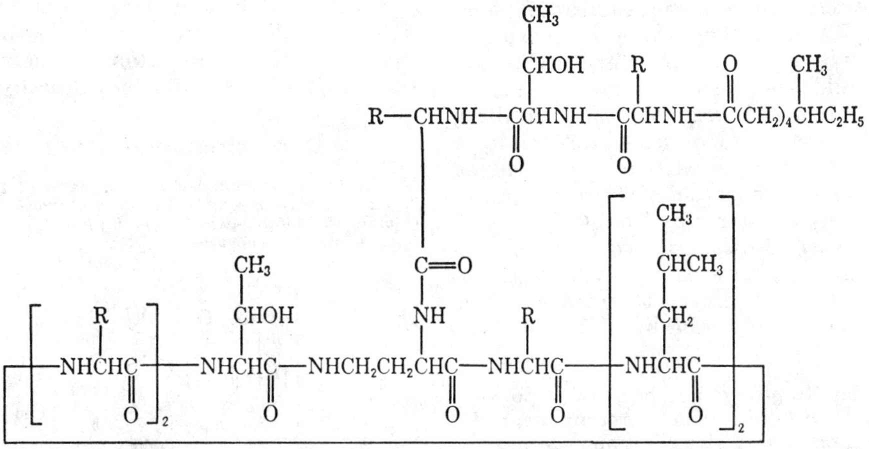

R = —CH₂CH₂NHCH₂SO₂ONa

at an alkaline pH. The dry powder is stable indefinitely.

Solubility—Freely soluble in water; slightly soluble in methanol; insoluble in acetone and ether.

Uses—Although indications for the use of Colistin Sulfate are the same as for polymyxin B (see page 1231), the former is preferred because of its lower toxicity. Colistin sulfate is especially effective in the

Sodium Colistimethate [$C_{58}H_{105}N_{16}Na_5O_{28}S_5$ = 1749.84] contains the pentasodium salt of the penta-(methanesulfonic acid) derivative of colistin A as the major component, with a small proportion of the pentasodium salt of the same derivative of colistin B. It conforms to the regulations of the federal Food and Drug Administration concerning antibiotic drugs (see page 1206).

Preparation—Purified colistin is treated with formaldehyde in aqueous solution, and the resulting colistin-formaldehyde complex (pentamethylolcolistin) is reacted with sodium bisulfite to generate the penta(methanesulfonate).

Description—White to slightly yellow, odorless, fine powder.

Solubility—Freely soluble in water; slightly soluble in methanol; insoluble in acetone and ether.

Uses—Since Sodium Colistimethate is water soluble, it is a suitable form of colistin for intramuscular injection. It has the same antibacterial spectrum as *Colistin* (above) against certain Gram-negative bacilli and it also elicits the same renal and neural toxic symptoms. The drug is especially useful in the treatment of infections caused by *Pseudomonas* species.

Dose—*Intramuscular*, the equivalent of **1.5 to 5 mg** of colistin per **Kg** of body weight daily; *usual*, the equivalent of **1 mg** of colistin per **Kg** of body weight 2 to 4 times a day.

Dosage Forms—for Injection USP: 30 and 150 mg.

Cycloserine USP

[D-(+)-4-Amino-3-isozazolidinone; Seromycin (*Lilly*)]

Cycloserine is a substance produced by the growth of *Streptomyces orchidaceus* or obtained by synthesis. It contains not less than 90.0% of $C_3H_6N_2O_2$ (102.09). Cycloserine conforms to the regulations of the federal Food and Drug Administration concerning antibiotic drugs (see page 1206).

Preparation—Cycloserine may be isolated from the fermentation of *Streptomyces garyphalus* or made synthetically as follows.

DL-Serine, converted to its methyl ester hydrochloride by Fischer esterification, is treated with ethyl iminobenzoate to give DL-2-phenyl-4-carbomethoxy-2-oxazoline which is reacted with hydroxylamine and sodium ethoxide. Acidification of the reaction mixture yields DL-2-phenyl-4-carbohydroxamido-2-oxazoline which is treated with hydrogen chloride in dry dioxane to give DL-α-benzamido-β-chloropropionohydroxamic acid. The hydroxamic acid is treated with 1 N alkali followed by acidification to form DL-4-benzamido-3-isoxazolidone which is treated with a concentrated solution of methanolic hydrogen chloride to give DL-β-(aminooxy)alanine methyl ester dihydrochloride. Reaction of the ester with potassium hydroxide forms DL-cycloserine. This racemate is resolved with D-tartaric acid to give D-cycloserine D-tartrate which is converted to Cycloserine by Amberlite IR-120 resin. US Pat. 2,773,878.

Description—A white to pale yellow, crystalline powder. It is odorless or has a faint odor. It is hygroscopic and deteriorates upon absorbing water. Its solutions are dextrorotatory.

Solubility—Freely soluble in water.

Uses—Cycloserine inhibits a wide variety of both Gram-positive and Gram-negative bacteria, including mycobacteria. However, Pseudomonas, Proteus and gonococci are resistant. It has been used successfully against stubborn urinary tract infections caused by streptococci, staphylococci, coliform bacteria and *Aerobacter aerogenes*. However, interest mainly centers upon its moderate usefulness in the therapy of tuberculosis resistant to other drugs; it is a "back-up" drug secondary to isoniazid, streptomycin, and aminosalicylic acid. It is commonly combined with other antituberculosis drugs. Resistance to cycloserine does develop.

Depending on the dose, toxic effects referable to the central nervous system occur in a large percentage of patients. These are reversible on discontinuance of therapy. Such effects are headache, vertigo, lethargy, behavioral changes, psychotic episodes, and convulsions. Central nervous system toxicity can be controlled by the administration of pyridoxine, anticonvulsants, sedatives, and tranquilizing agents. Toxic effects are minimized if blood levels of the drug do not exceed 25 to 30 mcg per ml.

Dose—**250 mg to 1 Gm** daily; *usual*, **250 mg** 2 times a day.

Dosage Forms—Capsules USP: 250 mg.

Demeclocycline NF

[7 - Chloro - 4 - (dimethylamino) - 1,4,4a,5,5a,6,11,12a - octahydro - 3,6,10, 12,12a- pentahydroxy- 1,11- dioxo-2- naphthacenecarboxamide; 7- Chloro-6 demethyltetracycline]

Demeclocycline contains not less than 97.0% of $C_{21}H_{21}ClN_2O_8$ (464.86), calculated on the anhydrous basis. Demeclocycline conforms to the regulations of the federal Food and Drug Administration concerning certification of antibiotic drugs (see page 1206).

For the structure, see *Demeclocycline Hydrochloride*.

Preparation—see *Demeclocycline Hydrochloride*.

Description—A yellow, crystalline powder. It is odorless and has a bitter taste. Its 1 in 100 solution has a pH of about 4.8.

Solubility—Sparingly soluble in water; soluble in alcohol; readily dissolves in dilute hydrochloric acid and in alkaline solutions.

Uses—See *Demeclocycline Hydrochloride*.

Dose—**150 to 900 mg** a day; *usual*, **600 mg** daily in 4 divided doses of 150 mg each or 2 divided doses of 300 mg each.

Dosage Forms—for Oral Suspension NF: an amount of demeclocycline equivalent to 900 mg of demeclocycline hydrochloride/60-ml container; Oral Suspension NF: an amount of demeclocycline equivalent to 75 mg of demeclocycline hydrochloride/5 ml.

Demeclocycline Hydrochloride NF

[7 - Chloro - 4 - (dimethylamino) - 1,4,4a,5,5a,6,11,12a - octahydro - 3,6,10,- 12,12a- pentahydroxy- 1,11- dioxo- 2- naphthacenecarboxamide Monohydrochloride; 7-Chloro-6-demethyltetracycline Hydrochloride; Demethylchlortetracycline Hydrochloride NF XII; DMCT; Ledermycin; Declomycin (*Lederle*)]

Demeclocycline Hydrochloride contains not less than 90.0% of $C_{21}H_{21}ClN_2O_8 \cdot HCl$ (501.32). Demeclocycline Hydrochloride conforms to the regulations of the federal Food and Drug Administration concerning certification of antibiotic drugs (see page 1206).

Preparation—An appropriate mutant strain of *Streptomyces aureofaciens* is grown in an appropriate liquid nutrient medium under controlled conditions of temperature, pH, and aeration. The harvested broth is acidified and filtered, and the antibiotic is isolated from the filtrate, either by solvent extraction or by chemical precipitation, and converted into the hydrochloride.

Description—Occurs as a yellow, crystalline powder. It is odorless and has a bitter taste. pH of 1 in 100 solution is about 2.5.

Solubility—1 Gm dissolves in about 90 ml of water and about 980 ml of alcohol; sparingly soluble in solutions of alkali hydroxides and carbonates; practically insoluble in acetone and chloroform.

Uses—Demeclocycline belongs to the tetracycline group and is the 6-desmethyl analog of *Chlortetracycline* (page 1211). It has a broad spectrum of activity similar to other members of the group, but its potency *in vitro* against most of the organisms susceptible to the group is equal to or greater than that of the other tetracycline compounds. It is better absorbed after oral administration than chlortetracycline and oxytetracycline, but not as well absorbed as tetracycline. Its half-life is about 12 hours, so that its duration of action is longer than that of tetracycline, chlortetracycline, or oxytetracycline. Because of its lower rate of excretion, its efficacy against urinary tract infections is compromised. In general, Demeclocycline has the same uses as the other tetracyclines. Also, the incidence and type of side effects encountered with this drug are similar to those of the other tetracyclines. However, photodynamic and photosensitivity reactions appear more frequently with Demeclocycline. Aluminum hydroxide preparations or milk should not be taken with the drug, since these interfere with its gastrointestinal absorption.

Dose—**150** to **900 mg** a day; *usual*, **600 mg** daily in 4 divided doses of 150 mg each or 2 divided doses of 300 mg each.

Dosage Forms—Capsules NF: 75 and 150 mg; Tablets NF: 75, 150, and 300 mg.

Erythromycin USP

[5 - (4 - Dimethylaminotetrahydro - 3 - hydroxy - 6 - methyl - 2 - pyranyloxy) - 6,11,12,13 - tetrahydroxy - 2,4,6,8,10,12 - hexamethyl - 9 - oxo - 3 (tetrahydro - 5 - hydroxy - 4 - methoxy - 4,6 - dimethyl - 2 - pyranyloxy)-pentadecanoic Acid, μ-Lactone; E-Mycin (*Upjohn*); Erythrocin (*Abbott*); Ilotycin (*Lilly*)]

ployed as a back-up drug for penicillin, when penicillin fails, and often in lieu of penicillin in mild infections, especially in pediatrics. It may be appreciably more active against Gram-positive organisms and definitely less active against coliform and enteric bacilli than are the tetracyclines or streptomycin. The drug is equally effective against both penicillin-sensitive and penicillin-resistant strains of staphylococci; it is also active against bacteria which have developed resistance to streptomycin. It has been shown to have *in vivo* activity against amebae, treponemes, and pinworms. The activity demonstrated by erythromycin against certain of the large viruses and rickettsia places this drug in the so-called "broad-spectrum" group, since it attacks three types of microorganisms (bacteria, rickettsia, and viruses) although showing a low activity against some of the important disease producing organisms of the Gram-negative group. Except for carbomycin, spiramycin, and oleandomycin, there is no cross resistance between erythromycin and other antibiotics. However, bacteria that are multiple-resistant to Erythromycin and one or more other antibiotics are becoming more frequent.

Erythromycin is particularly effective in medical and surgical infections caused by Gram-positive cocci, including staphylococci, streptococci, and pneumococci. It has been successfully employed in systemic infections caused by these organisms, including *pneumonia, empyema, meningitis, bacteremia, osteomyelitis,* and *wound infections.* The antibiotic is not particularly effective against *Str. faecalis* infections and is not uniformly curative in subacute bacterial endocarditis. Miscellaneous infections responding to Erythromycin therapy include *Vincent's stomatitis, granuloma inguinale, psittacosis,* the *diphtheria* carrier state, and micrococcic (staphylococcic) *enteritis* secondary to therapy with the tetracyclines. Local infections susceptible to Erythromycin include *impetigo, wound* and *burn infections, infected eczema,* and *sycosis vulgaris.* Because of the possibility of producing resistant strains of staphylococci, the indiscriminate topical use of Erythromycin should be avoided. A large number of staphylococci have already become resistant to the drug. Erythromycin is also moderately effective in the treatment of

Erythromycin contains not less than 85.0% of $C_{37}H_{67}NO_{13}$ (733.95), calculated on the anhydrous basis. It conforms to the regulations of the federal Food and Drug Administration concerning antibiotic drugs (see page 1206).

Description—White or slightly yellow crystals or powder. It is odorless or practically odorless, and is slightly hygroscopic. Its solutions in alcohol are levorotatory.

Solubility—1 Gm dissolves in about 1000 ml of water. It is soluble in alcohol, chloroform, ether, and acetone; moderately soluble in amyl acetate and ethylene dichloride.

Uses—Erythromycin has a spectrum of activity which closely resembles that of penicillin. It is em-

intestinal *amebiasis* and is reported to be of value in eradicating extraintestinal forms of the disease.

Untoward reactions attributable to Erythromycin therapy are uncommon and of little consequence. Nausea, vomiting, and, occasionally, diarrhea may occur, particularly with large doses. Serious systemic toxicity has not been observed and there are no absolute contraindications to the use of Erythromycin.

Erythromycin is adequately absorbed after oral administration. Peak plasma levels are attained in 1 to 4 hours following which the concentration declines sharply by the fourth to sixth hour. A single oral dose of 200 to 300 mg usually provides a plasma concentration of 0.6 to 0.8 mcg per ml. The antibiotic does not readily diffuse into the cerebrospinal fluid, but attains antibacterial concentrations in peritoneal and pleural fluids. Approximately 20% of administered Erythromycin is excreted in inactive form by the kidney. The antibiotic is concentrated in the liver and excreted in active form in the bile; the feces of patients given large oral doses of Erythromycin contain about 0.5 mg per Gm.

Dose—*Oral* or *intravenous*, 1 to 4 **Gm** daily; *usual, oral*, as the base or in the form of a suitable derivative, the equivalent of **250 mg** of erythromycin base every 6 hours; *usual, intravenous*, in the form of a suitable derivative, the equivalent of **250 mg** of erythromycin base, as a **0.1%** solution, every 6 hours.

Veterinary Dose—*Oral* dosage in nonherbivorous animals is about **4 mg** per **pound** of body weight per day administered in 3 or 4 divided doses.

Dosage Forms—Ointment: 10 mg/Gm; Ophthalmic Ointment: 5 mg/Gm; Tablets: 100 and 250 mg.

Erythromycin Estolate NF

[Erythromycin 2' - Propionate (Ester) Dodecyl Hydrogen Sulfate (1:1); Erythromycin Propionate Lauryl Sulfate; Ilosone (*Lilly*)]

Erythromycin Estolate $[C_{40}H_{71}NO_{14} . C_{12}H_{26}O_4S = 1056.41]$ contains not less than 60.0% of $C_{37}H_{67}NO_{13}$ (erythromycin), calculated on the anhydrous basis. Erythromycin Estolate conforms to the regulations of the federal Food and Drug Administration concerning certification of antibiotic drugs (see page 1206).

For the structure of *Erythromycin*, see page 1215.

Preparation—Erythromycin base is reacted with propionic acid anhydride in acetone solution to form the 2'-propionate ester which is then converted to its hydrochloride. The ester salt is then metathesized with sodium dodecyl sulfate.

Description—White, crystalline powder. It is odorless or practically odorless and is practically tasteless.
Solubility—Practically insoluble in water; soluble in alcohol, acetone, and chloroform.

Dose—The action and uses of this drug are similar to those of *Erythromycin* (page 1215). It is very insoluble in water, and it is more acid stable and less affected by the presence of food in the stomach than are other erythromycin preparations. Jaundice has occurred in patients medicated with the estolate, although the role of the drug has not been clearly established.

Dose—The equivalent of **250** to **500 mg** of erythromycin; *usual*, **250 mg** every 6 hours.

Dosage Forms—Capsules NF: the equivalent of 125 and 250 mg of erythromycin; for Oral Suspension NF: the equivalent of 1.50 Gm/60 ml and 3.75 Gm/150 ml of erythromycin; Tablets NF: the equivalent of 125 mg of erythromycin.

Erythromycin Ethylcarbonate USP

[Erythromycin 2'-(Ethylcarbonate); Ilotycin Ethyl Carbonate (*Lilly*)]

Erythromycin Ethylcarbonate $[C_{40}H_{71}NO_{15} = 806.01]$ contains not less than 77.5% of erythromycin $(C_{37}H_{67}NO_{13})$, calculated on the anhydrous basis. It conforms to the regulations of the federal Food and Drug Administration concerning antibiotic drugs (see page 1206).

Preparation—Erythromycin is esterified directly by reaction with ethyl chloroformate in acetone in the presence of an excess of sodium bicarbonate.

Description—It occurs as a white, crystalline, practically odorless and tasteless powder.
Solubility—Slightly soluble in water and cyclohexane; freely soluble in alcohol, methanol, acetone, chloroform, ether, and dioxane.

Uses—See *Erythromycin*. This ester is particularly suitable for flavored oral suspensions for pediatric use.
Dose—The equivalent of **1** to **2 Gm** of erythromycin daily; *usual*, **250 mg** every 6 hours.
Other Dose Information—For children under 36 Kg (80 pounds) of body weight, use ½ of the above dose.
Dosage Forms—for Oral Suspension USP: 1 Gm/10 ml and 2.4 Gm/60 ml.
Veterinary Dose—*Dogs*, 300 to 1800 mg daily in 2 to 4 divided doses; *Cats*, 200 mg daily in 2 to 4 divided doses.

Erythromycin Ethylsuccinate NF

[Erythromycin 2'-(Ethyl Succinate); Erythrocin Ethylsuccinate (*Abbott*) Pediamycin (*Ross*)]

Erythromycin Ethylsuccinate $[C_{43}H_{75}NO_{16} = 862.07]$ contains the equivalent of not less than 76.5% of $C_{37}H_{67}NO_{13}$ (erythromycin base), calculated on the anhydrous basis. Erythromycin Ethylsuccinate conforms to the regulations of the federal Food and Drug Administration concerning antibiotic drugs (see page 1206).

For the structure of *Erythromycin*, see page 1215.

Preparation—Erythromycin is esterified by reacting it with ethyl 3-chloroformylpropionate $[ClCOCH_2CH_2-CO_2Et]$ in dry acetone in the presence of sodium bicarbonate.

Description—White, odorless powder.
Solubility—Freely soluble in acetone and chloroform; soluble in 95% ethanol and benzene; sparingly soluble in ether; very slightly soluble in water.

Uses—Erythromycin Ethylsuccinate is relatively nonirritating to tissues and hence is well suited to intramuscular injection. It is relatively tasteless and hence is also used in flavored oral "suspensions" for pediatric use. Except as noted above, the actions and uses of Erythromycin Ethylsuccinate are essentially those of *Erythromycin* (page 1215).
Dose—*Usual, intramuscular*, **100 mg** every 4 to 12 hours; *oral*, **1** to **2 Gm** daily in divided doses.
Dosage Forms—Injection NF: 100 mg/2 ml, 500 mg/10 ml; for Oral Suspension NF: 1.2 Gm/30 ml and 2.4 Gm/60 ml; Tablets NF: 200 mg.

Erythromycin Gluceptate USP

[Erythromycin Glucoheptonate USP XVI; Ilotycin Glucoheptonate (*Lilly*)]

Erythromycin Gluceptate $[C_{37}H_{67}NO_{13} . C_7H_{14}O_8 = 960.13]$ contains not less than 60.0% of erythromycin $(C_{37}H_{67}NO_{13})$, calculated on the anhydrous basis. It conforms to the regulations of the federal Food and Drug Administration concerning antibiotic drugs (see page 1206).

Preparation—This erythromycin salt is prepared by dissolving erythromycin in an aqueous solution containing the proper amount of glucoheptonic acid and removing the solvent under reduced pressure.

Description—It occurs as a white powder which is odorless or practically odorless and slightly hygroscopic. Its 1 in 20 solution is neutral or slightly acid.
Solubility—Freely soluble in water, alcohol, and methanol; slightly soluble in acetone and chloroform; practically insoluble in ether.

Uses—See *Erythromycin*. This salt is particularly suited for intravenous administration. It is also used in dental cones.

Dose—*Intravenous*, the equivalent of **1** to **4 Gm** of erythromycin daily; *usual*, **250 mg** 3 or 4 times a day; *infusion*, **1 Gm** daily.

Other Dose Information—The intravenous dose should be administered slowly over a period of 20 to 60 minutes. By continuous infusion, 1 to 4 Gm of base per day (see the manufacturer's recommendations for diluting the sterile, dry material); in dental cones, 5 mg.

Dosage Forms—Sterile USP: 250 and 500 mg, and 1 Gm.

Erythromycin Lactobionate USP

[Erythrocin Lactobionate (*Abbott*)]

Erythromycin Lactobionate [$C_{37}H_{67}NO_{13}.C_{12}H_{22}O_{12}$ = 1092.25] contains not less than 60.0% of erythromycin ($C_{37}H_{67}NO_{13}$), calculated on the anhydrous basis. It conforms to the regulations of the federal Food and Drug Administration concerning antibiotic drugs (see page 1206).

Preparation—Using lactobionic acid, this erythromycin salt may be prepared as described above for the glucoheptonate.

Description—It occurs as white or slightly yellow crystals or powder, having a faint odor. Its 1 in 20 solution is neutral or slightly alkaline.

Solubility—Freely soluble in water, alcohol, and methanol; slightly soluble in acetone and chloroform; practically insoluble in ether.

Uses—The water solubility of this salt of erythromycin allows it to be given parenterally, either intravenously or intramuscularly. It has the same uses and actions as the erythromycin base (see *Erythromycin*). However, the parenteral route should be employed only if the patient cannot tolerate the base by the oral route.

Dose—*Intravenous*, the equivalent of **1** to **4 Gm** of erythromycin daily; *usual*, **250 mg** 3 or 4 times a day; *infusion*, **1 Gm** daily.

Dosage Forms—For Injection USP: 500 mg and 1 Gm.

Veterinary Dose—*Intravenously*, *Horses* and *Cattle*, **0.5** to **1.0 Gm** every 12 hours; *Swine*, **100** to **300 mg** every 12 hours; *Sheep*, **100** to **300 mg** every 12 hours. *Intramuscularly*, double intravenous dose. Use only until oral medication is possible.

Erythromycin Stearate USP

[Erythrocin Stearate (*Abbott*)]

Erythromycin Stearate [$C_{37}H_{67}NO_{13}.C_{18}H_{36}O_2$ = 1018.43] is the stearic acid salt of erythromycin, with an excess of stearic acid. It contains not less than 50.0% of erythromycin ($C_{37}H_{67}NO_{13}$), calculated on the anhydrous basis. It conforms to the regulations of the federal Food and Drug Administration concerning antibiotic drugs (see page 1206).

Preparation—This water-insoluble erythromycin salt is prepared readily by reacting erythromycin with the proper quantity of stearic acid in acetone solution and then diluting the solution with water to precipitate the salt.

Description—It occurs as white or slightly yellow crystals or powder. It is practically odorless and has a slightly bitter taste. Its saturated solution is alkaline to litmus.

Solubility—Practically insoluble in water; soluble in alcohol, methanol, chloroform, and ether.

Uses—The actions and uses of Erythromycin Stearate are identical to those of the base (see *Erythromycin*).

Dose—The equivalent of **1** to **4 Gm** of erythromycin daily; *usual*, **250 mg** 3 or 4 times a day.

Dosage Forms—Tablets USP: 100 and 250 mg.

Veterinary Dose—*Orally*, *average size dogs*, **100 mg** every 6 to 8 hours (for larger breeds and in fulminating infections dose may be doubled).

Gentamicin Sulfate USP

[Garamycin (*Schering*)]

Gentamicin Sulfate is the sulfate salt of the antibiotic substances produced by the growth of *Micromonospora purpurea*. Its potency is equivalent to not less than 590 mcg of gentamicin per mg, calculated on the anhydrous basis. Gentamicin Sulfate conforms to the regulations of the federal Food and Drug Administration concerning antibiotic drugs (see page 1206).

Gentamicin has been shown to be a mixture of two closely related pseudo-oligosaccharides (gentamicin C_1 and gentamicin C_2) with essentially identical specific rotations but significantly different melting points. Each component contains a 2-deoxystreptamine residue and a molecular formula established to the extent indicated by $C_{17-18}H_{34-36}N_4O_7$. Each also contains three amino groups, one *N*-methyl group, and one *C*-methyl group, and they are equally susceptible to *N*-acetylation. The mixed antibiotic combines readily with acids to form salts. For a resumé of structure studies, see Shaffner, Maehr.[4]

Preparation—Gentamicin (base) is recovered from a fermentation broth produced when submerged cultures of two recently isolated subspecies of *Micromonospora purpurea* are grown in a yeast extract-cerelose medium. US Pat. 3,136,704.

Description—A white to buff powder that is odorless. It is stable in light, air, and heat. It melts with decomposition between 200° and 250°.

Solubility—Soluble in water; insoluble in alcohol, acetone, and benzene.

Uses—Gentamicin Sulfate closely resembles *Neomycin Sulfate* (page 1219) in its antibacterial activity and toxicity. Thus it is quite active against most strains of *Klebsiella*, *Aerobacter*, *E. Coli*, and many strains of *Pseudomonas*. It is moderately active against some species of *Proteus* and most Group A beta hemolytic streptococci. It does not affect fungi, yeasts, or viruses. Its action against *Pseudomonas* is of especial interest, since species of that genus have become an important cause of surgical infections and they almost always invade burned skin. However, because of systemic toxicity, present systemic use is mainly limited to life-threatening infections caused by *Pseudomonas* and *Proteus*. Abscesses and infected cysts must be drained and scabs or crusts, such as those of impetigo contagiosa, must be removed prior to local application. The cutaneous sensitizing potential is low, but allergic skin reactions and photosensitivity have been reported. Systemic toxicity, which does not occur with topical application, include auditory and vestibular impairment and nephrotoxicity.

Dose—*Topically*, the equivalent of **0.1%** of gentamicin in a cream or ointment 3 or 4 times a day.

Other Dose Information—Apply to the affected area 3 or 4 times a day. For intramuscular use, 0.8 to 3 mg per Kg of body weight per day, in at least 3 divided doses. In the presence of Gram-negative bacillary sepsis, 5 mg per Kg may be used.

Dosage Forms—Cream USP: 1 mg/Gm; Injection: 40 mg/ml; Ointment USP: 1 mg/Gm.

Gramicidin NF

Gramicidin is an antibacterial substance produced by the growth of *Bacillus brevis* Dubos (Fam. *Bacillaceæ*). It may be obtained from tyrothricin.

Gramicidin has a potency of not less than 900 mcg of activity per mg. Gramicidin conforms to the regulations of the federal Food and Drug Administration concerning certification of antibiotic drugs (see page 1206).

The total composition of Gramicidin has yet to be determined. However, it has been shown to contain at least three cyclic polypeptides:

Gramicidin J_1—$C_{44}H_{65}N_9O_7$

┌L-Phe—D-Leu—D-Phe—L-Orn—L-Val—D-Orn—L-Pro┐

Gramicidin J_2—$C_{35}H_{56}N_8O_6$

┌D-Phe—D-Leu—L-Orn—L-Val—D-Orn—L-Pro┐

Gramicidin S—$C_{60}H_{92}N_{12}O_{10}$

┌L-Val—L-Orn—L-Leu—D-Phe—L-Pro┐
└L-Pro—D-Phe—L-Leu—L-Orn—L-Val┘

Description—It occurs as a white, or nearly white, odorless, crystalline powder. Melting range—not below 229°, when previously dried in vacuum at 60° for 3 hours. Specific rotation +3° to +7°.

Solubility—Soluble in alcohol; insoluble in water.

Uses—Gramicidin is active against Gram-positive organisms, except for the Gram-positive bacilli, and against certain Gram-negative organisms, such as the Neisseria. It is bacteriostatic to some organisms and bactericidal to others, especially in high concentrations. It is partially inhibited by serum and body fluids. It is effective only by topical application; not only is it ineffective systemically, but it is highly toxic. It should not be used for the irrigation of the paranasal sinuses. Oral gramicidin, however, has a very low order of toxicity; consequently, the drug may be incorporated into troches, lozenges, etc.

Gramicidin has essentially the same uses as *Tyrothricin* (page 1235). It is the active ingredient of tyrothricin, in which it is present as 20%, w/w.

Dose—*Topically* as **0.05%** solution.

Veterinary Use—*Topically* for upper respiratory tract, ear, eye, nose, and throat infections and for chronic mastitis for its activity against Gram-positive cocci. Use of drug not widespread.

Gramicidin, Neomycin Sulfate, and Polymyxin B Sulfate Ophthalmic Solution—see page 1220.

Griseofulvin—see page 1257.

Kanamycin Sulfate USP

[Kanamycin Sulfate (1:1); Kantrex (*Bristol*)

Kanamycin Sulfate contains an amount of kanamycin sulfate [$C_{18}H_{36}N_4O_{11} \cdot H_2SO_4 = 582.59$] equivalent to not

less than 75.0% of kanamycin [$C_{18}H_{36}N_4O_{11} = 484.51$] (the antibiotic activity of 750 mcg of kanamycin in each mg) and not more than 5.0% of kanamycin B sulfate, both calculated on the anhydrous basis. Kanamycin Sulfate conforms to the regulations of the federal Food and Drug Administration concerning antibiotic drugs (see page 1206).

Kanamycin base is 4,6-diamino-3-[(3-amino-3-deoxy-D-glucopyranosyl)oxy]-2-hydroxycyclohexyl 6-amino-6-deoxyglucopyranoside. It is produced solely by fermentation using *Streptomyces kanamyceticus*.

Description—White, odorless, crystalline powder.
Solubility—Freely soluble in water; insoluble in alcohol, acetone, ethyl acetate, and benzene.

Uses—Kanamycin, like neomycin, is active against Gram-negative organisms such as *Klebsiella, Aerobacter, Shigella, Salmonella, E. coli*, and many strains of *Proteus*. It is also effective against many Gram-positive bacteria, although the common ones such as streptococci and pneumococci are not inhibited at levels usually attained in body fluids. Most sensitive organisms can develop resistance to Kanamycin both *in vitro* and *in vivo*. Furthermore, there is almost complete cross-resistance with neomycin.

Systemic infections do not respond to oral therapy since Kanamycin is not absorbed from the gastrointestinal tract. However, parenteral administration has been effective in the treatment of respiratory tract and urinary tract infections. Gastrointestinal infections due particularly to *Salmonella* and *Shigella* have responded to oral administration of Kanamycin.

Ototoxicity is the most significant side effect resulting from the use of Kanamycin when given parenterally. Since this toxicity seems to be directly related to blood levels of the antibiotic, the recommended daily dose should not be exceeded. Frequent renal irritation has been observed, but this appears to be reversible on termination of therapy. Because of its toxicity, Kanamycin is not widely used, and its status is that of a second-order "back-up" drug.

Dose—*Oral*, the equivalent of **3** to **12 Gm** of kanamycin daily; *usual*, for *therapy in intestinal infections*, **1 Gm** 3 or 4 times a day; *usual*, for *preoperative preparation*, **1 Gm** every hour for 4 doses, then **1 Gm** every 6 hours for 36 to 72 hours. *Intramuscular*, on a body-weight basis, up to a total of not more than **1.5 Gm** daily for up to 5 days; *usual*, for *therapy in systemic infections*, **7.5 mg** per **Kg** of body weight 2 times a day.

Other Dose Information—The dose for preoperative preparation of the bowel is the same as that for intestinal infections.

Dosage Forms—Capsules USP: 500 mg; Injection USP: 75 and 500 mg/2 ml, 1 Gm/3 ml.

Lincomycin Hydrochloride USP

[Methyl 6,8-dideoxy-6-(1-methyl-4-*trans*-propyl-L-2-pyrrolidinecarboxamido)-1-thio-D-*erythro*-α-D-*galacto*-octopyranoside Monohydrochloride; Lincomycin Hydrochloride Monohydrate; Lincocin (*Upjohn*)]

Lincomycin Hydrochloride [$C_{18}H_{34}N_2O_6S \cdot HCl$ = 443.01] is the monohydrated hydrochloride salt of lincomycin, a substance produced by the growth of a member of the *lincolnensis* group of *Streptomyces lincolnensis* (Fam. *Streptomycetaceae*). It has a potency equivalent to not less than 790 mcg of lincomycin per mg, calculated on the anhydrous basis. Lincomycin Hydrochloride conforms to the regulations of the federal Food and Drug Administration concerning antibiotic drugs (see page 1206).

Description—A white or practically white, crystalline powder. It is odorless or has a faint odor and a bitter taste. It is stable in light and air. Its solutions are acid and are dextrorotatory.

Solubility—Freely soluble in water; soluble in dimethylformamide; very slightly soluble in acetone.

Uses—The antibacterial activity of Lincomycin closely resembles that of *Erythromycin* (page 1215). It has a rather broad spectrum of activity against Gram-positive organisms, especially staphylococci, pneumococci, pyogenic streptococci, and corynebacteria. However, it has little efficacy against enterococci, which are Gram-positive. Gram-negative cocci, such as gonococci and meningococci, are very little affected by the drug, and Gram-negative bacilli are unaffected. Lincomycin is used to treat infections of the respiratory and urinary tracts or of soft tissues when the infecting organism is appropriately susceptible. It also appears to be of benefit in some cases of osteomyelitis. Since there is no cross-resistance between penicillin and Lincomycin and infrequently between erythromycin and Lincomycin, the drug is useful when resistance to the other antibiotics emerges. Resistance to Lincomycin does develop, although slowly.

Lincomycin may cause nausea and vomiting, abdominal cramps, or diarrhea in some patients. Less frequently there may be headache, dizziness, malaise and aching, pruritus, rash, proctitis, vaginitis, or moniliasis. Jaundice, leukopenia, or neutropenia rarely occur.

Although Lincomycin is incompletely absorbed from the gut, oral administration provides adequate blood levels.

Dose—*Usual, oral,* the equivalent of **500 mg** of lincomycin 3 to 4 times a day; *intramuscular,* **600 mg** 1 to 2 times a day; *intravenous infusion,* **600 mg** in 8 to 12 hours.

Other Dose Information—The dose for infusion should be contained in no less than 250 ml of 5% dextrose solution or sodium chloride injection.

Dosage Forms—Capsules USP: 250 and 500 mg; Injection USP: 1, 2, and 10 ml; Pediatric Drops: 50 mg/ml; Syrup: 250 mg/5 ml.

Methacycline Hydrochloride NF

[4 - (Dimethylamino) - 1,4,4a,5,5a,6,11,12a - octahydro - 3,5,10,12,12a-pentahydroxy - 6 - methylene - 1,11 - dioxo - 2 - naphthacenecarboxamide Monohydrochloride; Rondomycin Hydrochloride (*Wallace*)]

Methacycline Hydrochloride [$C_{22}H_{22}N_2O_8 \cdot HCl$ = 478.89] has a potency of not less than 832 mcg of $C_{22}H_{22}N_2O_8$ (methacycline) per mg. Methacycline Hydrochloride conforms to the regulations of the federal Food and Drug Administration concerning certification of antibiotic drugs (see page 1206).

Preparation—5-Hydroxytetracycline is reacted with a halogenating agent such as *N*-chlorosuccinimide in an inert solvent to form 11a-chloro-5-hydroxytetracycline-6,12-hemiketal (I). Dehydration of (I) with liquid HF or some other acid, eg, perchloric, polyphosphoric, etc, yields 11a-chloro-6-methylene-5-hydroxytetracycline. Dechlorination at 11a may be accomplished by catalytic hydrogenation or by any of the usual reduction processes. The methacycline (base) thus obtained is dissolved in methanol and treated with HCl to form the official salt which is precipitated by the addition of ether. Purification is achieved through recrystallization from acidified (HCl) methanol or acetone. US Pat. 2,984,686.

Description—A yellow to dark yellow, crystalline powder. The pH of a 1% solution is between 2 and 3. It is odorless and has a bitter taste. It is unstable in light, nonhygroscopic, and stable at room temperature. It decomposes without melting at about 225°.

Solubility—Freely soluble in water; slightly soluble in alcohol; insoluble in ether and chloroform.

Uses—Methacycline has actions and uses essentially the same as those of *Chlortetracycline Hydrochloride* (page 1211). Organisms sensitive to Methacycline will be sensitive to any other tetracycline and *vice versa*. Likewise, the development of resistance is mutual among Methacycline and all other tetracyclines. Furthermore, any patient hypersensitive to another tetracycline will be allergic to Methacycline. Toxicity and side effects are those of other tetracyclines, but photosensitivity is more frequent than with tetracycline, chlortetracycline, or oxytetracycline. Thus the only advantage of Methacycline is its longer duration of action. The half-life is approximately 15 hours, which is slightly longer than that of *Demeclocycline* (page 1214). The long duration of action is in part due to a greater binding by plasma and tissue proteins, which binding diminishes the effective plasma level of the drug, and there is a greater lag between the initial dose and the achievement of an optimal concentration of free drug. Furthermore, the low rate of excretion results in a lower urine concentration than with the older tetracyclines, so that it is less effective in urinary tract infections. Methacycline should not be used in patients with impaired renal function.

Dose—*Usual,* **600 mg** (equivalent to 560 mg of methacycline base) daily in divided doses.

Dosage Forms—Capsules NF: 150 mg (equivalent to 140 mg of methacycline) and 300 mg (equivalent to 280 mg of methacycline); Oral Suspension NF: 75 mg (equivalent to 70 mg of methacycline)/5 ml.

Neomycin Sulfate USP

[Mycifradin Sulfate (*Upjohn*)]

Neomycin Sulfate is the sulfate of an antibacterial substance produced by the growth of *Streptomyces fradiæ* Waksman (Fam. *Streptomycetaceæ*). It contains an amount of neomycin sulfate equivalent to not less than 60.0% of neomycin base, calculated on the dried basis. It conforms to the regulations of the federal Food and Drug Administration concerning antibiotic drugs (see page 1206).

Neomycin consists almost entirely of a pair of

$C_{23}H_{46}N_6O_{13}$ epimers designated as Neomycin B and Neomycin C, and the ratio of B to C has been observed to vary widely among different production lots. The total structure and the common names of the component parts of Neomycin C are shown below. The structure of Neomycin B is reported to be identical except for the configuration of the indicated aminomethyl group.

Neomycin C

*Opposite configuration in Neomycin B.

Description—White to slightly yellow crystals or powder. It is odorless or practically odorless, and is hygroscopic. Its solutions are dextrorotatory. The pH of an aqueous solution, 33 mg in each ml, is between 5.0 and 7.5.

Solubility—1 Gm dissolves in about 1 ml of water; very slightly soluble in alcohol; insoluble in acetone, chloroform, and ether.

Uses—Neomycin Sulfate, an antibiotic with a broad antimicrobial spectrum of activity, is used topically and for its local antibacterial action in the lumen of the bowel. Parenteral therapy is contraindicated, unless the offending organism is not susceptible to other less toxic chemotherapeutic agents. Neomycin is effective against a variety of Gram-positive and Gram-negative bacteria and against acid-fast bacilli and actinomycetes. Consequently, the antibiotic is effective in a wide variety of local infections including *burns, wounds, ulcers, impetigo, infected dermatoses, furunculosis, otitis externa, conjunctivitis,* and *sty.* Orally, the drug has been used to produce intestinal antisepsis prior to large bowel surgery. Because of the rapid overgrowth of non-susceptible bacteria, oral neomycin therapy should not be continued for longer than 72 hours. Intramuscular therapy should be reserved for infections caused by *S. aureus, K. pneumoniae, H. influenzæ, E. coli,* and *Pseudomonas* and *Proteus* organisms which do not respond to other less toxic antibiotic and chemotherapeutic agents.

Although orally administered neomycin rarely causes systemic toxic effects, it frequently produces loose stools and nausea. Applied topically, the drug is well tolerated, relatively nonirritating, and has a low index of sensitivity. Injected parenterally, neomycin causes serious nephrotoxic and neurotoxic effects. The renal injury is usually reversible and is manifested by albumin and granular casts in the urine and an elevation of non-protein nitrogen in the blood; the neurological damage, irreversible injury to the eighth cranial nerve, is mainly auditory and may be additive to that produced by streptomycin. Because of the possibility of renal and auditory injury, parenteral injection and prolonged oral administration of neomycin are generally contra-indicated.

Neomycin is poorly absorbed from the gastrointestinal tract; an oral dose of 3 Gm produces a peak serum level of only 1 to 4 mcg per ml. About 97% of orally administered neomycin is eliminated unchanged in the feces. The antibiotic is readily absorbed after intramuscular injection; a dose of 1 Gm produces a peak serum level of 20 mcg per ml. Absorbed neomycin is rapidly excreted by the kidney in active form.

Dose—For *preoperative preparation,* the equivalent of **2.8 to 8.4 Gm** of neomycin base; *usual,* **700 mg** every hour for 4 doses, then every 4 hours for 24 to 72 hours.

Other Dose Information—For topical use, the ointment is applied to the affected area 2 or 3 times daily, or the drug can be used in isotonic sodium chloride solution (5 mg per ml) as a wet dressing, irrigation, or instillation. For preoperative disinfection of the colon, 1 Gm of neomycin is given orally every hour for 4 doses and then every 4 hours for 1 to 3 days.

Dosage Forms—Cream: 5 mg/Gm; Ointment USP: 5 mg/Gm; Ophthalmic Ointment: 5 mg/Gm; Oral Solution USP: 60 and 500 ml; Sterile; 0.5 Gm; Tablets USP: 500 mg (equivalent to 350 mg of neomycin base).

Veterinary Dose—Single *oral* dose of **2 Gm** given to the dog. Infused intramammarily in the cow as an ointment, **0.5 Gm** per infected quarter.

Neomycin Sulfate and Dexamethasone Sodium Phosphate Cream—see page 966.

Neomycin Sulfate, Polymyxin B Sulfate, and Gramicidin Ophthalmic Solution NF

[Neo-Polycin (*Dow*); Neosporin (*Burroughs-Wellcome*)]

Neomycin Sulfate, Polymyxin B Sulfate, and Gramicidin Ophthalmic Solution is a sterile isotonic solution of neomycin sulfate, polymyxin B sulfate, and gramicidin. It contains 90.0–130.0% of the labeled amounts of neomycin sulfate, polymyxin B sulfate, and gramicidin. It conforms to the regulations of the federal Food and Drug Administration concerning the certification of antibiotic drugs.

Uses—This mixture presents a broad spectrum of antibacterial activity which will be effective against most of the various microorganisms that cause superficial infections of the eye and lids. Not only is Neomycin a relatively broad spectrum antibiotic (see *Neomycin,* page 1219), but Polymyxin B acts against a wide variety of gram-negative organisms (see *Polymyxin B,* above) and Gramicidin is effective against many gram-positive organisms (see *Gramicidin,* page 1218). However, it must be remembered that it is sometimes necessary to employ concomitant systemic therapy to eradicate even superficial infections. Although each of the components has a low sensitizing potential, with three in the mixture, the probability of allergic reactions is multiplied.

Dose—*Topical,* 1 or 2 drops in the eye 2 to 4 times daily.

Dosage Forms—Solution NF: 2.8 mg, 5000 units, and 0.02 mg of each constituent/ml.

Neomycin Sulfate, Polymyxin B Sulfate, and Zinc Bacitracin Ointment NF

[Neo-Polycin (*Dow*); Neosporin (*Burroughs-Wellcome*)]

Neomycin Sulfate, Polymyxin B Sulfate, and Zinc Bacitracin Ointment contains not less than 90.0% of the labeled amounts of neomycin sulfate, polymyxin B sulfate, and zinc bacitracin. It conforms to the regulations of the federal Food and Drug Administration concerning the certification of antibiotic drugs.

Uses—This mixture combines the topical efficacy of *Polymyxin B* (see page 1231) against Gram-negative organisms with that of *Bacitracin* (see page 1209) against Gram-positive organisms and adds that of the relatively broad spectrum of antibacterial activity of *Neomycin* (see page 1219). Thus the mixture may be employed for the management of a wide variety of superficial infections. (Summarize the monographs for the individual components for the potential topical usefulness.) Where the identity and antibacterial sensitivity of the invading organism are known (as it should be), the appropriate single agent should be employed instead of this mixture, unless medical experience indicates that certain types of secondary infections or superinfections (overgrowth) susceptible to the mixture are quite probable. It must be remembered that superinfections are more likely to occur when broad spectrum antibiotics or mixtures are employed than when narrow spectrum agents are used. When there is a mixed infection, this mixture may be indicated. Although the sensitizing property of each component is low, the probability is compounded in the mixture.

Dose—*Topical*, to the affected area 2 to 5 times a day.

Dosage Forms—Ointment NF: 5 mg, 5000 units, and 400 units of each constituent/Gm, or 4.27 mg, 8000 units, and 400 units of each constituent/Gm.

Calcium Novobiocin NF

[Novobiocin Calcium Salt (2:1); Albamycin Calcium (*Upjohn*)]

Calcium Novobiocin $[C_{62}H_{70}CaN_4O_{22} \cdot 2H_2O = 1299.37]$ contains the equivalent of not less than 80.0% of novobiocin (as the free acid, $C_{31}H_{36}N_2O_{11}$), calculated on the dried basis. Calcium Novobiocin conforms to the regulations of the federal Food and Drug Administration concerning certification of antibiotic drugs (see page 1206).

The free acid, Novobiocin $[C_{31}H_{36}N_2O_{11} = 612.64]$, is chemically 7-[4-(carbamoyloxy)tetrahydro-3-hydroxy-5 - methoxy - 6,6 - dimethylpyran - 2 - yloxy] - 4-hydroxy - 3 - [4 - hydroxy - 3 - (3 - methyl - 2 - butenyl)benzamido]-8-methylcoumarin.

Description—White or practically white, crystalline powder, which is odorless or practically odorless. The pH of a saturated solution is between 6.5 and 8.5. The specific rotation is −50° to −58°.

Solubility—1 Gm dissolves in about 250 ml of water, 30 ml of alcohol, 450 ml of ether, and 1100 ml of chloroform.

Uses—Calcium Novobiocin has the same actions and uses as the sodium salt (see *Sodium Novobiocin*, below). However, the calcium salt is more stable in aqueous suspension, so that it is used primarily for oral administration in liquid form.

Dose—The equivalent of **250** to **500 mg** of novobiocin acid; *usual*, **250 mg** every 6 hours.

Dosage Forms—Oral Suspension NF; Syrup: 125 mg/5 ml.

Sodium Novobiocin NF

[Albamycin (*Upjohn*)]

Sodium Novobiocin $[C_{31}H_{35}N_2NaO_{11} = 634.62]$ contains the equivalent of not less than 80.0% of novobiocin (as the free acid, $C_{31}H_{36}N_2O_{11}$), calculated on the dried basis. Sodium Novobiocin conforms to the regulations of the federal Food and Drug Administration concerning certification of antibiotic drugs (see page 1206).

For the structural formula of novobiocin, see *Calcium Novobiocin*, this page. The chemical name for the free acid is also provided there.

Description—White or practically white, crystalline powder, which is odorless or practically odorless and hygroscopic. The pH is between 6.5 and 8.5 and the specific rotation is between −50° and −58°.

Solubility—Very soluble in water; freely soluble in alcohol, glycerin, and propylene glycol.

Uses—Novobiocin is mainly active against Gram-positive organisms; fortunately it is particularly active against *Staphylococcus pyogenes* var. *aureus*. It has little or no activity against most gram-negative organisms, but certain strains of *Proteus vulgaris* and coliform bacteria are moderately susceptible to the drug. It is only moderately active against Gram-negative cocci. Its use should be reserved for the treatment of infections caused by staphylococci that have been proved to be resistant to all other safe antibiotics or for other infections in the occasional patient that is allergic to all the common effective antibiotics. Since staphylococci readily become resistant to novobiocin, it is imperative that its use be limited by the above conditions, lest its usefulness as a drug-in-reserve be destroyed.

Novobiocin has a relatively high index of sensitization with both dermatologic and hematologic manifestations with leukopenia. The drug may also induce nausea and vomiting, diarrhea, abdominal pain, intestinal hemorrhage, vertigo, drowsiness, arthritis, conjunctivitis, alopecia, pneumonitis, and myocarditis.

The principal route of administration is oral, although intravenous or intramuscular injection may be used when oral therapy is not feasible. Intramuscular deposition is painful.

Dose—*Oral, intravenous*, or *intramuscular*, the equivalent of **1** to **2 Gm** of novobiocin acid daily in 4 divided doses; *usual, oral*, **250 mg** every 6 hours; *usual, intravenous* and *intramuscular*, **500 mg** every 12 hours.

Other Dose Information—For severe infections, 2 Gm per day in 4 divided doses may be given intravenously. It must be first dissolved in 5 ml of a suitable solubilizing agent and diluted to not less than 30 ml of an acceptable saline parenteral fluid. The intravenous dose should be given slowly in not less than 5 minutes.

Dosage Forms—Capsules NF: the equivalent of 250 mg of novobiocin; for Injection NF: the equivalent of 500 mg of novobiocin.

Veterinary Dose—In general, *intramuscular*, **10** to **30 mg** per **Kg** of body weight.

Nystatin—see page 1259.

Oleandomycin Phosphate NF

[Oleandomycin Phosphate (Salt), (1:1)]

Oleandomycin Phosphate [$C_{35}H_{61}NO_{12} \cdot H_3PO_4$ = 785.87] has a potency of not less than 775 mcg of oleandomycin base [$C_{35}H_{61}NO_{12}$ = 687.88] activity per mg. It conforms to the regulations of the federal Food and Drug Administration concerning certification of antibiotic drugs (see page 1206).

Description—It occurs as a white, practically odorless, crystalline powder. A 1 in 20 solution has a pH range between 3.0 and 6.0. Specific rotation (100 mg in 10 ml of methanol) −42° to −52°; specific rotation (same concentration in water) −24° to −36°.

Solubility—1 Gm dissolves in about 2.2 ml of water and 3 ml of alcohol; slightly soluble in ether.

Uses—The antibacterial spectrum, uses, and limitations of oleandomycin are very similar to those of *Erythromycin* (page 1215). It is about ¼ as potent as erythromycin. Cross-resistance to erythromycin occurs frequently, but Oleandomycin may often be effective in staphylococcal or other infections refractory to erythromycin. Oleandomycin Phosphate is not as well absorbed from the intestine as triacetyloleandomycin, hence the latter is generally preferred for oral use.

Dose—*Usual, intravenous*, **1 to 3 Gm** daily, in divided doses; *intramuscular*, **200 mg** every 6 to 8 hours.

Dosage Forms—Sterile NF: 200 mg.

Veterinary Use—Treatment of canine pyogenic dermatites.

Veterinary Dose—*Medium sized dogs*, **250 mg** (5 mg per ml in sterile water) by slow *intravenous* injection daily for 6 to 8 days.

Oxytetracycline

[4 - (Dimethylamino) - 1,4,4a,5,5a,6,11,12a - octahydro - 3,5,6,10,12,12a-hexahydroxy - 6 - methyl - 1,11 - dioxo - 2 - naphthacenecarboxamide; 5-Hydroxytetracycline; Oxytetracycline Dihydrate; Terramycin (*Pfizer*)]

Oxytetracycline [$C_{22}H_{24}N_2O_9 \cdot 2H_2O$ = 496.48] contains the equivalent of not less than 900 mcg per mg, calculated on the anhydrous basis. Oxytetracycline conforms to the regulations of the federal Food and Drug Administration concerning certification of antibiotic drugs (see page 1206).

Preparation—Oxytetracycline is produced by the growth of a selected strain of *Streptomyces rimosus* on a medium consisting of water, proteins, and nutrient salts. The submerged process (page 1207) is employed. When the fermentation has proceeded to the desired yield, the broth is filtered and the Oxytetracycline is precipitated, purified, and dried.

Description—A yellow, odorless, crystalline powder. It is stable in air, but exposure to strong sunlight causes it to darken. It deteriorates in solutions of pH below 2, and is rapidly destroyed by alkali hydroxide solutions. Its saturated solution is nearly neutral to litmus, having a pH of about 6.5. Specific rotation −207° to −216° (100 mg in 10 ml of 0.1 N HCl).

Solubility—1 Gm dissolves in about 2000 ml of water and about 100 ml of alcohol; it readily dissolves in dilute hydrochloric acid.

Uses—The antibiotic spectrum, actions and uses, absorption, fate and excretion, and doses of Oxytetracycline are essentially those of *Chlortetracycline* (page 1211). The relative susceptibilities of various microorganisms to Oxytetracycline are virtually the same as to chlortetracycline and tetracycline, with a few possible exceptions. Bacterial resistance to Oxytetracycline automatically accompanies resistance to chlortetracycline or tetracycline. Oxytetracycline is also used in the treatment of intestinal amebiasis; it removes both cysts and motile forms from the intestine and compares favorably with the arsenicals and halogenated quinolines. The absorption and disposition of Oxytetracycline is like that of chlortetracycline, but it is not bound to plasma proteins as extensively; its sojourn in the body is longer, the biologic half-life being about 10 hours. The gastrointestinal side effects from Oxytetracycline are greater than from the other two related antibiotics.

Dose—*Usual, oral*, **250 mg** 4 times a day; *intramuscular*, **250 to 500 mg**.

Dosage Forms—Injection NF: the equivalent of 50, 100, and 250 mg of anhydrous oxytetracycline/2 ml; for Oral Suspension: 1.5 Gm.

Veterinary Dose—**5 to 25 mg** per **pound** of body weight daily in 2 or 3 doses.

Calcium Oxytetracycline NF

[Calcium Terramycin (*Pfizer*)]

Calcium Oxytetracycline [$C_{44}H_{46}CaN_4O_{18}$ = 958.95] has a potency of not less than 865 mcg of oxytetracycline per mg, calculated on the anhydrous basis. Calcium Oxytetracycline conforms to the regulations of the federal Food and Drug Administration concerning certification of antibiotic drugs (see page 1206).

Calcium Oxytetracycline is a calcium chelate salt of

oxytetracycline. The primary site of chelation is reported to be that shown in the above structure.

Preparation—Aqueous solutions of oxytetracycline hydrochloride and calcium chloride are mixed and the product precipitates as the pH is adjusted to the neutral range. US Pats. 2,516,080 and 2,903,395.

Description—A yellow to light-brown, crystalline powder that is odorless and tasteless. It discolors in light and is sensitive to air oxidation. The pH of a 1 in 40 suspension is about 7.0.

Solubility—Insoluble in water in the neutral pH range; readily soluble in dilute acid (eg, stomach juice) with breakdown of the calcium chelate to yield free oxytetracycline. In strong aqueous acid the oxytetracycline so formed will degrade. Calcium oxytetracycline will also dissolve in excess aqueous caustic. In contrast to free oxytetracycline under such conditions, the calcium chelate is quite stable in the absence of oxygen.

Uses—The actions of Calcium Oxytetracycline are those of *Oxytetracycline* (page 1222). The compound is less soluble than oxytetracycline, and it lacks the disagreeable flavor of the hydrochloride, so that it is used in syrups and pediatric drops.

Dose—250 to 500 mg; *usual*, **250 mg** 4 times a day.

Dosage Forms—Oral Suspension NF: the equivalent of 125 mg of oxytetracycline/5 ml.

Oxytetracycline Hydrochloride USP

[5-Hydroxytetracycline Monohydrochloride; Terramycin Hydrochloride (*Pfizer*)]

Oxytetracycline Hydrochloride [$C_{22}H_{24}N_2O_9 \cdot HCl$ = 496.91] contains the equivalent of not less than 83.5% of $C_{22}H_{24}N_2O_9$, calculated on the anhydrous basis. Oxytetracycline Hydrochloride conforms to the regulations of the federal Food and Drug Administration concerning certification of antibiotic drugs (see page 1206).

Description—A yellow, crystalline powder. It is odorless, has a bitter taste, and is hygroscopic. It decomposes above 180°, and exposure to strong sunlight or to temperatures above 90° in moist air causes darkening, but no appreciable loss in potency. Its potency is affected in solutions of pH below 2, and is rapidly destroyed by alkali hydroxide solutions. The pH of a 1 per cent solution is about 2.5. Specific rotation −192° to −200° (100 mg in 10 ml 0.1 N HCl).

Solubility—1 Gm dissolves in 2 ml of water, but the solution becomes cloudy or turbid due to liberation of oxytetracycline base; 1 Gm dissolves in 35 ml of alcohol and 45 ml of methanol; less soluble in dehydrated alcohol; insoluble in chloroform and ether.

Uses—See *Oxytetracycline* (page 1222).

Dose—*Oral*, the equivalent of **1** to **4 Gm** of oxytetracycline daily; *usual*, **250 mg** 4 times a day; *intramuscular*, **200** to **500 mg** daily; *usual*, **100 mg** 2 or 3 times a day; *intravenous infusion*, **500 mg** to **2 Gm** daily; *usual*, **250** to **500 mg** in 1/2 to 1 hour 2 times a day.

Other Dose Information—Topically, as a 0.5% ophthalmic solution.

Dosage Forms—Capsules USP: the equivalent of 125 and 250 mg of oxytetracycline; for Injection USP: 250 and 500 mg; Ophthalmic NF.

Penicillin

History—During an inspection of some culture plates in the laboratory of St. Mary's Hospital, London, in 1928, Professor Alexander Fleming observed the lysis of staphylococcus organisms by a contaminating mold. Upon subculturing the mold he found in the broth a powerful, but nontoxic antibacterial substance. He gave it the name "penicillin" from the organism *Penicillium notatum* which caused the generation of the antibiotic.

The name "penicillin" now designates a number of antibiotic substances produced by the growth of *Penicillium notatum* or *Penicillium chrysogenum* Thom (Fam. *Aspergillaceæ*) or produced by other means. The better known natural penicillins are listed in Table I. Penicillins F, G, and X are also sometimes referred to as I, II, and III, respectively. In the discussion which follows, the term penicillin refers to penicillin G unless indicated otherwise. The unique properties of some of the other penicillins will be indicated in the appropriate sections.

Penicillin of commerce is largely pure crystalline G. It occurs in fermentation liquors together with variable amounts of K and F penicillins and doubtless smaller amounts of others, and is separated from the other penicillins during purification. Commercial practice suppresses to a certain extent the natural tendency of the mold to form penicillins other than the desired G by the incorporation of a precursor of G, namely phenylacetic acid or phenylacetamide or other substance containing the phenylacetyl radical, which is built directly into the penicillin G molecule. Penicillin G has the additional advantage of being much easier to crystallize than K or F.

Penicillin V is a modified penicillin, having C_6H_5-OCH_2 (phenoxymethyl) as the radical R in Table I. It is relatively stable in the presence of gastric acidity, soluble in the duodenal fluids, and orally effective without buffers.

As indicated below, penicillin is an acid. The potassium salt predominates in use, with the sodium salt next. Salts of the other alkali metals, alkaline earth metals, and aluminum have been prepared. They are all very soluble in water, but the heavy metal salts are but slightly soluble. The acid of penicillin is insoluble in water and is unstable.

Pure penicillin is white and crystalline. The yellow to brown color of the penicillin formerly found in commerce was due to pigments produced by the mold.

Penicillin in solution is very unstable at pH 5 or less and at 8 or above. Solutions of penicillin begin to deteriorate upon standing a few days, even in the cold. Penicillin is both bactericidal and bacteriostatic, particularly to Gram-positive bacteria. The Gram-negative bacteria (*E. coli*, *Salmonella*) can be inhibited by relatively high concentrations of penicillin. Certain amino acids and derivatives, such as methionine, threonine, and methionine sulfoxide, exert a synergistic effect with penicillin on these organisms. These amino acids antagonize the depressing effect of several other amino acids on penicillin action.

The penicillin resistance of many Gram-positive and Gram-negative bacteria is due to their elaboration of a penicillin-destroying enzyme, *penicillinase*. Penicillinase is produced by large numbers of bacteria and actinomycetes and converts penicillin into inactive *penicilloic acid* by liberation of a second carboxyl group. Resistance of bacteria to penicillin cannot be explained entirely on penicillinase production because many resistant organisms produce little or no penicillinase. By selection and cultivation in progressively higher concentrations of penicillin, highly resistant cultures can be developed from initially sensitive cultures. These may be mutants of the original culture or the result of colony selection. The development of "penicillin-fast" cultures is also encountered clinically.

Many penicillins, natural and semisynthetic, are now known. Systematically, the parent molecule is 4-thia-1-azabicyclo[3.2.0]heptane-2-carboxylic acid (I). The 3,3-dimethyl-7-oxo derivative of (I) is commonly known by the trivial name penicillanic acid (II), and the penicillins are 6-carboxamido derivatives of it (III):

I

Penicillanic Acid
II

Penicillins
III

Penicillins are variously named in the literature as derivatives of (I), (II), and (III) above. Nomenclature by (I) is purely systematic whereas that by (II) and (III) are trivial. As derivatives of (II), it is merely necessary to identify the specific 6-carboxamido group; as derivatives of (III), only the R of the 6-carboxamido group is identified. Examples:

3,3-Dimethyl-7-oxo-6-(2-phenylacetamido)-4-thia-1-azabicyclo-
[3.2.0]heptane-2-carboxylic Acid
6-(2-Phenylacetamido)penicillanic Acid
Benzylpenicillin (or Benzyl Penicillin)

6-[2-(Allylthio)acetamido]-3,3-dimethyl-7-oxo-4-thia-1-azabicyclo-
[3.2.0]heptane-2-carboxylic Acid
6-[2-(Allylthio)acetamido]penicillanic Acid
[(Allylthio)methyl]penicillin (or (Allylthio)methyl Penicillin)

Penicillins known differ in the nature of the radical R. Several of the natural penicillins are shown in Table I.

The introduction of various amines and amides into the medium in which the mold is developing leads to the production of biosynthetic penicillins in which the residues (precursors) comprise R. Phenylacetamide and phenylethylamine, for example, supply the radical

needed by the mold for synthesis of penicillin G. Dozens of biosynthetic *penicillins* have been prepared in this manner in an attempt to obtain compounds superior to penicillin G with respect to various physical, microbiological, or pharmacological properties. For example, penicillin O, which is obtained by growing the mold in a medium containing allylmercaptoacetic acid, has been introduced clinically because it is less allergenic. In 1958 methods were devised for preparing the penicillin nucleus, thus paving the way for a myriad of new (*semisynthetic*) penicillins that could not be formed biosynthetically. The objectives sought by this approach were three-fold: (1) increased acid stability; (2) resistance to penicillinase; and (3) increased breadth of antibacterial spectrum. All these goals have been achieved to some degree. For example, potassium alpha-phenoxyethyl penicillin, the first semisynthetic penicillin to become commercially available, was claimed to have greater acid stability and somewhat more resistance to penicillinase than penicillin G. However, the antibacterial spectra of the two compounds are similar. The availability of alpha-phenoxyethyl penicillin was of major importance in that it demonstrated that synthesis of new penicillins by the chemical addition of side chains to the nucleus was commercially feasible.

The antibacterial activities of the natural penicillins vary, by a small numerical factor, against any single organism. Thus, the effectiveness of penicillins G, F, X, and K against *S. aureus* NRRL B-313 are 1667, 1490, 845, and 2200 units per mg, respectively, and against a rough *B. subtilis* NRRL B-558 are 1667, 970, 1200, and 700 units per mg, respectively. However, some of the semisynthetic penicillins have a broad antibacterial spectrum and are effective against certain organisms that are not sensitive to the natural penicillins.

Cells undergoing partial inhibition are greatly enlarged and in the case of rod-shaped bacteria extremely long bizarre cells are observed, as though growth had proceeded without cell division. Various tinctorial and cultural changes are also noted. Penicillin is known to interfere with the synthesis of *N*-acetylmuramic acid mucopeptides and teichoic acids which are part of the cell wall material. Consequently, the growing protoplast cannot form a protective cell wall. Conditions favoring rapid growth of bacteria are best for the inhibitory action of penicillin. Under favorable conditions, penicillin exerts a direct bactericidal action, and successful penicillin therapy may be relatively independent of immunity mechanisms of the host.

Potency—The potency of penicillin is expressed in units per mg. *One International Unit is equivalent to the activity of 0.6 mcg of pure crystalline sodium penicillin G (sodium penicillin II) to which, by agreement between the United States and Britain, a potency of 1667 units per mg has been assigned.* See Table II.

Assay—See *Biological Testing* (page 642).

Uses—Penicillin is especially effective in the treat-

Table I—Some Natural Penicillins

Natural Penicillin	Radical (R)
Penicillin G	benzyl
Penicillin F	Δ² pentenyl
Penicillin dihydro-F	*n*-amyl
Penicillin K	*n*-heptyl
Penicillin O	(allylthio)methyl
Penicillin V	phenoxymethyl
Penicillin X	*p*-hydroxybenzyl
Penicillin N	D-4-amino-4-carboxybutyl
Penicillin S	γ-chlorocrotylmercaptomethyl
Penicillin BT	butylmercaptomethyl
Flavicidin	Δ³ pentenyl

Table II—Potencies of Penicillin Products

Drug	Units/mg
Benzathine Penicillin G	1211
Potassium Penicillin G	1595
Potassium Phenoxyethyl Penicillin	1476
Procaine Penicillin G	1009
Sodium Penicillin G Master Standard	1667
Sodium Penicillin V Master Standard	1695

ment of infections caused by Gram-positive bacteria, particularly against staphylococcal, streptococcal, pneumococcal, and clostridial infections. Penicillin is also of great value in the treatment of Gram-negative gonococcal and meningococcal infections. It is now the chief therapeutic agent in the treatment of both *gonorrhea* and *syphilis*. Penicillin is often life-saving in the treatment of subacute bacterial *endocarditis* when the causative organism is penicillin-sensitive. As much as 10 to 100 million units of penicillin may be injected daily in this disease. It is also used in the treatment of *diphtheria*, *anthrax*, and *Vincent's* infections and in *actinomycosis* and *leptospirosis*.

Penicillin is sometimes employed in combination with other agents. The results of such therapy are often, but not invariably, superior to those obtainable with penicillin alone. Combined therapy with streptomycin, bacitracin, or neomycin is frequently used. When it is administered with the tetracyclines, chloramphenicol, or the sulfonamides, antagonism may be noted if the microorganism is highly susceptible to penicillin when it is administered alone.

The number of bacteria and the quantity of pus appear to have only a minor influence upon the antibacterial action of penicillin, except when the organism produces penicillinase. Microorganisms exposed to subeffective concentrations of penicillin frequently develop resistance to the antibiotic. For example, in recent years the many strains of staphylococci isolated from clinical material are resistant. The incidence of penicillin-resistant strains of microorganisms is higher in hospitalized patients and hospital personnel in whom cross-infection is more prominent than in the community at large. *Acquired bacterial resistance is an important clinical problem, and therapy should be designed to minimize its development.*

Penicillin is practically nontoxic. However, hypersensitivity reactions occur in 10 to 12% of patients, depending on the type of preparation employed and the route of administration. The most common manifestation of this allergic response is a skin rash. Topical application to the skin may be followed by epidermal sensitivity in more than 10% of patients. The indiscriminate topical use of the drug is therefore discouraged, particularly because such induced sensitivity may preclude the subsequent use of the antibiotic in serious infections endangering the life of the patient. Like other antibiotics, penicillin can markedly alter the normal bacterial flora of man. As a result, superimposed infection by a penicillin-resistant microorganism may develop during the course of treatment and appropriate chemotherapy should be instituted as soon as possible.

Penicillin is given intravenously by continuous infusion only when it is imperative to maintain very high blood concentrations such as in the treatment of subacute *bacterial endocarditis*. For this purpose the soluble sodium or potassium salt of penicillin is employed.

Penicillin in the form of its sodium or potassium salt is rapidly absorbed from subcutaneous and intramuscular sites. The intramuscular route is preferred. The rate of absorption from intramuscular sites of injection may be markedly slowed by the use of repository (depot) preparations consisting of relatively insoluble salts of penicillin in a suitable vehicle. For example, therapeutic blood levels persist 12 to 24 hours after a single 300,000-unit dose of *Procaine Penicillin in Aqueous Suspension;* 24 to 48 hours after *Procaine Penicillin in Oil;* 48 to 96 hours after *Procaine Penicillin in Oil*

with Aluminum Stearate; and 1 week or more after *Benzathine Penicillin G.*

The absorption of penicillin G from the gastrointestinal tract is incomplete and irregular, but some other penicillins are well absorbed. To obtain the same blood concentrations as by the intramuscular route, 3 to 5 times the parenteral dose of penicillin G must be employed. Except for Benzathine Penicillin G and Penicillin V, penicillin should be ingested when the stomach is empty. Although hydrochloric acid in the gastric juice destroys penicillin, buffer agents have not proved to be necessary for successful oral medication. Sodium penicillin may be given in the form of oral tablets. Oral penicillin G therapy should never be relied upon alone in severe infections.

Penicillin does not readily penetrate the subarachnoid space from the blood stream; hence, in *meningitis* it may be advisable to use both the intrathecal and intramuscular routes. For intrathecal administration a soluble salt is used. Crystalline penicillin has an irritating effect when applied directly to the central nervous system. Symptoms following intrathecal administration include listlessness, headache, nausea, vomiting, respiratory difficulty, cyanosis, fall in blood pressure, thready pulse, muscular twitching, and convulsions. These are all reduced or eliminated by lowering the dose.

Penicillin in the form of an aerosol or a specially prepared powder may be used for inhalation therapy in some cases of *pneumonia* if it is felt necessary to enhance the local concentration of penicillin in the lungs over that of the blood and other tissues. From 3 to 6% of patients receiving penicillin by inhalation, it should be noted, manifest hypersensitivity reactions.

Troches have been used in treating *Vincent's stomatitis* and other penicillin-susceptible infections of the mouth. The use of penicillin troches for several days has produced a foul, black, hairy tongue, possibly due to a change in the normal flora of the mouth.

Penicillin is destroyed in the tissues. A substantial amount is excreted in the urine. Substances (See *Probenecid*, page 950) which interfere with renal tubular excretion of penicillin serve to enhance and prolong the effective blood levels of the antibiotic. Probenecid, in sufficient concentration in the blood, completely blocks the renal tubular secretion of penicillin into the tubular urine. This drug therefore markedly slows the excretion of the antibiotic because about 80% of the circulating penicillin reaches the tubules (the glomerular filtration rate is about 20% of the renal plasma flow and the antibiotic excreted in the glomerular filtrate is not reabsorbed by the tubules).

Ampicillin USP

[6 - (D - 2 - Amino - 2 - phenylacetamido) - 3,3 - dimethyl - 7 - oxo - 4 - thia - 1 - azabicyclo [3.2.0] heptane - 2 - carboxylic Acid; (D - α - Aminobenzyl) penicillin; Alpen (*Lederle*); Amcill (*Parke-Davis*); Omnipen (*Wyeth*); Penbritin (*Ayerst*); Polycillin (*Bristol*)]

Ampicillin is anhydrous or contains three molecules of water of hydration. It contains not less than 90.0% of $C_{16}H_{19}N_3O_4S$ (349.41), calculated on the anhydrous basis. It conforms to the regulations of the federal Food and Drug Administration concerning antibiotic drugs (see page 1206).

Preparation—6-Aminopenicillanic acid is acylated with D-(−)-glycine. US Pat. 2,985,648.

Description—White, needle-like crystals, or a white, crystalline powder. The crystals are birefringent and show extinction under polarized light. It is odorless, or has a faint odor characteristic of the penicillins. It occurs as the trihydrate, which is stable at room temperature.

Solubility—1 Gm dissolves in about 90 ml of water, 20 ml of methanol, 250 ml of absolute ethanol, 13 ml of dimethylacetamide, and less than 10 ml of dimethylsulfoxide; practically insoluble in ether, ethyl acetate, petroleum ether, benzene, and chloroform; it is not stable in aqueous solutions of alkali hydroxides and carbonates, and is decomposed by dilute solutions of mineral acids.

Uses—Ampicillin is the first commercial semi-synthetic penicillin to provide increased activity against Gram-negative bacteria. Ampicillin is useful in the treatment of infections due to sensitive strains of *Shigella, Salmonella, E. Coli, H. influenzae, Aerobacter,* and *P. mirabilis.* Its *in vitro* spectrum against Gram-positive cocci is similar to, but generally somewhat less effective than that of penicillin G, except that it is somewhat more effective against *Streptococcus faecalis.* It is poorly effective against penicillinase-producing organisms. Ampicillin is useful in the treatment of *urinary tract infections* caused by *E. coli, P. mirabilis,* nonhemolytic streptococci, and penicillin G-resistant enterococci. It is especially indicated in respiratory tract infections caused by *H. influenzae* and *D. pneumoniae* together. Since Ampicillin is excreted in the bile, it is valuable in treating biliary tract infections due to *E. coli* or penicillin-resistant salmonellae, shigella, or enterococci. Intestinal salmonellosis responds erratically. Ampicillin often effects a satisfactory response in meningitis in children in which the bacterium is meningococcus, pneumococcus, or *H. influenzae.* In mixed infections containing ampicillin-sensitive cocci and bacilli, Ampicillin may be preferred to a combination of penicillin G–streptomycin. Ampicillin causes the allergic reactions typical of other penicillins. Ampicillin is acid-resistant and it is well absorbed by the oral route. Ampicillin may be used in the anhydrous form or as the trihydrate.

Dose—1 to **4 Gm** daily; *usual,* **500 mg** 4 times a day.
Other Dose Information—For genitourinary and gastrointestinal tract infections, 500 mg; for respiratory tract infections caused by *H. influenzae,* 250 mg. When infections are severe, larger doses may be used. With stubborn infections treatment may require several weeks. Children, 100 mg per Kg of body weight daily, in equally divided doses at 6-hour intervals.

Dosage Forms—Capsules USP (equivalent to anhydrous ampicillin): 125, 250, and 500 mg; for Oral Suspension USP (equivalent to anhydrous ampicillin): 100 mg/ml, 1.5 Gm/15 and 60 ml, 2 Gm/20 and 80 ml, 3.75 Gm/150 ml, 4 Gm/80 ml, 7.5 Gm/150 ml.

Veterinary Dose—*Dogs* and *Cats,* **10 mg** per **Kg** of body weight 3 to 4 times daily.

Sodium Ampicillin USP

[Sodium 6 - (D - 2 - Amino - 2 - phenylacetamido) - 3,3 - dimethyl - 7 - oxo - 4 - thia - 1 - azabicyclo [3.2.0]heptane - 2 - carboxylate; D - α - Aminobenzyl) penicillin Sodium; Alpen-N (*Lederle*); Amcill S (*Parke-Davis*); Penbritin-S (*Ayerst*); Polycillin-N (*Bristol-Myers*)]

Sodium Ampicillin contains not less than 90.0% of $C_{16}H_{18}N_3NaO_4S$ (371.39) and not less than 845 mcg of ampicillin per mg. It conforms to the regulations of the federal Food and Drug Administration concerning antibiotic drugs (see page 1206).

Preparation—*Ampicillin* (above) is dissolved in a suitable organic solvent and precipitated as the sodium salt by the addition of sodium acetate.

Description—White to off-white, crystalline powder; hygroscopic.

Solubility—Very soluble in water and isotonic NaCl and dextrose solutions.

Uses—The actions of Sodium Ampicillin are those of *Ampicillin* (above). It is the form of Ampicillin that is employed for intramuscular and intravenous administration.

Dose—*Intramuscular* or *intravenous,* the equivalent of **1** to **14 Gm** of ampicillin daily; *usual,* **500 mg** 4 times a day.
Other Dose Information—Children, 25 to 50 mg per Kg daily, in equally divided doses at 6-hour intervals.

Dosage Forms—Sterile USP: 125, 250, and 500 mg, and 1 and 2 Gm.

Sodium Cloxacillin USP

[Sodium 6-[3-(o-Chlorophenyl)-5-methyl-4- isoxazolecarboxamido] - 3,3 - dimethyl-7-oxo-4 - thia - 1 - azabicyclo [3.2.0]heptane - 2 - carboxylate; Sodium Cloxacillin Monohydrate; Tegopen (*Bristol*)]

Sodium Cloxacillin [$C_{19}H_{17}ClN_3NaO_5S \cdot H_2O$ = 475.89] contains not less than 90.0% of $C_{19}H_{17}ClN_3NaO_5S$, calculated on the anhydrous basis. It conforms to the regulations of the federal Food and Drug Administration concerning antibiotic drugs (see page 1206).

Preparation—6-Aminopenicillanic acid is acylated with 3-(o-chlorophenyl)-5-methyl-4-isoxazolecarboxylic acid and the resulting cloxacillin (acid) is purified by recrystallizations and converted to the sodium salt.

Description—A white, odorless, crystalline powder having a bitter taste. It is stable in light and only slightly hygroscopic. Its aqueous solution is alkaline. It decomposes between 170° and 173°.

Solubility—Freely soluble in water; soluble in alcohol; slightly soluble in acetone and chloroform.

Uses—Sodium Cloxacillin is a penicillinase-resistant penicillin similar to *Sodium Oxacillin* (page 1228) and *Sodium Nafcillin.* Thus, its antibacterial spectrum against Gram-positive bacteria is like that of penicillin except it is broader by the margin of those strains or species that produce penicillinase. However, it is less active than penicillin G against non-penicillinase-producing bacteria, especially streptococci. It is not effective against Gram-negative organisms. Consequently, its use should be limited to treating infections caused by penicillinase-producing susceptible micro-organisms which are resistant to penicillin G. By thus limiting its use, the development of resistance to Cloxacillin is discouraged. Methicillin-resistant staphylococci are also sensitive to Cloxacillin, so that the drug is useful in treating infections which have become resistant to methicillin.

The adverse effects caused by Cloxacillin are virtually identical to those caused by other penicillins (see the general statement under *Penicillin*, page 1223). The incidence of allergic reactions is less than those caused by penicillin G, in part, perhaps, because the drug has not been in use as long. Rash and urticaria are the principal allergic manifestations. Not all patients allergic to penicillin G are sensitive to Cloxacillin, but cross-sensitization does occur. Cloxacillin may also cause occasional nausea, vomiting, abdominal discomfort, epigastric fullness, or diarrhea. Superinfections occasionally occur.

Cloxacillin is relatively stable in gastric acid, but absorption by the oral route is nevertheless erratic; the recommended dose is high enough to compensate for irregularity in the effected blood levels. Food in the stomach interferes with absorption.

Dose—1 to **6 Gm** daily; *usual*, **500 mg** to **1 Gm** 4 times a day.

Dosage Forms—Capsules USP: 125 and 250 mg; for Solution USP: 2 Gm/80 ml, 3.75 Gm/150 ml.

Sodium Methicillin USP

[Sodium 6 - (2,6 - Dimethoxybenzamido) - 3,3 - dimethyl - 7 - oxo - 4 - thia - 1 - azabicyclo [3.2.0] heptane - 2 - carboxylate; (2,6 - Dimethoxyphenyl) penicillin Sodium; Dimocillin-RT (*Squibb*); Staphcillin (*Bristol*)]

Sodium Methicillin contains not less than 90.0% of $C_{17}H_{19}N_2NaO_6S.H_2O$ (420.42). It conforms to the regulations of the federal Food and Drug Administration concerning antibiotic drugs (see page 1206).

Preparation—Fermentation-produced 6-amino-penicillanic acid is condensed with 2,6-dimethoxybenzoyl chloride in a suitable organic solvent and the resulting methicillin is precipitated as the sodium salt by the addition of sodium acetate.

Description—Fine, white, crystalline powder, odorless or having a slight odor.

Solubility—Freely soluble in water, methanol, and pyridine; slightly soluble in propyl and amyl alcohols, chloroform, and ethylene chloride; insoluble in acetone, ether, and benzene.

Uses—Sodium Methicillin is a semisynthetic penicillin which is highly resistant to penicillinase. It is not as effective as penicillin G in infections caused by *hemolytic streptococci, pneumococci, gonococci,* or penicillin G-sensitive *staphylococci.* It is effective against penicillin G-resistant *staphylococci. Restriction of its use to penicillin G-resistant staphylococci infections should minimize the development of Methicillin-resistant strains of bacteria.* Sodium Methicillin is well absorbed after intramuscular injection. The drug is relatively non-irritating to tissues, although there is sometimes more pain after its intramuscular injection than after similar injections of penicillin G.

Besides producing the well-known allergic reactions typical of all penicillins, the most serious effects of Sodium Methicillin reported thus far are several cases of depression of red bone marrow functions producing anemia, neutropenia, or granulocytopenia. These symptoms are reversible after prompt termination of therapy.

Dose—*Intramuscular,* **4** to **8 Gm** daily; *intravenous,* **4** to **16 Gm** daily; *usual, intramuscular* or *intravenous,* **1** to **2 Gm** 4 to 6 times a day.

Other Dose Information—The intramuscular dose for children is 25 mg per Kg of body weight every 6 hours. The adult dose for staphylococcal meningitis is 12 Gm per day.

Dosage Forms—for Injection USP: 1, 4, and 6 Gm.

Sodium Nafcillin USP

[Sodium 6-(2-Ethoxy-1-naphthamido)-3,3-dimethyl-7- oxo - 4 - thia - 1 - azabicyclo [3.2.0]heptane-2-carboxylate; 6 - (2 - Ethoxy - 1 - naphthyl)penicillin Sodium; Unipen (*Wyeth*)]

Sodium Nafcillin is anhydrous or contains one molecule of water of hydration. It contains not less than 90.0% of $C_{21}H_{21}N_2NaO_5S$ (436.47), calculated on the anhydrous basis, and not less than 855 mcg of $C_{21}H_{22}N_2O_5S$ per mg. It conforms to the regulations of the federal Food and Drug Administration concerning antibiotic drugs (see page 1206).

Preparation—6-Aminopenicillanic acid is acylated by treatment with 2-ethoxy-1-naphthoyl chloride in an anhydrous organic solvent containing triethylamine. An aqueous extract of this product is admixed with a water-immiscible solvent and nafcillin (acid) is precipitated by the addition of sulfuric acid. Sodium Nafcillin is precipitated by mixing ethanolic solutions of the acid and sodium ethylhexanoate. US Pat. 3,157,639.

Description—White to yellowish white powder having not more than a slight characteristic odor.

Solubility—Freely soluble in water; soluble in alcohol.

Uses—Nafcillin is resistant to penicillinase, and hence Sodium Nafcillin is used primarily for therapy of infections caused by penicillinase-producing *staphylococci* and other Gram-positive *cocci.* It is also effective against hemolytic streptococci, pneumococci, and gonococci; however, it is usually not used to treat infections caused by these bacteria unless they are part of a mixed infection with penicillin G-resistant staphylococci. It also suppresses the growth of *E. coli* and certain other organisms that cause urinary tract infections, and Nafcillin is sometimes used to treat such infections; however, after oral administration, especially, urine levels of the drug are generally lower than with some other penicillins or too erratic, so that parenteral administration or other penicillins may be preferred. In order to minimize the development of staphylococci resistant to Nafcillin, the drug should be reserved for the treatment of only those infections caused by penicillinase-producing bacteria.

Nafcillin is relatively stable in gastric acid and is absorbed from the gut, although somewhat erratically. For serious infections, initial therapy should be by parenteral administration. Untoward reactions to this drug appear to be similar to those shown by the other penicillins. It is irritating and may cause pain and an increase in serum transaminase activity after intramuscular injection. There may be cross-sensitivity between Nafcillin and other penicillins.

Dose—*Oral, intravenous,* and *intramuscular,* the

equivalent of **1** to **6 Gm** of nafcillin daily; *usual*, the equivalent of **500 mg** of nafcillin 4 to 6 times a day.

Dosage Forms—Capsules USP: 250 mg; Sterile USP: 500 mg.

Sodium Oxacillin USP

[Sodium 3,3 - Dimethyl - 6 - (5 - methyl - 3 - phenyl - 4 - isoxazolecarbox-amido) - 7 - oxo - 4 - thia - 1 - azabicyclo[3.2.0]heptane - 2 - carboxylate; (5-Methyl-3-phenyl-4-isoxazolyl)penicillin Sodium; Prostaphlin (*Bristol*); Resistopen (*Squibb*)]

Sodium Oxacillin contains not less than 90.0% of $C_{19}H_{18}N_3NaO_5S \cdot H_2O$ (441.44). It conforms to the regulations of the federal Food and Drug Administration concerning antibiotic drugs (see page 1206).

Description—Fine, white, crystalline powder, odorless or having a slight odor.

Solubility—Freely soluble in water, methanol, and dimethylsulfoxide; slightly soluble in absolute alcohol, chloroform, pyridine, and methyl acetate; insoluble in ethyl acetate, ether, benzene, and ethylene chloride.

Preparation—Fermentation-produced 6-amino-penicillanic acid is condensed with 5-methyl-3-phenyl-4-isoxazolyl chloride in a suitable organic solvent and the resulting oxacillin is precipitated as the sodium salt by the addition of sodium acetate.

Uses—This semisynthetic penicillin is highly resistant to penicillinase and is absorbed by the oral route of administration. Its actions and uses are nearly identical to those of *Sodium Nafcillin* (above). Like sodium methicillin and sodium nafcillin, it should be restricted to treatment of penicillin G-resistant *staphylococci* infections to minimize the development of resistant strains. Also, because of the variation in absorption after oral administration, oral Sodium Oxacillin is not the drug of choice for most serious infections such as bacteremia and osteomyelitis, but the drug may be given parenterally. However, it may be given orally after the infection is under control.

Allergenic effects are similar to the other penicillins, although cross reactions do not always occur. Oxacillin may also cause nausea, vomiting, diarrhea, fever, eosinophilia, hairy tongue, and, rarely, moniliasis. Because an increased plasma concentration of SGOT has occurred in a few cases, it is suggested that special attention be paid to the use of oxacillin in newborn infants and in patients with hepatic dysfunction. The presence of food in the stomach interferes with absorption.

Dose—*Oral, intramuscular,* or *intravenous,* **1** to **12 Gm** daily; *usual,* **500 mg** 4 to 6 times a day.

Other Dose Information—The oral dose is usually given 1 to 2 hours before meals. For *mild staphylococcic infections* for *adults and children over 40 Kg* the dose is 500 mg every 4 to 6 hours for at least 5 days; for *more serious staphylococcic infections*, 1 Gm every 4 to 6 hours; for *children under 40 Kg*, 50 to 100 mg per Kg of body weight daily in 4 divided doses for at least 5 days.

Dosage Forms—Capsules USP: 250 and 500 mg; for Injection USP: 250 and 500 mg and 1 Gm; for Solution USP: 5 Gm/100 ml.

Benzathine Penicillin G USP

[3,3 - Dimethyl - 7 - oxo - 6 - (2 - phenylacetamido) - 4 - thia - 1 - azabicyclo[3.2.0]heptane - 2 - carboxylic Acid Compound with *N,N* - Dibenzylethylenediamine (2:1); Benzathine Benzylpenicillin; *N,N'*-Dibenzylethylenediamine Dipenicillin G; Bicillin (*Wyeth*)]

Benzathine Penicillin G contains not less than 85.0% of $C_{32}H_{36}N_4O_8S_2 \cdot C_{16}H_{20}N_2 \cdot 4H_2O$ (981.21) and not less than 1050 Penicillin Units* per mg. It conforms to the regulations of the federal Food and Drug Administration concerning antibiotic drugs (see page 1206).

Description—A white, odorless, crystalline powder. Its saturated solution is slightly acid or is neutral to litmus, having a pH of 5.0 to 7.5.

Solubility—1 Gm dissolves in about 5000 ml of water and about 1000 ml of alcohol.

Uses—Benzathine penicillin has a low water solubility. Hence, upon intramuscular injection, it is released slowly and yields sustained blood levels of penicillin generally for 1 to 4 weeks. Its insolubility also renders it less susceptible to acid destruction in the stomach so that it may be administered orally without buffers. Its antibacterial activity and, hence its indications for use are those of the penicillin G base (see general statement, pages 1224 and 1225).

Dose—*Intramuscular,* **600,000** to **3,000,000 Units** 3 times a week to once a month; *usual,* **1,200,000 Units** once a month.

Dosage Forms—Sterile Suspension USP: 600,000 Units/ml, 1,200,000 Units/2 ml, 2,400,000 Units/4 ml, 3,000,000 Units/10 ml.

Potassium Penicillin G USP

[Potassium 3,3 - Dimethyl - 7 - oxo - 6 - (2 - phenylacetamido) - 4 - thia - 1 - azabicyclo[3.2.0]heptane-2-carboxylate; Potassium Benzylpenicillin; Crystalline Penicillin G Potassium; Benzylpenicillin; Pentids (*Squibb*); Pfizerpen (*Pfizer*)]

Potassium Penicillin G contains not less than 85.0% of $C_{16}H_{17}KN_2O_4S$ (372.49) and not less than 90.0% of

* One mg of Benzathine Penicillin G represents 1211 Penicillin Units (see footnote, USP page 523).

total penicillins, calculated as potassium penicillin G. It conforms to the regulations of the federal Food and Drug Administration concerning antibiotic drugs (see page 1206).

Description—Colorless or white crystals, or a white, crystalline powder. Odorless or practically so, and moderately hygroscopic. Dextrorotatory in solution. Decomposed by prolonged exposure to temperatures of about 100°, moisture accelerating decomposition. Not appreciably affected by air or by light. Its solutions deteriorate at room temperature, but solutions stored below 15° remain stable for several days. Rapidly inactivated by acids and alkalies, and also by oxidizing agents. The pH of an aqueous solution, 30 mg per ml, is between 5.0 and 7.5.

Solubility—Very soluble in water, saline TS, and dextrose solutions; soluble in alcohol (but is inactivated by this solvent), glycerin, and many other alcohols.

Uses—See *Penicillin* (pages 1224 and 1225).

Dose—*Oral* or *intramuscular*, **300,000** to **2,000,000 Units** daily; *usual, oral* or *intramuscular*, **500,000 Units** every 6 hours; *intravenous*, **2,000,000** to **40,-000,000 Units** daily; *usual*, **5,000,000 Units** 1 or 2 times a day.

Dosage Forms—for Injection USP; Sterile USP; Tablets USP: 100,000, 200,000, 250,000, 500,000, and 800,000 Units.

Veterinary Dose—A minimum of **2000 units** per **pound** of body weight, *intramuscularly*, every 3 to 4 hours in aqueous vehicle, and in oily vehicle every 12 hours.

Procaine Penicillin G USP

[3,3 - Dimethyl - 7 - oxo - 6 - (2 - phenylacetamido) - 4 - thia - 1 - azabicyclo-[3.2.0]heptane - 2 - carboxylic Acid Compound with 2 - (Diethylamino)ethyl *p*-Aminobenzoate (1:1); 2-(Diethylamino)ethyl *p*-Aminobenzoate Penicillin G; Procaine Benzylpenicillin; Crysticillin (*Squibb*); Duracillin (*Lilly*); Wycillin (*Wyeth*)]

Procaine Penicillin G [$C_{16}H_{18}N_2O_4S \cdot C_{13}H_{20}N_2O_2 \cdot H_2O$ = 588.73] has a potency of not less than 900 Penicillin Units* per mg (89.0%) and it contains not less than 85.0% of procaine penicillin G. It conforms to the regulations of the federal Food and Drug Administration concerning antibiotic drugs (see page 1206).

Preparation—An aqueous solution of sodium (or potassium) penicillin G is caused to undergo metathesis with an equimolar quantity of procaine hydrochloride. The precipitated Procaine Penicillin G is collected by filtration, washed, and dried.

Description—White, fine crystals or a white, very fine, microcrystalline powder. Odorless or practically so, and is not appreciably affected by air or by light. Its solutions are dextrorotatory, and the pH of a saturated solution is between 5.0 and 7.5. Rapidly inactivated by acids and by alkali hydroxides, also by oxidizing agents.

Solubility—1 Gm dissolves in 250 ml of water, about 120 ml of alcohol, and about 60 ml of chloroform.

Uses—Procaine Penicillin G has a relatively low

---

* See USP, page 523.

solubility; hence, upon intramuscular injection, it slowly releases the penicillin G and increases the duration of effective blood levels. For its uses see the general statement for *Penicillin* (pages 1224 and 1225).

Dose—*Intramuscular*, **300,000** to **1,200,000 Units**; daily; *usual*, **600,000 Units** 1 or 2 times a day.

Other Dose Information—The doses for *Procaine Penicillin G with Aluminum Stearate Suspension* and *Procaine Penicillin G and Sodium Penicillin G for Injection* are listed under the statements for these products, below.

Dosage Forms—Sterile Suspension USP (see below): 300,000 and 600,000 Units/ml, 600,000 Units/ 1 and 1.2 ml, 1,200,000 Units/2 ml, 2,400,000 Units/4 ml, 3,000,000 Units/10 ml; Sterile with Aluminum Stearate Suspension USP (see below): 300,000 Units/ 1 and 10 ml; Procaine Penicillin G and Sodium Penicillin G for Injection NF (see below): 400,000, 2,000,-000, and 4,000,000 Units/1-, 5-, and 10-dose containers.

Veterinary Dose—A minimum of **2000 units** per **pound** of body weight, *intramuscularly*, every 24 hours.

Sterile Procaine Penicillin G Suspension USP, is a sterile suspension in water for injection of procaine penicillin G and one or more suitable suspending or dispersing agents and buffers and, when packaged in a multiple-dose container, a suitable preservative. It contains not less than 90.0% of the labeled amount of Penicillin Units, the labeled amount being not less than 300,000 Units per ml. It may contain procaine hydrochloride in a concentration not exceeding 2.0%, and may contain one or more suitable stabilizers. It conforms to the regulations of the federal Food and Drug Administration concerning antibiotic drugs (see page 1206). *Description:* The pH is between 5.0 and 7.5.

Sterile Procaine Penicillin G with Aluminum Stearate Suspension USP [DepoPenicillin (*Upjohn*); Lentopen (*Wyeth*)] is a sterile suspension of procaine penicillin G in refined peanut oil or sesame oil that has been gelled with 2.0% of aluminum monostearate. It contains not less than 90.0% of the labeled amount of Penicillin Units, the labeled amount being not less than 300,000 Units per ml. It may contain suitable dispersing agents. It conforms to the regulations of the federal Food and Drug Administration concerning antibiotic drugs (see page 1206). *Uses:* The water repellency of the aluminum stearate retards the rate of dissolution of the procaine penicillin G. See general statement (page 1224). *Dose: Intramuscular, 300,000 to 1,200,000 Units* daily to 2 times a week; *300,000 Units* on alternate days.

Procaine Penicillin G and Sodium Penicillin G for Injection NF is a sterile, dry mixture of procaine penicillin G and sodium penicillin G and one or more suitable, harmless suspensing or dispersing agents. It contains not less than 90.0% of the labeled amount of penicillin units. It contains sodium penicillin G equivalent to not less than 50,000 units for each 300,000 units of procaine penicillin G. It conforms to the regulations of the federal Food and Drug Administration concerning certification of antibiotic drugs. *Dose: Usual, intramuscular, 400,000 units* 1 or 3 times daily as required.

Sodium Penicillin G NF

[Sodium 3,3 - Dimethyl - 7 - oxo - 6 - (2 - phenylacetamido) - 4 - thia - 1 - azabicyclo [3.2.0]heptane-2-carboxylate; Sodium Benzylpenicillin; Crystalline Penicillin G Sodium; Benzylpenicillin]

Sodium Penicillin G contains not less than 85.0% of $C_{16}H_{17}N_2NaO_4S$ (356.38), and not less than 90.0% of total penicillins, calculated as sodium penicillin G. Sodium Penicillin G conforms to the regulations of the federal Food and Drug Administration concerning certification of antibiotic drugs (see page 1206).

The structure is analogous to that for *Potassium Penicillin G*, page 1228.

Description—Occurs as colorless or white crystals, or as a white to slightly yellow, crystalline powder. It is odorless or practically so, and is moderately hygroscopic. Its solutions are dextrorotatory. It is relatively stable in air, but is inactivated by prolonged heating at about 100°, especially in the presence of moisture. Its solutions lose potency fairly rapidly at room temperature, but retain substantially full potency for several days at temperatures below 15°. Its solutions are rapidly inactivated by acids, alkali hydroxides, oxidizing agents, and penicillinase.

Uses—See the general statement, pages 1224 and 1225.

Dose—*Usual, oral* and *intramuscular*, **400,000 units** 4 times a day; *usual, intravenous*, **10,000,000 units** daily.

Dosage Forms—for Injection NF: 5,000,000 Units.

Veterinary Dose—A minimum of **2000 units** per **pound** of body weight, *intramuscularly*, every 3 to 4 hours in aqueous vehicle, and in oily vehicle every 12 hours.

Phenoxymethyl Penicillin USP

[3,3 - Dimethyl - 7 - oxo - 6 - (2 - phenoxyacetamido) - 4 - thia - 1 - azabicyclo-[3.2.0]heptane-2-carboxylic Acid; Penicillin V; Compocillin-V (*Abbott*); Pen-Vee (*Wyeth*); V-Cillin (*Lilly*)]

Phenoxymethyl Penicillin contains not less than 90.0% of $C_{16}H_{18}N_2O_5S$ (350.40) and not less than 1550 Penicillin Units* per mg of total penicillins as phenoxymethyl penicillin. It conforms to the regulations of the federal Food and Drug Administration concerning certification of antibiotic drugs (see page 1206).

Preparation—Phenoxymethyl Penicillin is a semisynthetic penicillin prepared by culturing the penicillium organism in the presence of 2-phenoxyethanol with an autolyzate of yeast as the source of nitrogen.

Description—White, odorless crystalline powder. The pH of a saturated solution is between 2.5 and 4.0.

Solubility—1 Gm dissolves in about 1200 ml of water, 9 ml of alcohol, and about 6 ml of acetone; insoluble in fixed oils.

Uses—The antibacterial spectrum of Phenoxymethyl Penicillin (penicillin V) is essentially that of penicillin G. Consequently, it shares the same uses (see general statement, page 1224), except that in several acute infections parenteral penicillin G is preferred initially to obtain rapid, high blood levels. Phenoxymethyl penicillin is inactivated less by gastric juice than are the other penicillins. Thus it may be administered orally without the use of buffers. Like penicillin G it may

cause allergic reactions, and it shows cross-sensitivity to the other penicillins. However, allergic reactions are much less common with administration of oral penicillin than with intramuscular forms.

Dose—**500 mg** to **2 Gm** daily; *usual*, **125 to 250 mg** (approximately 200,000 to 400,000 USP Units) 3 or 4 times a day.

Dosage Forms—Capsules USP: 125 and 250 mg (200,000 and 400,000 Units); for Oral Suspension USP: 1.5 Gm (2,400,000 Units)/5 ml, 2 Gm (3,200,000 Units)/80 ml, 3 Gm (4,800,000 Units/60 ml); Tablets USP: 125 and 300 mg (200,000 and 500,000 Units).

Veterinary Dose—*Oral, Dogs* and *Cats*, **200,000 to 500,000 units** at 6- to 8-hour intervals. Usually economically impractical in farm animals wherein recommended doses are: *Horses*, **10,000 to 20,000 units** per **Kg** of body weight; *Swine*, **27,000 units** per **Kg** of body weight; *Fowl*, **27,000 units** at least twice daily.

Potassium Phenoxymethyl Penicillin USP

[Potassium 3,3 - Dimethyl - 7 - oxo - 6 - (2 - phenoxyacetamido) - 4 - thia - 1-azabicyclo [3.2.0]heptane-2-carboxylate; Penicillin V Potassium; Ledercillin V-K (*Lederle*); Pen-Vee K (*Wyeth*) V-Cillin-K (*Lilly*)]

Potassium Phenoxymethyl Penicillin contains not less than 90.0% of $C_{16}H_{17}KN_2O_5S$ (388.49) and not less than 1380 Penicillin Units* per mg of total penicillins as phenoxymethyl penicillin. It conforms to the regulations of the federal Food and Drug Administration concerning antibiotic drugs (see page 1206).

Description—White, odorless, crystalline powder. The pH of an aqueous solution, 30 mg per ml, is between 4.0 and 7.5.

Solubility—Very soluble in water; insoluble in acetone; 1 Gm dissolves in about 150 ml of alcohol.

Uses and **Dose**—Oral Potassium Phenoxymethyl Penicillin provides faster and higher blood levels than phenoxymethyl penicillin. The absorption of the drug does not appear to be diminished if administered after meals. Its actions and uses are those of *Phenoxymethyl Penicillin* (this page).

Dose—**500 mg** to **2 Gm** (800,000 to 3,000,000 Units) daily; *usual*, **125 to 250 mg** (200,000 to 400,000 Units) 3 or 4 times a day.

Dosage Forms—Tablets USP: 125, 250, and 500 mg (200,000, 400,000, and 800,000 Units).

Potassium Phenethicillin NF

[Potassium 3,3-Dimethyl-7-oxo-6-(2-phenoxypropionamido)-4-thia-1-azabicyclo [3.2.0]heptane-2-carboxylate; Potassium (1-Phenoxyethyl)penicillin; Potassium Penicillin-152; Chemipen (*Squibb*); Maxipen (*Roerig*); Ro-Cillin (*Rowell*); Syncillin (*Bristol*)]

Potassium Phenethicillin occurs as crystalline potassium DL-α-phenoxyethyl penicillin and contains not less than 90.0% of $C_{17}H_{19}KN_2O_5S$ (402.52). It contains 55.0–75.0% of potassium L-α-phenoxyethyl penicillin.

---

* See USP page 493.

* See USP, page 526.

Potassium Phenethicillin conforms to the regulations of the federal Food and Drug Administration concerning certification of antibiotic drugs (see page 1206).

Preparation—Fermentation produced 6-aminopenicillanic acid is condensed with 2-phenoxypropionyl chloride in a suitable organic solvent to form phenethicillin which is then precipitated as the potassium salt by means of potassium acetate.

Uses—Potassium Phenethicillin is relatively stable in gastric acid and is used only for oral administration. Its spectrum of antibacterial activity and therapeutic uses are similar to those of penicillin G (see general statement, page 1224). However, for serious infections Phenethicillin is not indicated, parenteral penicillin being superior. Although Phenethicillin is slightly more active than penicillin G against penicillinase-producing staphylococci, the difference is not clinically significant.

Dose—125 to **500 mg**; *usual*, **125 to 250 mg** 3 times a day.

Dosage Forms—for Oral Solution NF: 1.5 Gm/60-ml container, 3.75 Gm/150-ml container; Tablets NF: 125 and 250 mg.

Polymyxin B Sulfate USP

[Aerosporin (*Burroughs-Wellcome*)]

Polymyxin B Sulfate is a substance produced by the growth of *Bacillus polymyxa* (Prazmowski) Migula (Fam. *Bacillaceæ*). It has a potency of not less than 6000 Units of polymyxin B activity per mg, calculated on the dried basis. It conforms to the regulations of the federal Food and Drug Administration concerning antibiotic drugs (see page 1206).

Preparation—The filtered broth from the fermentation step (see page 1207) is treated with a certified dye and the Polymyxin B–dye salt complex thus precipitated is collected by filtration, washed with water, and treated with an alcoholic solution of a lower aliphatic amine sulfate. The Polymyxin B Sulfate thus formed is filtered off, purified, and lyophilized.

There are several polymyxins each of which is an N-monoacylated decapeptide with seven of the amino acid residues in cyclic union. Polymyxin B is a mixture of polymyxin B_1 ($C_{56}H_{98}N_{16}O_{13}$) and polymyxin B_2 ($C_{55}H_{96}N_{16}O_{13}$) the only difference being in the composition of the N-acyl group:

$$L\text{-DAB-}L\text{-THR-}L\text{-DAB-}\overset{\overset{\displaystyle O}{\|}}{C}\text{-R}$$

$$\lceil L\text{-DAB-}L\text{-DAB-}L\text{-THR-}L\text{-DAB-}L\text{-DAB-}D\text{-PHE-}L\text{-LEU}\rceil$$

(DAB = 2,4-diaminobutyric acid)
Polymyxin B_1 R = (+)-6-methylheptyl
Polymyxin B_2 R = 6-methylhexyl

The close relationship between these polymyxins and the colistins (page 1212) is readily apparent. In fact, colistin A is polymyxin E_1 and colistin B is polymyxin E_2.

Description—A white to buff-colored powder. It is odorless or has a faint odor. Its solutions are slightly acid or are neutral to litmus, having a pH of 5 to 7.5.

Solubility—Freely soluble in water; slightly soluble in alcohol.

Uses—The *in vitro* and *in vivo* antimicrobial spectrum of activity of Polymyxin B Sulfate is restricted to Gram-negative bacteria, including *Aerobacter, Eberthella, Escherichia, Hemophilus, Klebsiella, Pasteurella,* *Pseudomonas, Salmonella, Shigella,* and *Vibrio*. Most strains of *Proteus* are unaffected by the antibiotic; some strains of *Neisseria* are also resistant, as are Grampositive bacteria. Bacteria initially sensitive to the antibiotic rarely acquire resistance to it. Substances which antagonize cationic surface-active agents, such as soap and lipositol, impair the action of the antibiotic.

Clinically, polymyxin is effective in the therapy of *pseudomonal bacteremia, meningitis,* and *urinary tract infections,* and of meningitis caused by other Gramnegative bacilli, such as *A. aerogenes, E. coli, K. pneumoniae,* and *H. influenzae*. The drug is also used topically for the treatment or the prevention of *local cutaneous and mucosal infections* caused by susceptible microorganisms, especially *Ps. aeruginosa*.

Polymyxin is readily absorbed when injected subcutaneously or intramuscularly. Peak levels are attained within 30 minutes to 2 hours after injection; the antibiotic is detectable in the serum for 12 hours or more. The drug does not gain access to the cerebrospinal fluid, and gastrointestinal absorption is slow and negligible; conventional oral doses do not yield detectable serum concentrations of the drug. The antibiotic is excreted by the kidney; a total of 60% of the administered drug can be recovered from the urine.

Polymyxin B Sulfate, when given parenterally, can adversely affect the nervous system and the kidney, especially if the total daily dose exceeds 3 mg (30,000 U) per Kg. Neurological disturbances are usually subjective and include dizziness, mild weakness, and paresthesias of the mouth, face, and the extremities. Symptoms are rarely severe when recommended doses are employed; but larger amounts have caused incoordination, ataxia, dysarthria, and dyssynergia. Nephrotoxic effects, with damage to the kidney glomerular and tubular epithelium, are manifested by albumin, red blood cells, leukocytes, and, occasionally, granular casts in the urine; in severe cases, oliguria and elevated level of serum nonprotein nitrogen are noted. No residual damage has been reported and all toxic effects usually clear within 4 days after the last dose of the drug.

Dose—*USP: Intramuscular,* up to **1,500,000 Units** daily; *usual, intramuscular,* **2500 to 5000 Units** per **Kg** of body weight 4 times a day; *intravenous,* up to **2,000,000 Units** daily; *usual, intravenous infusion,* **5000 to 10,000 Units** per **Kg** of body weight in 200 to 500 ml of 5% Dextrose Injection over a period of 60 to 90 minutes 2 times a day; *topically,* as an ointment containing **20,000 Units** in each **Gm,** or as a solution containing **10,000 to 25,000 Units** in each ml. *NF: Oral, usual,* **750,000 Units** 4 times a day.

Other Dose Information—Polymyxin B sulfate is given orally for infections of the intestinal tract, intramuscularly for systemic infections, intrathecally for infections of the meninges, and topically for local infections. The oral dose for adults and older children is 450,000 to 600,000 Units 4 times daily; for children up to 2 years of age, 150,000 to 300,000 Units 3 times daily. The intramuscular dose is administered as a 10% solution in 1% sterile procaine hydrochloride solution; it is ordinarily injected in three equal amounts at intervals of 6 to 8 hours. Intrathecally, the following doses are suggested: children under 2 years of age, 12,000 Units daily for 3 or 4 days, then 15,000 Units every other day; children over 2 years and adults, 30,000 Units daily for 3 or 4 days, then 30,000 Units every other day. The intrathecal solution should contain 30,000 Units in 1 ml of 0.9% sterile sodium chloride solution. For topical application, the drug, in sterile dry form, is dissolved in distilled water or isotonic sodium chloride solution to make a solution of 0.1 to 0.25% and used a drops, spray, wet dressing, or irrigation.

Dosage Forms—Ointment USP; Sterile USP: 500,000 Units; Tablets NF: 250,000 and 500,000 Units.

Veterinary Dose—**10,000 units** per **Gm** in ointments for local application.

Neomycin Sulfate, Polymyxin B Sulfate, and Gramicidin Ophthalmic Solution—see page 1220.
Neomycin Sulfate, Polymyxin B Sulfate, and Zinc Bacitracin Ointment—see page 1220.

Rolitetracycline NF

[4 - (Dimethylamino) - 1,4,4a,5,5a,6,11,12a - octahydro - 3,6,10,12,12a-pentahydroxy - 6 - methyl - 1,11 - dioxo - N - (1 - pyrrolidinylmethyl) - 2-naphthacenecarboxamide; Syntetrin (*Bristol*); Velacycline (*Squibb*)]

Rolitetracycline [$C_{27}H_{33}N_3O_8$ = 527.58] has a potency of not less than 900.0 mcg per mg, calculated on the anhydrous basis. Rolitetracycline conforms to the regulations of the federal Food and Drug Administration concerning antibiotic drugs (see page 1206).

Preparation—Tetracycline, formaldehyde, and pyrrolidine are mixed in an organic solvent. The required condensation occurs spontaneously with the Rolitetracycline crystallizing as it is formed. US Pat. 3,104,240.

Description—A light-yellow, crystalline powder having a characteristic, musty, amine-like odor. It decomposes between 162° and 165°.
Solubility—1 Gm dissolves in 0.8 ml of water; soluble in acetone; slightly soluble in absolute ethanol; very slightly soluble in ether.

Uses—The actions and uses of Rolitetracycline are the same as those of the other tetracyclines (see *Chlortetracycline Hydrochloride*, page 1211). However, it is more soluble than the other tetracyclines, so that it is not necessary to use a salt or to acidify solutions of the drug; consequently, solutions are nearly neutral and are less irritating to the tissues. Therefore, the drug is especially appropriate for parenteral administration. Its molecular potency is about the same as that of chlortetracycline, but, because of a higher molecular weight, somewhat higher doses are required. Toxicity is the same as with other tetracyclines. Since with parenteral administration it is easier to achieve toxic blood levels, care must be exercised in patients with renal or hepatic dysfunction and in pregnant women; the blood level should not exceed 15 mcg per ml.
Dose—*Usual, intramuscular,* **150** to **350 mg** every 12 hours; *intravenous infusion,* **350** to **700 mg** every 12 hours.
Dosage Forms—for Injection NF: 150, 350, and 700 mg.

Cephalothin

Cephalothin [$C_{16}H_{16}N_2O_6S_2$ = 396.45] is 3-(hydroxymethyl) - 8 - oxo - 7 - [2 - (2 - thienyl)acetamido]-5-thia-1-azabicyclo [4.2.0]oct-2-ene-2-carboxylic acid acetate.

For the structure, see *Sodium Cephalothin*.

Preparation—7-Aminocephalosporanic acid is N-acylated through condensation with 2-thiopheneacetyl chloride in an appropriate dehydrochlorinating environment. The starting acid may be prepared from the natural antibiotic, cephalosporin C, by either proton-catalyzed or enzymatic hydrolysis.

Uses and **Dose**—See *Sodium Cephalothin*.

Sodium Cephalothin USP

3 - (Hydroxymethyl) - 8 - oxo - 7 - [2 - (2 - thienyl)acetamido] - 5 - thia - 1 - aza-bicyclo[4.2.0]oct-2-ene-2-carboxylic Acid Acetate Sodium Salt; Keflin (*Lilly*)]

Sodium Cephalothin contains an amount of $C_{16}H_{15}$- $N_2NaO_6S_2$ (418.43) equivalent to not less than 85.0% of cephalothin ($C_{16}H_{16}N_2O_6S_2$), calculated on the anhydrous basis. It conforms to the regulations of the federal Food and Drug Administration concerning antibiotic drugs (see page 1206).

Preparation—*Cephalothin* (this page) may be converted into its sodium salt by interaction with sodium acetate in a suitable organic solvent.

Description—A white to off-white, practically odorless, crystalline powder that is dextrorotatory and moderately hygroscopic. It decomposes on heating.
Solubility—Freely soluble in water, saline TS, and dextrose solution; sparingly soluble in methanol; slightly soluble in alcohol; insoluble in most organic solvents.

Uses—Although Cephalothin is semisynthetic, it is classified as an antibiotic because of the fungal origin of the aminocephalosporanic acid nucleus. Its spectrum of antibacterial activity closely resembles that of the penicillins. It is not affected by penicillinase and hence is active against many penicillinase-producing strains against which penicillin G is ineffective. It is effective against penicillinase-producing staphylococci, beta-hemolytic streptococci, pneumococci, and various strains of Gram-negative bacteria, such as *E. Coli, P. mirabilis, A. aerogenes, H. influenzae, Klebsiella, S. typhosa,* and *Paracolobactrum.* Bacterial resistance to penicillin does not confer resistance to Cephalothin, so that Cephalothin can be used when penicillin fails. The drug should be reserved for treatment of only serious infections resistant to penicillin or in patients allergic to penicillin. Bacteremias, infections of the respiratory tract, and urinary tract infections may be treated with the drug.

Sodium Cephalothin may cause occasional urticaria, rash, eosinophilia, or fever; leukopenia or neutropenia are rare. Superinfections (overgrowth) may occur, especially with *Pseudomonas.* The drug is irritant and may cause pain, induration, or sterile abscesses.

Cephalothin is destroyed in the gastrointestinal tract and must be given parenterally. It is secreted into the urine by the renal tubular transport system and is also secreted into the bile.

Dose—*Parenteral,* the equivalent of **2** to **8 Gm** of cephalothin daily; *usual,* the equivalent of **500 mg** to **1 Gm** of cephalothin 4 to 6 times a day.
Dosage Forms—Sterile USP: 1 and 4 Gm.

Streptomycin

Streptidine
[1,1'-(2,4,5,6-tetrahydroxy-1,3-cyclohexylene)diguanidine]

Streptose

Streptobiosamine

N-Methyl-l-glucosamine

Streptomycin base

Streptomycin $[C_{21}H_{39}N_7O_{12} = 581.58]$ consists of the several antibiotic substances produced by the growth of *Streptomyces griseus* (Krainsky) Waksman et Henrici (Fam. *Actinomycetaceæ*), or each of the same substances produced by any other means. It is usually available as the sulfate $[(C_{21}H_{39}N_7O_{12})_2 . 3H_2SO_4 = 1457.40]$. It complies with the requirements of the federal Food and Drug Administration.

Streptomycin is an organic base, consisting of *N*-methyl-*l*-glucosamine and streptidine linked through the carbohydrate streptose. The overall structure is portrayed above.

Preparation—This antibacterial agent was isolated from soil by Waksman and his colleagues of Rutgers University in 1943.

Streptomycin is produced in organic or synthetic media, in surface or submerged cultures of an actinomycete, *Streptomyces griseus*, a mold-like organism with filaments (mycelium) of bacterial thickness.

Commercially, streptomycin is manufactured like penicillin, microbiologically in tank fermenters with aeration and agitation. The culture medium generally contains a complex nutrient-like meat extract or corn-steep liquor, glucose, an enzymatic digest of casein, and sodium chloride. Soya bean meal also is used. Maximum streptomycin potency is obtained in approximately 40 hours at 25°–28°. After pressure filtration, activated charcoal is added to the filtrate and the streptomycin eluted from the charcoal with acidified methanol. Further purification is achieved by solvent precipitations, or chromatographically, or by a combination of both methods.

Mutation work similar to that used in developing more potent strains of penicillin-producing fungi has also been applied to *Streptomyces griseus* with considerable success. Sometimes the actinomycete growth dissolves before it reaches maturity and this lysis is caused by a phage similar in its action to ordinary bacteriophages. Commercial streptomycin fermentations employ phage-resistant strains of *Streptomyces griseus*.

Description and Properties—The salts of streptomycin mentioned above are bitter, white to slightly pink or pale brownish granules or powder; odorless or nearly so; hygroscopic, and may deliquesce on exposure to air, but are not affected by air or light. Their solutions are levorotatory.

Streptomycin solutions are not precipitated by alkali hydroxides or carbonates (except that calcium carbonate may be precipitated in solutions of the double salt with calcium chloride) or by alkaloid precipitants such as iodine TS, mercuric-potassium iodide TS, or trinitrophenol TS.

Solubility—Very soluble in water; almost insoluble in alcohol, chloroform, and ether.

Uses—Streptomycin in low concentrations is bacteriostatic to a large number of Gram-negative and to some Gram-positive bacteria. It causes misreading of the genetic code and hence disrupts bacterial metabolism. It does not affect fungi, protozoa, or viruses.

Clinically, streptomycin is mainly employed in the treatment of a number of medical and surgical infections caused by Gram-negative organisms; it is frequently combined with penicillin in the treatment of infections caused by certain Gram-positive organisms and it may be occasionally used alone against susceptible Gram-positive organisms that are resistant to other antibiotics. The diseases in which streptomycin is effectively employed include *tuberculosis*, *tularemia*, *bacillary meningitides*, *bacteremias* caused by streptomycin susceptible bacilli or cocci, several *urinary tract infections*, *plague*, and *granuloma inguinale*. Administered alone or with sulfonamides or penicillin, it is also often of considerable value in the treatment of *peritonitis*, *subacute bacterial endocarditis*, *bacillary pneumonias*, *whooping cough* in infants, and *coccal infections refractory to other drugs*. Combined with one of the tetracyclines or sulfadiazine, streptomycin is effective in the treatment of *brucellosis*. *Chancroid* and *gonorrhea* respond to streptomycin, but penicillin is preferred. Given orally, streptomycin more effectively reduces the number of flora in the bowel than does any of the sulfonamides and may thus be used prophylactically prior to bowel surgery. Streptomycin is not effective in typhoid fever, bacillary dysentery, clostridial infections, syphilis, protozoal infections, mycoses, or viral infections.

Streptomycin has been extremely important in the treatment of tuberculosis, although isoniazid, particularly in combination with other agents, is now used more frequently in this application. Streptomycin and isoniazid are frequently employed in combination in the treatment of tuberculosis, especially when the disease is disseminated. Streptomycin exerts a definitely suppressive effect in the majority of cases of pulmonary as well as extra-pulmonary tuberculosis. The drug may be life-saving in the treatment of *miliary tuberculosis* or *tuberculous meningitis*. It should be emphasized that streptomycin is not a curative agent, and it does not in any way minimize the necessity for other established procedures in the management of the disease. Furthermore, only through the use of agents such as isoniazid, para-aminosalicylic acid, etc., which enable streptomycin to be used for long periods of times with minimal development of streptomycin-resistance, are the full potentialities of the antibiotic realized in the treatment of tuberculosis.

In addition to mycobacteria, many bacteria rapidly become highly resistant to streptomycin during the course of therapy, and several species can produce strains actually dependent upon the antibiotic. Since streptomycin was originally introduced into medicine, the number of streptomycin-resistant strains of bacteria has increased so greatly that at the present time the majority of strains of certain Gram-negative pathogens are resistant to the drug. Therefore, the antibiotic should be employed only in the treatment of those infections in which the pathogen is known to be streptomycin-susceptible. The possibility of the emergence of drug-resistant strains of bacteria during therapy also demands careful attention to the adequacy of the initial dose and to the maintenance schedule. The sulfonamides or other appropriate antibacterial agents are often combined with streptomycin to delay the emergence of drug-resistant bacteria, as well as to enhance the antibacterial action of the antibiotic.

The principal toxic effects of streptomycin are hypersensitivity and neurotoxicity, although mild malaise, muscular aching, and drug fever also frequently occur. Hypersensitivity may be natural or acquired, and it almost invariably occurs if therapy is prolonged and the dose is moderate to high. Neurotoxicity occurs chiefly to the eighth cranial nerve; it may not become apparent until sometime after therapy has been discontinued. Hearing loss may even result from small doses given only for a short period of time. Eighth nerve damage may result in either vestibular disturbances, which are frequent and often permanent, or auditory impairment, which occurs somewhat less frequently and is more often reversible than are vestibular disturbances. Dihydrostreptomycin causes more auditory impairment than vestibular disturbance; consequently, the two streptomycins were once combined in half-doses each, the therapeutic and toxic effects of the components of the mixture supposedly adding in such a way as to promote a slight increase in over-all therapeutic index. However, auditory impairment proved to occur more frequently with the combination than with full doses of streptomycin alone; consequently, the two drugs are no longer used in combination.

Streptomycin may be administered by any parenteral route but the *deep intramuscular* route is preferred.

Streptomycin Sulfate USP

[Streptomycin Sulfate (2:3); Strycin Sulfate (*Squibb*)]

Streptomycin Sulfate contains an amount of $(C_{21}H_{39}N_7O_{12})_2 \cdot 3H_2SO_4$ (1457.40) equivalent to not less than 65.0% of streptomycin base $[C_{21}H_{39}N_7O_{12} = 581.58]$ (the antibiotic activity of 650 mcg of the base per mg). It conforms to the regulations of the federal Food and Drug Administration concerning antibiotic drugs (see page 1206).

For the structure of streptomycin, see page 1233.

Description—A white or practically white powder. It is odorless or has not more than a faint odor. It is hygroscopic, but is stable toward air and light. Its solutions are acid to nearly neutral to litmus, and are levorotatory.

Solubility—Freely soluble in water; very slightly soluble in alcohol; practically insoluble in chloroform.

Uses—See *Streptomycin* (page 1233).

Dose—*Intramuscular*, the equivalent of **1 Gm** weekly to **2 Gm** daily of streptomycin; *usual*, **1 Gm** 2 to 7 times a week.

Other Dose Information—The drug is dissolved in isotonic dextrose or sodium chloride solution to yield a concentration of 100 to 200 mg of base per ml. The dose varies according to the severity of the infection and the susceptibility of the pathogen. The total daily dose varies from 1 to 4 Gm of base, taken in divided doses at 6- to 12-hour intervals; 500 mg every 6 hours is a common regimen. Except in the treatment of tuberculosis or subacute bacterial endocarditis, 7 to 10 days of treatment are generally sufficient. Other parenteral routes occasionally employed are the *sub-*

cutaneous, intravenous, intraperitoneal, and *intrapleural* routes. In meningitis, the drug is sometimes given *intrathecally* in doses of less than 1 mg per pound of body weight, not to exceed 50 mg, although neurotoxicity is more probably by this route. For pulmonary infections, solutions containing 50 to 100 mg per ml are sometimes administered as aerosols for inhalation. *Oral* ingestion is utilized only for local antibacterial effects in the gastrointestinal tract; 500 mg to 1.0 Gm is administered every 6 hours for 2 to 3 days. For *topical* application, a solution of streptomycin sulfate, 25 to 50 mg per ml, is employed, but cutaneous reactions and drug resistance are favored by this route, and the poor penetrability of the drug also discourages this use.

In tuberculosis, 0.5 to 1.0 Gm is given daily or twice weekly with PAS 12.0 Gm daily or isoniazid 300 mg daily. The streptomycin is injected intramuscularly and the PAS and isoniazid given orally.

Dosage Forms—Injection USP: 500 mg/1 and 1.25 ml, 1 Gm/2 and 2.5 ml, 5 Gm/10 and 12.5 ml.

Veterinary Dose—**5 mg** per **pound** of body weight *intramuscularly* in aqueous solution at 12 to 24-hour intervals for mammals.

Tetracycline USP

[4 - Dimethylamino - 1,4,4a,5,5a,6,11,12a - octahydro - 3,6,10,12,12a-pentahydroxy - 6 - methyl - 1,11 - dioxo - 2 - naphthacenecarboxamide; Achromycin (*Lederle*); Panmycin (*Upjohn*); Steclin (*Squibb*); Tetrac he (*Rachelle*); Tetracyn (*Roerig*)]

Tetracycline $[C_{22}H_{24}N_2O_8 = 444.45]$ contains, in each mg, the antibiotic activity of not less than 975 mcg of tetracycline hydrochloride $[C_{22}H_{24}N_2O_8 \cdot HCl = 480.91]$, calculated on the anhydrous basis. Tetracycline conforms to the regulations of the federal Food and Drug Administration concerning antibiotic drugs (see page 1206).

Preparation—Tetracycline is prepared by removal of the chloride atom from chlortetracycline by means of a hydrogenation procedure. At the Antibiotic Symposium held in Washington in October, 1953, the Heyden Chemical Corporation announced the isolation of tetracycline from a *Streptomyces sp.* found in a soil sample from Texas. Ultraviolet, infrared, and crystallographic studies have shown the fermentation product to be identical with that produced by catalytic hydrogenation. A study of blood concentrations following oral administration of various doses of tetracycline made by fermentation resulted in findings similar to those obtained with the synthesized product.

Description—A yellow, odorless, crystalline powder. It is stable in air, but exposure to strong sunlight causes it to darken. Its potency is affected in solutions of pH below 2, and is rapidly destroyed by alkali hydroxide solutions. Tetracycline is more soluble than chlortetracycline and within the physiological and moderately alkaline range of pH is more stable. Solutions of Tetracycline darken more rapidly than chlortetracycline but less than oxytetracycline. Specific rotation $-254°$ to $-270°$ (C = 1, 0.1 N HCl). pH of aqueous suspension (10 mg per ml) is between 3.0 and 7.0.

Solubility—1 Gm dissolves in about 2500 ml of water and about 50 ml of alcohol; freely soluble in dilute hydrochloric acid and alkali hydroxide solutions; practically insoluble in chloroform and ether.

Uses—The antibiotic spectrum, actions, absorption, fate and excretion, doses and uses of Tetracycline are essentially the same as those of *Chlortetracycline Hydrochloride* (page 1211). The relative susceptibilities and resistance of the various microorganisms are virtually identical for both drugs and for oxytetracycline, demeclocycline, and rolitetracycline. The gastrointestinal side effects from Tetracycline are less than those from the two related antibiotics. The duration of action of Tetracycline lies between those of chlortetracycline and oxytetracycline.

Dose—The equivalent of **10** to **40 mg** of tetracycline hydrochloride per **Kg** of body weight daily; *usual*, **2.5** to **5 mg** 4 times a day.

Dosage Forms—Oral Suspension USP: 100 mg/ ml, 125 mg/5 ml; for Oral Suspension USP: 1.5 Gm./ 30 ml.

Tetracycline Hydrochloride USP

[4 - (Dimethylamino) - 1,4,4a,5,5a,6,11,12a - octahydro - 3,6,10,12,12a - pentahydroxy - 6 - methyl - 1,11 - dioxo - 2 - naphthacenecarboxamide Monohydrochloride]

Tetracycline Hydrochloride contains not less than 90.0% of $C_{22}H_{24}N_2O_8$. HCl (480.91). It conforms to the regulations of the federal Food and Drug Administration concerning antibiotic drugs (see page 1206).

Description—A yellow, odorless, crystalline powder. It is moderately hygroscopic. It is stable in air, but exposure to strong sunlight in moist air causes it to darken. Its potency is affected in solutions of pH below 2, and is rapidly destroyed by alkali hydroxide solutions. Its 1 in 100 solution has a pH between 1.8 and 2.8. Specific rotation −250° to −263° (C = 1, 0.1 N HCl).

Solubility—1 Gm dissolves in 10 ml of water and about 100 ml of alcohol, the aqueous solution becoming turbid after some time because of hydrolysis; soluble in solutions of alkali hydroxides and carbonates; practically insoluble in chloroform and ether.

Uses—See *Tetracycline* (page 1234). Since the Hydrochloride is the more soluble form of Tetracycline, it is used for parenteral administration and in solutions for topical use.

Dose—*Oral*, **1** to **4 Gm** daily; *usual*, **250 mg** 4 times a day; *intramuscular*, **200** to **500 mg** daily; *usual*, **100 mg** 2 or 3 times a day; *intravenous*, **500 mg** to **2 Gm** daily; *usual*, *infusion*, **250** to **500 mg** in 1/2 to 1 hour 2 times a day; *topically*, **0.1** to **0.2 ml** of a **0.5**% solution applied to eyelid or conjunctiva.

Dosage Forms—Capsules USP: 50, 100, 125, and 250 mg; for Injection USP: 100, 250, and 500 mg; for Ophthalmic Solution NF: 25 mg/5 ml; Tablets NF: 50, 100, and 250 mg.

Veterinary Dose—*Parenterally, large animals*, **1** to **2 mg** per **pound** of body weight daily; *small animals*, **5 mg** per **pound** of body weight daily.

Tetracycline Phosphate Complex NF

[Panmycin Phosphate (*Upjohn*); Sumycin (*Squibb*); Tetrex (*Bristol*)]

Tetracycline Phosphate Complex has a potency of not less than 750.0 mcg per mg, as tetracycline hydrochloride, on the anhydrous basis. Tetracycline Phosphate Complex conforms to the regulations of the federal Food and Drug Administration concerning certification of antibiotic drugs.

Preparation—This relatively insoluble complex precipitates when a solution of tetracycline hydrochloride is treated with a solution of sodium metaphosphate. US Pat. 3,053,892.

Description—Yellow, odorless, fine, crystalline powder. The crystals are birefringent and show extinction under polarized light. Its pH in an aqueous suspension prepared by adding 10 mg per ml is between 2.0 and 4.0.

Solubility—Sparingly soluble in water; 1 Gm dissolves in about 30 ml of methanol, about 500 ml of absolute ethanol, and less than 10 ml of formamide, dimethylformamide, dimethylacetamide, and dimethylsulfoxide; very slightly soluble in acetone; practically insoluble in ether, ethyl acetate, petroleum ether, benzene, and chloroform.

Uses—The actions, uses, and toxicity of Tetracycline Phosphate Complex are identical to those of *Tetracycline* (page 1234). It has been claimed that oral Tetracycline Phosphate Complex yields faster and higher blood levels than with tetracycline or tetracycline hydrochloride. However, the effect, if any, is minor and does not in any way change the dosage schedule of this agent from that of tetracycline.

Dose—The equivalent of **250** to **500 mg** of tetracycline hydrochloride; *usual*, **250 mg** 4 times a day.

Dosage Forms—Capsules NF: 100, 250, and 500 mg.

Troleandomycin NF

[Oleandomycin Triacetate (Ester); Triacetyloleandomycin NF XII; Cyclamycin (*Wyeth*); TAO (*Roerig*)]

Troleandomycin [$C_{41}H_{67}NO_{15}$ = 813.99] is the triacetyl ester of oleandomycin. It has a potency of not less than 760 mcg per mg. It conforms to the regulations of the federal Food and Drug Administration concerning certification of antibiotic drugs (see page 1206).

For the structure of oleandomycin, see page 1222.

Preparation—Oleandomycin is triacetylated by reaction with acetic anhydride in the presence of pyridine.

Description—It occurs as a white, odorless, crystalline powder. A solution in diluted alcohol has a pH range between 7.5 and 9.0. The specific rotation of a solution in trichlorethylene (200 mg in 10 ml) −16° to −22°.

Solubility—1 Gm dissolves in about 10 ml of alcohol; slightly soluble in ether and water.

Uses—Identical to *Oleandomycin Phosphate* (page 1222); however, it is somewhat more completely absorbed from the gastrointestinal tract and thus has a longer duration of action and less frequent dosage may be used. Troleandomycin is converted in the body to oleandomycin.

Dose—**250** to **500 mg**; *usual*, **250 mg** 4 times a day.

Dosage Forms—Capsules NF: 125 and 250 mg; Oral Suspension NF: 125 mg/5 ml.

Veterinary Use—Treatment of canine pyogenic dermatitides.

Veterinary Dose—*Dogs*, medium sized, **250 mg** *orally* twice daily for 10 to 14 days.

Tyrothricin NF

Tyrothricin is an antibacterial substance produced by the growth of *Bacillus brevis* Dubos (Fam. *Bacteriaceæ*). It consists principally of gramicidin and tyrocidine, the tyrocidine usually being present as the hydrochloride. Tyrothricin has a potency of 900–1400 mcg in each mg. Tyrothricin conforms to the regulations of the federal Food and Drug Administration concerning certification of antibiotic drugs. (see page 1206).

The gramicidin component (10 to 20%) of Tyrothricin is neutral and is, itself, a mixture of at least three polypeptides (see *Gramicidin*, page 1218). The tyrocidine component (40 to 60%) is basic and has been fractionated into three polypeptides, tyrocidine A, B, and C, by counter-current distribution. Tyrocidine A ($C_{66}H_{87}N_{13}O_{13}$) has been shown to be:

```
     1          2          3          4          5
   L-Val——L-Orn——L-Leu——D-Phe——L-Pro
    |10         9          8          7          6|
   L-Tyr——L-Glu——L-Asp——D-Phe——L-Phe
```

Tyrocidine B ($C_{68}H_{88}N_{14}O_{13}$) is 6-L-tryptophanetyrocidin A and Tyrocidin C ($C_{70}H_{89}N_{15}O_{13}$) is 7-D-tryptophane tyrocidin B.

Preparation—Tyrothricin is produced by an aerobic spore-forming bacteria, *Bacillus brevis*, and the active material is extracted from the bacterial cells. Yields are highest in surface cultures in media containing complex nitrogen fractions such as casein digests, although smaller yields can be obtained on synthetic media, and also in submerged culture. The presence of biotin in the medium increases the yield of Tyrothricin. The whole culture is adjusted to pH 4.5, which precipitates the cells and debris and which then are separated and extracted with 95% ethanol. Amorphous tyrothricin is precipitated from the alcohol by the addition of 10 volumes of 1% NaCl. Yields as high as 3 Gm per liter are possible.

Tyrothricin consists of two crystallizable polypeptides, *gramicidin* and *tyrocidine* (see below), the former amounting to about 20% of the total.

Description—White, grayish white, or brownish white powder. Odorless, or nearly odorless, and almost tasteless.

Solubility—Practically insoluble in water; 1 Gm dissolves in about 15 ml of alcohol, usually leaving a small amount of residue; freely soluble in glacial acetic acid; slightly soluble in acetone; insoluble in chloroform and ether.

Uses—Tyrothricin is useful in the local treatment of a variety of superficial infections caused by susceptible Gram-positive bacteria including surgical and traumatic *wounds*, decubitus, traumatic and varicose *ulcers, infectious eczematoid dermatitis, pyoderma, impetigo, folliculitis, furunculosis*, and certain *dermatophytoses*. In addition, the antibiotic is used for the preparation of infected ulcers or granulating wounds prior to skin grafting. It is also effective in the various infections of the eye, nose, and throat, such as *acute conjunctivitis* and *keratoconjunctivitis*, resistant marginal *corneal ulcer*, and acute *rhinopharyngitis*. Tyrothricin is widely and successfully employed in *bovine streptococcal mastitis*, for which purpose it is introduced into the test canal.

Tyrothricin is ineffective when given orally and ineffective and *dangerous* when given intravenously; it is a potent hemolytic agent and should not be administered by any route which will permit it to come into contact with the blood stream. Local application of Tyrothricin, when correctly employed, is practically devoid of untoward reactions; healing of surface lesions is not delayed, and hypersensitivity reactions are practically unknown. Irrigation of the paranasal sinuses with Tyrothricin suspensions has resulted in *chemical meningitis* with serious sequelae and even death. Disturbance of olfactory sense has followed the application of the drug to the nasal mucosa.

Tyrothricin is used as a solution (in alcohol), as a spray, and as a troche. The concentration of antibiotic usually employed is 0.5 mg per ml or per Gm. Tyrothricin must be applied locally, *not intravenously or taken internally by mouth.*

Dose—*Topically*, to the skin and mucous membranes in dosage forms which contain **0.05 to 0.3%** of Tyrothricin.

Vancomycin Hydrochloride USP

[Vancocin (*Lilly*)]

Vancomycin Hydrochloride is a substance produced by the growth of *Streptomyces orientalis* (Fam. *Streptomycetaceae*). It has a potency equivalent to not less than 900 mcg of vancomycin per mg, calculated on the anhydrous basis. It conforms to the regulations of the federal Food and Drug Administration concerning antibiotic drugs (see page 1206).

The composition of vancomycin is still being researched. It has been shown to have a molecular weight of about 3300 and to contain about 7% nitrogen and 16% carbohydrate.

Preparation—Vancomycin is produced by the submerged fermentation process (page 1207). After purification, the base is reacted with HCl to form the soluble hydrochloride.

Description—Tan to brown, free-flowing powder, odorless and having a bitter taste.

Solubility—Freely soluble in water; insoluble in ether and chloroform.

Uses—Vancomycin is highly active against gram-positive cocci. It has proved valuable in the treatment of severe staphylococci infections. The development of resistance to Vancomycin is virtually unknown, and there is no cross-resistance from other antibiotics. This is extremely important, since staphylococci are capable of resisting all the previous major systemic antibiotics, and a "back-up" drug is needed. Streptococci and pneumococci infections have also been successfully treated with Vancomycin. Used systemically the drug may cause deafness, thrombophlebitis, skin rashes, and fever. Consequently, the drug is held in reserve for serious infections that are unresponsive to other antibacterial agents. Vancomycin is poorly absorbed from the gastrointestinal tract, so that it may be used orally against staphylococcal and enterococcal enteritis. However, severe enteritis often requires concomitant systemic therapy and hence parenteral administration. Vancomycin is irritating and may cause thrombophlebitis or pain at the site of injection.

Dose—*Intravenous*, **1 to 2 Gm** daily; *usual*, **500 mg** in 100 to 200 ml of an isotonic solution every 6 hours by slow infusion over a period of 30 minutes.

Other Dose Information—The usual oral dose is 500 mg to 1 Gm, up to a maximum of 4 Gm per day.

Dosage Forms—Sterile USP: 500 mg.

Viomycin Sulfate USP

[Viomycin (*Parke-Davis*); Vinactane Sulfate (*Ciba*); Viocin Sulfate (*Pfizer*)]

Viomycin Sulfate ($C_{25}H_{36}N_{12}O_8 \cdot xH_2SO_4$) is the sulfate salt of an antibacterial substance produced by the growth of *Streptomyces puniceus, Streptomyces floridae*, or *Actinomyces vinaceus*, or by other means. It contains an amount of viomycin sulfate equivalent to not less than 70.0% of viomycin, calculated on the anhydrous basis.

It conforms to the regulations of the federal Food and Drug Administration concerning antibiotic drugs (see page 1206).

Description—Fine, white or cream-white, odorless, crystalline powder.

Solubility—Very soluble in water; practically insoluble in methanol and chloroform.

Uses—Unlike other antibiotics, Viomycin is relatively more active against Mycobacteria than against any other genus of microorganisms. However, it is not as potent as streptomycin, and its toxicity is relatively greater. But, it is active against streptomycin- and isoniazid-resistant strains of tubercle bacilli, so that it finds uses as an *antituberculous agent* when the causative organisms become adamant to streptomycin or isoniazid. Because of its toxicity, viomycin should not be used for routine therapy of minimal or primary pulmonary tuberculosis, unless other therapy has failed. However, it may be used as an adjunct to the therapy of extra-pulmonary tuberculosis, pneumonic tuberculosis or progressive exudative tuberculosis with hematogenous lesions. It may also be employed prophylactically with chest surgery in tuberculous patients. Other antituberculous agents may and should be combined with viomycin.

Viomycin may cause renal damage, edema or fluid retention, allergic reactions, vertigo, electrocardiographic abnormalities, and partial loss of hearing. Toxic manifestations are fewer and less severe with intramuscular than with intravenous injection; thus the intramuscular route is mandatory. It is ineffective by the oral route.

Dose—*Intramuscular*, the equivalent of **4 to 14 Gm** of viomycin weekly; *usual*, **1 Gm** 2 times a day every third day.

Other Dose Information—A course of therapy is 4 to 6 months. 2 Gm daily for 1 month may be given, if necessary, only if laboratory facilities to monitor toxicity are fully available.

Dosage Forms—Sterile USP: 1 and 5 Gm.

Other Antibiotics

Calcium Amphomycin is a calcium salt of amphomycin, an amphoteric polypeptide antibiotic with surface-active characteristics which accumulates during the culture of *Streptomyces canus*. It conforms to the regulations of the federal Food and Drug Administration concerning antibiotic drugs (see page 1206). *Description and Solubility:* A white to pale buff powder that has a characteristic yeast-like odor and a slightly bitter taste; it is stable in light, slightly hygroscopic, and stable in powder form up to 2 years at room temperature. 1 Gm dissolves in 50–100 ml of water; slightly soluble in alcohol; insoluble in ether. *Uses:* Amphomycin is an effective antibacterial agent against most Gram-positive organisms but not against Gram-negative bacteria. It is toxic systemically, so that its use is limited to topical application to the skin. It causes cutaneous allergic responses in probably less than 1% of patients; the exact incidence of hypersensitivity is not known, because the drug is marketed in a product in which neomycin and hydrocortisone are also contained. *Dose: Topically*, as a cream containing 0.5% of the amphomycin base, to be applied to the affected area 3 times a day.

Calcium Chlortetracycline [Aureomycin Calcium (*Lederle*)] is $C_{22}H_{21}CaClN_2O_8$. Its precise structure has not been established. It conforms to the regulations of the federal Food and Drug Administration concerning antibiotic drugs (see page 1206). *Description and Solubility:* A white powder. Insoluble in water; it will dissolve in acid solutions (pH 2.8) or in solutions of alkalies or alkaline carbonates (pH 10). *Uses:* A relatively stable, soluble form of chlortetracycline for incorporation into drops or syrups, for patients who cannot take dry forms of the drug and for topical application. Its actions and uses are those of *Chlortetracycline Hydrochloride* (page 1211). However, the calcium interferes slightly with absorption, so that blood levels are somewhat lower than with the hydrochloride. *Dose:* Express in terms of the hydrochloride salt (page 1211) and is supposedly identical.

Cephaloridine [Loridine (*Lilly*)] is 1-[(2-carboxy-8-oxo-7-[2-(2-thienyl)acetamido]-5-thia-1-azabicyclo-[4.2.0]oct-2-en-3-yl)methyl]pyridinium hydroxide inner salt [$C_{19}H_{17}N_3O_4S_2$ = 415.50]. *Preparation:* An aqueous mixture of *Cephalothin* (page 1232), a thiocyanate, pyridine, and phosphoric acid is heated for several hours. On cooling, diluting with water, and adjusting the pH with mineral acid, a cephaloridine thiocyanate salt precipitates which is purified and converted to Cephaloridine by pH adjustment or by interaction with an ion-exchange resin. *Description and Solubility:* A white to slightly off-white powder that has a slight pyridine odor and a trace pyridine taste; prolonged exposure to light and heat (over 26°) should be avoided; degradation is evidenced by a darkening of the powder and a decrease in antibiotic potency; it is stable in air. 1 Gm dissolves in about 2 Gm of water at 30° and in about 3.2 Gm of water at 26°; insoluble in both chloroform and ether at 26°; its degradation is apparent in alcohol.

Uses: The actions and uses of Cephaloridine are those of *Sodium Cephalothin* (see page 1232). The minimal effective concentrations of either drug are virtually identical regardless of the microorganism, except that Cephaloridine is about twice as potent against enterococci. Patients allergic to penicillin G are usually not sensitive to Cephaloridine, but occasional cross-sensitivity occurs. Above a total daily dose of 4 Gm Cephaloridine may cause nephrotoxicity. Patients with impaired renal function should have their renal function monitored carefully. Cephaloridine may also cause itching, urticaria, skin rashes, and rarely nausea and vomiting. Superinfections, particularly to *Pseudomonas*, sometimes occur during treatment. *Dose: Intramuscular* or *intravenous*, 250 mg to 1 Gm 2 to 4 times a day; *usual*, 500 mg 3 times a day. On intramuscular injection Cephaloridine causes less pain than does cephalalothin.

Dihydrostreptomycin Sulfate USP XVI ($C_{21}H_{41}N_7O_{12}$). $3H_2SO_4$—A white or practically white powder. 1 Gm dissolves in about 0.5 ml of water; very slightly soluble in alcohol; practically insoluble in chloroform. *Uses:* It has the same antibacterial spectrum as *Streptomycin* (page 1233). However, it should be used only in those patients who cannot tolerate streptomycin, because auditory impairment or total deafness may be caused by relatively small doses of the drug administered for a short time. Dihydrostreptomycin ordinarily should not be injected intrathecally and it must never be administered intravenously. *Dose: Intramuscular*, 1.25 Gm to 2.5 Gm.

Doxycycline [Vibramycin (*Pfizer*)] is 4-(dimethylamino)-1,4,4a,5,5a,6,11,12a-octahydro-3,5,10,12,12a-pentahydroxy - 6α - methyl - 1,11 - dioxo - 2 - naphthacene-carboxamide [$C_{22}H_{24}N_2O_8$ = 444.43]. It conforms to the regulations of the federal Food and Drug Administration concerning antibiotic drugs (see page 1206). *Preparation:* 6 - Deoxy - 6 - demethyl - 6 - methylene - 5 - oxytetracycline, dissolved or suspended in an inert liquid such as methanol, is hydrogenated under the influence of catalytic amounts of noble metals such as rhodium or palladium to produce a mixture of the 6α and 6β epimers of 6-deoxy-5-oxytetracycline. The desired 6α compound is then isolated by chromatographic processes. US Pat. 3,200,149. *Description and Solubility:* A yellow, crystalline powder that is odorless and has a bitter taste; it is unstable in light, nonhygroscopic, and stable at room temperature; it melts with decomposition between 167° and 170°. Very slightly soluble in water, alcohol, and chloroform; insoluble in ether.

Uses: Doxycycline is a tetracycline with a consequent antibacterial spectrum like that of other tetracyclines (see *Chlortetracycline Hydrochloride,* page 1211). Its uses will be essentially the same, except the urine concentrations are lower, so that it is not as efficacious as the shorter-acting tetracyclines in the treatment of urinary tract infections. The low rate of excretion results in a long duration of action. The half-life is about 15 hours, which is approximately the same as that of methacycline. The toxicity of Doxycycline is that of tetracyclines in general, but photosensitization occurs more frequently than with tetracycline, chlortetracycline, or oxytetracycline. In the presence of impaired renal function, a shorter-acting tetracycline should be used. *Dose: Usual, initial,* 300 mg in two divided doses on the first day; *maintenance,* 100 mg twice a day. The manufacturer recommends an initial dose of 200 mg and a maintenance dose of 100 mg once a day, except twice a day in urinary tract infections; however, reliable medical opinion considers this schedule to be inadequate.

Hetacillin [*Bristol*] is 6-(2,2-dimethyl-5-oxo-4-phenyl-1-imidazolidinyl) - 3,3 - dimethyl - 7 - oxo - 4 - thia - 1 - azabicyclo[3.2.0]heptane-2-carboxylic acid ($C_{19}H_{23}N_3O_4S$). It conforms to the regulations of the federal Food and Drug Administration concerning antibiotic drugs (see page 1206). *Description and Solubility:* A fine, white to off-white, crystalline powder having a slight odor and a warm, slightly bitter taste; it melts between 170° and 180°. Slightly soluble in water; very slightly soluble in absolute ethanol.

Uses: Hetacillin is virtually identical to *Ampicillin* (page 1225) in its antibacterial spectrum and therapeutic uses. Its antibacterial potency is comparable. Like ampicillin, it is destroyed by penicillinase and hence is limited in usefulness in the treatment of infections caused by penicillinase producers. It appears to be degraded in the body to a lesser extent than ampicillin, so that somewhat higher plasma concentrations are reached after oral ingestion and are maintained at higher levels. Urine concentrations are also higher than with ampicillin. Hetacillin has prove to be effective in the treatment of *urinary tract infections* caused by various Gram-negative bacilli, bacteremia caused by *E. coli,* shigellosis, typhoid fever, other salmonellosis, and pneumonia caused by pneumococci or *Hemophilus.* The untoward effects of Hetacillin appear to be the same as those of ampicillin. At the time of this writing, Hetacillin is still an experimental drug, but there is no question but that it will be approved shortly for general clinical use. *Dose: Oral, intramuscular,* or *intravenous,* 250 mg to 2 Gm; *usual,* 500 mg to 1 Gm every 6 hours.

Mandelic Acid [α-Hydroxyphenylacetic Acid][C_6H_5CH-(OH)COOH]—Crystallizes as orthorhombic plates from water. Darkens on prolonged exposure to light. *Uses:* Urinary antiseptic. It is generally used with *Methenamine* (page 1182). Contraindicated in renal insufficiency. *Dose:* 3 Gm.

Chloroprocaine Penicillin O [Depo-Cer-O-Cillin (*Upjohn*] [$C_{13}H_{18}N_2O_4S_2 \cdot C_{13}H_{19}ClN_2O_2 \cdot H_2O$] is the 2-chloroprocaine salt of [(allylthio)methyl]-penicillin. It conforms to the regulations of the federal Food and Drug Administration concerning antibiotic drugs (see page 1206). *Description and Solubility:* Slender needles which melt between 89° and 81°; in the dry form it is stable at room temperature; in aqueous suspension it is stable at room temperature for 1

week and at refrigerator temperatures for 3 weeks. The following are a few of the solubility values determined by Weiss, *et al,*[5] in mg per ml at about 28°: water, 9.2; alcohol, >20; carbon tetrachloride, 0.60; chloroform, >20. *Uses:* Like procaine penicillin G, this antibiotic has a relatively low water solubility and hence is administered intramuscularly for its "depot" action. The blood levels of penicillin achieved are about equal to those from a similar depot of procaine penicillin G, but the duration of the penicillin O in the blood may exceed that of penicillin G by 30 to 100%. Patients sensitive to penicillin G may or may not be sensitive to penicillin O, so that care must be exercised in patients sensitive to penicillin G. *Dose: Intramuscular,* 300,000 to 600,000 Units once or twice daily.

Hydrabamine Phenoxymethyl Penicillin [Hydrabamine Penicillin V; Compocillin V (*Abbott*)] consists chiefly of the N,N'-bis[(1,2,3,4,4a,9,10,10a-octahydro-7-isopropyl-1,4a-dimethyl-1-phenanthryl)-methyl]ethylenediamine salt of phenoxymethyl penicillin [$C_{42}H_{64}N_2 \cdot 2C_{16}H_{18}N_2O_5S$], along with small quantities of dihydro and tetrahydro derivatives. It conforms to the regulations of the federal Food and Drug Administration concerning antibiotic drugs (see page 1206). The hydrabamine radical is commonly known by the trivial name dehydroabietyl. *Description and Solubility:* A fine, white, practically odorless powder. Sparingly soluble in acetone and chloroform; slightly soluble in benzene; practically insoluble in water and ether. *Uses:* This salt of phenoxymethyl penicillin is insoluble and hence is relatively resistant to acid attack in the gastric juice. It is used in the form of an aqueous suspension for oral administration. Phenoxymethyl penicillin is released in the gastrointestinal tract. See *Phenoxymethyl Penicillin* (page 1230) for actions and uses. *Dose: Usual,* 300,000 Units every 4 to 6 hours; 300,000 to 600,000 Units per day for prophylaxis of rheumatic fever.

Penicillin O Sodium [(Allylthio)methyl]penicillin.—[(Allylthio)methyl]penicillin. *Uses:* The antibacterial spectrum and uses of potassium salts of penicillin O are essentially the same as those of the soluble salts of penicillin G (see general statement, page 1224). Penicillin O is less sensitizing, but it may nevertheless often induce allergic reactions in many patients allergic to penicillin G, and care must be exercised in such patients. *Dose:* see *Potassium Penicillin G* (page 1228).

Sodium Dicloxacillin [Sodium Dicloxacillin Monohydrate; Dynapen (*Bristol*); Pathocil (*Wyeth*); Veracillin (*Ayerst*)] is sodium 6-[3-(2,6-dichlorophenyl)-5-methyl-4-isoxazolecarboxamido] - 3,3 - dimethyl - 7 - oxo - 4 - thia - 1 - azabicyclo[3.2.0]heptane - 2 - carboxylate [$C_{19}H_{16}Cl_2N_3$-$NaO_5S \cdot H_2O$ = 510.35]. *Preparation:* 6-Aminopenicillanic acid is acylated with 3-(2,6-dichlorophenyl)-5-methyl-4-isoxazolecarboxylic acid and the resulting dicloxacillin (acid) is purified by recrystallizations and converted to the sodium salt. *Description and Solubility:* A white to nearly white powder with a faint, characteristic odor; it melts between 222° and 225° with decomposition. Freely soluble in water; soluble in alcohol.

Uses: Sodium Dicloxacillin is a penicillinase-resistant penicillin with a spectrum of antibacterial activity that is nearly identical to that of *Sodium Cloxacillin* (page 1226), except that it is only ⅓ as potent against pneumococci. It is ⅓ to 1/15 as potent as penicillin G against non-penicillinase-producing Gram-positive cocci, but it is more than 100 times as potent against penicillinase-producers. It is not active against Gram-negative organisms. Thus it should be used to treat only those infections caused by penicillinase-producing bacteria which are resistant to penicillin G but sensitive to Dicloxacillin; in this way the development of bacteria resistant to Dicloxacillin will be less than if the drug is used indiscriminately. Allergic reactions to Dicloxacillin occur, but not as frequently as to penicillin G; patients sensitive to penicillin G or other penicillins are sometimes but not always sensitive to Dicloxacillin. Skin rash or urticaria are the most frequent type of reaction. The drug may also cause gastrointestinal disturbances. It is relatively acid resistant and is effective by the oral route although is absorbed somewhat erratically. *Dose:* 125 mg to 1 Gm; *usual,* 250 mg 4 to 6 times a day, to be taken on an empty stomach;

children under 40 Kg, 12.5 to 25 mg per Kg per day in 4 divided doses; *intramuscular*, 250 to 500 mg every 4 to 6 hours; as much as 1 Gm every 2 to 4 hours has been given.

Sodium Fusidate [Fucidin (*Leo*)] is the sodium salt of fusidic acid ($C_{31}H_{48}O_6$), a steroid antibiotic obtained from the fermentation broth of *Fusidium coccineum*. It conforms to the regulations of the federal Food and Drug Administration concerning antibiotic drugs (see page 1206). Fusidic acid is a trivial name for $3\alpha,11\alpha,16\beta$-trihydroxy-29-nor-8α, $9\beta,13\alpha,14\beta$-dammara-17(20),24-dien-21-oic acid 16 acetate. The parent saturated hydrocarbon, dammarane, is a 4,4,8, 14-tetramethyl-18-nor-5α,-cholestane. *Description and Solubility:* A white powder; the pK of the acid is 5.35; concentrated neutral sterile solutions are stable for several weeks, but concentrations below 0.1 mcg per ml are stable for only a few days; the drug is less stable in alkaline than in neutral or acid media. Freely soluble in water.

Uses: Although Sodium Fusidate is an antibiotic with a steroid structure, it has no hormonal action. It is active primarily against Gram-positive organisms with very low activity against Gram-negative bacteria and fungi. While it is effective against both penicillin-resistant and penicillin-sensitive strains of *Staphylococcus aureus*, these organisms develop resistance rather frequently to the antibiotic. Thus, it can be predicted that widespread use of this drug will commonly result in resistance. Resistance seems to occur less frequently to combinations of fucidin and penicillin than to either drug separately. No cross-resistance has been observed with any clinically used antibiotics. The only side effects are due to local irritation and these seldom necessitate discontinuance of treatment. *Dose:* 500 mg 3 times daily.

Antibiotic Antagonist

Penicillinase [Neutrapen (*Riker*)]—A bacterial enzyme that hydrolyzes penicillin to the inactive penicilloic acid. It is used for the adjunctive treatment of slowly developing or delayed penicillin reactions; it is no substitute for other recognized therapy for penicillin reactions. Penicillinase can in itself cause serious allergic responses. The enzyme is also used in microbiological procedures to destroy penicillin in blood cultures. *Dose: intramuscularly*, 800,000 units repeated at an interval of 3 to 7 days.

Miscellaneous Systemic Antibacterial Drugs

Aminosalicylic Acid USP

[4-Aminosalicylic Acid; PAS; Pamisyl (*Parke-Davis*); Parasal (*Panray*)]

Aminosalicylic Acid contains 98.5–100.5% of C_7H_7-NO_3 (153.14), calculated on the anhydrous basis.

Caution—Under no circumstances use a solution if its color is darker than that of a freshly prepared solution.

Preparation—This acid is prepared from *m*-aminophenol by a modification of the Kolbe-Schmitt reaction which involves heating the phenol under pressure with a source of carbon dioxide such as ammonium carbonate or potassium bicarbonate.

Description—A white, or nearly white, bulky powder· Darkens on exposure to light and air. Odorless, or has a slight acetous odor. Melts between 135° and 140° with decomposition. The pH of a saturated aqueous solution is between 3.0 and 3.7.

Solubility—1 Gm dissolves in about 600 ml of water and about 21 ml of alcohol; slightly soluble in ether; practically insoluble in benzene.

Uses—*Para*-Aminosalicylic Acid (PAS) is a bacteriostatic agent (*antibacterial*) remarkably selective for pathogenic strains of tubercle bacilli causing human *tuberculosis*. *In vitro*, tested against virulent human strains, PAS has nearly the same potency as streptomycin, but *in vivo* it is considerably less potent. Used alone in the treatment of tuberculosis, PAS may have a beneficial effect on the course of the disease, but it is definitely inferior to either the streptomycin (see *Streptomycin* (page 1233) and *Dihydrostreptomycin* (page 1237), or *Isoniazid* (page 1241)). However, in combination with doses of streptomycin or isoniazid, PAS enhances the clinical response to full doses of these agents, or it permits lower doses to be employed. Furthermore, and most importantly, it delays the emergence of streptomycin- or isoniazid-resistant strains of tuberculosis. Consequently, PAS is generally used in combination therapy; it is used alone only when the strain of tubercle bacillus is already resistant to other generally more effective agents, when sensitivity to other agents contraindicates their use, or when surgery is anticipated and it is desired to reserve the streptomycins for that time. Drug-resistance occurs as with streptomycin. PAS frequently causes epigastric discomfort, anorexia, nausea, and vomiting; aluminum hydroxide gel lessens the incidence of gastrointestinal symptoms. Occasionally, soft stools, diarrhea, and renal irritation occur. Rarely, dermatoses, drug fever, or leukopenia result from treatment with PAS. Salicylism does not occur. PAS is administered orally in a daily dose of 8 to 16 Gm, generally divided into four or more doses.

Dose—10 to 20 Gm daily; *usual*, 3 Gm 4 times a day.
Dosage Forms—Tablets USP: 500 mg.

Calcium Aminosalicylate NF

[Calcium 4-Aminosalicylate; Calcium Para-aminosalicylate; Parasal Calcium (*Panray*); Pasara Calcium (*Dorsey*)]

Calcium Aminosalicylate [$C_{14}H_{12}CaN_2O_6 \cdot 3H_2O$ = 398.39] contains 98.0–100.5% of $C_{14}H_{12}CaN_2O_6$ (344.34), calculated on the anhydrous basis.

Caution—Prepare solutions of Calcium Aminosalicylate within 24 hours of administration. Under no circumstances use a solution if its color is darker than that of a freshly prepared solution.

Preparation—This salt may be prepared by neutralizing *p*-aminosalicylic acid with lime, followed either by crystallization through evaporation and cooling or by precipitation with water-miscible solvents such as ethanol.

Description—White to cream-colored crystals or powder. Odorless, and has an alkaline, slightly bitter-sweet taste. Somewhat hygroscopic. Aqueous solutions slowly decompose and darken in color.

Solubility—1 Gm dissolves in about 7 ml of water, about 6 ml of methanol and about 12 ml of acetone; slightly soluble in alcohol.

Uses—See *Aminosalicylic Acid*. The calcium salt causes less gastric irritation than the free acid. It is used in lieu of the sodium salt (page 1240) when sodium intake is restricted. It has no advantage over the potassium salt (page 1240).

Dose—10 to 25 Gm daily in 4 divided doses; *usual*, 4 Gm 4 times a day.

Dosage Forms—Capsules NF: 500 mg; Tablets NF: 500, 580, and 690 mg.

Potassium Aminosalicylate USP

[Potassium 4-Aminosalicylate]

Potassium Aminosalicylate contains 98.0–101.0% of $C_7H_6KNO_3$ (191.23), calculated on the dried basis.

Caution—Prepare solutions of Potassium Aminosalicylate within 24 hours of administration. Under no circumstances use a solution if its color is darker than that of a freshly prepared solution.

Preparation—*Aminosalicylic Acid* (page 1239) is reacted with an equimolar quantity of potassium hydroxide and the resulting salt is purified by recrystallization.

Description—A white to cream-colored, crystalline powder. It is practically odorless and has a saline taste. Its solutions decompose slowly and darken in color.

Solubility—Freely soluble in water.

Uses—The actions and uses of Potassium Aminosalicylate are those of *Aminosalicylic Acid* (page 1239), except that the gastrointestinal symptoms resulting from irritation caused by the free acid appear to be less than when aminosalicylic acid is used. Ordinarily, the potassium salt has no advantages over the sodium salt (this page), except when sodium intake is to be restricted, or over the calcium salt (page 1239).

Dose—10 to 20 Gm daily; *usual*, 3 Gm 4 times a day.

Dosage Forms—Tablets USP: 500 mg and 1 Gm.

Sodium Aminosalicylate USP

[Sodium 4-Aminosalicylate; Sodium Para-aminosalicylate; (*Various Mfgs.*)]

Sodium Aminosalicylate [$C_7H_6NNaO_3 \cdot 2H_2O = 211.15$] contains 98.0–101.0% of $C_7H_6NNaO_3$ (175.12), calculated on the anhydrous basis.

Caution—Prepare solutions of Sodium Aminosalicylate within 24 hours of administration. Under no circumstances use a solution if its color is darker than that of a freshly prepared solution.

Preparation—This salt is ordinarily prepared by neutralizing the free acid with sodium hydroxide or sodium carbonate, and precipitating the sodium salt by the addition of ethanol.

Description—A white to cream-colored, crystalline powder. Practically odorless. Taste, sweet and saline. Aqueous solutions decompose slowly and darken in color. The pH of an aqueous 1:50 solution is between 6.5 and 8.5.

Solubility—1 Gm dissolves in about 2 ml of water; sparingly soluble in alcohol; very slightly soluble in ether and chloroform.

Uses—The actions and uses of Sodium Aminosalicylate are identical to those of *Aminosalicylic Acid* (page 1239), except that the incidence of gastrointestinal symptoms resulting from irritation caused by the free acid is less when the sodium salt is employed. The sodium salt has no advantage over either the calcium salt (page 1239) or the potassium salt (this page).

Dose—10 to 20 Gm daily; *usual*, 3 Gm 5 times a day.

Dosage Forms—Tablets USP: 500 and 690 mg and 1 Gm.

Calcium Benzoylpas NF

[Calcium 4-Benzamidosalicylate; Benzapas (*Dorsey*)]; [Therapas (*Barnes-Hind*)]

Calcium Benzoylpas contains 98.0–101.5% of $C_{28}H_{20}CaN_2O_8 \cdot 5H_2O$ (642.64), calculated on the anhydrous basis.

Preparation—4-Aminosalicylic acid is *N*-benzoylated by treatment with benzoyl chloride in a suitable dehydrohalogenating environment. The benzoylated acid is then dissolved in alkali and metathesized with a soluble calcium salt to precipitate the official salt.

Description—White or cream-colored, odorless, crystalline powder. It is tasteless at first but will develop a characteristic, slightly bitter taste which leaves a saccharin-like sweet aftertaste.

Solubility—Soluble in anhydrous methanol; 1 Gm dissolves in 50 ml but precipitates in the anhydrous form after standing; insoluble in water and ether.

Uses—Calcium Benzoylpas is an antitubercular drug with uses supposedly identical with those of *Aminosalicylic Acid* (page 1239), from which it is derived. However, it acts directly on the tubercle bacillus and not by biotransformation to aminosalicylic acid. It is advantageous in that it causes fewer gastrointestinal disturbances than aminosalicylic acid and, possibly, its salts; therefore, it is especially indicated for use in patients who cannot tolerate the aminosalicylates. It is also nearly tasteless and is hence more palatable than the aminosalicylates. It is poorly absorbed compared to aminosalicylic acid, so that plasma levels are lower following oral ingestion than with the aminosalicylates. The duration of action is longer than that of the aminosalicylates. Calcium Benzoylpas should be restricted to use in combination with other agents.

The toxic effects of Calcium Benzoylpas are qualitatively the same as those of *Aminosalicylic Acid* (page 1239). It may cause hypercalcemia in patients with impaired ability to excrete calcium.

Dose—*Usual*, 10 to 15 Gm daily in 2 or 3 divided doses.

Other Dose Information—The usual dose is generally consumed immediately after meals.

Dosage Forms—Tablets NF: 500 mg.

Dapsone USP

[4, 4'–Sulfonyldianiline; DDS; Avlosulfon (*Ayerst*)]

Dapsone contains 99.0–101.0% of $C_{12}H_{12}N_2O_2S$ (248.31), calculated on the dried basis.

Preparation—Benzene is condensed with sulfuric acid to yield phenyl sulfone $[(C_6H_5)_2SO_2]$ which is then nitrated by standard procedures to yield the 4,4'-dinitro derivative. Reduction with tin and HCl or with various other appropriate reductants yields Dapsone.

Description—White or creamy white, crystalline powder. Is odorless and has a slightly bitter taste.

Solubility—Very slightly soluble in water; freely soluble in alcohol; soluble in acetone and dilute mineral acids.

Uses—Dapsone has an antibacterial spectrum and mechanism of action similar to that of sulfanilamide (see *Sulfonamides*, page 1195), of which Dapsone was originally studied as a congener. Limited success against tuberculosis has been achieved with Dapsone, but it is far surpassed by other agents. However, Dapsone is a useful drug in the chemotherapy of *leprosy*. Except for promizole, each of the sulfones used in the treatment of this disease owes both its oral activity and toxicity to Dapsone released from the molecule. For this reason, Dapsone is the preferred sulfone, since it is cheaper than and equally efficacious to the other sulfones. Dapsone is of some limited value in the treatment of *malaria*, especially that caused by *P. falciparum*; it may be combined with other antimalarial drugs, especially pyrimethamine.

Dapsone may cause hemolytic anemia, methemoglobinemia, gastrointestinal upset, headache, nervousness, blurred vision, paresthesias and pruritus, hematuria or rash. However, careful initial grading of dose and rest periods avoids much of the toxicity.

Dose—*Usual, leprostatic, initial,* **25 mg** 2 times a week for 1 month, then increased by 25 mg per dose at monthly intervals to a maximum of **100 mg** 4 times a week; *suppressant for dermatitis herpetiformis,* **100 to 200 mg** daily.

Dosage Forms—Tablets USP: 100 mg.

Ethionamide USP

[2-Ethylthioisonicotinamide; Trecator S. C. (*Ives*)]

Ethionamide contains 98.0–102.0% of $C_8H_{10}N_2S$ (166.25), calculated on the anhydrous basis.

Preparation—2-Ethylisonicotinamide is dehydrated to the nitrile which is then reacted with hydrogen sulfide in the presence of triethanolamine. US Pat. 2,901,488.

Description—A bright yellow powder with a faint to moderate sulfide-like odor. It melts between 157° and 162°.

Solubility—Slightly soluble in water, chloroform, and ether; soluble in methanol; sparingly soluble in alcohol and propylene glycol.

Uses—Ethionamide is chemically related to *Isoniazid* (this page) and shares with it a usefulness against *tuberculosis*. However, Ethionamide is less potent and more toxic than Isoniazid, so that its general use should be avoided; rather, it should be used only when the usual combinations of streptomycin, aminosalicylic acid, and isoniazid are ineffective or cannot be tolerated. Ethionamide should be used only in combination with other primary antitubercular drugs and only after the microorganism has been shown *in vitro* to be susceptible to the drug. Resistance to the drug develops rapidly. Untoward effects include gastrointestinal distress (nausea, vomiting, anorexia), occasional hepatotoxicity, purpura, gynecomastia, possible damage to the inner ear, drowsiness, depression, peripheral neuropathy, acne and allergic dermatitides. Ethionamide may also enhance the toxicity of the drugs with which it is given in combination.

Dose—**500 mg** to **1 Gm** daily; *usual,* **250 mg** 3 times a day.

Other Dose Information—To be given with meals.

Dosage Forms—Tablets USP: 250 mg.

Isoniazid USP

[Isonicotinylhydrazine; Isonicotinic Acid Hydrazide; INH (*Lilly*); Niconyl (*Parke-Davis*); Nydrazid (*Squibb*); Tyvid (*Merrell*)]

Isoniazid contains 98.0–101.0% of $C_6H_7N_3O$ (137.14), calculated on the dried basis.

Preparation—It may be prepared by heating isonicotinic acid or its ethyl ester with anhydrous hydrazine. Isonicotinic acid may be synthesized by various oxidative processes starting with 4-methylpyridine.

Description—Colorless or white crystals, or a white, crystalline powder. Odorless. Slowly affected by exposure to air and light. Its solutions are practically neutral to litmus. Melts between 170° and 173°.

Solubility—1 Gm dissolves in about 8 ml of water and about 50 ml of alcohol; slightly soluble in chloroform and ether.

Uses—Isoniazid is the most potent and selective of the known *tuberculostatic antibacterial* agents, and it may also become known as the most effective agent in the therapy of tuberculosis. It has also been employed as a prophylactic for use in persons constantly exposed to tubercular patients. The fact that Isoniazid gains access to all organs and to all body fluids, including cerebrospinal fluid, renders the drug of special value in treating tuberculous meningitis and other extrapulmonary forms of the disease. Used alone, it is at least the equal of streptomycin in the therapy of tuberculosis. The drug may be employed alone when the patient is sensitive to the streptomycins or when the tubercle bacilli are streptomycin-resistant. When used alone, isoniazid-resistant strains of the mycobacterium may emerge, but the rapidity of emergence and the degree of resistance are less than with streptomycin. Used in combination with the streptomycins, it perhaps enhances the clinical response, it permits a lower dose of streptomycin, and it retards the emergence of streptomycin-resistant tubercle bacilli. The drug is generally employed in combination with streptomycin.

Untoward effects from Isoniazid are relatively few except in persons who are slow acetylators, when the dose must be lowered. The effects may include restlessness, insomnia, muscle twitching, hyperreflexia, and paresthesia. These neurological disorders result from competition with pyridoxine; pyridoxine administration suppresses the neurological disorders without antagonizing the antitubercular action. Intramuscular injections cause local irritation.

Dose—*Oral or intramuscular,* **300** to **500 mg** daily; *usual,* **300 mg** once a day.

Other Dose Information—Orally or intramuscularly, for adults 4 to 6 mg per Kg of body weight daily in two divided doses, and for children 10 to 20 mg per Kg of body weight in two divided doses. Doses greater than these should be employed with caution. It may be necessary to reduce the dosage if toxicity contravenes. The concentration employed for intramuscular injections is 100 mg per ml.

Dosage Forms—Injection USP: 10 ml; Syrup USP; Tablets USP: 50, 100, and 300 mg.

Nalidixic Acid NF

[1 - Ethyl - 1,4 - dihydro - 7 - methyl - 4 - oxo - 1,8 - naphthyridine - 3 - carboxylic Acid; NegGram (Winthrop)]

Nalidixic Acid contains 98.0–102.0% of $C_{12}H_{12}N_2O_3$ (232.24), calculated on the dried basis.

Preparation—2-Amino-6-methylpyridine is condensed with the diethyl ester of (ethoxymethylene)-malonic acid to yield the dicarbethoxyvinylamino derivative (I). Through the abstraction of ethanol, (I) cyclizes to ethyl 1,4-dihydro-7-methyl-4-oxo-1,8-naphthyridine-3-carboxylate (II) which, on ethylation with ethyl bromide and subsequent saponification, yields Nalidixic Acid.

(I) (II)

Description—A white to slightly yellow, odorless, crystalline powder. It melts between 225° and 231°.

Solubility—Practically insoluble in water; slightly soluble in alcohol; soluble in chloroform; very slightly soluble in ether; soluble in solutions of fixed alkali hydroxides and carbonates.

Uses—Nalidixic Acid is an antibacterial agent that is effective against Gram-negative organisms, including most *E. coli* (especially) several *Proteus, Aerobacter,* and *Klebsiella,* and a few *Pseudomonas.* It is difficult to achieve effective plasma levels and plasma protein inhibits activity, but the drug reaches effective concentrations in the urine, so that the drug is used for the treatment of urinary tract infections. The frequent success against *Proteus* infections is of major interest, since few strains of *Proteus* respond to other antibacterial drugs. Unfortunately, bacterial resistance to Nalidixic Acid develops rapidly, and escape from control is common. Effective drug combinations to delay

the emergence of resistance have yet to be worked out.

The majority of patients tolerate Nalidixic Acid without untoward effects. Nausea, vomiting, skin rashes, and urticaria are the most frequent side effects. Occasionally fever, photosensitivity, or eosinophilia occur. Headache, vertigo, drowsiness, malaise, disturbances of vision, muscle weakness, or myalgia may occur infrequently. Convulsions have occurred in patients with parkinsonism or cerebral vascular insufficiency and in children with excessive doses. Nalidixic Acid gives false positive tests for urine glucose.

Dose—*Usual,* **1 Gm** 4 times a day for 1 to 2 weeks. Thereafter, for prolonged treatment, the dose may be reduced to **500 mg** 4 times a day.

Dosage Forms—Tablets NF: 250 and 500 mg.

Nitrofurantoin USP

[1-[(5-Nitrofurfurylidene)amino]hydantoin; Furadantin or Macrodantin (*Eaton*)]

Nitrofurantoin contains 98.0–102.0% of $C_8H_6N_4O_5$ (238.16), calculated on the dried basis.

Caution—Nitrofurantoin is discolored by alkali and by exposure to light, and is decomposed upon contact with metals other than stainless steel or aluminum.

Preparation—5-Nitro-2-furaldehyde (I) readily undergoes condensation with 1-aminohydantoin (II) to yield Nitrofurantoin. (I) is synthesized by direct nitration of "2-furfural diacetate" [2-furanmethanediol diacetate (III), prepared by the addition reaction between 2-furaldehyde and acetic anhydride] followed by saponification to regenerate the formyl group which, had it not been so protected, would have been oxidized to carboxyl during the nitration. (II) may be synthesized by effecting the addition of cyanic acid to hydrazinoacetic acid (IV) to produce the 3-carbamoyl derivative (V) which cyclizes by dehydration to (II).

I II III

IV V

Description—Lemon-yellow, odorless crystals or fine powder. It has a bitter aftertaste.

Solubility—Very slightly soluble in water and alcohol; soluble in dimethylformamide.

Uses—Nitrofurantoin is effective against a majority of urinary tract pathogens including certain strains of *E. coli, Klebsiella, Proteus sp., Pseudomonas,* and *Aerobacter sp.* It is also effective against many staphylococci, streptococci, pneumococci, clostridia, and *B. subtilis.* It is indicated for the treatment of infections of the genitourinary tract: pyelonephritis, cystitis, prostatitis, and pyelitis.

Nausea and vomiting occur in an appreciable number of patients. It is claimed that the use of a "macrocrystalline" product diminishes the incidence and intensity of gastrointestinal upsets without affecting the potency. Hypersensitivity reactions also occur. A few cases of polyneuropathy and also hemolytic anemia have been reported. Neuropathies appear to be more likely to occur if there is renal insufficiency. A course of Nitrofurantoin ordinarily should not exceed 2 weeks and courses should be separated by rest periods.

Dose—200 to 400 mg daily; *usual*, **100 mg** 4 times a day.

Dosage Forms—Oral Suspension USP; Tablets USP: 50 and 100 mg.

Veterinary Uses—For treatment of urinary tract infections in small animals and infections in small animals and infectious tracheobronchitis in dogs and urinary tract infections in horses.

Veterinary Dose—1 to 2 mg per **pound** of body weight 3 times daily.

Pyrazinamide USP

[Pyrazinecarboxamide; Aldinamide (*MSD*)]

Pyrazinamide contains 99.0–100.5% of $C_5H_5N_3O$ (123.12), calculated on the anhydrous basis.

Preparation—Pyrazinamide may be prepared by the thermal decarboxylation of 2,3-pyrazinedicarboxylic acid to form the monocarboxylic acid which is then esterified with methanol and the resulting methyl ester is subjected to controlled ammonolysis. The starting acid is readily prepared from quinoxaline by oxidation with permanganate. US Pat. 2,149,279.

Description—A white to practically white, odorless or practically odorless, crystalline powder. It melts between 189° and 191°. Its aqueous solutions are neutral.

Solubility—1 Gm dissolves in about 67 ml of water, about 135 ml of chloroform, and about 1000 ml of ether; slightly soluble in alcohol.

Uses—Pyrazinamide is an antituberculosis drug more effective than aminosalicylic acid, cycloserine, or viomycin, but not streptomycin or isoniazid. It is generally administered along with isoniazid, which it potentiates. However, it is quite toxic and should be held in reserve until other therapy fails. It may cause hepatic damage, with or without jaundice, and death has occurred. All patients intended to be treated with this drug should have prior liver-function tests, which tests must also be repeated periodically during therapy. All patients must be hospitalized during treatment. Pyrazinamide also may cause retention of uric acid, anorexia, malaise, nervousness, nausea and vomiting, arthralgias, dysuria, and mild fever.

Dose—1 to 3 Gm daily; *usual*, **5 to 7.5 mg** per **Kg** of body weight 4 times a day.

Other Dose Information—The total daily dose should not exceed 3 Gm.

Dosage Forms—Tablets USP: 500 mg.

Sodium Glucosulfone Injection USP

[Disodium   1,1-[Sulfonylbis(p-phenyleneimino)bis[D-*gluco*-2,3,4,5,6-pentahydroxy-1-hexanesulfonate]; Promin Sodium (*Parke-Davis*)]

Sodium Glucosulfone Injection is a sterile solution of sodium glucosulfone in water for injection. It contains, in each ml, 384–416 Gm of sodium glucosulfone [$C_{24}H_{34}N_2Na_2O_{18}S_3$ = 780.71]. Sodium Glucosulfone Injection contains no added antimicrobial agents.

Preparation—Sodium Glucosulfone may be prepared by adding 4,4'-sulfonyldianiline (4,4'-diaminodiphenylsulfone) to an aqueous solution of sodium bisulfite and dextrose and heating until complete solution occurs. The reaction may be considered as involving a typical sodium bisulfite addition to the aldehyde group in dextrose followed by a double condensation involving the 1-hydroxyl groups in the dextrose-sodium bisulfite addition compound and one of the hydrogens in each of the amino groups of the sulfone.

The 4,4'-sulfonyldianiline is readily synthesized by refluxing a mixture of benzene and sulfuric acid under conditions such that the water of condensation is continuously removed, followed by 4,4'-nitration of the resulting diphenylsulfone and reduction of the nitro groups to amino.

Description—A clear, pale yellow liquid. The pH is between 5.0 and 6.5.

Uses—Glucosulfone sodium was the first sulfone to be tried clinically in the treatment of *leprosy*. Its introduction marked the beginning of a new era in the chemotherapy of leprosy. It is also an occasional adjuvant in the treatment of *tuberculosis*. It is converted to dapsone (see *Dapsone*, page 1241), to which it owes its activity. Its toxicity is like that of dapsone.

Dose—*Intravenous*, **5 to 12.5 ml** daily; *usual*, **5 ml** once a day for 6 days of each week.

Other Dose Information—At the conclusion of each 2-week period, treatment is interrupted for 1 week.

Dosage Forms—Injection USP: 12.5 ml.

Sodium Sulfoxone USP

[Disodium [Sulfonylbis(p-phenyleneimino)]di(methanesulfinate); Sulfoxone Sodium USP XV; Diasone Sodium (*Abbott*)]

$$NaO_2S\ CH_2NH - \bigcirc - \overset{\overset{O}{\|}}{\underset{\underset{O}{\|}}{S}} - \bigcirc - NHCH_2SO_2Na$$

Sodium Sulfoxone is a mixture of disodium sulfonylbis(p-phenyleneimino)di(methanesulfinate) [$C_{14}H_{14}N_2Na_2O_6S_3$ = 448.45] and suitable buffers and inert ingredients. It contains 73.0–81.0% of $C_{14}H_{14}N_2Na_2O_6S_3$, calculated on the dried basis.

Preparation—*p*-Chloronitrobenzene is treated with sodium sulfide and the resulting 4-nitro-4'-aminodiphenyl sulfide is treated with hydrochloric acid and tin to form 4,4'-diaminodiphenylsulfide. After acetylation with acetic anhydride, the resulting N,N'-diacetyl compound is oxidized to the sulfone with the aid of potassium dichromate and sulfuric acid. Deacetylation is accomplished hydrolytically under the influence of hydrochloric acid, and the resulting 4,4'-diaminodiphenylsulfone is then condensed with sodium formaldehyde sulfoxylate.

Description—A white to pale yellow powder, having a characteristic odor.

HOCH$_2$—C—C—C—C—CH—NH—◯—SO$_2$—◯—NH—CH—C—C—C—C—CH$_2$OH

Sodium Glucosulfone

Solubility—Very soluble in water, yielding a clear, pale yellow solution; slightly soluble in alcohol.

Uses—Sodium Sulfoxone is used as an *antibacterial agent* (leprostatic) in the treatment of *leprosy*. Clinical improvement is evident in practically every patient treated with sulfoxone or with other derivatives (see *Dapsone*, page 1241, and *Sodium Glucosulfone Injection*, page 1243) of 4,4′-diaminodiphenylsulfone, which is probably the active intermediate of all the effective aromatic sulfones. The course of therapy is an arduous one, and it may require one to several years to clear lesions or to arrest their development. Even so, the aromatic sulfones are superior to other agents used in the treatment of leprosy. The efficacies of the several aromatic sulfones in the treatment of leprosy are very nearly equal.

Sulfoxone and related aromatic sulfones cause a high incidence of hemolytic anemia of varying degrees of severity. Methemoglobinemia also commonly results from the use of such drugs. Gastrointestinal upsets such as anorexia, nausea, and vomiting sometimes occur. Drug rashes, leukopenia, and rarely neurological disorders have been observed.

Dose—**300 mg** to **1 Gm** daily; *usual*, **300 mg** 1 or 2 times a day.

Dosage Forms—Tablets USP: 300 mg.

Other Miscellaneous Systemic Antibacterial Drugs

Ethambutol [Myambutol (*Lederle*)] is (+)-2,2′-(ethylenediimino)di-1-butanol dihydrochloride [$C_{10}H_{24}N_2O_2 . 2HCl$ = 277.23]. *Preparation:* (±)-2-Aminobutanol is resolved via its tartrate and the (+)-enantiomorph is then condensed with 1,2-dichloroethane in an appropriate dehydrochlorinating environment. US Pat. 3,297,707. *Description and Solubility:* A white, crystalline powder that is essentially odorless and has a bitter taste; it is stable in light and heat but is hygroscopic when exposed to high relative humidities; it melts between 198° and 202°. Freely soluble in water; soluble in propylene glycol; slightly soluble in alcohol; insoluble in chloroform.

Uses: Ethambutol is a tuberculostatic drug which is effective against tubercle bacilli that are resistant to isoniazid or streptomycin. It acts only on proliferating cells, apparently by interfering with the synthesis of RNA. When used alone in the treatment of tuberculosis, the drug may clear the sputum of mycobacteria within 3 months in the majority of patients, but bacterial resistance occurs in 35% of cases, and relapses frequently occur. In combination with isoniazid or other tuberculostatic drugs relapses are uncommon. It may be used in lieu of aminosalicylic acid as a companion drug to isoniazid, or, when the bacillus is resistant to all of isoniazid, streptomycin, and aminosalicylic acid, Ethambutol in combination with one of the lesser tuberculostatic drugs, such as cycloserine, pyrazinamide, or ethionamide, may become the key drug in the management of tuberculosis. Ethambutol occasionally causes blurred vision and diminished visual acuity to green light; these effects disappear upon discontinuation of the drug. Multivitamins should be given concurrently with Ethambutol. *Dose:* 12.5 mg per kg 2 times a day for 8 to 12 months.

Phenyl Aminosalicylate [Pheny-PAS-Tebamin (*Purdue-Frederick*)] is phenyl 4-aminosalicylate ($C_{13}H_{11}NO_3$). *Description and Solubility:* Crystals that melt at 153°. Water: 0.7 mg per 100 ml; serum: 12 mg per 100 ml.

Uses: Phenyl Aminosalicylate has antibacterial actions and therapeutic uses identical to those of *Aminosalicylic Acid* (page 1239). It is converted nearly completely to aminosalicylic acid, partly in the gastrointestinal tract and partly after absorption into the body. It does not give rise to as high a blood level as aminosalicylic acid, but this may be compensated by doubling the dose. Its advantage is that is does not cause the gastrointestinal irritation that aminosalicylic acid and its salts do. The toxicity of Phenyl Aminosalicylate appears to be that of aminosalicylic acid; no toxicity to the phenol has been reported. *Dose:* 4 Gm 3 times a day with meals.

Sodium Nitrofurantoin [Furadantin Sodium (*Eaton*)] is the sodium derivative of 1-[(5-nitrofurfurylidene)amino]-hydantoin. *Description:* A yellow to orange-colored, dry, sterile powder. *Incompatibilities:* Do not use solutions containing methyl or propyl parabens, phenol, or cresol as preservatives, as these compounds cause it to be precipitated from solution. *Uses:* See *Nitrofurantoin* (page 1242). The sodium salt is used for intravenous injection. Indications for intravenous use are rare. *The drug must not be given intramuscularly. Dose: Intravenous*, 180 mg 2 times a day. For persons under 120 pounds, 3 mg per pound. Sodium nitrofurantoin is contained in a vial. The crystals must be dissolved just prior to use by adding 15 ml of a 5% Dextrose Injection USP or Sterile Water for Injection USP to the vial. This will permit withdrawal of 180 mg of nitrofurantoin, as the sodium salt, which is then further diluted for administration.

Antimalarials

Until the last three decades, malaria has been the world's greatest scourge, its steady accumulated toll far exceeding that of the more explosive plague. Even today probably over 200 million people are afflicted, and over a million die each year from malaria. Knowledge of mosquito control, insecticides, and antimalarials, however, have all but eradicated the disease in the more advanced countries, such as the United States; similar strides have been made in certain relatively undeveloped countries, so that malaria now ranks second to tuberculosis in many of these countries.

The export of cinchona from Peru in 1643 allowed the European countries and their colonies some means of suppressing the disease, and the introduction of Quinine in the 19th century improved therapy somewhat. However, great advances were not made until the introduction of Pamaquine in 1926 and Quinacrine (Atabrine) in 1930, as the result of screening by I. G. Farben of over 12,000 candidates. These synthetics did not immediately displace quinine. Only when the supplies of quinine were cut off in World War II did it become imperative to supply synthetic antimalarials to our armed forces in the Pacific and Mediterranean. The US Office of Scientific Research and Development coordinated a study of about 7000 new, and an equal number of old, synthetic compounds. Not only were the older German compounds "rediscovered," but several new and superior agents (especially Amodiaquine, Chloroquine, Pentaquine, and Primaquine) resulted. The British counterpart of this program brought forth *Chloroguanide*. The continued search in this field has yielded other antimalarials, but the pace has recently been slow. However, because of the emergence of resistant strains of plasmodia, the effectiveness of several of the "newer" agents is rapidly diminishing, so that not only are new drugs again being actively sought, but combinations of old drugs are on trial. In this connection, it is of interest that dapsone and various sulfonamides are being tried with renewed interest.

Malaria is caused by several species of the protozoan *Plasmodium*, of which *P. vivax* and *P. falciparum* are the most common. They all have complex life cycles involving both the anopheles mosquito and the erythrocyte of the human host. In vivax, a persisting tissue phase continues to infect the blood at intervals for many years. Thus, the ideal antimalarial not only should eradicate the microzoan from the blood, (ie, to "suppress" the clinical attack) but from the tissues as well, to effect a "radical cure." The several antimalarials differ in their point of interruption of the cycle of the parasite and in the type of malaria affected.

Amodiaquine Hydrochloride NF

[4-[(7-Chloro-4-quinolyl)amino]-α-(diethylamino)-o-cresol Dihydrochloride Dihydrate; Camoquin Hydrochloride (Parke-Davis)]

Amodiaquine Hydrochloride [$C_{20}H_{22}ClN_3O.2HCl.-2H_2O$ (464.82)] contains 97.0–103.0% of $C_{20}H_{22}ClN_3.2HCl$ (428.79), calculated on the anhydrous basis.

Preparation—4,7-Dichloroquinoline is condensed with 2-(diethylamino)methyl-4-aminophenol. The free base is isolated and converted into the dihydrochloride which is crystallized from an appropriate solvent.

Description—Yellow, crystalline powder. It is odorless and has a bitter taste.

Solubility—Soluble in water; sparingly soluble in alcohol; very slightly soluble in benzene, chloroform, and ether.

Uses—Amodiaquine is very similar to chloroquine (see *Chloroquine Phosphate*, below) in its *antimalarial* actions. Thus, it is capable only of eradicating the parasite from the erythrocytes, so that only malaria caused by *P. falciparum* can be cured, but only the *suppression of acute attacks* in the other types of malaria can be effected. Unfortunately, resistance to Amodiaquine occurs, and in some regions successful management of malaria caused by *P. falciparum* is achieved in less than 25% of cases. When there fails to be an unfavorable clinical response, quinine, pyrimethamine, or dapsone may be added, although authorities are as yet uncertain which of these or which combinations are best. Like quinacrine and chloroquine, amodiaquine is of value in the treatment of *lupus erythematosus* and *giardiasis*.

Amodiaquine may cause nausea, vomiting, diarrhea, sialorrhea, motor incoordination, spasticity, or convulsions.

Dose—*Usual, suppressive,* **520 mg,** the equivalent of 400 mg of amodiaquine base, every 2 weeks; *therapeutic,* **780 mg** to **1.3 Gm,** the equivalent of 600 mg to 1 Gm of amodiaquine base.

Dosage Forms—Tablets NF: 200 mg.

Chloroquine USP

[7-Chloro-4-[[4-(diethylamino)-1-methylbutyl]amino]quinoline; (Winthrop)]   Aralen

Chloroquine contains 98.0–102.0% of $C_{18}H_{26}ClN_3$ (319.88), calculated on the dried basis.

Preparation—A mixture of 4,7-dichloroquinoline and 4-amino-1-(diethylamino)pentane is heated at 160° to 170° for 4 to 5 hours.

Description—A white to slightly yellow, crystalline powder. It is odorless and has a bitter taste. It usually is in a partly hydrated form.

Solubility—Very slightly soluble in water; soluble in dilute acids, chloroform, and ether.

Uses—The actions and uses of Chloroquine are those of *Chloroquine Phosphate* (this page). In the phosphate and hydrochloride it is the Chloroquine base that is active, and doses of the salts are expressed in terms of the base.

Dose—See *Chloroquine Hydrochloride Injection* and *Chloroquine Phosphate.*

Chloroquine Hydrochloride Injection USP

[Aralen Hydrochloride (Winthrop)]

Chloroquine Hydrochloride Injection is a sterile solution of chloroquine in water for injection prepared with the aid of hydrochloric acid. It contains, in each ml, 47.5–52.5 mg of $C_{18}H_{26}ClN_3.2HCl$ (392.80).

For the structure of the base, see *Chloroquine.*

Description—A colorless liquid. Its pH is between 5.5 and 6.5.

Uses—The actions and uses of Chloroquine Hydrochloride are those of *Chloroquine Phosphate* (below), except that the hydrochloride lends itself better to solutions for intramuscular injection. The intramuscular route may be indicated in patients who cannot tolerate oral Chloroquine or in cerebral malaria, in which a very rapid response is desired. The toxicity is like that of the phosphate, even to the occurrence of gastrointestinal complaints; in addition, respiratory depression, hypotension, or shock may occur consequent to too rapid a rate of injection or after an overdose.

Dose—*Intramuscular,* **200 mg** to **1 Gm** for 1 day only; *usual,* **200** to **250 mg,** repeated in 6 hours if necessary.

Other Dose Information—Intramuscular, for malaria, initial, 160 to 200 mg of base, to be repeated within 4 hours if necessary; for extraintestinal amebiasis, 160 to 200 mg of base daily for 10 to 12 days. In the treatment of malaria, following the initial dose above the patient should be switched to oral Chloroquine (as the phosphate) if possible, and treatment continued until a course of about 1.5 Gm of base has been given in 3 days. If oral administration cannot be accomplished, a comparable intramuscular course of the hydrochloride may be given.

Dosage Forms—Injection USP: 5 ml.

Chloroquine Phosphate USP

[7 - Chloro - 4 - [[4 - (diethylamino) - 1 - methylbutyl]amino]quinoline Phosphate (1:2); SN 7618; Resochin; Nivaquine-B; 3377RP; Aralen Phosphate (Winthrop)]

Chloroquine Phosphate contains 98.0–102.0% of $C_{18}H_{26}ClN_3.2H_3PO_4$ (515.87), calculated on the dried basis.

For the structure of the base, see *Chloroquine.*

Preparation—Chloroquine phosphate is formed by the addition of concentrated phosphoric acid to a hot ethanol solution of the chloroquine base.

Description—A white, crystalline powder. Odorless. Bitter taste. Slowly discolors on exposure to light. Its aqueous solution has a pH of about 4.5. Melting ranges: 193° to 195° (usual form) or 215° to 218° (other form).

Solubility—Freely soluble in water; practically insoluble in alcohol, chloroform, and ether.

Uses—Chloroquine is employed both for the control of acute attacks of *vivax malaria* and for suppressive purposes. The drug is neither a prophylactic nor a radical curative agent in *vivax* malaria. In regions where *P. falciparum* is generally sensitive to Chloroquine, it is markedly effective in terminating acute attacks of *falciparum malaria* and usually brings about complete cure in this type of malaria. However, in some regions a high incidence of resistance exists, being as high as 89% in Vietnam, so that other drugs such as pyrimethamine, dapsone, or quinine may have preference. Resistant strains of *P. vivax* also occur. Chloroquine was once the most generally useful of all antimalarial agents, but it now appears that emerging resistance is relegating the drug to secondary status.

Although not useful in intestinal amebiasis, Chloroquine is an effective agent in the treatment of *amebic hepatitis*. Clinical response is usually as prompt and complete as response to emetine. Since Chloroquine is well tolerated, it has been recommended that it be employed routinely even in cases of amebiasis without demonstrable hepatic involvement. Chloroquine has also been employed with some success in *giardiasis, clonorchiosis, tapeworm* infestation, and *leishmaniasis*. Like quinacrine, it may also be of value in chronic discoid *lupus erythematosus* and *rheumatoid arthritis*. Chloroquine is quite effective in the treatment of *photoallergic reactions*. The drug has actions on the heart like quinidine and may be used as an antiarrhythmic when the standard drugs cannot be used.

Chloroquine is less toxic than quinacrine in man. The dose employed for the therapy of an acute malarial attack may cause mild transient headache, visual disturbances, gastrointestinal complaints (nausea and vomiting, other), and pruritus. Prolonged chronic medication for suppression of the disease causes few significant toxic reactions. Only rarely must the drug be discontinued because of intolerance. A small percentage of chronically treated individuals develop a lichenoid skin eruption which disappears rapidly when the drug is withdrawn. For this reason the drug is contraindicated in psoriasis, porphyria, or when other drugs that cause dermatoses are being given. Large doses given for a period of a year to uninfected human volunteers have caused the following toxic, but in no instance incapacitating, reactions: blurring of vision, bleaching of hair, diminution in T wave without evidence of cardiovascular impairment, mild skin eruptions, headache, and slight weight loss. Retinal damage from prolonged treatment with high doses also has been reported. Convulsions have occurred on the intensive dose schedule employed for the treatment of amebiasis.

Chloroquine is almost completely absorbed from the gastrointestinal tract and is usually administered orally. Chloroquine (as the hydrochloride) is given intramuscularly when it is necessary to resort to parenteral administration. The tissues bind chloroquine, although not quite to the same degree as quinacrine. It is degraded in the tissues to unknown breakdown products. The drug is slowly excreted in the urine.

Dose—*Usual, antimalarial, suppressive,* **500 mg** once

a week *therapeutic, initial,* **1 Gm,** then **500 mg** in 6 hours, and **500 mg** on the second and third days. *Anti-amebic* (for abscess only) **250 mg** 2 or 3 times a day for 2 weeks, up to a total dose of **11 Gm.** *Lupus erythematosus suppressant,* **250 mg** 2 times a day for 1 to 2 weeks, then **250 mg** daily.

Other Dose Information—The above treatment schedule for malaria usually cures *falciparum* malaria caused by sensitive strains. For *vivax* infection, the treatment of the acute attack must be followed by suppressive therapy (500 mg weekly).

Dosage Forms—Tablets USP: 125 and 250 mg.

Dapsone—see page 1241.

Hydroxychloroquine Sulfate USP

[2 - [[4 - [(7 - Chloro - 4 - quinolyl)amino]pentyl]ethylamino]ethanol Sulfate (1:1) Plaquenil (*Winthrop*)]

Hydroxychloroquine Sulfate contains 98.0–102.0% of $C_{18}H_{26}ClN_3O \cdot H_2SO_4$ (433.96), calculated on the dried basis.

Preparation—Hydroxychloroquine (base) is prepared by condensing 4,7-dichloroquinoline with N^1-ethyl-N^1-(2-hydroxyethyl)-1,4-pentanediamine. After isolation and purification, the base may then be dissolved in absolute ethanol or another suitable organic solvent and precipitated as the sulfate by reaction with an equimolar portion of sulfuric acid.

Description—White or nearly white, crystalline powder. Odorless, and has a bitter taste. Its solutions are acid to litmus, having a pH of about 4.5. It exists in two forms, the usual form melting at about 240° and the other form melting at about 198°.

Solubility—Freely soluble in water; practically insoluble in alcohol, chloroform, and ether.

Uses—Hydroxychloroquine is similar in action and uses to chloroquine (see *Chloroquine Phosphate* (above). It mainly attacks the erythrocytic phase of the *malaria* parasite (ie, it is a suppressant), and therefore is not radically curative for *P. vivax infections*. Like chloroquine, it is of use in the treatment of *lupus erythematosus* and *rheumatoid arthritis*. Toxicity is similar to that of chloroquine phosphate. Early claims that Hydroxychloroquine is less toxic are subject to challenge. Skin rashes occur with equal frequency with either drug.

Dose—**200 to 800 mg** daily; *usual,* **400 mg** once a day.

Other Dose Information—The official dose (above) is for the treatment of lupus erythematosus. 12.5 Gm can be given in a single dose for falciparum malaria. 400 mg may be given weekly for chronic suppression in endemic area. The drug has been given intravenously.

Dosage Forms—Tablets USP: 200 mg.

Primaquine Phosphate USP

[8-[(4-Amino-1-methylbutyl)amino]-6-methoxyquinoline Phosphate(1:2); (*Winthrop*)]

Primaquine Phosphate contains 98.0–102.0% of $C_{15}H_{21}N_3O \cdot 2H_3PO_4$ (455.34), calculated on the dried basis.

Preparation—2-Chloropentylamine is condensed with 8-amino-6-methoxyquinoline and the resulting primaquine base is reacted with a double molar quantity of phosphoric acid.

Description—An orange-red, crystalline powder. It is odorless and has a bitter taste. Its solutions are acid to litmus. Melts at about 200°.

Solubility—1 Gm dissolves in about 15 ml of water; insoluble in chloroform and ether.

Uses—Primaquine is an antimalarial which is very important for the *radical cure of relapsing vivax malaria*; it is not employed for suppressive therapy or for control of the acute clinical attacks of the disease. The incidence of serious untoward effects is low. In Caucasians, therapeutic doses of Primaquine are adequately tolerated. Mild to moderate abdominal cramps and occasional epigastric distress occur in some individuals. Mild anemia, cyanosis (methemoglobinemia), and leukocytosis may also be observed. At higher dose levels these symptoms are accentuated and leukopenia may be noted. Toxicity is not increased by concurrent administration of quinine or chloroquine, which are often given concurrently. However, quinacrine greatly enhances the toxicity of Primaquine and must not be given at the same time. Impairment of liver function has not been noted, even in patients with infectious hepatitis. Abdominal distress may be alleviated by antacids and by administration of the drug at mealtime. Untoward effects in Negroes are similar, but the incidence and degree of anemia and intravascular hemolysis are greater. A daily dose of 15 mg of primaquine (base) can be safely administered for 14 days to both Caucasian and non-Caucasian adults without special medical supervision. Larger doses are too toxic for those Negroes and other persons whose erythrocytes are deficient in glucose-6-phosphate dehydrogenase but usually can be administered to white subjects, who should be carefully supervised.

Dose—*Usual,* **26.3 mg,** the equivalent of 15 mg of primaquine base, once a day for 14 days.

Other Dose Information—The currently recommended dose of primaquine for the purpose of radical cure of relapsing *vivax malaria* (temperate zone variety) is 10 to 15 mg (base) daily for 14 days. 30 mg (base) a day should not be exceeded except that a daily dose of 30 to 45 mg (base) for 14 days may be necessary for radical cure of patients infected with the Chesson strain.

Dosage Forms—Tablets USP: 26.3 mg (15 mg of base).

Pyrimethamine USP

[2,4-Diamino-5-(*p*-chlorophenyl)-6-ethylpyrimidine; Daraprim (*Burroughs-Wellcome*)]

Pyrimethamine contains 99.0–101.0% of $C_{12}H_{13}ClN_4$ (248.72), calculated on the dried basis.

Preparation—Ethyl propionate is condensed with *p*-chlorophenylacetonitrile in the presence of sodium methylate. The resulting α-propionyl-*p*-chlorophenyl-acetonitrile (I) is then reacted with isoamyl alcohol to form the hemiacetal (II) which undergoes dehydration to α-(*p*-chlorophenyl)-β-ethyl-β-isoamyloxyacrylonitrile (III). (III) is then reacted with guanidine (IV) whereupon cyclization occurs due to (*a*) the liberation of isoamyl alcohol by condensation involving the imino hydrogen of guanidine and the isoamyloxy group of (III), and (*b*) an addition reaction involving an amino group of guanidine and the nitrile group of (III).

Description—A white, odorless, crystalline powder. Melting range 238° to 241°.

Solubility—Practically insoluble in water; 1 Gm dissolves in about 200 ml of alcohol and about 125 ml of chloroform; slightly soluble in acetone.

Uses—Pyrimethamine is chemically related to chloroguanide and is similar to it in mechanism of action. It antagonizes folic acid; thus the developing parasite cannot utilize nucleic acid precursors needed for growth. Its action in preventing the development of the erythrocytic phase of the parasite is slow, so that it is of little value in the suppression of acute attacks; rather it is used mainly as a *suppressive prophylactic* used for the prevention of clinical attacks by *P. vivax* and *falciparum* in regions where they are endemic. It also renders the parasites incapable of sporulating in the mosquito, so that the life cycle of the parasite is broken. In some regions, treatment with Pyrimethamine is successful in up to 90% of cases; the addition of quinine increases the success rate to about 95%. Pyrimethamine is also of use in the treatment of *Toxoplasmosis* and as an *immunosuppressive*.

The toxicity of pyrimethamine is low, but it may cause megaloblastic anemia and, less commonly, leukopenia as the result of antagonism of folic acid. This action has been used in the therapy of *polycythemia vera*.

Dose—**25 to 75 mg** per dose; *usual, suppressive,* **25 mg** once a week; *therapeutic,* **50 mg** once a day for 2 days.

Other Dose Information—About 10 weeks are required before a suppressive cure of vivax malaria is effected.

Dosage Forms—Tablets USP: 25 mg.

Quinacrine Hydrochloride USP

6 - Chloro - 9 - [[4 - (diethylamino) - 1 - methylbutyl]amino] - 2 - methoxy-acridine Dihydrochloride; Mepacrine Hydrochloride; Atabrine; SN 390; Chinacerin; Atabrine Hydrochloride (*Winthrop*)]

Quinacrine Hydrochloride [$C_{23}H_{30}ClN_3O . 2HCl . 2H_2O = 508.92$] contains 99.0–101.0% of $C_{23}H_{30}ClN_3O . 2HCl$, calculated on the anhydrous basis.

Preparation—2,4-Dichlorobenzoic acid is condensed in alkaline solution with *p*-anisidine, and the resulting product on treatment with phosphorus oxychloride is cyclized to methoxy-dichloro-acridine. This is heated with 2-amino-5-diethylaminopentane in phenol solution and the reaction mixture is added to acetone containing hydrochloric acid. Quinacrine is precipitated as the dihydrochloride while the phenol is held in solution by the acetone.

Description—Bright yellow, odorless, bitter, crystalline powder.

Solubility—1 Gm dissolves in about 35 ml of water; soluble in alcohol; almost insoluble in chloroform or acetone.

Uses—Quinacrine inhibits the erythrocytic stage of development of the malarial parasite (suppressive action) and controls clinical attacks. It is neither a true causal prophylactic agent (an agent lethal to sporozoites or succeeding exoerythrocytic stages of development) nor a radical curative agent (an agent lethal to both erythrocytic and exoerythrocytic parasites). It does not prevent relapses in *vivax malaria*. However, suppressive doses of the drug at times *may* cure *falciparum malaria*. The drug is more effective and less toxic than quinine, but less effective and more toxic than chloroquine.

Quinacrine has also been employed with some success in *amebiasis*, *giardiasis*, *tapeworm*, and *pinworm* infestations, and in selected patients with chronic discoid *lupus erythematosus*. It also possesses anticonvulsant activity in *petit mal*.

Quinacrine induces inflammatory responses when applied locally. When introduced into the pleural or peritoneal cavity, it causes fibrous thickening and sometimes adhesions. This action has proven to be useful in the management of recurring pleural or peritoneal neoplastic effusions secondary to metastatic carcinoma of the lung or breast or to lymphoma or mesothelioma. The fibrosis brings about symptomatic improvement by suppressing effusion, but it does not affect the underlying neoplastic disorder.

A small percentage of patients treated with quinacrine exhibit untoward effects. The yellow pigmentation of the skin which occurs in the majority of treated patients causes no symptoms and apparently no harm. Mild toxic effects include nausea, vomiting, abdominal cramps, headache, vertigo, excessive sweating, fever, pruritus, insomnia, myalgia, and arthralgia. Hallucinosis infrequently follows large doses. Ileus sometimes occurs. By intracavitary administration regional pain usually occurs; the fever that occurs is often greater than that resulting from systemic use. Dyspnea frequently results from instillation into the pleural cavity.

The following types of skin disorders, probably hypersensitivity reactions, occur in a small percentage of patients: "symmetrical eczematoid dermatitis," atypical lichen planus (New Guinea or jungle rot), and exfoliative dermatitis. Hepatitis, severe aplastic anemia, and agranulocytosis have been observed rarely. Toxic psychoses have been observed. Very large doses of Quinacrine stimulate the central nervous system. Concurrent administration of quinacrine greatly enhances the toxicity of pamaquine and pentaquine.

Quinacrine is readily absorbed from the gastrointestinal tract and from intramuscular and intracavitary sites of injection. Quinacrine is very slowly excreted in the urine and accumulates in the tissue on chronic administration.

Quinacrine is usually administered by mouth. Each dose is given with water after a meal. If the oral route cannot be employed, intramuscular injection is preferred over the intravenous route of administration.

Dose—*Usual*, **200 mg** with **300 mg** of sodium bicarbonate every 10 minutes for 4 doses.

Other Dose Information—The dose above is that as an anthelmintic. In the therapy of an acute clinical attack of malaria, 200 mg plus 1 Gm of sodium bicarbonate are given every 4 to 6 hours for 5 doses. Thereafter 100 mg is given 3 times daily for 6 days. For suppressive therapy in malarious areas, 100 mg is administered daily. For intracavitary administration, each 200 mg of drug is dissolved in 10 ml of effusate (or water), and the solution is instilled into the pool of ascitic or pleural fluid. Usually some effusate is removed prior to instillation. Initially 50 to 100 mg is given for pleural effusions and 100 to 200 mg for ascites. According to individual tolerance, 200 to 400 mg is given daily for 4 or 5 days for pleural effusions and 400 to 800 gm daily for 3 to 5 days for ascites.

Dosage Forms—Tablets USP: 100 mg.

Quinine Dihydrochloride NF

Quinine Dihydrochloride contains 98.0–100.5% of $C_{20}H_{24}N_2O_2 . 2HCl$ (397.35), calculated on the dried basis.

For the structure of quinine, see page 494.

Preparation—A quantity of hydrochloric acid sufficient to form the dihydrochloride is added to a hot aqueous solution of quinine monohydrochloride, and the dihydrochloride crystallizes out on concentrating.

Description—A white, odorless powder having a very bitter taste. It is affected by light. Its solutions are acid.

Solubility—Very soluble in water; soluble in alcohol; slightly soluble in chloroform; very slightly soluble in ether.

Uses—Quinine Dihydrochloride has the same actions and uses as *Quinine Sulfate* (below). Since the dihydrochloride is more than 100 times as soluble as the sulfate, it is more suited to preparations intended for parenteral use.

Dose—*Parenteral, usual*, **1 Gm.**

Dosage Forms—Injection NF: 250 mg/ml, 300 mg/10 ml, 500 mg/l and 1.5 ml, 1 Gm/2 ml.

Quinine Sulfate USP

[Quinine Sulfate (Salt) (2:1)]

Quinine Sulfate is the sulfate of an alkaloid [$(C_{20}H_{24}N_2O_2)_2 . H_2SO_4 . 2H_2O = 782.96$] obtained from the bark of *Cinchona officinalis* Linné (*C. ledgeriana* Moens) (Fam. *Rubiaceae*) or other species of *Cinchona*. It contains 99.0–101.0% of $(C_{20}H_{24}N_2O_2)_2 . H_2SO_4$, calculated on the dried basis.

For the structural formula of quinine, see page 494.

Preparation—The crude sulfate, obtained as described under *Quinine*, is recrystallized once or twice from hot water slightly acidified with sulfuric acid. Quinine Sulfate is the primary material for the preparation of all other quinine compounds.

Quinine Sulfate crystallizes from water with 8 moles of the solvent (16.2%), but loses about 1 mole of the water very rapidly. The salt official in the USP until the 11th Revision (and still official in many other countries) was the heptahydrate. However, even the latter readily loses all but 2 moles of H_2O at ordinary temperatures, with the result that the pharmacist, after having opened the container a few times, dispensed about 10% excess of the drug. This situation was corrected in USP XI by making the dihydrate official. This is stable under normal conditions of storage even at summer temperatures.

Description—White, fine, needle-like crystals, usually lusterless, making a light and readily compressible mass. It is odorless, and has a persistent, very bitter taste. Its solution in dilute hydrochloric or sulfuric acid is levorotatory. When exposed to light, Quinine Sulfate acquires a brown tint. A saturated solution is neutral or slightly alkaline to litmus.

Solubility—1 Gm dissolves in about 500 ml of water, 120 ml of alcohol, 35 ml of water at 100°, and about 10 ml of alcohol at 80°; slightly soluble in chloroform and ether; freely soluble in a mixture of 2 volumes of chloroform and 1 volume of dehydrated alcohol.

Incompatibilities—The free alkaloid is liberated from solutions of quinine sulfate by *alkalies*. A precipitation is caused by alkaloidal precipitants such as *tannic acid*, *iodides*, etc, and by *acetates, citrates, tartrates, benzoates*, and *salicylates*. For a full discussion see *Alkaloids*, page 491.

Uses—As an antimalarial drug, Quinine was largely replaced by less toxic and more effective drugs, except in areas where Quinine was available locally and was less expensive than the newer agents. However, the occurrence of resistance to the newer and usually superior antimalarial drugs has left a place for the use of Quinine. Quinine only has effects on the erythrocytic form of the plasmodia and hence is used only as a suppressive in the management of acute attacks of *vivax, malariae,* or *ovale* malaria. It may cure up to 50% of infections caused by *falciparum* plasmodia, but some strains are resistant. Quinine may be combined with pyrimethamine, but it appears to be antagonized by chloroquine.

Quinine was used as an *analgetic* and *antipyretic* in the same manner as the salicylates and related coal-tar analgetics. However, it lacks the antirheumatic action of the salicylates and is ineffective in gout. Quinine also is sometimes effective in auricular fibrillation, auricular flutter, and premature systoles, but quinidine is preferred for these arrhythmias. Quinine is both a *local anesthetic* and *sclerosing agent*, and it was once employed in the treatment of *varicose veins*, in the combination *Quinine and Urea Hydrochloride*. Quinine is an *oxytocic* and is occasionally employed to initiate labor. It enjoys some lay popularity as an abortifacient but is most unreliable in this regard. Quinine has an effect to suppress neuromuscular transmission. In the symptomatic treatment of a rare myopathy known as *myotonia congenita*, or Thomsen's disease, quinine is almost a specific. Quinine is also used as a diagnostic test for still another myopathy known as myasthenia gravis, in which syndrome the symptoms are markedly aggravaged by quinine but characteristically relieved by neostigmine. It occasionally benefits patients with spasmodic torticollis (torsion spasm) and also persons with nocturnal leg cramps. Quinine is a frequent constituent of bitter *tonics* and *stomachic* preparations. It is occasionally employed in rectal suppositories to relieve the pain of hemorrhoids, and also to relieve constipation. It use in "hair tonics" is irritational and has caused severe skin rashes in hypersensitive individuals.

A syndrome of toxic effects known as "cinchonism," follows the repeated use of full therapeutic doses of quinine. Mild cinchonism is characterized by tinnitus, headache, nausea, and slight disturbance of vision. In severe cinchonism the skin is hot and flushed, rashes are frequent, and the central nervous system is involved; headache, fever, vomiting, apprehension, excitement, confusion, delirium, and syncope are common. The emesis is due to a central action of quinine as well as to the local irritant action of the drug on the intestinal mucosa. In a few cases, renal damage and hypoprothrombinemia may occur. Agranulocytosis has rarely been observed. Transient ventricular tachycardia is noted in rare instances after massive acute overdosage. Although Quinine generally exerts vasodilator actions, retinal vasoconstriction, leading to loss of vision, has been described.

Quinine is readily absorbed from the gastrointestinal tract. The drug is only moderately concentrated in tissues and undergoes degradation particularly in the liver. Quinine and its degradation products are rapidly excreted in the urine and for this reason the drug must be given every 6 hours in order to maintain relatively constant plasma levels.

The drug is given after meals to minimize gastric irritation. Intramuscular and subcutaneous injections of quinine are painful and are frequently followed by local tissue injury. The intravenous route is rarely used and only in emergencies.

If Quinine Sulfate is dispensed in an aqueous medium, it is better to suspend it in syrup without using acid, with the addition of a little fluidextract of glycyrrhiza and a small quantity of ammonia water. Quinine salts are usually dispensed in capsules or tablets to conceal their nauseatingly bitter taste.

Dose—*Usual, therapeutic,* **300 mg** 3 times a day for 9 days.

Other Dose Information—Recent evidence indicates that in falciparum malaria the best curative results are obtained if treatment is continued for 13 days or longer.

Dosage Forms—Capsules USP: 125, 200, and 300 mg; Tablets USP: 300 mg.

Veterinary Dose—*Horses* and *Cattle,* **8** to **15 Gm;** *Dogs,* **300** to **600 mg.**

Other Antimalarials

Chloroguanide Hydrochloride USP XIV [Proguanil Hydrochloride BP, PhI; Paludrine (*Ayerst*); 1-(*p*-Chlorophenyl)-5-isopropylbiguanide hydrochloride; $C_{11}H_{16}ClN_5$.-HCl]—Colorless crystals or a white crystalline powder. Odorless. Bitter taste. Stable in air but slowly darkens on exposure to light. Melting range: 248° to 252°C. 1 Gm dissolves in about 75 ml water and about 30 ml alcohol. Insoluble in chloroform and ether. *Uses:* prophylaxis and suppression of malaria. In addition to being a potent schizonticide, it is lethal to actively developing pre-erythrocytic tissue forms of plasmodia and exerts unique sterilizing action on gametocytes of *P. falciparum*. However, its clinical value is seriously compromised by the development of chloroguanide-resistant strains of plasmodia. It undergoes degradation in the tissues, probably chiefly in the liver. *Dose:* 100 to 400 mg daily.

Quinine NF X—An alkaloid (see page 494) usually obtained from the bark of *Cinchona sp.* (Fam. *Rubiaceæ*). An odorless, white, microcrystalline powder having an intense, bitter taste. It is efflorescent in dry air (it occurs as a trihydrate) and is affected by light. 1 Gm dissolves in about 1560 ml water, 1 ml alcohol, 1 ml chloroform, and is soluble in ether. It melts at 57°C. *Uses:* antimalarial used in the same manner and dosage as quinine bisulfate. See *Quinine Sulfate* (page 1248 and this page).

Trimethoprim [Bactrim (Roche); Syraprim (Burroughs - Wellcome)] is 2,4 - diamino - 5 - (3, 4, 5 - trimethoxybenzyl)pyrimidine ($C_{14}H_{18}N_4O_3$). *Description:* Pale yellow crystals that melt between 195° and 197°. *Uses:*

Trimethoprim is both an antimalarial and antibacterial drug. As an antimalarial, it is employed especially against infections caused by *P. falciparum* which are resistant to other antimalarial agents. In many respects it resembles pyrimethamine. Like pyrimethamine, it is often used in combination with sulfonamides. As an antibacterial drug, it has a relatively broad spectrum, having activity against *Str. pyogenes, Staph. aureus, Str. pneumoniae, H. influenzae, K. pneumeniae, K. aerogenes, E. coli, Proteus sp., Salmonella sp., Shigella sp., Bordetella pertussis;* and *V. cholera.* Although it is claimed that resistance to the drug does not develop, resistance depends upon the species of bacterium, and considerable resistance has been reported to occur in those species that readily develop resistance to other antibacterial drugs, especially to sulfonamides. Trimethoprim is a folic acid antagonist. In combination with sulfonamides a remarkable supra-additivity occurs, so that both the Trimethoprim and sulfonamide may be used in small doses. Untoward effects include nausea and vomiting, malaise, and, rarely, rash. Care must be exercised in patients with renal impairment. *Dose:* In combination with a sulfonamide, 160 mg 2 times a day.

Amebacides

The incidence of amebiasis in the United States has been estimated to be from 5 to 20%, depending on the locality. Most infections are essentially asymptomatic, but the number of severe infections is still large.

Amebic infections generally remain confined to the intestines, where they may give rise to dysentery; but in an appreciable fraction of cases the amebae may locate elsewhere, especially in the liver. The chemotherapy of amebiasis thus must provide drugs to treat both the intestinal and extraintestinal forms of the disease. In addition, the ideal amebacide also is capable of eliminating amebic cysts from the intestine. No safe drug exists that will eradicate all of motile forms, cysts, and extraintestinal amebae, but judicious combined therapy can eliminate the parasite from all sites.

Bacitracin—see page 1209.

Carbarsone NF

[*p*-Ureidobenzenearsonic Acid; *N*-Carbamoylarsanilic Acid; (Lilly)]

OAs(OH)$_2$

NH—CO—NH$_2$

Carbarsone contains 97.5–101.0% of C$_7$H$_9$AsN$_2$O$_4$ (260.08), calculated on the dried basis.

Preparation—Carbarsone may be prepared by the action of sodium cyanate on arsanilic acid in the presence of hydrochloric acid.

It may also be made by heating sodium arsanilate with ethyl chloroformate, and then subjecting the resulting *N*-carbethoxyarsanilic acid to ammonolysis.

Description—A white, almost odorless, powder having an acid reaction and taste. It is reasonably stable in dry air. Its saturated solution is acid to litmus.

Solubility—Slightly soluble in water and alcohol; very slightly soluble in chloroform and ether; soluble in solutions of alkali hydroxides and carbonates.

Uses—Carbarsone is probably the most useful, potent, and safe *antiprotozoan* arsenical drug used in the therapy of *intestinal amebiasis.* Carbarsone therapy requires no special adjuvants, bed rest, or diet, which, along with its oral efficacy, render the drug valuable in the treatment of carriers and mild ambulatory cases. It is also capable of relieving severe acute cases of *amebic dysentery,* but it acts more slowly than emetine. In the intestinal tract, it acts directly against motile forms and decreases the number of cysts indirectly. It is ineffective in the therapy of extraintestinal amebiasis. The clinical usefulness and efficacy of Carbarsone and the hydroxyquinolines (see *Chiniofon, Iodochlorohydroxyquin,* and *Diiodohydroxyquin*) are very similar, but most authorities prefer to start with the hydroxyquinolines. Sometimes Carbarsone is alternated or given in combination with the hydroxyquinolines.

Carbarsone is also effective in the local treatment of *Trichomonas vaginalis vaginitis* and also has been used successfully in the therapy of *balantidial dysentery.*

Severe toxic reactions to the drug are uncommon, but diarrhea, loss of weight, polyuria, skin rashes, localized edema, and mild gastrointestinal distress are sometimes seen. Hepatitis and encephalopathy may occur; Carbarsone is contraindicated in the presence of hepatic or renal disease.

Dose—100 to 250 mg; *usual,* **250 mg** 2 or 3 times a day for 10 days.

Other Dose Information—Several courses may be repeated, provided that a 10-day rest follows each course. Rectally, the dose is 130 mg.

Dosage Forms—Capsules NF: 250 mg; Tablets NF: 250 mg.

Chloroquine Phosphate—see page 1245.

Diiodohydroxyquin USP

[Diiodohydroxyquinoline; Diodoquin; 5,7-Diiodo-8-quinolinol; 5,7-Diiodo-8-hydroxyquinoline; Floraquin (*Searle*); Yodoxin (*Glenwood*)]

OH

Diiodohydroxyquin contains 96.0–100.5% of C$_9$H$_5$-I$_2$NO (396.96), calculated on the dried basis.

Preparation—8-Quinolinol, prepared from quinoline via 8-quinolinesulfonic acid–NaOH fusion, is iodinated by treatment with iodine monochloride or with a solution of iodine in potassium iodide.

Description—A light yellowish to tan, microcrystalline powder. Wetted by water with difficulty. Odorless or nearly so. Stable in air. Melts with decomposition.

Solubility—Practically insoluble in water; sparingly soluble in alcohol and ether.

Uses—An amebacide similar to *Iodochlorhydroxyquin* (page 1252). It is effective in the treatment of intestinal forms of the disease but is ineffective in the treatment of extraintestinal amebiasis such as hepatic abscess. Bed rest is not required. It may be of value in cases of quinacrine-resistant *lambliasis* and in balantidial *dysentery.* It also may be used in the local and systemic treatment of a *Trichomonas vaginalis* vaginitis and infections caused by *Trichomonas hominis* (intestinalis). Like iodochlorhydroxyquin, it has also been used in the topical treatment of certain *pyo-*

genic and *fungal cutaneous infections.* Diiodohydroxyquin has a low order of toxicity, but iodine toxicoderma, chills, fever, mild to severe dermatitis, anal irritation, abdominal discomfort, diarrhea, and headache have been observed.

Dose—**650 mg to 2 Gm** daily; *usual,* **650 mg** 3 times a day for 20 days.

Dosage Forms—Tablets USP: 650 mg.

Emetine Hydrochloride USP

[Emetine Dihydrochloride]

Emetine Hydrochloride [$C_{29}H_{40}N_2O_4 \cdot 2HCl = 553.58$] is the hydrochloride of an alkaloid obtained from ipecac, or prepared by methylation of cephaëline, or prepared synthetically. It contains 98.0–101.5% of $C_{29}H_{40}N_2O_4 \cdot 2HCl$, calculated on the anhydrous basis.

History—Pelletier and Magendie, the celebrated French scientists, discovered this alkaloid in 1817.

Preparation—In the preparation of emetine finely ground ipecac is mixed with ammonia and then extracted with ether to remove the alkaloids. From the ether the alkaloids are extracted with dilute acid, the latter then being nearly neutralized with sodium hydroxide and shaken with ether or chloroform to remove impurities. The aqueous solution, which contains the alkaloids, is now made definitely alkaline with sodium hydroxide. This treatment precipitates emetine, while cephaëline, which is a phenolic base, remains in solution. The emetine is removed by extraction with ether and, after purification, it is converted into a hydrochloride. The cephaëline in the sodium hydroxide solution is precipitated by treatment with acid and then ammonia. This alkaloid is then converted to emetine by methylation with such substances as methyl sulfate or phenyltrimethylammonium hydroxide. By this process the yield of emetine from ipecac is substantially increased. It contains variable amounts of water of hydration.

Description—A white or very slightly yellowish, odorless, crystalline powder. It is affected by light. Its specific rotation is +21° in water.

Solubility—Freely soluble in water and alcohol.

Uses—The principal clinical use of Emetine Hydrochloride is for the treatment of *amebiasis.* It is concentrated and stored in the liver, and for that reason it has been used especially for *amebic hepatitis;* it is also of considerable value in the treatment of amebic abscesses in other locations. However, *Chloroquine Phosphate* (page 1245) is nearly as effective as emetine in the therapy of amebic hepatitis and is much less toxic; hence chloroquine has largely replaced it in the treatment of extraintestinal amebiasis. It is sometimes the practice to use Emetine and chloroquine concurrently. Occasionally, however, emetine may be life-saving. It rapidly relieves the symptoms of intestinal amebiasis by destroying motile amebae, but the percentage of

cures is below 15%, since cysts are little affected; consequently, other agents are not only safer but superior. Emetine may be used initially to control quickly severe intestinal ameba sis; the drug is then followed by treatment with other agents. It has no place in the therapy of mild ambulatory or chronic cases. The alkaloid is also useful in the treatment of *balantidiasis* and certain *liver fluke infestations.*

The incidence of toxic effects from emetine is very high, both by local and systemic administration. Diarrhea, nausea, and vomiting are frequent, as are also skeletal muscle weakness, stiffness, and aching. Sensory disturbances also occur. By far the most important toxic effects are cardiovascular; they include hypotension, precordial pain, dyspnea, tachycardia, and long-persisting electrocardiographic changes; electrocardiographic recordings at frequent intervals are necessitated.

The preferred route of emetine medication is subcutaneous. The intravenous route is contraindicated. A course of emetine should not continue for more than 10 days. The patient should be kept in bed, and carefully watched for toxic effects.

Dose—*Usual, subcutaneous,* **1 mg** per **Kg** of body weight, but not exceeding 65 mg, daily for 5 to 10 days.

Dosage Forms—Injection USP: 30 and 60 mg/ml.

Erythromycin—see page 1215.

Glycobiarsol NF

[(Hydrogen *N*-glycoloylarsanilato) oxobismuth; Milibis (*Winthrop*)]

Glycobiarsol contains 97.0–103.0% of $C_8H_9AsBi\text{-}NO_6$ (499.07), calculated on the dried basis.

Preparation—Glycobiarsol is synthesized from arsanilic acid. Treatment with monochloroacetic acid yields *N*-(chloroacetyl)arsanilic acid which, through alkaline hydrolysis and neutralization, is converted to sodium *N*-glycolylarsanilate. Reaction with bismuth nitrate in aqueous glycerin solution produces Glycobiarsol.

Description—An odorless, yellowish white to flesh-colored amorphous powder. Decomposes when heated.

Solubility—Very slightly soluble in alcohol and water; practically insoluble in benzene, chloroform, and ether.

Uses—Glycobiarsol is an *antiprotozoan* arsenical containing bismuth. It is employed in the therapy of *intestinal amebiasis;* it is not effective in the treatment of extraintestinal forms of the disease. Its efficacy is about the same as that of the other arsenicals. It has also been successfully used in the treatment of *trichomonal* and *monilial vaginitides.* It is poorly absorbed from the intestinal tract; consequently, side effects are few, but systemic arsenical poisoning with exfoliative dermatitis, hepatitis, or encephalopathy has been reported. The drug is contraindicated in the presence of hepatic or renal disease.

Dose—*Usual,* **500 mg** 3 times a day for 7 to 10 days.

Other Dose Information—The dose above is for amebiasis; for vaginitis, 250 mg by suppository.

Dosage Forms—Tablets NF: 500 mg.

Hexetidine—see page 1193.

Iodochlorhydroxyquin USP

[5-Chloro-7-iodo-8-quinolinol; Vioform (*Ciba*)]

Iodochlorhydroxyquin contains 93.0–100.5% of C_9H_5ClINO (305.50) (the 5-chloro-7-iodo-8-quinolinol isomer).

Preparation—This amebacide is made by chlorination of 8-quinolinol, dissolved in chloroform, with sulfuryl chloride [SO_2Cl_2] followed by iodination of the 5-chloro-8-hydroxyquinoline with iodine dissolved in alkali.

In the chlorination step, a dichloroquinoline is also formed. The 5-chloro-8-hydroxyquinoline is separated from the by-product by extraction with hot water. The desired product is readily soluble in hot water whereas the dichloroquinoline is not.

Description—A voluminous, spongy, yellowish white or brownish yellow powder having a slight, characteristic odor. It melts with decomposition at about 180° and is affected by light.

Solubility—Practically insoluble in water or alcohol; soluble in hot ethyl acetate and hot glacial acetic acid.

Uses—Iodochlorhydroxyquin is used in the treatment of *amebiasis* (page 1250). The drug is effective only in the intestinal phase, in which it attacks motile amebae and causes cysts to disappear, probably by eliminating trophozoites. Bed rest is not required. It is also effective as a *vaginal tract local anti-infective* in the treatment of *Trichomonas vaginalis* vaginitis, for which purpose it may be employed as a vaginal suppository or by insufflation; combination of oral with local administration yields superior results. It has also been applied locally in various forms for the treatment of various dermatitides, such as *seborrheic dermatitis, atopic dermatitis, pruritus ani* and *vulvae, eczema, impetigo,* and acute *psoriasis;* in these uses it is often combined with a glucocorticoid, such as hydrocortisone (see *Iodochlorhydroxyquin and Hydrocortisone* products, under *Dosage Forms,* below). Iodochlorhydroxyquin has also been applied as a dusting powder to cutaneous *wounds, ulcers,* and *burns.*

Toxic reactions to Iodochlorhydroxyquin are rarely serious; frequently a transient diarrhea and occasionally anal pruritus occur. Mild iodism and gastric distress occur in approximately 5% of patients.

Dose—*Intravaginal,* **250** to **500 mg** daily; *usual,* **250 mg** as vaginal suppository once a day; *topically,* as a **3**% ointment 2 or 3 times a day.

Other Dose Information—The course may be repeated after 7 to 10 days. Local dosage depends upon the infection and the form in which the drug is applied.

Dosage Forms—Cream USP: 3%; Ointment USP: 3%; Compound Powder NF (see below); Suppositories USP: 250 mg; Tablets NF: 250 mg; and Hydrocortisone Cream NF: 3% (iodochlorhydroxyquin) and 0.5 or 1% (hydrocortisone); and Hydrocortisone Lotion NF: 3% (iodochlorhydroxyquin) and 1% (hydrocortisone); and Hydrocortisone Ointment NF: 3% (iodochlorhydroxyquin) and 0.5 or 1% (hydrocortisone).

Compound Iodochlorhydroxyquin Powder NF—
Preparation: Mix lactic acid (25 Gm) with lactose (525 Gm), then add iodochlorhydroxyquin (250 Gm) and zinc stearate (200 Gm), and mix the Powder to make 1000 Gm.

Oxytetracycline—see page 1222.

Paromomycin Sulfate NF

[Paromomycin Sulfate; Humatin (*Parke-Davis*)]

Paromomycin Sulfate [$C_{23}H_{45}N_5O_{14} \cdot xH_2SO_4$] is the sulfate of an antibiotic substance or substances produced by the growth of *Streptomyces rimosus* var. *paromomycinus,* or by other means. It has a potency equivalent to not less than 675 mcg of paromomycin base [$C_{23}H_{45}N_5O_{14}$ = 615.64] per mg, calculated on the anhydrous basis. Paromomycin Sulfate conforms to the regulations of the Federal Food and Drug Administration concerning certification of antibiotic drugs (see page 1206).

Preparation—Paromomycin is isolated from fermentation broths by ion exchange adsorption and elution from the cation exchange resin IRC 50. After additional purification via a second IRC 50 column and finally an IRA 401-S column, the free base is converted to the sulfate, precipitated, and dried under vacuum.

Description—An off-white to light-yellow, amorphous powder that is odorless or practically odorless and has a slightly bitter taste. It is stable in light, stable but very hygroscopic in air, and stable but may experience some darkening of color in heat.

Solubility—1 Gm dissolves in 2 ml of water; insoluble in alcohol, chloroform, and ether.

Uses—Paromomycin is an antibacterial drug which is effective against various species of *Shigella* and *Salmonella* and strains of *E. coli.* It may be used to treat gastroenteritis or bacterial dysentery caused by these organisms, but the relapse rate is high and other antibiotics are more successful. However, it may be used to reduce the bacterial content of the intestine prior to surgery on the bowel or to rid the bowel of nitrogen-forming bacteria in patients with hepatic coma. It alters the ecology of the intestinal flora in such a way that the growth of intestinal amebae is discouraged and it also helps to prevent secondary infections that may follow or facilitate amebic invasion of the intestinal wall. Consequently, its principal use is in the treatment of *intestinal amebiasis.* It is of no value in treating hepatic or other extraintestinal amebic abscesses, because it is not well absorbed from the gut and also because it lacks a direct amebacidal action. It is not the drug of first choice in treating intestinal amebiasis, but it is indicated when the patient cannot tolerate the iodinated hydroxyquins.

Paromomycin often causes gastrointestinal hypermotility, nausea, and diarrhea, which generally appear on the second or third day of treatment. Occasionally the drug may cause headache, vertigo, vomiting, abdominal pain, or skin rash; overgrowth of enteric staphylococci and other pathogenic bacteria may occur, especially if treatment is prolonged. There is mutual cross-resistance to kanamycin and neomycin, and often to streptomycin. Although Paromomycin is poorly absorbed from the gut, there is potential nephrotoxicity, especially in the presence of renal disease. For this reason, the undesirability of prolonged diarrhea, and the danger of superinfection, treatment with Paromomycin should be of short duration.

Dose—The equivalent of **500 mg** to **1 Gm** of paromomycin; *usual,* **500 mg** every 6 hours taken with meals.

Dosage Forms—Capsules NF: 250 mg.

Other Amebacides

Arsthinol [2 - (3 - Acetamido - 4 - hydroxyphenyl) - 1,3,2 - dithiarsolane - 4 - methanol; 3 - Hydroxypropylene ester of 3-acetamido-4-hydroxydithiobenzenearsonous acid; Mercaptoarsenol; Balarsen (*Endo*)]. *Description and Solubility:* A white, odorless, microcrystalline powder that melts between 163° and 166°. 2.7 *w/v* in alcohol; very slightly soluble in water and ether. *Uses:* In the treatment of *intestinal amebiasis;* it compares favorably with the other arsenicals in this use. It is also of value in the treatment of yaws and certain other protozoal infections. *Dose:* 10 mg per Kg of body weight, with a maximum total dose of 500 mg daily. A course lasts 5 days.

Miscellaneous Antiprotozoal Drugs

Among the common protozoal infections that are endemic to the United States are amebiasis, trichomoniasis, syphilis,* and malaria, in decreasing order of incidence. Other protozoal infections, uncommon in the United States, nevertheless constitute serious public health and agricultural problems within the possessions and elsewhere. Until the advent of the antibiotics all the protozoal infections were managed very similarly, with heavy metals providing the backbone of therapy, except for malaria. However, the heavy metals are infrequently employed today in the treatment of syphilis and yaws and are not essential to the management of amebiasis or trichomoniasis. The amebacides and antimalarials are useful in the treatment of a number of other protozoal infections. The antimalarials and amebacides have been treated in separate sections above. The antisyphilitics are largely included among the antibiotics. Consequently, the drugs listed below are a miscellaneous group consisting of certain organometallic, arsenical, and nitrogenous compounds.

Amodiaquine Hydrochloride—see page 1245.

Antimony Potassium Tartrate—see page 1265.

Diiodohydroxyquin—see page 1250.

Iodochlorhydroxyquin—see page 1252.

Metronidazole USP

[2-Methyl-5-nitroimidazole-1-ethanol; Flagyl (*Searle*)]

Metronidazole contains 99.0–101.0% of $C_6H_9N_3O_3$ (171.16), calculated on the dried basis.

Preparation—2-Methyl-5-nitroimidazole is condensed with ethylene chlorohydrin by heating with a large excess of the chlorohydrin. After removing the surplus chlorohydrin, the residue is extracted with water and the extract is alkalinized and extracted with chloroform. Evaporation of the chloroform yields crude Metronidazole which is recrystallized from ethyl acetate. US Pat. 2,944,061.

Description—White to pale yellow, odorless, crystals or crystalline powder. It is stable in air, but darkens on exposure to light. It melts between 159° and 163°.

Solubility—Sparingly soluble in water, alcohol, and chloroform; slightly soluble in ether.

Uses—Metronidazole is a systemic trichomonacide which is highly effective in the treatment of infections caused by *Trichomonas vaginalis* in both the male and the female. Metronidazole is most efficacious by the oral route, but it may also be applied intravaginally. The drug appears to be specific for trichomonads; it is inactive against *Monilia albicans* and other organisms that cause vaginitis.

No serious reactions have been reported for the use of metronidazole. The most common untoward effect is nausea. Other untoward effects include diarrhea, unpleasant taste, urticaria, vaginal burning, rash, vertigo, headache, and insomnia. The urine sometimes turns a dark color. During Metronidazole treatment the patient should refrain from drinking alcoholic beverages, since Metronidazole is claimed to have an effect similar to *Disulfiram* (page 1087). Leukopenia has been reported, so that a blood count should be made, especially before a second course of the drug. In patients with blood dyscrasias great care must be exercised.

Dose—*Usual, oral,* **250 mg** 3 times a day in the female, or 2 times a day in the male, for 10 days; *vaginal,* **500 mg** once a day in addition to 250 mg orally 2 times a day.

Other Dose Information—The oral dose differential between males and females is based upon insubstantial evidence; 500 mg probably would suffice for either sex. However, the FDA has approved only the oral dose as stated above.

Dosage Forms—Suppositories USP: 500 mg; Tablets USP: 250 mg.

Quinacrine Hydrochloride—see page 1247.

Stibophen—see page 1268.

---

* Some authorities classify the treponema as bacteria, but there are equally cogent reasons for classifying them as protozoans.

Tryparsamide USP XVII

[Monosodium *N*-(Carbamoylmethyl)arsanilate]

$$H_2N-\overset{\overset{\displaystyle O}{\|}}{C}-CH_2NH-\!\!\!\!\bigcirc\!\!\!\!-\overset{\overset{\displaystyle O}{\|}}{As}\overset{OH}{\underset{ONa}{<}}\quad.1/2H_2O$$

Tryparsamide [$C_8H_{10}AsN_2NaO_4.\frac{1}{2}H_2O = 305.10$] contains an amount of arsenic (As) corresponding to 99.0–101.0% of $C_8H_{10}AsN_2NaO_4$ (296.09), calculated on the anhydrous basis.

Preparation—Arsanilic acid, suspended in water, is dissolved with just sufficient sodium bicarbonate; a moderate excess of 2-chloroacetamide is added and heat is applied until the reaction shown in the equation below is complete.

$$\underset{\text{Chloroacetamide}}{\overset{\text{OH}}{H_2NC_6H_4AsO.ONa}\xrightarrow{CH_2ClCONH_2}}$$
$$H_2NCOCH_2.HNC_6H_4AsO(OH)_2+NaCl$$

The tryparsamide (acid) so formed is dissolved in just sufficient sodium hydroxide solution, about 2 volumes of alcohol are added, and the salt is allowed to crystallize.

The arsanilic acid is prepared by heating aniline with arsenic acid. Chloroacetamide is obtained by cold ammonolysis of ethyl chloroacetate.

Description—White, odorless, crystalline powder. Is slowly affected by light. Its 1 in 20 solution in neutral to litmus.

Solubility—1 Gm dissolves in about 2 ml of water; slightly soluble in alcohol; insoluble in ether and chloroform.

Uses—Tryparsamide is an *antiprotozoan* and *trypanocidal* agent which once was also of occasional value in the treatment of central nervous system *syphilis*, especially early *paresis*, either prior to or subsequent to malariotherapy. It lacks the serious toxic effects of the arsphenamines but may cause severe damage to the optic nerve, sometimes resulting in blindness. It must not be used in patients with optic damage. Tryparsamide is also highly effective in certain trypanosomal diseases, especially, *African sleeping sickness*, but melarsoprol and non-arsenicals have largely replaced it, except in a few localities.

Dose—*Intravenous*, 1 to 3 Gm; *usual*, 3 Gm weekly up to a total dose of 20 to 45 Gm.

Dosage Forms—Sterile USP XVII.

Other Miscellaneous Antiprotozoal Drugs

Acetarsone NF XI [Stovarsol, Acetarsol] is 3-acetamido-4-hydroxybenzenearsonic acid [$C_8H_{10}AsNO_5$]. *Descriptive and Solubility:* A white, odorless powder. Slightly soluble in water; insoluble in alcohol; soluble in solutions of alkali hydroxides or carbonates forming the alkali salt of acetarsone. *Uses:* A *protozoacide* which was formerly used in the treatment of *amebic dysentery*. However, carbarsone is safer. Acetarsone is currently employed mostly in the treatment of *Trichomonas vaginalis* vaginitis in the form of a powder or vaginal suppository. *Dose: Usual, intravaginal,* 250 mg.

Antimony Sodium Tartrate—Colorless or whitish scales or powder containing not less than 96% $C_4H_4NaO_7Sb$ (BP allows 98–101%). Soluble in 1.5 parts of water, insoluble in alcohol. *Uses:* see *Antimony Potassium Tartrate* (page 1265). *Dose:* [2 to 8 mg; *emetic*, 30 to 60 mg; *intravenously*, 30 to 120 mg: unofficial].

Bismuth Sodium Triglycollamate USP XVI [Bismuth Sodium Nitrilotriacetate; Bistrimate (*Smith, Miller & Patch*)]—It is a double salt consisting of one molecule of

sodium bismuthyl triglycollamate and 3 molecules of disodium triglycollamate [$C_{24}H_{28}BiN_4Na_7O_{25}$]. It occurs as an odorless, white, crystalline powder. It is very soluble in water; insoluble in alcohol, acetone, benzene and ether. *Uses:* Still marketed for the treatment of syphilis, but it is obsolete. It has been used alone for certain forms of the disease but not for the curative therapy of early or active syphilis. It was not even the bismuth preparation of choice except when the more usual bismuth preparations could not be tolerated by the patient. The drug may be of value in *lupus erythematosus, lichen planus,* or *scleroderma*. The toxicity of Bismuth Sodium Triglycollamate is similar to that of the other bismuth compounds. In ordinary use it may cause gastrointestinal distress, dark stools, and a blue line along the gum margin. Larger doses may cause rashes, hepatitis, and evidence of central nervous disturbances. *Dose:* 400 mg 2 or 3 times daily, after meals.

Melarsoprol [2-[*p*-[(4,6-diamino-*s*-triazin-2-yl)amino]-phenyl]-1,3,2-dithiarsolane-4-methanol] [$C_{12}H_{15}AsN_6OS_2$]— A slightly cream or grayish-cream powder; slight odor; bitter taste. Insoluble in water, in alcohol, and in ether; slowly soluble in cold propylene glycol. It melts about 217° with decomposition. *Uses:* In the treatment of advanced trypanosomiasis. It has replaced all other arsenicals for this purpose. *Dose: Intravenous,* for adults, 3.6 mg per Kg of body weight daily for 3 days; for children, 1.8 mg per Kg of body weight daily for 3 days. The courses should be repeated after an interval of 10 days.

Pentamidine Dimethylsulfonate [4,4'-(Pentamethylenedioxy)dibenzamidine dimethanesulfonate]—A white or very faintly pink, granular powder that is practically odorless. *Purity:* equivalent to 63.2–64.2% of $C_{19}H_{24}N_4O_2$. It is slightly soluble in water and practically insoluble in alcohol, ether, chloroform, benzene, and ethyl acetate. A 5% aqueous solution has a pH of 4.6–6. It melts at 185–190°C. *Uses:* Antiprotozoal drug, as for pentamidine isethionate. See *Pentamidine Isethionate* (below). *Dose: intramuscularly,* 0.15 to 0.3 Gm.

Pentamidine Isethionate [Lomidine; 4,4'-(Pentamethylenedioxy)dibenzamidine diisethionate] [$C_{23}H_{36}N_4O_{10}S_2$]—It occurs as a hygroscopic, very bitter, crystalline material which melts at about 190°. It is soluble in water and glycerin; slightly soluble in alcohol. *Uses:* in the treatment of protozoal infections such as African trypanosomiasis and leishmaniasis. In veterinary medicine it is used to treat infections caused by *Babesia canis*. It also possesses local anesthetic activity, for which it is sometimes used. Side effects include hypotension, headache, vertigo, nausea and vomiting, convulsions and renal and liver damage. *Dose: Intramuscularly,* in man, 50 to 250 mg.

Sodium Stibogluconate—*Purity:* 30–34% of total antimony in a compound of indefinite composition. A complex containing pentavalent antimony, probably as the stibo ($-SbO_2$)group, in chemical union with sodium gluconate. The BP complex contains from 30 to 34% of antimony, and this corresponds approximately to one stibo group per sodium gluconate. It occurs as an odorless, colorless, amorphous powder. It is very soluble in water and insoluble in alcohol and ether. It is much less toxic than antimony sodium tartrate. *Uses:* in the treatment of leishmaniasis, employing a course of therapy of 6 daily injections of 6 ml each of a 30% solution; in the treatment of oriental sore, not more than 2 ml of a 30% solution being infiltrated around the edges of the lesions at one time. *Dose: intravenously or intramuscularly,* 0.6 to 2 Gm daily.

Sodium Suramin USP XVII [Bayer 205; Suramin; Hexasodium 8,8' - [Ureylenebis[*m* - phenylenecarbonylimino(4 - methyl - *m* - phenylene)carbonylimino]]di - 1,3,5 - naphthalenetrisulfonate] contains not less than 97.5% of $C_{51}H_{34}N_6Na_6O_{23}S_6$ (1429.19), calculated on the anhydrous basis. *Preparation:* 8-Amino-1,3,5-naphthalenetrisulfonic acid is condensed with *m*-nitro-*p*-toluoyl chloride in the presence of sodium acetate. The resulting nitro compound is reduced, and the amino compound is condensed with *m*-nitrobenzoyl chloride and the product is reduced to the corresponding amino compound which is then reacted with carbonyl chloride in the ratio of two moles of the former to one of the latter. The suramin acid thus obtained is neutralized with sodium hydroxide to produce the sodium salt. *Description and Solubility:* A white or slightly pink powder, which is odorless and has a slightly bitter taste; it is very hygroscopic and is affected by light; the pH of a solution is between 5.5 and 7.0. Soluble in water; slightly soluble in alcohol; insoluble in ether, chloroform, and benzene.

Uses: Suramin is one of the few nonmetallic compounds effective in the treatment of *trypanosomiasis.* Several species of African trypanosomes respond to the drug, but the Texan and South American species, *T. cruzi* (agent of Chagas' disease) does not respond. Suramin is also an effective agent for the treatment of *onchocerciasis.* It has also been effectively employed in the treatment of *pemphigus.* In a small percentage of patients Suramin may cause nausea and vomiting, shock, and loss of consciousness immediately after injection. Later, sensory disturbances (photophobia, paresthesias, etc), papular eruptions, and palpebral edema may occur. Still later, albuminuria, hematuria, and casts may occur. Hemolytic anemia and agranulocytosis are rare but possible. Since the drug is not absorbed from the gastrointestinal tract, it is given by slow intravenous administration. It is irritating upon intramuscular injection. *Dose: Usual, intravenous,* 1 Gm weekly, up to a total of 5 to 10 Gm. *Veterinary Use:* Prophylaxis and treatment of trypanosomiasis. *Veterinary Dose: Horses, prevention,* 2 Gm repeated at 10-day intervals; *treatment,* 7 to 10 mg per Kg of body weight; *Cattle, prevention,* 1 to 2 Gm; *treatment,* 12 mg per Kg of body weight.

Antidotes to the Heavy Metals

During the time when the use of arsenicals in war gases and in antiluetics was at its peak, no successful antidote to heavy metal poisoning existed, although the erratic sodium sulfoxylate antidote to mercury had been developed. Dimercaprol appeared at the end of the era of arsenical antiluesis, but the continued use of arsenic, antimony, and bismuth for other purposes has left a place for this agent. Because arsenic, antimony, and bismuth are still used, somewhat, in the treatment of protozoal infections, antidotes to the heavy metals are included here, rather than in a separate chapter. Calcium Disodium Edetate is discussed below because it is useful as an antidote to lead and several other heavy metals, even though such metals have no antimicrobial applications.

Calcium Disodium Edetate USP

[Calcium Disodium Ethylenediaminetetraacetate; Calcium Disodium (Ethylenedinitrilo)tetraacetate; Disodium [(Ethylenedinitrilo)tetraacetato] calciate (2-); Calcium Disodium Versenate (*Riker*)]

$$NaOOC-CH_2 \quad CH_2-COONa$$

Calcium Disodium Edetate is a mixture of the dihydrate and trihydrate of calcium disodium ethylenediaminetetraacetate (predominantly the dihydrate). It contains 97.0–102.0% of $C_{10}H_{12}CaN_2Na_2O_8$ [(anhydrous) 374.28], calculated on the anhydrous basis.

Preparation—Among other ways, the salt may be prepared by boiling an aqueous solution of disodium edetate (page 843) with slightly more than an equimolar quantity of calcium carbonate until carbon dioxide is no longer evolved, filtering while hot, and crystallizing.

Description—White, crystalline granules or white, crystalline powder. Is odorless, is slightly hygroscopic, and has a faint, saline taste. Is stable in air.

Solubility—Freely soluble in water.

Uses—Calcium Disodium Edetate is used primarily in the treatment of lead poisoning, but may be used for removing certain other heavy metals from the body. Since this agent already contains calcium, it is useless as an anticoagulant or for the treatment of hypercalcemia. The value of oral edetates in heavy-metal intoxication is disputed.

Dose—*Intravenous infusion,* up to **10 Gm** per course of treatment; *usual,* **1 gm** in 250 to 500 ml of isotonic solution over a period of 1 hour 2 times a day.

Other Dose Information—Usual, oral, 4 Gm in divided doses.

Dosage Forms—Injection USP: 5 ml; Tablets: 500 mg.

Deferoxamine—see page 844.

Dimercaprol USP

[British Anti-Lewisite; 2,3-Dimercapto-1-propanol; BAL in Oil (*Hynson*)]

$$CH_2-CH-CH_2$$
$$SH \quad SH \quad OH$$

Dimercaprol contains 97.0–100.5% of $C_3H_8OS_2$ (124.22) and not more than 1.5% of 1,2,3-trimercaptopropane ($C_3H_8S_3$).

Preparation—Dimercaprol is prepared as follows: A methanol solution of sodium hydroxide is saturated with hydrogen sulfide resulting in the formation of sodium hydrogen sulfide [NaSH]. 2,3-Dibromopropanol is added and the mixture heated at 40° under pressure.

2,3-Dibromopropanol is prepared by bromination of allyl alcohol.

Description—Colorless or almost colorless liquid. Offensive, mercaptan-like odor. Specific gravity: 1.242 to 1.244. Boiling point: about 122° (15 mm Hg) or about 116° (10 mm Hg).

Solubility—1 Gm dissolves in about 20 ml of water; soluble in alcohol, methanol, benzyl benzoate, and vegetable oils.

Uses—Dimercaprol in oil solution is an *antidote* used in the treatment of *arsenic, gold, and mercury poisoning.* The drug also may be of value in the treatment of antimony and bismuth poisoning. It is used in the treatment of lead poisoning only in conjunction with *Calcium Disodium Edetate* (above). The thiol groups of Dimercaprol compete with the physiologically essential —SH groups found in the tissues, and thus prevent combination of the toxic metals with these groups in the body. The combination of heavy metal and Dimercaprol is a stable compound which is rapidly excreted. The body is therefore rapidly freed of the toxic metals.

Dimercaprol is particularly useful in hemorrhagic encephalitis resulting from arsenotherapy, in arsenical or gold dermatitis, and possibly in postarsenical jaundice.

Dose—*Intramuscular,* **0.025** to **0.05 ml** (2.5 to 5 mg of dimercaprol) per **Kg**; *usual,* **0.03 ml** of a **10%** solution (3 mg of dimercaprol) per **Kg** of body weight,

6 times a day on the first 2 days, then 4 times a day on the third day, and 2 times a day for the next 10 days, if necessary.

Dosage Forms—Injection USP: 300 mg/3 ml.

Penicillamine USP

[D-(−)-3-Mercaptovaline; Cuprimine (MSD)]

$$CH_3-\underset{\underset{HS}{|}}{\overset{\overset{CH_3}{|}}{C}}-\underset{\underset{NH_2}{|}}{\overset{\overset{H}{|}}{C}}-COOH$$

Penicillamine contains 97.0–100.5% of $C_5H_{11}NO_2S$ (149.21), calculated on the dried basis.

Preparation—Penicillamine may be prepared by acid hydrolysis of penicillin. It is precipitated from the hydrolysis mixture as the mercuric salt which is then collected, suspended in water, and treated with hydrogen sulfide to liberate the free acid. Purification involves only recrystallization from water.

Description—A fine, white or practically white, crystalline powder, having a slight characteristic odor and a slightly bitter taste. It is relatively stable in both light and air. It melts at about 200° with decomposition.

Solubility—Freely soluble in water; slightly soluble in alcohol; insoluble in chloroform and ether.

Uses—Penicillamine is a chelating agent useful in the treatment of *Wilson's disease* (in which serum copper concentration is excessively high), and *lead, gold,* or *mercury poisoning*. It is especially useful in the long-term treatment of lead poisoning because of its oral efficacy, which the edetates lack.

The incidence of side effects is low; side effects most often appear shortly after therapy has begun. It may cause echymosis, dermatitis, eruptions of the mucous membranes, leukopenia, thrombocytopenia, agranulocytosis, fever, nephrosis, and lymphadenopathy.

Dose—1 to 5 Gm daily; *usual,* **250 mg** 4 times a day.

Dosage Forms—Capsules USP: 250 mg.

Other Antidotes to the Heavy Metals

N-Acetylpenicillamine [*N*-acetyl-3-mercaptovaline]— *Uses:* a chelating agent useful in the treatment of poisoning due to gold, lead, or mercury. Unlike penicillamine, it will not mobilize copper and hence is of no use in Wilson's disease. *Dose: orally,* 30 mg per kg of body weight per day, in 4 divided doses.

Antifungal Drugs

The fungi comprise five widely differing classes of primitive flora, including the bacteria; the variations in cell physiology and biochemistry are extreme among the fungi. Thus, the antifungal agents include a wide variety of chemical types of rather narrow antifungal spectrum. Broad spectrum antifungal agents in general are toxic and are irritants, as expected from their nonselectivity; however, many of these have a limited absorption through the epidermis and so may be employed in dermatologic preparations. Not all antifungal agents are fungicidal; certain of them may owe their efficacy to a keratolytic action.

In medical use the term fungus excludes the bacteria; the antibacterial agents have been treated earlier in this chapter.

Amphotericin B USP

[Fungizone (*Squibb*)]

Amphotericin B [$C_{46}H_{73}NO_{20}$ = 960.09] is a substance produced by the growth of *Streptomyces nodosus*. It has a potency of not less than 750 mcg of amphotericin B per mg, calculated on the anhydrous basis. Amphotericin B conforms to the regulations of the federal Food and Drug Administration concerning antibiotic drugs (see page 1206).

The structure is in the process of elucidation.[6] It is reported to be a polyene type of antibiotic containing mycosamine (3,6-dideoxy-3-amino-D-mannopyranose) as the nitrogen-contributing moiety.

Preparation—Amphotericin B is produced by the growth of selected strains of *Streptomyces nodosus* in an appropriate medium under controlled conditions of temperature, pH, and aeration. After extracting from the medium, the crude product is purified by treatment with various solvents at controlled acidity.

Description—Yellow to orange powder; odorless or practically so.

Solubility—Insoluble in water, anhydrous alcohol, ether, benzene, and toluene; soluble in dimethylformamide and dimethylsulfoxide; slightly soluble in methanol.

Uses—Amphotericin B has the widest spectrum of antifungal activity of any systemic antifungal drug. By the intravenous route is an extremely useful drug for the therapy of *systemic fungus diseases*, especially coccidiomycosis, cryptococcosis, systemic moniliasis, histoplasmosis, and North American blastomycosis. It is also used topically in the treatment of superficial monilial infections. It is incorporated with tetracyclines in products for oral administration, but expert medical opinion holds this combination to be unnecessary. It is not effective against viruses, protozoa, or bacteria. However, it is effective against some species of *leishmania*. Acquired resistance to the drug has not been observed. It is very poorly absorbed from the gastrointestinal tract. It is slowly excreted by the kidneys, and its duration of action may exceed 18 hours.

Amphotericin B may induce chills and fever, nausea and vomiting, diarrhea, abdominal "cramps," hemorrhagic gastroenteritis, headache, vertigo, pain in the vein injected, thrombophlebitis, anemia, purpura, cardiac arrest, ventricular fibrillation, skin rashes, renal damage, and other untoward effects. When given intrathecally it may cause grand mal convulsions, paralysis of the extremities, urinary retention, and other difficulties. Because of the potential seriousness of its toxic effects, the patient should always be hospitalized during a course of therapy.

Dose—*Intravenous,* **100** to **250 mcg** per **Kg** every 2 to 4 days to **1.5 mg** per **Kg** every other day; *usual,* by slow infusion of a 100 mcg-per-ml solution over a period of 6 hours; *initial,* **250 mcg** per **Kg** of body weight daily, then up to **1 mg** per **Kg** of body weight daily for 4 to 8 weeks. *Intrathecal,* **25 mcg,** increased to **500 mcg** every 2 to 4 days.

Dosage Forms—for Injection USP: 50 mg.

Anthralin—see page 773.

Candicidin NF

[Candeptin (*Schmid*)]

Candicidin is a substance produced by the growth of *Streptomyces griseus* Waksman and Henrici (Fam. Streptomycetaceae). Candicidin contains not less than 1000 mcg per mg. Candicidin conforms to the regulations of the federal Food and Drug Administration concerning certification of antibiotic drugs (see page 1206).

Candicidin is a polyene antibiotic reported to be a conjugated heptaene complex containing also residues of mycosamine and *p*-aminoacetophenone. It has been separated into three fractions designated A, B, and C. A is reported to be simply the sodium salt of B and both A and B are actively antifungal. Fraction C possesses little activity and is thought to be a degradation product. The antifungal activity of Candicidin is highly pH-dependent, maximal at 7.0 to 8.0.

Description—A yellow-green powder that has a fatty acid-type odor and a bitter taste. It is unstable in light in the UV range, unstable to moisture and sensitive to oxidation, and unstable to elevated temperatures. A 1% aqueous solution has a pH of 8 to 10.

Solubility—Insoluble in water, alcohol, chloroform, and acetone; soluble in a saturated solution of *n*-butanol in water, and in dimethyl sulfoxide.

Uses—Candicidin is an antibiotic with a rather broad spectrum of activity similar to that of amphotericin B. However, it is not active against filamentous fungi, including the ringworm varieties, and coccidioides. It is very active against *Monilia* (*Candida*) *albicans*, hence the origin of its name. The drug is used topically for the treatment of monilial infections of the skin and nails and in *monilial vaginitis*. Its status compared to amphotericin B and nystatin remains to be determined.

Candicidin is not absorbed from the gastrointestinal tract. Candicidin occasionally causes a mild irritation of the vulva. Irritation of the skin has not been reported. The drug may rarely cause an allergic reaction.

Dose—*Usual, vaginal,* **3 mg** inserted twice daily for 14 days.

Dosage Forms—Ointment NF: 0.06%; Suppositories NF: 3 mg.

Carbol-Fuchsin Solution NF

[Castellani's Paint; Pigmentum Magentae; Paint of Magenta; Paint of Fuchsine; Carfusin (*Rorer*)]

Basic Fuchsin	3 Gm
Phenol	45 Gm
Resorcinol	100 Gm
Acetone	50 ml
Alcohol	100 ml
Purified Water, a sufficient quantity,	
To make	1000 ml

Dissolve the basic fuchsin in a mixture of the acetone and alcohol, and add to this solution the phenol and resorcinol previously dissolved in 725 ml of purified water. Then add sufficient purified water to make the product measure 1000 ml. Mix thoroughly.

Description—A dark purple liquid which appears purplish red when spread in a thin film. Its specific gravity is between 0.990 and 1.050.

Uses—Carbol-Fuchsin Solution is an *antifungal* preparation, widely employed for topical application to superficial fungus infections of the skin. This preparation is of value in epidermophytosis interdigitalis pedum (*athlete's foot*) and is effective against *Tinea trichlophytina* (*ringworm*) and *Tinea imbricata* (*gogo* or *scaly ringworm* of the tropics). It should be used only in subacute or chronic dermatophytoses.

Dose—*Topically,* apply undiluted once or twice daily.

Benzoic Acid—see page 1316.

Butylparaben—see page 1176.

Chlorquinaldol—see page 1192.

Coal Tar—see page 774.

Creosote—see page 1192.

Cresol—see page 1176.

Diiodohydroxyquin—see page 1250.

Formaldehyde Solution—see page 1177.

Basic Fuchsin NF

[Basic Magenta]

Rosaniline Hydrochloride

Basic Fuchsin is a mixture of rosaniline and pararosaniline hydrochlorides.

Description—A dark green powder or greenish glistening crystalline fragments having a bronze-like luster, and not more than a faint odor.

Solubility—Soluble in water, alcohol, and amyl alcohol; insoluble in ether.

Uses—An ingredient in *Carbol-Fuchsin Solution* (see above).

Glycobiarsol—see page 1251.

Griseofulvin USP

[7 - Chloro - 2′,4,6 - trimethoxy - 6′β - methylspiro[benzofuran - 2(3*H*),1′- [2]-cyclohexene]-3,4′-dione; Fulvicin (*Schering*); Grifulvin (*McNeil*)]; Grisactin (*Ayerst*)

Griseofulvin [$C_{17}H_{17}ClO_6 = 352.77$] is a substance produced by the growth of *Penicillium griseofulvum* or by other means. It has a potency equivalent to not less than 900 mcg of $C_{17}H_{17}ClO_6$ per mg, calculated on the anhydrous basis. Griseofulvin conforms to the regulations of the federal Food and Drug Administration concerning antibiotic drugs (see page 1206).

Preparation—Griseofulvin is produced by the submerged process (page 1207) using selected strains of *Penicillium patulum*.

Description—White to creamy white, odorless powder, in which particles less than 4μ in diameter predominate.

Solubility—Soluble in acetone and chloroform; sparingly soluble in alcohol; very slightly soluble in water.

Uses—Griseofulvin is an effective agent in the treatment of superficial fungus infections. It is fungistatic and not fungicidal. Administered systemically, the drug is highly effective in the management of *tinea capitis, tinea corporis, tinea unguium* (onychomycosis) and the chronic form of *tinea pedis* caused by the dermatophytes, *Microsporon, Trichophyton,* and *Epidermophyton.* It also may be dramatically effective against *favus.* Infections caused by *T. rubrum* may respond, but relapses are frequent. Part of the reason for relapses is that some of the fungi, at least, grow in dead and dying squamous epithelial cells and their keratin residues. Since Griseofulvin does not kill but only arrests reproduction of the organism, it is necessary to continue medication long enough for the entire epidermis to be shed and replaced in order to remove reinfecting organisms. When there is hyperkeratosis, the time for desquamation may be long. Griseofulvin is probably deposited in the basal cells and is carried outwards into the epidermis as normal skin growth proceeds. This also makes for a long latency from the time medication is begun until evidence of improvement occurs. Although serious untoward reactions are infrequent, skin eruptions, leukopenia, allergic reaction, and headache are among the side effects reported. It is recommended that the drug be reserved for use in infections not amenable to conventional topical measures and for those in which the causative organism has been shown to be susceptible to its effect.

Griseofulvin may cause nausea and occasional vomiting; these may often be avoided by giving the drug with or shortly following a meal. Headache is also relatively frequent. Infrequently, lassitude and fatigue occur, and rarely there is mental confusion, motor incoordination and various manifestations of hypersensitivity (photosensitivity, serum sickness, or angioneurotic edema).

Dose—**500 mg** to **1 Gm** daily; *usual,* **250 mg**, 2 times a day.

Other Dose Information—The dose for children is 5 mg per pound of body weight administered as a single dose or in divided doses. For tinea capitis, 4 to 8 weeks may be required or a single dose of 3 to 4 Gm may be given; for tinea pedis, 4 weeks to several months are required; for tinea unguium, 4 months to a year are needed. Griseofulvin is also marketed in an ultrafine form, which is better absorbed and gives rise to considerably higher blood levels than the standard form. Consequently, the dose is reduced to about 50% of the standard form.

Dosage Forms—Capsules USP: 125 and 250 mg; Tablets USP: 125, 250, and 500 mg.

Veterinary Use—Before starting therapy, responsible organism should be identified by suitable culture techniques. The drug is useful in the treatment of superficial fungus infections caused by *Trichophyton mentagrophytes, rubrum, interdigitale, schoenleini, sulphureum* and *verrucosum,* and *Microsporum audouini, canis,* and *gypseum,* but is inactive against bacteria, *monilia, actinomycetes, neocardia, blastomycetes, coccidioides, histoplasma, cryptococcus,* and *aspergillus.*

Veterinary Dose—*Dogs* and *Cats,* oral, daily, in single or divided doses, up to 6 pounds of body weight, **125 mg**; 6 to 18 pounds, **250 mg**; 18 to 36 pounds, **500 mg**; 36 to 48 pounds, **750 mg**; 48 to 75 pounds, **1 Gm**. Involvement of skin and hair requires daily therapy for 3 to 4 weeks; onychomycotic lesions may require 3 to 4 months of continuous therapy.

Hexetidine—see page 1193.

Hydroxystilbamidine Isethionate USP

[2 - Hydroxy - 4,4 - stilbenedicarboxamidine Isethionate (1:2); 2 - Hydroxy-ethanesulfonic Acid 2-Hydroxy-4,4′-stilbenedicarboxamidine Compound (2:1), (*Merrell*)]

Hydroxystilbamidine Isethionate contains 95.0–105.0% of $C_{16}H_{16}N_4O \cdot 2C_2H_6O_4S$ (532.60), calculated on the dried basis.

Preparation—Dry hydrogen chloride is passed into a solution of 2-hydroxy-4,4′-vinylenedibenzonitrile and absolute ethanol in anhydrous ether whereby the nitrile groups are converted into iminoether hydrochlorides; ie, $-CN \rightarrow -C(OC_2H_5):NH \cdot HCl$. Treatment with excess alcoholic ammonia removes the HCl and effects ammonolysis at the ethoxy linkage, thus yielding the diamidine. This is then reacted in alcoholic solution with a double equimolar portion of isethionic acid to form the readily crystallizable diisethionate.

Description—It occurs as a fine, yellow, crystalline powder. It is odorless. It is stable in air but decomposes upon exposure to light. Its 1 in 100 solution has a pH between 3.3 and 5.3. It melts at about 280°.

Solubility—Soluble in water; slightly soluble in alcohol; and insoluble in ether.

Uses—Hydroxystilbamidine Isethionate vies with *Amphotericin B* (page 1256) the best available drug for the treatment of North American *blastomycosis.* It can eradicate severe pulmonary and systemic forms of the disease. Prior to the diamidines this disease was incurable. Today, treatment usually begins with amphotericin B because of lesser toxicity. It is effective against actinomycosis. It is of no use in histoplasmosis or Torula infections. It may be used in the treatment of *leishmaniasis* when antimonials cannot be used. It causes relief from pain in *multiple myeloma,* but it does not appear to affect the cause of the disease.

Upon injection, hydroxystilbamidine causes hypotension, tachycardia, dyspnea, flushing, sialorrhea, sweating, formication, vertigo, headache, nausea and vomiting, syncope, facial and palpebral edema, urinary and fecal incontinence may occur. These effects may be minimized by slow intravenous infusion. It is rarely given intramuscularly.

Dose—*Intravenous infusion,* **150** to **225 mg** daily to every other day to a total of **6 to 7 Gm**; *usual,* **225 mg** once a day.

Dosage Forms—Sterile USP: 225 mg.

Ichthammol—see page 774.

Iodine—see page 1180.

Iodochlorhydroxyquin—see page 1252.

Mercuric Oxide, Yellow—see page 1182.

Mercury, Ammoniated—see page 1182.

Methylrosaniline Chloride—see page 1178.

Nifuroxime NF

[(Z)-5-Nitro-2-furaldehyde Oxime; Microfur (*Eaton*)]

Nifuroxime, dried at 55° for 2 hours, contains 97.0–103.0% of $C_5H_4N_2O_4$ (156.10).

Caution: Do not use if darker than a medium tan.

Note: Nifuroxime will discolor upon contact with alkaline material and upon exposure to direct sunlight. Do not permit contact with metals other than stainless steel or aluminum.

Preparation—Nifuroxime is a typical aldehyde condensation product of 5-nitrofuraldehyde (I) and hydroxylamine (II). It is prepared in crude form by heating a mixture of the "diacetate" of (I) [see the discussion under Nitrofurantoin, page 1242] and the acid sulfate of (II) to 100°C. Conversion to the official *trans*(*anti*)-form is effected by dissolving in hot isopropyl alcohol containing hydrogen chloride.

Description—It occurs as a white to pale yellow crystalline powder when fresh. Upon standing it may become tan in color. It should not be used if darker than a medium tan.

Solubility—1 Gm is soluble in about 1 liter of water and about 25 ml of alcohol; very soluble in dimethylformamide.

Uses—Nifuroxime is a mild antifungal agent principally effective against infections caused by *Monilia* (Candida) *albicans*. At the present its use is restricted to the treatment of vaginal infections, for which it is combined with *Furazolidone* (page 1178).

Dose—See *Furazolidone and Nifuroxime Suppositories*, (page 1178) and the *Powder* (page 1178).

Nystatin USP

[Mycostatin (*Squibb*)]

Nystatin [$C_{46}H_{77}NO_{19}$ = 948.12] is a substance produced by the growth of *Streptomyces noursei* Brown, *et al.* (Fam. *Streptomycetaceæ*). It contains not less than 2000 Units of nystatin activity per mg. It conforms to the regulations of the Federal Food and Drug Administration concerning antibiotic drugs (see page 1206).

The structure of Nystatin has not been completely elucidated. Like erythromycin, it is known to be a macrocyclic lactone and may be included among the polyene antibiotics. It is also known to contain a mycosamine (a 3-amino-3,6-dideoxy-D-mannopyranose) moiety, an epoxy group, and an all-*trans* tetraene system.

Description—Yellow to light tan powder, having an odor suggestive of cereals. It is hygroscopic, and is affected by long exposure to light, heat, and air. The specific rotation is between 0° and +25°. The pH is between 6.5 and 8.0.

Solubility—Very slightly soluble in water; slightly to sparingly soluble in alcohol, methanol, *n*-propyl alcohol, and *n*-butyl alcohol; insoluble in chloroform, ether, and benzene.

Uses—Nystatin is active in vitro against a number of yeasts and molds, but its clinical usefulness thus far has been determined only in the treatment of *moniliasis*. Its local efficacy against monilial infections of the skin and mucous membranes have been firmly established, but it is not effective by the oral route against systemic monilial infections. The antibiotic is poorly absorbed from the gastrointestinal tract; consequently the residue in the feces suppresses intestinal moniliasis and may prevent the emergence of moniliasis superinfections resulting from oral therapy with broad spectrum antibiotics, although such superinfections are so infrequent that the routine "prophylactic" use of nystatin is not worthwhile. The Food and Drug Administration has declared combinations of Nystatin with other antibiotics to be ineffective. It does *not* prevent diarrhea from oral broad-spectrum antibiotics. Nystatin has been employed with variable success in the treatment of oral "thrush" (moniliasis).

Nystatin is relatively nontoxic, but nausea, vomiting, and diarrhea may occur with oral therapy.

Dose—*Oral*, 1,500,000 to 6,000,000 Units daily; *usual, oral*, as aqueous suspension or tablets, 500,000 Units 3 times a day; *usual, intravaginal*, as tablets, 100,000 Units 2 times a day; *topically*, as ointment or suspension, 2 to 4 times a day as required.

Dosage Forms—Ointment USP; for Oral Suspension USP: 2,400,000 Units/24 ml; Tablets USP: 500,000 Units (for oral administration), 100,000 Units (for intravaginal administration).

Parachlorophenol—see page 1185.

Penicillin—see page 1223.

Phenol—see page 1370.

Potassium Iodide—see page 872.

Potassium Permanganate—see page 1186.

Potassium Sorbate—see page 1317.

Resorcinol—see page 1187.

Resorcinol Monoacetate—see page 1188.

Salicylic Acid—see page 781.

Salicylanilide NF

[*N*-Salicylaniline; Salinidol (*Doak*)]

Salicylanilide, dried at 80° for 2 hours, contains 99.0–100.5% of $C_{13}H_{11}NO_2$ (213.24).

Preparation—Salicylanilide is readily prepared by heating an ester of salicylic acid, eg, methyl salicylate, with aniline.

Description—Odorless, white or slightly pink crystals which are stable in air. Melting range 136° to 138°.

Solubility—Freely soluble in alcohol, ether, chloroform, and benzene; slightly soluble in water.

Uses—Salicylanilide is an externally applied *antifungal* agent eight times as effective as undecylenic acid in the treatment of *tinea capitis* caused by *M. audouini*. It is not fungicidal but only fungistatic, and other local hygiene must be attended.

Dose—*Topically*, as a **3** to **5**% ointment applied to the scalp as required.

Selenium Sulfide—see page 1188.

Sodium Benzoate—see page 1189.

Sodium Hypochlorite Solution—see page 1189.

Sodium Hypochlorite Solution, Diluted—see page 1189.

Sodium Propionate NF

[Mycoban]

Sodium Propionate ($CH_3CH_2COONa . xH_2O$), dried at 105° for 2 hours, contains 99.0–100.5% of $C_3H_5NaO_2$ (96.06).

Preparation—This salt is prepared by neutralizing propionic acid with sodium carbonate or hydroxide and evaporating to crystallization or to dryness.

Description—Colorless, deliquescent (in moist air), transparent crystals or a granular, crystalline powder. It is odorless, or has a faint acetic-butyric odor.

Solubility—1 Gm dissolves in 1 ml of water or 24 ml of alcohol, or 0.65 ml of water at 100°.

Uses—Propionic acid and its soluble salts are fungistatic and bacteriostatic against a number of Gram-positive cocci. Clinically Sodium Propionate is used in the treatment of *otomycosis*. It is also used in the treatment of *epidermophytosis*, but it is not as effective as undecylenic acid, the zinc salt of which is often compounded with sodium propionate in antimycotic preparations. It is only fungistatic and not fungicidal, so that other hygiene must be emphasized. Sodium Propionate is often compounded with antibiotics or antiseptics. The propionates of calcium and sodium are marketed for use in preventing the molding of bread.

Dose—*Topically*, in dosage forms containing **5** to **10**% of Sodium Propionate.

Other Dose Information—Apply ointment or solution 3 to 4 times a day. Some topical solutions are marketed in strengths of 0.5 to 1%. To the ear apply 3 to 5 drops of a 0.5% solution 3 to 4 times a day.

Veterinary Uses—Sodium Propionate is effective in the early treatment of *ketosis* of cattle or as follow-up treatment after dextrose therapy of this disease.

Veterinary Dose—*Cattle*, **100** to **350 Gm.**

Sodium Thiosulfate USP

["Sodium Hyposulfite"; Antichlor; "Hypo"]

Sodium Thiosulfate [$Na_2S_2O_3.5H_2O = 248.18$] contains 99.0–100.5% of $Na_2S_2O_3$ (158.11), calculated on the anhydrous basis.

Preparation—The salt is readily prepared by dissolving sulfur in sodium sulfite solution and then crystallizing.

It is also prepared from the waste liquors obtained in the production of sodium sulfide, the liquors containing sodium carbonate and small amounts of sodium sulfite and sodium sulfate in addition to the sulfide. The concentration of the liquor is adjusted so that it will contain about 8% of Na_2S and 6% of Na_2CO_3 and then sulfur burner gas, containing about 7% of SO_2, is passed through the solution. Sodium Thiosulfate is produced according to the equation:

$$2Na_2S + Na_2CO_3 + 4SO_2 \rightarrow 3Na_2S_2O_3 + CO_2$$

The liquid is allowed to cool and the crystals of thiosulfate are removed by centrifuging.

Description—Large colorless crystals, or a coarse, crystalline powder. It is deliquescent in moist air, and efflorescent in dry air at a temperature above 33°. When rapidly heated it melts at about 48° and decomposes when heated much above 100°. It is decomposed by diluted acids, liberating sulfur dioxide with precipitation of sulfur. It slowly decomposes in aqueous solution, more rapidly when the solutions are heated. The aqueous solution is neutral or faintly alkaline to litmus and is a good solvent for the halogen salts of silver.

Solubility—1 Gm dissolves in 0.5 ml of water; insoluble in alcohol.

Incompatibilities—Sodium Thiosulfate *solutions* slowly deposit sulfur on standing. *Acids* decompose them with similar precipitation. In acid solutions, sodium thiosulfate has reducing powers, and is therefore incompatible with *oxidizing agents*. *Lead, silver*, and *mercurous salts* precipitate as thiosulfates. *Silver halides* are made soluble by sodium thiosulfate. *Bismuth subnitrate* is partially converted to metallic bismuth. *Ferric chloride* gives a transient violet color. Dry trituration with *oxidizing agents* such as potassium chlorate, potassium permanganate, or a nitrate may cause an explosion.

Uses—Sodium Thiosulfate is an *antifungal* agent for topical treatment of *Tinea versicolor, Tinea cruris*, and possibly most other dermatophytes. The action is probably attributable to the slow release of colloidal sulfur; some authorities recommend the prior application of vinegar or dilute acetic acid to promote the decomposition to yield sulfur.

Sodium Thiosulfate has an important use as an antidote in the treatment of cyanide poisoning, being used in conjunction with nitrites (see *Sodium Nitrite*, page 846). The eventual compound formed is thiocyanate. Sodium Thiosulfate is also an effective *antidote for iodine* preparations.

Its principal uses are in the arts and as an *antichlor* in paper manufacture. In photography, under the abbreviated name of "hypo," it is invaluable as a solvent for the unaltered silver chloride or bromide in the film after development.

Dose—*Intravenous*, **500 mg** to **2 Gm**; *usual*, **1 Gm** in a **5** to **10**% solution.

Other Dose Information—Topically, as a 25 to 50% solution applied to the affected area several times a day. The solution spreads better if the area has been previously wetted. Prior wetting with vinegar improves the local antifungal action.

Dosage Forms—Injection USP: 10 ml.

Veterinary Uses—Sodium Thiosulfate is used as a remedy for gastric and intestinal *flatulence* in horses and cattle and in the treatment of *arsenic, mercury, cyanide, and iodine poisoning* cases.

Veterinary Dose—*Horses* and *Cattle*, **15** to **16 Gm**; *Dogs*, **200 mg** to **1 Gm.**

Sorbic Acid—see page 1318.

Sulfur, Sublimed—see page 1272.

Thymol—see page 1190.

Tolnaftate USP

[*O*-2-Naphthyl-*N,m*-dimethylthiocarbanilate; Tinactin (*Schering*)]

Tolnaftate contains 98.0–102.0% of $C_{19}H_{17}NOS$ (307.42), calculated on the dried basis.

Preparation—*N* - Methyl - *m* - tolylamine is condensed with 2-naphthyl chlorothionoformate by refluxing an acetone solution of the reactants in the presence of sodium bicarbonate or another suitable dehydrochlorinating agent. Crude Tolnaftate precipitates on pouring the reaction mixture into water and is purified by recrystallization from ethanol. The starting formate ester is readily prepared by condensing 2-naphthol with thiophosgene. French Pat. 1,337,797.

Description—A white to creamy white, odorless, fine powder. It melts between 110° and 113°.

Solubility—1 Gm dissolves in 7 ml of acetone; freely soluble in chloroform; sparingly soluble in ether; slightly soluble in alcohol and methanol; practically insoluble in water.

Uses—Tolnaftate is useful for the treatment of superficial *mycoses of the skin* (*tinea pedis, tinea cruris, tinea corporus, tinea manuum*) caused by *Epidermophyton floccosum, Malassezia furfur,* and several species of *Microsporon* and *Trichophyton*. It is not effective alone against infections of the hair or nails. When *T. rubrum* is the infecting agent, relapses are common. Tolnaftate is administered only topically and may be unable to reach infections in hyperkeratotic lesions or in the normally thick horny layers of the palms or soles, so that a keratolytic should be employed concurrently or systemic treatment with Griseofulvin should be employed. No adverse effects caused by Tolnaftate have been reported; but sensitization to other ingredients of the commercial product has been observed.

Dose—*Topically* as a 1% cream, powder, or solution. *Other Dose Information*—To be applied to the affected area 2 times a day. Treatment usually lasts from 3 to 6 weeks.

Dosage Forms—Cream USP: 1%; Powder: 1%; Solution USP: 1%.

Triacetin NF

[Glyceryl Triacetate;   Enzactin (*Ayerst*);   Fungacetin (*Harvey*)]

$$CH_2—OCOCH_3$$
$$CH—OCOCH_3$$
$$CH_2—OCOCH_3$$

Triacetin contains 97.0–100.5% of $C_9H_{14}O_6$ (218.21), calculated on the dried basis.

Preparation—Triacetin is prepared by direct esterification of glycerin with acetic anhydride.

Description—It occurs as a colorless liquid which melts at −78° and boils between 258° and 260°.

Solubility—Soluble in 14 parts water; soluble in alcohol, benzene, chloroform, and ether.

Uses—Triacetin is an antifungal drug marketed for use in the treatment of superficial fungous infections of the skin, especially for Trichophyta, Epidermophyta, and Microspora. The hydrolysis of the ester by mycoenzymes releases acetic acid, and any antimycotic action is attributable to the drop in pH. It is fungistatic only and does not obviate other hygiene. Although triacetin is mildly effective *in vitro*, medical authorities are dubious of its clinical efficacy. It is thus strange that this drug has been promoted to official status.

Triacetin is odorless, stainless, and nonallergenic

Dose—*Topically*, to affected area twice daily as a **15%** aerosol, a **25%** cream, or a **33%** powder.

Dosage Forms—Aerosol NF: 150 mg/Gm in 85-Gm containers;   Cream NF: 25%;   Powder NF: 33.3%.

Undecylenic Acid NF

[10-Undecenoic Acid;   Undecenoic Acid;   Desenex Solution (*WTS*)]

$$CH_2=CH(CH_2)_8COOH$$

Undecylenic Acid contains 95.0–100.5% of $C_{11}H_{20}O_2$ (184.28).

Preparation—Undecylenic acid is best prepared by the destructive distillation of castor oil under reduced pressure. The glyceride of ricinoleic acid, the chief constituent of castor oil, is cleaved and rearranged by pyrolysis into undecylenic acid and *n*-heptaldehyde:

$$CH_3(CH_2)_5CH{\mid}CH_2CH=CH(CH_2)_7COOH$$
$$OH{\mid}$$

Ricinoleic Acid (as Glyceride)

$$\downarrow \Delta$$

$$CH_3(CH_2)_5CHO + CH_2=CH(CH_2)_8COOH$$

Description—A yellow liquid with a characteristic odor. Specific gravity 0.910 to 0.913. Congealing range not below 21°. Refractive index 1.4475 to 1.4485.

Solubility—Practically insoluble in water; miscible with alcohol, chloroform, ether, benzene, and with fixed and volatile oils.

Uses—Undecylenic Acid is an antifungal agent which is employed in the treatment of *dermatophytosis*, and *tinea capitis*. Since it is only fungistatic and not fungicidal, attention must be given to other hygiene, especially if the lesions are raw. Astringents assist in reducing the rawness and irritation; thus zinc, in the form of *Zinc Undecylenate* (below) is often incorporated into powders, ointments, or aerosols of Undecylenic Acid. *Compound Undecylenic Acid Ointment* (below) contains the zinc salt. Responses of athlete's foot to the drug are sometimes dramatic, but other times the infection persists despite treatment. The efficacy in the treatment of tinea capitis is generally poor, although sometimes the condition seems to respond readily.

Undecylenic Acid has a rank, rancid odor. It rarely causes irritation or sensitization.

Dose—*Topically* as a **1 to 10%** ointment as required.

Compound Undecylenic Acid Ointment NF contains 18.0–22.0% of $C_{22}H_{38}O_4Zn$ (zinc undecylenate) and 4.5–5.5% of $C_{11}H_{20}O_2$ (free undecylenic acid). *Preparation:* Melt polyethylene glycol ointment (750 Gm) on a water bath at a temperature of about 65° and add undecylenic acid (50 Gm) and zinc undecylenate (200 Gm). Remove from the water bath and stir until congealed and all ingredients are well mixed. *Note*—In order to provide a product of suitable consistency under various climatic conditions, proportions of polyethylene glycol constituents of polyethylene glycol ointment may be altered, or another suitable ointment base may be used. However, the proportion of active ingredients must not be varied.

Zinc Undecylenate NF

[Zinc 10-Undecenoate;   Zinc Undecenoate]

$$[CH_2=CH(CH_2)_8COO—]_2Zn$$

Zinc Undecylenate contains 98.0–102.0% of $C_{22}H_{38}O_4Zn$ (431.92), calculated on the dried basis.

Description—A fine, white powder.

Solubility—Practically insoluble in water and alcohol.

Uses—see *Undecylenic Acid* and *Compound Undecylenic Acid Ointment* (above).

Dose—*Topically* as a 20% ointment as required.

Other Antifungal Drugs

Acrisorcin [Akrinol (*Schering*)] is 9-aminoacridine 4-hexylresorcinol compound [$C_{25}H_{28}N_2O_2 = 388.49$]. *Preparation:* 9-Aminoacridine is combined directly with an equimolar quantity of 4-hexylresorcinol in a suitable solvent medium such as acetone. *Description and Solubility:* A pale-yellow powder that is odorless; it is moderately sensitive to light and sensitive to heat; it melts between 185° and 190°. Soluble in acetone, pyridine, and alcohol; sparingly soluble in hot water; insoluble in chloroform. *Uses:* Acrisorcin is employed in the treatment of *tinea* (pityriasis) *versicolor*, a fungal infection caused by *Malassezia furfur*. It is fungicidal, but permanent cures are not always effected. It occasionally may cause burning sensations, hives, erythematous vesicles, and blisters. Exposure to ultraviolet light may promote itching. *Dose: Topical*, as a 0.2% cream applied to the affected area 2 times a day following a vigorous wash of the infected skin. Treatment should be continued for at least 6 weeks.

Benzoic and Salicylic Acid Ointment USP XVI [Whitfield's Ointment]—An ointment consisting of benzoic acid (60 Gm), salicylic acid (30 Gm), and polyethylene glycol ointment (qs) to make 1000 Gm. *Uses:* It was formerly very widely employed as a keratolytic and fungistatic agent and is still frequently prescribed today, despite the advent of undecylenic acid. It is used in the treatment of epidermophytosis and ringworm of the scalp. Salicylic acid is the principal active ingredient (see *Salicylic Acid*, page 781). In veterinary use it is employed for the treatment of ringworm.

Calcium Undecylenate [Ingredient of Caldecort (*Strasenburgh*); Caldesene (*WTS*)] is $Ca(C_{11}H_{19}O_2)_2$.

Uses: An antifungal agent with actions resembling *Zinc Undecylenate* (page 1261). The undecylenate moiety has antifungal and weak antibacterial activity, and the calcium moiety has mild astringent activity. The drug is not promoted for use in the treatment of athlete's foot but rather for prophylaxis and treatment of diaper rash, intertrigo, prickly heat, and dyshidrosis and for its soothing action to relieve itching or burning skin sensations in minor cutaneous irritations. It is also combined with neomycin and hydrocortisone acetate for the purpose of suppressing fungal infections that complicate other dermatologic conditions. The principal side effect is a transient mild stinging at the site of application when the site is excoriated. *Dose: Topical*, as a 15% ointment or powder.

Chlordantoin (Sporostacin (*Ortho*)] is 5-(1-ethylpentyl)-3-(trichloromethylthio)hydantoin ($C_{11}H_{17}Cl_3N_2O_2S$). *Uses:* A fungicide, the use of which is limited to the topical treatment of monilial infections (moniliasis; candidiasis) of the vagina, skin, nails, or buccal mucosa. It may occasionally cause sensitization. *Dose: Topical*, to be applied to the affected area 3 times a day, except 2 times a day for 14 days when the cream is employed in vulvovaginal moniliasis.

Diamthazole Dihydrochloride [6-[2-(Diethylamino)-ethoxy]-2-(dimethylamino)benzothiazole dihydrochloride; Asterol (*Roche*)] [($C_{15}H_{23}N_3OS.2HCl$]—Crystals, freely soluble in water, alcohol, and methyl alcohol. A 5% aqueous solution has a pH of about 2. *Uses:* An antifungal agent possessing negligible activity against bacteria and the common nonpathogenic molds. It is not readily absorbed through the skin, although enough may be absorbed in infants to cause convulsions. For the local treatment of mycotic infections caused by *Trichophyton*, *Microsporon*, and *Monilia*. *Dose: topically*, twice daily in a 5% concentration.

Antiviral Agents

Despite intensive efforts to discover drugs that may be of value in the systemic treatment of virus infections, such infections have been singularly resistant to chemotherapy, except for those caused by certain of the large "viruses," which yield to a number of antibiotics and sulfonamides. The intracellular and intimate relation to nuclear metabolism of virus reproduction makes it difficult to destroy a virus without irreparable damage also to the host cell. Nevertheless, research on virustatic and virucidal drugs continues. The discovery that idoxuridine could suppress certain virus infections in experimental animals and the prophylactic effect of amantadine against certain viruses have engendered new hope that wide-spectrum systemic antiviral agents are on the way. However, as an antiviral agent, idoxuridine is thus far limited in man to the *topical* treatment of herpes simplex keratitis, an infection caused by a *large* virus. There is also a continuing strong interest in interferon. An interferon is a proteinaceous substance, produced in response to exposure to active or inactivated viruses, or even certain bacteria, which enables cells to become refractory to infection by other viruses which are not necessarily serologically related. Unfortunately, clinical successes with interferons have been confounded by their antigenicity. Consequently, there is great interest in substances, such as statolon, which can stimulate the *in vivo* production of interferons.

Many antiseptics and astringents are virucidal and may be used for purposes of disinfection of virus-contaminated objects or substances. Also, β-propiolactone and certain other substances are specifically employed to destroy the virus of serum hepatitis that may contaminate human blood products.

Amantadine Hydrochloride NF

[1-Adamantanamine Hydrochloride; Symmetrel (*Du Pont*)]

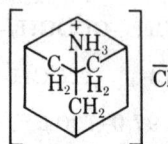

Amantadine Hydrochloride contains 98.5–101.5% of $C_{10}H_{17}N.HCl$ (187.71).

Preparation—Adamantane is brominated to the 1-bromo compound which is then reacted with acetonitrile in the presence of sulfuric acid to produce N-(1-adamantanyl)acetamide. Alkaline hydrolysis liberates amantadine (base) which is then reacted with hydrogen chloride in a suitable solvent to yield the official salt.

Description—A white or nearly white, odorless, crystalline powder. It has a bitter taste. It is stable in light, heat, and air. It does not melt up to 300°, but sublimes slowly.

Solubility—Freely soluble in water; soluble in alcohol and chloroform.

Uses—Amantadine prevents the entry of certain viruses into the cell. Once the virus has gained entry into the cell, the drug does not prevent viral replication and interference with cell function. Indeed, there is evidence that Amantadine actually facilitates viral replication. It is thus evident that the drug can only be of value when given prior to exposure to a virus. Although in tissue cultures Amantadine is effective against several types of virus, clinically the drug appears to be useful only as a *prophylactic against A_2 influenza virus (Asian flu)*. It protects approximately 50% of users. Failure, in part, is due to resistant strains. In some recipients infection is not prevented but symptoms are less severe. It is not effective against the B_2 virus, but, fortunately, B_2 is an infrequent cause of influenza. Since Amantadine is inferior to influenza vaccine as a prophylactic and is ineffective if taken after exposure to the virus, the use of the drug is limited mostly to persons who refuse vaccination or to situations in which the supply of vaccine is limited or there is too little time to complete a course of vaccination.

An experimental trial of Amantadine Hydrochloride in the treatment of patients with Parkinson's disease resulted in subjective or objective improvement of akinesia, rigidity, and tremor in two-thirds of a study group of 163 patients.

Amantadine may cause hyperexcitability, tremors, ataxia, slurring of speech, insomnia, lethargy, psychic depression, and vertigo. Less frequently, it may induce nausea and vomiting. There are indications that the drug may increase the incidence of measles. The drug is contraindicated in epileptics. Medicated persons should avoid driving or other tasks in which safety depends upon alertness.

Dose—*Usual*, **200 mg** per day, given as a single dose or in two divided doses.

Other Dose Information—For children 9 to 12 years of age, 100 mg twice a day; for children 1 to 9 years of age, 4 to 9 mg per Kg of body weight. The average duration of medication is 2 weeks, although it has been used for as long as 3 months.

Dosage Forms—Capsules NF: 100 mg; Syrup NF: 50 mg/5 ml.

Idoxuridine USP

[2'-Deoxy-5-iodouridine; IDU; Dendrid (*Alcon*) Herplex (*Allergan*); Stoxil (*SK&F*)]

Idoxuridine contains 98.0–101.0% of $C_9H_{11}IN_2O_5$ (354.10), calculated on the dried basis.

Preparation—Idoxuridine may be prepared by refluxing a solution of deoxuridine in aqueous mineral acid in the presence of iodine. Brit. Pat. 1,024,156. For the preparation of deoxuridine, see Ref. 7.

Description—White, practically odorless, crystalline powder. It turns black between 168° and 171°. A 0.1% aqueous solution has a pH of about 6. A 0.1% solution in distilled water and preserved with 1:50,000 thimerosal is stable at room temperature for over a year.

Solubility—Soluble in 0.2N NaOH; slightly soluble in water, 0.2N HCl, acetone, methanol, ethanol, dioxane, and ethyl acetate; practically insoluble in ether and chloroform.

Uses—Idoxuridine is an antimetabolite of thymidine. It may also be incorporated into desoxyribonucleic acid in lieu of thymidine, thus interfering with normal nuclear metabolism. It was first studied as an *antineoplastic* drug, and it may yet have usefulness as such. However, its *antiviral* activity has received the greater clinical scrutiny. At present its use is limited to the topical therapy of *herpes simplex keratitis;* the dendritic type responds readily, but the stromal type does not respond unless adrenal steroids are given concurrently. However, studies in both animals and man suggest that the drug may ultimately prove to be of value in the treatment of infections caused by both large and small viruses. Anterior uveitis and adenovirus conjunctivitis have been reported to respond to the drug.

Local treatment to the eye may occasionally cause reversible epithelial edema, inflammation, stinging, itching, or photophobia. It may interfere with the healing of deep lesions of the cornea. When applied to the cornea, Idoxuridine does not produce systemic toxicity. When given systemically, Idoxuridine may cause depression of bone marrow and alopecia.

The ointment does not require as frequent administration as the solution and hence is especially advantageous for use at night.

Dose—*Topically*, as a **0.5%** ointment 4 to 6 times a day, or **0.1 ml** of a **0.1%** solution every 1 to 2 hours, to the conjunctiva.

Other Dose Information—The above schedule is continued until the lesions no longer stain with fluorescein; thereafter, the intervals between applications may be doubled. The solution may be applied at 4-hour intervals if at each application 1 drop is instilled every minute for 5 minutes.

Dosage Forms—Ophthalmic Ointment USP: 0.5%; Ophthalmic Solution USP: 0.1%.

Other Antiviral Agents

Methisazone [Marboran (*Burroughs-Wellcome*)] is 1-methylindole-2,3-dione 3-thiosemicarbazone ($C_{10}H_{10}N_4OS$). *Description:* Crystals that melt at 245°. *Uses:* An antiviral drug shown to have protective value against smallpox and alastrim and may be of some benefit in eczema vaccinatum and vaccinia gangrenosa, especially in combination with gamma globulin. It appears to interfere with the synthesis of a protein required for assembly and morphogenesis of the virus. It does not affect replication of viral DNA or affect in RNA. The drug may cause nausea and vomiting and occasional reversible amnesia. *Dose:* 1.5 to 3.0 mg daily; as a prophylactic against smallpox, it must be given before the 8th or 9th day of the 12-day incubation period.

Cytarabine Hydrochloride [Cytosine Arabinoside Hydrochloride; 1-β-D-Arabinofuranosylcytosine Hydrochloride ($C_9H_{13}N_3O_5 \cdot HCl$); Cytosar (*Upjohn*)]. *Uses:* Cytarabine blocks the conversion of cytosine riboside to cytosine desoxyriboside and thereby impairs synthesis of DNA, by virtue of which action it has been used experimentally as an antiviral drug. In clinical trials it has been of benefit in the treatment of dendritic keratitis (caused by *Herpes simplex*), appearing to be effective even when idoxuridine is ineffective. Cytarabine has been found useful also in producing remissions in acute and chronic leukemia.

References

1. Johnson, Anker, and Meleney, *Science*, **102**, 376 (1945).
2. Porath, *Acta Chem. Scand.*, **6**, 1237 (1952).
3. Freaney and Allen, US Pat. 2,828,246.
4. Shaffner, M., 149th Am. Chem. Soc. Mtg., Detroit, Apr. 4–9, 1965, Abstr. of Papers, p. 9C.
5. Weiss, *et al*, *Antibiot. Chemotherapy*, **7**, 374 (1957).
6. *J. Am. Chem. Soc.*, **88**, 4228 (1966).
7. *J. Chem. Soc.*, **1958**, 3035.

68 | Parasiticides

Anthelmintics—pediculicides and scabicides

This chapter was prepared by

Ewart A. Swinyard, PhD, *Professor of Pharmacology, College of Pharmacy and College of Medicine, University of Utah, Salt Lake City, Utah 84112, and*
Stewart C. Harvey, PhD, *Associate Professor of Pharmacology, College of Medicine, University of Utah, Salt Lake City, Utah 84112*

The subject of parasiticides is an important part of pharmacology. In its broadest aspects, it includes the problem of eradication of all organisms which live within or upon man. However, discussion in this chapter will be limited to the anthelmintics and to those agents which are applied directly to the skin of the human host in the treatment of pediculosis and scabies.

Anthelmintics

The term anthelmintic frequently is restricted to drugs acting locally to expel parasites from the gastrointestinal tract. However, there are several types of worms which penetrate other tissues; drugs which act on these parasitic infestations are also known as anthelmintics. Furthermore, drugs that kill worms are commonly referred to as vermicides; those that affect the worm in such a manner that peristaltic activity or catharsis expels it from the intestinal tract are referred to as vermifuges. This arbitrary division serves no useful purpose since many anthelmintics manifest both actions, according to the dose employed. Therefore, the anthelmintics are more properly defined as drugs used to combat any type of helminthiasis.

The worm parasites of man belong to two phyla: *Nemathelminthes* (roundworms) and *Platyhelminthes* (flatworms). The roundworms include the hookworm, roundworm, whipworm, pinworm, *Strongyloides stercoralis*, *Trichinella spiralis*, and *Wuchereria bancrofti*. There are two common varieties of hookworm, *Necator americanus*, the American variety, and *Ancylostoma duodenale*, the European variety. They are cylindrical worms, 1 to 2 cm long, with two pairs of hooks near the mouth. They attach themselves to the mucosa of the duodenum and derive their nourishment by sucking blood from the surrounding blood vessels. The common roundworm, *Ascaris lumbricoides*, is the most prevalent of human helminths. They are 5 to 15 inches long, $\frac{1}{8}$ to $\frac{1}{4}$ inch in diameter, grayish to reddish in color, and inhabit the upper part of the small intestine; therefore, they are occasionally vomited up. The whipworm, *Trichuris trichiura*, is about 2 inches long and resembles a whip; it inhabits the cecum principally, but is also found in the lower part of the ileum and the appendix. The pinworm or threadworm, *Enterobius vermicularis*, is $\frac{1}{16}$ to $\frac{1}{2}$ inch long and inhabits the small intestine, cecum, and colon. *Strongyloides stercoralis* are only about $\frac{1}{12}$ inch long. They inhabit the duodenum chiefly, but may be found in the stomach, biliary passages, pancreatic ducts, and various parts of the intestinal tract. Infestation with *Trichinella spiralis* causes trichinosis, a condition which results from eating incompletely cooked pork infested with the larvae of the worm. When such meat is eaten, the cysts dissolve, the parasites mature, and a new crop of larvae develop which penetrate the intestinal mucosa and eventually lodge in the muscles. The most important filarial worm is *Wuchereria bancrofti*, which is transmitted by the bite of the mosquito. Symptoms result from the blocking of the lymphatic ducts with the adult worms.

The flatworms are of two types, segmented (cestodes) and nonsegmented (trematodes). The cestodes include the tapeworms and the trematodes include the flukes. Four common varieties of parasitic tapeworms are found in man; *Taenia saginata* (beef tapeworm), *Taenia solium* (pork tapeworm), *Diphyllobothrium latum* (fish tapeworm), and *Hymenolepis nana* (dwarf tapeworm). Except for the dwarf tapeworm, they are from 6 to 30 feet in length and may contain 3000 to 4000 segments, each segment being capable of producing hundreds of eggs. The dwarf tapeworm is only $\frac{1}{4}$ to $\frac{1}{2}$ inch in length, but consists of 150 to 200 segments. The larval stage of all tapeworms is spent in the muscles of the intermediate host, and human infection occurs through eating imperfectly cooked meat and fish. Three varieties of blood fluke inhabit the blood stream of man causing schistosomiasis: *Schistosoma haematobium*, *Schistosoma mansoni*, and *Schistosoma japonica*. These parasites cause epigastric distress, abdominal pain, anorexia, diarrhea with blood and mucus in the stools, enlarged and tender liver, pyrexia, and ascites. The intermediate host is either a fresh water snail or a fresh water mollusk. Transmission is by way of contaminated water.

Parasitic worms are harmful to the human host for a number of reasons. They deprive the host of food, they injure organs or obstruct ducts, they may elaborate substances toxic to the host, and they may provide a portal of entry for other organisms. It is desirable, therefore, even though the individual may be symptom-free, to eradicate the parasites as soon as they have been discovered.

Proper choice of the anthelmintic is important, as most drugs are more effective against some species than others. The older anthelmintics are more effective when there is no material in the intestinal tract. For this reason food is generally withheld for 24 hours before administering these drugs. A saline cathartic is given about one-half hour before the anthelmintic. An oil-base cathartic should not be used because it may increase the absorption of the anthelmintic and so increase its toxicity. The purgative is given again about one-half hour after the anthelmintic in order that the stupefied worms and the remaining drug be expelled. Many of the newer drugs require little or no change in the patient's normal routine. When the patient has a tapeworm infestation, a thorough examination of the stools produced by the second purgation is necessary. Unless the head of the worm has been expelled and identified, the worm will regenerate. Usually three specimens of stools are examined one week after administration of the anthelmintic. If ova or parasites are still present, the treatment should be repeated. All drugs which are poisonous to the worms are also poisonous to the patient. Therefore, the recommended methods of treatment for each drug should be followed carefully and the patient watched closely for the appearance of any untoward drug effects.

Antimony Potassium Tartrate USP

[Antimonyl Potassium Tartrate; Tartrated Antimony; Tartar Emetic; Stibii et Kalii Tartras]

KOOC.CH(OH).CH(OH).COO(SbO).½HO

Antimony Potassium Tartrate contains 99.0–103.0% of $C_4H_4KO_7Sb \cdot \frac{1}{2}H_2O$ (333.93).

History—Adrian Mynsicht, physician of the early seventeenth century, who invented *Elixir of Vitriol*, is also credited with having first discovered and used tartar emetic. Glauber in 1648 described in detail the process of preparing *Mynsicht's Emetic Tartar* as it was then called.

Preparation—This important antimonial compound may be made by dissolving a mixture of 10 parts of potassium bitartrate with 8 parts of antimony trioxide [Sb_2O_3] in 75 parts of boiling water, filtering while hot and allowing it to crystallize.

Description—Colorless, odorless, transparent crystals, or a white powder. The crystals effloresce upon exposure to air. Its solutions are acid to litmus.

Solubility—1 Gm is soluble in 12 ml of water and about 15 ml of glycerin, and about 3 ml of boiling water; insoluble in alcohol.

Incompatibilities—*Mineral acids*, when added to aqueous solutions of Antimony Potassium Tartrate, cause a precipitation of basic salts of antimony, with possibly some potassium bitartrate. *Alkali hydroxides* and *carbonates* of sufficient concentration precipitate antimony trioxide. Precipitation is retarded by citrates, tartrates, glycerin, and sugar. Many metallic salts form insoluble tartrates. Addition of *alcohol* to an aqueous solution may cause a precipitation. An insoluble tannate is formed with *tannic acid*. *Mercuric chloride* is reduced to calomel which precipitates.

Uses—Antimony Potassium Tartrate is used for the therapy of schistosomiasis and leishmaniasis, especially cases which are refractory to less toxic agents. It is also an *emetic*, chiefly by virtue of its irritant action on the gastrointestinal mucosa. Subemetic doses produce an *expectorant* action due to reflex stimulation of the salivary and bronchial glands. Toxic effects induced by Antimony Potassium Tartrate include pain at the site of injection, centrally induced emesis, liver or kidney damage, diarrhea, vertigo, cough, headache, arthralgia or myalgia, and cardiovascular changes (bradycardia, hypotension, circulatory collapse). Since these toxic effects are related to the content of antimony, they usually respond to dimercaprol.

Antimony Potassium Tartrate is used as a mordant in textile dyeing and also to disinfect gladioli.

Dose—*Usual, intravenous*, as a **0.5** to **1%** solution, *initial*, **40 mg**, repeated every 2 days, each dose increased by **20 mg** until **140 mg** is reached, then **140 mg** every other day for a total course-of-treatment dose of 2 **Gm**.

Veterinary Dose—*Expectorant*: *Cattle*, 1 to 5 **Gm**; *Horses*, **300 mg** to 2 **Gm**; *Sheep, Swine, and Goats*, **100** to **500 mg**; *Dogs*, 3 to **15 mg**.

Emetic: *Swine*, 1 to 2 **Gm**; *Dogs*, **100** to **300 mg**; *Cats*, **32** to **65 mg**.

Ruminatoric: *Cattle*, 8 to 10 **Gm**; *Sheep* and *Goats*, **300 mg** to 1 **Gm**.

Anthelmintic: *Horses*, 4 to 8 **Gm**.

Areca—see page 902.

Arecoline Hydrobromide—see page 902.

Bephenium Hydroxynaphthoate

[Alcopara (*Burroughs-Wellcome*)]

Bephenium Hydroxynaphthoate [$C_{17}H_{22}NO \cdot C_{11}H_7O_3$ = 443.55] is benzyldimethyl(2-phenoxyethyl)ammonium 3-hydroxy-2-naphthoate.

Preparation—1-Chloro-2-phenoxyethane is caused to condense with dimethylamine and the resulting dimethyl(2-phenoxyethyl)amine is quaternized with benzyl chloride. Metathesis with an aqueous solution of sodium 3-hydroxy-2-naphthoate yields the desired compound. US Pat. 2,918,401.

Description—A yellow to greenish-yellow powder which is odorless and has a somewhat bitter taste. It is stable in light and in air. It melts between 168° and 173°.

Solubility—Soluble in hot alcohol; insoluble in water.

Uses—Bephenium Hydroxynaphthoate is used in the treatment of hookworm infections. It is the anthelmintic of choice in *Ancylostoma duodenale* (hookworm) and is an alternative drug in *Necator americanus* (hookworm). It has also been reported to be of value in the treatment of common roundworm (ascaris) infections when they occur concomitantly with hookworms. Side effects are usually minimal and consist of nausea, vomiting, and diarrhea. The drug should be used with caution in hypertensive patients and others with labile blood pressure; it has mild ganglionic blocking action and if absorbed might cause a brief marked fall in blood pressure. Safety for use during pregnancy has not been established.

Dose—*Usual*, 5 **Gm** of granules (containing 4.33 Gm of bephenium hydroxynaphthoate equivalent to 2.5 Gm of bephenium ion) twice in one day. The dose may be repeated in a few days if necessary.

Dosage Forms—Granules: 5 Gm.

Chloroquine Phosphate—see page 1245.

Diethylcarbamazine Citrate USP

[*N,N*-Diethyl-4-methyl-1-piperazinecarboxamide Citrate (1:1); 1-Diethylcarbamoyl-4-methylpiperazine Dihydrogen Citrate; Hetrazan (*Lederle*)]

Diethylcarbamazine Citrate contains 98.0–100.5% of $C_{10}H_{21}N_3O \cdot C_6H_8O_7$ (391.32), calculated on the anhydrous basis.

Preparation—It may be prepared by acylating piperazine with diethylcarbamoyl chloride, and then methylating at the N^4-position by treatment with formaldehyde and formic acid. Treatment of the purified base with an equimolar portion of citric acid yields the official citrate.

Description—A white, crystalline powder. Odorless, or has a slight odor. Slightly hygroscopic. Melts between 135° and 138°.

Solubility—Very soluble in water; sparingly soluble in alcohol; practically insoluble in acetone, chloroform, and ether.

Uses—Diethylcarbamazine Citrate is the drug of choice for the treatment of *Wuchereria bancrofti*. In adequate dosage it rapidly clears the blood of the microfilariæ and it appears to be curative. The drug is also curative in the treatment of *loaiasis (loa loa)*. It is not of benefit in onchocerciasis; microfilariæ in the skin are removed, but adult forms survive and allergic reactions may be violent. The drug is not effective against adult hookworms, whipworms, tapeworms, or pinworms. Its value in filarial infections caused by *Acanthocheilonema perstans*, *A. streptocerca*, and *Mansonella ozzardi* is not established. Untoward reactions are frequent but not serious; they include headache, general malaise, weakness, joint pains, anorexia, nausea, and vomiting. Lymphatic swellings, leukocytosis, and eosinophilia are believed to be caused by dead filariæ.

Dose—*Usual*, **2 mg** per **Kg** of body weight 3 times a day for 1 to 3 weeks.

Other Dose Information—The drug is administered orally. For *Wuchereria bancrofti*, a dose of 2 mg per Kg is given 3 times daily for 1 to 2 weeks; however, there is evidence that a single dose of 20 mg per Kg may be effective. For loaiasis, a dose of 2 mg per Kg is given 3 times daily for 10 to 12 weeks. For ascariasis, a dose of 6 to 10 mg per Kg is given 3 times daily after meals for 7 to 10 days.

Dosage Forms—Syrup: 120 mg/5 ml; Tablets USP: 50 mg.

Veterinary Use—In the treatment of *ascariasis* in dogs and cats and *filiariasis* in dogs.

Veterinary Dose—*Dogs, anthelmintic*, **25 mg** per **pound** of body weight; *filiaricide*, **33 mg** per **pound** of body weight daily for 1 month; *Cats, anthelmintic*, **25 mg** per **pound** of body weight.

Emetine Hydrochloride—see page 1251.

Hexylresorcinol NF

[4-Hexylresorcinol; Crystoids (*MSD*)]

Hexylresorcinol [$C_{12}H_{18}O_2 = 194.28$], dried over silica gel for 4 hours, contains 98.0–100.5% of $C_{12}H_{18}O_2$.

Caution—Hexylresorcinol is irritating to the oral mucosa and respiratory tract and to the skin, and its solution in alcohol has vesicant properties.

Preparation—Resorcinol is heated with caproic acid [$CH_3(CH_2)_4COOH$] in the presence of zinc chloride as a condensing agent. The resulting caproylresorcinol is then heated with amalgamated zinc and hydrochloric acid (Clemensen's reduction) whereby the CO of the caproyl group is reduced to CH_2 yielding Hexylresorcinol.

Description—White, or yellowish white, needle-shaped crystals. It has a faint odor and a sharp, astringent taste, and produces a sensation of numbness when placed on the tongue. It acquires a brownish pink tint on exposure to light and air. It melts between 62° and 67°.

Solubility—1 Gm dissolves in about 2000 ml of water; freely soluble in alcohol, methanol, glycerin, ether, chloroform, benzene, and vegetable oils.

Uses—Hexylresorcinol is the alternate *anthelmintic* agent of choice (thiabendazole is preferred) in the treatment of *whipworm* infestations. It is also effective against *hookworm*, *ascaris*, *oxyuris*, and *dwarf tapeworm*. Due to its low toxicity, it can be used repeatedly at 3-day intervals. It is given in the adult dose of 1.0 Gm followed in 2 hours by a saline cathartic. Care should be taken that the pills containing the drug are swallowed whole or painful ulceration of the oral mucous membrane may result. The official *Hexylresorcinol Pills* (see below) are coated by a patented process, the gelatin coating being so tough that it cannot be readily broken even though chewed. Hexylresorcinol should not be dispensed in ordinary, hard gelatin capsules as these quickly become brittle, and may break in the mouth causing caustic burns.

Hexylresorcinol is a valued odorless and stainless *antiseptic*, commonly employed in a dilution of 1 : 1000. Hexylresorcinol also has a limited value as a *urinary antiseptic*.

Dose—*Usual*, **1 Gm**; may repeat at weekly intervals if necessary.

Other Dose Information—The usual dose for a child is 100 mg for each year of age.

Dosage Forms—Pills NF: 100 and 200 mg.

Veterinary Dose—*Anthelmintic: Small Puppies*, **200 mg**; *Large Puppies*, **400 mg**; *Mature Dogs* (10 to 20 pounds) **600 mg**; (20 pounds and over) **1 Gm**; *Urinary Antiseptic: Dogs*, **150** to **600 mg**; *Swine*, **3** to **4 Gm** for 50 pound pigs.

Lucanthone Hydrochloride USP

[1-[[2-(Diethylamino)ethyl]amino]-4-methylthioxanthen-9-one Monohydrochloride; (*Burroughs Wellcome*)]

Lucanthone Hydrochloride contains 98.5–100.5% of $C_{20}H_{24}N_2OS \cdot HCl$ (376.95), calculated on the anhydrous basis.

Preparation—*o*-Mercaptobenzoic acid is condensed with *p*-chlorotoluene giving a mixture of the 1-chloro-4-methyl and 1-methyl-4-chloro derivatives of thioxanthen-9-one. The mixture is then reacted with *N,N*-diethylethylenediamine under conditions such that only the 1-chloro-4-methyl derivative couples, thus yielding lucanthone base. The base is solvent extracted and reacted with an equimolar quantity of HCl.

Description—Yellowish orange, almost odorless powder. Has a bitter taste followed by a burning sensation. Readily stains the skin.

Solubility—1 Gm dissolves in about 110 ml of water, about 85 ml of alcohol, and about 20 ml of chloroform; insoluble in acetone and ether.

Uses—Lucanthone Hydrochloride is employed in the treatment of *schistosomiasis*. It is most effective against *S. haematobium*, less effective against *S. mansoni*, and relatively ineffective against *S. japonicum*. The drug prevents the formation of ova and ultimately destroys the parasite. Side effects, such as anorexia, nausea, and vomiting, are not uncommon. Convulsions, psychoses, and circulatory disturbances have also been reported. The ultimate value of Lucanthone in the management of schistosomiasis remains to be established.

Dose—10 to 20 mg per **Kg** of body weight for 1 to 3 weeks; *usual*, **5 mg** per **Kg** of body weight 3 times a day for 1 week.

Dosage Forms—Tablets USP: 200 mg.

Methylrosaniline Chloride—see page 1178.

Piperazine Calcium Edetate

[Calcium Piperazine (Ethylenedinitrilo)tetraäcetate; Perin (*Endo*)]

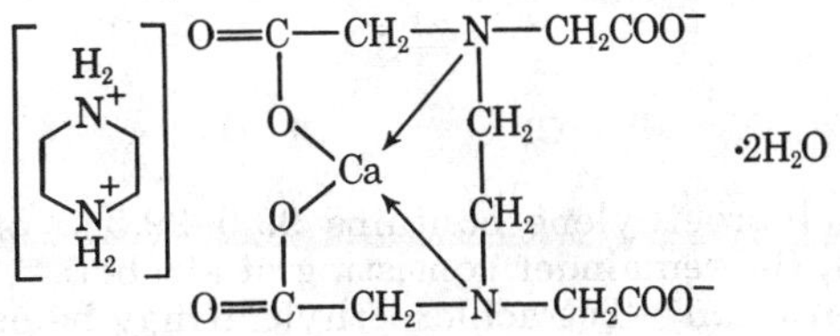

Piperazine Calcium Edatate [C$_{14}$H$_{24}$CaN$_4$O$_8$.2H$_2$O] is also well known as calcium piperazine ethylenediaminetetraacetate and as piperazine calcium edathamil.

Preparation—It is readily prepared by reacting edetic acid with calcium carbonate and piperazine. US Pat. 2,834,782.

Description—It occurs as crystals having a slightly salty taste. pH (20% aqueous solution) 4.3–5.4.

Solubility—Freely soluble in water; very slightly soluble in alcohol and chloroform; practically insoluble in ether.

Uses—Piperazine Calcium Edetate is used in the eradication of *pinworms* and *roundworms*. The effectiveness of the chelated form is of the same order as that of the citrate and tartrate salts of piperazine. It is well tolerated and free from toxic effects in the usual dosage.

Dose—*Usual*, *oral*, for *pinworms*, **75 mg** per **Kg** of body weight per day, administered at one time or in two divided doses for a period of 15 days; for *roundworms*, **100 mg** per **Kg** of body weight administered once or in two divided doses.

Dosage Forms—Syrup: 500 mg (of piperazine hexahydrate)/5 ml; Tablets: 500 mg.

Piperazine Citrate USP

[Piperazine Citrate (3:2) Hydrate; Antepar Citrate (*Burroughs-Wellcome*); Ascarex (*Savage*); Multifuge Citrate (*Bluline*); Pipizan Citrate (*MSD*)]

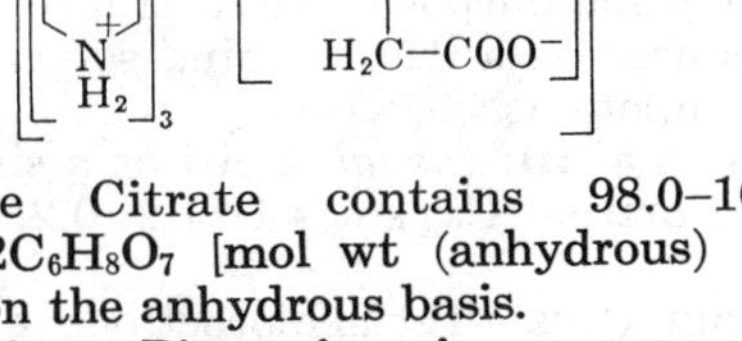

Piperazine Citrate contains 98.0–100.5% of (C$_4$H$_{10}$N$_2$)$_3$.2C$_6$H$_8$O$_7$ [mol wt (anhydrous) = 642.67], calculated on the anhydrous basis.

Preparation—Piperazine, in aqueous solution, is reacted with a ⅔ equimolar quantity of citric acid, and the resulting citrate is caused to crystallize.

Description—Occurs as white, crystalline powder, having not more than a slight odor. A 1 in 10 solution is acid to litmus, having a pH of 5 to 6.

Solubility—Soluble in water; insoluble in alcohol and ether.

Uses—Piperazine Citrate is the *anthelmintic* of choice for the treatment of infections caused by *pinworms* and *roundworms*. The drug is relatively nontoxic to humans and usually produces no side effects when administered in anthelmintic doses. The ingestion of excessively large amounts may produce urticaria or vomiting, blurred vision and general muscular weakness, which disappear when the drug is discontinued. Excessively prolonged or repeated treatment should be avoided.

Dose—Against *enterobius*, the equivalent of up to **2.5 Gm** of piperazine hexahydrate (C$_4$H$_{10}$N$_2$.6H$_2$O) daily; *usual*, **2 Gm** once a day for 7 days; against *ascaris*, up to **3.5 Gm** daily; *usual*, **3.5 Gm** once a day for 2 days.

Dosage Forms—Syrup USP: 500 and 550 mg/5 ml; Tablets USP: 275 and 500 mg.

Veterinary Use—The various piperazine salts are effective against most or certain species of roundworms, pinworms, hookworms, heartworms, and certain strongyles infecting domestic animals and cecal worms in chickens.

Veterinary Dose—The drug is administered at the rate of about **1 Gm** of the base per **10 pounds** of body weight in large animals and **50 mg** per **pound** of body weight in small animals regardless of the salt used.

Pyrvinium Pamoate USP

[6 - (Dimethylamino)- 2 - [2 - (2,5 - dimethyl - 1 - phenylpyrrol - 3 - yl)vinyl]- 1-methylquinolinium 4,4'-Methylenebis[3-hydroxy-2-naphthoate] (2:1); Povan (*Parke- Davis*)]

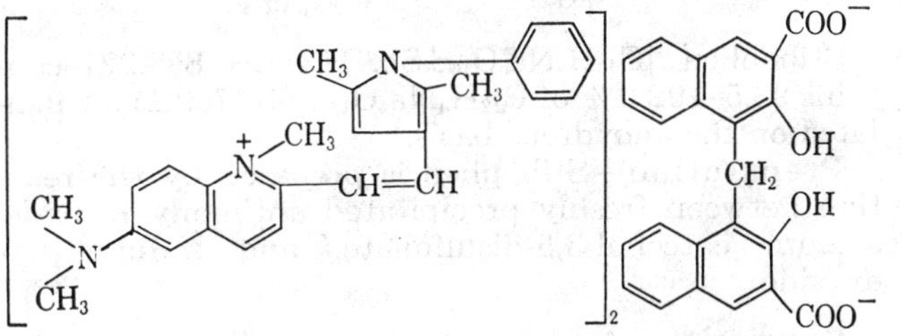

Pyrvinium Pamoate contains 96.0–104.0% of C$_{75}$H$_{70}$N$_6$O$_6$ (1151.43), calculated on the anhydrous basis.

Preparation—6 - (Dimethylamino) - 1 - methylquinaldinium methyl sulfate (I) is condensed with 2,5-dimethyl-1-phenyl-3-pyrrolecarboxaldehyde (II) by refluxing in methanol containing a small quantity of piperidine. The resulting crude pyrvinium methyl sulfate is purified by recrystallization from aqueous ethanol and then metathesized with disodium 4,4'-methylenebis[3-hydroxy-2-naphthoate]. The crude product is recrystallized from suitable solvents. I is readily prepared from 6-aminoquinaldine by various standard methylation procedures followed by quaternization with dimethyl sulfate. II may be prepared by condensing 2,5-dimethyl-1-phenylpyrrole with form-

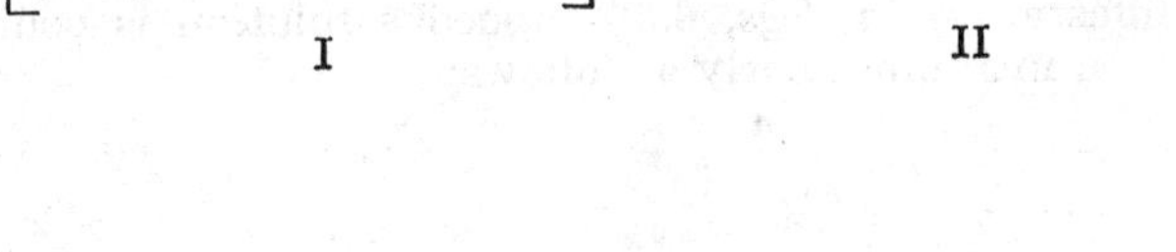

I

II

amide and degrading the resulting 3-carboxamide compound to the aldehyde.   US Pat. 2,515,912.

Description—Bright orange or orange-red to almost black, crystalline powder.

Solubility—Practically insoluble in water and ether; slightly soluble in chloroform and methoxyethanol; very slightly soluble in alcohol.

Uses—Pyrvinium Pamoate is the anthelmintic of choice for the treatment of pinworm (*Enterobius vermicularis*) infestations. An adequate single dose will clear 90 to 100% of infected patients within 2 weeks. It is also effective in the treatment of *strongyloides stercoralis* infestations. Pyrvinium Pamoate is well tolerated and causes few untoward effects. Nausea, vomiting, and transient photosensitization have been reported. The drug resembles a cyanine dye and colors the stools bright red.

There have been few reports of its use in children weighing less than 22 pounds.

Dose—*Usual*, the equivalent of **5 mg** of pyrvinium per **Kg** of body weight in a single dose.

Dosage Forms—Oral Suspension USP: 50 mg/5 ml; Tablets USP: 50 mg.

Quinacrine Hydrochloride—see page 1247.

Sodium Suramin—see page 1254.

Stibophen USP

[Pentasodium Bis[4,5-dihydroxy-*m*-benzenedisulfonato(4-)]antimonate(5-); Sodium Antimony Bis(pyrocatechol-2,4-disulfonate); Neoantimosan; Fuadin (*Winthrop*)]

Stibophen [$C_{12}H_4Na_5O_{16}S_4Sb.7H_2O$ = 895.22] contains 98.5–102.0% of $C_{12}H_4Na_5O_{16}S_4Sb$ (769.11), calculated on the anhydrous basis.

Preparation—Stibophen is prepared by the reaction between freshly precipitated antimony trioxide, sodium catechol-3,5-disulfonate, and sodium hydroxide.

Description—A white, odorless, crystalline powder. It is affected by light and is oxidized upon prolonged exposure of its solution to air; therefore, unused portions of its solution should be discarded. Its aqueous solution is alkaline and stable when autoclaved; however, prolonged storage should be avoided since this may cause its dissociation and resultant increasing toxicity. Owing to its phenolic character and the presence of sulfonic acid groups it is discolored by ferric iron.

Solubility—Freely soluble in water; practically insoluble in alcohol, ether, and chloroform.

Uses—Stibophen is an *antischistosomal* drug that is also useful in the therapy of leishmaniasis and granuloma inguinale. Treatment with Stibophen should be stopped if recurrent vomiting, albuminuria, intercurrent febrile infection, or blood dyscrasias occur. The use of Stibophen is contraindicated in the presence of severe liver, kidney, or cardiac insufficiency.

Dose—*Usual*, *intramuscular* or *intravenous*, **100 mg** on first day, then **300 mg** on alternate days, up to a total of **2.5 to 4.6 Gm.**

Dosage Forms—Injection USP: 300 mg/5 ml.

Veterinary Dose—For the treatment of heartworm infestation in *dogs*, **6.3%** aqueous solution is usually used intramuscularly as follows:

Body weight of dog		Daily dose for first 6 days, ml	Daily dose for second 6 days, ml	Daily dose after second 6 days, ml
Kg	lbs			
Under 10	22	0.5	1.0	1.0
10–15	22–35	1.0	1.5	1.5
15–20	35–44	1.0	1.5	2.0
20–25	44–55	1.5	2.0	2.0
Over 25	55	2.0	2.5	2.5

An interval of 1 day should elapse between each course of 6 successive injections. Each ml is equivalent to 8.5 mg of trivalent antimony.

Tetrachloroethylene USP

[Perchloroethylene; Tetrachlorethene; Ethylene Tetrachloride; Carbon Dichloride]

Tetrachloroethylene contains 99.0–99.5% of C_2Cl_4 (165.83), the remainder consisting of alcohol.

Preparation—Tetrachloroethylene may be prepared by several methods: (1) By the action of milk of lime on pentachloroethane [C_2HCl_5] whereby 1 molecule of HCl is split off. (2) By passing pentachloroethane vapors over strongly heated adsorbent carbon or over a metal chloride catalyst heated to about 300°. (3) By the addition of chlorine to acetylene.

Pure Tetrachloroethylene is relatively unstable, especially in the presence of moisture and, therefore, as in chloroform, 0.5 to 1% of alcohol is added to it as a preservative.

Description—A clear, colorless, mobile liquid, with a characteristic ethereal odor. It is not flammable, but is slowly decomposed by light and by various metals in the presence of moisture. Its specific gravity is between 1.603 and 1.615, indicating 99 to 99.5% of C_2Cl_4, and not less than 90% distils between 118° and 122°. It solidifies at about −22° and has a refractive index of 1.5018 at 20°.

Solubility—Practically insoluble in water; miscible with an equal volume of alcohol, with chloroform, ether, solvent hexane, and benzene; dissolves in most of the fixed and volatile oils.

Uses—Tetrachloroethylene is the anthelmintic of choice for the treatment of *Necator americanus* (hookworm) infestations and is also useful in the eradication of *Ancylostoma duodenale* (hookworm) infestations. It is also of some value against *oxyuriasis*, *whipworms*, and *flukes*. It is relatively nontoxic; however, depression, giddiness, inebriation, and rarely loss of consciousness have been reported. The patient should be kept at rest for 4 hours after the drug is administered. No alcohol should be taken before or for 24 hours after the drug. It is extensively used in veterinary medicine for the same purpose. Industrially, Tetrachloroethylene is used as a dry-cleaning solvent and in degreasing compounds.

Dose—3 to 5 ml; *usual*, 5 ml as a single dose.

Dosage Forms—Capsules USP: 0.2, 0.5, 1.0, 2.5, and 5 ml.

Veterinary Uses—Tetrachloroethylene is used as an *ascaricide* for swine; treatment of *stomach worms* in sheep; and in all species for the elimination of *nematodes*.

Veterinary Dose—*Pigs*, up to 100 pounds, **2.5 ml;** *Hogs*, **5 ml;** *Lambs*, **2.5 ml;** *Heavy Sheep*, **5 ml;** *Dogs* and *Cats*, **0.1 ml** per **pound** of body weight.

Thiabendazole USP

[2-(4-Thiazolyl)benzimidazole; Mintezol (*MSD*); Thibenzole (*Merck*)]

Thiabendazole contains 98.0–101.0% of $C_{10}H_7N_3S$ (201.25), calculated on the anhydrous basis.

Preparation—Ethyl pyruvate is brominated and the resulting 2-bromo ester is reacted with thioformamide whereby, through dehydration and dehydrobromination, cyclization occurs with the formation of ethyl 4-thiazolecarboxylate. This ester is then saponified and condensed with *o*-phenylenediamine in the presence of polyphosphoric acid to introduce the benzimidazole moiety. US Pat. 3,017,415.

Description—A white to practically white, odorless or practically odorless, tasteless powder. It is stable in light and is nonhygroscopic. It melts between 296° and 303°.

Solubility—Slightly soluble in acetone and alcohol; very slightly soluble in chloroform and ether; practically insoluble in water.

Uses—Thiabendazole is an *anthelmintic* agent which is recommended for the treatment of various roundworm infections of man. It is considered the drug of choice for cutaneous larva migrans (which results from the penetration of the human skin by larvae of the dog and cat hookworm), *Strongyloides stercoralis* (threadworm), and *Trichinella spiralis* (trichinosis). It is also useful in *roundworm, whipworm,* and *pinworm* infestations. No special diet or purgation is needed with Thiabendazole. Side effects usually include nausea, vomiting, vertigo, headache, and weakness. Leukopenia and crystalluria have also been reported. Since from $\frac{1}{3}$ to $\frac{1}{2}$ of patients are usually incapacitated for several hours after receiving the drug, the drug should be given on days when the patient does not have to go to school or to work. Patients on the drug should be cautioned not to engage in activities requiring mental alertness.

Dose—Up to **3 Gm** daily for 1 to 4 days; *usual*, **25 mg** per **Kg** of body weight 2 times a day for 2 days.

Dosage Forms—Oral Suspension USP: **500 mg/5 ml.**

Veterinary Dose—*Horses* (against the genera *Strongylus, Cyathostoma, Cylicobrachytus* and related genera, *Craterostomum, Oesophagodontus, Poteriostomum,* and *Oxyuris*) **1 Gm** per **50 pounds** of body weight; *Cattle* (against the genera *Haemonchus, Ostertagia, Trichostrongylus,* and *Cooperia*) **3 to 5 Gm** per **100 pounds** of body weight, followed by a second dose 1 to 2 weeks later; *Sheep* and *Goats* (against the genera *Trichostrongylus, Haemonchus, Ostertagia, Cooperia, Nematodirus, Bunostomum, Strongyloides, Chabertia* and *Oesophagostomum*) **1 Gm** per **50 pounds** of body weight.

Thymol—see page 1190.

Other Anthelmintics

Aspidium USP XVI [Male Fern; Male Shield Fern; Bear's Paw Root]—It consists of the rhizomes and stipes of *Dryopteris Filix-mas* (Linné) Schott, or of *Dryopteris marginalis* (Linné) Asa Gray. For standardization, the active constituents are assumed to be crude filicin. *Uses:* An anthelmintic in the form of the oleoresin. The oleoresin contains not less than 24% of crude filicin. It must be used with caution as it becomes a violent poison if allowed to remain in the alimentary tract until absorbed. It is usually administered after 12 to 24 hours of fasting and must be followed within a few hours by an active saline purge. Castor oil should never be used as the purge since it promotes absorption. *Dose:* 3 to 5 Gm of the oleoresin.

Butyl Chloride NF XII [*n*-Butyl Chloride; 1-Chlorobutane] contains not less than 99.0% of C_4H_9Cl (92.57). *Caution: Butyl Chloride is very flammable. Do not use where it may be ignited. Preparation:* It may be prepared by heating a mixture of *n*-butyl alcohol and hydrogen chloride in the presence of anhydrous zinc chloride which functions as a dehydrating agent. *Description and Solubility:* A clear, colorless, volatile liquid, having a characteristic, nonresidual odor; specific gravity, 0.880–0.885; distilling range, 77°–79°. Insoluble in water; miscible with dehydrated alcohol and ether. *Uses:* An *anthelmintic* for horses and dogs. *Veterinary Dose: Usual* (based on the weight of the animal), *Horses,* 15 to 90 ml; *Dogs,* 1 to 24 ml.

Carbon Tetrachloride NF XI [CCl₄ = 153.82]—A clear, colorless liquid which boils at about 77°. It is soluble in about 2000 volumes of water; miscible with alcohol, acetone, ether, chloroform, and benzene. *Uses:* A cheap and effective *anthelmintic* for the treatment of *hookworm* infestation. Inasmuch as carbon tetrachloride causes severe injury to the liver, if absorbed, care must be exerted that the drug be taken on an empty stomach and the ingestion of alcohol or fat avoided. The anthelmintic dose is 0.15 ml per year of age for children and from 2 to 3 ml for adults. It may be given in hard gelatin capsules or emulsified in skimmed milk. It is followed in 2 hours by a saline cathartic. Three weeks should elapse before a second dose is given.
Veterinary Uses: Carbon Tetrachloride is used to remove *hookworms* and *roundworms* in the dog and fox; *strongyloides, roundworms,* and *bot larva* from the horse; common stomach worms and *liver flukes* from sheep; and large intestinal roundworms from chickens. *Dose: Caution—Anthelmintic for adults, usual single dose, 3 ml. Veterinary Dose: Horses,* 25 to 50 ml for a 1000-pound animal; *Cattle,* 10 to 30 ml; *Sheep,* 1 ml per Kg for adults; *Dogs* and *Foxes,* average dose 0.3 ml per Kg of body weight; *Chickens,* 4 ml per Kg of body weight.

Chenopodium Oil NF X [American Wormseed Oil]—The volatile oil distilled from the fresh, above-ground parts of the flowering and fruiting plant of *Chenopodium ambrosioides* Linné, var. *anthelminticum* (Linné) A. Gray (Fam. *Chenopodiaceæ*). It contains not less than 65% (*w/w*) of ascaridol [$C_{10}H_{16}O_2$]. A pale yellow liquid having a peculiar, unpleasant odor and a bitter, burning taste. It dissolves in 8 volumes of 70% alcohol. It explodes when heated alone or with acids at 130–150°C. *Uses:* As an anthelmintic against hookworm, roundworm, and dwarf tapeworm. Employed as an emulsion, the oil first being mixed with twice its volume of olive oil. *Dose:* 1 ml as a single dose for adults. It has caused death in doses of 2 ml.

Diphenan BP [α-Phenyltolyl Carbamate] [$C_{14}H_{13}NO_2$]—A white crystalline powder almost insoluble in water and sparingly soluble in alcohol. *Uses:* An anthelmintic for threadworms. *Dose:* Infants up to 18 months, 125 mg; children up to 10 years, 250 mg; older children, 500 mg; adults, 500 mg to 1 Gm. These doses are given 3 times daily after meals for one week. A purgative is given at the end of the course of treatment.

Drocarbil NF XII [Arecolinium 3-Acetamido-4-hydroxybenzenearsonate; Arecoline *N*-Acetyl-4-hydroxy-*m*-arsanilate; $C_{16}H_{23}AsN_2O_7$ (430.29)] is the acetarsone salt of arecoline. It contains 34.0–36.5% of $C_8H_{13}NO_2$ (155.20), and 64.0–67.0% of $C_8H_{10}AsNO_5$ (275.09). *Preparation:* It is synthesized by proceeding through several intermediates beginning with *p*-chloroaniline and ending with 3-acetamido-4-hydroxybenzenearsonic acid which is treated with an equimolar quantity of arecoline. *Description and Solubility:* A nearly white or slightly yellow, odorless powder; stable at ordinary temperatures. Freely soluble in water. *Uses:* A *veterinary anthelmintic* useful in the treatment of tapeworm infestations in dogs and cats. *Veterinary Dose:*

Usual, to be determined by the veterinarian according to the species and need of the animal. *Dogs*, over 3 months of age, 18 mg per 8 pounds of body weight; *Cats*, over 1 year of age, 14 to 27 mg in milk. *Caution:* Drocarbil causes cardiac slowing and catharsis.

Pelletierine Tannate—A mixture in varying proportions of the tannates of the several alkaloids obtained from pomegranate, *Punica Granatum* Linné (Fam. *Punicaceæ*). It contains an amount of the alkaloids equivalent to not less than 20% as the hydrochloride. *Uses:* An anthelmintic used chiefly against the pork tapeworm. Highly toxic. Given only to robust adults. *Dose:* 0.25 Gm.

Phenothiazine NF XII [C₁₂H₉NS (199.28)] is thiodiphenylamine. *Caution: Animals should be treated with Phenothiazine only upon the advice of a veterinarian. Preparation:* Heat diphenylamine and sulfur at about 180° using a trace of iodine as a catalyst. Hydrogen sulfide is evolved and the crude Phenothiazine is purified by washing with carbon tetrachloride or similar solvent to remove the excess sulfur. *Description and Solubility:* A pale greenish yellow to dark greenish gray powder, granules, or flakes. It is tasteless and has a slight characteristic odor; it slowly oxidizes and darkens upon prolonged exposure to air; a freezing point (not less than 179°) is specified because its flakes melt about 3° lower than the material obtained by slow cooling. 1 Gm dissolves in about 75 ml of alcohol, 5 ml of acetone, and 20 ml of chloroform; usually incompletely soluble in ether and insoluble in water. *Uses:* Introduced into therapy as a urinary antiseptic and as a *veterinary anthelmintic* for the treatment of pinworm infestation. It has proved to be toxic, however, causing a severe anemia. It is still of value for the treatment of *helminthiasis* in sheep and other domestic animals. *Veterinary Dose: Usual* (based on the weight of the animal), *Horses* and *Mules*, 30 to 50 Gm; *Cattle*, 50 to 80 Gm; *Calves*, 24 to 40 Gm; *Swine*, 4 to 30 Gm; *Sheep* and *Goats*, 25 Gm; *Lambs* (up to 60 pounds), 15 Gm; *Chickens*, 500 mg.

Piperazine [Diethylenediamine] [C₄H₁₀N₂]—Forms colorless, hygroscopic crystals, melting at 105° when anhydrous. It boils at 145° to 146°, and is very soluble in water or glycerin, less soluble in alcohol, insoluble in ether. From water piperazine crystallizes with 6H₂O in colorless crystals called *Piperazine Hydrate*, melting at 44° and boiling between 125° and 130°. It is incompatible with salts of heavy metals, alkaloidal salts, also incompatible with acetanilid, phenacetin, and nitrites.

Uses and *Dose:* See *Piperazine Citrate* (page 1267).

Piperazine Adipate BP—Purity: not less than 98.5% of C₁₀H₂₀N₂O₄. The salt formed by reacting equimolar quantities of piperazine and adipic acid. An odorless, white, crystalline powder having a slightly acid taste. It is soluble in 18 parts of water and insoluble in alcohol. An aqueous solution (5%, *w/v*) has a pH range of 5 to 6. *Uses:* As for piperazine citrate. See *Piperazine Citrate* (page 1267). *Dose: Orally*, in the treatment of threadworm infestation, 1 to 2 Gm daily, in divided doses; as an ascaricide, 4.5 Gm as a single dose.

Piperazine Phosphate BP—The monohydrated salt formed by the interaction of equimolar quantities of piperazine and phosphoric acid. Purity: not less than 98.5% of C₄H₁₀N₂.H₃PO₄, calculated on the anhydrous basis. An odorless, slightly acid, white, crystalline powder. It is soluble in 60 parts of water and insoluble in alcohol. A 1% (*w/v*) aqueous solution has a pH range of 6 to 7. *Uses* and *Dose:* As for piperazine citrate. See *Piperazine Citrate* (page 1267).

Piperazine Tartrate [Monopiperazine Bitartrate] [C₄H₁₀N₂.C₄H₆O₆]—An anthelmintic formed by the reaction of equimolar portions of piperazine hexahydrate with tartaric acid. Very soluble in water. *Uses:* For the treatment of infections caused by pinworms (*Enterobius vermicularis*) and roundworms (*Ascaris lumbricoides*). *Dose: Orally*, adults and children, 50 mg/Kg body weight but not more than 2 Gm daily for a total of 14 days.

Pediculicides and Scabicides

Pediculicides are compounds effective in the treatment of pediculosis. Pediculosis in man is caused by three species of sucking lice known as *Pediculus humanus* variety *capitis*, the head louse, *Pediculus humanus* variety *corporis*, the body louse, and *Phthirus pubis*, the crab louse. These parasitic, wingless insects thrive where personal hygiene is neglected. The eggs (nits) of the body louse are attached to the fibers of clothing while those of the other two species are attached to hairs by a chitin-like cement. Cutting the hair short or shaving the area is helpful in destroying the eggs. The period of development from egg to adult is about 2 to 4 weeks. To be effective completely, an antipedicular agent must kill both parasites and eggs. Should the latter fail to be destroyed, repeated applications of the agent may be necessary to destroy the newly hatched lice.

Scabicides are compounds that are effective against *Sarcoptes scabiei*, the animal parasite that causes scabies in man. The parasite, a mite, thrives where personal hygiene is neglected. After copulation takes place on the surface of the skin, the female mite excavates a sinuous inward-sloping burrow in the corneous layer of the skin. The eggs are laid in the burrow and, after hatching, the larvae and nymphs may exit. To be effective completely, an antiscabious agent must kill both parasites and eggs. Should the latter fail to be destroyed, repeated applications of the antiscabious agent may be necessary. The life cycle from egg to adult parasite is from 8 to 15 days. Sulfur ointment has been a time-honored scabicide, but has now been replaced by more effective agents.

Since many agents possess both antipedicular and antiscabious properties, the pediculicides and scabicides are listed together.

Gamma Benzene Hexachloride USP

[Benzene Hexachloride;   γ-1,2,3,4,5,6-Hexachlorocyclohexane;   Lindane;   Gammexane;   BHC;   666;   Kwell (*Reed & Carnrick*)]

Gamma Benzene Hexachloride is the gamma isomer of hexachlorocyclohexane [C₆H₆Cl₆ = 290.83]. It contains 99.0–100.5% of C₆H₆Cl₆.

The accepted chemical name (hexachlorocyclohexane) is preferred to the official title in order to avoid possible confusion with hexachlorobenzene (C₆Cl₆). The compound is one of the nine theoretical stereoisomeric forms of 1,2,3,4,5,6-hexachlorocyclohexane. It has been shown to have the conformation and, in terms of equatorial-axial notation, becomes 1*e*,2*e*,3*e*,4*a*,5*a*,6*a*-hexachlorocyclohexane.

Preparation—Gamma Benzene Hexachloride is prepared by the chlorination of benzene in the presence of light. The reaction product is a mixture of stereoisomers containing from 10 to 15% of the insecticidally active gamma isomer which may be separated by solvent extraction processes.

Description—A white, crystalline powder having a slight musty odor.

Solubility—Practically insoluble in water; slightly soluble in ethylene glycol; 1 Gm dissolves in about 20 ml of dehydrated alcohol, about 3.5 ml of chloroform, and about 40 ml of ether.

Uses—Gamma Benzene hexachloride, a compound which exists in the form of nine stereoisomers, is widely used as an *arachnicide*. The gamma isomer, the form recognized by the USP and the one most active as an insecticide, finds application in medicine as a *scabicide* and *pediculicide*. As a scabicide, Gamma Benzene Hexachloride is employed in a 1% concentration in a vanishing cream or lotion. The mixture is applied in a thin layer over the entire cutaneous surface (15 to 25 Gm or ml for an adult) and is not removed for 24 hours. A single application often relieves pruritus within 24 hours and is usually adequate to eliminate the active parasites; a second or third application, at weekly intervals, may be required on rare occasions. The presence of secondary infections of the skin does not reduce its miticidal activity, but subsequent treatment with bactericides may be required to control such complications.

As a pediculicide, Gamma Benzene Hexachloride is effective in the treatment of *pediculosis pubis, capitis,* and *corporis*. Usually a single application of the 1% ointment eradicates the ectoparasite. Following treatment, all clothing and bed linen should be sterilized by boiling to prevent reinfestation; wool garments should be dry cleaned.

Gamma Benzene Hexachloride is not readily absorbed through intact skin and, when used locally in a 1% concentration, it is relatively nontoxic. Irritation, sensitization, or toxic effects from local application of the compound have not been reported. The compound is only slowly absorbed after oral ingestion. Nevertheless, poisoning from the accidental oral ingestion of insecticides containing Gamma Benzene Hexachloride has been reported.

Gamma Benzene Hexachloride may also be used in an inert base as a dusting powder (1%).

Toxicity—Toxic symptoms include excitation, hyperirritability, loss of equilibrium, clonic–tonic convulsion and late depression. Treatment of acute poisoning is the same as that for DDT; the drug remaining in the stomach and gastrointestinal tract is removed by lavage followed by a saline laxative; the hyperirritability and convulsions are controlled by large doses of pentobarbital.

Dose—*Topically,* 1% in cream or lotion, or in an inert base as a dusting powder.

Dosage Forms—Cream USP: 1%; Lotion USP: 1%/60 and 500 ml.

Benzyl Benzoate USP

[Zylate (*Upjohn*)]

Benzyl Benzoate contains 99.0–100.5% of $C_{14}H_{12}O_2$ (212.25).

Preparation—Benzyl Benzoate is one of the active constituents of Peruvian Balsam. It is also present in small quantities in other natural balsamic substances. The market supply of it, however, is produced synthetically by the esterification of benzoic acid with benzyl alcohol in a manner similar to the production of ethyl acetate.

This ester may also be prepared by transposition between sodium benzoate and benzyl chloride. The sodium benzoate is well mixed with about 1.5 mol equivalents of benzyl chloride; about 0.5% of a tertiary amine such as triethylamine, based on the weight of the benzyl chloride, is added and the mixture is heated at 120° to 140° for 1 hour. The amine functions as a catalyst and increases the speed of the reaction.

Description—A clear, colorless, oily liquid having a slight, aromatic odor and a sharp, burning taste. Its specific gravity is between 1.116 and 1.120, and it congeals at a temperature not below 18.0°. Refractive index 1.5680 to 1.5700. It boils at about 320° with some decomposition. Its solution in alcohol is practically neutral to moistened litmus paper.

Solubility—Practically insoluble in water or glycerin; miscible with alcohol, ether, or chloroform.

Uses—Benzyl Benzoate is applied externally in concentration of 10 to 30% as a scabicide. It is widely employed in the treatment of *scabies* and is also useful in the treatment of *pediculosis*. Severe skin irritation may occur in some patients. It is usually employed as *Benzyl Benzoate Lotion*.

Veterinary Uses—Applied in the treatment of sarcoptic and demodectic *mange* in the dog. The drug is toxic to cats.

Dose—*Topically,* as lotion over previously dampened skin of entire body, except face.

Benzyl Benzoate Lotion NF [Benzyl Benzoate Application] contains 26–30% (*w/w*) of $C_{14}H_{12}O_2$. *Preparation:* Mix triethanolamine (5 Gm) with oleic acid (20 Gm), add benzyl benzoate (250 ml), and mix. Transfer the mixture to a suitable container of about 2000-ml capacity, add purified water (250 ml), and shake the mixture thoroughly. Finally add the remaining purified water (500 ml), and again shake the mixture thoroughly. A Benzyl Benzoate Lotion, official in USP XIII, may also be prepared as follows: Shake saponated benzyl benzoate (275 ml) with water (250 ml) in a suitable container of about 2000-ml capacity, until the benzyl benzoate is well emulsified. Add the remaining water (475 ml), and again shake the mixture thoroughly.

Uses: This lotion is used for the treatment of *scabies*. It is applied with a brush after the entire body has been thoroughly scrubbed with soft soap and hot water. A second coat is applied when the first is dry and the lotion is left on the body for 24 hours. At the end of that time the body is again thoroughly bathed and dressed in clean clothes. Adults require from 120 to 180 ml; a child from 60 to 90 ml. Do not apply to the face. *Dose:* See *Benzyl Benzoate,* this page.

Betanaphthol—see RPS-13, page 1316.

Chlorophenothane USP

[1,1,1-Trichloro-2,2-*bis*(*p*-chlorophenyl)ethane; Dicophane; Gesarol; GNB; DDT; Neocid; SBLY]

Chlorophenothane contains 96.0–102.0% of $C_{14}H_4Cl_5$ (354.49).

Preparation—DDT was first prepared by Zeidler, a graduate student at the University of Strasbourg in 1874, by condensing chlorobenzene and chloral. The insecticidal properties of the compound were not discovered, however, until shortly before World War II. DDT is prepared commercially by condensing chloral and chlorobenzene in the presence of sulfuric acid. There are several grades of the product. Technical DDT is a mixture containing about 70% of *p,p'*-DDT and 30% *o,p'*-DDT. Purified DDT (aerosol DDT) is a purer grade containing a higher percentage of the *p,p'*-isomer. Medicinal DDT consists of this highly purified DDT, suitable for use in solution directly upon the skin.

Description—Colorless or white crystals, or a white to slightly off white crystalline powder. It is odorless or has a slight aromatic odor, and has a bitter taste. Stable in air. Slowly discolored by light. It congeals at a temperature not lower than 89°.

Solubility—Insoluble in water; 1 Gm dissolves in 40 to 60 ml of alcohol, 5 to 7 ml of boiling alcohol, about 2.5 ml of actone, 3.5 ml of chloroform, and about 4 ml of ether; the greater the purity the lower is its solubility in alcohol.

Uses—Chlorophenothane (DDT) is highly effective in *pediculosis;* it is effective against *head lice, body lice,* and *crab lice.* A simple, effective, and safe preparation is a mixture of 10% DDT powder with talc or any other suitable diluent. For the treatment of head or pubic lice, the powder is rubbed into the hair and allowed to remain for several days. For the treatment of body lice, the underclothes are dusted with the preparation. All contaminated clothing should be thoroughly laundered or dry cleaned to prevent reinfestation. One application is usually sufficient to control pediculosis, but treatment may be repeated after a week, if necessary.

DDT is not an effective miticide and should not be employed alone for the treatment of scabies. See also the chapter on *Pesticides*, page 1274.

Toxicity—When applied locally as a powder, the compound is nonirritating and is not absorbed through intact skin. However, when it is dissolved in organic solvents, appreciable percutaneous absorption occurs. The compound is only slowly absorbed from the gastrointestinal tract; absorption is greatly facilitated in the presence of fats and oils. The fatal oral dose of DDT for man is not known; a dose of 20 Gm has produced severe poisoning, but not death. The signs and symptoms of DDT poisoning in humans are vague and ill-defined; vomiting, numbness, and partial paralysis of the extremities, mild convulsions, loss of proprioception and vibratory sensation of the extremities, and hyperactive knee jerk reflexes are commonly observed. Treatment consists in gastric lavage followed by a saline laxative. Symptomatic therapy includes the judicious use of phenobarbital or pentobarbital to calm the patient.

DDT finds broad application in the fields of agriculture and public health and as a household insecticide.

Dose—*Topically*, **5** or **10%** (in an inert base as a dusting powder) 1 or 2 times a week.

Isobornyl Thiocyanoacetate-Technical

[Thanite; (*Hercules*)]

Isobornyl Thiocyanate-Technical is a yellow, oily liquid containing not less than 82% of isobornyl thiocyanoacetate [$C_{13}H_{19}NO_2S$ = 253.36].

Preparation—It may be prepared by treating isoborneol with chloroacetyl chloride and metathesizing the resulting ester with potassium thiocyanate. US Pats. 2,217,611–2,217,615.

Uses—Isobornyl Thiocyanoacetate-Technical is used as a pediculicide. In combination with dioctyl sodium sulfosuccinate it is used to eradicate both the adult and ova forms of crab, head, and body lice. It may irritate the skin of some individuals. It should never be applied near the eyes or on mucous membranes.

Dose—An emulsion [Bornate (*Wyeth*)] containing 5% Isobornyl Thiocyanoacetate-Technical and **0.6%** dioctyl sodium sulfosuccinate is applied externally in amounts of 30 to 60 ml, worked into a lather, and allowed to remain for 10 min. The preparation should then be washed off with bland soap and water. More than two such applications should be avoided.

Mercury Oleate—see page 1351.

Precipitated Sulfur USP

[Precipitated Sulphur; Lac Sulfuris; Milk of Sulfur]

Precipitated Sulfur contains 99.5–100.5% of S (32.06), calculated on the anhydrous basis.

Preparation—To a slurry of 1 part of lime and 10 parts of water, 2 parts of sublimed sulfur are added, thoroughly mixed, and the mixture is boiled with frequent agitation until all of the sulfur is dissolved. The reaction between the calcium hydroxide and sulfur is illustrated in the following equation:

$$12S + 3Ca(OH)_2 \rightarrow 2CaS_5 + CaS_2O_3 + 3H_2O$$

After allowing it to cool, the clear liquid is decanted through a filter, and the residue is washed with a little water and added to the filtrate. A slight excess of hydrochloric acid, calculated from the quantity of lime used, is added to the filtrate. The acid decomposes the calcium pentasulfide and the thiosulfate with the precipitation of sulfur, according to the following equation:

$$2CaS_5 + CaS_2O_3 + 6HCl \rightarrow 3CaCl_2 + 12S + 3H_2O$$

In actual practice the quantity of sulfur produced is only about ⅔ of the theoretical yield because considerable amounts of H_2S and SO_2 gas, which are initially formed in the reaction, rapidly escape from the solution.

Description—A very fine, pale yellow, amorphous or microcrystalline powder, odorless and tasteless.

Solubility—It has the same solubilities as Sublimed Sulfur, but it dissolves more quickly in carbon disulfide than other forms of sulfur. The USP makes use of this property to distinguish it from the other forms of sulfur. On shaking 1 Gm of Precipitated Sulfur with 5 ml of carbon disulfide it should dissolve quickly except for a small amount of insoluble material represented by the *Residue on ignition*.

Incompatibilities—Sulfur is sufficiently hydrophobic that it sometimes causes trouble in lotions where it tends to float on the surface. Among substances which have been shown to promote the wetting of sulfur and thus aid its dispersion are triethanolamine oleate and benzoin tincture. Trituration of the sulfur with a few drops of alcohol, glycerin, or a dilute solution of a wetting agent is also of some service.

Uses—Precipitated Sulfur is used in the form of the ointment. It is often preferred to the other forms in liquid mixtures because the particles are lighter and more easily suspended. Ointments made with it are smoother than those made with sublimed sulfur. Sulfur is an active *parasiticide* and is of value in the treatment of *ring worm infections, scabies,* and *pediculosis.* Full-strength USP ointment is suitable for these purposes. Sulfur is also actively *keratolytic* and, in the form of full strength official ointment or in combination with other keratolytic agents such as 2% salicylic acid, it is used in the treatment of skin disorders such as *psoriasis, seborrhea, eczema-dermatitis,* and *lupus erythematosus.* The percentage of sulfur in an ointment should be reduced in the event that a patient's skin shows intolerance. Precipitated sulfur is preferred for ointments because it makes a smoother ointment with a greater reactive surface. Prolonged use of sulfur may result in a characteristic dermatitis venenata.

Dose—*Topically,* as a **10%** ointment every night for 3 nights.

Sulfur Ointment USP, contains 9.5–10.5% of S. *Preparation:* Levigate precipitated sulfur (100 Gm) with mineral oil (100 Gm) to a smooth paste, and then incorporate with white ointment (800 Gm) to make 1000 Gm.

Sublimed Sulfur NF

[Sublimed Sulphur; Abric; Flores Sulfuris; Flowers of Sulfur]

Sublimed Sulfur, dried over phosphorus pentoxide for 4 hours, contains 99.5–100.5% of S (32.06).

Preparation—When vapors of sulfur are conducted into a chamber properly cooled, they are condensed in the form of a crystalline powder, which collects on the sides and bottom of the chamber. The yellowish powder is known as sublimed sulfur, or *flowers of sulfur. Ground roll sulfur* is sometimes sold as *flour of sulfur;* it is not identical in physical properties with the official sublimed sulfur.

Description—A fine, yellow, crystalline powder having a faint odor and taste.

Solubility—Practically insoluble in water; nearly insoluble in alcohol; 1 Gm dissolves slowly and usually incompletely (nonvolatile substances) in about 2 ml of carbon disulfide, about 150 ml of ether, or about 100 ml of olive oil.

Uses—Sublimed Sulfur has the same actions and uses as *Precipitated Sulfur* (above).

Veterinary Uses—When applied to the skin, sulfur is *antiparasitic, fungicidal,* and *keratolytic.* Sulfur in the form of a dust or as a dip or combined with cube or derris powder is effective in the control of cattle *lice,* goat *lice,* depluming *mites* and *chiggers* of poultry; and in sarcoptic, notoedric and otodectic *mange* in dogs and cats.

Other Pediculicides and Scabicides

Crotamiton BP [*N*-Ethyl-*o*-crotonotoluidide; *o*-CH₃-C₆H₄N(C₂H₅)COCH:CHCH₃; Eurax *(Geigy)*]—A sarcopticide specific in the topical treatment of scabies, and possessing nonspecific antipruritic action in a wide variety of dermatoses. It occurs as a light yellow, oily liquid with a faint fish odor and is stable to light and air. It is miscible with alcohol and slightly soluble in water. *Uses:* In the treatment of scabies. *Dose: Topically,* 30 Gm or ml of the 10% cream or lotion is applied to the entire body, excluding the head, by gentle massage. A second application 24 hours later is advised to assure complete eradication of the mites.

Sulfur, Washed NF X [Sulfur Lotum]—Purity: not less than 99.5% S. Prepared by mixing 100 Gm of sublimed sulfur with 100 ml of purified water and 10 ml of diluted ammonia solution. Set aside for 3 days and wash with purified water until the washings no longer impart a blue color to litmus. An odorless, tasteless, fine, yellow, crystalline powder. It is practically insoluble in water and alcohol but soluble in about 150 parts of ether. *Uses:* As for sublimed sulfur, but is the form employed for oral administration. *Dose: Orally,* 4 Gm.

Sulfurated Lime Solution NF XII [Solution of Oxysulfuret of Calcium; Vleminckx' Solution; Vleminckx' Lotion]—*Preparation:* Slake lime (165 Gm) with sublimed sulfur (250 Gm), and add the mixture gradually to boiling water (1750 ml). Boil this mixture, with frequent agitation, until it is reduced to 1000 ml, and maintain approximately this volume for 1 hour, while boiling, by the addition of water from time to time. Cool, filter, and pass sufficient water through the filter to make the product measure 1000 ml. The solution so prepared contains as its active ingredient calcium pentasulfide and in addition, calcium thiosulfate. *Description:* A clear, orange liquid having a slight odor of hydrogen sulfide; it is alkaline to litmus. *Incompatibilities: Mineral acids* decompose it with the liberation of hydrogen sulfide and elemental sulfur. See *Precipitated Sulfur* (page 1272). *Uses:* It is usually diluted with 9 volumes of water and used externally in the treatment of those conditions described under *Sublimed Sulfur* most frequently as a *scabicide.* A more concentrated lime sulfur solution, containing about 20% of sulfur and known as *Lime Sulfur Sublimed* is used, after suitable dilution, as an insecticide on plants. *Dose: For external use,* dilute with 9 volumes of water.

69 | Pesticides

Control of insects (insecticides, fumigants, and repellents), rodents,
fungi and bacteria, weeds and plants, and other agricultural pests—
precautionary information

This chapter was prepared by

Ara H. Der Marderosian, PhD, *Associate Professor of Pharmacognosy,*
Philadelphia College of Pharmacy and Science, Philadelphia, Pa.   19104

The use of pesticides continued unabated during
the years 1962–1969 with an increasing number of
products made available in recent years. Close on the
heels of these developments, many Federal laws were
enacted as concern for environmental pollution by
these agents continued. It should be stated at the
outset that while there are uncertainties in the use of
pesticides, the apparent hazards have not been shown
to be any greater today than a decade ago and the
advantages of increased food production and control
of some 27 diseases far outweigh their disadvantages.

To give some idea of the volume of organic pesticides used, the US production of these in 1965 totaled
some 877 million pounds.

Public interest in the protection of the Nation's
health and its resources has led to the expansion of
existing legislation and the firmer establishment of administrative procedures to regulate the marketing and
use of pesticides. The Federal Insecticide, Fungicide
and Rodenticide Act (FIFRA) specifically covers pest
products which are used in agriculture for the production and protection of food crops and meat animals;
products used in the home to control destructive,
disease-bearing, and nuisance insects, rodents, molds,
mildews, and bacteria; materials used in the general
environment to destroy unwanted fish and undesirable
wildlife; products to repel mosquitoes, ticks, lice, and
other vermin from the human body and from pets and
livestock; chemicals to control nematodes; agents
which modify and regulate plant growth (desiccants,
defoliants, etc); and chemicals used to control moles,
birds, predatory animals, and other forms of non-
rodent wildlife pests.

Because the FIFRA required that all pesticides, intended for shipment in interstate commerce, be registered with the US Secretary of Agriculture *before* shipment and the agriculture department was given control over all precautionary statements in the labeling
of pesticides, good enforceable standards were established for proper labeling. In addition, registration
could be withheld until data on efficacy, toxicity, and
chemical residues were made available. Thus, under
this dynamic statute of Federal law, with its registration and enforcement features, proper control could be
effected against untested, improperly labeled, or
adulterated pesticides.

However, it should be stated that the FIFRA provides no control over the actual user of the pesticide
product. It essentially leaves the user with the responsibility for reading and following label directions.
Herein lies the real danger in misuse and abuse of
potentially toxic materials. While some states have
regulatory controls over users and even their licensing,
others have none. It, therefore, behooves the pharmacist who may sell certain pesticides to become aware
of their proper use and hazard potential. He should,

at the minimum, provide adequate basic information
and be aware of how specific details may be obtained,
if the user requires or needs it. The pharmacist also
should be aware that many factors affect pesticides
efficacy, such as their chemical characteristics, rainfall, sunlight, humidity, type of surface applied to,
period of time involved, and amount of pesticide deposited. Further, it cannot be overemphasized that
while commercial processes (trimming, washing, cooking) remove most persistent residues, thorough home
washing of all vegetables is indicated at all times as a
final step.

Another important control over pesticide dispersal
is seen in the Food, Drug and Cosmetic Act which was
amended in 1954 to include pesticide chemicals.
Specifically, the Act deals with the safety of food materials on which pesticides have been used. The current law requires that the petitioner present the Food
and Drug Administration certain analytical and toxicity data, and the tolerances that are safe in order
that these can be practically applied when the material is used. The FDA is continuing research on
multiresidues in foods and new bioassay procedures.

Since the publication of *Silent Spring,*[1] enormous
public interest has centered on the potential hazards
of pesticide use and the pollution of our environment
by their residues. A great number of publications
have appeared which either tend to support the thesis
that the continued wide use of pesticides may be
hazardous (eg, Rudd[2]) and that biologic control based
on balanced ecology is preferable, or tend to support
the thesis that pesticides are an absolute necessity and
residue hazards do not really exist (eg, Whitten[3] and
McMillen[4]). It should be noted that during the past
few years enormous interest has centered on the contamination of our environment by all substances including pesticides. In fact the problem is of worldwide proportions because of the geopolitical nature of
the environmental system. Due to excellent analytical methods, perhaps more detailed information is
available on pesticidal contaminants than any other
pollutant. It may be stated with relative assurance
that most pesticides are biodegradable (including
some of the chlorinated hydrocarbons) and therefore
offer little problem. At least no side effects are known
from this class of pesticides.

However, under certain conditions, the persistent
chlorinated hydrocarbon insecticides (eg, DDT) and
others have caused problems in that they concentrate
in the food chain with consequent harmful effects on
wildlife and fish. A number of well-documented cases
may be found in the literature to substantiate the
death or debility of certain nontarget species. As far
as humans in the US and in other parts of the world
are concerned, studies show a body burden of from
10 to 20 ppm of chlorinated hydrocarbon pesticides

and their conversion products. Thus far, there is no hard evidence that long-term low-level exposure to pesticide residues has been harmful to human health. The few documented cases of fish-kills and the deleterious effects of DDT on birds have led to a widespread popular campaign against the use of this compound. In fact, Sweden barred the use of DDT in 1969 and the USDA has temporarily restricted the use of it in its own programs as of this same year. Much politics and hysteria have brought this state of affairs about and it remains to be seen which direction the continued use or banning of DDT will take in years to come. It can only be stated again at this point that it seems to be a necessary evil until something better becomes available.

Certainly, pesticide-monitoring programs on all phases of the environment should be continued; eg, extensive educational programs and licensing of pesticide users should be undertaken; persistent pesticides should be used minimally and replaced where possible with degradable materials as they become available; more ecological studies need to be conducted on the food-chain concentration factors and other relationships; and finally much more study is required on the ultimate effects of long-term low-level exposure to pesticides on humans, particularly the close scrutiny of any dose–response relationship of pesticide chemicals or derivatives suspected of being carcinogens. Whatever the import of the arguments presented, it seems obvious that synthetic pesticides will be around for quite some time with a slow, steady trend to biologic modes of control as ecologic research makes them available. Some trends are also seen in the direction of the development of more specific short-lived (biodegradable) synthetic pesticides. While it is difficult to predict what the eventual outcome will be, insect resistance being what it is, perhaps every available means will be pursued for many years to come. Put in another way, it is fortunate that there are a wide variety of methods available for pest control including all the synthetics and some of the newer developments; eg, radiation-induced sterility procedures, insect scent lures, juvenile hormones, biologic control, chemosterilants, repellents, etc. As indicated at a recent National Academy of Sciences symposium on the scientific aspects of pest control, the public is safe from either sudden or subtle poisoning by pesticides in the environment and an integrated pest-control approach (specific chemical and biologic techniques) is the trend of the future. It is interesting to note further that investigations are being undertaken to develop insecticide-impregnated containers for storing and shipping use. The wide variety of publications concerned with effects of pesticides on health and the environment (eg, Refs. 5–7) more than attest to the wide concern over the pesticide pollution problem. Investigations reported in these publications reveal some of the deleterious health effects of pesticides through accidents, and through residue accumulations, and even accumulations of pesticides in various organs of flora and fauna passed through the wide food chain of many organisms.

At the same time that these studies continue, the World Health Organization and the Food and Agriculture Organization of the United Nations press for wider use of pesticides to help raise the level of efficiency in agriculture in order that enough food can be produced to stem the tide of the demands of increases in birth rate throughout the world.

Beyond the use of pesticides simply to increase crop yields there exists a whole area of interest which focuses on the pest as a vector of disease. It is well known that insects such as chiggers, itch mites, ticks, and others transport disease to man directly or via foodstuffs and that mosquitoes, tsetse flies, rat fleas, and others are capable of directly injecting disease organisms into his blood stream. In addition, malaria control is effected through use of DDT to kill the mosquito vector of this disease.

Less well known is the fact that plant diseases are carried by the same or similar types of pests which, of course, must be eradicated to prevent loss of valuable plants.

Pest control enters even into areas where livestock must be protected against predatory animals such as coyotes, wolves, bobcats, and others.

While it is difficult to classify all pesticides chemically, it will be useful to list some of the major categories with a few examples in each class:

Organic Phosphorus Insecticides—Chorthion, Demeton, Malathion, Parathion, TEPP.
Carbamate Insecticides—Carbaryl.
Chlorinated Hydrocarbon Insecticides—Chlordane, DDT, Dieldrin, Endrin.
Botanical Insecticides—Pyrethrum, allethrin, rotenone, nicotine.
Rodenticides—Phosphorus, sodium fluoroacetate, thallium, warfarin, Raticide.
Fungicides—
Dithiocarbamates—Ferbam, Ziram, Maneb, Nabam.
Organic Mercury Compounds—Ethyl mercury phosphate, phenyl mercuric acetate.
Pentachlorophenol.
Herbicides—
Arsenicals (tri- and pentavalent arsenic)—Arsenic trioxide, sodium arsenite, Paris green.
Chlorophenoxy Herbicides—2,4,-D (2,4 dichlorophenoxyacetic acid), 2,4,5,-T (2,4,5 trichlorophenoxyacetic acid).
Dinitrophenols—DNOC (4,6 dinitro-*o*-creosol), isopropanolamine.

It should be stated that many of the chemical names given to pesticides are contractions of longer systematic nomenclature which usually serve as nonproprietary names. As with drugs, many proprietary names are featured.

General Suggestions to Pharmacists

The pharmacy is a logical source where one may obtain pesticide and pest control information. However, if the pharmacist desires to handle pesticides and build up a permanent patronage, he should acquaint himself with the common pest problems, with chemicals recommended, and how such materials should be used.

The pharmacist should also keep abreast of new laws which will influence the ways in which chemicals may be used legally. Particular attention should be placed on becoming familiar with the Pesticide Chemicals Amendment to the Food, Drug, and Cosmetic Act dealing with the safety determination needed on the residue of pesticides on raw agricultural commodities. This amendment is commonly known as the "Miller Bill" and was passed in 1954. The pharmacist should also study the Chemical Additives Amendment to that same Act passed in 1958 and fully effective in 1960.

With the above thought in mind, the following suggestions are offered for the control of weeds, insects, and plant diseases:

Contact the entomologist and plant pathologist of your State Agricultural Experiment Station. He will gladly identify insects or plant diseases which are unknown to you and provide the most up-to-date information. You should secure the available publications on weed, insect, and plant disease control from your experiment station. In addition, you should write the Office of Information, US Department of Agriculture, Washington, D.C., requesting a list of available publications. From this list you can order the publications which you need for your reference library.

Many states are holding annual one-half to one day district meetings of insecticide dealers, usually including dealers in four or five counties. Your county agricultural agent can advise you of such meetings and if there is a demand your county agent can probably secure assistance from the State Extension Service for such meetings. Such meetings are helpful in keeping you advised of the materials being recommended for use on the farm and of the new developments.

Since there are many dependable processors of pesticides, the average pharmacist will find it advantageous to obtain packaged materials for their sales. To aid them in contacting wholesalers, the guide known as ENTOMA, prepared and distributed by the Eastern Branch of the American Association of Economic Entomologists, will be found invaluable. It can be obtained by addressing George S. Langford, Department of Entomology, University of Maryland, College Park, Maryland.

For guidance on methods of rodent and predatory animal control, write to the US Fish and Wildlife Service, Department of the Interior, Washington, D.C. for information on the details of the new amendments to the Food, Drug, and Cosmetic Act, write to the Food and Drug Administration, Department of Health, Education and Welfare, Washington, D.C.

Control of Insects

Insects may be controlled through proper application of chemicals by means of suitable techniques.

Classification of Insect Control Chemicals

Insect control chemicals may be classified as insecticides, fumigants, repellents, and attractants.

Insecticides—Insecticides are often classified according to the type of action that results in destruction of the insect. Three broad categories, namely *stomach poisons*, *contact insecticides*, and *fumigants* are generally recognized. Among older insecticides such classification was rather distinct. However, with the new synthetic organic compounds, a single material often produces insecticidal action in all three ways. Certain materials are often selected and used, however, in such a manner as to accomplish control primarily by stomach, contact, or fumigating action.

Stomach Poisons—For control of insects by this method it is usually necessary to apply the insecticide to the food that they consume. Stomach poisons are widely used to control leaf-feeding insects or other pests of plants that will result in consumption of the surface-contaminated material. Stomach poisons are also used in specially prepared baits for controlling a variety of insects. With the rapid advances in employing systemic insecticides it is now feasible to destroy by stomach action certain insects which feed on plant juices or blood and tissues of animals, which in the past were considered vulnerable only to contact insecticides. Systemic insecticides are those chemicals which move in plants and animals from one location where applied to another location where the insect may be feeding. Some of the more widely used systemic insecticides include Systox (Demeton; *O,O*-diethyl-*O* (and *S*)-(2-ethylthioethyl)phosphorothioates), Meta Systox R, and Dimethoate (*O,O*-dimethyl *S*-(*N*-methylcarbamoylmethyl)phosphorodithioate. Stomach poisons include a variety of *arsenicals, fluosilicates, rotenone,* various *chlorinated hydrocarbons,* and the new *organic phosphates* and *carbamates.*

Contact Insecticides—Most of the insecticides in use today depend largely on contact action to destroy insects. *Pyrethrum, rotenone, oil emulsions, nicotine,* and *soaps* have been used for this purpose for many years. However, *chlorinated hydrocarbon* insecticides such as DDT, BHC, chlordane, dieldrin, endrin, etc and the *organic phosphates* such as parathion, TEPP, malathion, etc and the carbamates such as carbaryl (Sevin), are employed most extensively at this time. These contact insecticides are employed against chewing as well as sucking insects.

Fumigants—Fumigants are gases or vapors used for the control of insects, usually in enclosed spaces. The fumigants include *hydrocyanic acid, ethylene dichloride, carbon tetrachloride, methyl bromide, chloropicrin,* and many others. A number of the *chlorinated hydrocarbon* and *organic phosphorus* insecticides have sufficiently high vapor toxicity to cause marked fumigating action against insects particularly in enclosed spaces and in soils. Lindane, TEPP (tetraethylpyrophosphate), Phosdrin (2-carbomethoxy-1-methylvinyl dimethyl phosphate), Naled, and DDVP [2,2-dichlorovinyl dimethyl phosphate] are among the most active in this category.

Repellents—A variety of insect control chemicals possess repellent action. *Citronella* and *creosote* are examples of older materials. *Dimethyl phthalate, ethohexadiol,* and *diethyltoluamide* (see page 1300) are examples of materials more recently developed. Such materials often cause insects to avoid contact with treated surfaces. Repellency in a strict sense might vary greatly as to mode of action. Some insecticides such as pyrethrum have little or no repellent action except on contact. However, the action of *pyrethrum* is so rapid that the spraying of animals may cause flies and mosquitoes to leave after alighting and before biting. Actually DDT, a slow-acting insecticide, may repel insects from treated surfaces after the insects rest on the exposed surface for just a few minutes.

Attractants—The use of attractants to lure insects to poisons or traps has been employed as a means of control for many years. The attractants employed are usually favorite foods for the particular insect involved, such as *molasses, sugar,* or *milk* for houseflies, sugar or *grease* for ants, *bran* for cutworms, *bananas* for cockroaches, decaying *meats* for blowflies, and protein hydrolysate materials for tropical fruit flies such as the Mediterranean fruit fly. In some cases specific chemicals prove highly attractive. Notable examples are *methyl eugenol* for attracting males of the oriental fruitfly, a serious pest of fruits in some tropical areas and a synthetic substitute called "Gyplure" (*cis*-9-octadecene-1,12-diol 12-acetate) developed to replace a sex attractant material found in virgin Gypsy Moth females.

The Needs of Dealers in Insecticides

A recognition of the three important steps in insect control will explain the needs of dealers who wish to develop an insecticide trade and aid their communities in preventing losses by insects. These are: (1) recognition of the type of insect causing the damage, either from an examination of the insect or from the injury it produces, (2) provision of a remedy, based upon the action of various insecticides or other insect control chemicals and upon the life history, habits, and structure of the insect responsible, and (3) application of the remedy, for which the user is largely responsible, although the dealer should be in a position to provide instructions when necessary.

In addition to these three fundamental concepts the pharmacist should familiarize himself with the following information:

1. An understanding of the relative importance of different insects and the relation of the cost of treatment to the increase in value resulting therefrom to the product injured is necessary. Not infrequently the cost will exceed the damage that might be done. If the value of the product is small, the insect may not cause appreciable loss even though it may be conspicuously evident. Again, the damage may have been done before its recognition and the delayed treatment will not affect the insect or aid in preventing the damage.

2. A knowledge of the life history, and of the habits of the common insects is desirable, as all insect control methods are based on a knowledge of these things.

3. The ability to recognize the common insects is a great aid as it is the first step in providing suitable control. The county agents, federal entomologists, and the members of the staff of the respective State Agricultural Experiment Stations are usually available to aid in the identification of insect pests.

4. A knowledge of how insecticides kill, of the relation of types of mouth parts to the kind of insecticide to use, and when and how the material should be applied is useful.

5. A knowledge of the usual insect problems of a community will enable the dealer to carry in stock the insecticides likely to be needed. This will eliminate surplus stocks and will provide the materials which so often fill emergency needs.

6. A knowledge of the toxicity of an insecticide to warm-blooded animals, persistence of residues on plants or in animal tissues, hazard of the materials to bees, or fish and wildlife is important in order that advice can be given on precautions which should be taken in the use of certain chemicals. A wide variety of chemicals is in use today. They vary in their toxicity and hazards to different organisms. The degree of danger is not only governed by the inherent toxicity to higher animals and beneficial organisms in a lower category but also by the manner of use and extent of exposure. A highly toxic material properly applied in small amounts may be less hazardous than a material low in toxicity which is applied in large amounts. The variety of insect control chemicals is clearly apparent by mentioning some of the materials in wide use today. They include: arsenicals, nicotine compounds, various chlorinated hydrocarbon insecticides such as DDT, dieldrin, chlordane, toxaphene, BHC, aldrin, endrin, and heptachlor, and the insecticides grouped under the name *organic phosphates*, which at present includes *parathion, tetraethyl pyrophosphate (TEPP), malathion, dipterex, diazinon,* and the newer carbamates, which include Sevin (carbaryl, 1-naphthyl-*N*-methyl-carbamate) and others.

7. It is important to follow the recommendations for each locality. An insecticide effective in one region may not be in others.

8. It is well to understand the labels on trade-named preparations.

9. The knowledge of the essentials of a good insecticide, its effect on insects, and its availability and cost, will add to the quality of the dealer's service.

10. Those manufacturing and offering preparations such as insecticides, rodenticides, etc for sale on the open market, must familiarize themselves with the various regulations of the individual states where the products are being manufactured or are to be sold. If such products are shipped in interstate commerce, these preparations must also comply with the various federal regulations, especially the Federal Insecticide, Fungicide and Rodenticide Act, approved June 25, 1947, and enforced by the Pesticide Regulations Division, Agricultural Reesarch Service of the US Department of Agriculture, and the Food, Drug, and Cosmetic Act, including Public Law 518, an amendment often referred to as the Miller Pesticide Chemicals amendment.

Information on any insect problem is usually available through the county agricultural agent, the Department of Entomology of the State Agricultural Experiment Station, or the Entomology Research Division, Agricultural Research Service of the US Department of Agriculture, at Washington, D.C. Many of the manufacturers and formulators of insecticides have trained specialists in insect control that can also provide information on insect problems. Most state universities have pesticide, plant disease, and weed control specialists.

Mouth Parts and Relation to Insect Control—In general, insects have two kinds of mouth parts: chewing and sucking. An understanding of the mouth parts and how they relate to the use of different chemical insecticides will often aid in recommending a satisfactory insecticide treatment.

Chewing insects include the *grasshoppers, cockroaches, crickets, bird lice, beetles, slugs,* and *caterpillars.* Such insects have mandibles or jaws which enable them to cut off and take into their stomachs solid tissue. Consequently, an insecticide can be used which kills when taken into the stomach with food eaten by the insect. Most of the newer insecticides, however, are active both as contact and as stomach poisons.

Sucking insects include *plant bugs, leafhoppers, scale insects, aphids, fleas, mosquitoes, flies,* and *sucking lice* on animals. Such an insect punctures the plant or animals but does not take any of the surface tissue into its stomach; consequently, stomach poisons which have no contact action will be ineffective when applied to the surface. During recent years, however, a variety of compounds have been found which are absorbed through the roots, stems, or leaves and transported to various parts of the plant where the chemical is available to sucking insects or chewing insects that feed inside or on the plant or fruit. This class of compounds is referred to as systemics. Insecticides having systemic action offer great promise for controlling insects, and a number of such compounds are now being employed on both plants and animals.

Plants which have been attacked by chewing insects are frequently recognized by the appearance of the eaten areas. Some plant feeders eat the entire tissue as do *potato beetles;* others eat holes in leaves as do *flea beetles;* while some chewing insects skeletonize the leaves as do *slugs* and the *Mexican bean beetle.*

Sucking insects injure plants in different ways and it is often difficult to determine the kind of insect responsible for the damage unless specimens are available. Sucking insects or mites may remove the sap and cause the plant to "stand still," wilt, or drop its foliage; or they may deform the plant, causing the leaves or shoots to curl and become deformed. Some sucking insects, such as the *potato leafhopper* and *tarnished plant bug*, inject toxic secretions at the time of feeding, causing the death of plant cells while others—*plant lice, leafhoppers,* and *striped cucumber beetles*—may injure plants directly by feeding as well as through the transmission of plant diseases. Sucking insects may also affect animals by removing the blood, injecting toxic secretions, causing swelling and irritation, or carrying disease organisms.

Life History and Habits of Insects—In general, there are two types of metamorphosis or development among insects, known as incomplete and complete. Those with incomplete metamorphosis, such as aphids, grasshoppers, plant bugs, and scale insects, have only three stages in development: the *egg* or *embryo*, the *nymph* and the *adult* or *imago*. Insects with complete metamorphosis, such as beetles, butterflies, moths, flies, bees, ants, and wasps, have four stages in development.

In this type, the larva hatching from the egg has no resemblance to the adult, there being also an intermediate resting stage known as the *pupa*, during which remarkable changes in structure take place.

The interrelation of insects, where they hibernate, when they are actively feeding, where they lay their eggs, natural enemies which feed on destructive pests, etc, all have an important bearing on controls. The ant is essential to the life of the corn root aphid and cultural practices which eliminate the ant will likewise eliminate the aphid; the fact that anopheles mosquitoes often rest in homes and other sheltered areas explains the great success of residual type spray such as DDT and dieldrin for controlling malaria which such mosquitoes transmit; a knowledge of the preferred oviposition sites for grasshoppers permits surveys of egg abundance or abundance of newly hatched nymphs to forecast impending outbreaks of grasshoppers.

Methods of Insect Control

For convenience insect controls can be grouped as follows:

Natural Controls—Those which are usually present and which normally tend to hold insects in check.

1. *Natural Enemies*—Parasitic and predacious insects. Every insect is more or less hindered in its increase by other insects as well as by predacious birds, mammals, and other animal life. Although insect-eating birds and certain mammals are important, the insect parasites, predators, and insect diseases are usually the most important factors in natural insect control. In fact, it is probable that outbreaks of insects, such as the army worm, are often due not so much to favorable conditions for the pests as to unfavorable conditions for the insect parasites and predators which normally hold them in check. The use of a specific insecticide against a major pest on a crop might lead to a serious outbreak of a secondary pest because of the destruction of natural enemies which normally keep it in check, particularly if the pesticide chosen was largely ineffective against the secondary pest. Such an upset in the balance between destructive and useful insects is a problem of increasing concern in developing insect control chemicals.

2. *Weather and Topographic Influences*—Summer and winter temperatures, rainfall, soil and atmospheric humidity, and all similar natural factors have their effect on insects and their hosts. No definite statement can be made concerning the effect of these factors on all insects. A severe winter may be harmful to some insects such as those which winter in an exposed condition; on the other hand, such conditions may have little effect on insects which are well protected. Similarly, a severe winter may weaken trees and make them more susceptible to insect attack, or it may kill the fruit buds and deprive fruit-infesting insects of their food. However, it should be remembered that insects have a high reproductive capacity and the seasonal conditions, especially spring and early summer conditions, may aid insects in becoming destructively abundant even though they pass the winter few in numbers. On the other hand, an insect overwintering in large numbers may not be important the following season if the weather is not favorable for increase. In tropical, temperate, and frigid climates there are to be found insect pests peculiar to these areas due to their adaptation to prevailing weather and topographic influences. Topographic features, such as mountain ranges, act as rather effective barriers to insect migration. However, the great increase in the amount and speed of national and international travel and commerce during the last few decades has provided greater opportunities for hitch-hiking insect species to overcome such barriers.

Artificial Controls—Those which are scientific developments of man.

1. *Farm Practices*—Many of our most effective aids to insect control are those which may be called farm practices. These include rotations, cultivation, time of planting, time of harvesting, sanitation, good seed, good fertility, good planting conditions, and drainage. In general, it may be said that the practices recognized as the best garden, agronomic, orchard, greenhouse, or other farm practices, are likewise the best for holding insects in check. Certain insect problems are intensified however, because of changes in practices such as irrigation, prolonged fruiting periods, etc. It is generally recognized, for example, that supplemental irrigation, increased use of fertilizers

and the planting of higher yielding varieties of cotton have increased the boll weevil problem.

2. *Mechanical Devices*—Aside from devices for applying insecticides, there are mechanical devices of value in fighting insect pests. The house screens, fly swatters, insect-proof packages for cereals, and other contrivances may be included in this classification.

3. *Insecticides*—An insecticide may include any material used for the purpose of killing insects or of protecting crops, animals, or other property against insect attack. Insect repellents, fumigants, and attractants are considered insecticides in a broad sense. It is important to note that some insecticides may destroy only certain insect pests and are not effective against all insects.

4. *Parasiticides*—These substances kill animal parasites such as itch mites, ticks, etc.

5. *Sterilizing Agents*—The release of large numbers of insects treated by radioisotopes or chemicals to interfere with reproduction has produced high degrees of control of native populations with whom the sterilized individuals mate. Intensive research to extend this insect control concept is underway.

Application of Insecticides

How Insecticides Kill—An understanding of how insecticides affect insects will assist in explaining methods and timing of applications.

Stomach poisons kill by being taken into the stomach where they are acted upon by the digestive juices, absorbed through the stomach walls, and assimilated by the blood. Details of the mode of action which leads to the death of the insect are not too well known, even for our most common insecticides. However, much information is being obtained on the general nature of toxic action. Available information on the mode of action of the newer organic chemicals is discussed by Metcalf.[8]

Contact insecticides kill by direct or indirect contact with the insect. Sometimes the insecticide may penetrate directly through the body integument; in other cases it causes oxidation and suffocates the insect, dissolves the insect covering, or may prevent settling of the young, as in scale insects, when lime-sulfur has been used. Some contact insecticides are effective only when applied in the presence of the insect, a fact which explains the necessity of the proper timing of applications as well as the importance of directing the spray or dust to the insect itself. Other contact insecticides of the residual type may persist on the treated surfaces where insects rest, such as barn walls, leaves of plants, etc, and kill pests which contact the insecticide deposit.

Fumigants can be applied only in enclosed spaces. Fumigants surround the insect and, being in a gaseous state, readily enter the breathing pores of the insect and kill much as do all volatile insecticides.

Essentials of a Good Insecticide—There are certain important factors which have a definite bearing on the practicability of insecticides. These are: (1) insecticidal or killing properties, (2) effect on the plant or animal or environment being treated under varying conditions, (3) physical properties, such as color, odor, staining properties, adhesiveness, spreading properties, stability under varying seasonal and storage conditions, reaction with other insecticides or with fungicides, consistency, and cost of preparing suitable formulations, (4) availability, (5) cost, (6) safety in the hands of the user, (7) safety and palatability of the food products exposed to the insecticide, (8) ease of application, and (9) flammability or explosive character. All of these points must be kept in mind by those interested in insect control by the use of insecticides, whether researcher, manufacturer, dealer, or user.

Insecticide Formulations—Most of the contact and stomach insecticides cannot be used for insect control as manufactured. They must be compounded in a form that will permit the user to apply them directly or in a manner that requires simple mixing with water or some other diluent before application. Many insect repellents, however, are applied to the skin or clothing without being formulated. The fumigants are also used without special preparation before use.

Insecticides are generally employed in two ways—as dusts or as sprays.

Dust Preparations—Prepared dusts ready for use may contain from 1 to 20% of the active insecticide in a carrier such as talc, bentonite, or pyrophyllite. When the insecticide compound is a crystalline material such as DDT, it usually has to be ground to a fine state so that the finished product will readily flow from the dusting equipment and disperse readily. In dusts made from insecticide chemicals which are liquid, such as chlordane or parathion as examples, the concentration of the active material seldom can exceed 5% and still have good dusting qualities. Special conditioning agents may be necessary and special equipment might be required to make a satisfactory dust product. For this reason the ultimate user is seldom in position to make his own insecticidal dusts from the manufactured insecticide chemical.

Insecticide dusts are used for controlling pests on agricultural crops, in homes, on man, or on animals.

In some instances where it is desired to limit the drift of dust particles and to prevent particles from adhering to vegetation, dry preparations are prepared so that the particles are about the size of sugar granules. Such preparations, called "granular insecticides," are coming into use for treating soils for soil inhabiting pests and for certain other pests such as the European cornborer where the granules collect in whorls or leaf axilla and destroy the young larvae before they bore into the stalk. They are also employed to some extent for controlling mosquito larvae, sand fly larvae, and other insects affecting man. In general, however, dusts and granular insecticides are not used as extensively as are sprays.

Spray Preparations—Insecticidal sprays are formulated in three ways—as solutions, emulsions, or suspensions.

In preparing *solutions* the material may be dissolved in a suitable solvent such as crude or refined kerosene.

The solutions are then ready for use. Many insecticide preparations containing pyrethrum, DDT, Lethane, malathion, Thanite, chlordane, lindane, methoxychlor, etc for household use are distributed in solution form ready for application.

When employed as *emulsions*, the chemical is dissolved in a solvent in combination with an emulsifying agent. It is usually highly concentrated. Such concentrate is intended for dilution with water before use. DDT emulsion concentrates, for example, may contain 25% DDT, 65% xylene, and 10% of an oil-soluble emulsifying agent. Depending on the intended use this concentrate is added to water at rates varying from 1 part of concentrate to 4 or as much as 100 parts of water. Emulsion sprays are used widely in the agricultural field for controlling both plant and animal pests and for controlling household and industrial pests.

Suspensions are prepared in dry form similar to dusts but contain a wetting agent which makes it possible to prepare suspensions in water. These preparations in concentrate form are usually called wettable powders.

The wettable powders may contain from 15 to 75% of the active ingredient depending on the insecticide formulated.

Wettable powder concentrates (25–85%) are added to water for application at concentrations ranging from about 0.1 to 2.5% of the active ingredient. Wettable powder sprays are used on crops, livestock, and as barn sprays. Such sprays are particularly useful for application to plants that might be sensitive to the oils employed for emulsions or solutions.

Other Insecticide Preparations—Insecticides are employed in several other ways. Heat is used to produce vapors or smokes for dispensing lindane for insect control. This method is also employed for treating greenhouses with azobenzene and other insecticides for controlling pests.

One of the most widely used methods of dispensing insecticides is in aerosol form. The *aerosol bomb* developed just prior to and during World War II and employed by the military services has gained general favor by civilians. Millions of the aerosol "bombs" are now sold annually for dispensing insecticides in homes and industrial establishments for controlling flies, mosquitoes, and other household pests. Pyrethrum, allethrin, organic thiocyanates, DDT, and methoxychlor in various formulations are used most frequently as the insecticides. The insecticides are dissolved in liquefied gas such as Freon 12, plus a suitable solvent under pressure in the container. When applied, the Freon volatilizes instantly, leaving the insecticide and nonvolatile solvent suspended in the air as minute droplets which contact the insects present. Aerosols are also employed for applying insecticides in greenhouses. Methyl chloride may be substituted for the Freon for such uses.

The liquefied gas propellent is also being used to apply "wet aerosols" or so-called "self-propelled" sprays. The amount of nonvolatile solvent is increased so that the droplets are larger and will readily wet the surface treated. Such wet aerosol sprays are used for applying insect repellents to the skin or clothing or for applying insecticides as residual sprays for controlling various household insects.

The development of systemic insecticides for controlling plant and animal pests has led to other special methods of use. For control of cattle grubs in cattle boluses containing the insecticide are administered orally. In using plant systemics the treatment of soils prior to planting with a slurry of the insecticide is one of the methods of use.

Equipment for Applying Insecticides—Often failure to obtain satisfactory results with insecticide preparations is due to improper equipment for their application. A knowledge of the type of equipment to employ is therefore important to the supplier of insecticides. The equipment might vary in type from the small hand sprayers or even paint brushes for use in homes to large power sprayers for treating livestock, field crops, fruit or large shade trees. The use of airplanes and helicopters for insecticide dispersal is steadily increasing. The manufacturers of equipment, also county agents, entomologists, and agricultural engineers with state and federal governments, as well as suppliers of insecticides, are in a position to give advice on insect control equipment to the potential user.

Control of Household Pests and Insects Attacking Man

The pharmacist is often asked to provide materials or is asked to advise on the control of insects, ticks, and mites affecting man or those that are pests in homes or industrial establishments. Suggestions for the control of such arthropods are therefore presented below.

General Considerations

The most important measure to follow in minimizing insect problems in the home or on the person is to practice *sanitation* and *good housekeeping*. Many of the pests in homes and industrial establishments, including cockroaches, ants, and silverfish, depend on exposed foods or scraps of food for their existence. Cleanliness will therefore go a long way toward reducing the insect problem within homes, restaurants, and other buildings. Pantry pests, such as grain moths, and weevils of various kinds develop in flour, corn meal, dog biscuits, and many other food products. An open container of oatmeal or dog biscuits hidden away in a pantry for several months can produce hundreds of moths or other pests which may continue to emerge over a period of weeks or months. Obviously, the simplest and best solution for such a problem is to destroy the source of the infestation rather than to use insecticides repeatedly.

A homeowner might be alarmed, and rightly so, when an infestation of fleas is detected in his home. In most modern dwellings the odds are great that the source of the fleas is the cat or dog which has not had proper care. The householder can minimize the danger of flying pests such as mosquitoes and flies getting into the premises by maintaining screen doors and windows in proper condition and by closing any openings into the home. Poorly cared-for garbage containers can be responsible for serious fly problems by attracting adult flies and by providing places for fly breeding. A few tin cans or tire casings which catch rainwater can provide the moisture essential for mosquito breeding on the premises.

It is recognized, however, that in spite of proper precautions, every home owner is likely to be faced with insect problems which must be solved by applying insect control chemicals. In some cases, however, the solution is not simple. It may require knowledge of the habits of the pest, a thorough survey of the problem, and know-how to control the pests involved. Often it is not practical for the owner to attempt to do the job himself. In such circumstances the services of a licensed pest control operator should be sought. The National Pest Control Association is in a position to advise on qualified pest control firms in almost every city. County agents, entomologists in State Experiment Stations, and with the Federal Government are prepared to give advice and furnish publications which will be helpful in many cases.

For insect control in living quarters, in food-handling establishments, and on the person, the factor of safety in handling and applying toxic chemicals must be considered fully. Fortunately a number of efficient insecticides have low levels of hazard to man and animals, although no insecticide can be considered completely harmless. The petroleum oil solvent most commonly used as the carrier in household sprays is in itself sufficiently hazardous to cause toxic effects if the operator is careless in use and permits overexposure to it.

Foods and food utensils should not be left uncovered while insecticides are being used. Care is needed in handling and applying pesticides to avoid excessive inhalation or skin contact. All poisons should be stored so that they are inaccessible to children or where they cannot be mistaken for food. It must also be kept in mind that many preparations containing petroleum oil are flammable or the vapors are explosive.

While stressing necessary precautions, it must be kept in mind that the proper use of insecticides should not be discouraged. Many pests in and around homes are capable of transmitting diseases, and experience has shown that the disease hazard may be far greater than that of the chemicals needed to control the insects responsible for propagating an epidemic.

Ants—Several species of ants are pests in the home or around the premises. In the past, poison baits of various kinds containing *arsenicals*, *thallium*, or other poisons were used to destroy them. The use of thallium sulfate is no longer permitted as ant poison around the home due to its excessive toxicity. Such methods are still effective under certain conditions but the use of newer sprays or dusts provides more effective and more rapid results.

Efforts should be made to locate the colony and destroy it if possible, although inside buildings the colony often cannot be found or may be inaccessible for treatment. The use of suitable sprays applied to the point of runoff on runways and other surfaces where ants have been seen, and along baseboards, borders of floors, window frames, doorsills, and similar places will usually give satisfactory control, although follow-up treatments may be necessary. In general, the procedure for poisoning ants is similar to that for controlling roaches.

For ant control on lawns or in gardens, the best procedure is to locate the ant colony and apply chlordane, heptachlor, or dieldrin emulsion or wettable powder suspended in water. The material may be applied with a sprinkling can, sprayer, or any other convenient method of treatment. A concentration of 0.25% of these insecticides is suggested for treating individual mounds. The amount to apply varies with the size of the colony. A quart may be sufficient for small colonies or up to 3 gallons may be necessary for large fire ant colonies a foot high and 2 to 3 feet in diameter at the base. The surface of the mound or soil should be disturbed by raking and the material poured on and immediately around the nest. A 5 to 6% chlordane or a 1 to 2% dieldrin or heptachlor dust may also be used by raking into the surface of the nest and by distributing on the soil around the colony. A dust is generally less efficient than a spray material.

If the colonies are numerous on lawns or in gardens, it may be desirable to treat the entire area. For this purpose dilute the emulsifiable or wettable powder concentrate with water and apply at a rate of 2 to 4 pounds chlordane per acre or 1 to 2 pounds of dieldrin or heptachlor per acre. As much as 50 gallons of spray material may be required to obtain uniform distribution on an area the size of an acre.

Children and pets should not be permitted to play on the lawns until the area has been watered or rained upon and allowed to dry. It is advocated that the insecticide be washed off the vegetation and into the ground by sprinkling. This will not reduce the efficacy of the treatment.

Chlordane solution is the most widely used insecticide for ant control in homes or industrial establishments. Many ready-prepared oil sprays containing from 2 to 3% chlordane are being marketed. A 2% water spray can also be prepared with an emulsifiable concentrate.

Either a sprayer or paint brush is satisfactory for application of the chlordane solution. A 5% chlordane dust is also satisfactory for ant control although generally less desirable than a solution.

Dieldrin may be used for ant control in the home in the same manner described for chlordane, except that a 0.5% spray is recommended. It should be noted that dieldrin is generally considered too toxic for home-owner use for ant control.

Other Insecticides—Lindane as a 0.5% spray and synergized pyrethrum sprays may also be employed for ant control in homes. These insecticides are less effective than chlordane or dieldrin.[9]

Bed Bugs—The bed bug is effectively controlled by spraying thoroughly the bed frame, springs, edges, and ticking of mattresses with a 5% DDT oil spray or emulsion or with a 0.5% lindane spray. Cracks and crevices, and surfaces behind objects near the wall should also be treated. Bed bugs stay well hidden in such places. Spraying or painting the bed and other hiding places to the point of run off of the DDT solution will provide long lasting control. The treated mattress should be well aired before use.

The occurrence of DDT and lindane-resistant bed bugs has been reported from various parts of the world. Synergized pyrethrum solutions or a 1% malathion spray applied thoroughly as advocated for DDT may be used as substitutes. Several applications at intervals of a few weeks may be required for bed bug control with pyrethrum.

Chiggers—Chiggers or red bugs cause severe annoyance to many people. These mites are most common in southern and midwestern areas. Some individuals are particularly susceptible to chigger bites, especially if they have not previously been exposed to them.

The insect repellents, dimethyl phthalate, dimethyl carbate, diethyltoluamide, 2-ethyl-1,3-hexanediol, Indalone, and benzyl benzoate, when applied to clothing, are excellent to prevent attack by chiggers. The repellents may be applied by hand to the socks, inside cuffs of trousers and sleeves, and the edges of any other openings in the clothing. Additional application of the repellent to the skin on the legs and forearms and base of neck will increase the probability of complete protection. Chiggers seldom attack the exposed portion of the body and are killed or repelled while crawling over treated clothing or exposed skin.

Clothing may be made repellent by light spraying, by drawing the mouth of the bottle along the parts of cloth to be treated (cuffs, fly, etc), or by complete impregnation of the cloth. For more complete information on the use of insect repellents consult the publication by Smith, *et al.*[20]

Although the repellents are highly effective in providing protection against chigger attack, persons often become exposed in areas where they do not expect chiggers to be present. After chiggers attack, there is no known treatment of the bites that will destroy the toxic substance which causes the irritation, although certain local anesthetics such as Benzocaine will provide relief for several hours. A thorough soapy bath as soon as chigger irritation is noted, which may be within a few hours after exposure, will kill those attached and thus reduce the extent of irritation.

If chigger-infested areas are known it is possible to destroy the mites by applying insecticides. Chlordane, toxaphene, and lindane are effective for the purpose. The insecticides may be used as sprays or dusts. Wettable powder or emulsion sprays should be used. Use about 25 gallons per acre of a 1% chlordane or toxa-

phene spray or a 0.125% lindane spray. Dusts as a rule are slightly less effective than sprays but they are also satisfactory. Apply a 5% chlordane or toxaphene dust at the rate of 40 pounds per acre or a 1% lindane dust at the rate of 25 to 40 pounds per acre. Recent information on the control of chiggers is available.[10]

Cockroaches—The German, American, and brown-banded are the most common species found in homes and industrial establishments. Although the efficacy of different insecticides varies with the species, those in common use can be employed effectively in most instances.

Most aerosol formulas contain pyrethrum or allethrin plus DDT. Although intended primarily for flying insects, the aerosol bomb can be used fairly effectively for roach control if applied in considerable amounts directly into the hiding places or liberated heavily in closed rooms. A thorough spray or dust treatment is considered more effective and longer lasting. Many purchasers of aerosols expect roach control in the home by a light treatment. Such treatment, although satisfactory for flies, mosquitoes, and similar pests, is inadequate for good roach control.[11]

Boric Acid and Borax in finely powdered form, applied to hiding places and runways, are used for roach control, although they are less effective and slower to produce results than most other insecticides. The materials are also used in tablet form mixed with food baits which the roaches must eat. When well distributed in office buildings or rooms where there is little food for roaches, they often provide satisfactory control.

Chlordane sprays and dusts are widely used insecticides for roach control. Chlordane sprays, either oil base or prepared from an emulsifiable concentrate, should contain about 2% and dusts should contain about 5% of the insecticide. During the day, roaches usually remain well hidden in cracks, crevices, and behind objects. It is important to know where the roaches hide and where they run. The coarse, wet insecticide sprays are applied to these runways and hiding places so that the surface is wet to the point of runoff. A few puffs of a mist spray will not provide satisfactory control. A paint brush may be used to apply the solution instead of a sprayer, if desired. A dust should be blown directly into hiding places and placed along runways.

During recent years chlordane-resistant roaches have appeared in various parts of the country. This development has created local problems in obtaining satisfactory control and other insecticides must be employed.

DDT can be used successfully for roach control when applied thoroughly. It is not regarded as effective as chlordane. For adequate control, it is necessary to treat all hiding places and runways thoroughly with a 5% DDT spray or a 10% DDT dust.

Lindane as a coarse, wet 0.5% spray applied as suggested for chlordane is also an effective roach insecticide.

Pyrethrum sprays or dusts usually will provide satisfactory roach control. It is necessary, however, to treat with pyrethrum more often than with chlordane to obtain and maintain control. The use of synergists with this insecticide has made it more effective.

Sodium Fluoride has been used with success for many years, although it is generally less effective than the newer materials. It is used undiluted or in a powder containing not less than 50% of the active ingredient.

When chlorinated hydrocarbon resistance is encountered in roaches malathion as a 1 to 2% spray has proved to be an effective substitute. Diazinon (*o,o*-diethyl - *o* - (2 - isopropyl - 4 - methyl - 6 - pyrimidinyl)phosphorothioate) has also proved useful where roach resistance has been a problem. The residual life of malathion is generally less than that obtained with chlordane prior to the appearance of insecticide-resistant strains. More detailed information on the control of cockroaches is available.[11]

Fleas—Fleas are often pests in homes or even in lawns in some areas. Infestations are usually associated with the presence of cats, dogs, rats, or other animals. To prevent recurrence of fleas, the source of the trouble should be treated. For dogs use powders containing 5% DDT, 1% lindane, pyrethrum, or rotenone. For cats, only rotenone or pyrethrum insecticides are recommended, because these animals are very susceptible to toxic effects of chlorinated hydrocarbons. If the source of the fleas is rats, the host animals should be eliminated by following suitable rodent control measures. Actual flea control in homes is usually not difficult. A 5% DDT oil spray applied lightly to floors, rugs, or low furniture will usually provide adequate control. Bedding where dogs sleep should be removed and the area thoroughly cleaned and treated with DDT spray or dust. Ordinary household sprays containing pyrethrum may also be used in the manner described for DDT although several repeat treatments may be required.

In cases where fleas occur on lawns, in dog kennels, or in out-buildings, a 2.5% DDT wettable powder or a 5% emulsion spray applied to infested areas with an ordinary garden sprayer is suggested. About 1 to 2 gallons of spray per 1000 square feet is suggested. If plants are to be treated in the process, the wettable powder spray is advocated.

As with other household pests, fleas resistant to chlorinated hydrocarbon insecticides have been encountered. Malathion as well as Sevin (carbaryl) are excellent materials for the control of fleas in the home or in infested yards. More detailed information on the control of fleas is available.[12]

Flies—For most homes or industrial establishments flies which enter can be eliminated by using ordinary household sprays or aerosols. The most common ones consist of deodorized kerosene, about 0.1% pyrethrins or allethrin, 0.75% of a synergist such as piperonyl butoxide or sulfoxide and 1% DDT. Other formulations may contain 3 to 5% of Lethane or Thanite. Many variations in percentages of such insecticides are included in different formulations. Aerosol formulas often contain from 0.25 to 0.6% pyrethrins or allethrin, 0.8 to 1% of a synergist, and from 1 to 2% DDT or methoxychlor. Thanite or Lethane to the extent of 2% might be used in combination with a reduced amount of pyrethrins or allethrin. The method of using the sprays or aerosols is generally known and usually well described on the labels.

If flies are a serious problem on the premises other methods of control must be followed. DDT and other residual sprays of this type have become ineffective in many areas because resistance of flies to the insecticides has developed. During recent years the use of poison baits has become more widespread. Dry sugar containing 1% Bayer L 13/59, malathion, or Diazinon sprinkled around the premises where flies congregate has given good control. The use of these materials in sweetened liquid bait (syrup in sugar) sprinkled in such places has also been used with good success.

Malathion and Diazinon sprays used as residual treatments outdoors around homes, in livestock buildings (including inside dairy barns), and similar places have recently come into use. Although not as effective as DDT and other chlorinated hydrocarbon residual

insecticides, before resistance developed, these materials often provide good fly control up to several weeks after application. More detailed information on the control of flies is available.[13]

Itch Mite—Many preparations have been employed for controlling the itch mite, or *scabies*. One of the most successful has been the NBIN emulsion discussed for head louse control. DDT does not contribute to the control of the itch mite; but a preparation of this type with DDT omitted and diluted to contain about 11% benzyl benzoate and 2% Benzocaine will provide excellent control. It is important that all portions of the body be treated, and that a bath be delayed for about 12 hours after treatment. A second treatment may be needed after one week although one thorough treatment will usually eliminate the infestation.

Lice—Three kinds of lice attack man. These are the *body louse, head louse,* and the *crab (pubic) louse.* In the United States head louse and pubic louse infestations are more common than those of the body louse.

Body louse infestations can be controlled by regular changes of clothing and sterilization of all wearing apparel and bedding. When the use of insecticides is indicated, a thorough dusting of the clothing with 10% DDT dust is recommended. During recent years, however, the body louse has become resistant to DDT in many parts of the world. The Department of Defense has substituted 1% lindane dust for the DDT in such areas, although resistance to lindane is already suspected in areas where this insecticide has been used for several years. The Department of Defense and the World Health Organization are considering the adoption of a 1% malathion dust if final toxicological clearance is obtained. This substitute treatment if approved will provide a highly efficient material for louse control. Synergized pyrethrum dusts are also highly effective for body louse control. A formula known as MYL developed during World War II consisted of 0.2% pyrethrins, 2% *n*-butyl undecylenamide, 2% Benzocaine (ovicide), 0.25% of an antioxidant in a pyrophyllite carrier. Recent investigations have shown that the synergists piperonyl butoxide or sulfoxide are equally as effective as the *n*-butyl undecylenamide. It has also been found that allethrin is about as effective as pyrethrins in such formulations.

Head louse infestations are readily controlled with 10% DDT powder. One treatment applied to the hair on the head before bedtime will kill all motile stages of the lice, which may be brushed or washed out of the hair in the morning. Because DDT will not destroy the eggs and newly hatched lice will survive if the DDT is removed, the treatment should be repeated about once a week for two additional weeks. If the dust is permitted to remain in the hair without washing for two weeks, a single treatment will usually eliminate infestations. To be on the safe side, however, a second treatment within 7 to 10 days should be made.

NBIN—A liquid preparation developed during War II known as NBIN is exceptionally effective for controlling head lice. The material is prepared as a concentrate containing 68% benzyl benzoate, 12% Benzocaine, 6% DDT, and 14% Tween-80 emulsifier. This preparation is diluted at the rate of 1 part NBIN concentrate plus 5 parts water. Thorough saturation of the hair will eliminate the infestation. The Benzocaine kills the eggs so that a second treatment is not necessary. The DDT destroys the lice and has sufficient residual action to kill stray lice which may get on the head for a week or more after treatment. The treatment does not leave any visible residues in the hair. Pyrethrum powder discussed in connection with the control of the body louse is also an excellent control for head lice. If any members of the family have head louse infestations, it is important that all members be treated with the preparation chosen.

Crab louse infestations are effectively controlled with any of the preparations discussed under *head louse*. It is important that all hairy portions of the body be treated. For DDT two or three treatments at 7- to 10-day intervals are necessary. The NBIN solution diluted as indicated for the head louse will usually eliminate infestations. Although two treatments at 7- to 10-day intervals might be used for assurance of complete elimination.

Mosquitoes—Mosquitoes which occasionally enter homes can be killed easily with the type of space sprays and aerosols discussed in connection with fly control. Mosquitoes often breed in areas several miles from the places where they are serious nuisances. Community mosquito control programs are the only real solution to this problem. A house owner can in some cases temporarily control the pest on his own premises by thoroughly spraying vegetation and other resting places with DDT. The problem of achieving satisfactory mosquito control in a community is usually so complex and extensive that the help and advice of specialists is necessary.

Persons exposed to mosquitoes, biting gnats, and flies outdoors in connection with work or recreation can obtain relief by applying skin repellents. The most common individual repellents available on the market are diethyltoluamide, dimethyl phthalate, ethohexadiol (Rutgers 612), dimethyl carbate, and Indalone. Various combinations of these are also available. All of these materials used as directed on container labels will provide transient relief from insect attack.

In some circumstances treatment of the exposed skin alone is inadequate because the mosquitoes may also bite through clothing. The application of repellents to clothing by impregnation, by light spraying, or by hand will prevent attack. The same repellent materials intended for skin application may be used. Most of the repellents are plasticizers. They should not be applied to rayons and similar synthetic clothing.

Moths and Carpet Beetles—Every home owner is likely to encounter damage due to clothes moths or carpet beetles, often called "buffalo" moths. The damage caused by these insects to woolens and other items such as furs, materials made of animal hair, feathers, etc is very great.

For many years the fumigants, naphthalene and paradichlorobenzene, were the chief means of control. It takes a high concentration of vapor to kill clothes moths or carpet beetles however. Many pounds of these fumigants are needed to eliminate infestations in closets that are not tight or where the doors are opened too often to permit sufficient concentration of vapor. In using these fumigants add crystals, flakes, or balls at the rate of 1 pound per 100 cubic feet and make closets tight by sealing cracks and edges of doors. Since the gas is considerably heavier than air, the fumigant should be placed high in the closet. For protecting clothing, furs, etc in trunks, etc for long periods, add about 1 pound for an average size trunk.

In stuffed furniture it is often difficult to get the insecticide to the infestation. Fumigation in vaults by companies prepared to do such work may be necessary. The use of DDT, methoxychlor, chlordane, and lindane sprays as contact insecticides and as residual sprays is a great aid in controlling moth infestations in homes. All of these materials will kill the different stages on contact. DDT and methoxychlor are not highly effective as residual deposits, however, for killing carpet beetles which crawl over treated surfaces. Chlordane and lindane are superior for this purpose.

In using surface sprays to eliminate general infestations in a home use 5% DDT, 5% methoxychlor, 2% chlordane, or 0.5% lindane. Apply the spray to the edges of rugs, floor area between rug and wall, and baseboards. In closets, treat the entire floors—corners, walls, etc. Apply also behind pictures, radiators, and other hard to clean places. The entire rug may be sprayed with DDT or methoxychlor. Chlordane and lindane are not recommended for general treatments in homes because of possible excessive vapors or skin contact that might be hazardous. Limited spot treatment is advocated for these materials. Other materials such as fluoride solutions are also satisfactory for treatment of rugs and similar items. Directions on the label should be followed at all times.

Moth infestations are destroyed and woolen items effectively protected against subsequent infestations by treating with DDT or methoxychlor. These materials do not kill moths or carpet beetles rapidly or may not even kill at all but they are remarkably effective in preventing moth feeding. Clothing may be sprayed lightly with oil solutions or wet aerosol sprays and aired out and stored. Washable items may also be impregnated with an emulsion. A product called *EQ-53*, which contains DDT as the active ingredient, has been developed for this purpose. The material in emulsifiable concentrate form is diluted as directed on the container and the clothing soaked, rinsed, and dried. Additional information on the control of clothes moths and carpet beetles is available.[14]

Silverfish—For control of silverfish, use the chlordane, DDT, dieldrin, lindane, or pyrethrum sprays and dusts as advocated for cockroaches. Silverfish may be found in many places in the home—basement, attic, around books, and behind wall paper. They feed on the starch material used as glues or for sizing paper. More detailed information on the control of silverfish is available.[15]

Ticks—Ticks are serious pests in some areas. If the infested areas must be used, it is possible to kill the ticks by following the procedures suggested for area chigger control. In addition to the insecticides mentioned for chigger control, DDT sprays or dusts are also highly effective. Protection of individuals from tick attack, however, is fairly effective if clothing is thoroughly impregnated with certain repellents. Emulsions of Indalone (Butopyronoxyl USP XV), dimethyl carbate (dimethyl 5-norbornen-*cis*-2,3-dicarboxylate), dimethyl phthalate, diethyltoluamide, or benzyl benzoate may be used for such treatment.

Insecticides, Fumigants and Repellents

The number of insecticides and repellents currently in use has increased greatly during the past two decades. New synthetic compounds have come into use for many pests for which practical chemical control methods were unknown, and in some cases have largely replaced certain inorganic compounds and insecticides of plant origin. However, some of the more recently developed chemicals are being replaced by even newer materials because of the development of resistance by various insects to insecticides. This is a problem of major significance in insect control. The housefly, for example, has become resistant to DDT and to other chlorinated hydrocarbon insecticides within 5 to 10 years after they came into extensive use. Organic phosphorus insecticides were developed as substitutes but within a few years evidence of resistance to them became apparent. A wide variety of insects affecting man, livestock, fruits, vegetables, and cotton are resistant to one or more of the newer insecticides. Currently the resistant strains are still generally restricted to certain localities. However, authorities in insect control are generally agreed that such local resistance problems are likely to become more widespread with continued use of the materials.

The more widely employed insect control chemicals and their areas of use will be discussed briefly. The extensive literature on the many insecticides may be consulted for further details and the US Department of Agriculture, State Experiment Stations, the US Public Health Service, and manufacturers of specific insecticides are all prepared to provide more detailed information. See also the publication by Metcalf[1] and Brown.[16]

Common Insecticides

Allethrin (*dl*-2-allyl-4-hydroxy-3-methyl-2-cyclopenten-1-one esterified with a mixture of *cis* and *trans dl*-chrysanthemum monocarboxylic acids)—This synthetic pyrethrin-like compound has been developed as the result of basic studies on the complex composition of the active principles in pyrethrum insecticides. It has many of the desirable features of pyrethrum—high insecticidal activity with low toxicity to warm-blooded animals. In general allethrin is effective against the same insects as pyrethrum. For some species such as the *housefly* and the *body louse* it is equally as effective, but against others it is less effective than pyrethrum. At present it can be produced commercially at a cost somewhat lower than the cost of the pyrethrins (principal active ingredients in pyrethrum). This advantage in practical use is offset, however, due to the fact that the insecticidal activity of allethrin is not increased to the same degree as the pyrethrins when combined with synergists available at present.

The development of allethrin is of great significance however. It is now used in household sprays and aerosols as a substitute for pyrethrins or to supplement the pyrethrins. The Department of Defense is employing the insecticide in sprays and aerosols supplied to troops. Research has shown that allethrin is highly efficient for the control of lice affecting man. The availability of allethrin assures a supply of a pyrethrum-like insecticide in the event our source of supply of pyrethrum is cut off or greatly reduced as during World War II.

Arsenicals—The arsenicals including *Paris green* (an acetoarsenite of copper), *lead arsenate, calcium arsenate, calcium arsenite,* and *sodium arsenite* are among the older insecticides. Arsenicals are still employed to a limited extent as dusts and sprays for controlling a variety of *chewing insects*, for use as dips for *ticks* and other livestock pests, in poison baits for *fly* control or for controlling *cutworms*, and as larvicides for *Anopheles mosquitoes*. Due to the development and availability of many new insecticides equally as effective and often less hazardous to plants and animals the arsenicals are rapidly being replaced by other insecticides. However, due to boll weevil resistance to a number of chlorinated hydrocarbon insecticides, calcium arsenate has again come into considerable use for the control of this major pest of cotton.

Borax—This common chemical is employed to some extent for controlling *cockroaches*. It is a slow-acting stomach poison for roaches but is one of the least hazardous insecticides for this purpose. Borax is also employed for controlling *fly larvae* when applied to animal and vegetable refuse at a concentration of 1½ ounces of borax dissolved in 2½ gallons of water. The use of borax for this purpose, largely discontinued for a time, has been renewed to some extent since flies have become resistant to DDT and other chlorinated hydrocarbon insecticides.

Fluorine Compounds—*Sodium fluoride*, one of several fluorine compounds, has served a useful purpose for controlling *roaches* and *silverfish* in homes and industrial establishments. Largely replaced with chlordane for this purpose for a number of years, it is again being used to some extent against roaches that have become resistant to chlordane and DDT. The insecticide has also been employed for controlling lice on poultry as a powder or when dissolved in water and used as a dip. *Sodium fluosilicate* compounds are also used to a limited extent in baits for controlling certain vegetable pests, as *moth*-proofing compounds and other purposes. *Cryolite*, another fluorine insecticide, is used to control such garden pests as the *cucumber beetle, strawberry weevil, tomato worm,* and *blister beetles*. For additional information see the review of the fluorine compounds as insecticides by Carter and Busbey.[17]

Lime-Sulfur—Originally used as a *sheep dip* for the control of *mites* and *ticks*, lime-sulfur in liquid and dry form is now better known as a dormant spray for the control of *scale insects* and as a summer spray for the control of certain *plant diseases*. For the methods of using the lime-sulfur liquid concentrate, follow recommendations on the container. The dry lime-sulfur is not as effective for most purposes and if used as a dormant spray for the control of scale insects, it should be used as 1½ to 2 times the label strength. Dry lime-sulfur is more expensive than the liquid concentrate for dormant strengths but is easier to carry in stock and may be recommended when only a few plants are to be treated. Lime-sulfur is never recommended for use in cities or near buildings as it discolors paint.

Nicotine—This, the volatile liquid alkaloid of tobacco (*Nicotiana tabacum*), is a powerful insecticide; however, it is highly toxic to the nervous system of man and other animals. Nicotine extracts are usually obtained from the stems and refuse parts of tobacco. It is available in two forms, namely, free nicotine and nicotine sulfate. The latter is available mainly as an aqueous solution, containing 40% of nicotine. For the common garden sprays to control *aphids* (*plant lice*) and similar insects, the nicotine sulfate is the form commonly used although dusts containing nicotine sulfate are also available. It kills a wide range of both chewing and sucking insects. Soap or saponin* should always be used with nicotine sulfate unless combined with an alkaline solution such as Bordeaux mixture or lime-sulfur. This is needed to break down the chemical compound and liberate the nicotine, which is the active killing agent.

Nicotine is effective as a destructive agent for *plant lice* and also serves as an efficient stomach poison for some pests. It is water soluble, but should be kept in tightly stoppered containers as it decomposes very quickly. Nicotine, as used, does not injure the most delicate foliage. It is generally considered to be most effective as a contact insecticide when used during the warm part of the day.

Many trade-named insecticides contain nicotine in varying amounts and the directions on the container should be followed.

The following dilution table is for the 40% strength of nicotine sulfate:

Strength	To make 100 gallons	To make 1 gallon
1 : 500	1½ pints 40% nicotine sulfate	2 teaspoonfuls
1 : 800	1 pint 40% nicotine sulfate	1¼ teaspoonfuls
1 :1000	¾ pint 40% nicotine sulfate	1 teaspoonful
1 :1500	½ pint 40% nicotine sulfate	⅔ teaspoonful

Where soap is needed as a spreader, use 1 ounce (1 cubic inch to 1 gallon) or 4 to 5 pounds (or 1 ounce of saponin) for each 50 gallons. The usual dilution for most insects is 1 to 800, although a weaker or a stronger concentration is recommended for some insects.

Free nicotine is used for fumigating greenhouses because the nicotine is immediately volatilized.

Nicotine has lost much of its popularity in recent years, due to the introduction of new, synthetic chemicals having improved effectiveness and equal or greater safety.

Oil Sprays—Oils made from petroleum are among the insecticides that have been used for many years, chiefly as contact insecticides for *scale insects* and *mites* attacking plants. Oils will destroy other insects however, including *aphids, thrips, leafhoppers,* and *eggs* of certain *Lepidopterous species*.

There are two classes of oils used as insecticides: the *dormant oils* and *summer oils*. The dormant oils are applied to more hardy trees during the dormant period. The summer oils are used on fruit and vegetable crops during the growing season. The chief differences between the two types are the degree of refinement and their heaviness or viscosity, which determine in part the degree of phytotoxicity. The oils are applied as emulsions which permit dilution with water and more uniform distribution on the plants. The concentration of oil in the finished spray for citrus usually ranges from 1.66 to 2.0%. Small amounts of insecticides such as parathion added to the oil sprays increases their efficacy against various insects.

Pyrethrum—Pyrethrum is no longer official in the NF. The flowers and their use are discussed on page 1301. Pyrethrum, the

* Saponin is obtainable from Merck and Co.

first widely used insecticide, possesses unusually fast contact action against many insects causing paralysis in a few minutes. Its low mammalian toxicity and its rapid toxic action against many pests are features that are not present in the newer materials.

The active substances, pyrethrins I and II, occur in the oleoresin secretion of certain floral parts (achenes) of the closed or partially open flowers. A maximum of about 1.4% of pyrethrins has been adopted by the foremost manufacturers of pyrethrum insecticides.

Formerly, pyrethrum insecticides were prepared as dusts by using the finely ground flowers or were prepared and used as liquids by extracting the active ingredients from the flowers with special fractions of light petroleum oil, preferably odorless kerosene. Today manufacturers extract and concentrate the active ingredients in products containing about 20% pyrethrins. This concentrate is used to prepare the various preparations employed by the public including dusts, petroleum oil solutions, emulsion concentrates, wettable powders, and aerosol formulations.

Pyrethrum is still used as an ingredient in most household sprays and aerosols chiefly for its *knockdown* effects against insects. It is also used in dusts and liquid preparations for controlling a variety of garden pests and *fleas, lice,* and *ticks* on pets.

The continued prominent place of pyrethrum as an insecticide has been maintained chiefly because of the development of chemicals which when combined with pyrethrum have the remarkable property of increasing the insecticidal activity of the insecticide even though the material added alone has little or no insecticidal properties. This cooperative potentiation is known as *Synergism.*

These compounds include sesamin, piperonyl butoxide, sulfoxide, and others and are called "synergists." The development of these synergists has increased the range of activity of pyrethrins and at the same time permits reduction in the cost of formulas containing it.

"Synergised" pyrethrum combinations, although not so long-lasting as the chlorinated hydrocarbon insecticides, are used chiefly in household sprays and aerosols for *flies, mosquitoes,* and other *household pests,* in liquid and dust preparations for controlling *external parasites* on pets, as sprays for flies on dairy cattle, and as dusts and sprays for controlling certain *vegetable pests.* Synergised pyrethrum powders and liquids were employed extensively for a time in controlling *lice* attacking man during World War II. In view of the resistance to DDT acquired by body lice, pyrethrum preparations may again come into use for this purpose.

Rotenone—This is a useful botanical insecticide and represents the chief chemical constituent of derris (*D. elliptica* and *D. chinensis*) and cubé roots (species of *Lonchocarpus*) and other sources. Rotenone [$C_{23}H_{22}O_6$] is commercially available as such or in the form of derris and cubé roots, sold with assayed rotenone content usually on a 5% rotenone content.

Rotenone is incorrectly classified as a non-toxic insecticide. It can cause skin irritation. Its use for louse control on humans is not recommended since irritation is often produced, especially in the groin region. On internal administration in moderately large doses, especially in the presence of fatty foods, it is very toxic to higher animals. In general, however, rotenone insecticides are considered low in hazard. The relatively small amounts applied and rapid loss of toxic action results in minor residues on food crops.

Its paralyzing action on insects is slower than that of pyrethrum but more certain, with usually no recoveries. As a dry, crystalline powder, rotenone is odorless and relatively stable. It is soluble in alcohol, oils, chloroform, and carbon tetrachloride (used in the extraction from the crude drug and its quantitative determination). It is slightly soluble in water, but the aqueous sprays, particularly in the presence of alkaline soaps, quickly deteriorate and must therefore be prepared fresh before use.

Rotenone dusts at concentrations ranging from 0.75 to 1.0% are still widely used to control pests such as the *Mexican bean beetle, Cabbage worms, leaf hoppers,* and other insects attacking a variety of vegetables. It is especially useful for application to vegetables near the time for harvest when certain of the effective newer insecticides cannot be used because of potentially excessive residues.

Rotenone is also used for controlling insect parasites of animals. It is effective for controlling *cattle grubs,* and is employed also for *lice, fleas,* and *ticks* on pets and livestock.

Sulfur is widely used in insecticide preparations. It was formerly used for controlling such insects as *plant mites, fleahoppers* on cotton, *lice* on livestock, and *chiggers.* The new insecticides available today are far more efficient than sulfur for most insects. However, it is still one of the more effective insecticides for certain species of plant mites. Sulfur is also used in combination with many other insecticide dusts as a diluent. It serves a useful purpose in such combinations in controlling or preventing a buildup of mites and for the control of *plant diseases.* Sulfur is employed as a spray made from wettable sulfur or is used in wettable powder preparations containing other insecticides.

Thiocyanates—There are several organic chemicals, known as thiocyanates, on the market under trade names, which have proved rather successful as substitutes for pyrethrum and other contact insecticides, when used in sprays. The common thiocyanates are *lauryl thiocyanate(Lor),β-butoxy-β'-thiocyanodiethyl ether* (*Lethane*

384), *β-thiocyanoethyl esters of fatty acids* (*Lethane 60*), and *fenchyl* and *bornyl thiocyanoacetates.*

Lethane is the trade-marked name of synthetic aliphatic thiocyanate concentrates and is marketed by Rohm and Haas (Philadelphia, Pa.) as Lethane 384, Lethane 384 Special, and Lethane 60. *Thanite,* the thiocyanate of a secondary terpene alcohol, is marketed by the Hercules Powder Co. (Wilmington, Del.). Lethane and Thanite have been used extensively as household and livestock sprays for controlling *flies, mosquitoes,* and similar insects. They possess rapid paralytic action similar to pyrethrum. During World War II, when pyrethrum was not available for civilian use, the sprays served as satisfactory substitutes. The products are usually employed in oil base sprays in concentrations ranging from 2½ to 5%. Such sprays used on livestock should be applied as a light mist. On dairy cows about 1 to 2 ounces per cow applied at each milking will provide good control of blood sucking flies.

The thiocyanates have also come into use in aerosol formulations. They can be used to replace pyrethrum partly.

Other materials—A number of other insecticides that have been used as pesticides, but for limited purposes include: *Pentachlorophenol* (C_6Cl_5OH), widely used as a wood preservative to control termites, other wood infesting insects, and wood rots; *ryania* a plant product containing alkaloids is used to some extent for controlling corn borers and codling moths on apples; and *sabadilla* another plant product which is effective for controlling squash bugs, lygus bugs, and harlequin bugs.

Chlorinated Hydrocarbon Insecticides

The advances in insect control since about 1940 have been phenomenal because of the development and extensive use of a variety of chemical compounds broadly classified as synthetic chlorinated hydrocarbons. The use of this class of insecticides began with DDT which was first employed in Switzerland, but within a decade a number of new similar insecticides of comparable, or in some instances greater, insecticidal activity came into use. These materials, although effective against similar pests in many instances, vary in their usefulness for controlling insects. Insect species vary in their susceptibility to the different compounds. In addition a factor of great significance that limits the practical use of many insecticides, is the hazard associated with their use. Some of the insecticides possess long residual action—which may be of great advantage in controlling certain pests—but which is an objectionable feature when applied to food plants consumed by man and animals. Some of the materials are stored in fat or are excreted in milk of animals when the residues are consumed on forage treated for insect control or when the insecticides are applied to the animals for controlling pests. Such residues of some insecticides may persist for months while others are eliminated within a few days or weeks.

Obviously it is not possible in this chapter to discuss in detail the many uses for the various chlorinated hydrocarbon insecticides. The formulation to use, amount to apply, method and time of application, precautions that must be observed in avoiding harmful residues on the harvested crop, and many other aspects must be considered. Information on the uses for various insecticides on agricultural crops and livestock is available in condensed form in a Handbook issued by the US Department of Agriculture.[18] Only a brief discussion of the more important compounds in this class and their areas of use follows:

Aldrin (The *endo-exo* isomer of 1,2,3,4,10,10-hexachloro-1,4,4a,5,-8,8a-hexahydro-1,4:5,8-dimethanonaphthalene)—This compound is chemically and physically somewhat similar to dieldrin. It is almost equally toxic to the same kinds of insects and the acute toxicity to animals of the same general order, but it is much less persistent. Therefore, it does not possess the long residual action. Aldrin changes into dieldrin after application to soil or plants. This permits its use for controlling certain *pests on agricultural crops* when timed so that the residues disappear before harvest, but this feature limits its use where a persistent poison is needed.

Benzene Hexachloride (*BHC, Lindane, 666, Gammexane, Gexane*)—The insecticidal properties of this compound were discovered in France and England. The product as manufactured consists of a mixture of isomers. The gamma isomer is most active against insects, but the product sold to formulators may contain from 12 to 99% of the gamma isomer. The almost pure gamma isomer, called *lindane*, is recognized as a different insecticide from BHC, although all grades of BHC depend on the gamma isomer for insecticidal activity. Lindane, because of its purity, is most desirable where the musty odor of the cruder products is objectionable. It is also regarded safer from the standpoint of chronic toxicity because some of the other isomers present in the cruder grades are regarded more toxic chronically and are more persistent as residues on foods. It is the official (USP) form.

Gamma BHC is active against a wider variety of *insects, ticks*, and *mites* and is generally effective at lower dosages than is DDT. In practical insect control, however, it may or may not be more useful. The chief advantage of DDT over BHC in this regard is its longer residual action. BHC has wide uses for controlling *pests on cotton* and other crops where the odor is not a factor. Many food products retain the musty odor when exposed to BHC; therefore, its use on food and field crops is restricted. See also *Gamma Benzene Hexachloride*, page 1270.

Lindane is used in household sprays and dusts on livestock and other animals and for controlling some *pests on fruits and vegetables*. When *lice* resistant to 10% DDT powder appeared in Korea the Department of Defense substituted a 1% lindane dust for controlling this insect attacking man.

The acute oral toxicity of lindane to animals is somewhat higher than DDT, but when absorbed through the skin it is more toxic than DDT. Lindane possesses high insecticidal activity in vapor form. This property has resulted in certain restricted use for the compound in devices that generate vapors with the aid of heat.

Chlordane (*Velsicol 1068, CD-68, Octachlor, Octa-Klor*) (1,2,4,5,-6,7,8,8 - octachlor - 2,3,3a,4,7,7a - hexahydro - 4,7 - methanoindene)—This insecticide, developed in the United States, is a viscous amber-colored liquid, nearly odorless. It is readily soluble in a wide variety of solvents. Commercial preparations are available as solutions, emulsifiable concentrates, wettable powders, and dusts.

Chlordane is distinctly superior to DDT and gamma BHC for controlling a number of species of insects and is about equally as effective against others. The chief uses of chlordane are for controlling such household pests as *cockroaches* and *ants*, a variety of insects that live in soils such as *rootworms, ants*, and *wireworms*, and general feeders such as *grasshoppers*. Chlordane is also among the most effective of the available insecticides for controlling *lice, ticks*, and other *animal parasites*. In recent years resistance to chlordane has become widespread among cockroaches, and its use for this purpose has declined.

The insecticide has rather low acute oral and moderate dermal toxicity. It is reported to be highly toxic chronically, which limits its use under circumstances where foods might be contaminated.

Chlorbenside [*p*-chlorobenzyl sulfide]—This is a new miticide with limited use at present.

DDT (dichloro-diphenyl-trichloroethane; 1,1,1-trichloro-2,2-bis-(*p*-chlorophenyl)ethane)—This is a crystalline material, practically odorless, with low vapor pressure and high toxic action to a wide range of insects. One of its chief uses is in the field of medical entomology particularly for controlling *mosquito larvae and adults, flies, body lice, bedbugs*, and *fleas*. It is also of great value for controlling pests of livestock, farm crops, forest and shade trees and stored products. In spite of the development of a number of newer materials, DDT is still the leading insecticide in use today. It should be noted that the use of DDT is slowly declining due to its persistence and ubiquitous nature. Recent research has indicated its accumulation and storage in various members of the food chain with possible long-term deleterious results.

A disturbing feature in the long range use of this insecticide is the phenomenon of resistance that is appearing among a long list of insect pests. Flies, mosquitoes, body lice, bedbugs, codling moth, potato beetles, flea beetles, cabbage worms, leafhoppers are among the insects that have become resistant to DDT in many areas. However, many other insects are still controlled effectively with this insecticide after more than a decade of use.

DDT is formulated in many types of preparations—dusts, oil solutions, emulsions, wettable powders for suspension sprays, and as aerosols.

DDT has a relatively low acute toxicity to animals. The chief toxicity hazard is in prolonged consumption of residues in foods. Its persistence as residues and the tendency to store in fatty tissues of animals and to be excreted in the butter fat of milk leads to many restrictions in its use where foods or feed might be contaminated. See *Chlorophenothane* (page 1271).

Dieldrin (The *endo-exo* isomer of 1,2,3,4,10,10-hexachloro-6,7-epoxy - 1,4,4a,5,6,7,8,8a - octahydro - 1,4:5,8 - dimethanonaphthalene)—This is a white granular material. It is one of the most potent chlorinated hydrocarbons in use today. It controls a wider range of

pests than DDT. The main disadvantage of dieldrin is its rather high toxicity both orally and dermally as well as its high chronic toxicity to animals. It has properties similar to DDT in regard to its accumulation in fatty tissues of animals and its excretion in milk. These unfavorable features together with its high chronic toxicity have limited the use of dieldrin to a great extent.

The generally higher insecticidal action permits considerably lower rates of application than needed for satisfactory insect control with most of the other related insecticides. As a consequence, the practical hazards of use may not exceed those of many other chlorinated hydrocarbon insecticides.

Dieldrin insecticides are available principally as dusts and as emulsifiable and wettable powder concentrates. The formulations are used extensively for controlling *cotton insects, grasshoppers*, certain *soil insects, mosquitoes, cockroaches, ants*, and for treatment of fruits, vegetables, and forage when such use will not lead to residues on the harvested crops. Dieldrin is being employed in some parts of the world as a residual spray for *Anopheles mosquito* control where malaria is a serious problem.

Endrin   (1,2,3,4,10,10-hexachloro-6,7-epoxy-1,4,4a,5,6,7,8,8a-octahydro-1,4:5,8-*enda-endo*-dimethanonaphthalene)—Endrin is one of the newer chlorinated hydrocarbon insecticides which is highly effective against many pests, but it has high toxicity for man and animals. It is employed extensively for controlling most of the *cotton* and *tobacco insects*.

Ethyl 4,4′-dichlorobenzilate [Trademark: Chlorobenzilate]—This is a new acaricide–miticide with a growing popularity.

Heptachlor (1,4,5,6,7,8,8 - heptachloro - 3a,4,7,7a - tetrahydro - 4,7 - methanoindene)—This compound is a crystalline solid chemically related to chlordane. It is highly active against a wide range of insects. Its acute toxicity to animals is higher than that of chlordane, although the fact that its insecticidal activity is generally somewhat higher also permits lower rates of application in insect control.

Heptachlor is effective for controlling *soil insects*, and certain *pests attacking vegetables* and *fruits*. It is used for controlling certain ants, including the imported fire ant, a species of major importance in the southern states. Its usefulness was reduced drastically on January 19, 1960, when the Food and Drug Administration cancelled existing tolerances.

Methoxychlor (1,1,1-trichloro-2,2-*bis*(*p*-methoxyphenyl)ethane)—This insecticide has chemical and physical properties quite similar to DDT. It is generally less effective than DDT, although for some species of insects it is equally toxic. The chief advantage of methoxychlor over other chlorinated hydrocarbon insecticides is its low hazard to animals. It is satisfactory for controlling *flies* and other *household pests*, including clothes *moths, flies* and *lice* on livestock, *Mexican bean beetles*, and a variety of other *insects* attacking *fruit, vegetable*, and *forage crops*.

Methoxychlor is one of the few chlorinated hydrocarbon insecticides that is not readily stored in animal fat or excreted in milk when consumed as residues on forage crops. For this reason it is employed for controlling a number of insects on livestock feeds and forage. Until recent years it was also employed as a spray for controlling flies and lice on dairy cows. Small amounts of methoxychlor appear in milk, however, when applied to dairy cows and in view of the zero tolerance for this material in milk it is no longer recommended for this purpose.

TDE (dichloro-diphenyl-dichloroethane; 1,1-dichloro-2,2-bis(*p*-chlorophenyl)ethane)—The compound, chemically and physically similar to DDT, is useful against many of the same insects that are controlled by DDT but on the average is less effective. By ingestion TDE is considerably less toxic to animals than is DDT but has similar properties in regard to storage in fat and excretion in milk.

TDE is employed for controlling a number of *pests on vegetables and tobacco*. In the medical entomology field TDE is about equal to DDT against *mosquito larvae* but inferior against the adults.

Toxaphene ($C_{10}H_{10}Cl_8$)—This compound, developed in the United States, is the reaction product of chlorine with camphene. The structure of the compound is not known. The technical product, a waxy cream-colored material, consists of a mixture of chlorinated camphenes.

The chief uses of toxaphene are in the control of *cotton insects, ticks, lice and flies* on livestock, *armyworms, cutworms, grasshoppers, cabbage worms, plant bugs on alfalfa*, and a variety of other insects. One of the chief advantages of toxaphene over other chlorinated hydrocarbons is its low toxicity to honey bees. It is not used to a great extent against insects affecting man although quite effective against *mosquito larvae, ticks, chiggers*, and *fleas*.

The acute oral and dermal toxicity of toxaphene to animals is considerably higher than for DDT. Its chronic toxicity is reported to be somewhat lower than that of DDT. Toxaphene does not accumulate to any large extent in fat of livestock. It is one of the most toxic of the chlorinated hydrocarbon insecticides to fish.

Toxaphene is available principally as dusts, and as emulsifiable and wettable powder concentrates.

Miticides—A variety of synthetic organic insecticides are now in use for controlling mites on plants in addition to the older insecticides such as sulfur and the organic phosphates which are discussed below. Among the compounds used special mention is made of Ovex (*p*-chlorophenyl *p*-chlorobenzenesulfonate), Dimite (4,4'-dichloro-*alpha*-methylbenzhydrol), Aramite 2-(*p*-tert-butylphenoxy)-1-methylethyl 2-chloroethyl sulfite, and Kelthane, 1,1-bis(*p*-chlorophenyl)-2,2,2-trichloroethanol, which is receiving extensive usage on fruits and vegetables. These miticides may be used as dusts or sprays. They are often combined with other insecticide applications or in insecticide-fungicide applications.

Organic Phosphorus Compounds

A large variety of organic compounds of phosphorus possess high insecticidal activity. They are often referred to as organophosphorus compounds. Some of these compounds also have unusually high potency as miticides, and many are also extremely toxic to man and other warm-blooded animals.

A number of human fatalities in the United States and other parts of the world have occurred as a result of exposure to phosphate insecticides and many other persons have suffered ill effects. It is important, therefore, that the more toxic of these insecticides be handled with extreme caution and strictly in accordance with recommendations outlined by the manufacturer and federal and state agencies.

The reputation of the organic phosphorus insecticides is such that to the uninformed most compounds in this class are regarded as being dangerous to use. This is a misconception. The mammalian toxicity of some of the compounds is of a low order and they can be handled with no more danger than that associated with the use of a number of the synthetic chlorinated hydrocarbon insecticides which are employed without serious toxic reactions.

The organophosphorus compounds will control a wide range of pests and disease carriers. Certain of these compounds possess systemic action, a characteristic that offers great promise for controlling important insect pests of crops as well as livestock.

The organic phosphorus insecticides are used extensively, in many instances replacing in part, at least, some of the chlorinated hydrocarbons and older insecticides such as rotenone. This trend is due to several factors. Resistance to the chlorinated hydrocarbons by a number of pests has necessitated substitute materials possessing a different mode of insecticidal action. Several of the organic phosphorus compounds do not accumulate in meat and milk as readily as do certain chlorinated hydrocarbon insecticides when consumed as residues on forage crops.

The phosphorus insecticides have not been in use as long as the older materials and relatively few insects have become resistant to them. There is no assurance, however, that many pests will not in time become resistant to the phosphorus materials. A number of species of mites on plants became resistant within a few years, and, as already mentioned, the house fly has also developed resistance to certain organic phosphorus compounds. There is some evidence, however, that in some insect species, resistance to the phosphorus insecticides does not develop to the high level encountered among the chlorinated hydrocarbons.

Organic phosphorus insecticides generally destroy a wide range of insect species. Consequently, their use often kills many parasites, predators, and pollinating insects as well as the destructive pests.

The more widely used organic phosphorus insecticides are briefly described, and some of their more important uses are given. For more detail, the general references previously cited should be consulted.

Ciodrin (dimethyl phosphate of α-methylbenzyl-3-hydroxy-*cis*-crotonate)—An insecticide for control of animal parasites and for premises use.

Co-Ral [(Bayer 21/199) (*O*-(chloro-4-methylumbelliferone) *O*,*O*-diethylphosphorothioate)]—This compound is one of the newer organophosphorus insecticides that is gaining prominence as a systemic insecticide for controlling cattle grubs (Hypoderma spp.). It is a slightly brownish crystalline material with a weak pleasant odor. Co-Ral is best known at present for its systemic action for cattle grub control when applied as a dermal spray, but it is also an excellent contact insecticide. It is employed for fly control in barns and for application to livestock for the control of the screw-worm, lice, horn flies, and ticks. Co-Ral is moderate in toxicity being much less toxic than parathion but more toxic than malathion. When applied to livestock as a spray, it is employed in concentrations ranging from 0.25 to 0.5%.

Demeton—This is a mixture of *O*,*O*-diethyl *S* (and *O*)-2(ethylthio) ethyl phosphorothioates. A commercial product called Systox contains demeton. Demeton possesses systemic action. It is an amber-colored liquid with a somewhat unpleasant odor. Demeton is absorbed by plants when applied to foliage, to trunks of the plant, or to the seed. It is also taken up by the roots when mixed with soil. When absorbed by the plant, it becomes available to sucking insects such as plant lice, scale insects, leafhoppers, thrips, and the mites. It has also been shown experimentally to kill certain leaf-feeding lepidopterous larvae, larvae of fruit flies, and even boll weevils on cotton. It is employed in insect control on potatoes, apples, cotton, walnuts, and certain ornamental plants primarily as a foliage spray or dust. It possesses contact action, but its main action is systemic.

Demeton is regarded as one of the most desirable insecticides for controlling aphids on alfalfa because, through systemic action, the aphids are controlled without serious kill of the parasites and predators. This is an example of successful integration of an insecticide with biological control agents to obtain satisfactory control of insects. Demeton is in the same category as parathion and TEPP so far as mammalian toxicity is concerned. It must, therefore, be used with equal caution. The methyl analogue of demeton, called methyl-demeton, has also come into use as a systemic. It has insecticidal action similar to demeton. For certain aphids it seems to provide longer lasting control.

Diazinon [*O*,*O*-diethyl *O*(2-isopropyl-4-methyl-6-pyrimidinyl) phosphorothioate]—This compound, an amber-colored liquid with a somewhat objectionable odor in its technical form, is an excellent insecticide. It is less toxic than parathion but more so than malathion to warm-blooded animals. Diazinon is highly toxic to flies as a contact and residual spray as well as a stomach poison and is in use for controlling these insects both as sprays and in poison baits. It is also effective against aphids, mites, leafhoppers, the codling moth, fruitflies, cabbage worms, mosquitoes, roaches, and other insects.

Dibrom (1,2-dibromo-2,2-dichloroethyl dimethylphosphate) (Naled)—A broad-spectrum insecticide for both plant protection and premises use.

Dipterex [*O*,*O*-dimethyl 2,2,2-trichloro-1-hydroxyethylphosphonate]—This compound is a white solid without objectionable odor; it is somewhat soluble in water. The material also known as Bayer L 13/59 is used in poison baits for controlling flies. The toxicity of Dipterex to warm-blooded animals is reported to be of a low order.

EPN [*O*-ethyl *O*-*p*-nitrophenyl phenylphosphonothioate]—EPN, an amber liquid, is effective against a wide range of pests, including aphids, mites, scale insects, the European corn borer, mosquito larvae, boll weevil, pink bollworm, codling moth, plum curculio, and others. It is slightly less toxic to warm-blooded animals than parathion but merits the same degree of extreme caution in its use.

Guthion [*O*,*O*-dimethyl *S*-(4-oxo-3H-1,2,3-benzotriazine-3-methyl) phosphorodithioate]—This compound, also known as Bayer 17147, is a crystalline material relatively insoluble in water.

It has a wide spectrum of activity as a contact insecticide for the control of insect pests. It is generally more persistent on plants than other commonly used organophosphorus insecticides. The material is employed as a dust or spray. Although the toxicity of guthion is somewhat lower than parathion, it is in the class of highly toxic materials and must be handled with extreme precaution. Guthion is finding wide use for controlling cotton insects, particularly the boll weevil, which has become resistant to chlorinated hydrocarbon insecticides. Guthion is also highly effective for the control of fruit pests such as the plum curculio, codling moth, stink bugs, aphids, and mites.

Malathion—This phosphorus compound, *S*-[1,2-bis(ethoxycarbonyl)ethyl] *O*,*O*-dimethyl phosphorodithioate, as produced commercially, is a light amber liquid, having a sulfur-like odor. It is relatively low in toxicity to most warm-blooded animals and is active against a wide range of insects, although in general it is less effective than parathion or TEPP. The much lower toxicity to warm-blooded animals and rapid loss of residues on plants makes it an acceptable insecticide for many uses.

Malathion is used extensively for controlling insects on vegetables.

fruits, and cereal and forage crops as well as for controlling insects affecting man and animals. The residues disappear in a few days to two weeks, thus permitting application near the harvest period. The compound is available commercially as emulsifiable concentrates, wettable powders, and as dusts.

Parathion [*O,O*-diethyl *O-p*-nitrophenyl phosphorothioate]—This compound is a brownish liquid. It is highly active against most insects. Its use is restricted, however, by its high toxicity to man and animals. Parathion insecticides are available commercially as dusts and as emulsifiable and wettable powder concentrates for mixing sprays.

Parathion is especially useful for controlling aphids, spider mites, and scale insects but is also effective against many other insect pests, including leaf feeding insects, certain soil pests, corn borers, and mosquitoes. The insecticidal action is primarily by contact, but it also has powerful stomach action. Its vapor pressure and toxicity in vapor form are sufficiently high to result in marked fumigating action against some insects although the compound is not classed as a fumigant. Parathion is not excreted in milk or stored in tissues of animals when consumed as residues on feed crops. It is, therefore, of considerable interest for use on feed crops for insect control.

The hazards of parathion are so great that it is often advocated that the compound be used only by or under the supervision of persons who fully understand the precautions that should be followed in handling and applying the insecticide. There is danger in handling and mixing the insecticide. It is readily absorbed through the skin. When sprays are used without protective equipment, toxic reactions may result; also there is danger in prolonged exposure to the usual dusts or sprays.

Methyl Parathion—This is a compound closely related to parathion and has insecticidal and toxic properties somewhat similar to it. Methyl parathion is employed for controlling mites, aphids, thrips, and other insects, including such pests as the boll weevil.

Phorate [*O,O*-diethyl *S*-(ethylthiomethyl) phosphorothioate) Thimet]—A limited-use systemic insecticide.

Phosdrin [1-methoxycarbonyl-1-propen-2-yl dimethyl phosphate]—This compound, originally known as Shell OS-2046, is a relatively new organophosphorus compound that is finding a place for the control of a variety of agricultural pests. Phosdrin is a liquid material, miscible with water and quite volatile. The toxicity of phosdrin is high, and it must be employed with extreme precaution such as that required for parathion.

The insecticide destroys insects both as a contact and stomach poison. The residue disappears rather rapidly from treated plants which makes it particularly desirable for controlling pests on crops near the harvest time. The insecticide is useful for controlling such pests as aphids, mites, flea beetles, cutworms, and army worms.

Phosphamidon [2-chloro-2-diethylcarbamoyl-1-methylvinyl dimethyl phosphate]—Another phosphate gaining increased use.

TEPP [tetraethyl pyrophosphate]—This compound is present in the manufactured product to the extent of about 40%. It is a dark amber to colorless liquid, readily miscible with water, but not miscible with petroleum oils such as kerosene.

TEPP is rapidly hydrolyzed in the presence of water. Its insecticidal activity is, therefore, short lived after dilution. It is extremely toxic to insects, however, and will control such insects as aphids, spider mites, and thrips at low rates of application. The rapid loss of the toxicant after application makes this a valuable insecticide for use in controlling insects on food crops that are to be harvested within a few days.

The acute toxicity of TEPP to warm-blooded animals is somewhat higher than that of parathion. Therefore, it must be used with extreme caution.

Thimet [*O,O*-diethyl *S*-(ethylthio)methyl phosphorodithioate]—Thimet is a liquid material with an objectionable odor. It is relatively insoluble in water. It is one of the more toxic of the organophosphorus insecticides and must be handled with extreme caution. Thimet is primarily systemic in action and is readily absorbed by the roots of plants when applied to the seeds or when added to the soil. Thimet has had limited use for controlling aphids, spider mites, thrips, leafhoppers, and certain other insects on cotton and sugar beets.

Trolene [(Dow ET-57); Korlan (*O,O*-dimethyl *O*-(2,4,5-trichlorophenyl) phosphorothioate]—This compound, a crystalline material, is under development for use against a variety of insect pests affecting animals and plants. It is currently best known as a systemic for controlling cattle grubs. For this purpose it is administered by mouth in bolus form. The commercial product is known as Trolene or Dow ET-57. The same compound, less highly purified, has been designated by the name Korlan and is under development as a contact insecticide for controlling both plant and animal pests. The compound is low to moderate in toxicity to warm-blooded animals. The oral dosage rate for cattle grub control is 100 to 110 mg of Trolene per Kg of body weight of the host.

Other Organic Phosphorus Insecticides—The list of organic phosphorus insecticides coming into use for controlling plant pests or the pests and disease vectors attacking man is steadily growing. In addition to those already discussed, mention should be made of: **DDVP** [2,2-dichlorovinyl dimethyl phosphate]; **Delnav** [dioxathion; 2,3-*p*-dioxanedithiol *S,S*-bis(*O,O*-diethyl phosphorodithioate]; **Di-Syston** [*O,O*-Diethyl *S*-2-(ethylthio)ethyl phosphorodithioate]; **Ethion** [*O,O,O',O'*-tetraethyl *S,S'*-methylene bisphosphorodithioate]; **Romnel** [*O,O*-dimethyl *O*-(2,4,5-trichlorophenyl) phosphorothioate]; **Thiodan** endosulphan [6,7,8,9,10,10-hexachloro-1,5,5a,6,9,9a - hexahydro - 6,9 - methano - 2,4,3 - benzodioxathiepin-3-oxide]; and **Trithion** [(carbophenothion), *S*-(*p*-chlorophenylthio) methyl *O,O*-diethyl phosphorodithioate].

Carbamate Insecticides

The new group of synthetic organic insecticides classed as carbamates is becoming of increasing importance as the search for new insecticides continues. The carbamates, like the organic phosphorus compounds, inhibit insect cholinesterases. Their mode of action is sufficiently different, however, for them to be regarded as a separate class of compounds. The carbamates are having increased use for insect control. A material first called "Sevin" but now known as "carbaryl" is being developed for controlling a number of insects. However, it is highly toxic to bees.

The carbamates of most interest at the present time include **Dimetan** [5,5-dimethyl-3-oxo-1-cyclohexen-1-yl dimethylcarbamate]; **Isolan** [1-isopropyl-3-methyl-5-pyrazolyl dimethylcarbamate]; **Pyrolan** [3-methyl-1-phenyl-5-pyrazolyl dimethylcarbamate]; and **Carbaryl** [1-naphthyl *N*-methylcarbamate].

The carbamates of interest as insecticides are moderate to low in toxicity to higher animals.

The compound carbaryl is relatively low in mammalian toxicity. The compound is a crystalline solid, slightly colored, and nearly odorless. It is highly effective against a wide range of insects including codling moth, Mexican bean beetle, cabbage worms, gypsy moth, boll weevil, and pink bollworm. It is not highly effective against most insects of medical importance or against mites affecting plants. It is highly toxic to the honey bee.

New Methods of Insect Control—In order to reduce the dangers of persistent residues, extensive research is underway on new methods of insect control. Three experimental procedures are showing promise and should be discussed briefly here.

The first of these is the use of irradiation to destroy the breeding capacity of the insect. Certain insects breed only once, and when the female of such a species is mated with a sterile mate, that female will not produce fertile eggs. Advantage has been taken of this biological fact in controlling the screw worm—a serious pest of cattle in the southern United States. In this operation males are irradiated with controlled doses of radioactive cobalt and are then released in tremendous numbers in the areas to be protected. Preliminary results have been so promising that this procedure is being considered for use against other species of insects with the same biological characteristics.

A second new procedure is to distribute spores of organisms which are pathogenic for certain insect species only. A strain of spores, *Bacillus thuringiensis*, has been shown to have value in controlling a small number of insect species.

The third method is the use of certain of the silica aerogels which act on soft-bodied insects by desiccation. Since the silica aerogels are exceedingly low in toxicity to humans, residues may be insignificant.

Fumigants

Fumigants have and still are being used extensively for controlling a wide range of insects. Homes, industrial establishments, ships, and other structures may be fumigated to control household or structural pests. Large amounts of fumigants are employed to control pests in grains and woolens, in soil, and in living plants or plant products such as nursery stock, fruits, and vegetables.

The most comon fumigants and their uses are briefly discussed below. For more detail concerning fumigants consult articles by R. D. Chisholm, Randall Latta and M. C. Lane, and R. T. Cotton.[19]

Aluminum phosphide—A new pelletized source of phosphine plus fire retardant. Presently used widely in grain fumigation.

Carbon Disulfide (CS_2)—This is one of the older fumigants. It is a liquid having a clear to slightly yellow color and a disagreeable odor. The gas is heavy (about 2.6 times that of air). The chief disadvantage of carbon disulfide is its extreme explosiveness. It is also toxic to animals and lengthy exposure must be avoided.

To reduce its flammability, carbon disulfide is used in combination with carbon tetrachloride, usually in the ratio of 1 part carbon disulfide to 4 parts carbon tetrachloride. Carbon disulfide is most often used for *treatment of grains in storage bins*. It has limited use in emulsion form for controlling *soil infesting insects*.

Carbon Tetrachloride (CCl_4)—This is a liquid with heavy vapors (5 times that of air). This fumigant alone does not have extensive use because it does not possess a high degree of fumigating action to most insects. It is, however, used in combination with other fumigants, because the vapors are nonflammable; its use with such fumigants as carbon disulfide and ethylene dichloride reduces the fire hazard. It is employed also in combination with methyl bromide or ethylene dibromide to aid in the distribution of the vapors. Combinations of carbon tetrachloride and other fumigants are employed most extensively in *grain fumigation*. *Caution: Carbon tetrachloride can be toxic on inhalation.*

Chloropicrin, Trichloronitromethane (CCl_3NO_2)—This is a colorless liquid which causes intense irritation of the eyes and throat and induces vomiting. Chloropicrin is used chiefly as a *soil fumigant*. It may be injected in the soil in combination with xylene, carbon tetrachloride, or ethylene dichloride to help distribute the gas. It is also used in combination with certain other fumigants for *treating stored products* by sprinkling or spraying the infested materials. Since the gas is only slowly volatilized thorough airing after use is required.

D-D Mixture—This is a mixture of 1,3-dichloropropene and 1,2-dichloropropane. It is a dark colored liquid having a sharp disagreeable odor. The material is flammable and is highly toxic to humans. The chief use of D-D Mixture is for *soil fumigation* to control *nematodes*, etc. It is toxic to most plants and is therefore applied to the soil several weeks before planting the crop.

Dichloroethyl Ether (β,β'-dichloroethyl ether) ($C_4H_8Cl_2O$)—This is a colorless liquid with vapors 4.9 times as heavy as air. The fumigant is not explosive. The principal use for dichloroethyl ether is for *soil fumigation*. It is applied to lawns, gardens, and soils in green houses. The chemical may injure growing plants although grasses are less affected than are other plants; therefore the soil should be aerated before planting. It is most satisfactory for soils when plants are not growing.

Ethylene Dibromide (CH_2BrCH_2Br)—This is a colorless liquid, having a sharp chloroform-like odor. It is 6.5 times as heavy as air. There is no explosive hazard associated with its use, but it is highly toxic to humans. Prolonged breathing the vapors even at low temperatures should be avoided and if the liquid is spilled on clothing the clothing should be removed immediately.

Ethylene dibromide is highly effective for controlling many pests. It is useful *for treating soils*. For such use it may be emulsified with water and applied to the soil surface, or mixed into soil in a xylene or light petroleum oil solution. Certain fruits and vegetables are treated with the fumigant to destroy insect infestations, although there is often only a narrow margin of safety between the dosage that does not adversely affect the commodity and that required to destroy the insects. The fumigant is also effective against most *grain insects*. It is usually applied by spraying, in combination with other fumigants, on top of the grain in tight bins.

Ethylene Dichloride (CH_2ClCH_2Cl)—This is a colorless liquid. The vapors are 3.5 times as heavy as air. Although not flammable under most conditions of use it is a fire hazard and is often used in combination with carbon tetrachloride. Like most fumigants it is toxic to humans. Ethylene dichloride is used against a wide variety of pests especially *grain insects*. Emulsions of the chemical are also employed to destroy *soil insects*.

Ethylene Oxide ($\overline{CH_2CH_2}O$)—This is a gas at ordinary temperatures and is relatively light (1.5 times as heavy as air). Because the vapor readily forms an explosive mixture in air, it is usually combined with carbon dioxide to reduce the explosive hazard. An ethylene oxide-carbon dioxide mixture (ratio of 1 to 9) is available in metal cylinders. This gas is especially useful for fumigating insects in packaged cereals, bagged rice, tobacco, and clothing and furs in vaults. It leaves no odor or harmful residues in the products. It

may injure foods like nuts, and dried fruits or fresh fruits. It is also used in vaults for fumigating valuable *packaged documents*.

Hydrocyanic Acid (HCN)—This is a colorless gas lighter than air, with an odor of almond. It is perhaps the best known of the fumigants. HCN is deadly to most living things. Therefore, its use as a fumigant is extremely hazardous. Nevertheless it is widely used and when employed with necessary precautions it is one of the most useful fumigants available. The gas is liberated from cylinders under pressure or by the addition of sodium or potassium cyanide to sulfuric acid and water. Calcium cyanide as dusts or granules is also used and generates the gas slowly in moist air.

For many years HCN was used under tents to control *scale* and other *citrus pests*. Its use for this purpose has been discontinued because the California red scale developed resistance to the gas. HCN is used in warehouses and other industrial establishments, shops, homes, etc. to destroy *pests*. Certain foodstuffs and a wide range of non-foods may be treated in warehouses or special vaults for insect control.

Methyl Bromide (CH_3Br)—This is a colorless and almost odorless gas at ordinary temperatures with vapors about 3 times as heavy as air. The gas is non-flammable and is sometimes used as a fire extinguisher. The gas is highly toxic to humans; and the absence of odor and slow toxic action are characteristics which increase its hazard. Methyl bromide is among the most widely used fumigants. It destroys a wide range of *pests*. It is not highly toxic to most plants and leaves no objectionable odor in food. Since the chemical is a gas at ordinary temperatures it is applied from containers into which it has been compressed as a liquid. It readily vaporizes at temperatures ordinarily encountered in fumigating.

Some important uses of methyl bromide are for *fumigating warehouses, ships, railroad cars, residences, grains, living plants* shipped under quarantine regulations, *tobacco*, and many other products. The fumigant is also used to destroy *soil pests*. During World War II it was used successfully to *fumigate clothing of refugees and prisoners of war* to control *body lice*.

Naphthalene ($C_{10}H_8$)—This is a white crystalline material with vapors about 4.4 times as heavy as air, and a characteristic odor not unpleasant to most people. Naphthalene is perhaps the most commonly used fumigation for protecting clothing and furs from *moth* attack. It is used in flake form or as "moth balls."

Orthodichlorobenzene ($C_6H_4Cl_2$)—This is a colorless liquid with a strong characteristic odor. The vapors are about 5 times as heavy as air. Although it will burn, the chemical does not have a great explosive hazard. The chemical is toxic to animals and spillage on the skin or prolonged breathing of the vapors should be avoided. The fumigant is too toxic to plants to be used in soil where plants are to be grown. The chief use of orthodichlorobenzene is *to treat logs or timber* to destroy insect infestations. The chemical is also an effective *larvicide for flies*. It can be used successfully in emulsion form to destroy fly larvae in latrines or on carcasses of animals.

Paradichlorobenzene ($C_6H_4Cl_2$)—This is a white crystalline compound with a characteristic odor which at low temperature is not unpleasant. The vapors are 5 times as heavy as air. They are not explosive under most conditions.

Paradichlorobenzene crystals are used extensively in homes to destroy *moths*. Woolen clothing treated with the crystals and stored away in reasonably tight boxes will be well protected from moth attack.

Paradichlorobenzene is also used to control such insects as the *peach tree borer*. It is placed in a shallow trench about 2 to 4 inches from the base of the trunk and covered with soil.

Sulfur Dioxide (SO_2)—This is one of the oldest fumigants. The gas is formed by burning sulfur or it may be furnished in commercial cylinders. It has been replaced by other more desirable fumigants. The chief objections to its use are the tarnishing effects of the gas in moist air and its powerful bleaching action.

Insect Repellents

Repellent materials protect animals and plants from insect attacks by making the hosts objectionable or disguising the odor of the host.

New Insect Repellents—During World War II, troops on many fronts in tropical and semitropical regions employed repellents effectively in the preventive campaign to keep away mosquitoes and other annoying and disease-carrying insect pests. The problem here was to obtain not only compounds with effective staying powers and nonirritating properties when applied to the skin of man and animals, but also preparations without a pronounced, penetrating odor, as this was objectionable during scouting and patrolling or combat since it would aid the enemy by supplying information as to hide-outs, etc. During and since World War II over 10,000 chemical compounds have been tested by the US Department of Agriculture laboratory at Orlando, Florida. As a result of these studies a combination of three chemicals was developed for use by the military during World War II as a repellent for *flies*, *mosquitoes*, *chiggers*, *ticks*, and *gnats*. Since World War II other combinations were developed for use on the skin or for the treatment of clothing to protect individuals from attack by these pests and disease vectors.

USP XV recognized an *insect repellent* which was found quite effective by the Armed Service. It was formerly official as *Compound Dimethyl Phthalate Solution* (see page 1301) and consists of 60 parts of dimethyl phthalate, 20 parts ethohexadiol (Rutgers 612), and 20 parts of butopyronoxyl (Indalone). It is relatively non-irritating to the skin but somewhat irritating to mucous membranes and care must be taken when it is used to keep it away from the eyes.

A new insect repellent developed since World War II, called diethyltoluamide, has proved to be the most effective all-purpose individual repellent yet discovered, and has had several years successful use.

For detailed information on the use of insect repellents for application to the skin or clothing to protect individuals from attack by insects, ticks, and mites consult Smith, *et al.*[20]

Citronella and Other Mosquito Repellents—Oils of citronella, cedarwood, eucalyptus, pennyroyal, bergamot, cassia, cloves, wintergreen, and lavender are repellent, in a minor degree, to *mosquitoes* and similar annoying insects but are not nearly as effective as the new repellents referred to above.

A variety of repellents and repellent compositions are on sale for public use. In addition to Compound Dimethyl Phthalate Solution, ethohexadiol and dimethyl phthalate are each packaged as a single composition. These alone or in combination are compounded as emulsions, creams, or in semisolid stick form. Diethyltoluamide is also marketed as a single composition under various trade names. Most of these materials will provide excellent relief, for periods varying from 30 minutes to 2 hours or more, from attack by *mosquitoes*, *biting flies*, and *gnats*. For more details regarding repellents and their use against *mosquitoes*, *gnats*, *chiggers*, *ticks*, and other insects, refer to the section on pages 1280 to 1283.

Control of Rodents

The following compounds are commonly employed to control rodents. They are dangerous and must be handled with caution (see page 1300).

ANTU is the abbreviation for the chemical *alphanaphthylthiourea*, a wartime discovery, found to be useful primarily for the control of the Norway rat. It is not recommended for use against black rats or house mice, and is ineffective against all species of field rodents. From 2 to 5% ANTU is considered to be the proper amount for use in bait mixtures. It can kill dogs, cats, swine, and baby chicks, but its toxicity to humans is felt to be fairly low. Because of its specificity for Norway rats and its tendency to cause resistance, this poison is rapidly losing popularity, and is no longer being manufactured.

Arsenicals—Arsenic has been used in rat and mouse control for many years. At present the most popular forms of arsenic baits are: (1) Food type, solid baits usually containing 3 to 5% white arsenic (arsenic trioxide, arsenious acid) of a finely powdered grade, and (2) Solutions, usually aqueous with a so-called "lure," and possibly a sugar or syrup as an added food item together with 2 to 3½% of sodium arsenate or arsenite.

All arsenicals are toxic to humans and beneficial animals, and must be used with caution to prevent accidents. A frequent claim that rats and mice killed with arsenical preparations will be "embalmed," is unfounded.

Barium Carbonate—Barium Carbonate has been used with varying degrees of success for several years in rat and mouse control. It is moderately toxic, and 1 part of poison should be blended with 4 parts of palatable food bait to insure an effective mixture. Baits made with barium carbonate would be dangerous to pets or children, so must be placed where they cannot be found by animals other than rats and mice. This poison is losing in popularity to the newer and more effective toxic agents.

Compound 1080—This is the code number by which *sodium fluoroacetate* was known during the war. This poison deserves its reputation as being the most effective mammal poison yet discovered. The substance is so toxic, however, that it is available only to governmental agencies and experienced pest control operators. There is little reason to expect that baits containing "1080" will ever be suitable for sale to the general public. One reason for this is in its very high secondary poisoning danger. Cats and dogs, for example, may be killed readily by eating the carcasses of rodents which have died from the effects of "1080." Certain local governmental agencies have legislated against use of "1080" except under permit, even by licensed pest control operators. For further details, see Ward.[21]

Phosphorus—White or yellow phosphorus is available in the form of prepared baits for rat or mouse control. Often it is packaged as a low percentage paste for use in treating bread or other palatable rat food. Phosphorus is a dangerous poison which is toxic to all animals which eat it. Great care must be used in placing baits made with it.

Red Squill—Because of its relative safety for humans, pets, and domestic animals, properly standardized red squill powders and extracts are quite generally recommended poisons for rats. Red squill contains a strong emetic which causes humans and most species of domestic animals to void the poison promptly. Red squill is available on the open market in a variety of trade-named products. These are red squill "fortified" powders, standardized extracts, or prepared baits. All retail containers carry labels giving precise directions for use, which if followed are adequate to insure the highest degree of control of which the product is capable.

Red squill is not a mouse poison, and will rarely give satisfactory control of this species.

Red squill must not be confused with the white squill of the drug trade which is completely ineffective as a rat poison.

Rats cannot vomit so do not get rid of the poison once it is ingested. To prepare red squill for use as a rat poison, the bulbs which grow as a wild crop in the region around the Mediterranean Sea are harvested when from three to ten years of age. The bulbs are sliced into thin sections which usually are dried in the sun to form the "chips" of commerce. Upon reaching the eastern seaboard of the United States, the chips are ground to a commercial-size powder. The various lots of this powder are bioassayed to determine toxicity. To be acceptable for interstate sale in this country, the red squill powder must have a toxicity such that a dose of 400 mg of the powder, per kilogram of standard male rat body weight, will kill one-half of the test animals.

If the powder fails to have such toxicity, it is fortified by a process of extracting and blending until a "fortified" red squill with the required toxicity as stated is produced.

Poultry are quite resistant to squill. Dogs, cats, hogs, and other domestic animals either tend to refuse red squill baits, or usually vomit them rapidly. These characteristics combine to make red squill one of the safer poisons for use in areas where it is difficult to exclude pets and livestock. Red squill seems to have a reputation for complete safety which it does not deserve. Occasionally a cat, dog, or hog has been killed and other animals have survived only after a session of marked discomfort during which the poison is being eliminated. As a consequence, it is wise to warn against careless and indiscriminate exposure of red squill baits, where animals other than rats can reach them.

A new use of red squill is in so-called "tracking powders," which are dusted liberally along rat and mouse runways. In locations where the powder is not objectionable this procedure has promise.

Strychnine—Strychnine is another powerful poison but seldom used in rat baits because it is so readily detected by them. However, it is one of the best poisons to use for *field* and *house mice*, *prairie dogs*, *pocket gophers*, *ground squirrels* (sometimes called gophers in sections of the West where they are common), and similar animals and certain species of birds. Strychnine is available on the market both as the alkaloid and as the sulfate. While either may be used in baits, the alkaloid is recommended for coated baits. Strychnine sulfate, being more soluble, is the form usually recommended for soaked baits.

Strychnine has been used successfully for many years to control predatory animals such as coyotes. For information on this usage get in touch with the US Fish & Wildlife Service.

(a) *For English sparrows.* Mix ⅛ ounce of pulverized strychnine alkaloid with 1½ teaspoonfuls of gloss or laundry starch or wheat flour and moisten with sufficient cold water to make a paste of the consistency of thick cream. To this mixture add 3 fluidounces of boiling water and thoroughly mix. Pour this thin paste over 1 quart of small-kerneled wheat and stir the whole thoroughly until the poisoned paste is well distributed. Spread it out thinly and allow it to dry: then it may be stored in properly labeled jars for future use.

(b) *For rabbits and ground squirrels.* Mix 1 tablespoonful of gloss starch with ½ pint of cold water. Pour this into 1½ pints of boiling water and continue the boiling until the starch is clear. Mix 1 ounce of the strychnine alkaloid and 1 ounce of sodium bicarbonate and sift it over the hot starch liquid, stirring thoroughly. Then add ⅛ ounce of saccharin and stir. Pour this mixture over 12 quarts of oats, mixing until all of the grain is wet. Allow the grain to dry thoroughly before using.

(c) *For crows.* Put 2 tablespoonfuls of starch and 1 oz. of powdered strychnine alkaloid in 1½ pints of water and heat to boiling, stirring thoroughly after the starch begins to thicken. Pour this mixture over 20 quarts of shelled corn and stir until every kernel is coated. Spread out the grain and allow it to dry.

(d) *For field mice.* Mix 1 tablespoonful of gloss starch in 1 fluid-ounce of cold water. Add ¾ pint of boiling water and stir to make a thin clear paste. In another container mix 1 ounce of powdered strychnine alkaloid with 1 ounce of sodium bicarbonate and add to the starch paste, stirring to a smooth, creamy mass free of lumps. Stir in ¼ pint of heavy corn syrup and 1 tablespoonful of glycerin or petrolatum. Apply to 12 pounds of wheat, or preferably steam-crushed whole oats, and mix thoroughly to coat each kernel. Spread out the poisoned grain and allow it to dry. The steam-crushed oats bait is available ready-prepared through the US Fish and Wildlife Service.

(e) *For house mice.* The bait recommended for field mice may also be used for house mice. A simpler formula for the housewife is to mix ⅛ ounce of powdered strychnine alkaloid with an equal quantity of sodium bicarbonate and stir thoroughly into 1 quart or rolled oats or corn meal. This poison may be left in small open boxes in places out of reach of children or domestic animals where it will provide a permanent poison supply available to mice at all times.

Thallium Sulfate—Thallium sulfate (Tl_2SO_4) is a highly toxic, cumulative poison which must be used very carefully. Its use in ant control has been mentioned on page 1280. Formulas containing 3½–5% thallium sulfate appeared during the middle 1950's on the retail markets in the southern states for the control of cockroaches and ants. A number of poisonings of small children resulted, and in 1958, the state of Texas passed a law limiting the amount of thallium in a pesticide to 1% when it was to be sold for household use. Similar restrictive action was taken in 1960 by the US Department of Agriculture and in 1965, household use of all thallium formulations was dropped, except by government officials.

Thallium sulfate has a mild, metallic, alum-like taste which is not objectionable to rodents, so it has little repellent effect. It is a slow poison, and has some secondary poisoning danger, since predatory animals will feed on sick or dead rodents, and occasionally will eat enough poison in these carcasses to be killed thereby.

Thallium is absorbed by the intact skin, so should be handled in the concentrated form by experienced persons only.

Its use in controlling coyotes on the western plains has been discontinued.

Tributyl Tin Salts—A mixture of salts of tributyltin, which is a widely used antifoulant, fungicide, and bactericide, has recently been incorporated into a plastic-based cable coating which has proved in field tests to be about 95% effective in repelling rodent attack. Apparently, rodents cannot tolerate the taste and smell of tributyl tin and strictly avoid anything coated with it after a preliminary nibble. This has been developed by the M&T Chemicals Co. and field-tested by the Department of Interior's Wildlife Research Center.

Viruses—Rat viruses are not registered for use in the United States at present. Governmental agencies responsible for protecting human and animal health have recommended against the general sale of bacterial cultures for pest mammal control.

Warfarin (*WARF-42, Compound 42*) (3-(α-acetonylbenzyl)-4-hydroxycoumarin)—This chemical relative of dicoumarol is one of the newest of the rat and mouse poisons to be introduced into this coun-

try. It acts by causing a loss of clotting power of the blood, and the animals die of exhaustion caused by multiple hemorrhages. The product was the first successful anticoagulant rodenticide and was unique in that it had to be eaten repeatedly to cause death. For rats, the feeding time is usually from 3 to 10 days, and for mice a much longer period of daily feeding is needed. Fantastically low percentages of the poison in food are effective, and food baits now on the market contain 0.025–0.05% of the poison, and concentrates for making solutions of the sodium salt of warfarin containing 0.005% of warfarin equivalent are available. At these levels rats and mice do not detect the material in the baits and will continue to come back to eat or drink until too weak to do so.

Warfarin itself is a highly toxic poison, but the fact that it is needed at such low concentrations in baits and that these must be eaten repeatedly to cause symptoms makes it less likely to injure pets and children, than certain other poisons. It has had a good record of safety and is considered one of the less dangerous rat and mouse control materials.

Several other coumarin derivatives are available; eg, 3-(1-furyl-3-acetyl-ethyl)-4-hydroxycoumarin, known by the nonproprietary name coumafuryl and marketed under several tradenames (eg, Fumarin, Fumasol, Krumkil, Lurat, and Rat-A-Way). This was developed and produced by Amchem Products, Inc.

Zinc Phosphide [Zn_3P_2]—This is a phosphorus preparation which has found a definite place in a specialized rodent control problem in the United States. It is blended with a diluent to permit its easier use as a dusting powder over cut apples in the preparation of a highly effective orchard mouse bait. Just enough of the perishable bait is made to supply an afternoon's work, and it is placed by uncovering the mouse's tunnels and making a bait spot of two or three apple sections placed directly in the runway. This is repeated at several points in the trails around each orchard tree, and when properly done is quite effective. The same zinc phosphide blend can be used on other types of food bait for domestic rat or mouse control. It is dangerous to animals other than rats or mice, and should be handled carefully.

2-Pivalyl-1,3-indanedione (Pival)—This is another anticoagulant resembling warfarin very closely in formulation and method of use.

It is available in concentrates and prepared baits, as well as in solutions.

It must be used exactly in accordance with directions to be most effective.

2-Isovaleryl-1,3-indandione (Valone)—This poison and its salts provide another anticoagulant group of rat and mouse poisons. A trademarked product containing the calcium salt has been used as a "tracking powder."

2-Diphenylacetyl-1,3-indanedione (Diphenadione; Diphacinone)—This is the most toxic of the anticoagulants in use at present. While the other chemicals in this class are usually used in bait at 0.025% diphacinone is effective at 0.005%.

Other indanedione derivatives are available for the same use.

1,2,3,4,10,10 - Hexachloro - 6,7 - epoxy - 1,4,4a,5,6,7,8,8a - octahydro-1,4 : 5,8-*endo-endo*-dimethanonaphthalene (Endrin)—This is an insecticide which has found use as a ground spray to control orchard mice. A dosage rate of 2 pounds per acre is applied, and about ½ of the ground surface is treated. This practice has been questioned because it risks injury to livestock and wildlife, but has gained wide acceptance in apple growing areas of the eastern United States.

5 - (Alpha - hydroxy - alpha - 2 - pyridylbenzyl) - 7 - (alpha - 2 - pyridylbenzylidene)-5-norbornene-2,3-dicarboximide—This is known by the nonproprietary name Norbormide and is marketed under various tradenames; eg, Raticide, Raticate, and Shoxin. It was developed and produced by Tavolek Labs., Div., J&J. This dicarboximide compound is generally used in dry baits against Norway (brown or common) rats. It is fast acting and kills after a single feeding. It is virtually nontoxic to 15 common mammalian species found around farms (eg, cat, chicken, cow, dog, pig, etc). It is extremely stable and persistent in all baits and environments.

A great deal of study is underway to find chemicals which may be applied to plants and structures to repel rodents and thus protect without destroying the animals. Much progress has been made, and formulas which are both satisfactory and economical are expected to be introduced into commercial use before long.

Control of Fungi and Bacteria

Fungicides are chemical compounds used to prevent or retard the deleterious action of a varied group of plants, for the most part microscopic, devoid of green coloring matter and reproducing by spores.

These plants, known as fungi, are present throughout the world. They attack other living and dead plants, animals, human beings, and such diversified inanimate objects as foodstuffs, cloth, paper, lumber, paint, plastic coverings, and leather, to mention only a few of the substances affected.

Some fungicide materials are also toxic to bacteria but in general the term is limited to those materials used for protection against fungi. For many years fungicides have been used extensively in agriculture for the protection of crops.

The prevalence of fungi fluctuates with environmental conditions. Early historical and religious writings contain references to the blasting, blighting, rusting, or mildewing of the crops. From the dawn of civilization down to the present day there has been a constant battle between the agriculturist on one hand and the fungi on the other, with the environmental conditions swinging the balance to one side and then to the other. Prior to 1853 losses resulting from the attacks of fungi were accepted as inevitable since the true cause was not understood but in that year Anton de Bary established the parasitism of the fungi associated with the rust and smut diseases. This discovery, establishing the science of plant pathology, has been followed by an ever increasing number of investigations into the cause of plant diseases and by the development of a wide variety of materials used for the control of these diseases.

Fundamental Requirements of a Fungicide—To protect plants against the attack of fungi the compounds used must be toxic to the parasite yet relatively noninjurious to the host plant. These materials may be applied in either liquid or powder form. The process of applying substances in liquid form is termed spraying; that of applying them in powder form, dusting.

Irrespective of the method of application a fungicide, to be entirely satisfactory, must be

1. Capable of destroying the fungus.
2. Relatively noninjurious to the host plant.
3. Easy to apply.
4. Easy to prepare.
5. Reasonable in cost.

Types of Fungicidal Action—Fungicide materials are of varied composition and their exact mode of action against specific organisms is beyond the scope of this discussion. In general, however, all materials fall into two general categories; ie, (1) *protective* and (2) *eradicative*.

In the *protective type* the material does not necessarily kill the fungus spores but does prevent their germination. The various forms of elemental *sulfur* used as spray or dust are protective in their action against the spores of the apple scab fungus (*Venturia inaequalis*) and are widely used by commercial orchardists to prevent numerous infections from developing on the apple leaves and fruit. However, the same materials used against certain rust fungi are definitely eradicative in their action upon the rust spores. This diverse effect on different fungi is but one example of the complexity of the problem.

In the *eradicative type* the material kills the fungus and in this way stops the disease either before or soon after initial infection has occurred. The complex *calcium polysulfides* and certain organic mercury preparations, for example, have a definite eradicative effect upon the apple scab fungus. Unfortunately, most of the eradicative materials are rather caustic in their action and they can be used only under certain conditions since they are apt to produce injury often more serious in consequence than the disease they are being used to combat. However, whenever it is possible to use an eradicative type of fungicide without incurring serious injury to the plant, this procedure should be adopted

as it is productive of the most satisfactory control results.

Commonly Used Fungicides

It is realized that the pharmacist is not expected to have the detailed knowledge of a technically trained plant pathologist regarding the use of fungicide materials. However, he is frequently asked for advice and called upon to make recommendations regarding the control of diseases on household and garden plants.

The following list of commonly used materials should enable him to answer intelligently the majority of questions with which he is confronted. Requests for information concerning large-scale usage of fungicides should be referred to the State Agricultural Experiment Station or to the US Department of Agriculture.

Ammoniacal Copper Carbonate—A copper fungicide of especial value when a material is needed that does not discolor the foliage. It is water-soluble and is readily washed off by rain; but it has been employed for the control of *Botrytis* blight of begonia and for rose anthracnose and brown canker. Readily prepared in small quantities by dissolving 1 level teaspoonful of copper carbonate in 2 tablespoonfuls of ammonia water and adding 1 gallon of water.

Arasan—see *Tetramethylthiouram disulfide.*

Bichloride of Mercury—see *Corrosive Sublimate.*

Bioquin I—see *Copper 8-Quinolinolate.*

Bismuth Subsalicylate—Used at the rate of 1½ pounds per 100 gallons plus a spreader sticker, this material has given effective control of downy mildew (blue mold) of tobacco.

Bluestone—see *Bordeaux mixture.*

Blue Vitriol—see *Bordeaux mixture.*

Borax (*Sodium Tetraborate*)—Used as a prebedding dip (6 pounds borax in 30 gallons of water) for sweet potatoes to control black rot.

Bordeaux Mixture—A complex chemical compound resulting from the mixing of a dilute solution of copper sulfate with a dilute suspension of lime in water. Some of the mixtures commonly used are 8-8-100, 4-8-100, 4-6-100, 8-12-100, 4-16-100, and 12-24-100. In each case the first figure represents the pounds of powdered copper sulfate and the third figure represents gallons of water. Any quantity of these various mixtures may be prepared as long as the proper ratios are maintained. In general, the amount of lime should be equal to or greater than the amount of copper sulfate to prevent copper injury, but with some crops, as pecan and walnuts, excess lime causes injury and "*Low-Lime*" Bordeaux mixture, such as 4-2-100 is recommended.

Bordeaux mixture should not be used on peaches and sweet cherries during the growing season; and its use on apples, tomatoes, raspberries, cantaloupes, cucumbers, and watermelons is always attended by risk of injury. On the other hand Bordeaux mixture has proved to be of great value for the control of diseases on the following plants: aster, beet, begonia, blackberry, carnation, carrot, celery, cranberry, currant, dahlia, delphinium, geranium, gladiolus, grape, hollyhock, iris, ivy, lilac, lily, narcissus, pansy, peony, pepper, phlox, potato, rhododendron, rose, snapdragon, strawberry, and tulip.

Bordeaux mixture leaves a whitish spray deposit and it should not be used where such spray residue would be objectionable for aesthetic reasons. This residue should be washed off any edible portion of the plant before it is consumed to avoid eating unnecessary chemicals.

Various commercial forms of powdered Bordeaux mixture are available. They are easier to handle but are apt to lack the adhesive qualities of freshly prepared Bordeaux mixture.

Botran—This tradename and others (DCNA, Allisan) refer to *2,6-dichloro-4-nitroaniline*, which was developed in England. This substituted amine is formulated as a yellow, wettable powder used for spraying (75%) and for dipping (50%); it is also used as dust. It is generally used as a soil and foliar fungicide to control *Sclerotinia* mold, *Monilinia* rot, *Rhizopus* rot, *Sclerotium* and *Botrytus* mold, including storage or transit on vegetables, fruits, and ornamentals. It is almost nontoxic to rats but phytotoxic to strawberries, wilted leaf lettuce, astors, petunias, and some other greenhouse plants, and to some germinating seeds and annual seedlings. It is persistent on leaf surfaces for 1–2 weeks and involves low hazard generally.

Caution—Avoid inhalation of dust and spray mist; occasional cases of contact dermatitis have been reported.

Burgundy Mixture—A modified form of Bordeaux mixture is prepared by combining solutions of copper sulfate and sodium carbonate at the rates of 2 pounds of copper sulfate dissolved in 50 gallons, and 3 pounds of sodium carbonate in an additional 50 gallons of water.

Burgundy mixture is used mainly where the discoloration of foliage by Bordeaux mixture is objectionable.

Calcium Hypochlorite—The activity of this compound as a general disinfectant is based on its ability to release chlorine. The compound has been found helpful in the control of *Penicillium* bulb rot of lilies. In general, 5½ ounces of calcium hypochlorite (chlorine content from 20 to 27%) is mixed with each 50 pounds of packing soil.

Calomel—Calomel (mercurous chloride), containing approximately 85% of metallic mercury, has long been used as a seed and bulb disinfectant. It has been used to control diseases of gladiolus by dipping the corms for 1 minute in a solution containing 1 pound of mercurous chloride in 5 gallons of water. A weaker solution (3 ounces in 1 gallon) may be used but the corms then have to be dipped for 5 minutes.

Captan (*N-trichloromethylthio-4-cyclohexene-1,2-dicarboximide*)—A new organic fungicide used at the rate of 1 to 2 pounds per 100 gallons of water for control of diseases of fruits, vegetables, and ornamental plants. Excellent for summer spraying of apple trees. Do not use with lime or other strong alkali.

Ceresan—See *Ethyl Mercury Chloride*.

Ceresan M—See *Ethyl Mercury p-Toluenesulfonanilide*.

Ceresan New Improved—See *Ethyl Mercury Phosphate*.

Chloranil—See *Tetrachloroparabenzoquinone*.

C. O. C. S.—See *Copper oxychloride sulfate*.

Copper Oxalate—This compound has been used for the control of walnut bacteriosis, a bacterial disease prevalent in the Pacific Northwest. The general recommendation requires the use of 4 pounds of copper oxalate in 100 gallons of water.

Copper Oxychloride Sulfate—A copper preparation frequently used as a substitute for Bordeaux mixture on cherries, melons, and cucumbers to reduce risk of copper injury.

Copper Phosphate—This compound, containing approximately 44% of copper, has been used for the control of apple scab and pear leaf spot and potato diseases. It produces much less injury than Bordeaux mixture but is only mildly effective as a fungicide and is rarely used on apple and pear trees at present.

Copper 8-Quinolinolate—An organic copper compound (sold under the trade name *Bioquin 1*) is used for the control of the apple scab fungus, tomato foliage diseases, and as a seed treatment; generally recommended to be used at the rate of 1 pound to 100 gallons of water. *Zinc* and *magnesium compounds* of similar composition have also been tested as well as *8-hydroxyquinoline sulfate*, *8-quinolinol benzoate*, and *8-quinolinol*.

Copper Sulfate—In addition to being the principal ingredient of Bordeaux mixture, copper sulfate is frequently used as a general disinfecting solution, as a seed-treatment material, and as the essential component of many commercial copper fungicides.

Corrosive Sublimate—*Bichloride of mercury*, or corrosive sublimate, has long been used as a general disinfectant and as a seed treatment. The seeds are generally soaked in a 1 to 1000 solution for varying periods depending on the kind of seed. After treatment the seeds must be thoroughly washed. Care must be used to avoid using treated seed for human food or animal feed. Corrosive sublimate is a very poisonous compound and it must be used with proper precautions.

Cycloheximide [(*3* - [*2* - (*3,5* - *dimethyl* - *2* - *oxocyclohexyl*) - *2* - *hydroxyethyl*]*glutarimide; Acti-Dione-PM (-RZ, -BR, and -S); Acti-spray*]—This antibiotic-type compound is noncorrosive and is formulated as an oil solution, a wettable powder, and water-soluble tablets. It is generally used as a wound dressing for black knot fungus on plums and prunes and also for white pine blister rust, cedar apple rust, some turf fungi, and powdery mildew on ornamentals. Its toxicity varies according to formulation. It is highly toxic to rats with some phytotoxicity, particularly in producing some injury to fruit when used with flowable parathion. Injury has also been reported to sour cherry when the fruit was ¼ in. or less in diameter. In addition, early sprays may cause injury to tender foliage. It has some phytotoxicity to numerous rose cultivars. There are no particular hazards except with concentrated formulations. *Caution*—It will irritate the skin on prolonged contact.

Dexon [(*Chemagro*); *p-Dimethylaminobenzenediazo Sodium Sulfonate;* no common name]—It is a nonmercurial seed and seedling protectant. It is sensitive to light. Its principal formulations are a 70% wettable powder, a 2.5% dust, and a 5% granular preparation. It has general usage as a soil fungicide for the control of *Pythium* and *Aphanomyces* damping off and root and stem rot from *Pythium* and *Phytophthora*, particularly with vegetables, ornamentals, and turf. It is moderately toxic to birds, moderately to highly toxic to rats, but it is not generally phytotoxic as used. Its persistence is relatively short. *Caution*—Wear mask and gloves when treating seed or loading spreader.

Difolatan [(*Chevron*); *cis-N-[(1,1,2,2-tetrachloroethyl)thio]-4-cyclohexene-1,2-dicarboximide;* no common name]—This sulfenimide is a solid of low toxicity which is insoluble in water. It is formulated as an 80% wettable powder and a 7.5% dust. It is generally used as a fungicidal protectant–eradicant, particularly for the control of early and late blight on potatoes. It is slightly toxic to rats, fish, and birds. Foliage of some roses may be injured with this fungicide. It is persistent on plant surfaces for 7 to 10 days. No hazard occurs in its use.

It is not compatible with strongly alkaline materials. It should not be used in combination with or closely following oil sprays.

Dichlone—This organic spray preparation, sold under the trade name *Phygon XL*, has been found to be an effective substitute for both sulfur and copper in the control of the various fungus diseases of fruit trees. It is generally used at a dosage of ¾ to 1 pound to each 100 gallons of spray. It has also been employed dry as a seed treatment at rates varying from 1 to 4 ounces per 100 pounds of seed. *Caution*—One serious drawback to its use is the fact that the chemical may cause skin irritations.

Diphenyl—Used as a preservative for citrus in storage and transit.

Disodium Ethylenebisdithiocarbamate Hexahydrate—See *Nabam*.

Dithane D 14—See *Nabam*.

Dithane Z 78—See *Zineb*.

Dodine [(Am. Cyanamid); *N-Dodecylguanidine Acetate;* Cyprex, Melprex; Doquadine]—This agent is a fairly stable fungicide formulated as a 65% wettable powder and a protectant and eradicant–fungicide, particularly for apple and pecan scab, cherry leaf spot, sycamore anthracnose, and other tree diseases. It may cause foliage or fruit injury, particularly if applied at freezing or near-freezing temperatures. *Caution*—It may produce eye and skin irritation. If exposed, flush eyes for at least 15 min.

Dyrene [*2,4 - Dichloro - 6 - (o - chloroanilino) - s - triazine;* Kemate (*Chemagro*); no common name]—It is used as a foliar fungicide for the control of turf diseases, some vegetable diseases, berries, and gladiolus. It may be phytotoxic to some fruit and ornamentals and potentially hazardous to animals. It can cause skin irritation.

Elgetol—See *Sodium dinitro-ortho-cresylate*.

Ethyl Mercury Chloride, Ethyl Mercury p-Toluenesulfonanilide, and **Ethyl Mercury Phosphate**—These three organic mercury compounds are used for the treatment of seeds to prevent seed decay and seedling blights, and for the dipping of bulbs.

Caution—Since they all contain mercury they are poisonous compounds and the manufacturer's precautions covering their use must be strictly adhered to, particularly in regard to use of masks to prevent absorption of mercury through the respiratory tract. Do not use treated seed for food or feed.

Ferbam—This iron organic compound, *ferric dimethyldithiocarbamate*, is used extensively as a substitute for sulfur and copper compounds in the control of fungus diseases of fruit trees. It is employed as a specific for the control of the apple cedar rust. In the Pacific Northwest it is used instead of sulfur for the control of pear scab since it does not russet the fruit. Likewise, it is used for the control of the fungi causing apple scab, apple blotch, and bitter rot since it reduces the risk of spray injury and at the same time gives satisfactory control of these fungi.

It is also used for the control of tomato anthracnose, and is especially effective for the control of anthracnose leaf blight, downy mildew, and fruit rot of cucumbers and melons. It causes less leaf injury than copper compounds on tomatoes, cucumbers, and melons.

Caution—Ferbam is a flammable material and must not be mixed near an open flame. In mixing sprays the operator should avoid inhaling ferbam. It is not safe to apply ferbam just before or just after applications of Bordeaux mixture.

Fermate—See *Ferbam*.

Ferric Dimethyldithiocarbamate—See *Ferbam*.

Folpet [(*Stauffer*); (*N-Trichloromethylthio*)*phthalimide;* Phaltan; Rose and Garden Fungicide (*Ortho; Stauffer*)]—It is generally used as a protectant–eradicant fungicide for fruit, vegetables, ornamentals, and turf. It is especially good for black spot of rose. It is slightly more phytotoxic than captan. It is not recommended for apples before the 4th cover spray, it may burn grape leaves in hot, dry seasons, and it may also severely injure sweet cherry leaves and snapdragons. It has a low health hazard. Concentrated solutions may cause skin irritation.

Formaldehyde [Formalin (*Celanese*); D&P77 (*Allied*); Karsan (*Du Pont*)]—It is generally used in seed and plant bed treatments for damping off, in mushroom houses, vegetables, ornamentals, and a soil treatment for onion smut. It also possesses germicidal properties. Concentrated solutions can be phytotoxic to plants both on contact and when injected into soil. It is not persistent in that it breaks down quickly in soil and water. It can be very irritating on prolonged breathing and on contact with the skin.

Glyodin (*2-Heptadecylglyoxalidine acetate*)—An organic spray compound used by commercial growers to control cherry leaf spot. Also used combined with phenyl mercury sprays for commercial control of the apple scab fungus.

Hydroxymercurichlorophenol—See *Semesan*.

Lime-Sulfur Solution—A widely used spray material consisting of approximately 30% *calcium polysulfides* prepared by heating sulfur and lime together with appropriate quantities of water.

Lime-sulfur solution has proved especially effective for the control of the apple scab fungus, and has been used widely for the control of many other plant diseases. The water dilution for use during the growing season varies from 1 gallon of the concentrate for 50 gallons of spray to 1 gallon for 100 gallons. Used at a concentration of 12 gallons for 100 gallons of spray during the winter months lime-sulfur has long been used on peach trees for the combined control of San Jose scale and the leaf curl fungus.

Since the calcium polysulfides are apt to produce spray injury, lime-sulfur is being replaced by less injurious forms of sulfur and various organic materials in large-scale commercial spraying operations.

Ethoxyquin   [1,2-dihydro-6-ethoxy-2,2,4-trimethylquinoline]— Used as a fungicide dip on apples and pears.

Karathane [(*Rohm & Haas*); *2-(1-Methylheptyl)-4,6-dinitrophenol crotonate* and other nitrophenols or derivatives; Iscothan; no common name]—It is a dark-brown liquid available as a 25% wettable powder, a 48% liquid concentrate, and a dust. Its formulation is water soluble and therefore is washed off by rain. It is generally useful against powdery mildew on fruit, vegetables, and ornamentals. It also has miticidal properties. It is less effective than sulfur but safer on sulfur-sensitive plants. It exhibits low phytotoxicity except for the possibility of injury when sprayed in temperatures over 90°F. No hazards are involved when it is used as directed.

Karbam Black—See *Ferbam*.

Karbam White—See *Ziram*.

Krenite—See *Sodium dinitro-ortho-cresylate*.

Maneb (*Manganese ethylenebisdithiocarbamate*)—The manganese salt of dithiocarbamic acid is used at the rate of 1–2 pounds per 100 gallons of water for the control of potato, tomato, celery, carrot, and onion diseases. It has also been used to control grape black rot.

Mercaptobenzothiazole—Used on apples.

Mercuric Chloride—See *Corrosive Sublimate*.

Mercuric Oxide—See *Yellow Oxide of Mercury*.

Mercurous Chloride—See *Calomel*.

Mercurous Chloride and **Mercuric Chloride Mixture**—A mixture of 65% mercurous chloride, 32% mercuric chloride, and 3% of an activator substance has been used as a turf fungicide in the prevention of snow mold. The US Golf Association suggests the following dosage rates for each 1000 square feet of turf. In the spring, 2 ounces; summer, 3 ounces; and late fall, 4 ounces. To prevent injury the dosage should be reduced to 1 ounce during periods of humid, hot weather.

Nabam—When zinc sulfate and hydrated lime are added to disodium ethylenebis-dithiocarbamate, an extremely effective fungicide, called nabam or *Dithane D 14*, is formed. It finds extensive use in the commercial production of truck crops and has been especially valuable against the late blight (*Phytophthra infestans*) of tomatoes. It has also proved effective for the control of late blight of potatoes and has proved beneficial in the control of downy mildew on cabbage and cauliflower, and of leaf spot on pepper plants in seed beds. This material is sold as a liquid and the dosage varies from 1½ to 2 quarts per 100 gallons. One pound of zinc sulfate and one-half pound of hydrated lime are added in the order named after the dithiocarbamate salt has been added to the water.

Niacide A [*Niagara*]—It is composed of 35% ferbam, 24% manganous dimethyldithiocarbamate, 6.2% thiram, 1.2% manganous benzothiozylmercaptide, and 1.1% 2,2-dithiobisbenzothiazole. It is used for prebloom and early cover sprays for the control of scab and rusts on apples.

Panogen 15 [(*Morton*); *Cyano(methylmercuri)guanidine*; Panogen 43; Panospray 30; Pano-Drench 4; Morsodren]—This organic mercury compound is formulated as a 0.6% to 6.3% water-soluble solution. It is used as a dip for potato seed pieces and other seed treatments, soil drench for damping off of greenhouse plants, turf fungicide, and foliar spray for diseases such as *Botrytis* on ornamentals. It is highly toxic to rats and fish as such but since it is used primarily as a soil drench and seed treatment, it produces no great danger. It should not be used on mercury-sensitive plants such as roses and should not be applied to the turf in bright sunlight. *Caution*—It can be a hazard via the applicator because it can blister the skin on prolonged contact. It should be used only in well-ventilated areas.

Pentachlorophenol—Used as a wood preservative.

Phenylmercuric Compounds—This common name covers a host of phenylmercuric salts (eg, acetate, borate, chloride, lactate, oleate, monoethanol ammonium acetate, naphthenate, nitrate, propionate, salicylate, thiocyanate, triethanol ammonium lactate) marketed under such tradenames as Coromerc, Puratized Agricultural Spray, Puratized Apple Spray, Paraturf 10, Tag, PMAS, Quicksan, and Phix and produced by the following manufacturers: Gallowhur, Stecker, Vanderbilt, Ortho, Cleary, Merck, Wood Ridge, Guard, and Niagara. The organic mercury salts given here vary from slightly soluble to soluble in water. Some are used dry, others as sprays. These have general use as protectant and eradicant fungicides on apples, pears, and certain other fruits and also include use with lilies, gladiola bulbs, potato and sweet potato seed pieces, turf, and shade tree anthracnose. The phenylmercuric compounds can be moderately phytotoxic to many ornamentals and may cause injury when used full strength on wet fruit foliage, especially during or preceding high temperatures. Foliage injury, russeting, and reduced blossoms and fruit set may follow repeated use.

Caution—The concentrated solutions are poisonous and must be handled with great care. The mercury content of the spray prohibits its use on edible parts of the plant. These materials should only be used during the blossom period on apples. They must not be applied to trees previously sprayed with Ferbam or Bordeaux mixture.

Phybam-S [*Grace*]—This is a wettable powder formulation of 3% dichlone, 9.5% ferbam, and 71% elemental sulfur. It has general usage against apple scab, apple rust, and powdery mildew through petal fall. It causes less injury than dichlone used alone.

Phygon XL—See *Dichlone*.

Polyram [*Niagara*]—This is a mixture of 5.2 parts by weight (83.9%) of ammoniates of [ethylenebis(dithiocarbamato)] zinc with 1 part by weight (16.1%) ethylenebis [dithiocarbamic acid], bimolecular and trimolecular cyclic anhydrosulfides and disulfides. These dithiocarbamates are solids and are insoluble in most common solvents. They decompose under strongly basic or acidic conditions. It is available as an 80% wettable powder and several dusts. Moisture can cause deterioration. It is generally used as blight control on potatoes and tomatoes. It can control apple scab, cedar apple rust, sooty blotch, and fly speck and is also used on ornamentals. It has no known phytotoxicity and is persistent on plant surfaces for 10 to 14 days. This agent is compatible with chlorinated hydrocarbons, coppers, sulfurs, and phosphates except parathion oil sprays. Karathane or Diazinon should be added just before use. It is safer than lead arsenate on apples. It exhibits low hazard potential.

Potassium Permanganate—This general disinfectant is used at times as a dip for the control of certain diseases. A solution containing 1 ounce of potassium permanganate in 7½ gallons of water has been used for the control of the bacterial wilt disease of carnation plants. The cuttings are dipped in the solution for 10 minutes.

Potassium Sulfide—A solution of 3 ounces of this chemical in 10 gallons of water is used for the control of powdery mildews of various ornamental plants. Since some plants are injured it is advisable to test this spray on a few leaves before putting it to general use. The solution does not keep and a fresh solution must be prepared each time the spray is used.

Puratized Agricultural Spray—See *Phenyl Mercury Triethanol Ammonium Lactate*.

Puratized 806—See *Phenyl Mercury Formamide*.

Semesan—A pink soluble powder containing *hydroxymercurichlorophenol*, used to treat bulbs and seeds. Quantities used should be in accord with manufacturer's directions, and all label cautions must be followed.

Semesan Jr.—See *Ethyl Mercury Phosphate*.

Sodium Dinitro-ortho-cresylate (*Elgetol*, *Krenite*)—A caustic, amber liquid used only as a dormant spray for the control of certain diseases and insects. When used at the rate of 2 quarts in 100 gallons of spray it is an effective material to destroy the apple scab fungus over-wintering on the fallen leaves. The diluted spray used for this purpose should be applied at the rate of 400 to 600 gallons per acre. It is also used as a ground spray to destroy overwintering material of the asparagus rust and of peony leaf blotch and stem spot fungi.

Sodium o-phenylphenate—Used on a variety of fruits to increase storage life.

Spergon—See *Tetrachloroparabenzoquinone*.

Sulfur—The element sulfur has long been one of the standard fungicide materials and is still widely used to control a wide variety of plant diseases. Sulfur is sold as a dry powder ground to varying degrees of fineness, as a paste, or fused with clay (bentonite) and subsequently ground. Many special brands are available and each manufacturer claims special virtues for his particular product. They all depend for their effectiveness upon the inherent toxic property of sulfur in affecting the growth processes of the various fungi. The directions on the packages will be a guide to their use. Sulfur is one of the cheapest fungicide materials and will probably continue to be used extensively as spray or dust for many years to come.

Combined with lime and water and heated for a considerable period sulfur forms complex *polysulfides*. This reaction product called *lime-sulfur* has been described in a preceding paragraph. If sulfur is added to slaking stone lime and the only heat supplied is that of the stone lime combining with water, another type of spray called *self-boiled lime-sulfur* results. Properly prepared self-boiled lime-sulfur has a very low calcium polysulfide content and produces very little injury. Self-boiled lime-sulfur can be used with safety on peaches during the growing season whereas lime-sulfur used at that time would cause excessive injury to the trees.

TAG H L 331—See *Phenylmercuric Acetate*.

Tersan—See *Tetramethylthiuram Disulfide*.

Tetrachloroparabenzoquinone—This chlorinated quinone, sold under the trade name of *Spergon*, is widely used as a seed treatment to prevent decay of the seeds in the soil during periods unfavorable to their germination. Manufacturer's recommendations should be followed regarding dosage to be used with the different seeds. Do not use treated seed for food or feed.

Tetramethylthiuram Disulfide [Bis(dimethylthiocarbamoyl) disulfide]—A pink powder available in wettable and non-wettable forms under trade names of *Arasan* and *Tersan*. Used extensively as a seed treatment for the control of seed decay and damping off. Dosage for this purpose should be in accord with manufacturer's directions. Used also as a spray for the control of turf and lawn grass diseases, such as dollar spot and brown patch. Used with low-pressure sprinkler, 1 pound in 100 gallons of water will treat 6000 square feet. If pressure of 200 to 300 pounds is available the same coverage can be obtained by suspending 1 pound in 50 gallons of water. Do not use treated seed for food or feed.

Thiram—This is the common name for *tetramethylthiuram disulfide*, marketed as Arasan, Tersan, and Thylate by Du Pont, Pennwalt, Vineland, Merck, and Cleary. This dithiocarbamate solid is almost insoluble in water and relatively stable under storage except where exposed to air, heat, and moisture; these conditions hasten loss of strength. It is generally used as a vegetable seed treatment against rot, damping off, and onion smut. It is also useful as a fungicide on some fruit and turf. It is persistent on plant surfaces for 10 to 14 days and shows low hazard potential. It can be irritating to the nose, throat, and skin.

Yellow Cuprous Oxide—This material, containing 47 per cent of metallic copper, is sold under the trade name of *Yellow Cuprocide* and may be used as a spray or dust. Used at the rate of 1½ pounds per 100 gallons it is effective against celery blight, Alternaria blight of tomato, early and late blights of potato, anthracnose, downy mildew, and other leaf diseases of cucurbits and is recommended for a variety of vegetable crops wherever a copper spray is needed.

Yellow Oxide of Mercury—This yellow powder (*Mercuric Oxide*) has been used for the treatment of potato seed pieces prior to planting. The seed pieces are wet with a solution containing 1 pound of yellow oxide to 15 gallons of water. After treatment the seed pieces are dried before planting.

Zerlate—See *Ziram*.

Zinc Dimethyldithiocarbamate—See *Ziram*.

Zinc Ethylenebisdithiocarbamate—See *Zineb*.

Zinc Oxide—Used mainly as a seed treatment. One level teaspoonful per pound of seed is the dosage rate for radish seed while 3 level teaspoonfuls are recommended for each pound of spinach seed.

Zinc Sulfate—Zinc sulfate and hydrated lime, 8 pounds of each to 100 gallons of water, are used to prepare a spray called *zinc-lime* which is the zinc equivalent of Bordeaux Mixture. Zinc-lime is used extensively for the control of the bacterial spot disease of peaches. At least 5 applications at intervals of two weeks, starting at the time of petal fall, are required for the control of this troublesome disease. If the monohydrated form ($ZnSO_4 + H_2O$) is used instead of fully hydrated crystals ($ZnSO_4 + 7H_2O$) the quantity used may be reduced from 8 to 5 pounds. Zinc sulfate has been added (1 to 2 pounds per 100 gallons) to sprays containing lime and arsenate of lead to reduce arsenical spray injury. The advent of certain organic insecticides to replace arsenate of lead has reduced the need for this specialized use of zinc sulfate. The zinc-lime spray cannot be used on apples and pears without risk of serious russeting of the fruit.

Zineb—This compound, *zinc ethylenebisdithiocarbamate*, has also proved to be exceptionally effective in the control of potato and tomato late blight in Florida. It has not been much superior to copper compounds in the more northern tomato-growing sections. Zineb is less injurious to the tomato and potato plants than copper compounds, a factor of considerable importance in the South where numerous spray applications are required during the long growing season.

Zineb has also been used on cucumbers, muskmelons, and watermelons for downy mildew and anthracnose control, especially in Florida. The lack of injury on these plants is an especially valuable feature of this compound, since cucumbers and melons are extremely susceptible to copper injury. For the same reason this compound has proved of value for the control of cabbage and cauliflower diseases. It is sometimes used to control fire blight on apple and pear trees.

Zineb is used at the rate of 1½ to 2 pounds in 100 gallons of water. It has also been applied as a dust containing 8 to 10% of the fungicide.

Ziram—Ziram, *zinc dimethyldithiocarbamate*, is a white powder and does not leave an objectionable residue. At the rate of 1 to 2 pounds per 100 gallons it has found extensive use in the control of vegetable diseases (celery leaf blight, downy mildew of cucurbits, bean anthracnose, cabbage downy mildew, and squash black rot). Ziram has also been used for peach brown rot control, but is apt to produce leaf injury and fruit russet when used on apples, sour cherries, and pears. It is not an effective material for the control of potato or tomato late blight.

Antibiotics

Streptomycin—This antibiotic is marketed as the sulfate or nitrate under the tradenames Agrimycin 17, AG-Strep, and Phytomycin by Pfizer, Merck, and Olin Mathieson. It is formulated as a dry, wettable powder (sulfate) and liquid (nitrate). Its salts are very soluble in water. It has general use as an antibacterial against fire blight of apples and pears and similar infections on ornamentals including woody and herbaceous plants. It is persistent on plant surfaces for up to 4 months, but is considered of low general toxicity. It can produce allergenic reactions such as rashes, conjunctivitis, and bronchial asthma. This agent should not be applied following Bordeaux mixture and it is incompatible with lime sulfur, pyrethrane, and aldrin.

Relatively crude, denatured forms of streptomycin and oxytetracycline are being used to control many bacterial diseases of plants. Cycloheximide, under the name Actidione, is being used to control cherry leaf spot and dollar spot of turf. The agricultural use of these and other antibiotics is growing.

Control of Weeds and Plants*

Many herbicides are being used for weed control, and many others are being evaluated experimentally to determine their usefulness. Only those of current general interest and usefulness are described below.

Available information on the degree of toxicity of herbicides is listed in the descriptions of chemicals used for weed control. The symbol LD_{50} (lethal dose that kills 50% of the experimental animals) precedes each number that indicates relative toxicity. For example, the single acute oral dose for calcium cyanamide, $LD_{50} = 1400$ mg/Kg, indicates a relatively low oral toxicity. The larger the LD_{50} number, the less poisonous the herbicide.

All LD values listed in this guide are based on a single dose of material orally administered to animals, followed by observation of the treated animals for a definite period of time. However, these findings do not indicate the possible hazards that may arise from skin contact or inhalation of the substance or substances indicated. Likewise, these data do not accurately predict the toxicity of a formulation which may differ according to the solvent or diluent employed. A complete coverage of herbicides, covering basic principles and methods of weed control, precautions for safe use, and weed control under all possible field conditions is available.[22]

Phenoxy Compounds

Several compounds in this group, including 2,4-dichlorophenoxyacetic acid (2,4-D), 2,4,5-trichlorophenoxyacetic acid (2,4,5-T), 2-methyl, 4-chlorophenoxyacetic acid (MCPA), and 2,4,5-trichlorophenoxypropionic acid (silvex) are used as post-emergence selective herbicides to control broadleaved weeds in corn, small grains, sorghum, rice, flax, lawns, and to control brush and weeds in pastures, along roadsides, rights-of-way, and drainage and irrigation ditches. Some of the phenoxy compounds also may be applied to the surface of the soil as a pre-emergence treatment to control grasses and broadleaved weeds in corn and other crops.

Phenoxy compounds usually are formulated and marketed as two basic types. They are of low to intermediate oral toxicity ($LD_{50} = 375$ to 1200 mg/Kg) for the various formulations.

1. Salts

The most widely used salts of 2,4-D, MCPA, 2,4,5-T, and other phenoxy acids include such organic amine salts as diethanolamine, triethanolamine, alkanolamine, dimethylamine, triethylamine, isopropylamine, and others. These organic amine salt formulations are available chiefly as water-soluble liquids. The amine salt formulations are more phytotoxic per pound of acid equivalent than the other salt forms, and are more effective in controlling a wider range of weeds.

---

* This section on Herbicides is taken directly from Special Report 22-46 of the Agricultural Research Service, US Department of Agriculture, and is used with the approval of that agency.

Some of the phenoxy compounds also are commercially available as sodium and ammonium salt formulations. These compounds are available chiefly as water-soluble powders, but some of these herbicides also are available as water-soluble liquids. These salt formulations are satisfactory to use on easy-to-kill weeds, such as mustard, pigweed, and lambs-quarters, but they are less phytotoxic per pound of acid equivalent than the amine salts and are not as effective in controlling as wide a range of weeds.

The salt formulations of 2,4-D, MCPA, 2,4,5-T, and other phenoxy compounds are practically nonvolatile, and are much safer to use near valuable susceptible plants than ester formulations if spray drift is avoided.

2. Esters

(a) Relatively high volatile esters.—This type includes methyl, ethyl, isopropyl, butyl, amyl, and others known to possess relatively high vapor activity. These esters of 2,4-D, MCPA, 2,4,5-T, and other phenoxy compounds are liquids which, when properly formulated, form emulsions when mixed with water. Because they are highly volatile, they should not be used under high temperature conditions for weed control in areas adjacent to susceptible plants, such as cotton, tomatoes, grapes, flowers, and ornamentals. These volatile esters are more phytotoxic per pound of acid equivalent than the amine or other salts of 2,4-D, MCPA, and 2,4,5-T to most crops, annual weeds, and hard-to-kill weeds and brush, especially in the more arid regions and under conditions adverse to rapid plant growth. They penetrate leaves rapidly and their effectiveness is not reduced by rain unless it occurs immediately after application. If a range of rates of application is suggested, the esters should be applied at the lower rates and the amine or other salts at the higher rates.

(b) Relatively low volatile esters.—This type includes the butoxyethanol, butoxyethoxypropanol, capryl, ethoxyethoxypropanol, isooctyl, propylene glycol butyl ether, and other esters known to be low volatile. The low volatile esters are less hazardous than high volatile esters in areas adjacent to susceptible crops when temperatures are 95°F or less. When temperatures exceed 95°F, the vapors of both the high and low volatile esters will cause injury. Even under such high temperatures the low volatile esters are less hazardous to adjacent susceptible crops.

2,4-Dichlorophenoxyethyl Sulfate (Sesone)

This herbicide is formulated as the sodium salt and is a white crystalline powder that is soluble in water. When applied to moist soils, sesone is converted into a herbicide with properties similar to 2,4-D. It is effective as a pre-emergence herbicide for weed control in a number of crops. Unlike 2,4-D, however, sesone possesses little or no phytotoxicity as a foliage spray on most plants. Sesone, therefore, is much safer than 2,4-D as a pre-emergence treatment in areas where 2,4-D spray drift, or vapors of esters of 2,4-D, are hazardous to susceptible crops, such as cotton, grapes, tomatoes, and sugar beets. Sesone is not effective as a post-emergence foliage spray; therefore it must be applied to the soil before emergence of the weeds to give effective control. It has been effective as a post-planting spray for weed control in strawberries when applied before emergence of the weeds. The herbicide has been erratic in performance during periods of inadequate soil moisture.

Sesone is of relatively low toxicity (LD_{50} = 730 to 1400 mg/Kg) for rats.

Substituted Phenols

The dinitro alkyl phenols and chloro substituted phenols have been used widely as contact selective and nonselective post-emergence herbicides. They have also been used for selective pre-emergence weed control in a number of large-seeded crops, including peanuts, soybeans, lima beans, snapbeans, and cotton. The substituted phenols consist mainly of two types.

1. Dinitro Compounds

These include the parent compounds 4,6-dinitro-ortho-secondary-butylphenol (DNBP), 4,6-dinitro-ortho-secondary-amylphenol (DNAP), and 3,5-dinitro ortho cresol (DNC). They are not soluble in water but are soluble in oil and may be applied in an oil carrier, or emulsified with water and applied as an emulsion. The parent compounds are used for pre-emergence and nonselective post-emergence weed control. The salts of these compounds, including sodium, ammonium, various amines, and others, are water soluble, and are used for selective pre-emergence and post-emergence weed control in some crops.

The dinitro compounds are yellow dyes that impart a yellow coloration to clothes and skin. These compounds can be used for weed control without danger if precautions are taken to avoid inhaling the vapors or coming in contact with the spray drift or spray solution. When these materials are used as pre-emergence sprays, severe injury to the crop often results if extremely high temperatures occur in the 2-week period following treatment.

The dinitro compounds are highly toxic (LD_{50} = 26 to 45 mg/Kg) for rats.

2. Chloro Substituted Phenols

These include pentachlorophenol (PCP), which is soluble in oil but not in water, and its sodium salt (sodium pentachlorophenate), which is soluble in water. PCP is used as a fortifying agent in oil sprays for nonselective weed control. PCP in oil and sodium PCP in water are also used for selective pre-emergence weed control in several crops.

The pentachlorophenols are of relatively intermediate to high oral toxicity (LD_{50} = 50 to 500 mg/Kg for the various formulations) when fed to rats.

Carbamates

The carbamates at present include isopropyl N-phenylcarbamate (IPC), isopropyl N-(3-chlorophenyl)carbamate (CIPC), and 2-chloroallyl diethyldithiocarbamate (CDEC). They are relatively insoluble in water but are formulated with organic solvents as emulsifiable concentrates. The carbamates form emulsions with water and may be applied as either low- or high-gallonage sprays. They are effective as selective dormant post-emergence sprays for the control of annual grasses, chickweed, and some other broadleaved weeds in alfalfa and clovers. CIPC is less volatile than IPC and possesses greater residual weed control properties. Both are now being used effectively in some areas for pre-emergence weed control in cotton, snapbeans, lima beans, spinach, and certain other field and horticultural crops. The carbamates also are used as pre-planting sprays for weed control in canning peas and sugar beets.

CDEC is formulated as an emulsifiable concentrate. Prolonged contact with the skin will cause irritation. CDEC has shown promise for the pre-emergence control of certain weeds in several vegetable crops. It is more effective on weedy grasses than on broadleaved weeds; however, excellent control of henbit and moderate control of chickweed is obtained by pre-emergence treatments.

The carbamates are of relatively low oral toxicity (LD_{50} = 3000 to 5000 mg/Kg) for rats.

Substituted Urea Herbicides

The substituted urea herbicides nclude 3-(p-chlorophenyl)-1,1-dimethylurea (monuron); 3-(3,4-dichlorophenyl)-1, 1-dimethylurea (diuron); 3-(phenyl)-1,1-dimethylurea (fenuron), and 1-n-butyl-3-(3,4-dichlorophenyl)-1-methylurea (neburon), previously known as CMU, DCMU, PDU, and DMBU, respectively. These compounds are only slightly soluble in water. They are formulated as wettable powders or as liquids and must be applied as suspensions in high volumes of water. They are the first group of organic chemicals to possess sufficient residual properties to be used as soil sterilants. At present they are being used for nonselective weed control on noncultivated land. However, diuron and monuron also have shown considerable experimental promise and are being used as selective pre-emergence herbicides in cotton and certain other crops. Neburon has the least herbicidal activity and is least toxic of the substituted urea herbicides listed above to many crops, particularly perennial grasses.

The substituted urea herbicides are relatively low in oral toxicity (LD_{50} = 3400 to 7500 mg/Kg) for rats.

Trichloroacetic Acid (TCA)

There are several salts of trichloroacetic acid (TCA) being used as weed killers, including the ammonium and sodium salts. Sodium TCA is used most widely. It has shown varying degrees of effectiveness in controlling quackgrass, Bermudagrass, Johnsongrass, and other annual and perennial grasses. Best results are obtained when it is applied in combination with tillage and cultural practices. Sodium TCA also is being used as a pre-emergence spray for the control of annual grasses and several broadleaved weeds in flax, sugar beets, sugarcane, and certain other crops. The residual toxicity from high rates of TCA for the control of perennial grasses may disappear within a few weeks or may persist for a year or longer depending on the rate of application, soil type, temperature, and soil-moisture relations. Sodium TCA is highly soluble in water, somewhat caustic, and will corrode spray equipment.

TCA has low oral toxicity (LD_{50} = 5000 mg/Kg) for rats.

2,2-Dichloropropionic Acid (Dalapon)

This herbicide possesses properties somewhat similar to TCA. In contrast with TCA, when dalapon is applied to the foliage of grasses in the vegetative stages of growth, it is translocated from the leaves to the roots of most species. Dalapon has proved less erratic and more effective than TCA when applied as a foliage spray for the control of most of the annual grasses. It is much more effective on quackgrass, Bermudagrass, Johnsongrass, and other perennial grasses. The sodium salt of dalapon, which is highly soluble in water, is the most widely used formulation. Research indicates that it is most effective as a pre-emergence or post-emergence spray for controlling perennial grasses when applied in combination with tillage and cultural practices. Dalapon apparently possesses less residual toxicity than TCA; but further research is needed to determine the rate of disappearance of the herbicide from the soil. Dalapon* has shown promise in experiments for weed control in sugarcane, sugar beets, birdsfoot trefoil, alfalfa, and for spot treatment control of Johnsongrass and other grasses in cotton. It has given effective control of cattails and phragmites on irrigation and drainage canals.

Dalapon is low in oral toxicity (LD_{50} = 6590 to 8120 mg/Kg) for rats.

3-Amino-1,2,4-Triazole (Amitrol)

This herbicide is generally available as a water soluble white, crystalline powder. It has shown promise for control of Canada thistle, leafy spurge, quackgrass, Bermudagrass, sedges, horsetail rush, cattails, and tules, and several woody plants such as poison ivy, poison oak, white ash, and prickly ash. Amitrol† is translocated throughout the plant and affects the growing points, producing chlorosis and inhibition. It is quickly inactivated in most soils and appears promising for control of certain perennial weeds in apple and pear orchards and in cornland.

Amitrol is low in acute oral toxicity (LD_{50} = 15,000 mg/Kg) for mice. This chemical is the one responsible for the widely publicized seizure of cranberries in 1959. It is no longer used in cranberry culture.

N-1-Naphthylphthalamic Acid (NPA)

This chemical is formulated for experimental herbicidal use as the sodium salt, imide, and acid. The sodium salt of NPA is available as a wettable powder and as a liquid concentrate. Presently, NPA is being used for pre-emergence control of grasses and broad-leaved weeds in cucumbers, squash, cantaloupes, and other crops in the cucurbit group. It also has shown some promise for weed control in irrigated cotton in the West.

NPA has low oral toxicity (LD_{50} = 8200 mg/Kg).

3,6-Endoxohexahydrophthalic Acid (Endothal)

In research studies the disodium salt of this acid has shown promise for control of certain weeds in turf, alfalfa, sugar beets, and in certain other crops. It is being used as a pre-harvest aid, a general contact herbicide, and chemical defoliant.

Endothal has high oral toxicity (LD_{50} = 35 to 120 mg/Kg) for rats.

1,2-Dihydro-pyridazine-3,6-dione (Maleic Hydrazide, MH)

This chemical is formulated as a water-soluble sodium or di-ethanolamine salt for use as a herbicide. It has shown promise for control of several annual and perennial grasses when applied in combination with tillage and cultural treatments. It is being used also as a grass inhibitor to reduce mowing on areas such as roadsides. The chemical, however, has performed erratically both as a herbicide and as a grass inhibitor. Additional research is needed to determine the place of this compound in the field of weed control.

MH has low oral toxicity (LD_{50} = 5800 mg/Kg) for rats.

Phenyl Mercuric Acetate (PMA)

This herbicide is available in a number of formulations. It is sometimes impregnated on various carriers such as vermiculite, but PMA is also available as a liquid concentrate that must be diluted with water and applied as a spray. Most of the formulations presently available contain 10 per cent PMA by weight or approximately 1 pound of active ingredient per gallon of concentrate. PMA is an effective herbicide for selective control of crabgrass in lawns.

The compound is highly toxic to humans and warm-blooded animals and must be handled with care. Its oral toxicity for rats: LD_{50} = 27 mg/Kg. It is not used presently for weed control in cultivated crops.

Potassium Cyanate (KOCN)

This herbicide is a white, water-soluble powder, effective in controlling seedling weeds. It is used as a selective spray for weed control in onions, and to control crabgrass and chickweed in lawns. For best results against crabgrass, it should be applied when the crabgrass is small. The herbicide will often discolor lawn grasses at rates required to kill crabgrass, but the discoloration usually will disappear in 7 to 10 days.

KOCN has relatively low oral toxicity (LD_{50} = 780 mg/Kg) for rats.

Calcium Cyanamide (CaCN₂)

Calcium cyanamide is a water-soluble solid. It usually is formulated as a granulated solid or pulverized powder. The by-products of calcium cyanamide decomposition in acid soils possess both phyto-toxic and fertilizing properties. For this reason it is often used as a combination herbicide and crop fertilizer.

This chemical has long been used in tobacco plant beds as an herbicide for weed control and as a fertilizer. In recent years, it has been used with erratic performance for pre-emergence weed control in corn and in several horticultural crops. The herbicide is also being used as a temporary pre-planting soil sterilant for turf seedbeds. The chemical should be applied and worked into the soil surface at least 3 weeks before seeding lawns and other turf.

In some areas, calcium cyanamide is being used in turf renovation programs.

Calcium cyanamide has relatively low oral toxicity (LD_{50} = 410 mg/Kg) for rabbits.

Ammonium Sulfamate (NH₄SO₃NH₂)

This water-soluble, white, crystalline powder is most widely used for control of woody plants in areas adjacent to cotton, grapes, tomatoes, and other plants that are susceptible to the phenoxy compounds. It will prevent stumps from sprouting when applied to the cut surface, and will kill large trees and sprouting stumps when the crystals or concentrated solutions are used in cups (ax chips) made around the base of a tree or stump.

Ammonium sulfamate has relatively low oral toxicity (LD_{50} = 3900 mg/Kg) for rats.

Herbicidal Oils

Herbicidal oils usually are obtained in the distillation of petroleum and coal tar. Aromatic constituents usually have the greatest influence on their herbicidal properties. Recent research, however, has shown that a number of constituents of oils affect both total herbicidal activity and selectivity. Several herbicidal oils are known under a variety of names such as aromatic solvent, solvent naphtha, and petroleum naphtha. These oils vary widely in their herbicidal toxicity and selectivity depending on their origin and composition. One specific example is a petroleum-naphtha with A. P. I. gravity 49 to 50, boiling range 300° to 400°F, unsaturated compounds 0.5 to 1.0%, aromatic content 22 to 24%, sulfur compounds 0.25 to 0.30%, and a maximum aniline point to 128°F, which is being used extensively as a directed postemergence spray for control of seedling annual grasses and broadleaved weeds in cotton.

Stoddard solvent and light aromatic oils have been used extensively as selective herbicidal oils for weed control in crops of the carrot family. Nonselective herbicidal oils with high aromatic contents are being used effectively to control Johnsongrass on ditchbanks in the Southwest. Aromatic solvents also are being used to control aquatic weeds in irrigation canals and ditches in the Western States. Diesel oil, fuel oil, stove oils, and other oils are used as carriers for herbicides. Oil sprays usually are more effective than water sprays in wetting leaf surfaces and in penetrating waxy leaf surfaces. Oil-water emulsions fortified with dinitrophenols or chlorophenols are used rather extensively for control of annual weeds in orchards and alfalfa, as well as weeds on ditchbanks and other noncrop areas.

Herbicidal oils are relatively low in oral toxicity; for example, Stoddard solvent: LD_{50} = 2000 mg/Kg for rats.

Chlorates

A number of chlorates, including sodium and calcium, are used to control deep-rooted perennial weeds. They also are used for temporary and semipermanent soil sterilization to prevent growth of all types of vegetation. Sodium chlorate is used most extensively. It is a white, crystalline, water-soluble powder. Sodium chlorate can be applied in dry form by hand or with various types of spreaders, or as a spray using high-volume spray equipment.

Semipermanent soil sterilization in humid areas requires 500 to 2400 pounds of sodium chlorate per acre (3 to 12 pounds per square rod). In semiarid areas, 500 to 1000 pounds of the chemical per acre (3 to 6 pounds per square rod) are required for semipermanent soil sterilization. Sodium chlorate leaves the soil unproductive for 1 to 4 years, depending on the precipitation, prevailing temperatures, soil type, and other soil and climatic factors. For semipermanent sterilization, higher rates of application are required on the sandy soils of humid regions than on the heavy soils of lower rainfall areas. To kill all vegetation, higher initial rates of application are necessary on the heavy soils of arid regions than on soils of humid areas. Toxicity persists for longer periods in arid regions because there is less leaching and slower decomposition than in humid regions.

Sodium chlorate has low oral toxicity (LD_{50} = 7000 mg/Kg) for rats.

---

* Dalapon cannot be recommended (as of April 1, 1958) for use on birds-foot trefoil and alfalfa since evidence has not been developed to prove it will leave no residue or/and tolerances have not been set under Public Law 518.

† Amitrol cannot be recommended (as of April 1, 1958) for use in citrus orchards and on grapes since evidence has not been developed to prove it will leave no residue or/and tolerances have not been set under Public Law 518.

Caution. The manufacturer's directions for use of sodium chlorate should be followed carefully. This chemical, particularly in spray solutions, must be handled with extreme caution. Any inflammable materials, such as clothing, shoes, hay, wood, or weeds, that have dried after having been wet with a sodium chlorate solution become violently inflammable and even explosive. They can be ignited easily by friction, sparks, or even by the heat from the sun. *Serious injury or property damage* may result from carelessness or failure to observe caution.

Boron Compounds

A number of boron compounds, including borax, sodium pentaborate, boron trioxide, anhydrous sodium diborate, and mixtures of these compounds with 2,4-D, sodium chlorate, and/or a substituted urea compound are used to control deep-rooted perennial weeds, and for temporary and semipermanent soil sterilization to prevent growth of all vegetation. Boron compounds should be applied at rates of 2400 to 4800 pounds of borax equivalent per acre (15 to 30 pounds per square rod) for control of all vegetation and semipermanent soil sterilization in humid areas. In arid regions the rates required are usually higher—4800 to 6400 pounds per acre (30 to 40 pounds per square rod). The soluble borate compounds are effective at lower rates of treatment. Addition of 2,4-D, sodium chlorate, or a substituted urea herbicide to boron compounds will greatly influence the rate of application required for killing all vegetation. Boron compounds normally are applied as dry granular formulations, but mixtures of boron and 2,4-D, and boron and sodium chlorate, also are formulated for spray application.

Arsenicals

Arsenical herbicides include sodium arsenite, arsenic trioxide, arsenic pentoxide, disodium methylarsonate, and other formulations of arsenic acid. Sodium arsenite (the most commonly used arsenical) is used extensively to kill submerged aquatic weeds and as a semipermanent soil sterilant to control all vegetation on driveways, tennis courts, railroad rights-of-way, industrial storage sites, and on other nonagricultural areas inaccessible to animals. It leaves the soil unproductive for 1 to 4 years, depending on soil type and climatic conditions.

Areas frequented by livestock should not be treated with sodium arsenite because of hazard of poisoning: Sodium arsenite is highly toxic for mammals (LD_{50} = 10 to 50 mg/Kg) when administered orally.

2-Chloro-*N,N*-diallylacetamide (CDAA)

CDAA [1,3 - bis(2,2,2 - trichloro - 1 - hydroxyethyl)urea] is formulated as an emulsifiable concentrate. It has shown promise for pre-emergence control of weed grasses in soybeans, corn, and in certain other crops. CDAA is less effective on broadleaved weeds than on grasses. It often causes some temporary stunting of broadleaved weeds which opens the way to more effective control by timely cultivation. *CDAA may cause serious irritation to the eyes.* This hazard can be reduced by wearing goggles and rubber gloves during application.

Dichloral Urea (DCU)

DCU [1,3-bis(2,2,2-trichloro-1-hydroxyethyl)urea] is used for pre-emergence weed control in sugar beets. It is more effective for control of grasses than for broadleaved weeds. It is low in solubility and is formulated as a wettable powder.

DCU is claimed to have low oral toxicity.

Methyl Bromide

Methyl bromide applied at heavy rates as a volatile temporary soil sterilant will kill most weed seeds and plants. It has a boiling point of 38°F, and is sold in sealed cans as a liquid under pressure. When released at 68°F, it becomes a gas 3.2 times heavier than air. The gas must be released under an airtight cover for use as a soil sterilant. Confining the gas under an airtight cover for 24 hours is usually sufficient for weed control if soil in the treated area is moist and has been loosened to aid gas penetration. It is safe to plant crops 2 to 3 days after the airtight cover is removed. *Methyl bromide gas is poisonous to man and animals.* Effects of exposures within a 24-hour period are cumulative. Skin contact can produce severe burns. The gas is colorless with a slight, sweetish odor, and warning traces of other gases, such as chloropicrin, are sometimes added.

Methyl bromide is relatively toxic, having the power to be absorbed by the skin as well as by inhalation.

2,3-Dichloro-1,4-Naphthoquinone (Dichlone)

Dichlone is available as a dry, wettable powder that wets and disperses readily in water. It is used for control of blue-green and green algae in lakes and ponds. It mixes well with oil, is chemically stable, and, as an algicide, remains active in water with a pH up to 9 or 10.

Dichlone is relatively low in oral toxicity (LD_{50} = 1500 mg/Kg) for rats.

Rosin Amine D Acetate (RADA)

RADA is a water-soluble material that effectively controls freshwater algae in irrigation canals. It also prevents algae from forming on surfaces of such structures as humidification systems and irrigation installations.

Relatively New Compounds Available for Herbicidal Use

The new herbicides described in the following section have shown promise in preliminary tests, but further evaluations are necessary before recommendations for their use can be made.

(1) *4-(2,4-Dichlorophenoxy)butyric acid [4-(2,4-DB)] and 4-(2-methyl-4-chlorophenoxy)butyric acid [4-(MCPB)]* have shown promise for post-emergence control of broadleaved weeds in (*a*) cereals underseeded with certain forage legumes; (*b*) establishment of pure stands of forage legumes; (*c*) forage legume seed-production fields; (*d*) flax; and (*e*) other weed-crop situations. Legumes that are relatively tolerant to 4-(2,4-DB) include white clover, alsike clover, red clover, alfalfa, and birdsfoot trefoil. It is marketed as Butoxone (*Amchem*) and Butyrac (*Chipman*).

(2) *2-Chloro-4,6-bis(ethylamino)-s-triazine (simazin)* is a wettable powder with low solubility in water and in organic solvents. It is being tested for pre-emergence weed control in corn, transplanted tomatoes, and fruit crops. As a soil sterilant, simazin has been effective when applied at heavy rates. Simazine is marketed as Simazine 80WP (*Geigy*). It is used to control both broadleaf weeds and grasses in ornamentals, fruits, and corn, and for noncrop uses. It is not recommended that crops be planted the same season as application was made as injury may result. Several plants are sensitive to this chemical. See label cautions. Other substituted triazines are available.

Simazin has low oral toxicity (LD_{50} = 5000 mg/Kg) for mice.

(3) *2,3,6-Trichlorobenzoic acid (2,3,6-TBA)* and several other isomers of benzoic acid have shown promise as herbicides. The herbicide 2,3,6-TBA is translocated in plants and is effective against a number of weeds that other herbicides have failed to control. It has been used with some success as a pre-emergence spray for weed control in corn. It is effective as a post-emergence spray for the control of wild garlic, annual weed brome grasses, quackgrass, some species of brush, several perennial weeds, and certain other weeds that are serious pests in lawns and turf. It has residual herbicidal activity in the soil. One isomer of benzoic acid—*viz.*, 3-amino-2,5-dichlorobenzoic acid, marketed as Vegiben (*Amchem*)—is available and is used as a selective pre-emergence herbicide on vegetables, corn, and soybeans.

(4) *Ethyl di-n-propylthiocarbamate (EPTC)* has been used successfully in preliminary trials as a pre-emergence herbicide to control annual grasses and many broadleaved weeds in forage legume seedlings and in certain other field and horticultural crops. It remains active in the soil for short periods. EPTC is formulated as an emulsifiable concentrate, is stable, and apparently noncorrosive. It is marketed as Eptam (*Stauffer*).

(5) *3,5-Dimethyltetrahydro-1,3,5-2H-thiadiazine-2-thione (DMTT)* is a volatile soil sterilant that can be applied without the use of an airtight cover over the soil for control of weeds, soil fungi, and nematodes. It may be applied as a dry powder, or as a spray (wettable powder). After application in either form, the material is mixed into the soil to a depth of about 6 inches. Best weed control has resulted when this treatment has been followed by irrigation with at least 1 inch of water. A 21-day interval should elapse between time of treatment and planting crops.

(6) *Sodium N-methyldithiocarbamate dihydrate (SMDC)* is also a volatile soil sterilant that may be applied without the use of an airtight cover over the soil for control of weeds, soil fungi, and nematodes. The liquid may be applied in two ways: sprayed onto the soil surface, then soaked into the soil with water; or, mixed with the surface 6-inch layer of soil, followed by an application of water, thoroughly wetting the surface to provide a gas seal. A 7- to 14-day interval should elapse between treatment and the planting of crops.

Plant Regulators

Plant regulators are chemicals used to change the growth patterns of ornamentals, fruits, and vegetables, and now include a number of useful products. Gibberellic acid is used extensively on seeds to aid in uniform germination and growth and on grapes to increase size. Beta Napthoxyacetic acid, 2(2,4,5-trichlorophenoxy) propionic acid (Silvex), 2-methyl-4-chlorophenoxy acetic acid (MCPA), and a number of related chemicals are used to thin blossoms, to stop the premature drop of fruits or vegetables before harvest, to increase the uniformity of ripening, and for a wide variety of other purposes. 2,4-D, for example, when applied properly will increase the red color in potatoes, and other chemicals will produce pineapples of more uniform shape than untreated ones. This field of chemical usage is just getting well underway and would appear to have a future limited only by the necessity to prove that the uses will be safe, from both the toxicological and nutritional viewpoints.

Desiccants and Defoliants

Desiccants and defoliants are also becoming of increasing importance as mechanical harvesting gains popularity in farming. In the same way that removal of weeds by use of herbicides just before the combines are put into the fields to harvest wheat will prevent clogging of the machines with weed debris, the removal of cotton leaves with a chemical treatment aids mechanical harvesting of cotton and other leafy crops. Arsenic acid, pentachlorophenol and more complex chemicals such as S,S,S tributylphosphorotrithioate and S,S,S tributylphosphorotrithioite, and others are being used for this purpose. Since this section introduces a new area of the pesticide field not previously presented in this book, it is likely that there will be many questions. These should be addressed to the United States Department of Agriculture, the state Experiment Stations, or the manufacturers of the specific products. Questions on the legal status of any pesticides, including these new ones, should be sent to Director, Pesticides Regulation Division, Agricultural Research Service, US Department of Agriculture, Washington, D.C. 20250.

Control of Other Agricultural Pests

Other pesticides of importance to agriculture include products proposed and sold to control or repel predatory animals, pest birds, coarse or trash fish, reptiles and similar pests. A variety of chemicals, which have been discussed under other categories are employed with quite variable success. Strychnine and sodium fluoacetate are the most common predatory animal poisons, with the latter used almost entirely by state and federal trained hunters. Pest birds are fought with strychnine, endrin, and some of the highly toxic organic phosphates, with government crews supervising much of the operation. Fish poisoning is largely used for improving the habitat for sport fishing by removing undesirable species. Rotenone is the chemical most widely used.

Snake poisons and repellents are usually of questionable value, but there are a few products on the market with claims that they will drive snakes away. The active ingredients are usually the more toxic chlorinated hydrocarbons.

General Safety Factors

In the foregoing pages of this chapter many references have been made to insecticides and rodenticides of a highly poisonous nature, such as the following items: *strychnine, arsenic, sodium fluoride, compound 1080, Paris green, hydrocyanic acid, calcium cyanide, sodium cyanide, mercury bichloride, phosphorus, thallium sulfate, tetraethyl pyrophosphate, parathion, endrin, and others.*

While these substances are highly effective as pesticides, one should fully realize the problems involved in using such preparations. They may be hazardous for the operator who must prepare and apply the material. They are highly dangerous from the standpoint that pets, children, and others are likely innocently to find the material or come in contact with it sufficiently to become poisoned. Furthermore, fruits and vegetables which have been sprayed or treated with poisons may carry the residues to the consumer. Washing such fruits as apples and pears to remove excess residues is a common practice among fruit growers. Leafy vegetables such as cabbage, cauliflower, and lettuce are especially likely to carry insecticide poisons unless considerable care is exercised as the insecticides are applied. All users of pesticides should be cautioned to follow directions precisely, and to avoid keeping pesticides in cupboards and other places where foods or drugs are stored, or where they may be found by children, irresponsible persons, pets or livestock.

There are some states which have enacted legislation, or regulations have been issued through the state departments concerned, requiring that all white powders marketed as insecticides should be colored with certain specified colors. A colored powdered sodium fluoride or other insecticidal mixture is not apt to be mistaken for baking soda or flour, or other similar material which is used in the kitchen. The use of color is increasing slowly with other toxic agents and should decrease the danger of accident through mistaking a poison for a food.

Additional information on the emergency treatment of poisoning can be found in Chapter 100, *Poison Control* (page 1947).

Pharmacists and Pest Control—Throughout this chapter the pharmacist has been given an outline of the many products available for use in the control of insects, plant diseases, weeds and rodents, in order that he may more capably serve the community as a source of advice on this phase of public health. The mere reading of this chapter will not make him a pest control expert, however. Experience and special aptitudes are required in the successful pest control operator and carefully trained service men are available in this specialized field for handling the many problems concerned with the most efficient control of insects, fungi, weeds, and rodents, particularly in the cities, where protection of homes and commercial premises is of primary importance. In rural and farming areas sound advice on pest control problems is usually available through the County Agricultural Agent.

Requests for particular information on predatory animal, bird and fish poisons and on rodenticides and rodent control, however, should be addressed to the US Fish and Wildlife Service, US Dept. of the Interior, Washington, D.C.

The Safe Use of Economic Poisons

(Herbicides—Insecticides—Fungicides—Rodenticides)

The Pesticides Regulation Division of the US Department of Agriculture, to which is assigned the enforcement of the Federal Insecticide, Fungicide, and Rodenticide Act, in 1962 published certain warnings, cautions, and suggestions for antidotes in case of poisoning. This type of information[23] is required to appear on the labels of all packages of "pesticides," the name now generally applied to economic poisons, which have moved in interstate commerce.

When a product is "highly toxic" under the regulations, its label must carry the word "Poison" in red on a contrasting background, the skull, crossbones, and an antidote statement.

The extensive use today of various forms of pesticides in the home and on the farm has greatly increased the dangers that may arise from their improper use. The need to protect humans, pets, and other animals, as well as decorative and useful plants and trees, through proper precautionary labeling, is imperative.

Pesticides Official in USP

Diethyltoluamide USP

[*N,N*-Diethyl-*m*-toluamide]

$$CON(C_2H_5)_2$$

$$CH_3$$

Diethyltoluamide contains 95.0–103.0% of the meta isomer of $C_{12}H_{17}NO$ (191.28), calculated on the anhydrous basis.

Preparation—*m*-Toluic acid is treated with thionyl chloride to produce *m*-toluyl chloride which is then condensed with diethylamine to form the diethylamide. The crude product may be purified by recrystallization from diluted ethanol.

Description—It occurs as a colorless liquid, having a faint, pleasant odor. The specific gravity is not less than 0.9965 and not more than 1.0020. The refractive index is not less than 1.5200 and not more than 1.5235. It boils at about 111° under a pressure of 1 mm of mercury.

Solubility—Practically insoluble in water and glycerin; miscible with alcohol, isopropyl alcohol, ether, chloroform, and carbon disulfide.

Uses—Diethyltoluamide is employed principally as a mosquito repellent, although it is capable of repelling certain other insects. The agent generally is not used alone but rather is incorporated into creams and lotions.

Dose—*Topically*, as a **50** to **75**% solution in alcohol to skin and clothing.

Dosage Forms—Solution USP: 50 and 75%; Solution USP (pressurized containers): 15 to 25%.

Ethohexadiol USP

[Ethylhexanediol; 2-Ethyl-1,3-hexanediol; Rutgers 612]

$$CH_3—CH_2—CH_2—CH—CH—CH_2OH$$
$$OH \quad C_2H_5$$

Ethohexadiol contains 97.0–100.5% of $C_8H_{18}O_2$ (146.23).

Preparation—Ethohexadiol may be prepared by starting with commercially available *n*-butyraldehyde, three molecules of which condense under the catalytic influence of magnesium and aluminum ethoxides to yield 2-ethyl-1,3-hexanediol butyrate. Saponification of this ester with alcoholic alkali yields the free alcohol.

Description—Clear, colorless, oily liquid. Odorless or has only a slight odor. Specific gravity: 0.936 to 0.940.

Distilling range: 240° to 250°. Refractive index: 1.4465 to 1.4515.

Solubility—1 ml dissolves in about 50 ml of water; miscible with alcohol, chloroform, and ether.

Uses—Ethohexadiol is used as an *arthropod* or *insect repellant* and is applied topically to skin and clothing for this purpose.

Dose—*Topically*, to skin and clothing.

Other Pesticides

Arsenic Acid [H_3AsO_4]—A white hygroscopic powder. It is very soluble in water, soluble in alcohol or glycerin. In commerce it is usually available as a solution containing 75 to 80% H_3AsO_4. *Uses:* Basic material for the manufacture of arsenates, such as calcium and lead arsenates which are extensively used as insecticides, and also for the production of organic arsenicals. *Poisonous*.

Barium Carbonate [$BaCO_3$]—White powder. Insoluble in water; readily decomposed by acids with the evolution of carbon dioxide. *Uses:* A rat poison; used in the preparation of other barium compounds.

Butopyronoxyl USP XV [Indalone; Butyl 3,4-dihydro-2,2 - dimethyl - 4 - oxo - 1,2*H* - pyran - 6 - carboxylate]

[$OC(CH_3)_2CH_2COCH:CCOOC_4H_9$]—A yellow liquid, having a characteristic, aromatic odor, reasonably stable in air and slowly affected by light. It is insoluble in water but miscible with alcohol, chloroform, and ether. The refractive index is 1.4745–1.4755. *Uses:* Insect repellent. An ingredient in Compound Dimethyl Phthalate Solution USP XV.

Calcium Arsenate [$Ca_3(AsO_4)_2$]—White powder, slightly soluble in water; soluble in dilute acids. *Uses:* An insecticide, particularly useful against insects destructive to plants and trees. *Poisonous*.

Citronella Oil—Distilled from the leaves of *Cymbopogon Winterianus* and *Andropogon nadus* (Fam. *Gramineæ*). Habitat, Ceylon. Contains geraniol, citronellal, and a heptoic aldehyde. *Uses:* As a perfume in some soaps and as a mosquito repellent.

Dibutyl Phthalate BP, PhI—The normal butyl ester of *o*-benzenedicarboxylic acid. An odorless, clear, colorless, somewhat viscous liquid. It is soluble in 2500 parts of water and miscible with alcohol and ether. It has a Sp. Gr. of 1.043–1.048 and a refractive index, at 20°, of 1.492–1.495. It is thought to be slightly less effective as an insect repellent than dimethyl phthalate but is more effective against the trombidid mite, the insect vector of scrub typhus. *Uses:* As an insect repellent. *Dose:* A fortnightly application of about one fluidounce per set of clothes, rubbed in by hand.

p-Dichlorobenzene [$C_6H_4Cl_2$]—Colorless or white crystals with a characteristic odor. Melts at 53°. Boils at 174°, and sublimes at room temperature. Insoluble in water; freely soluble in alcohol, benzene, chloroform, and many other organic solvents. *Uses:* For killing moths and their larvae; for the preservation of woolen fabrics from moth attacks; also used against peach tree borers.

Dimethyl Phthalate USP XV, BP [Methyl phthalate; DMP]—The normal methyl ester of *o*-benzenedicarboxylic acid. Purity: not less than 98% $C_{10}H_{10}O_4$. A clear, colorless, oily liquid having a slight aromatic odor. It is stable in air but slowly affected by light. It is insoluble in water but miscible with alcohol, ether, and chloroform. Its refractive index is 1.5130–1.5170 at 20°. *Uses:* Insect repellent, particularly effective against harvest midges. Usually applied to the skin as a 35% lotion.

Lead Arsenate [approx. $PbHAsO_4$]—White, heavy powder, insoluble in water; soluble in nitric acid and in caustic alkalies. *Uses:* A constituent of various insecticides for larvae of gypsy moth, boll weevil, etc. *Poisonous.*

Parathion [Thiophos; Niran; Aphamite; Genithion; Mackathion; Alkron; Corothion; Penphos; Phos-kil; Vapophos; Plantthion; E-605; Compound 3422; DNTP; AAT; DPP; *O,O*-Diethyl *O*-*p*-nitrophenyl thiophosphate; $SP(OC_2H_5)_2(OC_6H_4NO_2)$]—Parathion is employed in agriculture as an organic phosphorus insecticide. Like various other organophosphorus compounds, parathion acts as an irreversible inhibitor of the enzyme cholinesterase. Hence, its muscarinic, nicotinic, and central neural effects are explained on the basis of the accumulated acetylcholine. Parathion is absorbed through the intact skin and all portals of the body. It is a potentially dangerous agent and death or serious illness may result in those who come in contact with it, if proper precautions are not employed to prevent its entrance into the body via the lungs, mouth, and skin. Toxic symptoms include headache, giddiness, blurred vision, weakness, nausea, cramps, diarrhea, and discomfort in the chest. Sweating, miosis, salivation, pulmonary edema, cyanosis, papilledema, convulsions, and coma are characteristic of more severe intoxication. Treatment consists of keeping the patient fully atropinized for as long as necessary, decontamination by washing the patient thoroughly with soap and water, removal of any ingested poison, artificial respiration with oxygen, hospitalization, and constant medical and nursing attention. Poisoning in persons who work with parathion may be prevented by constant, thoughtful care on the part of every operator and by the use of protective clothing and masks.

Pyrethrum Flowers NF X [Insect Flowers]—The dried flower heads of *Chrysanthemum cinerariaefolium* Visiani, of *C. coccineum* Willdenow (*C. roseum* Weber et Mohr), or of *C. marschallii* Ascherson (Fam. *Compositæ*). It yields not less than 0.5% of total pyrethrins, which are esters of the ketone-alcohol pyretholone with two acids. The pyrethrins are soluble in petroleum benzin, ether, alcohol, and several other organic solvents. *Uses:* Insecticide for its "knockdown" effect, since it is a contact poison for insects.

Rotenone [$C_{23}H_{22}O_6$]—Principal active constituent of derris root, cubé, etc. White, odorless crystals. Insoluble in water; soluble in alcohol, acetone, carbon tetrachloride, and many other organic solvents. *Uses:* Highly toxic to insects both by contact and through stomach, but practically nontoxic to man and animals; also toxic to fish (1 part in 20,000,000 kills gold fish in 3 hours).

Sodium Cyanide [NaCN]—White, amorphous pieces or granular powder. It is deliquescent and emits the odor of hydrocyanic acid. *It is very poisonous* and should be handled with great caution. *Uses:* An insecticide; used in the extraction of gold and silver in electroplating, and in the heat treatment of metals.

Sodium Fluoroacetate [Compound 1080; ($FCH_2.COONa$)]—A white powder soluble in water. It is extremely toxic to rodents and other small animals, including fowl, yet is practically tasteless to them in the dilutions employed (see *Pesticides*). The LD_{50} dose for wild Norway rats is 5 mg per Kg.

References

1. Carson, R., *Silent Spring*, Houghton-Mifflin, Boston, 1962.
2. Rudd, R. L., *Pesticides and the Living Landscape*, Univ. of Wisc. Press, Madison, 1964.
3. Whitten, J. L., *That We May Live*, Van Nostrand, Princeton, N. J., 1966.
4. McMillen, W., *Bugs or People*, Appleton-Century-Crofts, New York, 1965.
5. *The Effects of Pesticides on Fish and Wildlife*, US Dept. of Interior, 1965.
6. *Health Aspects of Pesticides* (Abstr. Bull.), US Dept. of Health, Education, and Welfare.
7. *Pesticides Monitoring Journal*, Fed. Comm. on Pest Control.
8. Metcalf, R. L., *Organic Insecticides, Their Chemistry and Mode of Action*, Interscience, New York and London, 1955.
9. *Ants in the Garden and How to Control Them*, US Dept. of Agr. Home & Garden Bull. No. 28, 1966, SR.
10. *Controlling Chiggers*, US Dept of Agr Home & Garden Bull. No. 137, 1967.
11. *Cockroaches and Their Control*, US Dept. of Agr. Leaflet No. 144, 1950.
12. *Controlling Fleas*, US Dept. of Agr. Home & Garden Bull. No. 121, 1967.
13. *The House Fly—How to Control It*, US Dept. of Agr. Leaflet No. 390, 1966.
14. *Clothes Moths and Carpet Beetles—How to Combat Them*, US Dept. of Agr. Home & Garden Bull. No. 24, 1953.
15. *Silverfish and Firebrats—How to Control Them*, US Dept. of Agr. Leaflet No. 412, 1966, SR.
16. Brown, A. W. A., *Insect Control by Chemicals*, Wiley, New York, 1951.
17. Carter and Busbey, *Plant Quarant. Mimeo E-466*, US Bur. of Entomol., 1939.
18. *Insecticide Recommendations of the Entomology Research Division for the Control of Insects Attacking Crops and Livestock*, Agr. Handbook No. 120, Entomol. Res. Div., US Dept. of Agr., Mar., 1960.
19. *Insects, The Yearbook of Agriculture*, US Dept. of Agr., 1952.
20. Smith, C. N., *et al, Use of Insect Repellents*, ARS-33-26, Agr. Res. Serv., US Dept. of Agr., Mar., 1957.
21. Ward, J. C., *J. APhA, Sci. Ed.*, **36,** 1427 (1946).
22. Suggested Guide for Weed Control, Agr. Handbook No. 332, Agr. Res. Serv., US Dept. of Agr., 1967.
23. *Interpretation with Respect to Warning, Caution, and Antidote Statements Required to Appear on Labels of Economic Poisons*, Govt. Circ., Title 7, Chap. 111, Interpretation 18, Rev. II, Sec. 362,116; reprinted from *Fed. Register* (Mar. 9, 1962).

70 | **Diagnostic Drugs**

Drugs used as x-ray contrast media—drugs used to test organ function—
drugs used to determine blood volume and hemopoietic function—
miscellaneous diagnostic drugs

This chapter was prepared by

Ewart A. Swinyard, PhD, *Professor of Pharmacology, College of Pharmacy and
College of Medicine, University of Utah, Salt Lake City, Utah 84112, and*
Stewart C. Harvey, PhD, *Associate Professor of Pharmacology, College of
Medicine, University of Utah, Salt Lake City, Utah 84112*

Diagnostic methods have become increasingly complex and frequently involve the use of drugs. For many years inorganic substances have been used for visualization of the gastrointestinal tract. More recently a variety of organic substances have been employed for visualization of the liver, gall bladder, urinary tract, bronchi, lungs, heart, blood vessels, and spinal canal. Drugs of varying chemical structure have been used for the study of blood flow, blood volume, and for the diagnosis of diseases such as pernicious anemia and myasthenia gravis. A number of radioactive substances have been introduced to measure organic function. These are discussed in Chapter 34, *Medical Applications of Radioisotopes*.

Although some drugs employed as diagnostic agents are innocuous, others possess pharmacologic activity and/or undesirable side actions. Indeed, no diagnostic test or drug is completely devoid of risk. Sudden death from anaphylactic reaction has followed the intravenous injection of such a relatively inert substance as dehydrocholic acid. Alarming pharmacological responses have been observed to follow the use of more active agents, such as Diodrast and similar compounds. Iodism quite commonly follows the use of diagnostic agents with a high iodine content. Therefore, it is generally agreed that the clinician should evaluate carefully the need of every test and should reserve diagnostic drugs for those situations where effective management of the patient depends upon their use.

Some of the more commonly employed diagnostic drugs are listed in this chapter. For convenience in presentation, they are divided according to use into four groups as follows: drugs used as x-ray contrast media, drugs used to test organ function, drugs used to determine blood volume and hemopoietic function, and drugs used for miscellaneous diagnostic tests.

Drugs Used as X-ray Contrast Media

Certain salts of heavy metals, such as barium and bismuth, and compounds containing iodine or bromine, are opaque to x-rays. By administering these preparations in various ways it is possible to visualize with the fluoroscope or to photograph by x-rays various structures such as the gastrointestinal tract, gall bladder and ducts, ureters and kidney pelvis, and uterus and fallopian tubes.

Hence, drugs described in this section help to reveal anatomic evidence of disease.

Drugs Used for Outlining the Gastrointestinal Tract

Previous to the introduction in 1910 of barium sulfate as a contrast medium, insoluble bismuth salts were used in roentgen examination of the gastrointestinal tract. Bismuth subcarbonate was preferred over the subnitrate because of its lower toxicity. In modern medical practice, barium sulfate has largely replaced the bismuth salts, because it is completely innocuous even when taken in very large doses, and it is inexpensive. Since the soluble barium salts are highly toxic, it is recommended that when barium sulfate is prescribed the title should be written out in full.

Barium Sulfate USP

[Synthetic or Artificial Barytes; Artificial Heavy Spar; Blanc Fixé; Permanent White]

Barium Sulfate contains 98.0–100.5% of BaSO₄ (233.40).

The USP adds the following special note to emphasize to both the physician and the pharmacist the danger from mistakes when prescribing this salt.

Caution—When Barium Sulfate is prescribed, the title always should be written out in full to avoid confusion with the poisonous barium sulfide or barium sulfite.

Other salts of barium, especially the sulfide, are employed for legitimate purposes and are frequently sold by the manufacturer or wholesale druggist, but they are so rarely prescribed by the physician that it is a safe rule never to dispense for human use any other salt than the *sulfate* even should the physician write for "Bar. Sulf."

Preparation—Barium Sulfate precipitates when an aqueous solution containing barium ion is mixed with a solution containing sulfate ion. It also can be obtained by suitable purification of native barium sulfate.

Description—A fine, white, odorless, tasteless, bulky powder, free from grittiness. Its suspension in water is neutral to litmus paper.

Solubility—Practically insoluble in water, solutions of acids and of alkalies, and organic solvents.

Uses—Medicinally, Barium Sulfate is used in roentgenography (page 550) for the purpose of making the intestinal tract opaque to the x-ray so that it may be photographed. As the amount required is large, 60 to 250 Gm (2 to 8 ounces), and as soluble salts of barium are extremely poisonous, it is highly important to be sure that the sulfate dispensed is of USP quality. When preparing Barium Sulfate mixtures for X-ray diagnosis, strain them through gauze or mix them well with the food, otherwise lumps of the salt may give false indication of an ulcer niche. The following suggestions are offered if specific directions are not given by the attending physician:

For the Roentgen-Ray Examination of the Stomach— The evening before the examination, the patient receives 1 fluid ounce of castor oil or other suitable cathartic. In the morning an ordinary portion of wheat-meal porridge, with which 2 ounces of Barium Sulfate has been well mixed, together with a little sugar and cream, is administered by mouth. The patient is then directed to abstain from further food. The examination is made 6 hours later.

For the Roentgen-Ray Examination of the Colon— An enema consisting of 16 ounces of mucilage of acacia, 3 pounds of condensed milk, and 8 ounces of Barium Sulfate is warmed to body temperature and injected into the rectum from a height of from 3 to 6 feet (90 to 180 cm). The examination is made with a fluoroscope while the injection is passing into the rectum.

Dose—*Usual*, oral, **200** to **300 Gm** in suitable suspension; *usual*, rectal, **400** to **750 Gm** in suitable suspension.

Bismuth Subcarbonate—see page 788.

Bismuth Subnitrate—see page 789.

Drugs Used for Outlining the Gall Bladder and Bile Ducts

(Cholecystography and Cholangiography)

Certain radiopaque substances are excreted in the bile and, hence, are used for visualization of the gall bladder (cholecystography) and bile ducts (cholangiography). They are generally organic iodine compounds that cast a shadow on the x-ray film. Since iodism, anaphylactic shock, and even death have been attributed to the use of iodine-containing contrast media, their use is not without some risk.

Calcium Ipodate NF

Calcium 3-[[(Dimethylamino)methylene]amino]-2,4,6-triiodohydrocinnamate; Oragrafin Calcium (*Squibb*)]

Calcium Ipodate contains 97.5–102.5% of $C_{24}H_{24}CaI_6N_4O_4$ (1233.99), calculated on the anhydrous basis.

Preparation—Calcium Ipodate may be prepared by precipitation using aqueous solutions of sodium ipodate and calcium chloride. The crude precipitate is recrystallized from a suitable solvent such as aqueous dimethylformamide. The preparation of *Sodium Ipodate* is described on page 1304.

Description—A white to off-white, fine crystalline powder that is odorless and has a chalky, very bitter taste. It should be stored at room temperature in a tightly closed container protected from light. It melts at 300° with decomposition.

Solubility—1 Gm dissolves in about 1700 ml of water; slightly soluble in alcohol, chloroform, and methanol.

Uses—Calcium Ipodate is a water-insoluble substance which contains 61.7% iodine and is used as a contrast media for cholangiography and cholecystography. The agent is rapidly absorbed from the gastrointestinal tract and excreted in the bile in sufficient quantity to outline the biliary ducts within 30 min after administration; optimal opacification of the ducts occurs 1 to 3 hours after ingestion. Maximal visualization of the gall bladder occurs 10 hours after administration of the salt. Untoward effects reported include abdominal cramping, diarrhea, nausea, vomiting, dysuria, urticaria, headache, heartburn, and epigastric pain. Although rare, hypotension and circulatory collapse have been reported. The drug is contraindicated in patients with severe renal disease and in patients known to be allergic to iodine.

Dose—*Usual*, **3** to **6 Gm** as a single dose given 10 to 12 hours before the examination.

Dosage Forms—for Oral Suspension NF: 3 Gm.

Iopanoic Acid USP

[Iodopanoic Acid; 3-Amino-α-ethyl-2,4,6-triiodohydrocinnamic Acid; Telepaque (*Winthrop*)]

Iopanoic Acid contains an amount of iodine (I) equivalent to 97.0–101.0% of $C_{11}H_{12}I_3NO_2$ (570.94), calculated on the dried basis.

Preparation—A mixture of *m*-nitrobenzaldehyde, butyric anhydride, and sodium butyrate is heated in xylene at reflux for 12 hours to effect a Perkin condensation yielding *m*-nitro-α-ethylcinnamic acid. The acid is extracted with aqueous alkali and then reduced with hydrogen in the presence of Raney nickel. The resulting *m*-amino-α-ethylhydrocinnamic acid is iodinated with iodine monochloride in an acetic acid solution and the crude Iopanoic Acid thus formed is purified by crystallization from ethyl acetate.

Description—A cream-colored powder. Tasteless or nearly so. Faint, characteristic odor. Affected by light. Melts with decomposition between 152° and 158°.

Solubility—Insoluble in water; soluble in alcohol, chloroform, and ether; soluble in solutions of alkali hydroxides and carbonates.

Uses—Iopanoic Acid is administered orally as a *radiopaque medium* in *cholecystography*. It is promptly absorbed from the gastrointestinal tract, concentrated in the gall bladder, and subsequently excreted in the bile. It is relatively free from undesirable reactions and has low toxicity. Occasionally, nausea and diarrhea and, rarely, dysuria have followed its administration. It is contraindicated in patients with acute nephritis and uremia. It should not be administered when disorders of the gastrointestinal tract exist which prevent absorption of the medium.

The usual regimen is to give the patient a fat-free evening meal following which the Iopanoic Acid is administered approximately 10 hours before the time scheduled for roentgenography. Immediately after the roentgen examination, the patient is given a high-fat meal and additional exposures are made in order to evaluate the contraction of the gall bladder and to visualize the patency of the extrahepatic ducts. When the latter structures are of particular interest, the dose of Iopanoic Acid may be increased to 5 or 6 Gm.

Dose—3 to 6 Gm; *usual*, 3 Gm.
Dosage Forms—Tablets USP: 500 mg.

Meglumine Iodipamide Injection USP

[Cholografin Methylglucamine Injection (*Squibb*)]

Meglumine Iodipamide Injection is a sterile solution of 3,3′-(adipoyldiimino)bis-2,4,6-triiodobenzoic acid in water for injection, prepared with the aid of methylglucamine. It contains 95.0–105.0% of the labeled amount of meglumine iodipamide [$C_{34}H_{48}I_6N_4O_{16}$ = 1530.21]. It may contain small amounts of suitable buffers and of calcium disodium edetate or disodium edetate as a stabilizer. Meglumine Iodipamide Injection intended for intravenous use contains no anti-microbial agents.

Preparation—As indicated above, the Injection is prepared by reacting the iodipamide acid moiety with a double equimolar portion of methylglucamine.

For the synthesis of 3,3′-(adipolydiimino)bis-(2,4,6-triiodobenzoic acid), see *Sodium Iodipamide Injection* (this page).

For the synthesis of methylglucamine, see *Meglumine Diatrizoate Injection* (page 1307).

Description—It is a clear, colorless to pale yellow, slightly viscous liquid. The pH is between 6.5 and 7.7.

Uses—Meglumine Iodipamide Injection is used in nonsurgical visualization of the biliary ducts, especially in patients with post-cholecystectomy syndrome; for cholecystography prior to surgery when the gall bladder has lost its power to concentrate bile; and in delineation of biliary structures in patients who are unable to ingest or absorb oral mediums. It is contraindicated in patients with hyperthyroidism or with severe renal or hepatic impairment.

Dose—*Usual, intravenous*, 20 ml of a 52% solution over a period of 10 minutes.

Sodium Iodipamide Injection USP

[Sodium 3,3′-(Adipoyldiimino)bis[2,4,6-triiodobenzoate] Injection; Cholografin Sodium (*Squibb*)]

Sodium Iodipamide Injection is a sterile solution of 3,3′-(adipoyldiimino)bis[2,4,6-triiodobenzoic] acid in water for injection prepared with the aid of sodium hydroxide. It contains 95.0–105.0% of the labeled amount of sodium iodipamide [$C_{20}H_{12}I_6N_2Na_2O_6$ = 1183.73]. It may contain small amounts of suitable buffers and of calcium disodium edetate or disodium edetate as a stabilizer. Sodium Iodipamide Injection intended for intravenous use contains no antimicrobial agents.

Preparation—Iodipamide may be prepared from benzoic acid by the following sequence of reactions: (*a*) nitration to 3-nitrobenzoic acid; (*b*) reduction by means of stannous chloride or various other reagents to 3-aminobenzoic acid; (*c*) iodination with iodine mono-chloride in acetic acid to the 2,4,6-triiodo derivative; and (*d*) acylation of the amino group by means of adipoyl chloride [$ClCO(CH_2)_4COCl$].

Description—Clear, colorless solution, the viscosity of which increases with the concentration.

Uses—Sodium Iodipamide, a radiopaque water-soluble organic iodine compound, is used for intravenous cholangiography and cholecystography. Because greater risks are involved when the intravenous route of administration is employed, this agent is used only in cases which do not give satisfactory results with orally administered drugs or in emergencies where immediate visualization is essential. A sufficient amount accumulates within 15 to 20 minutes to produce radiopacity of the hepatic and common bile ducts. Toxic reactions are not frequent and are usually mild; transient restlessness, sensations of warmth and pressure in the upper abdomen, and nausea and vomiting may occur. It should not be administered to individuals hypersensitive to iodine or to individuals with hyperthyroidism or impaired liver function.

Dose—*Intravenous*, 20 to 40 ml; *usual*, 40 ml of 20% solution administered over a period of 10 minutes.
Dosage Forms—4 Gm/20 ml.

Sodium Ipodate NF

[Sodium 3-[[(Dimethylamino)methylene]amino]-2,4,6-trriodohydrocinnamate; Oragrafin Sodium (*Squibb*)]

Sodium Ipodate contains 97.5–102.5% of $C_{12}H_{12}I_3N_2NaO_2$ (619.94), calculated on the anhydrous basis.

Meglumine Iodipamide

Preparation—3-Amino-2,4,6-triiodohydrocinnamic acid is condensed with *N,N*-dimethylformamide with the aid of iodomethanesulfonyl chloride. The reaction mixture is then poured into ice water which precipitates the 3-[[(dimethylamino)methylene]amino]-2,4,6-triiodohydrocinnamic acid. Neutralization of the acid with an equimolar portion of sodium hydroxide yields the sodium salt [*Chem. Ber.*, **93**, 2347 (1960)].

Description—A white to off-white, crystalline powder that is odorless. It should be stored at room temperature in a tightly closed container protected from light. It melts between 303° and 304° with decomposition.

Solubility—1 Gm dissolves in 5 ml of water.

Uses—Sodium Ipodate is a radiopaque media for the visualization of the gall bladder and biliary tract. Except that Sodium Ipodate is somewhat less rapidly absorbed from the gastrointestinal tract, is soluble in water, and contains slightly less iodine (61.4%), its actions, uses, onset, and duration of effects and contra-indications are similar to those for *Calcium Ipodate* (page 1303).

Dose—3 to 6 Gm; *usual*, **3 Gm** given 12 hours before examination.

Dosage Forms—Capsules NF: 500 mg.

Other Drugs Used for Outlining the Gall Bladder and the Bile Ducts

Iodoalphionic Acid NF XII [Pheniodol; 3-(4-Hydroxy-3,5-diiodophenyl)-2-phenylpropionic Acid; Priodax (*Schering*)], dried over phosphorus pentoxide for 4 hours, contains an amount of iodine equivalent to 98.0–102.0% of $C_{15}H_{12}I_2O_3$ (494.07). *Preparation:* The first step is the Perkin's reaction, a classical method for the preparation of α,β-unsaturated acids; *p*-hydroxybenzaldehyde is reacted with sodium phenylacetate in the presence of acetic anhydride at 180°. The second step, reduction of the unsaturated acid, is carried out by catalytic hydrogenation using Raney nickel catalyst. The last reaction, iodination of the phenolic nucleus, is best accomplished with iodine monochloride using a mixture of aqueous acetic acid and hydrochloric acid

as the solvent. Traces of free iodine are removed from the product by treatment with sodium sulfite. *Description and Solubility:* White crystals or a white or faintly yellow powder having a faint, characteristic odor and taste; stable in air, but slightly discolored on prolonged exposure to light; melting range, 160° to 164° with some decomposition. Insoluble in water; readily soluble in alcohol; soluble in ether; slightly soluble in benzene and chloroform. *Uses:* A *radiopaque medium* for cholecystography. It is claimed to cause less nausea, vomiting, and diarrhea than sodium iodophthalein. The drug is excreted primarily through the kidneys. It is contraindicated in acute nephritis, uremia, and acute disorders of the gastrointestinal tract. Side effects that may be encountered occasionally include pain on urination, nausea, vomiting, diarrhea, griping, headache, sensation of burning in the esophagus, generalized itching, dryness of the mouth, general weakness, and flatulence. *Dose: Usual, 3 Gm.*

Iophenoxic Acid USP XVI [α-Ethyl-3-hydroxy-2,4,6-triiodohydrocinnamic Acid; Teridax (*Schering*)] [$C_{11}H_{11}I_3O_3$] —A white or creamy white, crystalline powder which melts between 146° and 149°. It is very slightly soluble in water, freely soluble in alcohol and in ether, and soluble in chloroform. *Uses:* Used for cholecystography by oral administration. It usually produces a consistent and dense gall bladder shadow for the visualization of non-opaque stones and for observing the functional capacity of the gall bladder to concentrate and expel bile after a high fat meal. Iophenoxic Acid induces a low level of unpleasant side effects. Nausea, vomiting, and diarrhea are minimal, rarely severe. As with other systemically administered iodinated compounds, it should be used with extreme caution, if at all, in patients with advanced renal impairment. *Dose: Usual, 50 mg per Kg* of body weight orally.

Iodophthalein Sodium NF XI [$C_{20}H_8I_4Na_2O_4.3H_2O$] 3,3′,5,5′-Tetraiodophenolphthalein Sodium]—A blue-violet crystalline powder with a saline and astringent taste. One Gm dissolves in about 7 ml of water. It is slightly soluble in alcohol; insoluble in chloroform or ether. *Uses:* A *radiopaque medium* used in the roentgenographic examination of the gall bladder. Following the intravenous injection, or if decomposition is avoided, the oral administration, the substance appears in the normal gall bladder in sufficient concentration to cast a shadow to the roentgen ray. *Dose: Intravenous, 2 to 4 Gm; usual, 2 Gm.*

Drugs Used for Outlining Various Cavities

A number of radiopaque preparations are available which consist of iodine addition products of vegetable oils. These preparations are nonirritating and can be injected as contrast media into various cavities of the body such as the urinary and genital tracts, bronchi, fistulous tracts, and the spinal canal. Thus, they are useful in the x-ray diagnosis of gynecologic conditions, bronchial and pulmonary lesions, and tumors of the spinal cord. They are removed slowly from closed cavities and may give rise to foreign-body reactions; some reports indicate blood iodine level may be elevated for 2 to 4 years after the use of one of these agents. Other untoward reactions are characteristic of iodine compounds. Iodized oils are usually quite viscid, and for injection may be thinned by diluting with ethyl oleate or rendered miscible with water by emulsification.

Ethiodized Oil USP

[Ethiodol (*Fougera*)]

Ethiodized Oil is an iodine addition product of the ethyl ester of the fatty acid of poppyseed oil, containing 35.2–38.9% of organically combined iodine. It is sterile.

Preparation—Ethiodized Oil may be prepared by saponifying poppyseed oil and subjecting the resulting fatty acid to iodination and subsequent esterification with ethanol.

Description—A straw-colored to amber-colored, oily liquid.

Uses—Ethiodized Oil is a *contrast medium* used in hysterosalpingography, sialography, and visualization of sinus and fistulous tracts. It is contraindicated in acute parotitis and myelography. It should not be used for bronchography or in the presence of intra-uterine bleeding, pelvic infection, or pregnancy. Likewise, it should not be used in patients known to be sensitive to iodine. Except for pulmonary embolism resulting from accidental intravasation of the medium, side effects are minimal and of little consequence.

Dose—0.5 to 20 ml by *special injection; usual*, **10 ml.**

Other Dose Information—*Usual*, for *hysterosalpingography*, **6 ml**, slowly, under pressure (160 mm Hg) in increments of **1 ml**, preferably under fluoroscopic control.

Dosage Forms—Injection USP: 2 and 10 ml.

Iodized Oil NF

[Iodised Oil Viscous Injection; Lipiodol (*Fougera*)]

Iodized Oil is an iodine addition product of vegetable oil or oils, containing 38.0–42.0% of organically combined I (iodine). It is sterile.

Preparation—The methods of preparing Iodized Oil depend upon the addition of elemental iodine to the unsaturated fatty constituents of a vegetable oil, the resulting oil containing chemically saturated iodoglycerides. The oil most generally used is poppy seed oil.

Description—A thick, viscous, oily liquid, having an alliaceous odor and an oleaginous taste. It is light to dark brown in color, and on exposure to air and light it becomes darker due to liberation of iodine. Its specific gravity is about 1.35.

Solubility—Insoluble in water; soluble in ether, chloroform, or petroleum benzin; the NF requires that 1 ml of Iodized Oil should yield a clear solution with 10 ml of solvent hexane.

Uses—Iodized Oil is used as a *radiopaque medium* (myelographic), especially for outlining of internal cavities such as bronchi, spinal canal, fistulous tracts, paranasal sinuses, lacrimal ducts, uterus and tubes, otitic brain abscess, etc. Contraindications and side effects are similar to other iodine-containing radiopaque materials.

Dose—*Usual*, **1 to 30 ml** by special injection, and depending on procedure.

Dosage Forms—Injection: 1, 5, 10, and 20 ml.

Iophendylate Injection USP

[Ethyl 10-(Iodophenyl)undecanoate Injection;   Myodil;   Pantopaque (*Lafayette*)]

$$I-\underset{\text{(phenyl ring)}}{\bigcirc}-\overset{\displaystyle \underset{|}{CH_3}}{CH}-CH_2(CH_2)_7COOC_2H_5$$

Iophendylate Injection is a sterile mixture of isomers of ethyl iodophenylundecanoate. It contains 98.0–100.5% of $C_{19}H_{29}IO_2$ (416.35).

Preparation—This substance is reported to be manufactured as follows. Benzene is reacted with undecylenic acid forming a mixture of isomers of phenylundecylic acid. The mixture is iodinated and finally esterified with ethyl alcohol. After decolorization, the desired fraction is separated by distillation.

Description—A colorless to pale yellow, viscous liquid. Darkens on long exposure to air. Odorless or possesses a faintly ethereal odor. Specific gravity between 1.248 and 1.257. Refractive index between 1.5235 and 1.5255.

Solubility—Very slightly soluble in water; freely soluble in alcohol, benzene, chloroform, and ether.

Uses—This Injection is used as a *radiopaque medium* for myelography. It is commonly used for visualization of tumors or herniation of the intervertebral disc or other lesions compressing the spinal cord. It is absorbed at a rate of about 1 ml per year, varying with the condition of the tissues.

Dose—**0.5 to 16 ml**; *usual, intrathecal* or by special injection, **6 ml.**

Dosage Forms—Injection USP: 1, 3, 6, and 12 ml.

Propyliodone USP

[Propyl 3,5-Diiodo-4-oxo-1(4*H*)pyridineacetate; Dionosil (*Glaxco*)]

$$\underset{O}{\underset{\|}{\bigcirc}}\overset{N-CH_2COOCH_2CH_2CH_3}{\underset{I}{\overset{I}{}}}$$

Propyliodone contains 99.0–101.0% of $C_{10}H_{11}I_2NO_3$ (447.01), calculated on the dried basis.

Preparation—4(1*H*)-Pyridone, as the nitrate in aqueous solution, is iodinated by treating with a mixture of sodium iodide and sodium iodate in the presence of sulfuric acid. The basic 3,5-diiodo-4(1*H*)-pyridone thus formed is isolated and condensed with chloroacetic acid to yield 3,5-diiodo-4-oxo-1(4*H*) pyridineacetic acid which is then esterified with propyl alcohol.

Description—A white, or almost white, crystalline powder. It is odorless or has a faint odor. Melting range 187° to 190°.

Solubility—Practically insoluble in water; soluble in acetone, alcohol, and ether.

Uses—*Radiopaque medium* for bronchographic use. Direct instillation into the bronchi results in well-defined bronchograms for at least 30 minutes. It is usually eliminated from the lungs in 7 to 10 days. Propyliodone is contraindicated in patients with pulmonary emphysema or bronchiectasis.

Dose—**10 to 20 ml**; *usual, intrathecal,* **0.2 ml** per **Kg** of body weight, to a maximum of **20 ml.**

Dosage Forms—Sterile Suspension USP: 20 ml; Sterile Oil Suspension USP: 20 ml.

Other Drugs Used for Outlining Various Cavities

Chloriodized Oil USP XVI—The iodine monochloride addition product of vegetable oil or oils. *Purity:* 7.3–8.3% of organically combined chlorine and 26.0–28.0% of organically combined iodine. A clear, yellow, viscous, oily liquid, having a faint characteristic odor and an oleaginous taste. It may decompose on long standing or on exposure to heat and sunlight, becoming dark brown to black in color. Insoluble in water and alcohol; freely soluble in chloroform, ether, and fixed oils. *Uses:* For the visualization of all hollow structures. *Dose:* From 1 to 20 ml, depending on the size of the cavity to be visualized.

Sodium Anoxynaphthonate BP [The trisodium salt of 8-(4-anilino-5-sulfo-1-naphthylazo)-1-naphthol-3,6-disulfonic acid; Sodium Anazolene]—A blue or bluish-black powder; odorless and hygroscopic. Soluble, at 20°, in 30 parts of water; insoluble in alcohol, acetone, and chloroform. *Uses:* A dye used in the investigation of cardiac disease. *Dose:* Intravenous, 50 to 100 mg.

Drugs Used for Intravenous Pyelography and Angiography

Satisfactory x-ray pictures of the urinary tract, blood vessels, or heart may be obtained by the intravenous injection of soluble iodine compounds of low toxicity which are rapidly excreted in the urine. The inorganic iodide, sodium iodide, is too toxic for intravenous injection; however, there are organic iodine compounds available for this use. These same organic compounds may also be used for ureteral retrograde pyelography (direct injection into the renal pelvis through a ureteral catheter). One of these agents (Sodium Iothalamate

Injection) is intended specifically for angiocardiography and aortography, although satisfactory urograms may also be obtained.

Iodopyracet Injection NF

[3,5-Diiodo-4-oxo-1(4H)-pyridineacetic Acid 2,2'-Iminodiethanol (1:1) Compound Injection; Diodone Injection; Diodrast (*Winthrop*)]

Iodopyracet Injection is a sterile solution of iodopyracet in water for injection. It contains 95.0–105.0% of the labeled amount of $C_{11}H_{16}I_2N_2O_5$ (510.07).

Preparation—Pyridine is allowed to react with thionyl chloride at room temperature for a few days and the 4-pyridylpyridinium chloride hydrochloride thus formed is then hydrolyzed at 150° to yield 4(1H)-pyridone (I). Reaction of (I) with iodine monochloride or an acidified mixture of sodium iodide and sodium iodate introduces the two iodine atoms. Condensation of the resulting diiodopyridone with monochloroacetic acid in a dehydrochlorinating environment yields the acid moiety of Iodopyracet which is then neutralized with an equimolar portion of diethanolamine.

Description—A clear and nearly colorless liquid, neutral to litmus. Its specific gravity is about 1.19.

Uses—Iodopyracet is used as a *radiopaque medium* for intravenous urography. It has also been employed for intravenous venography, angiography, angiocardiography, cholangiography, and bronchography; however, its use for these purposes has declined in favor of the newer agents which contain three atoms of iodine in each molecule. The latter agents produce greater x-ray density and better contrast.

Dose—*Usual, intramuscular* and *intravenous*, **20 ml.**

Dosage Forms—Injection NF: 3.5 Gm/10 ml, 7 Gm/20 ml, 10.5 Gm/30 ml.

Meglumine Diatrizoate Injection USP

[1-Deoxy-1-(methylamino)glucitol 3,5-Diacetamido-2,4,6-triiodobenzoate (Salt) Injection; Cardiografin (*Squibb*); Gastrografin (*Squibb*); Renografin (*Squibb*)]

Meglumine Diatrizoate Injection is a sterile solution of 3,5-diacetamido-2,4,6-triiodobenzoic acid [$C_{11}H_9I_3N_2O_4$ = 613.92] in water for injection, prepared with the aid of methylglucamine. It contains 95.0–100.5% of the labeled amount of meglumine diatrizoate [$C_{18}H_{26}I_3N_3O_9$ = 809.14]. It may contain small amounts of suitable buffers and of calcium disodium

edetate or disodium edetate as a stabilizer. Meglumine Diatrizoate Injection intended for intravenous use contains no antimicrobial agents.

Preparation—As indicated above, the Injection is prepared by reacting equimolar quantities of diatrizoic acid and methylglucamine.

Diatrizoic acid may be prepared from benzoic acid by the following sequence of reactions: (*a*) nitration to the 3,5-dinitro acid; (*b*) reduction by means of stannous chloride or various other reagents to the corresponding diamino acid; (*c*) iodination with iodine monochloride in acetic acid to the 2,4,6-triiodo derivative; and (*d*) acetylation of the amino groups by means of acetic anhydride.

Methylglucamine may be prepared by treating glucose with hydrogen and methylamine under pressure and in the presence of Raney nickel.

Description—It is a clear, colorless to pale yellow, slightly viscous liquid. The pH is between 6.0 and 7.6.

Uses—Meglumine Diatrizoate, a radiopaque water-soluble organic iodine compound available in 30, 60, 76, and 85% solutions, is used for intravenous excretory urography, visualization of the cardiovascular system, and roentgenographic examination of the gastrointestinal tract. Following intravenous administration, excellent visualization of the renal collecting system is usually obtained within 15 minutes and adequate cystograms in 25 to 40 minutes. In concentrations of 30%, it is also satisfactory for retrograde pyelography. Meglumine Diatrizoate has been successfully used for contrast visualization of the cardiovascular system and yields satisfactory venograms, aortograms and peripheral, cerebral, and coronary arteriograms. For roentgenographic examination of the gastrointestinal tract, it is somewhat less satisfactory than the standard barium suspension. However, it may be used in patients who refuse or cannot tolerate barium and for demonstrating those lesions for which a solution of low viscosity is required.

The incidence of side effects after the intravenous use of Meglumine Diatrizoate is relatively low. Nevertheless, this agent should be used with the same precautions as attend the use of other organic iodine compounds. It should be used with caution in patients with severe hepatic or renal disease, hyperthyroidism or tuberculosis.

Dose—*Intravenous*, **25 to 50 ml**; *usual*, **25 ml** of a 76 to 85% solution.

Other Dose Information—Doses in addition to the official dose are as follows: retrograde pyelography, 15 ml of a 30% solution; peripheral arteriography, adult, 15 to 20 ml of a 60 to 76% solution injected into the femoral or subclavian artery; angiocardiography, 40 to 50 ml of an 85% solution; roentgenographic examination of the gastrointestinal tract, oral, adult, 30 to 90 ml of a 76% solution.

Dosage Forms—Injection USP: 85%/50 ml, 76%/ml, 60%/25 and 30 ml.

Meglumine Iothalamate Injection USP

[1-Deoxy-1-(methylamino)glucitol 5-Acetamido-2,4,6-triiodo-*N*-methyliso-phthalamate (Salt) Injection; Conray (*Mallinckrodt*)]

Meglumine Iothalamate Injection is a sterile solution of 5-acetamido-2,4,6-triiodo-*N*-methylisophthalamic acid [$C_{11}H_9I_3N_2O_4 = 613.92$] in water for injection, prepared with the aid of methylglucamine. It contains 95.0–105.0% of the labeled amount of meglumine iothalamate [$C_{18}H_{26}I_3N_3O_9 = 809.14$]. It may contain small amounts of suitable buffers and of calcium disodium edetate or disodium edetate as a stabilizer. Meglumine Iothalamate Injection intended for intravenous use contains no antimicrobial agents.

Preparation—As indicated above, the Injection is prepared by reacting equimolar quantities of iothalamic acid and methylglucamine. Iothalamic acid may be prepared by oxidizing *m*-xylene with potassium permanganate, condensing the resulting isophthalic acid with an equimolar quantity of methylamine, and iodinating by means of iodine monochloride in acetic acid.

Uses—Meglumine Iothalamate is used for *intravenous urography*. The agent is rapidly excreted by the kidneys; maximum radiographic density occurs in most instances within 3 to 8 minutes after injection. Since Meglumine Iothalamate contains 28.2% iodine, it is contraindicated in patients allergic to this substance and should be used with the same precautions as other iodine-containing diagnostic aids. It should be used very cautiously and only if absolutely necessary in patients with advanced renal disease, since excretion of the medium may be severely impaired.

Dose—*Usual, intravenous,* **30 ml** of a **60%** solution.

Dosage Forms—Injection USP: 60%/20, 30, and 50 ml.

Sodium Diatrizoate Injection USP

[Sodium 3,5-Diacetamido-2,4,6-triiodobenzoate Injection; Hypaque Sodium (*Winthrop*)]

Sodium Diatrizoate Injection is a sterile solution of 3,5-diacetamido-2,4,6-triiodobenzoic acid in water for injection, prepared with the aid of sodium hydroxide. It contains 95.0–105.0% of the labeled amount of sodium diatrizoate [$C_{11}H_8I_3N_2NaO_4 = 635.90$]. It may contain small amounts of suitable buffers and of calcium disodium edetate or disodium edetate as a stabilizer. Sodium Diatrizoate Injection intended for intravenous use contains no antimicrobial agents.

Description—Clear, colorless to pale yellow solution, the viscosity of which increases with the concentration.

Preparation—Diatrizoic acid is neutralized with an equimolar portion of sodium hydroxide. For the synthesis of diatrizoic acid, see under *Meglumine Diatrizoate Injection* (page 1307).

Uses—Sodium Diatrizoate Injection is used for intravenous urography. With normal kidney function adequate shadows are obtained within 5 minutes after injection. With impaired kidney function and delayed excretion, 30 minutes or more may be required. Sodium Diatrizoate should be used with the same precautions as for other organic iodine compounds and is contraindicated in severe liver disorders and in advanced renal impairment with severe uremia. Side effects are minimal and the agent rarely produces severe vascular reactions.

Dose—*Usual, intravenous,* **30 ml** of a **50%** solution.

Other Dose Information—The dose is administered over a period of 1 to 3 minutes.

Dosage Forms—Injection USP: 10 Gm/20 ml, 15 Gm/30 ml.

Sodium Iothalamate Injection USP

[Sodium 5-Acetamido-2,4,6-triiodo-*N*-methylisophthalamate Injection; Angio-Conray (*Mallinckrodt*)]

Sodium Iothalamate Injection is a sterile solution of 5-acetamido-2,4,6-triiodo-*N*-methylisophthalamic acid [$C_{11}H_9I_3N_2O_4 = 613.92$] in water for injection prepared with the aid of sodium hydroxide. It contains 95.0–105.0% of the labeled amount of sodium iothalamate [$C_{11}H_8I_3N_2NaO_4 = 635.90$]. It may contain small amounts of suitable buffers and of calcium disodium edetate or disodium edetate as a stabilizer. Sodium Iothalamate Injection intended for intravenous use contains no antimicrobial agents.

Description—Clear, colorless solution, the viscosity of which increases with the concentration.

Uses—Sodium Iothalamate Injection is used for intravascular angiocardiography and aortography. Since it is rapidly distributed throughout the vascular system and promptly excreted by the kidneys, incidental urograms also may be obtained and may provide additional diagnostic information in some cases. Untoward effects are usually transient and include flushing, nausea, vomiting, and a bitter taste. Infrequent severe reactions observed are respiratory difficulty and cardiovascular collapse. Since the drug is excreted by the kidneys, it is contraindicated in patients with renal impairment. It is also contraindicated in patients known to be sensitive to iodine preparations and in patients with severe cardiovascular disease.

Dose—*Usual, intravenous* or *intra-arterial*, **40 to 50** ml of a **66.8**% or an **80**% solution per **Kg** of body weight.

Dosage Forms—Injection USP: 16 Gm/20 ml, 16.7 Gm/25 ml, 33.4 and 40 Gm/50 ml.

Sodium Methiodal NF

[Sodium Iodomethanesulfonate; Sodium Monoiodomethanesulfonate; Skiodan (*Winthrop*)]

ICH₂SO₃Na

$$ICH_2SO_3Na$$

Sodium Methiodal, dried at 105° for 4 hours, contains 98.0–102.0% of CH_2INaO_3S (243.98).

Preparation—Methiodal Sodium is prepared by heating a mixture of iodoform, sodium carbonate, and sodium bisulfite in water until the iodoform disappears. The product separates from the mixture on chilling.

$$CHI_3 + NaHSO_3 + Na_2CO_3 \rightarrow ICH_2SO_3Na +$$
$$NaI + NaIO + CO_2$$

Description—A white, crystalline powder. It is odorless and has a slightly saline taste, followed by a sweetish after-taste. Decomposes on exposure to light, becoming yellow. Its solutions are neutral to litmus.

Solubility—Soluble in water; very soluble in methanol; slightly soluble in alcohol; practically insoluble in acetone, ether, and benzene.

Uses—Sodium Methiodal is used as a *radiopaque medium* for excretion *urography* or retrograde *pyelography*.

Dose—*Intravenous*, **10 to 30 Gm**; *usual*, **20 Gm** in 50 ml.

Dosage Forms—Injection NF: 10 and 20 Gm/50 ml, 40 Gm/100 ml.

Other Drugs Used for Intravenous Pyelography and Angiography

Iodopyracet Compound—A solution containing a mixture of the diethylamine and diethanolamine salts of 3,5-diiodo-4-oxo-1(4*H*)-pyridine-acetic acid. *Uses:* In urography, by intravenous injection or direct injection into the renal pelvis through a ureteral catheter. See *Iodopyracet Injection* (page 1307). *Dose:* 20 ml of either a 12.5% or a 50% solution.

Iodopyracet Concentrated—A 70% solution of the diethanolamine salt of 3,5-diiodo-4-oxo-1(4*H*)-pyridine-acetic acid. *Uses:* Visualization of the heart, aorta, superior vena cava, pulmonary artery and branches, coronary arteries, and other structures. *Not to be used for excretion urography*. Contraindicated in idiosyncrasy, hepatic disease, nephritis, and hyperthyroidism. Because of its many toxic side effects, iodopyracet concentrated should be used intravenously only in difficult diagnostic problems, and by skilled persons. See *Iodopyracet Injection* (page 1307). *Dose:* 30 to 45 ml of a 70% solution.

Sodium Iodomethamate NF XII [Disodium 1,4-Dihydro-3,5-diiodo-1-methyl-4-oxo-2,6-pyridinedicarboxylate; Iodoxyl; Neo-Iopax (*Schering*)], dried over phosphorus pentoxide in a vacuum desiccator for 24 hours, contains 50.5–52.5% of iodine (I), corresponding to not less than 98.0% of $C_8H_3I_2NNa_2O_5$ (492.91). *Preparation:* The acid of sodium iodomethamate is prepared by a series of reactions starting with ethyl oxalate and acetone. In the first step two distinct reactions occur: one molecule of ethyl oxalate condenses with each of the two methyl groups of acetone yielding an open-chain compound which cyclizes to *chelidonic acid* when boiled with concentrated hydrochloric acid; the conversion of chelidonic acid to *chelidamic acid* is accomplished by heating with excess ammonium hydroxide. The iodination step occurs readily at elevated temperatures. Methylation with dimethyl sulfate is carried out in the conventional manner. *Description and Solubility:* A white, odorless powder. 1 Gm dissolves in about 1 ml of water and about 100 ml of alcohol; insoluble in ether and chloroform.

Uses: A *radiopaque medium* in intravenous *urography* and retrograde *pyelography*. Systemic reactions occur uncommonly and are usually mild and fleeting. Intravenous use is contraindicated in patients with severe liver disorders, nephritis, and severe uremia, and it should be used with caution in cases of tuberculosis and hyperthyroidism. Caution must be exercised also in patients with any severe systemic disease. Preliminary liver and kidney tests are advisable in suspected cases. *Dose:* Usual, *intravenous* and by special injection, 10 Gm.

Drugs Used to Test Organ Function

The classic studies of Abel and Rowntree in 1909 demonstrated that parenterally administered phenoltetrachlorphthalein was excreted only in the bile, while phenolsulfonphthalein was excreted almost exclusively in the urine. These findings were promptly adopted by Rowntree and his associates as a means of testing liver and kidney function. The importance of these early observations is attested by the several drugs which are now commonly used to test organ function. Described in this section are those drugs used to test liver, kidney, and gastric function.

Sodium Iodide I 131 Capsules—see page 566.

Sodium Iodide I 131 Solution—see page 566.

Drugs Used to Test Liver Function

Unfortunately, available methods for estimating the extent of liver damage by various measurements of decreased liver function are still comparatively unsatisfactory. The liver itself has such a large reserve of functional capacity that most methods of determining decreased function do not reveal such a state until 70 to 90% of the liver cells have been damaged. Most liver function tests involve the intravenous injection of a standardized amount of substance, such as bilirubin, rose bengal, or sulfobromophthalein, agents which depend almost wholly on the liver for excretion. The rate of clearance of the substance from the plasma becomes a measure of the excretory capacity of the liver.

Indocyanine Green USP

[2-[7-[1,1-Dimethyl-3(4-sulfobutyl)benz[*e*]indolin-2-ylidene]-1,3,5-heptatrienyl]-1,1-dimethyl-3-(4-sulfobutyl)-1*H*-benz[*e*]indolium Hydroxide Inner Salt Sodium Salt; Cardio-Green (*Hynson*)]

Indocyanine Green contains 90.0–100.5% of $C_{43}H_{47}N_2NaO_6S_2$ (774.98), calculated on the dried basis.

Preparation—Indocyanine Green may be prepared

by reacting 1,1,2-trimethyl-3-(4-sulfobutyl)-1*H*-benz-[*e*]indolium hydroxide inner salt (I) with a bis(Schiff base) derived from glutaconic aldehyde. Acetic anhydride is used to favor the condensation and the acidic dye is ultimately neutralized with sodium hydroxide. The starting indolium compound (I) is readily prepared by heating 1,1,2-trimethyl-1*H*-benz[*e*]-indole with 4-hydroxy-1-butanesulfonic acid δ-sultone. The details for preparing this class of tricarbocyanine dyes are provided in US Pats. 2,251,286 and 2,895,955.

Description—A green powder or crystals which are odorless and tasteless. It is very hygroscopic. It decomposes gradually above 200°.

Solubility—Soluble in alcohol and methanol; soluble, but unstable, in water.

Uses—Indocyanine Green is used to determine *liver function*. The calculated amount of the diagnostic agent is injected into an arm vein. Twenty minutes after injection, 6 ml of venous blood is withdrawn from the opposite arm. After coagulation and centrifugation, the clear serum is read in a photometer at 800 to 810 mμ. A dye retention of less than 4% is found in healthy subjects. Following intravenous injection, Indocyanine Green is rapidly bound to plasma protein, quickly removed from the circulation by the liver, and excreted in the bile in unconjugated form. Failure to remove the dye, as indicated by serum levels in excess of 4%, is indicative of impaired hepatic function. No toxic effects of consequence have been reported. The safe use of this drug in pregnancy has not been established.

Dose—*Usual, intravenous, blood volume determination*, **5 mg** in **1 ml**; *hepatic function determination*, **500 mcg** per **Kg** of body weight.

Dosage Forms—Sterile USP: 10, 25, 40, and 50 mg.

Sodium Sulfobromophthalein USP

[4,5,6,7-Tetrabromo-3′,3″-disulfophenolphthalein Disodium Salt; Bromsulphalein R Sodium; Bromtetragnost; B.S.P.; Bromsulphalein (*Hynson*)]

Sodium Sulfobromophthalein contains 95.0–105.0% of $C_{20}H_8Br_4Na_2O_{10}S_2$ (838.00), calculated on the dried basis.

Preparation—Tetrabromophthalic anhydride, made by brominating phthalic anhydride in alkaline solution (sodium phthalate) and precipitating with acid, is condensed with phenol by a process similar to that used for fluorescein. The resulting phenoltetrabromophthalein is sulfonated by treatment with sulfuric acid, and the disulfonic acid so obtained converted into the sodium salt with sodium carbonate.

Description—A white, crystalline powder. It is odorless and has a bitter taste. It is hygroscopic.

Solubility—Soluble in water; insoluble in alcohol and acetone.

Uses—Sulfobromophthalein is used as a *diagnostic aid* for the determination of *liver function*. It is injected intravenously and 30 minutes later a sample of blood is drawn and the dye content of the alkalinized serum is compared with a series of standards. The normal liver excretes most of the dye within a period of 30 minutes.

Dose—*Usual, intravenous*, **5 mg** per **Kg** of body weight.

Dosage Forms—Injection USP: 3, 7.5, and 10 ml.

Other Drugs Used to Test Liver Function

Galactose [$C_6H_{12}O_6.H_2O$]—First prepared by Pasteur in 1856 from milk sugar. Occurs as a component of pectins, gums, and mucilages. Obtained by hydrolysis of milk sugar. Colorless or white crystals. Melts at 118° to 120°, 165° when anhydrous. $[\alpha]_D^{20}$ is +81°. Soluble in about 3.5 parts of water; soluble in pyridine; slightly soluble in alcohol. *Uses:* For diagnosing hepatic function. The patient takes 40 Gm. galactose in 420 ml tea in the morning and fasts until urine has been passed every hour for 4 hours. The sugar in the urine is then quantitatively determined.

Phenoltetrachlorophthalein [$C_{20}H_{10}Cl_4O_4$]—Formed by the condensation of phenol and tetrachlorophthalic acid or its anhydride. *Uses:* For the determination of the functional activity of the liver; excretion is determined by disappearance from the blood stream, excretion in the duodenum by means of a duodenal tube, or excretion in the stool. Sodium salt given intravenously; should not be given subcutaneously or intramuscularly. *Dose: Intravenously*, 5 mg per Kg of body weight.

Drugs Used to Test Kidney Function

The rate of excretion of a number of drugs in the urine has been proposed as a means of measuring the functional capacity of the kidney. Glomerular filtration rate can be measured by the renal plasma clearance of inulin, thiosulfate, mannitol, or endogenous creatinine. The inulin clearance is thought to be most reliable since mannitol is subject to some tubular reabsorption, thiosulfate to some tubular excretion and reabsorption, and endogenous creatinine to some tubular excretion. Effective renal plasma flow and tubular functional capacity can be measured by the use of sodium aminohippurate, iodopyracet, and iodohippurate. Because of the greater accuracy and facility of chemical methods for the determination of the compound, sodium aminohippurate is considered the drug of choice. Although the excretion of phenolsulfonphthalein is accomplished by the same mechanisms as the excretion of sodium aminohippurate, its plasma clearance averages about two-thirds of the effective renal plasma flow, and its toxicity prevents it use for the determination of functioning tubular capacity.

Aminohippuric Acid USP

[*N*-(4-Aminobenzoyl)glycine; PAH; PAHA; *p*-Aminohippuric Acid; *N*-(*p*-Aminobenzoyl)glycine]

Aminohippuric Acid contains 98.0–100.5% of $C_9H_{10}N_2O_3$ (194.19), calculated on the dried basis.

Preparation—It may be prepared by reacting *p*-nitrobenzoyl chloride with glycine and then reducing the *p*-nitro group with tin and hydrochloric acid.

Description—A white, crystalline powder. Discolors on exposure to light. Melting range between 197° and 199°.

Solubility—1 Gm dissolves in 45 ml of water, 50 ml of alcohol, and 5 ml of diluted hydrochloric acid; very slightly soluble in benzene, carbon tetrachloride, chloroform, and ether; freely soluble in solutions of alkali hydroxides or carbonates with some decomposition.

Uses—Aminohippuric Acid (PAH) is secreted into the urine by the renal tubules. The capacity of the tubules to transport this acid (the transport maximum or Tm) is limited and measurement of this Tm is employed as a *diagnostic aid in evaluating kidney function*. The Tm of PAH and other compounds such as iodopyracet, penicillin, and probenecid are mutually lowered since all employ the same excretory mechanism, ie, all compete for an essential intermediary in the tubular transport system. *Probenecid* (page 950), for example, lessens renal tubular transport of penicillin and thus maintains efficient blood levels of the antibiotic. Similarly, the excretion of other diagnostic agents, eg, phenolsulfonphthalein, may be depressed by PAH.

Known quantities (sufficient to produce 2 mg/100 ml of blood plasma) of PAH are administered intravenously to the patient. The urine formed during a definite but short period is collected and the average amount of PAH eliminated is calculated in mg/min. This value divided by the PAH plasma content in mg/ml is equivalent to the *effective renal plasma flow* in ml/min. The normal rate for men is 697 ± 136 ml/min and for women 594 ± 102 ml.

To determine *tubular excretory mass*, a sterile solution of the sodium salt of PAH is injected intravenously in a volume sufficient to "saturate" the capacity of the tubular cells to excrete PAH (above 60 mg per 100 ml of plasma), and the PAH content of the plasma is determined in mg/ml. The amount excreted in the urine is determined in mg/min, this value including both glomerular filtration and tubular excretion. The glomerular filtration rate, using *Mannitol* (page 937) is determined in mg/min. From the glomerular filtration rate and the PAH content per ml of plasma is calculated the amount of PAH that was filtered through the glomeruli in one minute (ml/min × mg/ml). Then the total number of mg/min excreted in the urine minus the amount filtered through the glomeruli per minute equals the amount of PAH in mg/min excreted by the tubules (tubular excretory mass or Tm).

Sodium Aminohippurate Injection USP

Sodium Aminohippurate Injection is a sterile solution of aminohippuric acid in water for injection prepared with the aid of sodium hydroxide. It contains 95.0–105.0% of the labeled amount of $C_9H_9N_2NaO_3$ (216.17).

For the structure of *Aminohippuric Acid*, see page 1310.

Preparation—Sodium *p*-aminohippurate is prepared by reacting *p*-aminohippuric acid with the theoretical amount of sodium hydroxide and adjusting the pH of the resulting solution to 7.0 to 7.2 by means of citric acid. The salt is not isolated from the solution.

Description—The pH of the Injection is between 7.0 and 7.6.

Uses—Diagnostic aid (kidney function). See *Aminohippuric Acid*.

Dose—*Usual, intravenous,* **2 Gm.**

Dosage Forms—Injection USP: 2 Gm/10 ml, 10 Gm/50 ml.

Mannitol—see page 937.

Phenolsulfonphthalein USP

[4,4'-(3*H*-2,1-Benzoxathiol-3-ylidene) diphenol *S,S*-Dioxide; Phenol Red; P. S. P.; Sulfonphthal]

Phenolsulfonphthalein contains 95.0–105.0% of $C_{19}H_{14}O_5S$ (354.38), calculated on the dried basis.

Preparation—Phenolsulfonphthalein may be made by fusing the anhydride of *o*-sulfobenzoic acid with phenol. The *o*-sulfobenzoic anhydride may be obtained by heating the acid with phosphorus pentoxide.

Description—A crystalline powder, varying in color from bright to dark red. It is stable in air.

Solubility—1 Gm dissolves in about 1300 ml of water and about 350 ml of alcohol; almost insoluble in chloroform and ether; freely soluble in solutions of alkali hydroxides and their carbonates.

Uses—Phenolsulfonphthalein is a *diagnostic aid* used for determining *kidney function*. When injected intramuscularly or intravenously, it begins to be excreted in patients with normal kidneys in from 5 to 10 minutes. In patients with deficient renal function, the first appearance of its secretion is delayed. In normal cases, after intramuscular injections, almost the total amount is excreted within 2 hours (from 60 to 80%). Failure to excrete nearly the full amount within 2 hours indicates a deficient functional activity, and the degree of this functional deficiency may be estimated by the proportionate amount excreted within 2 hours. The average normal eliminations after intravenous administration are from 35 to 45% in 15 minutes, from 50 to 65% in 30 minutes, and from 65 to 80% in the first hour.

From 20 minutes to half an hour before administering the test, the patient is given from 200 to 400 ml of water in order to insure free urinary excretion; otherwise delayed time of appearance may be due to lack of excretion.

Under aseptic precautions a catheter is introduced and the bladder is completely emptied, or the patient is allowed to empty it voluntarily. The time is noted, and 1 ml of a carefully prepared solution of the Phenolsulfonphthalein containing 6 mg to the ml is accurately administered intramuscularly into the lumbar muscles, or intravenously, by means of an accurately graduated syringe. Great care must be taken that all of the solution is injected.

The urine is allowed to drain into a test tube in which has been placed a drop of 25% sodium hydroxide solution, and the time of the appearance of the first faint pinkish tinge is noted.

In patients having no urinary obstruction, the catheter is withdrawn at the time of the appearance of the drug in the urine. If injection is made *intramuscularly*, the patient is instructed to void into a receptacle at the end of 1 hour and 10 minutes, and into a second receptacle at the end of the second hour. If injection is made *intravenously*, the patient is instructed to void into a receptacle at the end of 15 or 30 minutes or 1 hour.

When the passing of a catheter is disagreeable and no urinary retention is present, its use can be dispensed with and the time of appearance of the drug can be disregarded.

The urine collected is made alkaline with a 25% solution of sodium hydroxide and then diluted to 1 liter. The solution is thoroughly mixed and a small filtered portion taken to compare with the standard which is used for all of these estimations. Comparison is made in a colorimeter, a special form of which has been devised for this purpose.

Dose—*Usual, intramuscular* or *intravenous*, **6 mg.**

Dosage Forms—Injection USP (see below): 6 mg/ 1 ml.

Phenolsulfonphthalein Injection USP—*Preparation:* It may be prepared as follows, using proportional quantities of phenolsulfonphthalein and sodium bicarbonate for other concentrations:

To phenolsulfonphthalein (6 Gm) contained in a beaker of about 500-ml capacity, add water for injection (100 ml), then dissolve sodium bicarbonate (1.43 Gm), added in small portions, by stirring. Add sodium chloride (9 Gm), and boil the mixture gently until the volume of the solution has been reduced to about 70 ml. Filter through a pledget of sterile cotton into a suitable flask, and wash the filter with water for injection. Dilute to about 950 ml with water for injection, and test the solution for sensitiveness as directed in the USP. If necessary, adjust the solution so that it will conform to the test for sensitiveness by adding sufficient weak solution of sodium hydroxide. Then dilute with water for injection to 1000 ml, mix well, distribute into suitable containers, and sterilize. *Note:* The 1.43 Gm of sodium bicarbonate may be replaced by 17 ml of normal sodium hydroxide.

Sodium Indigotindisulfonate USP

[Disodium 3,3'-Dioxo[$\Delta^{2,2'}$-biindoline]-5,5'-disulfonate; Soluble Indigo Blue; Indigo Carmine]

Sodium Indigotindisulfonate contains 96.0–100.5% of sodium indigotindisulfonates, calculated on the dried basis as $C_{16}H_8N_2Na_2O_8S_2$ (466.36).

Preparation—Sodium Indigotindisulfonate is now exclusively produced synthetically. In the process now most generally used anthranilic acid (*o*-aminobenzoic acid) is the basic material. This acid is usually obtained from *phthalimide* which is made from the now inexpensive phthalic anhydride. The anthranilic acid is treated with chloroacetic acid to form phenylglycine-*o*-carboxylic acid. The latter is then fused with potassium or sodium hydroxide at 250° to 300° and the resulting indoxylacetic acid loses carbon dioxide to form *indoxyl*. The latter product is oxidized by air to *indigo blue*. Indigo carmine is prepared from indigo blue by sulfonating with sulfuric acid and neutralizing the SO_3H groups with sodium carbonate.

Description—A dusky, purplish blue powder, or blue granules with a coppery luster. It is affected by light. Sodium Indigotindisulfonate solutions have a blue or bluish purple color.

Solubility—1 Gm dissolves in about 100 ml of water; slightly soluble in alcohol; practically insoluble in most other organic solvents.

Uses—This dye is used in a *kidney function test*. The rate of excretion of the dye in the urine after injection (usually intravenously) is determined colorimetrically by comparison of the color of the urine with color standards. Indigo carmine is also employed as a *reagent*, as a *stain* for microscopic specimens, and as a *dye*.

Dose—*Usual, intramuscular*, **50 to 100 mg;** *usual, intravenous*, **40 mg.**

Dosage Forms—Injection USP: 40 mg/5 ml.

Sodium Iodohippurate I 131—see page 567.

Sodium Iodohippurate I 131 Injection—see page 567.

Other Drugs Used to Test Kidney Function

Hippuric Acid [Benzoylaminoacetic Acid; $C_6H_5CO.NH.CH_2.COOH$]—This acid is present in the urine of herbivorous animals, and in earlier times it was a source of benzoic acid which was obtained from it by hydrolysis. Colorless, or white, odorless crystals, melts at 187° to 188°. Soluble in about 250 parts water; slightly soluble in cold alcohol, but freely soluble in hot alcohol; soluble in aqueous solutions of sodium phosphate; very slightly soluble in ether or chloroform; insoluble in benzene. *Uses:* Sodium iodohippurate, a derivative of hippuric acid, is used as a contrast medium in x-ray examinations of kidneys and ureters.

Inulin [$(C_6H_{10}O_5)_n$]—A substance closely allied to starch except that is a levulan rather than a dextran. It is found in some of the plants belonging to the family *Compositæ*, eg, Inula, Taraxacum, Pyrethrum, Lappa, etc. It has also been found, according to Kraus, in plants of the *Campanulaceæ*, *Goodeniaceæ*, *Lobeliaceæ*, and *Stylidaceæ*. It differs from starch in the following particulars: it is colored yellow by iodine, does not gelatinize with water, and is not found in plants in the form of granules having concentric layers like starch. When hydrolyzed with acid, fructose is produced. *Uses:* Diagnostic agent for evaluation of glomerular filtration.

Iodohippurate Sodium [Sodium *o*-iodohippurate dihydrate; Hippuran; $C_9H_7INNaO_3.2H_2O$]—Contains 34.95% I. White crystalline powder; very soluble in water. *Uses:* Radiopaque agent for intravenous, oral, or retrograde urography. *Dose: Orally* or *intravenously*, 12 Gm.

Phloridzin [Phlorizin; Phlorhizin; $C_{21}H_{24}O_{10}$]—A glycoside from the root bark of the apple, pear, cherry, etc. *Uses:* It was used in malaria but of no value. It is used to produce experimental diabetes and to test the functional activity of the kidney. *Dose:* 0.005 Gm in 1 ml of 0.5% solution of sodium carbonate, by injection, for kidney test, but is dangerous.

Drugs Used to Test Gastric Function

In some clinical situations it is important to know whether the stomach can secrete hydrochloric acid. Proof of the absence of hydrochloric acid in the stomach is essential to the diagnosis of pernicious anemia and, in some circumstances, offers presumptive evidence of gastric cancer. On the other hand, the presence of hydrochloric acid contributes to the diagnosis of peptic ulcer and peptic esophagitis, which conversely can be virtually excluded by the demonstration of true achlorhydria.

Because the volume of acid secreted by the normal stomach covers the entire range of volume encountered in disease and because there is no sharp line of demarcation in the secretory capacity of the stomach variously diseased, the quantity of acid secreted even in response to a controlled stimulus is seldom of any diagnostic importance. Therefore, it is usually important only to establish the presence or absence of free hydrochloric acid in the stomach. The gastric stimulants described in this section are frequently of value for this purpose.

Alcohol—see page 1357.

Betazole Hydrochloride USP

[3-(2-Aminoethyl)pyrazole Dihydrochloride; Betazolium Chloride; Histalog (*Lilly*); *Sp.* Clorhidrato de Betazol]

Betazole Hydrochloride contains 98.0–101.0% of $C_5H_9N_3 \cdot 2HCl$ (184.07), calculated on the dried basis.

Preparation—Diethyl oxalate and acetone are condensed by refluxing in naphtha solution with sodium ethylate to yield acetonedioxalic ester (I). Cyclization to chelidonic acid (II) is effected by heating with concentrated hydrochloric acid. After purification, II is decarboxylated by heating in the presence of copper powder to yield 4-pyrone (III). III is then reacted with 100% hydrazine hydrate in the methanol, cooled to about −30°C, added to anhydrous ammonia in an autoclave containing Raney nickel, and subjected to catalytic reduction to yield betazole base (IV). After purification by vacuum distillation, the base is dissolved in cold alcohol and converted into the dihydrochloride by anhydrous HCl. Addition of ether to the alcoholic solution precipitates the salt which is collected, washed with ether, and dried.

Description—Occurs as a white, crystalline, nearly odorless powder. Its solutions are acid to litmus. The pH is about 1.5 for a 1 in 20 solution. It softens at a temperature not lower than 215°, and finally melts at a temperature not higher than 240°.

Solubility—Soluble in water; practically insoluble in chloroform.

Uses—Betazole Hydrochloride, a synthetic analog of histamine, is a *diagnostic aid*. It can be used in place of histamine in clinical tests of gastric function. The usual 0.5 mg per Kg of body weight dose of the drug produces a gastric response equal to that induced by the usual 0.01 mg per Kg dose of histamine base or 0.0275 mg per Kg of histamine phosphate. Although the incidence of side effects with betazole is much lower than with histamine, they are qualitatively similar. In addition, betazole produces no significant fall in blood pressure and only minimal increases in pulse rate. The drug should be used cautiously in patients with bronchial asthma. The effect of antihistaminic drugs in combating the side effects has not been determined.

Dose—*Subcutaneous*, 40 to 60 mg; *usual*, 50 mg.

Dosage Forms—Injection USP: 50 mg/ml.

Caffeine—see page 1155.

Caffeine and Sodium Benzoate—see page 1156.

Histamine Phosphate—see page 1142.

Pentagastrin

[Peptavlon (*Ayerst*)]

Pentagastrin is *N*-[*N*-[*N*-[*N*-(*N-tert*-Butoxycarbonyl - *β* - alanyl) - L - tryptophanyl] - L - methionyl] - L-aspartyl]-L-phenylalaninamide.

Description—A colorless or virtually colorless crystalline solid. Solutions are photosensitive and should be protected from light and stored at temperatures not exceeding 4°. It is recommended that the pH of the solvent be kept between 8 and 9 when small quantities of material are dissolved at one time.

Solubility—Almost insoluble in water, ethanol, ether, benzene, chloroform, and ethyl acetate; soluble in dimethylformamide and dimethylsulfoxide.

Uses—Pentagastrin is used to test gastric function in much the same way as histamine, Histalog, or Mecholyl. Pentagastrin, however, has the advantage of being relatively free from side effects.

Dose—*Usual, subcutaneous*, 6 mcg per Kg per hour; *continuous infusion*, 0.025 to 6.0 per Kg per hour.

Drugs Used to Determine Blood Volume and Hemopoietic Function

The estimation of blood volume is important in detecting impending shock and as a guide to the amount of plasma or other fluids to be used in order to avoid inadequate or excessive dosage. The determination of the circulating red blood cell volume and the measurement of the absorption of vitamin B_{12} are valuable in the diagnosis of megaloblastic anemia. Diagnostic agents used for these purposes are described herein.

Evans Blue USP

[C.I. Direct Blue 53;   T-1824]

Evans Blue contains 95.0–105.0% of $C_{34}H_{24}N_6Na_4$-$O_{14}S_4$ (960.82), calculated on the dried basis.

Preparation—It may be prepared by diazotizing *o*-tolidine and coupling the resulting diazo compound with 1-amino-8-naphthol-2,4-disulfonic acid.

Description—A green, bluish green, or brown powder; odorless. The dried product is hygroscopic. Exhibits a maximum absorbance at about 610 mμ.

Solubility—Very soluble in water; very slightly soluble in alcohol; practically insoluble in benzene, carbon tetrachloride, ether, and chloroform.

Uses—Evans Blue is a *diagnostic agent* employed in *blood volume estimation*. A known quantity of the dye is quantitatively injected into the blood stream. After

allowing time for thorough mixing, withdrawal of a sample of blood and determination of the concentration of the dye in the sample enables the clinician to calculate the volume of blood in the patient.

Dose—*Usual, intravenous*, the equivalent of **22.6 mg** of dried Evans blue.

Dosage Forms—Injection USP: 5 ml.

Miscellaneous Diagnostic Drugs

A number of drugs have useful diagnostic applications. Some agents, such as fluorescein sodium, guaiac, and congo red, are used primarily for diagnostic purposes, whereas other drugs exert major pharmacological actions which are described in other chapters of this text, but are also used more or less incidentally for certain specific diagnostic tests. Phentolamine, piperoxan, phenoxybenzamine, and tetraethylammonium chloride are used in the differential diagnosis of hypertension and pheochromocytoma. The vasoconstrictor ergot alkaloids are useful adjuncts in the determination of coronary function. Edrophonium chloride, quinine sulfate, and neostigmine are employed in the diagnosis of myasthenia gravis, and the latter drug is sometimes used in a pregnancy test. Sodium Phosphate P 32 is used for the diagnosis and localization of brain and intraocular tumors. Although most of these applications are mentioned in the monograph for each drug, they are mentioned here as a reminder of these uses.

Azuresin NF

[Azure A Carbacrylic Resin;   Diagnex Blue (*Squibb*)]

Azuresin is a complex combination of 3-amino-7-(dimethylamino)phenazathionium chloride, known as azure A dye, and a carbacrylic cationic exchange resin. It contains, in each Gm, 50–70 mg of the dye, calculated on the dried basis.

Preparation—The resin component is prepared by catalytic polymerization of a suitable carbacrylic monomer. The azure A dye component may be prepared by the method described for Methylene Blue on page 846 except that an equimolar mixture of *N,N*-dimethyl-*p*-phenylenediamine and *p*-phenylenediamine is employed instead of the former alone. In preparing the Azuresin, the resin component is mixed intimately with a solution of the dye whereupon the cationic component of the dye displaces proton from the resin, thus forming the dye salt of the resin. The structure of the dye component may be represented as follows:

Description—Occurs as moist, irregular, dark blue or purple colored granules. It has a slightly pungent odor.

Uses—Azuresin is used as an indicator for the detection of achlorhydria without the discomfort of intubation. A stimulant of gastric secretion (caffeine) is given one hour before administration of 2 Gm of the resin. If hydrochloric acid is secreted, the hydrogen ions displace the blue dye (azure A) from the resin. The azure A dye is absorbed and excreted in the urine within 2 hours after administration of the resin. The urine specimen collected 2 hours after administration of the resin is examined visually and the concentration of dye estimated as an indication of the presence or absence of free hydrochloric acid in the stomach. The concentration of azure A in the urine is estimated by means of a color comparator which is supplied with each test unit of the drug. Azuresin is of negligible toxicity and no cases of idiosyncrasy have been reported.

Dose—*Usual*, **2 Gm** preceded by **500 mg** of *Caffeine and Sodium Benzoate*.

Dosage Forms—for Injection: 500 mg.

Edrophonium Chloride—see page 900.

Methacholine Chloride—see page 901.

Metyrapone USP

[2-Methyl-1,2-di-3-pyridyl-1-propanone;   Metopirone (*Ciba*)]

Metyrapone contains 97.0–103.0% of $C_{14}H_{14}N_2O$ (226.28), calculated on the dried basis.

Preparation—Methyl-3-pyridyl ketone is electrolytically reduced to the corresponding pinacol, 2,3-bis (3-pyridyl)-2,3-butanediol (I). Heating (I) with a strong inorganic acid results in dehydration of the pinacol with subsequent rearrangement to form Metyrapone. Purification of the Metyrapone is accomplished by solvent crystallization (US Pat. 2,966,493).

Description—White to light amber, fine, crystalline powder, having a characteristic odor. Darkens on exposure to light.

Solubility—Soluble in methanol and chloroform; forms water-soluble salts with acids.

Uses—Metyrapone is a synthetic compound which has the unique ability to inhibit the 11-beta-hydroxylation in the biosynthesis of cortisol, corticosterone, and aldosterone. Hence, it is used to test for residual pituitary function. In the normal individual, Metyrapone blocks the enzymatic step which leads to cortisol and corticosterone synthesis, produces an intense stimulation of ACTH secretion, and induces a marked increase in the urinary excretion of 17-hydroxycorticosteroids. In patients with abnormal pituitary function, the ability to increase ACTH production is lacking and no significant increase in 17-hydroxycorticosteroids is seen. The drug is particularly valuable as a diagnostic aid in patients suspect of hypopituitarism and Cushings syndrome.

Dose—*Usual,* **750 mg** every 4 hours for 6 doses.
Dosage Forms—Tablets: 250 mg.

Neostigmine Bromide—see page 904.

Phenoxybenzamine—see page 909.

Phentolamine Hydrochloride—see page 909.

Phentolamine Mesylate—see page 909.

Quinine Sulfate—see page 1248.

Sodium Fluorescein USP

[Soluble Fluorescein; Resorcinolphthalein Sodium; Uranin; Uranine Yellow]

Sodium Fluorescein contains 98.5–100.5% of $C_{20}H_{10}Na_2O_5$ (376.28), calculated on the dried basis.

Preparation—It is prepared by heating 7 parts of resorcinol with 5 parts of phthalic anhydride at 195° to 200° until the mixture solidifies. The mass is then disintegrated and boiled with water to remove soluble impurities. The residue is treated with sodium hydroxide solution and filtered. From the filtrate the fluorescein is precipitated with acid, and, after purification by dissolving in sodium hydroxide and reprecipitating with acid, the fluorescein is dissolved in the required amount of sodium hydroxide solution and evaporated to dryness on a steam bath.

Description—An orange-red, odorless powder. It is hygroscopic. Its aqueous solution is strongly fluorescent even in extreme dilution; the fluorescence disappears when the solution is made acid, and reappears when the solution is again made alkaline.

Solubility—Freely soluble in water; sparingly soluble in alcohol.

Uses—Sodium Fluorescein in 2% aqueous solution has been used as an ophthalmic *diagnostic aid.* It is applied topically for the diagnosis of *corneal lesions* and the detection of minute *foreign bodies* embedded in the cornea. While a weak solution of fluorescein will not stain the normal cornea, ulcers or parts deprived of epithelium will become green and remain so for a time; foreign bodies will appear surrounded by a green ring; loss of substance in the conjunctiva is indicated by a yellow hue. Fluorescein also reveals defects or disease of the endothelium of the cornea, producing a deep coloration of the diseased area. It is also used to outline and demarcate *tumors,* particularly in the central nervous system.

In using Sodium Fluorescein in the eye, it is particularly important that the preparation be sterile and that no accidental contamination of the solution with *Pseudomonas aeruginosa* take place. A diseased or injured eye is readily infected with this organism which can cause blindness. Sodium Fluorescein, being anionic in character, is not compatible with effective preservatives such as benzalkonium chloride or substances known effective against *Pseudomonas aeruginosa,* such as Polymyxin B Sulfate. The solution is best used employing a unit-dose package or dispensed from a container which protects the contents from contamination. Another approach is to use paper strips impregnated with Sodium Fluorescein which are dried, heat-sterilized, and packaged in hermetically sealed unit-dose packets. One of these dipped into the lacrimal fluid of the eye to be examined releases enough of the highly soluble drug to permit examination of the eye for lesions or injury.

Dose—*Topically,* **0.1** to **0.3 ml** of a **2%** solution, to the conjunctiva.

Sodium Phosphate P 32—see page 567.

Tetraethylammonium Chloride—see page 850.

Other Miscellaneous Diagnostic Drugs

Congo Red USP XV [Disodium 3,3'-[4,4'-biphenylenebis(azo)]bis[4-amino-1-naphthalenesulfonate]; C. I. Direct Red 28] [$C_{32}H_{22}N_6Na_2O_6S_2$]—Dark red or reddish brown powder. It is odorless and decomposes on exposure to acid fumes. Its solutions have a pH of 8–9.5. 1 Gm dissolves in about 30 ml water but is only slightly soluble in alcohol. *Uses:* Diagnosis of amyloidosis, estimation of blood volume, determination of the functional capacity of the reticuloendothelial system, an antidote for roentgen sickness, an antitoxic substance against the toxins of diphtheria and botulinus, and as a vital stain. Severe allergic reactions or even sudden death occasionally occur following administration of average doses. *Dose: Intravenously,* 0.1 to 0.2 Gm as a 1% solution in water for injection.

71 | Pharmaceutical Necessities

Antioxidants and preservatives—coloring, flavoring, and diluting agents—
emulsifying and suspending agents—ointment bases—pharmaceutical
solvents—miscellaneous pharmaceutical necessities

This chapter was prepared by

Ewart A. Swinyard, PhD, *Professor of Pharmacology, College of Pharmacy and
College of Medicine, University of Utah, Salt Lake City, Utah 84112, and*
Stewart C. Harvey, PhD, *Associate Professor of Pharmacology, College of
Medicine, University of Utah, Salt Lake City, Utah 84112*

This chapter describes substances which are of little or no therapeutic value, but which are useful in the manufacture and compounding of various pharmaceutical preparations. Hence, they are referred to as pharmaceutical necessities. The substances described include antioxidants and preservatives; coloring, flavoring, and diluting agents; emulsifying and suspending agents; ointment bases; pharmaceutical solvents; and miscellaneous agents. For a more detailed review of the uses of these agents, the interested reader is referred to the various chapters in Part VIII of this book.

Antioxidants and Preservatives

An antioxidant is an agent which inhibits oxidation, and it is used to prevent rancidity of oils or fats or the deterioration of other materials through oxidative processes. A preservative is a substance which is added to some other preparation to prevent bacterial growth and subsequent spoilage of the preparation. Products with these qualifications find wide application in various pharmaceutical preparations such as biological products, emulsions, mucilages, ointments and bases, and sterile solutions.

Alcohol—see page 1357.

Ascorbyl Palmitate NF

[Ascorbic Acid Palmitate (ester); L-Ascorbic Acid 6-Palmitate]

$$CH_3CH_2(CH_2)_{12}CH_2COOCH_2CH$$

Ascorbyl Palmitate contains 95.0–100.5% of $C_{22}H_{38}O_7$ (414.54), calculated on the dried basis.

Preparation—Ascorbyl Palmitate may be prepared by condensing palmitoyl chloride with ascorbic acid in the presence of a suitable dehydrochlorinating agent such as pyridine.

Description—A white to yellowish white powder having a characteristic odor. It melts between 107° and 117°.

Solubility—Very slightly soluble in water and vegetable oils; freely soluble in alcohol.

Uses—Ascorbyl Palmitate is an *antioxidant* used in foods and pharmaceuticals. It is also used to prevent rancidity, to prevent the browning of cut apples, in meat curing, and in the preservation of canned or frozen foods.

Benzoic Acid USP

[Flowers of Benzoin; Flowers of Benjamin; Phenylformic Acid]

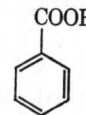

Benzoic Acid, dried over silica gel for 3 hours, contains 99.5–100.5% of $C_7H_6O_2$ (122.12).

Benzoic Acid is the simplest acid of the aromatic series. Although the acid is of minor significance as a medicinal agent, its derivatives and salts constitute an important group of valuable medicinal agents. Many local anesthetic agents have a benzoyl group in the molecule, eg, cocaine, procaine, etc.

Another group of benzoic acid derivatives, namely, the esters of *para*-hydroxybenzoic acid, are now extensively used for the preservation of syrups and a number of other pharmaceutical preparations. The esters most frequently used are the methyl, ethyl, propyl, butyl, and benzyl *para*-hydroxybenzoates. Three of these esters, the methyl and propyl, are official in the USP under the names of *Ethylparaben*, *Methylparaben*, and *Propylparaben*, respectively (pages 1177, 1184, and 1187).

Preparation—Benzoic Acid is found naturally in benzoin, Peru and tolu balsams, storax, and several other balsamic substances. It may be obtained from these by sublimation, but the yield is very small and all benzoic acid of commerce is made synthetically by several processes, of which the following are the most practical:

1. Boiling toluene is chlorinated to benzotrichloride, which yields benzoic acid when hydrolyzed under pressure, preferably in the presence of lime.

2. Phthalic anhydride, made by the oxidation of naphthalene in the vapor state with air in the presence of a suitable catalyst, is made into calcium phthalate by treatment with water and lime. The calcium phthalate is then heated with an excess of lime which results

in the formation of calcium benzoate and calcium carbonate as shown in the equation. The calcium benzoate, upon treatment with hydrochloric acid, yields benzoic acid.

3. Benzoic acid may also be prepared by direct oxidation of toluene or benzyl chloride [$C_6H_5CH_2Cl$] by means of chromic acid ($Na_2Cr_2O_7 + H_2SO_4$) or manganese dioxide and H_2SO_4.

Description—White needles or scale-like crystals. It is odorless or may have a slight benzaldehyde-like odor. It is somewhat volatile at moderately warm temperatures and is freely volatile in steam. It congeals between 121° and 123° and boils at 250°.

Solubility—1 Gm dissolves in about 300 ml of water, about 3 ml of alcohol, about 5 ml of chloroform, about 3 ml of ether, 20 ml of boiling water, and 1.5 ml of boiling alcohol; soluble in benzene and fixed and volatile oils; sparingly soluble in solvent hexane.

Incompatibilities—See *Sodium Benzoate* (page 1189).

Uses—Benzoic Acid is used medicinally as an *antifungal* agent chiefly in the form of Whitfield's Ointment. It is largely used for the manufacture of benzoates, sodium benzoate being the most important and extensively used *preservative* for canned foods as well as syrups and similar preparations.

Veterinary Uses—Mixed with salicylic acid in an ointment, it has been used to treat *ringworm*.

Benzyl Alcohol—see page 1066.

Chlorobutanol USP

[Chlorbutol; Chlorbutanol; 1,1,1-Trichloro-2-methyl-2-propanol; Acetone chloroform; Chloretone (*Parke-Davis*)]

$$CH_3-\underset{\underset{OH}{|}}{\overset{\overset{CH_3}{|}}{C}}-CCl_3$$

Chlorobutanol is anhydrous or contains not more than one-half molecule of water of hydration. It contains 98.0–100.5% of $C_4H_7Cl_3O$ (177.46), calculated on the anhydrous basis.

Preparation—Chloroform is caused to undergo chemical addition to acetone under the catalytic influence of powdered potassium hydroxide.

Description—Colorless to white crystals, of a characteristic, somewhat camphoraceous odor and taste. The anhydrous product melts at about 95°, while the hydrous form melts at about 76°. It boils with some decomposition at 165° to 168°.

Solubility—1 Gm dissolves in 125 ml of water, 1 ml of alcohol, or about 10 ml of glycerin; soluble in acetone, chloroform, ether, and volatile oils.

Identification—An aqueous solution treated with sodium hydroxide TS and iodine TS yields iodoform (derived from the acetone component of the product). When Chlorobutanol is mixed with sodium hydroxide solution and a few drops of aniline, and the mixture gently warmed, the disagreeable odor of phenylisocyanide (*poisonous*) is formed (this reaction being given by the chloroform portion of the product). Alcoholic potassium or sodium hydroxide decomposes it into alkali chloride and several organic decomposition products.

Labeling—The label indicates whether anhydrous or hydrous.

Incompatibilities—The anhydrous form must be used in order to prepare a clear solution in liquid petrolatum. It is decomposed by *alkalies*; *ephedrine* is sufficiently alkaline to cause its breakdown with the formation of ephedrine hydrochloride which will separate from a liquid petrolatum solution.

It is only slightly soluble in water, hence alcohol must be used to dissolve the required amount in certain vehicles.

A soft mass is produced by trituration with *antipyrine*, *menthol*, *phenol*, and other substances.

Uses—Chlorobutanol is used topically as a solution in clove oil as a *dental analgesic*. It has *local anesthetic* potency to a mild degree and has been employed as an anesthetic dusting powder (1 to 5%) or ointment (10%). Chlorobutanol, being *antibacterial*, is also serviceable as a *preservative* in solutions of epinephrine, posterior pituitary, etc. When administered orally, it has much the same therapeutic use as chloral hydrate. Hence, Chlorobutanol may be employed as a sedative and hypnotic. It has been taken orally to allay vomiting due to gastritis.

Veterinary Uses—Chlorobutanol is used as an *antiseptic* and *local anesthetic*; internally, it is used as a *sedative* and *hypnotic*. It appears to be of value in *gastritis* with persistent vomiting in dogs.

Dose—*Topically*, as a 25% solution in clove oil.

Other Dose Information—The dose by mouth is 300 mg to 1.0 Gm, given in tablets or capsules.

Veterinary Dose—*Horses*, 8 to 16 Gm; *Dogs*, **300 to 600 mg.**

Ethylenediamine USP

Ethylenediamine contains 97.0–100.5% of $C_2H_8N_2$ (60.10), calculated on a weight/weight basis.

Caution—Use care in handling Ethylenediamine because of its caustic nature and the irritating properties of its vapor.

Note—Ethylenediamine is strongly alkaline and may readily absorb carbon dioxide from the air to form a nonvolatile carbonate. Protect Ethylenediamine against undue exposure to the atmosphere.

Preparation—Ethylenediamine may be prepared by reacting ethylene dichloride with ammonia, then adding sodium hydroxide and distilling.

Description—A clear, colorless, or only slightly yellow liquid, having an ammonia-like odor and strong alkaline reaction. It is miscible with water and alcohol. Anhydrous ethylenediamine boils between 116° and 117° and solidifies at about 8°. It is volatile with steam. Ethylenediamine is a strong base and readily combines with acids to form salts with the evolution of much heat.

Uses—Ethylenediamine is used as a *pharmaceutical necessity* to stabilize *Aminophylline Injection*. Anhydrous Ethylenediamine is used as a solvent for albumin, casein, shellac, sulfur, etc. It is also used as an emulsifier, an inhibitor in antifreeze solutions, and in textile lubricants.

Ethylparaben—see page 1177.

Ethyl Vanillin—see page 1327.

Glycerin—see page 1359.

Methylparaben—see page 1184.

Phenol—see page 1370.

Phenylethyl Alcohol—see page 1331.

Phenylmercuric Nitrate—see page 1186.

Potassium Sorbate NF

[Potassium 2,4-Hexadienoate]

$$CH_3CH{=}CHCH{=}CHCOOK$$

Potassium Sorbate contains 98.0–101.0% of $C_6H_7KO_2$ (150.22), calculated on the dried basis.

Preparation—Sorbic Acid (this page) is reacted with an equimolar portion of potassium hydroxide. The resulting Potassium Sorbate may be crystallized from aqueous ethanol. US Pat. 3,173,948.

Description—White crystals or powder with a characteristic odor; decomposes at 270°.

Solubility—Soluble in alcohol; freely soluble in water.

Uses—Potassium Sorbate is a water-soluble salt of sorbic acid is used in pharmaceuticals to *inhibit the growth of molds and yeasts*.

Propylparaben—see page 1187.

Sassafras Oil—see page 1338.

Sodium Benzoate—see page 1189.

Sodium Bisulfite USP

[Sodium Hydrogen Sulfite; Sodium Acid Sulfite; Leucogen]

Sodium Bisulfite consists of sodium bisulfite [$NaHSO_3 = 104.06$] and sodium metabisulfite [$Na_2S_2O_5 = 190.10$] in varying proportions. It yields $58.5–67.4\%$ of SO_2.

Description—White or yellowish white crystals or granular powder having the odor of sulfur dioxide. It is unstable in air.

Solubility—1 Gm dissolves in 4 ml of water; slightly soluble in alcohol.

Uses—Sodium Bisulfite is used as an *antioxidant* and *stabilizing agent*. Epinephrine hydrochloride solutions may be stabilized by the addition of small quantities of the salt. It is also used as a reagent for the determination of aldehydes and ketones. Industrially it is employed as a disinfectant and *bleach* in dyeing, in paper making (to remove chlorine), in laundering (as a stripper or reducer), and in the coagulation of rubber latex. It is also useful for removing permanganate stains and for solubilizing certain dyes and other chemicals (see *Menadione Sodium Bisulfite*, page 1022).

Sodium Metabisulfite

Sodium Metabisulfite [$Na_2S_2O_5 = 190.10$] is sodium pyrosulfite.

Preparation—Sodium Metabisulfite is formed when sodium bisulfite undergoes thermal dehydration. It may also be prepared by passing sulfur dioxide over sodium carbonate.

Description—Colorless, prismatic crystals (or a white powder) having a sulfurous odor and an acid and saline taste. On exposure to air and moisture, it is slowly oxidized to sulfate with disintegration of the crystals. A solution in water is acid to phenol red and has the odor of sulfur dioxide.

Solubility—1 Gm dissolves in 2 ml of water, but is less soluble in alcohol.

Uses—Sodium Metabisulfite is a *reducing agent*. It is used in easily oxidized pharmaceuticals, such as epinephrine hydrochloride, phenylephrine hydrochloride, and ascorbic acid injections to retard their oxidation.

Sorbic Acid NF

[(*E,E*)-2,4-Hexadienoic Acid]

$$CH_3CH=CHCH=CHCOOH$$

Sorbic Acid contains $99.0–101.0\%$ of $C_6H_8O_2$ (112.13), calculated on the anhydrous basis.

Preparation—Sorbic Acid may be prepared by various processes. Among the more recent are (1) additive condensation of crotonaldehyde and ketene in the presence of boron trifluoride, and (2) dealkanolation and hydrolysis of a 3,5-dialkoxyhexanal dialkyl acetal under oxidative conditions. US Pat. 2,921,090.

Description—A free-flowing, white, crystalline powder, having a characteristic odor. It melts between 133° and 137°.

Solubility—Slightly soluble in water; soluble in alcohol and ether.

Uses—Sorbic Acid is a *mold and yeast inhibitor*. It is also used as a fungistatic agent for foods, especially cheeses.

Sulfur Dioxide USP

Sulfur Dioxide contains not less than 97.0%, by volume, of SO_2 (64.06).

Preparation—Sulfur Dioxide is prepared by burning sulfur or sulfides and by reacting a bisulfite or a sulfite with a strong acid.

Description—A colorless, nonflammable gas, with a strong, suffocating, odor characteristic of burning sulfur. One liter weighs 2.927 Gm at 760 mm of mercury pressure and 0°. It readily liquefies under pressure forming a colorless liquid with a density of approximately 1.5 Gm per ml and a boiling point of −10°.

Solubility—One volume of water dissolves approximately 36 volumes of Sulfur Dioxide at 760 mm and 20°; 1 volume of ethyl alcohol dissolves approximately 114 volumes under the same conditions; soluble in ether and in chloroform.

Note—*Sulfur dioxide is used most in the form of a gas in pharmaceutical applications, and is described herein for such purposes. However, it is usually packaged under pressure, hence the USP specifications (Water, Nonvolatile residue, and Sulfuric acid) are designed for the testing of its liquid form.*

Uses—The gas in the presence of moisture forms sulfurous acid which is a *bleaching agent*, *fungicide*, and *bactericide*. For this reason fruits are often exposed to the gas before drying to prevent darkening and the growth of molds and bacteria. The gas is also an *antioxidant* and a pharmaceutical necessity for *Injections*.

Thimerosal—see page 1190.

Other Antioxidants and Preservatives

Maleic Acid BP [Toxilic Acid; *cis*-Butenedioic acid]—*Purity:* not less than 99% of $C_4H_4O_4$ (116.07). *Preparation:* Benzene vapor is oxidized by passage over heated vanadium pentoxide. An odorless, white, crystalline powder having a strongly acid taste. It is soluble in 1.5 parts of water in 2 parts of alcohol, and in 12 parts of ether. It melts at 132–140°C. *Uses:* In the preparation of ergometrine maleate injection; as a rancidity retardant in fats and oils (1:10,000).

Propyl Gallate BP [Propyl 3,4,5-Trihydroxybenzoate]— A white to creamy-white crystalline powder; odorless; slightly bitter taste. Soluble in 1000 parts of water, and in 3 parts of alcohol. *Uses:* A preservative.

Sodium Formaldehyde Sulfoxylate [Sodium Hydroxymethanesulfinate; $HOCH_2SO_2Na.2H_2O$ (154.12)]—*Preparation:* Zinc dust is reacted with sulfur dioxide in the presence of formaldehyde and water to form a mixture of zinc formaldehyde sulfoxylate and zinc formaldehyde bisulfite according to the equation:

$$2Zn + 4SO_2 + 4CH_2O + 2H_2O \rightarrow$$
$$Zn(HOCH_2SO_2)_2 + Zn(HOCH_2SO_3)_2$$

Upon the addition of more sodium hydroxide, the zinc salts are converted to sodium salts, and further reaction with zinc dust under pressure reduces the bisulfite component to form more sulfoxylate. US Pat. 2,013,125. Colorless or white crystals. Soluble in water. *Uses:* Mercury antidote reducing corrosive mercuric chloride to insoluble mercurous salts, or metallic mercury. Also used as antioxidant in parenteral formulations. See *Mercury Bichloride* (page 1193) under *Antidotes. Dose:* 10 Gm in ½ glass of water swallowed or in 500 ml water administered with a stomach tube and first half of solution recovered by siphonage, the last portion remaining in stomach; 10 Gm in 150 ml of water for injection, *intravenously.* However, this compound is not nearly as effective as *Dimercaprol* (page 1255) in systemic mercury poisoning and is not to be preferred if Dimercaprol (BAL) is available.

Coloring, Flavoring, and Diluting Agents

The use of properly colored and flavored medicinal substances, although offering no particular therapeutic advantage, is of considerable importance psychologically. A water-clear medicine is not particularly acceptable to most patients and, in general, is thought to be quite inert. Many very active medicinal substances are quite unpalatable, and the patient may fail to take his medicine simply because the taste or appearance is objectionable to him. Even disagreeable medication can be given an attractive appearance and be made pleasing to the taste by the careful selection of the appropriate coloring, flavoring, and diluting agent. Therefore, the judicious use of these substances is important in securing patient cooperation in taking or using the prescribed medication.

There is no sharp line of demarcation which separates the various coloring, flavoring, and diluting agents. Indeed, it is possible to obtain all three qualities in a single agent. Nevertheless, it is convenient to divide these agents into three groups (on the basis of their primary use) and to discuss them separately in the following sections.

Coloring Agents

Coloring Agents[1-3] may be defined as compounds which are employed in pharmacy solely for the purpose of imparting color. They may be classified in various ways. They may be categorized as natural or synthetic; they may just as logically be categorized as inorganic or organic. For the purposes of this discussion two subdivisions are used: (1) *Natural Coloring Principles* and (2) *Synthetic Coloring Principles.* The members of these groups are used as colors for pharmaceutical preparations, cosmetics, and foods, as bacteriological stains, and as attractive colors to improve the appearance of pharmaceutical packages and literature.

Natural Coloring Principles

Natural coloring principles are obtained from the three kingdoms—mineral, plant, and animal. They are used primarily for artistic purposes, as symbolical adornments of natives, as colors for foods, drugs, and cosmetics, and for other psychological effects.

Mineral colors are frequently termed *pigments* and are used to color lotions, cosmetics, and other preparations, usually for external application. Examples are *Red Ferric Oxide* (page 1378) and *Yellow Ferric Oxide* (page 1378).

The term pigment is also applied generically to plant colors by phytochemists. Many vegetable drugs contain coloring principles which are only incidental to their composition, their principal use being for the therapeutic effect which is due to other constituents. The green leaf drugs containing chlorophyll (belladonna and digitalis), certain cathartic drugs (rhubarb and aloes), and many others are in this class. On the other hand, some vegetable drugs, such as cudbear and red saunders, are used almost exclusively for coloring. Most plant colors have now been characterized and synthesized, however, and those with the desirable qualities of stability, fastness, and pleasing hue are available commercially as synthetic products.

Animals have been a source of coloring principles from the earliest periods of recorded history. For example, *Tyrian purple*, once a sign of royalty, was prepared by air oxidation of a colorless secretion obtained from the glands of a snail (*Murex brandaris*). This dye is now known to be 6,6'-dibromoindigo, and has been synthesized, but cheaper dyes of the same color are available. Several insects produce dyes. Cochineal from *Coccus cacti* (page 1321) contains the bright red coloring principle, *carminic acid*, a derivative of anthraquinone.

Carminic Acid (from cochineal)

Synthetic Coloring Principles

The synthetic coloring principles date from 1856 when W. H. Perkin accidentally discovered *mauveine,* also known as *Perkin's purple,* while engaged in unsuccessful attempts to synthesize quinine. He obtained the dye by oxidizing aniline containing o- and p-toluidines as impurities. Other discoveries along this line followed soon after, and a major industry grew up in the field of coal-tar chemistry, which in its broadest sense includes research on synthetic medicinals.

The earliest colors were prepared from aniline and for many years all coal-tar dyes were called aniline colors, irrespective of their origin. The coal-tar dyes include more than a dozen well-defined groups among which are the *nitroso-dyes, nitro-dyes, azo-dyes, oxazines, thiazines, indigoids, anthraquinones, acridines, rosanilines, phthaleins, quinolines,* and others. These in turn are classified, according to their method of use, as *acid dyes* and *basic dyes,* or *direct dyes* and *mordant dyes.*

The chemistry of the above groups of dyes which have representatives useful in pharmacy and medicine is presented under the official representatives.

Uses—Most synthetic coloring principles are used in coloring fabrics and for various artistic purposes. They also find application as indicators, as bacteriological stains, and as reagents in microscopy, etc.

Many coal-tar dyes were originally used in foodstuffs and beverages without careful selection or discrimination between those which were harmless and those which were toxic and without any supervision as to purity or freedom from poisonous constituents derived from their manufacture.

After the passage of the Food and Drugs Act in 1906, the US Department of Agriculture established regulations by which a few colors came to be known as *permitted colors*. Certain of these colors may be used in foods, drugs, and cosmetics, but only after certification by the Food and Drug Administration that they meet certain specifications. From this list of permitted colors may be produced, by skillful blending and mixing, other colors that may be used in foods, beverages, and pharmaceutical preparations.

The word "permitted" is used in a restricted sense. It does not carry with it the right to use colors for purposes of deception, even though they be "permitted" colors; for all food laws have clauses prohibiting the coloring of foods and beverages in a manner so as to conceal inferiority or to give false appearance of value.

The certified colors are classified into three groups as follows: (1) FD&C dyes which may legally be used in foods, drugs, and cosmetics, (2) D&C dyes which may legally be used in drugs and cosmetics, and (3) External D&C dyes which may legally be used only in externally applied drugs and cosmetics. As the use status of these colors is still subject to change, the latest regulations of the FDA should be consulted to determine how they may be used.

The Coal-Tar Color Regulations specify that the term "externally applied drugs and cosmetics" means drugs and cosmetics which are applied only to external parts of the body and not to the lips or any body surface covered by mucous membrane. No certified dye, regardless of its category, may legally be used in any article which is to be applied to the area of the eye. The term "area of the eye," means the area enclosed within the circumference of the supra-orbital ridge and the infra-orbital ridge, including the eyebrow, the skin below the eyebrow, the eyelids and the eye-lashes, the conjunctival sac of the eye, the eyeball, and the soft areolar tissue that lies within the perimeter of the infra-orbital ridge.

The application of dyes to pharmaceutical preparations is an art that can be acquired only after an understanding of the characteristics of dyes and a knowledge of the composition of the products to be colored have been obtained. Specific rules for the choice or application of dyes to pharmaceutical preparations are difficult to formulate. Each preparation may present unique problems.

Preparations which may be colored include most liquid pharmaceuticals, powders, ointments, and emulsions. Some general hints may be offered in connection with solutions and powders, but desired results can usually be obtained only by a series of trials. In general, an inexperienced operator tends to use a much higher concentration of the dye than is necessary. The amount of dye present in any pharmaceutical preparation should be of a concentration low enough to prevent permanent staining of fabrics in the event that the preparation is spilled on them.

Liquids (Solutions)—The dye concentration in liquid preparations and solutions should usually come within a range of 0.0005% (1 in 200,000) and 0.001% (1 in 100,000), depending upon the depth of color wanted and the thickness of column to be viewed in the container. With some dyes, concentrations as low as 0.0001% (1 in 1,000,000) may have a distinct tinting effect. Dyes are most conveniently used in the form of stock solutions.

Powders—White powders usually require the incorporation of 0.1% (1 in 1000) of a dye to impart a pastel color. The dyes may be incorporated into the powder by dry blending in a ball mill or, on a small scale, with a mortar and pestle. When a dye is to be incorporated by trituration, place the calculated amount required in a mortar, add about an equal bulk of the powder, and mix the two intimately by trituration. Then add successive portions of the powder, from time to time, until the whole is added, and continue the trituration after each addition until the dye is intimately mixed with the powder. Powders may also be evenly colored by adding a solution of the dye in alcohol or some other volatile solvent having only a slight solvent action on the powder being colored. When this procedure is employed, add the solution in portions with thorough mixing after each addition, and then allow the solvent to evaporate from the mixture.

Many of the syrups and elixirs used as flavoring and diluting agents are colored. When such agents are used no further coloring matter is necessary. The use of colored flavoring agents is discussed in a subsequent section. However, when it is desired to add color to an otherwise colorless mixture, one of the following agents may be used:

Amaranth USP

[3-Hydroxy-4-[(4-sulfo-1-naphthyl)azo]-2,7-naphthalenedisulfonic Acid Trisodium Salt; C. I. Acid Red 27; FD & C Red No. 2]

Amaranth contains 94.0–100.5% of $C_{20}H_{11}N_2Na_3O_{10}S_3$ (604.48), calculated on the dried basis.

Description—A dark red-brown powder.

Solubility—1 Gm dissolves in about 15 ml of water; very slightly soluble in alcohol.

Uses—Amaranth is one of the red dyes certified for use in coloring foods, drugs, or cosmetics. It is also used for dyeing wool and silk, as an indicator in hydrazine titrations, and in color photography.

Amaranth Solution USP is a solution of amaranth in purified water. It contains, in each 100 ml, 0.9–1.1 Gm of with but a slight odor. *Uses:* Amaranth Solution is a *coloring agent* for coloring pharmaceutical preparations red, and for dyeing wool and silk. It provides the color for *Phenobarbital Elixir* (page 1082).

Compound Amaranth Solution NF—*Preparation:* Dissolve caramel (100 Gm) in purified water (500 ml), add amaranth solution (90 ml), alcohol (250 ml), and sufficient purified water to make the product measure 1000 ml, and mix well. *Alcohol Content:* From 22 to 25% of C_2H_5OH. *Uses:* A color for pharmaceuticals.

Caramel NF

[Burnt Sugar Coloring]

Caramel is a concentrated solution of the product obtained by heating sugar or glucose until the sweet taste is destroyed and a uniform dark brown mass results, a small amount of alkali, alkaline carbonate, or a trace of mineral acid being added while heating.

Description—A thick, dark brown liquid with the characteristic odor of burnt sugar, and a pleasant, bitter taste. Its specific gravity is not less than 1.30. One part dissolved in 1000 parts of water yields a clear solution having a distinct yellowish orange color which is not changed and no precipitate is formed after exposure to sunlight for 6 hours. When spread in a thin layer on a glass plate, Caramel appears homogeneous, reddish brown, and transparent.

Solubility—Miscible with water in all proportions and with dilute alcohol up to 55% by volume; immiscible with ether, chloroform, acetone, benzene, solvent hexane, or turpentine oil.

Uses—Caramel is used to produce a brown color in elixirs, syrups, and other preparations.

Cochineal NFXII

[Coccus; Red Scale Insect]

Cochineal consists of the dried female insects, *Coccus cacti* Linné (Fam. *Coccidæ*), enclosing the young larvæ.
Constituents—Cochineal owes its red color to a glucosidal anthraquinone, *carminic acid* (page 1319), which is present to the extent of 8 to 10% as an alkali carminate in the yolks of the eggs and the fatty parts of the insects. This substance may be precipitated by most metallic salts; aluminum hydroxide forms a metal complex, termed a lake, which is known as *carmine*. The red dye, carmine, is very soluble in ammonia water and advantage is taken of this fact in preparing a solution of carmine.

Cochineal also contains about 10% fat and about 2% of a wax, *coccerin*.

Uses—Cochineal is only used in pharmacy to impart a bright red color to various preparations.

Other Coloring Agents

Red Saunders NF X [Red Sandalwood]—The dried heart-wood of *Pterocarpus santalinus* Linné filius (Fam. *Leguminosæ*). It contains santalin, tannin, pterocarpin, and santal. *Uses:* Red coloring agent.

Rose [Red Rose Petals; French Rose; Rosa Gallica]—The dried petals of *Rosa Gallica*, collected just before the expansion of the flowers. It contains *quercitrin* and *quercitannic acid*. *Uses:* Chiefly for its odor and color.

Flavoring Agents

Flavor

The word flavor refers to a mixed sensation of taste, touch, smell, sight, and sound, all of which combine to produce an infinite number of gradations in the perception of a substance. The four primary tastes—*sweet, bitter, sour,* and *saline*—appear to be the result partly of physicochemical and partly of psychological action. Taste buds, located at various places in the mouth and on the tongue, contain very sensitive nerve endings which react, in the presence of moisture, with the flavors in the mouth and as a result of physicochemical activity electrical impulses are produced and transmitted via the seventh, ninth, and tenth cranial nerves to the areas of the brain which are devoted to the perception of taste. Some of the taste buds are specialized in their function, giving rise to areas on the tongue which are sensitive to only one type of taste. The brain, however, usually perceives taste as a composite sensation, and accordingly the components of any flavor are not readily discernible.

As mentioned above, taste is partly dependent on the ions which are produced in the mouth, but psychologists have demonstrated that sight and sound also play a definite role when certain reflexes become conditioned through custom and association of sense perceptions. Thus in the classic experiments of Pavlov demonstrating "conditioned reflexes," the ringing of a bell or the showing of a circle of light caused the gastric juices of a dog to flow although no food was placed before it, and much of the enjoyment derived from the eating of celery is due to its crunchy crispness as the fibrovascular bundles are crushed. The effect of color is just as pronounced; oleomargarine is very unpalatable to most people when it is uncolored, but once the dye has been incorporated gourmets frequently cannot distinguish it from butter.

A person suffering from a head cold finds his food much less palatable than usual because his sense of smell is impaired, and if the nostrils are held closed raw onions taste sweet and it is much easier to ingest castor oil and other nauseating medicines. The volatility of a substance is an important factor which is influenced by the warmth and moisture of the mouth since the more volatile a compound the more pronounced is its odor. The sense of smell detects very minute amounts of material and is usually much more sensitive in detecting the presence of volatile chemicals, but the tongue is able to detect infinitesimal amounts of some vapors if it is protruded from the mouth so that solution of the gases in the saliva may take place. In this manner traces of sulfur dioxide can be detected in the air since it dissolves in the saliva and creates a sour taste.

Flavors described as hot are those which exert a mild counterirritant effect on the mucosa of the mouth, those which are astringent and pucker the mouth contain tannins and acids which produce this effect by reacting with the lining of the mouth, and wines possess a bouquet due to the odor of the volatile constituents. Indian turnip (Jack-in-the-pulpit) owes its flavor largely to the stinging sensation caused by the minute acicular crystals of calcium oxalate which penetrate the mucous membrane. There is a definite threshold of taste for every substance which varies somewhat with the individual and with the environment. The experienced chef tastes his delicacies at the temperature at which they will be served since heat and cold alter the flavor of many preparations. Thus, lemon loses its sour taste entirely at an elevated temperature and other flavors become almost non-volatile, tasteless, and odorless when cooled sufficiently. In addition to the influence of temperature the sensitivity of each individual must be considered. For example, it has been determined by experiment that the amount of sugar that can just be detected by the average individual is about 7 mg. However, this amount cannot be tasted by some and it is definitely sweet to others.

The association of early sensations with various flavors creates in the child definite likes and dislikes which continue on into maturity. Thus, certain flavors may be associated with illness and nauseating medicines or some other childhood experience, and unless a person analyzes the tastes he encounters he can never approach the delight in his environment achieved by the epicurean.

Preservation of Flavors—Most monographs of official products contain specific directions for storage. Proper methods of storage are essential to prevent deterioration which in many instances results in destruction of odor and taste. Under adverse conditions undesirable changes occur due to one or a combination of the following: enzymatic activity, oxidation, change in moisture content, absorption of odors, activity of microorganisms, and effects of heat and light. In certain products some of the changes wrought by these factors are desirable, as when esters are formed due to the activity of enzymes and when blending and mellowing result from the interchange of the radicals of esters (*transesterification*). For a further discussion of preservation see *Antioxidants and Preservatives* (page 1316).

One method for protecting readily oxidizable substances, such as lemon oil, from deteriorating, and thus preserving their original delicate flavor, is to encapsulate them. The capsules containing the flavors are then enclosed in various packaged products (eg, powdered gelatins) which are deliciously flavored when the capsule is disintegrated by mixing and warming with water.

Correlation of Chemical Structure and Flavor— The compounds employed as flavors in vehicles vary considerably in their chemical structure, ranging from simple esters (methyl salicylate), alcohols (glycerin), and aldehydes (vanillin) to carbohydrates (honey) and the complex volatile oils (anise oil). Synthetic flavors of almost any desired type are now available on the market. These frequently possess the delicate flavor and aroma of the natural products and also the desirable characteristics of stability, reproducibility, and comparatively low cost. Synthetic products such as cinnamaldehyde and benzaldehyde, first officially recognized when several of the essential oils became scarce during war years, have been widely used.

There is a close relationship between chemical structure and taste. Much research has been undertaken to correlate molecular configuration and flavor, but only a start has been made. The degree of ionization and the type of ions produced in the saliva definitely influence the sensation interpreted by the brain, although many non-ionizing compounds (chloroform) have definite tastes. It is known also that an increase in the number of hydroxyl groups increases the sweetness of a compound (sucrose is sweeter than glycerin). This may be due in some instances to an increased solubility brought about by the entry of more polar groups into the molecule, since the less soluble a substance the less taste it has. In general, amines (amphetamine), amides (acetanilid), and other ammonia derivatives such as the alkaloids (strychnine) are bitter, and also lactones (santonin) and the glycosides (salicin), but certain imides (saccharin) and sulfamates (cyclamate) are intensely sweet. Alcohols, aldehydes, and esters are usually pleasant in flavor and possess agreeable odors, especially those with an aromatic nucleus. Unsaturation (eg, acrolein, $CH_2{=}CHCHO$) frequently bestows a sharp, biting odor and taste upon compounds and as a general rule substances which yield hydrogen ions (citric and other acids) in solution are sour.

Selection of Flavors[4,5]

The proper selection of flavors for disguising nauseating medicines aids in the ingestion and sometimes the absorption of the medicine by the patient. Occasion-

ally, sensitive patients have become sufficiently nauseated to vomit at the thought of having to take disagreeable medication, and it is particularly difficult to persuade children to swallow distasteful preparations. It is desirable to know the allergies and idiosyncrasies of the patient; thus, it is foolish to use a chocolate-flavored vehicle for the patient who dislikes the flavor or who is allergic to it, notwithstanding the fact that this flavor is generally acceptable.

Flavors, as used by the pharmacist in compounding prescriptions, may be divided into four main categories according to the type of taste which is to be masked, as follows:

1. *Salty Taste*—Cinnamon Syrup is the best vehicle for ammonium chloride, and other salty drugs such as sodium salicylate and ferric ammonium citrate according to Wright.[6] In a study of the comparative efficiency of flavoring agents for disguising salty taste, he compiled the following additional vehicles arranged in descending order of usefulness: Orange Syrup, Compound Sarsaparilla Syrup, Aromatic Eriodictyon Syrup, Citric Acid Syrup, Cherry Syrup, Cocoa Syrup, Wild Cherry Syrup, Raspberry Syrup, Glycyrrhiza Elixir, Aromatic Elixir, and Glycyrrhiza Syrup. The last named is particularly useful as a vehicle for the salines due to its colloidal properties and double sweetness due to glycyrrhizin and sucrose.

2. *Bitter Taste*—Cocoa Syrup NF V was found[6] to be the best vehicle for disguising bitter taste, then followed, in descending order of usefulness, Raspberry Syrup, Aromatic Eriodictyon Syrup, Cacao Syrup NF VI, Cherry Syrup, Cinnamon Syrup, Compound Sarsaparilla Syrup, Citric Acid Syrup, Licorice Syrup, Aromatic Elixir, Orange Syrup, Wild Cherry Syrup, and Licorice Elixir. This order was obtained using quinine bisulfate as the bitter agent.

3. *Acrid or Sour Taste*—Raspberry Syrup and other fruit syrups are especially efficient in masking the taste of sour substances such as hydrochloric acid. Acacia Syrup, Althea Syrup, and similar mucilaginous vehicles are best for disguising the acrid taste of substances, such as capsicum, since they tend to form a colloidal protective coating over the taste buds of the tongue. If the sour or acrid substance is present as a dispersed phase in an emulsion, these vehicles tend to form a film around each particle of the internal phase. Tragacanth, unlike acacia, may be used in an alcoholic vehicle. Glycyrrhiza vehicles cannot be used in the presence of acids for the glycyrrhizin is precipitated. Aromatic Elixir is also frequently useful.

4. *Oily Taste*—Castor Oil may be made palatable by mixing it with an equal volume of Aromatic Rhubarb Syrup or it may be mixed with Compound Sarsaparilla Syrup and then emulsified with a fine stream of soda water. Cod Liver Oil is effectively disguised by the addition of Wintergreen Oil or Peppermint Oil. Lemon, Orange, Almond, Coriander, Geranium, Cardamom, and Anise or combinations of these are useful. It is better to mix most of the flavor with the oil before emulsifying it, and then the small remaining quantity can be added after the primary emulsion is formed.

Those flavors which are most pleasing to the majority of people are associated with some stimulant of a physical or physiological nature. This may be a central nervous stimulant such as caffeine, which is the reason so many enjoy tea and coffee as a beverage, or it may be a counterirritant such as one of the spices which produce a "biting" sensation, or an agent which "tickles" the throat such as soda water. Sherry owes its sharp flavor to its acetaldehyde content and some of the volatile oils contain terpenes which are stimulating to the mucous surfaces.

Selection of Vehicles

Too few pharmacists realize the unique opportunity they have in acquainting physicians with a knowledge of how to increase both the palatability and efficacy of their prescribed medicines through the judicious selection of vehicles. Because of the training which a pharmacist receives, his knowledge of the characteristics of various pharmaceuticals and therapeutic agents and his technique and skill in preparing elegant preparations are well developed, so that he is admirably qualified to advise concerning the proper use of vehicles.

A large selection of flavors is available as well as a

choice of colors, so that one may prescribe a basic drug for a prolonged period, but by changing the vehicle from time to time, the taste and appearance are so altered that the patient does not tire of the prescription or show other psychological reactions to it.

Waters—These are the simplest of the vehicles and are available with several flavors. They contain no syrup, a fact to be considered at times, since syrup under certain circumstances may be undesirable. They are likewise nonalcoholic, another fact which frequently influences vehicle selection.

Elixirs—These have added sweetness which waters lack, and they usually contain alcohol, which imparts an added sharpness to the flavor of certain preparations, making the latter more pleasing to the taste.

Syrups—These vehicles, like elixirs, offer a wide selection of flavors and colors from which to choose. Their specific value, however, lies particularly in the fact that they are intensely sweet and do not contain any large quantity of alcohol, a combination which makes them of singular value as masking agents for the

class of saline drugs.

The statement of the late Dr. Bernard Fantus that "the best solvent is the best vehicle" helps to explain this situation. For instance, if one dissolves equal substantial quantities of potassium bromide in Aromatic Elixir and in Raspberry Syrup, the salty taste of the bromide will be intensified in the first instance while in the case of the syrup, the saltiness will be almost entirely lost. As a matter of fact, such a syrup, containing 10 to 15 grains of bromide to the teaspoonful, tastes as though one had added "a pinch" of salt to bring out the flavor of the syrup. This is explained by noting, first of all, the high solubility of these salts in water and their relative insolubility in alcohol. Thus, when one tastes the elixir preparation, the salt will have a tendency to flow into the solvent of choice, in this case the aqueous saliva, and consequently cause a marked increase in the resulting salty taste because of the increased concentration. On the other hand, the tendency for salt to redistribute itself from the aqueous syrup to the aqueous saliva will be far less pronounced. In addition, the sugar being somewhat more soluble in the saliva than is the salt, the predominating taste will be that of sweetness, thus masking the salty preparation to an unusual degree.

Vehicles consisting of a solution of pleasantly flavored volatile oils in syrup or glycerin (1:5000) have been successfully employed in producing uniform and stable preparations. These vehicles are prepared by adding 2 ml of the volatile oil, diluted with 6 ml of alcohol, to 500 ml of glycerin or syrup, which has been gently warmed. The solution is added a little at a time with continuous shaking, and then sufficient glycerin or syrup is added to make 1000 ml; and mixed well.

A listing of substances, most of them official, used as flavors, flavored vehicles, or as sweeteners, is given in Table I.

Table I—Flavoring Agents

Acacia Syrup	Glycyrrhiza Syrup
Anethole	Honey
Anise Oil	Iso-Alcoholic Elixir
Aromatic Elixir	Lavender Oil
Aromatic Elixir, Red	Lemon Oil
Benzaldehyde	Lemon Tincture
Benzaldehyde Elixir, Compound	Methyl Salicylate
	Myristica Oil
Calcium Cyclamate	Orange, Bitter, Elixir
Calcium Cyclamate and Calcium Saccharin Solution	Orange, Bitter, Oil
	Orange Flower Oil
	Orange Flower Water
Calcium Cyclamate and Calcium Saccharin Tablets	Orange Oil
	Orange Peel, Bitter
	Orange Peel, Sweet, Tincture
Calcium Saccharin	Orange Spirit, Compound
Caraway	Orange Syrup
Caraway Oil	Peppermint
Cardamom Oil	Peppermint Oil
Cardamom Seed	Peppermint Spirit
Cardamom Spirit, Compound	Peppermint Water
	Phenylethyl Alcohol
Cardamom Tincture, Compound	Raspberry Juice
	Raspberry Syrup
Cherry Juice	Rosemary Oil
Cherry Syrup	Rose Oil
Cinnamon	Rose Water
Cinnamon Oil	Rose Water, Stronger
Cinnamon Water	Saccharin
Citric Acid Syrup	Sarsaparilla Syrup, Compound
Clove Oil	
Cocoa	Sodium Cyclamate
Cocoa Syrup	Sodium Cyclamate and Sodium Saccharin Solution
Coriander Oil	
Dextrose	
Eriodictyon	Sodium Cyclamate and Sodium Saccharin Tablets
Eriodictyon Fluidextract	
Eriodictyon Syrup, Aromatic	
	Sodium Saccharin
Ethyl Acetate	Sodium Saccharin Tablets
Ethyl Vanillin	Sorbitol Solution
Fennel Oil	Spearmint
Ginger	Spearmint Oil
Ginger Fluidextract	Sucrose
Ginger Oleoresin	Syrup
Glycerin	Thyme Oil
Glycyrrhiza	Tolu Balsam Syrup
Glycyrrhiza Elixir	Vanilla
Glycyrrhiza Extract	Vanilla Tincture
Glycyrrhiza Extract, Pure	Vanillin
Glycyrrhiza Fluidextract	Wild Cherry Syrup

References

1. Fieser, L. F., *J. Chem. Ed.*, **7**, 2609 (1930).
2. Brooker, L. G. S., *et al*, *J. Am. Chem. Soc.*, **62**, 1116 (1940); **63**, 3192, 3203, 3214 (1941); **64**, 199 (1942).
3. Pauling, L., *Proc. Nat. Acad. Sciences*, **25**, 577 (1939).
4. Lankford, B. L., and Becker, C. H., *J. APhA*, *Sci. Ed.*, **40**, 77, 83 (1951).
5. Purdum, W. A., *J. APhA*, *Sci. Ed.*, **31**, 298 (1942); **32**, 103 (1943).
6. Wright, H. N., *J. Am. Med. Assoc.*, **108**, 959 (1937).
7. Ewing, C. O., *et al*, *J.APhA*, *Sci. Ed.*, **34**, 129 (1945).

Acacia Syrup—see page 1339.

Anethole USP

[*p*-Propenylanisole; Anethol; Anise Camphor]

$$CH_3O \!-\!\! \langle \rangle \!-\! CH\!=\!CHCH_3$$

Anethole [$C_{10}H_{12}O = 148.21$] is obtained from anise oil and other sources, or is prepared synthetically.

Preparation—Anethole is the principal constituent of anise and fennel oils and is usually obtained from these sources by fractionating and chilling the proper fraction whereby it crystallizes out.

Description—A colorless or faintly yellow liquid at or above 23°. It has the aromatic odor of anise and a sweet taste. It is affected by light. Its specific gravity is 0.983 to 0.988. It distils completely between 231° and 237° and congeals at not less than 20°. Refractive index: 1.5570 to 1.5610 at 25°. Anethole is practically optically inactive, and its alcohol solution is neutral to litmus.

Solubility—Slightly soluble in water; soluble in alcohol, acetone, benzene, petroleum benzin, and ethyl acetate; miscible with chloroform or ether; yields a clear solution with 2 volumes of alcohol.

Uses—A *flavoring agent*. The uses of Anethole are similar to those of anise oil. It is sometimes sold as *Synthetic* or *Artificial Anise Oil* for flavoring and is a licorice-like flavor used in *Diphenhydramine Hydrochloride Elixir*.

Anise Oil USP

[Aniseed Oil; Star Anise Oil]

Anise Oil is the volatile oil distilled with steam from the dried, ripe fruit of *Pimpinella anisum* Linné (Fam. *Umbelliferæ*) or from the dried, ripe fruit of *Illicium verum* Hooker filius (Fam. *Magnoliaceæ*).

Note—If solid material has separated, carefully warm the Anise Oil until it is completely liquefied, and mix it before using.

Constituents—The official Oil varies somewhat in composition, depending upon whether it was obtained from *Pimpinella anisum* or the star anise, *Illicium verum*. Anethole (*parapropenyl anisole*), officially recognized in the USP, is the chief constituent of both oils, occurring to the extent of 80 to 90%. *Methyl chavicol*, an isomer of anethole, and *anisic ketone* [$C_{10}H_{12}O_2$] are also found in both oils. Old samples of either Oil are likely to contain *anisic aldehyde* and *anisic acid*, formed by the oxidation of anethole; such samples congeal with greater difficulty than freshly distilled oil. *Acetaldehyde*, malodorous sulfurated products, and possibly traces of terpenes may be present in the first fractions of the Oil distilled from *Pimpinella Anisum*.

In addition to the compounds already mentioned, star anise oil contains *d-α-pinene*, *α-* and *β-phellandrene* in both *d-* and *l-* forms, *l-limonene, dipentene, p-cymene*, the sesquiterpenes *l-bisabolene* and *d-cadinene*, *α-terpineol, cineol, hydroquinone ethyl ether*, and traces of *safrol*. The congealing test of the USP depends upon the anethole content of the Oil and is thus a means of determining the quality of the sample. Anise Oil is usually shipped in lead containers and may thus become contaminated with that metal; hence the official test for heavy metals.

Description—Anise Oil is a colorless or pale yellow, strongly refractive liquid, having the characteristic odor and taste of anise. Specific gravity: 0.978 to 0.988. Optical rotation: from $-2°$ to $+1°$ in a 100-mm tube. Refractive index: 1.5530 to 1.5600 at 20°. Congealing temperature: not below 15°. (For details of this procedure see page 590.) Anise oil is soluble in 3 volumes of 90 per cent alcohol.

Uses—Anise Oil is extensively used as a *flavoring agent*, particularly for licorice candies. It may be given as a *carminative* in a dose of 0.1 ml.

Aromatic Elixir—see page 1341.

Aromatic Elixir, Red—see page 1341.

Benzaldehyde NF

[Artificial Essential Almond Oil]

Benzaldehyde contains 98.0–100.5% of C_7H_6O (106.13).

Preparation—Benzaldehyde may be synthesized by the interaction of benzal chloride with lime in the presence of water. Benzal chloride is obtained by treating boiling toluene with the proper amount of chlorine.

Synthetic benzaldehyde is free from hydrocyanic acid, but is liable to retain traces of chlorine compounds. *This product must not be confounded with nitrobenzene* (oil of mirbane) which has a somewhat similar odor and has been used for perfuming soap, polishing compounds, etc.

Description—A colorless, strongly refractive liquid, having an odor resembling that of bitter almond oil, and a burning aromatic taste. It is affected by light. Its specific gravity is 1.041 to 1.046. It boils at about 180°, solidifies at about $-56.5°$, and has a refractive index of 1.5440 to 1.5465 at 20°. Benzaldehyde is volatile with steam and on exposure to air it gradually oxidizes to benzoic acid. It reduces silver ammonium nitrate TS to metallic silver.

Solubility—Dissolves in about 350 volumes of water; miscible with alcohol, ether, chloroform, fixed and volatile oils.

Uses—Benzaldehyde is used in place of bitter almond oil for *flavoring* purposes; it is much safer than the latter because it contains no hydrocyanic acid. It is also extensively used in *perfumery* and in the manufacture of dyestuffs and many other organic compounds, such as aniline, acetanilid, mandelic acid, etc.

Compound Benzaldehyde Elixir NF—*Preparation*: Dissolve benzaldehyde (0.5 ml) and vanillin (1 Gm) in alcohol (50 ml); add syrup (400 ml), orange flower water (150 ml), and sufficient purified water, in several portions, shaking the mixture thoroughly after each addition, to make the product measure 1000 ml; then filter, if necessary, until the product is clear. *Alcohol Content:* From 3 to 5% of C_2H_5-OH. *Uses:* This is a useful vehicle for administering bromides and other salts, especially when a low alcoholic content is desired.

Calcium Cyclamate NF

Calcium Cyclohexanesulfamate; Sucaryl Calcium (*Abbott*)]

$$\left[\langle \rangle -NH-SO_2-OCaO-SO_2-NH-\langle \rangle \right] 2H_2O$$

Calcium Cyclamate [$C_{12}H_{24}CaN_2O_6S_2 . 2H_2O = 432.57$] contains 98.0–101.0% of $C_{12}H_{24}CaN_2O_6S_2$, calculated on the anhydrous basis.

Preparation—Cyclohexylamine is sulfonated with chlorosulfonic acid using carbon tetrachloride as the solvent. The crude cyclohexanesulfamic acid which precipitates is collected and purified by conversion to its pure soluble barium salt followed by treatment with the requisite amount of sulfuric acid to liberate the acid. Neutralization with calcium hydroxide or any other suitable basic calcium compound produces the calcium salt.

Description—White crystals or a white, crystalline, odorless powder. In dilute solution it is about 30 times as sweet as sucrose. Its solutions are neutral to litmus.

Solubility—1 Gm dissolves in about 4 ml of water, 1.5 ml of propylene glycol, and 60 ml of alcohol; practically insoluble in chloroform and ether.

Uses—Calcium Cyclamate is a synthetic, stable, *noncaloric sweetener* for use in the diet of diabetics and other patients who must restrict their intake of carbohydrates. It may be used in patients on a low-sodium diet. Cyclamate has been reported to soften the stool, induce photoallergic dermatitis, markedly reduce the intestinal absorption of lincomycin, and compete with other substances for binding sites on bovine plasma albumin. From 2 to 50% of cyclamate is metabolized to cyclohexylamine, the compound used to synthesize cyclamate. Cyclohexylamine has been shown to cause chromosomal breaks in human leukocytes *in vitro* and, when administered in massive doses directly into the bladder, to be carcinogenic. As a result of the latter observation, the Food and Drug Administration ruled in October, 1969, that cyclamates could no longer be used in foods and beverages. The pure liquid or solid forms of cyclamate are available as drugs, however, for use by diabetics and overweight persons.

Dose (unofficial)—1.25 ml (¼ teaspoonful) of a 15% solution (equivalent to about 2 teaspoonfuls of sugar).

Calcium Cyclamate and Calcium Saccharin Solution NF

[Compound Sucaryl Calcium Solution (*Abbott*)] contains 90.0–110.0% of the labeled amounts of $C_{12}H_{24}CaN_2O_6S_2.2H_2O$ (calcium cyclamate) and of $C_{14}H_8CaN_2O_6S_2.3\frac{1}{2}H_2O$ (calcium saccharin). The labeled concentration of calcium cyclamate is not less than 6.0% and is at least 10 times the labeled concentration of calcium saccharin. *Description:* Clear, colorless liquid having a sweet taste. A 1-ml portion of the Solution is equivalent in sweetening power to approximately 4.8 Gm (⅘ of a standard "cube") of sucrose. *Dosage Forms:* Solution NF: 6% (calcium cyclamate) and 0.6% (calcium saccharin).

Calcium Cyclamate and Calcium Saccharin Tablets NF [Compound Sucaryl Calcium Tablets (*Abbott*)] contain 90.0–110.0% of the labeled amounts of $C_{12}H_{24}CaN_2O_6S_2.2H_2O$ (calcium cyclamate) and of $C_{14}H_8CaN_2O_6S_2.3\frac{1}{2}H_2O$ (calcium saccharin). The labeled content of calcium cyclamate is at least 10 times the labeled content of calcium saccharin. *Description:* One Compound Calcium Cyclamate Tablet is equivalent in sweetening power to approximately 4 Gm (slightly less than 1 "tablet") of sucrose. *Dosage Forms:* Tablets NF: 50 mg (calcium cyclamate) and 5 mg (calcium saccharin).

Calcium Saccharin NF

[1,2-Benzisothiazolin-3-one 1,1-Dioxide Calcium Salt;   Calcium *o*-Benzosulfimide]

Calcium Saccharin $[C_{14}H_8CaN_2O_6S_2.3\frac{1}{2}H_2O = 467.49]$ contains 95.0–100.5% of $C_{14}H_8CaN_2O_6S_2$ (404.44), calculated on the anhydrous basis.

Preparation—Saccharin is reacted with a semimolar quantity of calcium hydroxide in aqueous medium and the resulting solution is concentrated to crystallization.

Description—White crystals or a white, crystalline powder. Odorless or has a faint aromatic odor, and an intensely sweet taste even in dilute solutions. In dilute solutions it is about 500 times as sweet as sucrose, hence 10 mg is equivalent in sweetening power to approximately 5 Gm (about 1 tablet) of sucrose.

Solubility—1 Gm dissolves in 1.5 ml of water.

Uses and Dose—See *Saccharin*.

Camphor Water—see RPS-13, page 436.

Caraway NF

[Carum; Caraway Seed; Caraway Fruit; Kümmel]

Caraway is the dried ripe fruit of *Carum Carvi* Linné (Fam. *Umbelliferæ*).

Constituents—This fruit contains about 5% of *volatile oil*, with a little *fixed oil* and other constituents.

Uses—It is used as a *flavor*. It has also been used empirically as a *carminative* and *stimulant*.

Caraway Oil NF [Oleum Cari] is a volatile oil distilled from the dried, ripe fruit of *Carum Carvi* Linné (Fam. *Umbelliferæ*). Caraway Oil yields not less than 50.0% (*v/v*) of $C_{10}H_{14}O$ (carvone). *Constituents:* The chief odoriferous component of the Oil is the ketone *d-carvone* [$C_{10}H_{14}O$], which is the optical isomer of the levorotatory variety occurring in Spearmint Oil. The remainder of the Oil consists mainly of the terpene *d-limonene* [$C_{10}H_{16}$], known in the earlier literature as "carvene." From 1 to 2% of a mixture of *dihydrocarvone* [$C_{10}H_{16}O$], *dihydrocarveol* [$C_{10}H_{17}OH$], and possibly *carveol* [$C_{10}H_{15}OH$] also is present, as well as traces of several other compounds. The *d*-carvone may be extracted from the Oil by means of its crystalline addition product with hydrogen sulfide; the ketone is then regenerated by means of alcoholic potassium hydroxide, and steam distilled. Carvone also forms a crystalline, water-soluble addition product with sodium sulfite, and this forms the basis of the official assay for the Oil. Sulfides are found in the aqueous distillate which comes over with the Oil, as are also several constituents which are ordinarily considered only to accompany destructive distillation products, as methyl alcohol, acetaldehyde, etc. *Description:* A colorless or pale yellow liquid, with the characteristic odor and taste of caraway. Specific gravity: 0.900 to 0.910. Angular rotation: from +70° to +80° in a 100-mm tube. Refractive index: 1.4840 to 1.4880 at 20°. 1 volume of the Oil is soluble in 8 volumes of 80% alcohol. *Uses:* This Oil, sometimes called *oil of kümmel*, is used in making caraway water and as a *flavor* and *carminative* in other pharmaceutical preparations.

Cardamom Seed NF

[Cardamomi Semen; Cardamom Fruit; Cardamom; Ceylon or Malabar Cardamom]

Cardamom Seed is the dried ripe seed of *Elettaria Cardamomum* (Linné) Maton (Fam. *Zingiberaceæ*). *Cardamom Seed should be recently removed from the capsule.*

Constituents—This valuable aromatic is imported from India. It contains a *volatile oil*, the yield of which is 1.3% from Malabar-Ceylon Seeds and 2.6% from Mysore-Ceylon Seeds. *Fixed oil* is present to the extent of 10%, also starch, mucilage, etc. Owing to the presence of the fixed oil, the Seeds are very difficult to powder alone, hence the practice in preparing compound powders containing Cardamom of mixing the other ingredients with it, so that they may absorb the oil. An oil of Cardamom which is a mixture of both volatile and fixed oils, is sometimes made by percolation with ether. This must not be confused with the official volatile oil.

Uses—It is used as a *flavor*. For many years it was empirically employed as an *aromatic*, *stomachic*, and *carminative*.

Cardamom Tincture, Compound—see page 1342.

Cherry Syrup—see page 1339.

Cinnamon NF

[Cinnamomum; Saigon Cinnamon; True Cinnamon; Saigon Cassia]

Cinnamon is the dried bark of *Cinnamomum loureirii* Nees (Fam. *Lauraceæ*).

Cinnamon contains, in each 100 Gm, not less than 2.5 ml of volatile oil.

Constituents—It owes its virtue to a volatile oil. There are also present tannin, mucilage, sugar, etc.

Uses—Cinnamon is used as a *flavoring agent*. Formerly, it was used empirically as a carminative.

Cinnamon Oil USP [Oleum Cinnamomi; Cassia Oil; Oil of Chinese Cinnamon] is the volatile oil distilled with steam from the leaves and twigs of *Cinnamomum cassia* (Nees) Nees ex Blume (Fam. *Lauraceæ*), rectified by distillation. It contains not less than 80.0%, by volume, of the total aldehydes of Cinnamon Oil. *Constituents:* There are two Cinnamon Oils in commerce: one procured from the Ceylon cinnamon (*Cinnamomum zeylanicum*), the other from the Chinese cinnamon (*Cinnamomum Cassia*). The latter (cassia oil) is now the only official one. The Chinese cinnamon is much the cheaper and more abundant of the two and will probably continue to be generally employed, notwithstanding the fact that the Ceylon product has the finer flavor. The value of cassia oil depends on the percentage of *cinnamaldehyde* (page 1337) which it contains. *Cinnamyl acetate* and *cinnamic acid* are also present, as well as small amounts of *phenylpropyl acetate* and the *methyl ether* of *orthocumaric aldehyde*, the latter a crystalline substance which deposits on aging. In the Ceylon Cinnamon Oil, cinnamaldehyde is the chief constituent, but *eugenol* is present to the extent of 4 to 10%. α-*Pinene, p-cymene, benzaldehyde, nonyl aldehyde, cuminaldehyde, hydrocinnamic aldehyde, l-linaloöl, caryophyllene,* and *phellandrene* have also been reported. Cinnamon leaf oil contains much eugenol and very little cinnamaldehyde, *safrol* and *benzaldehyde* being present as minor constituents. Moderate oxidation of the Oil yields the corresponding *cinnamic acid* [$C_9H_8O_2$], but more energetic oxidation yields *benzoic acid* [$C_7H_6O_2$]. Both the Ceylon and Chinese Cinnamon Oils have a slightly acid reaction. Ceylon Cinnamon Oil has a specific gravity between 1.023 and 1.040. It is readily soluble in alcohol, and contains between 65 and 75% of cinnamic aldehyde and from 4 to 8% of eugenol. When cooled to $-10°$ it remains clear, but at a lower temperature a solid portion separates from it. Chinese Cinnamon Oil (cassia oil) has similar properties, the marked difference being that its specific gravity is between 1.045 and 1.063, the aldehyde content being 80% or above, and that it contains no eugenol. The odor and taste are not quite so agreeable as that of the Ceylon variety. Since lead containers are usually used when the Oil is shipped from China, a test for *Heavy metals* is necessary. Ceylon Cinnamon Oil, when not very fresh, contains cinnamic acid in sufficient quantity to give a permanent cloudiness to cinnamon water made from it. *Description:* A yellowish or brownish liquid, becoming darker and thicker by age or exposure to the air, and having the characteristic odor and taste of cassia cinnamon. Specific gravity: 1.045 to 1.063. Angular rotation: from $+1°$ to $-1°$ in a 100-mm tube. Refractive index: 1.6020 to 1.6135 at 20°. *Solubility*—Soluble in an equal volume of alcohol, 2 volumes of 70% alcohol, and an equal volume of glacial acetic acid. *Uses:* Cinnamon Oil is used as a *flavor*. It was formerly employed empirically in a dose of 0.1 ml for flatulent colic.

Cinnamon Water—see page 1338.

Citric Acid Syrup—see page 1339.

Cocoa USP

Cacao USP XVI; Prepared Cocoa; Powdered Cocoa; Cocoa Powder; Medium Fat Cocoa]

Cocoa is a powder prepared from the roasted, cured kernels of the ripe seed of *Theobroma cacao* Linné (Fam. *Sterculiaceæ*).

Cocoa yields 10.0–22.0% of nonvolatile, ether-soluble extractive.

Preparation—The cocoa bean is dark colored as the result of a fermentation and roasting process which it undergoes. *Plain chocolate* consists of shelled cocoa beans (*cocoa nibs*) ground to a smooth paste which forms a hard cake when it cools because of the high fat content (50 to 58%).

Cocoa is the food prepared by pulverizing the residue remaining after part of the fat has been removed by expression from plain chocolate. Cocoa may be flavored by the addition of ground spice, ground vanilla bean, vanillin, ethylvanillin, coumarin, salt, and other flavors as long as they don't imitate the flavor of chocolate, milk, or butter. Three types of Cocoa are recognized depending on fat content: *breakfast cocoa* or *high fat cocoa* (22% minimum), *Cocoa* or *medium fat cocoa* (10 to 22%), and *low fat cocoa* (less than 10%).

Sweet chocolate is plain chocolate plus added sugar and flavor (usually vanilla).

Milk chocolate is a mixture of sweet chocolate and milk powder or other dairy product. Chocolate and the products described above contain the purines, theobromine and caffeine, and considerable quantities of fat (cocoa butter or theobroma oil), as well as protein and starch. These factors are lowered in sweet chocolate because of the large amount of added sugar (more than 50% of the final product).

Description—A weak reddish to purplish brown to moderate brown powder having a chocolate-like odor and taste, free from sweetness.

Uses—Cocoa is used as a food and pharmaceutically as a flavor in tablets, syrups, pill and tablet coatings, troches, etc.

Cocoa Syrup—see page 1339.

Coriander Oil USP

Coriander Oil is the volatile oil distilled with steam from the dried ripe fruit of *Coriandrum sativum* Linné (Fam. *Umbelliferae*).

Constituents—The alcohol *d-linaloöl* (formerly termed "*coriandrol*") is the chief constituent of this Oil, occurring in amounts varying from 60 to 80%. *l-Borneol* is also present; *acetic acid* occurs in the form of esters. Other oxygenated compounds reported to be present are *geraniol* and *decylic aldehyde*. *Pinene* is found in its *dl-α-, d-α-,* and *β*-modifications. Minute amounts of *p-cymene* and *dipentene* have been identified; both α- and γ-*terpinene* are also present. The presence of *terpinolene* and *phellandrene* is indicated, but has not been definitely established.

Description—A colorless or pale yellow liquid, having the characteristic odor and taste of coriander. Specific gravity: 0.863 to 0.875. Angular rotation: from $+8°$ to $+15°$ in a 100-mm tube. Refractive index: 1.4620 to 1.4720 at 20°.

Solubility—Soluble in 3 volumes of 70% alcohol.

Uses—The Oil is used as a flavoring agent. It was formerly employed empirically in a dose of 0.1 ml as *carminative* and *stomachic*.

Eriodictyon NF

[Consumptives' Weed; Mountain Balm; Yerba Santa]

Eriodictyon is the dried leaf of *Eriodictyon californicum* (Hooker et Arnott) Torrey (Fam. *Hydrophyllaceæ*).

Constituents—A bitter *resin, volatile oil, eriodictyonone* [$C_{16}H_{14}O_6$, also called *homoeriodictyol*], *fixed oil, tannin, gum,* etc.

Uses—Pharmaceutical necessity. It is used in the preparation of *Eriodictyon Fluidextract*.

Eriodictyon Fluidextract NF [Yerba Santa Fluidextract]—*Preparation:* Using Eriodictyon (in moderately coarse powder, 1000 Gm), prepare the Fluidextract by Process A (page 1591), using a mixture of 4 volumes of alcohol and 1 volume of water as the menstruum. Macerate the drug during 48 hours, then percolate at a moderate rate, and reserve the first 800 ml of percolate. *Alcohol Content:* From 57 to 62% of C₂H₅OH. *Uses:* A peculiar, aromatic *flavor,* used in syrups and elixirs, especially for masking the taste of bitter drugs like quinine. Because of its resinous character it requires an alkali to render it soluble in aqueous mixtures.

Eriodictyon Syrup, Aromatic—see page 1339.

Ethyl Acetate NF

$$CH_3COOC_2H_5$$

[Acetic Ether; Æther Vegetabilis; Æthylium Aceticum]

Ethyl Acetate contains 99.0–100.5% of $C_4H_8O_2$ (88.11).

Preparation—Ethyl Acetate is usually prepared by slowly mixing equal weights of alcohol and sulfuric acid, then adding a quantity of glacial acetic acid equivalent to that of the alcohol. After allowing the mixture to stand overnight it is slowly distilled. The distillate of crude ethyl acetate is washed with a small volume of cold dilute sodium carbonate solution to remove any free acetic acid that may have distilled over, and finally fractionally distilled to remove the water as well as ethyl ether which is usually formed also in this process.

Description—A transparent, colorless liquid with a fragrant and refreshing, slightly acetous odor, and a peculiar acetous, burning taste. Its specific gravity is 0.894 to 0.898. It distils between 76° and 77.5°.

Solubility—1 ml is soluble in about 10 ml of water; miscible with alcohol, acetone, ether, chloroform, fixed and volatile oils.

Uses—Ethyl Acetate is chiefly used as a *flavoring agent.* It is used industrially in artificial fruit essence, as a *solvent* for nitrocellulose varnishes and lacquers, in the manufacture of smokeless powder, and as a solvent in organic chemistry.

Ethyl Vanillin NF

[3-Ethoxy-4-hydroxybenzaldehyde; Bourbanal; Ethovan; Vanillal; Vanirome]

Ethyl Vanillin, dried over phosphorus pentoxide for 4 hours, contains 98.0–101.0% of $C_9H_{10}O_3$ (166.18).

Preparation—Ethyl Vanillin may be prepared by reacting *o*-ethoxyphenol with formaldehyde and *p*-nitrosodimethylaniline in the presence of aluminum and water.[1]

It may also be prepared by application of the Reimer-Tiemann reaction to *o*-ethoxyphenol.

Description—Fine white or slightly yellowish crystals. Odor and taste similar to vanillin. It is affected by light. Its solutions are acid to litmus. Melting range 76° to 78°.

Solubility—1 Gm dissolves in about 100 ml of water at 50°; freely soluble in alcohol, chloroform, ether, and solutions of fixed alkali hydroxides.

Uses—Ethyl Vanillin is used as a *flavor,* like vanillin, but is stronger. It also has value as a *preservative.*

Eucalyptus Oil NF

Eucalyptus Oil is the volatile oil distilled with steam from the fresh leaf of *Eucalyptus globulus* Labillardière or of some other species of *Eucalyptus* L'Heritier (Fam. *Myrtaceæ*). Eycalyptus Oil contains not less than 70.0% of $C_{10}H_{18}O$ (eucalyptol).

Constituents—The most important constituent of this Oil is *eucalyptol (cineol).* Other compounds present include *d-α-pinene, globulol, pinocarveol, pinocarvone,* and several aldehydes, *valeraldehyde, butyraldehyde, capronaldehyde,* and *d-myrtenal.*

Description—A colorless or pale yellow liquid, having a characteristic, aromatic, somewhat camphoraceous odor, and a pungent, spicy, cooling taste. Specific gravity: 0.905 to 0.925 at 25°. Refractive index: 1.4580 to 1.4700 at 20°. Soluble in 5 volumes of 70% alcohol.

Uses—Eucalyptus Oil is used as a *flavoring agent* and an *expectorant* in chronic bronchitis. It also has *bacteriostatic* properties. Some prescribers prefer *Eucalyptol* (see below) to the Oil.

Dose—(unofficial) **0.5 ml.**

Fennel Oil USP

[Oleum Fœniculi]

Fennel Oil is the volatile oil distilled with steam from the dried ripe fruit of *Fœniculum vulgare* Miller (Fam. *Umbelliferæ*).

Note—*If solid material has separated, carefully warm the Fennel Oil until it is completely liquefied, and mix it before using.*

Constituents—*Anethole* [$C_{10}H_{12}O$] is the chief constituent, occurring to the extent of 50 to 60%. The terpenes *d-α-pinene, camphene, α-phellandrene,* and *dipentene* are present in Galician oil; *methyl chavicol* may also be found. The ketone *d-fenchone* [$C_{10}H_{16}O$], an oily liquid with an intense camphoraceous odor and a bitter taste, is present in Galician oils, but absent in French and Macedonian oils. It is this compound which imparts a disagreeable taste to the oils in which it occurs. Much of the Oil in commerce is stated to be of Galician and Rumanian origin. Old samples of the Oil may contain *anisic aldehyde* and *anisic acid,* which are oxidation products of anethole, and traces of *acetaldehyde;* the latter substance can usually be detected by its odor. The quality of Fennel Oil is estimated by the official requirement for its congealing temperature.

Description—A colorless or pale yellow liquid, having the characteristic odor and taste of fennel. Specific gravity: 0.953 to 0.973. Angular rotation: from +12° to +24° in a 100-mm tube. Refractive index: 1.5280 to 1.5380 at 20°. The congealing temperature of Fennel Oil is not below 3°.

Solubility—Soluble in 8 volumes of 80% alcohol and in 1 volume of 90% alcohol.

Uses—Fennel Oil is used as a flavoring agent. It was formerly employed empirically in a dose of 0.1 ml as a *carminative.*

Glycyrrhiza USP

[Licorice Root; Liquorice Root; Sweetwood; Italian Juice Root; Spanish Juice Root]

Glycyrrhiza is the dried rhizome and roots of *Glycyrrhiza glabra* Linné, known in commerce as Spanish Licorice, or of *Glycyrrhiza glabra* Linné var. *glandulifera* Waldstein et Kitaibel, known in commerce as Russian Licorice, or of other varieties of *Glycyrrhiza glabra*

Linné, yielding a yellow and sweet wood (Fam. *Leguminosæ*).

Constituents—This well-known root contains 5 to 7% of the sweet principle *glycyrrhizin,* or *glycyrrhizic acid* which is 50 times as sweet as cane sugar. This was found by Roussin to exist in the root in combination with ammonia. The amount present in glycyrrhiza varies greatly and no official standard or assay has been adopted.

There is also present in Glycyrrhiza an oleoresinous substance to which its slight acridity is due. If alcohol or an alkali is used as a menstruum for the root and the preparation not treated to deprive it of acridity, it will have a disagreeable after-taste. For this reason the USP has adopted boiling water for its extraction in both the extract and the fluidextract.

Description—The USP provides descriptions of *Unground Spanish and Russian Glycyrrhizas, Histology,* and *Powdered Glycyrrhiza.*

Uses—Glycyrrhiza is valuable in pharmacy chiefly on account of the *sweet flavor.* It is one of the most efficient substances known for masking the taste of bitter substances, like quinine. Acids precipitate the glycyrrhizin and should not be added to mixtures in which Glycyrrhiza is intended to mask the disagreeable taste. Most of the imported licorice is used by tobacco manufacturers to flavor tobacco. It is also used in making candy.

Pure Glycyrrhiza Extract USP [Pure Licorice Root Extract]—*Preparation:* Moisten 1000 Gm of glycyrrhiza, in granular powder, with boiling water, transfer it to a percolator, and percolate with boiling water until the glycyrrhiza is exhausted. Add enough diluted ammonia solution to the percolate to impart a distinctly ammoniacal odor, then boil the liquid under normal atmospheric pressure until it is reduced to a volume of about 1500 ml. Filter the liquid, and immediately evaporate the filtrate until the residue has a pilular consistency. Pure Extract of Glycyrrhiza differs from the commercial extract in that it is almost completely soluble in aqueous mixtures. The large amount of filler used in the commercial extract to give it firmness renders it unfit to use as a substitute for the pure extract. *Description:* A black, pilular mass having a characteristic, sweet taste. *Uses:* A *flavoring agent.* One of the ingredients in *Aromatic Cascara Sagrada Fluidextract.*

Glycyrrhiza Fluidextract USP [Licorice Root Fluidextract; Liquid Extract of Liquorice]—*Preparation:* To 1000 Gm of coarsely ground glycyrrhiza add about 3000 ml of boiling water, mix, and allow to macerate in a suitable, covered percolator for 2 hours. Then allow the percolation to proceed at a rate of 1 to 3 ml per minute, gradually adding boiling water until the glycyrrhiza is exhausted. Add enough diluted ammonia solution to the percolate to impart a distinctly ammoniacal odor, then boil the liquid actively under normal atmospheric pressure until it is reduced to a volume of about 1500 ml. Filter the liquid, evaporate the filtrate on a steam bath until the residue measures 750 ml, cool, and gradually add 250 ml of alcohol and enough water to make the product measure 1000 ml, and mix. *Alcohol Content:* From 20 to 24%, by volume, of C_2H_5OH. *Uses:* A pleasant *flavor* for use in syrups and elixirs to be employed as vehicles and correctives.

Glycyrrhiza Elixir—see page 1341.

Glycyrrhiza Syrup—see page 1340.

Honey—see page 1378.

Hydriodic Acid Syrup—see page 1340.

Iso-Alcoholic Elixir—see page 1341.

Lavender Oil NF

[Lavender Flowers Oil]

Lavender Oil is the volatile oil distilled with steam from the fresh flowering tops of *Lavandula officinalis* Chaix ex Villars (*Lavandula vera* DeCandolle) (Fam. *Labiatæ*). It contains not less than 35.0% of esters calculated as $C_{12}H_{20}O_2$ (linalyl acetate).

Constituents—Lavender Oil is a product of considerable importance in perfumery. A fine grade is produced at Mitcham, England; in general, English oils command higher market prices than the French. *Linalyl acetate* is the chief constituent, occurring to the extent of 6 to 10% in English oils, though larger amounts have been reported by some investigators; up to 44% of this compound occurs in French oils. *Cineol* appears to be a normal constituent of the English oils, having been reported to occur to the extent of 23 to 32%; the French oil contains only traces. Free *linalool* is also an important compound, although present in only small amounts. Other constituents include the following: *amyl alcohol; d-borneol* (small, amount); *geraniol; lavandulol* ($C_{10}H_{18}O$); *nerol; acetic, butyric, valeric,* and *caproic acids* (combined as esters); traces of *d-pinene, limonene* (in English oils only), and the sesquiterpene *caryophyllene; ethyl n-amyl ketone;* an aldehyde (probably *valeric aldehyde*); and *coumarin.*

Spike Lavender oil is obtained by steam distillation from the wild plant *Lavandula latifolia* Vill. (*L. Spica* var. *B.* Linné). It is an inferior grade of lavender oil, having a somewhat camphoraceous odor, and is used largely as a soap perfume.

Description—This oil is a colorless or yellow liquid, having the characteristic odor and taste of lavender flowers. The Oil is soluble in 4 volumes of 70 per cent alcohol. Specific gravity: 0.875 to 0.888. Angular rotation: from −3° to −10° in a 100-mm tube. Refractive index: 1.4590 to 1.4700 at 20°.

Solubility—1 volume dissolves in 4 volumes of 70% alcohol.

Uses—The Oil is used primarily as a *perfume.* It was formerly used empirically in doses of 0.1 ml as an *aromatic* and *carminative.*

Lemon Oil USP

Lemon Oil is the volatile oil obtained by expression, without the aid of heat, from the fresh peel of the fruit of *Citrus Limon* (Linné) Burmann filius (Fam. *Rutaceæ*), with or without the previous separation of the pulp and the peel. The total aldehyde content, calculated as citral ($C_{10}H_{16}O$), is 2.2–3.8% for California-type Lemon Oil, and 3.0–5.5% for Italian-type Lemon Oil.

Note—Do not use Lemon Oil that has a terebinthine odor.

Constituents—From the standpoint of odor and flavor, the most noteworthy constituent is the aldehyde *citral,* which is present to the extent of about 4%. About 90% of *d-limonene* is present; small amounts of *l-α-pinene, β-pinene, camphene, β-phellandrene,* and *γ-terpinene* also occur. About 2% of a solid, nonvolatile substance called *citroptene, limettin,* or *lemon-camphor,* which is dissolved out from the peel, is also present. In addition, there are traces of several other compounds: *α-terpineol;* the *acetates* of *linalool* and *geraniol; citronellal, octyl* and *nonyl aldehydes;* the sesquiterpenes *bisabolene* and *cadinene;* and the ketone *methylheptenone.*

When fresh, the Oil has the fragrant odor of lemons. Because of the instability of the terpenes present, the

Oil readily undergoes deterioration by oxidation, acquiring a terebinthinate odor. This development may be retarded by the addition of 5% of alcohol and separation of any resulting sediment. Alternatively, 5% of either olive or cottonseed oil may be added, though possible incompatibilities may arise in the manufacture of certain preparations because of the presence of the fixed oil.

Italian Lemon Oil from Messina, a "hand-pressed" Oil, has always brought a premium price in the market, although the California Oil is now claimed to compare favorably with it in quality. The latter is produced with the aid of machines. (See page 505 for a discussion of the machine method of expression of the citrus oils.)

Originally, the Italian hand-pressed Oil was the only one which could meet the USP requirements. The Italian product contained 3.5 to 5.5% of citral, but the California Oil had a lower content of this constituent. The latter, however, contained certain unidentified substances which gave the product a distinctive flavor value lacked by the Italian Oil. The US Department of Agriculture recognized this fact and revised its standards, which were then adopted by the USP.

Lemon Oil produced by the machine method is much more yellow in color than the hand-pressed oil. The solid portion resulting from the process yields considerable *pectin*, which finds important uses in food products and in pharmacy.

Description—Lemon Oil is a pale yellow to deep yellow or greenish yellow liquid, with the characteristic odor and taste of the outer part of fresh lemon peel. Specific gravity: 0.849 to 0.855. Angular rotation: +57° to +65.6° in a 100-mm tube. Refractive index: 1.4738 to 1.4755 at 20°.

Solubility—Soluble in 3 volumes of alcohol, and miscible in all proportions with dehydrated alcohol, carbon disulfide, or glacial acetic acid.

Uses—As a *flavor* in the official preparations and in certain candies and foods.

Lemon Tincture USP

[Lemon Peel Tincture]

Lemon Tincture is prepared from lemon peel, which is the outer yellow rind of the fresh, ripe fruit of *Citrus Limon* (Linné) Burmann filius (Fam. *Rutaceæ*), by Process M (see page 1590), 500 Gm of the lemon peel being macerated in 900 ml of alcohol and the preparation being completed with alcohol to make the product measure 1000 ml. Use talc as the filtering medium.

The white portion of the rind must not be used, as the proportion of oil, which is found only in the yellow rind, is reduced and the bitter principle, *hesperidin*, introduced.

Alcohol Content—From 62 to 72% of C_2H_5OH.

Uses—This Tincture is used similarly to lemon oil as a *flavor*, its fineness of flavor being assured as it comes from the fresh fruit, and being an alcoholic solution it is more stable than the oil.

Methyl Salicylate USP

[Gaultheria Oil; Wintergreen Oil; Betula Oil; Sweet Birch Oil; Teaberry Oil; Artificial Wintergreen Oil; Synthetic Wintergreen Oil]

Methyl Salicylate [$C_6H_4(OH)COOCH_3 = 152.15$] is produced synthetically or is obtained by maceration and subsequent distillation with steam from the leaves of *Gaultheria procumbens* Linné (Fam. *Ericaceæ*) or from the bark of *Betula lenta* Linné (Fam. *Betulaceæ*). It contains 98.0–100.5% of $C_8H_8O_3$.

Note—Methyl Salicylate must be labeled to indicate whether it was made synthetically or distilled from either of the plants mentioned above.

In the USP, gaultheria oil, betula oil, and Methyl Salicylate are combined under the same title, as it is difficult to distinguish between them chemically, and practically the same tests apply to all. There are slight differences in the specific gravity and optical activity but these factors are not sufficiently characteristic to enable the detection of either in a mixture.

Preparation—Methyl Salicylate is found naturally in gaultheria and betula oils and in many other plants but the commercial product is usually synthetic, made by esterifying salicylic acid and with methyl alcohol in the presence of sulfuric acid and distilling.

Description—A colorless, yellowish, or reddish liquid, having the characteristic odor and taste of wintergreen. Specific gravity: synthetic, 1.180 to 1.185; from gaultheria or betula, 1.176 to 1.182. Refractive index: 1.5350 to 1.5380 at 20°. It boils between 219° and 224° with some decomposition. Both synthetic Methyl Salicylate and the oil from betula are optically inactive. Methyl Salicylate from gaultheria is slightly levorotatory, not exceeding −1.5° in a 100-mm tube.

Solubility—Slightly soluble in water; soluble in alcohol and glacial acetic acid.

Identification—1 drop mixed with 5 ml of water yields a deep violet color upon the addition of one drop of ferric chloride TS.

Incompatibilities—Methyl Salicylate is decomposed by *alkalies* to form methyl alcohol and a salicylate.

Uses—Methyl Salicylate is used as a pharmaceutical necessity and counterirritant. As a pharmaceutical necessity, it is used to flavor the official *Aromatic Cascara Sagrada Fluidextract*. As a *flavoring agent* it is equal in every respect to wintergreen oil or sweet birch oil. Care must be taken to select a product conforming to the official tests. As a counterirritant, it is applied to the skin in the form of a liniment; however, care should be exercised since salicylate is absorbed through the skin.

Caution—Because it smells like wintergreen candy, Methyl Salicylate is frequently ingested by children and has caused many fatalities. *Keep out of the reach of children*. See *Poison Control*, page 1947.

Dose—Topically, in lotions and solutions in **10** to **25**% concentration.

Myristica Oil NF

[Nutmeg Oil; East Indian Nutmeg Oil; West Indian Nutmeg Oil]

Myristica Oil is the volatile oil distilled with steam from the dried kernels of the ripe seed of *Myristica fragrans* Houttuyn (Fam. *Myristicaceæ*).

Constituents—The composition of the volatile oils of nutmeg and mace is practically identical, and no distinction is made between them in commerce. Nutmeg Oil is derived from the dried kernels of the seed; mace oil, from the dried exterior coating (arillode) of the thin, brown shell which contains the seed.

Nutmeg Oil contains 80% of *d-pinene* and *d-camphene*, 8% of *dipentene*, about 6% of the alcohols *d-borneol*, *geraniol*, *d-linaloöl*, and *terpineol*, 4% of *myristicin*, 0.6% of *safrol*, 0.3% of *myristic acid* free and as esters, 0.2% of *eugenol* and *isoeugenol* and traces of the alcohol *terpinenol-4*, a citral-like aldehyde, and several acids, all of which are present as esters. These include *formic*, *acetic, butyric,* and *octanoic* acids; also a monocarboxylic acid of the formula $C_{13}H_{18}O_3$.

Expressed Nutmeg Oil, known also as expressed Mace Oil, or *Nutmeg Butter,* is made by expressing nutmegs between hot plates, or macerating them in carbon disulfide, and distilling the liquid to get rid of the solvent. It has been reported as containing the glyceride of *myristic acid* [$C_{14}H_{28}O_2$]. It contains both fixed and volatile oil and is said to contain a toxic principle. *Nutmeg Butter* is an article of commerce in England, being used externally as a mild stimulant of pleasant odor, and in hair tonics.

Description—A colorless or pale yellow liquid, having the characteristic odor and taste of nutmeg. Specific gravity: East Indian Oil—0.880 to 0.910; West Indian Oil—0.854 to 0.880. Angular rotation: East Indian Oil—+8° to +30°; West Indian Oil—+25° to +45°. Both sets of values apply to determinations made in a 100-mm tube. Refractive index: East Indian Oil—1.4740 to 1.4880 at 20°; West Indian Oil—1.4690 to 1.4760 at 20°.

Solubility—Soluble in an equal volume of alcohol; the East Indian Oil is soluble in 3 volumes of 90% alcohol; the West Indian Oil is soluble in 4 volumes of 90% alcohol.

Uses—Myristica Oil is used primarily as a flavoring agent. It is used for this purpose in *Aromatic Ammonia Spirit* (see page 868). The Oil is also employed as a *flavor* in foods, certain alcoholic beverages, dentifrices, and tobacco; to some extent, it is also used in perfumery. It was formerly used as a *carminative* and *local stimulant* to the gastrointestinal tract in a dose of 0.03 ml. In overdoses it acts as a narcotic poison. This Oil is very difficult to keep and even if slightly terebinthinate is unfit for flavoring purposes.

Orange Oil USP

[Oleum Aurantii; Sweet Orange Oil]

Orange Oil is the volatile oil obtained by expression from the fresh peel of the ripe fruit of *Citrus sinensis* (Linné) Osbeck (Fam. *Rutaceæ*). The total aldehyde content, calculated as decanal, is 1.2–2.5%.

Note—Do not use Orange Oil that has a terebinthine odor.

Constituents—This Oil consists of *d-limonene* to the extent of at least 90%; in the remaining 5 to 10% are the odorous constituents, among which, in samples of American origin, are *n-decylic aldehyde, citral, d-linalool, n-nonyl alcohol,* and traces of *esters* of *formic, acetic, caprylic,* and *capric* acids.

In addition to most of these compounds, Italian-produced oil contains *d-terpineol, terpinolene, α-terpinene,* and *methyl anthranilate.*

Kept under the usual conditions Orange Oil is very prone to decompose, and rapidly acquires a terebinthine odor. It may be preserved by shaking it with one-eighth of its volume of distilled water, allowing it to separate, then removing the essential Oil, filtering rapidly if necessary, and mixing the filtered Oil with 95% alcohol in the proportion of 1 volume of the Oil to 7 volumes of alcohol.

It may also be preserved by adding 10% of its volume of olive oil. In this case, however, the presence of the fixed oil may result in incompatibilities in the filling of certain prescriptions or the manufacture of preparations.

Description—An intensely yellow, orange, or deep orange liquid, which possesses the characteristic odor and taste of the outer part of fresh sweet orange peel. Specific gravity: 0.842 to 0.846. Angular rotation: +94° to +99° in a 100-mm tube. Refractive index: 1.4720 to 1.4740.

Solubility—It is miscible with dehydrated alcohol and with carbon disulfide; it dissolves in an equal volume of glacial acetic acid.

Uses—It is used as a *flavoring agent* in elixirs and other preparations.

Orange Flower Oil NF

[Oleum Aurantii Floris; Neroli Oil]

Orange Flower Oil is the volatile oil distilled from the fresh flowers of *Citrus aurantium* Linné (Fam. *Rutaceæ*).

Constituents—The constituents of this Oil are *β-ocimene, l-α-pinene, l-camphene, dipentene, l-linalool, geraniol, farnesol, d-terpineol, phenylethyl alcohol, nerol, nerolidol, decylic aldehyde, jasmone, methyl anthranilate, indole, acetic esters of the alcohols* present, and traces of *esters of benzoic, phenylacetic,* and *palmitic acids.*

Description—A pale yellow, slightly fluorescent liquid, which becomes reddish brown on exposure to light and air. It has a distinctive, fragrant odor, similar to that of orange blossoms, and an aromatic, at first sweet, then somewhat bitter, taste. The Oil may become turbid or solid at low temperatures. Specific gravity: 0.863 to 0.880. Angular rotation: +1.5° to +9.1° in a 100-mm tube. It is miscible with an equal volume of alcohol and with about 2 volumes of 80% alcohol, the solution becoming cloudy on the further addition of alcohol of the same percentage. It is neutral to litmus paper. An alcoholic solution of the Oil has a *violet fluorescence.*

Uses—It is used as a flavor and perfume. Several less valuable varieties of the Oil are commercially known. These are designated as *Bigarade* (from the fresh flowers of the bitter orange, the ordinary neroli oil), *Portugal* (from the fresh flowers of sweet orange), and *Petit-grain* (from the leaves and young shoots of the bitter orange). The finest variety is known as *Petale.*

Orange Flower Water—see page 1338.

Bitter Orange Peel NF

[Aurantii Amari Cortex; Bitter Orange; Curaçao Orange Peel; Bigarade Orange]

Bitter Orange Peel is the dried rind of the unripe but fully grown fruit of *Citrus aurantium* Linné (Fam. *Rutaceæ*).

Constituents—The inner part of the peel from the bitter orange contains a volatile oil and the glycoside *hesperidin* [$C_{28}H_{34}O_{15}$]. This, upon hydrolysis in the presence of sulfuric acid, yields *hesperetin* [$C_{16}H_{14}O_6$], *rhamnose* [$C_6H_{12}O_5$] and D-glucose [$C_6H_{12}O_6$].

Uses—Bitter Orange Peel is employed as a *flavoring agent.* It has been used empirically in a dose of 0.6 to 2.6 Gm as a bitter tonic.

Sweet Orange Peel Tincture USP

[Tinctura Aurantii Dulcis]

Sweet Orange Peel Tincture is prepared from sweet orange peel, which is the outer rind of the non-artificially colored, fresh, ripe fruit of *Citrus sinensis* (Linné) Osbeck (Fam. *Rutaceæ*), by Process M (see page 1590). Macerate 500 Gm of the sweet orange peel (*Note—Exclude the inner, white portion of the rind*) in 900 ml of alcohol, and complete the preparation with alcohol to make the product measure 1000 ml. Use talc as the filtering medium.

The white portion of the rind must not be used, as the proportion of oil, which is only in the yellow rind, is reduced, and the bitter principle *hesperidin* is introduced.

Alcohol Content—From 62 to 72% of C_2H_5OH.

Uses—A *flavor*, used in syrups, elixirs, and emulsions. This Tincture was introduced to insure a delicate orange flavor direct from the fruit instead of depending upon orange oil which so frequently is terebinthinate and unfit for use. The Tincture keeps well.

Compound Orange Spirit USP

[Spiritus Aurantii Compositus]

Compound Orange Spirit contains, in each 100 ml, 25–30 ml of the mixed oils.

Orange Oil	200 ml
Lemon Oil	50 ml
Coriander Oil	20 ml
Anise Oil	5 ml
Alcohol, a sufficient quantity,	
To make	1000 ml

Mix the oils with sufficient alcohol to make the product measure 1000 ml.

Alcohol Content—From 65 to 70% of C_2H_5OH.

Uses—A *flavor* for elixirs. An alcoholic solution of this kind permits the uniform introduction of small proportions of oils and also preserves orange and lemon oils from rapid oxidation. These two oils should be bought in small quantities by the retail pharmacist, since the spirit is most satisfactorily made from oils taken from bottles not previously opened. This will insure that delicacy of flavor which should always be characteristic of elixirs.

Orange Syrup USP

[Syrupus Aurantii; Syrup of Orange Peel]

Orange Syrup contains, in each 100 ml, 450–550 mg of citric acid ($C_6H_8O_7$).

Sweet Orange Peel Tincture	50 ml
Citric Acid	5 Gm
Talc	15 Gm
Sucrose	820 Gm
Purified Water, a sufficient quantity,	
To make	1000 ml

Triturate the talc with the tincture and citric acid, and gradually add 400 ml of purified water. Then filter, returning the first portions of the filtrate until it becomes clear, and wash the mortar and filter with enough purified water to make the filtrate measure 450 ml. Dissolve the sucrose in this filtrate by agitation, without heating, and add enough purified water to make the product measure 1000 ml. Mix, and strain.

Note—*Do not use Orange Syrup that has a terebinthine odor or taste or shows other indications of deterioration.*

Alcohol Content—From 2 to 5% of C_2H_5OH.

Uses—A pleasant vehicle.

Peppermint USP

[Mentha Piperita; American Mint; Lamb Mint; Brandy Mint]

Peppermint consists of the dried leaf and flowering top of *Mentha piperita* Linné (Fam. *Labiatæ*).

Uses—Peppermint is the source of green color for Peppermint Spirit. The odor of fresh peppermint is due to the presence of about 2% of a volatile oil, much of which is lost on drying the leaves in air. Peppermint is widely cultivated both in the United States and Europe. It was formerly used as a carminative.

Peppermint Oil USP [Oleum Mentha Piperitæ] is the volatile oil distilled with steam from the fresh overground parts of the flowering plant of *Mentha piperita* Linné (Fam. *Labiatæ*), rectified by distillation and neither partially nor wholly dementholized. It yields not less than 5.0% of esters, calculated as menthyl acetate [$C_{12}H_{22}O_2$], and not less than 50.0% of total menthol [$C_{10}H_{20}O$], free and as esters. *Constituents:* This is one of the most important of the group of volatile oils. The chief constituent is *Menthol* (page 775) which occurs in the levorotatory form; its ester, *menthyl acetate*, is present in a much smaller amount. Other compounds which are present include the ketone *menthone, piperitone, α-pinene, l-limonene, phellandrene, cadinene, menthyl isovalerate, isovaleric aldehyde, acetaldehyde, menthofuran, cineol*, an unidentified *lactone* [$C_{10}H_{16}O_2$], and probably *amyl acetate*. *Dimethyl sulfide* and certain other constituents, objectionable from the standpoint of flavor, are largely removed by the steam distillation which is required for rectification. The higher the menthol content of an oil, usually the lower is its percentage of menthone. Peppermint Oil is distilled in large quantities in Michigan, Indiana, New York, and Ohio from cultivated plants. It is also produced in England, France, Italy, Russia, Spain, China, and Japan. The Japanese oil, which is distilled from *Mentha arvensis* var. *piperascens*, is the cheapest of all peppermint oils, but it is not suitable for all purposes because of the bitter taste which it possesses. Japanese peppermint oil contains 75 to 90% of menthol, of which 40 to 50% can be separated by freezing. Menthol from *Mentha arvensis* oil is now being obtained from Brazil, where the plant is extensively cultivated. The eleoptene or so-called "dementholized" oil has at times been substituted in whole or in part for the genuine Oil. It has been shown that the polariscope is an uncertain guide in determining the quality of a sample of Peppermint Oil. For this purpose it is necessary to assay one sample for its content of esters, calculated as menthyl acetate, and a second sample for its content of total menthol, free and as esters. *Description:* A colorless or pale yellow liquid, having a strong, penetrating odor of peppermint, and a pungent taste, followed by a sensation of cold when air is drawn into the mouth. Specific gravity: 0.896 to 0.908. Angular rotation: from $-18°$ to $-32°$ using a 100-mm tube. Refractive index: 1.4590 to 1.4650 at 20°. One volume dissolves in 3 volumes of 70 per cent alcohol. *Uses:* Peppermint Oil is a *flavoring agent, carminative, antiseptic*, and *local anesthetic*. It is also extensively used as a *flavor* in candy, chewing gum, etc.

Peppermint Spirit—see page 813.

Peppermint Water—see page 1338.

Phenylethyl Alcohol NF

[Phenethyl Alcohol; 2-Phenylethanol]

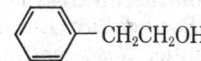

Phenylethyl Alcohol [$C_8H_{10}O$ = 122.17] occurs in a number of essential oils such as those of rose, neroli, hyacinth, carnation, and others. Because of its pleasant odor, it has long been employed as an ingredient in certain perfumes and flavors.

Preparation—Older methods include (1) reduction of ethyl phenylacetate with sodium and alcohol, and (2) catalytic (nickel) hydrogenation of phenylacetaldehyde. A more modern and very convenient method involves the chemical addition of ethylene oxide to phenyl magnesium bromide and hydrolysis of the resulting 2-phenylethoxy magnesium bromide.

Description—A colorless liquid with a rose-like odor and a sharp, burning taste. It solidifies at $-27°$, has a specific gravity between 1.017 and 1.020, and a refractive index at 20° between 1.5310 and 1.5340.

Solubility—1 Gm dissolves in 50 ml of water; very soluble in alcohol, fixed oils, glycerin, and propylene glycol; slightly soluble in mineral oil.

Identification—Oxidation with neutral potassium permanganate yields a filtrate containing potassium benzoate which responds to the identification tests for benzoate. Concentration of the filtrate and subsequent acidifications yields benzoic acid, identifiable through its melting point.

Uses—Phenylethyl Alcohol was introduced for use as an antibacterial agent in ophthalmic solutions but it is of limited effectiveness.

It is used in *flavors*, as a *soap perfume*, and in the preparation of synthetic oils of rose, lilac, hyacinth, jasmine, narcissus, neroli, lily of the valley, etc. It is also a valuable perfume fixative.

Pine Needle Oil NF

[Oleum Pini Pumilionis; Dwarf Pine Oil]

Pine Needle Oil is the volatile oil distilled with steam from the fresh leaf of *Pinus mugo* Turra and its variety *pumilio* (Haenke) Zenari (Fam. *Pinaceæ*). Pine Needle Oil contains 3.0–10.0%, by weight, of esters calculated as $C_{12}H_{20}O_2$ (bornyl acetate).

Constituents—This Oil is produced in the Austrian Tyrol; the yield of Oil from the needles and twigs is from 0.4 to 0.7%. It contains the terpenes *l-α-pinene*, *β-pinene*, *l-phellandrene*, *l-limonene*, *dipentene*, and possibly *sylvestrene* (though some authorities believe that the isomeric $Δ^3$-*carene*, not sylvestrene, is present), the ester *bornyl acetate*, and several unidentified terpene and sesquiterpene alcohols. The presence of the ketone *pumilone* [$C_8H_{14}O$] is now questioned.

Description—A colorless or yellowish liquid, having a pleasant, aromatic odor and a bitter, pungent taste. Specific gravity: 0.853 to 0.871 at 25°. Optical rotation: from −5° to −15.5° in a 100-mm tube at 25°. Refractive index: 1.4750 to 1.4800 at 20°.

Solubility—Dissolves in from 4.5 to 10 volumes of 90% alcohol, often with turbidity.

Uses—Pine Needle Oil is used chiefly as a *perfume and flavoring agent*. It is also employed as an inhalant in *bronchial infections*.

Raspberry Syrup—see page 1340.

Rose Oil NF

[Otto of Rose; Attar of Rose]

Rose Oil is the volatile oil distilled with steam from the fresh flowers of *Rosa gallica* Linné, *Rosa damascena* Miller, *Rosa alba* Linné, *Rosa centifolia* Linné, and varieties of these species (Fam. *Rosaceæ*).

Constituents—From the quantitative standpoint the chief components of Rose Oil are the alcohols *geraniol* [$C_{10}H_{18}O$] and *l-citronellol* [$C_{10}H_{20}O$]. The sesquiterpene alcohols *farnesol* and *nerol* occur to the extent of 1% and 5 to 10%, respectively. Together, the four alcohols constitute 70 to 75% of the Oil. *Phenylethyl alcohol*, which comprises 1% of the Oil, is an important odoriferous constituent. Other compounds present are *linaloöl*, *eugenol*, *nonyl aldehyde*, traces of *citral*, and two solid hydrocarbons of the paraffin series.

The finest grade of Oil is the Bulgarian, which is obtained from the damask Rose. French Rose Oil is prepared from *Rosa centifolia*, and differs from the Bul-

garian Oil in that it contains but little phenylethyl alcohol, which fact causes it to have an inferior quality of odor. Much of this constituent resides in the aqueous portion of the distillate because of the manner in which the operation is conducted in France. This produces, however, a Rose water of high grade.

The principal adulterants of Rose Oil are geraniol, citronellol, and phenylethyl alcohol, all of which raise the specific gravity and lower the melting point. In consequence of these peculiar factors paraffin wax and spermaceti are sometimes added as adulterants.

Description—Rose Oil is a colorless or yellow liquid, which has the characteristic odor and taste of Rose. At 25° this oil is a viscous liquid. Upon gradual cooling it changes to a translucent, crystalline mass, which may be easily liquefied by warming. Specific gravity: from 0.848 to 0.863 at 30° compared with water at 15°. Angular rotation: −1° to −4° in a 100-mm tube. Refractive index: from 1.4570 to 1.4630, at 30°. 1 ml of Rose Oil mixes with 1 ml of chloroform without turbidity. Upon the addition of 20 ml of 90% alcohol to this solution, the resulting liquid is neutral or acid to moistened litmus paper and deposits a crystalline residue within 5 minutes upon standing at 20°.

Uses—Rose Oil is principally used as a *perfume*. It is officially recognized for its use as an ingredient in Rose Water Ointment.

Stronger Rose Water NF

[Aqua Rosæ Fortior; Triple Rose Water]

Stronger Rose Water is a saturated solution of the odoriferous principles of the flowers of *Rosa centifolia* Linné (Fam. *Rosaceæ*), prepared by distilling the fresh flowers with water and separating the excess volatile oil from the clear, water portion of the distillate.

Note—Stronger Rose Water, diluted with an equal volume of purified water, may be supplied when *Rose Water* is required.

Description—Stronger Rose Water is a nearly colorless and clear liquid which possesses the pleasant odor and taste of fresh rose blossoms. It must be free from empyreuma, mustiness, and fungal growths.

Uses—This perfumed water is an ingredient in *Rose Water Ointment*. It is sometimes prepared extemporaneously from concentrates or from Rose Oil, but such water is not official and rarely compares favorably with the fresh distillate from Rose petals.

Rosemary Oil NF XII

Rosemary Oil is the volatile oil distilled with steam from the fresh flowering tops of *Rosmarinus officinalis* Linné (Fam. *Labiatæ*). It yields not less than 1.5% of esters calculated as bornyl acetate [$C_{12}H_{20}O_2$], and not less than 8% of total borneol [$C_{10}H_{18}O$], free and as esters.

History—Under the name *Aqua Reginæ Kungariæ* or *Hungary Water*, a spirit prepared from rosemary was very popular several centuries ago.

Constituents—The amount of esters, calculated as *bornyl acetate*, and of total *borneol*, respectively, varies somewhat with the geographic source of Rosemary Oil. Of the former, French oils contain from 1 to 4.9%; Spanish, 1 to 3.5%; English, 4.9%. Of the latter, French oils contain 8 to 11%; Spanish, 10 to 14%; English, 13.7%. *Cineol* is present to the extent of about 19 to 25%, depending on the source. The terpenes *d-* and *l-α-pinene*, *dipentene*, and *camphene*, and the ketone *camphor* also occur in this Oil, 17% of the latter constituent having been found in a sample of Sicilian origin.

Description—A colorless or pale yellow liquid, having the characteristic odor of rosemary, and a warm, camphoraceous taste. Specific gravity: 0.894 to 0.912. Optical rotation: from −5° to +10° in a 100-mm tube. Refractive index: 1.4640 to 1.4760 at 20°. The Oil is soluble in 1 volume of 90 per cent alcohol, by volume, but upon further dilution may become turbid.

Uses—Rosemary Oil is used as a *flavor* and *perfume*, chiefly in rubefacient liniments such as *Camphor and Soap Liniment*. The oil is rarely administered internally, but may be given in a dose of 0.1 ml.

Saccharin USP

[1,2-Benzisothiazolin-3-one 1,1-Dioxide;   Gluside;   o-Benzosulfimide]

Saccharin contains 98.0–101.0% of $C_7H_5NO_3S$ (183.19), calculated on the dried basis.

Preparation—Saccharin is made from toluene by the following series of reactions. First the toluene is reacted with chlorosulfonic acid to form the orthotoluenesulfonyl chloride. This is then reacted with ammonia to form the sulfonamide. The methyl group is then oxidized with dichromate yielding orthosulfamylbenzoic acid which, when heated, forms the cyclic imide, Saccharin.

Description—White crystals or a white crystalline powder. Odorless or has a faint aromatic odor. In dilute solution Saccharin is about 500 times as sweet as sucrose. Its solutions are acid to litmus. Melting range 226° to 230°.

Solubility—1 Gm dissolves in 290 ml of water and in 31 ml of alcohol, or in 25 ml of boiling water; slightly soluble in chloroform and in ether and is readily dissolved by dilute solution of ammonia, by solutions of alkali hydroxides, and by solutions of alkali carbonates with the evolution of CO_2; the hydrogen attached to the nitrogen is weakly acidic and reacts, therefore, with alkalies.

Uses—Saccharin is used as a sweetening agent in *Aromatic Cascara Sagrada Fluidextract*. It is an intensely sweet substance. A 60-mg portion of Saccharin is equivalent in sweetening power to approximately 30 Gm of sucrose. It is used as a *sweetening agent* in vehicles, canned foods, beverages, and in diets for diabetics to replace the sucrose. The relative sweetening power of Saccharin is increased by dilution.

Sarsaparilla Syrup, Compound—see RPS-13, page 445.

Sherry Wine—see page 1342.

Sodium Cyclamate NF

[Sodium Cyclohexanesulfamate; Sucaryl Sodium (*Abbott*)]

Sodium Cyclamate, dried at 105° for 1 hour, contains 98.0–101.0% of $C_6H_{12}NNaO_3S$ (201.22).

Preparation—The free acid is prepared as described above for the calcium salt. It is then neutralized with sodium hydroxide or any other suitable basic sodium compound.

Description—White crystals or as a white, crystalline powder. It is odorless. In dilute solutions it is about 30

times as sweet as sucrose. Its solutions are neutral to litmus.

Solubility—1 Gm dissolves in 5 ml of water and 24 ml of propylene glycol; practically insoluble in alcohol, chloroform, and ether.

Uses—Sodium cyclamate is a synthetic, stable, non-nutritive sweetening agent used as a substitute for sugar by diabetics and as a sweetening agent for oral forms of drugs. It is about 30 times as sweet as sugar. The limitations and untoward effects of Sodium Cyclamate are the same as those for *Calcium Cyclamate* (page 1324).

Sodium Cyclamate and Sodium Saccharin Solution NF [Sucaryl Sodium Solution (*Abbott*)] contains 90.0–110.0% of the labeled amounts of $C_6H_{12}NNaO_3S$ (sodium cyclamate) and of $C_7H_4NNaO_3S.2H_2O$ (sodium saccharin). The labeled concentration of sodium cyclamate is not less than 6.0%, and is at least 10 times the labeled concentration of sodium saccharin. *Description:* A clear, colorless liquid having a sweet taste. A 1-ml portion of the Solution is equivalent in sweetening power to approximately 4.8 Gm ($\frac{5}{6}$ of a standard "cube") of sucrose.

Sodium Cyclamate and Sodium Saccharin Tablets NF [Sucaryl Sodium Tablets (*Abbott*)] contain 90.0–110.0% of the labeled amounts of $C_6H_{12}NNaO_3S$ (sodium cyclamate) and of $C_7H_4NNaO_3S.2H_2O$ (sodium saccharin). The labeled content of sodium cyclamate is at least 10 times the labeled content of sodium saccharin. *Description:* 1 tablet is equivalent in sweetening power to approximately 4 Gm ($\frac{7}{10}$ of a standard "cube") of sucrose. *Dosage Forms:* Tablets NF: 50 mg (sodium cyclamate) and 5 mg (sodium saccharin).

Sodium Saccharin NF

[Sodium 1,2-Benzisothiazolin-3-one 1,1-Dioxide;   Saccharinum Sodicum Soluble Saccharin;   Soluble Gluside;   Sodium o-Benzosulfimide]

·2 H₂O

Sodium Saccharin [$C_7H_4NNaO_3S.2H_2O$ = 241.20] contains 98.0–101.0% of $C_7H_4NNaO_3S$ (205.17), calculated on the anhydrous basis.

Preparation—Saccharin is dissolved in an equimolar quantity of aqueous sodium hydroxide and the solution is concentrated to crystallization.

Description—White crystals or a white crystalline powder. Odorless or has a faint aromatic odor and an intensely sweet taste even in dilute solutions. It is about 500 times as sweet as sucrose, hence 15 mg is equivalent in sweetening power to approximately 7.5 Gm (about 1½ tablets) of sucrose. When in powdered form it usually contains about ⅓ the theoretical amount of water of hydration due to efflorescence.

Solubility—1 Gm dissolves in 1.5 ml of water and about 50 ml of alcohol.

Uses—Sodium Saccharin has the same uses as *Saccharin* but has the advantage of being more soluble in neutral solutions.

Application—**15 to 60 mg** as necessary.

Dosage Forms—Tablets NF: 15, 30, and 60 mg.

Sorbitol USP

[D-Glucitol; Sionin; Sorbit; D-Sorbitol; Sorbo (*Atlas*)]

Sorbitol contains 91.0–100.5% of $C_6H_{14}O_6$ (182.17), calculated on the anhydrous basis. It may contain small amounts of other polyhydric alcohols.

Preparation—Sorbitol is prepared commercially by the reduction (hydrogenation) of certain sugars such as glucose. One of the important processes is reported to consist of the following steps: (1) preparing the reaction slurry by dissolving the refined sugar in water and mixing with nickel catalyst; (2) continuous catalytic reduction of the sugar to sorbitol with hydrogen in a specially designed high pressure reactor system; (3) filtering off the spent catalyst from the solution and reprocessing it for return to the system; (4) purifying the solution by ion exchange and decolorizing it with activated carbon; and (5) concentrating the purified sorbitol solution in a vacuum evaporator and adjusting its concentration by adding demineralized water.

Description—White, hygroscopic powder, granules, or flakes, having a sweet taste. The usual form melts at about 96°.

Solubility—1 Gm dissolves in about 0.45 ml of water; slightly soluble in alcohol, methanol, and acetic acid.

Uses—Sorbitol is an *osmotic diuretic* given intravenously in 50% (*w/v*) solution to diminish edema, to lower cerebrospinal pressure, or to reduce intraocular pressure in glaucoma. It is also used as a laxative, sweetener, humectant, and, in 70% (*w/w*) solution, as a vehicle.

Dose (unofficial)—**50** to **100 ml** of a **50%** solution. As a *laxative*, **30** to **50 Gm** *orally*.

Sorbitol Solution USP is a water solution containing, in each 100.0 Gm, 69.0–71.0 Gm of total solids consisting essentially of D-sorbitol and a small amount of mannitol and other isomeric polyhydric alcohols. The content of D-sorbitol $[C_6H_8(OH)_6]$ in each 100.0 Gm is not less than 64 Gm. *Description:* A clear, colorless, syrupy liquid, having a sweet taste and no characteristic odor. It is neutral to litmus, and has a specific gravity of not less than 1.285 and a refractive index at 20° of 1.455 to 1.465. It is not to be injected.

Spearmint NF

[Mentha Viridis; Spearmint Leaves; Spearmint Herb; Mint]

Spearmint consists of the dried leaf and flowering top of *Mentha spicata* Linné (*Mentha viridis* Linné) (Common Spearmint) or of *Mentha cardiaca* Gerard ex Baker (Scotch Spearmint) (Fam. *Labiatæ*).

Uses—Spearmint is used as a flavoring agent. Fresh spearmint is used in preparing mint sauce, and also the well-known mint julep. The volatile oil is the only constituent of importance in this plant; the yield is from ½ to 1%.

Spearmint Oil NF [Oleum Menthæ Viridis] is the volatile oil distilled with steam from the fresh, over-ground parts of the flowering plant of *Mentha spicata* Linné (*Mentha viridis* Linné) (Common Spearmint) or of *Mentha cardiaca* Gerard ex Baker (Scotch Spearmint) (Fam. *Labiatæ*). It contains not less than 55.0%, by volume, of $C_{10}H_{14}O$ (carvone = 150.22). *Constituents:* The chief odoriferous constituent of this Oil is the ketone *l-carvone* $[C_{10}H_{14}O]$, which occurs to the extent of 35 to 66% in oils of American and German origin. Russian oil, however, contains only 5 to 10% of this substance. American oil also contains *dihydrocarveol acetate* $[CH_3COOC_{10}H_{17}]$, *l-limonene* $[C_{10}H_{16}]$, a small amount of *phellandrene* $[C_{10}H_{16}]$, and traces of *esters of valeric* and *caproic acids*. The *acetate of dihydrocuminic alcohol* $[CH_3-COOC_{10}H_{15}]$ is present in German oil. *Cineol* [eucalyptol,

$C_{10}H_{18}O$] occurs in both Russian and German oil. From 50 to 60% of the alcohol *l-linaloöl* $[C_{10}H_{18}O]$ is found in Russian oil. *Description:* A colorless, yellow, or greenish yellow liquid, having the characteristic odor and taste of spearmint. The Oil is soluble in 1 volume of 80% alcohol, but upon further dilution may become turbid. Specific gravity: 0.917 to 0.934. Angular rotation: from −48° to −59° in a 100-mm tube. Refractive index: 1.4840 to 1.4910 at 20°. *Uses:* Spearmint Oil is used primarily as a flavoring agent. It has also been used as a *carminative* in dose of 0.1 ml.

Sucrose USP

[Saccharum; Sugar; Cane Sugar; Beet Sugar]

Sucrose $[C_{12}H_{22}O_{11} = 342.30]$ is a sugar obtained from *Saccharum officinarum* Linné (Fam. *Gramineæ*), *Beta vulgaris* Linné (Fam. *Chenopodiaceæ*), and other sources. It contains no added substances.

For the structural formula, see page 470.

Preparation—Sucrose is prepared commercially from the sugar cane, beet root, and sorghum. Originally sugar cane was the only source; but at present the root of *Beta vulgaris* is largely used in Europe, and to an increasing degree in this country, for making sucrose.

The sugar cane is crushed and the juice amounting to about 80% is expressed with roller mills. The juice after "defecation" with lime and removal of excess of lime by carbonic acid gas, is run into vacuum pans for concentration and the saccharine juice is evaporated in this until it begins to crystallize. After the crystallization is complete, the warm mixture of crystals and syrup is run into centrifuges, in which the crystals of raw sugar are drained and dried. The syrup resulting as a by-product from raw sugar is known as *molasses*. Raw beet sugar is made by a similar process, but is more troublesome to purify than that made from sugar cane.

The refined sugar from either raw cane or beet sugar is prepared by dissolving the raw sugar in water, clarifying, filtering, and finally decolorizing the solution by passing it through bone-black filters. The water-white solution is finally evaporated under reduced pressure to the crystallizing point and then forced to crystallize in small granules which are collected and drained in a centrifuge.

For making troches, *confectioner's sugar* or *XXXX sugar*, a very finely powdered sugar, is now generally available. *Pulverized sugar*, as it is called, is not suitable for such a purpose. When sugar is crystallized in regular, large, monoclinic prisms, it is called *rock candy*, and has the specific gravity 1.606.

Ultramarine was formerly added by refiners to save the expense of using bone black. A sugar so blued is readily detected, for the syrup is slightly yellow, and a sediment is deposited.

When heated to 185° cane sugar melts into a viscid, colorless liquid, which on being suddenly cooled forms a transparent amorphous mass, called *barley sugar*. At a higher temperature between 204.4° and 215.5°, it loses 2 molecules of water, and is converted into a very thick, black liquid, called *caramel*, which is used largely for coloring aqueous or hydroalcoholic liquids and is official in the NF. At a still higher heat it yields combustible gases, carbonic acid, empyreumatic oil, and acetic acid, and there remains about one-fourth of its weight of charcoal, which burns without residue.

Cane and beet sugar are chemically and physically identical and therefore cannot be distinguished from each other in the refined product. Sucrose may be distinguished from dextrose by *Trommer's Test*, which consists in the use of copper sulfate and caustic potash.

If a solution of cane sugar is mixed with a solution of copper sulfate, and potassium hydroxide added in excess, a deep blue liquid is obtained, which on being heated deposits, after a time, a little red powder. A solution of dextrose, similarly treated, yields, by heat, a copious greenish precipitate, which rapidly changes to reddish orange, and eventually to dark red.

The sucrose content of *raw sugar*, syrups, and other preparations is usually evaluated polarimetrically.

Description—Colorless or white crystals, crystalline masses or blocks, or a white, crystalline powder. It is odorless, has a sweet taste, is stable in air, and its solutions are neutral to litmus. It melts with decomposition between 160° and 185°, and has a specific gravity of about 1.57. The specific rotation of Sucrose at 20° is not less than +65.9°. Unlike the other official sugars (dextrose, fructose, and lactose), Sucrose does not reduce Fehling's solution even in hot solutions. It also differs from these sugars in that it is darkened and charred by sulfuric acid in the cold. Sucrose is fermentable, and in dilute aqueous solutions it ferments into alcohol and eventually acetic acid, if carelessly exposed to warm, dustladen air.

Sucrose is hydrolyzed by dilute mineral acids, slowly in the cold, and rapidly on heating into one molecule each of dextrose and levulose. This process is technically known as "inversion" and the product is referred to as "invert sugar"; the term inversion being derived from the change, through the hydrolysis, in the optical rotation from dextro of the sucrose to levo of the hydrolyzed product. The enzyme *invertase* also hydrolyzes sucrose.

Solubility—1 Gm dissolves in 0.5 ml of water, 170 ml of alcohol, and in slightly more than 0.2 ml of boiling water; insoluble in chloroform and ether.

Uses—Sucrose is used principally as a pharmaceutical necessity for making syrups, confections, masses, troches, etc.

Intravenous administration of hypertonic solutions of Sucrose has been employed chiefly to initiate *osmotic diuresis*. Such a procedure is not completely safe and renal tubular damage may result, particularly in patients with existing renal pathology. Safer and more effective diuretics are available.

Syrup—see page 1340.

Tolu Balsam USP

[Tolu]

Tolu Balsam is a balsam obtained from *Myroxylon balsamum* (Linné) Harms (Fam. *Leguminosæ*).

Constituents—Tolu Balsam contains up to 80% of *resin*, about 7% of *volatile oil*, from 12 to 15% of free *cinnamic* and *benzoic acids*, and 0.05% of *vanillin*. The volatile oil is composed chiefly of *benzyl benzoate* and *benzyl cinnamate; ethyl benzoate, ethyl cinnamate*, a terpene called *tolene* (possibly identical with *phellandrene*), and the sesquiterpene alcohol *farnesol* have also been reported to be present.

Description—A brown or yellowish brown, plastic solid; transparent in thin layers and brittle when old, dried, or exposed to cold temperatures. It has a pleasant, aromatic odor resembling that of vanilla, and a mild, aromatic taste.

Solubility—Nearly insoluble in water and in solvent hexane; soluble in alcohol, chloroform, and ether, sometimes with slight residue or turbidity.

Uses—In the form of the syrup, it is used as a *vehicle* and stimulating *expectorant*. It is also an ingredient of *Compound Benzoin Tincture* (page 766).

Tolu Balsam Syrup NF [Syrup of Tolu; Tolu Syrup]—*Preparation:* Add tolu balsam tincture (50 ml, all at once) to magnesium carbonate (10 Gm) and sucrose (60 Gm) in a mortar, and mix intimately. Gradually add purified water (430 ml) with trituration, and filter. Dissolve the remainder of sucrose (760 Gm) in the clear filtrate with gentle heating, strain the syrup while warm, and add purified water (qs) through the strainer to make the product measure 1000 ml. Mix thoroughly. *Note:* Tolu Balsam Syrup may be made also in the following manner: Place the remaining sucrose (760 Gm) in a suitable percolator, the neck of which is nearly filled with loosely packed cotton, moistened after packing with a few drops of water. Pour the filtrate, obtained as directed in the formula above, upon the sucrose, and regulate the outflow to a steady drip of percolate. When all of the liquid has run through, return portions of the percolate, if necessary, to dissolve all of the sucrose. Then pass enough purified water through the cotton to make the product measure 1000 ml. Mix thoroughly. *Alcohol Content:* From 2 to 4% of C_2H_5OH. *Uses:* Used chiefly for its agreeable *flavor* in cough syrups. *Dose:* 10 ml (unofficial).

Tolu Balsam Tincture NF [Tolu Tincture]—*Preparation:* With tolu balsam (200 Gm), prepare a tincture by Process M (page 1590), using alcohol as the menstruum. *Alcohol Content:* From 77 to 83% of C_2H_5OH. *Uses:* A balsamic preparation employed as an addition to expectorant mixtures. Also used in the preparation of *Tolu Balsam Syrup. Dose:* 2 ml (unofficial).

Vanilla NF

[Vanilla Bean]

Vanilla is the cured, full-grown, unripe fruit of *Vanilla planifolia* Andrews, often known in commerce as Mexican or Bourbon Vanilla, or of *Vanilla tahitensis* J. W. Moore, known in commerce as Tahiti Vanilla (Fam. *Orchidaceæ*).

Vanilla yields not less than 12.0% of anhydrous extractive soluble in diluted alcohol.

Constituents—This valuable drug contains a trace of a volatile oil, fixed oil, 4% of resin, sugar, *vanillic acid*, and about 2.5% of *vanillin* (this page). The highest grade of Vanilla comes from Madagascar; considerable quantities of the drug are also produced in Mexico. In certain brands of vanilla-flavored ice cream tiny specks of Vanilla may be noted. Adulteration of Vanilla may be detected by determination of the lead number, which is a measure of the amount of Vanilla resins present. This procedure involves the precipitation of the lead soaps.

Assay—A sample is extracted with diluted alcohol, and the extract is evaporated to dryness. After suitable drying, the residue is weighed.

Uses—Vanilla is used as a flavor.
Note —Do not use Vanilla which has become brittle.

Vanilla Tincture NF [Extract of Vanilla]—*Preparation:* Add water (200 ml) to comminuted vanilla (cut into small pieces, 100 Gm) in a suitable covered container, and macerate during 12 hours, preferably in a warm place. Add alcohol (200 ml) to the mixture of vanilla and water, mix well, and macerate about 3 days. Transfer the mixture to a percolator containing sucrose (in coarse granules, 200 Gm), and drain; then pack the drug firmly, and percolate slowly, using diluted alcohol (qs) as the menstruum. If the percolator is packed with an evenly distributed mixture of the comminuted vanilla, sucrose, and clean, dry sand, the increased surface area permits more efficient percolation. This Tincture is unusual in that it is the only official one in which sucrose is specified as an ingredient. *Alcohol Content:* From 38 to 42% of C_2H_5OH. *Uses:* A *flavoring agent.* See the section on *Flavors*, beginning on page 1321.

Vanillin USP

[4-Hydroxy-3-methoxybenzaldehyde]

Vanillin contains 97.0–103.0% of $C_8H_8O_3$ (152.15), calculated on the dried basis.

Preparation—Vanillin may be obtained from vanilla, which contains from 2 to 3%. It is also found in many substances, and in the tissues of certain plants, in crude beet sugar, asparagus, and even in asafetida. The vanillin of commerce is made artificially, and, while chemically identical with the product obtained from the "vanilla bean," owing to the fact that the vanilla contains other odorous products, "flavoring preparations," made from vanillin, never equal in flavor the preparation in which vanilla alone is used. Vanillin is synthesized by oxidation processes from either coniferin or eugenol, by treating guaiacol with chloroform in the presence of an alkali, and by other methods. It is frequently adulterated. Some of the substances which have been detected are acetanilid, boric acid, benzoic acid, sugar, and coumarin.

Description—Fine, white to slightly yellow crystals, usually needlelike, having an odor and taste suggestive of vanilla. It is affected by light. Its solutions are acid to litmus. It melts between 81° and 83°.

Solubility—1 Gm dissolves in about 100 ml of water and about 20 ml of glycerin; 1 Gm dissolves in 20 ml of water at 80°; freely soluble in alcohol, chloroform, ether, and solutions of the fixed alkali hydroxides.

Identification—A cold saturated aqueous solution yields a blue color with ferric chloride. On heating, the color changes to brown, and on cooling a whitish precipitate forms. It is completely extracted from its ether solution by shaking with a saturated solution of sodium bisulfite, from which it is precipitated by acids. A cold solution of Vanillin yields a white precipitate with lead subacetate TS; this precipitate is sparingly soluble in hot water but soluble in acetic acid.

Incompatibilities—It combines with *glycerin*, forming a compound which is almost insoluble in alcohol. It is decomposed by *alkalies* and is slowly oxidized by the *air*.

Uses—Vanillin is used only as *flavor*. Solutions of it are sometimes sold as a synthetic substitute for vanilla for flavoring foods but it is inferior in flavor to the real Vanilla Extract.

Wild Cherry USP

[Prunus Virginiana; Wild Black Cherry Bark; Prunus Serotina]

Wild Cherry is the carefully dried stem bark of *Prunus serotina* Ehrhart (Fam. *Rosaceæ*), free of borke and preferably having been collected in autumn.

Constituents—Wild Cherry bark contains a glucoside of *d-mandelonitrile* [$C_6H_5.CHOH.CN$] known as *prunasin* (page 475), the enzyme *emulsin*, tannin, a bitter principle, starch, resin, etc. In the British Pharmacopœia and the English literature this drug has been termed "Virginian Prune"—a literal but incorrect translation of the older botanical name, *Prunus virginiana*.

Prunasin is hydrolyzed, in the presence of moisture and the enzyme emulsin, into glucose, benzaldehyde and HCN. This glycoside may also be obtained from *amygdalin*, the glycoside of bitter almond (page 475), by a special hydrolysis with yeast which removes only one glucose moiety from the gentiobiose in the amygdalin molecule. Thus amygdalin is prunasin β-linked to another glucose molecule.

Uses—Wild Cherry is used as a flavoring agent. It is an ingredient in *Wild Cherry Syrup*. As with bitter almond, contact with water, in the presence of emulsin, results in the production of benzaldehyde and hydrocyanic acid. All preparations of Wild Cherry should be made without heat, in order to avoid destruction of the enzyme which is responsible for the production of the free active principles.

Wild Cherry Syrup—see page 1340.

Water—see page 1338.

Water, Purified—see page 1338.

Other Flavoring Agents

Almond Oil, Bitter NF X [Volatile Bitter Almond Oil]—The volatile oil obtained from the dried kernel (deprived of fixed oil) of *Prunus Amygdalus* Batsch var. *amara* (DeCandolle) Focke (Fam. *Rosaceæ*), or from other kernels containing amygdalin, by maceration with water and subsequent distillation with steam. It contains not less than 80% of benzaldehyde, C_6H_5CHO, and the equivalent of 2–4% of hydrocyanic acid, HCN. It is produced as the result of the reaction of the enzyme emulsin on the glycoside amygdalin in the aqueous mixture of ground almond. *Caution:* not to be used for flavoring foods. The food flavor has had the HCN removed. *Uses:* Perfume for lotions, etc.

Anise NF IX [Anise Seed; European Aniseed; Sweet Cumin]—The dried ripe fruit of *Pimpinella Anisum* Linné. It contains about 1.75% of an official oxygenated volatile oil. *Uses:* Flavor, carminative. *Dose:* 0.5 Gm.

Bergamot Oil NF XI—The volatile oil obtained by expression from the rind of the fresh fruit of *Citrus Bergamia* Risso et Poiteau (Fam. *Rutaceae*). It yields not less than 36% of the esters calculated as linalyl acetate. *Uses:* A constituent of *Cologne Water* (formerly official as *Perfumed Spirit*), and is extensively used as a perfume in pomades, hair dressings, and toilet preparations for men.

Calcium Saccharate PhI [Calcium D-saccharate; Calcium D-glucarate]—*Purity:* the equivalent of 98.5–102% of $C_6H_8CaO_8.4H_2O$. The normal calcium salt of D-glucosaccharic acid. An odorless, tasteless, white, crystalline powder. It is very slightly soluble in alcohol and in cold water, slightly soluble in boiling water, and practically insoluble in ether and in chloroform. A saturated aqueous solution is neutral to litmus. *Uses:* A stabilizing agent in solutions of calcium gluconate for injection.

Cardamom Oil NF XII is the volatile oil distilled from the seed of *Elettaria Cardamomum* (Linné) Maton (Fam. *Zingiberaceæ*). *Constituents:* There is said to be little difference in composition between the Malabar-Ceylon and Mysore-Ceylon varieties of this Oil. These contain *d-α-terpineol* [$C_{10}H_{17}OH$] both free and as the acetate, from 5 to 10 per cent of *cineol* [$C_{10}H_{18}O$], and *limonene* [$C_{10}H_{16}$]. The Ceylon Oil, however, contains the alcohol 4-*terpineol* (4-carbomenthenol) [$C_{10}H_{17}OH$], the terpenes *terpinene* and *sabinene*, and *acetic* and *formic acids*, probably combined as esters. *Description:* A colorless or very pale yellow liquid and it possesses the aromatic, penetrating, and somewhat camphoraceous odor of Cardamom, and a persistently pungent, strongly aromatic taste. It is affected by light. Specific gravity: 0.917 to 0.947. Angular rotation: from +22° to +44° in a 100-mm tube. Refractive index: from 1.4630 to 1.4660 at 20°. *Solubility*—Miscible with alcohol; dissolves in 5 volumes of 70% alcohol. *Uses:* It is used as a *flavor*.

Compound Cardamom Spirit NF XII—*Preparation:* Mix cardamom oil (100 ml), orange oil (100 ml), cinnamon oil (10 ml), clove oil (5 ml), caraway oil (0.5 ml), and anethole (5 ml) with sufficient alcohol to make the product measure 1000 ml. *Alcohol Content:* From 68 to 74% of C_2H_5OH. *Uses:* A flavoring agent.

Ceylon Cinnamon NF XI, BP—The dried inner bark of the shoots of coppiced trees of *Cinnamomum zeylanicum* Nees (Fam. *Lauraceae*). It contains in each 100 Gm, not less than 0.5 ml of volatile oil. *Uses:* A *carminative* and *flavor*.

Cinnamaldehyde NF IX [Cinnamic aldehyde; Cinnamyl aldehyde] [$C_6H_5CH = CHCHO$]—A yellow, strongly refractive liquid having an odor resembling that of cinnamon oil, and a burning, aromatic taste. Its specific gravity is 1.048 to 1.052. It boils at about 250° with partial decomposition and solidifies at about −8°. It dissolves in about 700 parts of water and is miscible with alcohol, chloroform, ether, and with fixed or volatile oils. *Uses:* To replace natural oil as a flavor.

Civet [Civetta]—An odorous substance obtained from two animals of the genus *Viverra* which inhabit the East Indies. It is semisolid, unctuous, yellowish; becoming brown and thicker by exposure to air. It has a very strong, peculiar odor and a bitterish, acrid, and nauseous taste. It contains volatile oil, and resinous and other matters. *Uses:* In perfumery as a fixative.

Clove NF XI—The dried flower-bud of *Eugenia caryophyllus* (Sprengel) Bullock et Harrison (Fam. *Myrtaceae*). It contains, in each 100 Gm, not less than 16 ml of clove oil. *Uses:* An *aromatic* in doses of 0.25 Gm and as a condiment in foods.

Coriander NF XI, BP—The dried ripe fruit of *Coriandrum sativum* Linné (Fam. *Umbelliferæ*). It yields not less than 0.25 ml of volatile coriander oil from each 100 Gm. *Uses:* Seldom used alone, but is sometimes combined with other remedies, chiefly as a *flavor*. It is also used as a condiment and flavor in cooking.

Coumarin NF X [Cumarin; Tonka Bean Camphor] [$C_9H_6O_2$]—Colorless, prismatic crystals with a characteristic, fragrant odor and a bitter, aromatic, burning taste. It is slightly soluble in water but freely soluble in alcohol, ether, chloroform, and fixed oils. It melts at 68–70°C. *Uses:* A fixative, and perfume, having the odor known as new-mown hay.

Eucalyptol NF XII [Cineol; Cajeputol; $C_{10}H_{18}O$ (154.25)] is obtained from eucalyptus oil and from other sources. *Preparation:* Eucalyptol may be obtained from many volatile oils, and for that reason the name *cineol* is often preferred. It may be separated from the purified volatile oils by taking advantage of its property of forming crystals when subjected to a low temperature (its congealing temperature is not below 0°). *Description and Solubility:* A colorless, liquid, having a characteristic, aromatic, distinctly camphoraceous odor, and a pungent, cooling, spicy taste; specific gravity, 0.921 to 0.924 at 25°; boiling range, 174° to 177°. 1 volume is soluble in 5 volumes of 60% alcohol; miscible with alcohol, chloroform, ether, glacial acetic acid, and fixed or volatile oils; insoluble in water. *Uses:* Primarily as a *flavoring agent*. Locally it is employed for its *antiseptic* effect in inflammations of the nose and throat and in certain skin diseases. It is sometimes used by inhalation in bronchitis. *Dose:* 0.3 ml (unofficial).

Fennel NF X [Fennel Seed]—It is the dried ripe fruit of cultivated varieties of *Foeniculum vulgare* Miller (Fam. *Umbelliferæ*). It contains from 4–6% of an oxygenated volatile oil and 10% of a fixed oil. *Uses:* A flavor and carminative. *Dose: orally*, 1 Gm.

Ginger NF XII [Zingiber] is the dried rhizome of *Zingiber officianale* Roscoe (Fam. *Zingiberaceæ*), known in commerce as Jamaica Ginger, African Ginger, and Cochin Ginger. The outer cortical layers are often either partially or completely removed. *Constituents:* A pungent substance, *gingerol;* volatile oil (Jamaica Ginger, about 1%; African Ginger, 2 to 3%), containing the terpenes *d-camphene* and *β-phellandrene* and the sesquiterpene *zingiberene; citral, cineol,* and *borneol.* *Uses:* A flavoring agent. It was formerly employed in a dose of 600 mg as an intestinal stimulant and carminative in colic and in diarrhea. *Veterinary Dose: Horses* and *Cattle,* 8 to 30 Gm; *Sheep* and *Swine,* 4 to 8 Gm; *Dogs,* 300 mg to 1 Gm.

Ginger Oleoresin NF XII yields 18–35 ml of volatile ginger oil from each 100 Gm of Oleoresin. *Preparation:* Extract the oleoresin from ginger, in moderately coarse powder, by percolation, using either acetone, alcohol, or ether as the menstruum.

Glycyrrhiza Extract NF Licorice Root Extract; Licorice] is an extract prepared from the rhizome and roots of species of *Glycyrrhiza* Tournefort ex Linné (Fam. *Leguminosæ*). *Description:* Occurs as a brown powder or in flattened, cylindrical rolls or in masses. The rolls or masses have a glossy black color externally, and a brittle, sharp, smooth, conchoidal fracture. The Extract has a characteristic and sweet taste which is not more than very slightly acrid. *Uses:* A *flavoring agent*.

Glycyrrhizic Acid [Glycyrrhetinic Acid Glycoside; $C_{42}H_{62}O_{16}$] is a glycoside obtained from *Glycyrrhiza glabra*. Hydrolysis with acid splits it into 2 molecules of glucuronic acid and 1 molecule of glycyrrhetinic acid ($C_{30}H_{46}O_4$), the structure of which was elucidated in 1943 by Ruzicka, *et al.*[11, 12] *Description and Solubility:* Prisms or platelets with an intensely sweet taste. Freely soluble in hot water; soluble in hot dilute alcohol; insoluble in ether and dehydrated alcohol. *Uses:* A sweet flavor.

Isobutyl Alcohol [2-Methyl-1-propanol; Isopropylcarbinol] [$(CH_3)_2CHCH_2OH$]—Colorless, refractive liquid with an odor similar to amyl alcohol. Sp gr 0.806. Boils 108°C. Miscible with alcohol and ether. *Uses:* In manufacturing esters for fruit flavors.

Lavender [Lavandula]—The flowers of *Lavandula spica* (*Lavandula officinalis* or *Lavandula vera*). It contains a volatile oil with the principal constituent *l*-linalyl acetate. *Uses:* Perfume.

Lemon Peel USP XV, BP [Fresh Lemon Peel]—The outer yellow rind of the fresh ripe fruit of *Citrus Limon* (Linné) Burmann filius (Fam. *Rutaceæ*). It contains a volatile oil and hesperidin. *Uses:* As a flavor.

Lemon Peel, Dried BP—The dried, outer part of the pericarp of the ripe, or nearly ripe, fruit of *Citrus limon* Burm. It has an aromatic odor and an aromatic and bitter taste. It contains not less than 2.5% of volatile oil. *Uses:* As flavoring agent and as a bitter.

Myrcia Oil NF XI [Bay Oil; Oil of Bay]—The volatile oil distilled from the leaves of *Pimenta racemosa* (Miller) J. W. Moore (Fam. *Myrtaceæ*). It contains the phenolic compounds, eugenol and chavicol. *Uses:* In the preparation of Bay Rum as a *perfume*.

Myristica NF XI [Nutmeg]—The dried ripe seed of *Myristica fragrans* Houttuyn (Fam. *Myristicaceæ*), deprived of its seed-coat and arillode and with or without a thin coating of lime. *Uses:* Widely used flavor in foods; stimulating aromatic and *carminative*. Its dose is 0.5 Gm.

Orange Oil, Bitter NF X—The volatile oil obtained by expression from the fresh peel of the fruit of *Citrus Aurantium* Linné (Fam. *Rutaceæ*). It contains primarily *d*-limonene. It is a pale yellow liquid with a characteristic, aromatic odor of the Seville orange. If it has a terebinthinate odor it should not be dispensed. It is miscible with anhydrous alcohol and with about 4 volumes of alcohol. The refractive index is 1.4725–1.4755 at 20°. It differs little from *Orange Oil* (page 1330) except for the botanical source. *Uses:* As a flavor.

Orange Peel, Sweet USP XV—The fresh, outer rind of the non-artificially colored, ripe fruit of *Citrus sinensis* (Linné) Osbeck (Fam. *Rutaceæ*). The white, inner portion of the rind is to be excluded. It contains a volatile oil but no hesperidin, since the glycoside occurs in the white portion of the rind. *Uses:* As a flavor.

Orris NF X [Orris Root; Iris; Florentine Orris]—The peeled and dried rhizome of *Iris germanica* Linné, including its variety *florentina* Dykes (*Iris florentina* Linné), or of *Iris pallida* Lamarck (Fam. *Iridaceæ*). It contains about 0.1–0.2% of a volatile oil called orris butter, myristic acid, and the ketone irone. Irone provides the fragrant odor of orris. *Uses:* As a perfume.

Pimenta Oil NF XI [Pimento Oil; Allspice Oil]—The volatile oil distilled from the fruit of *Pimenta officinalis* Lindley (Fam. *Myrtaceæ*). *Uses:* As *carminative* and *stimulant* and also as a *condiment* in foods. The dose is 0.1 ml.

Sassafras NF XI—The dried bark of the root of *Sassafras albidum* (Nuttall) Nees (Fam. *Lauraceæ*). *Uses:* Used principally because of its high content of volatile oil which serves to disguise the taste of disagreeable substances. An infusion (*sassafras tea*) was formerly extensively used as a home remedy, particularly in the southern states. The dose is 10 Gm.

Sassafras Oil NF XI—The volatile oil distilled with steam from *Sassafras* (this page). *Uses:* As a flavor by confectioners, particularly in hard candies. Either the Oil or safrol is used as a *preservative* in mucilage and library paste, being far superior to methyl salicylate for this purpose. Since the Oil is *antiseptic*, it is sometimes employed in conjunction with other agents for local application in diseases of the nose and throat; safrol is also so used. The Oil may be given internally in a dose of 0.1 ml.

Diluting Agents

Diluting agents (vehicles) are indifferent substances which are used as solvents for active medicinals. They are of primary importance for diluting and flavoring drugs which are intended for oral administration, but a few such agents are specifically designed for diluting parenteral injections. The latter group is considered separately.

The expert selection of diluting agents has been an important factor in popularizing the "specialties" of manufacturing pharmacists. Since a large selection of diluting agents is available in a choice of colors and flavors, the practicing physician has an unusual opportunity to make his own prescriptions more acceptable to the patient. The best diluting agent is usually the best solvent for the drug. Water-soluble substances, for example, should be flavored and diluted with an aqueous agent and alcohol-soluble drugs with an alcoholic agent. Thus, the diluting agents presented herein are divided into three groups on the basis of their physical properties: aqueous, hydroalcoholic, and alcoholic.

Aqueous Diluting Agents

Aqueous diluting agents include aromatic waters, syrups, and mucilages. Aromatic waters are used as diluting agents for water-soluble substances and salts, but cannot mask the taste of very disagreeable drugs. Some of the more common flavored aqueous agents and the official forms of water are listed below.

Cinnamon Water NF XII

Cinnamon Water is a clear, saturated solution of cinnamon oil in purified water, prepared by one of the processes described under *Aromatic Waters* (page 1478).

Uses—A *flavored vehicle*.

Orange Flower Water NF

[Aqua Aurantii Florum;   Stronger Orange Flower Water;   Triple Orange Flower Water]

Orange Flower Water is a saturated solution of the odoriferous principles of the flowers of *Citrus aurantium* Linné (Fam. *Rutaceæ*), prepared by distilling the fresh flowers with water and separating the excess volatile oil from the clear, water portion of the distillate.

Description—This Water should be nearly colorless, clear, or only faintly opalescent; the odor should be that of the orange blossoms. It must be free from empyreuma, mustiness, and fungoid growths.

Uses—It is employed as a *vehicle flavor*, and *perfume* in syrups, elixirs, and solutions.

Peppermint Water NF

[Aqua Menthae Piperitae]

Peppermint Water is a clear, saturated solution of peppermint oil in purified water, prepared by one of the processes described under *Aromatic Waters* (page 1478).

Uses—A *carminative* and *flavored vehicle*. The dose is 15 ml.

Tolu Balsam Syrup—see page 1335.

Water USP

[Aqua]

Water is hydrogen monoxide ($H_2O = 18.02$).

Description and Properties—A clear, colorless liquid, practically odorless and tasteless.

Incompatibilities—When alcohol has been used as the solvent for many substances, such as free alkaloids, organic acids, volatile oils, or resins, the addition of Water or aqueous liquids to the *alcoholic solutions* will cause partial or complete precipitation of the dissolved substances. Water does not mix with *oils* unless an emulsifying agent is present.

Uses—In pharmacy, Water is used as a solvent (eg, in the extraction of vegetable drugs and in the manufacture of a few preparations used externally), as a precipitating agent, and for purifying certain water-insoluble products. Other more highly purified forms of water must be used in manufacturing finished pharmaceutical preparations and in filling prescriptions.

Purified Water USP

[Aqua Purificata]

Purified Water is water obtained by distillation or ion-exchange treatment.

Caution—Do not use Purified Water in preparations intended for parenteral administration. For such purposes, use Water for Injection, page 1343, *Bacteriostatic Water for Injection*, page 1343, *or Sterile Water for Injection*, page 1344.

Preparation—The Pharmacopeia does not describe a method for preparing Purified Water, simply establishing its degree of purity, but a former official process for Water, when prepared by distillation, is copied below. The pharmacist who is preparing sterile solutions, and must have freshly distilled water of exceptionally high grade, not only free from all bacterial or other microscopic growths but also free from the products of metabolic processes resulting from the growth of such organisms in the water, may advantageously follow this plan. The metabolic products are commonly spoken of as *pyrogens* and usually consist of complex organic compounds which cause febrile reactions if present in the solvent for parenteral medicinal substances. See *Pyrogens* (page 1524). Purified Water conforming to the USP requirements may also be prepared by one of the automatic stills described under *Distillation* (page

184) or by a deionizer such as that described in RPS-13 on page 704.

Distillation Process

Water	1000 Vol
To make	750 Vol

Distil the water from a suitable apparatus provided with a block-tin or glass condenser. Collect the first 100 volumes and reject this portion. Then collect 750 volumes and keep the distilled water in glass-stoppered bottles, which have been rinsed with steam or very hot distilled water immediately before being filled. The first 100 volumes are discarded to eliminate foreign volatile substances found in ordinary water and only 750 volumes are collected, since the residue in the still contains concentrated dissolved solids.

Description—A colorless, clear liquid, without odor or taste.

Uses—Purified Water must be used in the compounding of sterile pharmaceuticals applied externally, such as collyria and dermatological preparations, but these must be sterilized before use.

Whenever water is called for in official tests and assays, Purified Water must be used. Purified Water must also be used in compounding pharmaceutical preparations for internal (oral) administration.

Syrups Used as Diluting Agents

Syrups are useful as diluting agents for water-soluble drugs and act both as solvents and flavoring agents. The flavored syrups usually consist of simple syrup (85% sucrose in water) diluted with appropriate flavoring substances. *Glycyrrhiza Syrup* is an excellent vehicle for saline substances because of its colloidal properties, sweet flavor, and lingering taste of licorice. *Acacia Syrup* is valuable in disguising the taste of urea. Fruit syrups are especially effective for masking sour tastes. *Aromatic Eriodictyon Syrup* is the diluting agent of choice for masking the bitter taste of alkaloids.

Acacia Syrup NF

Acacia, granular or powdered	100 Gm
Sodium Benzoate	1 Gm
Vanilla Tincture	5 ml
Sucrose	800 Gm
Purified Water, a sufficient quantity,	
To make	1000 ml

Mix the acacia, sodium benzoate, and sucrose; then add 425 ml of purified water, and mix well. Heat the mixture on a steam bath until solution is completed. When cool, remove the scum, add the vanilla tincture and sufficient purified water to make the product measure 1000 ml, and strain if necessary.

Uses—Acacia Syrup is a *flavored vehicle* and *demulcent*.

Cherry Syrup USP

[Syrupus Cerasi]

Cherry Juice	475 ml
Sucrose	800 Gm
Alcohol	20 ml
Purified Water, a sufficient quantity,	
To make	1000 ml

Dissolve the sucrose in the cherry juice by heating on a steam bath, cool, and remove the foam and floating solids. Add the alcohol and sufficient purified water to make 1000 ml, and mix.

Alcohol Content—From 1 to 2% of C_2H_5OH.

Uses—Cherry Syrup is a pleasantly *flavored vehicle* which is particularly useful in masking the taste of saline drugs.

Citric Acid Syrup USP

[Syrup of Lemon]

Lemon Tincture	10 ml
Citric Acid, hydrous	10 Gm
Purified Water	10 ml
Syrup, a sufficient quantity,	
To make	1000 ml

Dissolve the citric acid in the purified water, and mix the solution with 950 ml of syrup. Add the tincture and enough syrup to make the product measure 1000 ml, and mix.

Note—Do not dispense Citric Acid Syrup if it has a terebinthine odor or taste or shows other indications of deterioration.

Alcohol Content—Less than 1% of C_2H_5OH.

Incompatibilities—This syrup has reactions characteristic of the acid which it contains. Hence it is not a suitable vehicle for alkaline ingredients such as *phenobarbital sodium* from which substance it precipitates phenobarbital.

Uses—It is employed solely as a pleasant vehicle, the formula making it possible to prepare extemporaneously and quickly a syrup having the flavor of lemon.

Cocoa Syrup USP

[Cacao Syrup; Chocolate-flavored Syrup; Chocolate Syrup]

Cocoa	180	Gm
Sucrose	600	Gm
Liquid Glucose	180	Gm
Glycerin	50	ml
Sodium Chloride	2	Gm
Vanillin	0.2	Gm
Sodium Benzoate	1	Gm
Purified Water, a sufficient quantity,		
To make	1000	ml

Mix the sucrose and the cocoa, and to this mixture gradually add a solution of the liquid glucose, glycerin, sodium chloride, vanillin, and sodium benzoate in 325 ml of hot purified water. Bring the entire mixture to a boil, and maintain at boiling temperature for 3 minutes. Allow to cool to room temperature, and add sufficient purified water to make the product measure 1000 ml.

Note—Cocoa containing not more than 12% of nonvolatile, ether-soluble extractive ("fat") yields a Syrup having a minimum tendency to separate. "Breakfast cocoa" contains over 22% of "fat."

Uses—Cocoa Syrup is employed as a pleasantly *flavored vehicle*. It should not be used for patients who dislike cocoa or are allergic to it.

Aromatic Eriodictyon Syrup NF

[Aromatic Yerba Santa Syrup; Syrupus Corrigens]

Eriodictyon Fluidextract	32	ml
Potassium Hydroxide Solution (1 in 20)	25	ml
Compound Cardamom Tincture	65	ml
Lemon Oil	0.5	ml
Clove Oil	1	ml
Alcohol	32	ml
Sucrose	800	Gm
Magnesium Carbonate	5	Gm
Purified Water, a sufficient quantity,		
To make	1000	ml

Dissolve the oils in the alcohol, add the fluidextract and the tincture, then the potassium hydroxide solution and 325 ml of purified water. Add the magnesium carbonate, shake the mixture, allow it to stand overnight, filter, and add sufficient purified water through the filter to make the liquid measure 500 ml. Pour this filtrate upon the sucrose contained in a bottle, and dissolve by placing the bottle in hot water, and agitating the contents frequently. Cool the solution, and add sufficient purified water to make the product measure 1000 ml.

Alcohol Content—From 6 to 8% of C_2H_5OH.

Incompatibilities—This syrup is alkaline in reaction due to the potassium hydroxide used in its manufacture. *Acids* are neutralized with usually a concurrent precipitation of the resins of the syrup. The tannin which it contains introduces the incompatibilities of that substance.

Uses—A pleasantly *flavored vehicle*, especially adapted to the administration of bitter substances like quinine.

Glycyrrhiza Syrup USP

[Licorice Syrup]

Glycyrrhiza Fluidextract........	250	ml
Fennel Oil......................	0.05	ml
Anise Oil......................	0.5	ml
Syrup, a sufficient quantity,		
To make....................	1000	ml

Add the oils to the fluidextract and agitate until mixed. Then add sufficient syrup to make the product measure 1000 ml, and mix.

Alcohol content—From 5 to 6% of C_2H_5OH.

Incompatibilities—The characteristic flavor of the syrup is destroyed by acids due to a precipitation of the glycyrrhizin.

Uses—A *flavored vehicle*, especially adapted to the administration of bitter or nauseous substances.

Raspberry Syrup USP

[Syrupus Rubi Idæi]

Raspberry Juice..................	475	ml
Sucrose........................	800	Gm
Alcohol........................	20	ml
Purified Water, a sufficient quantity,		
To make....................	1000	ml

Dissolve the sucrose in the raspberry juice by heating on a steam bath, cool, and remove the foam and floating solids. Add the alcohol and sufficient purified water to make 1000 ml, and mix.

Alcohol Content—From 1 to 2% of C_2H_5OH.

Incompatibilities—The juice from which this Syrup is prepared is required to contain not less than 1.5% of citric acid. The Syrup, therefore, has reactions characteristic of this acid, notably its incompatibility with alkaline substances.

Uses—Raspberry Syrup is a pleasantly *flavored vehicle* used to disguise the salty taste of saline medicaments.

Syrup USP

[Sirup; Simple Syrup]

Sucrose........................	850	Gm
Purified Water, a sufficient quantity,		
To make....................	1000	ml

Syrup may be prepared by using boiling water or, preferably, without heat, by the following process:

Place the sucrose in a suitable percolator the neck of which is nearly filled with loosely packed cotton moistened, after packing, with a few drops of water. Pour carefully about 450 ml of purified water upon the sucrose, and regulate the outflow to a steady drip of percolate. Return the percolate, if necessary, until all of the sucrose has dissolved. Then wash the inside of the percolator and the cotton with sufficient purified water to bring the volume of the percolate to 1000 ml, and mix.

Specific gravity—The specific gravity of Syrup is about 1.31.

Uses—Syrup is employed as a *sweet vehicle*, sweetening agent, excipient in pills, and as the basis for many flavored and medicated syrups.

Tragacanth Mucilage—see page 1348.

Wild Cherry Syrup USP

[Syrupus Pruni Virginianæ]

Wild Cherry, in coarse powder......	150	Gm
Glycerin........................	150	ml
Sucrose........................	675	Gm
Alcohol........................	20	ml
Water, a sufficient quantity,		
To make......................	1000	ml

Pack the wild cherry, previously moistened with 100 ml of water, in a cylindrical percolator, and add sufficient water to leave a layer of it above the powder. Macerate for 1 hour, then proceed with rapid percolation, using added water, until 400 ml of percolate is collected. Filter the percolate, if necessary, add the sucrose and dissolve it by agitation, then add the glycerin, the alcohol, and sufficient water to make the finished product measure 1000 ml. Strain the Syrup if necessary.

Wild Cherry Syrup may be made also in the following manner:

The sucrose may be dissolved by placing it in a second percolator as directed for preparing *Syrup*, above, and allowing the percolate from the wild cherry to flow through it and into a graduated vessel containing the glycerin and alcohol until the total volume measures 1000 ml.

It is to be noted that heat is avoided in the manufacture of this preparation, lest the enzyme emulsin be inactivated. If this should happen, the preparation would contain no free hydrocyanic acid, upon which its action as a sedative for coughs mainly depends. For a discussion of the chemistry involved, see *Wild Cherry* (page 1336).

Alcohol Content—From 1 to 2% of C_2H_5OH.

Uses—Wild Cherry Syrup is employed chiefly as a *flavored vehicle* for cough syrups.

Other Syrups Used As Diluting Agents

Hydriodic Acid Syrup NF XII contains, in each 100 ml, 1.3–1.5 Gm of HI (127.91). *Preparation:* Mix diluted hydriodic acid (140 ml) with purified water (550 ml), and dissolve dextrose (450 Gm) in this mixture by agitation. Add purified water (qs) to make the product measure 1000 ml, and filter. *Caution: Hydriodic Acid Syrup must not be dispensed if it contains free iodine, as evidence by a red coloration. Description:* A transparent, colorless, or not more than pale straw-colored, syrupy liquid; it is odorless and has a sweet, acidulous taste; specific gravity, about 1.18. Hydriodic acid is easily decomposed in simple aqueous solution (unless protected by hypophosphorous acid), free iodine being liberated, and if taken internally, when in this condition, it is irritating to the alimentary tract. The dextrose used in this syrup should be of the highest grade obtainable.

Incompatibilities: It possesses the reactions of the *acids* (page 1481) as well as those of the *Iodides* (see *Potassium Iodide*, page 872). Oxidizing agents liberate iodine; alkaloids may be precipitated. *Uses:* Traditionally employed as a *vehicle for expectorant* drugs. Its therapeutic properties are those of the iodides. *Dose: Usual,* 5 ml.

Mucilages Used as Diluting Agents

Mucilages are also suitable as diluting agents for water-soluble substances, and are especially useful for suspensions and emulsions.

The following mucilages used for this purpose are described in this chapter under *Emulsifying and Suspending Agents.*

Acacia Mucilage—see page 1347.

Hydroalcoholic Diluting Agents

Hydroalcoholic diluting agents are suitable for drugs soluble in either water or dilute alcohol. The most important agents in this group are the elixirs. These solutions contain approximately 25% alcohol. The numerous official *medicated* elixirs which have therapeutic activity in their own right are not included in this section. Listed below are the common, non-medicated elixirs which are used purely as diluting agents.

Aromatic Elixir USP

[Simple Elixir]

Compound Orange Spirit	12 ml
Syrup	375 ml
Talc	30 Gm
Alcohol,	
Purified Water, each, a sufficient quantity,	
To make	1000 ml

To the compound orange spirit add alcohol to make 250 ml. To this solution add the syrup in several portions, agitating vigorously after each addition, and afterwards add, in the same manner, the required quantity of purified water. Mix the talc with the liquid, and filter through a filter wetted with diluted alcohol, returning the filtrate until a clear liquid is obtained.

The compound spirit is used to ensure a uniform proportion of the several oils (ie, orange, lemon, coriander, and anise), in every lot of the elixir. The alcoholic solution also preserves the delicate flavor of the orange and lemon for a considerable time.

Alcohol Content—From 21 to 23% of C_2H_5OH.

Uses—A pleasantly *flavored vehicle*, employed in the preparation of many other elixirs. The chief objection to its extensive use is the high alcohol content (about 22%) which at times may counteract the effect of other medicines.

Cardamom Spirit, Compound—see page 1336.

Gentian Elixir—see RPS-13, page 448.

Gentian Elixir, Glycerinated—see RPS-13, page 448.

Iso-Alcoholic Elixir NF

[Iso-Elixir]

Low-Alcoholic Elixir
High-Alcoholic Elixir....of each a calculated volume

Mix the ingredients.

Low-Alcoholic Elixir

Compound Orange Spirit	10 ml
Alcohol	100 ml
Glycerin	200 ml
Sucrose	320 Gm
Purified Water, a sufficient quantity,	
To make	1000 ml

Mix the alcohol, glycerin, and 500 ml of purified water, add the compound orange spirit, agitate thoroughly from time to time, and let stand 24 hours. Filter this solvent mixture through a hard filter paper, returning, if necessary, the first portions of the filtrate until it passes through clear. Dissolve the sucrose in the filtrate by agitation or percolation, and add enough of the solvent mixture to make the product measure 1000 ml.

Alcohol Content—From 8 to 10% of C_2H_5OH.

High-Alcoholic Elixir

Compound Orange Spirit	4 ml
Saccharin	3 Gm
Glycerin	200 ml
Alcohol, a sufficient quantity,	
To make	1000 ml

Dissolve the compound orange spirit and the saccharin in 700 ml of alcohol, add the glycerin and sufficient alcohol to make the product measure 1000 ml, mix well, and filter.

Alcohol Content—From 73 to 78% of C_2H_5OH.

Adjustment of Iso-Alcoholic Elixir

Low-alcoholic elixir	High-alcoholic elixir	Suitable as vehicle for preparations of the following alcohol strengths
Undiluted	None	0–10%
4 volumes	1 volume	10–20%
3 volumes	1 volume	20–30%
2 volumes	1 volume	30–40%
1 volume	1 volume	40–50%
1 volume	2 volumes	50–60%
1 volume	3 volumes	60–70%
None	Undiluted	70% or more

Uses—Iso-Alcoholic Elixir is intended to serve as a general *vehicle* for various medicaments that require solvents of different alcohol strengths. When Iso-Alcoholic Elixir is specified in a prescription, the proportion of its two ingredients to be used is that which will produce a solution of the required alcohol strength.

The alcohol strength of the Iso-Alcoholic Elixir to be used with a single liquid galenical in a prescription is approximately the same as that of the galenical. When galenicals of different alcohol strengths are used in the same prescription, the Iso-Alcoholic Elixir to be used is to be of such alcohol strength as to secure the best solution possible. This will generally be found to be the average of the alcohol strengths of the several ingredients.

For nonextractive substances, the lowest alcohol strength of Iso-Alcoholic Elixir that will yield a perfect solution should be chosen.

Other Hydroalcoholic Diluting Agents

Red Aromatic Elixir NF XII [Red Elixir]—*Preparation:* Mix amaranth solution (14 ml) and aromatic elixir (986 ml). *Alcohol Content:* 20 to 23%. *Uses:* A red-colored, *flavored vehicle.*

Glycyrrhiza Elixir NF XII [Elixir Adjuvans; Licorice Elixir]—*Preparation:* Mix glycyrrhiza fluidextract (125 ml) and aromatic elixir (875 ml) and filter. *Alcohol Content:* 21 to 23%. *Uses:* A *flavored vehicle.*

Alcoholic Diluting Agents

Alcoholic diluting agents are useful for substances soluble in strong alcohols, or as flavors to be added in small quantities to syrups or elixirs. The alcohol content of these vehicles is approximately 50%. There are two types of alcoholic diluting agents: tinctures and spirits. Only nonmedicated tinctures and spirits are used as diluting agents.

Compound Cardamom Tincture NF

Cardamom Seed, in moderately coarse powder........................	**20 Gm**
Cinnamon, in fine powder..........	**25 Gm**
Caraway, in moderately coarse powder	**12 Gm**
To make......................	**1000 ml**

Prepare a tincture by Process M (page 1590), macerating the mixed powders in 750 ml of a mixture of 50 ml of glycerin and 950 ml of diluted alcohol, and completing the preparation by using first the remainder of the mixture of alcohol and glycerin prepared as directed above, and then diluted alcohol.

Note—Compound Cardamom Tincture may be colored with one or more colors (see page 1319).

Alcohol Content—From 43 to 47% of C_2H_5OH.

Uses—A useful vehicle because of its pleasant *flavor* and color.

Lemon Tincture—see page 1329.

Myrcia Spirit, Compound—see RPS-18, page 452.

Orange Spirit, Compound—see page 1331.

Orange Peel, Sweet, Tincture—see page 1330.

Peppermint Spirit—see page 813.

Wines

Wine, when generally referred to in pharmacy, means grape wine and is practically the only kind of wine used for pharmaceutical purposes.

There are three classes of wines: table wines, dessert wines, and appetizer wines. Members of these classes may be red or white, sweet or dry; they may be foreign or domestic.

Table wines are *Clarets, Burgundies, Rhines, Sauterne,* and a number of others; they contain up to 14% of alcohol by volume. Those consisting mostly of one grape are varietal wines, for example: *Zinfandel, Concord, Muscatel,* etc.

Dessert wines are more or less sweet wines which have been brandy strengthened principally for preservation; they contain up to 22% of alcohol by volume. Because of their higher alcohol content these wines are stable and usually better solvents and preservatives for most pharmaceutical purposes. The principal ones used in pharmacy are *Sherry, White* and *Red Port, Angelica,* and others. Most foreign ports come from Portugal and most imported sherry from Spain.

A third class of wines are appetizer or *aperitif wines,* the principal member being *Vermouth.* Sometimes sherry wine is included in this class although unlike vermouth it does not contain herbs or any natural flavoring materials. Most imported sweet vermouth comes from Italy and most of the imported dry vermouth from France.

Sparkling wines are still another special class of wines in which still dry table wines are made effervescent by re-fermenting them in closed containers or by artificially carbonating them. *Red* and *White Champagne,* and *Sparkling Burgundy* are some of these products.

There are many kinds of other wines not made from grapes but from apples, berries, and many other fruits, even some occasionally made from vegetables. All wines are made the same way in that they are fermented with cultivated yeast or spontaneously with natural yeast during which alcohol and CO_2 are produced principally, but many side reactions, producing numerous products, also occur during fermentation.

Wine as such, while not specifically rated as a medicine either as to its use as a vehicle or as an ingredient, has some therapeutic and physiological value in its action on digestive, respiratory, cardiovascular, and other reactions in the human body. While wine is not considered as a rich source of vitamins, Vitamins A, B, C, D, and others have definitely been identified in wines. As a food it furnishes nutriments such as sugars, amino compounds, and other body-building ingredients along with important minerals or inorganic elements essential for body building such as calcium, magnesium, manganese, iron, copper, zinc, cobalt, sodium, potassium, chlorides, and iodides.

The clarification or fining of wines is discussed in the chapter on *Separation* under *Clarification* and *Decoloration* (pages 387 and 389).

Other Alcoholic Diluting Agents

Sherry Wine NF XI [Vinum Xericum]—An alcoholic liquid obtained by fermenting the juice of sound, ripe grapes, fortifying with brandy, and containing *ca* 20% ethyl alcohol. *Uses:* Employed as a vehicle. It is more often used as a vehicle for medicinal ingredients than any other wine, not because it has more of any special medicinal value as such than other wines, but because of its general availability, its moderately high alcohol content, and its stability.

Diluting Agents for Injections

Injections are liquid preparations, usually solutions or suspensions of drugs, for parenteral use. Diluting agents used for these preparations are either aqueous or non-aqueous. The aqueous diluting agents include Water for Injection and electrolyte-containing solutions. Preparations of this type can be given by all parenteral routes of administration. The nonaqueous diluting agents are generally fatty oils of vegetable origin. These agents are used to dilute oil-soluble substances and to suspend water-soluble substances when it is desired to decrease the rate of absorption and, hence, prolong the duration of action of the latter substances. Preparations of this type are given intramuscularly. See *Injections*, page 1519.

Corn Oil USP

[Oleum Maydis;   Maize Oil]

Corn Oil is the refined fixed oil obtained from the embryo of *Zea Mays* Linné (Fam. *Gramineæ*).

Corn oil is expressed from the Indian corn embryos or germs which are separated from the grain in starch manufacture.

Description—A clear, light yellow, oily liquid with a faint characteristic odor and taste. Specific gravity: 0.914 to 0.921.

Solubility—It is slightly soluble in alcohol; miscible with ether, chloroform, benzene, and solvent hexane.

Uses—Its main official use is as a *solvent* and *vehicle for injections.* It is also used in making soaps, as an edible oil, and for burning. It is a semidrying oil and therefore unsuitable for lubricating or mixing with paint.

Cottonseed Oil USP

[Oleum Gossypii Seminis; Cotton Seed Oil; Cotton Oil]

Cottonseed Oil is the refined fixed oil obtained from the seed of cultivated plants of various varieties of *Gossypium hirsutum* Linné or of other species of *Gossypium* (Fam. *Malvaceæ*).

Preparation—This oil is made in the southern part of the United States on a very large scale where cotton is grown. The seeds contain about 15% of oil. The testæ of the seeds are first separated, and the kernels are exposed to powerful expression in hydraulic presses. The crude oil thus obtained has a bright red to blackish red color. It requires purification before it is suitable for medicinal or food purposes.

Description—A pale yellow, oily liquid with a bland taste. It is odorless or nearly so. Particles of solid fat may separate below 10° and the Oil solidifies at about 0° to −5°. Specific gravity 0.915 to 0.921.

Solubility—Slightly soluble in alcohol; miscible with ether, chloroform, solvent hexane, and carbon disulfide.

Identification—A red color develops when 2 ml of Cottonseed Oil is mixed in a test tube with 2 ml of a mixture of equal volumes of amyl alcohol and a solution of sulfur in carbon disulfide (1 in 100), and then heated for 5 to 15 minutes in a boiling saturated solution of sodium chloride (*Halphen test*).

Uses—Cottonseed Oil is official as a *solvent* and *vehicle for injections*. It is sometimes taken orally as a mild cathartic in the dose of 30 ml or more. Taken internally, digestible oils retard gastric secretion and motility and increase the caloric intake. Cottonseed Oil is also used in the manufacture of soaps, oleomargarine, lard substitutes, glycerin, lubricants, and cosmetics.

Ethyl Oleate

$$HC(CH_2)_7CH_3$$
$$\|$$
$$HC(CH_2)_7COOC_2H_5$$

Ethyl Oleate is $C_{20}H_{38}O_2$ (310.52).

Preparation—Among other ways, Ethyl Oleate may be prepared by reacting ethanol with oleoyl chloride in the presence of a suitable dehydrochlorinating agent.

Description—A pale yellow, oily liquid with a strong and disagreeable odor and taste. Its specific gravity is 0.869 to 0.874. It has an acid value not greater than 0.5 and an iodine value of 75 to 84. It is sterilized by heating at 150° for 1 hour. It has properties similar to those of almond and arachis oils, but is less viscous and more rapidly absorbed by the tissues. It boils between 205° and 208°.

Solubility—Insoluble in water; miscible with alcohol and ether.

Uses—Ethyl Oleate is used as a *vehicle* for certain parenteral preparations which are to be administered by the intramuscular route.

Peanut Oil USP

[Oleum Arachidis; Arachis Oil; Groundnut Oil; Nut Oil; Earth-Nut Oil]

Peanut Oil is the refined fixed oil obtained from the seed kernels of one or more of the cultivated varieties of *Arachis hypogæa* Linné (Fam. *Leguminosæ*).

Description—A colorless or pale yellow, oily liquid, with a characteristic nutty odor and a bland taste. Its specific gravity is between 0.912 and 0.920.

Solubility—Very slightly soluble in alcohol; miscible with ether, chloroform, and carbon disulfide.

Identification—The crystallized arachidic acid, obtained by saponification of Peanut Oil, precipitation with acid, and subsequent purification, melts between 73° and 76°.

Uses—Peanut Oil is used as a *solvent* in preparing oil solutions for injection (page 1523). It is a nondrying oil and is therefore not suitable for use in paints but it is used as a fuel for oil lamps and as a lubricant for machinery. It is also used for making liniments, ointments, plasters, and soaps, as a substitute for olive oil.

It is frequently used as an adulterant for olive oil.

Sesame Oil USP

[Teel Oil; Benne Oil; Gingili Oil]

Sesame Oil is the refined fixed oil obtained from the seed of one or more cultivated varieties of *Sesamum indicum* Linné (Fam. *Pedaliaceæ*).

Description—A pale yellow, almost odorless, oily liquid with a bland taste. Its specific gravity is between 0.916 and 0.921.

Solubility—Slightly soluble in alcohol; miscible with ether, chloroform, solvent hexane, and carbon disulfide.

Identification—1 ml of Sesame Oil shaken with a solution of 0.1 Gm of sucrose in 10 ml of hydrochloric acid for half a minute produces in the acid layer a pink color, which changes to red on standing (*difference from most other fixed oils*) (*Baudouin test*).

Uses—Sesame Oil is used as a *solvent* and *vehicle* in the official injections. It is used much like olive oil both medicinally and for food. It has replaced cottonseed oil in ammonia liniment, as it saponifies more readily and produces a more permanent and less sticky emulsion. It does not readily turn rancid. Sesame Oil is also used in the manufacture of cosmetics, iodized oil, liniments, ointments, and oleomargarine.

German sesame oil is a name given to *cameline oil*; from the seeds of *Camelina Sativa* (*Myagnim Sativum*).

Water for Injection USP

Water for Injection is water purified by distillation It contains no added substance.

Caution—Water for Injection is intended for use as a solvent for the preparation of parenteral solutions. For parenteral solutions that are prepared under aseptic conditions and are not sterilized by appropriate filtration or in the final container, first render the Water for Injection sterile and thereafter protect it from microbial contamination.

Description—It is a clear, colorless, odorless liquid.

Bacteriostatic Water for Injection USP

Bacteriostatic Water for Injection is sterile water for injection containing one or more suitable antimicrobial agents.

Note—Use Bacteriostatic Water for Injection with due regard for the compatibility of the antimicrobial agent or agents it contains with the particular medicinal substance that is to be dissolved or diluted.

Sterile Water for Injection USP

[Water for Parenterals]

Sterile Water for Injection is water for injection sterilized and suitably packaged. It contains no antimicrobial agent.

Description—It is a clear, colorless, odorless, liquid.

Uses—Sterile Water for Injection is used for the preparation of *all aqueous parenteral solutions*, including those used in *animal assays* (page 631). See page 1521 for a detailed discussion.

Emulsifying and Suspending Agents

An emulsion has been defined as an intimate mixture of two immiscible liquids by means of an intermediate agent. The intermediate agent which must be present in order to form a stable emulsion is called the emulsifying, dispersing, or stabilizing agent. Some of these agents are also used in suspensions. A suspension is defined as a dispersion containing finely divided insoluble material suspended in a liquid medium. The presence of a suspending agent is required to overcome agglomeration of the dispersed particles and to increase the viscosity of the medium so that the particles settle slowly. Emulsifying and suspending agents are used extensively in the formulation of elegant pharmaceutical preparations for oral, parenteral, and external use. For the theoretical and practical aspects of emulsions the interested reader is referred to pages 334 and 1492. More detailed information on the use of suspending agents is given on page 1475.

Acacia USP

[Gum Arabic]

Acacia is the dried gummy exudate from the stems and branches of *Acacia Senegal* (Linné) Willdenow or of other related African species of *Acacia* (Fam. *Leguminosæ*).

Constituents—This gum consists mostly of the calcium salt of *arabic acid* (arabin) which yields *arabinose*, galactose, and arabinosic acid when hydrolyzed.

Solubility—Acacia is insoluble in alcohol, but almost completely soluble in twice its weight of water at room temperature; the resulting solution flows readily and is acid to litmus.

Incompatibilities—*Alcohol or alcoholic solutions* precipitate acacia as a stringy mass when the alcohol amounts to more than about 35% of the total volume. Solution is effected by dilution with water. The mucilage is destroyed through precipitation of the acacia by *heavy metals*. *Borax* also causes a precipitation which is prevented by glycerin. Acacia contains calcium and, therefore, possesses the incompatibilities of this ion.

Acacia contains a *peroxidase* which acts as an oxidizing agent and produces colored derivatives of *aminopyrine, antipyrine, cresol, guaiacol, phenol, tannin, thymol, vanillin,* and other substances. Among the alkaloids affected are *atropine, apomorphine, cocaine, homatropine, hyoscyamine, morphine, physostigmine,* and *scopolamine.* A partial destruction of the alkaloid occurs in the reaction. Heating the solution of Acacia for a few minutes at 100° destroys the peroxidase and the color reactions are avoided.

Uses—In pharmacy, Acacia is extensively used as a *suspending agent* for the suspension of insoluble substances in water (pages 1496 and 1497), in the preparation of emulsions (pages 1492 to 1496), and for making pills and troches (page 1677).

It is used for its *demulcent* action in inflammations of the throat or stomach.

The osmotic pressure of solutions of Acacia is approximately the same as equal concentrations of serum protein. Consequently, Acacia has received clinical trial as a substitute for serum protein in the treatment of *shock* and as a *diuretic* in hypoproteinemic edema, but with the advent of dried stable preparations of human serum protein, the medicinal use of Acacia for this purpose has been condemned since it produces serious syndromes which may result in death.

Two kinds of powdered Acacia are used, one a coarse powder called *granulated*, the other *finely dusted*. The granulated dissolves more readily in water, because it has lost during desiccation only a part of its moisture, while in preparing "finely dusted" powder, the high heat used to dry it drives off nearly all water; also, the latter tends to form clumps as a result of hydration of some particles, which then retard access of water to others. When an especially pure solution is needed, selected tears of whole Acacia should be used. An exceptionally pure variety is *Flake Acacia*. It is prepared by dissolving clear and light-colored whole Acacia in water, filtering the solution, concentrating, and scaling the Acacia on glass plates. Its easy solubility and its absence of tendency to form "lumps" cause the coarse powder to be preferred for solutions, emulsions, etc.

Veterinary Dose—*Horses* and *Cattle*, 25 to 50 Gm; *Sheep* and *Swine*, 5 to 25 Gm; *Dogs*, 1 to 5 Gm; *Cats*, 500 mg to 2 Gm.

Agar USP

[Agar-Agar; Vegetable Gelatin; Gelosa; Chinese or Japanese Gelatin]

Agar is the dried, hydrophilic, colloidal substance extracted from *Gelidium cartilagineum* (Linné) Gaillon (Fam. *Gelidiaceæ*), *Gracilaria confervoides* (Linné) Greville (Fam. *Sphærococcaceæ*), and related red algæ (Class *Rhodophyceæ*).

Constituents—This substance consists chiefly of the calcium salt of a galactan mono(acid sulfate).

Solubility—Insoluble in cold water, but soluble in boiling water.

Incompatibilities—Like other gums, agar is dehydrated and precipitated from solution by *alcohol*. *Tannic acid* causes precipitation; *electrolytes* cause partial dehydration and decrease in viscosity of sols.

Uses—Agar is a common ingredient in a variety of proprietary cathartics, in some of which it may provide moisture and bulk to the intestinal contents. In mineral oil emulsions it acts as a stabilizer. The usual dose is 4 to 16 Gm once or twice a day.

It is also used in culture media for bacteriological work (see *Diagnostic Reagents*) and as a stabilizer in emulsions.

Veterinary Dose—*Dogs*, 2 to 8 Gm.

Alginic Acid

Alginic Acid (*Norgine*) is a colloidal, acidic substance (see *Sodium Alginate* below for composition) obtained from seaweeds such as fucus (bladderwrack). It is employed commercially as a sizing agent in the paper and textile industries and as a binder and emulsifying agent in a variety of applications.

Bentonite USP

[Wilhinite; Soap Clay; Mineral Soap]

Bentonite is a native, colloidal, hydrated aluminum silicate.

Occurrence—Bentonite is found in the Midwest of the United States and in Canada. Originally called *Taylorite* after its discoverer in Wyoming, its name was changed to Bentonite after its discovery in the Fort Benton formation of the Upper Cretaceous of Wyoming.

Description—A very fine, odorless powder with a slightly earthy taste, free from grit. The powder is nearly white, but may be pale buff or cream-colored.

The US Geological Survey has defined Bentonite as "a transported stratified clay formed by the alteration of volcanic ash shortly after deposition." Chemically it is $Al_2O_3.4SiO_2.H_2O$ plus other minerals as impurities. It consists of colloidal crystalline plates, of less than microscopic dimensions in thickness, and of colloidal dimensions in breadth. This fact accounts for the extreme swelling that occurs when it is placed in water, since the water penetrates between an infinite number of plates. A good specimen swells 12 to 14 times its volume.[7]

Solubility—Insoluble in water or acids, but it has the property of adsorbing large quantities of water, swelling to approximately twelve times its original volume, and forming highly viscous thixotropic suspensions or *gels*. This property makes it highly useful in pharmacy. Its gel-forming property is augmented by the addition of small amounts of alkaline substances, such as magnesium oxide. It does not swell in organic solvents.

Incompatibilities—*Acids* and *acid salts* decrease the water absorbing power of Bentonite and thus cause a breakdown of the magma. Suspensions are most stable at a pH above 7.

Uses—Bentonite is employed as a protective colloid for the stabilization of suspensions. It also has been used as an emulsifier for oil, as a base for plasters, ointments, and similar preparations.

Bentonite Magma USP—*Preparation:* Sprinkle bentonite (50 Gm), in portions, upon hot purified water (800 ml), allowing each portion to become thoroughly wetted without stirring. Allow it to stand with occasional stirring for 24 hours. Stir until a uniform magma is obtained, add purified water to make 1000 ml, and mix. The Magma may be prepared also by mechanical means such as by use of a blender, as follows: Place purified water (about 500 ml) in the blender, and while the machine is running, add bentonite (50 Gm). Add purified water to make up to about 1000 ml or up to the operating capacity of the blender. Blend the mixture for 5 to 10 minutes, add purified water to make 1000 ml, and mix. *Uses:* The Magma is employed as a *suspending agent* for insoluble medicaments.

Cetyl Alcohol—see page 1352.

Cholesterol USP

[Cholesterin]

Cholesterol [$C_{27}H_{46}O$ = 386.67] is cholest-5-en-3β-ol.

For the structural formula, see page 480.

It is a steroid alcohol widely distributed in the animal organism. In addition to cholesterol and its esters several closely related steroid alcohols have been found in the yolk of eggs, the brain, milk, fish oils, wool fat (10 to 20%), etc. These closely resemble it in properties. Cholesterol may therefore be regarded as a fundamental constituent of every animal cell and an essential nutrient factor. Fish oils constitute one of the principal sources of cholesterol. One of the more important methods of commercial production involves extracting the unsaponifiable matter in the spinal cord of cattle, with petroleum benzin.

Description—White or faintly yellow, almost odorless pearly leaflets or granules. It usually acquires a yellow to pale tan color on prolonged exposure to light or to elevated temperatures. Cholesterol melts between 147° and 150°, and has a specific rotation of −34° to −38° in dioxane.

Solubility—Insoluble in water; 1 Gm slowly dissolves in 100 ml of alcohol, and about 50 ml of dehydrated alcohol; soluble in acetone, hot alcohol, chloroform, dioxane, ether, ethyl acetate, solvent hexane, and vegetable oils.

Uses—It is largely used as an absorption base for the incorporation and emulsification of medicinal products in oils or fats. It is a *pharmaceutical necessity* for *Hydrophilic Petrolatum*. See the chapter on *Coarse Dispersions*, page 341.

Dioctyl Sodium Sulfosuccinate—see page 805.

Gelatin USP

[White Gelatin]

Gelatin is a product obtained by the partial hydrolysis of collagen derived from the skin, white connective tissue, and bones of animals. Gelatin derived from an acid-treated precursor is known as Type A and exhibits an isoelectric point between pH 7 and pH 9, while Gelatin derived from an alkali-treated precursor is known as Type B and exhibits an isoelectric point between pH 4.7 and pH 5.

Gelatin for use in the manufacture of capsules in which to dispense medicines, or for the coating of tablets, may be colored with a certified color, may contain not more than 0.15% of sulfur dioxide, and may have a lower gel strength than is specified in the USP monograph.

Regarding the special Gelatin for use in the preparation of emulsions, see under *Emulsions* (page 341).

Description—Sheets, flakes, or shreds, or a coarse to fine powder. It is faintly yellow or amber in color, the color varying in depth according to the particle size. It has a slight, characteristic bouillon-like odor. It is stable in air when dry, but is subject to microbic decomposition when moist or in solution.

Solubility—Insoluble in cold water, but swells and softens when immersed in it, gradually absorbing from 5 to 10 times its own weight of water; soluble in hot water, acetic acid, and hot mixtures of glycerin and water; insoluble in alcohol, chloroform, ether, and fixed and volatile oils.

Uses—Gelatin is largely used in pharmacy to coat pills and form capsules, and as a vehicle for suppositories. It is also recommended as an emulsifying agent. See *Pharmagel A* and *B* in the chapter on *Coarse Dispersions* (page 341), also *Suppositories* (page 1617), and *Absorbable Gelatin Sponge* (page 837).

Glyceryl Monostearate—see page 1353.

Lanolin, Anhydrous—see page 1351.

Methylcellulose USP

[Methocel (*Dow*); Cellothyl (*Warner-Chilcott*); Syncelose (*Blue Line*)]

Methylcellulose is a methyl ether of cellulose containing 27.5–31.5% of methoxy (OCH_3) groups, calculated on the dried basis. The viscosity of a solution containing 2 Gm of Methylcellulose in each 100 ml is 80–120% of that stated on the label for viscosity types of 100 centipoises or less; and 75–140% of that stated on the label for viscosity types higher than 100 centipoises.

Preparation—Methylcellulose is a cellulose ether made by the reaction of methyl chloride or of dimethyl sulfate on cellulose dissolved in sodium hydroxide. The cellulose methyl ether so formed is coagulated by the addition of some methanol or other suitable agent and centrifuged. Since cellulose has 3 hydroxyl groups per glucose residue, several methylcelluloses can be made, varying, among other properties, in their solubility and viscosity. Very useful types for pharmaceutical application contain from 1 to 2 methoxy radicals per glucose residue.

Description—A grayish white, fibrous powder or granules. Its aqueous suspensions are neutral to litmus. It is stable to alkalies and dilute acids.

Solubility—Insoluble in ether, alcohol, and in chloroform; soluble in glacial acetic acid, and in a mixture of equal parts of alcohol and chloroform; swells in water, producing a clear to opalescent, viscous colloidal solution; insoluble in hot water and saturated salt solutions. Salts of minerals acids and particularly of polybasic acids, phenols, and tannins coagulate solutions of Methylcellulose, but this can be prevented by the addition of alcohol or of glycol diacetate.

Uses—Methylcellulose is a synthetic substitute for the natural gums and has both pharmaceutic and therapeutic applications. Pharmaceutically, it is used as a *dispersing, thickening, emulsifying, sizing*, and *coating agent*. It finds use in nose drops, eye preparations, burn medications, cosmetics, tooth pastes, liquid dentrifices, hair fixatives, creams, and lotions. It functions as a protective colloid for many types of dispersed substances and is an effective stabilizer for oil-in-water emulsions.

Therapeutically, it is used as a *bulk laxative* in the treatment of *chronic constipation*. Taken with water, it forms a colloidal solution in the upper alimentary tract; this solution loses water in the colon, to form a gel which increases the bulk and softness of the stool. The gel is bland, demulcent, and non-irritating to the gastrointestinal tract. Once a normal stool develops, the dose should be reduced to a level adequate for maintenance of good function. Although Methylcellulose takes up water from the gastrointestinal tract quite readily, tablets of Methylcellulose have caused fecal impaction and intestinal obstruction when taken with a limited amount of water.

Dose (unofficial)—**1 to 4 Gm;** *usual*, **1 Gm** with water 1 to 4 times daily.

Veterinary Dose—*Dogs* and *Cats*, **1 to 4 Gm;** allow free access to drinking water.

Polyvinyl Alcohol

[Vinyl Alcohol Polymer]

$$\left[-CH_2CH-\atop\quad\;\;OH\right]_n$$

Preparation—Polyvinyl acetate is saponified in a methanol–methyl acetate solution in the presence of either mineral acid or alkali.

Description—White to cream-colored powder.
Solubility—Forms colloidal solutions with water.

Uses—Polyvinyl Alcohol is used as a *suspending agent* and *emulsifier*, either with or without the aid of a surfactant. It is also used for making water-soluble films.

Povidone NF

[Poly 1-(2-oxo-1-pyrrolidinyl)ethylene; 1-Vinyl-2-pyrrolidinone Polymer; Polyvinylpyrrolidone; PVP]

$$\left[-CH_2CH-\atop\quad N\diagdown_O\right]_n$$

Povidone is a synthetic polymer consisting of linear 1-vinyl-2-pyrrolidone groups, the degree of polymerization of which results in polymers of various molecular weights. It is produced commercially as a series of products having mean molecular weights ranging from about 10,000 to about 700,000. The viscosity of solutions containing 10% or less of Povidone is essentially the same as that of water; solutions more concentrated than 10% become more viscous, depending upon the concentration and the molecular weight of the polymer used. Povidone contains 12.0–13.0% of nitrogen, calculated on the dried basis.

Preparation—1,4-Butanediol is thermally dehydrogenated with the aid of copper to γ-butyrolactone which is then reacted with ammonia to form 2-pyrrolidinone. Addition of the latter to acetylene yields vinylpyrrolidinone (monomer) which is thermally polymerized in the presence of hydrogen peroxide and ammonia.

Description—A white to creamy white, odorless powder. It is hygroscopic.
Solubility—Soluble in water, alcohol, and chloroform; insoluble in ether.

Uses—Povidone is used as a *dispersing* and *suspending agent* in pharmaceutical preparations.

Propylene Glycol Monostearate

$$CH_3(CH_2)_{16}COOCH_2CHCH_3\atop\qquad\qquad\qquad\qquad\;\; OH$$

Propylene Glycol Monostearate $[C_{21}H_{42}O_3 = 342.57]$ is 2-hydroxypropyl stearate.

Preparation—Propylene Glycol Monostearate may be prepared by reacting propylene glycol with stearoyl chloride in a suitable dehydrochlorinating environment.

Description—Cream-colored wax. Melts at about 45°.
Solubility—Insoluble in cold, dispersible in hot, water; soluble in oils.

Uses—Propylene Glycol Monostearate is a *surfactant*. It is particularly useful as a dispersing agent for perfume oils or oil-soluble vitamins in water, and in cosmetic preparations.

Silicon Dioxide, Colloidal—See page 1372.

Sodium Alginate NF

[Algin; Manucol; Norgine; Kelgin (*Kelco*)]

Sodium Alginate is the purified carbohydrate product extracted from brown seaweeds by the use of dilute alkali. It consists chiefly of the sodium salt of alginic acid, a polyuronic acid composed of beta D-mannuronic acid residues linked so that the carboxyl group of each unit is free while the aldehyde group is shielded by a glycosidic linkage.

Description—A nearly odorless and tasteless, coarse of fine powder, yellowish white in color.

Solubility—Dissolves in water, forming a viscous, colloidal solution; insoluble in alcohol and in hydroalcoholic solutions in which the alcohol content is greater than about 30% by weight; insoluble in chloroform, ether, and acids when the pH of the resulting solution becomes lower than about 3.

Uses—Sodium Alginate is used as a thickening and emulsifying agent. This property makes it useful in the cosmetics, the rubber industry, and elsewhere. For example, it is used to impart smoothness and body to ice cream and to prevent formation of ice particles.

Sodium Carboxymethylcellulose—see page 803.

Sodium Lauryl Sulfate USP

[Irium; Duponol C (*Du Pont*); Gardinol WA (*Procter & Gamble*)]

Sodium Lauryl Sulfate is a mixture of sodium alkyl sulfates consisting chiefly of sodium lauryl sulfate $[CH_3(CH_2)_{10}CH_2OSO_3Na = 288.38]$. The combined content of sodium chloride and sodium sulfate is not more than 8%.

Preparation—The fatty acids of coconut oil, consisting chiefly of lauric acid, are catalytically hydrogenated to form the corresponding alcohols. The latter are then esterified with sulfuric acid (sulfated) and the resulting mixture of alkyl bisulfates (alkylsulfuric acids) is converted into a mixture of the sodium salts by reacting with alkali under controlled conditions of pH.

Description—Small, white or light yellow crystals having a slight, characteristic odor.

Solubility—1 Gm dissolves in 10 ml of water, forming an opalescent solution.

Incompatibilities—Sodium Lauryl Sulfate is compatible with soaps and alkalies, dilute acids, and calcium and magnesium ions. It reacts with *cationic surface-active agents* to cause precipitation and loss of value.

Uses—This anionic surface-active agent is employed as an emulsifying, detergent, and wetting agent in ointments, tooth powders, and other pharmaceutical preparations, and in the metal, paper, and pigment industries. See the chapters on *Medicated Applications* (page 1594) and *Coarse Dispersions* (page 330).

Note—Sodium Lauryl Sulfate conforming to the standards of the USP monograph is designed for external use only.

Sorbitan Monooleate

Sorbitan Monooleate is $C_{24}H_{44}O_6$ (428.61).

Preparation—Sorbitol (page 1333) is dehydrated to form a *hexitan* (cyclic hexitol anhydride) which is then esterified with an equimolar portion of oleic acid. See discussion under *Polysorbate 80*, page 1355.

Description—Amber viscous liquid.
Solubility—Dispersible in water; soluble in mineral oil.

Uses—Sorbitan Monooleate is a nonionic *surfactant* which is used as an emulsifying agent in the preparation of certain water-in-oil emulsions.

Stearic Acid—see page 1353.

Stearyl Alcohol USP

Stearyl Alcohol contains not less than 90.0% of stearyl alcohol $[C_{18}H_{38}O = 270.50]$, the remainder consisting chiefly of cetyl alcohol $[C_{16}H_{34}O = 242.45]$.

Preparation—Among other ways, stearyl alcohol may be prepared through the reducing action of lithium aluminum hydride on ethyl stearate.

Description—Stearyl alcohol occurs as white, unctuous flakes or granules having a faint, characteristic odor and a bland taste. It melts between 55° and 60°.

Solubility—Insoluble in water; soluble in alcohol, chloroform, ether, and vegetable oils.

Uses—Stearyl Alcohol is a surface-active agent used for emulsifying. It *stabilizes emulsions* and increases their ability to retain larger quantities of water. See *Hydrophilic Ointment* (page 1353), *Hydrophilic Petrolatum* (page 1352), and the chapters on *Coarse Dispersions* (page 339) and *Ointments* (page 1601).

Sterculia Gum—see page 803.

Tragacanth USP

[Gum Tragacanth; Hog Gum; Goat's Thorn]

Tragacanth is the dried gummy exudation from *Astragalus gummifer* Labillardière, or other Asiatic species of *Astragalus* (Fam. *Leguminosæ*).

Constituents—This gum consists of 60 to 70% bassorin, and 30 to 40% soluble gum (*tragacanthin*). The bassorin swells in the presence of water to form a gel and tragacanthin forms a colloidal solution. Bassorin, consisting of complex methoxylated acids, resembles pectin. Tragacanthin yields glucuronic acid and arbinose when hydrolyzed.

Description—Introduced into water, Tragacanth absorbs a certain proportion of that liquid, swells very much, and forms a soft adhesive paste, but does not dissolve. If agitated with an excess of water, this paste forms a uniform mixture; but in the course of one or two days the greater part separates, and is deposited, leaving a portion dissolved in the supernatant fluid. The finest mucilage is obtained from the whole gum or *flake* tragacanth. Several days should be allowed for obtaining a uniform mucilage of the maximum gel strength. Tragacanth is wholly insoluble in alcohol. A common adulterant is *Karaya Gum*, and the Pharmacopeia has introduced tests to detect its presence.

Uses—Tragacanth, in the form of a glycerite, affords an excellent *pill excipient;* the powder itself is often used to stiffen a pill mass and render it adhesive. It is also used as a *suspending agent* in lotions, mixtures, and in extemporaneous preparations and prescriptions. It is used with emulsifying agents largely to increase consistency and retard creaming. It is sometimes used as a *demulcent* in sore throat.

The jelly-like product formed when the gum is allowed to swell in water serves as a basis for pharmaceutical jellies, eg, *Ephedrine Sulfate Jelly*.

Other Emulsifying and Suspending Agents

Acacia Mucilage NF XII [Mucilage of Gum Arabic]—*Preparation:* Place acacia (in small fragments, 350 Gm) in a graduated bottle having a wide mouth and a capacity not greatly exceeding 1000 ml, wash the drug with cold purified water, allow it to drain, and add enough warm purified water, in which benzoic acid (2 Gm) has been dissolved, to make the product measure 1000 ml. After stoppering, lay the bottle on its side, rotate it occasionally, and when the acacia has dissolved strain the mucilage. *Acacia Mucilage may also be prepared as follows:* dissolve benzoic acid (2 Gm) in purified water (400 ml) with the aid of heat, and add the solution to powdered or granular acacia (350 Gm), in a mortar, triturating until the acacia is dissolved. Then add sufficient purified water to make the product measure 1000 ml, and strain if necessary. This second method is primarily for the extemporaneous preparation of Acacia Mucilage. *Uses:* Acacia Mucilage is a *demulcent* and a *suspending agent.* It is also employed as an *excipient* in making pills and troches, and as an *emulsifying agent* for cod liver oil and other substances. *Caution—Acacia Mucilage must be free from mold or any other indication of decomposition.*

Carbomer [Carboxypolymethylene; Carbopol (*Goodrich*)] is a polymer of acrylic acid cross-linked with allyl sucrose. *Description:* A white powder that is highly ionic and slightly acidic. It reacts with fatty amines to form thick and stable emulsions of oils in water. *Uses:* A thickening, suspending, dispersing, and emulsifying agent for pharmaceuticals, waxes, paints, and other industrial products.

Chondrus NF XI [Irish Moss; Carrageen]—The dried sun-bleached plant of *Chondrus crispus* (Linné) Stackhouse (Fam. *Gigartineæ*). *Uses:* Used principally as an emulsifying agent for liquid petrolatum and for cod liver oil. It is also a protective.

Malt—The partially germinated grain of one or more varieties of *Hordeum vulgare* Linné (Fam. *Gramineæ*) and contains amylolytic enzymes. Yellowish or amber-colored grains, having a characteristic odor and a sweet taste. The evaporated aqueous extract constitutes malt extract.

Malt Extract NF XI—The product obtained by extracting malt, the partially and artificially germinated grain of one or more varieties of *Hordeum vulgare* Linné

(Fam. *Gramineæ*). *Uses:* An infrequently used emulsifying agent.

Oleyl Alcohol NF IX—A mixture of aliphatic alcohols consisting chiefly of oleyl alcohol [(*Z*)-9-octadecen-1-ol]. It is a pale, yellow liquid having a faint characteristic odor and bland, mild taste. Specific gravity about 0.850. Melts between 13° and 19°. When strongly heated in air, it decomposes with the production of acrid vapors. Insoluble in water; soluble in alcohol, chloroform, ether, and vegetable oils. *Uses:* Similar to stearyl alcohol, but it does not raise the melting points of creams and lotions since it is a liquid at ordinary temperatures.

Quillaja NF IX, BP [Quillaja Bark, China or Murillo Bark, Panama Bark, Soap Bark]—The dried inner part of the bark of *Quillaja saponaria* Molina, and of other species of *Quillaja.* It is odorless with an acrid and astringent taste, the dust being strongly sternutatory. The dust contains two toxic saponins to which the drug owes its emulsifying properties. It is a violent local irritant, producing gastroenteritis. *Uses:* Formerly as an emulsifying agent in the form of a liquid extract or tincture, especially for creosote and tar preparations, for chloroform, and for small quantities of volatile oils.

Tragacanth Mucilage NF XII—*Preparation:* Mix glycerin (18 Gm) with purified water (75 ml) in a tared vessel, heat the mixture to boiling, discontinue the application of heat, add tragacanth (6 Gm) and benzoic acid (0.2 Gm), and macerate the mixture during 24 hours, stirring occasionally. Then add enough purified water to make the mixture weigh 100 Gm, stir actively until of uniform consistency, and strain forcibly through muslin. *Uses:* Tragacanth Mucilage is used pharmaceutically as a pill or troche *excipient*, and as a suspending agent for insoluble substances in internal mixtures. It is also a *protective* agent.

Ointment Bases

Ointments are semisolid preparations for external application, of such consistency that they readily may be applied to the skin by inunction. They should be of such composition that they soften, but not necessarily melt, when applied to the skin. Therapeutically, ointments function as protectives and emollients for the skin, but are used primarily as vehicles or bases for the topical application of more active medicinal substances.

Ideally, an ointment base should be compatible with the skin, stable, permanent, smooth and pliable, nonirritating, nonsensitizing, inert, able to absorb water or other liquid preparations, and able readily to release its incorporated medication. Since there is no single ointment base which possesses all these characteristics,

continued research in this field has resulted in the development of numerous new bases. Indeed, ointment bases have become so numerous as to require classification. Although ointment bases may be grouped in several ways, it is generally agreed that they can be classified best according to type (based on composition). Hence, the following four classes are recognized herein: oleaginous ointment bases, absorption ointment bases, emulsion ointment bases, and water-soluble ointment bases.

For completeness, substances are included which, although not used alone as ointment bases, contribute some pharmaceutical property to one or more of the various bases.

Oleaginous Ointment Bases

The oleaginous ointment bases include fixed oils of vegetable origin, fats obtained from animals, and semisolid hydrocarbons obtained from petroleum. The vegetable oils are used chiefly in ointments to lower the melting point or to soften the bases of higher consistency. These oils can be used as a base in themselves when a high percentage of powder is incorporated in a small amount of oil.

Animal fats, such as lard and suet, were the chief bases employed until the middle of the nineteenth century. The vegetable oils and the animal fats have two marked disadvantages as ointment bases: (1) the water-absorbing capacity is low; (2) they have a tendency to become rancid. Insofar as vegetable oils are concerned, the second disadvantage can be overcome

by hydrogenation; a process which converts many fixed oils into white, semisolid, lardlike fats, or into hard, almost brittle, waxes. Freshly prepared bases composed of vegetable oils or animal fats are said to be endodermic, since they are thought to possess a greater degree of penetration than the hydrocarbon bases.

The hydrocarbon bases comprise a group of substances with a wide range of melting points so that any desired consistency and melting point may be prepared with representatives of this group. They are stable, bland, chemically inert, and will mix with virtually any chemical substance. They do not release their medication with any degree of certainty and are thought to act primarily on the skin surface; hence, the hydrocarbon bases are epidermic in type.

White Ointment USP

[Unguentum Album; Unguentum Simplex; Ointment USP XI; Simple Ointment]

White Wax	50 Gm
White Petrolatum	950 Gm
To make	1000 Gm

Melt the white wax in a suitable dish on a water bath, add the white petrolatum, warm until liquefied, then discontinue the heating, and stir the mixture until it begins to congeal. See page 585 for allowable variations.

Uses—Emollient vehicle for other ointments.

Yellow Ointment, NF

[Unguentum Flavum; Unguentum Simplex; Simple Ointment]

Yellow Wax	50 Gm
Petrolatum	950 Gm
To make	1000 Gm

Melt the yellow wax in a suitable dish on a steam bath, add the petrolatum, warm until liquefied, then discontinue the heating, and stir the mixture until it begins to congeal. See page 585 for allowable variations.

Uses—Yellow Ointment is used as an emollient and as a vehicle for other ointments. Both White and Yellow Ointment are known as "Simple Ointment." White Ointment should be used to prepare white ointments and Yellow Ointment should be used to prepare colored ointments when Simple Ointment is prescribed.

Oleic Acid USP

[Oleinic Acid; Elaic Acid]

Oleic Acid is obtained from tallow and other fats, and consists chiefly of (Z)-9-octadecenoic acid [$CH_3(CH_2)_7$-$CH:CH(CH_2)_7COOH = 282.47$].

It usually contains variable amounts of the other fatty acids present in tallow such as linolenic and stearic acids.

Preparation—Oleic acid is obtained as a byproduct in the manufacture of the solid stearic and palmitic acids used in the manufacture of candles, stearates, and other products. The crude oleic acid is known as "red oil," the stearic and palmitic acids being separated by cooling the mixture and filtering.

Description—A water-white to pale yellow, oily liquid with a peculiar lard-like odor and taste. Its specific gravity is about 0.895 and it congeals at a temperature not above 10°. Pure Oleic Acid solidifies at 4°. At atmospheric pressure it decomposes when heated at 80° to 100°. On exposure to air it gradually absorbs oxygen, darkens, and develops a rancid odor.

Solubility—Practically insoluble in water; miscible with alcohol, chloroform, ether, benzene, and fixed and volatile oils.

Incompatibilities—Oleic acid reacts with *alkalies* to form soaps. *Heavy metals* and *calcium salts* form insoluble oleates. *Iodine solutions* are decolorized by formation of the iodine addition compound of oleic acid. Oleic acid is oxidized to various derivatives by *nitric acid, potassium permanganate*, and other agents.

Uses—Oleic Acid is used in the preparation of Benzyl Benzoate Lotion and Green Soap. It is also used as the basis for the oleates.

Technical grades of the acid are sulfonated to form *Turkey Red Oil*, which is extensively used as a detergent in textile dyeing.

Olive Oil USP

[Sweet Oil]

Olive Oil is the fixed oil obtained from the ripe fruit of *Olea europæa* Linné (Fam. *Oleaceæ*).

Preparation—It is obtained by crushing the recently collected ripe olives in a mill without breaking the putamen, then moderately pressing the pulpy mass. This produces the highest grade oil, known as *virgin oil*, "sublime oil," or "first expressed oil." The mass in the press is then mixed with water and again expressed with greater pressure, an oil of second quality resulting. Any oil remaining in the press cake is finally extracted with carbon disulfide, or the mass is thrown into large cisterns, mixed with water, and the oil allowed to separate. This is sometimes called "Pyrene oil," "bagasse oil," or "huile d'enfer." Many years ago it was difficult to obtain pure Olive Oil, but since the passage of the Food and Drugs Act it is unusual to find original packages labeled "olive oil" which do not contain Olive Oil. When bought in bulk or from unlabeled containers, cottonseed oil, colza oil, grapeseed oil, sesame oil, or other bland oils are not uncommonly found as adulterants. Large quantities of Olive Oil are imported from Italy and other countries bordering the Mediterranean, and it is produced to a limited extent in the Southern United States, chiefly in California. The finest European oil is imported from Leghorn.

Description—A pale yellow or light greenish yellow, oily liquid, having a slight characteristic odor and taste, with a faintly acrid aftertaste. Its specific gravity is 0.910 to 0.915.

Solubility—Slightly soluble in alcohol; miscible with carbon disulfide, chloroform, and ether.

Incompatibilities—Olive Oil is frequently used in external emulsion or liniment type preparations. When an emulsion is to be prepared, it is, of course, necessary to use the correct type and amount of emulsifying agent and to have the oil and aqueous phases present in suitable proportions.

Uses—Olive Oil is used in making cerates, ointments, liniments, and plasters. It is a bland, agreeable oil, well suited for *emollient* purposes and for food. The usual dose is 30 ml.

Veterinary Dose—*Dogs*, 15 to 60 ml; *Cats*, 4 to 30 ml.

Paraffin NF

[Paraffinum Durum; Paraffin Wax, Hard Paraffin]

Paraffin is a purified mixture of solid hydrocarbons obtained from petroleum.

Description—A colorless or white, more or less translucent mass, with a crystalline structure; it is slightly greasy to the touch. It is odorless and tasteless and congeals between 47° and 65°.

Solubility—Freely soluble in chloroform, ether, volatile oils, and most warm fixed oils; slightly soluble in dehydrated alcohol; insoluble in water and alcohol.

Identification—When strongly heated, Paraffin ignites with a luminous flame and deposits carbon. When heated in a dry test tube with an equal weight of sulfur, hydrogen sulfide is evolved and a black residue of carbon remains.

Uses—Paraffin is used to increase the consistency of some ointments.

Petrolatum NF

[Yellow Soft Paraffin; Amber Petrolatum; Yellow Petrolatum; Petroleum Jelly; Paraffin Jelly]

Petrolatum is a purified mixture of semisolid hydrocarbons obtained from petroleum. It may contain a suitable stabilizer.

Preparation—The "residuums," as they are termed technically, which are obtained by the distillation of petroleum, are purified by melting, usually treating with sulfuric acid, and then percolating through recently burned bone black or adsorptive clays; this abstracts the odor and modifies the color. Selective solvents are also sometimes employed to extract impurities.

The Petroleum Stabilizer—It has been found that the extent of purification required to produce *Petrolatum* NF and *Light Mineral Oil* NF quality removes antioxidants which are naturally present, and the purified product subsequently has a tendency to oxidize and develop an offensive odor. This is prevented by the addition of a minute quantity of α-tocopherol, or other suitable antioxidant, as now authorized by the NF. The use of this stabilizer in petroleum products is patented but the owners of the patent, the Sonneborn Co. of New York City, graciously offered to authorize its use, upon application, without the payment of royalties.

Description—An unctuous mass of yellowish to light amber color. It has not more than a slight fluorescence after being melted, and is transparent in thin layers. It is free or nearly free from odor and taste. It has a specific gravity of 0.815 to 0.880 at 60°, and it melts between 38° and 60°.

Solubility—Insoluble in water; almost insoluble in cold or hot alcohol and in cold dehydrated alcohol; freely soluble in benzene, carbon disulfide, chloroform, and turpentine oil; soluble in ether, solvent hexane, and in most fixed and volatile oils, the degree of solubility in these solvents varying with the composition of the petrolatum.

Uses—Petrolatum is used as a base for ointments. It is highly occlusive and therefore a good emollient but it may not release certain drugs readily.

White Petrolatum USP

[Petrolatum Album; White Petroleum Jelly; White Soft Paraffin]

White Petrolatum is a purified mixture of semisolid hydrocarbons obtained from petroleum, and wholly or nearly decolorized. It may contain a suitable stabilizer.

Preparation—It is prepared in the same manner as petrolatum, the purification treatment being continued until the product is practically free from yellow color. The product often sold for white petrolatum, made by mixing paraffin and liquid petrolatum, is not satisfactory for pharmaceutical purposes as it is granular and the liquid portion often separates. The USP test, describing the appearance of thin layers cooled to 0°C, excludes this variety.

Description—A white or faintly yellowish, unctuous mass. It is transparent in thin layers, even after cooling to 0°. Specific gravity 0.815 to 0.880 at 60°.

Solubility—Similar to that described under *Petrolatum*.

Uses—White Petrolatum is similar to yellow petrolatum in uses and characteristics but is often preferred because of its freedom from color. It is employed as a protective and as a base for ointments and cerates and to form the basis for burn dressings. See *Petrolatum Gauze* (page 765).

Spermaceti USP

[Cetaceum]

Spermaceti is a waxy substance obtained from the head of the sperm whale, *Physeter macrocephalus* Linné (Fam. *Physeteridæ*).

History—Spermaceti in the time of Shakespeare and previously was called *parmcety* and was largely used internally as well as in ointments and cerates. There was considerable mystery as to its real origin for many centuries. It was believed by some to be the sperm, by others to be the marrow, and by still others to be the brain substance of the whale. Some believed it to be a solidified form of the froth of foam of the sea.

Constituents—Spermaceti is a mixture of several constituents of which cetin, or cetyl palmitate [$C_{15}H_{31}$COOC$_{16}H_{33}$], predominates. When recrystallized from alcohol, *cetin* is obtained, while the mother liquor on evaporation deposits an oil, *cetin elain*, which when saponified yields *cetin elaic acid*, an acid resembling, but distinct from, oleic acid.

Preparation—Spermaceti is obtained by the forcible expression of the oleaginous material found in the head of the sperm whale to separate the liquid portion which is known as sperm oil, and which is a liquid wax. The solid fat is termed *cetin* (cetyl palmitate) and also belongs to the class of waxes.

Description—White, somewhat translucent, slightly unctuous masses with a crystalline fracture and pearly luster. It has a faint odor, a bland, mild taste, and is free from rancidity. Its specific gravity is about 0.94. It melts between 42° and 50°.

Solubility—Insoluble in water; practically insoluble in cold alcohol; slightly soluble in cold solvent hexane; soluble in boiling alcohol, ether, chloroform, and fixed and volatile oils.

Uses—Spermaceti is one of the solid fatty substances employed to give consistency and texture to cerates and ointments, as in the well-known *Cold Cream* and *Rose Water Ointment*.

Dose—*For external use*, topically as required.

Starch Glycerite NF

[Glyceritum Amyli; Starch Glycerin]

Starch	100 Gm
Benzoic Acid	2 Gm
Purified Water	200 ml
Glycerin	700 ml
To make about	1000 Gm

Rub the starch and the benzoic acid with the purified water in a porcelain dish until a smooth mixture is produced, then add the glycerin, and mix well. Heat the mixture on a sand bath to a temperature between 140° and 144°, with constant but gentle stirring until a translucent, jelly-like mass results, and then strain through muslin.

Starch Glycerite should be freshly prepared.

Uses—Starch Glycerite is an *emollient*. It is sometimes used as a substitute for fatty ointment vehicles and as a *pill excipient*.

Dose—*For external use*, *topically* as required.

White Wax USP

[Cera Alba; Bleached Beeswax; White Beeswax; Bleached Wax]

White Wax is the product of bleaching and purifying yellow wax that is obtained from the honeycomb of the bee [*Apis mellifera* Linné (Fam. *Apidæ*)].

Preparation—The color of yellow wax is discharged

by exposing it with an extended surface to the combined influence of air, light, and moisture. The process of bleaching is often conducted upon a large scale. The wax, previously melted, is made to fall in streams upon a revolving cylinder kept constantly wet, upon which it concretes, forming thin layers. These layers are spread upon linen cloths stretched on frames and exposed to the air and light, care being taken to wet and occasionally turn them. In a few days they are partially bleached; but to deprive the wax completely of color it is necessary to repeat the whole process one or more times. When sufficiently white, it is melted and cast into small circular cakes.

Description—A yellowish white, nearly tasteless, somewhat translucent solid with a faint, characteristic odor. It is free from rancidity. Melting range 62° to 65°. Specific gravity is about 0.95.

Solubility—Insoluble in water; sparingly soluble in cold alcohol; boiling alcohol dissolves the cerotic acid and a portion of the myricin, which are constituents of White Wax; completely soluble in chloroform, ether, and fixed and volatile oils; partly soluble in cold benzene and cold carbon disulfide; completely soluble in these liquids at about 30°.

Uses—White Wax is employed as a stiffening agent in many of the official preparations such as cerates, pastes, and ointments.

Yellow Wax NF

[Cera Flava; Beeswax; Yellow Beeswax]

Yellow Wax is the purified wax from the honeycomb of the bee, *Apis mellifera* Linné (Fam. *Apidæ*).

Constituents—Beeswax is a mixture of three different substances, which may be separated from one another by alcohol—*viz.*: (1) *myricin*, insoluble in boiling alcohol and consisting chiefly of *myricyl palmitate* [$C_{31}H_{63}(C_{16}H_{31}O_2)$] and *myricyl alcohol* [$C_{31}H_{63}OH$]; (2) *cerin* or *cerotic acid* [$C_{26}H_{52}O_2$], formerly called *cerin* when obtained only in an impure state, which is dissolved by boiling alcohol, but crystallizes out on cooling; (3) *cerolein*, which remains dissolved in the cold alcoholic liquid. This latter is probably a mixture of fatty acids, as indicated by its acid reaction to litmus paper.

Preparation—Yellow Wax is a natural secretion of bees. It is obtained on the large scale by first abstracting the honey from the combs by shaving off the ends of the cells, draining, and then placing them in centrifuges. The honey is rapidly whirled out, water is added, and the wax is thoroughly and quickly cleaned;

it is then melted and strained and run into flat dishes or molds to cool and harden.

Description—A yellow to grayish brown solid with an agreeable, honey-like odor, and a faint, characteristic taste. When cold it is somewhat brittle and when broken it presents a dull, granular, non-crystalline fracture. It becomes pliable from the heat of the hand. Its specific gravity is about 0.95 and it melts between 62° and 65°.

Solubility—Insoluble in water; sparingly soluble in cold alcohol; completely soluble in chloroform, ether, and fixed and volatile oils; partly soluble in cold benzene and carbon disulfide; completely soluble in these liquids at about 30°.

Uses—Yellow Wax is employed as a stiffening agent in many pharmaceutical preparations.

Other Oleaginous Ointment Bases

Lard NF X [Adeps; Prepared Lard]—The purified internal fat of the abdomen of the hog, *Sus scrofa* Linné var. *domesticus* Gray (Fam. *Suidæ*). It is a white, soft, unctuous mass having a faint odor and a bland taste, free from rancidity. It is insoluble in water but readily soluble in ether and chloroform. It consists of a mixture of stearin, palmitin, and olein, prepared by careful removal of membranes and adhering flesh and then rendered. *Uses:* As an ingredient in ointments. Must be protected from conditions favoring rancidity.

Lard, Benzoinated NF X [Adeps Benzoinatus]—Prepared by mixing 1000 Gm of lard with 10 Gm of Siam benzoin, rendered homogeneous by melting in a covered container at a temperature just under 60°C for 2 hours. The benzoin has the property of preventing or retarding rancidity and provides a pleasant vanilla-like odor. *Uses:* As an ingredient in ointments.

Linseed Oil NF X, BP [Flaxseed Oil; Raw Linseed Oil]—The fixed oil obtained from the dried ripe seed of *Linum usitatissimum* Linné (Fam. *Linaceæ*). Boiled linseed oil, that is, oil treated with a drier such as litharge and heated, must not be used as a drug. A yellow, oily liquid having a characteristic odor and a bland taste. When exposed to air, it gradually thickens, darkens in color, and acquires a more pronounced odor and taste. It has a sp gr of 0.925–0.935. It is a drying oil consisting mainly of linolein. *Uses:* In preparations such as liniments, pastes, medicinal soft soap, and saponated cresol solution. It has been used as a laxative in doses of 30–60 ml.

Mercury Oleate NF XI—A yellowish-brown substance of ointment-like consistency. It is insoluble in water and only slightly soluble in alcohol and ether, but is readily soluble in fixed oils. It is prepared by adding 25 Gm of yellow mercuric oxide to 75 Gm of oleic acid and heating the mixture at 50° until the mercuric oxide is dissolved. *Uses:* This oleate is used chiefly for the preparation of Mild Mercurial Ointment. Occasionally it is used as a parasiticidal application to the skin.

Absorption Ointment Bases

The term absorption is used here to denote the water-absorbing properties of these bases and not to describe their action on the skin. These bases are generally anhydrous substances which have the property of absorbing considerable quantities of water and still retaining their ointment-like consistency. Preparations of this type do not contain water as a component of their basic formula, but if water is incorporated, when and as desired, a water-in-oil emulsion results. Only two official products fall into this category.

Anhydrous Lanolin USP

[Adeps Lanæ; Wool Fat USP XVI; Refined Wool Fat]

Anhydrous Lanolin is lanolin that contains not more than 0.25% of water.

Constituents—Lanolin contains the sterols *cholesterol* [$C_{27}H_{45}OH$] and *oxycholesterol* as well as triterpene and aliphatic alcohols. About 7% of the alcohols are found in the free state, the remainder occurring as esters of the following fatty acids: *carnaubic, cerotic, lanoceric, lanopalmitic, myristic,* and *palmitic acids.* Some of these acids are found free. The emulsifying and emollient actions of lanolin are due to the alcohols which are found in the unsaponifiable fraction when lanolin is treated with alkali. Constituting approximately 50% of this fraction and known as *wool wax alcohols,* each 100 parts contains on the average 30 of *cholesterol,* 25 of *lanosterol,* 3 of *cholestanol (dihydrocholesterol),* 2 of *agnosterol,* and 40 of various other alcohols.

Anhydrous Lanolin although often considered with

the *fats*, is more accurately classified chemically as a *wax*.

Preparation—This substance is prepared by purifying the fatty matter (*suint*) obtained from the wool of the sheep. This natural wool fat contains about 30% of free fatty acids and fatty acid esters of *cholesterol* and other higher alcohols. The cholesterol compounds are the important constituents and, to secure these in a purified form, many processes have been devised. In one of these the crude wool fat is treated with weak alkali, the saponified fats and emulsions centrifuged to secure the aqueous soap solution, from which, on standing, a layer of partially purified wool fat separates. This product is further purified by treating it with calcium chloride and then dehydrating by fusion with unslaked lime. It is finally extracted with acetone and the solvent subsequently separated by distillation. Anhydrous Lanolin differs from Lanolin in that the former contains practically no water.

Description—A yellow, tenacious, unctuous mass having a slight, characteristic odor. It melts between 36° and 42°.

Solubility—Insoluble in water, but mixes without separation with about twice its weight of water; sparingly soluble in cold alcohol; more soluble in hot alcohol; freely soluble in ether and chloroform.

Uses—Anhydrous Lanolin is used as an ingredient of ointments, especially when a liquid is to be incorporated. It is included in some ointments of the NF, as it gives a distinctive quality to the ointment, at times increasing absorption of active ingredients and maintaining a uniform consistency for the ointment under most climatic conditions. However, Anhydrous Lanolin has been omitted from all ointments in the USP on the recommendation of dermatologists who have found that many patients are allergic to this animal wax.

A proprietary ointment vehicle, sold under the trade name *Eucerin*, is said to consist of 3% of the free alcohols from Anhydrous Lanolin, incorporated with petrolatum. A similar product is called *Aquaphor*. The claim is made that this vehicle will not reduce metallic oxides but is capable of suspending large proportions of water.

Hydrophilic Petrolatum USP

Cholesterol	30 Gm
Stearyl Alcohol	30 Gm
White Wax	80 Gm
White Petrolatum	860 Gm
To make	1000 Gm

Melt the stearyl alcohol, white wax, and white petrolatum together on a steam bath, then add the cholesterol, and stir until it completely dissolves. Remove from the bath, and stir until the mixture congeals.

Uses—This ointment is used as a *protective* and *water-absorbable ointment base*. It will absorb a large amount of water or aqueous solutions of medicating substances, forming a water-in-oil type of emulsion. See under *Ointments* (page 1601).

Other Absorption Ointment Bases

Hydroxystearin Sulfate NF IX [Sulfated Hydrogenated Castor Oil; SHCO]—A substance prepared by sulfating hydrogenated castor oil. It is a pale, yellow-brown, unctuous semisolid mass with a faint odor containing about 9% organically bound SO_3. Dispersible in water and glycerin. Miscible with propylene glycol, petrolatums, and fixed oils. *Uses:* A surface-active agent used in preparing hydrophilic ointment bases and other emulsions.

Emulsion Ointment Bases

Emulsion ointment bases are actually solid emulsions. These preparations can be divided into two groups on the basis of emulsion type: emulsion ointment base water-in-oil type and emulsion ointment base oil-in-water type. Bases of both types will permit the incorporation of additional amounts of water without reducing the consistency of the base below that of a soft cream. However, only oil-in-water emulsion ointment bases can be removed from the skin and clothing with water. Water-in-oil emulsions are better removed using oil.

Cetyl Alcohol NF

[1-Hexadecanol; Cetostearyl Alcohol; "Palmityl" Alcohol]

$$CH_3(CH_2)_{14}CH_2OH$$

Cetyl Alcohol [$C_{16}H_{34}O$ = 242.45] is a mixture of solid alcohols consisting chiefly of cetyl alcohol.

Cetyl Alcohol is an aliphatic solid alcohol.

Preparation—It may be obtained by saponification procedures from naturally occurring spermaceti in which it is present as *cetyl palmitate*.

Description—Unctuous, white flakes, granules, cubes, or castings, having a faint characteristic odor and a bland, mild taste. It melts between 45° and 50° and not less than 90 per cent distils between 316° and 336°.

Solubility—Insoluble in water; soluble in alcohol, chloroform, ether, and vegetable oils.

Uses—Similar to *Stearyl Alcohol* (page 1347). Cetyl Alcohol also imparts a smooth texture to the skin, and is widely used in cosmetic creams and lotions.

Cold Cream USP

[Petrolatum Rose Water Ointment USP XVI]

Spermaceti	125 Gm
White Wax	120 Gm
Mineral Oil	560 Gm
Sodium Borate	5 Gm
Purified Water	190 ml
To make about	1000 Gm

Reduce the spermaceti and the white wax to small pieces, melt them on a steam bath with the mineral oil, and continue heating until the temperature of the mixture reaches 70°. Dissolve the sodium borate in the purified water, warmed to 70°, and gradually add the warm solution to the melted mixture, stirring rapidly and continuously until it has congealed.

If the Ointment has been chilled, warm it slightly before attempting to incorporate other ingredients (see page 585 for allowable variations).

Uses—This USP preparation represents a variation of the formerly official Petrolatum Rose Water Ointment. It differs in that the fragrant rose oil and Stronger Rose Water have been omitted. It also resembles the long-established Rose Water Ointment (see below), differing only in the replacement of the Expressed Almond Oil or Persic Oil by an equal weight of Mineral Oil and omitting the fragrance. This change produces an ointment base which is not subject to rancidity like one containing a vegetable oil. Cold Cream is useful as an emollient, cleansing cream, and ointment base.

Glyceryl Monostearate NF

[Monostearin]

This ester is a mixture of variable proportions of glyceryl monostearate [$C_3H_5(OH)_2C_{18}H_{35}O_2 = 358.57$] and glyceryl monopalmitate [$C_3H_5(OH)_2C_{16}H_{31}O_2 = 330.52$].

Preparation—Among other ways, it may be prepared reacting glycerin with commercial stearoyl chloride.

Description—A white, wax-like solid or occurs in the form of white, wax-like beads, or flakes. It has a slight, agreeable, fatty odor and taste. It does not melt below 55°. It is affected by light.

Solubility—Insoluble in water, but may be dispersed in hot water with the aid of a small amount of soap or other suitable surface-active agent; dissolves in hot organic solvents such as alcohol, mineral or fixed oils, benzene, ether, and acetone.

Uses—A thickening and emulsifying agent for ointments. See under *Ointments* (page 1601).

Hydrophilic Ointment USP

Methylparaben	0.25 Gm
Propylparaben	0.15 Gm
Sodium Lauryl Sulfate	10 Gm
Propylene Glycol	120 Gm
Stearyl Alcohol	250 Gm
White Petrolatum	250 Gm
Purified Water	370 Gm
To make about	1000 Gm

Melt the stearyl alcohol and the white petrolatum on a steam bath, and warm to about 75°. Add the other ingredients, previously dissolved in the water and warmed to 75°, and stir the mixture until it congeals.

Uses—Hydrophilic Ointment is used as a *water-removable ointment base* for the so-called "washable" ointments.

Lanolin USP

[Adeps Lanæ Hydrosus; Hydrous Wool Fat]

Lanolin is the purified, fat-like substance from the wool of sheep, *Ovis aries* Linné (Fam. *Bovidæ*). It contains 25.0–30.0% of water.

Description—A yellowish white, ointment-like mass, having a slight, characteristic odor. When heated on a steam bath it separates into an upper oily and a lower water layer. When the water is evaporated a residue of *Lanolin* remains which is transparent when melted.

Solubility—Insoluble in water; soluble in chloroform and ether with separation of its water.

Uses—This substance is used largely as a vehicle for ointments, for which it is admirably adapted, on account of its compatibility with skin lipids. It absorbs aqueous liquids.

Rose Water Ointment NF

[Cold Cream; Galen's Cerate]

Spermaceti	125	Gm
White Wax	120	Gm
Almond Oil	560	Gm
Sodium Borate	5	Gm
Stronger Rose Water	25	ml
Purified Water	165	ml
Rose Oil	0.2	ml
To make about	1000	Gm

Reduce the spermaceti and the white wax to small pieces, melt them on a steam bath, add the almond oil, and continue heating until the temperature of the mixture reaches 70°. Dissolve the sodium borate in the purified water and stronger rose water, warmed to 70°, and gradually add the warm solution to the melted mixture, stirring rapidly and continuously until it has cooled to about 45°. Then incorporate the rose oil.

Rose Water Ointment must be free from rancidity. If the Ointment has been chilled, warm it slightly before attempting to incorporate other ingredients (see page 585).

History—This preparation was originated by Galen, the famous Roman physician–pharmacist of the 1st century A.D., and was known for many centuries by the name of *Unguentum* or *Ceratum Refrigerans*. It has changed but little in proportions or method of preparation throughout many centuries.

Uses—An *emollient* and *ointment base*.

Stearic Acid USP

[Cetylacetic Acid; Stearophanic Acid]

Stearic Acid is a mixture of stearic acid [$C_{18}H_{36}O_2 = 284.49$] and palmitic acid [$C_{16}H_{32}O_2 = 256.43$], which together constitute not less than 90.0% of the total content. The content of $C_{18}H_{36}O_2$ is not less than 50.0% of the total.

Preparation—It is usually prepared from tallow and similar fats by boiling them with soda lye, separating the glycerin and decomposing the resulting soap with sulfuric or hydrochloric acid. The stearic acid is subsequently separated from any oleic acid by cold expression. It is also prepared by the hydrogenation and subsequent saponification of *olein* (page 477). It may be purified by recrystallization from alcohol.

Description—A hard, white or faintly yellowish somewhat glossy and crystalline solid, or a white or yellowish white powder. It has an odor and taste suggestive of tallow. The official Acid melts at about 55.5° and should not congeal at a temperature below 54°. The pure Acid melts at 69° to 70°. Stearic Acid slowly volatilizes at 90°–100°.

Solubility—Practically insoluble in water; 1 Gm dissolves in about 20 ml of alcohol, 2 ml of chloroform, 3 ml of ether, 25 ml of acetone, or 6 ml of carbon tetrachloride; freely soluble in carbon disulfide; also soluble in amyl acetate, benzene, and toluene.

Incompatibilities—Insoluble stearates are formed with many *metals*. Ointment bases made with stearic acid may show evidence of drying out or lumpiness due to such a reaction when *zinc* or *calcium* salts are compounded therein.

Uses—Its chief use in pharmacy is in the preparation of sodium stearate which is the solidifying agent for the official glycerin suppositories, and for many other commercial products, such as toilet creams, solidified alcohol, etc.

Other Emulsion Ointment Bases

Wool Alcohols BP—Prepared by the saponification of the grease of the wool of sheep and separation of the fraction containing cholesterol and other alcohols. It contains not less than 30% cholesterol. A golden-brown solid, somewhat brittle when cold but becoming plastic when warm, with a faint characteristic odor. It has a smooth and shiny fracture. It is insoluble in water, moderately soluble in alcohol, completely soluble in 25 parts of boiling anhydrous alcohol, and freely soluble in ether, chloroform, and light petrolatum. Its melting point is not below 58°, its acid value is not more than 2, and its saponification value is not more than 12. Emulsions made with this material do not darken on the surface or acquire an objectionable odor in hot weather.

Uses: As an emulsifying agent for the preparation of water-in-oil emulsions; as a water absorbable substance in ointment bases; to improve the texture, stability, and emollient properties of oil-in-water emulsions.

Sodium Stearate USP XVI—A fine, white powder which is soapy to the touch. *Uses:* It is used as a solidifying substance in *Glycerin Suppositories.* Alkali stearates have also been used in the formulation of certain vanishing creams.

Water-Soluble Ointment Bases

Included in this section are those bases which are prepared from the higher ethylene glycol polymers known as Carbowax compounds. The Carbowaxes have a wide range in molecular weight. Those with molecular weights ranging from 200–700 are liquids; those above 1000 are wax-like solids. These compounds are water-soluble, nonvolatile, inert, unctuous agents. They do not hydrolyze or deteriorate and will not support mold growth. The properties which have been mentioned here, along with their ability to form an emollient base, account for their wide use in washable ointments.

Glycol Ethers and Derivatives

This special class of ethers has assumed considerable importance during the past two decades. Both mono- and poly-functional compounds are represented in the group. The simplest member is ethylene oxide [$\overline{CH_2CH_2O}$], the internal or cyclic ether of the simplest glycol, ethylene glycol [$HOCH_2CH_2OH$]. External mono- and di-ethers of ethylene glycol [$ROCH_2CH_2OH$ and $ROCH_2CH_2OR'$] are well known due largely to the Carbide and Carbon Chemicals Co., which has conducted much of the fundamental research in this field.

Preparation—In the presence of sodium hydroxide at temperatures of the order of 120° to 135° and under a total pressure of about 4 atmospheres, ethylene oxide reacts with ethylene glycol to form compounds having the general formula $HOCH_2(CH_2OCH_2)_nCH_2OH$ commonly referred to as condensation polymers and termed polyethylene (or polyoxyethylene) glycols. Other glycols besides ethylene glycol function in similar capacity, and the commercial generic term adopted for the entire group is polyalkylene (or polyoxyalkylene) glycols.

Nomenclature—It is to be noted that these condensation polymers are bifunctional; ie, they contain both ether and alcohol linkages. The compound wherein $n = 1$ is the commercially important diethylene glycol [$HOCH_2CH_2OCH_2CH_2OH$], and its internal ether is the familiar dioxane [$\overline{CH_2CH_2OCH_2CH_2O}$]. The mono- and di-ethers derived from diethylene glycol have the formulas $ROCH_2CH_2OCH_2CH_2OH$ and $ROCH_2CH_2OCH_2CH_2OR'$. The former are commonly termed *"Carbitols"* and the latter *"Cellosolves,"* registered trademarks belonging to the Carbide and Carbon Chemicals Co.

Polyethylene glycols are differentiated in commercial nomenclature by adding a number to the name which represents the average molecular weight. Thus, polyethylene glycol 400 has an average molecular weight of about 400 (measured values for commercial samples range between 380 and 420) corresponding to a value of n for this particular polymer of approximately 8. Polymers have been produced in which the value of n runs into the hundreds. Up to $n =$ approximately 15, the compounds are liquids at room temperature, viscosity and boiling point increasing with increasing molecular weight. Higher polymers are waxy solids and are termed commercially *Carbowaxes* (another Carbide and Carbon Chemicals Co. trademark).

It should be observed that the presence of the two terminal hydroxyl groups in the polyalkylene glycols makes possible the formation of both ether and ester derivatives, several of which are marketed products.

Uses—Because of their vapor pressure, solubility, solvent power, hygroscopicity, viscosity, and lubricating characteristics, the polyalkylene glycols or their derivatives function in many applications as effective replacements for glycerin and water-insoluble oils. They find considerable use as plasticizers, lubricants, conditioners, and finishing agents for processing textiles and rubber. They are also important as emulsifying agents and as dispersants for such diverse substances as dyes, oils, resins, insecticides, and various types of pharmaceuticals. In addition, they are frequently employed as ingredients in modern ointment bases and in a variety of cosmetic preparations.

Monographs presented here include those for *Octylphenoxy Polyethoxyethanol* (a mono-ether of a polyethylene glycol); *Polyethylene Glycols 300, 400, 1540, and 4000; Polyethylene Glycol Ointment; Polyoxyl 40 Stearate;* and *Polysorbate 80.* These are all polyoxyethylene compounds.

Octoxynol NF

[Polyethylene Glycol Mono[*p*-(1,1,3,3-tetramethylbutyl)phenyl] Ether; Octylphenoxy Polyethoxyethanol NF XII]

$$CH_3C(CH_3)_2CH_2C(CH_3)_2 - \langle\!\!\!-\!\!\!\rangle - O(CH_2CH_2O)_nH$$

Octoxynol is an anhydrous liquid mixture of mono-*p*-(1,1,3,3-tetramethylbutyl)phenyl ethers of polyethylene glycols in which *n* varies from 5 to 15, and which has an average molecular weight of 647, corresponding to the formula $C_{34}H_{62}O_{11}$.

Preparation—It may be prepared by reacting *p*-(1,1,3,3-tetramethylbutyl)phenol with ethylene oxide according to the general procedure described on this page.

Description—A clear, pale yellow, viscous liquid, having a faint odor and a bitter taste. Specific gravity between 1.059 and 1.068. Refractive index is about 1.4894. The pH of a 1 in 20 aqueous solution is between 7 and 9.

Solubility—Miscible with water, alcohol, and acetone; soluble in benzene and in toluene; insoluble in solvent hexane.

Uses—This substance is official as a pharmaceutical necessity in *Nitrofurazone Solution* where it functions as a surfactant. See *Polyethylene Glycol 400* below.

Polyethylene Glycol 300 NF

[Carbowax 300 (*Carbide & Carbon*)]

Polyethylene Glycol 300 is an addition polymer of ethylene oxide and water, represented by the formula $HOCH_2(CH_2OCH_2)_nCH_2OH$, where the average n varies from 5 to 5.75. It has an average molecular weight of 285–315.

Description—A clear, colorless or practically colorless, viscous liquid, having a slight, characteristic odor. Slightly hygroscopic. Specific gravity at 20° between 1.124 and 1.130. The pH of a 1:20 aqueous solution is between 4.0 and 7.0. A 25% aqueous solution is free from haze or turbidity.

Solubility—Miscible with water, alcohol, acetone, and other glycols; insoluble in ether and aliphatic hydrocarbons; soluble in aromatic hydrocarbons.

Uses—See *Polyethylene Glycol 400*. A pharmaceutical necessity for *Nitrofurazone Ointment* and *Solution*.

Polyethylene Glycol 400 USP

[Carbowax 400 (*Carbide & Carbon*)]

Polyethylene Glycol 400 is a polymer of ethylene oxide and water, represented by the formula $H(OCH_2CH_2)_nOH$, in which the average n varies from 8.2 to 9.1.

Description—A clear, colorless or practically colorless, viscous liquid, having a slight, characteristic odor. Slightly hygroscopic. Specific gravity 1.110 to 1.140.

Solubility—Miscible with water, alcohol, acetone, and other glycols; insoluble in ether and aliphatic hydrocarbons; soluble in aromatic hydrocarbons.

Uses—The polyethylene glycols possess a wide range of solubilities and compatibilities, which makes them useful in pharmaceutical and cosmetic preparations. Their blandness renders them highly acceptable for hair dressings, hand lotions, sun-tan creams, leg lotions, shaving creams, and skin creams. They are very useful constituents of ointments. For example, a peroxide ointment which is stable may be prepared using Carbowaxes, while oil-type bases inactivate the peroxide. Their use in washable ointments is discussed in the section on *Ointments* (page 1604). They are also used in making suppositories. hormone creams, etc. See *Polyethylene Glycol Ointment* (this page) and *Glycol Ethers* (page 1354).

Polyethylene Glycol 1540 NF

[Polyethylene Glycol 1300–1600; Carbowax 1540 (*Carbide & Carbon*)]

Polyethylene Glycol 1540 is an addition polymer of ethylene oxide and water, represented by the formula $HOCH_2(CH_2OCH_2)_nCH_2OH$, where the average n varies from 28 to 36. It has an average molecular weight of 1296–1648.

Description—A white, waxy, plastic material, having a consistency similar to beeswax, and having a slight, characteristic odor. Congealing range 42° to 46°. The pH of a 1:20 aqueous solution is between 4.0 and 7.0.

Solubility—1 Gm dissolves in about 1 ml of water, about 100 ml of absolute alcohol, and about 3 ml of chloroform; insoluble in ether.

Uses—See *Polyethylene Glycol 400*. A pharmaceutical necessity for *Nitrofurazone Ointment* and *Solution*.

Polyethylene Glycol 4000 USP

[Carbowax 4000 (*Carbide & Carbon*)]

Polyethylene Glycol 4000 is a polymer of ethylene oxide and water represented by the formula $H(OCH_2CH_2)_nOH$, in which the average n varies from 68 to 84.

Description—A pale, creamy-white, waxy solid or flakes resembling paraffin in appearance and texture. Practically odorless and tasteless. Congealing range 53° to 56°. The pH of a 1:20 aqueous solution is between 4.5 and 7.5.

Solubility—1 Gm dissolves in about 4 ml of water, 2.5 ml of alcohol, and 2 ml of chloroform; insoluble in ether.

Uses—Polyethylene Glycol 4000 is official as a pharmaceutical necessity. It is an ingredient in *Polyethylene Glycol Ointment* to which it imparts good consistency at ordinary temperature. See also preceding monographs.

Polyethylene Glycol Ointment USP—*Preparation*: Heat polyethylene glycol 4000 (400 Gm) and polyethylene glycol 400 (600 Gm) on a water bath to 65°. Allow to cool, and stir until congealed. If a firmer preparation is desired, replace up to 100 Gm of polyethylene glycol 400 with an equal amount of polyethylene glycol 4000. *Uses: A water-soluble ointment base.* See preceding monographs.

Polyoxyl 40 Stearate USP

[Polyoxyethylene 40 Monostearate; Stearethate 40; Myrj 52 (*Atlas*)]

Polyoxyl 40 Stearate is a mixture of the monostearate and distearate esters of mixed polyoxyethylene diols and the corresponding free glycols, the average polymer length being equivalent to about 40 oxyethylene units.

Preparation—This substance may be prepared by heating the corresponding polyethylene glycol with stearic acid, using the latter in equimolar proportion to the glycol.

Description—A waxy solid, light tan in color. Odorless or has a faint, fat-like odor. Congealing range between 39° and 44°.

Solubility—Soluble in water, alcohol, ether, and acetone; insoluble in mineral and vegetable oils.

Uses—Polyoxyl 40 Stearate contains ester and alcoholic linkages that impart to it both lyophilic and hydrophilic characteristics. It is thus very useful as a surfactant, emulsifier, and as an ingredient in the preparation of water-soluble ointment and cream bases. See *Glycol Ethers* (page 1354).

Polysorbate 80 USP

[Sorbitan Monooleate Polyoxyethylene (20) Derivative; Olethytan 20; Monitan (*Ives-Cameron*); Sorlate (*Abbott*); Tween 80 (*Atlas*)]

Polysorbate 80 is an oleate ester of sorbitol and its anhydrides copolymerized with approximately 20 moles of ethylene oxide for each mole of sorbitol and sorbitol anhydrides.

Preparation—This is one of a series of important nonionic surfactants (page 316) manufactured by the Atlas Powder Co. and marketed under the registered trademark *Tweens*. In general, these are prepared starting with a hexahydric aliphatic alcohol (a hexitol) by effecting the following: (1) elimination of one molecule of water to form a *hexitan* (cyclic hexitol anhydride); (2) partial esterification of the hexitan with a fatty acid such as oleic or stearic acid to yield a hexitan ester known commercially as a *Span*; and (3) condensation of the Span with ethylene oxide to yield the polyoxyethylene ether. In the preparation of Polysorbate 80, the hexahydric alcohol employed is sorbitol, the fatty acid is oleic acid, and approximately 20 moles of ethylene oxide are condensed with 1 mole of the sorbitan mono-oleate.

The total synthesis of Polysorbate 80 may be represented schematically as follows, but it is to be noted that all Spans and Tweens are *mixtures*:

Sorbitol →

Sorbitol Anhydride
(Sorbitan)

→

Sorbitan Mono-oleate
(a *Span*)

→ $H(OCH_2CH_2)_{n3}O$ — with $CH_2OCC_{17}H_{33}$, $O(CH_2CH_2O)_{n1}H$, $O(CH_2CH_2O)_{n2}H$

Polysorbate 80
(a *Tween*)

Description—A lemon- to amber-colored, oily liquid having a faint, characteristic odor, and a warm, somewhat bitter, taste. Specific gravity between 1.07 and 1.09; viscosity 345–445 centistokes at 25°; pH of 1:20 aqueous solution between 6 and 8.

Solubility—Very soluble in water, producing an odorless and nearly colorless solution; soluble in alcohol, cottonseed oil, corn oil, ethyl acetate, methanol, and toluene; insoluble in mineral oil.

Uses—Because of its excellent hydrophilic and lyophilic characteristics, this nonionic surfactant is very useful as an emulsifying agent in the preparation of pharmaceuticals, cosmetics, and other types of products. It is official as a pharmaceutic necessity for use in the preparation of *Coal Tar Ointment* and *Coal Tar Solution*. See *Glycol Ethers* (page 1354).

Other Water-Soluble Ointment Bases

Polyethylene Glycol 400 Monostearate USP XIV—A semitransparent, whitish, odorless, or nearly odorless mass. It is an ether, alcohol, and an ester. Melting range: 30° to 34°. Freely soluble in carbon tetrachloride, chloroform, ether, and petroleum benzin; slightly soluble in alcohol; insoluble in water. *Uses:* A nonionic surface-active agent for use in the preparation of creams, lotions, ointments, and similar pharmaceutical preparations, which are readily soluble in water.

Pharmaceutical Solvents

There has recently been a remarkable growth in the solvent industry. Over 300 solvents are now being produced on an industrial scale. Chemically, these include a great variety of organic compounds, ranging from hydrocarbons through alcohols, esters, ethers, and acids to the newer nitroparaffins. Their main applications are in industry and the synthesis of organic chemicals. Comparatively few, however, are used as solvents in pharmacy, because of their toxicity, volatility, instability, and flammability. The commonly used pharmaceutical solvents are described in this section.

Acetone NF

[Dimethyl Ketone; 2-Propanone; β-Ketopropane]

Acetone contains not less than 99.0% of C_3H_6O (58.08).

Caution—Acetone is very flammable. Do not use where it may be ignited.

Preparation—This liquid was formerly obtained exclusively from the destructive distillation of wood. The distillate, consisting principally of methanol, acetic acid, and acetone was neutralized with lime and the acetone was separated from the methyl alcohol, which constitutes the principal bulk in the wood spirit, by fractional distillation. Additional quantities of acetone were obtained by pyrolysis of the calcium acetate formed in the neutralization of the distillate.

Acetone is now largely obtained as a by-product of the butyl alcohol industry. This alcohol is formed in the fermentation of carbohydrates such as corn starch, molasses, etc, by the action of the bacterium *Clostridium acetobutylicum* (Weizmann fermentation) and Acetone is always one of the products formed in the process. It is also obtained by the catalytic oxidation of isopropyl alcohol, which is prepared from propylene resulting from the "cracking" of crude petroleum.

Description—A transparent, colorless, mobile, volatile, flammable liquid with a characteristic odor. It has a specific gravity of not more than 0.789, distils between 55.5° and 57°, and congeals at about −95°. Its aqueous solution is neutral to litmus.

Solubility—Miscible with water, alcohol, ether, chloroform, and with most volatile oils.

Identification—A warm 1:200 aqueous solution of acetone rendered alkaline with sodium hydroxide yields a yellow precipitate immediately upon the addition of iodine TS. On mixing 1 ml of a solution of Acetone (1 in 200) with 5 drops of sodium nitroferricyanide TS and 2 ml of sodium hydroxide TS, and adding a slight excess of acetic acid, a deep red color is produced which develops a bluish purple tint when the mixture is diluted with several volumes of water.

Uses—Acetone may be used as the menstruum in the preparation of oleoresins in place of ether. It is used as a *solvent* for dissolving fatty bodies, resins, pyroxylin, mercurials, etc, and also in the manufacture of many organic compounds such as chloroform, chlorobutanol, and ascorbic acid.

Alcohol USP

[Aethanolum; Ethanol; Ethyl Alcohol; Spiritus Vini Rectificatus; S. V. R.;
Spirit of Wine; Methylcarbinol]

Alcohol contains 92.3–93.8%, by weight, corresponding to 94.9–96.0%, by volume, at 15.56° (60°F), of C_2H_5OH (46.07).

History—The term alcohol is of Arabic origin, the word *Al-Kohl* being applied to the black antimony sulfide employed by the harem beauties to darken their eyebrows and eyelashes. The word in its original significance meant finely divided and is still used in this way in the term *alcoholized iron* which simply means finely divided iron.

Distillation was first practiced shortly after the beginning of the Christian Era in Alexandria, but no definite record occurs of strong alcoholic liquids prepared by distillation until Arnold of Villanova who wrote in the latter part of the thirteenth century and who called such a product *aqua vini* or *aqua vital* and extolled its virtues as "it strengthens the body and prolongs life." It is said that when Henry II invaded Ireland in the twelfth century the inhabitants were making and drinking a strongly alcoholic liquid which they called *uisgebeatha* (from the first half of which we get the name whisky) which is Gaelic for "water of life."

Preparation—The production of ethyl alcohol, ordinarily termed alcohol, depends on the decomposition (fermentation) of the saccharide dextrose into alcohol and carbon dioxide in the presence of *zymase*, an enzyme present in yeast cells.

$$C_6H_{12}O_6 \rightarrow 2C_2H_5OH + 2CO_2$$

Intermediate and complex reactions occur in this fermentation. In addition to *propyl, butyl,* and *amyl alcohol,* the following substances are reported as being produced at different stages of the process: *acetaldehyde, dihydroxyacetone, glyceric aldehyde, glycerin, methyl glyoxal,* and *pyruvic acid* and other organic compounds. On account of the cost, dextrose itself is not employed, but substances rich in starch, such as corn, rye, barley, and potatoes, are used instead. The starches must, however, first be gelatinized and then hydrolyzed to saccharides by the action of an amylase, such as *diastase,* an enzyme present in malt. This reaction is termed *saccharification* and may be represented by the equation:

$$\underset{\text{Starch}}{(C_6H_{10}O_5)_n} + n_2H_2O \xrightarrow{\text{(Diastase)}} \underset{\text{Maltose}}{n/2 C_{12}H_{22}O_{11}}$$

This equation shows the final reaction, but actually other reactions take place, for among the intermediate products formed are dextrins (*amylodextrin, erythrodextrin,* and *achroödextrin*) and maltose.

When the saccharification process has proceeded far enough, brewer's yeast is added. This supplies the enzyme *maltase* which converts the maltose into dextrose:

$$\underset{\text{Maltose}}{C_{12}H_{22}O_{11}} + H_2O \xrightarrow{\text{(Maltase)}} \underset{\text{Dextrose}}{2C_6H_{12}O_2}$$

In this country molasses is also used for the production of alcohol. Since, however, sucrose, the sugar present in molasses, is not directly fermentable it must first be changed to monosaccharides; this is accomplished with the catalytic aid of *invertase,* an enzyme also present in yeast.

$$\underset{\text{Sucrose}}{C_{12}H_{22}O_{11}} + H_2O \xrightarrow{\text{(Invertase)}} \underset{\text{Dextrose}}{C_6H_{12}O_6} + \underset{\text{Levulose}}{C_6H_{12}O_6}$$

The monosaccharides, dextrose and levulose, are then acted upon by zymase as described above. Alcohol is also produced commercially from sulfite liquors, whey, and cellulose pulp.

If a liquid in which alcoholic fermentation has occurred is not properly preserved or if the alcoholic content is very low, subsequent fermentation of a different character ensues in which the alcohol is converted into acetic acid through the influence of the microscopic organism known as *Mycoderma aceti.*

This reaction is also expressed in a simple form as:

$$\underset{\text{Alcohol}}{C_2H_5OH} + \underset{\text{Oxygen}}{O_2} \xrightarrow{\text{(Mycoderma Aceti)}} \underset{\text{Acetic Acid}}{CH_3COOH} + \underset{\text{Water}}{H_2O}$$

Here also intermediate reactions take place, *acetaldehyde* being one of the products formed.

The fermented liquid, containing about 15% of alcohol, is submitted to distillation using an efficient fractionating column, and thus a distillate containing 94.9% of C_2H_5OH, by volume, is obtained. For the production of higher concentrations of C_2H_5OH, as in *absolute alcohol,* the 95% product is dehydrated by special processes discussed under *Dehydrated Alcohol.*

Fusel Oil, which is a mixture of amyl, butyl, and propyl alcohols together with traces of other more complex organic substances, is produced from proteins present in the fermenting liquids from which Alcohol is distilled. It must be removed by distillation during the refining process; an official test is provided to make certain that it is not present in USP Alcohol.

Increasing amounts of ethyl alcohol are now being made from ethylene by converting it into ethyl hydrogen sulfate (or diethyl sulfate) and then hydrolyzing the ester.

Description—A transparent, colorless, mobile, volatile liquid with a slight, but characteristic odor and a burning taste. It boils at 78° but volatilizes even at a low temperature, and is flammable. When pure, it is neutral towards all indicators. The specific gravity of Alcohol at 15.56° (the US Government standard temperature for Alcohol) is not above 0.816, indicating not less than 92.3% of C_2H_5OH by weight or 94.9% by volume.

Solubility—Miscible with water, acetone, chloroform, ether, and many other organic solvents.

Incompatibilities—Alcohol and preparations containing a high percentage of alcohol will precipitate many inorganic salts from an aqueous solution. *Acacia* is generally precipitated from a hydroalcoholic medium when the alcohol content is greater than about 35%.

Strong *oxidizing agents* such as *chlorine, nitric acid, permanganate,* or *chromate* in acid solution react, in some cases violently, with alcohol to produce oxidation products.

Alkalies cause a darkening in color due to the small amount of aldehyde usually present in alcohol.

Uses—Alcohol is used in pharmacy principally for its solvent powers (page 257). It is also used as the starting point in the manufacture of many important compounds, like ether, chloroform, iodoform, etc. *Cologne Spirit* is a brand of Alcohol which is rectified particularly for perfumers' use. It is said to be made by diluting the ordinary alcohol with sufficient water to bring it to the strength of diluted alcohol, passing this through bone black, and then redistilling and concentrating it again to the proper strength in a rectifying column and still. Alcohol is also used as a fuel, chiefly in the denatured form (page 1358).

The pharmacist must be familiar with the regulations

for the handling of alcohol and alcoholic beverages, as established by the state in which he is doing business. These are in addition to the federal requirements and may be more restrictive than the national regulations.

Alcohol is a *depressant to the central nervous system* in the same manner as the general anesthetics. Medical use is made of this property by employing alcoholic beverages for the purposes of causing *sedation* and *sleep*. Alcoholic beverages and nutrient drinks (eggnogs, etc) are often used in convalescents to supply readily utilizable energy. They are also *carminative* and improve appetite and digestion. Alcohol is also used to test gastric function. Alcohol also has *antipyretic* activity when taken internally, in part due to the vasodilatation which it causes, allowing increased heat loss. Nevertheless, the value of alcohol in patients with *coronary arteriosclerosis* or *angina pectoris* is controversial. The analgesic effect of alcohol may mask the pain of cardiac ischemia and give the anginal or postcoronary patient a false sense of security. Alcoholic drinks are frequently taken to treat or abort "colds" and probably are effective by virtue of the combined effects of sedation, sleep, and vasodilatation in chilled cutaneous or mucosal surfaces.

Alcohol is sometimes administered intravenously for preoperative and postoperative sedation in patients in whom other measures are ineffective or contraindicated. The dose employed is 1 to 1.5 ml per Kg. The intravenous use of alcohol is a specialized procedure and should be employed only by one experienced in the technique of such use.

Externally, Alcohol has a number of medical uses. It is a solvent for the toxicodendrol causing *ivy poisoning,* and should be used to wash the skin thoroughly soon after contact. Alcohol (25%) is employed for bathing the skin for the purposes of *cooling* and *reducing fevers.* In high concentrations it is a *rubefacient* and an ingredient of many liniments. Alcohol (50%) is used to prevent sweating in *astringent* and *anhidrotic* lotions. It is also employed to cleanse and harden the skin and is helpful in preventing *bedsores* in bedridden patients. Alcohol (70% by weight) is a good *antiseptic* for the skin (*local anti-infective*) and also for instruments. Alcohol is also used as a *solvent* to cleanse the skin splashed with phenol. High concentrations of Alcohol are often injected into nerves and ganglia for the *relief of pain*, accomplishing this by causing nerve degeneration.

Denatured Alcohol

An act of Congress June 7, 1906, authorizes the withdrawal of alcohol from bond without the payment of internal revenue tax, for the purpose of denaturation and use in the arts and industries. Denatured alcohol is ethyl alcohol to which have been added such denaturing materials as to render the alcohol unfit for use as an intoxicating beverage. Denatured alcohol is divided into two classes, namely, *completely denatured alcohol* and *specially denatured alcohol*, prepared in accordance with approved formulas prescribed in Federal Industrial Alcohol Regulations 3.

Information regarding the use of alcohol and permit requirements may be obtained from the office of Director, Alcohol and Tobacco Tax Division, Internal Revenue Building, Washington 25, D.C. Federal regulation provides that completely and specially denatured alcohols may be purchased by properly qualified persons from duly established denaturing plants or bonded dealers. No permit is required for the purchase and use of completely denatured alcohol unless the purchaser intends to recover the alcohol.

Completely Denatured Alcohol—This term applies to ethyl alcohol to which have been added materials (methyl isobutyl ketone, pyronate, gasoline, acetaldol, kerosene, etc) of such nature that the products may be sold and used within certain limitations without permit and bond.

The number of completely denatured alcohol formulas authorized is somewhat limited and may vary from time to time depending upon the availability of suitable denaturants. The use of completely denatured alcohol dropped from 28,443,067 gallons in 1934 to 626,773 gallons in 1953. Most of this alcohol went into antifreeze preparations, industrial solvents, and ore flotation solutions.

Specially Denatured Alcohol—This alcohol is intended for use in a greater number of specified arts and industries than completely denatured alcohol and the character of the denaturant or denaturants used is such that specially denatured alcohol may be sold, possessed, and used only by those persons or firms that hold basic permits and are covered by bond.

Formulas for products using specially denatured alcohol must be approved prior to use by the Director, Alcohol and Tobacco Tax Division, Internal Revenue Service, Washington, D.C.

Uses—Approximately fifty specially denatured alcohol formulas containing combinations of more than ninety different denaturants are available to fill the needs of qualified users. Large amounts of specially denaturated alcohols are used as raw materials in the production of acetaldehyde, synthetic rubber, vinegar, and ethyl chloride; as well as in the manufacture of proprietary solvents and cleaning solutions. Ether and chloroform can be made from suitably denatured alcohols and formulas for the manufacture of Iodine Tincture USP, Green Soap Tincture NF, and Rubbing Alcohol NF are set forth in the regulations.

Specially denatured alcohols are also used as solvents for surface coatings, plastics, inks, toilet preparations, and external pharmaceuticals. Large quantities are used in the processing of such food and drug products as pectin, vitamins, hormones, antibiotics, alkaloids, and blood products. Other uses include supplemental motor fuel, rocket and jet fuel, antifreeze solutions, refrigerants, and cutting oils. Few products are manufactured today that do not require the use of alcohol at some stage of production. Specially denatured alcohol may not be used in the manufacture of foods or internal medicines where any of the alcohol remains in the finished product.

Rum may be denatured as *Specially Denatured Rum Formula No. 4,* by the addition of prescribed amounts of nicotine and methylene blue.

Diluted Alcohol USP

[Diluted Ethanol]

Diluted Alcohol is a mixture of alcohol and water containing 41.0–42.0%, by weight, corresponding to 48.4–49.5%, by volume, at 15.56°, of C_2H_5OH (46.07).

Diluted Alcohol may be prepared as follows:

Alcohol . . . . **500 ml**
Purified Water . . . . **500 ml**

Measure the alcohol and the purified water separately at the same temperature, and mix. If the water and the alcohol and the resulting mixture are measured at 25°, the volume of the mixture will be about 970 ml.

When equal volumes of alcohol and water are mixed together, a rise in temperature and a contraction of about 3% in volume take place. In small operations the contraction is generally disregarded; in larger operations it is very important. If 50 gallons of official alcohol are mixed with 50 gallons of water, the product will not be 100 gallons of Diluted Alcohol, but only 96¼ gallons, a contraction of 3¾ gallons. United States *Proof Spirit* differs from diluted alcohol and is stronger; it contains 50%, by volume, of absolute alcohol at 15.56° (60°F). This corresponds to 42.5% by weight, and has a specific gravity of 0.9341 at the same temperature. If spirits have a specific gravity lower than that of "proof spirit" (0.9341), they are said to be "*above proof*," if greater, "*below proof*."

Diluted Alcohol may also be prepared from the following:

Alcohol...........................   408 Gm
Purified Water...................   500 Gm

Rules for Dilution—The following rules are applied when making an alcohol of any required lower percentage from an alcohol of any given higher percentage:

I. By Volume—Designate the volume percentage of the stronger alcohol by V, and that of the weaker alcohol by v.

Rule—Mix v volumes of the stronger alcohol with purified water to make V volumes of product. Allow the mixture to stand until full contraction has taken place, and until it has cooled, then make up the deficiency in the V volumes by adding more purified water.

Example—An alcohol of 30% by volume is to be made from an alcohol of 94.9% by volume.—Take 30 volumes of the 94.9% alcohol, and add enough purified water to produce 94.9 volumes at room temperature.

II. By Weight—Designate the weight-percentage of the stronger alcohol by W, and that of the weaker alcohol by w.

Rule—Mix w parts by weight of the stronger alcohol with purified water to make W parts by weight product.

Example—An alcohol of 50% by weight is to be made from an alcohol of 92.3% by weight.—Take 50 parts by weight of the 92.3% alcohol, and add enough purified water to produce 92.3 parts by weight.

Description—Diluted Alcohol has the properties described for *Alcohol*, except its specific gravity is between 0.935 and 0.937 at 15.56°, indicating that the strength of C_2H_5OH corresponds to that given in the official definition.

Uses—Diluted Alcohol is used as a menstruum in making tinctures, fluidextracts, extracts, etc. Its properties have been already fully described in connection with the various preparations. Its value consists not only in its *antiseptic* properties, but also in its possessing the *solvent* powers of both water and alcohol. See *Alcohol*.

Nonbeverage Alcohol

Nonbeverage alcohol is tax-paid alcohol or distilled spirits used in the manufacture, by approved formula, of such medicines, medicinal preparations, food products, flavors, or flavoring extracts as are unfit for beverage purposes. Internal Revenue Service Regulations 29 provide that qualified holders of Special Tax Stamps who use tax-paid alcohol or distilled spirits in the types of products listed above, may file a claim for *alcohol tax drawback* or refund of a considerable part of the tax paid.

Amylene Hydrate NF

[*tert*-Pentyl Alcohol; Tertiary Amyl Alcohol; Dimethyl Ethylcarbinol]

$$CH_3CH_2.\overset{\overset{\text{OH}}{|}}{C}(CH_3)_2$$

Amylene Hydrate is 2-methyl-2-butanol [$C_5H_{12}O$ = 88.15].

Preparation—Amylene is mixed with 2 volumes of 60% H_2SO_4, both previously cooled to 0°, for about 1 hour; then neutralized with soda, distilled, and the first half of the distillate containing most of the amylene hydrate is treated with anhydrous potassium carbonate and redistilled.

The amylene is obtained along with isomerides by a reverse process, namely, the abstraction of H_2O from fusel oil by distilling it from a mixture containing also sulfuric acid or anhydrous zinc chloride.

Description—A clear, colorless liquid of camphoraceous odor. Its solution is neutral to litmus. Its specific gravity is between 0.803 and 0.807, and it distils completely between 97° and 103°.

Solubility—1 Gm dissolves in about 8 ml of water; miscible with alcohol, chloroform, ether, and glycerin.

Uses—A *sedative–hypnotic* which stands midway between chloral hydrate and paraldehyde in its depressant properties. The hypnotic dose is 1 to 4 Gm, administered in glycerin, but the drug is almost never used for the purpose of sedation or sleep. Its chief use is as a *pharmaceutical necessity* for *Tribromoethanol Solution* (page 1064).

Chloroform—see page 1056.

Ether—see page 1057.

Ethyl Acetate—see page 1327.

Glycerin USP

[1,2,3-Propanetriol; Glycerol]

$$\underset{\text{OH}}{CH_2}-\underset{\text{OH}}{CH}-\underset{\text{OH}}{CH_2}$$

Glycerin contains not less than 95.0% of $C_3H_8O_3$ (92.10).

Chemically, glycerin is the simplest trihydric alcohol. It is worthy of special note because the two terminal alcohol groups are primary whereas the middle one is secondary. Glycerol thus becomes the first polyhydric alcohol which can yield both an aldose (*glyceraldehyde*) and a ketose (*dihydroxyacetone*).

Esters of glycerin constitute important compounds. There are two isomeric classes of monoesters designated as *alpha* when a terminal OH is esterified and as *beta* when the middle OH is esterified. Similarly, there are two isomeric classes of diesters designated as α,α' when the two terminal OH's are esterified and as α,β when one terminal OH and the middle OH are esterified. In the triesters, all three OH's are esterified.

History—Glycerin was discovered by K. W. Scheele in 1779 but was more fully investigated by M. E. Chevreul who named it glycerin. It came into use in medicine and pharmacy about 1846, and was first obtained in this country, on a commercial scale, from the washings of lead plaster, by Robert Shoemaker of Philadelphia. In making the plaster, litharge, olive oil, and water were boiled together, whereby the olein of the oil was saponified.

Preparation—Glycerin is obtained in several ways.

1. By the saponification of fats and oils in the manufacture of soap.

2. By the hydrolysis of fats and oils through pressure and superheated steam. This process is the one most frequently used. It originated with R. A. Tilghman, of Philadelphia, and consists in subjecting fatty bodies to the action of water at a high temperature under pressure, whereby the fats, which are glyceryl esters (*glycerides*) of the fatty acids, are hydrolyzed into glycerin and fatty acids.

3. By the fermentation of beet sugar molasses in the presence of large amounts of sodium sulfite. Under these conditions a reaction, expressed as follows, takes place:

$$C_6H_{12}O_6 \rightarrow C_3H_5(OH)_3 + CH_3CHO + CO_2$$
Glucose   Glycerin   Acetaldehyde

4. Glycerin is now prepared in large quantities from propylene, a petroleum product. This hydrocarbon is chlorinated at about 400° to form allyl chloride, which is converted to allyl alcohol. Treatment of the unsaturated alcohol with hypochlorous acid [HOCl] yields the chlorohydrin derivative. Extraction of HCl with soda lime yields 2,3-epoxypropanol which undergoes hydration to glycerin.

Description—A clear, colorless, syrupy liquid with a sweet taste and not more than a slight, characteristic odor, which is neither harsh nor disagreeable. When exposed to moist air it absorbs water and also such gases as H_2S and SO_2. Its solutions are neutral. Its specific gravity is not below 1.249, corresponding to not less than 95% $C_3H_5(OH)_3$. It boils at about 290° under 1 atmos pressure, with decomposition, but can be distilled intact in a vacuum.

Solubility—Miscible with water, alcohol, and methanol; 1 Gm dissolves in about 12 ml of ethyl acetate and about 15 ml of acetone; insoluble in ether, mineral, volatile, or vegetable oils, chloroform, or other halogenated hydrocarbons.

Identification—Glycerin is identified by its yielding the intensely pungent unsaturated aldehyde *acrolein* when it is heated with powdered potassium bisulfate or with anhydrous magnesium sulfate.

Incompatibilities—An explosion may occur if Glycerin is triturated with strong *oxidizing agents* such as *chromium trioxide, potassium chlorate,* and *potassium permanganate.* In dilute solutions the reactions proceed at a slower rate forming several oxidation products. Iron is an occasional contaminant of Glycerin and may be the cause of a darkening in color in mixtures containing *phenols, salicylates, tannin,* etc.

With *boric acid* or *sodium borate,* Glycerin forms a complex, generally spoken of as glyceroboric acid, which is a much stronger acid than boric acid.

Uses—Glycerin is one of the most valuable products known to pharmacy by virtue both of its *solvent* and *preservative* properties. Glycerin is useful as a *humectant* in keeping substances moist, owing to its hygroscopicity. It is a valuable *emollient* in many skin diseases, and its agreeable taste and nonpoisonous properties adapt it for many purposes. Some modern ice collars and ice bags contain glycerin and water hermetically sealed within vulcanized rubber bags. The latter are sterilized by dipping in a germicidal solution and are stored in the refrigerator until needed.

Isopropyl Alcohol—see page 1181.

Methyl Isobutyl Ketone NF

[4-Methyl-2-pentanone]

$$(CH_3)_2CHCH_2COCH_3$$

Methyl Isobutyl Ketone contains not less than 99.0% of $C_6H_{12}O$ (100.16).

Preparation—Among other ways, Methyl Isobutyl Ketone may be prepared by reacting sodio acetoacetic ester with isopropyl bromide and treating the resulting 2-isopropylacetoacetic ester with dilute acid to saponify the ester and decarboxylate the resulting keto acid.

Description—A transparent, colorless, mobile, volatile liquid having a faint, ketonic and camphoraceous odor. It distills between 114° and 117°.

Solubility—Slightly soluble in water; miscible with alcohol, ether, and benzene.

Uses—Methyl Isobutyl Ketone is used as a *denaturant* for rubbing alcohol and also as a *solvent* for gums, resins, nitrocellulose, etc. It may be irritating to the eyes and mucous membranes, and, in high concentrations, narcotic.

Monoethanolamine NF

[2-Aminoethanol; Ethanolamine; Ethylolamine]

$$HOCH_2CH_2NH_2$$

Monoethanolamine contains 98.0–100.5% of C_2H_7NO (61.08).

Preparation—Monoethanolamine, one of the simpler and earliest known alkanolamines, is conveniently prepared by treating ethylene oxide with ammonia.

Description—A clear, colorless, moderately viscous liquid having a distinctly ammoniacal odor. It is affected by light. Specific gravity between 1.014 and 1.021. Distillation range 167° to 173°.

Solubility—Miscible in all proportions with water, acetone, alcohol, glycerin, and chloroform; immiscible with ether, solvent hexane, and fixed oils; dissolves many essential oils.

Uses—Monoethanolamine, a *solvent* for fats, oils, and many other substances, is a pharmaceutical necessity for *Thimerosal Solution.* It combines with fatty acids to form soaps which find application in various types of emulsions such as lotions, creams, etc. See *Thimerosal Solution,* page 1190.

Propylene Glycol USP

$$CH_3CHCH_2OH$$
$$|$$
$$OH$$

Propylene Glycol is 1,2-propanediol [$C_3H_8O_2$ = 76.10].

Preparation—Propylene is converted successively to its chlorohydrin (with HOCl), epoxide (with Na_2CO_3), and glycol (with water in presence of proton).

Description—A clear, colorless, viscous, and practically odorless liquid having a slightly acrid taste. Its specific gravity is 1.035 to 1.037 and it boils at about 190°. Completely distils between 184° and 189°. It absorbs moisture from moist air.

Solubility—Miscible with water, alcohol, acetone, and chloroform; soluble in ether; dissolves many volatile oils; immiscible with fixed oils.

Uses—Propylene Glycol is used as a *solvent, preservative,* and *humectant.* See *Hydrophilic Ointment,* page 1353.

Triethanolamine USP

Triethanolamine is a mixture of alkanolamines consisting largely of triethanolamine [$N(C_2H_4OH)_3$ = 149.19], containing some diethanolamine [$NH(C_2H_4OH)_2$ = 105.14] and monoethanolamine [NH_2-C_2H_4OH = 61.08]. It contains 97.0–103.0% of the labeled amount of alkanolamines, calculated as $N(C_2H_4OH)_3$.

Preparation—It is produced, along with some mono- and diethanolamine, by the action of ammonia on ethylene oxide.

Description—Colorless to pale yellow, viscous, hygroscopic liquid having a slight odor of ammonia. Its aqueous solution is very alkaline. Melts at 20° to 21°. Its specific gravity is between 1.1204 and 1.1284 and the refractive index 1.481 to 1.486 at 20°. Triethanolamine is a strong base and readily combines even with weak acids to form salts.

Solubility—Miscible with water or alcohol; soluble in chloroform; slightly soluble in ether or benzene.

Identification—(1) It yields a deep blue color with copper sulfate TS which is not discharged upon the addition of sodium hydroxide TS; (2) a carmine-red color is produced with cobalt chloride TS; (3) its vapors turn red litmus paper blue.

Uses—It is used in combination with a fatty acid, eg, oleic acid (see *Benzyl Benzoate Lotion*, page 1271), as an *emulsifier*. See *Monoethanolamine* (above).

Water—see page 1338.

Other Pharmaceutical Solvents

Alcohol, Dehydrated NF X, BP, PhI [Dehydrated Ethanol; Absolute Alcohol]—*Purity:* not less than 99% by weight of C_2H_5OH. It is a transparent, colorless, mobile, volatile liquid having a characteristic odor and a burning taste. It is hygroscopic, flammable and boils at about 78°C. It is miscible with water, ether, and chloroform. Its sp gr is not more than 0.798 at 15.56°C. *Uses:* Pharmaceutical solvent.

Coconut Oil NF IX [Cocoanut Oil; Copra Oil]—The fixed oil obtained by expression or extraction from the kernels of the seeds of *Cocos nucifera* Linné (Fam. *Palmæ*). A pale yellow to colorless liquid between 28° to 30°, a semisolid at 20°, and a hard, brittle, crystalline solid below 15°. It is odorless and tasteless or has a faint odor and taste characteristic of coconut. It must not be used if it has become rancid. Melting range: 22° to 25°. Sp gr 0.918 to 0.923. It is readily soluble in alcohol, ether, chloroform, carbon disulfide, and petroleum benzin, but is insoluble in water.

Ethyl Oxide NF XII [Solvent Ether] contains 96.0–98.0% of $C_4H_{10}O$ (74.12), the remainder consisting of alcohol and water. *Caution: Ethyl Oxide is solvent ether and must not be used for anesthesia. Ethyl Oxide is highly flammable. Do not use where it may be ignited. Description:* Agrees with the description and properties given under *Ether. Uses:* A reagent and solvent. See *Ether* (page 1057).

Glyceryl Triacetate NF X [Triacetin] [$C_3H_5(C_2H_3O_2)_3$]—*Purity:* not less than 98.5% $C_9H_{14}O_6$. A colorless, oily liquid with a slight, fatty odor, and a bitter taste. It is soluble in water and miscible with alcohol, ether, and chloroform. It has a refractive index of 1.4288–1.4296 and a sp gr of 1.154–1.158. *Uses:* As a solvent in some topical formulations.

Lauric Acid [$CH_3(CH_2)_{10}.COOH$]—It occurs as the glyceride in laurel oil, hence the name lauric acid, in coconut oil, and in some other vegetable oils or fats. White, crystalline powder having a slight odor of bay oil. Specific gravity about 0.87 at 50°. Melts at about 44°. Distillable without decomposition under reduced pressure. Insoluble in water; freely soluble in alcohol, ether, and benzene. *Ethyl laurate* is used as a vehicle for drugs in place of vegetable oils.

Methanol [Methyl Alcohol; Wood Alcohol] [CH_3OH]—A colorless, clear liquid. Flammable. Sp gr 0.790. Boils 64.1°C. Miscible with water and most organic solvents. Toxic. Ingestion may result in blindness. Vapors also may cause toxic reactions.

Methylated Spirit, Industrial BP [I. M. S.]—A mixture of 19 volumes of alcohol (95%) with 1 volume of approved wood naphtha, and is of the quality known as "66 O. P. Industrial Methylated Spirits." It can also be obtained at a strength of 74 O. P. and this quality is known as "Absolute Industrial Methylated Spirits." It is incompatible with iodine owing to the presence of acetone in the spirit. It has a sp gr not greater than 0.814 and complies with the description given under *Alcohol* (page 1357) but having in addition the odor of wood naphtha. *Uses:* For the storage of sterilized surgical instruments and hypodermic needles; in the preparation of various pharmaceuticals.

Paraffin, Chlorinated NF VIII [Chlorcosane]—A liquid paraffin which has been treated with chlorine. A light amber, clear, thick, oily liquid. Odorless and stable. *Uses:* Solvent for Dichloramine-T.

Petroleum Benzin NF X [Petroleum ether; Purified benzin]—A clear, colorless, volatile liquid having an ethereal or faint, petroleum-like odor and a neutral reaction. It is practically insoluble in water but miscible with ether, chloroform, benzene, and fixed oils. Its sp gr is 0.634–0.660. *Caution:* highly flammable, and its vapor, when mixed with air and ignited, may explode. *Uses:* Solvent for fats, resins, oils, and similar substances.

n-Propyl Alcohol [1-propanol] [$CH_3CH_2CH_2OH$]—Clear, mobile liquid. Sp gr 0.804. Boils 97° to 98°C. Miscible with water, alcohol, ether.

Miscellaneous Pharmaceutical Necessities

The agents listed in this section comprise a heterogeneous group of substances with both pharmaceutical and industrial applications. Pharmaceutically, some of these agents are used as diluents, enteric coatings, excipients, filtering agents, and as ingredients in galenical products considered in other chapters. Industrially, some of these agents are used in various chemical processes, in the synthesis of other chemicals, and in the manufacture of fertilizers, explosives, etc.

Acetic Acid USP

Acetic acid is a solution containing 36.0–37.0%, by weight, of $C_2H_4O_2$ (60.05).

Preparation—This acid is prepared by diluting with distilled water an acid of higher concentration, such as the 80% product, or more commonly glacial acetic acid, using 350 ml of the latter for the preparation of each 1000 ml of Acetic Acid.

Description—A clear, colorless liquid, having a strong characteristic odor and a sharply acid taste. Its specific gravity is about 1.045 and it congeals at about −14°. It is acid to litmus.

Solubility—Miscible with water, alcohol, and glycerin.

Identification—Acetic Acid responds to the *Tests for Acetate:* When acetates are warmed with sulfuric acid the odor of acetic acid is evolved. If acetic acid or an acetate is warmed with moderately dilute sulfuric acid and alcohol the characteristic odor of ethyl acetate is evolved. The addition of a solution of a ferric salt to a neutral solution of an acetate produces a deep red color which is destroyed by the addition of mineral acids.

For the identification of the acetate radical in acetate esters, the latter are heated with aqueous or alcoholic potassium or sodium hydroxide solutions, the organic base (alcohol or phenol) is removed by filtration, distillation, or extraction with an immiscible solvent, and the acetate is then identified by the above reactions.

Incompatibilities—*Silver* and *mercurous acetates* are only sparingly soluble. Other acetates, except those of the alkali metals, form less soluble basic salts by hydrolysis in aqueous solution. With *ferric salts*, a deep red color is produced indicating formation of ferric acetate which hydrolyzes to a colloidal ferric hydroxide.

Uses—Acetic Acid is used in pharmacy as a *solvent* and *menstruum*, and for making diluted acetic acid. The crude acetic acid, called *pyroligneous acid*, is sometimes put up under the name of *liquid smoke* and sold for the purpose of preserving meat, fish, etc, which are dipped therein and then dried, instead of subjecting them to the customary smoking process. This use of pyroligneous acid is prohibited by most food laws. Acetic Acid is also used as a starting point in the manufacture of many other organic compounds, eg, acetates, acetanilid, sulfa drugs, etc. It also finds many applications in the textile industry. It is official primarily as a *pharmaceutic necessity* for the preparation of *Aluminum Subacetate Solution* (page 770).

Diluted Acetic Acid NF

[Dilute Acetic Acid]

Diluted Acetic Acid is a solution containing, in each 100 ml, 5.7–6.3 Gm of $C_2H_4O_2$ (60.05).

Diluted Acetic Acid may be prepared as follows:

Acetic Acid..	**158 ml**
Purified Water, a sufficient quantity,	
To make......................	**1000 ml**

Mix the ingredients.

Note—This acid may also be prepared by diluting 58 ml of glacial acetic acid with sufficient purified water to make 1000 ml.

Description—Diluted Acetic Acid has essentially the same properties, solubility, purity, and identification reactions as Acetic Acid, but its specific gravity is about 1.008 and it congeals at about −2°.

Uses—Diluted Acetic Acid is *bactericidal* to many types of microorganisms and is occasionally used in 1% solution for surgical dressings of the skin. A 1% solution is also actively *spermatocidal*.

Diluted Acetic Acid is superior to *vinegar* as a menstruum, and is used in preparing Squill Vinegar because of its greater purity, more uniform strength, and freedom from color.

Veterinary Uses—Solutions of 1 part Diluted Acetic Acid to 3 parts of water have been recommended for infections in which *Actinomyces necrophorus* is a primary or secondary etiological organism (*calf diphtheria, necrotic stomatitis* of swine, *foot rot* and *leg ulceration* of sheep, *gangrenous dermatitis* of horses, *necrosis* of the anus and vulva of cattle).

Glacial Acetic Acid USP

[Acetum Acerrimum; Concentrated Acetic Acid; Crystallizable Acetic Acid; Ethanoic Acid; Vinegar Acid]

CH₃COOH

Glacial Acetic Acid contains 99.5–100.5%, by weight, of $C_2H_4O_2$ (60.05).

Preparation—This acid is termed "glacial" because of its solid glassy appearance when congealed. In one process it is produced by distillation of weaker acids to which has been added a water-entraining substance such as ethylene dichloride. In this method, referred to as "azeotropic distillation," (page 186) the ethylene dichloride distils out with the water before the acetic acid distils over, thereby effecting concentration of the latter.

In another process aqueous acetic acid is mixed with triethanolamine and heated. The acetic acid combines with the triethanolamine to form a triethanolamine acetate. The water is driven off first; then, at a higher temperature, the triethanolamine compound is broken up to yield Glacial Acetic Acid.

A greater part of the Glacial Acetic Acid now available is made synthetically from acetylene.

When acetylene is passed into acetic acid containing a metallic catalyst such as mercuric oxide, ethylidene diacetate is produced which yields, upon heating, acetic anhydride and acetaldehyde. Hydration of the former and air oxidation of the latter yields acetic acid.

The specific gravity of Glacial Acetic Acid (100%) is 1.0471 is 25°C and the specific gravity of 39% acetic acid is nearly the same, 1.0474, while 79, 80, 77, and 76% acids have exactly the same specific gravity. It will thus be seen that specific gravity cannot be relied upon as a criterion for strength. The glacial acid may, however, be distinguished from the 39% acid by the freezing temperature. The percentage of acetic acid, especially in concentrations of 96% and over, is also most conveniently determined from its freezing (congealing) temperature as given in the table at the end of this monograph.

Description—A clear, colorless, liquid with a pungent, characteristic odor. When well diluted with water, it has an acid taste. Its specific gravity is about 1.049. It boils at about 118° and congeals at a temperature not lower than 15.6°, corresponding to a minimum of 99.4% of CH₃COOH.

Solubility—Miscible with water, alcohol, acetone, ether, and glycerin; insoluble in carbon tetrachloride and in chloroform.

Identification—A 1:2 mixture with water responds to the tests under *Acetic Acid*.

Uses—Glacial Acetic Acid is an excellent *solvent* for fixed and volatile oils as well as for many other organic compounds. It also dissolves phosphorus, sulfur, and halogen acids. Medicinally, it is a *caustic* and *vesicant* when applied externally and is often sold under various disguises as a *corn solvent*. It is used industrially in the manufacture of acetate, acetanilid, acetophenetidin, and other acetyl compounds; also in the blending of textiles and the dyeing of silk.

It is official primarily as a *pharmaceutic necessity* for the preparation of *Aluminum Acetate Solution*.

Veterinary Uses—The daily application of Glacial Acetic Acid to *warts* (papillomatosis) or the base of the wart following their surgical removal has been recommended.

Congealing Temperatures of Various Concentrations of Acetic Acid

% Acetic Acid (CH₃COOH)	Congealing temp., °C	% Acetic Acid (CH₃COOH)	Congealing temp., °C
100.00	+16.75	97.00	11.81
99.90	16.57	96.80	11.48
99.80	16.28	96.60	11.16
99.70	16.05	96.40	10.83
99.60	15.84	96.20	10.50
99.50	15.65	96.00	10.17
99.40	15.47	93.50	8.15
99.30	15.29	90.34	3.11
99.20	15.12	85.60	−2.01
99.10	14.96	80.50	−7.80
99.00	14.80	76.30	−11.20
98.80	14.49	70.50	−16.70
98.60	14.17	62.50	−24.60
98.40	13.86	60.20	−20.40
98.20	13.55	40.40	−15.60
98.00	13.25	31.40	−12.10
97.80	12.96	19.70	−6.80
97.60	12.66	10.52	−3.20
97.40	12.37	6.10	−1.90
97.20	12.09	2.52	−0.80

Almond Oil—see page 767.

Aluminum

Aluminum [Al = 26.98] is the free metal in the form of finely divided powder. It may contain oleic acid or stearic acid as a lubricant. It contains not less than 95.0% of Al, and not more than 5.0% of *Acid-insoluble substances*, including any added fatty acid.

Description—A very fine, free-flowing, silvery powder free from gritty or discolored particles.

Solubility—Insoluble in water and alcohol; soluble in hydrochloric and sulfuric acids and in solutions of fixed alkali hydroxides.

Uses—A *protective*. An ingredient in *Aluminum Paste* (page 772).

Aluminum Monostearate USP

Aluminum Monostearate is a compound of aluminum with a mixture of solid organic acids obtained from fats, and consists chiefly of variable proportions of aluminum monostearate and aluminum monopalmitate. It contains the equivalent of 14.5–16.0% of Al_2O_3 (101.96).

Preparation—One method of preparing the salt is as follows. A 6% solution of stearic acid in alcohol is neutralized by adding the calculated quantity of a two per cent aqueous solution of potassium hydroxide. This hydroalcoholic solution of potassium stearate is then added, with stirring, to a 2½% aqueous solution of potassium alum. The white precipitate which forms contains free stearic acid and some aluminum distearate as well as the desired monostearate. It is washed with water until sulfate-free, then with large volumes of ethyl ether, and finally with large volumes of acetone, and then dried. The product thus obtained is still relatively crude and may be refined by boiling it with a large volume of 98% methanol and then filtering and washing the solid repeatedly with large volumes of acetone followed by ethyl ether and then acetone again. The Aluminum Monostearate thus refined melts at 195°C.

Description—Occurs as a fine, white to yellowish white, bulky powder, having a faint, characteristic odor.

Solubility—Insoluble in water, alcohol and ether.

Uses—Aluminum Monostearate is a *pharmaceutic necessity* used in the preparation of *Sterile Procaine Penicillin G with Aluminum Stearate Suspension* (see page 1229).

Strong Ammonia Solution NF

[Stronger Ammonia Water; Stronger Ammonium Hydroxide Solution; Spirit of Hartshorn]

Strong Ammonia Solution is a solution of NH_3 (17.03), containing 27.0–30.0% (*w/w*) of NH_3. Upon exposure to air it loses ammonia rapidly.

Caution—Use care in handling Strong Ammonia Solution because of the caustic nature of the Solution and the irritating properties of its vapor. Cool the container well before opening, and cover the closure with a cloth or similar material while opening. Do not taste Strong Ammonia Solution, and avoid inhalation of its vapor.

Description—A colorless, transparent liquid, having an exceedingly pungent, characteristic odor. It is miscible with alcohol. Even when well diluted it is strongly alkaline to litmus. Its specific about 0.90.

Uses—This liquid is used only for chemical and pharmaceutical purposes. It is used primarily in making ammonia water by dilution and as a chemical reagent. It is too strong for internal administration. It is an ingredient in *Aromatic Ammonia spirit* (page 868).

Barium Hydroxide Lime USP

Barium Hydroxide Lime is a mixture of barium hydroxide octahydrate and calcium hydroxide. It may contain also potassium hydroxide and may contain an indicator that is inert toward anesthetic gases such as ether, cyclopropane, and nitrous oxide, and that changes color when the Barium Hydroxide Lime no longer can absorb carbon dioxide.

Caution—Since Barium Hydroxide Lime contains a soluble form of barium, it is toxic if swallowed.

Description—White or grayish white granules. It may have a color if an indicator has been added.

Uses—See *Soda Lime*.

Boric Acid NF

[Boracic Acid; Orthoboric Acid]

Boric Acid contains 99.5–100.5% of H_3BO_3 (61.83), calculated on the dried basis.

Preparation—Lagoons of the volcanic districts of Tuscany formerly furnished the greater part of the Boric Acid and borax of commerce. Borax is now found native in California and some of the other western states; calcium and magnesium borates are found there also. Boric Acid is produced from native borax, or from the other borates, by reacting with hydrochloric or sulfuric acid.

Description—Colorless scales of a somewhat pearly luster, or crystals, but more commonly a white powder slightly unctuous to the touch. It is odorless and stable in the air. It volatilizes with steam.

Solubility—1 Gm dissolves in 18 ml of water or alcohol and 4 ml of glycerin; 1 Gm is soluble in 4 ml of boiling water and 6 ml of boiling alcohol; its solubility in water is increased by citric or tartaric acids.

Incompatibilities—In powders containing boric acid and *sodium bicarbonate*, a reaction occurs in the presence of moisture resulting in the liberation of carbon dioxide. *Water of crystallization* in another ingredient as, for example, an *alum*, may be the source of the trouble. Traces of *iron* in *boric acid* have sometimes caused a coloration when dispensed in powder mixtures containing phenol.

Trouble is sometimes experienced with prescriptions requiring the solution of more boric acid than is soluble in the specified volume. Since boric acid solutions are frequently used in the eye, it is essential that only clear solutions be dispensed. In combination with salicylic acid, boric acid is an *alkaloidal precipitant* through formation of an insoluble borosalicylate.

Uses—Boric Acid is used as a buffer, and it is this use that is officially recognized in the NF. Boric Acid is a very weak *germicide* (*local anti-infective*). However, its nonirritating properties make solutions of Boric Acid suitable for application to such delicate structures as the cornea of the eye. Aqueous solutions are employed as an eye wash, mouth wash, and for irrigation of the bladder. A 2.2% solution is isotonic with the lacrimal fluid. Solutions of Boric Acid, even if they are made isotonic, will hemolyze red blood cells. Boric Acid may also be employed as a dusting powder, when diluted with some inert material.

Although Boric Acid is innocuous when applied topically, *serious poisoning can result from oral ingestion* of as little as 5 Gm. Symptoms of Boric Acid poisoning are nausea, vomiting, abdominal pain, diarrhea, headache, and visual disturbance. The kidney may be injured and death may result. Its use as a preservative in beverages and foods is prohibited by national and state legislation. *There is always present the danger of confusing Boric Acid with dextrose when compounding milk formulas for infants. Fatal accidents have occurred.* For this reason Boric Acid in bulk is colored, so that it cannot be confused with dextrose.

Boric Acid is used to prevent discoloration of physostigmine solutions.

Dose (unofficial)—*Topically*, as required.

Calcium Hydroxide USP

[Slaked Lime; Calcium Hydrate]

Calcium Hydroxide contains 95.0–100.5% of Ca-(OH)$_2$ (74.09).

Preparation—Calcium Hydroxide is prepared by reacting freshly prepared calcium oxide with water.

Description—A white powder, possessing an alkaline, slightly bitter taste. It absorbs carbon dioxide from the air forming calcium carbonate. The solution exhibits a strong alkaline reaction.

Solubility—1 Gm dissolves in 630 ml of water and in 1300 ml of boiling water; soluble in glycerin and in syrup; insoluble in alcohol; the solubility in water is decreased by the presence of fixed alkali hydroxides.

Uses—Calcium Hydroxide is used in the preparation of *Calcium Hydroxide Solution*.

Calcium Hydroxide Solution USP

[Liquor Calcis; Lime Water; Aqua Calcariæ]

Calcium Hydroxide Solution is a solution containing, in each 100 ml, not less than 140 mg of Ca(OH)$_2$ (74.09).

Note—The solubility of calcium hydroxide varies with the temperature at which the solution is stored, being about 170 mg per 100 ml at 15°, and less at a higher temperature. The official concentration is based upon a temperature of 25°.

Preparation—Calcium Hydroxide Solution may be prepared as follows:

Calcium Hydroxide................	**3 Gm**
Purified Water...................	**1000 ml**

Add the calcium hydroxide to 1000 ml of cool, purified water, and agitate the mixture vigorously and repeatedly during 1 hour. Allow the excess of calcium hydroxide to settle. Dispense only the clear, supernatant liquid.

The undissolved portion of the mixture is not suitable for preparing additional quantities of Calcium Hydroxide Solution.

When lime water is exposed to air, which almost always contains CO_2, the calcium hydroxide is quickly converted into the insoluble carbonate.

Lime water is very extensively used in pharmacy; the object of keeping it over undissolved calcium hydroxide is to insure a saturated solution. Calcium hydroxide is but sparingly soluble in water and less soluble in hot water than in cold; when the solution is heated, a deposition of calcium hydroxide takes place which is redissolved on cooling.

Description—A clear, colorless liquid with an alkaline taste, and a strong alkaline reaction. It absorbs carbon dioxide from the air, a film of calcium carbonate forming on the surface of the liquid. When heated, it becomes turbid,

owing to the separation of calcium hydroxide, which is less soluble in hot than in cold water.

Incompatibilities—Calcium Hydroxide Solution precipitates *acetylsalicylic acid* from solution forming calcium acetylsalicylate. It precipitates most *alkaloids* from solutions of their salts. Many *metals* are precipitated as the hydroxide. *Mercuric salts* are precipitated as yellow mercuric oxide. *Calomel* is blackened by calcium hydroxide. Calcium Hydroxide Solution has the incompatibilities of the calcium salts, see *Calcium Bromide* (page 1090), and those of the hydroxides. See *Potassium Hydroxide* (page 779). For a discussion of its use in lotions and emulsions of the water-in-oil type see page 339.

Uses—This Solution is too dilute to be effective as a gastric antacid. It is employed *topically* as a *protective* in various types of lotions. The USP classes it as an *astringent*. It is often included in the diet of infants to insure adequate calcium intake.

Dose—*Topically*, in astringent solutions and lotions as required (see *Calamine Lotion*, page 770).

Veterinary Uses—Lime water is frequently used mixed with milk and fed to orphaned or young animals, and fed to dogs and cats in the treatment of *gastritis*.

Veterinary Dose—*Dogs*, 4 to 30 ml.

Calcium Pantothenate, Racemic—see page 1037.

Calcium Stearate NF

Calcium Stearate is a compound of calcium with variable proportions of stearic and palmitic acids [calcium stearate, $C_{36}H_{70}CaO_4 = 607.04$; calcium palmitate, $C_{32}H_{62}CaO_4 = 551.29$]. It contains the equivalent of 9.0–10.5% of CaO (calcium oxide).

Preparation—This insoluble soap may be prepared by precipitation from calcium chloride and the sodium salts of the mixed fatty acids (stearic and palmitic). The precipitate is collected and washed with water to remove the sodium chloride.

Description—A fine, white to yellowish white, bulky powder having a slight, characteristic odor. It is unctuous and is free from grittiness.

Solubility—Insoluble in water, alcohol, and ether.

Uses—Calcium Stearate is used as a *lubricant* in the manufacture of compressed tablets. It is also used as a conditioning agent in food and pharmaceutical products. Its virtually nontoxic nature and unctuous properties makes it ideal for these purposes.

Calcium Stearate is also used for waterproofing fabrics, cement, stucco, and explosives; as a releasing agent for plastic molding powders; as a stabilizer for polyvinyl chloride resins; as a lubricant; and in pencils and wax crayons.

Calcium Sulfate NF

[Gypsum; Terra Alba]

Calcium Sulfate is anhydrous [$CaSO_4 = 136.14$] or contains 2 molecules of water of hydration [$CaSO_4 \cdot 2H_2O = 172.17$]. When dried at 250° to constant weight, it contains 99.0–101.0% of $CaSO_4$.

Preparation—Calcium Sulfate may be prepared from natural sources or by precipitation from calcium chloride and a soluble sulfate.

Description—A fine, white to slightly yellow-white, odorless powder.

Solubility—Dissolves in diluted hydrochloric acid; slightly soluble in water (its solubility in water is increased by acids and ammonium chloride).

Uses—Calcium Sulfate is used as a *diluent* in the manufacture of compressed tablets. It is sufficiently inert that few undesirable reactions occur in tablets made with this substance. It is also used for making plaster casts and supports.

Industrial uses of Calcium Sulfate include the manufacture of artificial marble and plaster of paris; as a white pigment, filter or glaze in paints, enamels, pharmaceuticals, paper, insecticide dusts, water treatment, polishing powders, etc.

Carnauba Wax USP

Carnauba Wax is obtained from the leaves of *Copernicia cerifera* Mart. (Fam. *Palmae*).

Preparation—The wax consists chiefly of *myricyl cerotate* with smaller quantities of *myricyl alcohol, ceryl alcohol*, and *cerotic acid*. It is obtained by treating the leaf buds and leaves of *Copernicia cerifera*, the so-called *Brazilian Wax Palm*, with hot water.

Description—A light-brown to pale yellow, moderately coarse powder, possessing a characteristic bland odor, and free from rancidity. Its specific gravity is about 0.99. It melts between 81° and 86°.

Solubility—Insoluble in water; freely soluble in warm benzene; soluble in warm chloroform and toluene; slightly soluble in boiling alcohol.

Uses—Carnauba Wax is a pharmaceutic aid used as a *polishing agent* in the manufacture of tablets.

Cellulose Acetate Phthalate USP

Cellulose Acetate Phthalate is a reaction product of phthalic anhydride and a partial acetate ester of cellulose. When dried at 105° for 2 hours, it contains 19.0–23.5% of acetyl (C_2H_3O) groups and 30.0–36.0% of 36.0% of phthalyl (*o*-carboxybenzoyl, $C_8H_5O_3$) groups, calculated on the acid-free basis.

Preparation—Cellulose is esterified by treatment with acetic and phthalic acid anhydrides.

Description—A free-flowing, white powder. It may have a slight odor of acetic acid.

Solubility—Insoluble in water and alcohol; soluble in acetone and dioxane.

Uses—Cellulose Acetate Phthalate is used as an *enteric tablet coating material*. Coatings of this substance disintegrate due to the hydrolytic effect of the intestinal esterases, even when the intestinal contents are acid. *In vitro* studies indicate that Cellulose Acetate Phthalate will withstand the action of artificial gastric juices for long periods of time, but will readily disintegrate in artificial intestinal juices. Tablets coated with this material may be sealed with wax to improve water impermeability.

Cherry Juice USP

[Succus Cerasi]

Cherry Juice is the liquid expressed from the fresh ripe fruit of *Prunus cerasus* Linné (Fam. *Rosaceæ*). It contains not less than 1.0% of malic acid [$C_4H_6O_5$ = 134.09].

Preparation—Coarsely crush washed, stemmed, unpitted, sour cherries in a grinder so as to break the pits but not mash the kernels. Dissolve 0.1% of benzoic acid in the mixture, and allow it to stand at room temperature (possibly for several days) until a small portion of the filtered juice remains clear when mixed with one-half of its volume of alcohol and the resulting solution does not become cloudy within 30 minutes. Then press the juice from the mixture, and filter it.

Description—A clear liquid with an aromatic, characteristic odor, and a sour taste. It is affected by light. The color of the freshly prepared Juice is red to reddish orange. The pH is between 3.0 and 4.0, the refractive index is not less than 1.3500, and the specific gravity is between 1.045 and 1.075.

Uses—Cherry Juice is used to prepare *Cherry Syrup* (page 1339).

Citric Acid USP

$$CH_2.COOH$$
$$|$$
$$HO.C.COOH$$
$$|$$
$$CH_2.COOH$$

Citric Acid is anhydrous [$C_6H_8O_7$ = 192.13] or contains one molecule of water of hydration [$C_6H_8O_7.H_2O$ = 210.14]. It contains 99.5–100.5% of $C_6H_8O_7$, calculated on the anhydrous basis.

History—This Acid was first isolated from lemon juice by the famous Swedish pharmacist Scheele in 1784, after having discovered, in the preceding decade, several organic acids, among them lactic and tartaric acids.

Preparation—Citric Acid is found in many plants. It was formerly solely obtained from the juice of limes and lemons by a simple process, but one requiring careful manipulation. The boiling juice is first completely saturated with calcium carbonate (chalk or whiting) in fine powder, and the calcium citrate formed is allowed to subside. This is then washed repeatedly with water, and is then decomposed by dilute sulfuric acid. Insoluble calcium sulfate is precipitated, and the liberated citric acid remains in solution. This is carefully concentrated under reduced pressure and the solution transferred to other vessels to cool and crystallize.

Citric acid has been produced in considerable quantities in Hawaii from damaged or otherwise unusable "cull" pineapples.

Since about 1925 increasing quantities of the acid have been produced by fermentation of sucrose solution including molasses, by fungi belonging to the *Aspergillus niger* group. This process, often referred to as the *synthetic* process, was developed in this country, and now most of the acid used here as well as in many other countries is produced by this process. Theoretically the reaction proceeds as follows:

$$C_{12}H_{22}O_{11} + 3O_2 \rightarrow 2H_3C_6H_5O_7 + 3H_2O$$
Sucrose   Oxygen   Citric Acid   Water

but in practice there are deviations from this stoichiometric relationship. Many factors have to be taken into consideration and many precautions must be observed, such as careful selection of fungi, proper preparation of a nutrient medium containing small quantities of various inorganic salts, adjustment of the initial hydrogen ion concentration, prevention of contamination by other organisms, etc.

Citric acid contains one molecule of water of crystallization; it differs in this respect from tartaric acid, which contains none. The presence of this molecule of water of crystallization makes it valuable in the preparation of granular effervescent salts.

Description—Colorless, translucent crystals, or a white, granular to fine crystalline powder. It is odorless and has a strongly acid taste. The hydrous form of the Acid effloresces in moderately dry air, but is slightly deliquescent in moist air. It loses its water of crystallization at about 50°. Dilute aqueous solutions of Citric Acid are subject to molding (fermentation), oxalic acid being one of the fermentation products.

Solubility—1 Gm dissolves in 0.5 ml of water, 2 ml of alcohol, and about 30 ml of ether; freely soluble in methanol.

Incompatibilities—Citric acid reacts with *calcium* and *strontium* salts to produce sparingly soluble calcium citrate and strontium citrate. See also *Potassium Citrate* (page 872).

Uses—Citric Acid in solution is often used as a substitute for lemon juice. It is sometimes called *"salt of lemon"* which has led to confusion with some toxic oxalates which are also called by that name. When any inquiry is made for salt of lemon, its proposed use should be carefully investigated and in dispensing it the true name also should be placed upon the label.

Citric Acid is also known as *"sour salt,"* and is sold in small cartons bearing that label for use by Jewish cooks in preparing certain sour dishes. The dose is from 0.3 to 2 Gm (5 to 30 gr). It is rarely given in its free state, but is largely used in combination, in many solutions and syrups, and in making effervescent salts. Its aqueous solution, even when concentrated, is not very stable, as it develops fungoid growths.

Denatonium Benzoate NF

[Benzyldiethyl[(2,6-xylylcarbamoyl)methyl]ammonium Benzoate]

Denatonium Benzoate, dried at 105° for 2 hours, contains 99.5–101.0% of $C_{28}H_{34}N_2O_3$ (446.59).

Preparation—2-(Diethylamino)-2',6'-xylidide is quaternized by reaction with benzyl chloride. The quaternary chloride is then treated with methanolic potassium hydroxide to form the quaternary base which, after filtering off the KCl, is reacted with benzoic acid. The starting xylidide may be prepared by condensing 2,6-xylidine with chloroacetyl chloride and condensing the resulting chloroacetoxylidide with diethylamine. US Pat. 3,080,327.

Description—A white, odorless, crystalline powder. It has an intensely bitter taste. It melts between 166° and 170°.

Solubility—Soluble in water; freely soluble in alcohol and chloroform; sparingly soluble in acetone; practically insoluble in ether.

Uses—Denatonium Benzoate is used as a *denaturant* for ethyl alcohol.

Dextrose USP

[Anhydrous Dextrose; Dextrose Monohydrate; Glucose; D(+)-Glucose; α-D(+)-Glucopyranose; Medicinal Glucose; Purified Glucose; Grape Sugar; Bread Sugar; Cerelose; Starch Sugar; Corn Sugar]

Dextrose is a sugar usually obtained by the hydrolysis of starch. It contains one molecule of water of hydration [$C_6H_{12}O_6 \cdot H_2O$ = 198.17] or is anhydrous [$C_6H_{12}O_6$ = 180.16]. For the structure, see page 470.

Preparation—See *Liquid Glucose* (page 1367).

Description—Colorless crystals or a white, crystalline or granular powder. It is odorless, and has a sweet taste. Its specific rotation (anhydrous) is +52.5° to +53°. The attainment of constant rotation is hastened by boiling the solution, and is effected at once by the addition of a small quantity of ammonia or caustic soda. Hence in preparing the solutions of dextrose or lactose for determining their specific rotation the USP directs the addition of 0.2 ml of ammonia TS so that the rotation will become constant at once. Anhydrous dextrose melts at 146°. Dextrose slowly reduces alkaline cupric tartrate TS in the cold and rapidly on heating, producing a red precipitate of cuprous oxide (difference from *sucrose*).

Solubility—1 Gm dissolves in about 1 ml of water and about 100 ml of alcohol; more soluble in boiling water and boiling alcohol.

Uses—See *Dextrose Injection* (page 844). It is also used, instead of lactose, as a supplement to milk for infant feeding.

Dichlorodifluoromethane NF

CCl_2F_2

Dichlorodifluoromethane is CCl_2F_2 (120.91).

Preparation—Carbon tetrachloride is reacted with antimony trifluoride in the presence of antimony pentafluoride.

Description—A clear, colorless gas having a faint, ethereal odor. Its vapor pressure at 25° is about 4883 mm of mercury.

Uses—Dichlorodifluoromethane is used as a *propellant* (No. 12, see page 1736) in aerosols.

Dichlorotetrafluoroethane NF

$CClF_2CClF_2$

Dichlorotetrafluoroethane [$C_2Cl_2F_4$ = 170.92] is 1,2-dichlorotetrafluoroethane.

Preparation—Dichlorotetrafluoroethane may be prepared by reacting 1,1,2-trichloro-1,2,2-trifluoroethane with antimony trifluorodichloride [SbF_3Cl_2] whereupon one of the 1-chlorine atoms is replaced by fluorine. The starting trichlorotrifluoroethane may be prepared from hexachloroethane by treatment with SbF_3Cl_2. Henne, A. L., *Org. Reactions* II, 65 (1944).

Description—A clear, colorless gas having a faint, ethereal odor. Its vapor pressure at 25° is about 1621 mm of mercury. It usually contains 6–10% of its isomer, $CFCl_2$—CF_3.

Uses—Dichlorotetrafluoroethane is used as a *propellant* (No. 114 and 114a, see page 1736) in aerosols.

Ethylcellulose NF

Ethylcellulose is an ethyl ether of cellulose containing 44.0–51.0% of ethoxy [$-OC_2H_5$ = 45.06] groups, calculated on the dried basis. The viscosity of a 5% (*w/w*) solution of medium-grade Ethylcellulose, containing less than 46.5% of ethoxy ($-OC_2H_5$) groups, in a mixture of 60 parts of toluene and 40 parts of alcohol, by weight, is 90.0–110.0% of that stated on the label in centipoises. The viscosity of a 5% (*w/w*) solution of standard-grade Ethylcellulose, containing 46.5% or more of ethoxy ($-OC_2H_5$) groups, in a mixture of 80 parts of toluene and 20 parts of alcohol, by weight, is 90.0–110.0% of that stated on the label in centipoises, with the exception that the 7-centipoise viscosity grade may vary between 6.0 and 8.0 centipoises and the 4-centipoise viscosity grade may vary between 3.0 and 5.5 centipoises.

Preparation—Ethylcellulose is prepared by the same general procedure described on page 1345 for *Methylcellulose* except that ethyl chloride or ethyl sulfate is employed as the alkylating agent. The 45 to 50% of ethoxy groups in the official ethylcellulose corresponds to from 2.25 to 2.61 ethoxy groups per $C_6H_{10}O_5$ unit, thus representing from 75 to 87% of the maximum theoretical ethoxylation which is three ethoxy groups per $C_6H_{10}O_5$ unit.

Description—It occurs as a free flowing white powder. It forms films that have a refractive index of about 1.47. Its aqueous suspensions are neutral to litmus.

Solubility—The medium type is freely soluble in cyclohexane, methyl acetate, chloroform, and mixtures of aromatic hydrocarbons with alcohol; the standard type is freely soluble in alcohol, methanol, toluene, chloroform, and ethyl acetate; both types are insoluble in water, glycerin, and propylene glycol.

Uses—Ethylcellulose is used as a *pharmaceutic necessity*.

Gelatin—see page 1345.

Liquid Glucose USP

[Glucose; Starch Syrup; Corn Syrup]

Liquid Glucose is a product obtained by the incomplete hydrolysis of starch. It consists chiefly of dextrose [D(+) glucose, $C_6H_{12}O_6 = 180.16$] dextrins, maltose, and water.

Preparation—Liquid Glucose is obtained commercially by the action of very weak sulfuric acid or hydrochloric acid on starch.

One of the processes for the manufacture of glucose is as follows: The starch, usually from corn, is mixed with 5 times its weight of water containing less than 1% of hydrochloric acid, the mixture is heated to about 45°, and then transferred to a suitable lead-lined vessel into which steam is passed under pressure until the temperature reaches 120°. The temperature is maintained at this point for about an hour, or until tests show the complete disappearance of starch. The mass is then heated to volatilize most of the hydrochloric acid, sodium carbonate or calcium carbonate is added to neutralize the remaining traces of acid, the liquid is filtered, then decolorized in charcoal or boneblack filters, as is done in sugar refining, and finally concentrated in vacuum to the desired consistency.

Liquid Glucose, when made by the above process, contains about 30 to 40% of dextrose mixed with about an equal proportion of dextrin, together with small amounts of other carbohydrates, notably maltose. By varying the conditions of hydrolysis, the relative proportions of the sugars also vary.

If the crystallizable dextrose is desired, the conversion temperature is higher and the time of conversion longer. The term "glucose" as customarily used in the chemical or pharmaceutical literature usually refers to dextrose, the crystallizable product.

Dextrose can be obtained as a hydrate in small and laminated crystals from aqueous solution, and in anhydrous form in hard crystalline masses either from alcoholic solution or from very concentrated aqueous solution. It is less sweet than cane sugar. It is also less soluble in water, and much more soluble in alcohol. Strong mineral acids hardly act on dextrose, but rapidly destroy cane sugar. On the other hand, dextrose is destroyed by alkalies, whereas cane sugar forms definite compounds with alkalies called *sucrates*. When dissolved in water and subjected to prolonged ebullition, dextrose undergoes very little alteration. It is dextrorotatory in aqueous solution and is capable of undergoing vinous fermentation directly, without passing through any intermediate state.

The name "grape sugar" is sometimes applied to the solid commercial form of dextrose because the principal sugar of the grape is dextrose, although the fruit has never been used as a source of the commercial supply.

Description—A colorless or yellowish, thick, syrupy liquid. It is odorless, or nearly so, and has a sweet taste. Liquid glucose differs from sucrose in that it readily reduces hot alkaline cupric tartrate TS producing a red precipitate of cuprous oxide.

Solubility—Miscible with water; sparingly soluble in alcohol.

Uses—Liquid Glucose is used officially as a *diluent* in pilular extracts; commercially it has replaced glycerin in many pharmaceutical preparations. It is sometimes given *per rectum* as a *food* in cases where feeding by stomach is impossible. It should not be used in the place of dextrose for intravenous injection. It is a *pharmaceutic necessity* for *Cocoa Syrup* (page 1339).

Hydrochloric Acid USP

[Chlorhydric Acid; Muriatic Acid; Spirit of Salt]

Hydrochloric Acid contains 35.0–38.0%, by weight, of HCl (36.46).

History—This acid was first prepared commercially by Glauber in the 17th century by distilling sea salt with sulfuric acid, hence the name *spirit of salt* by which it was known for many years. Another common name for this acid is *muriatic acid*, meaning the acid from salt, the word *murea* being the Latin word for salt.

Preparation—Hydrochloric Acid is produced by the interaction of sodium chloride and sulfuric acid or by combining chlorine with hydrogen. It is obtained as a byproduct in the manufacture of sodium carbonate from sodium chloride by the Leblanc process in which common salt is decomposed with sulfuric acid. Sodium sulfate is formed, and hydrogen chloride gas is liberated. The latter is conducted into a tall tower filled with coke, called a coke scrubber, the ascending gas being met by a descending flow of water, which readily dissolves the gas.

Hydrochloric acid is also a by-product in the electrolytic production of sodium hydroxide from sodium chloride. The liberated chlorine is converted to hydrochloric acid either by heating with steam to 1000° (1832°F), in the presence of an excess of carbon or by directly combining it with hydrogen, which is also obtained in the electrolytic production of sodium hydroxide. Important quantities of hydrochloric acid also result as a byproduct in operations involving chlorination of hydrocarbons such as benzene.

The yellow color of the technical acid is due to the presence of traces of ferric iron. This grade of acid (muriatic) is used for soldering and is sometimes called for by plumbers and tinsmiths under the very old name of *spirit of salt*.

Description—A colorless, fuming liquid having a pungent odor. The fumes and odor disappear when it is diluted with 2 volumes of water. It is strongly acid to litmus even when highly diluted. Its specific gravity is about 1.18. It is miscible with water or alcohol.

Hydrochloric Acid is one of the strongest acids, being more highly ionized in aqueous solutions than most other acids. It attacks many metals with the evolution of hydrogen.

When diluted hydrochloric acid is boiled (see *Nitric Acid* also) a weak acid distils over first, and when a concentrated acid is boiled, chiefly hydrogen chloride gas is expelled first; in both cases an acid containing (when distilled at 760 mm) 20.2% HCl remains ultimately in the still, and this distils unchanged (azeotropic mixture) at 110° and has a specific gravity of 1.097 at 25°. This acid is usually designated *constant boiling hydrochloric acid.*

The white fumes, produced when the acid is exposed to the air, are caused by the gaseous acid dissolving in moisture in the air, to form visible droplets of solution, and also reacting with a trace of ammonia usually present, forming ammonium chloride.

Incompatibilities—Hydrochloric Acid presents the incompatibilities characteristic of the *Inorganic Acids* (page 1481). The chloride ion is precipitated by *lead* and *silver salts*. *Oxidizing agents* such as *potassium chlorate* liberate chlorine from hydrochloric acid and acidified solutions of chlorides.

Uses—This acid is a *pharmaceutic necessity* for preparing *Diluted Hydrochloric Acid* (page 795).

Hydroxypropyl Methylcellulose NF

[Propylene Glycol Ether of Methylcellulose]

Hydroxypropyl Methylcellulose is the propylene glycol ether of methylcellulose. The proportions of its hydroxypropyl and methyl groups, which are attached to the anhydroglucose rings of cellulose by ether linkages, may be varied to produce a range of characteristic properties. Hydroxypropyl Methylcellulose, previously dried at 105° for 2 hours, contains 19.0–30.0% of methoxy ($-OCH_3$), and 3.0–12.0% of hydroxypropoxy ($-OC_3H_6OH$). The viscosity of a solution containing 2 Gm of Hydroxypropyl Methylcellulose in each 100 Gm of solution is 80.0–120.0% of that stated on the label for viscosity types of 100 centipoises or less, and 75.0–140.0% of that stated on the label for viscosity types higher than 100 centipoises.

Preparation—Hydroxypropyl Methylcellulose may be prepared by direct hydroxypropylation of the appropriate grade of methylcellulose. The procedure is analogous to that described under *Methylcellulose*, page 1345, using 3-hydroxypropyl chloride as the subsequent halide for the additional condensation.

Description—It occurs as a white, fibrous or granular powder.

Solubility—Swells in water and produces a clear to opalescent, viscous, colloidal solution; insoluble in anhydrous alcohol, ether, and chloroform.

Uses—Hydroxypropyl Methylcellulose is used as a *suspending agent.*

Hypophosphorous Acid NF

Hypophosphorous Acid contains 30.0–32.0% of HPH_2O_2 (66.00).

Preparation—Hypophosphorous Acid is made by reacting calcium hypophosphite with sulfuric acid. To utilize fully the calcium hypophosphite, a slight excess of sulfuric acid is used which can be removed by the addition of barium hydroxide or carbonate. The acid obtained in this manner contains a small quantity of calcium sulfate. A purer acid is obtained by using barium hypophosphite instead of the calcium salt.

Description—A colorless or slightly yellow, odorless liquid. Its solution is acid to litmus even when highly

diluted. Its specific gravity is about 1.13. It is miscible with water or alcohol.

Incompatibilities—Hypophosphorous Acid is oxidized on exposure to air and by nearly all *oxidizing agents*. *Mercury, silver,* and *bismuth salts* are reduced partially to the metallic state as evidenced by a darkening in color. *Ferric compounds* are changed to ferrous.

Uses—Hypophosphorous Acid is used as a reducing agent in the formerly official Ferrous Iodide Syrup and in diluted hydriodic acid to prevent discoloration through the oxidation of the iodides by air. It is used to assist in the solution of the hypophosphites, especially calcium hypophosphite, in Compound Hypophosphites Syrup NF X (RPS-13, page 445). In addition to the official acid, a 50% acid is also available on the market.

Iron—see page 827.

Isopropyl Myristate

$$CH_3(CH_2)_{12}COOCH(CH_3)_2$$

Isopropyl Myristate is $C_{17}H_{34}O_2$ (270.46).

Preparation—Isopropyl Myristate may be prepared by reacting myristoyl chloride with isopropanol with the aid of a suitable dehydrochlorinating agent.

Description—A liquid of low viscosity that is practically odorless. It solidifies at about +3° and decomposes at 208°. It withstands oxidation and does not readily become rancid.

Solubility—Soluble in alcohol, acetone, chloroform, ethyl acetate, toluene, mineral oil, castor oil, and cottonseed oil; practically insoluble in water, glycerol, and propylene glycol; dissolves many waxes, cholesterol, and lanolin.

Uses—Isopropyl Myristate is used in cosmetics and topical medicinal preparations to enhance absorption through the skin.

Kaolin—see page 811.

Lactic Acid USP

[2-Hydroxypropionic Acid; Propanoloic Acid; Milk Acid]

Lactic Acid is a mixture of lactic acid ($C_3H_6O_3$) and lactic anhydride ($C_6H_{10}O_5$) equivalent to a total of 85.0–90.0%, by weight, of $C_3H_6O_3$ (90.08).

History—Lactic Acid, discovered by Scheele in 1780, is the acid formed in the souring of milk, hence the name *lactic*, from the Latin name for milk. It results from the decomposition of the lactose (milk sugar) in milk. This acid is also the acid present in sauerkraut and in pickled cucumbers.

Preparation—A solution of glucose or of starch previously hydrolyzed with diluted sulfuric acid is inoculated after the addition of suitable nitrogen compounds and mineral salts, with *Bacillus lactis*. Calcium carbonate is also added to neutralize the lactic acid as soon as it is formed, otherwise the fermentation stops when the amount of acid exceeds 0.5%. When the fermentation is complete, as indicated by failure of the liquid to give a test for glucose with Fehling's solution, the solution is filtered, and the filtrate is concentrated and allowed to stand. The calcium lactate that crystallizes out is decomposed with dilute sulfuric acid and filtered with charcoal. The lactic acid in the filtrate is extracted with ethyl or isopropyl ether, then the ether is distilled off and the aqueous solution of the acid concentrated under reduced pressures.

Other sources and methods for the manufacture of this Acid have been proposed from time to time but they are apparently not as economical as this.

Description—A colorless or yellowish, nearly odorless, syrupy liquid. It is acid to litmus. It absorbs water on exposure to moist air. When a dilute solution of Lactic Acid is concentrated to above 50%, lactic anhydride begins to form. In the official acid the anhydride amounts to about 12 to 15%. The specific gravity of Lactic Acid is about 1.206. The Acid decomposes when distilled under normal pressure but may be distilled without decomposition under reduced pressure.

Solubility—Miscible with water, alcohol, and ether; insoluble in chloroform.

Uses—Lactic Acid has a limited usefulness as a *spermatocide*. It is usually incorporated in a jelly base in the concentration of 1 to 2%. It is also used in baby milk formulas and as an *acidulant* in other food preparations. Technical grades, containing 22 to 50% of the acid are used in textile and leather manufacture.

Lactose USP

[4-*o*-β-D-Galactopyranosyl-α-D-glucose; Saccharum Lactis; Milk Sugar]

Lactose is a sugar obtained from milk. It is anhydrous $[C_{12}H_{22}O_{11} = 342.30]$ or contains one molecule of water of hydration $[C_{12}H_{22}O_{11}.H_2O = 360.32]$.

For the structural formula, see page 470.

Preparation—Sugar of milk is prepared by the addition of diluted hydrochloric acid to skim milk to precipitate the casein. After the removal of the casein by filtration, the reaction of the whey is adjusted to a pH of about 6.2 by the addition of lime and the remaining albuminous matter is coagulated by heating; this is filtered out and the liquid set aside to crystallize. Animal charcoal is used to decolorize the solution in a manner similar to that used in purifying sucrose.

Another form of lactose, known as *β-lactose*, is also available on the market. It differs in that the D-glucose moiety is β instead of α. It is reported that this variety is sweeter and more soluble than ordinary lactose and for that reason is preferable in pharmaceutical manufacturing where lactose is used. Chemically, β-lactose does not appear to differ from ordinary α-lactose. It is manufactured in the same way as α-lactose up to the point of crystallization, then the solution is heated to a temperature above 93.5° this being the temperature at which the *alpha* form is converted to the *beta* variety. The *beta* form occurs only as an anhydrous sugar whereas the *alpha* variety may be obtained either in the anhydrous form or as a monohydrate.

Description—White, hard, crystalline masses or a white powder. It is odorless, and has a faintly sweet taste. It is stable in air, but readily absorbs odors. Its solutions are neutral to litmus. The specific rotation of Lactose is between +54.8° and +55.5° when determined in a solution containing 10 Gm of Lactose previously dried to constant weight at 80°, and 0.2 ml of ammonia TS in each 100 ml of solution, using a 200-mm tube. See *Dextrose*.

Solubility—1 Gm dissolves in 5 ml of water and 2.6 ml of boiling water; very slightly soluble in alcohol; insoluble in chloroform or ether.

Uses—Lactose is a *diluent* largely used in medicine and pharmacy. Lactose is generally an ingredient of the medium used in penicillin production. It is extensively used as an addition to milk for infant feeding. It is an ingredient in *Compound Iodochlorhydroxyquin Powder*.

Magnesium Stearate—see page 763.

Meglumine USP

[1-Deoxy-1-(methylamino)glucitol; *N*-Methylglucamine]

$$HOCH_2-\overset{\overset{\displaystyle H}{|}}{\underset{\underset{\displaystyle OH}{|}}{C}}-\overset{\overset{\displaystyle H}{|}}{\underset{\underset{\displaystyle OH}{|}}{C}}-\overset{\overset{\displaystyle OH}{|}}{\underset{\underset{\displaystyle H}{|}}{C}}-\overset{\overset{\displaystyle H}{|}}{\underset{\underset{\displaystyle OH}{|}}{C}}-CH_2NHCH_3$$

Meglumine contains 99.0–100.5% of $C_7H_{17}NO_5$ (195.22), calculated on the dried basis.

Preparation—Meglumine may be prepared by treating glucose with hydrogen and methylamine under pressure and in the presence of Raney nickel.

Description—White to faintly yellowish white, odorless crystals or powder. It melts between 128° and 132°.

Solubility—Freely soluble in water; sparingly soluble in alcohol.

Uses—Meglumine is used in forming salts of certain pharmaceuticals, surface-active agents, and dyes. See *Meglumine Diatrizoate Injection* (page 1307), *Meglumine Iodipamide Injection* (page 1304), and *Meglumine Iothalamate Injection* (page 1308).

Microcrystalline Cellulose NF

Microcrystalline Cellulose is purified, partially depolymerized cellulose prepared by treating alpha cellulose, obtained as a pulp from fibrous plant material, with mineral acids.

Preparation—Cellulose is subjected to the hydrolytic action of 2.5 normal hydrochloric acid at the boiling temperature of about 105° for 15 minutes whereby amorphous cellulosic material is removed and aggregates of crystalline cellulose are formed. These are collected by filtration, washed with water and aqueous ammonia, and disintegrated into small fragments, often termed cellulose crystallites, by vigorous mechanical means such as a Waring blendor. US Pat. 3,141,875.

Description—A fine, white, odorless, crystalline powder. It consists of free-flowing, nonfibrous particles which may be compressed into self-binding tablets which disintegrate rapidly in water.

Solubility—Insoluble in water, dilute acids, and most organic solvents; slightly soluble in sodium hydroxide solution (1 in 20).

Uses—Microcrystalline Cellulose is used as a combination *binder–disintegrant* in the manufacture of compressed tablets. It is also used as a separatory medium in thin-layer and column chromatography. Microcrystalline Cellulose is also of value for the stabilization and emulsification of liquid and foam systems.

Light Mineral Oil NF

[Light Liquid Petrolatum NF XII; Light Liquid Paraffin; Light White Mineral Oil]

Light Mineral Oil is a mixture of liquid hydrocarbons obtained from petroleum. It may contain a suitable stabilizer.

Description—A colorless, transparent, oily liquid, free, or nearly free, from fluorescence. It is odorless and tasteless when cold, and develops not more than a faint odor of petroleum when heated. Its specific gravity is 0.818–0.880, and it has a kinematic viscosity of not more than 37 centistokes at 37.8°.

Solubility—Insoluble in water and alcohol; miscible with most fixed oils, but not with castor oil; soluble in volatile oils.

Uses—It should never be used for internal administration because of "leakage." It was intended for use as a solvent for nasal and throat medication but such use is now generally condemned. See *Mineral Oil* (page 804).

Nitrogen USP

Nitrogen contains not less than 99.0%, by volume, of N_2 (28.01).

Preparation—See page 416.

Uses—Nitrogen is used as a diluent for medicinal gases. Pharmaceutically it is employed to replace air in the containers of substances which would be adversely affected by air oxidation. Examples include its use with fixed oils, certain vitamin preparations, and a variety of injectable products.

Persic Oil NF

[Apricot Kernel Oil; Peach Kernel Oil]

Persic Oil is the oil expressed from the kernels of varieties of *Prunus armeniaca* Linné (Apricot Kernel Oil), or from the kernels of varieties of *Prunus Persica* Sieb. et Zucc. (Peach Kernel Oil) (Fam. *Rosaceæ*).

Description—A clear, pale straw-colored or colorless, almost odorless, oily liquid with a bland taste. Its specific gravity is between 0.910 and 0.923. It is not turbid at temperatures above 15°.
Solubility—Slightly soluble in alcohol; miscible with ether, chloroform, benzene, and solvent hexane.

Uses—Persic Oil was recognized by NF XI as an alternative for expressed almond oil, in preparing Rose Water Ointment; the two oils are very similar. The current NF, however, recognizes the use of only Almond Oil. Persic Oil is a vehicle.

Phenol USP

[Carbolic Acid]

Phenol contains 99.0–100.5% of C_6H_6O (94.11), calculated on the anhydrous basis.
Preparation—This valuable product belongs to a well-marked class of phenols of which it is the prototype. For many years it was made only by distilling crude carbolic acid from coal tar and separating and purifying the distillate by repeated crystallizations, but it is now prepared synthetically. One process involves treating benzene with fuming sulfuric acid to produce benzenesulfonic acid which is then converted to its sodium salt, fused with sodium hydroxide, and acidified with hydrochloric acid. The crude phenol is purified by distillation.

A more recent process utilizes chlorobenzene as the starting point in the manufacture of Phenol. The chlorobenzene is heated with sodium hydroxide solution at a temperature of 350° to 380° and at a pressure of 5000 psi. Under these conditions the chlorine atom is replaced by the —ONa group, producing sodium phenolate from which Phenol is obtained by acidification. Because of the possibility of forming other derivatives, careful control of the details of the process must be observed.

When perfectly pure, Phenol is devoid of the odor of cresol, but it has a peculiar, aromatic odor, which is not disagreeable.

Description—Colorless to light pink, interlaced, or separate, needle-shaped crystals, or a white or light pink, crystalline mass. It has a characteristic odor. When undiluted, it whitens and cauterizes the skin and mucous membranes. When gently heated, Phenol melts, forming a highly refractive liquid. It is liquefied by the addition of 10% of water. Its vapor is flammable. Phenol gradually darkens on exposure to light and air. The specific gravity of Phenol is 1.07 and it boils at 182°. It congeals at a temperature not lower than 39°.

Solubility—1 Gm dissolves in 15 ml of water; very soluble in alcohol, glycerin, chloroform, ether, and fixed and volatile oils; soluble in petrolatum and in about 70 parts of liquid petrolatum.
Incompatibilities—Phenol produces a liquid or soft mass when triturated with *camphor, menthol, acetanilid, acetophenetidin, aminopyrine, antipyrine, ethyl aminobenzoate, methenamine, phenyl salicylate, resorcinol, terpin hydrate, thymol,* and several other substances including some *alkaloids.* It also softens *theobroma oil* in suppository mixtures.

Phenol is soluble in about 15 parts of water; stronger solutions may be obtained by using as much glycerin as phenol. Only the crystallized Phenol is soluble in fixed oils and liquid petrolatum, the liquefied Phenol is not all soluble due to its content of water. *Albumin* and *gelatin* are precipitated by Phenol. *Collodion* is coagulated by the precipitation of pyroxylin. A sticky precipitate occurs in solution of *lead subacetate* but not in *lead acetate.* Phenol combines with *alkalies* to form soluble phenolates which slowly darken in color. It becomes pink in color through exposure to air; other *oxidizing agents* affect it in various ways. *Hydrogen peroxide* produces pyrocatechin, quinone, and hydroquinone; *permanganate* breaks it down to oxalic acid and carbon dioxide; *nitric acid* forms mono-, di-, or trinitrophenol; *nitrous acid* forms nitroso-phenol which finally becomes deep brown in color. Traces of *iron* in various chemicals such as *alum, borax,* etc, may produce a green color.

Uses—Phenol is *caustic,* a *disinfectant,* a *topical anesthetic,* and a pharmaceutical necessity as a *preservative* for Injections, etc. At one time widely used as a germicide and still the standard against which other antiseptics are compared, it has few legitimate uses in modern medicine. In full strength, a few drops of Liquefied Phenol may be used to cauterize small wounds, dog bites, snake bites, etc. Phenol is commonly employed as an *antipruritic,* either in the form of Phenolated Calamine Lotion (1%), Phenol Ointment (2%), or a simple aqueous solution (0.5 to 1%). Phenol has been used for sclerosing hemorrhoids, but more effective and safer drugs are available. A 5% solution in glycerin is used in simple earache. Crude carbolic acid is an effective, economical agent for disinfecting excrement. Phenol is of some therapeutic value as a *fungicide,* but more effective and less toxic agents are available.

Caution—The local application of a mixture of equal portions of Phenol and camphor, a preparation which gained wide publicity in the lay press for the treatment of *epidermophytosis* ("athlete's foot"), is potentially dangerous; serious local lesions can result, especially when it is applied to a moist skin. If accidentally spilled, Phenol should be removed promptly from the skin by swabbing with alcohol.

Liquefied Phenol USP [Liquefied Carbolic Acid] is phenol maintained in a liquid condition by the presence of 10.0% of water. It contains not less than 89.0%, by weight, of C_6H_6O. *Note—When phenol is to be mixed with a fixed oil, mineral oil, or white petrolatum, use crystalline Phenol, not*

Liquefied Phenol. Preparation: Liquefied Phenol may be prepared by the following method: Melt phenol (a convenient quantity) by placing the unstoppered container in a steam bath and applying heat gradually. Transfer the liquid to a tared vessel, weigh, add 1 Gm of purified water for each 9 Gm of phenol, and mix thoroughly. *Description:* A colorless liquid, which may develop a red tint upon exposure to air and light. It has a characteristic, somewhat aromatic odor. When undiluted it cauterizes and whitens the skin and mucous membranes. The specific gravity is about 1.065, and when it is subjected to distillation, the boiling temperature does not rise above 182°, which is the boiling temperature of Phenol. It partially solidifies at about 15°. *Solubility:* Miscible with alcohol, ether, and glycerin; a mixture of Liquefied Phenol and an equal volume of glycerin is miscible with water. *Uses:* Liquefied Phenol, a mixture of phenol 90% and purified water 10%, is a formulation which facilitates the dispensing of concentrated phenol. Its therapeutic uses are described above under Phenol. It is a *pharmaceutic necessity* for *Phenolated Calamine Lotion* (page 770).

Phenyl Salicylate—see page 1379.

Phosphoric Acid NF

[Orthophosphoric Acid; Acidum Ossium; Syrupy Phosphoric Acid; Concentrated Phosphoric Acid; Acidum Phosphoricum Solutum]

Phosphoric Acid contains 85.0–88.0%, by weight, of H_3PO_4 (98.00).

Preparation—Phosphorus is converted to phosphorus pentoxide [P_2O_5] by exposing it to a current of warm air, then the P_2O_5 is treated with water to form phosphoric acid. The conversion of the phosphorus to the pentoxide is caused to take place while the phosphorus, distilling from the phosphorus manufacturing operation, is in the vapor state.

A commercial grade of acid is made by the action of sulfuric acid on bone ash or calcium phosphate minerals. The crude acid so obtained is unfit for medicinal use unless it is properly purified.

Description—A colorless, odorless liquid of a syrupy consistency. Its specific gravity is about 1.71.

Phosphoric Acid of about 88% will frequently crystallize on prolonged cooling, the crystals having the composition $H_3PO_4.\frac{1}{2}H_2O$. The aqueous acid can be dehydrated by heating at 150°. At about 200° the acid gradually changes to pyrophosphoric acid, and at higher temperature it passes into metaphosphoric acid. The concentrated acid attacks porcelain when heated in it.

Phosphoric acid forms three series of salts: (1) *acid phosphates, biphosphates, monobasic phosphates,* or *primary phosphates* in which only one of the hydrogens is replaced by metal; (2) when two of the hydrogens are replaced by metal, the resulting salts are known as *dibasic phosphates* or *secondary phosphates;* these are often also referred to simply as *phosphates;* and (3) when all the three hydrogens are substituted by metals, *tribasic phosphates,* also known as *tertiary phosphates,* are formed. The monobasic alkali and alkaline earth phosphates are soluble in water and the solutions are acid to litmus and to phenolphthalein TS but neutral or only slightly acid to methyl orange. Dibasic and tribasic phosphates of all metals, excepting the alkali metals and ammonium, are practically insoluble in water. The soluble dibasic salts exhibit an alkaline reaction towards litmus and phenolphthalein and the tribasic alkali salts exhibit a still stronger alkaline reaction.

Solubility—Miscible with water or alcohol, with the evolution of heat.

Incompatibilities—The precipitation which sometimes occurs when phosphoric acid is mixed with *ferric chloride tincture* is generally due to the presence of pyrophosphoric acid, ferric pyrophosphate being precipitated in the form of an insoluble gelatinous precipitate.

Uses—Phosphoric Acid is used to make the diluted acid and several galenical preparations. Industrially it is used in dental cements and in beverages as an acidulant, also to rust proof metals before painting.

Diluted Phosphoric Acid NF [Dilute Phosphoric Acid] contains, in each 100 ml, 9.5–10.5 Gm of H_3PO_4 (98.00). *Preparation:* Diluted Phosphoric Acid may be prepared as follows: Mix phosphoric acid (69 ml) and purified water (qs) to make 1000 ml. *Description:* A clear, colorless, odorless liquid. Its specific gravity is about 1.057. It is miscible with water and alcohol. *Uses:* Diluted Phosphoric Acid is used as a *pharmaceutic necessity*. It has also been employed in *lead poisoning* and in other conditions in which it is desired to administer large amounts of phosphate and at the same time produce a mild acidosis. It is given in the dose of 60 ml daily (5 ml per hour) under carefully controlled conditions.

Potassium Phosphate, Monobasic—see page 1372.

Pumice NF

[Pumex]

Pumice is a substance of volcanic origin, consisting chiefly of complex silicates of aluminum, potassium, and sodium.

Description—Very light, hard, rough, porous, grayish masses or a gritty, grayish powder of several grades of fineness. Pumice is odorless, tasteless, and is stable in the air.

Solubility—Insoluble in water and is not attacked by acids or alkali hydroxide solutions.

The N. F. describes three powders:

Pumice Flour or *Superfine Pumice*—Not less than 97% passes through a No. 200 standard mesh sieve.

Fine Pumice—Not less than 95% passes through a No. 150 standard mesh sieve, and not more than 75% passes through a No. 200 standard mesh sieve.

Coarse Pumice—Not less than 95% passes through a No. 60 standard mesh sieve, and not more than 5% passes through a No. 200 standard mesh sieve.

Uses—Pumice is used as a *filtering* and *distributing medium* for pharmaceutical preparations. Industrially, it is used as an *abrasive* in metal polishes. It is also used in fireproofing and insulating materials. Because of its grittiness, powdered Pumice is used in certain types of soaps and cleaning powders and also as a *dental abrasive*.

Pyroxylin USP

[Soluble Guncotton]

Pyroxylin is a product obtained by the action of a mixture of nitric and sulfuric acids on cotton, and consists chiefly of cellulose tetranitrate [$(C_{12}H_{16}N_4O_{18})_n$].

Note—Pyroxylin available commercially is moistened with about 30% of alcohol or other suitable solvent. The alcohol or solvent must be allowed to evaporate from the Pyroxylin to yield the dried substance described in the Pharmacopeia. Pyroxylin moistened with alcohol or other solvent may be used in the tests set forth in the USP monograph, provided the weight of sample taken corresponds to the specified amount of dry Pyroxylin.

Preparation—Shönbein, in 1846, found that nitric acid acts on cotton and produces a soluble compound. It was subsequently proved that this substance, pyroxylin, or guncotton, belongs to a series of closely related nitrates in which the nitric acid radical replaces the hydroxyl of the cellulose formula. This is usually indicated by taking the double empirical formula for cellulose $C_{12}H_{20}O_{10}$ and indicating replacement of four of the OH groups thus:

$$C_{12}H_{20}O_{10} + 4HNO_3 \rightarrow C_{12}H_{16}O_6(NO_3)_4 + 4H_2O$$

Cellulose   Cellulose Tetranitrate

The pyroxylin used in preparing collodion is a varying mixture of the di-, tri-, tetra-, and pentanitrates, but is mainly tetranitrate. The hexanitrate is the true explosive guncotton, and is insoluble in ether, alcohol, acetone, or water.

Description—A light yellow, matted mass of filaments, resembling raw cotton in appearance, but harsh to the touch. *It is exceedingly flammable*, burning, when unconfined, very rapidly and with a luminous flame. When kept in well-closed bottles and exposed to light, it is decomposed with the evolution of nitrous vapors, leaving a carbonaceous residue.

Solubility—Insoluble in water; dissolves slowly but completely in 25 parts of a mixture of 3 volumes of ether and 1 volume of alcohol; soluble in acetone and glacial acetic acid, and is precipitated from these solutions by water.

Uses—Pyroxylin is a *pharmaceutic necessity* for *Collodion* (page 764). It has been used extensively by film manufacturers as the base upon which the sensitized emulsion is spread. It is now replaced to a great extent by cellulose acetate. The composition known as *celluloid*, which was once employed so largely for useful and ornamental articles, was made from Pyroxylin and camphor heated together under pressure.

Raspberry Juice USP

[Succus Rubi Idæi]

Raspberry Juice is the liquid expressed from the fresh ripe fruit of varieties of *Rubus idæus* Linné or of *Rubus strigosus* Michaux (Fam. *Rosaceæ*).

Raspberry Juice contains not less than 1.5% of acids calculated as citric acid [$C_6H_8O_7 . H_2O = 210.14$].

Preparation—It may be prepared as follows:

Express the juice from the washed, well-drained, fresh, ripe red raspberries. Dissolve 0.1% of benzoic acid in the expressed juice and allow it to stand at room temperature (possibly for several days) until a small portion of the filtered juice produces a clear solution when mixed with one-half of its volume of alcohol, the solution remaining clear for not less than 30 minutes. Strain the juice from the mixture or filter it, if necessary.

Description—A clear liquid with an aromatic, characteristic odor and a characteristic, sour taste. The freshly prepared juice is red to reddish orange. It is affected by light. Its specific gravity is between 1.025 and 1.045 and its pH is between 2.7 and 3.8. Its refractive index is not less than 1.3445.

Uses—Raspberry Juice is used in the preparation of *Raspberry Syrup USP* (page 1340), a *flavored vehicle*.

Monobasic Potassium Phosphate NF

[Potassium Biphosphate; Potassium Acid Phosphate; Potassium Dihydrogen Phosphate; Monopotassium Phosphate; Sorensen's Potassium Phosphate]

Monobasic Potassium Phosphate, dried at 105° for 4 hours, contains 98.0–100.5% of KH_2PO_4 (136.09).

Description—It occurs as colorless crystals or as a white, granular or crystalline powder. It is odorless and is stable in air. The pH of a 1 in 100 solution is about 4.5.

Solubility—Freely soluble in water; practically insoluble in alcohol.

Uses—Monobasic Potassium Phosphate is used as a component of various buffer solutions. Medicinally it has been used as a urinary acidifier.

Rosin NF

[Resina; Colophony; Georgia Pine Rosin; Yellow Pine Rosin]

Rosin is a solid resin obtained from *Pinus palustris* Miller, and from other species of *Pinus* Linné (Fam. *Pinaceæ*).

Constituents—According to a recent investigation, American rosin contains amorphous *sylvic acid* [$C_{20}H_{30}O_2$], α-, β-, and γ-*abietic acids* [$C_{20}H_{30}O_2$], γ-*pinic acid* (from which α- and β-pinic acids are gradually formed), and *resene*. Some authorities also include *pimaric acid* [$C_{20}H_{30}O_2$] as a constituent. French rosin is called *galipot*.

Description—Rosin occurs as sharply angular, translucent, amber-colored fragments, frequently covered with a yellow dust; fracture brittle at ordinary temperatures, shiny and shallow-conchoidal. The odor and taste are slightly terebinthinate. Rosin is easily fusible and burns with a dense, yellowish smoke. Specific gravity: 1.07 to 1.09.

Solubility—Freely soluble in alcohol, ether, benzene, glacial acetic acid, and fixed or volatile oils; soluble in dilute solutions of the fixed alkali hydroxides.

Uses—Rosin is a component of plasters, cerates, and ointments to which it adds adhesive qualities. Its principal industrial uses are in sizing, waterproofing, soap making, etc. Powdered Rosin is useful as an application to belts on machinery to prevent slipping.

Purified Siliceous Earth USP

[Terra Silicea Purificata; Purified Kieselguhr; Purified Infusorial Earth; Diatomaceous Earth; Diatomite]

Purified Siliceous Earth is a form of silica [SiO_2] consisting of the frustules and fragments of diatoms, purified by boiling with acid, washing, and calcining.

History and Occurrence—Large deposits of this substance are found in Virginia, Maryland, Nevada, Oregon, and California, usually in the form of masses of rocks, hundreds of feet in thickness. Under the microscope it is seen to consist largely of the minute siliceous frustules of diatoms. It must be carefully purified in a manner similar to that directed for *Talc* (page 1375), and thoroughly calcined. The latter treatment destroys the bacteria which are present in large quantities in the native earth.

Description—A very fine, amorphous, white, light gray, or pale buff, gritty powder. It absorbs about four times its weight of water without becoming fluid.

Solubility—Insoluble in water, acids, or in dilute solutions of alkali hydroxides.

Uses—Purified Siliceous Earth was introduced into the USP as a distributing and *filtering medium* for aromatic water but is better adapted for the filtration of elixirs. Like talc it may be used with no fear of its exerting an absorptive power upon active constituents. It is used in filter presses to form the *Filter-cel* sold commercially. The native infusorial earth is extensively used in metal polishing powders and pastes and as an absorbent for nitroglycerin to produce the explosive known as *dynamite*. It is difficult to obtain USP quality.

It is also used in the laboratory to test microscopes for absence of aberration; the many fine markings on the frustules of the diatoms should be sharply defined.

Colloidal Silicon Dioxide NF

Colloidal Silicon Dioxide is a submicroscopic fumed silica prepared by the vapor-phase hydrolysis of a silicon compound. It contains 99.0–100.5% of SiO_2 (60.09), calculated on the dried basis.

Description—It occurs as a light, white, nongritty powder of extremely fine particle size (about 15 mμ).

Solubility—Insoluble in water and acids (except hydrofluoric); dissolved by hot solutions of alkali hydroxides.

Uses—Colloidal Silicon Dioxide is used as a *tablet diluent* and as a *suspending* and *thickening agent* in pharmaceutical preparations.

Soda Lime USP

[Calx Sodica]

Soda Lime is a mixture of calcium hydroxide and sodium or potassium hydroxide or both.

It may contain an indicator that is inert toward anesthetic gases such as ether, cyclopropane, and nitrous oxide, and that changes color when the Soda Lime no longer can absorb carbon dioxide.

Description—White or grayish white granules. If an indicator is added, the Soda Lime may have a color. It absorbs carbon dioxide and water on exposure to air.

Uses—Soda Lime is neither a therapeutic nor a pharmaceutical agent. It is a *reagent for the absorption of carbon dioxide* in anesthesia machines, in oxygen therapy, and in metabolic tests. Because of the importance of the proper quality of Soda Lime for these purposes it has been made official and standardized in the USP and BP.

Sodium Carbonate USP

[Monohydrated Sodium Carbonate USP XVII]

Sodium Carbonate [$Na_2CO_3 \cdot H_2O = 124.00$] contains 99.5–100.5% of Na_2CO_3 (105.99), calculated on the anhydrous basis.

Preparation—The process for the manufacture of sodium carbonate was elaborated by Leblanc, a French apothecary, in 1784, and for over a century it supplied the civilized world with an inexpensive material for the low cost production of soap, glass, and many other necessities. Notwithstanding this great service, Leblanc died a pauper in a French asylum, due to his process having been seized by the Government during the Reign of Terror, without return or credit to the inventor. Although the *Leblanc Process* is not used in this country and is being superseded by other methods abroad, it is still interesting chemically. It consists of two steps: first, the conversion of common salt [NaCl] into sodium sulfate by heating it with sulfuric acid, and second, the decomposition of the sulfate by calcium carbonate (limestone) and charcoal (coal) at a high temperature to yield sodium carbonate and calcium sulfide. The carbonate is then leached out with water.

The *Solvay Process* for making sodium bicarbonate, given on page 793, has almost entirely replaced the Leblanc process. The bicarbonate is easily converted into carbonate by heating, and the carbon dioxide is returned to the process.

Sodium carbonate is also prepared by the electrolysis of sodium chloride, whereby sodium and chlorine are produced, the former reacting with water to produce sodium hydroxide and this solution treated with carbon dioxide to produce sodium carbonate. The process is most extensively used in localities where electric power is very cheap.

The cryolite process was also formerly used in the United States. Cryolite is a double fluoride of alumi-

num and sodium [$AlF_3 \cdot 3NaF$]. By heating it with chalk, calcium fluoride is formed, while the sodium and aluminum combine to form sodium aluminate, a weak salt, which is dissolved out by lixiviation. Carbon dioxide under pressure is passed into the solution, sodium carbonate and aluminum hydroxide are formed, and the latter, being insoluble, separates out.

Monohydrated Sodium Carbonate was first introduced into USP VIII because it is permanent in both moist and dry atmospheres, and is also free from the large amount of water of crystallization (63%), found in *sal soda* or ordinary sodium carbonate, which is the cause of the rapid efflorescence of this latter compound in a dry atmosphere. On account of its stability under variable conditions of atmospheric humidity the monohydrated salt is also preferable to the hygroscopic anhydrous product.

The monohydrated form is made by crystallizing a concentrated solution of sodium carbonate at a temperature above 35° (95°F), and stirring the liquid so as to produce small crystals. It contains about 15% of water of crystallization.

Soda ash is a term designating a commercial quality of anhydrous sodium carbonate. Its annual production is very large, and it enjoys a wide variety of applications, among which are the manufacture of glass, soap, and sodium salts; it is also used for washing fabrics.

Washing soda, or *Sal soda* is sodium carbonate with 10 molecules of water. It is in the form of colorless crystals which rapidly effloresce in the air.

Description—Colorless crystals or a white, crystalline powder. Stable in air under ordinary conditions. When exposed to dry air above 50° the salt effloresces, and at 100° becomes anhydrous. It is decomposed by weak acids forming the salt of the acid and liberating carbon dioxide. Its aqueous solution is alkaline to indicators (pH about 11.5).

Solubility—1 Gm dissolves in 3 ml of water and 1.8 ml of boiling water; insoluble in alcohol.

Incompatibilities—*Acids, acid salts,* and *acidic preparations* cause its decomposition. Most *metals* are precipitated as carbonates, hydroxides, or basic salts. *Alkaloids* are precipitated from solutions of their salts.

Uses—Sodium Carbonate is occasionally used topically for dermatitides as a lotion; it has been used as a mouthwash and a vaginal douche. It is used in the preparation of the sodium salts of many acids.

Sodium Hydroxide USP

[Caustic Soda; Soda Lye]

Sodium Hydroxide contains 95.0–100.5% of total alkali, calculated as NaOH (40.00), including not more than 3.0% of Na_2CO_3 (105.99).

Caution—Exercise great care in handling Sodium Hydroxide, as it rapidly destroys tissues.

History—This salt was originally called *mineral alkali* as contrasted with potassium hydroxide which was called *vegetable alkali* and ammonium hydroxide which was called *animal alkali*. The origin of these alkalies dates from a very early period, and the alkali carbonates and hydroxides are mentioned by Dioscorides. The word *lixivium* was a Roman term applied to the lye made from wood ashes. The term alkali is of Arabic origin and was first used in the 13th century.

Preparation—Sodium Hydroxide, commercially termed *caustic soda*, may be made by treating sodium carbonate with milk of lime, or by the electrolysis of a solution of sodium chloride as explained under *Potas-*

sium Hydroxide (page 779). It is now largely produced by the latter process.

Description—White, or nearly white, fused masses, small pellets, flakes, sticks, and other forms. It is hard and brittle and shows a crystalline fracture. Exposed to the air, Sodium Hydroxide rapidly absorbs carbon dioxide and moisture. It melts at about 318°. Its specific gravity is 2.13. When it is dissolved in water or alcohol, or when its solution is treated with an acid, much heat is generated. Its aqueous solutions, even when highly diluted, exhibit a strong alkaline reaction to indicators, and blacken calomel.

Solubility—1 Gm dissolves in 1 ml of water; freely soluble in alcohol or glycerin.

Incompatibilities—Exposed to air, it absorbs *carbon dioxide* and is converted to sodium carbonate. With *fats* and *fatty acids*, it forms soluble soaps; with *resins* it forms insoluble soaps. See *Potassium Hydroxide* (page 779).

Uses—Sodium Hydroxide is too alkaline to be of medicinal value. It is occasionally used in veterinary practice as a caustic, but is less popular than caustic potash. It is extensively used in pharmaceutical processes and is generally preferred to potassium hydroxide because it is milder, less deliquescent, and less expensive; in addition, less of it is required since 40 parts of it are equivalent to 56 parts of potassium hydroxide. It is a pharmaceutical necessity in the preparation of *Glycerin Suppositories* (page 779).

Industrially, caustic soda is widely used in numerous processes, among which is the manufacture of soap. To industrial consumers not too distant from manufacturing plants, caustic soda is now furnished as an approximately 50% solution. This is more economical as it saves the expense of evaporation to form the solid and the subsequent handling.

Veterinary Uses—Sodium Hydroxide has been used in a 2 to 5% solution as a *disinfectant* for farm buildings and animal quarters.

Sodium Stearate NF

Sodium Stearate consists chiefly of $C_{18}H_{35}NaO_2$ (sodium stearate = 306.47) and $C_{16}H_{31}NaO_2$ (sodium palmitate = 278.41).

Preparation—Stearic acid is reacted with an equimolar portion of sodium hydroxide.

Description—A fine, white powder, soapy to the touch. It usually has a slight, tallow-like odor. It is affected by light. Its solutions are alkaline to phenolphthalein TS.

Solubility—Slowly soluble in cold water and cold alcohol; readily soluble in hot water and hot alcohol.

Uses—Sodium Stearate is used in glycerin suppositories. It is also used in some toothpastes. It has been used topically in sycosis and other skin diseases.

Starch USP

[Amylum; Corn Starch]

Starch consists of the granules separated from the mature grain of *Zea Mays* Linné (Fam. *Gramineæ*).

Preparation—In making starch from corn, the germ must be separated mechanically and the cells then softened so as to permit the escape of the starch granules. This is generally done by permitting it to become sour and decomposed, stopping the fermentation before the starch is affected. Upon the small scale, starch may be made from wheat flour by making a stiff ball of dough and kneading it while a small stream of water trickles upon it. The starch is carried off with the water, while the *gluten* remains as a soft, elastic

mass; the latter may be purified and used for various purposes to which gluten is applicable. The quality of commercial starch largely depends upon the purity of the water used in its manufacture. Starch may be made from potatoes by first grating them, and then washing the soft mass upon a sieve, which separates the cellular substances and permits the starch granules to be carried through. The starch must then be thoroughly washed by decantation, and the quality of this starch also depends largely upon the purity of the water that is used in washing it.

Description—Irregular, angular, white masses or a fine powder, consisting chiefly of polygonal, rounded, or spheroidal grains up to 35 microns in diameter and usually with a circular or several-rayed central cleft. It is odorless, and has a slight, characteristic taste.

Solubility—Insoluble in cold water and in alcohol; when it is boiled with about 20 times its weight of hot water for a few minutes and then cooled a translucent, whitish jelly results; its aqueous suspension is neutral to litmus.

Identification—The most outstanding chemical characteristic of starch is the purplish blue or deep blue color it gives with iodine TS. The iodine is, however, loosely bound and is removed by solutions of sodium thiosulfate, sulfites, silver salts, etc. By hydrolysis with dilute minerals acids, starch is converted into dextrose (glucose).

Uses—Starch is used in a number of official preparations chiefly because of its absorbent properties; also as a *filler* or *diluent* in tablets and, in the latter, as a *disintegrator* (see *Tablets*). It is used externally as an *absorbent*, and is applied to the skin as a *dusting powder*. It is also used to make pastes for applying in skin diseases. See *Zinc Oxide Paste* (page 772).

Industrially Starch is consumed in large quantities in sizing and laundering of cotton fabrics and garments, in preparation of adhesives (mucilages), and in production of corn syrup and dextrose.

Starch is present in many drugs, and is an important constituent of many vegetable *foods*.

Starch, when moistened with diluted acids and heated, or through the action of diastase, or even when heated alone, is converted into *dextrin*, a substance resembling gum in appearance and properties. See page 1377.

Storax USP

[Liquid Storax; Styrax; Sweet Gum; Prepared Storax]

Storax is a balsam obtained from the trunk of *Liquidambar orientalis* Miller, known in commerce as Levant Storax, or of *Liquidambar styraciflua* Linné, known in commerce as American Storax (Fam. *Hamamelidaceæ*).

Constituents—The following constituents occur in both varieties of Storax: *styracin* (*cinnamyl cinnamate*), *styrol* (*phenylethylene*, C_8H_8), α- and β-*storesin* (the cinnamic acid ester of an alcohol called *storesinol*), *phenylpropyl cinnamate*, free *cinnamic acid*, and *vanillin*. In addition to these, Levant Storax contains *ethyl cinnamate, benzyl cinnamate*, free *storesinol, isocinnamic acid, ethylvanillin, styrogenin*, and *styrocamphene*. This variety of Storax yields from 0.5 to 1% of *volatile oil*; from this have been isolated *styrocamphene, vanillin*, the cinnamic acid esters of *ethyl, phenylpropyl, benzyl*, and *cinnamyl alcohols, naphthalene*, and *styrol*.

American Storax contains, in addition to the substances previously enumerated as common to both varieties, *styaresin* (the cinnamic acid ester of the alcohol *styresinol*, an isomer of storesinol) and *styresinolic acid*. It yields up to 7% of a dextrorotatory volatile oil, the composition of which has not been completely investigated. Styrol and traces of vanillin have been isolated from it.

Description—Storax is a semi-liquid, grayish to grayish brown, sticky, opaque mass, depositing on standing a heavy dark brown layer (Levant Storax); or a semi-solid, sometimes a solid mass, softened by gentle warming (American Storax). Storax is transparent in thin layers, has a characteristic odor and taste, and is more dense than water.

Solubility—Insoluble in water, but soluble, usually incompletely, in an equal weight of warm alcohol; soluble in acetone, carbon disulfide, and ether, some insoluble residue usually remaining.

Uses—It is an *expectorant* but is used chiefly as a local remedy, especially in combination with benzoin; eg, it is an ingredient of *Compound Benzoin Tincture* (page 766). It may be used, like benzoin, to protect fatty substances from rancidity.

Sucrose Octaacetate NF

Sucrose Octaacetate contains 98.0–100.5% of $C_{28}H_{38}O_{19}$ (678.60), calculated on the anhydrous basis.

Preparation—Sucrose is subjected to exhaustive acetylation by reaction with acetic anhydride in the presence of a suitable condensing agent such as pyridine.

Description—A white, practically odorless powder having an intensely bitter taste. It is hygroscopic. It melts not lower than 78°.

Solubility—Very soluble in methanol and chloroform; soluble in alcohol and ether; very slightly soluble in water.

Uses—Sucrose Octaacetate is a *denaturant* for alcohols. It is also used as an adhesive; for impregnating and insulating papers; and in lacquers and plastics.

Sulfurated Potash NF

[Hepar Sulfuris; Kalium Sulfuratum; Liver of Sulfur]

Sulfurated Potash is a mixture composed chiefly of potassium polysulfides and potassium thiosulfate. It contains not less than 12.8% of S (sulfur) in combination as sulfide.

Preparation—Sulfurated Potash may be prepared by thoroughly mixing 1 part of sublimed sulfur with 2 parts of potassium carbonate and gradually heating the mixture in a covered iron crucible until the mass ceases to swell and is completely melted. It is then poured on a stone or glass slab and, when cold, broken into pieces and preserved in tightly-closed bottles. When the heat is properly regulated during its production, the reaction is approximately represented by the equation:

$$3K_2CO_3 + 8S \rightarrow 2K_2S_3 + K_2S_2O_3 + 3CO_2$$

As this product rapidly deteriorates on exposure to moisture, oxygen, and carbon dioxide, it is desirable for the prescription pharmacist to secure it recently prepared to produce satisfactory preparations.

Description—Irregular pieces, liver-brown when freshly prepared, changing to a greenish yellow. It decomposes upon exposure to air. It has an odor of hydrogen sulfide and a bitter, acrid, and alkaline taste. Even weak acids cause the liberation of H_2S from Sulfurated Potash.

Solubility—1 Gm dissolves in about 2 ml of water, usually leaving a slight residue; alcohol dissolves only the sulfides.

Uses—Sulfurated Potash is extensively used in dermatologic practice, especially in the official *White Lotion* or *Lotio Alba* which appears on page 771. The equation for the reaction of the potassium trisulfide in preparing the lotion is as follows:

$$ZnSO_4 + K_2S_3 \rightarrow ZnS\downarrow + 2S\downarrow + K_2SO_4$$

The mixture of insoluble zinc sulfide and sulfur gives it the creamy white appearance and the potassium sulfate goes into solution.

Talc USP

[Talcum; Purified Talc; French Chalk; Soapstone; Steatite]

Talc is a native, hydrous magnesium silicate, sometimes containing a small proportion of aluminum silicate.

Occurrence and Preparation—Native talc, called *soapstone* or *French chalk*, is found in various parts of the world. An excellent quality is obtained from deposits in North Carolina. Deposits of a high grade of Talc, conforming to the USP requirements, are also found in Manchukuo (Manchuria). Native talc is usually accompanied by variable amounts of other mineral substances. These are separated from it by mechanical means, such as flotation or elutriation. The talc is then finely powdered, treated with boiling dilute hydrochloric acid, washed well, and dried.

Description—A very fine, white, or grayish white crystalline powder. It is unctuous to the touch, adhering readily to the skin, and is free from grittiness.

Uses—Purified Talc is used as a distributing and *filtering medium* in making medicated waters, elixirs, etc. Its medicinal value depends on its desiccant and lubricating effects.

When perfumed or medicated, it is also used extensively as a toilet powder under the name *talcum powder*. For toilet purposes it should be in the form of an impalpable powder, but when used as a filtering medium, a coarser powder has been considered preferable to prevent its passing through the pores of the filter paper. As a filtering medium, it may be used for all classes of preparations with no danger of adsorption and retention of active principles. It is preferred as a dusting powder when making hand-made suppositories. *It should not be used on surgical gloves since it is very irritating to the peritoneal cavity.*

Talc is used industrially as an electric and heat insulator, a filler for paper, and as a lubricant.

Tartaric Acid NF

[(+)-Tartaric Acid; L-Tartaric Acid; L-2,3-Dihydroxysuccinic Acid]

HOCHCOOH
|
HOCHCOOH

Tartaric Acid, dried over phosphorus pentoxide for 3 hours, contains 99.7–100.5% of $C_4H_6O_6$ (150.09).

History—This is one of the several organic acids discovered by Scheele, the famous Swedish apothecary, while investigating cream of tartar which had been known for many centuries.

Preparation—This important acid may be prepared from *argol*, the crude cream of tartar deposited on the sides of wine casks during the fermentation of grapes. Tartaric Acid is prepared by neutralizing a hot solution of argon with calcium carbonate, and decomposing the resulting insoluble calcium tartrate by sulfuric acid, which precipitates calcium sulfate and liberates the tartaric acid. The process, when thus conducted, furnishes only one-half of the tartaric acid. The other half may be procured by adding calcium chloride in excess and subsequent treatment of the precipitated calcium tartrate with sulfuric acid:

$$2KHC_4H_4O_6 + CaCO_3 \rightarrow$$
$$K_2C_4H_4O_6 + CaC_4H_4O_6 + H_2O + CO_2$$
$$K_2C_4H_4O_6 + CaCl_2 \rightarrow CaC_4H_4O_6 + 2KCl$$
$$CaC_4H_4O_6 + H_2SO_4 \rightarrow CaSO_4 + H_2C_4H_4O_6$$

Description—Large, colorless or translucent crystals, or a white granular to fine crystalline powder. It is odorless, has an acid taste and is stable in the air and its solutions are acid to litmus. This Acid is dextrorotatory and its specific rotation $[\alpha]_D^{20}$ in a 20% aqueous solution is about $+12°$.

Solubility—1 Gm dissolves in 0.8 ml of water, about 0.5 ml of boiling water, about 3 ml of alcohol, and about 250 ml of ether; freely soluble in methanol.

Identification—In solutions of *tartrates*, neutralized if necessary to litmus, silver nitrate produces a white precipitate. On adding just sufficient ammonia to dissolve the precipitate and warming the solution, metallic silver is deposited on the side of the test tube forming a mirror. On adding to a solution of a tartrate, previously acidified with acetic acid, one drop of ferrous sulfate TS, then a few drops of hydrogen peroxide TS, and finally an excess of sodium hydroxide, a purple or violet color is produced. Tartaric acid or tartrates are charred by concentrated sulfuric acid and the odor of burning sugar is emitted.

Incompatibilities—*Potassium* salts cause a precipitation of potassium bitartrate; with *potassium iodide*, hydriodic acid is formed and slowly liberates iodine. *Calcium* and *lead* salts form insoluble compounds with tartrates. Tartaric Acid is a mild reducing agent. Although the tartrates of many metals are insoluble, an excess of Tartaric Acid often produces a soluble complex.

Uses—Tartaric Acid is chiefly used as the acid ingredient of preparations in which it is neutralized by a bicarbonate, as in effervescent salts, and the free acid is completely absent or present only in small amounts in the finished product. It is also used in baking and jelly powders, and in making silver mirrors.

Theobroma Oil USP

[Cacao Butter; Cocoa Butter; Oil of Theobroma]

Theobroma Oil is the fat obtained from the roasted seed of *Theobroma cacao* Linné (Fam. *Sterculiaceæ*).

Preparation—The Oil is made by grinding the kernels of the "chocolate bean" and expressing in powerful, horizontal hydraulic presses. The yield is about 40%. It has also been prepared by dissolving the oil from the unroasted beans by the use of a volatile solvent.

Constituents—Chemically it is a mixture of stearin, palmitin, olein, laurin, linolein, and traces of other glycerides.

Description—A yellowish, white solid with a faint, agreeable odor and a bland (if obtained by extraction) or chocolate-like (if obtained by pressing) taste. It is usually brittle below 25°. Its specific gravity is between 0.858 and 0.864 at 100°/25°. Its refractive index is 1.4537 to 1.4585 at 40°.

Solubility—Slightly soluble in alcohol; soluble in boiling dehydrated alcohol; freely soluble in ether and chloroform.

Uses—Owing to its low fusing point and its property of becoming solid at a temperature just below the melting point, Theobroma Oil is valuable in pharmacy for making suppositories. See *Suppositories* (page 1617). In addition to this use, cocoa butter is an excellent emollient application to the skin when inflamed; it also is used in various skin creams, especially the so-called "*skin foods.*" It is also used in massage. Its adulterants are coconut oil and palm nut oil stearins; also stearin and tallow. It is an excellent source of stearic acid.

Thromboplastin USP

[Thrombokinase]

Thromboplastin is a powder or a liquid suspension that exhibits thrombokinase activity derived from the acetone-extracted brain and/or lung tissue of freshly killed rabbits. It may contain added sodium chloride and calcium chloride in suitable proportions. It is used in the form of a suspension for the determination of the prothrombin time and activity of the blood.

The thrombokinase activity is such that the addition of Thromboplastin gives a clotting time of 11 to 16 seconds with normal human plasma and the proper concentration of calcium ions.

Description—In the dry form, it is a buff-colored powder. In the liquid form, it is an opalescent or a turbid suspension from which some solid matter may be deposited on standing. It may have a characteristic odor of dried animal tissue. It may contain a suitable antibacterial agent.

Uses—Thromboplastin is a necessary reagent in the determination of prothrombin activity or prothrombin time of the plasma. It is active by virtue of its content of thrombokinase, a factor which is necessary, along with calcium ions, for the conversion of prothrombin to thrombin. It is used in the form of a suspension adjusted to a concentration such that in the standard prothrombin determination with normal human plasma and calcium concentration the clotting time lies between 11 and 16 seconds. It has also been used in surgery as a hemostatic to arrest hemorrhage, but it is little used for this purpose.

Titanium Dioxide USP

[Titanic Anhydride]

Titanium Dioxide contains 99.0–100.5% of TiO_2 (79.90), calculated on the dried basis.

Preparation—Titanium Dioxide may be prepared by adding ammonia or an alkali carbonate to a solution of titanyl sulfate ($TiOSO_4$). Titanic acid [$Ti(OH)_4$ or $TiO(OH)_2$] is precipitated and, after filtration and washing, is dried and ignited. It may also be prepared by neutralizing a solution of a titanium salt with sodium carbonate and then boiling with a large volume of water. Metatitanic acid [$TiO(OH)_2$] is precipitated and it yields the Dioxide on heating.

Description—A white, amorphous, tasteless, odorless, infusible powder. Its specific gravity is about 4. Its suspension in water (1 in 10) is neutral to litmus. When heated with sulfuric acid until fumes of SO_3 are liberated, the residue, dissolved in water, responds to the identification reactions for titanium.

Solubility—Dissolves in hot concentrated sulfuric acid and in hydrofluoric acid, rendered soluble by fusion with potassium bisulfate or with alkali hydroxides or carbonates; insoluble in water, hydrochloric acid, nitric acid, and dilute sulfuric acid.

Uses—Titanium Dioxide is used in lotions as a *protective* against sunlight and in dusting and face powders. It is also used as a white pigment in paints, lacquers, rubber, shoe creams, plastics, and is used in artificial teeth to whiten the yellow color of the plastic. Other industrial uses include the manufacture of enamels, glazes, linoleum, and artificial leather; as a mordant for textiles; and in paper as a filler.

Dose—*Topically*, as **15 to 25%** ointment or lotion as required.

Trichloromonofluoromethane NF

[Trichlorofluoromethane]

CFCl₃

Trichloromonofluoromethane is CCl₃F (137.37).

Preparation—Carbon tetrachloride is reacted with antimony trifluoride in the presence of a small quantity of antimony pentachloride. The reaction produces a mixture of CCl_3F and CCl_2F_2 which are readily separable by fractional distillation.

Description—A clear, colorless gas having a faint, ethereal odor. Its vapor pressure at 25° is about 796 mm of Hg. It boils at approximately 24°.

Solubility—Practically insoluble in water; soluble in alcohol, ether, and other organic solvents.

Uses—Trichloromonofluoromethane is used as a *propellant* (No. 11, see page 1736) in aerosols.

Zinc–Eugenol Cement NF

[Zinc Compounds and Eugenol Cement NF XI]

The Powder

Zinc Acetate	0.5 Gm
Zinc Stearate	1 Gm
Zinc Oxide	70 Gm
Rosin	28.5 Gm

Powder the rosin and incorporate it with about an equal weight of zinc oxide until thoroughly mixed. Sift the mixture on a sieve of not less than 100-mesh. Regrind the material which does not pass through the sieve with more of the zinc oxide and sift again; repeat the process until all of the material readily passes through the sieve. Thoroughly mix the zinc stearate and zinc acetate with a portion of the zinc oxide and pass through a 100-mesh sieve. Thoroughly mix the two mixtures with the remainder of the zinc oxide.

The Liquid

Eugenol	85 ml
Cottonseed Oil	15 ml

Thoroughly mix the liquids together in the proportions specified.

The Cement

To prepare the cement mix 10 parts of the Powder with 1 part of the Liquid to a thick paste immediately before use. *Note:* The amount of Liquid may be varied to give any desired consistency.

Description—*The Powder* is yellowish white to white in color. *The Liquid* is thin and colorless to weak yellow, having a strong aromatic odor of clove and a pungent, spicy taste. It is affected by light. Specific gravity 1.043 to 1.048. Refractive index 1.528 to 1.531 at 20°.

Solubility—*The Liquid* is miscible with alcohol, chloroform, and ether; only slightly soluble in water.

Uses—This Cement is employed in general dental practice as a *dental protective*, ie, as a pulp capping or a *temporary filling.*

Other Miscellaneous Pharmaceutical Necessities

Althea NF XI [Marshmallow Root]—The dried root of *Althaea officinalis* Linné (Fam. *Malvaceæ*), deprived of the brown corky layer and small roots. *Uses:* A demulcent and filler for pill masses; it is an ingredient in *Ferrous Carbonate Pills.*

Aralia NF XI [American Spikenard; Spignet]—The dried rhizome and roots of *Aralia racemosa* Linné (Fam. *Araliaceæ*). *Uses:* An ingredient of *Compound White Pine Syrup.*

Bismuth Oxychloride [Bismuthyl Chloride; Pearl White] [BiOCl]—It is a white, lustrous, crystalline powder; insoluble in water. *Uses:* Ingredient of face powders and pigments.

Calcium Fluoride [CaF₂]—Insoluble in water; slightly soluble in very dilute acids; dissolved by concentrated mineral acids. *Uses:* Used in the form of a lozenge as an aid in the prevention of dental caries where the fluorine content of the water is low. Also used in the manufacture of enamels, glass, and hydrofluoric acid. *Dose:* 2 mg a day for prevention of dental caries.

Carbon Disulfide [Carbon Bisulfide] [CS₂]—Prepared by heating powdered carbon with sulfur. A colorless or slightly yellow, clear, *very flammable* liquid. When freshly distilled it is almost odorless but it soon acquires a disagreeable odor. Sp gr 1.260. Boils at 46–47°. Slightly soluble in water, miscible with dehydrated alcohol, chloroform, and several other anhydrous solvents. Keep in tight containers in a cool place and *remote from flame. Uses:* Formerly used externally as a counterirritant in rheumatism and neuralgia. Industrially, it is used as a soil disinfectant, for fumigating cereal grains, and as a solvent for phosphorus in the manufacture of matches, but its principal use is in the manufacture of artificial silks.

Ceresin [Ozokerite; Earth Wax; Cerosin; Mineral Wax; Fossil Wax]—A hard, white odorless solid resembling spermaceti when purified, occurring naturally in deposits in the Carpathian Mountains, especially in Galicia. It is a mixture of natural complex paraffin hydrocarbons. Melts between 61° and 78°. Sp gr 0.91 to 0.92. Stable toward oxidizing agents. Soluble in 30% alcohol, benzene, chloroform, petroleum benzin, and hot oils. *Uses:* Substitute for beeswax; in dentistry for impression waxes; in the manufacture of candles, wax figures, waxed paper, polishes, insulators, and bottles for hydrofluoric acid.

Dextrin [British Gum; Starch Gum; Leiocom] [C₆H₁₀(O₅)ₙ]—Produced by the incomplete hydrolysis of starch with dilute acids, or by heating dry starch. White or yellow, amorphous powder. The white is practically odorless; the yellow has a characteristic odor. It is dextrorotatory. $[\alpha]_D^{20}$ generally above 200°. Soluble in 3 parts boiling water forming a gummy solution; less soluble in cold water; insoluble in alcohol and ether. Does not reduce Fehling's solution; gives a reddish brown color with iodine. *Uses:* Excipient for dry extracts and pills; for preparing emulsions and dry bandages; for thickening dye pastes and mordants used in printing fabrics; sizing paper and fabrics; manufacture of printers' inks and mucilage; in matches, and explosives.

Ethereal Oil NF IX—A volatile liquid consisting of equal volumes of heavy oil of wine and ether. It is a transparent, nearly colorless, volatile liquid, with an aromatic odor, and a pungent, refreshing, bitter taste. *Uses:* An ingredient in compound ether spirit.

Ethylenediamine Hydrate BP, PhI [H₂N.CH₂.CH₂.NH₂.H₂O]—*Purity:* the equivalent of 97.5–101.5% of

$C_2H_8N_2.H_2O$. A clear, colorless or slightly yellow liquid with an ammoniacal odor and characteristic alkaline taste. It is miscible with water and alcohol, soluble in 130 parts of chloroform, and slightly soluble in benzene and ether. It solidifies on cooling to a crystalline mass (mp 10°). It has a boiling point of 118–119°C and a sp gr of about 0.96. It is hygroscopic and absorbs CO_2 from the air. Aqueous solutions are alkaline to litmus. *Uses:* In the manufacture of aminophylline and in the preparation of aminophylline injections.

Ethylene Oxide $[CH_2\overset{\frown{O}}{-}CH_2]$—A colorless liquid below 12°. Sp gr 0.882 at 10°. Soluble in water, alcohol, and ether. Used by itself or as a mixture with 10 parts of carbon dioxide or Freon to fumigate foodstuffs and textiles and to sterilize thermolabile solids such as plastic materials (see page 1512).

Ferric Ammonium Sulfate [Ferric Alum] [$FeNH_4(SO_4)_2.12H_2O$]—An indicator in titrating halogens.

Ferric Oxide, Red NF IX—Red Ferric Oxide contains not less than 90% Fe_2O_3. It is made by heating native ferric oxide or hydroxide at a temperature which will yield a product of the desired color. The color is governed by the temperature and time of heating, the presence and kind of other metals, and the particle size of the oxide. A dark colored oxide is favored by prolonged heating at high temperature and the presence of manganese. A light colored oxide is favored by the presence of aluminum and by finer particle size. *Uses:* Imparting color to Neocalamine and cosmetics.

Ferric Oxide, Yellow NF IX—Yellow Ferric Oxide contains not less than 97.5% Fe_2O_3. It is prepared by heating ferrous hydroxide or ferrous carbonate in air at a low temperature. *Uses:* As for *Red Ferric Oxide* (above).

Ferrous Ammonium Sulfate [Mohr's Salt] [$Fe(NH_4)_2(SO_4)_2.6H_2O$]—A reducing agent for standardization of $KMnO_4$ and $K_2Cr_2O_7$.

Glass—The most important artificial silicate is glass. The composition of glass varies according to its application. Ordinary glass is made by heating a mixture of sand, limestone, and soda ash. In *hard* (Bohemian) *glass* the sodium carbonate is replaced by potassium carbonate. In *borosilicate glass* about 10 to 15% boric oxide is added with a corresponding reduction in the alkali metal and alkaline earth oxides. Because of its resistance to heat and water borosilicate glass is most used for chemical glassware. The use of lead oxide in the glass composition renders the glass softer and more brilliant, and, therefore, such glass is used for *cut-glass ware*. *Opal glass* is made by adding a white insoluble substance, such as bone ash or cryolite, to the fused glass. *Colored glass* is made by introducing into the fusion mixture oxides or carbonates of elements whose salts are colored, such as cobalt oxide, copper oxide, etc. *Amber glass* is made by the introduction of finely powdered carbon or iron sulfide into the fused mixture.

Honey NF XII [Mel; Clarified Honey; Strained Honey] is the saccharine secretion deposited in the honeycomb by the bee, *Apis mellifera* Linne (Fam. *Apidæ*). It must be free from foreign substances such as parts of insects, leaves, etc, but may contain pollen grains. *History:* Honey is one of the oldest of food and medicinal products. During the 16th and 17th centuries it was recommended as a cure for almost everything. *Constituents: Invert sugar* (62–83%), *sucrose* (0–8%), and *dextrin* (0.26–7%). *Description:* A thick, syrupy liquid of a light yellowish to reddish brown color. It is translucent when fresh, but frequently becomes opaque and granular through crystallization of dextrose. It has a characteristic odor and a sweet, faintly acrid taste. *Uses:* A sweetening agent and pharmaceutic necessity. It is employed in the preparation of the formerly official Ferrous Carbonate Mass. Its reducing action tends to maintain the iron in the ferrous state. It was also employed as a constituent of the formerly official Mercury Mass where it aided in dispersing the mercury and in preventing oxidation of the metal.

Hydriodic Acid, Diluted, NF XII contains, in each 100 ml, 9.5–10.5 Gm of HI (127.91), and 600 mg–1.0 Gm of HPH_2O_2 (66.00). The latter is added to prevent the forma- tion of free iodine. *Caution: Diluted Hydriodic Acid must not be dispensed or used in the preparation of other products if it contains free iodine. Preparation:* On a large scale, it is made by the interaction of iodine and hydrogen sulfide. The acid thus obtained is received in a mixture of water and the proper amount of hypophosphorous acid (to prevent the oxidation of HI to iodine by atmospheric oxygen). *Description and Solubility:* A colorless or not more than pale yellow, odorless liquid. Specific gravity, about 1.1. Miscible with water or alcohol. *Incompatibilities:* See *Incompatibilities of Inorganic Acids* (page 1481). *Uses:* In *Hydriodic Acid Syrup* (page 1340). The latter has been used as an expectorant. It is also used in the manufacture of inorganic iodides and disinfectants. The 57% acid is also used for analytical purposes, such as methoxyl determinations.

Hydrofluoric Acid—A solution of hydrogen fluoride gas [HF] in water. The acid of commerce usually contains 50 to 55% of HF. It is made by heating calcium fluoride with concentrated sulfuric acid in platinum or lead vessels. The HF is absorbed in water. Hydrogen fluoride is a colorless gas, very soluble in water or alcohol. The gas and its aqueous solutions are highly corrosive and *very poisonous*. They attack glass or any siliceous materials forming silicon tetrafluoride. Lead, platinum, and wax are not attacked by HF. Hydrofluoric acid is a colorless, or nearly colorless, fuming liquid. The acid is chiefly used for etching designs and various other markings on glass, for removing efflorescence on bricks and stone, or sand particles from metal castings. The object to be etched is first coated with a film of substance impervious to hydrogen fluoride, like wax, paraffin, or a so-called etching varnish. The desired markings are then cut through this coating by means of a sharp instrument and the object is exposed to hydrogen fluoride gas or dipped into its solution. Upon the removal of the coating the markings are etched upon the glass. When hydrogen fluoride gas is used the tracings are white and opaque whereas the solution forms transparent lines. *Storage:* Because of its corrosive action on glass, hydrofluoric acid is kept in bottles made of wax, gutta percha, or cakelite. In bulk it is stored in lead containers.

Hydrogen Sulfide [Sulfhydric acid; Sulfuretted hydrogen; Hydrosulfuric acid] [H_2S]—A colorless, poisonous gas. Disagreeable odor. It may prove fatal when inhaled in a concentration of 1 part per 200 parts of air. It behaves as a weak acid when dissolved in water. Its solutions precipitate the heavy metals as sulfides. See *Heavy Metals Test* (page 589).

Lead Monoxide NF X, BP [Litharge]—*Purity:* not less than 97% PbO. A heavy, yellowish or reddish powder. Its Sp gr is 9.5. On exposure to the air, it slowly absorbs moisture and carbon dioxide. It is odorless and tasteless. It is almost insoluble in water, to which, however, it imparts a faintly alkaline reaction; it is insoluble in alcohol. It is soluble in acetic acid, diluted nitric acid, and in warm solutions of the hydroxides of fixed alkalies. *Uses:* In the preparation of lead subacetate solution, lead plaster, and other pharmaceutical products.

Lime NF XII [Calx; Calcium Oxide; Quicklime; Burnt Lime; Calx Usta], when freshly ignited to constant weight, contains not less than 95.0 of CaO (56.08). *Preparation:* Lime (calcium oxide) is made by calcining *limestone* (a native calcium carbonate) in kilns with strong heat. *Description and Solubility:* Hard, white, or grayish white masses or granules, or a white or grayish white powder. It is odorless. Its solution is strongly alkaline. 1 Gm is soluble in about 840 ml of water and 1740 ml of boiling water; soluble in glycerin and syrup; insoluble in alcohol. *Uses:* In making mortar, whitewash, and various chemicals and products. It is an ingredient in *Sulfurated Lime Solution* (page 1273). In the USP, Calcium Hydroxide has replaced Lime, as it is more stable and more readily available of a quality suitable for medicinal use than the lime usually obtainable. Unless protected from air, Lime soon becomes unfit for use, due to the action of carbon dioxide and moisture in air. See *Calcium Hydroxide* (page 1364).

Lime, Chlorinated USP X [approx. CaClOCl with H_2O] Bleaching Powder; Chloride of Lime; Calcium Hypochlorite]—Made by absorbing chlorine in powdered, slaked lime. It is a white or grayish powder emitting, on exposure to air, the odor of chlorine. It is soluble in water, some insoluble matter (calcium carbonate, etc), usually being present. It contains not less than 35% available chlorine. Chlorinated lime is an unstable product which loses oxygen readily on exposure to moist air. It should be kept in tight containers. Chlorinated lime is extensively used for bleaching wood pulp and various fabrics, disinfecting drinking water and sewage, and manufacturing organic compounds. It was formerly used for making sodium hypochlorite solution by its reaction with sodium carbonate or sodium phosphate.

Mastic NF XI [Mastiche; Mastich; Mastix]—The concrete resinous exudation from *Pistacia Lentiscus* Linné (Fam. *Anacardiaceæ*). *Uses:* Used in the formerly official Aloe and Mastic Pills to modify the therapeutic action of the aloe. In the arts and in dentistry, it is employed to form a varnish.

Mercury NF XI, PhI [Quicksilver]—A bright, shiny, silvery white metal which is liquid at ordinary temperatures. *Uses:* Medicinally, mercury is used only for preparing *Mild Mercurial Ointment* and some other pharmaceutical preparations. Its vapors are extremely toxic and it should be used with care in a closed space.

Nitric Acid, Diluted USP VIII—Contains 10% *w/v* HNO_3. Prepared by diluting 105 ml of nitric acid with sufficient distilled water to make 1000 ml.

Nitrohydrochloric Acid NF IX [Chlorazotic acid; Aqua Regia]—Nitrohydrochloric acid is made by mixing 20% nitric acid with 80% hydrochloric acid in a dish or loosely stoppered container and allowing to stand at room temperature for about 15 hours or until gas is no longer evolved. The mixture should not be warmed to hasten the reaction or diluted before the reaction is complete:

$$HNO_3 + 3HCl \rightarrow NOCl + Cl_2 + 2H_2O$$

The acid should not be dispensed unless it immediately liberates iodine when 1 drop of the acid is added to 1 ml of an aqueous solution of potassium iodide (1 in 5). The acid is used by jewelers to dissolve gold. It has been used clinically in subchlorhydria and to increase bile flow. *Dose:* 0.2 to 0.3 ml, well diluted.

Nitrohydrochloric Acid, Diluted NF IX—This acid is made by diluting 22 ml of Nitrohydrochloric Acid to 100 ml with distilled water. It is less stable than the concentrated acid.

Palmitic Acid [Cetylic acid] [$CH_3(CH_2)_{14}COOH$]—It occurs as the glyceride in many oils and fats, particularly in palm oil from which the acid derives its name. White, crystalline scales. Sp gr about 0.85 at 62°. Melts at 63° to 64°. The commercial acid melts at a lower temperature, depending on the degree of its purity. It is insoluble in water, sparingly soluble in cold alcohol, freely soluble in hot alcohol, in ether, chloroform, and other alcohols.

Peach Oil—An oil resembling almond oil obtained from *Persica vulgaris* (Fam. *Rosaceæ*). See *Persic Oil* (page 1370).

Perchloric Acid [$HClO_4$] is available in aqueous solution in 70% concentration. It is a powerful oxidizer and may cause deflagration in contact with organic and other oxidizable substances. *Uses:* The acid is largely used in analytical chemistry, and its alkali salts, termed *perchlorates*, are used in explosives and the electroplating of metals. It is useful for the isolation and purification of bases, particularly alkaloids.

Phenyl Salicylate NF XI—The salicylic acid ester of phenol occurs as fine white crystals which melt between 41° and 43°. 1 Gm dissolves in 6500 ml of water and 6 ml of alcohol. It is very soluble in ether, chloroform, and in fixed and volatile oils. *Uses:* It was employed to coat solid dosage forms, eg, pills, forming an enteric product. It was formerly used for analgesia but in the intestine it is hydrolyzed to salicylic acid and phenol, the latter being quite toxic. It is used locally in sunburn preparations. *Dose:* 300 mg.

Potassium Carbonate NF XI [Vegetable Alkali; Salt of Tartar]—A white granular powder which is very soluble in water but insoluble in alcohol. *Uses:* Potassium Carbonate is too strong an alkali to be used internally. In large doses it is a caustic irritant. It is a pharmaceutical necessity in formerly official *Ferrous Carbonate Pills*. Industrially, Potassium Carbonate is used in the manufacture of soft soap and hard glass.

Potassium Dichromate [Potassium Bichromate] [$K_2Cr_2O_7$]—An official oxidizing reagent.

Sarsaparilla NF XI—The dried root of *Smilax aristolochiæfolia* Miller, known in commerce as Mexican Sarsaparilla; or of *Smilax regelii* Killip et Morton, known in commerce as Honduras Sarsaparilla; or of *Smilax febrifuga* Kunth, known in commerce as an Ecuadorian Sarsaparilla; or of undetermined species of *Smilax* Linné, variously known in commerce as Ecuadorian and Central American Sarsaparilla (Fam. *Liliaceæ*). *Constituents:* Sarsaparilla contains glycosides of the saponin group, *sarsasaponin* (*parillin*) and *smilasaponin* (*smilacin*) which are related structurally to the digitalis glycosides, and possess the steroid nucleus. When hydrolyzed with dilute acids, they split into sugars and the corresponding sapogenin. Sarsasaponin yields *sarsasapogenin* (*parigenin*) plus one rhamnose and two glucose molecules, and smilacin yields *smilagenin* plus sugar molecules. There are also present starch, resin, coloring matter, and volatile oil. *History:* This drug was first used in Europe in the 16th century as a much-vaunted remedy for syphilis. The origin of the name is in doubt. *Uses:* This agent is without pharmacological actions, and is not employed in modern therapeutics, although the laity is inclined to attribute certain therapeutic virtues to its use.

Soap, Hard NF XI [Soap; Castile Soap]—A whitish, hard solid which has a faint odor and is free from rancidity. Chemically, it is a sodium soap of oleic, palmitic, and coconut oil fatty acids. *Uses:* It is used in pill mases, in combination with resins, to render them soluble and to modify their harsh action.

Soda Lime BP—A mixture of sodium hydroxide, or sodium hydroxide and potassium hydroxide, with calcium hydroxide. It absorbs not less than 20% of its weight of carbon dioxide. It occurs as white or grayish-white granules, or it may be colored with an indicator to show when its absorptive power is exhausted. The indicator used should be inert with respect to its reactivity with ether, ethylene, cyclopropane, and nitrous oxide. Suitable indicators include phenolphthalein, potassium permanganate, and methyl violet. It is partially soluble in water and almost completely soluble in dilute acetic acid. *Uses:* To absorb carbon dioxide in a closed-circuit anesthetic apparatus, and to absorb acid gases such as phosgene in gas respirators.

Sodium Carbonate—Obtained by the action of heat on sodium bicarbonate and subsequent crystallization from water. *Purity:* 99 to 105% $Na_2CO_3.10H_2O$. It occurs as colorless, odorless, efflorescent, rhombic crystals with a strong alkaline taste. It is soluble in 2 parts of water at 20°C, and insoluble in alcohol. *Uses:* For washing textiles, bleaching linen and cotton, and as a general cleanser. It is too alkaline for medicinal use as an antacid.

Sodium Chlorate [$NaClO_3$]—Colorless and odorless crystals with a cooling saline taste. Soluble in water and in alcohol. It is a powerful oxidizing agent and should not be triturated with any combustible substance. Sodium chlorate is more soluble and contains a higher percentage of oxygen than potassium chlorate but because of its tendency to be hygroscopic in mixtures it is less desirable in dry explosives.

Sodium Formate [HCOONa]—White, deliquescent crystals or crystalline powder. Usually has a slight odor of formic acid. Melts at about 253°. At higher temperatures it decomposes into sodium oxalate and hydrogen, then into sodium carbonate. Soluble in about 1.3 parts water; soluble in glycerin; slightly soluble in alcohol. *Uses:* Sodium Formate has been employed as a constituent of salt mixtures to replace sodium chloride in salt-free diets. However, this use is completely irrational because sodium rather than chloride is the ion to be avoided in the conditions for which salt-free diets are prescribed, and this preparation contains sodium.

Sodium Glutamate [Sodium Acid Glutamate] [HOOC.-CH(NH₂).CH₂.CH₂.COONa]—White or nearly white, crystalline powder. Very soluble in water; sparingly soluble in alcohol. *Uses:* Imparts a meat flavor to foods.

Sodium Malate $[C_2H_3(OH)(COONa)_2.\frac{1}{2}H_2O]$—White, granular powder. Freely soluble in water. *Uses:* Its use in salt-free diets is irrational (see *Sodium Formate*, above). Formerly sold as *Eka Salt*.

Sodium Thioglycollate [Sodium Mercaptoacetate] $[HSCH_2COONa]$—Hygroscopic crystals which discolor on exposure to air or iron. Freely soluble in water; slightly soluble in alcohol. *Uses:* Reducing agent in Fluid Thioglycollate Medium for sterility testing.

Starch, Potato—From *Solanum tuberosum.* Granular powder consisting of starch grains of characteristic shape and appearance when examined microscopically.

Starch, Rice—From *Oryza sativa.* Prepared by heating rice with soda-lye, which dissolves the nitrogenous impurities and leaves pure starch, then adding a solution of borax to facilitate the separation of the starch from the gluten. It is used for making perfumes; also for the production of several of its salts, which are used to some extent medicinally.

Suet, Prepared NF IX [Mutton Suet]—Internal fat of the abdomen of the sheep, *Ovis aries* (Fam. *Bovidæ*), purified by melting and straining. A white, solid fat with a slight, characteristic odor and taste when fresh. It melts between 45° and 50° and congeals between 37° and 40°. Must be preserved in a cool place in tight containers. *Uses:* In ointments and cerates.

Sulfuric Acid NF X [Oil of Vitriol]—*Purity:* 94–98% H_2SO_4. It is a colorless, odorless liquid having an oily consistency. It is very caustic and very corrosive. It is miscible with water and with alcohol with the evolution of much heat. It has a sp gr of about 1.84. *Caution:* when diluting, the acid should be added to the diluent. Avoid contact with the skin as it produces severe burns. *Uses:* Pharmaceutical necessity where an active inorganic acid is required. It has been used topically as a caustic, but its use for this purpose is too dangerous.

Sulfuric Acid, Aromatic—This acid was official in the former Pharmacopeias, including the USP XI, in which the formula of its preparation was given as follows:

Sulfuric Acid	114 ml
Ginger Fluidextract	10 ml
Cinnamon Oil	1 ml
Alcohol, a sufficient quantity,	
To make	1000 ml

Add the sulfuric acid gradually, and with great caution, to 700 ml of alcohol, and allow the mixture to cool. Then mix with it the ginger fluidextract and the cinnamon oil, and add enough alcohol to make the product measure 1000 ml. The product was required to contain in each 100 ml an amount of free sulfuric acid and ethyl sulfuric acid equivalent to 19–21 Gm of H_2SO_4. This preparation, also known as *Elixir of Vitriol*, was devised by Dr. Adrian Mynsicht in the early part of the seventeenth century and has been used for diarrhea. *Dose:* 0.5 ml.

Sulfuric Acid, Diluted NF X—A solution in water containing, in each 100 ml, 9.5–10.5 Gm of H_2SO_4. A colorless, odorless liquid having an acid taste. It has a sp gr of about 1.067. *Uses:* Pharmaceutical necessity where a diluted inorganic acid is required. Has been used internally in gastric hypoacidity in a dose of 0.6–2.0 ml diluted in 200 ml of water and sipped through a glass tube to minimize injury to the teeth.

Sulfurous Acid—A solution of about 6% of SO_2 in water. It was official in the USP VIII. It possesses the characteristic odor of sulfur dioxide and an acid reaction. It oxidizes rather rapidly in the air forming sulfuric acid. It may be prepared by saturating water with sulfur dioxide. On a laboratory scale the sulfur dioxide is best prepared by treating sodium bisulfite or sodium sulfite with diluted sulfuric acid. *Uses:* In dentistry for bleaching teeth; antiseptic; in gastric fermentative processes, tonsillitis, and skin diseases. *Dose:* 2 ml.

Taraxacum NF XI [Dandelion Root; Lion's Tooth; Puff Ball]—The dried rhizome and root of *Taraxacum officinale* Weber (Fam. *Compositæ*). *Uses:* An obsolete drug of questionable activity which was formerly employed as a *cholagogue* and *diuretic*.

Thioglycollic Acid $[HS.CH_2COOH]$—Made by heating monochloroacetic acid with potassium or sodium hydrogen sulfide. A colorless liquid of a strong, unpleasant odor. Miscible with water, and soluble in alcohol. This acid is a very sensitive reagent for iron. Its salts, eg, antimony or bismuth sodium thioglycollates, are used as medicinal agents, and sodium thioglycollate is extensively used in the preparation of "thioglycollate culture medium" in bacteriologic work. Thioglycollates are used in both hair-waving preparations and depilatories, the type of action depending on concentration and pH.

72 | Adverse Effects and Interactions of Drugs

Pharmacogenetics—drug interactions—resistance transfer factors—
types of drug-induced diseases—adverse reaction reporting

This chapter was prepared by

Robert H. Moser, MD, *Col., MC, US Army, Chief, Department of Medicine,
Walter Reed General Hospital, Washington, D.C.   20012*

The physician and his patient are the beneficiaries of the most dramatic expansion of medical capability in the long history of medicine. But the rapid proliferation of medical knowledge has not been entirely benign. The reverses have been minor when contrasted to the advances, but negative effects cannot be ignored or derogated. This discussion involves one aspect of this problem—the emergence of what may be called "Diseases of Medical Progress" [1] or iatrogenic (Gk, *iatros,* physician) diseases.

Pertinent to this evolution of medical capability has been the improvement in quantity and quality of drugs. In the early days new drugs came in a trickle. There was time for the physician to become familiar with their virtues and idiosyncrasies. Soon the trickle became a stream. There was less time for study and reflection. The stream has now become a torrent; it is impossible for the physician to keep pace. One might say his little black bag runneth over.

It has been stated that drug-induced adverse effects are the price to be paid for more effective and better medicaments. There can be no quarrel with this statement; it is the *high* price that is of concern. The thalidomide disaster indicated how expensive it can be. [2,3]

By last count there were 2625 amelic and phocomelic children born in West Germany between 1958 and 1962. About 1000 of these deformed children will be obliged to remain under regular prosthetic care and supervision; 100 with the most serious deformities will remain under medical supervision the rest of their lives. Fortunately between 80 and 90% of the deformed children were in school by the end of 1967; 60 to 70% in regular schools.

From the financial aspect, the Health Ministry of West Germany has spent $2.8 million in research, treatment, rehabilitation, and developing facilities for the deformed children. This sobering catastrophe had the effect of catalyzing international concern about adverse effects of drugs, which had been a rather amorphous sentiment before thalidomide.

The deluge of new drugs has produced a widespread spirit of discontent with empiricism in therapeutics. The modern practitioner demands drugs that have proper credentials, and this has precipitated a virtual renaissance in drug investigation. Thus we have come to learn more of the wonders and hazards of contemporary therapeutic agents.

The demands of the clinician to know more about drugs are being met by increasing capability in the laboratory. New insight and appreciation of the complexities of drug effects have come from several diverse avenues of investigation. Percutaneous bi-opsy, electron microscopy, and immunofluorescent techniques have resulted in dramatic revelations; the mysteries of intracellular morphology and physiology in the living organism have begun to unfold. Often, we are able to observe the specific site of drug action within the cell and subcellular structures. In other areas techniques continue to be perfected for assay of blood and tissue levels of drugs, intermediate products, enzymes, and hormones.

The problems of adverse drug effects are many. Reduced to the simplest elements, when Drug A is introduced into the body, ultimately it or its metabolic products will be carried in blood and body fluids to bathe virtually all cells of the organism. The effects of Drug A become clinically perceptible only when the function of certain organs is modified by whatever mechanism, either beneficially or detrimentally, to the point of producing clinically perceptible changes. It is by these phenomena that we learn to characterize the nature of Drug A.

Yet as we focus attention upon the response of a specific organ (or organs) to this drug, we are inclined to forget that Drug A is also in contact with other tissues of the organism. Effects in these areas are not in immediate evidence, but subtle nefarious influences may be at work which become manifested clinically, at a much later date. Such long-range effects may never be correlated with the antecedent administration of Drug A. If Drugs B, C, D, E, F, etc are added, one begins to appreciate the endless combinations and permutations.

Studies of Adverse Reactions

The discovery of a significant adverse reaction follows a long but familiar pattern. Scattered unsubstantiated reports (hearsay, anecdote, word of mouth) are gathered, suggesting that a drug has caused a certain undesirable effect. Then begins the tedious process of painstaking retrospective analysis of many cases. Ultimately the suspected denominator—the provocative drug—is revealed. Then one must follow with a meticulously controlled prospective study which will involve provocative testing in animals and often in man before it can be proved that indeed it was the suspected drug that caused the difficulty. It is a tedious, frequently unrewarding process, but it is the only technique currently available.

This is a shadow world of pathophysiology where relation of cause to effect is at best difficult to assess. The still raging controversy over phenacetin and renal disease demonstrates the difficulty.

There are other problems. Perhaps the most careful, definitive study of adverse drug reactions is being conducted by Irey of the recently established Registry of Tissue Reactions to Drugs.[4] In reviewing the first 509 cases discussed in the new registry, Irey cited four principal areas of difficulty in his investigations:

1. Incomplete time-related drug and disease information.
2. Multiplicity of drugs administered in most cases.
3. Lack of an objective means of demonstrating a direct relationship between drug and reaction.
4. The limited number of reaction patterns of the body to the entire range of physical, chemical, and biologic causes of disease.

Following the appropriately rigid criteria established by the Registry, it was observed that in only 8% of the cases could a specific drug be definitely called the "causative" factor; in 40%, it was considered "probable;" in 32%, "possible;" in 15%, "coincidental;" and in 4%, "not related." The contribution of drug interactions to this complex milieu will be discussed later.[5]

The widely quoted adverse reaction studies of Cluff and associates[6,7] dramatically underscored the "iceberg" nature of the problem. This was an intensive prospective assault on the question conducted by highly motivated House Officers; 714 such patients were discovered during a 3-month period.

The results were rather astonishing; 13.6% of the patients admitted during this period suffered an adverse drug reaction. About 4% of all patients admitted to the general medical services were suffering an adverse drug reaction (admitting diagnosis). Of this group, 30.4% acquired *another* drug reaction during the course of hospitalization. The Cluff team observed a 4.2% incidence of reactions among those receiving 6–10 drugs; 24.2% with 11–15 drugs; 40% with 16–20 drugs; and 45% with 21 or more drugs!

Antimicrobial agents and cardiac drugs were implicated most often: 21.2% of all reactions each (42.4% total). Hypnotics and sedatives produced 13.0% of reactions; insulin, 8.9%; and antihypertensive drugs, 8.2%.

The clinical manifestations of adverse drug reactions were: gastrointestinal, 35.6%; neuromuscular, 15.8%; metabolic, 13%; cardiovascular, 11.6%; cutaneous, 10.3%; hematologic, 4.8%; renal, 3.4%; and multiple systems, 2.7%. Pulmonary and miscellaneous types of reactions accounted for about 1.4% each.

About 7% of all adverse drug reactions observed during this period of study were life-threatening or fatal; 5 deaths were attributed to adverse drug reactions.

Over two-thirds of the in-hospital adverse drug reactions were detected within 4 days after the causative drug had been started. Allergic reactions developed between the 5th to 10th day; some came on in an accelerated fashion. Nausea, vomiting, or diarrhea were the most common manifestations and occurred most frequently in women. Adverse drug reactions were more common in patients over 50; whites suffered more than blacks; women more than men. The average duration of hospitalization for patients with adverse drug reactions was 20.8 days, in contrast with a 14.3 day interval for all patients on the medical wards.

In another well-known study of adverse drug reactions performed by five cooperating medical school hospitals in the Philadelphia area (Hahnemann, Jefferson, Temple, Pennsylvania, and Women's), 772 adverse drug reactions were reported during a 24-month period of study by Durant.[8] Dermatologic and allergic reactions were most common, accounting

for 65% of all case reports. Penicillin was suspected in 101 reactions; phenobarbital and digitalis preparations in 21; and aspirin in 20.

The over-all incidence of adverse drug reactions was 0.49% of all hospitalized patients for the first year of the study and 0.41% for the second year. (It was during this study that the first demonstration of a positive Coombs test in patients taking cephalothin sodium was detected.)

The differences in incidence of adverse drug reactions between the studies of Cluff, Schimmel[9] (in which 10% of all hospitalized patients suffered adverse drug reactions), Durant, and others may be related to techniques of data gathering and definition of an "adverse drug reaction." Durant (in Philadelphia) and Koch–Weser[10] (at the Massachusetts General Hospital) required that for admission to their protocol a reaction must be "severe enough to be commented upon in the progress notes." (Those familiar with the mystique of the busy House Officer might consider this a chancy qualification.) Of course, this was not a determinant in the Cluff and Schimmel studies. Finally, Cluff and Schimmel utilized the prospective method while the other groups used the retrospective method.

Some Specific Problems

The problems of adverse drug reactions to placebos or spontaneously occurring symptoms cannot be discounted entirely, especially when minor reactions to drugs are being evaluated.[11] However, it may be equally safe to assume that for every patient who becomes sufficiently ill with an adverse drug effect to trek to an emergency room or a physician's office, there are perhaps 10 who will not.

The reasons are plentiful; the reaction may be quite mild, fear of loss of time from the job, etc are factors. At the present time there are many studies underway throughout the country to gather more meaningful data on this subject. These will be commented upon later.

The problem may be approached from another aspect. What is known of the role played by drugs in predisposing the organism to attack by microorganisms or degenerative disease? One example is the effect of long-term corticosteroids in predisposing the leukemia or lymphoma patient to systemic fungus infections.

A great deal has been heard about the so-called "opportunistic organisms" (perhaps a semantically poor euphemism), but it is appropriate here to mention *Candida albicans*. This is one of a group of saprophytes of limited pathogenicity under normal circumstances. *Candida* may emerge as a systemic infection and seed into many organs during or following broad spectrum antibiotic therapy with or without concomitant corticosteroids or immunosuppressives. This phenomenon has been related to suppression of susceptible enteric flora with disruption of the normal ecologic balance. This permits unaffected microorganisms to proliferate and often escape their enteric confines, at a time when normal defense mechanisms are all but paralyzed.

Another example is the devastating influence of prolonged corticosteroid therapy on the elderly patient who is somewhat immobilized by cardiovascular disease or arthritis. Accelerated demineralization is encouraged through the antianabolic effect of corticosteroids. This is a classic demonstration of exacerbation of a degenerative process by a drug. We start with one disease, and our treatment for it produces another disease.

Let us modify the question again. What is known of the effects of drugs on a previously diseased organ, with limited capability to metabolize or detoxify or otherwise cope with a drug given to treat another illness? The phenacetin controversy has been mentioned. The discussion here revolves around the status of analgesic compounds in the provocation of a variety of interstitial pyelonephritis and papillitis in a normal kidney. But what effect does phenacetin and/or aspirin and/or caffeine have upon a sick kidney, already poorly disposed to resist assault from either microorganism or nephrotoxic drug?

Finally, the phenomenon of delayed excretion of drugs or their active metabolites by a disease-damaged kidney must be considered. The unanticipated high blood levels introduce a whole new spectrum of toxic effects. And what happens to the diseased kidney, *per se*, if the drug which it has been reticent to excrete happens to be nephrotoxic and becomes superconcentrated in the surging countercurrents of the medullary interstitium?

Or, consider the patient with subclinical hepatic disease—a mild cirrhosis, if you will. What happens when he is given halothane or chlorpromazine or phenylbutazone—drugs known, occasionally, to be unkind to the normal liver?

Many examples could be cited wherein an organ with marginal function may be further insulted by a drug administered, most innocently, to treat another ailing system. The thought remains a continuing source of uneasiness in drug therapy.

The mechanisms of adverse drug reaction have been the subject of many taxonomies. One feasible classification is that modified from Long.[12]

1. Hypersensitivity (allergy)
2. Idiosyncrasy
3. Immunological injury
4. Enzyme induction (acceleration of drug metabolism)
5. Enzyme inhibition (inhibition of drug metabolism)
6. Carcinogenesis
7. Teratogenesis and mutagenesis

These will not be discussed in detail, but rather highlights will be presented.

Pharmacogenetics

Perhaps the most fascinating new dimension in drug reactions was the identification of a relationship between enzyme systems and drug effects. In 1959 Vogel[13] introduced the term *pharmacogenetics* into clinical medicine. This was defined as "the study of genetically determined variations that are revealed solely by the effects of drugs." The genetic aberration results in the absence or insufficiency of certain specific enzyme systems.

This mechanism (the revelation of smoldering enzyme insufficiencies) has already been cited as one major explanation of the extraordinary human variability in response to conventional doses of conventional drugs. Here we are discussing the effects of a single drug (A) on a patient with a congenital disorder of specific enzymes. One may ponder the possibilities of what might happen when Drug A inhibits or stimulates enzymes responsible for the metabolism of Drug B. A few notable examples will be cited.

The historical and classical prototype of a *pharmacogenetic* disease is the hemolytic anemia suffered by some members of certain ethnic groups—specifically, Mediterranean basin dwellers, rare Scandinavians, and Negroes, who have a quantitative or qualitative deficiency of glucose-6-phosphate dehydrogenase.[14] Brisk hemolysis may follow exposure to many common therapeutic agents (among these are the 4-aminoquinolines, certain sulfonamides, acetylsalicylic acid, the nitrofurantoins, the sulfones, aminosalicylic acid, phenacetin, acetanilid, propantheline, and the water-soluble analogs of vitamin K). Even the old nemesis, the Fava bean, continues to kill a few Sardinian children each year by triggering a catastrophic hemolytic anemia on the same basis.

The cause of this hemolysis is a genetically transmitted defect that results in varying degrees of deficiency (quantitative or qualitative) of this intra-erythrocytic enzyme. Such patients are normal clinically; they have no morphologic or physiologic abnormality of their red cells, until one of the provocative drugs is given. Then brisk hemolysis occurs. Parenthetically, deficiency of glucose-6-phosphate dehydrogenase has been cited as another cause of neonatal jaundice.

Glucose-6-phosphate dehydrogenase is somewhat of a problem in the chloroquine–primaquine antimalarial prophylaxis program in Southeast Asia.[15] Soldiers known to suffer clinical manifestations of this disorder are restricted from duty in endemic malarious areas.

"Blue soldiers"[16] suffer from congenital intraerythrocytic enzyme insufficiency. It was discovered that congenital heterologous methemoglobin reductase insufficiency can cause significant methemoglobinemia when such individuals are given routine antimalarial prophylaxis with chloroquine, primaquine, and dapsone (DDS), among other drugs.

Other red cell enzyme deficiencies of great subtlety have begun to emerge; these include aldolase, catalase, glutathione, hexokinase, glutathione reductase, phosphoglucomutase, ATP, pyruvate kinase, triose phosphatases, and isomerases. Almost every enzyme involved in Emden–Meyerhof cycle (anaerobic) glycolysis has come under scrutiny in the evaluation of the role of drugs capable of precipitating clinically significant hemolysis.

In a similar vein, another cause of kernicterus in the premature infant is related to immaturity of the neonatal liver. This organ is deficient in glucuronyl transferase and therefore feeble in its effort to conjugate bilirubin. Administration of sulfisoxazole or vitamin K analogs exaggerates this reaction.[17] Novobiocin may provoke jaundice in the newborn (and rarely in adults) by direct inhibition of glucuronyl transferase.[18] The "gray syndrome" of neonates may be related to a defect in chloramphenicol metabolism due to immaturity of hepatic microsomal enzymes.[19]

One might ask—do these adults have a marginal deficiency of glucuronyl transferase which becomes evident only when they are challenged with novobiocin? Is it congenital, or is it acquired as the result of a preceding episode of hepatic disease? At present, the answers are not known.

There are other equally fascinating pharmacogenetic diseases.

1. Hemoglobin Zurich[20]—If a certain Swiss family had not been given sulfonamide drugs, it is quite likely that this abnormal hemoglobin disease would have continued to escape detection. A frank hemolytic anemia developed after administration of sulfadi-

methoxine and sulfamethoxypyridazine to family members. A new hemoglobin with electrophoretic mobility between A and S was identified.

2. Hemoglobin H Disease[21]—Patients with this alpha thallasemia variant have hemoglobin which is a tetramer of four beta chains. Their erythrocytes appear normal until they are given sulfisoxazole; then a brisk hemolytic anemia may develop.

3. It is known that there is a variation in the ability of certain patients to metabolize isoniazid (INH), sulfamethoxazole, and hydralazine.[22] Such individuals are classified into phenotypes on the basis of their ability to acetylate these drugs. "Slow acetylators" have a deficiency of hepatic acetyl transferase. They maintain higher concentrations of unacetylated drugs for longer periods in body fluids than "rapid acetylators."

In the case of isoniazid it is not surprising that "slow acetylators" suffer a greater incidence of adverse drug reactions due to isoniazid than to the other group. Unduly sustained and elevated blood levels of isoniazid is the current explanation for the initiation of the sequence of events that causes the CNS damage and polyneuropathy found in slow acetylators of isoniazid. Fortunately, there is no difference in therapeutic responsiveness, and the development of resistance by the tubercle bacillus to isoniazid is similar in both phenotypes.

In another study, investigation of the monoamine oxidase antidepressive drug, phenelzine, revealed that significantly more severe adverse drug reactions were observed in a group of "slow acetylators" than in a group of "rapid acetylators."[23] Adverse drug reactions consisted of drowsiness, nausea, dizziness, and constipation—again related to sustained levels due to slow acetylation.

4. About 1 or 2% of patients have a congenitally determined clinical deficiency of plasma cholinesterase (pseudocholinesterase).[24] Five genotypes have been identified, characterized by either quantitative or qualitative insufficiencies. This malady will remain asymptomatic and undetected unless the patient is challenged with succinylcholine, usually upon the induction of anesthesia in prelude to surgery. The response is dramatic; a 2- to 3-min period of apnea will ensue. Of course, plasma cholinesterase is required to metabolize succinylcholine. Without this enzyme, unanticipated high serum levels of the drug will persist, with paralysis of the muscles of respiration.

5. It is suspected that increased susceptibility to dyskinesias subsequent to phenothiazine administration may be related to congenital enzyme insufficiencies.

6. Another curious interplay between drugs and enzymes exists in gout.[25] It is known that certain uric acid overproducers (as opposed to underexcretors) lack the enzyme hypoxanthine-guanine-phosphoribosyl-transferase (HGPTase). This is the basic lesion of the Nyham–Lesch syndrome. Without delving into the complex function of this salvage enzyme, it seems that a significant factor in the anti-uric acid effect of allopurinol depends on a plentiful supply of HGPTase.

Allopurinol appears to decrease the rate of *de novo* biosynthesis of purine. This function apparently is distinct from its better known action which is to inhibit hypoxanthine oxidase, an enzyme which catalyzes the oxidation of hypoxanthine to xanthine and xanthine to uric acid. Apparently the influence exerted by allopurinol to depress purine biosynthesis

contributes to its effectiveness to decrease uric acid serum levels.

In patients who suffer a relative deficiency of HGPTase, allopurinol will not decrease purine biosynthesis. It seems that HGPTase activity is necessary for allopurinol to exert its suppressive effect on purine synthesis. However, this effect of allopurinol is erratic; it did not suppress purine synthesis in several gouty patients who had normal uric acid production and normal HGPTase activity (underexcretors).

7. There are other inborn errors of metabolism which may alter the ability of afflicted individuals to effectively utilize or eliminate certain drugs. Hypophosphatemic vitamin D refractory rickets may be related to a defective receptor enzyme which has poor affinity for vitamin D.[26] This may interfere with transfer of vitamin D across the intestinal mucosa.

At the other extreme, patients who suffer excessive responses to conventional doses of vitamin D with resultant hypercalcemia and its nefarious sequelae, are suspected of having some other aberration of enzyme transport mechanisms.

Variations in pyridoxine responsiveness resulting in hypochromic microcytic anemia are suspected of being enzyme-insufficiency states. The porphyrinuric reactions to barbiturates are due to failure of regulatory mechanisms which result in overproduction of alpha aminolevulenic acid synthetase. This, in turn causes an excessive production of porphyrins which exceeds the ability of the marrow to employ them in the synthesis of heme. Porphyrins accumulate in the blood and can cause an exacerbation of acute intermittent porphyria.[27]

Drug-induced acute intermittent porphyrinuria attacks have also been related to sulfonamides, chloramphenicol, quinine, anticoagulants, tranquilizers, diethylstilbestrol, and oral contraceptives.

One could speculate on Wilson's Disease with defective or deficient ceruloplasmin, or hemochromatosis related to a defect which permits excessive iron to pass through the small intestine into the blood. Both of these may be related to enzymatic or carrier protein abnormalities. One might also wonder about the effect of drugs on other enzyme insufficiencies such as lactase in the small intestine, hydroxylase in the adrenal glands, and others.

Thus, if one reflects on the multitude of known enzyme systems, as well as those suspected as latent or subclinical, but not as yet identified, it could be predicted that many reactions now classified as idiosyncratic or even allergic will gradually be herded into the fold of pharmacogenetic disorders or acquired enzyme insufficiencies.

Drug Interactions*

One of the more complex, fascinating, and disturbing areas of pharmacology which has direct pertinence in any discussion of adverse drug reactions is *drug interactions*. Efforts to establish a feasible classification continue as new mechanisms are discovered.

Hartshorn[5] defines drug interaction as "The phenomenon which occurs when the effects of one drug are modified by the prior or concurrent administration of another (or the same) drug(s). Drug interactions may arise either from alteration of the absorption, distribution, biotransformation, or excretion of one

---

* For further information, see Table IV (page 1835) in Chapter 94, *The Prescription.*

drug by another or from combination of their actions or effects." He makes a distinction between interaction and incompatibility. The latter term is reserved for reactions which occur *in vitro*.

Irey[4] classifies drug interactions under several categories:

1. Interaction with other drugs (or themselves)
2. Interaction with endogenous physiologic chemical agents (eg, monoamine oxidase inhibitors and epinephrine)
3. Interaction with components of the diet (eg, MAOI with tyramine in cheese)
4. Interaction with chemicals used in diagnostic tests or the results of such tests (eg, oral contraceptives and glucose tolerance tests)

However, perhaps a more comprehensive classification is offered by Hartshorn.[28]

A. Chemical reactions between drugs
B. Pharmacodynamics
  1. Modification of intestinal absorption
    a. Alteration of pH
    b. Effect on transport systems
    c. Complex formation
    d. Miscellaneous
      i. Changes in circulation (eg, epinephrine and local anesthetics)
      ii. Precipitation (eg, procaine and penicillin)
  2. Displacement of drugs from storage tissue component
    a. Drug–drug
    b. Drug–endogenous substance (hormone or neurohormone)
  3. Modification of drug action at receptor site
    a. Physiological antagonism
    b. Competitive inhibition
    c. Nonequilibrium antagonism
    d. Noncompetitive antagonism
    e. Partial agonist
  4. Biotransformation
    a. Enzyme inhibitors
    b. Enzyme stimulators
    c. Complex mechanisms
  5. Alteration of excretion
    a. Change urinary pH
    b. Direct effect on kidney
    c. Complex reactions
C. Physiological factors affecting drug interactions
  1. Age
  2. Body temperature
  3. Nutritional state
  4. Pathological state
  5. Sex, species, genetics, strain, etc
D. Others
  1. Increase or decrease in synthetics
  2. Effect on transport mechanism (eg, insulin and glucose)

A detailed analysis of drug interactions is proper fare for textbooks of pharmacology. The text by Goldstein, et al[21] is recommended.

This discussion will be confined to enzyme induction (stimulation of enzymatic metabolism), enzyme inhibition (interference with enzymatic metabolism), and a few comments on drug excretion and residual drug effects. Examination of the chemical and physical mechanisms involved in drug interactions is beyond the scope of this chapter.

In many instances the actual mechanisms involved in known drug interactions have not been elucidated. An effort has been made to express the potential complexity with a simple Venn diagram. Fig. 502 shows the interaction between Drug A, Drug B, an enzyme system, and the end organ. Each of the overlapping segments could represent a site of modification of drug action. It must be realized that the areas of interaction may not be symmetrical, and—if one were to add circles representing more drugs, more enzyme systems, more end organs, intermediate drug metabolites, and the varieties of illness—the infinite complexity becomes almost overpowering.

Giving drugs to patients is not a simple business.

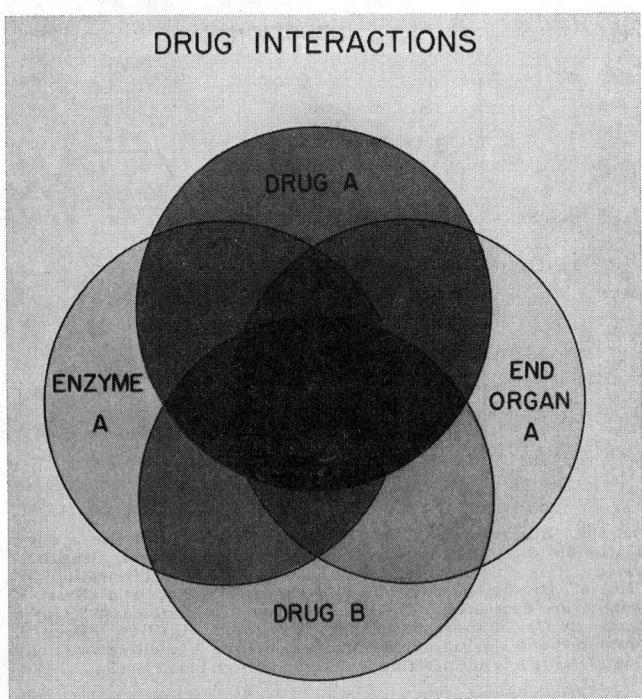

Fig. 502. A Venn diagram demonstrating the interaction of two drugs with each other, an enzyme system, and an end organ. The dark central area indicates the confluence of factors that influence drug actions. The addition of extra drugs, extra enzyme systems, end organs, and diseases can provide some visual conception of the complexity of drug interactions.

Enzyme Induction

Many drugs taken over a period of time can cause a marked acceleration of their own metabolism or can accelerate the metabolism of other drugs being administered concomitantly or subsequently. This effect is mediated through stimulation of drug metabolizing enzymes in liver microsomes. The process is called *enzyme induction*,[29-31] and it has become an important aspect of drug therapy.

Induction can lead to an escalating requirement for maintenance doses. There are several classic examples of this phenomenon; phenylbutazone self-induction is an example. In animal experiments increased daily doses were required to maintain plasma levels which inevitably declined. Coincidentally, with the highest doses, toxic effects such as vomiting, anorexia, and bloody stools were observed.[31]

The same phenomenon has been observed with probenecid, glutethimide, meprobamate, diphenhydramine, chlorcyclizine, and hexobarbital.[32] It is readily apparent that there are great difficulties in adjusting the dosage of a drug capable of causing enzyme induction. In the case of probenecid, it took approximately three weeks for enzyme induction to develop fully, and with it came a requirement to increase daily dosage to maintain satisfactory blood levels.

Of course, most drugs do not invoke enzyme induction. Nor is it known if all individuals are susceptible to enzyme induction by a specific drug. There is an evident need for a convenient test to determine whether or not enzyme induction is a potential problem before one decides upon long-term administration of any drug.

This brings us to another aspect of this effect. Not only may a drug accelerate its own metabolism, but it may affect others. The administration of

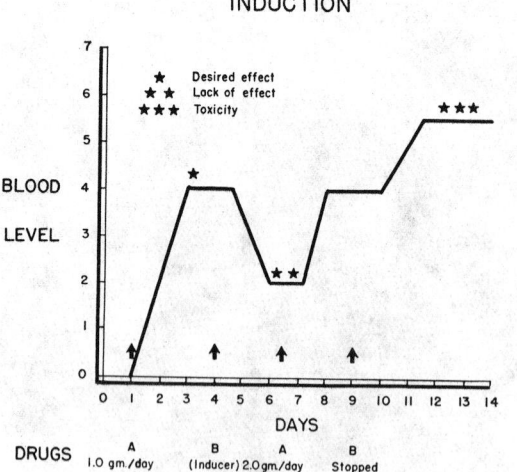

INDUCTION

★   Desired effect
★★   Lack of effect
★★★   Toxicity

BLOD
LEVEL

DAYS

DRUGS   A   B   A   B
1.0 gm./day   (Inducer) 2.0gm./day   Stopped

Fig. 503. Drug A is started at a conventional dose (1.0 Gm a day). By the 3rd day, "desired effect" is achieved. On day 4, Drug B is added; it is an "inducer" (*accelerates* metabolic deterioration) of Drug A. By the 6th day, blood levels (and therapeutic effect) of Drug A are decreased. The dose of Drug A is doubled (2.0 Gm a day). By Day 8, therapeutic effect is restored. On Day 9, Drug B, is stopped and the induction influence on Drug A is withdrawn. By Day 12, Drug A is manifesting toxicity (and high blood levels).

Drug A may stimulate hepatic microsomes to produce enzymes which accelerate the metabolic breakdown of Drug B. If this phenomenon is not appreciated and anticipated, it may result in lower than expected blood levels of Drug B.

In this idealized diagram (Fig. 503), we see that the patient is given Drug A in a conventional dose (1.0 Gm a day). After a few days an adequate clinical response is obtained. Then he is given Drug B (by the same or another physician). It happens that Drug B is capable of "inducing" enzymes that accelerate the metabolism of Drug A. In a few days (mysteriously) the previous benefit from Drug A has vanished. So the dose is doubled (2.0 Gm a day); within a few days, therapeutic levels are again achieved. If blood levels were determined, they would correlate with the clinical response. But now Drug B is withdrawn, and the stimulus to induction is gone; Drug A remains in the blood at twice the normal level, and we have a drug-intoxicated patient. If this all occurs without the physician appreciating the mechanism, he could develop paranoid delusions.

Thus, the importance of enzyme induction cannot be overemphasized. For example, in animals the hypnotic effect of hexobarbital, the muscle relaxant action of zoxazolamine, and the anticonvulsant action of diphenylhydantoin are almost completely abolished in dogs pretreated for several days with phenobarbital.[32] In each instance, phenobarbital exerts its effect by accelerating the metabolic degradation of the subsequently administered drug.

The remarkable ability of phenobarbital to stimulate drug metabolism in animals directed attention to the problem in man. The most extensive work also has been done in the acceleration of bishydroxycoumarin metabolism by phenobarbital.[31,33] There have been many clinical reports of this phenomenon where the dose of a coumarin drug had to be increased to maintain satisfactory anticoagulant activity, while conventional doses of phenobarbital were being given. Other drugs which are susceptible to enzyme induction by phenobarbital include warfarin, meprobamate, chlordiazepoxide, oral contraceptive agents, and

griseofulvin. This is a vast area which is rapidly expanding.

To repeat the cardinal principle: individual doses of drugs may be required that are quite toxic in an effort to maintain blood levels that were achieved with much lower doses earlier in the course of drug therapy. The corollary is equally as important: one may consider that a drug is ineffective, when the actual fact is that the blood levels are too low despite the administration of "proper" doses.

To repeat, we must devise simple tests to determine if *the* drug we are about to prescribe for *this* patient will cause induction (of itself, or some other drug(s) we intend to give at the same time). This should be a prime mission of clinical pharmacology.

Enzyme Inhibition

Perhaps a more familiar situation, which is antithetical to enzyme induction and accelerated drug metabolism, is *inhibition* of the metabolic breakdown of one drug by another with *potentiation* of effect.

This is illustrated in an idealized diagram (Fig. 504). Drug A is given in conventional dosage (1.0 Gm a day). A satisfactory blood level and therapeutic response is obtained. Then Drug B is given, which inhibits the metabolic degradation of Drug A. After a few days the blood level of Drug A rises, and toxic effects are noted. So Drug A is decreased (0.5 Gm a day), and soon the blood level has declined to normal levels, and evidence of toxicity regresses. Suddenly Drug B is withdrawn; the inhibiting effect upon the breakdown of Drug A is removed, and the blood level falls with a loss of therapeutic effectiveness. It is another situation designed to aggravate the clinician who is not aware of the mechanisms at play.

This is epitomized by the *persistence* of high blood levels of coumarin anticoagulants due to inhibition of breakdown metabolism by some rather common therapeutic agents such as phenyramidol, acetylsalicylic acid, tetracycline, streptomycin, thyroxine, methandrostenolone, phenylbutazone, oxyphenbutazone, chloral hydrate, quinine, and diphenylhydantoin.[32]

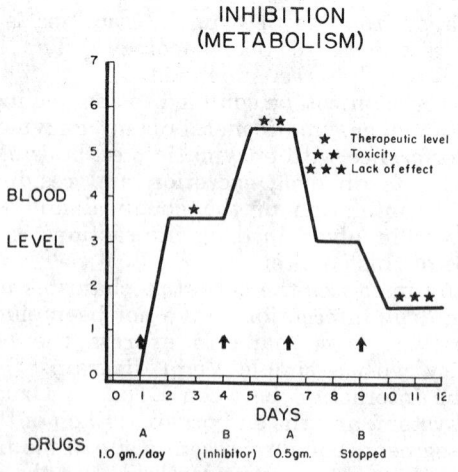

INHIBITION
(METABOLISM)

★   Therapeutic level
★★   Toxicity
★★★   Lack of effect

BLOOD
LEVEL

DAYS

DRUGS   A   B   B
1.0 gm./day   (Inhibitor) 0.5gm.   Stopped

Fig. 504. Drug A is started in a dose of 1.0 Gm a day. Therapeutic effect (and satisfactory blood levels) are attained by Day 2. On Day 4, Drug B is added; it happens to *inhibit* the metabolic deterioration of Drug A. By Day 5, excessive blood levels with toxicity are related to Drug A. On Day 6, the dose of Drug A is cut to 0.5 mg a day. By Day 7, the blood levels are again satisfactory and toxicity has gone. On Day 9, Drug B is stopped—the effect of inhibiting the breakdown of Drug A is gone. By Day 10, we have lower than therapeutic blood levels and loss of beneficial effect.

There are many other examples of this. Methandrostenolone will inhibit the metabolic breakdown of oxyphenylbutazone. Phenylbutazone, sulfadimethoxine, sulfaphenazole, and dicoumarol[34] will prolong blood levels of tolbutamide.

Mechanisms are complex. In some instances there is direct inhibition of the enzymes involved in metabolic breakdown. A classic example occurs with monoamine oxidase inhibitors.[1,35] Under normal circumstances monoamine oxidase destroys amines, such as catecholamines and serotonin. After a monoamine oxidase-inhibiting drug is given, of course, the metabolic breakdown of catecholamines is inhibited. If releasers of catecholamines are then given, an acute hypertensive crisis can occur, which may result in disastrous vascular complications.[35] Examples of catecholamine-releasers are: tyramine (ingested in the form of pickled herring, old cheddar cheese, or chianti wine), amphetamine, methamphetamine, reserpine, and guanethidine.

Parenthetically, Levine and Strauch[36] described a young man who developed paradoxical hypertension following intravenous administration of methyldopa. Under normal circumstances, methyldopa exerts its antihypertensive effect by interference with the transmission of adrenergic impulses by displacing norepinephrine from nerve endings and substituting relatively weak *false neurotransmitter* metabolites (alphamethyldopamine, alphamethylnorepinephrine). Thus, after a period of administration of methyldopa, formation of these metabolites generally results in a decrease in blood pressure.

However, intravenous administration of alphamethyldopamine[37] or alphamethylnorepinephrine paradoxically raises blood pressure. They produce their pressor effects by either of two mechanisms: (1) indirectly by release of norepinephrine or (2) directly by stimulation of adrenergic alpha receptors.

In view of this information, these authors suggested that the paradoxical pressor response to methyldopa in their patient was mediated by either excessive synthesis of pressor metabolites or supernormal sensitivity of end organs. "It seems unlikely that there were increased stores of norepinephrine. He was not taking MAO-inhibiting drugs. The clinical findings and urinary VMA excretions did not suggest pheochromocytoma."[36]

Another drug interaction phenomenon is related to the tricyclic antidepressants. Amitriptyline, desipramine, imipramine, and nortriptyline should never be given with or soon after MAOI drugs. One can get a severe atropine-like reaction with tremors, severe hyperpyrexia, clonic convulsions, delirium, and even death.[32]

The clinical capriciousness of patients receiving oral anticoagulant therapy is familiar. Even those who take their medications faithfully often have erratic prothrombin responses. Factors such as variation in the dietary intake of vitamin K, inhibition of vitamin K synthesis by intestinal bacteria (as would occur with broad spectrum oral antibiotic administration), or changes in intestinal dynamics (as in blind loop syndrome) have been implicated. In addition there are many disease states characterized by hepatic involvement that may inhibit synthesis of hepatic clotting factors (and thereby increase the patient's sensitivity to oral anticoagulants). And, of course, many *drugs* which modify anticoagulant-induced depression of prothrombin synthesis have been discovered.

To summarize, there are several mechanisms of drug interactions that can explain variation in anticoagulant response.

1. Drugs which alter availability of enteric vitamin K (antibiotics).
2. Drugs which accelerate coumarin metabolism (glutethimide, griseofulvin, barbiturates).
3. Drugs which inhibit coumarin metabolism (phenyramidol, chloral hydrate, acetylsalicylic acid).
4. Drugs which displace coumarin drugs from plasma binding sites (phenylbutazone).
5. Drugs which inhibit synthesis of prothrombin and other procoagulant factors.

There are other mechanisms whereby one drug can cause unanticipated high or sustained blood levels of another: (1) disease of the excretory organ can be exacerbated by Drug A, which then causes inhibition of excretion of Drug B; (2) physical displacement from albumin binding sites of Drug A by Drug B, to permit more free Drug A to circulate.

Drug Excretion

A prototype example of a drug affecting the excretion of another is phenylbutazone, which causes unusually high blood levels of acetohexamide (Dymelor) by inhibiting renal excretion of its active metabolite hydroxyhexamide.[38] Clinical hypoglycemia has occurred. Drugs known to inhibit excretion of penicillin by inhibition of tubular reabsorption are probenecid and zoxazolamine.

The effects of drugs upon tubular enzyme systems which then influence reabsorption and excretion of other drugs are just beginning to be explored.

Residual Drug Effects

Residual drug effects remain another enigmatic area. For example, reserpine continues to exert its influence in certain patients for several weeks after it has been discontinued. It may cause unpredictable responses to general anesthesia.[39,40] Reserpine may obscure the phentolamine test for pheochromocytoma for several weeks after it has been stopped. The persisting and progressive retinal damage induced by chloroquine will be discussed in later sections.

Elevated levels of protein-bound iodine were found in the sera of women who had received iophenoxic acid, a cholecystographic medium, up to seven years previously. Babies born several years after their mothers had ingested iophenoxic acid had extremely high levels of protein-bound iodine.[41]

These agents may lie dormant in fat depots for many years, apparently innocuous, but in curious contradiction to the usual tendency of the organism to rid itself of foreign substances. What other drugs are "stored" for prolonged periods? Do they exert adverse effects? Questions come easily; answers do not.

Resistance Transfer Factors[42–44]

A new dimension was integrated into the study of drug resistance by Watanabe.[43] He first described Resistance Transfer Factors (RTF), responsible for the transmission of specific antibiotic resistance from microorganism to microorganism. Resistance transfer factors are contained in episomes. These are non-chromosomal genetic determinants—packages of DNA which exist autonomously in cytoplasm and may become attached to chromosomes. Transmission of antibiotic resistance was first demonstrated in *Shigella*; now it has been demonstrated in various other Gram-negative enterobacteriaciae species (including *Escherichia, Salmonella, Citrobacteria*); also, *Klebsiella, Aerobacter, Serratia, Pasteurella, Pseudomonas,* and *Vibrio* have shown a genetic ability to transfer drug resistance. Recently a report of this phenomenon occurring in *Staphylococcus aureus* has appeared, the first Gram-positive organism implicated.

Sulfonamides were the first antibacterials against which RTF developed. Now tetracyclines, ampicillin, neomycin, kanamycin, and streptomycin must be included in this unfortunate category.

Schroeder, *et al,*[44] reviewed the problem of antibiotic resistance and transfer factors in *Salmonella* in the US; 22% of 400 strains were resistant to one or more antibiotics (streptomycin, 14.2%; tetracycline, 12.5%; sulfathiazole, 11.5%). Resistance was significantly more frequent in *Salmonella typhimurium* than in other serologic types. Of 52 strains exhibiting resistance to multiple drugs, 79% demonstrated RTF. However, this survey revealed no significant change in clinical incidence of resistant *Salmonella* organisms over the past five years.[44]

The cause is suspected to be related to widespread indiscriminant use of antibiotics in animal feeds. Low blood levels are achieved which are insufficient to kill microorganisms, yet permit them to develop RTF.

This mechanism is distinct from true chromosome-borne genetic resistance to antibiotics which accounts for most variations in species sensitivity to antibiotics. Mechanisms may be similar in episomes and chromosomes.

Drug-Induced Diseases by Systems

Now that we have seen something of the broad introductory area of drug-induced diseases, a logical question might be: What will be the ultimate effect of these new therapeutic endeavors? The answer must lie somewhere in the misty interface between philosophy and physiology.

The evolution of man is a continuing source of wonderment to students of physiology. Through the centuries of evolutionary metamorphosis, each challenge thrown at man by his environment was met by gradual genetic modulation that enabled him to survive. The species has arrived at the current state of advanced physiologic capability, admirably adapted to its environment. We can dig diamonds at 9000 ft in 123° heat and 100% humidity; we can spend a lifetime mining tin at 14,900 feet elevation; we can hike across the pole; and we can float weightless for 14 days in space.

But in the past few decades we have devised methods unprecedented in the entire previous experience of the species to challenge the adaptability of the organism. We have designed molecules unique to human physiology and insinuated them into blood and tissue by techniques that are also unique in physiologic experience. Intravenous, intramuscular, and subcutaneous injections; positive-pressure inhalation; rectal administration; and agents that facilitate passage of molecules through intact skin—all are unnatural modes of gaining access to the body. Add radiation—by x-ray, beta ray, gamma ray, and neutron, plus oxygen under greatly increased barometric pressure, and some others doubtlessly forgotten—and one begins to appreciate the magnitude and genius of man's conspiracy to bypass the conventional avenues for introducing new environmental factors to the physiology of man.

In the past we only had to cope with naive nature and unsubtle environment. And they were confined to the gastrointestinal tract, lungs, and occasionally the abraided skin, as avenues of access for alien materials to get at the core of man.

The implications of these ingenious tactics of assault, these strange man-made chemicals and emanations upon the beleaguered human mechanism are fascinating to contemplate. One could speculate that this incredibly resilient physiologic engine of ours is sufficiently advanced in design to be able to cope with all environmental transgressors. We have evolved defenses at all levels from the simplest reflex to the most complex immune reactions to meet the daily challenges of environment. And we have done very well in the matter of self-preservation.

Yet it is quite evident that some of these unprecedented therapeutic intrusions overtax the ability of the body to accommodate—and it will react with displeasure, if not violent rejection. And, of course, this is the heart of our thesis—drug-induced diseases.

Every new drug must be evaluated for efficacy and toxicity, and this is not an easy task. Only passage of time and acquisition of experience will determine the ultimate verdict. Firm pronouncements based on animal experimentation or fragmentary early clinical trials are premature and meaningless. Often it takes years before the full spectrum of efficacy or toxicity of a drug becomes evident. This poses an almost insoluble conundrum. If we are timid and withhold the drug, how will we ever gain the necessary clinical experience? If the agent is effective and safe, it would seem unfair to withhold it. But if the drug is ineffective or toxic, it would seem equally unfair to use it on patients. All that one can propose is prudence, caution, and reservation of final judgment until objective studies are completed.

Most of the data used to prepare the following sections of this chapter were obtained from case reports describing one or several patients; some are little better than clinical impressions. In the study of drug reactions, objective data are hard to come by; prospective studies are still comparatively rare. Few physicians have the inclination or forensic courage to challenge a patient with a drug suspected to be significantly toxic.

This is very close to the heart of the problem of adverse drug reaction reporting. There remains a critical need to derive realistic incidence figures for drug-induced diseases. More important, we must find means to identify *which patient* will respond adequately, poorly, or adversely to *which* drug. We are not interested in statistics, but rather in how the *individual* will respond.

Now let us proceed to some specifics. A detailed discussion of drug-induced diseases would require the space of a fair-sized book;[1] this presentation will highlight a few specific areas.

Dermatologic Reactions

Rostenberg and Fagelson[45] reviewed the literature from 1960 to 1964 to gather data on "life-threatening drug reactions." These were divided into four groups. Each will be discussed in turn.

Group 1 (*Stevens–Johnson Syndrome*)—These workers documented 23 cases with four deaths. Fourteen of this total and two of the deaths were related to sulfamethoxypyridazine. Carroll, *et al,*[46] reviewed their FDA data from 1957 to 1965 regarding case reports of Stevens–Johnson syndrome associated with long-term sulfonamides. Out of 116 reports received, only 27 presented sufficient information to implicate long-acting sulfonamides. The median time of appearance of the reaction was about the 10th day from the start of the drug; extremes were from the 2nd day to as late as 6 days after the drug had been discontinued. FDA has required that a warning regarding the possibility of Stevens–Johnson syndrome be published on the package inserts for sulfamethoxypyridazine and sulfadimethoxine.

Ten other drugs alone or in combination were cited in addition as probable etiologic factors in Stevens–Johnson syndrome. These included penicillin, antipyrine, phenolphthalein, quinine, mercury preparations, aspirin, phenylbutazone, chlorpropamide, anticonvulsants, antitoxins, vaccines, and deep irradiation.

Bianchine, et al,[47] raised some doubts concerning the indictment of long-acting sulfonamides in the genesis of Stevens–Johnson syndrome, especially sulfamethoxypyridazine. According to their data, penicillin, short-acting sulfonamides, phenolphthalein-containing preparations, and sedatives were more commonly associated with this severe mucocutaneous disorder than long-acting sulfonamides.

However, the prevalence of case reports in which sulfonamides have been suspected, in addition to the reports of hepatitis and blood dyscrasias related to long-acting sulfonamides, would make it prudent to suggest that all sulfonamide drugs be employed with circumspection.[48]

Group 2—*Toxic epidermal necrolysis* was found in 13 patients with 5 deaths; phenylbutazone accounted for 4 of the 13 cases.[45]

Group 3—*Systemic lupus erythematosus* was discovered in 16 patients; procainamide was involved in 6 of the 16 cases.[45]

Group 4—*Exfoliative dermatitis* was reported in 6 patients with 2 deaths. Aminosalicylic acid, diphenylhydantoin, griseofulvin, phenindione, and sulfamethoxypyridazine accounted for one patient each. Of the entire group, the sulfonamides were the most frequent offenders.[45]

Dermatitis medicamentosa continues to plague the dermatologists as new topical agents are introduced to challenge the resilience of the integument. Neomycin was the most common offender in a recent series.[49] This was followed by iodochlorhydroxyquin, thimerosal, tripelennamine, methapyrilene, and the topical anesthetics (benzocaine, cyclomethycaine, and dibucaine).

Photosensitivity reactions of the phototoxic and photoallergic varieties have been related to many drugs.[50] Among the most common offenders are coal-tar derivates, thiazides, sulfonamide compounds, chlorpromazine, demethylchlortetracycline, promethazine, oral hypoglycemic agents (chlorpropamide and tolbutamide), cyclamate (the artificial sweetener),[51] and furocoumarins.

Then there are some interesting random observations from the dermatology literature. Generalized pustular psoriasis due to the ingestion of potassium iodide continues to be described.[52] Shelley[53] reported 2 patients in whom systemic manifestations developed; these included hepatitis, fever, leukocytosis, hypoproteinemia, hypocalcemia, and elevations of serum transaminase and alkaline phosphatase. A challenge with 500 mg of orally administered potassium iodide reproduced typical attacks. In one patient, a single oral challenge with progesterone (5.0 mg) was followed

by a minor clinical attack of pustular psoriasis. Salicylates also appear capable of inducing similar adverse effects in susceptible individuals.[54] The numerous drugs capable of causing acneform eruptions will not be discussed.[55]

Electron microscopic examination and assay of extracts and residues of normal and involved skin from patients with chlorpromazine-induced discolorations revealed that the pigmentation was due to a combination of drug and melanin.[56]

The unfortunate experience with triparanol has been reviewed; complications included alopecia, change in skin color, and icthyosis, followed by the development of posterior subcapsular cataracts in 6 patients.[57] Of course, this drug has been withdrawn. Individual case reports of adverse dermatologic reactions related to specific drugs are legion.

Gastrointestinal Diseases

Ulcers caused by drugs continue to occupy a prominent status as iatrogenic diseases. Several years ago, notoriety was achieved by enteric-coated potassium chloride tablets, indicated as the culprit in the genesis of circumferential ulcers of jejunum and ileum.[58,59]

But there are many other old drugs residing in the physician's armamentarium which occasionally demonstrate their erosive personalities. These include salicylates[60] (especially aspirin; this is unrelated to physical form and seems to be a function of individual reaction),[61] phenylbutazone, reserpine, indomethacin,[62] histamine, caffeine, nicotinic acid, nitrofurantoin, and phenylephrine. The controversy over corticosteroid provocation of peptic ulcer remains incompletely resolved. Most clinicians feel that the relationship is often devastatingly real.[63] Gastrointestinal involvement with buccal ulcerations and inflammation of intestines is the chief expression of 5-fluorouracil toxicity.

Digitalis toxicity has been implicated as a rare contributory cause of nonocclusive hemorrhagic enteropathy.[64] In this unusual syndrome, there is extensive hemorrhagic necrosis involving the gastrointestinal mucosa. One finds mesenteric venous congestion but no occlusion of vessels, venous or arterial. This condition usually develops in a clinical setting of severe congestive heart failure, shock, and cardiac arrhythmias. Other manifestations of digitalis toxicity have been present in some of these cases. It has been suggested that the vasoconstrictor action of digitalis on hepatic and mesenteric veins may be a factor of importance.

The roster of drugs capable of causing jaundice continues to expand. The problem of separating drug-induced hepatitis from viral hepatitis remains vexing.[65] Popper and his associates[66] have attempted to classify hepatotoxic agents on the basis of their pathologic effect.

1. *Zonal injury*—characterized by carbon tetrachloride.
2. *Uncomplicated cholestasis*—exemplified by all anabolic steroids.
3. *Nonspecific drug hepatitis with or without cholestasis*—characterized by chlorpromazine and its congeners as the prototypes.
4. *Viral hepatitis-like reaction*—characterized by iproniazid, sulfonamides, and halothane.
5. *Drug-induced steatosis*—epitomized by the tetracyclines.[67–69]

When given in large doses by the intravenous route to pregnant young women with pyelonephritis, tetracycline has caused fatal steatosis. Liver pathology is dominated by cytoplasmic fat globules. This is similar to the steatosis of pregnancy (acute yellow atrophy) observed in the preantibiotic era.[70] Tetracycline retards protein synthesis, and it is suspected that steatosis follows in the wake of hepatic protein inhibition. Modification of indigenous flora by the antibiotic plays no part.

Since the early reports, hepatic steatosis has been observed following ingestion of oral tetracycline by *nonpregnant* women and in men with pre-existing liver disease. We have seen a tragic young soldier who returned from Vietnam severely burned. He contracted systemic melioidosis and was treated with large doses of intravenous tetracycline. He died of hepatic steatosis.

Other additions to the hepatotoxic rogues gallery included estrogens,[71] acetohexamide,[72] erythromycin estolate,[73,74] sulfamethoxazole,[75,76] sulfisoxazole,[77] trimethobenzamide,[78] sulfamethoxypyridazine,[79] colchicine,[80] mercaptopurine,[81] oxacillin,[82] tranylcypromine,[83] chlordiazepoxide,[84] prochlorperazine,[85] methoxyflurane,[86] thioridazine,[87] tannic acid (in barium sulfate enemas),[88] phenazopyridine,[89] chlorpropamide,[90] oral contraceptives,[91] and indomethacin.[92]

The status of halothane as a rare cause of severe hepatic failure has been studied. The National Halothane Study reviewed data on 856,000 patients undergoing general anesthesia and surgery in 34 institutions before and after appearance of reports on liver damage.[93,94]

On the basis of the most careful statistical analysis of mortality data, the death rate following halothane anesthesia was found to be lower than the over-all average and midway among the 5 general anesthetic practices. Massive hepatic necrosis was a rare complication occurring only 82 times (1 per 10,000 cases following surgery and anesthesia).

Thus, the very small hazard of hepatic necrosis is outweighed by its over-all safety record. Halothane is a superb anesthetic; it continues to be employed with circumspection and proper observation of contraindications. However, unexplained early postoperative fever or delayed onset of jaundice or abnormal liver function after exposure are ominous signs. In this situation, re-exposure is contraindicated. It is generally conceded that it is inadvisable to give repeated inductions with halothane over a short period of time.[95]

Recent interest has been focused on the phenomenon of sudden death due to hepatic failure occurring in children with rheumatoid arthritis receiving indomethacin.[92,96] Five documented cases have been found. The syndrome is characterized by an acute febrile illness with icterus, acidosis, and death occurring within 72 hours to 2 weeks. Duration of indomethacin therapy ranged from 1 month to more than 1 year. Other drugs were often administered simultaneously (steroids, salicylates, and antibiotics), but none of these has been known to cause hepatic necrosis. It would seem prudent *not* to give indomethacin to children.

Bunamiodyl has been observed to compete with sulfobromophthalein for excretion; this can cause false positive tests for sulfobromophthalein retention.[97]

Cholestyramine given to pruritus-ridden patients with primary biliary cirrhosis has been related to the appearance of calcium-containing gallstones; one patient had associated calcification of the head of the pancreas.[98] In nine patients thus far reported with this disorder, positive calcium balance has been detected while the patients were on cholestyramine.[99]

Occasional case reports of hepatoma related to long-forgotten administration of thorium dioxide as a contrast medium to illuminate the splenoportal system continue to appear.[100] Hepatoma related to heavy-metal injection for antisyphilis chemotherapy also has been reported.[101]

Acute hemorrhagic pancreatitis has been attributed to chlorthalidone, sulfamethoxazole, corticosteroids, indomethacin, and thiazide diuretics.[102]

Other gastrointestinal diseases include serum hepatitis acquired from pooled plasma fractions, especially fibrinogen, and kernicterus of the newborn subsequent to administration of vitamin K analogs or sulfisoxazole. The latter disorder is related to immaturity of the neonatal liver which lacks adequate stores of glucuronyl transferase. This enzyme is required to conjugate bilirubin to its secretable, more-soluble glucuronide. The drugs compete for the meager amount of enzyme and insoluble, unconjugated bilirubin piles up in the serum, seeps into the cerebrospinal fluid, and damages delicate neonatal cerebral tissue.[103]

The *gray syndrome* of newborns is related to a deficiency of hepatic enzymes needed to conjugate chloramphenicol. This clinical configuration results from high levels of unconjugated (free) chloramphenicol.[19,104] Malabsorption syndromes resulting from administration of aminosalicylic acid or oral antibiotics may produce broad or selective deficiency states (hypovitaminoses).[105]

Many investigators have described the complications of diuretic therapy in patients with ascites due to hepatic cirrhosis. Sherlock, *et al*,[106] analyzed patients on various combinations of low-sodium diet, chlorothiazide, spironolactone, furosemide, and ethacrynic acid: 75% had experienced mild serum electrolyte disturbances; in 26% this was severe. Hypocalcemia and hyponatremia occurred in about 40%; azotemia in 34%; hypochloremic alkalosis related to chloride loss in about 12%. Furosemide and ethacrynic acid were the most frequent offenders.

Methysergide maleate has been implicated as a cause of postprandial abdominal angina without other cardiac, vascular, and fibrotic complications.[107]

A final iatrogenic gastrointestinal disorder is pseudomembranous enterocolitis resulting from staphylococcal overgrowth following suppression of normal flora by tetracyclines and other broad spectrum antibiotics.[108]

Hematologic Disorders

Of all the areas of drug-induced disease, the literature on hematologic disorders is the most prodigious. The subject was reviewed in a series of brief articles by the members of the Hematology Panel of the Registry of Adverse Drug Effects; they will serve as the matrix of this discussion.

Beutler[109] divided drug-induced hemolytic anemias into three groups.

1. Those related to glucose-6-phosphate-dehydrogenase deficiency, in which the anemia is precipitated by "oxidant" drugs such as primaquine, nitrofurantoin, and acetanilid (this was discussed previously).
2. Hemolysis due to the development of antibodies to drugs such as stibophen, penicillin, quinine, quinidine, cephalothin, methyldopa, and phenacetin. This is a rather complex group, which will be discussed in greater detail.
3. Rarely, hemolytic anemia develops due to the persistence of unusually high blood levels of certain drugs because of impaired renal excretion.

Instances of hemolytic anemia due to minor blood-group incompatibilities (usually related to previous transfusions) continue to occur. An anti-Jk[b] reaction, in which antibodies were not detected until hemolysis occurred 8 days after the last transfusion, has been observed.[110]

In recent months there has been considerable interest in the subject of drug-induced, Coombs-positive reactions and hemolytic anemia.[111–113] Four varieties of this phenomenon have been identified. The oldest is related to penicillin.[111] When this drug is taken in high doses or conventional doses are given in the presence of renal insufficiency (which results in the acquisition and retention of high blood levels), penicillin may act as a hapten. In conjunction with a protein moiety it can provoke antibody production. The antigen–antibody complex may come to rest on the surface of the red blood cell (RBC), resulting in modification of surface characteristics. This results in a decreased RBC survival—frequently (but not invariably) culminating in frank hemolysis. A "broad spectrum" type of Coombs antibody test will be positive.

A second variety is that related to quinidine and stibophen.[112] To delineate this entity, a complement-specific Coombs test must be performed. Complement has been identified on the surface of the RBC which can be detected by anticomplementary Coombs sera. Of course, the same mechanism applies to the thrombocytopenic purpura, occasionally seen with quinidine and stibophen as described by Shulman, et al.[114] Again modification of surface lipoproteins increases the vulnerability to destruction by the reticuloendothelial system.

A third variety is that seen with alphamethyldopa.[115] In this condition the drug cannot be identified on the surface of the red cell, although specific anti-IGG Coombs sera will detect the presence of gamma globulin on the surface of the red cell. Thus, it is quite similar to autoimmune hemolytic anemia. It is almost as though the alphamethyldopa precipitates an autoimmune reaction.

Carstairs and co-workers[116] found 20% of patients taking alphamethyldopa to have a positive direct anti-IGG Coombs test. None developed hemolytic anemia, although several had mildly elevated reticulocyte counts. In all instances patients who developed Coombs positivity had been taking the drug for 5 or more months. This phenomenon occurred more commonly in patients receiving larger doses.

The same group of investigators later reported 25 of 30 patients in whom a frank hemolytic anemia developed in association with anti-IGG Coombs positivity. In most instances withdrawal of alphamethyldopa or the administration of corticosteroids terminated the anemia, but the positive Coombs test persisted for periods of 7 to 12 months.

The appearance of clinical hemolysis in a patient receiving alphamethyldopa certainly would make one suspect the drug. However, the relative rarity of the phenomenon must cause one to consider other etiologic factors. Of course, if a positive Coombs reaction develops during a course of treatment, it would be prudent to switch to another antihypertensive agent.

The fourth variety has been related to cephalothin (Keflin) and cephaloridine (Loridine).[117] This has been reported to cause a positive Coombs test in 40 to 75% of patients receiving long-term cephalothin, usually in high doses. Apparently, cephalothin binds with normal pre-existing plasma proteins (either regular plasma constituents or RBC membrane proteins). In-vitro studies with washed "cephalothinized" RBC mixed with anti-beta (non-gamma) Hyland reagent were invariably positive. In one series all patients had azotemia and hypoalbuminemia.

Molthan, et al,[117] suspect that a combination of high cephalothin blood concentrations (poor clearance), plus erythrocytes with increased sensitivity (due to uremic syndrome), may be factors in promoting Coombs positivity. Hypoalbuminemia may contribute to the problem since under normal circumstances the albumin fraction binds over 95% of circulating cephalothin. Thus, more free cephalothin may be available when hypoalbuminemia exists.

One may summarize the four mechanisms: penicillin, in which the drug acts as a haptene with the presence of an antigen–antibody complex on the RBC surface; stibophen and quinidine, in which a complement is identified on the RBC surface; alphamethyldopa, in which an anti-IGG globulin can be identified on the RBC surface; and cephalothin, in which there is a beta, non-antibody globulin on the RBC surface. The importance with regard to cephalothin resides in the fact that it may complicate blood-banking procedures when one is cross-matching on the minor side.

Erslev[118] reviewed cases of aplastic anemia collected by the Hematology Registry. He discussed the difficult problem of dissociating idiopathic cases from those caused by drugs. In about 44% of the cases of aplastic anemia, a drug could be identified as the cause. Chloramphenicol headed the list, accounting for about 20% of the cases in which a solitary drug could be cited definitely as the offending agent.

Best reviewed the experience of the American Medical Association Registry on Adverse Drug Reactions on the subject of chloramphenicol-associated blood dyscrasias.[119] A total of 408 patients had been reported to the Registry from 1953 to 1964, who were known to have received chloramphenicol during the year preceding the development of a non-neoplastic depression of blood-cell formation. In 40% of the patients, chloramphenicol was the only drug known to have been administered during the preceding 6 months. One other drug was mentioned in 19%, 2 in 13%, and 3 or more drugs had also been taken in 28%.

In 96% of the cases there was a strong suspicion that chloramphenicol was the causative agent of the aplastic anemia; in the remaining cases, chloramphenicol could not be excluded as the culprit.

Chloramphenicol can produce two varieties of bone marrow toxicity.[120] The first usually occurs during therapy; it is probably universal (occurring in greater or lesser degree in all chloramphenicol recipients) and related to dose. Such patients demonstrate an essentially normal cellular marrow, but it contains sideroblasts with cytoplasmic vacuoles. Such patients may have anemia but do not have associated leukopenia or thrombocytopenia. The disorder does not progress to aplastic anemia and regresses when chloramphenicol is withdrawn.

Most notorious is the second variety. This disorder has a delayed onset and is not dose-related; it represents an idiosyncratic reaction. These patients have an aplastic marrow with pancytopenia; death is a common sequela. The cases in Best's report fell into the latter category. It is important to know that as individual cases emerge they are not always easy to pigeonhole; often one cannot predict the outcome. From the best educated guess, Best says that the possibility of serious marrow toxicity occurs once in every 100,000 courses of therapy. In California, this was estimated at 1 in 60,000.

Perhaps the most critical and distressing aspect of this study was that chloramphenicol was prescribed for typhoid, paratyphoid, or Hemophilus influenzae meningitis (prime indications for its use), in only 6.6% of the fatal cases. It is true that chloramphenicol may also be indicated in specific, life-threatening acute or chronic Gram-negative rod infections (on the basis of *in-vitro* sensitivities), but with the later-generation antibiotics, this is a rare occurrence. Thus, in 93.4% of all fatal cases in the Registry, chloramphenicol was *not* indicated. Crosby[121] reminds us of the sobering fact that an estimated 8.0 million doses of chloramphenicol had been taken before this deadly relationship was established.

In the Registry cases, the initial reaction occurred in 10 days or less following the initial dose in 10% of cases; in 95 days or less in 50%. Ten per cent of patients went 260 days before aplastic anemia developed. The median time from discontinuation of the drug until clinical appearance of dyscrasia was 38 days.

A new dimension to the chloramphenicol story has been added with reports of acute myeloblastic leukemia that has emerged in patients who had aplastic anemia following chloramphenicol therapy.[122] It has been suggested that any agent that is severely myelo-toxic may also be a potential leukemogen.[120]

Fraumeni[123] reported a study of 151 patients who developed bone marrow depression following the use of *chloramphenicol* (124), *phenylbutazone* (24), or both (3). Leukemia was observed in three patients with bone marrow depression attributed to the use of chloramphenicol, but he felt that only one had characteristics suggesting a cause and effect relationship. He feels that current evidence is inadequate to state dogmatically that either drug is leukemogenic.

Crosby[121] advises that at least 20 cases have been called to his attention citing the emergence of acute myeloblastic leukemia from chloramphenicol-destroyed bone marrow.

Jensen and Roll[124] reported 50 patients who developed acute leukemia. They felt that three of these might have been related to phenylbutazone administration, but the available hard evidence precluded a definite statement. In another case, reported by Cassileth,[125] a patient with chlorpromazine-induced agranulocytosis developed a marked monocytosis; 18 months after complete recovery, acute leukemia developed.

Thus, a relationship between drug-induced bone marrow injury (whether the suspected agent is phenyl-butazone, chloramphenicol, or chlorpromazine) and the subsequent development of acute leukemia, is a matter of worrisome speculation. It cannot be dismissed lightly.

Other drugs implicated as rare causes of aplastic anemia include ethylmethylphenylhydantoin, other hydantoin anticonvulsants, sulfonamides, oral antidiabetic agents, phenylbutazone, insecticides, quinacrine, ethosuximide, and solvents.[118,126] The unfortunate shoe factory workers of northern Italy suffer an inordinate incidence of aplastic anemia and acute myeloblastic leukemia, which has been related to chronic inhalation of benzene fumes in pursuit of their livelihood.

Agranulocytosis was discussed by Huguley;[127] 382 cases were admitted to the Registry in which a single drug was held responsible for the illness. This is the most common adverse hematologic reaction to drugs.

Phenothiazines accounted for 128 of the 382 cases. Analgesics such as aminopyrine, dipyrone, phenyl-butazone, and oxyphenbutazone accounted for 48 cases of agranulocytosis. Chloramphenicol contributed 16; sulfanilamide, 20; thiouracil, 19; methimazole, 17; phenindione, 9.

Isolated case reports have appeared recording agranulocytosis alleged to be due to thioridazine,[128] chlorthalidone,[129] chlorpropamide,[130] vinblastine,[131] carbutamide, antimalarial therapy (with pyrimethamine, quinine, and DDS),[132,133] quinidine,[134] cephalothin,[135] and, perhaps, lincomycin.[136] Fatal agranulocytosis related to ethacrynic acid has appeared.[137]

Crosby and Kaufman[138] reviewed drug-induced thrombocytopenias. Offending drugs were divided into two groups: (1) those causing accelerated platelet destruction and (2) those depressing platelet production. More important drugs in the former category (which apparently mediate their effect through a sensitization mechanism) are quinidine, chlorothiazide, hydrochlorothiazide, acetazolamide, digitoxin, sulfisoxazole, and phenylbutazone. Oski and Naiman[139] described transient thrombocytopenia in 38 of 44 children who received live measles vaccine; it was maximal 3 days after the inoculation and there was no bleeding.

Depression of platelet production may be the first manifestation of a generalized bone marrow effect. Drugs implicated in this process include chloramphenicol, streptomycin, quinacrine, sulfamethoxypyridazine, arsphenamine, pyrimethamine, the anticonvulsants, (trimethadione and ethylmethylphenylhydantoin), potassium perchlorate, oral hypoglycemic agents, gold salts, phenylbutazone, and colchicine. Ristocetin has caused a dose-related direct toxic reaction on circulating platelets. Thrombocytopenia of the newborn has occurred when their mothers received thiazide diuretics in the last trimester of pregnancy; the mothers did not develop platelet deficiency.[140]

Case reports continue to appear confirming the relationship of anticonvulsive drugs and anti-folic acid agents to megaloblastic anemia.[141] Triamterene has precipitated a megaloblastic anemia due to folic acid antagonism.[142] Nitrofurantoin has caused a severe hemolytic anemia with megaloblastic erythropoiesis.[126]

Transient bone marrow depression related to methicillin was reported; this was quite significant since this reaction has not been observed during two decades of experience with penicillin G.[143]

Undesired adverse effects from conventional doses of anticoagulants continue to be reported: "purple toes,"[144] intramural hematoma of the bowel,[145] intestinal bleeding, epidural bleeding, peripheral gangrene, petechiae, and ecchymoses.[146] Femoral nerve entrapment by hematoma[147] and many other similar effects have been recorded. The potentiating and inhibiting effects of other drugs on coumarin derivatives have already been discussed.

Colchicine was related to the onset of vascular purpura in a patient with gout.[148] Bone marrow hypoplasia was attributed to chloramphenicol eye drops.[149] Pyrazinoic acid has caused a reversible sideroblastic anemia.[150] Sulfisoxazole has been related to a reversible Pelger–Huet anomaly of white blood cells.[151]

Cases of mesantoin-induced adenopathy simulating Hodgkin's disease were described again.[152] Diphenyl-hydantoin has caused a curious malignant lymphoma to appear. Adenopathy regressed when the drug was stopped, but subsequently a fatal malignant lymphoma developed.[153] One report told of the appearance of Reed–Sternberg cells on histologic examination of a lymph node from such a patient. A postvaccinal lymphadenitis simulating malignant lymphoma was reported in 9 of 20 cases of lymphadenitis.[154]

A normocytic normochromic anemia related to amphotericin B was reported.[155] Two patients receiving phenazopyridine hydrochloride developed methemoglobinemia and Heinz-body hemolytic anemia.[156] Administration of parenteral iron to 4 patients with paroxysmal nocturnal hemoglobinuria was associated with increased hemolysis.[157] Prilocaine, used to induce lumbar epidural block, caused methemoglobinemia in 7 patients.[158] Allopurinol, which inhibits xanthine oxidase, may cause depletion of this enzyme which plays an essential role in iron metabolism (mobilization of iron from hepatic stores and gastrointestinal iron absorption). Chronic ingestion of allopurinol may cause iron deficiency anemia.[159]

Hypersensitivity Phenomena

In March 1965 the Panel on Allergy of the Registry of Adverse Drug Reactions had collected 153 allergic reactions to drugs.[160] This represented an accumulation of about 18 months of reports. It is probably less than 1% of the cases that actually occurred in this period. In this group were 57 patients who manifested anaphylaxis by shock; severe respiratory depression, 29; serum sickness, 27; drug fever, 34. Penicillin accounted for 12 of the 57 cases of anaphylactic shock, 4 of the 29 respiratory depressions, 9 of the 27 serum sickness reactions, and 6 of the 34 drug fevers.

In one report oral penicillin G, 250,000 units, was suspected as the cause of anaphylactic shock and fatal ventricular tachyarrhythmia which culminated in death within 5 minutes. At postmortem a fresh anteroseptal infarct was discovered. A cause–effect relationship was impossible to establish.[161] Space precludes discussion of all drugs involved in anaphylaxis and serum sickness. However, a few recent admissions to the "anaphylactic club" are diphenhydramine hydrochloride,[162] cephalothin,[163] cephaloridine,[164] demethylchlortetracycline,[165] probenecid,[166] and iron dextran (given by the total-dose technique).[167] A generalized allergic reaction occurred in a patient who was given a second injection of bovine thyrotropin 2 years after the first.[168] Anaphylactoid reactions have been reported following intradermal testing for tetanus antitoxin sensitivity.[169] An anaphylactic reaction to dextran has been reported.[170] Polymyxin B given to a patient with generalized mastocytosis provoked a similar reaction.[171] Phenylbutazone was related to a sarcoid-like reaction in one patient[172] and the production of angiitis and periangiitis in another.[173]

Reports continue to describe the lupus erythematosus-like syndrome (SLE) precipitated by procainamide hydrochloride.[174–176] There have been at least 43 documented cases. Siegel, et al,[177] have observed a rising incidence of drug-induced SLE in New York City residents from 1957 to 1966. Drugs implicated in this series were taken for prolonged periods (1–12 years); they included diphenylhydantoin, hydralazine, isoniazid, and procainamide. Women were affected twice as frequently as men; the mean age for epileptic patients who developed diphenylhydantoin-induced SLE was 33.4; the mean age for cardiac patients who revealed procainamide-induced SLE was 60.7 years.

In another series of 258 cases of SLE, 12% had been treated with one of these drugs for longer than 3 months. Of 19 patients in whom the offending drugs were withdrawn, 18 had a remission of SLE; of 15 others who continued to receive the suspected agent, 6 had remissions.

In a group of 25 children receiving anticonvulsant drugs, 7 developed SLE.[178]

This entity bears clinical similarity to the hydralazine-induced SLE first described by Dustan and associates[179] and subsequently expanded by Alarcon-Segovia.[180] The mechanism remains obscure, but it is suspected that these drugs have the ability to unmask a lupus diathesis which has remained dormant. Other drugs have been implicated in the provocation of a lupus-like syndrome. These include other anticonvulsants (mesantoin, trimethadione, primidone),[181] aminosalicylic acid, penicillin, sulfonamides (acetazolamide, sulfisoxazole, sulfadiazine, sulfadimethoxypyridazine),[182] chlorpromazine, tetracycline, pyrazinamide, gold salts, methysergide, and griseofulvin.

A diffuse vasculitis resembling periarteritis nodosa was observed in 3 patients taking guanethidine.[183] Rosin[184] described a 53-year-old man with severe heart disease who developed a violent vasculitis with positive LE cell tests, while receiving procainamide. These tests became negative after the drug was withdrawn, but peripheral vasculitis and signs of intellectual derangement persisted. Gradual improvement occurred after amputation of gangrenous distal digits.

Most curiously, patients with idiopathic SLE—who for one reason or another receive procainamide—suffer no apparent exacerbation.[185]

A scan of the literature reveals that vasculitis has been attributed to such drugs as chlorpromazine, cyclobarbital, diphenylhydantoin, iodides, methylthiouracil, phenylbutazone, poison ivy extracts, sulfonamides, diphenhydramine,[186] and thiouracil. A necrotizing arteriolitis involving skin and kidneys occurred in a 62-year-old woman receiving hydrochlorothiazide.[187] The controversial issue regarding the ability of corticosteroids to provoke de novo vasculitis in patients with rheumatoid arthritis continues to be debated.

Reports of new drugs causing serum sickness continue to appear. A highly provocative paper, published by Karliner and Belaval,[188] described a 16.3% incidence of serum sickness reactions among 526 patients who had received antirabies hyperimmune globulin. Kaiser and associates[189] have reported 3 patients who developed immediate-type reactions involving the gastrointestinal tract following rabies duck embryo vaccine (DEV) administration. Perine, et al,[190] have reported Arthus-like reactions and delayed hypersensitivity in a man who had received DEV.

Edsall, et al,[191] found that prevailing antibody titers in 45 children seen for routine or emergency tetanus toxoid boosters was 43 to 2,500 times above that needed for minimal protection. In 22 other patients who developed allergic or Arthus-like reactions to the toxoid, antibody levels were above the threshold of protection. They contend that booster doses of toxoid "are being given with unnecessary and indeed excessive frequency; continuing to do this will produce a more highly toxoid sensitive population without adding significantly to the already high protection that the immunized population has against tetanus."[191]

Fardon[192] described a "severe urticarial-type systemic allergic reaction" to tetanus toxoid. Live measles vaccine has been related to generalized hypersensitivity reaction resembling Arthus-type phenomena.[193,194]

Without descending too deeply into the labyrinth of drug hypersensitivity, one must mention penicillin.[195] Penicillin has been discussed in the context of serum sickness and direct Coombs-positive hemolytic anemias, but it should be kept in mind that penicillin anaphylaxis still kills about 300 patients a year in this country. It probably saves 1,000 times that number.

Metabolic Diseases

Reports continue to appear describing thiazide-induced hyperglycemia.[196] Investigation of the antihypertensive agent, diazoxide, indicated that clinical diabetes mellitus could be precipitated in patients with previously normal glucose metabolism.[197] Phenformin-induced lactic acidosis continues to intrigue students of metabolism.[198,199] Severe hypoglycemic reactions in elderly patients receiving therapeutic doses of tolbutamide remains a minor therapeutic hazard.[200-203] Prolonged and profound hypoglycemia has been reported occasionally in patients who have taken other sulfonylurea drugs. This has occurred in patients receiving these medications for parkinsonism as well as for diabetes. Tolbutamide, chlorpropamide, and acetohexamide have been implicated as causes of hypoglycemia.

Usually the patients are elderly and it occurs during the initial period of sulfonylurea therapy; doses are usually in the conventional therapeutic range. In some instances, hypoglycemia persisted for 96 hours, with blood-glucose levels dipping to 9 mg/100 ml. This may persist despite food, or oral or intravenous glucose. If relief does occur, "premature" discontinuation of carbohydrate may result in rapid recurrence of hypoglycemia.

Many of these patients had associated hepatic or renal disease that conceivably might have interfered with the metabolism or excretion of the sulfonylureas. But this serious complication occurred in many other patients without such associated diseases. Therefore, other causes for this phenomenon have been sought.

Recent attention has been focused on the concomitant administration of other drugs. For example, sulfaphenazole and sulfadimethoxine are known to prolong the half-life of tolbutamide, but there are no reports of hypoglycemic reactions. There is convincing evidence that phenylbutazone will potentiate the hypoglycemic action of sulfonylurea compounds, especially acetohexamide.[204] This is produced by interfering with the renal excretion of the active metabolite, hydroxyhexamide. The conversion of acetohexamide to hydroxyhexamide was not affected, but a metabolic jam-up occurred resulting in higher levels of circulating acetohexamide and its active metabolite; this stimulated insulin release and blood-glucose levels fell.

It was proven that beta cells became hyperresponsive to other insulinogenic stimuli such as glucagon. Responsiveness of the beta cells to hyperglycemia was enhanced with continuous production of insulin, and this could account for the observation that glucose may provide only transient relief of sulfonylurea-induced hypoglycemia. Thus, it was demonstrated that phenylbutazone and probably sulfaphenazole and sulfadimethoxine act by interfering with the metabolism or excretion of acetohexamide and probably other sulfonylurea drugs.

Kotler, et al,[205] and others[206-209] have shown that

propranolol may induce severe hypoglycemia in diabetic patients receiving insulin. The mechanism is not clear.

A rather disconcerting report described detailed postmortem examinations on 20 sulfonylurea-treated diabetic patients and appropriate controls.[210] Microgranulomatous lesions, reminiscent of the hypersensitivity reactions seen with sulfonamides, were found in a higher percentage of sulfonylurea-treated patients than in diabetic controls who had received other forms of treatment. These lesions were not considered specific for sulfonylurea toxicity. There was "no correlation between the granulomatous lesions and clinical symptoms, laboratory abnormalities or cause of death." Myocarditis was found in 2 patients but was not considered cause of death.

Thonnard-Newmann[211] described a rising evidence of diabetes mellitus among hospitalized psychotic women (from 4.2 to 17.2%) in the 11 years since chlorpromazine had been introduced at his institution (1954). About 25% of women who had received 100 mg a day of chlorpromazine (or corresponding doses of another psychoactive phenothiazine) for a year or longer developed hyperglycemia and glycosuria. In 25% of these patients, remissions occurred either upon withdrawal or reduction in dose. It occurred more frequently in obese patients over 50 years of age and in paranoid schizophrenics.

Other fascinating dimensions of "drug-induced metabolic disorders" recently have been described.

Clinical and chemical signs of osteomalacia were observed in a patient who had ingested excessive amounts of aluminum hydroxide. This was related to profound phosphorus depletion; symptoms disappeared and serum calcium and phosphorus levels were restored to normal by discontinuing the aluminum hydroxide. Four years later, this patient suffered hyperparathyroidism due to an autonomously functioning adenoma. The authors postulated that the osteomalacia with low serum calcium and phosphate concentrations served as a stimulus for the development of secondary parathyroid hyperplasia; this, in turn, led to an autonomously functioning parathyroid adenoma.[212]

Triamterene employed alone or with a thiazide diuretic has produced sufficient hyperkalemia to result in electrocardiographic changes and death in one patient.[213]

Vivacqua, et al,[214] have described a syndrome of "selective" pituitary insufficiency secondary to the use of busulfan. It was characterized by severe weakness, lassitude, anorexia, weight loss, and hyperpigmentation of the skin. This syndrome developed in the course of long-term busulfan therapy for chronic granulocytic leukemia (1 patient) and agnogenic myeloid metaplasia (1 patient). Upon discontinuation of busulfan, pituitary–adrenal function returned to normal in both patients with regression of signs and symptoms.

It was suggested that replacement cortisone therapy may be indicated during periods of stress in such patients. Two other patients with polycythemia, receiving busulfan for long periods, did not reveal any clinical or laboratory evidence of pituitary-adrenal insufficiency.

Thyroid enlargement and hypothyroidism were observed in 3 children who were treated for seizures with aminoglutethimide. They had low protein-bound iodine (PBI) and butanol-extractable iodine (BEI) values, high thyroid uptake of I^{131}, and discharge of greater than 50 per cent of I[131] following administration of thiocyanate. This signified that there was a block in organic incorporation of iodine. This phenomenon was not observed in adults receiving aminoglutethimide.[215]

Two patients with hypercalcemia treated with intravenous phosphate buffer developed sudden precipitous falls in serum calcium. Both patients developed hypotension and acute renal failure. Bilateral renal cortical necrosis developed in one patient. The authors caution against using more than 50 mM of phosphate buffer intravenously as an initial dose in the treatment of severe hypercalcemia.[216]

In 60 patients with hyperlipoproteinemia treated with clofibrate, 5 developed elevated serum transaminase and serum creatine phosphokinase levels. Two patients experienced severe myalgia, stiffness, weakness, and malaise coincident with drug administration. Cessation of therapy resulted in prompt resolution of symptoms in both cases. An identical clinical syndrome reappeared when one of these patients was rechallenged with clofibrate. Three of the 60 patients had asymptomatic elevations in transaminase and creatine phosphokinase levels. In one instance, these abnormal elevations were clearly dose related. In some cases, transaminase levels became normal while clofibrate was continued, but creatine phosphokinase continued to be elevated throughout the period of treatment.

It was assumed, since creatine phosphokinase is absent from liver, that skeletal muscle was the major source of the elevated serum enzymes. The authors suggest that periodic examinations for muscle tenderness and dysfunction and frequent determinations of serum transaminase and creatine phosphokinase levels should be routine procedures for all patients receiving clofibrate.[217]

At this juncture, the hyperuricemia induced by thiazide diuretics and chlorthalidone,[218] the osteoporosis caused by prolonged heparin administration,[219] and the hypoaldosteronism related to prolonged heparin therapy will not be discussed.[220]

Also, the multitude of adverse effects related to corticosteroids will not be discussed. This is covered in depth by Newman.[221]

Ovulatory Suppressants

Some attention should be directed to the ovulatory suppressants, the so-called "progestational" agents. The incredibly widespread clinical use of "the pill" has been attended by a remarkable paucity of adverse effects in the 10 years since its introduction.[222-225] Yet there are some rumbles in paradise. There is ample evidence of frequent disturbance of hepatic function detectable in the laboratory, yet clinical manifestations have occurred rarely. It is felt that the estrogen component of some products (mestranol) causes effects similar to estradiol. This is manifested by damage to common pathways of biliary excretion with SGOT elevation, rise in BSP retention, but no alkaline phosphatase or bile acid elevation. Pruritus without jaundice has been observed.

Reports of interference with some coagulation factors and case histories of patients with thromboembolic complications continue to appear.[226-230] A study performed by Schrogie and colleagues[231] indicated that treatment with oral contraceptive agents decreases the hypoprothrombinemic response to bishydroxycoumarin. The rate of metabolism is accelerated through microsomal enzyme induction (as discussed earlier). Women taking oral contraceptives may require increased doses of bishydroxycoumarin in order to produce the desired anticoagulant effect. Reports of varying effects upon first-stage coagulation factors have appeared; they are most difficult to assess.[232]

It is suspected that oral contraceptives may also cause in-vitro activation of inactive precursors of one or more of the vitamin K-dependent clotting factors. Present studies show an increased activity of Factor X in plasma from patients treated with progestational agents. A possible explanation may reside in the fact that an increase in various lipid fractions is observed in women taking oral contraceptives.

Overabundance of certain saturated fatty acids will shorten plasma recalcification time. Thus, elevated levels of lipids may provide a surface upon which activation of the prothrombin complex factor may occur. Oral progestational agents may cause elevation of plasma triglycerides by increasing endogenous production and impairing removal of triglycerides. It is probable that the hormone combination activates an enzyme inhibitor in the circulation that hinders triglyceride clearance.

There has been some recent evidence to suspect that prolonged use of oral contraceptives has caused some other metabolic problems in addition to triglyceride elevation. These include hyperglycemia ("subclinical diabetes")[233] and elevated renin–aldosterone concentration, possibly contributing to hypertension.[234]

Progestational agents are known to cause elevation of PBI and depression of triiodothyronine uptake by erythrocytes.[235]

Shafey and Scheinberg[236] editorialized about the occurrence of migraine headaches in almost 50 women on progestational steroids. Three had temporary focal neurologic defects following the migraine attack. Appropriate antimigraine therapy was ineffective until the steroid was stopped. Abnormal electroencephalograms have been reported in women with headaches receiving oral contraceptives.[237]

New dimensions continue to be added to the lexicon of concern about oral progestational agents. Taylor, et al,[238] reported "a destructive type of atypical polypoid endocervical hypoplasia" in 13 women receiving progestin-like drugs. The median age was 25 years; norethynodrel with mestranol or norethindrone with mestranol were taken in 10 instances; 1 was receiving a sequential estrogen–progesterone preparation and 2 were "not sure" of the drug. Such lesions have the appearance of adenocarcinoma, but they are considered benign polyps. Thus far, it would seem that these lesions have been observed only in women taking oral contraceptives. The implication is not known; when polyps occur, the drugs should be stopped.

There are other reports citing hazards attributed to oral contraceptives. Hepatic vein thrombosis culminating in Budd–Chiari Syndrome and death has been attributed to oral contraceptives.[239] A case of infarction of the mid-gut has been related to the same drug combination.[240] Other phenomena related to these agents include: progressive pulmonary disease,[241] appearance of LE cells in peripheral blood,[242,243] galactorrhea,[244] melasma,[245] and benign intracranial hypertension.[246]

Other potentially serious effects are premature epiphyseal closure in young women and stimulation of pre-existing uterine fibromyomata.

The controversy over the role of oral contraceptives and thromboembolism continues to rage—unresolved. In a comprehensive review of the role of oral contraceptive agents and thromboembolic disease, Tausk says, "Notwithstanding large statistical data which seemed to disprove any cause or relationship between the occurrence of thromboembolic episodes in apparently healthy young women on the one hand and the use of oral contraceptives on the other, many physicians and other medical people do not entirely succeed in shaking off the suspicion that there might be a more than coincidental association."[232] Indeed, if such an association exists, it must be considered as a rare adverse effect.

The evidence thus far indicates that these drugs, which are unique in the history of pharmacology because of their far-reaching socioeconomic importance, have been impressively benign. Yet final judgment must be reserved. There are many of us who feel that at the present time the use of such agents may not be justified in societies where other methods of contraception are readily available and effective.

When the hazard of pregnancy and parturition outweighs the potential danger of the drug, the decision is simple. The religious, social, and economic aspects of widespread population control are beyond the scope of this section.

MAOI Effects

One of the more dramatic iatrogenic diseases to be observed in recent years should be mentioned again here; ie, the marked potentiation of catecholamine pressor activity by MAOI drugs.[247,248] This was discussed briefly under *Drug Interactions*.

This relationship was identified with the syndrome of hypertensive crisis characterized by encephalopathic headache, occasionally associated with cerebrovascular bleeding, which rarely proceeded to coma and death. It occurred very mysteriously after the subject had ingested cheese, pickled herring, chianti wine, or some other exotic food containing significant amounts of tyramine. The denominator was soon discovered to be the MAOI drugs. Similar hypertensive crises were associated with concomitant administration of a MAO inhibitor and a sympathomimetic amine.

Methyldopa may cause paradoxical hypertension without the concomitant use of MAO inhibitors.[249,250] The pressor reaction is mediated by excessive synthesis or supranormal sensitivity to the pressor metabolites of methyldopa (alphamethyldopamine and alphanorepinephrine). Parenteral guanethidine and reserpine may suddenly release large amounts of norepinephrine from tissue stores and increase blood pressure.

Hypotensive reactions have also been documented. It is now accepted dictum that it is unwise to prescribe antihypertensive agents such as alphamethyldopa for several weeks after administration of MAO inhibitors. MAO may be suppressed for a prolonged period with accumulation of large tissue stores of norepinephrine that are not available at nerve endings. Antihypertensive agents could result in significant sustained hypotension.

Johnson[251] recently described a curious case of a young nurse who took tranylcypromine after a capsule of dextroamphetamine and amytal. She suffered a temperature to 108° with semi-coma. She recovered in a few days after intensive supportive treatment.

Ocular Syndromes

Birge[252] listed 24 major drugs which were capable of causing ocular damage. Concentrating only on agents that caused retinal pathology, the list includes corticosteroids, chloramphenicol, streptomycin, chloroquine, quinacrine, quinidine, stramonium, high concentrations of oxygen (in premature infants),[253] and isoniazid (given intrathecally). Drugs which cause corneal and lenticular damage are even more numerous.

Most recent notoriety has been attained by phenothiazine drugs[254-256] and chloroquine.[257,258] It is estimated that about 30% of the patients on high-dosage, long-term phenothiazines will develop corneal and lenticular damage. In most series, the daily dose ranges from 300 to 1600 mg a day; the total dose is between 1,000 and 2,000 Gm. In addition to changes in cornea and lens, a significant number of patients develop a peculiar cutaneous pigmentation. Some become bronzed as if suntanned; others acquire a gray or violaceous pigmentation. Thus, we must add ocular and dermal changes[259] to the extrapyramidal dyskinesias, hypertensive crisis, cholestasis, and sudden death that have been attributed to phenothiazines.

To digress for a moment, the "sudden death" phenomenon in phenothiazine administration was investigated in 12 patients. All had collapsed suddenly; postmortem examinations failed to establish cause of death. Airway obstruction due to aspirated food was not a factor in this series. A review of electrocardiograms revealed 8 patients with abnormal tracings; there was one left bundle branch block with frequent ventricular premature contractions, one right bundle branch block, one atrioventricular block, and the remainder had ST–T abnormalities.[260]

Destructive lesions of the arteriocapillary bed of the subendocardium of the right and left atrial conduction bundle and papillary muscles (which were considered unique) were found in patients with sudden phenothiazine-related death. Less-extensive focal lesions were found in 70% of the *tranquilized* patients who died from other causes. They appeared similar to the *metabolic* vascular and myocardial lesions ascribed to catecholamines.

The indictment against long-term chloroquine as a cause of ocular problems[257,258] is even more striking than against phenothiazines. Corneal opacification associated with prolonged chloroquine administration is usually reversible when the drug is stopped. However, the retinopathy is relentless and insidious; it may not become clinically evident until months or years after the drug has been stopped.

Perhaps the most pernicious aspect of chloroquine retinopathy is that even after the drug is withdrawn, the pathologic process may continue. Rare instances of retinopathy have occurred with doses of 250 mg a day administered over a period of 6 months. Fortunately, most problems have developed in patients taking higher doses for a year or longer. The delay in onset and predilection for eye and skin are related to the affinity of chloroquine for melanin-bearing cells and slow rate of excretion.[261] Retinal lesions are associated with a central visual defect, pigmentary changes, and retinal edema. The insidious nature of the pathologic process is such that periodic electroretinography and visual field checks may be quite normal on the very day that "enough chloroquine is ingested and stored in the liver to give rise to ocular changes 3 to 6 months hence."[259]

It is pertinent to add that the current weekly

300-mg dose of chloroquine being given to the troops in Southeast Asia is without importance in this problem.[15] Perhaps even 200 mg a day for a period of 1 year is safe. However, it is quite probable that unless the 4-hydroxyquinolines are the *only* drugs that will arrest or suppress a particular connective tissue disorder (a rare situation), these drugs should not be used.

Pulmonary Diseases

Perhaps the most fascinating drug-induced pulmonary disease should be considered a metabolic disease. This is the apnea caused by succinylcholine, which was discussed briefly earlier.[24] This phenomenon may be related to a qualitative or quantitative deficiency of pseudocholinesterase, the enzyme required for rapid destruction of succinylcholine. It has been discovered that sensitivity to this drug is an inherited characteristic. Several genetic phenotypes are capable of producing this syndrome.

1. Individuals may be homozygous for a rare gene which produces an abnormal pseudocholinesterase, rather than a low level of normal enzyme. This qualitatively insufficient enzyme is less active than normal in hydrolyzing succinylcholine and is resistant to most cholinesterase inhibitors.
2. A second variety occurs in heterozygotes who possess a mixture of both normal and abnormal enzymes. Population surveys have indicated that succinylcholine-sensitive homozygotes occur in about 1 out of 2,800 individuals, while about 38 out of 1,000 of the general population are heterozygous.
3. Another genetic variant has been described in which the homozygote demonstrates a complete absence of serum pseudocholinesterase. This gene has been called the *violent pseudocholinesterase gene.*

A total of 5 different phenotypes have been identified. Of the 5 groups, it is the atypical homozygotes (who possess atypical enzymes of 2 varieties) which are succinylcholine sensitive. This is certainly a rare phenomenon, since Leahmann, *et al,*[262] studied over 80,000 patients given succinylcholine and did not discover a *single* case of succinylcholine-induced apnea.

It now seems likely that in some instances, combined administration of succinylcholine and an antibiotic may be responsible for serious respiratory compromise. Apnea has been reported to follow the use of succinylcholine, diphenhydramine, neomycin, streptomycin, polymixin B, kanamycin, sodium colistimethate,[263] and the quaternary ammonium germicides. Neostigmine reversed this reaction in a patient who had been given intramuscular kanamycin.[264]

Unanticipated death in status asthmaticus has prompted speculation that chlorpromazine and excessive use of nebulized isoproterenol may be at fault. Pertinent to this observation is a report by Van Meter and associates[265] of 17 patients who died of asthma. Two died within 5 minutes after an intramuscular injection of chlorpromazine, 50 mg. Other factors considered in the deaths were inadequate corticosteroid therapy (in those who had been on prolonged maintenance) and procedures which temporarily inhibited ventilation. These included tension pneumothorax, tracheostomy, tracheal intubation, and sedation with secobarbital. Fourteen of the patients were using nebulized isoproterenol; 9 in excessive amounts. In 7 patients, intermittent positive pressure was used to deliver the isoproterenol.

These authors coined the expression, *locked lung syndrome.* It is characterized by persistent wheezing, which becomes progressively more severe and then refractory to escalating doses of isoproterenol. Three of the 9 patients died after intensive hospital treatment. Further investigation revealed that many other refractory patients were using higher than recommended doses of nebulized isoproterenol. Treatment with all the usual forms of therapy (including corticosteroids) was ineffective, until isoproterenol nebulization was discontinued. The mechanism is not known; it is more than tachyphylaxis.

Keighley[266] described a similar experience in 3 patients who had personal or family histories of atopy. Airway obstruction was partially relieved with conventional therapy, including corticosteroids in high doses. But complete remission was not attained until all adrenergic aerosols were withdrawn. Subsequent challenge with aerosols containing isoproterenol again precipitated severe and protracted airway obstruction. Thus, isoproterenol used as an aerosol may actually induce severe, prolonged airway obstruction that is indistinguishable from a clinical attack of asthma. Further use of aerosol simply perpetuates the difficulty.

A study of iatrogenic pulmonary edema in surgical patients was reported by Adriani, *et al.*[267] They cited several causes:

1. Drugs causing incomplete cardiac emptying by depressing myocardial contractility (thiopental, local anesthetics, barbiturates, narcotics); drugs which cause tachycardia (atropine, epinephrine), and drugs which can cause persistent severe arrhythmias (cyclopropane, halothane).
2. Redistribution of blood from the periphery (vasoconstrictors, central stimulation).
3. Negative pressure on the airway (obstruction, bronchospasm).
4. Circulatory overload (blood, fluids, absorption of irrigating fluids).
5. Injury to the alveolar membranes by noxious inhalants, excretion of poisons (kerosene) and aspiration of gastric contents while attempting to evacuate the stomach in cases of poisoning. Circulatory overload and anesthetics which depress the myocardium, particularly when used in combination with potent vasoconstrictors, seem to be the most frequent offenders.

Another pulmonary hazard is related to lymphangiography. A fall in carbon dioxide diffusion capacity and decrease in pulmonary surfactant due to minute lipid emboli to the lungs occurs in almost every individual given intralymphatic oily contrast media. These are rare causes of clinical pulmonary complications.[268]

Diffuse interstitial pulmonary fibrosis has been described following busulfan therapy.[269] Several patients have developed severe bronchospasm following the inhalation of the mucolytic agent, acetylcysteine.[270] Allergic pulmonary infiltration, occasionally associated with pleural effusion and eosinophilia, has been caused by nitrofurantoin.[271,272] This simulated pulmonary edema in 2 patients.[273]

Strauss and Griffin[274] reported 2 patients with *nitrofurantoin-pneumonia;* one had 5 distinct episodes. This brings the total in the literature to 10 patients who suffered 28 bouts of pneumonia following the use of nitrofurantoin. Nicklaus and Snyder[275] reported a case of *noncardiac acute pulmonary edema* related to nitrofurantoin.

In both instances, pneumonia or acute pulmonary edema, the syndrome may start within a few hours after the ingestion of one or a few tablets. The pneumonia is usually located in the posterior bases of the lungs and resolves within hours of discontinuing nitrofurantoin.

Pulmonary infiltration and bronchospasm with eosinophilia was observed in a 69-year-old woman taking chlorpropamide.[276] Aspirin-induced asthma has been reported in patients with nasal polyps.[277]

Renal Diseases

The controversy regarding analgesic nephrotoxicity seems interminable.[278-282] Case reports continue to appear. Gilman[283] feels that "analgesic nephrotoxicity may not represent a single entity but may merely reflect the susceptibility of the kidney to a variety of chemical agents." The requirement for objective prospective studies is evident. The concern regarding the effects of analgesic compounds upon the previously damaged kidney was mentioned earlier.

It is axiomatic that in the patient with compromised renal function, drug dosage must be modified appropriately if the agent is metabolized or excreted by a renal route.[284] The kidneys are the principal route of elimination of most antimicrobal agents. Exceptions are the erythromycins, triacetyloleandomycin, novobiocin, and probably griseofulvin; these antibiotics are excreted through the biliary tract.

Antibacterial agents with "frequent" nephrotoxic effect are amphotericin B,[285,286] bacitracin, polymyxins B and E (colistimethate),[287] and ristocetin. "Occasional" nephrotoxicity is seen with kanamycin, neomycin, sulfonamides, and vancomycin. "Rare" nephrotoxic effects have been observed with viomycin, methenamine mandelate, and griseofulvin.[288]

Other antibacterial agents which are excreted via the kidneys which do not have a direct nephrotoxic effect are isonicotinic hydrazide (INH), aminosalicylic acid (PAS), and nalidixic acid.

Other drugs that can be added to the list include bismuth,[289] penicillamine (nephrotic syndrome),[290-292] phenindione (fatal nephropathy),[293] phenylbutazone (acute renal failure),[294] and organic mercurials.[295] Quinine sulfate has also been associated with acute renal failure in early pregnancy.[296] There have been 26 cases of nephrotic syndrome related to paramethadione and trimethadione.[297,298] Case reports have appeared describing nephrotic syndrome related to probenecid.[299]

Kunin[300] advised that antibiotics known to be excreted by the kidney be given in a conventional initial (loading) dose and thereafter reduced in amount ($1/2$ the loading dose) and administered at intervals equal to the serum half-life of the drug. Schedules are available. Some notoriously ototoxic drugs that are also nephrotoxic should be employed with great caution in the patient with damaged kidneys. High blood levels of penicillin are usually well tolerated; problems could arise incident to hyperkalemia since each million units of penicillin G contains 1.7 mEq of potassium.

Tetracycline serum levels may rise to remarkable heights in the presence of renal damage or oliguria; pre-existing azotemia may be exaggerated in the patient given high doses of tetracycline. Usual oral doses are well tolerated.

Nitrofurantoin-induced peripheral neuritis may occur with the high levels of the drug associated with impaired renal excretion. Intoxication with digoxin may occur if conventional doses are employed in the patient with decreased renal clearance.

The occurrence of acute renal failure following the administration of multiple doses of bunamiodyl sodium is thought to result from a combination of overdosage, hepatic derangement and hypotension.[301-304] Bunamiodyl sodium has been removed from the market. Iodoalphionic acid, iodopanoic acid, and sodium iodomethamate have also caused renal injury, but less frequently and with less severity than bunamiodyl.

The accumulation of evidence regarding methysergide-induced syndromes is continuing.[107,305,306] Over 50 cases of methysergide-induced retroperitoneal fibrosis with vascular and ureteral obstruction have been reported. This is a critically important diagnosis to establish since the retroperitoneal fibrosis may start to regress within 1 week after withdrawal of methysergide, even after it has been given for up to 6 years.

In addition, there is evidence that methysergide may cause vascular fibrosis with narrowing of the aorta, carotid, brachial, femoral, iliac, and mesenteric vessels. Symptoms of claudication have been noted after a few doses and have disappeared upon discontinuation of the drug. Patients taking methysergide should be advised to have examinations 3–4 times a year for observation for signs of cardiovascular involvement. Heart valve damage and pleuropulmonary fibrosis have also been observed. This syndrome has been compared to the hydralazine- and procainamide-induced connective tissue disorders. Methysergide maleate has been implicated as a cause of postprandial abdominal angina without other complications.[107]

Teratogenic Drugs

By inference, glutethimide, which contains the same glutarimide nucleus as thalidomide, is considered an undesirable drug for women of childbearing age.[307] However, it must be emphasized that there has been no documented evidence of human teratogenicity. Other drugs that contain the glutarimide nucleus are aminoglutethimide, bemegride and cycloheximide.

The teratogenic effect of antileukemic and antitumor drugs remains a source of continuing concern.[308,309] Aminopterin and amethopterin, folic acid antagonists, are notorious teratogenic and abortifacient agents. The use of 6-mercaptopurine has been attended by freedom from teratogenic effects.

Busulfan has been employed widely in chronic myelocytic leukemia; no reports of abnormal fetal development have appeared, even when the drug has been given during the first trimester. A woman given 6-mercaptopurine, splenic irradiation, and busulfan during the first several weeks of gestation delivered a baby with multiple congenital anomalies.[310] Busulfan can cause malformation and resorption in rats with predictable regularity.[308]

Nitrogen mustard used in treatment of Hodgkin's disease has a checkered record. There are many reports of its benign character when used during pregnancy. However, several investigators have shown that nitrogen mustard may exert teratogenic effects late in pregnancy, in contrast to antifolates and irradiation, which act early. Chlorambucil follows this rule as well.

Vinblastine has been given throughout pregnancy of women with Hodgkin's disease with no adverse effects on infants.[311] In hamsters, vinblastine and vincristine have caused fetal malformations and abortions (similar to colchicine). A similar phenomenon has been observed in pregnant rats given methylhydrazine.

Thus, *all* such drugs are suspect and are to be accorded great respect when used in pregnant women. It is a matter of critical judgment when the pregnant woman with leukemia or lymphoma becomes a candidate for chemotherapy. This subject has been reviewed in an excellent essay by Kalter.[309] This situation could represent the surface ripples of an enormous problem. Most teratologists believe that almost *any* drug may be teratogenic if administered to a pregnant woman in the right dose at the right time.

Before we leave this area, a slight digression would seem appropriate. There are several drugs which when given to the pregnant mother may cause adverse effects in the offspring. We have already mentioned the thrombocytopenic effect of thiazide diuretics.[140] We must add the enamel hypoplasia and staining of deciduous teeth that may occur in the baby born to a mother taking tetracycline. Maternal ingestion of progestins may cause masculinization of a female infant; iodides and thiourea compounds may result in congenital goiter.

Space does not permit discussion of drug-induced diseases that manifest themselves by signs and symptoms referable to the cardiovascular and central nervous systems. Also, not included in this panoramic overview are the antibiotic-induced, corticosteroid-induced, radiation-induced, surgically-induced disorders, or those related to diagnostic procedures, or psychiatric-neurologic disorders provoked by drugs.

Adverse Reaction Reporting

The reporting of adverse drug reactions has not been consistently good. Both the American Medical Association (AMA) and the Food and Drug Administration (FDA) became involved in the business of trying to obtain data on adverse drug reactions. The AMA had a potential information source of over 7,000 hospitals and 250,000 physicians. How many reports were received? The total as of December 1967 was 8,198. And the quality and accuracy of reports was often appalling. The original Registry on Blood Dyscrasias fed information back to the profession in the form of semiannual tabulations. These provided much helpful information. For example, knowledge of chloramphenicol and dipyrone toxicity was documented and facilitated through this mechanism.

Tabulations were prepared regularly until 1964 when it was decided that the data should be transferred to computer storage. Unfortunately, this conversion never came to fruition. Also, anticipated plans for free communication between the AMA and the FDA programs never achieved a working reality. Through both programs, it has been estimated that roughly 1 to 2% of adverse reactions that were occurring in the US were being reported.

The FDA continues to receive fragmentary reports from about 85 hospitals, mostly military and federal, throughout the country. The AMA Registry continues to invite reports from any physician who detects an adverse reaction. However, the Council on Drugs of the AMA is in the process of devising an elastic prototype program that will enable hospitals of every size and mission to establish ongoing studies on adverse drug reactions and drug utilization.

The author is a working member of this committee, and is assured that these labors are still in an early germination stage. Yet if such a program can be established, and the data gathering made painless— yet pertinent—so that physicians may be helped to learn more about drugs, it will be worth the effort.

Role of the Pharmacist

In this schema the pharmacist has an essential role. Under optimal circumstances he should be integrated into the therapeutic team as an active member. While the physician must make the ultimate decision regarding the choice of therapy, the pharmacist often can be of considerable help to the responsible physician in the effective and safe use of drugs.

The treatment of a patient includes too many variables beyond drug therapy. Social and psychologic perturbations, in addition to physiologic disruptions, combine to escalate the problems of "treatment" to a plane beyond consideration of drug therapy, *per se.* Nevertheless, the pharmacist has a vital role.

In the Walter Reed General Hospital, pharmacists are active members of the Therapeutic Agents Board (TAB) and the Drug Utilization and Adverse Drug Reactions Committee (DUADRC). Teams of pharmacists visit all wards of the hospital (twice each week) and contact individual ward officers to inquire about adverse drug reactions that have occurred. The pharmacists then complete Form FD 1639 from information derived from the patient's chart and by communication with the responsible ward officer.

The FDA forms are reviewed by the DUADR Committee (1 physician and 3 pharmacists); pertinent data are presented at the TAB meeting, and then copies of Form FD 1639 are forwarded to the FDA.

In the future it is anticipated that the committee will conduct drug utilization studies and ultimately drug efficacy studies.

In addition, the pharmacists maintain a ready file of FDA Adverse Reactions reports as a source of information for physicians. They maintain also current files of books and journals—available to physicians for immediate information on drugs (efficacy, interactions, toxicity).

Thus, the pharmacist—with his special interest in pharmacology—has become an essential, permanent member of the therapeutic team.

Role of the Physician

Despite the impotence of past efforts to obtain meaningful adverse-drug reaction data through physician-reporting techniques, information is abundantly available concerning drugs. It is recommended that every physician who treats patients subscribe to *The Medical Letter.*[311] For a modest cost per year (less for house officers), one is provided current, unbiased, candid information on new drug efficacy and toxicity. Add to the bookshelf *Drugs of Choice,*[312] *New Drugs* (the annual publication of the Council on Drugs of the AMA),[313] and a good, current pharmacology text. Another helpful addition to the bookshelf is the comprehensive *AMA Drug Evaluation* book.

Thus, significant steps are being taken toward meeting the challenge of new responsibility that accompanies increased capability. Our remarkable therapeutic arsenal is a tribute to the drug industry and the devoted chemists and pharmacologists of our schools. But neither AMA, FDA, or the industry can solve the problem completely.

A plea is directed to the physician on the firing line —the doctor who prescribes the drug. His predecessors had limited diagnostic and therapeutic resources. Some of the drugs they used were worthless, others dangerous; some were impure and unstandardized to the point of unpredictability. The few effective drugs were trusted allies whose strengths and weaknesses were well known. Modern pharmacology has brought this unhappy era to an end; today we enjoy the privilege of fine, powerful, well-standardized therapeutic weapons.

Now it is important to create an atmosphere of rational caution and critical evaluation, where each physician will pause before putting pen to prescription pad and ask himself, "Do I know enough about this drug to prescribe it? Does the possible benefit I hope to derive from this drug outweigh its potential hazard?"

This is not intended as therapeutic nihilism, but rather as *therapeutic rationalism*.

References

1. Moser, R. H., *Diseases of Medical Progress*, 3rd ed., Thomas, Springfield, Ill., 1969, p. xiii.
2. Mellin, G. W., and Katzenstein, M., *New Engl. J. Med.*, **267**, 1184 (1962).
3. *Hospital Tribune*, **2**, 2 (Mar. 11, 1968).
4. Irey, N., *Registry of Tissue Reaction to Drugs*, I, II, and III, Armed Forces Inst. of Pathol., Washington, D.C., 1968.
5. Hartshorn, E. A., *Drug Intelligence*, **2**, 57 (1968).
6. Cluff, L. E., *et al*, *Trans. Assoc. Am. Physicians*, **78**, 255 (1965).
7. Smith, J. W., *et al*, *New Engl. J. Med.*, **274**, 998 (1966).
8. Durant, T. M., *J. Am. Med. Assoc.*, **192**, 973 (1965).
9. Schimmel, E. M., *Ann. Internal Med.*, **60**, 100 (1964).
10. Koch-Weser, J., *Drug. Inform. Bull.*, **2**, 72 (July–Sep., 1968).
11. Reidenberg, M. M., and Lowenthal, D. T., *New Engl. J. Med.*, **279**, 678 (1968).
12. Long, J. W., *Drug Inform. Bull.*, **2**, 78 (July–Sep., 1968).
13. Vogel, F., *Ergeb. Inn. Med. Kinderheilk.*, **12**, 52 (1959).
14. Marks, P. A., and Banks, J., *Ann. NY Acad. Sci.*, **123**, 198 (1965).
15. Vivona, S., *Bull. World Health Organ.*, **25**, 267 (1961).
16. Cohen, R. J., *et al*, *Clin. Res.*, **16**, 301 (1968).
17. Lucey, J. F., and Dolan, R. G., *Pediat.*, **23**, 553 (1959).
18. Hargreaves, T., and Holton, J. B., *Lancet*, **I**, 839 (1962).
19. Sutherland, J. M., *Am. J. Diseases Children*, **97**, 761 (1959).
20. Frick, P. G., *et al*, *Blood*, **20**, 261 (1962).
21. Goldstein, A., *et al*, *Principles of Drug Action*, Hoeber, New York, 1968, p. 444.
22. Price-Evans, D. A., and White, T. A., *J. Lab. Clin. Med.*, **63**, 394 (1964).
23. Price-Evans, D. A., *et al*, *Clin. Pharmacol. Therap.*, **6**, 430 (1965).
24. Telfer, A. B. M., *et al*, *Brit. Med. J.*, **I**, 153 (1964).
25. Kelley, W. N., *et al*, *New Engl. J. Med.*, **278**, 287 (1968).
26. Wasserman, R. H., and Taylor, A. N., *Science*, **152**, 791 (1966).
27. Granick, S., and Mauzerall, D., *J. Biol. Chem.*, **232**, 1119 (1958).
28. Hartshorn, E. A., *Drug Intelligence*, **2**, 2 (1968).
29. Remmer, H., in Brodie, B. B., and Erdos, E. G., *Metabolic Factors Controlling Duration of Drug Action*, vol. 6, Macmillan, New York, 1962, p. 235.
30. Fouts, J. R., *Advan. Enzyme Regulation*, **1**, 225 (1963).
31. Burns, J. J., *et al*, *Ann. NY Acad. Sci.*, **123**, 273 (1965).
32. Melmon, K., *et al*, *Patient Care*, 1, 32 (Nov., 1967).
33. Goss, J. E., and Dickhaus, D. W., *New Engl. J. Med.*, **273**, 1094 (1965).
34. Kristensen, M., and Hansen, J. M., *Diabetes*, **16**, 211 (1967).
35. Goldberg, L. I., *J. Am. Med. Assoc.*, **190**, 456 (1964).
36. Levine, R. J., and Strauch, B. S., *New Engl. J. Med.*, **275**, 946 (1966).
37. Mason, A., *Lancet*, **I**, 1073 (1963).
38. Field, J. B., *et al*, *Diabetes*, **15**, 520 (1966).
39. Clark, R. B., and Maier, E. S., *GP*, **29**, 106 (1964).
40. *Brit. Med. J.*, **I**, 1033 (1961).
41. Mann, E. B., *Am. J. Roentgenol.*, **83**, 497 (1960).
42. Smith, D. H., *New Engl. J. Med.*, **275**, 625 (1966).
43. Watanabe, T., *Bacteriol. Rev.*, **27**, 87 (1963).
44. Schroeder, S. A., *J. Am. Med. Assoc.*, **205**, 903 (1968).
45. Rostenberg, A. J., and Fagelson, H. G., *J. Am. Med. Assoc.*, **194**, 660 (1965).
46. Carroll, O. M., *et al*, *J. Am. Med. Assoc.*, **195**, 691 (1966).
47. Bianchine, J. R., *et al*, *Am. J. Med.*, **44**, 390 (1968).
48. *Med. Letter Drug Therap.*, **8**, 13 (1966).
49. Epstein, E., *J. Am. Med. Assoc.*, **198**, 517 (1966).
50. Baer, R. L., and Harber, L. C., *J. Am. Med. Assoc.*, **192**, 989 (1965).
51. Lamberg, S. I., *J. Am. Med. Assoc.*, **201**, 747 (1967).
52. Shelley, W. B., and Kirschbaum, J. O., *Arch. Dermatol.*, **84**, 73 (1961).
53. Shelley, W. B., *J. Am. Med. Assoc.*, **201**, 1009 (1967).
54. Shelley, W. B., *J. Am. Med. Assoc.*, **189**, 985 (1964).
55. Hitch, J. M., *J. Am. Med. Assoc.*, **200**, 879 (1967).
56. Zelickson, A. S., *J. Am. Med. Assoc.*, **198**, 341 (1966).
57. Winkelman, R. R., *et al*, *Arch. Dermatol.*, **87**, 372 (1963).
58. Lawrason, F. D., *et al*, *J. Am. Med. Assoc.*, **191**, 641 (1965).
59. Brown, C. H., and Akin, N., *Cleveland Clin. Quart.*, **33**, 85 (1966).
60. Davenport, H. W., *New Engl. J. Med.*, **276**, 1307 (1967).
61. Leonards, J. R., and Levy, G., *Clin. Pharmacol. Therap.*, **8**, 400 (1967).
62. *The Medical Letter*, **7**, 98 (1965).
63. Roth, J. L. E., *J. Am. Med. Assoc.*, **187**, 418 (1964).
64. Gazes, P. C., *et al*, *Circulation*, **23**, 358 (1961).
65. Babior, B., and Davidson, C. S., *N. J. Med.*, **41**, 491 (1966).
66. Popper, H., *et al*, *Arch. Internal Med.*, **115**, 128 (1965).
67. Schultz, V. C., *et al*, *New Engl. J. Med.*, **269**, 999 (1963).
68. Kunelis, C. T., *et al*, *Am. J. Med.*, **38**, 359 (1965).
69. *Am. J. Med.*, **43**, 274 (1967).
70. Ober, W. B., and LeCompte, P. M., *Am. J. Med.*, **19**, 743 (1955).
71. Cappas, A., *Gastroenterol.*, **52**, 113 (1957).
72. Goldstein, M. J., and Rothenberg, A. J., *New Engl. J. Med.*, **275**, 97 (1966).
73. Fischer, H. W., and Koak, J. C., *Am. J. Med. Sci.*, **247**, 283 (1964).
74. Farmer, C. D., *et al*, *Gastroenterol.*, **45**, 157 (1963).
75. DuJovne, C. A., *et al*, *New Engl. J. Med.*, **277**, 785 (1967).
76. Macoul, K. L., *New Engl. J. Med.*, **275**, 39 (1966).
77. Freeze, J., and Siraganian, R., *New Engl. J. Med.*, **274**, 95 (1966).
78. Borda, I., and Jick, H., *Arch. Internal Med.*, **120**, 371 (1967).
79. Tisdale, W. A., *New Engl. J. Med.*, **258**, 687 (1958).
80. Carr, A. A., *Arch. Internal Med.*, **115**, 29 (1965).
81. Einhorn, M., and Davidsohn, I., *J. Am. Med. Assoc.*, **188**, 802 (1964).
82. Ten Pas, A., and Quinn, E. L., *J. Am. Med. Assoc.*, **191**, 674 (1965).
83. Bandt, C., and Hoffbauer, F. W., *J. Am. Med. Assoc.*, **188**, 752 (1964).
84. Abbruzzese, A., and Swanson, J., *New Engl. J. Med.*, **273**, 321 (1965).
85. *New Engl. J. Med.*, **277**, 255 (1967).
86. Klein, N. C., and Jeffries, G. H., *J. Am. Med. Assoc.*, **197**, 1037 (1966).
87. Barancik, M., *et al*, *J. Am. Med. Assoc.*, **200**, 175 (1967).
88. Lucke, H. H., *et al*, *Can. Med. Assoc. J.*, **89**, 1111 (1963).
89. Hood, J. W., and Toth, W. N., *J. Am. Med. Assoc.*, **198**, 1366 (1966).
90. Haunz, E. A., *et al*, *J. Am. Med. Assoc.*, **188**, 237 (1964).
91. Stoll, B. A., *et al*, *Brit. Med. J.*, **I**, 960 (1966).
92. Jacobs, J. C., *J. Am. Med. Assoc.*, **199**, 932 (1967).
93. *J. Am. Med. Assoc.*, **197**, 775 (1966).
94. *J. Am. Med. Assoc.*, **197**, 811 (1966).
95. *Am. J. Med.*, **45**, 589 (1968).
96. Kelsey, W. M., and Scharyi, M., *J. Am. Med. Assoc.*, **199**, 586 (1967).
97. Shotton, D., *et al*, *New Engl. J. Med.*, **264**, 550 (1961).
98. Wells, R. F., *et al*, *Am. J. Digest. Diseases*, **13**, 86 (1968).
99. Schaffner, F., *et al*, *Gastroenterol.*, **48**, 293 (1965).
100. Mackay, J. S., and Ross, R. C., *Can. Med. Assoc. J.*, **4**, 1298 (1966).
101. Wells, R. S., Lt. Col., US Army, Brooke General Hospital, Fort Sam Houston, Tex., Personal Communication, 1968.
102. Scott, N. M., in *Diseases of Medical Progress*, 3rd ed., Thomas, Springfield, Ill., 1968, p. 255.
103. Scott, N. M., in *Diseases of Medical Progress*, 3rd ed., Thomas, Springfield, Ill., 1968, p. 253.
104. Burns, L. E., *et al*, *New Engl. J. Med.*, **261**, 1318 (1959).
105. Levine, R. A., *Ann. Internal Med.*, **68**, 1265 (1968).
106. Sherlock, S., *et al*, *Lancet*, **I**, 1049 (1966).
107. Katz, J. N., and Vogel, R. M., *J. Am. Med. Assoc.*, **191**, 124 (1967).
108. Nemeth, E. T., and Feharj-Szinay, G., *Z. Ges. Inn. Med. Ihre Grenzgebiete*, **18**, 756 (1963).
109. Beutler, E., *J. Am. Med. Assoc.*, **187**, 143 (1964).
110. Kurtides, E. S., *et al*, *J. Am. Med. Assoc.*, **197**, 816 (1966).
111. Lai, M., *et al*, *J. Am. Med. Assoc.*, **198**, 483 (1966).
112. Croft, J. D., *et al*, *Ann. Internal Med.*, **68**, 176 (1968).
113. *New Engl. J. Med.*, **277**, 157 (1967).
114. Shulman, N. R., *Progr. Hematol.*, **4**, 222 (1966).
115. Lo Buglio, A. F., and Jandl, J. H., *New Engl. J. Med.*, **276**, 658 (1967).
116. Carstairs, K., *et al*, *Lancet*, **I**, 211 (1966).
117. Molthan, L., *et al*, *New Engl. J. Med.*, **277**, 123 (1967).
118. Erslev, A. J., *J. Am. Med. Assoc.*, **188**, 531 (1964).
119. Best, W. R., *J. Am. Med. Assoc.*, **201**, 181 (1967).
120. *New Engl. J. Med.*, **277**, 1035 (1967).
121. Crosby, W. H., Chief, Hematol. Serv., New Engl. Med. Ctr., Boston, Personal Communication, 1969.
122. Brauer, M. J., and Dameshek, W., *New Engl. J. Med.*, **277**, 1003 (1967).
123. Fraumeni, J. F., *J. Am. Med. Assoc.*, **201**, 828 (1967).
124. Jensen, M. K., and Roll, K., *Acta Med. Scand.*, **178**, 505 (1965).
125. Cassileth, P. A., *Am. J. Med.*, **43**, 471 (1967).
126. Barrett, O., in Moser, R. H., ed., *Diseases of Medical Progress*, Thomas, Springfield, Ill., 1968, p. 298.
127. Huguley, C. M., *J. Am. Med. Assoc.*, **188**, 817 (1964).
128. Rosenthal, D. S., *et al*, *J. Am. Med. Assoc.*, **200**, 81 (1967).
129. Klein, M., *J. Am. Med. Assoc.*, **184**, 310 (1963).
130. Stein, J. H., *et al*, *Arch. Internal Med.*, **113**, 186 (1964).
131. Nordlund, J. J., *et al*, *Ann. Internal Med.*, **69**, 581 (1968).
132. Rogoway, W. M., 6th Med. Ctr., Republic of Viet Nam, Written Communication, 1968.
133. Jones, T. C., and Cardamore, J. M., *Ann. Internal Med.*, **69**, 639 (1968).
134. Barzel, U. S., *J. Am. Med. Assoc.*, **201**, 325 (1967).
135. Finegold, S. M., *et al*, *Intersci. Conf. Antimicrobial Agents Chemotherap. 3rd*, Washington, 1963; abstracted in *Intern. Pharm. Abstr.*, **1**, 128 (Feb., 1964).
136. Brown, E. B., and Cunningham, C. E., *J. Am. Med. Assoc.*, **194**, 668 (1965).
137. Walker, J. G., *Ann. Internal Med.*, **64**, 1303 (1966).
138. Crosby, W. H., and Kaufman, R. M., *J. Am. Med. Assoc.*, **189**, 417 (1964).
139. Oski, F. A., and Naiman, J. L., *New Engl. J. Med.*, **275**, 352 (1966).
140. Rodriguez, S. U., *et al*, *New Engl. J. Med.*, **270**, 881 (1964).
141. Hamfelt, A., *et al*, *Acta Med. Scand.*, **177**, 549 (1965).
142. Lieberman, F. L., and Bateman, J. R., *Ann. Internal Med.*, **68**, 168 (1968).
143. Levitt, B. H., *et al*, *Clin. Pharmacol. Therap.*, **5**, 301 (1964).
144. Feder, W., and Auerbach, R., *Ann. Internal Med.*, **55**, 911 (1961).
145. Kramer, R. A., and Hill, R. L., *Arch. Internal Med.*, **113**, 213 (1964).
146. Nalbandian, R. M., *et al*, *J. Am. Med. Assoc.*, **192**, 603 (1964).
147. Susens, G. P., *et al*, *Ann. Internal Med.*, **69**, 575 (1968).
148. Sinaly, N. P., *Ann. Internal Med.*, **60**, 471 (1964).
149. Rosenthal, R. L., and Blackman, A., *J. Am. Med. Assoc.*, **191**, 136 (1965).
150. McCurdy, P. R., *et al*, *Ann. Internal Med.*, **64**, 1280 (1966).
151. Kaplan, J. M., and Barrett, O., *New Engl. J. Med.*, **277**, 421 (1967).
152. Doyle, A. P., and Hellstrom, H. R., *Ann. Internal Med.*, **59**, 363 (1963).
153. Garus, R. A., *et al*, *Ann. Internal Med.*, **69**, 557 (1968).
154. Hartsock, R. J., *J. Am. Med. Assoc.*, **198**, 41 (1966).

155. Brandriss, M. W., *et al, J. Am. Med. Assoc.*, **189**, 663 (1964).
156. Greenberg, M. S., and Wong, H., *New Engl. J. Med.*, **271**, 431 (1964).
157. Mengel, C. E., *et al, Blood*, **26**, 74 (1965).
158. Daly, D. J., and Davenport, J., *Brit. J. Anaesthesiol.*, **36**, 737 (1964).
159. *J. Am. Med. Assoc.*, **200**, 39 (1967).
160. *Tabulation of Reports Compiled by the Panel of Allergy of the Registry of Adverse Reactions*, Council on Drugs, Am. Med. Assoc., Chicago, Mar., 1965.
161. Bernreiter, M., *J. Am. Med. Assoc.*, **197**, 324 (1966).
162. Lauderdale, W. H., *et al, Internal Med.*, **14**, 693 (1964).
163. Kabius, S. A., *et al, J. Am. Med. Assoc.*, **193**, 175 (1965).
164. Kaplan, K., and Weinstein, L., *J. Am. Med. Assoc.*, **200**, 75 (1967).
165. Pollen, R. H., *New Engl. J. Med.*, **271**, 673 (1964).
166. Helleke, N. A., *J. Am. Med. Assoc.*, **193**, 740 (1965).
167. Clay, B., *et al, Brit. Med. J.*, **I**, 29 (1965).
168. Sherman, W. B., and Werner, S. C., *J. Am. Med. Assoc.*, **190**, 244 (1964).
169. Reisman, R. E., *et al, Ann. Internal Med.*, **59**, 883 (1963).
170. Getgen, J. H., and Speiggle, W., *Arch. Internal Med.*, **112**, 168 (1963).
171. Craps, L., *Arch. Dermatol.*, **87**, 2 (1963).
172. Goldstein, G., *Ann. Internal Med.*, **59**, 97 (1963).
173. Edelstein, J. M., *Am. Heart J.*, **69**, 573 (1965).
174. Kaplan, J. M., *et al, J. Am. Med. Assoc.*, **192**, 444 (1965).
175. Paine, R., *J. Am. Med. Assoc.*, **194**, 23 (1965).
176. Bodman, S. F., *et al, J. Am. Med. Assoc.*, **201**, 35 (1967).
177. Siegel, M., *et al, Arthritis Rheumat.*, **10**, 407 (1967).
178. Lee, S. L., Am. Rheumat. Assoc. Mtg., 1967; to be published.
179. Dustan, H. P., *et al, Circulation*, **18**, 644 (1958).
180. Alarcon-Segovia, D., *et al, New Engl. J. Med.*, **272**, 462 (1965).
181. Ahuja, G. K., and Schumacher, G. A., *J. Am. Med. Assoc.*, **198**, 669 (1966).
182. Cohen, P., and Gardner, F. A., *J. Am. Med. Assoc.*, **197**, 817 (1966).
183. Dewar, H. A., and Peaston, M. J. T., *Brit. Med. J.*, **II**, 609 (1964).
184. Rosin, J. M., *Am. J. Med.*, **42**, 625 (1967).
185. Prockop, L. D., *Arch. Neurol.*, **14**, 325 (1966).
186. Davenport, P. M., and Wilhelm, R. E., *Arch. Dermatol.*, **92**, 577 (1965).
187. Kjellbo, J., *et al, Lancet*, **I**, 1034 (1965).
188. Karliner, J. S., and Belaval, G. S., *J. Am. Med. Assoc.*, **193**, 359 (1965).
189. Kaiser, H. B., *et al, J. Am. Med. Assoc.*, **193**, 369 (1965).
190. Perine, P. L., *et al, J. Am. Med. Assoc.*, **205**, 559 (1968).
191. Edsall, G., *et al, J. Am. Med. Assoc.*, **202**, 17 (1967).
192. Fardon, D. F., *J. Am. Med. Assoc.*, **199**, 125 (1967).
193. McNair-Scott, T. F., and Bonanno, D. E., *New Engl. J. Med.*, **277**, 248 (1967).
194. Buser, F., *New England J. Med.*, **277**, 250 (1967).
195. Van Arsdel, P. P., Jr., *J. Am. Med. Assoc.*, **191**, 238 (1965).
196. Dollery, C. T., *et al, Lancet*, **II**, 735 (1962).
197. Kvam, D. C., and Staunton, H. C., *Diabetes*, **13**, 639 (1964).
198. Ewy, G. A., *et al, Ann. Internal Med.*, **59**, 878 (1963).
199. Proctor, D. W., *et al, Brit. Med. J.*, **1**, 216 (1967).
200. Gardner, P., *et al, J. Am. Med. Assoc.*, **186**, 991 (1963).
201. Spurny, O. M., *et al, Arch. Internal Med.*, **115**, 53 (1965).
202. Bauer, H. G., *Metabolism*, **14**, 220 (1965).
203. Wadia, R. S., *et al, J. Assoc. Physicians (India)*, **15**, 575 (1967).
204. Field, J. B., *et al, New Engl. J. Med.*, **277**, 889 (1967).
205. Kotler, M. N., *et al, Lancet*, **II**, 1389 (1966).
206. Reveno, W. S., *et al, Lancet*, **I**, 920 (1968).
207. Sussman, K. E., *et al, Lancet*, **I**, 626 (1967).
208. Simpson, T., *Lancet*, **I**, 508 (1967).
209. Mackintosh, T. S., *Lancet*, **I**, 104 (1967).
210. Bloodworth, J. M. B., and Hamui, G. J., *Diabetes*, **10**, 90 (1961).
211. Thonnard-Newmann, E., *Am. J. Psychiat.*, **124**, 978 (1968).
212. Ludwig, G. D., *et al, J. Am. Med.*, **43**, 136 (1967).
213. Cohen, A. B., *Ann. Internal Med.*, **65**, 521 (1966).
214. Vivacqua, R. J., *et al, Ann. Internal Med.*, **67**, 380 (1967).
215. Rallison, M. L., *et al, J. Clin. Endocrinol. Metab.*, **27**, 265 (1967).
216. Shackney, S., and Hasson, J., *Ann. Internal Med.*, **66**, 906 (1967).
217. Langer, T., and Levy, R. T., *New Engl. J. Med.*, **279**, 856 (1968).
218. Bryant, J. M., *et al, Am. J. Med.*, **33**, 408 (1962).
219. Griffith, G. C., *et al, J. Am. Med. Assoc.*, **193**, 91 (1965).
220. Wilson, I. D., and Goetz, F. C., *Am. J. Med.*, **36**, 635 (1964).
221. Newman, S., in *Diseases of Medical Progress*, 3rd ed., Thomas, Springfield, Ill., 1969, p. 361.
222. Kleiner, G. J., *et al, New Engl. J. Med.*, **273**, 420 (1965).
223. Bakke, J. L., *Brit. Med. J.*, **I**, 631 (1965).
224. Larsson-Cohn, U., and Stenram, U., *J. Am. Med. Assoc.*, **193**, 422 (1965).
225. Boake, W. C., *et al, Ann. Internal Med.*, **63**, 302 (1965).
226. Ask-Upmark, E., *Acta Med. Scand.*, **179**, 463 (1966).
227. *Reports of Suspected Adverse Reactions*, Food & Drug Admin., Dept. of Health, Education and Welfare, Washington, Dec., 1964, p. 30.
228. *Brit. Med. J.*, **II**, 187 (1968).
229. *Can. Med. Assoc. J.*, **98**, 1117 (1968).
230. *Lancet*, **I**, 962 (1968).
231. Schrogie, J. J., *et al, J. Clin. Invest.*, **46**, 1114 (1967).
232. Tausk, M., in Meyler, L., and Peck, H. M., eds., *Drug-Induced Diseases*, vol. 3, Excerpta Medica Foundation, Amsterdam, 1968, p. 183.
233. Kalhoff, R. K., *et al, Diabetes*, **17**, 307 (1968).
234. Laragh, J. H., *et al, J. Am. Med. Assoc.*, **201**, 918 (1967).

235. Hollander, C. S., *et al, New Engl. J. Med.*, **269**, 501 (1963).
236. Shafey, S., and Scheinberg, P., *Ann. Internal Med.*, **65**, 863 (1966).
237. West, J., and West, E. D., *Lancet*, **I**, 1180 (1966).
238. Taylor, H. B., *et al, J. Am. Med. Assoc.*, **202**, 637 (1967).
239. Clubb, A. W., and Giles, C., *Brit. Med. J.*, **I**, 252 (1968).
240. Brennan, N. F., *et al, New Engl. J. Med.*, **279**, 1213 (1968).
241. Oakley, C., *et al, Lancet*, **I**, 890 (1968).
242. Pinstone, B. L., *Lancet*, **I**, 1153 (1968).
243. Schleicher, E. M., *Lancet*, **I**, 821 (1968).
244. Bolognese, R. J., *et al, J. Am. Med. Assoc.*, **199**, 42 (1967).
245. Hammer, C. J., *Northwest Med.*, **67**, 251 (1968).
246. Elin, M., *et al, Obstet. Gynecol.*, **31**, 685 (1968).
247. Blackwell, B., *Lancet*, **II**, 849 (1963).
248. Brownlee, G., and Williams, E. W., *Lancet*, **I**, 669 (1963).
249. Van Rossum, J. M., *Lancet*, **I**, 950 (1963).
250. Levine, R. J., and Strauch, B. S., *New Engl. J. Med.*, **275**, 946 (1966).
251. Johnson, J. F. III, Lecture, St. Luke's Hospital Seminar, Pasadena, Calif., Dec. 4, 1968.
252. Birge, H. L., *Am. J. Med. Sci.*, **247**, 223 (1964).
253. Fujikura, T., *Am. J. Obstet. Gynecol.*, **90**, 854 (1964).
254. Siddall, J. R., *Arch. Ophthalmol.*, **74**, 460 (1965).
255. Mathalone, M. G., *Diseases Nervous System*, **29**, 29 (1968).
256. DeLong, S. L., *Diseases Nervous System*, **29**, 19 (1968).
257. Gildes, C. L., and Henderson, J. W., *Am. J. Med. Sci.*, **248**, 230 (1965).
258. Rothermich, N. O., *Ann. Internal Med.*, **61**, 1203 (1964).
259. Zelickson, A. S., *J. Am. Med. Assoc.*, **198**, 341 (1966).
260. Richardson, H. L., *et al, J. Am. Med. Assoc.*, **195**, 254 (1966).
261. *New Engl. J. Med.*, **275**, 730 (1966).
262. Leahmann, H., *et al, Brit. Med. J.*, **I**, 1116 (1963).
263. Parisi, A. F., and Kaplan, M. H., *J. Am. Med. Assoc.*, **194**, 289 (1965).
264. Ream, C. R., *Ann. Internal Med.*, **59**, 384 (1963).
265. Van Meter, T. E., Jr., *J. Am. Med. Assoc.*, **199**, 31 (1967).
266. Keighley, J. F., *Ann. Internal Med.*, **65**, 985 (1966).
267. Adriani, J., *et al, Surgery*, **61**, 183 (1967).
268. MacDonald, H. R., and Hess, R., in *Diseases of Medical Progress*, 3rd ed., Thomas, Springfield, Ill., 1969, p. 779.
269. Leake, E., *et al, Lancet*, **II**, 432 (1963).
270. Bernstein, I. L., and Ausdenmoore, R. W., *Diseases Chest*, **46**, 469 (1964).
271. Muir, D. C. F., and Stanton, J. A., *Brit. Med. J.*, **I**, 1072 (1963).
272. Robinson, B. R., *J. Am. Med. Assoc.*, **189**, 239 (1964).
273. Murray, M. J., and Kronenberg, R., *New Engl. J. Med.*, **273**, 1185 (1965).
274. Strauss, W. G., and Griffin, L. M., *J. Am. Med. Assoc.*, **199**, 765 (1967).
275. Nicklaus, T. M., and Snyder, A. B., *Arch. Internal Med.*, **276**, 368 (1967).
276. Bell, R. J. M., *Lancet*, **I**, 1249 (1964).
277. Salvaggio, J. E., *et al, J. Am. Med. Assoc.*, **188**, 323 (1964).
278. Plass, H. F. R., *Ann. Internal Med.*, **60**, 111 (1964).
279. Young, J. V., *et al, Ann. Internal Med.*, **62**, 727 (1965).
280. Shelley, J. H., *Clin. Pharmacol. Therap.*, **8**, 427 (1967).
281. Farriss, B. L., and Knochel, J. P., *Military Med.*, **132**, 341 (1967).
282. Gault, M. H., *et al, Can. Med. Assoc. J.*, **98**, 619 (1968).
283. Gilman, A., *Am. J. Med.*, **36**, 167 (1964).
284. *The Medical Letter*, **7**, 69 (1965).
285. Takacs, F. J., *et al, Ann. Internal Med.*, **59**, 716 (1963).
286. Butler, W. T., *et al, Ann. Internal Med.*, **61**, 175 (1964).
287. Beirne, G. J., *et al, J. Am. Med. Assoc.*, **202**, 62 (1967).
288. Kunin, C. M., *Registry of Adverse Drug Effects*, Am. Med. Assoc., Chicago, July 14, 1966.
289. Czerwinski, N. A., and Ginn, H. E., *Am. J. Med.*, **37**, 969 (1964).
290. Adams, D. A., *et al, Am. J. Med.*, **36**, 330 (1964).
291. Rosenberg, L. E., and Hayslett, J. P., *J. Am. Med. Assoc.*, **201**, 608 (1967).
292. Jaffe, I. A., *et al, Am. J. Med.*, **69**, 549 (1968).
293. Galea, E. G., *et al, Lancet*, **I**, 920 (1963).
294. Richardson, J. H., and Alderfer, A. H., *New Engl. J. Med.*, **268**, 809 (1963).
295. Freeman, R. B., *et al, Ann. Internal Med.*, **57**, 34 (1962).
296. Lang, P. A., and Jones, C. C., *J. Am. Med. Assoc.*, **188**, 464 (1964).
297. Talamo, R. C., and Crawford, J. D., *New Engl. J. Med.*, **269**, 15 (1963).
298. Heyman, W., *J. Am. Med. Assoc.*, **202**, 893 (1967).
299. Sokol, A., *et al, J. Am. Med. Assoc.*, **199**, 43 (1967).
300. Kunin, C. M., *J. Am. Med. Assoc.*, **202**, 204 (1967).
301. Sannen, F. J., *et al, Arch. Internal Med.*, **113**, 241 (1964).
302. Wennberg, J. E., *et al, J. Am. Med. Assoc.*, **186**, 461 (1963).
303. Fink, H. E., Jr., *et al, J. Med. Sci.*, **247**, 201 (1964).
304. Harrow, B. R., and Sloane, J. A., *Am. J. Med. Sci.*, **249**, 26 (1965).
305. Utz, D. C., *et al, J. Am. Med. Assoc.*, **191**, 983 (1965).
306. Conley, C. E., *et al, J. Am. Med. Assoc.*, **198**, 808 (1966).
307. *The Medical Letter*, **4**, 61 (1962).
308. Murphy, M. L., in Wilson, J. W., and Warkany, J., eds., *Teratology, Principles and Techniques*, Chicago Univ. Press, Chicago, 1965, p. 145.
309. Kalter, H., in Seigler, P., and Moyer, J. H. III, eds., *Animal and Clinical Pharmacologic Techniques in Drug Evaluation*, vol. 2, Year Book, Chicago, 1967, p. 123.
310. Diamond, I., *et al, Pediatrics*, **25**, 85 (1960).
311. *The Medical Letter*, 305 E. 45th St., New York, N.Y. 10017.
312. Modell, E. F., *Drugs of Choice 1968–69*, Mosby, St. Louis, 1968.
313. *New Drugs*, Council on Drugs, Am. Med. Assoc., Chicago, 1967.
314. *AMA Drug Evaluation*, Am. Med. Assoc., Chicago: to be published.

73 | Introduction of New Drugs

Drug legislation—evaluation of new drugs—application to the FDA—
obstacles to the evaluation of drugs—problems of drug selection—drug
obsolescence

This chapter was prepared by

Ewart A. Swinyard, PhD, *Professor of Pharmacology, College of Pharmacy
and College of Medicine, University of Utah, Salt Lake City, Utah 84112*

Most drugs used in primitive medicine were obtained from plants. These naturally occurring substances were employed in the form of infusions, decoctions, or poultices, and came into medicine by way of an accident or the herb doctor. The plants used as drugs were fairly innocuous and relatively free from toxic effects or were so toxic that their lethal effects were well known.

Drugs used in 19th-century medicine were naturally occurring substances extracted ready-made from plants, animals, or minerals. The active principles were isolated and came into medicine largely on an empirical basis. For example, opium and morphine were used in the control of pain, digitalis and other cardiac glycosides in the management of cardiac failure and edema, and quinine in the treatment of malaria. Although these agents are still used today, they were first used in man without prior laboratory evaluation.

With the explosive development of new methods of organic chemistry in the last decades of the past century and the first decades of the present century, it became possible to elucidate the structures of the pharmacologically active natural products and to synthesize either the active principle or a modified molecule which retained the pharmacological properties of the parent substance. Subsequently, efforts were directed toward the synthesis of molecules in which the pharmacologic properties of the original natural product were preserved or present to a more pronounced degree, while toxic side effects were reduced. The latter led to the synthesis of agents with novel structures, the pharmacologic properties of which were determined by study in laboratory animals.

This approach proved very fruitful and led to thousands of new and potent synthetic drugs. The discovery of aspirin as an analgesic was the result of attempts to improve on the properties of the plant constituent salicylic acid. The local anesthetic procaine evolved from attempts to synthesize a simple molecule retaining the structural features of the alkaloid cocaine.

Numerous analgesics were discovered in attempts to synthesize simple compounds structurally related in various ways to the alkaloid morphine. Efforts to find a substitute for quinine in the treatment of malaria led to the discovery of atabrine and a number of other effective antiplasmodial compounds. The study of the pharmacologic properties of synthetic antimalarials led unexpectedly to the antihistamines and, eventually, to the discovery of an entirely novel kind of drug, the antihistamine tranquilizers. Thus, two important modern drug discoveries, antihistamines and tranquilizers, really stem from an old traditional remedy, quinine.

Drug Legislation

The original Food and Drugs Act of 1906 contained no provision for the control over the introduction of new drugs. This act provided that drugs moving in interstate commerce were not to be adulterated or misbranded.[1] The pharmaceutical industry took the initiative in the preclinical testing of candidate drugs in laboratory animals. Over a period of 30 years these laboratory tests for efficacy and toxicity were consistently improved.

The first specific legislation directed at drug safety was triggered by a tragedy—the marketing of a sulfanilamide elixir in diethylene glycol. This resulted in a modification of the Food, Drug and Cosmetic Act in 1938 to require firms planning to market a new drug product to submit a new drug application. This act provided that, before a drug could be approved for marketing, it must be shown to be safe when used as directed on the label. It was not necessary to show that the claims for efficacy were valid.[2]

From 1938 until the early 1960's drugs were introduced into medicine in ever increasing numbers. Many of these man-made drugs were highly selective in their effects and altered body physiology in very discrete ways. The pharmaceutical industry recognized the remarkable selectivity contained within many of these agents and developed innumerable ingenious pharmacological tests to reveal their profile of action prior to their first clinical use in man. Despite these advances, another drug tragedy—the thalidomide affair—led to the enactment by Congress in 1962 of the Kefauver–Harris amendments to the Food, Drug and Cosmetic Act.[3]

The most significant provisions of the Kefauver–Harris Amendments of 1962 were those which require that all drugs be proved effective as well as safe for their intended uses. To accomplish this the new legislation made four basic changes in the Food, Drug and Cosmetic Act.[4]

1. All experimental drug studies must be registered in the form of a "Notice of Claimed Investigational Exemption for a New Drug" (IND).
2. Manufacturers must submit data in a New Drug Application (NDA) format supporting efficacy of the product as well as safety.
3. Consideration of efficacy in addition to safety led to greater emphasis on labeling which, as defined by the Food and Drug Administration (FDA), includes the package inserts.
4. Advertising for prescription products was brought under the general supervision and surveillance of the FDA.

In addition to these four basic changes, the amendments also provided that drugs introduced between 1938 and 1962 on the basis of safety alone must be re-evaluated to establish if clinical evidence supports the manufacturers' claims for clinical effectiveness.

The Food and Drug Administration (FDA) had neither the manpower nor the breadth of scientific and medical knowledge necessary to carry out this latter assignment. Therefore, the FDA solicited the aid of the National Academy of Sciences—National Research Council (NAS—NRC)—to conduct this review.[5] Accordingly, in July 1966 the Academy signed a contract with the FDA to undertake an evaluation of all drugs for which New Drug Applications had been approved between 1938 and 1962. This enormous study was organized by Dr. Keith Cannon—former Chairman of the National Research Council's Division of Medical Sciences—with an advisory committee under the chairmanship of Dr. William S. Middleton— Dean Emeritus of the University of Wisconsin School of Medicine, and chairman of the National Research Council's Drug Research Board.

For this study the guidelines were drafted by an ad hoc group under the chairmanship of Dr. Alfred Gilman—Professor and Chairman of the Department of Pharmacology, Albert Einstein College of Medicine —and the categories of drug usage by an ad hoc committee guided by Dr. Walter Riker—Professor and Chairman of the Department of Pharmacology, Cornell University Medical Center. The actual evaluation was conducted by 27 panels of experts, the membership of which was known only to their colleagues.

In July of 1966 the industry was invited by the FDA to submit presentations and supporting data for all therapeutic claims for drugs that it wished to have evaluated by the Academy. A total of 237 pharmaceutical firms submitted presentations on some 3600 drug formulations. The recommended therapeutic indication for each formulation was reviewed by the panels (a few drugs were reviewed by as many as 10 or 15 panels) and the product classified as follows: "effective," "probably effective," "possibly effective," and "ineffective." In some cases a fifth category was employed: "effective, or probably effective, but ——."

Over 10,000 independent judgments were required to complete the task. These recommendations were then forwarded to the FDA for review. Subsequently, they were transmitted to the manufacturers involved with the New Drug Applications. At the same time, an announcement was published in the *Federal Register* inviting interested parties to a meeting to discuss the FDA's position on the NAS–NRC recommendations.

The above historical review points up the evolution which has taken place in drug legislation. It also provides a background for the consideration of how new drugs are marketed today.

Evaluation of New Drugs

Today the discovery, development, and marketing of a new drug is a time-consuming costly procedure. It has been estimated that it takes a minimum of four years to market a novel agent. The various steps which must be followed in the development of a new drug have been the subject of a number of reviews[6-8] and are illustrated in Fig. 505.

Selection of Area—The development of a new drug usually begins with a decision made by the Scientific Advisory Board of a pharmaceutical company. This decision is based on numerous scientific and economic factors, including the need for a drug in a particular illness, the potential market for the drug, the scientific data which justify exploratory

research, and the scientific aptitude of the company's research staff.

When the decision is made to create a drug for use in a particular disease state, virtually all departments within the company become involved in its development, including the biological research (pharmacology and toxicology), chemical research, quality control, pharmaceutical product development, research administration, and legal departments. This multifaceted approach is frequently so complex as to require computer facilities in order to control and process the vast amount of data accumulated during drug development. For this reason this discussion will largely be restricted to the chemical, biological, and clinical aspects of drug development and little mention will be made of the many legal problems and those associated with product formulation and product, package, and label design.

Source and Characterization of New Drugs— Hundreds of products may be made in an effort to find a novel new agent. These substances may be created by chemical synthesis, fermentation processes, or isolation from natural products. After discovery of a new material with potential drug activity, isolation and purification of the active principle must be accomplished prior to initial chemical, physical, and biological characterization.

Chemical and physical characterization of a new purified substance is greatly facilitated by the many sophisticated instruments that are now available to the chemist. Instruments and techniques such as infrared, ultraviolet, and nuclear magnetic resonance spectroscopy, x-ray diffraction, optical rotatory dispersion, mass spectrometry, polarography, titrimetry, and other technological advances have tremendously improved the exactness and speed with which structural formulas can be determined. Structural formulas which ten years ago required the combined efforts of four or five chemists and their associates for three or four years can now be revealed in two or three short months.

Chemical and physical characterization of substances isolated from natural sources may stimulate chemists to synthesize the naturally occurring materials. This leads to the possibility of synthesizing other substances chemically related to the isolated material.

When an adequate amount of material has been characterized and its purity assured, it is subjected to a series of biological tests designed to detect therapeutic activity in a number of areas. Most of these screening procedures are conducted in the intact animal. However, *in vitro* tests are employed to detect antibiotic activity and tissue culture techniques to detect possible antitumor or antiviral activity.

Many "screening procedures" are employed by the pharmacologist in his search for new drugs. Such procedures usually provide the first clue that a particular compound has some therapeutic activity. Thousands of compounds are screened routinely but only a very small number of encouraging leads are discovered. Those which exhibit some favorable activity are administered in varying amounts and in various forms to different species of laboratory animals to ascertain their approximate toxic dose and the type of toxicity induced. Useful drugs should exert a therapeutic effect in a dose range which is devoid of toxic effects and has little influence on normal body processes.

The data accumulated are reviewed at appropriate

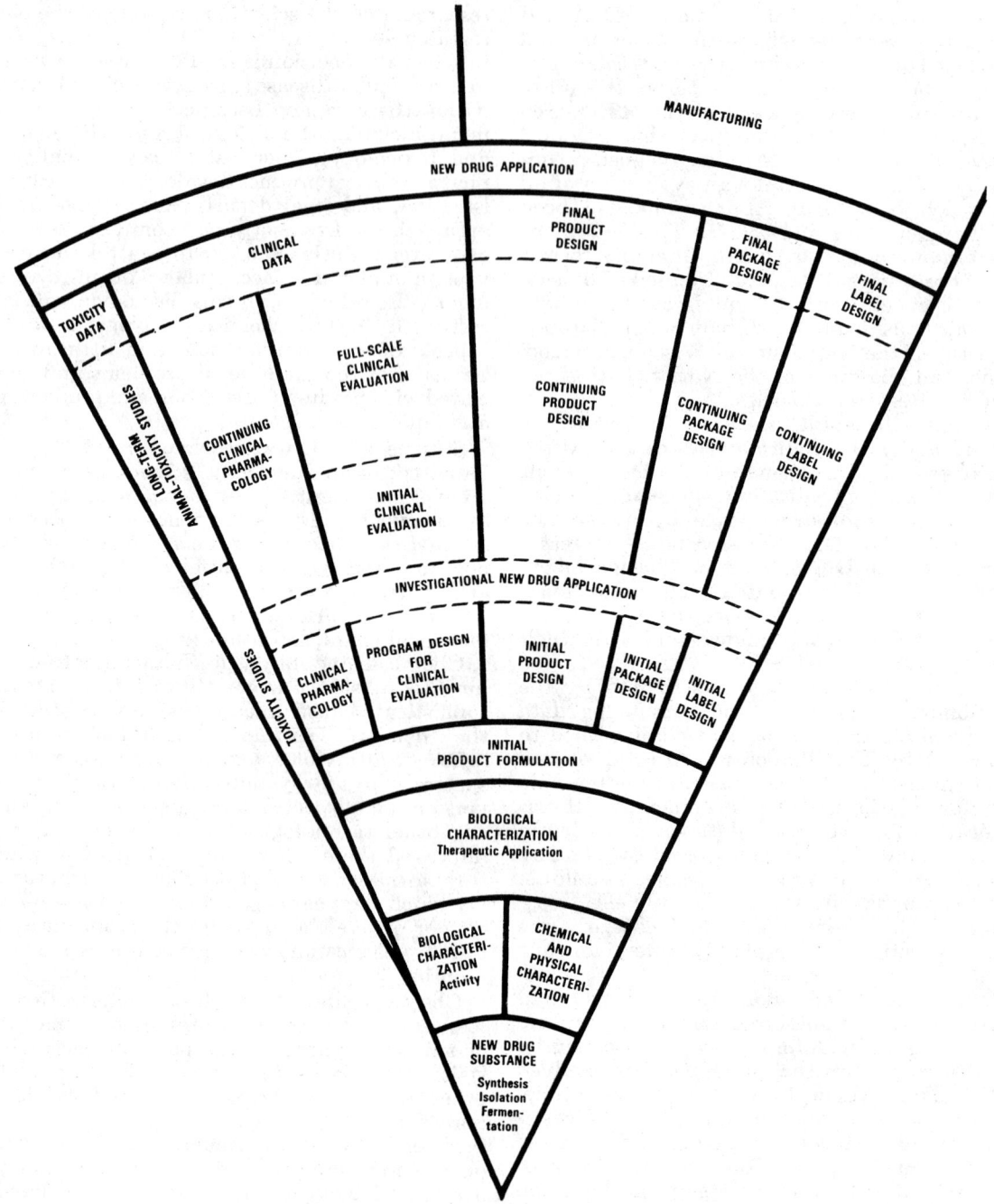

Fig. 505. The steps involved in the development of a new drug (courtesy, Lilly).

intervals by the company's Scientific Advisory Board. Based on such review the most promising agent is recommended for more definitive biological study.

The determination of acute toxicity is prerequisite to more definitive tests in experimental animals. This is usually expressed as the LD50 (lethal dose to 50% of the animals). Further extensive studies on a specific pharmacological activity make it possible to determine an ED50 (effective dose for 50% of the animals). The ratio between these two values (LD50/ED50) provides the first indication of "margin of safety" or "therapeutic ratio" of the drug.

A large margin of safety in experimental animals is a desirable property since it suggests the drug may be safely used in man. At this time subacute toxicity studies are also initiated in an effort to determine dose range when the drug is administered chronically and to reveal possible effects on growth rate and organ function. Any deviation from the growth rate in control animals is considered an undesirable feature. Likewise, adverse effects on renal, hepatic, or bone marrow function may terminate further investigation of the drug. Some animals are usually sacrificed at the end of 30 days' drug administration and their tissues subjected to careful microscopic examination by a trained pathologist. Metabolic studies may be conducted simultaneously in order to ascertain the mechanism of action and the fate of the drug in animals.

An important part of pharmacology is the study of drug absorption, distribution, and excretion. The distribution and concentration of the drug in various organs must be determined. The ultimate fate of the drug must also be ascertained. It is important to know the route by which the drug is excreted and whether it is eliminated from the body unchanged or is changed into some other form. Such studies will often reveal clues as to what might be expected when the drug is used in patients on other medication. This subject is treated more fully in Chapter 42, *Drug Absorption, Action, and Disposition*, page 727.

Application to the FDA

Upon completion of the screening procedures, acute and subacute toxicity studies, and preliminary metabolic experiments, the company's Scientific Advisory Board again reviews all experimental data and decides whether the drug is sufficiently promising to warrant clinical trial. If an affirmative decision is made, application to do so must then be made to the FDA.

Investigational New Drug Application—This is submitted to the FDA on a special form (FDA form 1571). The compilation of the data required for this form, a "Notice of Claimed Investigational Exemption for a New Drug" (IND), is a time-consuming procedure. The filing of the IND informs the FDA that studies of the efficacy and safety of the drug in man will be initiated. The IND is a very important communication between the pharmaceutical manufacturer and the FDA and should include the following information:

1. A description of the chemistry and the biologic activity (toxicology in animals and pharmacological actions) of the drug.
2. Specifications of the dosage form to be given to man.
3. Details of all quality control measures employed to assure exact reproducibility of manufacture and identification of all ingredients, qualitatively and quantitatively.
4. A description of all manufacturing equipment, manufacturing facilities, and manufacturing procedures employed.
5. The names and qualifications of, and the facilities available to, each investigator who will participate in the initial studies (Phase 1).
6. A statement (FDA form 1572) signed by each investigator which (a) confirms his understanding of the nature of the drug he will study; (b) guarantees supervision of every aspect of the study by himself or one or more named associates who are directly responsible to him; (c) describes the facilities available to him; and (d) confirms his understanding that the drug will be administered only to volunteers or patients to whom a full disclosure has been made of the actions of the drug, the purpose of administering it, and the benefits to be derived from the study, and from whom an informed written consent has been obtained for the administration of the drug.
7. Protocols of the doses of the drug to be administered per day, the route and duration of its administration, and the specific clinical observations and laboratory examinations to be performed.
8. A copy of the detailed data sheet supplied to each investigator prior to his initiation of the study.

Studies of new drugs in man are divided into three phases: Phase 1 is the initial cautious trial in normal man; Phase 2 deals with more detailed observations of drug effects in normal patients and initial trials in disease states; and Phase 3 consists of broad clinical trials designed to ascertain whether the drug is of clinical benefit in the disease state or syndrome for which effectiveness is to be claimed. Clinical pharmacologists generally direct Phase 1 and 2 studies within a hospital setting, whereas Phase 3 studies, which usually overlap the latter part of Phase 2, are directed by physicians within the pharmaceutical company and utilize the services of clinicians who have specialized in the particular illness and are attached to a university medical center, teaching hospital, or private clinic.

The Phase 1 study usually involves a comparatively small number of normal human volunteers and is primarily concerned with the determination of biologic activity in man and effects on such target organ systems as the liver, kidney, bone marrow, and heart. Observations on the metabolism of the drug may also be made during Phase 1. These are performed to ascertain the manner in which the drug is handled metabolically by human subjects, as well as the amount and kind of excretion products produced as a consequence of this metabolism. (Such metabolism studies in humans can be utilized in the intelligent selection of proper animal species for the chronic toxicity studies which may be needed if the drug is subjected to Phase 3 studies.) Dosage-range studies are also initiated in Phase 1, but the determination of safe dosage range may continue over into the Phase 2 part of the clinical trial.

Phase 1 studies may be of relatively short duration for new drugs which are related chemically and biologically to drugs of known activity in man. On the other hand, these studies may be quite extensive when completely unrelated novel drugs are under investigation.

In Phase 2, studies are extended to include the initial therapeutic trials on a limited number of patients suffering from the disease entity or syndrome for which the drug is expected to be useful. Clinical protocols are constructed setting forth the duration of drug administration, the clinical observations, and the results of any laboratory determinations which were done. These initial observations are critical in the development of a new drug. The data obtained from this small number of patients, and those obtained in the Phase 1 studies are evaluated by the company's Scientific Advisory Board and a decision is made relative to the advisability of subjecting the drug to the more intensive and extensive studies required in Phase 3.

If the data suggest that the drug should be subjected to Phase 3 studies, long-term chronic toxicity studies in laboratory animals are initiated, a final dosage form is selected, and plans are made to carry out a broad clinical trial. The FDA expects that the duration of chronic toxicity studies in laboratory animals (one rodent and one non-rodent species) be as long as the contemplated duration of administration to man.

The routes of administration of the drug that are to be used in man are employed in toxicity studies in experimental animals. The drugs under evaluation are given for a *minimum* period of 13 weeks, and observations are made of the animals' behavioral and metabolic responses. In addition, the clinical laboratory tests later to be performed in human trials are performed on the animals. At the end of the required experimental period, the animals are sacrificed and their internal organs examined both grossly and microscopically.

The data obtained in these procedures are analyzed and presented for review to the FDA. At this time special animal studies are initiated to determine the effect of the new drug upon the reproductive and fertility processes, as well as its potential for inducing abnormalities in the developing fetus. Once again the decision must be made whether to proceed further with studies of the drug.

During the early clinical studies in man the chemical manufacturing, quality control, and pharmaceutical research divisions have usually completed their assessments of dosage forms and stability of the drug under investigation. At this point, immediately preceding the initiation of broad clinical trials (Phase 3), the final dosage form is selected.

The monitor of the clinical trial (usually a physician employed by the pharmaceutical company) now prepares a new clinical data sheet which incorporates the information obtained to date and develops new protocols for the desired additional investigations. He also selects those clinical investigators who will be invited to participate in the study. Since the data presented in the NDA pertain to the specific formulation of the drug used in the Phase 3 trials and for which approval for marketing is being sought, the complete manufacturing process for the drug substance, as well as for the various dosage forms, must be fixed at this time.

In Phase 3, the construction of the clinical protocol, the selection of patients, the treatment regimen to be followed, and the measurements to be made should be designed to satisfy two judgments: (1) Is the drug safe? and (2) Is the drug effective? The word "safe" in this connotation cannot mean absolutely safe; otherwise, there would be few if any new drugs marketed.

The adverse effects must be weighed against the therapeutic benefits. If it is a lifesaving agent or is palliative in a serious condition for which there is no effective remedy, a definite hazard is tolerable, certainly much beyond the degree which would be acceptable for a drug useful only for controlling a symptom amenable to other drugs. Thus, each drug presents an individual problem involving a variety of factors.

It is well known that infants and children react differently to drugs than adults. The incompletely developed enzyme systems of the infant may result in an altered metabolism of drugs or, conversely, drugs may have a greater effect on the incompletely developed enzymatic processes of the infant than of the adult. Therefore, if the new drug has a therapeutic application in infants and children, Phase 3 studies must be designed to show safety and effectiveness in the various age groups.

It is impossible to predict in advance the number of clinical case reports which may be necessary to demonstrate that the test drug is safe and effective for the proposed indications. In some instances only a few well-controlled detailed case reports may suffice, whereas in others several thousand may be required. Again, this is governed by the disease state for which efficacy is claimed and the nature of the claims for the drug under investigation.

New Drug Application—Upon the completion of all the pharmacology studies (long-term toxicity, effects on fertility and reproduction, and special studies in immature animals) and all three phases of the clinical studies, the company's Scientific Advisory Board must make a decision as to whether the data have satisfactorily demonstrated safety and efficacy of the test drug when used under the recommended conditions. The company then submits to the Food and Drug Administration a New Drug Application (NDA). This is usually an extensive document; many submissions run over 100 2-in. volumes of material.

On the basis of information provided in the NDA, the safety and effectiveness of the drug are evaluated by the FDA staff. If the studies are adequate in number, well conducted, and clearly reported, the FDA should have all the necessary information for prompt approval of the NDA. This is rarely the case. Supplementary laboratory and clinical studies and frequent conferences between representatives of the pharmaceutical company and the FDA are often necessary before the NDA is approved. Once approved, however, the manufacturer can proceed to make this new drug available through the normal channels of distribution for prescription drugs.

Obstacles to the Evaluation of Drugs

The definitive evaluation of candidate new drugs is compromised by a number of obstacles; the major ones include the limitations of both laboratory screening procedures and animal toxicity tests, the extrapolation of laboratory data to man, and the powerful placebo and its effect.

Limitations of Screening Procedures—The ultimate objective of the routine screening of chemical agents in animals is to sort out those drugs which may prove valuable in the prevention or treatment of specific disease entities. The prediction of possible clinical usefulness is based on the ability of the candidate drug to alter, in laboratory animals, the experimentally induced or naturally occurring counterpart of the particular disease entity, or to modify *normal* tissue or organ function in such a way as to suggest an effect of value in human pathological states. Unfortunately, experimental pharmacology has not yet reached the point where the majority of the principal diseases which occur in man can be simulated reliably in animals.

Even the most dependable laboratory tests, such as the analgesic and antiepileptic screening devices, have inherent weaknesses which are occasionally revealed when candidate drugs with novel chemical structures are subjected to clinical trial. The inadequacies of present techniques are emphasized by the fact that many of the drugs widely employed in neurology and psychiatry today did not originate as a result of correct predictions from planned laboratory investigations but were "discovered" only after they had been tried clinically for some other reason. Numerous reviews and conference reports[9–12] have emphasized the need for more reliable screening techniques.

What is the best method for screening drugs for a particular activity? This is a frequent question for which there is no definitive answer; nevertheless, it is of sufficient importance to warrant some consideration. Drug effects can be studied in the test tube, on isolated cells, tissues, and organs, as well as on intact animals.

Many basic pharmacologic problems can be approached at several biologic levels, whereas others can be studied more directly. For example, blood pressure is the sum of numerous factors and drugs which lower blood pressure can be studied at various biologic levels: central nervous system, autonomic ganglia, sympathetic neuroeffector cells, carotid sinus, peripheral blood vessels, or intact normal animals. On the other hand, anti-infective agents can be studied more directly; drugs which inhibit streptococcus *in vitro* will usually inhibit the organism *in vivo*. When the drug effect can be studied at several biologic levels, the particular preparation and screening procedures selected, more often than not, are determined by the skills and prejudices of the experimenter. Be that as it may, there are several criteria which characterize an ideal screening procedure and by which one might evaluate the usefulness of a particular procedure.

Ideally, a drug screen should discern potent new agents. It is one thing to choose a screen because of its theoretical significance or because it may reveal some basic information about a disease entity; it is quite another to select a screen on actual ability to uncover useful new drugs. An ideal screen is simple, rapid, and sorts out potent compounds which have the same order of potency in humans. A screening procedure which yields a high percent of false positives —ie, selects compounds which are active in the laboratory but inactive in the clinic—is a useless screen. Likewise, a screening procedure which yields a high percent of false negatives—ie, fails to detect compounds in the laboratory which are subsequently shown to be active in the clinic—is a useless screen.

An ideal screen is efficient, reveals a minimum number of false positives and false negatives and accurately ranks active agents. These criteria suggest that it might be worthwhile to test an occasional discard clinically in order to see whether the screen is completely dependable. Indeed, one wonders how many active compounds have been "missed" through the use of screening procedures which are not completely reliable.

What are some of the major obstacles to the routine screening of drugs?

● The first obstacle is that the etiology of many diseases for which drug treatment is sought is not completely understood. For example, knowledge of the cause of epilepsy is still incomplete and is largely classified on the basis of the electrical activity of the brain and overt symptoms. Therefore, therapy on the basis of etiology is not yet possible. Yet the fact that this disorder is characterized by certain functional disturbances which can be reproduced in animals allows for a fairly reasonable approach to the symptomatic therapy of this disorder, and drug treatment is directed toward control of the seizures rather than removal of the cause.

Useful antiepileptic agents can be detected on the basis of their anticonvulsant properties in animals, despite the fact that the mechanisms of the various forms of experimentally induced seizures in laboratory animals may have little in common with the causes of epilepsy in man. Therefore, even when the etiology of a particular human disease is unknown, one attempts to induce alterations in laboratory animals which simulate the primary functional disturbance of the disorder in order to devise a screening test for detecting agents which might prove useful in the symptomatic control of the disease in man.

● A second obstacle is that it is difficult to produce the exact counterpart of many human disabilities in laboratory animals, even when the causes are known. For example, in the field of pain, the comprehensive review by Beecher[12] emphasizes the fact that the reflex response to a noxious stimulus, commonly used in the measurement of experimental pain variously evoked in laboratory animals, is quite different from the pathologic pain in man with its associated psychic components. Although some investigators have devised screening techniques for analgesics which combine anxiety or fear with experimental pain, it is quite unlikely that this contrived situation approximates the real state which arises when pathologic pain or trauma is experienced in man.

This very familiar example serves to illustrate the fact that it is rarely possible to duplicate accurately in laboratory animals a particular human syndrome or disease. Hence the experimental pharmacologist is frequently forced to adopt another line of action. He can adopt as a model a drug that is already successful in clinical therapeutics and then attempt to duplicate, in other chemical structures, the profile of pharmacologic effects of the model. The objective of this type of screening is not to find a novel therapeutic agent but to find a drug that will be preferable to the model compound, for any of a number of well-known reasons, including safety, potency, duration of action, minimal side effects, patient acceptability, cost, etc.

This approach prompts many investigators to emphasize the importance of a battery of tests and profiles of action rather than a single procedure. Although such an approach is essential, it is limited in that it is not directed toward the challenging new fields of therapy for which novel drugs are not yet available.

● A third obstacle is the fact that the goals of drug therapy for many diseases have not been clearly defined. This is particularly true in the case of mental diseases such as schizophrenia. Thus, it is difficult to obtain a clear picture of the nature of the psychologic effects which the ideal "psychotherapeutic" drug should produce. Even if the pharmacologist's armamentarium included a wide range of tests which could be used reliably to select drugs with various specific psychologic effects, it would still be difficult to decide which of these drugs might be beneficial in schizophrenia. Progress in this area might be made, however, by defining the goals of therapy in the same manner as in other fields of experimental therapeutics.

Once the primary psychologic disorders which characterize schizophrenia are sorted out, therapy can then be directed toward their amelioration. Until the primary functional disturbances in schizophrenia and in other mental diseases have been disclosed with certainty, progress in this area will be slow. However, the value of basic neuropharmacologic techniques should not be overlooked. For example, not a single phrenotropic drug known today is devoid of some classical effect on the nervous system, such as analgesic, anticonvulsant, sedative, potentiative, skeletal muscle relaxant, central hypotensive, or antiemetic. Whether these pharmacologic effects are merely side actions or whether they are related to the primary desiderata of drug action against clinical psychoses has yet to be established. Nevertheless, a battery of tests based on these classical neuropharmacologic actions has proven a valuable adjunct to the laboratory detection of more effective agents.

● A fourth obstacle is one which concerns the experimental design used in the laboratory tests. This obstacle usually results from failure to devote sufficient time to the proposed experiment to assure that the profile of action of the candidate drug is covered in its entirety. Thus, some workers confine their observations to the effect of a single dose for a particular endpoint. On the other hand, many drugs exhibit their characteristic effects in human patients only after a period of chronic administration. Therefore, it would appear equally important to screen drugs for pharmacologic activity after chronic administration. This suggestion is supported by the fact that some clinically useful agents, for example, many vitamins and hormones, exert little useful effect when administered in a single dose; whereas other drugs (eg, morphine) become less effective when administered frequently. Therefore, it would appear desirable to study in laboratory animals the pharmacologic effects induced by the chronic administration of the drug.

Chronic studies, in addition to revealing valuable information on tolerance and cumulative potentialities of the drug, might reveal valuable therapeutic agents which otherwise would be missed.

● A fifth obstacle is one concerned with the proper laboratory evaluation of drug mixtures. Despite the attention given drug mixtures by drug manufacturers and clinicians, comparatively few of them have been subjected to laboratory study prior to clinical use. The mixtures and doses employed are selected on the basis of trial and error or on the basis of impressions gained from previous clinical experience with the individual agents. This potentially dangerous procedure is encouraged by the complex nature of the problem and the lack of a simple and reliable laboratory method for the evaluation of combined drug effects. For those interested in the theory of drug interactions and the difficulties encountered in the laboratory testing of drug mixtures, the scholarly review by Loewe[13] is recommended.

Limitations of Animal Toxicity Tests—There is no sharp line of demarcation between drug screening and the determination of drug toxicity. Indeed, the initial acute toxicity studies on a candidate drug usually either precede or progress simultaneously with the search for pharmacologic activity. On the other hand, the subacute and long-term toxicity studies are initiated only after the agent has been demonstrated to possess desirable properties in man.

All laboratory toxicity studies and associated pathologic observations are directed toward a single objective: the safe use of the candidate drug in man. This objective has never been fully realized for at least three reasons:

1. The results of acute toxicity experiments are often incorrectly related to man.
2. Available laboratory tests are either not generally reliable or are incapable of detecting certain types of toxicity.
3. Several laboratory tests which can demonstrate particular types of toxicity when conducted in a particular species are frequently carried out in the wrong laboratory animal.

Each one of these topics is worthy of extensive development, but this discussion will be limited to a few pertinent examples.

Many factors influence the LD50 of a drug, including the species and strain of animal employed. Since different species of animals and even various strains of the same species differ widely in sensitivity to drugs, the LD50 should be determined in at least three species of animals, one of which should be a nonrodent. If all of the LD50's are of the same order of magnitude, it is usually safe to assume a similar LD50 for man. If, however, there is a wide variation of LD50's among species of test animals, the estimation of the probable LD50 for man is much more hazardous. In such cases a more reliable estimate may be obtained by also taking into consideration man's position in the phylogenetic scale in relation to the test animal and/or the biochemical and metabolic similarities of man with the test animal.

It is well known that even routine toxicity studies may give highly variable results when conducted under certain environmental situations. For example, when mice are employed as test animals for certain sympathomimetic amines, Chance[14] has shown that the LD50 is several times higher for singly confined animals than for aggregated mice. This observation has been confirmed by many investigators and emphasizes the fact that even rodents are responsive to their social environment. It also suggests that certain types of acute toxicity studies should be done both with individually isolated animals and with uniform groups of animals housed together under similar conditions.

It should be mentioned that interpretations based on the slope of the dosage–mortality curves are frequently neglected or ignored. The slope of the dosage–mortality curve is a measure of the change in mortality which occurs with a change of dosage. Very "flat" curves indicate that occasional instances of extreme susceptibility to the chemical may be expected, perhaps even at the levels of proposed use. On the other hand, a "steep" curve indicates little variability and consequently permits a better estimate of safe dosage.

In general, compounds which have a flat dose-response curve and/or a marked delay in the onset of symptoms are frequently quite toxic upon long-term ingestion. For example, diethylene glycol is a substance which in most species of animals gives rise to a "flat" dose–response curve. This flatness was reflected in the human-poisoning cases with diethylene glycol in which some individuals died from relatively small doses, whereas others survived comparatively large doses. In contrast to diethylene glycol, the dose–response curve of gonyaulax toxin, a toxin occurring occasionally in clams and mussels, is so "steep" that a quarter of the LD50 can be eaten with almost no risk or fatality. These observations point up the weaknesses which occur when even routine toxicity measurements are used merely as tools for estimating the LD50.

Available laboratory tests are incapable of detecting certain types of toxic manifestations which occur in man. This is emphasized by the data of Zbinden[15] shown in Table I. This table shows that at least 22 of the 45 most frequently recorded untoward effects are unlikely to be recognized in an animal experiment. In addition, available laboratory tests are either weak or entirely lack the ability to reveal the potentiality of the candidate drug for causing serious skin disorders and liver and bone marrow disturbances. It is possible but not definitely proven that these toxicities

Table I—The Most Frequent Untoward Reactions to Drugs[15,a]

Side effect[b]	No.	Side effect[b]	No.
Drowsiness	426	Skin rash	29
Nausea	211	Anorexia	23
Dizziness	198	Depression	23
Sedation	176	Increased appetite	21
Dry Mouth	133	Tremor	21
Nervousness	98	Perspiration	21
Epigastric distress	98	Dermatitis	19
Headache	91	Increased energy	18
Vomiting	83	Vertigo	16
Weakness	61	Palpitations	16
Nasal stuffiness	57	Blurred vision	16
Hypertension	57	Lethargy	15
Insomnia	56	Nocturia	15
Fatigue	55	Excitation	14
Constipation	54	Abdominal distention	14
Tinnitus	49	Frequent bowel	
Weight gain	39	movement	14
Hypotension	38	Flatulence	14
Dryness of nasopharynx	38	Stiffness	13
Heartburn	38	Urticaria	13
Diarrhea	30	Tachycardia	13

^a Observed in 11,115 patients treated with 77 different drugs or drug combinations; summarized from 86 recent drug-evaluation papers.

a Observed in 11,115 patients treated with 77 different drugs or drug combinations; summarized from 86 recent drug-evaluation papers.
b Side effects for the detection of which there is no satisfactory animal model available are shown in *italics*.

are hypersensitivity reactions peculiar to man and cannot be induced in laboratory animals.

Some types of toxicity which can be detected if the drug is administered to a particular species may be missed if the experiment is conducted in the wrong laboratory animals. For example, it is well known that methemoglobin is not readily induced in monkeys, rats, and rabbits; suspect candidate drugs should be tested in the cat or dog, species known to produce this response similar to man.

The data in Table I and the examples cited above indicate that available toxicity tests leave much to be desired. Even multiple determinations of LD50 in several animal species cannot always be relied upon to estimate the LD50 in man. The effect of environment on toxicity is frequently neglected and little attention is given to the implications of the slope of dose–mortality curves on toxicity. Many of the commonly encountered untoward effects in man cannot be detected with available laboratory techniques, and certain types of toxicity may be missed if the drug is tested in the wrong animal species.

Extrapolation of Laboratory Data to Man— There is often a large measure of uncertainty when one attempts to project to man the results obtained in laboratory animals. The extent of uncertainty is often inversely proportional to our understanding of the mechanisms involved. It is generally agreed that in certain pharmacologic areas results obtained in laboratory animals can be used reliably to predict the pharmacologic effect in man. Such areas include the effect of drugs on neuromuscular transmission, impulse conduction in nerve, diuresis, blood pressure, etc.

The high reliability with which extrapolations between phylogenetic levels can be made in the case of the above discrete examples results from the fact that a great deal is known concerning the functional basis of the observed effects; consequently, tests used to identify drugs effective in these areas have become highly selective. On the other hand, extrapolations from animal to man in less clearly defined areas of pharmacology are more difficult. To cite an extreme example, extrapolation based on the effects of drugs on more complex and less understood functions in laboratory animals, such as behavior, are less reliable than those based on the actions of drugs on an identifiable enzyme system at the cellular level.

Many examples could be cited to illustrate the difficulties encountered when extrapolating animal data to man. Limitations of space dictate that this discussion be restricted to a brief consideration of the problems encountered when relating animal terato-genic and toxicity studies to human patients.

The major obstacle to the clinical interpretation of teratogenic studies in laboratory animals is the large number of false-positive results obtained in laboratory animals with many well-established medications, such as insulin, penicillin, streptomycin, salicylates, pheno-barbital, and others. It has even been shown that nicotine[16] and caffeine[17] are teratogenic in animals. This has led to the suggestion that more attention should be given to the effect of the candidate drug on fetal mortality. In general, agents which kill the fetus at doses tolerated by the mother will also tend to deform the offspring if given in a lower dose. The reliability of extrapolating this observation to man remains to be established.

The extrapolation of chronic toxicity results to man appears to be compromised by at least two major factors: (1) nonspecific consequences of the experi-mental procedure and (2) species differences. Three dose levels are required in chronic toxicity experi-ments: a high dose which is expected to produce obvious signs of toxicity; a low dose which will be tolerated without obvious toxic effects; and an inter-mediate dose. Abrams and co-workers[18] have pointed out that the toxicologist must distinguish between the toxic manifestations of the drug and those tissue changes which are nonspecific consequences of the experimental procedure.

Organ functions are limited in their ability to respond to noxious stimuli, and organ change due to general overloading with the drug is not uncommon. Such overloading is frequently accompanied by mal-nutrition which is known to induce a variety of organ changes, particularly of the hemopoietic system, lymphatic system, adrenals, liver, kidney, and repro-ductive system. These changes are frequently in-distinguishable from those directly related to the drug and complicate extrapolation of such data to man.

Species differences account for many of the limita-tions of animal toxicity studies. In many cases species differences can be explained by differences in metabolism. It is important to remember that drug absorption, distribution, and penetration through membranes depends on the physicochemical properties of the agent and therefore is essentially the same in various species. Important differences are known to occur in the pathway of metabolism and rate of inactivation. Therefore, drug metabolism studies should be instituted at an early stage of drug investiga-tions and chronic toxicity studies done in animal species which metabolize the drug similar to man.

These examples emphasize the importance of a thorough understanding of the comparative functional biology of both laboratory animals and man. They also suggest that when possible, new drugs should be tested in laboratory animals which respond to the drug in a manner similar to man. It is clearly evident that the pharmacologic, teratogenic, and toxicologic properties of drugs as determined in laboratory animals can be applied reliably only to those clinical situations which clearly correspond.

The Powerful Placebo— Drug administration is more than the introduction of a drug into the body. It represents the culmination of the physician–patient relationship. The physician prescribes a drug in anticipation that it will induce the expected salutary effect. The patient desperately desires the drug to be effective and shares the physician's expectation that it will produce the desired effect. Thus, drug administration takes place under circumstances char-acterized by biased expectations and enhanced sug-gestability on the part of both physician and patient.

Health and disease are greatly influenced by psychic and emotional factors. Symptoms of psychosomatic origin are just as "real" as those resulting from minor, organic causes. Similarly, psychic responses to drugs and psychic modifications of drug action represent real phenomena.

All reactions to drug administration that arise from the act of taking the drug and that are unrelated to the pharmacologic actions of the drug are known as *placebo effects*. An inert chemical substance used as a drug is called a *placebo* (Latin "I shall please"). Thus, any and every drug administered to a conscious patient elicits a placebo effect superimposed on a pharmacologic effect. This complicates drug evalua-tion in man and dictates that all clinical studies be designed to enable the clinical pharmacologist to distinguish between the placebo and pharmacologic effects of drugs.

The placebo effect is powerful, universal, either desirable or undesirable, consistent yet variable, and capable of mimicking drug effects. Few would deny the ability of the placebo to influence pain, anxiety, or other "subjective" effects in certain individuals. The ability of placebos to affect "objective" phenomena, such as vomiting, or to produce unwanted side effects is also recognized. Lesser known, however, is the fact that placebos can mimic certain pharmacologic aspects of active drugs, such as time course, cumulative effect, carry-over effect, and efficacy dependent upon the severity of the symptom. Examples will be cited to illustrate three of the more important of these effects. Readers interested in a more detailed analysis of these phenomena are referred to the following reviews.[19-21]

● The first example illustrates the effect of suggestion. If a physician warns a patient that certain toxic manifestations may occur following drug administration or if the patient has heard about untoward actions occurring from this medication, the patient may then anticipate effects other than the beneficial ones for which the drug is given. This is illustrated by the report of Pincus[22] on the side effects produced by oral contraceptive agents. In order to determine the cause of a number of annoying symptoms such as headache, nausea, dizziness, and abdominal pain, Pincus administered the contraceptive pill to three groups of Puerto Rican women.

A group of women using conventional methods of birth control was selected from the same native population and divided into two subgroups. One group received placebo pills, the other received contraceptive pills. Both groups were advised to continue with the same contraceptive practices they had been using but were admonished to note any adverse effects. They were told that the pills had to be tested to see if they were suitable for continued use. A third group of women, selected from a different town, were given the contraceptive pills without any admonition. Table II shows the results of this experiment. It may be seen that the side effects noted were due to the admonition and not to the drug. The study further demonstrated that the incidence of side effects declined to a very low level with continued use of the drug in large groups of women.

Table II—Placebo Side Effects in the Trial of an Oral Contraceptive[22]

Group	No. of patients	Cycles No.	Reactions[a] %
No admonition, drug	15	48	6.3
Admonition, drug	13	30	23.3
Admonition, placebo	15	41	17.1

[a] Includes complaints of physical ill-being, such as nausea, vomiting, headache, vertigo, gastrointestinal distress, and malaise.

● The second example reflects the fact that a placebo has a time–effect relationship. Lasagna and co-workers[23] studied the effects of aspirin or a placebo on postpartum pain; 128 patients were studied in an obstetrical ward during the five-day period after delivery. Identical-appearing capsules of aspirin or a placebo were administered at random to any patients requesting medication for pain. All patients were interviewed by the same technician under double-blind

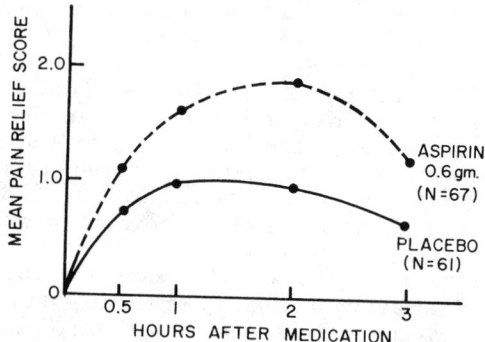

Fig. 506.   Mean pain relief scores after placebo or aspirin in patients suffering from postpartum pain (courtesy, Lasagna, *et al*[23]).

conditions immediately prior to medication, and ½, 1, 2, and 3 hr after medication.

Four arbitrary categories of pain were employed and each patient given a pain relief score for each interview after medication. The sum of all scores for all patients at a given interview point was then divided by the number of patients to give a mean pain relief score for each time interval after medication.

The data obtained are shown in Fig. 506 from which it may be seen that there is a similarity in the shape of the curves for those patients receiving aspirin and for those receiving a placebo. The two treatments differed considerably in efficacy. The mean total pain relief score for aspirin the first 3 hr after medication was 5.91 ± S.E. of 0.35; for the placebo it was 3.45 ± 0.44. This difference was found to be significant at the 0.01 level. At least two important points are illustrated by these data: (1) placebo medication elicits a time–effect relationship and (2) the placebo itself relieved pain in a significant number of patients.

● The final example illustrates that efficacy is inversely related to the severity of a given complaint. In the previously described postpartum-pain study, Lasagna and co-workers[23] plotted the per cent of patients completely relieved of slight to moderate pain or severe to very severe pain by placebo medication against time. The results are shown in Fig. 507. The percentage of patients reporting complete relief of pain at some time during the 3-hour test period was 57% and 21% for the slight–moderate group and severe–very severe group, respectively. This difference is significant at the 0.01 level. The aspirin data were similarly analyzed and also indicate a lessened efficacy in patients with greater pain. Thus the efficacy of placebos, like the efficacy of active drugs, is inversely related to the intensity of the symptom.

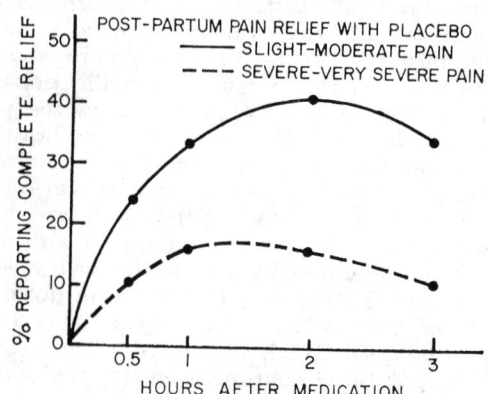

Fig. 507.   Relationship between reported severity of pain and analgesic efficacy of placebo (courtesy, Lasagna, *et al*[23]).

There are certain implications in these examples as regards the evaluation of new drugs.

1. Placebo controls are not always necessary or desirable. If a useful drug is already available, and the question is whether or not a new drug is superior, a placebo control is inappropriate; the clinical study should be designed to compare the toxicity and efficacy of the old drug and the new. On the other hand, if the new drug is to be tested for a clinical condition for which there is no known therapy, a placebo control is indispensable.

2. Uncontrolled studies that claim therapeutic benefit because of "peak effects," "cumulative effects," or persistent benefit after cessation of treatment should be interpreted cautiously.

3. The placebo effect is not an "all or none" phenomenon.

4. The placebo time–effect relationship should be taken into consideration when deciding upon times when data are to be collected in controlled clinical trials.

5. Selection of patients presenting severe therapeutic challenges may lessen the necessity for or the importance of placebo controls.

Adherence to these and other principles enables the clinical pharmacologist to distinguish between the placebo and pharmacological effects of new drugs.

Problems of Drug Selection

Every new drug introduced into medicine further complicates the unique and difficult position assumed by the physician when he selects the best drug to treat a particular illness. His position is unique in that he assumes the responsibility of selecting the least toxic and most efficacious agent for the patient's condition with the full knowledge that it will ultimately be the patient who will pay for this medication. His position is difficult in that he must select one agent from among the several thousand that are available to him.

In addition to the usual routine pharmacological knowledge of the agent, it is the physician's responsibility to know how the medication selected will interact with other medication that might be indicated or with medication the patient might already be taking. The task of drug selection is further complicated by a number of general problems only four of which, namely, drug names, generic equivalency, drug combinations, and drug-induced diseases, will be mentioned here.

Drug Names—By the time a new drug becomes generally available to the physician, it already has several names. A "drug" refers to the active ingredient in a "drug product," such as a tablet, capsule, or other dosage form that is administered to the patient.

First, a drug is given a *chemical name* which describes its structure by standard chemical nomenclature.

Second, a *code number* is assigned to the chemical for use during chemical, biological, and early clinical studies.

Third, it receives a *nonproprietary name* (frequently incorrectly referred to as a generic name) which is often a contraction of the chemical name but which may also indicate the chemical class of drug to which it belongs. The US Adopted Names Council, composed of representatives from the American Medical Association, US Pharmacopeia, National Formulary, and Food and Drug Administration, recommends nonproprietary names of all new drugs. The US Adopted Name (USAN) is developed according to a number of guiding principles, which are broken down into general and specific rules. The general rules say that a name should be:

1. Useful primarily to health practitioners.
2. Short, easy to pronounce, easy to recognize and recall.
3. Such that it reflects pharmacologic, chemical, or other characteristics and relationships of actual practical value to the user.
4. Free of conflict with other drug names and neither confusing nor misleading.

5. A name of established usage if it conforms reasonably well to the other guiding principles.

Since 1962 the FDA must approve all nonproprietary names.

Fourth, the drug is given a *trademarked name* (brand name) designated by a superscript® at the end of the name, indicating that this name has been registered with the US Patent Office. Only the registrant may use the trademarked name for the particular drug; it is this name which distinguishes a particular product from those of competitors.

Considerable confusion results from the common practice of granting multiple brand names for a single chemical entity. Random selection of a few commonly used drugs from the *Merck Index* (8th ed., 1968) shows the number of brand names as follows: diphenhydramine, 13; chloramphenicol, 45; chlorpromazine, 16; meperidine hydrochloride, 26; meprobamate, 64; phenobarbital, 22; prednisone, 29; vitamin B_{12}, 82. The possibilities for confusion and misunderstanding among all members of the health profession are readily apparent. For example, instead of using the name "prednisone" he may use a word such as Juvason, Meticorten, Deltasone, Decortin, Decortisyl, Dekortin, Di-Adreson, Dacortin, Mostacortin, Deltisone, Colisone, Paracort, Ancortone, Cortancyl, Decortancyl, Ultracorten, Bicortone, Delta-Cortelan, Ultracortene, Deltra, Deltacortone, or Delta Prenovis.

To avoid such confusion most authorities recommend that physicians prescribe by nonproprietary name and indicate in parenthesis the manufacturer of the product desired. This procedure has a number of factors in its favor: it encourages accurate recognition of the drug; it uses the name which is employed in current medical literature; it eliminates the burden of memorizing multiple names; and it circumvents the problem sometimes encountered where different names are used for the same drug promoted for different uses. For example, Benadryl is promoted as an antihistaminic, whereas Dramamine is the name used for the same active agent promoted as an anti-motion-sickness remedy. Finally, it should be emphasized that prescribing by nonproprietary name and designating the manufacturer in parenthesis still leaves the choice of the particular agent in the hands of the physician.

Generic Equivalency—The several years required to develop a novel new drug for market drastically reduces the profitable patent life of the agent. Furthermore, as soon as the patent has expired, other companies are free to produce this same drug under their own trade name. The availability of drugs under both a nonproprietary (generic or branded generic) name and a variety of tradenames focused attention on the price differential between products supposedly containing the same chemical entity. This price differential was further brought out in the government drug hearings which revealed that in some instances the pharmacist paid several hundred per cent more for a particular item than the government or a hospital. Numerous instances were cited showing a similar price differential in favor of products available by generic name.

The original Food and Drugs Act of 1906 charged the United States Pharmacopeia (USP) and the National Formulary (NF) with the responsibility of establishing standards for drugs; therefore, it was a logical next step to assume that generic products were also equivalent in efficacy.

Many of the factors in the formulation and manufacture of dosage forms which affect the efficacy of the product have been reviewed in detail.[24,25] To cite but three examples, a commonly used filler, dicalcium phosphate, was found to depress the blood concentration of tetracycline;[26] particle size has been reported to affect the absorption of the sulfa drugs, griseofulvin, and insulin;[27] tablet hardness has been shown to be inversely related to absorption.[28] Isolated clinical reports also indicate that results obtained with certain nonproprietary products are inferior to those obtained with a trademarked product. For example, clinical results with various nonproprietary brands of prednisone,[29] cortisone,[30] tolbutamide,[31] and phenylbutazone[32] have been reported to be inferior in certain respects to results obtained with the respective trademarked product.

The now classical chloramphenicol studies done by Parke, Davis Company brought this controversy into sharp focus. These data showed that nonproprietary brands of chloramphenicol, sampled on the US market after certification by government laboratories, are not clinically equivalent to Chloromycetin. Similar results were obtained by the FDA and, subsequently, their approval of generic chloramphenicol products was withdrawn. These observations suggested that some drugs may be "generically equivalent" but "therapeutically nonequivalent." The pros and cons of this interpretation have been discussed in a number of publications.[33-35] For an extensive list of references, the interested reader is referred to the *Bibliography on Biopharmaceutics*.[36]

There is a tendency to minimize the importance of variations in therapeutic equivalence among drug products. For example, it has been reported that there are only "17 such drugs out of a total of perhaps 3000 single entities in general use today."[37]

The absolute number of drugs that are known to be "therapeutically nonequivalent" is of little importance, since the number of suspect drugs may vary enormously as newer methods of study are developed and information on this important subject is accumulated.

It is important, however, to recognize that such a phenomenon does occur and to design tests to verify therapeutic availability of formulated products prior to marketing. This demands increased information not only on the pharmacology and toxicology of drugs *per se*, but also on the biologic availability and rate of *in vivo* release of the active ingredient from the drug formulations to be used in man. Beckett and Tucker,[38] have devised an *in vivo* test based on urinary excretion data to determine the degree to which a formulation becomes biologically available. These workers[39] have also suggested the following guidelines be observed when testing biologic availability:

1. Use a panel of closely supervised human subjects, acting as their own controls, for comparative tests on drugs and drug formulations. (Animal data and/or *in vitro* tests are not acceptable as sole evidence for the efficacy of a product in humans.)
2. Compare the performance of the product in humans with that of a single and identical dose of the drug in a nonformulated form, preferably in aqueous solution. Estimate the variability of drug release relative to normal biologic variation in response to the drug.
3. Determine the total availability of the drug and the rate at which it becomes available from the preparation to the biologic system.
4. Determine the effects of storage and batch to batch variation of the product, not only on the chemical stability of the drug but also on the biologic availability and rate of release of the drug from the formulated product to the biologic system.

In the case of prolonged or sustained-release preparations these investigators suggested an additional requirement, namely

5. Compare the performance of the product with that of a divided but identical total dose of the drug in a nonformulated form.

The ultimate proof of equivalent efficacy must come from clinical results. However, much can be learned from *in vivo* studies in healthy human subjects. Ideally, target tissue concentration would be more indicative of therapeutic equivalency. Since such studies are virtually impossible in healthy human subjects, blood and urine level data are generally equated with therapeutic efficacy. Thus, if two preparations are generically equivalent and yield similar blood absorption and urinary excretion curves for the active ingredient after administration, they are assumed to be therapeutically equivalent and to elicit similar pharmacologic effects. Until such tests have been conducted and the information made available, the physician would be well advised to restrict his prescribing of suspect drugs to brands which have survived the test of time.

Drug Combinations—Many effective new drugs are eventually made available in combination with one or more other drugs. A recent national prescription audit indicated that 200 prescription drugs accounted for 67% of all prescription orders filled. Of these 200 most frequently prescribed drugs, 40% (80) were mixtures of two or more drugs.

There are few rational reasons for the administration of two or more drugs in a fixed-dose combination (see also Chapter 42). Physicians who prescribe this kind of medication sacrifice the ability to individualize the dosage of each ingredient to the specific needs of the patient in favor of a supposedly economic factor; ie, a price advantage from two or more ingredients in a single formulation. This is more theoretical than practical, since most drug mixtures are trademarked products, are based on empiricism rather than clinical confirmation, and have not been subjected to an *in vivo* study of drug interaction.

The following example emphasizes the latter two points. Amphetamine depresses the appetite and is sometimes used in the control of food intake. Proprietary diet control formulations often include a barbiturate in the same tablet or capsule to counteract the central excitant effects of the amphetamine. One would expect the barbiturate in such combinations to stimulate drug metabolism and to increase the rate of destruction of amphetamine. This suggests that perhaps the same end-result could be obtained merely by a lower dose of amphetamine and no barbiturate at all. When considered in this light it is apparent that the irrational use of drug mixtures exposes the patient to several drugs needlessly, each of which may cause toxic or allergic effects.

Drug-Induced Diseases—The introduction of hundreds of new proprietary and prescription drugs has undoubtedly made people in the US the most medicated population in the world. Expenditures for proprietary home remedies amount to nearly $2 billion,[40] and nearly 1 billion new and refill prescription orders were filled in 1967.[34] All this medication is for a population of only 200 million people. Hospital studies show that patients receive an average of 10 potent drugs per stay—some receive as many as 20 or more. There are many reasons to believe that such multiple drug use is as great or even greater on an outpatient basis.

Excessive self-medication is responsible for many ills. It is questionable whether the benefits derived from self-medication with proprietary home remedies outweigh the potential harm they do. They are responsible for many poisonings (by accident or suicidal intent), they cause allergic and other adverse reactions, and their use often delays proper medical attention to serious illness.

The excessive use of prescription drugs also presents a real problem. It is not unusual for a patient to see several medical specialists for wholly unrelated reasons. Likewise, it is not uncommon for a patient to save a drug prescribed for one illness and use it on another occasion or by another member of the family. The seriousness of this situation is reflected by a recent study in three Boston hospitals covering 13,868 consecutive uses of drugs among 1,400 patients.[41] About 6% (900 reports) of all drugs administered resulted in adverse drug reactions. Adverse drug reactions were believed to be directly responsible for eight deaths and to be a major factor but not the specific cause of the death of 26 others.

It is experiences of this kind which have led health scientists to speak of "drug-induced diseases" and "iatrogenic diseases." Iatrogenic diseases (Gk *iatros* = physician) are those caused by physicians prescribing drugs irrationally and for trivia. The magnitude of this problem is not known. However, the high frequency of adverse drug reactions suggests that the problem may be far more extensive than is presently recognized.

What does all this mean? It means that no drug in use today is completely and thoroughly understood. Consequently, physicians are obliged to use drugs about which additional, pertinent information is needed. There are inherent risks in doing so but these are risks which must be taken in order to obtain the benefits afforded by modern drugs. It means also that the pharmacist of today is obliged to keep drug records on his patients. He should record not only all drugs they receive, but also instances of known drug sensitivities, idiosyncracies, and other unusual responses. Such information, passed on to the physician at the appropriate time, might save a life.

Drug Obsolescence

The introduction of a new prescription drug is usually received by an overly enthusiastic response by prescribing physicians. Hopeful of providing their patients with the latest medication and perhaps of helping patients who are not doing as well as might be expected on existing medication, physicians accept at face value claims for new drugs and prescribe them freely. The widespread clinical use of such new agents naturally results in reports of untoward effects and limitations which had either not been observed or occur so infrequently as to escape detection in early limited clinical trials. Thus, the initial enthusiasm is replaced by a skeptical attitude toward the safety and efficacy of the new agent. As more detailed clinical information accumulates, however, the new drug either falls into obscurity or assumes its well-earned place in the physician's armamentarium.

The pharmaceutical industry budgeted $476.2 million in 1967 for research. This research was directed toward the improvement of existing drugs, the development of more effective drugs than those now available, and the discovery of new agents for illnesses for which there are no drugs effective. Such highly competitive research efforts markedly shorten the life of new drugs.

The effects of "planned obsolescence" may be seen from a study done by Arthur D. Little, Inc. for the members of the Pharmaceutical Manufacturers Association. Products introduced into the market prior to 1951 showed a declining sales trend from 1951 to 1960. Thus, the older prescription products accounted for a continuously smaller percentage of the total prescription market. The data indicate that new prescription drugs reach peak demand the first and second year after the year of introduction, and decline in popularity thereafter. For example, products introduced in 1953 accounted for 16% of sales in 1954, but declined in per cent of sales each year thereafter; by 1960 (six years from introduction) these agents accounted for only 4.7% of sales. Furthermore, in each year from 1956 to 1960 over 50% of sales were for products introduced into the market within the past five or six years.

These data show that prescription drugs, in general, have a relatively short period of market eminence. They also confirm the product obsolescence pattern within the pharmaceutical industry and underscore the dynamic nature of new-drug competition within the ethical pharmaceutical field.

Despite the numerous problems confronting the pharmaceutical industry in the development of new drugs and the numerous unsolved problems in the health sciences, the effect of concerted efforts toward improving the general health of the nation is readily apparent. Today the standard of health care in the United States is one of the highest in the world. Statistics indicate that in 1967 the death rate of newborns was the lowest in history and that life expectancy reached 70.5 years, the highest ever attained in this country. This represents an increase of ten full years in life expectancy over what existed in 1937.

In 1967 the pharmaceutical industry clinically tested more than 1300 new drugs.[42] Many of these are for illnesses and conditions for which no effective drug is currently available. This tremendous effort is even more remarkable when it is noted that only 9.5¢ of every health dollar was spent for prescription drugs as compared to 11.5¢ in 1957.

It is generally agreed that these advances resulted from medical and drug research supported by voluntary health agencies, the National Institutes of Health of the US Public Health Service, and the pharmaceutical industry. It is to be hoped that an equal amount of progress and support will be forthcoming in the future.

References

1. Pettit, W., *Manual of Pharmaceutical Law*, Macmillan, New York, 1957, p. 97.
2. Hodges, R., *FDA Papers*, **1**(6), 27 (July-Aug., 1967).
3. "Federal Food, Drug and Cosmetic Act, as amended," *Code of Federal Regulations, Title 21*, US Government Printing Office, Washington, 1963.
4. Ley, H. L., Jr., *J. Clin. Pharmacol./J. New Drugs*, **8**, 3 (1968).
5. Goddard, J. L., *FDA Papers*, **2**, 7 (Mar., 1968).
6. "Clinical Testing: Symposia of the New Drug Regulations," *FDA Papers*, **1**, 21 (Mar., 1967).
7. Barron, B. A., and Bukantz, S. C., *Arch. Intern. Med.*, **119**, 547 (1967).
8. *Tile and Till*, **54**, Nos. 1, 2, 3, and 4 (1968).
9. Van Winkle, W., Jr., *et al*, *J. Am. Med. Assoc.*, **126**, 958 (1944).
10. Leake, C. D., *et al*, *J. Am. Med. Assoc.*, **127**, 244 (1945).
11. Craver, B. N., *Ann. NY Acad. Sci.*, **64**, 463 (1956).
12. Beecher, H. K., *Pharmacol. Rev.*, **9**, 59 (1957).
13. Loewe, S., *Arzneimittel-Forsch.*, **3**, 285 (1953).
14. Chance, M. R. A., *J. Pharmacol. Exptl. Therap.*, **87**, 214 (1946).
15. Zbinden, G., *J. New Drugs*, **6**, 1 (1966).
16. Nishimura, H., and Nakai, K., *Science*, **127**, 877 (1958).
17. Nishimura, H., and Nakai, K., *Proc. Soc. Exptl. Biol. Med.*, **104**, 140 (1960).
18. Abrams, W. B., *et al*, *J. New Drugs*, **5**, 199 (1965).
19. Pepper, O. H. P., *Am. J. Pharm.*, **117**, 409 (1945).
20. Gold, H., *Cornell Conferences on Therapy*, vol. 2, Macmillan, New York, 1947, p. 1.
21. Wolf, S., *Pharmacol. Rev.*, **11**, 689 (1959).

22. Pincus, G., *Science,* **153,** 493 (1966).
23. Lasagna, L., *et al, J. Clin. Invest.,* **37,** 533 (1958).
24. Nelson, E., *Clin. Pharmacol. Therap.,* **3,** 673 (1962).
25. Delgado, J. N., and Cosgrove, F. P., *Texas State J. Med.,* **59,** 1008 (1963).
26. Boger, W. P., and Gavin, J. J., *New Engl. J. Med.,* **261,** 827 (1959).
27. Levy, G., *Am. J. Pharm.,* **135,** 78 (1963).
28. Schulert, A. R., and Weiner, M., *J. Pharmacol. Exptl. Therap.,* **110,** 451 (1954).
29. Keller, W., *Pharmazie,* **15,** 56 (1960).
30. Rosenheim, M. L., and Ross, E. J., *Lancet,* **2,** 1371 (1958).
31. Carter, A. K., *Can. Med. Assoc. J.,* **88,** 98 (1963).
32. Searl, R. O., and Pernarowski, M., *Can. Med. Assoc. J.,* **96,** 1513 (1967).
33. Lowenthal, W., *MCV Quart.,* **3**(2), 113 (1967).

34. Goddard, J. L., *J. Clin. Pharmacol./J. New Drugs,* **8,** 205 (1968).
35. Hollister, L. E., *et al, J. Clin. Pharmacol./J. New Drugs,* **8,** 69 (1968).
36. *Bibliography on Biopharmaceutics,* Pharmaceutical Manufacturers Assoc., 1155 15th St., N.W., Washington, D.C. 20005.
37. Reese, K. M., *Chem. Eng. News,* **46,** 61 (Jan. 29, 1968).
38. Beckett, A. H., and Tucker, G. T., *J. Pharm. Pharmacol.,* **S18,** 72 (1966).
39. Beckett, A. H., and Tucker, G. T., Symposium, "The Influence of Formulation on the Absorption of Drugs," *27th Intern. Congr. Pharm. Sci.,* Montpellier, France, 1967.
40. Smith, M. C., *Principles of Pharmaceutical Marketing,* Lea & Febiger, Philadelphia, 1968, p. 228.
41. Stone, F. L., and Brown, J. H. U., *J. APhA,* **NS8,** 438 (1968).
42. *PMA Newsletter,* **10,** 3 (July 26, 1968).

Part VII

BIOLOGICAL PRODUCTS

Bernard Witlin, DSc, *Professor of Microbiology, Philadelphia College of Pharmacy and Science, Philadelphia, Pa. 19104*

Immunity—antigens and antibodies—types of immunity—
hypersensitivity—control of biological products—biological licenses—
classification of biological products

This chapter was prepared by

Bernard Witlin, DSc, *Professor of Microbiology, Philadelphia College of
Pharmacy and Science, Philadelphia, Pa. 19104*

A biological product is one which has been obtained directly from, or has been derived from, living matter —animals, plants, or microorganisms. It has become customary to apply a more restrictive meaning to the term, so that these products may be adequately distinguished from pharmaceutical preparations (including organic and inorganic chemicals and plant extracts). Thus, with only a very few exceptions, biologicals are essentially either antigens or immune antibodies.

Antigens are high molecular weight foreign substances which induce antibody formation when injected into or beyond the epithelial tissue of an animal. For the most part they are protein, but may be polysaccharides. Most proteins are good antigens which possess many reactive groups or radicals and tend to differ markedly between species. Antigens may be "organized" as in the case of bacteria, or "unorganized" as in the case of the white of egg or serum protein.

Antibodies are formed in cells of the lymphoid series, which appear to develop into plasma cells when subjected to suitable antigenic stimulation. *In vivo* as well as *in vitro* experiments indicate that antibodies are synthesized *de novo* from free amino acids rather than from more complex precursors. The antibody-producing cells are situated in various organs, notably the spleen and lymph nodes. The former are particularly active following intravenous or intraperitoneal injection of antigen, the latter after subcutaneous or other local injection.

A theory of immune response must explain two salient features of the process. The first is sensitization. Upon first exposure to a germ or other antigen, several days may be required before an individual achieves peak production of antibodies.

On subsequent exposure, however, the body appears to remember the first trial and is ready to produce the appropriate antibody. This secondary response is fast and massive, often peaking within a few hours.

At present, there are two divergent theories of immune response. In need of explanation is the extraordinary specificity of the immune reaction. All data support the idea that each antibody is good for only one antigen and each antigen stimulates the production of only one antibody. The body may remember exposure to one flu virus yet be unprepared for the virus' first cousin.

One of the two basic theories of immunity takes the chemical approach, the other a more biological approach.

The chemical theory—called the template theory—holds that the antigen particle absorbed by the leukocyte somehow takes the place of the mRNA* produced by the genes. The antigen serves as the specific mold for its own antibodies, which pass into the bloodstream to combine with and neutralize any antigen still at large.

Later modifications of the theory postulate an essential role for large amoeba-like cells called macrophages. These engulf the antigen particles, break them into fragments, and pass the fragments on to leukocytes. Leukocytes have been shown in time-lapse microphotographs to crowd around macrophages. The larger cells appear to form tubular connections with the leukocytes, and material is seen flowing from macrophage to leukocyte.

Antigen fragments, by themselves often not antigenic, can be found in the body joined to a form of RNA. Tiny amounts of these complexes persist, apparently indefinitely.

The hypothesis is that the macrophage synthesizes the RNA and combines it with the antigen fragments before passing the complex to the leukocytes. The leukocytes behave as if the RNA–antigen molecule were its own mRNA. After the primary response is over, small amounts of the complex are stored, possibly in the liver. Another exposure to the same antigen releases these molecules, which then act as super antigens, stimulating the faster, more massive secondary response.

The biologists declare that the theory is not in full agreement with modern concepts of genetic action. Antibodies are proteins and protein patterns must be read off DNA by mRNA. The biological or clonal theory is sometimes also called the selective theory.

An antigen, be it virus, bacterium, poorly matched blood cell, organic chemical toxin, or whatever foreign macromolecule, makes its way into the bloodstream and encounters a form of white blood cell called a leukocyte which absorbs it.

Like all nuclei, the nucleus of the leukocyte contains strands of deoxyribonucleic acid (DNA)-bearing genes. In the normal operation of the nucleus certain of these genes are inactive. Certain others serve as templates for the building of molecules of messenger ribonucleic acid (mRNA). The mRNA migrates out of the nucleus into the cytoplasm of the cell, where it attaches itself to a kind of cellular workbench called a ribosome. There it serves in its turn as a template for the construction of protein molecules. Each gene makes a specific form of mRNA, and each mRNA makes a specific protein. In this way the function of the cell and ultimately of the whole organism is controlled by the gene.

The clonal theory rests on the belief that the bloodstream contains a vast variety of leukocytes. For every possible antigen there is a small group of leukocytes bearing the necessary active genes for the production of an appropriate antibody.

---

* Messenger ribonucleic acid.

An incoming antigen floats in the bloodstream until it runs across one of these appropriate leukocytes. The meeting stimulates intensive cell division by the leukocyte until a group, or clone, of daughter cells is formed; it proceeds to produce the needed antibody.

A residue of the daughter cells remains after primary response. This residue makes subsequent recognition of the antigen more likely, thus faster.

This theory meets the requirements of genetics. The DNA is indeed the source of the antibody's design. The clonal theory in fact has held the inside track for a while because of its agreement with genetics. But it faces its own contradiction, and a large one. There are millions of naturally occurring proteins which could be antigenic to a given organism. There are millions more synthetic antigens possible, and some already have been proved able to induce immune response. How can an organism afford to be ready for all of them?

Genetic capacity is after all finite, even if vast. With all the great and small machinery of the body to control, how can so much of this capacity be given over to defenses with an extremely low likelihood of ever being used?

There has to be a better explanation than either theory. The best answer may well lie between the two.

Role of Biologicals in the Development of Immunity

A biological product is analogous:

To a virus (see page 1426) if prepared from or with a virus or agent actually or potentially infectious, without regard to the degree of virulence or toxicogenicity of the specific strain used.

To a therapeutic serum (see page 1426), if composed of whole blood or plasma or containing some organic constituent or product other than a hormone or an amino acid, derived from whole blood, plasma, or serum, and not intended for ingestion.

To a toxin or antitoxin, if intended, irrespective of its source of origin, to be applicable to the prevention, treatment, or cure of disease or injuries of man through a specific immune process.

By law "trivalent organic arsenicals" have been included under the jurisdiction of the same governmental agency (Department of Health, Education, and Welfare, also see page 1421).

Any product prepared from or with the aid of a biological product whose use or intended use is applicable to diagnosis, evaluation of the degree of susceptibility or immunity, diagnosis, prevention, treatment, or cure of diseases or injuries in man is considered as being a "biological." This is irrespective of the recommended mode of administration or application. (See also *Federal Control of Biological Products*, page 1421, and definition of "biological," page 1426.)

The effectiveness of biological products in modern use depends upon their ability to elicit an immune response, or to supply certain antibodies as such. Biologicals are used to prevent or to treat certain infectious diseases; consequently, an understanding of the processes of immunology is a requisite in helping to explain why this group of products holds such an important place in the practice of medicine.

Immunity may be most simply described as a state of nonsusceptibility to infection. The reactions which take place between infecting microorganisms and the host are quite complex, and the degree and speed with which the invaders may do harm depend completely upon the resistance or lack of resistance (which may be attributed to the age, sex, race, etc) of the host. It is not possible to differentiate sharply between states of immunity and of susceptibility since these terms are entirely relative. The virulence of the bacteria, viruses, or fungi, and the level of resistance offered by the body tissues and cells are of the utmost importance in determining the outcome of any given infection. As a result of the development of an adequate level of immunity, the host adapts itself to the presence of foreign proteins, displays marked resistance to the invasive powers of the infecting microorganisms, or is capable of protecting itself against the deleterious action of their toxic products.

Infection

When the natural barriers of the body fail to prevent the entrance of microorganisms, infection may result if such organisms are pathogenic. During the initial stage the organisms pass through the mucous surfaces and proceed to a regional lymph gland where they begin to proliferate. Then, through the normal clearing action of the blood, they accumulate in the reticulo-endothelial systems, in the liver and spleen, for example. Proliferation, however, continues in the lymph glands, and at this point the disease may be considered to be in the so-called incubation phase. If the condition is serious, the blood stream is reinvaded with resulting bacteremia, and now the invaders are carried to many other areas previously uninfected. Clinical illness becomes manifest, and if the host is incapable of withstanding the attack, the disease progresses, and may even terminate fatally.

Under more favorable conditions the host has adjusted itself to the presence of foreign proteins, and inflammation—which is an immune process—has set in. Leukocytes have been mobilized, and the production of antibodies has begun. Some body-tissues and blood cells have been destroyed in the process, but the clearing mechanisms are speeded up, and eventually the bacteremia disappears. The remaining infection for a time persists only in isolated foci, in the liver, spleen, or in scattered lymph nodes. At this stage the patient probably is not capable of infecting others. Finally, when all foci of infection are eliminated, the host is, of course, free of infection, and complete recuperation follows.

It is important to point out that in some individuals an infection may be so mild that the disease never reaches the clinical stage (subclinical infection). Antibodies, however, may be produced, and in a sufficient amount so that the individual will become immune to possible future infections by the same species of microorganism. In routine immunological studies, protective antibodies to a variety of infections are found in individuals who have never had a clinically recognized case of the disease in question. This is the case, particularly, with many of the viral diseases. At the same time, it must be kept in mind that the degree of immunity possessed is the determining factor in successful resistance against future exposures. It is known that a level of immunity may be entirely effective against a moderate contact with a given disease, yet become ineffective in the event of exposure to an overwhelming dose of infective organisms. Other factors relating to the general level of health contribute, along with specific immune substances, to the resistance offered against invading pathogenic microorganisms.

Antigens and Antibodies

Antibodies or protective agents of various kinds (eg, antitoxins, agglutinins, bacteriolysins, precipitins) may be found in the body of normal individuals. Due to a transference of specific antibodies through the placenta or during nursing (colostrum in milk), a congenital passive temporary immunity may be established in the newborn. The presence of natural antitoxins and of antibacterial antibodies may occur in the young and old as they develop as a result of response of the body to external environmental stimuli.

Antibodies develop in response to infection (active disease) or to the invasion by an agent (antigen) foreign to the blood and tissues of the animal injected. The substance or agent possessing the power of causing the production or formation of antibodies or protective substances is known as an antigen (antibody-producer).

Antibody formation is induced more effectively by the direct injection of an antigen in the tissues, either subcutaneously, intracutaneously, or intramuscularly. However, sensitizing substances which play an important role in anaphylaxis, which is related to immune phenomena, may develop as a result of ingestion, dermal contact, or even of inhalation of provoking agents. The antibodies produced are generally specific for the antigen which caused their production and are usually demonstrable in the blood serum and other body fluids. The antibodies are particularly associated with the globulin fractions of the serum proteins.

The generic term applicable to a wide variety of substances which are antagonistic to or capable of neutralizing the antigens responsible for their production is *antibodies*. These include antitoxins, agglutinins, lysins, and precipitins. The general classification of antibodies is determined by the phenomena that follow their interaction with antigens.

If bacteria or other cells containing a given antigen are clumped together after the antibody–antigen interaction, the antibody is termed an *agglutinin*. If clouding, with flocculent precipitation of antigen-containing particles occurs, the antibody is referred to as a *precipitin*. If cells or particles containing the antigen break down and dissolve, the antibody is called a *lysin*. In similar fashion, if a toxin is neutralized or made nontoxic as a result of combination with an antibody, such a substance is called an *antitoxin*. Finally, an increased susceptibility to phagocytosis is induced by a so-called *opsonin*. Other antibodies may be bacteriostatic, bactericidal, or virucidal. Many common diagnostic tests are based on antigen-antibody reactions. Clinically, antibodies are distinguished as being antibacterial (or antiviral), and as being antitoxic. Specific antibodies are reactive only against the substance which stimulated their production.

Most circulating antibodies occur in the globulin fraction of the proteins contained in the blood serum. Blood cells and platelets are practically devoid of antibody content. The antitoxins are localized principally in the pseudoglobulin fraction; thus, high degrees of purification and concentration are made possible. Efforts at refinement of any circulating antibody aim to isolate those fractions of highest antibody titer. Some antibodies, of course, are found to be intimately bound with tissue cells. This is believed to be especially true of those related to the allergies, in which case the antigen–antibody manifestations are highly localized.

Types of Immunity

There are three types of normal protection against infectious disease:

1. *Nonsusceptibility* represents an absolute protection against particular diseases and is associated with species characteristics.

2. *Natural resistance*, an individual matter, is relatively nonspecific and variable. It is determined by physiologic conditions that are subject to variation from one individual to another and within a single individual at different times.

3. *Natural immunity* is attributed to antibodies present or appearing without obvious external stimulus.

However, if protection is acquired accidentally or artificially, it is called *acquired immunity*. Acquired immunity is attributed to antibodies produced or received at some time after birth. The two general types of acquired immunity are commonly spoken of as *active acquired immunity* and *passive acquired immunity*.

The scheme shown below illustrates the main categories into which the various kinds of immunity may be arbitrarily classified.

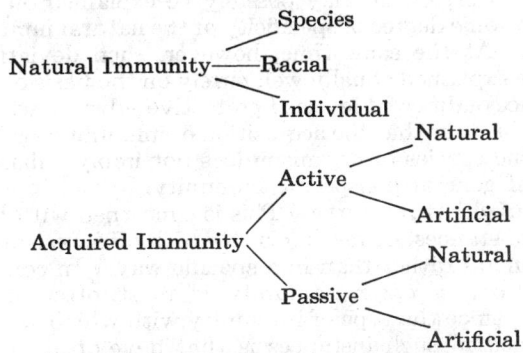

More complete treatments of this phase of immunology are available in numerous textbooks on the subject. It will, however, be helpful to spend some time in reviewing the principal aspects of acquired immunity since it is in this field of medicine that biologicals play their most important role.

Natural Immunity—This is a state of immunity that is innate or inherited in the body cells of the host. The body may possess natural immunity under normal conditions without having had the opportunity to generate specific antibodies as a result of a previous infection. Individuals in good health are endowed with a high level of such natural immunity. General good health also implies healthy body tissues, skin, and mucous membranes—all important bacterial barriers—of good quality, leukocytes in plentiful supply and properly active, and so forth. The kind and quality of the bacterial flora in the large intestine and in the upper respiratory tract, including the oral cavity, undoubtedly play some part in resisting invasion by other species of microorganisms capable of producing infection. Similarly, the gastric juice, as a result of acidity and digestive properties, is to a marked degree bactericidal and capable of destroying many species of harmful bacteria and viruses which may be ingested during eating and drinking. In addition, the intestinal enzymes help to set up a valuable secondary guard.

It is a well-recognized fact that levels of resistance to certain infectious diseases vary considerably among species, races, and even among individuals as to age and sex. Some ninety diseases, like tuberculosis, anthrax, psittacosis, and rabies, occur in both man and animals alike. There are other human diseases, however, such as syphilis, measles, leprosy, gonorrhea, mumps, typhoid fever, dysentery, whooping cough, etc, which, insofar as is known, do not affect animals. Further, there are differences in resistance among races; for example, certain races of man are notably more susceptible to tuberculosis than are others. The resistance of individuals in a given community also may vary greatly, although it must be recognized, at the same time, that some of this apparent difference possibly can be attributed to a certain amount of acquired immunity which had developed as a result of previous contact. Attention must also be given to predisposing factors such as nutritional well being and excessive fatigue which must be taken into account in any attempt to explain differences in resistance.

The distinction between natural and acquired immunity, however, is more often based on whether the state of nonsusceptibility is normally present in the host, or has been acquired by one method or another, rather than on specificity. It is obvious, too, that differences in immunity between individuals among a population, not previously exposed to a given infective species of organism, may possibly be explained on the basis of some degree of specificity of the natural immune bodies. At the same time, however, such deviations may be explained equally well purely on the basis of the existence of different levels of protective substances. It should be clear that the acquisition of immunity against a specific species of organism does not imply enhancement of general nonspecific immunity.

Acquired Immunity—This is concerned with factors, substances, or mechanisms which offer resistance in a general rather than in a specific way. In contradistinction, *acquired* immunity is most often more specific, since the type of immunity with which we are concerned in such instances is that developed in response to a specific stimulus. Acquired immunity is a kind which the individual develops in response to the introduction of foreign substances, or which he acquires in the form of immune substances produced in another individual or in another species. This brings us, therefore, to the two arbitrary classes of acquired immunity, namely, active and passive.

Active Acquired Immunity—Resistance of this kind may be acquired in one of several ways:

1. By having the disease.
2. By single or repeated exposure to sub-infectious doses of the disease organism, or
3. By being treated (usually by injection) with the modified disease organisms or their derivatives (vaccination).

When resistance is developed following active contact with disease organisms under normal conditions the resulting immunity is termed *natural acquired immunity*. Immunity produced by vaccination following the injection of toxins, attenuated toxins (toxoids), allergenic products, or live, attenuated, or killed microorganisms or their products is designated as being *artificially acquired*. The end products in both instances are presumed to be the same. Natural acquired immunity is developed slowly, depending upon many factors, including the antigenicity of the organisms or their derivatives in the case of artificially induced immunity, and on the duration or, at times, repetitiveness of the disease in the event immunity results from natural exposure.

The duration of active immunity is quite variable, in some cases being rather brief; but in others, such as immunization against yellow fever, protection lasts many years, and in some cases, may last for life.

It might be emphasized at this point that in the study of biological products we are concerned for the most part with induced immunization with antigenic materials, including vaccines, antigens, and toxoids.

Passive Acquired Immunity—It has already been mentioned that it is possible for the host to acquire a state of immunity against a given infection as a result of the injection of immune bodies which have been pro-

duced in another individual, or even in another species. This kind of immunity is commonly referred to as *passive immunity*. The kinds of biologicals which are used to provide passive immunity are limited to prophylactic and therapeutic sera obtained from animals or humans, such as antitoxins, certain antiviral sera, convalescent sera, concentrated and refined human sera, and immune serum globulins prepared from human placental extracts. Theoretically, in this instance the individual who receives antitoxin or an immune serum merely serves as the recipient, and antibodies thus received, as long as they are present in sufficient amounts, are capable of rendering a considerable degree of protection.

The immunity provided by these means is not long-lasting, and it is known that such antibodies leave the body tissues and fluids of the host within a comparatively short time. Thus, the administration of diphtheria antitoxin to a patient who has diphtheria will offer protection during the critical period when help is most urgently needed, but would not be suitable for the development of lasting immunity to this disease.

Hypersensitivity—The biologicals which occasionally give trouble are mostly limited to those derived from animal serums. Protein sensitization encompasses a variety of states of hypersensitivity which may become manifest in varying degrees in the form of serum sickness, anaphylaxis, allergy, drug and food idiosyncrasies, and the like.[1]

Protein sensitization is closely related to other immunization processes, and the general mechanisms involved are quite similar. Essentially, a state of hypersusceptibility to a given protein results from an antigen-antibody response. Specifically, such reactions are concerned with so-called foreign proteins. As a general rule an animal's own protein, or that from another individual of the same species, is not capable of eliciting an antibody response.

The structure of the protein molecule is highly complex. It is made up of a variety of chemical units which, in turn, contain the elements carbon, hydrogen, oxygen, nitrogen, and very often sulfur. When protein is hydrolyzed with acids, or digested with suitable enzymes, simpler proteins—such as the proteoses and albumoses—result. If the process is carried to completion, a further breakdown proceeds through the polypeptides, peptides, and ultimately to building units, the amino acids. The latter are no longer proteins as such, and, therefore, are not capable of producing foreign protein reactions.

Protein sensitization or hypersensitiveness may appear in many ways, but is most dramatically manifest in the phenomenon known as *anaphylaxis*. This development of an abnormal sensitivity may be demonstrated experimentally in the following manner. An initial dose of a foreign protein such as horse serum or egg white may be injected into a guinea pig or rabbit. After a suitable incubation period, usually ten to twelve days, when a second dose is injected symptoms appear which result primarily from contractions of the involuntary or smooth muscles. In the guinea pig this affects particularly the smooth muscle fibers of the bronchi, producing marked respiratory distress, frequently followed by death. In the rabbit the reaction apparently centers in the smooth muscle fibers in the walls of the arterial system of the lungs. The circulation through the lungs is stopped, and the animal dies as a result of general oxygen starvation. The animal is said to be "sensitized" by the first injection, and the second dose of the same protein is called the "shocking dose." Although this phenomenon is readily produced in animals, very fortunately anaphylaxis is observed only infrequently in humans.

Serum sickness is likewise a manifestation of protein sensitization, and is encountered fairly frequently by the physician. In its most usual form serum sickness appears within 10 to 13 days after the injection of a serum derived from animal species. It is characterized by the formation of a rash, urticaria, skin eruptions, edema or swelling, joint pains, and sometimes by a slight fever. Infrequently serum sickness assumes a form resembling shock. This type of reaction occurs usually after the first dose of the serum, and develops only in those individuals who possess a sensitivity to horse serum. Fortunately, a natural sensitivity to horse serum is very rare. Most individuals are not normally sensitive to horse serum and may be given antitoxin or products derived from the horse without any immediate or severe reactions. Subsequent injections, however, particularly after a long interval, should be given only after ascertaining that the patient is not sensitive. This may be determined by a skin test or by the injection of a minute amount.

Before administering antitoxins it is customary for the physician to inquire into the history of the patient to determine whether or not antitoxins may have been given some time earlier. It is also important to ascertain whether the patient has a history of asthma. Sensitiveness can be readily determined by making a preliminary skin test using very small quantities of a dilution of the antitoxin to be administered. This is usually carried out by making an intradermal injection, and if the patient is found to be sensitive a noticeable reaction appears within one-half hour in the nature of an area of redness and the development of a wheal around the site of injection.

The administration of an antitoxin to those who show a positive reaction must be carried out very carefully, usually beginning with a very small dose and gradually increasing this at regular intervals until a larger amount may be administered without causing perceptible reaction. Doses are subsequently increased until the required therapeutic amount has been administered.

Federal Control of Biological Products

Biologicals are classified in accordance with their ability to produce immunity in the individual through the stimulation of antibody formation (*active immunization*) or by transferring preformed antibodies which were produced in another individual of the same species or in an animal of another species (*passive immunization*).

The distribution and sale of medicinal products are controlled by regulations imposed by federal and state laws, and at times are further regulated by additional legal requirements which have been established by the health departments of some of the larger cities. For certain classes of products government control extends either directly or indirectly to the actual manufacture of such preparations, this being the case notably for biologicals, antibiotics, and narcotics. Advertising and certain other phases of promotion must comply with requirements as set forth under Section 502(n) of the Federal Food, Drug and Cosmetic Act. It may be of some interest to review briefly the relationships which exist between the several important regulatory groups and the classes of products with which they are concerned.

Pharmaceutical preparations are regulated under the provisions of the Federal Food, Drug and Cosmetic Act, approved in basic form on June 25, 1938.* Numerous amendments have been promulgated since this date. This Act essentially has to do with interstate commerce, and specifically prohibits shipment between states of adulterated or misbranded foods, drugs, devices, and cosmetics. Special requirements are imposed to control new drugs; Section 505 of the Act states that no person shall introduce or deliver for introduction into interstate commerce any new drug unless a new drug application has been allowed to become effective with respect to such drug.

Insulin and insulin derivatives must comply with specifications outlined in Section 506 of the Act.[2] These require that master lots of insulin and insulin derivatives must be certified by the Food and Drug Administration. The initial request for certification must be accompanied by a full statement of the facilities and controls used to maintain the identity, strength, quality, and purity of each batch. Subsequent requests for certification of individual master lots require detailed data pertaining to identity, quantities involved, lot numbers, results of assay, etc, and the submission of representative samples.

All antibiotic and antibiotic-containing drugs must meet special requirements under Section 507, which provides for the certification of batches of drugs composed wholly or partly of any kind of an antibiotic or any derivative thereof. As in the case of insulin, requests for certification must be accompanied by detailed data describing results of potency, toxicity, sterility, and other tests, and by representative samples.

Another group of products requiring certification are the coal-tar colors used in drugs, foods, and cosmetics. Because of alleged potential carcinogenic properties, the use of many so-called coal-tar colors previously accepted is now prohibited. Still another very important class of pharmaceutical products, namely, the narcotics, is rigidly regulated by a separate Act known as the Harrison Narcotics Law. For more detailed information, see Chapter 101, *Laws Governing Pharmacy.*

The production and sale of biological products are controlled under licenses issued by the Department of Health, Education and Welfare after approval is received and recommendations made by the Division of Biologics Standards. The latter is one of eleven separate Institutes or Divisions of the National Institutes of Health located in Bethesda, Maryland. Producers of biologicals must comply fully with the Regulations for the Sale, Barter, or Exchange of Any Virus, Therapeutic Serum, Toxin, Antitoxin or Analogous Product. These regulations[3] have been issued under Section 351 of the Public Health Service Act (Public Law 410, 78th Congress), approved July 1, 1944. Prior to this time the manufacture and sale of biologicals were controlled under an earlier Act approved July 1, 1902.

Section 351 (a) provides that:

"No person shall sell, barter, or exchange, or offer for sale, barter, or exchange in the District of Columbia, or send, carry, or bring for sale, barter, or exchange from any State or possession into any other State or possession or into any foreign country, or from any foreign country into any State or possession, any virus, therapeutic serum, toxin, antitoxin, or analogous product, or arsphenamine or its derivatives (or any other trivalent organic arsenic compound), applicable to the prevention, treatment, or cure of diseases, or injuries of man, unless (1) such virus, serum, toxin, antitoxin, or other product has been propagated or manufactured and prepared at an establishment holding an unsuspended and unrevoked license, issued by the Secretary as hereinafter authorized, to propagate or manufacture, and prepare such virus, serum, toxin, antitoxin, or other product for sale in

---

* The original Food and Drug Act was enacted June 30, 1906.

the District of Columbia, or for sending, bringing, or carrying from place to place aforesaid; and (2) each package of such virus, serum, toxin, antitoxin, or other product is plainly marked with the proper name of the article contained therein, the name, address, and license number of the manufacturer, and the date beyond which the contents cannot be expected beyond reasonable doubt to yield their specific results. The suspension or revocation of any license shall not prevent the sale, barter, or exchange of any virus, serum, toxin, antitoxin, or other product aforesaid which has been sold and delivered by the licensee prior to such suspension or revocation, unless the owner or custodian of such virus, serum, toxin, antitoxin, or other product aforesaid has been notified by the Secretary not to sell, barter, or exchange the same."

The Act also provides that standards, designed to insure the continued *safety, purity,* and *potency* of licensed products, shall be prescribed in regulations issued by the Surgeon General of the Public Health Service and approved by the Secretary of the Department of Health, Education and Welfare.

Biological Licenses—There are two forms of licenses: establishment and product. To obtain a license for any establishment of biological products dealing in interstate commerce, the manufacturer makes application to the Director, Division of Biologics Standards, on forms prescribed for such purposes, and in the case of an application for a product license, submits data derived from laboratory and clinical studies which demonstrate that the manufactured product meets prescribed standards of safety, purity, and potency, a full description of manufacturing methods, data establishing stability of the product through the dating period, sample(s) representative of the product to be sold, bartered or exchanged or offered, sent, carried or brought for sale, barter or exchange, summaries of results of tests performed on the lot(s) represented by the submitted sample(s), and specimens of the labels, enclosures and containers proposed to be used for the product. An application for license is not considered as filed until all pertinent information and data have been received from the manufacturer by the Division of Biologics Standards.

Licenses are issued by the Secretary on recommendation of the Surgeon General of the US Public Health Service. This is done only after inspection of the establishment and examination of the product for which a product license is desired and upon a determination that the establishment and the product meet the standards prescribed in the regulations. Additional product licenses are issued only upon examination of the product and a determination that the product meets the standards prescribed in the regulations.

A biological product (eg, a trivalent organic arsenical) undergoing development, but not yet ready for a product license, may be shipped or otherwise delivered from one state or possession into another state or possession, for purposes of controlled investigation, only in accordance with regulations under Section 505 of the Federal Food, Drug and Cosmetic Act, as amended, and provided that such material is not offered for sale, barter, or exchange.

The Surgeon General recommends to the Secretary that an establishment or product license be suspended or revoked whenever he finds, after notice and opportunity for hearing, that

1. Public Health Service inspectors after reasonable efforts have been unable to gain access to an establishment or a location for the purpose of carrying out the inspection required at least once a year under the regulations.
2. Manufacturing of products or of a product has been discontinued to an extent that a meaningful inspection cannot be made.
3. The establishment or any location thereof, or the product for which the license has been issued fails to conform to the standards prescribed (safety, purity, and potency).

Summary Suspension—Whenever the Surgeon General has reasonable ground to believe that an establishment or product for which a license has been issued fails to conform to the standards prescribed in the regulations in this part, and that by reason of such failure and of failure of the manufacturer to take prompt corrective measures on notice thereof, the distribution or sale of a licensed product would constitute a danger to health, or that the establishment and manufacturing methods have been so changed as to require in order to protect the public health a new showing that the establishment or product meets the standards prescribed in the regulations in this part, he may recommend to the Secretary that the license for the establishment or the product be summarily suspended and the manufacturer be required (a) to notify the selling agents and distributors to whom such product or products have been delivered of such suspension, (b) to furnish complete records of such deliveries and notice of suspension, and (c) to show cause within 60 days or such other period as may be specified in the order why the license should not be revoked.

Review Board—In matters involving the safety, purity, and potency of licensed products or products for which an application for license is pending, the reports of inspection and laboratory examinations, together with any pertinent data the establishment may submit must be passed upon by a special board of three officers appointed by the Surgeon General for that purpose. The board reports its findings to the Surgeon General who forwards the report, together with his findings and recommendations to the Secretary.

A manufacturer whose application for a license has been denied, or whose establishment or product license has been summarily suspended, without prior opportunity for hearing, may appeal from such denial or suspension and shall be entitled to a hearing thereon before a review body. The Surgeon General, upon review of the record, may affirm, reverse, or modify the findings of the review board, or may direct the taking of further testimony, and shall forward his determinations and recommendations to the Secretary.

An establishment or product license, previously suspended or revoked may be reissued or reinstated upon a showing of compliance with required standards and upon such inspection and examination as may be considered necessary by the Director of the Division of Biologics Standards.

An establishment or product license, excluding a location or locations that fail to comply with prescribed standards, may be issued without further application and concurrently with the suspension or revocation of the license for noncompliance at the excluded location or locations.

Classification of Biological Products

For Active Immunization:	**Human Blood and Derivatives:**
Bacterial Vaccines	Whole Blood
Bacterial Antigens	Rh₀(D) Immune Globulin
	Plasma
Multiple Antigen Preparations	Radioiodinated (^{131}I) Albumin
	Normal and Immune Serums
Viral and Rickettsial Vaccines	Packed Red Cells
Toxoids	Grouping Serums
For Passive Immunization:	Anti Rh Typing Serums
Antitoxins	**Allergens:**
Antivenins	Allergenic Extracts
Therapeutic Immune Serums	Proteins
Diagnostic Agents:	**Miscellaneous:**
Toxins	Venoms, Pyrogens
Tuberculin	
Virus Antigens	
Proteins	

Foreign Products—Any biological product or trivalent organic arsenical propagated or manufactured and prepared in any foreign country and intended for sale, barter, or exchange is refused entry by collectors of customs unless produced in an establishment holding an unsuspended and unrevoked license and a license for the product. Unlicensed products intended solely for purposes of controlled investigation are admissible only if in accord with applicable regulations under Section 505 (i) of the Federal Food, Drug and Cosmetic Act, as amended.

The most recent list of licensed establishments[4] includes about 300 firms or laboratories among which are 18 foreign laboratories. Several licensees are state or city health departments. About 25 laboratories are licensed to manufacture vaccines, toxoids, antitoxins, and other analogous biologicals, ranging from a few products to many.

Establishment Inspection—Inspections, with or without notice, are made by an officer who has special knowledge of the methods used in production and control of biological products. The inspector calls upon the active head of the establishment, interrogates him and other personnel as may be necessary, examines in detail the entire establishment, obtains and sends to the Division adequate samples of all licensed products, and makes recommendations as indicated by the inspection.

Records—Detailed and complete records must be kept as directed for all biological products as to sterilization, cultures, reference samples, animal necropsy, recall, and of divided responsibility (if two or more establishments participate) in the manufacture of a product.

Animals Used for Production—Animals used in production of biological products must be kept under competent daily inspection and preliminary quarantine for a period of at least 7 days before use. Animals of the equine genus infected with glanders and those of the bovine genus infected with tuberculosis must be eliminated during quarantine period. In case of infection with foot-and-mouth disease, glanders, tetanus, anthrax, gas gangrene, equine infectious anemia, or equine encephalomyelitis among animals intended for use or used for the production of biological products, the manufacturer must immediately notify the Division.

Human Blood Donors—Only those persons may serve as a source of the whole blood for use in preparing a licensed product whose physical condition is such that the withdrawal of the desired amount of blood will not endanger their health and who are certified by a qualified doctor of medicine as being free of disease transmissible by blood transfusion as far as can be determined from the donor's personal history, from physical examination, and such clinical tests as appear necessary for each donor on the day upon which the blood is withdrawn from the donor except that this requirement may be modified by the Division if the licensed product is processed by a method which insures the destruction or complete removal of the causative agent of such disease.[5] In addition, blood may be collected incidental to the expulsion of the human placenta, and from the placenta itself. Only those women may serve as donors who are certified by a licensed physician as being free of those diseases in which the causative agent may be present in the blood and not killed or removed by the processing method. Also, the donor shall be free of diseases which in the opinion of the certifying physician might have significant harmful effects on the recipient. The processing method used for the separation of the globulin fraction in preparing Immune Serum Globulin (Human) must have been demonstrated to be capable of producing a final product free of the agent(s) of viral hepatitis.

Labeling—The following items must appear on the label affixed to each container of a product capable of bearing a full label:

1. The proper name of the product.
2. Name, address, and license number of manufacturer.
3. Lot number.
4. The expiration date.

The label affixed to the outside carton must include, in addition to the proper name and the items required on the label of the final container, the following:

1. The preservative used and its concentration.
2. The volume of the contents, if a liquid, or the weight, if a solid, and the potency or dosage if more than one strength is dispensed.
3. The recommended storage temperature.
4. The words "Shake Well," or equivalent, when indicated by the character of the product.
5. The dose and route of administration recommended or reference to such directions in an enclosed circular.
6. The source of the product when a factor for safe administration.
7. Minimal potency of product expressed in terms of official standard of potency or, if potency is a factor and no standard of potency has been prescribed, the words "No US standard of potency."

If two or more establishments participate in the manufacturing process, the name, address, and license number of each must appear on the label of the final container, if capable of bearing a full label, and on the outside label.

Official Titles—The titles of the biologicals described in the separate monographs appearing in this and following chapters are those prescribed by the National Institutes of Health. In paragraph 73.51 of the Public Health Service Regulations, relating to labeling, it is stated that the *proper name*, which is considered to be the *official name* or title, shall appear on each container label in the exact form designated in the product license. Further, this name must be given precedence in position and prominence over any trademark or tradename used.

Some slight deviations are permissible in the case of very lengthy titles, such as those required for polyvalent vaccines, for example. The proper or official name for a catarrhal type vaccine, for instance, becomes unreasonably unwieldy in the designated form of Bacterial Vaccine Made From Pneumococci (10,000 million each, Types I, II, V and VII), 40,000 million, Streptococci (viridans, hemolytic, indifferent) 15,000 million, H. influenzae, Type b, 2500 million and M. catarrhalis, 2500 million. The indiscriminate use of names other than those official with the National Institutes of Health may lead to confusion. This is particularly true for the wide variety and combinations of the diphtheria and tetanus toxoids marketed in fluid and in adsorbed forms. Diphtheria Toxoid, as a further example, in addition to being available in so-called fluid form, may also be purchased in three forms: as the adsorbed product, namely, alum precipitated; aluminum hydroxide adsorbed; and aluminum phosphate adsorbed. The USP, to save space and in monographs describing several similar products as one, sometimes employs titles differing somewhat from the NIH official titles.

Standards—No lot of any licensed product may be released by the manufacturer prior to the completion of tests for conformity with the standards applicable to such product.

Complete descriptions of potency tests when applicable and all other pertinent tests are described in separate Minimal Requirements. The latter are detailed instructions which are issued by the Division of Biologics Standards to cover each individual product for which an official standard of potency exists. Other detailed information relating to licensed products and to general test requirements is published from time to time in the *Federal Register*.

Potency—Tests for potency are made on each lot only after completion of those processes of manufacture which may affect the potency of the final product. The tests shall consist of either *in vitro* or *in vivo* tests, or both, which have been specifically designed for each product.

Identity and Safety—The content of a final container of each filling of each lot is tested for identity and for safety either after the labels have been affixed to the final container or affixed, both outside and inside, to the multiple container storage receptacle just prior to its sealing for storage purposes. However, exceptions to this procedure may be authorized by the Division of Biologics Standards of the NIH to apply when the volume of the final container is very large and when more than one lot is processed each day.

The identity test is specific for each product in a manner which will adequately identify it and distinguish it from any other product being processed in the same laboratory. In general, identity is established either through the physical or chemical characteristics of the product, inspection by macroscopic or microscopic methods, specific cultural tests, or *in vitro* or *in vivo* immunological tests.

In general, the safety test consists of the parenteral injection of the maximal volume tolerated, but not more than 0.5 ml into mice weighing approximately 20 Gm each and 5.0 ml into guinea pigs weighing approximately 350 Gm each. When the injections are made into at least two animals of each species, neither significant symptoms nor death should result during an observation period of not less than 7 days. Variations from this test, either in the volume injected or in the species of test animal used, is made whenever required because of the human dose level demanded of the product or because of any individual demands of the product itself.

Sterility—Samples from final containers selected at random after each filling from each lot of each product are tested for sterility. The random sampling is made in such a manner that all stages of the filling from the bulk container have equal change of being represented. The number of final filled containers to be tested is determined by the total number contained in the lot. In any test of this kind where one is dealing with a nonhomogeneous attribute, that is sterile or nonsterile, special attention must be given to the effect of sampling error on the general level of confidence which may be given to final test results.[6]

Purity—The purity of a product includes its relative freedom from residual moisture and pyrogenic substances whenever these are factors of significance in the safe use of the product. The relative freedom from residual moisture is determined by a procedure which accurately measures the amount of uncombined water or other volatile liquid present in the finished product. The relative freedom from pyrogenic substances is determined by the intravenous injection into normal rabbits of not less than 3.0 ml/Kg of body weight.

Tests for safety, purity, and potency applicable to the product are completed for each lot of any licensed product prior to its release by the manufacturer, and samples of any lot of any licensed product may at any time be required to be sent to the Division for examination. All ingredients used in a licensed product and any diluent provided as an aid in the administration of the product must meet generally accepted standards of purity and quality. Any preservative used must be sufficiently nontoxic so that the amount present in the recommended dose of the product will not be toxic to the recipient, and in the combination used shall not denature the specific substances in the product below the minimal acceptable potency within the dating period when stored at the recommended temperature.

Except as otherwise provided by regulation, no liquid serum or antitoxin may contain more than 20% total solids. Licensed products may not be combined with other licensed products, whether therapeutic, prophylactic, or diagnostic, except as a license is obtained for the combined product. Licensed products may not be combined with nonlicensable therapeutic, prophylactic, or diagnostic substances except as a license is obtained for such combination.

Glass used in the container of a licensed product intended for administration by injection must be colorless and fully transparent. The quality of the glass and of the closure used is such as not to hasten the deterioration of the licensed product or render it less suitable for the use intended within the dating period.

Dating Period and Date of Manufacture—The dating period is determined with reference to the date of manufacture:

1. For products for which an official standard of potency exists or which are subject to official potency tests, the last date of satisfactorily passing a potency test.
2. For products for which no official standard of potency exists or which are not subject to official potency tests: (a) the date of removal from the animal in case of animal products; (b) the date of extraction in the case of products used for specific desensitization; (c) the date of solution in cases of venoms; and (d) the date of cessation of growth in case of other products.
3. For products which are submitted to the Division for approval prior to release, the date of official release notice.

Dating Period for Products in Cold Storage—The dating period may be determined with reference to the period of issue from cold storage, *provided*, that, except as may be otherwise prescribed for individual products, the date of such issue is not more than 6 months after the date of manufacture and the product is kept constantly at a temperature not exceeding 10 °C, or not more than 1 year after the date of manufacture if the product is kept constantly at a temperature not exceeding 5 °C, or not more than 2 years if the product is kept constantly at a temperature not exceeding 0 °C.

Added Preservatives—Bacterial vaccines and other biologicals containing particulate matter, as for example, the alum precipitated toxoids, must be handled throughout the manufacturing process by aseptic methods. These products are heat labile and, therefore, cannot be subjected to heating for purpose of sterilization. Other products in which the active materials are soluble, for example bacterial antigens,* fluid toxoids, antitoxins, etc, may be sterilized by filtration through suitable filters (Berkefeld, Mandler, Seitz, sintered glass, Millipore, etc). Although all these precautions are taken it has been found advisable to add a bacteriostatic agent in the last stages of handling as an additional safeguard against contamination. The small amount of antiseptic present produces no deleterious effect. The most commonly used preservatives are phenol, 0.5%, and thimerosal (Merthiolate),

---

* A *soluble* bacterial vaccine is called a bacterial antigen.

1:10,000 or 1:20,000. Some limited use is made of one or more of the ρ-hydroxybenzoic acid esters.

Dried Products—The use of rapid freezing, with rapid dehydration from the frozen state under high-vacuum lyophilization offers a practical method for the preservation of the maximal biological activity of antitoxins, antiserums, plasma, and other biological products. In the marketed package, the dried biological product is placed in one sterile container and sterile Water for Injection, or other suitable diluent, in another, the latter being used to dissolve the dry product. Lyophilization maintains the potency of biological products over longer periods than those specified for identical liquid preparations.

Care in Dispensing—In dispensing biological products the pharmacist must recognize that he is dealing with preparations, most of which are intended for injection subcutaneously, intramuscularly, intravenously, or by some other parenteral route. It is, therefore, of paramount importance that the sterile condition and potency of the preparations be maintained until they are actually injected. Sterility is assured by the processes used in the manufacturing establishments, and no product is released until repeated tests have shown it to be safe in this respect. The pharmacist contributes to the maintenance of potency of the product and insures safety to the patient by observing proper requirements. The label should be carefully examined for specific instructions as to the required temperature at which the product should be maintained, the expiration date, and other essential information pertaining not only to the product but also to the particular lot. All products must be dispensed in the unopened containers in which they were placed by the manufacturer. Freezing temperatures should be avoided, except in the cases of live, attenuated virus vaccines—smallpox, poliomyelitis, measles, and mumps.

Biologics (USP Standards)—For pharmacopeial purposes, the term "biologics" refers to those products that must be licensed under the federal Public Health Service Act of 1944, as amended, and that comply with Public Health Service Regulations, Part 73, pertaining to federal control of these products, as administered by the Division of Biologics Standards of the National Institutes of Health.

The pharmacopeial standards for *Biologics* conform to the Public Health Service Regulations in covering those aspects of identity, purity, potency, and packaging and storage that are of particular interest to pharmacists and physicians responsible for the purchase, storage and use of biologics (the requirements of these regulations are given in preceding pages of the chapter). Vehicles and added substances suitable for biologics are those named in the Public Health Service Regulations. Containers for biologics intended to be administered by injection meet the requirements for *Containers for Injections* under *Injections* (USP, page 798); the volumes in such containers meet the requirements for *Volume in Container* under *Injections* (USP, page 798) and, in addition, provide such other information as the Public Health Service Regulations require.

References

1. Wilson, G. S., and Miles, A. A., *Topley and Wilson's Principles of Bacteriology and Immunity*, 4th ed., Williams & Wilkins, Baltimore, 1957.
2. *Federal Register*, **19** (July 8, 1954).
3. *US Public Health Service Regulations—Title 42, Part 73* (PHS Publ. No. 437); revised Jan., 1967.
4. *Biological Products* (PHS Publ. No. 50); revised Jan. 1, 1967.
5. *Technical Methods and Procedures of the American Association of Blood Banks*, 4th ed., Am. Assoc. of Blood Banks, Chicago, 1966.
6. Knudsen, L. F., *J. APhA, Sci. Ed.*, **38**, 322 (1949).

75 | Immunizing Agents

Products for active immunization: bacterial vaccines; toxoids; viral vaccines; rickettsial vaccines—products for passive immunization: antitoxoids, immune serums, and antivenins (animal); immune serums and blood derivatives (human)

This chapter was prepared by

Bernard Witlin, DSc, *Professor of Microbiology, Philadelphia College of Pharmacy and Science, Philadelphia, Pa. 19104*

The term *biological* as applied to *biologics* or to *biological products* is defined in the Public Health Service Act,* which states that "Biologic Product means any virus, therapeutic serum, toxin, antitoxin, or analogous product applicable to the prevention, treatment, or cure of diseases or injuries in man."

These classes of substances are further defined as;

1. A *virus* is a product containing the minute living cause of an infectious disease and includes but is not limited to filterable viruses, bacteria, rickettsia, fungi, and protozoa.

2. A *therapeutic serum* is the product obtained from the blood of an animal or of man by removing the clot components and the blood cells and not intended for ingestion.

3. A *toxin* is a product containing a soluble substance poisonous to laboratory animals or to man in doses of 1 ml or less (or equivalent in weight) of the product, and having the property, following the injection of nonfatal doses into an animal, of causing to be produced therein another soluble substance which specifically neutralizes the poisonous substance and which is demonstrable in the serum of the animal thus immunized.

The immunizing biologicals as a general class may best be reviewed when considered as two main categories, namely, those which produce *active* immunity and those which confer a *passive* type of immunity. The first type when administered stimulates the production of specific antibodies. The second type merely transmits antibodies which have been formed in the same or in another species.

Products for Active Immunization

Bacterial Vaccines

The term *vaccine* has often been confused with antitoxins and with serums. The word vaccine† was originally given to the material used for immunization against smallpox, this being a glycerinated suspension of lymph tissue obtained from the vesicles of calves inoculated with vaccinia, or cowpox. Later its meaning was extended to include all antigenic materials made from viruses, and in later years to those made from bacteria and rickettsiae as well. It has become particularly important for all persons who are called upon to dispense or to use biologicals to have a clear understanding of official terminology‡ relating to this class of products.

Another point of confusion arises with respect to proper differentiations between vaccines and antigens. The word antigen is, of course, generic, and as such would cover all antigenic materials including vaccines, toxoids, and even such products as tuberculin, Schick toxin, allergenic extracts, and the diagnostic proteins. In order to comply strictly with the definition specified by the Division of Biologics Standards of the National Institutes of Health, and which definition also takes into account labels and labeling requirements, it is necessary to point out that when dealing with a product made from bacteria, a *bacterial vaccine* is the official designation for a *suspension* of whole bacteria whether they be killed or attenuated; but when the antigenic material, derived from bacteria, is in the form of a solution consisting of the soluble components of bacteria, such a product is then officially called a bacterial *antigen*. Bacteriophage, for example, is thus classified as a bacterial antigen and the same connotation holds for any soluble product prepared from bacteria disrupted by any one of numerous agents capable of producing lysis.

Some comments may be in order also on the methods used for naming bacterial vaccines. If, for example, a product consists of a mixture of suspensions of *Staphylococcus aureus* and *Streptococcus hemolyticus*, the official name becomes "Bacterial Vaccine made from Staphylococcus aureus and Streptococcus hemolyticus." Immediately following this title appears the count of each species contained in 1 ml. On the other hand a product comprising solubilized staphylococci, that is, staphylococci lysed by bacteriophage or by some other suitable means, would be designated as a "Bacterial Antigen made from Staphylococcus aureus."

Classes—Bacterial vaccines, as stated above, are sterile suspensions of killed or attenuated bacteria in physiological salt solution. They contain a preservative such as phenol or thimerosal (Merthiolate). Bacterial vaccines are divided into two main classes: (1) *stock vaccines* and (2) *autogenous vaccines*. Autogenous bacterial vaccines are those prepared from the patient's own infection. The offending species of organisms obtained from the lesion or the blood of the individual are used for the preparation of the bacterial vaccine. Stock bacterial vaccines are those prepared from stock cultures maintained in the laboratory and which consist of strains capable of stimulating production of immunity.

A *simple* bacterial vaccine is one made from only a

---

* Public Law 410, 78th Congress HR 4624 (58 Stat. 682); approved July 1, 1944; Sec. 73.1, amended Nov. 3, 1961 (26 FR 10355), includes trivalent organic arsenicals.

† Derived from the Latin word, *vacca*, meaning cow.

‡ Designated by the Division of Biologics Standards of the National Institutes of Health.

single species of microorganism. A *mixed* bacterial vaccine is one containing two or more different species of bacteria, eg, triple vaccine, made from typhoid bacillus, paratyphoid A bacillus, and paratyphoid B bacillus. A *monovalent* bacterial vaccine is one containing but a single strain or species of organism. A *polyvalent* bacterial vaccine is one prepared from more than one species of organisms which may be obtained from many different sources.

Preparation—The first step in preparing bacterial vaccines is to obtain a culture medium most suitable for the growth of species of the organisms from which the vaccine is to be prepared.

In mixed bacterial vaccines the individual species of organisms are isolated and secured in pure form and then cultured separately to obtain sufficient organisms for the preparation of the vaccine. The suspensions of the different species are later mixed together. Freshly isolated organisms are almost invariably of the "S" type (smooth colony variation when cultured) but in continued subculture tend to degenerate into the "R" type (rough variation). "R" variants have been found to be valueless as protective antigens. Stock vaccines are therefore made of recently isolated cultures; where this is impracticable, the cultures are kept so that they retain their full antigenic value. Stock cultures

Table I—Packaging, Storage, and Expiration Date Information

	Storage, °C	Expiration date,[a] months		Storage, °C	Expiration date,[a] months
Products for Active Immunization			Smallpox Vaccine USP		
Bacterial Vaccines			Liquid	i	3
BCG Vaccine USP	b	6	Dried	i	18
Cholera Vaccine USP	2–8	18	Yellow Fever Vaccine USP	j	12
Pertussis Vaccine USP	2–8[c]	18	*Rickettsial Vaccines*		
Pertussis Vaccine, Adsorbed USP	2–8[c]	18	Rocky Mountain Spotted Fever		
Plague Vaccine USP	2–8	18	Vaccine USP	2–8	18
Typhoid Vaccine USP	2–8	18	Typhus Vaccine USP	2–8	18
Typhoid and Paratyphoid Vaccine NF	2–8	18	**Products for Passive Immunization**		
Toxoids			*Antitoxins (Animal)*		
Diphtheria Toxoid USP	2–8	24	Botulism Antitoxin USP	2–8	36
Diphtheria Toxoid, Adsorbed USP	2–8	24	Diphtheria Antitoxin USP	2–8	12–48[k]
Tetanus Toxoid USP	2–8	24	Gas Gangrene Antitoxin	2–8	60
Tetanus Toxoid, Adsorbed USP	2–8	24	Tetanus Antitoxin USP	2–8	12–48[k]
Multiple Antigens			Tetanus and Gas Gangrene Antitoxin		
Diphtheria and Tetanus Toxoids USP	2–8	24	NF	2–8[l]	12–48[k]
Diphtheria and Tetanus Toxoids, Adsorbed USP	2–8	24	*Immune Serums (Animal)*		
			Antipneumococcic Serum	2–8	12
Diphtheria and Tetanus Toxoids and Pertussis Vaccine USP	2–8	18	Antirabies Serum USP	2–8	24
Diphtheria and Tetanus Toxoids and Pertussis Vaccine, Adsorbed USP	2–8	18	*Antivenins (Animal)*		
			Crotaline Antivenin, Polyvalent USP	m	n
Viral Vaccines			*Immune Serums (Human)*		
Adenovirus Vaccine	2–8	6	Measles Immune Serum (Human)		
Influenza Virus Vaccine USP	2–8	18	Liquid	2–8	12
Mumps Vaccine	2–8	18	Dried	2–8	60
Poliomyelitis Vaccine USP	2–8	6	Measles Immune Globulin USP		
Poliovirus Vaccine, Live Oral USP	d	12[e]	Liquid	2–8	36
Poliovirus Vaccine, Live, Oral, Monovalent	f	g	Dried	2–8	60
			Mumps Immune Serum (Human)		
Poliovirus Vaccine, Live, Oral, Trivalent	f	g	Liquid	2–8	12
			Dried	2–8	60
Measles Virus Vaccine, Inactivated USP	2–8[c]	12	Pertussis Immune Globulin USP	2–8	36
			Pertussis Immune Human Serum USP XVI		
Measles Virus Vaccine, Live, Attenuated	2–8[h]	12	Liquid	2–8[o]	12
Mumps Vaccine, Live, Attenuated	2–8	12	Dried	2–8[o]	60
Rabies Vaccine USP			Rh₀ Immune Globulin (Human)	2–8	6
Liquid	2–5	6	Scarlet Fever Immune Serum (Human)		
Dried	2–5	18	Liquid	2–8	12
			Dried	2–8	60

[a] After date of manufacture or date of issue.
[b] Preserve in hermetic containers, preferably of Type I glass, at a temperature not exceeding 5°C.
[c] Avoid freezing.
[d] Preserve in single-dose or multiple-dose containers at temperature recommended by manufacturer.
[e] When stored at freezing temperatures.
[f] Store at freezing temperature. Note that vaccines containing sorbitol remain fluid above −14°C. After thawing, agitate to insure homogeneity of contents prior to use. Once the temperature of vaccine rises above 0°C, or after the bottle has been opened, the contents must be used within 7 days, during which period the vaccine must be stored no higher than 10°C.
[g] If maintained in frozen state: 2 years after date of manufacture or 1 year after date of issue; if maintained no higher than 10°C and issued as a liquid: 7 days after date of issue.
[h] Preserve in single-dose containers, preferably of Type I glass.

[i] Preserve and dispense in the containers in which it was placed by manufacturer: liquid vaccine, during storage and in shipment, preferably below 0°C and never exceeding 5°C; dried vaccine, not exceeding 25°C.
[j] Preserve in nitrogen-filled, flame-sealed ampuls, preferably below 0°C, but never above 5°C, throughout the dating period. Preserve during shipment in suitable container adequately packed in solid carbon dioxide, or provided with other means of refrigeration, to insure a temperature constantly below 0°C.
[k] Excess of potency: 20%, 1 year; 30%, 2 years; 40%, 3 years; 50%, 4 years.
[l] Preserve preferably at the lower limit. Dispense in unopened glass container in which it was placed by the manufacturer.
[m] Preserve in single-dose containers and avoid exposure to excessive heat.
[n] Excess of potency: 10%.
[o] Preserve preferably at the lower limit. Dispense in unopened container in which it was placed by the manufacturer.

are most often maintained in a lyophilized state.

Generally, the cultures are allowed to incubate for 24 hours at a suitable temperature. Young cultures are most desirable for preparing bacterial vaccines, but occasionally it may be necessary to extend the incubation period for 48 to 72 hours or until growth occurs in sufficient amount. This is especially true in preparing autogenous and stock bacterial vaccines from some of the higher forms of bacteria. At the end of the particular period of incubation the bacteria are harvested under aseptic conditions by pouring sterile isotonic salt solution on the solid

Table II—Immunization Requirements for International Travelers Leaving from the US or Canada

S – Smallpox
t – Typhoid/Paratyphoid
C – Cholera
T – Typhus
Y – Yellow Fever
D – Diphtheria
P – Plague

o – Required by country

x – Recommended by country and U.S. Public Health Service

Country	S	t	C	T	Y	D*	P
Afghanistan	o	x		x		x	x
Algeria	x	x				x	x
Argentina	o	x				x	
Australia	o	x				x	
Austria	x	x				x	
Bahama Islands		x				x	
Barbados		x				x	
Belgium	x	x				x	
Bermuda		x				x	
Bolivia	o	x		x	x	x	
Brazil	x	x			x	x	
British Guiana	x	x			x	x	
Burma	o	x	x			x	x
Ceylon	o	x	x		x	x	x
Chile	o	x				x	
China	x	x	x	x		x	x
Colombia	o	x		x	x	x	
Costa Rica	o	x			x	x	
Cuba		x				x	
Denmark	x	x				x	
Ecuador	o	x		x	x	x	
Egypt	x	x				x	x
El Salvador	o	x			x	x	
Finland	x	x	x			x	
France	x	x				x	
French Morocco	x	x				x	
Germany	x	x				x	
Ghana	o	x			x	x	
Great Britain	x	x				x	
Greece	x	x				x	
Guatemala	o	x			x	x	
Haiti	o	x				x	
Honduras	o	x			x	x	
India	x	x	x		x	x	x
Indonesia	x	x	x			x	x
Iran	o	x		x		x	
Iraq	x	x	x			x	
Ireland	x	x				x	
Israel	o	x				x	
Italy	x	x				x	
Jamaica	x	x				x	

Country	S	t	C	T	Y	D*	P
Japan	x	x				x	
Lebanon	o	x				x	
Luxembourg	x	x				x	
Mexico	o	x				x	
Netherlands	x	x				x	
Netherlands East Indies	x	x				x	x
New Zealand	o	x				x	
Nicaragua	o	x			x	x	
Norway	x	x				x	
Pakistan	x	x	x		o	x	x
Panama Canal Zone	o	x			x	x	
Paraguay	o	x				x	
Peru	x	x		x	x	x	
Philippines	o	x				x	
Portugal	x	x				x	
Puerto Rico	x	x				x	
Saudi Arabia	o	x	o	x		x	
South Africa	x	x			x	x	
Spain	x	x				x	
Sweden	x	x				x	
Switzerland	x	x				x	
Syria	o	x				x	
Thailand		x	x			x	x
Trinidad and Tobago	x	x			x	x	
Tunisia	x	x		x		x	
Turkey	x	x				x	
Uruguay	o	x				x	
Venezuela	o	x			x	x	
Virgin Islands		x				x	
Yugoslavia	x	x		x		x	

All immunizations, with the exception of yellow fever, may be obtained from a private physician. Smallpox and cholera vaccinations *must be certified* by the local or state health officer of the area in which the immunizing physician practices, or by an officer of the Public Health Service. Yellow fever inoculations are given to the public at specific stations of the United States Public Health Service. To find out where these stations are located, write to the Department of Health, Education, and Welfare, U. S. Public Health Service, Washington, D. C.

For full information on the number of months or years an immunization certificate remains valid, check with your travel agent or your local Public Health officer.

TRAVELERS MUST HOLD A CERTIFIED SMALLPOX VACCINATION CERTIFICATE BEFORE RE-ENTERING THE UNITED STATES.

★ Canada only—Only Shick test positive persons with negative control test should be immunized.

media and then gently shaking or scraping until all the microorganisms have been suspended. If scraping is necessary, removal of excessive amounts of the culture medium is avoided. If bouillon or other liquid medium is used, the suspension is centrifuged at high speed, the supernatant liquid discarded, and the sediment containing the bacteria is suspended in sterile saline solution, shaken well, again centrifuged, the supernatant washings discarded, and the sediment again resuspended in sterile saline solution. The salt solution suspension of bacteria, in either case, is examined by means of a stained smear for purity, and is transferred into a sterile flask, bottle, or tube with or without sterile beads. If clumped, the container is shaken by some mechanical device or by hand (on a small scale) to break up the clumps and to form a uniform suspension. Bacterial vaccines are standardized by estimating the number of bacteria in each milliliter of suspension or by measuring turbidity by comparing against an artificial standard, usually a suspension of very finely divided Pyrex glass particles. Suitable standards can also be prepared from other finely divided insoluble substances.

After the concentration of bacteria per ml has been determined the suspension is diluted by adding sterile physiological salt solution, so as to bring the content to the equivalent of 1,000,000,000/ml or to any other number desired. The organisms are then killed by the addition of a suitable germicide or by heating at a minimal temperature and time of exposure which have been determined to be adequate to kill the bacteria. In most instances this is 60°C for ½ to 1 hour.

The use of ultraviolet irradiation for inactivating bacterial and viral vaccines has been recommended by Levinson, et al,[1] for the production of more highly potent antigenic preparations.

A suitable preservative is added and the bulk suspension is tested, according to the requirements of the Division of Biologics Standards of the National Institutes of Health, for identity, safety, and sterility; and, in addition, some vaccines are tested for toxicity. Antigenicity or potency tests are performed when applicable.

Uses—As antigenic agents capable of producing active immunity, some of the bacterial vaccines have proved of great value, especially in prophylaxis. The prophylactic use of typhoid vaccine and pertussis vaccine are outstanding examples. The employment of

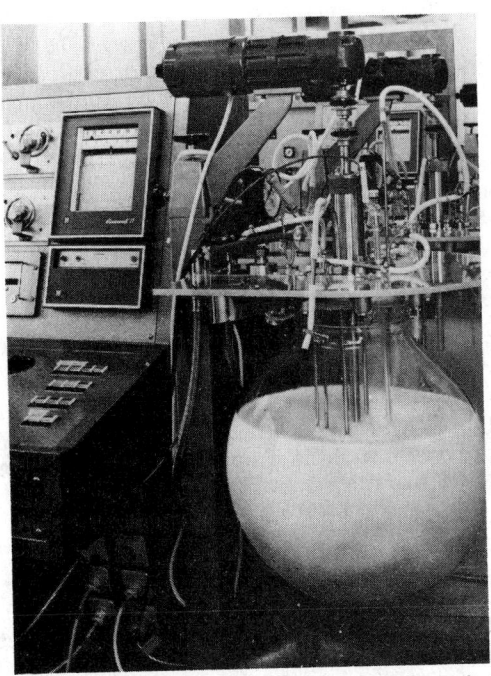

Fig. 509.   Closeup of a portion of the equipment shown in Fig. 508.

bacterial vaccines in the treatment of disease has been extensive mainly in chronic infectious diseases, and infrequently in the acute stages. No general statement can be made of their value in this connection, except that subacute and chronic cases seem to be more amenable to treatment. Some apparently have given much more favorable results than others. Specific indications are mentioned under the individual products following.

Information pertaining to required and recommended immunization for foreign travel is available from the US Public Health Service.[2]

BCG Vaccine USP

[Bacillus Calmette-Guérin Vaccine]

BCG Vaccine is a dried, living culture of the bacillus Calmette-Guérin strain of *Mycobacterium tuberculosis* var. *bovis*. The culture is grown in a suitable medium from a seed strain of known history that has been maintained to preserve its capacity for conferring immunity. BCG Vaccine is free from other organisms, and contains a suitable stabilizer. It contains no antimicrobial agent. Its production and distribution are subject to federal regulations (see *Biologics*, page 1425).

Note—*Preferably use the Vaccine within 2 hours after its reconstitution, and discard any unused portion after that period.*

Description—White to creamy white, dried mass having the characteristic texture of material dried in the frozen state.

Dose—*Usual, intradermal,* **0.1 ml** of reconstituted Vaccine; *percutaneous,* **1 drop** of reconstituted Vaccine, on surface of skin, administered by the multiple-pucture method.

Dosage Forms—in amounts sufficient for 10 or 50 doses, depending upon route of administration and on package size.

Cholera Vaccine USP

Cholera Vaccine is a sterile suspension, in isotonic sodium chloride solution or other suitable diluent, of

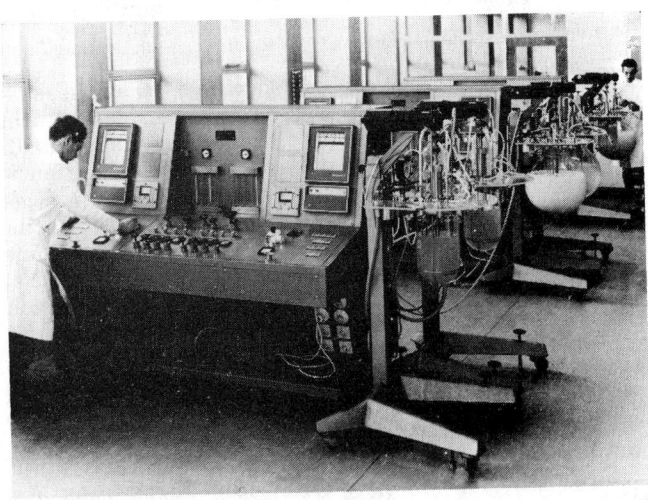

Fig. 508.   Incubation of cultures for production of bacterial vaccines (courtesy, Honeywell).

killed cholera vibrios (*Vibrio choleræ*). It is prepared from equal portions of suspensions of cholera vibrios of the Inaba and Ogawa strains. The Inaba strain used possesses an antigenic value not less than that of NIH Inaba strain 35-A-3, and the Ogawa strain possesses an antigenic value not less than that of NIH Ogawa strain 41. At the time of manufacture Cholera Vaccine contains, in each ml, approximately 8 billion cholera organisms. It contains a suitable antimicrobial agent. Its production and distribution are subject to federal regulations (see *Biologics*, page 1425).

Description—Turbid, whitish liquid, nearly odorless or having a faint odor due to the preservative.

Dose—*Usual, subcutaneous* or *intramuscular*, **0.5 ml,** and then **1 ml** 4 weeks later; **1-ml** reinforcing dose repeated every 6 months if necessary.
Dosage Forms—1.5 and 20 ml.

Pertussis Vaccine USP

[Whooping-cough Vaccine]

Pertussis Vaccine is a sterile bacterial fraction or suspension of killed pertussis bacilli (*Bordetella pertussis*) of a strain or strains selected for high antigenic efficiency. It has a potency of 12 protective units per total immunizing dose based on the US Standard Pertussis Vaccine. Its production and distribution are subject to federal regulations (see *Biologics*, page 1425).

Description—More or less turbid, whitish liquid, nearly odorless or having a faint odor due to the preservative.

Dose—*Usual, subcutaneous*, 3 injections of **0.5** or **1 ml,** at least 4 weeks apart.
Dosage Forms—7.5 ml.

Adsorbed Pertussis Vaccine USP

[Pertussis Vaccine, Alum Precipitated; Pertussis Vaccine, Aluminum Hydroxide Adsorbed; Pertussis Vaccine, Aluminum Phosphate Adsorbed]

Adsorbed Pertussis Vaccine is a sterile bacterial fraction or suspension, in a suitable diluent, of killed pertussis bacilli (*Bordetella pertussis*) of a strain or strains selected for high antigenic efficiency and precipitated or adsorbed by the addition of aluminum hydroxide, or aluminum phosphate, and resuspended. It has a potency of 12 protective units per total immunizing dose based on the US Standard Pertussis Vaccine. It contains not more than 850 mcg of aluminum in the volume stated in the labeling to constitute one injection. Its production and distribution are subject to federal regulations (see *Biologics*, page 1425).

Description—Markedly turbid, whitish liquid. Is substantially odorless or may have a faint odor due to the preservative.

Dose—*Usual, intramuscular*, 3 injections of **0.5** or **1 ml,** at least 4 weeks apart.
Dosage Forms—7.5 ml.

Plague Vaccine USP

[Vaccinum Pestis; Haffkine's Vaccine; Plague Bacillus Vaccine; Anti-Plague Vaccine]

Plague Vaccine is a sterile suspension, in isotonic sodium chloride solution or other suitable diluent, of killed plague bacilli (*Pasteurella pestis*) of a strain selected for high antigenic efficiency. It contains, in each ml, approximately 2 billion plague bacilli. Its production and distribution are subject to federal regulations (see *Biologics*, page 1425).

Description—Turbid, whitish liquid, nearly odorless or having a faint odor due to the preservative.

Dose—*Usual, intramuscular*, 2 injections of **0.5 ml,** at least 4 weeks apart, then **0.2 ml** 4 to 12 weeks later.
Dosage Forms—2 and 20 ml.

Typhoid Vaccine USP

Typhoid Vaccine is a sterile suspension or solid containing killed typhoid bacilli (*Salmonella typhosa*) of a strain selected for high antigenic efficiency. Its production and distribution are subject to federal regulations (see *Biologics*, page 1425).

Description—More or less turbid, whitish fluid, nearly odorless or having a faint odor due to the preservative.

Dose—*Usual, subcutaneous*, 2 or 3 injections of **0.5 ml,** at least 4 weeks apart.
Dosage Forms—1.5, 5, 10, and 20 ml; and 50-ml size for jet-injector use only.

Typhoid Vaccine, Dried (Acetone-Inactivated)

Typhoid Vaccine, Dried (Acetone-Inactivated) is a dried preparation which, upon reconstitution, contains no more than 10^9 killed *Salmonella typhosa* (Ty-2 strain) organisms per ml. After propagation the bacteria are suspended in $0.02M$ phosphate buffered saline and precipitated by addition of acetone. Inactivation is completed by heating at 37°C for 24 hours. Upon reconstitution, each ml of the final product contains no more than 0.02 mg total nitrogen. The filled vials are placed in a vacuum-drying chamber to remove the acetone and moisture and then stoppered under vacuum.

The diluent for reconstitution is sterile $0.02M$ phosphate (sodium) buffer at pH 7.2 to 7.3 in isotonic saline containing 0.5% phenol as a preservative.

Its production and distribution are subject to federal regulations (see *Biologics*, page 1425).

Dose—*Usual, subcutaneous*, two injections of **1 ml,** at least 4 or more weeks apart.
Dosage Forms—To yield 1 ml when reconstituted.

Typhoid and Paratyphoid Vaccine

[Typhoid—Paratyphoid A and B Vaccine; T. A. B. Vaccine]

Typhoid and Paratyphoid Vaccine is a sterile suspension, in buffered, isotonic sodium chloride solution or other suitable diluent, of killed typhoid bacilli (*Salmonella typhosa*) of a strain selected for high antigenic efficiency, killed paratyphoid "A" bacilli (*Salmonella paratyphi*), and killed paratyphoid "B" bacilli (*Salmonella schottmülleri*). The paratyphoid strains are smooth strains having complete antigenic structure. Typhoid and Paratyphoid Vaccine contains, in each ml, approximately 1 billion typhoid organisms and approximately 250 millions of each of the paratyphoid organisms. It contains, in each ml, not more than 55 mcg of total nitrogen. It may contain a suitable preservative. Typhoid and Paratyphoid Vaccine complies with the requirements of the US Public Health Service. Its production and distribution are subject to federal regulations (see *Biologics*, page 1425).

Description—More or less turbid, whitish fluid, nearly odorless or having a faint odor due to the preservative.

Dose—*Usual, subcutaneous*, three injections of **0.5 ml**, at least 7 days apart.

Dosage Forms—1.5, 5, 7.5, 15, and 20 ml.

Other Bacterial Vaccines

There are available, of course, other bacterial vaccines which have not been mentioned in the foregoing. These would include, for example, vaccines made from species of *Staphylococci*, or *Streptococci*, singly and in combination. There are vaccines of *E. coli*, of *Brucella abortus*, and of *Neisseria* (gonococci). Mixed vaccines containing *Staphylococci, Streptococci, Diplococci, K. pneumoniae, N. catarrhalis*, and *H. influenzæ* have been used extensively in the past for the prevention and for the treatment of secondary respiratory infections.

While none of these vaccines is described in the USP or in the NF, the production and distribution of all such biologicals are subject to federal regulations (see *Biologics*, page 1425).

On the other hand, there are no official methods available for measuring the antigenicity of this group of vaccines and, consequently, the labels of products falling into this category must bear the statement, "No US Standard of Potency."

Frequently use is made of vaccines for purposes other than eliciting the formation of specific antibodies. Typhoid Vaccine, for example, is used to some extent as a pyrogenic agent in fever therapy, and, as a matter of fact, it is believed that a significant part of the beneficial results of vaccine therapy in general stems from nonspecific effects.

Toxoids

Toxoids are detoxified toxins. Certain bacterial species, notably those which produce so-called exotoxins, when grown in liquid media yield filtrates which are potently toxic. Two such bacterial species are *C. diphtheriæ* and *Cl. tetani*. Their toxins when suitably detoxified are strongly antigenic. It is believed that the exotoxins of these species are largely responsible for the pathological changes which are produced during the course of infections by the diphtheria or tetanus organisms.

Preparation—In the preparation of either diphtheria or tetanus toxoids only strains which are capable of producing potent toxins are used. The filtrates, obtained from the cultures, are detoxified by the addition of formaldehyde plus incubation at approximately 40°C for periods of a month or longer. Only toxins meeting rigid standards with respect to toxicity may be used in producing toxoids.

Within recent years methods have been developed for the purification of the toxoids along with subsequent concentration (Fig. 510). Concentrated forms are especially desirable for the preparation of the multiple antigens, and have resulted in products which can be given in reduced volume. The toxoids used for immunization against diphtheria and against tetanus are available both in unprecipitated form, usually designated as fluid, and in precipitated or adsorbed form. Precipitation may be accomplished by the addition of alum solution, aluminum hydroxide or aluminum phosphate. The toxoids in common use are available as single or as multiple antigens, the latter being offered as mixtures of tetanus and diphtheria toxoids, fluid, and precipitated, or adsorbed with aluminum hydroxide or with aluminum phosphate, and with or without pertussis vaccine.

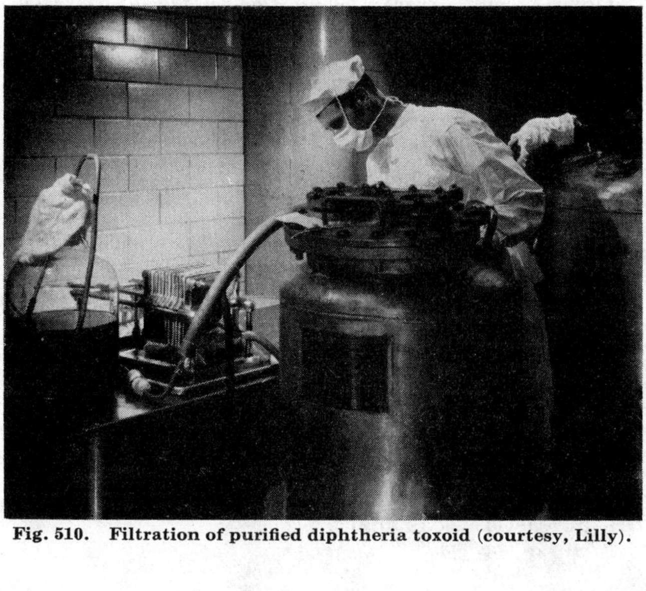

Uses—The precipitated and adsorbed forms of the toxoids are claimed to yield higher levels of immunity on the assumption that the depot effect persists over a much longer period. Such precipitated or adsorbed toxoids are relatively insoluble, and when injected the insoluble mass persists for some time before becoming completely absorbed. A fairly high incidence of so-called sterile abscesses follows the use of precipitated and adsorbed toxoids. As a rule these are of no important consequence.

In a massive immunization program involving mainly infants and young children it is possible that an artificially induced primary immunity is apt to wane and even disappear. Also, the disease may extend itself to those in higher age groups who were not immunized. Therefore, control procedure must be concerned with maintaining an immunity, once it is established, by giving booster doses and also with the immunization of a wider age group than that previously considered.

Diphtheria—In areas of increased diphtheria prevalence, inoculation or reinoculation of all children through high-school age who have not been so treated within the 3 years immediately preceding is recommended. Older children and adults should be inoculated with caution and preferably only after Schick testing.

Adolescents, and especially adults, who have been exposed to diphtheria should not only be Schick tested but they also should be subjected to the Schick control test. Reactors to the latter are generally not actively immunized as they usually possess either actual or latent immunity and frequently such individuals give marked reactions to toxoid. At present, plain diphtheria toxoid is the preparation of choice for adolescents and adults who are Schick-positive.

In general, use of the Schick test to determine the immune status of children prior to immunization is not

Fig. 510. Filtration of purified diphtheria toxoid (courtesy, Lilly).

necessary since it is known that practically all such young children are Schick-positive. Furthermore, there is little need for a post-immunization Schick test since, with the recommended schedule, essentially 100% of those injected become Schick-negative. Time devoted to an additional injection, such as the Schick test, may be used more profitably in the administration of additional toxoid. From the standpoint of the practicing physician who may want to know the Schick reaction of a specific patient, there may be some indication for applying the test.

The clinical protection afforded against diphtheria by active immunization is impressive. The protection is not absolute, as is the case with all active immunization procedures, but decreases in proportion to the interval elapsing since inoculation. The incidence of clinical diphtheria among those immunized is about 10 to 15% of that among nonimmunized individuals. Furthermore, clinical diphtheria is usually milder in immunized than in nonimmunized persons.

There is no doubt as to the value of artificial active immunization as a prophylactic measure. This is well demonstrated by the correlation between widespread active immunization and the accentuated decline in the number of deaths due to diphtheria. It is felt that communities which maintain rates of active immunization of 35% or more of the children under 5 years of age, plus 50% of children of school age, are free from the danger of significant outbreaks of diphtheria. There is evidence, however, that as diphtheria has diminished in incidence through the years and carriers of virulent diphtheria bacilli have tended to disappear, there has been a reduction in the acquisition of natural immunity by the population, particularly by the age group under 10 years. To compensate for this reduction, it is essential that artificial active immunity be increased.

Tetanus—The tetanus toxoids, used only for active immunization, possess great prophylactic value in the limited field of their usefulness. They are also employed for the active immunization of horses in the commercial production of tetanus antitoxin. Their use is practical and safe.

Active immunization against tetanus is highly advocated in allergic individuals and those who are hypersensitive to horse serum, in hunters, public utility workers in field duty, those in military service, farmers, horsemen, veterinarians, children, and others whose occupation and duties continually expose them to injuries favorable for the development of tetanus infection.

Probably the largest field for the practical use of Tetanus Toxoid is in military service especially during mechanized warfare and bombing. Hall[3] reported a detailed study of immunization with tetanus toxoid in the US Navy since 1934. Tetanus immunization with toxoid has been adopted by the French, Italian, British, and American armies.

Evidence indicates that the markedly low incidence of clinical tetanus among the Allied troops in World War II was due to the fact that most of them were actively immunized with tetanus toxoid. Glenn[4] in a report on tetanus concluded that the protection of the American soldier against tetanus by active immunization with tetanus toxoid during World War II is one of the most successful projects yet demonstrated in the field of preventive medicine. He further stated, present-day mortality rates indicate that the disease is best controlled by prevention rather than by any known therapy of a curative nature.

Diphtheria Toxoid USP

[Diphtheria Vaccine (FT); Diphtheria Prophylactic; Diphtheria Anatoxin; Anatoxin-Ramon]

Diphtheria Toxoid is a sterile solution of the formaldehyde-treated products of growth of the diphtheria bacillus (*Corynebacterium diphtheriæ*). It contains not more than 0.02% of residual free formaldehyde. Its production and distribution are subject to federal regulations (see *Biologics*, page 1425).

Description—Clear, brownish yellow, or slightly turbid liquid, having a faint, characteristic odor.

Dose—*Usual, intramuscular* or *subcutaneous*, 3 injections of **0.5** or **1 ml,** at least 4 weeks apart, and a fourth, reinforcing dose 6 to 12 months later.
Dosage Forms—7.5 and 15 ml.

Adsorbed Diphtheria Toxoid USP

[Diphtheria Toxoid, Alum Precipitated; Diphtheria Toxoid, Aluminum Hydroxide Adsorbed; Diphtheria Toxoid, Aluminum Hydroxide Precipitated; Diphtheria Toxoid, Aluminum Phosphate Adsorbed; Diphtheria Vaccine (ATP); Diphtheria Vaccine (PTAP)]

Adsorbed Diphtheria Toxoid is a sterile suspension of diphtheria toxoid precipitated or adsorbed by the addition of alum, aluminum hydroxide, or aluminum phosphate to a formaldehyde-treated solution of the products of growth of the diphtheria bacillus (*Corynebacterium diphtheriæ*). Its production and distribution are subject to federal regulations (see *Biologics*, page 1425).

Description—Turbid, white, slightly gray or slightly pink suspension.

Dose—*Usual, intramuscular*, 2 injections of **0.5** or **1 ml,** at least 4 weeks apart, and a third, reinforcing dose 6 to 12 months later.
Dosage Forms—0.5, 1.5 and 5 ml.

Tetanus Toxoid USP

[Tetanus Vaccine]

Tetanus Toxoid is a sterile solution of the formaldehyde-treated products of growth of the tetanus bacillus (*Clostridium tetani*). Its production and distribution are subject to federal regulations (see *Biologics*, page 1425).

Description—Clear colorless to brownish yellow, or slightly turbid liquid having a characteristic odor, or an odor of formaldehyde.

Dose—*Usual, intramuscular* or *subcutaneous*, 3 injections of **0.5** or **1 ml,** at least 4 weeks apart.
Dosage Forms—0.5, 1.5, 7.5, and 15 ml.

Adsorbed Tetanus Toxoid USP

[Tetanus Toxoid, Alum Precipitated; Tetanus Toxoid, Aluminum Hydroxide Adsorbed; Tetanus Toxoid, Aluminum Hydroxide Precipitated; Tetanus Toxoid, Aluminum Phosphate Adsorbed]

Adsorbed Tetanus Toxoid is a sterile suspension of tetanus toxoid precipitated or adsorbed by the addition of alum, aluminum hydroxide, or aluminum phosphate to a formaldehyde-treated solution of the products of growth of the tetanus bacillus (*Clostridium tetani*). Its production and distribution are subject to federal regulations (see *Biologics*, page 1425).

Description—Turbid, white, slightly gray or slightly pink suspension.

Dose—*Usual, intramuscular*, 2 injections of **0.5** or **1, ml.** at least 4 weeks apart.

Dosage Forms—0.5, 1, 1.5, 5, and 7.5 ml.

Multiple Antigens

Reference has been made to the use of multiple antigens which obviously eliminates the need for two or three separate immunization courses. The mixture containing diphtheria and tetanus toxoids along with pertussis vaccine is particularly appealing to pediatricians and, of course, to mothers. Infants and young children tolerate these highly antigenic mixtures surprisingly well.

Diphtheria and Tetanus Toxoids USP

[Diphtheria and Tetanus Toxoids Combined; Diphtheria and Tetanus Vaccine; Diphtheria–Tetanus Prophylactic]

Diphtheria and Tetanus Toxoids is a sterile solution prepared by mixing suitable quantities of fluid diphtheria toxoid and fluid tetanus toxoid. The potency and the proportions of the toxoids are such as to provide an immunizing dose of each toxoid in the total dosage prescribed in the labeling. It contains not more than 0.02% of residual free formaldehyde. Its production and distribution are subject to federal regulations (see *Biologics*, page 1425).

Description—Clear, colorless to brownish yellow or very slightly turbid liquid, having a characteristic odor.

Dose—*Usual, intramuscular or subcutaneous,* 2 injections of **0.5** or **1 ml,** at least 4 weeks apart, and a third, reinforcing dose 6 to 12 months later.
Dosage Forms—7.5 and 15 ml.

Adsorbed Diphtheria and Tetanus Toxoids USP

[Diphtheria and Tetanus Toxoids Combined, Alum Precipitated; Diphtheria and Tetanus Toxoids Combined, Aluminum Hydroxide Adsorbed; Diphtheria and Tetanus Toxoids Combined, Aluminum Hydroxide Precipitated; Diphtheria and Tetanus Toxoids Combined, Aluminum Phosphate Adsorbed; Diphtheria and Tetanus Toxoids Combined, Aluminum Phosphate Precipitated]

Adsorbed Diphtheria and Tetanus Toxoids is a sterile suspension prepared by mixing suitable quantities of adsorbed diphtheria toxoid and adsorbed tetanus toxoid, each having been precipitated or adsorbed by the same precipitating or adsorbing agent, which agent may be alum, aluminum hydroxide, or aluminum phosphate. The potency and the proportions of the toxoids are such as to provide an immunizing dose of each toxoid in the total dosage prescribed in the labeling. Its production and distribution are subject to federal regulations (see *Biologics*, page 1425).

Description—Turbid, white, slightly gray or slightly pink suspension.

Dose—*Usual, intramuscular,* 2 injections of **0.5** or **1 ml,** at least 4 weeks apart, and a third, reinforcing dose 6 to 12 months later.
Dosage Forms—1 and 5 ml.

Adsorbed Tetanus and Diphtheria Toxoids USP

[Tetanus and Diphtheria Toxoids Combined, Alum Precipitated (For Adult Use); Tetanus and Diphtheria Toxoids Combined, Aluminum Hydroxide Adsorbed (For Adult Use); Tetanus and Diphtheria Toxoids Combined, Aluminum Hydroxide Precipitated (For Adult Use); Tetanus and Diphtheria Toxoids Combined, Aluminum Phosphate Adsorbed (For Adult Use)]

Adsorbed Tetanus and Diphtheria Toxoids is a sterile suspension of adsorbed diphtheria toxoid and adsorbed tetanus toxoid prepared by mixture in such proportions that each dose contains a specified quantity of tetanus toxoid, and a specified smaller quantity of diphtheria toxoid. Its production and distribution are subject to federal regulations (see *Biologics*, page 1425).

Description—Turbid, white, slightly gray or cream-colored suspension.

Dose—*Usual, for immunization of adolescents and adults, primary immunization, intramuscular,* 2 injections of **0.5** or **1 ml** at least 4 weeks apart, and a third injection 6 to 12 months later; *booster dose,* **0.1** to **0.5 ml.**
Dosage Forms—0.5 and 5 ml.

Diphtheria and Tetanus Toxoids and Pertussis Vaccine USP

[Diphtheria and Tetanus Toxoids and Pertussis Vaccine Combined; Diphtheria, Tetanus, and Pertussis Vaccine; Diphtheria–Tetanus–Whooping-cough Prophylactic]

Diphtheria and Tetanus Toxoids and Pertussis Vaccine is a sterile suspension of killed pertussis bacilli (*Bordetella pertussis*), in a mixture of diphtheria toxoid and tetanus toxoid. The components are combined in such proportions as to yield a mixture which meets the antigenic and other requirements of each separate component. Its production and distribution are subject to federal regulations (see *Biologics*, page 1425).

Description—More or less turbid, whitish to light yellowish or brownish liquid having a faint odor due to the toxoid components, the preservative, or both.

Dose—*Usual, subcutaneous or intramuscular,* 3 injections of **0.5** or **1 ml,** as specified in the labeling, at least 4 weeks apart, and a fourth, reinforcing dose 12 months later.
Dosage Forms—1.5 and 7.5 ml.

Adsorbed Diphtheria and Tetanus Toxoids and Pertussis Vaccine USP

[Diphtheria and Tetanus Toxoid, Alum Precipitated, and Pertussis Vaccine, Combined; Diphtheria and Tetanus Toxoids and Pertussis Vaccine Combined, Alum Precipitated; Diphtheria and Tetanus Toxoids and Pertussis Vaccine Combined, Aluminum Hydroxide Adsorbed; Diphtheria and Tetanus Toxoids and Pertussis Vaccine Combined, Aluminum Hydroxide Precipitated; Diphtheria and Tetanus Toxoids and Pertussis Vaccine Combined, Aluminum Phosphate Adsorbed; Diphtheria and Tetanus Toxoids and Pertussis Vaccine Combined, Aluminum Phosphate Precipitated]

Adsorbed Diphtheria and Tetanus Toxoids and Pertussis Vaccine is a sterile suspension of the precipitate obtained by treating a mixture of diphtheria toxoid, tetanus toxoid, and pertussis vaccine with alum, aluminum hydroxide, or aluminum phosphate. The components are combined in such proportion as to yield a mixture containing an immunizing dose of each in the total dosage prescribed in the labeling. Its production and distribution are subject to federal regulations (see *Biologics*, page 1425).

Description—Markedly turbid, whitish liquid; nearly odorless or having a faint odor due to the preservative.

Dose—*Usual, intramuscular,* 3 injections, usually of **0.5** or **1 ml.,** at least 4 weeks apart, and a fourth, reinforcing dose 12 months later.
Dosage Forms—1.5 and 7.5 ml.

Viral Vaccines

Many of the infectious diseases of man, animals, and of plants are caused by the so-called filtrable viruses. These species of organisms are so small as to be capable of passing through membrane filters which readily retain bacteria and other larger forms of microorganisms. Some of the better known diseases caused by viruses are the common cold, chicken pox, dengue, herpes labialis (fever blister), herpes zoster (shingles), influenza, lymphogranuloma venereum, measles, mumps, poliomyelitis, encephalitis, psittacosis (parrot fever), rabies, smallpox, and yellow fever.

It is of some interest to point out that among the earliest developed of our present biological products are the vaccines used in the prevention of smallpox and of rabies. The production of influenza vaccine received its greatest impetus during World War II.

The methods of production and of testing of virus vaccines are considerably more elaborate and tedious than those necessary for the preparation of bacterial vaccines. For detailed information one may refer to textbooks on biological products.

Adenovirus Vaccine

The production of Adenovirus Vaccine is very similar to that outlined on page 1437 for the preparation of Poliomyelitis Vaccine. Such vaccine shall consist of an aqueous preparation of one or more adenoviruses grown in monkey kidney tissue cultures inactivated by a suitable method. Where more than one type of virus is used in the preparation of the vaccine, approximately equal proportions of each type shall be combined.

Only those strains of virus may be used that (1) produce a vaccine meeting safety and potency requirements, (2) that never had any passage in malignant cells of human or animal origin, and (3) that have been maintained in monkey kidney cultures for at least ten passages prior to use.

It is particularly important that all phases of the preparation of adenovirus vaccine, including personnel and facilities, shall be isolated from any other activities in the laboratories dealing with any other pathogenic virus.

Extraneous protein capable of producing allergenic effects in human subjects shall not be added to the final virus production medium. If animal serum is used at any stage, its calculated concentration in the final medium shall not exceed 1 part in 1,000,000.

Its production and distribution are subject to federal regulations (see *Biologics*, page 1425).

Description—A clear liquid, reddish tinged if an indicator is used in the growth phase of its production. It contains a suitable preservative.

Dose—1 ml as specified in labeling.
Dosage Forms—5 ml.

Influenza Virus Vaccine USP

[Influenza Virus Vaccine, Types A and B; Influenza Vaccine; Inactivated Influenza Vaccine]

Influenza Virus Vaccine is a sterile, aqueous suspension of suitably inactivated influenza virus prepared from the extra-embryonic fluid of influenza virus-infected chick embryo. The strains of influenza virus used in the preparation of this Vaccine are those designated by the Division of Biologics Standards of the National Institutes of Health. Influenza Virus Vaccine may contain an adsorbant such as calcium phosphate or protamine. Its production and distribution are subject to federal regulations (see *Biologics*, page 1425).

This product is not to be confused with the bacterial influenza vaccine (*H. influenzæ*) which is often present as a component of mixed vaccines recommended for the prevention or treatment of respiratory infections. Its first extensive use occurred during World War II

Table III—Survey of Vaccines Against Important Human Viral Infections[5]

Virus	Vaccine status	
	Existing[a]	Developmental-experimental
Smallpox	Live	Live, further attenuated; killed
Rabies	Killed; live	Killed, cell-culture-grown
Arbovirus		
Yellow fever	Live	None
WEE, EEE, VEE[b]	Killed (animal)	Live (animal); killed (man)
Japanese B encephalitis	Killed	Killed, cell-culture-grown; live, cell-culture-grown
RSSE[c]	Killed (Soviet)	Killed, cell-culture-grown
Kyasanur forest	None	Killed (ineffective)
Dengue	None	Live
Rift Valley fever	None	Killed, cell-culture-grown
West Nile	None	Live, cell-culture-grown
Respiratory complex		
Influenza A and B	Killed; live (Soviet)	Killed, purified; killed, viral subunits
Influenza C	None	None
Adenovirus	Killed[d]	Killed, viral subunits; live
Parainfluenza 1, 2, and 3	None	Killed, purified and concentrated; live
Respiratory syncytial	None	Killed, purified and concentrated; live
Mycoplasma pneumoniae (bacterial)	None	Killed
Rhinovirus	None	Killed; live
Reovirus	None	None
Enterovirus		
Poliovirus	Killed; live	None
ECHO and Coxsackie	None	None
Systemic myxoviruses[e]		
Rubeola (measles)	Live; killed	Killed, viral subunits
Mumps	Killed; live	None
Rubella (German measles)	None	Live
Herpes virus group		
Herpes simplex	None	Killed
B virus	None	Killed
Cytomegalovirus	None	None
Varicella zoster	None	None
Infectious mononucleosis	None	None
Hepatitis	None	None

[a] Now licensed in the US.
[b] Western, Eastern, and Venezuelan equine encephalomyelitis viruses.
[c] Russian spring–summer encephalitis.
[d] Removed from commercial distribution because of oncogenicity of most serotypes.
[e] Rubella family position not established.

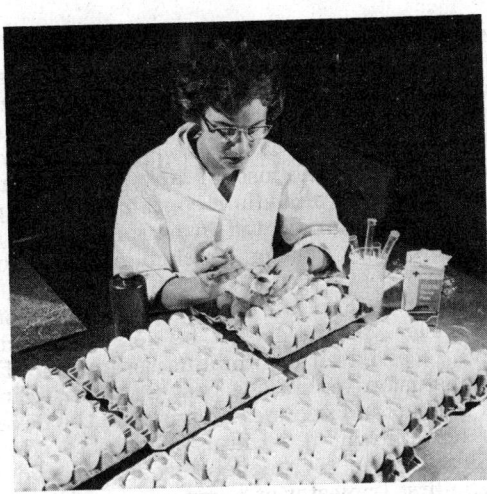

Fig. 511. Fertile eggs inoculated with influenza virus (courtesy, Du Pont).

by the Armed Services, and after undergoing almost yearly changes in formula it continues to be a required item in the immunization schedules established for personnel of the Army, Navy, and Air Force.

Preparation—For production of the vaccine, the various strains of influenza virus are grown in the chorio-allantoic membrane of incubated fertile hen eggs (Fig. 511). The morphology of the virus has been studied with the aid of the electron microscope. There are several methods of concentrating the virus from the infected allantoic fluid: hemagglutination, adsorption on calcium phosphate, alcohol precipitation, and by ultracentrifugation. The amount of virus is standardized by the hemagglutination method and by the mouse protection test. The potency or antigenicity of each killed virus component is expressed in terms of CCA (chick cell agglutinating) units.

Description—Slightly turbid (opalescent) liquid, which may have a slight yellow or reddish tinge and may have an odor due to the preservative. The potency of each lot is determined by its power to stimulate the formation of specific virus-neutralizing antibodies in mice. The potency is expressed in terms of the chicken red-cell agglutination titer (as "CCA units" in each ml).

Uses—Influenza virus vaccine is used as a specific immunizing agent against influenza virus, Types A, A₁, A₂, and B.

Dose—*Usual, intramuscular* or *subcutaneous*, 2 injections of **0.5** or **1 ml,** 2 months apart.

Dosage Forms—1, 5, and 10 ml.

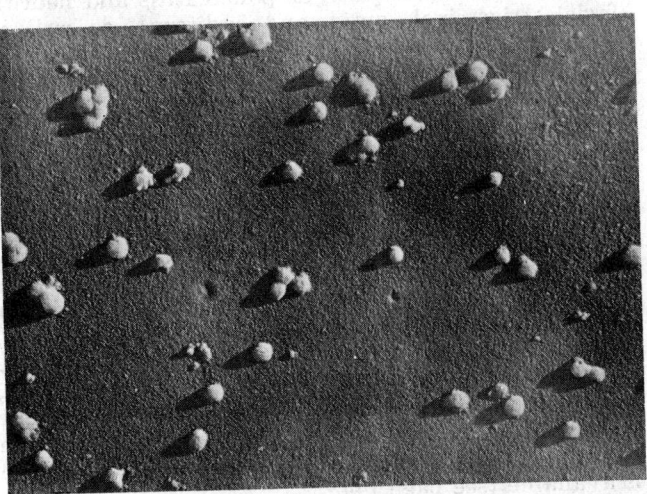

Fig. 512. Photomicrograph of influenza virus.

Inactivated Measles Virus Vaccine

Inactivated Measles Virus Vaccine is a killed preparation (usually formaldehyde inactivated) of measles virus, Edmonston strain.[6] The virus may be propagated either in chick embryo tissue culture or in money kidney tissue culture in an appropriate medium under aseptic conditions. If chick embryo tissue culture is used for the cultivation of measles virus, the embryonated eggs used as source shall be derived from flocks certified to be free of *Salmonella pullorum,* avian tuberculosis, fowl pox, Rous sarcoma, avian leukosis and all other adventitious agents known to be pathogenic for chickens. If the embryonated eggs are procured from flocks that are not so certified, tests must be performed to demonstrate that the virus pool is free from all such agents prior to inactivation of the measles virus. If monkey kidney tissue culture is used for the cultivation of measles virus, only monkeys in overt good health, that have reacted negatively to tuberculin at the start of the prescribed quarantine period, may be used for the production of vaccine.

Measles vaccine contains a suitable preservative and may or may not be alum precipitated. No extraneous protein, capable of producing allergenic effects upon injection into human subjects, is added to the final virus production medium. If animal serum is used at any stage, its calculated concentration in the final medium does not exceed 1 part per million. Antibiotics suitable for inhibiting bacterial growth during production of the virus may be used in minimum concentration in the tissue culture medium employed, and if penicillin is used, not more than 200 USP Units/ml may be added.

Its production and distribution are subject to federal regulations (see *Biologics,* page 1425).

Other Requirements—The inactivated vaccine is tested in cortisone-stressed healthy monkeys and in various tissue culture systems to demonstrate the absence of viable viruses. Additional animal, tissue culture, and *in vitro* tests are performed to demonstrate the absence of B virus, lymphocytic choriomeningitis, SV₄₀, *Mycobacterium tuberculosis* and all other possible microbial contaminants. Chemical analysis is made to insure that maximum levels of residual protein nitrogen (<0.02 mg/dose) and alum (<15 mg/dose) are not exceeded. The potency of the finished vaccine is standardized in animals by comparison with standard reference vaccines.

Dose—The recommended dosage for persons 8 months old or older is a series of three injections of 0.5 ml each, given at approximately montly intervals.

Other Dose Information—This vaccine should be administered either by the *subcutaneous* or *intramuscular* routes. Alum precipitated vaccine should be administered only by the intramuscular route, preferably using a dry needle technique. In order to assure adequate serologic response to vaccination, only children 8 months of age or older should be immunized, since children 7 months old or younger almost always have sufficient maternal measles antibody to interfere with the immunizing capacity of the vaccine.

Precautions—According to the Ad Hoc Advisory Committee on Measles Control to the Surgeon General of the USPHS[7] this vaccine is not contraindicated in (1) pregnancy; (2) leukemia, lymphomas, and other generalized malignancies; or (3) therapy which depresses resistance such as steroids, irradiation, alkylating agents, and antimetabolites.

The Committee on the Control of Infectious Diseases of the American Academy of Pediatrics states that immunization procedures should be deferred in the presence of acute respiratory disease or other active infections.[8]

Dosage Forms—0.5 ml.

Live Attenuated Measles Virus Vaccine USP

Live Attenuated Measles Virus Vaccine is a sterile preparation derived from a strain of measles virus found suitable for human immunization but grown for purposes of vaccine production on cultures of either chicken-embryo tissue or canine renal tissue. It may contain suitable antimicrobial agents. Its production and distribution are subject to federal regulations (see *Biologics*, page 1425).

Attenuated Live Measles Virus Vaccine is a living, attenuated measles virus vaccine prepared from the Edmonston strain of measles developed by Enders, *et al.*[9] A single dose of the living, attenuated vaccine confers immunity against the natural disease of measles (rubeola). It is not effective in the prevention of German Measles (rubella).

Description—Solid having the characteristic appearance of substances dried from the frozen state. Undergoes loss of potency on exposure to sunlight.

Dose—*Usual, intramuscular* or *subcutaneous,* **0.5 ml.**

Other Dose Information—The vaccine in a dose of **0.5 ml,** is injected *subcutaneously* into the upper arm. Each 0.5 ml dose of vaccine must contain no less than 1000 $TCID_{50}$ (tissue culture infective doses, fifty) of measles virus expressed in terms of the assigned titer of a reference measles virus supplied by the National Institutes of Health. Immune serum globulin (human) having a predetermined measles neutralizing antibody content [Measles Immune Globulin (Human)] and administered in a dose of 0.01 ml/pound of body weight, is injected immediately thereafter into the deltoid muscle of the opposite arm. The administration of the immune serum globulin *after* the vaccine reduces the severity of the reaction without blocking the immunizing effect since the virus is permitted to infect the cells of the injection site prior to the distribution of measles antibody from the injection of the immune serum globulin. In order to assure adequate serologic response to vaccination, it is recommended that only children 9 months of age or over be immunized. The majority of children 6 to 7 months old or younger still retain measles neutralizing antibody of maternal origin. It has been found that children who showed the presence of maternal antibody at the time of vaccination did not respond serologically or clinically to the vaccine, whereas when the maternal antibody was lost, they became fully susceptible to the immunizing capability of the vaccine.[10,11] Infants who had no maternal antibody at the time of the first vaccination and who responded serologically to it, still retained the antibody titer 7 to 9 months later but were not responsive to a second dose of vaccine, as indicated by the absence of both a clinical and serologic response.[10,11] Though the duration of immunity is not yet known, satisfactory levels of neutralizing antibody have been maintained for at least 2.5 years.[12] The actual duration of immunity can only be determined from repeated observations of vaccinated individuals in the future.

Contraindications—Measles vaccination is contraindicated in individuals with leukemia.[13] The presence of brain damage in an infant is likewise an indication for delay in starting active immunization procedures until after a year of age.[14] Any febrile respiratory illness or other active infection is reason for delaying live virus measles vaccination, except when the physician believes that withholding the vaccine entails even greater risk.

A small number of persons are extremely allergic to egg proteins and may show severe reactions to injections of a vaccine prepared from chick embryos.[15-18] Possible reactors should be sought by careful questioning as to the presence of allergy to egg, chicken meat, or chicken feathers. The use of any vaccine prepared from virus grown in a medium containing chick protein is absolutely contraindicated in persons with a history of hypersensitivity to egg, chicken meat, or chicken feathers.

Precautions—For full effectiveness, administration of the measles vaccine should be deferred in children who have received either immune serum globulin or a blood transfusion within the past 6 weeks. Since the effect of live, attenuated measles virus on the developing fetus is not known, it is advisable not to administer this living vaccine to pregnant women, certainly not during the first trimester of pregnancy. If live measles vaccine is to be administered to children with cystic fibrosis, a history of tuberculosis, or with any condition involving stress, it is imperative that immune serum globulin be given immediately thereafter.

Dosage Forms—in an amount sufficient to yield 0.5 ml of vaccine upon being reconstituted.

Mumps Vaccine

Mumps vaccine is a sterile aqueous suspension of suitably concentrated and inactivated mumps virus prepared from the allantoic fluid of embryonated chicken eggs infected with mumps virus by the method described by Habel.[19] Only one strain of mumps virus is used, since all isolated strains appear to be the same immunologically.

Its production and distribution are subject to federal regulations (see *Biologics*, page 1425).

Development—Mumps, as it is clinically manifest in children, generally causes little or no permanent damage; hence, it has seldom been considered as a serious disease. More recently, however, there is an accumulating feeling that some of the complications occurring in later life, such as meningoencephalitis and eighth nerve damage—rare as they are—may have had their beginning as a result of mumps. Complications in adolescent and adult groups are much more frequent and severe orchitis in the male has the highest incidence and is most feared. Oöphoritis has been reported as occurring in about 5% of adult females with mumps. Other complications, such as pancreatitis and neuritis (facial, trigeminal, optic, and auditory), as well as secondary infections, occur less frequently.

Eagles,[20] in a report of a four-year study involving 2500 cases in military personnel, noted an incidence of epididymo-orchitis in 25.5%, meningoencephalitis in 2.6%, presternal edema in 1.2%, and other complications with still lower incidence.

Description—Slightly opalescent liquid, which may have a slight yellow or reddish tinge and may have an odor due to the preservative.

Dose—The recommended immunizing dose for children and adults is two injections of **1.0 ml** each, administered either *subcutaneously* or *intramuscularly.* The interval for optimal immunization is not known, but 1 to 4 weeks between injections is suggested. The vaccine used for immunization is too strong for skin testing. For this purpose Mumps Skin Test Antigen is available (see page 1448).

Dosage Forms—2 and 10 ml.

Live Attenuated Mumps Vaccine

Live Attenuated Mumps Vaccine is a living, attenuated mumps virus vaccine prepared from the Jeryl Lynn (B level) strain, named after the patient from whom the virus was initially recovered. According to the general procedures of Enders, the virus used to prepare the vaccine is grown in cell cultures of chick embryos. Its production and distribution are subject to federal regulations (see *Biologics*, page 1425).

Reconstitution—Prior to reconstitution, store the vaccine in a refrigerator at 2° to 8°C. Protect from sunlight. To reconstitute, inject all the diluent in the syringe into the vial of lyophilized vaccine and agitate to ensure thorough mixing. Draw back entire contents into the syringe and inject total volume of restored vaccine subcutaneously. Each dose of reconstituted vaccine contains not less than 5000 $TCID_{50}$ of mumps virus vaccine expressed in terms of the assigned titer of the NIH reference mumps vaccine. Use only the diluent supplied and reconstitute the vaccine just before using. If not used immediately, return the reconstituted vaccine to the refrigerator at 2° to 8°C. Discard after 8 hours.

Uses—Live attenuated Mumps Virus Vaccine induces protective antibodies in essentially all non-immune recipients, provides protection against natural mumps in most cases, and has not been shown to cause significant systemic or local reactions. Evidence indicates that the mumps virus infection initiated by the vaccine is not contagious.

The vaccine is indicated for immunization of infants over 1 year of age, children, and adults. It is not recommended for infants less than 1 year old because they may retain maternal mumps neutralizing antibodies which may interfere with the immune response.

Since about 28 days are required for antibodies to develop, the vaccine cannot be used to prevent mumps after exposure. Antibodies induced by the vaccine persist for at least 2 years without substantial decline, and the pattern of antibody closely resembles that observed for natural mumps, although the antibody level is significantly lower than that following the natural infection. If this pattern continues, it will provide a basis for expectation that immunity following the vaccine will be permanent.

Contraindications—Do not give Live Attenuated Mumps Virus Vaccine to pregnant women; at this time the effects on fetal development are not known. Do not give this vaccine to persons sensitive to eggs, chicken, chicken feathers, or neomycin. The vaccine is prepared from an attenuated strain of mumps virus grown in a chick embryo cell culture medium containing 25 mcg per dose of neomycin.

Because their normal defense mechanisms are suppressed, patients suffering with leukemia, lymphomas, and other generalized malignancies should not receive this vaccine. For the same reason withhold it from children receiving corticosteroids, irradiation, alkylating agents, or antimetabolites. Also, the vaccine is contraindicated in any patient known to have a gamma globulin deficiency.

Any active infection is reason for delaying mumps vaccination unless not doing so involves a greater risk to the patient. Do not administer the vaccine with other vaccines, but allow 1 month to elapse between elective immunizations.

Dose—The dose of vaccine, 0.5 ml, is the same for all: children 12 months and older, adolescents, and adults. The vaccine should be given at least 1 month before or after other elective immunizations.

Dosage Forms—0.5 ml.

Poliomyelitis Vaccine USP

[Poliomyelitis Vaccine (Inactivated)]

Poliomyelitis Vaccine is a sterile suspension of inactivated poliomyelitis virus of Types 1, 2, and 3. The virus strains are grown separately in primary cultures of monkey kidney tissue, and after inactivation are combined in suitable proportions.

No extraneous protein, capable of producing allergenic effects upon injection into human subjects, is added to the final virus production medium. If animal serum is used at any stage, its calculated concentration in the final medium does not exceed 1 part per million. Suitable microbistatic agents may be used during the production.

Its production and distribution are subject to federal regulations (see *Biologics*, page 1425).

The work of Enders and his associates revolutionized the immunological and epidemiological study of poliomyelitis. With their development of tissue culture technique, a method was devised for the first time which would permit the cultivation of poliomyelitis virus in other than central nervous tissue; in this case monkey kidney tissue-culture is now routinely used. Using this technique, Salk was successful in preparing a vaccine containing representatives of all three types of polioviruses.

The trivalent vaccine contains the Mahoney, MEF-1, and Saukett strains representing types 1, 2, and 3 polioviruses, respectively. The virus-containing monkey kidney tissue-cultures are incubated to allow maximal production of the virus. After filtration capable of removing bacteria, the filtrates are inactivated with an appropriate concentration of formaldehyde.

Exhaustive tests are performed to determine thoroughness of inactivation, to assure freedom from *M. tuberculosis* and *lymphocytic choriomeningitis* virus, and bacterial and mold contamination. The tests designed to assure complete absence of any remaining viable virus are quite extensive, using the so-called roller-tube, tissue culture technique (Fig. 513). This is supplemented by additional safety tests performed on monkeys. Finally, appropriate tests are conducted to measure antigenicity.

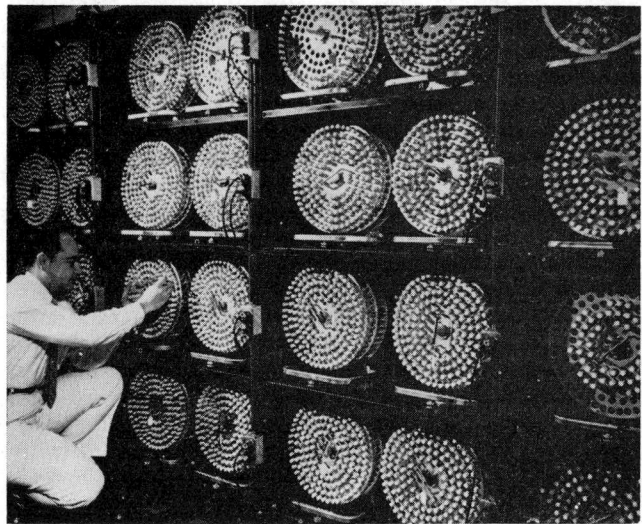

Fig. 513. Tissue culture roller tubes for poliomyelitis vaccine safety test (courtesy, Lilly).

Evaluation of each lot is based on the examination of protocols which include data pertaining to manufacture and control, supplemented by tests conducted in the laboratories of the Division of Biologics Standards. Poliomyelitis Vaccine is available also in mixture with Diphtheria and Tetanus Toxoids and with Pertussis Vaccine.

Description—Clear, reddish-tinged liquid, which may have a slight odor due to the preservative.

Dose—*Usual, subcutaneous,* 2 injections of **1 ml,** 4 to 6 weeks apart, then **1 ml** at least 7 months later.
Dosage Forms—1 and 9 ml.

Live Oral Poliovirus Vaccine USP

[Poliomyelitis Vaccine (Oral)]

Live Oral Poliovirus Vaccine is a preparation of one or a combination of the three types of live, attenuated polioviruses that have been grown separately in primary cultures of monkey kidney tissue. The vaccine is free from any known microbial agent other than the attenuated poliovirus or polioviruses declared in the labeling. Its production and distribution are subject to federal regulations (see *Biologics*, page 1425).

Note—See also the monographs on *Monovalent Live Oral Poliovirus Vaccine* and *Trivalent Live Oral Poliovirus Vaccine*.

Description—Is generally frozen but, in liquid form, is clear and colorless, or may have a yellow or red tinge.

Dose—*Usual,* the volume indicated in the labeling as representing one dose, at intervals of 6 to 8 weeks, of each type of the monovalent vaccine, followed in 8 to 12 months by one dose of the trivalent vaccine; or the volume representing two doses, 6 to 8 weeks apart, of the trivalent vaccine, followed in 8 to 12 months by a third dose.

Dosage Forms—in various strengths, such that the amount representing one dose varies from 2 drops to 2 ml, in volumes from 0.5 to 10 ml.

Monovalent Live Oral Poliovirus Vaccine

Monovalent Live Oral Poliovirus Vaccine is available as 3 separate monovalent vaccines indicated for the prevention of poliomyelitis caused by polioviruses types 1, 2, and 3. Each of the attenuated strains of poliovirus is propagated separately in monkey kidney cells, shown by exhaustive tests to be free of all known bacterial, fungal, or viral contaminants. Thus far, only the attenuated poliovirus strains of Sabin have been accepted by the Surgeon General of the US Public Health Service, although a great deal of work with other attenuated strains (known as the Lederle or Cox and Koprowski strains) has been carried out in various countries of the world. For a review of the development and status of living, oral, poliovirus vaccine, see Refs. 21–27.

A vaccine which may be given orally is especially attractive because of economy and ease of administration, making it ideally suitable for mass vaccinations. Of greater importance is the fact that the living, oral vaccine confers an immunity in the intestinal tract, which we know today is the location in which naturally occurring poliomyelitis infections originate. There is increasing evidence, too, that immunity conferred by a living, oral vaccine is longer lasting than that produced by the killed vaccine, and that vaccination in this manner more nearly approaches the process of immunization following natural exposure to the disease.

Its production and distribution are subject to federal regulations (see *Biologics*, page 1425).

Description—It is propagated in monkey kidney tissue-culture. The monovalent vaccine strains are marketed as a 2-ml dose wherein a stabilizing vehicle such as sorbitol is used, and also as a 2-drop dose product wherein tissue-culture maintenance medium is the final diluent. In either case the poliovirus concentration in the monovalent strain dose ranges from $10^{5.3}$ to $10^{5.7}$ TCID$_{50}$ (200,000 to 500,000 Tissue Culture Infective Doses, Fifty). To qualify for license from the National Institutes of Health, the monovalent vaccines when administered orally as a single dose, as recommended, must induce type specific neutralizing antibodies (from less than 1:4 before vaccine treatment to 1:16 or greater after vaccine treatment) in 80% or more of susceptible persons, as determined by clinical trials of adequate statistical design.

Administration—It is to be administered *orally* under the supervision of a physician. *Under no circumstances should the vaccine be administered parenterally.* It is recommended that the monovalent vaccines be administered in the order of type 1, type 3, and type 2, with an interval of 6 weeks or more between each dose. This procedure tends to minimize the possibility of interference among the three vaccine virus types and to provide a better opportunity for maximum antibody and intestinal immune response. Immunity is induced to each type of poliovirus within at least 4 weeks following its administration.

Dosage—Vaccine containing sorbitol: **2 ml,** *orally,* single administration. Vaccine without sorbitol: **2 drops,** *orally,* single administration.

1. Infants. Immunization should be initiated between 6 weeks and 3 months of age and subsequent doses given according to the following schedule:

Number of doses	Type	Interval from previous dose
First	1	. . .
Second	3	6 weeks
Third	2	6 weeks
Fourth	Trivalent	6 months or longer

2. All Others (including community use):

Number of doses	Type	Interval from previous dose
First	1	. . .
Second	3	6 weeks
Third	2	6 weeks

While the need for booster doses in children and adults has not yet been clearly established, a booster dose of trivalent vaccine should be considered every 2 to 4 years, or under threat of an epidemic.

Contraindications and Precautions—There are no known contraindications to oral poliovirus vaccines. This includes conditions previously of concern such as tonsillectomy, tooth extraction, pregnancy, penicillin hypersensitivity, therapy with steroids, agammaglobulinemia, diphtheria and tetanus toxoids and pertussis vaccine combined inoculation, smallpox vaccination, and others.

Because the efficacy of orally administered live poliovirus vaccine depends on multiplication of the virus in the intestinal tract, it follows that immunization should be postponed if there is persistent diarrhea or vomiting.

Other viruses, such as enteroviruses and polioviruses, may interfere with the desired response. The vaccine is not effective in cases of existing and/or incubating poliovirus infection.

Dosage Forms—1- and 10-dose vials.

Trivalent Live Oral Poliovirus Vaccine

Trivalent Live Oral Poliovirus Vaccine is indicated for the prevention of poliomyelitis caused by types 1, 2, and 3 polioviruses.

Its production and distribution are subject to federal regulations (see *Biologics*, page 1425).

Description—This is a mixture of the three polioviruses which have been propagated separately in monkey kidney tissue-culture. The final vaccine is marketed both as a 2-ml dose, wherein a stabilizing vehicle such as sorbitol is used as the diluent, and also as a 2-drop dose product wherein tissue-culture maintenance medium is the final diluent. The latter product is especially proficient for use in mass immunization programs. In either case each immunizing dose contains less than 5 mcg of each of the antibiotics—streptomycin, neomycin, and nystatin. The potency is expressed, in terms of the amount of virus contained in the recommended dose, as tissue culture infective doses ($TCID_{50}$). The approximate concentration of poliovirus for each strain in a single immunizing dose expressed logarithmically is: type 1, $10^{5.9}$ $TCID_{50}$; type 2, $10^{5.0}$ $TCID_{50}$; type 3, $10^{5.7}$ $TCID_{50}$. To qualify for license from the National Institutes of Health, the trivalent vaccine when administered orally in 2 separately spaced doses, as recommended, must induce type specific neutralizing antibodies for all 3 poliovirus types (from less than 1:4 before vaccine treatment, to 1:16 or greater after vaccine treatment) in 90% or more of susceptible persons, as determined by clinical trials of adequate statistical design.

Administration—This is to be administered orally under the supervision of a physician. *Under no circumstances should this vaccine be administered parenterally.* The dose may be dispensed in a teaspoon or in a cup. Infants and small children may receive the vaccine directly from a graduated dropper. Alternatively, the 2-drop dose may be administered mixed with liquids such as distilled water, tap water containing no free chlorine, Syrup USP or milk, or adsorbed on any one of a number of substances such as bread, cake, or cube sugar.

Immunization of the newborn (under 6 weeks of age) is not recommended, primarily because a varying proportion of such infants may be refractory.

Dose—*Usual, initial immunization,* children and adults: Vaccine containing sorbitol, 2 doses of **2 ml** each, administered *orally* at least 8 weeks apart; vaccine without sorbitol, 2 doses of **2 drops** each, administered *orally* at least 8 weeks apart.

Usual, initial immunization, Infants: immunization of infants may be initiated between 6 weeks and 6 months of age, but should be repeated at 10 to 12 months. If 1 dose each of monovalent types 1, 2, and 3 vaccines was used for initial immunization, a single dose of Trivalent Vaccine should be administered at 10 to 12 months of age. If initial immunization was with Trivalent Vaccine, one dose of Trivalent Vaccine should be administered at 10 to 12 months of age.

Other Immunization—The initial immunization schedule is recommended when the history of previous immunization is negative, unknown, in doubt, or when only the killed (Salk type) vaccine has been given. Where there is incomplete or uncertain previous immunization with Monovalent Oral Poliovirus Vaccines, two doses of Trivalent Vaccine at an interval of 8 weeks should be administered. This Vaccine can be used if the individual has previously received oral immunization against only one or two monovalent types.

Booster Immunization—One dose of **2 ml** administered *orally*. While the need for booster doses in children and adults has not yet been clearly established, a booster dose of Trivalent Vaccine should be considered every 2 to 4 years, or under threat of an epidemic.

Contraindications and Precautions—There are no known contraindications to oral poliovirus vaccines, including conditions previously of concern, such as tonsillectomy, tooth extraction, pregnancy, penicillin hypersensitivity, therapy with steroids, agammaglobulinemia, diphtheria and tetanus toxoids and pertussis vaccine combined inoculation, smallpox vaccination, and others. The clinical judgment of the responsible physician should prevail in all cases.

Because the efficacy of orally administered live poliovirus vaccine depends upon multiplication of the virus in the intestinal tract, it follows that immunization should be postponed if there is persistent diarrhea or vomiting.

Other viruses, such as enteroviruses and polioviruses, may interfere with the desired response. The vaccine is not effective in cases of existing and/or incubating polio virus infection.

Dosage Forms—0.5- and 2-ml vials, 20-drop vial, 1-dose disposable pipette.

Rabies Vaccine USP

Rabies Vaccine is a sterile preparation, in liquid or in dried form, of killed, fixed virus of rabies. The virus is obtained from the brain tissue of rabbits, or from duck embryos, that have been infected with fixed rabies virus. [The virus obtained from the brain tissue of rabbits is attenuated or killed, and that obtained from duck embryos is killed.] Its production and distribution are subject to federal regulations (see *Biologics*, page 1425).

Description—Liquid Vaccine is a turbid, white to brownish suspension having a slight odor due to the preservative. Dried Vaccine is a white to straw-colored amorphous pellet, which may or may not become fragmented when shaken.

Dose—*Usual, subcutaneous,* the labeled dose once a day for 14 to 21 days.

Dosage Forms—packages containing 7 individual doses.

Smallpox Vaccine USP

Smallpox Vaccine contains the living virus of vaccinia (cowpox) that has been grown in the skin of a vaccinated bovine calf, or in the membranes of the chick embryo. It is available in dried and in liquid form. Its production and distribution are subject to federal regulations (see *Biologics*, page 1425).

The present vaccine is essentially the same as the original Jenner vaccine, except that calf lymph is used instead of human lymph and bacterial contamination is successfully controlled by the use of glycerin and ripening. It is supplied in capillary tubes.

Description—The liquid vaccine is a grayish, turbid suspension which may have a slight odor due to the preservative. The dried vaccine is a yellow to reddish-brown pellet, which may or may not become fragmented when shaken.

Uses—The event which first foreshadowed the modern development of active immunization to infection was Jenner's use of the virus of vaccinia, or cowpox, to produce active immunity to smallpox. The practice has changed little since his day. Protection is relatively complete but does not last indefinitely, and revaccination is necessary. The first vaccination may be carried out early in life, any time after the umbilicus has healed. It is usually postponed until after the third

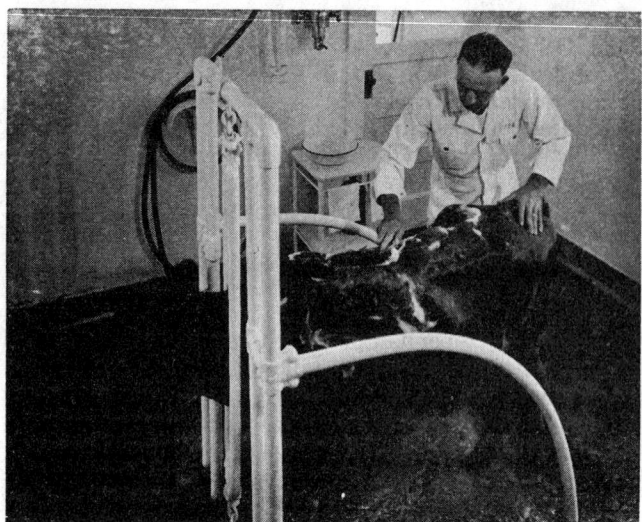

Fig. 514. Calf being prepared for vaccinia inoculation (courtesy, Lilly).

month and is preferably carried out during the cooler months, when the vaccine is less susceptible to deterioration and there is less likelihood of secondary infection. Vaccination should be repeated at the time of entrance into school and again in early adult life. All persons exposed directly or indirectly to smallpox should be vaccinated or revaccinated immediately, unless they have had smallpox.

The *vaccination technique* involves the deposition of the vaccine in the deeper layers of the epidermis without drawing blood. Vaccination by multiple pressure on a small area of skin over the deltoid is preferred;

no dressing need be applied. Children with eczema should not be vaccinated or come into contact with recently vaccinated persons. After revaccination, examination should be made at 3rd and 9th days to determine whether reaction is of primary, vaccinoid or early (immediate) type. An early reaction is difficult to interpret. If in doubt, revaccinate. If no reaction is obtained, always revaccinate.

Dose—*Usual, percutaneous,* contents of one capillary tube, or 1 drop of the reconstituted Vaccine, by the multiple-puncture method.

Dosage Forms—Liquid Vaccine: 1, 5, and 10 capillary tubes; Dried Vaccine: 10 and 100 immunization doses.

Yellow Fever Vaccine USP

Yellow Fever Vaccine is an attenuated strain of living yellow fever virus, selected for high antigenic activity and safety. It is prepared by the culturing of the virus in the living embryo of the domestic fowl (*Gallus domesticus*), from which a suspension is prepared, processed with aseptic precautions, and finally dried from the frozen state, and sealed under dry nitrogen. It is sterile, and contains no human serum and no antimicrobial agent. Its production and distribution are subject to federal regulations (see *Biologics*, page 1425).

Yellow Fever Vaccine is reconstituted, with *Sodium Chloride Injection* (see page 842) containing no bacteriostatic agent, just prior to use.

Description—Slightly dull, light-orange colored, flaky or crustlike desiccated mass.

Dose—*Usual, subcutaneous,* **0.5 ml.**
Dosage Forms—5- and 20-dose ampuls.

Rickettsial Vaccines

The rickettsiae are small Gram-negative microorganisms, intermediate between bacteria and viruses, which live within the cells of their host. The only filtrable member of the group is that causing Q fever. The rickettsial diseases are transmitted to man by insects including ticks, lice, fleas, and mites.

The organisms attack the endothelium of the arterioles and arterial capillaries, giving rise to proliferation and necrosis. There is also perivascular infiltration of round cells. The changes occur principally in the vessels of the skin, central nervous system, and myocardium. The lesions appear as microscopic swellings. They may produce thrombosis and hemorrhage.

Table IV—Diseases Caused by Rickettsiae

Disease	Organism	Vector
Typhus Group		
Epidemic typhus	*R. prowazekii*	Louse
Endemic (murine) typhus	*R. typhi*	Flea
Spotted Fever Group		
Rocky Mountain spotted fever	*R. rickettsii*	Tick
South American spotted fever	*R. rickettsii*	Tick
Fièvre boutonneuse	*R. conorii*	Tick
South African tick-bite fever	*R. conorii*	Tick
Tsutsugamushi Disease Group		
Tsutsugamushi disease (scrub typhus)	*R. tsutsugamushi*	Mite
Q Fever Group		
Australian Q fever	*Coxiella burnetii*	Tick
American Q fever	*Coxiella burnetii*	Tick

The diseases caused by rickettsiae may be divided into four groups: typhus, spotted fever, tsutsugamushi disease, and Q fever. The Weil-Felix agglutination reaction, formerly employed for differentiation of the rickettsiae, has now been superseded by complement-fixation tests.

Rocky Mountain Spotted Fever Vaccine USP

Rocky Mountain Spotted Fever Vaccine is a sterile, aqueous suspension of inactivated *Rickettsia rickettsii* that has been prepared by growing the virus in the embryonic tissues of the domestic fowl (*Gallus domesticus*). It may be purified by chemical treatment. It contains an antimicrobial agent. Its production and distribution are subject to federal regulations (see *Biologics*, page 1425).

A vaccine has been developed but enjoys only limited use. Fortunately, several of the broad spectrum antibiotics such as chloramphenicol and chlortetracycline are almost specific in their effects in the treatment of Rocky Mountain spotted fever, so that this disease is no longer feared by the physician called upon to treat it.

The acute infectious disease known as Rocky Mountain spotted fever, or as tick fever, is caused by *Rickettsia rickettsii*. It is transmitted by the tick family Ixodidæ. In the Rocky Mountain and Pacific Coast states, the wood tick is the principal vector; in the East and South, the dog tick. The disease is primarily an endangiitis, especially of the peripheral blood vessels.

Description—A slightly turbid, white or slightly reddish, liquid.

Dose—*Usual, subcutaneous,* 3 injections of **1 ml** at intervals of 7 to 10 days.

Dosage Forms—3 ml.

Typhus Vaccine USP

[Epidemic Typhus Vaccine USP XIV]

Typhus Vaccine is a sterile suspension of the killed rickettsial organisms of a strain or strains of epidemic typhus rickettsiae (*Rickettsia prowazeki*) selected for antigenic efficiency. Typhus Vaccine consists of refined material derived from an aqueous suspension of the infected yolk sac membrane, and the rickettsiae are killed by means of a suitable chemical agent. Its production and distribution are subject to federal regulations (see *Biologics*, page 1425).

There are two kinds of typhus, epidemic and that classified as endemic or murine. Epidemic (louseborne) typhus is an acute infectious disease caused by *Rickettsia prowazekii*. It does not occur in the United States. Epidemic typhus is transmitted by the body louse, either by the introduction of infected louse feces through the louse bite or other small abrasions or by inhalation of dust containing dry louse feces.

Endemic (murine) typhus is an acute infectious disease caused by *Rickettsia typhi*. It is transmitted to man by the rat flea and occurs in the southern portion of the United States, Africa, Asia, and parts of South America.

Description—A slightly turbid, colorless or reddish tinged liquid having a slight odor related to the method of purifying the rickettsial suspension.

Dose—*Usual, subcutaneous,* 2 injections of the labeled dose (**0.5 or 1 ml**), at least 4 weeks apart.

Dosage Forms—1, 2, 10, and 20 ml.

Products for Passive Immunization

Preparation—Antibodies are made available commercially either as purified antitoxins or as immune sera. Antibodies to be used therapeutically are usually produced by active immunization of an animal, such as the horse (Fig. 515) or the rabbit. The serum, after collection, is processed in such a way as to concentrate the antibody-containing fraction and to eliminate or modify, insofar as possible, all other protein fractions. Sterile solutions of the purified antitoxic substances are termed *antitoxins*. Against some infections, *human convalescent* or *human immune serum* is used. The chief antitoxins are those for diphtheria, tetanus, and gas gangrene.

Basic Requirements—The basic requirements of antiserums or antitoxins are (1) proper specificity, (2) high potency, (3) maximal concentration and purification, (4) adequate dosage, and (5) administration by the proper route.

Uses—The antitoxins continue to be widely used in the immediate prophylaxis and treatment of gas gangrene, tetanus, and diphtheria, although the duration of immunity established by the injection of antitoxins or immune serums is not as lasting as that induced by

the injection of appropriate antigens. Thus, the proper use of diphtheria and of tetanus toxoids to produce an active immunity to these two diseases is much to be preferred; but after a susceptible individual has become exposed, there is not sufficient time for active immunity to develop, and reliance must be placed on antitoxins or immune serums conferring passive immunity.

The number and variety of immune serums currently in use has decreased markedly with the advent of the antibacterial drugs such as the antibiotics and sulfonamides.

Administration—Absorption of antibody following subcutaneous injection is slower than after intramuscular or intravenous injection. Therefore antitoxin for prophylaxis is best given subcutaneously, whereas for therapy the other routes are preferred. The first therapeutic dose is often given intravenously for rapid effect. The duration of adequate passive immunity following a single dose is 7 to 30 days or more, depending on the size of the dose. After previous injections of serum from the same animal, the antibody is eliminated more rapidly.

Since the antibodies given to provide passive immunity are themselves proteins usually derived from the serum of other than the human species, they may act as antigens in the human body, inducing allergy or hyper-

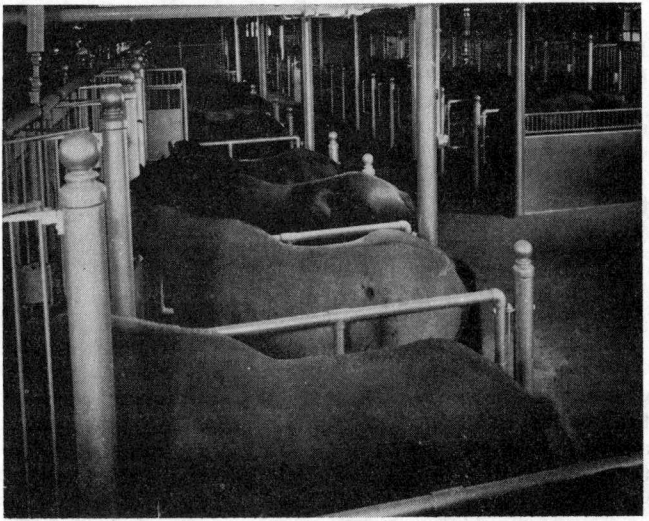

Fig. 515. Horses used for diphtheria antitoxin production (courtesy, Lilly).

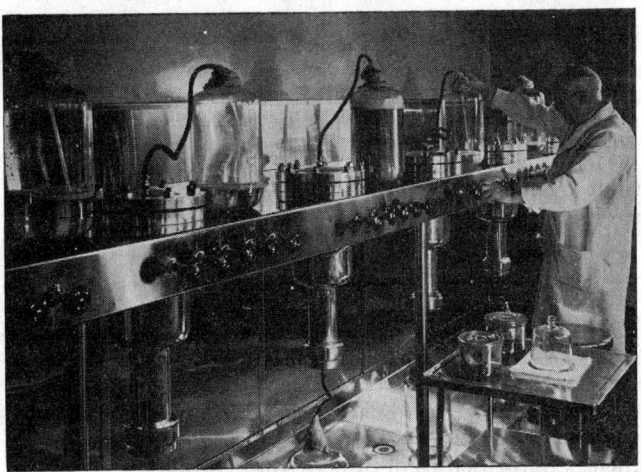

Fig. 516. Sterilizing antitoxins by bacterial filtration.

sensitivity. As a rule, the manifestations of hypersensitivity to serum preparations are mild and without danger. However, cases are on record in which fatal anaphylactic shock has followed a single injection or even an intradermal skin test. Fatalities after second injections are very rare, although alarming symptoms may occur. Every care and caution should be exercised in the administration of serums, but the possibility of anaphylaxis is not to be compared with the danger incurred in withholding serum from cases in which it is indicated.

All patients who are to receive therapy of this type should be questioned about previous serum injections (including toxin-antitoxin) or ingestion of horseflesh. A history should also be obtained as to symptoms of asthma, hay fever, or hives, since patients having such symptoms are likely to be sensitive to many proteins, including horse serum. Persons sensitive to horse protein(s), should never be given serum products. Skin and ophthalmic tests have been employed in an effort to detect those patients who will have unfavorable reactions to serum therapy. Unfortunately, such tests are not infallible. Patients with positive tests may have no systemic reaction on administration of serum, and patients with negative tests may have serious reactions.

Antitoxins (Animal)

Botulism Antitoxin USP

[Botulinum Antitoxin]

Botulism Antitoxin is a sterile solution of the refined and concentrated antitoxic antibodies, chiefly globulins, obtained from the blood of healthy horses that have been immunized against the toxins produced by both the type A and type B and/or type E strains of *Clostridium botulinum*. It contains not more than 20.0% of solids and contains a suitable antimicrobial agent. Its production and distribution are subject to federal regulations (see *Biologics*, page 1425).

Description—Transparent or slightly opalescent liquid, nearly colorless, and nearly odorless or having an odor due to the preservative.

Dose—*Usual, intravenous,* **20,000** to **43,000 units,** repeated at 2- to 4-hour intervals as necessary.

Dosage Forms—20,000 or 21,500 units including all strains in each vial.

Diphtheria Antitoxin USP

[Serum Antidiphthericum]

Diphtheria Antitoxin is a sterile solution of the refined and concentrated proteins, chiefly globulins, containing antitoxic antibodies obtained from the blood serum or plasma of a healthy animal, usually the horse, that has been immunized against diphtheria toxin. It has a potency of not less than 500 antitoxin units per ml [based on the NIH Standard Diphtheria Antitoxin]. Its production and distribution are subject to federal regulations (see *Biologics*, page 1425).

Description—Transparent or slightly opalescent liquid, nearly colorless, and nearly odorless or having an odor due to the preservative.

Uses—Diphtheria Antitoxin is a *specific therapeutic agent* against *diphtheria.*
Dose—*Intramuscular* and *intravenous, prophylactic,* **1000** to **10,000 units;** *therapeutic,* **10,000** to **80,000 units;** *usual, prophylactic,* **1000 units.**
Dosage Forms—1000, 10,000, 20,000, and 40,000 units.

Tetanus Antitoxin USP

[Serum Antitetanicum]

Tetanus Antitoxin is a sterile solution of the refined and concentrated proteins, chiefly globulins, containing antitoxic antibodies obtained from the blood serum or plasma of a healthy animal, usually the horse, that has been immunized against tetanus toxin or toxoid. It has a potency of not less than 400 antitoxin units per ml [based on the NIH Standard Tetanus Antitoxin]. In the liquid state, either as distributed or following reconstitution from the cryodesiccated product as directed in the labeling, it contains not more than 20.0% of solids. Its production and distribution are subject to federal regulations (see *Biologics*, page 1425).

Description—Transparent or slightly opalescent liquid, faint brownish, yellowish, or greenish in color, and nearly odorless or having an odor due to the preservative.

Dose—*Usual, intramuscular* or *subcutaneous, prophylactic,* **1500** to **10,000 units;** *therapeutic,* **10,000** to **100,000 units.**
Dosage Forms—1500, 3000, 5000, 10,000, 20,000, and 40,000 units.

Gas Gangrene Antitoxin

Gas Gangrene Antitoxin is a sterile solution of antitoxic materials produced from the blood plasma of hyperimmunized horses. Gas Gangrene Antitoxin Polyvalent (Globulin-Modified) (*Lederle*), has the following composition:

10,000 units *Clostridium welchii* (*Cl. perfringens*) antitoxin
10,000 units *Vibrion septique* (*Cl. septicum*) antitoxin
3,000 units *B. histolyticus* (*Cl. histolyticum*) antitoxin
1,500 units *B. oedamatiens* (*Cl. novyi*) antitoxin and
1,500 units *B. sordelli* (*Cl. oedematoides*) antitoxin.

The product contains a suitable preservative. Its production and distribution are subject to federal regulations (see *Biologics*, page 1425).
Uses—A specific therapeutic agent for use against gas gangrene.
Dose—*Usual, therapeutic,* initial dose is **4 vials.** This dose may be repeated every 2 hours if required. A total therapeutic dose may require as many as 20 vials.
Dosage Forms—Vial containing 1 therapeutic dose.

Tetanus and Gas Gangrene Antitoxins NF

Tetanus and Gas Gangrene Antitoxins is a sterile solution of antitoxic substances obtained from the blood of healthy animals which have been immunized against the toxins of *Clostridium tetani, Clostridium perfringens,* and *Clostridium septicum.* Each package of the Antitoxins contains not less than 1500 units of tetanus antitoxin and not less than 2000 units of each of the other component antitoxins. Tetanus and Gas Gangrene Antitoxins complies with the requirements of the

United States Public Health Service. Its production and distribution are subject to federal regulations (see *Biologics*, page 1425).

Description—Transparent or slightly opalescent liquid of a faint brownish, yellowish, or greenish color, nearly odorless or having an odor due to the presence of a preservative; it may have a slight granular deposit. It must be free from harmful substances detectable by animal inoculation and must not contain an excessive proportion of preservative (not more than 0.5% of phenol or 0.4% of cresol, if either of these is used).

Uses—A *specific prophylactic agent* against *tetanus* and *gas gangrene* caused by one or more of species of organisms mentioned in the definition.
Dose—*Usual, parenteral, prophylactic,* the contents of one or more packages.
Dosage Forms—Vial containing 1 therapeutic dose.

Other Antitoxins (Animal)

In addition to the gas gangrene antitoxins marketed as bivalent, trivalent, and pentavalent mixtures, some limited use is made of monovalent gas gangrene antitoxins available as individual antitoxins prepared from each of the five species which were used in Pentavalent Gas Gangrene Antitoxin NF X (ie, *Clostridium per-fringens*, *Clostridium septicum*, *Clostridium oedematiens* (Novyi), *Clostridium bifermentans* (Sordelli), and *Clostridium histolyticum*).

Other antitoxins, whose production and distribution are all subject to federal regulations (see *Biologics*, page 1425), include Botulism Antitoxin, Dysentery Antitoxin (Shigella), and Staphylococcus Antitoxin. All of these are prepared and standardized in a manner similar to that used in the preparation of the antitoxins described in this section on page 1442 and they meet similar standards.

Gas-Gangrene Antitoxin (Welchii) [Gas-Gangrene Antitoxin (Perfringens)]—Gas-Gangrene Antitoxin (Welchii) is a preparation from native serum containing the antitoxic globulins or their derivatives that have the specific power of neutralizing the alpha toxin formed by *Clostridium Welchii*. *Description:* Almost colorless or very faintly yellow liquid free from turbidity; almost odorless except for the odor of any added bactericide. *Identification:* Specifically neutralizes the alpha toxin formed by *Clostridium Welchii*, rendering it harmless to susceptible animals. *Potency:* Not less than 1500 Units per ml. *Dose:* Intramuscular or intravenous, prophylactic, 10,000 Units; therapeutic, not less than 30,000 Units. *Storage:* Store in refrigerator between 2° and 10°.

Immune Serums (Animal)

Antirabies Serum USP

Antirabies Serum is a sterile solution containing antiviral substances obtained from the blood serum or plasma of a healthy animal, usually the horse, that has been immunized against rabies by means of vaccine. It contains a suitable antimicrobial agent. Its production and distribution are subject to federal regulations (see *Biologics*, page 1425).

Description—Transparent or slightly opalescent liquid, faint brownish, yellowish, or greenish in color, and nearly odorless or having a slight odor due to the preservative.

Use—Treatment of individuals exposed to rabies infection.
Dose—40 to **120 units** per Kg; *usual, intramuscular,* **70 units** per Kg of body weight as a single dose.
Dosage Forms—1000 units.

Antipneumococcic Serum

Antipneumococcic Serum is obtained from the blood of an animal which has been immunized with cultures of a pneumococcus (*Diplococcus pneumoniæ*) of one of the types for which a serum has been prepared and which has been standardized or has been released by the Division of Biologics Standards, the National Institutes of Health. It must be prepared from healthy animals, and must be free from harmful substances detectable by animal inoculations. It may not contain an excessive amount of preservative. The potency of Antipneumococcic Serum shall be expressed in units of protective antibody, and the unit shall be that established by the Division of Biologics Standards, the National Institutes of Health. The specific type or types of pneumococcus represented shall be declared on the label.

Its production and distribution are subject to federal regulations (see *Biologics*, page 1425).

Description—Yellowish, clear, opalescent, or slightly turbid liquid.

Dose—*Usual, therapeutic,* **20,000 to 100,000 units.**
Dosage Forms—Vial containing 1 therapeutic dose.

Other Immune Serums (Animal)

Other immune serums prepared in animals include Antibrucella Serum, Antierysipeloid Serum, Anti H. Influenzae Type B Serum, Anti Rocky Mt. Spotted Fever Serum, Antitularemic Serum, and Antipertussis Serum.

The production and distribution of all of these serums are subject to federal regulations (see *Biologics*, page 1425).

For the interested student, details regarding general methods of preparation and standardization may be obtained from the Division of Biologics Standards, the National Institutes of Health, US Public Health Service, Washington, D.C.

Antivenins (Animal)

Polyvalent Crotaline Antivenin USP

[Antivenin (Crotalidæ) Polyvalent; North and South American Antisnakebite Serum]

Polyvalent Crotaline Antivenin is a sterile preparation derived by drying a frozen solution of specific venom-neutralizing globulins obtained from the serum of healthy horses immunized against venoms of four species of pit vipers, *Crotalus atrox, Crotalus adamanteus, Crotalus durissus terrificus,* and *Bothrops atrox* (Fam. *Crotalidæ*). Its production and distribution are subject to federal regulations (see *Biologics*, page 1425).

Description—Solid, exhibiting a honeycomb-like structure when viewed microscopically, and light cream in color. It is standardized by biological assay on mice, in terms of its potency for neutralizing the venoms of *Crotalus atrox* (Western Diamondback), *Crotalus terrificus* (South American rattlesnake) and *Bothrops atrox* (South American Fer de Lance).

Use—Polyvalent Crotaline Antivenin is a *specific therapeutic agent* against the venomous bites of certain species of pit vipers.

Dose—**10** to **100 ml**, followed by **10 ml** every ½ to 2 hours as necessary; *usual, intramuscular* or *intravenous*, **10 ml** of reconstituted Antivenin.

Veterinary Dose—For average size dogs, 1 to 5 syringes *intramuscularly* or *subcutaneously*, according to species of snake and size and condition of victim. The smaller the animal the more antivenin is required.

Dosage Forms—in a kit containing the equivalent of 10 ml of reconstituted Antivenin, with the accessories needed for its administration.

Spider-Bite Antivenin

[Antivenin (*Latrodectus mactans*); Black Widow Spider Antivenin]

Spider-Bite Antivenin is prepared from the blood serum of horses immunized against the venom of the black widow spider (*Latrodectus mactans*).

Description—A solid, having the characteristic appearance of substances dried from the frozen state. It is standardized by biological assay in mice in terms of its potency for neutralizing the venom of *Latrodectus mactans*.

Uses—Spider-Bite Antivenin is a *specific therapeutic agent* against the venomous bites of the black widow spider.

Dose—*Intramuscular*, **2.5 ml,** in the region of the deltoid muscle.

Dosage Forms—A kit containing a vial of freeze-dried antiserum and a vial of sterile diluent to reconstitute the contents of the serum vial to 2.5 ml.

Immune *Serums (Human)*

There are available a number of disease specific immune serums derived from humans. These are prepared from the blood of humans who have recovered from known attacks of the disease for the treatment of which the serum is to be used. Six such serums are described in the following.

Globulin, Immune Serum—see page 822

Measles Immune Serum (Human)

Measles Immune Serum (Human) is sterile serum obtained from the blood of healthy donors who have recovered from measles.

Its production and distribution are subject to federal regulations (see *Biologics*, page 1425).

Description—A transparent or slightly opalescent liquid, faint brown, yellow, or green in color. It is nearly odorless or has an odor due to the preservative. It must be free from harmful substances detectable by animal inoculation, and must not contain an excessive amount of preservative.

Dose—*Usual, prophylactic,* **10 ml**; *therapeutic,* **20 ml,** repeated as necessary.
Dosage Forms—0.5 ml.

Plasma Protein Fraction—see page 820

Mumps Immune Serum (Human)

Mumps Immune Serum (Human) is a sterile serum obtained from the blood of healthy donors who have recovered from an attack of mumps.

Its production and distribution are subject to federal regulations (see *Biologics*, page 1425).

Description—Transparent or slightly opalescent liquid, faint brown, yellow, or green in color. It is nearly odorless or has an odor due to the preservative; it must be free from harmful substances detectable by animal inoculation. It must not contain an excessive amount of preservative.

Dose—*Usual, prophylactic,* **10 ml**; *therapeutic,* **20 ml,** repeated as necessary.

Pertussis Immune Globulin USP

[Pertussis Immune Globulin (Human)]

Pertussis Immune Globulin is a sterile solution of globulins derived from the blood plasma of adult human donors who have been immunized with pertussis vaccine. It contains 15–18 Gm of protein per 100 ml, of which not less than 90.0% is globulin. It may contain glycine as a stabilizing agent. Its production and distribution are subject to federal regulations (see *Biologics*, page 1425).

Description—Transparent or slightly opalescent liquid, nearly colorless and nearly odorless. May develop a slight, granular deposit during storage.

Uses—This immune serum is used for the treatment or prevention of *pertussis*.

Dose—*Usual, intramuscular, prophylactic,* **1.25** to **2.5 ml,** repeated 1 or 2 times at 1-week intervals; *therapeutic,* **1.25** to **2.5 ml,** repeated 1 or 2 times at 1-day intervals.

Dosage Forms—1.25 and 1.5 ml.

Pertussis Immune Human Serum USP XVI

[Pertussis Immune Serum (Human)]

Pertussis Immune Human Serum is the liquid or dried serum of blood obtained from donors who have recovered from pertussis and who for the preceding 7 or more days have been without fever or other active clinical manifestation of the disease. Pertussis Immune Human Serum is suitably irradiated with ultraviolet light, and contains a suitable preservative. Its production and distribution are subject to federal regulations (see *Biologics*, page 1425).

Description—A transparent or slightly opalescent liquid, having a yellow or deep pink color. It is nearly odorless or has an odor due to the preservative. The dried serum has a yellow, creamy, or pink color.

Uses—This immune serum is used for the treatment or prevention of *pertussis*.

Dose—20 to 100 ml; *usual, prophylactic (intramuscular* and *intravenous*), **20 ml** at 1- to 2-day intervals for 3 doses; *usual, therapeutic (intramuscular),* **20 ml**; *usual, therapeutic (intravenous),* **60 ml**.

Scarlet Fever Immune Serum (Human)

Scarlet Fever Immune Serum (Human) is a sterile serum obtained from the blood of healthy donors who have recovered from an attack of scarlet fever. Its production and distribution are subject to federal regulations (see *Biologics*, page 1425).

Description—A transparent or slightly opalescent liquid, faint brown, yellow, or green in color. It is nearly odorless or has an odor due to the preservative; it must be free from harmful substances detectable by animal inoculation. It must not contain an excessive amount of preservative.

Dose—*Usual, prophylactic,* **10 ml;** *therapeutic,* **20 ml,** repeated as necessary.
Dosage Forms—10 and 20 ml.

Tetanus Immune Globulin USP

[Tetanus Immune Globulin (Human)]

Tetanus Immune Globulin is a sterile solution of globulins derived from the blood plasma of adult human donors who have been immunized with tetanus toxoid. It contains 10–18 Gm of protein per 100 ml, of which not less than 90.0% is globulin. It may contain glycine as a stabilizing agent. Its production and distribution are subject to federal regulations (see *Biologics*, page 1425).

Description—Transparent or slightly opalescent liquid, practically colorless and practically odorless. May develop a slight granular deposit during storage.

Dose—*Usual, intramuscular, prophylactic,* **250 units;** *therapeutic,* **3000 to 10,000 units** as a single dose.
Dosage Forms—250 units of tetanus antitoxin.

Immune Blood Derivatives (Human)

Globulin, Immune Serum—See page 822

Measles Immune Globulin USP

[Measles Immune Globulin (Human)]

Measles Immune Globulin is a sterile solution of globulins derived from the blood plasma of normal, adult human donors. It is prepared from immune serum globulin that complies, after dilution if necessary, with the measles antibody requirements of the US Public Health Service. It contains 10–18 Gm per 100 ml, of which not less than 90.0% is gamma globulin. Its production and distribution are subject to federal regulations (see *Biologics*, page 1425).

Source Material—The source of this globulin is blood, plasma, or serum from human donors determined at the time of donation to have been free of causative agents of diseases that are not destroyed or removed by the processing method, as determined by the donor's history and from such physical examination and clinical tests as appeared necessary for each donor at the time the blood was obtained.

Preparation—The globulin must be prepared by a method that (1) has been shown to be capable of concentrating tenfold from source material at least two different antibodies, (2) does not affect the integrity of the globulins and is capable of consistently yielding a product which is safe for subcutaneous and intramuscular injection, and (3) will not transmit viral hepatitis.

Final Product—The final product must be a 10 to 18% solution of globulin containing 0.3 *M* glycine and a preservative.

Potency—Each lot must contain no less than the minimum levels of antibodies for diphtheria and measles as follows: (1) the product shall contain no less than 2 units of diphtheria antitoxin per ml, adjusted for dilution from the 16.5% solution, and (2) each lot of final product shall contain a measles antibody level of 0.5 times the level of a reference measles serum furnished by the Division of Biologics Standards of the National Institutes of Health.

Uses—It is recommended for simultaneous administration with Attenuated Live Measles Virus Vaccine to minimize the incidence and severity of rash and fever.

Dose—*Usual, intramuscular, prophylactic,* **0.25 ml** per **Kg** of body weight; *modification,* **0.02 to 0.05 ml** per **Kg.**
Dosage Forms—2 and 10 ml.

Rh₀ (D) Immune Globulin (Human)

Rh₀ Immune Globulin (Human) is a sterile concentrated solution of specific gamma globulin (IgG) containing Anti-Rh₀ (D) antibody obtained from carefully screened human plasma by a cold alcohol method of fractionation. It contains 15% ($\pm$1.5%) Anti-Rh₀ (D) antibody contained in serum globulin, approximately 2.9 mg/ml of sodium chloride, and 15 mg/ml of glycine, preserved with thimerosal 1:10,000.

Description—Transparent or slightly opalescent liquid, nearly colorless and nearly odorless.

Dose—*Usual, intramuscular,* **1 ml,** to the immunized Rh-negative mother within 72 hours of delivery of an Rh-positive baby or following a miscarriage.
Dosage Form—1 ml.

Other Immune Serum Globulins

There are available other immune serum globulins licensed by the National Institutes of Health and recommended for the prophylaxis and treatment of specific diseases. These are prepared from the blood of healthy donors who have recovered from known attacks of the diseases for which the product is to be used.

The production and distribution of all such products are subject to federal regulations (see *Biologics*, page 1425).

The methods of preparation, description, etc, are similar to those used in the manufacture of Immune Serum Globulin.

These include Antihemophilic Globulin, Mumps Immune Serum Globulin, Pertussis Immune Globulin, Poliomyelitis Immune Globulin, and Tetanus Immune Globulin.

Other important, nonimmune blood and blood fractions or derivatives from human sources include:

Normal Human Serum Albumin—See page 819.
Iodinated I 131 Serum Albumin—See page 563.
Citrated Whole Human Blood—See page 816.
Packed Human Blood Cells—See page 817.
Fibrin Foam—See page 837.
Fibrinogen—See page 830.
Normal Human Plasma—See page 820.
Thrombin—See page 831.

More than 100 establishments hold licenses to prepare Citrated Whole Human Blood and one of these, namely the American National Red Cross, draws upon more than 50 regional blood centers.[28]

References

1. Levinson, *et al*, *J. Am. Med. Assoc.*, **125**, 531 (1944); *J. Infect. Diseases*, **78**, 69 (1946).
2. *Immunization Information for International Travel* (USPHS Publ. No. 384), rev. July, 1967. Available from USPHS, Epidemiology and Research Analysis Section, Foreign Quarantine Program, National Communicable Disease Center, Atlanta, Ga. 30333.
3. Hall, W. W., *Ann. Internal Med.*, **14**, 565. (1940)
4. Glenn, F., *Ann. Surg.*, **124**, 1030 (1946).
5. Hilleman, M. R., *Science*, **164**, 507 (1969).
6. Enders, J. F., *et al*, *New Engl. J. Med.*, **263**, 153 (July 28, 1960).
7. Ad Hoc Advisory Committee on Measles Control: Statement on the status of Measles Vaccines. *J. Am. Med. Assoc.*, **183**, 13 (Mar. 30, 1963).
8. Report of the Committee on the Control of Infectious Diseases, American Academy of Pediatrics, Evanston, Ill., 1961.
9. Enders, J. F., *et al*, *New Engl. J. Med.*, **263**, 153 (July 29, 1960).
10. Stokes, J., Jr., *et al*, *Am. J. Public Health*, **52**, 29 (Feb. 1962).
11. Reilly, C. M., *et al*, *New Engl. J. Med.*, **265**, 165 (July 27, 1961).
12. Stokes, J., Jr., *et al*, *New Engl. J. Med.*, **267**, 222 (Aug. 2, 1962).
13. Mitus, A., *et al*, *Am. J. Diseases Children*, **103**, 413 (March, 1962).
14. Report of the Committee on the Control of Infectious Diseases, 1961 Red Book, American Academy of Pediatrics, Evanston, Ill., p. 2.
15. Sprague, H. B., and Barnard, J. H., *U. S. Navy Med. Bull.*, **45**, 71 (July, 1945).
16. Ratner, B., and Untracht, S., *J. Am. Med. Assoc.*, **132**, 899 (Dec. 14, 1946).
17. Ratner, B., and Untracht, S., *Am. J. Diseases Children*, **83**, 309 (March, 1952).
18. Curphey, T. J., *J. Am. Med. Assoc.*, **133**, 1062 (Apr. 12, 1947).
19. *Public Health Report*, **61**, 1655 (1946).
20. Eagles, A. Y., *Arch. Internat. Med.*, **80**, 374 (1947).
21. *WHO Chronicle*, **14**, No. 4, 137 (Apr., 1960).
22. *WHO Chronicle*, **14**, No. 4, 142 (Apr., 1960).
23. Cox, H. R., *et al*, *Brit. Med. J.* **2** (Oct. 3, 1960).
24. Sabin, A. B., *J. Am. Med. Assoc.*, **171**, (7), 99/863–104/867 (Oct. 17, 1959).
25. Melnick, J. L., *et al*, *J. Am. Med. Assoc.*, **171**, (9), 1165 (Oct. 31, 1959).
26. First International Conference on Live Poliovirus Vaccines (Washington, D.C., June 22–26, 1959). Papers Presented. Pan American Health Organization, Scientific Publication No. 44.
27. Second International Conference on Live Poliovirus Vaccines (Washington, D.C., June 6–10, 1960). Papers Presented. Pan American Health Organization, Scientific Publication No. 50.
28. *Biological Products—Establishments Licensed for the Preparation and Sale of Viruses, Serums, Toxins, and Analagous Products, and the Trivalent Organic Arsenic Compounds* (USPHS Publ. No. 50), US Dept. of Health, Education, and Welfare, Washington, D.C., rev. Jan. 1, 1957.

This chapter was prepared by

Bernard Witlin, DSc, *Professor of Microbiology, Philadelphia College of Pharmacy and Science, Philadelphia, Pa. 19104*

Antigens may be useful in a number of ways for determining the state of immunity. They may be injected into the patient to detect the presence of neutralizing antibodies, or to ascertain sensitivity induced by infection with the organism from which the given antigen was obtained. The number of biologicals available for this purpose is relatively small.

Labeling—The package labels for these diagnostic antigens are required to provide certain specified information including the following: a designated product name; the lot number; the expiration date; the manufacturer's name, license number, and address; and for the tuberculins, the strength in terms of the equivalent of NIH reference standard per ml.

Blastomycin USP

Blastomycin is a sterile, standardized liquid concentrate of the soluble growth products developed by the fungus *Blastomyces dermatidis*, when grown in the mycelial phase on a synthetic medium. It contains suitable antimicrobial agents and a red dye certified for use in drugs by the federal Food and Drug Administration. Its production and distribution are subject to federal regulations (see *Biologics*, page 1425).

Description—A clear, red-amber liquid.
Solubility—Miscible with water.

Uses—Blastomycin is a *diagnostic aid* (dermal reactivity indicator) for the detection of North American Blastomycosis (Gilchrist's disease). Blastomycin is also available as a tine (see page 1450).
Dose—*Usual, intradermal,* **0.1 ml** of a **1:100** dilution.

Table I—Packaging, Storage, and Expiration Date Information

	Storage, °C	Expiration date,[a] months
Blastomycin USP	2–8	24
Coccidioidin USP	2–8	36
Diphtheria Toxin, Diagnostic USP	2–8	12
Diphtheria Toxin, Diagnostic, Inactivated USP	2–8	12
Lymphogranuloma Venereum	2–8	36
Mumps Skin Test Antigen	2–8	18
Histoplasmin USP	2–8	24
Trichinella Extract USP	2–8	18
Tuberculin, Old USP (Undiluted)	2–8	60
Tuberculin, Old USP (Diluted)	2–8	12
Tuberculin, Purified Protein Derivative USP	2–8	60
Tuberculin, Tine Test	Room temp.	24

[a] After date of manufacture or date of issue.

Dosage Forms—USP 0.01 ml, to be diluted with 1 ml of the accompanying diluent.

Coccidioidin USP

Coccidioidin is a sterile solution containing the by-products of growth of the fungus *Coccidioides immitis*. It contains a suitable antimicrobial agent. Its production and distribution are subject to federal regulations (see *Biologics*, page 1425).

Description—A clear, practically odorless or amber-colored liquid.

Uses—Coccidioidin is a *diagnostic aid* (dermal reactivity indicator) for the detection of coccidiomycosis (San Joaquin Fever). Sensitivity to Coccidioidin develops and will produce a skin reaction 10 to 21 days after infection. This sensitivity apparently persists for life, except in the terminal stages of the illness when anergy appears. Coccidioidin is also available as a tine test (see page 1450).
Dose—*Intradermal,* **0.1 ml** of a **1:10,000** to **1:10** dilution; *usual,* **0.1 ml** of a **1:100** dilution.
Dosage Forms—USP: 1 ml (10 tests) of a 1:10 dilution and 1 ml (10 tests) of a 1:100 dilution.

Diagnostic Diphtheria Toxin USP

[Diphtheria Toxin for Schick Test; Schick Test Toxin]

Diagnostic Diphtheria Toxin is a sterile solution of the toxic products of growth of the diphtheria bacillus (*Corynebacterium diphtheriæ*). Its production and distribution are subject to federal regulations (see *Biologics*, page 1425).

Description—Transparent liquid.

Uses—The *Schick Test* is performed to ascertain susceptibility to diphtheria. It may be applied two months to one year after active immunization against diphtheria to determine the establishment of immunity. It is also used as a screening test in persons six years of age or older who have not previously been immunized. Because older children and adults tend to exhibit unpleasant reactions after immunizing procedures, it is advisable to immunize only known susceptibles in these groups. Children under six are immunized without previous testing, because of the high percentage who are susceptible and the low incidence of reactions.

For the test, 0.1 ml of the Schick Test Solution (containing diphtheria toxin) is injected intradermally on the flexor surface of the forearm. Because of the frequency of pseudoreactions due to sensitivity to diphtheria bacillus protein, it is advisable to make an intradermal injection of 0.1 ml of Schick Control Solution (see *Inactivated Diagnostic Diphtheria Toxin* below) in the other arm. The Control Solution is made from the same lot of toxin as the Test Solution, but it has been heated sufficiently to destroy the toxin while leaving uninjured the substances responsible for pseudoreactions.

A positive reaction will occur only at the site of injection of the Test Solution. It means *susceptibility* to diphtheria. Absence of reaction is best read on the fourth or fifth day (if no control has been used, reading on the seventh day may help eliminate errors due to pseudoreactions). It is characterized by redness and infiltration which appear in 24 to 36 hours and persist 4 or 5 days. The reaction gradually disappears, leaving a persistent desquamating area of brownish pigmentation.

A pseudoreaction will occur at the sites of injection of both the Test Solution and the Control Solution. It appears earlier than the true positive reaction and usually disappears in 48 hours, leaving no pigmentation. It is occasionally seen in persons who have natural antitoxin.

The positive-combined reaction is one in which the positive reaction and a pseudoreaction overlap. Doubtful reading should be interpreted as positive. Children with positive or positive-combined reactions are susceptible to diphtheria. Sometimes a negative Schick test will be accompanied by a positive control; such individuals are immune.

Dose—*Usual, intradermal,* **0.1 ml.**

Inactivated Diagnostic Diphtheria Toxin USP

[Schick Test Control; Schick Control]

Inactivated Diagnostic Diphtheria Toxin is diagnostic diphtheria toxin that has been inactivated. Its production and distribution are subject to federal regulations (see *Biologics*, page 1425).

Description—Transparent liquid.

Uses—See *Diagnostic Diphtheria Toxin.*
Dose—*Usual, intradermal,* **0.1 ml.**

Histoplasmin USP

Histoplasmin is a sterile, standardized liquid concentrate of the soluble growth products developed by the fungus *Histoplasma capsulatum*, when grown in the mycelial phase on a synthetic medium. It contains a red dye certified for use in drugs by the federal Food and Drug Administration. Its production and distribution are subject to federal regulations (see *Biologics*, page 1425).

Description—Clear, amber to red liquid. The *Histoplasmin, Tine Test* unit consists of a stainless steel disc, with four tines or prongs 2 mm long, attached to a plastic handle. The tines have been dipped in a solution of Histoplasmin, containing approximately 4% acacia (Gum Arabic) and 8% lactose as stabilizers, and then dried. The entire unit has been sterilized by ethylene oxide gas and the protected portion will remain sterile as long as the plastic cap remains in place. Approximately 0.13 mcg thimerosal/tine is present as a preservative.
Solubility—Miscible with water.

Uses—This is an intradermal test for the detection of reactivity of the skin to histoplasmin.
Dose—*Usual, intradermal,* **0.1 ml** of 1:100 dilution.

Lymphogranuloma Venereum Antigen USP

L.G.V. [Antigen]

Lymphogranuloma Venereum Antigen is a sterile suspension of the inactivated agent of *Miyagawanella*

lymphogranulomatis that has been prepared by growing the organism in the embryonic tissues of the domestic fowl (*Gallus domesticus*). It contains an antimicrobial agent. Its production and distribution are subject to federal regulations (see *Biologics*, page 1425).

Description—A slightly turbid, whitish liquid.

Uses—Lymphogranuloma Venereum Antigen is a *diagnostic aid* (dermal reactivity indicator) for the detection of lymphogranuloma venereum (Frei test). A positive test is reasonable proof of either a healed or an active lymphogranuloma venereum infection.
Dose—*Usual, intradermal,* **0.1 ml.**
Dosage Forms—1 ml (10 tests), accompanied by 1 ml of a control suspension.

Mumps Skin-Test Antigen

Recovery from mumps, whether the classical parotitis or the more obscure systemic type of infection, produces a lasting immunity. This immunity causes specific skin hypersensitivity to the virus which may be detected by intradermal injection of mumps skin-test antigen.

Preparation—Mumps Skin-Test Antigen is prepared in the same manner as Mumps Vaccine except it is more dilute. The vaccine should not be used for skin testing.

Uses—The Mumps Skin-Test Antigen may be employed at any age for *determining susceptibility to mumps*. It is particularly useful during and after adolescence to identify those who should be protected against the disease and its complications which so frequently develop in this age group. Because of the relatively long incubation period of mumps, there is time to apply the test after exposure and to vaccinate individuals requiring protection. As a matter of fact, the test itself produces some increase in immunity. However, active immunization with mumps vaccine or repeated tests do not affect the skin reaction.

The test is performed by injecting 0.1 ml of Mumps Skin-Test Antigen intracutaneously. A control test is not necessary. The reaction should be examined in 24 to 36 hours. An area of erythema 1.5 cm or more in diameter, with or without induration, indicates immunity. Conversely, a negative reaction indicates susceptibility to infection. Pseudopositive reactions may develop in the presence of hypersensitivity to egg protein.

Trichinella Extract USP

Trichinella Extract is an aqueous extract of the killed, washed, defatted, and powdered larvae of *Trichinella spiralis*, usually obtained from inoculated rodents. It consists of the water-soluble antigens of the larvae in a buffered saline solution, which contains 0.40% of phenol as an antimicrobial agent. Its production and distribution are subjected to federal regulations (see *Biologics*, page 1425).

Note—No official standard of potency exists.

Preparation—The production method of Bozicevich[1] is used.

Description—Clear solution, which may have a slight odor due to the preservative.
Contraindications and Precautions—A survey of the literature has failed to reveal any ill effects from the application of this test. If allergic phenomena should appear, the test should not be further employed. Any allergic symptoms may be controlled by the administration of epinephrine.

Technique of the Test—The flexor surface of the forearm is swabbed with alcohol and allowed to dry. With a clean, sterile syringe and needle (27 gauge, ⅜ in.) 0.05 to 0.10 ml of Trichinella Extract is injected intracutaneously. A control injection of diluent Saline Solution Control is made in the same manner on the contralateral arm. The areas should be observed for 24 hr.

Interpretation of the Test—A positive reaction to the intracutaneous test is of the immediate type and appears usually within 15 to 20 min after the injection of the antigen. In rare cases there may be a delayed reaction which does not reach its height before 24 hr. Judgment must be used in interpreting the reaction. The formation of a wheal, the diameter of which exceeds that of the control wheal by 3 mm or more, with or without pseudopodia, represents a positive reaction to the test.

Limitations of the Test—The skin test does not become positive until about the second week of infection.[2] A few apparently normal individuals give positive skin tests. This may be due to: (1) a previously unrecognized trichinosis, (2) infestation with other parasites, (McCoy, *et al*, reported that a proportion of persons infected with *Trichuris trichuria* gave positive skin tests with trichina antigen[3]), and (3) indication that the patient may harbor either a clinical infection with trichinella or a latent and healed infection without clinical significance. Thus, a positive trichinella test is only suggestive of clinical trichinosis and should be confirmed by further clinical observations or by biopsy. Eosinophilia may be present in other conditions, including allergy, so that even the combination of eosinophilia and a positive skin test is not sufficient in an obscure clinical condition for a diagnosis of active trichinosis. After the usual latent period, however, a negative trichinella skin test does enable the physician to rule out trichinosis. Therefore, this test should be applied in many cases of chronic or subacute febrile conditions which present a symptomatology similar to that of trichinosis.[4]

Uses—Trichinella Extract is a *diagnostic aid* (dermal reactivity indicator) for the detection of trichinosis (trichiniasis). The test becomes positive during the acute phase of the disease, whereas serologic tests do not become positive until 4 or more weeks.

Dose—*Usual, intradermal,* **0.1 ml.**

Dosage Forms—USP: 1 ml.

Old Tuberculin USP

[Concentrated Tuberculin; Crude Tuberculin; Tuberculin-Koch; Tuberculinum Pristinum]

Old Tuberculin is a sterile solution of the concentrated, soluble products of growth of the tubercle bacillus (*Mycobacterium tuberculosis*) adjusted to the standard potency by addition of glycerin and isotonic sodium chloride solution. Its final glycerin content is approximately 50%. Old Tuberculin in diluted form suitable for injection is prepared in a buffered diluent. Its production and distribution are subject to federal regulations (see *Biologics*, page 1425).

Description—Clear, brownish liquid, which is readily miscible with water and has a characteristic odor.

Uses—Tuberculin is used chiefly for *diagnosis of tuberculous infection,* principally in the form of the Mantoux or intradermal test. Occasionally it is used therapeutically; initial doses are extremely small and are increased gradually as in a series of hyposensitizing

doses in allergy. Proper therapeutic use requires considerable skill and experience.

Old Tuberculin is prepared by boiling, filtering, and concentrating a bouillon culture of tubercle bacilli. Earlier preparations varied in potency, but it is now possible to standardize the antigenicity of tuberculin in such a way as to assure equal potency of all manufactured lots.

One milliliter of standard Concentrated Human Old Tuberculin is sometimes referred to as 1000 mg OT; 1 ml of a 1:10 dilution (0.1 ml OT + 0.9 ml saline) would then contain 100 mg. Similarly, a 1:100 dilution would contain 10 mg/ml, and so on. Such dilutions should be prepared fresh every two weeks.

The *Mantoux test* may be performed by injecting intracutaneously 0.1 ml of a 1:1000 dilution of Old Tuberculin. The injection is usually made in the flexor surface of the forearm. A positive reaction consists of infiltration and hyperemia about the site; it appears in a few hours, reaches its maximum in about 48 hours, and ordinarily disappears in 6 to 10 days.

Old Tuberculin also may be administered intracutaneously by pressing a 9-point applicator (Fig. 517), that has had tuberculin applied onto the points, over a previously cleaned site on the belly muscle or the forearm (also see following page).

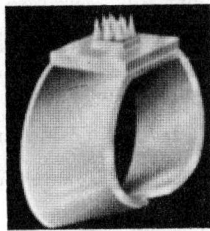

Fig. 517. Disposable multiple-puncture vaccinator (courtesy, Lincoln).

If the test is negative but there is still reason to suspect tuberculosis, it may be in order to repeat the test using 1:100 OT. Many physicians hesitate to use the 1:1000 dilution until after they have obtained a negative test with a 1:10,000 dilution. Otherwise this larger dose might be followed by necrosis and scar formation. Very occasionally, when caution is highly desirable, the initial dose is with 1:100,000 OT. If this is negative, it is followed by 1:10,000, and if still negative, by 1:1000 OT.

A positive reaction means only that the patient has had contact with the tubercle bacillus; it is not an indication of clinical activity. It is of great significance before the age of two, but after that its importance diminishes. About 90% of adults have positive reactions. On the other hand, a negative reaction is very significant in ruling out tuberculosis. It must be recalled, however, that the test may become negative in very advanced progressive tuberculosis and in the presence of certain other diseases, such as measles.

Dose—*Intradermal,* **0.1 ml** of a **1:10,000** to **1:100 dilution;** *usual,* **0.1 ml** of a **1:1000 dilution.**

Purified Protein Derivative of Tuberculin USP

[Tuberculin PPD; Tuberculin Purified Protein Derivative]

Purified Protein Derivative of Tuberculin is a sterile, soluble, purified product of growth of the tubercle bacillus (*Mycobacterium tuberculosis*) prepared in a special liquid medium free from protein. Its production and distribution are subject to federal regulations (see *Biologics*, page 1425).

Note—Do not use solutions of Purified Protein Derivative of Tuberculin that have been prepared for longer than 3 days.

Description—A whitish, amorphous powder, readily soluble in water. Is supplied usually in tablet form.

Dose—*Intradermal*, **0.01** to **5 mcg** in **0.1 ml** of solution; *usual*, **0.1 mcg** in **0.1 ml** of solution.

Tuberculin, Tine Test

The Tuberculin, Tine Test is an intradermal test for the detection of tuberculin sensitivity. It has been standardized by comparative studies, utilizing 0.05 mg US Standard Old Tuberculin (5 International Units) or 0.0001 mg US Standard (5 International Units) by the Mantoux technique. The reliability appears to be comparable to the standard Mantoux test.

The Tine Test unit is disposable, thereby eliminating the need for special equipment such as syringes and needles.

Its production and distribution are subject to federal regulations (see *Biologics*, page 1425).

Description—Each unit consists of a stainless steel disk, with four tines or prongs 2 mm long, attached to a plastic handle. The tines have been dipped with Old Tuberculin USP. The entire unit has been sterilized by ethylene oxide gas and will remain sterile until removed from its individual container. A test unit may exhibit a yellow or brown colored deposit on the stainless steel disk and/or the base of the plastic holder. This deposit is not rust but excess Old Tuberculin USP left by the dipping process and does not adversely affect the reliability of the test. No preservative is added.

Precautions—Tuberculin testing should be done with caution in persons with active tuberculosis. However, activation of quiescent lesions is not to be expected.

Directions for Use—To give accurate, standardized tuberculin testing, the volar surface of the upper one-third of the forearm over a muscle belly, is the preferred site. The skin must be clean and dry. It may be cleansed with alcohol, acetone, ether, or soap and water. Other skin areas are less reliable and quantitatively do not bear the same significance to the standardized test.

To remove the Tuberculin, Tine Test unit, hold the plastic protective base in one hand, and with the other hand, use a twisting, pulling motion on the white plastic handle—grasp the patients arm firmly with one hand,

stretch the skin of the forearm tightly, and apply the disk with the other hand. Hold momentarily (1 second) and withdraw. Sufficient pressure should be exerted so that the four puncture sites, and a circular depression of the skin from the plastic base, are visible. *The Tine Test unit should never be reused.* Local care of the skin is not necessary.

Reading the Reaction—Tests should be read at 48 to 72 hours. Erythema is to be ignored; extent of induration is the sole criterion. It is important that the indurated area be measured precisely, by close examination under adequate light and by thorough palpation. Identification of the application site is usually easy because of the distinct four point pattern. Two mm or more of palpable induration around one or more puncture sites is equivalent to 5 mm or more by the standard intradermal (5 tuberculin units of 0.0001 mg PPD) Mantoux test. This may be considered positive until further diagnostic procedures are accomplished.

Other Licensed Diagnostic Substances

Other licensed diagnostic substances for dermal tests include Blastomycin, Coccidioidin, Histoplasmin, and Scarlet Fever Streptococcus Toxin for Dick Test. Some of these items are also available dried onto prongs (tines) for skin testing (Fig. 517). Information regarding the official requirements for these products may be obtained from the Division of Biologics Standards, the National Institutes of Health, US Public Health Service, Washington, D.C.

In addition to the diagnostic substances for dermal tests, the National Institutes of Health also license numerous other biological diagnostic agents which are intended for the performance of laboratory tests; these include Blood Grouping Serums (see page 823), singly and combined, a variety of Anti-Rh Typing Serums (see page 823). Included also are Anti-Human Serum, Anti-Human Precipitin Serum, Anti-Influenza Virus Serum for the Hemagglutination Inhibition Test, and Pneumococcus Typing Serum.

References

1. Bozicevich, *J. Public Health Rept.*, **53**, 2130 (1938).
2. Schapiro, M. M., Crosby, B. L., and Sickler, M. M., *J. Lab. Clin. Med.* **23**, 681 (Apr., 1938).
3. McCoy, O. R., Miller, J. J., Jr., and Friedlander, R. D., *J. Immunol.*, **24**, 1 (Jan., 1933).
4. Augustine, D. L., *New Engl. J. Med.*, **216**, 463 (Mar. 18, 1937).

77 | Allergenic Extracts

Signs and symptoms of allergy—diagnosis of allergy—preparation of
allergenic extracts for testing and treatment—filling the allergy
prescription—federal licensure

This chapter was prepared by

George L. Phillips, MS, *Director of Pharmacy Service, University of Michigan
Hospital, Ann Arbor, Mich. 48104*

Unusual susceptibility or hypersensitivity in humans to any offending substance is commonly termed an *allergy*. The offending substance is called an *allergen*. Concentrated solutions of the allergen, for diagnosis or treatment, are known as *allergenic extracts*. Unfortunately the complex immunochemical aspects of allergy are not nearly as simple as these definitions. A discussion of immunology and protein chemistry as they relate to allergy is beyond the scope of this chapter but may be reviewed in standard text books.[1,2]

Signs and Symptoms—The signs and symptoms of allergy, often termed clinical manifestations, are legion. These symptoms range from the swollen nasal mucous membranes of hay fever to the complex afflictions of the bronchi and lungs encountered in bronchial asthma. Other common and diverse signs are hives, migraine, gastrointestinal disturbance, eczema, and dermatitis.

Diagnosis—The diagnosis of allergy depends principally on the use of allergenic extracts which are applied to the patient's skin. Three general methods of application are followed.

The *cutaneous* or *scratch test* is accomplished by scarifying or making small abrasions on the skin of the patient's back and applying a small amount of the concentrated scratch test extract. A positive reaction is indicated by swelling and redness at the point of application. The size and appearance of the reaction is a measure of the degree of sensitivity.

Intracutaneous or *intradermal testing* is performed by injecting the test extract between layers of skin and observing the reaction in the same fashion as described in the scratch test. Intracutaneous extracts are usually less concentrated as the reaction is more profound. The intracutaneous test is more sensitive and often detects sensitivity that may be obscure in the scratch test. Many and varied testing extracts are required and often as many as one hundred extracts must be tried before the offending ones are discovered.

Patch testing is a diagnostic procedure similar to scratch testing. The patch test is a contact test. A small square (¼ or ½ in.) of 4-ply gauze or blotting paper is soaked in the liquid allergen to be tested and is applied directly to the skin (inner or outer surface of the forearm or the back).

Ointments may be put on the square intact. Powders may be moistened with distilled water or isotonic physiological saline and then applied. Solids, insoluble in water may be tested as saturated solutions in suitable solvents. The gauze is permitted to dry before being placed on the skin in order to eliminate the action of the solvent on the skin.

Insoluble substances of a resinous character and solid substances may be applied directly to the skin.

Correlation of the test results with the patient's history is of prime importance in determining treatment.

If the patient is sensitive to foods, clothing, nail polish, and other items that may be avoided then alternate treatment is seldom required. Sensitivity to air-borne substances such as pollens, dusts, and molds, may necessarily require desensitization by injecting, intracutaneously, serial dilutions of extracts of the offending materials. Immunity lasting several months or even years may be built up in this manner.

Preparation of Allergenic Extracts

The preparation of allergenic extracts involves the same precautions as those required for the preparation of other injections (see page 1519). Terminal sterilization of the extract in the final container is impractical since the extracts are thermolabile. It follows that rigid aseptic conditions must be maintained throughout the preparation as sterilization is accomplished by filtration and subsequent aseptic packaging.

In the preparation of allergenic extracts the original material should be altered as little as possible. The cruder preparation is more likely to contain the allergenic portion. Allergenic extracts are stable if refrigerated and remain potent for at least one year. It is better to prepare quantities of extracts sufficient to last for at least one year so as to avoid subjecting the patient to changes in extracts during the normal seasonal treatment period.

The following general procedures are usually applicable to the preparation of all extracts: (1) grinding, (2) defatting, (3) extraction, (4) clarification, (5) dialysis, (6) concentration, (7) sterilization, (8) sterility testing, and (9) standardization. In certain cases some of these steps are omitted and, in others, portions of the procedures must be modified.

Grinding—The material to be extracted is ground or subdivided to increase the surface area and break up cell membranes since efficient extraction depends upon the state of subdivision. Three general methods are commonly used to reduce materials to a finely divided condition. Materials containing a small amount of moisture may be rapidly ground in the type of equipment commonly referred to as a "blender." Blenders are available at most appliance stores.

Materials containing a large amount of moisture may be broken up and extracted in a juice-extracting machine. An ordinary household food or meat grinder might serve the same purpose but with decreased efficiency.

The third method of grinding or comminution is by cutting with scissors or shears. Certain resistant materials must be subdivided in this fashion. These materials include animal hairs, feathers, kapok, silk, and synthetic fabrics.

Defatting—Materials to be extracted are defatted to obtain clear final extracts and to prevent emulsification during the extraction process. Foods with a large amount of moisture usually do not require defatting. Ethyl oxide is most commonly used for defatting but other organic solvents such as toluene and xylene are sometimes employed. The defatting procedure is carried out most effectively by shaking the material to be defatted with successive portions of ether using sufficient quantity to cover the material. The ether layer is decanted before adding a fresh portion of ether. Under ordinary conditions three portions of ether will defat sufficiently. The defatting procedure should be carried out at room temperature taking the usual precautions with ether to avoid flames and sparks.

All pollens must be defatted and it is advisable to save the ether extract and concentrate it by evaporation. The extractive is useful as a patch-testing material and for oral pollen oil treatment of plant oil contact dermatitis. The pollen oil is usually diluted with peanut or olive oil before using. It is more efficient and convenient to defat a complete shipment of pollen at one time. After the successive ether extractions the pollen is freed of the organic solvent in the open air, dried over calcium chloride, and sealed in a sterile glass container. When thus completely dry and defatted, the pollen will retain potency indefinitely.

Some materials contain large amounts of irritating oils, resins, and waxes. Examples are coffee, tea, cocoa, cottonseed, pepper, mustard, and ginger. In defatting these materials it is advisable to use three different solvents such as toluene, alcohol, and ether and to wash or extract with three separate portions of each. Removal of the volatile solvents may be hastened by using a fan or air blower.

Extraction—Extraction removes the active allergenic substances from the material and incorporates them into the solvent. The active fractions are proteins and polysaccharides which are soluble in alkaline solution. They may be extracted with a buffered saline solution at a pH of 8. Extraction is usually carried out in a wide-mouthed bottle which can be capped tightly and agitated, preferably on a shaking machine. While extracting, bottles should lie on their sides to expose a

greater surface. Extracting menstruums include the following:

1. **Buffered Saline**

Sodium Chloride A. R.	5.0 Gm
Monobasic Potassium Phosphate A. R.	0.36 Gm
Dibasic Sodium Phosphate A. R., anhydrous	7.0 Gm
Phenol Crystals	4.0 Gm
Water for Injection USP, to make	1000.0 ml

Adjust the final pH to 8 if necessary with either sodium hydroxide or hydrochloric acid. Sterilize by filtration through a sterile microporous cellulose membrane filter (see page 1512 for details) and package in sterile vials or bottles of suitable capacity.

2. **Coca's Solution**

Sodium Chloride A. R.	5.0 Gm
Phenol Crystals	5.0 Gm
Sodium Bicarbonate A. R.	2.5 Gm
Water for Injection USP, to make	1000.0 ml

Follow procedure outlined under No. 1.

3. Glycerinated Coca's Solution
4. Isotonic Sodium Chloride Solution
5. Tenth Normal Sodium Hydroxide Solution
6. Sodium Bicarbonate Solution
7. Glycerin Saline Solution
8. Alcohol Saline Solution
9. Dextrose Solution 5%
10. Dextrose Saline Solution

All of the extracting fluids listed must be maintained sterile and pyrogen free. Solutions No. 3 through No. 10 require the addition of a bacteriostatic agent such as 0.5% phenol.

Extraction is carried out by macerating the material to be extracted in the extracting fluid for 24 to 72 hours at room temperature with occasional shaking. If mold growth interferes with extraction at room temperature in certain preparations, they may be extracted at normal refrigerator temperatures to prevent mold formation. Extraction is improved by shaking on a machine for 30-minute periods several times during the extraction period. Bacterial fermentation may be arrested by adding 2 ml of toluene as an additional bacteriostatic agent.

The advantages of using the buffered extracting fluid are: (1) It neutralizes both acids and alkalies, resisting change from the pH of 8, which is optimum for extraction. (2) It neutralizes acids and alkalies which may prove irritating in the final extract.

Clarification—After the material has been extracted, the solvent containing the active ingredients must be separated from the inactive material. Clarification, or preliminary filtration is carried out to remove excess suspended materials which might clog the bacteriological filters used later to sterilize the solution.

The following procedures may be used singly or in combination to achieve the desired result. Materials to be extracted, especially foods, may vary from one batch to the next. Therefore the steps required may also vary. Some of the procedures that may be employed include:

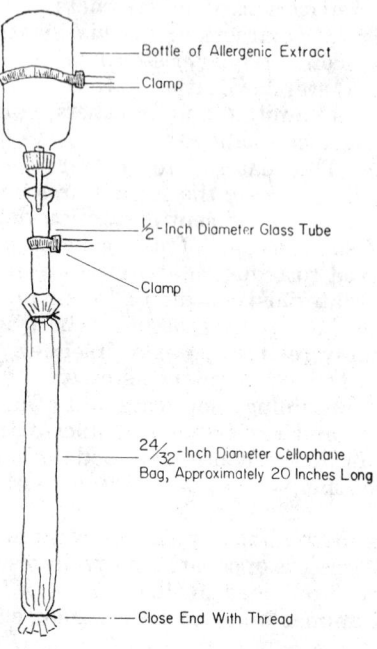

Fig. 518.   Concentration apparatus.

1. Coarse filter paper.
2. Cotton pledget in funnel.
3. Büchner suction funnel covered with coarse filter paper.
4. Centrifugation and decanting the supernatant fluid.
5. Allowing to stand overnight in refrigerator.
6. Freezing in ice tray compartment followed by thawing.
7. Filtration through cheesecloth.

Dialysis—The purpose of dialysis is to rid the extract of irritating substance and coloring material which might stain the skin of the patient. The following substances seem to give universally positive reactions unless dialyzed: house dust, mustard, potato, spinach, and beet.

Dialysis is accomplished by suspending the extract in a cellophane tube* about 3 feet long and immersing the tube in buffered saline. The buffered saline dialyzing fluid is changed every 8 hours and dialysis is usually complete after 3 changes. The buffered saline dialyzing fluid is the same formula as used for extracting. If the volume of the extract increases in the cellophane tube during dialysis, it may be concentrated to original volume by suspending the tube in air and allowing the extract to concentrate to the original volume after dialysis is completed.

Concentration—The purpose of concentration is to obtain a large amount of the active ingredient in a small volume of the extract. Most finished extracts represent a tenfold concentrate of the original volume used in extracting. The concentrating process usually takes two to three days. The same cellophane tubing described under dialysis is used for concentrating. Fig. 518 shows the concentration apparatus. A 3- to 4-inch length of ½-inch glass tubing, with the ends slightly flared, is tied to the open end of the cellophane tube and this serves as a funnel for pouring into the tube. The glass tube also serves as a means for clamping the tube onto a ring stand or other support necessary to suspend the cellophane tube in the air for drying. A fan blowing air onto the cellophane tube will hasten evaporation or concentration. To facilitate filling the cellophane bag, a bottle of the proper size containing the extract is inverted above the bag so that a glass tube inserted into a cork in the neck of the bottle runs directly into the glass tube holding the cellophane bag. Constant refilling of the cellophane bag is thus attained with a minimum amount of attention required.

Sterilization—Allergenic extracts are thermolabile and are sterilized most readily by filtration through a sterile microporous cellulose membrane filter. This type of disposable membrane filter is available in many porosities and sizes from a variety of companies including Millipore.† These membrane filters have other advantages including disposability of the filter pad and extremely low loss of antigenic principles on the filter. Filters of 0.222-μ porosity usually will sterilize the extract on the first filtration. Some extracts tend to clog the membrane filters and require an overlay of a coarser filter. All of the filter suppliers are cooperative in providing information to assist with special filtration problems.

Sterility Testing—Sterility tests for both aerobic and anaerobic organisms should be performed on the finished extracts. Either brain heart infusion with 0.1% agar or thioglycollate medium with 0.1% agar makes a suitable testing medium for both aerobes and anaerobes.‡ The sample to be tested should be shaken well down into the medium in the test tube. The lower portion of the medium simulates anaerobic conditions. Absence of mold contamination may be verified by testing with *Sabouraud's* medium.

Standardization—The potency of allergenic extracts is measured in a number of different systems.

Table I—Equivalents of Dilution Extract

1 ml of a 1:50 dilution extract (*w/v*) is equal to:
1. 20,000 Pollen Units
2. 20,000 Noon Units
3. 10,000 P. N. (Protein Nitrogen) Units
4. 0.26 mg Total Nitrogen (N)
5. 26,000 Total Nitrogen Units

Table II—Equivalents of Extracted Pollen

0.001 mg of extracted pollen is contained in:
1. 1 ml of a 1:1,000,000 dilution extract (*w/v*)
2. 1 Noon Unit
3. 1 Pollen Unit
4. 0.5 P. N.[a] Units or Cooke P. N.[a] Units
5. 0.000,013 mg Total Nitrogen
6. 1.3 Total Nitrogen Units

[a] Protein Nitrogen.

The preceding tables will prove helpful in comparing these methods. Most of these relationships are derived from clinical experience and are not necessarily universally applicable owing to variations in materials and techniques.

There are no accurate chemical methods for determination of allergic potency. Most clinicians agree, however, that the protein nitrogen content of an extract corresponds rather closely with its clinical potency. The micro-Kjeldahl method is used to determine total nitrogen and protein nitrogen content of the extract.

The experimental development of gas-chromatographic methods of analysis for amino acids has revealed possible new avenues for the standardization of allergenic extracts. It may prove possible to standardize batch-to-batch production of allergenic extracts by analyzing amino acid content, either free or derived from the proteins present. Preliminary investigation of this method has shown promise. Further evaluation will need to be done to show if there is correlation between specific amino acid content and actual biological activity of the extract.

Types of Allergenic Extracts

The following specific directions will serve to illustrate how the general procedures are combined in the actual preparation of extracts. The allergenic extracts are discussed in the following order:

1. Hairs, danders, insects, powders
2. Dusts
3. Horse serum
4. Pollens
5. Foods
6. Animal proteins
7. Sea foods
8. Egg
9. Milk
10. Foods containing irritants
11. Fungi

Since a given volume of extracting menstruum will take up only a certain amount of the active ingredient of a substance, it is necessary to extract with a fairly large volume and then concentrate the resulting solution to a smaller volume. This smaller volume of extract will then contain all of the active allergenic ingredient. In order not to have excessive sodium chloride and phenol in the final concentrated extract only that amount which should be in the final volume of the concentrated extract is used. The finished scratch extract will always contain 50% glycerin as a preservative. Propylene glycol may be used in place of glycerin for its greater bacteriostatic effect.

In the following preparation methods it will be noted that the materials have been grouped together according to their physical properties which of course affect ex-

---

* Cellophane tubing for this purpose is available from Visking; see page 2023.
† See page 1512.
‡ All of these media are available from Difco.

traction. For the preparation of items not listed these same physical conditions or properties need to be considered in setting up extraction methods.

Hairs, Danders, Insects, Powders

Camel	Horse	Orris Root
Cat	Rabbit	Caddis fly
Cattle	Feathers	May fly
Goat	Kapok	Brewer's Yeast
Dog	Silk	Pyrethrum
Hog	Tobacco	

Preparation of Scratch Testing Material— Scratch testing materials (final concentration 1:5) are prepared from the above hairs, danders, insects, and powders as follows:

1. Cut hairs, feathers, kapok, and silk into fine pieces with scissors. Powder tobacco, orris root, and others in blender.
2. Defat three times with ether. Cover material contained in a beaker with ether, stir well, and allow to stand for five minutes. Decant ether after final application and dry material in air.
3. To a sterile 32-ounce screw capped wide-mouthed bottle add:

Scratch Testing Extract

Defatted Material.................	14.0 Gm
Glycerin or Propylene Glycol........	35.0 ml
Buffered Saline.....................	70.0 ml
Water for Injection.................	244.0 ml
Toluene...........................	1.0 ml

Note that 350 ml is prepared to insure collection of 250 ml when filtered.

4. Extract at room temperature for 72 hours. Shake on machine for at least two 30-minute periods each day.
5. Filter through coarse paper and collect 250 ml.
6. Concentrate to 50 ml in cellophane tube as discussed under general directions.

Preparation of Intracutaneous and Treatment Material—The formulas given here are for the preparation of concentrated stock solutions (final concentration 1:50), convenient for storage, and *further dilution is imperative* prior to using these extracts for intradermal testing or treatment.

Intracutaneous and Treatment Extract

Defatted Material.................	4.0 Gm
Sterile Buffered Saline..............	196.0 ml
Toluene..........................	1.0 ml

Use same procedure as for scratch material through step No. 5 then as follows· Sterilize by filtration and fill into 50-ml capacity, sterile Type 1, glass, multiple-dose vials. Stopper and seal the vials, test for sterility, and label.

Suggestions for collection of material in this group are as follows. Cut hair is not always a good source of the allergen to which the patient is sensitive. More often it is the epithelial debris (danders or dandruff) which is the important factor. Combing and brushing the animal over a paper will yield the epithelial material which contains a large quantity of the allergen required to make good testing and treatment material.

Freshly plucked feathers are not allergenic. Something related to the aging process or some external factor which is introduced through time and usage causes the feathers to become allergenic. The effective material in feathers seems to be closely related to the house dust allergen. The best source of feather dust is stuffing from used pillows and down comforters which may be obtained from a renovating company.

Kapok allergen is obtained from kapok seed fibers.

Two factors in silk should be considered when making testing material. The silk sericin acts as the glue which sticks the fibers together. The sericin is water soluble and can be removed from the silk by serial washing with soap and water. The silk sericin rather than the other part, the fibroin, which is insoluble, is considered to be the portion which causes trouble in silk-sensitive patients. Therefore to obtain silk extract for testing, unwashed sericin containing silk should be obtained from a silk processing firm. Unbleached silk cocoons are another source of the silk sericin.

Dusts

House Floor Dust	Thresher Dust
Mattress Dust	Autogenous Dust
Mill Dust	

In preparing house dust extracts a more representative preparation is obtained if dusts from several sources are pooled and the extract made from the pooled material. Dust should be obtained from houses containing no dogs, cats, or other animals. Old cotton linters, employed as stuffing from used mattresses, contain the most potent quantity of house dust antigen. This material may be obtained from a bedding renovating company.

Preparation of Intracutaneous Testing and Treatment Material—The following steps are employed for the preparation of dust extracts:

1. Defat the dust three times with ether.
2. Air dry the dust then make the following mixture

Defatted Dust.....................	100.0 Gm
Toluene..........................	2.0 ml
Sterile Buffered Saline.............	400.0 ml

3. Extract, following directions under preceding group.
4. All dusts but house dust, filter through paper. For house dust place mixture in juice extractor and centrifuge off solvent, then filter through paper.
5. Place in cellophane tube and dialyze for 24 hours against buffered saline changing the dialysate three times during the dialysis. Mark tube at original volume.
6. Concentrate to original volume by allowing cellophane tube to hang in air. Use fan to hasten process if desired.
7. Adjust pH if necessary to range of 5.5 to 8.5 with sodium hydroxide or hydrochloric acid.
8. Sterilize by filtration. Transfer to sterile storage vials. Test for sterility and label.

Preparation of Scratch Testing Material—This is prepared from dust as follows:

Scratch Testing Extract

Defatted Dust.....................	100.0 Gm
Glycerin or Propylene Glycol........	25.0 ml
Toluene..........................	2.0 ml
Buffered Saline.....................	50.0 ml
Water for Injection USP............	325.0 ml

Proceed as for intracutaneous material up to step No. 5.

5. Place in cellophane tube and dialyze 24 hours against a mixture containing: 2.5% glycerin, 10% buffered saline, and 87.5% purified water. Change dialysate three times. Mark original volume on tube.
6. Concentrate to one-tenth of original volume before dialysis. Store in suitable sterile screw-capped bottle. Label.

Horse Serum

Obtain nondespeciated horse serum from state biological laboratories.

Scratch Testing Extract

Horse Serum...........................	50%
Glycerin.................................	50%

Intracutaneous Testing Extract

Horse Serum	4.0 ml
Sterile Buffered Saline	196.0 ml

Add the horse serum to the sterile buffered saline, sterilize by filtration, and transfer to suitable sterile Type I serum vials. Test for sterility and label.

Note—Dilute to 1:500 or 1:5000 before using for intradermal testing.

Pollens

Alder (tag)	Bermuda grass	Sagebrush (biennial)
Birch (paper)	Kentucky blue-grass	Sagebrush (common)
Box elder		Kochia
Maple (mixed)	Orchard grass	Russian thistle
Mountain cedar	Redtop	Western waterhemp
Cottonwood poplar	Timothy	Wormwood (tall)
	Plantain (English)	Shadscale
Elm (American)	Burweed marsh elder	Lambs quarters
Hickory (shell-bark)		Pigweed
	Cocklebur	Mesquite
Oak (mixed)	Ragweed (giant)	Mulberry (paper)
Sycamore	Ragweed (short)	
Walnut (black)	Ragweed (western)	
Willow (black)		

Most makers of allergenic extracts purchase the pollens from botanical houses who specialize in pollen collection. The most important factor at the time of collection is prompt dehydration of the pollen. Calcium chloride or hot air is usually employed in the dehydration process. Some pollen may have as high as 40% moisture content at the time of collection. There may be great variation in the antigenic potency of pollen from one year to the next.

Nitrogen content is regarded as an indication of potency of a pollen, but the protein nitrogen content is considered the most important factor. When pollen is allowed to retain its moisture content, the total nitrogen remains the same, but some of the protein nitrogen is converted to nonprotein nitrogen. Each pollen sample should contain no greater than 5% of foreign material such as dirt, gravel, and insect material. Pollens vary in cost depending on ease of collection, preparation, and similar factors. When purchasing large amounts of pollens it is wise to obtain bids from the various botanical suppliers.

Several common pollens are shown in Fig. 519.

Pollen Scratch Testing Extract

Pollen, defatted	10.0 Gm
Glycerin or Propylene Glycol	25.0 ml
Toluene	1.0 ml
Sterile Buffered Saline	50.0 ml
Water for Injection	415.0 ml

Mix the ingredients in a sterile 32-ounce screw-capped bottle. Extract for 72 hours at room temperature. Shake on machine for two 30-minute periods each day during extraction period. Filter through coarse fluted paper. Concentrate to 50 ml in cellophane tube. Store in sterile 2-ounce screw-capped bottle. For dispensing scratch extracts a 5-ml dropper or applicator bottle is sufficient to last the average allergist from 1 to 3 months.

Pollen Intracutaneous Testing and Treatment Extract (1:50)

Pollen	8.0 Gm
Toluene	1.0 ml
Sterile Buffered Saline	392.0 ml

Mix and extract as under scratch material but omit concentration and then proceed as follows. Filter through coarse paper, then sterilize by filtration. Package in sterile 50-ml Type I glass vials. Test for sterility and label.

Foods with Low Moisture Content

Oat	Corn (meal)	Avocado
Rice	Navy bean	Peanut
Rye	Coconut (dry)	Almond
Wheat	Buckwheat	Pecan
Barley	Mushroom (dried)	Walnut

These foods usually contain about 5% moisture. Powder the food in a blender, then defat with ether or toluene. Toluene has the advantage of removing the water in case the food is to be stored for long periods.

Scratch Testing Extract

Food, defatted	150.0 Gm
Sterile Buffered Saline	75.0 ml
Glycerin or Propylene Glycol	25.0 ml
Butyl para-hydroxybenzoate (10% alcoholic solution)	0.5 ml
Water for Injection	500.0 ml

Follow scratch procedure listed under pollens. If wheat or rye should become pigmented during the extraction process, dialyze against buffered saline until clear. Other grains usually do not discolor.

Intracutaneous Testing Extract

Food, defatted	5.0 Gm
Toluene	1.0 ml
Sterile Buffered Saline	245.0 ml

Follow intracutaneous procedure listed under pollens. In the preparation of intracutaneous extracts of oat, rice, wheat, rye, and barley the addition of 0.6 Gm of ascorbic acid to the formula prevents oxidation and subsequent discoloration.

Foods with High Moisture Content

Grapefruit	Carrot	Cantaloupe
Orange	Celery	Squash
Lettuce	Apple	Onion
Pineapple	Apricot	Asparagus
Sweet potato	Peach	Cabbage
Potato	Pear	Broccoli
Tomato	Strawberry	Lemon
String bean	Beet	Cauliflower
Pea	Spinach	

Remove outer peel from grapefruit, orange, and lemon before juicing. Mustard, beet, potato, and spinach must be dialyzed before concentrating.

Scratch Testing Extract

1. Extract juice.
2. Filter through paper and obtain 500 ml.
3. Add 25 ml glycerin or propylene glycol and mix thoroughly.
4. Add 0.5 ml of 10% alcoholic solution of butyl para-hydroxybenzoate and mix thoroughly.
5. Concentrate to 50 ml in a cellophane tube.
6. Package in 2-ounce screw-capped bottle and label.

Intracutaneous Testing Extract

1. Dilute the freshly extracted juice 1:10 with sterile buffered saline.
2. Filter through paper.
3. Sterilize by filtration.
4. Test for sterility and label.

Animal Protein

Beef	Lamb
Chicken	Pork

Obtain fresh whole blood from a local abattoir. Collect the blood as it drains from the animal in a sterile bottle containing the specific amount of Anticoagulant

Solution USP. Allow the citrated blood to stand in the refrigerator overnight during which time the cells should settle leaving the supernatant plasma. Hemolysis may occur if the plasma is not separated from the cells within 48 hours. Carefully remove the quantity of plasma required and proceed as follows:

Scratch Testing Extract

Plasma............................ 25 ml
Glycerin........................... 25 ml

Mix thoroughly and package in sterile two-ounce screw-capped bottles.

Intracutaneous Testing Extract

Plasma........................... 20.0 ml
Sterile Buffered Saline.............. 180.0 ml

Mix thoroughly and sterilize by filtration. Package in 50-ml sterile Type I glass vials. Test for sterility and label.

Sea Foods

Clam	Shrimp	Smelt
Oyster	Salmon	Perch
Lobster	Whitefish	

Dry fish protein suitable for the preparation of sea-

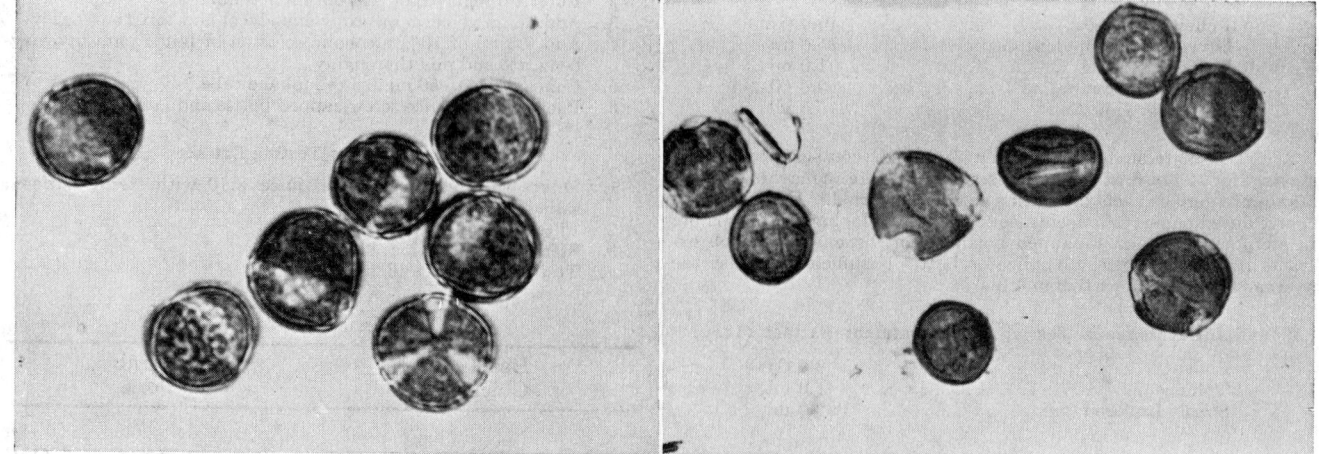

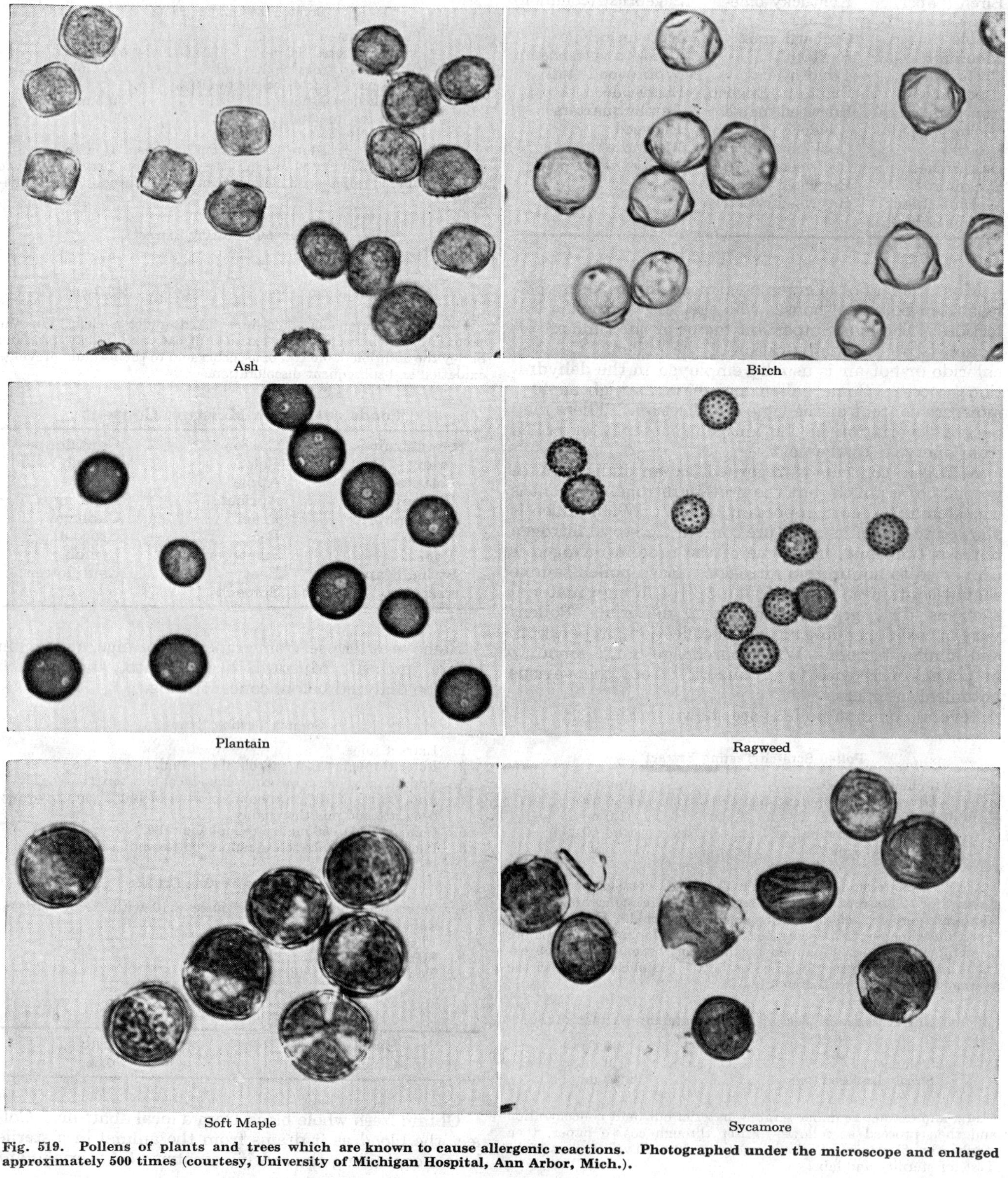

Fig. 519. Pollens of plants and trees which are known to cause allergenic reactions. Photographed under the microscope and enlarged approximately 500 times (courtesy, University of Michigan Hospital, Ann Arbor, Mich.).

food testing extracts may be obtained from Hollister-Stier, Wilkinsburg, Pa. Usually only scratch material is prepared for testing for sensitivity to this group.

Scratch Testing Extract

Fish Protein........................	1.0 Gm
Sodium Hydroxide Solution N/10.....	20.0 ml
Sterile Buffered Saline...............	5.0 ml
Glycerin or Propylene glycol.........	25.0 ml

Add the fish protein to the sodium hydroxide solution contained in a sterile 2-ounce screw-capped bottle. Allow to stand with occasional shaking for 72 hours. Then add the buffered saline and the glycerin and mix thoroughly.

Egg

Wash a whole egg thoroughly, then immerse in 50% isopropanol for 3 hours. Aseptically insert a large gauge needle through the egg shell and aspirate the egg white with a large sterile syringe.

Scratch Testing Extract

Egg white............................	25 ml
Propylene glycol......................	25 ml

Mix thoroughly and place in a sterile 2-ounce screw-capped bottle.

Intracutaneous Testing Extract (1–1000)

Egg white........................	0.2 ml
Sterile Buffered Saline...............	199.8 ml

Mix thoroughly and sterilize by filtration. Package in sterile Type I glass serum vials. Test for sterility and label.

Milk

It is generally agreed that the lactalbumin fraction of milk is the most important allergenically.

Defat fresh skim milk twice with ether using a separatory funnel. To 600 ml of the defatted milk, add one rennin or junket tablet and incubate at 37°C for 90 minutes. This procedure produces a casein curd and supernatant fluid containing the lactalbumin fraction. Filter off the curd, saving the filtrate, then proceed as follows.

Scratch Testing Extract

Add 25 ml of propylene glycol to 500 ml of the milk curd filtrate. Mix thoroughly and dialyze overnight against buffered saline in a cellophane tube. Then concentrate to 50 ml by air drying the cellophane tube and contents. Package in a sterile 2-ounce screw-capped bottle.

Intracutaneous Testing Extract

Dilute 10 ml of the milk curd filtrate with 90 ml of sterile buffered saline. Sterilize by filtration and package in sterile Type I glass serum vials. Test for sterility and label.

Foods Containing Irritants

Coffee	Cottonseed	Mustard
Tea	Pepper	Ginger
Cocoa		

This group is made up of substances containing a large amount of resins, volatile oils, and other irritating substances which might cause universal positive reactions unless removed. The irritants are removed by extracting three times with each of the following: toluene, isopropanol, and ether, in the order given. Then scratch and intracutaneous extracts are prepared from the defatted material using the same procedures as described under foods with low moisture content (page 1489).

Fungi

In certain geographic areas of the world fungi cause the majority of all allergenic reactions and are responsible to varying degrees in almost all sections. Of the approximately eighty thousand different species of fungi, less than one dozen are normally required for testing and treatment of the allergy patient.

In preparing fungus extracts, either pure or mixed, proper identification is of prime importance in order to obtain potent extracts. Classification of fungi, including methods of identification, can be found in standard texts on the subject.

Media for Culturing Fungi—Solid media are generally conceded to be best for raising fungi or molds. This medium may be prepared as follows:

Culture Medium for Fungi

Protein Casein Hydrolysate Mixture..	15.0 Gm
Agar.............................	6.0 Gm
Purified Water....................	300.0 ml

Heat the water to boiling and dissolve the protein hydrolysate. Then dissolve the agar and sterilize this mixture by autoclaving at 121°C for 20 minutes. This media should be poured while still hot into sterile Petri dishes, covered, and placed in a refrigerator until needed.

The protein casein hydrolysate mixture used to prepare the culture medium listed previously may consist of:

Protein Casein Hydrolysis Mixture

Sodium Chloride...............	11.4	Gm
Calcium Carbonate..............	3.8	Gm
Calcium Phosphate, Dibasic.....	1.9	Gm
Potassium Phosphate, Dibasic....	8.5	Gm
Ferrous Sulfate, Exsiccated.......	0.095	Gm
Thiamine HCl..................	0.0057	Gm
Riboflavin....................	0.0057	Gm
Niacinamide...................	0.038	Gm
Ascorbic Acid..................	0.19	Gm
Citric Acid, Anhydrous..........	5.6	Gm
Dextrose, Anhydrous............	778.6	Gm
Protolysate...................	189.9	Gm

Mixed Fungus Intracutaneous Extract

1. Expose a Petri dish of protein hydrolysate medium for approximately 12 minutes from the top of a high building. Collect samples on different plates on several days so that a representative group of prevalent air-borne fungi will be obtained.

2. Cover the plates and incubate at room temperature for three weeks or until fungi cover the entire culture plate. It is important to obtain the spore fraction, and growth is observed until sporulation occurs. Sporulation may be stimulated if necessary by scratching the mycelium of the surface colonies with a sterile nichrome wire loop. A potent extract of mixed fungus depends on the presence of the following fungi:

Alternaria	Hormodendrum	Penicillium
Aspergillus	Monilia	Brewer's Yeast
Helminthsporium	Mucor	

Identification of these fungi should be made by the signs described in botanical texts.

3. When sporulation has occurred and the listed fungi identified, cover the plate with ether for 24 hours.

4. Remove cover from plate and allow ether to evaporate.

5. When plate is completely dry, add 10 ml of Coca's Solution to each plate. Leave plates in refrigerator at 35° to 40° F for 48 hr, agitating frequently.

6. Pool supernatant fluid from plates and sterilize by filtration. Package in sterile Type I glass serum vials. Test for sterility and label.

Mixed Fungus Scratch Testing Extract

Mix the intracutaneous extract with an equal portion of propylene glycol and package in a sterile screw-capped bottle. The intracutaneous extract may be concentrated in a cellophane tube for preparing more potent scratch extracts.

Individual intracutaneous or scratch extracts may be prepared in the same fashion as mixed fungus by transplanting spores or whole isolated colonies to a different plate to harvest a pure culture. Ex-

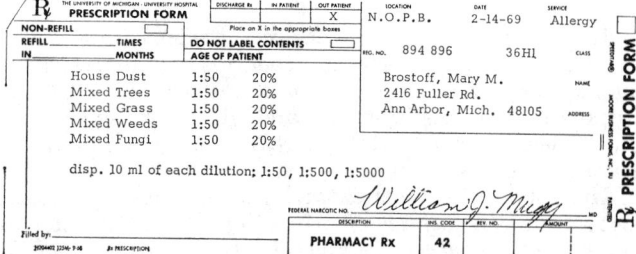

NON-REFILL			DISCHARGE Rx	IN PATIENT	OUT PATIENT	LOCATION	DATE	SERVICE
					X	N.O.P.B.	2-14-69	Allergy

Place an X in the appropriate boxes

REFILL	TIMES	DO NOT LABEL CONTENTS		REG. NO.		CLASS
IN	MONTHS	AGE OF PATIENT		894 896	36 Hl	

					NAME
House Dust	1:50	20%	Brostoff, Mary M.		
Mixed Trees	1:50	20%	2416 Fuller Rd.		
Mixed Grass	1:50	20%	Ann Arbor, Mich. 48105		ADDRESS
Mixed Weeds	1:50	20%			
Mixed Fungi	1:50	20%			

disp. 10 ml of each dilution: 1:50, 1:500, 1:5000

William J. Mugg

FEDERAL NARCOTIC NO.				NO.
DESCRIPTION	INS. CODE	REV. NO.	AMOUNT	

Filled by:

PHARMACY Rx   42

Fig. 520. Typical allergy prescription (courtesy, University of Michigan Hospital, Ann Arbor, Mich.).

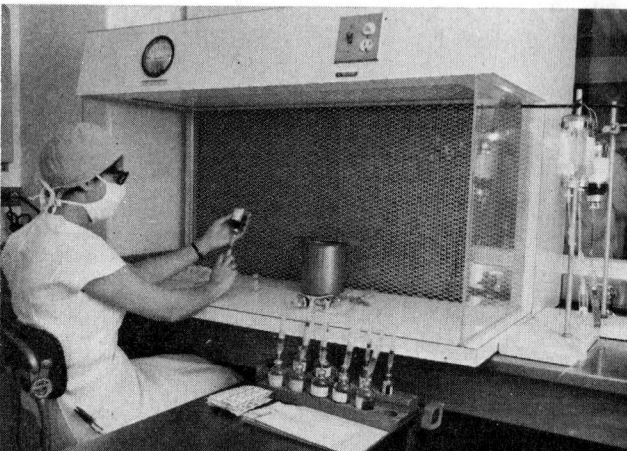

Fig. 521. Pharmacist filling allergy prescriptions. Concentrated intracutaneous extracts are mixed according to the allergist's prescription (courtesy, University of Michigan Hospital, Ann Arbor, Mich.).

traction from the plate is then carried out in the same fashion as for mixed fungus.

Repository Extracts

For quite some time allergists have been clinically investigating repository extracts for the treatment of hay fever and asthma as well as prophylactic treatment for anaphylaxis due to insect bites from bees and wasps and other stinging insects. Under ideal conditions sufficient total allergenic units would be injected at one time to protect the patient for the entire season. The extract is then released slowly from the injection site to provide the prolonged protection.

Repository extracts have been prepared by various methods such as:

1. Stable emulsions of aqueous allergenic extracts in mineral oil or vegetable oil.
2. Pyridine extracted alum precipitated extracts.

New dosage forms of this type are subject to US FDA regulations where they apply.

Filling the Allergy Prescription

As previously mentioned the allergist clinician determines the program of treatment for the patient based on the results of the scratch and intracutaneous tests correlated with the patient's history. If desensitization to a specific protein or proteins seems indicated then treatment will consist of an extract of the offending protein injected subcutaneously. Sometimes a single extract is injected but more frequently a mixture of extracts is necessary. A patient allergic to one pollen will usually manifest sensitivity to other pollens from botanically closely allied plants. Therefore it is common practice for the allergist to prescribe "mixed trees"

or "mixed weeds." The composition of these mixtures would then vary according to the pollens prevalent in the patient's geographical environment.

The pharmacist should fill the allergy prescription (Fig. 520) under a semi-sterile hood or shield taking all of the precautions required for aseptic technique. The rubber diaphragms of the extract storage vials should be disinfected with a cotton swab saturated with isopropanol 50% or ethanol 70%. Sterile 5-ml syringes are used for withdrawing the extracts from the stock bottles and then for making the dilutions. (See Fig. 521.) The most concentrated solution is prepared as follows:

Allergenic Extract 1:50

Mixed Fungus, 1:50, 30%	3.0 ml
Giant Ragweed, 1:50, 20%	2.0 ml
House Dust, 1:50, 50%	5.0 ml

This mixture constitutes the 1:50 extract. Serial dilutions are prepared from this initial bottle as follows:

Initial Extract Mixture	1.0 ml
Sterile Buffered Saline	9.0 ml

Thus the 1:500 extract is prepared and the 1:5000 in similar fashion using the 1:500 extract as starting material.

Overage to the extent of 10 to 20% may be added to the original bottle if more than the 9 ml (10 ml minus 1 ml) is required in the most concentrated bottle.

The most convenient vial for dispensing the allergy prescription is the Type I glass vial similar to that manufactured by Wheaton,* under the trade name of "Twentieth Century Line." These vials may be obtained in two neck finishes and several different capacities. A good grade of rubber stopper for allergens is the 124 stock manufactured by West.* These stoppers are available in pink, white, yellow, and green shades. Some clinicians prefer to color code the various dilutions of the allergenic extracts and the colored stopper serves this purpose. Aluminum foil closures plus the Fermpress closing tool may also be obtained from West. See page 1525 for a full description of these items.

Labels should be typewritten giving patient's name, components of extract, and date of preparation. Since the allergy prescription must be stored under refrigeration, label varnish or scotch tape over the label helps maintain legibility for identification.

Federal Licensure

The manufacturing or compounding of allergenic products intended for interstate sale, export, or import, must be carried out in laboratories that have been licensed as required by Section 351 of the Public Health Service Act. The provisions of this act do not prohibit compounding of allergenics which would be dispensed on a prescription when dispensing and administration is intended for use within the state of origin.

For a complete discussion of the Federal licensing requirements the reader should refer to Public Health Service publications No. 437 and No. 50 which are available from the Division of Biologics Standards, National Institutes of Health, Bethesda, Md. 20014.

References

1. Boyd, W. C., *Fundamentals of Immunology*, 3rd ed, Interscience, New York, 1956.
2. Wilson, G. S., and Miles, A. A., *Topley and Wilson's Principles of Bacteriology and Immunity*, 4th ed, Williams and Wilkins, Baltimore, 1957.

* See page 2023.

Part VIII

PHARMACEUTICAL PREPARATIONS and THEIR MANUFACTURE

EDITOR

Robert E. King, PhD, *Professor of Industrial Pharmacy,*
Philadelphia College of Pharmacy and Science, Philadelphia, Pa. 19104

78 | Classification

This chapter was prepared by

John E. Hoover, BSc, *Managing Editor, Remington's Pharmaceutical Sciences,*
Middletown, Ohio 45042

The various classes of pharmaceutical preparations are discussed in Part VIII. Each discussion begins with a definition of the class, followed by the official description of the manufacturing processes with appropriate explanations. The various theoretical considerations involved in the preparation of these dosage forms are treated in Part II, *Pharmaceutics*, pages 75–394.

The USP and NF include, under the heading *Pharmaceutical Preparations*, definitions for the officially recognized dosage forms. They present the general principles involved in the manufacture of some of them, particularly on a small scale. This and other information given bears on the use of official substances in extemporaneous compounding of nonofficial dosage forms.

The *formula* and detailed information for each official preparation is presented in Part VI, *Pharmaceutical and Medicinal Agents*, where the monograph of the most important ingredient of the formula is given. Cross references indicate where related monographs may be found.

The following table classifies pharmaceutical preparations recognized in pharmacopeias and other official and nonofficial compendia. The order of presentation is the same as that followed in the chapters of this Part.

Definitions of Other Forms of Medication

Application	A preparation for external use
Auristilla	A preparation for internal medication of the ear
Bacillula	A rod-shaped lozenge
Bacillum	A bougie
Balneum	A bath for general application
Bolus	A large pill (over 5 gr)
Bougie	An instrument or form of medication for insertion into the urethra or other body cavity
Buginarium	A nasal bougie
Cerates	Unctuous substances which owe their name to the presence of wax
Cereolus	A urethral bougie
Charta	A medicated paper
Chartula	A folded paper containing powder
Chartula Amylacea	A cachet sheet
Chrisma	A salve
Clyster	An enema
Collunarium	A nose wash
Collutorium	A mouth wash
Collyrium	An eye wash
Confection	A sweetened mass; see also *Conserve* and *Electuarium*
Conserve	A confection of fresh medicinal agents
Cordial	A sweetened alcoholic preparation
Cremor	A cream
Curatio	A dressing
Decoction	A liquid preparation made by boiling vegetable substances with water
Dental Liniments	Liquid preparations which are applied to the gums for their local stimulant and anesthetic effect
Effervescent Salts	Powders or granules composed of medicinal ingredients, tartaric and citric acids, and sodium bicarbonate
Electuarium	A confection of dried medicinal agents
Embrocation	A liniment
Enema	A rectal injection—a clyster
Escharotic	A caustic application
Essence	A spirit
Foment	An aqueous preparation to be applied on a woolen cloth while hot
Fotus	See *Foment*
Fluidglycerates	Similar to Fluidextracts—contain about 50% glycerin and no alcohol
Gelatin	A semisolid gelatinous preparation for internal or external use
Globule	A sphere of sugar
Glycerinum	A glycerite
Granula	An effervescing granular salt
Granule	A sugar pellet impregnated with medicinal matter
Gutta	A drop
Haustus	A draught
Infused Oils	Oil solutions of the soluble constituents of plants
Infusion	A liquid preparation made by extracting vegetable substances with either hot or cold water (the drug is not subjected to the boiling process as in *Decoction*)
Insufflation	A snuff
Inunction	An ointment to be applied with friction
Irrigation	A liquid used for flushing an area
Lamel, Lamella	A glycerogelatin disk for use in the eye
Lavatio	A mouth wash
Ligamentum	A bandage
Linctus	A viscous liquid to be sipped slowly or licked
Litus	A fluid preparation applied by means of a brush
Lohoch	A linctus
Masses	The preliminary stage of pill making—a moist adhesive mass containing the active ingredient, the diluent, and the excipient
Medicated Pencils	A plastic mass, dried in the form of cylinders, for the direct application of medicinal agents to the skin
Moxa	A cone of combustible matter used for cauterization by burning
Mull	High fusion ointments on muslin
Oculentum	An ointment for the eye
Oleate	A liquid or semisolid product formed by reacting alkaloids, basic oxides, or hydroxides with oleic acid
Oleum Infusum	Oil solutions of plant constituents
Orbicule	A sphere of sugar
Oxymel	Acid–honey preparations
Parogenum	Petroxolin
Parvule	A small sugar-coated pill
Pastille	A form of lozenge. Also a combustible cone of aromatic drugs used for fumigation
Pessum or Pessarium	A pessary—a medicated vaginal suppository
Pigmentum	A medicinal preparation to be applied by means of a brush
Pilula Comprimata	A compressed pill or tablet
Pilula Enterica	An enteric pill
Plasma	A nonfatty unctuous preparation
Pomatum	A fat saturated with odorous principles
Potus or Potion	A draught
Rotula	A globule or orbicule
Sericum Oleatum	Oiled silk
Sinapismus	A blister
Solvella	Solution-tablets dissolved in water for external use
Species	Herbal tea
Stili Medicamentorum	See *Medicated Pencils*
Stilus Dissolubilis	A pencil containing a caustic or an astringent
Stilus Unguentis	A salve pencil—cooling, antiseptic, or astringent
Stupe	A cloth wrung out of hot water and sprinkled with a counterirritant, as turpentine-stupe
Tea	See *Species*
Tela	A tissue
Vapor	Steam—plain or medicated
Vapor siccus	A dry inhalation
Vinegar	Solutions of the active principles of drugs in diluted acetic acid
Vinum	See *Wine*
Wine	Preparations similar to tinctures and using wine as the menstruum

79 | Formulation

Consideration of the physical and chemical problems inherent in the
formulation of dosage forms for new pharmaceuticals

This chapter was prepared by

Thomas J. Macek, PhD, *Director of Revision, The United States Pharmacopeia,*
Bethesda, Md. 20014

In medical practice it is rare for a drug substance to be administered as the pure chemical compound itself. Drugs are almost always administered in some kind of formulation. These may be as simple as solutions in water. More often, however, they are complex mixtures containing a selected chemical derivative of the drug compound, in proper physical form, together with excipients, diluents, stabilizers, preservatives, or a variety of other components. This complexity is not intentional, but rather is determined by the composition and nature of the dosage form and the properties of the drug compound in the formulation environment or drug delivery system.

In recent times great emphasis has been placed on the importance of formulations with the recognition that they can significantly influence the physiologic availability of drugs. It is becoming increasingly evident that the rate of dissolution or release of the drug from the formulation is of paramount importance, and that even minor changes unknowingly can greatly influence this property in some cases.

By this criterion all formulations of the same drug may not be equivalent to each other even though conforming to accepted and published general standards of chemical and physical quality. Indeed, some formulations even differ in this respect from lot to lot. When one considers such characteristics along with all of the possible chemical and physical interactions that can occur between the drug compound and the "inert" components, even with the container components at a molecular level, formulation systems sometimes become much more complex than we ever could have imagined.

The high degree of uniformity, the physiologic availability and the therapeutic quality which is expected of modern medicinal products usually is the result of considerable effort and expertness on the part of formulation pharmacists. These qualities are attained by careful selection and control of the quality of the various ingredients employed, by appropriate manufacture according to well-defined processes, and most important, by adequate consideration of the many variables which may influence the compositions, the stability, and the utility of the product.

In dealing with the formulation of new products, as the variety and complexity of materials and techniques have increased, it has become necessary to apply the best research methods and tools in order to develop, produce, and control the potent, stable, and effective dosage forms which make up our modern medical armamentarium.

In addition to the basic disciplines of chemistry and microbiology, pharmacodynamics and toxicology, and analysis and physical measurements, the research pharmacist today has need for specialized areas of other sciences.

Chemical kinetics is invaluable for a thorough understanding of the conditions influencing degradation and chemical change; application and interpretation of rate studies by means of the Arrhenius equation have been useful in the prediction of stability. The composition and usefulness of some formulations have been influenced markedly by colloid chemistry. A knowledge of various newer physiological concepts and the use of tagged compounds have contributed to a better understanding of drug absorption and excretion.

The physics of solids and gases, experiment planning and data interpretation with the aid of statistics, the methods of radioactive tracer techniques to study homogeneity and a variety of other problems, and even the principles of engineering all contribute to the solution of problems encountered in the formulation of modern drugs and the development of processes for their production.

Invariably, very little is known about many of the properties and especially the subtle chemical reactivity of new drugs when the research pharmacist is first called on to prepare suitable dosage forms. This is true for synthetic organic compounds of known chemical structure as well as for partially purified extractives from natural sources, where structure may only be partly understood, if at all. At this stage of development one of the principal tasks of the research pharmacist, therefore, is to acquire the necessary data and information relating to these properties. This must be done before he can proceed intelligently to carry out subsequent operations of preparative pharmacy.

A consideration of some of these factors will be useful immediately. It should be recognized, however, that at times important properties or changes in new drug formulations evade identification until the products are stored or even used for considerable periods of time. Frequently such changes are not discovered until more discriminating test methods are developed and applied.

Therapeutically active compounds frequently are unstable or are chemically reactive. If one keeps this premise in mind, detailed study of the properties of new drugs takes on greater significance. Information obtained as a result of the study of these properties becomes useful indeed. Intimate knowledge of the various characteristics of compounds and of various classes of compounds then contributes greatly to the experience required to anticipate difficulty and to forsee problems that may arise later during the course of distribution, storage, or use of the dosage forms. Such insight not only assures the production and consumption by the patient of drugs at optimum potency but also has far-reaching economic and legal implications. The decomposition or extensive recall of substandard products is a wasteful, expensive procedure, not at all relished by the manufacturer and all others involved.

Physical Properties

It is the purpose of this chapter to consider some of the more unusual and unexpected problems which may arise in the formulation of new drugs. While formulation difficulties are more frequently encountered with liquid preparations, they are not uncommon with solids. Many concern incompatibility and stability.

In dealing with new drugs one frequently works with compounds and materials whose properties and optimum conditions for use are not yet well known. This is unlike working with most diluents, excipients, solvents, and other additives commonly employed in the formulation. The latter generally are quite well standardized and usually are of known or more or less predictable behavior. But they, too, can change in properties and thereby affect formulations.

The kind of problem that may be encountered in formulation often can be related to the physical properties of materials, and especially of the new drug itself. Certainly, physical properties of a new drug can influence the size of the product, methods of handling during manufacture, overage additions, label requirements, conditions of packaging and storage, etc.

A detailed consideration of the physical properties of the new drug therefore is of first importance. In view of this, some important properties are considered in the following sections together with selected examples to illustrate some of the problems.

Physical Form

More than half of the formulations of new drugs in any given period of time are likely to be compressed tablets and dry-filled capsules. For such use one prefers to work with a solid form of the drug if possible and a great majority of new therapeutic materials are made available in the solid form.

However, they may be amorphous or crystalline, anhydrous or of varying degrees of hydration, and the particles may be of varying hardness, shape, and size, of varying density, and in some special instances, of varying activity and stability. The physical form thus can be of considerable importance in relation to ease or difficulty of formulation, and as regards stability and biological activity.

As an example, let us consider the problem with the antibiotic *novobiocin*. In tablets and capsules novobiocin generally is used as the sodium salt. This form is active orally. It is unstable in solution, however, and cannot be employed in liquid formulations without serious decomposition.

Insoluble forms of novobiocin are much more stable, and it has been shown[1] that the insoluble amorphous form of novobiocin acid is absorbed in dogs and in man following oral administration; however, the crystalline form of novobiocin acid is not. Furthermore, unless special precautions are taken to maintain the solid in suspension in the amorphous state by the addition of materials to suppress crystallization, amorphous novobiocin slowly converts to a crystalline form. The formulation becomes less and less absorbable and finally loses therapeutic effectiveness entirely.

In this particular case the microbiological assay of the suspension product, because it is conducted at concentration levels at which the antibiotic is in solution, did not change. The compound was stable chemically. Even the appearance of the product remained unchanged, but yet biological activity had been altered drastically purely by change in physical state.

In recent years the effect of the physical form, or the polymorphic state, on the availability of drugs from formulations has been studied intensively. Among other antibiotics, the anhydrous form of ampicillin has been reported to give earlier and higher blood level peaks in dogs and in man than the trihydrate form.

In another study[2] a close correlation was noted between the rate of hydrolysis of several chloramphenicol esters and their rate of intestinal absorption. When administered orally in finely divided suspensions both the palmitate ester and the stearoyl glycolate ester produced good blood levels in humans, but the benzoate ester was poorly absorbed. It was subsequently observed that the blood levels with the palmitate ester generally were higher than from the stearoyl glycolate ester.

Still more recently,[3] however, it was found that chloramphenicol palmitate occurred in two physical forms. Of these, Form B gave higher blood levels after oral administration of a suspension than did Form A, a polymorph distinguishable from the former by x-ray diffractometry. Indeed the blood levels could be decreased proportionally as the concentration of Form B was decreased in the oral suspension.

Adding surfactant to improve wetting, or varying the particle size of the absorbable Form B up to about 25 μ had little effect on the blood levels attained. In this case the physical or polymorphic form was of much greater significance for absorption than was particle size.

In the case of *penicillin G*, amorphous forms of the sodium and potassium salts, even when obtained by the simple expedient of evaporation from solution, have proved much less stable than their crystalline counterparts. Crystalline potassium penicillin and crystalline procaine penicillin can withstand dry heat for several hours without significant decomposition. Under similar conditions the amorphous forms would lose considerable activity.

This property is important if one is interested in depositing penicillin on a solid, as in tablet coating. Application from solution in a volatile solvent obviously would lead to greater instability, whereas deposition of a suspension of the crystalline form, even though in a very fine state of subdivision, would be expected to result in greater stability.

In the presence of acetate buffer, zinc combines with *insulin* to form an extremely insoluble complex of the protein. This complex can be obtained either as an amorphous precipitate or as crystals, depending on the pH. The amorphous precipitate is known as *semilente insulin*. It is rapidly absorbed following intramuscular or subcutaneous injection and has a short duration of action. The large crystalline solid, known

Table I—Sieve Size Information

US sieve size	Wire diam. in.	Opening in in.	μ^a
30	0.0130	0.0232	590
40	0.0098	0.0165	420
60	0.0064	0.0098	250
80	0.0047	0.0070	177
100	0.0040	0.0059	149
200	0.0021	0.0029	74
325	0.0014	0.0017	44
625 theoretical	...	...	20
1,250 theoretical	...	...	10
2,500 theoretical	...	...	5
12,500 theoretical	...	...	1

^{a} 1 μ is 0.001 mm.

as *ultra-lente insulin*, is much more slowly absorbed and has a longer duration of action. The chemical composition of both forms is identical. The difference in rate of absorption and activity resides mainly in the difference in physical form.

A physical mixture of 70% of the crystalline ultra-lente and 30% of the amorphous semi-lente provides a composition known as *lente insulin* which is intermediate in duration of action, thus meeting the needs of most diabetics. Here then, is another example of physical form determining the rate of absorption and the duration of action. Recognition and proper use of such forms enables the research pharmacist to prepare new formulations of greater therapeutic usefulness and better patient acceptability.

Particle Size

Powdered solids of commerce generally obtained by pulverization consist of aggregations of smaller particles. Sometimes the degree of fineness of such powders is stated, as in official monographs, in descriptive terms such as coarse powder, fine powder, very fine powder, etc. These terms also may refer to some standard sieve size. For many chemical powders and for many new drugs these methods for describing powder fineness frequently prove inadequate. For one thing, the powders under scrutiny, especially those deliberately made fine by special precipitation or crystallization procedures, may fall outside the range of conventional sieve sizes. The actual size of individual particles, and not agglomerates, may be more pertinent to the problem. The powder fineness and variations in uniformity of fineness, particularly in the subsieve ranges, substantially can affect the physical quality of the dosage forms prepared from these powders. In suspensions, especially, agglomerates are disrupted by mixing or milling, and the individually dispersed particles are free to move about and to form new associations, some good, others troublesome. The latter may involve changes in viscosity, excessive settling, creaming or caking, poor syringeability, and defective injectability. The flow properties of such dispersions are useful in their characterization, as are particle-size measurements on the dispersed solid itself. The physical state of a suspension is determined largely by the nature of the new associations of the dispersed solid. In some cases variations in particle size may even affect physiologic activity. An understanding of the effect of particle size on all of the properties of a new drug formulation often, therefore, may be of considerable importance. Several examples may help illustrate.

In repository injection products one generally might anticipate a slower rate of dissolution from suspensions of larger particles and a greater prolongation of effect. As a rule this has been true; an even further slowing in rate of absorption can be obtained by subcutaneous implantation of an insoluble or very slowly soluble pellet. This has been practiced extensively in the veterinary field. In the case of *procaine penicillin*, however, a solid micronized to below 5-μ particle size gave much better prolongation of effect as determined by maintenance of blood levels than larger crystals. This required a special vehicle, however, comprising peanut or sesame oil gelled with 2% or more of aluminum monostearate.[4]

In this case the gel-like structure of the vehicle and its highly thixotropic quality contributed substantially toward further reduction in rate of solution of the suspended solid. The micronized solid proved better than coarser particles in such form, suggesting actual physical entrapment of the very small particles within tiny cells of the hydrophobic structural network of the gel. Such entrapment reduced the rate at which the solid dissolved in tissue fluids. A similar oil–aluminum monostearate preparation of vitamin B_{12} in fine particle size prolonged plasma levels in man for up to 27 days.[5]

In another study[6] particle size and specific surface of procaine penicillin proved to be the two most critical parameters for the preparation of aqueous parenteral suspensions for repository effect. Here it was found desirable to control the specific surface of the solid in excess of 10,000 cm^2/Gm and to control the particle size to a relatively broad distribution. The highly thixotropic aqueous suspensions containing between 40 and 70% of such solid not only were more injectable through hypodermic needles but also formed compact, spherical depots on injection into the muscle. These depots accounted for the prolonged therapeutic response observed.

The need for fine solid particles for use in the preparation of suspensions of the adrenocortical steroids was made necessary by the unusual application of such products in the eye. Ophthalmic application of fluids containing suspended solid was without precedent, but the finely divided solid had to be prepared sterile and suspended aseptically in a sterilized vehicle. Particle size also proved important in preparations of suspensions of the adrenocortical steroids for injection into the joint. Large crystals left the patient with a feeling of sand or gritty particles in the injected area; on the other hand, suspensions made with extremely fine particles, usually below 10 μ, were much better tolerated.

The effect of particle size on the systemic properties of medicinals given by inhalation aerosol has been investigated.[7] Indeed, the particle size of such aerosols must be rigidly controlled between 0.5 and 4 μ for optimum penetration into the bronchial tree.

Beginning with the observation that several microcrystalline sulfonamide compounds were better and more rapidly absorbed orally than were ordinary larger particles, the study of the dissolution properties of drugs and their significance in drug absorption has attained considerable attention in recent years. The microcrystalline sulfonamide particles provided a much greater surface for dissolution than similar macro particles. The surface was more easily wetted by the solvent, and the particles therefore dissolved at a faster rate, yielding solutions of higher concentration. Similarly, a correlation between particle size, rate of dissolution, and oral absorption of drugs such as griseofulvin, chloramphenicol, tolbutamide, spironolactone, medroxyprogesterone acetate, sulfisoxazole, and aspirin has been described. Analogous behavior has been experienced with the nonsteroidal anti-inflammatory

Table II—Particle Size Measurement

Method	Useful limits
Sieve	Above 40 μ
Optical microscope	0.25–100 μ
Electron microscope	0.004–1 μ
Gas adsorption	0.002–20 μ
Sedimentation[a]	1–50 μ
Light-scattering, light-blockage, change in electrical resistance[b]	1–100 μ

[a] Includes Sharples Air Sedimentation, Micromerograph, Andreason Pipette.
[b] Coulter Counter, Royco Counter.

compound, indomethacin, an organic acid of low water solubility. On the other hand, with nitrofurantoin,[8] it was discovered that there was an optimal average crystal size of about 150-mesh, which reduced emesis in dogs while still permitting ample urinary excretion of this antibacterial agent for efficacy in urogenital tract infections.

Rate of dissolution of an active ingredient can be altered adversely, however, by improper choice of tablet or capsule ingredients and by other formulation factors despite the use of solids of appropriate fineness.[9] Because of compaction during tablet manufacture or capsule filling, hydrophobicity imparted by tablet lubricants, adsorption of air on the particle surface, a surface charge, etc, fine particles often may prove more slowly soluble than larger particles. These properties, therefore, must be recognized and treated appropriately in the course of good formulation.

An unusual example of retardation of dissolution time was reported for aluminum aspirin in a basic aqueous medium due to the formation of a basic water-insoluble aluminum compound on the surface of the drug solid. The formation of this film was prevented by the addition of the sequestrant EDTA.[10]

The importance of particle size, rate of dissolution, and formulation properties on drug absorption and therapeutic effectiveness are dramatically illustrated in a report of inactive Prednisone Tablets USP XVI. Despite adequate disintegration, the sample was without therapeutic effect, which was explainable by its poor dissolution.[11]

Differences in physiological activity between the free and colloidal forms of elements such as sulfur, silver, gold, bismuth, and mercury, or their inorganic salts, can be attributed, at least in part, to the smaller particle size of the colloidal form. In the field of entomology this behavior is well known since the effectiveness and toxicity of many insecticides depend on their fineness of particle-size subdivision.

Crystal Form

It is well known that a given chemical substance sometimes may exist in more than one crystal form, depending on conditions under which crystallization occurred. It is also well known that crystals change from one form into another. In the case of sulfur, for example, crystallization in the *monoclinic* system occurs at temperatures above 95.6°C, but at lower temperatures, the element crystallizes in the *rhombic* form. The temperature at which a crystal changes from one form to another is termed its *transition* temperature. Rhombic sulfur is metastable above, and monoclinic sulfur is metastable below, the transition point. Both forms, however, can be obtained in the metastable state, and the transformation to the stable form may vary greatly, taking place at an extremely slow rate sometimes or quite rapidly at other times. However, the transition will occur eventually, and the velocity of the transformation can be influenced in a number of different ways.

New drug compounds sometimes are obtained in crystal forms that prove metastable in the final formulation, especially of the suspension type. The form obtained from crystallization solvents need not necessarily be the one best suited for aqueous systems, or even for solid formulations. Transformation to a more stable state in aqueous suspensions sometimes may be accompanied by significant growth in particle size, change in viscosity, excessive sedimentation, or even caking. Any one of these changes is objectionable and may, in fact, lead to physically deteriorated products. Furthermore, it is usually not possible to predict changes in crystal form in advance, and the existence of a more stable modification may not be recognized until a transformation actually takes place. The research pharmacist must do everything possible to assure that such changes will not occur in suspension products once distributed for marketing and use by the patient.

Changes in crystal form have been observed by the author and others[12,13] in suspensions of cortisone acetate. Such changes also have occurred in suspensions of hydrocortisone acetate and undoubtedly occur quite frequently in many other pharmaceutical suspensions but go unrecognized. Sometimes, microscopic examination will reveal alterations in crystal form, particularly if there has been a simultaneous increase in particle size or if the crystals involved are quite different in appearance.

Other ways for studying such changes employ x-ray diffraction and hot-stage microscopy. Differential thermal analysis and differential scanning colorimetry likewise can provide useful information.

In the case of cortisone acetate at least five different crystal forms have been distinguished by x-ray. Under anhydrous conditions Forms 1 and 3 have been obtained as microcrystalline solids with particles predominantly less than 10 μ in size. These forms are stable under anhydrous conditions and can be used in solid formulations, including tablets and ointments comprising an anhydrous base. Aqueous suspensions of these forms, although acceptable when first made, invariably revert to a hydrated Form 5 crystal on standing. Recrystallization has occurred more readily when the suspension was exposed to a rapid change from a warm to a cool temperature. Recrystallization invariably is accompanied by crystal growth, excessive settling of the larger particles, and their welding together to form a solid caked layer on the bottom of the container if left undisturbed.

To preserve Form 5, which can be crystallized in the presence of water, it has been necessary to avoid drying and to employ the solid in the formulation of products in the form of a wet cake. Another solution of the problem of crystal reversion is to employ additives, gums, or dispersion stabilizers to suppress crystallization. This is more often possible in oral suspensions than in suspensions intended for use in the eye or by injection.

More recently, a crystalline form of cortisone acetate was described similar to anhydrous Form 3. It was found stable in aqueous suspensions, provided the particles were maintained in the 40–60 μ range. Four phases of each of the *tert*-butylacetate esters of hydrocortisone and prednisolone have been described.[14]

The dissolution rate behavior of the polymorphic forms of sulfathiazole and methylprednisolone has been reported,[15] as have been the heats of transition.[16] The polymorphic forms of chloramphenicol palmitate and stearate were studied by IR spectrophotometry.[17]

In the formulation of a new product the research pharmacist is confronted with the delicate problem of determining in a short time if his suspension is in a stable physical state. In the absence of knowledge of the stable form it is wise to subject the product to extremes of temperature and motion and even to do this in rapid succession, with an aim toward inducing a change in crystal form, if such change is to occur. Thus, alternate storage of a suspension product between 50° and 5°C, sometimes freezing, is extremely useful in judging the stability of the crystal form of the suspended solid. If crystal forms other than that used in suspension are available, samples of the product should be seeded with such forms during this treatment.

Very often a new compound may occur in several different crystal habits, all apparently stable in suspension, but one may be preferred for pharmaceutical use over the others. Thus, procaine penicillin has been obtained as prismatic, rodlike crystals, and as flat, scalelike platelets. Both crystals are of the same form as determined by x-ray diffraction; the platelets are produced in the presence of a protective colloid during crystallization. The plateletlike crystal has exhibited advantages for the preparation of sterile, dry penicillin formulations where bulk and injectability were a troublesome problem. The theory of coarse suspension formulation and problems of pharmaceutical suspensions relating to crystal properties recently have been reviewed.[18]

Bulk Control

In the interest of convenience to the patient it sometimes becomes necessary to alter the bulk of a new drug to provide a more acceptable size of a solid dosage form. Thus, a 250-mg dose of a bulky compound may require a No. 0 gelatin capsule, but a No. 1 would be more acceptable.

The bulk of a powder can be defined as the sum of the true bulk (ie, the volume occupied by 1 Gm of the densest solid form) and the variable free air space. Alteration in bulk therefore involves changing the free air space by variation of the size and shape of the particles by physical (milling, screening, bulk rolling, and wetting) or chemical (crystallization) methods. Milling tends to make particles more spherical, thus generally lowering bulk, provided that an excess of air is not also adsorbed by the finer powder.

Screening may produce a fraction of powder with lesser bulk, while that portion retained on the screen usually has a higher bulk. Compression rolling, or compaction, of powders functions to reduce the air space, as does dry compression (slugging) on a tablet machine. When the slugs or masses produced by compression rolling are subsequently milled, more spherical particles are produced having a lesser bulk. Sometimes the bulk of a powder can be reduced appreciably simply by subjecting the powder to a vacuum to remove excess air. If the material is stable, it can be moistened with a solvent in which it has partial solubility. The solvent is removed by drying at a slightly elevated temperature, frequently yielding a dry powder of somewhat greater density.

The control of bulk by chemical means involves alterations in conditions of crystallization or precipitation to yield more dense solids. A number of variables such as temperature, concentration of reactants, rate of addition and agitation, duration of digestion, and choice of solvent may be altered in attempts to obtain the desired bulk. Seeding also is important, as is rate of cooling.

Frequently the research pharmacist is confronted with the problem of making suitable dosage forms of bulky materials administered in large daily doses. If it is not feasible to administer the large dose, eg, 5 Gm, or more per day, as tablets or capsules, consideration usually is given to the preparation of liquid dosage forms, either ready-made or for extemporaneous preparation at time of use by the patient. Such formulations have been required for some antacids, adsorptive resins, and sulfonamide–antibiotic mixtures. Often, a dry form of product is required for reasons of stability as well as bulk. Dry forms of several antibiotics have been prepared in such form for pediatric use because of a child's inability to swallow capsules or tablets.

A more bulky material often is desired for use in ready-made suspensions where excessive settling may be a problem, or a greater degree of thixotropy is wanted. Here again, the method of precipitation or crystallization of the material may be pertinent. A more bulky powder can be obtained by milling to a more finely divided state, or even precipitation in the final vehicle may be worthy of study. There is much to be said for the use of wet-cakes in preparing suspensions. Such techniques are practiced to a large extent in fields outside of pharmacy, as in the preparation of pigments for the manufacture of paints.

Sometimes the appearance of greater bulk is desired in suspensions having only small amounts of insoluble solids, as with some of the more potent, insoluble steroids. Uniformity of dosage then becomes a problem requiring a product that does not settle rapidly. The use of materials to increase viscosity, where applicable, or to increase density of the suspending vehicle is of considerable value in such situations.

Solubility

Only three types of solutions are generally encountered in pharmaceutical new drug formulations. These are (1) solutions of solids in liquids, which comprises the most important category; (2) solutions of liquids in liquids; and (3) solutions of gases in liquids. The variety of pharmaceutically useful solvents is limited, especially for oral or parenteral use. In dealing with new drugs, either in solid or liquid form, it is desirable and useful to learn something of approximate solubility early in the course of experimentation.

When a solution is in equilibrium with a solid at a given temperature, the solution is said to be saturated; the concentration of the solute in that solution is known as the solubility at that temperature. In dissolving a solid in a liquid it is necessary for the crystal lattice of the solid to break down into the molecules and ions of which it is built. A factor of great importance in this breakdown is the high dielectric constant of the solvent and the polarity of both the solvent and solute molecules. In the case of sodium chloride, water, which is highly polar and has a high dielectric constant, supplies the energy required to fracture the ionic bonds and the salt dissolves. The ions derived from sodium chloride fill the volume of the solvent until the solution becomes saturated. In most cases heat is absorbed during the process of dissolving a salt; if there is interaction between ions and solvent, heat may be evolved. The mechanism of this interaction or solvation is not well understood. It is worth noting, however, that hydroxyl derivatives such as water, glycols and alcohols, and organic acids are the best salt solvents, followed by ammonia and amines. This list is in order of decreasing polarity of the solvents.

Because of its ionic character sodium chloride also is very polar and therefore dissolves most readily in water. Other organic compounds possess polarity but not to so great an extent as the inorganic electrolyte, sodium chloride, and therefore differ in their solubility. Nonpolar solvents such as hydrocarbons, although poor for polar solutes, usually dissolve other materials

Table III—Solubility (Gm/100 ml) of Phenobarbital in Water–Glycerin–Ethanol Mixtures[a] at 25°C[19]

Ethanol	Glycerin					
	0%	10%	20%	30%	60%	80%
0%	0.12	0.19	0.20	0.21	0.37	0.66
10%	0.19	0.22	0.30	0.37	0.84	1.59
20%	0.30	0.42	0.57	0.83	2.11	4.13
30%	0.64	0.93	1.35	1.89	4.45	...
60%	5.33	7.47	9.19	11.23	14.25	...
80%	11.56	13.58	16.27	...	...	...

[a] Mixtures represent % by volume. Where the sum of the percentages of ethanol and glycerin mixtures does not equal 100, the difference is water

of low polarity including fixed oils and hydrocarbons.

There are several ways for determining solubility. The principal method is to agitate the solvent with an excess of the powdered solute until there is no further change in concentration. Sufficient time should be allowed for equilibrium to become established. However, in dealing with small quantities of precious or expensive new drugs it is often necessary to determine solubility with as little solute as possible. In such cases the careful technique of adding small, accurately weighed increments (milligrams) of solute to a small, weighed quantity of solvent until no more dissolves probably is most expeditious and provides reasonably accurate solubility information.

A solvent may cause no permanent change in the solute or it may react with the solute and thereby solubilize as a result of contact with it (eg, inorganic or organic acids or bases and some organic solvents). In dealing with new compounds of low solubility it is desirable to approach the saturation concentration by stirring an excess of solute with solvent and also by allowing a warm solution containing excess solute to cool and reach equilibrium at the desired temperature. Frequently a difference in solubility by these two methods may be a clue to an unsuspected reaction of solute with solvent or a change in phase resulting from passage through a transition temperature to which the system had been heated. A marked difference in solubility also may be indicative of a strong tendency for supersaturation. This occurrence has been quite commonly observed among the adrenocortical steroids, for example.

Supersaturation probably occurs because the submicroscopic crystals, which would normally be the first to deposit, have a higher solubility than larger particles of the solute, and the process of crystallization has difficulty in getting started. When a supersaturated solution is seeded with a larger particle or crystal of the solute, the amount of solute in excess of saturation may crystallize immediately. In this connection it is also interesting to note that if a mixture of large crystals and very small ones is allowed to stand, the small

Table IV—Solubility of Sucrose in Water–Ethanol Mixtures at 25°C[23]

Ethanol vol. %	Sucrose gm/100 ml
0	90
10	85
20	80
30	70
40	60
50	50
60	40
70	25
80	10

crystals tend to disappear and the larger ones increase in size. Occasionally this phenomenon can be observed in pharmaceutical suspensions such as the aqueous suspensions of the adrenocortical steroids. This behavior also serves as a basis for rendering fine precipitates such as barium sulfate more suitable for filtration in quantitative analytical procedures.

The solubility of new drugs in mixtures of solvents containing even as few as two components is not easily estimated from data of solubility of the compound in each of the pure solvents alone. It is best determined by actual experimentation; yet mixtures of two, three, or more solvents are very common and are of vital importance to pharmaceutical formulation. Except for water or a fixed oil, none of the useful solvents are administered orally or by injection as is; they are always administered in some form of solvent mixture. One generalization may be useful. If a solute has good solubility in an alcohol or a polyhydroxy compound alone (eg, glycerin or propylene glycol) and limited solubility in water, addition of one or more of the hydroxy compounds invariably will improve its solubility in the aqueous mixture.[19-22] The reverse also is generally true. If a solute has good solubility in water but limited solubility in alcohol or a polyhydroxy compound, addition of the latter will decrease solute concentration in the aqueous mixture.[23] The latter problem has particular significance in the formulation of soluble aerosol products using liquefied fluorinated hydrocarbon propellants. These possess low polarity, are poorly miscible with many pharmaceutical solvents and in addition, limit the solubility of new drugs in the solvent–propellant systems. See also the chapter on *Aerosols*, page 1729.

An interesting use of an approximate dielectric constant to blend solvent systems for new drug formulation has been described by Moore[24] and applied in solubility studies with secobarbital.[25] Others also have examined the correlation between solubility and dielectric constants in pharmaceutical systems.[26] Several other points may prove helpful with problems regarding solubility. If there is structural similarity between solute and the solvent or solvent mixture, solubility is likely to be greater. Solvation or hydrogen bonding increases solubility, often above predicted values, and may be imparted by the addition of appropriate solvents to a mixture. Thus, polar groupings such as OH, CHOH, CH_2OH, COOH, NH_2, and SO_3H, generally increase solubility of organic compounds in water, whereas nonpolar or weakly polar additives reduce solubility. The greater the number of carbon atoms in a homologous series, the more the members become like the hydrocarbons from which they were derived. Introduction of halogens into compounds tends to reduce solubility; branching of chains generally increases solubility. Finally, because a solvent must disrupt molecular association to dissolve, solid compounds of high molecular aggregation, or compounds with high melting points, are generally more difficult to dissolve, as are many polymers or compounds of high molecular weight.

Occasionally in new drug formulation some use can be made of the observation that like structures may dissolve in a given solvent more or less independently of the concentration of the other. Thus, one finds that a saturated aqueous solution of cortisone will also dissolve a significant amount of hydrocortisone and perhaps even a third steroid such as prednisolone.

In some problems of formulation, particularly with slightly soluble salts, it may be desirable to reduce solubility of the compound. In any system in which solid is in equilibrium with its solution, the solubility product is determined by the product of its ion concentrations. If one of the ions involved is added as a different, more soluble salt, the solubility product is exceeded. Consequently, a portion of the first compound will be precipitated. In other words, a compound having an ion in common with a slightly soluble salt decreases the solubility of the latter by means of the common-ion effect. The extent of the repression of solubility can be calculated if the concentration of the common ion in excess is known.[27]

The repression of the solubility of a new drug by the common-ion effect may have great practical significance in improving the stability of some formulations. The principle has been applied, for example, in stabilization of aqueous suspensions of procaine penicillin by the addition of procaine hydrochloride.

Rate of solubility of new drugs may be an important consideration. A marked difference was found in the rate with which several different salts of theophylline dissolved at hydrogen-ion concentrations analogous to those encountered after oral administration. These studies tended to explain the reasons for the clinical differences observed with these salts. The blood levels after oral administration were higher and more prolonged for the choline and isopropanolamine salts than for the ethylenediamine salt. This difference apparently was attributed to the differences observed in the rate of solution of each compound.[28] Since this early work, the dissolution rate and influence on absorption of a great many drug compounds have been similarly studied.

Generally, rate of solubility of most soluble materials can be increased by *lyophilization*. Rate of solution or dispersion of a number of pharmaceutical gums and suspending agents also was increased markedly by lyophilization. These included sodium carboxymethylcellulose, Veegum, polyethylene glycol 6000, acacia, tragacanth, sodium alginate, bentonite, agar, and pectin.[29] Gelatin or mannitol have been used in lyophilization of active medicinals for a long time either to provide a good structural form or "plug" in the lyophilized product. They thus aid substantially in increasing the rate of solution of this dosage form.

Wetting of Solids

The preparation of suspensions of insoluble new drugs involves some consideration of "wettability." The process also may be of concern in wet granulation of insoluble compounds for tablet compression (page 1655). *Wetting* is a process by which a liquid comes in contact with a solid particle to form a solid–liquid interface. Three things can happen. The liquid can spread over the solid, displacing adsorbed gases and wetting the solid completely. The liquid does not spread over the solid but remains as a drop or lens (nonwetting). The liquid spreads partially, forming a junction at the solid with a finite contact angle. The last situation occurs most frequently, and the concept of the *contact angle*, or wetting angle, has been developed as a means of measuring the spreading of liquid over solid surfaces. If the liquid is water and spreads over the solid surface easily, the contact angle is less than 90° and the solid is said to be hydrophilic. In wetting the solid the liquid has to displace substantial quantities of air adsorbed on the surface of the powder in order to wet that surface. A solid is said to be hydrophobic if it is not easily wet by water because the solid–air

Table V—Suppression of Solubility of Procaine Penicillin by Procaine Hydrochloride

% Procaine HCl Added	Procaine Penicillin, Gm/L
0	5.9
0.5	3.4
1.0	2.1
2.0	1.6
3.0	1.5

interface cannot be readily displaced; the resulting contact angle is greater than 90°. Similarly, when hydrophilic solids are immersed in nonpolar solvents or oils, the surface contains adsorbed moisture and is in effect analogous to a water surface that is not easily wet by oil.

The wetting of a solid surface can be altered one way or the other by the use of additives, generally termed *wetting agents*. These are compounds which, when added to water or other liquid, favor the replacement of the solid–air interface by a solid–liquid interface. To be efficient, the wetting agent must (1) concentrate at the solid–liquid interface and thus reduce the contact angle (reduce liquid–solid interfacial tension) and (2) diffuse rapidly to the solid–liquid interface from the bulk of the liquid. Most wetting agents are of the type which facilitate the wetting of solids by water or aqueous solutions. Some of these, therefore, are useful in formulation of pharmaceutical suspensions, although the list is not large because of toxicity limitations, especially for use in parenterals.[30]

Some wetting agents increase the affinity of solids for oil rather than for water. This phenomenon is made use of in the paint industry in the "flushing" of inorganic pigments that are more easily ground in water rather than in the dry state or with organic solvents. These agents (eg, fatty amines or fatty quaternary ammonium salts) appear to function by adsorbing on the particle surface with the hydrophilic group attached to the solid and the hydrophobic group directed outward into the aqueous phase. The net effect is that the particles are more hydrophobic than before and, thus, become more easily wetted by oil or other low-polar liquids. This, too, can be made use of in some formulations involving a fatty or oleaginous vehicle.

A number of substances such as sodium hexametaphosphate, polyvinyl alcohol, and sodium carboxymethylcellulose are often used with wetting agents in commercial detergents. They function to improve the dispersion or deflocculation of solid particles and thus prevent redeposition of the solid on the articles being washed. Use of similar compounds in the preparation of pharmaceutical suspensions is not without precedent as indicated by the following composition for a parenteral suspension of cortisone acetate.

Cortisone acetate, microfine	25 mg
Polysorbate 80 (wetting agent)	4 mg
Sodium CMC (detergent synergist)	5 mg
Sodium chloride (for isotonicity)	9 mg
Benzyl alcohol (preservative)	9 mg
Water for injection, to make	1 ml

Flow, Cohesiveness, and Compressibility

Inasmuch as compressed tablets comprise the most important dosage form of new drugs, this chapter would be incomplete without brief mention of some of the physical properties important to their manufacture. The physics of tablet compression has been the subject of extensive studies by Higuchi and Busse and their associates.[31]   However, with the introduction of equipment for compression coating, multilayer compression, and high-speed tablet compression, it appears that greater attention needs to be given to those physical properties of tablet granulations having to do with free flow, cohesiveness, and compressibility.

A discussion of the significance of the *angle of repose* has been presented by DallaValle.[32] The angle of repose is defined as the base angle of the cone formed when a powdered or granular material falls freely on a flat surface from an orifice.   Measurements of this property with a tablet granulation were reported by Nelson.[33]

More recently, other studies failed to produce a correlation between the tangent of the angle of repose and flow rate.[34] The effect of glidants on flow rate and angle of repose also has been studied.[35]

It appears that free flow depends on the frictional forces that exist between particles making up the granulation, the distribution of the size of the particles within that granulation, the amount of lubricants or other additives, and probably also on other factors. All of these characteristics are dependent on the components of the granulation and on the drug, particularly if present in major proportion. The flow of solids also has been treated in terms of Jannssen's equation which relates to the pressure exerted by material as it flows in straight-sided bins and hoppers.[36]

In studies reported by Jaffe and Foss[37] an attempt was made to correlate cohesiveness of materials on direct compression into tablets with crystal habit, amount of water of crystallization, and other properties. It was interesting to note that only substances crystallizing in the cubic system showed a general pattern of tablet formation on direct compression. Water of crystallization functioned as a "built-in" binding agent facilitating compression, while removal of this water prevented tablet formation.   Density was not a significant factor in altering tablet hardness, but the latter appeared to be related directly with molecular aggregation, or cohesiveness, of various solids as judged by their boiling points.

Wolff and Kaplan[38] suggested a scheme for testing the compression characteristics of various individual tablet ingredients and new drugs as an aid to formulation.   Test slugs of the materials were formed from 40-mesh powder in a uniform manner on a flat-faced punch, ½ in. in diameter, with the die cavity of the tablet machine (Stokes Model F Single-punch) set at a depth of ½ in. The ejected slug was carefully examined for fill weight, ratio of cavity volume to compressed volume (ie, compressibility), ejection difficulty (ie, binding), lamination (ie, cohesiveness), sticking, hardness, and disintegration.   Sticking was defined as adhesion of powder to either the upper or lower punch; binding represented adhesion of powder to the die wall. For additional information, see Chapter 87, page 1649.

Organoleptic Properties

Modern medicine requires that pharmaceutical formulations of new drugs appeal to the patient. Preparations therefore must look pleasing and if not flavored should at least be free of objectionable odor and taste.   With this in mind, in formulation of new drugs the research pharmacist now employs attractive shades of color for tablets and fluids, hard-gelatin capsules in complementary two-color schemes, highly polished sugar coatings, mildly medicinal perfumes for creams and lotions, and very often, immediate containers of plastic, metal, and other materials designed for utility and attractiveness.   Sometimes these supplementary agents cause considerable difficulty. A few of the problems will be considered in the next section.

Taste and smell are both chemical senses. For a substance to arouse a sensation of taste it must be dissolved, either taken in solution or dissolved in the saliva.   Herein lies the key to handling materials with objectionable taste.   If a new drug cannot be masked with flavoring agents, or the taste cannot be hidden within a coated tablet or capsule, it may be necessary to produce derivatives having a lower solubility and, consequently, a more appropriate taste.

Thus, while narcotine hydrochloride is extremely bitter, the less soluble narcotine base is practically tasteless.   Hydrocortisone alcohol is bitter, but the acetate, though not very much less soluble, is without taste.   Similarly, amitriptyline hydrochloride, a water-soluble salt, possesses a marked anesthetic taste, whereas the insoluble pamoate is tasteless.   Cyproheptadine hydrochloride is bitter, but cyproheptadine base is not.   Propionyl erythromycin lauryl sulfate has approximately $\frac{1}{12}$ the solubility of propionyl erythromycin, is practically tasteless, and is useful for the formulation of oral suspensions.   The base itself, on the other hand, is quite unpleasant.

Sometimes taste can be altered by physical coating. This technique has been used for producing tasteless vitamins (Mercote) and is the basis for the microencapsulation of drug compounds by the NCR process (see page 1676).   Chloramphenicol palmitate is less soluble and more palatable than chloramphenicol and is used in a pediatric dosage form.

Aftertaste usually is due to the continued action of the stimulating agent, which, having entered the taste pore, is removed with difficulty by the saliva or even by rinsing the mouth.   Finally, there are a few compounds, of which quinine is an example, which are secreted in the saliva even hours after being swallowed.

Smell is very closely related to taste and is a much more sensitive perception.   Fortunately, smell can be altered more readily with perfumes and aromatics than taste.   In this connection it should be noted that quite often mild, hardly recognizable odor principles such as watermelon, vanilla, and grapefruit do much more in masking some objectionable odors than can be accomplished with highly aromatic compositions.

Chemical Properties

The study of the relationship between chemical structure and physiological activity has led to the synthesis of a host of valuable therapeutic compounds, but new drugs comprise many different kinds of structures, some quite selective and specific in action, others where the relationship is more broad.   In certain instances specificity of structure is of such fundamental importance that even optical isomers differ in their pharmacological activity.   On the other hand many compounds possess multiple actions and can undergo substantial modification without serious loss of activity, as with local anesthetics or the morphine nucleus.   In these cases changes in molecular configuration may alter certain actions but not others.

Regardless of the kind of structure or type of action, it behooves the research pharmacist to formulate new drugs in a manner that will best preserve structural configuration and total composition. Further, it is necessary to preserve stability not only at the time of formulation but also for substantial periods of time afterwards.   Very often this is not easily done.   Structures possessing drug action in many instances are labile or reactive compounds, capable of changes detectable only by the most discriminating study, changes which can go unnoticed chemically or even physiologically for long periods of time.

The problems of stability of pharmaceutical dosage forms, because of complexity or otherwise, thought of through the years only in qualitative terms, now must be considered quantitatively. Newer compounds are more potent and generally are administered as single entities. Former organoleptic criteria of instability have had to be scrapped in favor of modern methods involving precise chemical and biological analysis. Controls adequate to preserve the characteristics of a new drug and data to support any conclusions on stability of its formulations are even required by law. Quantitative stability data therefore form an integral part of the application for governmental approval of any new drug composition.

The term *incompatibility* has been used in pharmacy for many years to designate a combination of two or more ingredients possessing antagonistic properties in either a therapeutic, chemical, or physical sense. As regards the latter, this term generally referred to changes that were readily observable immediately, or shortly after, compounding. Such changes involved nondescript precipitation in otherwise clear liquids, precipitation due to chemical reaction, evolution of a gas, changes in color or clarity, explosive reactions, and even questions of immiscibility or insolubility of active components. There is no more general term than "instability" to include also those modifications that are not readily discernible. A large part of this section, therefore, will deal with changes involved in new drug formulation under the broad general heading of instability. A new drug is considered to be substandard or unstable if it does not conform immediately or even after storage to the normal limits established by the "Standards of Strength" provided by official compendia, FDA requirements, or recognized quality standards established by pharmaceutical manufacturers for control purposes within their own plants.

Changes Principally Involving the New Drug

A brief consideration of some of the more prominent reactions accounting for the instability of new drug compounds will be useful. Obviously, some compounds would not undergo any significant decomposition if kept dry and away from air in a sealed container, although there are exceptions even to this, but unfortunately they are not used in medicine in this form. We must therefore consider, for purposes of this discussion, that the new drug is in some kind of formulation environment, combined with suitable excipients, solvents, or pharmaceutical additives.

Hydrolysis—This destructive process is probably most frequently encountered in formulation of new drugs. It occurs with sugars, esters, amides, lactones, nitriles, salts of a weak acid and a strong base, thioesters, thiohalides, and polymeric materials, among others. A few drug compounds which may undergo decomposition by hydrolysis are procaine, sulfonamides, chlorothiazide, barbituric acid derivatives, aspirin, some alkaloids, hydrocortisone phosphate, and penicillin; formulation ingredients include gelatin, sucrose, sodium acetate, flavoring oils, chlorobutanol, to name a few. In this connection extensive kinetic studies have been reported recently for the hydrolysis of an imidazoline,[39] the cationic ester, *dl*-α-phenyl-2-piperidylacetate

(Ritalin, *Ciba*);[40] the preservative, chlorobutanol;[41] the antibiotics, streptovaricin[42] and chloramphenicol, both in water[43] and in water–propylene glycol systems;[44] the local anesthetics, procainamide, procaine, and benzocaines;[45] the alkaloid, homatropine;[46] and alkaloidal salts, homatropine methylbromide and atropine methylbromide;[47] and the adrenocortical steroid ester, hydrocortisone phosphate.[48]

From a kinetic standpoint hydrolysis reactions are *second-order* reactions because the rate is proportional to the concentration of two reactants. However, in solutions, since water is usually present in excess and therefore at relatively constant concentration, experimentally, the reactions are frequently treated as *monomolecular*, or *first-order*, reactions. This simplification permits calculation of the extent of decomposition under precise experimental conditions by less-complicated means. Extrapolation of the rate to room temperature conditions provides exceedingly useful stability information and data for judging the conditions necessary for optimum stability.

The rate of hydrolysis depends primarily on temperature and a catalyst, the most important being hydrogen ions or hydroxyl ions. In the case of solids the amount of moisture present also is important. The hydrolytic process is dependent on pH. Usually there is a pH of minimum decomposition, at which the catalytic effect of hydrogen ions and hydroxyl ions is approximately equal. The use of buffers of sufficient capacity to maintain optimum pH often helps to improve stability of the compound. Sometimes, however, the pH for optimum stability may not be best in regard to solubility, irritation, or toxicity and therapeutic use. In such cases a compromise in pH and buffer concentration may be necessary somewhere between the region of optimum stability and clinical utility. Occasionally, the salt used as buffer may exhibit a specific ion effect promoting decomposition, but this is quite rare. The stability of penicillin is claimed to be better with citrate buffer than with phosphate buffer, for example. Actually, such stabilization may be due to the sequestering action of citrate ion for trace metals. Hydrolytic changes are sometimes induced by bacteria or enzymes so that care needs to be exercised in this regard.

Hydrolytic decomposition often can be avoided by use of the drug in an insoluble form, or, if water-soluble, by preparation of a solid dosage form. Insoluble chlorothiazide is perfectly stable in neutral aqueous suspension, for example, but solutions of the sodium salt at pH 10 decompose quite rapidly. However, a sterile lyophilized form of the sodium salt is much more stable and is useful for the extemporaneous preparation of solutions for injection.[49] Frequently, the replacement of water by substantial quantities of some other solvent such as alcoholic or polyhydroxy solvent mixtures aids substantially in avoiding hydrolysis in solutions. As an example, replacement of part of the water by sorbitol improved hydrolytic stability of an acetylsalicylic acid suspension.[50] A similar scheme combined with the solubility-suppressing effect of added procaine hydrochloride was employed to reduce hydrolytic cleavage of procaine penicillin in aqueous suspension formulations.[51] Elimination of moisture in dry solids, or the preparation of mixtures with dry buffer salts, can help stabilize solid compounds normally subject to hydrolysis. Hydrolytic decomposition of aspirin in the solid state has been studied.[52] Higuchi and his associates have inhibited the hydrolysis of aromatic esters in solution by the formation of various molecular complexes.[53] Thus, hydrolytic decomposition of procaine hydrochloride and tetracaine hydrochloride was decreased substantially by the addition of caffeine. Both caffeine and a synthetic homolog, 1-ethyltheobromine, stabilized benzocaine through molecular complex formation.

More recently, the stabilization of esters to alkaline hydrolysis was reported to be improved by the micellular structure of anionic surfactants and to acid hydrolysis by the micellular structure of cationics. The charge on the micelle surface and depth of penetration of the ester within the micelle appeared to be critical factors.[54]

Oxidation—In formulation of new drugs this process of decomposition is equal in importance to hydrolysis. In fact, if one considers the numerous changes, especially discoloration, that occur in pharmaceutical products without measurable chemical change, the problems arising from the oxidation process are manifold and usually quite troublesome.

Chemically, oxidation consists of the loss of electrons; reduction is the opposite, or gain of electrons. The oxidative process may involve atmospheric oxygen directly, as when formaldehyde reacts with a mole of oxygen to produce formic acid. Oxidation also may occur by loss of electrons and without the addition of oxygen in the final product, as when ferrous chloride oxidizes to ferric chloride. Both types of reactions are important, but those involving atmospheric oxygen are more frequently encountered in new product research. Oxidation reactions may involve both aqueous and oily formulations. Oxidative decomposition occurs with aldehydes, alcohols, phenols, unsaturated compounds, sugars, alkaloids, fatty acids, and others. Drug compounds subject to oxidation include vitamin A, ascorbic acid, streptomycin, neomycin, morphine, resorcinol, epinephrine, prednisolone, glucose, benzyl alcohol, flavoring oils, oleyl alcohol, and unsaturated fats and oils. A series of publications appeared recently on the kinetics of the photo-oxidation of a series of phenothiazine derivatives.[55]

The oxidation reaction depends on several factors including temperature, oxygen concentration in the liquid, catalysts present, and the concentration of the oxidizable component. In sealed containers a reduction in the rate of oxidation can be observed by lowering the temperature. Catalysts are of great importance. The pH of the formulation sometimes is critical since a great number of oxidation–reduction processes depend on concentration of hydrogen or hydroxyl ion. Light often accelerates an oxidative process; storage of products in dark containers frequently does much to preserve stability. Photochemical changes many times involve the formation of other reactive compounds or free radicals which function to propagate the decomposition, once started. Similar events, termed *autoxidation*, may even occur in the absence of light when susceptible materials such as fats or oils are stored in the presence of air. The autoxidation of phenolic compounds is of special significance in new drug formulation since many pharmacologically active structures are phenols. Epinephrine and isoproterenol are examples. Heavy-metal ions are important catalysts. Cupric ion or ferric ion accelerate the oxidation of ascorbic acid, for example. Frequently, only trace quantities of metal ions occurring as impurities in the water or other ingredients may be sufficient to cause an increased rate of decomposition. Thus, inconsistent stability of ascorbic acid in different samples of commercial sorbitol solutions was attributed to variations in trace metals contamination of the latter.[56]

The oxygen concentration in solution is a factor in many cases and often depends on the temperature of storage or the solvents employed. Oxygen becomes more soluble in water as the temperature lowers, so that oxygen-dependent reactions can sometimes proceed more rapidly at lower temperatures employed for storage. Ascorbic acid is appreciably more stable to oxidation when dissolved in 90% propylene glycol or in Syrup USP than in water, presumably because of lower oxygen concentration in these vehicles.

It should be noted that decomposition by oxidation often is a complicated process, with over-all rate dependent on several of the factors involved. Preparations sensitive to oxidation are stabilized by the removal of oxygen and by the addition of substances to inhibit the process. *Nitrogen-flushing* of parenteral solutions sealed in ampuls is of considerable aid in this regard. Carbon dioxide gas also is employed, although it may sometimes cause change in the pH of the solution.

A wide variety of reducing agents, and compounds to sequester metals and inhibit chain reactions, have been employed for stabilization, but relatively few are acceptable for parenteral products. Frequently, best results are obtained by combinations of several agents. Thus, concentrated aqueous solutions of dihydrostreptomycin, equivalent to 500 mg of the base per ml, have been stabilized against discoloration by oxidation with a combination of sodium bisulfite and sodium formaldehyde sulfoxylate as reducing agents, sodium citrate as a sequestrant, and adjustment of the pH to 7.5 for optimum buffer effect.[57] Detailed kinetic studies have been reported for the oxidative decomposition of prednisolone[58] and for injection solutions of sodium sulfadiazine.[59] The rate of oxygen consumption in the latter solutions was found to be directly related to the ability of added reducing agent to deter color formation. Sodium sulfite alone, and a combination of sodium formaldehyde sulfoxylate and ascorbic acid, were employed.[60]

Racemization—In this process optically active substances lose their optical activity without structural change. If the *enantiomorphs* possess different degrees of physiological action, such change results in reduced therapeutic effect. Studies on the acid-catalyzed racemization[61,62] and base-catalyzed racemization of epinephrine have shown that these changes are first-order. In the studies conducted at a higher pH there was further difficulty with low solubility of the epinephrine and with autoxidation.[63] The cause of racemization in compounds is not fully understood but may involve formation of an activated complex and a *Walden-type inversion*. Racemization of *l*-hyoscyamine to form atropine was found to proceed rapidly in alkaline solutions, while in acid solutions no racemization could be demonstrated after several years of storage at room temperature. Racemization occurred when the solutions were heated, however.[64]

Polymerization—This problem, which involves reaction of two or more identical molecules, is not of great significance but occasionally causes difficulty in formulation of new products. A classic example of this type of change involves polymerization of formaldehyde to form paraformaldehyde, which crystallizes from solution. Loss, on standing, of solubility of gelatin capsules, hardened with small quantities of formaldehyde, also may be due to polymeric decomposition. The darkening of solutions of glucose by heat has been attributed to polymerization of 5-hydroxymethylfurfural, a decomposition product.[65] Similar changes have been noted with other sugar-containing compounds such as streptomycin.

Isomerization—This process involves the change of one structure into another having the same empirical formula but with different properties in one or more respects. A recent example of an apparent decomposition of vitamin A during storage of aqueous multivitamin drops was reported.[66] In this study all-trans-vitamin A was found to isomerize to a mixture containing not only all-trans- and 2-cis-vitamin A but also significant quantities of 6-mono-cis- and 2,6-di-cis-isomers, which were biologically less active.

Decarboxylation—This decomposition involves the evolution of carbon dioxide from the carboxylic acid group of a substituted aromatic acid. An example of such a decomposition is encountered in aqueous solutions of p-aminosalicylic acid, especially on heating.

Enzymatic Decomposition—Chemical decomposition, some of formulations by enzymatic processes though not frequent, may occur as the result of bacterial contamination or by enzymes introduced with drugs from natural sources. Even gums such as acacia contain oxidases and peroxidases capable of reducing the stability of some preparations. These enzymes can be destroyed by heating to 80–100°C, but such treatment is deleterious to the mucilage. Liquefaction of gelatin solutions as a result of enzyme action from bacteria has been reported by Barr and Tice,[67] who also have shown that various microorganisms such as *Pseudomonas aeruginosa, Aspergillus niger, Penicillium niger,* and *Monilia albicans* can grow in unpreserved solutions or dispersions of nonionic surfactants containing fatty acids. These organisms produce esterases which hydrolyze the fatty acid from the surfactant molecule. Extensive decomposition of surfactant by this means may result in loss of the desirable emulsifying or solubilizing properties of the surfactant. Several agents, such as sorbic acid, phenylmercuric salts, and benzalkonium chloride, are effective in preserving against contamination of the sorbitan partial fatty ester and polyoxyethylene ester types, but various phenolic preservatives, commonly used in solutions of these surfactants, such as the esters of p-hydroxybenzoic acid, complex with the polyether groupings and become ineffective.

Accidental contamination of penicillin solutions by organisms producing the enzyme *penicillinase* can cause very rapid deterioration of antibiotic activity. Rancidity in fatty substances frequently has been attributed to bacterial contamination. The addition of preservatives, heat treatment, or sterilization represent methods for overcoming instability due to these causes.

Other Changes—Other reactions which may involve a new drug itself in decomposition are molecular rearrangement, deamination, and photolytic changes. Certain amino acids have been reported to be *deaminated* under the influence of ultraviolet light. The *photolysis* of the antibiotic fumagillin has also been reported.[68] An *elimination* reaction may occur as shown by Higuchi and Reinstein, involving the formation of anhydrovitamin A from vitamin A alcohol or its acetate.[69] *Transesterification* is sometimes encountered when methyl esters are in contact with ethyl alcohol or other ethyl esters. Loss of activity of a formulation is not uncommon because of volatility of active components; solids such as chloral hydrate and chlorobutanol sublime. Spontaneous decomposition with gas formation has been observed with amyl nitrite.[70] The reaction is stabilized by the addition of solid acid adsorbents.[71] In some cases loss of activity may occur as a result of adsorption of the active component on surfaces of a plastic container, a stopper, or even on a suspended solid. The latter was reported with prednisolone in aqueous suspensions of magnesium trisilicate.[72] The binding of benzoic acid, p-aminobenzoic acid, and aspirin was reported with nylon syringes but not with polyethylene or polystyrene.[73] It should be kept in mind, however, that adsorbates of medicinal agents can be very useful materials in some uses, and there are many examples of their use. The adsorption described here refers to undesirable or unsuspected changes that sometimes occur in the formulation of new drugs.

Changes Involving Other Drug Ingredients

Newer drugs more and more frequently are being prepared as formulations of single entities. Incompatibilities of the kind encountered between active ingredients of multicomponent formulations a decade or more ago, therefore, are becoming less frequent. There are exceptions, of course, because some products are formulated primarily as mixtures. Multivitamin and vitamin–mineral compositions are good examples and represent an economically important group of products. Not unexpectedly, however, they exhibit numerous problems with instability, some of which are still not fully understood. Consequently, numerous studies continue to be reported year after year on vitamin stability problems, either singly or in combinations.

The classic instability of thiamine hydrochloride in dry compositions was aided considerably by the introduction of the less soluble and less hygroscopic salt, thiamine mononitrate.[74] The need for an acidic stabilizer such as tartaric acid was eliminated when thiamine mononitrate was used in multivitamin tablets and capsules. This deletion alone helped to stabilize calcium pantothenate, an acid-sensitive vitamin. The later introduction of pantothenyl alcohol further assisted with this problem. The dicetylsulfate salt of thiamine, produced in Japan but not yet available in the US, also is reputed to be a more stable, non-hygroscopic form, suitable for use in dry formulations but not in solutions because of poor solubility.[67] Although the discoloration which occurs when niacinamide and ascorbic acid are mixed dry has been known for some time, the interaction between these substances has now been studied in solution. The yellow color is due to a complex which forms in a 1:1 ratio and is pH dependent.[75] The reduction of cyanocobalamin by ascorbic acid was first reported in 1949.[76] Several methods have been described to lessen the rate of decomposition. These include the addition of sorbitol to the aqueous vehicle, addition of traces of iron to stabilize the cyanocobalamin (although this is detrimental to the ascorbic acid), and the use of adsorbates of cyanocobalamin.

A reasonably stable liquid formulation of the otherwise mutually incompatible ingredients—ascorbic acid, cyanocobalamin, and ferrous gluconate—has been described. The formulation employs 70% sorbitol, either alone or with added glycerin, as a vehicle, thus lending credence to the use of solvents in place of water to improve stability.[77] Various aspects of the thiamine–cyanocobalamin incompatibility have been considered by several authors.[78–82]

Despite the numerous problems various ways have been devised for producing multivitamin and vitamin–mineral combinations having acceptable stability in both solid and liquid form. Much of this is due to the ingenuity and resourcefulness of research pharmacists in developing special granulating methods, coating techniques, solvent systems, and more useful derivatives. An outstanding contribution in this regard was the use of a gelatin matrix to coat emulsified vitamins A and D to produce thereby a stable, dry form of these fat-soluble vitamins for use in tablets and capsules.

Another incompatibility occurring between active components of a formulation involved decomposition of prednisolone when combined dry with antacids, particularly aluminum hydroxide, in compressed tablets. The side chain of the prednisolone molecule is extremely sensitive to air oxidation at pH 6 and above. The addition of an acid component such as aspirin aided considerably in stabilizing prednisolone in such a combination but undoubtedly also decreased the therapeutic usefulness of the antacid. The problem was solved in much better fashion by physical separation when prednisolone and aluminum hydroxide were placed, respectively, in the core and coating of multiple-compressed tablets.

The antagonism between anionic hexachlorophene and cationic quaternary ammonium compounds has been found to be due to a relatively insoluble complex which forms at approximately equimolar concentrations of the components of the mixture. Under such conditions there is also a maximum loss of antibacterial activity.[83] A similar reaction between hexylresorcinol and quaternary ammonium compounds also has been recognized. Hexylresorcinol also was found to be decomposed by reaction with aldehydes present in flavor oils.

Changes Involving Formulation Additives

A great many problems in new drug formulation arise because of chemical interactions between substances added as stabilizers, preservatives, or pharmaceutical excipients to improve pharmaceutical form. Certain of these interactions even involve the new drug itself. The great irony of this situation is that in most cases useful formulations would not be possible without the additives. Actually, a large number of the interactions have been recognized only within the last few years. Once identified, however, suitable alternatives can usually be found to circumvent the problems involved.

Stabilizers—Sodium bisulfite, or sulfite ion, is an extremely effective and useful stabilizer whose application in oxygen-sensitive pharmaceutical systems is well known. Unlike many other potent reducing compounds this agent yields a colorless water-soluble salt when it is itself oxidized. This is a principal attribute. Unfortunately, bisulfite is a reactive ion. It adds at double bonds, reacts with aldehydes and certain ketones, and also has been involved in more specific decomposition reactions such as destruction of the thiamine molecule by the so-called "bisulfite cleavage." Many of the reactions with bisulfite are irreversible, and the resulting sulfonic acids frequently are biologically inactive.

A degradation of epinephrine induced by bisulfite has been reported recently,[84] which later was shown to involve the hydroxybenzyl alcohol portion of the molecule. Nucleophilic addition of sulfite at the asymmetric, secondary alcohol carbon atom yielded a sulfonic acid with simultaneous loss of bisulfite and optical activity of epinephrine.

Other sympathomimetic drugs such as Methadren and Synephrine, and also compounds such as salicyl alcohol, all of which are o- or p-hydroxybenzyl alcohol derivatives, as well as p-hydroxybenzyl alcohol itself, reacted with bisulfite in like manner. m-Hydroxy compounds such as Neosynephrine and salicylamide, as well as m-hydroxybenzyl alcohol, did not react; p-aminobenzyl alcohol showed reactivity. Chloramphenicol, a p-nitrobenzyl alcohol derivative, also reacted with bisulfite, but this degradation was complicated by side reactions, possibly involving simultaneous nitro reduction by the bisulfite ion.[85] The stabilization of epinephrine to sulfite attack has been studied by Riegelman.[86]

The addition of bisulfite to carbonyl functions occurring in adrenocortical steroid molecules is quite well known. Fortunately, such additions are reversible, depending on pH, so that no loss in biological activity is involved as a result of this reaction. Indeed, this addition has been useful in solubilizing structures such as hydrocortisone-21-aldehyde as the aldehyde–bisulfite addition complex.

The addition of bisulfite to the 3-keto position of ring A in the steroid nucleus may result in loss of biological activity, however, with some compounds.

The aldehyde group in the streptomycin molecule probably also is involved in a similar addition of bisulfite when this stabilizer is employed as an antioxidant. Generally, such addition occurs at acid pH, the aldehyde being regenerated as the pH increases to the alkaline range.

Preservatives—The methyl and propyl esters of p-hydroxybenzoic acid have been employed in combination as compatible, nontoxic preservatives for pharmaceutical liquids and creams for many years. However, since 1950, a number of investigators have observed the inactivation of these agents in the presence of several nonionic surfactants and vegetable gums. deNavarre,[87] and Barr and Tice[88] suggested that the loss of activity might be due to the formation of a complex between the preservative and the surfactant. In this connection the tendency of phenols to form molecular complexes with polyethers present in polyethylene polymers was noted separately by others.[89,90] This led Kostenbauder[91] to study the reaction quantitatively using a dialysis technique in which a high degree of interaction between Tween 80 and the methyl and propyl esters of p-hydroxybenzoic acid was observed. The macromolecular complex did not dialyze, permitting measurement of the freely dialyzable p-hydroxybenzoate. The amount of binding depended on the concentration of the reactants but was substantial at ordinary use levels. At a concentration of 5% Tween 80, for example, only 22% of the added methyl ester and 4.5% of the added propyl ester remained in solution in the unbound or dialyzable form. The mechanism of binding appeared to be the same as that responsible for solubilization of the preservative by micelle formation involving the Tween. It was further shown[91] that the p-hydroxybenzoates could be employed efficiently as preservatives, provided higher concentrations were used to offset that quantity bound by the nonionic surfactant.[92] The effect of surfactants on activity of phenolic-type germicides and preservatives was reviewed recently by Evans and Dunbar.[93]

Using equilibrium dialysis, studies also were conducted to determine the degree of association of methyl and propyl p-hydroxybenzoates with other macromolecules that are useful in pharmaceutical formulations. Some interaction was found with polyethylene glycol, methylcellulose polyvinylpyrrolidone and gelatin but was considerably less than that observed with nonionic surfactants, eg, Tween 80. No significant interaction was observed with carboxymethylcellulose or tragacanth.[94] The efficacy of the combination of 0.2% methyl and 0.05% propyl esters of p-hydroxybenzoic acid as a suitable preservative for gum tragacanth jellies was confirmed with bacteriological studies by Taub, et al.[95] Further studies of the interactions between phenolic preservatives and polysorbate 80,[96] and of methylrosaniline and tetracaine with polysorbate 80,[97] have been reported. Sorbic acid, as well as the esters of parahydroxybenzoic acid, were found to react with nonionic macromolecules (Tween 80, Myrj 52) but not with polyethylene glycol 4000–6000 or their esters.[98]

The complexing tendencies of methylcellulose have also been studied.[99] This polymer was found to interact with several compounds in roughly the following decreasing order: p-hydroxybenzoic acid, p-aminobenzoic acid, methyl p-hydroxybenzoate, propyl p-hydroxybenzoate, and butyl p-hydroxybenzoate. Some of these interactions are important in view of the increased use of methylcellulose in ophthalmic solutions. Complexation of methylcellulose also was found with highly surface-active compounds such as tetracaine and dibutoline sulfate, both of which are used in ophthalmology.[100]

In other studies two quaternary ammonium compounds, cetylpyridinium chloride and benzalkonium chloride, were shown to be bound in significant amounts by Tween 80,[101] and solutions of chlorobutanol containing Tween 20 were reported to have less preservative action than solutions of chlorobutanol alone.[102] Complexation of methyl and propyl p-hydroxybenzoates also has been found with polyethylene glycol 4000 and 6000, and with dimethylurea, which is sometimes used as a solubilizer. Sorbic acid and boric acid did not complex with the glycols, however.[103] Finally, binding of preservatives such as p-hydroxybenzoic acid, the methyl and propyl esters, sorbic acid, phenol, and 4-chloro-3-methylphenol has been reported with nylon barrels employed in disposable hypodermic syringes.[104]

Mercurial preservatives in some cases react with constituents in certain types of rubber stoppers used for vials of sterile solutions. Other preservatives such as chlorobutanol, p-chloro-phenylethyl alcohol, phenylethyl alcohol, methylparaben, and benzyl alcohol also are lost to the rubber closure in varying amounts depending on the composition of the elastomer and the storage conditions.[105] The sorption of benzyl alcohol by rubber stoppers caused deflocculation of a suspension, known to the author, with subsequent sedimentation and caking of the product. The problem was corrected by changing to a butyl stopper with which benzyl alcohol did not react. Mercurials have also been observed to react with polyethylene containers

employed for nasal sprays, sometimes with deposition of a black film. Propylparaben has been shown to have an affinity for nylon employed in packaging.[106]

Suspending and Dispersing Agents—*Polyelectrolytes* are finding increasingly greater use as suspending, dispersing, and binding agents in pharmaceutical systems. Anionic water-soluble compounds such as sodium carboxymethylcellulose, pectin, alginic acid, and other hydrocolloids, although generally considered chemically inert, frequently enter into liquid formulations where they can undergo reaction with drug compounds. A study of the interaction of several such structures indicated that binding of the drug ions occurred on dissolved polyelectrolytes frequently even before the formation of visible haze or precipitation. Carboxymethylcellulose thus formed complexes with cationic molecules such as quinine, Benadryl, procaine, and Pyribenzamine. It also complexed with the positively charged antibiotics, neomycin and kanamycin. The interaction of carageenin and other hydrocolloids with many medicinal agents, including alkaloids, promazine, chlorpromazine, reserpine, meprobamate, and antihistaminic agents, was reported in a series of studies by Graham, et al.[107] In some instances the complexation was an aid to stability, as with the CMC–neomycin adduct. The possibility of utilizing complexes of positively charged drugs with nondiffusible polyelectrolytes for slow release has been described,[108] although this idea has not yet found widespread usage. Graham, however, reported that the injection of a carageenin–promazine hydrochloride complex into rabbits released free promazine to the bloodstream up to 6 days after the administration whereas the free form disappeared in 24 hr. Suggestions also have been made for utilizing polyelectrolytes for the reverse process of increasing the rate of absorption of ionic drugs. This phenomenon is largely explainable on the basis of the *Donnan Membrane Theory*, wherein a salt of the nondiffusible polyelectrolyte (eg, sodium CMC) functions to drive a salt of a drug (eg, sodium salicylate) through the cell membrane at an increased rate of transfer.[109]

Phenolic compounds in general were found to interact with polyvinylpyrrolidone, polyethylene glycol 6000, and polypropylene glycol 1200. These included phenol, resorcinol, tannic acid, and β-naphthol, all frequently employed in dermatological preparations. Interaction in these cases resulted in the formation of a haze or the separation of oil or a precipitate.[110] Polyvinylpyrrolidone strongly complexes elemental iodine to yield a water-soluble powder containing both iodide ion and available iodine. Such a powder has had considerable use as a germicide and antiseptic.

Apart from complexation reactions with drugs, other problems may sometimes be encountered with "inert" suspending ingredients of formulations. Polyvalent ions such as calcium form insoluble salts with sodium alginate and carageenin, both strongly charged anionic polyelectrolytes. Because of their charge these latter hydrocolloids also react with positive groupings of proteins when used together. By such reaction large polymers are formed which become less soluble with increasing size until either a gel structure or precipitation occurs. Thus, carageenin and albumen, or a high-isoelectric-point gelatin, form a precipitate or a haze, depending on the order of addition. Carageenin and guar gum, another anionic hydrocolloid, when used together, result in a large increase in viscosity.

An unexpected instability has been observed with neutral solutions of Carbopol 934, a hydrophilic suspending and thickening agent. When exposed to light, such solutions or gels of this material undergo oxidative degradation with loss of viscosity. The change has been retarded by addition of a sequestering agent (ETDA), thus indicating that trace metals catalyze the oxidation. Ionic antioxidants such as sodium bisulfite could not be employed for stabilization because the electrolyte caused deswelling of the polymer and a lowering of viscosity.[111]

Viscosity stability of tragacanth solutions on extended storage was found greatly affected by pH and was decreased below pH 4 or above pH 6. Maximum stability of viscosity occurred at a pH close to 5. Thus, physical characteristics and settling of solids in suspensions containing tragacanth as a thickening agent might be expected to change drastically if viscosity of the product was altered on standing as a result of change in pH.[112]

Dyes—Because they are used in very low concentration to color pharmaceuticals, certified dyes are often treated as inert materials, and their potential chemical reactivity frequently has been overlooked. Several reports have appeared recently concerning the reactivity of certified dyes with different pharmaceutical materials. Sugars such as dextrose, lactose, and sucrose were found to increase the rate of fading of FD&C Blue No. 2, but the sugar alcohols, mannitol and sorbitol, were without effect unless they contained traces of strong reducing catalysts. Except for nordihydroguiaretic acid, the addition of antioxidants did not appreciably retard the rate of fading of the dye in the presence of a reducing sugar such as dextrose.[113]

Further study demonstrated chemical interaction between the quaternary ammonium compounds (cetylpyridinium chloride, benzalkonium chloride, and others) and FD&C Red No. 1, FD&C Blue No. 1, and D&C Yellow No. 10. Insoluble complexes were formed, although regions of miscibility between the reactants could be designated by means of phase diagrams.[114]

Retention of color of six certified dyes (FD&C Blue No. 2, Yellow No. 5, Red No. 1, Red No. 4, Green No. 1 and D&C Orange No. 3) in 1% aqueous solutions of various nonionic surfactants (Tween 20, Brij 35, Igepal CA-710, Myrj 52, and Pluronic F-68) was studied. Fading of color was noted in almost every case during storage for 14 days at 48°C.[115]

Solid Excipients and Lubricants—Even in the apparent dry state one may encounter difficulties involving a new drug. Such problems as discoloration and decomposition of compressed tablets containing aspirin, acetophenetidin, and caffeine, especially in the presence of codeine phosphate, are quite well known. The effect of different USP talcs on the stability of aspirin in tablets also was described.[116] It also is generally agreed that magnesium and calcium stearate are poor lubricants for aspirin tablets because they accelerate decomposition. The strong adsorption of cyanocobalamin on talc precludes the use of this material as a lubricant or diluent for this vitamin. Cetylpyridinium chloride also is irreversibly adsorbed by talc, as shown by both chemical and bacteriological tests.[117]

Miscellaneous—Reference has already been made to special problems that arise with containers and closures (see page 1473). The clarity of parenteral solutions has been of much concern to the pharmaceutical industry for many years. Many reasons have been given for the development of trace precipitates and haze in ampuls and ampul vials, for example. The manufacturers of both glass and closures have made considerable progress in supplying materials of greater resistance and inertness for use with parenteral products. Nevertheless,

problems still arise at times which cannot be attributed to changes other than those involving the container or closure. Today, perhaps as a direct result of new methods for detection, the particulate contamination of parenterals is a high-priority problem.[118]

The sorption of water by rubber closures used for injections and haze formation from rubber closures are problems that have been examined recently.[119] According to these studies, haze from stoppers is due mainly to the formation of colloidal solutions of zinc salts or sulfur. Zinc oxide is a common closure ingredient, and zinc stearate is employed during the moulding operation in closure manufacture. Sulfur also is an ingredient of most closure compositions and has the peculiar property of "blooming" (rising to the surface) as closures are stored. Other insoluble materials sometimes used in closure manufacture, such as barium sulfate and clay, can be expected to form colloidal solutions if extracted from the closure by the product. Both sodium bisulfite and acetic acid were found to prevent haze formation in parenterals since these agents are capable of precipitating the colloidal particles. Furthermore, sodium bisulfite reacts with sulfur, and acetic acid with zinc salts, to form soluble derivatives.

Silicone films have been employed on glass vials for the purpose of improving drainage, particularly with suspension products. These usually are applied by a process which involves curing the silicone film to the glass surface at temperatures in excess of 200°C for one or more hours. Silicone films are generally quite stable at acidic pH but are unstable at alkaline pH after prolonged standing,[120] and may contribute substantially to particulate matter contamination.

Finally, the microbiological contamination of medical preparations is receiving considerable attention by manufacturers and regulatory agencies. Much of this stems from studies in Sweden which reported several serious eye disorders following the use of a contaminated eye ointment, and Salmonellosis in more than 200 persons from thyroid tablets contaminated with Salmonella organisms.

General Comments

The formulation of new drugs into suitable dosage forms calls for the application of a broad knowledge of the properties of materials, both physical and chemical. The solution of problems encountered in formulation, however, presents the pharmaceutical scientist with the finest opportunity for the application of scientific training, diverse skills, and of creative aptitudes.

References

1. Mullins, J. D., and Macek, T. J., *J. APhA, Sci. Ed.*, **49**, 245 (1960).
2. Glazko, A. J., *et al, Antibiot. Chemotherapy*, **8**, 516 (1958).
3. Aguiar, A., *et al, J. Pharm. Sci.*, **56**, 847 (1967).
4. Buckwalter, F. H., and Dickison, H. L., *J. APhA, Sci. Ed.*, **47**, 661 (1958).
5. Arnold, A., *et al, Am. J. Clin. Nutr.*, **10**, 56 (1962).
6. Ober, S. S., *et al, J. APhA, Sci. Ed.*, **47**, 667 (1958).
7. Robillard, E., *et al, Can. Med. Assoc. J.*, **86**, 362 (1962).
8. Paul, H. E., *et al, J. Pharm. Sci.*, **56**, 882 (1967).
9. Levy, G., *et al, J. Pharm. Sci.*, **52**, 1039, 1047, 1139 (1963).
10. Levy, G., and Procknal, J. A., *J. Pharm. Sci.*, **51**, 294 (1962).
11. Campagna, F. A., *et al, J. Pharm. Sci.*, **52**, 605 (1963).
12. Macek, T. J., US Pat. 2,671,750 (Mar. 9, 1954).
13. Magerlein, B. J., *et al, US Pat. 2,828,319 (Mar. 25, 1958); US Pat. 2,841,599 (June 1, 1958).
14. Biles, J. A., *J. Pharm. Sci.*, **52**, 1066 (1963).
15. Higuchi, W. I., *et al, J. Pharm. Sci.*, **56**, 200 (1967).
16. Guillory, J. K., *et al, J. Pharm. Sci.*, **56**, 72 (1967).
17. Anderson, C. M., *Australasian J. Pharm.*, **47**, 544 (1966).
18. Heistand, E. N., *J. Pharm. Sci.*, **53**, 1 (1964); Frederick, K. J., *Ibid*, **50**, 531 (1961).
19. Krause, G. M., and Cross, J. M., *J. APhA, Sci. Ed.*, **40**, 137 (1951).
20. Peterson, C. F., and Hopponen, R. E., *J. APhA, Sci. Ed.*, **42**, 540 (1953).
21. Osol, A., and Pines, C. C., *J. APhA, Sci. Ed.*, **41**, 634 (1952).

22. Barr, N., and Tice, L., *Am. J. Pharm.*, **129**, 332 (1957).
23. Reber, L. A., *J. APhA, Sci. Ed.*, **42**, 192 (1953).
24. Moore, W. E., *J. APhA, Sci. Ed.*, **47**, 855 (1958).
25. Moore, W. E., *J. Pharm. Sci.*, **51**, 391 (1962).
26. Parnta, A. An., *et al*, *J. Pharm. Sci.*, **51**, 704 (1962).
27. Kolthoff, I. M., and Sandell, E. B., *Textbook of Quantitative Inorganic Analysis*, Macmillan, New York, 1936, p. 51.
28. Nelson, E., *J. APhA, Sci. Ed.*, **46**, 607 (1957).
29. Lachman, L., and Chavkin, L., *J. APhA, Sci. Ed.*, **46**, 412 (1957).
30. Macek, T. J., *J. Pharm. Sci.*, **52**, 694 (1963).
31. Higuchi, T., *et al*, *J. APhA, Sci. Ed.*, **41**, 93 (1952); **42**, 194 (1953); **43**, 344, 596, 685, 718 (1954); **44**, 223, 494 (1955); **45**, 51, 354, 482, (1956); **49**, 35 (1960).
32. Dalla Valle, J. M., *Micromeritics*, 2nd ed., Pitman Publ. Corp., New York, 1948, p. 150.
33. Nelson, E., *J. APhA, Sci. Ed.*, **44**, 435 (1955).
34. Sumner, E. D., *et al*, *J. Pharm. Sci.*, **55**, 1441 (1966).
35. Gold, G., *et al*, *J. Pharm. Sci.*, **55**, 1291 (1966).
36. Rudd, J., *Modern Packaging*, 209 (Mar., 1954).
37. Jaffe, J., and Foss, N. E., *J. APhA, Sci. Ed.*, **48**, 26 (1959).
38. Wolff, J. E., and Kaplan, L. L., Unpublished report read before Pharmacy Subsection, AAAS, Washington, D.C., Dec., 1958.
39. Stern, M. J., *et al*, *J. APhA, Sci. Ed.*, **48**, 641 (1959).
40. Siegel, S., *et al*, *J. APhA, Sci. Ed.*, **48**, 431 (1959).
41. Nair, A. D., and Lach, J. L., *J. APhA, Sci. Ed.*, **48**, 390 (1959).
42. Garrett, E. R., *J. APhA, Sci. Ed.*, **48**, 169 (1959).
43. Higuchi, T., and Marcus, A. D., *J. APhA, Sci. Ed.*, **48**, 530 (1959).
44. Marcus, A. D., and Taraszka, A. J., *J. APhA, Sci. Ed.*, **48**, 77 (1959).
45. Marcus, A. D., and Baron, J., *J. APhA, Sci. Ed.*, **48**, 85 (1959).
46. Patel, J. L., and Lemberger, A., *J. APhA, Sci. Ed.*, **47**, 878 (1958).
47. Patel, J. L., and Lemberger, A. P., *J. APhA, Sci. Ed.*, **48**, 106 (1959).
48. Marcus, A. D., *J. APhA, Sci. Ed.*, **49**, 383 (1960).
49. Charnicki, W. F., *et al*, *J. APhA, Sci. Ed.*, **48**, 656 (1959).
50. Blaug, S. M., and Wesolowski, J. W., *J. APhA, Sci. Ed.*, **48**, 691 (1959).
51. Swintosky, J. V., *et al*, *J. APhA, Sci. Ed.*, **45**, 37 (1956).
52. Lecson, L. J., and Mattocks, A. M., *J. APhA, Sci. Ed.*, **47**, 329 (1958).
53. Higuchi, T., *et al*, *J. APhA, Sci. Ed.*, **44**, 521 (1955); **45**, 290 (1956); **46**, 32, 36 (1957).
54. Riegelman, S., Paper read before the Scientific Section, APhA, Cincinnati, Ohio, Aug., 1959.
55. Fujisawa, S., and Kawabata, S., *Yakugaku Zasshi*, **86**, 504, 510, 514, 708, 714 (1966).
56. Bartilucci, A. J., *et al*, *J. APhA, Sci. Ed.*, **46**, 627 (1957).
57. Macek, T. J., and Hanus, E. J., US Pat. 2,657,171 (Oct. 27, 1953).
58. Guttman, D. E., and Meister, P. D., *J. APhA, Sci. Ed.*, **47**, 773 (1958).
59. Swartz, C. J., and Autian, J., *J. APhA, Sci. Ed.*, **47**, 490 (1958).
60. Swartz, C. J., and Autian, J., *J. APhA, Sci. Ed.*, **47**, 649 (1958).
61. Schroeter, L. C., and Higuchi, T., *J. APhA, Sci. Ed.*, **47**, 426 (1958).
62. Kisbye, J., and Schou, S. A., *Dansk Tidsskr. Farm.*, **25**, 185 (1951).
63. Kisbye, J., *Dansk Tidsskr. Farm.*, Suppl. No. 2, 156 (1956).
64. Schou, S. A., and Mørch, J., *Report on the Stability of Pharmaceutical Preparations*, Copenhagen, 1959, p. 25.
65. Webb, N. E., *et al*, *J. APhA, Sci. Ed.*, **47**, 101 (1958).
66. Lehman, R. W., *et al*, Paper read before the Scientific Section, APhA, Cincinnati, Ohio, Aug., 1959.
67. Barr, M., and Tice, L. F., *J. APhA, Sci. Ed.*, **46**, 442, 445 (1957).
68. Garrett, E. R., and Eble, T. E., *J. APhA, Sci. Ed.*, **43**, 385, 536 (1954).
69. Higuchi, T., and Reinstein, J. A., *J. APhA, Sci. Ed.*, **48**, 155 (1959).
70. Yunker, M. H., *et al*, *J. APhA, Sci. Ed.*, **47**, 613 (1958).
71. Yunker, M. H., and Higuchi, T., *J. APhA, Sci. Ed.*, **47**, 621 (1958).
72. Chulski, T., and Forist, A. A., *J. APhA, Sci. Ed.*, **47**, 553 (1958).
73. Kim, H. K., and Autian, J., Paper read before the Scientific Section, APhA, Cincinnati, Ohio, Aug., 1959.
74. Macek, T. J., *et al*, *J. APhA, Sci. Ed.*, **39**, 365 (1950).
75. Guttman, D. E., and Brooke, D., *J. Pharm. Sci.*, **52**, 941 (1963).
76. Gakenheimer, W. C., and Feller, B. A., *J. APhA, Sci. Ed.*, **38**, 660 (1949).
77. Gerber, C. F., *et al*, *J. APhA, Sci. Ed.*, **46**, 635 (1957).
78. Feller, B. A., and Macek, T. J., *J. APhA, Sci. Ed.*, **44**, 662 (1955).
79. Ravin, L. J., and Doerge, R. F., *J. APhA, Sci. Ed.*, **48**, 425 (1959).
80. Blitz, M., *et al*, *J. APhA, Sci. Ed.*, **43**, 651 (1954).
81. Mukherjee, S. L., and Sen, S. P., *J. Pharm. Pharmacol.*, **11**, 26 (1959).
82. Gambier, A. S., and Rahn, E. P., *J. APhA, Sci. Ed.*, **46**, 134 (1957); **47**, 356 (1958).
83. Walter, G. R., and Gump, W. S., *J. Pharm. Sci.*, **51**, 770 (1962).
84. Schroeter, L. C., *et al*, *J. APhA, Sci. Ed.*, **47**, 723 (1958).
85. Higuchi, T., and Schroeter, L. C., *J. APhA, Sci. Ed.*, **48**, 535 (1959).
86. Riegelman, S., and Fischer, E. Z., *J. Pharm. Sci.*, **51**, 206, 210 (1962).
87. deNavarre, M. G., *J. Soc. Cosmetic Chemists*, **8**, 68 (1957).
88. Barr, M., and Tice, L. F., *J. APhA, Sci. Ed.*, **46**, 442 (1957).
89. Higuchi, T., and Lach, J. L., *J. APhA, Sci. Ed.*, **43**, 465 (1954).
90. Guttman, D., and Higuchi, T., *J. APhA, Sci. Ed.*, **45**, 659 (1956).
91. Patel, N. K., and Kostenbauder, H. B., *J. APhA, Sci. Ed.*, **47**, 289 (1958).
92. Pisano, F. D., and Kostenbauder, H. B., *J. APhA, Sci. Ed.*, **48**, 310 (1959).
93. Evans, W. P., and Dunbar, S. F., *Soc. Chem. Ind. (London) Monograph*, **19**, 169 (1965).
94. Miyawaki, G. M., *et al*, *J. APhA, Sci. Ed.*, **48**, 315 (1959).
95. Taub, A., *et al*, *J. APhA, Sci. Ed.*, **47**, 235 (1958).
96. Patel, N. K., and Foss, N. E., *J. Pharm. Sci.*, **53**, 94 (1964).
97. Hurwitz, A. R., *et al*, *J. Pharm. Sci.*, **52**, 893 (1963).
98. Blaug, S. M., and Ahsan, S. S., *J. Pharm. Sci.*, **50**, 138, 441 (1961).
99. Tillman, W. J., and Kuramoto, R., *J. APhA, Sci. Ed.*, **46**, 211 (1957).
100. Swan, K. C., *Arch. Ophthalmol.*, **33**, 378 (1945).
101. DeLuca, P. P., and Kostenbauder, H. B., Paper read before the Scientific Section, APhA, Cincinnati, Ohio, Aug., 1959.
102. Deeb, E. N., and Boenigk, J. W., *J. APhA, Sci. Ed.*, **47**, 807 (1958).
103. Lach, J. L., *et al*, *J. APhA, Sci. Ed.*, **46**, 615 (1957).
104. Marcus, E., *et al*, *J. APhA, Sci. Ed.*, **48**, 457 (1959).
105. Lachman, L., *et al*, *J. Pharm. Sci.*, **51**, 224 (1962).
106. Kapadia, A. J., *et al*, *J. Pharm. Sci.*, **53**, 28 (1964).
107. Graham, H. D., *et al*, *J. Pharm. Sci.*, **50**, 483 (1961); **51**, 988 (1962); **52**, 192, 964 (1963).
108. Cavallito, C. J., and Jewell, R., *J. APhA, Sci. Ed.*, **47**, 165 (1958).
109. Higuchi, T., *et al*, *J. APhA, Sci. Ed.*, **43**, 646 (1954).
110. Guttman, D., and Higuchi, T., *J. APhA, Sci. Ed.*, **45**, 659 (1956).
111. Schwartz, T. W., and Levy, G., *J. APhA, Sci. Ed.*, **47**, 442 (1958).
112. Schwartz, T. W., *et al*, *J. APhA, Sci. Ed.*, **47**, 695 (1958).
113. Kuramoto, R., *et al*, *J. APhA, Sci. Ed.*, **47**, 175 (1958).
114. Lachman, L., *et al*, *J. APhA, Sci. Ed.*, **47**, 871 (1958).
115. Scott, M. W., *et al*, Paper read before the Scientific Section, APhA, Cincinnati, Ohio, Aug., 1959.
116. Gold, G., and Campbell, J. A., *J. Pharm. Sci.*, **53**, 52 (1964).
117. Batyios, N. A., and Brecht, E. A., *J. APhA, Sci. Ed.*, **46**, 524 (1957).
118. "Liquid-Borne Particle Metrology," *NY Acad. Sci. Monograph*, To be published.
119. Milosovich, G., and Mattocks, A. M., *J. APhA, Sci. Ed.*, **46**, 350, 377 (1957).
120. Meyst, M., *Pharm. Weekblad.*, **90**, 869 (1955); **92**, 561 (1957).

80 | Solutions, Emulsions, and Suspensions

Aqueous solutions—sweet or other viscid aqueous solutions—
nonaqueous solutions—emulsions—suspensions

This chapter was prepared by

M. Pernarowski, PhD, *Professor of Pharmaceutical Chemistry, Faculty of Pharmaceutical Sciences, The University of British Columbia, Vancouver 8, British Columbia, Canada*

Solutions, emulsions, and suspensions were first prepared by the priests of the ancient religions and the apothecaries of the now-dead empires. They dissolved or suspended a wide variety of unpalatable (but, on occasion, therapeutically effective) medicinal agents and dispensed them to the sick. Incantations and methods and times of administration were often more important than product elegance or acceptability. Although the basic characteristics of these dosage forms have not changed, modern technology has altered many of the properties of these preparations to the point that they can no longer be compared with those described in ancient manuscripts. They may be compared with the newer dosage forms (eg, tablets and injections) but such a comparison has no real meaning because each has its own specific advantages and disadvantages. Bulkiness of these liquid forms and, in some cases, their disagreeable taste and lack of stability are compensated for by their homogeneity, prompt action, and ease of administration.

The preparation of the various forms described herein requires special skills and, often, the liquid form is the only type of preparation that the pharmacist is asked to compound in this era of prepackaged pharmaceuticals. Certain simple prescriptions are a mixture of two or more specialties and a knowledge of the properties of each is essential if the final preparation is to retain the elegance, stability, and acceptability inherent in the parent pharmaceuticals.

Three general classes of liquid preparations will be considered in this chapter. These, in their broadest sense, are solutions, suspensions, and emulsions. However, in each of these categories, there are a number of preparations that are considered elsewhere. In general, these are the liquids that are intended for ophthalmic or parenteral use or are prepared by maceration or percolation. The appropriate chapters (see the index) should be consulted for a discussion of the preparation and characteristics of these particular dosage forms.

Aqueous Solutions

The major ingredient in most of the dosage forms described in this section is water. Water is used both as a vehicle and as a solvent for the desired flavoring or medicinal ingredients. Its tastelessness, freedom from irritating qualities, and lack of pharmacological activity make it ideal for such purposes. However, it does provide a favorable environment for many chemical reactions, supports the growth of microorganisms when contaminated, and, in its purified forms, adds to the cost of producing the pharmaceutical preparation.

A solution is a homogeneous mixture that is prepared by dissolving a solid, liquid, or gas in another liquid and represents a group of preparations in which the molecules of the solute or dissolved substance are dispersed among those of the solvent. This definition includes a wide variety of preparations and differs from that in USP XVIII. The latter definition is given under the subsection entitled *Solutions*. Solutions may also be classified on the basis of physical or chemical properties, method of preparation, use, physical state, number of ingredients, and particle size. The narrower definition herein limits the solvent to water and excludes those preparations that are sweet and/or viscid in character. This section includes, therefore, those pharmaceutical forms that are designated as *Waters*, *Aqueous Acids*, *Solutions*, *Douches*, *Enemas*, *Gargles*, *Washes*, and *Juices*. It should be pointed out that the definition for the pharmaceutical preparation called solution differs from the physical chemist's definition of solution given in Chapter 19, page 246.

This section, and the chapter as a whole, must be considered as part of a broad subject that is based on principles presented in several chapters of Part II.

Waters

The official waters include the four solvent waters official in USP and the aromatic or medicated waters. Water, as H_2O, is described in detail in Chapter 28 on *Inorganic Pharmaceutical Chemistry*, page 402. The student should also refer to Chapter 71 on *Pharmaceutical Necessities*, page 1338, for further information on the ingredients in aromatic waters and their use, not only in the preparation of the official waters but also in the formulation of syrups, tinctures, and similar pharmaceutical forms.

Water—Two of the four solvent waters described in the USP are used in the preparation of parenterals. *Water* and *Purified Water* are suitable solvents for the ingredients in other official solutions. In general, *Water* is recommended for those preparations intended for external use only. *Purified Water* must be used for all other pharmaceutical operations and preparations and, as needed, in all the tests and assays of the compendia. The individual monographs specify the type of water required for the preparation of each official solution. In the production of specialties, economics may dictate the use of the cheaper form. However, the dissolved substances in such water may react with the active ingredients to produce a product that is pharmaceutically undesirable. For example, the water may comply with the specifications in the USP but, if it is used to prepare *Diluted Alcohol*, the resulting solution may be turbid or may contain a precipitate consisting of insoluble calcium and magnesium salts. It is for this reason that *Purified Water* should be used in the compounding of the majority of liquid preparations.

The major impurities in water are calcium, iron, magnesium, manganese, silica, and sodium. The cations are usually combined with the bicarbonate, sulfate, or chloride anions. "Hard" waters are those that contain the calcium and magnesium cations. Bicarbonates are the major impurity in the "alkaline" waters.

Demineralizing processes will efficiently and economically remove most of the major impurities in water. One such process is shown in Fig. 522. Hydrogen zeolite (H_2Z), a cation exchanger, first converts bicarbonates, sulfates, and chlorides to their respective acids.

$$\left.\begin{array}{c} CaSO_4 \\ MgSO_4 \\ Na_2SO_4 \end{array}\right| + H_2Z \rightarrow \left.\begin{array}{c} Ca \\ Mg \\ Na_2 \end{array}\right| Z + H_2SO_4$$

$$\left.\begin{array}{c} Ca(HCO_3)_2 \\ Mg(HCO_3)_2 \\ 2NaHCO_3 \end{array}\right| + H_2Z \rightarrow \left.\begin{array}{c} Ca \\ Mg \\ Na_2 \end{array}\right| Z + 2H_2CO_3$$

Carbonic acid decomposes to carbon dioxide (which is removed by aeration in the decarbonator) and water.

The anion exchanger unit may contain either a weakly basic or a strongly basic anion resin. These resins adsorb sulfuric, hydrochloric, and nitric acids. Chemical reactions may involve complete adsorption or an exchange with some other anion.

$$H_2SO_4 + A \rightarrow A \cdot H_2SO_4$$

If the resin contains a hydroxyl radical, water is formed during the purification process.

$$H_2SO_4 + 2AOH \rightarrow A_2SO_4 + 2H_2O$$

Weakly dissociated carbonic and silicic acids can be removed only by strongly basic anion resins.

$$H_2SiO_3 + 2AOH \rightarrow A_2SiO_2 + 2H_2O$$

Unit capacity varies with the nature of the installation but it is possible to process as much as 15,000 gal of water/min.[1]

Aromatic Waters—Aromatic waters, known also as medicated waters, are defined in the USP as "clear, saturated aqueous solutions (unless otherwise specified) of volatile oils or other aromatic or volatile substances." The compendium further states that their odors and tastes are similar to those of the drugs or volatile substances from which they are prepared, and the preparations should be free from empyreumatic (smoke-like) and other foreign odors. They are used principally as flavored or perfumed vehicles. The volatile substances from which aromatic waters are to be made should be of pharmacopeial quality or, in the case of nonofficial preparations, of the best quality if the finest flavors are to be obtained.

Aromatic waters may be prepared by one of two official processes.

Distillation—Distillation represents the most ancient and frequently the most satisfactory method for making this class of preparations. However, it is the slowest and the most expensive of the two methods. The USP gives the following directions:

"Place the odoriferous portion of the plant or drug from which the aromatic water is to be prepared in a suitable still with sufficient purified water, and distil most of the water, carefully avoiding the development of empyreumatic odors through the charring or scorching of the substances. Separate the excess of the oil from the distillate, and preserve or use the clear water portion, filtering if necessary."

Different authorities give different directions for the preparation of aromatic waters by distillation. For fresh drugs the proportions range from one part of drug to two of distillate, to two parts of drug to one part of distillate. For dried drugs such as cinnamon, anise, dill, caraway, and fennel the proportion is one part of drug to ten parts of distillate. In the case of dried leaf drugs such as peppermint, the proportion is

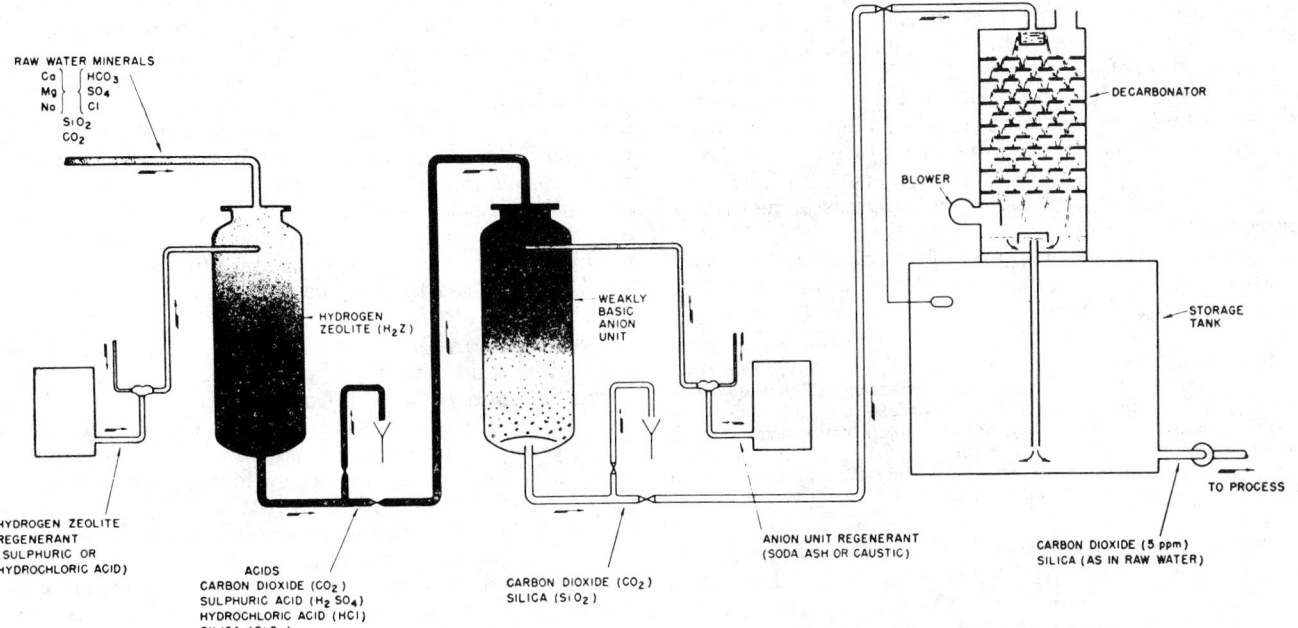

Fig. 522. The process of demineralization with weakly basic anion exchangers (courtesy, Crane).

three parts of drug to ten parts of distillate. Metallic distillation apparatus is usually employed, sometimes using a current of steam passed through the still from the outside. The drug should be contused or coarsely ground. Most distilled aromatic waters acquire an unpleasant empyreumatic odor as soon as they are distilled. This passes off gradually upon exposure to air, if care has been taken not to expose the drug to the action of direct heat during distillation. If precautions are not taken to protect the drug from partial burning, the odor of the carbonized substance will be noticeable in the distilled aromatic water. To avoid this difficulty, the drug should be placed in a partially filled round-bottomed copper wire cage, which is placed in the still to thus avoid any contact of the substance with the heated surface. The meshes of the cage are coarse enough to permit the free passage of vapors and boiling water. If the volatile principles in the water are delicate and present in small quantities (eg, as in orange flower and rose waters), the distillate is returned several times to the still with fresh portions of flowers, thus giving rise to the commercial terms *double distilled*, *triple distilled*, or *quadruple distilled*, according to the number of redistillations. This process is called *cohobation*.

The NF states that Orange Flower Water and Stronger Rose Water are to be made by distillation.

Solution—The following procedure is officially recognized:

"Shake 2 Gm or 2 ml (if a liquid) of the volatile substance (suitably comminuted if a solid) with 1000 ml of purified water in a container of sufficient capacity, and repeat the shaking several times during a period of about 15 minutes. Set the mixture aside for 12 hours or longer, filter through wetted filter paper, and add purified water through the filter to make the product measure 1000 ml."

In terms of time and equipment this method is more convenient than that described above. However, the making of medicated waters by agitation with an excess of volatile oil, permitting the excess to remain and drawing off the water as required, is not recommended. Volatile oils may deteriorate through exposure to light and air and, because of this, may yield unsatisfactory aromatic waters.

Certain waters are prepared by dissolving well-defined substances in purified water. Camphor Water NF XI is a saturated solution of camphor in purified water. Chloroform Water NF XI is prepared by adding enough chloroform to purified water (in a dark amber-colored bottle) to maintain a slight excess after the mixture has been thoroughly agitated. The latter water is used as a sedative in cough, asthma, and colic mixtures and as a vehicle for administering active ingredients.

The USP permits the use of an alternate solution method for the preparation of aromatic waters. This method is given below:

"Thoroughly incorporate the volatile oil (or the suitable comminuted volatile solid) with 15 Gm of talc or with a sufficient quantity of purified siliceous earth or pulped filter paper. Add 1000 ml of purified water, and thoroughly agitate the mixture several times during 10 minutes. Then filter the mixture, returning the first portions, if necessary, to obtain a clear filtrate, and add purified water through the filter to make the product measure 1000 ml."

This is the process most frequently employed since the water can be prepared promptly, only 10 minutes of agitation being required. The use of talc, purified siliceous earth, or pulped filter paper greatly increases the surface of the volatile substance, insuring more rapid saturation of the water. These dispersing substances also form an efficient filter bed which produces a clear solution. They are also unreactive.

Magnesium carbonate was formerly used for this purpose, but its slight solubility and basic nature produced an alkaline water which precipitated alkaloids and similar chemical substances. Calcium phosphate, kaolin, pumice, charcoal, precipitated chalk, and similar substances have also been suggested, but these likewise are objectionable. The calcium ions, present in water which has dissolved a minute quantity of the very slightly soluble phosphate (or other slightly soluble calcium salts), form insoluble salts with many anions. Charcoal and other adsorbent substances tend to remove odoriferous principles.

Other methods have been suggested for the preparation of aromatic waters. These are based on the use of soluble concentrates or on the incorporation of solubilizing agents such as Polysorbate 80 or Tween 20 (*Atlas*). However, such preparations are susceptible to mold growth and, in concentrations higher than 2%, impart an objectionable oil taste.[2-4] The British Pharmacopoeia and the British Pharmaceutical Codex permit the use of aqueous alcoholic solutions of the volatile oil for the preparation of the aromatic water. These concentrated waters contain 20 ml of volatile oil per liter of solution and sufficient alcohol to produce an ethanol content of about 53% *v/v*. The aromatic water is prepared by diluting this type of solution with 39 times its volume of water. In general these methods yield aromatic waters that are slightly inferior in quality to those prepared by the official processes.

Concentrated waters may be prepared in the following manner: Dissolve 20 ml of the volatile oil in 600 ml of 90% alcohol. Add sufficient water in successive small portions to produce 1000 ml of solution. Shake vigorously after each addition. Add 50 Gm of purified talc, shake occasionally for several hours, and filter. Five concentrated waters are official in either BP 1968 or BPC 1968. These are Anise BPC (in which the volume of alcohol is increased to 700 ml), Caraway BPC, Cinnamon BPC, Dill BPC, and Peppermint BP.

Incompatibilities—The principal difficulty experienced in the compounding of prescriptions containing aromatic waters is due to a "salting out" action of certain ingredients, such as very soluble salts, on the volatile principle of the aromatic water. A replacement of part of the aromatic water with purified water is permissible when no other function is being served than that of a vehicle. Otherwise a dilution of the product with a suitable increase in dosage is indicated. Cooper and Brecht[5] have suggested that this salting out action of soluble salts may be used in the evaluation of aromatic waters. The method is based on the determination of the amount of standard sodium citrate solution required to produce cloudiness in the aromatic water.

Preservation—Aromatic waters will deteriorate with time and should, therefore, be made in small quantities and protected from intense light and excessive heat. Deterioration may be due to volatilization, decomposition, or mold growth and will produce solutions that are cloudy and have lost all traces of their agreeable odor. Distilled water is usually contaminated with mold-producing organisms. *Recently* distilled and boiled water should, therefore, be used in the preparation of medicated waters. No preservative should be added to medicated waters. If they become cloudy or otherwise deteriorate, they should be discarded.

Stronger Rose Water acquires a musty odor when stored in tightly closed containers over long periods of time. The NF states that the odor of this water is best preserved by allowing a limited access of fresh air to the container. Cotton plugs exclude foreign matter but, at the same time, permit air to enter the container.

Aqueous Acids

The official inorganic acids and certain organic acids, although of minor significance as therapeutic agents, are of great importance in chemical and pharmaceutical manufacturing. This is especially true of acetic, hydrochloric, nitric, and sulfuric acids. The three latter acids, because of their relative completeness of ionization, are termed strong acids. These acids, and especially the latter two, are very caustic and corrosive.

The inorganic acids are generally divided into two groups: (1) the *hydracids*, which contain no oxygen, eg, hydriodic, hydrobromic, hydrochloric, and hydrofluoric acids and (2) the oxygen-containing acids, eg, hypophosphorous, nitric, phosphoric, and sulfuric acids.

Percentage Strengths—Many of the more important inorganic acids are available commercially in the form of concentrated aqueous solutions. The percentage strength varies from one acid to another and depends on the solubility and stability of the solute in water and on the manufacturing process. Thus, the official Hydrochloric Acid contains from 35 to 38% by weight of HCl, whereas Nitric Acid contains from 67 to 71% by weight of HNO_3 and Sulfuric Acid contains from 94 to 98% by weight of H_2SO_4.

Because the strengths of these concentrated acids are stated in terms of % by weight, it is essential that specific gravities also be provided if one is to be able to calculate conveniently the amount of absolute acid contained in a unit volume of the solution as purchased. The mathematical relationship involved is given by the equation $M = V \times S \times F$, wherein M is the mass in Gm of absolute acid contained in V ml of solution having a specific gravity S and a fractional percentage strength F. As an example, Hydrochloric Acid containing 36.93% by weight of HCl has a specific gravity of 1.1875. Therefore, the amount of absolute HCl supplied by 100 ml of this hydrochloric acid solution is given by:

$$M = 100 \times 1.1875 \times 0.3693 = 43.85 \text{ Gm HCl}$$

Commercially, the specific gravities of liquids are often given on the arbitrary Baumé scale. In instances where this is the only kind of specific gravity data provided, it is necessary first to calculate the true specific gravity from the Baumé degree figure. Tables relating the percentage strengths of acids to specific gravity and to the Baumé degree are usually provided in commercial handbooks of chemistry and physics.

Incompatibilities—Although many of the reactions characteristic of acids offer opportunities for incompatibilities, only a few are of sufficient importance to require more than casual mention. Acids and acid salts decompose carbonates with the liberation of carbon dioxide and, in a closed container, sufficient pressure may be developed to produce an explosion. Inorganic acids react with salts of organic acids to produce the free organic acid and a salt of the inorganic acid. If insoluble, the organic acid will be precipitated. Thus, salicylic acid and benzoic acid are precipitated from solutions of salicylates and benzoates. Boric

acid is likewise precipitated from concentrated solutions of borates. By a similar reaction, certain soluble organic compounds are converted into an insoluble form. Sodium phenobarbital, for example, is converted into phenobarbital which in aqueous solution will precipitate.

The ability of acids to combine with alkaloids and other organic compounds containing a basic nitrogen atom is utilized in preparing soluble salts of these substances.

It should be borne in mind that certain fluidextracts, syrups, tinctures, and other pharmaceutical preparations may contain free acid which causes these preparations to exhibit the incompatibilities of the acid.

Acids also possess the incompatibilities of the anions which they contain, and in the case of organic acids, these are frequently of prime importance. These are discussed under the specific anions.

Diluted Acids—The diluted acids are aqueous solutions of acids, of a strength suitable for internal administration or for the manufacture of other preparations. The USP does not recognize any diluted acids (except as reagents). Diluted acids official in the NF are 10% *w/v* in strength except Diluted Acetic Acid which is 6% *w/v*.

The strengths of the official undiluted acids are expressed as percentages weight in weight whereas the strengths of the official diluted acids are expressed as percentages weight in volume. It therefore becomes necessary to consider the specific gravities of the concentrated acids when calculating the volume required to make a given quantity of diluted acid. The following equation will give the number of ml required to make 1000 ml of diluted acid:

$$\frac{\text{Strength of diluted acid} \times 1000}{\text{Strength of undiluted acid} \times \text{sp gr of undiluted acid}}$$

Thus, if one wishes to make 1000 ml of Diluted Hydrochloric Acid using Hydrochloric Acid which assays 36.22% HCl (sp gr 1.18), the amount required is

$$\frac{10 \times 1000}{36.22 \times 1.18} = 234 \text{ ml}$$

One of these diluted acids, Diluted Hydrochloric Acid, is used in the treatment of achlorhydria. However, it may irritate the mucous membrane of the mouth and attack the enamel of the teeth. The usual dose is 5 ml, well diluted with water. In the treatment of achlorhydria no attempt is made to administer more than a relief-producing dose. The normal pH of the gastric juice is 0.9 to 1.5 and, in order to attain this level, particularly in severe cases of gastric malfunction, somewhat larger doses of Diluted Hydrochloric Acid would be required. Because of the disadvantages of this gastric acidifier, Glutamic Acid Hydrochloride is often recommended for the treatment of gastric hypoacidity. This substance is a solid and can be administered without causing the irritation observed with solutions of acids.

Many therapeutically active substances have acidic properties. Some (eg, aminosalicylic, ascorbic, folic, and salicylic) are designated as acids; others (eg, phenobarbital, phenylbutazone, and tolbutamide) are named in such a way that their acidic properties are not readily recognized. Substances that fall into these two categories should not be confused with the aqueous acids described in this section. The latter acids (eg, diluted acetic, hydriodic, and phosphoric) are usually classified as pharmaceutical necessities and possess few therapeutically significant properties.

Solutions

This category originally included all aqueous solutions of nonvolatile substances except those forming separate distinctive classes, such as syrups, infusions, and decoctions. The solutions of ammonia, of hydrogen peroxide, and of a few other volatile substances were exceptions.

The USP definition for this type of dosage form places emphasis on the aqueous solution. However, no solvent is specified in many of the monographs in the compendia. Preparations of this type are available only under a trademarked name or are solutions which in themselves represent the usual commercial form. An example of this type of preparation is Benzethonium Chloride Solution NF. The USP definition for this class of pharmaceuticals is:

"Solutions are liquid preparations that contain one or more soluble chemical substances usually dissolved in water. They are distinguished from Injections, for example, because they are not intended for administration by infusion or injection. The solute is usually nonvolatile. Solutions are used for the specific therapeutic effect of the solute, either internally or externally. They vary widely as to composition, method of preparation, strength, potency, mode of administration, use, and dosage."

Solvents, solubility, and general methods for the incorporation of a solute in a solvent are discussed in Chapter 19 on *Solutions and Phase Equilibria*, page 246. Solutions are usually bottled automatically by utilizing equipment of the type shown in Fig. 523.

Preparation—A specific method of preparation is given in the compendia for most solutions. These procedures fall into three main categories.

Simple Solution—Solutions of this type are prepared by dissolving the solute in a suitable solvent. The solvent may contain other ingredients which stabilize or solubilize the active ingredient. Calcium Hydroxide Solution USP (Lime Water), Formaldehyde Solution

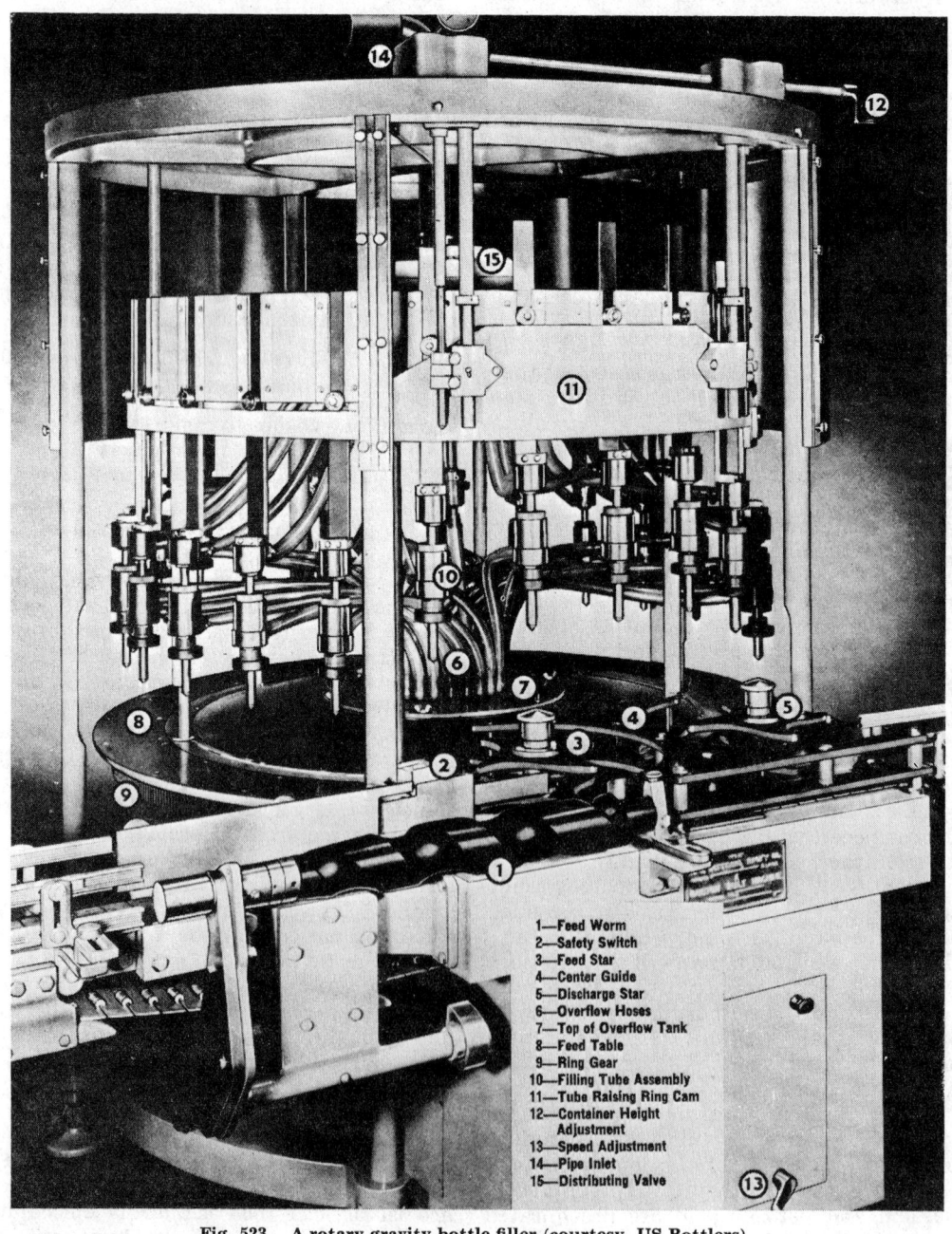

1—Feed Worm
2—Safety Switch
3—Feed Star
4—Center Guide
5—Discharge Star
6—Overflow Hoses
7—Top of Overflow Tank
8—Feed Table
9—Ring Gear
10—Filling Tube Assembly
11—Tube Raising Ring Cam
12—Container Height Adjustment
13—Speed Adjustment
14—Pipe Inlet
15—Distributing Valve

Fig. 523.   A rotary gravity bottle filler (courtesy, US Bottlers).

USP, and Strong Iodine Solution USP (Lugol's Solution) are examples of solutions that are prepared in this way.

Calcium Hydroxide Solution contains, in each 100 ml, not less than 140 mg of $Ca(OH)_2$. The solution is prepared by vigorously agitating 3 Gm of calcium hydroxide with 1000 ml of cool, purified water. Excess calcium hydroxide is allowed to settle out and the clear, supernatant liquid is dispensed.

An increase in solvent temperature usually implies an increase in solute solubility. This rule, however, does not apply to calcium hydroxide. At 15°C, 1 Gm dissolves in 780 ml of water; at 25°C in 714 ml of water, and at 80°C, in 3000 ml of water. The official solution is prepared at a temperature of 25°C.

Solutions containing hydroxides react with the carbon dioxide in the atmosphere.

$$OH^- + CO_2 \rightarrow HCO_3^-$$

$$OH^- + HCO_3^- \rightarrow CO_3^- + H_2O$$

$$Ca^{++} + CO_3^- \rightarrow CaCO_3$$

Calcium Hydroxide Solution should, therefore, be preserved in well-filled, tight containers, at a temperature not exceeding 25°C.

Formaldehyde Solution contains not less than 37.0%, by weight, of CH_2O. The USP recommends the addition of methanol to the solution in order to prevent the polymerization of the formaldehyde.

Strong Iodine Solution contains, in each 100 ml, 4.5–5.5 Gm of iodine, and 9.5–10.5 Gm of potassium iodide. It is prepared by dissolving 50 Gm of iodine in 100 ml of purified water containing 100 Gm of potassium iodide. Sufficient purified water is then added to make 1000 ml of solution.

One Gm of iodine dissolves in 2950 ml of water. However, solutions of iodides dissolve large quantities of iodine. Strong Iodine Solution is, therefore, a solution of polyiodides in excess iodide.

$$I^- + nI_2 \rightarrow I^-_{(2n-1)}$$

Doubly charged anions may also be formed.

$$2I^- + nI_2 \rightarrow I^=_{(2n-2)}$$

Strong Iodine Solution is classified as an antigoiterogenic. The usual dose is 0.3 ml 3 times a day.

Solution by Chemical Reaction—These solutions are prepared by reacting two or more solutes with each other in a suitable solvent. An example of a solution of this type is Aluminum Subacetate Solution USP.

Aluminum sulfate (160 Gm) is dissolved in 600 ml of cold water. The solution is filtered and precipitated calcium carbonate (70 Gm) is added, in several portions, with constant stirring. Acetic acid (160 ml) is slowly added and the mixture is set aside for 24 hr. The product is filtered and the magma on the Buchner filter is washed with cold water until the total filtrate measures 1000 ml.

The solution contains pentaquohydroxo- and tetraquodihydroxoaluminum (III) acetates and sulfates dissolved in an aqueous medium saturated with calcium sulfate. The solution contains a small amount of acetic acid. It is stabilized by the addition of not more than 0.9% boric acid.

The reactions involved in the preparation of the solution are given below. The hexaquo aluminum cations are first converted to the nonirritating $[Al(H_2O)_5(OH)]^{++}$ and $[Al(H_2O)_4(OH)_2]^+$ cations.

$$[Al(H_2O)_6]^{+++} + CO_3^- \rightarrow [Al(H_2O)_5(OH)]^{++} + HCO_3^-$$

$$[Al(H_2O)_6]^{+++} + HCO_3^- \rightarrow [Al(H_2O)_5(OH)]^{++} + H_2O + CO_2$$

As the concentration of the hexaquo cations decreases, secondary reactions involving carbonate and bicarbonate occur.

$$[Al(H_2O)_5(OH)]^{++} + CO_3^- \rightarrow [Al(H_2O)_4(OH)_2]^+ + HCO_3^-$$

$$[Al(H_2O)_5(OH)]^{++} + HCO_3^- \rightarrow [Al(H_2O)_4(OH)_2]^+ + H_2CO_3$$

The pH of the solution now favors the precipitation of dissolved calcium ions as the insoluble sulfate. Acetic acid is now added. The bicarbonate which is formed in the final stages of the procedure is removed as carbon dioxide.[6]

Aluminum Subacetate Solution is used in the preparation of Aluminum Acetate Solution USP (Burow's Solution). The latter solution contains 15 ml of glacial acetic acid, 545 ml of Aluminum Subacetate Solution, and sufficient water to make 1000 ml. It is defined as a solution of aluminum acetate in approximately 5%, by weight, of acetic acid in water. It is stabilized by the addition of not more than 0.6% boric acid.

Solution by Extraction—Drugs or pharmaceutical necessities of vegetable or animal origin are often extracted with water or with water containing other substances. Preparations of this type may be classified as solutions but, more often, are classified as extractives. These are described in detail in Chapter 84.

Douches

A douche is an aqueous solution which is directed against a part or into a cavity of the body. It functions as a cleansing or antiseptic agent. An *eye douche*, used to remove foreign particles and discharges from the eyes, is directed gently at an oblique angle and is allowed to run from the inner to the outer corner of the eye. *Pharyngeal douches* are used to prepare the interior of the throat for an operation and to cleanse it in suppurative conditions. Similarly, there are *nasal douches* and *vaginal douches*. Douches are usually directed to the appropriate body part by using bulb syringes. These are described in Chapter 99 on *Health Accessories*.

Douches are most frequently dispensed in the form of a powder with directions for dissolving in a specified quantity of water, usually warm. However, tablets for preparing solutions are available (eg, Dobell's Solution Tablets) or the solution may be prepared by the pharmacist. If powders or tablets are supplied, they must be free from insoluble material, in order to produce a clear solution. Tablets are produced by the usual processes but any lubricants or diluents used must be readily soluble in water. Boric acid may be used as a lubricant and sodium chloride is normally used as a diluent. Tablets deteriorate on exposure to moist air and should be stored in airtight containers.

Preparations of this type may contain alum, zinc sulfate, boric acid, phenol, or sodium borate. The ingredients in one douche are alum (4 Gm), zinc sulfate (4 Gm), liquefied phenol (5 ml), glycerin (125 ml), and water (a sufficient quantity to make 1000 ml of solution). Sodium borate (borax, sodium tetraborate) is used in the preparation of Compound Sodium Borate Solution NF XI (Dobell's Solution). A solution of sodium borate in water is alkaline to litmus paper. In the presence of water, sodium metaborate, boric acid, and sodium hydroxide are formed.

$$Na_2B_4O_7 + 3H_2O \rightarrow 2NaBO_2 + 2H_3BO_3$$

$$NaBO_2 + 2H_2O \rightarrow NaOH + H_3BO_3$$

The official solution contains sodium borate, sodium bicarbonate, liquefied phenol, and glycerin. The reaction between boric acid and glycerin is given in the section on *Washes*.

Douches are not official as a class of preparations but several substances in the USP and NF are frequently employed as such in weak solutions, eg, Benzalkonium Chloride USP is used in various douches and Compound Sodium Borate Solution NF XI is used as a nasal or pharyngeal douche.

Vaginal or urethral douches are occasionally referred to as Irrigations. These solutions may have an antiseptic, astringent, or soothing action and are prepared immediately before use by dissolving the medicament in the required amount of water. One example of such a preparation is Irrigation of Lactic Acid BPC 1963. This solution contains 3.75 ml of lactic acid in every 600 ml of aqueous product.

Enemas

Enemas are rectal injections employed to evacuate the bowel, to influence the general system by absorption, or to affect locally the seat of disease. They may possess anthelmintic, nutritive, sedative, or stimulating properties, or they may contain radiopaque substances for roentgenographic examination of the lower bowel. Enemas are usually given at body temperature in quantities of 1 to 2 pints injected slowly with a syringe. If they are to be retained in the intestine, they should not be used in larger quantities than 6 fluid ounces for an adult.

Starch enema may be used either by itself or as a vehicle for other forms of medication. A thin paste is made by triturating 30 Gm of powdered starch with 200 ml of cold water. Sufficient boiling water is added to make 1000 ml of enema. The preparation is then reheated to obtain a transparent liquid.

Barium sulfate enema contains 120 Gm of barium sulfate, 100 ml of acacia mucilage, and sufficient starch enema to make 500 ml.

Sodium chloride, sodium bicarbonate, sodium monohydrogen phosphate, and sodium dihydrogen phosphate are used in enemas. These substances may be used alone, in combination with each other, or in combination with irritants such as soap. Enema of Soap BPC 1963 is prepared by dissolving 50 Gm of soft soap in sufficient purified water to make 1000 ml of enema. Fleet Enema, a commercially available enema containing 16 Gm of sodium acid phosphate and 6 Gm of sodium phosphate in 100 ml, is marketed as a single-dose disposable unit.

Gargles

Gargles are aqueous solutions used for treating the pharynx and nasopharynx by forcing air from the lungs through the gargle which is held in the throat. Many gargles must be diluted with water prior to use. Although mouth washes are considered as a separate class of pharmaceuticals, many are used as gargles, either as is or diluted with water.

Phenol Gargle is official in BP 1968. It contains 50 ml of Phenol Glycerin (16% *w/w* phenol and 84% *w/w* glycerin), 10 ml of Amaranth Solution (1% *w/v* in chloroform water), and water to 1000 ml.

Washes

A mouthwash is an aqueous solution which is most often used for its deodorant, refreshing, or antiseptic effect. It may contain alcohol, glycerin, synthetic sweeteners, and surface-active, flavoring, and coloring agents. Commercial preparations contain such local anti-infective agents as hexetidine and cetylpyridinium chloride. They may be either acidic or basic in reaction and, in some instances, are fairly effective in reducing bacterial concentrations and odors in the mouth for short periods of time.

The products of commerce (eg, Cepacol, Listerine, Micrin, Scope, etc) vary widely in composition. Compound Sodium Borate Solution NF XI (Dobell's Solution) is used as an antiseptic wash. Antiseptic Solution and Mouthwash are described in NF XII. The latter wash contains sodium borate, glycerin, and potassium bicarbonate. The reactions which take place when these substances are dissolved in water are given below.

Compound Sodium Chloride Mouth Wash is described in BPC 1968. It is a solution of 15% *w/v* sodium chloride and 10% *w/v* sodium bicarbonate in peppermint water.

Juices

A juice is prepared from fresh ripe fruit, is aqueous in character, and is used in making syrups which are employed as vehicles. The freshly expressed juice is preserved with benzoic acid, and is allowed to stand at room temperature for several days, until the pectins which are naturally present are destroyed by enzymatic action, as indicated by the filtered juice yielding a clear solution with alcohol. Pectins, if allowed to remain, would cause precipitation in the final syrup.

Cherry Juice and Raspberry Juice are official in the USP. Concentrated Raspberry Juice included in BPC 1968 is prepared from the clarified juice of raspberries. Pectinase is stirred into pulped raspberries and the mixture is allowed to stand for 12 hr. The pulp is pressed, the juice is clarified, and sufficient sucrose is added to adjust the weight per ml at 20°C to 1.050–1.060 Gm. The juice is then concentrated to one-sixth of its original volume. Sufficient sulfurous acid or sodium metabisulfite is added to preserve the juice.

Artificial flavors have now replaced many of the natural fruit juices. Although they lack the flavor of the natural juice, they are more stable and are easier to incorporate into the final pharmaceutical form.

Juices expressed from fresh plants and evaporated were formerly known as *Inspissated Juices*.

Sweet or Other Viscid Aqueous Solutions

Solutions which are sweet or viscid include Syrups, Honeys, Mucilages, and Jellies. All of these preparations are viscous liquids or semisolids. The basic sweet or viscid substances giving body to these preparations are sugars, polyols, or polysaccharides (gums).

Syrups

Syrups are concentrated solutions of a sugar such as sucrose in water or other aqueous liquid. When purified water alone is used in making the solution of sucrose, the preparation is known as *syrup*, or *simple syrup*. In addition to sucrose, certain other polyols, such as glycerin or sorbitol, may be added to retard crystallization of sucrose or to increase the solubility of added ingredients. When the aqueous preparation contains some added medicinal substance, the syrup is called a *medicated* syrup. A *flavored* syrup is one which is usually not medicated, but which contains various aromatic or pleasantly flavored substances and is intended to be used as a vehicle or flavor for prescriptions.

Flavored syrups offer unusual opportunities as vehicles in extemporaneous compounding and are readily accepted by both children and adults. Because they contain no or very little alcohol, they are the vehicle of choice for many of the drugs that are prescribed by pediatricians. Their lack of alcohol makes them superior solvents for water-soluble substances.

Syrups possess remarkable masking properties for bitter and saline drugs. Glycyrrhiza Syrup has been recommended for disguising the salty taste of bromides, iodides, and chlorides. This has been attributed to its colloidal character and to its double sweetness—the immediate sweetness of the sugar and the lingering sweetness of the glycyrrhizin. This syrup is also of value in masking bitterness in preparations containing the B complex vitamins. Acacia Syrup, because of its colloidal character, is of particular value as a vehicle for masking the disagreeable taste of many medicaments. Raspberry Syrup is one of the most efficient flavoring agents and is especially useful in masking the taste of bitter drugs. Many factors, however, enter into the choice of a suitable flavoring agent. Literature results are often contradictory and there appears to be no substitute for the taste panel. The literature on this subject has been reviewed by Meer,[7] and this reference and Chapter 71 on *Pharmaceutical Necessities* should be consulted for further information on the flavoring of pharmaceuticals.

In manufacturing syrups the sucrose must be carefully selected and a purified water, free from foreign substances, and clean vessels and containers must be used. The operation must be conducted with care so as to avoid contamination, if the products are to be stable preparations.

It is important that the concentration of sucrose approach but not quite reach the saturation point. In dilute solutions sucrose provides an excellent nutrient for molds, yeasts, and other microorganisms. In concentrations of 65% by weight or more, the solution will retard the growth of such microorganisms. However, a saturated solution may lead to crystallization of a part of the sucrose under conditions of changing temperature.

When heat is used in the preparation of syrups, there is almost certain to be an inversion of a slight portion of the sucrose.

$$\underset{\text{Sucrose}}{C_{12}H_{22}O_{11}} \xrightarrow{\text{H}_2\text{O}} \underset{\text{Invert sugar}}{2C_6H_{12}O_6}$$

Sucrose solutions rotate polarized light to the right but, as hydrolysis proceeds, the optical rotation falls and becomes negative when the reaction is complete. This reaction is termed *inversion* because *invert sugar* (dextrose plus levulose) is formed. The speed of inversion is greatly increased by the presence of acids; the hydrogen ion acts as a catalyst in this hydrolytic reaction. Invert sugar is more readily fermentable than sucrose and tends to darken in color. Nevertheless its two reducing sugars are of value in retarding the oxidation of other substances.

Invert Syrup is described in the BPC 1968. The syrup is prepared by hydrolyzing sucrose with hydrochloric acid and neutralizing the solution with calcium or sodium carbonate. The sucrose in the 66.7% *w/w* solution must be at least 95% inverted. The monograph states that invert syrup, when mixed in suitable proportions with syrup, prevents the deposition of crystals of sucrose under most conditions of storage.

The levulose formed during inversion is sweeter than sucrose and therefore the resulting syrup is sweeter than the original syrup. The relative sweetness of levulose, sucrose, and dextrose are in the ratio 173: 100:74. Thus invert sugar is 1/100 (173 + 74) ½ = 1.23 times as sweet as sucrose. The levulose formed during the hydrolysis is also responsible for the darkening of Syrup. It is sensitive to heat and darkens readily, particularly in solution. When syrup or sucrose is overheated, it caramelizes. See *Caramel* (page 1320).

At one time blue dyes, such as ultramarine and Prussian Blue, were added to sugar to cover up the yellow tint which resulted from certain impurities. Today the processing and quality of sugar have been so improved that dyes are not employed. The white crystalline variety, known commercially as *granulated sugar*, is most frequently used in making syrup. A more detailed description of the processes involved in the production of sucrose is given in Chapter 71 on *Pharmaceutical Necessities*, page 1334. The sugar should be dry, or an allowance made for the moisture content, to ensure proper concentration in the syrup.

Preparation—Syrups are prepared in various ways, the choice of the proper method depending on the physical and chemical characteristics of the substances entering into the preparation. Four methods which are employed may be summarized as follows: (1) solution with heat; (2) agitation without heat; (3) addition of a medicating liquid to syrup; and (4) percolation.

Solution with Heat—This is the usual method of making syrups when the valuable constituent is neither volatile nor injured by heat, and when it is desirable to make the syrup rapidly. The sucrose is usually added to the purified water or aqueous solution and heated until solution is effected, then strained, and sufficient purified water added to make the desired weight or volume. If the syrup is made from an infusion, a decoction, or an aqueous solution containing organic matter, it is usually proper to heat the syrup to the boiling point to coagulate albuminous matter; this is separated subsequently by straining. If the albumin or other impurities were permitted to remain in the syrup, fermentation would probably be induced in warm weather. Saccharometers are very useful in making syrups by the hot process in cases where the proper specific gravity of the finished syrup is known. The saccharometer may be floated in the syrup while boiling, and thus the exact degree of concentration determined without waiting to cool the syrup and having to heat it again to concentrate it further. When taking a reading of the specific gravity of the hot syrup allowance must be made for the variation from the official temperature (specific gravities in the USP are taken at 25 °C).

Excessive heating of syrups at the boiling temperature is undesirable since more or less inversion of the sucrose occurs with an increased tendency to ferment. Syrups cannot be sterilized in an autoclave without some caramelization. This is indicated by a yellowish or brownish color resulting from the formation of caramel, by the action of heat upon sucrose.

The formula and procedure given for Acacia Syrup NF (page 1339) illustrate this method of preparation.

Agitation without Heat—This process is used in those cases where heat would cause the loss of valuable volatile constituents. In making quantities up to 2000 ml or 2 quarts the sucrose should be added to the aqueous solution in a bottle of about twice the size required for the syrup. This permits active agitation and rapid solution. A "five-pint," glass-stoppered tincture bottle is well adapted for the making of 1000 ml of syrup by this process. The stoppering of the bottle is important, as it prevents contamination and loss during the process. The bottle should be allowed to lie upon its side when not being agitated. Glass-lined tanks with mechanical agitators, especially adapted to the dissolving of sucrose, are used for making syrups in large quantities.

The formula and procedure given for Ferrous Sulfate Syrup NF (page 826) illustrate this method of preparation.

Addition of a Medicating Liquid to Syrup—This method is resorted to in those cases in which fluid extracts, tinctures, or other liquids are added to syrup to medicate it. Syrups made in this way usually develop precipitates since alcohol is often an ingredient of the liquids thus used, and the resinous and oily substances dissolved by the alcohol precipitate when mixed with the syrup, producing unsightly preparations. A modification of this process, frequently adopted, consists of mixing the fluidextract or tincture with the water, allowing the mixture to stand to permit the separation of insoluble constituents, filtering, and then dissolving the sucrose in the filtrate. It is obvious that this procedure is not permissible when the precipitated ingredients are the valuable medicinal agents.

The formula and procedure given for Aromatic Eriodictyon Syrup NF (page 1339) illustrate this method of preparation.

Percolation—In this procedure, purified water or an aqueous solution is permitted to pass slowly through a bed of crystalline sucrose, thus dissolving it and forming a syrup. A pledget of cotton is placed in the neck of the percolator and the water or aqueous solution added. By means of a suitable stopcock the flow is regulated so that drops appear in rapid succession. If necessary, a portion of the liquid is repassed through the percolator to dissolve all of the sucrose. Finally, sufficient purified water is passed through the cotton to make the required volume.

To be successful in using this process, care in several particulars must be exercised: (1) the percolator used should be cylindrical or semicylindrical, and cone-shaped as it nears the lower orifice; (2) a coarse granular sugar must be used, otherwise it will form into a compact mass, which the liquid cannot permeate; (3) the purified cotton must be introduced with care. If pressed in too tightly, it will effectually stop the process; if inserted too loosely, the liquid will pass through the cotton rapidly and the filtrate will be weak and turbid (from imperfect filtration); it should be inserted completely within the neck of the percolator, since a protruding end, inside the percolator, up through the sucrose, will permit the last portions of water to pass out at the lower orifice without dissolving all of the sucrose. For specific directions see *Syrup* (page 1340). The process of percolation is applied on a commercial scale for the making of official syrups as well as those for confectionary use.

Percolation is permitted as an alternate method for the preparation of Syrup USP (page 1340), Wild Cherry Syrup USP (page 1340), and Tolu Balsam Syrup NF (page 1335).

Preservation—Syrups should not be made in larger quantities than can be used within a few months, except in those cases where special facilities can be employed for their preservation. A low temperature is the best method of preservation for syrups. The USP suggests that syrups be kept at a temperature not above 25°. Concentration without supersaturation is also a condition favorable to preservation. The USP states that syrups may contain preservatives to prevent bacterial and mold growth. Preservatives such as glycerin, methylparaben, benzoic acid, and sodium benzoate may be added, particularly when the concentration of sucrose in the syrup is low. Any attempt to restore syrups which have been spoiled through fermentation by heating them and "working them over" is reprehensible.

A simple and yet effective method of preserving syrups, especially adapted to fruit syrups, is as follows: A number of bottles are provided which hold not more than a pint each. The bottles are thoroughly cleaned and kept hot by immersion in boiling water until ready for use, and a sufficient number of good corks, which have been thoroughly soaked in hot, distilled water, and of the proper size for the bottles, should be at hand. The syrup should be heated to the boiling point (strained, if necessary, and reheated), and poured into the hot bottles until they are filled to the brim. The corks are inserted by forcibly pressing them into the necks of the bottles, thereby displacing a small portion of the syrup, and tied down with twine or wired in place. Then, while the necks of the bottles are still hot (and before the syrup can contract in volume through cooling) they are dipped into melted paraffin contained in a suitable vessel. By this method the organisms which produce fermentation are destroyed by the heat, and no air, carrying new contamination, can find its way to the syrup, as the bottles are hermetically sealed.

The official syrups should be preserved in well-dried bottles, preferably those which have been sterilized. These bottles should not hold more than is likely to be required during four to six weeks and should be completely filled, carefully stoppered, and stored in a cool, dark place.

Syrups Prepared from Juices

Blackberry syrup, pineapple syrup, and strawberry syrup may be prepared by following the directions given in the USP for Cherry Syrup (page 1339). Syrup of Black Currant BPC 1968 is prepared in a similar manner but with certain modifications. The pectin in the juice is destroyed with pectinase. The syrup is prepared from 700 Gm of sucrose and 560 ml of clarified juice and is preserved with sulfurous acid or sodium metabisulfite. The addition of a dye is permitted, provided it complies with the pertinent British regulations.

Honeys

Honeys are thick liquid preparations somewhat allied to the syrups, differing in the use of honey, instead of syrup, as a base. They are unimportant as a class of preparation today but at one time, before sugar was available and honey was the most common sweetening agent, they were widely used. BPC 1968 lists two preparations containing honey. The first, Oxymel, or "acid honey," is a mixture of acetic acid (150 ml), purified water (150 ml), and honey (sufficient to produce 1000 ml of product). Squill Oxymel contains squill, water, acetic acid, and honey and is prepared by a maceration process.

Mucilages

The official mucilages are thick, viscid, adhesive liquids, produced by dispersing gum in water, or by extracting with water the mucilaginous principles from vegetable substances. The mucilages are all prone to decomposition, and should never be made in larger quantities than can be used immediately, unless a preservative is added. Both Acacia Mucilage NF XII and Tragacanth Mucilage NF XII contain benzoic acid.

The former mucilage may be prepared by placing 350 Gm of acacia in a graduated bottle, washing the drug with cold purified water, allowing it to drain, and adding enough warm purified water, in which 2 Gm of benzoic acid has been dissolved, to make the product measure 1000 ml. The bottle is then stoppered, placed on its side, rotated occasionally, and the product is strained when the acacia has dissolved.

Tragacanth Mucilage is prepared by mixing 18 Gm of glycerin with 75 ml of water, heating the mixture to boiling, discontinuing the application of heat, adding 6 Gm of tragacanth and 0.2 Gm benzoic acid, and macerating the mixture for 24 hr. Sufficient purified water is then added to make the mixture weight 100 Gm. The mucilage is strained forcibly through muslin.

Mucilages are used primarily to aid in suspending insoluble substances in liquids; their colloidal character and viscosity help them prevent immediate sedimenta-

tion. Examples include sulfur in lotions, resin in mixtures, and oils in emulsions. Both tragacanth and acacia are either partially or completely insoluble in alcohol. Tragacanth is precipitated from solution by alcohol, but acacia, on the other hand, is soluble in diluted alcoholic solutions. A 60% solution of acacia may be prepared with 20% alcohol, and a 4% solution of acacia may be prepared even with 50% alcohol.

The viscosity of tragacanth mucilage is reduced by acid, alkali, and sodium chloride, particularly if the mucilage is heated. It shows maximum viscosity at a pH of 5.[8] Acacia is hydrolyzed by dilute mineral acids to arabinose, galactose, aldobionic and galacturonic acids. Its viscosity is low but is maintained over a wide pH range.

Several synthetic mucilage-like substances such as *polyvinyl alcohol, methylcellulose, carboxymethylcellulose,* and related substances, are used as mucilage substitutes. Methylcellulose (page 1345) is widely used as a bulk laxative since it absorbs water and swells to a hydrogel in the intestine in much the same manner as *psyllium* or *karaya gum.* The synthetic gums are nonglycogenetic and may be used in the preparation of diabetic syrups. Several formulas for such syrups, based on sodium carboxymethylcellulose, have been proposed.[9]

Jellies

The NF defines Jellies under Gels and states that they are a class of gels in which the structural coherent matrix contains a high portion of liquid, usually water. They are similar to mucilages, in that they may be prepared from gums similar to those used for mucilage, but they differ from the latter in having a jelly-like consistency. A whole gum of the best quality rather than a powdered gum is desirable in order to obtain a clear preparation of uniform consistency. Tragacanth is the gum used in the preparation of Ephedrine Sulfate Jelly NF XII. These preparations may also be formulated from acacia, chondrus, gelatin, carboxymethylcellulose, and similar substances, with water.

Jellies are used as lubricants for surgical gloves, catheters, and rectal thermometers. Therapeutic vaginal jellies are available and certain jelly-like preparations are used for contraceptive purposes. The latter preparations often contain surface active agents to enhance the spermatocidal properties of the jelly. Aromatics, such as methyl salicylate and eucalyptol, are often added to give the preparation a desirable odor.

Although Gels and Jellies are defined together in the NF, these products differ characteristically in their physical properties. The Gels are closely related to the Magmas and are, therefore, considered elsewhere in this chapter.

Nonaqueous Solutions

It is difficult to evaluate fairly the importance of nonaqueous solvents in pharmaceutical processes. That they are important in the manufacture of pharmaceuticals, is an understatement. However, pharmaceutical preparations, and, in particular, those intended for internal use, rarely contain more than minor quantities of the toxic solvents that are common to the manufacturing or analytical operation. For example, the industry uses large quantities of chloroform in some operations but the solvent is of only minor importance

with respect to the final product. One ml of chloroform dissolves in about 200 ml of water and the solution so formed finds some use as a vehicle (see the section on *Waters*). This solvent is also found in a number of cough syrups and, in one formulation, is present in a concentration of 2 grains per fluid ounce of syrup. Solvents such as acetone, benzene, and petroleum ether should not be ingredients in preparations intended for internal use.

The products of commerce may contain solvents such

as ethanol, glycerin, propylene glycol, certain oils, and liquid paraffin. Preparations intended for external use may contain methanol, isopropyl alcohol, polyethylene glycols, various ethers, and certain esters. A common practice is to mix water into many preparations which are classified as nonaqueous in character. One example of this is in the preparation of elixirs. Although the lines between aqueous and nonaqueous preparations tend to blur in those cases where the solvent is water soluble, it is possible to categorize a number of products as nonaqueous. This section is, therefore, devoted to four groups of nonaqueous solutions; the first includes the alcoholic or hydroalcoholic solutions, examples of these being elixirs and spirits; the second, the ethereal solutions, an example being the collodions; the third, the glycerin solutions, as exemplified by the glycerites; and lastly, the oleaginous solutions, as represented by the liniments, medicated oils, oleovitamins, sprays, and toothache drops.

Although the above list is self-limiting, a wide variety of solvents are used in various pharmaceutical preparations. Solvents such as glycerol formal, dimethylacetamide, glycerol dimethylketal, and dimethyl sulfoxide have been recommended for many of the products produced by the industry.[10,11] However, the toxicity of many of these solvents is not well established and, at least in one case, that of dimethyl sulfoxide, therapeutic claims have been made for the substance. Its use has been suggested for the treatment of bursitis and allied conditions. However, the observed side-effects are of such significance that the clinical trials on the substance have been suspended. The toxicity of formulations containing this or similar solvents should not only be determined but also reported to the FDA before the product is marketed.

A basic definition for the term *solution* has been given in a previous section of this chapter. The theory of solution is presented in Chapter 19, page 246.

Collodions

Collodions are liquid preparations containing pyroxylin (a nitrocellulose) in a mixture of ethyl ether and ethanol. They are applied to the skin by means of a soft brush or other suitable applicator and, when the ether and ethanol have evaporated, leave a film of pyroxylin on the surface. The official medicated collodion, Salicylic Acid Collodion USP, contains 10% *w/v* of salicylic acid in Flexible Collodion USP and is used as a keratolytic agent in the treatment of corns and warts. Collodion USP and Flexible Collodion USP are water-repellent protectives for minor cuts and scratches. Collodion is made flexible by the addition of castor oil.

Elixirs

The USP defines elixirs as follows:

"Elixirs are clear, sweetened, hydroalcoholic liquids intended for oral use. They contain flavoring substances and, in the case of medicated elixirs, active medicinal agents. Their primary solvents are alcohol and water, with glycerin, sorbitol, and syrup sometimes used as additional solvents and/or sweetening agents. They are prepared by simple solution or admixture of the several ingredients.

"They are used either as vehicles (eg, *Aromatic Elixir*) or for the therapeutic effect of the medicinal substance that they contain (eg, *Diphenhydramine Hydrochloride Elixir* and *Phenobarbital Elixir*)."

This definition, therefore, divides the elixirs into two groups, those that are used as flavors and vehicles in prescriptions and those that are classified as the medicated elixirs. However, the distinction between the two is not quite as clear as the definition implies. The pharmacist may be required to use a medicated elixir as a vehicle for other drugs. This is particularly true of the elixirs of commerce and the student should be able to recognize those products that fall into this category of pharmaceutical preparations.

Elixirs contain ethyl alcohol. However, the alcoholic content will vary greatly, from elixirs containing only a small quantity, to those that contain a considerable portion as a necessary aid to solubility. For example, Aromatic Elixir USP contains 21 to 23% C_2H_5OH; Compound Benzaldehyde Elixir NF, on the other hand, contains 3 to 5% C_2H_5OH.

Elixirs may also contain glycerin and syrup. These may be added to increase the solubility of the medicinal agent or for sweetening purposes. Some elixirs contain propylene glycol. Claims have been made that this solvent is a satisfactory substitute for both glycerin and alcohol. Sumner,[12] in his paper on terpin hydrate preparations, summarized the advantages and disadvantages of this solvent and suggested several formulations with therapeutic characteristics superior to those of the elixir described in the NF (page 875).

One usual dose of the elixir (5 ml) contains 85 mg of terpin hydrate. This substance is used in bronchitis in doses of 125 to 300 mg as an expectorant. The elixir is, therefore, ineffective for the treatment of bronchitis. However, the elixir is used as a vehicle for the drugs in many commercially available cough syrups. These may contain dextromethorphan hydrobromide, codeine phosphate, chlorpheniramine maleate, pyrilamine maleate, ammonium chloride, creosote, chloroform, and a wide variety of other drugs with expectorant and antitussive properties.

Two of the four formulations described in Sumner's paper are given below.

Formulation 1

Terpin Hydrate	6.0 Gm
Lemon Tincture	5.0 ml
Orange Tincture	5.0 ml
Sodium Saccharin	0.5 Gm
Propylene Glycol	65.0 ml
Glycerin	15.0 ml
Sorbitol Solution, USP, a sufficient quantity, To make	100.0 ml

Dissolve the terpin hydrate in the propylene glycol and the glycerin which have been heated to 50°C. Dissolve the sodium saccharin in the tinctures and add to the solution of terpin hydrate at 25°C. Add sufficient sorbitol solution to make the product measure 100 ml.

Formulation 2

Terpin Hydrate	6.0 Gm
Orange Oil	0.1 ml
Benzaldehyde	0.005 ml
Sorbitol Solution USP	10.0 ml
Propylene Glycol	40.0 ml
Alcohol	43.0 ml
Purified Water, a sufficient quantity, To make	100.0 ml

Dissolve the terpin hydrate in the propylene glycol and sorbitol solution which have been heated to 50°C. Add the oil and the benzaldehyde to the alcohol and mix with the terpin hydrate solution at 25°C. Add sufficient purified water to make the product measure 100 ml.

Both of these elixirs contain 300 mg of terpin hydrate per 5 ml, a minimal quantity of alcohol, and flavoring agents which adequately mask the taste of propylene glycol.

Although alcohol is an excellent solvent for some drugs, it does accentuate the saline taste of bromides and similar salts. It is often desirable, therefore, to substitute some other solvent that is more effective in masking such tastes for part of the alcohol in the formula. In general, if taste is a consideration, the formulator is more prone to utilize a syrupy rather than a hydroalcoholic vehicle.

An elixir may contain water and alcohol soluble ingredients. If such is the case, the following procedure is indicated:

Dissolve the water soluble ingredients in part of the water. Add and solubilize the sucrose in the aqueous solution. Prepare an alcoholic solution containing the other ingredients. Add the aqueous phase to the alcoholic solution, filter, and make to volume with water.

Sucrose increases viscosity and decreases the solubilizing properties of water and so must be added after primary solution has been carried out. A high alcoholic content is maintained during preparation by adding the aqueous phase to the alcoholic solution. Elixirs should always be brilliantly clear. They may be strained or filtered and, if necessary, subjected to the clarifying action of purified talc or siliceous earth.

One of the elixirs official in the NF, Iso-Alcoholic Elixir (page 1341), is actually a combination of two solutions, the one containing 8 to 10% ethanol and the other containing 73 to 78% ethanol. The elixir is used as a vehicle for various medicaments that require solvents of different alcohol strengths. For example, the alcohol strength of the elixir to be used with a single liquid galenical is approximately the same as that of the galenical. When different alcohol strengths are used in the same prescription, the elixir to be used is the one that produces the best solution. This is usually the average of the alcohol strengths of the several ingredients. For nonextractive substances, the lowest alcohol strength of elixir that will produce a clear solution should be used.

Incompatibilities—Since elixirs contain alcohol, incompatibilities of this solvent are an important consideration during the formulation process. Alcohol precipitates tragacanth, acacia, and agar from aqueous solutions. Similarly, it will precipitate many inorganic salts from similar solutions. The implication here is that such substances should be absent from the aqueous phase or should be present in such concentrations that there is no danger of precipitation on standing.

If an aqueous solution is added to an elixir, a partial precipitation of ingredients may occur. This is due to the reduced alcohol content of the final preparation. Usually, however, the alcohol content of the mixture is not sufficiently high to cause separation. As vehicles for tinctures and fluidextracts, the elixirs generally cause a separation of extractive matter from these products due to a reduction of the alcohol content.

Many of the incompatibilities between elixirs and the substances combined with them are due to the chemical characteristics of the elixir *per se* or of the ingredients in the final preparation. Thus certain elixirs are acid in reaction while others may be alkaline and will, therefore, behave accordingly.

A closely related group of preparations are the *cordials*. These are pleasantly flavored and are intended for internal administration. However, they are no longer official and, therefore, require no particular emphasis.

Glycerites

Glycerites are solutions or mixtures of medicinal substances in not less than 50% by weight of glycerin. Most of the glycerites are extremely viscous and some of them are of a jelly-like consistency. Few of the glycerites are extensively used.

Glycerin is a valuable pharmaceutical solvent forming permanent and concentrated solutions not otherwise obtainable. Some of these solutions are used in their original form as medicinal agents while others are used to prepare aqueous and alcoholic dilutions of substances which are not readily soluble in water or alcohol. One of the glycerites, Phenol Glycerin BPC 1968, is diluted with glycerin to form the pharmaceutical preparation, Phenol Ear-Drops BPC 1968.

Phenol Glycerin BPC 1968

Phenol	160 Gm
Glycerin	840 Gm

Dissolve the phenol in the glycerin.

Phenol Ear-Drops BPC 1968

Phenol Glycerin	40 ml
Glycerin, a sufficient quantity,	
To make	100 ml

Add the glycerin to the glycerite.

Water should not be added to this preparation. It reacts with the phenol to produce a preparation which is caustic and, consequently, damaging to the area of application.

Starch Glycerite NF, an emollient, contains starch (100 Gm), benzoic acid (2 Gm), purified water (200 ml), and glycerin (700 ml).

Glycerites are hygroscopic and should be stored in tightly closed containers.

Inhalations and Inhalants

Inhalations

These preparations are so used or designed that the drug is carried into the respiratory tree of the patient. The vapor or mist reaches the affected area and gives prompt relief from the symptoms of bronchial and nasal congestion. The USP defines Inhalations in the following way:

"Inhalations are drugs or solutions of drugs administered by the nasal or oral respiratory route for local or systemic effect. Examples in this Pharmacopeia are *Epinephrine Inhalation* and *Isoproterenol Hydrochloride Inhalation*. Nebulizers are suitable for the administration of inhalation solutions only if they give droplets sufficiently fine and uniform in size so that the mist reaches the bronchioles.

"This class includes also volatile and powdered medicaments and aerosols that are administered by the respiratory route with the aid of appropriate mechanical devices."

As stated in the pharmacopeia, particle size is of major importance in the administration of this type of preparation. The various types of mechanical devices that are used in conjunction with inhalations are described in some detail in Chapter 99, *Health Accessories*. It has been reported in the literature that the optimum particle size for penetration into the pulmonary cavity is of the order of ½ to 7 microns. Fine mists are produced by pressurized aerosols and hence possess basic advantages over the older nebulizers. In addition to this, metered aerosols deliver more uniform doses than those obtained with the older mechanical devices. The literature[13,14] and Chapter 90 on *Aerosols*, page 1729, should be consulted for further details on this subject.

The term *Inhalation* is used commonly by the layman to represent preparations intended to be vaporized with the aid of heat, usually steam, and inhaled. Benzoin Inhalation BPC 1968 contains benzoin, storax, and alcohol. The vapors from a preparation containing 1 teaspoonful of the tincture and 1 quart of boiling water may be inhaled. The device known as a *vaporizer* is used with a number of commercially available preparations of this type.

The official Inhalations contain epinephrine, isoproterenol hydrochloride, or isoproterenol sulfate.

Inhalants

A companion preparation, the Inhalant, is described in the NF. The definition therein is as follows:

"Inhalants are drugs or combinations of drugs which, by virtue of their high vapor pressure, can be carried by an air current into the nasal passage where they exert their effect. The device making possible the administration of an inhalant is known as an *inhaler*. An example of such a product is *Propylhexedrine Inhalant*, which contains the volatile sympathomimetic, propylhexedrine.

"Another group of products also known as inhalants or insufflations (but none of which is currently official in the NF) consists of finely powdered or liquid drugs that are carried into the respiratory passages by the use of special devices. Such devices include the low-pressure "aerosol" containers, which hold a solution or suspension of the drug in a liquefied propellant such as a fluorine- or fluorine and chlorine-substituted hydrocarbon. When released through a suitable spray nozzle, a metered dose of the inhalant is propelled into the respiratory tract of the patient. (See also *Aerosols*)."

The official preparation is described as consisting of cylindrical rolls of suitable fibrous material impregnated with propylhexedrine, usually aromatized, and contained in a suitable inhaler.

Liniments

Liniments are solutions or mixtures of various substances in oil, alcoholic solutions of soap, or emulsions. They are intended for external application and should be so labeled. They are applied with rubbing to the affected area and, because of this, were once call *embrocations*. The dental liniments, which are no longer official, are solutions of active substances and are rubbed into the gums. Most dentists question their usefulness and, consequently, this type of preparation is relatively unimportant as a pharmaceutical form.

Liniments are usually applied with friction and rubbing of the skin, the oil or soap base providing for ease of application and massage. Alcoholic liniments are used generally for their rubefacient, counterirritant, mildly astringent, and penetrating effects. Such liniments penetrate the skin more readily than do those with an oil base. The oily liniments, therefore, are milder in their action but are more useful when massage is required. Depending on the ingredients in the preparation, such liniments may function solely as protective coatings. Liniments should not be applied to skin areas that are bruised or broken.

Camphor and Soap Liniment NF XII is classified as a rubefacient.

Camphor and Soap Liniment NF XII

Green Soap	120 Gm
Camphor, in small pieces	45 Gm
Rosemary Oil	10 ml
Alcohol	700 ml
Purified Water, a sufficient quantity,	
To make	1000 ml

Dissolve the camphor and rosemary oil in the alcohol, add the green soap and stir or agitate until the mixture is clear. Add sufficient purified water to make the product measure 1000 ml, mix, set it aside in a cool place for 24 hr, and filter.

Calamine Liniment

Calamine	80 Gm
Zinc Oxide	80 Gm
Olive Oil	500 ml
Calcium Hydroxide Solution, a sufficient quantity,	
To make	1000 ml

Mix the calamine and the zinc oxide with the olive oil. Gradually add, with constant agitation, sufficient calcium hydroxide solution to make the product measure 1000 ml.

Other liniments contain antipruritics, astringents, emollients, and analgesics and are classified on the basis of the active ingredient in the formulation. Dermatologists prescribe products of this type but only those containing the rubefacients are extensively advertised and used by consumers for treatment of minor muscular aches and pains.

Oleovitamins

Oleovitamins are fish liver oils diluted with edible vegetable oil or solutions of the indicated vitamins or vitamin concentrates (usually vitamins A and D) in fish liver oil. The definition is sufficiently broad to include a wide variety of marketed products.

The indicated vitamins are unstable in the presence of rancid oils and, therefore, these preparations, and in particular, Oleovitamin A, should be stored in small, tight containers, preferably under vacuum or under an atmosphere of an inert gas, protected from light.

Spirits

Spirits, popularly known as essences, are alcoholic or hydroalcoholic solutions of volatile substances. Like the aromatic waters, the active ingredient in the spirit may be a solid, liquid, or gas. The genealogical tree for this class of preparations begins with the distinguished pair of products, Brandy (*Spiritus Vini Vitis*) and Whisky (*Spiritus Frumenti*), and ends with a wide variety of products that comply with the definition given above. Physicians have debated the therapeutic value of the former products and these are no longer official in the compendia.

Many of these spirits are used internally for their medicinal value, several are used medicinally by inhalation, while a large number are used as flavoring agents. The latter group provides a convenient and ready means of obtaining the volatile oil in the proper quantity. For example, a spirit or spirit-like preparation may be used in the formulation of aromatic waters or other pharmaceuticals that require a distinctive flavor.

Spirits should be stored in tight, light-resistant containers, and in a cool place. This prevents evaporation and volatilization of either the alcohol or the active principle.

Preparation—There are four classic methods for the preparation of this official group: These are *simple solution, solution with maceration, chemical reaction,* and *distillation*.

Simple Solution—This is the method by which the majority of spirits are prepared. No special skill is required but a great deal of conscientious care must be used in the selection of the volatile oils. Filtration is sometimes necessary to obtain a product of the desirable brilliancy.

No specific directions are given in the compendia for the preparation of the spirits of the volatile oils. However, former editions recommended that 65 ml of the volatile oil be dissolved in sufficient alcohol to make 1000 ml of spirit. This quantity of volatile oil is less than that recommended in the British Pharmaceutical Codex 1968. This publication lists several such spirits and directs that 100 ml of the volatile oil be combined with sufficient alcohol to make 1000 ml of solution.

Alcoholic solutions of volatile principles as employed in pharmacy may be regarded as a development of the perfume industry. It was discovered that alcoholic solutions of volatile oils possessed more delicate and fragrant odors than the pure oil itself, and as more aromatic principles were discovered or synthesized, experimentation resulted in the production of innumerable blends to satisfy every individual desire.

The formula and procedure given for Aromatic Ammonia Spirit NF illustrate this method of preparation.

Aromatic Ammonia Spirit NF

Ammonium Carbonate, in translucent pieces....	34 Gm
Strong Ammonia Solution....................	36 ml
Lemon Oil.............................	10 ml
Lavender Oil...........................	1 ml
Myristica Oil..........................	1 ml
Alcohol................................	700 ml
Purified Water, a sufficient quantity	
To make.............................	1000 ml

Dissolve the ammonium carbonate in the strong ammonia solution and 195 ml of purified water by gentle agitation, and allow the solution to stand for 12 hours. Dissolve the oils in the alcohol, contained in a graduated bottle or cylinder, and gradually add the ammonium carbonate solution and enough purified water to make the product measure 1000 ml. Set the mixture aside in a cool place for 24 hours, occasionally agitating it, and then filter, using a covered funnel.

The spirit is a respiratory stimulant and is administered by inhalation of the vapor as required. It is marketed in suitable tight, light-resistant containers but is also available in a single-dose glass vial wrapped in a soft cotton envelope. The vial is easily broken; the cotton acts as a sponge for the spirit.

Ammonium carbonate is a mixture of ammonium bicarbonate and ammonium carbamate (NH_2COONH_4). The carbamate reacts with water to form the carbonate.

$$NH_2COONH_4 + H_2O \rightarrow 2NH_4CO_3$$

An ammonium carbonate solution is, therefore, a solution of ammonium bicarbonate and ammonium carbonate in water. However, it decomposes in water, the decomposition products being ammonia, carbon dioxide, and water. The stability of the spirit is improved by the addition of strong ammonia solution. This represses the hydrolysis of ammonium carbonate and, in this way, decreases the loss of dissolved gases.

Solution with Maceration—In this procedure, leaves of the drug are macerated in purified water to extract water-soluble matter. They are then expressed, and the moist macerated leaves are added to a prescribed quantity of alcohol. The volatile oil is added to the filtered liquid. Peppermint Spirit NF is made by this process. Peppermint Spirit BPC 1968 differs from the official product in that it is a solution of the volatile oil in alcohol only. The concentration of volatile oil in the final product is about the same but the official preparation possesses a green color. The ready availability of soluble chlorophyll and other coloring agents has led to the frequent suggestion that a more uniform product could be obtained through their use. However, these agents cannot be used in preparing the official article.

The formula and procedure given for Peppermint Spirit NF (page 813) illustrate this method of preparation.

Chemical Reaction—No official spirits are prepared by this process. Ethyl nitrite is made by the action of sodium nitrite on a mixture of alcohol and sulfuric acid in the cold. This substance is then used to prepare Ethyl Nitrite Spirit, a product which is no longer official.

Distillation—Brandy and Whisky are made by distillation. The latter product is derived from the fermented mash of wholly or partially germinated malted cereal grains and the former from the fermented juice of ripe grapes.

Incompatibilities—Spirits are, for the most part, preparations of high alcoholic strength and do not lend themselves well to dilution with aqueous solutions or liquids of low alcoholic content. The addition of such a solution invariably causes a separation of some of the material dissolved in the spirit, the evidence of separation being a turbidity which, in time, may disappear as distinct layering occurs. Salts may be precipitated from their aqueous solutions by the addition of spirits due to their lesser solubility in alcoholic liquids.

Some spirits show incompatibilities peculiar to the ingredients which they contain. For example, Aromatic Ammonia Spirit NF cannot be mixed with aqueous preparations containing alkaloids (eg, codeine phosphate). An acid–base reaction (ammonia–phosphate) occurs and, if the alcoholic content of the final mixture is too low, codeine will precipitate out of solution.

Sprays

Sprays are solutions of various drugs in oily or aqueous vehicles and are applied to the mucous membrane of the nose and throat by means of an atomizer or nembulizer. The spray device should produce relatively coarse droplets if the action of the drug is to be restricted to the upper respiratory tract. Fine droplets tend to penetrate farther into the respiratory tract than is desirable.

Many of the older sprays contained menthol, thymol, camphor, methyl salicylate, and ephedrine dissolved in light liquid petrolatum. The use of light liquid petrolatum as a vehicle has, however, been severely criticized. There are two basic reasons for this. The first relates to the danger of lipoid pneumonia from the use of these oily preparations. Other reports have indicated that such sprays retard the normal ciliary activity on the nasal mucosa. In addition to this, the basic formulations have been criticized because of the instability of ephedrine in light liquid petrolatum.[15]

On the basis of the above reports, aqueous sprays which are isotonic with nasal secretions and of approximately the same pH are to be preferred. Such sprays may contain antibiotics, antihistamines, vasoconstrictors, alcohol, and suitable solubilizing and wetting agents. The pharmacist will handle many commercial preparations that comply with the basic definition given above and that help to alleviate the nasal congestion due to the common cold. For example, one of these contains chlorpheniramine maleate, phenylephrine hydrochloride, and gramicidin. Another is described as an isotonic, buffered (pH 6.2), aqueous solution containing phenylephrine hydrochloride, phenylpropanolamine hydrochloride, pheniramine maleate, and chlorobutanol. Most of the highly advertised sprays are marketed either in standard dropper bottles or in plastic squeeze units.

Ayerst Laboratories market a throat spray containing anise oil (0.6%), cassia oil (0.1%), pyrilamine maleate (0.05%), antipyrine (0.3%), methyl salicylate (0.05%), menthol (0.1%), sodium caprylate (0.5%), alcohol (1%), glycerol (2%), and methylrosaniline chloride. The "Spray-O-Mizer" squeeze bottles are a convenient device for delivering this spray into the throat cavity.

Toothache Drops

Toothache drops are preparations used for the temporary relief of toothache by application of a small pledget of cotton saturated with the product into the tooth cavity. Clove oil and mixtures of phenol with camphor or creosote are probably the most frequently used toothache remedies. When phenol, creosote, or volatile oils are dissolved in paraffin to which a few filaments of cotton have been added, and the mixture molded into sticks, a preparation referred to as *dental wax* is formed.

These preparations are no longer recognized by either of the compendia. Furthermore, dentists do not recommend the use of toothache drops if the patient has ready access to adequate dental services. The preparations may damage the gums and produce complications more severe than the original toothache. However, many areas do not have adequate dental services and the pharmacist will, of necessity, handle these preparations. If such is the case, the pharmacist should warn the patient of the possible hazards associated with the use of these products.

Toothache Drops NF XI contain 25 Gm of chlorobutanol in sufficient clove oil to make the product measure 100 ml. Another formulation contains creosote (50 ml), clove oil (50 ml), and chloroform (50 ml).

Emulsions

An emulsion is a two-phase system and is prepared by combining two immiscible liquids, one of which is uniformly dispersed throughout the other and consists of globules that have diameters equal to or greater than those of the largest colloidal particles. The globule size is, of course, critical and must be such that the system achieves a maximum of stability. However, even under the best of conditions, separation of the two phases will occur unless a third substance, an *emulsifying agent*, is incorporated into the original product. The basic emulsion must, therefore, contain three components but the products of commerce may consist of a number of therapeutic agents dissolved in either of the two phases of the preparation.

Most emulsions are so prepared as to incorporate an aqueous phase into a nonaqueous phase (or *vice versa*). However, it is possible to prepare emulsions that are basically nonaqueous in character. For example, McMahon, *et al*,[16] investigated the emulsifying effects of twelve anionic and five cationic surfactants on the nonaqueous immiscible system, glycerin and olive oil. They observed that certain amines and three cationic agents produced stable emulsions of this system. This broadening of the basic definition for the term *emulsion* is evident in the USP.

"An emulsion is a two-phase system in which one liquid is dispersed in the form of small globules throughout another liquid. The dispersed liquid is known as the internal phase, whereas the dispersion medium is known as the external or continuous phase. When oil is the dispersed phase and an aqueous solution is the continuous phase, the system is designated as an oil-in-water (O/W) emulsion. Conversely, when water or an aqueous solution is the dispersed phase and oil or oleaginous material is the continuous phase, the system is designated as a water-in-oil (W/O) emulsion."

The USP continues the definition by describing and discussing the effects of various emulsifying agents. These substances fall into three broad groups.[17]

Natural Emulsifying Agents—These substances may be derived from either animal or vegetable sources. Examples of those obtained from the former source are gelatin, egg yolk, casein, wool fat, and cholesterol. Acacia, tragacanth, chondrus, and pectin are representative of those obtained from vegetable sources.

Finely Divided Solids—Examples of emulsifying agents of this type are bentonite, magnesium hydroxide, aluminum hydroxide, and magnesium trisilicate.

Synthetic Emulsifying Agents—This group may be further subdivided into the anionic, cationic, and nonionic agents. Examples of these three types of emulsifying agents are, in order of presentation, sodium lauryl sulfate, benzalkonium chloride, and polyethylene glycol 400 monostearate.

Many of these emulsifying agents are described in

greater detail in Chapter 71 on *Pharmaceutical Necessities*, page 1344.

The NF suggests that only O/W emulsions are suitable for oral use because these are water-miscible and thus their oiliness is masked. This compendium gives specific directions for the preparation of emulsions utilizing gelatin as an emulsifying agent. These preparations are based on either types A or B gelatin. Type A gelatin is prepared from acid-treated precursors and is used at a pH of about 3.2. It is incompatible with anionic emulsifying agents such as the vegetable gums. The following formula is recommended:

Gelatin (Type A)	8.0 Gm
Tartaric Acid	0.6 Gm
Flavor as desired	
Alcohol	60.0 ml
Oil	500.0 ml
Purified Water, to make	1000.0 ml

Add the gelatin and the tartaric acid to about 300 ml of purified water, allow to stand for a few minutes, heat until the gelatin is dissolved, then raise the temperature to about 98°, and maintain this temperature for about 20 minutes. Cool to 50°, and add the flavor, the alcohol, and sufficient purified water to make 500 ml. Add the oil, agitate the mixture thoroughly, and pass it through a homogenizer or a colloid mill until the oil is completely and uniformly dispersed.

This emulsion cannot be prepared by trituration or by the use of the usual stirring devices.

Type B gelatin is prepared from alkali-treated precursors and is used at a pH of about 8.0. It may be used with other anionic emulsifying agents but is incompatible with the cationic types. If the emulsion contains 50% oil, 5 Gm of Type B gelatin, 2.5 Gm of sodium bicarbonate, and sufficient tragacanth or agar should be incorporated into the aqueous phase so as to yield 1000 ml of product of the required viscosity.

The emulsion type (O/W or W/O) is of lesser significance if the final preparation is to be applied to the skin. If there are no breaks in the skin, a W/O emulsion can be applied more evenly since the skin is covered with a thin film of sebum. The latter substance favors the oily phase and contributes to the ease of application. The choice of emulsion type will, however, depend on many other factors. This is particularly true for those preparations which have basic cosmetic characteristics. It may be advantageous to formulate an O/W emulsion if ease of removal is an important consideration to the patient.

Very few emulsions are now included in official compendia and the BPC 1968. Mineral Oil Emulsion is described in the NF. The BPC 1968 lists Liquid Paraffin

Emulsion, Liquid Paraffin and Magnesium Hydroxide Emulsion, Liquid Paraffin and Phenolphthalein Emulsion, and Liquid Paraffin Emulsion with Cascara. This, however, should not lead the student to the conclusion that emulsions are a relatively unimportant class of pharmaceuticals. While it is true that few preparations carry the term *emulsion* in their titles, they are of great significance as bases for other types of preparations, particularly in the dermatological and cosmetic areas. Academically, they illustrate the importance of the relationship between the theory and practice of emulsion technology and, practically, they possess a number of important advantages over other liquid forms. These are listed in the literature[18] and may be summarized in the following way.

1. In an emulsion, the therapeutic properties and the spreading ability of the constituents are increased. At times, however, this may be a disadvantage. The NF's description of this class of preparation contains a statement that illustrates this point. It is reported therein that water-soluble antiseptics are more active but also potentially more irritating when incorporated into an O/W emulsion.

2. The unpleasant taste or odor of the oil can be partially or wholly masked by the process of emulsification. Secondary masking techniques are available to the formulator but these must be used with caution. If flavors and sweetening agents are added to the emulsion, only minimal amounts should be used in order to prevent the nausea or gastric distress that results on ingestion of larger quantities of these formulation aids.

3. The absorption and penetration of medicaments are more easily controlled if they are incorporated into an emulsion.

4. Emulsion action is more prolonged and the emollient effect is greater than that observed with comparable preparations.

5. Water is not only an inexpensive diluent but is a good solvent for the many drugs and flavors that are incorporated into the emulsion.

The aqueous phase of the emulsion favors the growth of microorganisms and, because of this, a preservative is usually added to the product. Mixtures of methylparaben and propylparaben and alcohol are suitable for this purpose. The latter substance is added to the external phase (O/W emulsions) in a concentration of 12 to 15%, based on the volume of water being incorporated into the preparation.

An emulsion can be diluted with the liquid that constitutes or is miscible with the external phase. The diluting liquid will, however, decrease the viscosity of the preparation and, in certain instances, will invert the emulsion. The latter phenomena may occur if the emulsifier-in-water method (see below) is used to prepare the emulsion.

Preparation

The theory of emulsion preparation is discussed in Chapter 24 on *Coarse Dispersions*, page 334. Emulsification techniques are outlined in detail by Becher[19] and by Griffin, *et al.*[20, 21] The following procedures are those suggested by Griffin and his coworkers.

The formulator must first determine the physical and chemical characteristics of the active ingredient. He must know the following:

1. Structural formula
2. Melting point
3. Solubility
4. Stability
5. Dose
6. Specific chemical incompatibilities

It is also necessary, at this stage, to decide upon the type of emulsion required. Washable emulsions are of the O/W type; nonwashable, the W/O type. In general, O/W emulsions contain over 70% water.

W/O emulsions will usually contain higher concentrations of oils and waxes.

Experimental formulations may be prepared by the following procedure:

1. Group the ingredients on the basis of their solubilities in the aqueous and nonaqueous phases.

2. Determine the type of emulsion required and calculate an approximate HLB value.

3. Blend a low HLB emulsifier and a high HLB emulsifier to the calculated value. For experimental formulations, use a higher concentration of emulsifier (eg, 10–30% of the oil phase) than that required to produce a satisfactory product. Emulsifiers should, in general, be chemically stable, nontoxic, and suitably low in color, odor, and taste. The emulsifier is selected on the basis of these characteristics, on the type of equipment being used to blend the ingredients, and on the stability characteristics of the final product. Emulsions should not coalesce at room temperature, when frozen and thawed repeatedly, and at elevated temperatures of up to 50°C. Mechanical energy input varies with the type of equipment used to prepare the emulsion. The more the energy input, the less the demand on the emulsifier. Both process and formulation variables can affect the stability of an emulsion.[22]

4. Dissolve the oil-soluble ingredients and the emulsifiers in the oil. Heat, if necessary, to approximately 5° to 10°C. over the melting point of the highest melting ingredient or to a maximum temperature of 70° to 80°C.

5. Dissolve the water-soluble ingredients (except acids and salts) in a sufficient quantity of water.

6. Heat the aqueous phase to a temperature which is 3° to 5°C higher than that of the oil phase.

7. Add the aqueous phase to the oily phase with suitable agitation.

8. If acids or salts are employed, dissolve them in water and add the solution to the cold emulsion.

9. Examine the emulsion and make adjustments in the formulation if the product is unstable. It may be necessary to add more emulsifier, to change to an emulsifier with a slightly higher or lower HLB value, or to use an emulsifier with different chemical characteristics.

Becher[19] described four methods of preparation based on the mode of addition of the ingredients.

Emulsifier-in-Water Method—The emulsifying agent is dissolved in the water and the oil is added, with agitation, to the aqueous solution. An O/W emulsion is produced but inversion (to a W/O emulsion) will take place if more oil is added to the preparation.

Emulsifier-in-Oil Method—The emulsifier is dissolved in the oil. The mixture may be added directly to the water to form an O/W emulsion or water may be added to the mixture to form a W/O emulsion. The Emulsifier-in-Oil Method is the *Continental Method* for the preparation of emulsions and is used to prepare Mineral Oil Emulsion NF (page 804).

Soap Method—This method may be used to prepare those emulsions which are stabilized by soaps. The fatty acid part of the "soap" is dissolved in the oil; the alkaline part, in the water. Soap forms at the interface when the two phases are brought together. This method may be used to prepare either O/W or W/O emulsions.

Alternate Addition Method—The emulsion is prepared by adding water and oil alternately to the emulsifying agent. This is the so-called *English Method* for the preparation of emulsions. The emulsifying agent (eg, acacia) is first triturated with twice its weight of water. Small quantities of oil are now added to the mucilage. The mixture is triturated for several minutes and, if it becomes too viscous, a small quantity of water is added to the primary emulsion. The remaining oil, active ingredients, and water are then incorporated into the preparation.

Equipment

When emulsions are prepared, a certain amount of energy must be expended to form an interface between the oily and aqueous phases. Emulsification equipment includes, therefore, a wide variety of agitators, homogenizers, colloid mills, and ultrasonic devices. Becher,[19] Griffin *et al*,[21] and Peck, *et al*,[23] have evaluated the emulsification equipment used by pharmacists and drug manufacturers. These publications should be consulted for further details on the use of such apparatus for the preparation of emulsions and related products.

Agitators—Ordinary agitation or shaking may be used to prepare the emulsion. This method is frequently employed by the pharmacist, particularly in the emulsification of the easily dispersed, low-viscosity oils. Under certain conditions, intermittent shaking is considerably more effective than ordinary continuous shaking. Continuous shaking tends to break up not only the phase to be dispersed but also the dispersion medium and, in this way, impairs the ease of emulsification. Laboratory shaking devices may be used for the small-scale production of emulsions. However, Clayton[24] claims that shaking is an inferior method for the production of emulsions "because, as the emulsion becomes more perfect, the smashing action between the relatively heavy and light particles becomes more feeble, whereas the smashing forces should be increased."

The mortar and pestle are widely used by the prescription pharmacist in the extemporaneous preparation of emulsions. This equipment has very definite limitations because its usefulness depends largely on the viscidity of the emulsifying agent. A mortar and pestle cannot be used to prepare an emulsion if the emulsifying agent lacks viscidity (eg, gelatin solutions). These emulsifying agents will produce stable emulsions only if other types of equipment are used to mix the ingredients and the agent together.

Small electric mixers may be used to prepare emulsions at the prescription counter. These mixers will save time and energy and product satisfactory emulsions when the emulsifying agent is acacia or agar. However, these mixers cannot be used if the emulsifying agent is gelatin.

The commercially available *Waring Blendor* disperses efficiently by means of the shearing action of rapidly rotating blades. This mixer transfers large amounts of energy and incorporates air into the emulsion. If an emulsion is first produced by using a blender of this type, the formulator must remember that the emulsion characteristics obtained in the

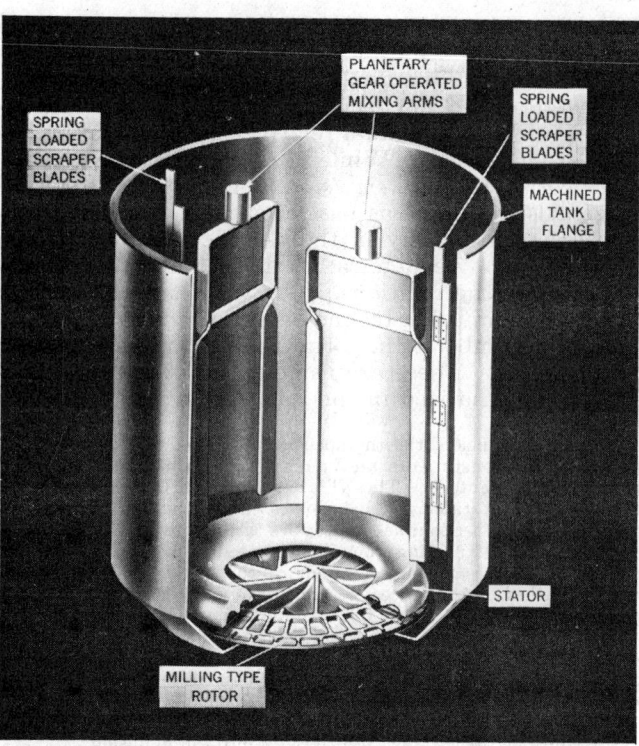

Fig. 525. Standard paste-type dispersall mixer with "cupped-rotor" milling element and double-rotating mixing arm circulating element (courtesy, Abbe Engineering).

laboratory will not necessarily be duplicated by the production-size agitators.

Production-size agitators include high-powered propeller shaft stirrers immersed in a tank or self-contained units with propeller and paddle systems. The latter units are usually so constructed that the contents of the tank may be either heated or cooled during the production process. Baffles are often built into a tank and these increase the efficiency of agitation. Two mixers manufactured by the same company are shown in Figs. 524 and 525.

Colloid Mills—The principle of operation of the colloid mill is the passage of the mixed phases of an emulsion formula between a stator and a high-speed rotor revolving at speeds of 2000–18,000 rpm. The clearance between the rotor and the stator is adjustable, usually from 0.001 in. upward. The emulsion mixture, in passing between the rotor and stator, is subjected to a tremendous shearing action which effects a fine dispersion. Two of the many types of colloid mills on the market are shown in Figs. 526 and 528. The operating principle is the same for all but each manufacturer incorporates specific features which result in changes in operating efficiency. The shearing forces applied in the colloid mill may result in a temperature increase within the emulsion. It may be necessary, therefore, to cool the equipment when the emulsion is being produced.

Homogenizers and Viscolizers—In the viscolizer and the homogenizer, the mixed phases are passed between a finely ground valve and seat under high pressure. This, in effect, produces an atomization which is enhanced by the impact received by the atomized mixture as it strikes the valve head. This type of apparatus operates at pressures of 1000–5000 lb/sq in. and produces some of the finest dispersions obtainable in an emulsion.

Homogenizers may be used in one of two ways: (1) the ingredients in the emulsion are mixed and then

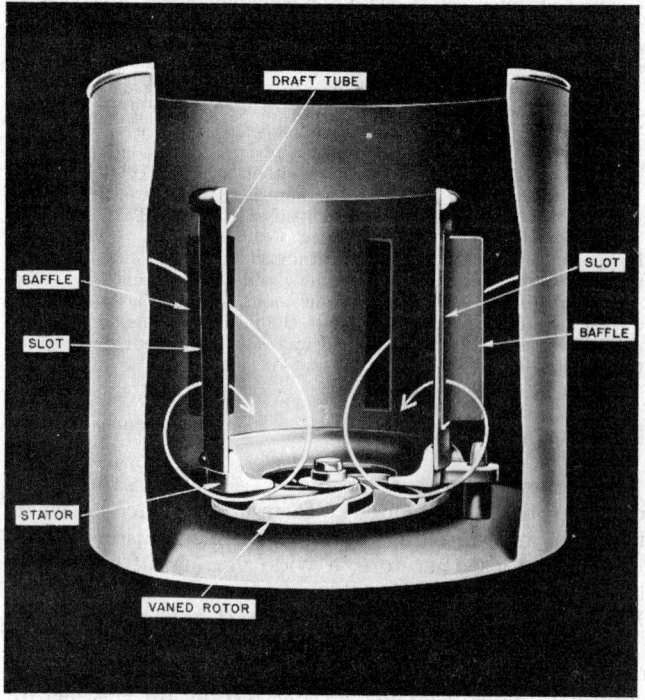

Fig. 524. Standard slurry-type dispersall mixer with vaned-rotor "mixing" element and slotted draft-tube circulating element (courtesy, Abbe Engineering).

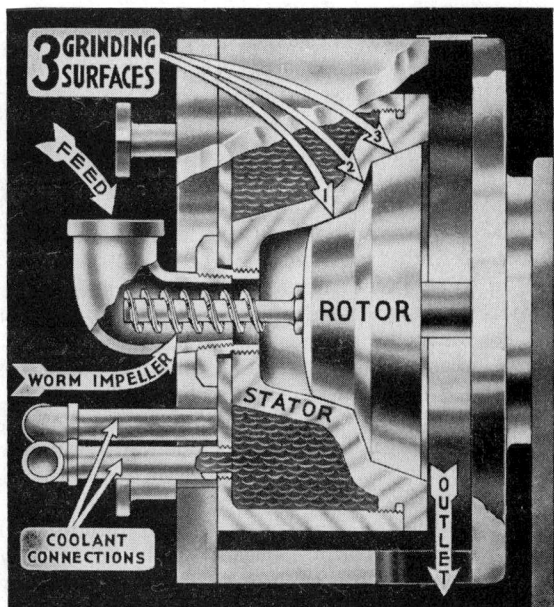

Fig. 526. A colloid mill shown in cross section (courtesy, Tri-Homo).

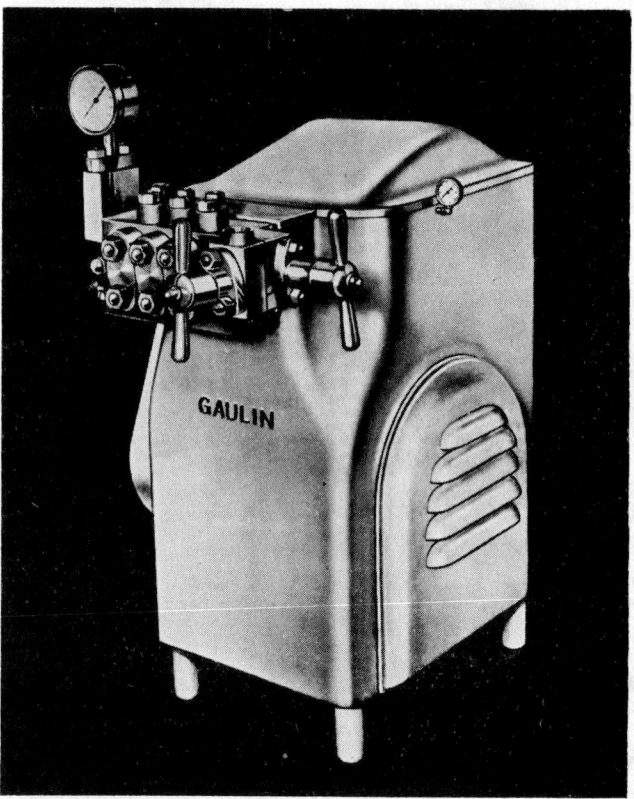

Fig. 529. Two-stage homogenizer (courtesy, Manton Gaulin).

passed through the homogenizer to produce the final product; or (2) an emulsion is prepared in some other way and is then passed through a homogenizer for the purpose of decreasing the particle size and obtaining a greater degree of uniformity and stability.

Two-stage homogenizers (Fig. 529) are so constructed that the emulsion, after treatment in the first valve system, is conducted directly to another where it receives a second treatment. A single homogenization may produce an emulsion which, although its particle size is small, has a tendency to clump or form clusters. Emulsions of this type exhibit increased creaming tendencies. This is corrected by passing the emulsion through the first stage of homogenization at a high pressure (eg, 3000–5000 lb/sq in.) and then through the second stage at a greatly reduced pressure (eg, 1000 lb/sq in.). This breaks down any clusters formed in the first step.

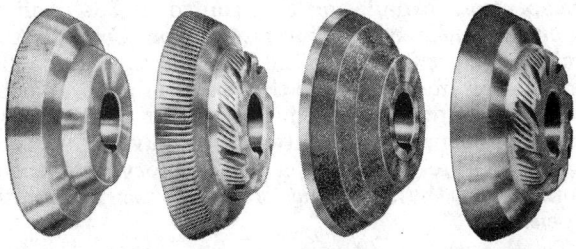

Fig. 527. Types of rotors used in colloid mills. These may be smooth (for emulsification of most emulsions), serrated (for the emulsification of ointments and very viscous products), or of vitrified stone (for the emulsification of paints and pigment dispersions) (courtesy, Tri-Homo).

Fig. 528. The Premier colloid mill, a gravity flow, vertical colloid mill with only one moving member, the rotor. Adjustment of clearance between the rotor and stator can be made from 0.001 in. upward. Speeds range from 3600 to 17,600 rpm for this type of mill, which may be used for the even and uniform distribution of the ingredients in a wide range of pharmaceutical products.

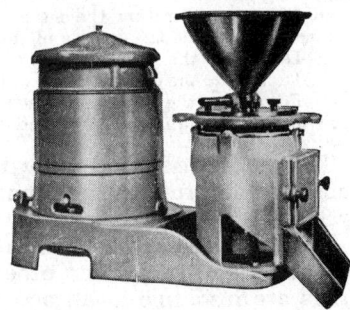

For small-scale extemporaneous preparation of emulsions, the inexpensive *hand homogenizer** is particularly useful. It is probably the most efficient emulsifying apparatus available to the prescription pharmacist. The two phases, previously mixed in a bottle, are hand pumped through the apparatus. Recirculation of the emulsion through the apparatus will improve its quality.

A homogenizer does not incorporate air into the final product. Air may ruin an emulsion because the emulsifying agent is preferentially adsorbed at the air/water interface. This is followed by an irreversible precipitation termed *denaturization*. This is particularly prone to occur with protein emulsifying agents.

Homogenization may spoil an emulsion if the concentration of emulsifying agent in the formulation is less than that required to take care of the increase in surface area produced by the process.

The temperature rise during homogenization is not very large. However, temperature does play an important role in the emulsification process. An increase in temperature will reduce the viscosity and, in certain instances, the interfacial tension between the oil and the water. There are, however, many instances, particularly in the manufacturing of cosmetic creams and ointments, where the ingredients will fail to emulsify properly if they are processed at too high a temperature. Emulsions of this type are first processed at an elevated temperature and then homogenized at a temperature not exceeding 40°C.

The Marco Flow-Master Kom-bi-nator (Fig. 530) employs a number of different actions, each of which takes the ingredients a little further along in the process of subdividing droplets until complete homogenization results. The machine is equipped with a pump

* Hand homogenizers are available from Medical Times (see page 2023).

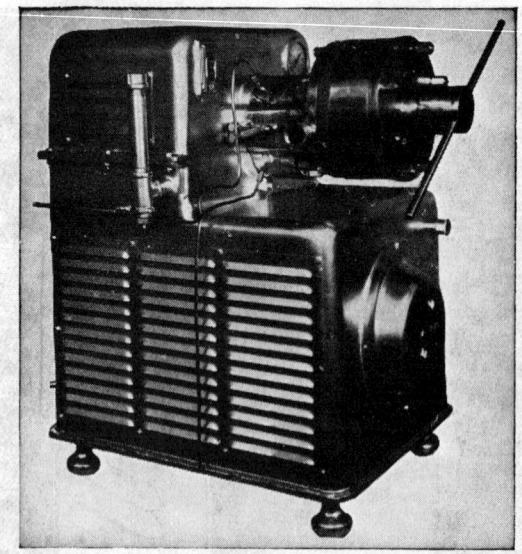

Fig. 530. Marco Flow-Master Kom-bi-nator combines the functions of a homogenizer and a colloid mill (courtesy, Marco).

which carries the liquid through the various stages of the process. In the first stage, the ingredients are forced between two specially designed rotors (gears) which shoot the liquid in opposite directions in a small chamber and, in this way, mixed thoroughly. These rotors also set up a swirling action in the next chamber into which the liquid is forced and swirled back and forth in eddies and cross currents. The second stage is a pulsing or vibrating action at rapid frequency. The product then leaves this chamber,

goes through a small valve opening, and is dashed against the wall of the homogenizing chamber. Pressure is applied but is not as great as that used in other types of homogenizers. Pressure is accurately controlled by adjusting devices on the front of the machine, and temperature is controlled by passing coolants through the stators.

Ultrasonic Devices—The preparation of emulsions by the use of ultrasonic vibrations is also possible. An oscillator of high frequency (100,000–500,000/sec) is connected to two electrodes between which is placed a piezoelectric quartz plate. The quartz plate and electrodes are immersed in an oil bath and, when the oscillator is operating, high-frequency waves flow through the fluid. Emulsification is accomplished by simply immersing a tube containing the emulsion ingredients into this oil bath. Considerable research has been done on ultrasonic emulsification, particularly with regard to the mechanism of emulsion formation by this method. Limited data indicates that these devices will produce stable emulsions only with liquids of low viscosity. The method is not, however, practical for large-scale production of emulsions.

Special techniques and equipment will, in certain instances, produce superior emulsions. Scott[25] describes a shock-cooling method for manufacturing emulsions containing waxes, fats, and other low-melting solids. Peck, *et al*,[23] claim that the homogenizer described in their paper produced a significant decrease in particle size and, therefore, a better emulsion. Ultrasonic devices have been evaluated and compared to a colloid mill by Singiser and Beal.[26] Jass[22] cooled a W/O cream emulsion rapidly and showed that such cooling produced a more stable product.

Suspensions

The physical chemist defines the word "suspension" as a two-phase system consisting of a finely divided solid dispersed in a solid, liquid, or gas. The pharmacist accepts this definition and can show that a variety of dosage forms fall within the scope of the preceding statement. There is, however, a reluctance to be all-inclusive and it is for this reason that the main emphasis is placed on solids dispersed in liquids. In addition to this, and because there is a need for more specific terminology, the pharmaceutical scientist differentiates between such preparations as Suspensions, Mixtures, Magmas, Gels, and Lotions. In a general sense, each of these preparations represents a suspension but the state of subdivision of the insoluble solid varies from particles which gradually subside on standing to particles which are colloidal in nature. The lower limit of particle size is approximately 0.1 micron and it is the preparations containing dispersed solids of this magnitude or greater that are pharmaceutically defined as suspensions.[27,28]

Certain authors also include liniments and the newer sustained-release suspensions in any discussion of this particular subject.[29] The former preparations are now usually considered as solutions although a number of older liniments were, in fact, suspensions. The sustained-release suspensions represent a very specialized class of preparation, and as such, are discussed in more detail in the Chapter 89 on *Prolonged-Action Pharmaceuticals*, page 1699. Some insoluble drugs are also administered in aerosol form. One example of such a

preparation is dexamethasone phosphate suspended in a propellant mixture of fluorochlorocarbons.[30] More detail on aerosols is available in Chapter 90, page 1729.

Suspension formulation and control is based on the principles outlined in Chapters 23 on *Colloidal Dispersions*, page 319, and 26 on *Rheology*, page 359. Formulation involves more than suspending a solid in a liquid. A knowledge of the behaviour of particles in liquids, of suspending agents, and of flavors and colors is required to produce a satisfactory suspension. Chong[31] lists the following procedure for formulating suspensions.

1. Determine the ionic character of the drug.
2. Determine the ionic character of each of the other ingredients in the formula. If possible, use nonionic ingredients.
3. Determine the density of the drug and the size of the largest particle to be suspended. At this point, select the most suitable suspending agent.
4. After incorporating the suspending agent and the bulk ingredients, determine the density of the suspension medium.
5. Determine the sedimentation force of the particles.
6. Determine the concentration of the suspending agent.
7. Formulate the suspension medium and check its rheological behavior before adding the powdered drug.

This publication and other references[32–35] should be consulted for further information on the theory and practice of suspension formulation.

Preparations such as those mentioned above possess certain advantages over other dosage forms. Some drugs are insoluble in all acceptable media and must, therefore, be administered as a tablet, capsule, etc, or as a suspension. Because of its liquid character, the latter preparation insures some uniformity of dosage but does present some problems in the maintenance of a consistent dosage regimen. Disagreeable tastes can be covered by the use of a suspension of the drug or a derivative of the drug, an example of the latter being the drug chloramphenicol palmitate. Suspensions are also chemically more stable than solutions. This is particularly important with certain antibiotics and the pharmacist is often called upon to prepare such a suspension just prior to the dispensing of the preparation. In addition to this, a suspension is an ideal dosage form for those patients who have difficulty swallowing tablets or capsules. This factor is of particular importance in the administration of drugs to children.

Suspensions should possess certain basic properties. The dispersed phase should settle slowly and should be readily re-dispersed on shaking. They should not cake on settling and the viscosity should be such that the preparation pours easily. As with all dosage forms, there should be no question as to the chemical stability of the suspension. Lastly, the suspension must be acceptable to the patient on the basis of its taste, color, and cosmetic qualities, the latter two factors being of particular importance in preparations intended for external use.

Gels

Pharmaceutical terminology is, at best, confusing and no two authors will classify Gels, Jellies, Magmas, Milks, and Mixtures in the same way. The NF describes Gels as a special class of pharmaceutical preparations but does consider Jellies under the same heading. The latter preparations usually contain water soluble active ingredients and are, therefore, considered in another part of this chapter. The USP definition for Gels is given below.

"Gels are suspensions, in a water medium, of insoluble drugs in hydrated form wherein the particle size approaches or attains colloidal dimensions. *Aluminum Hydroxide Gel* is an example of such a product. Gels are almost identical with milks in their nature except that their particle size is somewhat smaller, and they require a label statement that they are to be well shaken before each use."

In addition to the active ingredient, Aluminum Hydroxide Gel USP may contain peppermint oil, glycerin, sorbitol, sucrose, saccharin, and various preservatives. This list of ingredients is not all-inclusive but is based on information found in the monographs for the above preparation and for Aluminum Phosphate Gel NF. Incorporation of these substances and the active ingredient into the pharmaceutical is based on the general rules for suspension formulation, such rules being given in previously cited references or in standard textbooks on pharmaceutics.[36]

Generally, if left undisturbed for some time, gels may become semisolid or gelatinous. With some gels, small amounts of water may separate on standing.

Lotions

Lotions are usually liquid suspensions or dispersions intended for external application to the body. They may be prepared by triturating the ingredients to a smooth paste and then cautiously adding the remaining liquid phase. High-speed mixers or homogenizers produce better dispersions and are, therefore, the tools of choice in the preparation of larger quantities of lotion. Calamine Lotion USP is the classical example

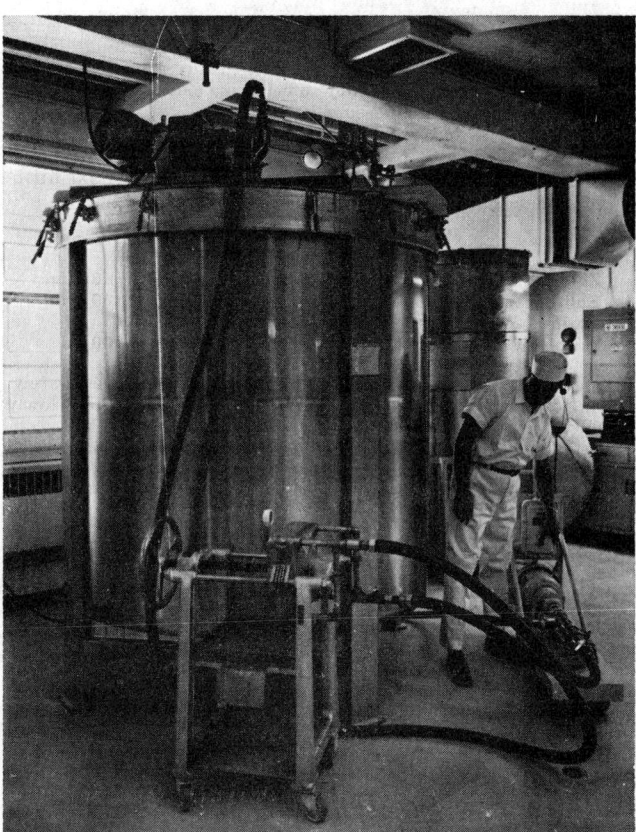

Fig. 531. This 5000-liter stainless steel tank is used in the final stages of production of an antacid suspension. The suspension is made to volume with filtered water, mixed, and pumped directly to an automatic bottle filler situated on a lower floor (courtesy, S K & F Montreal, Que.).

of this type of preparation and consists of finely powdered, insoluble solids held in more or less permanent suspension by the presence of suspending agents and/or surface-active agents. Many investigators have studied Calamine Lotion and this had led to the publication of many formulations, each possessing certain advantages over the others but none satisfying the collective needs of all dermatologists. The formula for the official lotion is given on page 770.

Phenolated Calamine Lotion USP (page 770) contains 10 ml of liquefied phenol in sufficient calamine lotion to make the product measure 1000 ml. Haberle[37] claims that formulations containing Avicel R* and carboxymethylcellulose settle less than do the official preparations.

Calamine Lotion

Calamine	8 Gm
Zinc Oxide	8 Gm
Glycerin	2 ml
Avicel R Gel	2 Gm
Carboxymethylcellulose	2 Gm
Calcium Hydroxide Solution, a sufficient quantity,	
To make	100 ml

Phenolated Calamine Lotion

Calamine	8 Gm
Zinc Oxide	8 Gm
Glycerin	2 ml
Avicel R Gel	2 Gm
Carboxymethylcellulose	2 Gm
Liquified Phenol	1 ml
Calcium Hydroxide Solution, a sufficient quantity,	
To make	100 ml

* Avicel R is the brand name for the hydrated microcrystalline cellulose marketed by *Am. Viscose.*

Mix 45 Gm of Avicel R with 55 Gm of water in a suitable electric mixer. This gel is used in the preparation of the calamine lotion. Mix the calamine and the zinc oxide with the glycerin, the gel and the carboxymethylcellulose. Add sufficient calcium hydroxide solution to make the product measure 100 ml.

Suspensions may also be formed by chemical interaction in the liquid. White Lotion NF is an example of this type of preparation.

White Lotion NF

Zinc Sulfate	40 Gm
Sulfurated Potash	40 Gm
Purified Water, a sufficient quantity	
To make	1000 ml

Dissolve the zinc sulfate and the sulfurated potash separately, each in 450 ml of purified water, and filter each solution. Add slowly the sulfurated potash solution to the zinc sulfate solution with constant stirring. Then add the required amount of purified water, and mix.

Sulfurated potash is a solid of variable composition but is usually described as $K_2S_3 \cdot K_2S_2O_3$. The chemical reaction which occurs when the sulfurated potash solution is added to the zinc sulfate solution is given below.

$$ZnSO_4 \cdot 7H_2O + K_2S_3 \cdot K_2S_2O_3 \rightarrow ZnS\downarrow + S_2\downarrow + K_2SO_4 + K_2S_2O_3 + 7H_2O$$

This lotion must be freshly prepared and does not contain a suspending agent. Bentonite Magma has been used in some formulations. Coffman and Huyck[38] attempted to stabilize the lotion and modify its viscosity by using dioctyl sodium sulfosuccinate. Their formula possessed few advantages over the official lotion but the publication does include a detailed discussion of the chemistry and the problems involved in the preparation of a suitable product.

The NF recognizes a second type of lotion. These are emulsions of the O/W type stabilized by a surface-active agent. Benzyl Benzoate Lotion NF is an example of this type of preparation. Lastly, some lotions are clear solutions and, in fact, the active ingredient of one official lotion, Dimethisoquin Hydrochloride Lotion NF, is a water-soluble substance. However, one unofficial formulation for this lotion lists dimethisoquin hydrochloride, menthol, and zinc oxide as active ingredients and the preparation thus becomes a suspension.

Lotions are usually applied without friction. Even so, the insoluble matter should be very finely divided. Particles approaching colloidal dimensions are more soothing to inflamed areas and are more effective in contact with infected surfaces. A wide variety of ingredients may be added to the preparation to produce better dispersions or to accentuate the cooling, soothing, drying, or protective properties of the lotion. Bentonite is a good example of a suspending agent used in the preparation of lotions. Methylcellulose or sodium carboxymethylcellulose will localize and hold the active ingredient in contact with the affected site. A formulation containing glycerin will keep the skin moist for a considerable period of time. The drying and cooling effect may be accentuated by the addition of alcohol to the formula.

Dermatologists frequently prescribe lotions containing anesthetics, antiseptics, astringents, germicides, protectives, or screening agents, to be used in treating or preventing various types of skin diseases and dermatitis. Antihistamines, benzocaine, calamine, resorcin, steroids, sulfur, zinc oxide, and zirconium oxide are common ingredients in unofficial lotions. The value of various active ingredients and the methods for incorporating these into suitable pharmaceutical forms are outlined in various publications.[39-41] In many instances the cosmetic aspects of the lotion are of great importance. Many lotions compare badly with cosmetic preparations of a similar nature. A discussion of the cosmetic elegance of dermatological preparations may be found in a paper by Witten and March.[42] The manufacture of fine lotions to meet the specialized needs of the dermatologist provides the pharmacist with an excellent opportunity to demonstrate his professional competence.

Lotions tend to separate or stratify on long standing, and they require a label directing that they be shaken well before each use. All lotions should be labeled "For External Use Only."

Magmas and Milks

Magmas and milks are aqueous suspensions of insoluble, inorganic drugs and differ from gels mainly in that the suspended particles are larger. When prepared, they are thick and viscous, and because of this, there is no need to add a suspending agent to the preparation.

Bentonite Magma USP (page 1345) is prepared by simple hydration. Two procedures are given in the compendium for the preparation of this product.

Magmas may also be prepared by chemical reaction. Magnesium hydroxide is prepared by the hydration of magnesium oxide.

$$MgO + H_2O \rightarrow Mg(OH)_2$$

Milk of Magnesia USP (page 791) is a suspension of magnesium hydroxide containing 7.0–8.5% $Mg(OH)_2$. It has an unpleasant alkaline taste. This taste can be masked with 0.1% citric acid and 0.05% of a volatile oil or a blend of volatile oils. The citric acid reduces the alkalinity of the preparation.

Milk of Bismuth NF (page 788) contains bismuth hydroxide and basic bismuth carbonate in suspension in water. The Magma is prepared by reacting bismuth subnitrate with nitric acid and ammonium carbonate with ammonia solution and then mixing the resulting two solutions.

The following reactions occur during the preparation of the magma.

$$(NH_4)_2CO_3 \rightarrow 2NH_4^+ + CO_3^=$$
$$NH_3 + H_2O \rightarrow NH_4^+ + OH^-$$
$$2BiO^+ + CO_3^= \rightarrow (BiO)_2CO_3\downarrow$$
$$BiO^+ + OH^- \rightarrow BiO(OH)\downarrow$$

If the insoluble substance is freshly precipitated by mixing hot, dilute solutions, there is only slight sedimentation on standing. This characteristic of magmas is sometimes enhanced by passing the product through a colloid mill.

For the most part, magmas are intended for oral use, although Bentonite Magma is used primarily as a suspending agent for insoluble substances either for local application or for internal use. All magmas require a label directing that they be shaken well before use. Freezing must be avoided.

Mixtures

The official mixtures are aqueous liquid preparations which contain suspended, insoluble, solid substances and are intended for internal use. The insoluble substance does not make the mixture very viscous and the particles may be held in suspension by the use of suitable suspending or thickening agents. This class was originally introduced to secure uniformity in the formulas of certain well-known and largely used preparations. Frequently the term *mixture* is applied loosely to aqueous preparations of every description. The term *shake mixture* is often used for liquid preparations which contain insoluble ingredients and must, therefore, be shaken before use. The USP does not recognize the term and the NF does not attempt to define this class of pharmaceuticals. The term *suspension* is now used to describe a number of similar preparations.

The pectin and the tragacanth in Kaolin Mixture with Pectin NF (page 811) act as suspending agents. An alternate formula, based on Veegum (*Vanderbilt*) and sodium carboxymethylcellulose, has been proposed.[43]

Kaolin Mixture with Pectin

Veegum	0.88 Gm
Sodium Carboxymethylcellulose	0.22 Gm
Purified Water	79.12 Gm
Kaolin	17.50 Gm
Pectin	0.44 Gm
Saccharin	0.09 Gm
Glycerin	1.75 Gm

Add the Veegum and the sodium carboxymethylcellulose to the water with continuous stirring. Add, with mixing, the kaolin. Mix the pectin, the saccharin, and the glycerin and add to the suspension. A preservative and a flavoring agent may be added to the product.

Brown Mixture NF XII contains glycyrrhiza fluidextract, antimony potassium tartrate, paregoric, alcohol, glycerin, and water. A precipitate is formed when the major ingredients in the formula, glycyrrhiza fluidextract and paregoric, are combined.

The insoluble material in mixtures must be in a very finely divided state and it must be uniformly distributed throughout the preparation. This is accomplished by the use of colloid mills, special methods of precipitation, and suspending agents. There are three main reasons for having the insoluble substances in as fine a state of subdivision as possible.

1. The more nearly the colloidal state is approached by protectives, such as kaolin, magnesium trisilicate, and magnesium phosphate, the more active they become as adsorbents and protectives when in contact with inflamed surfaces.

2. Finely divided particles are suspended more readily and settle out much more slowly than large particles, thus enabling the patient to obtain uniform doses of suspended substances. Homogeneous mixtures are especially desirable when administering medication to form an evenly distributed, soothing, protective coating on the gastrointestinal tract.

3. The palatability of many preparations is enhanced by the use of colloidal suspending agents.

Mixtures containing suspended material should have a "Shake Well" label affixed to the container in which they are dispensed.

Official Suspensions

The USP and NF place particular emphasis on the term suspension by providing specific definitions for a wide variety of oral, parenteral, and ophthalmic preparations that are formulated in such a way that an insoluble substance is suspended in a liquid at some stage of the manufacturing or dispensing process. The USP definition begins as follows:

"Suspensions are preparations of finely divided, undissolved drugs dispersed in liquid vehicles. Powders for suspension are preparations of finely powdered drugs intended for suspension in liquid vehicles. An example of the ready-to-use type is *Trisulfapyrimidines Oral Suspension*, in which the three sulfapyrimidines are already sus-

pended in a liquid, flavored vehicle in a form suitable for oral administration. *Tetracycline for Oral Suspension* is finely divided tetracycline mixed with suspending and dispersing agents. It is intended to be diluted with the prescribed volume of purified water and mixed before it is dispensed by the pharmacist for oral administration to the patient."

Neither this definition nor the monographs give specific directions for the preparation of the suspension although pharmacopeias usually permit the addition of suitable flavoring agents, suspending agents, preservatives, and certified color additives. One procedure for the preparation of the commonly used *Trisulfapyrimidines Oral Suspension* is given below.[43]

Trisulfapyrimidines Oral Suspension

Veegum	1.00 Gm
Syrup USP	90.60 Gm
Sodium Citrate	0.78 Gm
Sulfadiazine	2.54 Gm
Sulfamerazine	2.54 Gm
Sulfamethazine	2.54 Gm

Add the Veegum, slowly and with continuous stirring, to the syrup. Incorporate the sodium citrate into the Veegum-syrup mixture. Premix the sulfa drugs and add to the syrup. Stir and homogenize. Add sufficient 5 per cent citric acid solution to adjust the pH of the product to 5.6. A preservative and a flavoring agent may be added to the product.

Methods of preparation for these formulations which contain several active ingredients and are being produced in large quantities tend to be more complex than that given above. Sinutab Pediatric Suspension* contains 162.5 mg acetaminophen, 12.5 mg of phenylpropanolamine hydrochloride, and 10 mg of phenyltoloxamine citrate in each 5 ml of product. The other ingredients in the suspension are sugar, glycerin, sodium carboxymethylcellulose, Avicel R, Veegum, sorbitol solution, polysorbate 80, a coloring agent, sodium benzoate, sodium cyclamate, sodium saccharin, a flavoring agent, citric acid, and sodium citrate. The method of preparation for this suspension is as follows:

1. Dissolve the sugar in hot water. Mix, strain, and divide this syrup into three portions:
    Portion A–Add the syrup to a mixture of glycerin and sodium carboxymethylcellulose. Mix.
    Portion B–Mix the Avicel R, in three stages, with the syrup.
    Portion C–Add the Veegum to the syrup. Mix and viscolize.
2. Add Portion A to Portion B. Mix and viscolize.
3. Combine Portion C with the mixture prepared in Step 2 to produce a pink, opaque suspension with a characteristic odor and taste.
4. Mix the polysorbate 80 with the sorbitol solution; combine this with the suspension prepared in Step 3. Add the active ingredients, the preservative, and the sweetening, coloring, and flavoring agents. Mix and viscolize.

It must be emphasized, however, that the above procedures are an abbreviated version of those used by the manufacturer. For example, the procedure states that Veegum is added to syrup and viscolized. The manufacturing instructions are much more detailed. The manufacturer gives a mixing time, the operating characteristics of the viscolizer (lb/sq in.), and the specifications which must be met before the mixture is used in the next step of the procedure. Similar details are given for all the steps in the manufacturing process.

Certain drugs are chemically unstable when suspended in water; others will remain stable in suspension for only a short period of time. Both types are usually prepared by the pharmacist from dry formula-

---

* The information herein was supplied by Warner-Chilcott Laboratories, Toronto, Ontario, the manufacturers of the suspension.

tions. An example of the latter type of product is barium sulfate suspension. This suspension is used in roentgenographic or fluoroscopic examinations of the gastrointestinal tract. Joynt and Zuck[44] claim that the formulation given below is readily suspended prior to use and will remain stable for at least 12 hr.

Barium Sulfate Suspension

Barium Sulfate USP	100 Gm
Methocel 50 (*Dow**)	0.5 Gm
Compound Calcium Cyclamate Solution NF	4.5 ml
Flavor	1.0 ml

Blend the barium sulfate with the Methocel 50. Add the flavor and the compound calcium cyclamate solution dropwise with continuous mixing in a suitable mixer.

The flavoring agent may be a 2.25% alcoholic solution of raspberry flavor (*Magnus**) or a 3% alcoholic solution of coconut custard flavor (*Intern. Flavors**).

Suspensions intended for parenteral and ophthalmic use are also described in the USP. For a discussion of these suspensions, reference should be made to chapters 83 on *Ophthalmic Solutions*, page 1545, and 82 on *Parenteral Preparations*, page 1519. The USP continues its description of suspensions as follows:

"By its very nature, the particulate matter of a suspension tends to settle slowly from the liquid vehicle in which it is dispersed, since its density is almost always greater than that of the liquid vehicle. In some cases, an added inert suspending agent is permitted to retard such sedimentation by increasing vehicle density, viscosity, or yield value. In one, *Sterile Procaine Penicillin G with Aluminum Stearate Suspension*, a thixotropic gel exists which retards sedimentation.

"It is important that suspensions be shaken well before each use to insure a uniform distribution of solid in the vehicle, and thereby, uniform and proper dosage.

"Suitable preservatives should be included to protect the preparations from bacterial and mold contamination."

References

1. *Handbook on Demineralizing*, Cochrane Div., Crane Co., King of Prussia, Pa., 1966.

* See page 2023.

2. Monte-Bovi, A. J., *J. APhA, Pract. Ed.*, **11,** 107 (1950).
3. Monte-Bovi, A. J., *J. APhA, Pract. Ed.*, **12,** 565 (1951).
4. Steen, C. V., Marcus, A. D., and Benton, B. E., *J. APhA, Pract. Ed.*, **13,** 180 (1952).
5. Cooper, B. F., and Brecht, E. A., *J. APhA, Sci. Ed.*, **41,** 394 (1952).
6. Discher, C. A., *Modern Inorganic Pharmaceutical Chemistry*, John Wiley, New York, 1964, p. 503.
7. Meer, T., *Flavoring Pharmaceutical Preparations*, Smith Kline & French Laboratories, Selected Pharmaceutical Research References, manuscript Number 4, February 11, 1957.
8. Schwarz, T. W., *et al*, *J. APhA, Sci. Ed.*, **47,** 695 (1958).
9. Martin, E. W., *Husa's Pharmaceutical Dispensing*, Mack Publishing Company, Easton, 1959, p. 211.
10. Spiegel, A. J., and Noseworthy, M. M., *J. Pharm. Sci.*, **52,** 917 (1963).
11. Brown, V. K., *et al*, *J. Pharm. Pharmacol.*, **15,** 688 (1963).
12. Sumner, E. D., APhA, NS8, 250 (1968).
13. Porush, I., *et al*, *J. APhA, Sci. Ed.*, **49,** 70 (1960).
14. Young, J. G., *et al*, *J. APhA, Sci. Ed.*, **49,** 72 (1960).
15. Pernarowski, M., and Chatten, L. G., *J. APhA, Sci. Ed.*, **44,** 526 (1955).
16. McMahon, J. D., *et al*, *J. Pharm. Sci.*, **52,** 1163 (1963).
17. Sprowls, J. B., *Prescription Pharmacy*, J. B. Lippincott, Philadelphia, 1963, p. 189.
18. Burlage, H. M., *et al*, *Physical and Technical Pharmacy*, McGraw-Hill, New York, 1963, p. 539.
19. Becher, P., *Emulsions: Theory and Practice*, Reinhold, New York, 1965, p. 267.
20. Griffin, W. C., *et al*, *Drug Cosmetic Ind.*, **102,** 41 (1967).
21. Griffin, W. C., *et al*, *Drug Cosmetic Ind.*, **102,** 52 (1967).
22. Jass, H. E., *J. Soc. Cosmetic Chemists*, **18,** 591 (1967).
23. Peck, G. E., *et al*, *J. APhA, Sci. Ed.*, **49,** 75 (1960).
24. Clayton, W., *The Theory of Emulsions and Their Technical Treatment*, 3rd ed., Blakiston, Philadelphia, 1935, p. 294.
25. Scott, M. W., *J. Pharm. Sci.*, **53,** 208 (1964).
26. Singiser, R. E., and Beal, J. M., *J. APhA, Sci. Ed.*, **49,** 482 (1960).
27. Hiestand, E. N., *J. Pharm. Sci.*, **53,** 1 (1964).
28. Polderman, J., *Am. J. Hosp. Pharm.*, **19,** 611 (1962).
29. Burlage, H. H., *Physical and Technical Pharmacy*, McGraw-Hill, New York, 1963, p. 518.
30. Bickerman, H. A., and Itkin, S. E., *J. Am. Med. Assoc.*, **184,** 533 (1963).
31. Chong, C. W., *J. Soc. Cosm. Chem.*, **14,** 123 (1963).
32. Martin, A. N., *J. Pharm. Sci.*, **50,** 513 (1961).
33. Samyn, J. C., *J. Pharm. Sci.*, **50,** 517 (1961).
34. Oldshue, J. Y., *J. Pharm. Sci.*, **50,** 523 (1961).
35. Frederick, K. J., *J. Pharm. Sci.*, **50,** 531 (1961).
36. Martin, E. W., *Husa's Pharmaceutical Dispensing*, 6th ed, Mack Publishing Company, Easton, 1965, p. 219.
37. Haberle, J. E., *Am. J. Hosp. Pharm.*, **25,** 180 (1968).
38. Coffman, H. L., and Huyck, C. L., *Am. J. Hosp. Pharm.*, **20,** 132 (1963).
39. Ebling, F. J., *J. Pharm. Pharmacol.*, 13 Supplement, 23 T (1961).
40. Jarrett, A., *J. Pharm. Pharmacol.*, 13 Supplement, 35 T (1961).
41. Hadgraft, J. W., *J. Pharm. Pharmacol.*, 13 Supplement, 43 T (1961).
42. Witten, V. H., and March, C. H., *Drug Cosmetic Ind.*, **93,** 794 (1963).
43. Kalish, J., *Drug and Cosmetic Ind.*, **94,** 279 (1964).
44. Joynt, B. P., and Zuck, D. A., *Hosp. Pharm.*, **20,** 201 (1967).

81 | Sterilization

Sterilization indicators—sterility testing methods—laminar flow—
sterilization methods (steam under pressure, dry heat, filtration, gases,
radiation, aseptic handling, and alternate methods)

This chapter was prepared by

John H. Brewer, PhD, *Senior Microbiological Consultant, Becton, Dickinson
& Co., Rutherford, N.J. 07070, and*
G. Briggs Phillips, PhD, *Director, Becton, Dickinson Research Center, Becton,
Dickinson & Co., Rutherford, N.J. 07070*

The pharmaceutical manufacturer and the hospital pharmacist are constantly called on to prepare or produce sterile pharmaceutical preparations, particularly those for injection. A thorough understanding of definition of terms commonly used in such endeavors is necessary before an adequate discussion of this subject can be presented.

Sterility is the absence of life and there is no compromise with this term. An object is either sterile or contaminated. Statistical concepts enter the picture, however, when there is need to verify the sterility of a batch of treated materials by taking a sample that is submitted to sterility testing. In actual practice the doctor may speak of a "sterile" area or a "partially sterile" technique, when he really means an *aseptic technique* (one that is free of organisms that might produce sepsis) but he does not necessarily mean sterile.

From the point of view of the pharmacist or the pharmaceutical manufacturer, however, terms related to sterility, asepsis, etc, must be precisely denoted and clearly understood:

Sterilization—inactivation or removal of all viable organisms.
Disinfectant—a substance used on inanimate objects to render them noninfectious; a disinfectant may be an antiseptic or a germicide.
Germicide—anything that kills germs.
Bactericide—anything that kills bacteria.
Antiseptic—a substance used to prevent sepsis, usually applied to animate objects; an antiseptic may work by actually killing organisms or by merely preventing their multiplication.
Bacteriostatic agent—a substance that prevents the multiplication of organisms. Such materials are usually employed as preservatives in pharmaceutical preparations.

In recent years a long list of factors, including the increased use of antibiotics and the requirement that ophthalmic solutions be sterile, have focused attention on pharmacists and the pharmaceutical industry with regard to product sterility and have increased the need to apply the principles of sterilization over a broad industrywide basis. These principles receive increased use because standards for many nonsterile pharmaceuticals now require certification of the absence of *Salmonella, Escherichia coli, Staphylococcus aureus,* and *Pseudomonas,* as well as control over the total microbial load in materials.

The hospital pharmacist is commonly called on to produce or supervise the preparation of sterile compresses, gauze packs or other surgical dressings, parenteral solutions, as well as the preparation of official and nonofficial injections in ampuls and vials of both oleaginous and aqueous materials. Also, recently, it has become commonplace for pharmacists to aseptically fill syringes with injectables and to repackage other fluids and tablets on a semiproduction basis.

It is not sufficient simply to accomplish sterilization; in addition, during subsequent handling, sterility must be maintained. Because microorganisms are highly ubiquitous, materials in unprotected environments easily may become contaminated. Therefore, great care should be observed in the removal of stoppers or closures, and equipment used in the preparation of sterile solutions should be kept in closed containers or wrapped in paper in a manner known to protect the sterility.

Pharmaceutical materials may be rendered sterile by a number of physical or chemical means. These include exposure to heat (dry or moist), ultraviolet light, ionizing radiation, or gases such as ethylene oxide, propylene oxide, or formaldehyde; addition of sterilant chemicals; or passage through one of a number of types of filters that remove all bacteria. In addition, it is commonplace to use combinations of sterilization methods when full treatment with one method causes product deterioration.

There are four major considerations in the sterilization and subsequent use of pharmaceutical materials:

1. Application of an adequate sterilization treatment.
2. Verification, by appropriate means, that the materials in each batch are actually sterile.
3. Protection of the sterile material by its packaging and during storage.
4. Delivery, opening, and use of the sterile material without the entrance of contamination.

In relation to these points certain facts about microorganisms themselves also must be kept in mind. Some bacteria multiply in the refrigerator; others at temperatures as high as 60°C. Bacteria vary in their oxygen requirements from the strict *anaerobes* that cannot tolerate oxygen to *aerobes* that demand it. Slightly alkaline growth media will support the multiplication of many microorganisms while others flourish in acid environments. Many bacteria can grow in concentrated pharmaceutical preparations. Some microorganisms have the ability to utilize nitrogen and carbon dioxide from the air and thus can actually multiply in distilled water.

In general, however, most pathogenic bacteria have rather selective cultural requirements, with optimum temperatures of 30°–37°C at a neutral pH. Contaminating yeasts and molds can develop readily in dextrose and other sugar solutions. Because many sugars cannot be sterilized by heating to high temperatures for long periods of time, dangerous contamination and subsequent untoward reactions in patients may result as a consequence if sterilization of such solutions is not achieved.

Actively growing bacteria are, for the most part, vegetative forms with little resistance to heat and chemical germicides. However, some forms of bacteria have the ability when they stop multiplying to assume a *spore* or hibernation state. These spore forms are very resistant to heat as well as to many disinfectant solutions that would normally kill the vegetative forms. Among these are those that cause anthrax, tetanus, and gas gangrene. Many of the spore forms of bacteria found in dust are not disease-producing but may give rise to high-temperature reactions upon injection. Therefore, successful sterilization under practical conditions is evaluated on the ability to kill the spore forms of bacteria.

The official requirements for sterilization are presented in considerable detail under *Sterilization* (page 830) and under *Sterility Tests* (page 851) in the USP. Equivalent information is also found in the NF. The section in the USP (page 846) entitled *Microbial Limit Tests* also will be of interest to pharmacists.

Sterilization Indicators

Of the several emerging concepts about sterilization and sterility testing, the most important seem to be:[1]

1. The best assurance of sterilization probably results when the process is one that from past experience is known to be effective, when it is performed with adequate monitoring and control of all physical and chemical parameters and repeated frequently and regularly with little run-to-run variation.
2. Adequate sterilization conditions are best arrived at by studies and data revealing the *rates* at which inactivation of microorganisms is taking place during the treatment process.
3. Biological indicators are of great value both in establishing and monitoring sterilization cycles.

For the above, the importance of the role of sterilization indicators is obvious. Strictly speaking, there could be said to be physical, chemical, and biological type indicators. However, it is probably much better to think of the physical factors (measurements of time, temperature, relative humidity, pressure, vacuum, gas concentration, etc) as elements of *process control* rather than indicators.

Even with chemical indicators, their applicability should be considered carefully. Some of these indicators are in reality small melting-point tubes. The most satisfactory and generally available chemical indicators are those for heat sterilization procedures. Here, however, an important point is that while most indicators will show whether or not a particular temperature was reached, most do not indicate the length of exposure to that temperature.

Some heat sterilization indicators, including one particularly popular in England, depend on the progressive oxidation of a chromate solution at autoclave temperatures. A color change indicates not only that the proper temperature was reached but also that the time of heating was sufficient. With regard to chemical indicators for sterilization processes, excluding the use of steam under pressure, some tapes and indicators show merely that the articles have been in a moist, hot chamber. However, these cannot be relied on for more information. One chemical indicator for ethylene oxide has been incorporated into a strip bearing bacterial spore indicators.*

---

* Available from BBL (see page 2023).

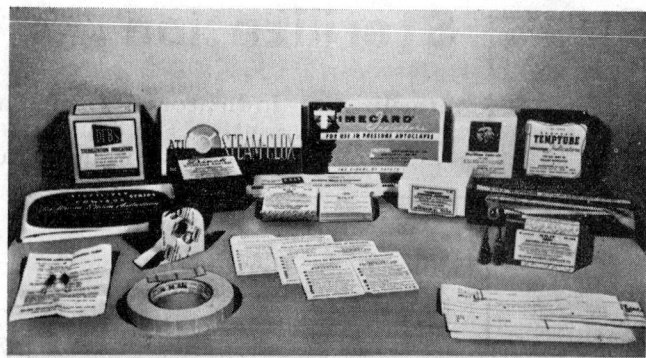

Fig. 532. A number of sterilizer indicators and controls that are commercially available.

In the final analysis there is no substitute for the use of *biological* indicators, as exemplified by the use of prepared bacterial spores. Although a variety of biological indicators are available, care must be exercised to select one appropriate to the sterilization process. Fig. 532 shows some of the various types of sterilization indicators that are available commercially. Fig. 533 shows how one firm includes a spore strip with a chemical indicator between the ribs of the rubber plunger stoppers of syringes used for sterility controls in ethylene oxide sterilization cycles.[2]

The use of biological indicators involves the following steps:

1. Selection
2. Production of the indicator
3. Preparation and calibration of the carrier system
4. Placement
5. Retrieval after the sterilization treatment
6. Assay of biological indicators

Each of these steps will be discussed in detail. Steps 1, 2, and 3 are obviously easily accomplished through the use of commercially available biological spore indicators that meet the criteria established for the particular sterilization method employed.

A number of microorganisms have been employed for biological indicators. *Clostridium novyi* was long used in the sterilization of catgut sutures. *Clostridium sporogenes* has been used for many years in the canning industry. *Bacillus subtilis* var. *niger* (*B. globigii*) is widely used both in Europe and America as a wet- and dry-heat and ethylene oxide sterilization indicator. *Bacillus pumilus*[3] is often used for radiation sterilization, in addition to *Streptococcus radiodurans*.[4] Recently, the use of a radiation sterilization indicator employing *Streptococcus faecium* has been suggested.[5]

We have found that the use of *Bacillus stearothermophilus* spores most adequately meets the needs as a sterilization indicator. The use of *B. stearothermophilus* (NIH No. 7953) has been approved by the

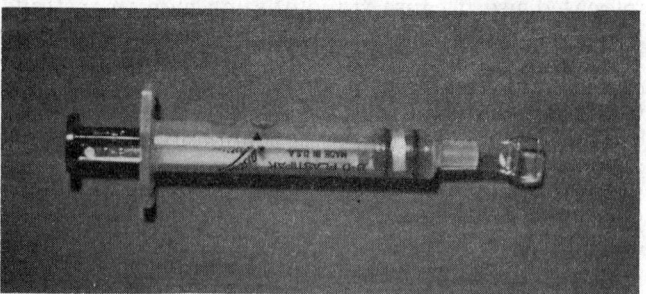

Fig. 533. Sterility indicator syringe with spore strip between the ribs of the plunger stopper (courtesy, BD & Co.).

Table I—Probabilities for Sterility Testing of Items with Assumed Levels of Contamination

"True" % contamination	Probability of designated positives out of 10 samples tested										
	0	1	2	3	4	5	6	7	8	9	10
0.1	0.990	(total = 0.010)									
0.5	0.960	(total = 0.040)									
1.0	0.904	0.091	0.004	0.000	0.000						
2.0	0.817	0.167	0.015	0.001	0.000						
5.0	0.599	0.315	0.075	0.010	0.001						
10.0	0.349	0.387	0.194	0.057	0.011	0.001					
20.0	0.107	0.268	0.302	0.201	0.088	0.026	0.005	0.001			
30.0	0.028	0.121	0.233	0.267	0.200	0.103	0.037	0.009	0.001		
40.0	0.006	0.040	0.121	0.215	0.251	0.201	0.111	0.042	0.011	0.001	
50.0	0.001	0.010	0.044	0.117	0.205	0.246	0.205	0.117	0.044	0.010	0.001

National Institutes of Health (NIH) as a sterilizer control for use in licensed establishments. Its use meets the requirements of the USPHS Regulations, Part 73, revised July 28, 1961. It is an obligate thermophile and will not grow at the official NIH and USP Sterility Test incubation temperature of 30° to 35°C; its temperature of growth is between 55° and 65°. In addition to this high-temperature requirement, *B. stearothermophilus* seems to be an ideal test spore because it is nonpathogenic, nontoxic, nonpyrogenic, and is, therefore, esthetically acceptable as a biological indicator.[6]

Bacterial spores used as biological indicators may be dried onto the items that are to be sterilized or onto glass, metal, plastic, or paper strips that are placed in or on the items. In some cases the spores are dried on the inside bottom of test tubes to facilitate the later addition of culture broth. The practice of drying the spores onto small strips of filter paper is the most common method.

One rather unique indicator for use in monitoring sterilization by autoclaving is a sealed ampul containing bacteriological culture medium with an indicator and a standardized suspension of heat-resistant *B. stearothermophilus* spores.[7] The ampul is placed within the load and, following sterilization, is incubated at the optimum temperature for the control organism. If growth occurs within 48 hr, it is obvious that sterilization was not attained. Another indicator employing positive spore controls is a strip of paper impregnated with *B. stearothermophilus* spores, culture media, and an indicator. In use it is placed in the sterilizer, usually in a pack, and after autoclaving is transferred from its envelope to a tube of sterile water and incubated. If sterilization has not occurred, the original purple medium will become turbid and yellow.

Sterility Testing Methods

After applying one or more of the methods of sterilization, there are several techniques for determining whether or not the particular lot of material is sterile. The only method for determining the sterility of any one lot of a pharmaceutical preparation with 100% assurance would be to run a total sterility test, ie, to test every ampul or vial in the lot without opening the container. This can only be done, however, using sterile culture media that will support growth of a portion of the known species of bacteria and fungi. Obviously, because of the destruction involved, a total sterility test using every container in the lot cannot be run and other measures must be employed to certify the sterility of the product.

To illustrate more specifically how low levels of

contamination in treated lots of medical items may escape detection by the usual sterility test procedures, Tables I and II show some representative probabilities.[1] The data are calculated from the binomial expansion employing certain assumed values of percent contamination with large lot sizes (>5000) and include standard assumptions with regard to the efficiency of recovery media, etc.

In Table I the probability data are calculated for lots with various degrees of assumed contamination when 10 random samples/lot are tested. Opposite each "true" contamination figure the table indicates the probability of obtaining all negative growth tubes from 1, 5, or 10 positive tubes when a total of 10 samples from a lot are cultured. For example, a lot that has one in each 1000 items contaminated (0.1% contamination) could be passed as satisfactory (by showing no positive samples from the 10 tested) in 99 tests out of 100. When the true contamination rate is 5%, all 10 culture tubes are expected to remain sterile in 60 of each 100 lots tested. Even at the 10% contamination level, contamination would be detected only 2 out of 3 times.

Table II shows the degree of improvement that can be made in the validity of sterility tests by increasing sample size. It is clear that for contamination levels as low as 0.1%, increasing the sample size from 10 to 20, or even to 100, has a relatively small effect in improving the probability of accepting lots. Even a sample size of 500 would result in erroneously accepting a lot 6 times out of 10. On the other hand, if we were dealing with a lot contaminated to the extent of 10%, then by testing 100 samples the probability of passing it would be reduced to a theoretical zero.

Experience shows that many of the problems of sterilization cycles and sterility testing arise from lots with from 1 to 5% contamination. As shown in Table II, with a 5% true contamination and a sample size of 20 items, lots would be passed as sterile 36%

Table II—Relationship of Probabilities of Acceptance of Lots of Varying Assumed Degrees of Contamination to Sample Size

Number of samples Tested (*n*)	Probability of no positive growth tubes					
	"True" % contamination of lot					
	0.1	1	5	10	15	20
10	0.99	0.91	0.60	0.35	0.20	0.11
20	0.98	0.82	0.36	0.12	0.04	0.01
50	0.95	0.61	0.08	0.007		
100	0.91	0.37	0.01	0.00		
300	0.74	0.05				
500	0.61	0.01				

of the time. In this instance increasing the sample size to 50 gives a substantial improvement.

The information in Table II may be viewed in another way. If, for the probability values shown for each different sample size, we select that value which approximates P = 0.05 (95% confidence level), it is clear that using 20 samples will discriminate only contamination levels of 15% or more. If the 20 tubes show no growth, the lot could, of course, be sterile but we would have no way of knowing this from the test.

To put it another way, from such a test we could state only that it is unlikely that the lot would be contaminated at a level higher than 15%. Similarly, a satisfactory test using 50 samples would not indicate sterility at the 95% confidence level, but would only indicate that the lot is not contaminated by more than 5%. Finally, on a theoretical basis, a lot contaminated to the extent of 1% when 500 samples are tested would be erroneously accepted only once in 100 tests; or conversely, a satisfactory test indicates at a 99% confidence level that it is sterile—or at least not contaminated more than 1%.

It is apparent from the above that additional sterilization verification methods must be employed. The use of biological spore indicators is the most frequent method of improving the verification of sterilization processes and for providing an adequate margin of safety.

There are many factors involved in the sterility test that have not yet been entirely resolved; therefore, one must also seek other means to assure the sterility of products in addition to the usual sterility test. Some of these methods, in addition to the use of positive spore controls, involve the use of recording instruments to indicate that the sterilizing temperature and required exposure time (and moisture concentration when appropriate) has been reached and maintained.

Great care must be exercised in eliminating the bacteriostatic properties of the product being tested in order that false *negatives* not be obtained. The USP has attempted to eliminate the problem by suggesting that products that are bacteriostatic or fungistatic, when tested as directed, shall be treated with a suitable inactivating agent, either prior to culturing or by inclusion of the inactivating agent in the sterility test medium. An even better method involves the use of membrane filters. This method not only is appropriate for substances that possess bacteriostatic or fungistatic activity, but also can be used for the sterility testing of oils, ointments, and certain non-bacteriostatic substances not readily soluble in culture media.

Where possible, the substance is dissolved or suspended in a sterile fluid and the resulting solution or suspension is passed through a sterile bacteria-retaining membrane, that then is subjected to the sterility test. Where this form of preparation is inappropriate, the substance or object is rinsed with sterile fluid, that then is passed through the filter.

A suitable unit consists of a closed reservoir and a receptacle between which a properly supported membrane of appropriate porosity is placed. A membrane generally suitable for sterility testing has a porosity of $0.45 \pm 0.02\mu$, a diameter of approximately 47 mm, and a flow-rate of 55 to 75 ml of water/min at a pressure of 70 cm of mercury. The unit should be assembled and sterilized prior to use. Where the sample to be tested is an oil, sterilize the membrane

separately, and after thorough drying, assemble the unit, using aseptic precautions.

The successful use of this technique requires skill and the frequent use of positive and negative controls. One should occasionally use known contaminated solutions containing very few (approximately 10 cells in the total volume involved) of varying types of microorganisms to confirm the adequacy of the techniques being used. Full instructions, including information on the diluting fluids to be used, are included under *Sterility Tests* in the USP.

Whenever possible, it is recommended that sterility testing be done in accord with the methods outlined in the USP. Table III summarizes information from these methods relating to sterility test media, temperature and length of incubation, numbers of samples to test, etc. Emphasis is put on the inclusion of biological indicators in sterilization loads. Of course, for small pharmacies and where limited amounts of materials are sterilized, the numbers in Table III become prohibitive. In the case of small lots of this nature it is recommended that the test consist of not less than 10% of the items. Biological indicators, however, should be used with every sterilization load.

Laminar Flow

A new procedure for producing dust-free areas was discovered by Whitfield in 1961.[8] It is called *laminar flow*. In principle, the entire body of air within a confined area moves with uniform velocity along parallel flow lines. By employing prefilters and then high-efficiency filters, this sterile air sweeps all dust from the chamber or hood through the open side. The velocity of the air should be 90 ± 20 fpm. Laminar air flow devices can be vertical or horizontal; they can be actual rooms or cabinets or benches.

Almost from the beginning of the laminar flow era it was evident that this technique would find wide biomedical application. In addition to its use in sterilization and sterility testing, laminar flow devices have found application in hospitals (both in surgical theaters and in patient rooms), in veterinary medicine and animal care, and in problems of spacecraft sterilization. While there is no doubt of the value of laminar air flow for providing improved environmental control for such applications, it is important that proper attention be paid to its manner of use.[9]

Enough is now known concerning the advantages of laminar air flow for sterility testing, for aseptic assembly and filling operations, and for use in other aspects related to sterilization that its use can be recommended strongly. Probably the use of filtered laminar flow air should be considered mandatory for any new sterilization or sterility testing facility. However, like any other useful technique, the realization of the best advantages and the selection of the best type of laminar flow equipment can only follow an understanding of a few of the basic principles and some of the experiences of others. The following few paragraphs are intended to give the reader some basic information and background data.

For the most satisfactory environment for sterility testing and aseptic assembly operations, some type of laminar flow cabinet or bench is essential. If possible, each cabinet or bench should be located in a separate, small, clean room having a filtered air supply. The selection of the type of cabinet to use will depend on the operation itself. For most sterility testing operations, horizontal laminar air flow units appear to be

Table III—Procedural Details for Sterility Tests

Class of product	Type of sterilization	Form of biological indicator if used	Description of sample	No. of units required per lot	Medium	Temperature of incubation	No. of days of incubation
A	Not sterilized in final container	None	Product as received	30	Fluid Thioglycollate	30° to 35°	14[a]
				30	Soybean-Casein Digest	20° to 25°	14[a]
B	I—Sterilized by steam under pressure	None	Product—Liquid	20	Fluid Thioglycollate	30° to 35°	7
			Solid	20	Fluid Thioglycollate	30° to 35°	10
		Attached indicator	Attached indicator	10	Optimal[b]	Optimal[b]	7
			Product—Liquid	10	Fluid Thioglycollate	30° to 35°	7
			Solid	10	Fluid Thioglycollate	30° to 35°	10
		Incorporated indicator, or simulated product	Product containing indicator	10	Optimal[b]	Optimal[b]	7
	II—Sterilized by other means	None	Product	20	Fluid Thioglycollate	30° to 35°	14
				20	Soybean-Casein Digest	20° to 25°	14
		Attached indicator	Attached indicator	10	Optimal[b]	Optimal[b]	7
			Product	10	Fluid Thioglycollate	30° to 35°	10
				10	Soybean-Casein Digest	20° to 25°	10
		Incorporated indicator, or simulated product	Product containing indicator	10	Optimal[b]	Optimal[b]	7

[a] 7 days, if membrane filtration is used.
[b] Medium and temperature of incubation optimal for the type of microorganisms used as the biological indicator.

superior to vertical flow hoods because the air movement is less likely to wash organisms from the operators hands or equipment into the sterility test media. Fig. 534 shows the sterility testing of syringes in a horizontal laminar air flow hood. Fig. 535 shows an outward convergent flow hood, called the Minibench (*BD & Co.*), that is convenient for many pharmaceutical uses and for sterility testing.

The major disadvantage of the horizontal laminar air flow units is that any airborne particulate matter generated in the units is blown directly out into the room and against the technical personnel. In situations where infectious material is involved or where one must prevent contamination of the environment with a powder or drug, use of specifically designed

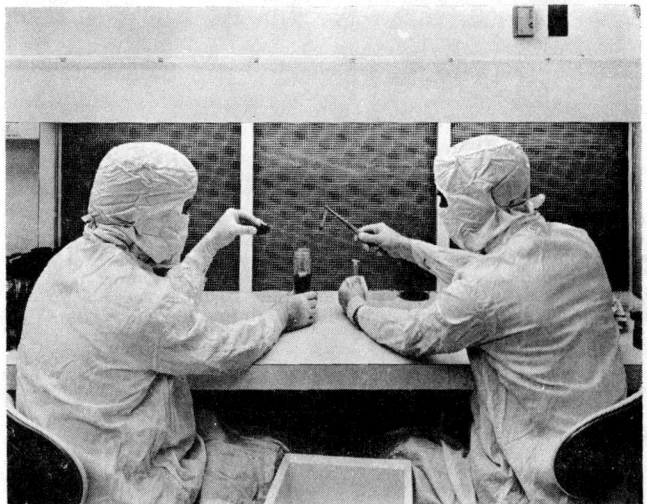

Fig. 534. Sterility testing of plastic disposable syringes in a horizontal laminar air flow bench (courtesy, BD & Co.).

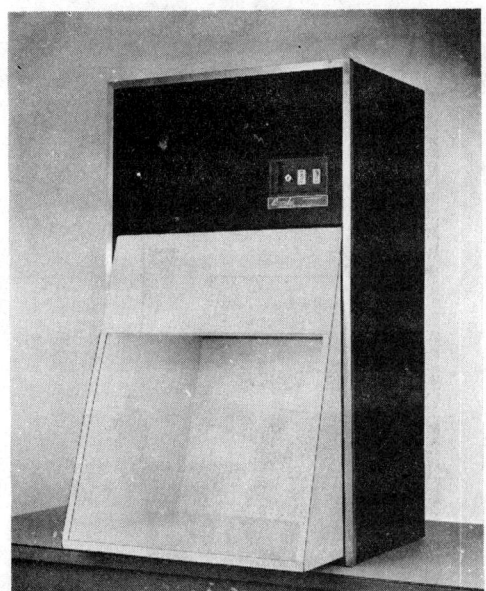

Fig. 535. Convergent laminar air flow Minibench for sterility testing and aseptic assembly operations (courtesy, BD & Co.).

laminar *down flow* units is recommended. Recently, such down flow units have become available that do an excellent job of providing both product and personnel protection. Such a unit is shown in Fig. 536.

To achieve maximum benefit from laminar air flow, one must first realize that the filtered air flow itself does not remove microbial contamination from the surface of objects. Thus, it is still necessary to reduce the microbial load on the outside of materials used in sterility testing to avoid false laboratory results.

Laminar flow will do an excellent job of maintaining the sterility or cleanliness of an article bathed in the air flow; however, the sterility testing procedure must create the least possible turbulence within the hood. Moreover, an awareness of the turbulent air patterns created by the operation is necessary to avoid critical operations in turbulent zones. To illustrate how effectively airborne particles are washed from an environment by laminar air flow, Table IV shows the distance various size particles will travel horizontally before falling three feet.

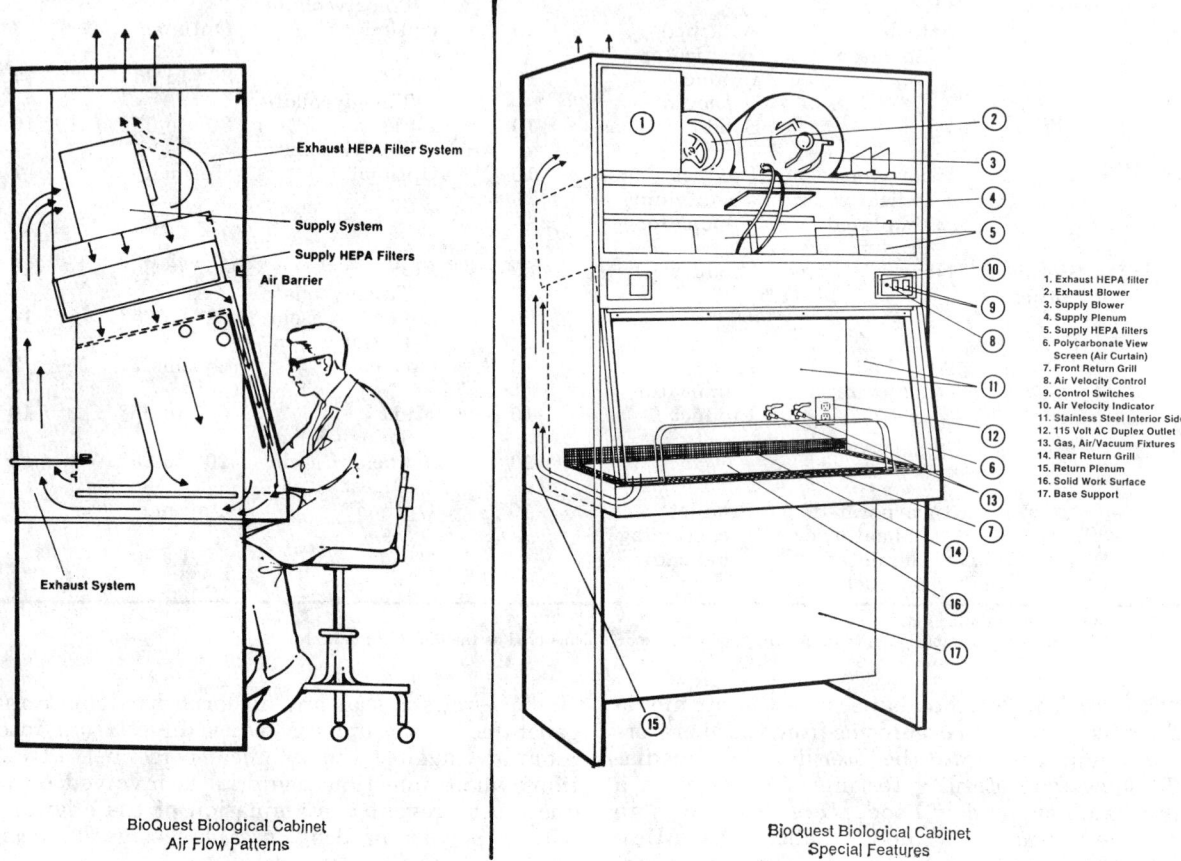

**BioQuest Biological Cabinet
Air Flow Patterns**

**BioQuest Biological Cabinet
Special Features**

1. Exhaust HEPA filter
2. Exhaust Blower
3. Supply Blower
4. Supply Plenum
5. Supply HEPA filters
6. Polycarbonate View Screen (Air Curtain)
7. Front Return Grill
8. Air Velocity Control
9. Control Switches
10. Air Velocity Indicator
11. Stainless Steel Interior Sides
12. 115 Volt AC Duplex Outlet
13. Gas, Air/Vacuum Fixtures
14. Rear Return Grill
15. Return Plenum
16. Solid Work Surface
17. Base Support

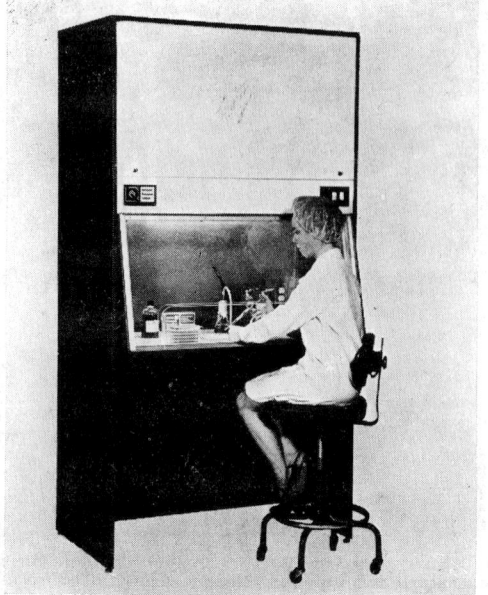

Fig. 536. Sketch (*above*) and photograph (*left*) of a biological cabinet with vertical, recirculating laminar flow cabinet and HEPA filtered exhaust. HEPA filtered air is supplied to the work area at 90 ± 20 fpm. Air flow patterns in combination with a high-velocity curtain of air form a barrier at the front access opening which protects both the work and the worker from airborne contamination (courtesy, BioQuest).

Laminar flow clean benches should supply Class 100 air as defined in Federal Standard 209a.[10] They must be tested periodically to ascertain that they are functioning properly. An air velometer should be used at regular intervals to check the air flow rates across the face of the filter, smoke tests are useful in visualizing air flow patterns, and a particle analyzer can be used to check the quality of the air.

The filters of each laminar air flow device should be tested and certified at the time of purchase and installation as well as each time new filters are installed. Although it is possible to use a tracer microorganism for this evaluation, it is probably better to employ the dioctylphthalate (DOP) test.[11] This standard acceptance test determines the validity of the filter and its seal using DOP smoke (mean particulate diameter of 0.3μ) and a light-scattering aerosol photometer. The smoke, at a concentration of 80–100 mg/liter, is introduced into the plenum of the unit, and the entire perimeter of the filter face is scanned with the photometer probe at a sampling rate of 1 ft³/min. A reading of 0.01% of the upstream smoke concentration is considered a leak.

Table IV—Settling Rates of Sand and Clay Particles (sp gr, 2.65) in Laminar Air Flow

Particle diameter μ	Approximate floating distance (ft) of particles while falling 3 ft in cross drafts of 60 fpm	90 fpm
104	1.1	1.66
76	2.0	3.1
53	4.3	6.4
40	7.5	11.3
20	30.0	45.0
10	120.0	180.0
2	>750.0	>1100.0

In addition to the routine air flow measurements and filter efficiency testing, biological testing should be done on a more or less continuous basis to monitor the effectiveness of the laminar air flow systems. Microbial air sampling and the use of agar settling plates are useful in monitoring these environments. Phillips[12] evaluated horizontal laminar flow hoods by tabulating the number of "false positives" appearing in sterility test media over a period of time. These results showed very low numbers of "false positives" (Table V).

Sterilization Methods

This discussion will be limited to the methods of sterilization from the point of view of the pharmacist or small hospital pharmacy, as well as those that could be employed by the large hospital pharmacy or the pharmaceutical manufacturer.

Steam Under Pressure

Heat is the most generally used method of sterilization. Moist heat in the form of saturated steam under pressure (autoclaving) is perhaps the most reliable method for the destruction of all forms of microorganisms. According to Perkins[13] the cause of death in sterilization by moist heat is quite different from that encountered in dry-heat processes. In brief, death by moist heat is the result of coagulation of some protein in the cell; death by dry heat is primarily an oxidation process.

Table V—False Positives Occurring in a Laminar Flow Hood

Product	Number of units sterility tested	Number of false positives	% false positives
Syringes	9793	2	0.02
Needles	4676	2	0.04
Misc.	306	0	0

The simplest form of an autoclave available is the home pressure cooker (Fig. 537) which, with an electrical hot plate or other arrangement for heating, is very suitable for use in the smaller laboratory. One advantage of the type shown in this figure is that it has a one-piece pressure regulator that is very simple to use. It also has an interlocking lid with an automatic safety fuse. This type is available in 2½- to 16-qt sizes.

Fig. 538 is a sketch of a typical gravity or downward displacement autoclave. These depend on the difference in density of air and steam, air being heavier and displaced to the bottom of the chamber and out as steam is admitted near the top. It is customary of such units to sense the temperature at the drain point to assure that no more air is moving out of the system. Fig. 539 shows a typical modern-day hospital autoclave.

Although the pressure cooker may serve in the small pharmacy or hospital laboratory for steam sterilization, it is not automatic and requires a great deal of attention in order to sterilize materials properly. For the larger hospital pharmacy and for the pharmaceutical manufacturer, conventional autoclaves

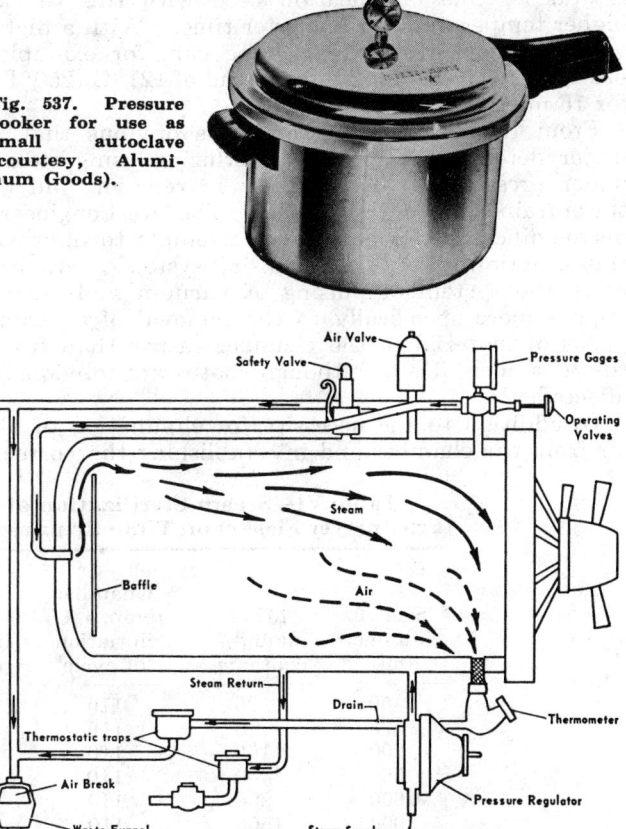

Fig. 537. Pressure cooker for use as small autoclave (courtesy, Aluminum Goods).

Fig. 538. Longitudinal cross-section of a downward displacement sterilizer showing essential parts and a flow pattern for the movement of steam and air (courtesy, Wilmot-Castle).

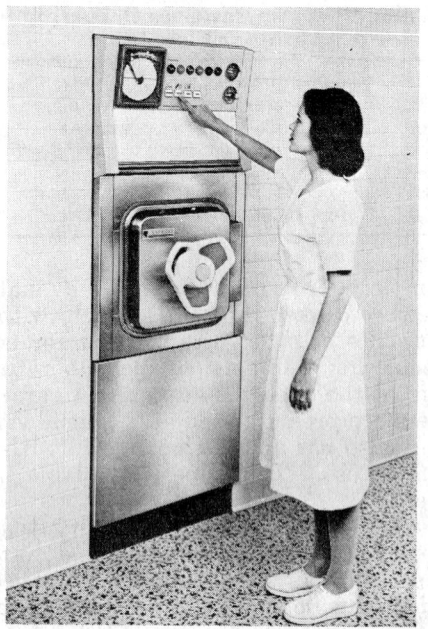

Fig. 539. Typical hospital steam sterilizer with automatic controls (courtesy, Am. Sterilizer).

are recommended. Models are available in a wide range of sizes, from about 12 in. in diameter to 6 ft or larger in diameter (Figs. 540–542).

Several improved methods for steam sterilization have been developed in recent years. The first of these, originally developed by British workers, was the high-vacuum steam sterilization method.[14] This method involves the evacuation of the chamber to 15 mm absolute pressure within 4 min before the steam is added. One modification used with this was a higher temperature for a shorter time. With a high-vacuum, high-pressure cycle one can, for example, use 135°C (275°F) for 3 min instead of 121°C (250°F) for 15 min.[15]

From the above discussion it is obvious that a major deterrent to chamber sterilizing using steam under pressure is the difficulty in removing all of the entrained and entrapped air. The latest engineering modification for autoclaves attempts to improve this situation by providing pulsing systems. Apparently the system of pulsing of vacuum and steam applies more specifically to the removal of air from packs of material in the chamber rather than from the chamber itself, although both are obviously affected.

In addition to the necessity for elimination of all air from the chamber and in establishing the correct autoclave temperature, it is also necessary to consider how long after reaching the required temperature the material should be held to achieve sterility. For small volumes (up to 250-ml flasks) a minimum of 20 min will suffice, whereas larger volumes will require a longer heating period before all of the solution has reached 121°C. Up to 55 min of heating at 121°C (for 8 liters in a standard Pyrex bottle) may be required for the solution to be sterilized. Tables VI and VII, based on the sterilizations of liquids in Erlenmeyer flasks, will give adequate examples of the need to lengthen cycle time due to container size and number of containers/load.[16]

Regardless of the type of autoclave, the arrangement of the load in the chamber is of the utmost importance. All packages must be arranged loosely so that the steam may permeate the innermost parts (Fig. 540). When large vessels of dressings or other articles are sterilized, they should be placed on their side so that a path is provided for the escape of air. Automatic autoclaves may be obtained complete with thermocouples for measuring the temperature in various locations and with automatic timers that measure the time of sterilization, beginning when the appropriate temperature is reached, and automatically turn off at the end of the sterilizing period. In some of the large autoclaves made for sterilizing parenteral solutions, outside jackets are equipped with cooling water

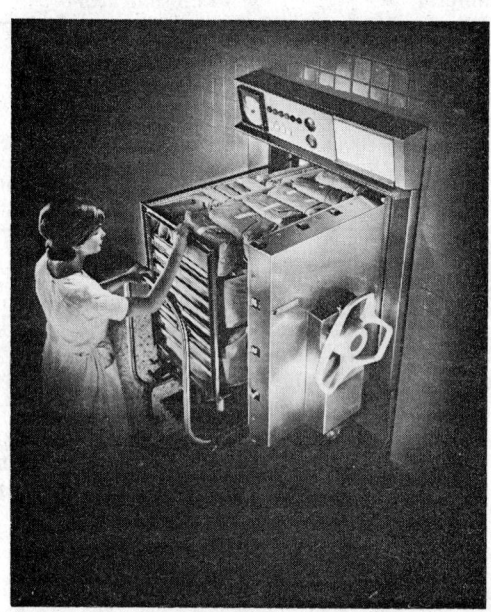

Fig. 540. Large hospital sterilizer with automatic controls showing a method of loading the chamber (courtesy, Am. Sterilizer).

Table VI—Steam Sterilization of Liquids—Effect of Volume/Container (Erlenmeyer Flasks) on Time Required To Reach 121°C (Single Container Load)[16]

Size of container (ml)	Ml of liquid/ container	Chamber temp. (°C) initiation of cycle	Liquid temp. (°C) at initiation of cycle	Min for chamber to reach 121°C	Min for center of liquid to reach 121°C	Total time (min) of cycle
50	25	110	25	2	4	14
125	75	110	25	2	5	15
200	150	110	25	3	7	17
500	400	110	25	3	10	20
1000	800	110	25	3	14	24
2000	1500	110	25	6	19	29
3000	2500	110	25	7	25	35
5000	4500	110	25	8	33	43
6000	5500	110	25	8	44	54

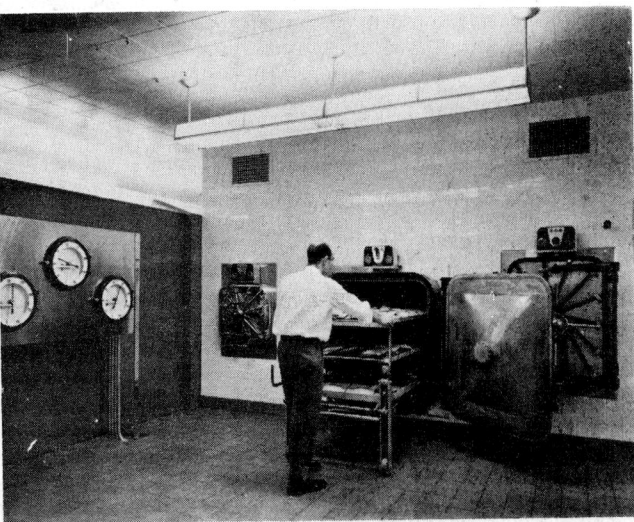

Fig. 541. Large autoclaves with indicating thermometer and automatic controls for use in hospital pharmacy (courtesy, Clinical Center, NIH).

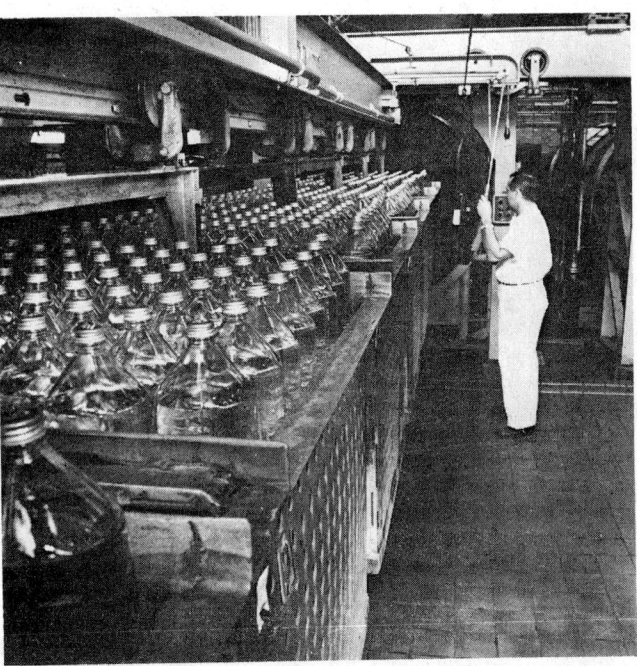

Fig. 542. Large commercial steam sterilizer for the sterilization of large volumes of intravenous solutions (courtesy, Abbott).

that will cool the load so that it may be removed from the autoclave after a much shorter period of time (Fig. 542).

There are both advantages and disadvantages associated with all types of autoclaves and a definitive discussion of them is beyond the scope of this chapter. However, for anyone faced with the initial purchase of an autoclave, prior detailed study of these points as outlined in appropriate texts would be in order.[17]

Dry Heat

Many materials such as dry glassware, petroleum jelly, mineral oils, greases, waxes, and talcum powder cannot withstand sterilization by moist heat and therefore can be sterilized dry in a hot-air oven (Figs. 543 and 544). Such ovens are usually thermostatically controlled and are either electric or gas fired. They should be constructed to provide proper circulation of inside air so that there is no layering of the hot air that would cause overheating in some sections and less than sterilizing temperatures in other sections.

In more elaborate models fans are employed to circulate the hot air, whereas in less expensive models baffling and the method of application of the heat are depended on to secure adequate distribution.

It is difficult, if not impractical, to establish a single temperature–time relationship for dry-heat sterilization. However, some temperature–time figures commonly mentioned for the sterilization of hospital supplies in current texts on sterilization are:

170°C (340°F)–1 hr
160°C (320°F)–1 or 2 hr
150°C (300°F)–2.5 hr
140°C (285°F)–3 hr*

---

* This chapter does not include a discussion of the kinetics of dry-heat sterilization. For those interested in a more basic understanding of this subject, including the new knowledge brought about by research on the dry-heat sterilization of spacecraft, reference is made to Lawrence and Block[17] and to work sponsored by the National Aeronautics and Space Administration.[18,19]

Table VII—Steam Sterilization of Liquids—Effect of Volume/Container and Number of Containers on Time Required for Liquid To Reach 121°C[16,a]

L of liquid/ container	No. of containers/ load	Chamber temp. (°C) at initiation of cycle	Liquid temp. (°C) at initiation of cycle	Min for chamber to reach 121°C	Min for center of liquid to reach 121°C	Total time (min) of cycle
0.5	30	27	29	10	19	29
1.0	20	27	26	12	34	44
1.5	15	56	26	12	36	46
2.0	10	46	27	13	37	47
2.5	10	66	26	15	40	50
3.0	8	46	26	15	43	53
3.5	6	46	26	12	50	60
4.0	5	43	26	12	52	62
4.5	5	44	26	14	58	68
5.0	5	46	26	15	60	70
5.5	5	42	26	17	60	70
6.0	4	42	26	15	62	72

 a Chart or external thermometer readings reflect the temperature of the chamber, not the load. Variations in load and equipment necessitate the use of a temperature-sensing device in the center of the load. Consequently a thermocouple and potentiometer or similar device shall be used to determine the sterilization cycle. Once the cycle has been established there is no need to use thermocouples for daily use. It is recommended, however, that the cycle be checked once every 2 weeks.

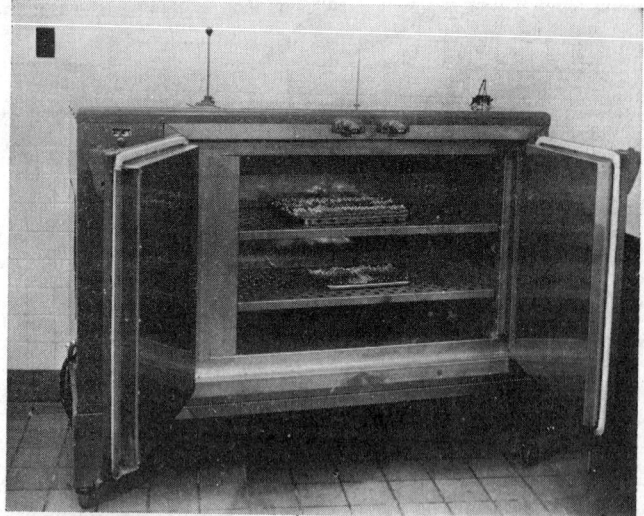

Fig. 543. Small electric hot-air sterilizer for use in hospital pharmacy (courtesy, Clinical Center, NIH).

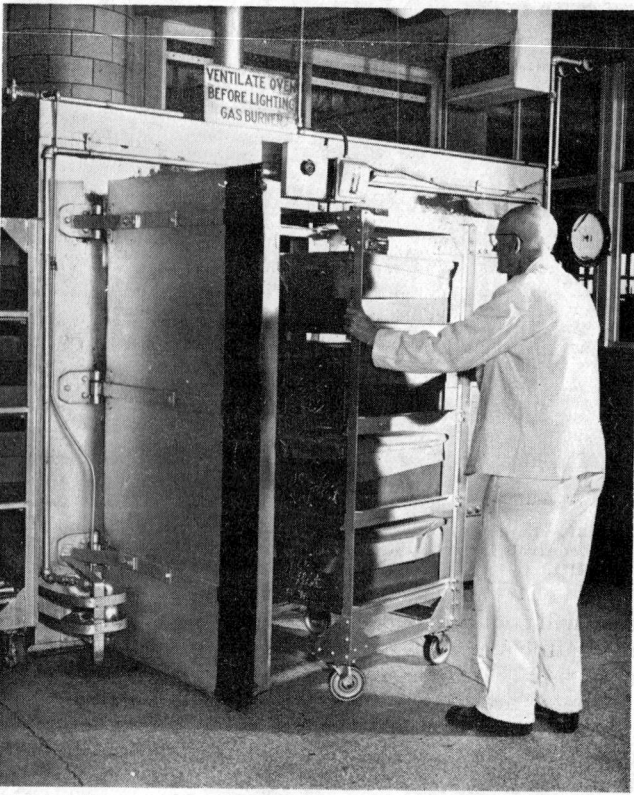

Fig. 544. Large gas-fired sterilizing oven (courtesy, Parke-Davis).

For products that will not tolerate these high temperatures, such as the sulfonamides, experimentation employing live spores as controls may indicate that a lower temperature than 140°C for a longer period of time will adequately sterilize the product. For example, one standard used for the dry-heat sterilization of interplanetary spacecraft is 125°C for 24 hr.[20]

In the sterilization of powders that will not withstand the usual hot-air sterilizing temperatures because of lower melting points, it is necessary to determine what combination of time and temperature are necessary to destroy the most resistant of the organisms. This can be done by the use of dummy packages containing spores of a resistant strain of bacteria (eg, *Clostridium sporogenes*) placed in every ft³ of oven space.

When the sterilization parameters have been established, routine sterilization should be monitored by the sterility testing of these control packages, plus the testing of regular samples of the product in compliance with USP requirements. In the case of *Cl. sporogenes* the spore controls are planted in thioglycollate medium and incubated at 30°–35°C. There is good assurance of sterility if all of the culture tests are found to be sterile.

Normally such spore controls cannot be used in buildings that are under license from the NIH for biological products, because their regulations strictly forbid the use of spore-forming anaerobes in such facilities. This method of testing, however, is an excellent one and is employed with the approval of the Food and Drug Administration (FDA) in many installations.

In the sterilization of solutions in oil, for example, BAL (dimercaprol), a similar technique employing spores is followed. BAL in 10% solution in peanut oil may be sterilized in a hot-air oven at 160°C for 2 hr. Since it is possible to have as high as 100,000 spores/ml in peanut oil and still have it pass the standard sterility test, very little reliance can be placed on the sterility testing of oils, without employing special techniques.

Therefore, control ampuls made of amber glass are prepared to differentiate them from the regular ampuls of clear glass. In these, spores are suspended in polyethylene glycol that will withstand a sterilizing temperature of 170°C and yet be readily miscible with culture media and thus allow the spores to germinate. These amber-colored control ampuls should be spotted throughout the oven and after the sterilization period they should be tested for sterility, along with ampuls from the regular lot, to ensure the sterility of the entire lot.

In both of these techniques, due to variation in the individual load caused by changing air currents, it is necessary to place controls in each run. The test samples should be identified with specific positions in the oven to allow readjustment of the louvres or resterilization of any part of the load in which the spore controls were not killed.

Heating over a direct flame is a satisfactory method of dry-heat sterilization that is satisfactory for forceps, needles, metal spatulas, and other instruments of this type. The process involved is the direct incineration of the organisms. This method is used to sterilize the lips of beakers, test tubes, flasks, and similar objects by applying the flame directly for approximately 5 sec. The process is often not satisfactory because very often the parts will overheat and in the case of metallic instruments the temper may be destroyed, or in the case of glassware it may become too hot and break.

The direct flame is used, however, for sterilizing contaminated materials such as small pledgets of cotton or for disinfecting the nichrome or platinum loop used in transferring bacterial cultures. This method should *not* be used for sterilizing greasy or oily materials because the spattering in the flame will tend to spread contamination rather than eliminate it.

Filtration

For solutions that cannot be heated, sterilization is usually accomplished by filtration employing one of the several bacterial filters that are available. In the smaller pharmaceutical laboratory Pasteur, Chamberland, small Seitz, or Berkefeld-type filters have been employed traditionally (Figs. 545–547). These filters work by virtue of the interlacing pores either of fused porcelain, sintered glass, or metal, or a combination of cellulose and asbestos fibers. Bacteria become entrapped in these pores and are thus removed from the solution.

Since gravity filtering by these means would be very slow, vacuum or pressure or both are usually employed to make the solution move more rapidly through the filter. In the smaller laboratory, vacuum is usually employed, although airborne bacteria may enter if the joint between glass and stopper is not tight. The recent tendency for both small and large filter operations is to use membrane filters.

The need for the different types of bacteria-removing filters is understood when it is realized that some pharmaceuticals are readily adsorbed by one type of filter and not by another. Some solutions that might be adsorbed by the Seitz type of asbestos pad may be run through a porcelain or sintered glass filter without difficulty. When bacteria-removing filters are used for sterilization of a pharmaceutical product, a sterile technique must be maintained throughout the operation and the filters, together with all of the assembly, with the exception of the tank in which the bulk solution is first placed, must be sterilized before use. Most bacteria-removing filters are sterilized by heat in either a completely assembled setup or they are aseptically assembled after sterilization in a clean room or laminar air flow apparatus.

Seitz Filters—The Seitz type of filter is available in sizes ranging from the small Swinny syringe filter (Fig. 545) to the larger plate-type filter (Fig. 547). The Seitz pads are available in several porosities that make them quite valuable in the "polishing" of solutions (ie, a final filtration to impart a brilliant, sparkling clarity) as well as in the removal of bacteria. One of the disadvantages of this type of filter is that occasionally fibers get in the solution unless the filter is backed with nylon mesh or sintered stainless steel.

Several laboratory-size filters are slightly larger than the Swinny filter. These are valuable when only a few hundred milliliters are to be processed. When

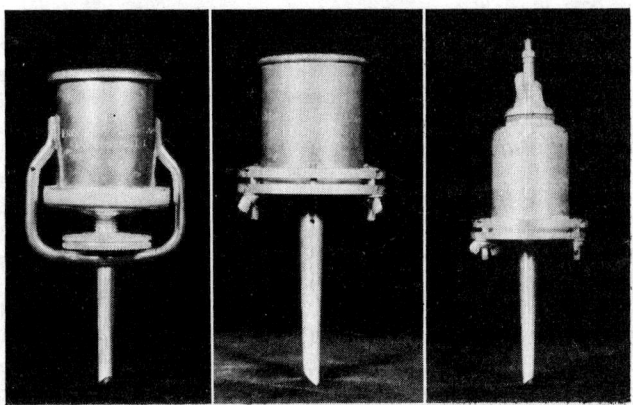

Fig. 546. Three models of small laboratory Seitz filters. *A* and *B*: for vacuum; *C*: for pressure or vacuum (courtesy, Hercules).

larger volumes are to be filtered, a Seitz filter (Fig. 546) may be employed. This is particularly valuable for a large hospital pharmacy or a small production laboratory. The Seitz filter pads are relatively inexpensive and new pads are inserted each time the apparatus is used.

Porcelain Filters—Another type of filter is that made from unglazed porcelain. The general principle of assembly is shown in Fig. 548. The simplest laboratory setup (Fig. 549) illustrates the construction and assembly of an all-porcelain-type filter element as utilized in conjunction with an assembly for vacuum filtration. This particular assembly, including the filter element, is often utilized for the handling of pharmaceutical, biological, and bacteriological preparations that can be damaged by metallic contact.

The disadvantage of porcelain or sintered glass-type filters is that the pores become plugged with organisms

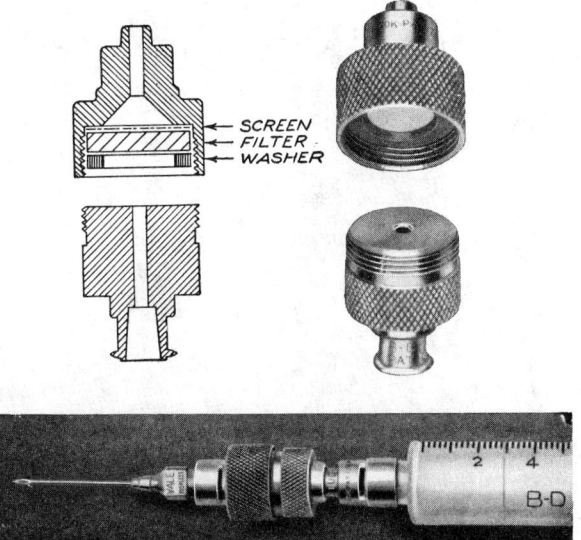

SCREEN
FILTER
WASHER

Fig. 545. *Below:* Swinny filter attached to syringe; *above:* the Swinny filter adapter separated and in cross section (courtesy, BD & Co.).

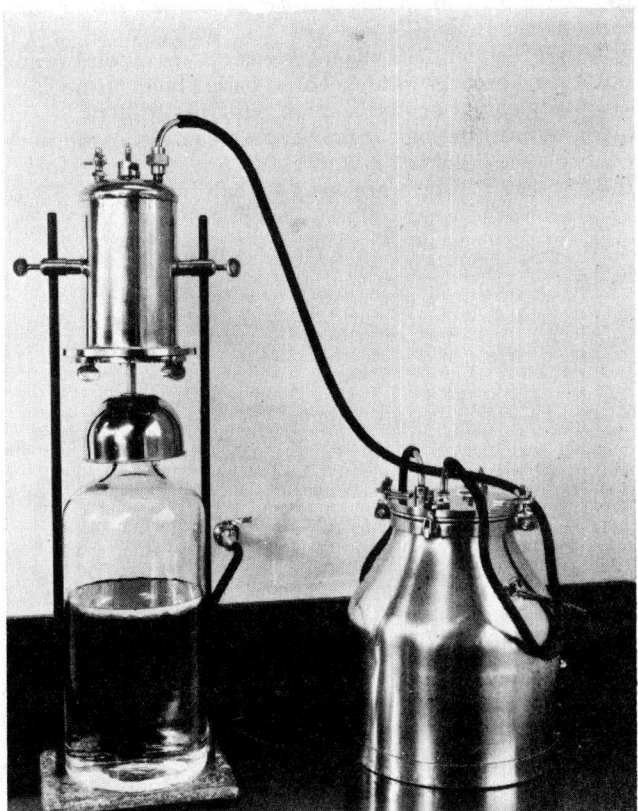

Fig. 547. Seitz filter with pressure tank (16-L capacity) (courtesy, Hynson).

and debris and must be cleaned with strong acids or burned out at high temperatures. In these cases the porosity size may change so that they no longer remove the bacteria. These filters should be tested from time to time by employing a test organism such as *Serratia marcescens* that is readily identifiable. Users of porcelain filters are encouraged to obtain directions for their care and use from the manufacturer.

Membrane Filters—In recent years ultrafiltration methods have become increasingly popular. This has been due mainly to the increased refinement of the various membranes. For the most part, cellulose and derivations of cellulose are the most commonly employed materials in these filters. Currently, a large number of distinct pore size grades are available, ranging from 8μ downward to 0.22μ.

The liquid to be sterilized is forced through the membrane filter by a variety of methods such as vacuum, forced pressure, or centrifugation. Approximately 80% of the total filter volume is composed of the pores. Thus, the filter acts primarily as a simple screen. It retains on its surface all particles whose size exceeds the filter pore size. The particles, on being deposited, adhere to the filter in virtually a single microscopic plane. This action is due mostly to the combined forces of gravity and van der Waals forces. Because of this random settling, little overlapping occurs and the filter itself may be subjected directly to such analytical procedures as counting, sizing, weighing, culturing, or staining.

Membrane filtration has the decided advantage of filtering at a flow rate of at least 40 times faster than other filtering procedures having a similar particle size retention capability. However, such filters are obviously subject to clogging by small particles in solutions being filtered.

Many types of filter membranes have been shown to be soluble in ketones, nitroparaffins, esters, and various alcohols. They are also susceptible to the action of strong alkalies. Newer type membranes, however, are available that have been especially designed for the sterilization and microfiltration of alcohol–base biological materials, reactive monomers, concentrated acids and alkalies, and other "exotic" fluids. Such filters are said to exhibit only a 15 to 25% swelling in very strong solvents but without an effect on the filtration efficiency. They may be sterilized by autoclaving or by exposure to dry heat at 200°C (400°F). Pore sizes currently available for the Solvinert (*Millipore*) filter are 1.5, 0.5 and 0.25μ.

Being necessarily thin and frequently subjected to pressure differential, the membrane filter is somewhat brittle. A number of supporting filter holders are available, however, to add more strength to the filter. Most commonly used are stainless steel screens, silver screens, glazed porcelain, porous carbon discs, sintered glass, and porous earthenware.

Aside from the quantitative procedures, large-scale application is found in the production of biological preparations, hormones, and enzymes. Membrane filter equipment may be placed easily in the hospital pharmacy, being small in size and readily portable. Larger equipment such as that used in the manufacturing of pharmaceuticals and other industrial purposes is also available. Figs. 550–553 show apparatus for small- and large-scale use.

Gases

Gaseous sterilization may be defined as the destruction of all living microorganisms with a chemical in a gaseous or vapor state. The concept of such sterilization is quite old. The ancient burning of incense, purification in smoke of articles during epidemics, and dissemination of odors from spices were all attempts to purify or render harmless objects suspected of being unclean. Lister's technique of spraying phenol in the air of operating rooms was, indeed, a form of gaseous disinfection. The burning of sulfur candles and fumigation with formaldehyde in sickrooms likewise represented attempts at gaseous sterilization.

There are many occasions when solid materials may not be sterilized by either moist or dry heat because of damage or destruction to the material or product. The use of chemical sterilization with gaseous agents frequently avoids these problems and, since gases by nature dissipate when unconfined, the problem of removal is readily solved. Use of these gaseous agents

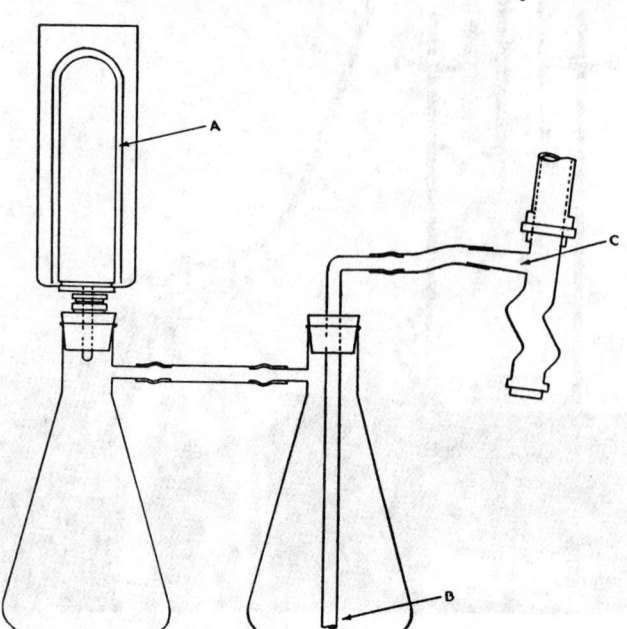

Fig. 548.   **Vacuum filtration assembly.**

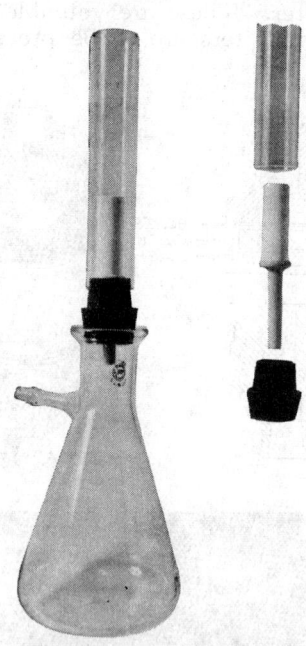

Fig. 549.   **Expanded view of microporous porcelain filter elements for laboratory use** (courtesy, Selas).

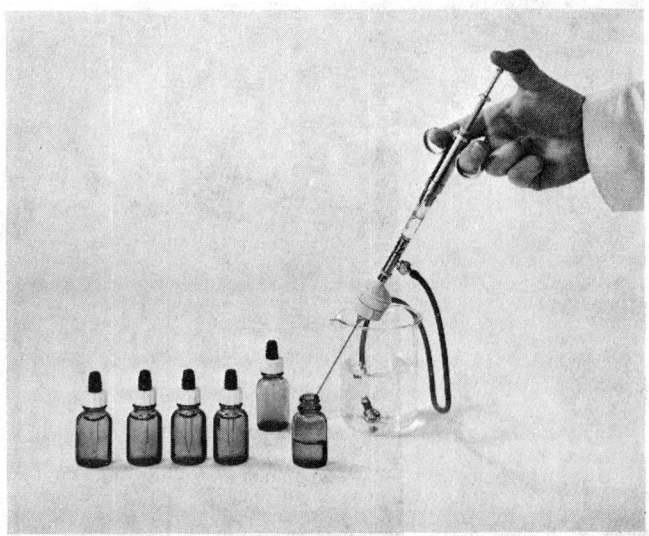

Fig. 550. Use of a membrane filter holder and a Cornwall pipet syringe for dispensing measured volumes of sterilized fluids (courtesy, Millipore).

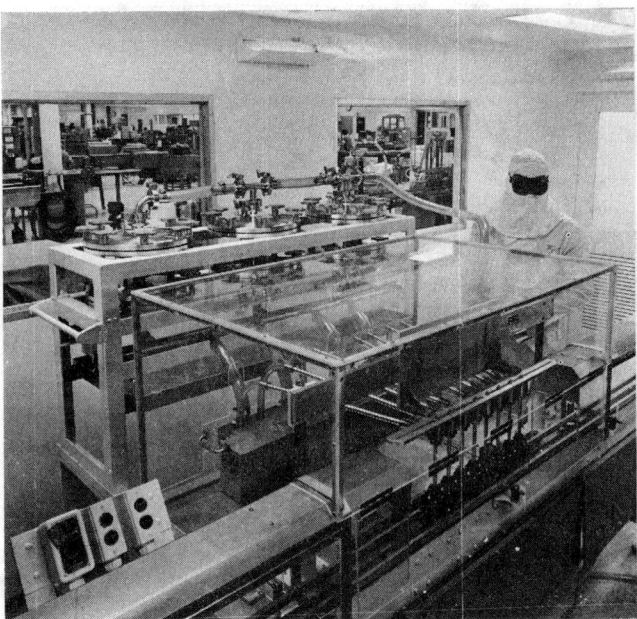

Fig. 552. Eight-head bottle-filling machine that uses three parallel-connected high-volume sterilizing filter holders (courtesy, Wyeth and Millipore).

has solved many difficulties encountered in the sterilization of certain biologicals, foodstuffs, cotton, wool, laboratory equipment, and more recently a large number of plastic disposable syringes, needles, and tubing sets.

A variety of vapors and gases possess germicidal properties. Among these are ethylene oxide, formaldehyde, propylene oxide, β-propiolactone, ozone, chloropicrin, peracetic acid, and methyl bromide. When these agents are employed in closed systems and under controlled conditions of temperature and humidity, excellent decontamination can result. Under controlled conditions, and with specific limitations, some of these can be used as sterilizing agents.

Formaldehyde, formerly used for sickroom disinfection, has in the past been employed as a satisfactory sterilant by making use of pressure cookers. Gaseous

formaldehyde is generated either by dripping formaldehyde solution into potassium permanganate or the holding of the entire load at 56°C with paraformaldehyde, whereby sterilization occurs in several hours. Such chamber loads are usually left overnight. A disadvantage of this type of formaldehyde sterilization is the difficulty in removing residuals of the compound following its use.

Vacuum, extensive airing, heat, and neutralization are the methods most often used to remove polymerized formaldehyde deposits (Figs. 554 and 555). Recently, there has been renewed interest in formaldehyde sterilization due to the availability of a highly purified form of paraformaldehyde that apparently increases the ease of production of the gas and reduces the problems of residuals. Heating of this polymer results in the release of pure formaldehyde gas with little or no waste. In England, a sterilization proce-

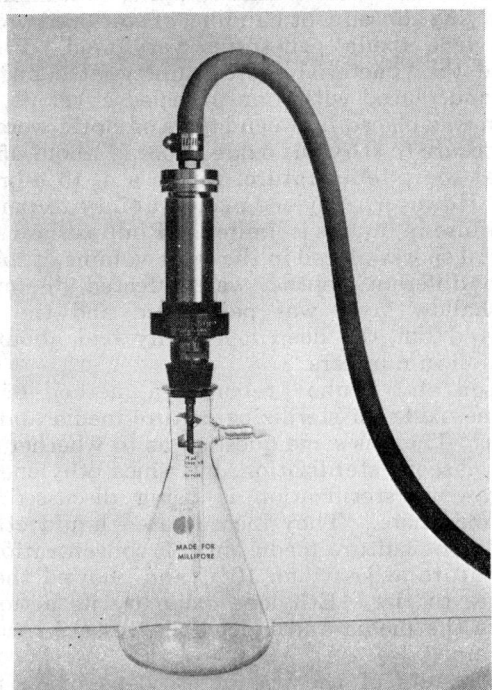

Fig. 551. Pressure filter apparatus for sterilizing moderate volumes of liquids (courtesy, Millipore).

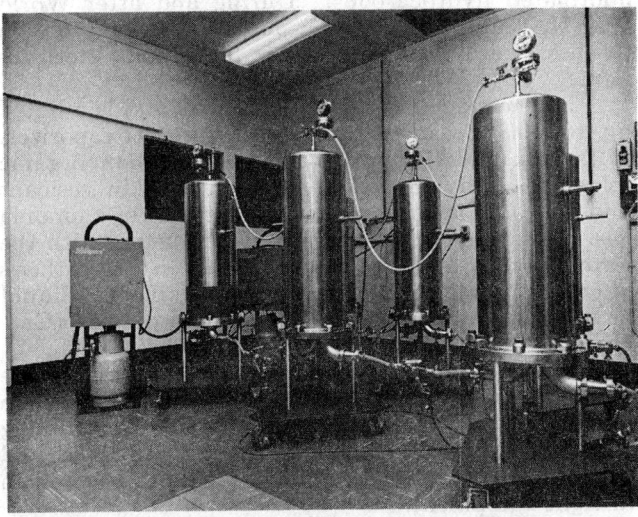

Fig. 553. In-place sterilization large-scale membrane filtering equipment. Banks of multiplate filters are sterilized before use with ethylene oxide. Portable sterilizer console (*left*) contains vacuum pump and automatic controls for sterilization cycle and tank of sterilizing gas (courtesy, MSD).

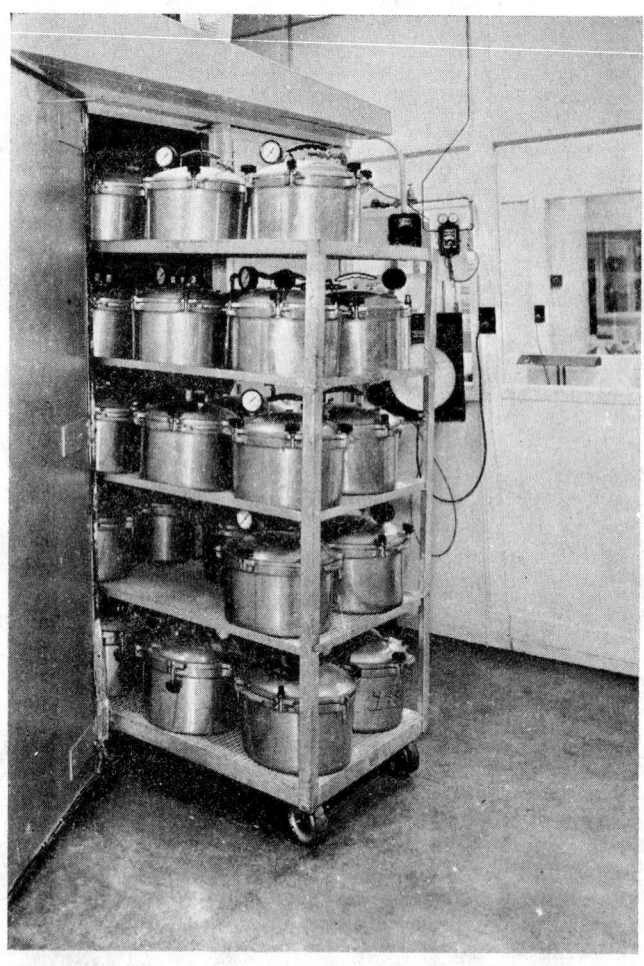

Fig. 554. Rack of pressure cookers in which plastic parts have been placed with paraformaldehyde and which have been evacuated previous to being placed in a low-temperature oven at approximately 60°C (courtesy, Abbott).

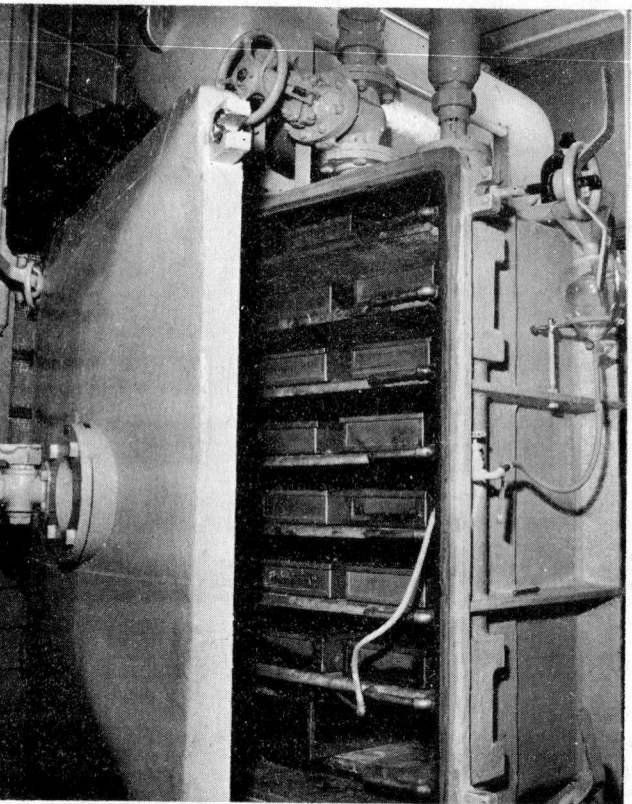

Fig. 555. Devine drying oven equipped with means for introducing formalin onto potassium permanganate in the generating box shown in the bottom of the dryer. This type of equipment is particularly suitable since it can be thoroughly evacuated (courtesy, Lilly).

dure involving the injection of formaldehyde into a steam chamber held at 80°C and at a reduced pressure has been reported to be successful.[21]

In addition to the use of formaldehyde, ethylene oxide (ETO) is often employed either in the form of a pure gas or in combination with carbon dioxide or fluorinated hydrocarbons. During and after World War II, Phillips and Kaye[22] published extensively on the use of ethylene oxide vapor for gaseous sterilization.

Ethylene oxide freezes at −111.3°C and is a liquid up to 10.8°C, at which temperature it vaporizes. It is miscible with water and all common organic solvents. Ethylene oxide can act as a skin vesicant and has an inhalation toxicity about that of ammonia gas. It is a cyclic ether or epoxy compound with the formula shown on page 1378. It is used in the synthesis of other organic chemicals and is available as a liquid or in a 10% mixture with 90% carbon dioxide (Carboxide*) or in a 12% mixture with Freon.†

Ethylene oxide is highly flammable and may explode violently when mixed with air; with 90% carbon dioxide it is not combustible and in this form is gaining widespread use. The gas is readily diffusible and because of its penetrating ability it must be used in airtight equipment.

Some of the things that have been successfully

sterilized with ethylene oxide are medical and biological preparations, dry foods and cereals in burlap bags, catgut, pancreatin, papain, plastic equipment parts and bottle closures, antibiotics, plaster bandages, culture media, books and hospital bedding, eggs, spices, foodstuff, heavy equipment, and soil.[23] Often material can be sterilized in final shipping containers, thus simplifying subsequent handling of sterilized products.

Ethylene oxide penetrates very well. Phillips[24] showed that bacterial spores impregnated on cotton cloth and placed within an unsealed envelope, which in turn was placed between layers of cloth, were killed by exposure to ethylene oxide vapor at about 450 mg/liter, at room temperature, within a 4- to 6-hr exposure. However, ethylene oxide's ability to penetrate and diffuse in liquids is limited. Phillips showed that bacterial spores placed in the same volume of solution, but in different depths, were affected dissimilarly. The shallow layer was penetrated and the spores destroyed but the deep layer only had about 50% reduction in numbers.

Wilson and Bruno[25] reported a method of using ethylene oxide for sterilizing culture media and other liquids. There is some question as to whether or not this is gaseous sterilization, but since ethylene oxide and gaseous sterilization is being discussed, it is mentioned here. They incorporated liquid ethylene oxide in the culture media, in 1% concentration at a temperature of less than 10°C and allowed the temperature to rise. Ethylene oxide by its action will sterilize the media and indeed the vessel in which it is contained.

The results of the use of ethylene oxide in the pharmaceutical industry have been so successful that commercial equipment is now available that may be

---

* Source: Carbide and Carbon.
† Source: Pa. Eng.

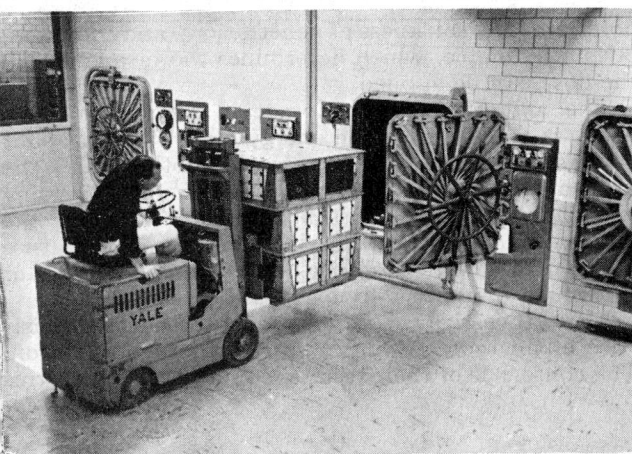

Fig. 556.   Bank of ethylene oxide sterilizers for plastic syringes, needles, and tubing sets (courtesy, BD & Co.).

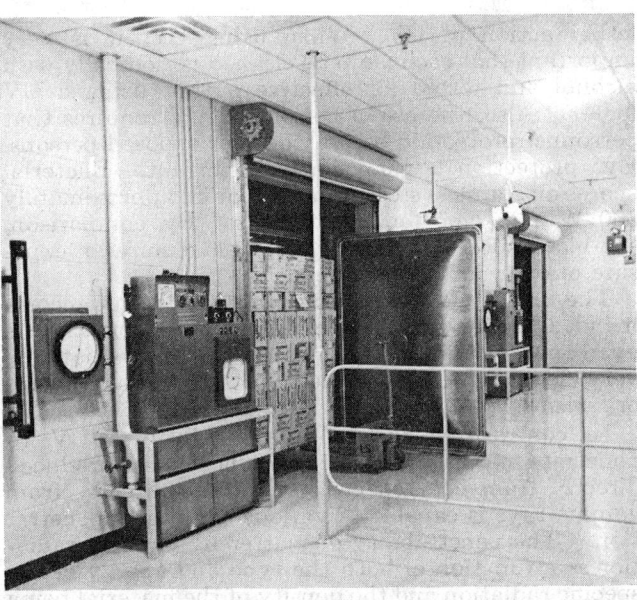

Fig. 557.   Large (1000 ft³) chamber used with 100% ethylene oxide for the sterilization of plastic syringes (courtesy, BD & Co.).

used either for steam autoclaving or for sterilizing with ethylene oxide (see Fig. 556).   The advantage of these sterilizers is that a combined method of operation, using steam in the jacket and Carboxide or ethylene oxide–Freon gas in the chamber, is employed. The combined method of operation is advantageous in certain types of work in that it becomes practical to use shorter exposure periods because of the temperature coefficient of the gas and more rapid diffusion at higher temperatures.   A large industrial sterilizer utilizing 100% ethylene oxide is shown in Fig. 557.

Carboxide is commercially available in 30- and 60-lb cylinders.   To admit gas to the chamber, it is only necessary to connect the cylinder to the chamber inlet valve by means of flexible metal tubing.   When using this method with autoclaves of less than 30 ft³ in volume, the gas should be admitted first to an expansion tank to insure a uniform concentration of ethylene oxide in the chamber.

The use of ethylene oxide requires an awareness of the possible retention of the gas or the formation of residual byproducts in materials being treated. Articles such as rubber and plastic tubing will adsorb ethylene oxide gas upon gaseous sterilization.   It is very important that such articles not be used until they have been detoxified by airing at room temperature for at least 5 days.

Hoffman and Warshowsky[26] presented a thorough discussion on the use of β-propiolactone (BPL) as a sterilizing agent.   They showed that BPL vapor, when applied under conditions of maximum effectiveness, is approximately 25 times more active as a disinfectant than formaldehyde gas, about 4000 times more active than ethylene oxide, and 50,000 times more active than methyl bromide.   They further state that the fact that BPL is many times more effective than ethylene oxide does not imply that it should be used as a substitute in all situations.   Ethylene oxide has good penetration properties and is effective at moderately low humidities; this is not true of BPL.   On the other hand, formaldehyde and ethylene oxide are not effective at low temperatures; BPL is effective at 10°C and below.

The use of BPL is limited at the present time to decontaminating rooms, chambers, and buildings. It must be used with caution because it is an irritant to the eyes and mucosa; good ventilation is necessary after its use.   At present, because of these and other factors, it is not recommended for use in pharmaceutical applications.

Radiation

Radiation is generally classified as (1) electromagnetic or (2) particulate.   Electromagnetic radiation, comprised of photons of energy, includes ultraviolet, gamma, X, and cosmic radiation.   Particulate or corpuscular radiation includes a formidable list of particles but, for the purpose of this discussion, will be limited to beta particles or electrons, as produced in the linear accelerator.

The principles of sterilization by irradiation, as made possible by advances in radiobiological research, have been known since the early 1940's.[27]   Artificially produced ultraviolet (UV) radiation in the region of 2537 Å has been used for its germicidal activity for more than 30 years.[28]   This region of the UV spectrum has been shown to possess the greatest activity in destroying microorganisms.   While germicidal UV has been used for many years in the pharmaceutical industry in the maintenance of aseptic areas and rooms, only rarely can it be used satisfactorily as a sterilizing agent.

Inactivation of microorganisms by UV is principally a function of radiant energy dose: the application of an effective radiation intensity over a proper interval of time.   However, dose requirements for different microorganisms vary widely.   Vegetative bacteria are most susceptible while bacterial spores appear to be 3–10 times as resistant to inactivation.   Of utmost importance, as a limiting factor, is the fact that fungal spores may be 100 to 1000 times more resistant to UV than vegetative bacteria.

Even with adequate dose, however, the requirements for proper application of germicidal UV in most pharmaceutical situations are such as to discourage its use for *sterilization* purposes.   On the other hand, UV as an ancillary germicidal agent can often fill a very useful function.   For example, UV lamps can help to maintain the sterility of products or surfaces following a sterilization treatment.

The principal disadvantage to the use of germicidal UV is its limited ability to penetrate.   The 2537 Å wavelength radiation is screened out by most materials.   This means that clumps of organisms, and those protected by dust or debris can easily escape the lethal action of UV. When using UV, it is very important that each lamp be cleaned periodically with alcohol and tested for effective output using a UV meter. Also, the use of germicidal UV requires that personnel protection be provided for exposed persons. Eye protection is particularly important. Bacterial spores on stainless steel surfaces require approximately $800\mu W$ min/cm^2 for inactivation. By comparison, the black spores of *Aspergillus niger* require an exposure of over $5000\mu W$ min/cm^2.[28]

The use of UV as a sterilizing agent is not recommended unless the basic problem of penetration is overcome and unless the material to be irradiated is very clean and free of crevices that can protect microorganisms.

In contrast to the relative inability of UV to penetrate materials, ionizing radiation as produced directly from charged electrons and indirectly from gamma rays is capable of various degrees of penetration. The penetrability of matter by ionizing radiation is a function of both the type and energy of the specific radiation and the density of the material being irradiated. Due to their charge and mass, corpuscular radiation such as beta particles have significantly shorter mean ranges in matter than electromagnetic radiation of equivalent energy; ie, a 1 mev gamma ray has a range more than 80 times as great as a 1 mev electron in water before being completely dissipated. The importance of material density as a factor in radiative energy absorbance cannot be stressed too strongly.

The interaction of charged particles with matter causes both ionizations and excitations. Ionization of matter results in the formation of ion pairs which are comprised of the negatively charged ejected orbital electrons and positively charged counterpart ions. The intensity of ionization is referred to as specific ionization (ie, ion pairs/distance mean path) and is a function of the linear energy transfer (LET) of the specific ionizing particle. The LET is defined as the energy lost/μ of path of the ionizing particle.

Charged particles such as electrons interact directly with matter causing ionization, whereas electromagnetic radiation causes ionization through various mechanisms that result in the ejection of an orbital electron to which a specific amount of energy from the incident gamma ray is transferred. These ejected electrons then behave similarly to beta particles in ionization reactions. Thus, both corpuscular and electromagnetic radiation (ie, high-energy gamma and x-rays) are considered as ionizing radiation and differ from UV radiation in this respect.

One theory of the mechanism by which high-energy radiation affects microorganisms concerns the formation of free radicals. Orbital electrons of an atom are dislodged by the accelerated particles and reunite with ionized molecules to form an unstable chemical structure. In the radiolysis of water the free radicals can combine to form hydrogen peroxide, resulting in damage to the cell. Another theory involves the direct action of the radiation on a vital structure of the cell, such as the chromosomal nucleoprotein. Probably a combination of both effects is present, causing complete and irreversible inactivation of microorganisms.

Requirements for sterilization by ionizing radiation involve the consideration of the following factors: the dose, or the amount of radiation that is absorbed by the material; the energy level available, which along with the bulk density of the material will determine the thickness of penetration; and the power output available, which determines the rate at which the dose can be applied.

The unit of radiation dosage is the roentgen (r), which is equivalent to an energy absorption of about 84 ergs/Gm in air. More recently another unit—the rad—has become widely used in radiation processing applications. The rad is arbitrarily defined as the absorption of 100 ergs/Gm, independent of the nature of the irradiated substance. Sterilization doses, for convenience, are usually expressed in megarads.

Many investigators have studied the relative resistance of microorganisms to sterilization by radiation. The consensus of their results is that vegetative forms

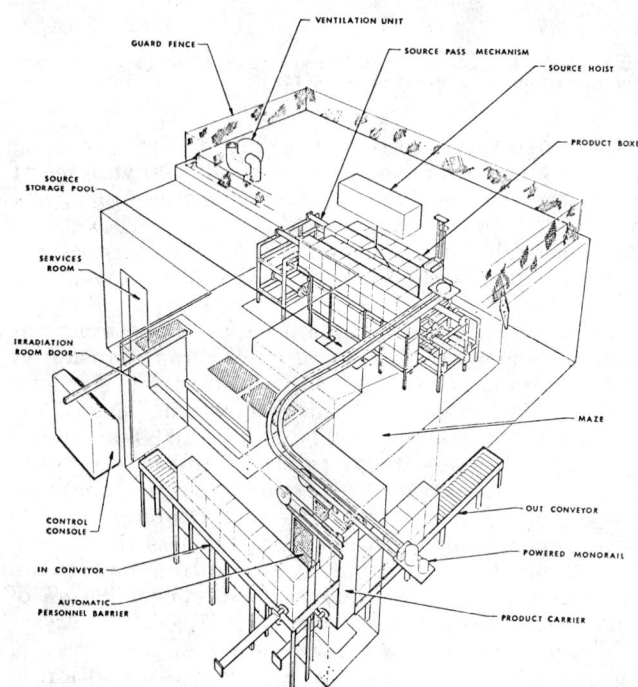

Fig. 558.   500,000-curie cobalt-60 medical products irradiator (courtesy, Atomic-Canada).

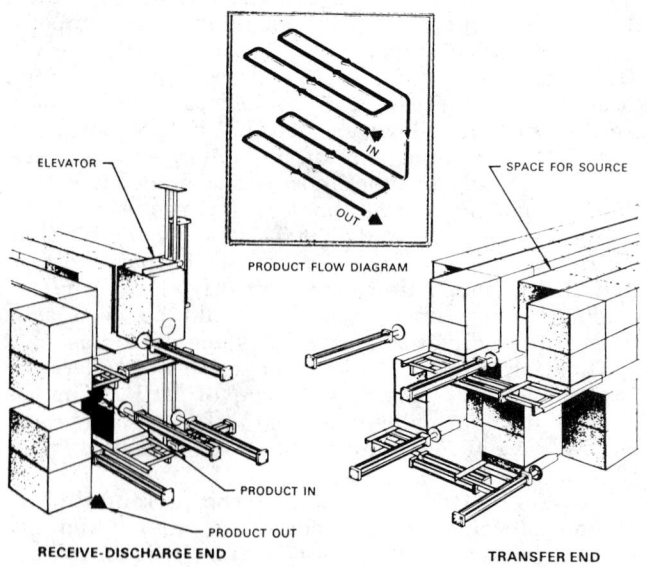

Fig. 559.   Mechanisms for passing medical goods through the cobalt-60 irradiator (courtesy, Atomic-Canada).

are most sensitive, followed by molds, yeasts, spore-formers, and viruses in decreasing order of sensitivity. It is generally agreed that a radiation dose of about 2.4 megarads is sufficient to kill the most resistant microorganisms with an adequate safety factor under most conditions.[3]

The sources of gamma rays used for radiosterilization are usually waste fission products and radioisotopes such as cobalt-60 and cesium-137. Modern sterilization facilities used by pharmaceutical and medical device firms generally utilize cobalt-60 and are designed to hold up to 2,000,000 curies of radioactive source material. Fig. 558 shows a modern cobalt-60 radiosterilization facility and Fig. 559 is an industrial sterilization plant.

Electron accelerators may be of the electrostatic type such as the van der Graaff accelerator in which negative electricity is carried by a continuous belt to a hollow dome where the electrons are removed and accumulated. The electrons are then discharged through a vacuum column where they are accelerated by a series of magnetic fields. The electron beam is then spread over the conveyor carrying the product to be sterilized. In the linear accelerator electrons are emitted from a cathode source at the top of the column. The electrons are accelerated by means of microwaves traveling down the accelerator tube. Fig. 560 shows the control panel of a linear accelerator.

Ionizing radiation has been used successfully for the sterilization of such items as hospital supplies, vitamins, antibiotics, steroids, hormones, bone and tissue transplants, and medical devices such as plastic syringes, needles, surgical blades, plastic tubing, catheters, prostheses, petri dishes, and sutures. There is no doubt about the effectiveness of this process as a sterilization method. However, the main disadvantage at present is the high cost of equipment and installation which makes the process practical only for high volumes of materials such as commercial products produced by the pharmaceutical and medical device industries.

Aseptic Handling

Although not actually a sterilization process, one other technique should be mentioned at this time; ie, aseptic handling or manipulation. A typical example of its use is found in the compounding of prescriptions that will not withstand sterilization by one of the previously described processes but in which all of the ingredients are available in a sterile form.

In such cases sterility must be maintained throughout the operation and it is necessary to use sterile equipment and material. Therefore, all containers and general apparatus such as beakers, graduates, pipettes, spatulas, mortars, and pestles should be sterilized by one of the previously mentioned processes. Such work should be conducted only by an operator who fully recognizes the possibility of contamination by faulty technique. This subject and a fuller description of technique involved is given in detail in the chapter on *Parenteral Preparations*, page 1519. The use of laminar flow devices for aseptic handling is discussed on pages 1504 and 1529.

Alternate Methods

Some pharmaceutical preparations cannot tolerate the high temperature of dry-heat or steam sterilization nor can they be sterilized by filtration. In such cases it is necessary to resort to some less reliable method such as fractional sterilization or heat at temperatures below 121°C, either with or without bacteriostatic agents. Such techniques may be classed as alternate methods of sterilization.

The method of *fractional sterilization*, also known as *Tyndallization*, can be applied to substances that are nutritive in nature and contain no bacteriostatic or inhibitory agents. Sterilization by this procedure is accomplished by heating the material in free-flowing steam for 1 hr, and then placing the material in an incubator so that the bacterial spores present can germinate. The material is heated again the following day to kill the vegetative bacteria. This process is carried out three times to complete the Tyndallization.

A second alternate method of sterilization is to heat the material to some temperature below 100°C (boiling) in the presence of a chemical agent. This is usually done by employing spores in containers similar to those used for the product being sterilized. After the heating period it is necessary to test these spores

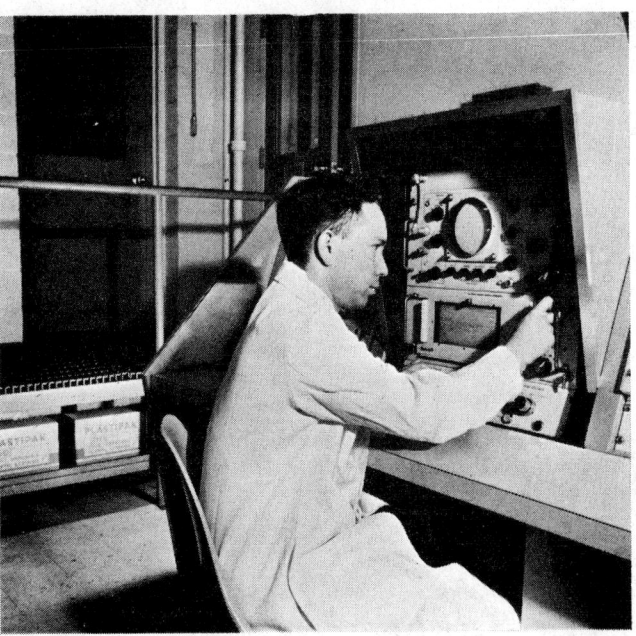

Fig. 560. Control panel of a linear accelerator, showing conveyor carrying products to be sterilized to the shielded target area (courtesy, BD & Co.).

and, if they are found to be sterile, it is an indication that the time and temperature employed produced sterilization of the product.

Instruments, hypodermic syringes, and needles can be rendered aseptic by boiling for 15 min. However, if spores are present, sterility cannot be guaranteed. *Sterilization* by boiling is no longer an acceptable method.

References

1. Brewer, J. H., and Phillips, G. B., *Bull. Parenteral Drug Assoc.*, **22**, 157 (1968).
2. Brewer, J. H., and Arnsberger, R. J., *J. Pharm. Sci.*, **55**, 57 (1966).
3. Borick, P. M., and Fogarty, M. G., *Appl. Microbiol.*, **15**, 785 (1967).
4. Anderson, A. W., *et al*, *Food Technol.*, **10**, 575 (1956).
5. Christensen, E. A., and Sehested, K., *Acta Pathol. Microbiol. Scand.*, **62**, 448 (1964).
6. Brewer, J. H., and McLaughlin, C. B., *J. Pharm. Sci.*, **50**, 171 (1961).
7. Brewer, J. H., *et al*, *Bacteriol. Proc.*, 61 (1956).
8. Whitfield, W. J., *A New Approach To Clean Room Design*, VC-37 Instruments, TID-4500, 16th ed., 1962.
9. Phillips, G. B., and Brewer, J. H., in *Developments in Industrial Microbiology*, vol. 9, Am. Inst. of Biol. Sci., Washington, D.C., 1968, p. 105.
10. *Clean Room and Work Station Requirements, Controlled Environment*, Federal Standard No. 209A, Gen. Serv. Admin., Specifications Activity, Printed Mater. Supply Div., Washington, D.C.

11. Steinberg, S. B., *Air Engr.*, 14 (July, 1966).
12. Phillips, G. B., *Sterility Testing Environment: Equipment and Facilities*, to be published in *Adv. Ind. Microbiol.* (1969).
13. Perkins, J. J., in Reddish, G. F., ed., *Antiseptics, Disinfectants, Fungicides and Sterilization*, Lea & Febiger, Philadelphia, 1954, p. 656.
14. Bowie, J. H., *Hosp. Engr.*, **11**, 74 (1957).
15. Penikett, E. J. K., *Can. Med. Assoc. J.*, **85**, 886 (1961).
16. *NASA Standard Procedures for the Microbiological Examination of Space Hardware*, (NHB 5340.1A). Natl. Aeronautics & Space Admin., Washington, D.C., Oct., 1968.
17. Lawrence, C. A., and Block, S. S. *Disinfection, Sterilization and Preservation*, Lea & Febiger, Philadelphia, 1968.
18. Bruch, C. W., in Florkin, M., and Dollfus, A., eds., *Live Sciences and Space Research, II*, North Holland Publ. Co., Amsterdam, 1964, pp. 357–371.

19. Koesterer, M. G., *Develop. Ind. Microbiol.*, **6**, 268 (1964).
20. Bruch, C. W., *Spacecraft Sterilization Technology* (NASA SP-108), Natl. Aeronautics & Space Admin., Washington, D.C., 1966, pp. 207–229.
21. Alder, V. G., *et al*, *J. Clin. Pathol.*, **19**, 83 (1966).
22. Phillips, C. R., and Kaye, S., *Am. J. Hyg.*, **50**, 270 (1949).
23. Kaye, S., *J. Lab. Clin. Med.*, **35**, 823 (1950).
24. Phillips, C. R., *Bacteriol. Proc.*, 23 (1950).
25. Wilson, A. T., and Bruno, P., *J. Exptl. Med.*, **91**, 449 (1950).
26. Hoffman, R. K., and Warshowsky, B., *Appl. Microbiol.*, **6**, 358 (1958).
27. Proctor, B. E., *et al*, *Res. Reps. on US Quartermaster Contract Proj.*, July 1942–June 1943, Dept. Food Technol., Mass. Inst. Technol., 1943, p. 217.
28. Phillips, G. B., and E. Hanel, Jr., *Use of Ultraviolet Radiation in Microbiological Laboratories*, (P.B. 147 043). US Library of Congress, Washington, D.C., listed in *US Govt. Res. Rept.*, **34** (2), 122 (Aug., 19, 1960).

82 | Parenteral Preparations

History—administration—accumulation and selection of components—production facilities and procedures—quality control—packaging and labeling

This chapter was prepared by

Kenneth E. Avis, DSc, *Professor of Pharmaceutics, College of Pharmacy, The University of Tennessee, Memphis, Tenn. 38103*

Parenteral preparations are those pharmaceutical dosage forms which are administered under or through one or more layers of the skin or mucous membrane. The term "parenteral" is derived from two Greek words, *para enteron*, meaning beside the intestine. Parenteral preparations are introduced directly into the body fluid systems composing the intra- or extracellular fluid compartments, the lymphatic system, or the blood circulatory system.   Since the highly efficient protective barriers of the skin and mucous membranes are circumvented, the introduction of microorganisms or toxic agents is very dangerous.   Because of this, it is imperative that parenteral preparations be as nearly perfect as possible with respect to purity, freedom from toxicity, and freedom from contamination.   Therefore, great care must be taken to maintain near-perfect quality standards in the manufacture of these preparations.   No effort may be spared in making these products the very best pharmaceutical preparations.

History

Sir Christopher Wren was probably the first person to inject successfully drugs into the veins of living animals, in about the year 1657.[1]   From a very crude beginning, the technique for intravenous injection and a knowledge of the implications thereof developed slowly during the next century and a half.   During the first half of the 19th century, the subcutaneous route of administration was being developed.   In 1855 Dr. Alexander Wood of Edinburgh described what was probably the first subcutaneous injection of drugs for therapeutic purposes using a true hypodermic syringe.

The latter half of the 19th century brought an increasing concern for safety in the administration of parenteral solutions, largely because of the work of Robert Koch and Louis Pasteur.   While Charles Chamberland was developing both hot-air and steam sterilization techniques and the first bacteria-retaining filter (made of unglazed porcelain), H. Nordtmeyer was developing a filter made of kieselguhr (the Berkefeld filter), and Stanislaus Limousin was developing a suitable container, the all-glass ampul.   Shortly after the beginning of the 20th century, attention focused on the disturbing chills and fever which often followed the intravenous injection of drugs.   In the middle 1920's Dr. Florence Seibert provided proof that this reaction was caused by potent products of microbial growth which could be eliminated from water by distillation and from glassware by heating at elevated temperatures.   These developments provided the foundation for an increasing use of parenteral routes for the administration of drugs.

The 5th edition of the National Formulary (NF)

contained the first official standards for parenterals in the United States.   In 1926 six injectable solutions became official under the classification of "Ampuls." The current NF contains 91 monographs and the USP 165 monographs under the category of "Injections." Thus, the number of parenteral preparations has grown rapidly, signifying their present importance among therapeutic dosage forms.

Administration

Injections may be classified in five general categories: (1) solutions ready for injection, (2) dry, soluble products ready to be combined with a solvent just prior to use, (3) suspensions ready for injection, (4) dry, insoluble products ready to be combined with a vehicle just prior to use, and (5) emulsions.   These injections may be administered by one or more routes, such as, intravenous, subcutaneous, intradermal, intramuscular, intraspinal, intracisternal, and intrathecal.   The nature of the product will determine the particular route of administration that may be employed.   Conversely, the desired route of administration will place requirements on the formulation.   For example, suspensions would not be administered directly into the blood stream because of the danger of insoluble particles blocking capillaries.   Solutions to be administered subcutaneously would require strict attention to tonicity adjustment, otherwise irritation of the plentiful supply of nerve endings in this anatomical area would give rise to pronounced pain.   Injections intended for intraspinal, intracisternal, and intrathecal administration require the highest purity standards because of the sensitivity of nerve tissue to irritant and toxic substances.

As with all dosage forms, injections possess certain advantages and disadvantages when compared with other dosage forms.   If immediate physiological action is needed from a drug, it usually can be provided by an intravenous injection.   Modification of the formulation or another route of injection can be used to slow the onset and prolong the action of the drug. The therapeutic response of a drug is more readily controlled by parenteral administration since the irregularities of intestinal absorption are circumvented. Also, since the drug normally is administered by a professionally trained person, it may be confidently expected that the dose was actually and accurately administered.   Drugs can be administered parenterally when they cannot be given orally because of the unconscious or uncooperative state of the patient, or because of inactivation or lack of absorption in the intestinal tract.   Among the disadvantages of this dosage form are the requirement of asepsis at administration, the real or psychological pain factor, and the difficulty in correcting an error, should one be made. In the latter situation, unless a direct pharmacological antagonist is immediately available, correction of an error may be impossible. One other disadvantage is that daily or frequent administration poses difficulties, either for the patient to visit a professionally trained person or to learn to inject himself.

Parenteral Combinations

When a large volume of an electrolyte or a nutrient is being administered intravenously to a patient, the attending physician often prescribes the addition of one or more other parenteral preparations as a means of reducing the number of injections the patient must endure.

Until recently, the pharmacist usually has had little or no knowledge of the events transpiring at the patient's bedside, being called upon only to dispense the required preparations individually. However, physicians and nurses have become increasingly aware of the precipitates, colors, and other visible changes which sometimes occur when certain preparations are combined.

As pharmacists have been queried concerning these happenings, an awareness has gradually developed of the widespread occurrence of visible as well as invisible physical, chemical, and therapeutic incompatibilities when certain drugs are added to intravenous fluids.

The development of a precipitate or a color change when preparations are combined is an immediate warning that an alteration has occurred. Such a combination should not be administered to the patient because the solid particles may occlude the blood vessels, the therapeutic agent may not be available for absorption, or the drug may have been degraded into toxic substances. Moreover, in other instances changes not visually apparent may have occurred which could be equally or more dangerous to the welfare of the patient.

A number of charts have been compiled recently, based almost exclusively on the visible changes that can be observed when two or more preparations are combined.[2,3] Such charts are valuable as guides to visible incompatibilities, but they are subject to constant change as a modification is made in a commercial product or new products appear on the market.

Such variations as the order of mixing, the proportions in the mixture, or the period of time that the combination is held before use may also alter the results. Some attempts have been made to utilize a more basic approach by emphasizing the role of pH[4,5] and reaction rates[6] in predicting or describing the extent of degradation.

The pharmacist is the professionally trained person best qualified to predict the likelihood of incompatibilities from the combination of two or more preparations. Ideally, no combination should be used unless it has been thoroughly evaluated to be sure that it is compatible from the physical, chemical, and therapeutic aspects, not only in generic but in specific commercial forms.

Since this is almost an impossible task and at present has been done on few, if any, drug combinations, such combinations should be avoided. Actually, combinations will continue to be prescribed. Therefore, the pharmacist should become involved with these problems and should seek information to

make decisions adequately on the propriety of administering combinations of parenteral therapeutic agents.

General Requirements

The inherent requirement for the very best quality and reliability for parenteral preparations places a high moral and professional responsibility on the pharmacist accountable for their manufacture. While these requirements are very demanding, they can be accomplished, as attested to by the large number of injectable products manufactured each year. What is required?

1. The manufacturer must possess and apply high moral and professional ethics. He must not permit himself to entertain even the thought of using inferior techniques or ingredients in the manufacturing process. The proper attitude of the person responsible for the preparation of the product is its most vital ingredient.
2. He must use to full measure the pharmaceutical training that he has received. The challenges to his knowledge will be many and varied.
3. He must employ the specialized techniques required for the manufacture of sterile preparations with alertness and sound judgment. These techniques must be subjected to continuous, critical review for faults, omissions, and improvements.
4. He must use ingredients of the highest quality obtainable. At times, ingredients may require special purification beyond that of the commercial supply. This will normally require that cost factors be given second place in importance.
5. He must establish the stability and effectiveness of the product. Variation in techniques and ingredients may alter the results as compared with those found elsewhere. Therefore, stability and effectiveness cannot be taken for granted, even when the data have been obtained from a highly reliable source.
6. He must establish a rigid control program to assure the quality of the product and the repetition of valid production procedures. This involves evaluation of all ingredients, vigilant control of all steps in the production procedure, and careful evaluation of the finished product.

Injections are rarely prepared in a retail pharmacy because of the lack of adequate facilities necessary to prepare a reliable and safe product.

In some hospital pharmacies injections or irrigating fluids are manufactured, but in an increasing number aseptic processing is being utilized primarily in the combining of various added drugs to intravenous solutions for the individual patient. The vast majority of injectable products used clinically are prepared by the pharmaceutical industry.

General Process

The preparation of a parenteral product may be considered to encompass four general areas as follows: (1) accumulation and selection of the components, (2) production facilities and procedures, (3) control, and (4) packaging and labeling. The components of the product to be accumulated and selected include vehicles, solutes, containers, and closures. Production includes the sequential steps of preparing and controlling the environment, cleaning the containers and equipment, preparing the product, filtering the solution, filling containers with the product, sealing the containers, and sterilizing the product. Control includes the evaluation of the components, determination that the production had been executed within prescribed requirements, and conduction of necessary evaluative tests on the finished product. The final area of packaging and labeling includes all the steps necessary to properly identify the finished product and enclose it in such a manner that it is safely and properly prepared for sale and delivery to the user. In the following sections, these four areas and appropriate subtopics will be discussed in detail.

Components and Containers

The establishment of specifications with respect to the quality of each of the components of an injection is of vital importance. These specifications will be coordinated with the requirements of the specific formulation and will not necessarily be identical for a particular component if used in several different formulations.

The most stringent requirements normally will be encountered with aqueous solutions, particularly if the product is to be sterilized at an elevated temperature where reaction rates will be greatly accelerated. Modification of aqueous vehicles to include a glycol, or replacement with a nonaqueous vehicle, will usually reduce reaction rates and the stringency of ingredient specifications. Dry preparations pose relatively few reaction problems but may require rigid physical specifications for some ingredients to ensure the desired solution or dispersion characteristics when the vehicle is added.

Containers and closures are herein considered components of the product because they are in prolonged intimate contact with the product and may contribute substances or remove ingredients from the product.

Vehicles

The component present in the largest quantity in most liquid preparations is the vehicle. A vehicle normally has no therapeutic activity and is nontoxic. However, it is of great importance in the formulation since it presents to body tissues the form of the active constituent for absorption. Absorption normally occurs most rapidly and completely when a drug is presented to body tissues in the form of an aqueous solution. Modification of the vehicle with water-miscible liquids or substitution with water-immiscible liquids normally decreases the rate of absorption. Absorption from a suspension may be affected by such factors as the viscosity of the vehicle, its capacity for wetting the solid particles, the solubility equilibrium produced by the vehicle, and the distribution coefficient between the vehicle and aqueous body systems.

The vehicle of greatest importance for parenteral products is water. Water of suitable quality for parenteral administration must be prepared by distillation. Only by this means is it possible to adequately separate various liquid, gas and solid contaminating substances from the pure water.

Distillation of Water

In general, a still consists of a boiler (evaporator) containing the raw water (distilland), a source of heat to vaporize the water in the evaporator, a headspace above the level of distilland with condensing surfaces for refluxing the vapor and thereby returning non-volatile impurities to the distilland, a means for eliminating volatile impurities before the hot-water vapor is condensed, and a condenser for removing the heat of vaporization, thereby converting the water vapor to a liquid distillate.

It should be apparent that the specific construction features of a still and the process specifications will markedly affect the quality of distillate obtained from a still.[7] Those required for producing high-purity water, such as Water for Injection USP, must be considerably more stringent than those required for Purified Water USP. Among the factors that must be considered are:

1. The quality of the raw water will affect the quality of the distillate. If it is required that the raw water be first deionized or even distilled, a considerably higher quality final distillate will be obtained.
2. The size of the evaporator will affect the efficiency. The evaporator should be large enough to provide a low vapor velocity, thus reducing entrainment of distilland either as a film on vapor bubbles or as separate droplets.
3. The baffles (condensing surfaces) determine the effectiveness of refluxing. They should be designed to efficiently remove entrainment at optimal vapor velocity, collecting and returning the heavier droplets contaminated with distilland.
4. Redissolving of volatile impurities in the distillate reduces purity. Therefore, volatile impurities should be separated efficiently from the hot-water vapor and eliminated by aspirating to the drain or venting to the atmosphere.
5. Contamination of the vapor and distillate from the metal parts of the still can occur.[8] Present standards for high-purity stills are that all parts contacted by the vapor or distillate should be constructed of metal coated with pure tin, of 304 or 316 stainless steel, or chemically resistant glass.

Design features of a still also influence its efficiency of operation, relative freedom from maintenance problems, or the extent of automatic operation. Considerations relative to such features include the following:

1. The removal of solids from raw water by filtration, deionization, or distillation will reduce the frequency of cleaning required for the evaporator. Deionizing columns are prone to extensive contamination with microbial growth and pyrogens. Frequent sterilization of the columns may be necessary.
2. The drainage of the evaporator frequently during operation and at the end of a cycle of use will reduce the deposit of scale in the boiler. This may be done automatically or manually.
3. The utilization of process steam is usually the most economical source of heat for the evaporator, although electric or gas heaters may be more practical, particularly for small stills.
4. The utilization of a portion of the cooling water from the condenser as distilland after it has been heated by the heat of vaporization from the distillate conserves energy consumption. Its utilization to aspirate volatile constituents from the vapor train conserves the consumption of water.
5. The installation of a conductivity meter cell in the distillate line provides a continuous measure of the ionic quality of distillate being produced. Connection to an automatic discharge valve permits discharge of subquality water before it is collected in the storage tank.

It is apparent that stills can be constructed to produce varying qualities of distillate. They may also be constructed of varying size, rated according to the volume of distillate that can be produced per hour of operation under optimum conditions. Only stills designed to produce high-purity water may be considered for use in the production of Water for Injection USP.

One commercial conventional still* features metal construction coated with pure tin and a Spanish Prison Baffle system for the preparation of high-purity water. These stills are available from 1 to 30 gal/hr capacity with a variety of automatic features. Another commercial line of high-purity stills is constructed of chemically resistant glass.† Extremely low metallic recontamination occurs in such stills. They are available in capacities from 1.4 to 11.4 liters/hr.

Another commercial line of stills, known as Ultrapure,‡ has been redesigned recently to feature all 304 stainless steel construction with the production

---

* Supplier: *Barnstead.*
† Supplier: *Corning.*
‡ Supplier: *Am. Sterilizer.*

and delivery of the distillate under low pressure. This permits installation with the storage tank located above the still. These stills are available in capacities from 5 to 30 gal/hr with a variety of automatic features.

Compression Distillation—The vapor compression still, primarily designed for the production of large volumes of distillate, requires a brief discussion because of its distinctive features, as shown in Fig. 561. To start, the feed water is heated in the evaporator to boiling. The vapor produced in the tubes is separated from entrained distilland in the separator and is conveyed to a compressor which compresses the vapor and raises its temperature to approximately 224°F. It then flows to the steam chest where it condenses on the outer surfaces of the tubes containing distilland, thereby the vapor is condensed and drawn off as distillate while giving up its heat to bring the distilland in the tubes to the boiling point.

Once the process has started, little energy is required except for the operation of the compressor. Therefore, this method is a very efficient process, being conservative in both energy and water consumption, since almost all of the water consumed is converted to distillate. With properly constructed parts, high-purity water can be produced by such a still.[9]

Vapor compression stills are available in capacities from 50 to 2800 gal/hr.* In addition to their use by the pharmaceutical industry, they are utilized extensively by military and governmental installations for the production of potable water from sea and brackish well water.

Water for Injection USP

This is a high-purity water intended to be used as a vehicle for other preparations. Sterile Water for Injection USP is described in a separate monograph and differs in that it is intended as a packaged and sterilized product.

Storage—Water for Injection should be used immediately. This is usually not possible since the quantity required in production must be accumulated from the operation of a still for a period of time. When storage of water is necessary, the conditions for storage and subsequent delivery to the point of use must meet strict standards. Otherwise, recontamination may occur. To prevent such recontamination,

Water for Injection should be collected in a scrupulously clean, closed system; that is, the outlet from the condenser should be connected directly to a storage tank. All inlet and outlet connections should be sealed. Such a system is shown in Fig. 562. To allow for changes in pressure during filling and emptying of the tank, an outlet should be provided through a filter so constructed that microorganisms and chemical vapors will be prevented from entering the tank. The material of construction for the tank and connecting lines should be of chemically resistant glass, of metal parts with a heavy internal coating of pure tin, or of 304 or 316 stainless steel. Polyvinyl chloride plastic tubing and pipe lines are more likely to contribute contamination, although this plastic is sometimes used because of its lower cost. In addition, polyvinyl chloride softens at a temperature of about 70°C, rendering the piping useless at temperatures above this point.

Although water vapor should be expected to be sterile, contamination of distillate can occur even with a closed collection system. Therefore, during the period of storage, which should not exceed 24 hr, the water must be kept under conditions which will prevent the growth of microorganisms. This is normally done by maintaining the water at an elevated temperature or by the use of ultraviolet light. In the former instance, a steam coil is introduced into the storage tank and the water is held at a temperature of about 80°C. The water will, therefore, be hot when used. This may be an advantage in reducing solution time of certain solutes and heating time of the finished solution, if autoclaved. However, the formula must allow for the shrinkage which will occur on cooling. The use of ultraviolet light in water storage tanks is relatively new but has been reported as being very successful.[7] The water in this case is held at room temperature.

If relatively small quantities of Water for Injection are to be collected and stored, they may be collected in clean, sterile bottles made of chemically resistant

---

* Supplier: *Aqua-Chem.*

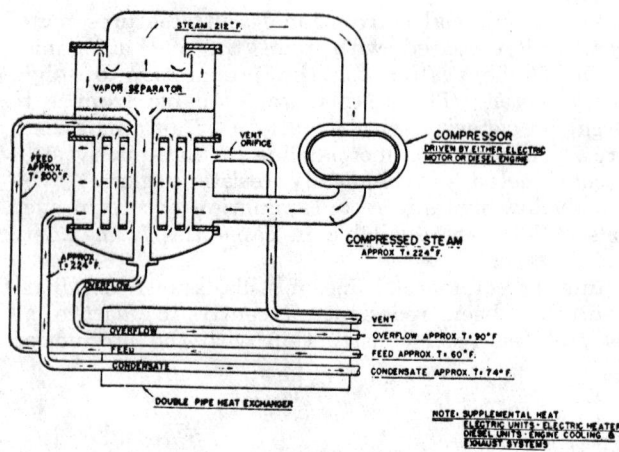

Fig. 561. Vapor compression still.

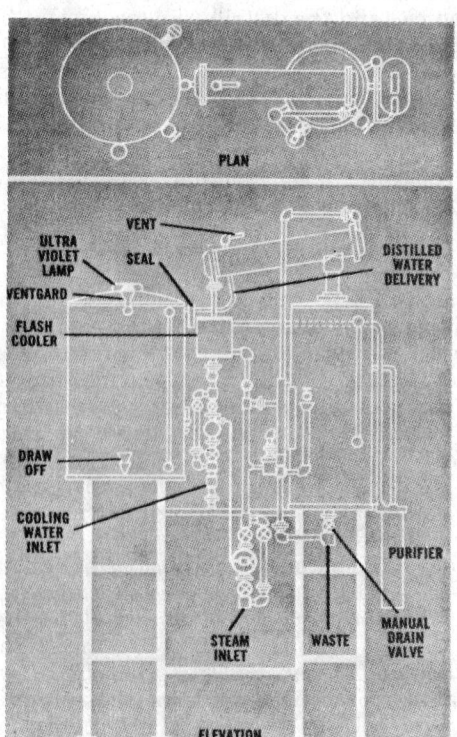

Fig. 562. Still and sealed-water storage system (courtesy, Barnstead).

glass. These containers then may be sealed and stored at a temperature of 80°C or under refrigeration to prevent the growth of microorganisms, or they may be sterilized by autoclaving and kept until needed.

Purity—The USP monographs provide standards of purity for Water for Injection and for Sterile Water for Injection. A few of these standards require comment.

Sterile Water for Injection must meet the requirements of the USP Sterility Test, but Water for Injection need not since it is to be used in a product which will be sterilized. Both must meet the requirements of the USP Pyrogen Test (page 644).

The limits for total solids varies in the two monographs. For the sterile form it may be as much as 20, 30, or 40 ppm, according to the ratio of surface area of the container to unit volume of water. The larger the surface area of the glass container per unit volume of water, the greater the amount of glass constituents that may be leached into the water, particularly during the elevated temperature of steam sterilization.

The Water for Injection monograph stipulates a maximum of 10 ppm of total solids. This is generally considered to be much too high to assure a quality of water that would permit stable formulation of many drugs. A relatively few metallic ions present can often render a formulation unstable. Therefore, it is common practice to set a limit of 0.1 ppm or less of ionic contaminants expressed as sodium chloride.

Ionic contaminant level is not the same as total solids, the former being a measurement of only the ionic content, while the latter is a measurement of undissociated constituents as well. The ionic content of water can be measured very easily by means of a conductivity meter, and is frequently used as an indication of the purity. The results are expressed in one of three terms; namely, as sodium chloride ions, as resistance in ohms or megohms, or as conductance in micromhos. Ohms and mhos have a reciprocal relationship to each other, but they are related to ppm sodium chloride by an experimentally determined curve. To give one point of comparison, 0.1 ppm sodium chloride is equal to approximately 1.01 megohms and 0.99 micromhos. It should be mentioned that, although frequently implied, conductivity measurements give no direct indication of pyrogen content of water since pyrogens are undissociated organic compounds.

Water for Injection may not contain an added substance. Sterile Water for Injection may contain a bacteriostatic agent when in containers of 30-ml capacity or smaller. This restriction is designed to prevent the administration of a large quantity of a bacteriostatic agent that probably would be toxic in the accumulated amount of a large volume of solution, even though the concentration was low.

Types of Vehicles

Aqueous Vehicles—Certain aqueous vehicles are recognized officially because of their valid use in parenteral formulations. Often they are used as isotonic vehicles to which a drug may be added at the time of administration. The additional osmotic effect of the drug may not be enough to produce any discomfort when administered. These vehicles include: Sodium Chloride Injection, Ringer's Injection, Dextrose Injection, Dextrose and Sodium Chloride Injection, and Lactated Ringer's Injection.

Water-Miscible Vehicles—A number of solvents which are miscible with water have been used as a portion of the vehicle in the formulation of parenterals. These solvents are used primarily to effect solubility of certain drugs and to reduce hydrolysis. The most important solvents in this group are ethyl alcohol, polyethylene glycol of the liquid series, and propylene glycol. Ethyl alcohol is used particularly in the preparation of solutions of cardiac glycosides and the glycols in solutions of barbiturates, certain alkaloids, and certain antibiotics. Although occasionally used for intravenous administration, such preparations are usually given intramuscularly.

These solvents, as well as nonaqueous vehicles, have been reviewed by Spiegel and Noseworthy.[10]

Nonaqueous Vehicles—The most important group of nonaqueous vehicles are the fixed oils. The USP provides specifications for such a vehicle. A few of these requirements need to be discussed. The fixed oils must be of vegetable origin in order that they may be metabolized, will be liquid at room temperature, and will not become rancid rapidly. The first specification eliminates oils of mineral origin and the latter two, those of animal origin. To be liquid at room temperature, a fixed oil must contain esters of unsaturated fatty acids. However, excessive unsaturation will produce tissue irritation. Therefore, the USP stipulates upper and lower limits to the iodine value for the oil. The development of rancidity must be prevented by the inclusion of antioxidants such as tocopherol, natural constituent of many fixed oils. The USP also prescribes an upper limit for free fatty acids in order to minimize the degree of tissue irritation. Other specifications are included primarily to detect adulteration. The oils most commonly used are corn oil, cottonseed oil, peanut oil, and sesame oil. It should be noted that the official monographs for some of these oils provide for greater latitude than the specifications required for the use of the oil as a vehicle for a parenteral. Therefore, parenteral vehicle oils must be select oils or specially purified to meet the more stringent requirements. Fixed oils are used particularly as vehicles for certain hormone preparations. These and other nonaqueous vehicles, such as ethyl oleate, isopropyl myristate and benzyl benzoate, may be used provided they are safe in the volume administered and do not interfere with the therapeutic efficacy of the preparation or with its response to prescribed assays and tests. The label also must state the name of the vehicle so that the user may beware in case of known sensitivity or other reactions to it.

Solutes

The requirements for purity of the medicinal compound used in an injection often make it necessary to undertake special purification of the normal chemical grade available. In a few instances, a special parenteral grade of a compound is available, for example, ascorbic acid freed from all traces of copper contamination. For most compounds no such grade is commercially available. As a general rule, the best chemical grade obtainable should be used, but further purification may be necessary. It should be obvious that, if a few ppm of ionic contaminants in Water for Injection may cause stability problems, a similar level of contamination in the solute itself may, likewise, cause stability problems. Metallic catalysis of chemical reactions is one of the most important problems.

Other factors to be considered with respect to the quality of solutes include: freedom from microbial contamination, freedom from pyrogenic contamination, solubility characteristics as determined by the chemical or physical form of the compound, and freedom from gross dirt.

Added Substances—The USP includes in this category all substances added to a preparation to improve or safeguard the quality of the product. An added substance may effect solubility, as does sodium benzoate in Caffeine and Sodium Benzoate Injection, or provide patient comfort, as do substances added to make a solution isotonic. They may enhance the chemical stability of a solution, as do antioxidants, inert gases, chelating agents, and buffers, or they may preserve a preparation against the growth of microorganisms. The term "preservative" is sometimes applied only to those substances which prevent the growth of microorganisms in a preparation. This term should not be so limited but should include all substances that act to retard or prevent the chemical, physical, or biological degradation of a preparation.

While added substances may prevent a certain reaction from taking place, they may induce others. Not only may visible incompatibilities occur, but hydrolysis, complexation, oxidation, and other invisible reactions may decompose or otherwise inactivate the therapeutic agent. Therefore, added substances must be selected with due consideration and investigation of the effect of the substance on the total formulation.

Antimicrobial Agents—The USP states that antimicrobial agents in bacteriostatic or fungistatic concentrations must be added to preparations contained in multiple-dose containers. They must be present in adequate concentration at the time of use[11] to prevent the multiplication of microorganisms inadvertently introduced into the preparation while withdrawing a portion of the contents with a hypodermic needle and syringe. Among the compounds most frequently employed, with the concentration limit prescribed by the USP, are: phenylmercuric nitrate and thimerosal 0.01%, benzethonium chloride and benzalkonium chloride 0.01%, phenol or cresol 0.5%, and chlorobutanol 0.5%. The above limit is rarely used for phenylmercuric nitrate, being most frequently employed in a concentration of 0.002%. Methyl p-hydroxybenzoate 0.18% and propyl p-hydroxybenzoate 0.02% in combination, and benzyl alcohol 2% are also frequently used. In oleaginous preparations, no antibacterial agent commonly employed appears to be effective. However, it has been reported that hexylresorcinol 0.5%[12] and phenylmercuric benzoate 0.1%[13] are moderately bactericidal.

Antimicrobial agents must be studied with respect to compatibility with all other components of the formula. In addition, their activity must be evaluated in the total formula. It is not uncommon to find that a particular agent will be effective in one formulation but ineffective in another. This may be due to the effect of various components of the formula on the biological activity or availability of the compound; for example, the binding and inactivation of esters of p-hydroxybenzoic acid by macromolecules such as Polysorbate 80[14] or the reduction of phenylmercuric nitrate by sulfide residues in rubber closures. A physical reaction encountered is that bacteriostatic agents are sometimes removed from solution by rubber closures.[15] These facts establish the principle that antimicrobial agents must be evaluated for their activity in the total formula to assure their activity when needed, normally at the time of use.

Buffers—Buffers are used primarily to stabilize a solution against the chemical degradation that would occur if the pH changed appreciably. Buffer systems employed should normally have as low a buffer capacity as feasible in order not to disturb significantly the body buffer systems when injected. In addition, the buffer range and the effect of the buffer on the activity of the product must be evaluated carefully.[16] The acid salts most frequently employed as buffers are citrates, acetates, and phosphates.

Antioxidants—Antioxidants are frequently required to preserve products because of the ease with which many drugs are oxidized. Sodium bisulfite 0.1% is most frequently used. The use of sulfites as antioxidants has been reviewed by Schroeter.[17] Acetone sodium bisulfite, sodium formaldehyde sulfoxylate, and thiourea are also sometimes used. The sodium salt of ethylenediaminetetraacetic acid has been found to enhance the activity of antioxidants in some cases, apparently by chelating metallic ions that would otherwise catalyze the oxidation reaction.

Pyrogens

Pyrogens are not predetermined components of parenteral preparations, but they may be present as unwanted contaminants. If they are present, the product may have to be discarded since it is very difficult to remove them without adversely affecting the product. The only safe and proper way to manage pyrogen contamination is to keep it out of the product. Presence of pyrogens, therefore, is indicative of an improperly prepared product.

Pyrogens cause a febrile reaction in human beings. Other symptoms include chills, pains in back and legs, and malaise. While pyrogens are rarely fatal, they produce significant discomfort for the patient. On the other hand, pyrogens have been shown to induce a general nonspecific resistance to microorganisms[18] and, on this basis, have been used therapeutically.

Pyrogens are products of the growth of microorganisms. The most potent pyrogenic substances are produced by Gram-negative bacteria, but Gram-positive bacteria and fungi also produce pyrogenic substances. The potency varies with the species producing it. Chemically, pyrogenic material has been shown to be lipid in nature, sometimes containing phosphorus, and is attached to a polysaccharide or a protein or both. When so complexed, it is a weak antigen.[18] A tolerance to pyrogens will develop in man and susceptible animals.

Pyrogens can be destroyed by heating at high temperatures. The recommended procedure for depyrogenation of glassware and equipment is heating at a temperature of 250°C for 45 min. It has been reported that 650°C for 1 min or 180°C for 4 hr will likewise destroy pyrogens. The usual autoclaving cycle will not do so. Although heating with strong alkali solutions will destroy pyrogens, the usual washing cycles, including detergent treatment, cannot be relied on to completely eliminate pyrogens from glassware. Heating with oxidizing agents, such as hydrogen peroxide, will destroy pyrogens. It has been reported that anion exchange resins will adsorb pyrogens from water.[19] However, the most reliable method for the elimination of these substances from water is distillation. Pyrogenic substances are not volatile and thus will remain in the distilland. The only method available for consideration for the removal of pyrogenic substances from solutions is filtration through asbestos filters. This method is quite limited, however, since asbestos fibers remove the pyrogen by adsorption and the same physical phenomenon may act to remove chemical constituents as well. In addition, since the mechanism of action is adsorption, once the fibers of asbestos are saturated, the remaining pyrogenic material will pass through the filter. In-process destruction of pyrogens in pharmaceutical preparations may be accomplished sometimes by careful heating with dilute alkali, dilute acid, or mild oxidizing agents.

Sources of Pyrogens—Pyrogens may enter a preparation by any means that will introduce living or dead microorganisms or the products of their growth. Perhaps the greatest potential source of such contamination is the water used in products. However, proper distillation will provide pyrogen-free water. Another potential source of contamination is equipment. Pyrogenic materials adhere strongly to glass surfaces in particular, but also to the surface of other equipment. Reusing containers, as is often practiced in hospitals, is a dangerous and a significant source of pyrogenic contamination. Residues of solutions in used bottles often become bacterial cultures from septic patients or the environment. Such bottles will be heavily contaminated with pyrogens. Even washed bottles left wet and exposed to the atmosphere may contain sufficient nutrients for microorganisms to grow. Since drying does not destroy pyrogens, they may remain in equipment for long periods of time. Adequate washing accompanied by dry heat depyrogenation will render contaminated equipment suitable for use.

The solute also may be a source of pyrogens. Solutes may be crystallized or precipitated from aqueous liquids containing pyrogenic contamination. In the process pyrogens may be trapped within the particle layers. In such cases the solute must be purified by recrystallization, precipitate washing, or other means to eliminate the pyrogens.

The manufacturing process also must be carried out with great care and as rapidly as possible to minimize the risk of microbial contamination. Preferably, no more product should be prepared than can be completely processed within one working day, including sterilization. By far the best procedure is to prevent the introduction of pyrogens rather than to attempt to remove them, a task which well may be virtually impossible.

Containers

Containers are an integral part of the formulation of an injection and may be considered a component, for there is no container that is totally insoluble or does not in some way affect the liquid it contains, particularly if the liquid is aqueous. Therefore, the selection of a container for a particular injection must be based on a consideration of the composition of the container, as well as of the solution, and the treatment to which it will be subjected.

Plastic

Thermoplastic polymers are being considered and a few are being used as the container material for selected sterile products, particularly ophthalmic solutions. However, it is generally conceded that thermoplastic compounds have not been studied sufficiently to prove their nonreactivity, or to establish a definite reactivity pattern to define their safety for the packaging of injections.

Autian has thoroughly reviewed the use of plastic materials in pharmaceutical practice.[20] He and others have shown that extractives are obtained from thermoplastic materials and, with certain polymers, sorption (absorption and/or adsorption) of drug molecules or ions may occur.[21] The latter is observed in particular with polyamides such as nylon.

The lack of sufficiently high standards in the manufacture of plastics and the fact that the lower-cost polymers cannot be sterilized by thermal methods are also deterrents to their use. These and other problems are receiving concentrated attention. It seems reasonable to expect that eventually thermoplastic materials will be used for containers of selected injectable preparations. At present, however, the use of these materials is limited largely to components of disposable injection units where contact with the solution is brief.

For ophthalmic preparations the flexibility of the low-density polyethylene polymer provides a significant use characteristic, making it possible to squeeze out and administer one or more drops of the preparation. Therefore, several ophthalmic formulations have been adapted to plastic containers.[22]

When thermoplastic containers are used for sterile solutions, the empty container must be sterilized by means of ethylene oxide or ionized radiations and filled aseptically with a sterile solution. Considerable attention is being given to the small amount of ethylene oxide residue in plastics after sterilization and its potential toxic effects.[23] See Chapter 91 on *Plastics*.

Glass

Glass is employed as the container material of choice for most injections. It is composed principally of silicon dioxide with varying amounts of other oxides such as those of sodium, potassium, calcium, magnesium, aluminum, boron, and iron. The basic structural network of glass is formed by the silicon oxide tetrahedron.[24] Boric oxide will enter into this structure, but most of the other oxides do not. The latter are only loosely bound, are present in the network interstices, and are relatively free to migrate. These migratory oxides may be leached into a solution in contact with the glass, particularly during the increased reactivity of thermal sterilization. The oxides thus dissolved may hydrolyze to raise the pH of the solution, catalyze reactions, or enter into reactions. In a manner as yet uncertain, some glass compounds will be attacked by solutions and, in time, dislodge glass flakes into the solution. Disturbing reactions such as these can, however, be minimized by the proper selection of the glass composition.

Types—The USP has aided in this selection by providing a classification of glass; namely, Type I, a borosilicate glass; Type II, a soda-lime treated glass; Type III, a soda-lime glass; and NP, a soda-lime glass not suitable for containers for parenterals. Type I glass is composed principally of silicon dioxide and boric oxide, with low levels of the nonnetwork-forming oxides. It is a chemically resistant glass (low leachability) also having a low thermal coefficient of expansion. Type II and Type III glass compounds are composed of relatively high proportions of sodium oxide and calcium oxide. This makes the glass chemically less resistant. Both of these types melt at a lower temperature, are easier to mold into various shapes, and have a higher thermal coefficient of expansion than Type I. While there is no one standard formulation for glass among manufacturers of these USP type categories, Type II glass usually has a lower concentration of the migratory

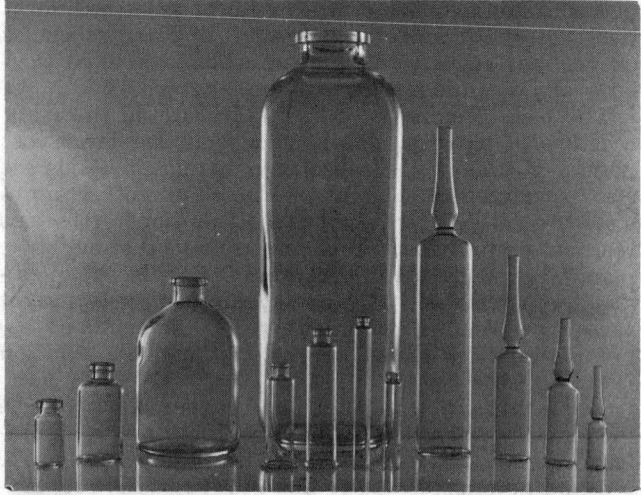

Fig. 563. Various types of ampuls and multiple-dose vials for parenterals (courtesy, Kimble).

oxides than Type III. In addition, Type II glass has been treated under controlled temperature and humidity conditions with sulfur dioxide to dealkalize the internal surface of the container. While it remains intact, this surface will substantially increase the chemical resistance of the glass. However, repeated exposures to sterilization procedures and to alkaline detergents will break down this dealkalized surface and expose the soda-lime compound. Therefore, Type II glass containers may be considered to be of relatively good chemical resistance for only one use.

The glass types are determined from the results of two tests provided by the USP, the Powdered Glass Test and the Water Attack Test. The latter is used only for Type II glass and is performed on the whole container, because of the dealkalized surface. The former test is performed on powdered glass, which exposes internal surfaces of the glass compound. The results are based upon the amount of alkali titrated by 0.02 N sulfuric acid after an autoclaving cycle with the glass sample in contact with a special distilled water.[25]

Care must be used in selecting the glass type to be used for a particular injectable product.[26] In general, Type I glass will be suitable for all products, although sulfur dioxide treatment is sometimes used for a further increase in resistance. Because cost must be consid-

ered, one of the other less expensive types may be acceptable. Type II glass may be suitable, for example, for a solution which is buffered, has a pH below 7, or is not reactive with the glass. Type III glass will usually be suitable principally for anhydrous liquids or dry substances.

Physical Characteristics—Examples of the physical shape of glass ampuls and vials are illustrated in Fig. 563. Commercially available containers vary in size from 0.5 to 1000 ml. Sizes up to 100 ml may be obtained as ampuls and vials, and larger sizes as bottles. The latter are used mostly for intravenous and irrigating solutions. Smaller sizes are also available as cartridges. Ampuls and cartridges are made by being drawn from glass tubing. The smaller size vials, drawn from tubing, have recently become obtainable. The making of tubing is illustrated in Fig. 564. Other vials and bottles are made by molding. Containers made by drawing from tubing are generally optically clearer and have a thinner wall than molded containers (see Fig. 563). Molded containers are more uniform in external dimensions and are stronger. Therefore, larger containers are made by molding.

Easy-opening ampuls that permit the user to break off the tip of the ampul at the neck constriction without the use of a file are marketed under the names Color-Break* and Score-Break.† An example of a modification of container design to meet a particular need is the double chambered vial, under the name Univial,‡ designed to contain a freeze-dried product in one chamber and solvent in the other. Other examples are wide-mouth ampuls with flat or rounded bottoms to facilitate filling with dry materials or suspensions, and various modifications of the cartridge for use with disposable dosage units.

Glass containers must be strong enough to withstand the physical shocks of handling and shipping and the pressure differentials that develop, particularly during the autoclave sterilization cycle. They must be able to withstand the thermal shock resulting from striking temperature changes during processing, for example, when the hot bottle and contents are removed from the autoclave at the end of the sterilization cycle. Therefore, a glass having a low coefficient of thermal expansion is necessary. The glass container also must be transparent to permit inspection of the contents. Preparations which are light sensitive must be protected by placing them in amber glass containers or by enclosing flint glass containers in opaque cartons labeled to remain on the container during the period of use. Silicone coatings are sometimes applied to containers to produce a hydrophobic surface, where the adherence of a heavy, costly suspension would cause an appreciable loss.

The size of single-dose containers is limited to 1000 ml by the USP and multiple-dose containers to 30 ml, unless stated otherwise in a particular monograph. Multiple-dose vials are limited in size to reduce the number of punctures for withdrawing doses and the accompanying risk of contamination of the contents. As the name implies, single-dose containers are opened with aseptic care and the contents used at one time. The integrity of the container is destroyed when opened so that the container cannot be closed again. A multiple-dose container is designed so that more than one dose can be withdrawn at different times, the container

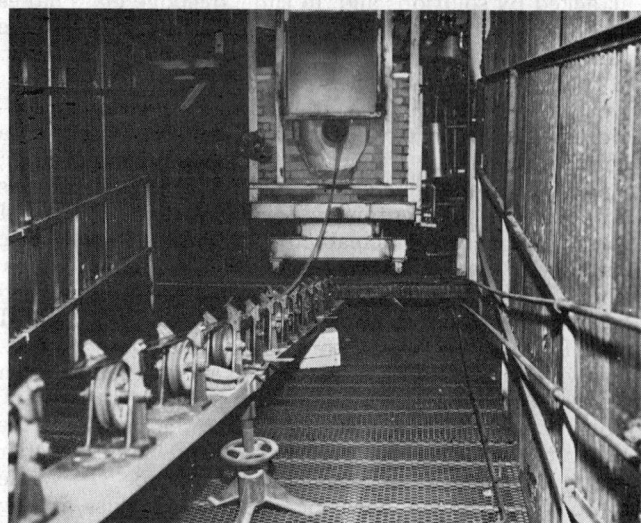

Fig. 564. Tubing being formed from molten glass in brick tank (courtesy, Wheaton).

* Supplier: *Kimble.*
† Supplier: *Wheaton.*
‡ Supplier: *Univial.*

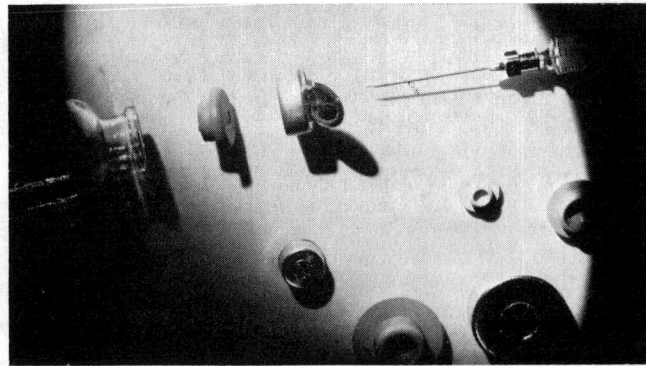

Fig. 565. Extended view of sealing components for a multiple-dose vial (courtesy, West).

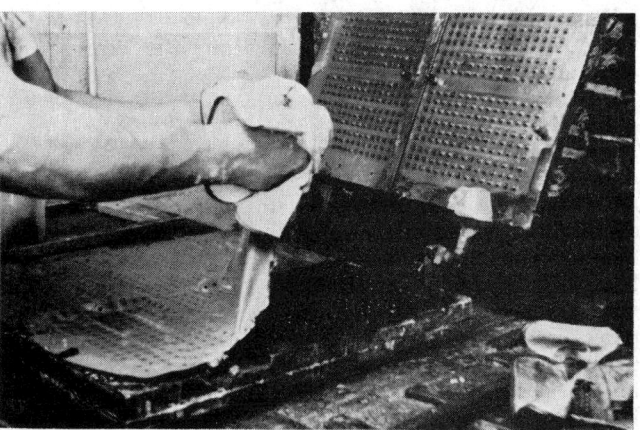

Fig. 566. Removing a sheet of rubber closures from a mold (courtesy, Carron).

maintaining a seal between uses. It should be evident that with full aseptic precautions, including sterile syringe and needle for withdrawing the dose and disinfection of the exposed surface of the closure, there is still a substantial risk of introducing contaminating microorganisms and viruses into the contents of the vial. Because of this risk, the USP requires that all multiple-dose vials must contain an antibacterial agent. However, there is no effective antiviral agent available for such use. Therefore, in spite of the advantage of flexibility of dosage provided the physician by a multiple-dose vial, the greater safety of single-dose, disposable administration units has caused their use to increase rapidly during recent years.

Rubber Closures

In order to permit the introduction of a needle from a hypodermic syringe into a multiple-dose vial and provide for resealing of the vial as soon as the needle is withdrawn, each vial is sealed with a rubber closure held in place by an aluminum band. Fig. 565 illustrates how this is done. This principle is also followed for single-dose containers of the cartridge type, except that there is only a single introduction of the needle to make possible the withdrawal or expulsion of the contents.

Rubber closures are composed of several ingredients,[27] the primary ones being natural rubber (latex), a synthetic polymer, or a combination of natural rubber and a synthetic polymer. Other ingredients include a vulcanizing agent, usually sulfur; an accelerator, one of several active organic compounds such as 2-mercaptobenzothiazole; an activator, usually zinc oxide; fillers, such as carbon black or limestone; and various other ingredients such as antioxidants and lubricants. These ingredients are compounded together and then vulcanized in the desired shape, making use of molds under high pressure and temperature. Fig. 566 shows the molding of rubber closures.

Rubber closures must have sufficient elasticity to provide a snug fit between the closure and the lip and neck of the vial and must spring back to close the hole made by the needle immediately on withdrawal. They must not be so hard that they are highly resistant to the insertion of the needle, and they must not frag-

ment as the hollow needle passes through them. Ideally, they should be completely nonreactive with the solution and its ingredients and should provide a complete barrier to vapor transfer. These qualities are not perfectly met by any rubber compound now available. It is, therefore, essential to determine the compatibility of the rubber compound with each preparation with which it is to be used.[28,29] In addition to the physical tests of elasticity, hardness, fragmentation, and vapor transfer, the closures should be exposed to the product for prescribed periods of time at designated temperature and humidity conditions. The effect on the product of extractives from the rubber compound or loss of ingredients from the product to the closure should be determined analytically.[30]

The physical shape of a closure may be seen in Fig. 566. Most closures have a lip and a protruding flange that extends into the neck of the vial or bottle. Many disk closures are now being used, particularly in the high-speed packaging of antibiotics. Slotted closures are used on freeze-dried products to make it possible to insert the closure part way into the neck of the vial during the drying phase of the cycle. Partial insertion provides protection from contamination while providing a passageway for the escape of water vapor from the drying product. The plunger type is used to seal one end of a cartridge. At the time of use, the plunger expels the product by a needle inserted through the closure at the other end of the cartridge.

Special design closures are available for use with large volume intravenous and irrigating solutions under hospital conditions. The closure is designed with a flange and has a permanent hole for adapters of administration sets or an opening for pouring. The lip of the closure extends over the lip of the bottle and down over the outside to grip the flask neck firmly. A flexible lip extends upward and makes contact with a cover cap. The flexible lip permits venting during the autoclaving cycle, but during the cooling phase, as a vacuum is produced within the bottle, the flexible lip makes a seal against the cap. The cap is pulled down tight by the vacuum to seal the bottle. These closures and caps are intended to be reused.

Production Facilities

A product having components of the best quality quickly may become totally unacceptable if the environment in which it is processed is contaminated or if the

manufacturing procedure is not carried out properly. Therefore, the production facilities and the procedure used in processing the product must meet standards adequate for the task to be accomplished. The nearer these standards approach perfection, the better and safer should be the product.

Arrangement of Area

The production area normally should be divided into five sectional areas: the clean-up area, the preparation area, the aseptic area, the quarantine area, and the finishing or packaging area. All of these areas should be designed and constructed for effective ease of cleaning, efficient operation, attractiveness, and comfort of personnel. The extra requirements for the aseptic area are designed to provide an environment where an injection may be exposed to the environment for brief periods during subdivision from a bulk container to the individual dose containers without becoming contaminated. Contamination of concern includes dust, lint, and microorganisms. Such contaminants are normally found floating in the air, lying on counters and other surfaces, on clothing and body surfaces of personnel, in the exhaled breath of personnel, and deposited on the floor. The design and control of an aseptic area is directed toward so reducing the presence of these contaminants that they are no longer a hazard to aseptic filling. Although the aseptic area must be adjacent to the other areas so that an efficient flow of components may be achieved, it must be arranged so that it is separated from the other areas in order that an aseptic condition may be maintained. This normally involves sealed partitions, often glass-paneled for greater visibility and light. Entrances into the aseptic area should only be through security doors that require passage through an airlock so designed that both doors cannot be opened at the same time. Figs. 567 and 569 show an arrangement of an aseptic area modified to provide a service area for the areas of maximum security, the aseptic filling areas.

Flow Plan—In general, the components for a parenteral product will flow from the stockroom, either: (1) to the preparation room, as for ingredients of the formula, or (2) to the clean-up area, as for containers

and equipment. See Fig. 569 for a process flow diagram. After proper processing in these areas, the components will flow into the security of the aseptic area for filling of the product in appropriate containers. From there the product will pass into the quarantine area where it will be held until all necessary tests have been performed. If the product is to be sterilized in its final container, the passage normally will be interrupted after the product leaves the aseptic area for subjection to the sterilization process. After the results from all tests are known and the product has been found effective and safe, it will pass to the finishing area for final labeling and packaging. There are sometimes variations from this flow plan to meet the specific needs of an individual product or to conform to available facilities.

Clean-Up Area—The clean-up area will be constructed to withstand moisture, steam, and detergents. The ceiling, walls, and floor should be constructed of impervious materials so that moisture will run off and not be held. These areas should be adequately exhausted so that the heat and humidity will be removed for the comfort of personnel. Precautions must be taken to prevent the accumulation of dirt and the growth of microorganisms, especially in the presence of high heat and humidity. While this area does not need to be aseptic, it must be cleanable and kept clean. Since it is not aseptic, precautions must be taken to prevent carrying contaminants into the aseptic area.

Preparation Area—In the preparation area the formula is compounded and preparation is made for the filling operation, such as assembling equipment. Adequate sink and counter space must be provided. Although it is not essential that this area be aseptic, control over it should be more stringent than in the clean-up area. Cabinets and counters should, preferably, be constructed of stainless steel. They should fit snugly to walls and other furniture so that there are no catch areas for dirt to accumulate. Ceiling, walls, and floor should be sealed. One of the "spray-on-tile" finishes with a vinyl or epoxy sealing coat provides a continuous surface free from all holes or crevices. All

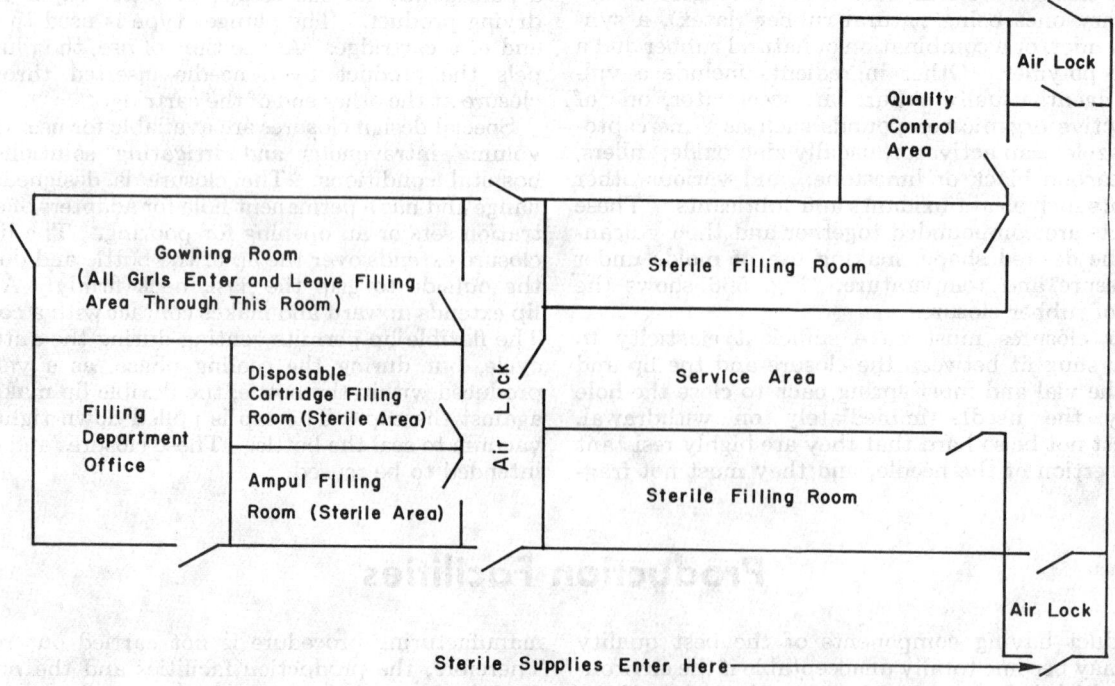

Fig. 567. Floor plan of an aseptic filling area with its service area (courtesy, Wyeth).

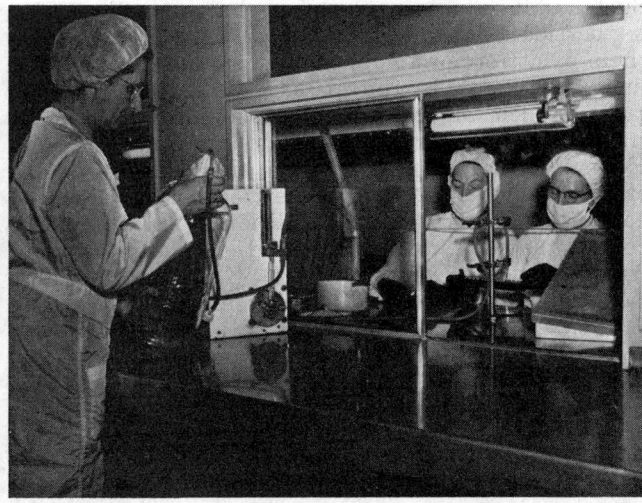

Fig. 568. View from service area with pipetting machine and stock bottle retained outside of aseptic filling area (courtesy, Wyeth).

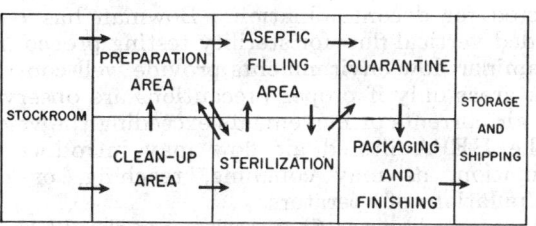

Fig. 569. Process flow diagram.

such surfaces can be washed at regular intervals to keep them thoroughly clean. Fig. 570 illustrates such an area.

Aseptic Area

The aseptic area requires construction features which have been designed for maximum security. The ceiling, walls, and floor must be sealed so that they not only may be washed but also treated with an antiseptic wipe or spray before each use. Some prefer the use of germicidal paint, such as Fungi-Chek,* which provides germicidal action as long as it is on the wall. All counters should be constructed of stainless steel and hung from the wall so that there are no legs to accumulate dirt where they rest on the floor. All light fixtures, utility service lines, and ventilation fixtures should be recessed in the walls or ceiling to eliminate ledges, joints, and other locations for the accumulation of dust and dirt. As much as possible, tanks containing the compounded product and mechanical equipment should remain outside the aseptic area and the product should be fed into the area through hose lines. Fig. 568 shows such an arrangement. Mechanical equipment that must be located in the aseptic area should be housed as completely as possible within a stainless steel cabinet in order to seal the operating parts and their dirt-producing and accumulating tendencies from the aseptic environment. Mechanical parts that will contact the parenteral product should be demountable so that they can be sterilized. In some cases, where the amount of product to be handled is small, a hood is used with armholes through which an operator works. The hands of the operator are inserted through armlets fitted at the wrist or into sterile rubber gloves. The inside of the hood is cleansed thoroughly and treated with an antiseptic. A hood may be either an adjunct to an aseptic area to further increase the degree of security, or it may serve as the aseptic area. In the latter case, the hood is located in a larger room, perhaps the preparation room.

Personnel entering the aseptic area should enter only through an airlock. Although convictions differ somewhat, it is generally agreed that they should be attired in sterile gowns with sterile hats, masks, and foot covers. Movement within the room should be minimal

* Supplier: *Chas. Bowman.*

during a filling procedure, and in and out movement should be prohibited. The requirements for preparation of the room and for the personnel may be relaxed somewhat if the product is to be sterilized in a sealed container. Some are convinced, however, that it is better to have one standard procedure meeting the most rigid requirements.

Laminar Flow Environments—A marked improvement in the environmental control of aseptic areas has been made possible by the development of laminar flow enclosures. Laminar air flow provides a total sweep of a confined area because the entire body of air moves with uniform velocity along parallel lines, with a minimum of eddies, originating through a HEPA (high efficiency particulate air) filter occupying one entire side of the confined area. Therefore, it bathes the entire area with very clean air (particles of 0.3μ removed with 99.97% or better efficiency) sweeping away contaminates.

The arrangement for the direction of air flow can be horizontal (see Fig. 571) or vertical, and may involve a confined area such as a work bench or an entire room. The minimum effective air velocity is considered to be 100 ± 10 ft/min.[31]

It must be borne in mind that any contamination introduced upstream from such as equipment, arms of the operator, or leaks in the filter will be blown downstream. In the instance of horizontal flow this may be to the critical working area, the face of the operator, or across the room.

Should the contaminate be, for example, penicillin powder or viable microorganisms, the danger is apparent. For operations involving such contaminants a vertical system is much more desirable with the air flowing out through perforations in the counter top or along the edge of the counter where it can be

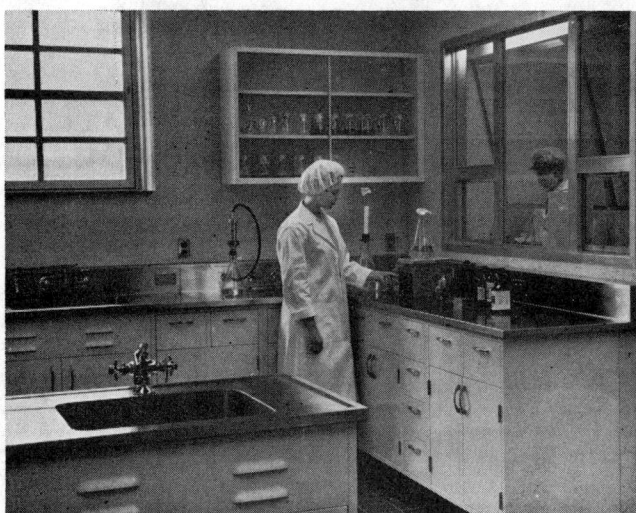

Fig. 570. A preparation area adjacent to an aseptic filling area (courtesy, The University of Tennessee College of Pharmacy).

directed for decontamination. Bowman has recommended vertical flow for sterility testing procedures.[32]

Laminar flow environments provide well-controlled work areas only if proper precautions are observed.[33] Any air currents or movements exceeding the velocity of the HEPA-filtered air flow may introduce contamination, as may coughing, reaching, or other manipulations of operators.

Therefore, laminar flow work areas should be protected by being located within controlled environments. Personnel should preferably be attired for aseptic processing as described below. All movements and processes should be carefully planned to avoid the introduction of contamination upstream of the critical work area. Checks of the air stream should be performed initially and at regular intervals to be sure no leaks have developed through or around the HEPA filters.

In addition to the horizontal or vertical work benches, modules suspended above filling lines and other processes to provide a vertical bathing of the process line with HEPA-filtered air are finding application in pharmaceutical manufacturing (see Fig. 572). Such installations provide added protection within a controlled environment.

Work benches and other types of laminar flow enclosures are available from several commercial sources.*

Air Cleaning

The air in these areas can be one of the greatest sources of contamination. It need not be, however, because several methods are currently available for providing clean air essentially free from dirt particles and microorganisms.

To provide such air, it must be thoroughly cleaned of all contaminants. Ideally, this may be done by a series of treatments. The air from the outside is first passed through a prefilter, usually of glass wool, to remove large particles. It then passes through a filter capable of removing particles of 0.3μ with an efficiency of 99.97% or better, a HEPA filter.† Then it is treated by passage through an electrostatic precipitator.‡

---

* Suppliers: *Air Control; Baker; Contamination Control; Controlled Environment; Edcraft; DCA; Envirco; Laminaire; Matthews Res.*
    † Suppliers: *Am. Air; Cambridge.*
    ‡ Suppliers: *Am. Air; Electro-Air; Sturtevant.*

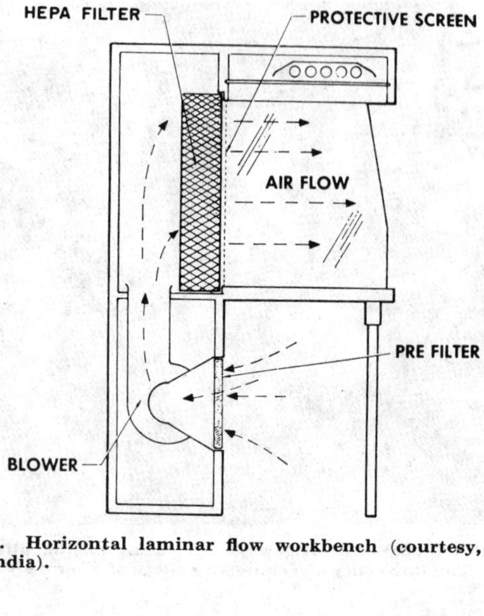

Such a unit induces an electrical charge on all remaining particles in the air, irrespective of size, and removes them by attraction to oppositely charged plates. The final treatment is the passage around ultraviolet lamps; their antibacterial action aids in rendering the air free from any viable microorganisms that may have eluded the filters. Less than ideal systems eliminate one or more of these treatments. For the comfort of personnel, air conditioning and humidity control should be incorporated into the system. Another available system, the Kathabar system,§ cleans the air of dirt and microorganisms by washing it in an antiseptic solution and, at the same time, controls the humidity. The clean, aseptic air is introduced into the aseptic area under positive pressure. Positive pressure prevents outside air from rushing into the aseptic area through cracks, temporarily open doors, or other openings.

Ultraviolet Radiation

Ultraviolet lamps should be installed in at least the clean-up area, the preparation area, and the aseptic area to aid in the control of microorganisms in the air. Even if it were possible to sterilize the air entering this entire area, it would soon be contaminated from organisms carried in on the shoes of personnel, wheels of trucks, etc, and from the skin, hair, and breath of personnel. Therefore, continual antibacterial action is needed. This may be obtained through the action of ultraviolet light rays.

Ultraviolet rays are irritating to the skin and particularly the eyes of human beings. Therefore, personnel in the area must be protected from direct exposure to ultraviolet light. This is usually accomplished by installing fixtures on the wall about 7 ft from the floor with a deflector that directs the rays above the heads of personnel. Convection currents carry the

---

§ Supplier: *Surface Combustion.*

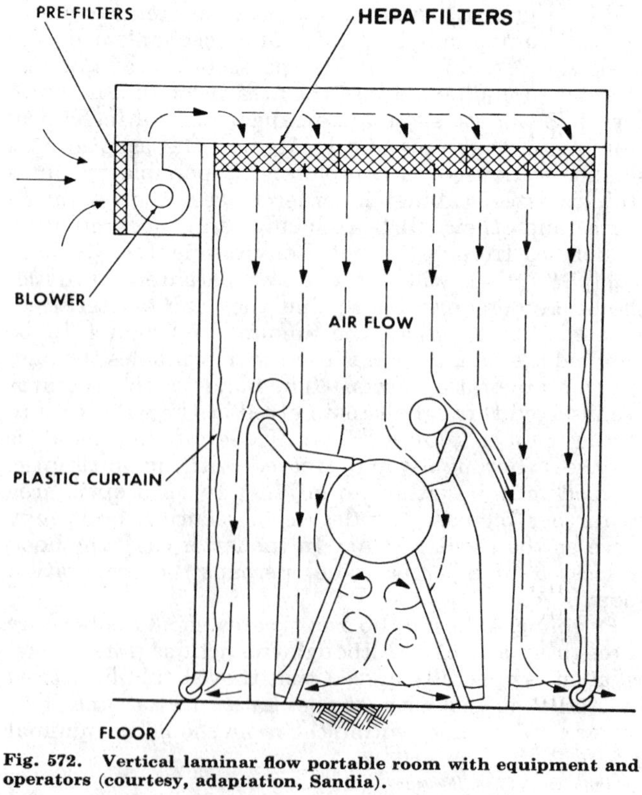

Fig. 571. Horizontal laminar flow workbench (courtesy, adaptation, Sandia).

Fig. 572. Vertical laminar flow portable room with equipment and operators (courtesy, adaptation, Sandia).

air in the room past the light source, whereby micro-organisms are irradiated. The viable bacterial content of the air is thereby reduced, although it cannot be assumed to have been sterilized. Care must be taken that surfaces of the ceiling, walls, or objects do not reflect sufficient ultraviolet light to cause irritation of personnel. The degree of reflection of ultraviolet wavelengths by various objects is different from that of visible light. Further protection of personnel may be had, if necessary, by providing clothing to cover the skin and ultraviolet absorbing goggles to protect the eyes.

Direct irradiation of a room when personnel are not present is a valuable means of reducing bacterial counts on working surfaces and floors. Local irradiation is also highly desirable within hood-type fixtures over filling, filtering, and bottling operations, or anyplace where additional protection from contamination is needed, provided the product is not adversely affected by ultraviolet rays. Ultraviolet light rays travel in straight lines only; therefore, objects in the path of the light beam cast shadows with resultant lack of irradiation in the shadow area. Also, these rays do not penetrate most materials. Therefore, its antibacterial effect is only exerted on the surface of materials, with the principle exceptions of air and very pure water. With these limitations must be included the fact that although bacteria may be killed by irradiation with ultraviolet light for a sufficient time at an effective intensity, it has been found that certain bacteria have grown after exposure to supposedly lethal irradiation. This attenuating rather than killing effect was found by subjecting the organisms to certain conditions after irradiation,[34] such as special nutrients, change in pH, darkness, and daylight.

The best practical source of ultraviolet light rays is the cold-cathode mercury vapor lamp. This lamp emits a high proportion of ultraviolet rays at the 253.7 mμ wavelength. A special glass is used for the tube so that the rays will pass to the outside. This glass will gradually change in crystal structure with use so that passage of the rays is gradually reduced. Such lamps, therefore, rarely burn out as do visible light lamps but gradually reach an emission level which is ineffective. These lamps also must be kept clean, for dust and grease will drastically lower the effective emission. It is generally stated that an irradiation intensity of 20 μw/cm^2 is required for effective antibacterial activity.

Maintenance of the Aseptic Area

One of the most important aspects in the control of environmental contamination in the aseptic area is the care and maintenance. This work should not be done in a haphazard manner by the general maintenance crews, but rather by crews given special instruction and under the supervision of personnel trained in the care of aseptic areas. In general, the cleaning and maintenance should be done after the completion of the day's work with an interval of quietude before the beginning of another aseptic operation. All maintenance equipment should be selected for its effectiveness and freedom from lint-producing tendencies and should be reserved for use in the aseptic areas only.

Personnel

Personnel selected to work on the preparation of a parenteral product must be neat, orderly, and reliable.

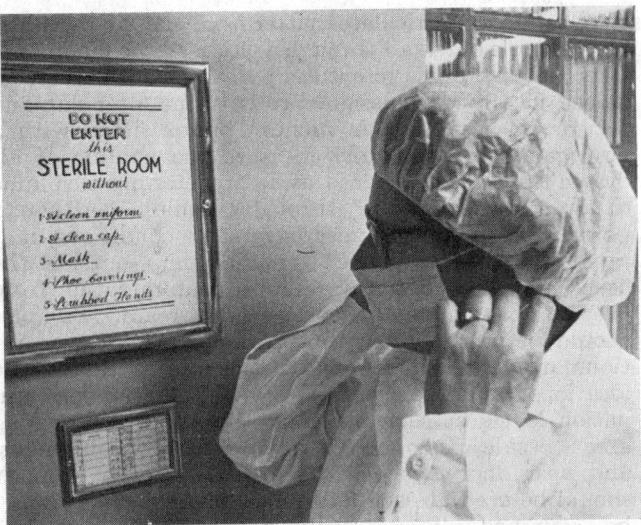

Fig. 573. Operator preparing to enter aseptic filling room (courtesy, Lederle).

They should receive physical examinations at regular intervals to be sure that they are not carriers of an infectious organism. If they show symptoms of a head cold or other illness, they should not be permitted in the aseptic area until recovery is complete. They must receive intensive instruction in the principles of aseptic processes. They also must be made to appreciate the vital part that every movement they make has in determining the reliability of the final product. Supervisors should be selected with particular care. They must be individuals who understand the particular requirements of aseptic procedures and who are able to obtain the full participation of other employees in fulfilling these exacting requirements.

The attire prescribed for personnel varies from one manufacturing facility to another. However, uniforms should be freshly laundered for each day. For use in the aseptic area, it is generally agreed that uniforms should be sterile. This means that fresh, sterile uniforms should be used after every break period, or whenever the individual returns to the aseptic area. In some plants this is not required if the product is to be sterilized in its final container. The uniform usually consists of dresses for women and coveralls for men, hats to completely cover the hair, face masks, and cloth or plastic boots (Fig. 573). Sterile rubber gloves also may be required for some operations. However, thorough scrubbing of the hands with a hexachlorophene soap is considered by some to be adequate and less cumbersome.

Lint is also a problem in these areas. Although cotton uniforms are usually more comfortable, Dacron uniforms are essentially lint free and are reasonably comfortable. Air showers are sometimes directed on personnel entering the processing area to blow loose lint from the uniforms.

Environmental Control Tests

In spite of the elaborate precautions taken by pharmaceutical manufacturers to provide satisfactory conditions for the proper processing of parenterals, the air may become laden with bacteria or other particles with subsequent contamination of the product. For this reason suitable environmental control tests should be performed at regular intervals.

Two air sampling techniques will be described to illustrate what can be done. The first method involves a collection of particulate matter from the air by drawing a sample of the air through a clean, sterile membrane filter of bacterial retentive porosity. The filter is placed in a holder* designed to hold the filter flat and to prevent leakage. A vacuum pump, fitted with a flow gauge to accurately measure the volume of air drawn through the filter, draws a predetermined volume of air, frequently 10 ft³, through the filter. Although portable units are very useful in some conditions, it is preferable to locate the vacuum pump outside the aseptic area in order to minimize contamination from the pump and the discharge air stream. Samples should be taken, preferably during an aseptic operation, at planned locations in the aseptic area. The locations should be chosen to reveal potential contamination levels at such places as the filling and sealing area, beside personnel, next to moving equipment, and near doorways or other openings. A new filter should be used at each location. The filters then may be examined microscopically for particulate matter, such as lint and dust, or placed on culture media and incubated for the detection of microorganisms.

To eliminate the dehydrating effect on microorganisms, the air sample may be drawn into a measured volume of nutrient broth in an impinger. Organisms in the broth then may be collected by filtration on a membrane filter and incubated. In order to be meaningful, such a test must be conducted at planned intervals, with standards set from experience to decide the level of contamination permissible.

A second method involves the exposure of nutrient agar culture plates to the settling of microorganisms from the air. If pathogenic microorganisms are particularly of interest, blood agar plates may be needed. With this method also, the locations for the collection of the samples should be planned carefully. Such a plan is illustrated in Fig. 574. The exposure period should be planned and should be uniform each time in order that comparisons may be meaningful. The exposure period may vary as deemed needful for given circumstances, but a period of one hour or more may be required to collect one microorganism under conditions of use in a well-controlled aseptic area.

Results from these tests are very valuable for informing cleaning and production personnel of the level of contamination. This may be used to encourage them to continue the good technique required to maintain the permissible level. The results may also serve to indicate failures in air cleaning equipment or the

* Suppliers: *Gelman; Millipore.*

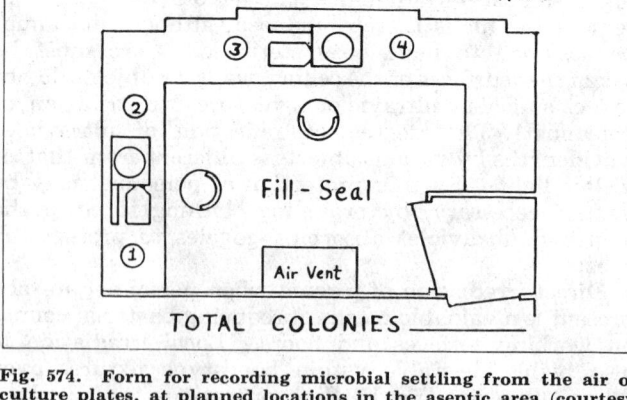

Fig. 574. Form for recording microbial settling from the air on culture plates, at planned locations in the aseptic area (courtesy, Hynson).

presence of personnel who may be disseminating large numbers of bacteria without apparent physical ill effects.

Another test which is much more stringent is to fill and seal sterile fluid thioglycollate medium or trypticase soy broth in sterile ampuls under the same conditions used for an aseptic fill of a product. The entire lot of ampuls is then incubated and examined subsequently for the appearance of growth of microorganisms. Such growth is indicative of contamination from the environment, including the equipment. It also may be used as a measure of the efficiency of a particular operator. Since this is a total sterility test, it is the best indication of the efficiency of the aseptic filling process.

Several instrumental methods are currently being utilized to obtain particle counts from a measured volume of air as a means of indicating the level of particle contamination in the environment. These instruments operate on the principle of the measurement of light scattered from particles passed through the optical system.† They can be adjusted to measure particles of a broad or narrow range of particle size. Difficulty has been experienced in obtaining consistent results, but their automatic electronic features make them useful for routine monitoring of an environment.

Standards for clean rooms[35] have been developed by the General Services Administration of the US Government based on standard methods for their evaluation[36] developed by the American Society for Testing and Materials.

† Suppliers: *B&L; Dynac; Royco.*

Production Procedures

Cleaning Containers and Equipment

Containers and equipment coming in contact with parenteral preparations must be meticulously cleaned. It is obvious that if this were not so, all other precautions to prevent contamination of the product would be useless. It also should be obvious that even new, unused containers and equipment will be contaminated with such debris as dust, fibers, chemical films, and other materials arising from such sources as the atmosphere, cartons, the manufacturing process, and human hands. Much greater and more dangerous contamination must be removed from previously used containers

and equipment before they will be suitable for reuse. Equipment should be rigidly reserved for use only with parenteral preparations and, where conditions dictate, only for one type product in order to reduce the risk of contamination.

A variety of devices are available for the cleaning of containers for parenteral products. These will vary in complexity from a single jet tube for rinsing by hand one inverted container with distilled water at a time, to complex, automatic washers capable of processing several thousand containers an hour. The selection of the particular type to be used will be determined largely by the physical type of containers, their condi-

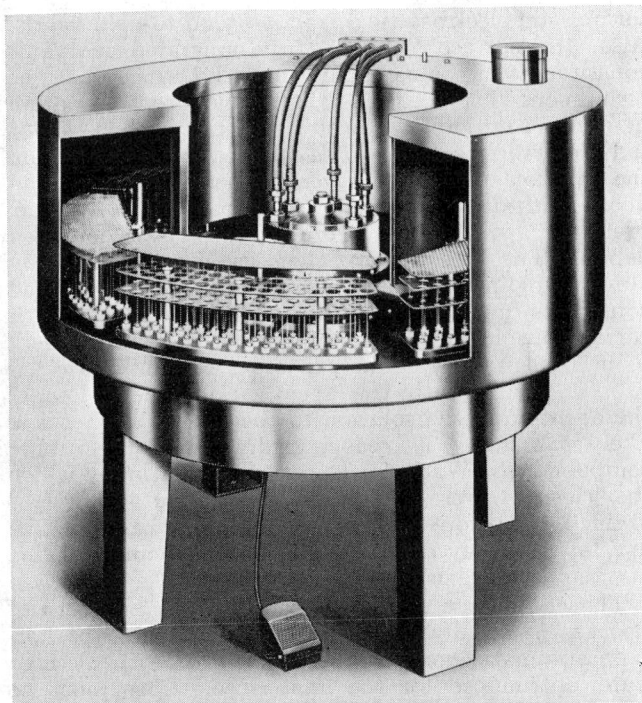

Fig. 575. Rotary rinser for ampuls (courtesy, US Bottlers).

and pressure, and for a long enough period, to remove contaminants from the previous use. Such contaminants may be microbiological, pyrogenic, chemical, or physical and may be extremely difficult to remove completely. Therefore, the desirability of reusing containers for parenteral preparations should be considered cautiously. In all cases, the final rinse must be of very clean distilled water and/or air. To be adequately clean, the distilled water and the air may require filtration to remove particulate matter and oleaginous contaminants accumulated from the processing equipment or from the pipes through which it passed.

Machinery for Containers—The machinery available for cleaning large numbers of containers embodies the above principles but varies in the mechanics by which it is accomplished. In one approach, the jet tubes are arranged on arms like the spokes of a wheel, which rotate around a center post through which the treatments are introduced. An operator places the unclean containers on the jet tubes as they pass the loading point and removes the clean containers as they complete one rotation. Such a machine is pictured in Fig. 575. Another machine has a row of jet tubes across a con-

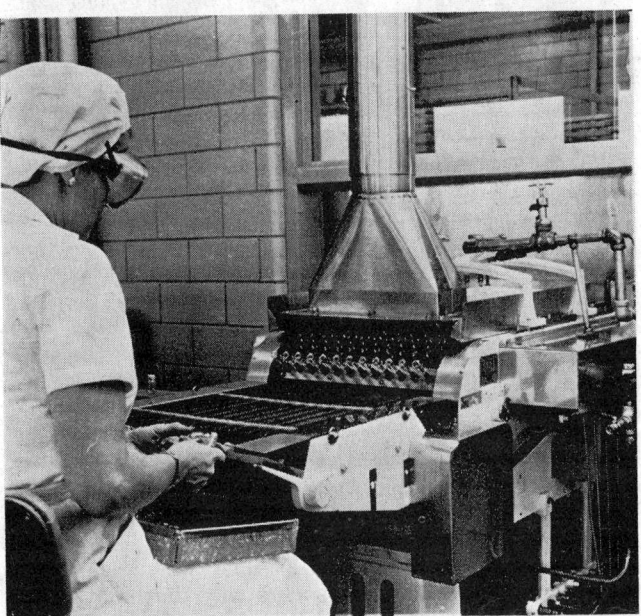

Fig. 576. Conveyor rinser discharging clean vials in preparation area (courtesy, Schering).

tion with respect to contamination, and the number of containers to be processed in a given period of time. It is also possible to clean a small number of ampuls or vials by boiling them in a cleaning solution. Ampuls can be made to fill with solution as the residual air within them contracts after removal of the heat, the tips being inverted and submerged. Rinsing can be accomplished in the same manner.

Characteristics of Machinery—Regardless of the type of cleaning machine selected, certain fundamental characteristics are required.

1. The liquid or air treatment must be introduced in such a manner that it will strike the bottom of the inside of the inverted container, spread in all directions, and smoothly flow down the walls and out the opening with a sweeping action. The pressure of the jet stream should be such that there is minimal splashing, and the flow should be such that it can leave the container opening without accumulating and producing turbulence inside. Splashing may fail to clean all areas and turbulence may redeposit loosened debris. Therefore, direct introduction of the jet stream within the container with control of the flow of the jet stream is required.

2. The container must receive a concurrent outside rinse.

3. The cycle of treatment should provide for a planned sequence with alteration of very hot and cool treatments. The final treatment should be an effective rinse with good quality distilled water followed by an optional clean air blast.

4. All metal parts coming in contact with the containers and with the treatments should be constructed of stainless steel or some other noncorroding and noncontaminating material.

Treatment Cycle—The cycle of treatments to be employed will vary with the condition of the containers to be cleaned and the desires of the individual processor. In general, no detergent treatment is used if the containers are new. This is based on the assumption that most of the debris is loose and can be removed by a rinsing action. However, a thermal shock sequence in the cycle is usually employed to aid, by expansion and contraction, in the loosening of debris that may be adhering to the container wall. Some processors recommend only an air rinse for new containers.

For containers that are to be reused, an adequate hot detergent treatment is essential. This treatment must be introduced at a sufficiently high temperature

veyor belt. The belt moves the row of containers past the treatment stations and discharges the clean containers on the opposite end of the machine, preferably through a wall into a clean room. Two operators are required for this machine (Fig. 576). A cabinet-type washer permits loading the containers on a rack of jet tubes. The rack is pushed inside the cabinet during the cleaning cycle. This type of machine permits handling a variety of sizes and types of containers quite easily, but the number of containers handled in a given period of time is relatively small. Fig. 577 shows a machine of this type. A machine designed to process a large number of containers, particularly bottles and larger size containers, employs a conveyor chain to draw rows of jet tubes through a long tunnel where the treatments are introduced. The clean containers are returned to the loading point for removal.*

---

* Supplier: *Better Built.*

The disadvantage common to all of the above types of machines is that they require the individual handling of each container for loading and unloading. A type which overcomes this disadvantage is the rack-loading washer. Racks are prepared to fit over the open ends of ampuls or vials as they are found in shipping cartons. Inverting the carton permits the containers to be transferred from the carton to the washer without handling the individual containers. A battery of jet tubes is arranged to enter each container positioned in the rack. The clean containers may be removed in the rack and transferred to a box for dry-heat sterilization and storage (see Fig. 578). Another type of rack-loading washer employs an entirely different principle. Containers are filled and emptied by centrifugal force as they are spun with the openings facing the center during filling and away from the center during emptying.* The tank in which the containers are submerged is alternately filled with solution and emptied to complete the cycle. More details of the industrial washing of glassware have been given by Barclay.[37]

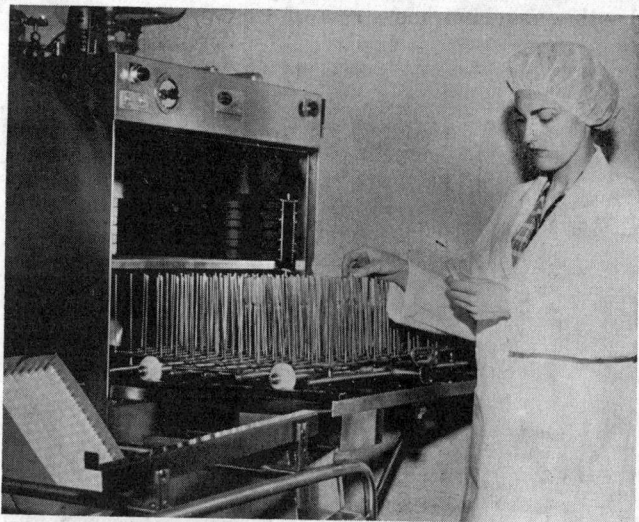

Fig. 577. Cabinet washer being loaded with ampuls (courtesy, The University of Tennessee College of Pharmacy).

Handling after Cleaning—The wet, clean containers must be handled in such a way that contamination will not be reintroduced. A wet surface will much more readily collect contaminants than will a dry surface. In addition, microorganisms are more likely to grow in the presence of moisture. Therefore, it is preferable, if not required, that containers be dry-heat sterilized in a stainless steel box that will protect the containers from contamination during storage after sterilization. Doubling the heating period will also assure destruction of pyrogens, especially likely to be present on reused containers. If it is proved that sterilization is not essential, the containers should be dried and stored where they will be protected from contamination until used. In some instances it may be acceptable to briefly drain the clean containers and immediately fill them with the product. The latter method eliminates the need for storage of the clean container, but it also eliminates the sterilizing and depyrogenating step of the dry-heat treatment, often a vital step. Therefore, it should be used only where a sterile pyrogen-free container is not essential.

Closures—Rubber closures are coated with lubricant from the molding operation. In addition, the rough

surface and electrostatic attraction tend to hold debris. Also, the surface "bloom" from migrated inorganic constituents of the compound must be removed. The recommended procedure calls for vigorous agitation in a hot solution of a water softener such as 0.5% sodium pyrophosphate. The closures are removed from the solution and rinsed several times with water and finally with distilled water. The rinsing is to be done, preferably, with a spray in order to flush away loosened debris. The closures are then usually sterilized by autoclaving in Water for Injection and stored in closed containers until ready for use. At times this step is carried out in a solution of the bacteriostatic agent to be used in the product, in order to equilibrate the rubber closure with the agent. Subsequent loss of the agent from the solution to the closure is then less likely to occur. To reduce hydration of the rubber compound, the Water for Injection or solution in which the closures were immersed during autoclaving is drained off before storage. If the closures must be dry for use, they may be subjected to vacuum drying at a temperature in the vicinity of 100°C.

The equipment used for washing large numbers of closures is usually an agitator or horizontal basket-type automatic home washing machine, with distilled water introduced for the final rinse. Care must be taken, however, to control the abrading action on the closures that the vigorous agitation of the washer may produce.

Equipment—Details of certain prescribed techniques for the cleaning and preparation of equipment, as well as of containers and closures, have been presented elsewhere.[38] Here, a few points will be emphasized.

Stainless steel equipment should be disassembled as much as possible to provide access to internal structures. All parts should be scrubbed thoroughly with a stiff brush using an effective detergent, paying particular attention to joints, crevices, screw threads, and other structures where debris is apt to collect. Exposure to a stream of clean steam will aid in dislodging residues from the walls of stationary tanks, spigots, pipes, and similar structures. Thorough rinsing with distilled water should follow the cleaning steps. Large stationary tanks should be protected as much as possible from contamination after cleaning but should be rinsed thoroughly again with distilled water prior to reuse.

Glassware should be thoroughly scrubbed and rinsed. Where possible, all openings should be covered with aluminum foil and dry-heat sterilized. It is sometimes recommended that dichromate cleaning solution be used on glassware. While this solution will effectively clean glassware of traces of organic residues, it should be used cautiously since the dichromate ion adheres strongly to the glass surface and is completely removed only with great difficulty. Should any remain, it may be transferred to the product subsequently made in the glassware and produce detrimental effects.

Rubber tubing, rubber gaskets, and other rubber parts may be washed in a manner such as described for rubber closures. Thorough rinsing of tubing must be done by passing distilled water through it. If more rigorous treatment is required for new tubing or parts, it has been suggested that the tubing should be soaked in 10% sodium hydroxide solution for 24 hr, rinsed thoroughly, boiled for 1 hr in 1% hydrochloric acid solution, and rinsed thoroughly with distilled water. Rubber tubing must be left damp when preparing for sterilization by autoclaving.

---

* Supplier: *BBL.*

Product Preparation

The basic principles employed in the compounding of the product do not vary from those used routinely by qualified pharmacists. However, selected aspects will be mentioned for emphasis. All measurements should be made as accurately as possible and should be checked by a second qualified person. Although most liquid preparations are made by volume, where possible they should be made by weight, with the weight experimentally determined from the required volume. This method is more accurate since no consideration need be given to the temperature of the components. In addition, measurements by weight normally can be performed more accurately than those by volume.

Care must be taken that equipment is not wet enough to significantly dilute the product or, in the case of anhydrous products, to cause a physical incompatibility. The order of mixing of ingredients may significantly affect the product, particularly those of large volume where attaining homogeneity requires considerable mixing time. For example, the adjustment of pH by the addition of a dilute acid may cause excessive local reduction in the pH of the product so that adverse effects are produced before the acid can be dispersed throughout the entire volume of product.

Parenteral dispersions, including colloids, emulsions, and suspensions, provide particular problems. These have been reviewed by Macek[39] and by Nash.[40] In addition to the problems of achieving and maintaining proper reduction in particle size under aseptic conditions, the dispersion must be kept in a uniform state of suspension throughout preparative, transfer, and subdividing operations.

The formulation of a stable product is of paramount importance. Certain aspects of this have been mentioned in the discussion of components of the product. Exhaustive coverage of the topic is not possible within the limits of this text, but further coverage is provided in Chapter 79, page 1463. It should be mentioned here, however, that thermal sterilization of parenteral products increases the possibility of chemical reactions. Such reactions may progress to completion during the period of elevated temperature in the autoclave, or be initiated at this time but continue during subsequent storage. Assurance of attainment of stability in a product requires a high order of pharmaceutical knowledge and responsibility.

Filtration

After a product has been compounded, if it is a solution, it must be filtered. The primary objective of filtration is to clarify a solution. A high degree of clarification is termed "polishing" a solution. This term is applied when particulate matter down to approximately 2 μ in size is removed. A further step, removing particulate matter down to 0.2 μ in size, would eliminate microorganisms and would accomplish "cold" sterilization. A solution having a high degree of clarity conveys the impression of high quality and purity, desirable characteristics for a parenteral solution.

Filters are thought to function by one or, usually, a combination of the following: (1) sieving or screening, (2) entrapment in tortuous passageways, and (3) electrostatic attraction. When a filter retains particles by sieving, the particles are retained on the surface of the filter. Entrapment occurs when a particle, smaller than the dimensions of the passageway (pore), be-

comes lodged in a turn or ledge of the passageway. Electrostatic attraction causes particles opposite in charge to that of the surface of the filter pore to be held or adsorbed to the surface. It should be noted that increasing or prolonging the force behind the solution may tend to sweep particles held by entrapment or electrostatic charge through the pores and into the filtrate.

The contact between a solution and a filter is very intimate. Therefore, minute effects of a filter on a solution may be magnified to considerable significance, particularly on the first portion of the solution passing through a filter. This can be demonstrated readily by passing a solution of methylene blue through an asbestos pad filter. The first portion of the filtrate will be entirely colorless, but subsequent portions of the filtrate will become increasingly blue in color. This indicates that adsorption had at first occurred, but that methylene blue molecules passed through the filter after the filter fibers had become saturated. The adverse effect of a filter on a solution sometimes can be

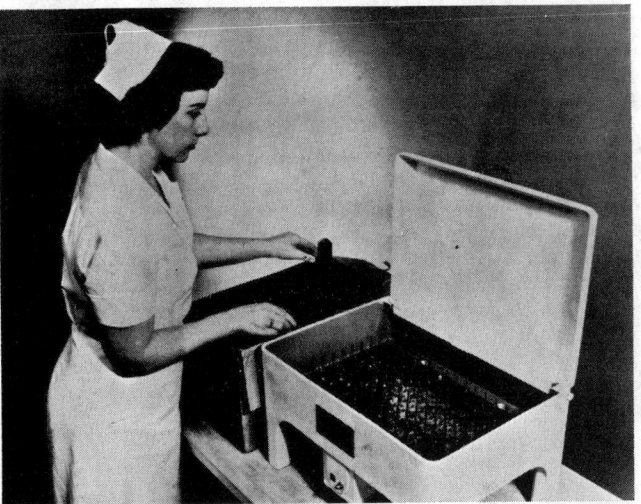

Fig. 578. Metromatic rack-loader washer being loaded directly from container carton (courtesy, Price).

eliminated or reduced by treating the filter prior to use, for example, with hydrochloric acid solution to neutralize alkaline constituents of the filter.

Of the common filters used for parenteral solutions, the asbestos pad* is the most reactive. Unglazed porcelain,† sintered glass,‡ and cellulose ester membranes§ are less likely to be reactive. The characteristics of these filters are considered in more detail in Chapter 81, page 1510. Various other factors to be considered in the selection of a filter for use with a parenteral solution include the flow rate required, loss of vehicle by evaporation or absorption, and cleanability.[41] The last is of principal concern when the filter is designed to be reused rather than when the entire filter medium is discarded after use. However, fittings holding and supporting the disposable filter may be difficult to clean. Cleaning problems with reusable filters may make it desirable to retain them for use with one type of solution only. Even so, cleaning will require considerable care and effort to prevent residues from a previous use from contaminating a subsequent filtrate. Specific techniques for cleaning some

---

* Suppliers: *Ertel; Hercules; Hormann; Republic.*
† Supplier: *Selas.*
‡ Suppliers: *Corning; Kimble.*
§ Suppliers: *Gelman; Millipore; Schleicher.*

filters have been reported;[38] others may be found in the literature of the supplier.

Filling

During the filling of containers with a product, the most stringent requirements must be exercised to prevent contamination, particularly if the product has been sterilized by filtration and will not be sterilized in the final container. Under the latter conditions it is usually called an "aseptic fill." During the filling operation, the product must be transferred from a bulk container and subdivided into dose containers. This operation exposes the product to the environment, equipment, and manipulative technique of the operator. In addition, the open container is exposed to the environment during filling and until it can be sealed. Therefore, this operation is carried out in the aseptic filling area where maximum protection is provided. Additional protection may be provided by filling in a laminar flow workbench within the aseptic area.

Normally, the compounded product is in the form of either a liquid or a solid. A liquid is more readily uniformly subdivided and introduced into a container having a narrow mouth than is a solid. Mobile, non-sticking liquids are considerably easier to transfer and subdivide than viscous, sticky liquids. The latter require heavy-duty machinery for rapid production filling.

Although many devices are available for filling containers with liquids, certain characteristics are fundamental to them all. A means is provided for repetitively forcing a measured volume of the liquid through the orifice of a delivery tube which is introduced into the container. The size of the delivery tube will vary from that of about a 20-gauge hypodermic needle to a tube 1 in. or more in diameter. The size required is determined by the physical characteristics of the liquid, the speed of delivery desired, and the inside diameter of the neck of the container. The tube must enter the neck of the container and deliver the liquid

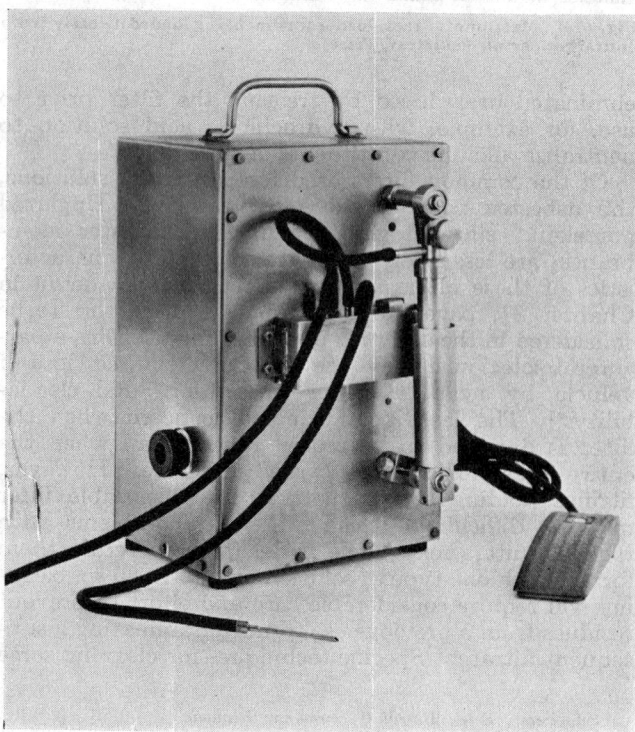

Fig. 579. Filling machine employing piston valve and stainless steel syringe (courtesy, Chase-Logeman).

well into the neck to eliminate spillage, allowing sufficient clearance to permit air to leave the container as the liquid enters. The delivery tube should be as large as possible in diameter in order to reduce the resistance to the flow of the liquid. For smaller volumes of liquids, the delivery is usually obtained from the stroke of the plunger of a syringe, forcing the liquid through a two-way valve providing for alternate filling of the syringe and delivery of mobile liquids. A sliding piston valve would be used for heavy, viscous liquids. For large volumes the quantity delivered is usually measured in the container by the level of fill in the container, the force required to transfer the liquid being provided by gravity, a pressure pump, or a vacuum pump.

The narrow neck of an ampul limits the clearance possible between the delivery tube and the inside of the neck. Since a drop of liquid normally hangs at the tip of the delivery tube after a delivery, the neck of an ampul will be wet as the delivery tube is withdrawn, unless the drop is retracted. Therefore, filling machines should have a mechanism by which this drop can be drawn back into the lumen of the tube.

Since the liquid will be in intimate contact with the parts of the machine through which it flows, these parts must be constructed of nonreactive materials such as borosilicate glass or stainless steel. In addition, these parts should be easily demountable for cleaning and for sterilization.

Liquids—The filling of a small number of containers may be accomplished with a hypodermic syringe and needle, the liquid being drawn into the syringe and forced through the needle into the restricted opening of the container. A device for providing greater speed of filling is the Cornwall Pipet.* This device has a two-way valve between the syringe and the needle and a means for setting the stroke of the syringe so that the same volume will be delivered each time.

Mechanically operated instruments substitute a motor for the operator's hand in the previous devices described. Thereby, a much faster filling rate can be achieved. By careful engineering, the stroke of the syringe can be repeated precisely; and so, once a particular setting has been calibrated to the delivery, high delivery precision is possible. However, the speed of delivery, the expansion of rubber tubing connecting the valve with the delivery tube, and the rapidity of action of the valves can affect the precision of delivery. A filling machine employing a two-way valve assembly is shown in operation in Fig. 568. One employing a piston valve is shown in Fig. 579. Stainless steel syringes are usually employed with viscous liquids because glass syringes are not strong enough to withstand the high pressures developed during delivery.

Fig. 580 illustrates the filling of large-volume bottles by means of a pressure pump filler. As the delivery tube is lowered into the bottle, the rubber sealer is pressed against the lip of the bottle and the pressure opens a pinch valve. This permits the liquid to flow into the container until it reaches the overflow tube. The operator then raises the delivery assembly, automatically closing the pinch valve. The level of fill is governed by the position of the overflow tube in the container. Any liquid drawn into the overflow tube is returned to the reservoir. It is obvious that the accuracy of fill will vary since it is determined by the height of the liquid in the bottle. It is customary to plan a liberal excess with such filling operations.

* Supplier: *BD & Co.*

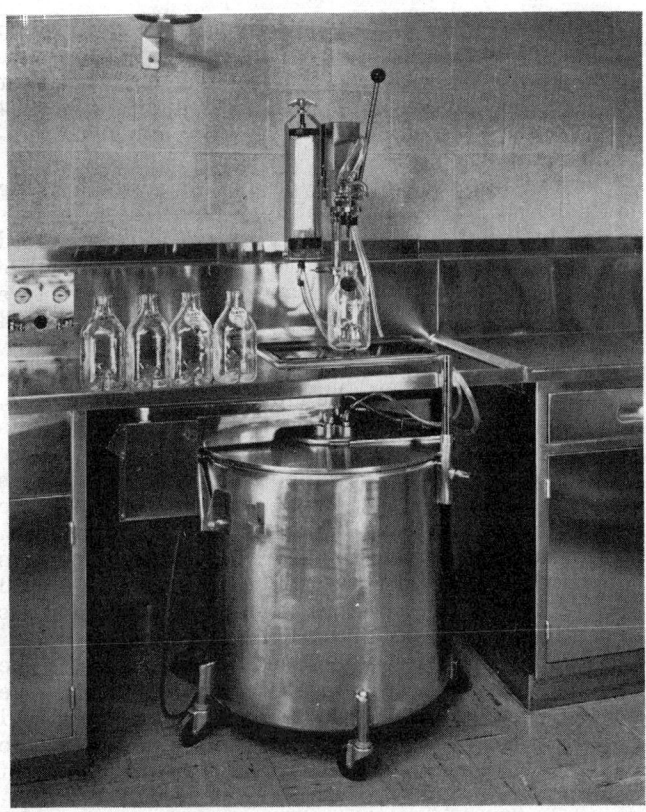

Fig. 580. A pressure pump filler for liter solution bottles in a hospital (courtesy, Am. Sterilizer).

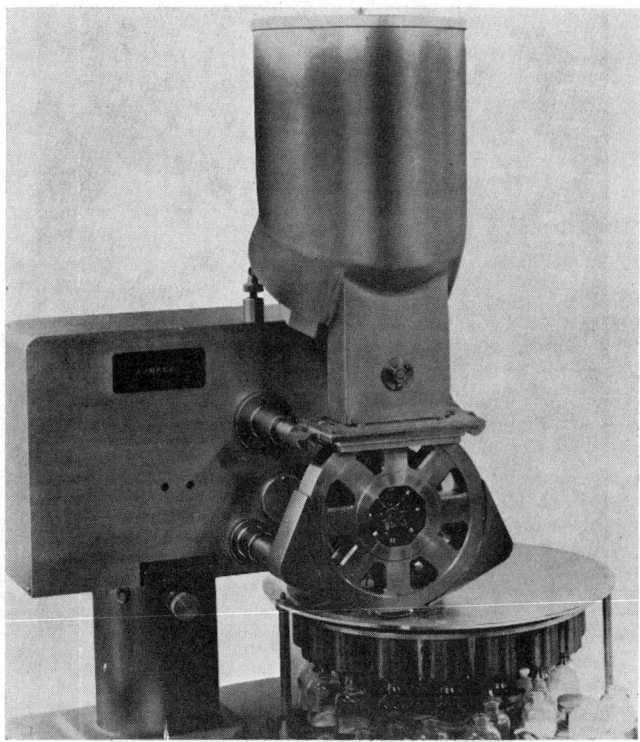

Fig. 581. Accofil vacuum powder filler (courtesy, Perry).

The USP states that "each container . . . is filled with a volume in slight excess of the labeled 'size' or that volume which is to be withdrawn." A table of suggested excess volumes is given in the USP.

Solids—Sterile solids, such as antibiotics, are more difficult to subdivide evenly into containers than are liquids. The rate of flow of solid material is slow and irregular. Even though a container with a larger diameter opening is used to facilitate filling, it is difficult to introduce the solid particles, and the risk of spillage is ever present. The accuracy of the quantity delivered cannot be controlled as well as with liquids. Because of these factors, the tolerances permitted for the content of such containers must be relatively large. Suggested tolerances will be found in the USP.

Many sterile solids are subdivided into containers by individual weighing. A scoop is usually provided to aid in approximating the quantity required, but the quantity filled into the container is finally weighed on a balance. This is a slow process. When the solid is obtainable in a granular form so that it will flow more freely, other methods of filling may be employed. In general, these methods involve the measurement and delivery of a volume of the granular material which has been calibrated in terms of the weight desired. In a machine, shown in Fig. 581, an adjustable cavity in the rim of a wheel is filled by vacuum and the contents held by vacuum until the cavity is inverted over the container. The solid material is then discharged into the container by the use of sterile air. Another machine employs an auger in the stem of a funnel at the bottom of a hopper. The granular material is placed in the hopper. By controlling the size of the auger and its rotation, a regulated volume of granular material can be delivered from the funnel stem into the container. Such a machine is shown in Fig. 582.

Sealing

Ampuls—Filled containers should be sealed as soon as possible to prevent the contents from being contaminated by the environment. Ampuls are sealed by melting a portion of the glass neck. Two types of seals are normally employed, either tip-seals (bead-seals) or pull-seals. Tip-seals are made by melting enough glass at the tip of the neck of an ampul to form a bead and close the opening. Such seals can be

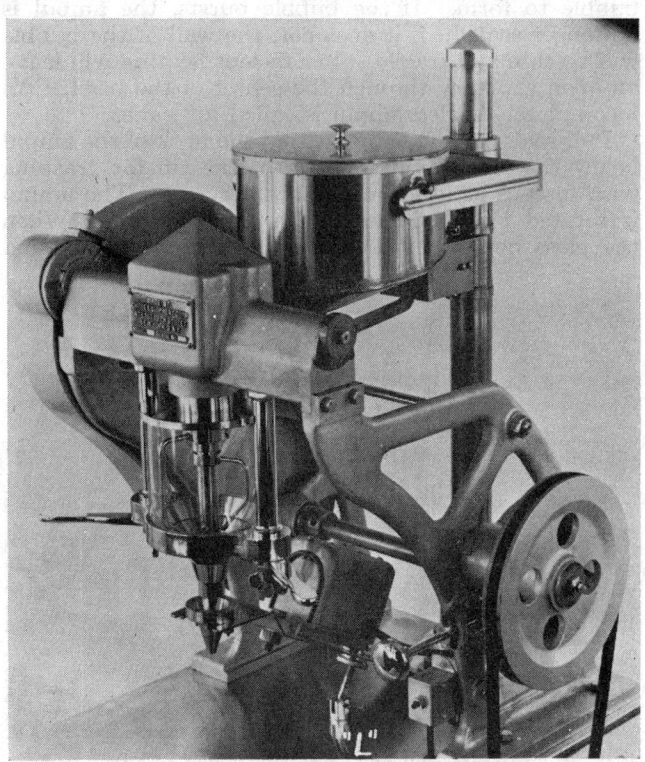

Fig. 582. Auger-type powder filler (courtesy, Chase-Logeman).

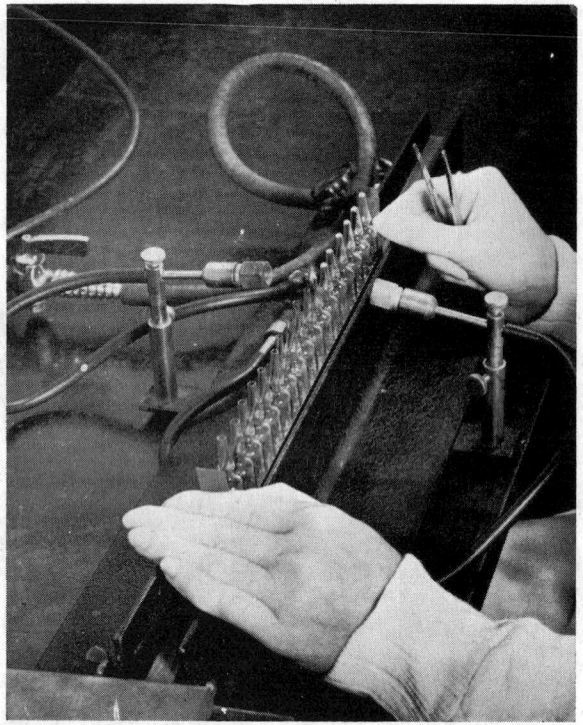

Fig. 583. Ampuls being sealed in a crossfire of a Bunsen burner (courtesy, Hynson).

made rapidly in a high-temperature gas–oxygen flame. To produce a uniform bead, the ampul neck must be heated evenly on all sides. This may be accomplished by means of burners on opposite sides of stationary ampuls (see Fig. 583) or by rotating the ampul in a single flame. Care must be taken to properly adjust the flame temperature and the interval of heating to obtain complete closing of the opening with a bead of glass. Excessive heating will result in expansion of gases within the ampul against the soft bead seal and cause a bubble to form. If the bubble bursts, the ampul is no longer sealed; if it does not, the wall of the bubble will be thin and fragile. Insufficient heating will leave an open capillary through the center of the bead. An incompletely sealed ampul is called a "leaker."

Pull-seals are made by heating the neck of the ampul below the tip, leaving enough of the tip for grasping with forceps or other mechanical devices. The ampul is rotated in the flame from a single burner. When the glass has softened, the tip is grasped firmly and

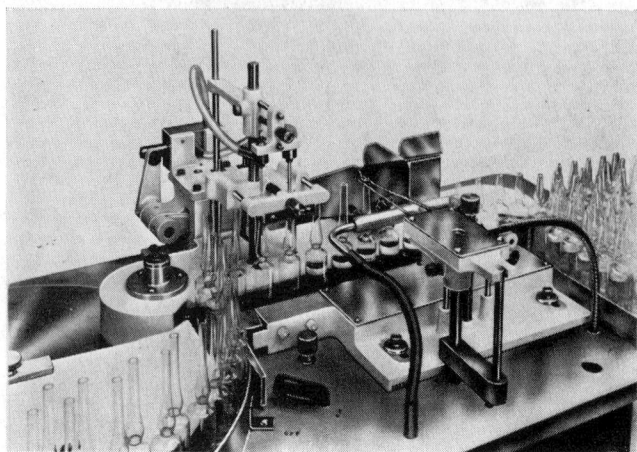

Fig. 584. Automatic filling and pull-sealing of ampuls (courtesy, Cozzoli).

pulled quickly away from the body of the ampul, which continues to rotate. The small capillary tube thus formed is twisted closed. Pull-sealing is slower, but the seals are more sure than tip-sealing. Fig. 584 shows a machine combining the steps of filling and pull-sealing ampuls.

Powder ampuls or other types having a wide opening must be sealed by pull-sealing. Were these ampuls sealed by bead-sealing, the very large bead produced would induce glass strain with subsequent fracture at the juncture of the bead and neck wall. Fracture of the neck of ampuls during sealing also may occur if wetting of the necks occurred at the time of filling. Also, wet necks increase the frequency of bubble formation. If the product in the ampul is organic in nature, wet necks will also result in unsightly carbon deposits from the heat of sealing.

In order to prevent decomposition of a product, it is sometimes necessary to displace the air in the space above the product in the ampul with an inert gas. This is done by introducing a stream of the gas, such as nitrogen or carbon dioxide, during or after filling with the product. Immediately thereafter the ampul is sealed before the gas can diffuse to the outside.

Vials and Bottles—These are sealed by closing the opening with a rubber closure (stopper). This must be accomplished as rapidly as possible after filling and with reasoned care to prevent contamination of the contents. The large opening makes the introduction of contamination much easier than with ampuls. Therefore, a means should be provided to keep these containers covered except for the few seconds required for filling and for the actual introduction of the rubber closure. In Fig. 585 the entire procedure is being performed within a closed hood in an aseptic room.

The closure must fit the mouth of the container snugly enough so that its elasticity will permit adjustment to

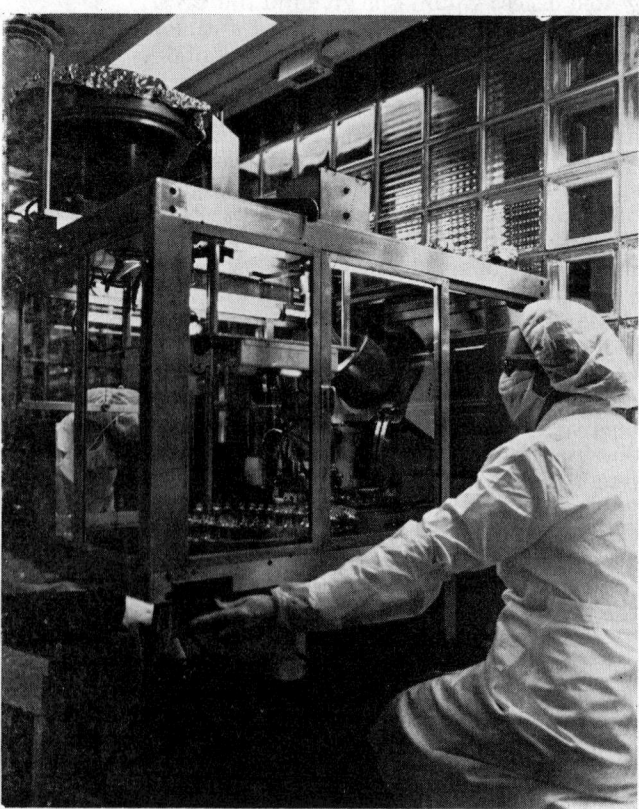

Fig. 585. Filling and stoppering vials within a closed hood in an aseptic room (courtesy, Lederle).

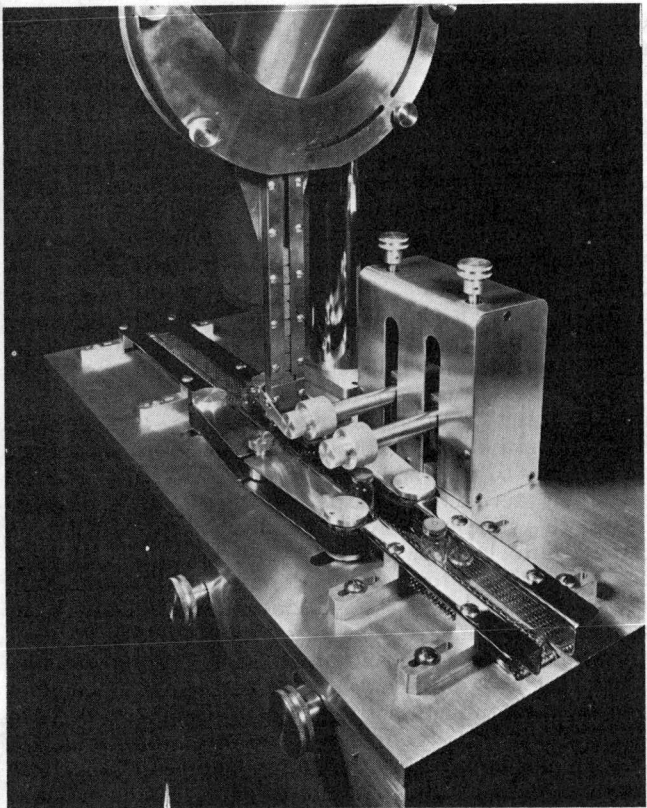

Fig. 586. Mechanical device for inserting rubber closures in vials (courtesy, Perry).

slight irregularities in the lip and neck of the container. However, it must not fit so snugly that it is difficult to introduce into the neck of the container. When rubber closures are to be inserted mechanically, the surface of the closure is often halogenated to give it less friction. Thus, it is possible to convey the closure through a shute to the place where it is positioned over a vial and then inserted by a plunger or some other pressure device. Mechanical stoppering has been developed in recent years because of the need for high-speed production. An example of such a mechanical device is shown in Fig. 586. Closures may also be inserted aseptically with sterile forceps or directly with hands encased in sterile rubber gloves, as shown in Fig.

587. In a modification of this technique, rubber closures may be picked up and then inserted into a vial by means of a tool connected to a vacuum line. Such a procedure is shown in Fig. 588.

Rubber closures are held in place by means of aluminum caps. The aluminum cap covers the closure and is crimped under the lip of the vial or bottle to hold the closure in place (see Fig. 565). The closure cannot be removed without destroying the aluminum cap. Therefore, an intact aluminum cap is proof that the closure has not been intentionally or unintentionally removed. Such confirmation is necessary to assure the integrity of the contents as to sterility and other aspects of quality. The aluminum caps are so designed that the outer layer of double-layered caps, or the center of single-layered caps, can be removed to expose the center of the rubber closure without disturbing the band which holds the closure in the container. Rubber closures for use with intravenous administration sets must have a permanent hole through the closure. In such cases, a thin rubber disk overlayed with a solid aluminum disk is placed between an inner and outer aluminum cap. A seal of the hole through the closure is thereby provided. These are called triple-layered aluminum caps.

Single-layered aluminum caps may be applied by means of a hand crimper known as the Fermpress.* Double- or triple-layered caps require greater force for crimping; therefore, heavy-duty mechanical crimpers are required.†

Sterilization

Whenever possible, the parenteral product should be sterilized after being sealed in its final container and within as short a time as possible after the filling and sealing has been completed. Since this usually involves a thermal process, due consideration must be given to the effect of the elevated temperature upon the stability of the product. Many products, both

---

* Suppliers: *West; Wheaton.*
† Suppliers: *Alcoa; United Shoe; West; Wheaton.*

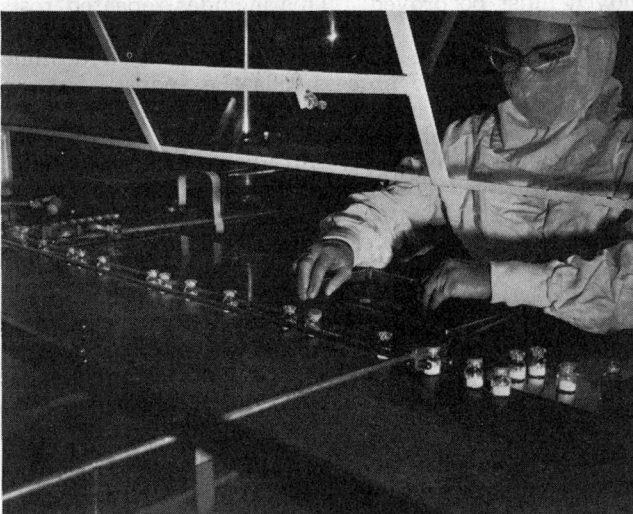

Fig. 587. Inserting rubber closures in vials by hand under aseptic conditions (courtesy, Abbott).

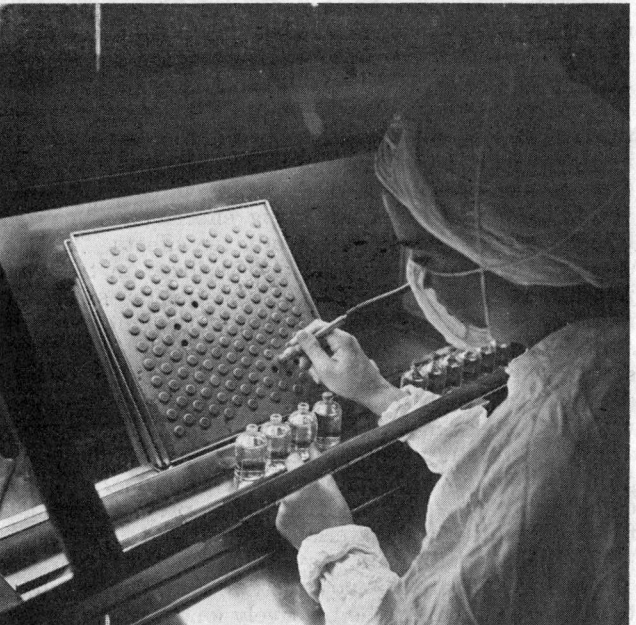

Fig. 588. Inserting rubber closures in vials by means of a tool connected to a vacuum line, under aseptic conditions (courtesy, Abbott).

pharmaceutical and biological, will be adversely affected by the elevated temperatures required for thermal sterilization. Such products must, therefore, be sterilized by a nonthermal method. Most thermolabile solutions may be sterilized by filtration through bacteria-retaining filters. Subsequently, all operations must be carried out in an aseptic manner so that contamination will not be introduced into the filtrate. To perform such an aseptic procedure is difficult, and the degree of its accomplishment is always uncertain. Colloids, oleaginous solutions, suspensions, and emulsions that are thermolabile may require a process in which each component is sterilized and the product is formulated and processed under aseptic conditions. Because of the ever-present risk of a momentary or prolonged lapse in aseptic control during an aseptic process, and the dangerous condition that could result, sterilization of a product in its final container (terminal sterilization) is preferred.

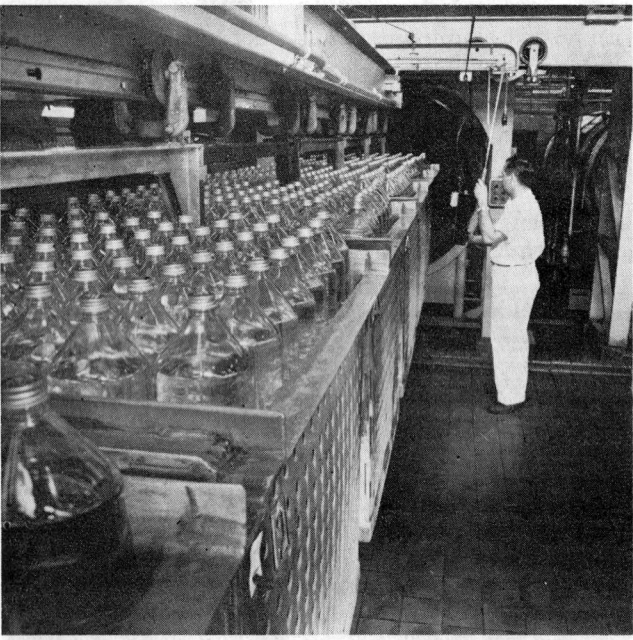

Fig. 589. A large autoclave being loaded with liter bottles of solution (courtesy, Abbott).

Some of the newer nonthermal methods of sterilization are finding important application to components of injections and to administration devices. Certain dry solids such as penicillin, streptomycin, polyvitamins, and certain hormones are being effectively sterilized by ionized radiations without adverse effects. Catgut sutures are now being routinely sterilized in the final package by this method. Administration sets, disposable needles and syringes, and other plastic and stainless steel equipment and components are being sterilized by ionizing radiations and by gaseous ethylene oxide sterilization. Generally speaking, however, neither of these methods may be used for liquid preparations without adverse effects on the product, and gaseous sterilization cannot be used where a glass container or other impervious barrier prevents the gas from permeating the material.

Dry-heat sterilization may be employed for a few dry solids that are not adversely affected by the high temperatures and for the relatively long heating period required. This method is most effectively applied to the sterilization of glassware and metalware. After sterilization, the equipment will be sterile, dry and, if

the sterilization period is approximately doubled, pyrogen free.

Saturated steam under pressure (autoclaving) is the most commonly used and probably the most effective method for the sterilization of aqueous liquids or substances that can be reached or penetrated by steam. Fig. 589 shows large baskets containing liter bottles of solution being loaded into an autoclave for sterilization. It is ineffective in anhydrous conditions, such as within a sealed ampul containing a dry solid or an anhydrous oil. Since the temperature employed in an autoclave is lower than that for dry-heat sterilization, equipment made of materials such as rubber and polypropylene may be sterilized. As mentioned previously, some injections will be adversely affected by the elevated temperature required for autoclaving. Sometimes the use of an autoclave designed to permit a rapid rise to sterilizing temperature and rapid cooling after the sterilizing hold period will make it possible to use this method. For example, Dextrose Injection can be autoclaved without adverse effects if the total heating period is reduced by the use of a rapid heating and cooling cycle. Other products that will not withstand autoclaving temperatures may withstand marginal thermal methods such as Tyndallization or Inspissation. These methods may be rendered more effective for some injections by the inclusion of a bacteriostatic agent in the product.

It should be obvious that all materials subjected to sterilization must be protected from subsequent contamination to maintain their sterile state. Therefore, materials subjected to autoclaving must be wrapped or covered so that microorganisms may not gain access when removed from the autoclave. Equipment and supplies are most frequently wrapped with paper and tied or sealed with special autoclave tape. The wrapping must permit penetration of steam during autoclaving but screen out microorganisms when dry. A double wrapping with lint-free parchment paper within and kraft paper without is probably best. Synthetic fiber cloth such as nylon or Dacron also may be used for the inner wrapping. The openings of equipment subjected to dry-heat sterilization are often covered with silver–aluminum foil or with metal or glass covers. Cellulose wrapping materials are adversely affected by the high temperatures of dry-heat sterilization.

The effectiveness of any sterilization technique employed must be proved. This includes repeated tests with materials and equipment assemblies purposely contaminated with resistant spores to determine whether or not the process kills the spores. Proven methods must be carried out under the strict supervision of personnel thoroughly familiar with the technique and its limitations. Sterilizing indicators must also be employed as evidence that the proven technique has been repeated.

Further details concerning methods of sterilization and their application will be found in Chapter 81, page 1507. In addition, the USP provides suggestions concerning the sterilization of injections and related materials.

Freeze-Drying

Freeze-drying (lyophilization) is a process of drying in which water is sublimed from the product after it is frozen.[42]

The particular advantages of this process are that biologicals and pharmaceuticals which are relatively unstable in aqueous solution can be processed and filled into dosage containers in the liquid state, taking advantage of the relative ease of processing a liquid; dried without elevated temperatures, thereby eliminating adverse thermal effects; and then stored in the dry state in which there are relatively few stability problems.

Further advantages include the fact that freeze-dried products are often more soluble and/or more rapidly soluble, dispersions are stabilized throughout the shelf life of the product, and products subject to degradation by oxidation have enhanced stability because the process is carried out in a vacuum.

However, the increased time and handling required for processing and the cost of the equipment limits the use of this process to those products which have significantly enhanced stability if stored in the dry state.

The fact that ice will sublime at pressures below 3 mm Hg has been a long-established laboratory principle. Its application to the freeze-drying of clinical materials occurred more recently through the work of Flosdorf.[43] The extensive program for the freeze-drying of human plasma during World War II provided the impetus for the rapid development of the process.

Freeze-drying essentially consists of the following:

1. Freezing an aqueous product at a temperature below its eutectic temperature.[44]
2. Evacuating the chamber, usually below 0.1 Torr (100 μ Hg).
3. Subliming ice on a cold condensing surface at a temperature below that of the product, the condensing surface being within the chamber or in a connecting chamber.
4. Introducing heat to the product under controlled conditions, thereby providing energy for sublimation at a rate designed to keep the product temperature below its eutectic temperature.

Fig. 590 shows such a system. The product may be frozen on the shelf in the chamber by circulating refrigerant (usually Freon, ammonia, or ethylene glycol) from the compressor through pipes within the shelf. After freezing is complete, which may require several hours, the chamber and condenser are evacuated by the vacuum pump, the condenser surface having been previously chilled by circulating refrigerant from the large compressor.

Heat is then introduced from the shelf to the product by electric resistance coils or by circulating hot water or hot glycol. The process continues until the product is dry (usually 1% or less moisture), leaving a spongelike matrix of the solids originally present in the product, the input of heat being controlled so as not to degrade the product.

For most pharmaceuticals and biologicals the liquid product is sterilized by filtration and then filled into the dosage container aseptically. The containers must remain open during the drying process, therefore, they must be protected from contamination during transfer from the filling area to the freeze-drying chamber, while in the freeze-drying chamber, and at the end of the drying process until sealed.

Chambers may be equipped with hydraulic or rubber diaphragm internal-stoppering devices designed to push slotted rubber closures into the vials to seal while the chamber is still evacuated, the closures having been partially inserted immediately after filling so that the slots were open to the outside.

If internal stoppering is not available or containers such as ampuls are used, filtered, dry air or nitrogen must be introduced to the chamber at the end of the process to establish atmospheric pressure. Then the containers must be removed and sealed under aseptic conditions. If the product is very sensitive to moisture, the environmental humidity must also be controlled until it is sealed.

Factors Affecting the Process Rate—The greater the depth of the product in the container, the longer will be the drying process. Therefore, a product to be frozen by placing the container on a refrigerated shelf (plug freezing) should be filled to a planned, limited depth. If a large volume of solution must be processed, the surface area may be increased and the depth decreased by freezing the solution on a slant or while rotating the container on an angle (shell freezing) in a liquid refrigerant bath, such as dry ice and alcohol.

The actual driving force for the process is the vapor pressure differential between the vapor at the surface where drying of the product is occurring (the drying

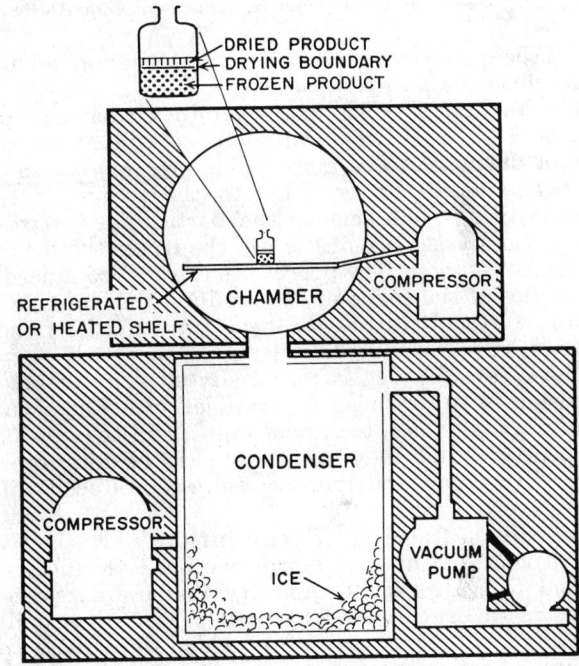

Fig. 590. Essential components of a freeze-drying system.

boundary) and the vapor pressure at the surface of the ice on the condenser. The latter is determined by the temperature of the condenser as modified by the insulating effect of the accumulated ice. The former is determined by a number of factors, including:

1. The rate of heat conduction through the container and the frozen material, both usually relatively poor thermal conductors, to the drying boundary while maintaining all of the product below its eutectic temperature.
2. The impeding effect of the increasing depth of dried porous product above the drying boundary.
3. The temperature and heat capacity of the shelf itself.

This may be visualized by referring to Fig. 590.

The passageways between the product surface and the condenser surface must be wide open and direct for effective operation. Therefore, the condensing surfaces in large freeze-driers are usually in the same chamber as the product. Evacuation of the system is necessary to reduce the impeding effect that collisions with air molecules would have on the passage of water molecules. However, the residual pressure in the system must be greater than the vapor pressure of the

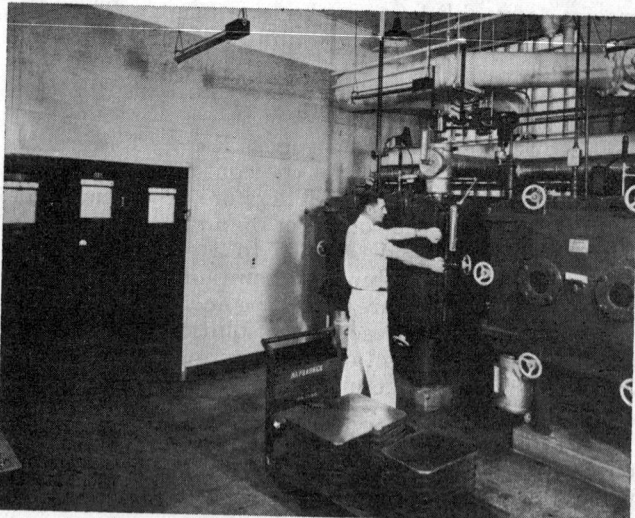

Fig. 591. Freeze-drying equipment (courtesy, Parke-Davis).

ice on the condenser or the ice would be vaporized and pulled into the pump.

The amount of solids in the product, their particle size, and their thermal conductance will affect the rate of drying.[45] The more solids present, the more impediment will be provided to the escape of the water vapor. The smaller the particle size, particularly the crystal size of the ice, the faster the drying generally will be. The poorer the thermal conducting properties of the solids in the product, the slower will be the rate of transfer of heat through the frozen material to the drying boundary.

The rate of drying is essentially slow, most often requiring 24 hr or longer for completion. The actual time required, the rate of heat input, and the product temperatures that may be utilized must be determined for each product and then carefully reproduced with successive processes.[46]

Factors Affecting Formulation—The active constituent of many pharmaceutical products is present in such a small quantity that if freeze-dried alone its presence would be hard to detect visually. Therefore, substances are often added to increase the amount of solids present.

Some consider it ideal for the dried product plug to occupy essentially the same volume as that of the original solution. To achieve this, the solids content of the original product must be between approximately 10 and 25%. Among the substances found most useful for this purpose, usually as a combination,

are sodium or potassium phosphates, citric acid, tartaric acid, gelatin, and carbohydrates such as dextrose, mannitol, and dextran.

Each of these substances contributes appearance characteristics to the plug, such as whether dull and spongy or sparkling and crystalline, firm or friable, expanded or shrunken, and uniform or striated. Therefore, the formulation of a product to be freeze-dried must include consideration not only of the nature and stability characteristics required during the liquid state, both freshly prepared and when reconstituted before use, but the characteristics desired in the dried plug.

Modifications in the Process and Equipment—In some instances a product may be frozen in a bulk container or in trays rather than in the final container and then handled as a dry solid. This may be desirable when large volumes of a product are processed.

Heat may be introduced to all sides of the product by radiation from infrared sources, rather than only from the bottom as with conductive heating. While this generally increases the rate of drying, there are at least two major disadvantages to radiant heating of pharmaceuticals; these are (1) multiple containers produce shadowing with resultant blockage of the radiations and (2) the dried material on the outside of the frozen product may be scorched easily by the heat as drying progresses.

When large quantities of material are processed it may be desirable to utilize ejection pumps in the equipment system. These draw the vapor into the pump and eject it to the outside, thereby eliminating the need for a condensing surface. Such pumps are expensive and usually practical only in large installations.

Available freeze-driers* range in size from small laboratory units to large industrial models such as those shown in Fig. 591. Their selection requires consideration of such factors as tray area required, volume of water to be removed, whether or not aseptic processing will be involved, is internal stoppering required, will separate freezers be used for initial freezing of the product, and the degree of automatic operation desired.[47]

Freeze-drying is now being utilized for research in the preservation of human tissue and is finding increasing application in the food industry. Progress on new developments is being made in both the process and the equipment.

---

* Suppliers: *Hull; Industrial Dynamics; NRC; Repp; Stokes; Thermovac; Virtis.*

Quality Control

The importance of undertaking every possible means to be assured of the quality of the finished product cannot be overemphasized. Every component and every step of the manufacturing process must be subjected to intense scrutiny to be confident that quality is attained in the finished product. The responsibility for supervising this is a grave one, and lapses of requirements or short cuts in procedure may not be permitted. Such responsibility applies wherever parenteral preparations are manufactured.

The principles of quality control are basically the same for the manufacture of any pharmaceutical.

These are discussed beginning on page 1762. During the discussion of the preparation of injections, mention was made of numerous quality requirements for components and manufacturing processes. Here, only certain tests characteristically applicable to parenteral preparations will be discussed.

Sterility Test

All lots of injections in their final containers must be tested for sterility. The USP prescribes the requirements for this test for official injections. The

Food and Drug Administration uses these requirements as a guide for testing unofficial sterile products. The official test has acknowledged limitations in the information that it can provide. Therefore, it should be noted that this test is not intended as a thoroughly evaluative test for a product subjected to a sterilization method of unknown effectiveness. It is intended primarily as a check test on the repetition of a previously proved sterilization procedure, or to give assurance of its continued effectiveness. A discussion of sterility testing is given on page 1503.

It should be noted that a "lot" with respect to sterility testing is that group of product containers which has been subjected to the same sterilization procedure. For containers of a product which have been sterilized by autoclaving, for example, a lot would constitute those processed in a particular sterilizer cycle. For an aseptic filling operation, a lot would constitute all of those product containers filled during a period when there was no change in the filling assembly or equipment and which is no longer than one working day or shift.

Pyrogen Test

The presence of pyrogens in parenteral preparations is evaluated by a qualitative fever response test in rabbits. The USP test is described on page 644. Rabbits are used as test animals because they show physiologic response to pyrogenic substances similar to that by man. While a minimum pyrogenic dose (MPD), the amount just sufficient to cause a positive USP Pyrogen Test response, may sometimes produce uncertain test results, a content equal to a few times the MPD will leave no uncertainty. Therefore, the test is valid and has remained first in choice since introduced by Seibert[48] in 1923. It should be understood that not all injections may be subjected to the pyrogen test since the medicinal agent may have a physiologic effect on the test animal such that any fever response would be masked. Therefore, the pyrogen test is performed primarily on vehicles.

Clarity Tests

The USP does not provide specifications for a clarity test. It contains only the following statement:

Good pharmaceutical practice requires also that each final container of Injection be subjected individually to a physical inspection, whenever the nature of the container permits.

The development of test procedures to meet this general requirement is the responsibility of the manufacturer.

The objective of the clarity inspection is to prevent the distribution and use of parenterals which contain particulate matter that may be psychologically or actually harmful to the recipient. Solutions to be introduced intravenously require the most critical evaluation.

Until recently, concern about particulate matter in parenteral solutions was limited largely to the psychological effect on the user in that the presence of visible "dirt" would suggest that the product was of inferior quality. With the report of Garvan and Gunner,[49] a new assessment of the significance of particles in solutions to be introduced into the blood stream has been undertaken. While data defining the extent and risk of toxic effects is still rather

nebulous, it has been shown that particles of lint, rubber, insoluble chemicals, and other foreign particulate matter can produce emboli in vital organs of animals[50] and man.

A study of the size distribution of particulate matter in commercial intravenous solutions showed that the number of particles increased approximately logarithmically with decreasing size.[51] The counts were made with a Coulter Counter,* a resistance-type counter. This finding would suggest that a count made at an arbitrarily chosen size could be used to predict the number of particles at another size.

Particles may also be counted and examined microscopically by collection on the surface of a membrane filter,[52] a method that permits identification of the particles as well as a count. Methods of particulate evaluation such as these are performed on a sample from a container. Such methods cannot be utilized for the in-line evaluation of every container produced commercially, but may be used for quality-control sampling of the process.

The particle size that should be of particular concern has not been determined but it has been suggested that, since erythrocytes have a diameter of approximately 4.5μ, particles of more than 5μ should be the basis for evaluation.[53] This is a considerably smaller particle than can be seen with the unaided eye; approximately 50μ is the lower limit unless the Tyndall effect is utilized, whereby particles as small as 10μ may be seen by the light scattered from them.

This new concern over the presence of particulate matter in parenteral products will eventually lead to the development of new standards of evaluation and new refinements in processing techniques. Whatever form they take, the patient will be the recipient of cleaner and better products as a result of the continuing search for technological improvement.

Meanwhile, the product units from the production line will be inspected individually by human inspectors under a good light, baffled against reflection into the eye, against a black and a white background. Although this inspection is subject to the limitations in the size of particles that can be seen, the variation in visual acuity from inspector to inspector, the emotional state of the inspector, eye strain and fatigue, and other personal factors that will affect what the inspector sees, it does provide a means for eliminating the normally few units which contain visible particles and it is a check on the repetition of the standard clean processing procedure established for that product.

Leaker Test

Ampuls that have been sealed by fusion must be subjected to a test to determine whether or not a passageway remains to the outside. If such a passageway remains, all or a part of the contents of the ampul may leak to the outside and spoil the package, or microorganisms or other contaminants may enter. Changes in temperature during storage cause expansion and contraction of the ampul and contents, and will accentuate interchange if a passageway exists.

A leaker test is usually performed by producing a negative pressure within an incompletely sealed ampul while the ampul is entirely submerged in a deeply colored dye solution.[54] Most often, approximately a 1% methylene blue solution is employed. The test

---

* Supplier: *Coulter*.

may be performed by subjecting the ampuls to a vacuum in a vacuum chamber, the ampuls being submerged in a dye bath throughout the process. Another procedure frequently employed is to simply autoclave the ampuls in a dye bath. A modification of this is to remove them from the autoclave while hot and quickly submerge them in a cool bath of dye solution. After carefully rinsing the dye solution from the outside, color from the dye will be visible within a leaker. Leakers are, of course, discarded.

Vials and bottles are not subjected to a leaker test because the sealing material is not rigid. Therefore, results from such a test would be meaningless.

Safety Test

The National Institutes of Health requires of most biological products routine safety testing in animals. Under the new Kefauver-Harris Amendments to the Federal Food, Drug, and Cosmetic Act, most pharmaceutical preparations will now be required to be tested for safety. Because it is entirely possible for a parenteral product to pass the routine sterility test, pyrogen test, and chemical analyses and still cause unfavorable reactions when injected, a safety test in animals is essential to provide additional assurance that the product does not have unexpected toxic properties. Safety tests in animals are discussed in detail in the USP.

Packaging and Labeling

A full discussion of the packaging of parenteral preparations is beyond the scope of this text. It is essential, of course, that the packaging should provide ample protection for the product against physical damage from shipping, handling, and storage and should protect light-sensitive materials from ultraviolet radiation.

Packaging—The USP states certain other requirements for the packaging and storage of Injections:

The volume of injection in single-dose containers provides the amount specified for parenteral administration at one time and in no case is more than sufficient to permit the withdrawal and administration of one liter.

Preparations intended for intraspinal, intracisternal, or peridural administration are packaged only in single-dose containers.

Unless otherwise specified in the individual monograph, no multiple-dose container contains a volume of Injection more than sufficient to permit the withdrawal of 30 ml.

Injections labeled for veterinary use are exempt from packaging and storage requirements concerning the limitation to single-dose containers and the limitation on the volume of multiple-dose containers.

Labeling—The labeling of an injection must provide the physician or other user with all of the information needed to assure the safe and proper use of the therapeutic agent. Since all of this information cannot be placed on the immediate container and be legible, it may be provided on accompanying printed matter.

The labeling requirements of the USP for Injections are as follows:

The term "labeling" designates all labels and other written, printed, or graphic matter upon an immediate container of a preparation or upon, or in, any package or wrapper in which it is enclosed,

except any outer shipping container. The term "label" designates that part of the labeling upon the immediate container.

The label states the name of the preparation; in the case of a liquid preparation, the percentage content of drug or amount of drug in a specified volume; and in the case of a dry preparation, the amount of *active* ingredient. The volume of liquid to be added to prepare an injection or suspension from a dry preparation may be given in the labeling. Also, the label indicates the name of the manufacturer or distributor and an identifying lot number. The lot number is capable of yielding the complete manufacturing history of the specific package, including any single manufacturing, filling, and sterilizing operations.

The container is so labeled that a sufficient area of the container remains uncovered for its full length or circumference to permit inspection of the contents.

The labeling of packages of immediate containers indicates the vehicle used in the Injection, if other than water for injection, identifying it by name with an official preparation or, otherwise, giving its composition, and stating the constituents and the percentage of them present; the names and proportions of all substances added to increase stability or usefulness; and the expiration date, where required by the individual monograph.

Injections intended for veterinary use are labeled to that effect.

Preparations labeled for use as irrigation solutions meet the requirements for Injections other than those relating to volume, and, in addition, bear label statements to the effect that such solutions are not intended for injection.

References

1. Griffenhagen, G. B., *Bull. Parenteral Drug Assoc.,* **16**(2), 12 (1962).
2. Patel, J. A., and Phillips, G. L., *Am. J. Hosp. Pharm.,* **23**, 409 (1966).
3. Pelissier, N. A., and Burgee, S. L., Jr., *Hosp. Pharm.,* **3**, 15 (Jan., 1968).
4. Sr. Mary Virginia, *Hosp. Pharm.,* **2**, 7 (Aug., 1967).
5. Parker, E. A., *et al, Bull. Parenteral Drug Assoc.,* **21**, 197 (1967).
6. Carlin, H. S., and Perkins, A. J., *Am. J. Hosp. Pharm.,* **25**, 271 (1968).
7. Everett, N. A., *Bull. Parenteral Drug Assoc.,* **15**(5), 1 (1961).
8. Beck, W. D., *et al, Materials Protection,* **6**(6), 50 (1967).
9. Saylor, H. M., *Bull. Parenteral Drug Assoc.,* **19**, 132 (1965).
10. Spiegel, A. J., and Noseworthy, M. M., *J. Pharm. Sci.,* **52**, 917 (1963).
11. Sykes, G., *J. Pharm. Pharmacol.,* **10**, 40T (1958).
12. Eisman, P. C., *et al, J. APhA, Sci. Ed.,* **42**, 659 (1953).
13. Bandelin, F., and Tuschoff, J., *Bull. Parenteral Drug Assoc.,* **11**(3), 16 (1957).
14. Pisano, F. D., and Kostenbauder, H. B., *J. APhA, Sci. Ed.,* **48**, 310 (1959).
15. Lachman, L., *et al, J. Pharm. Sci.,* **52**, 244 (1963).
16. Windheuser, J. J., *Bull. Parenteral Drug Assoc.,* **17**(5), 1 (1963).
17. Schroeter, L. C., *J. Pharm. Sci.,* **50**, 891 (1961).
18. Todd, J. P., *Pharm. J.,* **185**, 53 (July 16, 1960).
19. Whittet, T. D., *J. Pharm. Pharmacol.,* **8**, 1034 (1956).
20. Autian, J., *J. Pharm. Sci.,* **52**, 1, 105 (1963).
21. Autian, J., *Bull. Parenteral Drug Assoc.,* **22**, 276 (1968).
22. Mullins, J. D., *Bull. Parenteral Drug Assoc.,* **22**, 38 (1968).
23. O'Leary, R. K., and Guess, W. L., *J. Pharm. Sci.,* **57**, 12 (1968).
24. Subrahmanyam, S. V., and Majeske, J. P., *Am. J. Pharm.,* **129**, 222 (1957).
25. Greene, J. F., and Hinson, A. L., *Bull. NF Comm.,* **17**(2), 48 (1949).
26. Majeske, J. F., *Bull. Parenteral Drug Assoc.,* **16**(4), 1 (1962).
27. Garvey, B. S., *Bull. Parenteral Drug Assoc.,* **16**(1), 1 (1962).
28. Portner, P. E., *Bull. Parenteral Drug Assoc.,* **14**(1), 17 (1960).
29. Lachman, L., *et al, J. Pharm. Sci.,* **52**, 244 (1963).
30. Hopkins, G. H., *J. Pharm. Sci.,* **54**, 138 (1965).
31. Whitfield, W. J., *et al, Reprint SC-R-64-145A,* Sandia Corp., Albuquerque, N.M, 1964.
32. Bowman, F. W., *Bull. Parenteral Drug Assoc.,* **22**, 57 (1968).
33. Beck, R. P., *Bull. Parenteral Drug Assoc.,* **22**, 222 (1968).
34. Weatherwax, R. S., *J. Bacteriol.,* **72**, 329 (1956).
35. *Federal Std. No. 209a,* General Services Admin., Washington, D.C. 20407, Aug. 10, 1966.
36. *F 25-63T,* Am. Soc. for Testing & Materials, Philadelphia, 1963.
37. Barclay, E. S., *Am. J. Pharm.,* **129**, 313 (1957).
38. Avis, K. E., *et al, Am. J. Hosp. Pharm.,* **18**, 223 (1961).
39. Macek, T. J., *J. Pharm. Sci.,* **52**, 694 (1963).
40. Nash, R. A., *Drug Cosmetic Ind.,* **97**, 843 (1965); **98**, 39 (1966).
41. Avis, K. E., *Am. J. Pharm.,* **129**, 410 (1957).
42. *Ann. NY Acad. Sci.,* **85**, 501–734 (1965).
43. Flosdorf, E. W., *et al, J. Immunol.,* **50**, 21 (1945).
44. Lachman, L., *et al, J. Pharm. Sci.,* **54**, 1342 (1965).
45. MacKenzie, A. P., *Bull. Parenteral Drug Assoc.,* **20**, 101 (1966).
46. Gross, H. M., *Drug Cosmetic Ind.,* **75**, 468 (1954).
47. Thompson, T. N., *Bull. Parenteral Drug Assoc.,* **19**, 33 (1965).
48. Seibert, F. B., *Am. J. Physiol.,* **67**, 90 (1923).
49. Garvan, J. M., and Gunner, B. W., *Med. J. Australia,* **2**, 1 (July 4, 1964).
50. Gross, M. A., *Drug Intelligence,* **1**, 12 (1967).
51. Vessey, I., and Kendall, C. E., *Analyst,* **91**, 273 (1966).
52. Trasen, B., *Bull. Parenteral Drug Assoc.,* **22**, 1 (1968).
53. Groves, M. J., *J. Pharm. Pharmacol.,* **18**, 161 (1965).
54. Artz, W. J., *et al, J. Pharm. Sci.,* **50**, 258 (1961).

83 | Ophthalmic Solutions

Anatomy and physiology of the eye—administration—preparation—
properties—sterilization—preservation—packaging—application and
use—contact lenses and their solutions

This chapter was prepared by

Dwight L. Deardorff, PhD, *Professor of Manufacturing Pharmacy, College of
Pharmacy, University of Illinois, Chicago, Ill. 60612*

Ophthalmic solutions are sterile aqueous or oily solutions of alkaloids, alkaloidal salts, antibiotics, sulfonamides, steroids, enzymes, antihistamines, dyes, metabolic antagonists, or other substances. Such solutions are intended for instillation into the cul-de-sac, that is, the space between the eyeball and the eyelids.

Ophthalmic solutions may be used either as drops (eye drops) or as washes (eye lotions). The effects desired from this medication include anesthetic, anti-infective, anti-inflammatory, miotic, mydriatic, cycloplegic, hypotensive, astringent, or antiseptic action. It may also function as a lubricant or as a substitute for tears.

Pain—In addition to therapeutic effects, topical application of medications to the eye may have the effect of discomfort, pain, or actual tissue damage. These potential effects should be kept in mind by the pharmacist. Riegelman and Vaughan[1] have pointed out that there are potential causes of pain directly related to the properties of the drug itself. These include the surface-active and protein-denaturation reactions of many of the local anesthetics, heavy metal salts, and quaternaries at high concentrations. Superficial corneal damage may result. This response may be cumulative, each additional instillation increasing the damage and concomitant pain.

The possibility of pain caused by the vehicle is discussed in later sections.

Frequency of Use—Many pathological conditions of the eye require both local and systemic administration of drugs. A general examination of the eye typically requires instillation of a variety of medicinal preparations which may be diagnostic or therapeutic in nature. This means that a given multiple-dose container of medication may be used with many patients during a single day, and if contaminated may have a widespread effect.

Anatomy and Physiology of the Eye[2-6]

The human eye is an excellent subject for the topical administration of drugs. The basis of this can be found in the anatomical arrangement of the surface tissues and in the permeability of the cornea. Since time immemorial, medicinals have been "instilled" into the eye. The protective operation of the eyelids and lacrimal system is such that there is rapid removal of material instilled into the eye, unless the material is chemically and physiologically compatible with surface tissues. This means that an understanding of the anatomy and physiology of the eye is needed for proper formulation and use of ophthalmic medicinals (Figs. 592[7] and 593[7]).

Eyelids—Between the anterior surface of the eyeball and the outside world there is interposed an ante-

chamber which serves two purposes: mechanical protection of the globe and creation of an optimum milieu for the cornea. The eyelids form the outer wall of this antechamber and the conjunctiva its lining. It is lubricated and kept fluid-filled by the secretions of the lacrimal glands and other glands. The antechamber has the shape of a narrow cleft directly over the front of the eyeball, with pocket-like extensions upward and downward. The pockets are called the superior and inferior fornix (vault), and the entire space the cul-de-sac (bottom of the bag). The elliptical opening between the eyelids is called the palpebral fissure.

Eyeball—The human eyeball (bulbus, globe) is approximately spherical. Its wall is composed of three concentric layers or tunics.

1. The outer fibrous tunic.
2. A middle vascular tunic—the uvea or uveal tract, consisting of the choroid, the ciliary body, and the iris.
3. A nervous tunic—the retina.

The outer tunic is tough, pliable, but only slightly stretchable. In its front portion—the portion facing the outside world—the fine structure of the outer tunic is so regular and the water content so carefully adjusted that it acts as a clear transparent window (the cornea). Over the remaining two thirds the fibrous coat is opaque (the "white" of the eye) and is called the sclera. It ordinarily contains very few blood vessels.

The eyeball houses an optical apparatus that causes inverted reduced images of the outside world to form on the retina which is a thin translucent membrane. The optical apparatus consists, in sequence, of the cornea, the pupil, and the crystalline lens, with layers of clear fluid or gel-like material interposed between the solid structures. The pupil, a round centric hole in a contractile membranous partition (called the iris), acts as the variable aperture of the system. The crystalline lens is a refractive element with variable power controlled and supported by a muscle incorporated in the ciliary body. The choroid is the metabolic support for the retina.

The optical function of the eye calls for the stability of its dimensions which is provided partly by the fibrous outer coat; more effective as a stabilizing factor is the intraocular pressure which is in excess of the pressure prevailing in the surrounding tissues. This intraocular pressure is the result of a steady production of specific fluid, the aqueous humor, which originates from the ciliary processes* and leaves the eye by an intricate system of outflow channels. The resistance encountered during this passage and the rate of aqueous production are the principal factors determining the level of the intraocular pressure. In addition to this

---

* Ciliary processes: fin-like inward projections of the ciliary body.

hydromechanical function, the aqueous humor acts as a carrier of nutrients, substrates, and metabolites for the avascular tissues of the eye.

The bones of the skull join to form an approximately pyramid-shaped housing for the eyeball, called the orbit. The open bases of the orbits face the outside world.

Conjunctiva—The conjunctival membrane covers the outer surface of the white portion of the eye and the inner aspect of the eyelids. In most places it is loosely attached and thereby permits free movement of the eyeball. This makes possible subconjunctival injections. Next to the cornea the conjunctiva is the most exposed portion of the eye.

Lacrimal System—The conjunctival and corneal surfaces are covered and lubricated by a film of fluid secreted by the conjunctival and the lacrimal glands. The secretion of the lacrimal gland, the tears, is delivered through a number of fine ducts into the conjunctival fornix. The secretion is a clear, watery fluid containing 0.7% protein and the enzyme lysozyme. Small accessory lacrimal glands are situated in the conjunctival fornices. Their secretion suffices for lubrication and cleansing under ordinary conditions and for maintaining a thin fluid film covering the cornea and conjunctiva (the precorneal film). The main lacrimal gland is called into play only on special occasions. The sebaceous glands of the eyelids secrete an oily fluid. This helps to prevent overflowing of tears at the lid margin and reduces evaporation from the exposed surfaces of the eye by spreading over the tear film.

Spontaneous blinking occurs 10–20 times a minute. Each blink replenishes the fluid film by pushing a thin layer of fluid ahead of the lid margins as they come together. The excess fluid is directed into the lacrimal lake—a small triangular area lying in the angle bounded by the innermost portions of the lids. The

skin of the eyelids is the thinnest in the body and folds easily, thus permitting rapid opening and closing of the palpebral fissures. The movement of the eyelids includes a narrowing of the palpebral fissures in a zipper-like action from the lateral canthus toward the medial canthus.* This aids the transport or movement of fluid toward the lacrimal lake.

The tears are drained from the lacrimal lake by two small tubes—the lacrimal canaliculi. The minute orifices of the latter—the puncta lacrimalia—may be seen on the margin of each lid close to the medial canthus. The lacrimal canaliculi lead into the upper part of the nasolacrimal duct, the roomy beginning of which is called the lacrimal sac. The drainage of tears into the nose does not depend merely on gravity. Fluid enters and passes along the lacrimal canaliculi by capillary attraction aided by aspiration caused by a contraction of a muscle embedded in the eyelids. When the lids close, as in blinking, contraction of the muscle causes dilation of the upper part of the lacrimal sac and compression of its lower portion. Tears are thus aspirated into the sac, and any which have collected in its lower part are forced down the nasolacrimal duct toward its opening into the nose. As the lids open, the muscle relaxes. The upper part of the sac then collapses and forces fluid into the lower part, which at the same time is released from compression. Thus, the act of blinking exerts a suction—force—pump action in removing the tears from the lacrimal lake and emptying them into the nasal cavity. Lacrimation is induced reflexly by stimulation of nerve endings of the cornea or conjunctiva. The reflex is abolished by anesthetization of the surface of the eye, and by disorders affecting its nerve components.

The normal cul-de-sac is usually free of pathogenic organisms and often found sterile. The sterility may be due partly to the action of lysozyme in the tears, which normally destroys saprophytic organisms, but has little action against pathogens. More effective in producing sterility may be the fact that the sterile

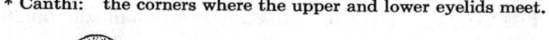

*Canthi: the corners where the upper and lower eyelids meet.

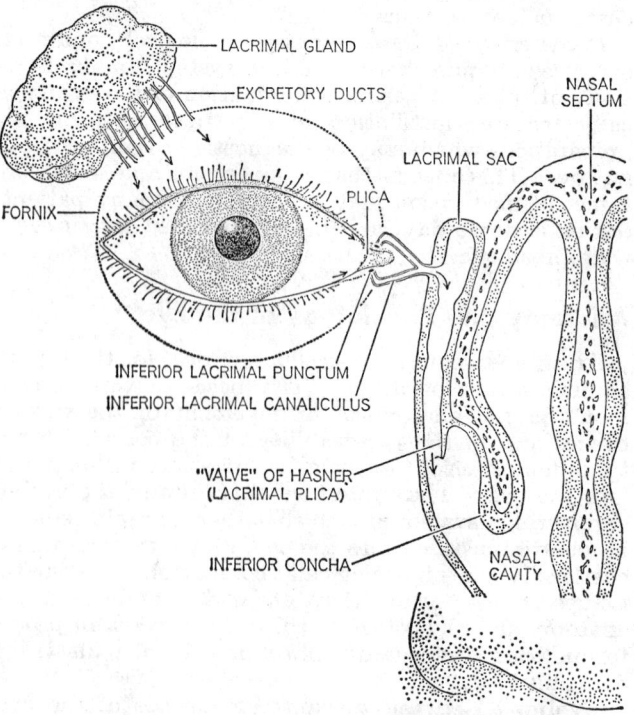

Fig. 592. The eye: vertical section (courtesy, Botelho[7]).

Fig. 593. Nasolacrimal duct (courtesy, Botelho[7]).

tears constantly wash the bacteria, dust, etc, down into the nose. In certain diseases the lacrimal gland, like other glandular structures in the body, undergoes involution, with the result that the lacrimal fluid becomes scanty. Furthermore, changes in the conjunctival glands may lead to alteration in the character of the secretion so that quality as well as quantity of tears may be abnormal. This may lead to symptoms of dryness, burning, and general discomfort and may interfere with visual acuity.

Cornea—The cornea is from 0.5 to 1 mm in thickness. Its three principal layers lie in the following order (from the front backwards):

1. Corneal epithelium.
2. Substantia propria (stroma).
3. Corneal endothelium.

The cornea is transparent to ordinary diffuse light, largely because of a special laminar arrangement of the cells and fibers and because of the absence of blood vessels. The essential factor is probably the well-ordered arrangement of the collagen fibers in the corneal laminae. The important point about this transparency is not that there is but little loss of light by absorption, which merely affects the luminosity of the retinal image, but that the amount of light scattered is small, which adds to the sharpness of the retinal image.[5] Scattering is due to the presence of particles of different refractive index from that of the matrix material. Cloudiness of the cornea may be due to any one of several factors including excess pressure in the eyeball as in glaucoma; scar tissue, as due to injury or infection; or deficiency of oxygen or excess hydration such as may occur during the wearing of improperly fitted contact lenses. A wound of the cornea usually heals as an opaque patch which would be a permanent disability unless it is located in the periphery of the cornea.

The chief refraction of light for the eye occurs at the outer surface of the cornea where the index of refraction changes from that of air (1.00) to that of corneal substance (1.38). Any alteration in its shape or transparency interferes with the formation of a clear image, therefore, any pathologic process, however slight, may interfere seriously with the resolving power or visual acuity of the eye. The normal corneal surface forms a perfect reflecting surface, and any defect in it can be detected at once by the disturbances of this mirror reflection.

The outer surfaces of the cornea and of the conjunctiva are kept moist by the tears and the secretion of the glands inbedded in the conjunctiva. The protein content of the tears helps to give them a low surface tension and enables them to wet the epithelial surface more perfectly.

The normal cornea possesses no blood vessels except at the corneoscleral junction. The cornea, therefore, must derive its nutrition by diffusion and must have certain permeability characteristics. In addition to the nutrient supply that comes in through the blood vessels at the corneo-scleral junction the cornea receives nourishment from the fluid circulating through the chambers of the eye and also from the air. The fact that the cornea is devoid of blood vessels is an important feature in surgical grafting. The corneal nerves do not supply all forms of sensation to the cornea. Pain and cold are well supplied. The pain fibers have a very low threshold which makes the cornea one of the most sensitive portions of the body's surface. It is now generally agreed that the cornea

possesses a true sense of touch; nerve endings supplying the sensation of heat are lacking.

The corneal epithelium provides an efficient barrier against bacterial invasion. Unless its continuity has been broken by an abrasion (a traumatic opening or defect in the epithelium) pathogenic bacteria, as a rule, cannot gain a foothold. Trauma, therefore, plays an important part in most of the infectious diseases of the cornea which occur exogenously. Any foreign body which either scratches the cornea or lodges and becomes imbedded in the cornea is of serious moment because of the role it may play in permitting pyogenic bacteria to gain a foothold.

Small foreign bodies on the cornea may be missed unless good focal illumination and a magnifying loupe is available. A means of detecting abrasions on the corneal surface is afforded by staining the cornea with fluorescein. In one technique 1 or 2 drops of a sterile 2% aqueous solution of sodium fluorescein are instilled into the cul-de-sac, and after allowing a few seconds for staining to occur, the excess is washed out with sterile normal saline or sterile boric acid solution. If there is an abrasion of the epithelium, the underlying layer stains a brilliant green, so that even pinpoint abrasions show up quite clearly. Abrasion may occur during tonometry, that is, during the measurement of ocular tension with a tonometer. Care must be used in applying the device to the cornea to avoid abrasion of the cornea. Corneal abrasions sometimes result from wearing contact lenses. Every corneal abrasion is subject to infection.

Absorption through the Cornea—As stated previously, the therapeutic effect of many topically administered (instilled) drugs is contingent upon their absorption from the cul-de-sac into the eye. Drugs which are administered by instillation and which must penetrate into the eye enter primarily through the cornea, as it is a much more effective route into the eye than the conjunctiva and underlying sclera.

The conjunctiva contains many blood vessels and lymphatic vessels. The blood vessels usually dilate when irritation is set up by a foreign body, a microbial infection, or by chemical means. Of the drug molecules which penetrate into the conjunctiva a large proportion enters the blood stream where they may cause undesirable systemic reactions. Below the conjunctiva lies the sclera, which water-soluble drugs penetrate with ease and which lipoid-soluble drugs penetrate with difficulty.

A good many of the molecules of the active drug which have been instilled do not penetrate the eyeball but instead are washed into the nasal cavity by the lacrimal drainage system. It should be noted that systemic effects, sometimes of major significance, have been reported following the topical instillation of cycloplegics,[8,9] miotics,[10,227] sympathomimetics, anticholinesterases, and steroids.[11]

Most ophthalmic solutions are so formulated as to mix readily with the lacrimal fluids and spread over the surfaces of the cornea and conjunctiva. With the usual technique of instillation the major portion of the drug is deposited in the lower fornix. Capillarity, diffusional forces, and the blinking reflex are the forces that bring about the incorporation of the drug in the precorneal film from which it penetrates into and through the cornea.

Experiments with solutions of the strongly fluorescent sodium fluorescein indicate that the constituents of eye drops remain in visible contact with the cornea as long as 5 to 6 minutes. The work of Cogan, *et al*,[12–15]

Swan and White,[16] and others indicates that a substance will pass through the cornea most easily if it has a biphasic solubility, that is, if it is soluble both in fat and in water.

The epithelium and the endothelium are rich in lipoids. The stroma is poor in lipoids and is of an aqueous nature. The epithelium is said to contain a hundred times as much lipoid material as the stroma. The epithelium and endothelium will be penetrated relatively readily by material which is lipoid soluble. Penetration of the stroma is more feasible in general with water-soluble material. One way to have biphasic solubility is to have a material which can exist in an equilibrium situation containing both fat-soluble and water-soluble moieties.

Many ophthalmic drugs are weak bases and are applied to the eye in aqueous solutions of their salts. The free base and the salt will be in an equilibrium which will depend on the pH and on the individual characteristics of the compound. To aid in maintaining storage stability and solubility, the medication may be acidic at the moment of instillation but usually the neutralizing action of the lacrimal fluid will convert it instantaneously to the physiological pH range (approximately pH 7.4) at which there will be enough free base present to begin the penetration of the cornea.

Kinsey[2] has described the following concept for the transfer of a weak base, eg, the alkaloid homatropine, through the intact cornea. As it is used clinically, a solution of homatropine hydrobromide contains homatropine ions (positive R_3NH^+), bromide ions, undissociated homatropine hydrobromide, and a small amount of the homatropine free base (undissociated R_3N). The ratio undissociated/dissociated particles depends on the prevailing pH. At a pH of 6.0, for example, the ratio of the amount of dissociated homatropine to the undissociated portion has been estimated as being about 1000 to 1. When a drop of this solution is placed on the cornea, the undissociated free base penetrates the epithelium because of its lipoid solubility. The dissociated remainder cannot penetrate the epithelium to any extent as it is not fat soluble. Once inside the epithelium the undissociated free base immediately dissociates to a degree. Again the homatropine will exist in both the dissociated and undissociated forms. The dissociated moiety will then tend to penetrate the stroma because it is water soluble, whereas the undissociated fraction cannot penetrate to any extent. At the junction of the stroma and endothelium the same process that took place at the outer surface of the epithelium must again occur. Finally, the dissociated homatropine leaves the endothelium for the aqueous humor. Here it can readily diffuse to the iris and the ciliary body, the site of its pharmacological action. In each of these four steps the substance is able to penetrate because of the difference in solubility of the two forms in which it exists. The process of transfer will not be limited by the exhaustion of the amount of homatropine present in any one form since, as soon as one molecule of either form (dissociated or undissociated) leaves the layer, redissociation or reassociation takes place and the process continues as before.

Maurice has written a comprehensive review on the permeability of the cornea.[17,18] The cornea can be penetrated by ions to a small, but measurable, degree. Under comparable conditions, the permeabilities are similar for all ions of small molecular weight, which suggests that the passage is through the extracellular spaces. The diameter of the largest particles which can pass across the cellular layers seems to be in the range 10–25 Å. Increase in the permeability of the cellular layers can be produced by experimental techniques which involve slight manipulations such as touching the cornea, or instilling solutions differing in tonicity from that of the body fluids, or even stirring the solution in contact with the corneal surface.

Administration

Reasons for Instillation

In many instances only topical effects are desired and drugs are administered for local effect without need for penetration into the eyeball. Examples are medication for superficial anti-infective effects as in inflammation of the conjunctiva.

The drugs which penetrate into the eye when administered topically are, in general, alkaloids, most corticosteroids, and some local anesthetics. Fluorescein and the sulfonamides penetrate to some degree. These drugs penetrate as far as the ciliary body and therefore are used when given in this way to treat the anterior segment of the eye. For example, the use of topically administered corticosteroids is indicated only for inflammation of the anterior portion of the uveal tract.

Systemic administration in general does not accomplish as much as topical administration in the treatment of the anterior segment of the eye. The blood–aqueous barrier constituted of the blood vessel wall and various thicknesses of the ocular tissues prevents certain drugs from reaching the anterior segment in therapeutic concentrations if administered systemically. Some drugs may do so only if administered systemically in quantities that would cause harm in other parts of the body.

In the inflamed eye permeability of the blood–aqueous barrier is increased, allowing some drugs administered systemically to reach the anterior chamber of an inflamed eye in therapeutic quantities.

Comparison of Instilled Preparations[6]

In addition to ophthalmic solutions, suspensions and ointments can be topically administered by instillation.

Solutions are the most commonly used type of preparation for the local medication of eyes. They are easily instilled and rarely cause adverse reactions. The vehicle does not cause interference with vision and does not interfere with regeneration of the corneal epithelium. Their chief disadvantage is that they do not remain in contact with the eye as long as desired so it may be necessary to instill the solution at relatively frequent intervals in order to achieve therapeutic results.

Oily solutions such as for medicaments which are incompatible with water are infrequently used. The only official ophthalmic solution using oil is that of isoflurophate.

Suspensions of corticosteroids are used to some extent. They are stated to have the advantage of more extended action and the disadvantage that it is difficult to avoid the presence of a few particles which are large enough to cause irritation.

Ointments are frequently used. They have the advantages of more prolonged contact and effect, hardly any irritation on initial installation, slower movement into lacrimal ducts, greater storage stability, and less likelihood of contamination problems. Their disadvantages are that they produce a film over the eye and thereby blur vision; and they may interfere with the firm attachment of new corneal epithelial cells to their normal base.

Other Nonsystemic Modes of Administration

Packs—These are sometimes used to give prolonged contact of the solution with the eye. A cotton pledget is saturated with an ophthalmic solution and this pledget is inserted into the superior or inferior fornix. Packs are commonly used to produce maximal mydriasis. In this case the cotton pledgets can be, for example, saturated with phenylephrine solution.

Iontophoresis—This procedure keeps the solution in contact with the cornea in an eyecup bearing an electrode. Diffusion of the drug is effected by difference of electrical potential.[20]

Subconjunctival Injections[6]—Subconjunctival injections are frequently used to introduce medications which, if instilled, either do not penetrate into the anterior segment or penetrate too slowly for the desired effect. The drug is injected underneath the conjunctiva and probably passes through the sclera and into the eye by simple diffusion. The most common use of subconjunctival injection is for the administration of antibiotics in infections of the anterior segment of the eye. Subconjunctival injections of mydriatics and cycloplegics are also used to achieve maximal pupillary dilation or relaxation of the ciliary muscle. If the drug is injected underneath the conjunctiva and the underlying Tenon's capsule in the more posterior portion of the eye, effects on the ciliary body, choroid, and retina can be obtained.

Retrobulbar Injections[6]—Drugs administered by retrobulbar injection may enter the globe in essentially the same manner as the medications given subconjunctivally. The orbit is not well vascularized and the possibility of significant via-blood stream effects of retrobulbar injections is very remote. In general, retrobulbar injections are given for the purpose of getting medications into the posterior segment of the globe and to affect the nerves and other structures in the retrobulbar space.

Preparation

Precautions

Records indicate that there are more law suits instituted against pharmacists on the basis of ophthalmic solutions than any other class of prescriptions. Solutions for use in the eye should be prepared with meticulous care because its mucous membranes are very sensitive, particularly if they are already inflamed, eg, when the eyes are traumatized by accident, disease, or surgery. The instillation of eye drops may create problems much more serious than is often realized.

The NF states:

"The sterility of solutions applied to the injured eye is of the greatest importance. Sterile preparations in special containers for individual use on one patient should be available in every hospital, office, or other installation where accidentally or surgically traumatized eyes are treated."

Riegelman and Vaughan stated:[22]

"The use of a contaminated solution on an eye may result in serious infection and loss of the eye. An injured eye has even less resistance to infection than the blood-stream so that at least the same precautions should be taken in preparing ophthalmic solutions as in preparing solutions for intravenous use."

As an aid in safeguarding this class of preparation, many pharmacists are providing a special department for use only in preparing ophthalmic products. The department is frequently segregated from the rest of the prescription section. A special set of utensils and a separate set of ingredients is held for use in this department only. The availability of small, low-cost laminar-flow hoods should aid this trend.

A series of three articles by Riegelman and Vaughan is of particular value.[1,21,22] Other general articles along this line have been written by Anderson,[23] Cadwallader,[24] and others.[25,26]

Accuracy—Accidental substitution of one type of drug for another can have serious consequences, as for example the substitution of a mydriatic for a miotic. The miotic pilocarpine is used in glaucoma to increase the rate of outflow of aqueous humor and thus reduce intraocular pressure. If atropine were accidentally used in certain types of glaucoma, the dilation of the eye would block the aqueous outflow and could cause an acute attack of glaucoma. Surgical intervention may be required to save the eye if the use of atropine antagonists is unable to reverse the mydriasis. This type of accident may seem to be quite unlikely, but in filtration of solutions of ophthalmic drugs, for example, unless special precautions are taken, some drugs may remain in the filter system and be carried into the succeeding solution being filtered. This gives the basis for the recommendation that there are several sets of filters, one for each type of ophthalmic drug.

Scopolamine (hyoscine) is usually used in a 0.2% solution. Accidental use of a 1% solution has been known to cause severe systemic toxicity. Murphy, et al,[27] emphasized the need to pay particular attention to substances which carry several moles of water of hydration. For example, Zinc Sulfate USP contains almost 50% water by weight; the use of the fully effloresced salt would almost double the intended concentration of the active ingredient and would produce a highly irritating eye solution.

Cleanliness and Sterility—Cleanliness and sterility are of the utmost importance in the proper preparation of eye solutions. Official cognizance has been taken of the danger of infection by the drafting of federal regulations in 1953,[28] and later, requiring manufacturers and dispensers of eye medicaments to prepare sterile solutions to which suitable preservatives have been added. The US Food and Drug Administration (FDA) statement is as follows:

"Investigations by pharmaceutical manufacturers, physicians, and the Food and Drug Administration have revealed that liquid preparations for ophthalmic use contaminated with viable microorganisms have been responsible for serious eye injuries and, in some cases, loss of vision. The Administration has conducted a survey and has found that is is the consensus of informed medical opinion that such preparations should be sterile. It is evident that liquid preparations offered or intended for ophthalmic use, including cosmetic-type preparations for cleansing the eyes and contact-lens solutions, purport to be of such purity and quality as to be suitable for safe use in the eye. The Administration concludes that such preparations fall below their professed standard of purity or quality and may be unsafe for use if they are not sterile. Accordingly such liquid preparations offered or intended for ophthalmic use that are not sterile may be regarded as adulterated within the meaning of section 501 (c) of the Federal Food, Drug, and Cosmetic Act and, further, may be misbranded within the meaning of section 502 (j) of the act.

"Liquid ophthalmic preparations packed in multiple-dose containers should (1) contain one or more suitable and harmless substances that will inhibit the growth of microorganisms, or (2) be so packaged as to volume and type of container and so labeled as to duration of use and with such necessary warnings as to afford adequate protection and minimize the hazard of injury resulting from contamination during use."

"Eye cups, eye droppers, and other dispensers intended for ophthalmic use should be sterile and may be regarded as falling below their professed standard of purity or quality if they are not sterile. They should be so packaged as to maintain sterility until the package is opened and be so labeled on or within the retail package, as to afford adequate directions and necessary warnings to minimize the hazard of injury resulting from contamination during use."

Thus since 1953 the FDA has considered a nonsterile ophthalmic solution as being adulterated and misbranded. Although, in a legal sense, this regulation has been stated to affect only manufacturers and repackers, the compounding pharmacist bears an obligation to take adequate measures to assure sterility of his ophthalmic preparations.[29] This development in federal policy came especially from reports of loss of eyes from corneal ulcerations due to the use of medications contaminated by *Pseudomonas aeruginosa*.

The American Medical Association (AMA) has also recognized the need for sterility in ophthalmic medication as shown by the following statement in 1953 by its then Council on Pharmacy and Chemistry:[19,44,137]

"Before accepting any solution or suspension for ophthalmic use, the Council requires that the manufacturer submit protocols to show that adequate tests for sterility are made before any release of any batch of finished product."

The NF states:

"Ophthalmic solutions are sterile solutions, essentially free from foreign particles and suitably compounded and dispensed for instillation into the eye. Preparation of an ophthalmic solution involves careful consideration of such factors as the inherent toxicity of the drug itself, isotonicity value, the need for buffering agents, the need for a preservative (and if needed, its selection), sterilization, and proper packaging."

Sodium fluroescein solutions are of particular importance because they have been frequently found to be contaminated, and because of their use in injured eyes.

The NF states:

"Sodium fluorescein solutions should be dispensed in a sterile, single-use container or in the form of a sterile impregnated paper strip. The strip releases a sufficient amount of the drug for diagnostic purposes when touched to the eye being examined for a foreign body or a corneal abrasion. Contact of the paper with the eye can be avoided by leaching the drug from the strip on to the eye with the aid of sterile water or sterile sodium chloride solution."

pH—It is essential that careful consideration be given to the acidity of the solution. This has a substantial effect on the steps taken to attain initial sterility and to maintain subsequent self-sterilization, while at the same time giving adequate attention to other factors which include the solubility, stability, irritation, and therapeutic effect.

Position of Ophthalmologist

The above complex situation has led to a great increase in the commercial production of sterile ophthalmic medication. There is thus some basis for the following statement by Ellis and Smith:[6]

"Within a few years, most of the prescribed ophthalmic medications will be prepared by a pharmaceutical manufacturer. Although the purists may argue that the physician has thus been forced to standardize his dosage, the advantages of commercial ophthalmic preparations seem to outweigh their disadvantages. Stability, uniformity, and sterility characterize these products."

Position of the Dispensing Pharmacist

The dispensing pharmacist will desire to maintain adequate facilities for the preparation of sterile ophthalmic solutions. By doing so he can prepare not only products which are available commercially but he can also prepare products which are not available

commercially due to stability considerations, which are not available in the formulation and packaging desired by the physician, or which are temporarily not available for other reasons.

The dispensing pharmacist must recognize that because of the length of time required to carry out batch methods, prescriptions cannot, in general, be filled by commercial batch procedures. The following sections will endeavor to explain both the factors involved in batch production and in the extemporaneous preparation of a single prescription, and will state the recommendations for extemporaneous preparation of ophthalmic solutions made by Riegelman and Sorby.[32] It should be noted that both a batch system and an extemporaneous system will find a place in many of the larger dispensing services in hospitals, and in certain prescription pharmacies which fill relatively large numbers of ophthalmic prescriptions.

Extemporaneous Procedures

Riegelman and Sorby[32] give the following comprehensive statement of recommended extemporaneous procedures:

Recommended Extemporaneous Procedures

I. Solutions Intended for Application to Traumatized Eyes—(1) With the exception noted below, all drugs used in eyes traumatized by accident or at surgery should be compounded with 2% boric acid solution. Sodium fluorescein and the sulfonamides should be compounded in purified water. All solutions intended for use during surgery should be filtered free of lint or other particulate matter and should be prepared without the addition of a preservative, since all preservatives at bactericidal concentrations are irritating to the inner structure of the eye. Two-tenths per cent of sodium bisulfite may be added to the boric acid solution of physostigmine, epinephrine, or phenylephrine in order to minimize discoloration due to oxidation.

(2) All such solutions should be dispensed in small containers (5 to 10-ml glass bottles with screw caps) for single-patient use only.

(3) The closed bottle, plus a separate dropper, should be packaged in a container that can be autoclaved.

(4) This unit should be autoclaved for fifteen minutes at 121°. To prevent the cap from rupturing, the autoclave should be allowed to return slowly to atmospheric pressure before being opened.

II. Solutions Intended for Applications to the Eyes with an Intact Corneal Epithelium—

(1) Such solutions may be packaged in multiple-dose containers for general patient and office use.

(2) Stock bottles of sterile purified water, isotonic sodium chloride solution, 2% boric acid solution, and phosphate buffer at pH 6.8, to which preservatives have been added, should be available for the compounding of prescriptions to be used in the intact eye. Alkaline drugs should be compounded in the preserved water. Pilocarpine salts for home use should be compounded in the phosphate buffer. All other drugs should be compounded in normal saline, or preferably in 2 per cent boric acid solution.

(3) If the antibacterial agent selected for use as a preservative is sufficiently heat-stable, it should be added during the compounding of the stock vehicle.

(4) All stock vehicles should be stored in sealed containers of moderate volume, such as 120- or 240-ml prescription bottles, depending on the rate at which they are to be used.

(5) The sealed bottles of stock vehicles should be sterilized in an autoclave for fifteen minutes at 121° and the autoclave be allowed to return slowly to atmospheric pressure before the bottles are removed. An alternative sterilizing procedure is to boil the preservative-containing stock solution for at least 30 minutes. The cooled solutions should be agitated sufficiently to redisperse any coagulated methylcellulose which may have been added.

(6) All intermediate containers, final containers, and closures should be treated by boiling, or sterilized with a suitable disinfectant, and then rinsed thoroughly with sterile or freshly boiled water.

(7) If extraneous suspended particles or excessive amounts of lint are introduced accidentally during compounding, the solution should be clarified with equipment that has been cleaned and sterilized as indicated above.

(8) Bacterial filtration procedures may be employed, but precautions should be taken to prevent transfer of a therapeutically active amount of previously filtered drugs into subsequent ophthalmic solutions. A suitable antibacterial agent must still be added to the solution to eliminate, insofar as possible, the hazards of chance contamination during use.

(9) Once the seal of the stock bottle has been broken, the vehicle should be discarded or resterilized after 24 hours. If gravity flow from a large bottle is used, extreme care should be taken to prevent its contamination, and the outlet tube, which may make contact with the final container, should be sterilized frequently and shielded from exposure when not in use.

(10) It should be borne in mind that the criteria for use of ophthalmic solutions for home and office use are vastly different. In the latter circumstances, contaminated solutions have resulted in transfer of the organisms to treated patients.

Preparations packaged in multiple-dose containers for office or clinic use should be sterilized in the final container or by an effective aseptic technique which assures equivalent sterility. They should be resterilized at weekly intervals or replaced if necessary. If possible, prescriptions formulated for home use also should be sterilized by autoclaving the final package.

Properties

Stability

The rate of deterioration of a solution depends on the nature of the active drug, modified by the pH of the solution, the temperature to which it is subjected, and in certain instances by the amount of oxygen and ultraviolet light to which it is exposed.

The NF suggests dispensing salts of physostigmine and epinephrine in a 1.9% boric acid vehicle containing 0.1% sodium sulfite. It states that sodium sulfite has limited stability in this vehicle.

Higuchi, et al,[30,31] have shown that a degradation of epinephrine and other drugs, which are p- or o-hydroxybenzyl derivatives, is induced by the addition of bisulfite. A sulfonic acid derivative is formed which seems to possess little or no activity.

Riegelman and Vaughan[21,32] compiled the material in Table I. They point out that the relative stability of various ophthalmic drug solutions has an important bearing on formulation, methods of preparation, and storage. A neutral pH may be desired for comfort, autoclaving may be needed for sterility, etc. Many of the active ophthalmic drugs contain ester linkages. This includes local anesthetics, cycloplegics, and many of the miotics. If these substances are hydrolyzed, such as by autoclaving, the resulting compounds are not effective. At a fixed temperature the rate of decomposition depends on the pH. In most instances one can expect a drug to be 100 times more stable at pH 5.0 than at pH 7.0. This, of course, depends on the association characteristics of the compound and on the relative stability of its free base and cation.

Higuchi, et al,[33] studied the ester hydrolysis of procaine[33] and tetracaine[21] and found them to have almost identical rates of deterioration. Tetracaine possesses local anesthetic activity at the lower pH; procaine is topically active only when the pH is above 6.8, and

Table I—Stability of Selected Ophthalmic Drugs
(*Time for 50% Decomposition*)

Drug	pH 5.0		pH 6.8	
	25°C	120°C	25°C	120°C
Procaine and tetra- caine	19 yr	36 hr	...	10 min
Atropine	130 yr	60 hr	2 yr	1 hr
Pilocarpine	S[a]	>24 hr	66 day	34 min
Physostigmine	S	~1 hr[b]	6 mo	<10 min
Phenylephrine	S	>2 hr	...	...
Chlorobutanol	40 yr	~2.5 hr	1 yr	<5 min
Homatropine	14 yr	10 hr	0.4 yr	<10 min

[a] S: several years.
[b] When properly buffered, methylamine is formed during the hydrolysis. It shifts the pH to more alkaline values, and thereby increases the rate of hydrolysis.

is inactivated by autoclaving. Riegelman and Vaughan[21] state that the similarity of the hydrolysis rates might have been anticipated from the similarity of their chemical structures, and by analogy they conclude that Proparacaine (Ophthaine) and Benoxinate (Dorsacaine) have similar stability characteristics.

The work of Kondritzer, et al,[34,35] and of Patel and Lemberger[36] was used to predict the stability of atropine and homatropine, respectively. Pilocarpine, homatropine, and physostigmine are progressively less stable than atropine.[21,32]

The above work by Riegelman and Vaughan[21,32] is in general agreement with the conclusions of Morrison and Truhlsen[37,38] and of Murphy, et al,[27] and support the statements in the USP and NF that a great many ophthalmic solutions will remain adequately stable when autoclaved at 121°C for 15 minutes if they have been prepared in 1.9% boric acid solution.

Hydrogen-Ion Concentration

The general principle of buffer solutions has been explained in Chapter 20 on *Ionic Solutions and Electrolytic Equilibria*, page 283. In the case of eye solutions special emphasis is placed on the advisability of buffering to specific pH values in order to provide greater serviceability of the solution in several respects, as discussed below.

In 1947 Hind and Goyan[39] made an important contribution to ophthalmology by emphasizing the importance of hydrogen-ion concentrations and buffer systems in the preparation of ophthalmic solutions, giving consideration to buffer systems, buffer capacity, hydrogen-ion concentration, osmotic effect, chemical stability, and equilibrium concentration of the free base. In their original report they classified ophthalmic drugs according to their physical and chemical properties as they were known at that time. This resulted in five groups with a special buffered isotonic vehicle for each group. Changes in knowledge and perspective have modified some of their original conclusions.

The hydrogen-ion concentration of an ophthalmic solution has a substantial effect on the therapeutic action, comfort of the patient, stability, and solubility.

The proper control of pH may greatly increase physiological and therapeutic activity. Many drugs, especially alkaloidal salts, are most active therapeutically at pH levels that favor the undissociated free base.

The greatest comfort or the least irritation for the patient should be found at the normal pH of approximately 7.4, but comfort is usually stated to be adequate in the pH range 6 to 8.

Many essential ingredients are substantially unstable when stored at a neutral or slightly alkaline pH, which might be recommended for reasons other than stability, such as for maximum therapeutic effect and minimum irritation.

Some essential ingredients are not sufficiently soluble at the pH which would be an optimum from the standpoint of therapeutic effect and comfort.

Most of the active ingredients used in ophthalmic solutions are salts of weak acids and have a low buffer capacity. This indicates in general both a need for addition of a buffering agent and a probability of ease of buffering. These concepts are supported by the work of Hind and Goyan summarized in Fig. 594[39] and by the analogous results of Riegelman and

Vaughan.[1] The titration curves show that, for most of the drugs studied, only a small amount of alkali is required to shift the pH of the unbuffered solutions to the alkaline range.   There the preparation is subject to hydrolysis and inactivation.

Therapeutic Effect—It has been stated in previous sections that the free base must be present in equilibrium in order to penetrate and have therapeutic effect.   These statements are based particularly on the work of Swan and White in 1942.[16] For many drugs we have the greatest activity at pH levels which favor the formation of the free base by hydrolysis of the ionized salt.   This refers to a pH of 7 or above and applies especially to alkaloidal salts.   The free alkaloidal base is more lipoid soluble and can thus penetrate more readily into the cornea.   The mechanism of penetration was described in a previous section.

In 1953 Floyd, et al,[41] reviewed the earlier results and attempted to evaluate their clinical significance. They applied two drops of 1% pilocarpine hydrochloride solution of known pH to each eye tested and measured the miotic response.   The reactions to solutions prepared at two different pH levels were compared.   The pH levels were 4.0–4.2 and 6.6–7.4.   The buffers in each comparison were (1) sodium bicarbonate, (2) boric acid–borate, or (3) phosphate.   That is, the same ion species in differing proportions were used to give the two different hydrogen-ion concentrations in each comparison.   Less than 0.5% of the molecules were in the free base form in the more acidic solutions, 40–60% were in the free base form in the less acidic solutions.

In every case the miotic effect was greater for the less acidic solutions.   However, the differences were usually not statistically significant, and in no case were judged to be of practical significance.   All observations were compatible with the view that the buffer capacity of the tears is operative and highly effective in adjusting the pH of a drug solution to prevailing conditions.   That is, the neutralizing capacity of the tears was able to increase greatly the percentage of free base available for absorption.

Riegelman and Vaughan carried out a similar experiment.[1] They used 10 patients and dilated their eyes with 10% phenylephrine hydrochloride.   This fixed the iris in the fully dilated position so that the pupillary light reaction was eliminated.   Their reactions to a boric acid solution of 1% pilocarpine hydrochloride (pH 4.2) were compared with the reactions to the same alkaloid in a Sørensen phosphate buffer solution (pH 6.6).   Photographs were taken and the pupil size determined from the enlarged image.   The differences between the effects of the two solutions were statistically insignificant.

It seems that vehicles with a nearly physiological pH have no clearcut clinical superiority over more acid vehicles of low buffer capacity.   The above experiments are particularly valuable because pilocarpine hydrochloride solutions are believed to possess the greatest resistance to neutralization of all the common

ophthalmic drugs as indicated by Fig. 594.   Therefore, this conclusion would appear to have wide application.[21] A different approach was used by Boberg-Ans, et al.[42] Instillation of the medicated solution was preceded by a drop of borax solution (pH 9.2).   They reported normal effects from solutions of ½ to ¹⁄₂₀ the usual concentrations.

In regard to the treatment of diseased eyes Hosford and Hicks[43] have considered the pH of tear fluid and the use of buffer solutions for the eye.   They refer to the characteristic pH which is often developed in tear fluid as the result of a diseased condition and for treatment they recommend a solution of the opposite pH, as acid for alkaline and alkaline for acid.   For example, they refer to the fact that in injuries to the cornea, the pH of the tears shifts to the alkaline side, 8.0 to 8.4, and accordingly treatment with an acid solution is suggested. Similarly, corneal ulcers are associated with an increase in alkalinity, and again an acid solution is helpful, but not to the extent observed in corneal injuries.   Vernal catarrh shows a marked shift to a pH of about 8.0 to 8.4, and an acid buffer is considered more advantageous than a simple solution of weakly dissociated acid.   It will neutralize alkalinity without producing undesirable symptoms caused by a pH below 6.6.   It does not stimulate the production of more alkali.   Where the deviation from normal is marked, or where the causative organism is unknown or a mixed infection is present, a buffer of about pH 7.3 is recommended.   These authors point out also that pneumococci cannot live under a pH of 7.0 and, therefore, a logical treatment would be with a solution having an acid reaction. Staphylococci and streptococci tend to form acid and may, therefore, be treated to advantage with an alkaline solution.

If an eye wash is to be used in cases of acid splash, a mild isotonic sodium bicarbonate solution is indicated, whereas for counteracting the effect of an irritation caused by alkalies a mild acid eye wash, such as an isotonic boric acid solution (1.9%), would be of greater service.

Comfort—Comfort usually can be controlled satisfactorily in extemporaneous preparations by use of weak or mild buffering such as by a vehicle of 1.9% boric acid, which together with certain alkaloids (see below) is usually stated to have a mild buffering effect. Comfort is possible because of the additional buffer capacity of tear fluid.   As previously stated, tears are a buffer system of electrolytes and proteins.   One may assume the usual case of the instillation of a small volume (1 to 2 drops) of a solution, in a vehicle of low buffer capacity, of an active ingredient which is weakly acidic.   In most such instances the lacrimal fluid buffers such an added solution very quickly to a pH approximating the normal pH range.[13] Additional lacrimal fluid is available immediately from the primary lacrimal glands if needed.   This fluid will dilute the added medication if the medication is somewhat irritating.   The lacrimal fluid will flow copiously and flush out the medication if there is substantial irritation.   Reasonable comfort is usually attained.

The pH of the normal tear (lacrimal) fluid is approximately 7.4, with variations according to ailment. The actual pH of the thin film of tears in contact with the surface of the eye may be somewhat higher such as 7.4 to 8.0 because of loss of carbon dioxide to the atmosphere.[40] It is commonly believed that an uncomfortable condition exists when the pH is under 6 or over 8, but that the eye is more sensitive to acid than to alkaline solutions.

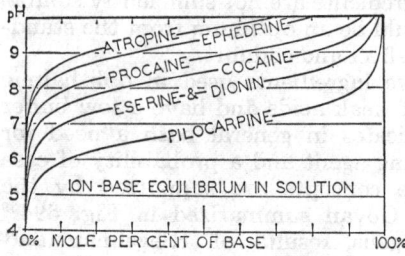

Fig. 594. Ion base equilibrium in solutions of salts of certain ophthalmic drugs (courtesy, Ref. 39).

Table II

Microliters of 0.01 N NaOH added	pH of 0.1 ml	
	1% Atropine sulfate solution	1% Pilocarpine hydrochloride solution
0	4.15	4.30
2	6.01	4.79
4	7.18	5.15
6	7.51	5.28
8	7.80	5.40
10	7.98	5.49

Trolle-Lassen[45] stated that the eye will tolerate isotonic solutions which are more alkaline than the tear fluid, better than isotonic solutions which deviate on the acid side. He found that solutions of pH 7.3 and 9.7 will irritate the eye in 1% of the cases and that solutions of pH 5.8 and 11.4 will irritate in 99% of the cases. The buffer capacity was not defined.

The buffer capacity of the tear fluid is not sufficient from the standpoint of comfort for a few strongly acidic drugs, for example, pilocarpine hydrochloride (and nitrate) and epinephrine bitartrate. It is necessary then to use a solution buffered to give the best compromise between the several factors. Usually in this situation a pH of 6.8 will be used. This pH was recommended by Hind and Goyan[39] and Riegelman.[1] The latter made an experimental comparison of the neutralization of solutions of atropine sulfate and pilocarpine hydrochloride by sodium hydroxide solution. The results are given in Table II.[1] One may make an arbitrary assumption as to the acid neutralizing power of tears and assume that the normal tears would be roughly equivalent to 8 to 10 microliters of 0.01 N sodium hydroxide. Here neutralization of two drops of 1% atropine sulfate (0.1 ml) gave a pH of 7.4 or higher. However, a similar titration of 1% pilocarpine hydrochloride gave a pH of approximately 5.5 and the pH would have been lower if the pilocarpine hydrochloride had been more concentrated as would often be the case.

Hind and Goyan originally suggested that the pain and irritation caused by certain eye drops were related to the concentration of the free base in the solution. Riegelman[1] states that this is not a general case. If it were, an acidic solution of an alkaloidal salt should become more irritating as it is made less acidic. However, when pilocarpine hydrochloride (2–4%) is prepared in a phosphate buffer with a pH of 6.8, the solution is much less irritating than when the compound is dissolved in boric acid solution, even though the phosphate solution contains more than 100 times the concentration of free base. It would seem then that the pain and irritation are caused by the acidity of the eye solution when it is instilled and that their duration depends on the amount of tears required to bring the pH within the normal range.

Stability—Stability is usually best for alkaloidal salts at a pH of 2 to 3. At this pH the solutions, if strongly buffered, would be irritating and less effective therapeutically. In addition, at a pH of 2 to 3, if unbuffered and stored in glass, the drug may slowly undergo hydrolysis as a result of alkali leached from the glass and if autoclaved substantial hydrolysis can occur in a short time. A pH of 4.7, as obtained with 1.9% boric acid, is often satisfactory.

One of the major exceptions to the above statement is pilocarpine hydrochloride.[22] It has been shown that a pH of 6.8 is needed for reasonable comfort. At this pH

pilocarpine is not stable enough for normal shelf life or for autoclaving. It has been suggested that pilocarpine hydrochloride for use in the home on an uninjured eye be prepared at a pH of 6.8 by sterile filtration, not by autoclaving, and have an expiration date of 1 month to take care of the shelf-life problem. The technical problems of sterilization by sterile filtration should be carefully considered before adopting this procedure. The same compound for use with injured eyes should be left unbuffered or dissolved in 1.9% boric acid solution at a pH of 4.7, and autoclaved. The fact that it would give more irritation would have to be accepted. Recent work by Anderson and FitzGerald[46] suggests that pilocarpine eye drops may be more stable than found by Riegelman.

Boric acid is shown above to be increasingly recommended as a vehicle. A 1.9% solution is useful with alkaloids which are weaker acids than boric acid (pK_a 9.2). Riegelman has stated that it is not a strong enough acid to be ideal for this purpose,[32] and mentions the additional value of EDTA which lies in a pK_a^3 of 6.2 and which has some buffering action in the pH range 6 to 8. This means that EDTA acts as a supplement to boric acid from the standpoint of buffering. The NF states that boric acid solutions do not possess buffering capacity.

Some formulations use isotonic saline as a vehicle, omit a buffer, accept a pH of 2 to 3 for the solution (due to the active ingredient), and assume that the product will be used before alkalinity from a glass container becomes a problem.

Solubility—At pH 7.4, many drugs are not appreciably soluble in water; most alkaloidal salts may precipitate as the free alkaloid at this pH. For example, Hind and Goyan[39] state that precipitation of the free base has been observed at a pH of 7.4 in 1% solutions of phenacaine hydrochloride, tetracaine hydrochloride, ethyl hydrocupreine hydrochloride, and dibucaine hydrochloride.

Buffered Solutions—Hind and Goyan[39] divided most of the drugs which are used in ophthalmic practice into two groups, one to be dispensed in a 1.9% boric acid solution with a pH about 4.7; the other in a modified Sørensen phosphate buffer solution with a pH about 6.8 (see Table III). The boric acid solution is isotonic. They adjusted their phosphate solutions with sodium chloride to be isotonic with blood serum, namely, with a freezing point of −0.52°. This is also the approximate freezing point of tear fluid. An earlier estimate of the freezing point of tear fluid was −0.80°.

The buffer solutions are as follows:

Boric Acid Solution

Boric Acid, crystals.. 19 Gm
Sterile Preserved Water,* sufficient to make.............1000 ml

Sørenson Phosphate Stock Solutions

Monobasic Sodium Phosphate Solution

Monobasic Sodium Phosphate, anhydrous
(NaH_2PO_4)..................... 8.00 Gm
Sterile Preserved Water, sufficient
quantity to make............... 1000 ml

Dibasic Sodium Phosphate Solution

Dibasic Sodium Phosphate, Anhydrous
(Na_2HPO_4)..................... 9.47 Gm
Sterile Preserved Water, sufficient
quantity to make............... 1000 ml

---

* See *Preservation*, page 1569.

Table III—Sørensen Phosphate Buffer Solutions

Monobasic sodium phosphate solution, ml	Dibasic sodium phosphate solution, ml	Resulting buffer solution, pH	NaCl to render isotonic, Gm
90	10	5.91	0.52
80	20	6.24	0.51
70	30	6.47	0.50
60	40	6.64	0.49
50	50	6.81	0.48
40	60	6.98	0.46
30	70	7.17	0.45
20	80	7.38	0.44
10	90	7.73	0.43
5	95	8.04	0.42

Since monobasic sodium phosphate is available only in the monohydrated form, 9.208 Gm must be used, instead of 8.00 Gm of the anhydrous form.

The USP states that the boric acid vehicle is suitable for salts of the following substances:

Benoxinate	Phenylephrine	Proparacaine
Cocaine	Piperocaine	Tetracaine
Dibucaine	Procaine	Zinc

and that the phosphate vehicle is recommended for salts of the following substances:

Atropine	Eucatropine	Pilocarpine
Ephedrine	Homatropine	Scopolamine

At the suggested pH of 6.8, solutions of the salts of the latter bases are reported to lose only between 10 and 20% of their activity in 30 days.[44] Thus some activity is sacrificed but not sufficient to alter materially the usefulness of the solutions, if they are not too old. The NF states that solutions of eucatropine, homatropine, pilocarpine, and scopolamine salts exhibit limited stability in the phosphate vehicle.

Penicillin solutions, containing about 5000 units/ml, are sometimes prescribed for the treatment of the eye. Such solutions should preferably be buffered at a pH about 6.5, and kept in a refrigerator. Molinas and Welch[47] have shown that commercial crystalline penicillin solutions show no significant loss in potency (less than 15%) after 7 days at a pH between 6.0 and 6.5, and at a temperature of 15° or less, the lower the temperature the better. They report over 15% loss of potency with solutions prepared at a pH between 5.12 and 5.8. At a critical pH of 4.5 and below, stability is greatly impaired. Unbuffered solutions, even with an initial pH of 6.2 to 6.6, undergo greater loss in potency than do properly buffered solutions.

Caution—Many patients using penicillin solutions in the eye develop sensitivity and other localized penicillin reactions. These reactions occur frequently on the second or third day of use and especially when the solution has not been kept in a refrigerator. It is therefore important to instruct the patient to keep the penicillin solution in the refrigerator.

Solutions containing sodium propionate are best dispensed at a pH 7.2. Fluorescein sodium solutions (pH 9.0) must be prepared with sterile water (see page 1315). All highly alkaline drugs are best dispensed unbuffered.

For a 5% solution of sulfathiazole sodium the following vehicle is recommended.[48]

Boric Acid	0.43 Gm
Sodium Borate	4.20 Gm
Sterile Preserved Water, sufficient to make	1000 ml

For sodium salts of the sulfonamides, Hind and Szekely[49] published a formula which was tested and found satisfactory as a vehicle for the following drugs: sulfadiazine sodium 5%, sulfacetamide sodium 30%, sulfathiazole sodium 5%, sulfisoxazole diethanolamine 4%.

The Sulfonamide (Sodium salt)	qs
Phenylmercuric Nitrate	1:25,000
Sodium Sulfite, anhydrous	0.1%
Sterile Water	qs

The inclusion of sodium sulfite retards the discoloration of the solutions. The use of sodium metabisulfite has been discussed by Clarke.[50]

It is suggested that all stock solutions used in this work be stored in hard-glass containers not exceeding 100 ml and be kept under refrigeration. All equipment for measuring, mixing, and filtration should be sterilized.

While numerous other buffer solutions have been proposed, those which formerly were most generally used for the preparation of collyria are referred to as Gifford's Buffer Solutions.[51,52] They are based upon the work of Atkins and Pantin[53] and consist of a stock acid solution and a stock alkaline solution. Combinations of the former with small quantities of the latter provide solutions of varying pH to meet any given need and are sometimes used as the solvent in the preparation of eye solutions.

The formulas given below represent Gifford's solutions with some additional stock solution ratios being added to provide uniform pH increments. Some of the pH readings have been corrected to give what appear to be more nearly the true values to the nearest decimal. See Table IV.

Boric acid crystals should be used if possible. Since it is difficult to maintain the sodium carbonate in

Gifford's Stock Buffer Solutions

Stock Acid Solution

Boric Acid	12.4 Gm
Potassium Chloride	7.4 Gm
Sterile Preserved Water	1000 ml

Stock Alkaline Solution

Sodium Carbonate, Anhydrous	21.2 Gm
Sterile Preserved Water	1000 ml

its anhydrous state, the monohydrated form may be used, making allowance for molecular weight (24.8 Gm monohydrated sodium carbonate is equivalent to 21.2 Gm anhydrous sodium carbonate). The

Table IV—Gifford's Buffer Solutions

ml of stock acid solution	ml of stock alkaline solution	pH of resulting buffer solution	Solution number
30	0.00	5.0	Acid No. 1
30	0.05	6.0	Acid No. 2
30	0.10	6.2	
30	0.15	6.4	
30	0.20	6.6	
30	0.30	6.8	
30	0.60	7.0	
30	1.00	7.2	
30	1.50	7.4	Alkaline No. 1
30	2.00	7.6	
30	3.00	7.8	
30	4.00	8.0	Alkaline No. 2
30	8.00	8.6	

Table V—Sodium Acetate—Boric Acid Buffer Solutions

ml of sodium acetate solution	ml of boric acid solution	pH of resulting solution
...	100	5
5	95	5.7
10	90	6.05
20	80	6.3
30	70	6.5
40	60	6.65
50	50	6.75
60	40	6.85
70	30	6.95
80	20	7.1
90	10	7.25
100	5	7.4
100	...	7.6

buffer solutions are conveniently based on 30-ml (1-ounce) units and should be prepared in such quantities as will provide accuracy in the measurement of the stock alkaline solution. Graduated pipets should be a part of the equipment for the preparation of these solutions. The pH should be checked as a matter of protection against any possible errors because of the ultimate use of the solutions. The methods of determinating pH have been discussed in Chapter 20 on *Ionic Solutions and Electrolytic Equilibria.*

Gifford's Buffer Solutions are no longer advocated as vehicles for the preparation of ophthalmic solutions as they are hypertonic. They are listed here for reference purposes as they are used in a number of commercial ophthalmic solutions.[116]

For the dispensing pharmacist pHydrion papers are recommended for a simple colorimetric method of determining pH by the use of paper treated with indicator solution. When wetted with the solution whose pH is to be tested it will give a definite color which is compared with a color chart. The pHydrion paper is supplied in two different sets, a wide range paper and a short range paper. If the pH of a solution is entirely unknown the wide range paper which covers a pH from 1 to 11 is used first. When the pH of the unknown solution has been approximately determined, the short-range paper, which covers two pH units or less is used. The color obtained is compared with the color standard supplied. Relatively good readings are obtained. This complete assembly of pH papers is very useful for quick pH determinations.

Investigators in Germany[54] have suggested the use of a sodium acetate–boric acid buffer as a vehicle for ophthalmic drugs. Two isotonic stock solutions are prepared. They are sterilized in an autoclave, using hard-glass containers, and they are stored in a cool place. These solutions should not be kept longer than 3 months.

Sodium Acetate—Boric Acid Stock Solutions

Sodium Acetate Solution, Alkaline Stock Solution pH 7.6
Sodium Acetate, NF 3 mol H_2O............ 20 Gm
Sterile Preserved Water, sufficient quantity to make............................... 1000 ml
Boric Acid Solution, Acid Stock Solution pH about 5
Boric Acid, crystals...................... 19 Gm
Sterile Preserved Water, sufficient quantity to make............................... 1000 ml

Combinations of definite volumes of these stock solutions provide solutions of different pH values. See Table V. Both stock solutions are isotonic, ie, 2% sodium acetate solution corresponds to a 0.9% sodium chloride solution. A 1.9% boric acid solution is also isotonic, as stated before. The combination of two isotonic solutions results in isotonicity unless they interact.

This buffer covers a wide range of compatibility and its buffer capacity is claimed to be 10% greater than that of the phosphate buffer solution.

The USP includes a statement in the monograph on *Silver Nitrate Ophthalmic Solution:*

"Silver Nitrate Ophthalmic Solution is a solution of silver nitrate in a water medium.... The solution may be buffered by the addition of sodium acetate."

No quantities or specific directions are given. The above solution, either pH 5.7 or pH 6.05 lends itself very well for such a "buffered water medium." The use of this *Sodium Acetate–Boric Acid Buffer* is highly recommended particularly since the USP lists the pH of the *Silver Nitrate Ophthalmic Solution* as between pH 4.5–6.0. Other pH levels, such as pH 6.75, are suggested for alkaloidal salts, in place of Sørensen's Phosphate Buffer, pH 6.8.

In regard to making the most highly accurate computations of the tonicity of solutions it should be noted that the relative proportions of a drug existing in ionic and nonionic forms will depend on the hydrogen-ion concentration.

Isotonic Solutions

If a solution is placed in contact with a membrane that is permeable to molecules of the solvent but not to molecules of the solute (a semipermeable membrane), the movement of solvent through the membrane is called osmosis. If a solution of greater solute concentration is in contact with the other side of the membrane, the solvent will tend to pass into the more concentrated solution until equilibrium has been established. The pressure required to prevent this movement is called the osmotic pressure. It is defined as the excess pressure, or pressure greater than that above the pure solvent, which must be applied to the solution to prevent the passage of the solvent through a perfect semipermeable membrane. The

concentration of a solution with respect to effect on osmotic pressure is related to the number of "particles" of solute in solution and thus is affected by the degree of ionization.

Body fluids, including blood and lacrimal fluid, have an osmotic pressure corresponding to that of a 0.9% solution of sodium chloride. Thus, a sodium chloride solution of this concentration is said to be iso-osmotic with physiologic fluids. The term isotonic, meaning equal tone, is commonly used interchangeably with iso-osmotic although the former term must be used with reference to some body fluid, and iso-osmotic is actually a physical term which compares the osmotic pressure (or other colligative property), of two liquids, either of which may not be a physiologic fluid, or which may be a physiologic fluid only in certain circumstances. For example, a solution of boric acid which is iso-osmotic with both blood and lacrimal fluid is isotonic only with the lacrimal fluid as this solution causes hemolysis of red blood cells because the molecules of boric acid pass freely through the erythrocyte membrane regardless of concentration. A solution is isotonic with a living cell if there is no net gain or loss of water by the cell, or other change in the cell, when in contact with that solution. Solutions with a lower osmotic pressure than body fluids or a 0.9% sodium chloride solution are commonly referred to as hypotonic; solutions having a greater osmotic pressure are termed hypertonic.

Tonicity is often stated as "isotonicity value," the tonicity in terms of a sodium chloride solution. Isotonicity values may be determined by freezing-point measurements and recalculated as osmotically equivalent weights or percentages of sodium chloride. These values should not be confused with true isotonic concentrations which are defined in terms of specific biological systems. It is permissible to use such values where the intended use of the solution is such that it will not significantly modify blood plasma, and where experience indicates that similar preparations have proved to be satisfactory.

In most cases when a solution is iso-osmotic with 0.9% sodium chloride, it will also be isotonic with body fluids. Only in special cases, as when the biologica, membrane does not act as an ideal semipermeable membrane, does the relationship between iso-osmoticity and isotonicity break down, as discussed in Chapter 19.

A knowledge of colligative properties of solutions is essential for one to understand fully the principles involved in rendering intravenous solutions isotonic with blood serum, or ophthalmic solutions isotonic with lacrimal fluid. Solutions thus adjusted produce less shock and much less irritation than those which are hypotonic or hypertonic, and present-day practice recognizes the desirability of making the necessary adjustments wherever possible.

Inasmuch as the problem resolves itself into an adjustment of the tonicity value of the solution to be injected into the vein or instilled into the eye, it would appear that some convenient method of learning the tonicity value would be desirable for routine use in preparing isotonic solutions. Osmotic-pressure measurements are made only with comparatively great difficulty and, as a rule, are not as accurate as measurements of the other colligative properties of solutions which, as pointed out in Chapter 19, can be used to predict the magnitude of the osmotic pressure. Determinations of vapor-pressure lowering are also impractical because of the elaborate apparatus required. The boiling-point elevation may be determined but the readings are especially sensitive to changes in barometric pressure. In the case of an aqueous solution the molal boiling-point elevation for a nonelectrolyte is considerably less than the freezing-point depression, thus not lending itself to as great accuracy as the latter. Accordingly, of the four related properties of solutions, the freezing-point depression, which is quite readily measured with a fair degree of accuracy, is most frequently used in determining the tonicity value of a solution.

The results of investigations by Lund and co-workers[55] indicate that the freezing point of normal, healthy human blood is −0.52°C and not −0.56°C, as previously assumed.* Inasmuch as water is the medium in which the various constituents of blood are either suspended or dissolved in this method, it is assumed that *any aqueous solution* freezing at −0.52°C is *isotonic with blood.* Now it is only rarely that an aqueous solution to be injected intravenously has a freezing point of −0.52°C and to attain to this freezing point it is necessary either to add some other therapeutically inactive solute if the solution is hypotonic (freezing point above −0.52°C) or to dilute the solution if it is hypertonic (freezing point below −0.52°C). The usual practice is to add either sodium chloride or dextrose to adjust hypotonic intravenous solutions to isotonicity. Certain solutes, including ammonium chloride, boric acid, urea, glycerin, and propylene glycol, cause hemolysis even when they are present in a concentration that is iso-osmotic; such solutions obviously are not isotonic. See Table VI and page 1555.

In a similar manner solutions intended for ophthalmic use may be adjusted to have a freezing point identical with that of lacrimal fluid, namely, −0.52°C.* Ophthalmic solutions with higher freezing points are usually made isotonic by the addition of boric acid or sodium chloride.

In laboratories where the necessary equipment is available, the method usually followed for adjusting hypotonic solutions is to determine the freezing-point depression produced by the ingredients of a given prescription or formula, and then to add a quantity of a suitable salt which is calculated to lower the freezing-point to −0.52°C, whether the solution is for intravenous injection or ophthalmic application. A final determination of the freezing-point depression may be made to verify the accuracy of the calculation. If the solution is hypertonic, it must be diluted if an isotonic solution is to be prepared, but it must be remembered that some solutions cannot be diluted without impairing their therapeutic activity. For example, solutions to be used for treating varicose veins require a high concentration of the active ingredient (solute) to make the solution effective. Dilution to isotonic concentration is not indicated in such cases.

The problem of adjusting a solution to isotonicity has been studied by many investigators, who have published extensively on the subject and recommended procedures that in most instances are essentially equivalent in effect. The report by Husa and Rossi[56] provides a synopsis of the earlier methods which have been used in preparing isotonic solutions, and a valuable bibliography is given. Certain papers are recommended for further reading.[57-72]

Calculations Based on Freezing Points

As explained in the preceding section, freezing-point data often may be employed in solving problems of isotonicity adjustment. Obviously, the utility of such data is limited to those solutions where the solute does not penetrate the membrane of the tissue, eg, red blood cells, with which it is in contact. In such cases, Table VI, giving the freezing-point depression of solutions of different concentrations of various substances, provides information essential for solving the problem.

For most substances listed in the table the concentration of an isotonic solution, ie, one that has a freezing point of −0.52°C, is given. If this is not listed in the table, it may be determined with sufficient accuracy by

---

* See discussion of *Reliability of Freezing-Point Data* in this chapter.

Table VI—Sodium Chloride Equivalents, Freezing-Point Depressions, and Hemolytic Effects of Certain Medicinals in Aqueous Solution

	0.5% E	0.5% D	1% E	1% D	2% E	2% D	3% E	3% D	5% E	5% D	%	E	D	H	pH
Alum (potassium)			0.18				0.15		0.15		6.35	0.14		24*	3.4
Amantadine HCl	0.31	0.090	0.31	0.180	0.31	0.354					2.95	0.31	0.52	91	5.7
Aminophylline				0.10^d											
Ammonium carbonate	0.70	0.202	0.70	0.405							1.29	0.70	0.52	97	7.7
Ammonium chloride			1.12								0.8	1.12	0.52	93	5.0
Ammonium lactate	0.33	0.093	0.33	0.185	0.33	0.370					2.76	0.33	0.52	98	5.9
Ammonium nitrate	0.69	0.200	0.69	0.400							1.30	0.69	0.52	91	5.3
Ammonium phosphate, dibasic	0.58	0.165	0.55	0.315							1.76	0.51	0.52	0	7.9
Ammonium sulfate	0.55	0.158	0.55	0.315							1.68	0.54	0.52	0	5.3
Amobarbital sodium			0.25	0.14			0.25				3.6	0.25	0.52	0	9.3
d-Amphetamine HCl											2.64			98	5.7
Amphetamine phosphate			0.34	0.20			0.27	0.47			3.47	0.26	0.52	0	4.5
Amphetamine sulfate			0.22	0.13			0.21	0.36			4.23	0.21	0.52	0	5.9
Amylcaine HCl			0.22				0.19				4.98	0.18		100	5.6
Antimony potassium tartrate			0.18				0.13		0.10						
Antipyrine			0.17	0.10			0.14	0.24	0.14	0.40	6.81	0.13	0.52	100	6.1
Apomorphine HCl			0.14	0.08											
Ascorbic acid				0.11^b							5.05		0.52^b	100*	2.2
Atropine methylbromide			0.14				0.13		0.13		7.03	0.13			
Atropine sulfate			0.13	0.075			0.11	0.19	0.11	0.32	8.85	0.10	0.52	0	5.0
Bacitracin			0.05	0.03			0.04	0.07	0.04	0.12					
Barbital sodium			0.30	0.17			0.29	0.50			3.12	0.29	0.52	0	9.8
Benzalkonium chloride			0.16				0.14			0.13					
Benztropine mesylate	0.26	0.073	0.21	0.115	0.15	0.170	0.12	0.203	0.09	0.242					
Benzyl alcohol			0.17	0.09^c			0.15								
Bethanechol chloride	0.50	0.140	0.39	0.225	0.32	0.368	0.30	0.512			3.05	0.30		0	6.0
Bismuth potassium tartrate			0.09				0.06		0.05						
Bismuth sodium tartrate			0.13				0.12	0.11			8.91	0.10			
Boric acid			0.50	0.29							1.9	0.47	0.52	100	4.6
Brompheniramine maleate	0.10	0.026	0.09	0.050	0.08	0.084									
Butacaine sulfate			0.20	0.12			0.13	0.23	0.10	0.29					
Caffeine and sodium benzoate			0.26	0.15			0.23	0.40			3.92	0.23	0.52	0	7.0
Caffeine and sodium salicylate			0.12	0.12			0.17	0.295	0.16	0.46	5.77	0.16	0.52	0	6.8
Calcium chloride			0.51	0.30							1.70	0.53	0.52	0	5.6
Calcium chloride (6 H$_2$O)			0.35	0.20							2.5	0.36	0.52	0	5.7
Calcium chloride, anhydrous			0.68	0.39							1.3	0.69	0.52	0	5.6
Calcium disodium edetate	0.21	0.061	0.21	0.120	0.21	0.240	0.20	0.357			4.50	0.20	0.52	0	6.1
Calcium gluconate			0.16	0.09			0.14	0.24							
Calcium lactate			0.23	0.13			0.12	0.36			4.5	0.20	0.52	0	6.7
Calcium levulinate			0.27	0.16			0.25	0.43							
Calcium pantothenate											5.50			0	7.4
Camphor				0.12^d											
Carbachol				0.21^c											
Chloramine-T											4.10			100*	9.1
Chloramphenicol				0.06^d											
Chloramphenicol sodium succinate	0.14	0.038	0.14	0.078	0.14	0.154	0.13	0.230	0.13	0.382	6.83	0.13	0.52	Partial	6.1
Chlordiazepoxide HCl	0.24	0.068	0.22	0.125	0.19	0.220	0.18	0.315	0.17	0.487	5.50	0.16	0.52	66	2.7
Chlorobutanol (hydrated)			0.24	0.14											
Chloroprocaine HCl	0.20	0.054	0.20	0.108	0.18	0.210									
Chloroquine sulfate	0.10	0.028	0.09	0.050	0.08	0.090	0.07	0.127	0.07	0.195					
Chlorpheniramine maleate	0.17	0.048	0.15	0.085	0.14	0.165	0.13	0.220	0.09	0.265					
Chlortetracycline HCl				0.06^d											
Chlortetracycline sulfate			0.13	0.08			0.10	0.17							
Citric acid			0.18	0.10			0.17	0.295	0.16	0.46	5.52	0.16	0.52	100*	1.8
Cocaine HCl			0.16	0.09			0.15	0.26	0.14	0.40	6.33	0.14	0.52	47	4.4
Codeine phosphate			0.14	0.08			0.13	0.23	0.13	0.38	7.29	0.12	0.52	0	4.4
Cupric sulfate			0.18				0.15			0.14	6.85	0.13		trace*	3.9
Cyclizine HCl	0.20	0.060													
Cyclophosphamide	0.10	0.031	0.10	0.061	0.10	0.125									
Demecarium bromide	0.14	0.038	0.12	0.069	0.10	0.108	0.08	0.139	0.07	0.192					
Dexamethasone sodium phosphate	0.18	0.050	0.17	0.095	0.16	0.180	0.15	0.260	0.14	0.410	6.75	0.13	0.52	0	8.9
Dextroamphetamine HCl	0.34	0.097	0.34	0.196	0.34	0.392					2.64	0.34	0.52		
Dextroamphetamine phosphate			0.25	0.14			0.25	0.44			3.62	0.25	0.52	0	4.7
Dextroamphetamine sulfate	0.24	0.069	0.23	0.134	0.22	0.259	0.22	0.380			4.16	0.22	0.52	0	5.9
Dextrose			0.16	0.09			0.16	0.28	0.16	0.46	5.51	0.16	0.52	0	5.9
Dextrose (anhydrous)			0.18	0.10			0.18	0.31			5.05	0.18	0.52	0	6.0
Dibucaine HCl				0.07^c											
Diethanolamine	0.31	0.089	0.31	0.177	0.31	0.358					2.90	0.31	0.52	100	11.3
Dihydrostreptomycin sulfate			0.06	0.03			0.05	0.09	0.05	0.14	19.4	0.05	0.52	0	6.1
Dimethpyrindene maleate	0.13	0.039	0.12	0.070	0.11	0.120									
Dimethylsulfoxide	0.42	0.122	0.42	0.245	0.42	0.480					2.16	0.42	0.52	100	7.6
Diperodon HCl	0.15	0.045	0.14	0.079	0.13	0.141									
Diphenhydramine HCl				0.12^d											
Echothiophate iodide	0.16	0.045	0.16	0.090	0.16	0.179									
Edathamil disodium	0.24	0.070	0.23	0.132	0.22	0.248	0.21	0.360			4.44	0.20	0.52	0	4.7
Emetine HCl				0.06				0.17		0.29					
Ephedrine HCl			0.30				0.28				3.2	0.28		96	5.9
Ephedrine sulfate			0.23	0.13			0.20	0.35			4.54	0.20	0.52	0	5.7
Epinephrine bitartrate			0.18	0.104			0.16	0.28	0.16	0.462	5.7	0.16	0.52	100*	3.4
Epinephrine hydrochloride			0.29	0.16^b			0.26				3.47	0.26			
Ergonovine maleate				0.09^c											
Erythromycin lactobionate	0.08	0.020	0.07	0.040	0.07	0.078	0.07	0.115	0.06	0.187					
Ethyl alcohol											1.39			100	6.0
Ethylene diamine				0.25^b											
Ethylmorphine HCl			0.16	0.09			0.15	0.26	0.15	0.43	6.18	0.15	0.52	38	4.7
Eucatropine HCl				0.11^d											
Fluorescein sodium			0.31	0.18			0.27	0.47			3.34	0.27	0.52	0	8.7
d-Fructose											5.05			0*	5.9
Furtrethonium iodide	0.24	0.070	0.24	0.133	0.22	0.250	0.21	0.360			4.44	0.20	0.52	0	5.4
Galactose											4.92			0	5.9
Glycerin				0.20^c							2.6			100	5.9
Gold sodium thiomalate	0.10	0.032	0.10	0.061	0.10	0.111	0.09	0.159	0.09	0.250					
Hexafluorenium bromide	0.12	0.033	0.11	0.065											

Table VI—Continued

	0.5%		1%		2%		3%		5%		At isotonicity^e				
	E	D	E	D	E	D	E	D	E	D	%	E	D	H	pH
Hexamethonium tartrate	0.16	0.045	0.16	0.089	0.16	0.181	0.16	0.271	0.16	0.456	5.68	0.16	0.52		
Hexobarbital sodium				0.15^c											
Histamine Di HCl	0.40	0.115	0.40	0.233	0.40	0.466					2.24	0.40	0.52	79*	3.7
Histamine phosphate				0.15^c											
Holocaine HCl			0.20	0.12											
Homatropine hydrobromide			0.17	0.10			0.16	0.28	0.16	0.46	5.67	0.16	0.52	92	5.0
Homatropine methylbromide			0.19	0.11			0.15	0.26	0.13	0.38					
Hyaluronidase	0.01	0.004	0.01	0.007	0.01	0.013	0.01	0.020	0.01	0.033					
Hydroxyamphetamine HBr				0.15^d							3.71			92	5.0
Hydroxystilbamidine isethionate	0.20	0.060	0.16	0.090	0.12	0.137	0.10	0.170	0.07	0.216					
Imipramine HCl	0.20	0.058	0.20	0.110	0.13	0.143									
Intracaine HCl											4.97			85	5.0
Iodophthalein sodium				0.07^c							9.58			100	9.4
Kanamycin sulfate	0.08	0.021	0.07	0.041	0.07	0.083	0.07	0.125	0.07	0.210					
Lactic acid											2.30			100*	2.1
Lactose			0.07				0.08		0.09		9.75	0.09		0*	5.8
Lidocaine HCl				0.13^c											
Lincomycin HCl	0.16	0.045	0.16	0.090	0.15	0.170	0.14	0.247	0.14	0.400	6.60	0.14	0.52	0	4.5
Lobeline HCl				0.09^b											
Magnesium chloride			0.45								2.02	0.45		0	6.3
Magnesium sulfate			0.17	0.10			0.15	0.26	0.15	0.43	6.3	0.14	0.52	0	6.2
Mannitol											5.07			0*	6.2
Maphenide HCl	0.27	0.075	0.27	0.153	0.27	0.303	0.26	0.448			3.55	0.25	0.52		
Menadione sodium bisulfite											5.07			0	5.3
Menthol				0.12^d											
Meperidine HCl				0.13^c							4.80			98	5.0
Mepivacaine HCl	0.21	0.060	0.21	0.116	0.20	0.230	0.20	0.342			4.60	0.20	0.52	45	4.5
Merbromin				0.08^b											
Mercuric cyanide			0.15				0.14		0.13						
Mersalyl				0.06^b											
Metaraminol bitartrate	0.20	0.060	0.20	0.112	0.19	0.210	0.18	0.308	0.17	0.505	5.17	0.17	0.52	59	3.8
Methacholine chloride				0.19^d							3.21			0	4.5
Methadone HCl				0.10^c							8.59			100*	5.0
Methamphetamine HCl				0.22^d							2.75			97	5.9
Methdilazine HCl	0.12	0.035	0.10	0.056	0.08	0.080	0.06	0.093	0.04	0.112					
Methenamine			0.23				0.24				3.68	0.25		100	8.4
Methitural sodium	0.26	0.074	0.25	0.142	0.24	0.275	0.23	0.407			3.85	0.23	0.52	78	9.8
Methoxyphenamine HCl	0.26	0.075	0.26	0.150	0.26	0.300	0.26	0.450			3.47	0.26	0.52	96	5.4
p-Methylaminoethanolphenol tartrate	0.18	0.048	0.17	0.095	0.16	0.190	0.16	0.282	0.16	0.453	5.83	0.16	0.52	0	6.2
Methyldopate HCl	0.21	0.063	0.21	0.122	0.21	0.244	0.21	0.365			4.28	0.21	0.52	Partial	3.0
N-Methylglucamine	0.20	0.057	0.20	0.111	0.18	0.214	0.18	0.315	0.18	0.517	5.02	0.18	0.52	4	11.3
Methylphenidate HCl	0.22	0.065	0.22	0.127	0.22	0.258	0.22	0.388			4.07	0.22	0.52	66	4.3
Monoethanolamine	0.53	0.154	0.53	0.306							1.70	0.53	0.52	100	11.4
Morphine HCl			0.15				0.14								
Morphine sulfate			0.14	0.08			0.11	0.19	0.09	0.26					
Nalorphine HCl	0.24	0.070	0.21	0.121	0.18	0.210	0.17	0.288	0.15	0.434	6.36	0.14	0.52	63	4.1
Naphazoline HCl			0.27	0.14^d			0.24				3.99	0.22		100	5.3
Neoarsphenamine											2.32			17	7.8
Neomycin sulfate			0.11	0.06			0.09	0.16	0.08	0.232					
Neostigmine bromide			0.22	0.12^c			0.19								
Neostigmine methylsulfate			0.20	0.12^c			0.18		0.17		5.22	0.17			
Nicotinamide			0.26	0.15			0.21	0.36			4.49	0.20	0.52	100	7.0
Nicotinic acid			0.25	0.14^c											
Nikethamide				0.10^b							5.94			100	6.9
Oxophenarsine HCl											3.67			trace*	2.3
Oxymetazoline HCl	0.22	0.063	0.22	0.124	0.20	0.232	0.19	0.335			4.92	0.18	0.52	86	5.7
Oxyquinoline sulfate	0.24	0.068	0.21	0.113	0.16	0.182	0.14	0.236	0.11	0.315					
d-Pantothenyl alcohol	0.20	0.053	0.18	0.100	0.17	0.193	0.17	0.283	0.16	0.468	5.60	0.16	0.52	92	6.8
Papaverine HCl			0.10	0.06											
Pargyline HCl	0.30	0.083	0.29	0.165	0.29	0.327	0.28	0.491			3.18	0.28	0.52	91	3.8
Penicillin G, potassium			0.18	0.10			0.17	0.29	0.16	0.46	5.48	0.16	0.52	0	6.2
Penicillin G, procaine				0.06^d											
Penicillin G, sodium			0.18	0.10			0.16	0.28	0.16	0.46					
Pentobarbital sodium				0.15^c											
Phenacaine HCl				0.09^d											
Pheniramine maleate				0.09^d											
Phenobarbital sodium			0.24	0.14			0.23	0.40			3.95	0.23	0.52	0	9.2
Phenol			0.35	0.20							2.8	0.32	0.52	0*	5.6
Phentolamine mesylate	0.18	0.052	0.17	0.096	0.16	0.173	0.14	0.244	0.13	0.364	8.23	0.11	0.52	83	3.5
Phenylephrine HCl			0.32	0.17^d			0.30				3.0	0.30		0	4.5
Phenylpropanolamine HCl			0.38								2.6	0.35		95	5.3
Physostigmine salicylate			0.16	0.09											
Physostigmine sulfate				0.08^d											
Pilocarpine HCl			0.24	0.14			0.22	0.38			4.08	0.22	0.52	89	4.0
Pilocarpine nitrate			0.23	0.13			0.20	0.35			4.84	0.20	0.52		
Piperocaine HCl				0.12^d											
Polyethylene glycol 300	0.12	0.034	0.12	0.069	0.12	0.141	0.12	0.216	0.13	0.378	6.73	0.13	0.52	53	3.8
Polyethylene glycol 400	0.08	0.022	0.08	0.047	0.09	0.098	0.09	0.153	0.09	0.272	8.50	0.11	0.52	0	4.4
Polyethylene glycol 1500	0.06	0.015	0.06	0.036	0.07	0.078	0.07	0.120	0.07	0.215	10.00	0.09	0.52	4	4.1
Polyethylene glycol 1540	0.02	0.005	0.02	0.012	0.02	0.028	0.03	0.047	0.03	0.094					
Polyethylene glycol 4000	0.02	0.004	0.02	0.008	0.02	0.020	0.02	0.033	0.02	0.067					
Polymyxin B sulfate			0.09	0.05			0.06	0.10	0.04	0.12					
Polysorbate 80	0.02	0.005	0.02	0.010	0.02	0.020	0.02	0.032	0.02	0.055					
Polyvinyl alcohol (99% hydrol.)	0.02	0.004	0.02	0.008	0.02	0.020	0.02	0.035	0.03	0.075					
Polyvinylpyrrolidone	0.01	0.003	0.01	0.006	0.01	0.010	0.01	0.017	0.01	0.035					
Potassium acetate	0.59	0.172	0.59	0.342							1.53	0.59	0.52	0	7.6
Potassium chlorate											1.88			0	6.9
Potassium chloride			0.76	0.44							1.19	0.76	0.52	0	5.9
Potassium iodide			0.34	0.20							2.59	0.34	0.52	0	7.0
Potassium nitrate			0.56								1.62	0.56		0	5.9
Potassium phosphate			0.46	0.27							2.08	0.43	0.52	0	8.4
Potassium phosphate, monobasic			0.44	0.25							2.18	0.41	0.52	0	4.4

Table VI—Continued

	0.5% E	0.5% D	1% E	1% D	2% E	2% D	3% E	3% D	5% E	5% D	At isotonicity[e] %	E	D	H	pH
Potassium sulfate			0.44								2.11	0.43		0	6.6
Pralidoxime chloride	0.32	0.092	0.32	0.183	0.32	0.364					2.87	0.32	0.52	0	4.6
Procainamide HCl			0.22	0.13			0.19	0.33	0.17	0.49					
Procaine HCl			0.21	0.12			0.19	0.33	0.18		5.05	0.18	0.52	91	5.6
Prochlorperazine edisylate	0.08	0.020	0.06	0.033	0.05	0.048	0.03	0.056	0.02	0.065					
Promazine HCl	0.18	0.050	0.13	0.077	0.09	0.102	0.07	0.112	0.05	0.137					
Propiomazine HCl	0.18	0.050	0.15	0.084	0.12	0.133	0.10	0.165	0.08	0.215					
Propylene glycol											2.00			100	5.5
Pyrathiazine HCl	0.22	0.065	0.17	0.095	0.11	0.123	0.08	0.140	0.06	0.170					
Quinacrine methanesulfonate				0.06[c]											
Quinine bisulfate			0.09	0.05			0.09	0.16							
Quinine dihydrochloride			0.23	0.13			0.19	0.33	0.18		5.07	0.18	0.52		
Quinine hydrochloride			0.14	0.08			0.11	0.19							
Quinine and urea HCl			0.23	0.13			0.21	0.36			4.5	0.20	0.52	64	2.9
Resorcinol											3.30			96	5.0
Scopolamine HBr			0.12	0.07			0.12	0.21	0.12	0.35	7.85	0.11	0.52	8	4.8
Scopolamine methylnitrate			0.16				0.14		0.13		6.95	0.13			
Secobarbital sodium			0.24	0.14			0.23	0.40			3.9	0.23	0.52		
Silver nitrate			0.33	0.19							2.74	0.33	0.52	0*	5.0
Silver protein, mild			0.17	0.10			0.17	0.29	0.16	0.46	5.51	0.16	0.52	0	9.0
Silver protein, strong				0.06[d]											
Sodium acetate			0.46	0.267							2.0	0.45	0.52		
Sodium acetazolamide	0.24	0.068	0.23	0.135	0.23	0.271	0.23	0.406			3.85	0.23	0.52		
Sodium aminosalicylate											3.27			0	7.3
Sodium benzoate			0.40	0.23							2.25	0.40	0.52	0	7.5
Sodium ascorbate											3.00			0	6.9
Sodium bicarbonate			0.65	0.375							1.39	0.65	0.52	0	8.3
Sodium biphosphate (H₂O)			0.40	0.23							2.45	0.37	0.52	0	4.1
Sodium biphosphate (2 H₂O)			0.36								2.77	0.32		0	4.0
Sodium bismuth thioglycollate	0.20	0.055	0.19	0.107	0.18	0.208	0.18	0.303	0.17	0.493	5.29			0	8.3
Sodium bisulfite			0.61	0.35							1.5	0.61	0.52	0*	3.0
Sodium borate			0.42	0.24							2.6	0.35	0.52	0	9.2
Sodium cacodylate			0.32				0.28				3.3	0.27		0	8.0
Sodium carbonate, monohydrated			0.60	0.346							1.56	0.58	0.52	100	11.1
Sodium cephalothin	0.18	0.050	0.17	0.095	0.16	0.179	0.15	0.259	0.14	0.400	6.80	0.13	0.52	Partial	8.5
Sodium chloride			1.00				1.00	1.73	1.00	2.88	0.9	1.00	0.52	0	6.7
Sodium citrate			0.31	0.18			0.30	0.52			3.02	0.30		0	7.8
Sodium colistimethate	0.16	0.045	0.15	0.087	0.14	0.161	0.14	0.235	0.13	0.383	6.85	0.13	0.52	0	8.4
Sodium iodide			0.39	0.23							2.37	0.38	0.52	0	6.9
Sodium lactate											1.72			0	6.5
Sodium lauryl sulfate	0.10	0.029	0.08	0.046	0.07	0.068	0.05	0.086							
Sodium metabisulfite			0.67	0.39							1.38	0.65	0.52	5*	4.5
Sodium methicillin	0.18	0.050	0.18	0.099	0.17	0.192	0.16	0.281	0.15	0.445	6.00	0.15	0.52	0	5.8
Sodium nafcillin	0.14	0.039	0.14	0.078	0.14	0.158	0.13	0.219	0.10	0.285					
Sodium nitrate			0.68								1.36	0.66		0	6.0
Sodium nitrite			0.84	0.48[b]							1.08	0.83		0*	8.5
Sodium oxacillin	0.18	0.050	0.17	0.095	0.16	0.177	0.15	0.257	0.14	0.408	6.64	0.14	0.52	0	6.0
Sodium phenylbutazone	0.19	0.054	0.18	0.104	0.17	0.202	0.17	0.298	0.17	0.488	5.34	0.17	0.52		
Sodium phosphate			0.29	0.168			0.27	0.47			3.33	0.27	0.52	0	9.2
Sodium phosphate, dibasic (2 H₂O)			0.42	0.24							2.23	0.40	0.52	0	9.2
Sodium phosphate, dibasic (12 H₂O)			0.22				0.21				4.45	0.20	0.52	0	9.2
Sodium propionate			0.61	0.35							1.47	0.61	0.52	0	7.8
Sodium salicylate			0.36	0.21							2.53	0.36	0.52	0	6.7
Sodium succinate	0.32	0.092	0.32	0.184	0.31	0.361					2.90	0.31	0.52	0	8.5
Sodium sulfate, anhydrous			0.58	0.34							1.61	0.56	0.52	0	6.2
Sodium sulfite, exsiccated			0.65	0.38											
Sodium sulfobromophthalein	0.07	0.019	0.06	0.034	0.05	0.060	0.05	0.084	0.04	0.123					
Sodium tartrate	0.33	0.098	0.33	0.193	0.33	0.385					2.72	0.33	0.52	0	7.3
Sodium thiosulfate			0.31	0.18							2.98	0.30	0.52	0	7.4
Sodium warfarin	0.18	0.049	0.17	0.095	0.16	0.181	0.15	0.264	0.15	0.430	6.10	0.15	0.52	0	8.1
Sorbitol (½ H₂O)											5.48			0	5.9
Streptomycin-calcium chloride				0.11[c]											
Streptomycin HCl			0.17	0.10[c]			0.16		0.16						
Streptomycin sulfate			0.07	0.04			0.06	0.10	0.06	0.17					
Sucrose			0.08	0.05			0.09	0.16	0.09	0.26	9.25	0.10	0.52	0	6.4
Sulfacetamide sodium			0.23	0.13			0.23	0.40			3.85	0.23	0.52	0	8.7
Sulfadiazine sodium			0.24	0.14			0.24	0.38			4.24	0.21	0.52	0	9.5
Sulfamerazine sodium			0.23	0.13			0.21	0.36			4.53	0.20	0.52		
Sulfapyridine sodium			0.23	0.13			0.21	0.36			4.55	0.20	0.52		
Sulfathiazole sodium			0.22	0.13			0.20	0.35			4.82	0.19	0.52	0	9.9
Tartaric acid											3.90			75*	1.7
Tetracaine HCl			0.18	0.10			0.15	0.26	0.12	0.35					
Tetracycline HCl			0.14	0.08[d]			0.10								
Theophylline				0.02[b]											
Theophylline sodium glycinate											2.94			0	8.9
Thiamine HCl											4.24			87*	3.0
Thiethylperazine maleate	0.10	0.030	0.09	0.050	0.08	0.089	0.07	0.119	0.05	0.153					
Thiopental sodium				0.16[c]											
Thiopropazate DiHCl	0.20	0.053	0.16	0.090	0.12	0.137	0.10	0.170	0.08	0.222					
Thioridazine HCl	0.06	0.015	0.05	0.025	0.04	0.042	0.03	0.055	0.03	0.075					
Triethanolamine	0.20	0.058	0.21	0.121	0.22	0.252	0.22	0.383			4.05	0.22	0.52	100	10.7
Trifluoperazine DiHCl	0.18	0.052	0.18	0.100	0.13	0.144									
Trimeprazine tartrate	0.10	0.023	0.06	0.035	0.04	0.045	0.03	0.052	0.02	0.061					
Trimethadione	0.23	0.069	0.23	0.133	0.22	0.257	0.22	0.378			4.22	0.21	0.52	100	6.0
Trimethobenzamide HCl	0.12	0.033	0.10	0.062	0.10	0.108	0.09	0.153	0.08	0.232					
Tripelennamine HCl				0.13[d]											
Tropicamide	0.10	0.030	0.09	0.050											
Tryparsamide				0.11[c]											
Tubocurarine chloride				0.08[c]											
Urea			0.59	0.34							1.63	0.55	0.52	100	6.6
Urethan				0.18[b]							2.93			100	6.3
Valethamate bromide	0.16	0.044	0.15	0.085	0.15	0.168	0.14	0.238	0.11	0.324					
Vancomycin HCl	0.06	0.015	0.05	0.028	0.04	0.049	0.04	0.066	0.04	0.098					

Table VI—Continued

	0.5%		1%		2%		3%		5%			At isotonicity[e]			
	E	D	E	D	E	D	E	D	E	D	%	E	D	H	pH
Viomycin sulfate			0.08	0.05			0.07	0.12	0.07	0.20					
Xylometazoline HCl	0.22	0.065	0.21	0.121	0.20	0.232	0.20	0.342			4.68	0.19	0.52	88	5.0
Zinc sulfate			0.15	0.09			0.13	0.23	0.12	0.35	7.65	0.12	0.52		

[a] The unmarked values were taken from the publications of Hammarlund and co-workers.[64, 73-75]
[b] Adapted from the values of Lund, et al.[55]
[c] Adapted from the values of the British Pharmaceutical Codex, 1954 and 1959 eds.
[d] Obtained from several sources.
[e] E: sodium chloride equivalents; D: freezing-point depressions, °C; H: hemolysis, %, at the concentration which is iso-osmotic with 0.9% NaCl, based on freezing-point determination or equivalent test; pH: approximate pH of solution studied for hemolytic action; *: change in appearance of erythrocytes and/or solution (see Refs. 74 and 75).

simple proportion using, as the basis for calculation, that figure which most nearly produces an isotonic solution. Actually the depression of the freezing point of a solution of an electrolyte is not absolutely proportional to the concentration but varies according to dilution; for example, a solution containing 1 Gm of procaine hydrochloride in 100 ml has a freezing-point depression of 0.12 °C, whereas a solution containing 3 Gm of the same salt in 100 ml has a freezing-point depression of 0.33 °C, *not* 0.36 °C (3 × 0.12°). Since the adjustment to isotonicity need not be absolutely exact, approximations may be made. When it is recalled that for many years an 0.85% solution of sodium chloride, rather than the presently employed 0.90% concentration, was widely accepted and proved to be eminently satisfactory as the isotonic equivalent of blood serum, it is apparent that minor deviations are not of great concern. Also, formerly a 1.4% solution of sodium chloride was considered to be isotonic with lacrimal fluid and found to be relatively tolerable when applied to the eye. Nevertheless, adjustments to isotonicity should be as exact as practicable.

As a specific illustration of the manner in which the data in the table may be used, suppose it is required to calculate the quantity of sodium chloride needed to make 100 ml of a 1% solution of calcium disodium edetate iso-osmotic with blood serum. Reference to the table indicates that the 1% solution provides for 0.12° of the necessary 0.52 °C of freezing-point depression required of an iso-osmotic solution, thus leaving 0.40° to be supplied by the sodium chloride. Again referring to the table, 0.52 °C is found to be the freezing-point depression of a 0.9% solution of sodium chloride and by simple proportion it is calculated that a 0.69% solution will have a freezing-point depression of 0.40 °C. Assuming additivity of the freezing-point depressions, a solution of 0.69 Gm of sodium chloride and 1 Gm of calcium disodium edetate in sufficient water to make 100 ml will be iso-osmotic with blood serum.

Likewise, to render a 1% solution of boric acid isotonic with lacrimal fluid by the addition of sodium chloride, one would proceed with the calculation as follows:

Freezing-point depression of lacrimal fluid.............	0.52°C
Freezing-point depression of 1% boric acid solution......	0.29°C
Freezing-point depression to be supplied by sodium chloride..	0.23°C
Freezing-point depression of a 0.9% solution of sodium chloride..	0.52°C

Therefore

$$0.52:0.9 = 0.23:x$$

$$0.52x = 0.207$$

x = 0.4% sodium chloride to be incorporated with 1% boric acid to produce a solution which will be isotonic with lacrimal fluid.

Similarly, should a solution contain more than one ingredient, the sum of the respective freezing points

of each ingredient would be determined and the difference between this sum and the required freezing point would represent the freezing point to be supplied by the added substance.

The preceding calculation can be expressed in the form of an equation, as follows:

$$x = \frac{(0.52° - a) \times c}{b}$$

where

x = Gm of adjusting solute required for each 100 ml of solution.
$0.52°$ = Freezing-point depression of blood serum or lacrimal fluid.
a = Freezing-point depression of given ingredients in 100 ml of solution.
b = Freezing-point depression of c Gm of adjusting substance per 100 ml.
c = Gm of adjusting solute per 100 ml, producing a freezing-point depression of b.

L Values—In dilute solutions, the expression for freezing-point depression may be written as:

$$\Delta T_f = Lc$$

in which ΔT_f is the freezing-point depression in °C, L is a constant, and c is the molar concentration of the drug. L_{iso} is defined as the specific value of L at a concentration of drug which is isotonic with blood or lacrimal fluid. Values of L have been calculated for a number of drugs by Goyan, et al;[58] average L_{iso} values have been determined by Wells[76] and are presented in Table VII.

If the freezing-point depression of a drug is not available, it may be calculated with sufficient accuracy by use of the equation:

$$\Delta T_f = L_{iso} \times \frac{w \times 1000}{M \times v}$$

in which w is the weight of solute in grams, M is the molecular weight of the solute, and v is the volume of the solution in milliliters.

Table VII—Average L_{iso} Values

Type of compound	L_{iso}	Examples
Nonelectrolytes	1.9	Sucrose, camphor
Weak electrolytes	2.0	Boric acid, phenobarbital
Di-divalent electrolytes	2.0	Magnesium sulfate, zinc sulfate
Uni-univalent electrolytes	3.4	Sodium chloride, phenobarbital sodium
Uni-divalent electrolytes	4.3	Sodium sulfate, atropine sulfate
Di-univalent electrolytes	4.8	Zinc chloride, calcium chloride
Uni-trivalent electrolytes	5.2	Sodium citrate, sodium phosphate
Tri-univalent electrolytes	6.0	Aluminum chloride
Tetraborates	7.6	Sodium borate

For example, suppose one wishes to determine the freezing-point depression of a 3% *w/v* solution of phenobarbital sodium. This drug, a uni-univalent electrolyte, has an L_{iso} value of 3.4; its molecular weight is 254. Substituting into the equation,

$$\Delta T_f = 3.4 \times \frac{3 \times 1000}{254 \times 100} = 0.40$$

For a more complete discussion of the use of L values, the reader is referred to the book by Martin.[77]

Effect of Solvents—Besides water, certain other solvents are frequently employed in nose drops, ear drops, and other preparations to be used in various parts of the body. Liquids such as glycerin, propylene glycol, or alcohol may compose part of the solvent. In solving isotonicity adjustment problems for such solutions it should be kept in mind that while these solvent components contribute to the freezing-point depression they may or may not have an effect on the "tone" of the tissue to which they are applied, ie, an *iso-osmotic* solution may not be *isotonic*. It is apparent that in such cases, the utility of the methods described above or, for that matter, of any other method of evaluating "tonicity" is questionable.

Reliability of Freezing-Point Data—While the freezing point of blood was formerly assumed to be −0.56 °C, Lund, *et al*,[55] reported that in consequence of ice being disengaged in freezing-point determinations as ordinarily performed the observed freezing point of blood is low; according to them the correct freezing point is −0.52 °C. The same investigators found the freezing point of a 0.9% solution of sodium chloride to be correspondingly low; the correct freezing point in this case is also −0.52 °C. Presumably all solutions commonly considered to be isotonic with blood will freeze, when a correction for disengaged ice is applied, at −0.52 °C. It is apparent, therefore, that there is no need to change the isotonic concentration, if the reference temperature for both blood and the solution under consideration is always the same, and provided that the *method* of determining the freezing point is the same. Also, there appears to be no objection to using freezing-point data for solutions of other than isotonic concentration if the method of determining the freezing point is the same in all cases, since any differences that may be obtained when another method is used (such as that of Lund *et al*[55]), will probably be proportional to concentration.

In a discussion of the significance of freezing-point data it is to be noted that there are some discrepancies in the literature concerning freezing points of solutions. An exact determination of freezing point is actually a difficult experiment, one which calls for the control of several variables which are commonly neglected, of which disengagement of ice is one. It is not possible at this time to select unequivocal freezing-point data for most of the solutions listed in Table VI included in this chapter. The comprehensive and valuable data of Lund, *et al*,[55] referred to above, actually represent in most instances measurements of vapor pressure which have been *calculated* to corresponding freezing-point depressions; it would seem to be desirable to have confirmatory evidence based on actual measurements of freezing point, determined more accurately than has generally been the case, before revisions of existing data are made. In the case of boric acid, which enters into the composition of some collyria, there is the further variable, reported by Lund and his associates, that a sterilized solution freezes at a higher temperature than a freshly prepared, unsterilized solution of the same

strength; specifically, a freshly prepared solution containing 2.85% of boric acid was found to freeze at the same temperature (−0.82 °C) as a 3.1% solution which had been sterilized under pressure.

Earlier in this section it was stated that at one time lacrimal fluid was considered to have the same osmotic pressure as a 1.4% solution of sodium chloride, the freezing point of which was found to be, by the usual method of determination, −0.80 °C. The experiments of Krogh, *et al*,[78] have indicated that lacrimal fluid has the same osmotic pressure as blood and that instead of assuming that the freezing point of solutions isotonic with lacrimal fluid is −0.80 °C it should be the same as that of blood, namely, −0.52 °C. Accordingly, the procedure for adjusting solutions to isotonicity with lacrimal fluid is qualitatively and quantitatively the same as the procedure for adjusting solutions to isotonicity with blood.

Hemolysis and Other Changes in Erythrocytes in Certain Iso-Osmotic Solutions*

Studies involving hemolysis of erythrocytes have included work by the following investigators:

1. Husa and co-workers on such frequently used ingredients as glycerin and boric acid (Adams[79]), amino acids and sugars (Grosicki[80]), urea and urea derivatives (Easterly[81]), zinc sulfate and other inorganic salts (Hartman[82]), salts of organic acids (Cadwallader[83, 84]), alkaloidal salts (Thomasson[85]), salts of gluconic acid (Ansel[86]), monohydric and polyhydric alcohols (Zanowiak[87]), local anesthetics (Marcus[88]), sympathomimetic amine salts and phenothiazine derivatives (Winters[89]), water-soluble organic iodine compounds (Schnell[90]), and compounds such as procaine hydrochloride which cause hemolysis even in the presence of 0.6% NaCl, which used independently prevents hemolysis (Shaw[91]). The work by Husa and co-workers was summarized, in part, by Cadwallader.[92, 93]

2. Ansel on the influence of polyethylene glycols on the hemolytic activity of phenolic preservatives[94] and on chlorhexidine diacetate;[95] and by Ansel and co-workers on other antibacterial preservatives (Cadwallader[96]), quaternary ammonium salts (Cadwallader[97]), and the influence of dimethyl sulfoxide on the hemolytic activity of phenol (Leake[98]).

3. Cadwallader on water–glycerin and water–propylene glycol[99] and Cadwallader and co-workers on various solvent systems, the effect of temperature and of various substances on hemolysis in water–glycerin and water–propylene glycol systems (Wickliffe and Smith[100]), water–propylene glycol (Smith[101]), and water–dimethyl sulfoxide (Drinkard[102]).

4. Hammerlund and co-workers on the iso-osmotic concentrations of 161 substances for which they had previously reported sodium chloride equivalents (Pedersen-Bjergaard[74]) and on 45 additional substances (Van Pevenage[75]). See Table VI.

5. Ansel, who reported on the response of human erythrocytes to commercial parenteral solutions having the osmotic equivalent of at least 0.6% sodium chloride. A number of solutions for which isotonicity was claimed caused hemolysis or marked change in appearance of the red blood cells.[103]

As an example of a different approach, Setnikar and Temelcou[104] chose to avoid hemolysis and to study the tonicity of injectable solutions by measuring variations of red cell volume. They state that while the hemolytic method can demonstrate very clearly the difference between solutes which are diffusible through the membrane of red cells and those which are not, it is not so easy to determine the isotonic concentration because, for this purpose, it is necessary to start from the premise that for all solutes there is a single ratio between isotonic concentration and hemolytic concentration, whereas it has been shown that, on the contrary, this ratio may vary from 1.4 to 3.1.

Hammarlung and Pedersen-Bjergaard state that there is no distinct pattern indicating the predom-

---

*Hemolysis is discussed here because of its relationship to isotonicity. The hemolytic properties of ophthalmic solutions are believed to be of no clinical significance.

inance of any single main mechanism of penetration of the erythrocyte by the solute and solvent which results in hemolysis of the erythrocyte.[74] It appears to be a combination of factors such as pH, lipoid solubility, the molecular and ionic size of the particles, or the inhibition of cholinesterase in the cell membrane. There are other complex forces which also may play a role because of their possible denaturing actions on the plasma membrane protein; substances such as alcohol and urea are known to rupture hydrogen bonding; low surface-tension forces may denature proteins; and acids, alkalies, and oxidizing agents often change the structure of proteins, owing, in part, to their effects on benzene ring structures, such as those present in the amino acids and histidine.

The picture is still incomplete, but some grouping of compounds has been done by Setnikar and Temelcou,[104] who give the following classification based on their studies of erythrocyte volume:

Group 1—Substances whose iso-osmotic concentration is isotonic; eg, NaCl, KCl, sodium thiosulfate, sodium borate, sodium propionate, sodium benzoate, sodium barbital, sorbitol, dextrose (for rabbit erythrocytes).
Group 2—Substances which do not exert any osmotic pressure; eg, urea, succinic dinitrile, antipyrine, aminophylline, ethanol, propylene glycol, sodium pentobarbital, polysorbate 80.
Group 3—Substances whose isotonic concentration is higher than their iso-osmotic concentration; eg, dextrose (for human erythrocytes), glycine, sodium salicylate.
Group 4—Substances which increase the permeability of the erythrocyte membrane to NaCl; eg, procaine HCl, adiphenine HCl, ethanol, propylene glycol (at concentrations greater than 10–20%), polysorbate 60.
Group 5—Substances with a pronounced hemolytic action; eg, saponin, sulfuric esters of methylandrostenediol and of testosterone.
Group 6—Substances which exert a protective action similar to that exerted by dextrose as regards the increase in permeability caused by procaine; eg, dextrose, sorbitol.
Group 7—Substances precipitating proteins; eg, ZnSO₄ and all precipitants of proteins.

The *in vitro* studies of the hemolysis of erythrocytes by iso-osmotic solutions usually mix a large amount of solution with a small amount of blood, with a ratio perhaps 100:1.[74] Hammarlund and Pederson-Bjergaard state that this proportion of solution to blood and tissue fluids is not very often obtained in the body, therefore the danger of hemolysis is usually much less than is indicated by the *in vitro* studies. They studied the hemolytic properties of a few strongly hemolytic substances in the completely reversed proportion of solution to blood volume of 1:10 and found no hemolysis. Thus, factors in the consideration of the use of isotonic solutions vs iso-osmotic solutions are the quantity and proportions of the substances used and the rapidity and ease of the dilution of the medicinal solution by the body fluids. The situation at the moment of injection should be considered.

Tonicity of Ophthalmic Solutions

An isotonic ophthalmic solution causes less discomfort than one that is hypotonic or hypertonic; it may, indeed, have a soothing rather than an irritating effect on the eye.

During the period prior to 1950 the majority of ophthalmic solutions were adjusted to a tonicity equivalent to approximately 1.4% sodium chloride when isotonicity was desired. More recently the trend has been to prepare these solutions to be iso-osmotic with 0.9% sodium chloride solution. However, some current textbooks on ophthalmology still give the isotonicity equivalent as 1.4% sodium chloride and the dispensing pharmacist may find it necessary to inform

the physician as to the true value. It has been customary to state that ophthalmic solutions should be exactly isotonic with tears. However, in the extemporaneous preparation of a single prescription the manipulation required to attain isotonicity often makes it much more difficult to prepare a sterile solution in a reasonable amount of time.

It has been found that in the typical occasional administration of small quantities of ophthalmic solutions as drops, the eye can tolerate a fairly wide range of tonicity before any pain or discomfort is observed. Moreover, there is a still wider concentration range in which discomfort is moderate and exists for only a very short time without damage to the tissues of the eye. The range of concentration permitted, in terms of sodium chloride, has been reported as 0.6–1.5%,[105] 0.6–2.0%,[78] and 0.5–2.0%.[106] The USP states that the range can be 0.6–1.5% without marked discomfort. The NF gives the limits as 0.6–2.0%. Lund, *et al*,[107] attempted to grade the response to solutions showing varying degrees of osmotic imbalances. Their results are listed in Table VIII. As another approach, Trolle-Lassen[45] reported the proportion of subjects who experienced irritation at particular sodium chloride concentrations. He found that about half of his series of healthy subjects experienced irritation if the sodium chloride concentration was reduced to 0.4% or increased to 1.8% and that with concentrations of 0.7% or 1.4% only about 1 in a 100 experienced irritation. It is evident that accurate adjustment is unnecessary in many cases. The British Pharmaceutical Codex (1968) does not require the addition of sodium chloride or other substances to adjust the tonicity of hypotonic ophthalmic solutions.

Sodium sulfacetamide has been used in ophthalmology quite extensively for more than two decades in concentrations from 10% to 30%. Weaker concentrations do not give the desired antibacterial action. Fenton[108] used concentrations of sodium sulfacetamide of 2.5% to 30% on 20 individuals. Concentrations below 5% were painless but as concentration was increased more pain was felt by more subjects until at 12.5% some pain was felt by all but one subject. Based on measurements of freezing point he stated that a 3.5% solution is approximately isotonic with a 0.9% solution of sodium chloride, a 10% solution with 3% sodium chloride, and a 30% solution with 9% sodium chloride. However, clinical experience shows that the 30% solution gives discomfort for only a short time, and does not damage the tissues when used as recommended. Maurice[17] has studied the effect of radioactive Na²⁴Cl on rabbits' eyes. He concluded that sodium chloride solutions in concentrations up to 10% should not cause any damage to the eye due to deviation from isotonicity. However, Krishna, *et al*,[109] state that isotonic saline seems to interfere with the regeneration of corneal epithelium.

Table VIII—Response to Various Concentrations of Sodium Chloride

Response	% sodium chloride
Very disagreeable after ½ min	2.0
Somewhat disagreeable after 1 min	1.5
Perceptibly disagreeable after 1 min	1.3
Completely indifferent after a long time	1.2
	0.8
Perceptibly disagreeable after 1 min	0.6

Table IX—Common Ophthalmic Solutions

Drug	Concentration
Antazoline Phosphate	0.5%
Atropine Sulfate	4%
Benoxinate Hydrochloride	0.4%
Benzalkonium Chloride	1:3000
Carbachol	1.5%
Cocaine Hydrochloride	4%
Cyclopentolate	2%
Epinephrine Bitartrate	2%
Epinephrine Hydrochloride	2%
Fluorescein Sodium	2%
Homatropine Hydrobromide	4%
Hydroxyamphetamine Hydrobromide	1%
Lidocaine Hydrochloride	2%
Neostigmine Bromide	2.5%
Phenylephrine Hydrochloride	0.25%
Physostigmine Salicylate	0.5%
Physostigmine Sulfate	0.5%
Pilocarpine Hydrochloride	2%
Pilocarpine Nitrate	3%
Scopolamine Hydrobromide	1%
Tetracaine Hydrochloride	0.5%

Table X—Permitted Ophthalmic Concentrations

Drug	Concentration
Carbachol	3%
Homatropine Hydrobromide	5%
Lidocaine Hydrochloride	4%
Neostigmine Bromide	5%
Phenylephrine Hydrochloride	2.5%
Pilocarpine Hydrochloride	5%
Pilocarpine Nitrate	5%

When an ophthalmic solution is to be used as an eye lotion (eye wash) it is much more essential to prepare an isotonic solution. A much larger volume of fluid is used and dilution by tears is not likely to suitably adjust the tonicity. Irritation may be severe with either markedly hypertonic or hypotonic solutions. In the administration of eye drops several times a day for months or years it is desirable to use a nonirritating solution if possible and isotonicity is one of the requirements.

Adjustment of Tonicity—The USP states that

"Since most drugs used in ophthalmic practice have large molecular weights, they usually can be added to isotonic sodium chloride solution or some other isotonic vehicle in amounts up to 3% without causing the osmotic pressure to increase to painful levels."

Table IX gives illustrations of commonly used ophthalmic solutions[19] which can be prepared in a 0.9% sodium chloride vehicle (or vehicle of equivalent tonicity, as 1.9% boric acid) without exceeding the limit of 1.5% set by USP XVII on sodium chloride equivalence. In instances where a solution can be used with a tonicity value up to approximately 2% Table X gives the permitted concentrations.

Riegelman has recommended a 0.8% sodium chloride vehicle, or its osmotic equivalent, as a stock vehicle.[1]

Drugs occasionally used in higher concentration, such as phenylephrine hydrochloride (10%) and pilocarpine hydrochloride or nitrate (6%) may employ as a vehicle either sterile distilled preserved water or a solution of lesser tonicity value than discussed above.

It is comparatively simple to adjust a hypotonic solution so that it will possess the same isotonicity value as lacrimal fluid, and for this purpose either boric acid or sodium chloride may be used. As previously indicated, such solutions are preferably prepared so as to have the same freezing point as tear fluid, namely— 0.52°, when they will also possess the same osmotic pressure as well as other colligative properties of tear fluid.

A solution containing 1.9% boric acid is isotonic with tear fluid, which helps to explain the suggestion usually offered when a saturated 5% solution of boric acid is sold, namely, to dilute the solution with about an equal volume of water for use as an eye wash. Such a diluted solution more nearly approaches isotonicity

with resulting increase in comfort when the solution is used. On the other hand the saturated solution of boric acid is stable while the weaker solution often shows signs of mold growth. Consequently, the former usually has been kept as a stock solution. The current preference for preserved solutions permits use of the 1.9% boric acid solution as a stock solution.

Generally speaking, the adjustment to isotonicity is of secondary importance when buffered solutions are used as vehicles in the extemporaneous preparation of eye drops. However, if irritation is too great due to gross deviation from isotonicity, accurate calculations for tonicity value can be carried out taking the freezing-point depression of the medicinal substance and the buffered vehicle into consideration. Hammarlund and Pedersen-Bjergaard published a table for determining the volume of solution containing the drug which upon dilution to 30 ml with an isotonic ophthalmic vehicle will give a 1% isotonic solution. Their data for some commonly used drugs are listed in Table XI.[110] For more detailed information the reader is referred to the original article.

Example 1:

A prescription calls for:

Atropine Sulfate .... 0.3 Gm
Sterile Preserved Water qs .... 60.0 ml

M.Ft.Collyr. isotonic and buffered S.A.
Sig: For Office Use.

This order is for a 0.5% solution of atropine sulfate. According to Table XI, 0.3 Gm of atropine sulfate dissolved in 4.3 ml of sterile preserved water will produce a 1% isotonic solution when diluted to 30 ml with an isotonic vehicle. For 30 ml of 0.5% solution, half the quantities of atropine sulfate and sterile preserved water would be used, but for 60 ml of 0.5% solution the same quantities as for 30 ml of 1% solution are required.

Therefore, to fill this prescription order, 0.3 Gm of atropine sulfate should be dissolved in 4.3 ml of sterile preserved water and diluted with isotonic preserved Sørensen's pH 6.8 phosphate buffer to 60 ml.

For more than one active ingredient in solution the quantity of water to be used is calculated for each ingredient separately. The values thus obtained are added, the total amount of sterile preserved water is then used to dissolve the active ingredients, and finally sufficient isotonic, buffered preserved solution (diluting solution) is used to make the required volume.

Example 2:

A prescription calls for:

Epinephrine Hydrochloride 0.5%
Zinc Sulfate 0.3%
Sterile Preserved Water qs to make .... 30 ml

M. Ft. Collyr. isotonic

In this example the active ingredients are given in percentage. The ideal vehicle is 1.9% boric acid solution. Reference to the table for isotonic solution values shows the following:

Epinephrine hydrochloride 0.3 Gm (1%) will make 9.7 ml of an isotonic solution when dissolved in sterile preserved water. Zinc sulfate 0.3 Gm will make 5 ml of an isotonic solution with sterile water.

Therefore, the quantities called for in this prescription will make 4.85 ml and 1.5 ml isotonic solutions resp. Dissolve the salts in sufficient sterile preserved water to make 6.35 ml and add sufficient 1.9% preserved boric acid solution to make 30 ml. The resulting solution is isotonic.

Since it is practically impossible to measure the required volumes accurately, it is feasible, in this instance, to use 6.35 ml of sterile preserved water as the total solvent for these two drugs. Exact adjustment to isotonicity is sacrificed, but the manipulations involved may introduce contamination. Graduated pipets, previously sterilized, are necessary for this work.

When isotonicity alone is desired, the calculations for adjustment are very simple by using the freezing-point depression method (see pages 1556–1561). A different approach is the use of the so-called sodium chloride equivalent method. The sodium chloride equivalent is defined as that weight of sodium chloride which will produce the same osmotic effect as one equal weight unit of the substance in question (Table VI). Thus, if the sodium chloride equivalent of boric acid is 0.5 at 1% concentration, it means that 1 Gm of boric acid in solution will produce the same freezing-point depression as 0.5 Gm of sodium chloride or a 1% boric acid solution is equivalent in colligative properties to a 0.5% solution of sodium chloride. For a 1.9% boric acid solution, ie, at isotonicity, the sodium chloride equivalent is 0.47, corresponding to 0.9% sodium chloride solution, (1.9×0.47).

Examples for calculations, using the sodium chloride equivalent method.

Example 1:

Homatropine Hydrobromide........................ 1%
to make collyr. isotonic........................... 60 ml

0.6 Gm of homatropine hydrobromide is required. 1 Gm or 1% of the drug is equivalent in osmotic effect to 0.17 Gm or 0.17% resp. of sodium chloride.

$$0.17 \times 0.6 = 0.102 \text{ Gm (sodium chloride)}$$

60 ml of an isotonic sodium chloride solution contains	0.54 Gm sodium chloride
0.6 Gm homatropine hydrobromide is equivalent to	0.102 Gm sodium chloride
	0.438 Gm sodium chloride

Therefore, 0.438 Gm of sodium chloride must be added to make 60 ml of a 1% homatropine hydrobromide solution isotonic with tear fluid. The same calculations may be carried through using percentage calculations. 1% of homatropine hydrobromide corresponds to 0.17% sodium chloride in colligative properties.

Thus, 0.9% minus 0.17% = 0.73% must be added, 0.73% of 60 ml = 0.438 Gm of sodium chloride to be added.

If boric acid is to be used as the adjusting substance the calculations have to be carried out one step further. There is no "boric acid equivalent," but the sodium chloride equivalent of boric acid at 1% concentration is 0.5, meaning that 1 Gm of boric acid (or 1%) corresponds in colligative properties to 0.5 Gm of sodium chloride (or 0.5%). Using the result obtained in Example 1, which was 0.438 Gm of sodium chloride to be added, it now follows that the sodium chloride equivalent of boric acid must be divided into the amount of sodium chloride or expressed as an equation:

$$1 \text{ Gm boric acid: } 0.5 \text{ Gm sodium chloride} = x \text{ Gm:} 0.438 \text{ Gm}$$
$$x = 0.876 \text{ Gm boric acid to be added}$$

For a prescription containing more than one active drug, the calculations for sodium chloride are carried out separately, the obtained quantities are added, and then the total is deducted from the 0.9% amount. Using the same example as in a previous determination the prescription reads as follows:

Example 2:

Epinephrine Hydrochloride........................ 0.5%
Zinc Sulfate.................................... 0.3%
Sterile Preserved Water qs, to make................ 30 ml

M.Ft.Collyr. isotonic S.A.

Sodium chloride equivalent of epinephrine HCl is 0.29
Sodium chloride equivalent of zinc sulfate is 0.15

150 mg epinephrine hydrochloride	~43.5 mg sod. chloride
90 mg zinc sulfate	~13.5 mg sod. chloride
Total ingredients are equivalent to	~57 mg sod. chloride

0.9% of 30 ml	270 mg sodium chloride
	57 mg
	213 mg

213 mg of sodium chloride must be added to make the solution (example 2) isotonic with tear fluid. Since boric acid is the adjusting substance of choice for the above solution 426 mg should be used (0.5 divided into 213 mg).

The sodium chloride equivalents are not always directly proportional to the concentration of the solute. This is due to interionic attraction which changes with greater concentration. The authors of this publication[73] based their work on freezing-point depression and vapor pressure lowering data. Most of the original work was carried out by a group of Danish investigators, who were instrumental in ascertaining the accurate freezing point of lacrimal fluid.[111]

It should be mentioned that still other methods are available for the adjustment of isotonic solutions. One which is used in many European countries is the "Graphic Method for Use in the Adjustment to Isotonic Solutions." In this method the percentage concentration of the substance to be made isotonic is read as the abscissa of a graph and the Gms of sodium chloride to add per 100 ml of solution or grains of sodium chloride/fluid ounce are read as the ordinate. For commonly used substances graphs have been published. The Danish Pharmacopeia (1948) includes similar graphs. Numerous other publications also refer to these graphs. For routine use in adjusting to isotonicity the freezing-point depression tables and the sodium chloride equivalent tables have been found very satisfactory.

The ophthalmologist does not necessarily prescribe buffered and isotonic collyria, but he does expect that clarity and sterility be achieved.

Surface Activity

Surface-active agents are often called wetting or penetrating agents. Because of these qualities, they have been suggested for use in vehicles recommended for ophthalmic drugs.[112] They have been shown to cause increased penetration into the cornea and other ocular tissues in certain formulations.

However, they may interact with other ingredients and reduce their effectiveness. This has been reported for *p*-hydroxybenzoic acid esters and polysorbate 80;[113] it is implicit in the selection of such compounds to neutralize antimicrobial preservatives, described in a later section, but is not, of course, restricted to bactericides and related compounds. Inclusion of surface-active substances can markedly reduce the drop-volume from a given dropper, and so can alter the volume of drug administered.[114]

Only those wetting agents which have been found suitable for ophthalmic use should be employed and then only when sufficiently diluted so as not to cause any damage to the ocular tissue. Local ophthalmic use of wetting agents is permissible only when directed by a physician who is familiar with their possible toxic properties.[115]

The agent most commonly used is benzalkonium chloride. The fact that this agent acts also as a preservative favors its selection (see page 1570). Other surfactants used are: benzethonium chloride, myristyl-gamma-picolinium chloride, polysorbate 20, polyoxyl 40 stearate, alkyl aryl polyether alcohol, polyoxypropylene-polyoxyethylenediol,[116] dioctyl sodium sulfosuccinate, and, especially, polysorbate 80. Much more work must be done to determine the usefulness of surface-active agents in ophthalmology and to find compounds that are devoid of the irritation which is so often encountered with surface-active substances.

Viscosity

The USP states:

"A suitable grade of methylcellulose (1% if the viscosity is 25 centipoises, or 0.25% if 4000 centipoises) or equally suitable thickening agent occasionally is added to ophthalmic solutions to increase the viscosity and aid in holding the drug in contact with the tissue. Although difficulty may be encountered in sterilization or filtration, the thickened ophthalmic solution must be free from visible particles."

Only a few of the suspending agents used in pharmacy have the proper optical clarity, refractive index, and lack of drug reaction to be useful as agents to increase the viscosity of ophthalmic solutions. Polyethylene glycol, polyvinyl alcohol, polyvinylpyrrolidone, hydroxypropylmethylcellulose, carboxymethylcellulose,

Table XI—Volumes of Water for Isotonicity[a]

Drug (1% or 0.3 Gm)	Water needed for isotonicity, ml	Drug (1% or 0.3 Gm)	Water needed for isotonicity, ml
Alcohol	21.7	Phenobarbital sodium	8.0
Ammonium chloride	37.3	Physostigmine salicylate	5.3
Amobarbital sodium	8.3	Pilocarpine hydrochloride	8.0
Amphetamine phosphate	11.3	Pilocarpine nitrate	7.7
Amphetamine sulfate	7.3	Piperocaine hydrochloride	7.0
Antipyrine	5.7	Polymyxin B sulfate	3.0
Apomorphine hydrochloride	4.7	Potassium chloride	25.3
Ascorbic acid	6.0	Potassium nitrate	18.7
Atropine methylbromide	4.7	Potassium phosphate, monobasic	14.7
Atropine sulfate	4.3	Procainamide hydrochloride	7.3
Bacitracin	1.7	Procaine hydrochloride	7.0
Barbital sodium	10.0	Scopolamine hydrobromide	4.0
Bismuth potassium tartrate	3.0	Scopolamine methylnitrate	5.3
Boric acid	16.7	Secobarbital sodium	8.0
Butacaine sulfate	6.7	Silver nitrate	11.0
Caffeine and sodium benzoate	8.7	Silver protein, mild	5.7
Calcium chloride	17.0	Sodium acetate	15.3
Calcium chloride (6 H_2O)	11.7	Sodium bicarbonate	21.7
Chlorobutanol (hydrated)	8.0	Sodium biphosphate, anhydrous	15.3
Chlortetracycline sulfate	4.3	Sodium biphosphate	13.3
Cocaine hydrochloride	5.3	Sodium bisulfite	20.3
Cupric sulfate	6.0	Sodium borate	14.0
Dextrose, anhydrous	6.0	Sodium iodide	13.0
Dibucaine hydrochloride	4.3	Sodium metabisulfite	22.3
Dihydrostreptomycin sulfate	2.0	Sodium nitrate	22.7
Ephedrine hydrochloride	10.0	Sodium phosphate	9.7
Ephedrine sulfate	7.7	Sodium propionate	20.3
Epinephrine bitartrate	6.0	Sodium sulfite, exsiccated	21.7
Epinephrine hydrochloride	9.7	Sodium thiosulfate	10.3
Ethylmorphine hydrochloride	5.3	Streptomycin sulfate	2.3
Fluorescein sodium	10.3	Sulfacetamide sodium	7.7
Glycerin	11.7	Sulfadiazine sodium	8.0
Holocaine hydrochloride	6.7	Sulfamerazine sodium	7.7
Homatropine hydrobromide	5.7	Sulfapyridine sodium	7.7
Homotropine methylbromide	6.3	Sulfathiazole sodium	7.3
Hyoscyamine sulfate	4.7	Tetracaine hydrochloride	6.0
Neomycin sulfate	3.7	Tetracycline hydrochloride	4.7
Oxytetracycline hydrochloride	4.3	Viomycin sulfate	2.7
Penicillin G, potassium	6.0	Zinc chloride	20.3
Penicillin G, sodium	6.0	Zinc sulfate	5.0
Pentobarbital sodium	8.3		

[a] Table of "Isotonic Solution Values" showing volumes in ml of solution that can be prepared by dissolving 300 mg of the specified drug in sterile water. The addition of an isotonic and/or buffered vehicle (commonly referred to as diluting solution) to make 30 ml yields a 1% solution.

methylcellulose,[116] and hydroxypropyl ethyl cellulose[117] are presumably all in this category, judged by their commercial use.[116] The most thoroughly investigated representative of these is methylcellulose.

Swan[118,119] first reported the use of methylcellulose (4000 cps viscosity type) solutions as a bland vehicle for ophthalmic medicaments, as a substitute for natural secretions in cases of keratoconjunctivitis sicca, and as an emollient and cohesive solution to be used with contact lenses and gonioscopic prisms. He stated that acacia, tragacanth, and gelatin had been the most widely used for this purpose but have the disadvantages that they have high refractive indexes, are chemically unstable, and are good media for the growth of microorganisms.

Methylcellulose solutions also may be used:

1. To increase therapeutic response.
2. To replace deficient tear secretions such as are found, for example, in many postmenopausal women and many men over 50 years of age.
3. After tonometry, with 0.1% ephedrine sulfate added to the methylcellulose solution.
4. As a protective lubricant in the postnucleation socket for the prosthesis.
5. As a protective medicament for various pathologic conditions of the cornea.

6. To relieve the discomfort in band form keratitis, in endothelia epithelial dystrophy, and in old, healed trachomatous pannus.[120]

Swan[118] reported that tetracaine and dibutoline sulfate, for example, are adsorbed by the methylcellulose sufficiently to retard their penetration of tissue. More recent research has shown the need for awareness of the possibility of interaction between such macromolecular substances and other ingredients, such as the parabens.[121,122]

Mueller and Deardorff[123] have studied the effect of methylcellulose on the therapeutic response of patients to homatropine hydrobromide. They found that a buffered aqueous solution containing 0.25% homatropine hydrobromide produced no cycloplegic or mydriatic response in any of nine subjects. The addition of 1% methylcellulose reduced accommodation to 20% and caused a pupillary dilation from 3.0 to 7.0 mm.

By comparing the effect of a plain solution with that of one containing 1% methylcellulose (4000 cps) on each eye of the same subject, Mueller and Deardorff found little or no difference in the response at the 1.0% homatropine level. At concentrations of 0.25, 0.50, and 0.75% homatropine hydrobromide, however, the increased contact time obtained with the more viscous, methylcellulose-containing solution resulted in greater therapeutic response than obtained for a given concentration of homatropine hydrobromide in a vehicle which was the same composition except that it did not contain methylcellulose. Analogous studies have been carried out on pilocarpine[124] and on scopolamine.[120]

In many cases the amount of medication in a more viscous preparation can be reduced as compared to the quantity used in an aqueous solution. Sulfacetamide sodium is used as a 30% solution in a buffered aqueous vehicle. When methylcellulose or an analogous compound is added, the concentration of the drug may be reduced to 10%.

Its routine use poses a number of problems, especially in extemporaneous preparations. Solutions containing methylcellulose, when subjected to heat sterilization, will show coagulation of the methylcellulose since the cellulose derivative is less soluble in water at elevated temperatures. Upon cooling the solution it will tend to redissolve and may or may not be completely dispersed. It has been reported that residue of undissolved particles has been found in such solutions. Filtration of methylcellulose solutions is commonly stated to be difficult or impossible; however, it is desirable, and Madden and Piecoro[125] describe a procedure using a 0.45-μ Millipore bacterial filter membrane.

Mims[126] found that a concentration of 0.33% methylcellulose 4000 cps was most satisfactory as a tear substitute, while concentrations of 0.25, 0.5, or 1% proved either too thin or too thick.

Bergy[127] reviewed the use of methylcellulose in ophthalmic solutions, presented several formulas, and discussed the pharmaceutical technique used in preparing methylcellulose solutions.

Scigliano[128] recommended the following methylcellulose vehicle for alkaloidal salts used in ophthalmology.

Methylcellulose 4000 cps	0.33 Gm
Sodium chloride	0.45 Gm
Hind and Goyan's Phosphate Buffer, pH 6.8	50.00 ml
Benzalkonium chloride 1:25,000, to make	100.00 ml

The solution is prepared by heating one-third of the total volume of the solvent to 70°C. The methylcellulose is allowed to soak in this solution for 30 minutes. The remainder of the solvent is added after it has cooled to 4°C.

As Campbell, et al,[129] have shown, the viscosity of methylcellulose generally increases as the pH increases. These authors found that a buffer low in total salt concentration, such as the Sørensen system, is preferable to the Gifford buffer because it has less influence on the viscosity of the final solution. High concentrations (over 1.4%) of sodium chloride increase the viscosity of methylcellulose solutions.

Solutions containing methylcellulose tend to form a crust on the eyelids, which, however, can be wiped off easily. The effect of methylcellulose on the internal structure of the eye is not completely known.

Krishna and Brow[109] describe a 1.4% polyvinyl alcohol ophthalmic vehicle which they believe to be possibly superior to methylcellulose. It will prolong contact time and reduce surface tension without interfering with the regeneration of corneal epithelium, gives a satisfactory optical system, is compatible with many of the usual ophthalmic ingredients, can be filtered through a 0.22-μ Millipore bacterial filter membrane, and can be autoclaved without coagulation.

Manufacturers of ophthalmic solutions add methylcellulose or analogous macromolecular compounds to many (almost 50%[116]) of their preparations. In summary, there seems to be a place in ophthalmology for agents that increase the viscosity of ophthalmic solutions. The principal contraindication is in ophthalmic solutions which are to be used in surgery. This is probably in the nature of a general precaution as they are not definitely known to be nonirritating to the internal structures of the eye.[109,130,131]

Clarity

All solutions for use in the eye should be brilliantly clear and free from foreign particles, fibers, and filaments. This has been recommended from a safety and a medico-legal point of view.

Extemporaneous procedures are likely to use a sintered-glass filter funnel, filter paper, or cotton.

The use of a glass, sintered-disk Buchner funnel is admirably adapted to this work since there are no loose fibers to be washed into the final solution as may happen when certain other forms of filters are used. There is no loss through absorption by the filter disk.

Filter paper is the next filtering medium of choice. A hard-surfaced paper should be used to eliminate unnecessary filaments in the filtrate and to provide for greater clarity of the final solution. Unless a sufficiently hard grade of paper is used, the filtrate may contain more particles than the unfiltered solution. An adequate hard-filter-surfaced paper is Whatmann No. 54, or Schleicher and Schuell (S & S No. 576). These are available from laboratory supply houses.

If cotton is used as a filtering medium, only the highest grade, long-staple cotton should be employed. If the filtrate is returned through the cotton once or twice, the few loose short fibers first washed out will become enmeshed in the long cotton fibers. This provides a suitable filter bed which is very difficult to obtain when most of the fibers are short. Only a small pledget of cotton should be used to prevent absorption of an excessive amount of solution. Particular care should be observed in rinsing the cotton to see that the rinse liquid is applied so that it will function efficiently and not just pass through the filter at one point.

As is indicated in the section on sterility of ophthalmic solutions, it is important that the equipment used in filtration be completely clean; and if permanent filters are used such as the sintered-glass type, consideration should be given to the use of different filters for mydriatics, miotics, and other categories because of the possibility of absorption and retention of the drug by the filter disk. It should be noted that filters previously used for medicines such as syrups and not thoroughly cleaned could mean the addition of many microorganisms to the ophthalmic solution.

Solutions which are subjected to sterile filtration or bacterial filtration as described under sterilization would have all other particles removed and would not need filtration specifically from the standpoint of clarity.

Sterilization

Ophthalmic solutions are required to be sterile when prepared, and great care must be exercised subsequently to prevent contamination in use. The common methods of sterilization are moist heat under pressure, bacterial filtration, and use of chemicals. The USP states:

"All ophthalmic solutions should be sterile as dispensed, but it is imperative that those used in the traumatized eye or during surgery be sterile. While sterilization by autoclaving in the final container is preferable, the method of attaining sterility is determined primarily by the character of the particular product (see *Sterilization*, page 1501).

"Mention has been made of the fact that buffering certain drugs near the physiological pH range makes them quite unstable at high temperature. This must not be overlooked. The decision must be made whether to use a lower and less desirable pH from the physiologic standpoint, or to mix the previously sterilized drug solution and sterile buffer solution by aseptic technique. With the exception of basic salts of weak acids such as sodium fluorescein or sodium sulfacetamide, solutions of all of the common ophthalmic drugs in 1.9% boric acid can be autoclaved at 121° for 15 minutes without serious effect on their therapeutic activity.

"The use of a bacteria-retaining filter, while it avoids the use of heat, poses some technical difficulties, and the filter often retains some of the drug even after washing. This may then contaminate a subsequent product unless great care is taken or a separate filter is reserved for each ophthalmic drug."

Dangers of Nonsterile Medication

The possibility of serious ocular infections resulting from the use of contaminated ophthalmic solutions has been amply documented in the literature. Table XII[132] summarizes part of the reports which have been made on the types of infections and microorganisms, the variety of medications involved, and the source of medication or the location. Other reports have listed contamination found in solutions of ethylmorphine, cocaine, dibucaine, tetracaine, homatropine, and other compounds, other organisms have been listed as contaminants.

Pseudomonas aeruginosa (*B. pyocyaneus; Pseudomonas pyocyanea; Blue pus bacillus*)—This is a very dangerous and opportunistic organism which grows well on most culture media and produces both toxins and antibacterial products. The latter tend to kill off other contaminants and allow the *Ps. aeruginosa* to grow in pure culture. This Gram-negative bacillus also grows readily in ophthalmic solutions which may become the source of extremely serious infections of the cornea.

The danger to eyesight from infections by this organism has been recognized for many years; reports have included those by Herbert,[133] Cooper,[134] McCulloch,[135] Theodore and Feinstein,[136,137] King,[138] Vaughn,[139] and Cassady.[140] Cassady stated that infections due to *Ps. aeruginosa* are more frequent now because penicillin disturbed the balance between cocci and bacilli. Species of *Pseudomonas* have the ability to adapt to wide changes in environment and these adaptations probably include changes in resistance to chemicals.[141-143] A major preventive action took place in 1953, as indicated above in the references.

Fisher and Allen reported[144] that the mechanism of corneal destruction by *Ps. aeruginosa* is apparently the formation of an enzyme which has collagenase activity and affects collagen of the cornea. This might help to explain the reports of Lepard[145] and Joy[146] that *Ps. aeruginosa* migrates so rapidly to inaccessible locations that topical therapy is usually not effective. An effort has been made by LaBorde, *et al*,[147] to prepare a *Pseudomonas* vaccine.

As one example of a widespread problem Riegelman, *et al*,[106] reported on eight cases of corneal ulceration due to *Ps. aeruginosa*. These cases had occurred in the San Francisco Bay area during the previous year. A careful review of the details of the cases resulted in the firm opinion that most of the infections occurred during the treatment of an abraded cornea. This may be treatment by a physician in his office, emergency treatment room, clinic, surgery, or hospital ward. It may also occur in self-treatment in an industrial plant; for example, the use of penicillin eye drops.[148] During the treatment of the relatively large numbers of patients seen each day in these offices by physicians, one patient with an eye grossly contaminated with *Ps. aeruginosa* organisms could be the cause of a number of infected solutions. A freshly opened sterile ophthalmic solution thereby can be converted into a potent source of contamination. As *Ps. aeruginosa* is a common inhabitant of human skin, the contaminating bacteria could come from the physician, the nurse, the patient, or the air.

A sterile ophthalmic solution in a multiple-dose container can be contaminated in a number of ways unless precautions are taken. For example, if a dropper bottle

Table XII—Contaminated Eye Drops Reported in the Literature

Source or location	Contaminant found	Collyria	Remarks
Pharmacies	Various	1% Atropine Sulf.	10 out of 25 St. Louis pharmacies dispensed contaminated collyria
Hospital	*Ps. aeruginosa*	Fluorescein, Eserine, etc.	5 out of 18 corneal ulcers traced to eye drop contamination
Hospital	*Ps. aeruginosa*	Fluorescein	26 out of 26 hospital collyria contaminated
Industrial infirmary	*Ps. aeruginosa*	Fluorescein	4 eyes believed lost due to contaminated collyria
Industrial infirmary	*Ps. aeruginosa*	Silver Proteinate	Contaminated collyria caused loss of sight
Eye clinic	*Proteus vulgaris*	2% Pilocarpine	Contaminated although preserved with 1:5000 Zephiran
Eye clinic	Gram neg. rods, *Pseudomonas*, *Staphylococcus*	Fluorescein	5 out of 9 collyria found contaminated
Ophthalmologist's office	Gram neg. rods, fungi, *Pseudomonas*	Fluorescein	15 out of 31 collyria found contaminated
Veterinarian's office	*Ps. aeruginosa*	Fluorescein	Contaminated solution caused loss of sight in 2 dogs

is used, the tip of the dropper while out of the bottle can touch the surface of a table or shelf if laid down, or can touch the eyelid or eyelash of the patient during administration. If the "drop-tainer" (see page 1574) type of bottle is used, the dropper tip can touch an eyelash, or the cap while removed to permit administration can have its edge touch a table or finger and that edge can touch the dropper tip as the cap is replaced. Separate droppers if stored in a drawer or on a shelf between uses can easily become contaminated in some way and may require cleaning just prior to use.

One may assume the solution contains the most effective antimicrobial known but the next use of the contaminated solution may occur before enough time has elapsed for all of the organisms to be killed. Here the still-living organisms can find their way through an abrasion into the corneal stroma. Once in the corneal stroma, the residual traces of antimicrobial agents are neutralized by tissue components and the organisms find an excellent culture medium for rapid growth and dissemination throughout the cornea and the anterior segment of the eye.

Tap water is often contaminated with *Ps. aeruginosa*. A study of the sources of bacterial contamination of eye solutions shows that the greatest source of bacteria is probably the improperly stored distilled water used in their preparation.[149] This emphasizes the need for the use of sterile distilled water in compounding ophthalmic solutions. Contaminated eye solutions may produce the most serious type of corneal ulcer encountered in ophthalmology.

Other Organisms—*Bacillus subtilis* may produce a serious abscess when it infects vitreous humor. The pathogenic fungus considered of particular importance in eye solutions is *Aspergillus fumigatus*. Other fungi or molds may be harmful by accelerating deterioration of the active drugs.

With regard to viruses, as many as 42 cases of epidemic keratoconjunctivitis were caused by one bottle of virus-contaminated tetracaine solution.[150] Virus contamination is particularly difficult to control because none of the preservatives now available is virucidal. Moreover, viruses are not removable by filtration. However, they are destroyed by autoclaving. The pharmacist and physician have not been made adequately aware of the dangers of transmitting virus infection via contaminated solutions. This is particularly pertinent to the adenoviruses (Types III and VIII) which are now believed to be the causative agents of viral conjunctivitis such as epidemic keratoconjunctivitis.

While a pharmacist may never see a patient with a corneal ulcer due to contaminated eye drops, every possible measure must be taken to prevent them since they are such devastating infections. Accidental conjunctivitis is more common, but less dangerous, than the pseudomonal corneal infection.[106]

Types of Sterilization

Steam Under Pressure—Sterilization by moist heat under pressure (121°) is the method of choice unless the chemical nature of one or several of the ingredients of the solution forbids the use of heat. It is commonly stated to kill all living organisms, including spores and viruses. However, Steiger-Trippi[151] states that, with the exception of combustion, there is no procedure which guarantees the destruction of all microorganisms. One of his examples was an actinomycetes which could be destroyed only by a 15–20-min exposure to saturated steam at 140°C. This, of course, supports the usual recommendation that contamination be held to as low a level as feasible, even if sterilization by steam under pressure is to be carried out. Procedural breakdowns are very rare, and a number of devices are available as aids to evaluation of the procedure, depending to some extent on the equipment used. Small autoclaves are available as discussed by Murphy, *et al*,[27] and more recently low-cost pressure cookers (Presto: *Sears*) have become available which are heated by a self-contained electrical heating unit and automatically controlled by a thermostat.

This type of sterilization can be carried out with the ophthalmic solution present in the final container. The total time required in the autoclave or pressure cooker depends on several factors including the capacity of the heating element and the size and number of the containers being sterilized but is usually no more than ½ hour for ophthalmic solutions in small containers in a pressure cooker. When a dropper bottle is used as the final container, it is usually preferable to package the dropper closure separately from the container for the medication. The container should be closed with a screw cap with a suitable liner, such as rubber.

Murphy, *et al*,[27] describe a practical method in considerable detail. They point out that pressure must be reduced slowly to prevent bursting of bottles and that the solutions can be preserved for a greater period of time by storage in the frozen state. Here sufficient air space should be provided in the bottle for expansion of the solution as it freezes.

Bacterial Filtration—Bacterial filtration has the advantage that it is done at room temperature and does not cause or accelerate decomposition by heating. However, it has several substantial disadvantages. It does not remove or destroy viruses and, as pointed out in an earlier section, this can be significant.

The other disadvantages are principally connected with the selection and use of equipment. They tend to rule out the method for extemporaneous compounding. However, the method can be used quite effectively when carried out routinely by experienced workers, as in a commercial batch preparation system.

The method involves transfer into the final containers after passage through the filter itself. Thus, sterilization is not carried out in the final container and there is a greater possibility of a breakdown in the sterile procedure. Filtration uses positive or negative pressure. Negative pressure is usually the more familiar to the worker and the more feasible from the standpoint of equipment. However, it offers considerable opportunity for entrance of contaminants into the system. Positive pressure filtration is often best done using nitrogen gas as a source of pressure. This is not convenient in most extemporaneous situations.

Facilities for bacterial filtration include equipment for sterilization by steam under pressure, as an autoclave, or equivalent equipment, for sterilization of the filtration equipment and of the drugs and chemicals which are not harmed by the treatment. It is essential to note that unless great care is taken small amounts of drug can be trapped in the filtration assembly. It is particularly important to separate the mydriatics and cycloplegics from the miotics and to separate these types of drugs from the other ophthalmic drugs. For example, Sollman[152] states that epinephrine in a 1:400,000,000 solution produces a definite mydriatic effect on the excised iris.

The application of filtration procedures to the

extemporaneous preparation of sterile ophthalmic solutions has been proposed by several workers.[29,136,138,153-156] Several types of equipment are available for small-scale work, as described in Chapter 81. Particular interest has been shown in the Swinny adapter fitted on a syringe,[111] and in the Millipore Swinnex disposable filter units. Empty sterile plastic "squeeze" containers and sterile plastic filtration units can be purchased directly from the manufacturers.* As usage increases, they will no doubt become available from wholesalers. They permit extemporaneous preparation of ophthalmic solutions which have a strong probability of being sterile if the work is carried out under aseptic conditions. The NF states that they should be used whenever possible, provided caution is exercised in selection, assembly, and use. A supplementary device can permit automatic refilling of the syringe. The filter membrane is replaced after each use of the filter, thus reducing the hazard of chemical or biological contamination.

In extemporaneous compounding such filtration can be a useful supplement to the use of chemical sterilization. This procedure affords a greater probability that the prescription will be sterile at the time of initial use and is applicable only where it is not feasible to sterilize by moist heat under pressure. Because of the technical difficulties of the filtration method, it should be used only under the close supervision of an individual whose technique has been shown to be of high quality by repeated evaluation, including sterility tests which are valid in the presence of the chemical antimicrobials.

Chemical Sterilization—In the present state of the art this method is, of necessity, widely used in the extemporaneous compounding of ophthalmic solutions. Therefore, it is necessary that careful attention be given to its shortcomings. It does not destroy viruses. It often requires considerable time to destroy bacteria and may be quite ineffective.

While testing for sterility is relatively difficult because of the presence of the antimicrobials, this in itself is not a reason for using steam under pressure or bacterial filtration for sterilization, as the addition of chemical antimicrobials is usually required as a supplement to these methods of sterilization.

In using this method the glassware should be as nearly sterile as possible; all solutions should be made with sterile distilled water, and the solution should be dispensed in a sterile container. Facilities for autoclaving are desirable for sterilizing equipment and containers. Several authors have recommended methods of this type.[49,157-162]

Preservation

Antimicrobials are required except when contraindicated. They are to be omitted in solutions intended for instillation or injection into the chambers of the eye (in the course of intraocular surgery). Most preservatives are irritating to the lining of the anterior chamber of the eye. It is recommended that the ophthalmic solutions used for intraocular (intracameral) use be packaged in sterile single-use or single-dose containers, as distinguished from multiple-dose containers. Solutions for such purposes are autoclaved and used on one patient only. This removes the need for an antimicrobial preservative of any kind. It has also been recommended that the same precautions be taken with ophthalmic solutions that are to be instilled into the conjunctival sac of injured eyes.

With the above exceptions the presence of an antimicrobial preservative is required even if the ophthalmic solution is sterilized by other means such as by autoclaving or bacterial filtration. This requirement is made because multiple-dose containers may easily become contaminated in use. It should be noted that in this instance rather rapid self-sterilization is necessary. In addition, one should note that the use of these chemicals does not alter the need to use very clean and careful technique in making and packaging ophthalmic solutions.

Attributes Desired

A suitable antimicrobial preservative or mixture of preservatives should possess as many as possible of the following properties:[27,49,163]

1. *Broad Spectrum*—It should have a wide bacteriostatic (fungistatic, etc) and preferably a bactericidal (fungicidal, etc) activity against organisms which have been found to be present in and are undesirable in ophthalmic solutions. This specifically includes known virulent-resistant strains of *Ps. aeruginosa* (*B. pyocyaneus*).

2. *Continuing Activity*—It should maintain such activity under normal conditions of autoclaving, storage, and contamination during use and preferably under less favorable circumstances.

3. *Rapid Action*—After such a solution has been contaminated during use it is important that the preservative resterilize the solution quickly. It should have the ability to carry out this resterilization in less than 1 hour's time.[49,164]

4. *Nonallergenic and Nonsensitizing*—It should not have any allergenic or sensitizing tendencies. For some medications such as pilocarpine hydrochloride this may well refer to usage over a period of many years.

5. *Nontoxic and Nonirritating*—It should be nontoxic and nonirritating to ocular tissues in the concentrations and frequencies used and should, specifically, produce no damage to the corneal epithelium.

6. *Compatibility*—It should be chemically and pharmacologically compatible with the other ingredients and should not significantly alter the pH and tonicity of the system.

7. *Stability*—It should be chemically stable and not undergo discoloration.

8. *Inactivation*—It should be readily possible to neutralize or inactivate the preservative for testing purposes.

9. *Solubility*—It should be readily and adequately soluble in the appropriate vehicles.

No single antimicrobial agent or mixture of agents is known which will satisfactorily meet all of the above conditions for all ophthalmic solutions. In formulating for batch production it is necessary to select the proper antimicrobial by suitable experimentation aided by theoretical consideration[165] and this often leads to the use of more than one agent. In extemporaneous compounding this experimentation is rarely feasible and it is necessary to select from a group of stock vehicles in most cases.

While protecting the patient against infection is the primary concern, guarding the medication from the growth of microorganisms also tends to maintain the potency of the dosage form.

Evaluation

The evaluation of antimicrobial preservatives is especially aimed at *Ps. aeruginosa*. Because of the incidence and seriousness of *Ps. aeruginosa* infections arising from the use of contaminated ophthalmic solutions, various workers have investigated the antibacterial agents employed as preservatives in such preparations. The findings of these workers have been partly contradictory. The usual types of *in vitro* procedures employed in evaluating the effectiveness of an antibacterial agent have been challenged. A recent report by Kohn, *et al*,[164] is a valuable aid to the selec-

---

Wheaton (polyethylene containers) and *Millipore* (Swinnex filter units).

Table XIII—Sterilizing Times against *Ps. aeruginosa*
(10⁸) for Chemical Agents Commonly Employed as
Preservatives in Ophthalmic Solutions

Chemical agents	Conc	Sterilizing time
Chlorobutanol	0.7%	9 hr
	0.5%	12 hr
Benzalkonium chloride	0.02%	45 min
	0.01	9 hr
Thimerosal	0.02%	6 hr
	0.01%	9 hr
Methylparaben and	0.2%	
propylparaben	0.04%	3 hr
Methylparaben and	0.18%	
propylparaben	0.02%	6 hr
Phenylmercuric nitrate	0.01%	6 hr
	0.005%	6 hr
Phenylethyl alcohol	0.5%	>24 hr
Polymyxin B sulfate	2000 units/ml	12 hr
	1000 units/ml	18 hr

tion of a preservative, and supports earlier work carried out by Lawrence[166] and by Riegelman.[167] A weakness of most of the reports on this subject has been the failure to recognize the importance of *in vivo* confirmation of *in vitro* results and the need for rapid action in self-sterilization occurring subsequently to contamination during use.

Until recently, most workers employed a dilution technique to differentiate between the bactericidal and bacteriostatic activities of antibacterial agents. The basis for this procedure is the dilution of the preservative to a concentration below the concentration known to have a significant antibacterial effect. If growth of the bacteria occurred after inoculation of this diluted solution into subcultured medium, the antibacterial agent was considered to, possibly, possess bacteriostatic activity. If growth did not appear, the antibacterial agent was reported as possessing bactericidal properties.

The above concept is not considered completely valid at present. As Klarmann has reported,[168] in some of the dilution techniques, a quantity of the antibacterial agent may be transferred to the subculture medium in a concentration that will produce stasis, and some may become affixed to the cell walls or cells, initially producing stasis. Therefore, a bacteriostatic effect may be produced and misinterpreted for a bactericidal effect. Another disadvantage of the dilution technique is that living bacteria present may be diluted to an infinite concentration and may not grow in the subculture medium.

It is essential to attain complete inactivation or inhibition of the antimicrobial agent in the evaluation procedure. This is the principle employed by Lawrence[166] and by Riegelman, *et al.*[167] Until recently, investigators had not attempted to correlate the results attained using the *in vitro* procedure with an *in vivo* test. As pointed out by Riegelman, *et al,*[167] an *in vivo* test has several advantages and becomes an important consideration in procedures used for the evaluation of antibacterial agents employed as preservatives in ophthalmic solutions.

The purpose of an *in vivo* study is to prove that the procedure for measuring the efficiency of antibacterial agents is valid, that is, that the bacteria are not capable of growing in the subculture medium, and accordingly are also not capable of producing an ocular infection *in vivo*; and that the inactivating media utilized are adequate. Inactivation of the antimicrobial

agent[164] was usually attained by the addition of compounds such as Polysorbate 80 or lecithin.

In the *in vivo* method[164] two contact time periods were used for each antibacterial agent–bacteria mixture studied. The contact time periods were selected from the findings of the *in vitro* experiments. The first contact time period selected was the longest period of time which still showed growth of the bacteria in the subculture medium. The other time selected was the contact time period immediately following the first contact time period. Obviously, the latter contact time period would have shown no growth of the bacteria in the subculture medium. The first exposure period was used to prove that when growth of *Ps. aeruginosa* occurs in the subculture medium, an infection could also be produced in a rabbit's eye. The second contact time period was used to fulfill the purpose of the *in vivo* experiment.

The antibacterial agent–bacteria mixture was injected intracorneally into a rabbit's eye. At the first contact time period selected the injection was given into one eye of each of two rabbits. At the next contact time, another intracorneal injection was given into the other eye of each of the same two rabbits. A third rabbit received an injection of the sterile antibacterial solution (positive control) in one eye and an injection of the diluted bacteria (negative control) in the other eye. The rabbits were observed for a period of seven days for evidence of ocular infections. Most eyes infected with *Ps. aeruginosa* were completely closed within 7 days after the injection.

The results of the *in vivo* experiments were in agreement in all instances with the results of the *in vitro* experiments. Those solutions which produced growth following transfer into subculture media produced ocular infections. Those which did not produce growth did not produce ocular infection.

An antibacterial agent intended for use as a preservative in ophthalmic solutions should have quick-acting bactericidal activity. There is no generally accepted definition for the term "quick-acting." An antibacterial agent was considered to possess quick-acting bactericidal activity against *Ps. aeruginosa* if the sterilizing time of that agent was 1 hour or less under the test conditions.

Types

Research on antimicrobial agents for ophthalmic solutions has repeatedly involved benzalkonium chloride, chlorobutanol, and phenylmercuric nitrate in addition to some compounds which have been used to a lesser extent.[169–177] The greatest amount of study has been carried out with benzalkonium chloride. The literature studies usually have not dealt with mixtures of two or more antimicrobial agents except in the case of the parabens. However, use of mixtures of these agents has been frequent in commercial preparations (currently, almost 50%[116]) and is expected to increase in extemporaneous compounding, as is indicated by the statements from the USP and the NF quoted below. As stated above, most of the published studies have not shown careful proof of neutralization or inactivation of the antimicrobial in the testing procedure. In addition, most of the published reports have not described a search for effect in a short time such as one hour. This relatively quick action is needed for resterilization, particularly in eye clinics.

Quaternary Ammonium Germicides—The NF states that benzalkonium chloride is frequently used as an antimicrobial in ophthalmic solutions in a concentration of 0.01%, but that it is not invariably satisfactory. In concentrations tolerated by the tissues of the eye, it, like chlorobutanol, phenylethyl alcohol, and phenylmercuric nitrate, is ineffective against some strains of *Ps. aeruginosa*. In addition, it is not compatible with anionic drugs, nonionic surfactants in high concentrations, salicylates, or nitrates. It may be effective against the resistant strains of *Pseudomonas* if addition is made of polymyxin B sulfate in a concentration of 1000 USP units per ml.

Resistant strains of *Ps. aeruginosa* have been made sensitive to benzalkonium chloride by the inclusion of 0.01 to 0.1% of disodium ethylenediaminetetraacetate (EDTA) which is a chelating agent for metals. This type of combination was initiated by MacGregor and Elliker[178] using an alkyl dimethylethyl benzyl ammonium chloride.

From the very extensive studies on the effect of benzalkonium chloride, it may be concluded that:

1. It is effective against certain strains of *Ps. aeruginosa*[157,160,161,163,166] but not against others.[167,179]

2. Its irritativeness to ocular tissues critically depends on concentration and on the specific circumstances of the test procedure.[157,158,160,161,180,181]

3. The drug is characterized by definite compatibilities and incompatibilities.[182,183]

Practically important is its compatibility with phosphate buffers, pilocarpine hydrochloride, and physostigmine sulfate.

The studies have used concentrations ranging from 1 in 100,000 up to 1 in 500. The concentration most commonly used is 1 in 10,000.[116] The concentration of choice is probably 1 in 5000, based on the work of Kohn, *et al*,[164] or 1 in 7500.[184] It is occasionally used in a higher concentration as 1 in 3000 for the special purpose of aiding the penetration of a drug which otherwise will not penetrate. A 1:1000 benzalkonium chloride solution is very irritating to the human conjunctiva, and produces edema and desquamation. A 1:3500 solution produces some conjunctival and corneal changes which are reversible.[158]

Strains of *Ps. aeruginosa* known to be resistant to benzalkonium chloride were rapidly killed by a solution of benzalkonium chloride 1 in 10,000 containing 0.01% disodium ethylenediaminetetraacetate. Possibly in the resistant strains a metal has been incorporated into the cell constituents which is removed by the inclusion of the chelating agent. Riegelman states that 0.1% EDTA is itself an active pseudomonacidal agent.[32] Monkhouse and Groves recommend 0.013% benzalkonium chloride with 0.1% EDTA, but do not find EDTA to be pseudomonacidal.[184]

A recent comprehensive study by Kohn, *et al*,[164] summarized in Table XIII, indicates that benzalkonium chloride is the most rapid in a action of the several agents studied. In this study a mixture of Polysorbate 80 and lecithin was used as a neutralizing or inactivating agent in testing.

About 50% of the commercial ophthalmic solutions use benzalkonium chloride, often with other antimicrobial agents, as EDTA.[116]

Other Quaternary Ammonium Germicides — Other quaternaries that have been used in ophthalmic solutions include benzethonium chloride (0.025%) and cetylpyridinium chloride (0.02%), and myristyl-gamma-picolinium chloride.[116] The following compounds have been reported by Kohn, *et al*,[185] as being more rapidly active than benzalkonium chloride. These compounds have been evaluated in ophthalmic solutions only for antipseudomonas activity.

1. Alkyl dimethyldichlorobenzyl ammonium chloride
2. Lauryl dimethylbenzyldimethyl ammonium chloride
3. Cetyl dimethylbenzyl ammonium chloride
4. Alkyl trimethyl ammonium chloride

Lawrence[163] (Table XIV) has reported on compatibilities and incompatibilities of quaternary ammonium germicides with ophthalmic drugs.

Substituted Alcohols and Phenols—The USP states that chlorobutanol is used in a concentration of 0.5% as an alternate to benzalkonium chloride, but that it hydrolyzes to form hydrochloric acid with resultant decrease in the pH of its solutions. This decomposition occurs rapidly during heating and slowly even at room temperature in unbuffered solutions that are neutral initially.

Chlorobutanol 0.5% was first introduced into all collyria used or dispensed at the Massachusetts Eye and Ear Infirmary in 1926 and has been in continuous use since that time.[27] Collyria containing it have been repeatedly instilled into the anterior chamber at the time of intraocular surgery, without any instance of endothelial damage or other ill effects upon the tissues within the eye. It has been used in miotics for many years by hundreds of glaucoma patients without a sin-

Table XIV—Compatibilities and Incompatibilities of Quaternary Ammonium Germicides with Ophthalmic Drugs

Drugs	Concentrations used
Compatibilities	
Acetate buffer	1:5000
Alkaloids	1:25000
Atropine	1:5000; 1:10000
Boric acid	1:5000
Bromides	1:10000
Carcholin	1:5000
Cocaine	1:5000; 1:10000
Compound "75-G"[a]	1:50000
Cortisone	1:10000
Ephedrine	1:10000
Epinephrine	1:5000
Eserine	1:3000; 1:5000
Eucatropine	1:5000; 1:10000
Fluorescein[a]	1:5000; 1:10000
Homatropine	1:5000; 1:10000; 1:100000
Hyaluronidase	1:3000
Hydrobromides	1:10000
Methylcellulose	1:5000; 1:50000
Neo-Synephrine	1:5000
Penicillin	1:5000
Phenazolin	1:5000
Physostigmine	1:1000; 1:5000
Pilocarpine hydrochloride	1:3000; 1:5000; 1:10000
Pontocaine (tetracaine)	1:3000; 1:3500; 1:5000; 1:10000
Procaine	1:3000; 1:10000
Rose bengal	1:5000
Scopolamine	1:5000; 1:10000
Zinc sulfate	1:1000; 1:10000; 1:50000
Incompatibilities[b]	
Boric acid[b]	1:5000
Fluorescein[b]	1:3000; 1:5000
Pilocarpine nitrate	1:5000
Salicylates	1:5000
Silver nitrate	1:5000
Silver proteinates	1:5000
Sulfathiazole sodium	1:5000
Nitrates	1:5000

[a] Schieffelin and Company brand of a basic ester of substituted phenylacetic acid with spasmolytic, mydriatic, and cycloplegic activities.

[b] Reported by some to be compatible and by others incompatible.

gle instance of sensitization being specifically attributed to it. It was also recommended by such early workers in this area as Gershenfeld and Tomkins[186] and Taub and Luckey.[187]

Murphy, et al,[27] prepared 0.5% solutions of chlorobutanol in 100-ml bottles in citric acid–sodium phosphate buffers with pH ranging from 2.6 to 8.0, and autoclaved them at 121°C for periods ranging from 5 to 20 minutes. After autoclaving the solutions gave positive tests for chloride ion and showed decrease in pH, presumably due to hydrolysis of the chlorobutanol. The hydrolysis at an initial pH of 5.0 was 2.4% for 5 minutes autoclaving and 7.7% for 20 minutes autoclaving. The final pH was 4.8 and 4.3 respectively. Hydrolysis was less at lower initial pH values but increased sharply for pH values of 6.0 and above.

In the more acid pH range, up to pH 6, autoclaving did not inactivate the antibacterial effect of chlorobutanol. When neutral or alkaline solutions of sufficiently high buffering capacity were autoclaved in the presence of chlorobutanol, the antibacterial effect of the latter was definitely impaired. It was presumed that the chlorobutanol had been hydrolyzed by heat at these higher pH values.

Chlorobutanol is stated to be effective against both Gram-positive and Gram-negative organisms, including *Ps. aeruginosa*, and some fungi. It is broadly compatible with other ingredients. Acid solutions are stable except for the limitation stated above.

A number of disadvantages have been reported. Chlorobutanol is decomposed in alkaline solutions, therefore, it is incompatible with alkaline buffers and sodium sulfacetamide.[157] It can have 90% stability for 45 days at pH 5–6 at 45–55°C.[188] Its decomposition in aqueous solution at 115° during a 30-minute heating period at pH 5 and at pH 6 were calculated to be 13% and 58%, respectively.[189] It is incompatible with silver nitrate.[190] Kohn, et al,[164] reported it to be slow-acting. It is slow to dissolve in water at room temperature. It dissolves more rapidly when heated but this hastens decomposition. It is neutralized or inactivated by 10% Tween 20 in nutrient broth.

Its combination with phenylethyl alcohol (0.5% of each) is reported[191] to be more effective against *Ps. aeruginosa*, *Staphylococcus aureus*, and *Proteus vulgaris* than either antimicrobial singly. In addition, solution of the chlorobutanol in phenylethyl alcohol permits dissolving the chlorobutanol in water without the use of heat.

Almost 25% of the commercial ophthalmic solutions use chlorobutanol, sometimes with EDTA.[116]

Other Substituted Alcohols and Phenols—Phenylethyl alcohol (0.5%) has been investigated repeatedly but is generally reported as being moderate in its effect. Kohn, et al,[164] and Murphy, et al,[27] believe it to be very inferior as an antibacterial preservative against *Ps. aeruginosa*. It may have value in combination with chlorobutanol as stated above.

The following compounds of this type have also been suggested for use in ophthalmic solutions:[32]

1. Parachlorometaxylenol (0.03%)
2. Parachlorometacresol (0.05%) (NF XII)
3. Phenoxy ethanol (0.3%)
4. Phenylethyl alcohol 0.1% (with phenol 0.25%)
5. Phenylethyl alcohol (0.5% with phenol 0.25%) is suggested by Riegelman for use with sodium fluorescein (pH 9.0)[32]

Organic Mercurials—The NF states that *Phenylmercuric Nitrate* or *Acetate*, 0.002%, should be used instead of benzalkonium chloride for salicylates and

nitrates, and in solutions of salts of physostigmine and epinephrine that contain 0.1% sodium sulfite.

It is used in concentrations from 0.002 to 0.004%.[116] It is sometimes ineffective against *Ps. aeruginosa*. It has the advantage over some of the other organic mercurials in that it is not precipitated by a slightly acid pH but is described as being slow in bactericidal action,[164] and as giving sensitization reactions.[27] Riegelman states that it is not an adequate preservative for sodium fluorescein. Brown[192] agrees, and finds that EDTA reduces its effectiveness. Kohn, et al,[164] reported its neutralization by Polysorbate 80 and lecithin in thioglycollate medium. Lawrence[163] (Table XV) summarized its compatibilities and incompatibilities with ophthalmic drugs. It is incompatible with bromides, hydrobromides,[49] and sulfadiazine sodium.[48] Physiological sodium chloride solutions are compatible with phenylmercuric nitrate 0.004%, but higher concentrations of sodium chloride may show a tendency to undergo precipitation.[49]

Phenylmercuric acetate is used in concentrations of of 0.001–0.002%.[116]

Thimerosal (Merthiolate) is used in concentrations of 0.005–0.01%. It is reported as slow in action by Kohn.[164]

Abrams[193] reported the development of iatrogenic mercury deposits in the crystalline lens (mercurialentis) resulting from the use of miotic eye drops containing phenylmercuric nitrate 0.004% 3 times a day for 3 to 6 years. No impairment of vision has been found, but the yellowish brown discoloration of the lens capsule is of a permanent nature.

Hess and Speiser[174,175] reported the activities of phenylmercuric borate and of thimerosal at four pH values. The borate (cationic) was much more effective in alkaline solution and the salicylate (anionic) more effective in acidic solution. Their effects on Gram-positive and Gram-negative organisms were described as identical.

About 20% of the commercial ophthalmic solutions use organic mercurials, usually thimerosal or phenylmercuric acetate.[116]

Esters of Parahydroxybenzoic Acid—This usually refers to mixtures of methylparaben and propylparaben. These are commonly used as mixtures in order to obtain a greater effect, such as methylparaben 0.18% and propylparaben 0.02% (see page 1184). They are reported to give ocular irritation[39,48] and to be slow in their antimicrobial action, by Kohn, et al,[164] who also report their inactivation by Polysorbate 80 in nutrient broth. They are more fungistatic than bacteriostatic.[194–196]

Antibiotics—*Polymyxin B Sulfate* has been recommended by the USP as a supplement to benzalkonium chloride as described in an earlier section. Riegelman states that there is no known instance of *Ps. aeruginosa* being resistant to polymyxin B sulfate, and that there are no known sensitivity reactions. Kohn, et al,[164] report it as being only slowly effective against *Ps. aeruginosa*. They used lecithin in nutrient broth to inactivate this compound. Because of the possibility of *Ps. aeruginosa* becoming resistant to polymyxin B sulfate, Riegelman recommends that the use of polymyxin B sulfate be reserved for the treatment of known *Ps. aeruginosa* infections. It is not a broad spectrum bactericide and additional antibacterial agents must be added to overcome its shortcomings in respect to Gram-positive organisms.[106]

Other Compounds—The greatest effort which has been made to identify other compounds of value for

Table XV—Compatibilities and Incompatibilities of Phenylmercuric Nitrate with Ophthalmic Drugs[163]

Compatibilities[a]	
Cocaine	Procaine
Dionin	Syntropan
Metycaine	Fluorescein
Nupercaine	Sulfisoxazole diethanolamine
Optochin	Sodium sulfacetamide
Phenacaine	Sodium sulfadiazine
Pontocaine	Sodium sulfathiazole
	Zinc

Incompatibilities[b]	
Atropine	Eucatropine
Ephedrine	Homatropine
	Pilocarpine

[a] Compatible when prepared in phosphate buffer pH 5.0 containing; boric acid—2%; phenylmercuric nitrate—1:25,000; distilled water.
[b] However, compatible when prepared in phosphate buffer pH 6.8 containing: sodium acid phosphate, anhydrous: 4 Gm; disodium phosphate, anhydrous: 4.73 Gm; benzalkonium chloride: 1:10,000; sodium chloride: 4.3 Gm; distilled water: qs, 1,000 ml.

this purpose is probably the work carried out by Kohn, et al.[185] They studied 51 chemical substances, believed not to have been previously employed as preservatives in ophthalmic solutions, for their effectiveness against 13 different strains of *Ps. aeruginosa*. *In vitro* and the important *in vivo* methods were employed. Care was taken to use adequate inactivating media. The main purpose was to learn if the sterilizing times were as short as or shorter than for benzalkonium chloride 0.02%; thus, the work did not include a study of toxicity, ocular irritation, stability, and compatibility with ophthalmic drugs and vehicles. 37 quaternary ammonium compounds were investigated of which only six were satisfactory:

1. Intexsan LB [alkyl dimethyl dichlorobenzyl ammonium chloride].
2. Intexsan MB [alkyl dimethylbenzyl ammonium chloride].
3. DMBC [lauryl dimethylbenzyl dimethyl ammonium chloride].
4. Cetol [cetyl dimethylbenzyl ammonium chloride].
5. Dichloran [dimethyl dichlorobenzyl ammonium chloride].
6. Arquad 16 [alkyl trimethyl ammonium chloride].

The eight amphoteric surfactants studied were all found to be inadequate. The three iodophors were all satisfactory:

1. Virac [(*N*-methyl heptyl colomino-formyl methyl)pyridinium chloride, containing coupled iodine; in liquid form and containing 0.6% available iodine].
2. Betadine [polyvinyl pyrrolidone-iodine complex; in liquid form and containing 1% available iodine].
3. Biopal VRO [iodine-nonyl phenoxypolyoxyethylene ethanol complex; in liquid form and containing 20% available iodine].

The other compounds investigated were Agosan, colistin, and chlorhexidine. Agosan (partially polymerized silver mannuride) was unsatisfactory. Colistin [Coli-Mycin S (*Warner-Chilcott*)] and chlorhexidine [Hibitane; the diacetate salt of bis(*p*-chlorophenyl diguanide)hexane] were satisfactory. Several workers have recommended that colistin be avoided as an antimicrobial preservative for the same reason that this recommendation is made for polymyxin B sulfate —its therapeutic use for *Pseudomonas* infections of the eye.

In evaluating this work by Kohn, et al, note should be taken of the summary of their work on the common ophthalmic preservatives.[164] Table XIII shows a marked difference between benzalkonium chloride 0.02% and all other systems tested, including benz-

alkonium chloride 0.01%. The work reported in the second paper lists only compounds and concentrations equal to or superior to benzalkonium chloride in speed of action. It may be that other systems of the compounds listed by Kohn would be inferior to benzalkonium chloride 0.02% but superior to all other compounds in common use at present.

In addition, the Kohn report does not touch on the addition of the EDTA type of compound to these systems, or, with the exception of the parabens, on the possible benefits from using more than one antimicrobial agent.

Chlorhexidine has been studied to a considerable extent following a report by Davies, *et al*, who reported on it as a new antimicrobial agent of high potency.[197] Preliminary studies were reported on by Anderson and Storch,[198] Jeffs,[199,200] and Mitchell, *et al*.[201] Graham[202] stated that it is effective against both Gram-negative and Gram-positive organisms, has a relatively low toxicity, causes no conjunctival irritation up to 0.05% for the diacetate and up to 0.2% for the gluconate. Anderson, *et al*,[203] report that chlorhexidine acetate 0.005%, and benzalkonium chloride 0.004% (with thimerosal 0.001%), were both superior to benzalkonium chloride (0.004, 0.013, and 0.02%) and chlorobutanol 0.25% (with phenylethanol 0.3%), in regard to bactericidal activity against *Ps. aeruginosa*. The activity of chlorhexidine is enhanced by the presence of EDTA.[204] Parker, *et al*,[205] state that it has a wide antimicrobial spectrum but that it is incompatible with bicarbonates, phosphates, borates, sulfates, fluorescein, and physostigmine. Foster[171] reports that its activity is diminished by serum and other organic matter, especially of a lipid nature, it is less active in the presence of ophthalmic medicaments than in plain saline, and it is possible to increase the resistance of *Ps. aeruginosa* to chlorhexidine by subculture on media containing this compound. A number of other papers describe its value when used in ophthalmic solutions.[177,206–217] However, its study has not been restricted to ophthalmic solutions.[218]

Combinations of Antimicrobial Agents—It is often desirable to use more than one antimicrobial agent in a given ophthalmic solution, but information on effective combinations is limited. The following combinations have been used in a number of commercial products.[116] They are listed in order of decreasing frequency of use.

1. Benzalkonium chloride with EDTA, especially with 0.01% of each
2. Benzalkonium chloride with chlorobutanol, phenylethyl alcohol, or phenylmercuric nitrate, sometimes with EDTA in addition
3. Chlorobutanol with EDTA or with parabens
4. Thimerosal with EDTA or with parabens
5. Phenylmercuric nitrate with EDTA
6. Phenylethyl alcohol with parabens

One may assume that these combinations have been proved to be effective for the particular combination of ingredients, container and closure, method of sterilization, etc, used in that particular product. However, one may not safely assume that the stated combination of antimicrobials would be effective if any change is made in any of the other factors listed. Each system must be independently evaluated.

Packaging

Eye lotions to be used as washes are usually dispensed in volumes from about 4–6 ounces. Often an eye cup is packaged with them. The patient should be instructed as to the proper use and care of the eye cup.

Eye drops for home or office use, for instillation into eyes with intact corneas, are packaged in multiple-dose containers usually ranging from 4–60 ml. They may be dispensed in a glass dropper bottle with the dropper either inserted or packaged separately, or in a so-called Droptainer (*Alcon*) (see page 1568), a plastic container which will dispense a drop of medication when the bottle is inverted and gently squeezed.

Ophthalmic solutions used for traumatized eyes and during surgery must be dispensed in sterile, single-use containers. "Minims" are sterile disposable units of ophthalmic solutions in plastic.

Fluorescein sodium is also available in the form of a sterile impregnated paper strip. The strip releases a sufficient amount of the drug for diagnostic purposes when touched to the eye. This is recommended as the method of administration because of the greater assurance of sterility.

It is also recommended that ophthalmic solutions to be applied as drops should be dispensed in small units, usually not larger than 15 ml and preferably smaller. A 7.5-ml container is a convenient size for the dispensing of eye solutions. Use of small containers shortens the time the medication will be kept by the patient and minimizes the number of exposures to contamination.

It is important when using dropper bottles to clean both the bottle and dropper prior to use. While the outer surface of the dropper may appear clean, the inner dropper surface, as well as the entire bottle, should be adequately rinsed with detergent solution, followed by sterile distilled water. This is done to remove talcum or other particulate matter which may be present during the manufacture of a dropper bottle.

It should be noted that in some cases polyethylene dropper tubes are used instead of glass tubes. These do not withstand autoclaving and are unsatisfactory from this standpoint.

A new multiple-dose glass container for eye drops has been developed.[219] It has two polypropylene screw caps: one attaching a silicon rubber teat to the container and the other covering the teat. It can be autoclaved and its design reduces the probability of the contamination of its contents during use.

The plastic "squeeze" containers are available from several commercial sources and can be purchased in a sterile condition, as mentioned in an earlier section. While such packages are appealing to the pharmacist and the physician, they possess certain definite deficiencies and hazards in use. The solution may be incompatible with the plastic. Due to their opaque appearance they cannot be effectively inspected for clarity and a change or precipitate formation in the solution is not easily observed.

The most generally available types are made from the low melting form of polyethylene and cannot be autoclaved. Recently, however, a high-melting type of polyethylene has become available and, while these bottles suffer in their ease of flexing, it has been stated that they can be autoclaved if left slightly opened.[220] Here, one should keep in mind the type of precautions needed when considering the use of plastic containers instead of glass.[221] The statement that they can be autoclaved may refer only to lack of visible change;[222] however, autoclaving may alter the physical properties of the plastic and thereby affect the permeation, leaching, and sorption properties of the container. Volatile components such as chloro-butanol may be lost.[223] Radiation sterilization may also affect the physical properties of the plastic. Each individual drug–plastic system should be evaluated.

The NF states that plastics used in containers for ophthalmics frequently contain residues from the polymerization process, plasticizers, stabilizers, antioxidants, pigments, and lubricants. Factors such as plastic composition, processing and cleaning operations, contacting media, inks, adhesives, absorption, adsorption, and permeability of preservatives, and conditions of storage may also affect the suitability of a plastic for a specific use. Evaluation of such factors should be made by appropriate additional specific tests to determine the suitability of a plastic for use as a container for ophthalmics. Such tests include injections into mice and instillation into rabbits' eyes of extracts of the container material.

They are stated to have the great advantage that contamination is kept at a minimum, unless the patient becomes rather careless in handling the container.

However, each time the container is used a portion of the liquid wets the outer surface of the dropper insert. After the drop breaks away and the patient or physician releases the pressure on the package, the remaining liquid is returned to the inside of the container. If this outer surface is contaminated by contact with an infected eyelid, or other foreign object, it is possible that some portion of the contaminant will thereby gain entrance into the fluid contents. It seems, however, that a dropper from a dropper bottle is more likely to become contaminated by carelessness than the dropper insert of a so-called droptainer.

Application and Use

In using an eye dropper the user should not allow the dropper to touch the eye or any other object lest the soiled dropper contaminate the solution. Droppers should be boiled before being used or equivalent precaution should be taken. It should be recognized that if a contaminated dropper is returned to the solution after use, it will contaminate the solution immediately. Any ophthalmic solution should be discarded if it is cloudy or discolored or contains foreign particles.[117] Attention should be given to the hazard of drug crystals in the eye from any ophthalmic solution if the drug crystallizes on the lip of the bottle or the dropper tip.[117]

Some physicians are using autoclaved disposable plastic straws or tooth picks to transfer the medication to the eye of the patient. An alert pharmacist can offer his colleagues in ophthalmology the service of packaging and sterilizing these ancillary disposable materials.

If the physician uses this method of drug instillation, he may desire the prescription packaged in an ordinary prescription bottle, as a dropper bottle would not be required, and it would be difficult to prevent contamination of the dropper from a dropper bottle while using the above technique.

Eye Cups—Ophthalmologists generally frown upon the use of an eye cup. When used, it frequently spreads the infection over the eye being treated and often transfers it to the other eye if used on both eyes, as is so often the case. Furthermore, several members of the same family may use the same eye cup without presterilization and thus spread the infection. The patient is likely also to return the solution to the bottle after use.

Because of the danger of contamination from droppers and especially from eye cups some doctors recommend the application of the solution to the eyes by dropping it from a pledget of absorbent cotton upon which the solution has been poured, with precautions for cleanliness.

In summary, it is the professional obligation of the pharmacist to instruct patients in the proper use and care of eye cups and eye droppers as well as the other modes of application. He should also support the use of relatively small containers and of disposable application devices where possible.

It should be noted that ophthalmic solutions should be dispensed with an expiration date not more than 30 days after the opening of the original package and the lip or dropper insert of the so-called droptainer must remain covered with the screw cap after use.

Contact Lenses and Their Solutions

This subject was reviewed by Krezanoski, *et al*,[224] and by Blaug.[225] As early as 1827 Sir John Herschel used a refractive device blown of glass which fitted over the eyeball but did not touch the cornea to protect the cornea from contact with infected lids. He used an unspecified "gelatinous substance" to fill the cup of the lens between the lens and the eye.

The term "contact lens" was first used by Dr. A. Eugen Fick in 1887 to designate this type of device. Fick used a 2% solution of grape sugar to fill the space between the lens and the eye.

In 1892 Professor Dor suggested use of physiological saline for this purpose. This was used principally until about 1939.

These large fluid-filled lenses were called "scleral lenses" because the rims rested on the sclera, not on the cornea. In using the scleral lens the filling solution was a necessary part of the optical system. As wearing continued the lens and the filling solution blocked normal respiration and the corneal tissues gradually became less transparent. For some wearers this "fogging" occurred as early as 30 minutes after the lenses were inserted in the eye. Other complaints were rainbow formations around sources of light, tearing, and pain. The scleral lens did interfere with the normal metabolism of the cornea and sclera.

In 1939 Hind suggested some substitutes for physiologic saline solution.

In 1948 Tuohy introduced the plastic corneal microlens. This lens was a light weight optically clear plastic and could be mounted on the cornea without pain as it did not contact the cornea. A properly fitted microlens will float freely on the precorneal fluid and mucous secretions. Therefore, the term "contact lens" is a misnomer. The microlens is easier to manipulate than the scleral lens, more comfortable to wear, and not particularly visible to other individuals. The average patient can wear this type of lens a full day. At the present time several million people wear contact lenses in the United States.

Two types of solutions are recommended for cleaning and treating the contact lens. These are referred to respectively as a wetting solution and a soaking solution. Advice on their use is an important professional pharmaceutical service.[225] Blaug points out that some individuals occasionally use a third solution which is formulated for more rigorous cleansing. If this is done it is still essential to condition the lenses with a wetting solution before insertion in the eyes.[225]

A recommended procedure for caring for contact lenses including the use of the two solutions is as follows:

1. Prior to any contact with the lenses the patient's hands should be thoroughly scrubbed and dried with a clean towel.
2. Remove lenses and apply wetting solution freely to clean away epithelial and sebaceous deposits accumulated during wearing. Rub between fingers for at least 1 full minute.
3. Rinse with water and examine for optical clarity by looking through the lens. Repeat cleaning with wetting solution if the lens is not optically clear.
4. Place lenses in soaking solution for storage to prevent dehydration and to permit dissolution of adsorbed deposits.
5. When lenses are to be worn again remove them from the soaking solution after scrubbing the hands. Rub wetting solution over the surface of the lens and without rinsing the lens insert it on the eye. A coating of wetting solution protects the lens surface from smudging upon contact with the lids or fingers during mounting.

The essential functions of a well formulated wetting solution are:

1. To convert the hydrophobic lens surface to a hydrophilic one, to wet the lens,
2. To provide a viscous protective coating over the lens surface so that the lens does not come in direct contact with the finger during insertion; this prevents transfer of oily sebaceous deposits normally present on the skin to the lens surface,
3. To provide lubrication between the lid and lens surface and, in turn, the desired cushioning effect between the lens and corneal surface,
4. To aid in cleaning the lens after its removal from the eye, and
5. To stabilize the lens on the fingertip to facilitate insertion.

Although some patients can tolerate a dry lens, most contact lens wearers will complain of eye irritation and an uncomfortable "foreign body" sensation unless some means is provided to wet the lens before it is inserted.

The wetting solution is generally formulated to contain a cellulose derivative to increase its viscosity. It should be isotonic, sterile and adequately self-sterilizing. It should be noted that some viscous ingredients may inactivate the antimicrobial preservative.

In formulating a wetting solution one must consider the limits of the natural built-in buffer capacity of tear fluid, just as in designing ophthalmic solutions containing medication. A wetting solution which is only weakly buffered can have a pH between 5 and 9. If it is strongly buffered the pH should approximate 7.4.

The standard criterion for a wetting solution is its suitability for direct ocular instillation in the undiluted form on a continuing day to day use schedule without any irritation to the ocular tissue. If a wetting solution cannot pass this test, it should not be used with contact lenses even when directions state that it be washed off with water before the contact lens is inserted.

It is obvious that this so-called wetting solution has detergent properties.

One reason that the solution is called a wetting solution is that the plastic lenses are hydrophobic and resist wetting with water.

The microlenses are usually made from polymethylmethacrylate or other ester polymers of methacrylic acid because of the nearly ideal optical characteristics of these plastics.

While saliva is an excellent wetting agent, its use is condemned by the medical profession because of the overall nonhygienic aspects and the possibility of eye infection.

Soaking Solution—The functions of the hydrating or soaking solution are:

1. To aid in cleaning the lens of tenacious ocular secretions after the lens is removed from the eye,
2. To prevent eye infection by a contaminated lens, and
3. To maintain the state of hydrated equilibrium which the lens achieves while it is being worn.

When the lens is removed from the eye, it will have on its surface various proteinaceous, oily, and sebaceous matter.   If these substances are not removed they will greatly reduce wettability and optical clarity.   In addition, if this material is not removed promptly and the lens is allowed to dry out, a scum will form which is very difficult to remove even with special buffing instruments.

Placing the lenses in water while they are not being worn is not a satisfactory alternative.

Tap water contains mineral contaminants which would react with some of the material on the surface of the lens and the reaction products would be quite difficult to remove.

Use of distilled water would not be satisfactory because it is neither sterile or self-sterilizing.

Clifton and Hall suggest an antimicrobial system consisting of benzalkonium chloride 0.004% and chlorobutanol 0.3%.

While the lenses are in the eye they are totally immersed in tear fluid and contain perhaps 1.5% water. It is desirable that they be stored in an aqueous medium in order to maintain hydration.

The selection of a soaking container is of importance. It should be easy to clean, should have labeled compartments for the right and left lens, and should be leakproof at all altitudes.   It should not exert pressure on the lenses; it should have sufficient capacity so that the lenses will float freely in an adequate quantity of material; and it must be made of a material that will not leach out into the solution and interact with the lenses.

The directions for care of lenses stipulate thorough scrubbing of the hands.   It should be noted that most commercial hand cleansers are formulated in such a way that it is difficult to rinse all of the residue off the hands after washing.   This applies particularly to the hexachlorophene preparations as they are meant to accumulate as a residue on the hands.   Any such residue may smudge the hands and it is recommended that one use a type of hand cleanser specially formulated for this purpose.

References

1. Riegelman, S., and Vaughan, D. G., Jr., *J. APhA, Pract. Ed.*, **19**, 474 (1958).
2. Adler, F. H., *Physiology of the Eye, Clinical Application*, 4th ed., Mosby, St. Louis, 1965.
3. Adler, F. H., *Textbook of Ophthalmology*, 7th ed., Saunders, Philadelphia, 1962.
4. Best, C. H., and Taylor, N. B., *Physiological Basis of Medical Practice*, 8th ed., Williams & Wilkins, Baltimore, 1966.
5. Davson, H., and Eggleston, M. G., *Principles of Human Physiology*, 14th ed., Lea & Febiger, Philadelphia, 1968.
6. Ellis, P. P., and Smith, D. L., *Handbook of Ocular Therapeutics and Pharmacology*, Mosby, St. Louis, 1963.
7. Botelho, S. Y., *Sci. Am.*, 80 (Oct., 1964).
8. Heath, W. E., *Brit. Med. J.*, **2**, 608 (1950).
9. Weiss, D. I., and Shaffer, R. N., *Arch. Ophthalmol.*, **68**, 727 (1962).
10. Anderson, R. A., *Australasian J. Pharm.*, **47**, S8 (1966).
11. Burch, P. G., and Migeon, C. J., *Arch. Ophthalmol.*, **79**, 174 (1968).
12. Cogan, D. G., *et al*, *Arch. Ophthalmol.*, **31**, 408 (1944).
13. Cogan, D. G., and Hirsch, E. O., *Arch. Ophthalmol.*, **32**, 276 (1944).
14. Cogan, D. G., and Kinsey, V. E., *Arch. Ophthalmol.*, **27**, 466 (1942).
15. Cogan, D. G., and Kinsey, V. E., *Arch. Ophthalmol.*, **27**, 696 (1942).
16. Swan, K. C., and White, N. G., *Am. J. Ophthalmol.*, **25**, 1043 (1942).
17. Maurice, D. M., *J. Physiol.*, **112**, 367 (1951).
18. Maurice, D. M., *Ophthalmol. Lit.*, **7**, 3 (1953).
19. *New and Nonofficial Remedies*, Lippincott, Philadelphia, 1953, p. xl.
20. Tower, P., *Arch. Ophthalmol.*, **41**, 730 (1949).
21. Riegelman, S., and Vaughan, D. G., Jr., *J. APhA, Pract. Ed.*, **19**, 537 (1958).
22. Riegelman, S., and Vaughan, D. G., Jr., *J. APhA, Pract. Ed.*, **19**, 665 (1958).
23. Anderson, R. A., *Australasian J. Pharm.*, **48**, S90 (1967).
24. Cadwallader, D. E., *Am. J. Hosp. Pharm.*, **24**, 32 (1967).
25. McCowan, J. R., and Husa, W. J., *J. APhA, Sci. Ed.*, **45**, 474 (1956).
26. Smith, G., *J. Indian Pharm. Manuf.*, **6**, 135 (1967).
27. Murphy, J. T., *et al*, *Arch. Ophthalmol.*, **53**, 63 (1955).
28. *Federal Register*, **18**(11), 351 (Jan. 16, 1953).
29. Parrott, E. L., *et al*, *J. APhA, Pract. Ed.*, **14**, 645 (1953).
30. Higuchi, T., and Schroeter, L. C., *J. APhA, Sci. Ed.*, **48**, 535 (1959).
31. Schroeter, L. C., *et al*, *J. APhA, Sci. Ed.*, **47**, 723 (1958).
32. Martin, E. W., ed., *Husa's Pharmaceutical Dispensing*, 6th ed., Mack Publ. Co., Easton, Pa., 1966.
33. Higuchi, T., *et al*, *J. APhA, Sci. Ed.*, **39**, 405 (1950).
34. Kondritzer, A. A., and Zvirblis, P., *J. APHA, Sci. Ed.*, **46**, 531 (1957).
35. Zvirblis, P., *et al.*, *J. APhA, Sci. Ed.*, **45**, 450 (1956).
36. Patel, J. L., and Lemberger, A. P., *J. APhA, Sci. Ed.*, **47**, 878 (1958).
37. Morrison, W. H., *Am. J. Ophthalmol.*, **37**, 391 (1954).
38. Morrison, W. H., and Truhlsen, S. M., *Am. J. Ophthalmol.*, **33**, 357 (1950).
39. Hind, H. W., and Goyan, F. M., *J. APhA, Sci. Ed.*, **36**, 33 (1947).
40. Hind, H. W., and Goyan, F. M., *J. APhA, Sci. Ed.*, **38**, 477 (1949).
41. Floyd, A., *et al*, *J. APhA, Sci. Ed.*, **42**, 333 (1953).
42. Boberg-Ans, J., *et al*, *Brit. J. Ophthalmol.*, **43**, 670 (1959).
43. Hosford, G. N., and Hicks, A. M., *Arch. Ophthalmol.*, **13**, 14 (1935).
44. *New Drugs*, Am. Med. Assoc., Chicago, 1967, p. 334.
45. Trolle-Lassen, T., *Pharm. Weekblad.*, **93**, 148 (1958).
46. Anderson, R. A., and FitzGerald, S. D., *Australasian J. Pharm.*, **48**, S108 (1967).
47. Molinas, S., and Welch, H., *J. APhA, Sci. Ed.*, **36**, 41 (1947).
48. Kostenbauder, H. B., *et al*, *J. APhA, Sci. Ed.*, **42**, 210 (1953).
49. Hind, H. W., and Szekely, I. J., *J. APhA, Pract. Ed.*, **14**, 644 (1953).
50. Clarke, P. A., *J. Indian Pharm. Manuf.*, **5**, 167 (1967).
51. Gifford, S. R., *Arch. Ophthalmol.*, **13**, 78 (1935).
52. Gifford, S. R., and Smith R. D., *Arch. Ophthalmol.*, **9**, 227 (1933).
53. Atkins, W. R. G., and Pantin, G. F. A., *Biochem. J.*, **20**, 102 (1926).
54. Neuwald, F., *et al*, *Pharm. Ztg. Ver. Apotheker-Ztg.*, **102** (40 & 51/52) (1957); **103**(12) (1958).
55. Lund, C. G., *et al*, *The Preparation of Solutions Iso-osmotic with Blood, Tears, and Tissue*, Danish Pharmacopoeial Commission, Einar Munksgaard, Copenhagen, 1947.
56. Husa, W. J., and Rossi, O. A., *J. APhA, Sci. Ed.*, **31**, 270 (1942).
57. Goyan, F. M., *J. APhA, Sci. Ed.*, **47**, 783 (1958).
58. Goyan, F. M., *et al*, *J. APhA, Sci. Ed.*, **33**, 74 (1944).
59. Goyan, F. M., and Johnson, R. D., *J. Pharm. Sci.*, **52**, 390 (1963).
60. Goyan, F. M., and Reck, D., *J. APhA, Sci. Ed.*, **44**, 43 (1955).
61. Goyan, F. M., *et al*, *J. Pharm. Sci.*, **50**, 684 (1961).
62. Greco, S. J., *J. APhA, Pract. Ed.*, **13**, 340 (1952).
63. Hammarlund, E. R., *J. APhA, NS5*, 324 (1965).
64. Hammarlund, E. R., *et al*, *J. Pharm. Sci.*, **54**, 160 (1965).
65. Hind, H. W., *et al*, *J. APhA, Sci. Ed.*, **36**, 413 (1947).
66. Johnson, R. D., *et al*, *J. Pharm. Sci.*, **54**, 1176 (1965).
67. Baggesgaard-Rasmussen, H., and Jerslev, B., *J. Pharm. Pharmacol.*, **7**, 967 (1955).
68. Sprowls, J., *J. APhA, Pract. Ed.*, **10**, 348 (1949).
69. Sprowls, J., *J. APhA, Pract. Ed.*, **14**, 216 (1953).
70. Szekely, I. J., and Goyan, F. M., *J. APhA, Sci. Ed.*, **41**, 30 (1952).
71. Szekely, I. J., *et al*, *J. APhA, Sci. Ed.*, **41**, 32 (1952).
72. White, A. I., and Vincent, H. C., *J. APhA, Pract. Ed.*, **8**, 406 (1947).
73. Hammarlund, E. R., and Pedersen-Bjergaard, K., *J. APhA, Sci. Ed.*, **47**, 107 (1958).
74. Hammarlund, E. R., and Pedersen-Bjergaard, K., *J. Pharm. Sci.*, **50**, 24 (1961).
75. Hammarlund, E. R., and Van Pevenage, G. L., *J. Pharm. Sci.*, **55**, 1448 (1966).
76. Wells, J. M., *J. APhA, Pract. Ed.*, **5**, 99 (1944).
77. Martin, A. N., *et al.*, *Physical Pharmacy*, 2nd ed., Lea & Febiger, Philadelphia, 1969.
78. Krogh, A., *et al*, *Acta Physiol. Scand.*, **10**, 88 (1945).
79. Husa, W. J., and Adams, J. R., *J. APhA, Sci. Ed.*, **33**, 329 (1944).
80. Grosicki, T. S., and Husa, W. J., *J. APhA, Sci. Ed.*, **43**, 632 (1954).
81. Easterly, W. D., Jr., and Husa, W. J., *J. APhA, Sci. Ed.*, **43**, 750 (1954).
82. Hartman, C. W., and Husa, W. J., *J. APhA, Sci. Ed.*, **46**, 430 (1957).
83. Cadwallader, D. E., and Husa, W. J., *J. APhA, Sci. Ed.*, **47**, 703 (1958).
84. Cadwallader, D. E., and Husa, W. J., *J. APhA, Sci. Ed.*, **47**, 705 (1958).
85. Thomasson, C. L., and Husa, W. J., *J. APhA, Sci. Ed.*, **47**, 711 (1958).
86. Ansel, H. C., and Husa, W. J., *J. APhA, Sci. Ed.*, **48**, 516 (1959).
87. Zanowiak, P., and Husa, W. J., *J. APhA, Sci. Ed.*, **48**, 565 (1959).
88. Marcus, D., and Husa, W. J., *J. APhA, Sci. Ed.*, **48**, 569 (1959).
89. Winters, E. P., and Husa, W. J., *J. APhA, Sci. Ed.*, **49**, 709 (1960).
90. Schnell, L. A., and Husa, W. J., *J. Pharm. Sci.*, **51**, 904 (1962).
91. Shaw, M. A., and Husa, W. J., *J. Pharm. Sci.*, **51**, 929 (1962).
92. Cadwallader, D. E., *Am. J. Hosp. Pharm.*, **21**, 22 (1964).
93. Cadwallader, D. E., and Husa, W. J., *Am. J. Pharm.*, **129**, 393 (1957).
94. Ansel, H. C., *J. Pharm. Sci.*, **54**, 1159 (1965).
95. Ansel, H. C., *J. Pharm. Sci.*, **56**, 616 (1967).
96. Ansel, H. C., and Cadwallader, D. E., *J. Pharm. Sci.*, **53**, 169 (1964).
97. Cadwallader, D. E., and Ansel, H. C., *J. Pharm. Sci.*, **54**, 1010 (1965).
98. Ansel, H. C., and Leake, W. F., *J. Pharm. Sci.*, **55**, 685 (1966).
99. Cadwallader, D. E., *J. Pharm. Sci.*, **52**, 1175 (1963).
100. Cadwallader, D. E., *et al*, *J. Pharm. Sci.*, **53**, 927 (1964).
101. Smith, B. L., and Cadwallader, D. E., *J. Pharm. Sci.*, **56**, 351 (1967).
102. Cadwallader, D. E., and Drinkard, J. P., *J. Pharm. Sci.*, **56**, 583 (1967).
103. Ansel, H. C., *Am. J. Hosp. Pharm.*, **21**, 25 (1964).
104. Setnikar, I., and Temelcou, O., *J. APhA, Sci. Ed.*, **48**, 628 (1959).
105. Lipschutz, H., *Klin. Monatsbl. Augenb.*, **82**, 87 (1929).
106. Riegelman, S., *et al*, *J. APhA, Pract. Ed.*, **16**, 742 (1955).
107. Lund, C. G., *et al*, *The Preparation of Solutions Iso-osmotic with Blood, Tears, and Tissue*, Heinemann, London, p. 173; through Train, D., *Pharm. J.*, **159**, 447 (1947).
108. Fenton, A. H., *Pharm. J.*, **166**, 6 (1951).
109. Krishna, N., and Brow, F., *Am. J. Ophthalmol.*, **57**, 99 (1964).

110. Hammarlund, E. R., and Pedersen-Bjergaard, K., *J. APhA, Pract. Ed.*, **19**, 39 (1958).
111. Lund, C. G., *et al, Contributions from the Danish Pharmacopeia Commission*, vol. 2, Einar Munksgaard, Copenhagen, 1947.
112. Feldman, J. B., *et al, Arch. Ophthalmol.*, **40**, 668 (1948).
113. Pisano, F. D., and Kostenbauder, H. B., *J. APhA, Sci. Ed.*, **48**, 310 (1959).
114. Heard, D. D., *Pharm. J.*, **196**, 318 (1966).
115. Leopold, I. H., *Arch. Ophthalmol.*, **34**, 99 (1945).
116. *Ophthalmology Prescription Handbook*, 2nd ed., Browning Med. Publ., Pasadena, Calif., 1968.
117. Lofholm, P. W., *J. APhA*, NS8, 497 (1968).
118. Swan, K. C., *Arch. Ophthalmol.*, **33**, 378 (1945).
119. Swan, K. C., *Arch. Ophthalmol.*, **41**, 253 (1949).
120. Blaug, S. M., and Canada, A. T., Jr., *Am. J. Hosp. Pharm.*, **22**, 662 (1965).
121. Miyawaki, G. M., *et al, J. APhA, Sci. Ed.*, **48**, 315 (1959).
122. Tillman, W. J., and Kuramoto, R., *J. APhA, Sci. Ed.*, **46**, 211 (1957).
123. Mueller, W. H., and Deardorff, D. L., *J. APhA, Sci. Ed.*, **45**, 334 (1956).
124. Haas, J. S., and Merrill, D. L., *Am. J. Ophthalmol.*, **54**, 21 (1962).
125. Madden, E. E., Jr., and Piecoro, J. J., Jr., *Am. J. Hosp. Pharm.*, **22**, 195 (1965).
126. Mims, J. L., Jr., *Arch. Ophthalmol.*, **46**, 664 (1951).
127. Bergy, G. A., *Am. Profess. Pharmacist*, **18**, 341 (1952).
128. Scigliano, J. A., *Bull. Am. Soc. Hosp. Pharm.*, **9**, 55 (1952).
129. Campbell, W. J., *et al, J. APhA, Pract. Ed.*, **16**, 38 (1955).
130. Anderson, D. L., and Shea, M., *Am. J. Ophthalmol.*, **51**, 1200 (1961).
131. Fleming, T. C., *et al, Arch. Ophthalmol.*, **61**, 565 (1959).
132. Dale, J. K., *et al, J. APhA, Pract. Ed.*, **20**, 32 (1959).
133. Herbert, H., *Ophthalmol. Rev.*, **20**, 339 (1901).
134. Cooper, E. L., *Arch. Ophthalmol.*, **28**, 180 (1942).
135. McCulloch, J. C., *Arch. Ophthalmol.*, **29**, 924 (1943).
136. Theodore, F. H., and Feinstein, R. R., *Am. J. Ophthalmol.*, **35**, 656 (1952).
137. Theodore, F. H., and Feinstein, R. R., *J. Am. Med. Assoc.*, **152**, 1631 (1953).
138. King, J. H., Jr., *Am. J. Ophthalmol.*, **36**, 1389 (1953).
139. Vaughan, D. G., *Am. J. Ophthalmol.*, **39**, 55 (1955).
140. Cassady, J. V., *Am. J. Ophthalmol.*, **48**, 741 (1959).
141. Beloian, A., and Koski, T., *J. Assoc. Offic. Agr. Chemists*, **47**, 804 (1964).
142. Brown, M. R. W., and Richards, R. M. E., *J. Pharm. Pharmacol.*, **16**, 51T (1964).
143. Richards, R. M. E., and Brown, M. R. W., *J. Pharm. Pharmacol.*, **16**, 360 (1964).
144. Fisher, E., Jr., and Allen, J. H., *Am. J. Ophthalmol.*, **46**, 249 (1958).
145. Lepard, C. W., *Arch. Ophthalmol.*, **28**, 180 (1942).
146. Joy, H. H., *Arch. Ophthalmol.*, **27**, 1135 (1942).
147. LaBorde, H. F., and deFajardo, C. L., *J. Bacteriol.*, **90**, 290 (1965).
148. Klein, M., and Millwood, E. G., *Trans. Ophthalmol. Soc.*, **75**, 515 (1955).
149. Rabe, C. C., *et al, J. APhA, Pract. Ed.*, **16**, 36 (1955).
150. Thygeson, P., *Am. J. Ophthalmol.*, **32**, 951 (1949).
151. Steiger-Trippi, K., *Am. J. Hosp. Pharm.*, **21**, 11 (1964).
152. Sollman, T., *A Manual of Pharmacology*, 8th ed., Saunders, Philadelphia, 1957, p. 369.
153. Altbach, H., and Mazzapica, F., *Bull. Am. Soc. Hosp. Pharm.*, **12**, 456 (1955).
154. Crisafi, R. C., *J. APhA*, NS4, 548 (1964).
155. Hammarlund, E. R., *J. APhA*, NS4, 542 (1964).
156. Johnson, W. F., *J. APhA, Pract. Ed.*, **16**, 40 (1955).
157. Heller, W. M., *et al, J. APhA, Pract. Ed.*, **16**, 29 (1955).
158. Hogan, M. J., *Calif. Med.*, **71**, 414 (1949).
159. Krause, W. O., *et al, Am. Profess. Pharmacist*, **19**, 905 (1953).
160. Scigliano, J. A., and Skolaut, M. W., *Bull. Am. Soc. Hosp. Pharm.*, **11**, 37 (1954).
161. Skolaut, M. W., *Bull. Am. Soc. Hosp. Pharm.*, **5**, 172 (1948).
162. Yalon, J. M., *Am. Profess. Pharmacist*, **16**, 360 (1950).
163. Lawrence, C. A., *Am. J. Ophthalmol.*, **39**, 385 (1955).

164. Kohn, S. R., *et al, J. Pharm. Sci.*, **52**, 967 (1963).
165. Garrett, E., *J. Pharm. Pharmacol.*, **18**, 589 (1966).
166. Lawrence, C. A., *J. APhA, Sci. Ed.*, **44**, 457 (1955).
167. Riegelman, S., *et al, J. APhA, Sci. Ed.*, **45**, 93 (1956).
168. Klarmann, E. G., *Ann. NY Acad. Sci.*, **53**, 123 (1950).
169. Brown, M. R. W., and Norton, D. A., *J. Soc. Cosmetic Chemists*, **16**, 369 (1965).
170. Foster, J. H. S., *Manuf. Chemist Aerosol News*, **36**, 45 (May, 1965).
171. Foster, J. H. S., *Manuf. Chemist Aerosol News*, **36**, 43 (June, 1965).
172. Foster, J. H. S., *J. Indian Pharm. Manuf.*, **3**, 281 (1965).
173. Foster, J. H. S., *J. Indian Pharm. Manuf.*, **3**, 317 (1965).
174. Hess, H., and Speiser, P., *J. Pharm. Pharmacol.*, **11**, 650 (1959).
175. Hess, H., and Speiser, P., *J. Pharm. Pharmacol.*, **11**, 694 (1959).
176. Richards, R. M. E., *Australasian J. Pharm.*, **48**, S86 (1967).
177. Richards, R. M. E., *Australasian J. Pharm.*, **48**, S96 (1967).
178. MacGregor, D. R., and Elliker, P. R., *Can. J. Microbiol.*, **4**, 499 (1958).
179. *New and Nonofficial Drugs*, Lippincott, Philadelphia, 1964, p. 176.
180. Klein, M., *et al, J. Pharm. Pharmacol.*, **6**, 725 (1954).
181. Swan, K. C., *Am. J. Ophthalmol.*, **27**, 1118 (1944).
182. Lawrence, C. A., *Surface Active Quaternary Ammonium Germicides*, Academic, New York, 1950.
183. Valko, E. I., and DuBois, A. S., *J. Bacteriol.*, **47**, 15 (1944).
184. Monkhouse, D. C., and Groves, G. A., *Australasian J. Pharm.*, **48**, S70 (1967).
185. Kohn, S. R., *et al, J. Pharm. Sci.*, **52**, 1126 (1963).
186. Gershenfeld, L., and Tomkins, D., *Am. J. Pharm.*, **111**, 385 (1939).
187. Taub, A., and Luckey, W. H., *J. APhA, Sci. Ed.*, **32**, 28 (1943).
188. Patwa, N. V., and Huyck, C. L., *J. APhA*, NS6, 373 (1966).
189. Nair, A. D., and Lach, J. L., *J. APhA, Sci. Ed.*, **48**, 390 (1959).
190. Goldstein, S., *J. APhA, Pract. Ed.*, **14**, 498 (1953).
191. Deeb, E. N., and Boenigk, J. W., *J. APhA, Sci. Ed.*, **47**, 807 (1958).
192. Brown, M. R. W., *J. Pharm. Sci.*, **57**, 389 (1968).
193. Abrams, J. D., *Trans. Ophthalmol. Soc.*, **83**, 263 (1963).
194. Gerrard, H. N., *et al, J. Pharm. Pharmacol.*, **14**, 103 (1962).
195. Hugo, W. B., and Foster, J. H. S., *J. Pharm. Pharmacol.*, **16**, 209 (1964).
196. Sokol, H., *Drug Std.*, **20**, 89 (1952).
197. Davies, G. E., *et al, Brit. J. Pharmacol.*, **9**, 192 (1954).
198. Anderson R. A., and Stock, B. H., *Australasian J. Pharm.*, **39**, 1110 (1958).
199. Jeffs, P. L., *Australasian J. Pharm.*, **40**, 218 (1959).
200. Jeffs, P. L., *Australasian J. Pharm.*, **43**, 1031 (1962).
201. Mitchell, J. A., *et al, Australasian J. Pharm.*, **42**, 1284 (1961).
202. Graham, P. A., *Brit. J. Ophthalmol.*, **44**, 761 (1960).
203. Anderson, K., *et al, Australasian J. Pharm.*, **48**, S80 (1967).
204. Brown, M. R. W., and Richards, R. M. E., *Nature*, **207**, 1391 (1965).
205. Parker, M. S., *et al, Soap Perfumery Cosmetics*, **39**, 371 (1966).
206. Anderson, K., *et al, Pharm. J.*, **138**, 593 (1964).
207. Anderson, R. A., *Australasian J. Pharm.*, **44**, S32 (1963).
208. Anderson, R. A., *Australasian J. Pharm.*, **45**, S35 (1964).
209. Anderson, R. A., *Australasian J. Pharm. Sci. Suppl.*, S25 (1965).
210. Brown, M. R. W., *et al, Pharm. J.*, **192**, 8 (1964).
211. Crompton, D. O., *Australasian J. Pharm.*, **43**, 1020 (1962).
212. Hess, H., *Soap Perfumery Cosmetics*, **38**, 955 (1965).
213. Hugo, W. B., and Foster, J. H. S., *J. Pharm. Pharmacol. (Suppl.)*, **16**, 124T (1964).
214. Hugo, W. B., and Longworth A. R., *J. Pharm. Pharmacol.*, **16**, 655 (1964).
215. Lawrence, C. A., *J. APhA, Sci. Ed.*, **49**, 731 (1960).
216. Polack, A. E., *Australasian J. Pharm.*, **48**, S64 (1967).
217. Wiseman, D., *J. Pharm. Pharmacol.*, **16**, 56T (1964).
218. Hugo, W. B., and Longworth, A. R., *J. Pharm. Pharmacol.*, **18**, 569 (1966).
219. Christensen, K., and Garup, K., *Am. J. Hosp. Pharm.*, **25**, 524 (1968).
220. Bing, G. H., *Australasian J. Pharm.*, **48**, S10 (1966).
221. Guess, W. L., *et al, Am. J. Hosp. Pharm.*, **24**, 495 (1967).
222. Polack, A. E., *Australasian J. Pharm.*, **48**, S104 (1967).
223. Russell, J., and Stock, B. H., *Australasian J. Pharm.*, **47**, S37 (1966).
224. Krezanoski, J. Z., *et al, J. APhA*, NS2, 417 (1962).
225. Blaug, S. M., *Am. J. Pharm. Educ.*, **31**, 74 (1967).

84 | Extraction and Extractives

Maceration—percolation—digestion—infusion—decoction—tinctures—fluidextracts—extracts—resins—oleoresins—finishing, packaging, and storing

This chapter was prepared by

George Motoasca, BS, *Manager, Product Development Department, S. B. Penick & Company, New York, N.Y. 10007, and*
George C. Walker, PhD, *Head, Department of Pharmacy, Faculty of Pharmacy, University of Toronto, Toronto 5, Ontario, Canada*

Extraction

Extractives are pharmaceutical preparations obtained from plant and animal tissues with the aid of solvents and standardized extraction procedures. These preparations, some of which were recorded in the literature as early as the 2nd century AD by the famous Greek physician Galen, contain active principles which have been separated as much as possible from inert constituents.

For many centuries extractives called *galenicals* (decoctions, fluidextracts, infusions, solid and semisolid extracts, and tinctures) were obtained from *plants* and were firmly established in pharmaceutical and medical practice. In the last few decades, however, substances with therapeutic utility have also been obtained from *animals* by extraction. And now, in more recent years, because many active principles from both plants and animals have been isolated, synthesized, and obtained as purified products of precisely known potency and stability, extractives are infrequently prescribed by the physician.

Crude drug extraction comprises those operations which have for their object the separation of desired principles from drugs by treating them with a suitable solvent called the *menstruum*. *Extraction* differs from solution in the fact that the presence of insoluble matter is implied in the former and the soluble constituents must therefore be *extracted* or separated, by appropriate methods, from those which are insoluble. The principal modes of extraction employed in pharmacy at present are as follows: (1) maceration, (2) percolation, (3) digestion, (4) infusion, and (5) decoction.

The processes of particular importance at this time, insofar as official texts are concerned, are those of maceration and percolation. Most pharmacopeias and formularies, including the United States Pharmacopeia (USP), National Formulary (NF), British Pharmacopeia (BP), British Pharmacopoeial Codex (BPC), and Pharmacopoea International is (PhI), refer to similar processes for removal of active principles.

The methods for obtaining the active constituents were the logical outcome of a consideration of the nature of the plant or animal tissue, the nature of the active principle, and the ease of solution of the principles. These methods and procedures, or modifications of them, find wide use in phytochemical and biochemical research, forensic chemistry, and the extraction of volatile oils, in addition to their use in preparing extracted pharmaceutical products. Constituents isolated from plant, animal, or microbial substances may use one, or a combination, of the extraction processes, but all involve similar basic extraction principles and use similar solvent systems with suitable modification. The principles underlying immiscible solvent systems and countercurrent distribution are used in refined extraction procedures.

Maceration

The process of maceration, which is of ancient origin, consists simply of extraction by soaking the properly comminuted drug or substance in the menstruum until the cellular structure is thoroughly penetrated and the soluble portions are softened and dissolved. The usual method is to introduce the drug into a bottle with the solvent or menstruum, stopper it tightly, and agitate it occasionally for a period ranging from 2 to 14 days; pour off the liquid; express the residue to avoid loss; and filter the mixed liquids. An advantage is sometimes gained by suspending the ground drug, tied in a bag, in the upper part of the menstruum. The drugs are macerated in definite quantities of menstruum, which consists of alcohol of various strengths, ether, ether and alcohol, or other specified solvent. A definite period of time is specified for the maceration, and agitation is directed for some tinctures. The liquid is separated by straining or expressing from the insoluble residue, and, after having been allowed to settle, it is filtered. Evaporation during filtration is to be avoided as much as possible.

Maceration has no advantages over percolation in making most liquid preparations from vegetable drugs, except in the hands of the careless or unskilled. If an operator possesses no knowledge whatever of the process of percolation, it is safer to use the maceration process, for here no particular skill or judgment is necessary; the soaking process is completed in due time, and the separation of the absorbed liquid, while laborious and sloppy, at least has the merit of leaving the tincture uniform in strength. Even if the process of expression is not thoroughly performed, and waste results through the smaller yield, the finished preparation properly represents the drug. On the other hand, in percolation, if the operator, through careless packing, has failed to exhaust the drug thoroughly with the amount of menstruum used, a portion of the activity of the drug remains in the residue, which is thrown out, and the preparation is thus deficient in strength. The maceration process must be used in the extraction of some drugs, notably those containing little or no cellular structure such as benzoin, aloe, styrax, tolu, etc.

Maceration is usually conducted at a temperature of from 15° to 20°C.

A substance such as myrrh, which contains primarily resin, gum, and volatile oil, would be difficult to manage by the percolation process since the resin and volatile oil would be extracted by a menstruum of alcohol leaving the gum behind as a sticky, amorphous mass, which would tend to choke the percolator. Tincture of Myrrh NF, Compound Benzoin Tincture USP, and others of this nature are thus prepared by Process M involving maceration, filtering, and washing of the residue on the filter. Due to the difficulty of extracting completely, in some cases, the active constituent(s) with one maceration, the process is repeated with the same or different solvents, or with different quantities of the solvent. Such processes have been referred to as double maceration, triple maceration, and repeated maceration.

Percolation

Percolation, or *lixiviation*, is the extraction process in which a granulated or powdered drug is deprived of its constituents by the descent of a suitable solvent through it. The importance of this process cannot be overestimated, as the progress made in pharmacy in America during the last century was largely due to the study and development of percolation, and the introduction of preparations which are the direct outgrowth of the process.

History—The practice of exhausting wood ashes of their soluble constituents by pouring water on them after their introduction into a conical-shaped wooden vessel, called a lye hopper, is an ancient one, and the process is still practiced and known as lixiviation. It is known that about 1813 a sort of percolator was used by Dumont in decolorizing syrups with charcoal in the refining of sugar and that in the Cafetiére de Dubelloy a similar outfit was used in the preparation of coffee, but the first attempt on record to apply the principle to powdered drugs was made by Count Real. In about the year 1815 M. Robiquet subsequently made some experiments to determine the power of ether as a solvent in extracting the fixed oil from the bitter almond. It was reserved, however, for the Boullays of Paris, in 1833, to apply the ideals of Real and Robiquet to drugs and medicinal substances in general, and to them belongs the credit of first demonstrating the value of the process of percolation in its pharmaceutical applications. The researches of the Boullays at once attracted the attention of American pharmacists, and the labors of Duhamel, Procter, Grahame, Squibb, Diehl, Oldberg, and others during the last century led to the widespread adoption of the process. For a very complete history of percolation, see an article written by Couch.[1]

Principle of Action—*When a powder placed in a cylindrical vessel with a porous diaphragm below is treated from above with a liquid capable of dissolving a portion of its substance, that portion of the fluid first in contact, in passing downward, exercises its solvent power on the successive layers of the powder, until saturated, and is impelled downward by the combined force of its own gravity and that of the column of liquid above it, minus the capillary force with which the powder tends to retain it.*

The physical forces playing an important part in percolation are *gravitation, viscosity, adhesion, friction, osmosis, capillarity, surface tension,* and *solution.* If the quantity of liquid added is not more than enough to satisfy the capillarity of the powder, no liquid will pass the diaphragm; but the careful addition of liquid on the top displaces that absorbed in the powder without mixing materially with it and takes its place to be, in turn, displaced by a fresh portion of liquid. The instrument used to hold the powder is called a *percolator;* the liquid poured on top of the powder, the *menstruum;* the liquid coming from the percolator impregnated with the soluble principles, the *percolate;* and the residual drug remaining in the percolator after the extraction of the soluble constituents, the *marc.*

Small-Scale Percolation

In order to understand thoroughly the process of percolation as applied to powdered drugs, it must be remembered that the soluble principles of vegetable substances are in a hard and dry condition and are generally contained in cells which are more or less disintegrated by the process of grinding. If the soluble principles could be separated from the insoluble cellular substance and deposited in the interstices of the ground particles, percolation would be rapid, for the descending column of liquid would immediately dissolve the soluble principles while the insoluble substances would remain in the percolator. But the powdering of the drug only partially separates the soluble principles from the insoluble, and the finest dust of the powder always contains a larger proportion of the soluble principles than of the insoluble substance because the latter, often being largely ligneous, offers the greatest amount of resistance to disintegration. Hence the first portion of the percolate is usually the most dense, the most highly colored, and contains the largest proportion of the soluble principles. This is because the first portion of menstruum, in its descent through the powder, has the first opportunity to come in contact with the largest proportion of the soluble principles, which are to be found in the finer dust scattered through the powder, and in the thoroughly disintegrated particles, which offer but slight resistance to the passage of the menstruum. In every well-conducted experiment in percolation it will be noticed that, as the operation proceeds, each succeeding portion of percolate is less highly colored and less active than the one preceding it; in the case of drugs containing easily dissolved coloring matter, an examination of the percolate will show that the shading is very marked, the lowest portion being very dense and dark colored, the upper portion almost colorless, while in the intermediate liquid the gradations of the tint are clearly perceptible.

Shape of the Percolator—In the USP of 1880 the shape and size of the cylindrical percolator preferred for pharmacopeial operations were for the first time definitely fixed (Fig. 595A). There can be no question that the glass cylindrical percolators (Fig. 595B) commonly furnished by the manufacturers are proportionately too

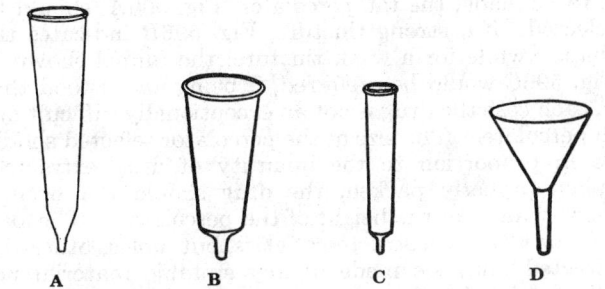

Fig. 595. Shape of percolators. (*A*) official; (*B*) glass cylindrical; (*C*) Oldberg; (*D*) conical.

broad for use in percolating drugs for fluidextracts where the quantity of drug is large in proportion to the quantity of menstruum; for ordinary tinctures, where the conditions are reversed, they answer admirably. The inference is obvious; the pharmacist should have percolators not only of different sizes, but also of different shapes. Fig. 595C shows the narrow percolator first recommended by Prof. C. Lewis Diehl but commonly known as the *Oldberg percolator*. The studies on percolation during the last half century have been directed toward simplifying the process, and the elaborate apparatus of Count Real and others has been replaced by the ordinary percolator and funnel. The conical percolator of the USP is understood to be a glass funnel (Fig. 595D).

Judgment is required in selecting a percolator for an operation. In making a fluidextract a comparatively narrow percolator should be chosen because it is desirable that the menstruum should traverse a higher column of powder, for every drop of the menstruum must be economically applied. The rate of flow of the percolator is thereby proportionally diminished, the percolate becomes saturated more rapidly, and thus the operation is more easily controlled, provided the limit has not been exceeded. *The character of the drug influences the limit.* For instance, one which contains a

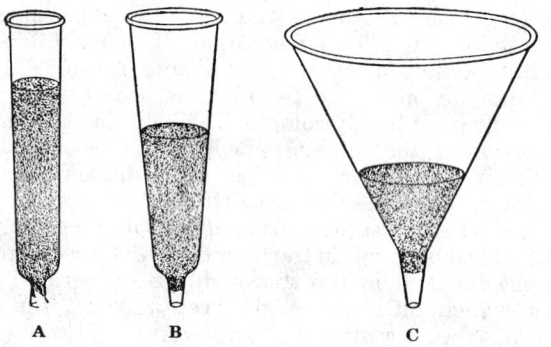

Fig. 596. Different types of percolators, each packed with 200 Gm of powder. (A) narrow; (B) ordinary; (C) conical.

large quantity of soluble matter, like kino, could not be successfully percolated in a narrow percolator because the percolate would soon become so dense that it would cease to descend. In making tinctures and weaker preparations a wider percolator is to be preferred because the quantity of menstruum is greatly in excess of the amount necessary to exhaust the drug and more rapid action is desirable. Figs. 596A, 596B, and 596C show three percolators of the same height, but of very different shapes. Exactly the same weight of powder is represented in each. The great difference in the height of the columns of powder will be readily noticed, and the necessity for judgment in selecting percolators is illustrated. If a fluidextract from the drug is to be made, the tall percolator, Fig. 596A, should be selected; if a strong tincture, Fig. 596B indicates the shape; while for a weak tincture, the funnel shown in Fig. 596C would be preferred, it being understood that in each case the drug is not an exceptionally difficult one to percolate. The size of the percolator selected should be in proportion to the quantity of drug extracted. When properly packed, the drug should not occupy more than ⅔ of the height of the percolator. The percolator is best constructed of glass, but, unless otherwise directed, may be made of any suitable material not affected by the drug or menstruum. Metallic percolators are required for hot percolation.

Comminution—The degree of comminution proper for each substance must depend on the physical structure of the drug, the ease with which the menstruum dissolves the active or desirable constituents, the length of time required to exhaust the powder, and the relative proportion of menstruum to drug. Nux vomica and ignatia are drugs having a tough, horny structure, in which the soluble constituents are embedded. If these drugs are to be quickly exhausted of their soluble principles, they must be in fine powder. On the other hand, gentian and rhubarb are drugs which part easily with their active constituents because their structure is loose and quickly penetrated by the menstruum. Therefore, these may be exhausted readily when in coarse powder. The relative proportion of menstruum to drug also has a bearing in determining the fineness of the powder, for it is clear that if a fluidextract is to be made in which 100 volumes shall represent 100 parts by weight of the drug, the powder should be a finer one than would be required for a tincture where 100 volumes are used to exhaust 10 parts by weight of the drug. In all cases, whether coarse or fine powder is directed, the powder should conform to the specifications of the USP for that degree of fineness and should be uniformly mixed. The object of this is to permit the uniform descent of the liquid, for fine particles offer more resistance to the passage of the menstruum than coarse ones; if the powder is not uniform, and the finer particles are deposited upon one side of the percolator, imperfect exhaustion may occur through the passage of the greater portion of the menstruum down the channel of least resistance; ie, through the coarser particles.

Botanical drug houses normally have available crude drugs ground for percolation (GFP) for specific percolation conditions.

For a complete discussion of this subject see the chapter on *Particle Phenomena*, page 349.

Moistening of the Powder—The general rule in percolation is to moisten the powder, and there are very few instances in the official processes where it is not directed. The object of moistening the powder is very apparent. If a perfectly dry sponge is held in the hand and a gentle stream of water poured on it, it will be noticed that very little water is absorbed by it; but if the sponge is thoroughly soaked, and all of the water squeezed out that possibly can be removed, the sponge will greedily absorb water. Vegetable drugs are substances which in their natural state contain moisture; however the process of desiccation has hardened and dried the tissues, so that they absorb moisture very slowly, and when compressed, as they are when packed in a percolator, the resistance is still greater. If a dry powder, like ground orange peel, is tightly packed in a glass percolator and water poured on it, it will be noticed that the water will penetrate the powder only a short distance. Its further passage is prevented by the particles which are immediately in contact with the water, which have become swollen to such a degree that they press tightly against the sides of the percolator, and thus entirely overcome the force of gravity and the penetrating power of the water. If, on the other hand, the powdered orange peel is moistened *with sufficient water to satisfy its tendency to swell, before it is packed* in the percolator, the addition of water is followed by its slow percolation through the mass without stoppage, and the utility of moistening the powder is thus proved.

The special cases in which the powder should not be moistened are those in which the addition of menstruum would produce adhesiveness and cause the powder to form lumps that could not be easily penetrated, those in which the moistened powder would offer too little resistance to the passage of the menstruum, and those in which the menstruum is too volatile or too flammable to render moistening desirable or safe. An instance of the first case is found in the so-called cold percolation of sugar in making syrups; instances of the second and third cases, in the preparation of the oleoresins where ether is used as the menstruum. In a small operation the moistening may be best accomplished by adding the menstruum to the ground drug contained in a relatively large, shallow dish, the drug being rubbed between the hands to secure uniformity. On a large scale a covered power mixer may be used. The drug also may be placed in a wooden trough or on a clean cement floor, the menstruum added, and the mixing done with a shovel. The latter plan may serve for aqueous menstruums, as in the percolation of cascara sagrada, but would not be economical if the menstruum is alcoholic.

Packing the Powder—The directions of earlier pharmacopeias with regard to this important part of the process of percolation varied continually. Where the degree of pressure was immaterial, no special directions were given. Where there was a likelihood of too much pressure being exerted, so that percolation would cease before it should, the directions were, "pack it moderately"; on the other hand, if there was danger of the operator allowing the menstruum to pass through too rapidly, so that the drug would not be exhausted of its active principles, the directions were, "pack firmly." Due to the introduction of Type Processes the USP has omitted this valuable aid to the beginner and it is necessary for each operator to determine for himself the degree of pressure to apply in packing the drug. Before beginning to pack the powder the throat of the funnel or of the percolator must be obstructed by a loose plug of absorbent cotton or a deeply notched cork (Fig. 597), or by some other method. Care should be taken not to moisten the cotton or cork with water unless the menstruum is aqueous, because if the drug to be percolated is resinous, the first portions of percolate which come through will be precipitated by the water in the cotton or on the cork. Instances have occurred where the percolation has been stopped from this cause. Where the notched cork is used, it is well to place over the top of the cork, when it is in place, a small circle of scored filtering paper (Fig. 598). This must be slightly larger in diameter than the cork, and the edges are therefore deflected up the sides.

The moistened powder should be deposited carefully in the percolator in layers, each succeeding layer being packed according to the requirements, "moderately" or "firmly," as the case may be, care being taken to use the same degree of pressure with each layer. Fig. 599 shows a convenient utensil for packing a percolator. It should be made of hard wood, preferably lignum vitæ; for the narrow percolators a longer packer must be used. The skill used in this part of the process will be proved by the manner in which the menstruum permeates the moistened powder. If the descent is regular and uniform, it will be shown in a glass percolator by the line marking the descent of the menstruum being perfectly horizontal. If the line is irregular, it is easy to point out just where the pressure was insufficient or too great. Fig. 600A shows loose and irregular packing, too much pressure being made on the right side, the menstruum descending on the left side more rapidly and escaping unsaturated. Fig. 600B illustrates a perco-

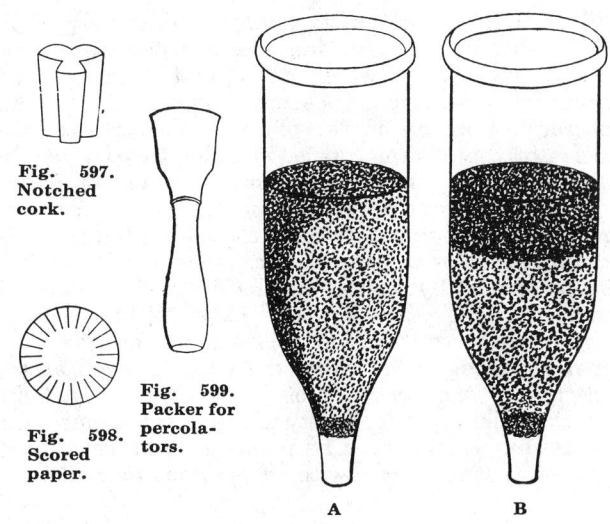

Fig. 597. Notched cork.

Fig. 598. Scored paper.

Fig. 599. Packer for percolators.

Fig. 600. Percolator (*A*) improperly and (*B*) properly packed.

lator which has been properly packed, the liquid descending uniformly.

Pretreatment of the Ground Drug—In certain cases, for the sake of longer stability or for other reasons, it is necessary first to remove the waxes and fixed oils from the ground drug. A preliminary extraction with petroleum benzin is commonly performed on ergot, digitalis, and certain other drugs.

Adding the Menstruum—When the last portion of moistened powder is introduced into the percolator, a sheet of filtering paper, scored at the edges and slightly larger in diameter than the surface of the powder (Fig. 598), should be laid on it, for the purpose of causing an even distribution of the menstruum. A weight of some kind is usually placed on the paper to keep it from floating out of place. Clean pebbles, a bottle stopper, or a small glass funnel may be used, but Fig. 601 shows a glass percolator weight, originally molded for this purpose by the Whitall Tatum Co. It is easily cleaned, not readily broken, and does not take up much room. Where the percolator is large enough to hold the whole of the menstruum, it may be at once added carefully. When this is not the case, and the menstruum must be added in divided portions, care must be observed to follow with the succeeding portion before the first has entirely disappeared, otherwise fissures may appear in the powder and the menstruum will, of course, seek the outlet offering the least obstruction and will leak through the fissures instead of percolating through the powder. This is more apt to occur in percolating very fine powders than in percolating coarse ones, although it is liable to take place in either. Where a large quantity of menstruum is required, a contrivance for continually suppling the menstruum should be used, in the form of an inverted bottle or flask, or any of the methods for continuous washing may be employed. The use of rubber tubing attached to the outlet, as illustrated in Fig. 603, and then bent with an upward curve so that the upper bend is above the level of the packed drug but the outlet below the percolator orifice, will prevent the drug from becoming dry should the operator fail to pour on additional menstruum.

Previous Maceration—This is recommended when the structure of the powder is tough, the soluble principles are not easily extracted by the menstruum, or a comparatively large quantity of powder is to be exhausted by a small quantity of menstruum. It is obvious that maceration is going on constantly while the menstruum is traversing the powder during its gradual descent, and when the amount of menstruum is more than sufficient to exhaust the drug, previous maceration is merely a waste of time. Nevertheless, the experts of the Pharmacopeia, in order to prevent the possibility of an unskilled or ignorant operator failing to exhaust a drug with the quantity of menstruum directed, have adopted in most cases the precaution of ordering previous maceration for a short time. This is best performed by moistening the drug, introducing it loosely into the percolator, and covering it closely to prevent loss by evaporation. This course has the additional advantage of allowing the drug to swell at the same time. A cover made of sheet rubber (Fig. 602), with a circular opening, is very useful in this connection. No attempt should ever be made to produce fluidextracts on the small scale without previous maceration.

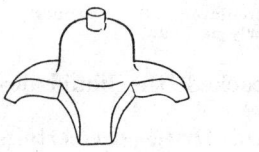

Fig. 601. Percolator weight.

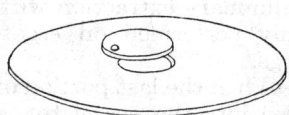

Fig. 602. Sheet rubber cover.

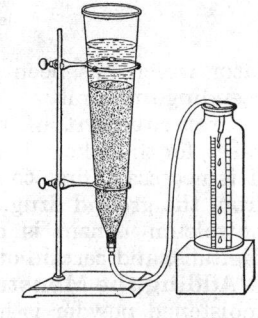

Fig. 603. Official percolation.

Finishing the Process—The official directions are frequently definite in fixing the quantity of percolate to be received from a given quantity of powder, but the oft-repeated direction to "percolate to exhaustion" at once raises the question of when a drug is exhausted of its activity. This question can be answered properly only by knowing beforehand the active principles of the drug. A few examples will sufficiently illustrate this. The activity of nux vomica, opium, and cinchona resides in the bitter alkaloids; hence, the *absence of bitterness* in the percolate in such cases indicates exhaustion. Cochineal and saffron are valued in pharmacy for nothing but the coloring matter contained in them; hence, the *absence of color* in the percolate shows the close of the process. Nutgall, kino, krameria, etc, contain tannin, and this is the only valuable principle; the *absence of astringency* in the percolate in these cases, therefore, shows the operator that percolation may be stopped. For even greater assurance that the drug is exhausted a qualitative test indicating residual *alkaloid* content, a color determination for colored materials, or a test for *tannins* may be conducted. The exhaustion of *resins* in drugs may be known by the absence of precipitation when the percolate is dropped into water. Where two or more active principles exist in a drug, the latter is not exhausted until the percolate is free from all of them. *The intelligent practice of the process of percolation, therefore, requires an accurate knowledge of the constituents and physical properties of medicinal substances.*

The Menstruum—The heterogeneous composition of plant and animal tissue necessitates the selection of a solvent system that will remove as completely as possible the desired constituents with a minimum of inert matter. Plant tissue contains many types of material, eg, carbohydrate, coloring matter, gum, inorganic salt, oil and fat, resinous matter, starch, tannin, and volatile oil, in addition to active constituents and other metabolic products. A maximum of active constituent(s) and a minimum of undesirable constituents in the finished extract are obviously desirable, and the selection of the proper solvent or combination of solvents aids in attaining these. Much research has therefore been done in securing the solvent systems used in the extracted preparations of the various official compendia.

Inert matter and active principles extracted from a given tissue vary in amount with the type of menstruum used. Therefore, a difference in intensity of physiological activity, or even a different response, is possible from extractions obtained with different solvents. Extraction of plant or animal tissue therefore requires considerable care in the selection of the menstruum.

Oils and fats may be removed, if necessary, by preliminary extraction with such solvents as hexane, petroleum benzin (petroleum ether), diethyl ether, and others.

The solvents, and the preparations resulting from their use, have varied widely. Wines were used in earlier years as extraction menstrua and were gradually replaced by the more efficient and less variable alcohol. Monographs for medicated wines appeared in USP VIII and NF IV, but the Brussels Conference of 1902 advised against their continued recognition because of the lack of uniformity in commercial wines. Wine of Ipecac is a typical example and if this preparation is requested, Tincture of Ipecac is now used.

Infused oils were solutions in oil of the soluble constituents of plant tissue, principally those containing alkaloids and volatile oils. NF V provided a monograph on Infused Oils and Compound Oil of Hyoscyamus is a typical example.

Fluidglycerates were intended to be of the same drug strength as fluidextracts but were prepared by extracting the plant drugs with glycerin and water as the menstruum. NF VI and NF VII provided a general process for drugs that did not require an acid or alkaline menstruum.

About 50% glycerin was used and no alcohol. Fluid glycerates of cascara, licorice, rhubarb, and hydrastis were once official.

Acetic Fluidextracts or *Fluidacetracts* were the titles proposed in earlier years for fluidextracts made by extracting plant drugs with acetic or diluted acetic acid of various strengths. Vinegar of Squill was official in the earlier compendia.

Vinegars were originally solutions of the active principles of plant drugs in vinegar, but they have been replaced almost completely by tinctures and fluidextracts. The variability in the quality and composition of vinegar as a solvent resulted in its replacement by diluted acetic acid. Typical illustrations are the Squill Vinegar NF X and Squill Vinegar BPC 1968, both of which are prepared by maceration with diluted acetic acid. Acetic acid has proved to be a most useful solvent and preservative in phytochemical and biochemical research, in addition to its frequent inclusion in solvent systems for extraction purposes (both plant and animal tissues).

Pure water, as such, finds use primarily in the preparation of the infusion and decoction (qv) and certain aqueous extracts (see *Extracts*). *Inspissated plant juices* were made by contusing fresh plant tissue, expressing the juice, heating to remove green coloring matter and to coagulate albumen, filtering, evaporating, restoring green color, and evaporating to a soft extract. They may be regarded as aqueous extracts.

The introduction of alcohol and mixtures of alcohol and water, with or without auxiliary solvents, resulted in the development of the more useful preparations, the *tincture* and the *fluidextract* (liquid extract). Water, alcohol, or mixtures of water and alcohol are the solvents commonly used for the preparation of extracts of plant drugs, although other solvents of proved value still may be used. Aromatic Ammonia Spirit was used in NF IX as the menstruum in the preparation of Ammoniated Guaiacum Tincture, and Ether Spirit is still used for the percolation of lobelia in the preparation of Ethereal Tincture of Lobelia BPC 1968.

Various substances such as glycerin, alkalies, and acids have been included in the solvent where the properties of these additives have been found necessary from experimental observation for the successful preparation of the extract in question. Acids such as acetic, hydrochloric, and tartaric are useful, and ammonium hydroxide solution is used frequently where alkali is required. The adjustment of pH of the solvent, or of the finished product, may be necessary in order to extract the particular principle desired or to give stability to the finished preparation.

Alcohol as the solvent of choice in the extraction of plant substance has many virtues. It has low toxicity internally, a selective action in dissolving the majority of active constituents while leaving behind inert material, and low latent heat of evaporation. It also improves the stability of solutions due to its solvent and preservative action, and minimizes hydrolysis.

The use of specially denatured alcohol is desirable and economical in the extraction process when the preparation is not intended for internal use and the solvent is completely removed by evaporation or distillation. The USP in its General Notices under Denatured Alcohol specifies that:

"In the manufacture of pharmacopeial preparations in which alcohol is used only as a solvent and does not remain in the finished product, alcohol especially denatured by the addition of volatile substances, in accordance with federal statutes and regulations of the Internal Revenue Service, may be substituted but the preparations so made must be identical with those prepared by the processes given in the monographs and must conform to the pharmacopeial standards set forth."

The BP and BPC provide similar regulations and permit the use of an Industrial Methylated Spirit (19 volumes of alcohol 95% and 1 volume of approved wood naphtha).

A solvent such as methanol is of particular value in the extraction of active constituents from plant tissue but is of no use in the preparation of an extracted liquid for internal or external use due to its toxicity.

The PhI in its General Notices under Nomenclature states that:

"In descriptions of ethanolic extracts, the nature of the solvent shall not be mentioned. When other solvents are used, the name of the solvent shall be mentioned. The consistency of the extract shall always be given."

Similar regulations, except for the requirement as to consistency, apply to tinctures.

Water is the solvent of choice from the standpoint of economy, and where experimentation has shown it to be satisfactory it is used. It does have disadvantages. Its solvent properties are less effective generally for organic constituents of most potent plant drugs. In addition, water extracts more undesirable constituents such as proteins, pectins, tannins, coloring matter, sugars, starches, and gums. Water requires more heat than alcohol during evaporation, as for example, in the preparation of pilular extracts. Long periods of heating promote hydrolysis and further decomposition. Plant tissues swell in the presence of water, and extraction may or may not be facilitated. Alcoholic menstruums on the other hand produce less tissue swelling than water and strong alcohol produces little, if any, swelling.

Water as a solvent also has the disadvantage that its solvent properties vary from time to time, and the miscellany of extractive matter which is always obtained produces a colloidal suspension rather than a true solution. These unstable products may continue to deposit extracted matter slowly on standing (pitching) due to hydrolytic, enzymatic, or other action, and the formation of insoluble compounds; or they may show precipitation on dilution with water or other solvent. Some of the undesirable features of water as a solvent are reflected in the earlier infusions and decoctions.

In the preparation of aqueous extracts, alcohol is frequently added to the finished product as a preservative. The BP uses the preservative action of chloroform by specifying chloroform water as the menstruum for the extraction of Liquorice Liquid Extract, and in the vehicle for Fluidglycerates (qv), though it was subsequently removed by evaporation.

Glycerin is a good solvent for many water-insoluble substances. Lack of toxicity and some preservative action, depending on concentration, enhance its useful properties. The inclusion of glycerin in aqueous or alcoholic menstruums for the extraction of plant tissue is widespread, principally because of its ability to dissolve undesirable matter and prevent its subsequent precipitation. Fluidextract of Wild Cherry NF X, which is prepared with a menstruum of glycerin and water (1:2), illustrates the usefulness of glycerin in preventing the precipitation of tannin and tannin oxidation products resulting from the extraction of tannin by the solvent combination. Other examples include Compound Tincture of Gentian NF XI and Fluidextract of Taraxacum NF XI, for which menstruums of alcohol, glycerin, and water are specified. The use of glycerin as a solvent in Fluidglycerates was referred to previously. It is also used in the preparation of allergenic extracts either in the extraction medium, or as the vehicle, or part of the vehicle, in the finished product. Its solvent properties, preservative action, lack of toxicity, and miscibility with tissue fluid are useful in such preparations.

The effect of surface-active agents in solvent systems has been studied. Butler and Wiese[2] investigated the use of a number of nonionic surface-active agents on the efficiency of the extraction of alkaloids from belladonna leaf, hyoscyamus, cinchona, and ipecac using official extraction procedures. The wetting agent was introduced into the preliminary moistening menstruum for each percolation in a concentration equivalent to 20 mg % of the final volume of the fluidextract. All percolations using the wetting agents consistently extracted more alkaloids than were extracted in control percolations.

Brochmann-Hanssen[3] extracted cinchona and ipecac using a simplified constant-temperature maceration technique with a mechanical shaker. A variety of anionic, cationic, and nonionic surface-active agents were used at concentrations varying between zero and 3%. Alkaloid content was determined as well as pH and surface tension. It was found that the addition of synthetic surface-active agents increased the rate of extraction of alkaloidal drugs. Alcoholic solutions of nonionic surfactants showed little or no increase in yield over that obtained with the solvent alone. Anionic agents precipitated alkaloids and therefore were not suitable, while cationic agents as the salts of mineral acids increased the yields of alkaloids significantly.

Srivastava and Chadha[4] employed both percolation and mechanical agitation processes to extract belladonna herb with a menstruum of 70% alcohol and water, to which was added 0.2% Tween 20 (*Atlas*) or 0.2% Tween 80 (*Atlas*). Both surfactants potentiated the solvent effect of the ethanol–water menstruum. Extraction was more complete and more rapid. Tween 20 appeared to be superior to Tween 80 when percolation was used while Tween 80 gave better results with mechanical agitation.

Absorbed Menstruum—The amount of menstruum which a powder will absorb and retain after percolation ceases can never be accurately predetermined. If it is important to know beforehand the percentage of menstruum capable of being absorbed, a practical trial should be made on the small scale, using the same powder and menstruum.

Substances possess very different capacities for retaining menstruums. Those having a light, spongy structure hold more than hard, ligneous drugs, and even the same drug will often vary in its capacity in this respect, while the amount of moisture present in the drug before it is percolated is never a constant quantity, varying sometimes as much as 8–20%. The advantages of percolation over maceration are very apparent in respect to the character of the liquid left in the exhausted residue or marc. In maceration the liquid left in the residue is finished tincture. In percolation it is merely menstruum, the active portions of the drug having been dissolved in the preceding percolate. In large operations, from an economical point of view, it is desirable to recover absorbed menstruums when the residues contain sufficient alcohol to make it worth the necessary time and labor.

Controlling the Flow of the Percolate—The necessity for some method of controlling the flow of the percolate is apparent. In simple percolation this is effected by the degree of pressure used in packing the moistened drug. Judgment and experience are absolutely necessary to guide the operator. Various mechanical expedients have been used to accomplish the same purpose. For the control of the flow of percolate by the official method (Fig. 603), the neck of the funnel-end should be rather short and should gradually and regularly become wider toward the orifice so that a perforated cork, bearing a short glass tube, may be tightly wedged into it.

The glass tube, which must not project above the inner surface of the cork, should extend 3–4 cm beyond the outer surface of the cork and should be provided with a closely fitting rubber tube, at least ¼ longer than the percolator itself and ending in another short glass tube whereby (when it is desired to interrupt the percolation) the rubber tube may be so suspended that its orifice shall be above the surface of the menstruum in the percolator, a rubber band or wire loop holding the tube in position.

In metallic percolators, stopcocks or spigots have been employed. It is possible to improvise a control of the flow by employing a narrow homeopathic vial, having a ⅛-in. hole in the side, ½ in. from the bottom, and passing it through a perforated cork fitting tightly in the neck of the percolator. By pulling the vial down, the hole is stopped by the encircling cork; by

pushing it up, the hole is exposed so that the percolate runs through the vial and thus the flow may be regulated. Fig. 604 illustrates a very useful method of controlling the flow of a percolate. This "sprinkler controller" was specially made, but if not available, the well-known sprinkler, made of white metal, used for liquid dentifrice bottles may be employed. The flow of liquid can be controlled perfectly by its use.

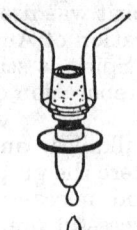

Fig. 604. Stopper for percolation control.

Rate of Flow—The success of the process of percolation largely depends on the regulation of the flow of the percolate. If this is too rapid, incomplete exhaustion will result; if this is too slow, valuable time is wasted and considerable loss of menstruum occurs from evaporation. For fluidextracts, tinctures, and other preparations made by percolation, using 1000 Gm of powder, the rate of flow should not exceed 5 ml/min. For official preparations definite rates of flow are prescribed. The terms used with their official meanings are:

slowly—1 ml/min
at a modern rate—1–3 ml/min
rapidly—3–5 ml/min

The proper rate of flow should vary with the quantity and character of the drug employed and the density of the menstruum.

Methods of Supporting Percolators—The ordinary retort stands are often used to support small percolators. The one shown in Fig. 603 is suitable, particularly if the ring is covered with rubber. Pieces of rubber tubing may be split down one side and then slipped

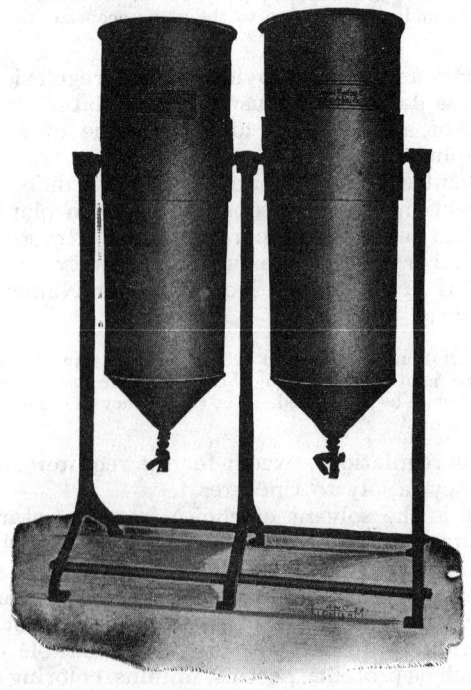

Fig. 605. Percolators suspended from a rack.

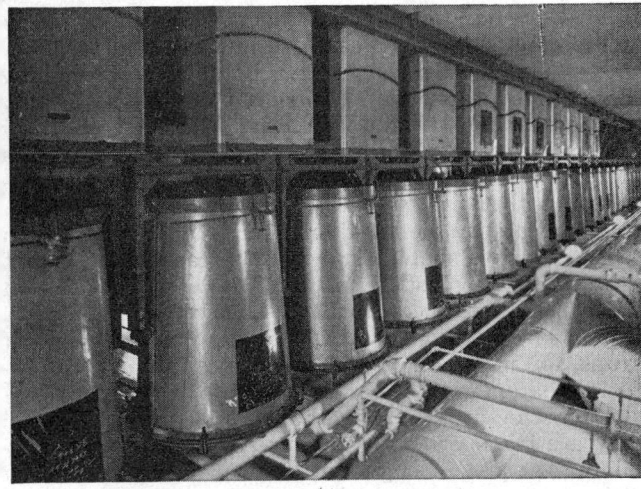

Fig. 606. Percolation of fluidextracts (courtesy, Lilly).

over the metal ring. Large percolators stand on tables or are suspended as illustrated in Figs. 605 and 606.

Sugar Percolation—The principle of percolation is also extensively applied to the solution of sucrose (sugar) in the preparation of syrups. For this purpose the ordinary percolator may be used but special percolators have also been devised. See *Syrups* (page 1485).

Receiving Bottles—A series of bottles of various sizes should be reserved for use in receiving percolates. Bottles with comparatively wide necks are to be preferred for receiving bottles. A strip of adhesive plaster may be pasted on the side and accurately measured quantities of water poured in, carefully marking the height of each addition (Fig. 609).

Fractional Percolation—This term, employed by Prof. C. Lewis Diehl and others, defines percolation when applied to two successive portions of powder, the principle of action being identical with that of repercolation.

Repercolation—This, as its name indicates, is the process of percolating substances with percolates, or, as defined by Dr. E. R. Squibb, the author of the process, "the successive application of the same percolating menstruum to fresh portions of the substance to be percolated." The principal object of repercolation is to effect the saving of alcohol and alcoholic menstruums by accomplishing the saturation of the menstruums, as nearly as possible, by passing the unsaturated or weaker per-

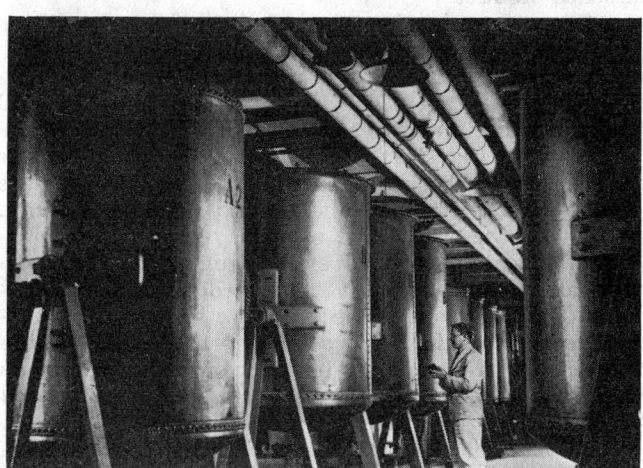

Fig. 607. Giant percolators, each holding 1½ tons of drug (courtesy, MSD).

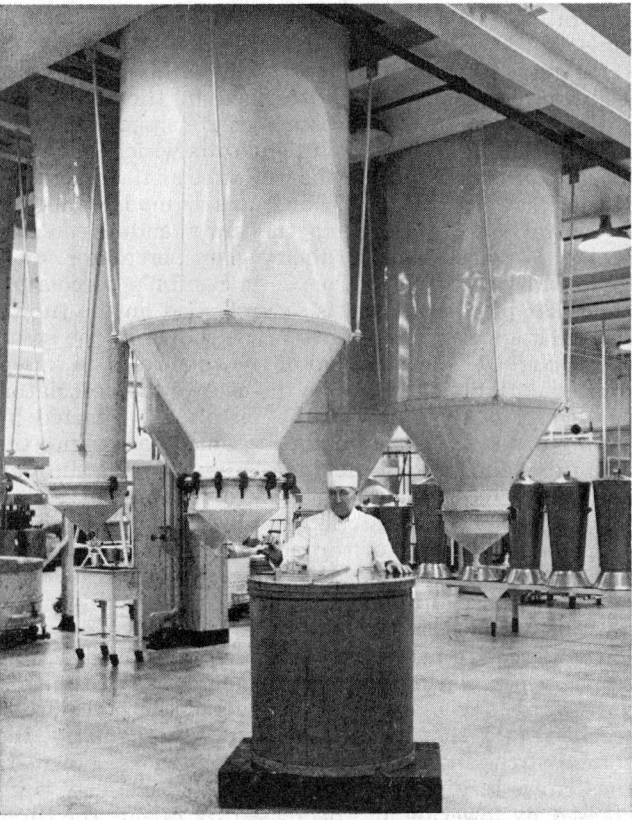

Fig. 608. Battery of gravity percolators. The large ones in the foreground are charged through openings in the mezzanine floor above the percolators. The small stainless percolators in the background, used for small quantities, are charged in the usual manner (courtesy, Upjohn).

colate from one portion of the drug through another portion, and again passing the unsaturated or weaker percolate from this second portion through a third portion. The fact that no heat is required to concentrate the percolate in the manufacture of fluidextracts is one of the special advantages of repercolation. The weak percolate from this last portion is generally set aside, to be used in succeeding operations on the same drug in the place of fresh menstruum. This process is useful only in those operations where the relative proportion of menstruum used is small, as in the fluidextracts and similar concentrated preparations. Practical illustrations may be seen by referring to Process C, under *Fluidextracts* (page 1591).

Well-Tube Percolator—An excellent method of percolation (Fig. 610), which was used by Squibb was based on the principle of drawing water from a well automatically as fast as it accumulates. This is effected by the use of a well tube placed in the center of an ordinary jar or pot and held in its place by the powdered drug which is packed around it. The menstruum is poured on the drug, and, after percolating through, collects in the well tube, from which it is drawn off by an ingeniously constructed siphon. The illustration clearly shows the method of using this

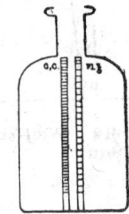

Fig. 609. Receiving bottle for percolates.

apparatus. It may be used for large or small operations.

Double-Tube Percolator—This differs from the well-tube percolator just described in the use of an ordinary percolator, the absence of the siphon, and the substitution of a simple, straight tube which is free to move up and down inside the well tube at the discretion of the operator. Fig. 611 illustrates its mode of action. A central well tube having the lower end irregularly broken is placed in an ordinary glass percolator, on a tuft of absorbent cotton, or, as in Squibb's percolator, a circular piece of muslin is securely tied on the tube a short distance from the bottom, as shown in the small cut in Fig. 611, and the end of the tube rests on a perforated cork fitting tightly in the neck of the percolator. The control of the flow of the percolate is effected by raising or lowering the small tube which passes into the well tube, and which is held in place by passing through the perforated cork in the neck of the percolator already mentioned, or through a perforated rubber nipple slipped over the end, or through a piece of rubber tubing. If previous maceration is directed, the narrow tube may be pushed up until the upper orifice is above the level of the menstruum, and of course above the level of the percolate in the well tube. When it is desirable to begin percolating, the tube is gently rotated with a downward movement until the level of the percolate is reached, and then percolation proceeds regularly, the course of the menstruum being indicated as shown by the arrows in Fig. 611. The rapidity of the flow is increased by lowering and decreased by raising the tube.

Large-Scale Percolation

Ordinary glass percolators cannot be used for large-scale manufacture and stainless steel or glass-lined equipment replaces the usual experimental glassware. Almost all of today's extracts, in their various forms, are made by firms specializing in extracts of vegetable drugs. The modern pharmacist has neither the time, the equipment, nor the special facilities for the manufacture and control of medicinal extracts comparable with those which can be made by the larger pharmaceutical firms. For large-scale operations, tax-free denatured alcohol is also available for many extractions and this materially reduces the cost.

In some cases the crude drugs are grown on farms owned or directly controlled by a firm having special

knowledge and interest in producing the highest quality of the drug. In other cases technically trained men, among them pharmacists and botanists, accompany the gatherers into the fields and woods to obtain only the best quality of crude material. This is especially true in the case of such widely used drugs as cascara sagrada bark, hyoscyamus leaves, ipecac root, podophyllum, digitalis, and belladonna.

Botanical suppliers bringing in crude drugs from other countries should, and in most cases do, conduct close pharmacognostic and chemical determinations on the drugs to insure conformity with accepted standards. Importers and drug collectors are in a position to select drugs, for instance, of high alkaloid content or of superior characteristics in other respects.

After the drugs are gathered and properly dried they are transported to warehouses to await the decision of the pharmacognosist or pharmacist as to their ultimate use. If required for an extract, either solid, pilular, powdered, fluid, or tincture, or for the preparation of an active ingredient such as an alkaloid or glycoside, the crude drugs are transferred to mills or cutters (see *Powders*, page 1626) where they are reduced to the necessary state of fineness for the proper extraction of the active medicinal ingredients.

The general rule or practice is to mix and pack drugs as soon as they are milled. In some cases, particularly in items having volatile oils as one of their active constituents, eg, ginger, pepper, buchu, or capsicum, the finely ground or powdered drug is milled directly into the percolator containing the specified menstruum.

Percolators, in large-scale manufacture, vary considerably in size. Leaves and herbs usually can be packed into very large percolators, as high as 12 to 16 ft and up to 6 or 8 ft in diameter. Roots, barks, and seeds, due to their greater density and in many cases difficulty in extraction, must be packed into smaller percolators.

Power mixers are used to moisten many drugs with the appropriate menstruum.

Following moistening, the drug is conveyed to the percolator and covered with the appropriate solvent or menstruum. Specially denatured alcohols of a formula authorized by the Federal Statutes and Regulations of the Internal Revenue Service may be used in many cases where alcohol or hydroalcoholic menstruum is prescribed as the official solvent. Permission is given by both the USP and NF to replace alcohol in official menstruums by suitable denatured alcohols in those cases in which all of the alcohol is removed from the finished product.

After macerating for the prescribed time percolation is allowed to proceed and, when the drug is exhausted, the percolate is transferred to tinned copper, stainless steel, or glass-lined stills with capacities up to 1000 gal and operating under a vacuum of from 27.5 to 29 in. of mercury (Fig. 612). The transfer of the percolate to the still is accomplished under controlled pressure which permits the still operator to regulate the rate of flow to the still. The solvent, removed by distillation, is again used to cover the drug until tests prove that all medicinally active or the desired ingredients have been removed. The percolate in the still is further reduced, under high vacuum, until all traces of the solvent are removed. The concentrated extract is then ready to be made into either a solid or powdered extract or a fluidextract in the usual manner.

The marc, or exhausted drug, with its retained menstruum, is transferred, by means of conveyors, to a continuous rotary dryer for the recovery of alcohol, or dry steam, under 60 to 70 lb pressure (corresponding

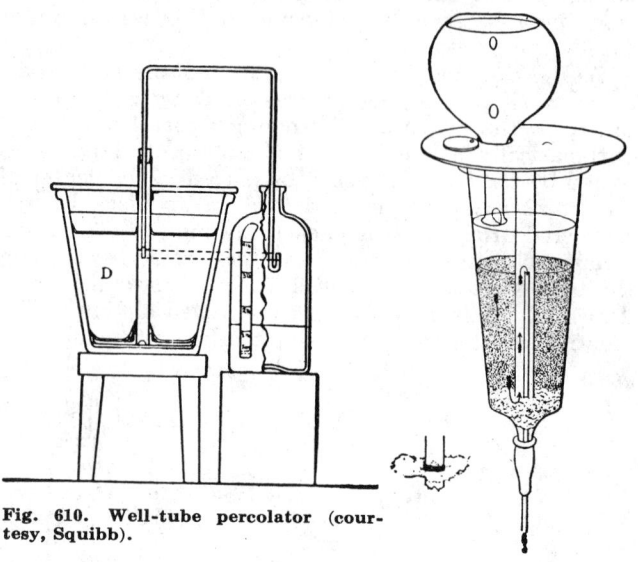

Fig. 610. Well-tube percolator (courtesy, Squibb).

Fig. 611. Double-tube percolator.

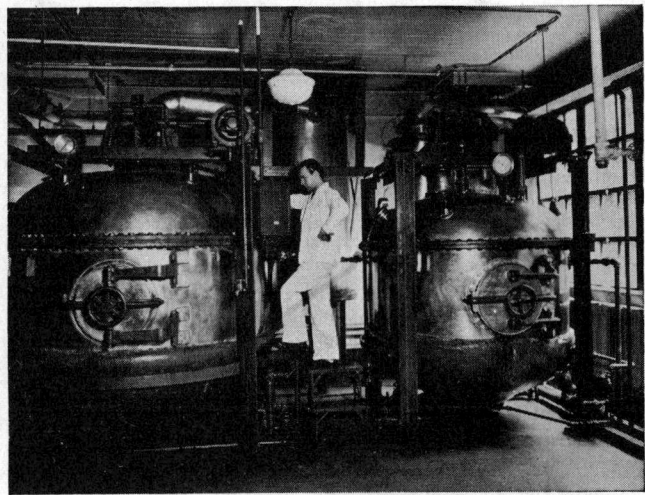

Fig. 612.   Large copper stills (courtesy, Lilly).

to about 155°), is introduced into the bottom of the percolator, which is in turn connected with a condenser, and the alcohol thus recovered.   From either process, the almost dry marc is conveyed to an incinerator where it is utilized as a source of heat for low-temperature and low-pressure operations.

New or combination types of extraction by percolation are being experimented with by American and foreign manufacturers.   One, a continuous rotary extractor, is similar in action to the combination extraction and solvent recovery apparatus described later under *Percolation with Hot Extraction.*   Another process (countercurrent) is also similar, except that the drug is not agitated while in contact with the menstruum.   Both operations are based on the principle of repercolation as defined by Squibb.   The freshly powdered drug first comes into contact with nearly saturated percolate, and the menstruum first comes into contact with the nearly exhausted drug.   The advantage of this type of extraction lies in the fact that the proportion of menstruum to that of drug can be accurately controlled so that almost 100% extraction can be achieved in a minimum of time.

Lloyd Extractor—The Lloyd extractor, which may be compared, in efficiency and character, to a Soxhlet extraction apparatus, cannot be employed where mixed solvents are used.   The varying boiling points of hydroalcoholic mixtures make it impractical in such cases.

Pressure Percolator—Percolation by pressure has sometimes been employed.   All forms of apparatus are based on the same principle—that of forcing the menstruum through the powder at a greater rate of speed than it would pass if it depended alone on gravity. This is only applicable under special conditions but is being employed in special extraction operations with the advantage of economy of time.   The complete extraction of the drug must be carefully checked. Fig. 613 illustrates a large-scale plant currently in operation.   Five batteries, each consisting of three percolators in series, are located in the section shown.   These percolators, designed and developed by the Upjohn Co., are charged from the mezzanine floor above them. The menstruum enters at the top of the first percolator under pressure and after passing through the column of drug emerges from the bottom.   It is piped to the top of the second percolator.   This process is repeated in the third of the series and the percolate is collected in the receiver (center foreground).   Any prescribed rate of flow of the percolate can be obtained by regulating

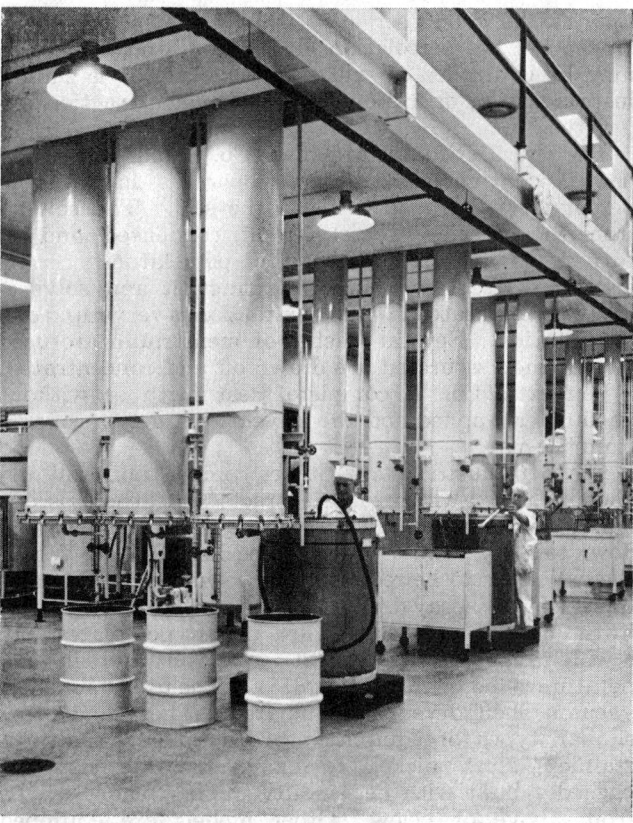

Fig. 613.   Pressure percolators (courtesy, Upjohn).

the rate of flow of the extract at the bottom of the third column.   Drums located beneath each percolator permit bleeding, which assures complete permeation of the drug and prevents channeling.

Percolation with Hot Extraction—In some cases it is desirable to exhaust drugs with hot menstruums. Lewin's extraction apparatus is shown in Fig. 614. The lower vessel is a still; immediately above it is the percolator having three movable sieves for the reception of the substance to be extracted; above the perco-

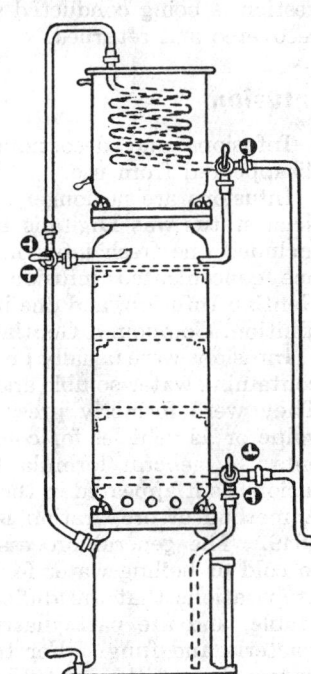

Fig. 614.   Hot extraction apparatus.

lator is the condenser. By the use of the three-way stopcocks, the percolation, distillation, and extraction may be controlled at will. This percolator is similar in principle of operation to the Soxhlet extraction apparatus.

The F. J. Stokes Machine Co. builds a steam-heated continuous-extraction apparatus in which a percolator is suspended inside the still. The solvent from the percolate is distilled off, condensed, and returned as menstruum to the percolator. Stokes also markets a combination extraction and solvent-recovery apparatus in which extraction is very rapid due to agitation. Several washes of menstruum are used which when saturated are drawn off and concentrated. When extraction is complete, heat, with or without vacuum, is applied and the solvent is largely recovered from the marc.

Fig. 616 illustrates the Stokes combination still and vacuum dryer which takes extracts and other viscous liquids from the liquid state, through the plastic stage, down to a dry powder which can be discharged. Where the extract is to be reduced to a powder, one means of doing so is by spray drying. This is especially workable in the case of aqueous and low-alcohol percolates with a wide range of solids content. Exposure to high temperature is momentary (Fig. 615). The use of auxiliary vacuum shelf dryers is eliminated. These and other similar types of equipment are supplied in copper, stainless steel, nickel, or monel metal. They are ruggedly built with heavy-duty mixing blades driven from above or below. Other models are equipped with vacuum filters for solutions that crystallize, cooling belts, centrifugal entrainment separators, etc.

Digestion

Digestion is that form of maceration which consists of the application of *gentle heat* to the substance which is being treated. It is used in those cases where a moderately elevated temperature is unobjectionable, the heat increasing the solvent powers of the menstruum. If the solvent or menstruum is readily volatilized at the temperature employed, it is necessary to attach a reflux condenser to the vessel in which the digestion is being conducted so that the solvent may be recovered and returned.

Infusion

Infusions and decoctions have almost completely disappeared from use.

Infusions are no longer official; the last to lose official status was Digitalis Infusion NF IX. BP 1953 included one fresh infusion and BP 1968 retains only one concentrated infusion, Concentrated Compound Gentian Infusion, and one infusion prepared from it by dilution, Compound Gentian Infusion.

Infusions were usually prepared from vegetable drugs containing water-soluble and easily extracted principles. They were formerly prescribed either for their own value or as vehicles for combinations of other ingredients. A general formula for the preparation of infusions as it appeared in the NF IX is presented below. A method of preparation is also outlined in the BPC 1949. The general process of exposing a plant drug to cold or boiling water for a period of time results in preparations that are difficult to standardize, are unstable, and are particularly susceptible to attack by bacteria and fungi. For these reasons it is necessary to use them within 12 hours of preparation.

General Formula for Infusions

The Drug, coarsely comminuted............	50 Gm
Water, a sufficient quantity,	
To make.............................	1000 ml

Moisten the drug in a suitable vessel, preferably of earthenware and provided with a cover, with 50 ml of cold water and allow it to stand for 15 min. Then add 900 ml of boiling water, cover the vessel tightly, and allow it to macerate during 30 min. Then strain the mixture, and pass enough water through the strainer to make the Infusion measure 1000 ml. If the activity of the Infusion is affected by the temperature of boiling water, cold water should be used.

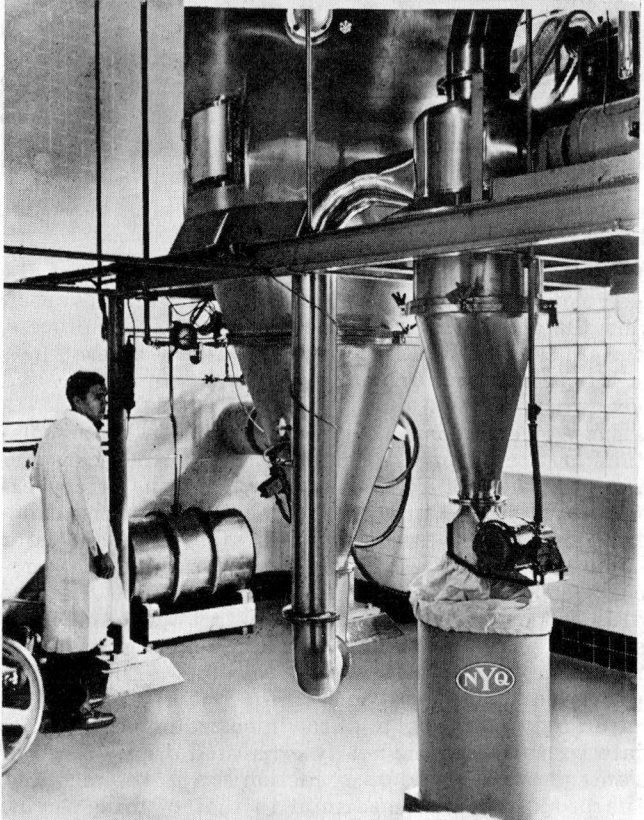

Fig. 615. Spray dryer (courtesy, Penick).

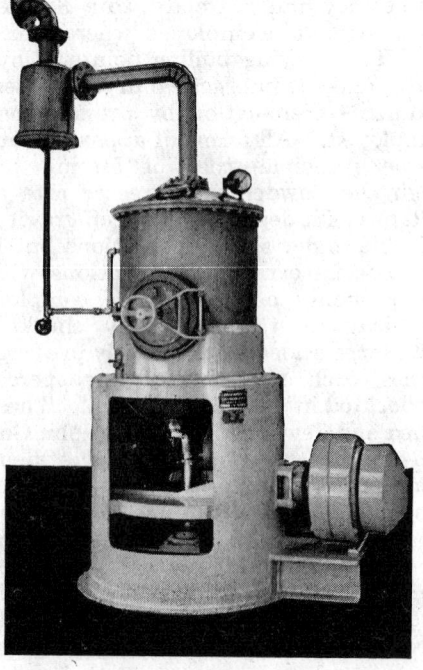

Fig. 616. Stainless steel combination still and vacuum dryer, steam jacketed.

Most fresh infusions are prepared with boiling water, but where the constituents of the drug are readily extracted, cold water may be used, as for example with quassia and calumba. The drug is not subjected to the boiling process.

In order to overcome some of the disadvantages of fresh infusions, concentrated infusions were introduced by the BP. These are actually liquid extracts, and the BPC 1968 defines them as "liquid extracts, prepared by modified percolation or maceration processes, which, after dilution with water, resemble in potency and aroma the corresponding fresh infusions." The dilution ratio is generally 1 volume of concentrate and 7 volumes of purified water. The BP still specifies that the infusion prepared from the dilution be dispensed within 12 hours since the alcoholic content of diluted concentrates has little preservative action.

Decoction

The general process for decoctions as described in the USP XII is given below. The process was used primarily for vegetable drugs containing water-soluble and heat-stable constituents since the method involves boiling the drug with water for a given period of time.

General Formula for Decoctions

The Drug, coarsely comminuted..............	50 Gm
Water, a sufficient quantity,	
To make...............................	1000 ml

Place the drug in a suitable vessel provided with a cover, pour upon it 1000 ml of cold distilled water, cover it well, and boil the mixture for 15 min. Then allow it to cool to about 40°C, express, strain the expressed liquid, and pass enough cold distilled water through the strainer to make the product measure 1000 ml.

Extractives

The treatment accorded the solution of the active constituents from a maceration or percolation process determines the nature of the finished product, that is whether it is to be a tincture, fluidextract, or extract. In general, these preparations may be simply classified on the basis of the strength or consistency of the final product.

If the solution of the active principles is a comparatively dilute one, that is, the active principles are low in concentration, the liquid is referred to as a tincture. A tincture is usually of such strength that ten parts by volume of the finished preparation is equivalent to one part by weight of the crude drug. A more concentrated liquid preparation is referred to as a fluidextract (liquid extract) and is usually of such a strength that one part by volume of the preparation is equivalent to one part by weight of the crude drug. Further concentration of a solution of the active principles by evaporation or distillation, generally at a low temperature or under reduced pressure, to a soft consistency or to dryness, results in the products classified by the USP as (1) semiliquids or liquids of syrupy consistency; (2) plastic masses, known as pilular or solid extracts (soft extracts); and (3) dry powders known as powdered extracts (Dry Extracts BP).

Tinctures

The USP defines tinctures as follows:

Tinctures are alcoholic or hydroalcoholic solutions prepared from vegetable materials or from chemical substances.

The definition of the NF differs only in the inclusion of the word "animal," and thus reads "from animal or vegetable drugs or from chemical substances."

The increasing use of pure, active principles isolated from crude drugs, or prepared by synthesis has resulted in decreasing use of plant extracts. Nevertheless, tinctures that are stable over long periods of time are of value where therapy requires use of a preparation of comparatively low potency and large dose.

A number of tinctures, fluidextracts, and extracts are required for use in the preparation of other pharmaceutical products. They are referred to as pharmaceutical, or pharmaceutic, necessities. Examples are Pure Glycyrrhiza Extract in the preparation of Aromatic Cascara Fluidextract (Glycyrrhiza Syrup USP),

Sweet Orange Peel Tincture (Orange Syrup USP), Beef Extract (Beef, Iron and Wine NF XI), Sarsaparilla Fluidextract (Compound Sarsaparilla Syrup NF XI), and Vanilla Tincture (Acacia Syrup NF).

The USP specifies as follows:

The proportion of drug represented in the different tinctures is not uniform but varies according to the established standards for each. Tinctures of potent drugs essentially represent the activity of 10 Gm of the drug in each 100 ml of tincture, the potency being adjusted following assay. Most other tinctures represent 20 Gm of the respective drug in each 100 ml of tincture. Compound tinctures are made according to long-established formulas, and the two official tinctures of fresh drugs, *Lemon Tincture* and *Sweet Orange Peel Tincture*, are made to represent 50 Gm of the respective drugs in each 100 ml of tincture.

The NF specifications for tinctures are similar to those outlined by the USP (except for Lemon Tincture and Sweet Orange Peel Tincture, as noted above). The NF points out that the activity requirements conform in principle to the recommendation of the International Protocol as adopted at Brussels, and with international standards. The International Protocol provided for 10% drug strength in tinctures of potent or therapeutically active drugs and 20% strength for other tinctures. The PhI states in its General Notices on Galenicals that "Tinctures of potent drugs, for which no proportion of active principles has been fixed, shall be of a strength of 10% by weight." There is practical conformity to this agreement in the USP and NF, but a few exceptions to the general rule exist where past experience has shown this to be desirable, for example, Strong Iodine Tincture (7 Gm per 100 ml), Iodine Tincture (2 Gm per 100 ml), and in the Lemon and Sweet Orange Peel Tinctures (50 Gm per 100 ml). In view of a recommendation made by the International Protocol that the name Tincture not be used for simple solutions of chemical substances, the BP adopted the name "Solution (Liquor)" for use in naming simple solutions of chemical substances; that is, Weak Iodine Solution has the official synonym Iodine Tincture. (Strong Iodine Solution, however, does not have Strong Iodine Tincture as an official synonym.) The PhI in its General Notices under Nomenclature specifies that the name of a tincture shall not be given to simple solutions of chemical substances.

Provision is made by the BP for modifications in the preparation of Lemon Tincture and Orange Tincture in tropical and subtropical parts where fresh peels cannot be obtained.

The USP directs that tinctures be prepared as follows:

The general processes to be employed for the manufacture of tinctures, unless otherwise directed in the individual monographs, are as follows:

Process P—Carefully mix the ground drug or mixture of drugs with a sufficient quantity of the prescribed solvent or solvent mixture to render it evenly and distinctly damp, allow it to stand for 15 min, transfer it to a suitable percolator, and pack the drug firmly. Pour on enough of the prescribed solvent or solvent mixture to saturate the drug, cover the top of the percolator and, when the liquid is about to drip from the percolator, close the lower orifice, and allow the drug to macerate for 24 hr or for the time specified in the monograph. If no assay is directed, allow the percolation to proceed slowly, or at the specified rate, gradually adding sufficient solvent or solvent mixture to produce 1000 ml of tincture, and mix (see page 1590 for definitions of flow rates, under *Fluidextracts*). If an assay is directed, collect only 950 ml of percolate, mix this, and assay a portion of it as directed. Dilute the remainder with such quantity of the prescribed solvent or solvent mixture as calculation from the assay indicates is necessary to produce a tincture that conforms to the prescribed standard, and mix.

Process M—Macerate the drug with 750 ml of the prescribed solvent or solvent mixture in a container that can be closed, and put in a warm place. Agitate it frequently during 3 days or until the soluble matter is dissolved. Transfer the mixture to a filter, and when most of the liquid has drained away, wash the residue on the filter with a sufficient quantity of the prescribed solvent or solvent mixture, combining the filtrates, to produce 1000 ml of tincture, and mix.

The processes of percolation and maceration as described by the USP and NF are, with the one or two exceptions in phraseology, identical.

Under Tinctures the BP includes General Processes for Maceration and Percolation. The processes are similar to those provided in the USP and NF. The maceration process employs the whole of the menstruum and a maceration period of 7 days. The percolation process uses a premoistening time of 4 hours before packing in the percolator and a collection of ¾ of the volume required for the finished tincture.

The PhI provides a general section on Tinctures and indicates that they may be prepared by maceration or by percolation.

The directions for the percolation process are similar to those provided in the BP and include the 4-hour preliminary moistening time (USP moistening time is 15 minutes), followed by the packing of the percolator and the 24-hour maceration period. Percolation is allowed to proceed until ⅘ of the required amount has been collected in the case of finished tinctures where no assay is provided and dilution made with menstruum to the required volume. In the case of tinctures for which an assay has been provided, percolation is continued until ¾ of the required amount has been collected and dilution is made to the required volume following assay.

The maceration process of the PhI for Tinctures is in general similar to the maceration process of the USP and the BP. It uses a maceration period of 5 days with ¾ of the prescribed menstruum, and the pressed marc is washed with sufficient menstruum to produce the required amount of tincture. The mixed liquids are clarified by subsidence or by filtration.

It is interesting to observe that the PhI provides monographs for 11 tinctures, 7 of which are prepared with the percolation process and a standard menstruum of Dilute Ethanol (70% *v/v* ethanol).

Preparation of Tinctures by Solution or Dilution—The following USP and NF tinctures are made by solution or dilution of active medicament: Iodine USP, Strong Iodine NF XI, Nitromersol NF, Thimero-sal NF, Ferric Chloride Tincture NF XI and Ferric Citrochloride Tincture NF XI.

The BP prepares five tinctures by dilution of the more concentrated Liquid Extract (Colchicum, Hyoscyamus, Ipecacuanha, Nux Vomica, and Stramonium) and two by dilution of a stronger Tincture (Weak Ginger and Camphorated Opium).

NF VI and NF VII permitted the preparation of a tincture by solution or dilution provided the tincture so prepared met all the official requirements. The dilution of a fluidextract to produce a tincture is, however, not generally permissible since the manufacturing procedures are often sufficiently different from those specified for the corresponding tinctures that dilution of the fluidextracts yields tinctures which vary from the official products in quantities of extracted matter and in alcoholic content. The PhI provides under its General Notices on Galenicals that "tinctures shall be prepared by maceration or percolation or, in certain cases, by dissolving an official extract of definite strength."

Fluidextracts

The BP, BPC, and PhI designate fluidextracts as Liquid Extracts. Fluidextracts are not frequently prescribed today, and if such medication is required, the tincture is more useful by virtue of its larger dose. Use of fluidextracts is confined primarily to the manufacture of other pharmaceuticals where plant extracts may have some therapeutic application, eg, the preparation and manufacture of expectorant mixtures, syrups, elixirs, tonics, vehicles, and flavoring agents. They are more concentrated preparations than tinctures and may be used for making diluted preparations. Reference to the dilution method for tinctures has already been made.

Fluidextracts are defined by the USP and NF as "liquid preparations of vegetable drugs, containing alcohol as a solvent or as a preservative, or both, and so made that each ml contains the therapeutic constituents of 1 Gm of the standard drug that it represents." The general introduction to the subject of fluidextracts is similar in the USP and NF. The USP specifies that fluidextracts be made by percolation using the menstruum specified in the particular monograph. Manufacture by the usual process calls for concentration of the more diluted portion of percolate by evaporation or distillation.

The PhI does not include monographs for fluidextracts but states under its General Notices on Galenicals the following:

Liquid Extracts of potent drugs, for which the proportion of active principles has not been fixed shall be prepared in such a way that one part by weight of the liquid extract represents one part by weight of the drug, and that Tinctures and liquid extracts of potent drugs, for which the proportion of active principles has been fixed shall, if necessary, be brought to the required strength by the addition of ethanol of the appropriate strength.

The time of maceration and the rate of flow during percolation may be varied to compensate for peculiarities in extraction and in some cases accomplish partial rejection of nonactive constituents. In all cases, the maceration and rate of flow are designed to extract insofar as is practicable the medicinally active or important constituents from the specified quantities of drugs, but the time and rate specified may be varied to accomplish this purpose when larger or smaller quantities of drug are being treated.

A cylindrical percolator is usually the best type for making fluidextracts, but for use with drugs that swell considerably in the menstruum a conical percolator may be preferred.

The rate of flow of the percolate is directed in such terms as: "percolate slowly," "percolate rapidly," and "percolate at a moderate rate." With reference to the extraction of 1000 Gm of drug, percolate slowly means a rate not exceeding 1 ml of percolate per minute; percolate rapidly means a rate of 3 to 5 ml per minute; percolate at a moderate rate means a rate of 1 to 3 ml per minute.

The NF XI provides five processes for the preparation of fluidextracts: (A) percolation with an alcoholic menstruum, (B) percolation with two menstruums, (C) fractional or divided percolation, (D) percolation with a menstruum of boiling water, and (E) pressure percolation. The processes are described as follows:

Process A. This process is used for preparing fluidextracts, which are made with menstruums of alcohol or of mixtures of alcohol and water, by ordinary percolation.

Carefully mix 1000 Gm of the ground drug with a sufficient quantity of the prescribed menstruum to render it evenly and distinctly damp. This usually requires from 600 ml to 800 ml of menstruum. Allow the dampened drug to stand for about 15 min, then pack it firmly in a suitable percolator, and pour on sufficient menstruum to saturate the drug and leave a stratum above. When the liquid is about to drop from the percolator, close the lower orifice, cover the percolator, and allow the drug to macerate for about the prescribed period of time. Then proceed with the percolation at the specified rate, adding fresh menstruum as needed until the drug is practically exhausted of its active principles. Reserve the first 850 ml of percolate (unless otherwise directed in the formula), recover the alcohol from the percolate subsequently collected, and concentrate the residue to a soft extract at a temperature not exceeding 60°. Dissolve this extract in the reserved percolate, and if no assay is directed, add enough of a mixture of alcohol and water to make the fluidextract measure 1000 ml and contain the required proportion of C_2H_5OH. Mix thoroughly. If the fluidextract being prepared is to be adjusted to a standard, assay a portion of the reserved percolate in which the soft extract has been dissolved, and dilute the remainder of the volume determined as necessary by calculation from the assay, using a sufficient quantity of an alcohol and water mixture to provide the required proportion of C_2H_5OH. Mix thoroughly.

Process B. This process is used in preparing fluidextracts, portions of the menstruums for which contain, in addition to alcohol, or a mixture of alcohol and water, definite quantities of other components such as an acid or glycerin, the two menstruums being successively employed.

Carefully mix 1000 Gm of the ground drug with a sufficient quantity of Menstruum I (containing the special ingredient) to render it evenly and distinctly damp. From 600 ml to 800 ml of menstruum is usually required. Allow the dampened drug to stand for about 15 min, then pack it firmly in a suitable percolator, and pour on the remainder of Menstruum I. When the liquid is about to drop from the percolator, close the lower orifice, cover the percolator, and allow the drug to macerate for the prescribed period of time. Then proceed with the percolation at the specified rate, and when the first menstruum has disappeared from the surface of the drug, use Menstruum II as needed until the drug is exhausted of its active principles. Reserve the first 850 ml of percolate, recover the alcohol from the percolate subsequently collected, and evaporate the residue to a soft extract at a temperature not exceeding 60°. Dissolve this extract in the reserved percolate, and if no assay is directed, add enough of a mixture of alcohol and water to make the fluidextract measure 1000 ml and contain the required proportion of C_2H_5OH. Mix thoroughly. If the fluidextract being prepared is to be adjusted to a standard, assay a portion of the reserved percolate in which the soft extract has been dissolved, and dilute the remainder to the volume determined as necessary by calculation from the assay, using a sufficient quantity of an alcohol and water mixture to provide the required proportion of C_2H_5OH. Mix thoroughly.

Process C. *Fractional or Divided Percolation.* This process is used for preparing fluidextracts, the constituents of which are injured by heat, or as an alternative for Process A or B, or in case suitable facilities for distillation and concentration are lacking. When Process C is used to prepare a fluidextract directed to be made by Process B, Menstruum I is used throughout the percolation.

Divide 1000 Gm of the ground drug into three portions, consisting of 500 Gm, 300 Gm, and 200 Gm. Mix the first portion (500 Gm) with sufficient of the prescribed menstruum to render it evenly and distinctly damp, transfer the dampened powder to a suitable percolator, the capacity of which should not greatly exceed the bulk of the moist drug when packed firmly, and allow it to stand for about 15 min. Then pack the drug in the percolator, saturate it with the menstruum, and allow it to macerate for the prescribed period of time. Then proceed with the percolation, first collecting and reserving 200 ml of percolate, and afterwards collecting five successive 300-ml portions of percolate, numbering them in the order in which they are obtained.

Dampen the second portion (300 Gm) of the drug with a sufficient quantity of the first of the 300-ml portions of percolate from the preceding lot of drug, and carry out the percolation as just directed for the first lot, except use the five 300-ml portions of percolate from the first lot of drug as menstruum in the order in which they were received, followed, if necessary, by sufficient fresh menstruum to supply the following portions of percolate: reserve the first 300 ml of percolate, and then collect five successive 200-ml portions, numbering them in the order in which they are collected.

Now dampen the third portion (200 Gm) of the drug with a sufficient quantity of the first numbered portion of percolate from the second lot of drug, and proceed with the percolation as before, using as the menstruum the 200-ml portions of percolate from the second lot of drug in the order received. If no assay is directed, collect and reserve 500 ml of percolate. Mix the three reserved percolates from the three lots of drug to make 1000 ml of fluidextract.

If the fluidextract being prepared by Process C is to be adjusted to a standard, collect and reserve only 420 ml of percolate from the third portion of drug instead of the 500 ml directed above. Mix the three reserved percolates from the three lots of drug, and assay a portion of the mixture. Dilute the remainder to the volume determined as necessary by calculation from the assay, using a sufficient quantity of an alcohol and water mixture to provide the required proportion of C_2H_5OH. Mix thoroughly.

Process D. This process is used for preparing fluidextracts with boiling water as the menstruum, alcohol being added as a preservative to the concentrated percolate.

To 1000 Gm of the coarsely ground drug add about 3000 ml of boiling water, mix well, and allow it to macerate in a suitable, covered metallic percolator for 2 hr. Then allow the percolation to proceed at the specified rate, gradually adding boiling water until the drug is exhausted. Evaporate the percolate on a water bath, or in a vacuum still, to the volume specified, cool, add the alcohol, and allow the mixture to stand in a stoppered container for several days. Then decant the clear liquid, filter the remainder into the decanted liquid, and wash the residue on the filter with a sufficient quantity of a mixture of alcohol and water to make the fluidextract measure 1000 ml and contain the required proportion of C_2H_5OH. Mix thoroughly.

Process E. This process is a modification of Process C, and can be used as an alternative for Processes A, B, or C. The percolation is conducted on a column of drug much greater in length than in diameter.

To 1000 Gm of the ground drug add a sufficient quantity of the prescribed menstruum to render it evenly and distinctly damp. Allow the dampened drug to stand for about 15 min, then pack it into a cylindrical percolator or series of such percolators joined together and having a total length sufficient to insure practically complete extraction of the drug by the collection of 1000 ml of percolate. Saturate the drug at a slow rate by forcing the menstruum through under pressure. Allow the drug to macerate for the prescribed period and proceed with percolation under pressure, at the rate specified for the other type processes, adding fresh menstruum as needed. It is necessary to work out conditions of percolation for each drug. The alcohol content of the percolate from some drugs will exceed the limit specification in the monograph; therefore, in those cases it is desirable to reduce the alcohol content of the menstruum accordingly.

Extracts

The USP and NF definitions for extracts are almost identical. The USP definition is as follows:

Extracts are concentrated preparations of vegetable or animal drugs obtained by removal of the active constituents of the respective drugs with suitable menstrua, evaporation of all or nearly all of the solvent, and adjustment of the residual masses or powders to the prescribed standards.

Three forms of extracts are recognized: semiliquid or those of syrupy consistency; plastic masses, known as pilular or solid extracts; and dry powders known as powdered extracts. These extracts provide concentrated forms for use in a number of solid or semisolid pharmaceutical preparations. The USP points out that pilular and powdered extracts of any one drug are interchangeable medicinally, but that each has its pharmaceutical advantages. The plastic or semisolid extracts are designated pilular extracts because they are of such consistency that they could be used in pill masses and conveniently shaped into finished pills. They are used in ointments and suppositories, and to facilitate their use in these preparations, the degree of concentration is directed to be that of a pilular consistency. Powdered extracts, on the other hand, are more useful where incorporation into a powdered mass or mixture is required, as in capsules, powders, or tablets. Semiliquid extracts or extracts of a syrupy consistency find use also as concentrates in the manufacture of pharmaceuticals. They are more difficult to define and less useful because they are more variable, ie, semiliquid or syrupy. Pilular extracts are semiliquid or syrupy extracts to which has been added sufficient inert diluent to produce a pilular consistency. Less variation on storage would be expected from a powdered extract than from a syrupy or pilular extract and recommended storage conditions for the latter should be observed.

Syrupy and solid extracts of many official and unofficial plant drugs are marketed as concentrates for reconstitution with an appropriate solvent. It is important to note that the solvent for reconstitution is specific in nature and variation can only result in an inferior product. In fact, variation from a specified solvent can cause incompatibility and instability in finished pharmaceutical preparations which utilize the resulting extract.

Extracts are prepared for the most part by the percolation process. The extracted liquid is concentrated by distillation under reduced pressure as directed in the monograph. The use of heat is to be avoided where possible because of the injurious effect of prolonged heating on active constituents. The menstruum may be more strongly alcoholic than that used in preparing the corresponding fluidextract or tincture since it is desirable to minimize or reduce the extraneous matter. Permission is granted by the USP and NF for the use of specially denatured alcohol in the extraction process since it is completely removed by distillation or evaporation (see page 1586). The rate of percolation, and other factors important in the percolation process, as outlined under *Fluidextracts*, should be followed carefully.

Extracts are adjusted to the prescribed strength or standard by the addition of diluents. The NF directs the use of liquid glucose as the diluent for pilular extracts and starch dried at 100°C for powdered extracts, but permits the use of other diluents as follows: malt extract and/or glycerin or glucose for pilular extracts; sucrose, lactose, powdered glycyrrhiza, magnesium carbonate, magnesium oxide, calcium phosphate, the finely divided marc remaining after the extraction of the drug, or other inert, nontoxic diluents for powdered extracts. Magnesium carbonate and magnesium oxide are not to be used in the preparation of powdered extracts of hysocyamus and belladonna. The use of chlorophyll or caramel is permitted in order to produce in a powdered extract a color corresponding to the normal color of the extract (green or brown) since the addition of starch, lactose, or other white or light-colored matter tends to lighten the natural color. The use of the coloring agent should be minimized.

A number of vegetable or animal drugs contain oily or fatty matter which must be removed in order to secure a satisfactory finished product. The NF permits the use of any suitable method for defatting either the drug or the extract itself and recommends two methods for treating the extract. Method I involves the addition of solvent hexane at the point where the extract is dried with a portion of starch. The mixture is stirred well several times over a period of 2 hours. Decantation or draining is followed by a repetition of the process with a smaller quantity of hexane, and again for a third time. The powder is dried and adjusted to the prescribed strength or quantity.

Method II involves the addition of slightly acidified water (about 0.05% hydrochloric acid or about 0.2% of tartaric acid) at a temperature of about 80°C to the soft extract or crude drug represented. When cold, the oily or fatty matter is discarded from the surface and the water layer retained. The extract is treated twice in this manner, and the combined water liquids evaporated to a soft extract at a temperature not exceeding 70°C. Starch is added and the mixture dried and completed in the usual manner.

The elimination of fat in Nux Vomica Liquid Extract BP is done by adding hard paraffin to the hot concentrated percolate, maintaining the liquid at 60°C and shaking vigorously. The hard paraffin rises and solidifies and the liquid extract is decanted.

Resins

Natural resins are referred to in Chapter 30 on *Natural Products*, page 507. They are solid preparations collected as exudates from plant substances. Mastic NF XI and Rosin NF are typical examples.

Prepared resins are made by percolating the powdered drug with an alcoholic menstruum, concentrating the percolate, and precipitating the resin by adding the concentrated percolate to hot water or acidified water. The following prepared or "galenical" resin is official: Podophyllum Resin USP.

Oleoresins

The oleoresins are liquid preparations, consisting of natural oils and resins extracted from vegetable substances by percolation with a menstruum of acetone or ether, which may be subsequently recovered. Alcohol is presented as an alternative for acetone or ether in the preparation of Ginger Oleoresin NF. The choice between ether and acetone may be a matter of cost or of using acetone in place of the more explosive ether. Acetone is superior to ether in making Capsicum Oleoresin NF XI.

The oleoresins were formerly classified with fluidextracts but differ from them with respect to solvent, yield, and in not bearing a uniform ratio of drug to finished extract. They are, however, in the broad sense of the term, extracts, and the BP still retains Extract of Male Fern, while the USP and PhI refer to the preparation as an oleoresin.

Oleoresins are prepared, in general, by percolating the powdered drug, contained in a cylindrical percolator provided with a cover and a receptacle suitable for volatile liquids, with the menstruum specified, until exhausted. The greater part of the liquid is recovered by distillation and the residue exposed in a shallow dish for spontaneous evaporation until the remaining solvent has been removed. A continuous extraction apparatus is useful for the extraction process and is specified in some cases in the monograph, for example, Capsicum Oleoresin BPC. The use of specially denatured alcohols is permitted as in the case of *Extracts* (page 1591).

Finishing, Packaging, and Storing

Extraction using any solvent or combination of solvents provides extractive matter of varying amount and the extract or solution is generally unstable due to the presence of suspended and colloidal matter. Deposition of such suspended matter in tinctures and fluidextracts occurs over a period of time, days, or even months, and has been referred to as sedimentation, precipitation, or pitching. Tinctures are more stable than fluidextracts as far as sedimentation is concerned. Pitching is influenced by many factors, eg, the nature of the extraction process, the concentration of the extract, the solvent system, the temperature, variation in solvent properties during extraction, hydrolysis, and enzyme activity. The formation of precipitates resulted in the official directions stating that:

A fluidextract that tends to deposit sediment may be aged or filtered or the clear portion decanted, provided the resulting clear liquid conforms to the pharmacopeial standards.

Other methods refer to clarification by subsidence and decantation, or by filtration, or by a combination of the two. The insoluble substance which settles out is almost always inert but this should be determined in order that activity is not lost. The PhI points out that tinctures whose active principles alter with time should be renewed every year; for example, Aconite, Belladonna, Hyoscyamus, and Stramonium.

Packaging and storage conditions are important; both the USP and NF recommend that tinctures and fluidextracts be preserved in tight, light-resistant containers and that exposure to direct sunlight and to excessive heat be avoided. Preservation, packaging, storage, and labeling regulations are presented in both official compendia under *General Notices*.

Absorption and loss of moisture have deleterious effects on semiliquid, pilular or powdered extracts, and oleoresins, affecting both the potency and the physical condition. Storage becomes particularly important with such preparations and a temperature below 30°C is preferable. Certain oleoresins may separate on standing and it may be necessary to warm and mix thoroughly before using.

References

1. Couch, J. F., *Am. J. Pharm.*, **91**, 16 (1919).
2. Butler, W. J., and Wiese, G. A., *J. APhA, Sci. Ed.*, **42**, 382 (1953).
3. Brochmann-Hanssen, E., *J. APhA, Sci. Ed.*, **43**, 27 (1954).
4. Srivastava, G. P., and Chadha, T. N., *J. Pharm. Sci.*, **52**, 299 (1963).

85 | Medicated Applications

Ointments—cataplasms—cements—cerates—contraceptives—creams—
dressings—glycerogelatins—pastes—plasters—suppositories

This chapter was prepared by

Louis C. Zopf, DSc, *Dean, College of Pharmacy, University of Iowa, Iowa City,
Iowa   52240, and*
Seymour M. Blaug, PhD, *Professor of Pharmacy, University of Iowa,
Iowa City, Iowa   52240*

Ointments

Ointments are semisolid preparations for external application of such consistency that they may be readily applied to the skin by inunction. They should be of such composition that they soften but not necessarily melt when applied to the body. They serve as vehicles for the topical application of medicinal substances and also function as protectives and emollients for the skin.

The *ointment base* usually constitutes the major portion of the pharmaceutical preparation and, therefore, may influence the efficacy of the incorporated medicinal substances.

For many years ointments were limited by definition and through use to mixtures of fatty substances. The present concept of this type of preparation is much broader. Today, in addition to such oleaginous mixtures, are included preparations of greater efficiency possessing the same general consistency but with an entirely different appearance. They may be entirely free of oleaginous substances *per se*. In many instances they are emulsions of fatty or wax-like materials with comparatively high proportions of water. These emulsions may be either of the water-in-oil (W/O) or oil-in-water (O/W) type depending primarily upon the selection of the emulsifying agent. Such semisolid emulsions are also referred to as *creams*.

Ideal Base

Among the properties which an ideal ointment base should possess are:

1. Does not retard wound healing.
2. Low sensitization index.
3. Pharmaceutical elegance.
4. A low index of irritation.
5. Nondehydrating.
6. Nongreasy.
7. Neutral in reaction.
8. Good keeping qualities.
9. Compatible with common medicaments.
10. Efficient release of medicament at site of application.
11. Washability (easily removed with water).
12. Minimum number of ingredients.
13. Ease of compounding.

Trends

Fats of animals and man and mixtures of such fats with resins, waxes, powdered herbs and minerals are among the earliest drugs employed by man.[1] Fat of animals, as well as that of man, was believed to have special medicinal virtue.

These various fats were by no means the only dermatological vehicles in ancient Babylon-Assyria and Egypt. Honey, wax, gums, and resins were also employed; these required a considerable amount of skill in compounding. A greaseless ointment was included among the formulas of the Papyrus Ebers (page 9) this consisting of Hartshorn beaten up with incense and flour and mixed with sweet ale.

Mucilages and balsams obtained from various plants often were used as well as oils, and combinations of these together with wax were also classified as ointments. The *rose cerate* or ointment (cold cream) of Galen was an early departure from the entirely fatty type of preparation.

Until the end of the eighteenth century there was little change in the preparation or evaluation of ointments but then the effects of scientific study began to reveal new substances, and this stimulated the development of new ideas. Lard was introduced as the chief ingredient in the first official ointment.[2] The addition of suet, wax, or spermaceti was permitted to give it the consistency of butter.

Because of the instability of lard it was replaced in later revisions of the USP with Benzoinated Lard, a product possessing a pleasant odor and the stimulating and antiseptic properties of the balsamic resin which also delayed the development of rancidity.

Schacht in 1858 introduced glycerite of starch, a translucent jelly, prepared by the action of glycerin on starch when heated in certain proportions and to certain temperatures. This type of preparation was adopted by the British Pharmacopœia in 1867 and the United States Pharmacopœia of 1880 (Sixth Revision).

Petrolatum under the name *Cosmoline* was introduced as an ointment base substance by Dr. A. W. Miller in 1873. Petrolatum was adopted in the United States Pharmacopœia of 1880. The rediscovery in 1885 of the therapeutic value of lanolin by the pharmacologist Oscar Liebrich brought the recognition of Adeps Lanæ Hydrosus (Lanolin) in the Seventh Revision (1893) and, subsequently, the addition of Adeps Lanæ (Anhydrous Lanolin) in the United States Pharmacopœia VIII (1905).

The early use of wool fat and lard and their property of absorbing or emulsifying considerable amounts of water led indirectly to the investigation of hydrophilic or water numbers for other substances.[3,4]

Due to its physical property of hardness and stability at relatively high temperatures, stearic acid was used as a substitute for wax as early as 1876. In recent investigations of cosmetic, pharmaceutical, and dermatologic preparations, stearic acid and a host of stearates are being used as emulsifying agents in ointments and also for improving their appearance and consistency.

Classification

Ointments can best be classified according to type (based on composition).

A. **Oleaginous Ointment Base**
1. Anhydrous
2. Does not absorb water readily (hydrophobic)
3. Insoluble in water
4. Not water removable

B. **Absorption Ointment Base**
1. Anhydrous
2. Will absorb water (hydrophilic)
3. Insoluble in water
4. Most are not water removable

C. **Emulsion Ointment Base**

Emulsion Ointment Base W/O
1. Hydrous
2. Will absorb water
3. Insoluble in water
4. Not water removable
5. Water-in-oil emulsion

Emulsion Ointment Base O/W
1. Hydrous
2. Will absorb water
3. Insoluble in water
4. Water removable
5. Oil-in-water emulsion

D. **Water-Soluble Ointment Base**
1. Anhydrous
2. Will absorb water
3. Soluble in water
4. Water removable
5. Greaseless

Based on their penetration, Goodman[5] divides ointment bases into three classes:

1. *Epidermic ointments* are those which demonstrate no, or at the most very slight, power of penetration into the skin. Preparations of this type are used when epidermal therapy is desired and especially where an emollient protective is indicated. In this group are placed the bases which contain petrolatum, waxes, and their combinations.
2. *Endodermic ointments* are those which possess some power of penetration into the deeper layers of the skin. Most of them have a somewhat lower melting point, approaching the temperature of the skin, and contain vegetable oils, lard, anhydrous lanolin, lanolin, and/or combinations of these. They are useful when an inflammatory action is indicated or where subepidermal therapy is desired.
3. *Diadermic ointments* are those which penetrate the skin thus offering a better opportunity for absorption of the medicament. Ointments of the emulsion type and the water-soluble bases belong to this group. They may permit a sufficient amount of absorption to demonstrate some systemic effects.

Polano, Bonsel, and Van der Meer[6] offer evidence that this classification of bases is not sound. They have shown that absorption does occur from petrolatum and lard bases particularly when applied to damaged epithelium. Absorption can and does occur from any ointment base, depending not only on the composition of the base, but also on the condition of the skin and on many other factors which are discussed in the preceding paragraphs on penetration. Polano concludes that when it is desired to have a drug penetrate into the skin, this effect may probably be most easily obtained by applying O/W emulsions and hydrogenated fats. The difficulty is in knowing when penetration is desirable. It is obvious that a topical anesthetic must penetrate to the nerve fibers, but should antibiotics for topical use get into the blood stream?

Types

Lane and Blank[7] have arbitrarily selected the following classification for all dermatologic vehicles, including ointments, according to whether their action on the skin is aqueous, oily, or that of an organic solvent:

A. **Vehicles which act as aqueous mixtures:**
1. Water
2. Shake lotions, eg, a mixture of zinc oxide and water
3. Gels of hydrophilic colloids, eg, bentonite jelly or surgical lubricant

B. **Vehicles which act as oils:**
1. Water-immiscible oils, eg, olive oil or petrolatum
2. Water-miscible oils, eg, anhydrous wool fat
3. Oil-in-water emulsions, eg, vanishing creams
4. Water-in-oil emulsions, eg, hydrous wool fat
5. Pastes, eg, a mixture of starch and petrolatum
6. Collodions

C. **Vehicles which act as powders:**
1. Hydrophilic powders, eg, starch
2. Hydrophobic powders, eg, talc or zinc stearate

D. **Vehicles which act as organic solvents:**
1. Water-miscible solvents, eg, alcohol or acetone
2. Water-immiscible solvents, eg, ether

Percutaneous Absorption

Medicaments may penetrate into and through the skin by the following avenues:[8]

1. Between the cells of the stratum corneum.
2. Through the walls of the hair follicles.
3. Through the sweat glands.
4. Through the sebaceous glands.
5. Through the cells of the stratum corneum.

These regions are shown in Fig. 617.

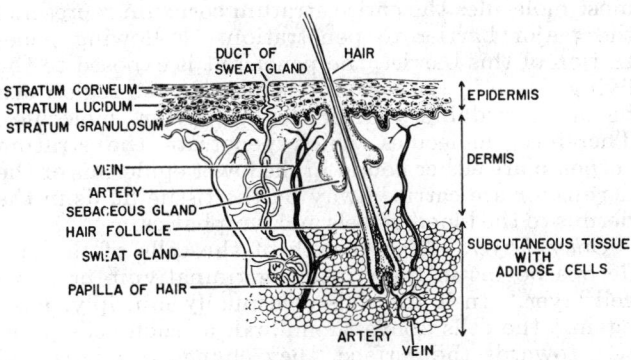

Fig. 617. Vertical section of human skin.

A discussion of the factors that affect percutaneous absorption of medicaments follows.

Skin Structure

The structure of human skin is very complex. This discussion is limited to the following parts of the skin and their effect on absorption: epidermis, hair follicles and sweat glands, and sebaceous glands.

Epidermis—The external or outer surface of the skin, the epidermis, is the site of application of medicated applications. The epidermis varies from a thickness of about 1 mm on the palms of the hands and soles of the feet to about 0.1 mm on parts of the face and body. It is covered with a discontinuous surface film of emulsified lipids.[8] This lipid film usually has a pH on the acid side, from about 4.5 to 6.5, depending on the region tested. It is sometimes referred to as the "acid mantle" of the skin. Jacobi and Heinrich[9] give a good descriptive account of the acid mantle. The epidermis is usually divided into five layers:

1. Stratum corneum (horny layer).
2. Stratum lucidum ("barrier zone").
3. Stratum granulosum (granular layer).
4. Stratum malpighii (prickle cell layer).
5. Stratum germinativum (basal cell layer).

These layers are formed by the cells that evolve from the basal layer and proliferate or push up from below. In the lower layers of the epidermis the cells are more densely packed than those in the stratum corneum.

Stratum Corneum—This horny layer is made up of several layers of flattened, keratinized cells (horny layer is 10–50 μ thick) which are constantly being shed and constantly being replaced by the cornification of the cells moving up from the lower layers.[10] The stratum corneum provides mechanical protection owing to its tough, durable properties.

Stratum Lucidum—This is a thin, membrane-like layer which has been called a "barrier zone" since it is reported[11,12] to act as a barrier to the transfer of water across the skin. There is intense sulfur activity in this region as demonstrated by a high sulfhydryl content. The sulfur-containing amino acids are probably utilized in this area in the synthesis of keratin.[13] Tregear[14] feels that the fully formed keratin layer of the stratum corneum is the main barrier to skin penetration. He questions the existence of a barrier zone at the base of the stratum corneum since, if such a layer is present, one would expect a more critical change of permeability when the outer layers of the skin are removed by stripping. It seems likely that the entire keratin layer provides the skin barrier, with the lower layers of the epidermis offering more resistance to the penetration of medicaments due to the denser packing of the cells in these layers.[15,16] For most molecules the entire stratum corneum represents the major barrier to penetration. Following penetration of this barrier, the penetrant is exposed to the living tissue in the dermis. This aqueous region can be a formidable barrier for nonpolar molecules. Therefore, molecules which penetrate the stratum corneum are either bound in the lower epidermis or the dermis, or are carried away by the tissue fluids in the dermis to the blood vessels and lymphatics.

Other Layers—The growth of the cells of the epidermis begins in the stratum germinativum or basal cell layer. In it the cells continually multiply, push against the cells above them, and, as such cells progress towards the surface, they change in shape and composition until they become horny cells of the stratum corneum.

Immediately below the epidermis is the dermis, known also as the true skin. Though the epidermis and dermis are well bound together to form a single entity, they are unlike morphologically. The dermis is mainly a network of collagen and elastin fibers, packed densely and with relatively few cells, in a colloidal ground substance consisting mainly of gelatinous mucopolysaccharides.[10] This tissue layer contains blood and lymph vessels, hair follicles, sebaceous glands, sweat glands, and muscle and nerve fibers.

Hair Follicles and Sweat Glands—There is evidence to suggest that the route of entry of medicaments into and through the skin is the epidermis itself rather than the appendages of the skin—ie, the hair follicles and sweat glands.[8,17,18] However, it is not known conclusively whether medicaments penetrate through the cells and/or between the cells of the stratum corneum. Clearly, the hair follicles and sweat glands of the skin represent potential parallel paths of the epidermis, through which penetrants may diffuse. There are reasons for believing that they are not important routes. In man, there are three times as many sweat glands per unit area of palm or sole skin as elsewhere,[19] yet palmar skin is less permeable to penetrants, except water, than the rest of the body.[20]

The penetration of materials down hair follicles has been reported.[21] If one assumes that penetration per unit area of epithelium is similar within and outside the hair follicle, skin penetration in man should be largely via the exposed epidermis, since only a small fraction of the available epithelium is in the hair follicles. Using pig skin, Tregear[22] showed that tri-*n*-butyl phosphate penetrated equally well whether or not the area included hair follicles.

Sebaceous Glands—These glands, located in the dermis and emptying into the hair follicle canal, do not play a significant role in the percutaneous absorption of medicaments.

Passive Diffusion

Tregear[23] offers three reasons for believing that the movement of molecules across the skin is by passive diffusion:

1. The impermeability of the skin remains long after the skin has been removed from the animal.[24]
2. Fick's law is obeyed (the rate of diffusion is proportional to the driving force, the difference in concentration between penetrant on the skin and in the skin), except by substances which are likely, on chemical grounds, to react with the skin surface.
3. Evidence[14–16] has been reported that the diffusional resistance is in the stratum corneum. Two possible exceptions to this are sodium ions and water which may be actively absorbed.[25,26]

Drug Solubility Characteristics

The lipid/water partition coefficient, as postulated in the Meyer–Overton theory, is actually important for the absorption of substances through the skin. Treherne[17] found a direct relationship between the ether/water partition coefficients of a series of radio-tagged substances and their permeability through excised skin. He suggested that a partition coefficient of unity might be the optimum for penetration. Stoughton, *et al*,[27] found a similar correlation between permeability through excised skin and ether/water partition coefficients for a series of nicotinic acid derivatives. Higuchi[28] also pointed out the importance of the thermodynamic properties of a medicament as it relates to its percutaneous absorption. These include the thermodynamic activity of the drug in the vehicle and in the skin-barrier phase, and the diffusion coefficient of the drug in the vehicle and skin-barrier phase. Drugs that are very soluble in a vehicle will probably exhibit slower rates of penetration than that exhibited by drugs which are less soluble in the vehicle. McKenzie and Aitkinson[29] related the activity of betamethasone and 23 esters of betamethasone to the lipid/water solubilities of the esters. Greater activity was shown by compounds possessing some lipid solubility plus a moderate aqueous solubility.

Using the vasoconstrictor technique developed by McKenzie and Stoughton[30,31] as an index of the percutaneous absorption of steroids, Katz and Shaikh[32] studied the correlation between the relative percutaneous absorption of a number of topical corticosteroids and the simple physical properties of solubility and partition coefficient. They correlated the experimentally determined physical properties of the corticosteroids with the McKenzie–Stoughton activity index of human skin vasoconstriction. Results indicate that the efficiency of percutaneous absorption may be a function of the physical constants of solubility and partition coefficient. This suggests that increases in topical corticosteroid anti-inflammatory activity produced by molecular modifications are in great measure proportional to changes in solubility and partition coefficients.

Poulsen, *et al*,[33] studied the effect of topical vehicle composition on the *in vitro* release of fluocinolone acetonide and its acetate ester. Steroid release was found to be a function of its concentration, solubility in the vehicles, and partition coefficient between vehicles and receptor phase (isopropyl myristate). Using vehicles containing propylene glycol and water, and gelled with Carbopol 934, they obtained maximum release from the vehicles containing the minimum amount of propylene glycol necessary to dissolve the steroid completely. One would expect the release rate to be highest when the vehicle was saturated with the steroid, since the thermodynamic activity of the drug increases up to saturation of the vehicle. Using other concentrations of propylene glycol the release rate decreased due to a change in the solvent property of the vehicle; ie, at high propylene glycol concentrations the vehicle was no longer saturated with the steroid, and at low propylene glycol concentrations the steroid was not completely soluble in the vehicle.

Medicament Concentration

Higuchi[28] developed relationships for systems where the rate-controlling step to absorption is in the skin and for systems where it is in the applied phase. In systems where the rate-controlling step is in the skin and the vehicle containing the penetrant does not appreciably affect the skin, the following approximate relationship was established for an idealized system between the steady state rate of penetration (dq/dt) and various properties of a fairly water-soluble penetrant:

$$\frac{dq}{dt} = (P.C.) \frac{(\text{Conc. of drug}) \, DA}{L}$$

where ($P.C.$) is the effective distribution coefficient of the penetrant between the vehicle and the barrier of the skin, (Conc. of drug) is the concentration of penetrant in the vehicle, D is the effective average diffusivity of the penetrant in the barrier phase, A is the effective cross-section area, and L is the effective thickness of the barrier phase. According to this equation the effective partition coefficient ($P.C.$) of the penetrant and its diffusivity (D) in the barrier phase are the main characteristics of the penetrant which determine its rate of entry through the skin. The important variable in the permeability constant $[(P.C.) \times (D)]$ is the effective partition coefficient since the diffusivity of a substance of similar molecular weight and shape usually differs only slightly, whereas the partition coefficient is an extremely sensitive function of molecular structure and size. For these systems, formulation variables are not directly important, the only significant factor involving the vehicle being the thermodynamic activity of the penetrating agent contained in it. The thermodynamic activity in the vehicle and the release rate from the vehicle increase up to saturation, for a given vehicle.

In systems where the rate-controlling step is in the applied base (ie, where the vehicle contains fine insoluble drug in suspension and where $C_s < A$), large concentration gradients develop in the applied phase. The amount of drug released from such suspension-type ointments is not directly proportional to concentration but is proportional to the square roots of the concentration of drug per unit volume (A), drug solubility (C_s) in the vehicle, diffusion constant (D) of the drug molecule in the vehicle, and time (t). The instantaneous rate of absorption at time t is dQ/dt:

$$\frac{dQ}{dt} = \sqrt{\frac{ADC_s}{2t}}$$

For these systems, skin properties are not directly important. The drug concentration in the base, the diffusion coefficient of the drug molecule, and the solubility of the drug in the base are the important factors. The rate of release of drug from such preparations can be regulated by controlling A, D, and C_s. A, the drug concentration, can be varied; D, the diffusion coefficient, is inversely proportional to the viscosity of the vehicle (Stoke-Einstein equation) (hence, it can be assumed that a decrease in the viscosity would yield an increased diffusion coefficient for the drug in the vehicle); and C_s can be varied, if a partly aqueous base in employed, by changing the effective pH of the vehicle for insoluble acidic and basic drugs or by addition of complexing agents or cosolvents.

Skin Hydration

Water is well sorbed by protein and protein degradation products contained in the outer skin. Singer and Vinson[34] compared the water-binding properties of the stratum corneum of the neonatal rat at various relative humidities with the data obtained by Blank[35] for human callus. They found that the water uptake at various relative humidities is almost identical for these tissues, suggesting that animal and human corneous tissue respond similarly with respect to the important property of water-binding capacity. In the temperature range tested (7–$49°$), the amount of water bound by corneum is a direct function of the relative humidity at each temperature and not of the absolute amount of moisture in the atmosphere. Hence, the relative moisture saturation of the air, and not the absolute amount of moisture in the air, determines the water content of the stratum corneum.

According to Higuchi,[28] the transfer properties of the several layers of the skin are probably strongly influenced by the presence of water. He demonstrated this, *in vitro*, using certain artificial membranes. At very high humidity (nearly 100%), the permeability of glyceryl monostearate was dependent on water activity, whereas, at very low humidity it was relatively insensitive to relative humidity.

Shelmire[36] also emphasized the importance of hydration of the stratum corneum when discussing the penetration of the skin by a medicament. Hydration may physically alter the skin tissue and also result in changes both in the diffusion coefficient and activity coefficient of the penetrating medicament, thereby increasing its rate of passage through the skin.

Wurster and Kramer[37] studied the absorption of three salicylate esters through the forearm of human subjects under hydrous and anhydrous skin conditions. The olive oil/water distribution coefficients of the esters varied from 7.7 for glycol salicylate to 1170 for ethyl salicylate. The absorption of all three esters was greater when a hydrous skin condition was maintained, the greatest increase in the penetration rate being shown by the ester with the smallest oil/water distribution coefficient. The same authors[37] studied the absorption of methyl salicylate through ether-defatted and nondefatted skin. They found a decrease of 27% in the total salicylate absorption following the defatting of the skin surface. The decrease in absorption may be due to disruption of the lipid pathway through which the salicylate normally diffuses. The decrease may also be due to partial dehydration produced by ether extraction of lipid-soluble materials and other substances responsible for the water-holding capacity of the skin.[38]

It follows that ointments containing water available for hydration of the keratin layer, such as oil-in-water emulsion bases, are likely to increase percutaneous penetration of certain medicaments. Conversely, bases which would tend to dehydrate the stratum corneum, or do not maintain hydration of the skin surface, would decrease percutaneous absorption. Shelmire[39] found that drugs soluble in oil and water did not penetrate when incorporated in a polyethylene glycol vehicle. Michelfelder and Peck[40] also found that a polyethylene glycol base was not a suitable vehicle for a water-soluble medicament, pyribenzamine hydrochloride, as far as penetration was concerned.

Ointment bases which leave occlusive films on the skin surface, such as petrolatum and water-in-oil emulsion bases, will induce hydration through sweat accumulation at the skin–vehicle interface. However, the degree of occlusion obtainable with ointments is likely to be small when compared with that obtained when a plastic film such as Saran wrap (*Dow*) is used to cover the skin. McKenzie and Stoughton[30] showed that the minimal effective concentration of certain steroids (dexamethasone, triamcinolone acetonide, and fluocinolone acetonide) is reduced by a factor of 100 when the site of application is occluded.

The Vehicle

Ointment bases have been classified according to their supposed effect on the penetration of medicaments through the skin (see *Classification of Ointments*, page 1595). It is now apparent that other factors such as the thermodynamic activity, diffusivity and solubility of the medicament in the base and in the skin,[28] and the degree of hydration of the skin[36,37] are of greater importance than the base itself in influencing penetration of a medicament into and/or through the skin. Conflicting reports concerning the importance of the vehicle in percutaneous absorption may be related to the fact that many absorption studies are carried out in animals whose skin permeability differs considerably from that of man.[41]

Peck, *et al*,[40,42] using the antiwhealing effect as a criterion for absorption of pyribenzamine hydrochloride from various vehicles, found that the best results were obtained with water-miscible emulsion bases. Shelmire[37] demonstrated that diffusion to the skin surface of an oil-soluble drug was greatest from a petrolatum vehicle. He also found that polyethylene glycol vehicles can provide a relatively high surface concentration of water-insoluble drugs with little

percutaneous absorption. Michelfelder and Peck[38] also found that a polyethylene glycol base is not a suitable vehicle for a water-soluble drug, as far as penetration is concerned. Since polyethylene glycol vehicles do not maintain hydration of the skin surface, it is understandable why water-soluble medicaments are not transferred readily to the skin surface.

Skin Condition

Differences between vehicles with regard to rate of drug penetration, as described above, become minor when the skin is in an abnormal state. Epidermal damage such as that caused by cuts, scratches, and blisters, or in eczema, enables medicaments to pass readily into and through the epidermis.[8] Using sarin (isopropoxymethylphosphoryl fluoridate) tagged with ^{32}P, Blank, *et al*,[43] demonstrated by autoradiography, as well as by chemical determination of extracts of the dermis, a striking increase in permeability following a superficial scratch extending just barely through the skin barrier. Similar data were obtained for trauma by adhesive tape stripping and puncture wounds.

Miscellaneous Factors

Several other factors may influence the percutaneous absorption of medicaments; the site of application, the length of time such application remains in contact with the skin, the amount of inunction used in applying the medicated application, and skin temperature.

Drugs which penetrate the stratum corneum do so most readily where the outer keratic layer is thin. Marzulli[44] showed that tri-*n*-butyl phosphate penetrated plantar skin *in vitro* much more slowly than skin from other regions. Blank, *et al*,[45] showed that excised scrotal skin was more permeable than abdominal skin to salicylic acid, hydrogen sulfide, or water vapor.

In general, the quantity of drug absorbed is proportional to the time the vehicle is in contact with the skin. Malkinson[46] showed that the rate of penetration of a medicament decreases with time as the tissues become saturated with the drug.

MacKee, *et al*,[47] and Peck, *et al*,[42] showed that, in general, the longer the period of inunction, the greater is the amount of drug absorbed.

In a sparsely haired mammal such as man, skin temperature varies greatly with environmental conditions. The temperature coefficient of penetration rate has been measured for several substances and ranges between 1.4 and 3.[48] Thus, in cold weather, penetration through a man's exposed skin should fall while in hot weather it should rise. Blank, *et al*,[49] reported that the rate of penetration of sarin increases approximately twofold for a 10° rise in temperature.

Ointment Bases

Oleaginous Bases

The term oleaginous bases includes the early ointments, which consisted almost entirely of vegetable and animal fats, as well as those containing petroleum hydrocarbons.

Fats and Fixed Oil Bases—Fixed oils of vegetable origin have frequently been employed as vehicles for the application of topical medication. Commonly

employed are olive, cottonseed, sesame, persic, and other oils.

Since the animal fats and vegetable oils are mixtures of the glycerides of fatty acids they undergo changes on exposure to light, air, and elevated temperatures causing decomposition with a resulting undesirable rancid odor. Antioxidants and other preservatives are therefore indicated.

Ointments of this type are emollient since they form

an occlusive covering on the skin, thereby inducing hydration through sweat accumulation at the skin–ointment interface. Hydration restores suppleness to dry skin.

Lard, the purified internal fat of the abdomen of the hog, was extensively employed as one of the early vehicles. Benzoinated Lard, prepared by the addition of 1% Siam Benzoin, is preferred because of better keeping qualities. Siam Benzoin contains balsamic acids (chiefly benzoic acid), coniferyl benzoate, and vanillin. The former serve as antioxidants and pre-servatives while the latter imparts a pleasant odor. Lard and lard-containing vehicles are mainly of his-torical interest since they are rarely used in modern dermatologic therapy.

Hydrocarbon Bases—Hydrocarbon bases include ointments prepared from petrolatum, or liquid petrola-tum, with wax or other stiffening agents. The official White Ointment of the USP is typical.

Petrolatum NF (Petroleum Jelly) is a tasteless, odorless, unctous, yellowish to light amber solid with a melting point of 38–60°C. It is frequently employed without modification for external application. White Petrolatum USP (White Petroleum Jelly) is petrolatum wholly or nearly decolorized. It is preferred when a white or translucent ointment is desired. It is to be noted that there is a wide range in the melting point for petrolatums. It is generally preferable to obtain a product which melts in the upper temperature limits.

The petrolatum type of base has a high index of com-patibility with the majority of substances most fre-quently prescribed in ointment form. They serve primarily as occlusive coverings for the skin, vehicles for ophthalmic ointments, and for antibiotics that are unstable in the presence of water; ie, bacitracin and the tetracyclines. White and yellow ointments are relatively stable to normal climatic temperature changes. The official compendia permit variation in the amounts of petrolatum and wax, to maintain a suitable consistency at extreme climatic conditions, as long as the proportion of active ingredient is not altered.

Bases of this kind are decreasing in favor because they are greasy and are difficult to remove from the skin and clothing. Hydrocarbon ointments have an advantage over oleaginous bases prepared from animal fats and vegetable oils in that they do not become rancid. Cold Cream USP (Petrolatum Rose Water Ointment USP XVI) possesses this advantage over the time-tried Rose Water Ointment which for years has been prepared from a vegetable oil, expressed almond oil or persic oil being recommended.

Oleaginous vehicles are occlusive and induce hydra-tion of the stratum corneum (horny layer of the epider-mis) through sweat accumulation. The control of hydration of the stratum corneum is important to the maintenance of the smooth and soft texture of the healthy skin surface. Oleaginous vehicles may be used solely for their physical effect on the skin surface such as the control of hydration. Other factors are involved in maintaining the hydration of the stratum corneum. Wheatley[50] has studied the role of skin lipids in maintaining normal skin emolliency.

Plastibase (Squibb), also called Jelene, is a combina-tion of mineral oils and heavy hydrocarbon waxes, having a mol. wt. of approximately 1300, the large proportion of which are liquid and are retained in what is believed to be a matrix of submicroscopic interstices.

Plastibase is a soft, unctuous, colorless, jelly-like substance. It melts at 90–91°C and maintains a desirable consistency over a wide temperature range (−15° to 60°). This means that it will not liquefy at temperatures occurring in tropical climates and will not harden excessively when exposed to relatively low tem-peratures.[51]

Plastibase has been used in place of petrolatum as an ingredient of the bases for several official and unofficial ointments. Ointments thus prepared have been com-pared over a period of several months with the same ointments containing petrolatum. Except in a very few instances, an ointment was obtained with Plasti-base which was superior in appearance, ease of applica-tion, and stability at elevated temperature to the official ointment bases.[52]

On the basis of *in vitro* studies, Plastibase appears to permit a greater release of the incorporated drug, when exposed to an O/W interface, than petrolatum. This would indicate that higher concentration of the drug in the tissue fluids would be obtained from Plastibase.[51]

Plastibase dissolves such substances as menthol, methyl salicylate, and camphor with the result that ointments containing these chemicals become too soft. Likewise, coal tar produces an ointment too soft to prevent separation. Plastibase does not lend itself to the incorporation of waxes as stiffening agents because it is difficult to cool the resulting mixture to a smooth consistency.[51]

Silicones—Silicones are synthetic polymers in which the basic structure is not carbon, as in the usual type of synthetic polymers, but an alternate chain of silicon and oxygen atoms (eg, —O—Si—O—Si—O—Si). See page 768. Depending on the number and type of organic groups attached to the silicon and the method of preparation, the material may be a liquid, resin, or rubber.

Silicones used by the pharmaceutical and cosmetic industries are generally dimethylpolysiloxane [D. C. 200 fluid (*Dow-Corning*); L-45 (*Union Carbide*)], methylphenylpolysiloxane [Dow Corning 555 fluid], and a stearyl ester of dimethylpolysiloxane [Dow Corning F-157]. All are insoluble in water and are water repellent. Dimethylpolysiloxanes are clear fluids available in a wide range of viscosities. They are widely used in protective creams and lotions. Two emulsion formulations containing dimethylpolysil-oxanes are shown below.

Silicone Gibson Base[53]

Cetyl Alcohol	15.0	Gm
Sodium Lauryl Sulfate	1.0	Gm
Dimethylpolysiloxane Polymer (1000 cps)	40.0	Gm
Purified Water	43.0	Gm
Methylparaben	0.25	Gm
Propylparaben	0.15	Gm

Warm the aqueous mixture of the sodium lauryl sulfate and the parabens to 75° and slowly add it to the warmed (25°) cetyl alcohol-silicone mixture. Stir the ointment until it congeals.

Vanisil Silicone Ointment[54]

Stearic Acid (Pearlstearic)	10.0	Gm
Synthetic Japan Wax	2.0	Gm
Dimethylpolysiloxane Polymer (1000 cps)	20.0	Gm
Potassium Hydroxide	0.5	Gm
Methylparaben	0.025	Gm
Propylparaben	0.015	Gm
Distilled Water	67.5	Gm

Mix in the customary manner.

Methylphenylpolysiloxane has the typical charac-teristics of dimethylpolysiloxane except for solubility in alcohol. Methylphenylpolysiloxane is soluble in 95% alcohol and is more compatible with organic substances than dimethylpolysiloxane. It is used in protective formulations, suntan lotions, hair sprays, and shave lotions. The stearyl ester of dimethylpolysiloxane is also compatible with a wide range of organic materials but is a waxy semisolid which makes it suitable for use in stick preparations such as lipsticks and lip pomades.[55]

Lesser[56] and Pail and Todd[55] have published reviews of the applications of silicones in pharmacy and medicine and in dermatologic and cosmetic formulations.

Silicone fluids are practically inert physiologically and appear to be essentially nontoxic.[57] Clinical studies[58] have shown silicones to be nonirritant when applied to the skin. Silicone ointments are being used in the management of dermatologic disorders in which protection from moisture is indicated.

Shaw and Crowe[59] and Lubowe[60] reported on the effectiveness of silicone fluids, as skin protectives, when incorporated in various dermatologic vehicles. Shaw and Crowe[59] found the most effective protection was provided by a mixture of 30% silicones in petrolatum alone. The nonsilicone commercial protective ointments were of little value against soap and hot water and soluble cutting oil exposures. Repeated washings disclosed the fact that all the protective ointments can be removed with soap and water after varying lengths of time, indicating the need for reapplication as required for any particular activity.

Steigleder and Raab[61] studied the water-repellent properties of a number of ointments including White Petrolatum, Hydrophilic Petrolatum, Zinc Oxide Ointment, Hydrophilic Ointment, and Olive Oil (all in the current USP), plus two silicone-containing ointments. They claim that the addition of silicones makes no difference in the water-repellent properties of White Petrolatum USP on the skin; They rated it as affording the best protective effect.

The chief difficulty in formulating ointments that afford protection against aqueous solutions is that of providing a film which resists soap and water yet is readily removable by surfactant solutions. One approach is to provide a film that cannot be removed easily by soap and water but only by a special remover. The approach generally used is to emulsify the silicones or other hydrophobic film-formers so that when the protective ointment is properly applied an "invisible" protective film is left on the skin. In addition to a silicone or silicones, a protective ointment or cream may contain film-forming agents such as polyvinylpyrrolidone, polyvinyl alcohol, and the cellulose derivatives.

Absorption Bases

The word absorption is used to denote the hydrophilic or water-absorbing properties of such bases and not to describe their action when applied to the skin. Absorption bases are generally anhydrous bases which have the property of absorbing several times their weight of water forming emulsions and still retaining their ointment-like consistency. These bases have found a definite place in pharmacy as well as cosmetology. Cosmetologists sometimes use absorption in a different vein, referring to the absorption of the base itself. Pharmaceutically speaking, this is not generally inferred although absorption of ointment bases has been demonstrated.

Absorption bases vary in their composition but for the greater part they are mixtures of animal sterols with petrolatum. Combinations of cholesterol and/or

other suitable lanolin fractions with white petrolatum are marketed under the name of absorption bases; *Eucerin* and *Aquaphor* were among the earlier commercial bases of this type.

The ability to absorb water to form W/O emulsions is the outstanding characteristic of Anhydrous Lanolin USP. A study of the literature reveals disagreement as to which fraction endows lanolin with this property. Our knowledge of the chemistry of lanolin, even at this date, remains incomplete. The composition of lanolin has been reviewed by Conrad.[62] Malmstrom[63] reported there is no indication that the free, combined or total cholesterol had an effect on the water absorption power of lanolin, and concluded that the water absorption properties were due to the composition of the mixture.

Bertram[64] attributed the emulsifying properties of lanolin to the high-molecular-weight diesters of hydroxyacids. Tiedt and Truter[65] concluded that lanolin esters were not capable of forming emulsions themselves. They attributed the emulsifying property to the free alcohols in lanolin. They also found that mixtures of the alcohols were better emulsifiers than a pure single alcohol.

Lanolin is a complex mixture of chemical compounds. Many of the lanolin components have been separated and transformed to materials more versatile than the parent product. In addition to the lanolin alcohols and absorption bases there are now available lanolic acid compounds, dewaxed or liquid lanolins, acylated lanolins, ethoxylated lanolins, hydrogenated lanolins, transesterified lanolins, lanolin esters, and other lanolin derivatives. Examples of products that fall into these categories are given by Wagner[66] and by Conrad and Maso.[67] The development, production, properties, and uses of liquid lanolin are discussed by Clark.[68]

Zopf Emollient Cream

White Petrolatum	41.0 Gm
Microcrystalline Wax	3.0 Gm
Fluid Lanolin*	10.0 Gm
Sorbitan Monooleate†	4.75 Gm
Polysorbate 80‡	0.25 Gm
Purified Water	41.0 Gm

Warm the aqueous dispersion of sorbitan monooleate and polysorbate 80 to 75° and add slowly to the melted wax, white petrolatum, fluid lanolin phase. Stir until congealed.

Hoch Formula (*Malmstrom*)

Phase A

Fluid Lanolin*	5.0 Gm
Castor Oil	35.0 Gm
Sorbitan Monostearate§	2.0 Gm
Mineral Oil	36.70 Gm
Stearic Acid	4.0 Gm
Propylparaben	0.20 Gm

Phase B

Polyethylene 20 Sorbitan Monostearate‖	1.0 Gm
Triethanolamine	0.90 Gm
Methylparaben	0.20 Gm
Purified Water	15.0 Gm

Heat phase A to 78° and phase B to 70°. Add phase B to phase A and stir until cooled to 25°.

The Zopf Emollient Cream, developed in the University of Iowa Pharmacy Laboratories, has undergone clinical evaluation in the Department of Dermatology, of the University of Iowa Hospitals, where it

---

* Lantrol (*Malmstrom*).
† Span 80 (*Atlas*).
‡ Tween 80 (*Atlas*).
§ Glycolmul "S" (*Glyco*).
‖ Glycosperse "S-20" (*Glyco*).

was found acceptable as an emollient preparation. The Hoch formula is another example of the use of a fluid lanolin preparation. However, this preparation is an O/W emulsion making it easier to remove from the skin and clothing than the Zopf Emollient Cream which is a W/O emulsion.

Hydrophilic Petrolatum USP

Cholesterol	30 Gm
Stearyl Alcohol	30 Gm
White Wax	80 Gm
White Petrolatum	860 Gm
To make	1000 Gm

Melt the stearyl alcohol, white wax, and white petrolatum together on a steam bath, then add the cholesterol and stir until it completely dissolves. Remove from the bath, and stir until the mixture congeals.

Hydrophilic Petrolatum USP is an absorption-type base. The formula differs from that which was introduced in the USP XIII in that the original formula contained 1% cholesterol and 15% anhydrous lanolin. Anhydrous lanolin was deleted and cholesterol increased because the dermatologists have evidence that some patients exhibit allergies to anhydrous lanolin.

A review[69] of the literature of reported instances of lanolin sensitivity yields a total of about 100-odd cases reported over a period of 30 years and from several countries. This seems to indicate that lanolin is not a potent sensitizer, yet it continues to be suspect by some dermatologists. However, Hjorth and Trolle-Lassen[70] made a detailed study of lanolin sensitivity and reported an impressive incidence of sensitivity to lanolin among patients with eczema. Sulzberger, et al[71] patch-tested 19 patients sensitive to lanolin with components and derivatives of the latter. They concluded that the allergen was in the aliphatic fraction of the alcoholic component.

The increase in cholesterol in the present formula gives a product which is capable of absorbing large quantities of water and the deletion of the anhydrous lanolin, it has been found, does not detract from the pharmaceutical elegance of the preparation.

Inclusion of the white wax and stearyl alcohol in the formula adds firmness to the base in addition to increasing the heat stability of the preparation, stearyl alcohol also increases the water absorption properties of the base.[3,4] Preparations of this type do not contain water as a component of their basic formula, but if water is incorporated, when and as desired, a water-in-oil W/O emulsion results.

The British Pharmacopœia contains an absorption base under the title Wool Alcohols Ointment (*Unguentum Alcoholium Lanæ*).

Wool Alcohols Ointment BP

Wool Alcohols	60 Gm
Hard Paraffin	240 Gm
White or Yellow Soft Paraffin	100 Gm
Liquid Paraffin	600 Gm

Melt together and stir until cold.

Wool alcohols[72] is the crude mixture of steroid and triterpene alcohols prepared by treating anhydrous lanolin with alkali and separating the fraction containing cholesterol and other alcohols. It is claimed that the water-in-oil emulsions formed are preferred to those made with anhydrous lanolin since they do not darken on the surface and no objectionable odor is detectable in hot weather. Five per cent of wool alcohol blended with soft paraffin permits up to three times as much water to be incorporated.

These bases were developed because it was desirable to have a product to which water or a solution of medicinal substances in water could be added easily. Many workers have demonstrated that antiseptic substances exercise little or no bacteriostatic or germicidal effect when incorporated into a fatty base. Li and Kuever[73] demonstrated that when an aqueous solution of phenylmercuric nitrate was added to an absorption base it exhibited distinctly higher antiseptic potency than when incorporated in White Ointment USP. Laug, et al,[74] in measuring the effect of particle size of calomel on the cutaneous penetration of mercury on rabbits and rats, found the oil-in-water (O/W) type of vehicle to exhibit the largest storage of mercury in kidney tissue.

These results can probably be attributed to the differences in the water content of the various bases since the importance of hydration to the percutaneous absorption of medicaments has been established.[75,76]

Aquabase Ointment*

Cholesterol	30 Gm
Cottonseed Oil	30 Gm
White Petrolatum	940 Gm
To make	1000 Gm

Heat the white petrolatum and cottonseed oil to 145°C. Remove from heat, add the cholesterin and stir until almost congealed. Then pour into jars.

Absorption bases such as Aquabase Ointment are used as vehicles for ophthalmic ointments and for antibiotics that are unstable in the presence of water such as bacitracin and the tetracyclines.

Absorption bases generally have a high index of compatibility toward the majority of medicaments used topically. As a class they are relatively heat stable. They can be utilized in their anhydrous form or emulsified with the addition of water where emolliency is desired. These bases, however, still possess the undesirable property of greasiness but they are more readily removable from the skin than the oleaginous bases.

Some commercially available absorption bases are Aquaphor (*Duke*), Hydrotex (*Texas Pharmacal*), and Polysorb (*Fougera*).

Emulsion Bases

Products coming under this classification are also known as hydrophilic or *water removable ointment bases*. The term "hydrophilic" means "having or denoting a strong affinity for water." Though it is possible to incorporate additional water into these preparations the term is perhaps more appropriate for absorption bases. Water removable as used here refers to the ease with which these bases and resulting ointments can be removed from the skin and clothing with water. This term is descriptive of one of their outstanding advantages. The term emulsion base is correctly used since these preparations are solid emulsions and similar products have long been used as cosmetic creams.

The availability of a number of newer organic compounds for use as wetting agents, dispersing agents, emulsifiers, penetrants, emollients, detergents, hardeners, preservatives, etc., have given a much greater degree of flexibility to ointment formulation. In the field of surface active agents which perform such function as wetting, emulsifying, dispersing, and solubilizing, there are a number of choices. Surface-active

---

* From the Formulary of the University of Iowa Hospitals.

agents may be ionic or nonionic. The ionic types are either anionic or cationic, depending upon whether the characteristically surface-active portion of the compound lies in the anion or cation. For example, in soap the anion (oleate) is the effective portion of the molecule and soap is therefore classified as an anionic surfactant.

Nonionic surface-active agents depend chiefly on hydroxyl groups and ether linkages (polyhydric alcohol anhydrides and polyoxyethylene chains) to create the hydrophilic action. Polysorbate 80 and Polyoxyl 40 Stearate, official in the USP represent such surface-active agents.

Generally, the nonionic agents are widely used in dermatological and pharmaceutical preparations. Ionic surface-active agents exhibit a particle charge, hence are sensitive to the presence of other ions. Thus, soaps (anionic agents) are ineffective in hard water due to the presence of divalent cations in the water. Cationic agents, on the other hand, are not stable in the presence of anionic agents including soap. Since nonionic agents do not ionize, they are comparatively insensitive to hard water, electrolytes, and ionic surface active agents. Furthermore, nonionic surface-active agents are generally less toxic and less irritating than ionic agents.

Other advantages of nonionic surface-active agents are their virtual neutrality, stability to freezing, stability to electrolytes, and ease of use.[77] Moore and Bell[78] point out that nonionic emulsifiers based on fatty acids—ie, Polysorbate 80 and Polyoxyl 40 Stearate—are limited in use by the comparative lack of stability of the ester linkage to hydrolysis. They cite reasons for preferring nonionic emulsifiers based on ethoxylated fatty alcohols [Brij-type surface-active agents (*Atlas*)] to other emulsifying agents. A more complete discussion of emulsifiers is given by de Navarre.[79]

Many dermatologic and cosmetic preparations contain amine soaps as emulsifying agents. These anionic emulsifiers are preferred to potassium and sodium soaps because they yield emulsions having relatively low pH's, being in the region of 8.0. Triethanolamine $[N(C_2H_4OH)_3]$ is generally used, along with a fatty acid, to produce the fatty acid amine soap. Triethanolamine usually contains small amounts of the mono- and diethanolamines. It combines stoichiometrically with fatty acids. Semisolid O/W bases containing triethanolamine soaps are generally prepared by dissolving the triethanolamine in water and then adding this to the oil phase, with stirring. A typical formula for such a base is given by de Navarre:[80]

Stearic Acid	18.0 Gm
Cetyl Alcohol	4.0 Gm
Triethanolamine	2.0 Gm
Glycerin	5.0 Gm
Distilled Water	71.0 Gm

Coal Tar Ointment USP contains a surface-active agent, Polysorbate 80, which serves a dual purpose. It functions as a dispersing agent and also aids in the removal of the ointment from the skin. See the formula below.

Coal Tar Ointment USP

Coal Tar	10 Gm
Polysorbate 80	5 Gm
Zinc Oxide Paste	985 Gm
To make	1000 Gm

Blend the coal tar with the polysorbate 80, and incorporate the mixture with the zinc oxide paste.

A compound known as *Lanette Wax* has been used extensively in England as a component of emulsion bases. There is some discrepancy in the literature regarding the composition of this material but generally it is agreed that it is a partially phosphated or sulfated mixture of cetyl and lauryl alcohols. It is a light cream-colored product with a melting point of approximately 50°C. It is self-emulsifiable with water, giving an oil-in-water (O/W) emulsion with fixed oils, fats and waxes. It may be closely approximated by mixing together 9 parts of cetyl alcohol and 1 part of sodium lauryl sulfate.

In general the formulas for water removable ointment bases contain an aqueous phase, an emulsifying agent and an oleaginous phase. The water phase of different formulas varies from 10 to 80% of the total base. Most bases of this group will permit the incorporation of additional water or medicinal solutions without reducing the consistency of the ointment below that of a soft cream. Glycerin, propylene glycol, or a polyethylene glycol is generally included with the aqueous phase to serve as a humectant for the finished ointment; these substances being hygroscopic in nature have a tendency to reduce water loss through evaporation and to lend a general softness to the creams. The addition of certain alcohols to emulsion base formulas also adds stability to the emulsion, and imparts a smooth and velvety feel to the skin surface. One of these alcohols, stearyl alcohol, a solid, also increases the consistency of the ointment, permitting the incorporation of more liquid components. Due to their ability to become hydrated such alcohols assist in water retention of emulsion bases. Cetyl alcohol has the lowest optimum concentration and stearyl alcohol causes the greatest potentiation of the water number of petrolatum.[4] The "*water number*"[3] is defined as the largest amount of water which 100 Gm of an ointment base or fat will hold at normal temperature (20°C). The fatty acid esters of sorbitan and mannitan greatly increase the water number of petrolatum and are also excellent emulsifying agents.[81] It has been demonstrated that some of the normal alkyl alcohols (C_{20} to C_{30}), constituents of the natural waxes, have water potentiating properties. The C_{20} alcohol causes the greatest water potentiation and the C_{24} alcohol has the lowest optimum concentration.[82] The cetyl alcohol content of emulsions should range from 1 to 5% depending on the composition of the individual formula;[83] 1% is suggested for use in vanishing creams.

The oleaginous phase may contain one or more of the following or similar ingredients: petrolatum, fats, waxes, organic alcohols, polyglycol esters, or other grease-like substances. These substances are emulsified with the aqueous phase through the action of the surface-active agent. The selection of the emulsifier is important since it is desired to produce an O/W emulsion. A few such agents are the alkali soaps, alkyl sulfates, amine soaps, polyglycol esters, alkyl aryl sulfates, quaternary ammonium compounds, etc. These newer emulsifying agents, plus many others, aid in dispersing fats and waxes in water and increase the stability of ointments.

Hydrophilic Ointment USP

Methylparaben	0.25	Gm
Propylparaben	0.15	Gm
Sodium Lauryl Sulfate	10	Gm
Propylene Glycol	120	Gm
Stearyl Alcohol	250	Gm
White Petrolatum	250	Gm
Purified Water	370	Gm
To make about	1000	Gm

Melt the stearyl alcohol and the white petrolatum on a steam bath, and warm to about 75°. Add the other ingredients, previously dissolved in the water and warmed to 75°, and stir the mixture until it congeals.

Hydrophilic Ointment USP is an emulsified base possessing a relatively high degree of compatibility and therapeutic efficiency as proved by *in vitro* and *in vivo* tests.[84] Inclusion of a petrolatum phase was found desirable for smoothness and "slip" and for its softening effect upon the residual film of ointment as applied to the skin. It has been indicated that emulsified bases containing petrolatum as one of the components lose less water, on the average, than those which contain no petrolatum.[85] This amount of petrolatum does not interfere with the release of medicinal agents. The sodium lauryl sulfate serves as the emulsifier while the stearyl alcohol acts as an adjuvant emulsifier and adds to the physical property of hardness. Hydrophilic Ointment USP XV contained polyoxyl 40 stearate, a nonionic surface-active agent, as the emulsifying agent. However, in the Manufacturing Laboratory at the University of Iowa College of Pharmacy, it was discovered that when bacitracin or phenol was incorporated in the USP XV base, a marked softening of the base occurred. Fennell, *et al*,[86] developed a lotion vehicle using polyoxyl 40 stearate as the emulsifying agent. The results of their compatibility tests indicated that the vehicle was incompatible with resorcinol, tannic acid, and Peru balsam. With phenol the vehicle was thinned considerably, and on standing a separation of water occurred. Salicylic acid also thinned the vehicle. For this reason the USP XIV formula for Hydrophilic Ointment was re-adopted in USP XVI.

The propylene glycol which is present in the product assists in obtaining a more intimate dispersion of soap, oils, greases, and other such substances in water. Due to its hygroscopicity, it absorbs and retains moisture from the air thus acting as a humectant in the ointment. Hydrophilic Ointment USP XIII softened considerably upon levigation. Substituting propylene glycol for glycerin in the 14th Revision removed this difficulty and also permitted the incorporation of benzoic and salicylic acids which were incompatible with the USP XIII product. Greatest stability to heat tests was displayed with emulsion bases when the aqueous phase was maintained at 36 to 40%.[87]

In a study by Chakravarty, *et al*,[87] it was shown that a number of pharmaceutical compounds interact with polyoxyl 40 stearate to form soluble and insoluble complexes. This complex formation may be responsible for the observed incompatibilities occurring with Hydrophilic Ointment and other formulations containing polyoxyethylene-type surface-active agents.

Many formulas of similar composition may prove efficacious as emulsion ointment bases but simplicity of manufacture, minimum number of ingredients, stability, water removability, and low index of sensitivity to the base or its components are all of paramount consideration. Materials used in formulating emulsion-bases and the general formulation of emulsions are discussed by de Navarre.[88]

The usual method of preparation involves melting the grease-like materials and waxes in one container, heating the water with the water-soluble components (which usually includes the emulsifier) in another container, and mixing both at the same temperature, 75°C. Stirring is continued until a smooth cream results and the temperature has been reduced to approximately 30°C. Passage of the ointment while it is still warm

through either a colloid mill or homogenizer always improves the product.

Thomssen[89] and others point out that there are several factors which must be considered in the preparation of emulsion bases. The quality and quantity of ingredients, the order of mixing, the speed and type of mixing, the temperature at which the emulsion is made, and choice of emulsifier are all equally important. Another very important factor is the pH of the finished ointment base. Preferably, it should have a pH of 5.5 to 7.

Bases of this group present a product of cosmetic-like appearance. This fact, together with their ease of application and simplicity of removal, produces a psychological effect on the patient which is desirable and insures better patient cooperation resulting in more efficacious therapy. Many people object to the greasy feel and general uncleanliness of the oleaginous ointments.

Damaged and diseased epithelium is assured of a moist application through the use of these ointments. A living cell is a moist cell. Release of the medicinal agent is enhanced by virtue of a water phase being present and the effect of the surface tension reducing property of the emulsifier and adjuvant agents included in the base.

Keratolytic effects have been demonstrated in a shorter length of time with the use of emulsion bases than with the petrolatum or nonemulsified type.[90]

Unpublished studies from the laboratory of the College of Pharmacy of the University of Iowa, using rats as test animals, demonstrate absorption of phenol red and strychnine sulfate from Hydrophilic Ointment and no absorption of the same substances from simple ointment. Phenol red (5% in Hydrophilic Ointment) was applied to a shaved area and allowed to remain for a period of 6 hr. Urine collected during this period gave positive tests for phenol red. Ointments containing 1 and 5% of strychnine sulfate applied to the rat in the same base gave definite early symptoms of strychnine absorption. The symptoms consisted of muscular twitching and a very high degree of peripheral sensitivity indicated by the manner in which the animal responded to the slightest touch. Tests using white ointment as the base were negative. Other workers[91–94] claimed that oil-in-water emulsion bases promote percutaneous absorption of drugs due to either the presence of surface active agents or the water miscibility of the base.

Emulsion bases are subject to water loss and have a tendency to develop mold growth. Propylene glycol has a greater power to inhibit mold growth than glycerin but it is generally desirable to add a preservative to such water-containing ointment bases.

Several O/W emulsion bases are commercially available under a variety of tradenames. Cetaphil (*Texas Pharmacal*), Neobase (*Burroughs Wellcome*), Unibase (*Parke, Davis*), Vanibase (*Warren-Teed*), Dermovan (*Texas Pharmacal*), and Phorsix (*Texas Pharmacal*) are examples of such bases.

Beeler's Base[95]

Cetyl Alcohol	15 Gm
White Wax	1 Gm
Propylene Glycol	10 Gm
Sodium Lauryl Sulfate	2 Gm
Water	72 Gm

Melt the cetyl alcohol and white wax in the propylene glycol on a water bath and heat to about 65°C. Dissolve the sodium lauryl sulfate in the water and heat on a water bath to about 65°C. Slowly add the oil phase to the well-stirred water phase and continue stirring on the water bath for about 10 min. Remove from the bath and continue stirring to the point of congealing.

U. C. H. Base*

Cetyl Alcohol	6.4 Gm
Stearyl Alcohol	5.4 Gm
Sodium Lauryl Sulfate	1.5 Gm
White Petrolatum	14.3 Gm
Mineral Oil	21.4 Gm
Water	50.0 Gm

Melt the alcohols together over a water bath at 65°C, add the sodium lauryl sulfate and stir well. Next add the white petrolatum and the liquid petrolatum and continue to heat the mixture until completely melted. Cool to room temperature and add the water slowly with constant mixing.

Anhydrous Emulsion Bases—Anhydrous emulsifiable solid-mixtures have been suggested as a means of producing emulsions extemporaneously as needed for prescription use.[96] One important consideration is that such a product be available as a powder or granular material so it can be accurately weighed and conveniently handled. This type of product is prepared by melting the ingredients together on a water bath and stirring vigorously until the preparation is completely solidified and a granular product results. It is not to be construed that all formulas employed as hydrophilic ointments lend themselves to this treatment when deprived of their water phase.

Solid-Mixture A

Stearyl Alcohol	53.0 Gm
Cetyl Alcohol	7.0 Gm
Polyethylene Glycol 400	38.6 Gm
Sodium Lauryl Sulfate	1.4 Gm
	100 Gm

Solid-Mixture B

Stearyl Alcohol	64.7 Gm
Cetyl Alcohol	8.6 Gm
Polyethylene glycol 1000 Monostearate†	13.0 Gm
Polyethylene glycol 1540†	8.7 Gm
Wool Fat	5.0 Gm
	100 Gm

Melt the ingredients together and stir until complete solidification. Continued stirring is necessary to insure complete mixing of the ingredients, and for the production of a granular product.

Physical Properties of the Solid-Mixtures: They are white to yellowish white coarsely white granular powders, slightly soluble in water but completely soluble in alcohol and benzene. Their melting point range is from 56° to 68°C.

Preparation of Base A: Melt 50 Gm of solid-mixture A, heat it to 70–75°C, and add it to 50 Gm of water at the same temperature. Stir until the emulsion begins to solidify and cools to 40°C.

Preparation of Base B: The method is the same as that used for base A except that the amounts of solid-mixture B and water are 40 Gm and 60 Gm, respectively. Overheating should be avoided when solid-mixture B is melted as it darkens at temperatures above 75°C.

Physical Properties of the Bases: The bases are white, semisolid oil-in-water emulsions of ointment-like consistency. They are nongreasy and washable with water. The emulsions are stable up to 55–60°C. Base A has a better sheen than base B; both exhibit good lubricity when applied to the skin.

The British Pharmacopeia[97] and the British Pharmaceutical Codex[98] give formulas for emulsifying waxes which are used in formulating emulsifying ointments. Such ointments are capable of emulsification with water to form O/W emulsions.

Emulsifying Wax BP

Cetostearyl Alcohol	90.0 Gm
Sodium Lauryl Sulfate	10.0 Gm
Purified Water	4.0 ml

---

* University of California Hospital.
† Carbowax polyethylene glycols (*Union Carbide*).

Emulsifying Ointment BP

Emulsifying Wax	30.0 Gm
Liquid Paraffin	20.0 Gm
White Soft Paraffin	50.0 Gm

Similar formulas are available in the British Pharmaceutical Codex[98] under the titles Cetrimide Emulsifying Wax (and Ointment) and Cetomacrogol Emulsifying Wax (and Ointment). Cetrimide consists essentially of tetradecyltrimethylammonium bromide; hence, Cetrimide Emulsifying Ointment can be used as a vehicle for the incorporation of cationic and nonionic medicaments. Cetomacrogol is polyethylene glycol 1000 monocetyl ether, a nonionic surfactant. Therefore, Cetomacrogol Emulsifying Ointment can be used as a vehicle for the incorporation of anionic, cationic, and nonionic medicaments.

Water-Soluble Bases

Soluble ointment bases include those bases which are prepared from the higher ethylene glycol polymers known as polyethylene glycol compounds. Arbitrarily included are the semisolid preparations produced through the use of bentonite, colloidal magnesium aluminum silicate, pectin and sodium alginate. Carbopol is also discussed under this classification.

Carbowax Polyethylene Glycol Compounds— The trade name "Carbowax" is applied to the waxlike, solid polyethylene glycols having a molecular weight above 1000. Structurally, they have the general formula $HOCH_2(CH_2OCH_2)_xCH_2OH$. They are water-soluble, nonvolatile, unctuous compounds, and this feature, combined with their inertness and ability to form an emollient base, recommends them as major ingredients in washable vehicles. They do not hydrolyze or deteriorate and they will not support mold growth.[99]

Patch tests have proved that these compounds are innocuous, being closely comparable in skin irritation to other products commonly used in ointments and cosmetics.[100] Extensive clinical tests on patients have further substantiated their low incidence of sensitization. Studies have shown[101] no evidence of irritation from a base containing 50% polyethylene glycol when applied to either the normal or the diseased skin of 86 clinical dermatologic patients.

Polyethylene glycol compounds 1500, 1540, 4000, and 6000 are of interest in ointment and lotion formulations. Polyethylene glycol 1500 is a soft waxy solid, similar in consistency to petrolatum, with a melting point 40° to 45°. Polyethylene glycol 1540 is a solid of the consistency of beeswax and is intermediate in physical properties between the 1500 and 4000 glycols. Polyethylene glycol 4000 with a melting point of 50° to 55° is most useful as a component of ointment bases for, in addition to the general property of being an emulsifying and dispersing agent, it also adds to the consistency of the base. Both the 4000 and 6000 compounds are nonhygroscopic. Polyethylene glycol 6000, a hard, translucent, waxy solid, has a melting point of 58° to 62°.

Polyethylene glycol 1500, as such, can be used as a vehicle for the topical application of medicinal substances. However, it is generally desirable to use one of the higher molecular weight compounds blended with one of the lower molecular weight (200 to 700) liquid polyethylene glycols for ointment formulation.

Polyethylene Glycol Ointment USP

Polyethylene Glycol 4000	500 Gm
Polyethylene Glycol 400	600 Gm

Heat the two ingredients on a water bath to 65°. Allow to cool and stir until congealed. If a firmer preparation is desired, replace up to 100 Gm of the polyethylene glycol 400 with an equal amount of polyethylene glycol 4000.

Note—If 6–25% of an aqueous solution is to be incorporated in polyethylene glycol ointment, replace 50 Gm of the polyethylene glycol 4000 with an equal amount of stearyl alcohol.

Polyethylene glycol ointment is completely water soluble and nonstaining to bed linens and clothing. If a firmer preparation is desired not more than 100 Gm. of Polyethylene Glycol 400 may be replaced by an equal amount of Polyethylene Glycol 4000. The high degree of solubility of Polyethylene Glycol Ointment precludes the addition of aqueous solutions in excess of 5–8% of the total formula. As noted in the monograph above, stearyl alcohol may be substituted for a portion of polyethylene glycol 4000 when it is desired to incorporate larger amounts of aqueous solutions.

On patients with normal skin and with dermatitis, greater absorption of an insoluble dye (phenolsulfonphthalein) occurred when the dye was incorporated in P.E.G. Ointment USP XIV than from an oleaginous base.[102] The absorption of the insoluble dye was greater through an inflamed or oozing surface than through the normal intact skin. This increase in absorption may range to as high as 12 times greater absorption from the water-soluble base in eczematous skin than from the oleaginous vehicle on normal skin.

However, this marked increase in absorption may not occur with all medicaments incorporated in a water-soluble base. Penetration and absorption are not wholly dependent upon the vehicle. The solubility of the medicament and the condition of the skin may markedly alter the degree of penetration and absorption. According to Shelmire[103] and Wurster,[104] the hydration of the stratum corneum is one of the most important factors in the penetration of skin by a medicament. Therefore, vehicles containing water available for hydration of the horny layer would seem to be desirable. Conversely, vehicles such as Polyethylene Glycol Ointment, which are anhydrous and nonocclusive and also tend to dehydrate the stratum corneum, would decrease percutaneous absorption. This may be desirable where a relatively high surface concentration of drug with little percutaneous absorption is required.

Polyethylene glycol can be incorporated as a component of emulsified bases.[105,106] It has an adjuvant action as an emulsifier and improves the factor of water removability of the emulsion.

The addition of an ester of polyethylene glycol to any of the polyethylene glycol ointments yields a water-removable, emulsifiable ointment base which requires no other levigating agent for the incorporation of different types of drugs.[107] The formula can be represented as:

Emulsifiable Glycol Ointment Base (Base G)

Polyethylene Glycol 400 Monostearate	26.0 Gm
Polyethylene Glycol 400	37.0 Gm
Polyethylene Glycol 4000	37.0 Gm

Mix and melt the glycols at about 65°C. Then stir while cooling to about 40°C. Melt the polyethylene glycol 400 monostearate at about 40°C, add the liquid to the glycol mixture with stirring until a uniform ointment is obtained.

Base G can also be prepared extemporaneously by levigating the polyethylene glycol 400 monostearate and adding polyethylene glycol ointment to it.

Water (10–15%) can be incorporated in Base G.

Surfactants and water can be added to a polyethylene glycol ointment without impairing the water removability of the base. Base III represents a typical formula of this type.

Base III[101]
(Hydrous)

Polyethylene Glycol 4000	50.0 Gm
Polyethylene Glycol 400	40.0 Gm
Sorbitan Monopalmitate*	1.0 Gm
Water	9.0 Gm

Warm the sorbitan monopalmitate and the polyethylene glycols together on a water bath to 70°C and add the water heated to the same temperature. Stir until congealed.

This hydrous base is a glossy, white semi-solid, which has a more cosmetic appearance than the anhydrous bases. It will withstand temperatures of 42°C and gives no indication of appreciable water loss when allowed to stand at room temperature in an open container for several weeks. It is compatible with most of the common therapeutic agents used in ointments such as *zinc oxide, sulfur, coal tar, Peruvian balsam, ammoniated mercury, ichthammol*, etc. Its stability is not markedly impaired by the addition of aqueous solutions up to 10% of the total weight of the product.

The consistency of this base may be altered by changing the ratio of the two polyethylene glycols. For example, if the 50:40 ratio represented in the formula is changed to a 56:34, the resulting product is more firm and consequently tolerates the addition of a larger quantity of liquid medicament or medicinal solution. On the other hand, a vehicle less firm in consistency and particularly suitable for the incorporation of insoluble powders can be prepared by increasing the proportion of the liquid polyethylene glycol with a corresponding reduction of the solid.

Sorbitan monopalmitate which appears in this formula as an emulsifying agent is a nonionic, surface-active agent, and hence has a low index of sensitization. Two other emulsified bases in which polyethylene glycol is incorporated have the following formulas:

Modified Landon-Zopf Base

Polyethylene Glycol 4000	20.0 Gm
Stearyl Alcohol	34.0 Gm
Glycerin	30.0 Gm
Water	15.0 Gm
Sodium Lauryl Sulfate	1.0 Gm

Heat the polyethylene glycol 4000, stearyl alcohol, and glycerin on a water bath to 75°C. Add in small quantities, with stirring, to the water which contains the sodium lauryl sulfate and has previously been heated to 75°C. Continue with moderate stirring until the base has congealed.

Canadian Formulary Base

Polyethylene Glycol 4000	11.2 Gm
Stearyl Alcohol	20.8 Gm
Glycerin	17.0 Gm
Sodium Lauryl Sulfate	0.6 Gm
Water	50.4 Gm

Heat the polyethylene glycol 4000, stearyl alcohol, and glycerin on a water bath to 70°C. Add the water which contains the sodium lauryl sulfate and has previously been heated to 70°C and stir until the base congeals.

Base IV[108]

Polyethylene Glycol 4000	42.5 Gm
Polyethylene Glycol 400	37.5 Gm
1,2,6-Hexanetriol	20.0 Gm

Heat polyethylene glycol 4000 with the 1,2,6-hexanetriol on a water

---

* Span 40 (*Atlas*).

bath at 60 to 70°. Add this melt to polyethylene glycol 400 at room temperature with vigorous stirring. Stir occasionally until solidification takes place. The melting point of this base is 51.7°.

This modified base is compatible with all important ointment ingredients. The solvent power of the 1, 2, 6-hexanetriol increases the compatibility of polyethylene glycols with drugs and improves the stability of the ointments.

The solubilizing effect of certain medicaments such as salicylic acid, benzoic acid, and phenol on P.E.G. Ointment is probably due to the interaction between these medicaments and the high molecular weight polyethylene glycols.[109] The preservative for ointments containing the high molecular weight polyethylene glycols must be carefully chosen since both methyl and propyl *p*-hydroxybenzoate, commonly used as preservatives in dermatologic formulations, have been shown to interact with polyethylene glycols 4000 and 6000.[110] Also, several cases of paraben sensitivity have been reported[111,112] among patients with chronic dermatitis.

Pectin NF—Pectin (page 811) is a carbohydrate product obtained from the inner rind of citrus fruit or apple pomace. Pectins are water-soluble colloids which form a gel capable of absorbing large quantities of water.

Pectin is usually referred to by a grade number. This number corresponds to the number of pounds of sugar required to form a satisfactory jelly with 1 lb of pectin. Fantus and co-workers[113] found that pectin products gave phenomenal results in the treatment of bedsores and stubborn ulcers. Evans[114] suggests the use of pectin base as a vehicle for tannic acid and sulfadiazine preparations. The NF IX contained two pectin products under the title of Pectin Paste and Thin Pectin Paste. Benzoic acid was used as the preservative.

Glyceryl Monostearate NF (page 1353)—Glyceryl monostearate is one of the polyhydric alcohol esters which have been widely used in cosmetic and ointment bases. The name is somewhat misleading as the commercial emulsifiers under this heading are mixtures of the mono- and diglyceryl esters of stearic acid. It is not, as has been so frequently stated, an emulsifying agent for the production of O/W emulsions since glyceryl monostearate is oil soluble and favors the formation of water-in-oil emulsions. Combinations of it, however, with soaps or sapamine salts are used to form oil-in-water emulsions. Glyceryl monostearate, like the stearates of many other alcohols, has the desirable property of a high melting point (56° to 58°C) and serves as a good emulsifying agent. The glyceryl monostearate emulsions generally contain rather high water phases, usually above 60%. Fiero and Dutcher employed 45 different polyhydric alcohol esters and found glyceryl monostearate to be among those producing superior ointment bases. It has the disadvantage of being incompatible with acidic substances.

There are three types of glyceryl monostearate:

1. *Glyceryl Monostearate NF, nonemulsifying* (page 1353). This is useful as a stabilizing and thickening agent in conjunction with other emulsion constituents.

2. *Glyceryl Monostearate, self-emulsifying.* This product is most commonly used for the production of creams and lotions. It is admixed with soap (usually sodium stearate), which imparts the self-emulsifying properties to it. It is incompatible with acids, alkalies, and electrolytes.

3. *Glyceryl Monostearate, acid-emulsifying.* This product consists of the ester plus an auxiliary emulsifier not destroyed by acids or electrolytes.

Glyceryl Monostearate Base

Mineral Oil	10.0 Gm
White Petrolatum	30.0 Gm
Glyceryl Monostearate S. E.	10.0 Gm
Cetyl Alcohol	5.0 Gm
Glycerin	5.0 Gm
Water	40.0 Gm

Cellulose Derivatives—Certain derivatives of cellulose such as methylcellulose [Methocel (*Dow*)] and hydroxyethyl cellulose [Cellosize (*Union Carbide*)] form colloidal solutions which in many respects resemble the gums and mucilages but are not as vulnerable to fungal or bacterial attack. Methylcellulose is dispersible in cold water. Heating will produce coagulation in rather concentrated solutions. Hydroxyethyl cellulose is more soluble at elevated temperatures so that the viscosity of aqueous solution decreases slightly on warming. It is a good protective colloid for aqueous dispersions of oils, waxes, and pigments.

Pharmaceuticals containing relatively high concentrations of methylcellulose, such as water-soluble ointments, jellies, etc, will frequently form stiff gels at slightly elevated temperatures. This may make it difficult to extrude such products from a tube.

A number of different grades of methylcellulose are now available which have a higher gel point than plain methylcellulose. These compounds are hydroxypropyl-methylcelluloses and are designated as Methocel 60 HG, Methocel 65 HG, Methocel 70 HG, and Methocel 90 HG.[115] The number refers to the approximate gel point of a 2% solution in degrees centigrade.

Lubricating Jelly[116]

Methocel 90 HC 4000	1.0 Gm
Carbopol 934[117]	0.3 Gm
Sodium Hydroxide qs pH 7.0	
Propylene Glycol	20.0 ml
Methylparaben	0.15 Gm
Purified Water, qs	100.0 ml

Add the Methocel slowly to 40 ml of hot water (80–90°) and agitate for 5 minutes. After cooling, store the solution overnight in a refrigerator. Dissolve the Carbopol 934 in 20 ml of water. Add a 1% sodium hydroxide solution slowly with cautious stirring to avoid incorporation of air. Add sufficient sodium hydroxide solution to adjust the pH to 7.0 (about 12 ml are required) and then water to make a total volume of 40 ml. Dissolve the methylparaben in the propylene glycol. Mix the Methocel, Carbopol, and methylparaben solutions using caution to avoid the incorporation of air.

Sodium Carboxymethyl Cellulose is the correct chemical name for another cellulose derivative but because of the awkward length of the name it is frequently referred to as *carboxymethyl cellulose* or *CMC*. It is an anionic compound and therefore can be used as a thickening or stabilizing agent for suspensions and for ointments of the emulsion type where the emulsifying agent is of the anionic or nonionic type. Any of these cellulose derivatives can be used to stabilize ointment formulas but it is important to remember that they are commercially available in various viscosity types and with various degrees of substitution.[118]

Sodium Alginate NF (page 1346).—This is a hydrophilic colloid which is compatible with small amounts of alcohol, glycerin, polyglycols, wetting agents, and solutions of alkali carbonates. It functions satisfactorily under acid or alkaline conditions within the pH range of 4.5–10. It is possible to make sodium alginate solutions into semi- or firm gels by the addition of small amounts of soluble calcium salts, ie, calcium gluconate, calcium tartrate, and calcium citrate. Ions of the alkaline earth metals and the various heavy metals will thicken or gelatinize sodium alginate solutions when present in low concentrations, while in high concentrations they will precipitate them. A 2.5% solution of sodium alginate is a satisfactory inert diluent for greaseless and other type ointments.

Huston and associates[119] experimented with several substances to obtain a satisfactory jelly base which would be stable, water-soluble, and compatible with a large number of medicaments. A base prepared according to the following formula was found compatible with sulfathiazole, Phemerol, Metaphen, ichthammol, phenol, boric acid, benzalkonium chloride, and Merthiolate:

Universal O/W Ointment Base

Calcium Citrate	0.05 Gm
Sodium Alginate	3.00 Gm
Methylparaben	0.20 Gm
Glycerin	45.00 Gm
Distilled Water, sufficient,	
To make	100.00 Gm

Dissolve the calcium citrate and the methylparaben in the water. Mix the glycerin with the sodium alginate to form a smooth paste. Add the aqueous mixture to this and stir until a smooth, stiff preparation is obtained. Set aside for several hours until thickening is complete.

This base has been found to be stable for over a year at room temperature both as the base and as the medicated jelly. It can be sterilized by autoclaving and has a pH of 6.3.

The propylene glycol ester of alginic acid [Kelcoloid (*Kelco*)] is a water-soluble colloid which may be used in aqueous solutions or ointments in which the pH is below 7. It is compatible with rather high concentrations of phenol and organic acids such as acetic, citric, and tartaric. It is also compatible with materials such as starches, natural and synthetic gums, oils, fats and waxes, various glycols, and other synthetic organic substances currently employed in the emulsion type and water-soluble lotions and ointments. In concentrations of 1 to 3% it may be employed as a bodying agent and thickener in ointments and creams.

Bentonite USP (page 1345)—Bentonite, a colloidal hydrated aluminum silicate, is insoluble in water but when mixed with 8 to 10 parts of water it swells to produce a slightly alkaline gel resembling petrolatum. The consistency of the product may be regulated by varying the amounts of water added. Ointments prepared from bentonite and water alone are found to be slightly drying and unstable on standing. Addition of a humectant (glycerin, sorbitol, etc) in amounts up to 10% will retard this action. Ointments prepared from bentonite do not encourage mold growth. They have the advantage of not spreading to the hair when applied to the scalp.

Hollander and McClanahan[120] describe a hydrophilic base containing bentonite for which they claim therapeutic value when used alone and which is compatible with a wide range of drugs.

Hollander and McClanahan Base

Petrolatum	32.0 Gm
Bentonite	13.0 Gm
Sodium Lauryl Sulfate	0.5 Gm
Water	54.0 Gm
Methylparaben	0.1 Gm

Allergic reactions to this base are said to be rare. Petrolatum is included in the base to prevent the formation of a hard-dry crust which cracks and shrinks causing friction dermatitis, as is the case with bentonite gels alone.

Darlington and Guth[121] report that the pH of bentonite bases may be adjusted by means of buffer mixtures and the buffering effect is less transient in the acid range. The *in vitro* activity of ammoniated mercury was enhanced by incorporation in acid-buffered bentonite bases. They point out that a desirable property of bentonite is its avid sorption for other substances, both organic and inorganic. They believe the activity of medicinals to be increased by combination with bentonite because they are carried on many microscopic particles. This encourages adherence and penetration of medicinals when applied in the form of ointments or creams.

Barr and Guth[122] prepared six bentonite ointment bases using five cation-saturated bentonites (Na, K, Ca, Mg, and H bentonites) and Volclay bentonite (which contains all 5 cations) as major constituents of the bases. Anti-infective ointments were then prepared using these various bentonite bases as vehicles. These ointments showed greater antibacterial activity, *in vitro*, than their respective USP and NF ointments. Sulfathiazole, phenol, and ammoniated mercury showed greater activity when incorporated in an H bentonite base than when these drugs were incorporated into the other bentonite bases.

Colloidal Magnesium Aluminum Silicate*—This is an inorganic emulsifier, suspending agent, and thickener. It is derived from a naturally occurring mineral base by a refining process. Veegum dispersions are slightly alkaline and are compatible with about 20 to 30% of ethyl alcohol, isopropyl alcohol, acetone, and similar solvents. Glycols such as glycerin and propylene glycol are compatible at 40 to 50% concentration. The viscosity of Veegum suspensions increases with age and elevated temperatures. One to 4% has been successfully employed for the stabilizing of lotions and creams.

M.G.H. Ointment Base†

Polyethylene Glycol 200 Monostearate	15.0 Gm
Veegum	2.5 Gm
Polysorbate 80	1.0 Gm
Methylparaben	0.1 Gm
Water, Purified	81.4 ml

Lotion Vehicle[123]

Veegum	1.0 Gm
Sodium Carboxymethylcellulose (med. visc.)	0.85 Gm
Water	90.15 ml
Glycerin	3.0 Gm
Dioctyl Sodium Sulfosuccinate (1% solution)	5.0 Gm

Mix all dry materials with water and glycerin in a Waring blender for one minute. Remove from blender and add the dioctyl sodium sulfosuccinate.

The properties of clays and their uses in pharmaceutical systems are discussed by Barr.[124]

Carbopol 934[117]—This is a fluffy, white, free-flowing acid polymer which disperses readily in water to yield an acid solution of low viscosity. When the acid solution is neutralized with a suitable base (sodium bicarbonate, sodium hydroxide, etc), a clear, stable gel results. Carbopol 934 is inert physiologically and is neither a primary irritant nor a sensitizer.

The thickening efficiency of Carbopol 934 can be employed in the preparation of such pharmaceuticals as creams, ointments, lotions, suspensions, and emul-

---

* Veegum (*Vanderbilt*).
† Massachusetts General Hospital Formulary.

sions.[125] In using Carbopol 934, the polymer should first be added slowly to water using moderate to high speed agitation and then neutralized to form the final gel.

Carbopol 934 exhibits excellent compatibility with materials frequently incorporated in pharmaceutical formulations. Soluble salts, both monovalent and polyvalent, cause a decrease in viscosity of Carbopol 934 mucilages.

The following formulas[126] illustrate the use of Carbopol 934 in a cold cream and a hand lotion formula.

Cold Cream

Spermaceti	6.0	Gm
Beeswax	6.0	Gm
Carbopol 934	10.0	Gm
Sodium Carbonate	4.75	Gm
Rose Water	5.0	ml
Rose Oil	0.02	ml
Expressed Almond Oil	56.0	Gm
Distilled Water	20.0	ml

Hand Lotion

Propylene Glycol	24.75	ml
Triethanolamine	1.0	ml
Water	12.0	ml
Oleic Acid	1.5	Gm
Polyethylene Glycol 400 Monostearate	10.5	Gm
Silicone Fluid, D.C. 200	10.0	ml
Carbopol 934, 2% mucilage	50.0	Gm

Sulfated hydrogenated castor oil (or SHCO) is a semisolid, water-dispersible substance which was used alone as an ointment base or as an ingredient of hydrophilic emulsion bases. It was official in NF IX and is seldom used in dermatologic preparations.

Preparation of Ointments

Ointments are prepared by two general methods: (1) mechanical incorporation and (2) fusion. The choice of method depends upon the medicament and the physical properties of the constituents of the base.

Preparation by Incorporation—Mechanical incorporation performed by trituration in a mortar, or on a glass slab with a spatula, is more frequently used by the pharmacist than any other method. The medicaments being incorporated into a base are frequently insoluble in the base and it is necessary, therefore, to reduce them to an impalpable powder. The fineness of powder cannot be overemphasized. Best results can be obtained by using a small portion of the base and gradually incorporating the powder to form a very smooth nucleus which can then be incorporated with less effort with the remainder of the base and with the assurance of a smooth homogeneous ointment.

It may be advantageous to use a small amount (approximately 5%) of an oil or an oil-miscible substance as a levigating agent when preparing oleaginous ointments. Generally, the base itself can be used as the levigating agent. The use of glycerin, propylene glycol, mineral oil, etc as levigating agents may yield a product that is too soft. When large amounts of powders such as starch and zinc oxide are to be incorporated into White Petrolatum to make a paste, a portion of the petrolatum can be melted and used as the levigating agent.

Water-soluble salts such as alkaloidal salts can be dissolved in a small volume of water before being incorporated in an ointment base. If the base is oleaginous, the aqueous solution can be incorporated in an equal weight of anhydrous lanolin before being incorporated in the base.

Some of the more polar constituents in ichthammol and in Peru balsam tend to "bleed out" or separate from nonpolar ointment bases such as petrolatum or White Ointment. These constituents can be solubilized in the oleaginous base by mixing the Peru balsam or ichthammol with an equal weight of castor oil or anhydrous lanolin before incorporating them in the base.

Ointment Slab—The preparation of ointments by this method requires a ground-glass plate and two 5- or 6-in. full blade stainless steel spatulas. Hard rubber or tested plastic spatulas should be used when there is a possibility of a reaction between the steel spatula and the constituents of an ointment, such as the incorporation of mercury salts and iodine. In preparing an ointment by this technique the spatula should be held so that it acts as a roller passing over any particles in the ointment. A slight twist of the wrist is required at the end of each stroke in order to reverse the position of the spatula, a technique quickly mastered with a little practice. It is a matter of convenience to use two spatulas, one for the actual mechanics of levigating, the other as an instrument to remove stubborn, adhering particles or accumulating ointment from the manipulating spatula. Slightly warming the base sufficiently to soften it expedites the operation of incorporating insoluble powders, and where soluble materials are used hastens the procedure. The pharmacist should avoid overheating emulsified water-containing bases as this results in water loss which in turn alters the consistency of the base, and increases the percentage of medicinal substance accordingly.

Mortar and Pestle—Mortars are preferred by some pharmacists for the preparation of all ointments although generally this method is used when a liquid is to be incorporated or where the quantity of finished ointment is not conducive to good manipulation on a slab. The use of a mortar and pestle is preferred when incorporating substances with a water-containing base since the percentage of ointment exposed to the air is much less by this method, and the possibility of water loss by evaporation, due either to friction or thinness of film, is reduced.

It seems superfluous to mention that ointments should be thoroughly levigated, must be free of gritty particles, and possess an unctuous feel and "slip" as well as possess the additive factor of pharmaceutical elegance. In no other type of pharmaceutical preparation is the pharmacist's professional skill, exactness, and manual dexterity so vividly revealed.

Mechanical Mixers—When ointments are prepared in lots of 5 lb or more it is desirable to use a mechanical mixer. The ordinary laboratory type of electric mixer will serve for the 1- to 5-lb quantities. The use of larger mixers, such as the Hobart and change-can mixers shown in Figs. 618 and 619, is desirable for lots of 25 lb or more. Thorough mechanical agitation of ointments insures a uniform distribution of medicinal substances. Ointments prepared in large amounts and particularly those containing gritty particles are passed through a mill to insure further uniformity and absolute smoothness. The most common ointment

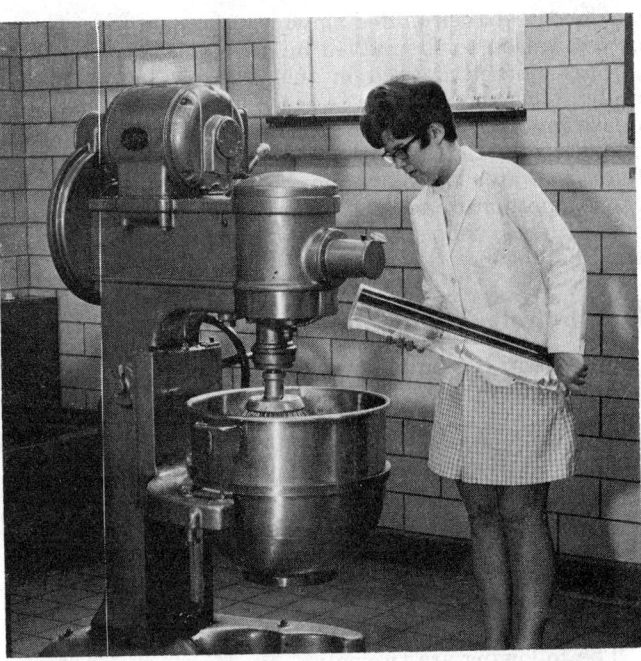

Fig. 618. Adding water to an ointment base in a Hobart mixer (courtesy, University of Iowa).

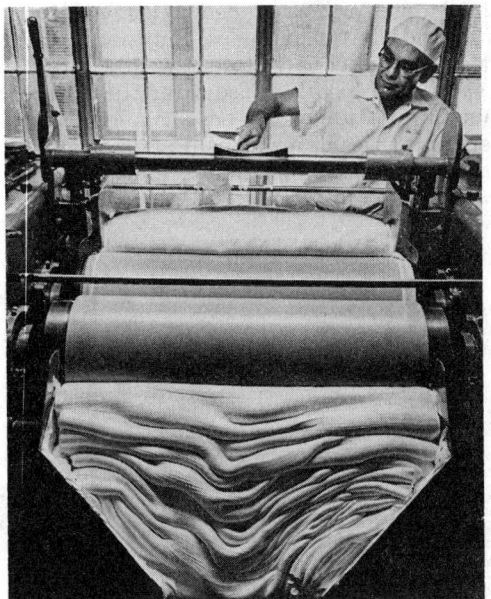

Fig. 620. Processing an ointment through a roller mill to insure a smooth, homogeneous product. The rollers may be water cooled so that melted material introduced as a liquid will emerge as an ointment (courtesy, Lilly).

mill is made on the principle of a paint mill used in reducing pigments in oils. They are available with water-cooled jackets which reduce the heating of the plates due to friction and the subsequent melting of the ointments during this operation. An example of this type of mill is shown in Fig. 620.

The roller mill with its variable speed rollers, is faster than the paint mill type and enjoys considerable use. Laboratory-size roller mills (Fig. 621) are useful for processing small batches of ointment.

In large-scale manufacturing the fine powders are generally sifted into the melted or softened base and stirred slowly until congealed. In some commercial

laboratories a concentrate of the powder and a portion of the base is prepared which is run through the mill several times and then thoroughly incorporated with the remainder of the base without further milling.

Preparation by Fusion—When wax, spermaceti, or other hard, fusible bodies are to be incorporated with soft, oleaginous materials, they are melted on a water bath to avoid excessive temperatures, beginning with the material possessing the highest fusion point and adding the other ingredients in order of decreasing values, until the softer oleaginous and perhaps liquid ingredients have all been thoroughly incorporated by stirring. The ointment should be stirred until it con-

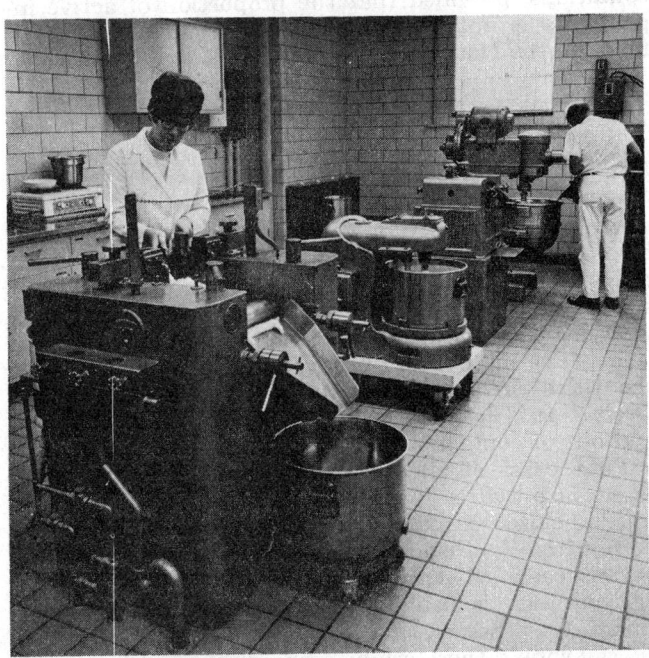

Fig. 619. Dermatologic manufacturing equipment. *Left to right:* Kent 3-roller mill, Day change-can mixer, Kent roller mill, and Hobart mixer (courtesy, University of Iowa).

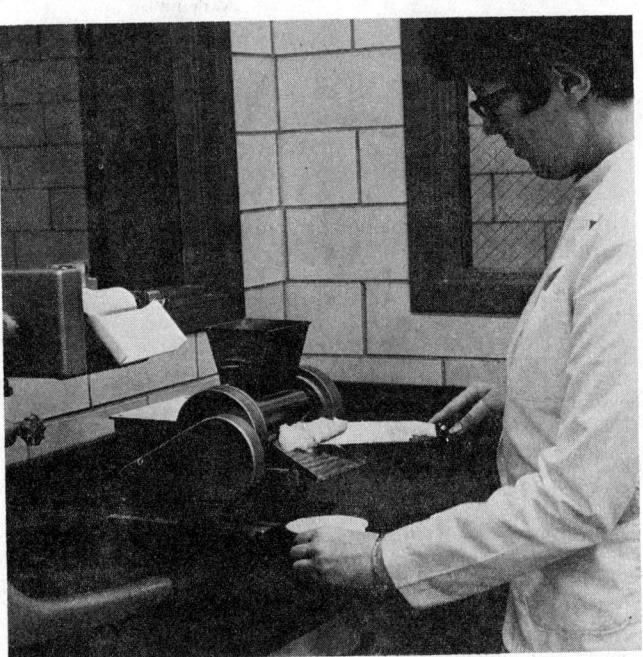

Fig. 621. Milling a small batch of ointment with an ASRA roller mill. To the left is an Erweka 3-roller mill with a detachable motor unit (courtesy, University of Iowa).

geals to insure a homogeneous preparation. It is recommended that stirring be continued until a uniform, thick product is obtained. Powdered medicaments should be incorporated after the base congeals, using a small portion of the base as a levigating agent. If larger quantities of aqueous liquids are to be incorporated with melted oleaginous materials, as in the preparation of Cold Cream USP, the liquid should be warmed and then added slowly with constant stirring or trituration to the melted mixture.

This method is used in the preparation of Hydrophilic Ointment USP. Where there is an aqueous phase involved it is advisable to keep the temperature of both this and the oleaginous phase at a minimum to avoid water loss by evaporation but not so low as to cause a premature separation or congealing of any of the constituents, thus interfering with the formation of a good emulsion.

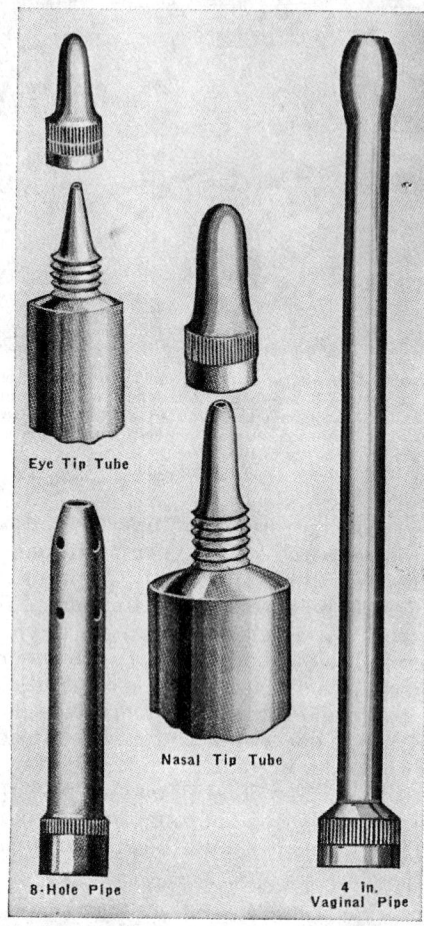

Fig. 622.   Special tips for ointment tubes (actual size).

Ophthalmic Ointments

Ointments for application to the eyelids should be prepared from specially selected and finely powdered chemicals.

The ointment vehicles should also be of the finest quality and the ointments should be dispensed in 1- or 2-dram collapsible tinplated tubes, fitted with a pointed nozzle (Fig. 622).

A number of ointments are regularly prescribed for this special use. Most frequently petrolatum, white or yellow ointment, or a bland absorption base is used as the vehicle.

The following are typical:

Atropine Sulfate Ointment, 1%.
Chloramphenicol Ointment, 0.85%.
Dibucaine Ointment, 0.5%.
Isofluorophate Ointment, 0.025%.
Phenacaine Hydrochloride Ointment, 1 or 2%.
Phenacaine (1%) and Epinephrine (2% of a 1 to 1000 solution of Epinephrine Hydrochloride) Ointment.   Use 10% of wool fat.
Yellow Mercuric Oxide Ointment, 0.5, 1, and 2%.
Sulfacetamide Sodium Ointment, 10%.
Sulfisoxazole Diethanolamine Ointment, 4%.
White's Ointment ⎰ Mercury Bichloride—1 part to 3000.
                ⎱ Sodium Chloride—5 parts to 3000.
Zinc Sulfate Ointment, 0.5%.

Permissible Alteration of Formulas—The US Pharmacopeia authorizes the modification of the official formulas under certain conditions. The statement is as follows: "In preparing *ointments*, the proportions of the substance constituting the base may be varied to maintain a suitable consistence under different climatic conditions, provided that the proportion of active ingredients is not varied." A similar authorization is made in the National Formulary.

Dispensing of Ointments

Maxims—When dispensing ointments, the following points should be observed.

1. They should always be homogeneous, smooth, and free from grittiness.
2. They should never be dispensed if they have the slightest evidence of rancidity or mold.
3. Ointments containing free acid, iodine, mercury, or tannin should not be levigated with a steel spatula because of the chemical action on the metal.
4. In removing the ointment from a stock jar always scrape it from the surface. Digging into the ointment leaves a greater surface exposed, thus increasing the possibility of rancidity, mold, and water loss.
5. Ointments on prescriptions are usually directed by weight; one-half ounce of ointment may or may not fill a "half-ounce jar" completely.
6. Water-containing ointments should be dispensed in moderate amounts in glass containers with good closures.
7. Use a spatula or finishing blade for the sake of appearance and to avoid contact of the ointment with the cap or cap-liner.

Preserving Stocks of Ointments—Ointments which contain animal or vegetable oils may sometimes be preserved from rancidity by the addition of balsamic resins or benzoic acid. The absorption, emulsion, and soluble type ointments are best preserved against mold growth by the addition of esters of *p*-hydroxybenzoic acid. The methyl and propyl esters are official under the titles *Methylparaben* and *Propylparaben*, respectively. It is desirable to keep ointments in a cool place and out of contact with light and air if possible.

Four cases of allergic contact sensitivity to alkyl esters of *p*-hydroxybenzoic acid were detected during routine closed-patch tests on 91 patients with chronic dermatitis.[112] Fisher[127] and Shamberg[111] also reported cases of paraben sensitivity. Sensitivity to one paraben is usually associated with cross-sensitivity to other parabens. Patients with paraben allergy should therefore be advised to avoid using any preparation to which parabens have been added.

Most ointments containing water should not be unduly exposed to the air, since the evaporation of water from these ointments completely changes their character and makes them unusable.

Ointment Containers—Ointment jars are available in clear, opal, amber, and green glass. The clear glass jars are perhaps the least preferable. The modern ointment jars have been standardized as to size and improved from the standpoint of availability of the entire contents. Straight-sided jars are the rule. They are available in standard sizes ½ oz to 8-oz capacity. Composition tops are attractive and with proper liners form a dust-free closure. Opal-like plastic ointment jars which are very light in weight are available in ½-oz to 16-oz capacity.

Filling and Finishing Ointments in Jars—Some skill is required to fill a jar with ointment neatly and deftly by using a spatula. The surface should be slightly lower than the edge of the jar to prevent the lid from touching the ointment. This is accomplished by taking advantage of the flexibility of the blade of a steel spatula. The spatula is forced across the ointment jar resting it on the top of the jar on both sides and at the same time pressing it into the ointment. This operation is repeated several times, turning the jar slightly each time, with the result that the surface is made perfectly smooth and slightly concave, although to all appearances it is straight. Another finish is made by holding a spatula at a slight downward angle, with its tip at the center of the jar and its edge resting on the jar. By slowly rotating the jar in short jerky movements a depression with a cartwheel effect is made which makes a good finish.

Collapsible Tubes—The most desirable container in which to dispense ointments is the collapsible tin tube. An ointment in a jar is frequently exposed to dust and is almost invariably removed from the jar by means of the finger. Both of these conditions are undesirable and unsanitary. In addition, the jar method of dispensing constantly exposes the ointment, over an extended surface, to the action of the air and frequently to the effect of light. Most commercial ointments are supplied in tubes.

For eye ointments, tubes with nozzle-like outlets are obtainable which facilitate the application of the product. Other tubes fitted with special nozzle-like ends permit the dispensing of ointments for application to the nasal passages, to the rectum, or to the vagina (Fig. 622).

In filling the tubes with a soft ointment in prescription work, a method which has given much satisfaction because of its cleanliness, rapidity, and simplicity is as follows: Place the finished ointment in the center of a piece of strong paper of sufficient size (for an ounce of ointment use a sheet about 8 by 10 inches), fold the paper so that the edges meet, with the ointment inside, place a pencil on the top fold, and slowly roll it toward the ointment. This causes the ointment to form into a cylinder, and, when this is of a smaller diameter than the tube, roll it over on the remainder of the paper so as to form a paper tube with the ointment inside. Now slip this into the collapsible tube, always holding the tube by the tip so as not to crush it, and start to fold over the protruding end of the paper tube. When the ointment has thus been forced completely into the metal tube, bring the edges of the tube together by flattening the open end and, with the tube resting upon a firm surface, hold the flattened edges together firmly with the index finger of the left hand and slowly withdraw the paper with the other hand. This leaves the ointment inside and the tube is ready to be closed permanently.

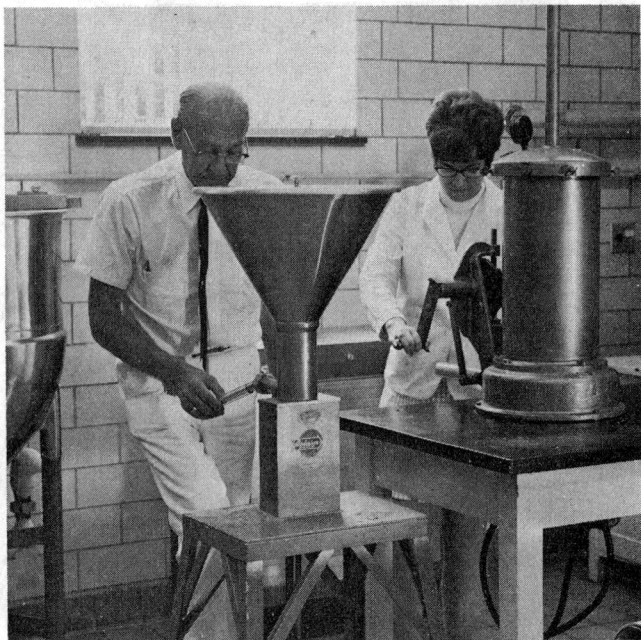

Fig. 623. Filling ointment tubes with the Anderson foot-operated cream and ointment filler (*left*) and the Colton hand filler (*right*) (courtesy, University of Iowa).

It has been suggested that the paper be cut off and left inside the tube, but its withdrawal seems preferable.

A spatula may also be placed firmly against the edges of the open end of the tube with the roll of ointment inside and a steady pull on the paper then forces the ointment neatly into the tube. The cap end of the tube should be open during this process of filling and closing.

In closing a tube, care must be taken to see that it is not filled too full; it should be folded over at least twice.

The capacity of each size of tube can be readily ascertained by a trial with petrolatum and this information may then become a permanent record for the prescription department.

Fig. 623 shows the use of hand- and foot-operated ointment fillers which are useful when a number of tubes are to be filled with the same preparation. Fig. 624 shows a Colton hand-operated tube closer which closes and folds the end of a tube.

Special pliers for closing tubes are obtainable at small

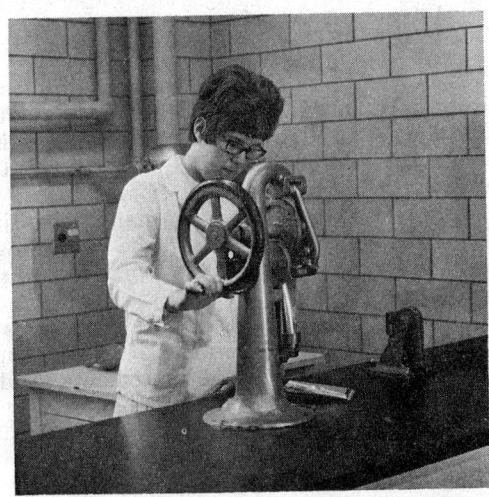

Fig. 624. Closing an ointment tube with a Colton hand-operated tube closure (courtesy, University of Iowa).

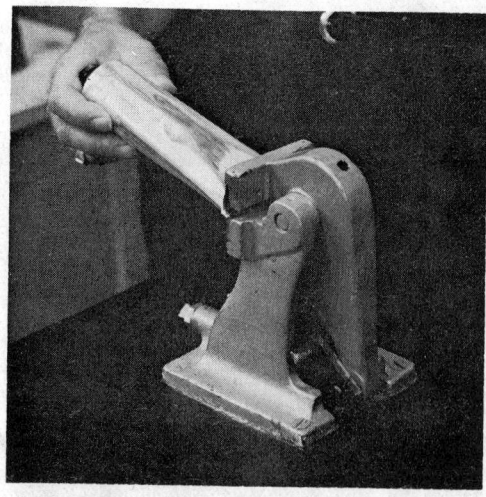

Fig. 625. Placing a metal clip over the folded end of an ointment tube using a foot-operated Colton crimper (courtesy, University of Iowa).

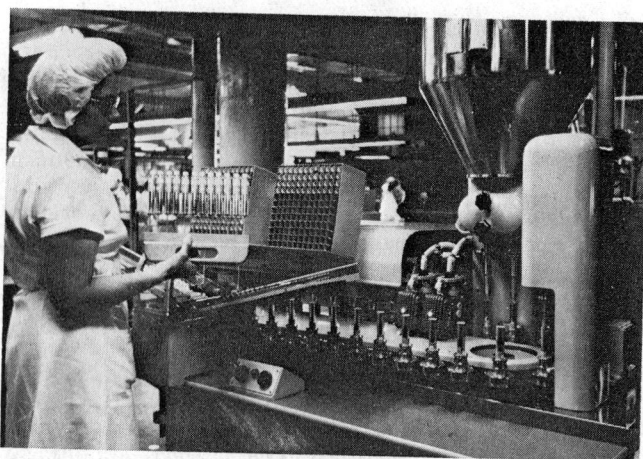

Fig. 626. Feeding prelabeled tubes into a machine which air-cleans and vacuums each tube, fills it with a measured amount of ointment, and crimps the base to seal the tube at a rate of 120 tubes/min (courtesy, Lilly).

cost, but the back of the heavy spatula is quite as effective as the more expensive devices. In using a spatula, hold the filled tube in the left hand on a counter with the open end to the right. Run the blade lightly along the tube to flatten it slightly; when near the end, increase the pressure and, when within a quarter of an inch from the opening, hold the spatula firmly and raise the tube, laying it over upon itself. Repeat this a second time and the tube is closed. A hard metal clip can be clamped over the fold to prevent the contents from being forced from the end when pressure is applied to the tube. These clips are not expensive and may be readily attached with the aid of a small vise, although many forms of machines are also available for the purpose (Fig. 625). On the large scale, tubes are also being sealed after filling by the use of cement or special folding and corrugation so that clips are not needed.

Fig. 626 shows a machine which automatically fills and crimps tubes of various sizes at a rate of 120/min.

Labeling Collapsible Tubes—One difficulty always experienced is in the labeling of the tubes. If the label is to be attached, the tube may be dipped in compound benzoin tincture or in a regular lacquer and afterward allowed to dry. It is always desirable, if labels are applied, to use them in strip form so as to encircle the tube completely and help prevent their coming off. Labels should be attached at the very top of the tube so that they will not be destroyed until the tube is practically empty. Solution of sodium silicate has also been used on tubes to cause the labels to stick. At best, however, labels are not very satisfactory, as the tube is likely to be completely rolled upon itself as the last of the ointment is used and the label soiled or destroyed. Some pharmacists use a pasteboard box to hold the tube and carry the label, while the tube itself is stamped in the tin with the prescription number, using a numbering machine or scratching it upon the shoulder of the tube with a sharp instrument. This will permit the identification of the prescription and its renewal, even if the box is lost. In large-scale operations for substances such as creams, toothpaste, shaving soap, etc, the label is printed or embossed on the tube itself and is thus permanently attached.

Other Medicated Applications

Cataplasms (Poultices)

Poultices are soft, semiliquid, external applications which either stimulate a body surface or alleviate an inflamed area by supplying medicating substances in the presence of heat and moisture. For many centuries they have been made from hot water and linseed meal or other cohesive materials which maintain intimate contact with the skin, at the same time remaining hot and moist; they are one of the oldest of recorded pharmaceutical preparations.

Poultices theoretically tend to draw infectious material from diseased tissues because of the absorptive and hygroscopic character of the ingredients used, eg, kaolin and glycerin. None is now official.

Cements

Cements are dental preparations employed primarily as temporary protective coverings for exposed pulps. They are also used for holding medicinal agents in tooth cavities and for rebasing of dentures. The dentist prepares the cement extemporaneously by mixing together a powder consisting of very finely powdered rosin, zinc oxide, and other metallic salts with a liquid consisting of either eugenol or clove oil mixed with a bland oil. Zinc acetate and other metallic salts accelerate the setting time. The consistency of the cement may be altered by varying the amount of liquid.

Cerates

Cerates are unctuous substances which owe their name to the presence of wax (*cera*). They are of such consistency that they may be easily spread, at ordinary temperatures, upon muslin or similar material with a spatula, and yet not so soft as to liquefy and run when applied to the skin. They are mostly used as dressings for inflamed surfaces, and are generally made with oil, lard, or petrolatum for a basis, with sufficient beeswax to give the desired consistency. Paraffin, spermaceti, and rosin have also been used to raise the melting points of oils and fats in the formulation of Cerates.

Cerates are made by *fusion*. See under *Ointments* (page 1608). The use of this type of preparation is practically obsolete. *Galen's Cerate* (a rose water ointment), is one of the oldest known pharmaceutical preparations, but in consistency it is more like an ointment than a cerate. No preparation is recognized by either the US Pharmacopeia or National Formulary under the title Cerate, although a modification of Galen's Cerate is official in the NF under the title of *Rose Water Ointment* (page 1353).

Contraceptives *

When protection from pregnancy is considered advisable, contraceptives are used to prevent passage of active spermatozoa from the vagina into the uterus. This is accomplished mechanically by occlusive devices, such as diaphragms, which lengthen the route which the spermatozoa must travel to reach the os, thereby assuring extensive exposure to a spermicidal jelly or cream when these are used in conjunction with such devices. Contraceptive jellies and creams act as chemical agents immobilizing the spermatozoa with which they come into contact. They are designed to melt or dissolve and spread without leakage over the entire surface of the vagina, cervix, and exposed surfaces of occlusive devices that may be conjunctively employed. Because of their consistency they also have an obstructive function. Certain accessory devices are used with these, such as inserters and extractors for the diaphragms, and syringe applicators for the jellies and creams. In control of conception acceptability probably plays a greater role in the use and therefore the effectiveness of a prescription than in most fields of medicine. The esthetic block or reluctance towards various methods differs with different users, and variation of method by a single user is often found to lead to greater acceptability and consequently a higher degree of protection.

When contraceptive preparations are prescribed, the physician should warn that there must be strict adherence to his directions. To do otherwise invites decrease in expected effectiveness. No one method can be guaranteed as being 100% effective, although a high degree of protection can be expected if the patient has been properly examined and informed by the physician.

Criteria for Acceptability of Contraceptive Agents, Syringe Applicators, and Nozzles

For guidance in reviewing contraceptive products, the Advisory Committee on Contraceptives of the Council on Drugs of the American Medical Association has proposed the following criteria. These have been adopted by the Council but it should be emphasized that they may be changed from time to time. As the experience of the committee and the Council grows, improvements may appear desirable.

1. The use of the word "contraceptive" need not be limited to materials which will prevent conception on every occasion of use.

2. Evidence shall be furnished that use of the material decreases the incidence of pregnancy. This evidence may be secured in connection with occlusive devices unless the manufacturer's advertising is directed chiefly toward the use of the jelly or cream without such devices. It is desirable that each case reported should be observed for at least 12 months, and that the minimum of 75 patient-years of experience should be reported. If cases are excluded from the series on the basis of their being irregular users, the number excluded and the nature of the evidence justifying their exclusion should be stated.

*The materials presented in this section has been abstracted from issues of *New and Nonofficial Drugs*, American Medical Association, Chicago, Ill., 1962–1964.

3. Evidence shall be submitted that 100 or more couples have used the material on 6 or more occasions without subjective injury.

4. Evidence shall be submitted that 12 or more women have received vaginal applications of the recommended dosage on 21 successive days without subjective irritation or injury and without evidence of physical damage shown on speculum examination by a physician with special experience in this field. Inspection of the vagina once a week should be done as a protection to the patient in case the jelly proves to be irritating.

5. The quantitative formula from which the contraceptive mixture is prepared shall seem to the Advisory Committee to be safe and, presumably, effective.

6. The consistency shall be satisfactory to the committee. It shall not show separation into more liquid and more solid portions visible to the naked eye.

7. Evidence shall be submitted that the consistency is not substantially changed after storage for 12 months at 27°C.

8. The consistency shall be reasonably uniform from batch to batch.

9. The spermicidal time of the contraceptive material as measured by the method of Brown and Gamble (*Human Fertil.*, 5, 97 [Aug.] 1940) with proportions of material, isotonic solution of sodium chloride, and semen of 1:4:5 shall be 30 min or less as measured by the average of 4 or more tests.

10. The use of jellies or creams suggested by the manufacturer need not be limited to use in conjunction with an occlusive device.

11. If a syringe applicator or nozzle is furnished for use in connection with the jelly or cream, it shall be sufficiently translucent to permit the detection of air which might lead to inadequate dosage.

If a perfume is used, a quantitative statement of ingredients is desired.

Criteria for Acceptability of Contraceptive Diaphragms or Caps

1. The advertising and direction of the manufacturer should make it clear that contraceptive diaphragms are intended for use in conjunction with a spermicidal jelly or cream.

2. The manufacturer's advertising must not state or imply that the appropriate diaphragm can be chosen without the aid of a physician.

3. Evidence must be submitted that the diaphragm will last under ordinary conditions of contraceptive use for 12 months or more without perforations or other defects.

4. With each diaphragm should be packed directions warning the user not to expose it to ordinary oils or greases, unless evidence is submitted that the material of which the diaphragm is made is not damaged by these substances.

5. The design shall be satisfactory to the committee.

6. The directions packed with each diaphragm shall include instructions to the user to inspect the diaphragm from time to time for holes or tears and discard the diaphragm if one is present.

The planned Parenthood Federation of America[128] offers a very general estimate of the clinical effectiveness of the various contraceptive methods by placing them in the following order:

1. Oral contraceptive medications.
2. Diaphragm or cervical cap with a cream or jelly. Condom.
3. Aerosol foam.
4. Cream or gel designed to be used alone.
   Vaginal tablets.
   Suppositories.
   Sponge and foam.
   Rhythm.
   Coitus interruptus.
5. Douche

Oral Tablets—Certain steroid compounds, usually a mixture of progestogen and estrogen, inhibit conception when taken orally by the female from the 5th through the 24th day of each menstrual cycle.

Contraceptive Capsules and Suppositories— Capsules and suppositories provide a convenient method for introducing obstructive and spermicidal material into the vagina with the advantage of freedom from the need of apparatus. The solid material introduced must be converted to a jelly or liquid form in order to cover the requisite area; hence prompt liquefaction is important. For some suppositories this results from a melting point below the temperature of the body. For others the active material is enclosed in a gelatinous shell which melts or opens when exposed to body temperature and moisture. The time required should be under 10 min, and the users should be instructed to allow this time to elapse before intercourse. A douche should *not* be taken within 6 hr after ejaculation.

To insure further protection, physicians may advise the concurrent use of an occlusive device such as a diaphragm (concerning which see general statement).

Specialties

Lorophyn Suppositories (Eaton)—Suppositories (2 Gm) hermetically sealed in metal foil each containing:

Phenylmercuric acetate	0.02%
Methylparaben	0.1
Methylbenzethonium chloride	0.2
Sorbitan sesquioleate	5.0
20-Dendro palmitic acid	14.68
Polyethylene glycol 1000	80.00%

Contraceptive Jellies and Creams—Jellies and creams for contraceptive use are introduced into the vagina, usually with an occlusive diaphragm or cervical cap, not more than 12 hr before sexual intercourse. When so used, a portion of the dose of jelly or cream may be placed within the vagina and between the occlusive device and the cervix. The jelly or cream is usually inserted by a special plunger-type of device. The remainder of the jelly or cream should then be placed in the cervical area of the vagina adjacent to the occlusive device. Jellies and creams may also be used without an occlusive device, but this may result in a lower degree of protection. Some users find this technique definitely more acceptable, sufficiently so to outweigh the differential in fertility rate. When so used the jelly or cream is introduced into the vagina within an hour before intercourse by a syringe applicator. The recommended dose varies but is usually approximately 5 ml. To allow adequate time for chemical immobilization, the occlusive device should not be removed nor should a douche be taken within 6 hr after ejaculation.

As most of the contraceptive diaphragms are made of rubber, which will deteriorate if exposed to greases, the jellies and creams used should not contain greasy substances.

Applicators are designed for ready filling from the container of contraceptive jelly or cream and for delivery under moderate pressure of the recommended dose (usually 5 ml) into the upper vagina. They should be transparent, to permit detection of air which might lead to inadequate dosage, and, if made of glass, should be sufficiently thick walled to make breaking while in the vagina extremely improbable. The end should be blunt, and sufficiently large to prevent entry into the urethra.

Specialties

Note—The following contraceptive creams and jellies are available with or without applicators. Applicators are usually of transparent plastic designed for ready filling from the container of cream or jelly and for delivery of the recommended dose into the upper vagina.

Contra Creme (*Res. Supplies*)—63.5-Gm collapsible tubes. A stearic acid cream having a pH of 7.3, packaged from the formula:

Phenylmercuric acetate	0.06%
Triethanolamine	0.06
Glycerin	2.50
Glycol monostearate	3.50
Stearic acid	12.00
Water, to	100.00%

Contra Applicator

Cooper Creme (*Whittaker*)—75-Gm collapsible tubes. A white, nongreasy, water-miscible stearate cream having a pH of 7.3 prepared from the formula:

Trioxymethylene	0.04%
Sodium oleate	0.67
Stearic acid	23.04
Trihydroxyethylamine	7.91
Dioctyl sodium sulfosuccinate	0.50
Hydrous aluminum silicate	2.34
Perfume (compounded oil of lavender)	qs
Water, to	100.00%

Cooper Creme Dosimeter.

Delfen Vaginal Cream (*Ortho*)—70-Gm collapsible tubes. Contains 5% nonylphenoxypolyethoxyethanol (spermicidal agent) in an oil-in-water emulsion at pH 4.5.

Delfen Vaginal Foam—20-Gm aerosol with or without applicator.

Emko Vaginal Foam (*Emko*)—30-Gm aerosol with applicator. Contains 8% nonylphenoxypoloxyethylene ethanol and 2% benzethonium chloride.

Immolin Cream-Jel (*Schmid*)—75-Gm collapsible tubes containing 5% methoxypolyoxyethyleneglycol 550 laurate (spermicidal agent) in a cream-jel emulsion base.

Koromex Cream (*Holland-Rantos*)—Collapsible tubes (78 Gm) containing a water-soluble stearic acid emulsion having a pH of 4.2 to 4.4 prepared from the formula:

Stearic acid	20.00%
Cetyl alcohol	1.00
Glycerin	5.00
Boric acid	2.00
Oxyquinoline benzoate	0.02
Phenylmercuric acetate	0.02
Polyoxyalkalene sorbitan monostearate	3.00
Sorbitan monoöleate	5.00
Perfume	0.015
Butyl *p*-hydroxybenzoate	0.02
Water, to	100.00%

Koromex Jelly—Collapsible tubes (85,128, or 142 Gm) containing a water-soluble jelly having a pH of 4.6, prepared from the formula:

Boric acid	2.00%
Oxyquinoline benzoate	0.02
Phenylmercuric acetate	0.02
Glycerin	10.00
Gum acacia	0.60
Tragacanth	2.50
Perfume	0.015
Butyl *p*-hydroxybenzoate	0.02
Water, to	100.00%

Koromex Vaginal Applicator

Lactikol Creme (*Durex*)—Collapsible tubes (56.5, 85, or 116 Gm) containing a water-dispersible cream having a pH of 4.9, prepared from the formula:

Glyceryl monoricinoleate	1.5
Sodium lauryl sulfate	0.6
p-Triisopropylphenoxypolyethoxyethanol	1.25
Sodium chloride	6.0
Glycerin	8.0
Glyceryl monostearate	7.5
Stearic acid	15.0
pH adjusted with lactic acid.	

Lactikol Jelly—Collapsible tubes (62.5, 93.5, or 128 Gm) containing a water-soluble jelly having a pH of 4.15, prepared from the formula:

Glyceryl monoricinoleate	1.0
Sodium lauryl sulfate	0.2
p-Triisopropylphenoxypolyethoxyethanol	1.25
Sodium chloride	6.0
Methyl-*p*-hydroxybenzoate	0.2
Glycerin	5.0
Acacia	1.0
Karaya	1.0
Tragacanth	2.7
pH adjusted with lactic acid.	

Lactikol Metri-Dose Applicator

Lactikol Plunger Applicator

Lanteen Jelly (*Esta*)—Collapsible tubes (42.5 and 85.35 Gm) containing a water-dispersible jelly having a pH of 5.2, prepared from the following formula:

Ricinoleic acid	0.50%
Hexylresorcinol	0.10
Sodium benzoate	0.20
Chlorothymol	0.0077
Tragacanth	1.73
Starch	0.97
Hydrochloric acid	0.043
Calcium hydroxide	0.026
Perfume	0.013
Water, to	100.00%

Lanteen Applicator

Lorophyn Jelly (*Eaton*)—Collapsible tubes (92 Gm) containing a water-soluble jelly having a pH of 7.5, prepared from the formula:

Phenylmercuric acetate	0.05%
Methylparaben	0.05
Polyethylene glycol of monoisooctyl phenyl ether	0.3
Glycerin	8.0
Sodium borate	3.0
Purified Irish Moss	0.72
Tragacanth	1.8
Water, to	100.00%

Lorophyn Jelly Applicator

Lygel Vaginal Applicator

Marvosan Creme (*Tablax*)—Collapsible tubes (70.8 Gm) containing a stearic acid cream having a pH of 7.45, prepared from the formula:

Paraformaldehyde	0.1%
Triethanolamine	1.96
Methylparaben	0.1
Propylparaben	0.1
Propylene glycol	5.4
Glycerin	6.3
Sodium oleate	0.5
Stearic acid	29.8
Perfume	0.07
Water, to	100.00%

Marvosan Applicator

Ortho-Creme (*Ortho*)—78 and 121 Gm collapsible tubes. A non-fatty stearic acid cream having a pH of 6, prepared from the formula:

Stearic acid	24.00%
Cetyl alcohol	0.50
Glycerin	8.00
Ricinoleic acid	0.75
Sodium lauryl sulfate	0.28
Boric acid	2.00
Triethanolamine	0.25
Perfume	0.05
Water, to	100.00%

Ortho-Gynol Vaginal Jelly—85 and 142 Gm collapsible tubes. A water-soluble jelly formed from tragacanth and acacia, having a pH of 4.5, prepared from the formula:

Tragacanth	3.00%
Acacia	0.53
Glycerin	5.00
Boric acid	3.00
Ricinoleic acid	0.75
Propyl ester of parahydroxybenzoic acid	0.05
Oxyquinoline sulfate	0.025
Perfume	0.025
Water, to	100.00%

The consistency is indicated by a 50–55 mm dart penetration at 40°C when tested with the Braun dart penetrometer.

Ortho Vaginal Applicator

Preceptin Vaginal Gel (*Ortho*)—Collapsible tubes (3 oz) containing a spermicidal vaginal gel with ricinoleic acid and p-diisobutyl-phenoxyethoxyethanol in a base of synthetic gel forming agents. Designed for conception control without a diaphragm.

Ramses Vaginal Jelly (*Schmid*)—Tubes (85 and 143 Gm) containing a water-soluble jelly (pH 4.5) prepared from the formula:

Dodecaethylene glycol monolaurate	5.00%
Boric acid	1.00
Alcohol	5.00

Carboxymethylcellulose	2.50
Glycerin	7.00
Butyl parahydroxybenzoate	0.02
Perfume	0.01
Water, to	100.00%

Ramses Vaginal Applicator

Veritas Kreme (*Veritas*)—Collapsible tubes (70.8 ad 134.6 Gm) containing a stearic acid cream having a pH of 7.45, prepared from the formula:

Paraformaldehyde	0.1%
Triethanolamine	1.96
Methylparaben	0.1
Propylparaben	0.1
Propylene glycol	5.4
Glycerin	6.3
Sodium oleate	0.5
Stearic acid	29.8
Perfume	0.07
Water, to	100.00%

Veritas Applicator and Veritas Plunger Applicator

Contraceptive Diaphragms—As diaphragms cannot be designed to form a junction with the vaginal wall or cervix which will prevent the passage of an organism of the size of a spermatozoon, a spermicidal jelly or cream should be prescribed for use with them.

The appropriate size of diaphragm (varying from 50 to 105 mm in diameter) must be chosen for each user. It should be as large as is comfortable, large enough to extend easily over the cervix, anchoring posteriorly in the posterior fornix and anteriorly behind the symphysis. The appropriate size may change after a delivery and during the postpartum months. Satisfactory fitting is not possible in some cases of variant anatomy of the soft parts (this does not refer to bony structure).

The diaphragm and jelly or cream should be inserted before intercourse (not more than 12 hours before) and left in place until 6 hours or more after ejaculation (not more than 36 hours). Rubber diaphragms should not be exposed to fatty substances and should be inspected from time to time for holes or tears.

Specialties

Note—Contraceptive diaphragms are made of latex rubber covering a circular spring. The external diameter usually varies in gradations of 5 mm from 50 to 100 mm.

Cooper Latex Diaphragm (*Whittaker*)
Durex Diaphragm (*Durex*)
Koromex Diaphragm (*Holland-Rantos*)
Lanteen Diaphragm (*Esta*)
Ortho Diaphragm (*Ortho*)
Ramses Diaphragm (*Schmid*)

Contraceptive Diaphragm Inserters—Inserters are designed to stretch the circular spring of a contraceptive diaphragm into a long oval and to furnish a handle with which it may be inserted into the vagina and guided beyond the cervix. To some users they have the esthetic appeal that they minimize digital contact with jelly or cream, or genitals.

Specialties

Durex Diaphragm Introducer (*Durex*)
Ortho Diaphragm Introducer (*Ortho*)
Ramses Diaphragm Introducer (*Schmid*)

Contraceptive Fitting Rings—To enable the physician to test the size of contraceptive devices needed for a given patient, circular coiled springs of the various sizes have been prepared without the thin rubber diaphragm. As these have thick rubber coatings, repeated sterilization by boiling is possible without deterioration.

Durex Fitting Rings (*Durex*)
Ramses Fitting Rings (*Schmid*)

Creams

Both the USP and the NF include preparations under this title. The term cream is most frequently applied to a soft cosmetic type of preparation. Creams of the oil-in-water type include preparations such as foundation creams, hand creams, shaving creams, etc. Creams of the water-in-oil type include cold creams, emollient creams, etc. Pharmaceutically, creams are solid emulsions containing suspensions or solutions of medicinal agents for external application. Generally, preparations of this type should come under the classification of ointments. Specifically they belong to the emulsion type bases. The term cream has also been used in referring to suspensions of medicinal agents for internal use (Bismuth Magma NF).

Dressings

Dressings are external applications resembling ointments in consistency, but remaining semisolid at body temperature; they liquefy at 50 °C and remain pliable in thin films below 28 °C. *Paraffin Dressing*, formerly official in the NF VI, was employed as an air-excluding, soft, pliable, analgesic, splint-like covering for surfaces denuded by burns.

Petrolatum Gauze USP is absorbent gauze saturated with white petrolatum. It is a sterile preparation and may be prepared by adding, under aseptic conditions, molten, sterile, white petrolatum to dry, sterile, absorbent gauze, previously cut to size, in the ratio of 85 Gm of petrolatum to each 20 Gm of gauze. Petrolatum Gauze is employed as a protective.

A *surgical dressing* is any material used as a covering, protective, or support for a diseased part. This class of materials is discussed in Chapter 97 on *Surgical Supplies*.

Glycerogelatins

Glycerogelatins are plastic masses, composed of gelatin, glycerin, water, and a medicament suitable for application in dermatological practice. They are applied by first melting and then painting on the surface with a brush. The temperature at which they are applied should not be so high that it is painful.

General Formula for Glycerogelatins

Glycerinated Gelatin	300 Gm
Glycerin	250 Gm
Distilled Water	350 ml
Medicinal Substance, in fine powder	100 Gm
To make	1000 Gm

Mix the medicinal substance thoroughly with the glycerin (or dissolve it in the glycerin), add the water, and incorporate this mixture with the glycerinated gelatin, previously melted on a water bath. Continue the heat, and stir until a homogeneous mixture is obtained; then pour it into chilled molds, and allow it to congeal. The amount of glycerinated gelatin may be decreased and the amount of glycerin and of water be increased to produce a mass of softer consistency and lower melting point. They may also be made starting with glycerin and granulated gelatin or Pharmagel A or B.

Glycerinated Gelatin

Gelatin	500 Gm
Glycerin	500 Gm
Water, a sufficient quantity	
To make	1000 Gm

Table I—Absorptive Power of Powders

Powder	% ointment strength	% of water absorbed
Zinc oxide	50	2.2
Starch	50	3.3
Magnesium carbonate, "cosmetic"	10	3.6
Talc, purified	30	3.9
Kaolin, heavy	50	4.0
Titanium dioxide	50	4.2
Yeast, dried and powdered	40	4.4
Aluminum stearate	30	4.7

Pour upon the gelatin sufficient distilled water to cover it, allow it to stand for one hour, pour off the water, and allow the gelatin to drain for a few minutes. Then transfer it to a dish, add the glycerin, and heat on a water bath until the gelatin is dissolved. Strain the solution while hot, transfer it to a tared dish, and heat it on a water bath until the product weighs 1000 Gm. When the mass has cooled, cut it into pieces.

The official Zinc Gelatin is a product of this type.

Pastes

Dermatologic pastes are ointment-like preparations employed in the practice of dermatology. They are usually stiffer, less greasy, and more absorptive than ointments due to a higher proportion of powdered ingredients such as starch, zinc oxide, calcium carbonate, and talc in the base. Pastes absorb serous secretions and are preferred for acute lesions having a tendency to ooze. They are less penetrating and less macerating than ointments.

Rae[129] studied the absorptive powers of different powders incorporated in a water-soluble ointment base, using as an index the amount of water absorbed by the ointment in 24 hours through a water-permeable cellulose film. Of special interest to the pharmacist are the data found in Table I.

Plasters

Plasters are substances intended for external application, made of such materials and of such consistency as to adhere to the skin and thereby attach a dressing. The purpose of the plaster is (1) to afford protection and mechanical support, (2) to furnish an occlusive and macerating action and to bring medication into close contact with the surface of the skin.

The base of the older form of plaster was the reaction product of litharge and oil. This was known as *diachylon plaster* (lead oleate plaster), and in a modified form is still employed. This type of mass requires the application of heat in spreading and in applying the plaster to the skin. Such a plaster mass has now been largely supplanted by a plaster made with a base of gum caoutchouc (rubber).

India rubber plaster mass, according to the nature of the plaster and its purpose, is a compound of gums, such as galbanum and olibanum, with waxes, resins, fats, and excipients such as Burgundy pitch, together with proper medication, and absorbent fillers, incorporated to complete the mass. The making of the India rubber plaster mass requires the use of extensive apparatus for the grinding and preparation of the rubber and gums, the mixing of the mass, and the final spreading upon cloth. Plasters are spread on cotton, felt, linen, muslin, silk, "moleskin," and paper. When perforated cloth is used, the product is called a "porous" plaster.

The lead and resin type of plaster mass must be

heated in order that it may adhere to the skin. In contrast, plasters made with an India rubber base are adhesive at the temperature of the body, hence ready for application without further treatment. The plaster mass, while adhesive, can be removed without the disturbance of the skin tissues.

Adhesive plasters consisting of vinyl resin, plasticizers, and other chemical additives have been developed. A vinyl chloride resin base yields an elastic-plastic film backing to the adhesive mass. The newer adhesive masses possess a very low incidence of irritation and excellent ability to remain adhered under severe conditions of moisture, heat, and other environmental factors. In use, this type of elastic-plastic adhesive is resistant to staining from all types of dirt and soil, lubricating greases, vegetable oils, lipstick, catsup, mustard, etc. When soiled, it is easily cleaned by washing with ordinary soap and water. In addition, constant contact with soap and water or water alone, over long periods of time will not adversely affect the plaster, since it is waterproof and water repellent. These newer adhesive plasters are available in colors such as flesh, striped, etc.

Modern plasters are practically all machine made. The official formulas are chiefly intended to serve as standards for manufacturers to insure uniformity of products. The spreading of plasters by the pharmacist was at one time an important service, requiring technical skill and experience. However, today, plaster spreading at the prescription counter is practically unknown. Those interested in it historically will find it discussed in the older textbooks of pharmacy.

Many forms of medicated plasters are still supplied by the manufacturers cut to a size of 5 × 7½ in., with a face cloth and a back cloth made porous. The porosity is considered a mechanical advantage in that it prevents the plaster from slipping from the point of application, each opening serving as a stop. Porous plasters are far more comfortable than the non-porous.

In dispensing plasters made with an India rubber base, the user should be instructed as to the methods of applying, which are, in brief, that the part to which the plaster is to be applied should be dry and clean. This, of course, can be accomplished by the ordinary method with soap and water, or with alcohol or other cleansing agents. Cleansing the skin is important, as it removes the skin coating and allows close contact with the plaster and quick absorption of the medicinal agent. Having applied the plaster, it should be rubbed until it conforms perfectly to the skin. The user should be instructed that if the cloth on the adhesive side of the plaster adheres too closely it can easily be removed by wetting it, in which case the plaster should be wiped dry before applying.

Removing Plasters—The removal of the rubber base plaster can be done easily and simply. The ordinary method is to lift one corner and pull the plaster off with a quick jerk. This is at times painful. A better method is to wet a sponge or a little piece of cotton with ether, benzin, or another suitable solvent, raise one corner of the plaster, squeeze the sponge or cotton, and allow the solvent to trickle between the skin and the plaster. The plaster may then be slowly and gently removed without injury to the skin.

Suppositories

Suppositories are solid dosage forms, usually medicated, for insertion into the rectum, vaginal cavity, or the urethral tract. After insertion they may melt or undergo dissolution in the secretions of the cavity. A variety of shapes and sizes are in actual use (Fig. 627). Suppositories may vary in weight, depending on the quantity of medicament incorporated in the base.

Types

Rectal Suppositories—The USP[130] describes rectal suppositories for adults as follows:

"(They) are tapered at one or both ends and usually weigh about 2 Gm each."

Infant rectal suppositories are usually about one-half the weight of adult suppositories.

About 1% of all new prescriptions written in 1967 were for rectal suppositories.[131] Rectal suppositories and ointments sold o-t-c for the relief of minor pain and itching associated with hemorrhoids account for sales of approximately $20 million a year.

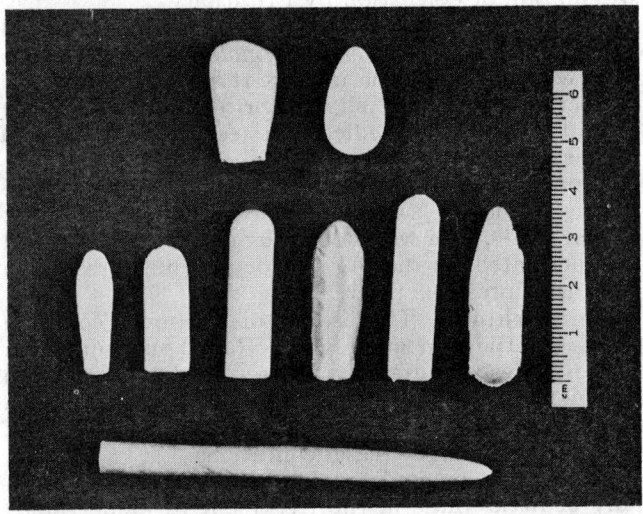

Fig. 627. Shapes and sizes of suppositories. *Top:* vaginal suppository and vaginal tablet; *middle:* infant and adult rectal suppositories; *bottom:* urethral suppository.

Vaginal Medications—The term medications is used rather than suppositories to denote the fact that this group includes vaginal preparations such as tablets or "inserts," creams, douche powders, aerosols, and gels. Vaginal medications account for less than 1% of all new prescriptions written.

The USP[130] describes vaginal suppositories as follows:

"(They) are usually globular or oviform and weigh about 5 Gm each."

Vaginal tablets are specially shaped tablets, made by compression, which generally undergo dissolution in the vaginal cavity. They are usually used in the treatment of *Trichomonas vaginitis.** A plastic inserter is usually supplied with vaginal tablets to enable the patient to place the tablet in the upper region of the vaginal tract.

Urethral Suppositories (Bougies) and Inserts—These are pencil-shaped dosage forms having the following approximate dimensions: diameter (5 mm); length (50 mm, female; 125 mm, male); and weight (2 Gm, female; 4 Gm, male).

Urethral suppositories are rarely prescribed and account for a very small percentage (<0.01%) of new

---

* Flagyl and Floraquin Vaginal Inserts (*Searle*) are examples of such tablets.

prescriptions.   A urethral insert* containing nitro-furazone is still in use.

Medicaments

Common constituents of o-t-c suppositories are those which provide astringent, local anesthetic, anti-pruritic, antiseptic, emollient, and vasoconstrictor effects.   Drugs commonly used are:

Astringents—bismuth salts, zinc oxide, tannic acid
Local Anesthetics—benzocaine, dibucaine, diperodon, tetracaine
Antipruritics—menthol, phenol, local anesthetics
Antiseptics—benzethonium chloride, boric acid, phenylmercuric nitrate, hexachlorophene, phenol
Emollients—cod liver oil, lanolin, castor oil, petrolatum
Vasoconstrictors—ephedrine sulfate

Therapeutic Uses

Suppositories are generally used where a local effect is desired, such as the soothing of surface tissue or the stimulation of defecation by irritation.

Vaginal suppositories and inserts are generally used locally against *Trichomonas vaginalis*, although drugs inserted into the vagina may exert systemic action.[132]

Rectal and urethral suppositories are also used for the introduction of medicaments to be absorbed into the circulatory system.

Suppositories may be particularly important where a drug cannot be tolerated orally, where the patient cannot swallow, or where the drug may be decomposed or inactivated by the pH and/or enzymes present in the gastrointestinal tract.

Hemorrhoids—This is one of the most common diseases of the anorectal region.   Rectal ointments and suppositories are used by the self-medicating public for the relief of minor pain and itching associated with hemorrhoids or for the symptomatic treatment of simple inflammatory rectal conditions.

It should be pointed out that suppositories are probably of little value in the treatment of hemorrhoids since, after insertion in the anus, the suppository slips into the rectum, thus passing the anus, the site of the pain and itching.

A patent[133] was issued in 1962 for suppositories so shaped that they would not be propelled upward or expelled downward after insertion into the anus, thereby presenting their medication to the diseased area.   The suppository is designed with a bulbous head, a stem, and a tail or base which is held at the anal opening, preventing upward propulsion.

Other Anorectal Itching—This can also be caused by parasitic infestation (pinworms), psoriasis, and seborrheic dermatitis of the anorectal region or may follow the use of some of the broad spectrum antibiotics.

Rectal Absorption

Some of the factors affecting drug absorption from rectal suppositories are:

1.   Anorectal physiology
2.   Drug solubility
3.   Drug concentration and particle size
4.   Suppository base (ie, melting point, solubility, and chemical reactivity)

Reigelman and Crowell,[134] Schanker,[135] Schwarz,[136] and others[137,138] discuss the rectal absorption of drugs.

Ano-Rectal Physiology—The terminal portion of the intestinal tract, the rectum, is about 150 mm in

length and terminates in the anus.   When drained of fecal matter the rectum contains a small amount of aqueous fluid with a pH of about 7.2 but of very low buffering capacity.   Thus, the pH of this fluid may be determined by the drug or drugs dissolved in it.   Schanker[135] reported the pH of the colon to be about 6.8, while Kakemi, *et al*,[137] suggest that the rectal absorbing surface has a pH of about 5.4, similar to the pH of the intestine reported by Hogben, *et al*.[139]   Such an acidic zone exists only at the rectal mucosa which separates the lumen from the plasma.   Like the other regions of the intestinal tract, the rectal epithelium is lipoidal in nature; hence, it is preferentially permeable to unionized drugs.   Kakemi, *et al*,[137] studied the absorption of sulfonamides from the rat rectum and found that the absorption rates of the drugs increased, reached a maximum, and then decreased, with increasing pH values.   The absorption rates were maximal at pH's corresponding to the isoelectric points of the sulfonamides, thus indicating that the absorption rate of sulfonamide from the rat rectum depends on the degree of ionization of the drug, being highest for the undissociated form.

The lower, middle, and upper hemorrhoidal veins surround the rectum.   The lower vein (located near the anal sphincter) and the middle vein (which receives blood from the capillary network around the middle region of the rectum) drain directly into the inferior vena cava, thus bypassing the liver.   The upper hemorrhoidal vein passes into the hepatic portal system.   Hence, some of the drug administered rectally bypasses the liver (where drugs may undergo modification in activity).[140]   The amount of drug absorbed directly into the general circulation depends on where the drug is released in the rectum.   If the suppository remains in the lower part of the rectum, a greater proportion of drug will enter the inferior vena cava and general circulation than will enter if the suppository moves to the upper regions of the rectum where the upper hemorrhoidal veins (which lead to the liver) predominate.

Drug Solubility—Allawalla and Riegelman[141] studied the relationship between drug solubility and its release from lipid and water-dispersible bases.   They conclude that a drug which is very soluble in a lipid base, and present in low concentration, will have little tendency to diffuse into the small volume of fluid present in the rectum.   Drugs which are only slightly soluble in the lipid base and present at near saturation levels will readily partition into the aqueous rectal fluid.   Thus, one would expect water-soluble salts like the soluble barbiturates to be readily absorbed from a cocoa butter base.   Therefore, as shown by Riegelman and Crowell,[134] the transport of drug from suppository base to rectal fluid is probably the rate-limiting step in the path of the drug to its site of action.   In the case of water-soluble suppository bases, if one assumes that the base undergoes rapid dissolution in the aqueous rectal fluid, the rate-limiting step in absorption would be the transport of the drug through the rectal mucosa.

Another factor of importance in determining the release of drug from a suppository base to the rectal mucosa is the physical state of the base.   Additional drug is released from a suppository base when the base liquefies or undergoes dissolution in the rectum since, at this point, release is no longer limited to the areas of the solid suppository in contact with the rectal fluid.[142]

Higuchi,[143] in his paper on percutaneous absorption, suggests that the penetration of a drug through the barrier phase (the epidermis of the skin or the mucosa

---

* Furacin Urethral Inserts (*Eaton*).   The base is composed of glyceryl monolaurate and polyoxyethylene-4-monostearate.

of the rectum) is proportional to a permeability constant which quantifies such factors as transfer of drug from base to barrier phase and diffusion of drug through the barrier. The transfer of drug from the base is related to the solubility of the drug in the base, and the diffusion through the barrier is related to the lipid (barrier phase)/water partition coefficient of the drug. Kakemi, et al,[137] calculated the permeability constants for several sulfonamides and correlated them with the absorption velocity constants of the sulfonamides as determined through the rat rectum. They concluded that the rectal absorption of sulfonamides is related to their diffusion through the lipoid barrier in the rectum, which is related to the lipid/water partition coefficient of the drug.

Drug Concentration and Particle Size—Riegelman,[134,141] demonstrated that the diffusion of drug from a suppository base is a function of the drug's concentration as well as its solubility in the base. Since transport across the rectal mucosa is a simple diffusion process, the rate of absorption will increase with drug concentration in the rectal fluid. However, one should keep in mind that the rate is also a function of the drug's degree of ionization and is highest for the undissociated form.

If a drug of limited water solubility is suspended in a suppository base, the particle size of the suspended drug will influence its release to the rectal fluid since the dissolution rate of the drug in the rectal fluid would be proportional to its particle size (Noyes–Whitney equation, pages 1701 and 1714).

Suppository Base—The melting point of a lipid suppository base or the solubility and dissolution rate of a water-soluble base influences the release of the drug and its absorption rate if one relates these physical properties to the solubility of the drug incorporated in the base. A water-soluble drug incorporated in a lipid suppository base will be released readily to the rectal fluid, if the base melts rapidly after insertion in the rectum. If the lipid base does not melt readily at body temperature, the release of drug will be retarded and the onset of action may be delayed. If a water-soluble base does not undergo rapid dissolution in the rectal fluid, the onset of action of any drug incorporated in the base will be slowed. Since the quantity of rectal fluid is very small, water-soluble suppository bases (page 1620) dissolve slowly after insertion in the

rectum. The disintegration times of some polyethylene glycol suppository bases are shown in Table V.

Interactions reported[144,145] between the high-molecular-weight polyethylene glycols and some medicaments may result in a drug complex which differs from the free drug with respect to its ability to penetrate the lipoidal rectal mucosa. Kakemi, et al,[137] reported a reduction in the absorption of some unionized sulfonamides incorporated in various water-soluble suppository bases. They attributed this to a decrease in the polarity of the aqueous phase on the addition of the water-soluble base, which results in a decrease in the lipid/water partition coefficient of the drug.

The addition of surfactants to lipid suppository bases as solubilizers and emulsifiers may affect the rectal absorption of a drug incorporated in the base. Kakemi, et al,[138] studied the effect of various types of surface-active agents on the rectal absorption of sulfisoxazole from cocoa butter, in rabbits. They found that, in general, low concentrations of surface-active agents accelerated drug absorption while high concentrations ($<5\%$) reduce it. The authors suggest that the increase in drug absorption at low concentrations of surface-active agents is due to an acceleration in the release of the drug from the lipid base to the dissolution medium, while the decrease observed at higher concentrations of surface-active agents may be due to entrapment in micelles. Also, surface-active agents may have direct effects on the rectal mucosa similar to those reported by Nissim[146] on the gastrointestinal mucosa.

Rectal Dosage

No fixed rule can be established concerning the relation between the oral and rectal dose of a drug, although one would expect the rectal dose to be at least equal to the oral dose. The assumption that the rectal dose of a drug is double its oral dose is not based on sound therapeutics. The rectal dose depends on the drug, whether it's being used for local or systemic effects, the dissociation characteristics of the drug, the lipid/water partition coefficient of the unionized drug, and the physical and chemical characteristics of the suppository base in which the drug is incorporated.

Vehicles for Suppositories—Three types of sup-

Table II—Suppository Vehicles[a]

Vehicle	Composition	Melting range (°C)	Congealing range (°C)
Lipid vehicles			
Cocoa butter	Triglycerides of oleic, palmitic and stearic acids	30–35	
Cotomar[b]	Partially hydrogenated cottonseed oil	35–39	
Hard butter S-70-XX[c]	Triglycerides	36.5	32
Suppository base G[d]	Branched saturated fatty alcohols (C_{10}–C_{18})	31–39	
Suppositol H, S, T & R[e]	Hydrogenated coconut oil triglyceride	34–38.5	
Wecobee W, R, S, M & FS[f]	Triglycerides derived from coconut and palm kernel oils	31.7–40.5	30–34
Witepsol H12, H15, W35,[g] S55, E75 & ES	Triglycerides of C_{12}–C_{18} fatty acids	32–44	29–34
Water dispersible vehicles			
Polyethylene glycols,[h] 1000, 1540, 4000 & 6000	Linear polymers of ethylene oxide	38–49	
Myrj 52[i]	Polyoxyl 40 Stearate USP	38–43	
Tween 61[i]	Polyethylene-4-sorbitan monostearate	35–39	

[a] For complete names and addresses of the manufacturers of these vehicles, see *Manufacturers Index*, page 2023. [b] *Procter & Gamble*. [c] *Best Foods*. [d] *Carnes* (four bases are available with differing melting ranges). [e] *Fritz Wetz* (four types vary in melting range with H the lowest and R the highest melting products). [f] *Drew* (different types vary in melting range and in narrowness of the melting range). [g] *Riches-Nelson* (different types vary in melting range, but all have a narrow melting range). [h] *Union Carbide* (blends of various polymers are used to formulate suppository bases). [i] *Atlas*.

positories, with respect to the vehicle or base used, are recognized:

1. The first type is prepared with *theobroma oil* or cacao butter (more commonly called cocoa butter) as the diluent and vehicle. Theobroma oil is an ideal vehicle or base for suppositories intended to melt when inserted into the rectum or other body cavities. It is a bland, nonirritating fat, pressed from ground cacao beans, and possessing the remarkable quality of maintaining its firmness, even exceptional hardness for a fatty substance, to within a few degrees of the body temperature, when it readily melts to a liquid, without passing through an appreciable softening stage. The melting point of theobroma oil is from 30° to 35°C (86° to 95°F).

It is rarely necessary to raise the melting point of cacao butter by the addition of wax, spermaceti, etc, except in the warmest summer weather, or when phenol, camphor, chloral hydrate, the volatile oils, or similar substances form the medicating ingredients.

2. The second type is water-soluble or water-miscible. One example is prepared by mixing the aqueous solution or suspension of the medicament with *glycerin* and *gelatin*. This type of suppository does not melt at the body temperature but slowly dissolves in the secretions of the mucous membrane. They are usually employed to provide a continuous medicating or germicidal action. *Polyoxyethylene glycols* and their derivatives are also miscible with the aqueous secretions of the mucous membrane and are ideal for water-soluble substances. Insoluble drugs can be suspended in polyethylene glycol bases.

3. The third type, represented by glycerin suppositories, or soap suppositories shaped from *castile soap*, is not expected to melt or dissolve completely but to perform its function in part mechanically, and in part by dissolving and producing some irritation. Their chief value is as a stimulation to peristalsis, through their presence in the rectum, and they are largely used for small children to avoid the use of a laxative.

A large number of suppository vehicles are used in Europe. Table II lists those used or available in the US. A more complete listing of these vehicles is given by Anschel and Lieberman.[147,148]

Preparation

This class of preparations is usually manufactured on a large scale with the aid of elaborate machinery but the pharmacist is occasionally called upon to prepare them in the pharmacy. Suppositories are prepared by hand rolling, by molding (fusion process), and by cold compression.

Rolled (Hand-made) Suppositories—These represent the simplest process, provided climate or weather conditions make it applicable. In warm countries or in hot summer weather one of the other methods should be used. This process possesses an advantage over the molding process in that no complications arise from the use of heat and no provision need be made for excess material, since the entire mass is divided into the desired number of suppositories.

The following general process may be employed:

General Process

Take the prescribed quantity of the medicinal substances and a sufficient quantity of grated theobroma oil. Reduce the medicating ingredients to a fine powder, or, if composed of extracts, soften with diluted alcohol and rub until a smooth paste is formed; the correct amount of grated theobroma oil is then added, and a mass resembling a pill mass is made by thoroughly incorporating the ingredients with a pestle, sometimes with the aid of a small amount of wool fat. When the mass has become plastic under the vigorous kneading of the pestle, it is quickly loosened from the mortar with a spatula, pressed into a roughly shaped mass in the center of the mortar, and then transferred with the spatula to a piece of filter paper which is kept between the mass and the hands during the kneading and rolling procedure. By quick, rotary movements of the hands, the mass is rolled to a ball which is immediately dropped to a pill tile. Here a suppository cylinder is formed by rolling the mass upon the tile with a flat board, partially aided by the palm of the other hand, if weather conditions permit. The suppository pipe will frequently show a tendency to crack in the center, developing a hollow core. This is due to the fact that the mass has not been kneaded and softened sufficiently, with the result that the pressure of the roller board is not carried uniformly throughout the mass but is exerted primarily upon the surface only.

The length of the cylinder usually corresponds to about four spaces on the pill tile for each suppository, thus making the piece, when cut, practically a finished suppository except for the shaping of the point. When the cylinder has been cut into the proper number of pieces with a spatula, the conical shape is given it by rolling *one end* upon the tile with a spatula, or in some cases even by shaping it with the fingers, so as to produce a rounded point.

With practice, excellent rolled, or handmade, suppositories can be made. This method has the substantial merit of requiring very little apparatus, but considerable skill is needed to produce suppositories equaling in finish those which are molded (Fig. 627). In the various stages described above, the suppository mass may become tacky or sticky. A careful manipulator will be able to prevent this by the manner in which the mass is handled.

Molded Suppositories (Fusion Process)—The capacity of each mold in use at the prescription counter, in terms of theobroma oil, must first be determined. This is done by molding plain theobroma oil and weighing the suppositories. This weight should be recorded and used in calculating the formula for subsequent suppositories. Now calculate the amount of theobroma oil required to make suppositories of the desired weight, taking into consideration the weight of the medication to be incorporated, and

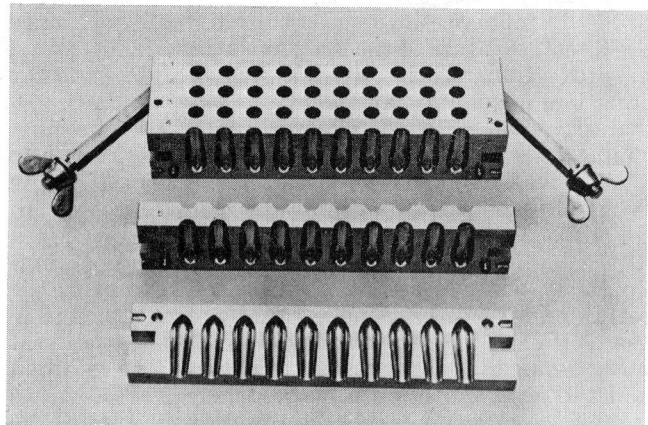

Fig. 628. Rectal suppository mold (courtesy, ChemiPharm).

also planning for enough additional medication and theobroma oil for at least one extra suppository. This is necessary to provide for the waste in pouring the suppositories, some mass always sticking to the dipper and other excess portions being cut from the top of the mold.

Suppository molds are available for the preparation of rectal and vaginal suppositories of various sizes (1–5 Gm) and shapes (torpedo, cylindrical, oval, double cone, etc). Molds are made of aluminum alloy, brass, or are plated. They are available with anywhere from six to several hundred cavities (Fig. 628).

The Density of Medication—If the medicinal substance has a density of approximately that of theobroma oil, the weight of medication may replace an equal weight of the oil. If, however, the medication is heavier, it will replace a proportionally smaller amount of oil.

For instance, tannic acid has a density of 1.6 as compared with theobroma oil. If the suppositories were to carry 0.1 Gm each, a dozen would require 1.2 Gm. This is divided by 1.6, the comparative density of tannic acid, which indicates that 1.2 Gm of tannic acid will replace only 0.85 Gm of theobroma oil, not 1.2 Gm, and proportionally more base must be taken to provide sufficient diluent for 12 suppositories.

It is always possible to determine the density of a medicinal substance, in relation to theobroma oil, if the information is not available, by mixing the amount for one suppository with a little melted oil, pouring it into a suppository mold and carefully filling the mold with plain theobroma oil. The cooled suppository is then weighed and the weight of the medication subtracted from it. This will indicate the amount of

Table III—Density Factors for Theobroma Oil Suppositories[a]

Medication	Factor
Acid, boric	1.5
Acid, benzoic	1.5
Acid, gallic	2.0
Acid, salicylic	1.3
Acid, tannic	1.6
Aloin	1.3
Alum	1.7
Aminophylline	1.1
Aminopyrine	1.3
Barbital	1.2
Belladonna extract	1.3
Bismuth carbonate	4.5
Bismuth salicylate	4.5
Bismuth subgallate	2.7
Bismuth subnitrate	6.0
Borax	2.0
Camphor	2.0
Castor oil	1.0
Chloral hydrate	1.3
Chrysarobin	1.5
Cocaine hydrochloride	1.3
Copper sulfate	2.5
Digitalis leaf	1.6
Eucalyptus oil (minims)[b]	1.0
Galls (powdered)	1.9
Glycerin	1.6
Ichthammol	1.1
Iodoform	4.0
Lead acetate	2.5
Lead iodide	10.0
Menthol	0.7
Morphine hydrochloride	1.6
Opium	1.4
Peruvian Balsam[b]	1.1
Phenol[b]	0.9
Phenyl salicylate[b]	1.0
Podophyllum Resin	1.3
Potassium bromide	2.2
Potassium iodide	4.5
Protein silver	1.6
Paraffin	1.0
Phenobarbital	1.2
Procaine	1.2
Quinine hydrochloride	1.2
Red mercuric iodide	4.0
Reduced iron	12.5
Resorcinol	1.4
Salol[b]	1.0
Santonin	1.3
Sodium bromide	2.3
Spermaceti	1.0
Sulfanilamide	1.7
Sulfathiazole	1.6
Sulfonal	1.5
Sulfur	1.6
White wax	1.0
Witch hazel fluidextract	1.1
Zinc oleate	1.1
Zinc oxide	4.0
Zinc sulfate	2.8

[a] Davis, H., *Bentley's Textbook of Pharmaceutics*, 5th ed, Williams & Wilkins, Baltimore, 1949; Büchi, J., *Pharm. Acta Helv.*, **20**, 403 (1949).
[b] Density adjusted taking into account white wax in mass.

theobroma oil used and from these data the density of the medication can be calculated.

Table III indicates the density, as compared with theobroma oil, of many substances commonly used in suppositories. Some of these factors are only approximate since many chemicals vary somewhat in density with the method of manufacture.

Having finely powdered the medicinal ingredients, if vegetable drugs or chemicals, and having softened extracts when present, weigh the total amount of theobroma oil needed and melt it in a casserole with a gentle heat. Incorporate the medicinal substances intimately with about an equal weight of the melted theobroma oil on an ointment slab, using a spatula and, when uniformly mixed, transfer the uniform mixture to the remainder of the melted theobroma oil, which has been cooled to the correct temperature, which is almost that of the solidifying point. Stir until all is again uniformly melted, avoiding all excess of heat, and pour at once.

Pouring the Mass—The melted mass should be poured into a chilled mold, lightly lubricated with mineral oil or green soap tincture. It should be vigorously stirred with a spatula immediately before the pouring begins: indeed, when heavy powders are directed, the stirring must not cease during the pouring, or the last suppositories will contain a larger proportion of the heavy powder than those which were first made. In pouring, each opening in the mold may be exactly and uniformly filled or the openings may all be overflowed so that the tops run together on the mold. In the latter case allow the mold to stand on the counter until the mass on top has solidified, then cut off the excess with a spatula. The mold is then placed in the freezing compartment of a refrigerator, and when sufficiently hardened the suppository will be found to have contracted slightly so that light pressure on the base of each suppository will cause it to loosen in the mold and readily drop out when the mold is open. If the suppository does not readily drop from the mold after it is opened, apply a quick, firm pressure with the thumb, first to the base, and if this does not free it, try pressing the point. Never apply continued pressure. It will melt the suppository. It is also desirable to cool the thumb, by placing it on the ice for a moment, before giving the quick, firm pressure. The novice almost invariably makes the mistake of opening the divided molds too soon (before the limit of contraction is reached); the suppository sticks to the mold, and splitting ensues.

The beginner often fails when starting with the fusion method due to the use of too much heat. When it is remembered that a theobroma oil suppository mass melts at the temperature of the body and that the least possible heat should be used, the dispenser soon learns to keep entirely away from a direct flame and use only a lukewarm water bath.

Many combinations are decomposed or separated from the base by overheating. This is notably the case with ichthammol, tannic acid, and with the extracts of opium, belladonna, stramonium, etc.

Polymorphism of Theobroma Oil—Theobroma oil, like many triglycerides, exhibits polymorphism.[149] That is to say, it can exist in several crystal forms, each with a different melting point. Polymorphism is much more pronounced in a relatively simple and chemically homogeneous triglyceride like theobroma oil than in more complex mixtures.

The polymorphic character of theobroma oil can cause great difficulty in making suppositories by the fusion method, as can be demonstrated by the following experiment. Theobroma oil is melted and brought to a relatively high temperature, say 60–70°C. It is then poured into molds and quickly chilled in a refrigerator. If the suppositories are now removed shortly after they have congealed, they will be found to melt at a temperature below 30°C and it is impossible to handle them. Such suppositories will melt at room temperature in the summer, and the patient in trying to insert them has trouble since they liquefy in the fingers. If, on the other hand, the theobroma oil is melted carefully at a temperature only a very few degrees above its melting point and at once poured into molds and congealed, the suppositories melt at a much higher temperature and can be handled easily. The experienced pharmacist knows the theobroma oil properly melted has a slight "sheen" rather than being perfectly clear. Using care in melting it permits crystallization nuclei of the more stable and higher melting point β crystals to remain in the liquid. This, on chilling, encourages the crystallization of the β form.

Hot theobroma oil rapidly chilled undergoes super-cooling and, when it does congeal, forms only α crystals. These melt at a very low temperature. Since this is a metastable condition, there is a slow transition from the α to the β' form and finally to the stable β form with the highest melting point. This takes considerable time in the solid state, although suppositories poured from overheated theobroma oil will, after several days, exhibit a normal melting point.

There are, of course, other reasons why theobroma oil should not be overheated; such as, sedimentation of suspended solids and excessive contraction on chilling, leaving a depression in the base.

Ingredients Which Soften Theobroma Oil— Chloral hydrate, and other substances which dissolve in theobroma oil, will produce a significant lowering of the melting temperature of the oil, particularly when high concentrations of medicament are used. As the concentration of soluble medicament is increased, the melting temperature of the suppository mass decreases until the eutectic point is reached. Addition of more medicament will increase the melting temperature of the suppository mass up to the melting point of the medicament. The molal freezing-point depression of theobroma oil has been estimated as about 12–14°C.[150,151]

Chloral hydrate has a very pronounced effect on the melting temperature of theobroma oil since its hypnotic dose may range from 0.5–1.0 Gm per suppository. Del Pozo and Cemeli[152] obtained cooling curves for pure theobroma oil and for theobroma oil containing 20% chloral hydrate. Pure theobroma oil, when melted at 35°C, solidified at 22°C. However, with the chloral hydrate in the base the suppository solidified at 8°C, a depression of 14°C in the solidification point, which agrees with the estimated molal freezing-point depression for theobroma oil.

Waxes, such as white wax or spermaceti, with high melting temperatures, must be added to a suppository mass whenever the melting point of the theobroma oil is lowered below ambient temperature by the medicament. Approximately 4–6% of white wax or 20–25% of spermaceti should raise the melting temperature of theobroma oil sufficiently to prepare a solid suppository. Lesser amounts of wax will give wax–theobroma oil mixtures which have lower melting temperatures than the theobroma oil.

Some of the lipid suppository vehicles shown in Table II, such as Witepsols, possess melting charac-

teristics superior to theobroma oil, making them useful as vehicles for medicaments which depress the melting temperature of theobroma oil. Del Pozo and Cemeli[152] found that 20% chloral hydrate in Witepsol H15 had only a slight effect on the melting and the solidification temperature of the base.

Other difficulties in molding suppositories are easily overcome by the exercise of judgment and knowledge of physical laws. A defect frequently seen in the finished cocoa butter suppository is that the surface is not always perfectly smooth. This may arise from several causes. Sometimes ridges are seen traversing the suppository. These are usually produced by overcautiousness, the operator pausing in pouring the melted mass into the mold, then pouring in a little more, then pausing again, and so on. On removing the suppository, a ridge will be found at each spot where a pause was made. The remedy for this is to keep on pouring steadily when this part of the process is reached. Other defects are pitting, causing an imperfection in points of the suppositories. This pitting is usually caused by drops of water which have not been shaken out of the mold before pouring the melted mass. Still another defect is a depression in the center of the base of each suppository. This is due to not overflowing the molds so as to leave an excess of mass upon the top and it is intensified by pouring the mass when too warm. In all cases there should be a little more mass than will fill the molds; after cooling, the excess may be cut off if desired. The most perfect suppositories, however, are those which have been poured slightly more than full, leaving a rounded top, but all must be uniform. As this is difficult it is usually the custom to cut off all bases even with the top of the mold, to make all suppositories alike.

Water-Soluble and Water-Miscible Suppositories—Early work with polyethylene glycol polymers was performed in Germany. Bochmuhl, Middendorf, and Starcy[153] received patents in Germany and the United States in 1937 for a polyethylene oxide polymer and ricinoleic acid mixture with water which they suggested as a suppository base. The polymer itself, called "Postonal" in Germany, "Scurol" in France, and "Carbowax" in the United States, was developed as a suppository base by Middendorf.[154] In 1949, two English workers also suggested the use of a polyethylene glycol base in suppositories.[155]

Collins, et al,[156] developed the polyethylene glycol suppository bases shown in Table IV.

In the preparation of the polyethylene glycol suppositories, both the mold and cold compression methods were found suitable. The method of incorporation of the medicinal substances does not differ greatly from that employed when using cocoa butter, however, special precautions to insure a dry mold must be taken because of the solubility of this type of base in water. Attempts to prepare a hand-rolled suppository using these bases were unsuccessful.

Base A is a low-melting base which would be useful if a relatively rapidly disintegrating base is desired. This base may require refrigeration during the summer months.

Base B is a more stable formulation and can be used if the suppository is to be subjected to extreme storage conditions.

Base C was formulated to accommodate those substances which have a definite lowering effect on the melting point of the polyethylene glycols.

Base D contains water, which will facilitate incorporation of water-soluble, polyethylene glycol-insoluble substances.

These bases should be regarded as general suggestions since it may be found necessary to modify these formulas to meet variations in the amounts and combinations of medicinals added.

Fourteen drugs commonly administered in suppository form were readily incorporated in the four bases. Of these, sulfonamides, chloral hydrate, ichthammol, Peru balsam, and tannic acid reduced the melting point of the polyethylene glycol bases. Therefore a base containing a high percentage of the higher molecular weight polyethylene glycols such as Base C is recommended.

An *in vivo* determination of disintegration time of polyethylene glycol suppositories and those prepared with cocoa butter was made by inserting a suppository containing 0.5 Gm of barium sulfate in a human subject. The disintegration process was recorded by taking x-ray photographs every 5 min or less. The results are shown in Table V. The patients reported no feeling of discomfort from the polyethylene glycol suppositories. Polyethylene glycol suppositories are also nongreasy and are stable at room temperature.

Gross and Becker[157] developed another water-soluble, high melting point suppository base with high percentage medicinal release in a short time interval. This base consists of polyoxyethylene 30 stearate,* water, white wax, and Aerosol OT. They recommend

Table IV—Carbowax Polyethylene Glycol Bases

Base A:	Polyethylene glycol 1000	96%
	Polyethylene glycol 4000	4%
Base B:	Polyethylene glycol 1000	75%
	Polyethylene glycol 4000	25%
Base C:	Polyethylene glycol 1540	70%
	Polyethylene glycol 6000	30%
Base D:	Polyethylene glycol 6000	50%
	Polyethylene glycol 1540	30%
	Water and medication	20%

the percentage of wax be varied according to the physical and chemical nature of the incorporated material so as to maintain a 50° melting point.

Compatibility and storage tests were carried out with specific drugs in the following categories: astringents, alkaloids, antibiotics, and barbiturates. These tests indicate a long possible shelf life for medicinal suppositories made with this base.

Ward,[158] in a study of water-miscible suppository bases, used a polyoxyethylene derivative of sorbitan monostearate† as a suppository base. This nonionic surface-active agent is dispersible in water and body fluids and its melting temperature approximates body temperature. By modifying the surface-active agent with other materials, a more rapidly melting suppository base was prepared.[159]

The surface-active properties of polyoxyethylene-4-sorbitan monostearate permit the formation of an emulsion with body fluids. This emulsion spreads in the body cavity and in time releases the incorporated medication. Eckert and Muhlemann[160] reported that, *in vitro*, water-soluble drugs dispersed in W/O emulsions are not as available as the same drugs dispersed in anhydrous vehicles.

Polyoxyl 40 stearate,‡ a nonionic surface-active agent, is a white solid with a melting range slightly above body temperature. It can also be used to prepare water-miscible suppositories.

Theobroma oil suppository bases can be modified by the addition of surfactants, particularly when aqueous

---

* Myrj 51 (*Atlas*).
† Tween 61 (*Atlas*).
‡ Myrj 52 (*Atlas*).

solutions are to be incorporated in the base. The addition of 8–10% anhydrous lanolin to theobroma oil enables the formulator to incorporate up to 25% water (a W/O emulsion is formed).

In using surface-active agents as suppository bases or as additives in theobroma oil bases, the formulator must be aware of the possible interaction between a medicament and the surface-active agent in the base. Such interactions have been reported[161–163] between nonionic surface-active agents and pharmaceuticals. The drug complex which forms may differ from the uncomplexed drug with respect to its solubility, partition coefficient, and ability to penetrate the rectal mucosa.

Compressed Suppositories—The compression method for making suppositories is applicable primarily to theobroma oil. Basically, the method involves mixing the drug with grated theobroma oil, forcing the mixture into a suppository mold, and extruding the molded suppositories. On an industrial scale, hydraulically operated, motor-driven, cold-compression suppository machines are used. These machines are capable of producing about 150 suppositories/min.

Table V—Disintegration Time of Suppositories

Base	X-ray disintegration time, min
Polyethylene glycol 1000	15
Cocoa butter	3
Base B	40

The suppository base used in the compression method must be plastic enough to flow into the mold under pressure and to solidify when the pressure is removed. Aside from theobroma oil, very few materials fit these requirements. Collins, *et al*[154] were able to prepare polyethylene glycol suppositories by cold compression.

Glycerinated Gelatin Suppositories—These are used chiefly as vaginal suppositories for the local application of antibacterial agents, bismuth salts, zinc oxide, etc. Medicinal substances may be incorporated by dissolving or suspending them in enough water to make 10% of the total weight, then adding the glycerin, followed by the Pharmagel A or B, and mixing carefully so as not to incorporate air. The mixture is heated in a water bath until the gelatin is dissolved, then poured into chilled nonlubricated molds and allowed to stand until congealed. When glycerinated gelatin suppositories are to be used rectally, the gelatin content may have to be increased to 25–30% to make a firmer suppository.

Either Pharmagel A or B may be used, depending on the properties of the medication added. If optimum results are to be achieved, the proper type gelatin must be used. For example, ichthammol is known to be incompatible with acids so Pharmagel A (made from an acid-treated precursor) should not be used. Mild silver protein suppositories made with Type A gelatin undergo shrinkage because they contain protein which is anionic. Boric acid suppositories made with Type B gelatin become sticky due to the presence of acid in an alkali-treated gelatin. The importance of choosing the proper type of gelatin is clearly indicated by these examples.

Suppositories destined for long storage should have some preservative added (pages 1184, 1187). The USP provides the following general formula:

Glycerinated Gelatin Suppositories

The Medicinal Substance, the prescribed quantity.....
Purified Water, a sufficient quantity, to make........ 10 Gm
Gelatin, granular............................... 20 Gm
Glycerin....................................... 70 Gm

Weigh the medicinal substance into a tared container, add purified water to make a total of 10 Gm, and dissolve or mix, depending upon the solubility of the medicinal substances. Add the glycerin, and mix well. To the mixture add the gelatin, mix carefully to avoid incorporating air, and heat on a steam bath until the gelatin is dissolved. Pour the melted mixture into chilled molds, and allow to congeal.

Glycerinated gelatin suppositories should not be confused with Glycerin Suppositories NF, which are prepared with glycerin, sodium stearate (gelling agent), and water. Glycerin suppositories are used only as bowel evacuants; hence, medicaments should not be incorporated in them.

Storage of Suppositories—Suppositories made with theobroma oil or with other low-melting ingredients must be stored in a cool place, preferably a refrigerator.

Suppositories are usually dispensed in partitioned boxes which hold the suppositories in an upright position. Boxes are available for rectal and vaginal suppositories. Because of the hydroscopicity of glycerin, glycerinated gelatin and glycerin suppositories should be stored in tightly closed glass containers and kept in a cool place.

References

1. Urdang, G., *What's New*, Abbott Laboratories, 1942.
2. *United States Pharmacopeia* of 1820.
3. Casparis, P., and Meyer, E. W., *Pharm. Acta Helv.*, **10**, 101, 163 (1935).
4. Halpern, A., and Zopf, L. C., *J. APhA*, **36**, 101 (1947).
5. Goodman, H., *J. APhA, Pract. Ed.*, **3**, 7, 243 (1942).
6. Polano, M. K. *et al*, *Skin Therapeutics*, Elsevier Publ. Co., Amsterdam, 1952, p. 167.
7. Lane, C. G., and Blank, I. H., *Am. Profess. Pharmacist*, **13**, 357 (1947).
8. Griesemer, R. D., *J. Soc. Cosmetic Chemists*, **11**, 79 (1960).
9. Jacobi, O., and Heinrich, H., *Proc. Sci. Sect. Toilet Goods Assoc.*, **21**, 6 (May 1954).
10. Wells, F. V., and Lubowe, I. I., *Cosmetics and the Skin*, Reinhold, New York, 1964, pp. 8–12.
11. Rothman, S., *J. Lab. Clin. Med.*, **28**, 1305 (1943).
12. Blank, I. H., *J. Invest. Dermatol.*, **12**, 259 (1953).
13. Selby, C. C., *J. Invest. Dermatol.*, **29**, 131 (1957).
14. Tregear, R. T., *Physical Functions of Skin*, Academic Press, New York, 1966, p. 21.
15. Kligman, A. M., *The Epidermis*, Academic, New York, 1964, p. 387.
16. Scheuplein, R. J., *J. Invest. Dermatol.*, **45**, 334 (1965).
17. Treherne, J. E., *J. Physiol.*, **133**, 171 (1956).
18. Tregear, R. T., *J. Soc. Cosmetic Chemists*, **13**, 145 (1962).
19. Szabo, G., *Advan. Biol. Skin*, **3**, 1 (1962).
20. Mali, J. W. H., *J. Invest. Dermatol.*, **27**, 451 (1955).
21. Choman, B. R., *J. Soc. Cosmetic Chemists*, **11**, 127 (1960).
22. Tregear, R. T., *J. Physiol.*, **156**, 303 (1961).
23. Tregear, R. T., *Physical Functions of Skin*, Academic, New York, 1966, p. 11.
24. Ainsworth, M., *J. Soc. Cosmetic Chemists*, **11**, 69 (1960).
25. Buettner, K. J. K., *J. Appl. Physiol.*, **14**, 269 (1959).
26. Dirnhuber, P., and Tregear, R. T., *J. Physiol.*, **152**, 58 (1960).
27. Stoughton, R. B., *et al*, *J. Invest. Dermatol.*, **35**, 337 (1960).
28. Higuchi, T., *J. Soc. Cosmetic Chemists*, **11**, 85 (1960).
29. McKenzie, A. W., and Aitkinson, R. M., *Arch. Dermatol.*, **89**, 741 (1964).
30. McKenzie, A. W., and Stoughton, R. B., *Arch. Dermatol.*, **86**, 608 (1962).
31. McKenzie, A. W., *Arch. Dermatol.*, **86**, 611 (1962).
32. Katz, M., and Shaikh, Z. I., *J. Pharm. Sci.*, **54**, 591 (1965).
33. Poulsen, B. J., *et al*, *J. Pharm. Sci.*, **57**, 928 (1968).
34. Singer, E. J., and Vinson, L. J., *Proc. Sci. Section Toilet Goods Assoc.*, **46**, 29 (1966).
35. Blank, I. H., *J. Invest. Dermatol.*, **18**, 433 (1952).
36. Shelmire, J. B., *Arch. Dermatol.*, **82**, 24 (1960).
37. Wurster, D. E., and Kramer, S. F., *J. Pharm. Sci.*, **50**, 288 (1961).
38. Wurster, D. E., *Am. Perfumer Cosmetics*, **80**, 21 (1965).
39. Shelmire, J. B., *J. Invest. Dermatol.*, **26**, 105 (1956).
40. Michelfelder, T. J., and Peck, S. M., *J. Invest. Dermatol.*, **19**, 237 (1952).
41. Tregear, R. T., *Physical Functions of Skin*, Academic, New York, 1966, p. 23.
42. Peck, S. M., *et al*, *Invest. Dermatol.*, **14**, 177 (1950).
43. Blank, I. H., *et al*, *J. Invest. Dermatol.*, **30**, 187 (1958).
44. Marzulli, F. N., *J. Invest. Dermatol.*, **37**, 387 (1962).
45. Blank, I. H., *et al*, *J. Invest. Dermatol.*, **36**, 337 (1961).
46. Malkinson, F. D., *J. Invest. Dermatol.*, **31**, 19 (1958).
47. MacKee, G. M., *et al*, *J. Invest. Dermatol.*, **6**, 43 (1945).
48. Tregear, R. T., *Physical Functions of Skin*, Academic, New York, 1966, p. 15.
49. Blank, I. H., *et al*, *J. Invest. Dermatol.*, **29**, 299 (1957).
50. Wheatley, V. R., *Proc. Sci. Sect. Toilet Goods Assoc.*, **40**, 17 (1963).
51. Foster, W., *et al*, *J. APhA, Sci. Ed.*, **40**, 123 (1951).
52. Jones, E. R., and Lewicki, B., *J. APhA, Sci. Ed.*, **40**, 509 (1951).
53. Plein, J. B., and Plein, E. M., *J. APhA, Sci. Ed.*, **42**, 19 (1953).
54. Plein, J. B., and Plein, E. M., *Bull. Am. Soc. Hosp. Pharmacists*, **13**, 38 (1956).
55. Pail, D., and Todd, C. W., *Am. Perfumer Cosmetics*, **77**, 162 (1962).
56. Lesser, M. A., *Drug Cosmetic Ind.*, **72**, 616 (1953).
57. Burkhard, C. A., *et al*, *Chem. Rev.*, **41**, 137 (1947).
58. Schoog, M., *C. A.*, **45**, 10487 (1951).
59. Shaw, J. M., and Crowe, F. W., *AMA Arch. Dermatol.*, **71**, 379 (1955).
60. Lubowe, I. I., *J. Soc. Cosmetic Chemists*, **6**, 19 (1955).
61. Steigleder, G. K., and Raab, W. P., *J. Invest. Dermatol.*, **38**, 129 (1962).
62. Conrad, L. I., *Am. Perfumer Essential Oil Rev.*, **64**, 177 (1954).
63. Malmstrom, I. W., *J. Soc. Cosmetic Chemists*, **1**, 241 (1949).
64. Bertram, S. H., *J. Am. Oil Chemists' Soc.*, **26**, 454 (1949).
65. Tiedt, J., and Truter, E. V., *Chem. Ind. (London)*, 403 (May 1952).
66. Wagner, H., *Am. Perfumer Aromat.*, **75**, 23 (1960).
67. Conrad, L. I., and Maso, H. F., *Am. Perfumer Cosmetics*, **77**, 97 (1962).
68. Clark, E. W., *Am. Perfumer Cosmetics*, **77**, 89 (1962).
69. Newcomb, E. A., *J. Soc. Cosmetic Chemists*, **17**, 149 (1966).
70. Hjorth, N., and Trolle-Lassen, C., *Trans. St. John's Hosp. Dermatol. Soc. (London)*, **49**, 127 (1963).
71. Sulzberger, M. B., *et al*, *J. Invest. Dermatol.*, **20**, 33 (1953).
72. *The British Pharmaceutical Codex*, The Pharmaceutical Press, London, 1963, p. 890.
73. Li, Ping-Lu, and Kuever, R. A., *J. APhA*, **27**, 12, 1217, 1221 (1938).
74. Laug, E. P., *et al*, *J. Pharmacol. Exptl. Therap.*, **89**, 42 (1947).
75. Shelmire, J. B., *J. Invest. Dermatol.*, **26**, 105 (1956).
76. Wurster, D. E., and Kramer, S. F., *J. Pharm. Sci.*, **50**, 288 (1961).
77. Wells, F. V., and Lubowe, I. I., *Cosmetics and the Skin*, Reinhold, New York, 1964, p. 556.
78. Moore, C. D., and Bell, M., *Am. Perfumer Cosmetics*, **77**, 81 (1962).
79. de Navarre, M. G., *The Chemistry and Manufacture of Cosmetics*, Van Nostrand, Princeton, N.J., 1962, p. 106.
80. *Ibid*, p. 129.
81. Halpern, A., and Squealia, N., *J. APhA, Sci. Ed.*, **38**, 290 (1949).
82. Halpern, A., and Wilkins, W. J., *J. APhA, Sci. Ed.*, **38**, 283 (1949).
83. *Cetyl Alcohol Pure*, Givaudan-Delawanna, Inc., New York, 1945, p. 5.
84. Zopf, L. C., *et al*, *J. APhA, Pract. Ed.*, **6**, 365 (1945).
85. Cataline, E. L., *et al*, *J. APhA, Pract. Ed.*, **11**, 36 (1950).
86. Fennell, J. R., *et al*, *J. APhA, Pract. Ed.*, **17**, 794 (1956).
87. Chakravarty, D., *et al*, *Drug Std.*, **25**, 137 (1957).
88. de Navarre, M. G., *The Chemistry and Manufacture of Cosmetics*, Van Nostrand, Princeton, N. J., 1962, pp. 122–132.
89. Thomssen, E. G., *Drug Cosmetic Ind.*, **56**, 720 (1945).
90. Strakosch, E. A., *Arch. Dermatol. Syph.*, **1** (47), 16 (1946).
91. Laug, E. P., *et al*, *J. Pharmacol. Exptl. Therap.*, **89**, 52 (1947).
92. Strakosch, E. A., and Clark, W. G., *Am. J. Med. Sci.*, **205**, 610 (1943).
93. Zeutlin, H. E. C., and Fox, C. L., *J. Invest. Dermatol.*, **11**, 161 (1948).
94. Gemmell, D. H. O., and Morrison, J. C., *J. Pharm. Pharmacol.*, **10**, 167 (1958).
95. Beeler, E. C., *Bull. Natl. Formulary Comm.*, **11**, 27 (1943).
96. Bhatia, V. N., and Zopf, L. C., *J. APhA, Pract. Ed.*, **10**, 410 (1949).
97. *The British Pharmacopeia*, The Pharmaceutical Press, London, 1968, pp. 372, 373.
98. *The British Pharmaceutical Codex*, The Pharmaceutical Press, London, 1963, p. 1169.
99. *"Carbowax" Compounds and Polyethylene Glycols*, Union Carbide Corp., New York, 1946, p. 3.
100. McClelland, C. P., and Bateman, R. L., *J. APhA, Pract. Ed.*, **10**, 30 (1949).
101. Meyers, D. B., *et al*, *J. APhA, Pract. Ed.*, **11**, 32 (1950).
102. Nadkarni, M. V., *et al*, *Arch. Dermatol. Syph.*, **64**, 294 (1951).
103. Shelmire, J. B., *Arch. Dermatol.*, **82**, 24 (1960).
104. Wurster, D. E., *Am. Perfumer Cosmetics*, **80**, 21 (1965).
105. Landon, F. W., and Zopf, L. C., *J. APhA, Pract. Ed.*, **4**, 251 (1943).
106. *"Carbowax" Polyethylene Glycols for Pharmaceuticals and Cosmetics*, Union Carbide Corp., New York, 1959, p. 14.
107. Goldstein, S. W., *J. APhA, Pract. Ed.*, **15**, 41 (1954).
108. Collins, A. D., and Zopf, L. C., *Am. Profess. Pharmacist*, **22**, 691 (1956).
109. Higuchi, T., and Lach, J. L., *J. APhA, Sci. Ed.*, **43**, 615 (1954).
110. Lach, J. L., *et al*, *J. APhA, Sci. Ed.*, **46**, 615 (1957).
111. Shamberg, I. L., *Arch. Dermatol.*, **95**, 626 (1967).
112. Wuepper, K. D., *J. Am. Med. Assoc.*, **202**, 127 (1967).
113. Fantus, B., and Dynievicz, H. A., *J. APhA*, **28**, 548 (1939).
114. Evans, C. H., *J. APhA, Pract. Ed.*, **3**, 235 (1942).
115. *Methocel Handbook*, The Dow Chemical Co., Midland, Mich., 1958.
116. Levy, G., and Schwarz, T. W., *Drug Cosmetic Ind.*, **81**, 601 (1957).
117. *Carbopol 934*, B. F. Goodrich Chemical Co., Cleveland, 1957.
118. *Cellulose Gum, Sodium Carboxymethylcellulose*, Hercules, Inc., Wilmington, Del., 1966.
119. Houston, M. J., *et al*, *Can. Pharm. J.*, **82**, 32 (Sept. 15, 1949).
120. Hollander and McClanahan, *J. Invest. Dermatol.*, **11**, 127 (1948).
121. Darlington, R. C., and Guth, E. P., *J. APhA, Sci. Ed., Pract. Ed.*, **11**, 82 (1950).
122. Barr, M., and Guth, E. P., *J. APhA, Sci. Ed.*, **40**, 13 (1951).
123. *Veegum Technical Bulletin #53*, R. T. Vanderbilt Co., New York, p. 6.
124. Barr, M., *J. APhA*, **NS4**, 180 (1964).
125. Swafford, W. B., and Nobles, L. W., *J. APhA, Pract. Ed.*, **61**, 171 (1955).
126. Nobles, L. W., *Drug Cosmetic Ind.*, **77**, 280, 281 (1956).
127. Fisher, A. A., *Cutis*, **3**, 498 (1967).
128. *Methods of Contraception in the United States*, Planned Parenthood Federation of America, Inc., New York, 1963.
129. Rae, J., *Brit. J. Dermatol.*, **59**, 338 (1947).
130. *The United States Pharmacopeia*, 17th rev., Mack Publishing Co., Easton, Pa., 1965, p. 793.

131. *National Prescription Audit*, R. A. Gosselin and Co., Inc., Dedham, Mass., 1967.
132. Robinson, G. D., *J. Obstet. Gynaecol. (Brit. Empire)*, **32,** 496 (1928).
133. Gordon, M. G., US Pat. 3,126,887 (Sept. 1962).
134. Riegelman, S., and Crowell, W. F., *J. APhA, Sci. Ed.*, **47,** 115 (1958).
135. Schanker, L. S., *J. Pharmacol. Exptl. Therap.*, **126,** 283 (1959).
136. Schwarz, T. W., in *American Pharmacy*, 6th ed, Lippincott, Philadelphia, 1966, pp. 312–218.
137. Kakemi, K., *et al*, *Chem. Pharm. Bull.*, **13,** 861, 976 (1965).
138. Kakemi, K., *et al*, *Chem. Pharm. Bull.*, **15,** 172 (1967).
139. Hogben, C. A., *J. Pharmacol. Exptl. Therap.*, **125,** 275 (1959).
140. Bucher, K., *Helv. Physiol. Pharmacol. Acta*, **6,** 821 (1948).
141. Allawala, N. A., and Riegelman, S., *J. APhA, Sci. Ed.*, **42,** 267 (1954).
142. Eckert, V., and Muhlemann, H., *Pharm. Acta Helv.*, **33,** 649 (1958).
143. Higuchi, T., *J. Soc. Cosmetic Chemists*, **11,** 85 (1960).
144. Higuchi, T., and Lach, J. L., *J. APhA, Sci. Ed.*, **43,** 465 (1954).
145. Lach, J. L., *et al*, *J. APhA*, **10,** 615 (1957).
146. Nissim, J. A., *Nature*, **187,** 305 (1960).
147. Anschel, J., and Lieberman, H. A., *Drug Cosmetic Ind.*, **97** (3), 341 (1965).
148. Anschel, J., and Lieberman, H. A., *Drug Cosmetic Ind.*, **97** (4), 507 (1965).
149. Baily, A. E., *Melting and Solidification of Fats*, Interscience, New York, 1950.
150. Riegelman, S., in Sprowls, J. B., *American Pharmacy*, 5th ed, Lippincott, Philadelphia, 1960, Chap. 19, p. 356.
151. Peterson, C. F., in Sprowls, J. B., *Prescription Pharmacy*, Lippincott, Philadelphia, 1963, Chap. 7, p. 232.
152. Del Pozo, A., and Cemeli J., *Galenica Acta*, **7,** 137 (1954).
153. German Pat. 650,000 (1937); US Pat. 2,149,005 (1937).
154. Middendorf, L., *C. A.*, **33,** 4742 (1939).
155. Gilliam, R. W., and Tomlension, J. E., *Pharm. J.* **162,** 472 (1949).
156. Collins, A. P., *et al*, *Am. Profess. Pharmacist*, **23,** 231 (1957).
157. Gross, H. M., and Becker, C. H., *J. APhA, Sci. Ed.*, **42,** 498 (1953).
158. Ward, W. C., *J. APhA, Sci. Ed.*, **39,** 265 (1950).
159. US Pat. 2,469,618 (1949).
160. Eckert, V., and Muhlemann, H., *Pharm. Acta Helv.*, **33,** 649 (1958).
161. Ahsan, S. S., and Blaug, S. M., *Drug Std.*, **28,** 95 (1960).
162. Blaug, S. M., and Ahsan, S. S., *J. Pharm. Sci.*, **50,** 138 (1961).
163. Blaug, S. M., and Ahsan, S. S., *J. Pharm. Sci.*, **50,** 441 (1961).

86 | Powders

Particle size reduction, classification, and measurement—mixing of powders—powders as a dosage form

This chapter was prepared by

Alvin Felmeister, PhD, *Associate Professor of Pharmacy, College of Pharmacy, Rutgers University, Newark, N.J. 07104*

Although there is no official definition of powders, this term generally refers to those pharmaceutical dosage forms that are made up of more or less finely divided, dry, solid material. The particle size of such powders may vary from the very fine, as in aerosols and insufflations, to the coarse, as in effervescent granules and some crude drug preparations. However, it should be noted that, in addition to constituting a class of pharmaceutical preparations, powders also serve as the starting point for other important dosage forms including tablets, capsules, and suspensions. While the use of powders as a dosage form has declined, the use of finely divided solid material in pharmaceutical manufacturing has become increasingly important.

With this has come the recognition of the influence of the particle size of these materials on the physical, chemical, and biological properties of the dosage form. The current literature is replete with studies that have served to establish relationships between particle size and dissolution, absorption, and therapeutic efficacy of drugs, particularly for those that are poorly or slowly soluble. Griseofulvin is probably the most dramatic and best documented example, although other equally important examples can be cited, such as the corticosteroids, insulins, and sulfonamides.

The influence of particle size on the physical and chemical properties of drugs and drug products also has been studied extensively. Flow properties, suspendibility, and compressibility of powders have all been related to particle size or surface area. The viscosity of suspensions have been modified by simply changing particle size or the charge on the particles. Furthermore, in a number of instances, chemical stability has been shown to be decreased markedly by the concomitant increase in surface area that results with particle size reduction. This is particularly true when the materials are sensitive to air oxidation or hydrolysis following water adsorption. Fincher[1] and Lees[2] have recently reviewed much of the literature in these areas.

Thus, since the importance of particle size in relationship to its influence on many properties of drugs and drug products has been well established, the methods of reducing, measuring, and controlling particle size must be considered of equal importance.

Particle Size Reduction

Comminution in its broadest meaning is the mechanical process of reducing the size of particles or aggregates. Thus, it embraces various operations such as cutting, slicing, chopping, rasping or grating, contusion, grinding, pulverizing, milling, micronizing, microatomizing, ball-milling, trituration, etc, depending primarily on the type of equipment or procedure employed. Some operations are performed primarily on crude drugs or vegetable materials, others on chemical substances. Vegetable substances offer varying degrees of resistance to comminution depending on the proportion and toughness of their ligneous fiber and the amount and kind of cellular tissue. Chemical substances vary in melting point, brittleness, hardness, and moisture content, all of which affect the ease of pulverization. As a result, many different machines and processes are employed to accomplish particular objectives.

Specifications for the finished product may differ depending on their end use. A granular, coarse, or fine powder may be required, or it may be necessary to reduce substances to specified particle size ranges, often in the micron, or subsieve, size. Special techniques and equipment are required to accomplish this, as well as to measure the state of subdivision.

Manual Methods and Equipment

Most of the comminution operations which were once used in pharmacy are rarely employed by the community pharmacist today. In the era when crude drugs and glandular materials were popular, the pharmacist had to prepare these substances in a proper state for extraction, or to reduce them to a powder. Now the pharmacist rarely employs the small-scale operations of cutting, chopping, rasping or grating, and the knives, cutters, graters and heavy contusion mortars have been largely supplanted by the prescription mortar and pestle, spatula, and on occasion the muller and slab with which most comminution and mixing procedures are presently conducted. With these, the pharmacist can reduce granular or crystalline chemicals to a fine powder or he can blend or mix several components into the homogeneous mixture required to assure uniformity of dosage in extemporaneously compounded prescriptions. If necessary, these techniques also can be used to reduce compressed tablets to a fine powder suitable for use in prescriptions.

The manually operated procedures usually employed by the prescription pharmacist today are *trituration, pulverization by intervention,* and *levigation.*

Trituration—This term refers to the process of reducing substances to fine particles by rubbing them in a mortar with a pestle. The term also designates the process whereby a mixture of fine powders is intimately mixed in a mortar. The circular mixing motion of the pestle on the powders contained in a mortar results in blending them and in also breaking up soft aggregates of powders. By means of the application of pressure on the pestle, crushing or grinding also can be effected.

When granular or crystalline materials are to be incorporated into a powdered product, these materials

1626

are comminuted individually and then blended together in the mortar.

Pulverization by Intervention—This is the process of reducing the state of subdivision of solids with the aid of an additional material which can be removed easily after the pulverization has been completed. This technique is often applied to substances which are gummy and tend to reagglomerate or which resist grinding. A prime example is camphor which cannot be pulverized easily by trituration because of its gummy properties. However, on the addition of a small amount of alcohol or other volatile solvent, this compound can be reduced readily to a fine powder. Similarly, iodine crystals may be comminuted with the aid of a small quantity of ether. In both instances the solvent is permitted to evaporate and the powdered material is recovered.

Levigation—In this process a paste is first formed by the addition of a suitable nonsolvent to the solid material. Particle size reduction is then accomplished by rubbing the paste in a mortar with a pestle or on an ointment slab using a spatula or muller. When using the muller and slab the circular and figure 8 motion of the muller (see Fig. 629) serves to both grind and mix the product. Levigation is generally used by the pharmacist to incorporate solids into dermatologic and ophthalmic ointments and suspensions.

The *levigating agent* is selected on the basis of its ability to form a smooth paste with the substance to be levigated, and on its compatibility in the product. Water, for example, could not be used as the levigating agent with a substance intended to be incorporated into an oleaginous ointment base; light mineral oil is the liquid of choice in such instances. In a number of instances a small portion of the ointment base itself may be used as the levigating agent.

Regardless of the agent selected, only an amount sufficient to form a plastic paste should be employed. Excessive amounts of levigating agent may adversely affect the viscosity or consistency of the finished product and actually increase the effort required to levigate the powder.

The Mortar and Pestle—These are the most frequently used utensils in small-scale comminution. Mortars made of various materials and in diverse shapes are available and while these are often used interchangeably the different kinds of mortars have specific utility in preparing or grinding different materials.

The classic mortar was designed for the heavy pounding required in *contusion* of crude drugs. These mortars

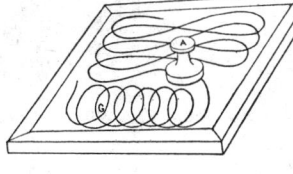

Fig. 629. Slab and muller.

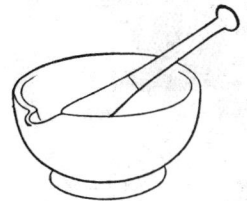

Fig. 630. Porcelain mortar and pestle.

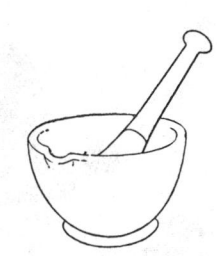

Fig. 631. Wedgwood mortar and pestle.

and pestles were made of cast iron, brass, bell metal or stainless steel. Generally, the crude drug was placed in the mortar and reduced to smaller particles by striking it with a succession of blows with the pestle. Wooden and marble mortars were once used similarly in contusing fresh roots and leaves. Contusion mortars are rarely used today.

Modern mortars and pestles are usually prepared from Wedgwood ware, porcelain or glass. Figs. 630 and 631 illustrate the conventional shapes for earthenware mortars. While pharmacists often use different mortars interchangeably, each type has a preferential range of utility which makes its use more efficient. Glass mortars, for example, are designed primarily for use in preparing solutions and suspensions of chemical materials in a liquid. They also are suitable for preparing ointments which require the reduction of soft aggregates of powdered materials or the incorporation of relatively large amounts of liquid. Glass also has the advantage of being comparatively nonporous and of not staining easily and thus is particularly useful when substances such as flavoring oils or highly colored substances are used. Glass cannot be used for comminuting hard solids.

Wedgwood mortars are well suited for comminution of crystalline solids or for the reduction in particle size of most materials used in modern prescription practice. They are capable of adequately powdering most substances which are available only as crystals or hard lumps. However, Wedgwood is relatively porous and will stain quite easily. A Wedgwood mortar is available with a roughened interior which aids in the comminution process but which requires meticulous care in washing since particles of the drugs may be trapped in the rough surface and cause contamination of materials subsequently comminuted in the mortar.

Porcelain mortars are very similar to Wedgwood except that the exterior surface of the former is usually glazed and thus less porous than the Wedgwood mortar. Porcelain mortars may be used for comminution of soft aggregates or crystals but is more generally used for the blending of powders of approximately uniform particle size.

Pestles are made of the same material as the mortar. Pestles for Wedgwood or porcelain mortars are available with hard rubber or wooden handles screwed into the head of the pestle (Fig. 632). The wooden handles have an unfortunate tendency to work loose from the head of the pestle and many pharmacists formerly employed a fused mixture of three parts beeswax and one part of orange shellac as a cement to affix the handle tightly to the head. Also available are one-piece Wedgwood pestles which avoid entirely the problem of loose handles. Pestles made entirely of porcelain are objectionable, because they are easily broken.

Pestles and mortars should not be interchanged. The efficiency of the grinding or mixing operation depends largely on a maximum contact between the surfaces of the head of the pestle and the interior of the mortar. The pestle should have as much bearing on the interior surface of the mortar as its size will permit. A pestle which does not "fit" the mortar will result in a waste of labor.

Spatulas—These are used during the comminution and trituration process to loosen the powdered material as it becomes packed on the inner sides of the mortar. Many materials will pack easily under the pressure exerted by the pestle and unless the compacted mass is frequently loosened, the work is hampered.

Spatulas are available in a variety of sizes and materials. The modern powder spatula, used in weighing or during the trituration of powders in a mortar, is made of stainless steel and has a balanced handle (Fig. 633). The weight of the handle is sufficient to overcome the weight of the blade, so that when the spatula is placed on the prescription counter, the blade will not touch the surface of the counter. The blade of a powder spatula is generally 4 inches long and is flexible enough to bend and conform to the inner curve of the mortar.

Fig. 634 shows a solid hard rubber spatula used when corrosive materials capable of reacting with steel are handled. Rubber spatulas are also useful in manipulating materials which are sensitive to metals.

Spatulas with oversize blades, up to 10 inches in length and 1 inch wide, are also available for use in preparing ointments on slabs and for use with oversized mortars capable of handling upward of a kilogram of powders. The broad blade simplifies the manipulation of an ointment on a slab and an experienced pharmacist can prepare a thoroughly uniform and smooth ointment with such a spatula in a very short time.

Pill knives or pill spatulas are also available. These differ from powder spatulas in possessing a shorter and thicker steel blade which is almost inflexible. Such spatulas are useful in working with masses used in preparing pills, troches or very stiff pastes.

Power Equipment—Although the community pharmacist rarely needs motor-driven mills, it is sometimes expedient to employ small-scale power comminuting machinery in grinding or pulverizing crude drug samples or in processing batches of powders of moderate size. The research pharmacist or hospital pharmacist who prepares pilot batches may also find such machinery convenient to his needs.

Many of the pieces of equipment described in the following sections are available in laboratory size suitable for use in a pharmacy. The familiar household blenders, such as the Waring Blendor, and small laboratory mills such as Wiley and Raymond laboratory mills (Figs. 635 and 636) are particularly useful in small-scale operations. Small mechanical mortars such as the Electromagnetic Laboratory Micromill and the Automatic Universal Mortar Grinder (both available from *Geoscience**) are also useful additions to the pharmacy or laboratory for the grinding of small quanties of material.

Small-scale laboratory models of comminuting machinery used in research and product development should be chosen with care and forethought. Ideally, small capacity counterparts of production scale machinery used in pilot plant operations should differ

from the larger machinery only with respect to capacity. Unfortunately, this is not always achieved, and the results obtained with the small scale operation often are not reproduced in production.

Mechanical Methods and Equipment

The requirements for grinding or milling machinery for use in the pharmaceutical industry depend to a large extent on the size and diversity of the manufacturer's operation. Few companies manufacture only one dosage form; the majority produce a variety of types of medication. The size of the operation often has greater influence in selecting the types of machines purchased than does the type of products manufactured.

Small manufacturers demand a much greater degree of versatility and portability in the machines they purchase than do larger producers. The former will look for types of equipment which can be adapted to a number of operations and be useful in the manufacture of several dosage forms. The larger manufacturers, on the other hand, generally prefer to select the equipment best suited for a specific purpose in a particular stage of their production cycles. This is due partly to a more generous budget, but also to the fact that the size of their operations allows them to make continuous use of a piece of equipment for one operation even if it is designed to do more than that specific job.

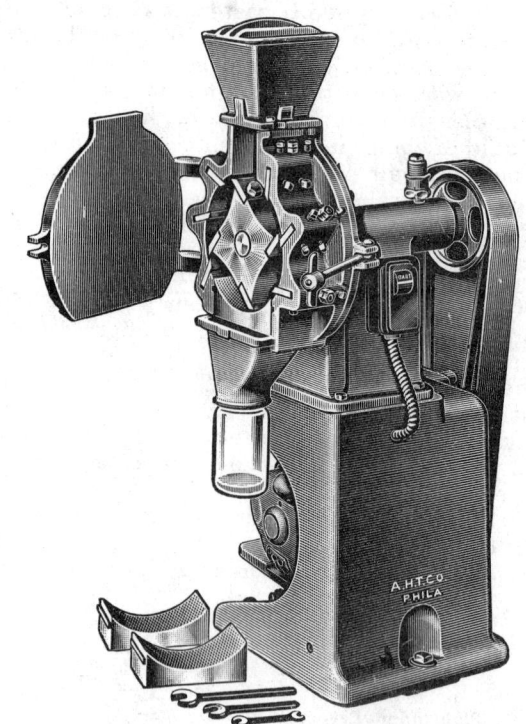

Fig. 635.   The Wiley laboratory mill (courtesy, Thomas).

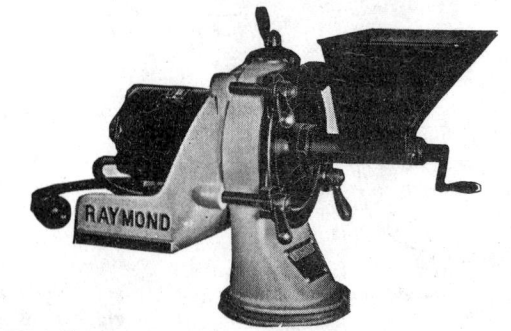

Fig. 636.   The Raymond laboratory mill (courtesy, Raymond).

---

* See *Manufacturers Index*, page 2023.

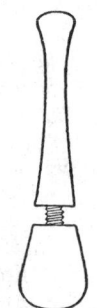

Fig.   632. Pestle with head screwed into handle.

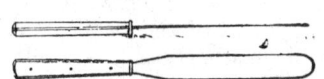

Fig. 633.   Balanced handle spatula.

Fig. 634.   Solid hard rubber spatula.

Contrasting these two situations, the smaller manufacturer demands a wide range of usefulness from his equipment even though a piece of machinery is not the most efficient for each process, while the larger manufacturer does not consider versatility as a primary factor but bases his selection of machinery on whether a particular machine is best suited for a specific stage of production.

Generally, the machinery used in pharmaceutical production should be of stainless metal construction because the reactive materials used in medicine are easily deteriorated or contaminated. Other desirable features which machinery should possess are easy disassembly or change-over for the purpose of obtaining a wide range of particle sizes, as well as facilitating thorough cleaning to prevent cross-contamination among different batches. Dust-free operation, durability, simplified construction and operation, a minimum of necessary adjustments, and large hopper or feeder capacities are important considerations in selecting comminution machinery. Ability to maintain continuous production of specified particle size ranges within narrow limits is also of importance. Finally, since most manufacturers have to process many materials having a diversity of physical properties, and thus varied degrees of grindability, it is of primary significance that comminuting machines should be capable of handling almost every type of material efficiently.

Large-scale comminution equipment may be divided into three main classes:

1. *Coarse crushers* (eg, jaw; gyratory; and roll crushers).
2. *Intermediate pulverizers* (eg, rotary cutters; disk, hammer, and chaser mills).
3. *Fine grinding mills* (eg, ball, vibrating ball, rod, buhrstone, hammer, colloid, and fluid energy mills; high-speed mechanical, screen, and centrifugal classifiers).

Machines used in the first category are ordinarily employed where the size of the feed material is relatively large, ranging from 1½ to 60 inches in diameter. Those used in the third category are limited to feed materials of less than 1 inch in diameter and grind these materials down to particles ranging from fractions of a micron upwards to 50 microns.

Coarse Crushers—Equipment in this category includes several types, differing in their mode of action and construction. The *Jaw Crusher* has a swinging jaw which moves back and forth against a stationary surface with which it forms a V-shaped chamber, wide at the top and narrow at the bottom. The crushing takes place within this chamber. The charge is introduced at the top and as the swinging jaw moves out, the charge slips down where it is crushed as the jaw moves back into the chamber. On the next outward movement of the jaw, the material passes farther down into the chamber until it is finally discharged at the bottom. The width of the discharge opening is adjustable and controls the size of the product. The jaws are essentially flat but in some models they may be corrugated or curved to concentrate the pressure on relatively small areas and reduce clogging.

Another type of crusher is the *gyratory crusher*. It has a central head or crusher element which has a rolling motion similar to a man sitting firmly while his shoulders describe a circle. As it gyrates, its edges come into close contact with the wall of the chamber while at another spot, 180° away, a maximum gap forms, into which the charge slips. At the next half gyration, the gap is reduced and the material in it is crushed by the pressure. Gyratory crushers are said to be superior to jaw crushers because they are rotary machines rather

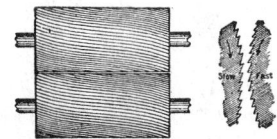

Fig. 637. Grooved rollers, side and end views.

than reciprocating ones. The strain on the former is less, the power consumption is steadier, and the capacity per unit of discharge area is larger.

Roll crushers operate by simple crushing or a combination of crushing and cutting. In its simplest form this mill consists of two rollers revolving in the same direction at different rates of speed. This principle has been developed and improved in modern milling, so that now a wide variety of roller mills are available. The rollers may be of steel, stainless steel, chilled iron, porcelain, or other ceramic material. Roll crushers may utilize two or more smooth, corrugated, ribbed or saw-toothed rollers (Fig. 637), or even a single specially cut roller, set either vertically or horizontally. They are used to crush a wide variety of materials ranging from stone to chemicals, and can be adjusted, by changing the distance between the rollers, to give a wide range of particle sizes.

Screw crushers utilize a two-bladed screw to crush and force material through a screen in the bottom of a trough.

Disk and *cone crushers* utilize a shaft on which is mounted a crushing head which is either cone- or disk-shaped. Operating either vertically or horizontally, the head grinds the material in a manner similar to the gyratory crusher; the movement is eccentric and approaches the periphery at one point and separates at another.

Intermediate Pulverizers—Much of the equipment employed for intermediate pulverizing can be adapted for coarse crushing and in some instances even fine pulverizing. A wide variety of equipment types are utilized.

Hammer mills include a wide variety of crushing and shredding devices that operate by impact rather than positive pressure or conventional grinding. The major advantage of impact milling over grinding methods is the low heat input and the high capacity obtainable. Since there is virtually no friction between material and moving surfaces, the only energy required is that which accelerates the particles to impact velocity. Temperature increases in the material being ground is thus reduced to minimum levels. Two types of hammer mills are used: one has stationary or rigid hammers mounted on a disk or plate, and the other has swinging hammers mounted on the disk or revolving drum by means of a pin. The whole is enclosed within a chamber. The bottom part of the chamber contains a grid or removable screen through which the material must pass. On the upper part is the feed hopper. As the material enters the chamber, the rapidly rotating hammers strike against it and break it into smaller fragments. These are swept downward against the screen where they undergo additional "hammering" action until they are reduced to a size small enough to pass through the openings and out. Oversize particles are hurled upward into the chamber where they also undergo further blows by the revolving hammers.

Edge runners, or chaser mills, consist of a vertical shaft to which is attached a horizontal one by means of a bevel gear and pinion. At the ends of the vertical shaft are attached heavy steel or granite wheels which rotate around the vertical shaft as well as about their own axis. The wheels rotate in this fashion within a station-

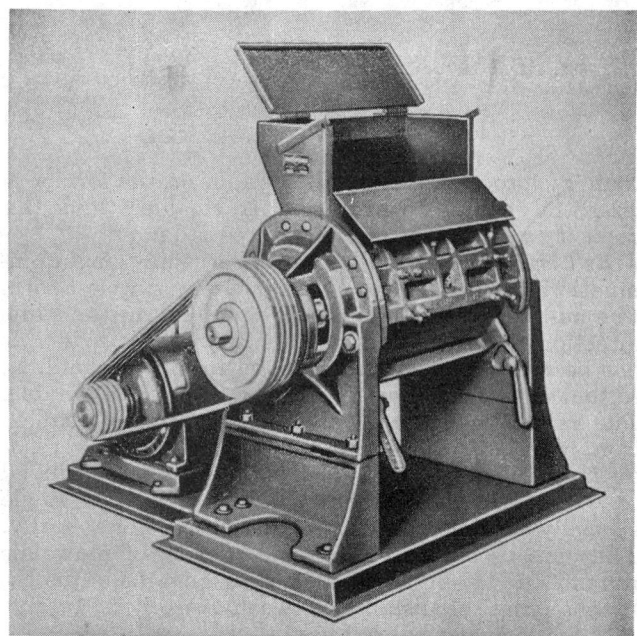

Fig. 638. Abbé cutter with V-belt and motor drive, mounted on unit bed plate.

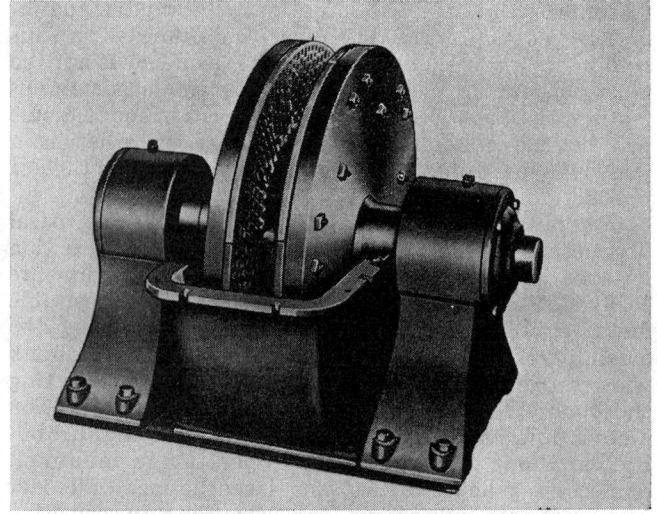

Fig. 639. Sprout-Waldron double attrition mill.

ary pan that holds the charge. Some models have the pan rotate while the wheels remain stationary. Though these machines occupy more space and have a smaller output than other mills, their upkeep is small and they require a minimum of attention during operation.

Cutter Mills—An example of a cutter mill is seen in Fig. 638. The Abbé Rotary Cutter contains five blades attached to a cylinder which revolves in a circular case upon the inside surface of which are fastened 6 blades; the blades are straight but are set at a slight angle, so that a "shearing action" is exerted on the substance to be cut. The bottom of the cases consists of a perforated plate, which can be replaced, and as the blades revolve a portion of the cut substance drops through the perforations. What remains is carried around and again subjected to the action of the cutters. By selecting suitable perforated plates the product may be cut coarser or finer as required.

Fine Grinding Mills or Pulverizers—The numerous types of fine grinding equipment available generally employ one of three basic operations or a combination of these operations.

1. *Attrition*—This involves breaking down of the material by a rubbing action between two surfaces. The procedure is particularly applicable to the grinding of fibrous materials where a tearing action is required to reduce the fibers to powder.

2. *Rolling*—This uses a heavy rolling member or centrifugal force to crush and pulverize the material. Theoretically, only a rolling-crushing type of action is involved, but in actual practice some slight attrition takes place between the face of the roller and the bed of the mill.

3. *Impact*—This involves the operation of hammers (or bars) at high speeds. These strike the lumps of material and throw them against each other or against the walls of the containing chamber. The impact causes large particles to split apart, the action continuing until small particles of required size are produced. In some instances high-velocity air or centrifugal force may be utilized as the impacting force.

Attrition Mills—These mills consist of either stones or steel grinding plates which revolve in opposite directions or one plate or stone remains stationary while the other one revolves. There are both horizontal and vertical types available.

The Bogardus Mill is constructed on a very ingenious principle. The grinding surfaces are two horizontal chilled iron plates, the lower one revolving, the upper one stationary; both have corrugations with sharp edges, arranged concentrically. The peculiarity of this mill is that the centers of the grinding plates are not directly over each other, but the center of the lower plate is placed a few inches to one side. By this arrangement the substance to be ground is caught by the ring edges of the revolving plate and dashed against the cutting edges of the stationary upper plate at an angle. The total effect of this action is simultaneous incision and crushing.

The Sprout-Waldron double runner attrition mill (Fig. 639) is an example of a mill which utilizes two rotating discs revolving in opposite directions. The particle size reduction is controlled by varying the speed at which the discs revolve, the space between the discs, and the size and number of ridges and indentations in the face of the discs.

The Buhrstone Mill is very extensively employed in drug milling. There are two kinds, termed, respectively, under runners and upper runners. The principle on which this type of mill operates is that of reducing the substance to particles by the friction and contusion of the substance contained in a contracted space formed by a rapidly revolving stone disk, brought into close contact with a similar disk which is stationary. In the under runners the upper stone is stationary and the lower stone revolves, the upper stone having a central circular opening through which the substance is fed, as shown in Fig. 640. In the upper runners the lower stone is stationary, the upper stone being perforated as in the under runners. In both, the moving

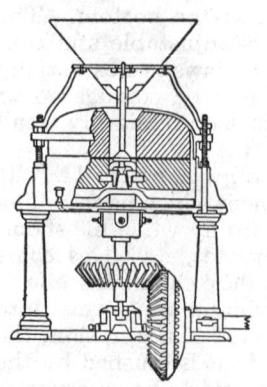

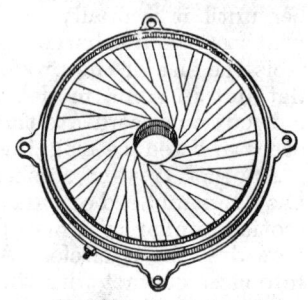

Fig. 641. Buhrstone.

Fig. 640. Under runner buhrstone mill.

stones revolve horizontally. The stone used must be very hard. The surfaces of the millstones are crossed with "furrows," which pass from the center to the circumference, as shown in Fig. 641. The object of the furrows is to provide a means for the passage of the ground particles to the outer circumference and to the trough. This is accomplished through the centrifugal force and current of air caused by the rapid revolution of the stone in motion. The fineness of the powder is regulated by raising or lowering one of the stones. Fig. 640 illustrates one type of buhrstone mill—Munson's under runner. There are also mills with stones rotating in a vertical position. The ground drug coming from a buhrstone mill requires bolting or sifting to separate the coarse particles which are then returned to the mill for regrinding.

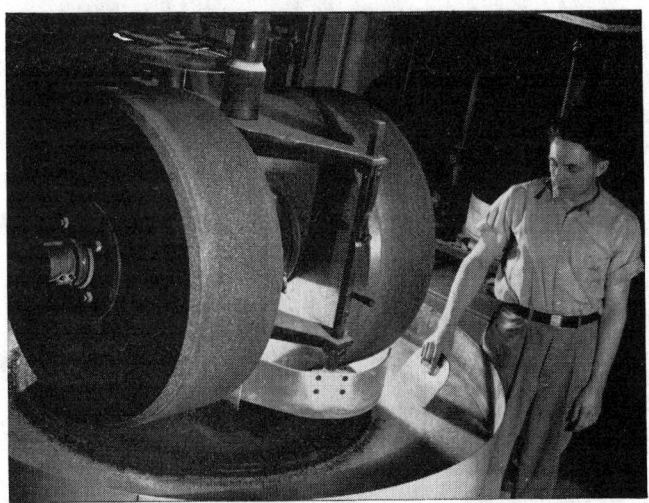

Fig. 642. Chaser mill (courtesy, MSD).

Chaser Mills are so called because two heavy granite stones, mounted vertically like wheels and connected by a short horizontal shaft, are made to revolve or *chase* each other upon a granite base (Fig. 642). The stones are discoid, and the grinding surfaces are the circumferential edges of the stones and the surface of the granite base; an iron cylinder, called a "curb," surrounds the circular base, and a "scraper," made of iron and adjusted at an angle, is connected with the shaft. It is evident that if the substance to be powdered is delivered upon the granite base in the path of the rapidly revolving stones it must speedily be reduced to powder, not only on account of the crushing weight of the heavy stones, but also because of the attrition caused by the outer edge of the stone traveling through a longer distance than the inner edge. In practice chasers are enclosed in a tight box or small room with airtight doors and the substance to be powdered is fed in from the top by an elongated funnel, the spout of which delivers the material immediately upon the path of the stones. The height of the curb may be increased by pasting heavy paper around it, and the fineness of the powder is influenced by the height of the curb. The revolution of the chasers produces an upward current of air; this carries over the lighter particles, which fall outside the curb and are subsequently collected as a fine powder. Those particles which are larger are, of course, heavier and cannot rise to the height of the curb, but fall back under the stones to be reground. In this way refractory substances can be reduced to very fine powder. Chasers are more largely employed in making "dusted" or very fine powders than any other form of pulverizing apparatus.

Pebble or Ball Mills, sometimes called "pot mills" or "jar mills," are operated on the principle of attrition and impact, the grinding being effected by placing the substance in jars or cylindrical vessels, lined with porcelain or a similar hard substance and containing "pebbles" or "balls" of flint, procelain, steel, or stainless steel. These cylindrical vessels revolve horizontally on their long axis and the tumbling of the pebbles or balls over one another and against the sides of the cylinder effects pulverization with a minimum loss of material. The advantage of such mills is that they afford a large grinding surface within a limited space. They are cleaner than many mills, economical, and because of the simplicity of their construction, require a minimum of maintenance. Much depends, however, on the hardness of the pebble, since these are continually striking against each other while in action. As a consequence these mills are not suitable for the preparation of chemicals where contamination by traces of porcelain or stone is objectionable. Such mills are adapted for grinding hygroscopic substances, extracts, and expensive chemicals. Fig. 643 shows a sectional view of a single jar mill. Fig. 644 illustrates a double jar mill. In this type of mill the jars are usually arranged parallel to the axis of revolution, but they are sometimes constructed with the jars at right angles. This produces a much more violent action than the stan-

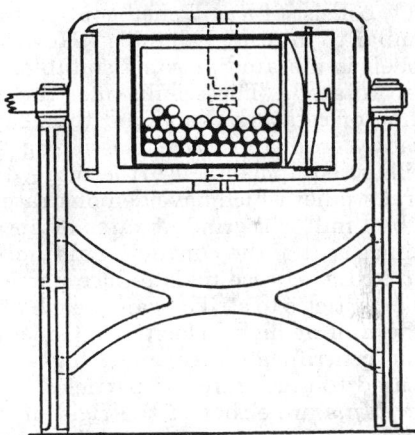

Fig. 643. Single jar mill.

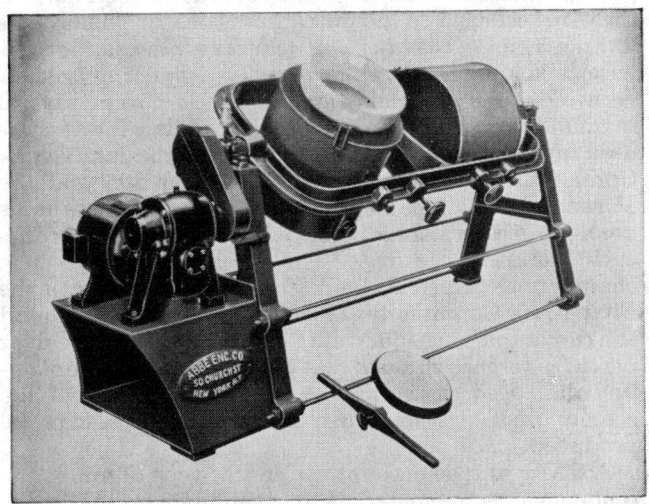

Fig. 644. Abbé double jar mill with roller chain and gear motor drive.

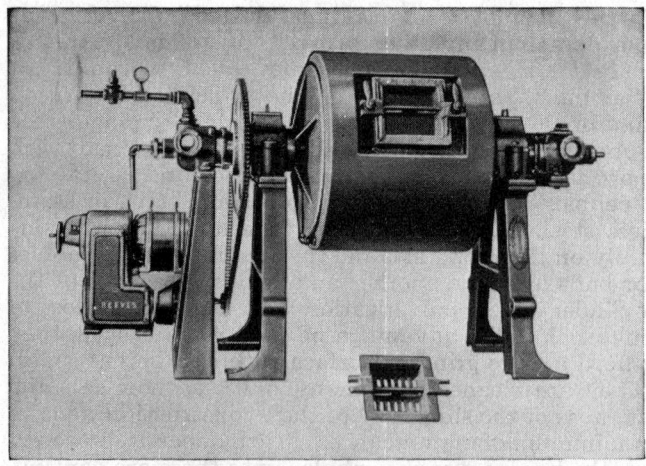

Fig. 645. Abbé pebble or ball mill with roller chain connecting to variable-speed motor; jacketed for heating or cooling with special stuffing boxes for operating mill under pressure or vacuum.

dard arrangement. The number of jars may be increased as needed in units of two or three. The advantage of multiplying the jars is that four, six, or a dozen different substances may be ground at one time. This type of mill may also be purchased with variable-speed motor, special stuffing boxes for operating the mill under pressure or vacuum, and special jacket for temperature regulation (see Fig. 645).

Vibrating Ball Mills, which also combine attrition and impact, consist of a mill shell containing a charge of balls similar to rotating ball mills. However, in this case the shell is vibrated at some suitable frequency, rather than rotated. These mills offer the advantage of being free of rotating parts, and thus can be integrated readily into a particle classifying system or other ancillary equipment. Furthermore, there have been several studies which have demonstrated that the vibrating ball mill will grind at rates often as high as 20 to 30 times that of the conventional tumbling mill.[3]

Impact Mills—These mills reduce particle size by causing the particles to strike against each other or the sides of the mill at high velocities. Generally a mechanical or centrifugal force, or a high-velocity air stream is used to accelerate the particles.

Hammer Mills are either of the rigid or the swing-hammer type. They are mostly combined with a fan and cyclone for collecting the material. When the ground product is sifted or air separated and the tailings are returned to the mill automatically, the process is known as *a closed-circuit grinding process;* otherwise it is known as an *open-circuited grinding process.*

Swing-hammer mills are available from several manufacturers. The most popular mills of this class used in the pharmaceutical industry are the Fitzpatrick Comminuting Machine, the Micro-Atomizer, and the Tornado Mill. The hammers, or disks, in these mills are mounted on a shaft by means of a pin which permits each hammer to swing. The whole is enclosed in a chamber. A screen at the bottom of the chamber of the Fitzpatrick Comminutor (Fig. 646), or mounted around the rim of the Tornado Mill (Fig. 647), permits the finer particles to pass through and be collected. By controlling the speed of the mill and varying the size of the screen used, a wide range of particle sizes may be produced.

A disadvantage encountered in this type of mill is the tendency of some materials to accumulate on the screen and block the passage of the reduced particles. This is particularly true with resinous materials. In such

instances the addition of small pieces of dry ice to the feed material reduces the temperature of the material and the comminution chamber and also reduces the incidence of build-up on the screen. Jacketed models of the Fitzpatrick mill are available to permit low-temperature pulverizing of volatile or resinous materials.

The Abbé Impact Grinding Mill (Fig. 648) is designed to grind and pulverize a wide variety of materials quickly, uniformly, and economically. The material is fed to the feed hopper, where it automatically drops by means of a shaker feed into a secondary hopper in the door of the mill. A slide gate in the feed hopper regulates the flow of material. If desired, the material may be introduced directly into the secondary hopper. The material enters the grinding chamber at the center of the mill and is advanced by centrifugal force generated by the rotor. The rotor is provided with beaters, toward its periphery, where the material is broken up

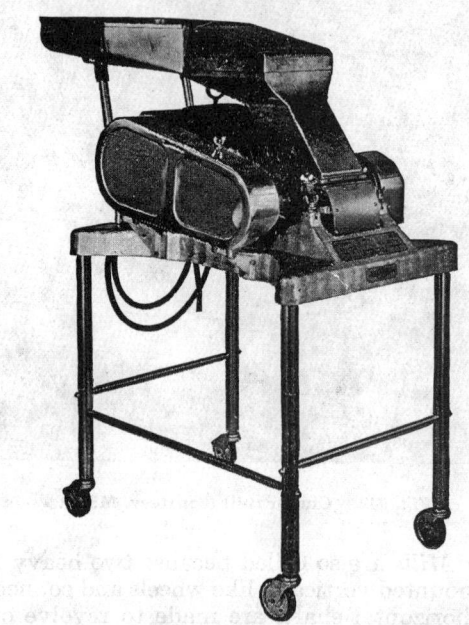

Fig. 646. The Fitzpatrick Model D comminuting machine.

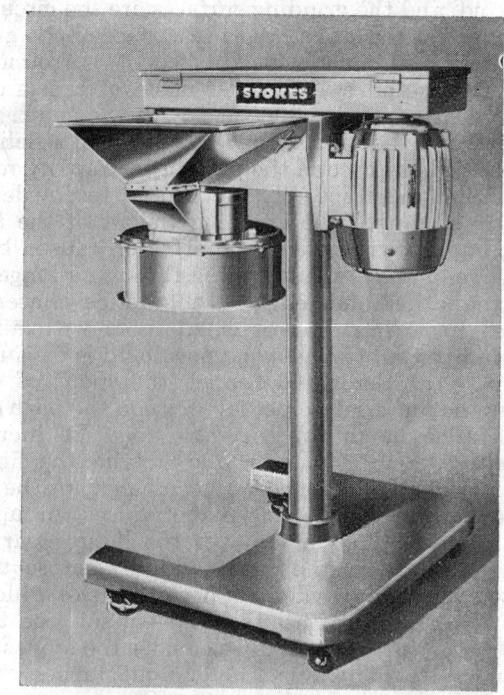

Fig. 647. The Tornado mill (courtesy, Stokes).

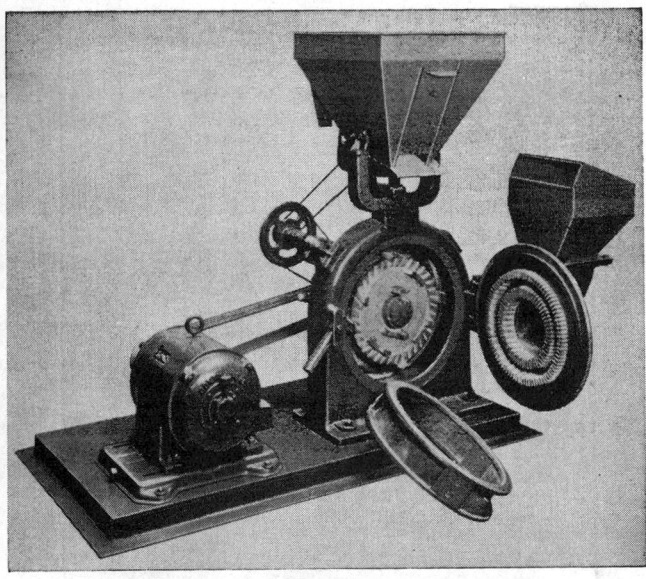

Fig. 648. Abbé impact grinding mill.

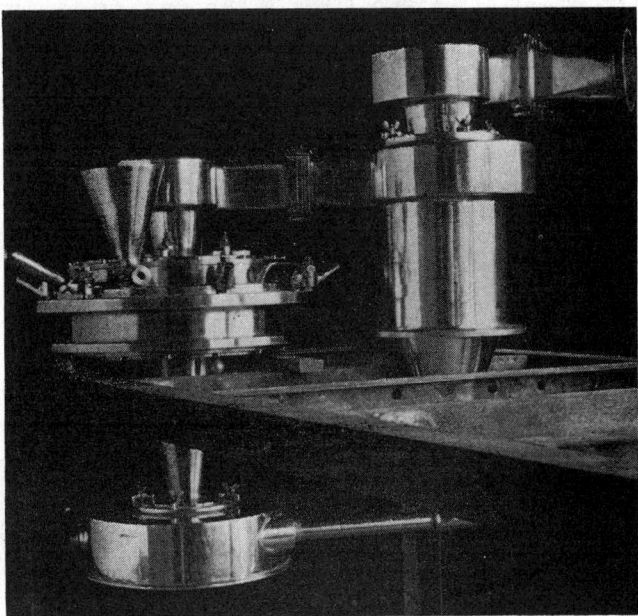

Fig. 650. Micronizer reduction mill.

by impact against the rapidly rotating beaters and the teeth on the grinding rings mounted on the door and the inside face of the mill casing. The rotor is carefully balanced for operation at high speeds. Reduction from a coarse material to the finest powder in only one pass through the mill is made possible because of the design of the toothed concentric rings which give a large grinding surface. The grinding teeth of the rotor together with the stationary grinding rings form practically a closed mill from which the material cannot escape until reduced to such fineness as to allow passage through the narrow space between the rings and the toothed surfaces of the rotor. For fine powder a circular sieve or screen is placed around the rotor. The hinged door permits quick cleaning and changing of screens. The pulverized material drops through the bottom of the mill into a bin or container.

Fluid energy mills are used for pulverizing and classifying extremely small particles of many materials. The mills have no moving parts, grinding being achieved by subjecting the solid material to streams of high velocity elastic fluids. The fluids employed are usually air, steam or an inert gas. The technique employs compressed gas introduced into the grinding chamber by means of jets. The material to be pulverized is exposed to the streams of air or gas and is swept into violent turbulence by the sonic and supersonic velocity of the streams. The particles are accelerated to relatively high speeds and when they collide with each other the impact causes violent fracture of the particles.

A schematic representation of one type of fluid energy mill is shown in Fig. 649. The elastic grinding fluid is introduced through nozzles in the lower portion of the mill under pressures ranging from 25 to 300 pounds per square inch.

The high pressure fluid is converted to either sonic or supersonic jet streams as it expands in the lower portion. In this way, a rapidly circulating flow of gas is generated in the hollow, doughnut-shaped mill. A Venturi feeder introduces the coarse material into the mill and the particles enter into the jet stream of rapidly moving gas. The raw material is quickly pulverized by mutual impact in the reduction chamber. As the fine particles form they are carried upward in the track. Particles are simultaneously ground and classified in this process. The smaller particles are entrapped by the drag of gas leaving the mill and are carried out to a collecting chamber or bag. Centrifugal force at the top of the chamber stratifies the larger, heavy particles and their greater momentum carries them downward and back to the grinding chamber.

Several variants of the fluid energy mill are available. Fig. 650 illustrates the Micronizer Reduction Mill which has a horizontally positioned "track" or grinding and classifying chamber. These mills are available in a variety of sizes. A laboratory model Jet-O-Mizer is shown in Fig. 651. Another laboratory model which is available in several sizes in portrayed in Fig. 652. This Gem Fluid Energy Mill is produced by the Helme Products, Inc. in Helmetta, N.J. The Gem Mill operates on the same principle of high-speed particle impaction except that it employs two diametrically opposed fluid energy jets in which the particles are caused to collide in the grinding or impact chamber.

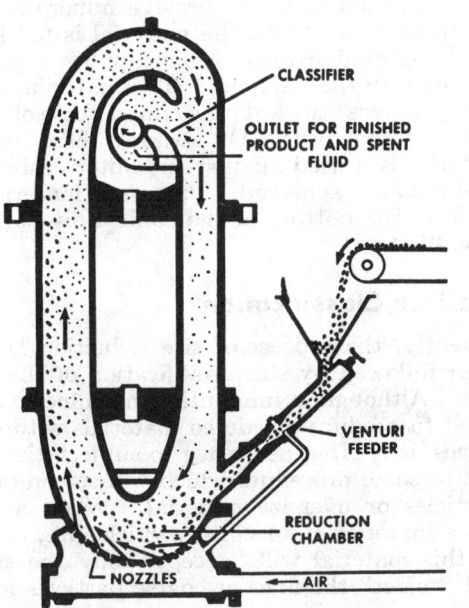

CLASSIFIER

OUTLET FOR FINISHED PRODUCT AND SPENT FLUID

VENTURI FEEDER

REDUCTION CHAMBER

NOZZLES — AIR

Fig. 649. The Jet-O-Mizer Fluid Energy mill (courtesy, Fluid Energy).

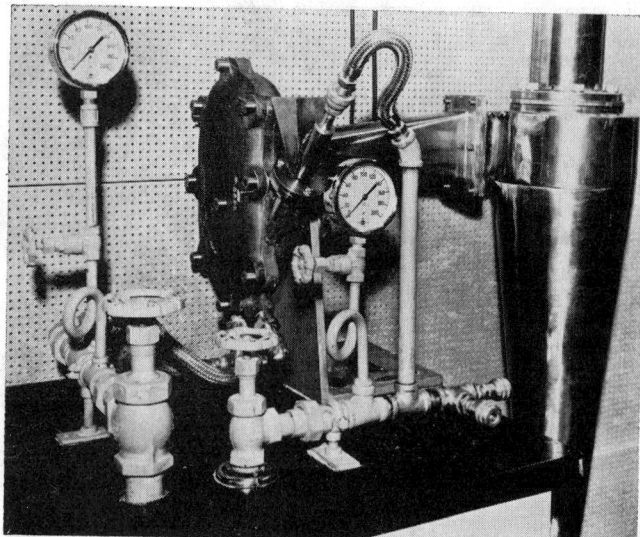

Fig. 651. Laboratory-size Jet-O-Mizer (courtesy, Fluid Energy).

Since contamination of the particles is always a danger, the Gem Mill is available with interchangeable chamber liners of urethane rubber, teflon, nylon, ceramic, or stainless steel.

The major advantage of the fluid energy mill lies in the fact that virtually no heat is generated in the material which is finely pulverized. The cooling effect of the grinding fluid as it expands in the grinding chamber more than compensates for the moderate heat generated during the grinding process. Pharmaceuticals such as antibiotics, enzymes or other heat sensitive materials may be ground to an extremely fine state with virtually no loss of activity due to heat. Another advantage in the use of these mills is the rather narrow range of particle sizes produced. When precise control of particle size is an important factor in the process, the grinding accomplished in a fluid energy mill produces very narrow ranges of particles with a minimum of effort.

One major disadvantage is found in the necessity of controlling the feeding of the coarse, raw material into

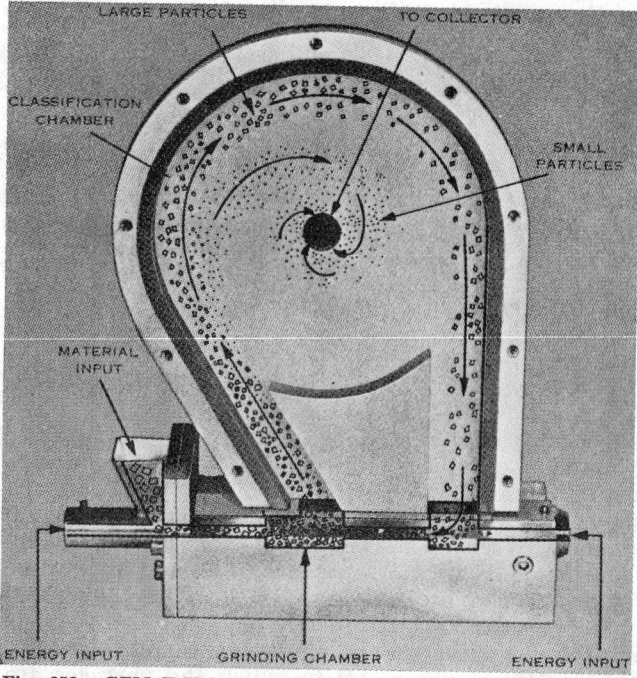

Fig. 652. GEM T-X laboratory mill (courtesy, Helme Products, Inc.).

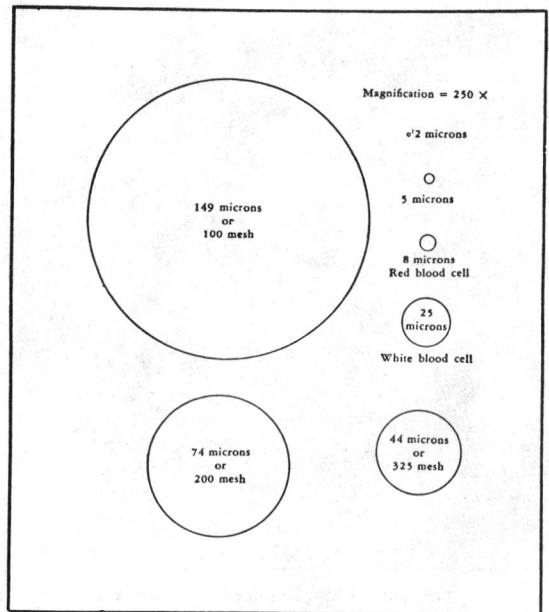

Fig. 653. Diagram of relative sizes.

the jet stream. Often the feeding device will become clogged by a clump of material and special feeding devices must be built to produce a uniform rate of feed.

The diagram of relative particle sizes in Fig. 653 is included to enable the reader to visualize the relative magnitude of particles which are produced by ordinary comminution methods and are classified by mesh size, in comparison with particles in the micron ranges produced by the jet mills.

The introduction of multiple jets and the redesigning of the grinding and classifying sections have served to improve the degree of uniformity of the fluid and material mix, and to simplify the processes of returning the oversize particles to the grinding zone as well as the collection of the final product. A comparison between these redesigned units and the simple fluid energy mills is made by Temperley and Blythe.[4]

Centrifugal-Impact Pulverizers also have been found to be effective for the reduction of the particle size of a wide variety of materials ranging from very soft organic chemicals to hard abrasive minerals. Basically, in these pulverizers, the material is fed into the center of a spinning rotor which applies a high centrifugal force to the particles. The material, thus accelerated, moves toward the impactor set at the periphery of the rotor. On striking these impactors the material is hurled against the outer casing where final reduction is achieved. Processed material is removed from the bottom of the conical discharge hopper (Fig. 654).

Particle Size Classification

Frequently, the process of size reduction is accompanied or followed by size classification of the ground material. Although comminuting machinery may be controlled to produce powdered materials within specified ranges, it is often necessary to subject the ground material to some procedure which will screen out very fine particles or oversize material. When a process requires a material of specified particle size, classification of this material will "accept" only the specified size and "reject" the fines or coarse particles for additional processing. Size classification also may be applied to particle size analysis, in which the proportion of each size of particle in a sample is determined and the data utilized to control raw materials or the quality of the manufactured product.

Techniques and Equipment

The basic processes generally employed for classification or fractionation of fine solid particles are *sieving, sedimentation* and *elutriation*. The techniques such as cyclone separation, electrostatic separation, and felvation are in the main modifications or combinations of these three basic processes.

Sieving—In this technique, particles of a powder mass are placed on a screen made up of uniform apertures. By application of some type of motion to the screen, the particles smaller than the apertures are made to pass through. The sieve motion generally is either (a) horizontal, which tends to loosen the packing of the particles in contact with the screen surface, permitting the entrapped subsieve particles to pass through or (b) vertical, which serves to agitate and mix the particles as well as to bring more of the subsieve particles to the screen surface.

The principle problems associated with this technique are lack of uniformity of apertures (this is a particular problem in mesh sizes below 120); "blinding" of the openings by oversize or irregular particles; and inefficient presentation of the particles to the screen surface. The use of horizontal and vertical screening motions, airjets, sudden periodic reversal of the sieve motion, and continuous cycling all have been used in an attempt to eliminate these problems.

The hand sieve is the simplest of devices used, all material passing through the sieve being accepted, while that remaining on the sieve is rejected for reprocessing. The frames of hand sieves are round, oval, square, or rectangular. Covered sieves, or drum sieves, have tight covers for the top and bottom. These may be purchased from any laboratory supply house. Sieves should be so constructed that they may be readily cleaned and the wire or cloth gauze replaced. One such screen is shown in Fig. 655. By loosening the Allen screws on four sides, the wire or cloth screen may be removed and replaced. It is held in place by rods along the frame which fit tightly as the screws are tightened. It is highly desirable to make sieve frames of stainless steel, which is less reactive than most other metals.

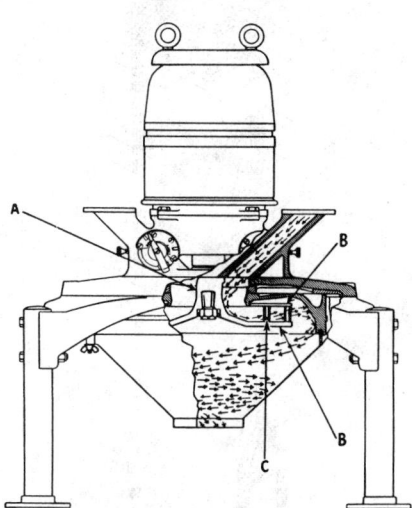

Fig. 654. CentriMil, a centrifugal impact mill, available in models ranging from 2 to 250 hp. *A:* **Spinning rotor;** *B:* **rotor hub discs;** *C:* **impacters (courtesy, Entoleter).**

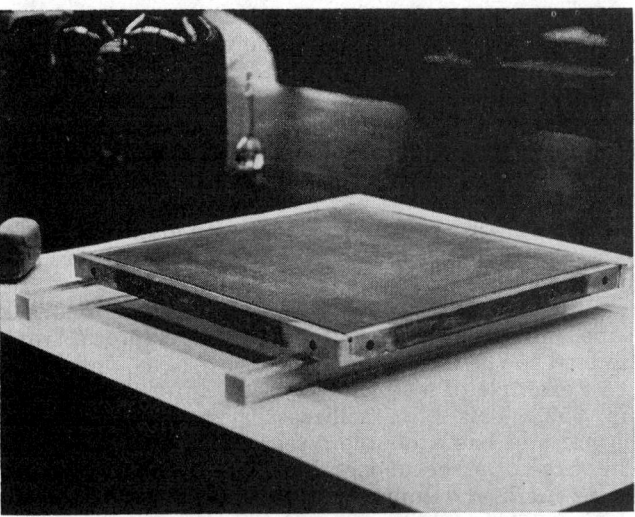

Fig. 655. Stainless steel sieve (courtesy, MSD).

Fig. 655 shows the proper positioning of the sieve in use. Note that it is raised from the surface of the laboratory bench by two plastic rods about 1¼ inches square. The plastic may be easily cleaned.

In research or development laboratories it is customary to have a sieve table with a top of stainless steel or plastic-impregnated birch wood. A hole is cut in the top of this table which just accommodates the sieves. A stainless steel pan is placed under the sieve on a shelf to catch the sieved powder. A quantity of powder may be placed on the table top and worked through the sieve with a muller (Fig. 629). Under this shelf it is convenient to have a rack to hold sieves, each stamped with its size and held in an upright position like books on a library shelf. Stainless steel channels at the top and bottom of this cabinet hold the sieves in the upright position.

A very important point, which must not be overlooked after sifting substances, is the need for thorough mixing of all portions of the sifted powder, in order that each part of the finished powder may have a uniform composition. In small-scale operations this may be easily effected with a spatula or mortar and pestle; in larger-scale operations special apparatus, as considered in the section on *Mixing of Powders,* is required.

Obviously, manually operated screens are suitable only for classifying small batches of materials, and then only within the limits imposed by the size of the openings in the screen selected. For continuous operations, the screens are attached to mechanical devices which supply the energy required to shake the particles through the openings in the screen and also prevent accumulation of fines within the openings as this tends to clog them and slow down the operation. Sieves may be used either in a sequence of sizes through which the material must pass or singly in the required size.

An example of a mechanical sieve shaker which utilizes a sequence of screen sizes is shown in Fig. 656. This apparatus is useful in obtaining size analysis data under controlled conditions. The sample is placed in the top of the nest of standard sieves arranged in a descending order. The length of time and force of vibration to which the sample is subjected may be preset by variable time and voltage controls. The controlled vibration causes the powder particles to pass through the sieves, each fraction coming to rest in the sieve through which it cannot pass. For the purpose of analysis, the weight of each fraction is determined and the percentage calculated.

The Sonic Sifter (*Allen-Bradley* *) is a laboratory sifter that utilizes sonic oscillation to classify particles. A mechanical pulse action is used to reduce blinding and agglomeration in the subsieve sizes. This combination of sonic and mechanical agitation permits dry sifting down to 10 μ. Standard sieves are available for this unit from 3½ to 400 mesh and in precision sizes from 150 to 10 μ.

Industrial-size mechanical sieves are manifold in design and capacity, and include the gyratory, circular rotatory, vibrating, shaking, and revolving sifters. In gyratory sifters the motion is in a single horizontal plane, but may vary from circular to reciprocal from the feed to the discharge end.

An example of a gyrating type of sifter is shown in Fig. 657. This sifter utilizes a gyratory hand sieve motion and has a double screen in its sifting frame. The screen on the underside of the frame is of very coarse mesh and supports a number of rubber balls, which in their motion keep the sieve pores open by coming in contact with the screen which is fastened to the upper side of the sifting frame. The frame is equipped with a number of beveled crossbars which tend to deflect the balls upward so that they tap the upper screen. This action may be likened to that of tapping the fingers against the under side of a sieve, but at the rate of 300 taps per minute. Fig. 658 illustrates the principle upon which it operates. The inclined sifting box which encloses the sifting frame is equipped with three spouts, one as a feeder, one for the purpose of carrying off the sifted powder, and the third for carrying off the coarse particles.

The circular sifter also confines the screen motion to a horizontal plane, but in this case the total motion applied to the sieve is circular. The Sprout-Waldron Gyro-Whip is an example of such a sifter. In this sifter the material enters the top and spreads over the first sieve. Some of the finer particles drop through and are discharged into the "throughs" channel. The remaining powder moves to the next sieve in order, the process is repeated until complete separation is accomplished (Fig. 659).

The Sweco Vibro-Energy Separator (Fig. 660) combines a vibrating screen with the circular motion of the rotary sieves for the purpose of increasing efficiency.

* See *Manufacturers Index*, page 2023.

This separator provides clean separation and accurate sizing in a wide range of mesh sizes from very large to as fine as 325 mesh. It can separate a variety of materials in the wet or dry states at high speed because the spiral travel of the particles spreads them over the entire screening surface.

Nonrotating vibrating screens also serve to fractionate powders efficiently and are frequently used because of their simplicity of design and general adaptability.

Centrifugal screening is utilized in the Symons V-Screen developed by Nordberg. Here the equipment is pushed through a spinning vertical wire cloth cylinder. Sharp cuts in particle size can be obtained with this equipment.

Wet Screening—The addition of water is sometimes employed to dissolve out any unwanted binders, remove fines or surface contamination, and to reduce surface forces, particularly in micro-mesh sieves, that

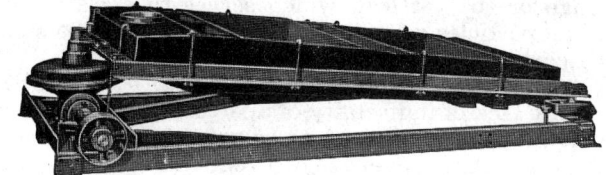

Fig. 657. Rotex sifter.

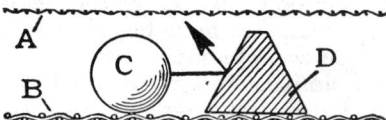

A—The Sifting Cloth
B—The Coarser Ball Support Screen
C—The Ball of Solid Rubber
D—The Inclined Surface Deflecting the Ball Upward

Fig. 658. Rotex cloth-cleaning system.

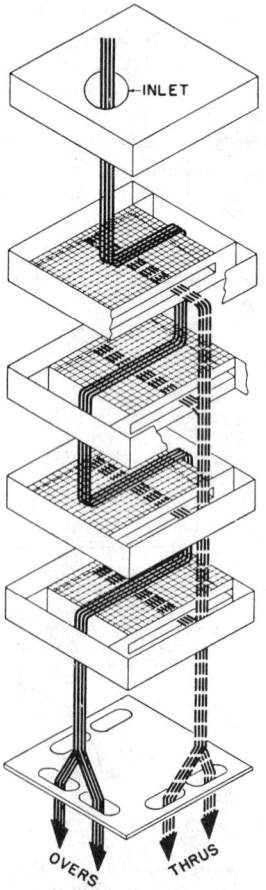

Fig. 659. Gyro-Whip sifter (courtesy, Sprout-Waldron).

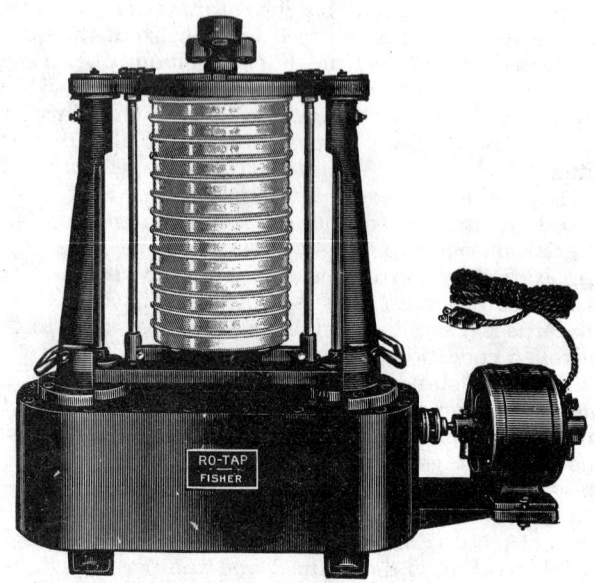

Fig. 656. Ro-Tap sieve shaker (courtesy, Fisher).

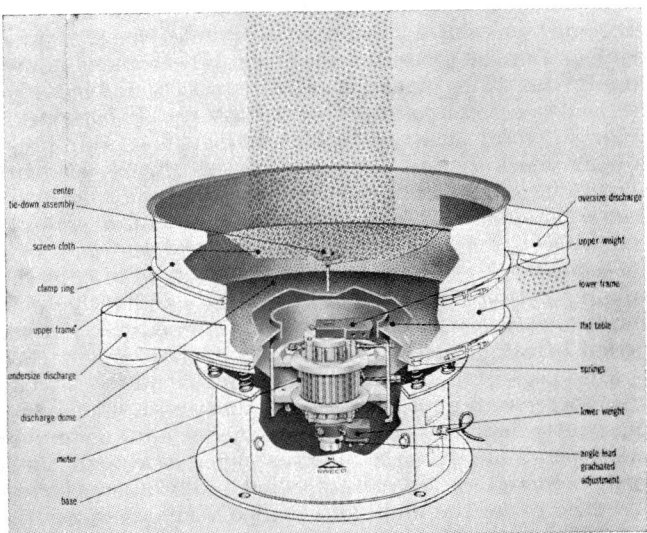

Fig. 660. Sweco Vibro-Energy Separator (courtesy, Southwestern).

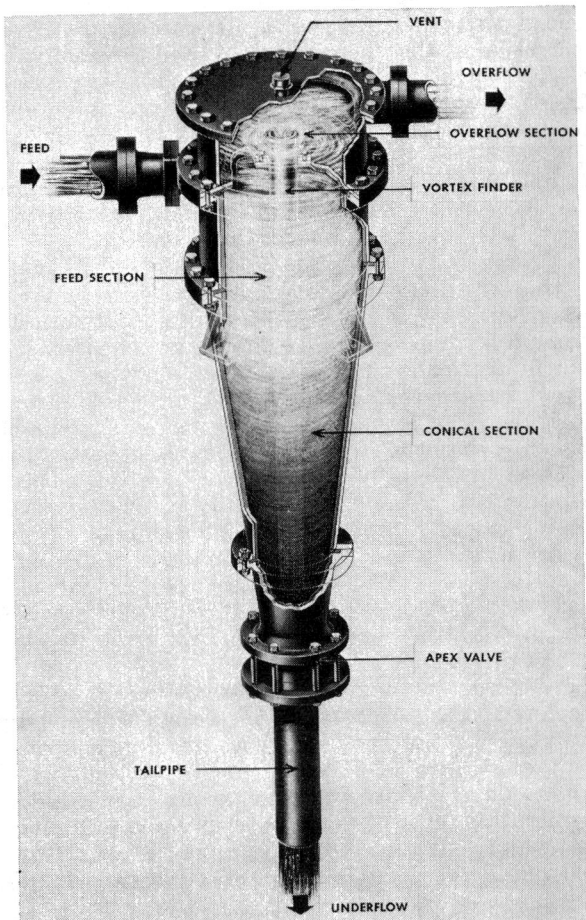

Fig. 661. DorrClone, a hydrocentrifugal classifier (courtesy, Dorr-Oliver).

oppose the flow of particles through the sieve. Some hydrophobic substances which resist wetting by water may be wet screened by the use of organic liquids such as petroleum ether, acetone, or alcohol. Wet screening may be accomplished by spraying both the screen surface and the material as it is fed onto the screen or by feeding a slurry of material directly onto the screen.

Sedimentation—This method employs the settling of particles in a liquid of a relatively low density, under the influence of a gravitational or centrifugal field. In free settling (ie, no particle–particle interference) the particles are supported by hydraulic forces and their fall can be described by Stokes' law. However, in most real situations particle–particle interference, nonuniformity, and turbulence are all present, resulting in more complex settling patterns. With centrifugation, entrainment of particles in the currents produced by other particles may also interfere with fractionation.

Gravitational settling chambers are often used for large-scale separation of relatively coarse particles in the range of 100 μ. Centrifugal devices are useful for the separation of much smaller particles (5–10 μ).

Elutriation—In this process the particles are suspended in a moving fluid. In vertical elutriation at any particular velocity of the fluid, particles of a given size will move upwards with the fluid, while larger particles will settle out under the influence of gravity. In horizontal elutriation a stream of suspended particles is passed over a settling chamber. Particles which leave the stream are collected in the bottom of the chamber. Normally, for all elutriation techniques, both undersize and oversize particles appear in each fraction and recycling is required if a clean cut is desired.

Centrifugal elutriation is basically the same process, except in this case the fluid stream is caused to spin so as to impart a high centrifugal force to the suspended particles. Those particles which are too large to follow the direction of flow separate out on the walls or bottom of the elutriator or cyclone. The finer particles escape with the discharge stream. Separation down to about 5 μ can be achieved with this technique.

The DorrClone (*Dorr-Oliver*) shown in Fig. 661 is an example of a centrifugal type classifier. The feed enters tangentially into the upper section. Centrifugal forces in the vortex throw the coarser particles to

the wall where they collect and then drop down and out of the unit. The fine particles move to the inner spiral of the vortex and are displaced upward and finally out of the top of the unit.

The Sharples Super Classifier (Fig. 662) is another example of a centrifugal classifier useful for the high-speed separation of fine particles. It has a capacity of about 250 lb/hr and operates at an air flow of about 100 cu ft/min at a maximum rotor speed of about 15,000 rpm.

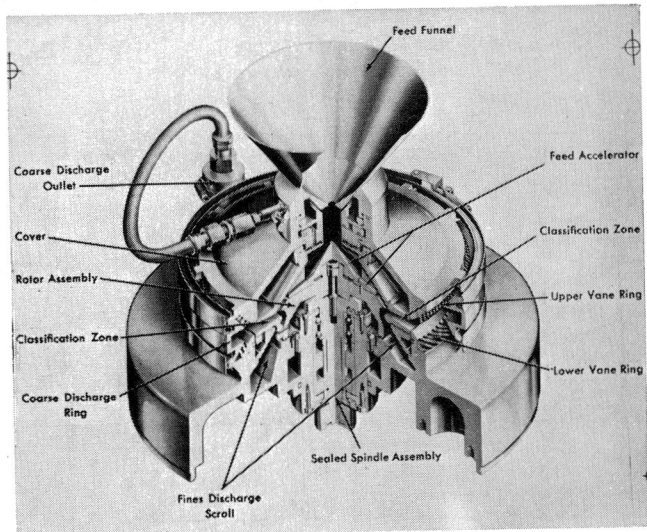

Fig. 662. The Sharples K-8 Super Classifier (courtesy, Sharples).

Inertial elutriators, which utilize an abrupt change in direction of the fluid stream to produce separation, are effective down to about 200 mesh. However, as with other elutriators a clean cut cannot usually be obtained without recycling.

Felvation is a unique process that combines elutriation and sieving along with a varying fluid flow rate and a turbulent fluidized bed to achieve particle separation.[5] The particles are fluidized within the felvation column. By gradually increasing the fluid flow rate the very fine particles are brought up to and then through a sieve surface set into the upper section of the column. These fines are subsequently filtered out of the fluid stream. A further increase in the fluid flow rate causes larger and larger particles to move through the sieve. The final stage is reached when particles just larger than the sieve aperture are elutriated up to the sieve. Because of the way in which the particles are presented to the sieve, very little blinding of the openings occur. Furthermore, since the sieve need only serve as a "go, no go" gauge and not as a supporting surface for the powder, a relatively small sieve surface is required. Thus the more uniform but more expensive electroform sieves, even down to a 10-μ size, can be utilized in this process.

Screening Surfaces—A number of factors must be considered in the selection of screening surfaces. Primary consideration is given to the size and shape of the aperture opening, selection of which is determined by the particle size that is to be separated. In addition, consideration must be given to wire diameter or thickness which influences such properties as stretch, breakage, degree of blinding, and sieve capacity and efficiency as well as the weave or hole pattern, and composition of screening surface. The screens commonly used in pharmaceutical processing include *wovenwire screen, bolting cloth, closely spaced bars,* and *punched plates.* Silk and other textiles are used in producing the very fine *bolting cloths* which are used in screening pigments and a few ultrafine pharmaceuticals. They are relatively weak and require careful handling and light loading. *Punched plates* are used for coarse sizing. Their holes may be round, oval, square, or rectangular. They are sturdy and withstand rough service. Sizes of these in common use range upward from ¼ inch.

Most screening, however, is accomplished with woven wire screens ranging in size from those with 400 openings to the inch to screens with 4 inch square openings or larger. There are numerous types of woven wire screens including the plain, twilled and braided weave. An example of the plain and twilled weave is shown in Figs. 663 and 664.

Two standard ways are commonly used to designate the size of screens with square openings: *the open space* and *the mesh.* The open space is measured from the inner edge of one wire to the inner edge of the neighboring wire; thus, space openings are independent of wire diameter. Mesh is the number of openings per linear mesh, and is measured from the center of one wire to the center of the next wire. In contrast to space openings, mesh depends on wire diameter. For example, a 16 mesh sieve may have a space opening ranging from 0.0032–0.0582 in., depending on the thickness of the wire.[6]

In order to avoid ambiguity and to clearly specify a sieve size, standards were established. Unfortunately, different countries and industries adopted their own standards. In the US, the two common standards are the Tyler Standard and US Standard Sieves. In both these series the sieve number refers to the number of openings per linear inch. For most purposes, screens from the two series are interchangeable, though in a few instances the number designation are different. Since these numbers do not define the size of the openings the Bureau of Standards has established specifications for *Standard Sieves*, as given in Table I. These specifications also establish tolerances for the evenness of weaving, as irregularities from careless weaving might permit much larger particles to pass the sieve

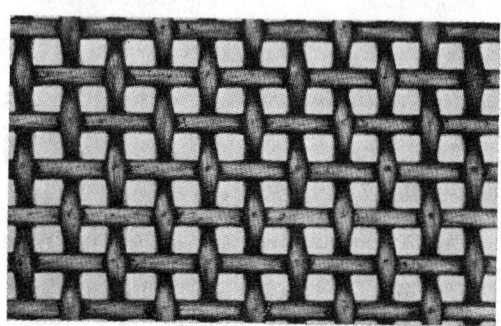

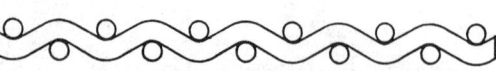

Fig. 663.   Plain weave screen.

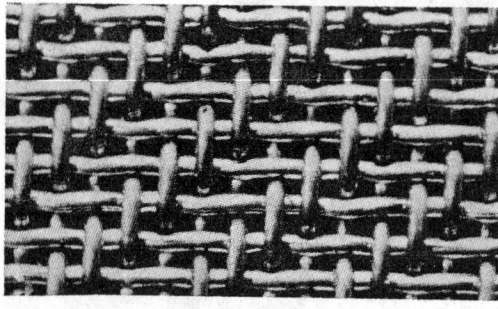

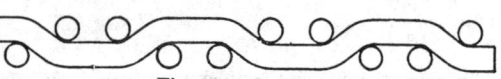

Fig. 664.   Twilled weave screen.

Table I—Nominal Dimensions of Standard Sieves

No.	Sieve opening mm	Sieve opening μ	Permissible variation in average opening, %	Permissible variation in maximum opening, %	Wire diameter, mm
2	9.52	9520	±3	+ 5	2.11 to 2.59
4	4.76	4760	±3	+10	1.14 to 1.68
8	2.38	2380	±3	+10	0.74 to 1.10
10	2.00	2000	±3	+10	0.68 to 1.00
20	0.84	840	±5	+15	0.38 to 0.55
30	0.59	590	±5	+15	0.29 to 0.42
40	0.42	420	±5	+25	0.23 to 0.33
50	0.297	297	±5	+25	0.170 to 0.253
60	0.250	250	±5	+25	0.149 to 0.220
70	0.210	210	±5	+25	0.130 to 0.187
80	0.177	177	±6	+40	0.114 to 0.154
100	0.149	149	±6	+40	0.096 to 0.125
120	0.125	125	±6	+40	0.079 to 0.103
200	0.074	74	±7	+60	0.045 to 0.061

than would be indicated. The standard sieves used for pharmaceutical testing are of wire cloth (not twilled) from brass, bronze, copper, steel, Monel, Inconel, pure nickel, or other suitable material, and are not coated or plated.

Standard sieves should never be mishandled. Forcing a powder through the sieve cloth by means of a spatula, for example, is likely to distort the size of the openings, particularly in the finer mesh screens, and thus lead to erroneous results. Sieves or wire screen cloth are often used to break up lumps or, as in tablet manufacture, to break down a granulation mass, but this is not the purpose for Standard sieves. Less expensive sieves or wire cloth held in suitable frames may be obtained for size-reduction operations and retained specifically for that purpose.

The fineness of powders is expressed in the USP in descriptive terms which correspond to the number assigned to a standard sieve as shown in Table II.

Determining Uniformity of Fineness—For determining uniformity of degree of fineness of powdered drugs and chemicals, the following process may be used, employing standard testing sieves which meet the requirements set forth above.

For *very coarse, coarse,* and *moderately coarse powders,* place from 25 to 100 Gm of the powder to be tested upon the proper standard testing sieve with a tightly fitting receiving pan and cover. Shake the sieve in a rotary horizontal direction and vertically by tapping on a hard surface for not less than 20 minutes or until no appreciable number of particles pass through the sieve. Weigh accurately the amount remaining on the sieve and in the receiving pan.

In the case of *fine* or *very fine powders,* proceed as for *coarse* or for *moderately coarse powders,* but shake the sieve for at least 30 minutes or until no appreciable number of particles pass through the sieve.

In the case of *oily or other powders which tend to clog* the openings, carefully brush the screen at intervals during the test. Break up lumps which form during the sifting test. Do not increase the fineness of the powder during the sieve testing.

Mechanical Sieve Shaker—The fineness of a powdered drug or chemical may be determined also by screening through standard sieves in a mechanical sieve shaker which reproduces the circular and tapping motion given to testing sieves in hand sieving, but with a uniform mechanical action, following the directions provided by the manufacturer of the shaker.

The Ro-Tap Sieve Shaker (Fig. 656) is a mechanical device which duplicates the shaking and tapping described in the USP and it, or a similar mechanical shaker, may be used in determining the uniformity of fineness in official powders.

Particle Size Measurement

Except for the case of regular-shaped particles such as perfect cubes and spheres, which can be completely described by a single measurement (ie, length of a side and diameter, respectively), particle size must be de-

fined. Often some linear dimension (generally referred to as the diameter), measured in a fixed direction, is used to describe irregular particles. However, it should be noted that the diameter determined will be a function of the method used to make the measurement. For example, if rod-shaped particles are measured by sieving the observed diameter will be a function only of the breadth of the particle. If these same particles are measured by sedimentation, the diameter will be a function of the particle mass and settling time, and will be calculated on the basis of the diameter of a sphere which would settle at the same rate.

The surface area of a particle is often of interest and can be calculated from a linear dimension or determined directly by permeability or gas adsorption techniques. However, the calculated surface area may differ markedly, depending on the method used for the measurement. For example, particles with very fine surface pores will generally show a larger surface area when measured by gas adsorption than by microscopy or sieving methods. Thus, in measuring particle size it is important to first select the parameter that is related to the ultimate use of the product, and then select the method that will measure this parameter.

Certainly more useful information would be gained if the particle size of a powder used in a suspension were determined by sedimentation than microscopy, or if the total surface area of the particle were the critical factor in its application (an adsorbant), a permeability or gas adsorption method would no doubt be more useful than sieving or sedimentation.

Sampling—While it is assumed in any particle size determination that the sample analyzed is representative of the total material, often this is not the case. A wide difference in the size measured may result if sufficient attention is not given to this phase of the analysis; ie, to obtaining a truly representative sample.[7] Generally, in sampling large batches of powder a series of grab samples are obtained at random from various parts of the material and then combined into one large sample. This large sample is mixed uniformly, and single samples of convenient size are taken at random. Numerous special techniques and pieces of equipment have been devised for obtaining these samples.[8] Particle size determination is made on these samples.

Analysis of Data—Since powders of particles consist of varying size, no single particle size can completely describe such a system. Thus, particle size distribution or a mean size or other characteristic of central tendency must be utilized. In describing the distribution, generally the frequency of the particles measured in a particular size range are plotted against the mean particle size in each range. This may be represented by a histogram or, by drawing a smooth curve through the points, as a distribution curve (Fig. 665). In this case the curve describes a normal or symmetrical distribution. However, most particulate material cannot be described by a normal distribution curve. The resultant curves are usually skewed as shown in Fig. 666. Such distributions can be better represented by the logarithm of the diameters; ie, a Log Normal Distribution, which permits the calculation of a mean size and standard deviation.

Cumulative frequency curves, in which the percentage of particles in a particular size range are plotted against the particle size, are also useful to characterize powders and to locate median values. The usefulness of such curves can generally be further increased by use of semilog plots which often result in a straight-line relationship. Detailed information concerning

Table II—Classification of Powders by Fineness

Classification of powder	Vegetable and animal drugs			Chemicals		
	Nominal designation no.[a] of powder	Fineness limit[b] %	Sieve no.	Nominal designation no.[a] of powder	Fineness limit[b] %	Sieve no.
Very coarse	8	20	60			
Coarse	20	40	60	20	60	40
Moderately coarse	40	40	80	40	60	60
Fine	60	40	100	80	100	80
Very fine	80	100	80	120	100	80

[a] All particles of the powder pass through a sieve of the nominal designation.

[b] Limit of the percentage that passes through a sieve of the size designated.

the treatment of particle size data can be found in the literature.[9–13]

Microscopy—Microscopic techniques have been classified as one of the most accurate of *direct* methods (ie, methods in which the actual dimensions of particles are directly measured, as contrasted with *indirect* methods which are based on measuring some other property of the particles which is related to their size). Microscopic techniques are useful in that particles are sized directly and individually, rather than being grouped statistically by some other means of classification.

The method is rather tedious and other limitations are found in the techniques required for preparation of the slides and in the maximum resolution which sets the lower limits of particle size measurement using visible light. White light can resolve particles within the range of 0.2 to 100 μ. This lower limit can be decreased to about 0.1 μ by the use of ultraviolet light and to about 0.01 μ by the use of the ultramicroscope. The electron microscope finds its greatest usefulness in particle size measurements in the range of 0.2 to 0.001 μ.

While microscopic methods for particle size determination are time consuming, tedious, and generally require more skill than some of the other techniques, they do offer a number of advantages. They supply information about the shape and thickness that cannot be obtained by other methods and, in addition, supply a permanent record through the use of photomicrographs.

Sedimentation—The settling rate of particles in a fluid (generally water or air) is the basis for this technique. Generally, the observed rate of fall is related to the particle size via Stokes' law and an equivalent diameter is calculated. However, there are a number of limitations in the application of this relationship that should be considered: Stokes' law describes the settling rate of a single, freely falling, hard, spherical particle under conditions such that the resistance to fall is purely viscous. Thus, aggregation, turbulence, particle distortion, or slip will result in deviations from Stokes' law and under such conditions some modification of the basic equation is necessary in order to describe mathematically the rate of fall.

Sedimentation balances are available which provide a means of directly weighing particles at selected time intervals as they fall in a liquid system. For continuous observations, automatic recording balances are also available.

Fig. 667 illustrates a commercially available instrument called a Micromerograph which utilizes the principle of sedimentation in an air column. This instrument and others related to it in principle offer more rapid determinations than those which utilize a liquid medium. There are, however, serious uncertainties in the method which must be taken into consideration. Deviations from Stokes' law and impaction of particles against the inner wall of the settling chamber are sources of possible error.

The Carey and Stairmand photosedimentometer[14] photographs the tracks of particles as they fall in a dispersion medium. The size determination is derived from the length of the photographic track, which is an indication of the distance traveled by the particles, and the time of exposure of the photograph.

Various equipment for the determination of sedimentation rates are described by Cadle.[15] A critical review of the design and operation of sedimentation methods including pipette, hydrometer, photosedimentation balance techniques can be found in a series of articles by Kaye.[16]

Elutriation—This technique, in contrast to sedimentation techniques, utilizes a moving stream of fluid to separate out particles of a particular size. By varying the fluid velocities step-wise the sample may be separated into fractions. The amount in each fraction then can be determined and the size limits calculated by the use of the Stokes' equation or measured directly by microscopy. Generally, water or air is used as the elutriating medium. Air elutriation usually will

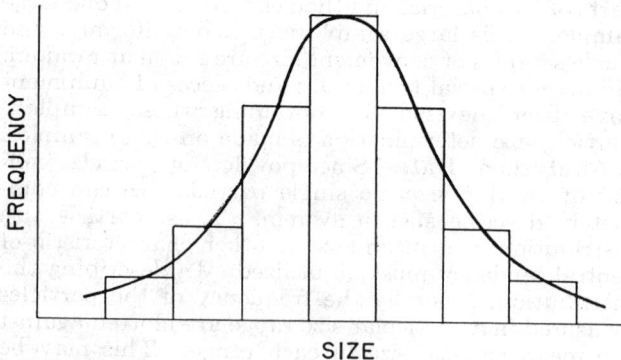

Fig. 665. Symmetrical particle size distribution curve.

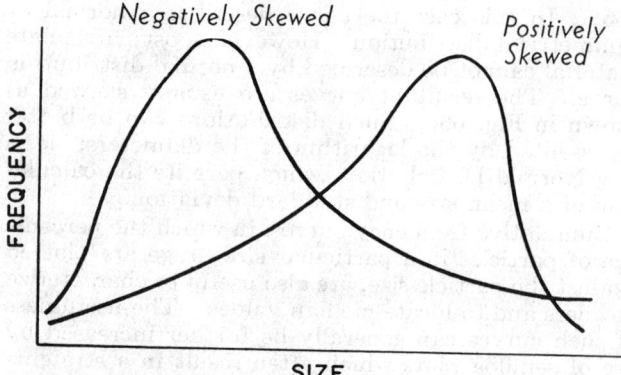

Fig. 666. Asymmetrical particle size distribution curves.

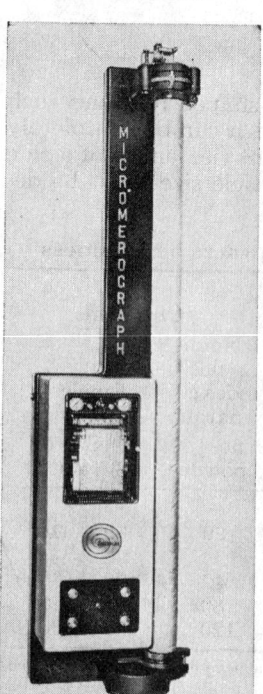

Fig. 667. The Sharples Micromerograph (courtesy, Sharples).

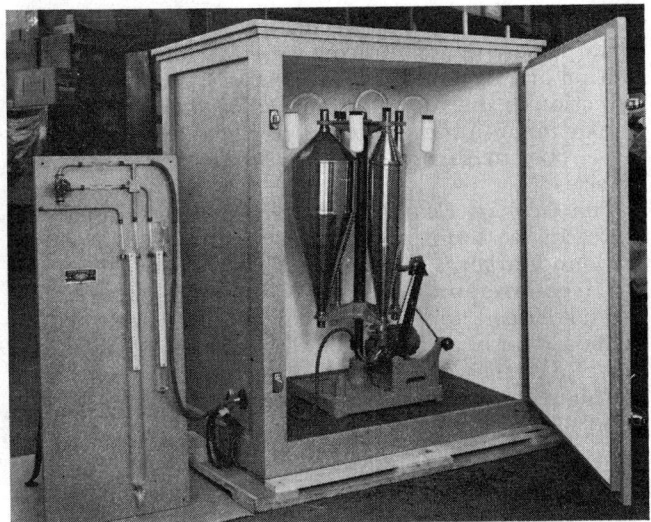

Fig. 668. Amico roller particle size analyzer (courtesy, Am. Instrument).

give a sharper fractionation in a shorter time than will water elutriation. Both, however, have the advantage over gravitational sedimentation of providing sized fractions. The Roller Particle Size Analyzer is an example of an air elutriator (Fig. 668).

Centrifugal elutriators, both air and water, are also useful to classify finely powdered solids. These generally extend the particle size range and improve the sharpness of the cut.

Certain fine cosmetic powders are prepared by air elutriation. The powder is blown into the atmosphere of a large closed cabinet. Baffle shelves are then interposed at various elevations in the cabinet, the finest powder is caught by the top shelf, and the remaining particles are distributed on the lower shelves in an increasing concentration gradient.

Sieving—This is one of the simplest and probably the most frequently used method for determining particle size distribution. The technique basically involves size classification followed by the determination of the weight of each fraction.

One major difficulty associated with this method is the production of screens with uniform apertures, particularly in the very fine mesh sizes. As a result the practical lower limit for woven-wire mesh screens is about 43 μ (325 Mesh). However, with the introduction of electroformed screens, sieves capable of analyzing particles in the 5-μ range are now available.

Sieve analysis, where applicable, offers a number of advantages over the other methods. It is rapid, requires very little skill, the equipment is relatively inexpensive, and can be adapted readily to give a series of size fractions. However, since it compares particles on the basis of geometric similarity much as do the microscopic techniques, it may not always give the information on particle size distribution that is most applicable to the use of the particular material. Therefore, it should not be selected on the basis of ease and simplicity only.

Adsorption of Gases—The methods described previously yield particle sizes that are based on gross dimensions. In cases where surface pores and irregularities are important to the properties of the powder, the use of an adsorption technique should be considered.

Adsorption of a solute from solution or of a gas at low temperatures onto powdered material serves as a measure of the particle surface area, generally reported as specific surface (area/unit mass). The most common adsorption technique is the adsorption of nitrogen at low temperatures. The volume of this gas adsorbed by a powdered sample is determined as a function of gas pressure, and an appropriate plot is prepared. The point at which a monomolecular layer of adsorbate occurs is estimated from the discontinuity that shows in the curve. The specific surface area then can be calculated from a knowledge of the volume of gas required to achieve this monolayer, and the area/molecule occupied by the gas, its molecular weight, and density. Frequently, more complex expressions such as the Brunauer, Emmett, and Teller (BET) equation must be used to describe the surface adsorption of some materials, and to determine the volume of gas required to produce an adsorbed monolayer. The surface properties of a number of pharmaceuticals have been investigated by this technique.[17,18]

Permeability—When a gas or liquid is allowed to flow through a powdered material, the resistance to this flow is found to be a function of such factors as specific surface of the powder, area of the bed, pore space, pressure drop across the bed, and viscosity of the fluid. This resistance can be described, and specific surface calculated by the Kozeny-Carmen equation which relates these factors. This method, while it does not provide a size distribution analysis, does offer a rapid and convenient means of size estimation that is useful for some industrial operations.

Commercially available instruments which measure the rate of flow of a gas through a powder bed under controlled pressure differential are available. The Fisher Sub-Sieve Sizer permits the reading of average particle size directly. The Blaine permeameter produced by Precision Scientific Company in Chicago utilizes the principle of filling the void spaces in a powder with mercury and then weighing it. The void fraction is calculated from the known density of mercury at different temperatures.

The calculations involved in permeability techniques are often complicated and yield only an average size of particles. In measuring particles in the subsieve ranges, rather large deviations may be encountered. With larger mesh sizes, some good agreement is found between the results obtained by techniques employing permeability and microscopy particularly if the powders are made up of spherical or near-spherical particles.

Impaction and Inertial Techniques—The laws which govern the trajectories of particles in fluid streams are utilized in several methods of particle size measurement. Impaction devices are based on the dynamics of deposition of fine particles in a moving air stream when directed past obstacles of defined geometric form, or when forced from a jet device onto a plane surface.

The *cascade impactor*, described by Pilcher and his co-workers[19] forces particle-laden air at a very high speed and fixed rate through a series of jets (each smaller than the preceding one) onto glass slides; impaction takes place in a series of stages. The velocity of the air stream and the particles suspended in it are increased as they advance through the impactor. As a result, the particles are classified by impaction on the different slides, with the larger particles on the top slides and the smaller ones on the downstream slides. Fig. 669 illustrates the principle of the cascade impactor. The exact size of impacted particles on each slide must subsequently be determined. Size analyses may be ob-

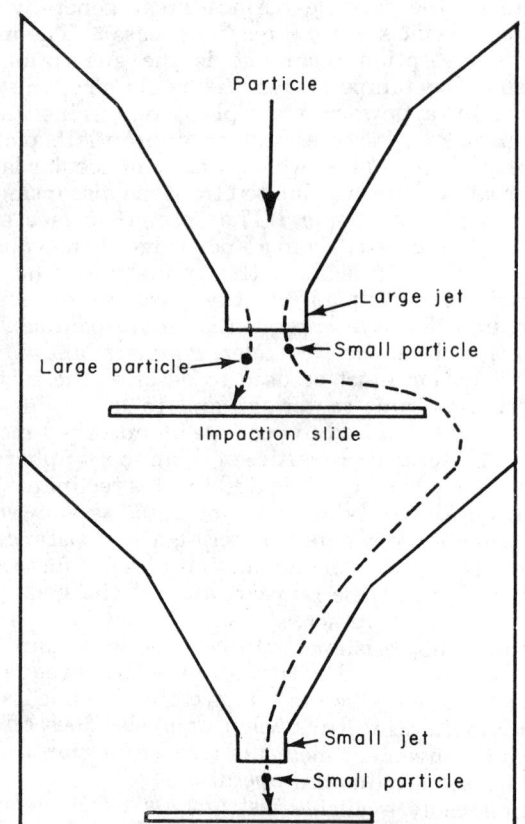

Fig. 669. The principle of the cascade impactor (adapted from Pilcher, J. M., et al, Proc. Chem. Specialties Mfgs. Assoc. Ann. Meeting, 1955, 74).

tained directly by theoretical treatment or prior calibration of the instrument.

Tillotson[20] has described an instrument based on inertial principles similar to those of the cascade impactor. This instrument may be adapted for automatic readout of size distribution by means of light scattering techniques and electronic counters. The method is claimed to provide complete particle size distribution data in a few minutes.

Automatic Particle Size Counters—The Coulter Counter, HIAC Counter, and Gelman Automatic Particle Counter represent three examples of automatic counting equipment.

The *Coulter Counter* will determine the particle volume distribution of material suspended in an electrolyte-containing solution. A table of size ranges of several methods compared with the Coulter principle is shown in Fig. 670. Details of this instrument may be found in Chapter 41, *Instrumental Methods of Analysis*.

The *HIAC Counter* measures the size distribution of particles suspended in either liquids or gases. The standard models will measure sizes from 2 to 2500 μ at pressures up to 3000 psi. Basically, in this instrument

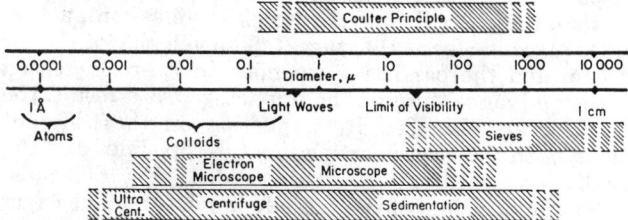

Fig. 670. Size range of Coulter method compared with coverage of sieve, sedimentation, and microscopic methods, and overlap of electron microscope and centrifuge ranges (courtesy, Coulter).

the particles pass a window one-by-one. Each particle as it passes, depending on its size, interrupts some portion of a light beam. This causes an instantaneous reduction in the voltage from a photodetector which is proportional to the size of the particle. Several counting circuits with preset thresholds tally the particles by size.

The *Gelman Counter* uses the principles of light-scattering to count particles in the air in the range of 0.5 μ and larger.

Miscellaneous Methods—Numerous other methods have been applied to particle size determination including x-ray and electron diffraction and ultrasonic techniques. Further information on these and other methods can be found in texts on particle size determination.[8,21]

Mixing of Powders

The mechanism of mixing powders involves convection (the random motion of large groups of particles) and diffusion (the random motion of individual particles) within the system. Thus, mixing can be considered to be a random shuffling-type operation involving both large and small particle groups and even individual particles. However, it should be noted that the use of random motion to achieve random distribution assumes that no other factors influence this distribution.

This is rarely if ever the case in practice. Instead, a variety of properties of the powders being mixed influence this approach to complete randomness. For examples, large differences in particle size tend to cause demixing, generally with the coarse particles moving toward the bottom of the mixer and the fine particles toward the top. Density differences also tend to promote segregation with the heavier particles settling toward the bottom. These two factors may balance each other to some extent if the coarse particles are less dense than the fine particles.

Particle shape also influences this approach to randomness. Elongated particles, because they move less freely through the mixture than symmetrically shaped particles, resist mixing. Stickiness or slipperiness of the particles also must be considered. As might be expected, the stickier the material the less readily it mixes and demixes. Electrostatic forces on the particle surface also can produce marked effects on the mixing process, and in fact may produce sufficient particle-particle repulsion to make random mixing impossible.

Large-Scale Mixing Equipment—The ideal mixer should produce a complete blend rapidly with as gentle as possible a mixing action to avoid product damage and demixing. It should be easily cleaned and discharged, be dust-tight, and require low maintenance and low power consumption. All of these assets generally are not found in any single piece of equipment, thus requiring some compromise in the selection of a mixer.

Rotating Shell Mixers—The drum-type, cubical-shaped, double-cone, and twin-shell blenders are all examples of this class of mixers. Drum-type blenders with their axis of rotation horizontal to the center of the drum are used quite commonly. These, however, suffer from poor crossflow along the axis. The addition of baffles or inclining the drum on its axis increases crossflow and improves the mixing action. Cubical- and polyhedron-shaped blenders with the rotating axis set at various angles also are available. However, in the latter, because of their flat surfaces, the powder is subjected more to a sliding than a rolling action, a motion which is not conducive to the most efficient mixing.

Double-cone blenders, an important class of rotating shell or tumbling mixers, were developed in an attempt to overcome some of the shortcomings of the previously discussed mixers. Here, the mixing pattern provides a good crossflow with a rolling rather than a sliding motion. Normally, no baffles are required so that cleaning is simplified. The twin-shell blender is another important tumbling-type blender. This blender combines the efficiency of the inclined drum-type with the intermixing that occurs when two such mixers combine their flow. The Zig-Zag blender, an extension of the twin-shell blender, provides efficient continuous precision blending (Fig. 671).

Fixed-Shell Mixers—The ribbon mixer, one of the oldest mechanical solid–solid blending devices, exemplifies this type of mixer. The ribbon mixer consists of a relatively long troughlike shell with a semicircular bottom. The shell is fitted with a shaft on which are mounted spiral ribbons, paddles, or helical screws, alone or in combination. These mixing blades produce a continuous cutting and shuffling of the charge by circulating the powder from end to end of the trough as well as rotationally. The shearing action that develops between the moving blade and the trough serves to break down powder agglomerates. However, ribbon mixers are not precision blenders; in addition, they suffer from the disadvantage of being more difficult to clean than the tumbler-type blenders and of having a higher power requirement.

Sigma-blade and *planetary paddle* mixers are also used for solid–solid blending, although most generally as a step prior to the introduction of liquids. Mixers with high-speed impeller blades set into the bottom of a vertical or cylindrical shell have been shown to be very efficient blenders. This type of mixer, in addition to its ability to produce precise blends, serves also to break down agglomerates rapidly. The mechanical heat buildup produced by this mixer within the powder mix, and the relatively high power requirement are often drawbacks to this use of this type of mixer.

Muller mixers are a specialized class of mixers, useful for heavy duty operations requiring high shearing forces. The mulling action is a shearing mechanism, and is the closest to the type of mixing achieved by the hand-operated mortar and pestle. *Vertical impeller mixers*, which have the advantage of requiring little floor space, employ a screw type of impeller which constantly overturns the batch (Fig. 672). The fluidized mixer is a modification of the vertical impeller type. The impeller is replaced by a rapidly moving stream of air fed into the bottom of the shell. The body of the powder is fluidized and mixing is accomplished by circulation and overtumbling in the bed (Fig. 673).

Generally, when precision solid–solid blending is required, the rotating twin shell or the double cone type blenders are recommended.[22] However, the fluidized bed and high-speed impeller mixers certainly deserve consideration. Recently, Baines and Cope[23] compared the blending efficiency of three basic types of solid–solid blenders, the rotating cone, ribbon, and

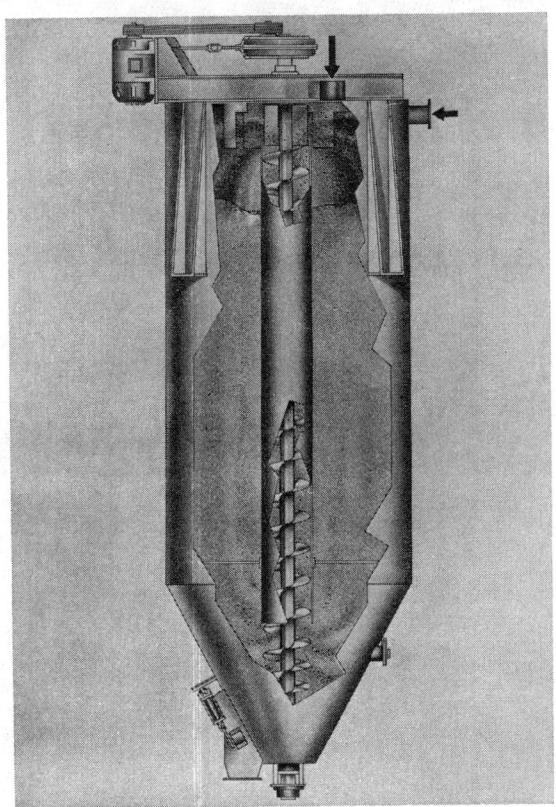

Fig. 672. Sprout-Waldron vertical mixer.

high-speed impeller blenders, by following the development of a red pigment added to talc or calcium carbonate. They reported a faster rate of color development (a measure of mixing) with the impeller mixer than with either the ribbon or cone mixer. In addition the intensity of the color reached at equilibrium was considerably higher with the impeller mixer. They also noted that an appreciable quantity of undispersed pigment was present in the final mixture from both the ribbon and cone blender. In their ranking of the production of evenness of blend, they rated the high-speed blender the best, the ribbon blender second, and the rotating cone as the poorest.

Small-Scale Mixing Equipment—The pharmacist most generally employs the mortar and pestle for the small-scale mixing usually required for prescription compounding. However, the use of spatulas and sieves also may be utilized on occasion. The mortar and pestle method combines comminution and mixing in a single operation. Thus, it is particularly useful where some degree of particle size reduction as well as

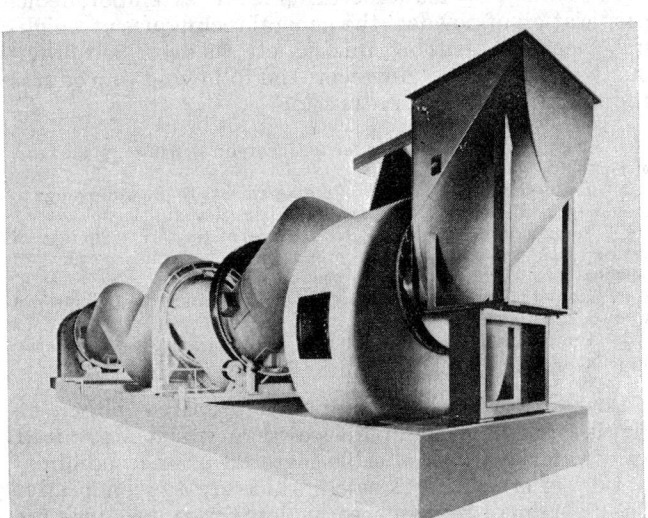

Fig. 671. Zig-zag continuous solid blender, available in capacities up to 3600 cu ft/hr (courtesy, Patterson-Kelley).

mixing is required as in the case of mixtures of crystalline material.

The blending of powders with a spatula on a tile or paper, a relatively inefficient method, is sometimes used for small quantities of powders often as an auxiliary blending technique or when the compaction produced by the mortar and pestle technique is undesirable.

Sieving is usually employed as a pre- or post-mixing method to reduce loosely held agglomerates and to increase the over-all effectiveness of a blending process.

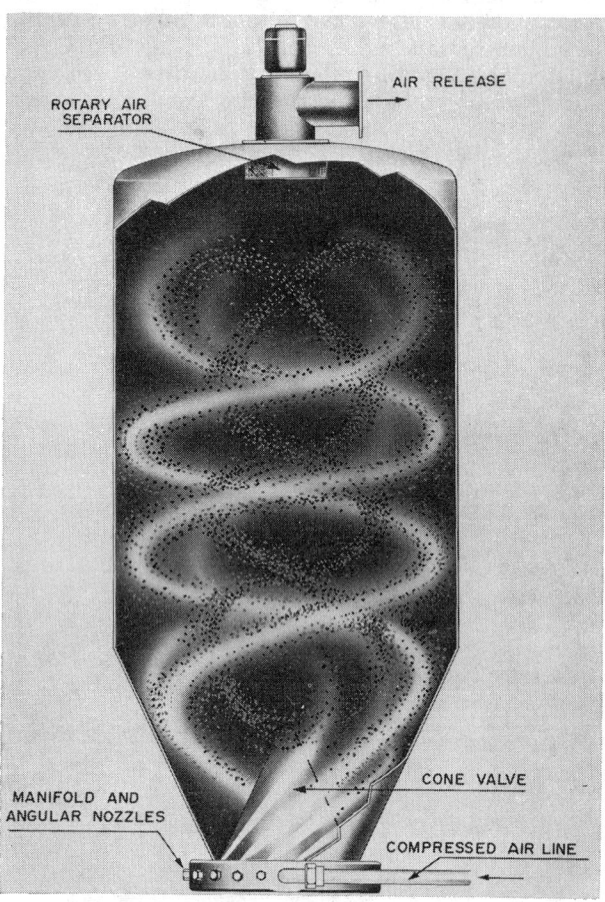

Fig. 673. Air Mix mixer (courtesy, Sprout-Waldron).

When used alone as a solid–solid blending technique, several passes through the sieve are required to produce a reasonably homogeneous mix.

Powders as a Dosage Form

Historically, powders represent one of the oldest dosage forms. They are a natural outgrowth of man's attempt to prepare crude drugs and other natural products in a more conveniently administered form. However, with declining use of crude drugs and increasing use of many highly potent compounds, powders as a dosage form have been replaced largely by capsules and tablets.

Advantages

In certain instances powders possess advantages and thus still represent a portion (although small) of the solid dosage forms currently being employed.

Flexibility—Since most medicines are available in a finely divided dry state, the prescriber has a wide selection of drugs, combinations, and dosage range.

Stability—The shelf life of many materials, such as aspirin and penicillin, is extended by dispensing in a dry powdered state rather than as a solution.

Rapid Therapeutic Effect—The rapid attainment of therapeutic blood levels, as well as the rapid adsorptive properties of finely divided powders, are directly related to the large surface area of these products.

Ease of Administration—When solid medication must be given to patients, especially young children who have difficulty in swallowing capsules or tablets, dry powder simply may be placed directly on the tongue and washed down with water. More commonly, the powder is first mixed or dissolved in water, milk, or flavored liquid prior to administration. If infants and patients find the taste of the medication unpleasant, flavor may be incorporated into the powder during compounding or the powder may be incorporated into soft, sweetened food such as applesauce.

Disadvantages

The chief disadvantages of powders as a dosage form are (1) they are time consuming to prepare and (2) they are not well suited for the dispensing of many unpleasant tasting, hygroscopic, or deliquescent drugs.

Bulk powders have another serious disadvantage when compared with divided and individually weighed powders—inaccuracy of dose. The dose is influenced by many factors including size of measuring spoon, density of powder, humidity, degree of settling, fluffiness due to agitation, and personal judgment. Not only do patients measure varying amounts of powder when using the same spoon but they often select one differing in size from that specified by their physician.

In some studies, attempts were made to duplicate bulk powder measurements with one person using the same spoon. The results varied widely. With several persons, the measurements differed from one to another by as much as a factor of four. Therefore, when the dose of a bulk powder is to be measured by the patient, it should contain only nontoxic substances so that wide variations in the dose will not adversely affect him. The use of bulk powders as a dosage form for potent drugs can have serious consequences.[24]

Extemporaneous Techniques

In both the manufacturing and extemporaneous preparation of powders the general techniques of weighing, measuring, sifting, mixing, etc, as described previously are applied. However, the following procedures should receive special attention.

1. Use of geometric dilution for the incorporation of small amounts of potent drugs.
2. Reduction of particle size of all ingredients to the same range to prevent stratification of large and small particles.
3. Sieving when necessary to achieve mixing or reduction of agglomerates, especially in the preparation of dusting powders or powders into which liquids have been incorporated.
4. Heavy trituration, when applicable, to reduce the bulkiness of a powder.
5. Protection against humidity, air oxidation, and loss of volatile ingredients.

Powders are most commonly prepared either as divided powders and bulk powders which are mixed with water or other suitable material prior to administration, or as dusting powders which are applied locally. They also may be prepared as dentrifices, products for reconstitution, insufflations, aerosols, and other miscellaneous products.

Divided Powders

Divided powders (*chartula* or *chartulae*) are dispensed in the form of individual doses and are generally dispensed in papers, properly folded. They also may be dispensed in metal foil, small heat-sealed plastic bags, or other containers.

Dividing Powders—After the weighing, comminuting, and mixing of ingredients are completed, the powders must be accurately divided into the prescribed number of doses. In order to achieve accuracy consistent with the other steps in the preparation, *each dose should be weighed individually* and transferred to a powder paper. Generally, the number of powder papers corresponding to the number of doses being prepared are arranged on the counter as shown in Fig. 674. The weighed powders are transferred from the balance to the individual papers. Following the completion of this step the powder papers are folded.

Folding Powders—The operations of folding powder papers are illustrated in Fig. 675. Care in making the several folds, and experience gained by repetition, are necessary to obtain uniformity when the powders are finally placed in the box for dispensing. Deviation from any of the three main folds will result in powders of varying height being formed and variations in the folded ends will likewise be noticeable when the powders are placed side by side.

All of the powder papers for the prescription being filled should be creased by folding down a margin on the top, care being observed that the fold is straight and uniform in all of the papers (Fig. 675*A*). About six papers may be folded at once, but if the number becomes too large, it will lead to variations in the depth of the fold. For a standard 3- by 4-in. powder paper, the fold should be about ½ in. wide. For other powder papers it should be in proportion. The papers then should be placed on the counter as indicated in Fig. 674, having them uniformly arranged and as close together as is convenient.

After the powder has been distributed over the papers as described, the additional folds are made as follows. The lower edge of the paper is lifted and folded over until it lies exactly in the crease of the original top fold (Fig. 675*B*) which is then pressed down over this lower edge (Fig. 675*C*). The top of the paper, as it now appears, is folded toward the operator until it exactly divides the folded paper in the center (Fig. 675*D*). The three folds mentioned will so regulate the height of the powders in a low-style powder box that they will just protrude slightly, thus making it possible to pick out one powder with the fingers without disturbing the others. For the old-style boxes having greater depth the final fold should be adjusted to make the powder at least even with the edge of the box.

When the individual powder paper has been folded lengthwise, it is picked up in both hands by the ends and pressed down over the ends of the box so that both ends are turned over exactly the same length. At the same time the end of the box is pressed in slightly so that the powder when finally completed will fit and slide evenly in the box (Fig. 675*E*).

The turned ends are simultaneously and firmly pressed between the thumb and finger to complete the folding. The top of the powder paper, at the center, should not be creased with the fingers or with a spatula, as the "roll edge" adds materially to the appearance of the finished box of powders, and creasing may unnecessarily cake the powder. However, where a large number of powders must be placed in a comparatively small box, creasing may help.

As the powders receive their final fold they are preferably placed on the counter in a row with the long fold toward the dispenser. When all are folded they may be assembled in one hand, with the lengthwise folds uppermost and toward the operator, and placed in the box. It is sometimes more convenient to place the powders into the box one at a time, using the forefinger of the hand holding the box to keep the inserted powders in place.

Some pharmacists prefer to alternate the folds, having one forward and one backward, and some even prefer to turn every other powder upside down to lessen the likelihood of the powders springing from the box when a powder is removed. This occurs most frequently when the powder is bulky and it is possible to adjust this partially by tapping the assembled powders down first from one side or end and then from the other to effect a more uniform distribution of the powder.

An attractive addition to the powder paper is to have the name of the pharmacist printed on the paper in such a position that when folded it will appear uniformly on the edge of all powders. The folded edge of the powder must not be creased. Powder papers, so printed, can be more readily folded with even ends than plain paper since the printed edge serves as a guide in folding.

Another suggestion to add to the attractiveness of folded powders is to hold the powders in place by a small strip of paper pasted to the shoulders of the powder box. This narrow strip of paper carries the name of the firm and acts as a seal to the powders, the protection to the customer being similar to that provided by a bottle cap when used on liquid prescription.

Packaging Divided Powders—Specially manufactured paper and boxes are available for dispensing divided powders.

Powder Papers—Four basic types of powder papers are available.

1. Vegetable parchment, a thin semiopaque moisture-resistant paper.
2. White bond, an opaque paper with no moisture-resistant properties.
3. Glassine, a glazed, transparent moisture-resistant paper.
4. Waxed, a transparent waterproof paper.

Hygroscopic and volatile drugs can be protected best by use of a waxed paper, double wrapped with a bond paper to improve the appearance of the completed powder. Parchment and glassine papers offer limited protection for these drugs.

A variety of sizes of powder papers are available. The selection of the proper size depends on the bulk of

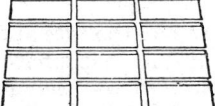

Fig. 674. Arrangement of powder papers

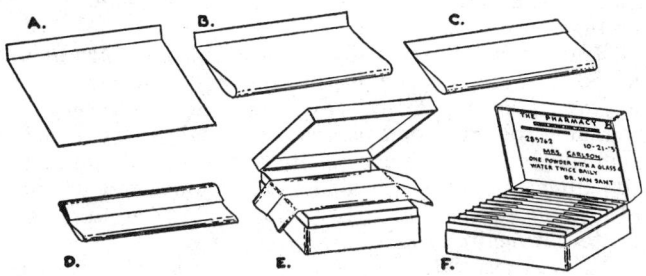

Fig. 675. Folding powder papers.

each dose and the dimensions of the powder box required to hold the number of doses prescribed.

Powder Boxes—Various types of boxes are supplied in several sizes for dispensing divided powders. The hinged-shoulder boxes shown in Fig. 676 are the most popular and have the advantage of preventing the switching of lids with the directions for use when several boxes of the same size are in the same home. The prescription label may be pasted directly on top of the lid or inside the lid. In the latter case the name of the pharmacy is lithographed on top of the lid.

Special Problems

The incorporation of volatile substances, eutectic mixtures, liquids, and hygroscopic or deliquescent substances into powders presents problems that require special treatment.

Volatile Substances—The loss of camphor, menthol, and essential oils by volatilization when incorporated into powders may be prevented or retarded by the use of heat-sealed plastic bags or by double wrapping with a waxed or glassine paper inside of bond paper.

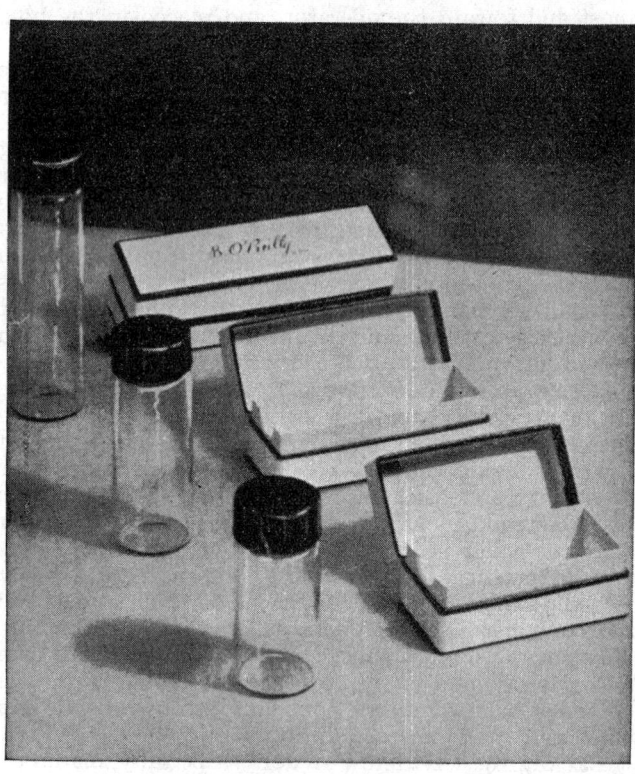

Fig. 676. Powder boxes with hinged lids are shown on the right.

Eutectic Mixtures—Liquids result from the combination of phenol, camphor, menthol, thymol, antipyrine, acetophenetidin, acetanilid, aspirin, salol, and related compounds at ordinary temperatures. These so-called eutectic mixtures may be incorporated into powders by the addition of an inert diluent. Magnesium carbonate or light magnesium oxide are the most commonly used and most effective diluents for this purpose, although kaolin, starch, bentonite, and other absorbents have been recommended. In 1952 a German patent was granted for the use of silicic acid to prevent eutexia with aspirin, phenyl salicylate, and other troublesome compounds. The incorporation of about 20% silicic acid (particle size, 50 μ) prevented

liquefaction even under the compression pressures required to form tablets.[25]

In handling this problem each eutectic compound should be first mixed with a portion of the diluent and gently blended together, preferably with a spatula on a sheet of paper. Generally, an amount of the diluent equal to the eutectic compounds is sufficient to prevent liquefaction for about two weeks. Deliberate forcing of the formation of the liquid state, by direct trituration, followed by absorption of the moist mass, will also overcome this problem. This technique requires the use of more diluent than the previously mentioned methods but offers the advantage of extended product stability. Thus the technique is useful for dispensing a large number of doses that normally would not be consumed over a period of one or two weeks.

Liquids—In small amounts, liquids may be incorporated into divided powders. Magnesium carbonate, starch, or lactose may be added to increase the absorbability of the powders if necessary. When the liquid is a solvent for a nonvolatile heat-stable compound, it may be evaporated gently on a water bath. Lactose may be added during the course of the evaporation to increase the rate of solvent loss by increasing the surface area. Some fluidextracts and tinctures may be treated in this manner, although the use of an equivalent amount of a powdered extract, when available, is a more desirable technique.

Hygroscopic and Deliquescent Substances—Substances which become moist because of their strong affinity for moisture in the air may be prepared as divided powders by the addition of inert diluents such as magnesium carbonate. Double wrapping is desirable for further protection.

Certain extremely deliquescent compounds such as potassium thiocyanate, lithium bromide, and potassium acetate cannot be satisfactorily prepared as powders. The pharmacist should recommend that they be dispensed in solution.

Bulk Powders

Bulk powders may be classified as (1) oral powders, (2) dentifrices, (3) douche powders, (4) dusting powders, (5) insufflations, and (6) triturations.

Oral Powders—These are generally supplied as *finely divided powders* or as *effervescent granules*.

The finely divided powders are intended to be suspended or dissolved in water or mixed with soft foods, eg, applesauce, prior to administration. Antacids and laxative powders are frequently administered in this form.

Effervescent granules contain sodium bicarbonate and either citric acid, tartaric acid, or sodium biphosphate, in addition to the active ingredients. On solution in water carbon dioxide is released as a result of the acid–base reaction. The effervescence from the release of the carbon dioxide serves to mask the taste of salty or bitter medications.

Granulation is generally accomplished by producing a moist mass, forcing it through a coarse sieve, and drying it in an oven. The moisture necessary for massing the materials is readily obtained by heating them sufficiently to drive off the water of hydration from the uneffloresced citric acid. The completed product must be dispensed in tightly closed glass containers to protect it against the humidity of the air.

NF VII gave the following general directions for the preparation of granular effervescent salts:

General Formula for Effervescent Salts

"The citric acid directed in the formulas shall be in effloresced crystals and be powdered just before using. The sodium bicarbonate directed in the formulas shall be in powder and dry; if kept in a cool, dry atmosphere, it will not require drying. All other ingredients should be dried at a temperature of 100° to 110°C until they cease to lose weight, and then be powdered and passed through a No. 60 sieve.

"As atmospheric dampness, if present, will be absorbed by the finished salt and will destroy the effervescent character of the product, it is important that these preparations be made and kept in a relatively dry atmosphere.

"The proportions of tartaric acid and citric acid may be varied, if necessary, to produce the proper consistency, but their combined acidity must be equivalent to the acidity in the official formula.

"**Directions for Granulating in an Oven**—Prepare the citric acid and the other ingredients of the formula as directed above; intimately mix the powders, without trituration, adding the citric acid last; spread the resulting product evenly, about 10 mm. thick, on a sheet of paper on a canvas tray, glass plate, or in a shallow porcelain or enameled dish; and place it in an oven heated to a temperature between 95° and 105°C.

"Allow the powder to remain in the oven, without stirring, until it becomes moist and acquires the proper consistency, about that of dough; then force the mass immediately through a No. 6 tinned-iron sieve, and dry the product at a temperature not exceeding 50°C. When it is dry, pass the granular product through a No. 6 tinned-iron sieve, and transfer it immediately to dry bottles or containers; seal them tightly.

"**Directions for Granulating on a Water Bath**—If a small quantity of the salt is to be prepared, transfer the powders, mixed as directed above, to a double boiler heated by water actively boiling, the inner dish being in contact with the water. When the pasty mass acquires the proper consistency, as described in the previous process, force it immediately through a No. 6 tinned-iron sieve, and dry the product at a temperature not exceeding 50°C. Promptly pass the dry granules through a No. 6 tinned-iron sieve and transfer to a dry container, which should then be tightly sealed."

In the manufacturing laboratory the mixture is usually heated in a shallow, enameled, jacketed steam kettle until moist, forced through a No. 6 sieve by mechanical means, and the moist granules are dried in a vacuum dryer. The mixture may also be heated until moist in a pill-coating pan, the heat being applied to the exterior of the revolving pan.

Effervescent powders may be prepared also by adding small amounts of water to the dry salts in order to obtain a workable mass. The mass is dried and ground to yield the powder or granule. Care must be utilized in this procedure to ensure that the reaction which occurs in the presence of water does not proceed too far before it is stopped by the drying process. Should this happen, the effervescent properties of the product will be destroyed.

Recently, other preparative techniques have been reported for effervescent powders. Coletta and Kennon[26] used a fluidized bed procedure in which the powders are blended and then suspended in a stream of air in a Wurster chamber. Water is sprayed into the chamber resulting in a slight reaction and an expansion of the particles to form granules ranging in size from 10 to 30 mesh. This approach apparently offers a number of advantages over the older techniques. The extent of reaction and particle size are controlled during the manufacture. A drying oven, trays, and even grinding devices are not required. Furthermore, the technique lends itself to a continuous as well as a batch operation.

The heat generated from the blending and mixing operation also has been used to mass the powders by causing the release of the water of hydration from the citric acid. The massed materials can be dried and sieved through a coarse sieve. This technique thus eliminates the need of an external heat source or a granulating solution.[27]

Dentifrices—These may be prepared in the form of

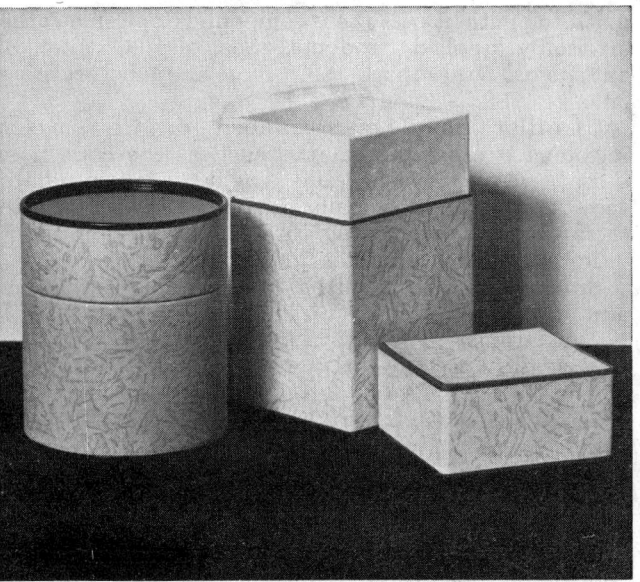

Fig. 677. Bulk powder boxes.

a bulk powder, generally containing a soap or detergent, mild abrasive, and an anticariogenic agent. These products are considered in more detail in Chapter 95 on *Dental Services*, page 1847.

Douche Powders—These products are completely soluble and are intended to be dissolved in water prior to use as antiseptics or cleansing agents for a body cavity. They are most commonly intended for vaginal use, although they may be formulated for nasal, otic, or ophthalmic use. Generally, since aromatic oils are included in these powders, they are passed through a No. 40 or 60 sieve to eliminate agglomeration and to insure complete mixing. Dispensing in wide-mouth glass jars serves to protect against loss of volatile materials and permits easy access by the patient. Bulk powder boxes as shown in Fig. 677 may be used for dispensing douche powders, although glass containers are preferred because of the protection afforded by these containers against air and moisture.

Dusting Powders—These are locally applied nontoxic preparations that are intended to have no systemic action. They always should be dispensed in a very fine state of subdivision to enhance effectiveness and minimize irritation. When necessary, they may be micronized or passed through a No. 80 or 100 sieve.

Extemporaneously prepared dusting powders should be dispensed in sifter-top packages. Commercial dusting powders are available in sifter-top cans, sterile envelopes (Steripak products of *Lilly*), or pressure aerosols. The latter, while generally more expensive than the other containers, offer the advantage of protection from air, moisture, and contamination, as well as convenience of application. Foot powders and talcum powders are currently available as pressure aerosols.

Dusting powders are applied to various parts of the body as lubricants, protectives, absorbents, antiseptics, antipruritics, antibromodrosis agents, astringents, and antiperspirants.

While in most cases dusting powders are considered nontoxic, absorption of boric acid through large areas of abraded skin has caused toxic reactions in infants. Accidental inhalation of zinc stearate powder has led to pulmonary inflammation of the lungs of infants. The pharmacist should be aware of the possible dangers when the patient uses these compounds as well as other externally applied products. See also Chapter 43 on *Topical Drugs*, page 763. Note the label warnings on page 1988.

Insufflations—These are finely divided powders introduced into body cavities such as the ears, nose, throat, tooth sockets, and vagina. An insufflator (powder blower) is usually employed to administer these products. However, the difficulty in obtaining a uniform dose has restricted their general use.

Specialized equipment has been developed for the administration of micronized powders of relatively potent drugs. The Norisodrine Sulfate Aerohaler Cartridge (*Abbott*) is an example of such a product. In the use of this Aerohaler, inhalation by the patient causes a small ball to strike a cartridge containing the drug. The force of the ball shakes the proper amount of the powder free, permitting its inhalation.

Pressure aerosols have also been employed as a means of administering insufflations, especially for potent drugs. This method offers the advantage of excellent control of dose, through metered valves, as well as product protection.

Triturations—These are dilutions of potent powdered drugs, prepared by intimately mixing them with a suitable diluent in a definite proportion by weight. They were at one time official as 1–10 dilutions. The pharmacist sometimes prepares triturations of such poisonous substances as strychnine sulfate, arsenic, mercury bichloride, atropine, etc, in a convenient concentration using lactose as the diluent, for use at the prescription counter. These medicinal substances are

more accurately and conveniently weighed by using this method.

Tablets of potent materials manufactured for the express purpose of affording a convenient means of incorporating potent agents are supplied under the name of *Dispensing Tablets* (page 1650).

References

1. Fincher, J. H., *J. Pharm. Sci.*, **57**, 1825 (1968).
2. Lees, K. A., *J. Pharm. Pharmacol.*, **15**, 43T (1963).
3. Smith, E. A., *Chem. Ind.*, 1436 (Aug. 19, 1967).
4. Temperley, H. N. V., and Blythe, G. E. K., *Nature*, **219**, 1218 (1968).
5. Kaye, B. H., and Jackson, M. R., *Powder Technol.*, **1**, 43 (1967).
6. Goldberg, S. A., and Walter, W., *Chem. Eng.*, **66** (3), 107 (1959).
7. Lieberman, A., *Chem. Eng.*, **74**, 164 (Apr. 24, 1967).
8. Cadle, R. D., *Particle Size Determination*, Interscience, New York, 1955, pp. 55–92.
9. *Information Circular #7224*, Bureau of Mines, Washington, D.C.
10. Schumann, R., Jr., *Tech. Paper #1189*, Am. Inst. Mining Met. Engrs., 1940.
11. Gaudin, A. M., *Trans. Am. Inst. Mining Met. Engrs.*, **73**, 253 (1926).
12. Resin, R., and Rammler, E., *J. Inst. Fuel*, **7**, 29 (1933).
13. Irani, R. R., and Callis, C. F., *Particle Size: Measurement, Interpretation and Application*, Wiley, New York, 1963.
14. Carey, W. F., and Stairmand, C. J., *Trans. Inst. Chem. Engrs. (London)*, **16**, 57 (1938).
15. Cadle, R. D., *Particle Size Determination*, Interscience, New York, 1955, pp. 208–261.
16. Kaye, B. H., *Chem. Eng.*, **73**, 242 (Nov. 7, 1966).
17. Swintosky, J. V., et al, *J. APhA, Sci. Ed.*, **38**, 210 (1949).
18. Haines, B. A., and Martin, A. N., *J. Pharm. Sci.*, **50**, 756 (1961).
19. Pilcher, J. M., et al, *Proc. Chem. Specialties Mfrs. Assoc. Ann. Meeting*, 66 (1956).
20. Tillotson, D., *Aerosol Age*, **3** (5), 41 (1958).
21. Orr, C., Jr., and DallaValle, J. M., *Fine Particle Measurement*, Macmillan, New York, 1959.
22. Fischer, J. J., *Chem. Eng.*, **67**, 107 (Aug. 8, 1960).
23. Baines, R. G., and Cope, G., *J. Soc. Cosmetic Chemists*, **19**, 225 (1968).
24. Capper, K. R., and Smith, G., *Pharm. J.*, **184**, 447 (1960).
25. *Selected Pharmaceutical Research References* (SK&F), **3**, 7 (1963).
26. Coletta, V., and Kennon, L., *J. Pharm. Sci.*, **53**, 1524 (1964).
27. Murray, R. B., *J. Pharm. Sci.*, **57**, 1776 (1968).

87 | Tablets, Capsules, and Pills

Compressed tablets—tablet formulas—molded tablets or tablet
triturates—hard and soft gelatin capsules—pills—other solid dosage
forms

This chapter was prepared by

Robert E. King, PhD, *Professor of Industrial Pharmacy, Philadelphia College
of Pharmacy and Science, Philadelphia, Pa. 19104*

Tablets

Tablets may be defined as solid pharmaceutical
dosage forms prepared by compressing or molding.
They have been in widespread use since the latter part
of the 19th century. They still remain the most popular of all the medicinal preparations intended for oral
use. Advantages of tablet preparation to the manufacturer include simplicity and economy in fabrication, stability, and convenience in dispensing and
shipping. The advantages to the consumer include
accuracy and compactness of dosage, portability, and
blandness of taste.

History

In Arabian manuscripts written by al-Zahrawi during
the latter half of the 10th century, tablet molds, formed
by engraving suitable hollow impressions in two facing
pieces of ebony, wood, ivory, or grinding stone, are
described. At least 1000 years ago the weight of
tablets was controlled. al-Zahrawi recommended that
in preparing tablets of an exact weight, a small portion of kneaded material should be placed into the
mold while soft and if it was found to be lighter than
the required weight, the engravings were widened
gradually until the pressed tablet reached the required
weight. The molds were painted with an oily material
which probably served as a lubricant to prevent the
tablets from sticking in the molds.[1]

Brockedon is credited with introducing tablet
fabrication in England.[2] About 1872 John Wyeth and
his brother in conjunction with Henry Bower designed
a machine that materially reduced the cost of compression. The tablets compressed with this machine
were made commercially available.[3] John Wyeth and
Brother of Philadelphia are believed to have been the
first to use the term *compressed tablet*.[4] By 1894, tablets for almost every known disease were sold in the
European and American markets. In the United
States in 1895 Joseph P. Remington devised a machine
for making tablets based on the Remington pill press
made in 1875. (Fig. 678). Remington's machine was
made of cast steel. The base had two countersunk depressions, with a short post (C) in the center of each;
a lenticular depression was made in the upper surface
of each post. A steel cylinder (B) having a central
aperture of the same diameter as the post was placed
over the post in the depression, the proper quantity of
powder was introduced, and the plunger (A), which
had a corresponding lenticular depression on its lower
surface, was placed on the powder and was struck a
quick blow with a mallet. The powder was thereby
compressed, and the tablet adhered to the cylinder

when it was lifted from the lower post. By holding the
cylinder over a box and tapping the plunger lightly the
tablet was forced out and dropped into the box.

Since the latter part of the 19th century, increasing
attention has been given to the manufacture of compressed tablets. Although the basic approach has remained the same from a mechanical point of view, the
technology has undergone great improvement.[5] The
physical and chemical characteristics of compressed
materials, as well as their subsequent disintegration
and dissolution, form the subject for an increasing
number of papers appearing in the current literature.[6-8]

Definitions

Although tablets are most frequently discoid in form,
they also may be round, oval, oblong, cylindrical, or
triangular. They are divided into two general classes,
depending on whether they are made by compression
or by molding. The various tablet types and abbreviations commonly employed in referring to them
are listed below.

Compressed Tablets (CT)

These tablets are formed by compression and contain no special
coating. They are made from powdered, crystalline, or granular
materials, alone or in combination with binders (adhesive substances), disintegrators (substances facilitating the breakup of tablets
after administration), lubricants (materials preventing sticking of the
tablets to the punches and dies), and fillers (inert diluents). They
are formed into many shapes and sizes.

Sugar-Coated Tablets (SCT)—These are compressed tablets containing a sugar coating. Such coatings are beneficial in covering up
medicinals possessing objectionable tastes or odors, and in protecting
sensitive medicinals subject to deterioration.

Film-Coated Tablets (FCT)—These are compressed tablets which
are covered with a thin layer or film of a water-soluble material. A
number of polymeric substances with film-forming properties are
used for this purpose. Film coating imparts the same general
characteristics as sugar coating with the added advantage of a
greatly reduced time required for the coating operation.

Enteric-Coated Tablets (ECT)—These are compressed tablets
coated with substances that resist solution in gastric fluid but disintegrate and release their medication in the intestine.

Chocolate-Colored Tablets (CCT)—The abbreviation CCT
indicates a chocolate-colored tablet. Originally, chocolate was used
as a coloring material and the same designation referred to "chocolate-

Fig. 678. Remington's tablet machine.

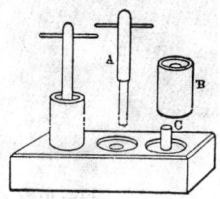

coated tablets." Iron oxides, standardized as to color, are now available and largely replace chocolate for this purpose.

Multiple Compressed Tablets (MCT)—These are compressed tablets made by more than one compression cycle.

Layered Tablets—Such tablets are prepared by compressing additional tablet granulation on a previously compressed tablet. This operation may be repeated a number of times to produce a multi-layered tablet.

Press-Coated Tablets—Such tablets are prepared by feeding a previously compressed tablet into a special tablet machine and compressing another layer around this preformed tablet. In this manner one can make a compressed tablet in which incompatible ingredients may be kept in separate layers. It has all the advantages of the compressed tablet, ie, slotting, monogramming, speed of disintegration, etc, while retaining the attributes of the sugar-coated tablet in masking the taste of medication in the internal layers.[9,10] An example of a press-coating tablet machine is the Manesty Drycota machine (Fig. 679).

Buccal or Sublingual Tablets—These are small, flat, oval tablets intended to be inserted in the buccal pouch, or beneath the tongue where the active ingredient may be directly absorbed through the mucosa.

Molded Tablets or Tablet Triturates (TT)

TT originally referred to tablet triturates, made from moist materials on a triturate mold which gave them the shape of cut sections of a cylinder. Such tablets must be completely and rapidly soluble. Tablet triturates are now usually made by compression on a tablet machine.

Dispensing Tablets (DT)—These tablets provide a convenient quantity of a potent drug that can be incorporated readily into powders, liquids, and other preparations at the dispensing counter. They should never be dispensed as such since these tablets contain very large and sometimes lethal doses of the potent drug.

Hypodermic Tablets (HT)—Hypodermic tablets are those made in a tablet triturate mold and formerly were intended for use in making hypodermic preparations for injection. Traditionally, these tablets are made with absolute cleanliness and in a form that is completely and rapidly soluble in an aqueous vehicle. Since stable parenteral solutions for most drugs are now available, this solid dosage form is used for oral medication. However, they continue to have characteristics similar to those that were made and used for parenteral purposes.

Compressed Tablets (CT)

In order for medicinal substances with or without diluents to be made into solid dosage forms with pressure, using available equipment, it is necessary that the material, either in crystalline or powdered form, possess a number of physical characteristics. These characteristics include the ability to flow freely, cohesiveness, and lubrication. Since most materials have none or only some of these properties, methods of tablet formulation and preparation have been developed to impart these desirable characteristics to the material which is to be compressed into tablets.

The basic mechanical unit in all tablet-compression equipment includes a lower punch which fits into a die from the bottom and an upper punch, having a head of the same shape and dimensions, which enters the die cavity from the top after the tableting material fills the die cavity. The tablet is formed by pressure applied on the punches and is subsequently ejected

from the die. The weight of the tablet is determined by the volume of the material which fills the die cavity. Therefore, the ability of the granulation to flow freely into the die is important in insuring an uniform fill, as well as the continuous movement of the granulation from the source of supply or feed hopper. If the tablet granulation does not possess cohesive properties, the tablet after compression will crumble and fall apart on handling. As the punches must move freely within the die and the tablet must be readily ejected from the punch faces, the material must have a degree of lubrication to minimize friction and to allow for the removal of the compressed tablets.

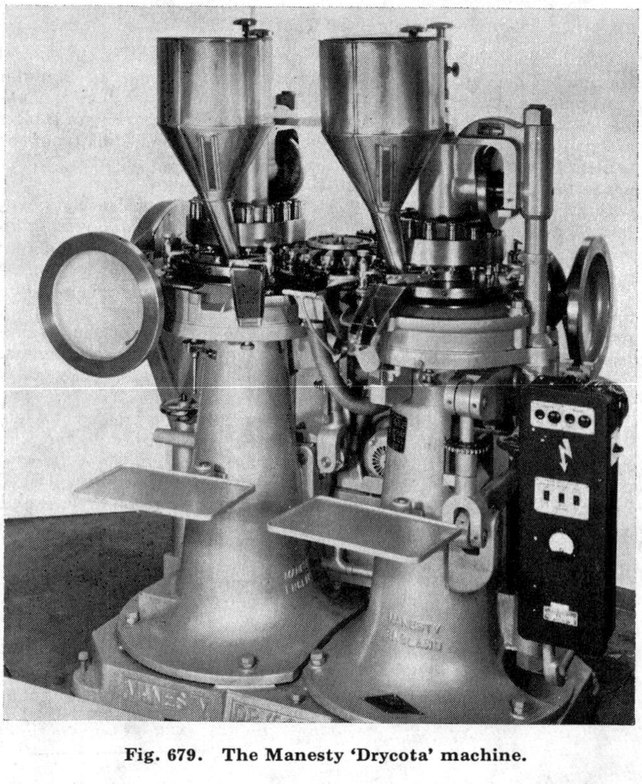

There are three general methods of tablet preparation: (1) the wet-granulation method; (2) the dry-granulation method; and (3) direct compression. The method of preparation and the added ingredients are selected in order to give the tablet formulation the desirable physical characteristics allowing the rapid compression of tablets. After compression the tablets must have a number of additional attributes such as appearance, hardness, disintegration ability, and uniformity which are also influenced both by the method of preparation and by the added materials present in the formulation. In the preparation of compressed tablets the formulator must also be cognizant of the effect which the ingredients and methods of preparation may have on the availability of the active ingredients and hence the therapeutic efficacy of the dosage form.[11–13] See Chapter 42 on *Drug Absorption, Action and Disposition*, page 727, and Chapter 79 on *Formulation*, page 1463.

Tablet Ingredients

In addition to the active or therapeutic ingredient, tablets contain a number of inert materials. The latter are known as additives or "adds." They may be classified according to the part they play in the finished tablet. The first group contains those which help to impart satisfactory compression characteristics to the formulation. These include (1) diluents, (2) binders, and (3) lubricants. The second group of added substances helps to give additional desirable physical characteristics to the finished tablet. Included in this group are (1) disintegrators, (2) colors, and in the case of chewable tablets, (3) flavors, and (4) sweetening agents.

Fig. 679. The Manesty 'Drycota' machine.

Diluents

Frequently the single dose of the active ingredient is small and an inert substance is added to increase the bulk in order to make the tablet a practical size for compression. Compressed tablets of dexamethasone contain 0.75 mg steroid per tablet, hence it is obvious that another material must be added to make tableting possible. Diluents used for this purpose include dicalcium phosphate, calcium sulfate, lactose, kaolin, mannitol, sodium chloride, dry starch, and powdered sugar. Mannitol is used extensively as the diluent for chewable tablets because of its pleasant taste, chemical stability, and lack of hygroscopicity.[14] Crystalline sorbitol being directly compressible and highly water soluble, also offers advantages as a diluent for chewable tablets. Most tablet formulators tend to use consistently only one or two diluents selected from the above group in their tablet formulations. Usually these have been selected on the basis of experience and cost factors. However, in the formulation of new therapeutic agents the compatibility of the diluent with the drug must be considered. For example, calcium salts used as diluents for the broad spectrum antibiotic tetracycline have been shown to interfere with the drug's absorption from the gastrointestinal tract.[15] The combination of amine bases with lactose, or amine salts with lactose in the presence of an alkaline lubricant, results in tablets which discolor on aging.[16,17]

Binders

Agents used to impart cohesive qualities to the powdered material are referred to as binders or granulators. They impart a cohesiveness to the tablet formulation which insures the tablet remaining intact after compression, as well as improving the free flowing qualities by the formulation of granules of desired hardness and size. Materials commonly used as binders include starch, gelatin, and sugars as sucrose, glucose, dextrose, molasses, and lactose.[18,19] Natural and synthetic gums which have been used include acacia, sodium alginate, extract of Irish moss, panwar gum, ghatti gum, mucilage of isapol husks, carboxymethylcellulose, methylcellulose, polyvinylpyrrolidone, Veegum, and larch arabogalactan.[20-26] Other agents which may be considered binders under certain circumstances are polyethylene glycol, ethylcellulose, waxes, water, and alcohol.[27]

The quantity of binder used has considerable influence on the characteristics of the compressed tablets. The use of too much binder or too strong a binder will make a hard tablet which will not disintegrate easily and which will cause excessive wear of punches and dies. Materials which have no cohesive qualities of their own will require a stronger binder than those with these qualities. Alcohol and water are not binders in the true sense of the word; but because of their solvent action on some ingredients such as lactose and starch, they change the powdered material to granules and the residual moisture retained enables the materials to adhere together when compressed.

Binders are used both as a solution and in a dry form depending on the other ingredients in the formulation and the method of preparation. The same amount of binder in solution will be more effective than if it were dispersed in a dry form and moistened with the solvent. By the latter procedure the binding agent is not as effective in reaching and wetting each of the particles within the mass of powders.[28] Each of the particles in a powder blend has a coating of adsorbed air on its surface, and it is this film which must be penetrated before the powders can be wetted by the binder solution. Since powders differ with respect to the ease with which they can be wetted, it is preferable to incorporate the binding agent in solution. By this technique it is often possible to gain effective binding with a lower concentration of binder.

Using the direct compression method for preparing tablets (see page 1659) requires a material present that acts as a dry binder. This use has been described for microcrystalline cellulose, amylose, and polyvinylpyrrolidone.[29-31] It has been postulated that microcrystalline cellulose is a special form of cellulose fibril in which the individual crystallites are held together largely by hydrogen bonding. The disintegration of tablets containing the cellulose occurs by breaking the intercrystallite bonds by the disintegrating medium.

Starch Paste—Corn starch is widely used as a binder. The concentration may vary from 10 to 20%. It is usually prepared as it is to be used.

Starch Paste

Starch	1 part by weight
Purified water, qs,	
To make	10 parts by weight

Place starch in a suitable container, slowly add the cold water, stirring continuously to avoid the formation of lumps. Heat slowly in a water bath with continued stirring until a translucent paste results. Allow to cool.

Gelatin Solution—Gelatin is generally used as a 10–20% solution; gelatin solutions should be freshly prepared as needed and used while warm or they will solidify.

Gelatin Solution

Gelatin	1 part by weight
Purified water, qs,	
To make	10 parts by weight

Cover the gelatin with cold water and allow the gelatin to soak in a covered container until it is hydrated. Heat gently on a water bath with agitation until the gelatin is dissolved. Add sufficient water to make up to final weight and stir well.

Glucose Solution—Generally a 25–50% solution is used. Glucose does not dry out well and is therefore not suitable where the tablets are subject to humid conditions. These solutions are not true 25 and 50% solutions since the corn syrup contains only approximately 80% solids.

Glucose Solution

Colorless corn syrup (glucose)	25 parts by weight
Purified water, qs,	
To make	100 parts by weight

Weigh out the corn syrup and sufficient purified water to dissolve it. Stir well and make up to weight; strain through muslin if necessary.

Ethylcellulose—This is insoluble in water. It is used effectively as a binder when dissolved in alcohol, or as a dry binder in a granulation which is then wetted with alcohol. As a binder in solution it is usually used as a 5% solution. It is widely used as a binder for moisture-sensitive materials.

Ethylcellulose Solution

Ethylcellulose	5 parts by weight
S.D. 3A alcohol (anhydrous), qs,	
To make	100 parts by weight

Stir the ethylcellulose in the denatured alcohol until the gum is dissolved; make up to final weight.

It will be noted that binder solutions are usually made up to weight rather than volume. This is to enable the formulator to determine the weight of the solids which have been added to the tablet granulation in the binding solution. This becomes part of the total weight of the granulation and must be taken into consideration in determining the weight of the compressed tablet which will contain the stated amount of the therapeutic agent.

Lubricants

Lubricants have a number of functions in tablet manufacture. They improve the rate of flow of the tablet granulation, prevent adhesion of the tablet material to the surface of the dies and punches, reduce interparticle friction, and facilitate the ejection of the tablets from the die cavity. Lubricants have been differentiated into three groups based on their ability to carry out the functions mentioned above.[32] These three groups are as follows.

1. **Glidants**—Acting as flow regulators, they improve the flow properties of the granules in the feed hopper. These materials are not generally deformed significantly under the pressure of the tableting machine. Examples of glidants are talc, starch, lycopodium, magnesium stearate, calcium stearate, boric acid, sugar, and sodium chloride.

2. **Antiadhesives or Antisticking Agents**—These prevent adhesion of the tablet surface to dies and punches during compression. Such materials are easily deformed under pressure. Examples of antisticking agents are paraffin, stearic acid, cocoa butter, and soaps.

3. **Lubricants**—These reduce interparticular friction during compression and friction between tablet and die wall during ejection. Examples of lubricants are talc, magnesium stearate, and calcium stearate.

The addition of the proper lubricant is highly desirable if the material to be tableted tends to stick to the punches and dies. Immediately after compression most tablets have the tendency to expand $\frac{1}{1000}$ or $\frac{2}{1000}$ in. and will bind and stick to the side of the die. The choice of the proper lubricant will effectively overcome this.

The method of adding a lubricant to a granulation is important if the material is to perform its function satisfactorily. The lubricant should be finely divided by passing it through a 100-mesh nylon cloth onto the granulation. In production this is called "bolting" the lubricant. After adding the lubricant the granulation is tumbled or mixed gently to coat the individual granules without breaking them down to finer particles. The quantity of lubricant varies, being as low as 0.1%, and in some cases as high as 5%. Lubricants have been added to the granulating agents in the form of suspensions or emulsions.[33] This technique serves to reduce the number of operational procedures and thus reduce the processing time.

In selecting a lubricant, proper attention must be given to its compatibility with the drug agent. Perhaps the most widely investigated drug is acetylsalicylic acid. Different talcs varied significantly on the stability of aspirin.[34] Talc with a high calcium content and a high loss on ignition was associated with increased aspirin decomposition. From a stability standpoint, the relatively acceptability of tablet lubricants for combination with aspirin was found to be as follows: hydrogenated vegetable oil, stearic acid, talc, and aluminum stearate.[35]

The primary problem in the preparation of a water-soluble tablet is the selection of a satisfactory lubricant. Soluble lubricants reported to be effective include boric acid, sodium benzoate, a mixture of sodium benzoate and sodium acetate, sodium chloride, leucine, and Carbowax 4000.[36–38] However, it has been suggested that formulations used to prepare water-soluble tablets may represent a number of compromises between compression efficiency and water solubility.[39] Greater insight into the mechanism of action and evaluation of tablet lubricants has resulted from a number of studies carried out at the University of Wisconsin.[40–43]

Disintegrators

A disintegrator is a substance, or a mixture of substances, added to a tablet to facilitate its breakup or disintegration after administration. The active ingredient must be released from the tablet matrix as efficiently as possible to allow for its rapid dissolution. Materials serving as disintegrants have been chemically classified as starches, clays, celluloses, algins, or gums.[44]

The most popular disintegrators are corn and potato starch which have been well-dried and powdered. Starch has a great affinity for water and swells when moistened, thus facilitating the rupture of the tablet matrix.[45] However, others have suggested that its disintegrating action in tablets is due to capillary action rather than swelling; the spherical shape of the starch grains increases the porosity of the tablet, thus promoting capillary action.[46] Starch, 5%, is suggested, but if more rapid disintegration is desired, this amount may be increased to 10 or 15%. Although it might be expected that disintegration time would decrease as the percentage of starch in the tablet increased, this does not appear to be the case for tolbutamide tablets. In this instance, there appears to be a critical starch concentration for different granulations of the chemical.[47] When their disintegration effect is desired, starches are added to the powder blends in the dry state. Starch pastes which are useful as binding agents will generally not be effective as disintegrating agents.

In addition to the starches a large variety of materials have been used and are reported to be effective as disintegrators. This group includes Veegum HV,[48] methylcellulose, agar,[49] bentonite,[50] cellulose and wood products,[51,52] natural sponge,[53] cation-exchange resins,[54,55] alginic acid,[56] guar gum,[57] citrus pulp,[58] and carboxymethylcellulose.[59] In a study evaluating the effect on disintegration times of compressed tablets containing surfactants, Aerosol QT and Aerosol MA were found to be the most effective of the 21 surface-active agents tried.[60] Sodium lauryl sulfate in combination with starch also has been demonstrated to be an effective disintegrant. In some cases the apparent effectiveness of surfactants in improving tablet disintegration is postulated as being due to an increase in the rate of wetting.[62]

The disintegrating agent is usually mixed with the active ingredients and diluents prior to granulation. In some cases it may be advantageous to divide the starch into two portions; one part is added to the powdered formula prior to granulation, and the remainder is mixed with the lubricant and added prior to compression.[63] Incorporated in this manner the starch serves a double purpose; the portion added to the lubricant rapidly breaks the tablet down to granules, and the starch mixed with the active ingredients disintegrates the granules into smaller particles. Veegum has been shown to be more effective as a disintegrator in sulfathiazole tablets when most of the quantity is added after granulation and only a small amount before granulation.[64] Likewise, the montmorillonite clays were found to be good tablet disintegrants when added to prepared granulations as powder. They are much less effective as disintegrants when incorporated within the granules.[65]

Factors other than the presence of disintegrators can affect significantly the disintegration time of compressed tablets. The binder, tablet hardness, and the lubricant have been shown to influence the disintegration time.[66,67] Thus, when the formulator is faced with a problem concerning the disintegration of a compressed tablet, the answer may not lie in the selection and the quantity of the disintegrating agent alone.

The evolution of carbon dioxide is also an effective way to cause the disintegration of compressed tablets. Tablets containing a mixture of sodium bicarbonate and an acidulant such as tartaric or citric acid will effervesce when added to water. Sufficient acid is added to produce a neutral or slightly acidic reaction when disintegration in water is complete. One drawback to the use of the effervescent type of disintegrator is that such tablets must be kept in a dry atmosphere at all times during manufacture, storage, and packaging.

Coloring Agents

Colors in compressed tablets serve functions other than making the dosage form more esthetic in appearance. Color helps the manufacturer to control the product during its preparation, as well as serving as a means of identification to the user. The wide diversity in the use of colors in solid dosage forms makes it possible to use color as an important category in the identification code developed by the AMA to establish the identity of an unknown compressed tablet in situations arising from poisoning.[68]

Any of the approved certified water-soluble FD&C dyes, mixtures of the same, or their corresponding lakes may be used to color tablets. A color lake is the combination by absorption of a water soluble dye and a hydrous oxide of a heavy metal resulting in an insoluble form of the dye. In some instances multiple dyes are used to give a purposeful heterogeneous coloring in form of speckling to compressed tablets. The dyes available do not meet all the criteria required for the ideal pharmaceutical colorants.[69] The photosensitivity of several of the commonly used colorants and their lakes has been investigated, as well as the protection afforded by a number of glasses used in packaging tablets.[70-75] Another approach for improving the photostability of dyes has been in the use of ultraviolet-absorbing chemicals in the tablet formulations with the dyes.[76] Colorimetric methods for testing color stability of tablets have been described.[77,78]

The most common method of adding color to a tablet formulation is to dissolve the dye in the binding solution prior to the granulating process. Another approach is to adsorb the dye on starch or calcium sulfate from its aqueous solution; the resultant powder is dried and blended with the other ingredients. If the insoluble lakes are used, they may be blended with the other dry ingredients. Frequently during drying, colors in wet granulations migrate, resulting in an uneven distribution of the color in the granulation. After compression the tablets will have a mottled appearance due to the uneven distribution of the color. Migration of colors may be reduced by drying the granulation slowly at low temperatures and stirring the granulation while it is drying. The affinity of several water-soluble anionic certified dyes for natural starches has been demonstrated; in these cases this affinity should aid in preventing color migration.[79] Other additives have been shown to act as dye migration inhibitors. Tragacanth (1%), acacia (3%), attapulgite (5%), and talc (7%) were effective in inhibiting the migration of FD&C Blue No. 1 in lactose.[80] In using dye lakes the problem of color migration is avoided since the lakes are insoluble. Prevention of mottling can be helped also by the use of lubricants and other additives which have been colored similarly to the granulation prior to their use. The problem of mottling becomes more pronounced as the concentration of the colorants increase. Color mottling is an undesirable characteristic common to many commercial tablets.

Flavoring Agents

Generally, flavoring is not considered to be necessary in the formulation of compressed tablets. However, chewable tablets and lozenges often require flavoring and sweetening. The flavors may be sprayed as an alcoholic solution onto the dry granules prior to compression, or the so-called dry flavors may be used and blended with the other tablet constituents.

In addition to the sweetness which may be afforded by the diluent of the chewable tablet, eg, mannitol or lactose, artificial sweetening agents may be used. The combination of ten parts of sodium cyclamate to one part of saccharin has been recommended for obtaining a potentiation of sweetness and minimizing the bitter taste of saccharin evident when the latter is used alone.[81] Another advantage offered by the synthetic sweetening agents is that their use reduces the bulk volume considering the quantity of sucrose required to produce the same degree of sweetness. Being present in small quantities, they do not markedly affect the physical characteristics of the tablet granulation.

Tablet Characteristics

Compressed tablets may be characterized or described by a number of specifications. These include the diameter size, shape, thickness, weight, hardness, and disintegration time. The diameter and shape depend on the die and the punches selected for the compression of the tablet. Generally, tablets are discoid in shape, although they may be oval, oblong, round, cylindrical, or triangular. Their upper and lower surfaces may be flat, round, concave, or convex to various degrees. The concave punches (used to prepare convex tablets) are referred to as shallow, standard, and deep cup, depending on the degree of concavity (see Figs. 691 and 692). The tablets may be scored in halves or quadrants to facilitate breaking if a smaller dose is desired. The top or lower surface may be embossed or engraved with a symbol or letters which serve as an additional means of identifying the source of the tablets. These characteristics along with the color of the tablets tend to make them distinctive and identifiable with the active ingredient which they contain.

The remaining specifications assure the manufacturer that the tablets do not vary from one production lot to another. In the case of new tablet formulations their therapeutic efficacy is demonstrated through clinical trials and it is the manufacturer's aim to reproduce the same tablet with the exact characteristics of the tablets which were used in the clinical evaluation of the dosage form. Therefore, from the control viewpoint these specifications are important for reasons other than physical appearance.

Tablet Hardness

The resistance of the tablet to chipping, abrasion, or breakage under conditions of storage, transportation, and handling before usage depends on its hardness. A commonly used rule of thumb describes a tablet to be of proper hardness if it is firm enough to break with a sharp snap when it is held between the second and third fingers and using the thumb as the fulcrum, yet doesn't break when it falls on the floor. For control purposes a number of attempts have been made to quantitate the degree of hardness.

A small and portable hardness tester was manufactured and introduced in the mid-thirties by the Monsanto Chemical Co.[82] It is now distributed by the F. J. Stokes Co. and may be designated as either the Monsanto or Stokes hardness tester. The instrument measures the force required to break the tablet when the force generated by a coil spring is applied diametrically to the tablet. The force is measured in kilograms and when used in production, hardness of 4 Kg is considered to be minimum for a satisfactory tablet.

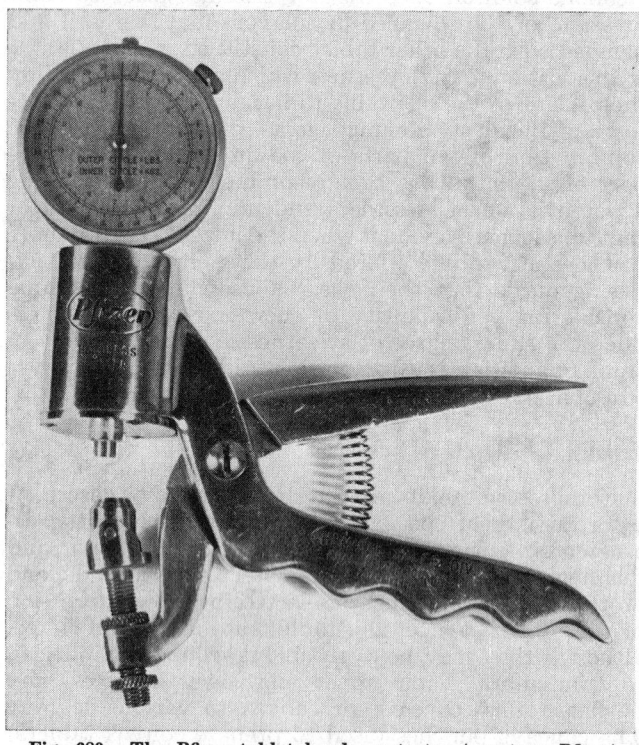

Fig. 680.   The Pfizer tablet hardness tester (courtesy, Pfizer).

The Strong-Cobb hardness tester introduced in 1950 also measures the diametrically applied force required to break the tablet.[83] In this instrument the force is produced by a manually operated air pump. As the pressure is increased, a plunger is forced against the tablet placed on anvil. The final breaking point is indicated on a dial calibrated into 30 arbitrary units. The hardness values of the Stokes and Strong-Cobb instruments are not equivalent. Values obtained with the Strong-Cobb tester were found to be 1.6 times those of the Stokes tester.[84]

A modification of the Strong-Cobb hardness tester has been proposed by workers at the Abbott Laboratories. The plunger and anvil of the tester have been redesigned to measure the tablet characteristic called tablet fracture.[85] This method is claimed to simulate the widely used manual method of measuring the hardness of tablets by the force required to break a

tablet when it is placed between the first two fingers and the thumb.

The most recently introduced instrument is the Pfizer hardness tester which operates on the same mechanical principle as ordinary pliers.[86] The force required to break the tablet is recorded on a dial and may be expressed as either kilograms or pounds of force. In an experimental comparison of testers the Pfizer and the Stokes testers were found to check each other fairly well. Again the Strong-Cobb tester was found to give values 1.4–1.7 times the absolute values on the other instruments.[87] See Fig. 680.

Hardness determinations are made throughout the tablet runs to determine the need for pressure adjustments on the tableting machine. If the tablet is too hard, it may not disintegrate in the required period of time; if it is too soft, it will not withstand the handling during packaging and shipping operations.

Another approach to the measurement of tablet hardness is the use of the Roche friabilator.[88] Rather than a measure of the force required to crush a tablet, the instrument is designed to evaluate the ability of the tablet to withstand abrasion in packaging, handling, and shipping. A number of tablets are weighed and

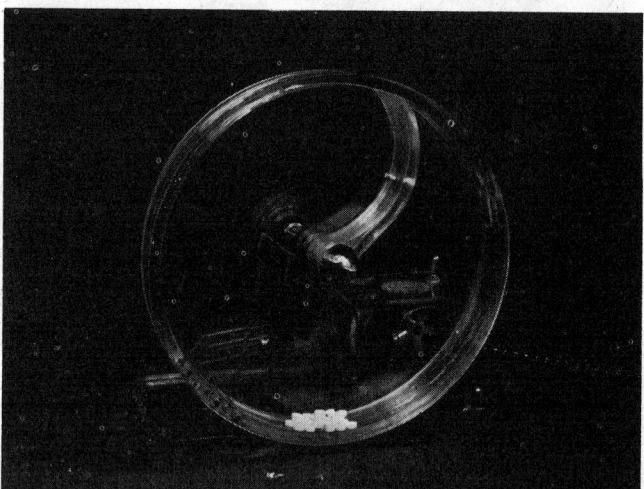

Fig. 681.   The Roche friabilator (courtesy, Hoffman-La Roche).

placed in the tumbling apparatus where they are exposed to rolling and repeated shocks resulting from free-falls within the apparatus. After a given number of rotations the tablets are weighed and the loss in weight indicates the ability of the tablets to withstand this type of wear (Fig. 681).

A similar approach is taken by many manufacturers when they evaluate a new product in the new market package by sending the package to distant points and back using various methods of transportation. The condition of the product on its return indicates its ability to withstand transportation handling.

Tablet Thickness

The thickness of the tablet from production run to production run is carefully controlled. Thickness can vary with no change in weight due to difference in the density of the granulation and the pressure applied to the tablets, as well as the speed of tablet compression. Not only is the tablet thickness important in reproducing tablets identical in appearance but also to insure that every production lot will be usable with selected packaging components. If the tablets are thicker than specified, a given number no longer may be contained in the volume of a given size bottle. Tablet thickness is determined with a caliper such as the Ames thickness gauge, which measures the thickness in millimeters. A plus or minus 5% may be allowed, depending on the size of the tablet.

Tablet Weight

The volumetric fill of the die cavity determines the the weight of the compressed tablet. In setting up the tablet machine the fill is adjusted to give the desirable tablet weight. The weight of the tablet is the quantity of the granulation which contains the labeled amount of the therapeutic ingredient. After the tablet machine is in operation the weights of the tablets are checked routinely to insure that proper weight tablets are being made. The USP suggests tolerances for the average weight of uncoated compressed tablets. Twenty tablets are weighed individually and the average weight is calculated. The variation from the average weight in the weights of not more than two of the tablets must not differ by more than the percentage listed below; no tablet differs by more than double that percentage.

Average Weight	Percentage Difference
130 mg or less	10
More than 130 mg and including 324 mg	7.5
More than 324 mg	5

Content Uniformity

In order to ensure that every tablet contains the amount of drug intended with little variation among tablets within a package, the official compendia have introduced the content uniformity test. With increased emphasis on drug efficacy and physiological availability, the content uniformity test has been extended to monographs on all capsules and all coated and uncoated tablets intended for oral administration where the range of sizes of the dosage form available includes a 50 mg or smaller size, in which case the test is applicable to all sizes (50 mg and larger and smaller) of that capsule or tablet. An exception is made in those cases where the assay method proves impracticable for the accurate determination of the drug content of individual dosage units.

Where a requirement of *Content uniformity* is specified in the individual monograph, select a sample of 30 tablets. Assay 10 of these individually as directed in the *Assay* in the monograph, unless otherwise directed under *Content uniformity*. If the amount of active ingredient in a single tablet is less than that required in the *Assay*, adjust the degree of dilution of the solutions and/or the volume of aliquots so that the concentration of the final solution will be of the same order as that obtained in the *Assay* provided in the monograph. See also the first paragraph under *Procedures*, under *Test and Assays* (USP, page 5). The requirements are met if the content of each of not less than 9 of the tablets is within the limits of 85% and 115% of the average of the tolerances specified in the potency definition in the monograph, and if the content of none of the tablets falls outside the limits of 75% and 125% of that average. If the content of not more than 2 tablets falls outside the limits of 85% and 115%, assay each of the remaining 20 tablets. The requirements are met if the content of each of the additional 20 tablets falls within the limits of 85% and 115% of the average of the tolerances specified in the potency definition in the individual monograph.

Tablet Disintegration

It is generally recognized that the *in vitro* tablet disintegration test does not necessarily bear a relationship to the *in vivo* action of a solid dosage form. To be absorbed, a drug must be in solution and the disintegration test is a measure only of the time required under a given set of conditions for a group of tablets to disintegrate into particles. In the present disintegration test the particles are those which will pass through a 10-mesh screen. In a comparison of disintegration times and dissolution rates or initial absorption rates of several brands of aspirin tablets, it was found that the faster absorbed tablets had the longer disintegration time.[89] Regardless of the lack of significance as to the tablets' *in vivo* action, the test provides a means of control in assuring that a given tablet formula is the same as regards disintegration from one production batch to another.

Exact specifications are given for the test apparatus in as much as a change in the apparatus can cause a change in the results of the test. The apparatus consists of a basket rack holding six plastic tubes, open at the top and bottom; the bottom of the tubes is covered with 10-mesh screen. The basket rack is immersed in a bath of suitable liquid, held at 37°C. The rack moves up and down in the fluid at a specified rate. The volume of the fluid is such that on the upward stroke the wire mesh remains at least 2.5 cm below the surface of the fluid and descends to not less than 2.5 cm from the bottom on the downward stroke. Tablets are placed in each of the six cylinders along with a plastic disk over the tablet. The plastic disks have a density which enables them to float above the tablets. The end-point of the test is indicated when the tablets have passed through the screen. The plastic disks help to force any soft mass which forms through the screen.

For compressed uncoated tablets the testing fluid is water at 37°C. If more than two tablets fail to disintegrate, 12 tablets must be used. Of the 18 tablets then tested, 15 must have disintegrated within the given period of time. The conditions of the test are varied somewhat for coated tablets, buccal tablets, and sublingual tablets. For the exact conditions of the test see the USP.

Dissolution Test

Like the disintegration test above, the dissolution test for measuring the time required for a given drug in a solid dosage form to go into solution under a specified set of conditions is an *in vitro* test. It is intended to provide a step towards the evaluation of the physiological availability of the drug. It is not designed to measure the safety or effectiveness of the dosage form being tested. As stated previously, both safety and effectiveness of a specific dosage form must be demonstrated initially by means of appropriate *in vivo* studies and clinical evaluation. A number of official monographs include this test as one of the standards.

Methods of Preparation

Wet-Granulation Method

The most widely used and most general method of tablet preparation is the wet-granulation method. Its popularity is due to the increased probability that the granulation will meet all the physical requirements for the compression of good tablets. Its chief disadvantages are the number of separate steps involved, as well as the time and labor necessary to carry out the procedure, especially on the large scale. The steps in the wet method are (1) weighing, (2) mixing, (3) granulation, (4) screening the damp mass, (5) drying, (6) dry screening, (7) lubrication, and (8) compression. The equipment involved depends on the quantity or size of the batch. The active ingredient, diluent, and dis-

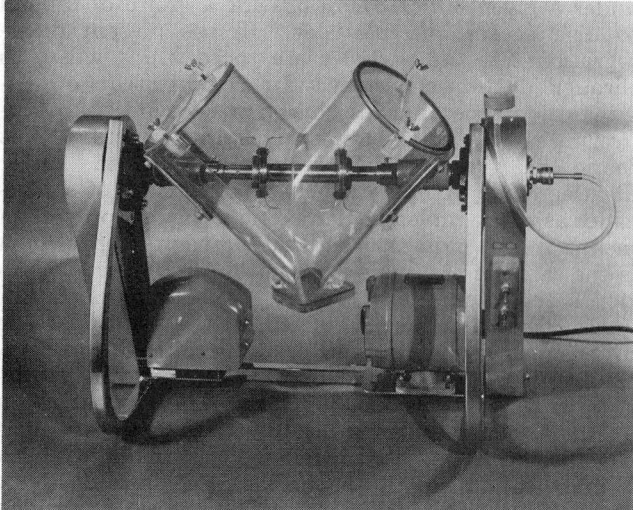

Fig. 682. Twin-shell blender for solids or liquid–solids blending (courtesy, Patterson-Kelley).

integrator are mixed or blended well. For small batches the ingredients may be mixed in stainless steel bowls or mortars. Small-scale blending also can be carried out on a large piece of paper by holding opposite edges and tumbling the material back and forth. The powder blend may be sifted through a screen of suitable fineness to remove or break up lumps. This screening also affords additional mixing. The screen selected should always be of the same type of wire or cloth that will not affect the potency of the ingredients through interaction. For example, the stability of ascorbic acid is deleteriously affected by even small amounts of copper, thus care must be taken to avoid contact with copper or copper-containing alloys.

For larger quantities of powder the Patterson-Kelley twin-shell blender and the double-cone blender offer means of precision blending and mixing in short periods of time (Fig. 682). Twin-shell blenders are available

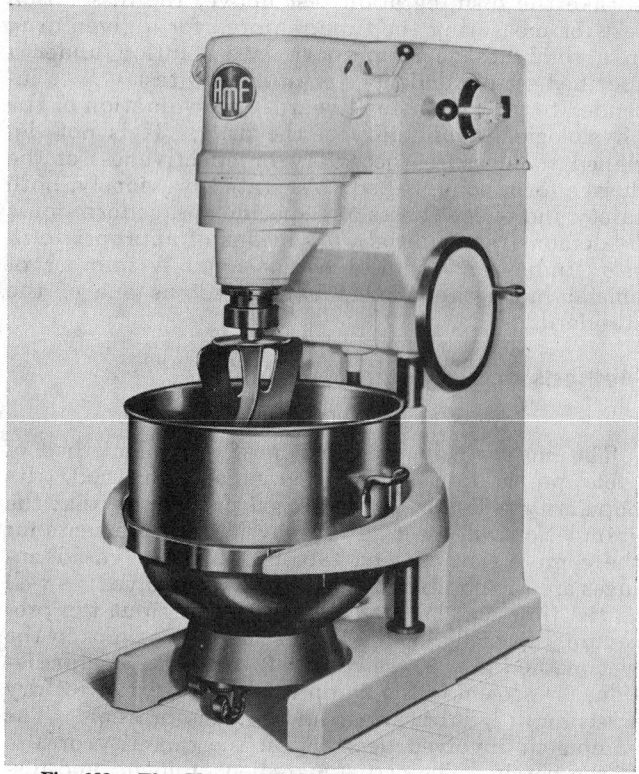

Fig. 683. The Glen powder mixer (courtesy, Am. Machine).

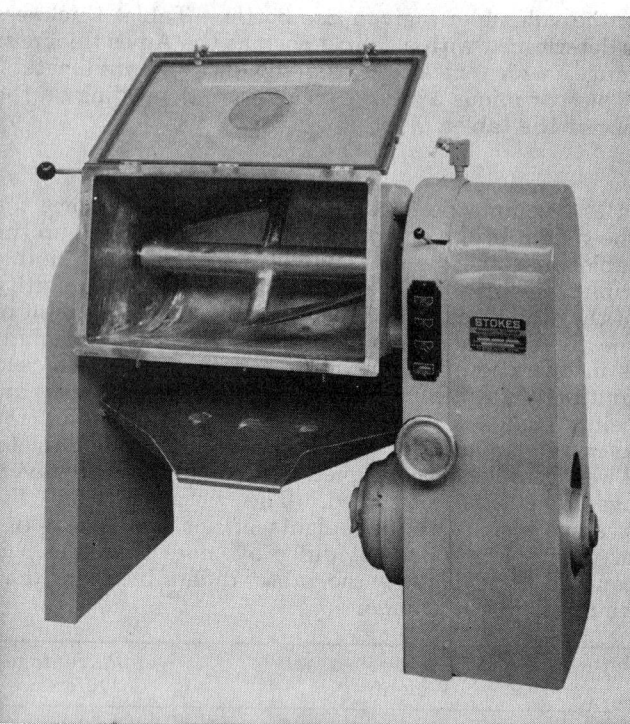

Fig. 684. Mass mixer for granulations (courtesy, Stokes).

in many sizes from laboratory models to large production models. Blenders of the vertical shaft type, eg, the Glen mixer and the Hobart mixer, have served this function in the pharmaceutical industry for many years (Fig. 683). On a large scale, ribbon blenders are also frequently employed and may be adapted for continuous production procedures.

Solutions of the binding agent are added to the mixed powders with stirring. The powder mass is wetted with the binding solution until the mass has the consistency of damp snow or brown sugar.[90] If the granulation is overwetted, the granules will be hard, requiring considerable pressure to form the tablets, and the resultant tablets may have a mottled appearance. If the powder mixture is not wetted sufficiently, the resulting granules will be too soft, breaking down during lubrication and causing difficulty during compression. For larger quantities mass mixers of the sigma blade type have been widely used in the pharmaceutical industry (Fig. 684). Twin-shell blenders are also constructed to permit the binding solution to be sprayed on the powder blend for granulation following the mixing operation.

The wet granulation is forced through a 6- or 8-mesh screen. Small batches can be forced through by hand using a manual screen. For larger quantities one of several comminuting mills suitable for wet screening can be used. These include the Stokes oscillator, the Colton rotary granulator, the Fitzpatrick comminuting mill, or the Stokes tornado mill. For tablet formulations where continuous production is justified, extruders such as the Reitz* extructor have been adapted for the wet-granulation process. The extruder consists of a screw mixer with a chamber where the powder is mixed with the binding agent and the wet mass is gradually forced through a perforated screen forming threads of the wet granulation. The granulation is then dried by conventional methods. A semiautomatic continuous process using the Reitz extructor has been described for the preparation of the

* See *Manufacturers Index*, page 2023.

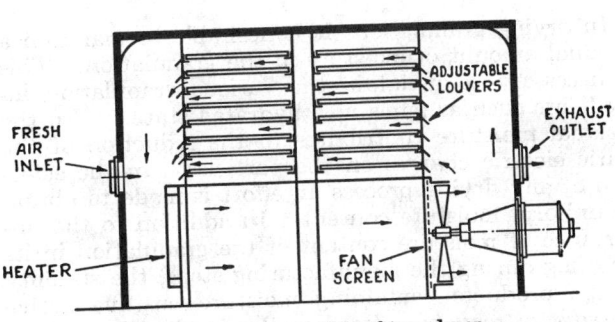

Fig. 687. Cross section of tray dryer.

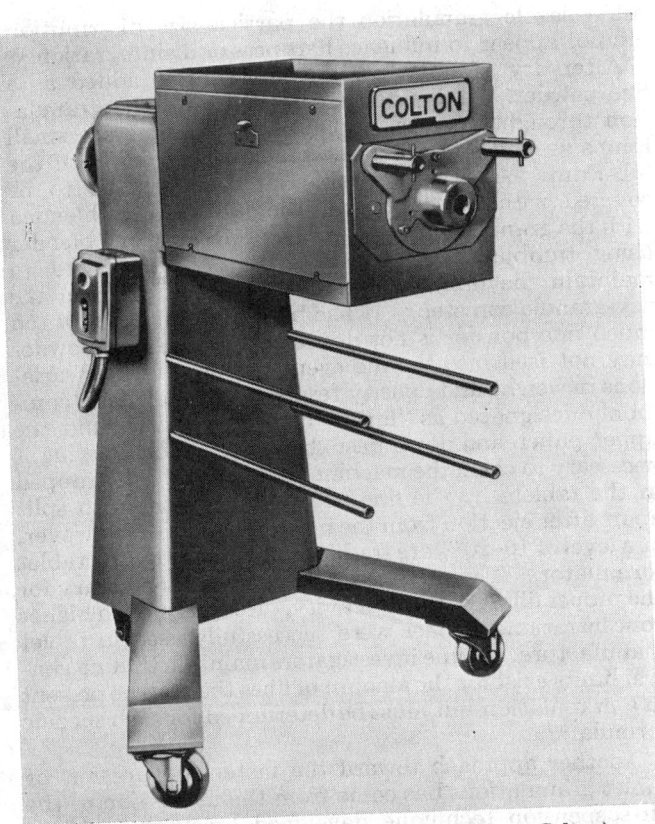

Fig. 685. Rotary granulator and sifter (courtesy, Colton).

antacid tablet Gelusil (*Warner-Lambert*).[91] See Figs. 686 and 688.

Moist material from the granulator is placed on large sheets of paper on shallow wire trays and placed in drying cabinets with a circulating air current and thermostatic heat control. While tray drying is the most widely used method of drying tablet granulations, other methods are being introduced with success. Notable among these are fluid bed dryers. In drying tablet granulations by fluidization the material is suspended and agitated in a warm air stream while the granulation is maintained in motion. Drying tests comparing the fluidized bed and a tray dryer for a number of tablet granulations indicated that the former was 15 times faster than the conventional method of tray drying. In addition to the decreased drying time the fluidization method is claimed to have other advantages such as better control of drying temperatures, decreased handling costs, and the opportunity to blend lubricants and other materials into the dry granulation directly in the fluidized bed.[92,93] See Fig. 688.

The application of radio-frequency drying and infrared drying to tablet granulations has been reported as successful for the majority of granulations tried.[94-96] These methods readily lend themselves to continuous granulation operations. The study of drying methods for tablet granulations led to the development of the the Rovac dryer system by Ciba pharmacists and engineers.[97] See Fig. 689. The dryer is similar in appearance to the cone blender except for the heating jacket and vacuum connections. By excluding oxygen and using the lower drying temperatures made possible by drying in a vacuum, opportunities for degradation of the ingredients during the drying cycle are minimized. A greater uniformity of residual moisture content is achieved because of the moving bed, the controlled temperature, and the controlled time period of the drying cycle. Particle-size distribution can be controlled by varying the speed of rotation and drying temperature as well as by comminuting the granulation to the desired granule size after drying.

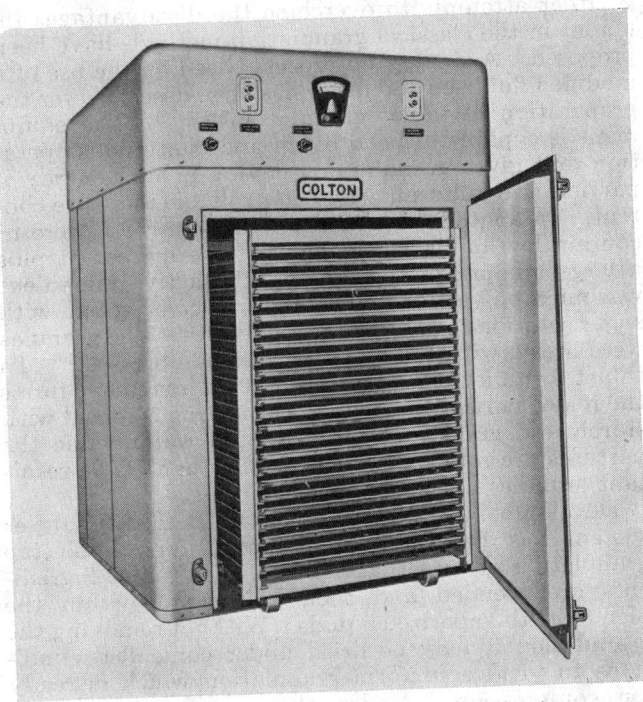

Fig. 686. Tray dryer oven (courtesy, Colton).

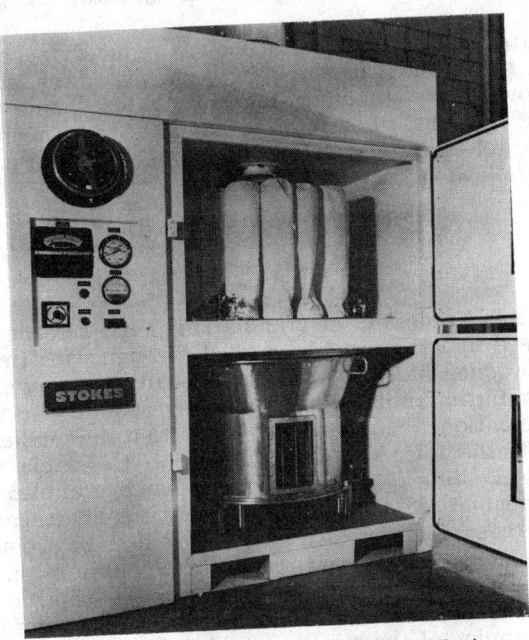

Fig. 688. Fluid bed dryer (courtesy, Stokes).

In drying granulations it is desirable to maintain a residual amount of moisture in the granulation. This is necessary to maintain the various granulation ingredients such as gums in a hydrated state. Also the residual moisture contributes to the reduction of the static electric charges on the particles. In the selection of any drying process an effort is made to obtain an uniform moisture content. In addition to the importance of moisture content of the granulation in its handling during the manufacturing steps, the stability of the products containing moisture-sensitive active ingredients may be related to the products' moisture content.[98]

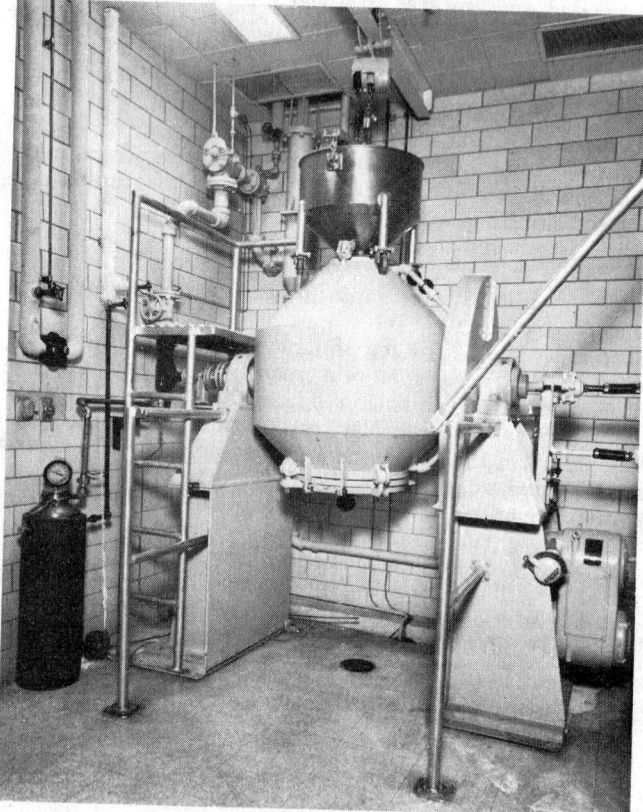

Fig. 689. Rovac dryer (courtesy, Ciba).

After drying, the granulation is reduced in particle size by passing it through a smaller mesh screen. Following dry screening the granule size tends to be more uniform. For dry granulations the screen size to be selected depends on the diameter of the punch. The following sizes are suggested.

> Tablets up to $\frac{3}{16}$-in. diam, use 20-mesh
> Tablets $\frac{7}{32}$ in. to $\frac{5}{16}$ in., use 16-mesh
> Tablets $1\frac{1}{32}$ in. to $1\frac{3}{32}$ in., use 14-mesh
> Tablets $\frac{7}{16}$ in. and larger, use 12-mesh

For small amounts of granulation, hand screens may be used and the material passed through with the aid of a wooden block. With larger quantities, any of the comminuting mills with screens corresponding to those just mentioned may be used. Note that the smaller the tablet, the finer the dry granulation to enable more uniform filling of the die cavity; large granules give an irregular fill to a comparatively small die cavity. In the case of compressed tablets of sodium bicarbonate, lactose, and magnesium trisilicate, a relationship has been demonstrated to exist between the particle size of the granulated material and the disintegration time and capping of the resultant tablets.[99] Although for a

sulfathiazole granulation the particle-size distribution did not appear to influence hardness or disintegration.[100]

After dry granulation, the lubricant is added as a fine powder. It is usually screened onto the granulation through 100-mesh nylon cloth to eliminate small lumps as well as to increase the covering power of the lubricant. As it is desirable for each granule to be covered with the lubricant, the lubricant is blended with the granulation very gently, preferably in a blender using tumbling action. Gentle action is desired to maintain the uniform granule size resulting from the dry-granulation step. It has been maintained that too much fine powder is not desirable because fine powder may not feed into the die evenly; as the result, variations in weight and density result. Fine powders, commonly designated as "fines," also blow out around the upper punch and down past the lower punch, making it necessary to clean the machine frequently. Air trapped in the tablets by the fine powder causes them to split apart after ejection from the machine. Fines, however, at a level of 10–20% are traditionally sought by the tablet formulator. The presence of some fines is necessary for the proper filling of the die cavity. Recently, even higher concentrations of fines were successfully used in tablet manufacture. Some investigators maintain that no general limits exist for the amount of fines that can be present in a granulation but must be determined for each specific formula.[101]

Another approach toward the faster preparation of tablet granulations has come from the utilization of the air-suspension technique developed by Wurster.[102–104] In this method particles of an inert material, or the active drug, are suspended in a vertical column with a rising air stream; while the particles are suspended, the common granulating materials in solution are sprayed into the column. There is a gradual particle buildup under a controlled set of conditions resulting in a tablet granulation which is ready for compression after addition of the lubricant. In addition to its use for the preparation of tablet granulations this technique also has been proposed for the coating of solid particles as a means of improving the flow properties of small particles (see page 1686).

Other attempts to overcome the disadvantages inherent in the classical granulation methods have been proposed. A single-step process based on the use of a modified fluidized bed dryer has been described for the preparation of tablet granulations.[105,106] The equipment is capable of both batch and continuous operation and gives granulations having a high degree of particle size uniformity and controllable moisture content. In another approach for tablets which were to contain low milligram potency of the ingredient plus a large amount of the diluent, the active ingredient was micropulverized and coated in a coating pan with sugar solution to give uniform granules. The granules were mixed with the lubricant and compressed.[107] In tablet formulations where the active ingredient forms the major portion of the tablet, the drug is mixed with starch and gums and sprayed with water while the particles are rotating in the coating pan. The resultant granules are mixed and compressed.[108]

Developmental experience with the Rovac dryer system has indicated its potential for a one-step granulation process (page 1655). The tablet ingredients are blended and then granulated within the blender with vaporized liquids. Without removing the granulation it may be dried under controlled conditions to yield a uniform granulation which is ready for compression. Under these circumstances the entire granulation process time can be reduced from a period of days to one of hours.[109,110]

Dry-Granulation Method

When tablet ingredients are sensitive to moisture or are unable to withstand elevated temperatures during drying, and when the tablet ingredients have sufficient inherent binding or cohesive properties, slugging may be used to form granules. This method is referred to as dry granulation, precompression, or the double-compression method. It eliminates a number of steps but still includes (1) weighing, (2) mixing, (3) slugging, (4) dry screening, (5) lubrication, and (6) compression. The active ingredient, diluent (if one is required), and part of the lubricant are blended. One of the constituents, either the active ingredient or the diluent, must have cohesive properties. Powdered material contains considerable amount of air; under pressure this air is expelled and a fairly dense piece is formed; the more time allowed for this air to escape, the better the tablet or slug.

When slugging is used, large tablets are made as slugs because fine powders flow better into large cavities. Also, producing large slugs decreases production time; ⅞ to 1 in. are the most practical sizes for slugs. Sometimes to obtain the pressure which is desired the slug sizes are reduced to ¾ in. The punches should be flat faced. The compressed slugs are comminuted through the desirable mesh screen either by hand, or for larger quantities through the Fitzpatrick or a similar comminuting mill. The lubricant remaining is added to the granulation, blended gently, and the material is compressed into tablets. Aspirin is a good example where slugging is satisfactory. Other materials such as aspirin combinations, acetophenetidin, thiamine hydrochloride, ascorbic acid, magnesium hydroxide, and other antacid compounds may be treated similarly.

Results comparable to those accomplished by the slugging process are also obtained by compacting mills. In the compaction method the powder to be densified passes between high-pressure rollers which compress the powder and remove the air. The densified material is reduced to a uniform granule size and compressed into tablets after the addition of a lubricant. Excessive pressures which may be required to obtain cohesion of certain materials may result in a prolonged dissolution rate.[111] Compaction mills available include the Chilsonator made by Fitzpatrick and the Compactor Mill available through Allis-Chalmers.

Direct Compression

As its name implies, direct compression consists of compressing tablets directly from powdered material without modifying the physical nature of the material itself. Formerly, direct compression as a method of tablet manufacture was reserved for a small group of crystalline chemicals having all the physical characteristics required for the formation of a good tablet. This group includes chemicals such as potassium salts (chlorate, chloride, bromide, iodide, nitrate, permanganate), ammonium chloride, and methenamine. These materials possess cohesive and flow properties which make direct compression possible.

Since the pharmaceutical industry is constantly making efforts to increase the efficiency of tableting operations and to reduce costs by utilizing the smallest amount of floor space and labor as possible for a given operation, an increasing amount of attention is being given to this method of tablet preparation.[112,113] Also, this method should produce tablets of faster dissolution rates because no colloidal binders such as gelatin or starch are used to surround the granules. Approaches being used to make this method more universally applicable include the introduction of formulation additives capable of imparting the characteristics required for compression, and the use of force-feeding devices to improve the flow of powder blends.

For tablets in which the drug itself constitutes a major portion of the total tablet weight, it is necessary that the drug itself possess those physical characteristics required for the formulation to be compressed directly. Direct compression for tablets containing small amounts of therapeutic ingredients frequently can be used by formulating with a suitable diluent. Among the diluents commercially available at the present time are the following: anhydrous lactose (*Sheffield*); dicalcium phosphate dihydrate, unmilled (*Victor*); pregranulated calcium sulfate; Dri-Tab (*Nulomalene*), a mixture of sucrose powder and invert sugars; spray-dried lactose (*Foremost*); and spray-dried mannitol.[114-116] Spray-dried solutions of lactose and mannitol give materials consisting of spherical aggregates of small particles which have good flow and compression characteristics. Spray-dried lactose tends to discolor due to the presence of 5-(hydroxymethyl)-2-furaldehyde.[117,118] The sugar, amylose (*Staley*), is reported to have characteristics that lend themselves to its use as a dry binder. Since it requires about 10–12% moisture for optimum compression, it may be unsuitable for use with drugs subject to hydrolytic decomposition. Other additives under intensive investigation in the formulation approach to direct compression include the use of colloidal silica [(Cab-O-Sil (*Cabot*) or Quso (*Phila. Quartz*)] as a flow-promoting agent; cellulose [Solka-Floc (*Brown*)] and microcrystalline cellulose [Avicel (*Am. Viscose*)] which have lubricating properties as well as flow-promoting properties.[119]

Forced-flow feeders are mechanical devices available from pharmaceutical equipment manufacturers designed to deaerate light and bulky material. Mechanically they maintain a steady flow of powder moving into the die cavities under moderate pressure. They attempt to minimize air entrapment and consequently capping in the finished tablet. By increasing the density of the powder, an higher uniformity in tablet weights is obtained.

The gradual improvement of formulation additives and development of mechanical feeding devices for the high-speed rotary tableting machines indicate the acceptance of direct compression as the preferred method for the future. Of all the methods, direct compression is the most adaptable to automation. Interest in direct compression is also stimulating basic research on the flowability of powders with and without the presence of additives.[120,121] Direct compression formulas are included in the formula section found on page 1668.

Related Drying Processes

Spray Drying—A number of tableting additives suitable for direct compression have been prepared by the drying process known as spray drying. The method consists of bringing together a highly dispersed liquid and a sufficient volume of hot air to produce evaporation and drying of the liquid droplets. The feed liquid may be a solution, slurry, emulsion, gel, or paste, provided it is pumpable and capable of being atomized. As shown in Fig. 690, the feed is sprayed into a current of warm filtered air. The air supplies the heat for evaporation and conveys the dried product to the collector; the air is then exhausted with the moisture.[122] As the liquid droplets present a large surface area to the warm air, local heat and transfer coefficients are high.

The spray-dried powder particles are homogeneous, approximately spherical in shape, nearly uniform in size, and frequently hollow. The latter characteristic results in low bulk density with a rapid rate of solution. Being uniform in size and spherical, the particles possess good flowability. The design and operation of the spray dryer can vary many characteristics of the final product, such as particle size and size distribution, bulk and particle densities, porosity, moisture content, flowability, and friability.[123] Among the spray-dried materials available for direct compression formulas are lactose, mannitol, and flour.[124] Another application of the process in tableting is spray drying the combination of tablet additives as the diluent, disintegrant, and binder. The spray-dried material is then blended with the active ingredient or drug, lubricated, and compressed directly into tablets.[125]

Since atomization of the feed results in a high surface area, the moisture evaporates rapidly. The evaporation keeps the product cool and as the result the method is applicable for drying heat-sensitive materials. Among heat-sensitive pharmaceuticals successfully spray-dried are the amino acids; antibiotics as aureomycin, bacitracin, penicillin, and streptomycin; ascorbic acid; cascara extracts; liver extracts; pepsin and similar enzymes; protein hydrolysates; and thiamine.

Frequently, spray drying is more economical than other processes since it produces a dry powder directly from a liquid and eliminates other processing steps as crystallization, precipitation, filtering or drying, particle size reduction, and particle classifying. By the elimination of these steps, labor, equipment costs, space requirements, and possible contamination of the product are reduced. Intrinsic factor concentrate obtained from hog mucosa previously was prepared at Lederle Laboratories using a salt precipitation process, followed by a freeze-drying.[126] By utilizing spray drying it was possible to manufacture a high-grade material by a continuous process. The spherical particles of the product facilitated its subsequent blending with vitamin B_{12}. Similar efficiencies have been found in processes producing magnesium trisilicate and dihydroxy aluminum sodium carbonate; both chemicals are widely used in antacid preparations.[127]

Encapsulation of chemicals also can be achieved using spray drying equipment. The process is useful in coating one material on another in order to protect the interior substance or to control the rate of its release. The substance to be coated can either be liquid or solid, but must be insoluble in a solution of the coating material. The oil-soluble vitamins, A and D, can be coated with a variety of materials as acacia gum to prevent their deterioration. Flavoring oils and synthetic flavors are coated to give the so-called dry flavors.

Spray Congealing—Also called spray chilling, spray congealing is a technique similar to spray drying. It consists of melting solids and reducing them to beads or powder by spraying the molten feed into a stream of air or other gas. The same basic equipment is used as with spray drying although no source of heat is required. Either ambient or cooled air is used depending on the freezing point of the product. For example, monoglycerides and similar materials are spray congealed with air at 50°F. A closed-loop system with refrigeration cools and recycles the air. Using this process, drugs can be dissolved or suspended in a molten wax and spray congealed; the resultant material then can be adapted for a prolonged-release form of the drug.

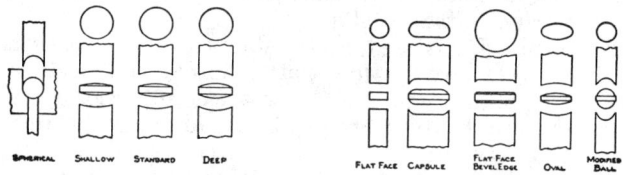

Fig. 691. Concave punches.   **Fig. 692. Specially shaped punches.**

Among the carbohydrates used in compressed tablets, mannitol is the only one which possesses high heat stability. Mannitol melts at 167°C and either alone or in combination with other carbohydrates can be fused and spray-congealed. Selected drugs have been shown to be soluble in these fused mixtures, and the resultant spray-congealed material possesses excellent flow and compression characteristics.[128]

Tablet Machines

As mentioned previously, the basic mechanical unit in tablet compression involves the operation of two steel punches within a steel die cavity. The tablet is formed by the pressure exerted on the granulation by the punches within the die cavity, or cell. The tablet assumes the size and shape of the punches and die used. While round tablets are more generally used, shapes such as oval, capsule-form, square, triangular, or other irregular shapes may be used. Likewise, the curvature of the faces of the punches determines the curvature of the tablets. The diameters generally found to be satisfactory and frequently referred to as standard are as follows: $3/16$ in., $7/32$ in., $1/4$ in., $9/32$ in., $5/16$ in., $11/32$ in., $7/16$ in., $1/2$ in., $9/16$ in., $5/8$ in., $11/16$ in., and $3/4$ in. Punch faces with ridges are used for compressed tablets scored for breaking into halves or fourths, although it has been indicated that variation among tablet halves is significantly greater than among intact tablets.[129] Tablets, engraved or embossed with symbols or initials, require punches with faces embossed or engraved with the corresponding designs. See Fig. 693, page 1661. The use of the tablet sometimes determines its shape; effervescent tablets are usually large, round, and flat, while vitamin tablets are frequently prepared in capsule-shaped forms. Tablets prepared using deep-cup punches appear to be round and when coated take on the appearance of pills. Veterinary tablets often have a bolus shape and are much larger than those used in medical practice.

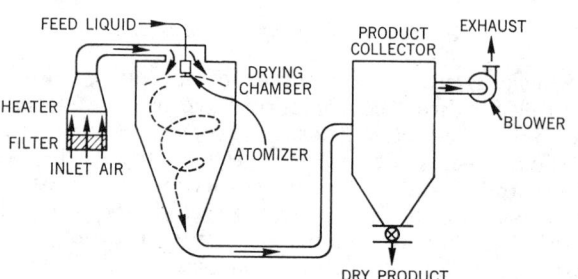

Fig. 690. Typical spray-drying system (courtesy, Bowen Eng.).

The quality-control program for punches and dies, frequently referred to as tooling, instituted by large pharmaceutical companies emphasize the importance of their care to modern pharmaceutical production.[130] To produce physically perfect compressed tablets, an efficient punch and die program must be set up. Provisions for inspection of tooling, parameters for cost per product determination, product identification, and tooling specifications must all be considered.[131] Regardless of the size of the tableting operation, the attention which must be given to the proper care of punches and dies should be noted. They must be

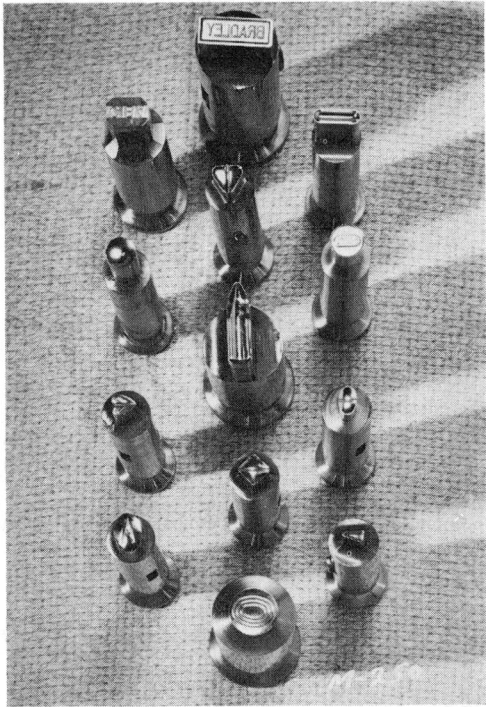

Fig. 693. Collection of punches (courtesy, Stokes).

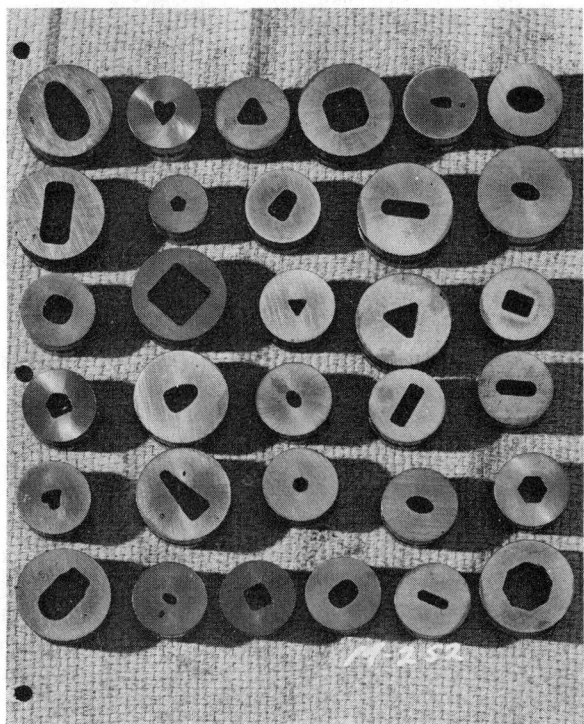

Fig. 694. Collection of dies (courtesy, Stokes).

Table I—Single-Punch Tablet Machines

Machine model	Maximum diameter of tablets, in.	Tablets per min	Maximum depth of fill, in.
Stokes equipment[a]			
Eureka[b]	½	75	⁷⁄₁₆
Model E	½	85–130	½
Model F	¾	60–95	1¹⁄₁₆
Model T	2	20–60	1¼
Model R[c]	3	14–16	2
Manesty equipment[d]			
Hand Machine	½	100	⁷⁄₁₆
Model E 2	½	85	⁹⁄₁₆
Model F 3	⅞	85	1¹⁄₁₆

[a] See *Manufacturers Index*, page 2023.
[b] Available as hand or power models.
[c] Widely used for veterinary boluses.
[d] American representatives: Thomas Eng. See *Manufacturers Index*, page 2023.

highly polished and kept free from rust and imperfections. In cases where the material pits or abrades the dies, chromium-plated dies have been used. Dropping the punches on hard surfaces will chip their fine edges. When the punches are in the machine, the upper and lower punches should not be allowed to contact each other. Otherwise, a curling or flattening of the edges will result which is one of the causes or capping. This is especially necessary to observe in the case of deep-cup punches.

When the punches are removed from the machine, they should be washed thoroughly in warm soapy water and dried well with a clean cloth. A coating of grease or oil should be rubbed over all parts of the dies and punches to protect them from the atmosphere. They should be stored carefully in boxes or paper tubes.

Single-Punch Machines

The simplest tableting machines available are those having the single-punch design. A number of models are available as outlined in Table I. While the majority of these are power driven, several hand-operated models are available. Compression is accomplished on a single-punch machine as shown in Fig. 695. The feed shoe filled with the granulation is positioned over the die cavity which then fills. The feed shoe retracts and scrapes all excess granulation away from the die cavity. The upper punch lowers to compress the granulation within the die cavity. The upper punch retracts and the lower punch rises to eject the tablet. As the feed shoe returns to fill the die cavity, it pushes the compressed tablet from the die platform. The weight of the tablet is determined by the volume of the die cavity; the lower punch is adjustable to increase or

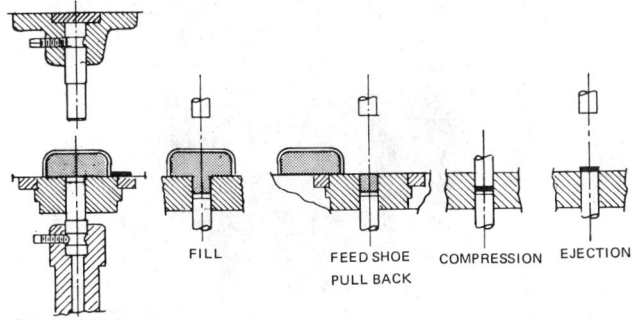

FEED SHOE OVER DIE   FILL   FEED SHOE PULL BACK   COMPRESSION   EJECTION

Fig. 695. Formation of tablet on single-punch machine (courtesy, Cherry-Burrell).

decrease the volume of granulation, thus increasing or decreasing the weight of the tablet.

For tablets having diameters larger than ½ in., sturdier models are required. This is also true for tablets requiring a high degree of hardness as in the case of compressed lozenges. The heavier models are capable of much higher pressures and are suitable for slugging.

Operation of Single-Punch Machines

In installing punches and dies in a single-punch machine insert the lower punch first by lining up the notched groove on the punch with the lower punch setscrew and slipping it into the smaller bore in the die table; the setscrew is not tightened as yet. The lower punch is differentiated from the upper punch in that it has a collar around the punch head. Slip the die over the punch head so that the notched groove (with the widest area at the top) lines up with the die setscrew. Tighten the lower punch setscrew after seating the lower punch by pressing on the punch with the thumb. Tighten the die setscrew,

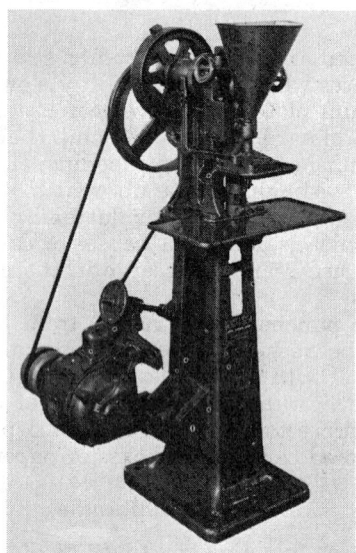

Fig. 696. Model E, single-punch machine (courtesy, Stokes).

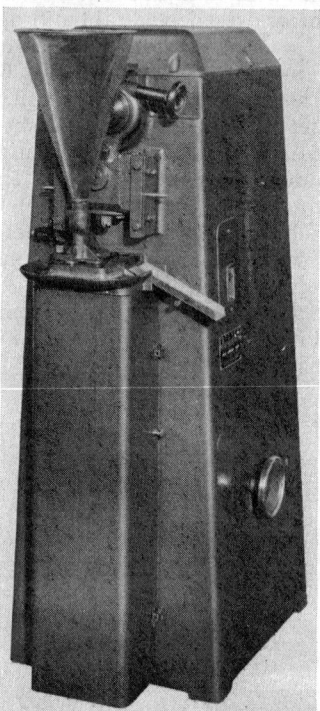

Fig. 697. Model F, heavy-duty single-punch machine for tablets requiring heavy pressure (courtesy, Stokes).

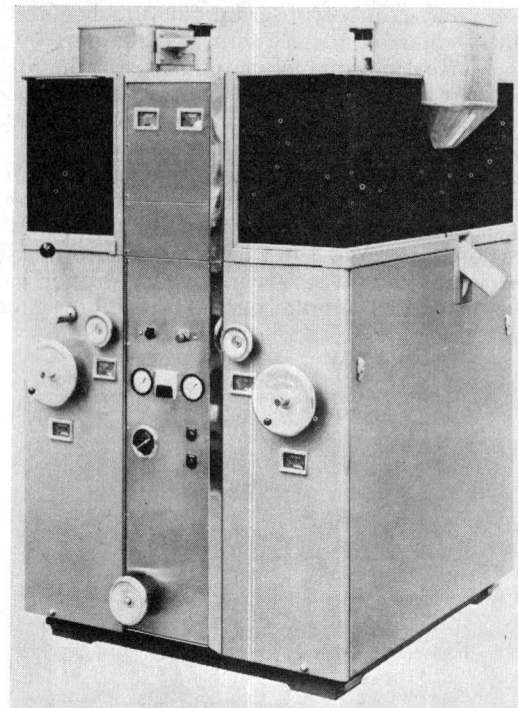

Fig. 698. Model 565-1, Ultra Press, double-sided rotary compacting press designed to produce at speeds over 10,000 tablets/min (courtesy, Stokes).

making certain that the surface of the die is flush with the die table. Insert the upper punch, again lining up the grooved notch with the upper punch setscrew. To be certain that the upper punch is securely seated, turn the machine over by hand with a block of soft wood or wad of cloth between the upper and lower punches. When the punch is seated, tighten the upper punch setscrew. Adjust the pressure so that the upper and lower punches will not come in contact with each other when the machine is turned over. Adjust the lower punch so that it is flush with the die table at the ejection point. Install the feed shoe and hopper.

After adding a small amount of granulation to the hopper, turn the machine over by hand and adjust the pressure until a tablet is formed. Adjust the tablet weight until the desired weight is obtained. The pressure will have to be altered concurrently with the weight adjustments. It should be remembered that as the fill is increased the lower punch moves further away from the upper punch and more pressure will have to be applied to obtain comparable hardness. Conversely, when the fill is decreased, the pressure will have to be decreased. When all the adjustments have been made, fill the hopper with granulation and turn on the motor. Hardness and weight should be checked immediately and suitable adjustments made if necessary. Periodic checks should be made on the tablet hardness and weight during the running of the batch at 15–30-min intervals.

When the batch has been run off, turn off the power and remove loose dust and granulation with the vacuum cleaner. Release the pressure from the punches. Remove the feed hopper and the feed shoe. Remove the upper punch, the lower punch, and the die. Clean all surfaces of the tablet machine and dry well with clean cloth. Cover surfaces with thin coating of grease or oil prior to storage.

As tablets are thrown from the machine after compression, they are usually accompanied with powder and uncompressed granulation. To remove this loose dust, the tablets are passed over a screen, which may be vibrating, and cleaned with an air blast or with a vacuum line.

Rotary Tablet Machines

For increased production the rotary machines offer the greatest advantages. A head carrying a number of sets of punches and dies revolves continuously while the tablet granulation runs from the hopper, through a feed frame, and into the dies placed in a large, steel plate revolving under it. This method promotes a uniform fill of the die and therefore an accurate weight for the tablet. Compression takes place as the upper and lower punches pass between a pair of rollers. This action produces a slow squeezing effect on the material in the die cavity from the top and bottom and so gives a chance for the entrapped air to escape. The lower punch lifts up and ejects the tablet. Adjustments for tablet weight and hardness can be made without the use of tools while the machine is in operation. Fig. 699 shows the tooling in a 16-station rotary press in the positions of a complete cycle to produce 1 tablet/set of tooling. One of the factors which contributes to the variation in tablet weight and hardness during compression is the internal flow of the granulation within the feed hopper.[132]

On most rotary machine models there is an excess pressure release which cushions each compression and relieves the machine of all shocks and undue strain. The punches and dies can be readily removed for inspection, cleaning, and for inserting different sets to produce a great variety of sizes and shapes. It is possible to equip the machine with as few punches and dies as the job requires and thus economize on installation costs. For types of rotary machines available, see Table II.

Operation of Rotary Machines

Before inserting punches and dies, make certain that the pressure has been released from the pressure wheel. The die holes should be cleaned thoroughly, making certain that the die seat is completely free of any foreign materials. Back off all die locks and loosely insert dies into the die holes, then tap each die securely into place with a fiber or soft metal rod through the upper punch holes. After all the dies have been tapped into place, tighten each die lockscrew progressively and securely. As each screw is tightened the die is checked to see that it does not project above the die table. Insert the lower punches through the hole made available by removing the punch head. Turn the machine by hand until the punch bore coincides with the plug hole. Insert each lower punch in its place progressively. Insert the upper punches by dropping them into place in the head. Each punch (upper and lower) should be coated with a thin film of mineral oil before inserting them into the machine. Adjust the ejection cam so that the lower punch is flush with the die table at the ejection point.

After insertion of the punches and dies adjust the machine for the tablet weight and hardness. The feed frame should be attached to the machine along with the feed hopper. Add a small amount of the granulation through the hopper and turn over the machine by hand. Increase the pressure by rotating the pressure wheel until a tablet is formed. Check the weight of the tablet and adjust the fill to provide the desired tablet weight. Most likely more than one adjustment of the fill will be necessary before obtaining the acceptable weight. When the fill is decreased, the pressure must be decreased to provide the same hardness in the tablet. Conversely, when the fill is increased, the pressure must be increased to obtain comparable hardness.

Fig. 699. Tooling for a 16-station rotary press showing positions of the cycle required to produce 1 tablet/set of tooling (courtesy, Cherry-Burrell).

Table II—Rotary Tablet Machines

Machine model	Tool sets	Maximum diameter of tablets, in.	Tablets per min	Maximum depth of fill, in.
Cherry-Burrell[a]				
No. 216	16	$5/8$	1180	$3/4$
No. 240	16	$7/8$	640	$1 3/16$
No. 250	12	$1 1/4$	480	$1 1/8$
No. 260	25	$1 3/16$	1450	$1 3/8$
	31	1	1800	$1 3/8$
	33	$1 5/16$	1910	$1 3/8$
	43	$5/8$	2500	$1 3/8$
No. 270	18	2	325	$2 3/4$
	25	$1 3/8$	450	$2 3/4$
Stokes equipment[a]				
Model B-2	16	$5/8$	350–650	$1 1/16$
Model BB-2	27	$5/8$	750–1400	$1 1/16$
	33	$7/16$	950–1700	$1 1/16$
	37	$7/16$	1050–1900	$1 1/16$
Model D-3	16	$1 5/16$	190–350	$1 3/16$
Model DS-3	15	$1 3/16$	180–335	$1 1/16$
Model DD-2	23	$1 3/16$	240–720	$1 3/8$
	31	$1 5/16$	325–975	$1 1/16$
Manesty equipment[a]				
Model B3B	16	$5/8$	700	$1 1/16$
	23	$7/16$	1000	$1 1/16$
Model BB3B	27	$5/8$	1520	$1 1/16$
	33	$7/16$	1850	$1 1/16$
	39	$7/16$	2180	$1 1/16$
Model D3B	16	1	500	$1 3/16$
Model D3RY	16	1	600	$1 3/16$
	23	$5/8$	900	$1 3/16$
Deltapress	16	1	600	$1 3/16$
	23	$5/8$	900	$1 1/16$
Model DX2	13	$1 1/4$	520	$1 1/16$
	16	1	640	$1 1/16$
	20	$5/8$	800	$1 1/16$
Model RS2	14	$2 1/2$	210	2
	19	$1 7/8$	284	2

[a] See *Manufacturers Index*, page 2023.

Fill the hopper with the granulation and turn on the power. Check tablet weight and hardness immediately after the mechanical operation begins and make suitable adjustments, if necessary. Check these properties routinely and regularly at 15–30-min intervals while the machine is in operation. When the batch has been run, turn off the power. Remove the hopper and the feed frame from the machine. Remove loose granulation and dust with a vacuum line. Remove all pressure from the wheel. Remove the punches and dies in the reverse order of that used in setting up the machine. First, remove the upper punches individually, then the lower punches, and finally the dies. Wash each punch and die in alcohol and brush with a soft brush to remove adhering material. Dry them with a clean cloth and cover them with a thin coating of grease or oil before storing.

High-Speed Rotary Tablet Machines

The rotary tablet machine has gradually evolved into models capable of compressing tablets at high production rates. This has been accomplished by increasing the number of stations, ie, sets of punches and dies, in each revolution of the machine head, improvement in feeding devices, and on some models the installation of dual compression points. In Fig. 702, the drawing shows a rotary machine having dual compression points. Rotary machines having dual compression points are referred to as double rotary machines, and those with one compression point, single rotary. In the diagram, half of the tablets are produced 180° from the tablet chute. They travel the outside perimeter and discharge with the second tablet production. While these models are mechanically capable of operating at the production rates shown in Table III, the actual speed still depends on the physical characteristics of the tablet granulation and the rate which is consistent with compressed tablets having satisfactory physical characteristics. Various styles of feeding devices to improve the flow of the granulation into the die cavities are illustrated in Fig. 703.

Multilayer Rotary Tablet Machines

The rotary tablet machines also have been developed into models capable of producing multiple-layer tablets; the machines are able to make one-, two-, or three-layer tablets. Stratified tablets offer a number of advantages. Incompatible drugs can be formed into a single tablet by separating the layers containing them with a layer of inert material. It has permitted the formulation of time-delay medication and offers a wide variety of possibilities in developing color combinations which give the products identity.[133]

Table III—High-Speed Rotary Tablet Machines

Machine model	Tool sets	Maximum diameter of tablets, in.	Tablets per min	Maximum depth of fill, in.
Cherry-Burrell[a]				
No. 246	33	5/8	1584–4686	3/4
	41	7/16	1968–5822	3/4
	49	7/16	2352–6958	3/4
No. 247	33	5/8	3480	3/4
	41	7/16	4300	3/4
	49	7/16	5150	3/4
Stokes equipment[a]				
No. 513-2	35	5/8	800–3200	1 1/16
	45	7/16	1050–4200	1 1/16
No. 533	27	1 3/16	800–1900	1 1/16
No. 540	35	5/8	800–2400	1 1/16
	41	7/16	950–2700	1 1/16
No. 551	51	7/16	1250–3750	1 1/16
No. 552	51	7/16	1250–5000	1 1/16
No. 565-1	65	7/16	3500–10,000	1 1/16
No. 565-2	53	5/8	2900–8100	1 1/16
No. 580-1	45	7/16	2100	1 1/16
No. 580-2	35	5/8	1600	1 1/16
Manesty equipment[a]				
Betapress	16	5/8	1500	1 1/16
	23	7/16	2160	1 1/16
Rotapress	37	1	3550	1 3/16
	45	5/8	4320	1 1/16
	55	7/16	5280	1 1/16
Mark II	45	5/8	8182	1 1/16
	55	7/16	10,000	1 1/16

[a] See *Manufacturers Index*, page 2023.

Originally the tablets were prepared by a single compression method. The dies were filled with the different granulations in successive layers and the tablet was formed by a single compression stroke. The separation lines of the tablets prepared by this method tended to be irregular. In the machines now available for multilayer production the granulation receives a precompression stroke after the first and second fill, which lightly compacts the granulation and maintains a well-defined surface of separation between each layer. The operator is able to eject either precompressed layer with the machine running at any desired speed for periodic weight and analysis checks.

Another development in the rotary compression machines has been the compression coating machines which are described in Chapter on *Coating of Tablets, Capsules, and Pills*, page 1681.

Capping and Splitting of Tablets

The splitting or capping of tablets is one of great concern and annoyance in tablet making. It is quite difficult to detect while the tablets are being processed but can be detected easily by vigorously shaking a few in the cupped hands. A slightly chipped tablet does not necessarily mean the tablet will cap or split.

There are many factors that may cause a tablet to cap or split:

1. Excess "fines" or powder which traps air in the tablet mixture.
2. Deep markings on tablet punches. Many designs or "scores" on punches are too broad and deep. Hairline markings are just as appropriate as deep, heavy markings.
3. Worn and imperfect punches. Punches should be smooth and buffed. Nicked punches will often cause capping.
4. Worn dies. Dies should be replaced or reversed. Dies that are chrome-plated or have tungsten carbide inserts wear longer and give better results than ordinary steel dies.

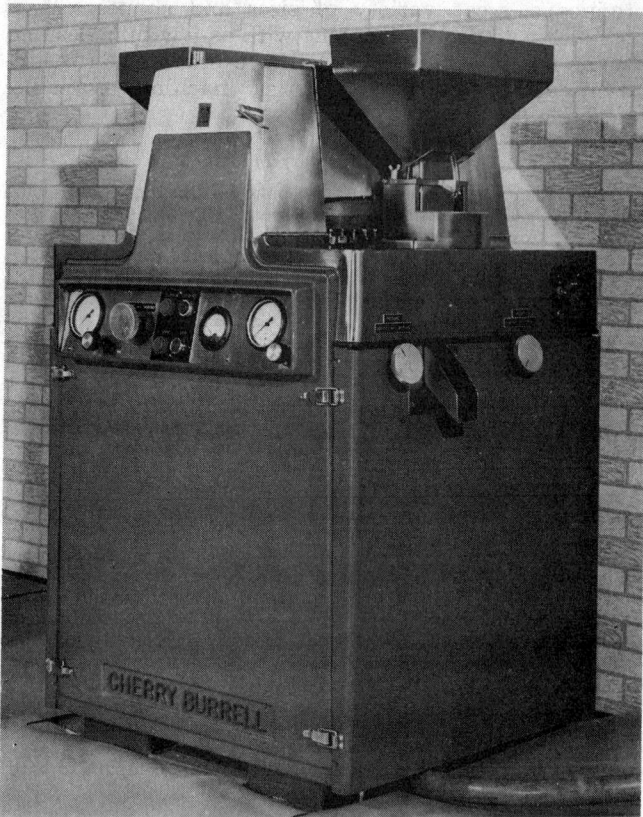

Fig. 700. Model 246, high-speed rotary machine (courtesy, Cherry-Burrell).

5. Too much pressure. By reducing the pressure on the machines the condition may be corrected.
6. Unsuitable formula. It may be necessary to change the formula. The diluents may be wrongly proportioned. For example, lactose, starch, or other fillers may be in excess and should be adjusted in the formula.
7. Moist and soft granulation. This type of granulation will not flow freely into the dies, thus giving uneven weights and soft or capped tablets.
8. Poorly machined punches. A set of punches used on rotary machines should be accurately machined to 0.005 in. Uneven punches are detrimental to the tablet machine itself and will not produce tablets of accurate weight. One punch out of alignment may cause one tablet to split or cap on every revolution.

A remedy for capping in many cases is to dampen the mixture slightly with water, alcohol, alcohol and water, glucose solution, or other suitable solution prior to compressing, providing no incompatibility is involved.

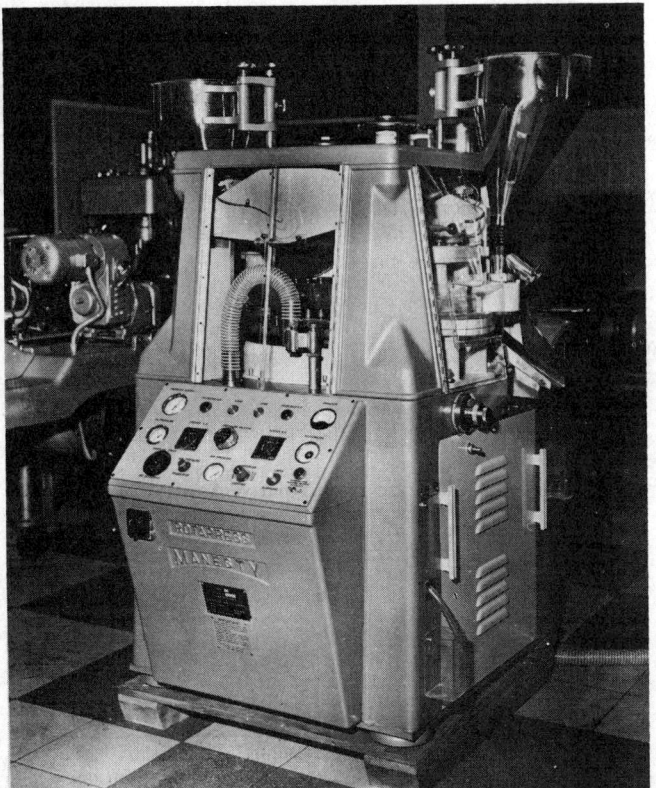

Fig. 701. Mark II Rotapress machine with 55 stations (courtesy, Manesty).

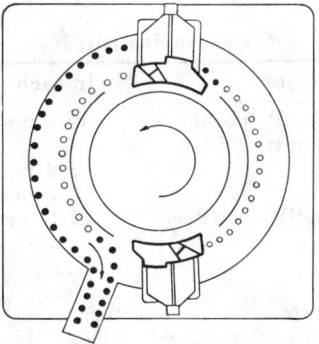

Fig. 702. The movement of tablets on die table of a double rotary press (courtesy, Cherry-Burrell).

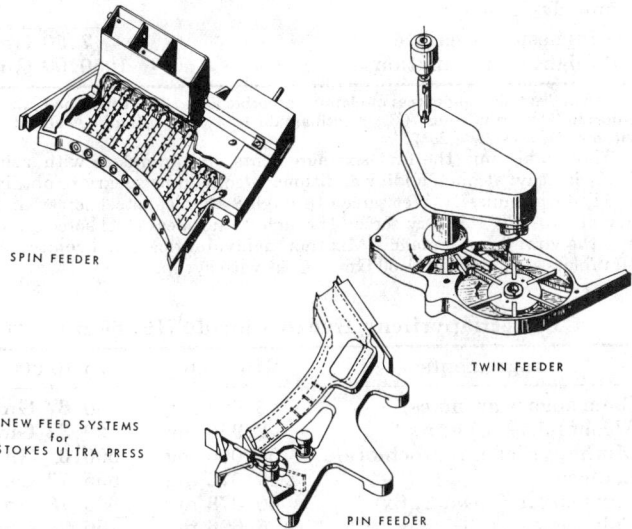

SPIN FEEDER

TWIN FEEDER

NEW FEED SYSTEMS
for
STOKES ULTRA PRESS

PIN FEEDER

Fig. 703. Feeding devices designed to promote flow of granulations for high-speed machines (courtesy, Stokes).

Contamination Control

While quality control procedures used by the pharmaceutical industry for many years have stressed the importance of cleanliness of equipment and facilities for the manufacture of drug products, the penicillin contamination problem has resulted in renewed emphasis to this aspect of manufacturing. Penicillin, either as an airborne dust or residual quantities remaining in equipment, is believed to have contaminated unrelated products in sufficient concentrations to cause allergenic reactions in individuals, hypersensitive to penicillin, who received these products. This resulted in the industry spending thousands of dollars to change or modify buildings, manufacturing processes, equipment, and standard operating procedures to eliminate penicillin contamination.

With this problem has come renewed emphasis on the dust problem, material handling, and equipment

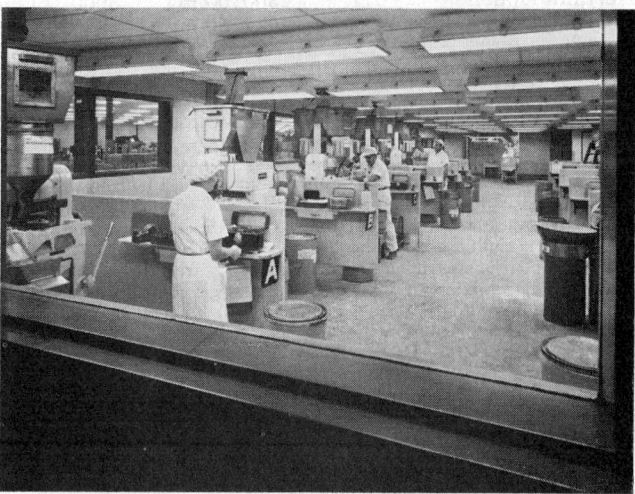

Fig. 704. Tablet compression department (courtesy, MSD).

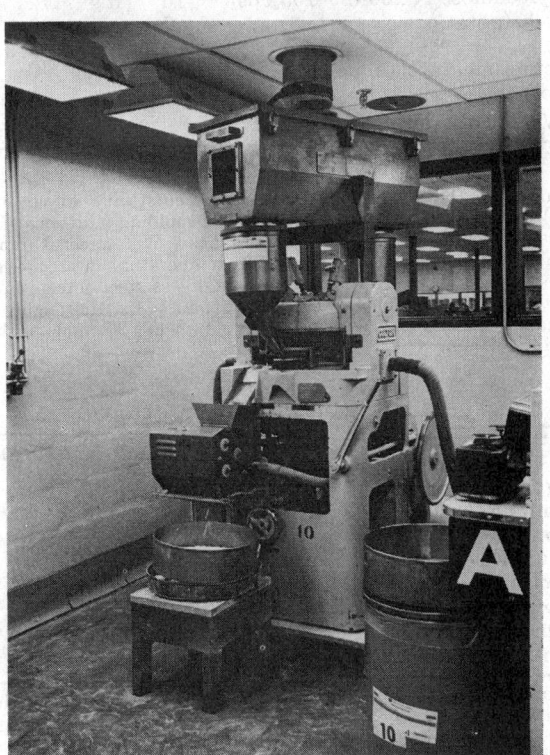

Fig. 705. 41-Punch compressing machine (courtesy, MSD).

cleaning in dealing with drugs, especially potent chemicals. Any process utilizing chemicals in powder form can be a dusty operation; the preparation of compressed tablets and encapsulation fall in this category. Fig. 705 illustrates a number of methods utilized to control the airborne contamination problem in tablet compression. The granulation for the 41-station compressing machine is prepared on the floor above and delivered to an isolated machine by means of a closed hopper system. A vacuum line attached to the press removes dust-laden air and excess powder from the vital press areas above and below the die table adjacent to the pressure rolls, cam tracks, punches, dies, and head drive gear. A second vacuum line removes all excess dust from the compressed tablets as they come from the machine.

This represents but one example of the industry's efforts to conform with the intent of current good manufacturing practice as defined by the Food and Drug Administration (see page 1762).

Tablet Formulations

Wet Granulation Method

CT Acetaminophen, 300 mg

Ingredients	In each	In 10,000
Acetaminophen	300.00 mg	3000.0 Gm
Polyvinylpyrrolidone	22.50 mg	225.0 Gm
Lactose	61.75 mg	617.5 Gm
Alcohol 3A—200 proof	4.50 ml	45.0 L
Stearic acid	9.00 mg	90.0 Gm
Talc	13.50 mg	135.0 Gm
Corn starch	43.25 mg	432.5 Gm

Blend acetaminophen, polyvinylpyrrolidone, and lactose together; pass through a 40-mesh screen. Add the alcohol slowly and knead well. Screen the wet mass through a 4-mesh screen. Dry granulation at 50°C overnight. Screen the dried granulation through a 20-mesh screen. Bolt the stearic acid, talc, and corn starch through 60-mesh screen prior to mixing by tumbling with the granulation. Compress using 7/16-in. standard concave punch. 10 tablets should weigh 4.5 Gm (courtesy, Abbott).

CT Ascorbic Acid USP, 50 mg

Ingredients	In each		In 7000	
Ascorbic Acid USP (powder No. 80)[a]	55	mg	385	Gm
Lactose	21	mg	147	Gm
Starch (potato)	13	mg	91	Gm
Ethylcellulose N 100 (80–105 cps)	16	mg	112	Gm
Starch (potato)	7	mg	49	Gm
Talc	6.5	mg	45.5	Gm
Calcium stearate (impalpable powder)	1	mg	7	Gm
Weight of granulation			836.5	Gm

[a] Includes 10% in excess of claim.

Granulate the above first three ingredients with ethylcellulose (5%) dissolved in anhydrous ethyl alcohol adding additional anhydrous alcohol to obtain good wet granules. Wet screen through 8 stainless steel screen and dry at room temperature in an air-conditioned area. Dry screen through 20 stainless steel screen and incorporate the remaining three ingredients. Mix thoroughly and compress. Use a flat beveled, 1/4-in. punch. 20 tablets should weight 2.39 Gm.

Chewable Antacid Tablets

Ingredients	In each	In 10,000
Magnesium trisilicate	500 mg	5000 Gm
Aluminum hydroxide, dried gel	250 mg	2500 Gm
Mannitol	300 mg	3000 Gm
Sodium saccharin	2 mg	20 Gm
Starch paste, 5%	qs	qs
Oil of peppermint	1 mg	10 Gm
Magnesium stearate	10 mg	100 Gm
Corn starch	10 mg	100 Gm

Mix the magnesium trisilicate and aluminum hydroxide with the mannitol. Dissolve the sodium saccharin in a small quantity of purified water, then combine this with the starch paste. Granulate the powder blend with the starch paste. Dry at 140°F and screen through 16-mesh screen. Add the flavoring oil, magnesium stearate, and corn starch; mix well. Age the granulation for at least 24 hours and compress using 5/8-in. flat-face bevel-edge punch (courtesy, Atlas).

Chewable Pediatric Aluminum Aspirin Tablets

Ingredients	In each	In 10,000
Aluminum aspirin	100.00 mg	1000.00 Gm
Sodium cyclamate	2.00 mg	20.00 Gm
Talc	8.00 mg	80.00 Gm
Corn starch	12.50 mg	125.00 Gm
CMC (high viscosity), 2% solution	qs	qs
Flavors and color	qs	qs

Mix aluminum aspirin, sodium cyclamate and color. Granulate with sufficient quantity of carboxymethylcellulose solution. Pass through a suitable screen and dry at 105°F. Pass dried granulation through a 20-mesh screen; add talc, corn starch, and flavor, mixing well. Compress using 1/2-in. standard concave punch (courtesy, Abbott).

CT Hexavitamin NF

Ingredients	In each		In 7000
Ascorbic Acid USP (powder)[a]	82.5 mg		577.50 Gm
Thiamine Mononitrate USP (powder)[a]	2.4 mg		16.80 Gm
Riboflavin[a]	3.3 mg		23.10 Gm
Nicotinamide USP (powder)[a]	22.0 mg		154.00 Gm
Starch	. . .		97.40 Gm
Lactose	. . .		41.20 Gm
Zein	. . .		45.00 Gm
Vitamin A acetate:	6250	U	
Vitamin D₂[a] (use Pfizer crystalets medium granules containing 500,000 U vitamin A acetate and 50,000 U vitamin D₂/Gm).	625	U	87.50 Gm
Magnesium stearate			7.50 Gm
Weight of granulation			1050.00 Gm

[a] Includes following excess of claim: ascorbic acid 10%, thiamine hydrochloride 20%, riboflavin 10%, nicotinamide 10%, and vitamin A acetate–vitamin D₂ crystalets 25%.

Thoroughly mix the first six ingredients and granulate with zein (10% in ethyl alcohol, adding additional alcohol if necessary to obtain good wet granules). Wet screen through 8 stainless steel screen and dry at 110–120°F. Dry screen through 20 stainless steel screen and add the vitamin crystalets. Mix thoroughly, lubricate and compress. 10 tablets should weigh 1.50 Gm. Coat with syrup.

CT Methapyrilene Hydrochloride NF, 50 mg

Ingredients	In each	In 10,000
Cane sugar (granules)	3.067 mg	30.67 Gm
Alcohol 3A—190 proof	2.938 mg	29.38 Gm
Methapyrilene hydrochloride	50.000 mg	500.0 Gm
Lactose	59.572 mg	595.72 Gm
Cane sugar (powder, 6x)	60.378 mg	603.78 Gm
Talc	6.696 mg	66.96 Gm
Stearic acid, powder	1.728 mg	17.28 Gm

Dissolve the sugar granules in 0.30 gal of water and add the alcohol. Charge methapyrilene hydrochloride, lactose, and powdered sugar into a suitable mixer. Add the syrup alcohol solution to the mass. Granulate through No. 3 band on the Fitz mill. Dry at 105°F. Sift dry granulation through 16-mesh screen. Lubricate by the addition of talc and stearic acid and mix well. Compress using a $\frac{5}{16}$-in. concave punch (courtesy, Abbott).

CT Sulfathiazole

Ingredients	In each	In 7000
Sulfathiazole (powder)	502 mg	3514 Gm
Magnesium stearate		
Starch	130 mg	910 Gm
Starch paste		qs
Weight of granulation		4424 Gm

Use a bisected flat-face $\frac{7}{16}$-in. punch. 10 tablets should weigh 6.46 Gm.

CT Theobromine–Phenobarbital

Ingredients	In each		In 7000	
Theobromine	325	mg	2275	Gm
Phenobarbital	33	mg	231	Gm
Starch	39	mg	273	Gm
Talc	8	mg	56	Gm
Acacia (powder)	8	mg	56	Gm
Stearic acid	0.7	mg	4.9	Gm
Weight of granulation			2895.9	Gm

Prepare a paste with the acacia and an equal weight of starch. Use this paste for granulating the theobromine and phenobarbital. Dry and put through a 12-mesh screen, add the remainder of the material, mix thoroughly, and compress into tablets, using a $\frac{13}{32}$-in. concave punch. 10 tablets should weigh 4.13 Gm.

CT Thiamine Hydrochloride USP, 10 mg

Ingredients	In each	In 7000	
Thiamine Hydrochloride USP[a]	11 mg	77	Gm
Milk sugar (powder)	390 mg	2730	Gm
Tartaric acid (powder)[b]	5 mg	35	Gm
Starch paste		qs	
Sterotex		4.55	Gm
Weight of granulation		2846.55	Gm

[a] Includes 10% in excess of claim.
[b] To adjust pH to 4.5.

Mix ingredients, except the sterotex, and granulate with starch paste. Dry and screen to 14–16-mesh. Lubricate. Use a standard-cup bisected $\frac{13}{32}$-in. punch. 10 tablets should weigh 4.08 Gm.

CT Dried Yeast NF

Ingredients	In each	In 7000	
Dried yeast (powder)	0.5 Gm	3500	Gm
Sugar (powder)		340.2	Gm
Acacia (powder)		20.8	Gm
Alcohol		173	Gm
Glycerin		178	Gm
Water		32	Gm
Weight of granulation		4014.71	Gm

Mix the powdered dry yeast, powdered acacia, and sugar. Put through a 20-mesh screen. Granulate with a mixture of the alcohol, glycerin, and water. Spread on trays, put in a tablet dryer, and heat at 140°F for about 3 hr only. If further drying is required, do this in the open. Put through a 16-mesh screen and compress into tablets, using a $\frac{7}{16}$-in. punch. 10 tablets should weigh 5.75 Gm.

CT Thyroid

Ingredients	In each	In 7000
Thyroid USP	33 mg	231 Gm
Milk sugar	57 mg	399 Gm
Acacia (powder)	11 mg	77 Gm
Starch paste		qs
Starch (powder)	11 mg	77 Gm
Weight of granulation		784 Gm

Mix the thyroid, milk sugar, and powdered acacia together, and granulate with the starch paste. Force through a 8-mesh screen while wet, dry at moderate temperature, and force through a 14-mesh screen. Add the powdered starch, mix, and compress. Use a standard $\frac{1}{4}$-in. punch. 10 tablets should weigh 1.26 Gm.

Dry Granulation Method

CT Acetylsalicylic Acid

Ingredients	In each	In 7000	
Acetylsalicylic Acid (crystals 20-mesh)	0.325 Gm	2275	Gm
Starch		226.8	Gm
Weight of granulation		2501.8	Gm

Dry the starch to a moisture content of 10%. Thoroughly mix this with the acetylsalicylic acid. Compress into slugs. Grind the slugs to 14–16-mesh size. Recompress into tablets, using a $\frac{13}{32}$-in. punch. 10 tablets should weigh 3.575 Gm.

CT Folic Acid USP, 5 mg

Ingredients	In each	In 10,000
Folic Acid USP	5.00 mg	50.00 Gm
Starch	15.00 mg	150.00 Gm
Milk sugar (powder)	149.00 mg	1418.00 Gm
Talc	18.00 mg	180.00 Gm
Stearic acid	0.20 mg	2.00 Gm
Weight of granulation		1800.00 Gm

Mix all ingredients thoroughly. Compress into slugs. Grind and screen to 14–16-mesh granules. Recompress into tablets, using $\frac{1}{4}$-in. concave punch. 10 tablets should weigh 1.80 Gm.

CT Methamphetamine Hydrochloride USP, 2.5 mg

Ingredients	In each	In 10,000
Methamphetamine hydrochloride	2.50 mg	25.00 Gm
Starch	45.00 mg	450.00 Gm
Milk sugar (powder)	97.00 mg	970.00 Gm
Talc	35.50 mg	355.00 Gm
Weight of granulation		1800.00 Gm

Mix all ingredients thoroughly. Compress into slugs. Grind and screen to 14–16-mesh granules. Recompress into tablets, using $\frac{5}{16}$-in. concave punch. 10 tablets should weigh 1.80 Gm.

CT Sodium Phenobarbital

Ingredients	In each		In 7000	
Phenobarbital sodium	65	mg	455	Gm
Milk sugar (granular, 12-mesh)	26	mg	182	Gm
Starch	20	mg	140	Gm
Talc	20	mg	140	Gm
Magnesium stearate	0.3	mg	2.1	Gm
Weight of granulation			919.1	Gm

Mix all the ingredients thoroughly. Compress into slugs. Grind and screen to 14–16-mesh granules. Recompress into tablets, using a $\frac{9}{32}$-in. concave punch. 10 tablets should weigh 1.3 Gm.

CT Vitamin B-Complex

Ingredients	In each	In 10,000
Thiamine mononitrate[a]	0.733 mg	7.33 Gm
Riboflavin[a]	0.733 mg	7.33 Gm
Pyridoxine hydrochloride	0.333 mg	3.33 Gm
Calcium pantothenate[a]	0.400 mg	4.00 Gm
Nicotinamide	5.000 mg	50.00 Gm
Milk sugar (powder)	75.200 mg	752.00 Gm
Starch	21.900 mg	219.00 Gm
Talc	20.000 mg	200.00 Gm
Stearic acid (powder)	0.701 mg	7.01 Gm
Weight of granulation		1250 Gm

[a] Includes 10% in excess of claim.

Mix all the ingredients thoroughly. Compress into slugs. Grind and screen to 14–16-mesh granules. Recompress into tablets, using a ¼-inch concave punch. 10 tablets should weigh 1.25 Gm.

Sufficient tartaric acid should be used in these tablets to adjust the pH to 4.5.

Direct Compression Method

CT Ascorbic Acid USP, 250 mg

Ingredients	In each	In 10,000
Ascorbic Acid USP (Merck, fine crystals)	255.000 mg	2550.00 Gm
Microcrystalline cellulose[a]	159.375 mg	1593.75 Gm
Stearic acid	8.500 mg	85.00 Gm
Colloidal silica[b]	2.126 mg	21.25 Gm
Weight of granulation		4250.00 Gm

[a] Avicel-PH-101.
[b] Cab-O-Sil.

Blend all ingredients in a suitable blender. Compress using ⁷⁄₁₆-in. standard concave punch. 10 tablets should weigh 4.25 Gm (courtesy, FMC).

Chewable Ascorbic Acid Tablets

Ingredients	In each	In 10,000
Ascorbic Acid USP (Pfizer, fine granular)[a]	72.58 mg	725.8 Gm
Sodium Ascorbate USP (Pfizer, granular)	217.52 mg	2175.2 Gm
Orange flavor (dry)	4.20 mg	42.0 Gm
Sodium Cyclamate NF	5.40 mg	54.0 Gm
Sodium Saccharin NF	0.60 mg	6.0 Gm
Microcrystalline cellulose[b]	96.00 mg	960.0 Gm
Mannitol NF	180.00 mg	1800.0 Gm
Stearic acid	15.00 mg	150.0 Gm
Magnesium stearate	3.00 mg	30.0 Gm
FD&C Yellow #6 lake	3.00 mg	30.0 Gm
Colloidal silica[c]	2.70 mg	27.0 Gm
Weight of granulation		6000.0 Gm

[a] Includes 7% in excess of claim.
[b] Avicel-PH-101.
[c] QUSO F-22 or Cab-O-Sil.

Blend all ingredients except lubricants for 30 min in Patterson-Kelley twin-shell blender. Add the lubricants and blend for an additional 15 min. Compress using ⁷⁄₁₆-in. standard concave punch. 10 tablets should weigh 6 Gm (courtesy, FMC).

Chewable Antacid Tablets

Ingredients	In each	In 10,000
Aluminum hydroxide and Magnesium carbonate, co-dried gel[a]	325 mg	3250 Gm
Mannitol NF (granular)	675 mg	6750 Gm
Microcrystalline cellulose[b]	75 mg	750 Gm
Corn starch	30 mg	300 Gm
Calcium stearate	22 mg	220 Gm
Flavor	qs	qs

[a] Reheis F-MA-11.
[b] Avicel.

Blend all ingredients in a suitable blender. Compress using ⅝-in. flat-face bevel-edge punch (courtesy, Atlas).

Chewable Multivitamin Tablets

Ingredients	In each	In 10,000
Vitamin A USP (dry, stabilized form)	5000 USP units	50 million units
Vitamin D (dry, stabilized form)	400 USP units	4 million units
Ascorbic Acid USP	60.0 mg	600 Gm
Thiamine Hydrochloride USP	1.0 mg	10 Gm
Riboflavin USP	1.5 mg	15 Gm
Pyridoxine Hydrochloride USP	1.0 mg	10 Gm
Cyanocobalamin USP	2.0 mcg	20 mg
Calcium Pantothenate USP	3.0 mg	30 Gm
Niacinamide USP	10.0 mg	100 Gm
Mannitol NF (granular)	236.2 mg	2362 Gm
Corn starch	16.6 mg	166 Gm
Sodium Saccharin NF	1.1 mg	11 Gm
Magnesium stearate	6.6 mg	66 Gm
Talc USP	10.0 mg	100 Gm
Flavor	qs	qs

Blend all ingredients in a suitable blender. Compress using ⅜-in. flat-face bevel-edge punch (courtesy, Atlas).

CT Ferrous Sulfate

Ingredients	In each	In 7000
Ferrous Sulfate USP (crystalline)	0.325 Gm	2275 Gm
Talc		0.975 Gm
Sterotex		1.95 Gm
Weight of granulation		2277.93 Gm

Grind to 12–14-mesh, lubricate, and compress. Coat immediately to avoid oxidation to the ferric state with 0.410 gr of tolu balsam (dissolved in alcohol) and 0.060 gr of salol and chalk. Use a deep concave 11⁄32-inch. punch. 10 tablets should weigh 3.25 Gm.

CT Methenamine

Ingredients	In each, Gm	In 7000, Gm
Methenamine (12- to 14-mesh crystals)	0.325	2275
Weight of granulation		2275

Compress directly, using a ⁷⁄₁₆-in. punch. 10 tablets should weigh 3.25 Gm.

CT Phenobarbital USP, 30 mg

Ingredients	In each	In 10,000
Phenobarbital	30.59 mg	305.9 Gm
Microcrystalline cellulose[a]	30.59 mg	305.9 Gm
Spray-dried lactose	69.16 mg	691.6 Gm
Colloidal silica[b]	1.33 mg	13.3 Gm
Stearic acid	1.33 mg	13.3 Gm
Weight of granulation		1330.0 Gm

[a] Avicel-PH-101.
[b] QUSO F-22.

Screen the phenobarbital to break up lumps and blend with microcrystalline cellulose. Add spray-dried lactose and blend. Finally add the stearic acid and colloidal silica; blend to obtain homogeneous mixture. Compress using ⁹⁄₃₂-in. shallow concave punch. 10 tablets should weigh 1.33 Gm (courtesy, FMC).

Molded Tablets or Tablet Triturates (TT)

Tablet triturates are small disklike masses of molded powders weighing 30 to 250 mg (½ to 4 gr) each. The base consists of lactose, β-lactose, mannitol, dextrose, or other rapidly soluble materials. It is desirable in making tablet triturates to prepare a solid dosage form which is rapidly soluble, and as the result they are generally softer than compressed tablets.

This type of dosage form is selected for a number of drugs because of a rapidly dissolving characteristic. Nitroglycerin in many concentrations is prepared in tablet triturate form since the molded tablet rapidly dissolves when administered by placing under the tongue. Potent alkaloids and highly toxic drugs used in small doses are prepared as tablet triturates which can serve as dispensing tablets to be used as the source of the drug in compounding other formulations or solutions. Narcotics in the form of hypodermic tablets are made as tablet triturates because they rapidly dissolve in sterile water for injection prior to administration. In a study evaluating diluents for hypodermic tablets containing morphine salts, either mannitol or lactose containing sodium metabisulfite was satisfactory for maintenance of the physical stability and solubility of the tablet triturates.[134]

Tablet triturates are made by forcing a moistened blend of the drug and diluent into a mold, extruding the formed mass, which is allowed to dry. This method is essentially the same as it was when introduced by Fuller in 1878.[135] Hand molds may vary in size but the method of operation is essentially the same. Molds consist of two plates made from polystyrene plastic, hard rubber, nickel-plated brass, or stainless steel. The mold plate contains 50–500 carefully polished perforations. The other plate is fitted with a corresponding number of projecting pegs or punches which fit the perforations in the mold plate. The mold plate is placed on a flat surface, the moistened mass is forced into the perforations, and the excess is scraped from the top surface. The mold plate is placed over the plate with the corresponding pegs and lowered. As the plates come together, the pegs force the tablet triturates from the molds.

Formulation

In developing a formula it is essential that the blank weight of the mold which is to be used is known. To determine this, the weight of the diluent which exactly fills all the openings in the mold is determined by experiment. This amount of diluent is weighed and placed aside. The total amount of the drug required is determined by multiplying the number of perforations in the plate used in the previous experiment by the amount of drug desired in each tablet. The comparative bulk of this medication is now compared with that of an equal volume of diluent and that quantity of diluent is removed and weighed. The drug and the remaining diluent are mixed by trituration, and the resulting triturate is moistened and forced into the openings of the mold. If the perforations are not completely filled, more diluent is added, its weight noted, and the formula written from the results of the experiments.

It is also permissible in the development of the formula to weigh the quantity of medication needed for the number of tablets represented by the number of perforations in the mold, triturate with a weighed portion (more than ½) of the diluent, moisten the mixture, and press it into the perforations of the mold. An additional quantity of the diluent is immediately moistened and also forced into the perforations in the plate until they are completely filled. All excess diluent is removed, the trial tablets are forced from the mold, then triturated until uniform, moistened again if necessary, and remolded. When these tablets are thoroughly dried and weighed, the difference between their total weight and the weight of medication taken will indicate the amount of diluent required and accordingly supply the formula for future use for that particular tablet triturate.

For proper mixing procedures of the medication with the diluent see Chapter 86 on *Powders*, page 1626.

Preparation

The mixed powders are moistened with a proper mixture of alcohol and water, although other solvents or moistening agents such as acetone, petroleum benzin, and various combinations of these may be used in specific cases; the agent of choice depends on the solvent action which it will exert on the powder mixture. Often the moistening agent is 50% alcohol, but this concentration may be increased or decreased depending on the constituents of the formula. Care must be used in adding the solvent mixture to the powder. If too much is used, the mass will be soggy, will require a long time to dry, and the finished tablet will be hard and slowly soluble; If the mass is too wet, shrinkage will occur in the molded tablets; and finally, a condition known as creeping will be noticed. Creeping is the concentration of the medication on the surface

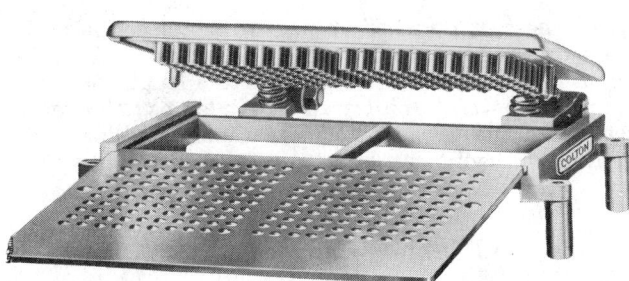

Fig. 706. Tablet triturate mold (courtesy, Colton).

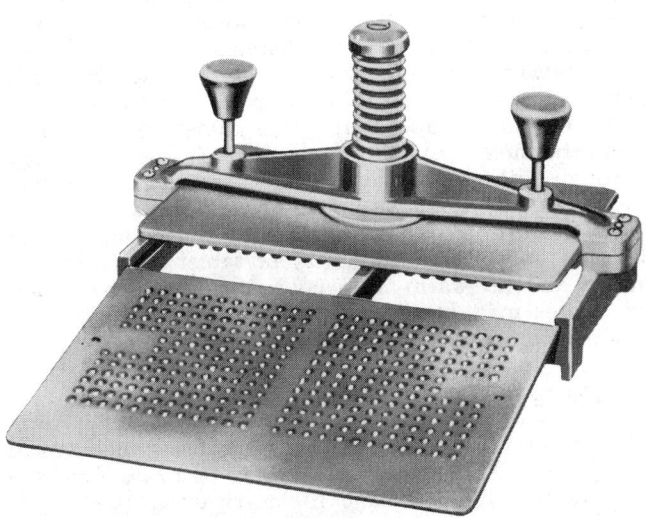

Fig. 707. Tablet triturate mold (courtesy, Colton).

of the tablet caused by capillarity and rapid evaporation of the solvent from the surface. Because molded tablets by their very nature are quite friable, an inaccurate strength in each tablet may result from creeping if powder is lost from the tablet's surface. On the other hand, if an insufficient amount of moistening agent is used, the mass will not have the proper cohesion to make a firm tablet. The correct amount of moistening agent can only be determined initially by experiment.

Hand Molding Tablet Triturates

In preparing hand-molded tablets place the mold plate on a glass plate. The properly moistened material is pressed into the perforations of the mold with a broad spatula exerting uniform pressure over each opening. The excess material is removed by passing the spatula at an oblique angle with strong hand pressure over the mold to give a clean, flat surface. The material thus removed should be placed with the remainder of the unmolded material.

The mold with the filled perforations should be reversed and moved to another clean part of the plate where the pressing operation with the spatula is repeated. It may be necessary to add more material to fill the perforations completely and uniformly. The

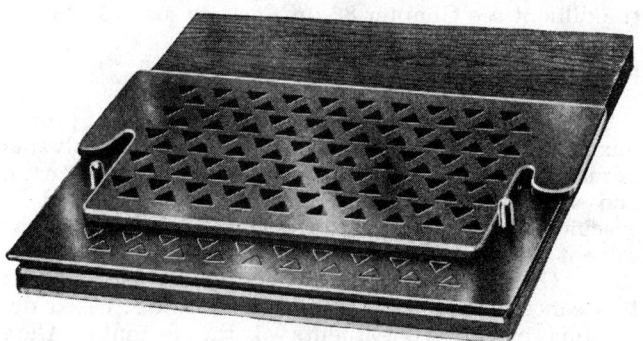

Fig. 708. Tablet triturate mold for special shapes and sizes (courtesy, Colton).

mold should be allowed to stand in a position so that part of the moistening agent will evaporate equally from both faces. While the first plate is drying, another mold can be prepared. As soon as the second mold has been completed, the first mold should be sufficiently surface dried so that the pegs will press the tablets from the mold with a minimum of sticking.

To remove the tablets from the mold, place the mold over the peg plate so that the pegs and the perforations are in juxtaposition. The tablets are released from the mold by hand pressure, which forces the pegs through the perforations. The ejected tablets are spread evenly in single layers on silk trays and dried in a clean, dust-free chamber with warm, circulating air. If only a small quantity of tablet triturates are made and no warm-air oven is available, the tablet triturates may be dried to constant weight at room temperature.

Machine Molding Tablet Triturates

Tablet triturates also can be made using mechanical equipment. The automatic tablet triturate machine illustrated in Fig. 709 makes tablet triturates at a rate of 2500/min. For machine molding, the powder mass need not be as moist as for plate molding since the time inter-

val between forming the tablet and pressing them is considerably shorter. The moistened mass passes through the funnel of the hopper to the feed plates below. In this feed plate are four holes having the same diameter as the mouth of the funnel. The material fills one hole at a time and when filled revolves to a position just over the mold plate. When in position the weighted pressure foot lowers and imprisons the powder. At the same time a spreader in the sole of the pressure foot rubs it into the mold cavities and evens it off so that the triturates are smooth on the surface and are of uniform density. When this operation is completed, the mold passes to the next position, where it registers

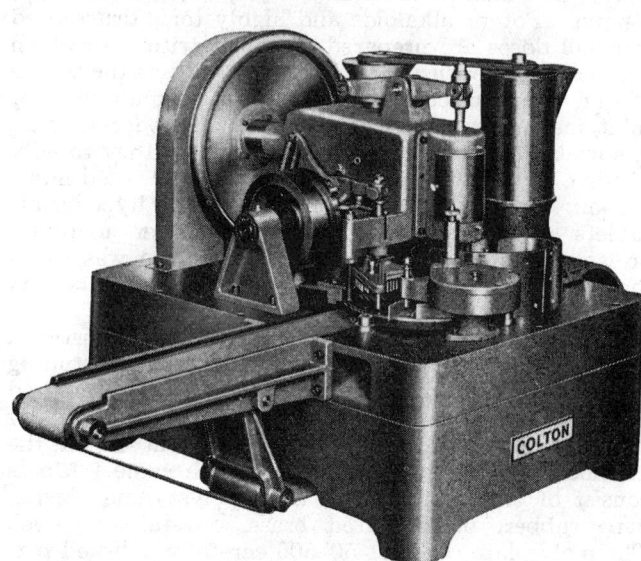

Fig. 709. Automatic tablet triturate machine (courtesy, Colton).

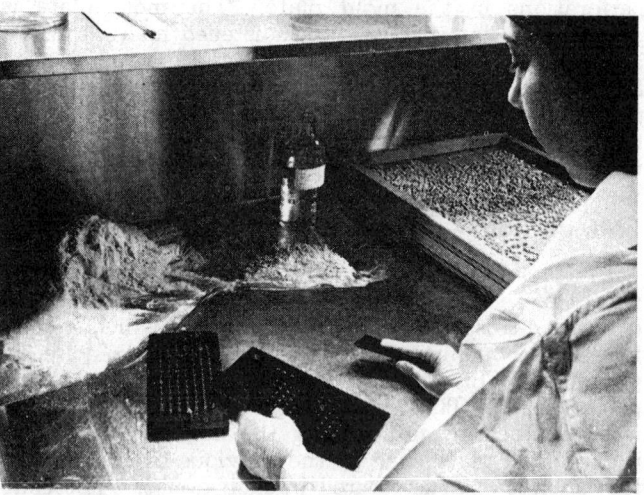

Fig. 710. Hand molding tablet triturates (courtesy, MSD).

with a nest of punches or pegs which eject the tablets from the mold plate onto a conveyor belt. The conveyor belt is sometimes extended to a length of 8 or 10 ft under a battery of infrared drying lamps to hasten the setting of the tablets for more rapid handling. This method of drying can be used only if the drug is chemically stable to these drying conditions.

Compressed Tablet Triturates

Frequently, tablet triturates are prepared on compression tablet machines using flat-face punches.

When solubility and a clear solution are required, water-soluble lubricants must be used to prevent sticking to the punches (page 1652). The granulations are prepared as directed for ordinary compressed tablets; lactose is generally used as the diluent.[136,137] Generally, tablet triturates prepared by this method are not as satisfactory as the molded type regarding their solubility and solution characteristics.

Capsules

Capsules are solid dosage forms in which the drug is enclosed in either a hard or soft, soluble container or shell of a suitable form of gelatin. The gelatin capsule was invented by Mothes, a French pharmacist in 1833. During the following year DuBlanc obtained a patent for his soft gelatin capsules. In 1848 Murdock patented the two-piece hard gelatin capsule. Although development work has been done on the preparation of capsules from methylcellulose and calcium alginate, gelatin because of its unique properties remains the primary composition material for the manufacture of capsules.

The encapsulating of medicinal agents remains a popular method for administering drugs. Capsules are tasteless, easily administered and easily filled either extemporaneously or in large quantities commercially. They permit the physician to prescribe the exact medication needed by the patient in a readily assimilable form. They are also gaining in popularity as the preferred method for administering new therapeutic agents for evaluation in initial clinical trials. The use of the capsule form eliminates the presence of numerous additives, as would be the case with tablets, which may influence the absorption of the drug and consequently the clinical response obtained. The preference of some patients for capsules has prompted pharmaceutical manufacturers to market the product in capsule form even though the product has already been produced in tablet form.

Hard Gelatin Capsules

The hard gelatin capsule, also referred to as the dry-filled capsule (DFC), consists of two sections, one slipping over the other, thus completely surrounding the drug formulation. Its shape is illustrated in Fig. 712. These capsules are filled by introducing the powdered material into the longer end or body of the capsule and then slipping on the cap. Hard gelatin capsules are made largely from gelatin, FD&C colorants, and sometimes an opacifying agent; the USP permits the gelatin for this purpose to contain 0.15% sulfur dioxide to prevent decomposition during manufacture. Gelatin capsules contain 12–16% water, but the water content can vary depending on the storage conditions. When the humidity is low, the capsules become brittle; if stored at high humidities, the capsules become flaccid and lose their shape. Storage in high temperature areas can also affect the quality of hard gelatin capsules. Gelatin capsules do not protect hygroscopic materials from atmospheric water vapor as moisture can diffuse through the gelatin wall.[138]

Both Eli Lilly & Co. and Parke, Davis & Co. have equipment for preparing empty hard gelatin capsules. With this equipment stainless steel pins, set in plates, are dipped into the gelatin solution, which must be maintained at a uniform temperature and an exact degree of fluidity. If the gelatin solution varies in viscosity, it will correspondingly decrease or increase the thickness of the capsule wall. This is important since a variation of not more than $\frac{1}{1000}$ in. is sufficient to make either a loose or a tight joint. When the pins have been withdrawn from the gelatin solution, they are thoroughly dried in kilns through which a strong blast of filtered air with controlled humidity is forced. Each capsule is stripped, trimmed to uniform length, and joined, the entire process being mechanical. A capsule-making machine installed in Lilly's capsule manufacturing plant is illustrated in Fig. 711.

Capsules are supplied in a variety of sizes. The hard, empty capsules (Fig. 712) are numbered from 000, the largest size which can be swallowed, to 5, which is the smallest. Larger sizes are available for use in veterinary medicine. In Fig. 712 the approximate capacity in grains for capsules from 000 to 5 is indicated, although this will vary because of the different densities of powdered drug materials. The No. 5 capsule in the illustration shows the base (*A*) and cap (*C*) separated.

Commercially filled capsules have the conventional oblong shape illustrated with the exception of capsule products by Eli Lilly & Co. and Smith, Kline & French. In these cases each company uses a distinctly different shaped capsule. For Lilly products, capsules are used in which the end of the base is tapered to give the capsule a bulletlike shape. Products encapsulated in this form are called *Pulvules*. The Smith, Kline &

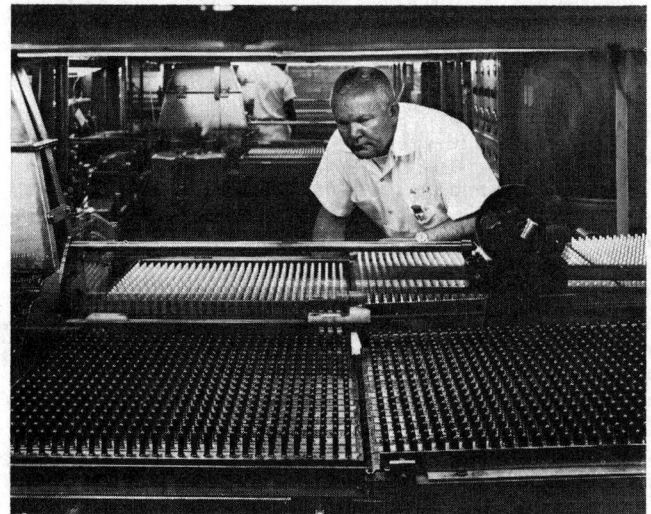

Fig. 711. Manufacture of gelatin capsules (courtesy, Lilly).

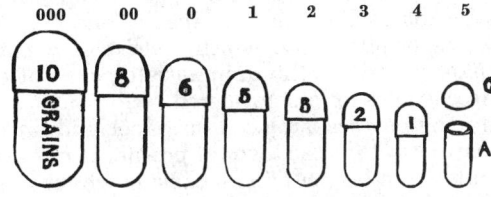

Fig. 712. Hard gelatin capsules showing relative sizes and average capacities.

French capsule appears to be different as both the ends of the cap and body are angular, rather than round.

A new type of empty gelatin capsule has become available to the pharmaceutical industry. It is called the *Snap-Fit* capsule, and it permits the joining and locking together the cap and body portions after filling. A pair of matched locking rings have been formed into the cap and body portions of the capsule. The presence of these rings provides the means by which the capsules are locked together. Prior to filling, these capsules are slightly longer than regular capsules of the same size. When the locking rings are engaged after filling, their length is equivalent to that of the conventional capsule.

It is usually necessary for the pharmacist to determine the size of the capsule needed for a given prescription through experimentation. The experienced pharmacist, having calculated the weight of material to compose a single capsule, will often select the correct size immediately. If the material is powdered, the base of the capsule is filled and the top is replaced. If the material in the capsule proves to be too heavy after weighing, a smaller size must be taken and the test repeated. If the filled capsule is light, it is possible that more can be forced into it by increasing the pressure or, if necessary, some of the material may be placed in the cap. This is not desirable as it tends to decrease the accuracy of subdivision and it is much better to select another size, the base of which will hold exactly the correct quantity. The base of an empty capsule is accurate to at least $\frac{1}{1000}$ in. and a fairly uniform pressure can be applied. In prescription filling it is wise to check the weight of each filled capsule.

In addition to the transparent, colorless, hard gelatin capsule, capsules are also available in various transparent colors such as pink, green, reddish-brown, blue, yellow, and black. If they are used, it is important to note the color as well as the capsule size on the prescription so that in the case of renewal the refilled prescription will duplicate the original. Colored capsules have been used chiefly by manufacturers to give a specialty product a distinctive appearance. Titanium dioxide is added to the gelatin to form white capsules, or to make an opaque colored capsule. In addition to color contrasts, many commercial products in capsules are given further identification by markings which may be either the company's name, a symbol on the outer shell of the capsule, or by banding. More recently, several manufacturers have marked capsules with special numbers based on a coded system to permit exact identification by the pharmacist or the physican.

Manual Filling Methods

When filling capsules on prescription, the usual procedure is to mix the ingredients by trituration, reducing them to a fine and uniform powder. The principles and methods for the uniform distribution of an active medicinal agent in a powder mixture are discussed in Chapter 86 on *Powders*, page 1626. Granular powders do not pack readily in capsules and crystalline materials, especially those which consist of a mass of filamentlike crystals as the quinine salts, are not easily fitted into capsules unless powdered.

Usually the powder is placed on paper and flattened with a spatula so that the layer of powder is not greater than about $\frac{1}{8}$ the length of the capsule which is being filled. This helps to keep both the hands and capsules clean. The cap is removed from the selected capsule

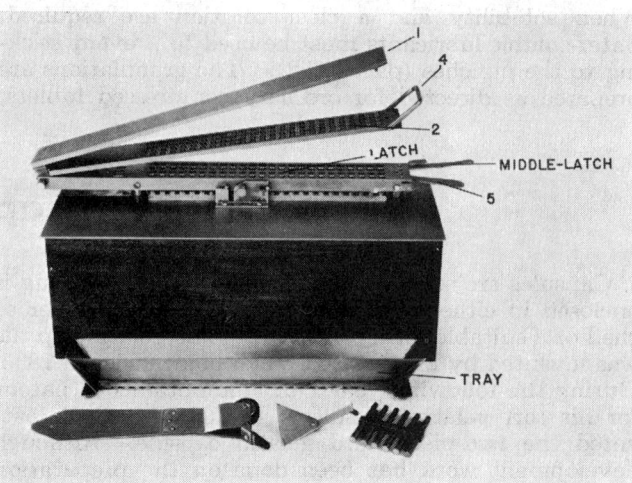

Fig. 713. Hand-operated capsule machine (courtesy, Chemi Pharm).

and held in the left hand; the body is pressed repeatedly into the powder until it is filled. The cap is replaced and the capsule is weighed. In filling the capsule the spatula is helpful in pushing the last quantity of the material into the capsule. If each capsule has not been weighed, there is likely to be an excess or a shortage of material when the specified number of capsules have been packed. This condition is adjusted before dispensing the prescription.

Machine Filling Methods

A number of manual filling machines and automatic capsule machines are available for increasing the speed of the capsule filling operation. Fig. 713 illustrates a capsule filling machine which was formerly known as the Sharp and Dohme machine. This equipment is now available through *ChemiPharm*. Many community pharmacists find this a useful piece of apparatus and some pharmaceutical manufacturers use it for small-scale production of specialty items. The machine fills 24 capsules at a time with the possible production of 2000/day. Entire capsules are placed in the machine by hand; the lower plate carries a clamp which holds the capsule bases and makes it possible to remove and replace the caps mechanically. The plate holding the capsule bases is perforated for three sizes of capsules. The powder is packed in the bases; the degree of accuracy depends on the selection of capsule size and the amount of pressure applied in packing. Other models with production capacities up to 2000 capsules/hr are available.

The hand-operated machine illustrated in Fig. 714 is known as the Cap-Fill machine and fills 36 capsules with each operation.* It also accommodates three capsule sizes. Its principle of operation is similar to that of the Sharp and Dohme machine.

Numerous other devices are used for capsule filling on a large scale; they are operated on the same principle as the manual machines, namely filling the base of the capsule. Most automatic equipment operates on the principle whereby the base of the capsule is filled and the excess is scraped off. Therefore the active ingredient is mixed with sufficient volume of a diluent, usually lactose or mannitol, which will give the desired amount of the drug in the capsule when the base is filled with the powder mixture. The manner of operation of the machine can influence the volume of the

---

*Cap-Fill Products Co.

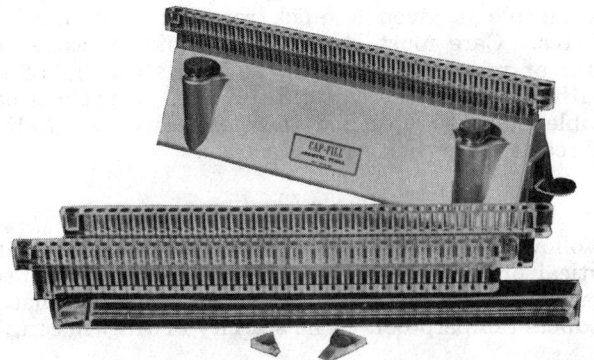

Fig. 714. Capsule filling machine made of leucite and aluminum (courtesy, Cap-Fill).

powder which will be filled into the base of the capsule; therefore, the weights of the capsules must be checked routinely as they are filled.

A semiautomatic capsule filling machine manufactured by Parke, Davis & Co. is illustrated in Figs. 715 and 716. The Type 8 capsule-filling machine performs mechanically under the same principle as the hand filling of capsules. This includes (1) separation of the cap from the body; (2) filling the body half; and (3) rejoining the cap and body halves.

Empty capsules are taken from the bottom of the capsule hopper into the magazine. The magazine gauge releases one capsule from each tube at the bottom of each stroke of the machine. Leaving the magazine, the capsules drop onto the tracks of the raceway and are pushed forward to the rectifying area with a push blade. The rectifier block descends, turning the capsules in each track, cap up, and drops them into each row of holes in the capsule holding ring assembly.

As the capsules fall into the holding ring, the cap half has a seat on the counter bore in each hole for the top ring. The body half is pulled by vacuum down into the bottom ring. When all rows in the ring assembly are full, the top ring, filled with caps only, is removed and set aside for later assembly. The body halves are now located in the bottom ring, ready for filling.

The ring holding the body halves is rotated at one of 8 speeds on the rotary table. The drug hopper is swung over the rotating ring and the auger forces drug powder into the open body cavities. When the ring has made a complete revolution and the body halves have been filled, the hopper is swung aside. The cap-holding ring is placed over the body holding ring and the assembly is ready for joining. The capsule-holding ring assembly is placed on the joiner and the joiner plate is swung down into position to hold the capsules in the ring. The peg ring pins are entered in the holes of the body holding ring and tapped in place by the air cylinder pushing the body halves back into the cap halves.

The holding ring assembly is now pushed by hand back onto the peg ring away from the joiner plate, thus pushing the capsules out of the holding ring assembly. The joined capsules then fall through the joiner chute into the capsule receiver box. The capsule receiver box screens the excess powder from the capsules and delivers them to any convenient container.

Many companies use the Type 8 capsule-filling equipment because of its ease of operation, low cost, and extreme flexibility. A Type 8 capsule filling machine will produce approximately 200,000 capsules/day. This, of course, depends upon the operator and

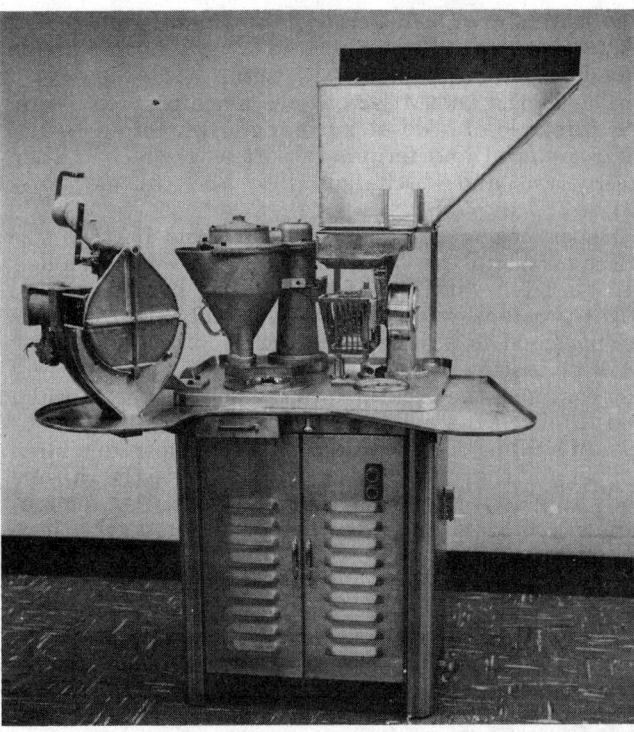

Fig. 715. Type 8 capsule-filling machine (courtesy, Parke-Davis.)

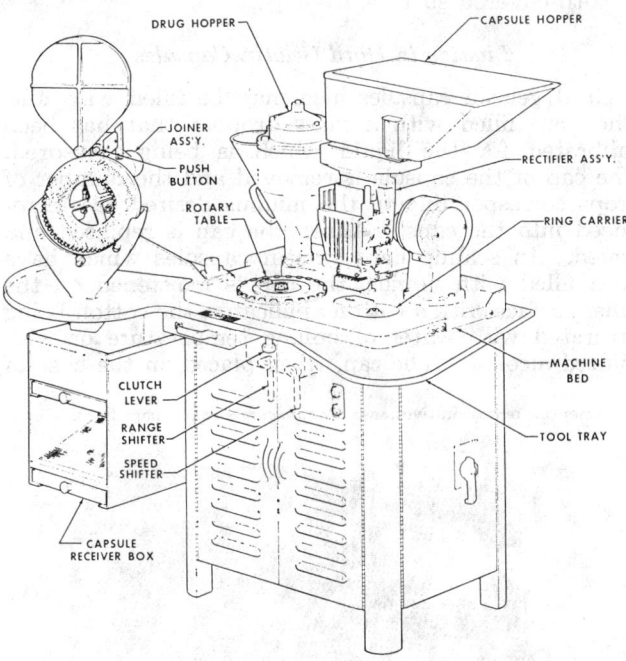

Fig. 716. Schematic of Type 8 capsule-filling machine (courtesy, Parke-Davis).

the type of material being filled. For this machine, a mathematical model has been developed that describes the effect of selected physical powder properties, as well as mechanical operating conditions on the capsule filling operation.[139] While the Type 8 capsule-filling machine has been in existence for many years, recent modifications have been made to this machine to improve the capsule-filling operations.

There are several pieces of equipment available that are classified as automatic capsule-filling machines. These are automatic in the sense that one operator can handle more than one machine. In this category are the Italian-made Zanasi (*United Shoe**) and MG-2 (*Supermatic**) models plus the West German-made Hoefliger & Karg models (*Amaco**).

The Zanasi and MG-2 capsule machines operate on the principle of a dosater coming down into a bed of drug material and forming a soft slug which is then transferred and discharged into the capsule body (Figs. 717 and 718).[140]

Depending on the flow properties and particle size of the product to be filled, the Hoefliger & Karg models can be fitted with one of three filling heads: (1) an auger-type dosing unit for powder and small particles having good flow properties; (2) compression filling units consisting of plungers which reciprocate rapidly and compress the product into the body of the capsule; and (3) disc-type units in which the filling device consists of a filling funnel which is discharged from a large hopper and the material drops directly into the capsule body to give capacity fill. The latter is used for materials as coarse grain powder or pellets. The economic justification for using automatic equipment is that one operator may be able to handle three machines and thus reduce the manhours required to produce the same number of capsules per day.

All capsules, whether they have been filled by hand or by machine, will require cleaning. Small quantities of capsules may be wiped individually with cloth. Larger quantities are rotated or shaken with crystalline sodium chloride. The capsules are then rolled on a cloth-covered surface.

Liquids in Hard Gelatin Capsules

Hard gelatin capsules also may be filled with oils. They are filled with a glass dropper that has been calibrated for the liquid which is being measured. The cap of the capsule is removed and the number of drops corresponding to the minims desired are introduced into the capsule base; the cap is replaced and sealed. In sealing hard gelatin capsules which have been filled with liquids, the cap is moistened on the inner surface with a cotton applicator, the cotton being saturated with water of boiling temperature or with diluted alcohol. The cap, when placed on the base of

---

* American representatives; see *Manufacturers Index*, page 2023.

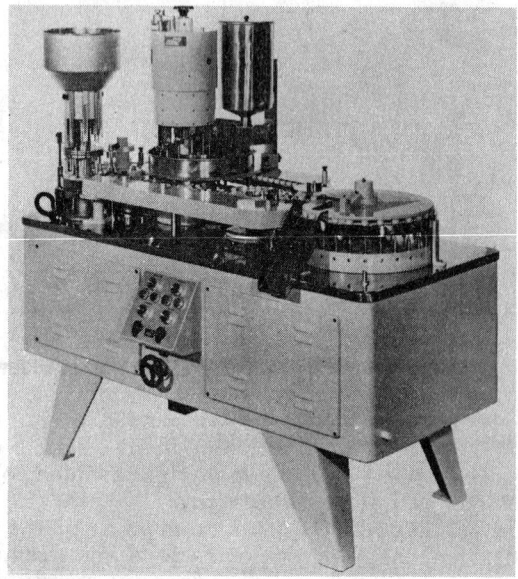

Fig. 717. MG-2, aromatic capsule-filling machine (courtesy, Supermatic).

the capsule is given a quick rotary motion until it adheres. Care must be taken to avoid an excess of water or moistening the cap beyond about ½ of its length, otherwise the cap will collapse. Gelatin is not soluble in cold water and therefore imperfect sealing will result unless hot water is used.

Capsule Banding

Following worldwide distribution of many pharmaceutical products, a problem arose which made it necessary for the manufacturer to make encapsulated products tamperproof. The scarcity of drugs in certain

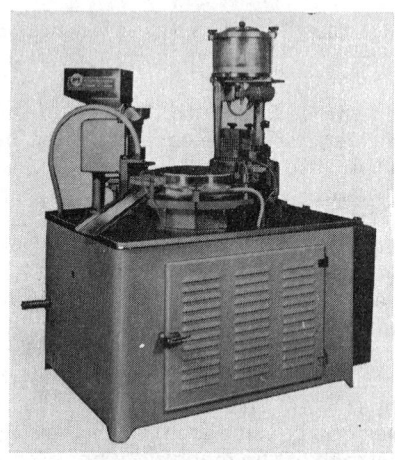

Fig. 718. Hoefliger & Karg automatic capsule-filling machine (courtesy, Amaco).

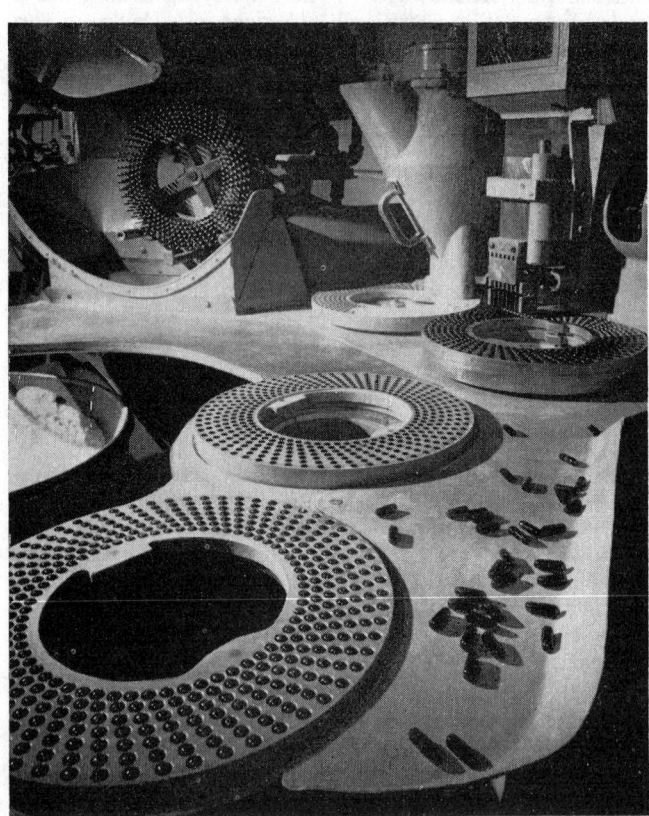

Fig. 719. Closeup of equipment for filling hard gelatin capsules. The empty gelatin capsules feed from the hopper and are pulled into the capsule ring by vacuum. The operator splits the ring which removes all the capsules in one operation. The half of the ring containing the bottom part of the capsules is placed under a filling hopper and the powdered ingredients added. The two halves of the ring are put together, then the capsules are closed by a blast of air, and removed by a series of metal pegs, upper left, corresponding to the holes in the capsule ring (courtesy, Upjohn).

foreign countries resulted in the unethical removal of the contents of capsules, refilling them with an inert material, and reselling both the refilled capsules and the material which had been removed. To prevent this, many capsules are now made tamperproof by sealing the capsule with a clear, colorless band of gelatin around the capsule joint. Opening the capsule will result in its destruction and it will not be possible to reassemble it. Colored gelatin bands around capsules have been used for many years as a trade mark by Parke, Davis & Co. for their line of capsule products, *Kapseals*.

Weight Variation

The USP provides the following requirements with respect to variation in the weight of hard capsule contents.

Weigh collectively 20 intact capsules, and calculate the average gross weight. Taking each capsule individually, balance it against weights representing 90% and 110% of the average, respectively; if each capsule weighs between 90% and 110% of the average gross weight, the sample meets the requirements.

If not all of the capsules fall within the aforementioned limits, weigh the 20 capsules collectively and individually, and remove the contents of each capsule with the aid of a small brush or pledget of cotton. Weigh the emptied shells collectively and individually, and calculate for each capsule the net weight of its contents by subtracting the weight of the shell from the respective gross weight. Determine the average net weight by subtracting the weight of the 20 emptied shells from the gross weight of the 20 capsules. Determine the difference between the net weight and the average weight; the sample meets the requirements if (1) not more than two of the differences are greater than 10% of the average and (2) in no case is the difference greater than 25%.

If more than 2 but less than 7 capsules deviate from the average between 10% and 25%, determine the net weights of an additional 40 capsules, and determine the average content of the entire 60 capsules. Determine the 60 deviations from the new average: in not more than 6 of the entire 60 capsules does the difference exceed 10% of the average, and in no case does the difference exceed 25%.

In addition to the specification for weight variation, monographs for certain capsule dosage forms may have a dissolution time specification. In these cases apparatus and procedure similar to that described in the official compendia for compressed tablets are used. Also, capsules that have been treated to resist solution in the gastric fluid meet the requirements for disintegration of enteric-coated tablets.

Soft Elastic Capsules

The soft elastic capsule (SEC) is a soft, globular, gelatin shell containing sufficient glycerin to retain permanent flexibility. As obtained commercially, these shells are hermetically sealed to prevent the walls from collapsing. The end which is to be opened for filling is elongated so that when it is cut off, sufficient gelatin is provided for the sealing. Where the suspending vehicle or solvent can be an oil, soft gelatin capsules provide a convenient and highly acceptable dosage form.

Elastic capsules are also made and filled by several commercial processes. In each of these the gelatin shell is plasticized by a polyol such as glycerin, although in finished form the capsules appear to be rather hard and firm.

Empty soft elastic capsules are made in much the same manner as hard capsules for the extemporaneous filling by the pharmacist. To fill, cut off the elongated end and insert the liquid with a glass dropper, avoiding the soiling of the edges. Finally seal the aperture with a hot gelatin solution which must possess definite characteristics to be satisfactory. If the melted tips do not supply enough sealing solution, the following formula may be used to prepare an additional quantity. Combine the following ingredients based on weight: gelatin, 10 parts; acacia, 1 part; glycerin, 10.4 parts; and water, 16.7 parts. Heat the mixture on a water bath for 12 hours, maintaining the consistency by the addition of water as required. For the commercial production of gelatin capsules, a number of processes are employed. Commercially filled soft gelatin capsules may be elliptical, oblong, or round in shape. Some sugar-coated tablets are quite similar in appearance to soft gelatin capsules. The essential differences are that the soft gelatin capsule has a seam at the point of closure of the two halves, and the contents can be liquid, paste, or powder. The sugar-coated tablet will not have a seam but will have a compressed core.

Plate Process

In this method a set of molds is used. A warm sheet of prepared gelatin is laid over the lower plate and the liquid is poured on it. A second sheet of gelatin is carefully put in place and this is followed by the top plate of the mold. The set is placed under the press where pressure is applied to form the capsules which are washed off with a volatile solvent to remove any traces of oil from the exterior. This process has been adapted and is used for encapsulation by the Upjohn Co.[141] The sheets of gelatin may have the same color or different colors.

Rotary Die Process

In 1933 the rotary die process for elastic capsules was perfected by Robert P. Scherer.[142] This process made it possible to improve the standards of accuracy and uniformity of elastic gelatin capsules and globules.

The rotary die machine is a self-contained unit capable of continuously and automatically producing finished capsules from a supply of gelatin mass and filling material which may be any liquid, semiliquids, or paste that won't dissolve gelatin. Two continuous gelatin ribbons, which the machine forms, are brought into convergence between a pair of revolving dies and an injection wedge. Accurate filling under pressure and sealing of the capsule wall occur as dual and coincident operations; each is delicately timed against the other. Sealing also severs the completed capsule from the net. The principle of operation is shown in Fig. 721. See also Fig. 720.

By this process the content of each capsule is measured individually by a single stroke of a pump so accurately constructed that plunger travel of 0.025 in. will deliver 1 ɱ (apoth). The Scherer machine contains banks of pumps so arranged that many capsules may be formed and filled simultaneously. All pumps are engineered to extremely small mechanical tolerances and to an extremely high degree of precision and similarity. All operations are controlled on a weight basis by actual periodic checks with a group of analytical balances. Individual net-fill weights of capsules resulting from large-scale production vary no more than ±1 to 3% from theory depending upon the materials used.

The rotary die process makes it possible to encapsulate heavy materials such as ointments and pastes. In this manner solids can be milled with a vehicle and filled into capsules. Where it is desirable to have a high degree of accuracy and a hermetically sealed product, this form of enclosure is ideally suited.

The modern and well-equipped capsule plant is

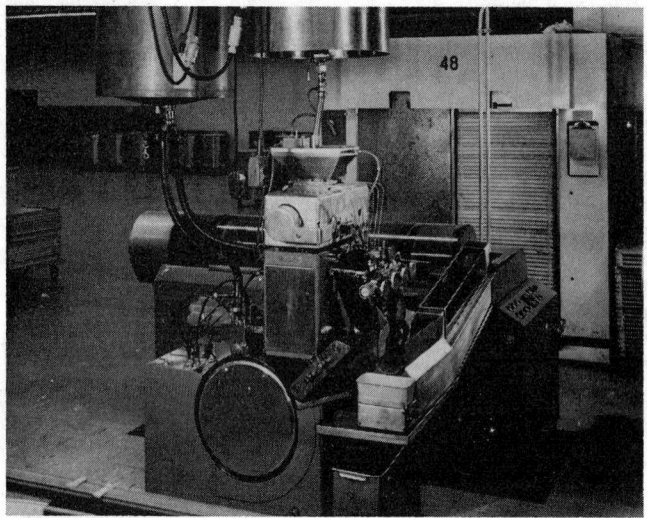

Fig. 720.   Scherer soft elastic capsule machine (courtesy, Scherer).

completely air conditioned, a practical necessity for fine capsule production. Its facilities and operations include the availability of carbon dioxide at every exposed point of operation for the protection of oxidizable substances before encapsulation. Special ingredients also have been used in the capsule shell to exclude light wavelengths which are destructive to certain drugs.

Norton Capsule Machine

This machine produces capsules completely automatically by leading two films of gelatin between a set of vertical dies. These dies as they close, open, and close, are in effect a continual vertical plate forming row after row of pockets across the gelatin film. These are filled with medicament and, as they progress through the dies, are sealed, shaped, and cut out of the film as capsules which drop into a cooled solvent bath.

Accogel Capsule Machine

The most recent and major advance in pharmaceutical capsule manufacture was made in 1948 when the Accogel machine and process were developed in the

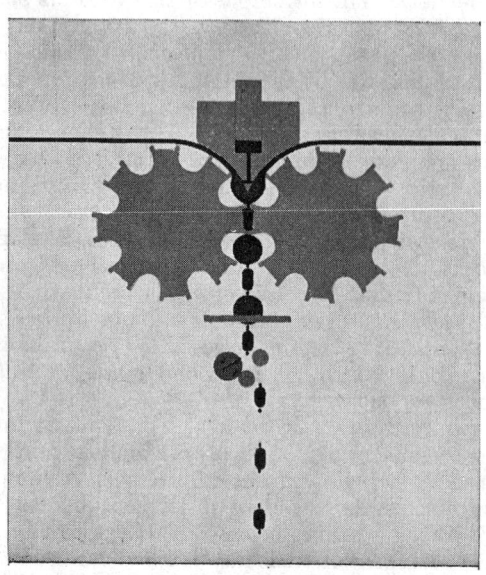

Fig. 721.   Rotary die elastic capsule filler.

Lederle Laboratories Div. of the American Cyanamid Co. The Accogel, or Stern machine, uses a system of rotary dies but is unique in that it is the only machine that can successfully fill dry powder into a soft gelatin capsule (Fig. 722). The machine is available to the entire pharmaceutical industry by a lease arrangement and is used in many countries of the world. The machine is extremely versatile, not only producing capsules with dry powder but also encapsulating liquids and combinations of liquids and powders. By means of an attachment, slugs or compressed tablets may be enclosed in a gelatin film. The capsules can be made in a variety of colors, shapes, and sizes.

Weight Variation

The USP provides the following requirements with respect to variation in the weight of soft capsule contents.

Weigh collectively 20 intact capsules, and calculate the average gross weight. Taking each capsule individually, balance it against weights representing 90% and 110% of the average, respectively; if each capsule weighs between 90% and 110% of the average gross weight, the sample meets the requirements.

For soft gelatin capsules that do not meet the requirements of the test for gross capsule weight, determine the net weight of the contents of individual capsules as follows: Weigh the intact capsules individually to obtain their gross weights, taking care to preserve the identity of each capsule. Then cut open the capsules by means of a suitable clean, dry cutting instrument such as scissors or a sharp open blade, and remove the contents by washing in a suitable solvent. Allow the occluded solvent to evaporate from the shells at room temperature over a period of about 30 minutes, taking precautions to avoid uptake or loss of moisture. Weigh the individual shells, and calculate the net weight of the contents.

Microencapsulation

As a technology, microencapsulation is placed in the section on capsules only because of the relationship in terminology to mechanical encapsulation described above. The topic could also have been included in a discussion of coating procedures. Essentially, microencapsulation is a process or technique by which thin coatings can be applied reproducibly to small particles of solids, droplets of liquids, or dispersions, thus forming microcapsules. It can be differentiated readily from other coating methods in the size of the particles involved; these range from several tenths of a micron to 5000 μ in size.[143]

A number of microencapsulation processes have been disclosed in the literature. Some are based on chemical processes and involve a chemical or phase change; others are mechanical and require special equipment to produce the physical change in the systems required. Many of the systems available have been summarized and described by Herbig.[144]

Among the processes applied to pharmaceutical problems is that developed by the National Cash Register Co. (NCR). The NCR process is a chemical operation based on phase separation or coacervation techniques. In colloidal chemistry coacervation refers to the separation of a liquid precipitate, or phase, when solutions of two hydrophobic colloids are mixed under suitable conditions.

The NCR process utilizing phase separation or coacervation techniques consists of three steps: (1) formation of three immiscible phases, a liquid manufacturing phase, a core material phase, and a coating material phase; (2) deposition of the liquid polymer coating on the core material; and (3) rigidizing the coating, usually by thermal, cross-linking or desolvation techniques, to form a microcapsule.

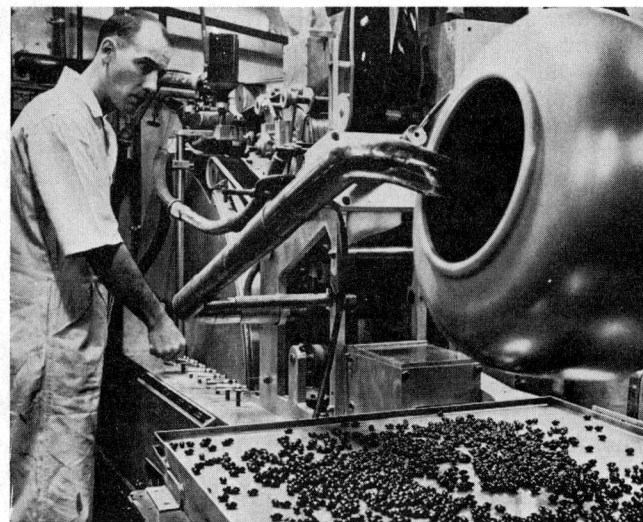

Fig. 722. Stern encapsulating machine for making dry-filled powder capsules, Lederle).

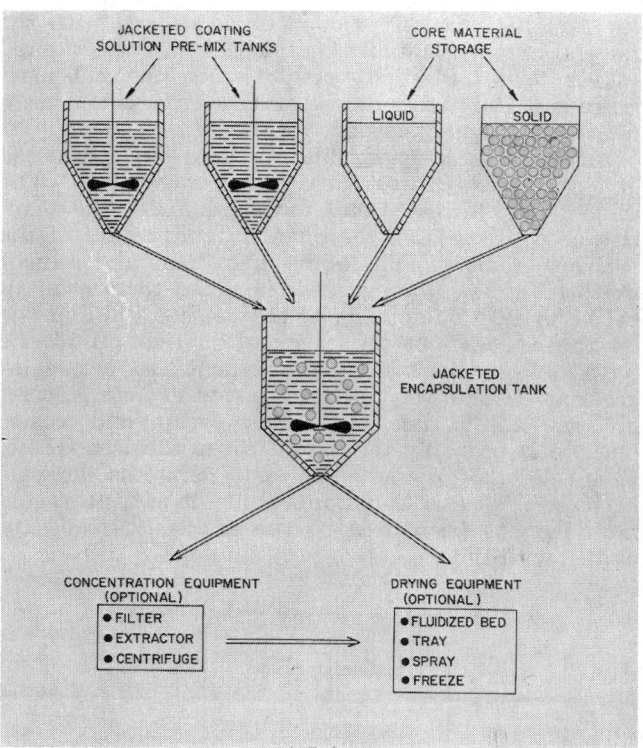

Fig. 723. Production installation for microencapsulation process (courtesy, NCR).

In Step 2, the deposition of the liquid polymer around the core material occurs only if the polymer is absorbed at the interface formed between the core material and the liquid vehicle phase. In many cases physical or chemical changes in the coating polymer solution can be induced so that phase separation (coacervation) of the polymer will occur. Droplets of concentrated polymer solution will form and coalesce to yield a two-phase liquid–liquid system. In cases where the coating material is an immiscible polymer or insoluble liquid polymer, it may be added directly. Also monomers can be dissolved in the liquid vehicle phase and be subsequently polymerized at the interface.[145]

Equipment required for microencapsulation by this method is relatively simple; it consists mainly of jacketed tanks with variable speed agitators. Fig. 723 shows a typical flow diagram of a production installation.

A number of coating materials have been used successfully; examples of these include gelatin, polyvinyl alcohol, ethylcellulose, cellulose acetate phthalate, and styrene maleic anhydride. The film thickness can be varied considerably depending on the surface area of

the material to be coated and other physical characteristics of the system. The microcapsules may consist of a single particle or clusters of particles. After isolation from the liquid manufacturing vehicle and dried, the material appears as a free-flowing powder. The powder is suitable for formulation as compressed tablets, hard gelatin capsules, suspensions, and other dosage forms.

The process provides answers for problems such as masking the taste of bitter drugs, a means of formulating prolonged action dosage forms, a means of separating incompatible materials, a method of protecting chemicals against moisture or oxidation, and a means of modifying a material's physical characteristics for ease of handling in formulation and manufacture.[146]

Pills

Pills are small, round solid dosage forms containing a medicinal agent and are intended for oral administration. Pills were formerly the most extensively used oral dosage form, but they have been largely replaced by compressed tablets and capsules. Substances which are bitter or unpleasant to the taste, if not corrosive or deliquescent, can be administered in this form if the dose is not too large.

Formerly pills were made extemporaneously by the community pharmacist whose skill at pill making became an art. However, pills which are now used in pharmacy are prepared on a large scale with mechanical equipment. The pill formulas of the NF were largely introduced for the purpose of establishing standards of strength for the well-known and currently used pills. Hexylresorcinol Pills NF consist of hexylresorcinol crystals covered with a rupture-resistant coating

that is dispersible in the digestive tract. It should be noted that the official hexylresorcinol pills are prepared by a patented process, the gelatin coating being sufficiently tough that it can not be readily broken, even when chewed. Therefore the general method for the preparation of pills given below does not apply to hexylresorcinol pills.

Preparation of Mass

In preparing pills the first step consists of making the pill mass. The ingredients in the pill mass include the active drug, the diluent or filler, and the excipient. The selection of the diluent and excipient is important in that they give the essential characteristics of adhesiveness, firmness, and plasticity to the mass. The mass must be sufficiently adhesive and firm to retain its shape, yet be soft enough to be worked with the fingers, or with suitable equipment, into the desired pilular form. Plasticity results when the pill mass possessing the proper degree of adhesiveness and firmness is thoroughly kneaded.

Among the common diluents used are powdered glycyrrhiza, starch, hard soap, and tragacanth. The diluent gives increased bulk to the pill mass; the quantity used depends on the quantity and nature of the active ingredient. The active ingredient and diluent are blended and the excipient is added to form a cohesive mass. The quality of the finished pill depends on the selection of the excipient in relation to the physical characteristics of the diluent and active ingredient. Commonly used excipients include glucose, glycerin, acacia mucilage, simple syrup, and water. Glucose is probably the closest to an ideal excipient. It is colorless, very adhesive, and maintains the pills in a soft, plastic condition. Pills in which acacia mucilage has been used as the excipient frequently harden with time.

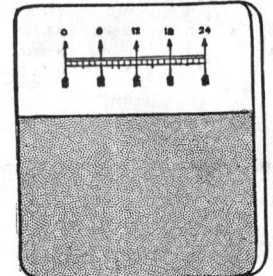

Fig. 724. Pill tile.

The ingredients of the pill mass must be thoroughly kneaded; for small quantities a mortar and pestle may be used. The ingredients are well blended with the operator using as much weight on the pestle as he can exert. The excipient is added as needed to give the proper degree of plasticity. On a large scale, mechanical equipment is used to give the same degree of thorough kneading.

Formerly pill masses represented an official class of preparations under the Latin name of *Massa*. The pill masses were given official recognition because they were kept in bulk by pharmacists for the extemporaneous preparation of pills.

Rolling the Pills

The pill mass is placed on a glass pill tile and rolled into a cylinder or pipe with a smooth flat board. When the pill pipe has been rolled to the proper length, it is placed over the scale on the pill tile. The place to cut each pill is indicated with a spatula, making only a slight depression in the mass. When the pills have been marked, the pill pipe is cut into the desired number of pills. The pieces of mass are rolled into globular form between the fingers. After the pills have been rolled into the desired form with the fingers, they may be further smoothed using a flat board.

To prevent the pill cylinder from sticking to the tile

or board, an absorbent powder is dusted on the surface. This may be rice flour, powdered magnesium carbonate, lycopodium, powdered althaea, powdered glycyrrhiza, or starch.

When pills were a popular dosage form, there were a number of manual pill machines available to make larger quantities of pills more quickly. They were devised to cut the pill pipe into equal sections and subsequently to roll the segments into perfectly round pills. Manual pill machines can be seen in many pharmaceutical museums.

Pill-Making Machines

Most pills manufactured today are made on equipment similar to the machines illustrated in Fig. 725. The machine on the left makes the mass homogeneous and passes the kneaded mass in the shape of balls to the machine on the right, known as the automata. The automata works the mass into a pill cylinder and divides the piping into pieces of uniform size and weight.

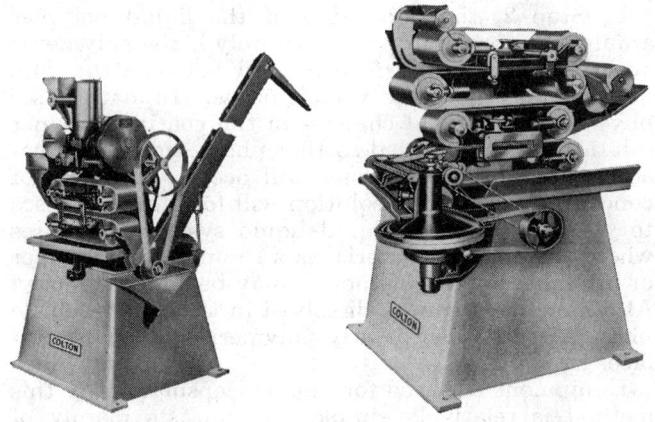

Fig. 725. Automatic pill machine (courtesy, Colton).

By the time the pieces leave the machine they have been rolled into perfect spheres. The automatic pill machine can produce 2-gr pills at the rate of 100,000/hr.

Another method for the preparation of pills which has been proposed but not used extensively is the drop method.[147] In Scandinavian countries it has been used for the preparation of vitamin A and D pills. In this method the active ingredients are dissolved or emulsified in material having a suitable congealing point. In the molten or liquefied state they are added as drops to a liquid in which they are insoluble and which has a specific gravity lower than the formed drops. The drops fall slowly through the liquid assuming a round spherical shape due to the surface tension of the melt, and the drops are congealed due to the temperature of the liquid at the end of their passage. Formerly the method was limited to fatty materials but has been applied recently to water-soluble or dispersible materials.[148] Uniform and exact dosage is the chief advantage claimed for the method.

Therapeutic agents are also being compressed in spherical form on tablet machines and when coated, these tablets resemble pills (page 1653).

Other Solid Dosage Forms

Troches

These forms of oral medication, also known as *lozenges* or *pastilles*, are discoid-shaped solids containing the medicinal agent in a suitably flavored base. The base may be a hard sugar candy, glycerinated glycerin, or the combination of sugar with sufficient mucilage to give it form. Troches are placed in the mouth where they slowly dissolve, liberating the active ingredient. The drug involved can be an antiseptic, local anesthetic, antibiotic, antihistaminic, antitussive, analgesic, or a decongestant.[149]

Formerly troches were prepared extemporaneously by the pharmacist. The mass is formed by adding water slowly to a mixture of the powdered drug, powdered sugar, and a gum until a pliable mass is formed. Powdered acacia in 7% concentration gives sufficient adhesiveness to the mass. The mass is rolled out and the troche pieces cut out using a cutter, or else the mass is rolled into a cylinder and divided. Each piece is shaped and allowed to dry before dispensing.

If the active ingredient is heat stable, it may be prepared in a hard candy base. Syrup is concentrated to the point where it becomes a pliable mass, the active ingredient is added, and the mixture is kneaded while warm to form a homogeneous mass. The mass is gradually worked into a pipe form having the diameter desired for the candy piece and the lozenges cut from the pipe and allowed to cool. This is an entirely mechanical operation with equipment designed for this purpose.

If the active ingredient is heat labile, it may be made into a lozenge preparation by compression. The granulation is prepared in a manner similar to that used for any compressed tablet. The lozenge is made using heavy compression equipment to give a tablet which is harder than usual as it is desirable for the troche to dissolve or disintegrate slowly in the mouth. In the formulation of the lozenge the ingredients are chosen which will promote its slow-dissolving characteristics. Compression is gaining in popularity as a means of making troches and candy pieces because of the increased speeds of compression equipment. In cases where holes are to be placed in troches or candy pieces, core rod tooling is used. Core rod tooling includes a rod centered on the lower punch around which the troche is compressed in the die cavity. The upper punch has an opening in its center for the core rod to enter during compression. It is evident that maximum accuracy is needed to provide alignment as the narrow punches are inserted into the die.

Cachets

Related to capsules, inasmuch as they provide an edible container for the oral administration of solid drugs, cachets were formerly used in pharmacy. They varied in size from $3/4$ to $1/8$ in. in diameter and consisted of two concave pieces of wafer made of flour and water. After one section was filled with the prescribed quantity of the medicinal agent, they were tightly sealed by moistening the margins and pressing firmly together. When moistened with water, their character was entirely changed; they became soft, elastic, and slippery. Hence, they could easily be swallowed by floating them on water.

Pellets

The term pellet is now applied to small, sterile cylinders about 3.2 mm in diameter by 8 mm in length, which are formed by compression from medicated masses. Whenever prolonged and continuous absorption of testosterone, estradiol, or desoxycorticosterone is desired, pellets of these potent hormones may be used by implantation (page 1918).

References

1. Hamarneh, S. K., *J. APhA, Pract. Ed.*, **21**, 90 (1960).
2. Brockedon, W., Brit. Pat. 9977 (Nov. 8, 1843).
3. Wood, J. R., *Tablet Manufacture*, Lippincott, Philadelphia, 1906, p. 11.
4. Anon., *Chemist Druggist*, **25**, 519, 567 (1883).
5. Foote, P. A., *Bull. Univ. Wisconsin* (Dec., 1928).
6. Evans, A. J., and Train, D., *A Bibliography of the Tabletting of Medicinal Substances*, The Pharmaceutical Press, London, 1963.
7. Evans, A. J., *A Bibliography of the Tabletting of Medicinal Substances*, 1st Suppl., The Pharmaceutical Press, London, 1964.
8. Lachman, L., *et al.*, *Industrial Pharmacy*, Lea & Febiger, Philadelphia, 1970.
9. Mitchell, K. A., *Mfg. Chemist*, **26**, 107 (1955).
10. Robinson, C. W., *Mfg. Chemist*, **26**, 164 (1955).
11. Levy, G., *J. Pharm. Sci.*, **52**, 1039 (1963).
12. Levy, G., *et al*, *J. Pharm. Sci.*, **52**, 1047 (1963).
13. Levy, G., and Gumtow, R. H., *J. Pharm. Sci.*, **52**, 1139 (1963).
14. Daoust, R. G., and Lynch, M. J., *Drug Cosmetic Ind.*, **93**, 26 (1963).
15. Boger, W. P., and Gavin, J. J., *New Eng. J. Med.*, **261**, 827 (1959).
16. Costello, R., and Mattocks, A., *J. Pharm. Sci.*, **51**, 106 (1962).
17. Duvall, R. N., *et al*, *J. Pharm. Sci.*, **54**, 607 (1965).
18. Nelson, E., *et al*, *J. APhA, Sci. Ed.*, **46**, 257 (1957).
19. Donaghy, L. S., *Drug Cosmetic Ind.*, **83**, 304 (1958).
20. Griffen, J. C., and Huyck, C. L., *J. APhA, Sci. Ed.*, **44**, 251 (1955).
21. Lehrman, G. P., and Skauen, D. M., *Drug Std.*, **26**, 120 (1958).
22. Patel, R. P., and Rana, A. S., *Indian J. Pharm.*, **19**, 4 (1957).
23. Nazareth, M. R., *et al*, *J. Pharm. Sci.*, **50**, 564 (1961).
24. Joshi, S. B., *et al*, *Pharmaceutist*, **10**, 12 (1964).
25. Patel, R. P., and Shah, A. B., *Ind. J. Pharm.*, **27**, 76 (1965).
26. Patel, R. P., and Alex, R. M., *Pharmaceutist*, **12**, 13 (1966).
27. Miller, B., and Chavkin, L., *J. APhA, Sci. Ed.*, **43**, 486 (1954).
28. Chavkin, L., *Drug Cosmetic Ind.*, **75**, 466 (1954).
29. Reier, G. E., *Dissertation Abstr.*, **25**, 2933 (1964).
30. Kwan, K. C., and Milosovich, G., *J. Pharm. Sci.*, **55**, 340 (1966).
31. Prescott, F., *Drug Cosmetic Ind.*, **97**, 497 (1965).
32. Munzel, K., First Industrial Symposium, Univ. of Wisconsin, Land O'Lakes, Wis., June, 1959.
33. Appino, J. B., *et al*, *Drug Std.*, **27**, 193 (1959).
34. Gold, G., and Campbell, J., *J. Pharm. Sci.*, **53**, 52 (1964).
35. Kornblum, S. S., and Zoglio, M. A., *J. Pharm. Sci.*, **56**, 1569 (1967).
36. Sperandio, G. J., and DeKay, H. G., *J. APhA, Pract. Ed.*, **10**, 572 (1949).
37. Sperandio, G. J., and DeKay, H. G., *J. APhA, Sci. Ed.*, **41**, 245 (1952).
38. Israsena, N., and Chavkin, L., *The Composition and Manufacture of Compressed Soluble Tablets*, Thesis, Columbia Univ., College of Pharmacy, May, 1957.
39. Strickland, W. A., *Drug Cosmetic Ind.*, **85**, 318 (1959).
40. Higuchi, T., *et al*, *J. APhA, Sci. Ed.*, **42**, 194 (1952).
41. Nelson, E., *et al*, *J. APhA, Sci. Ed.*, **43**, 596 (1954).
42. Strickland, W. A., Jr., *et al*, *J. APhA, Sci. Ed.*, **45**, 51 (1956).
43. Strickland, W. A., Jr., *et al*, *J. APhA, Sci. Ed.*, **49**, 35 (1960).
44. Feinstein, W., and Bartilucci, A. J., *J. Pharm. Sci.*, **55**, 332 (1966).
45. Patel, N. R., and Hopponen, R. E., *J. Pharm. Sci.*, **55**, 1065 (1966).
46. Curlin, L. C., *J. APhA, Sci. Ed.*, **44**, 16 (1955).
47. Commons, K. C., *et al*, *J. Pharm. Sci.*, **57**, 1253 (1968).
48. Gross, H. M., and Becker, C. H., *J. APhA, Sci. Ed.*, **41**, 187 (1952).
49. Firouzabadian, A., and Huyck, C. L., *J. APhA, Sci. Ed.*, **43**, 248 (1954).
50. Granberg, C. B., and Benton, B. E., *J. APhA, Sci. Ed.*, **48**, 648 (1949).
51. Fakouhi, T. A., *et al*, *J. Pharm. Sci.*, **52**, 700 (1963).
52. Bequette, R. J., and Huyck, C. L., *Drug Cosmetic Ind.*, **81**, 166 (1957).
53. Crisafi, R. C., and Becker, C. H., *J. APhA, Sci. Ed.*, **47**, 363 (1958).
54. Webster, A. R., to Genatosan, Ltd., Brit. Pat. 791,281 (Feb. 26, 1958).
55. Van Abbe, N. J., and Rees, J. T., *J. APhA, Sci. Ed.*, **47**, 487 (1958).
56. Gerding, T. G., and DeKay, H. G., *Drug Std.*, **23**, 132 (1955).
57. Eatherton, L. E., *et al*, *Drug Std.*, **23**, 42 (1955).
58. Kavarana, H., and Burlage, H. M., *Am. Profess. Pharmacist*, **21**, 346 (1955).
59. Kennon, L., and Swintosky, J. V., *J. APhA, Sci. Ed.*, **47**, 396 (1958).
60. Cooper, B. F., and Brecht, J. T., *J. APhA, Sci. Ed.*, **46**, 520 (1957).
61. Ward, J. B., and Trachtenberg, A., *Drug Cosmetic Ind.*, **91**, 35 (1962).
62. Ingram, J. T., and Lowenthal, W., *J. Pharm. Sci.*, **57**, 187 (1968).
63. Silver, J. A., and Clarkson, R., *Manufacture of Compressed Tablets*, F. J. Stokes Machine Co., Philadelphia, 1947, p. 23.
64. Nair, A. D., and Bhatia, V. N., *J. APhA, Sci. Ed.*, **46**, 131 (1957).
65. Wai, K., *Dissertation Abstr.*, **25**, 6550 (1965).
66. Kwan, K. C., *et al*, *J. APhA, Sci. Ed.*, **46**, 236 (1957).
67. Holstius, E. A., and DeKay, H. G., *J. APhA, Sci. Ed.*, **41**, 505 (1952).
68. Hefferren, J. J., *J. Am. Med. Assoc.*, **182**, 1145 (1962).

69. Swartz, C. J., and Cooper, J., *J. Pharm. Sci.*, **51**, 89 (1962).
70. Urbanyi, T., *et al*, *J. APhA, Sci. Ed.*, **49**, 163 (1960).
71. Lachman, L., *et al*, *J. APhA, Sci. Ed.*, **49**, 165 (1960).
72. Lachman, L., *et al*, *J. Pharm. Sci.*, **50**, 141 (1961).
73. Everhard, M. E., and Goodhart, F. W., *J. Pharm. Sci.*, **52**, 281 (1963).
74. Swartz, C. J., *et al*, *J. Pharm. Sci.*, **51**, 326 (1962).
75. Swartz, C. J., *et al*, *J. Pharm. Sci.*, **50**, 145 (1961).
76. Lachman, L., *et al*, *J. Pharm. Sci.*, **51**, 321 (1962).
77. Raff, A. M., *J. Pharm. Sci.*, **53**, 380 (1964).
78. Goodhart, F. W., *et al*, *J. Pharm. Sci.*, **56**, 63 (1967).
79. Zografi, G., and Mattocks, A. M., *J. Pharm. Sci.*, **52**, 1103 (1963).
80. Jaffe, J., and Lippmann, I., *J. Pharm. Sci.*, **53**, 441 (1964).
81. Endicott, C. J., and Gross, H. M., *Drug Cosmetic Ind.*, **85**, 175 (1959).
82. Smith, F. D., and Grosch, L., US Pat. 2,041,869 (May 29, 1936).
83. Albrecht, R., US Pat. 2,645,936 (July 21, 1953).
84. McCallum, A., *et al*, *J. APhA, Sci. Ed.*, **44**, 83 (1955).
85. Endicott, C. J., *et al*, *J. Pharm. Sci.*, **50**, 343 (1961).
86. Michel, F., US Pat. 2,975,630 (Mar. 21, 1961).
87. Fairchild, H. J., and Michel, F., *J. Pharm. Sci.*, **50**, 966 (1961).
88. Shafer, E. G. E., *et al*, *J. APhA, Sci. Ed.*, **40**, 114 (1956).
89. Levy, G., *J. Pharm. Sci.*, **50**, 388 (1961).
90. Clarkson, R., *Drug Cosmetic Ind.*, **66**, 270 (1950).
91. Snyder, H. T., *et al*, APhA Convention, Ind. Pharm. Sect., Dallas, Tex., Apr., 1966.
92. McAteer, P. J., APhA Convention, Ind. Pharm. Sec., Las Vegas, Nev., March, 1962.
93. Scott, M. W., *et al*, *J. Pharm. Sci.*, **52**, 284 (1963).
94. Patel, B. N., *et al*, *J. APhA, Sci. Ed.*, **38**, 247 (1949).
95. Patel, B. N., *et al*, *J. APhA, Sci. Ed.*, **38**, 250 (1949).
96. Patel, B. N., *et al*, *J. APhA, Sci. Ed.*, **38**, 245 (1949).
97. Cooper, J., *et al*, *J. Pharm. Sci.*, **50**, 67 (1961).
98. Scott, M. W., *et al*, *J. Pharm. Sci.*, **52**, 994 (1963).
99. Forlano, A. J., and Chavkin, L., *J. APhA, Sci. Ed.*, **49**, 67 (1960).
100. Higuchi, T., *et al*, *J. APhA, Sci. Ed.*, **42**, 194 (1953).
101. Tucker, S. J., and Hays, H. M., *J. APhA, Sci. Ed.*, **48**, 362 (1959).
102. Wurster, D. E., *J. APhA, Sci. Ed.*, **48**, 451 (1959).
103. Wurster, D. E., National Pharmaceutical Research Conference, Land O'Lakes, Wis., June, 1959.
104. Wurster, D. E., *J. APhA, Sci. Ed.*, **49**, 82 (1960).
105. Scott, M. W., *et al*, *J. Pharm. Sci.*, **53**, 314 (1964).
106. Rankell, A. S., *et al*, *J. Pharm. Sci.*, **53**, 320 (1964).
107. Tuerck, P. A., *et al*, *J. APhA, Sci. Ed.*, **49**, 344 (1960).
108. Tuerck, P. A., *et al*, *J. APhA, Sci. Ed.*, **49**, 347 (1960).
109. Lachman, L., and Sreydan, W. L., Jr., US Pat. 2,877,159 (Mar. 10, 1959).
110. Cooper, J., *et al*, US Pat. 2,857,313 (Oct. 21, 1958).
111. Kovac, G. M., *Drug Cosmetic Ind.*, **91**, 171 (1962).
112. Kovac, G. M., *Drug Cosmetic Ind.*, **91**, 297 (1962).
113. Milosovich, G., *Drug Cosmetic Ind.*, **92**, 557 (1963).
114. Gunsel, W. C., and Lachman, L., *J. Pharm. Sci.*, **52**, 178 (1963).
115. Batuyios, N., *J. Pharm. Sci.*, **55**, 727 (1966).
116. Cohn, R., *et al*, APhA Convention, Ind. Pharm. Sect., Dallas, Tex., Apr., 1966.
117. Brownley, C., and Lachman, L., *J. Pharm. Sci.*, **53**, 452 (1964).
118. Duval, R. N., *et al*, *J. Pharm. Sci.*, **54**, 1196 (1965).
119. Fox, C. D., *et al*, R., *Drug Cosmetic Ind.*, **92**, 161 (1963).
120. Gold, G., *et al*, *J. Pharm. Sci.*, **57**, 667 (1968).
121. Gold, G., *et al*, *J. Pharm. Sci.*, **57**, 2153 (1968).
122. Stalbaum, R. H., *Drug Cosmetic Ind.*, **100**, 47 (Feb., 1967).
123. Newton, J. M., *Mfg. Chemist*, **37**, 33 (1966).
124. Morris, R. M., *Dissertation Abstr.*, **26**, 3880 (1966).
125. Raff, A. M., *et al*, *J. Pharm. Sci.*, **50**, 76 (1961).
126. Anon., *Mfg. Chemist*, **33**, 137 (1962).
127. Anon., *Drug Cosmetic Ind.*, **102**, 86 (Feb., 1968).
128. Kanig, J. L., *J. Pharm. Sci.*, **53**, 188 (1964).
129. Chafetz, L., and Hodges, J. R., *Am. J. Hosp. Pharm.*, **22**, 382 (1965).
130. Swartz, C. J., *et al*, *J. Pharm. Sci.*, **51**, 1181 (1962).
131. Mathison, H. R., *Drug Cosmetic Ind.*, **99**, 52 (Sept., 1966).
132. Raff, A. M., *et al*, *J. APhA, Sci. Ed.*, **44**, 290 (1955).
133. Tsevdos, T. J., *Drug Cosmetic Ind.*, **78**, 38 (1956).
134. Scigliano, J. A., *et al*, *J. APhA, Sci. Ed.*, **39**, 627 (1949).
135. Kebler, L. F., *J. APhA, Pract. Ed.*, **3**, 820 (1914).
136. Sperandio, G. J., and DeKay, H. G., *J. APhA, Pract. Ed.*, **10**, 572 (1949).
137. Sperandio, G. J., and DeKay, H. G., *J. APhA, Sci. Ed.*, **41**, 245 (1952).
138. Strickland, W. A., and Foss, M., *J. Pharm. Sci.*, **51**, 1002 (1962).
139. Reier, G., *et al*, *J. Pharm. Sci.*, **57**, 660 (1968).
140. Stoyle, L. E., Jr., APhA Convention, Ind. Pharm. Sect., Dallas, Tex., Apr., 1966.
141. Anon, *Drug Cosmetic Ind.*, **82**, 606 (1958).
142. Hosman, P. S., *Drug Cosmetic Ind.*, **73**, 768 (1953).
143. Bakan, J. A., National Ind. Pharm. Res. Conf., Land O'Lakes, Wisconsin, 1966.
144. Herbig, J. A., "Microencapsulation," *Encyclopedia of Chemical Technology*, vol. 13, 2nd ed., Wiley, New York, 1967, pp. 436–456.
145. Baken, J. A., Eastern Regional IPT Sect., Acad. of Pharm. Sci., Philadelphia, Pa., 1968.
146. *Microencapsulation of Pharmaceuticals*, National Cash Register Co., Dayton, Ohio, 1966.
147. Aktieselpkapt Ferrosan, Brit. Pat. 402,611 (Dec. 7, 1933).
148. Bjornsson, S., and Miller, O. H., *J. APhA, Sci. Ed.*, **45**, 618 (1956).
149. Richard, G., *et al*, *Drug Cosmetic Ind.*, 45 (Aug., 1966).

88 | Coating of Tablets, Capsules, and Pills

History and introduction—coating equipment and materials—
preparation of coating solutions and powders—sugar coating—special
coating procedures—film coating—process automation—compression
coating—enteric coating—laminated tablets and pills—removal of coating

This chapter was prepared by

Louis C. Schroeter, PhD, *Assistant Manager, Pharmacy Research, The Upjohn
Company, Kalamazoo, Mich. 49001*

Pill coating has been a pharmaceutical technique for well over ten centuries: Rhazes (850–932 A.D.) employed a mucilage coating for pills in the ninth century; Avicenna (980–1037 A.D.) is credited with the introduction of silver and gold pill coatings (*121*).* The coating of pills with finely powdered talcum, called "pearl coating," was at one time popular (*33*). Gelatin coating of pills was introduced by Garot in 1838 (*102*). The first sugar-coated pills that acquired much repute in the United States were those imported from France about 1842 (*14*). Warner, a Philadelphia pharmacist, was among (*8*) the first to manufacture sugar-coated pills in the United States in 1856 (*13*). The coating of pills with tolu was first recommended about 1860 (*68*). In 1884, Unna (*6*) introduced enteric coating with keratin-coated pills. Fantus (*28*) in 1918 introduced sugar- and tolu-coated granules.

The first pills coated were handled singly and by crude methods. Pills were picked up one at a time, either on the point of a needle or with a pair of forceps, and dipped into the coating solution. Later the pills were held at the end of small tubes by suction while one-half of the pill was dipped, the process was then reversed and the other half dipped. Such dipping of pills failed to give a perfectly smooth coating (*33*).

Compressed tablets have been in existence for over a century. Just as tablet manufacture evolved from the manufacture of pills so tablet coating evolved from pill coating. Manual coating techniques were replaced by methods employing a mechanically revolving coating pan.

The invention of machines to make compressed tablets stimulated other farsighted investigators to attempt compression coating. Noyes (*9*) in 1896 was the first to be granted a patent for an "apparatus for sugar-coating pills." The literature indicates that it was not until 1953, 57 years later, that the first compression-coated commercial tablet was placed on the market. This technique is discussed in the section on *Compression Coating* (page 1688).

Still another method of coating tablets was patented by Wurster (*207*) in 1953. In brief, this process involves the coating of various materials in a chamber by moving an air stream upward past the materials with sufficient force to suspend them continuously therein, and introducing the coating solution into the air stream prior to its contact with materials. Instead of the tablets being tumbled in a coating pan they are tumbled in a current of air.

The processes and techniques employed in the coating of tablets and pills have been surrounded with more or less secrecy (*155*). Tablet and pill coating has been

identified as a manual art (*103*). However, as the extensive bibliography indicates, there is considerable literature on the subject. There has been much scientific investigation of enteric coatings, and in recent years, a scientific approach has been applied to the preparation of specially prepared dosage forms to achieve certain definite results such as the sustained action of a drug or the protection of ingredients from each other or from the atmosphere. In the background of the actual coating process there is a large field of investigation in studying the properties of substances to be used in coatings; it is here, especially, that a truly scientific approach may be made. In recent years there has been some attempt in industry to standardize coating procedures and in some cases to apply automation techniques in tablet coating. Koren and Benton (*155*) tried to develop a standardized method of tablet coating and emphasized that it is especially important that the liquids and solids used in coating solutions be combined in a definite ratio, thereby eliminating the guesswork in the most variable part of tablet coating. Spaulding (*248*) describes machinery installed at Parke, Davis and Co. which allows automatic control of the "jogging cycle," ie, where the coating pans are started and stopped to effect uniform drying of coated tablets. Lachman and Cooper (*3*) have described an electronically programmed film-coating process for tablets. This automated pan-coating method eliminates the human element from film coating, thereby producing more uniform and reproducible coatings. Pharmaceutical scientists are devoting more attention (*41–43, 46, 105*) to the challenge of designing automatic coating procedures; selected examples are discussed in the section on *Process Automation.*

Reasons for Coating Dosage Forms—In the book, *Ingredient X* (*1*), the author points out that dosage forms and ballistic missiles have much in common—both are delivery systems. Tablets, capsules, and pills are the form in which a measured dose of drug is delivered to the target site—the area in the gastrointestinal tract where drug absorption takes place. The coating applied to such dosage forms must not affect the efficiency with which the drug is delivered to the target site. Dosage forms are coated for one or more of the following reasons:

1. To protect the ingredients against the atmosphere. Oxygen or carbon dioxide of the atmosphere may react chemically with the drug in the presence of moisture, the medicinal substance may absorb moisture and hydrate, or the drug may react chemically with the water vapor of the air.
2. To mask unpleasant taste and odor.
3. To improve the appearance of uncoated tablets and pills.
4. To control the site of action of the drug. Enteric coating renders the dosage form insoluble in the stomach and soluble in the intestine. There are many reasons for the enteric coating of medicaments, and a discussion of these is given in that section (page 1689).

---

* Italicized numbers in parentheses refer to Bibliography on page 1696.

Table I—Capacities of Coating Pans

Weight of tablet	Average punch and die size	24-In. pan	36-In. pan
60 mg	7/32	200,000	500,000
300 mg	3/8	80,000	180,000

Some dosage forms are laminated in such a way that sustained or prolonged release of the medicaments is achieved. Some drugs, eg, hexylresorcinol, are caustic and must not be permitted to contact oral mucosa.

5. To prevent incompatibilities when two or more medicaments are incorporated into the same dosage form. The drugs, in the presence of moisture, may interact during the granulation process. Preparation of separate granulations or the application of an offending component as a laminated layer during the coating are means to circumvent this.

Coating Equipment

Various authors (34,152,157,176) have described large-scale coating equipment while others (40,132,202) have described small-scale coating equipment. The equipment of a coating department includes coating pans; polishings pans; a hot-air system including a heating unit, fan blower, and duct system; an exhaust system; steam-jacketed cooking kettles; compressed-air or electric stirrers; pails and other metallic vessels; ladles and powder scoops; paddles for counting tablets and pills; humidity-controlled drying ovens; scales and balances; trucks with tiered, removable, screened shelves for drying; a workbench; and storage space for incoming materials, finished products, and stock solutions and powders. Air conditioning of the coating rooms is highly desirable.

Coating Pans—These are generally constructed of stainless steel. They are available in many sizes among which are those having a diameter of 12, 16, 18, 24, 30, 36, 42, and 48 in. Recently some giant dough-nut-shaped coating pans, which handle the volume of a dozen regular commercial-size pans, have made their appearance. The capacity of the pan required for a particular coating operation depends on the size of the pills or tablets, the number of units to be coated, and the thickness of the coating to be applied. In some

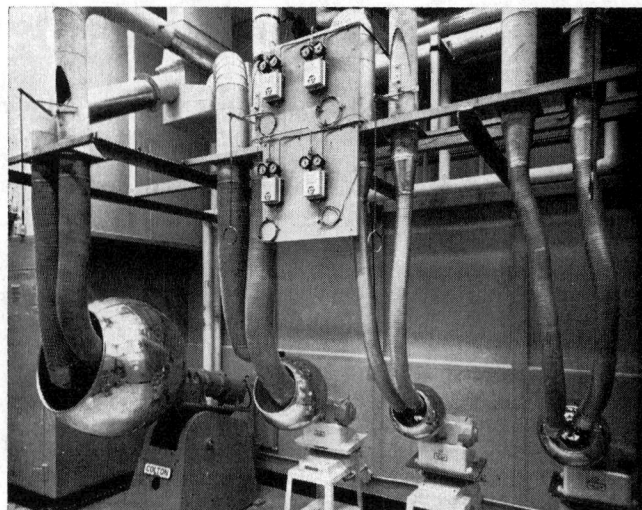

Fig. 727. Part of a coating development laboratory (courtesy, Upjohn).

coating operations the volume occupied by the tablets may increase by 50% or more during the coating operation; hence adequate allowance for this increase in volume must be made. The maximum capacity of various pans for some tablets is shown in Table I. The figures refer to uncoated tablets compressed with deep concave punches.

Fig. 726 shows a row of production-size coating pans each having a diameter of 36 in. The portable stand, seen in the photograph, allows ready transference of the coating solutions from the room where they are prepared to the coating room. Fig. 727 shows part of a coating development laboratory; to the right of the photograph are two stainless steel pans, each having a diameter of 12 in. while to the left are stainless steel pans having diameters of 18 and 36 in., the latter being used for pilot-plant batches. The latter units all have variable-speed controls. Fig. 728 shows the unique side-vented Accela-Cota pan-coating machine in which 100% of the drying air is pulled through the tumbling bed of tablets. It is reported that the machine provides significant improvements in coat quality and reduces drying times.

Polishing Pans—Probably the most widely used polishing pans are drum-shaped canvas pans made by stretching the fabric over a metal frame. However, frequently a galvanized coating pan lined with canvas strips and impregnated with a wax solution is used (Fig. 729). Some bench-type units, such as those shown in Fig. 727, have interchangeable coating and polishing pans. Since colors stain the canvas linings, it is necessary to have one polisher for white coatings, one for pastel shades, and one for darker colors.

Hot-Air and Exhaust Systems—A large volume of low-velocity air must be supplied to the coating pans after each application of coating solution in order to facilitate the rapid removal of water or nonaqueous solvent used. The temperature of the air should be about 120°F with a relative humidity of 35% (103), but there are differences of opinion. The pans shown in Fig. 726 are serviced with a controlled air blast with variable temperature control; the temperature of the air can be varied from room temperature to about 180°F. The standard type of fan blower of sufficient size to supply the necessary air blast to the pans is required; the size will depend on the number of coating pans to be serviced. About 120 to 150 cfm of hot air is necessary. Each drop pipe from the horizontal

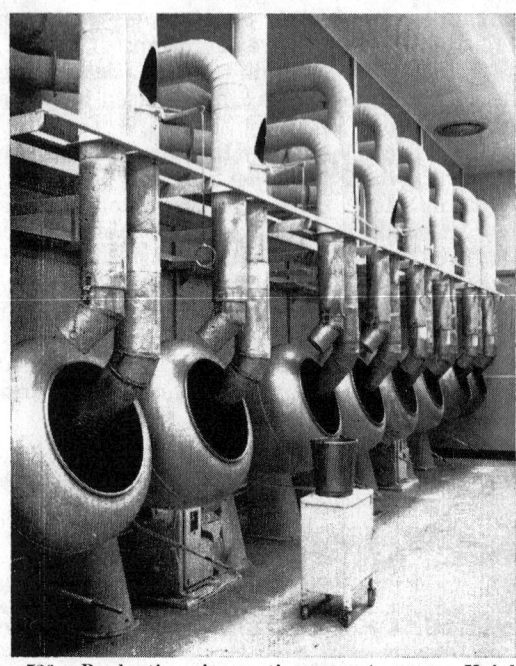

Fig. 726. Production-size coating pans (courtesy, Upjohn).

air duct should be about 6 in. in diameter and should be equipped with a damper to enable the coater to vary the volume of air delivered to the pan on which he is working.

The exhaust system can be constructed similarly to the hot-air system. To be efficient, the lift of the suction in the exhaust pipe must be greater than that of the pressure of the hot air in the hot-air pipe. An exhaust system serves two useful purposes; (1) it removes fine powder generated when the tablets grind against each other during the coating operations, and (2) it rapidly removes organic solvents used in enteric-coating operations.

Cooking Kettles—The various aqueous solutions used in tablet coating require heat and efficient stirring in their preparation. The cooking kettles should be situated near a workbench which has adequate room for filing formulas and desk space for current "tickets" or formulas. For stirring solutions in the kettles compressed-air stirrers are probably best but electric stirrers may be used. The cooking kettles should be situated near a sink which is serviced with hot, cold, and deionized or distilled water or the kettles should be serviced with their own water supplies and drainage systems.

Coating Solutions and Powders

Coating solutions and powders are subject to considerable variation from one coating department to another, and much of the information is still of a secre-

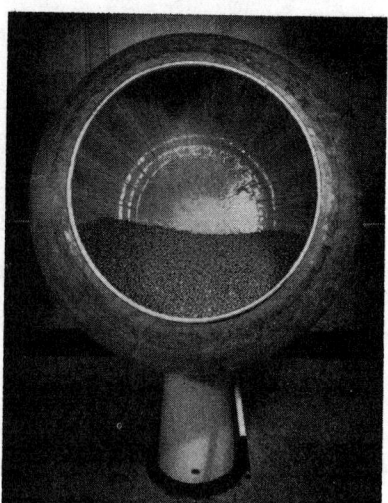

Fig. 729. Polishing pan for capsules and tablets. This pan, which is canvas lined, is rotated and a solution of wax is sprayed on the tablets. Through contact with both the canvas in the tub and other tablets, a high gloss is obtained which adds to the physical appearance of the finished tablet (courtesy, Upjohn).

tive nature in the industry. Many formulas appear in the literature (*15,18,33–36,50,115,144,145,149,152,155, 157,176*) for subcoating, finishing, and polishing solutions and powders, and before one attempts tablet coating it would be wise to study these in detail. Typical formulas only are indicated below and a specific coating task may require entirely different choices of solutions and powders.

The following subcoating solutions are recommended in the literature:

Syrup with Gelatin (*33*)		Special Syrup (*36*)	
Powdered acacia...	0.454 Kg	Acacia..........	0.454 Kg
Gelatin..........	0.538 Kg	Corn syrup......	0.454 Kg
Granulated sugar..	6.810 Kg	Syrup USP.......	3.785 L
Water..........	6.151 L		

Patented solutions or suspensions suitable for subcoating are as follows:

1. 200 parts sugar to 2–7 parts hydroxyethylcellulose to 0.5–3 parts titanium dioxide in aqueous media (*249*).
2. 200 parts sugar to 2–7 parts sodium carboxymethyl cellulose to 0.5–3 parts titanium dioxide in aqueous media (*250*).
3. A gelatin and sugar solution is the proportion of 1½–4½ parts by weight gelatin to 1 part by weight sugar (*251*).

The following subcoating powders are recommended:

White Coating Powder (*33*)		White Coating Powder (*36*)	
Powdered sugar...	39.55 Kg	Precipitated chalk....	16 Kg
Powdered acacia...	5.84 Kg	Powdered starch.....	2 Kg
		Powdered sugar......	2 Kg

The following smoothing syrups are recommended:

Heavy White Syrup (*33*)		Heavy White Syrup (*36*)	
Powdered sugar...	22.70 Kg	Powdered sugar....	2.72 Kg
Precipitated calcium carbonate..	7.94 Kg	Syrup USP........	3.78 L
Potato starch.....	1.13 Kg		
Plain syrup.......	22.71 L		

For coloring, suitable certified dyes usually are dissolved in syrup and applied in different strengths. A hot mixture of color syrup and Syrup USP are mixed beginning with a proportion of about 1 part color syrup and 5 parts Syrup USP, then gradually increasing the amount of color syrup until it is full strength or the desired shade is attained (*36*).

For polishing the following are recommended:

Suspension for Polishing (*144*)	
Bareco 190 wax (a microcrystalline wax)...........	15%
Tween 80..	0.75–1.0%
Carbon tetrachloride.............................	qs

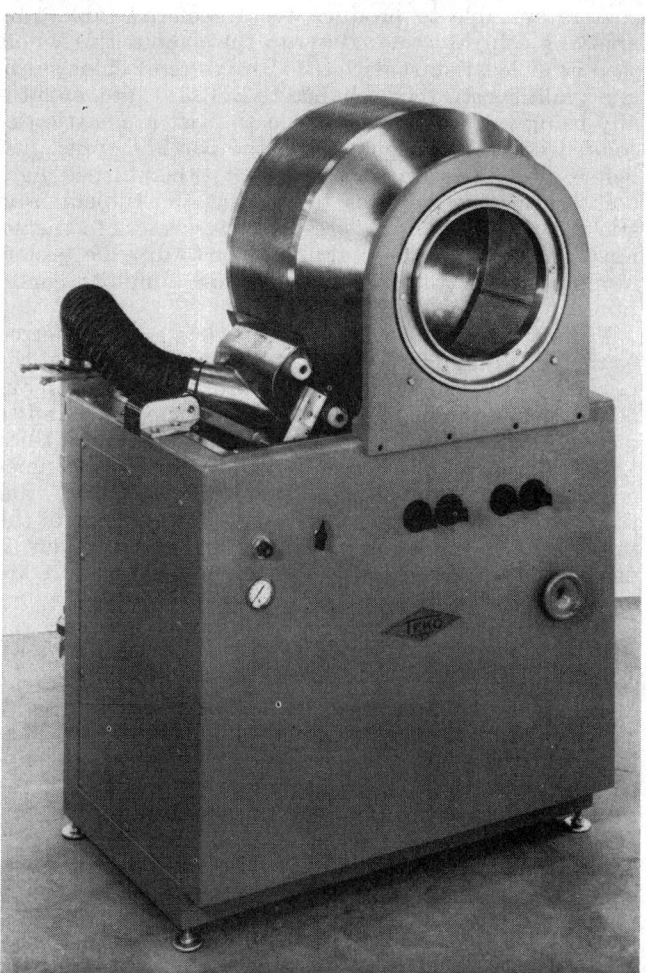

Fig. 728. The Accela-Cota, a side-vented coating pan (courtesy, Thomas Eng.).

Wax Mixture (*145*)		Polishing Wax	
Bareco 190 wax	50%	Carnauba wax	3 Kg
Carnauba wax	50%	Paraffin	2 Kg
		Beeswax	2 Kg

White (*33*) also recommends using a solution of carnauba wax with a small amount of white wax dissolved in chloroform; about 6.5 Gm of the solid combination are used for 50,000 300-mg tablets.

Sugar Coating

Tablets to be coated should be compressed with high convex faces and with as thin an edge as possible, and at the same time conform to good proportions. The thinner the edge of the tablet the easier it is to cover the corners with the coating. The tablets should be screened to remove loose powder and broken tablets before they are placed in the coating pans.

The Composition of Sugar Coatings—A large number of commercial sugar coatings on various tablets were analyzed by Stephensen and Smith (*177*). They found that sugar coatings usually comprise four layers:

1. *An undercoating* which frequently consists of a gum, dextrin, or gelatin layer which forms a bond between the tablet and the outer layers of the coating. In some cases—particularly when the tablets contain very hygroscopic substances—a thin layer of a water-insoluble varnish such as shellac is first applied to prevent absorption of moisture.

2. *An opaque zone* consisting usually of sugar with white insoluble powders. The qualitative examination of a number of commercial coatings has shown that the substances most frequently used in forming this white opaque layer include the following: starch, talc, calcium carbonate, magnesium oxide, and magnesium carbonate.

3. *A translucent zone* consisting almost entirely of sugar usually encloses the opaque layer giving a smooth appearance to the tablet.

4. *A glaze*, usually a very thin layer of white beeswax or carnauba wax or a mixture of these waxes, which gives the coating an attractive polish. The water-soluble matter in 17 samples examined ranged from 51–91.6%. By means of quantitative determinations for reducing sugars following inversion with acid they showed that the water-soluble matter agreed closely with the proportion of sugar, calculated as sucrose, present in the coatings.

General Description of the Process—Before taking up in detail the various steps in coating tablets the processes will be explained briefly. The steps involved in sugar coating may be subdivided into the following: (1) waterproofing and sealing, (2) subcoating, (3) rounding or smoothing, (4) coloring and finishing, and (5) polishing. Often the waterproofing and sealing step is omitted but, with sensitive substances such as vitamin mixtures, it must be included. (See page 1685.) Subcoating involves alternately wetting the tablets with subcoating solution and when partially dry sprinkling with dusting powder. This causes the tablets to be rapidly filled out. Rounding or smoothing involves applications of heavy syrup so that a hard, smooth surface is produced. Coloring and finishing involves the application of thinner, colored syrup in order to build up the tablet further and obtain the desired shade of color. Polishing involves rolling the tablets with wax or the application of a wax solution or suspension in order to give the finished tablets a high gloss.

Subcoating—As the tablets revolve in the coating pan, enough subcoating solution is added to cover all the tablets, the tablets are stirred well by hand and run until the tablets become tacky; subcoating powder is then applied until there are no wet tablets showing. The use of an excess of dusting powder is to be avoided since this will roll in the pan and affect the smoothness of the succeeding coat. Should excess powder accumulate, it will appear at the back of the pan and can be scooped out with a piece of white cardboard. The air blast is turned on until the coating is dry. The process is repeated until the edges are sufficiently covered. When the subcoating is completed, it is advisable to remove the tablets from the pan and screen them. The pan should be washed at this stage also.

Smoothing and Rounding—While the tablets are revolving in the pan, sufficient warm smoothing syrup to cover the tablets is added. The quantity of syrup should be sufficient to loosen previous applications so that the tablets will tend to cluster or adhere to the pan. However, stirring should be maintained to prevent clustering. When the tablets are rolling freely, air is blown on them until they are dry. A dusting powder may or may not be used during this stage. Usually the tablets are rounded until certain specified dimensions are attained.

Coloring and Finishing—As indicated before, the color is built up gradually to prevent a mottled or spotted appearance in the final product. In the beginning, syrups of low color intensity are used; the color intensity of the syrup is gradually increased until finally the desired shade is attained. The syrups should be used fairly warm (about 120°F initially). Sufficient syrup to cover the tablets is added while the tablets are rolling; the syrup is distributed by manual stirring. The tablets are allowed to roll for 3 or 4 min, then the air blast is turned on. The air should be just warm enough to dry the tablets. The tablets should not be allowed to roll too long between applications since the sugar will be ground off the tablets. A large number of applications of syrups having different concentrations of dye are usually necessary. However, some expert coaters are able to produce evenly colored tablets by applying a highly colored syrup throughout this whole step or at least start with a 1:1 mixture of color syrup and plain syrup, then, change to 2:1, 3:1, etc, eventually using full strength. When the last application of colored syrup has been applied the pan is stopped just before the tablets are dry. The pan is then turned manually every few minutes to prevent the tablets from sticking together and to present new surfaces to the atmosphere. It will take about ½ hr to dry the tablets in a stationary coating pan under low humidity conditions.

Polishing—The sugar-coated tablets are transferred to the polishing pan. The pan is set in motion and the polishing solution is added at the rate of about 3–4 fl oz/50,000 tablets. The tablets may be stirred by hand to distribute the solution. A second and possibly a third application of about 2 fl oz should be made. Sometimes a fine grade of talc, in small quantity, is applied after the organic solvent has evaporated; the addition of the talc improves the luster obtained. When no solvent is used for the wax, pieces of the wax or wax mixture are allowed to roll with the tablets.

Difficulties and Some of Their Causes—Uneven thickness in the coating is due usually to faulty subcoating which, in turn, may be caused by adding the dusting powder before the tablets have become tacky or using too little or too much powder or syrup. Failure to screen the tablets and wash the pan after the subcoating may cause small particles to adhere to the tablets. An uneven surface is usually caused by not carrying out the smoothing coating far enough. A spotted coating is generally caused by moisture working out, which in turn is due to the tablets not being dry before the next application of syrup is made. If one tablet has picked the surface of another, or if the tablets are stuck together in pairs or groups, the cause is usually insufficient stirring and improper use of the air blast (*36*). Prolonged storage of coloring syrups at high temperature may result in the formation of significant amounts of glucose which prolongs the drying time for the color coat. Bennett and Hess (4) suggest that color syrup be tested for glucose content prior to use.

More extensive treatments of the processes of tablet coating are given by various authors (11,12,14,18,33, 34, 36, 50, 80, 85, 89, 98, 103, 147, 148, 151, 152, 155, 157,176–178).

Waterproofing and Sealing—Some tablets, due to their contents, require care in coating to prevent the water in the subcoating solution from penetrating the tablet. Such water, if allowed to remain in the "core" tablet, would eventually diffuse through the coating causing discoloration and a mottled appearance. Also, the water may be a medium for undesirable reactions among the ingredients of the compressed tablet or as in the case of penicillin, eg, may cause partial destruction of the drug. In other cases it is desirable to exclude air from contact with the compressed tablet as much as possible; hence a film is formed around the compressed tablet initially to exclude as much air as possible.

Probably the most commonly used waterproofing and sealing agent is arsenic-free *shellac* (151,152,155,176). Koren and Benton (155) used 150 ml of a solution, containing 4 lb of arsenic-free shellac in 1 gal of alcohol, for approximately 15,000 tablets weighing 3900 Gm. Clarkson (176) recommends one or two applications of a solution containing 6 lb of arsenic-free shellac in 1 gal of denatured alcohol and indicates that the addition of ½–1 oz of castor oil per pint of shellac solution will plasticize it and reduce the tackiness. If more than three coats of shellac are applied, the disintegration time may be increased too much and it must be remembered that shellac has good enteric properties if applied in a film of sufficient thickness.

Newer substances which have been applied are the silicones. Organosilicon halides such as $MeSiCl_3$ are gases and may be applied as such (166). Tablets may be provided with a silicone coating which giv s them a gloss and smooth finish. Such coated table s are stated (165,196) to maintain a clear, unspotted a pearance, even in the presence of high humidity for a long time. Although the coatings are claimed to repel water, the disintegration time is stated to be not materially altered. Such coatings may be applied to tablets or capsules by allowing the vapors of the silicone resin to contact them or, preferably, by applying the silicone resin as a solution. The silicone fluids are said to be practically inert physiologically and appear to be essentially nontoxic (196). A patented waterproofing process (16) utilizes acetone solutions containing 20% w/v polyethylene glycol 6000 and 1–3% w/v cellulose acetate phthalate or 20% w/v glyceryl monostearate and 2% w/v cellulose acetate phthalate. Ida, et al (94,101,191) describe a sealing coat composed of amphoteric polyvinylpyridine-acrylic acid polymers which yield a protective film that is insoluble in water but soluble in acid.

Sometimes a sealing coat is applied over the top of another coating. For example, three applications of a solution of glyceryl monostearate, 25 parts, and beeswax, 75 parts, in carbon tetrachloride was recommended to be applied on top of an enteric coating of cellulose acetate phthalate (205).

Special Procedures

The use of insoluble colorants in the sugar coating of tablets has been described by Tucker (20,23). The method has two distinct advantages over the use of water-soluble dyes: tablets cannot be overcolored; color does not have to be applied to perfectly smoothed tablets in order to achieve uniform distribution. The Tucker procedure involves three basic phases:

1. The tablet is given two coats of acacia, using gelatin solution as the adhesive to give the tablet sufficient strength to withstand chipping and cracking in the coating pan and at the same time remove the sharp edges of the tablet. Since colorant is added to the adhesive, the coloring begins immediately.
2. The tablet is sealed with one coat of a gum or resin cast from a suitable solvent.
3. The tablet is finished off using a pigment coating suspension.

Typical coating and undercoating formulations follow.

Typical Coating Formulation

Stock suspension, ingredients

Purified water	250.00 ml
Dioctyl sodium sulfosuccinate	0.01 Gm
Insoluble colorant	1–15.00 Gm
Titanium Dioxide USP	0–100.00 Gm
Syrup USP	500.00 ml

Coating suspension

Stock suspension	100.00 Gm
Coating syrup qs ad	500.00 ml

Undercoating Formulations

Gelatin adhesive solution

Gelatin USP	800 Gm
Purified water	6500 ml
Acacia USP	600 Gm
Sucrose USP	9500 Gm

Undercoating adhesive suspension

Stock suspension	10–20%
Gelatin adhesive solution	80–90%

The tablets are placed in a conventional coating pan. Undercoating adhesive suspension is applied to the rolling tablets until they are evenly and completely wetted. When the mass becomes tacky, acacia powder is dusted on the tablets in the usual fashion. This procedure is repeated again. The tablets are sealed with a gum or resin cast from a suitable solvent, eg, a 4-lb cut of shellac diluted with an equal quantity of isopropyl alcohol—one coat is usually sufficient. Coating suspension is then applied—generally, 25 coats are sufficient. The tablets are finished off and polished in the usual fashion.

The finished product retains the same pharmaceutical elegance as when made by conventional methods, yet has a coating of approximately one-half the thickness. Coating may be accomplished in about one-half the usual time. Tucker (23) pointed out that the use of insoluble pigments in titanium dioxide–syrup suspension rather than dye shows the following advantages:

1. Coating can be applied immediately following the rounding coats in many cases, thereby eliminating the smoothing coats.
2. Time and number of coats required to apply the coloration are reduced.
3. Color can be matched easily from lot to lot.
4. Tablets cannot be overcolored.
5. New and different shades of color are available.
6. Excellent light stability has been attained with many of the pigments.

Film Coating

Certain basic drawbacks of sugar coating, the most significant being the very lengthy coating time necessary, led to the investigation of other types of tablet coatings. A coating procedure involving the use of cellulosic high polymers was reported by Doerr, et al (192). This method involved shellac-sealing the tablets and then applying several coats of hydroxyethyl-cellulose or sodium carboxymethylcellulose as 5% solutions in 50% v/v alcohol, followed by wax polishing. United States patents were issued for this process in 1957 (29).

Film-coating theory and practice have been reviewed by Banker (106); fundamental mechanical and physicochemical properties of films as affected by plasticization, solvents, film additives, and other factors are discussed in detail.

Film-type coatings have been investigated intensively during the past decade as evidenced by the selected sample of recent patent publications (128,130,137,141, 154,158,162,179,206,208,210,249,250). A comprehensive discussion of all these references is not possible within the confines of this chapter; therefore, comments will be limited to unique applications or properties of this type of coating. The Wurster air-suspension coating apparatus (207) has been widely adopted in the pharmaceutical industry for coating drug particles of widely varying sizes and shapes (107). Drug particles are suspended or fluidized in the air stream, while coating materials are introduced into the air stream in a fine spray. Fig. 730 shows one of the several configurations of a 12-in. Wurster column. Enteric film coats may be applied by the Wurster air suspension technique (72,120).

Long (19) has described a patented film-coating solution of sodium carboxymethylcellulose and shellac which does not significantly change its disintegration time on aging. Winters and Deardorff (37) reported that zein formed suitable film-type coatings. The best formulas for the coating solution were those containing 15% zein in 91% isopropanol and an additive which was usually 3% of a surfactant such as Tween 20, Tween 80, Span 20, or Span 80. Ahsan and Blaur (38) used solutions containing 5% polyvinyl-pyrrolidone and 2% polyethylene glycol 600 with or without 5% acetylated monoglyceride in 70% ethanol. A number of different compositions for film-type coatings were described in a British Patent Specification assigned to Abbott Laboratories (39). The coating solutions used in the examples contained cellulose acetate phthalate and polyethylene glycol 4000 or 6000 with or without added substances such as beeswax, castor oil–stearic acid, corn oil–cocoa butter, mineral oil–lanolin, sesame oil–cetyl alcohol, propylene glycol–paraffin, or castor oil–beeswax; a mixture of glyceryl monostearate and cellulose acetate phthalate and a mixture of polyethylene glycol and ESA resin (a stearic acid modified phthalic acid glyceride condensation product) were also cited. Angsusingh and Chavkin (233) reported on coatings prepared from a basic lipophilic mixture containing 3 parts of hydrogenated castor oil (Castorwax) and 1 part of acetylated monoglycerides (Myvacet 500) and made hydrophilic by the addition of either polyethylene glycol 400 monostearate or polyethylene glycol 400 distearate in proportions of 5–50% of the total coating solution. Although the report indicated that these coatings would be useful for timed disintegration, some of the formulas would appear suitable for rapidly dissolving film coatings.

The advantages of film coatings are:

1. Considerable saving in labor and coating materials with subsequent reduced coating costs.
2. The resulting tablets retain substantially their original shape, hence grooves and emblems initially present in the compressed tablet are retained.
3. Effective covering of bitter taste and bad odor.
4. Improved stability over sugar-coated tablets.
5. Increased resistance to abrasion.
6. Increased luster of tablets when the compressed tablet has little or no luster.
7. Little or no increase in disintegration time by *in vitro* test methods.
8. The process adds little to the tablet weight or volume, hence a reduction in packaging costs.
9. The weight variation among the finished tablets is decreased compared with sugar-coated tablets (192).

Process Automation

Spray-Pan Method—Anderson and Sakr (41) have described a new method of coating tablets using a revolving coating pan in which the coating materials are applied in solution or suspension, as a spray from a centrifugal disc atomizer. Addition of coating materials may be controlled at a rate which allows even deposition on the tablet. Dry powders need not be used; the process is therefore dust-free. The standard coating pan is used to support the tablet bed. The coating materials are sprayed onto the revolving tablets in a controlled manner from a centrifugal disc atomizer.

The apparatus is shown in Fig. 731. The spinning disc (4) for the laboratory model is 2 in. in diameter; it is driven counterclockwise by a variable-speed motor. The disc is surrounded by a rectangular stainless steel shield (5) open towards the coating pan, with an aperture (7) of variable width to allow spraying of fluids with different spray characteristics. Changing the size of the aperture and the position of the disc relative to the pan permits control of the spray. Ideally, the spray should fall only on the rolling tablets in a line from front to back of the pan. The shield is designed to collect excess coating fluid (80% of spray) which is circulated back to the thermostatically controlled feed reservoir (1) by means of a pump (8). Coating materials are fed onto the center

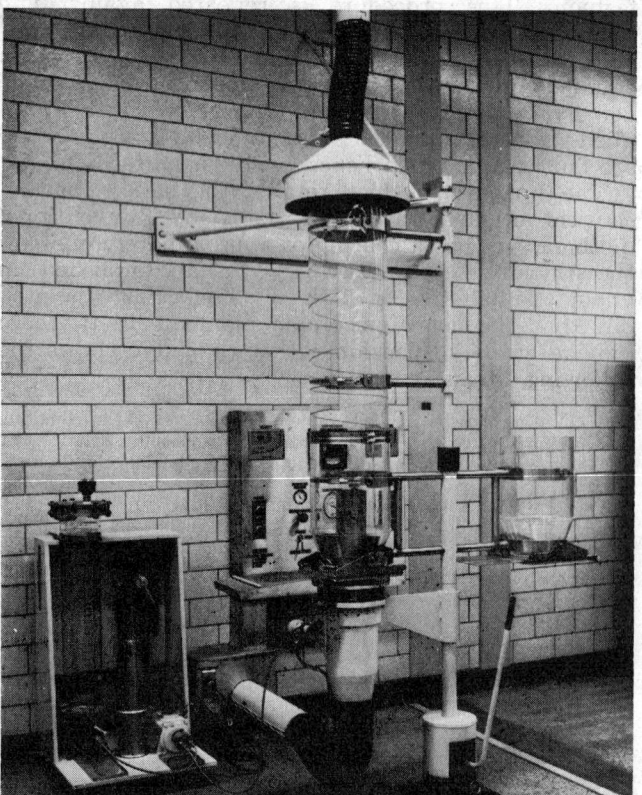

Fig. 730. Wurster air-suspension coating apparatus (courtesy, Upjohn).

of the spinning disc through an intermediate reservoir (3) which eliminates the pulsing flow from the pump (2). The pump controls the feed rate in conjunction with the size of the nozzle on the intermediate reservoir.

Anderson and Sakr used a 16-in. bench-type coating pan revolving at 30 rpm and receiving 15–20-ft³/min air supply at 60°. For a disc speed of 8000 rpm and feed rate of 100–150 ml/min the following operation cycle was used: spray, 1–1½ min; tumble only, 1 min without air; blown hot air, 1–2 min with tumbling. This cycle was repeated until the desired coated weight was attained.

Using this method, tablets could be coated with syrup or gelatin syrup alone; *subcoating and dusting powder were not used.* Tablets were also coated using titanium dioxide syrup, calcium carbonate syrup, kaolin syrup, barium sulfate syrup or acacia syrup suspension, and finished with syrup; *dusting powder was not applied.* The finished coated tablet weight was double the uncoated weight. When suspensions were used, two-thirds of the weight of coat was supplied by the suspension, syrup contributing the remainder. Anderson and Sakr demonstrated that tablets coated by the spray-pan method consistently have a coefficient of weight variation of less than 4%,

and close to that of the cores. This remarkable precision is only rarely achieved by the standard method of coating. This difference between the two methods of coating is caused by the use of free powder in the subcoating stage in the standard method. Anderson and Sakr demonstrated that the need is better met by using a liquid suspension applied in atomized form.

Other attempts to improve on the pan coating of tablets have been restricted to automation of the stages in the method. Kwan (85) has described an automated process to study drying of coatings. Butensky (80) also employed an automated process and confirmed experimentally the experience of tablet coaters that it is the powder–liquid additions and ratios, coupled with drying rates, which lead to the difficulties of the standard method.

The spray pan method has been suggested by Anderson and Sakr for uniform, controlled addition of coating materials at a known rate, without the hand mixing used in the traditional method. While spraying may be accomplished by pressure atomizers, the centrifugal disk is the simplest type of atomizer and is easily used and cleaned—high pressures are not required; and it can be used with fluids of widely varying properties over a wide range of feed rates. This gives greater possibility of controlled variation in application conditions and of producing sprays of uniform droplet size.

Programmed Automated Process—Lachman and Cooper (3,46) described in detail the design and operation of a programmed automated process for tablet coating. While this method is designed for film coating, it is nonetheless worth describing in some detail for it removes the human factor from this kind of coating operation. It may provide a glimpse of the future for all coating and many other pharmaceutical operations. The Lachman–Cooper apparatus is shown in Fig. 732. The coating pans are fitted with four stainless steel baffles 90° apart to provide desired tumbling action of tablets wetted with the film-coating fluids. The dusting powder (talc) is suspended in the coating liquid to eliminate the dusting step. The *spray suspension* is applied with a spray gun (Nordson) which gives an airless spray. The coating process is controlled by a perforated tape

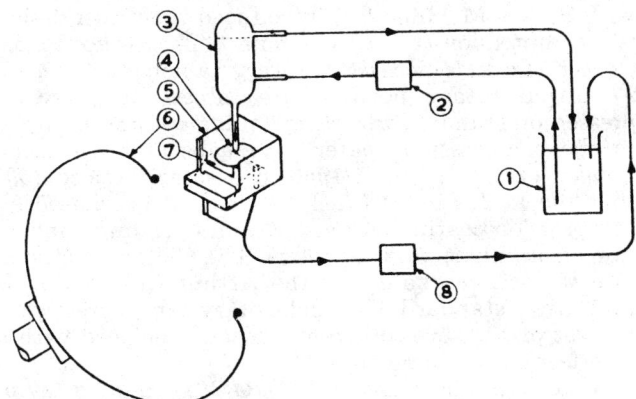

Fig. 731. Spray-pan coating process. *1:* feed reservoir; *2:* metering pump; *3:* intermediate reservoir; *4:* spinning disc; *5:* stainless steel shield; *6:* coating pan; *7:* aperture; *8:* pump (courtesy, Anderson and Sakr[41]).

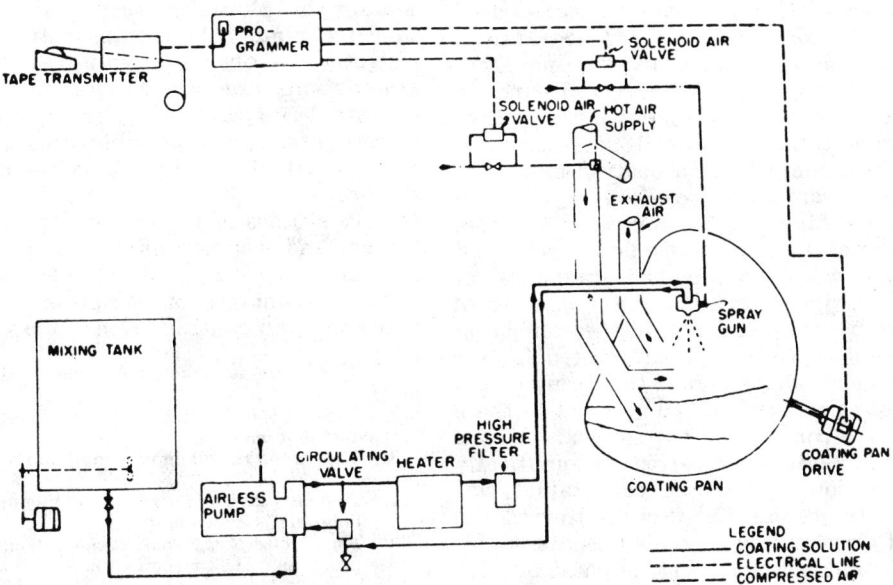

Fig. 732. The design and equipment for the programmed automated coating operation (courtesy, Lachman and Cooper[3]).

traveling at a certain distance per unit time and transmitting its signals through a tape transmitter to the necessary relays in the programmer to activate the several components of the coating cycle, which include:

1. Switching on the coating-pan motor to start pan rotation.
2. Regulating the pneumatic solenoid to open and close the automatic spray gun.
3. Controlling a pneumatic solenoid to activate a single-acting air cylinder that opens and closes the damper on the forced hot air duct.
4. Activating a latching relay to terminate the coating operation.

Freund Apparatus—This is a Japanese automatic sugar-coating machine produced by the Freund Industrial Co. of Tokyo and distributed in the US and Canada by Gardner Laboratory of Bethesda, Md. The Freund apparatus uses existing coating pans, pan drier units, and dry air systems. Spraying and drying operations are regulated by timers. The coating material is maintained at 60–75° and constantly pumped through the feed line by means of a gear pump and returned to the supply tank. The coating material is applied as a slurry using a spray gun.

Compression Coating

The usual pan-coating process for tablets requires skill and practice; however, this method has certain disadvantages: it is time consuming and expensive; the effect of moisture must be overcome by waterproofing, and this protective coat frequently delays disintegration of the finished tablets; the tablet to be pan-coated is usually compressed comparatively hard since it has to withstand the vigorous rolling and tumbling in the coating pan, and this hard "core" in the finished coated tablet may delay disintegration and decrease *in vivo* availability of the medicament.

As stated in the introduction, a few farsighted investigators attempted compression coating or "press-coating" according to British terminology (*217*). Since tablets are readily made by compression, it appeared to follow logically that tablets could be coated by compression techniques. After a lapse of more than 65 years since the first attempt (*9*), many pharmaceutical houses are marketing compression-coated tablets. Cooper and Pasquale (*47*) listed 29 manufacturers who market a total of 98 different compression-coated tablets. The first compression-coated tablet was Darstine Bromide, 50 mg, Stratalets, marketed in the fall of 1953 by Sharp and Dohme (*209*). The second product was Praducil, marketed early in 1954 by Evans Medical Supplies Ltd., of England (*218*).

The patent granted to Noyes (*9*) in 1896 described a crude machine which compressed a coating onto core tablets. The patent granted to Noyes (*10*) a year later described a crude machine which compressed the core tablets and coated them in one continuous cycle. In 1917 Stokes (*27*) described a modified rotary tablet machine which was capable of applying a coating of powder to a tablet by compression. In the confection industry, patents (*66,74,78*) have been granted for the design of machines for coating gum. Centering of the core tablet was not considered very important in these patents, provided the core tablet was convex. It was claimed that good centering occurred automatically during the compression step if the core tablet was relatively thick in the center and tapered toward the edges. Kilian, of Germany, was granted a patent (*77*) in 1937 for a compression-coating apparatus. He emphasized the importance of the exact centering of the core tablets relative to the coating powder, thus dis-

agreeing with previous investigators regarding their claim of automatic centering. However, because the core tablets were required to have a small circular depression with Kilian's early process, the tablets produced did not have a conventional appearance.

In 1951 Whitehouse (*217*) at Evans Medical Supplies Ltd., began investigations to improve compression-coating equipment, particularly the centering device (*49,52*). About the same time (*53*) work was going on at Sharp and Dohme which led to the commercial feasibility of compression coating. Originally, Evans Medical Supplies Ltd. worked with Manesty Machines Ltd. to improve the coating machines, but the two companies dissolved their agreement (*55,59*). Other patents (*60,228*) of interest in this field are cited.

Compression-coating machines of various designs have been commercially available. The Manesty Dry Cota is a combined tablet-making and compression-coating machine. This machine consists basically of two rotary tablet presses of the D-3 type coupled by a single drive shaft and special transfer device in such a manner that core tablets can be compressed and coated in one continuous cycle (*47*). The Kilian Prescoter is a dual purpose, single rotary compressing machine designed for the production of ordinary compressed tablets as well as compression-coated tablets (*47,59*). In the summer of 1955 the F. J. Stokes Machine Co. introduced their own design of a compression-coating machine. The Stokes Press-Coater is a modified BB-2 rotary tablet press with a 27-station rotary head. Core tablets are precompressed on standard tableting equipment and then fed to the compression coater by means of a vibrating hopper (*47*). In July, 1956, it was announced (*53*) that the F. J. Stokes Machine Co. had purchased all compression coating patents (*73*) and pending applications from Sharp and Dohme. The Colton Compression Coater, marketed by the Arthur Colton Co., is basically a standard 33-punch rotary tablet press with one set of pressure rolls removed and replaced with a core-feeding mechanism (*47*).

A few publications (*47,83,84,234*) and a symposium (*87*) have been concerned with compression-coating machine operation and the pharmaceutics of coating tablets by compression. Cooper (*47*) pointed out that there has been too little attention given to solving the pharmaceutical problems associated with this technique of overabsorption with mechanical gadgetry. Problems involved in obtaining suitable granulations are often quite difficult, but not insurmountable. Granulations must possess a homogeneity of particle size, compressibility, and a degree of lubrication not usually required in conventional tablet manufacture. Lachman, *et al* (*42,43*), have conducted extensive studies of the factors influencing core concentration and weight uniformity in compression-coated tablets.

The advantages of compression coating over conventional pan coating are as follows:

1. The process is entirely anhydrous so that waterproofing is unnecessary.
2. The core tablets can be compressed softer than usual, especially in the dual-unit machine.
3. The coated tablets have a more uniform and rapid disintegration rate.
4. There is a saving in time and coating materials.
5. Polishing is unnecessary.
6. The surface of the coating can be engraved or embossed with clearer and sharper markings than obtainable with film-coated tablets.
7. Some of the machines produce tablets having coatings of uniform thickness.

8. The weight and volume variation of the finished tablets is much less than for pan-coated tablets.

9. Compression coating can be used for odd shapes such as square or doughnut-shaped tablets.

Special pharmaceutical problems may be solved by means of compression coating. For example, water-sensitive drugs such as penicillin may be coated under essentially anhydrous conditions (*218*) and incompatible drugs can be separated readily by incorporating one of the drugs in the core tablet and one of the drugs in the coating. Special types of tablets may be prepared by compression-coating methods. For example, enteric-coated tablets (*109,234,235,251*), repeat-action tablets, and prolonged-action tablets have been prepared in compression-coated forms (*47*).

Coated Powders, Granules, or Pellets—As early as 1918 Fantus (*28*) investigated the coating of tiny granules and powder with insoluble substances. He mentioned that the medication, so coated, might be administered in the form of a powder or granules, or preferably in the form of compressed tablets. The literature appears to contain no further reference to the application of this technique in pharmacy until Consolazio (*159*) was granted a patent in 1949 for salt tablets which were made to dissolve very slowly after ingestion by coating them with a thin film of cellulose acetate or cellulose nitrate. Polymers may be applied to the salt granules either before or after compression (*119*).

Allan (*221*) describes the coating of antimalarial salts with fatty or waxy substances in amounts sufficient to inhibit leaching out of the salt due to atmospheric moisture but insufficient to inhibit *in vivo* absorption. Probably the first tablet claimed to give sustained action and containing coated granules was marketed in the United States (*212*). Apparently the coating of pellets with shellac has been one approach since one commentator (*211*) stated that when shellac-coated, medication-containing pellets are compressed into tablets, the coating often cracks and the patient gets double or even triple doses of the drug. However, other coating agents have been used which apparently circumvent most of these difficulties (*90,226*). The technique also can be used to increase the stability of moisture-sensitive powders (*91*). No attempt has been made to cover the literature in this field which is quite extensive and considered outside the scope of this section of the chapter.

Enteric Coating

Definition—An enteric coating is one that resists the action of stomach fluids and disintegrates or dissolves in the intestines.

Reasons for Enteric Coating—These are:

1. To prevent gastric digestion or decomposition of a drug such as a glandular product or an antibiotic, eg, erythromycin.
2. To prevent nausea and vomiting caused by a drug, eg, emetine, atabrine, and diethylstilbestrol.
3. To prevent dilution of the drug before reaching the intestine, eg, intestinal antiseptics and anthelmintics.
4. To prevent hindrance of gastric digestion by the drug, such as by alkaline medicaments.
5. To give delayed action of the drug, eg, barbiturates, amphetamine, and aspirin.
6. To deliver the medication to the intestinal tract for optimum absorption in the duodenum and jejunum (*97,111,202*). Each drug should be considered individually; recent evidence (*7*) indicates that certain combination drugs such as thiazide–potassium chloride may cause intestinal irritation or ulceration if administered in the form of enteric-coated tablets.

Requirements of a Good Enteric Coating—These are:

1. It must be nontoxic.
2. It and its degradation products, if any, must be physiologically inactive.
3. It must not disintegrate in the stomach in the duration of time that the enteric-coated dosage form may be expected to remain in the stomach.
4. It must disintegrate or dissolve in the intestines, thereby releasing the enclosed medicament (*200*).

Theory and Investigation of Enteric Coatings—There is a difference in pH in going from the stomach to the intestine, but this is usually not from an extremely acid to a strongly alkaline state. Fresh gastric juice as it is secreted by the glands contains from 0.5 to 0.6% hydrochloric acid (*125*); one source states that after a test meal the normal stomach has a pH of 1.67, and even when all the acid is combined with protein, the pH is 3.0 (*88*). After an overnight fast the volume of gastric secretion and concentration of acid depends on the condition of the subjects or patients (*180,182*). In a group of 147 patients without history of gastric disease or pernicious anemia, after a protein meal, 65% of the cases had gastric contents with pH values ranging from 1.5 to 2.5, and 86% had gastric contents with pH values ranging from 1.5 to 3.5. A great deal of evidence (*24,26,30–32,44,45,61,65*) indicates that the intestinal contents usually range from pH 3.6 to 7.9, and the observations indicate that the extreme range on the acid side (less than pH 7) is greater than the extreme range on the alkaline side (greater than pH 7). Wruble (*69*), as early as 1935, stated that: "Recent investigations have definitely indicated that our earlier notions regarding the acidity and alkalinity of the stomach and small intestine, respectively, are erroneous. More often the small intestine is slightly acid in reaction and the pH of the stomach will doubtless vary over a considerable range because of regurgitation and the other factors already enumerated."

The disintegration or dissolution of an enteric coating in the intestinal tract usually depends on one or more of the following factors:

1. The presence of acidic groups in the enteric substance cause it to be insoluble in the low-pH environment of the stomach but soluble in the intestinal tract due to the higher (but usually not alkaline) pH of the media there.
2. The enteric substance may be susceptible to hydrolysis which may be catalyzed by certain intestinal enzymes—the hydrolysis of susceptible linkages may aid in the disintegration of the enteric film.
3. Agents such as bile salts and cholesterol may aid in the formation of complexes and in the emulsification of fats, fatty acids, and waxes, when used as enteric substances, thus promoting disintegration of the coating.
4. The coating may act as a semipermeable membrane allowing diffusion of the medicament through the coating.
5. Hygroscopic substances may be included in the coating, and these swell in the presence of moisture, thus causing the coating to disperse.
6. Chemical reactions may occur, thus aiding disruption of the coating (*131,188,194,202*).

The first factor outlined under (1) has in the past been the most important one and will be discussed further. The degree of ionization of a weak acid depends upon two factors—the pH of the solution and the relative strength of the acid as indicated by its pK_a value. Consider the general equation:

$$R{-}COOH + OH^- \rightleftharpoons R{-}COO^- + H_2O$$

The position of this equilibrium is determined by two main factors: the dissociation constant of the acid, $R{-}COOH$ (sometimes expressed as the negative logarithm of the K_a value, namely the pK_a) and the pH of the medium. At low pH values, usually below pH

2 or 3, practically all the acid will be in the undissociated form. Most high-molecular-weight acids in their undissociated form have very low water solubilities. As the pH is raised, the equilibrium shifts more and more to the right causing the formation of more and more of the ionized form, R—COO⁻. In general the weak acid will be almost 100% ionized when the pH of the final solution is two pH units higher than the pK_a of the weak acid, and the weak acid will be almost nonionized when the pH of the final solution is two pH units lower than the pK_a of the weak acid (188). The ionized forms of most acids are water-soluble. Wruble (69) showed that ammoniated shellac coatings started to dissolve at pH 6.4, and Malm, et al (172), showed that the particular cellulose acetate phthalate which they used began to dissolve at pH 5.7 to 5.8. For polyacidic polymers such as cellulose acetate phthalate, a third factor must be taken into consideration and that is the percentage of free carboxyl (or other acidic) groups on the polymer molecule. For example, Hiatt (104) stated that those cellulose acetate phthalates having a free carboxyl (COOH) content between 9 and 15% by weight are most preferable for enteric coating. Similarly, Wagner, et al (93), showed that the minimum pH at which starch acetate phthalates dissolve depends on the percentage of free carboxyl groups on the polymer molecule. Hence, such polyacidic polymers will dissolve when there are a sufficient number of acidic groups and when these groups are ionized to a sufficient extent.

Other factors are important also in the disintegration or dissolution of an enteric coating. These are:

1. The thickness and uniformity of the coating.
2. The packing or density of the coating.
3. The strength of the bond between the coating and the tablet surface.
4. The brittleness of the coating and the presence or absence and type of plasticizer.
5. The presence or absence, type, and amount of dusting powder used with the coating solution (202,205).

It is difficult to compare data on different enteric coatings reported in the literature since the authors did not specify the amount of enteric substance applied to or retained by each tablet, the amount of dusting powder applied per tablet, the thickness and weight of the coating, and some measure of variation involved in the above measurements and in the disintegration times reported. It should be emphasized that such measurements are indispensable to a valid *in vitro* comparison of any two or more enteric coatings. Valid *in vitro* comparisons of different enteric coatings can be made by plotting the various variables involved. For example, one can plot the following variables for the coatings under consideration.

1. Initial average disintegration time vs average weight of coating.
2. Initial average disintegration time vs average thickness of coating on the side of the tablet.
3. Initial average disintegration time vs average weight of enteric substance applied per tablet.
4. Resistance time of the enteric coated tablets to Simulated Gastric Fluid (SGF) the average disintegration time of the enteric coated tablets (in Simulated Intestinal Fluid (SIF).)

In most cases the data can be fitted by equations for the straight line, namely $y = ax$ or $y = ax + b$, or by a simple power series of the type $y = ax + bx^2$. Hence, the positions of the lines and the slopes of the lines can be compared. An excellent enteric coating would be one which yields lines of very low slope in plots of types 1, 2, and 3, plus lines of very high slope in plots of type 4. The errors and variability involved in the measurements are readily shown on such plots by using bars on either side of the plotted points to mark off 95% confidence intervals about the average values. A coated product should have satisfactory proof of the *in vivo* availability of the medicament and clinical efficacy of the product. However, before the coated products are tested in the clinic, comparisons can be made by *in vitro* and animal tests. The most satisfactory screening tests, however, would be those in which some objective clinical response or clinical pharmacological quantity such as blood level or urinary excretion data were correlated with the laboratory-measured quantities such as *in vitro* disintegration time, weight or thickness of coating, and amount of enteric substance or other coating agent applied per dosage unit. The point has been stressed previously, however, that the physical characteristics of the coating and the amounts of the ingredients used are probably as important as the nature of the enteric substance.

The emptying time of enteric-coated dosage forms from the stomach is important also. Bukey and Brew (64) studied the time required for various sizes and shapes of enteric-coated tablets and pills to leave the stomachs of human subjects. The smallest dosage unit they studied was a coated pill with a diameter of 3.9 mm. The largest dosage unit was a rectangular tablet, 12.5 × 8.5 × 3.5 mm. They administered a total of 367 pills, tablets, and capsules to a total of 96 subjects. They reported that the largest number of dosage forms passed out of the stomach in 4 hr, but that the average emptying time was 5.9 hr. Other conclusions drawn from the study were as follows:

1. The size and shape of the dosage unit (in the size range studied) had no effect on the length of time it remained in the stomach.
2. The same subject did not react uniformly toward this type of medication with respect to stomach emptying time.
3. The emptying time may be influenced by the diet.
4. The type of coating had no effect on the length of time the coated units remained in the stomach.

In a later study Bukey and Brew (81) studied the effect of diet on the stomach emptying time of coated tablets. They reported that diets containing a large proportion of carbohydrate or cellulose were more conducive to rapid passing of the tablets from the stomach, whereas diets high in fat content tended to cause the tablets to be retained longer in the stomach. The quantity of food consumed had no apparent effect on the time the tablets remained in the stomach, but an excess of fluid seemed to retard the passing of the tablets. The range of average emptying times reported was from 2.7 hr on a cellulose diet at breakfast to 8.5 hr on a fat diet at dinner.

Crane and Wruble (96) made approximately 1000 roentgenographic and roentgenoscopic observations on 116 individuals ranging from 18 to 30 years of age. They reported that approximately 15% of the enteric-coated tablets remained intact within the stomach for a period of at least 9–10 hr. Calculations made from the data in this study indicate that 174, or 79%, of 220 enteric-coated tablets administered to 87 subjects emptied from the stomach after an average time of 3.6 hr; the standard deviation was 1.5 hr. Thirty-five tablets, or 16%, remained intact in the stomach for at least 9 or 10 hr, and 11 tablets, or 5%, disintegrated in the stomach.

Blythe (100) reported that the time it took a coated tablet to pass through the pylorus varied from a few minutes up to 12 hr. The average emptying time was 1.5 hr. He theorized that there would be less physiologic impediment to the passage of small coated pellets or granules through the pylorus and reported that subsequent studies proved the theory to be correct. He reported that the small coated pellets soon spread along the digestive tract. Similarly, Feinblatt and Ferguson (123) presented roentgenographic data which showed that 16 min after the ingestion of small coated granules to human subjects the granules had moved out of the stomach and become dispersed throughout the small intestine.

There is some doubt, however, about the accuracy of measuring the stomach-emptying time of tiny coated pellets by roentgenographic methods. Results reported by Feinblatt and Ferguson (123) are distinctly different than has been reported after animal studies with test meals. For example, Rosenthal and Nasset (126) showed that two different carbohydrate test meals emptied from the stomachs of rats at first-order rates. In these studies 50% of the food emptied after 107 min following ingestion of one meal and after 46 min following ingestion of the other meal. Addition of protein to the carbohydrate meals did not change the two emptying rates.

Composition of Enteric Coatings—A large number of enteric substances have been investigated. As indicated above, few comparisons have been made on a valid basis. The previous edition of this chapter (225) contains a very comprehensive listing of over 160 literature references on enteric coatings—there are 60 entries representing an even larger number of actually different enteric substances which have been tested. Of these, only the following groups— fats, fatty acids, waxes and mixtures, shellac, ammoniated shellac, and cellulose acetate phthalates—are utilized commercially to a considerable extent. For details of the individual studies the reader is referred to various reviews by other authors (58,110,127,129, 131,142,151,152,156,176,203,205).

An interesting development in the enteric-coating field was the report of Blubaugh, et al (234), that a satisfactory enteric compression-coated tablet could be prepared using a granulation containing 20% triethanolamine cellulose acetate phthalate, 79% lactose, and 1% magnesium stearate. Careful control of the amount of water added and the amount of kneading during granulation was required to achieve the desired results.

Laminated Coating

The word lamina means a thin layer or flake. In one sense, most coated tablets are laminated since they have layers of different composition. However, the terms laminated tablet or pill are generally reserved for those in which one drug or group of drugs is the "core" tablet and another drug or group of drugs is in one or more layers or coatings about the "core."

One of the earliest, if not the earliest, published examples of a laminated tablet was that patented by Kirk (56). This patent described a tablet of an intestinal disinfectant or other medicinal substance surrounded by an enteric coating and having an external coating which contained a spice or other substance adapted to stimulate secretion of hydrochloric acid by the stomach. A patent (118) was granted to Bickenheuser for the manufacture of a tablet with an annular effervescent portion and a thinner central portion of a medicament which is not readily soluble, such as aspirin, with a separating layer of soluble material such as glucose or a gum. Similarly, a Dutch patent (183) described a pressed tablet consisting of a kernel containing a disinfectant and surrounded by a layer containing a substance which cuts mucus for the purpose of adapting the latter for the disinfection.

Various laminated commercial tablets have made their appearance during the past few years. Many of these are marketed as repeat-action tablets in which an inner core tablet contains one dose of the medicament(s) and an outer layer contains a second dose of the same medicament(s). The two doses of medicament are separated by an enteric coating. The outer layer of medicament is usually sugar coated. Upon ingestion, the sugar coating dissolves and the first dose of medicament is released relatively rapidly, in most cases while the dosage form is in the stomach. The inner dose is not released until the remaining enteric-coated tablet has passed into the intestine. The major difficulty with the effectiveness of such dosage forms is the variable stomach emptying time for the relatively large-sized enteric-coated cores (100). This same type of "all-or-none" response with respect to stomach emptying time is not a problem when the coated units are very small (100). Patent literature (54,136) describes a variety of unique laminated tablets.

An Australian patent specification (140) described a laminated pill or tablet with the outer layer being soluble in the patient's mouth and containing beneath it a taste-indicating layer which informs the patient to swallow the tablet in order to obtain benefit from the inner core of medicament. A commercial product of this type is Isufranol (Winthrop), which has an outer layer of isoproterenol hydrochloride intended for sublingual absorption; a middle lemon (flavor-timer) layer; and an inner core of phenobarbital, benzylephedrine hydrochloride, and theophylline intended for release after the tablet is swallowed.

A United States patent (232) described laminated tablets which were prepared by applying coatings containing aspirin, phenacetin, caffeine, and/or an antihistaminic to waterproofed centers or cores. The latter were prepared by rotating compressed tablets containing a water-insoluble salt of penicillin in a coating pan in the presence of a ball made out of a mixture of peanut oil and corn starch.

Still another type of laminated tablet employing a new principle has been marketed (213). The "core" tablet contains amphetamine held to a polyacidic substance by ionic bonds and this is coated with an external layer containing caffeine. On administration, the external caffeine layer is stated to disintegrate rapidly, while the inner "core" allows only a slow release of the amphetamine.

Special Procedures for Vitamin Products

Every new vitamin product presents formulation problems for the solution of which no definite generalizations can be made since the effect of each ingredient of the product must be evaluated.

Incompatibilities of certain vitamins with some diluents and with other vitamins constantly appear and must be circumvented or prevented. For example, a rapid loss in vitamin B_{12} activity in the presence of ascorbic acid was reported (161). The greater stability of vitamin B_1 in the presence of ferrous gluconate than in the presence of iron peptonate or ferric ammonium citrate and the somewhat greater stability of thiamine mononitrate than thiamine hydrochloride in iron-containing preparations at pH 4.0 has been discussed (160). The fact that both white light and riboflavin promote the cleavage of folic acid and that riboflavin is very sensitive to light and undergoes irreversible decomposition on irradiation with ultraviolet rays or visible light (189) must be taken into consideration. Also, the hygroscopicity of crystalline vitamin B_{12} (*190*) and the ease of oxidation of vitamin A must be taken into account during formulation. These interactions and many others constantly present problems. Generalizations are difficult since concentration plays an important role. A small amount of one vitamin may be compatible with a small amount of another vitamin in a tablet provided there is enough of a third ingredient to keep them separated fairly well. However, if the concentrations of the vitamins are raised to high levels, such as in a therapeutic vitamin product, the problems may be entirely different. Vitamin–mineral combinations may present problems since not all vitamins are compatible with all the desired minerals. For example, it is known that ascorbic acid is inactivated on contact with copper ion. Also, some vitamins and minerals are most stable in acidic aqueous media, while other vitamins and minerals are most stable in neutral or alkaline aqueous media. Since water may enter the manufacturing process at some point, these factors must be considered.

A number of methods have been utilized to prevent or circumvent these difficulties. Some of these methods will be considered. Bogin (*173*) formed an emulsion from gelatin, the salt of a polyacidic polymer such as cellulose acetate phthalate, vitamins A and D, and water, with or without a plasticizer such as sugar or a sugar alcohol; this emulsion was run off in thin sheets, dried and the dried product comminuted, washed free of vitamin oil liberated during the grinding, and used as granules or put into gelatin capsules. Similarly, Taylor (*113*) protected vitamin A and Goett, *et al* (*193*), protected crystalline vitamin A acetate by incorporating them into gelatin beadlets using glucose, honey, or invert sugar as plasticizers. Such products can be used in compressed tablets or in coatings. Tablets containing vitamins from cod liver oil may be protected with a sugar or gelatin coating and also by an antioxidant such as hydroquinone (*62,117,138*). Oxidation of some vitamins may be prevented by dissolving the vitamins or their derivatives in a volatile solvent and mixing the solution with olive, linseed, or coconut oil, then stirring in a carrier which is insoluble in the solvent, evaporating the solvent from the mass and pressing the dried residue into tablets (*133*). Slugging instead of wet granulating may solve some of the problems. For example, Compton and Nicholls (*135*) incorporated B-complex vitamins with materials containing milk proteins and formed slugs which then were broken up into granules; the granules then were used to make tablets in the usual way. A derivative of a vitamin may be more stable than the original natural vitamin. For example, panthenol, the alcohol analog of pantothenic acid, is considerably more stable than pantothenate in acidic solutions at pH 3 to 5 and yet displays qualitatively and quantitatively the same vitamin activity (*150*). Puetzer (*139*) described new water-insoluble derivatives of thiamine which are useful in vitamin tablets. A Japanese patent (*181*) described the formation of a "solid colloid," by mixing an ether solution of cod liver oil with starch, evaporating the solvent *in vacuo*, and molding the product by compression into pills which were sugar coated. A number of recent patents have described methods for coating vitamins (*146,153,167–169,227,229,236*) and minerals (*170*) so as to increase their stability or decrease bitter tastes in various formulations. Generally these procedures involve coating small particles of the vitamin or mineral with a fatty or waxy material; however, improved stability may be obtained with vitamins imbedded in zein or hydrophilic carriers (*174,184*).

A problem pointed out by Termansen (*178*) was that pills containing vitamins A and D and made with a solid fat foundation had a hydrophobic surface and did not form a good bond with a hydrophilic sugar coating. He found that a thin layer of monostearin between the pill and the sugar and gelatin coating corrected this difficulty.

Other methods which have been utilized are:

1. Granulating with nonaqueous solvents.
2. Making 2- and 3-part granulations separately and combining them before compression.
3. Laminating some of the vitamins onto a tablet by a coating procedure, thus protecting them and preventing reaction with ingredients in the "core" tablet.
4. Placing compatible vitamins and minerals in one capsule or coated pill and inserting this into a larger capsule containing other desired constituents.

Testing of Coated Dosage Forms

Methods of testing coated dosage forms fall into five main classes:

1. *In vitro* disintegration tests.
2. *In vitro* dissolution-rate tests.
3. *In vivo* disintegration tests.
4. Physiological availability studies (in animal and man).
5. Clinical testing.

Examples of each of these will be discussed and the importance and limitation of each stressed.

In Vitro Disintegration Tests

An *in vitro* disintegration test for enteric-coated tablets is described in the USP. The Simulated Gastric Fluid TS has a pH of about 1.2 and is an aqueous solution containing pepsin and hydrochloric acid. The Simulated Intestinal Fluid TS has a pH of 7.5 ± 0.1 and is an aqueous solution prepared from monobasic potassium phosphate, sodium hydroxide, pancreatin, and water. In simplified form the requirements are that the enteric-coated tablets should withstand the Simulated Gastric Fluid TS for 1 hr and essentially disintegrate in the Simulated Intestinal Fluid TS within a period of time equal to the time specified in the monograph for the uncoated tablets plus 2 hr. Hence, for most tablets the time limit in the latter fluid is 2.5 hr, but for some tablets the time limit is 4 hr. When the tablets are in the Simulated Intestinal Fluid TS, each tube is provided with a slotted and perforated cylindrical plastic disk 9.5 ± 0.15 mm thick and 20.7 ± 0.15 mm in diameter. See the USP, page 932.

Prior to this test method becoming official, many different testing fluids were described in the literature (*21,22,40,51,75,111,122,132,134,143,185,200,240*). Not only has there been a great variation in the types of fluids used but also in the method of agitation (*22,40,48,111,116,122,175,185,241*), the temperature of the solutions, and the disintegration end-points (*40,111,175,199*). Many types of disintegration apparatus have been described; a few are cited here (*40,48,111,116,122,175,247*). In general the procedures of the *in vitro* disintegration tests for enteric-coated products have involved leaving the samples in a simulated gastric fluid for an arbitrary length of time, then transferring them to a simulated intestinal fluid, and noting the length of time required for disintegration.

In vitro disintegration tests are indispensable in research on coated products and for the purpose of quality control. As Kanig (*204*) pointed out: "At best it would seem advisable that a combination of standardized *in vivo* and *in vitro* tests be made on the same coating, and a uniform means of interpolating results from both would present a truer picture of the coating's relative efficiency. It is obvious that it is difficult, if not impossible, for human subjects to be utilized in a repeated quality control procedure of testing during large-scale production. For this reason it is of added importance that an established and standardized *in vitro* testing method be utilized as an additional check in the manufacturing laboratory."

In light of present knowledge, *in vitro* disintegration tests alone should not be used to predict what will happen to the coated dosage units in the human being or animals unless one first establishes a correlation between the *in vitro* and *in vivo* test results. The data obtained from both types of tests should be treated mathematically and statistically, and the relationship between the *in vitro* and *in vivo* results shown graphically or by an equation. A example of such a correlation is that of Wagner, *et al* (186), who related the disintegration times of certain enteric-coated tablets in the small intestine of the dog with the disintegration times of tablets from the same lots in artificial intestinal fluids, pH 6.9. Wagner, *et al* (108), reported that an *in vitro* test in simulated gastric fluid served to predict the period of time which tablets coated with styrene–maleic acid copolymer, dibutyl phthalate, and talc resisted stomach contents of human subjects.

Another useful preliminary screening test for enteric substances was reported by Antonides and DeKay (199). This method is based upon the weight of films of the substance lost when the films are placed separately in artificial gastric fluid and artificial intestinal fluid. A statistical method was applied to the data obtained.

Too often it is assumed that if a product is not enteric coated it is not necessary to carry out disintegration tests for control and research purposes. References (86,175,187,231) indicate that in some instances ordinary compressed tablets, sugar-coated tablets, and film-coated tablets have passed through the gastrointestinal tract and appeared in human feces. It is important to point out that one *can* make "sugar coatings" and "film coatings" as well as "compressed tablets" which are more resistant to *in vivo* disintegration than many enteric-coated tablets and other dosage units which do function in the intended manner.

Bruns and Huyck (195) reported disintegration times of 28 commercially available coated tablets (most of them sugar-coated tablets) obtained by use of the method which is now official in USP XVIII. Studies by Steinberg, *et al* (230), using x-ray visualization of tablets containing radiopaque pellets, have shown that agitation in the stomach is of a low order of magnitude. Substantially higher disintegration times may be encountered *in vitro* than those obtained using the USP *in vitro* apparatus.

In Vitro Dissolution-Rate Tests

In vitro dissolution-rate studies of enteric-coated tablets can yield a great deal of useful information about the efficiency of the coating. Determination of the dissolution profile in acid fluid serves to detect leaching of the drug from the coated tablet due to imperfections or nonuniformity of the coating. Dissolution-rate studies of coated and uncoated tablets in simulated intestinal fluid may be used to evaluate the effect of coating in the release of drug from the tablet matrix or granules. *In vitro* dissolution-rate studies of coated tablets may be conducted by sampling the dissolution

medium at various times and assaying the aliquot for drug content (5). The automated dissolution-rate method of Schroeter and Wagner (2) is especially well suited for continuously monitoring the dissolution fluid for long periods of time. Levy (63) has emphasized the importance of using physiologically realistic agitation intensities in conducting dissolution tests of dosage forms. Morrison and Campbell (79) have pointed out that available evidence suggests that no single dissolution rate test can be applied to all drugs.

In Vivo Disintegration Tests

In vivo disintegration tests which have been utilized may be categorized in two main classes—direct and indirect methods. Among the direct methods, roentgenography and roentgenoscopy have been the most commonly used. Roentgenography is preferred since a permanent record is obtained and since the exposure to x-rays is less than in the roentgenoscopic or fluoroscopic method (76). Lozinski and Diver (57) introduced the use of roentgenoscopy with barium sulfate tablets and the barium meal to follow the path of enteric-coated tablets through the stomach and into the intestine. However, they administered enteric-coated sodium salicylate tablets with the enteric-coated barium sulfate tablets and determined intestinal disintegration by means of a test for salicylate in the subject's urine. The fact that some tablets leave the stomach before others, even though they are all of the same size, complicates this method. Bukey and Brew (64) apparently were the first to report the use of roentgenography; they followed the path of a large number of enteric-coated dosage forms through the gastrointestinal tract of human subjects. The roentgenographic technique was used by many other investigators (68,71,75,81,82,95–97,99,111,124,134,143, 186,199). A number of other investigators (92,96,199– 201) used roentgenoscopy alone or in combination with roentgenography.

The advantages of these tests are as follows: (1) they provide a relatively simple method to determine the stomach emptying time of the coated units, and hence the effect of the size of the dosage units on the stomach emptying time can be investigated; (2) they provide a reasonably good estimate of the part of the gastrointestinal tract where disintegration of the dosage units takes place. If the latter is found to be considerably distal to the duodenum for a certain type of coating, this knowledge may preclude the use of that coating for drugs known to be absorbed from the stomach or the upper parts of the intestinal tract only.

The disadvantage of these tests is that observed disintegration in the gastrointestinal tract does not guarantee that the drug will be absorbed (197). In some cases the dosage unit may be distal to the normal site of absorption for the contained drug, and hence the percentage of the dose absorbed may be considerably less than would be possible with a different dosage unit. Each coated product should preferably be individually studied for such effects.

Another type of direct *in vivo* disintegration test was described by Gruber, *et al* (235). They attached a string by means of an impervious glue to the enteric dosage unit. The tablets were then swallowed by the subject and withdrawn after fixed periods of time to be examined visually or photographed. They reported that 20 in. of string was required for the stomach while 30 in. of string allowed the tablet to pass into the intestine. Metal rings were attached to the string near the tablet to permit x-ray determination of the position in the gastrointestinal tract.

The indirect *in vivo* disintegration tests which have been described in the literature have utilized radioactive, urine, and saliva indicators. Use of radioactive indicators to test enteric coatings was introduced by Lark-Horovitz and Leng (*112,114*). Their method was based on the use of radioactive ^{24}NaCl, the radiations of which are detected by a Geiger counter. The radioactive Na, mass 24, which has a half-life of 14.8 hr, is used in only very small quantities. Hence, the method is not dangerous. Capsules containing the radioactive salt were enteric-coated along with ordinary salt capsules and then separated using a Geiger counter. The capsules were administered and their path in the stomach and intestines was followed with a movable counter. By using a second stationary counter mounted in a lead shield, the entry of radioactive ^{24}Na into the blood (after disintegration of the enteric coating) was determined by measuring the activity in the hand of the subject. A plot was made of counts per minute vs time in hours. While the capsule was intact, the activity in the hand was zero or a relatively constant value due to background. When the capsule dissolved, a rapid increase of activity in the tissues was observed by a rapid increase in the counts per minute detected by the counter in the hand. The method has one definite advantage, ie, any leak or permeability of the coating before the coating actually disintegrates or dissolves is detected within a few minutes by the activity in the hand. Roentgenography or roentgenoscopy usually will not detect such slow release or a leak. The method has one definite disadvantage when applied to human subjects, ie, the exact site of disintegration cannot be established (*163*).

In an attempt to overcome this disadvantage of the radioactive indicator method, Peterson, *et al* (*163*), introduced a modification. They administered small pills containing radioactive ^{24}NaCl and gentian violet to rats and determined the time of disintegration by detecting the radiation in the rat's tail with a shielded Geiger counter. The animal was sacrificed, its abdomen opened, and the exact site of disintegration established by locating the gentian violet stain. Obviously, their modification is limited to animal studies.

Couvreur, *et al* (*198*), investigated cellulose acetate phthalate enteric coatings using radioactive ^{131}I alone and in combination with roentgenography using barium sulfate as the opaque substance. They reported that a dose of 10 microcuries of ^{131}I was capable of being detected satisfactorily in human subjects.

Wruble (*40*) introduced the so-called "double-check" tablets containing methylene blue and calcium sulfide. They were intended to function as follows: if the tablet disintegrated in the stomach, the acid reacted with the calcium sulfide giving rise to eructations of hydrogen sulfide; if the tablet resisted stomach contents and disintegrated in the intestines, the urine was colored blue; if neither effect was observed, it was concluded that the tablet passed through the gastrointestinal tract unchanged. Bukey and Bliven (*76*) stated that this method leads to erroneous interpretations of results because of the relatively small amount of hydrogen sulfide liberated and its solubility in stomach fluids.

Gruber, *et al* (*235*), used both direct and indirect methods to test a compression-coated enteric tablet. One of their indirect methods depended on the administration of enteric iodide tablets followed by assays for the iodide in the saliva.

Physiological Availability Studies

Physiological availability studies in animals and man have been performed for many years, but in recent years greater emphasis has been placed upon them. It was pointed out in an editorial (*197*) that "there could be a great difference between disintegration and absorption times, depending on what part of the intestine the drug had reached." Chapman, *et al* (*214*), stated that "both the pharmaceutical industry and regulatory bodies appear to have made more progress in developing methods for the determination of the ingredients of tablets than for assessing their physiological availability." A satisfactory physiological availability study (*187*) is one in which (1) the percentage of the dose of the drug administered which is available to the tissues is determined or (2) the amount of drug available to the tissues from a given dose of drug in one dosage form is compared with the amount of drug available to the tissues from the same dose administered in a control form (such as a compressed tablet or as a solution). When comparisons are made, the best control is really a solution of the drug in aqueous media. If this is possible, all considerations of disintegration time are eliminated. However, if the dose of drug under consideration is not soluble in a reasonable volume of water or, if for reasons of stability, etc, a solution would not be a normal method of administration of the drug, a rapidly disintegrating compressed tablet would provide a suitable control dosage form.

When blood concentration C is plotted against time t, following oral administration of a drug which is absorbed in the gastrointestinal tract, the curve rises to a maximum and falls off exponentially. Under certain conditions (*237*) the total amount of drug absorbed, y, is given by:

$$y = k_2 V \int_{t=0}^{t=\infty} C dt$$

where y is the amount of drug absorbed; V is the volume of distribution of the drug in the body; and k_2 is the elimination rate constant. The integral is equal to the area under the blood-level curve. If the same subjects are administered a drug in two different dosage forms in a cross-over experiment, one can determine whether the same amount of drug was available from each form by comparing the areas under the blood-level curves. The difficulty in applying this equation is that a sufficient number of blood-level determinations must be made following each dose on each subject to get a reasonably true representation of the actual blood-level curve. In cases where the drug undergoes metabolic transformation as well as urinary excretion, other terms sometimes have to be introduced (*237,238*). Wagner and Nelson (*17*) have described equations which permit one to prepare per cent absorbed-time plots directly from suitable blood- and/or urinary-excretion data following oral administration of a drug without knowing the volume of distribution V. Such *in vivo* per cent absorbed-time plots provide the optimum data for correlation with per cent released-time plots derived from *in vitro* dissolution-rate testing.

If the drug is stored in the tissues or metabolically transformed to some extent, one must show by a separate study that the urinary excretion parallels the amount of drug absorbed. For example, Oser, *et al* (*187*), showed that the urinary excretion of certain water-soluble vitamins parallels the quantity consumed (in completely available form), provided normal subjects are employed and that at the time of the tests they consume an adequate diet. For the purpose of calculating the degree of vitamin availability, comparison was made between the urinary excretion after taking the test dose and that following the oral administration of an aqueous solution of the pure vitamin.

The first physiological availability study done on a coated product was that reported by Wruble (70). He administered both uncoated and enteric-coated sodium salicylate tablets to eight subjects. A complete 48-hr specimen of urine was collected in each case and analyzed for salicylate after hydrolyzing the salicyluric acid. The average recovery following the ingestion of 15 gr of salicylate was approximately 30% of the dose, and the results indicated close agreement between the quantities of salicylate excreted following administration of the coated and the uncoated tablets. Swintosky and Blythe (67) employed urinary excretion data to determine availability of salicylate from enteric and uncoated tablets.

The study of Oser, *et al* (187), was quite extensive. They reported: "It has been demonstrated that vitamin availability may be reduced even in tablets or capsules which disintegrate *in vitro* and *in vivo*, and that one vitamin may be completely available for absorption while another is only partly available." Chapman, *et al* (214,243,244), reported data which indicated that tablets which did not disintegrate *in vitro* in 60 min (30 min in simulated gastric juice, pH 1.6, and 30 min, or until disintegrated, in simulated alkaline juice, pH 8.0) were not completely available to the human subject as judged by urinary excretion of riboflavin. The same authors reported similar results when sodium *p*-aminosalicylate was used as the tracer substance (246) and only sugar-coated tablets were tested. Middleton, *et al* (252), have demonstrated a close relationship between *in vitro* disintegration time and dissolution rate ($T_{50\%}$) for various sugar-coated riboflavin tablets. Both procedures correlated with physiological availability as measured by urinary riboflavin excretion. There is uncertainty in extrapolating such data and applying it to drugs other than those tested. Morrison and Campbell (25) reported that enteric-coated salicylate tablets with *in vitro* disintegration times as long as 213 min were fully available *in vivo*, whereas a riboflavin preparation with an *in vitro* disintegration time of 128 min was only 41% available *in vivo*. There are even greater mistakes made when it is assumed that physiological variations such as the pH of the intestines will affect coated dosage forms more than it will affect uncoated dosage forms (242).

Each drug and each coated dosage form is an individual problem. For example, even in the water-soluble vitamin field Johnson and Berger (239) showed that there was no statistical differences in the total fecal excretion of ^{60}Co-labeled vitamin B_{12} when it was administered to groups of human subjects in aqueous solution or in four different coated forms, the most heavily coated of which was designed for 7-hr release in the lower small intestine. Similarly, Endicott and Kirchmeyer (215) presented evidence that tablets requiring considerably more than 1 hr to disintegrate *in vitro* by the previous official test (USP XV-NF X) may still be satisfactory drug sources in the human body. They pointed out that "the two drugs studied by Chapman, *et al*, were both only slightly soluble in gastric juice" and "this insolubility in gastric juice would contribute to the results obtained *in vivo*." They also pointed out that "it may well be desirable to sacrifice a certain amount of 'availability' in order to

gain such advantages as (1) protecting a drug from the acid of the stomach, (2) covering a bitter taste so that it is more acceptable to the patient, (3) releasing the drug over a period of time so that the effect from one tablet will be prolonged for several hours instead of a short time, and (4) to protect the gastrointestinal tract from corrosive or nauseous substances."

Some reports have appeared in the literature concerning blood levels achieved after administration of enteric dosage forms. Kirby, *et al* (223), reported erythromycin serum concentrations following administration of acid-resistant tablets. Japanese investigators (245) claimed the blood level of Benadryl plateaued for 5–6 hr following administration of the drug in acid-resistant tablets. Tarnowski (216) pointed out that shellac-coated *p*-aminosalicylic acid granules progressively change in *in vitro* and *in vivo* disintegration behavior releasing drug much slower as they age at room temperature. There have been favorable blood-level studies reported for sustained-action products, as discussed on page 1709.

Clinical Testing

Clinical testing of coated dosage forms is an integral part of their proper evaluation. *In vitro* disintegration tests, *in vivo* disintegration tests, and physiological availability studies are essential research tools, but if the coated dosage form is to be used in the treatment of a specific disease or diseases then clinical testing is necessary also. The difficulty with clinical testing is that in many cases it is difficult to get good, objective end-points and data which can be analyzed and treated statistically. Blind, cross-over clinical trials which include suitable placebo and/or control dosage forms in the study are desirable for objective evaluation of the test preparation. Although criticism has been made by the medical profession about many coated dosage forms (242), the main difficulty stems from the fact that few adequately controlled studies have been made from which to draw conclusions, and the latter should not be made until the data are adequate. As pointed out previously, each drug and each coated dosage form is an individual problem and should be treated as such. In any given chemotherapeutic field thousands of compounds are screened and tested before a few become marketable drugs. There have been relatively few clinical tests on coated dosage forms, some being favorable and some others, unfavorable; just because a few tests have been unfavorable does not mean that we should stop research in this important area.

A few of the clinical papers on coated products (excluding sustained-action oral dosage forms which are reviewed in the next chapter) will be cited. Kupfer, *et al* (219), administered to each of 18 patients one 250-mg tablet of acetazolamide (Diamox) and 250 mg of the same drug in the form of an enteric-coated capsule every 12 hr. The authors reported this regimen reduced ocular tension for the 12 hr, whereas the effect of the tablet alone lasted for only about 6 hr. Tatge, *et al* (220), tested enteric-coated aminometramide (Mictine) and reported that this dosage form "may provide a safe and useful addition to the diuretic armamentarium." Sprecker (222) administered enteric-coated acetylsalicylic acid (Ecotrin) to 32 arthritic patients with histories of gastric intolerance to aspirin. Thirty of the 32 patients reported neither gastrointestinal disturbances nor any other side effects. Frye, *et al* (224), tested enteric-coated tablets of dithiazanine. They reported the dosage form was an effective trichuricide and that the patients showed no signs of intolerance. When the same drug was given in gelatin capsules, nausea and vomiting occurred.

Removal of Coating from Coated Tablets

The removal of coating from coated tablets which are considered unsuitable for release by control laboratories is sometimes necessary. An older method of doing this was to place the tablets in a pan, cover them with water, and stir them until the edges of the tablets began to appear. The water was then poured off and the tablets covered with denatured alcohol to absorb the excess water. After the alcohol was drained off the tablets were placed in a coating pan and dried under the air blast.

Another procedure (164) involved the removal of the coating with 45% isopropyl alcohol, after which 91% isopropyl alcohol was added to stop removal of the coating. The latter was added until the tablets were no longer sticky and then hot air was applied to the rolling tablets. It was claimed that the process required from 1 to 1½ hr, approximately 1 gal of 45% isopropyl alcohol, and somewhat more than 1 gal of 91% isopropanol for 60 to 80 lb of coated tablets.

A third method (171) for removing coatings has been reported. Nearly an equal weight of rejected coated tablets of a size different from those to be washed was selected so that a simple screening would separate the two sizes of tablets. The rejected tablets were rotated in a heated coating pan while the tablets from which the coating was to be removed were soaked in water until the coating was removed to the desired extent. The water was drained off and the washed tablets transferred to the coating pan and allowed to roll until dry. The heated rejected tablets absorbed the residual water from the washed tablets.

Stephensen and Smith (177) attempted to remove sugar coatings from commercial tablets with the intention of analyzing the coatings. They concluded that no simple or generally applicable method for the removal of sugar coatings from tablets had been found, but they suggested two methods which can be applied to a wide range of tablets. One method was to heat the tablets in an oven at 105°C for 5–15 min and drop them into alcohol. The coating in some cases could be removed immediately by pressing the tablets between the thumb nail and first finger. The other method was to expose the tablets to an atmosphere saturated with moisture until the coating could be scraped from the tablet.

Bibliography

1. Schroeter, L. C., *Ingredient X*, Pergamon Press, New York, 1968.
2. Schroeter, L. C., and Wagner, J. G., *J. Pharm. Sci.*, **51**, 957 (1962).
3. Lachman, L., and Cooper, J., *J. Pharm. Sci.*, **52**, 490 (1963).
4. Bennett, H. W., and Hess, F. T., *J. Pharm. Sci.*, **52**, 608 (1963).
5. Schroeter, L. C., et al, *J. Pharm. Sci.*, **51**, 865 (1962).
6. Unna, *Pharm. Zentralhalle*, **25**, 577 (1884); through *Fortschr. Med.*, **15**, 507 (1884). *Brit. Med. J.*; through *J. Am. Med. Assoc.*, **14**, 4 (Apr. 4, 1885). *Am. J. Pharm.*, **57**, 338 (1885).
7. Pomeranz, M. A., et al, *J. Am. Geriat. Soc.*, **14**, 200 (1966).
8. Sonnendecker, G., and Griffenhagen, G. B., *J. APhA, Pract. Ed.*, **18**, 486 (1957).
9. Noyes, P. J., US Pat. 568,488 (Sept. 29, 1896).
10. Noyes, P. J., US Pat. 582,794 (May 18, 1897).
11. Martin, E. W., ed., *Husa's Pharmaceutical Dispensing*, Mack Publ. Co., Easton, Pa., 1959, pp. 93–101.
12. Tucker, S. J., and Rednick, A. B., *J. APhA, Sci. Ed.*, **49**, 738 (1960).
13. Warner, W. R., Jr., *Am. J. Pharm.*, **74**, 32 (1902).
14. Wiegand, T. S., *Am. J. Pharm.*, **74**, 33 (1902).
15. Wood, J. R., *Tablet Manufacture*, Lippincott, Philadelphia, 1906, p. 85.
16. Abbott Labs., Brit. Pat. Spec. 764,342 (Dec. 28, 1956).
17. Wagner, J. G., and Nelson, E., *J. Pharm. Sci.*, **52**, 610 (1963).
18. Grosh, D. M., *Merck Report*, **20**, 181 (1911).
19. Long, S. (Upjohn Co.), US Pat. 3,043,747 (July 10, 1962).
20. Tucker, S. J., and Rednick, A. B., *J. APhA, Sci. Ed.*, **49**, 738 (1960).

21. Scoville, W. L., *J. APhA*, **4**, 1241 (1915).
22. Toplis, W. G., *Am. J. Pharm.*, **87**, 518 (1915).
23. Tucker, S. J., et al, *J. APhA, Sci. Ed.*, **47**, 849 (1958).
24. McClendon, J. F., *Am. J. Physiol.*, **38**, 191 (1915).
25. Morrison, A. B., and Campbell, J. A., *J. APhA, Sci. Ed.*, **49**, 473 (1960).
26. Long, J. H., and Fenger, F., *J. Am. Chem. Soc.*, **39**, 1278 (1917).
27. Stokes, F. J., US Pat. 1,248,571 (Dec. 4, 1917).
28. Fantus, B., *J. APhA*, **7**, 249 (1918).
29. Doerr, D. W., et al (Univ. of Ill. Found.), US Pats. 2,816,061 and 2,816,062 (Dec. 10, 1957).
30. McClendon, J. F., et al., *J. Am. Med. Assoc.*, **75**, 1638 (1920).
31. Myers, F. J., and McClendon, J. F., *J. Biol. Chem.*, **41**, 187 (1920).
32. Okada, S., and Arai, M., *J. Biol. Chem.*, **51**, 135 (1922).
33. White, R. C., *J. APhA*, **11**, 345 (1922).
34. Stokes, F. J., *Tablet and Pill Coating*, F. J. Stokes Co., Philadelphia, 1900.
35. Rose, E. S., *Am. J. Pharm.*, **96**, 590 (1924).
36. Rose, E. S., *Am. J. Pharm.*, **97**, 71 (1925).
37. Winters, E. P., and Deardorff, D. L., *J. APhA, Sci. Ed.*, **45**, 125 (1956); ibid, **47**, 608 (1958).
38. Ahsan, S. S., and Blaur, S. M., *Drug. Std.*, **26**, 29 (1958).
39. Abbott Labs., Brit. Pat. Spec. 762,229 (Nov. 28, 1956).
40. Wruble, M. S., *Am. J. Pharm.*, **102**, 318 (1930).
41. Anderson, W., and Sakr, A. M., *J. Pharm. Pharmacol.*, **18**, 783 (1966).
42. Lachman, L., et al, *J. Pharm. Sci.*, **52**, 379 (1963).
43. Lachman, L., et al, *J. Pharm. Sci.*, **55**, 958 (1966).
44. Bollman and Mann, *Proc. Staff Meet., Mayo Clinic*, **5**, 68 (1930).
45. Vérzar and von Kúthy, *Biochem. Z.*, **230**, 451 (1931).
46. Lachman, L., *Mfg. Chemist Aerosol News*, **37**, 35 (1966).
47. Cooper, J., and Pasquale, D., *Pharm. J.*, **181**, 397 (1958).
48. Weyland, J., *Apoth. Ztg.*, **46**, 470 (1931); through *Yearbook APhA*, **20**, 180 (1931).
49. Robinson, C. W., *Chemist Druggist*, 214 (Feb. 24, 1954).
50. Gjaldbaek, J. K., and Irgang, M., *Dansk Tidsskr. Farm.*, **6**, 201 (1932); through *C. A.*, **27**, 5146 (1933).
51. Husa, W. J., and Magid, L., *J. APhA*, **21**, 1030 (1932).
52. Evans Medical Supplies, Ltd., Brit. Pat. Spec. 744,799 (1956).
53. Anon., *Drug Trade News*, 9 (July 16, 1956).
54. Millar, J. F., et al (Charles E. Frosst & Co.), US Pat. 2,991,226 (July 4, 1961).
55. Mitchell, K. A., *Mfg. Chemist*, 107 (Mar., 1955).
56. Kirk, W. J., US Pat. 1,881,197 (Oct. 4, 1933); through *C. A.* **27**, 566 (1933).
57. Lozinski, E., and Diver, G. R., *J. APhA*, **22**, 143 (1933).
58. Wagner, J. G., et al, *J. APhA, Sci. Ed.*, **49**, 133 (1960).
59. Robinson, C. W., *Mfg. Chemist*, 164 (Apr. 1955).
60. Wolff, J. E. (Merck & Co.), US Pat. 2,757,124 (July 31, 1956).
61. Vérzar, F., *Nutr. Abstr. Rev.*, **2**, 441 (1933).
62. Nitardy, F. W., US Pat. 1,879,762 (Sept. 27, 1933); through *C. A.*, **27**, 374 (1933).
63. Levy, G., *J. Pharm. Sci.*, **52**, 1039 (1963).
64. Bukey, F. S., and Brew, M., *J. APhA*, **23**, 1217 (1934).
65. Carr, W. G., et al, *J. Clin. Invest.*, **14**, 893 (1935).
66. DeLong Gum Co., Brit. Pat. 439,534 (Dec. 9, 1935).
67. Swintosky, J. V., and Blythe, R. H., *Drug Std.*, **28**, 5 (1960).
68. Bukey, F. S., and Brew, M., *J. APhA*, **24**, 291 (1935).
69. Wruble, M. S., *J. APhA*, **24**, 570 (1935).
70. Wruble, M. S., *J. APhA*, **24**, 1074 (1935).
71. Bukey, F. S., and Rhodes, P., *J. APhA*, **24**, 567 (1935).
72. Singiser, R. E., and Lowenthal, W., *J. Pharm. Sci.*, **50**, 168 (1961).
73. US Pats. 2,700,938 (Jan. 1955) and 2,727,473 (Dec. 1955). See also Brit. Pat. Spec. 739,711 (Merck & Co.) (Nov. 2, 1955) and Ref. 60.
74. Peterson, C. E., US Pat. 2,044,748 (June 16, 1936).
75. Defelice, L. F., *Rev. Farm. (Buenos Aires)*, **78**, 453 (1936); through *C. A.*, **31**, 15535 (1937).
76. Bukey, F. S., and Bliven, C. W., *J. APhA*, **25**, 119 (1936).
77. Kilian, Brit. Pat. 464,903 (Apr. 27, 1937).
78. Peterson, C. E., US Pat. 2,087,675 (July 20, 1937).
79. Morrison, A. B., and Campbell, J. A., *J. Pharm. Sci.*, **54**, 1 (1965).
80. Butensky, I. S., *Automatic Coating of Tablets*, PhD Thesis, Univ. of Michigan, 1962, 201 pp.
81. Bukey, F. S., and Brew, M., *J. Lab. Clin. Med.*, **22**, 918 (1937).
82. Mills, L. M., *J. APhA*, **26**, 479 (1937).
83. Tsevdos, T. J., *Drug Cosmetic Ind.*, **78**, 38 (1956).
84. Windheuser, J., and Cooper, J., *J. APhA, Sci. Ed.*, **45**, 542 (1956).
85. Kwan, K. C., *Coating of Tablets with Syrup*, PhD Thesis, Univ. of Michigan, 1962, 138 pp.
86. Wynn, V., and Landon, J., *J. Pharm. Pharmacol.*, **15**, 123 (1963).
87. Wolff, J. E., et al, *Symposium on Compression Coating*, presented at 4th Pan-American Congress of Pharmacy and Biochemistry, Washington, D.C., Nov. 3–9, 1957.
88. Howell, W. H., *A Textbook of Physiology*, 13th ed., Saunders, Philadelphia, 1938, pp. 821, 849, 852, 858.
89. Tucker, S. J., et al, *J. APhA, Sci. Ed.*, **47**, 849 (1959).
90. Svedres, E. V. (Smith Kline & French International Co.), S. African Pat. 2741 (1953).
91. American Cyanamid Co., Brit. Pat. Spec. 756,082 (1956).
92. Leyton, C., and Peñafiel, M., *Anales Quim. Farm. (Chile)*, 23 (1938); through *C. A.*, **33**, 2282 (1939).
93. Wagner, J. G., et al, *J. APhA, Sci. Ed.*, **48**, 244 (1959).
94. Ida, T., et al, *J. Pharm. Sci.*, **51**, 1061 (1962).
95. Worton, A. G., et al, *J. APhA*, **27**, 21 (1938).
96. Crane, A. W., and Wruble, M. S., *Am. J. Roentgenol. Radium Therapy*, **39**, 450 (1938).
97. Goorley, J. T., and Lee, C. O., *J. APhA*, **27**, 379 (1938).
98. Rednick, A. B., et al, *J. Pharm. Sci.*, **50**, 174 (1961).
99. Bukey, F. S., and Klemme, C. J., *J. APhA*, **28**, 87 (1939).
100. Blythe, R. H., *Drug Std.*, **26**, 1 (1958).
101. Sugimoto, N., and Ida, T., US Pat. 3,041,243 (June 26, 1962).

102. Kremers, E., and Urdang, G., *History of Pharmacy*, Lippincott, Philadelphia, 1940, pp. 20, 319.
103. Chilson, F., *Drug Cosmetic Ind.*, **47**, 441 (1940).
104. Hiatt, G. D., US Pat. 2,196,768 (Apr. 9, 1940).
105. Mody, D. S., et al, *J. Pharm. Sci.*, **53**, 949 (1964).
106. Banker, G. S., *J. Pharm. Sci.*, **55**, 81 (1966).
107. Coletta, V., and Rubin, H., *J. Pharm. Sci.*, **53**, 953 (1964).
108. Wagner, J. G., et al., *J. APhA*, *Sci. Ed.*, **49**, 128 (1960).
109. Swintosky, J. V. (Smith Kline & French Labs.), US Pat. 2,971,889 (Feb. 14, 1961).
110. Lesser, M. A., *Drug Cosmetic Ind.*, **49**, 151 (1941).
111. Maney, P. V., and Kuever, R. A., *J. APhA*, *Sci. Ed.*, **30**, 276 (1941).
112. Lark-Horovitz, K., and Leng, Herta, R., *Nature*, **147**, 580 (1941).
113. Taylor, H. F., US Pats. 2,218,591 and 2,218,592 (Oct. 22, 1941).
114. Lark-Horovitz, K., and Leng, Herta, R., *J. APhA*, *Sci. Ed.*, **31**, 99 (1942).
115. Andersson, C. J., and Toft-Madsen, C. J., *Farmac. Tid.*, **52**, 252 (1942); *Chem. Zentr.*, II, 1152 (1942); through *C. A.*, **37**, 6089 (1943).
116. Schiffmann, R. Y., and Mirimanoff, A., *Pharm. Acta Helv.*, **17**, 141 (1942).
117. Vastagh, G., *Pharm. Zentralhalle*, **83**, 481 (1942); *Chem. Zentr.*, I, 59 (1943); through *C. A.*, **38**, 30919 (1944).
118. Bickenheuser, F. J., US Pat. 2,312,381 (Mar. 2, 1943).
119. Moeller, W. C., and Smith, L. A. (Parmelee Co.), US Pat. 2,955,982 (Oct. 11, 1960).
120. Wisconsin Alumni Research Foundation, Brit. Pat. Spec. 899,900 (1962).
121. Urdang, G., *What's New*, 5, (1943); through *J. APhA*, **34**, 135 (1945).
122. Abbott, A. H. A., and Allport, N. L., *Quart. J. Pharm. Pharmacol.*, **16**, 183 (1943); *Pharm. J.*, **151**, 52 (1943); *Chemist and Druggist*, **140**, 122 (1943).
123. Feinblatt, T. M., and Ferguson, E. A., Jr., *New Engl. J. Med.*, **256**, 331 (1957).
124. Brenner, J., *Pharm. Acta Helv.*, **18**, 283 (1943).
125. Best, C. H., and Taylor, N. B., *The Living Body: A Text in Human Physiology*, Henry Holt, New York, 1944, p. 232.
126. Rosenthal, S., and Nasset, E. S., *J. Nutr.*, **66**, 91 (1958).
127. Kläui, H., *Schweiz. Apoth. Ztg.*, **95**, 153 (1957); through *C. A.*, **51**, 12429d (1957).
128. Endicott, C. J., and Martin, W. T. (Abbott Labs.), Can. Pat. 643,311 (June 19, 1962).
129. Lyman, R. A., ed., *American Pharmacy*, Lippincott, Philadelphia, 1945, pp. 440–442.
130. Abbott Labs., Brit. Pat. Spec. 899,053 (1962).
131. Thompson, H. O., and Lee, C. O., *J. APhA*, **34**, 135 (1945).
132. Thompson, H. O., and Lee, C. O., *J. APhA*, **34**, 138 (1945).
133. Blumenthal, R. G., Brit. Pat. 568,691 (Apr. 17, 1945); through *C. A.*, **41**, 4278d (1947).
134. Junager, S. A., *Arch. Pharm. Chemi*, **53**, 425 (1946); through *Pharm. Abstr.*, **13**, 51 (1947).
135. Compton, W. A., and Nicholls, R. S., US Pat. 2,406,741 (Sept. 3, 1946); through *C. A.*, **41**, 254b (1947).
136. Hosler, W. W. (Strong, Cobb & Co.), Can. Pat. 512,355 (1955).
137. Tanabe Seiyaku Co., Brit. Pat. Spec. 888,131 (1962).
138. Sandell, E., *Farm. Revy.*, **45**, 697 (1946); through *C. A.*, **41**, 563d (1947).
139. Puetzer, B., US Pat. 2,397,903 (Apr. 2, 1946); through *C. A.*, **40**, 3858 (1946).
140. Winthrop-Stearns, Inc., Australian Pat. 206,852 (Apr. 4, 1957).
141. Zagnoli, R. C. (Abbott Labs.), Can. Pat. 651,929 (Nov. 6, 1962).
142. Osol, A., Farrar, G. E., et al, *The Dispensatory of the United States of America*, 24th ed., Lippincott, Philadelphia, 1947, p. 1178.
143. Bauer, C. W., and Masucci, P. E., *J. APhA*, *Sci. Ed.*, **37**, 124 (1948).
144. Kelley, W. C., *J. APhA*, *Sci. Ed.*, **37**, 332 (1948).
145. Kelley, W. C., *J. APhA*, *Sci. Ed.*, **37**, 253 (1948).
146. Koff, A. (Hoffmann-La Roche), US Pat. 2,080,292 (Mar. 5, 1963).
147. Rowell, T. H., *Drug Cosmetic Ind.*, **63**, 309 (1948).
148. Rowell, T. H., *Drug Cosmetic Ind.*, **63**, 458 (1948).
149. Nakao, K. Japan. Pat. 174,948 (June 24, 1958); through *C. A.*, **43**, 6791d (1949).
150. Rubin, S. H., *J. APhA*, *Sci. Ed.*, **37**, 502 (1948).
151. Rowell, T. H., *Drug Cosmetic Ind.*, **64**, 300 (1949).
152. Rowell, T. H., *The Art of Coating Tablets*, Baudette, Minn., 1949.
153. Merck & Co., Brit. Pat. Spec. 922,697 (1963).
154. Millar, J. F., and Lindner, G., Can. Pat. 652,743 (Nov. 20, 1962).
155. Koren, J. A., and Benton, B. E., *J. APhA*, *Sci. Ed.*, **38**, 267 (1949).
156. Lyman, R. A., ed., *Pharmaceutical Compounding and Dispensing*, Lippincott, Philadelphia, 1959, pp. 78–80.
157. Little, A., and Mitchell, K. A., *Tablet Making*, Northern Publ. Co. Ltd., Liverpool, England, 1949, pp. 53, 54, 82, 87.
158. Abbott Labs., Brit. Pat. Spec. 907,309 (1962).
159. Consolazio, W. V., US Pat. 2,478,182 (Aug. 9, 1949); through *C. A.*, **43**, 8619h (1949).
160. Taube, A., et al, *J. APhA*, *Sci. Ed.*, **38**, 119 (1949).
161. Gakenheimer, W. C., and Feller, B. A., *J. APhA*, *Sci. Ed.*, **38**, 660 (1949).
162. Abbott Labs., Brit. Pat. Spec. 907,310 (1962).
163. Peterson, C. F., et al, *J. APhA*, *Sci. Ed.*, **39**, 607 (1950).
164. Curlin, L. C., *J. APhA*, *Sci. Ed.*, **39**, 112 (1950).
165. Yen, E. C., and Stirn, F. E., US Pat. 2,512,192 (June 20, 1950).
166. Pierce, J. A., US Pat. 2,500,770 (Mar. 19, 1950); through *C. A.*, **44**, 4608f (1950).
167. Rosenberg, A., US Pat. 2,973,266 (Feb. 28, 1961).
168. Stoyle, L. E., et al (Merck & Co.), US Pat. 3,037,911 (June 5, 1962).
169. Stoyle, L. E., et al (Merck & Co.), Can. Pats. 646,134 and 646,135 (Aug. 7, 1962).
170. Stoyle, L. E., et al (Merck & Co.), Can. Pat. 641,311 (May 15, 1962).
171. Herreygers, F. W., *J. APhA*, *Sci. Ed.*, **40**, 218 (1951).
172. Malm, C. J., et al, *J. APhA*, *Sci. Ed.*, **40**, 520 (1951).
173. Bogin, H. H., US Pat. 2,553,544 (May 22, 1951).
174. Ratish, H. D., and Hochberg, M. (Nopco Chemical), US Pat. 3,067,105 (Dec. 4, 1962).
175. Hinkel, C. L., *Am. J. Roentgenol Radium Therap.*, **65**, 575 (1951).
176. Clarkson, R., *Tablet Coating*, Drug and Cosmetic Industry, New York, 1951.
177. Stephensen, D., and Smith, D. S., *J. Pharm. Pharmacol.*, **3**, 547 (1951).
178. Termansen, J. B., *Arch. Pharm. Chemi*, **58**, 727 (1951); through *C. A.*, **46**, 3213f (1952).
179. Völker, T., and Wenzel, F. (Rohm & Haas GmbH), US Pat. 3,070,509 (Dec. 25, 1962).
180. Levin, E., et al, *J. Lab. Clin. Med.*, **38**, 828 (1951).
181. Takahashi, K., Japan. Pat. 5947 (Oct. 2, 1951); through *C. A.*, **47**, 3529b (1953).
182. Bernstein, R. E., *J. Lab. Clin. Med.*, **40**, 707 (1952).
183. N. U. Syndicat voor Chemische en Pharmaceutische Industrie, Dutch Pat. 71,113 (Nov. 15, 1952); through *C. A.*, **47**, 4560 g(1953).
184. Jespersen, E. (Knud Abildgaard), Can. Pat. 645,607 (July 24, 1962).
185. Dequeker, R., *Pharm. Tijdschr. Belg.*, **29**, 97 (1952); through *C. A.*, **48**, 953g (1954).
186. Wagner, J. G., et al, *J. APhA*, *Sci. Ed.*, **47**, 681 (1958).
187. Oser, B. L., et al, *Ind. Eng. Chem.*, *Anal. Ed.*, **17**, 405 (1945).
188. Albert, A., *Pharmacol. Rev.*, 4, 136 (1952).
189. Scheindlin, S., et al, *J. APhA*, *Sci. Ed.*, **41**, 420 (1952).
190. Macek, T. J., and Feller, B. A., *J. APhA*, *Sci. Ed.*, **41**, 285 (1952).
191. Ida, T., et al, *J. Pharm. Sci.*, **50**, 592 (1961).
192. Doerr, D. W., et al, *Compressed Tablet Coatings: Cellulosic High Polymers*, presented at the APhA Convention, Salt Lake City, 1953.
193. Goett, E. J., et al, US Pat. 2,643,209 (June 23, 1953).
194. Higuchi, T., et al, *J. APhA*, *Sci. Ed.*, **42**, 157 (1953).
195. Bruns, L. G., and Huyck, C. L., *Drug Cosmetic Ind.*, **83**, 602 (1958).
196. Lesser, M. A., *Drug Cosmetic Ind.*, **72**, 616 (1953).
197. *New Engl. J. Med.*, Edit. Sect., **254**, 963 (1956).
198. Couvreur, A., et al, *Les Enrobes Modernes Des Drageés Et Des Pilules*, a partial translation distributed by Distillation Products Industries, Div. of Eastman Kodak Co., 1958.
199. Antonides, H. J., and DeKay, H. G., *Drug Std.*, **21**, 205 (1953).
200. Bauer, C. W., and Geraughty, R. J., *J. APhA*, *Pract. Ed.*, **14**, 504 (1953).
201. Stoklosa, M. J., and Ohmart, L. M., *J. APhA*, *Pract. Ed.*, **14**, 507 (1953).
202. Hawkins, D. B., and Thompson, H. D., *J. APhA*, *Sci. Ed.*, **42**, 424 (1953).
203. Ratcliff, J. D., *Collier's*, 71, (Mar. 14, 1953).
204. Kanig, J. L., *Production and Testing of Enteric Coatings*, presented before the Pharmaceutical Development Committee, ADMA Research and Development Section, Westchester Country Club, Rye, N.Y., Nov. 5, 1953.
205. Klemme, C. J., *Drug Allied Ind.*, 14, (Dec., 1953).
206. Abbott Labs., Australian Pat. Spec. 63,726 (1960).
207. Wurster, D. E., US Pat. 2,648,609 (Aug. 11, 1953).
208. Endicott, C. J., et al (Abbott Labs.), S. African Pat. Spec. 2477 (1962).
209. *Darstine Bromide, 50 mg, Stratalets*, Sharp & Dohme, Inc., Philadelphia, 1953.
210. Johnson, R. H. (Upjohn Co.), Can. Pat. 651,043 (Oct. 23, 1962).
211. Anon., *Drug Trade News*, Manuf. Sect., 44 (Mar. 29, 1954).
212. *Amsustain Tablets*, Key Corp., Miami, 1954.
213. *Stimalose "Durabond" Tablet* (Brochure), Irwin-Neisler Co., Decatur, Ill., 1954.
214. Chapman, D. G., et al, *J. APhA*, *Sci. Ed.*, **43**, 297 (1954).
215. Endicott, C. J., and Kirchmeyer, F. J., *Drug Std.*, **24**, 193 (1956).
216. Tarnowski, C. E., *Am. Rev. Tuberc. Pulmonary Diseases*, **76**, 159 (1957).
217. Whitehouse, R. C., *Pharm. J.*, 85 (Jan. 30, 1954).
218. Advertisement, Evans Medical Supplies, Ltd., England, *Pharm. J.*, Inset i (Feb. 20, 1954).
219. Kupfer, C., et al, *Am. J. Ophthalmol.*, **40**, 673 (1955).
220. Tatge, W. A., et al, *Am. J. Med. Sci.*, **232**, 175 (1956).
221. Allan, L. V. (Imperial Chemical Industries), US Pat. 3,082,154 (Mar. 19, 1963).
222. Sprecker, A. G., *Am. Practitioner Dig. Treat.*, **7**, 1801 (1956).
223. Kirby, W. M., et al, *Antibiot. Chemotherapy*, **3**, 473 (1953).
224. Frye, W. W., et al, *Am. J. Trop. Med. Hyg.*, **6**, 890 (1957).
225. Remington's Pharmaceutical Sciences, 13th ed., Mack Publ. Co., Easton, Pa., 1965, p. 604.
226. Svedres, E. V., S. African Pat. 18,934 (Mar. 1, 1954).
227. Hochberg, M., and Ely, C. (Nopco Chemical), US Pat. 3,067,104 (Dec. 4, 1962).
228. Thomas Kerfoot & Co. Ltd., Brit. Pat. Spec. 743,222 (Jan. 11, 1956).
229. Rosenberg, A. (Commercial Solvents Corp.), Can. Pat. 638,301 (Mar. 13, 1962).
230. Steinberg, W. H., et al, *J. Pharm. Sci.*, **54**, 747 (1965).
231. Council on Pharmacy and Chemistry, AMA, Statement by the Secretary on Evaluation of Enteric Coatings (May 12, 1954).
232. Buckwalter, F. H., and Granatek, A. P. (Bristol Labs.), US Pat. 2,768,115 (Oct. 23, 1956).
233. Angsusingh, S., and Chavkin, L., *Tablet Coatings for Timed Disintegration*, presented at the AAAS Meeting, Pharmacy Section, New York, Dec., 1956.
234. Blubaugh, F. C., et al, *J. APhA*, *Sci. Ed.*, **47**, 857 (1958).
235. Gruber, C. M., et al, *J. APhA*, *Sci. Ed.*, **47**, 863 (1958).
236. Koff, A. (Hoffmann-La Roche), US Pat. 3,080,293 (Mar. 5, 1963).
237. Teorell, T., *Arch. Intern. Pharmacodyn.*, **57**, 205 (1937).
238. Dominguez, R., and Pomerene, E., *Proc. Soc. Exptl. Biol. Med.*, **60**, 173 (1945).
239. Johnson, P. C., and Berger, E. S., *Clin. Res. Proc.*, **4**, 234 (1956).
240. Brindamour, N. E., and DeKay, R. G., *Drug Std.*, **23**, 10 (1955).
241. Crisafio, R., et al, *Drug Std.*, **23**, 1 (1955).

242. Dragstedt, C. A., Report to the Council on Drugs, *J. Am. Med. Assoc.*, **168,** 1652 (1958).
243. Chapman, D. G., and Campbell, J. A., *Can. J. Biochem. Physiol.*, **33,** 753 (1955).
244. Chapman, D. G., *et al*, *Can. Med. Assoc. J.*, **76,** 102 (1957).
245. Hasegawa, J., and Ikeda, K., *J. Pharm. Soc. Japan*, **75,** 359 (1955); through *C. A.*, **49,** 10585*h* (1955).

246. Chapman, D. G., *et al*, *J. APhA, Sci. Ed.*, **45,** 374 (1956).
247. Meneses, Maria, F. L., and Huyck, C. L., *Drug Std.*, **23,** 17 (1955).
248. Spaulding, J., *Drug Cosmetic Ind.*, **79,** 766 (1956).
249. Spradling, A. B. (Upjohn Co.), US Pat. 2,693,436 (1954).
250. Spradling, A. B. (Upjohn Co.), US Pat. 2,693,437 (1954).
251. Srinivas, R., *et al*, *J. Pharm. Sci.*, **55,** 335 (1966).
252. Middleton, E. J., *et al*, *J. Pharm. Sci.*, **53,** 1378 (1964).

Prolonged–Action Pharmaceuticals

Benefits and possible limitations of long-acting drugs—oral products—
gastrointestinal absorption—terminology—drug elimination rate—types
and construction—evaluation of major types—reviews on long-acting
drugs—parenteral products—pellet absorption—solution absorption—
dispersion absorption—reviews on long-acting parenteral products

This chapter was prepared by

Berton E. Ballard, PhD, *Associate Professor of Pharmacy and Pharmaceutical
Chemistry, University of California, San Francisco Medical Center, San Francisco,
Calif. 94122, and*
Eino Nelson, PhD, *late Professor of Pharmaceutics and Medicinal Chemistry,
School of Pharmacy, State University of New York at Buffalo, Buffalo, N.Y.
14214*

The last 20 years has seen the introduction of a large
number of products by pharmaceutical manufacturers that are intended to provide prolonged therapeutic action after administration. These products
are variously described as being "sustained release,"
"timed release," "prolonged action," "long-acting," or
by similar terms implying an extended period of action
for a given drug in some special dosage form. This
chapter reviews and considers the intended use, terminology, and factors involved in the design, construction, and evaluation of this type product. Since
the efficiency and, in some cases, practicability of long-
acting oral products depends on the gastrointestinal
tract as an absorption site, some factors influencing
drug absorption are briefly reviewed also.

Benefits and Possible Limitations of Long-Acting Drugs

It is evident that products intended to provide for
extended action of drug from a single dose may be considered "convenience dosage forms" by virtue of
eliminating the necessity for dosage several times during
the day. However, therapeutic benefits also may be
obtained, providing the products act as claimed. For
example, Lipowski,[1] whose patents describe the construction of a dosage form wherein a number of small
beads containing the dose of drug with several thicknesses of coating are used, discusses the desirability of a
slow and constant supply of drug to the organism.
Further, Blythe,[2] whose patent describes a dosage
form similar to Lipowski's,[1] points out that nocturnal
seizures associated with epilepsy may be controlled by
incorporation of the proper drug into the dosage form.
He also mentions control of the level of sleep throughout the entire period of sleep, the control of enuresis,
the control of incidence of migraine headache on
awakening, and elimination of undesirable side effects as
benefits obtained from properly designed timed-release
dosage forms. The administration of a long-acting
antibacterial product capable of maintaining effective
serum levels during the sleeping hours has distinct
benefit to an ill person if for no other reason than
eliminating the necessity of interruption of sleep to take
medication. Another advantage of these products is
in prevention of missed doses because of a patient's
forgetfulness.[3] Long-acting products, then, are a

therapeutically significant advance in dosage form
design and should be considered as being more than
"convenience dosage forms."

There may be several possible undesirable consequences of administering long-acting drugs. One is
concerned with the possible lack of precision of dosage.[4] Some long-acting dosage forms exist as laminated tablets. Part of the tablet is designed to release
some drug in the stomach, thus exposing an enteric-
coated core. When this core reaches the intestine, the
hope is that another dose will be released in 3 or 4
hours. The problem is that stomach retention time
for enteric-coated tablets is variable ranging from 0.5
to over 7 hours.[5] Stomach-emptying rate depends
upon the volume of the meal, which may be taken
prior or along with the dose, the meal's chemical composition, and other factors.[6] Also, there may be less
flexibility in giving fractional doses.[7]

The long-acting product may not release the drug
as completely or efficiently as the non-long-acting form
due to poor product design or other factors.[4,8,9] Some
drugs (eg, *p*-aminosalicylic acid) are more effective or
at least as effective in treating tuberculosis when given
as a single dose rather than in divided doses. Riboflavin is another drug which is probably no more
effective in a long-acting form.[4]

In the case of accidental poisoning, a long-acting
product may make the effective administration of an
antidote difficult.[10] Because of developmental and
production costs, many long-acting products are more
expensive for the patient than equivalent amounts of
the drug given in divided doses with non-long-acting
dosage forms.[11] Under certain conditions, if a prolonged-release dosage form is given too frequently, undesirably high blood levels of drug may result due to
the repetition of the loading dose. This point will be
discussed later. Levy[12] lists other possible limitations
of long-acting drug products.

Recent federal regulations govern prolonged-action
dosage forms. Any drug offered or intended for delayed or prolonged action or release, repeat action,
sustained or controlled release, or similar type of action
or release, is a new drug, and a new-drug application
is required for such a product to demonstrate that it
is properly made and controlled to release the active
components at a safe rate, and rate at which the drug
will have its intended effect(s).[13]

Oral Products

Gastrointestinal Absorption

Absorption Processes—Many factors are involved in the absorbability and rate of absorption of drugs from the gastrointestinal tract (some of the discussion in this section is pertinent for the section on *Parenteral Products*, page 1714).* The mechanisms by which drug transfer takes place across the membranes at the absorption sites are generally considered to be of two types. Absorption is spoken of as occurring by *passive transfer* or by *active transport*. Passive transfer may also be referred to as *absorption by free diffusion*. As a result of the fundamental studies[14-18] on absorption conducted by the research group headed by Brodie at the National Institutes of Health, it can be stated that most substances that would be considered drugs are absorbed passively.

In passive absorption the rate with which drug leaves the absorption site and enters the circulation directly depends on the concentration of drug at the absorption site. Therefore, as absorption proceeds, the rate becomes progressively slower. Theoretical consideration of the kinetics of drug absorption, distribution, and excretion discussed by Theorell[19] indicate, among other things, that when drug is absorbed passively, the peak concentration of drug in the blood stream reached from a given dose is directly proportional to the dose. Hence, doubling the dose should result in a doubled peak blood level. (Sometimes, however, because extent of plasma protein binding changes with concentration, this may not be observed even if the process is passive.) Frequently, pharmacological investigation of drug absorbability will include studies of this type to determine whether or not absorption is passive. However, due to physical chemical considerations of drug solubility in fluids at the absorption sites, the results of such tests may falsely indicate a non-passive absorption process. Passive absorption indicates also that the driving force for passage of a drug across absorbing membranes is the concentration gradient across the membrane. This is in accord with Fick's law of diffusion (see under *Passive Transport*, in Chapter 42, *Drug Absorption, Action, and Disposition*.

When absorption studies indicate that absorption rate is independent of concentration at the absorption site, this observation is taken to be indicative of a transport process in absorption. Some substances absorbed by transport processes are glucose and some other sugars, iron, some amino acids, and some vitamins. Materials may be also absorbed by a combination of transport and diffusion processes.

Absorption Sites—The entire gastrointestinal tract, including the stomach, small intestine, and large intestine, is capable of absorbing drugs. However, wide variation in absorption rate may be observed, for example, when comparing rate of absorption from the stomach to that in the intestine or from the small intestine to large intestine. One reason for the apparent superiority of the intestines as a site for absorption as compared to the stomach is due to the increased surface area for absorption presented by the intestinal surface. Another reason is concerned with physical–chemical properties of the drugs themselves as will be

discussed later (see this page). The small intestine with its villi present a large surface for absorption. It has been estimated[6,20] that the absorptive area of the human small intestine is about 4,500 M², or roughly the area of a football field. The normal peristaltic movements of the intestine facilitate absorption by transfer of materials to contact with the surface of the villi from whence absorption takes place. The same movements facilitate solution of drugs if they are initially in the intestine in the solid state.

The stomach may also be an important absorption site depending on the physical–chemical nature of the drug and the pH of stomach fluids in the normal state which will be discussed in more detail later. The fact that the stomach empties into the intestine (and that many drugs will be absorbed both from the stomach and intestines, although at different rates), is one factor that makes it difficult to gain a quantitative understanding of absorption since stomach emptying time is involved.

Physical–Chemical Properties and Absorbability—As a result of the studies by Brodie's research group[14-18] mentioned earlier, many important factors involved in absorption are now quite well understood. These studies have resulted in what may be referred to as a *pH-partition theory* for drug absorption.

In general terms, according to the pH-partition theory, the absorbability of drugs is favored when they are present in uncharged form at the absorption site and possess an intrinsic partition coefficient favoring oil in an oil–water system. These observations are based on researches made by workers studying permeability of membranes that indicated the existence of a lipoid-like barrier through which materials must pass in penetrating membranes. Since charged (ionized) materials are oil insoluble in general, those properties of drugs favoring their existing in fluids at absorption sites in the uncharged (unionized) form favor their absorption.

Weakly acidic drugs will exist in the stomach in the undissociated form, and hence their absorption will be favored from this acidic environment. Weakly basic drugs will exist at the same site as cations, hence charged and poorly absorbed. In the neutral or slightly alkaline intestine the reverse can be expected to be true. Degree of difference in absorbability at the two sites will depend on the relative acidic or basic strength of the drugs as well as the oil solubility of the undissociated form. The degree to which a weakly acidic drug is ionized may be easily calculated. Expressing the degree of ionization in per cent, then:

$$\% \text{ ionized} = \frac{[A^-]}{[HA] + [A^-]} \times 100 \qquad (1)$$

where $[A^-]$ is the molar concentration of the anion and $[HA]$ of the undissociated acid. Since the dissociation constant for a weak acid is defined by

$$K_a = \frac{[H^+][A^-]}{[HA]} \qquad (2)$$

where K_a is the dissociation constant and $[H^+]$ the hydrogen-ion concentration; substituting for $[A^-]$ in Eq. 1 after rearranging Eq. 2 yields

$$\% \text{ ionized} = \frac{100}{1 + \frac{[H^+]}{K_a}}$$

---

* The chapter on *Drug Absorption, Action, and Disposition* also deals with the interrelationships of absorption, distribution, metabolism, storage and excretion of drugs and the physicochemical properties of body tissues and drugs.

or using pH and pK$_a$ ([H^+] = 10^{-pH}; K$_a$ = 10^{-pK_a}):

$$\% \text{ ionized} = \frac{100}{1 + 10^{pK_a - pH}} \quad (3)$$

For example, aspirin which has a pK$_a$ of about 3.4 would exist at a stomach pH of say 2.0 in largely the undissociated form since substitution of these values of pK$_a$ and pH in Eq. 3 yields a value of 4 for percentage ionized. Assuming that aspirin is in the intestine at a pH of 7, it is easily calculated that aspirin at this site is more than 99.9% in the ionic form. According to the pH-partition theory, then, aspirin should be absorbed more rapidly from the stomach than from the intestine. It should be remembered that the absorbing surface of the intestine is very large and that this factor would tend to reduce the difference in absorbability from the two sites, depending on the length of intestine in contact with aspirin in solution. It should be remembered that although only the undissociated form is absorbed, the equilibrium between dissociated and undissociated acid is preserved by formation of more undissociated acid from dissociated acid as the former material leaves the absorption site.

The expression corresponding to Eq. 3 for weakly basic drugs is easily derived to be

$$\% \text{ ionized} = \frac{100}{1 + 10^{pH - pK_a}} \quad (4)$$

Further extension of the implications of the pH-partition theory to drug absorption involves pointing out that the driving force in a drug absorption by a passive diffusion process is the concentration difference between drug at the absorption site and concentration in the fluids in which it circulates in the body. Even with substances that are as soluble in blood as they are in gastric or intestinal fluids, a strong driving force to cause absorption exists because of the large volume of blood and other fluids of distribution compared to the volume of either gastric fluid or intestinal fluid. A given amount of drug may exist in a relatively concentrated solution in intestinal fluid, and yet when the same amount of drug enters blood, the blood concentration will be of low order. For substances that show a change in solubility with pH of medium in which they are contained, the pH-partition theory is of direct concern. The solubility of a weak acid may be calculated by[21]

$$S = S_0 \left(1 + \frac{K_a}{H^+}\right) = S_0(1 + 10^{pH - pK_a}) \quad (5)$$

and a weak base may be calculated by[21]

$$S = S_0 \left(1 + \frac{H^+}{K_a}\right) = S_0(1 + 10^{pK_a - pH}) \quad (6)$$

where S is the solubility in any convenient units, K_a is the dissociation constant for the acid or protonated base, S_0 the water solubility of the weak acid or base, and [H^+] is the hydrogen ion concentration of the medium. If the membrane through which the drug must pass is permeable only to undissociated acid or unprotonated (uncharged) base, equal concentrations of these species will exist on each side of the membrane. The ratio of Eq. 5 or 6 written for either the pH of gastric or intestinal fluid and the pH of blood is indicative of the driving force for absorption based on pH gradient. For example, if the ratio

$$R = \frac{1 + 10^{pH_b - pK_a}}{1 + 10^{pH_g - pK_a}} \quad (7)$$

is considered for the weak acid, aspirin, where pH$_b$ is the pH of the blood, 7.2, and pH$_g$ is the pH of gastric fluid, about pH 2.0, it will be seen that the pH gradient, stomach to blood, favors aspirin's absorption since this material has a pK$_a$ of about 3.4, and the ratio has a value much greater than 1.

$$R = \frac{1 + 10^{7 - 3.2}}{1 + 10^{2 - 3.2}} = \frac{1 + 10^{3.8}}{1 + 10^{-1.2}} \cong 10^{3.8}$$

A similar calculation for aspirin in the intestine at pH 7.0 indicates that the ratio is around 1. From this site the driving force for absorption will be due to the difference between the volume of blood and volume of intestinal fluid as mentioned earlier. Similar calculations made for basic substances indicate the reverse situation will be true, ie, absorption should proceed more rapidly from the intestine than from the stomach.

The research papers of Brodie's group[14-18] are excellent reading for the serious student of drug absorption.

Solution Rate Theory and Drug Absorption—It is not a well-recognized fact that drug absorption is at many times markedly influenced by the time necessary for the drug to dissolve at the absorption sites. Studies have indicated that in the case of weakly acidic and basic drugs the salt form used may be very important.[22] The surface area presented to the dissolution medium by the drug is also an important factor.[23] For example, consider the absorbability of a free acid vs its sodium salt: even though gastric fluid has the same capacity to dissolve phenobarbital as it does to dissolve sodium phenobarbital, the latter material will initially dissolve in this fluid at a rate about 800 times as fast. This means that gastric fluid will be almost instantaneously saturated with phenobarbital when the sodium salt is taken. Absorption removes drug from gastric fluid or it passes to the intestines, meaning that the dissolving sodium phenobarbital is able to keep gastric fluid saturated and absorption rate at a maximum. Free phenobarbital precipitates, of course, in this acidic medium, but the freshly precipitated crystals present a large surface area to the medium which is another factor helping to keep phenobarbital titer high in gastric fluid. This sequence of events does not occur with phenobarbital itself, and absorption rate is much slower. The sequence of events in the dissolution of sodium phenobarbital is essentially the same in intestinal fluids. Differences in rate of dissolution of all potassium and sodium salts of slightly soluble weak acids may be observed to occur when their rates are compared to the respective free acids.

If a series of different salts of the same acid are prepared and their dissolution rates studied, it will be observed that the rates are markedly different. In the case of theophylline, these differences were related to blood levels in clinical trials.[22]

Finely powdered tetracycline is absorbed much more rapidly than the same drug in a pellet of limited surface area.[23] The difference is attributable to the increased surface area obtained when particle size is reduced.

Quantitative understanding of the influence of salt form and surface on drug absorption may be gained by examining the Noyes–Whitney solution rate law which in its reduced form describes *in vivo* dissolution of drugs. The equation has the form

$$\frac{da}{dt} = kAC_s \quad (8)$$

where da/dt is the dissolution rate, k is a constant whose value depends on the amount of agitation and other factors, A is the surface area, and C_s is the concentration of the drug in a thin layer of fluid adjacent to the dissolving drug which is called the diffusion or boundary layer. It is immediately seen from Eq. 8 that rate is directly proportional to surface area. The C_s term is important when considering dissolution of salts of weak acids or bases in mediums that have a limited capacity for the free acid or base. With a salt, C_s has a high value. For example, even in gastric fluid, the pH of the diffusion layer would be essentially that of a saturated solution of sodium phenobarbital in water. Consequently, C_s would be nearly equal to the solubility of sodium phenobarbital in water. With phenobarbital itself, C_s would have the same value as its water solubility. A similar discussion is appropriate for weak bases and their salts dissolving in mediums of limited capacity for the free base.

Dosage Form Effects—The dosage form used may have important effect on the availability of a drug for absorption. Their influence on rate of absorption is, of course, the basis for many long acting products. However, substantial amounts of drug may be eliminated in the feces in some cases, indicating that all of the dose was not available to the patient. This occurrence is as serious a matter as if the preparation contained less than the labeled amount of active ingredient. Some work has been done to assess the effect of nondelayed release coatings on tablets.[24-27] Studies such as these are very pertinent to the evaluation of long-acting products.

Terminology

As mentioned in the introduction, long-acting oral products have been described by a variety of terms. It seems reasonable to classify these products in the following three types:

1. Sustained release
2. Prolonged action
3. Repeat action

A sustained-release product may be considered one in which a drug is initially made available to the body in an amount sufficient to cause the desired pharmacological response as rapidly as is consistent with the properties of the drug determining its intrinsic availability for absorption; and one which provides for maintenance of activity at the initial level for a desirable number of hours in excess of the activity resulting from the usual single dose of drug. To maintain a given level of activity, the net effect of product construction and physiological factors is such that drug becomes available for absorption at a constant rate, which rate is equal to the activity disappearance rate in the body after absorption. For drugs whose activities are directly proportional to concentration in the blood, blood concentration may be substituted for pharmacological activity in this definition.

Prolonged-action products may be considered to be those in which a drug is initially made available to the body in an amount either sufficient to, or not dangerously or undesirably in excess of, the amount needed to cause the desired therapeutic response; these products also provide for replacement of the drug at some rate which gives a measurable increase in the length of time activity may be noted for the preparations when compared to the usual single dose.

A repeat-action preparation may be considered one that provides for a usual single dose of drug and is so constructed to provide another single dose at some later time after administration.

As in the case of true sustained-release products, pharmacological activity may be substituted for by

blood concentration in the definitions of prolonged-release and repeat-action products when appropriate.

A sustained-release product may not be a suitable form for the administration of drugs that are needed in the night as well as day hours since repeated dosing could lead to undesirably high body levels if the level, for example, from the second dose is initially superimposed on the level that resulted from the first dose. However, many drugs are used either only during the day hours or only in the night hours, hence there is a definite place in therapeutics for this type of product. With a drug used during both day and night hours, sustained release products are practical when the drug has an intrinsically high disappearance rate in the body. This factor would eliminate the need for concern regarding accumulation on repeated dosing. For example, penicillin G, which is extremely rapidly eliminated and which is needed in 24-hour dosage, is a drug in which concern for accumulation is unnecessary.

Sustained release as defined here is difficult to achieve, and most products presently on the market should be considered as being of the prolonged-action type.

The relationships between the concentration or activity of drug and time resulting from a usual single dose, a sustained-release dose, and a prolonged active dose is depicted in Fig. 733. The situations portrayed for the sustained-release product and the prolonged-re-

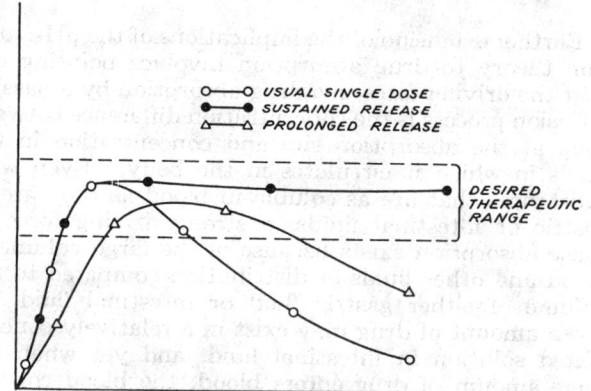

Fig. 733. Relationships between drug activity and time.

lease product are idealized. These curves should be considered types which would be found if, for example, the blood concentrations were determined in a number of test subjects and the mean values at various times were used to prepare the curves. Even in this case, the plotted points usually would indicate only the trend depicted by the curves shown. Individual values would vary widely from the mean values because people show great variation in their ability to absorb and metabolize and/or excrete drug even when administered in ordinary dosage forms. There is no reason to think that this variation will be compounded by properly constructed long-acting dosage forms.

From the foregoing discussion, it should be clear on theoretical grounds that to maintain a reasonably constant drug blood concentration over an extended time, the first dose should contain both the rapidly absorbed loading and delayed-release forms of the drug, while the second and succeeding doses should contain *only* the necessary amount of the delayed-release form of the drug. From a practical standpoint, however, it is desirable to limit the prescribed dosage form to a single package or unit. For example, a prolonged-release sulfaethidole suspension with half of the dose in a rapidly absorbed form and the other half in a delayed-release form was administered such that the first dose was twice the amount given every 12 hours thereafter for 5 consecutive doses. Under these conditions a reasonably constant blood concentration was maintained over approximately 72 hours. The average cumulative amount of free drug excreted in the urine vs time was constant over the same time period, which confirms the uniformity of drug absorption.[28]

Drug Elimination Rate—A Factor in Design and Efficiency

Elimination of drugs commences immediately with their absorption. Depending on the drug, the individual, and the individual's physiological state, wide variations are observed in the rate of this elimination. A measure of elimination rate is a drug's half-life (time for a 50% decrease in blood or body concentration) which may be as short as 23 seconds for a drug such as epinephrine[29] or as long as 2.5 years for a certain organic iodine compound used as an x-ray contrast medium.[30]

Drug elimination is usually by means of conversion by the body to an inactive or less active product or elimination of unchanged drug by the kidney. Other pathways such as the lungs may exist for elimination, but most drugs are eliminated by either one or both of the first mentioned processes.

When drug concentration in blood is determined as a function of time and the data plotted on semilogarithmic graph paper, it will usually be observed that in the postequilibrative and post-absorptive phases of drug elimination a straight line will be obtained on such a plot. The linearity of the plot implies that the mathematical relationship given as Eq. 9 describes the process.

$$C = C_0(\exp[-kt]) \tag{9}$$

In Eq. 9, C is the concentration at any time, C_0 is the zero time concentration, k is the rate constant in reciprocal time for the elimination process, and t is time. The rate constant, k, is equal to $0.693/t_{1/2}$ where $t_{1/2}$ is the half-life previously mentioned. Eq. 9, by analogy to chemical kinetics,[31] describes a first-order removal process. The rate constant K (and corresponding $t_{1/2}$) is the sum of the rate constants for the separate processes responsible for active drug removal. Thus, in the following scheme:

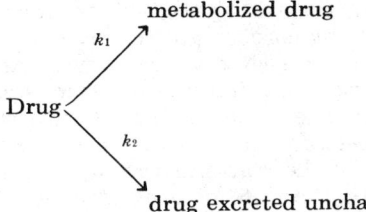

the over-all removal rate constant, k, referred to above is the sum of k_1 and k_2 which are the individual rate constants for the processes depicted. If another process or even several more processes were involved in removal, the over-all rate constant, k, would be the sum of those shown and the constants for the other processes involved.

With wide variations likely to be encountered in drug elimination time, the design of long-acting products is necessarily very much concerned with this factor. An equation has been proposed[32] and checked in actual experiments with d-amphetamine[33] to estimate

the maintenance dose in sustained release products. In the equation

$$Am = \frac{0.693\,bh}{t_{1/2}} \tag{10}$$

Am is the maintenance dose, b is the product of the usual single dose and the fraction of the blood level resulting from this single dose desired to be maintained, h is the number of hours of maintenance desired, and $t_{1/2}$ is the half-life of the drug. In the application of this equation to d-amphetamine,[33] it was found, for example, that the usual maintenance dose contained in certain types of sustained release products of this drug was in excess of that required. The clinical observations were in agreement with the calculation.

The extension in action time, which occurs when the dose of a drug is increased, may also be calculated. Letting C_e be the minimum effective concentration of drug in the body and C_0 the maximum concentration resulting from the usual dose, Eq. 9 may be written in the form

$$C_e = C_0(\exp[-0.693\,t^0/t_{1/2}]) \tag{11}$$

where t^0 is the time needed for the maximum drug concentration from the usual dose to fall to the minimum effective concentration. Assuming that the dose is doubled and that this dose results in a maximum level of $2\,C_0$, Eq. 9 may be written again as

$$C_e = 2\,C_0(\exp[-0.693\,t'/t_{1/2}]) \tag{12}$$

where t' is the time in which body concentration falls to the minimum effective concentration from the doubled dose. Equating Eqs. 11 and 12 and solving for $t' - t^0 = \Delta t$, ie, the length of time by which the minimum effective concentration will be extended, yields

$$\Delta t = t_{1/2} \tag{13}$$

or the time in which a minimum effective level will be extended will be equal to the half-life of the drug when a doubled dose is given.

Treating the more general case wherein n times the usual dose is given yields

$$\Delta t = (3.32 \log n)t_{1/2} \tag{14}$$

as the formula for calculating the increase or decrease in action time from larger or smaller doses, respectively.

Types and Construction

Coated Slow-Release Beads—Lipowski[1] described the first preparation of this type. In his first patent he described the division of the dose of medicinal into about 10 groups of pellets, about 1 to 2 mm in diameter. The first group of the 10 had one coating of material resistant to gastric and/or intestinal fluids, the second, two coats, and so forth. He specified a total thickness for the 10 coats of about $1/10$ mm. The coated pellets were mixed and taken as the dose. Coating materials mentioned were cellulose esters and ethers with or without added resins, fats, keratin, and gluten.

The construction of the Spansule® type brand of encapsulated coated pellets intended to provide sustained release of contained drugs has been described by Blythe.[2] According to the patents cited, the total dose is divided into 3 to 9 parts; one part of any given dose so divided consisting of drug intended to establish initial therapeutic level and the remaining parts being the sustained release dose. A given dose, later to be subdivided into the 3 to 9 parts consists of from 50 to 500 small pellets or beads of drug and excipients. Blythe states it is practical to divide the dose into 4 equal parts; one part consisting of uncoated beads, the next part with a coating which should on the average resist disintegration for 3 hours, the next with a 6-hour coating, and the last with a 9-hour coating. The patent describes an example wherein this scheme was applied to make 15-mg sustained-release capsules of d-amphetamine sulfate which were claimed to have established initial desired body level in about ½ hour and to have maintained this level for about 11 hours.

The nucleus of each bead was stated to be either the confectioner's nonpareil seeds in the 12 to 40-mesh size range or the drug itself and sucrose made into such beads. Coating of the beads was described as being performed in coating pans and presumably these were of the conventional type. When a given weight of coating material was applied to a batch of beads, the coatings varied within a range of 30 to 40% on either side of the median coating. These values represent the variation in median thicknesses of the coatings.

The Blythe patent mentioned a number of materials as being satisfactory for coatings. Included in this listing were mixtures of beeswax, carnauba wax, or bayberry wax with glyceryl monostearate. Other substances mentioned as coatings were as follows: stearic acid, palmitic acid, glyceryl myristate, cetyl alcohol, and similar substances that could be expected to be slowly dissolved or digested or to act as semipermeable membranes through which drug can diffuse when the preparations are ingested. The method suggested for applying coatings was to prepare 3 to 25%, by weight, solutions of the materials dissolved in carbon tetrachloride and to spray them on the granules with this coating mixture heated to about 60°C.

Preparation of prolonged-release beads are described in another patent.[34] In this patent a coating as such is not applied over the drug, but rather the drug is mixed with a material such as shellac in order to provide a mass from which drug is leached out when the beads are in contact with fluid at the absorption site. Preparation of small cylindrically shaped, slow-release pellets by extruding mixtures of drug and materials such as zein or kafirin for encapsulation is described by Rosenthal.[35] Wagner describes preparations of small beads with a pH-sensitive coating[36] for use in preparing long-acting pellets.

There are many products consisting of coated beads, granules, or pellets contained in hard gelatin capsules or compressed into tablets presently being marketed. Table I contains a summary of these. In Table I and in other tables listing products mentioned later, classification by product type is on the basis of descriptions given in advertising literature, in published literature wherein products were evaluated, and/or by examination of products. This information is limited in many cases, and the classification should be considered tentative. The coating materials used in these products may be assumed to be fats and waxes, polymeric substances sensitive to small changes in pH of gastrointestinal fluids, shellac, or various mixed or independently applied mixtures of these materials or others mentioned.

The principle involved in dividing a dose of drug into many small bodies as described by Lipowski[1] is theoretically quite sound. Gastrointestinal absorption of drugs is, in general, quite erratic. In many cases erratic absorption is due to variations in release of drug

from the dosage form. Division of the dose into many parts increases the probability that an effective dose of the drug will be made available for absorption, and, hence, properly designed long-acting products can be expected to make gastrointestinal absorption more regular and predictable. Some of the more recent developments in microencapsulation techniques have been reviewed by Sirine.[37] Solids, liquids, and gases have been encapsulated; however, most of the research has been done with liquids. Some possible wall materials include gelatin, polyvinyl alcohol, and ethylcellulose. Some newer long-acting products employ this principle.

Tablets with Slow-Release Cores—The preparation of one tablet of this type is described in the patent by Cooper and Windheuser.[38] The tablet described consists of a core containing the therapeutically active material evenly mixed in a mixture of substances nonabsorbable from the gastrointestinal tract but capable of slow dissolution or loss of drug by leaching therein, and an outer layer which is compressed onto the core and which also contains therapeutically active material as well as excipients, binders, and lubricants.

In one example given in the patent tripelennamine hydrochloride is added to a molten mass of carnauba wax and stearyl alcohol. The mass is stirred until solidified and then reduced to granules by passing through a 16-mesh screen. After lubrication with magnesium stearate the granules are compressed to form the cores. A compression coating for these cores is described as being made by mixing tripelennamine hydrochloride with carbowax 6000, lactose, confectioner's sugar, and talcum. After sieving, this mixture of powders is granulated with a mixture of acacia and tragacanth in alcohol (50%), passed through a sieve, and dried at about 40°C. After a final sieving the material is pressed around the cores in a press-coating machine. For the tripelennamine hydrochloride tablet described, the ratio of drug content, core to coat, was 2 to 1.

In another example, cores are described as being prepared by coating nonpareil beads with the active ingredient and then adding shellac coatings to these coated beads in a sufficient number such as to meet the desired disintegration time requirement. These coated beads are then mixed with core granules prepared in a manner similar to that described in the first example and compressed into cores.

Hermelin describes another method of producing prolonged-action tablets based on their possessing a slow-dissolving core.[39] In this invention the drug and inert filler are repeatedly wetted with, and dried after, an application of a mixture of glaze, stearic acid, and castor oil. The granules formed with these materials are compressed into cores. These cores are coated with more of the glaze mixture and kaolin, dried, and coated with the dose of drug intended to supply the initial dose. A final coat of sugar is described as being desirable.

Preparation of tablets of materials made in a manner somewhat similar to the cores described above, only using shellac by itself as the dissolution retarding material, is described in another patent.[40] The beads prepared according to this patent which are compressed into tablets are also described as being usable as a sustained release product after encapsulating.

Table II lists products of the type containing slow dissolving cores.

Repeat-Action Tablets—Strictly speaking, this type of product is not of the prolonged-action type

Table I—Long-Acting Products Containing Coated or Slow-Release Beads

Product	Active ingredient(s)	Manufacturer[a]	Product	Active ingredient(s)	Manufacturer[a]
Aerolate Capsules (Sr. & Jr.)	theophylline	Fleming	Hispril Spansule Capsule	diphenylpyraline HCl	SK&F
Amodex Timed Capsule	d-amphetamine HCl and amobarbital	Fellows-Testagar	Measurin Tablet	acetylsalicylic acid	Chesebrough-Ponds
Artane Sequels Capsule	trihexyphenidyl HCl	Lederle			Glenbrook
Bamadex Sequels Capsule	d-amphetamine SO₄ and meprobamate	Lederle	Meprospan	meprobamate	Wallace
			Mol-Iron Chronosule Capsule	molybdenum sesquioxide & ferrous SO₄	White
Benzedrine Spansule Capsule	dl-amphetamine SO₄	SK&F			
Bronchobid Duracap	theophylline, pseudoephedrine HCl, & butabarbital	Meyer	Neo-Corovas Tymcaps	pentaerythritol tetranitrate	Amfre-Grant
			Nitrospan	nitroglycerin	USV
Combid Spansule Capsule	isopropamide iodide & prochlorperazine maleate	SK&F	Ornade Spansule Capsule	chlorpheniramine maleate, phenylpropanolamine HCl, & isopropamide iodide	SK&F
Compazine Spansule Capsule	prochlorperazine maleate	SK&F			
Contac Capsule	atropine SO₄, scopolamine HBr, hyoscyamine SO₄, phenylpropanolamine HCl, & chlorpheniramine maleate	Menley & James	Pathilon Sequels Capsule	tridihexethyl chloride	Lederle
			Pavabid Plateau Capsule	papaverine HCl	Marion
			Pentritol Tempules	pentaerythritol tetranitrate	Armour
Corovas Tymcaps Capsule	pentaerythritol tetranitrate and secobarbital	Amfre-Grant	PERKe One Capsule	d-amphetamine SO₄	Ascher
Dexalme-S Duracap	d-amphetamine SO₄ & secobarbital	Meyer	PERKe Two Capsule	d-amphetamine SO₄ & amobarbital	Ascher
Dexamyl Spansule Capsule	d-amphetamine SO₄ & amobarbital	SK&F	PERKe Three Capsule	d-amphetamine SO₄, phenobarbital, atropine SO₄, thyroid, & aloin	Ascher
Dexedrine Spansule Capsule	d-amphetamine SO₄	SK&F			
Diamox Sequels Capsule	acetazolamide	Lederle	Prydon Spansule Capsule	belladonna alkaloids	SK&F
Diphetamine Granucaps	d & dl-amphetamine SO₄	Tutag	Prydonnal Spansule Capsule	belladonna alkaloids & phenobarbital	SK&F
Diphylets Capsule	d-amphetamine	Tutag	Pyma Timed Capsule	pyrilamine maleate, chlorprophenpyridamine maleate, prophenpyridamine maleate & phenylephrine HCl	Fellows-Testagar
Ectasule Timsules (Sr. & Jr.)	ephedrine & amobarbital	Fleming			
Ekko Capsules (Sr. & Jr.)	diphenylhydantoin	Fleming	Pymadex Timed Capsule	pyrilamine maleate, chlorprophenpyridamine maleate, prophenpyridamine maleate, phenylephrine HCl, & d-amphetamine HCl	Fellows-Testagar
Equanil L-A Capsule	meprobamate	Wyeth			
Eskabarb Spansule Capsule	phenobarbital	SK&F			
Eskaserp Spansule Capsule	reserpine	SK&F			
Eskatrol Spansule Capsule	d-amphetamine SO₄ & prochlorperazine maleate	SK&F	Quadamine Granucaps	d-amphetamine SO₄, amobarbital, vitamins, & minerals	Tutag
Evrodex-Plus Unitemp Capsule	d-amphetamine & amobarbital	Evron	Seco-8 Capsule	secobarbital sodium	Fleming
Evrodex Unitemp Capsule	d-amphetamine SO₄	Evron	Sinsule Capsule	chlorpheniramine maleate, phenylephrine HCl, & methscopolamine nitrate	Bentex
Feosol Spansule Capsule	exsiccated ferrous SO₄	SK&F			
Ferro-Sequels Capsule	ferrous fumarate & dioctyl sodium sulfosuccinate	Lederle	Teldrin Spansule Capsule	chlorpheniramine maleate	SK&F
Fortespan	vitamins A, B₁, B₂, B₆, B₁₂, C, D, nicotinamide, & pantothenic acid	SK&F	Tetrasule Timesule Capsule	pentaerythritol tetranitrate	Arnar-Stone
			Thorazine Spansule Capsule	chlorpromazine HCl	SK&F

[a] For complete names and addresses, see page 2023.

according to the definitions used here. However, an extension of action occurs because of the provision made to release a second dose of drug sometime after the effect of the first dose wears off. In this type tablet a core containing the repeat dose is prepared in much the same manner as the usual enteric-coated tablet (see Chapter 88, page 1689). The core then serves either as the base to which the initial dose is applied by usual

Table II—Tableted Products with Slow-Release Cores

Product	Active ingredient(s)	Manufacturer[a]	Product	Active ingredient(s)	Manufacturer[a]
Ambar Extentabs	methamphetamine HCl & phenobarbital	Robins	Gynetone Repetabs Tablet	ethinyl estradiol & methyltesterone	Schering
Aminophylline Dura-Tab	aminophylline	Wynn	Histadur Dura-Tab	chlorpheniramine maleate	Wynn
Butibel R-A Prestabs Tablets	sodium butabarbital & belladonna alkaloids	McNeil	Homatal Dura-Tab	homatropine methyl bromide & phenobarbital	Wynn
Butiserpazide-25/50 Prestabs Tablets	butabarbital, hydrochlorothiazide, & reserpine	McNeil	Mestinon Timespan Tablet	pyridostigmine Br.	Roche
Butiserpine R-A Prestabs Tablet	sodium butabarbital & reserpine	McNeil	Metamine Sustained	trolnitrate PO$_4$	Pfizer
Butizide-25/50 Prestabs Tablets	butabarbital & hydrochlorothiazide	McNeil	Metamine with butabarbital Sustained	trolnitrate PO$_4$ & butabarbital	Pfizer
Centerex Tablet	acetaminophen, acetophenetidin, caffeine, phenylpropanolamine HCl, phenyltoloxamine citrate & dextromethorphan HBr	Warner Lambert	Naldecon Tablet	phenylpropanolamine HCl, phenylephrine HCl, phenyltoloxamine citrate, & chlorpheniramine maleate	Bristol
Clistin R-A Tablet	carbinoxamine maleate	McNeil	Nebralin Tablet	pentobarbital & mephenesin	Dorsey
Dimetane Extentabs	brompheniramine maleate	Robins	Normacid Tablet	betaine HCl & pepsin	Stuart
Dimetapp Extentabs	brompheniramine maleate, phenylephrine HCl, & phenylpropanolamine HCl	Robins	Numa Dura-Tab	theophylline, ephedrine HCl, & butabarbital	Wynn
			Priscoline Lontabs	tolazoline HCl	Ciba
			Pyribenzamine Lontabs	tripelennamine HCl	Ciba
Donna Extentabs	belladonna alkaloids	Robins	Quinidex Extentabs	quinidine SO$_4$	Robins
Donnagesic Extentabs	atropine SO$_4$, hyoscyamine SO$_4$, phenobarbital, codeine PO$_4$, & hyoscine HBr	Robins	Stental Extentabs	phenobarbital	Robins
			Tri-Span Tablet	N-acetyl-p-aminophenol, pyrilamine maleate, caffeine, ephedrine SO$_4$, & phenylpropanolamine HCl	Vick
Donnatal Extentabs	hyoscyamine SO$_4$, atropine SO$_4$, hyoscine HBr, & phenobarbital	Robins	Vio-Dex Timelets	d-amphetamine SO$_4$, phenobarbital, vitamins A acetate, B$_1$, B$_2$, B$_6$, C, D$_2$, niacinamide, calcium panthothenate, & d-alphatocopheryl acid succinate	Rowell
Drixoral	dexbrompheniramine maleate & d-isoepherine SO$_4$	Schering			
Enzypan Tablet	pepsin, pancreatin, & ox-bile	Norgine			
Feosol Tablet	ferrous SO$_4$	SK&F			

[a] For complete names and addresses, see page 2023.

coating techniques, or it serves as the core of a press-coated tablet in which the initial dose is applied by pressing.

Tableted Mixed-Release Granules—The preparation of tablets containing not only granules made by usual methods (carrying the initial dose of drug) but also granules containing drug either coated with slowly digestible or poorly soluble materials or mixed with solution retarding additives offers a method of achieving prolonged action. Hamada[41] describes the preparation of one tablet of this type. According to his invention, granules of quinidine gluconate are prepared in the usual manner, using sugar and starch as excipients. These granules are intended to supply the initial dose of drug. Another set of granules is prepared by mixing quinidine gluconate with hydrogenated castor oil, heating the mixture to liquefy it and stirring to obtain a homogenous mixture, and, after cooling, forcing the mixture through sieves to obtain the granules. The two sets of granules are lubricated and compressed into tablets. A number of waxes, fatty acids, and hydrogenated oils are mentioned as being usable in place of the hydrogenated castor oil mentioned above.

A patent issued to Syedres[42] about two years before the Hamada patent[41] describes the preparation of sustained-release tablets of several drugs including d-amphetamine sulfate, procaine penicillin, and amobarbital by making the slow-release granules of these drugs, using glyceryl monostearate, glyceryl distearate, glyceryl monopalmitate, mixtures of some of these glyceryl esters and beeswax, or a mixture of stearic acid and cetyl alcohol as the dissolution retarding material. A noteworthy feature of this patent is that it describes the preparation of sustained-release tablets by the process set forth, using the free bases of dibenzyline or amphetamine which are liquid at room temperature.

The preparation of ethylcellulose coated beads for incorporation into tablets to provide for sustained effect of contained drug has also been described.[43] Beads prepared with this coating are claimed to be elastic enough so that the delaying action of the coat will not be affected by the process of compression into tablets.

Examination of other commercially available tablets utilizing the mixed granules principle under discussion in this section indicates that the slow-release granule portions may contain drug absorbed on inert material.

Table III—Tablets of Mixed-Release-Rate Granules

Product	Active ingredient(s)	Manufacturer[a]
Amsustain	d-amphetamine SO$_4$	Key
Belladenal Spacetabs	belladonna alkaloids with phenobarbital	Sandoz
Bellergal Spacetabs	belladonna alkaloids, ergotamine tartrate, & phenobarbital	Sandoz
Du-Oria	methamphetamine HCl & reserpine	Ascher
Geroniazol TT Tablet	pentylenetetrazol & nicotinic acid	Philips-Roxane
Hyasorb	potassium penicillin G	Key
Nitroglyn	nitroglycerin	Key

[a] For complete names and addresses, see page 2023.

In other cases it appears that more than one set of slow-release granules is incorporated in a given tablet. In still other cases the slow-release granules are dyed to give a speckled appearance to the tablet. A complete description of many of these products cannot be given because patents have not yet been issued for them.

Table III lists products of the type under discussion here.

Multiple-Layer Tablets—Modern, multiple-layer tablet compression machines have made this type of prolonged-action dosage form possible. These machines allow the incorporation into one tablet of 2 or 3 separate layers of granulation which may be made to release drug at different rates. Preparing prolonged-release tablets with these machines is not necessarily just another more elegant way of preparing solid dosage forms containing mixed-release-rate granules of the type described previously. For example, one layer may be made firm enough to remain intact during most of the time of its passage through the intestine, while dissolving slowly from its exposed faces in the course of this passage. If the layer is cylindrical in shape with a large diameter to height ratio, its surface area will remain nearly constant as it dissolves, meaning that drug will be released at a constant rate and the requirements for sustained-release met. In a design of this type the other layer is easily constructed to disintegrate rapidly after ingestion, thus providing the initial dose of medication. In three-layer tablets the third layer is either a sustaining or immediate-release source of drug.

Hermelin[44] describes the preparation of a two-layer sustained-release tablet. The sustained-release layer is made from granules prepared by mixing drug with shellac as previously disclosed.[40] The immediate-release layer contains granulation prepared in the usual manner. It is not disclosed in the patent[44] whether or not the sustained-release layer is intended to remain intact during passage through the intestine as described above.

Table IV contains a list of long-acting multiple-layer tablets.

Porous Inert Carriers—According to the advertising literature distributed by the manufacturer (Abbott Laboratories) of products of this type, the tablet is a small plastic pellet containing thousands of small passages which are filled with a "channeling agent" and drug. The channeling agent is claimed to attract fluids of the gastrointestinal tract which then dissolve the drug. Drug presumably diffuses from the passages to fluids in contact with the pellet and thence, after diffusion to the absorbing membrane, is absorbed. The inert plastic pellet is excreted, unchanged, in the

Table IV—Multiple-Layer Tablets

Product	Active ingredient(s)	Manufacturer[a]
Obedrin-LA Tablet	methamphetamine HCl, pentobarbital, ascorbic acid, thiamine mononitrate, riboflavin, & niacin	Massengill
Peritrate Sustained Action	pentaerythritol tetranitrate	Warner-Chilcott
Sul-Span Tabs	sulfaethylthiadiazole	SK&F
Tedral SA Tablet	theophylline, ephedrine HCl, & phenobarbital	Warner-Chilcott

[a] For complete names and addresses, see page 2023.

feces. The construction details of products of this or of a similar type are given in one patent.[45] Table V lists products based on this principle.

Ion-Exchange Resins—Extended action from preparations of drug bound on ion-exchange resin is presumed to result from the slow rate of the displacement reaction when drug–resin complex contacts gastrointestinal fluids and the ionic constituents are dissolved therein. The displacement reaction from drug–resin complex may be described by Eq. 15 where a sulfonic acid type cation-exchange resin combined with a basic drug (eg, a primary amine) is contacted by intestinal fluid:

$$(R-SO_3{}^- \ H_3\overset{+}{N}-R') + (X^+ \ Y^-) \rightleftharpoons$$
Amine drug resinate

$$(R-SO_3{}^- \ X^+) \ + \ (H_3\overset{+}{N}-R' \ Y^-) \quad (15)$$

$$\downarrow$$

Absorption

where X^+ is H^+, Na^+ or another cation, and Y^- is Cl^- or another anion. The situation depicted in Eq. 15 would also hold for an acidic drug bound to an anion exchange resin only with the chloride or other anion being the ion causing drug displacement. Preparation of drug–ion-exchange complexes are described in several patients.[46-48] Drug in solution in excess of or less than the amount required by stoichiometric considerations is contacted with a suitable resin displacing the cation or anion, whichever the case may be, from the resin. After washing with distilled or deionized water, the resin may be suspended in a liquid vehicle free of exchangeable ions or lightly dried for incorporation into other dosage forms. Table VI lists products of this type.

Slightly Soluble Salts or Complexes—The preparation of salts or complexes of active drugs that are only slightly soluble in gastrointestinal fluids may pro-

Table V—Inert Porous Solids as Drug Carriers

Product	Active ingredient(s)	Manufacturer[a]
Desoxyn Gradumet Tablet	methamphetamine HCl	Abbott
Fero-Grad-500	ferrous SO$_4$ with vitamin C	Abbott
Fero-Gradumet	ferrous SO$_4$	Abbott
Pramet	ferrous SO$_4$ with multi-vitamins & minerals	Abbott
Tral Gradumet	hexocyclium methylsulfate	Abbott
Tral Gradumet with Phenobarbital	hexocyclium methylsulfate with phenobarbital	Abbott

[a] For complete names and addresses, see page 2023.

Table VI—Ion-Exchange Resin Long-Acting Products

Product	Active ingredient(s)	Manufacturer[a]
Biphetamine Capsule	d- and dl-amphetamine on cation-exchange resin	Strasenburgh
Histionex Capsule	phenyltoloxamine on cation-exchange resin	Strasenburgh
Ionamin Capsule	phenyl tert-butylamine on cation-exchange resin	Strasenburgh
Rezipas	p-amino-salicylic acid on anion-exchange resin	Squibb
Tussionex Tablet	phenyltoloxamine & hydrocodone on cation-exchange resin	Strasenburgh

[a] For complete names and addresses, see page 2023.

duce a compound that results in prolonged action when taken orally in an appropriate dosage form.

The preparation of salts of tannic acid and therapeutically active amines has been described by Cavallito and Jewell.[49] The amine tannates were prepared by mixing methyl, ethyl, or propyl alcohol solutions of the amine and Tannic Acid NF in 20% excess, diluting the mixture with ice water to complete precipitation of the tannate, and, finally, collecting and washing the precipitate. The preparation of quinidine galacturonate is described by Halpern, et al.[50] In their procedure stoichiometric quantities of polygalacturonic acid and quinidine base were mixed in hydroalcoholic solution and the salt recovered by removal of the solvent under reduced pressure. Long-acting oral products that may be considered to be of the type under discussion here are listed in Table VII.

Liquid Preparations—These products may incorporate prolonged—release principles discussed previously. For example, the liquid preparation may be a suspension of drug on ion-exchange resin.

Robinson and Svedres[51] describe the preparation of slow-release granules of drug for incorporation into liquid preparation. In one example given in this patent, sulfamethylthiadiazole is mixed with hydrogenated castor oil dissolved in chloroform at about 60°C. The mixture is spray dried, and particles of drug mixed with wax having an average diameter of about 20 microns are obtained. These particles are suspended in a suitable aqueous medium. Another method of preparing slow-release particles for suspension is described by Grass and Robinson.[52] Here, after an initial preparation of particles mixed with a dissolution retarding material, the particles are coated with a similar material but of lower melting point. The particle size of the slow-release granules from the procedure described is in the range of 25 to 100 microns.

Patents have been issued based on administration of sulfonamides in an oil emulsion to obtain enhanced and prolonged action.[53]

Long-acting liquid products are listed in Table VIII.

Miscellaneous Types—Several manufacturers make long-acting oral products for distribution by the smaller pharmaceutical companies under the private labels of the latter companies.[54] These products will in most cases be of types that have already been discussed here.

Evaluation of Major Types

Ideally, evaluation of long-acting products should be done by properly designed trials in humans, where actual measurements of drug concentration or drug activity are compared to the concentrations or activity resulting from the usual single dose administered in solution or in a rapidly disintegrating tablet. However, such measurements are not possible in many cases, either because the usual dose of drug results in body drug concentrations that are lower than those which can be measured by known means or because measurements of activity, if this is the alternate or preferred assessment method, cannot be clearly defined. Information of a quantitative nature may be obtained from urinary excretion measurements, but this procedure is only applicable when unchanged drug is excreted or when, in the case of drug modified in the body prior to excretion in the urine, the metabolism of the drug is well understood.

As a result of these considerations, many products have been evaluated by clinical trials in which the subjective observations of the clinician or patients are the bases for judgment.

In assessments wherein subjective observations of, or in some cases even objective measurements by, clinicians or patients are the bases for judgment, it is extremely important that adequate controls be employed. For example, assume that it were desired to test the efficiency of a long-acting preparation of an anorectic agent to cause weight loss in obese patients and that the test was conducted by administering one dose per day in the morning and weighing the subjects once a week to determine whether or not a significant weight loss occurred. Assume, further, that the majority of the subjects did show a weight-loss rate which could be considered significant. The results of a test conducted under these conditions does not even allow the conclusion that the drug used is an anorectic agent, let alone that it is long-acting. In order to determine whether or not the drug itself is an anorectic agent with certainty, it would be necessary to divide the group of patients into two groups, giving one group a placebo of exactly the same appearance as the dosage form of anorectic agent and at an appropriate time switching preparations in the groups without the

Table VII—Slightly Soluble Salts or Complexes

Product	Active ingredient(s)	Manufacturer[a]
Atratan Tablet	atropine tannate	Neisler
Cardioquin	quinidine polygalacturonate	Purdue-Frederick
Rynatan Tabule Durabonded	phenylephrine tannate, pyrilamine tannate, & chlorpheniramine tannate	Neisler
Synatan Tabule	d-amphetamine tannate	Neisler
Unitensen Tablet	cryptenamine tannate	Neisler

[a] For complete names and addresses, see page 2023.

Table VIII—Long-Acting Liquid Preparations

Product	Active ingredient(s)	Manufacturer[a]
Lipo-Diazine	sulfadiazine	Donley-Evans
Lipo-Gantrisin Acetyl	N¹-acetylsulfisoxazole	Roche
Lipo-Triazine	sulfamethazine, sulfamerzine, & sulfadiazine	Donley-Evans
Ryntanan Suspension	phenylephrine tannate, pyrilamine tannate, & chlorpheniramine tannate	Neisler
Sul-Spansion	sulfaethylthiadiazole	SK&F
Tussionex Suspension	phenyltoloxamine & hydrocodone on cation-exchange resin	Strasenburgh

[a] For complete names and addresses, see page 2023.

knowledge of the patients and clinician. Weighings would be carried on continuously during the tests and the data collected subjected to appropriate statistical tests in order to determine significance and level of confidence in differences found. The necessity for such a procedure arises from the fact that suggestion is important consciously or unconsciously to subjects. The mere fact that patients could be told that they were participating in a test to determine whether or not a certain drug was capable of helping them to lose weight would cause some to react to the placebo. Another clinician conducting the same test would obtain different individual results because of differences in patients' attitude toward him or his toward them. Assume now that the test was conducted properly, and statistical tests did show a significant difference in weight loss rate at a high level of confidence. These data do not allow the claim that the product itself is long-acting. The ability of the product to produce extended action would have to be established by tests wherein one group was given the long-acting preparation in the morning and placebos before the noon and evening meals and the other group given the drug in a nonextended action form, but with placebo design before each of the 3 meal times. This scheme assumes that 3-times-a-day dosage is usual with the particular anorectic agent used. Even if no statistically significant difference could be shown in weight-loss rate in the two different dosage schemes, it would still be difficult to claim that the product was long acting. The drug may possess an intrinsically long half-life, and the usual 3-times-a-day dosage actually could be unnecessary. Further, the long-acting product may have released all of the dose immediately and as a result caused prolongation of activity by virtue of heavy dosage according to the calculations made previously. The existence of this possibility would require careful statistical evaluation of side effects produced in the groups.

The lack of complete objectivity in many clinical evaluations of long-acting products has been pointed out.[55] The hazards in interpretation of uncontrolled experiments have been discussed.[56,57]

Frederik and Cass[58] comment on some of the factors complicating the clinical evaluation of sustained-release drugs, and show examples of drug administration schedules designed to evaluate the efficacy, duration of action, and release rates of such products.[59] Levy[12] discusses several criteria for evaluating oral prolonged-release pharmaceuticals.

In vitro release tests are often used in connection with evaluation of long-acting products. Some of these tests attempt to simulate conditions *in vivo*, but as it has been pointed out by Blythe[60] and Campbell, *et al*,[61] the results of such tests are meaningless unless correlated with quantitative *in vivo* measurements, even though they are valuable for manufacturing control purposes.

Lack of adequate evidence of efficient performance coupled with the well-recognized erraticity of drug absorption from the gastrointestinal tract resulted in some unfavorable comment concerning long-acting products.[62] However, it should be pointed out again that properly designed long-acting dosage forms could be expected to decrease erraticity in absorption. The National Academy of Sciences–National Research Council has been studying the efficacy of drug products marketed from 1938 to 1962. Some long-acting products are included in this study.[63]

Encapsulated Slow-Release Beads—Since dosage forms of this type have been marketed for a longer time and are probably more widely used than any other single type of long-acting product, a relatively large number of trials have been reported.

It has been reported by *in vivo* roentgenographic studies—utilizing pellets or beads prepared in the usual manner for this type preparation except they contain radiopaque materials such as barium sulfate in the cores—that a wide dispersion of a capsule's contents may occur after ingestion. Green[64] presents serially taken roentgen traces after ingestion of capsules of this type. His plates show a wide dispersion of the beads in the gastrointestinal tract after 1 hour. Results of similar studies by other workers are also reported.[65] These studies establish that the planned dispersion of the dose does occur to some extent at least.

Clinical studies of a number of therapeutic classes of drugs contained in this type of dosage form report generally favorable results. However, in many cases, the interpretation of results of the studies should be tempered with due recognition to the subjective nature of the measurements and lack of adequate control comparisons.

In clinical tests using about 400 subjects exhibiting various types of allergic distress, Green[64] found that the antihistaminic drug chlorpheniramine, formulated into sustained-release capsules of the type under discussion here, gave excellent symptomatic relief to 66% of the subjects when they were given a 12-mg dose in sustained capsules, taken every 12 hours. This investigator remarked that the incidence of side effects to the dosage form and scheme was unusually light and, further, that patient acceptance was excellent because of the convenience of dosage. A similar patient response to the convenience of dosage has also been reported by Mulligan.[66] In another study with the same sustained-release preparation of chlorpheniramine, Bancroft[67] reports statistically significant differences in relief of allergic distress when results using this preparation were compared to results obtained using the usual 3-times-a-day dosage with another antihistaminic drug, tripelennamine hydrochloride, and other dosage forms. Symptomatic relief during the night was especially good with the sustained-release preparation. Similar results comparing the same sustained-release product to usual tablet dosage have been reported by Rogers[68] and by Bresler.[69]

A number of long-acting preparations of *d*-amphetamine intended mostly for use in the treatment of obesity through appetite depression are available. As judged by weight loss rate, Gelvin, *et al*,[70,71] report one of such preparations was at least as effective as the same dose in tablets, given 3 times a day. Other clinical studies have been reported with this type preparation used either alone or with amobarbital or prochlorperazine for weight control or for other therapeutic reasons.[72–77] A few data on amphetamine blood levels from sustained-release and usual single tablet dosage are also reported.[78]

Since long-acting oral products of *d*-amphetamine are so widely used and are available from several sources, Campbell and his co-workers[33] proposed criteria for the evaluation of these products based on a comparison of urinary excretion of *d*-amphetamine from the sustained-release dose to that resulting from the fractional dose incorporated in these preparations to establish initial body level of drug at a therapeutically effective value. Coincidence of excretion rates in the two cases and their maintenance at the initial value from the sustained-release product for the advertised action period indicated a satisfactory product. In this preliminary study one product met the criteria with respect to constancy of excretion rate at the level resulting from the fractional dose, but this rate was sustained for more than twice as long as the 11 or 12 hours usually desired with this particular drug. These quantitative measurements were in agreement with complaints of the subjects concerning their difficulty in sleeping the evening following morning ingestion of the sustained-release product. In a later study, using 8 commercial products, Shenoy, et al,[79] found widely different results for the same dose of drug in the several preparations tested. Substantial amounts of drug were unavailable from absorption from 3 of the preparations tested, no constant release rate was found with others, and only one product exhibited constant rate release at the desired level while maintaining full availability for absorption of the contained dose. These results emphasize the fact that the wide variation in results may be obtained with different products containing exactly the same dose of drug when assayed by the usual chemical means. These results also indicate the necessity for physiological assays on special dosage forms.

Several clinical and quantitative evaluations of encapsulated, coated-bead sustained-release products containing belladonna alkaloids have been reported. The efficiency of a preparation of this type in depressing basal gastric acid secretion of patients with peptic ulcer and chronic hypertrophic gastritis has been reported by Berkowitz.[80] The preparation produced achlorhydria in 23 of the 25 patients tested. The average duration of achlorhydria in 21 of these patients was about 140 minutes. Dosage at 8-hour intervals was found satisfactory for the average ulcer patient using the sustained release preparation.

An excellently controlled and analyzed evaluation of the same sustained release belladonna alkaloid preparation is reported by Reese, et al.[81] Quantitative assessment was made here by noting the decrease in volume of saliva secreted following a standard stimulatory procedure after ingestion of standard preparations, sustained-release preparation, and placebo. The results of these tests indicated that dosage with the sustained-release preparation caused the same response as 3-times-a-day dosage, but eliminated the decrease in response found preceding, and increase in response found following, ingestion of the drug in the latter scheme. The results of the tests in respect to the "smoothing out" of the response curve are in keeping with one of the objectives of sustained-release dosage. The criterion proposed by Campbell, et al,[33] for d-amphetamine long-acting products is met by this product when depression in salivary response is interpreted in the same manner as urinary excretion rate.

Other evaluations of the sustained-release dosage form of belladonna alkaloids of the type under discussions here have been made.[82-84]

Results of clinical tests using long-acting, encapsulated coated beads of other drugs have also been reported. Among these are tests with secobarbital for sleep management,[85-89] pentaerythritol tetranitrate,[65,90-92] iron,[93,94] chlorpromazine for schizophrenic patients,[95] papaverine for peripherial vascular ischemia,[96] and other drugs or combinations.[97-101]

A number of newer products utilize the microencapsulation technique to effect prolonged drug release. Following ingestion of the tablet or capsule, the dosage form breaks down into tiny coated spheres. Moisture within the gastrointestinal tract penetrates the membrane, and slowly dissolves the solid drug. Drug molecules then diffuse through the intact membrane. The process has been called microdialysis. After the solid in the cell is dissolved, the drug concentration within the cell and its release rate begin to decrease. According to Bachman[102] with PERKē capsule products, if the dialyzing membrane had constant permeability, the rate of drug release would fall to such a low value as to be therapeutically useless even though as much as 30 to 40% of the drug was still contained within the cell. However, the membrane covering the microcells is so formulated that it imbibes water and swells at a precisely controlled rate with an accompanying increase in membrane permeability and drug release rate. These two effects balance one another so that the rate of drug release tends to remain constant over the desired time interval. The release of drug from this type of product depends upon moisture and is relatively independent of pH, enzymatic activity, or agitation in the tract. Some prolonged-release aspirin products employ this principle,[103-106] as well as a product designed to treat allergic rhinitis.[107]

Tablets with Slow-Release Cores—In an evaluation of prolonged-action tablets of Mestinon bromide for the treatment of myasthenia gravis, Schwab, et al,[108] found an average duration of action of about 6 hours. This contrasted markedly to the necessity of frequent dosage (1- to 3-hour intervals) when the drug was given in the usual single dose dosage form. Approximately 85% of the patients participating in the tests continued to use the prolonged-release preparation in preference to the usual dosage scheme. The investigators reporting this work were of the opinion that the greatest value of the prolonged-action tablets was in eliminating the need for frequent interruptions of sleep to take medication. However, wide individual variation in response to the slow-release tablets was observed.

Another clinical study using a prolonged-release dosage form of methamphetamine and phenobarbital for management of obese patients is reported by Marks.[109] In this study administration of drug was in conjunction with diet instructions. A generally favorable response to the treatment with respect to weight loss was reported. However, no control comparisons using placebo and single-dose dosage were made.

Simon[110] reports clinical symptomatic and in vivo x-ray studies using tablets of tripelennamine in the former and sodium iodomethane sulfonate in the latter study. Both sets of tablets were constructed in the same manner except for the contained drugs, and two basic formulations were used. In vitro release from each set of tablets was nearly identical, and in the preferred formulation of the two tested x-ray examination showed remnants of radiopaque material present in the bowel at 8 hours with no material remaining at 10 hours. It was judged by this investigator that excellent symptomatic relief of hay fever symptoms was obtained for 8 to 12 hours in 100% of the patients.

An evaluation of sustained-action tablets constructed with cores of free p-aminosalicylic acid surrounded by buffered p-aminosalicylic acid is described by Small and co-workers.[111] Para-aminosalicylic acid is given in large doses, and gastrointestinal disturbances are frequent with the usual dosage forms. These investigators found that administration of the sustained action tablets to patients experiencing gastrointestinal discomfort with sodium p-aminosalicylic acid solution or buffered tablets was followed by a substantial increase in tolerance to the drug. Drug serum levels from the sustained action tablets were judged to be satisfactory.

In an evaluation of tablets containing benzyl penicillin and designed to provide long-lasting penicillin blood levels, Ballon, et al,[112] found that, in the majority of patients given this preparation, therapeutic levels were maintained for 12 hours. However, these levels, while therapeutically effective, were of low order. The results obtained could be interpreted to indicate that substantial amounts of the drug contained in the dosage form were not physiologically available. A clinical comparison between this tablet and intramuscular procaine penicillin is also reported.[113]

Clinical trials with a 12-mg isothipendyl tablet—whose long-acting properties are based on its possessing, in addition to a slow dissolving core and an initial dose layer of drug, a booster dose between the outer layer and core—have been reported by Spielman.[114] This clinician reported very good results in about 78% of the patients taking the preparation for symptomatic relief of allergic disorders. In about 90% of those responding this well, the preparation was effective for about 12 hours. No comparison was made to the usual dosage scheme.

Long-acting tablets of triethanolamine trinitrate biphosphate have been reported to have resulted in an improvement on the condition of about 78% of 103 patients suffering from angina pectoris.[115]

Repeat-Action Tablets—This kind of dosage form is planned to give the same general type of result as obtained with two individual doses of drug, and there is no need for an extended discussion here. It should be pointed out, however, that since these preparations contain enteric-coated cores, and, since there are extremely wide variations in stomach emptying time of such bodies,[5,116-118] results from these products may be expected to be very unpredictable.

Tableted Mixed-Release Granules—A fairly large number of drugs contained in this type of dosage form in its various modifications have been studied. In comparing a preparation of this type containing nitroglycerin to sublingual nitroglycerin for control of angina pectoris by means of cardiographic recordings, Mann[119] found that the average duration of effect from sublingual dosage was 18 minutes, which duration of effect contrasted markedly to an average of 343 minutes with the sustained-release tablets. However, in an evaluation of a large number of vasodilator drugs used for treatment of the same condition, Russek, et al,[120] judged results obtained with the same preparation disappointing. In testing another long-action preparation containing nitroglycerin, it was found that about 40% of a group of patients suffering from angina pectoris were able to get along with a greatly decreased use of sublingual tablets if dosed with the sustained-release preparation.[121]

Beck and co-workers[122] and Cobe[123] have reported on their evaluations of a long-acting benzyl penicillin preparation. The long-acting tablets each contained 125,000 units of penicillin, and drug was given in 500,000-unit doses. In both studies it was found that 9 hours after drug administration measurable blood levels of penicillin could be found. In both studies this was not the case when the same dose of phenoxymethyl penicillin was given in a regular tablet and in Cobe's study[123] when the same dose of benzyl penicillin was given in a buffered tablet. However, when the same preparations were evaluated in a government laboratory,[124] it was judged that the prolongation of activity with the long-acting preparation was insignificant and appeared to result from delayed absorption of the product. Peak penicillin levels were lower with the long-acting product than those obtained with

phenoxymethyl penicillin and buffered benzyl penicillin tablets.

An evaluation of a combination of an antispasmodic drug and a sedative in a long-acting dosage form is described by Steigmann, et al.[125] The patients involved in the study suffered from various gastrointestinal disturbances. In about half of these patients symptoms disappeared after dosage with the preparation once in the morning and once in the evening. No cross comparisons were made with the drug combination in its usual dosage form. The results obtained with this particular long-acting preparation were in accord with results obtained in other work, using the same preparation in the same type of study.[126-128]

Combinations of an antacid and antisecretory drug in a dosage form of the type used in the studies discussed above have been clinically studied.[129,130] Satisfactory results were obtained with the preparation. No nonprolonged-release preparation was used as a control. Other studies with the same type dosage form have also been reported.[131,132]

Other drugs contained in tablets of the mixed-release-rate granule type that have been used in clinical trials include quinidine gluconate[133] and nicotinic acid.[134]

Multiple-Layer Tablets—Several evaluations of this type product have been reported. Hirshleifer[135] studied the usefulness of pentaerythritol tetranitrate in angina pectoris with a product of this type. The particular preparation used contained 20 mg of drug with provision made to be released immediately after ingestion and 60 mg intended to dissolve slowly over a period of 8 hours. It was found that the frequency of anginal attacks were reduced and that nitroglycerin requirements were also reduced on the 2-tablet-a-day dosage schedule used. No control comparisons with nonprolonged-release dosage forms or placebo prolonged-release dosage forms, constructed in the manner of the true prolonged form, but containing the usual dose of drugs, were made. Hirshleifer[135] comments on the reassuring nature of prolonged acting dosage forms for anginal patients because of the tendency for such dosage forms to alleviate the anxiety which may precipitate the attacks of pain characteristic of this disease. Another similar study with the same prolonged-release pentaerythritol tetranitrate tablets is reported by Samuels.[136]

Two-layer prolonged-release tablets of sulfaethylthiadiazole were used by Sablosky[137] to determine the nature of the drug blood level vs time curve. The blood level resulting from a 4-Gm dosage showed a slightly reduced decay rate when compared to the decay rate reported in another publication, using nonsustained-release dosage forms of the same drug.[138] Other blood-level data from administration of this drug in the same sustained-release form are also reported.[60] Clinical evaluations of the same product also have been made.[139,140]

Porous Inert Carriers—Evaluations of a product of this type containing hexocyclium methylsulfate are reported by Kasich and Fein[141] and Kasich.[142] Basis for evaluation was the duration of increase in gastric pH in duodenal ulcer patients from the long acting as compared to the usual dosage form of the drug. Extension of activity was observed with the long-acting dosage form. Drugs formulated in these carriers include ferrous sulfate,[143] l-hyoscyamine,[144] and quinidine.[145,146]

Ion-Exchange Resins—A first approximation to the release rate of drug bound on ion-exchange resin allows an interesting assignment of products of this type to the class of prolonged-release products discussed earlier in this chapter in connection with types of release. In Eq. 15 presented earlier (page 1707), the release of drug from resin was shown to be dependent on the availability of cations (in the example used) to displace the cationic drug from the resin. The number of cations in the gastrointestinal environment is much greater than the number of drug cations bound to the resin in most cases of drug administration. This means that Eq. 15 can be written as

$$(R-SO_3^- \ H_3\overset{+}{N}-R') \rightleftharpoons R-SO_3^- + H_3\overset{+}{N}-R' \quad (16)$$

$$\downarrow$$

Absorption

since the concentration of cations, shown as (X^+Y^-) in Eq. 15, would remain essentially constant during the displacement reaction. Furthermore, if absorption of drug is relatively rapid after displacement from the resin, Eq. 16 can be written

$$(R-SO_3^- \ H_3\overset{+}{N}-R') \overset{K}{\rightarrow} R-SO_3^- + H_3\overset{+}{N}-R' \quad (17)$$

$$\downarrow$$

Absorption

Eq. 17 portrays a first-order chemical reaction for release of drug from the resin.[55] The equation describing the rate of this release is

$$\frac{d(R-SO_3^- \ H_3\overset{+}{N}-R')}{dt} = -K(R-SO_3^- \ H_3\overset{+}{N}-R') \quad (18)$$

and the concentration of drug remaining on the resin at any time will be given by

$$(R-SO_3^- \ H_3\overset{+}{N}-R') =$$
$$(R-SO_3^- \ H_3\overset{+}{N}-R')^0 \ (exp \ [-Kt]) \quad (19)$$

where $(R-SO_3^- \ H_3\overset{+}{N}-R')^0$ is the concentration of resin with drug at 0 time, K is the first-order rate constant for the displacement reaction, and t is time. As a consequence of Eq. 18 and 19, rate of release of drug from the resin will constantly decrease; as an additional consequence, only prolonged release, and not the constant rate release required for sustained release, can occur. Actually, due to the physical and physical chemical nature of ion-exchange resins, the release rate is even more complex than that described by Eq. 18, but this equation is a first approximation to release. In any event, rate decreases with time instead of remaining constant. A discussion of the kinetics of release from ion-exchange resins is available.[147]

Quantitative *in vivo* evaluation of both anionic and cationic drugs on anion and cation-exchange resins, respectively, has been reported. Abrahams and Linnell[148] presented blood-level curves of creatinine after the ingestion of this material as a marker material both bound to an ion-exchange resin and unbound. Initial absorption rate was decreased when drug on resin was ingested. Sufficient data are not included to judge whether or not the depression in levels and prolongation of action was concomitant with a marked reduction in physiological availability in the case of the resin preparation.

A more valid assessment of *in vivo* release and physiological availability of drugs on ion-exchange res-

ins has been reported by Chapman and co-workers.[149] In the case of creatinine there was no evidence of prolonged effect after comparing excretion rates following ingestion of drug resinate and plain drug. Administering drug as the resinate resulted in a marked decrease in physiological availability for absorption. With aspirin resinate there was no loss in availability for absorption but there was no evidence of significant prolonged release. With two commercial amphetamine products there was a slight loss in physiological availability and in the case of one product the excretion rate curve resulting from ingestion of drug resinate was superimposable on the curve resulting from ingestion of the drug in solution. Prolongation of release resulted with the other sample in accordance with the definition of the type of release adopted in this chapter. In the case of the two amphetamine resinates that showed different *in vivo* release behavior, it was not possible to demonstrate a significant difference in rate of release by *in vitro* procedures. It had been previously reported that *in vitro* and *in vivo* results with creatinine resinate correspond.[148]

Limited *in vivo* excretion tests with riboflavin-5'-phosphate complexed with an anion-exchange resin and blood-level evaluations of phenoxymethyl penicillin bound on the same type resins are reported by Brudney.[150] These tests indicate some prolongation of *in vivo* release from the drug-resin complexes.

Evidence for prolongation of effect from drug resinates is contained in work reported by Becker and Swift[151,152] conducted to determine reduction in toxicity when drug is combined with ion-exchange resin. Using cation-exchange resin in two different mesh sizes and drug as soluble salts, these workers found 1.2- to 12-fold decreases in toxicity when the LD50 of drugs on resins were compared to the LD50 of the unbound materials. Drugs studied included amphetamine, pyribenzamine, phenyltoloxamine, pyrilamine, and others. Furthermore, the time required to produce death was lengthened when drug was combined with resin prior to ingestion. It is implicit in these results that a prolongation of release of drug occurred by virtue of the combination with resin. However, it should be pointed out that since lethal or greater doses were given, there is no assurance that release rates under these conditions necessarily would be the same as the release rate with doses in therapeutic ranges. The displacement of drug from resin depends on the concentration of exchangeable ions at the absorption site. Large doses could be expected to cause a depletion in the number of these ions, which would result in a decrease in exchange rate. It also should be pointed out that all of the drug may not be displaceable from the resin.

Becker[153] and Becker and Hayes[154] have been able to demonstrate that oral codeine analgesia can be prolonged in the rat when codeine is bound to an ion-exchange resin. Measurements were made with a standard analgesiometric technique. A clinical comparison in humans of codeine and tuazolone resinates to other oral analgesic is reported by Cass, *et al.*[155]

Clinical investigations using appetite-suppressing drugs[148,156,157] and antitussives or analgesics[158-161] bound to ion-exchange resins have been reported. These reports are generally favorable to the use of drug resinates. Additional observations on the use of drug resinates have been made.[162,163]

Slightly Soluble Salts or Complexes—The largest number of products available in this form are those in which therapeutically active amines are combined with tannic acid. Garrett[164] has reported clinical trials on about 700 patients using *d*-amphetamine tannate. He reports that prolonged activity resulted from once-a-day administration and that a minimum of side effects were noted. No control comparison with the more commonly used salts of *d*-amphetamine was made. Such a control comparison is especially important with this drug since its half-life in humans is about 9 hours.[33] Another clinical study using a mixture of sympathomimetic amines and an antihistamine as tannates is reported by Kile.[165] This investigator reported that the product had a definite therapeutic advantage in about 80% of the patients used in the study. Side effects occurred in about 2% of the group. No control comparisons were made to these drugs in their usual dosage forms.

A clinical study with regard to the absorption, electrocardiographic effect, and antiarrhythmic properties of quinidine polygalacturonate is reported by Shaftel and Halpern.[166] Both dogs and man were used in the study. A sustained rate of absorption was noted in dogs on high dosages but was not noted in humans with therapeutic quantities of the composition. The pattern of absorption of the polygalacturonic acid salt of quinidine was similar to quinidine sulfate. However, the polygalacturonate was well tolerated by the patients since unfavorable side reactions did not occur. It was judged that the composition should be useful in cardiac patients who have been denied the benefit of quinidine in other forms because of the occurrence of local gastrointestinal distress. In another study on this composition Halpern, *et al*,[167] reports that its availability for absorption from the gastrointestinal tract appeared to be more uniform than the conventional inorganic salt of quinidine. Other studies with this compound have been reported.[168-170]

An evaluation of the dihydrocodeinone salt or complex of pectinic acid has been described by Brittain.[171] As a postoperative analgesic the composition was judged to have provided adequate relief of pain for periods up to three times that usually provided by morphine, meperidine, and similar analgesics. Side effects were reported as being slight. No control comparison to the usual salts of dihydrocodeinone was made.

Liquid Preparations—While certain long-acting preparations discussed under other headings (eg, *Ion-Exchange Resins*) may be administered in a liquid dosage form, there are other preparations that are unique in this classification.

Magnitude and duration of sulfaethylthiadiazole blood levels from a long-acting liquid preparation of this drug have been compared to those resulting from administration of the same drug in tablets.[138] Approximately the same maximum blood levels were obtained from both preparations, but they were somewhat prolonged with the liquid preparation. Other studies reporting sustained blood levels with the same preparation have also been presented.[67,149,172,173] Design considerations of *in vivo* and *in vitro* studies on the same product are discussed by Robinson and Swintowsky.[28] Several clinical reports on the use of the product have been published also.[174-178]

Long-acting liquid preparations consisting of sulfonamides suspended in lipid emulsions are based on the observation reported by Fienstone and co-workers[179] that simultaneous administration of oil with sulfonamides increased and prolonged blood levels of the drug. Studies have been made to compare blood levels resulting from ingestion of products made to exploit this absorption enhancement to the blood levels resulting from administration of the drugs in aqueous suspension. Results of trials comparing a lipid emulsion of N^1-acetylsulfisoxazole to an aqueous suspension of the same drug are reported by Svenson, *et al*.[180] Administration of the drug in the lipid emulsion resulted in markedly increased and prolonged levels of sulfisoxazole. A noncomparative blood-level study using the same preparation is reported by Krugman.[181] In another report the results of studying this preparation as well as lipid emulsions and aqueous suspensions of triple sulfonamides and sulfadiazine are given.[182] In this last report higher and more prolonged levels were obtained with the lipid emulsions of N^1-acetylsulfisoxazole and triple sulfonamides. With sulfadiazine the peak blood levels obtained were higher using the lipid emulsion but they were not as sustained as the levels resulting from administration of the aqueous suspension with diet. Additional observations on the use of lipid emulsion of sulfonamides have been reported by Stephens and Hendrickson,[183] Krugman and Frieden,[184] and Hagler, *et al*.[185]

Evaluations of work on the effect of oils on the absorption of sulfonamides should be made with recognition of the possible effect of an important variable on the results reported. It has been clearly shown by Reinhold, *et al*,[186] and Boyd and Dingwall[187] that blood levels of sulfonamides are markedly influenced by the particle-size distribution of the drug in the dosage form. Decreasing particle size increases surface area for a given weight of drug and in accordance with Eq. 8 increases solution rate of drug at the absorption sites and thereby in turn increases absorbability. Sulfonamides being only slightly soluble, and consequently slow dissolving, are subject to being rate-limited in absorption by the rate of the solid to solution step at the sites in accordance with the work on particle-size effect cited.[186,187] In the work cited with lipid emulsions[53,179-185] no mention is made of steps taken to control or characterize particle size distribution in the preparations compared. Difference in particle-size distribution in the products compared could cause the results reported.

Methods of in vitro Evaluation

No long-acting products are official in the current editions of the USP or NF. The standard disintegration time tester is valueless for evaluation of these products without modification, since the performance of such products depends upon release of drug into solution rather than fragmentation as required in the standard disintegration time test. In the NF one General Test describes an *in vitro* test procedure for time-release tablets and capsules. "The procedure is presented for its value as a routine control test method and is not intended to establish official specifications for any preparation recognized in the monographs section of this National Formulary." A caution appears which states: "This *in vitro* method is not designed to assure or measure safety or effectiveness, both of which must be determined through comprehensive *in vivo* studies and clinical evaluation. From the *in vivo* test data and clinical evaluation, however, suitable *in vitro* release limits may be established." It is obviously impractical for a manufacturer to submit each batch of his sustained-release product to a physiological assay. However, by careful calibration of a standardized *in vitro* method with results of appropriate physiological assays during the product development stage, the manufacturer should be able to exercise adequate control in subsequent production lots. A review[55] on long-acting products gives a summary of *in vitro* test methods; therefore only brief mention of the methods proposed will be made here.

The *in vitro* method used in the Food and Drug Laboratories is described by Lazarus and Cooper.[55] In this method the dosage form or its contents are placed in a glass tube fitted with a sintered glass filter above the bottom inlet and with a side neck for the outlet. Capsule contents are mixed with carborundum and placed in the body of the tube. Glass wool is used to retain tablets. Dissolution fluid at 37°C is pumped through the tube which is immersed in a constant temperature bath also held at 37°C. Samples of the dissolution fluid, which is initially simulated gastric fluid followed by simulated intestinal fluid, are withdrawn periodically for assay. Several methods are used wherein the USP disintegration tester is modified to provide a dissolution rate rather than disintegration time test. These have been described by Cooper,[188] Royal,[189,190] Campbell and Theivagt,[191] and Vliet.[192] Souder and Ellenbogen[193] describe a method for use with coated granules or bead-type products and apply it to *d*-amphetamine sustained-release capsules. Samples are placed in appropriately sized bottles containing gastric or intestinal fluids, and these are immersed in a constant temperature bath which contains mechanical devices to hold and rotate the bottles. Bottles are removed at appropriate times, and all beads larger than 40 mesh remaining are removed and assayed for drug content. Sjögren and Ervik[194] describe a method of determining drug-release rates from sustained-release tablets containing ephedrine hydrochloride or quinidine bisulfate in a plastic matrix.

It has been pointed out by Wagner[195] and others[196,197] that it is possible to describe *in vitro* release of drugs from long-acting products by relatively simple mathematical expressions.

Reviews on Long-Acting Drugs

Reviews on this subject have been published by Lang,[198] Grief and Eisen,[199] Lazarus and Cooper,[55,200] Stempel,[201,202] Campbell and Morrison,[203,204] Nelson,[4] Polli and Ravin,[205] Ravin and Bernardo,[206] and Shangraw.[207] In other reviews the pharmacological and clinical considerations[208] and pharmaceutical considerations[209,210] of prolonged-action products are discussed. An extensive evaluation of a number of anticholinergic drugs in both usual and long-acting dosage forms has been reported by Asher.[211]

Parenteral Products

Administration of drugs by the parenteral route is often employed in research and clinical practice for a sustained action of drug effect. But, as Wagner[212] has stated,

"There appears to be much less known about absorption from... various sites of (parenteral) administration than is known about absorption from the gastrointestinal tract or about percutaneous absorption. Despite the fact that the early testing of drugs in animals is mainly by parenteral routes of administration, and that many millions of dollars worth of parenteral products are sold annually for use in man, there has been very little good research done on the factors effecting absorption of drugs from parenteral sites of administration."

The discussion which follows will cover many physical, chemical, pharmacological, and physiological factors which may affect drug absorption after parenteral administration with particular emphasis on sustained-action medication. The history and merits of parenteral drug administration have already been mentioned elsewhere[213-215] (see Chapter 82 on *Parenteral Preparations*, page 1519). For convenience these factors will be considered under the headings of (1) drug pellet absorption, (2) solution absorption, and (3) parenteral dispersion absorption.

Pellet Absorption

The development and use of drug pellets in medical practice was initiated by Lafarge in 1861.[216] The technique was rediscovered in 1932,[217] 1936,[218] and 1937.[219] Deanesly and Parkes[219] stated, "It has now become clear that the chief problem in substitution therapy with hormone preparations is so to arrange administration as to imitate the steady continuous activity of the normal glands and avoid alternation of deficiency and wasteful excess of the hormone." In effect, the release of hormone from the pellet implant should mimic as nearly as possible hormone production in the normal gland. In recent years the clinical use of implanted pellets in human medicine has declined because of the development of effective oral dosage forms and parenteral solutions and suspensions. The three pellets which are official in the NF are listed in Table IX. The physical, chemical, and biological factors affecting pellet absorption will be discussed in the sections that follow.

Physical and Chemical Factors—Factors involved in the *in vivo* dissolution or absorption rate of a solid implanted pellet of drug can be better understood by expanding the Noyes–Whitney solution rate law given by Eq. 8 to the form shown here:

$$\bar{R} = \frac{k \bar{A} D S}{\delta} \tag{20}$$

where $\bar{R}$ is the mean absorption rate of a neutral organic drug from the pellet, k is a proportionality constant, $\bar{A}$ is the mean area of the pellet over the time interval of absorption, D is the drug's diffusion coefficient in the body fluids, S is the solubility of the neutral drug, and δ is the thickness of the diffusion or boundary layer around the pellet.

Solid Surface Area—In the earliest description of the pellet implantation technique, the investigators found that the drug's absorption rate was directly proportional to the area of the solid in direct contact with the body fluids at the site.[217] Subsequently, several absorption equations were proposed which were based solely on pellet geometry. These equations alone, however, could not be used to predict absorption rates of the

Table IX—Pellets in the NF

Desoxycorticosterone Acetate Pellets
Estradiol Pellets
Testosterone Pellets

solids since the equations did not have terms in them to account for the physical and chemical properties of the drugs used.[220] The pellet implantation technique is a valuable one in drug absorption studies since the variable of solid surface area can be readily measured and controlled. By contrast, the effective area of a mass of injected drug crystals exposed to the body tissues cannot be readily measured and controlled. The effective area of injected drug crystals depends on such factors as the distribution of particle sizes in the preparation and the technique of injection. On the other hand, the effective area of a pellet in contact with the body tissues can be measured before and after implantation by merely inspecting the solid directly. As a disk-shaped solid pellet is dissolved into body fluids at the implantation site, its dimensions are constantly changing with time; and due to the resulting area changes, the observed absorption rate initially would be greater than the rate later. To correct for these area changes, Eq. 20 has been defined in terms of a mean absorption rate, $\bar{R}$, and a mean area, $\bar{A}$.[221]

The Diffusion Coefficient—According to Eq. 20 and those that follow, the absorption rate of a solid drug is directly proportional to D, the diffusion coefficient of the drug molecule in solution. In this case one can think of the diffusion coefficient as a measure of the resistance to free diffusion of the drug molecule in the body fluids. According to the Einstein–Stokes equation,[222] the diffusion coefficient of a neutral molecule may be approximated by

$$D = k'T/6\pi\eta r \tag{21}$$

where k' and π are constants, T is the absolute temperature, η is the viscosity of the medium, and r is the radius of the diffusing molecule. At a given temperature all the terms except r in Eq. 21 are constant. Considering only spherical or near spherical molecules, experiments have shown that those with high molecular weights (large radii) have smaller diffusion coefficients than molecules having low molecular weights (small radii). As a consequence, the lower-molecular-weight molecules with larger values for D also would have more rapid absorption rates per unit area as defined by Eq. 20.

Solubility—From Eq. 20 a drug's absorption rate is directly proportional to its solubility in the fluid medium surrounding the pellet. A drug's solubility, S, at a particular temperature depends on many factors. Among these factors are its intrinsic solubility at a given temperature, S_0, its pK_a, the pH of the medium immediately adjacent to the solid, the polymorphic or solvate form of the drug, and others.

Although Eq. 20 applies to solid neutral organic drugs, it may be generalized to include solid organic weak acids or weak bases. Substitution of Eq. 5 into Eq. 20 yields for a solid monobasic weak acid

$$R/\bar{A} = \frac{kDS_0}{\delta}\left[1 + \frac{K_a}{(H^+)_d}\right] \tag{22}$$

And substitution of Eq. 6 into 20 yields for a solid monoacidic weak base

$$\bar{R}/\bar{A} = \frac{kDS_0}{\delta}\left[1 + \frac{(H^+)_d}{K_a}\right] \tag{23}$$

where the term $(H^+)d$ refers to the hydrogen-ion concentration of the diffusion layer surrounding the solid. Note that this may *not* necessarily be the same as the hydrogen-ion concentration of the body fluids such as the blood, serum, or lymph. In experimental subcutaneous measurements in Sprague–Dawley rats, the diffusion layer pH (or pH_d) has ranged from a low of 3.57 to a high of 9.00, depending on the drug used, while the pH of the rat blood was of the order of pH 7.3–7.4.[220] Although the present discussion bears directly upon parenteral absorption, one should realize that the diffusion layer pH may have an important influence on solid drug solubility and dissolution rate in the gastrointestinal tract or elsewhere in the body.

In addition to the influences of pH and pK_a on solubility, the drug's physical form may greatly affect solubility and drug availability to the animal. For example, the antibiotic, novobiocin, is a weak dibasic acid. When an aqueous solution of the sodium salt is acidified, an amorphous precipitate of novobiocin free acid results. This amorphous or noncrystalline form is metastable and converts upon standing to a crystalline form. The amorphous form is at least ten times more soluble in 0.1 N hydrochloric acid than is the crystalline form. No pellet implantation studies have been reported using this drug, but Mullins and Macek[223] found that when the amorphous and crystalline acids were separately administered orally to dogs, plasma levels of the drug were detected only with the amorphous form.

Some drugs show polymorphic character and have one or more distinct crystalline forms or types. The different crystalline forms of the same compound usually have different melting points, solubilities, and other physical properties such as density and refractive index. The importance of polymorphism on drug solubility and absorption rate may be seen in the following example. The water solubilities of two polymorphic forms of 6 α-methylprednisolone have been measured at 37°C, and form II had 1.2 times the water solubility of the more stable form I.[224] When these two forms were made into pellets and implanted subcutaneously into Sprague–Dawley rats, form II had 1.7 times the absorption rate of form I. While the agreement between the ratio of the water solubilities to the absorption rates was only approximate, this fact does point out the importance of polymorphism in drug absorption studies.[220] Brandstätter–Kuhnert[225] has emphasized that about one in every three organic compounds exhibits polymorphic behavior. Of 16 sex hormones listed in a recent edition of the Austrian Pharmacopeia, 11 are polymorphic. For example, testosterone, diethylstilbestrol, and estradiol have two forms, each with distinct melting points. Estrone has three forms, while progesterone has five polymorphs, two of which, the α (mp 128°–133°C) and the β (mp 121°C) forms, are official in the NF.

Although the use of different drug polymorphs provides investigators with one means of varying drug absorption rate due to solubility differences among the various forms, another important means of modifying drug solubility and absorption rate is by the use of drug solvates. Shefter and Higuchi[226] have pointed out that the tendency of many drugs to form adducts provide pharmaceutical investigators with a powerful tool in effecting rapid dissolution of highly insoluble substances. When some drugs are crystallized from aqueous or organic solvents, they may form hydrates or solvates having definite chemical composition and distinct physical properties apart from that of the nonsolvated form. The hydration of an anhydrous drug, G, in water may be represented by the equation

$$G_{solid} + xH_2O_{liquid} \rightleftharpoons [G(H_2O)_x]_{solid} \tag{24}$$

Anhydrous glutethimide, for example, melts at 83°C;

Table X—Selected Physical Properties and Absorption Rate Data on Prednisolone TBA Phases[228]

Crystal modification	Melting point (°C)	Number of animals	Absorption rate[a] initial area (mg/hr/cm²) × 10³	Crystallizing solvent
Phase I (anhydrous phase)	244–249	5	1.8_4 ($\pm0.4_2$)	20% Ethanol–water
Phase II (monoethanol solvate)	145	6	8.7_0 ($\pm0.9_1$)	90–95% Ethanol–water
Phase IV (hemiacetone solvate)	226–230	6	2.2_0 ($\pm0.6_9$)	Acetone

[a] Absorption rate followed by the 95% confidence interval in parentheses.

and when it is crystallized from water, a hydrated form with a melting point of 68°C precipitates. *In vitro* the dissolution behavior of these two forms in a 13.4% (w/v) ethanol–water mixture was also different as Fig. 734 shows. The maximum solubility level attained with the anhydrous form was 1.6 times greater than the solubility of the hydrated form at 25°C.[226]

The pellet implantation technique also has been used to study the absorption rates of drug solvates. Biles[227] has reported on some of the physical properties of the anhydrous and two solvated forms of prednisolone *tert*-butyl acetate (TBA). Samples of these forms were compressed into pellets and subcutaneously implanted into Sprague–Dawley rats. A summary of the results of this experiment is found in Table X. There was no significant difference in absorption rate between the anhydrous and hemiacetone solvate phases of prednisolone TBA, but there was over a fourfold enhancement of the absorption rate when the monoethanol solvate, Phase II, is compared to the anhydrous Phase I.

Shefter and Higuchi[226] have commented quite correctly that:

"It is apparent that the appropriate selection of the most suitable crystalline modification, whether arising from polymorphic differences or as a result of solvate complex formation, can often significantly increase the medicinal value of a given drug in a particular dosage form... Since molecular complexes of this type are readily produced, particularly by relatively insoluble drugs, this approach may often provide the answer for those products which are poorly available because of slow rates of dissolution."

Thus, any factor that might affect total drug solubility such as drug pK, diffusion layer pH, presence of drug polymorphs, or solvates may affect solid drug absorption rate sometimes to a large degree.

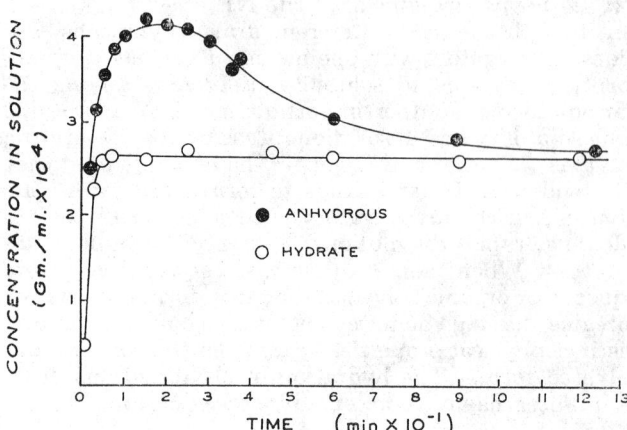

Fig. 734. The dissolution of anhydrous and hydrated glutethimide in 13.4% ethanol solution at 25°C (after Shefter, E., and Higuchi, T.[226]).

Diffusion Layer Thickness—According to Eq. 20 the absorption rate of a solid drug is inversely proportional to the thickness of the diffusion layer, δ. When the fluid movement surrounding the solid drug is slow and nonturbulent, as most likely is the case with body fluids at the site of implantation, the diffusion layer thickness may be estimated by

$$\delta = (\eta L/v\rho)^{0.5} \qquad (25)$$

where η is the viscosity of the medium surrounding the solid, L is the linear dimension of solid surface exposed to the medium, v is the stirring velocity of the medium, and ρ is the density of the medium.[229] Substitution of Eq. 25 into Eq. 20 and rearranging gives

$$\bar{R}/\bar{A} = k\,D\,S\,(v\rho/\eta L)^{0.5} \qquad (26)$$

From Eq. 26 it is clear that the observed absorption rate of an implanted solid will be increased if the stirring velocity, v, of the medium surrounding the pellet is increased, while the absorption rate will decrease if the viscosity of the medium is increased. The density term, ρ, would be constant at any given body temperature. The dimensional term, L, may be considered to remain nearly constant since experimentally only small amounts of drug were allowed to be removed from the pellets. Too much weight loss distorts the shape of the pellets, and Eq. 20 and those based on it become less exact.

Other Factors—Other physical factors that have been suggested to affect implanted drug absorption rates are pellet density (hardness), crystal size used in making the pellet, and the influence of diluents, as follows:

Density—The densities of pellets made of pure drug depend upon the compression pressure used in making them. Since absorption rate is directly proportional to the area of the pellet exposed to the body fluids at any time, pellet density *per se* should have no effect on absorption rate.[230]

Crystal Size—Experiments *in vivo* have shown that the size of drug crystals used in the manufacture of pellets of pure drug seem to have no effect on pellet absorption rate. Probably the best explanation for this observation is that the diffusion layer thickness as defined by Eq. 25 is large, particularly under the conditions where stirring velocity or movement of body fluids at the implantation site is small. Such a diffusion layer probably is thick enough to mask minor surface imperfections due to crystal size differences or other reasons.[230]

Diluents—While pellet density and the size of the crystals used in pellet manufacture apparently have no effect on absorption rate, the addition of a diluent to the formulation does have an effect. There are many types of diluents and their modes of action are different in either enhancing or retarding drug absorption from implants. Unfortunately, there are no general rules available for predicting absorption rates of a given drug-diluent mixture.[230]

Biological Factors—Several biological factors which have been suggested may affect drug absorption rate from implants. Among them are phagocytosis, physiological need for the drug or animal's sex, encapsulation, animal's age, species difference, "ghost" formation, the site of implantation, and body temperature. There is no evidence that the process of phagocytosis need occur during implant absorption. And neither physiological need for the drug nor animal's sex seems to effect absorption rate.[230] When drug pellets are allowed to remain *in situ* a week or longer, a fibrous tissue capsule tends to form about the solids. In an effort to explain the slow absorption rates of certain solids some authors have stated that the capsule might well be responsible for the drug's poor availability. Others state that the well-vascularized capsule had no observed effect on drug absorption rate. Unfortunately, no carefully controlled experiment has resolved the point, but what little evidence there is seems to indicate that encapsulation has little or no effect on solid drug absorption rate. In most cases the rate-limiting step in solid drug absorption is the dissolution process and not the passage of drug in solution through the biological membranes surrounding the pellet.

Both animal age and species differences have been reported to have an influence on implant absorption rates. The differences observed may well be due to differences in body temperature, composition of fluids at the site, and animal physical activity, or movement of body fluids at the absorption site.[230] Pellets implanted for an extended time often acquire a ghost, that is, the microscopic pores of the solid surface become occluded with a proteinaceous material. If the implant is then placed in a suitable solvent, the drug will dissolve away leaving the insoluble ghost residue usually having the shape of the original pellet. However, available evidence seems to show that the ghost has no effect on the absorption rate of solid drugs.[230]

Two biological factors that could have a large influence on solid drug absorption rate are the following: variations in implantation site in animals as well as variations in body temperature. According to Eq. 26 any increase in stirring velocity of the medium surrounding the solid should increase the drug absorption rate. It would seem that the implantation site should influence absorption rate because the agitation or stirring velocity may differ at different sites. One clinician[231] suggested that the patient should massage the skin region over the site of the steroid implant to enhance the rate of drug absorption.

In recent years there has been an increased interest in the use of hypothermia in medicine. This technique involves the cooling of a person below his normal body temperature of 37°C. The use of hypothermia has found application in heart, brain, and other types of surgery. This technique, among others, also has been considered seriously for use on space explorers because their oxygen and food requirements would be less.[232,233] From a physical–chemical standpoint one might expect that the lowering of body temperature would affect the absorption rates of parenterally administered solid drugs. Inspection of the right-hand side of Eq. 20 shows that the three terms, the diffusion coefficient, D, the solubility, S, and the diffusion layer thickness, δ, all should be affected by the animal's temperature and the body fluids surrounding the solid. Temperature would have an influence on each of these three terms and would differ in each case. For example, the diffusion coefficient (Eq. 21) decreases as the absolute temperature is lowered because D is directly proportional to T. The diffusion coefficient is also inversely proportional to the viscosity of the fluid medium. If the temperature of the animal is reduced, the viscosity

of its body fluids becomes greater with the result that the diffusion coefficient and absorption rate are reduced. Solubility of nearly all organic solids decreases as temperature is lowered, which would also result in a decreased absorption rate. Also, the diffusion layer thickness would become larger as the body temperature is reduced. A decrease in temperature would cause an increase in the viscosity, η, term in Eqs. 25 and 26. The net result is a decrease in absorption rate as body temperature is reduced. The influence of temperature on increasing or decreasing solid drug absorption rate from implanted pellets has been shown in quantitative animal experiments.[234,235] Folkman and Long[236] have demonstrated the usefulness of implanted silicone rubber capsules as carriers for prolonged drug therapy. They state that both the surface area of the capsule, as well as the storage temperature of the capsule prior to implantation, appear to govern the rate of drug release. Subdermal implantation of silicone rubber capsules containing either estrogen or the synthetic progestin, megestrol acetate, results in slow and constant release of the drug for prolonged time periods.[237] Such implants are under clinical trial for human fertility control.

The fact that parenteral solid drug absorption rate depends in part on body temperature makes this a variable which should be considered when drugs are tested preclinically on mammals having body temperatures different from humans. Furthermore, the human body temperature may vary over a wide range. Murphy and Faul[238] have found, for example, that aged persons may suffer from hypothermia during periods of cold weather. Of eight old people admitted to the hospital, the three that lived had body temperatures ranging from 29.4 to 32.2°C.

Solution Absorption

As seen from the previous section, the absorption rate of such solid dosage forms as pellet or crystal implants depends largely on the solid's physical and chemical properties and the properties of the solution immediately surrounding it. As a rule, absorption is rate-limited by the rate of solution of the solid into the biological fluids surrounding it. The influences that blood and lymph flow near the implant have on its absorption rate are minor and were considered negligible. However, the absorption rates of parenterally administered drugs dissolved in aqueous or nonaqueous solvents by such routes as the subcutaneous or intramuscular ones are much more sensitive to regional blood and lymph flow. Details of normal blood and lymph flow in and around the many possible parenteral injection sites may be found in standard texts.[239] The details of the mechanism of absorption or transport of drugs or ions in solution through biological membranes in general is a subject of intensive research today and one may refer to several excellent reviews on the subject.[214,240–242] The present discussion deals only with a qualitative outline of some of the physical and biological factors that may influence parenteral absorption of drugs already in solution. For this purpose, drug solutions intended for parenteral use may be divided into those which are administered in aqueous and nonaqueous media.

Aqueous Media

Most drugs given parenterally in aqueous solution produce their therapeutic effect quite rapidly. When they are given intravenously, the onset of action may occur within seconds, as in the case of the ultra-short-acting barbiturates used as anesthetics. Subcutaneous and intramuscular injections, while not so fast acting as the intravenous type, still produce a fairly prompt response if the drug is in aqueous solution. Prompt onset of action by reason of therapeutic blood levels is usually accompanied by fairly rapid drug inactivation and excretion or both. This may make frequent injections necessary for a sustained effect. Even if frequent injections are given, the blood level over a period of time may show a number of peaks and valleys, which is often objectionable. A parenteral preparation providing a sustained therapeutic effect following a single injection is frequently desirable and offers advantages; patients receiving such an injection are spared the unpleasantness and inconvenience of frequent injections, and the busy physician or nurse is assured that the patient is under continuous therapy.

Absorption Sites—When an aqueous drug solution is injected subcutaneously, for example, the absorption of small ions or molecules appears to occur primarily through the capillary walls and only a small fraction of the absorption occurs via the lymphatic system.[183] However, in the case of macromolecules, such as those found in snake venoms, it is believed that lymphatic drainage primarily accounts for their removal from the "bite" or injection site.

A sustained action may be obtained when the drug solution is given as a continuous infusion or drip by the intravenous or subcutaneous routes. With careful supervision such a procedure may be continued over several hours or days. Detailed discussions of some of the procedures involved with the continuous infusion technique may be found in technical publications available from manufacturers of these products.[243,244] One may prolong parenteral absorption of drugs in aqueous solution by mechanical or physical and pharmacological means.

Mechanical or Physical Means of Drug Prolongation—Drug solution absorption may be modified by the use of tourniquets or pressure cuffs, application of cold, changes in body movement, viscosity and osmotic effects of the vehicle, and changes in the concentration and volume of the injected solution.

Tourniquet—An early example of the use of a tourniquet in prolonging "drug" absorption is found in the treatment of snake bites. If a victim has been bitten on an extremity, the venom may spread by two routes. In the rare cases where the snake injects the venom directly into a large blood vessel, it will spread throughout the body and death may occur quickly. Usually, however, the venom is injected into an intramuscular or a subcutaneous site. The venom spreads from these sites by the lymphatic circulation, and it moves slowly, particularly if there is little or no muscular movement. Part of the suggested medical treatment calls for the victim to lie down and to apply a tourniquet a few inches above or proximal to the region of the bite. It should be tight enough to retard lymphatic and some venous flow but not enough to interfere with arterial flow to the limb. Eventually, the venom will reach the venous circulation from the upper thorax. If the spread from the injection site is thus delayed enough, the liver can metabolize the venom without having it swamp the liver's detoxifying mechanisms.[245-247]

In the early days of parenteral penicillin G therapy the sodium or calcium salts had to be frequently administered so as to maintain adequate blood levels. Single doses had to be given about every four hours to

offset the rapid excretion of the drug.[248] Carlinfanti and Morra[249] proposed that an aqueous penicillin solution could be injected subcutaneously into the thigh or arm and a rubber tourniquet could be applied to delay the venous and lymphatic drainage. These authors remarked that the pressure must be light so as not to cause discomfort in the limb. Although the technique did prolong the penicillin serum level, it had the disadvantage that the dose released to the general circulation could not be easily controlled.

Work with aqueous solutions of radioactive sodium chloride, $^{24}NaCl$, has shown the influence of the application of a tourniquet to a limb upon the clearance or disappearance of drug from subcutaneous and intramuscular injection sites. The decrease of radioactive counts with time could be measured by placing a Geiger–Müller tube over the injection site. After the injection of $^{24}NaCl$ solution intramuscularly, for example, a normal clearance or disappearance rate of radioactive material could be seen. When a tight tourniquet was applied to the limb, however, the counts per minute remained nearly constant. When the tourniquet was removed some minutes later, the clearance rate was increased over the normal rate. This increase was attributed to reactive hyperemia or congestion which follows when an organ's blood supply is obstructed for a time. The increase of clearance rate of $^{24}NaCl$ is probably due to a net flow of fluids into the capillaries from the perivascular spaces.[250-254]

It should be pointed out that the mode of clearance of ^{24}Na ion from an intramuscular injection differs from that previously discussed for snake venoms. Stone and Miller,[255] who studied the clearance of ^{24}Na ion from the dog's gastrocnemius muscle, concluded that the lymphatic system of the dog's leg played no significant role in its clearance. Virtually all the radiosodium ion could be accounted for in the femoral vein blood, while the amount of the ion recovered from the thoracic duct lymph was not greater than 1.1% of the injected amount.

Application of Cold—Before the advent of depot penicillin salts like procaine penicillin G, several investigators proposed that solutions of penicillin G could be retarded in their absorption by applying an ice pack over the intramuscular injection site.[256-258] By using this cooling technique they found a significant saving in the amount of penicillin required for each patient. The retarded absorption rate was attributed to a decrease in the circulation in and around the site of the intramuscular injection.[256,257] One would also expect that the diffusion coefficient and consequently the absorption rate for penicillin anion would be decreased by the lowered temperature in accordance with Eqs. 21 and 27.

However, application of cold may give rise to practical problems in parenteral therapy. In civilian disasters such as the 1942 Coconut Grove fire in Boston and in military encounters such as in the Italian campaign during World War II, some of the injured were subjected to extreme cold conditions. Their peripheral circulation was reduced by a combination of shock and cold. Absorption of subcutaneous or intramuscular injections of morphine sulfate often was greatly delayed over normal. The result was that the victim who had received multiple injections might experience a delayed morphine poisoning as much as 7 to 8 hours after the drug administration.[259,260] Under these conditions the recommended treatment was to give the drug intravenously, if possible, or give it intramuscularly (not subcutaneously) low in some extremity and apply massage to the injection site to enhance absorption rate. If signs of poisoning develop, a tourniquet should be placed above the morphine depot to slow absorption rate.

Franke, et al,[254] showed that the clearance rate of intramuscularly administered radioactive sodium chloride, ^{24}NaCl, from the hamstring muscles of dogs decreased compared to controls when an ice–salt mixture was applied over the injection site. Curiously enough, when radiant heat was applied to the region over the injection site, a decrease in the clearance rate of radiosodium over normal conditions was also observed. They concluded that the status of skin vessel dilation alone was not an adequate criterion of the effective circulation in the muscle. Miller and Wilson[253] injected radiosodium chloride solution intradermally and found likewise that reflex vasoconstriction due to the application of cold water led to a decrease in the clearance rate of ^{24}Na ion, but reflex vasodilation produced by hot-water packs resulted in little or no increase in the clearance rate. With intradermal studies Braithwaite and co-workers[261] found that environmental temperature did influence clearance rates of ^{24}Na ion.

Body Movement—It is generally reported that exercise or other muscular activity increases the clearance rates of intramuscular injections of ^{24}NaCl.[252] Although body movement has a net effect in increasing ^{24}Na ion clearance, one problem is that the conditions of "exercise" must be carefully defined in order to obtain reproducible results. Barcroft and Swan[262] have stated that although the mean blood flow through the calf, for example, is greater after than before rhythmic exercise there are wide variations in blood flow between the relaxation and contraction phases. To complicate the picture further, individuals with high emotional tone such as those with apprehension and hyperthyroidism also show higher clearance rates for ^{24}Na ion than normal individuals following intramuscular administration.[265]

Results similar to those obtained in intramuscular studies were found with subcutaneous injections of radiosodium ion into the human leg.[264] Braithwaite and co-workers[261] showed that there were variations in absorption rates of ^{24}NaCl solutions administered intradermally into various regions of a normal individual. The absorption rate from abdominal skin was 3% per minute, from the chest 5.7% per minute, and from the forearm 7.8% per minute. Such variations in absorption rate at different intradermal sites could be attributed to differences in body movement and circulation at the injection site.

Viscosity or Tonicity—Addition of water-soluble or water-miscible agents may modify the biological response to aqueous parenteral solutions markedly. Prescott and co-workers[266] conducted acute toxicity studies on mice by subcutaneously injecting streptomycin sulfate solutions of differing compositions. They held the injection volume of all solutions constant but varied the concentration of streptomycin sulfate and the added agent systematically. Agents added to the streptomycin sulfate solution were glycine, sodium glucuronate, sodium α-keto glutarate, sodium pyruvate, glycerin, and propylene glycol. Prescott, et al,[266] found, for example, that there was 8% survival in mice when 10 mg of streptomycin sulfate in water alone was injected. Survival was increased to 20% when 5 mg (0.27 M) glycine was added to the above formula, and 100% when 75 mg (4 M) glycine was added. They found similar trends in per cent survival with the other agents. In other studies[267] these workers found that

the use of 35% (v/v) aqueous glycerin as the solvent also decreased the acute toxicities in mice of subcutaneously administered streptomycin sulfate, isoniazid, and various mixtures of these two drugs as compared to the aqueous solutions of these drugs.

In this connection Brigham and Nielsen[268] noted that in mice the subcutaneous acute toxicities of aqueous solutions of streptomycin and dihydrostreptomycin sulfates were reduced when small amounts of calcium pantothenate were added to the aqueous media. The chronic toxicities of all of the preparations, however, were virtually identical by their method of analysis.[268] Acute toxicity studies in general are more sensitive to dosage form effects than are chronic toxicity studies. In tracer studies Madison and Christian[269] observed that the subcutaneous absorption rates of radiosodium chloride (^{22}NaCl and ^{24}NaCl) in water was reduced when concentrations of sucrose were increased up to 2M.

The role that nonelectrolytes such as glycerol and sucrose play in reducing acute toxicity or absorption rates of cations like streptomycin and sodium ions is due in part to changes they impart to the viscosity of the solvent system, and in part to their osmotic pressure effects. Robinson and Stokes[222] point out that *in vitro* all ions are reduced in mobility when in the presence of added nonelectrolytes. Different ions are affected differently by a given nonelectrolyte, and there is a fair correlation between the size of the ion and the extent of its retardation. With sodium ion, for example, the *in vitro* ion mobility in 10% aqueous sucrose solution was 81% of that found in water at 25°C, and in 20% sucrose ion mobility fell to 62%. Similar reductions of ion mobility were found in 10 and 20% glycerol.[222] Eastland[270] has cited other examples of the influence of viscosity on the absorption rate of parenteral products.

The addition of a weak or strong electrolyte such as an amino acid or calcium ion to a drug ion in solution should reduce drug-ion mobility partly by the viscosity effect previously mentioned and partly by interionic forces between the drug ion and the added ion or ions. In addition to the pure viscosity effects the presence of a hypertonic solution at the injection site would lead to a net flow of body fluids toward this site. Thus, a solvent drag effect, or the net flow of fluids toward the injection region, could account for part of the observed decrease in absorption rate.

Concentration and Volume—According to Fick's law of diffusion in one direction

$$\left(\frac{da}{dt}\right)' = -AD\frac{dc}{dx} \qquad (27)$$

where $(da/dt)'$ is the clearance rate of the drug, and dc/dx is the concentration gradient. The clearance, or absorption rate, of a diffusing molecule is directly proportional to the area, A, of the solution exposed to the absorbing membrane, the diffusion coefficient, D, and the concentration gradient, or the difference between the drug's concentration at the injection site and its concentration in the blood flowing past the injection site. A drug's concentration in the blood is usually assumed to be very small compared to that at the injection site because of the drug's dilution in the fluids of distribution, metabolism, and excretion. Thus, one might expect to find that if the area of the injected solution exposed to the absorbing membrane is held constant, the amount absorbed per unit area would be greater for the more concentrated solution. One of the problems presented in any discussion of drug absorption from solution is that the shape or area of the injected solution often varies. When the shape of the injected solution is spherical, for example, its area is proportional to the two-thirds power of the volume. When the same volumes are injected, the spherical shape would have the smallest area of all possible shapes. As can be seen from Eq. 27, clearance or absorption rates of a drug is directly proportional to its area exposed to the absorbing membrane, as well as its concentration in solution. Warner and co-workers[271] showed what the influence of both of these factors, volume and concentration, had on the clearance rate of radiosodium ion. Into the same subject, they injected 1 ml of a radiosodium solution into the gastrocnemius muscle of one leg. Then they injected into the other gastrocnemius muscle the same amount of radioactivity, but varied the volume of the vehicle. They found that the rate of clearance of ^{24}NaCl in the subject was greater for the smaller volumes than with the larger one. Apparently, the decrease in area exposed to the absorbing membrane was more than compensated for by the increase in drug concentration. When identical volumes were used on each leg in the same subject, the clearance rates at both sites were practically identical. The relatively long diffusion path for ^{24}Na ion from the center of the injection bubble might also be a rate-limiting factor. Schriftman and Kondritzer[272] conducted a similar experiment with intramuscular injections of atropine solutions. They reduced injection volume from 0.1 to 0.025 ml and at the same time increased the drug concentration from 2 to 8 mg/ml. They noted that the solution with the smaller volume (higher drug concentration) showed a greater per cent decrease in the amount of atropine remaining in the muscle after 10 minutes. However, when they held the concentration of atropine constant, and varied the volumes administered from 0.05 to 0.1 ml, the smaller volume was cleared more rapidly. On the other hand, when the volume was held constant, and the concentration was varied, the solution having the lower concentration was cleared more rapidly; Fick's law of diffusion alone does not explain these findings.

Pharmacological Means of Drug Prolongation—Schou[214] has suggested that delays in subcutaneous absorption of some drugs could be due to liberated histamine or 5-hydroxytryptamine at the injection site. When histamine solution alone is injected intradermally or subcutaneously, the capillaries dilate, the permeability of their walls increase, and local edema results. Edema indicates that the net flow of fluid peripherally to the injection region is greater than inward. When histamine was added to a solution of sodium sulfacetamide, for example, there was a decrease in the subcutaneous absorption rate of the sulfonamide as compared to a solution containing no histamine.[273] The mechanism for the delay of subcutaneous absorption produced by histamine is not at present known. Like some other drugs, atropine is capable of releasing histamine,[263] which may explain some of the findings of Schriftman and Kondritzer[272] discussed previously. Evidence that atropine has a local retarding action at the site of a subcutaneous or intramuscular injection was further borne out in the studies by Ramachandran and Ågren.[274] They found that when radioactive di*iso*propylfluorophosphate, D^{32}FP, and atropine were administered together at the same injection site, the absorption rate of D^{32}FP fell considerably as compared to when D^{32}FP was administered alone. The rate of absorption of carrier-free ^{32}P-labeled inorganic phosphate was also reduced by adding atropine. The

presence of histamine, however, does not always decrease absorption rate. McGirr[251] noted that the clearance rate of ^{24}NaCl from an intramuscular and intradermal site was increased by the addition of histamine.

An older technique for prolonging the action of drugs given by injection is to incorporate epinephrine hydrochloride[251] or a similar agent with the drug in solution. This approach is still often used with local anesthetics to slow down the removal of drug from the limited area where needed. The use of epinephrine for this purpose is unsatisfactory where a drug is being used for its systemic action. In such cases the amount of epinephrine required would produce rather profound and undesirable systemic effects.

Nonaqueous Media

Although water is the solvent of choice for the preparation of parenteral products, it often cannot be used because of the limited solubility of a given drug in water, or because of possible hydrolytic reactions between the solvent and the drug. Tables XI and XII list the official parenteral drugs in the NF and USP having a nonaqueous solvent as a vehicle. Reese[275] has pointed out that one of the major problems facing the industrial pharmacist is the solubilization of organic compounds. A good organic solvent for a drug may not necessarily be the best vehicle for its parenteral use. Reese lists the physical, chemical, and biological factors to consider in selecting nonaqueous solvents intended for parenteral use.

Some of the desirable physical properties of the vehicle listed by Reese[275] are that it should be clear and colorless, preferably without odor or taste, particularly if it, or its metabolites, is excreted via the lungs or

Table XI—Parenteral Drugs in the NF Having a Nonaqueous Solvent as a Vehicle

Digitoxin Injection (5–50% alcohol)
Dromostanolone Propionate Injection (oil)
Erythromycin Ethylsuccinate Injection
  (polyethylene glycol 400)
Estradiol Benzoate Injection (oil)
Estradiol Cypionate Injection (oil)
Estradiol Dipropionate Injection (oil)
Estrone Injection (oil)
Fluphenazine Enanthate Injection (vegetable oil)
Menadione Injection (oil)
Methocarbamol Injection (polyethylene glycol 300)
Nandrolone Decanoate Injection (sesame oil)
Nandrolone Phenpropionate Injection (oil)
Progesterone Injection (suitable solvent)

Table XII—Parenteral Drugs in the USP Having a Nonaqueous Solvent As a Vehicle

Aurothioglucose Injection (suitable vegetable oil)
Deslanoside Injection (10% alcohol)
Desoxycorticosterone Acetate Injection (vegetable oil)
Diethylstilbestrol Injection (suitable vegetable oil)
Digoxin Injection (10% alcohol)
Dimercaprol Injection (benzyl benzoate and vegetable oil)
Sterile Epinephrine Suspension (oil)
Estradiol Valerate Injection (suitable vegetable oil)
Hydroxyprogesterone Caproate Injection (suitable
  vegetable oil)
Sterile Procaine Penicillin G with Aluminum Stearate
  Suspension (refined peanut oil or sesame oil)
Sterile Propyliodone Oil Suspension (peanut oil)
Testosterone Cypionate Injection (suitable vegetable oil)
Testosterone Enanthate Injection (suitable vegetable oil)
Testosterone Propionate Injection (suitable vegetable oil)

Table XIII—Nonofficial Parenteral Nonaqueous Solvents[a]

Solvent	Appearance	Solubility	Specific gravity	Boiling point
1,3-Butylene glycol	Colorless, viscous liquid	Soluble in water and alcohol	1.005	204°C
N,N-Dimethyl-acetamide	Clear liquid	Miscible with water and alcohol and very soluble in organic solvents and mineral oil	0.943	165.5°C
Dioxanes: 2,2-Dimethyl-1,3-dioxolane-4-methanol	Colorless liquid, practically odorless	Miscible with water, alcohol, esters, aliphatic and aromatic hydrocarbons, and nearly all other organic solvents	1.064	82–83°C
Ethyl carbonate	Colorless liquid, pleasant ethereal odor	Immiscible with water, but miscible with alcohol and ether	0.975	126°C
Ethyl lactate	Colorless liquid, with characteristic odor	Miscible with water, alcohol and ether	1.042	154°C
Glycerol formal	Colorless, odorless liquid of low viscosity	Miscible with water	...	...
Glycofurol®	Colorless liquid	Miscible with water, and soluble in ethanol and glycerin	1.078	80–155°C
N-(β-Hydroxy-ethyl)-lactamide	Clear, colorless syrupy liquid	Miscible with water	1.192	...
Isopropyl myristate	...	Oil miscible and water immiscible	0.852	...

[a] Adapted from data in Spiegel, A. J., and Noseworthy, M. M.[276]

saliva. A liquid vehicle should remain so over a 0–50°C temperature range. If it is solid, the vehicle should remain so up to 45–50°C. In any event the vehicle should have a low vapor pressure so that ampuls containing it may be easily sealed by heat. The solvent should regain its normal properties after freezing and thawing. The pH of the aqueous solution should be compatible with the pharmaceutical and biological system or have low buffer capacity. The solvent or final dosage form should have such a viscosity that it is easily injectable. Finally, the vehicle should be miscible with both water and plasma, as well as with other common pharmaceutical solvents used in parenteral formulations.

Some of the desirable chemical properties of a parenteral solvent are that it should be stable at the high temperatures commonly used for accelerated storage conditions or heat sterilization. It should be unaffected by oxygen, light, or metals, or else be easily stabilized. Also, it should not react chemically with the ingredients in the formulation, and it should have stability over the pH range of 2 to 9.

Some of the desirable biological properties are that the vehicle should be easily sterilized by some common method. It should not readily support the growth of microorganisms, or else it should be easily preserved. The vehicle and its metabolites should have low acute and chronic toxicities in the amounts normally used in parenteral products. The vehicle should also conform to any Federal Food and Drug Administration requirements. The vehicle and metabolites should be pharmacologically inert, nonirritating, and nonsensitizing. Finally, the vehicle must be pharmacologically compatible with the drug and not interfere with its action or unduly delay the response of the drug.

Obviously, no known vehicle could fulfil all these requirements. However, such a compilation serves as a useful checklist for evaluating the suitability of any solvent proposed for parenteral use. Commonly used nonaqueous solvents for parenteral products are fixed oils (see Chapter 30 on *Natural Products*, page 476). Spiegel and Noseworthy[276] have reviewed the use of nonaqueous solvents in parenteral products and pointed out some of the problems associated with the use of fixed oils. They state that while the toxicity of these oils is low, some may elicit allergic responses in sensitive patients. These oils may give rise to local tissue reactions such as cyst formation, foreign body granulomas, and sometimes nerve injury. Further, fixed oils may be poor solvents for some drugs. Since these oils are not water miscible, they cannot be used in products for intravenous use unless they have been emulsified first. There have been attempts in recent years to expand the list of therapeutically and pharmaceutically acceptable vehicles for parenteral products. While none of the solvents listed in Table XIII are as yet official, many promise to be useful adjuncts for formulation. Spiegel and Noseworthy[276] point out, however, that such solvents should be used only if a definite need is established and that any formulation containing a nonaqueous solvent is potentially a new entity and must be thoroughly tested before its release.

Dosage Form Effects

As early as 1936 Deanesly and Parkes[277] reported on the influence of dosage form on the biological activity of some sex hormones. In one experiment they dissolved 2 mg of testosterone into different volumes of arachis oil, a fixed oil (see Table XIV). They administered these solutions subcutaneously to castrated male rats in 10 equal daily injections. The animals were killed one day after the last injection, and the weights of their prostate glands and seminal vesicles at the end of the

Table XIV—Effectiveness of 2 Mg Testosterone in Different Amounts of Arachis Oil[277,a]

Total volume of oil (cm³)	Average weight of	
	Prostate (mg)	Seminal vesicles (mg)
2.0	61	27
5.0	183	118
10.0	219	163

[a] 10 rats in second group, 5 in others.

experiment were taken as a measure of the physiological availability of the testosterone. They found that the biological response to the solutions as measured by organ weight was greatest for the largest volume of oil, or the lowest concentration of steroid. In another experiment they dissolved 10 mg of androsterone into the vehicles: olive oil, arachis oil, castor oil, and propylene glycol. The average prostate and seminal vesicle weights for the rats are shown in Table XV. These authors also cited earlier work which showed that the activity of testosterone varied according to the kind of oil in which it was dissolved. Testosterone dissolved in mineral oil, for example, was inactive biologically.[278] Thus, the biological response to steroids appears to depend in part on the volume of the vehicle, and in part on the kind of vehicle used.

More recently, Honrath, *et al*,[279] also demonstrated that the intensity of the biological activity of certain sex hormones could be greatly affected by the volume of the solvent used. They prepared separate solutions containing testosterone and testosterone propionate in 0.2 or 0.8 ml of sesame oil. Each of the four solutions was injected as a single dose subcutaneously into castrated male rats. The weight changes of the seminal vesicles and ventral prostate glands were followed over 15 days. Table XVI shows the approximate weights of the seminal vesicles at the end of 10 days. A similar weight trend was followed by the ventral prostate. Testosterone dissolved in 0.2 ml sesame oil showed a more prolonged and intense action than that dissolved in 0.8 ml of oil. When the same experiment was repeated using testosterone propionate, the reverse trend in biological effect was noted. The 0.8-ml solution now gave the more intense action compared to the 0.2-ml solution.[279] The work by Deanesly and Parkes[277] and Honrath, *et al*,[279] is presented in some detail, because they illustrate how important dosage form can be in affecting a given biological response. Their work also underscores some of the problems and pitfalls in the designing and screening of parenteral prolonged-acting drug products which employ nonaqueous solvents. Deanesly and Parkes[277] stated that in work comparing male hormone compounds the techniques employed must be carefully standardized. No doubt dosage form effects such as the ones previously mentioned may explain discrepancies observed in the experimental results from different laboratories.

Table XV—Effectiveness of 10 Mg Androsterone in 2 ml of Various Media[277,a]

Medium	Average weight of	
	Prostate (mg)	Seminal vesicles (mg)
Olive oil	78	18
Arachis oil	133	21
Castor oil	149	19
Propylene glycol	199	37

[a] 5 rats in each group.

The nature of drug release from nonaqueous solvents which are water miscible often differs greatly from those which are water immiscible. Deanesly and Parkes[277] found that androsterone was more than two times more effective in stimulating organ growth when administered in the water-miscible propylene glycol vehicle than in the water-immiscible olive oil vehicle (see Table XV). They suggested[219] that the steroid was probably precipitated after the injection when the propylene glycol was diluted with body fluids with the result that a crystalline mush formed at the injection site. A commercial preparation of estradiol in aqueous propylene glycol was designed to utilize this principle. After dilution in the body fluids at the intramuscular site, the water-insoluble estradiol precipitates in the tissues resulting in a prolonged effect.[280] Local anesthetic drugs precipitate in the subcutaneous region when injected with a water-miscible solvent.[281] Ekwall[282] has cited unpublished work on the spreading of a carcinogen from the site of a subcutaneous injection in mice by the use of a fluorescence microscope. When lipophilic liquid petrolatum was the solvent, the fluorescent oil drops remained unchanged for long periods. The carcinogen diffused from the oil so slowly that no fluorescence was observed in the surrounding tissue fluids. However, an increased fluorescence was observed in the subcutaneous fatty tissue. This indicated that at least a part of the carcinogen was concentrated there.

Table XVI—Approximate Seminal Vesicle Weight at the End of 10 Days[279]

Weight of steroid dissolved in different volumes of sesame oil	Seminal vesicle weight (mg/100 Gm Rat)	
	0.2 ml Oil	0.8 ml Oil
Testosterone 5 mg	28	10
Testosterone propionate 5 mg	58	140

When lipophilic–hydrophilic solvents were used, the spreading mechanism was of a different type. If the solvent employed was a polyglycol, the dissolving power of which rapidly diminished on dilution with body fluids, some of the carcinogen precipitated as crystals near the injection site.[282] Once drug crystals form, the mechanism of their absorption would be governed by many of the factors outlined in the preceding section on pellet absorption and the following section on parenteral dispersion absorption.

In summary, differences in biological effects arising from the parenteral use of nonaqueous solvents may be due to one or more of the following factors:

1. The area of the solution in contact with the absorbing membrane may not be constant for repeated injections of a given volume of solution.
2. The absorption rates of different vehicles may vary.
3. A drug's absorption rate from vehicles may vary because of differences in viscosity among them.
4. The drug's partition coefficient between the nonaqueous vehicle and the body fluids may differ from one vehicle to another.
5. The target organ's growth or response rate may be different according to the time course of drug or active metabolite concentrations in the body fluids.
6. The rate of metabolism and excretion of the drug, and the rate of excretion of its active metabolites, may depend on the drug release from the solvent used.
7. The miscibility of the solvent and the solute solubility in the body fluids may affect the mechanism of drug absorption.

Dispersion Absorption

Macek[283] notes that as a general rule, when biological activities are equal, it is more desirable and economical

Table XVII—Parenterals in the NF Having Suspended Drug

Sterile Betamethasone Sodium Phosphate and Betamethasone Acetate Suspension
Sterile Desoxycorticosterone Pivalate Suspension
Sterile Estradiol Suspension
Sterile Methylprednisolone Acetate Suspension
Sterile Progesterone Suspension
Sterile Testosterone Suspension

Table XVIII—Parenterals in the USP Having Suspended Drug

Aurothioglucose Injection (suitable vegetable oil)
Sterile Benzathine Penicillin G Suspension
Cholera Vaccine
Sterile Corticotropin Zinc Hydroxide Suspension
Sterile Cortisone Acetate Suspension
Adsorbed Diphtheria Toxoid
Adsorbed Diphtheria and Tetanus Toxoids
Diphtheria and Tetanus Toxoids and Pertussis Vaccine
Adsorbed Diphtheria and Tetanus Toxoids and Pertussis Vaccine
Sterile Epinephrine Suspension (oil)
Sterile Hydrocortisone Acetate Suspension
Sterile Hydrocortisone t-Butyl Acetate Suspension
Influenza Virus Vaccine
Isophane Insulin Suspension
Insulin Zinc Suspension
Extended Insulin Zinc Suspension
Prompt Insulin Zinc Suspension
Protamine Zinc Insulin Suspension
Sterile Medroxyprogesterone Acetate Suspension
Adsorbed Pertussis Vaccine
Pertussis Vaccine
Plague Vaccine
Poliomyelitis Vaccine
Sterile Prednisolone Acetate Suspension
Sterile Procaine Penicillin G Suspension
Sterile Procaine Penicillin G with Aluminum Stearate Suspension (refined peanut oil or sesame oil)
Sterile Propyliodone Oil Suspension (peanut oil)
Sterile Propyliodone Suspension
Rabies Vaccine
Smallpox Vaccine
Adsorbed Tetanus Toxoid
Adsorbed Tetanus and Diphtheria Toxoids
Sterile Triamcinolone Acetonide Suspension
Typhoid Vaccine
Typhus Vaccine

to search for water-soluble derivatives of new drugs intended for parenteral administration than it is to formulate the physically less stable parenteral dispersions such as colloids, emulsions, and suspensions. However, in some cases where water-soluble derivatives of slightly soluble compounds have been prepared, reduced pharmacological activity is observed when they are administered parenterally.[284]

Formulation of parenteral dispersions is often unavoidable when:

1. No adequate substitute is available for the pharmacologically active agent (eg, biological products like serum albumin, the insulins, and the natural oil form of vitamin K).
2. The drug is unstable when dissolved in aqueous solution (eg, the slightly soluble procaine and dibenzylethylenediamine salts of penicillin G).
3. A sustained-action depot preparation is desired (eg, the depot vitamin B$_{12}$, steroid, and insulin preparations).
4. An intravenous parenteral product contains a water-immiscible oil (eg, the oil-in-water emulsion of natural vitamin K, Sterile Phytonadione Emulsion USP, or parenteral fat emulsions).

Thompson[285] and others[286] have stated that it is possible with almost any drug which is to be administered parenterally to design a sustained- or prolonged-action preparation based on one or more of several mechanisms. Some of these have already been discussed in connection with pellet or solution absorption. The mechanisms involve the use of

1. Viscous water-miscible vehicles such as gelatin, dextrans, or polyvinylpyrrolidone (PVP).
2. Water-immiscible vehicles like oil as such or thickened with substances like aluminum monostearate.
3. Solid pellets.
4. Thixotropic "pellets."
5. Vasoconstrictors.
6. Insoluble derivatives.

Because of practical problems, usually the best method for preparing sustained-action medication involves the use of an insoluble derivative of the drug suspended in an aqueous or oily medium. Many factors which could affect drug absorption from suspensions have been mentioned previously in connection with drug pellets and drug solutions. Suspensions, however, have properties of their own which might influence drug absorption rate.

Physical Properties—A few physical properties of importance for suspensions are related to possible changes in the crystals making up the suspension, the use of pharmaceutical adjuvants, and rheological behavior. See Tables XVII and XVIII for parenterals in the NF and USP having suspended drug.

Crystal Changes—One problem often encountered by the formulator in preparing physically stable and therapeutically effective parenteral suspensions is that of controlling possible crystal changes with time. The crystal modification in the finished formulation may or may not involve changes in the crystal habit. The crystal habit refers to the external shape of a crystal, which depends on the relative sizes of the various crystal faces and upon the interfacial angles. For example, crystals in a formulation may change their size while not changing their habit because of the cycling or variations of shelf temperature. The resulting crystal size change could depend on many factors including the magnitude and frequency of the shelf temperature cycles, the slope of the temperature–solubility curve for the solid, and the rate of solution and the rate of crystallization for the solid. Crystal changes may also involve a change of crystal habit resulting in the formation of one or more polymorphic and solvate forms of the drug. Such changes often have an important bearing on the particle-size distribution of the parenteral formulation.[287] Work cited in connection with the influence of drug polymorphism and solvate formation on the absorption rates of pellet implants also indicates how important these factors might be on drug crystal availability. Macek[283] gives an example involving the formulation of a parenteral suspension of cortisone acetate. When the dry, premilled solid cortisone acetate of the wrong crystal form was rapidly suspended in an aqueous vehicle by mechanical agitation, and then allowed to stand undisturbed for a time, a conversion to the more stable form occurred, resulting in an unacceptable formulation which showed crystal growth and caking. There are many examples which could be cited where differences in particle size of crystals in the suspension affect the onset and duration of the desired biological response.[288–290]

Adjuvants—The formulation of parenteral dispersions often requires the use of pharmaceutical adjuvants such as surfactants, hydrocolloids, and other agents which aid in the manufacture and stability of parenteral dispersions. These agents must meet most of the requirements set forth for parenteral nonaqueous solvents that

Table XIX—Some Agents Used in Parenteral Dispersions[a]

Surfactants	Hydrocolloids	Other
Emulphor EL-620	Sodium carboxy-methylcellulose	Aluminum mono-stearate
Lecithin	Gelatin (nonantigenic)	Polyethylene glycol 300
Pluronic F-68 (polyethylene-polypropylene nonionic)	Methylcellulose	Propylene glycol
	Polyvinyl-pyrrolidone	Silicone antifoam
		Sorbitol
Polyoxyethylene sorbitan mono-laurate	Sodium alginate (nonantigenic)	
Polysorbate 80 USP (Tween 80)		
Sorbitan trioleate (Span 85)		

[a] Adapted from Macek, T.[283]

were discussed previously. In addition, adjuvants used in parenteral dispersions must be nonantigenic, non-pyrogenic, and nonhemolytic in the concentrations commonly used. Table XIX, adapted from data in an article by Macek[283] shows a partial listing of some of the agents used in commercial parenteral dispersions. The role that some of these adjuvants might play in prolonging drug release from the injection site has only been incompletely studied and should be the subject of further research.

Rheological Behavior—Although the physical properties of the individual suspended crystals affect the drug's physiological availability, the physical properties of the suspension as a whole influence the product's usefulness and availability. The work of Ober and co-workers[291] well illustrates how the parenteral product formulator can control the physical properties of the suspension to achieve a prolonged-action product. These investigators were concerned with formulating an intramuscular depot procaine penicillin G product. They knew from earlier work that the retarded absorption of procaine penicillin G seemed to depend on two factors, namely, (1) the low water solubility of the procaine salt compared with that of the sodium or potassium salts and (2) the formation of a compact drug depot within the muscle. Their problem was to design a product that was fluid enough to pass through a hypodermic needle, yet would "set up" as a compact depot in the muscle tissue.

This type of preparation has been called a "thixotropic pellet" to distinguish it from the solid pellets described previously.[285] Also, they had to devise suitable *in vitro* and *in vivo* methods to evaluate the effectiveness of these formulations. Among the physical factors of the drug suspension which they studied were the rheological structural breakdown point, the particle-size distribution of the crystals making up the suspension, the specific surface of the powders used in the suspension, and the per cent solids in the suspension.

The science of rheology concerns itself with the study of the properties and behavior of flowing substances such as suspensions. Certain suspensions show thixotropic behavior, which means that when they are shaken or stirred vigorously they become more fluid in their consistency and flow more readily than when they stand for some time. When a thixotropic suspension is stirred very slowly, it initially shows a nearly infinite viscosity. Yet, when it is stirred or shaken more vigor-

ously, its viscosity is reduced and the suspension begins to flow. The point at which the viscosity of the suspension suddenly becomes reduced, or the suspension structure begins to break due to an increase in stirring rate (rate of shear), is called the structural breakdown point. A thixotropic suspension has two advantages: (1) Under storage conditions the preparation is stabilized by its structure and high viscosity and (2) when the suspension is shaken prior to use, it can become fluid enough to pass through a hypodermic needle. Once the suspension reaches the site in the muscle the suspension structure reforms and a compact depot or "thixotropic pellet" results. Diffusion of the excess water in the product away from the injection site may also make a more compact depot.[287]

Because of the many test suspensions that had to be studied, it was impractical for Ober, *et al*,[291] to carry out extensive animal studies. They developed an *in vitro* technique for determining whether or not a compact depot was formed after drug injection. They injected 600,000 units of procaine penicillin G suspension into a 2% gelatin gel. Those suspensions having structural breakdown point (T) values in excess of 100,000 dyne-cm gave spherical depots in gelatin which resembled those found in muscle tissue of sacrificed rabbits. Pastelike suspensions having high penicillin dosage, but which lacked a T value of 100,000 dyne-cm, gave no spherical depot at all.

For a formulation to be practical there must be little chance that needle plugging will occur during its injection. Ober and co-workers[291] designed an instrument to measure needle plugging tendency *in vitro*. They found that suspensions having T values greater than 1,000,000 dyne-cm either due to high specific surface (S_w) or per cent solids or both, tended to give rise to excessive needle plugging. Further, they found that formulations having S_w values less than 10,000 cm²/Gm also tended to plug needles. Many of the interrelationships among the factors contributing to a successful prolonged-acting parenteral procaine penicillin G product are summarized in Fig. 735.

Thus, an acceptable formulation could result if the specific surface of the crystals used was between 10,000 and 30,000 cm²/Gm. Below 10,000 cm²/Gm, the formulation tended to plug a 20-gauge hypodermic needle. Above 30,000 cm²/Gm, the manufacturing problems of milling and handling of the powders became increasingly difficult. When the specific surface was 30,000 cm²/Gm, the per cent solids in the formulation could be varied from about 50 to 75% and still have an acceptable depot formulation. The particle-size distribution of the powder had to be a broad rather than a narrow one. For example, the powders tested were blends of three to one mixtures of micronized to milled samples. Finally, the rheological structural breakdown point, T, of the suspension could be between the 100,000 to 1,000,000 dyne-cm range. Less than 100,000 dyne-cm the spherical depots found by experience to give a sustained-action product were not formed. Above 1,000,000 dyne-cm, the preparation was difficult to inject.

Another illustration of how physical properties of a suspension as a whole may influence drug availability can be seen from the extensive work of Buckwalter and Dickison.[292] They studied the influence of drug particle size and the nature of the vehicle on the degree of absorption of intramuscular procaine penicillin G suspensions. They followed the blood levels of the drug in rabbits after the administration of procaine penicillin G in different vehicles. Some of their observations were that larger crystals of drug suspended in water, sesame oil, and peanut oil tended to delay absorption of drug and prolong the blood levels. However, in peanut and sesame oils gelled with 2% aluminum monostearate, the micronized form of the drug exhibited a more prolonged effect as seen from the rabbit blood-level values. In human studies the small particles of procaine penicillin G suspended in peanut oil gelled with 2% aluminum monostearate showed more delayed absorption than five other formulations. Frederick[287] suggested that this was probably due to the incipient depot formation brought about by the aluminum monostearate and was a result of the marked cementing action of the fine particles.

Crystal Type—Buckwalter and Dickison[292] also noted that the type of procaine penicillin crystals used had a profound effect on their absorption rates as measured by rabbit blood-level studies. They compared the blood levels of formulations prepared from small and large crystal types crystallized from propanol, crystals from an acetone–water mixture, and water precipitated crystals all ground to the same mesh size. Although the authors did not suggest this explanation for their results, the differences they observed among crystals precipitated from different solvents might well have been due to polymorphic or solvate formation changes in the penicillin crystals. However, this explanation can only be tentative, because Macek[293] states that procaine penicillin G can be crystallized as prismatic, rod-like needles and as flat, scalelike platelets. Both crystals are of the same form by x-ray diffraction examination. The plateletlike crystal has been shown to be superior for the preparation of sterile, dry penicillin formulations.

Biological Factors—An important factor affecting parenteral suspension absorption rate is that of body movement (stirring) at the injection site. The importance of this factor alone may be appreciated by considering a few selected examples from the clinical literature.

When procaine penicillin G preparations were undergoing clinical trials, the influence of body movement on drug absorption was studied. Robinson[294] administered an intramuscular injection of procaine penicillin G suspension (small particle size) with peanut oil and 2% (w/v) aluminum monostearate as the vehicle. She noted that the serum levels of the two active and three moderately active ambulatory patients were often higher initially than those of the sedentary patients. Twenty-four hours later the serum levels of the ambulatory patients tended to be lower than those of the sedentary patients. She concluded that the high levels found soon after injection might be due to increased massage of the injection site which released penicillin into the bloodstream early.[294] The rapid excretion of the penicillin from the bloodstream and the more rapid solution rate of the solid particles due to the activity of the patients accounted for the lower levels later on. It is worth noting that with certified lots of commercial preparations of procaine penicillin G suspended in oil gelled with aluminum monostearate irregular absorption has been found. Taggart and co-workers[295] frequently observed that after receiving a single injection, some patients failed to show measurable blood concentrations on one or more successive days only to be followed by measurable penicillin concentrations on succeeding days. However, they made no attempt to correlate blood level results with body activity data.

Boger, *et al*,[296] found the degree of body movement influenced the duration of effective penicillin blood level. They administered 300,000 units of procaine penicillin G suspended in oil intramuscularly to patients with lobar pneumonia, and to ambulatory control patients. Massage of the injection site was avoided. They found that in the group of ten pneumonia patients that the mean duration of penicillin plasma concentrations above 0.039 units per ml was 33 hours, and in the nine ambulatory patients the mean was 12 hours.

The report by Boger, *et al*,[296] prompted the Finnish workers Savolainen and Tommila[297] to extend their previous studies to include tests with certain penicillin preparations on outpatients or healthy working subjects in one group, and on hospital patients in another group. Single injections of 600,000 units of two commercially available products, F_1 and D_1, containing an aqueous suspension of procaine penicillin G, were made into the gluteal region. The mean peak serum levels attained at 1 to 2 hours for the ambulatory patients was more than twice as high as that for the hospital patients (see Table XX). Particularly high serum concentrations were found in those ambulatory subjects who played active games like basketball or tennis during the experiment. The authors stated that it was probable that the muscular movement in walking and running promoted absorption of penicillin from the gluteal region. The high serum concentrations after exertion could have been predicted since Eqs. 25 and 26 show for solids like implanted pellets or injected crystals that the observed absorption rate should be increased if the stirring velocity, v, of fluids surrounding the solid is increased due to muscular movement or massage of the injection site. With a greater absorption rate it is reasonable to expect to find a high serum penicillin concentration after exertion.

Lukash and Frank[298] also studied the variables of body movement and site of injection as they might influence the intramuscular absorption of depot benza-

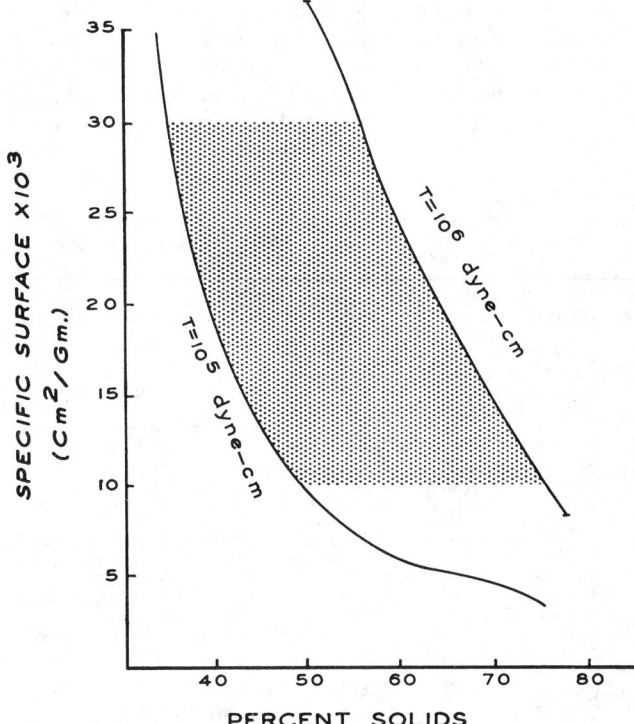

Fig. 735. Procaine penicillin G formulations having a broad particle-size distribution and values of specific surface, per cent solids, and *T* values falling within the shaded region form suspensions which can be readily injected, form spherical depots, and are clinically effective for prolonged-action therapy.[291]

thine penicillin G. The two sites were the traditional upper, outer quadrant of the gluteal region, referred to by these investigators as the "posterior site," and an anterior gluteal region on the lateral thigh referred to as the "anterior site." The test groups were Navy recruits. One group was in active training, while the other was hospitalized. The more active group had longer penicillinemia than the less-active, hospitalized group, but only with the posterior site of injection. Lukash and Frank[298] state that the responsible factor in determining the duration of penicillinemia may not necessarily be due to activity *per se*, but rather to specific movements at the injection site, whether it be muscular or mechanical, or both.

A final example illustrating the importance of injection site and body movement on drug absorption rate may be seen in the report by Stalnaker[299] who discussed the "lumpy insulin area syndrome." In 15 of 105 patients with diabetes mellitus, improper injection technique by the patients was a major factor in poor control of their disease. A diabetic patient not taught the correct way to inject insulin into himself could easily deposit the correct dosage too deeply (intramuscularly) or not deep enough (intradermally or into

Table XX—Mean Penicillin Concentrations in Sera of Hospital Patients and in Outpatients or Healthy Working Subjects During 24 Hours after a Single Intramuscular Injection of 600,000 Units of Commercial Preparations F₁ and D₁ Containing Procaine Penicillin G in Aqueous Suspension[297]

Preparation (strength)	Number of patients	Mean maximum concentration[a] U/ml serum	Mean concentration[a] at 24 hours U/ml serum
F₁ (outpatients)	11	0.72 (0.28)	0.13 (0.03)
F₁ (hospital patients) (350,000–360,000 U/ml)	10	0.29 (0.05)	0.15 (0.02)
D₁ (outpatients)	8	0.58 (0.18)	0.22 (0.03)
D₁ (hospital patients) (300,000–360,000 U/ml)	10	0.28 (0.09)	0.09 (0.02)

[a] Standard deviation indicated in parentheses.

the subcutaneous fat). Insulin not properly injected in the subcutaneous region, where normal absorption could take place, may become temporarily trapped, resulting in areas of lumpiness or swelling. This lumpiness tends to occur when injections were given into the same region for several days. As a result the patient's blood glucose would remain high despite a seemingly adequate insulin dosage. The attending physician might assume that the patient was resistant to treatment or the daily dosage was not high enough. The insulin dosage might be increased in an attempt to control the disease. However, if the patient should exercise or traumatize the lumpy area, insulin could be suddenly released into the system resulting in an insulin reaction. If this occurs, the insulin dosage would be promptly reduced. The result would be a vicious cycle which might be repeated several times before the difficulty was recognized.

Administration of drugs by the intramuscular route sometimes has been accompanied by tissue injuries and complications. Some causes of tissue damage may be attributable to improper injection technique, the drug product itself, or mechanical injury of tissue due to improper needle point geometry.[300-302] Table XXI lists

Table XXI—Sizes of Intramuscular Lesions after Antibiotic Injections into 10 Rabbits[300]

Substance injected	Mean size of necrosis and inflammation (cm)				
	2 days	4 days	7 days	18 days	40 days
Chloramphenicol succinate	6.8	4.8	3.9	2.8	2.8
Chloramphenicol vehicle	3.5	3.0	2.3	0.5	0.3
Tetracycline	4.8	4.9	5.5	2.5	1.6
Tetracycline vehicle	3.1	2.0	2.6	0.8	0.5
Oxytetracycline	3.5	3.2	2.4	0.6	0.5
Oxytetracycline vehicle	3.4	2.2	2.5	0.8	0.7
Penicillin	3.6	2.4	1.1	0.6	0.3
Penicillin vehicle	1.5	1.2	0.0	0.0	0.0
Saline (control)	1.0	0.7	0.0	0.0	0.0

a number of antibiotic preparations and the mean size of regions that showed necrosis and inflammation in muscle tissue of rabbits. What influence tissue damage may play in affecting absorption rates of intramuscularly administered drugs is not well known at present.

Reviews on Long-Acting Parenteral Products

A general review on biopharmaceutical considerations involved in long-acting parenteral products administered subcutaneously or intramuscularly has appeared.[235] Current developments in human fertility regulation and control have been reviewed by Swyer,[303] Segal,[304] and Diczfalusy.[305] Powell[306] reviewed long-acting antimalarial parenteral products.

The parenteral route of drug administration is an important one both for the preclinical screening and evaluation of drugs and the clinical use of drug products in human and veterinary medicine. Rational design of sustained-action parenterals depends upon many factors including the physical, chemical, and pharmacological properties of the drug and its adjuvants. Physiological factors such as injection site, body movement, and body temperature at the site all may play an important role in drug availability of such products.

References

1. Australian Pat. 109,438; Brit. Pat. 523,594.
2. US Pat. 2,738,303; Brit. Pats. 742,097 and 765,086.
3. Jenkins, B. W., *GP*, **9**(6), 66 (1954).
4. Nelson, E., *Clin. Pharmacol. Therap.*, **4**, 283 (1963).
5. Blythe, R. H., *et al*, *Am. J. Pharm.*, **131**, 206 (1959).
6. Davenport, H. W., *Physiology of the Digestive Tract*, 2nd ed., Yearbook, Chicago, 1966.
7. Kresnicka, R. D., *Hosp. Topics*, **45**(4), 73 (1967).
8. Ballard, B. E., *Am. J. Pharm. Educ.*, **32**, 938 (1968).
9. Asker, A. F., and Becker, C. H., *J. Pharm. Sci.*, **55**, 90 (1966).
10. Winek, C. L., *et al*, *Lancet*, **2**, 155 (1967).
11. Hollister, L. E., *New Engl. J. Med.*, **266**, 281 (1962).
12. Levy, G., *J. APhA*, NS4, 16 (1964).
13. *Federal Register*, **32** (Sep. 6, 1967).
14. Shore, P. A., *et al*, *J. Pharmacol. Exptl. Therap.*, **119**, 361 (1957).
15. Hogben, C. A. M., *et al*, *J. Pharmacol. Exptl. Therap.*, **120**, 540 (1957).
16. Schanker, L. S., *et al*, *J. Pharmacol. Exptl. Therap.*, **120**, 528 (1957).
17. Schanker, L. S., *et al*, *J. Pharmacol. Exptl. Therap.*, **123**, 81 (1958).
18. Hogben, C. A. M., *et al*, *J. Pharmacol. Exptl. Therap.*, **125**, 275 (1959).
19. Theorell, T., *Arch. Intern. Pharmacodyn.*, **57**, 205, 226 (1937).
20. Texter, E. C., *et al*, *Physiology of the Gastrointestinal Tract*, Mosby, St. Louis, 1968, p. 207.
21. Krebs, H. A., and Speakman, J. C., *J. Chem. Soc.*, **1945**, 593 (1945).
22. Nelson, E., *J. APhA*, *Sci. Ed.*, **46**, 607 (1957); **47**, 297 (1958); **48**, 96 (1959).
23. Nelson, E., *J. APhA*, *Sci. Ed.*, **48**, 96 (1959).
24. Chapman, D. G., *et al*, *J. APhA*, *Sci. Ed.*, **43**, 297 (1954).
25. Chapman, D. G., and Campbell, J. A., *Can. J. Biochem. Physiol.*, **33**, 753 (1955).
26. Chapman, D. G., *et al*, *J. APhA*, *Sci. Ed.*, **45**, 374 (1956).
27. Chapman, D. G., *et al*, *Can. Med. Assoc. J.*, **76**, 102 (1957).
28. Robinson, M. J., and Swintosky, J. V., *J. APhA*, *Sci. Ed.*, **48**, 473 (1959).

29. Filbert, M. G., and Weller, J. M., *Proc. Soc. Exptl. Biol. Med.*, **101**, 294 (1959).
30. Astwood, E. B., *Trans. Assoc. Am. Physicians*, **70**, 183 (1957).
31. Schwartz, M. A., and Nelson, E., *Husa's Pharmaceutical Dispensing*, 6th ed., Mack Publ. Co., Easton, Pa., 1966, p. 440.
32. Nelson, E., *J. APhA, Sci. Ed.*, **46**, 572 (1957).
33. Campbell, J. A., *et al, Can. Med. Assoc. J.*, **81**, 15 (1959).
34. US Pat. 2,809,918.
35. US Pat. 2,895,880.
36. US Pat. 2,897,121.
37. Serine, G., *Drug Cosmetic Ind.*, **101**, 56 (Sep., 1967).
38. US Pat. 2,887,438.
39. US Pat. 2,736,682.
40. US Pat. 2,809,916.
41. US Pat. 2,895,881.
42. US Pat. 2,793,979; S. African Pat. 18934/54.
43. US Pat. 2,853,420.
44. US Pat. 2,809,916.
45. S. African Pat. 4070/56.
46. S. African Pats. 966/53, 3211/58, 3486/58, 3487/58, and 3599/58.
47. Brit. Pat. 744,096.
48. Can. Pats. 518,324; 567,738; and 538,810.
49. Cavallito, C. J., and Jewell, R., *J. APhA, Sci. Ed.*, **47**, 165 (1958).
50. Halpern, A., *et al, Am. J. Pharm.*, **130**, 190 (1958).
51. US Pat. 2,805,977.
52. US Pat. 2,875,130.
53. US Pats. 2,238,973 and 2,867,565.
54. Feldmann, E. G., *J. APhA*, NS9, 8 (1969).
55. Lazarus, J., and Cooper, J., *J. Pharm. Pharmacol.*, **11**, 257 (1959).
56. Laurence, D. R., *Quantitative Methods in Human Pharmacology and Therapeutics*, Pergamon, London, 1959.
57. Modell, W., *J. Am. Med. Assoc.*, **167**, 2190 (1958).
58. Frederik, W. S., and Cass, L. J., *J. New Drugs*, **5**, 138 (1965).
59. Cass, L. J., and Frederik, W. S., *Curr. Therap. Res.*, **7**, 673, 683 (1965).
60. Blythe, R. H., *Drug Std.*, **26**, 1 (1958).
61. Campbell, J. A., *et al, Can. Med. Assoc. J.*, **77**, 602 (1957).
62. Dragstedt, C. A., *J. Am. Med. Assoc.*, **168**, 1652 (1958).
63. *J. APhA*, NS9, 46 (1969).
64. Green, M. A., *Ann. Allergy*, **12**, 273 (1954).
65. Feinblatt, T. M., and Ferguson, E. A., *New Engl. J. Med.*, **254**, 940 (1956); **256**, 331 (1957).
66. Mulligan, R. M., *J. Allergy*, **25**, 358 (1954).
67. Bancroft, C. M., *Ann. Allergy*, **15**, 297 (1957).
68. Rogers, H. L., *Ann. Allergy*, **12**, 266 (1954).
69. Bresler, R. R., *Penn. Med. J.*, **58**, 1231 (1955).
70. Gelvin, E. P., *et al, Am. J. Digest. Diseases*, **20**, 307 (1953).
71. Gelvin, E. P., *et al, N. Y. State J. Med.*, **54**, 1340 (1954).
72. Cohen, J. J., *GP*, **10** (6), 43 (1954).
73. Banghart, H. E., and Warter, P. J., *Am. Practitioner Dig. Treat.*, **5**, 867 (1954).
74. Pohlman, A. D., *J. Clin. Exptl. Psychopath.*, **18**, 159 (1957).
75. Shapiro, R. P., and Michaile, K. I., *Intern. Record Med. Gen. Pract. Clin.*, **169**, 638 (1956).
76. Roe, J. F., *Am. Practitioner Dig. Treat.*, **6**, 394 (1955).
77. Katzman, B., *Obstet. Gynecol.*, **6**, 652 (1955).
78. Gallagher, N. I., and Knight, W. A., Jr., *J. Chronic Diseases*, **8**, 244 (1958).
79. Shenoy, K. G., *et al, Drug Std.*, **27**, 77 (1959).
80. Berkowitz, D., *Gastroenterology*, **30**, 608 (1956).
81. Reese, D. R., *et al, Am. J. Digest. Diseases*, **4**, 220 (1959).
82. Thomson, T. J., *Glascow Med. J.*, **36**, 423 (1955).
83. Burness, S. H., *Am. J. Digest. Diseases*, **22**, 111 (1955).
84. Santor, D., *J. Med. Soc. New Jersey*, **54**, 53 (1957).
85. Roberts, E., *Am. J. Med. Sci.*, **227**, 609 (1954).
86. Shoemaker, D. M., *Antibiot. Med. Clin. Therapy*, **3**, 318 (1956).
87. Burket, L. C., *Am. J. Med. Sci.*, **229**, 22 (1955).
88. Messeloff, C. R., *Hospitals*, **29**, 122 (1955).
89. Rosen, E., and Swintosky, J. V., *J. Pharm. Pharmacol.*, **12**, 237T (1960).
90. Roberts, J. T., *Clin. Med.*, **4**, 1375 (1957).
91. Berry, J. W., and Roach, T. C., *Circulation*, **17**, 1041 (1958).
92. Cole, R. E., and Goldbert, R. I., *Curr. Therap. Res.*, **9**, 551 (1967).
93. Pote, H. H., *Intern. Rec. Med.*, **171**, 87 (1958).
94. Middleton, E. J., *et al, New Engl. J. Med.*, **274**, 136, 162 (1966).
95. Sugerman, A. A., and Rosen, E., *Clin. Pharmacol. Therap.*, **5**, 561 (1964).
96. Stern, F. H., *J. Am. Geriatrics Soc.*, **15**, 386 (1967).
97. Blake, A. D., Jr., *Clin. Med.*, **5**, 773 (1958).
98. Morrison, S., *Am. J. Gastroenterol.*, **29**, 519 (1958).
99. Jacoby, M. G., *et al, Diseases Nervous System*, **19**, 431 (1958).
100. Elia, J. C., *Curr. Therap. Res.*, **9**, 472 (1967).
101. Wagner, J. G., *et al, J. Pharmacol. Exptl. Therap.*, **129**, 101 (1960).
102. Bachman, E., B. F. Ascher Co., Inc., Nov. 18, 1966, private communication.
103. Bell, S. A., *et al, J. New Drugs*, **6**, 284 (1966).
104. O'Reagen, T., *Drug Cosmetic Ind.*, **98**, 35 (Apr., 1966).
105. Rotstein, J., *et al, J. Clin. Pharmacol.*, **7**, 917 (1967).
106. Gotoff, S. P., *et al, J. Pediatrics*, **73**, 127 (1968).
107. Bercher, P. R., *et al, Curr. Therap. Res.*, **9**, 379 (1967).
108. Schwab, R. S., *et al, J. Am. Med. Assoc.*, **165**, 671 (1957).
109. Marks, L., *Am. J. Gastroenterol.*, **30**, 518 (1958).
110. Simon, S. W., *Ann. Allergy*, **17**, 50 (1959).
111. Small, M. J., *et al, Am. Rev. Tuber. Pulmonary Diseases*, **77**, 184 (1958).
112. Ballon, H. C., *et al, Can. Med. Assoc. J.*, **79**, 751 (1958).
113. Malkin, S., *Can. Med. Assoc. J.*, **81**, 553 (1959).
114. Spielman, A. D., *Ann. Allergy*, **16**, 242 (1958).
115. Fuller, H. L., and Kassel, L. E., *Antibiot. Med.*, **3**, 322 (1956).
116. Bukey, F. S., and Brew, M., *J. APhA*, **23**, 1217 (1934).
117. Bukey, F. S., and Brew, M., *J. Lab. Clin. Med.*, **22**, 918 (1937).
118. Crane, A. W., and Wruble, M., *Am. J. Roentgenol. Radium Therapy*, **39**, 450 (1938).
119. Mann, H., *J. Mt. Sinai Hosp., N. Y.*, **23**, 279 (1956).
120. Russek, H. I., *et al, Am. J. Med. Sci.*, **229**, 46 (1955).
121. Plotz, M., *Am. Practitioner Dig. Treat.*, **9**, 903 (1958).
122. Beck, G. J., *et al, Antibiot. Med. Clin. Therapy*, **4**, 84 (1957).
123. Cobe, H. M., *Antibiot. Med. Clin. Therapy*, **4**, 149 (1957).
124. Welch, H., *et al, Antibiot. Med. Clin. Therapy*, **4**, 278 (1957).
125. Steigmann, F., *et al, Am. J. Digest. Diseases*, **4**, 534 (1959).
126. Bargen, J. A., *Gastroenterology*, **30**, 703 (1956).
127. Kadish, A. H., *Am. Practitioner Dig. Treat.*, **7**, 2006 (1956).
128. Lichstein, J., and Mayer, J. D., *J. Chronic Diseases*, **9**, 394 (1959).
129. Guth, P. H., and Allen, R., *Am. J. Gastroenterol.*, **32**, 360 (1959).
130. Weiss, S., *et al, Am. J. Gastroenterol.*, **30**, 316 (1958).
131. Miller, J., *Ann. Allergy*, **16**, 135 (1958).
132. Bernstein, A., and Simon, F., *Angiology*, **9**, 197 (1958).
133. Bellet, S., *et al, A. M. A. Arch. Inter. Med.*, **100**, 750 (1957).
134. O'Reilly, P. O., *et al, Can. Med. Assoc. J.*, **80**, 359 (1959).
135. Hirshleifer, I., *Angiology*, **9**, 31 (1958).
136. Samuels, S. S., *N. Y. State J. Med.*, **58**, 130 (1958).
137. Sablosky, L., *Antibiot. Med. Clin. Therapy*, **4**, 729 (1957).
138. Viek, N., *et al, J. Urol.*, **77**, 777 (1957).
139. Kennelly, J. M., Jr., and McDonald, D. F., *J. Urol.*, **81**, 222 (1959).
140. Henderson, W. H., *Antibiot. Med. Clin. Therapy*, **5**, 470 (1958).
141. Kasich, A. M., and Fein, H. D., *Am. J. Digest. Diseases*, **3**, 12 (1958).
142. Kasich, A. M., *Schweiz. Z., Path. Bakt.*, **21**, 354 (1958).
143. Israels, M. C. G., and Simmons, A. V., *Lancet*, **1**, 1297 (1967).
144. Dotevall, G., and Walan, A., *Acta Med. Scand.*, **178**, 759 (1965).
145. Ditlefsen, E.-M. L., and Loken, H. F., *Acta Med. Scand.*, **179**, 333 (1966).
146. Cullhed, I., *et al, Acta Med. Scand.*, **179**, 401 (1966).
147. Kitchener, J. A., *Ion-exchange Resins*, Methuen & Co., Ltd., London, 1957, Chap. 4.
148. Abrahams, A., and Linnell, W. H., *Lancet*, 1317 2, (1957).
149. Chapman, D. G., *et al, Can. Med. Assoc. J.*, **81**, 470 (1959).
150. Brudney, N., *Can. Pharm. J.*, **92**, (5), 45 (1959).
151. Becker, B. A., and Swift, J. G., *Federation Proc.*, **17**, 348 (1958).
152. Becker, B. A., and Swift, J. G., *Toxicol. Appl. Pharmacol.*, **1**, 42 (1959).
153. Becker, B. A., *Federation Proc.*, **17**, 187 (1958).
154. Becker, B. A., and Hayes, E. E., *Proc. Soc. Exptl. Biol. Med.*, **99**, 17 (1958).
155. Cass, L. J., *et al, Am. J. Med. Sci.*, **238**, 529 (1959).
156. Freed, S. C., *et al, Ann. Internal Med.*, **44**, 1136 (1956).
157. Freed, S. C., and Hays, E. E., *Am. J. Med. Sci.*, **238**, 55 (1959).
158. Chan, Y. T., and Hays, E. E., *Am. J. Med. Sci.*, **234**, 207 (1957).
159. Cass, L. J., and Fredrick, W. S., *Ann. Internal Med.*, **49**, 151 (1958).
160. Cass, L. J., and Fredrick, W. S., *New Engl. J. Med.*, **259**, 1108 (1958).
161. Townsend, E. H., Jr., *New Engl. J. Med.*, **258**, 63 (1958).
162. Newbold, G., *Brit. Med. J.*, **1**, 1303 (1957).
163. Margulies, H., *Brit. Med. J.*, **1**, 1531 (1957).
164. Garrett, T. A., *Clin. Med.*, **3**, 1185 (1956).
165. Kile, R. L., *Antibiot. Med. Clin. Therapy*, **5**, 578 (1959).
166. Shaftel, N., and Halpern, A., *Am. J. Med. Sci.*, **236**, 184 (1958).
167. Halpern, A., *et al, Antibiot. Chemotherapy*, **9**, 97 (1959).
168. Schwartz, G., *Angiology*, **10**, 115 (1959).
169. Gerstenblith, T., *et al, N.Y. State J. Med.*, **66**, 701 (1966).
170. Goldberg, W. M., and Charrabarti, S. G., *Can. Med. Assoc. J.*, **91**, 991 (1964); **92**, 138 (1965).
171. Brittain, G. J. C., *Lancet* **2**, 544 (1959).
172. Daeschner, C. W., *et al, J. Pediat.*, **50**, 531 (1957).
173. Foltz, E. L., *J. Pharmacol. Exptl. Therap.*, **119**, 145 (1957).
174. Dickstein, B., *J. Albert Einstein Med. Center*, **5**, 114 (1957).
175. McClellan, M., *Ohio State Med. J.*, **54**, 41 (1958).
176. Dougan, H. T., *Virginia Med. Monthly*, **85**, 15 (1955).
177. Bishoff, R. J., *Antibiot. Med. Clin. Therapy*, **3**, 399 (1956).
178. Farquhar, J. D., *J. Pediat.*, **50**, 190 (1957).
179. Fienstone, W. H., *et al, J. Bacteriol.*, **39**, 47 (1940).
180. Svenson, S. E., *et al, Antibiot. Med.*, **2**, 148 (1956).
181. Krugman, S., *Ann. N. Y. Acad. Sci.*, **69**, 399 (1957).
182. Daeschner, C. W., *et al, Am. J. Diseases Children*, **93**, 370 (1957).
183. Stephens, L. J., and Hendrickson, W. E., *J. Lancet*, **75**, 437 (1955).
184. Krugman, S., and Frieden, F., *J. Pediat.*, **50**, 16 (1957).
185. Hagler, S., *et al, J. Pediat.*, **48**, 588 (1956).
186. Reinhold, J. G., *et al, Am. J. Med. Sci.*, **210**, 141 (1945).
187. Boyd, E. M., and Dingwall, R. W., *Am. J. Med. Sci.*, **213**, 549 (1947).
188. Cooper, J., *Drug Cosmetic Ind.*, **81**, 312 (1957).
189. Royal, J., *Drug Std.*, **26**, 41 (1958).
190. Royal, J., *Drug Std.*, **27**, 1 (1959).
191. Campbell, D. G., and Theivagt, J. G., *Drug Std.*, **26**, 73 (1958).
192. Vliet, E. B., *Drug Std.*, **27**, 97 (1959).
193. Souder, J. C., and Ellenbogen, W. C., *Drug Std.*, **26**, 77 (1958).
194. Sjögren, J., and Ervik, M., *Acta Pharm. Suecica*, **1**, 219 (1964).
195. Wagner, J. G., *Drug Std.*, **27**, 178 (1959).
196. Wiegand, R. G., and Taylor, J. D., *Drug Std.*, **27**, 165 (1959).
197. Soliva, M., and Speiser, P., *Pharm. Acta Helv.*, **41**, 176 (1966).
198. Lang, E., *Schweiz. Apoth. Zeitung*, **96**, 773 (1958).
199. Grief, M., and Eisen, H., *Am. Profess. Pharmacist*, **25**, 93 (1959).
200. Lazarus, J., and Cooper, J., *J. Pharm. Sci.*, **50**, 715 (1961).
201. Stempel, E., *J. APhA, Pract. Ed.*, **20**, 334, 393 (1959).
202. Stempel, E., *Drug Cosmetic Ind.*, **98**, 44 (Jan., 1966); **98**, 36 (Feb. 1966).
203. Campbell, J. A., and Morrison, A. B., *Practitioner*, **183**, 758 (1959).
204. Campbell, J. A., and Morrison, A. B., *J. Am. Med. Assoc.*, **181**, 102 (1962).
205. Polli, G. P., and Ravin, L. J., *J. Pharm. Sci.*, **56**, 781 (1967).
206. Ravin, L. J., and Bernardo, P. D., *J. Pharm. Sci.*, **57**, 1075 (1968).
207. Shangraw, R. F., *Hosp. Pharm.*, **2**(10), 19 (1967).

208. Wilson, A., *Pharm. J.*, **183**, 191 (1959); *J. Pharm. Pharmacol.*, **11**, 44T (1959).
209. Edkins, R. P., *Pharm. J.*, **183**, 192 (1959); *J. Pharm. Pharmacol.*, **11**, 54T (1959).
210. *Modern Med.*, **27**, 229 (Mar. 15, 1959).
211. Asher, L. M., *Am. J. Digest. Diseases*, **4**, 260 (1959).
212. Wagner, J. G., *J. Pharm. Sci.*, **50**, 359 (1961).
213. Griffenhagen, G. B., *Parenteral Drug Assoc. Bull.*, **16**(2), 12 (1962).
214. Schou, J., *Pharmacol. Rev.*, **13**, 441 (1961).
215. Conley, B. E., *Parenteral Drug Assoc. Bull.*, **16**(5), 30 (1962).
216. Howard-Jones, N., *J. Hist. Med.*, **2**, 201 (1947).
217. Shelesnyak, M. C., and Engle, E. T., *Anat. Record*, **53**, 243 (1932).
218. Shear, M. J., *Am. J. Cancer*, **26**, 322 (1936).
219. Deanesly, R., and Parkes, A. S., *Proc. Roy. Soc.* (*London*) *Ser. B.*, **124**, 279 (1937).
220. Ballard, B. E., and Nelson, E., *J. Pharmacol. Exptl. Therap.*, **135**, 120 (1962).
221. Ballard, B. E., and Nelson, E., *Am. J. Vet. Res.*, **23**, 678 (1962).
222. Robinson, R. A., and Stokes, R. H., *Electrolyte Solutions*, 2nd ed, Academic Press, New York, 1959, pp. 12, 308.
223. Mullins, J. D., and Macek, T. J., *J. APhA, Sci. Ed.*, **49**, 245 (1960).
224. Higuchi, W. I., *et al, APhA Preprints of Papers, Las Vegas, Nevada.* A-IV, Mar. 26–29, 1962; *J. Pharm. Sci.*, **52**, 150 (1963).
225. Brandstätter–Kuhnert, M., *Ost. Apoth. Ztg.*, **13**(19), 297 (1959).
226. Shefter, E., and Higuchi, T., *J. Pharm. Sci.*, **52**, 781 (1963).
227. Biles, J., *J. Pharm. Sci.*, **52**, 1066 (1963).
228. Ballard, B. E., and Biles, J., A., *Steroids*, **4**, 273 (1964).
229. Jost, W., *Diffusion in Solids, Liquids, Gases*, Academic Press, New York, 1952, p. 78.
230. Ballard, B. E., and Nelson, E., *J. Pharm. Sci.*, **51**, 915 (1962); **53**, 1414 (1964).
231. Kearns, W. M., *J. Urol.*, **47**, 587 (1942).
232. Anderson, K. N., *Today's Health*, **41**, 20 (1963).
233. Schaefer, K. E., ed, *Bioastronautics*, Macmillan, New York, 1964, p. 125.
234. Ballard, B. E., *et al, J. Pharm. Sci.*, **53**, 424 (1964).
235. Ballard, B. E., *J. Pharm. Sci.*, **57**, 357 (1968).
236. Folkman, J., and Long, D. M., Jr., *J. Surg. Res.*, **4**, 139 (1964); *Dow Corning Center for Aid to Medical Research Bull.*, **5**, 9 (1963); *Ann. N.Y. Acad. Sci.*, **111**, 857 (1964).
237. Segal, S. J., *New Engl. J. Med.*, **279**, 364 (1968).
238. Murphy, E., and Faul, P. J., *J. Irish Med. Assoc.*, **53**, 4 (1963).
239. Abramson, D. I., ed, *Blood Vessels and Lymphatics*, Academic Press, New York, 1962.
240. Edelman, I. S., *Ann. Rev. Physiol.*, **23**, 37 (1961).
241. Kedem, O., and Katchalsky, A., *J. Gen. Physiol.*, **45**, 143 (1961).
242. Schanker, L. S., *Pharmacol. Rev.*, **14**, 501 (1962).
243. *Parenteral Administration*, Abbott Laboratories, North Chicago, Ill., 1959.
244. *Handbook on Parenteral Therapy*, Cutter Laboratories, Berkeley, Calif., 1961.
245. Boys, F., and Smith, H. M., *Poisonous Amphibians and Reptiles*, Charles C Thomas, Springfield, Ill., 1959.
246. Driesbach, R. H., *Handbook of Poisoning: Diagnosis and Treatment*, 2nd ed, Lange Medical Publications, Los Altos, Calif., 1959, pp. 329–330.
247. Russell, F. E., *J. Am. Med. Assoc.*, **177**, 903 (1961).
248. Elias, W. F., *Parenteral Drug Assoc. Bull.*, **10**(1), 15 (1956).
249. Carlinfanti, E., and Morra, F., *Lancet*, **1**, 521 (1947); *Schweiz. Med. Wochschr.*, **77**, 1235 (1947).
250. Kety, S. S., *Am. J. Med. Sci.*, **215**, 352 (1948).
251. McGirr, E. M., *Clin. Sci.*, **11**, 91 (1952).
252. McGirr, E. M., *Brit. Med. Bull.*, **8**, 192 (1951–1952).
253. Miller, H., and Wilson, G. M., *Brit. Heart J.*, **13**, 227 (1951).
254. Franke, F. R., *et al, Proc. Soc. Exptl. Biol. Med.*, **74**, 417 (1950).
255. Stone, P. W., and Miller, W. B., *Proc. Soc. Exptl. Biol. Med.*, **71**, 529 (1949).
256. Trumper, M., and Hutter, A. M., *Science*, **100**, 432 (1944).

257. Trumper, M., and Thompson, G. J., *J. Am. Med. Assoc.*, **130**, 627 (1946).
258. Gilbert, R. A., *et al, Johns Hopkins Hosp. Bull.*, **84**, 245 (1949).
259. Beecher, H. K., *J. Am. Med. Assoc.*, **124**, 1193 (1944).
260. Beecher, H. K., *Ann. Surg.*, **117**, 825 (1943).
261. Braithwaite, F., *et al, Brit. J. Plastic Surg.*, **4**, 38 (1951).
262. Barcroft, H., and Swan, H. J. C., *Sympathetic Control of Human Blood Vessels*, Edward Arnold, London, 1953, pp. 47–49.
263. Paton, W. D. M., *Pharmacol. Rev.*, **9**, 269 (1957).
264. Campbell, J. A., *et al, Radioisotope Techniques. Proceedings of the Isotopes Techniques Conference*, Oxford, July, 1951, sponsored by the Atomic Energy Research Establishment, Vol. 1, Her Majesty's Stationery Office, London, 1953, p. 212.
265. Cooper, F. W., Jr., *et al, Surg. Gynecol. Obstet.*, **88**, 711 (1949).
266. Prescott, B., *et al, Antibiot. Chemotherapy*, **8**, 27 (1958).
267. Prescott, B., *et al, Antibiot. Chemotherapy*, **8**, 81, 255 (1958).
268. Brigham, R. S., and Nielsen, J. K., *Antibiot. Chemotherapy*, **8**, 122 (1958).
269. Madison, W. L., and Christian, J. E., *J. APhA, Sci. Ed.*, **39**, 689 (1950).
270. Eastland, C. J., *J. Pharm. Pharmacol.*, **3**, 942 (1951).
271. Warner, G. F., *et al, Circulation*, **8**, 732 (1953).
272. Schriftman, H., and Kondritzer, A. A., *Am. J. Physiol.*, **191**, 591 (1957).
273. Schou, J., *Acta Pharmacol. Toxicol.*, **15**, 43 (1958).
274. Ramachandran, B. V., and Ågren, G., *Acta Pharmacol. Toxicol.*, **20**, 339 (1963).
275. Reese, D. R., *Parenteral Drug Assoc. Bull.*, **16**(5), 11 (1962).
276. Spiegel, A. J., and Noseworthy, M. M., *J. Pharm. Sci.*, **52**, 917 (1963).
277. Deanesly, R., and Parkes, A. S., *Lancet*, **1**, 837 (1936).
278. Miescher, K., *et al, Schweiz. Med. Wschr.*, **66**, 310 (1936).
279. Honrath, W. L., *et al, Steroids*, **2**, 425 (1963).
280. Goodhart, R. S., ed., *Modern Drug Encyclopedia and Therapeutic Index*, 9th ed., Donnelley, New York, 1963, p. 52.
281. Kopacova, L., *Bratislava Univ. Farm. Fak.*, **11**, 177 (1965).
282. Ekwall, P., *Acta Unio Intern. Contra Cancrum*, **10**(3), 44 (1954).
283. Macek, T. J., *J. Pharm. Sci.*, **52**, 694 (1963).
284. Lange, W. E., and Stein, M. E., *J. Pharm. Sci.*, **53**, 435 (1964).
285. Thompson, R. E., *Parenteral Drug Assoc. Bull.*, **14**(3), 6 (1960).
286. Bauman, J., *et al*, US Pat. 2,902,408.
287. Frederick, K. J., *J. Pharm. Sci.*, **50**, 531 (1961).
288. Meier, R., and Tschopp, E., *Arch. Exptl. Pathol. Pharmakol.*, **226**, 532 (1955).
289. Bates, R. W., and Loury, C., *Proc. Soc. Exptl. Biol. Med.*, **73**, 576 (1950).
290. Klette, H., US Pat. 2,895,875.
291. Ober, S. S., *et al, J. APhA, Sci. Ed.*, **47**, 667 (1958).
292. Buckwalter, F. H., and Dickison, H. L., *J. APhA, Sci. Ed.*, **47**, 661 (1958).
293. Macek, T. J., in *Remington's Pharmaceutical Sciences*, 14th ed., Mack Publ. Co., Easton, Pa., 1970, p. 1466.
294. Robinson, J. M., *J. Michigan State Med. Soc.*, **48**, 337 (1949).
295. Taggart, S. R., *et al, Am. J. Syphilis*, **33**, 515 (1949).
296. Boger, W. P., *et al, Am. J. Med. Sci.*, **215**, 250 (1948).
297. Savolainen, T., and Tommila, V., *Ann. Med. Exptl. Biol. Fenniae*, **33**, 345 (1955).
298. Lukash, W. M., and Frank, P. F., *Am. J. Med. Sci.*, **246**, 429 (1963).
299. Stalnaker, J. H., *Northwest Med.*, **62**, 438 (1963).
300. Hanson, D. J., *GP*, **27**, 109 (1963).
301. Pitel, M., and Wemett, M., *Am. J. Nursing*, **64**, 104 (1964).
302. Lindenmeyer, R. S., "Correlation of Needle Point Geometry with Coring and Sharpness," *Parenteral Drug Assoc. Bull.* (*Suppl.*), Technical Report 101, Manufacturing Process Laboratories, Inc., New York City, N.Y., 1959.
303. Swyer, G. I. M., *J. Reprod. Fert.*, **14**, 295 (1967).
304. Segal, S. J., *New Engl. J. Med.*, **279**, 364 (1968).
305. Diczfalusy, E., *Am. J. Obstet. Gynecol.*, **100**, 136 (1968).
306. Powell, R. D., *Clin. Pharmacol. Therap.*, **7**, 48 (1966).

90 | Aerosols

Mode of operation—propellants—containers—valves—actuators or buttons—dip tubes—packaging—applications—testing

This chapter was prepared by

John J. Sciarra, PhD, *Director, Graduate Division, and Professor of Pharmaceutical Chemistry, College of Pharmacy, St. John's University, Jamaica, N.Y. 11432*

The aerosol dosage form for the application of therapeutically active ingredients represents one of the major advances which has occurred in pharmaceutical technology during the past decade. Since the aerosol dosage form is convenient to use and allows for a greater degree of flexibility in administering medicinal agents than other dosage forms, its use has become widespread and has extended to almost all types of pharmaceutical and medicinal preparations.

Definitions—The term "aerosol" is used to denote various systems ranging from systems of a colloidal nature[1] to systems consisting of "pressurized packages."[2] Aerosols have been defined by Whytlaw-Gray and Patterson[3] as colloidal systems consisting of very finely subdivided liquid or solid particles dispersed in and surrounded by a gas. Originally, the term aerosol referred to liquid or solid particles having a specific size range, but this concept is falling into disuse. Sinclair[4] indicated that these particles should be smaller than 50 microns (μ) in size and generally less than 10 μ.

While the above definition is generally regarded as the classical one, a more recent definition includes as aerosols those products which depend on the power of a liquefied or a compressed gas to expel the contents from the container. This is slightly different from the definition by a subcommittee of the Chemical Specialities Manufacturers Association (CSMA), which states:[5]

"A self-contained sprayable product in which the propellent force is supplied by a liquefied gas. Includes space, residual, surface coating, foams, and various other types of product; but does not include gas-pressurized products such as whipping cream. The term aerosol as used here is not confined to the scientific definition."

One current system for the classification of aerosol products is based on particle size as follows:

1. *Space sprays,* which dispense the active ingredients as a finely divided spray with the particles no larger than 50 μ in diameter.
2. *Surface-coating sprays,*[6] which dispense larger particles, generally produce a wet or coarse spray, and are used to coat surface with a residual film.
3. *Aerated sprays,* which dispense shaving cream, whipping cream, and similar products.

While the term aerosol is used in this chapter to indicate these systems, other terms such as "pressurized package," "pressurized packaging," and "pressurized product," have also been used to describe these types of products.

History—While the development of the pressurized package as it is known today is of rather recent origin, the atomization of particles for use in aerosol therapy is not new. Such devices as burning sulfur candles to disinfect the air, spraying operating rooms with germicidal materials, and inhalation of the smoke of asthma powder are early, still useful, examples of aerosol therapy. When the physician recommends that his patient go to the beach and partake of the benefits

of salt air, he is suggesting, perhaps unknowingly, the therapeutic use of the tiny salt particles in the air produced by the atomization forces of the breakers.[7]

As early as 1899 Helbing and Pertsch[8] suggested means of propelling confined substances through use of liquids such as methyl and ethyl chloride. In 1901, 1902, and 1939 Gebauer[9-11] was issued patents describing the use of pressurized packages for dispensing medicinal agents such as tannic acid and ethyl chloride. In fact the use of ethyl chloride as a local anesthetic is considered by many to be the forerunner of the present-day aerosol.[12] Several antiseptic solutions[13] and perfume aerosols[14-17] were developed using carbon dioxide as the propellant.

Other chemical agents were investigated during the 1930's as possible propellants, including fluorinated chlorohydrocarbons which were originally developed as refrigerants.[18] One of these materials, dichlorodifluoromethane, was used by Goodhue and Sullivan[19,20] as the propellant in their aerosol insecticide which they developed for the US Department of Agriculture. They developed a light, portable aerosol dispenser that was capable of producing a fine spray of insecticidal ingredients which remained suspended in air for relatively long periods of time. These were used by the Armed Forces during World War II to combat the various insects which caused disease among overseas troops. The aerosol was packaged in a high-pressure cylinder of heavy steel construction[21] and had a vapor pressure of 70 pounds per square inch gauge (psig) at 70°F.* Interstate Commerce Commission regulations necessitated a heavy, bulky steel container for the shipment of these products.

Following World War II newer propellants, valves, and containers were developed so that a spray possessing the proper particle size could be produced using a pressure of 35–40 psig. An amendment to the regulations of the Interstate Commerce Commission in 1947 made possible the use of a thin-walled container by permitting a pressure of 40 psig at 70°F in essentially a "beer-type" container. Other container developments included the use of stainless steel and aluminum as well as glass and plastic.

Another area of development essential to the success of the aerosol package concerned the valve. Various valves were developed in order to dispense the product in the form of a fine stream, a fine mist, a coarse spray, or solid stream. Another development included the metered valves which are essential for medicinal aerosols. These valves make it possible to dispense quantities of medication ranging from 50 mg to as much as 1 oz accurately.

---

*The term psig represents the uncorrected gauge pressure and is to be distinguished from psia (pounds per square inch absolute) that is corrected to include atmospheric pressure (14.7 psig).

While dichlorodifluoromethane was the first fluorinated hydrocarbon to be used as a propellant, its pressure of approximately 70 psig at 70°F limited its use. However, with the availability of low-pressure propellants such as trichloromonofluoromethane and dichlorotetrafluoroethane, products can be developed having even lower vapor pressures. Recent advances in propellant technology include the use of compressed gases as well as hydrocarbons.

The first aerosols for consumer use appeared in the United States in 1947. At that time the aerosol insecticide was essentially the only aerosol product available. From 1947 to date the aerosol industry has grown from a total production of about 5½ million units per year and only one product, to a production of over 2½ billion units a year in 1968 representing aerosol products varying from insecticides, hair sprays, perfumes, colognes, paints, and room deodorants to pharmaceuticals, medicinals, cosmetics, and many specialty items.[22] These figures represent the nonfood-type aerosols.

The growth of pharmaceutical and medicinal aerosols, while not very impressive as to total units produced, nevertheless has been phenomenal. In 1968 over 50 million units of medicinal and pharmaceutical aerosol products were produced in the United States. This total included a variety of over 60 different aerosol products ranging from local anesthetics, first-aid products, antibacterial sprays, spray-on bandages, and protective ointments to medicinal aerosols intended for treatment of asthma, angina pectoris, and migraine headaches.[23-25] When it is noted that less than 1 million units of these products were produced in 1952, the newness of the development and the increased interest in this area are quickly realized.

Several other developments took place which enabled one to develop additional aerosol products. These developments involved systems for the physical separation of product from propellant as found in the piston-type container and later in the plastic bag type. Other systems were based on the "venturi" principle.[26] In 1968 a system was developed which allowed for the simultaneous dispensing of two incompatible ingredients. This system, termed "co-dispensing," resulted in the development of "hot" shave foams[27] and is currently under investigation for additional uses.

Advantages—One of the main reasons for the rapid and widespread acceptance of the aerosol dosage form for the administration of therapeutically active agents is that it affords many and distinct advantages to the user. These advantages have been described by various investigators.[7,28-33]

The pressure package is convenient and easy to use. Medication is dispensed in a ready-to-use form at the push of a button. There is generally no need for further handling of the medication. Since the medication is sealed in a pressure container, there is no danger of contamination of the product with foreign materials, and at the same time the contents can be protected from the deleterious effects of both air and moisture. Easily decomposed drugs such as epinephrine, vitamins, and penicillin, lend themselves to this type of package. When one considers the danger of contamination of unused topical, ophthalmic, ear, nose, and throat, preparations, the importance of this advantage is obvious. Sterility is always an important consideration with certain pharmaceutical and medicinal preparations. While initial sterility is generally no problem to the manufacturer, there is concern for the maintenance of the sterility of the package during use as for example,

in ophthalmic preparations. When necessary, the aerosol package can be prepared under sterile conditions and sterility can be maintained throughout the life of the product. For those products requiring regulation of dosage, a metered valve can be used. While this is no more accurate than the administration of oral dosage forms, it is advantageous when used with topical preparations since indiscriminate use and overuse of the product can be avoided. In addition, when used with expensive products such as some steroids and antibiotics, savings can be achieved by the user as compared to the use of other topical preparations such as ointments, creams, or lotions. The aerosol dosage form allows for the dispensing of the product in the most desirable form; spray, foam, or semisolid. Depending on the nature of the product, the characteristics of the spray or foam can be changed to insure the proper and most efficient use of the medication.

Other advantages of the aerosol package specific to topical aerosols and to those intended for inhalation will be indicated in a later portion of this chapter.

Mode of Operation

It is convenient to discuss the operation of aerosols by first classifying them into various categories. Several classifications have been used for aerosol preparations and are generally based on the nature of the product.[34] Other classifications are based not only upon the nature of the concentrate but also upon the nature of the propellant.

For the purpose of this chapter, aerosols may be classified as follows:

Liquefied-gas systems
    Two-phase
        Space spray
        Surface-coating spray
        Dispersion or suspension
    Three-phase
        Two-layer
        Foam
            Stabilized
            Quick-breaking
Compressed-gas systems
    Solid stream dispensing
        Insoluble inert gas
    Foam dispensing
        Soluble inert gas
    Spray dispensing
        Soluble inert gas
        Insoluble inert gas
Separation of propellant from concentrate systems
    Piston type
    Flexible bag type
    Atomizer type

Liquefied-Gas Systems

Liquefied gases have been widely used as propellants for most aerosol products. These compounds are useful for this purpose since they are gases at room temperature and atmospheric pressure. However, they can be easily liquefied by lowering the temperature (below the boiling point) or by increasing the pressure. The compounds chosen generally have boiling points below 70°F and vapor pressures between 13.4 and 85 psia at 70°F. When a liquefied gas propellant is placed into a sealed container, it immediately separates into a liquid and a vapor phase. Since these materials are liquefied gases, some of the molecules will leave the liquid state and enter the vapor state. As molecules enter the vapor state, a pressure gradually develops. As the number of molecules in the vapor state increases, the pressure will also increase. An equilibrium is soon attained between the number of molecules changing from a liquid to a vapor and from a vapor to a liquid. The pressure at this point is referred to as the vapor pressure and is characteristic for each propellant at any given temperature. This vapor pressure is exerted equally in all directions and is independent of the quantity present. The pressure exerted against the liquid phase is sufficient to push the latter up a dip tube and against the valve. When the valve is opened, the liquid phase is emitted and comes into contact with the warm air at atmospheric pressure. The liquid propellant immediately reverts to the vapor state since its boiling point is substantially below room temperature. As the contents of the container are expelled, the volume within the container occupied by the vaporized propellant is increasing causing a temporary fall in pressure. However, as soon as the pressure decreases, a sufficient number of molecules change from the liquid state to the vapor state and restore the original pressure. When a compressed gas is used as the propellant, the relationship is quite different and there is a drop in pressure as the contents are used.

Two-Phase System[35]—This is the simplest of all aerosol systems. It consists of a solution or a suspension of active ingredients in liquid propellant or a mixture of liquid propellant and solvent. Both a liquid and vapor phase are present, and when the valve is depressed, liquid propellant containing dissolved active ingredients and other solvents are released. Depending on the nature of the propellants used, the quantity of propellant present, and the valve mechanism, a fine mist or wet spray is produced due to the large expansion of the propellant at room temperature and atmospheric pressure.

A *space spray* generally contains from 2 to 20% active ingredients and from 80 to 98% propellant. While the pressure of space sprays is in the range of 30 to 40 psig, the particles which are produced are from less than 1μ to 50μ. These particles remain suspended in air for relatively long periods of time. Space insecticides, room deodorants, and vaporizer sprays are examples of this type of system. A *surface-coating*

Table I—Numerical Designation of Fluorinated Hydrocarbon Propellants[a]

Chemical name	Chemical formula	Designation
Trichloromonofluoromethane	CCl_3F	11
Dichlorodifluoromethane	CCl_2F_2	12
Monochlorodifluoromethane	$CHClF_2$	22
Dichlorodifluoroethane	$CClF_2CClF_2$	114
Chloropentafluoroethane	$CClF_2CF_3$	115
Asychlorodifluoroethane	CCl_2FCF_3	114a
Monochlorodifluoroethane	CH_3CClF_2	142b
Difluoroethane	CH_3CHF_2	152a
Octafluorocyclobutane	$\overline{CF_2CF_2CF_2CF_2}$	C-318

[a] These propellants are available as Freon (Du Pont), Genetron (Allied), Isotron (Pennsalt), and Ucon (Union Carbide).

spray (a relatively wet or coarse spray) can be achieved by decreasing the amount of low-boiling propellants and increasing the ratio of active ingredients and solvents. The product concentrate can vary from 20 to 75% and the propellant from 25 to 80%. Particles are produced ranging in size from over 50μ to 200μ. Products as hair sprays, residual insecticides, perfumes, colognes, paints, protective coatings, and topical sprays are formulated in this manner. These products are intended to coat a surface with active ingredients and as such, a wet spray is desirable. The pressure of this system is generally lower than the space spray.

Fig. 736 shows a cross section of a typical space or surface-coating aerosol spray.

The propellants widely used for these aerosol systems consist of Propellants 11, 12 and 114 (Table I). Combinations of Propellant 12/11 and Propellant 12/114 are used to achieve the desired results as to spray characteristics. Other combinations include a mixture of fluorinated hydrocarbons and hydrocarbons. In certain instances the nature of the product will determine the propellant combination. Dispersion or suspension sprays are similar to space and surface coating sprays in that they are two phase systems where the active ingredients are suspended, rather than dissolved in the liquid phase. Depending upon the relative amounts of high boiling and low boiling propellants and other liquids, particles are produced in the same range as obtained with either space or surface coating sprays.

Three-Phase System—These are useful in that they allow for the greater use of liquid components not miscible with the propellants. Water is not miscible with liquefied-gas propellants and in many instances presents a problem since active ingredients are soluble in water. These problems have been overcome to a large extent by use of the three-phase system. Depending on the nature of the formulation, one of the following two systems may be employed.

Two-Layer System[34]—In this system the liquid propellant, the vaporized propellant, and the aqueous solution of active ingredients make up the three phases. Since the liquid propellant and water are not miscible, the liquid propellant will separate as an immiscible layer. When this propellant is of the fluorocarbon type, being denser than water, it will fall to the bottom of the container. Hydrocarbons, on the other hand, are lighter than water, and when used in this manner will float on top of the aqueous layer. A typical three-phase aerosol system is shown in Fig. 737. A spray is produced by the mechanical action of an exceedingly small valve orifice through which the liquid is forced by the vapor pressure of the propellant. The vapor

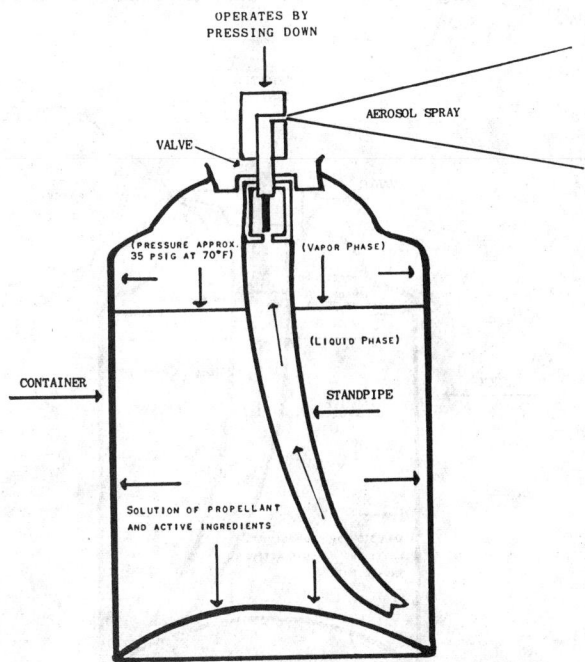

Fig. 736. Cross section of a typical space or surface-coating aerosol spray.

layer is continuously replaced by vapors from the liquid layer of propellant. None of the liquefied gas propellant is introduced into the aqueous solution while it is being ejected and, therefore, the breakup of the stream is due chiefly to the action of the "mechanical breakup actuator." This system generally operates at a pressure of about 15–20 psig and utilizes about 5–10% propellant. The propellants used are of the fluorocarbon and hydrocarbon type. In order to promote the vaporization of the propellant, glass chips or porous pot fragments are sometimes used. Mothproofing sprays and household cleaners exemplify this system.

A modification of this system involves replacement of the aqueous solution with a hydroalcoholic component.[36] The propellants which are used consist of a mixture of fluorocarbons and hydrocarbons such as butane, isobutane, and propane. An important characteristic of this system is that the propellant layer can be adjusted by varying the components so its specific gravity almost equals but does not exceed that of the hydroalcoholic phase. The propellant floats on top of the hydroalcoholic phase and, when shaken, is easily dispersed. When the valve is depressed, sprays are produced of varying characteristics depending on the nature of the formulation. A specially designed valve is also necessary to achieve the desired degree of atomization.

This system is one form of what is generally referred to as "water-based" aerosols. In some cases, water is used as the solvent together with either Propellant 12, butane, or a mixture of propellants. Depending on the nature of any surfactants which may be present, the product can be delivered as a spray or foam. These will be covered in greater detail in another portion of this chapter.

Many of the present-day insecticides and room deodorant aerosols have been reformulated from the original solvent- or oil-based products to the less-expensive water-based type. While these products tend to produce somewhat larger particles than that produced with solvent-based products, nevertheless these newer products are effective.

Foam System—Foam aerosols, which are often classified separately, consist of three-phase systems wherein the liquid propellant, which normally does not exceed 15% by weight, is emulsified with the propellant. When the valve is depressed, the emulsion is forced through the nozzle and, in the presence of warm air and at atmospheric pressure, the entrapped propellant reverts to a vapor and whips the emulsion into a foam. The use of a dip tube is optional with this type of system and, when present, the container is designed for upright use. For those containers where the dip tube is omitted, the container must be inverted prior to use. Foam valves have been developed which are applicable to both types of packages. Foam products operate at a pressure of about 35 to 40 psig at 70°F and generally contain about 6–10% propellant. A typical foam-type aerosol can be seen in Fig. 738. Shave creams and shampoos, as well as several topical pharmaceuticals, have been formulated as foam aerosols. Generally, Propellant 12/114[37] or a blend of propane/isobutane is used for foam aerosols. Other foam aerosols make use of the hydrocarbon propellants.

Several other developments in this area involve the development of the "quick-breaking" foam, non-aqueous foam, and water-based aerosols. These will be covered in a later portion of this chapter.

Compressed-Gas Aerosols

Compressed gases are used to dispense the product as a solid stream, wet spray, or foam. These aerosol products utilize an inert gas such as nitrogen, carbon dioxide, or nitrous oxide as the propellant. As the name indicates, the gas is compressed in the container, and it is the expansion of the compressed gas which provides the push or the force necessary to expel the contents from the container. This is somewhat similar to the action of the liquefied-gas aerosols except that there is little or no reservoir of gas so that as the contents of the container are expelled, the volume of the gas will increase causing a drop in pressure according to Boyle's law.

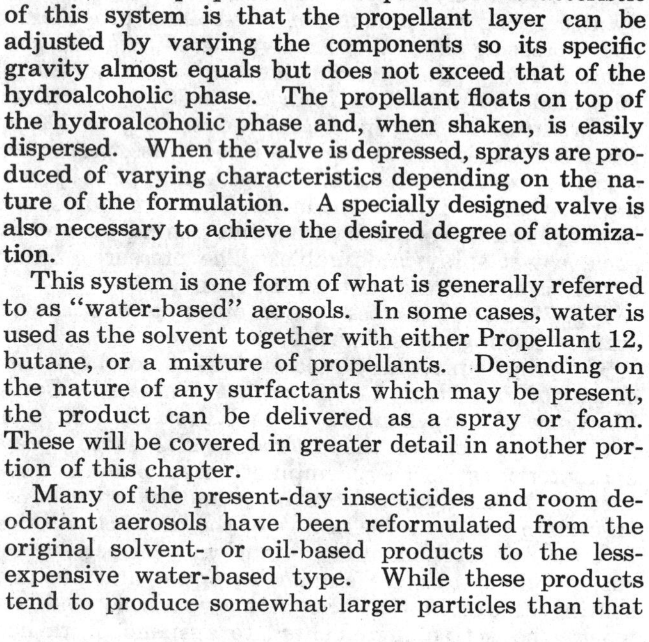

Fig. 737. **Three-phase glass aerosol.**

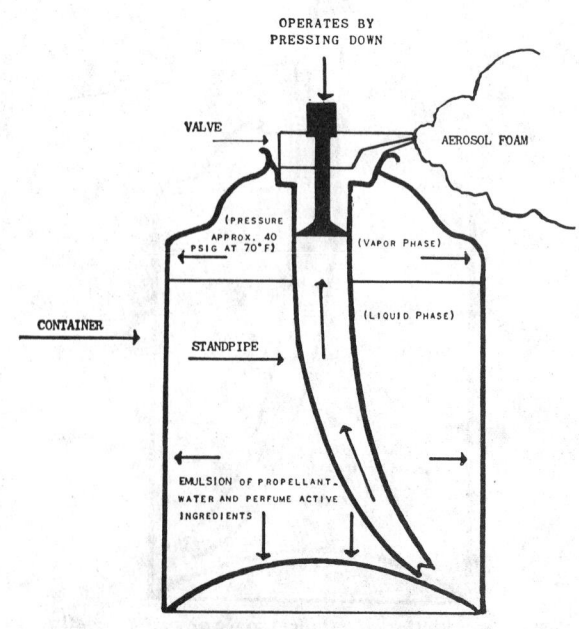

Fig. 738. **Foam-type aerosol.**

$$P = k\frac{1}{V}$$

where P = pressure and V = volume of gas. At constant temperature this law can be expressed as

$$P_1V_1 = P_2V_2$$

This enables one to calculate the drop in pressure as the contents of a compressed-gas aerosol are used.

Solid-Stream Dispensing—Nitrogen is used as the propellant for this type of product. The concentrate is generally semisolid in nature, and since the gas is insoluble and immiscible with the concentrate, the product is dispensed in its original form. Fig. 739 shows a typical compressed-gas aerosol. This system is applicable to the dispensing of dental creams, hair dressings, ointments, creams, cosmetic creams, vitamins, foods, and other products. Since there is no liquefied gas present, compressed-gas aerosols operate at a substantially higher initial pressure of 90–100 psig at 70°F. This higher initial pressure is necessary to insure adequate pressure for the dispensing of most of the contents from the container. The amount of product retained in the unit after exhaustion of the pressure varies with the viscosity of the product and loss of pressure due to seepage of gas during storage. Since the concentrate is generally semisolid in nature and the dispensing characteristics depend largely on the viscosity of the product and the pressure within the container,[38] the viscosity of the product concentrate must be adjusted accordingly.

Foam Dispensing—Soluble compressed gases such as nitrous oxide and carbon dioxide can be used to produce a foam when used with emulsion products. This system is typical for whipped creams and toppings. When this system is used, the gas dissolved in the concentrate will be emitted and cause a whipping of the emulsion into a foam. In order to facilitate the formation of a foam this system is shaken prior to use in order to disperse some of the gas throughout the product concentrate.

Spray Dispensing—This system is similar to a space or surface spray except that a compressed gas is used as the propellant. Since these gases do not possess the dispersing power of the liquefied gases, a mechanical breakup actuator is used. The product is dispensed as a wet spray and is applicable to solutions of medicinal agents in aqueous solvents. Webster[39] has investigated the use of some of the soluble compressed gases as propellants for products requiring a fine spray. This system generally is more compatible with aqueous than with nonaqueous liquids.

Another compressed-gas aerosol system is unique in that it makes use of three variables, namely the viscosity of the product, the orifice of the valve, and the pressure within the container to dispense the product as a fast moving "jet" stream, which becomes self-agitating if it is directed into milk or water.[40] In this process a compressed gas is used to dispense the product as an aerated foam into a liquid diluent. As the foam comes into contact with the diluent, the gases trapped within the foam expand, resulting in a complete mixture of the concentrate with the diluent. At the present time the system is used principally in the dispensing of food and beverage concentrates.[41]

Other Systems

Piston Type—Since it is difficult to completely empty the contents of a semisolid from an aerosol container, a piston-type aerosol system has been developed. This utilizes a polyethylene piston fitted into an aluminum container. The concentrate is placed into the upper portion of the container. The pressure from nitrogen (about 90–100 psig) or a liquefied gas such as Propellant 12 pushes against the other side of the piston; when the valve is opened, the product is dispensed. The piston scrapes against the sides of the container and dispenses most of the product concentrate.[42]

The piston-type aerosol system, termed "MiraFlo" (*Am. Can*) is shown in Fig. 740. This system has been successfully used to package cheese spreads, cake decorating icings, and ointments. Since the products which use this system are semisolid and viscous, they are dispensed as a lazy stream rather than as a foam or spray. This system is limited to viscous materials since limpid liquids, such as water, alcohol, etc, will pass between the wall of the container and piston.

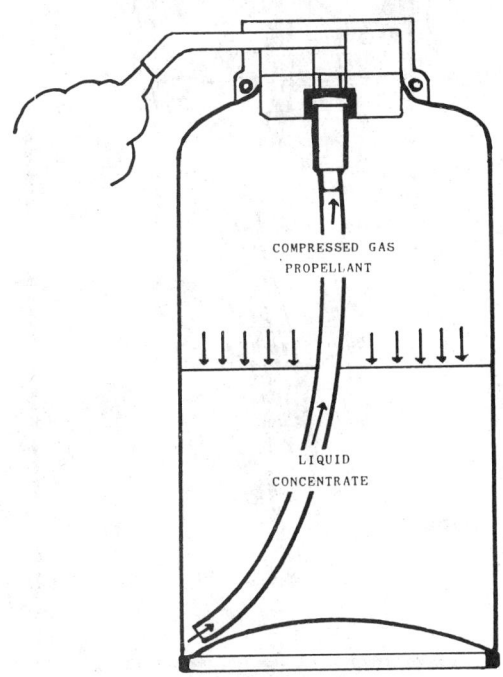

Fig. 739. Compressed-gas aerosol.

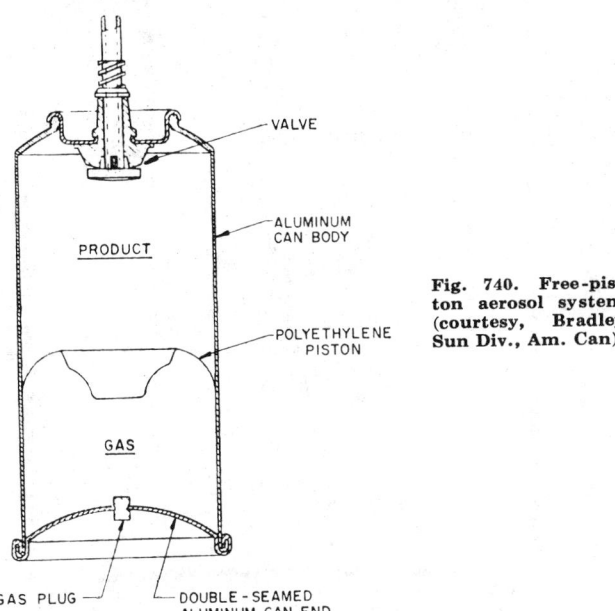

Fig. 740. Free-piston aerosol system (courtesy, Bradley Sun Div., Am. Can).

Plastic Bag Type—This system consists of a collapsible plastic bag fitted into a standard, three-piece, tinplate container as shown in Fig. 741. The product is placed within the bag and the propellant is added through the bottom of the container. Since the product is placed into a plastic bag, there is no contact between the product and the container wall except for any product which may escape by permeation through the plastic bag.

Limpid liquids, such as water, can be dispensed either as a stream or fine mist depending on the type of valve used, while semisolid substances are dispensed as a stream.[43] In order to prevent the gas from pinching the bag and preventing the dispensing of product, the inner plastic bag is accordion pleated. The Sepro

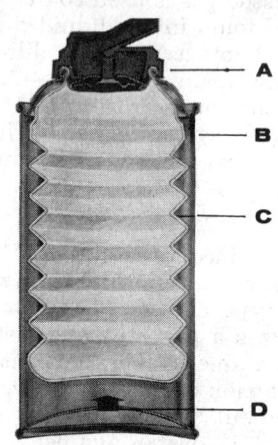

Fig. 741. Plastic bag aerosol system (Sepro). *A:* valve; *B:* standard three-piece tin-plate container; *C:* plastic bag; *D:* gas filling port (courtesy, Continental Can).

container (*Continental Can*), as this system is called, can be used for a variety of different pharmaceutical and nonpharmaceutical systems.

Venturi-Based Systems—Two systems have been developed which depend on the venturi principle. Vaporized propellant is allowed to flow past a small capillary opening which connects with the product to be sprayed.

In use, the product concentrate is added to the outer container, which need not be a pressure container, and then the valve with propellant cartridge is inserted. When the specially designed actuator is depressed, propellant vapor escapes from the propellant chamber. In doing so, it creates a "venturi" effect, drawing up some of the product. It is at this point that mixing of propellant vapor and product takes place. The vaporized propellant then aids in carrying the product through the actuator where it is dispersed into the proper type of spray.

Depending on the type of system used, the propellant cartridge can be made of aluminum,[44] as shown in Fig. 742, or glass[45,46] as shown in Fig. 743. The operation of the Innovair system (Fig. 743) is as follows:

Out of Operation

The container is hermetically sealed: the pressure valve prevents outflow of the propellant. The air inlet prevents passage of the liquid and exposure to the atmosphere.

In Process of Spraying

By actuating the pushbutton the 3 exits mentioned above will be opened: the valve allows the propellant to pass which, when flowing through the venturi, produces a vacuum. By means of the dip-tube the air inlet connects the spray chamber of the venturi nozzle with the container holding the liquid. This same air inlet, in

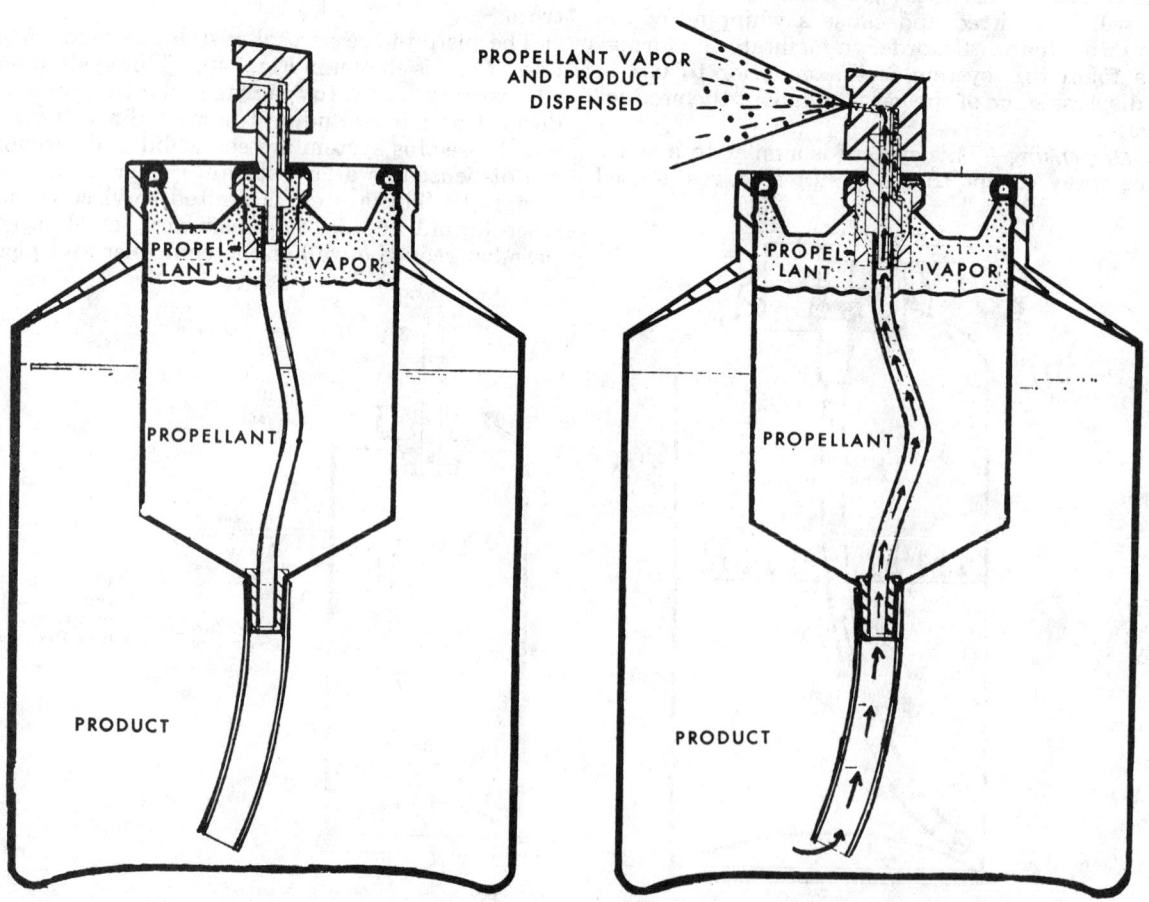

Fig. 742. Pre-Val system. *Left:* rest position; *right:* dispensing position (courtesy, Precision Valve).

opening, compensates for the pressure difference between the atmosphere and the vacuum created in the container by the exit of the liquid.

The outer container holds the product to be sprayed at atmospheric pressure. An inner cartridge contains the propellant under pressure maintained by the pressure valve. The latter is fixed in the actuator which comprises a pushbutton together with the venturi suction and spray micronozzle.

While there are some differences between these two systems, they are based on the same principle. These systems can be used to dispense aqueous and other liquids. Their chief advantages involve the lack of chilling effect since no liquefied propellant is dispensed and the product alone can be sprayed.

Co-Dispensing System—A great deal of time and effort has been expended during the past ten years toward the development of a system which would dispense a warm foam. While several attachments and fitments were developed for use with aerosol shave creams in order to produce a warm foam, none of these met with success. Many of them were electrically heated or had to be immersed or filled with hot water. The foam would then be heated by passing through these warm fitments.

In 1968 a system was developed which produced a hot foam as a result of an oxidation–reduction reaction.[47,48] In order to separate the two reactants until the time of use, a co-dispensing system, as shown in Fig. 744, was developed.[49]

This unit is inserted into a regular aerosol container and crimped in place in the usual manner. The oxidizing agent, which generally is hydrogen peroxide, is placed in the inner container. A reducing agent, such as potassium sulfite, potassium thiosulfate, or thiourea and a pyrimidine derivative, is mixed with the emulsion formulation and placed into the outer container.

When used, a measured amount of each component is dispensed and allowed to mix in the valve. An

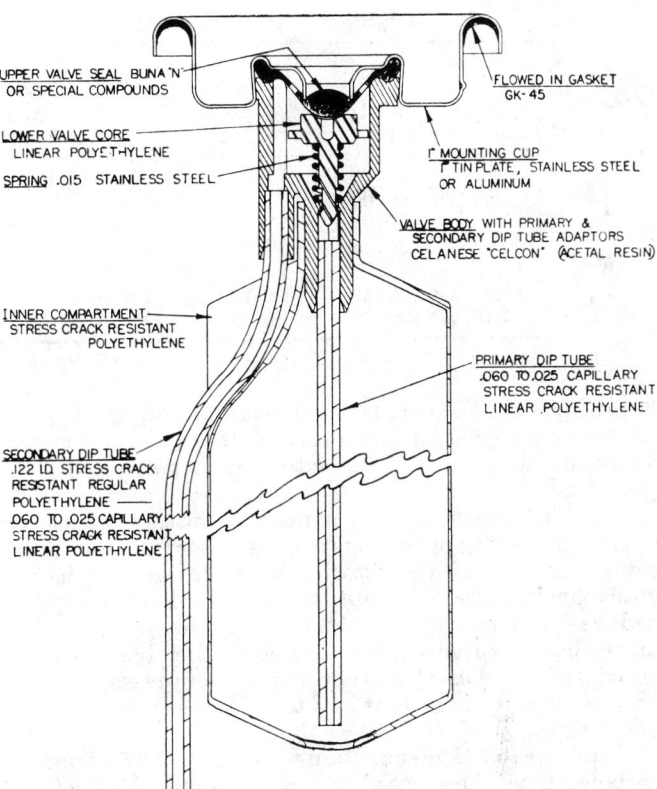

Fig. 744. Co-Dispensing system (courtesy, Oil Equipment).

exothermic reaction results with the liberation of sufficient calories to heat the foam. This is discussed in greater detail elsewhere in this chapter.

This system has been used to dispense a hair conditioner and can be used for a variety of pharmaceutical products where heat may be desired or where incompatible ingredients may be present.

Propellants

The propellant is generally regarded as the "heart" of the aerosol package. In addition to supplying the necessary force to expel the product, it must also act as a solvent and diluent and has much to do with determining the characteristics of the product as it leaves the container. Various chemical compounds have been used as aerosol propellants.

Compounds useful as propellants can be classified as follows:

Liquefied gases
    Fluorinated chlorinated hydrocarbons (halocarbons)
    Chlorinated hydrocarbons
    Hydrocarbons
Compressed gases

Liquefied Gases

The liquefied gas compounds have found widespread use as propellants since they are extremely effective in dispersing the active ingredients into a fine mist or foam depending on the form desired. In addition they are relatively inert and nontoxic. They have the added advantage that the pressure within the container remains constant when liquefied gases are used as propellants. Of the two types of liquefied gases used, the fluorinated hydrocarbons have found greater use since they are nonflammable as contrasted to the flammable hydrocarbons. The hydrocarbons are advantageous, however, since they are less expensive than the

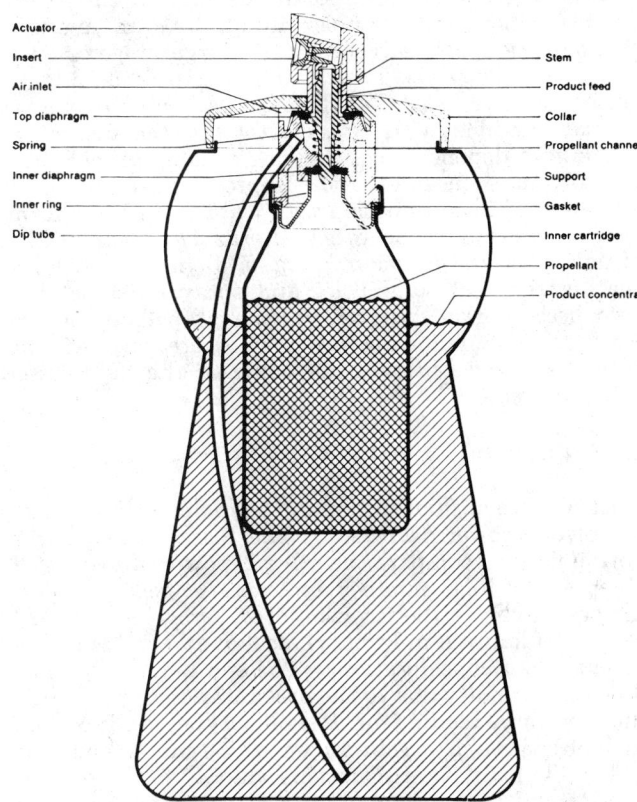

Fig. 743. Innovair system (courtesy, Geigy).

Table II—Physicochemical Properties of Fluorinated Hydrocarbons

Propellant	Mol wt	Boiling point		Liquid density, Gm/ml		Vapor pressure, psig[a]		Solubility of propellant in water, % w/w, 70°F	Solubility of water in propellant, % w/w, 70°F
		°F	°C	70°F	130°F	70°F[b]	130°F[c]		
11	137.38	74.7	23.7	1.485	1.403	2.6	24.3	0.140	0.009
12	120.93	−21.6	−29.8	1.325	1.191	70.2	181.0	0.040	0.008
114	170.93	38.4	3.6	1.468	1.360	12.9	58.8	0.013	0.007
115	154.48	−37.7	−38.7	1.309	...	103.0	252.1	0.006	...
152a	66.05	−11.2	−24.0	0.911	0.813	61.7	176.3	0.320	0.170
142b	100.50	15.1	−9.4	1.119	1.028	29.1	97.3	0.140	0.054
C-318	200.00	21.5	−5.9	1.515	...	25.4	92.0	...	0.014

[a] psig + 14.7 = psia.   [b] 70°F = 21.1°C.   [c] 130°F = 54.4°C.

fluorocarbons. Hydrocarbons have found increased use for shave foams and other water-based aerosols. They are used to a lesser extent with solvent-based products.

Liquefied gases provide a nearly constant pressure during packaging operations and have a large expansion ratio. Several of the fluorinated hydrocarbons have an expansion ratio of about 240, that is, 1 ml of liquefied gas will occupy a volume of approximately 240 ml if allowed to vaporize. Dimethylether has a value of over 350. On the other hand, compressed gases expand only to the extent of 3 to 10 times their original volume.

Fluorinated Hydrocarbons—Several of the fluorocarbons have been used as propellants. In fact a majority of commercial aerosol products make use of these materials as propellants.[50] These propellants are primarily derived from methane, ethane, and cyclobutane and are prepared by replacing one or more of the hydrogens of these compounds with chlorine and/or fluorine.

Some of the commonly used propellants may be prepared as follows:[51]

$$2C\,Cl_4 + 3HF \xrightarrow{catalyst} C\,Cl_3F + C\,Cl_2F_2 + 3HCl$$

Propellant 11 is separated from Propellant 12 by fractionation. Propellant 114 can be prepared from perchloroethylene according to the following reaction:

$$C\,Cl_2 = C\,Cl_2 + Cl_2 + 4HF \xrightarrow{catalyst} C\,ClF_2CClF_2 + 4HCl$$

The physicochemical properties of these compounds are of prime importance in the formulation and manufacture of aerosol products. The solvent power, stability, and reactivity of the propellants must be known and understood. Just as one considers the properties of some of the usually encountered nonaerosol liquids such as ethanol, glycerin, and acetone, so should the propellant be considered.

Nomenclature—In order to refer easily to the fluorinated hydrocarbons a relatively simple system of nomenclature was developed some time ago by the refrigeration industry. A numerical designation is used to identify each propellant.[52]

1. All propellants are designated by three digits. When the first digit is zero, the propellant is designated by two digits.
2. The first digit is one less than the number of carbon atoms in the compound. Where there are only 2 digits, zero is understood to be this figure and indicates a methane derivative (1 + 0). When this digit is 1, the propellant is an ethane derivative.
3. The second digit is one more than the number of hydrogen atoms in the compound.
4. The last digit represents the number of fluorine atoms.
5. The number of chlorine atoms in the compound is found by subtracting the sum of the fluorine and the hydrogen atoms from the total number of atoms which can be added to saturate the carbon chain.

6. In the case of isomers each has the same number and the most symmetric one is indicated by the number alone. As the isomers become more and more asymmetric, the letter a, b, c, etc, follows the number.
7. For cyclic compounds, a C is used before the number. The use of this system can be exemplified as follows: Propellant 114 is an ethane derivative, has no hydrogens, and contains 4 fluorine atoms. Since 6 atoms are required to saturate the carbon chain, of necessity there must be 2 chlorine atoms. These can be arranged in two different ways; however, since there is no letter following the numerical designation, the symmetrical structure refers to Propellant 114.

Propellant 114   **Propellant 114a**

Table I indicates the chemical name and numerical designation of several liquefied-gas propellants. Propellants 11, 12, and 114 have been admitted to the NF.

Physical Properties—Table II shows some of the more useful physicochemical properties of these propellants.

From a *solubility* standpoint the fluorinated hydrocarbons, which are nonpolar in nature, are miscible with most nonpolar solvents over a large range of temperatures. They also are capable of dissolving a large number of materials. For the most part the propellants are not miscible with water although the degree of miscibility depends on the individual propellants. A cosolvent such as ethanol, isopropanol, or acetone, must be used in conjunction with water in order to form a clear solution. The other alternative involves the formation of an emulsion. Fig. 745 shows charts indicating the best solubilities and spray patterns that have been worked out for various propellant–alcohol systems. The following order of decreasing solvent power has been observed for some of the fluorinated hydrocarbons:[53]

Propellant 21 > 11 > 113 > 22 > 12 > 114

As the degree of fluorination of the molecule increases, the solvent power decreases. The Kauri-Butanol test is often used to compare the solvent power of industrial solvents. A high number indicates a good solvent. The test involves the titration of 20 Gm of a standard solution of kauri-gum in butyl alcohol at 77°F with the solvent under consideration. The end-point is reached when the turbidity due to the precipitation of the kauri-gum prevents reading of 10-point type (approx. 0.4 cm high) through a solution in a 250-ml Erlenmeyer flask. Typical Kauri-Butanol values for the propellants and some commonly used solvents are given in Table III. Another system which can be used to

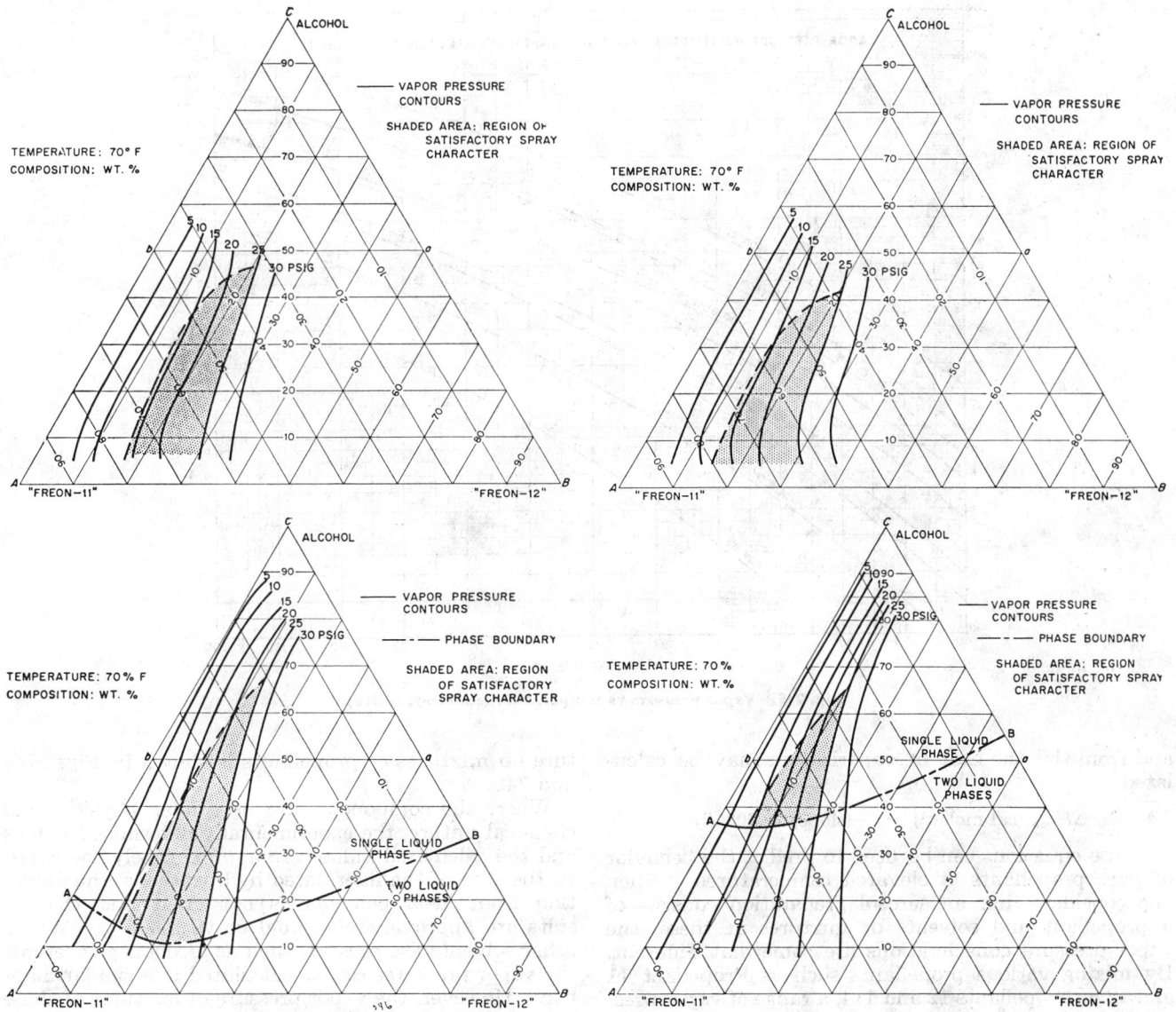

Fig. 745.   Properties of Propellant 12 and Propellant 11 in ethyl alcohol solutions.   I: 100%; II: 95%; III: 90%; IV: 85% by volume (courtesy, Du Pont).

predict the miscibility of various substances was developed by Hildebrand.[54,55]   As the difference between the solubility parameter of two substances decreases, the compounds become more miscible finally resulting in mutual solubility.   Several of these values are indicated in Table III.

One of the most important physicochemical properties of a propellant is its *vapor pressure*, which may be defined as the pressure exerted by a liquid in equilibrium with its vapor.   When the vapor pressure exceeds atmospheric pressure, boiling and vaporization take place.   However, if the vaporized molecules are prevented from leaving the container (by placing the propellant into a sealed container), they will fill the head space and eventually cause an increase in pressure. The pressure developed at equilibrium is the vapor pressure.   The vapor pressure of a liquefied gas is independent of the quantity used but is influenced by temperature changes.   This effect can be seen readily in Fig. 746.   Assuming ideal behavior for the liquefied gas, the effect of temperature on the vapor pressure can be calculated from the following equation:

$$\log P = -\frac{\Delta H_{vap}}{2.303\,RT}$$

where P = vapor pressure, ΔH = heat of vaporization, R = gas constant (generally 1.987 cal deg^{-1} mole^{-1}), and T = absolute temperature.

Since

$$\ln P = -\frac{\Delta H_{vap}}{RT} + C$$

a plot of the log P vs $1/T$ should yield a straight line

Table III—Kauri-Butanol Value and Solubility Parameter of Several Propellants and Solvents

Compound	Kauri-Butanol value	Solubility parameter
Propellant 11	60.1	7.5
Propellant 12	18.0	6.5
Propellant 114	11.8	6.2
Ethyl ether	..	7.3
Ethyl alcohol	..	12.7
Water	..	22.0
Ethylene glycol	..	14.0
Carbon tetrachloride	112.5	8.6
Methylene chloride	136.2	9.7
Chloroform	208.0	9.3

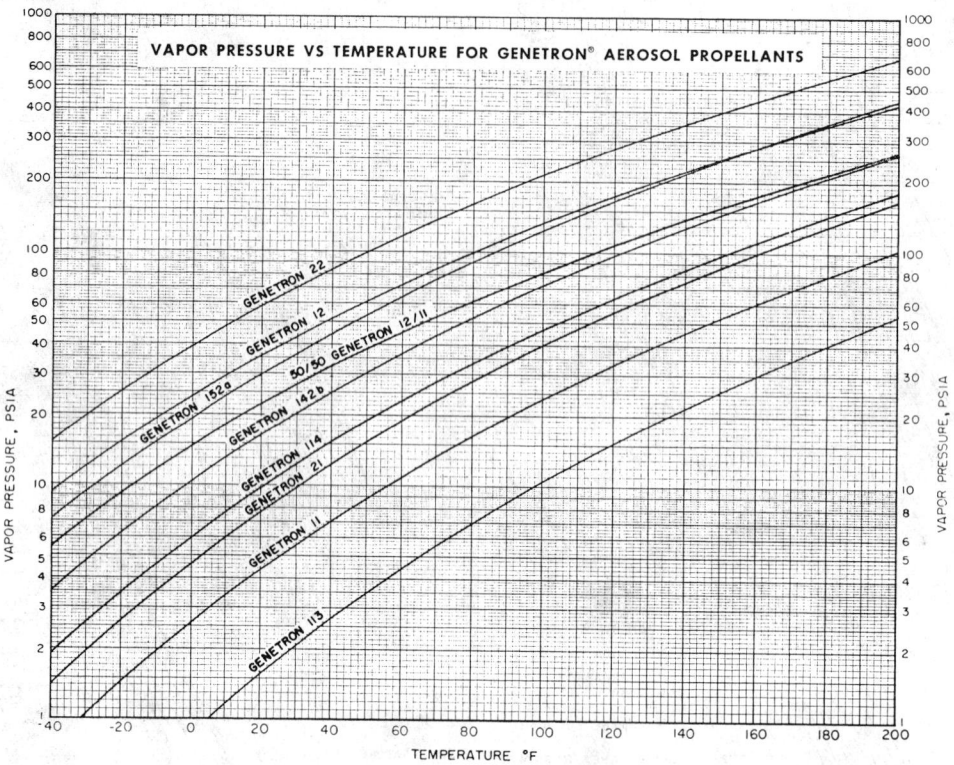

Fig. 746.   Vapor pressure vs temperature (courtesy, Allied).

and from this the heat of vaporization may be calculated.

$$\Delta H_{vap} \text{ (cal mole}^{-1}) = -(\text{slope)} (2.303\ R)$$

These equations can be used to predict the behavior of pure propellants at elevated temperatures. When one considers that an aerosol preparation consists of a propellant and solvents or mixtures of these, the vapor-pressure considerations are somewhat different. By mixing various propellants such as Propellant 11 and 12 or Propellants 12 and 114, a range of vapor pressures are obtained as seen in Fig. 747. The vapor pressure of a mixture of propellants may be calculated from Raoult's law, which states that the "vapor pressure of a solution is dependent upon the vapor pressure of the individual components. For ideal solutions, the vapor pressure is equal to the sum of the mole fractions of each component present times the vapor pressure of the pure compound at the desired temperature." Mathematically this law may be expressed as

$$p_A = \frac{n_A}{n_A + n_B}\, p_A{}^\circ = N_A p_A{}^\circ$$

where p_A = partial vapor pressure of Component A, $p_A{}^\circ$ = vapor pressure of pure Component A, n_A = moles of Component A, n_B = moles of Component B, and N_A = mole fraction of Component A.

Similarly,

$$p_B = \frac{n_B}{n_B + n_A}\, p_B{}^\circ = N_B p_B{}^\circ$$

The total vapor pressure of the system is obtained by

$$VP = p_A + p_B$$

When the mole fraction of one component is large, the other component has a small mole fraction and as such it does not appreciably affect the vapor pressure. This approaches ideal behavior. The effect of tempera-

ture on mixtures of propellants is shown in Figs. 748 and 749.

Where the components are of similar physical and chemical nature, the experimentally determined values and the calculated values are approximately the same. In the case of the fluorinated hydrocarbons, the deviation from ideal behavior is not great and the results are approximately equal or within 5%. Where other solvents are present, such as alcohols or acetone, the vapor pressures can be calculated in a similar manner. However, the vapor pressure of mixtures of these solvents and propellants deviates a great deal from ideal behavior and there is significant difference between the actual and theoretical values. Flanner[56] determined the vapor pressure of many systems consisting of mixtures of various propellants and solvents. Some of the results of these studies are seen in Figs. 750–753. Flanner indicated that four factors contribute to this positive deviation:

1. Internal pressure of the two components in the propellant–solvent mixture.

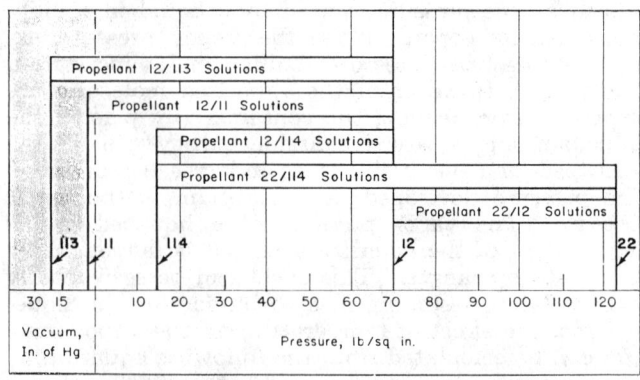

Fig. 747.   Range of pressures obtainable at 70°F with various propellants.

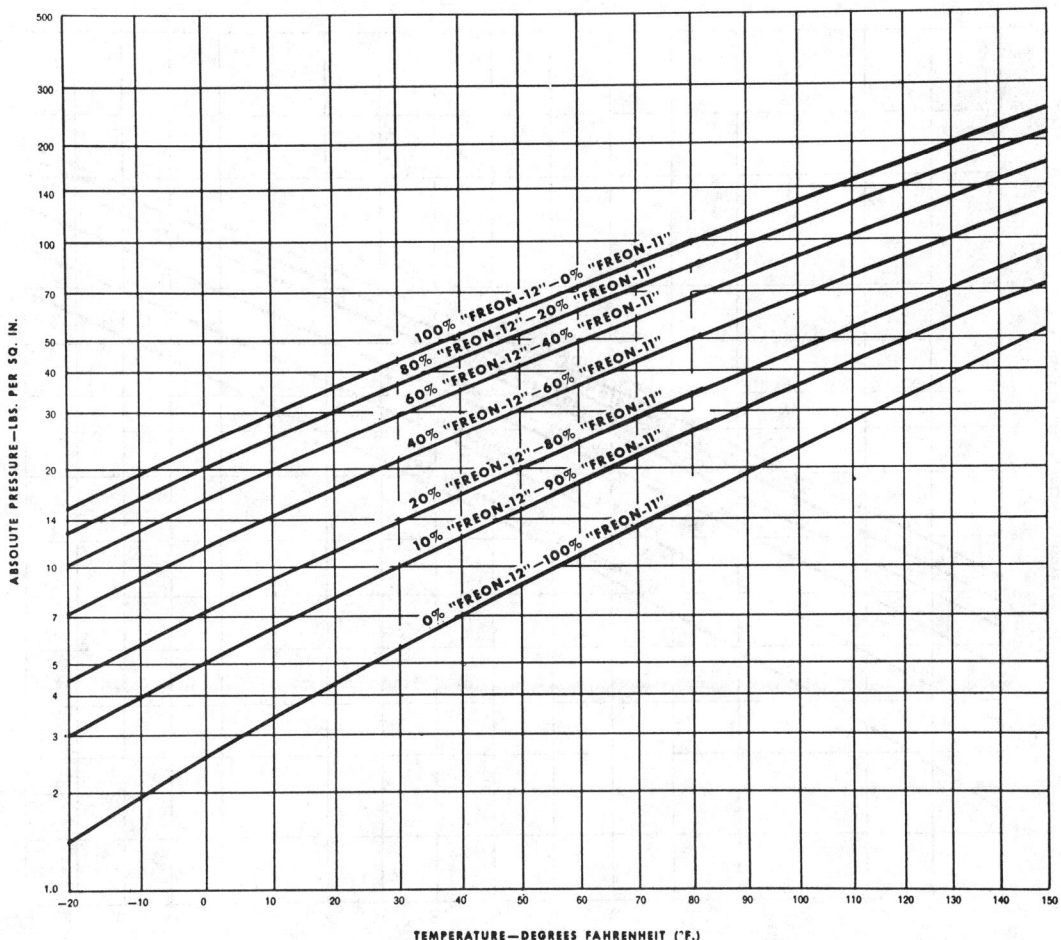

Fig. 748. Vapor pressure–temperature relationship of Propellant 12/11 (courtesy, Du Pont).

2. Polarity.
3. Length of the hydrocarbon chain or analogous grouping.
4. Association in the liquid phase of either component.

The *density* of the propellants is an important consideration in the formulation of aerosol products. Depending on the method of manufacture, fluorinated hydrocarbons are treated on a volume or weight basis. The density varies from 0.911 to 1.513 Gm/ml for the commonly encountered propellants. Generally, as the number of fluorine atoms increases, the density increases. There is a gradual decrease in density with an increase in temperature. Depending on the size of the container, the density of propellant in the vapor state may also be an important factor. The density of materials used as propellants is given in Table II.

Chemical Properties—The fluorinated hydrocarbons have found widespread use as aerosol propellants since they are generally considered to be chemically inert. From the viewpoint of formulation the only chemical property that need be considered is hydrolysis. The addition of fluorine to a carbon atom generally results in increased stability. However, in a propellant such as trichloromonofluoromethane there is the possibility of hydrolysis with the formation of hydrochloric acid. The hydrolysis rate of several propellants is seen in Table IV. Propellant 11 is not used with aqueous products since hydrolysis will take place. Propellant 114 is generally used as a replacement.

One additional reaction which has been studied involves the reaction between Propellant 11 and ethanol. Sanders found this to be a free-radical

reaction which required the presence of a catalyst.[57] The resulting products, acetaldehyde and acetal, are corrosive to metal containers and may cause puncturing. This led to the development of Propellant 11-S which is Propellant 11 containing a small amount of nitromethane which acts as an inhibitor for this reaction.

Chlorinated Hydrocarbons—Several chlorinated hydrocarbons have been used as propellants or in combination with other propellants in various type aerosols. Vinyl chloride, methylene chloride, and trichloroethane, have been used. They are especially useful in insecticidal sprays, certain hair sprays and room deodorants. When used, they generally replace or decrease the concentration of Propellant 11 resulting in a less expensive package. Vinyl chloride has

Table IV—Rate of Hydrolysis of Several Propellants[a]

(Gm propellant hydrolyzed/liter of water/year)

	1 Atmos pressure—86°F			
Compound	Water	Water + steel	Water + copper	Sodium carbonate 1%
Propellant 11	0.005	19.0	0.18	0.12
Propellant 12	0.005	0.8	0.005	0.04
Propellant 21	0.01	5.2	0.38	330
Propellant 114	0.005	1.4	0.005	0.01
Propellant 22	0.01	0.14	0.02	220

[a] *Note:* The hydrolysis rate of Propellant C-318 was found to be 2.2 mg/L of 10% sodium hydroxide solution/year.

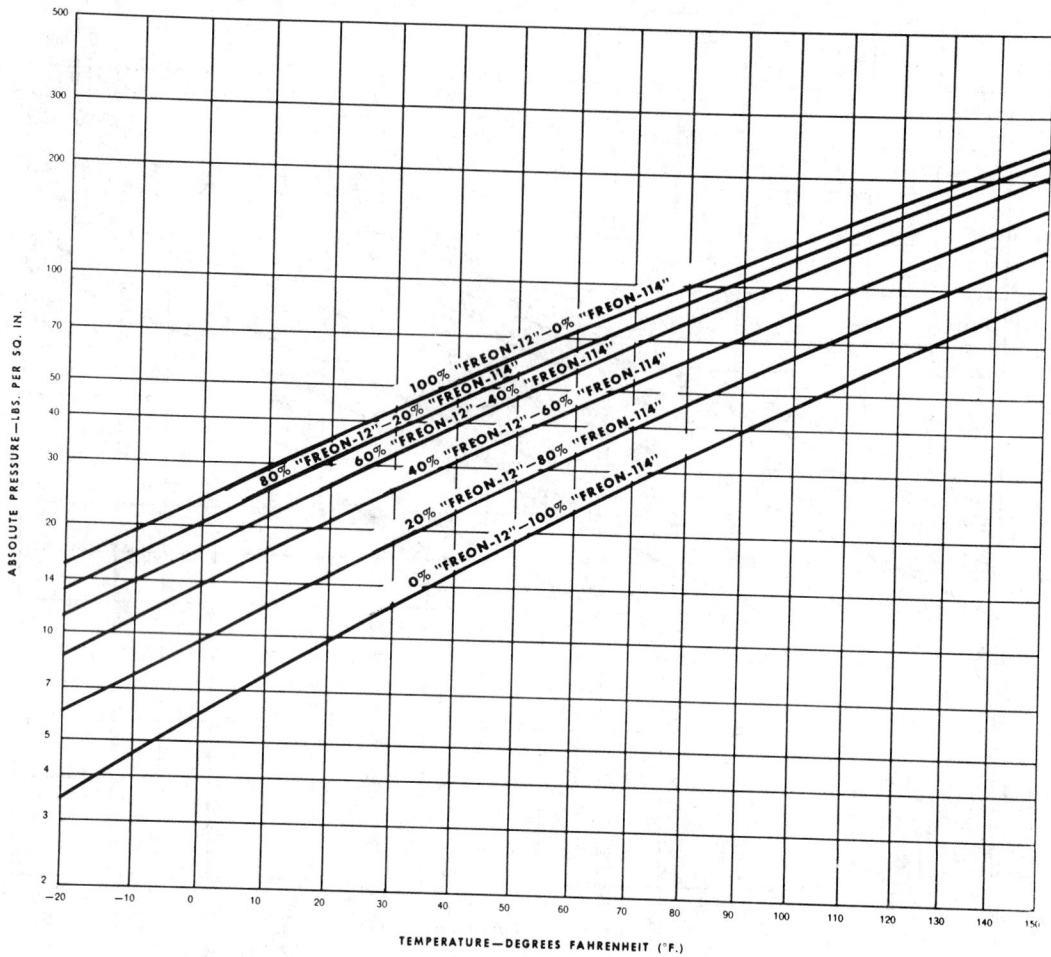

Fig. 749. Vapor pressure–temperature relationships of Propellant 12/114 (courtesy, Du Pont).

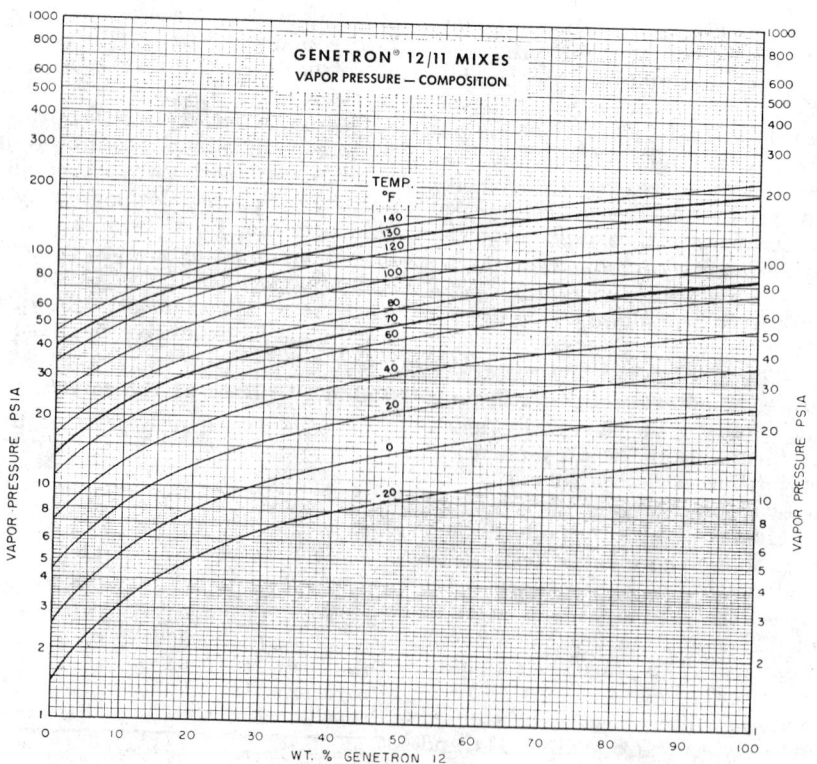

Fig. 750. Vapor pressure–composition of Propellant 12/11 (courtesy, Allied).

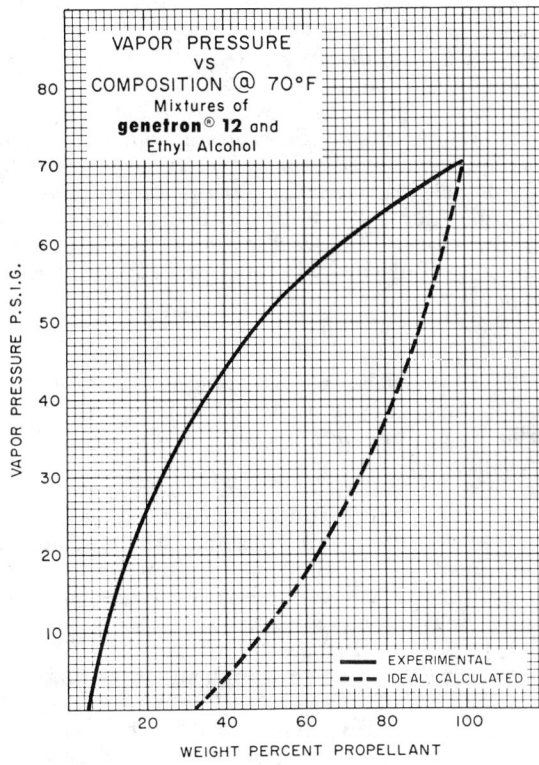

Fig. 751. Vapor pressure vs Propellant 12–ethyl alcohol mixture at 70°F (courtesy, Allied).

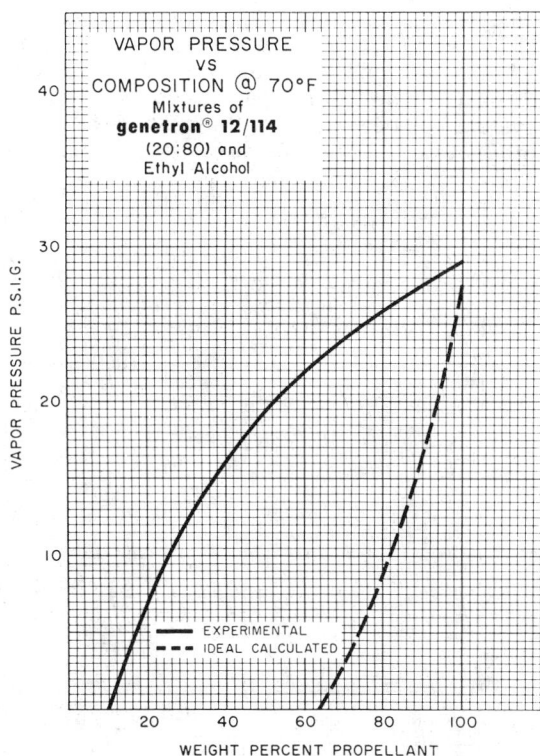

Fig. 752. Vapor pressure vs Propellant 12/11–ethyl alcohol mixture at 70°F (courtesy, Allied).

found greater use in foreign countries rather than the United States. The latter two chemicals find use as solvents for various aerosol products. However, they have not been utilized to date for pharmaceutical or medicinal aerosols.

Hydrocarbons—While the hydrocarbon propellants have not been utilized to date for pharmaceutical aerosols, they have been used for shave creams, shampoos, room deodorants, and household cleaners. While their low-order toxicity makes them suitable for use, their flammability limits their use.

By mixing the hydrocarbon with varying quantities of fluorinated hydrocarbon it is possible to decrease the flammability hazard. For example, Reed[52] noted that a mixture of 45% Propellant 12, 45% Propellant 11, and 10% by weight isobutane produced a propellant having a vapor pressure of approximately 35 psig at 70°F. The advantage of using hydrocarbons is their greater range of solubility and lower cost compared to fluorinated hydrocarbons.

The hydrocarbon propellants are produced from petroleum by distillation. They are purified to remove all possible impurities, especially unsaturated hydrocarbons which are prone to chemical reaction.

Table V shows some of the more important physical properties of the hydrocarbons.

The hydrocarbons have several properties which make them useful as propellants in addition to possessing the proper vapor pressure (see Fig. 754). They have a density of less than 1 and are not miscible with water. This makes them useful in the formulation of three-phase (two-layer) aerosols. Being lighter than water, the hydrocarbon will float on top of the aqueous layer. In this way the hydrocarbon serves to push the contents out of the container. Since they are not halogenated, they would possess better solubility characteristics than the fluorinated hydrocarbons. However, as indicated previously, their use is limited due to their flammability.

Finally, it should be indicated that the hydrocarbons are further characterized by their extreme chemical stability. They are not subject to hydrolysis, making them useful with water-based aerosols. They will react with the halogens, but only under severe conditions.

Compressed Gases[58]

The compressed gases such as nitrogen, nitrous oxide, and carbon dioxide have been used as aerosol propellants. Depending on the nature of the formulation and the valve design, the product can be dispensed as a

Table V—Physical Properties of the Hydrocarbon Propellants

Propellant	Propane	Isobutane	n-Butane
Chemical formula	$CH_3CH_2CH_3$	$(CH_3)_2CHCH_3$	$CH_3(CH_2)_2CH_3$
Molecular weight	44.1	58.1	58.1
Boiling point, °F	−43.9	13.6	30.9
Freezing point, °F	−275	−229	−211
Vapor Pressure (psia)			
70°F	124.7	45.7	30.7
130°F	274.7	110.7	80.7
Liquid density (Gm/ml) 68°F	0.5005	0.5788	0.5571

fine mist, foam, or semisolid. However, unlike the liquefied gases, the compressed gases possess little, if any, expansion power and will produce a fairly wet spray and foams which are not as stable as liquefied-gas foams. This system has been used for the most part to dispense food products and for non-foods to dispense the product in its original form as a semisolid. Compressed gases have been used in products such as dental creams, hair preparations, ointments, and aqueous antiseptic and germicidal aerosols.

Since compressed gases are utilized in the gaseous state and not in the liquid state, a higher initial pressure is required as well as a relatively larger head space than liquefied-gas aerosols. While the pressure of a liquefied-gas aerosol remains constant during use, a drop in pressure is noted during use of a compressed-gas aerosol. This drop in pressure can be calculated by application of the ideal gas laws:

$$PV = nRT$$

where P = pressure in atmospheres, V = volume in liters, n = moles of gas (Gm/mol wt), R = gas constant (0.08205 liter atmos deg $^{-1}$ mole $^{-1}$), and T = absolute temperature.

The initial pressure of a compressed-gas aerosol is usually about 90 psig and occupies a volume of about 15–25% of the container volume. As the contents of the container are expelled, the volume of head space increases with a corresponding decrease in pressure according to Boyle's law.

The physical and chemical properties of the compressed gases are not as vital to formulation as the properties of the liquefied gases.[59] These gases are, for the most part, chemically inert and do not react with the product concentrate. In the case of nitrogen there is no solubility of the gas in the product, whereas nitrous oxide and carbon dioxide are soluble to a certain extent. Table VI indicates this solubility. Mixtures of nitrous oxide and carbon dioxide have been used as propellants for whipped creams and toppings[60] and also for several veterinary emulsion products. The solubility of carbon dioxide in certain beverage food products is advantageous in that a slight degree of

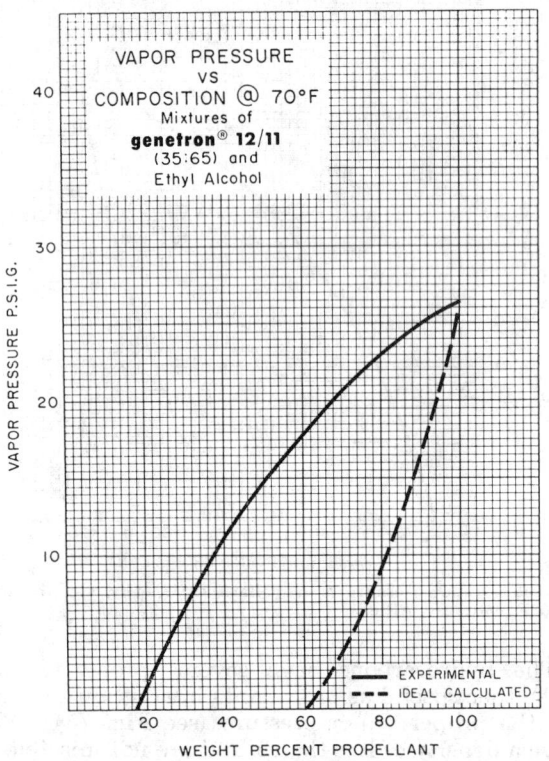

Fig. 753. Vapor pressure vs Propellant 12/114–ethyl alcohol mixture at 70° (courtesy, Allied).

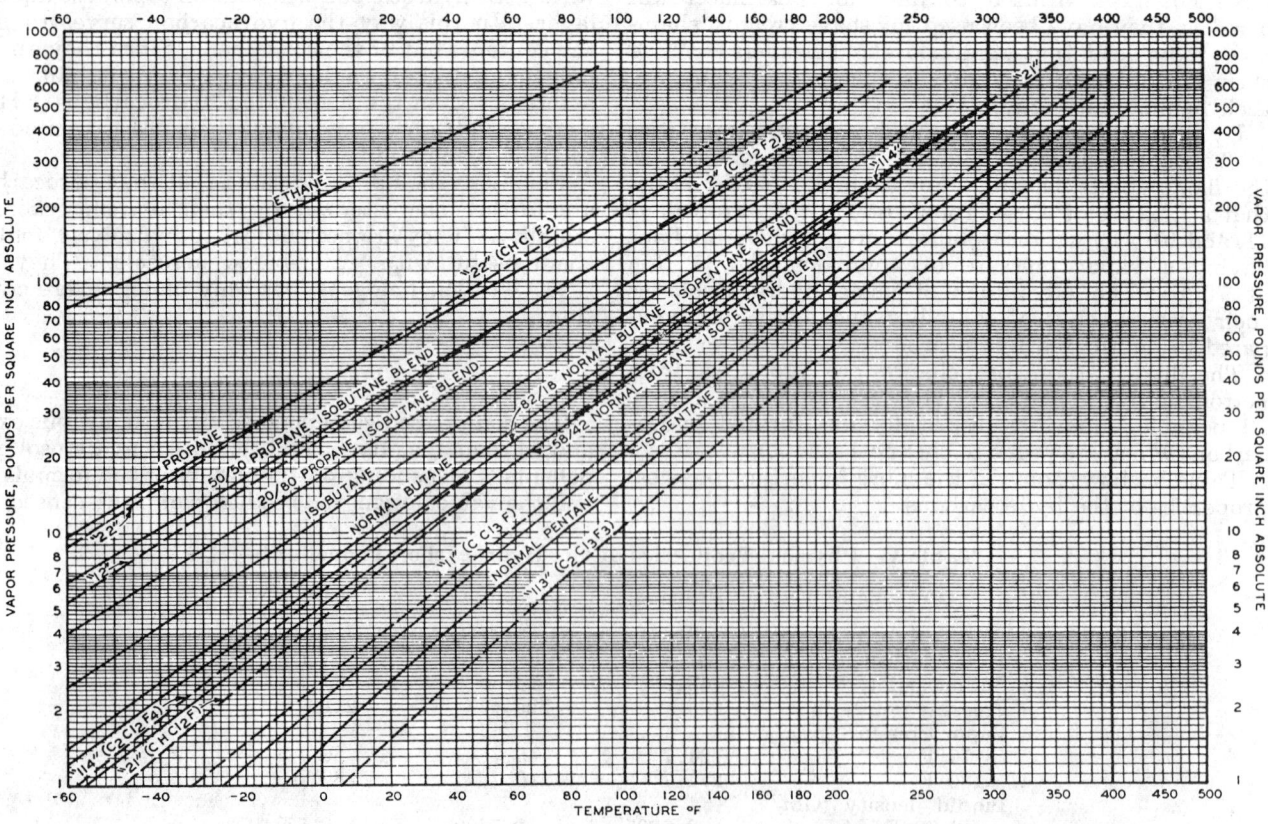

Fig. 754. Vapor pressure of several hydrocarbons (courtesy, Phillips Petroleum).

Table VI—Solubility of Some Gases in Water at 25°C and 1 Atmos Pressure of the Gas[a]

Gas	Solubility[b]
Nitrogen	0.0143
Nitrous oxide	0.5961
Carbon dioxide	0.759
Argon	0.0310

[a] *Handbook of Chemistry and Physics*, 49th ed., Chemical Rubber Publ. Co., Cleveland, Ohio, 1968–1969, p. B-172.

[b] Bunsen coefficient $= \dfrac{ml(STP)}{Atmos\text{-}ml}$ (liters of gas measured at standard conditions, dissolved in 1 L of water).

carbonation can be obtained.[41] Since these gases are generally inert and replace the air trapped in the head space, the stability of drugs is sometimes increased.[30,61]

A serious drawback to the use of these gases as propellants is loss of propellant through product misuse or leakage of propellant. Once the propellant is lost, the package becomes inoperative.

Propellant Blends

In order to achieve greater versatility as well as lower cost, a series of propellant blends have been developed for a variety of different uses.[62–66] These blends consist of mixtures of fluorinated hydrocarbons with other fluorinated hydrocarbons, hydrocarbons with other hydrocarbons, and compressed gases with other compressed gases. In addition, blends of fluorinated hydrocarbons with hydrocarbons and/or compressed gases are also used to achieve special effects. Table VII indicates some of the commonly used propellant blends. Blends are used for a variety of reasons, including (1) proper vapor pressure, (2) solubility, (3) taste—in the case of food aerosols, (4) reduction of cost, (5) reduction of flammability, and (6) proper density.

Flammability and Toxicity Considerations

Aerosol products are intended for spraying into large enclosed areas or application as a foam. As such, both the flammability and the toxicity are important. In addition, for pharmaceutical and medicinal aerosols, the inhalation effects as well as the topical effects must be determined. The flammability and toxicity ratings of several of the commonly used propellants are shown in Table VIII.

The fluorinated hydrocarbons do not present any flammability hazards; in fact they will extinguish a

Table VII—Propellant Blends

Components	Composition %	Vapor pressure 70°F, psig	Density 70°F, Gm/cc
Propellant 12/114	70:30	56.1	1.368
	25:75	30.4	1.434
	10:90	20.2	1.455
	20:80	27.1	1.441
	45:55	42.8	1.405
	55:45	48.4	1.390
Propellant 12/11	50:50	37.4	1.412
	35:65	27.0	1.435
	30:70	23.4	1.444
Propellant 12/11/isobutane	45:45:10	38.0	1.320
Propane/isobutane	16:84	46.0	0.554[a]
Propellant 12/11/vinyl chloride	20:45:35	36.0	1.190

[a] At 60°F.

Table VIII—Flammability and Toxicity of Propellants

Propellant	Flammability[a]	Toxicity[b]	Max. allowable conc., ppm
11	nonflammable	5A	1000
12	nonflammable	6	1000
114	nonflammable	6	1000
115	nonflammable	6	1000
152a	5.1–17.1	5A	..
142b	9.0–14.8	5A[c]	..
C-318	nonflammable	6[d]	1000
Propane	2.3–7.3	5B	1000
Butane	1.8–8.4	5B	1000
Isobutane	1.6–6.5	5B	1000
Nitrogen	nonflammable	6	..
Carbon dioxide	nonflammable	5	5000
Nitrous oxide	nonflammable	..	..

[a] Vol % in air.
[b] Underwriters' Laboratory Rating System.[67]
[c] Probable value.
[d] Preliminary value.

flame by excluding oxygen. The hydrocarbons are flammable and will form explosive mixtures with air. It is for this reason that caution must be exercised during the manufacture of these products. The compressed gases are not flammable and can be handled safely.

The toxicity of the propellants must be considered from the viewpoint of inhalation and topical application. Reed reviewed the toxicity considerations for propellants.[67] As noted from the Underwriters Laboratory (UL) ratings, the propellants are relatively nontoxic. When one considers that sulfur dioxide is given a rating of 1, ammonia, 2, and carbon tetrachloride, 3, with maximum allowable concentration of 10 ppm, 100 ppm, and 25 ppm, respectively, the safety of these materials can be ascertained quickly. Since the liquefied gas propellants will not support life, precautions must be taken to ensure an adequate air supply. This is of greater concern to a manufacturer than the user.

During 1968 several deaths were reported, apparently due to the deliberate inhalation of large quantities of fluorinated hydrocarbons. These involved teenagers who were using certain aerosol products known to contain only propellant. Death resulted from freezing of the trachea and the larynx, and from asphyxiation brought about by depletion of oxygen in the lungs. This is a practice which certainly should be discouraged and the aerosol industry is currently engaged in a public education program.

Skin sensitization to the propellants should be considered since many products are applied topically. There have been no reported cases of skin sensitization and rabbit-eye tests have indicated their lack of sensitization.[67] Dunne[68] and Broderick and Flanner[69] reported the possible chilling effect of liquefied gases when applied to the skin.

Containers

The following aerosol containers have been used to package aerosol products:

Metal
  Tin-plated steel
    Side-seam (three-piece)
    Two-piece or drawn
  Aluminum
    Two-piece
    Extruded
  Stainless steel

Glass
  Uncoated
  Plastic-coated
Synthetic resins and plastics

The original aerosol container was a "heavy-walled" steel container which was heavy, bulky, and expensive.

Metal

Tin-Plated Steel—In order to produce an aerosol container which was light and relatively inexpensive, tin-plated steel was used for aerosol containers. This resulted in the large scale production of aerosol containers.

Side-Seam—Following this, the beer can type was developed and finally led to the present-day three-piece container. This container consists of a body and two ends. The body is seamed longitudinally and the bottom is flanged and joined by a double-seaming operation. The top is pressed into shape and curled into a 1-in. opening and attached to the body in a similar manner to the attachment of the bottom. This makes for an exceptionally strong container and is available in sizes varying from 3 to 24 oz.

The tin plate which is used consists of steel base coated with varying thicknesses of tin. For example, a 25# tin plate indicates that ¼ lb of tin has been used to coat both sides of steel in a base box (a base box consists of 112 sheets, 20 × 14 in.). A 50#, 75#, and 100# tin plate is available in a hot-dipped plate.[70] In many instances the body of the container is made to have a certain thickness of tin and the ends would have another thickness. This is done in order to obtain increased stability in the container.

For certain products the tin affords sufficient protection so that no further treatment is necessary. Hair lacquers generally can be packaged in this type of container. However, the addition of water and other corrosive ingredients or other substances which will attack tin require a container having an additional protective coating. This coating is usually organic in nature and may consist of an oleoresin, phenolic, vinyl, or epoxy coating. The liner (single or double coat) is added to the container prior to fabrication, that is, it is applied to the flat sheets of tin plate.

During the fabrication process the coating may become scratched and therefore become a potential source of corrosion. This is one of the reasons for the examination of all containers prior to use. A spray coating is applied to the side seam following fabrication in order to further protect the product.

Several processes which were developed recently allow for a complete spraying of the inside of the container with an organic coating following fabrication. This produces a continuous coat of organic compound giving added resistance to the container.

Two-Piece or Drawn—In 1946 a two-piece container became available. The body was made of black iron formed from 100-lb deep-drawn sheet stock by a multiple-die drawing process. The bottom was concave and double-seamed into place. The opening was made to hold the standard 1-in. valve. The organic coating was generally applied by a spray process following fabrication. They are available in 6- and 12-oz capacity.

Aluminum—These containers first became available in 1954. They are produced by an impact extrusion process so that the container is seamless. This will give added strength to the container. A variety of different aluminum aerosol containers ranging in size from 15 ml to 45 fl oz are available. While aluminum is less reactive than other metals used in can manufacture, added resistance can be obtained by coating the inside of the container with organic materials such as epoxy, vinyl, and phenolic resins.

Stainless Steel—These containers have been developed mainly for use in perfume and medicinal aerosols. When Propellant 12 is used as the propellant, a stronger than usual container is needed. These containers are relatively expensive and are available in sizes ranging from 5 to 30 ml.

Glass—The first aerosols produced were packaged in glass containers. For pharmaceuticals and medicinals, glass is preferred due to the absence of incompatibilities, as well as for its esthetic value. The use of glass containers is limited to those products having a lower pressure and lower percentage of propellant. Glass aerosols have found use in the packaging of many perfumes, colognes, cosmetics, pharmaceuticals, and medicinals. While glass is basically stronger than most metallic aerosol containers, a potential hazard is present if, and when, the container is dropped with subsequent breakage. However, the danger involved can be compared somewhat to the hazard involved in the use of carbonated beverages in the home. Two types of glass aerosol containers are available. The uncoated glass container has the advantage of decreased cost and high clarity. The contents can be viewed at all times. The plastic-coated glass containers are protected by a coating which prevents the glass from shattering in the event of breakage. In one type the coating is bonded to the glass and becomes an integral part of the container. In another type, the coating fits over the glass container.

Synthetic Resins and Plastics

Attempts have been made over a number of years to develop a suitable plastic material which can be used to fabricate plastic aerosol containers. Some of the problems involved are concerned with moisture-vapor transmission through the plastic as well as the seepage of volatile oils and other ingredients. This has been somewhat controlled through the use of special resins and plastics. To date, plastic containers have been of limited use for aerosols. Fig. 755 shows a representative number of aerosol containers.

Valves

Probably the most basic part of any aerosol or pressurized package is the valve mechanism through which the content of the package is emitted. Together with the formulation, the valve determines the performance of a pressurized package. The interaction of these two is such that one cannot readily be discussed without reference to the other.

The primary purpose of the valve is to regulate the flow of product from the container. It provides a means of discharging the desired amount when needed and prevents loss at other times. The valve also exerts a major effect on the character of the dispensed product. For example, a product formulated to produce a foam can be dispensed as a spray or as a wet stream by the use of different actuators or push buttons on the valve. The selection of proper propellants also governs whether a foam, spray, or wet stream will be produced.

Spray Valves

Since the spray valve is the most commonly used valve, it will be discussed in detail. A cross-sectional view of one such valve mounted on a glass aerosol bottle is shown in Fig. 756. It may be noted that the core, B, is seated in a snugly fitting rubber valve seat, C. The two orifices, I, are 180° apart and extend through the walls of the core into groove K which

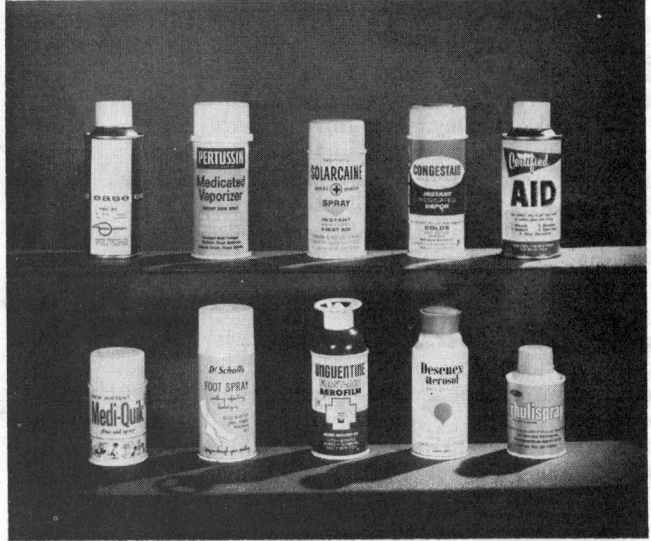

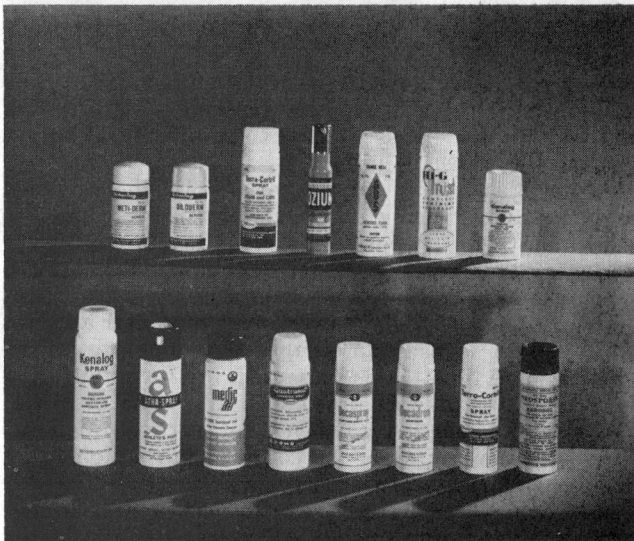

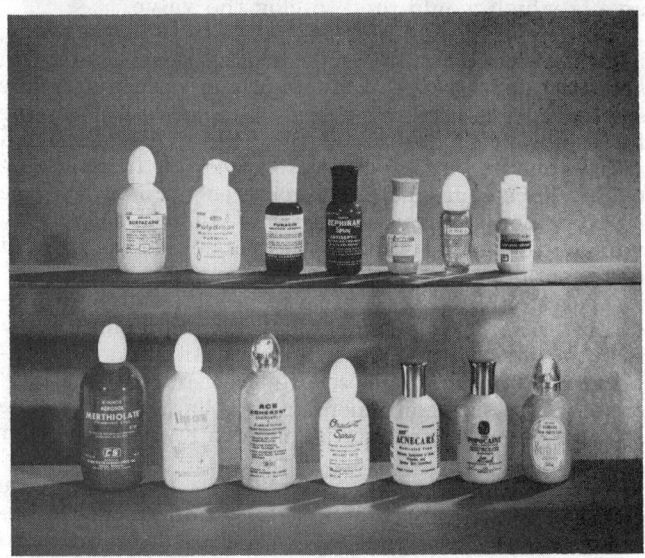

Fig. 755. Typical aerosol containers. *Top:* two-piece and three-piece, tin-plated; *middle:* aluminum; *bottom:* glass.

circles the lower end of the core. Valve seat C is a snug fit in valve cup D to which is attached the dip tube F. Gasket H provides a seal between the valve and the bottle. All of these parts are held together and to the bottle by a ferrule A which has been curled under the lip of the bottle. The actuator, E, carries or has formed in it the spray orifice and also provides a means for operating the valve. If the actuator is pushed at E, the core will be tilted and deflected from the seat at the lower left-hand corner. The groove will be uncovered and will allow the pressurized product to rise through the dip tube, pass through the orifices, rise through the core, and spray out through the terminal orifice. When finger pressure is removed from E, the core snaps back to the closed position due to the elasticity of the rubber seat.[71]

Actuator Button—The actuator button is usually made of polyethylene. Its design, including that of its orifice, depends on its end use. For example, in the case of a spray-type valve, a small (0.020 in.) external orifice is used as compared with a foam-type valve (0.300 in.). The diameter of the orifice is a factor in the determination of spray rate of the valve.

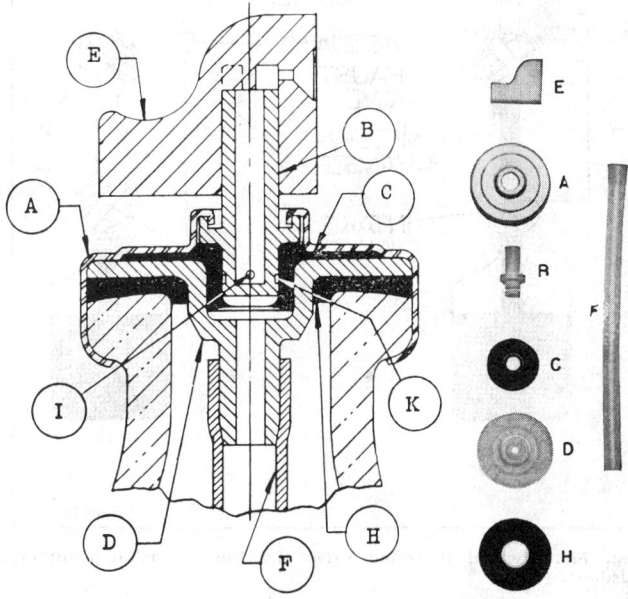

Fig. 756. Aerosol valve (courtesy, Risdon).

Elastomeric Seal—This part of the valve must be made of a material that is unaffected chemically by the product. It must not swell or deteriorate so as to cause leakage or malfunctioning of the valve.

Internal Orifice—The spray rate of the valve is determined largely by the diameter of the internal orifice. Some valves are so designed as to contain two or three internal orifices.

Expansion Chamber—All spray valves have a similar series of orifices with communicating passages (expansion chambers) and a shutoff point. Orifice diameters may range from 0.010 in. to 0.040 in. The size and number of orifices affects the spray rate and, in the case of sprays, the particle size of the product. When the propellant solution passes through the first orifice, the pressure drop is great enough to cause the liquefied propellant to expand and begin to boil. Passage through subsequent orifices results in a further expansion and violent boiling which atomizes the liquid product being swept along with the rapidly expanding gas stream.

Foam Valves

Valves for foam or aerated products usually have only one expansion orifice, the one at the seat. Following this is a single expansion chamber which serves as a delivery nozzle or applicator. It is sufficiently large in volume to permit immediate expansion of the pressurized product to form the familiar ball of foam. As demonstrated earlier, the same formulation will be discharged as a solid stream when dispensed with a valve and actuator having small orifices and expansion chambers. Under these latter conditions, the ball of foam will begin to develop where the stream impinges on a surface. This rather interesting performance is utilized in some pressurized surgical soaps on the market.

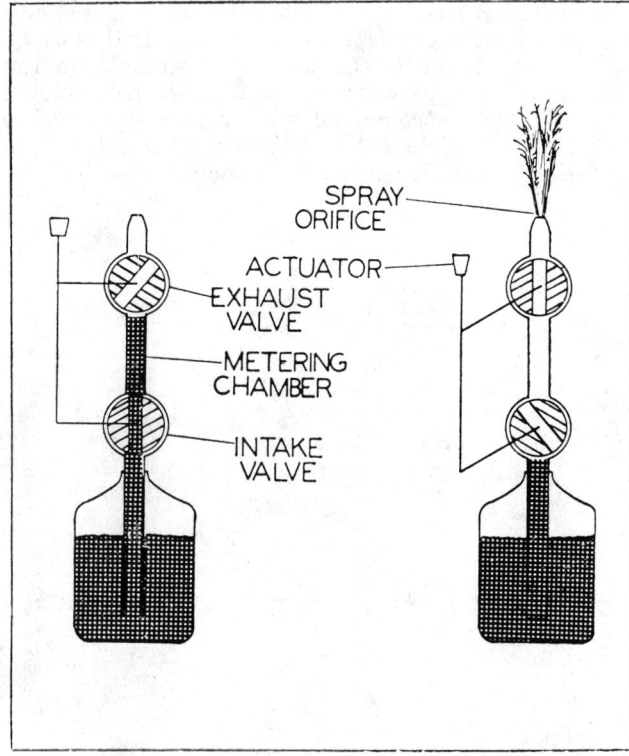

Fig. 757. Typical metering valve showing operation (courtesy, Risdon).

Because of their large openings foam valves may lend themselves for use with viscous materials such as syrups, creams, and ointments.

After a foam product such as shaving cream has been used a small accumulation of foam often will be seen on the end of the actuator. This buildup is not due either to leakage or slow shutoff of the valve, but rather to the expansion of the residual formulation in the actuator.

Metering Valves

Valves that deliver a measured quantity of spray at each actuation are called metering valves. The metering action is obtained by admitting the pressurized product into a metering chamber during either the up or the down stroke of the valve and releasing it during the reverse stroke and simultaneously isolating the bulk of the liquid phase within the dispenser (Fig. 757). The volume of the chamber in which the isolated portion is held determines the quantity of spray per shot. However, trade practice has been to take no account of the specific gravity of the product–propellant mixture

and to list valves with different capacities as being capable of delivering a certain number of milligrams per shot, eg, 50 mg, 100 mg, etc.

Aside from delivering predetermined doses and thus minimizing overdosage of active compounds, metering valves offer still another safety feature from the standpoint of aerosol packages for medical uses: they prevent the discharge of large volumes of comparatively high-pressure gas into body cavities. This is particularly true for nasal and oral applications.

Several other systems for the dispensing of metered quantities of aerosol products are available but of limited use. One such system makes use of a flexible rubber bag which has been fitted over a dip tube and fixed to the valve housing. By a series of different openings, the bag is filled with product and then emptied. The size of the bag determines the size of the dose dispensed.[72] A rigid inner cup can also be used as a metering chamber.[73] The product is directed into the cup and then dispensed. Since the reproducibility of the amount dispensed with each actuation of the valve depends on the degree to which the bag is filled each time, this system is not too satisfactory for use with small doses.

Special-Application Valves

Valves have been developed for several specific applications. While most of the valves previously described are used primarily with liquefied-gas aerosols, they can also be used with compressed gases. Where viscous liquids or semisolids are to be dispensed, larger sized orifices must be used.

Vapor Tap—This consists of a small hole placed into the valve housing and allows for the escape of a small quantity of vaporized propellant along with the product. This gives a greater degree of dispersion to the emitted spray as well as cleaning the valve orifices following discharge. However, since a greater amount of propellant is used as compared to non-vapor tap systems, care must be exercised during formulation of the product to take this into account. One may also note a change in spray pattern from start to finish due to the change in propellant composition which takes place as the contents are used. Vapor tap valves are used with powder aerosols, water-based aerosols, and aerosols containing suspended materials and other agents which would tend to clog the valve.

Co-Dispensing Valves—A variety of valves have been developed for this special use. Several of them are intended for use in the upright position[74] while some are to be used inverted.[75] One valve is available for use in either position. All of the valves are fitted with a plastic bag which is used to hold the oxidizing agent. The components are metered from each of the compartments through orifices of different size. By varying the size of some of these openings the ratio of one reactant to another can be changed.

Transfer Valves—Several valves, termed "mother–daughter" or "male–female," are available and allow for the easy transfer of aerosol product from one container to another. These are used primarily to fill small purse-size containers from a larger can. The stem of one of the valves is made to fit into the other valve and effect a transfer of product.

Valves For Use At Any Angle—Valves for use either in the upright or inverted position are also available. Several designs have been used in order to achieve an aerosol that will operate properly when held in any direction.

Actuators or Buttons

The actuator provides a rapid and convenient means for releasing the contents from a pressurized container. It provides the additional functional use in allowing the product to be dispensed in the desired form; that is, a fine mist, wet spray, foam, or solid stream. Mechanical breakup actuators are used for three-phase or compressed-gas aerosols. In addition, special actuators are available for use with pharmaceutical and medicinal aerosols which allow for the dispensing of products into the mouth, nose, throat, vagina, and eye. Several of these actuators and applicators are illustrated in Fig. 758.

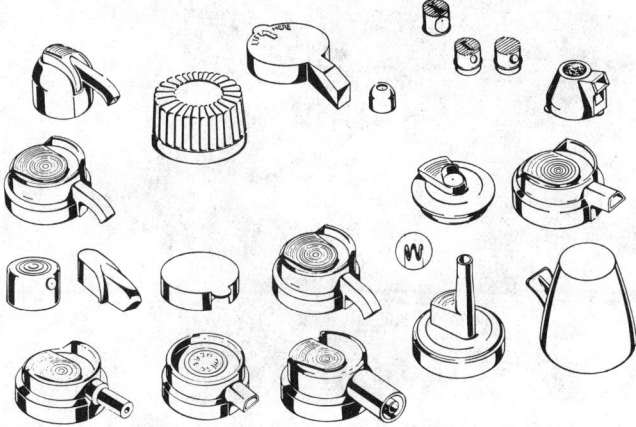

Fig. 758. A variety of spray, foam, and solid-stream actuators (courtesy, Precision Valve).

Dip-Tubes

An additional component which should be considered with the valve is the dip-tube. The dip-tube serves several purposes:

1. It conveys the liquid from the bottom of the container to the dispensing valve at the top.
2. It prevents the propellant from escaping without dispensing the contents of the package (when used according to directions).

The dip-tube comes into intimate contact with both product and propellant and therefore should be resistant to both physical and chemical attack. Polyethylenes and nylon have been found to possess many desirable properties making them useful for this purpose. However, since the dip-tube is stretched to fit tightly on the valve housing, it is possible that on standing the polyethylene or nylon will crack or breakdown at this point, rendering the product useless since it cannot be dispensed. This has been overcome through the use of specially developed polyethylene or polypropylene compounds.

The tube should extend almost to the bottom of the container. If the tube is too short, all of the product will not be dispensed, while a tube touching the bottom of the container will tend to block the passage of liquid. In this connection, most of the materials used for dip-tubes tend to elongate when immersed in certain solvents and propellants for long periods of time. This elongation should be anticipated when determining the length of the dip-tube.

Packaging

Two methods have been used to package aerosol products. Unlike non-aerosol products, part of the manufacturing of necessity takes place during the filling operation. The propellant and product concentrate must be brought together in such a way to insure uniformity of product.

Depending on the nature of the product concentrate, the aerosol can be filled by a cold-filling or a pressure-filling process. There are advantages and disadvantages to both methods, and there are many factors which must be considered before deciding upon which process to use. Since this is a rather specialized procedure, commercial filling facilities are available.

Cold-Fill Process—By lowering the temperature of a propellant below its boiling point, the propellant can be handled as a liquid at atmospheric pressure. The concentrate and propellant are chilled to low temperatures. The propellant is chilled to temperatures of about −30–40°F. The concentrate is generally cooled to below 0° in order to reduce loss of propellant during the filling operation. In practice the chilled concentrate is poured into the chilled container and the propellant is added. Sufficient time is allowed for the propellant to partially vaporize in order to expel the air in the container. The valve is crimped onto the container, which is placed into a water bath, and the contents are heated to 130°F to check for leaks and strength of container.

In the laboratory a dry ice–acetone bath is used to attain these temperatures. Refrigeration equipment is used for the large-scale production of aerosols. Fig. 759 illustrates equipment which can be used for laboratory filling of aerosols.

Pressure-Fill Process—By handling the propellant in a closed system it is possible to fill aerosol products at room temperature. The product concentrate is placed into the container and the valve is sealed in place. The propellant is forced through the valve orifice under pressure. Following this, the container is immersed in a water bath at 130°F in a manner similar to the cold-fill process. An apparatus capable of filling aerosols by this method can be seen in Fig. 760.

Another variation of this method of filling is referred to as "under-the-cap filling." In this method the product concentrate is added to the container and the valve fitted into place but not sealed. Then a plunger type fitting seals against the outer rim of the container, the valve is lifted and a vacuum is drawn on the system. The propellant is allowed to flow into the container. The valve is then dropped into place and sealed. While this method is faster than other methods, there is of necessity a greater loss of propellant; however, an efficient propellant-reclaimer system reduces the loss to a minimum.

Provisions must be made for evacuation of air which may be trapped in the container during the filling oper-

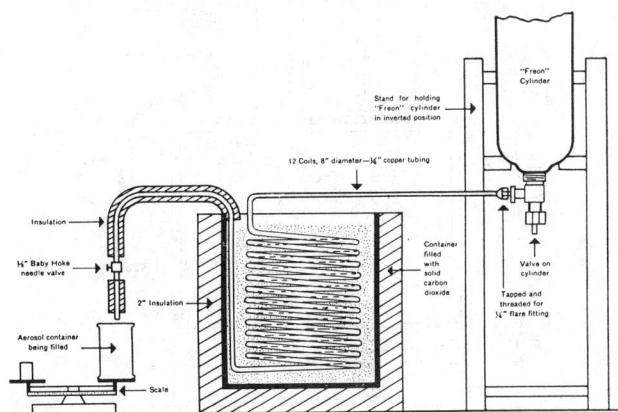

Fig. 759. Laboratory cold loading of aerosol container (courtesy, Du Pont).

ation. This is especially true for the pressure-filling process.

In cold filling, sufficient time elapses between the time the propellant is added and the valve crimped into place to allow for displacement of some of the air by the vaporized propellant. This can be accomplished by use of a vacuum crimper at the time the valve is crimped onto the container.

Another method involves the purging of air from the container by the addition of a small amount of propellant prior to the sealing of the container with the valve. The propellant vaporizes and displaces the air.

According to Dalton's law of partial pressures, the total pressure, P, will be equal to the sum of the pressure due to air, p_1, and the vapor pressure of the propellant, p_2.

$$P = p_1 + p_2$$

Where the total pressure is close to the ICC regulations, air may result in excessive pressure.

The pressure-filling technique can be used with most types of aerosol products. At first, the pressure-filling process was considerably slower than the cold-fill process, however, present-day pressure-filling equipment is comparable and sometimes faster than cold-filling procedures. Aqueous and emulsion aerosols cannot be filled by the cold-fill process since the product will freeze at these low temperatures. Hydrocarbons must be filled by the pressure process since in the cold process an excessive amount of propellant will be released into the air and may reach explosive concentrations. The use of these two methods has been fully discussed elsewhere.[76] Some of the production equipment used to add the propellant to aerosols is shown in Figs. 761 and 762.

Compressed-gas aerosols are filled by the pressure-fill process except that the propellant is added as a gas.

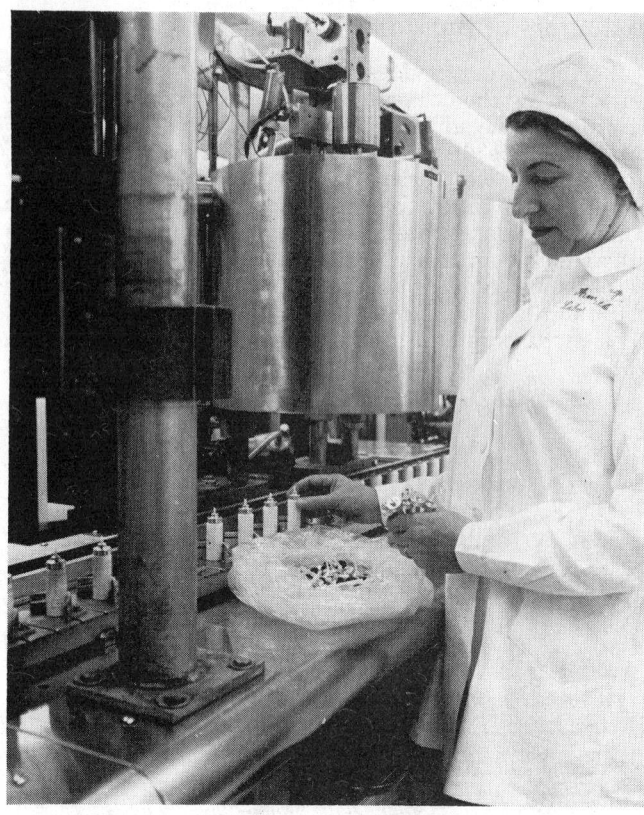

Fig. 761. **Hand placement of aerosol valves into filled containers (courtesy, Armstrong Labs).**

The propellant is not metered but is simply injected through the valve until a predetermined equilibrium pressure has been reached with the container. If the compressed gas used as a propellant is insoluble in the product, such as nitrogen, shaking during the propellant filling is not necessary. If the compressed gas is soluble in the product, the filling is accompanied by vigorous shaking in order to aid in its solution. Filling of compressed-gas aerosols in the laboratory is shown in Fig. 763.

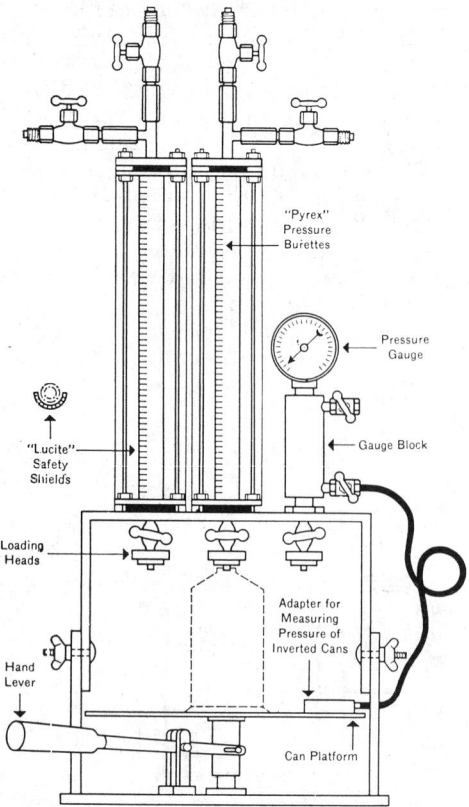

Fig. 760. **Apparatus for pressure loading aerosol containers in the laboratory (courtesy, Du Pont).**

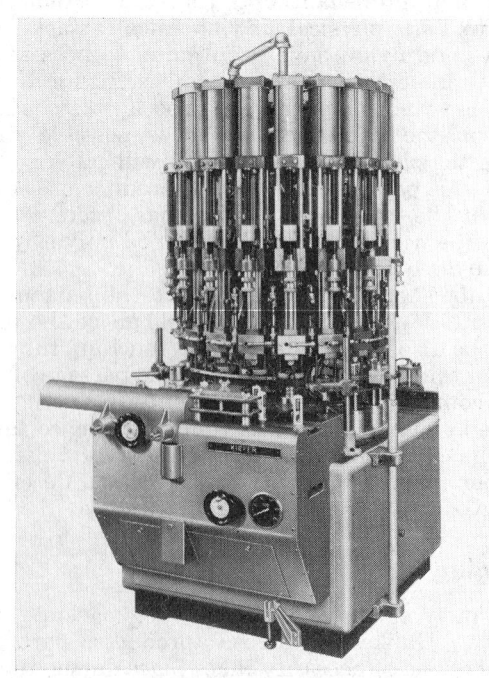

Fig. 762. **Rotary propellant filler (courtesy, Cherry-Burrell).**

Applications

Aerosol technology has been applied to the formulation of products containing therapeutically active ingredients. Since the considerations involved in the formulation of aerosols intended for inhalation therapy differ from those concerned with topical preparations, it is advisable to define further these aerosols.[77]

A pharmaceutical aerosol may be defined as an aerosol product containing therapeutically active ingredients dissolved, suspended, or emulsified in a propellant or a mixture of solvent and propellant and intended for topical administration or for administration into one of the body cavities such as the ear, rectum, and vagina.

Medicinal aerosols may be defined as those aerosol products containing therapeutically active ingredients dissolved or suspended in a propellant or a mixture of a solvent and a propellant and intended for administration as fine, solid particles or liquid mists via the respiratory system or the nasal passages. They are intended for local action in the nasal areas, throat, and lungs, as well as for prompt systemic effect when absorbed from the lungs into the bloodstream (inhalation therapy). The particle size must be considerably below 50 μ and, in most instances, should be below 10 μ and preferably between 3 and 6 μ for maximum therapeutic response.

Other definitions have been advanced to differentiate pharmaceutical and medicinal aerosols from other aerosols. Kanig[78] defines these aerosols as "those which are administered internally or externally and which have a therapeutic effect in the cure or alleviation of any human or animal disease or condition."

According to the NF and the USP; "Aerosols are pressurized dosage forms containing one or more active ingredients which upon actuation give a fine dispersion of liquid and/or solid materials in a gaseous medium." Several aerosol products have been admitted to the USP and NF.

Pharmaceutical Aerosols

The development of topical aerosol preparations has expanded rapidly during the past several years. Some of these applications include local anesthetics, antiseptics, germicides, and first-aid preparations, body rubs, dermatological products, foot preparations, spray-on protective films, vaporizers, and many others.[79,80] These preparations have met with widespread acceptance, chiefly due to their many advantages over non-aerosol products. In addition to the advantages found in all aerosols, these aerosols possess several distinct advantages of their own.

The irritation produced by the application of an ointment or cream over an abraded area of the skin is reduced and sometimes eliminated by the aerosol. These preparations are more economical since they can be easily applied in a thin layer with no waste due to the use of a cotton swab or other applicators. This may result in faster absorption and more efficient use of medication.[81] Since the package is sealed, there is no danger of contamination of the unused portion of the medication. The cooling effect of liquefied-gas aerosols may be desirable in certain skin conditions.[82]

Pharmaceuticals may be formulated as aerosols utilizing solutions, suspensions, emulsions, powders, and semisolid preparations.

Solutions—Solutions are the simplest of all aerosol products to formulate. They consist of propellant and active ingredients dissolved directly in the propellant or a mixture of propellant and a solvent which is miscible with the propellant. Ethyl alcohol has been used to the greatest extent for this purpose since it is relatively free from dermal toxicity and miscible with propellants in all proportions. Geary[83] describes the use of ternary systems consisting of water, propellant, and cosolvents. Other cosolvents which may be useful include acetone, hexadecyl alcohol, glycols, glycol ethers, and polyglycols. Porush has indicated some of the considerations of importance in pharmaceutical aerosols.[84]

These preparations are formulated using 50–90% propellant and 10–50% of active ingredients and cosolvent. Foot preparations, local anesthetics, dermatological preparations (containing a variety of active ingredients including steroids, antibiotics, and astringents), and spray-on protective films are representative of this system.

Dispersions or Suspensions (Powder Aerosols)—These aerosols are similar to solution aerosols except that the active ingredients are suspended or dispersed throughout the propellant or propellant and solvent

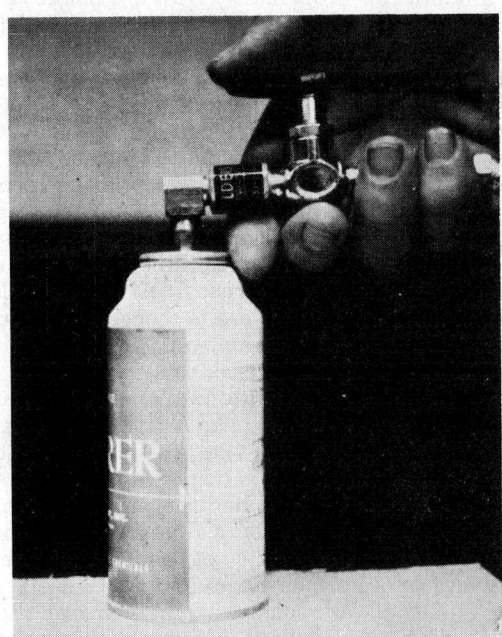

Fig. 763. Filling head for compressed gases (courtesy, Builders).

phase. This system is useful with antibiotics, steroids, and other difficultly soluble compounds. Some of the problems associated with the formulation of this system include agglomeration, caking, particle-size growth, and valve clogging. Some of these problems have been overcome through the use of lubricants such as isopropyl myristate,[85] light mineral oil, and other substances which provide slippage between particles of the compound as well as lubricating component parts of the valve. Surfactants have also been used to disperse the particles. The use of dispersing agents such as sorbitan trioleate, several Spans and Tweens (*Atlas*), and corn oil were found by Thiel, *et al*, to be useful in keeping the suspended particles from agglomerating.[86] Thought should also be given to the particle size as well as the moisture content of the powder. The moisture content should be kept below 300 ppm and the propellants and solvents must be dried by passing them through a drying agent. The particle size should remain in the micron range and should be between 1 and 10 μ.[87] A simple aerosol powder consists of:

Zinc stearate   10.00
Talc, 325-mesh   89.00
Isopropyl myristate   0.75
Perfume   0.25

To pressurize:

Powder concentrate   15
Propellant 12/11 (35:65)   85

This is useful as a body talc. A recent patent describes "a self-propelled powder aerosol system" consisting of about 85% powder and 15% propellant.[87] The propellant is absorbed by the powder (containing inert drying agent) resulting in essentially a dry system. The pressure is sufficient to expel the powder.

Since this system causes a bursting of the particles emitted from the actuator, it is difficult to control the deposition of the particles. This has been overcome to some extent by the use of a metered valve. This system has been used to apply antiperspirants and insecticidal dusts.

Emulsions—An emulsion system is useful for a great variety of products. Since it contains a relatively small amount of propellant (7–10%), there is little if any chilling effect. Active ingredients which may be irritating if inhaled can be used as a foam. Depending on the nature of the formulation and the manner in which the product is to be used, the foam is aqueous or nonaqueous and can be stable or quick breaking.

Emulsions can be dispensed from an aerosol container as a spray, stable foam, or quick-breaking foam depending on the type of valve used and the formulation. There are two types of emulsions which can be formulated for use in an aerosol. A W/O emulsion is one in which the water phase is dispersed throughout the oil phase; an O/W emulsion is one in which the water is the continuous phase.

If the product concentrate is dispersed throughout a propellant, the system behaves similar to a W/O emulsion. However, since the propellant is in the external phase, the product is dispersed as a wet stream rather than as a foam. When the propellant is in the internal phase (O/W), then a foam will be produced. The consistency and stability of the foam can be modified by choice of surfactant and solvents used.

Many of the water-based aerosols are of the W/O type where the propellant is in the external phase. Stable shave cream foams, on the other hand, are produced by keeping the propellant in the internal phase.[89]

The stable foam is similar to a shaving cream formulation into which therapeutically active ingredients are incorporated. The foam is dispensed and rubbed into the skin or affected area. By substituting glycols and glycol derivatives for the water in an emulsion, a nonaqueous foam is obtained.[90] The foam stability can be varied by the choice of surfactant, solvent, and propellant. It has been suggested that these foams are applicable to ointment bases, rectal and vaginal medication, and burn preparations.

A recent development in foam technology included the formulation of a thermal foam.[48] Heat is generated according to the following reaction:

$$H_2O_2 + SO_3^- \rightarrow H_2O + SO_4^-$$

Depending on the quantity of each reactant, temperatures as high as 175°F can be attained in a matter of seconds. The heat produced by reacting hydrogen peroxide with potassium sulfite or a mixture of potassium sulfite and potassium thiosulfate is shown in Fig. 765.

A quick-breaking foam allows for application of medication conveniently and efficiently.[92,93] In certain instances the product was dispensed as a foam which quickly collapsed. This was useful in covering large areas with no rubbing necessary to disperse the medication. These quick-breaking foams consist of alcohol, surfactant, water, and propellant in the following proportions:

Ethanol   46.0–66.0%
Surfactant   0.5– 5.0%
Water   28.0–42.0%
Propellant   3.0–15.0%

The surfactant can be nonionic, anionic, or cationic and should be soluble in one of the miscible solvents, but not in both. Several of the nonionic emulsifying waxes have been found to be advantageous in this type of formulation. A comprehensive study of foams has been given by Richmond and Shangraw.[94] The dispensing of foams has been indicated by Mace and Carrion.[95]

Semisolid Preparations—These preparations are formulated in the usual manner and depend on nitrogen to push the contents from the package. Viscosity plays an important role, and some of the factors involved in the dispensing of this type of product has been indicated by Mina.[96] The piston-type and flexible bag-type systems are finding use for these products. Creams and ointments are best packaged using these systems.

Much has been written as to the types of aerosol products available and to future aerosol products which will be useful.[97–100] The many advantages to the use of aerosols for pharmaceuticals makes many products likely candidates for this type of administration.

Medicinal Aerosols

The first pressurized package containing therapeutically active ingredients intended for internal administration was introduced in 1955. This consisted of a solution of epinephrine hydrochloride in water–ethyl alcohol and a fluorinated hydrocarbon propellant.[101] Soon thereafter, isoproterenol hydrochloride was administered in a similar manner. Many workers investigated the effectiveness of these compounds when given in this manner and found them to be acceptable to both physician and patient[102–109] in bringing about relief from the symptoms of asthma and other similar conditions. Others investigated the use of adrenocorticosteroids alone and in combination with isoproterenol with remarkable results.[110,111] Ergotamine tartrate has been administered by inhalation in treating the symptoms of migraine headache.[112–116]

The effectiveness of drugs administered by aerosol therapy has been confirmed by Dautrebande[117–119] and other investigators. Most of their studies were concerned with determining not only the effectiveness of the compound but the particle size responsible for maximum therapeutic response.

It is beyond the scope of this chapter to discuss the effect of particle size on therapeutic response and the physiology of the respiratory system. These effects have been indicated by Kanig[120] and Sciarra and Lynch.[121]

The particle size of aerosol preparations intended for administration to the lungs for either local or systemic activity should be between 3 and 6 μ. Most aerosol preparations in this class produce particles in the range

Table IX—Particle Size of Isoproterenol and Epinephrine Aerosol Suspensions

Mass median diameter, μ	Mass of particles with diameters		
	<5 μ, %	<7 μ, %	<10 μ, %
3.5	70	88	98
2.7	78	92	99
2.9	77	92	99
3.5	73	93	100

of 0.5 to 10 μ. However, over 99% are below 10 μ and most of them are in the optimum particle-size range. Table IX shows a typical size analysis for epinephrine and isoproterenol aerosols.[122]

Medicinal aerosols have been developed as solutions[101] or as dispersions.[123] Both systems have been used successfully to dispense the medication. The problems associated with the formulation of medicinal aerosols consisting of a suspension of active ingredients have been discussed elsewhere. The use of metered valves is imperative in order to maintain accurate and constant dosage. The development of these aerosols and the testing involved has been indicated by Porush[122] and Young.[124]

There are many advantages to the administration of medicinal agents by inhalation. Response to drugs administered by inhalation is prompt, faster in onset of activity compared with response to drugs given orally and with most drugs approaches intravenous therapy in rapidity of action. Drugs which are normally decomposed in the gastrointestinal tract can be safely administered by inhalation. The use of the self-pressurized aerosol package makes inhalation therapy simple, convenient, and acceptable compared to the use of atomizers and nebulizers, which are bulky and require cleaning. Several medicinal aerosols are shown in Fig. 764. Table X indicates the composition of several medicinal aerosols.

Testing

Since the techniques as well as the type of testing required of aerosol products is quite different from the usual test methods used in the pharmaceutical industry, attention should be given to this subject. Several test methods have been included in the NF.[125]

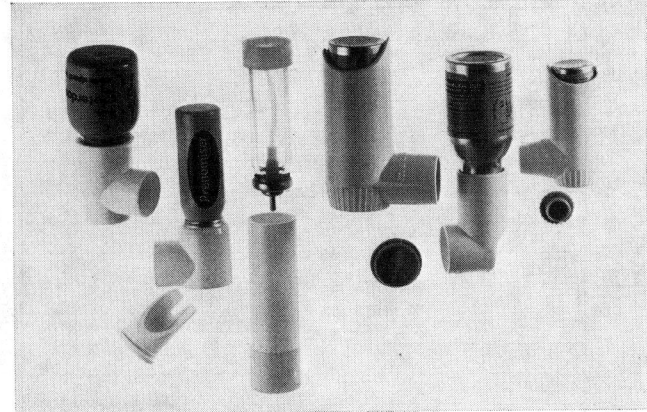

Fig. 764. Medicinal aerosols with oral applicators.

These include a method for delivery rate, leak testing, and pressure testing.

Delivery Rate—Select not less than 4 containers, and actuate each for 2 to 3 sec. Remove the caps and covers, weigh each accurately, and immerse in a constant-temperature bath until the internal pressure is constant at a temperature of 25 ± 1°, determining the pressure as directed under *Pressure Testing*. Remove the containers from the bath, remove the excess moisture by blotting with a paper towel, actuate each container for 5.0 sec (accurately timed by use of a stopwatch), and weigh each container again. Return the containers to the constant-temperature bath, and repeat the foregoing procedure three times for each container. Calculate the average delivery rate, in grams per second, for each container.

Leak Testing—Select not less than 4 containers, and immerse in a constant-temperature water bath maintained at 55 ± 1°, unless another temperature is specified in the individual monograph. Allow the containers to stand in the bath for 30 min, observing at 5-min intervals; no bubbles emanate from the valve area or any parts of the container.

Pressure Testing—Select not less than 4 containers, remove the caps and covers, and immerse in a constant-temperature bath until the internal pressure is constant at a temperature of 25 ± 1°. Remove the containers from the bath, shake well, and remove the actuator and water, if any from the valve stem. Place each container in an upright position, and determine the pressure in each container by placing a prepressurized gauge on the valve stem, holding firmly and actuating the valve so that it is fully open. The gauge should be of a calibration approximating the expected pressure and should be fitted with an adaptor appropriate for the particular valve stem dimensions. Read the pressure directly from the gauge.

Other test procedures which can be used to determine the spray rate, density, solids content, and other characteristics of aerosols are available from the CSMA.[5]

Table X—Several Medicinal Aerosols

Product	Manufacturer	Active ingredients	Type of system
Aero-Meter	Rexall	Epinephrine bitartrate	Suspension
Asthma-Meter	Rexall	Epinephrine	Solution
Asthma-Nefrin	Thayer	Epinephrine HCl (racemic)	Solution
Bronkometer	Breon	Phenylephrine HCl Isoetharine methansulfonate Thenyldiamine HCl	Solution
Medihaler-Duo	Riker	Isoproterenol HCl	Suspension
Medihaler-Epi	Riker	Epinephrine bitartrate	Suspension
Medihaler-Ergotamine	Riker	Ergotamine tartrate	Suspension
Medihaler-Iso	Riker	Isoproterenol sulfate	Suspension
Mistometer Isuprel	Winthrop	Isoproterenol HCl	Solution
Nebair	Warner-Chilcott	Isoproterenol HCl Thonzonium bromide	Solution
Norisodrine Aerotrol	Abbott	Isoproterenol HCl	Solution
Primatene-Mist	Whitehall	Epinephrine	Solution
Respihaler Decadron Phosphate	MSD	Dexamethasone 21-phosphate	Suspension
Respihaler Prodecadron	MSD	Dexamethasone 21-phosphate Isoproterenol sulfate	Suspension
Vaponefrine Metermatic	USV	Epinephrine HCl (racemic)	Solution
Vapo-N-Iso	USV	Isoproterenol sulfate	Solution

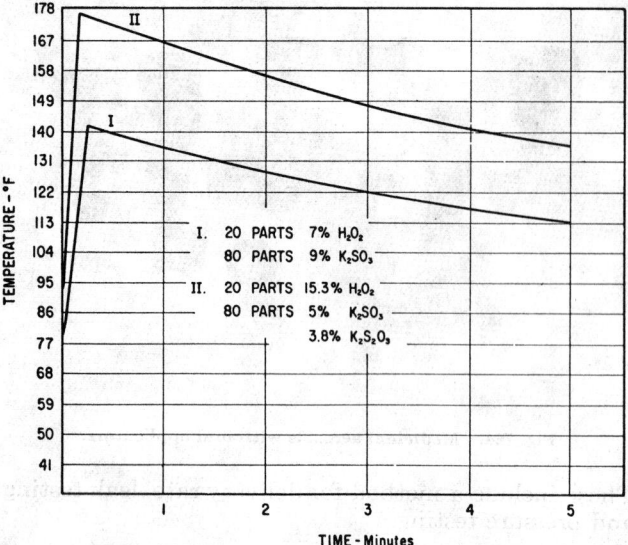

Fig. 765. Heat production: H₂O₂ reacted with K₂SO₃ and K₂S₂O₃ (courtesy, Du Pont).

Methods for the determination of particle-size distribution have been described by Kanig,[120] Grim,[126] and Sciarra.[127]

The moisture content of the propellant as well as the finished product is extremely important as the presence of moisture may decrease the stability of the product as well as cause corrosion in the container. A modified Karl Fisher titration method is used for this purpose.[125]

With products under pressure, special care must be taken in order to obtain a representative sample of the aerosol. Several methods have been advanced for this purpose. One method collects the sample by dissolving the sprayed material in a suitable solvent,[122] while other methods are based on transferring a sample to another pressure vessel and carrying out the analysis directly in the sampling container.[128] The NF describes the following method:

Sampling Apparatus—The apparatus described herein is employed, where indicated in the individual monograph, to obtain a sample from metered-dose containers.

The apparatus is illustrated in the accompanying diagram (Fig. 766). It consists of an intake system, comprised of the aerosol adapter (*A*), firing adapter (*B*), and intake tube (*C*, approximately 5 × 15 cm drawn to 8 mm at one end); a delivery tube to which is attached a sintered-glass dispersion bubbler (*D*); and a collection chamber (*E*, gas-washing bottle) which contains an absorbing solution. The aerosol adapter has tapered inlet holes drilled through its center to provide an airtight seal and against which the aerosol valves can be actuated, delivering quantitatively their sprays into the intake tube. To avoid loss of the drug into the atmosphere when the self-pressurized unit is discharged, air is drawn through the intake system into the collection chamber and absorbing solution by means of a suitable air pump. Alternately, an apparatus embodying the principle of the assembly described and illustrated may be used.

Additional tests which can be used for aerosols are available from several other sources.[129–132]

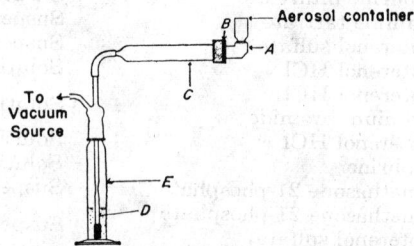

Fig. 766. Sampling apparatus for metered-dose aerosols (courtesy, NF XIII).

Regulations

The Interstate Commerce Commission (ICC) regulates the shipment of aerosol products. The regulations are concerned primarily with pressure and flammability restrictions on certain types of containers. The provisions of the Food, Drug, and Cosmetic Act as well as the Federal Hazardous Substances Act are applicable to aerosol products. Additionally, there are various state and local laws which control the sale of many of these products. The following pressure restrictions are currently in effect:

Nonspecification containers*	140 psig at 130°F
2P Specification	140–160 psig at 130°F
2Q Specification	160–180 psig at 130°F

The reader is referred to the actual regulations for other restrictions which may exist.

* These apply to metal containers which are fabricated from tin-plated steel. The specifications apply to the wall thickness and method of fabrication. The figures given represent the maximum pressure the container must withstand without bursting or showing evidence of leakage, distortion or other defects.

References

1. Ostwald, W., *Kolloid-Z.*, **1**, 332 (1906).
2. Sciarra, J. J., in Sprowls, J. B., *Prescription Pharmacy*, Lippincott, Philadelphia, 1963, p. 242.
3. Whytlaw-Gray, R. W., and Patterson, H. S., *Smoke*, Edward Arnold & Co., Ltd., London, 1932.
4. Sinclair, D., *Handbook on Aerosols*, Atomic Energy Commission, Washington, D. C., 1950, p. 64.
5. *Glossary of Terms Used in the Aerosol Industry*, Aerosol Guide, Chemical Specialties Manufacturers Assoc., New York, Mar., 1966, p. 25.
6. *Package for Profit*, Du Pont, Wilmington, Del., 1968, pp. 6–8.
7. Sciarra, J. J., *Aerosol Age*, **1** (5), 14 (1956).
8. Helbing, H., and Pertsch, G., US Pat. 628,463 (1899).
9. Gebauer, C. L., US Pat. 668,815 (1901).
10. Gebauer, C. L., US Pat. 711,045 (1902).
11. Gebauer, C. L., US Pat. 2,171,501 (1939).
12. Shepherd, H. R., *Aerosols: Science and Technology*, Interscience, New York, 1961, p. 2.
13. Mobley, L. K., US Pat. 1,378,481 (1921).
14. Moore, R. W., US Pat. 1,378,866 (1903).
15. Lemoine, D. R., US Pat. 532,194 (1926).
16. Rotheim, E., US Pat. 1,800,156 (1931).
17. Rotheim, E., US Pat. 1,892,750 (1933).
18. Midgley, T., Jr., *et al*, US Pat. 1,926,396 (1933).
19. Goodhue, L. D., and Sullivan, W. N., US Pat. 2,321,023 (1943).
20. Goodhue, L. D., *Ind. Eng. Chem.*, **34**, 1456 (1942).
21. Shepherd, H. R., *Aerosols: Science and Technology*, Interscience, New York, 1961, p. 1.
22. *The Aerosol Pressure Products Survey for 1968*, Chemical Specialties Manufacturers Assoc., New York, 1969.
23. Sciarra, J. J., *Aerosol Age*, **6** (12), 65 (1961)
24. Sciarra, J. J., *Kosmetik-Parfum-Drogen-Rondschau*, **11** (12), 171 (1961).
25. Barr, M., *Soap Chem. Specialties*, **34**, 86 (1958).
26. Roth, W., US Pat. 3,289,949 (1966).
27. *Soap Chem. Specialties*, **44** (4), 111 (1968).
28. Barr, M., *J. APhA, Pract. Ed.*, **19**, 675 (1958).
29. Bloom, C., *Aerosol Age*, **8** (12), 52 (1963); **9** (1), 36 (1964).
30. Pomerantz, E., *Drug Cosmetic Ind.*, **83**, 431 (1958).
31. Finch, J. W., *Med. Times*, **88**, 1029 (1960).
32. Freedman, T., *Postgrad. Med.*, **20**, 667 (1956).
33. Blaug, S., *Aerosol Age*, **13** (12), 46 (1968).
34. Eaton, S. E., US Pat. 2,728,495 (1955).
35. Sciarra, J. J., *J. APhA, Pract. Ed.*, **19**, 672 (1958).
36. Clapp, C., *Aerosol Technicomment*, **5**, 3 (1962).
37. Spitzer, J. G., *et al*, US Pat. 2,655,480 (1953).
38. Mina, F. A., *Chem. Specialties Mfrs. Assoc. Proc. Ann. Meeting*, **45**, 72 (1958).
39. Webster, R. C., *Aerosol Age*, **6** (6), 20 (1961).
40. Fox, I., and Palley, S., US Pat. 2,977,231 (1961).
41. Sciarra, J. J., *Chem. Specialties Mfrs. Assoc. Proc. Mid-Year Meeting*, **49**, 60 (1963).
42. Schultz, R. S., *Soap Chem. Specialties*, **38**, 127 (1962).
43. Irland, L. F., and Kinnavy, J. W., *Drug Cosmetic Ind.*, **101** (2), 42 (1967).
44. *Aerosol Age*, **11** (1), 29 (1966).
45. Roth, W., US Pat. 3,289,949 (1966).
46. *Aerosol Age*, **12** (10), 58 (1967).
47. Moses, R. E., and Lucas, R., US Pat. 3,341,418 (1967).
48. Boden, H., *Aerosol Age*, **13** (3), 19 (1968).
49. Lewis, W. D., US Pat. 3,325,056 (1967).
50. Reed, W. H., *Am. Perfumer*, **70**, 70 (1957).
51. Reed, F. T., in Shepherd, H. R., *Aerosols: Science and Technology*, Interscience, New York, 1961, pp. 237–238.
52. Reed, F. T., in Herzka, A., *International Encyclopaedia of Pressurized Packaging*, Pergamon, London, 1966, p. 133.

53. Herzka, A., and Pickthall, J., *Pressurized Packaging*, 2nd ed., Academic, New York, 1961, p. 36.
54. Hildebrand, J. H., and Scott, R. L., *Solubility of Nonelectrolytes*, 3rd ed., Reinhold, New York, 1950, pp. 47, 274.
55. Bower, F. A., and Palmer, F. S., in Shepherd, H. R., *Aerosols: Science and Technology*, Interscience, New York, 1961, p. 500.
56. Flanner, L., *Vapor Pressures of Solvents and Propellant Mixtures*, Allied Chemical Corp., New York, 1963.
57. Sanders, P. A., *Chem. Specialties Mfrs. Assoc. Proc. Mid-Year Meeting*, **46**, 66 (1960).
58. Sciarra, J. J., in Sprowls, J. B., *Prescription Pharmacy*, Lippincott, Philadelphia, 1963, p. 270.
59. Kleniewski, A., *Aerosol Age*, **13** (9), 40; (10), 63; (11), 40 (1968).
60. Herzka, A., and Pickthall, J., *Pressurized Packaging*, 2nd ed., Academic, New York, 1961, p. 177.
61. Kalish, J., *Drug Cosmetic Ind.*, **81**, 441 (1957).
62. Scott, R., and Terrill, R., *Soap Chem. Specialties*, **38** (1), 142 (1962).
63. Scott, R., and Terrill, R., *Aerosol Age*, **7** (1), 18 (1962).
64. "*VC*" *Mixes*, General Chem. Div., Allied Chem. Corp., New York.
65. Sciarra, J. J., *Paint Varnish Prod.*, **53**, 47 (1963).
66. Sciarra, J. J., *Paint Varnish Prod.*, **54**, 51 (1964).
67. Reed, F., *Am. Perfumer*, **75**, 42 (1960).
68. Dunne, T. F., *Aerosol Age*, **4** (5), 36 (1959).
69. Broderick, G. F., and Flanner, L. T., *Chem. Specialties Mfrs. Assoc. Proc. Mid-Year Meeting*, **51** (1965).
70. Johnsen, M. A., *Aerosol Age*, **7** (6), 20; (7), 29; (8), 39; (9), 39 (1962).
71. *The Risdon GB Valve*, Risdon Mfg. Co., Naugatuck, Conn. 06770.
72. *Drug Cosmetic Ind.*, **93** (4), 471 (1963).
73. Meshberg, P., *Aerosol Age*, **12** (5), 37 (1967).
74. Boden, H., *Freon Aerosol Report*, A-74, Du Pont, Wilmington, Del., 1968.
75. *Soap Chem. Specialties*, **44** (4), 111 (1968).
76. Herzka, A., in Herzka, A., *International Encyclopaedia of Pressurized Packaging*, Pergamon, London, 1966, pp. 620–645.
77. Sciarra, J. J., in Herzka, A., *International Encyclopaedia of Pressurized Packaging*, Pergamon, London, 1966, p. 574.
78. Kanig, J., *Aerosol Age*, **6** (5), 35 (1961).
79. Sciarra, J., *Aerosol Age*, **12** (12), 65 (1967).
80. Mintzer, H., in Martin, E. W., ed., *Husa's Pharmaceutical Dispensing*, 6th ed., Mack Publ. Co., Easton, Pa., 1966, pp. 359–397.
81. Fuller, A., et al, *Quart. J. Pharm. Pharmacol.*, **15**, 127 (1942).
82. Yontef, R., *Med. Times*, **86**, 1544 (1958).
83. Geary, D., *Chem. Specialties Mfrs. Assoc. Proc. Ann. Meeting*, **46**, 135 (1959).
84. Porush, I., in Shepherd, H., *Aerosols: Science and Technology*, Interscience, New York, 1961, pp. 387–393.
85. Parisse, A., *Aerosol Age*, **12** (5), 33 (1967).
86. Thiel, C., et al, US Pat. 3,014,844 (1961).
87. Kanig, J. L., and Cohn, R. M., *Proc. Sci. Sect. Toilet Goods Assoc.*, **37**, 19 (1962).

88. Gunning, P., and Rink, D., US Pat. 3,081,223 (1963).
89. Yakubik, J., *Drug Cosmetic Ind.*, **95** (1), 36 (1964).
90. Sanders, P., *Aerosol Age*, **5** (11), 33 (1960).
91. Sanders, P. A., *Drug Cosmetic Ind.*, **99** (2), 56; (3), 57 (1966).
92. Wallace, T., Jr., *Am. Perfumer*, **75**, 85 (1960).
93. Cooper, G. K., *Aerosol Age*, **12** (4), 32; (5), 71 (1967).
94. Richmond, D. M., and Shangraw, R. F., *Aerosol Age*, **11** (5), 36; (6), 30; (7), 28; (8), 39; (9), 45; (10), 32; (11), 28 (1966).
95. Mace, H., and Carrion, C., *Aerosol Technicomment*, **11** (3) (1968).
96. Mina, F., *Chem. Specialties Mfrs. Assoc. Proc. Ann. Meeting*, **45**, 72 (1958).
97. Sciarra, J. J., and Eisen, H., *Am. Perfumer*, **77**, 57 (1962).
98. Graham, J., *Drug Cosmetic Ind.*, **87**, 36 (1960).
99. Prussin, S., *Drug Cosmetic Ind.*, **84**, 584 (1959).
100. Blaug, S., et al, *Am. J. Hosp. Pharm.*, **24**, 603 (1967).
101. Porush, I., and Maison, G., US Pat. 2,868,691 (1959).
102. Kallos, P., and Kallos-Deffner, L., *Intern. Arch. Allergy Appl. Immun.*, **15**, 343 (1959).
103. Miller, R., et al, *Diseases Chest*, **28**, 309 (1955).
104. Kaufman, J., et al, *Am. J. Med.*, **10**, 442 (1951).
105. Freedman, T., *Postgrad. Med.*, **20**, 667 (1956).
106. Grater, W., and Shuey, C., *Southern Med. J.*, **51**, 1600 (1958).
107. Harris, M., *Postgrad. Med.*, **23**, 170 (1958).
108. Seltzer, A., *Med. Ann. District Columbia*, **27**, 131 (1958).
109. Swartz, H., *Ann. Allergy*, **8**, 488 (1950).
110. Bickerman, H., and Itkin, S., *J. Am. Med. Assoc.*, **184**, 533 (1963).
111. Norman, P. S., and Winkenwerder, W. L., *J. Allergy*, **36**, 284 (1965).
112. Harris, M., *Western Med.*, **2**, 234 (1961).
113. Meyers, L., and Craft, G., *NY State J. Med.*, **62**, 2191 (1962).
114. Speed, W., *Am. J. Med. Sci.*, **240**, 97 (1960).
115. Finch, J., *Med. Times*, **88**, 1029 (1960).
116. Blumenthal, L., and Fuchs, M., *Med. Ann. District Columbia*, **30**, 10 (1961).
117. Dautrebande, L., *Physiol. Rev.*, **32**, 214 (1952).
118. Dautrebande, L., *Microaerosols*, Academic, New York, 1962, p. 86.
119. Dautrebande, L., *Arch. Intern. Pharmacodyn.*, **129**, 455 (1960).
120. Kanig, J., *J. Pharm. Sci.*, **52**, 513 (1963).
121. Sciarra, J. J., and Lynch, V., *Drug Cosmetic Ind.*, **86**, 752 (1960).
122. Porush, I., et al, *J. Pharm. Sci.*, **49**, 70 (1960).
123. Thiel, C., et al, US Pat. 3,014,844 (1961).
124. Young, J., et al, *J. Pharm. Sci.*, **49**, 72 (1960).
125. *National Formulary XIII*, Mack Publ. Co., Easton, Pa., 1970, p. 772.
126. Grim, W., et al, *Aerosol Age*, **13** (3), 22 (1968).
127. Sciarra, J., et al, *J. Soc. Cosmetic Chem.*, in press.
128. Tuesley, S., and Sciarra, J., *J. Pharm. Sci.*, **57**, 488 (1968).
129. Root, M., *J. Soc. Cosmetic Chem.*, **9**, 105 (1958).
130. Yeomans, A., *J. Econ. Entomol.*, **49**, 415 (1956).
131. Sciarra, J., in Lachman, L., et al, *Industrial Pharmacy*, Lea & Febiger, Philadelphia, 1970, p. 605.
132. Sciarra, J., *Aerosol Age*, **13** (1), 51 (1968).

91 | Plastics

Nature of high polymers—plastics in use—plastic evaluation procedures

This chapter was prepared by

Harold H. Bryant, PhD, *Director, Huntingdon Research Center, Inc.,*
Baltimore, Md. 21204

In pharmacy and medicine the term *plastics* refers to a group of organic polymers, usually synthetic, which are molded, cast, extruded, drawn, or laminated into various forms. The term, however, is not very definitive and does not give any more specific information about a material than does the term *metal*. The public acceptance of plastics in the ready-to-use and disposable medical and pharmaceutical devices has in general been more rapid than the dissemination of knowledge about them. This is perhaps largely due to the very rapid introduction of so many plastic products of such widely diverse chemical composition.

The introduction of plastics into the field of pharmacy and medicine has taken place essentially in the past decade. The reluctance to introduce materials of unknown potential harmful effects into the practice of medicine can be readily understood. However, the tremendous versatility of selected plastic formulations when fabricated into low-cost single-use items has now been recognized. Syringes, needles, tubings, prosthetic devices, and many other therapeutic aids are available in individual packages, sterile and ready for use. The convenience of these aids to the physician and the fact that single use avoids the possible transfer of infection has led to the very rapid advent of plastic devices.

The introduction of these items, however, has not been without difficulties. The complexity of the usual plastic formulation when viewed in the light of the myriad of pharmaceutical preparations suggests immediately that each use of a plastic for a given device, or as a package material for a particular drug, must be "proved" to be suitable by appropriate tests.

The introduction of plastics into the realm of packaging material for pharmaceutical preparations must be undertaken with the greatest of care. There are many factors which enter into the picture here that are not present in the short-term one-use device, such as the single-use syringe or tubing. The length of time that the medicament and the container are in contact introduces such problems as leaching of material from the plastic into the drug, or absorption or adsorption of a significant portion of the active ingredient of the drug preparation into or onto the plastic, thus removing it from use. Other factors which are of concern in the area of drug packaging applications of plastic materials are rates of diffusion through the plastic, effects of pH, solvents, concentration, temperature and chemical structure of the plastic material itself. These points are considered in further detail in the latter part of the chapter.

The following is the American Society for Testing and Materials (ASTM) definition for plastics:

"A plastic is a material that contains as an essential ingredient an organic substance of large molecular weight, is solid in its finished state, and at some stage in its manufacture or in its processing into finished articles can be shaped by flow."

The term *resin* should not be confused with the term *plastics*. It usually refers to the essential ingredient, a high-molecular-weight polymer, before processing and fabrication.

The more common plastics include acrylics, alkyds, cellulosics, epoxy resins, phenolics, polyamides, polyesters, polyfluorocarbons, polyolefins, polystyrene, silicones, and vinyl plastics. Some procedures have been developed to assure suitability of formulation of these for pharmaceutical or medical applications. The protocol of tests set forth later in this chapter has been found very useful and reliable in ascertaining such suitability.

The use of plastics as containers for food has been a matter of interest to the Food and Drug Administration (FDA) and industry for sufficient time so that a number of publications have appeared stating which plasticizers and other substances may or may not be used for such items. This has led to a false sense of security on the part of some surgical suppliers and pharmaceutical packaging designers. They felt that since certain formulations met the food requirements they were satisfactory for labeling as Medical Grade, whereas when imbedded in the tissues of the body, they caused reactions.

The USP provides certain sterility and toxicity requirements for plastic tubing assemblies used in blood collection and transfusion. Requirements for plastic containers have also been studied. Minimal requirements for classification and testing of plastics to be used in medicine will be found in the USP and the NF. These must be supplemented by appropriate "use" tests.

Plastic prosthetics of a wide variety have appeared within the past few years. Vascular grafts[1] of plastics have proven to be at least of limited success and this has encouraged development of other materials and procedures. Among the materials used are nylon, Orlon, Dacron, Teflon, and others.

The growing pig has proved to be a most useful experimental animal for testing these grafts. The time of appearance of calcification between the filaments of the yarn in the graft materials in the pig was found to be 6 to 8 months, as opposed to 4 to 5 years in the dog. Tests have consisted for the most part of replacement of a section of the descending aorta with a like length of the prosthetic graft material with an equivalent internal diameter. The physical characteristics of the synthetic graft material, such as porosity, have been found to be more significant than the differences in the plastic materials from which they are made.

Numerous other applications of plastics in surgery include their use as tissue adhesives, replacement aortic valves, ventriculovenous shunts in the treatment of hydrocephalus patients, and even experimental replacement of the bladder. In all surgical applicaions, compatibility with the tissues of the body is of paramount importance. The changes which may take place in the composition and physical characteristics of the plastic over a period of time are also of critical concern.

Nature of High Polymers

There are over 50 distinctly different types of plastics.[2] The characteristics of any given formulation can be varied over a wide range depending on the basic resin in the mixture and other agents such as plasticizers, stabilizing agents, accelerators, fillers, colorants, and antistatic agents.

A finished product composed of plastics is seldom made of a pure polymer but represents a very complex mixture. Sometimes a second polymer is joined to the first to form a plastic substance. The product is then called a copolymer. In general, however, the particular plastics material is identified by the polymers or high-molecular-weight substances in the plastic as for instance polyvinyl chloride, polypropylene, or polyfluorocarbons.

Plastics can be of synthetic or natural origin; most are of the former but a few occur naturally, as for example rubber, gutta percha, and some types of vegetable waxes. The molecules of plastic are composed principally of carbon, hydrogen, oxygen, and nitrogen.

The silicones represent an exception; they consist of chains of alternate silicon and oxygen atoms.[3] The chains can be modified by various organic side groups attached to the silicon atoms or by crosslinking the molecular chains to give materials ranging in physical form from rigid resin to very thin inert fluids (see page 1756).

The plastics are generally classified into two broad groups in accordance with their response to thermal heat. Most plastics are either *thermoplastic* (remeltable) or *thermosetting* (nonremeltable). The thermoplastic material is usually rigid at normal temperatures but will soften upon application of heat and can be reformed under pressure. Thermosetting materials, on the other hand, will undergo chemical and physical changes under the influence of heat or catalysts and become infusible and insoluble.

Most plastic materials, as has been indicated, contain in addition to the polymer ingredients which give certain specific desired properties either of a chemical or physical nature. For each type of additive there are literally hundreds of choices.

Plasticizers—These are materials added to a resin to improve flexibility or to facilitate compounding. Vinyl dispersions of only the resin and the plasticizer are known as *plastisols*.[4] If the dispersing liquid contains volatile components, the dispersion is termed an *organosol*. A plastisol may be converted into an organosol by addition of thinners as volatile liquids. Generally speaking, plasticizers for plastisols are divided into two classes, the monomeric and the resinous types. The monomeric type is typified by such compounds as the phthalate esters (di-2-ethyl-hexyl, dicapryl, etc), and phosphate esters (tricresyl, triacetyl, etc), adipate esters, sebacate esters, and others. The compounds are high-boiling liquids of relatively low viscosity. Resinous plasticizers are compatible resins, usually of the linear polyester type. Their use is indicated in medical and therapeutic applications where migration and extraction of the plasticizer must be avoided. There are instances where a mixture of the

monomeric and resinous plasticizers is used in blends to obtain the desired end product. Plasticizers for organosols of vinyls, polar compounds which have some solvent action on the resin, frequently are the preferred dispersants.

Stabilizers—These form a second important class of ingredients which are added to plastisols to protect against chemicals released, such as hydrochloric acid from vinyl chloride polymer. They act as color stabilizers and protect against light. Inorganic oxides, salts of inorganic bases with weak acids, complex organometallic compounds, and various glycidyl compounds are widely used as stabilizers in vinyl polymers. Lead compounds which are pigments and soaps are also useful because the lead chloride formed in the process of stabilization does not detract from the water resistance of the polymer. Maleic acid is typical of a class of compounds used to stabilize against color developments in the vinyls.

Accelerators are, as the name implies, substances which accelerate polymerization of the resin.

Antioxidants are included in plastic material to retard oxidation. Examples are phenolic materials such as hydroquinone, aryl amines, sulfur compounds such as dilaurylthiodipropionate, and many others. The antioxidant is selected according to the type of plastic formulation.

Fillers are relatively inert materials added to plastics to modify strength, permanence, and working properties, or to lower cost. Examples range from glass, asbestos, and synthetic fibers to metal or even wood flour. For use in medicine, care must be exercised in the selection and use of fillers.

Colorants are frequently added and care must be exercised to insure against leachability, as has occurred in some instances.

Antistatic and **"slip" agents** are also added, especially for therapeutic device material to reduce adherence of dust and fine plastic chips. An example is calcium stearate.

The additives discussed are examples of the more important elements to be found in a formulation, but their listing here serves primarily to illustrate the complexity of the study of plastics composition. Plastics as a group can be seen to exhibit a wide range of physical, chemical, and biological properties. Some are relatively inert both biologically and chemically. Others are readily attacked by many organic solvents with the release of substances which exhibit a variety of biological effects. The release of a substance or substances from a plastics material, either into a medicament contained therein or into the body tissues from an indwelling tube or prosthesis, may be considered to constitute adulteration or "drug" administration.

Plastics in Use

There are at least 17 major classes of plastics, each with several subdivisions. The increased use of many of these as containers for various pharmaceutical preparations and for devices used in therapeutic procedures makes familiarity with some of the more common types desirable. The following classes are not necessarily in order of importance but are representative of those used to manufacture pharmaceutical and therapeutic devices.

Acrylics—This class includes the polymethacrylates, polyacrylates, and copolymers of acrylonitrile. There are many variations in this class, mainly concerned with the combinations of methacrylate and acrylate esters, as well as acrylonitrile. They are characterized by clarity and unusual optical properties, low specific gravity, low water absorption, good electrical resistivity, excellent weatherability, and fair tensile strength. Their heat resistance is low and care should be taken to keep them below temperatures of 200 °F, where they tend to soften.

Familiar examples of this class of material are Plexiglas and Lucite as well as fibers of acrylonitrile Orlon, Zefran, and others.

Cellulosics—The members of this class are available in a very wide range of physical characteristics. Cellulose acetate propionate and cellulose acetate butyrate are important examples. Plasticizers frequently used with the cellulose acetate butyrate include butyl and higher phthalate esters and esters of adipic, azelaic, and sebacic acids.

Epoxy Resins—Epoxy resins are produced by the reaction between epichlorohydrin and bisphenol.[5]

Two broad classes are available: solid resins and liquid resins. The former are modified with other resins and unsaturated fatty acids to make coating materials, the latter with curing agents such as diamine, dibasic anhydrides, polyamides, and polysulfides for adhesives.

The liquid resins are preferred for adhesives and plastics end uses. These liquids are converted to solid resins by reacting with amine or acid anhydride hardeners.

The epoxy resins have found a prominent place in fabrication of the single-use devices being produced for therapeutic uses. If thoroughly cured, they are very inert but experience has demonstrated that thorough curing is essential to their safe use.

Polyamides—Nylon is the generic designation for a class of polyamides containing repeating amide groups (—CONH—) connected to methylene units (—CH₂—) in the structure of the polymer. Other types of polyamides are derived from casein, the ureas, melamines, and other natural protein substances which contain the amide groups. The latter are composed of more complex polymer structure and have different properties.

There are a variety of nylons which are made by condensing a diamine with a dibasic acid. The numbers Nylon 6, Nylon 66, and Nylon 610 designate the polymer according to the number of carbon atoms in the segments of the diamine and dibasic acid from which they are made.

The nylons are thermoplastic and melt at temperatures above 400 °F forming very viscous liquids. They are characterized by good chemical resistance to most solvents and chemicals with the exception of strong solutions of certain mineral acids, phenolic compounds, and strong oxidizers. They are not attacked by fungi, insects, or rodents and can be easily sterilized at steam temperatures.

Nylon is suitable for many uses such as tubings, syringes, and adapters.

Polyesters—The esterification reaction between polyhydric alcohols and polybasic acids produces a class of materials known as polyester resins. The term *polyester* is for the most part used for linear polyesters derived from dihydric alcohols and dibasic acids.

The polyesters are thermosetting and have good physical properties.

Alkyds—Structurally the alkyd resins are modified polyesters. They are prominent in paint and other surface-finishing products.

Polyfluorocarbons—The original member of this class was the tetrafluoroethylene polymer *Teflon*, but there are now a large group of fluorocarbon resins available.

Most of the fluorocarbons are homo- and copolymers of tetrafluoroethylene, trifluorochloroethylene, hexafluoropropylene, and vinylidene fluoride.[2]

The polyfluorocarbons exhibit high softening points, excellent electrical resistance, inertness to chemical attack over a wide range of temperatures, low moisture absorption and permeability, and high strength properties.

Teflon, the well-known member of this class, is available in at least 11 types. There are two basic resins TFE (tetrafluoroethylene) and FEP (fluorinated ethylene, propylene).

The fluorocarbon resins of the Teflon group are subject to attack by active sodium and fluorine and by application of extreme heat and pressure. Strong organic acids and bases, boiling aqua regia, chlorine, bromine, and iodine have no effect.

Teflon has low surface energy and thus is nonadhesive and slippery. These surface characteristics coupled with inertness, both chemically and with body tissues, permit these materials to be used in prosthetic devices, tubings, and films in the body.

Polyolefins—There are two well-known members of this group, the polyethylenes and the polypropylenes. The polyolefins as a group are one of the most widely used plastics; production reached the 1.5 billion pound mark in 1961. They are prepared from ethylene and propylene, respectively.

Polyethylene—The properties of polyethylene vary according to molecular weight and type: low-density or branched, and high-density or linear. The linear type is more crystalline, more heat resistant, and stiffer than the low-density or conventional type. Both have low water absorption, excellent electrical resistance, high resistance to most solvents and chemicals, and are tasteless and odorless. They are thus well suited to many applications where only moderate to low heat exposure will be encountered.

Polypropylene—The polymer of propylene is lighter than polyethylene, yet it is much stiffer and more heat resistant with the same chemical and electrical resistance. This material is available as the highly crystalline isotactic polypropylene and the higher impact grades of atactic and syndiotactic types. The isotactic type has a well-ordered atom arrangement in the chain, while the atactic is less well ordered.

The polypropylenes withstand boiling water or steam temperatures, and devices made of this material can be autoclaved for sterilization.

Polystyrene—This polymer is one of the oldest and most used plastics. While at present the major use is as the 100% polystyrene resin, there is a continuing increase in use of the impact type made with the copolymers containing acrylonitrile and butadiene.

In the field of pharmaceutics and therapeutics, it has enjoyed a wide use for fabrication of containers, syringes, and so forth. Polystyrene has a relatively low heat resistance and is attacked by a number of chemical agents. It will not support mold or mildew, is rodentproof and imparts no odor or taste to foods.

Silicones—The silicones are among the more interesting of the newer materials to be introduced in the field of plastics with many applications helpful in therapeutics. Preparations range from rigid resins to inert fluids. The silicones as a class exhibit thermal and oxidative stability at high temperatures (400–500 °F or higher), retention of flexibility at temperatures as low as −110 °F or lower, prevention of things sticking ogether, suppression of foam, and they are remarkably inert. These characteristics and others mean that the silicones are destined for a significant role in the pharmaceutical and medical fields.

Chemically, silicones consist of chains of alternate silicon and oxygen atoms. These chains can be modified to get the desired physical properties by various organic side groups attached to the silicon atoms or by crosslinking of the molecular chains.

The nonadhesive characteristic of the silicone material gives it a great advantage in tubings where adherence to body exudates or tissues may be a problem. The ability to prevent sticking has led to the wide use of the fluid silicones as release agents in syringes, molds, and other medical and pharmaceutical equipment.

Silicone resins are available which may be formed in place or in forms which then can be used as prosthetic devices. The record to date would indicate that for the most part the silicones are remarkably compatible with the tissues of the body as indwelling implants.

Vinyl Plastics—The term *vinyl* comes from the radical CH_2=CH—, which has many derivatives. The versatile vinyl plastics are used to prepare materials ranging from soft, flexible sheeting to rigid, hard pipe. Several derivatives of the CH_2=CH— radical are employed, such as vinyl chloride (CH_2=$CHCl$) and vinyl acetate (CH_2=$CHOCOCH_3$). In the polymer forms there are two other derivatives, polyvinyl alcohol and polyvinyl acetals. Still another member of the family is vinylidine chloride (CH_2=CCl_2). With this group of vinyl compounds a great many polymers are made as homopolymers of themselves or as copolymers with other vinyl derivatives or other monomeric materials. The copolymers of vinyl chloride with vinyl acetate are the most common. Polyvinyl acetals are made by condensation of the polyvinyl alcohol with aldehydes, eg, formaldehyde or butyraldehyde.

The polyvinylidene chloride resins are better known as *Saran*. Resins of this type are for the most part copolymers of vinylidene chloride with vinyl chloride, acrylonitrile, and acrylate esters. These polymers are characterized by their high temperature resistance, with softening points ranging from 70° to 180°C or

higher. Other outstanding characteristics are their high solvent and chemical resistance, low water absorption and moisture permeability, and nonflammability. They are also odorless and tasteless.

The wide variety of polyvinyl chloride resins with their range of physical properties has led to the development of many applications of this material in the fields of pharmacy and medicine.

The polyvinyl alcohols are interesting because they are soluble in water but are not attached by less-polar organic compounds such as aliphatic and aromatic hydrocarbons. They are used as film packets for detergents and other materials where release of the contents is by dissolution of the polyvinyl alcohol.

The high concentration of additives found in the polyvinyl chloride formulations gives rise to possible problems of leaching from the material when in contact with drugs or tissues. However, the greater portion of tubings in use today in therapeutic procedures are of the vinyl plastics class.

Newer Plastics—Other members of the plastics family which should be discussed are the polycarbonates and polychloroethers. Lexan (General Electric) and Merlon (Mobay) are polycarbonates, while Penton (Hercules) is a polychloroether.

The polycarbonates are formed by condensation of polyphenols such as Bisphenol-A with phosgene. The polymers are transparent thermoplastics, with high strengths and high temperature resistance. They can be heat or solvent sealed, facilitating fabrication procedures. The polycarbonates have hardness properties similar to those of metals and are being used to replace metals in numerous industrial applications.

The polychloroethers such as Penton are made by partial chlorination of pentaerythritol and polymerization of the intermediate chloro-oxetane monomer in the presence of an ionic catalyst. The resulting polymer contains about 46% chlorine by weight.

The solid polyurethanes have recently attracted significant attention in the development of implantable prostheses in the body. One of the group, known as segmented polyurethane, has proven to be especially promising in heart-assist devices, catheters, and other like applications.

Plastic Evaluation Procedures

The wide range of biological, chemical, and physical properties exhibited by plastics as a group necessitates a careful consideration of applicable testing procedures.

The use of plastics in the field of pharmaceutics and therapeutics can be divided into two broad categories. The first and most extensive use is as containers. The use here is logically divided again into two groups: containers for oral or topically applied drugs and containers for injectables. Closely related to this group are the syringes and tubings used to administer the injectables. Obviously, the use of such drug–plastic combinations must of necessity be substantiated by appropriate specific tests, in addition to those suggested below for plastics evaluation.

The second area of use, or type of use, of plastics is as tubings or devices which will be in contact with nonepithelial tissues of the body. Drainage tubings, intravenous feeding tubings, catheters in contact with abraded tissues, or even stomach tubes indwelling

postoperatively are examples of such use. Also included in this category are the permanently indwelling prostheses such as vascular grafts, supportive cartilage replacements, breast prostheses, and pacemakers.

Physicochemical Tests

Assuming that a given resin is nontoxic, the use of a pure polymer should be relatively free of problems. However, as almost all plastics in use are not pure polymers but are composed of many and varied additives making up a formulation, the important criterion becomes one of freedom from migration or leaching of the constituent substances. As has been pointed out, any migration of a substance from a container into a food or drug contained therein constitutes an adulteration, a food additive, or a drug additive.

The presence in plastic formulations of many substances, including metals, is tolerable if these are bound so that they will not be extracted during use applications.

The first step in the evaluation of a plastic formulation is the extraction of the material with several menstruums and chemical determinations made on the extracts to ascertain the type and extent of extractants.

There are several menstruums used for evaluation of food package plastics including water, 3% sodium chloride in water, 3% sodium bicarbonate in water, 3% acetic acid in water, 3% lactic acid in water, 20% sucrose in water, and lard or a vegetable oil. The solvents used for evaluation of plastics for pharmaceutic and therapeutic uses have included 0.9% sodium chloride in water, 5% ethyl alcohol in 0.9% sodium chloride in water, sesame or cottonseed oil, and polyethylene glycol 400.[6]

The extraction temperatures used are selected to conform to both the physical stability and expected "use history" of the device. Three temperatures are normally used: 50°C for 72 hr, 70°C for 24 hr, or 121°C for 1 hr. The standard overlay concentration is 10 Gm of plastic to 50 ml of menstruum, with the material not to exceed 3 mm in thickness.

Among the determinations which have been found useful are heavy metals, including barium and cadmium as well as lead; chloride and sulfate ions; and ammonium ions and oxidizable substances. These along with a determination of the amount of residue both on drying and by ignition give a good index of the stability of the plastic material.

More refined procedures using spectroscopic, chromatographic, electrochemical, and even radiochemical techniques aid in detecting and identifying substances coming from the plastic.

Inasmuch as it has been impossible so far to correlate chemical analyses with toxicity, the formulation must be proved nontoxic and compatible with body tissues by appropriate pharmacological procedures using live animals.

Biological Tests

The procedures hereinafter set forth have been used extensively in the evaluation of plastics formulations intended for use in pharmacy and medicine and have been themselves further evaluated by a collaborative study by several laboratories with eventual inclusion in the USP.[7]

Systemic toxicity is based on the use of extracts. Tissue toxicity or irritant activity is based on intracutaneous injection of the extracts and on implantation of strips of the plastic, usually in the paravertebral muscle of the rabbit for a period of time. Pyrogenicity is determined using 10 Gm of plastic in 200 ml of pyrogen-free saline, heated to not less than 85°C for 1 hr, with the eluate being used in the standard USP Pyrogen Test Procedure.

Acute Systemic Toxicity—Extracts of the plastic material are made using four solvents and a temperature compatible with the heat resistance of the formulation up to 121°C. If the formulation in its "use" will never be exposed to a temperature of 121°C, a lower temperature of extraction may be used, as for instance with items which are to be sterilized by gas or irradiation, used once, and discarded. As set forth above, the three temperatures selected for inclusion in the USP Test Procedure are 50°C for 72 hr, 70°C for 24 hr, or 121°C for 1 hr. The material, however, should have been exposed to all conditions which are to be encountered in its fabrication and processing for use. Thus, a material intended for sterilization by irradiation must have been so exposed before a valid evaluation can be made.

The material, not exceeding 3 mm in thickness, is covered with an extraction menstruum in a Pyrex container closed with a Teflon or polypropylene screwcap.

Ten grams of the plastic is covered with 50 ml of extraction menstruum. If the material is a filament or a thin sheet material, an adjustment of the quantity of material is made based on surface area. For those plastics which will be exposed to a wide variety of menstruums, such as syringes, containers, and closures, the following four menstruums were selected for extraction use: 0.9% sodium chloride, 5% ethyl alcohol in 0.9% sodium chloride, sesame or cottonseed oil, and polyethylene glycol 400.

For plastics intended for more limited-use exposure, such as indwelling tubings, the use of 0.9% saline and the vegetable oil should be sufficient. Positive and negative known control plastic formulations may be prepared and run simultaneously to prove the adequacy of the extraction and the sensitivity of the test animals.

The preparations are agitated, the extracts collected and injected into healthy albino mice weighing 17–23 Gm. Animals of comparable weight are used for the control. The saline and alcoholic saline extracts are injected 1.0 ml intravenously. The oil is injected 1.0 ml intraperitoneally, and the polyethylene glycol is given at a level of 10,000 mg/kg intraperitoneally. The animals are observed for 72 hr to 7 days for evidence of toxic effects.

The 1.0-ml doses are equivalent to injecting the total substance extracted from 10 Gm of plastic/kg of body weight.

Irritant Tests—These consist of intracutaneous, intraocular, and dermal applications.

Intracutaneous Reactivity—The presence of a toxic or irritating extractant in eluates from plastics can be detected easily by injection of the menstruums intracutaneously into thin-skinned rabbits. In practice ten 0.2-ml intracutaneous blebs are formed by injecting each of the four menstruums. These are paralleled by ten like control blebs. The saline, alcoholic saline and vegetable oil are injected undiluted; the polyethylene glycol 400 is diluted with 0.9% saline to contain 24 mg of polyethylene glycol in the 0.2-ml bleb.

Any increased tissue erythema, swelling, or necrosis within 72 hr gives evidence of the presence of toxic extracts.

Other methods—The 0.9% saline eluate may be instilled in the lower conjunctival sac of the rabbit's eye as a further study. Also, dermal application of all four of the eluates may be useful to determine the reactivity of intact skin to the irritant.

Implantation Tests—The most significant acute test for possible leachable tissue toxicants in material subject to contact with body tissues is observed by imbedding the material in the appropriate tissue. The "full-strength" plastic is in direct contact with the tissue, with all of its extractive juices.

The tissues used are subcutaneous, intramuscular, and cerebral. The reactivities subcutaneously and intramuscularly are illustrated in a paper by the author.[8] As a general rule, less reaction is noted subcutaneously than intramuscularly perhaps because of the better circulation and exchange of fluids, which reduces the concentration of extracted toxic material.

The implanted sections are approximately 1.0–1.5 mm in diameter and 8–10 mm in length. They may be cut and sterilized or they may be cut from within the plastic material just before imbedding. The imbedding is accomplished quite easily using a prepared 13-gauge needle and trochar and with the animal under pentobarbital anesthesia. The cerebral implants are made through 4-mm trephined openings.

The optimal duration of acute implantation is 72 hr to 7 days. The lowest grade reactions may, however, be missed at 7 days. There has been no instance in the author's experience where a reaction was present at 7 days which was not detectable at 3 days.

The reactive materials can be detected easily by gross examination subcutaneously and intramuscularly as the reaction material about the implants is easily seen. The intramuscular implants are examined for reaction about the cross section of the center of the implant as slight pressure necrosis may be seen at the ends. The cerebral implant sites are always evaluated histopathologically as the appearance of the tissue and reactant material is so similar to the eye.

As a standard procedure, four subcutaneous or intramuscular test material implants are made in a rabbit, paralleled by two positive and two negatively reacting controls. In the cerebral implantation procedure two rabbits each receive two test strips and one negative control strip. Those substances which show a reaction in the acute implantation test also tend to exhibit toxicity and/or tissue reactivity with the vegetable oil extract.

For chronic effects a similar design of implantations is made and allowed to remain in place for not less than 90 days. They are then removed and examined both grossly and histopathologically. There are substances which will elicit a significant fibrosis adjacent to the material with no evidence of tissue toxicity.

The data collected during the collaborative study indicated that there were occasions when a given material exhibited a reaction intramuscularly but not subcutaneously for reasons previously discussed. In view of this the USP calls for intramuscular implantation only. The tests specified in the USP are set forth in Table I.

Pyrogenicity Test—The freedom of a given plastic formulation from pyrogenic effects can best be determined by covering a 10-Gm sample of the material with 200 ml of pyrogen-free 0.9% saline and heating to not less than 85°C for 1 hr. The temperature of the supernate is adjusted to 37°C and injected in the USP pyrogen test procedure.

The USP sets forth a pyrogen test procedure for *Transfusion and Infusion Assemblies*, wherein the saline is passed through the tubing in preparation for the test. It is felt that a greater concentration of material and a more vigorous extraction or elution of the possible pyrogens, as would be obtained in the heating procedure above, is desirable.

Blood Compatibility Test—The gross compatibility of a plastic substance with whole blood is evaluated with an eluate of the material with USP Acid Citrate Dextrose (ACD), Formula A, for 24 hr at 45°C. Five grams of the plastic is covered with 25 ml of the ACD. After exposure for 24 hr the ACD is used to preserve freshly drawn rabbit blood for 14 days in the refrigerator. Comparison of the amounts of hemoglobin in the plasma of the test preparation and a control gives an index of gross compatibility with red blood cells. Also of importance is the ability of the ACD to prevent clotting of the blood after exposure to the plastic.

A second test preparation is made by overlaying 5 Gm of the plastic with 25 ml of freshly drawn ACD-preserved rabbit blood and holding in the refrigerator for a similar length of time. The same observations are made as with the eluate above.

It should be noted that these are not survival tests but rather gross compatibility tests. If the plastic is satisfactory here, it can be further evaluated by suitable survival tests.

Nonantigenicity Tests—The problem of sensitization to a given plastic formulation is one which must be given careful attention. The test which has been used is an adaptation of that set forth in the USP, using male guinea pigs.

The sensitizing solution is prepared by eluting the test material for 24 hr at 45°C with 0.9% saline and either cottonseed or sesame oil. If the material is to be sterilized by steam, the sensitizing solution is prepared by autoclaving for 1 hr at 121°C.

Five male guinea pigs weighing 420–480 Gm each receive 6 ml of the sensitizing solution intraperitoneally on the second, fourth, and sixth days of each of two successive weeks. If both the saline and oil eluates are to be used, the animals receive 3.0 ml of each at each injection.

The animals are held for 30–37 days following the last injection and challenged with 3 ml of a similarly prepared 0.9% saline sensitizing solution, given intravenously, at a rate of 2 ml/min. The animals are

Table I—Classification of Plastics

Plastic classes[a]						Tests to be conducted			
I	II	III	IV	V	VI	Test material	Animal	Dose	Procedure[b]
x	x	x	x	x	x	Extract of *Sample* in *Sodium Chloride Injection*	Mouse	50 ml/Kg	A (i.v.)
x	x	x	x	x	x		Rabbit	0.2 ml/animal at each of 10 sites	B
	x	x	x	x	x	Extract of *Sample* in *1 in 20 Solution of Alcohol in Sodium Chloride Injection*	Mouse	50 ml/Kg	A (i.v.)
	x	x	x	x	x		Rabbit	0.2 ml/animal at each of 10 sites	B
		x		x	x	Extract of *Sample* in *Polyethylene Glycol 400*	Mouse	10 Gm/Kg	A (i.p.)
				x	x		Rabbit	0.2 ml/animal at each of 10 sites	B
		x	x	x	x	Extract of *Sample* in *Sesame Oil*[c]	Mouse	50 ml/Kg	A (i.p.)
			x	x	x		Rabbit	0.2 ml/animal at each of 10 sites	B
		x			x	Implant strips of *Sample*	Rabbit	4 strips/animal	C

[a] Tests required for each class are indicated by "x" in appropriate columns.
[b] Legend: A (i.p.)—Systemic Injection Test (intraperitoneal); A (i.v.)—Systemic Injection Test (intravenous); B—Intracutaneous Test (intracutaneous); C—Implantation Test (intramuscular implantation).
[c] *Cottonseed Oil* (see page 1343) may be used instead of *Sesame Oil*.

carefully observed during the injection and for 30 min thereafter for any of the symptoms indicative of anaphylaxis, such as licking the nose or rubbing the nose with the forefeet, ruffling of hair, weakness, labored breathing, sneezing or coughing, or retching.

A similar group of guinea pigs which has been given the sensitizing solution is injected intracutaneously with the sensitizing solution to determine if a local or tissue sensitization has developed. The reaction, if there is one, should not exceed that observed in a like control group of animals which had not received the sensitizing solution.

Cardiovascular Tests—Inasmuch as certain plastic formulations have been shown to have leachable constituents which will significantly affect the coronary flow rate and force of contraction of the heart, appropriate evaluation of a plastic substance intended for use in a cardiovascular device is imperative.

The perfusion of the isolated heart with a perfusion fluid, prepared using a saline extract of the plastic in the Anderson and Craver modification of Langendorf's procedure, has served very well.

Embryological Reaction—If a plastic material is to be used in devices intended for use particularly in connection with infants and pregnant women, toxic or teratogenic effects may be detected by injection of extracts of the material into the yolk of fertile eggs prior to incubation.[9] This method supplements but does not replace observations in other species or in other tests as those previously discussed. One hundred eggs are injected with 0.1 ml of the extract, paralleled by a significant number of control eggs, both uninjected and injected with control saline. The percentage hatch observed in the test and control groups as well as abnormalities of embryos gives an indication of toxicity. The important advantage here is the fact that there is no placental barrier to modify the drug effects.

Drug–Plastic Evaluations—It is abundantly clear from the previous considerations that plastics are not necessarily inert and basically safe to use, but rather are a very complex and varied group of materials. As has already been pointed out, each application of a plastic to a specific use in pharmacy or medicine must be a "law unto itself" and such tests as are pertinent and necessary must be performed to assure compatibility and safety of use. Extensive reviews of the problems of drug-plastic applications are presented in two articles by Autian[10,11] and the student is referred to these for further discussion.

The several phases of drug–plastic evaluation which have been found useful in assessing a particular plastic are permeation, leaching, adsorption and absorption, chemical reactivity, and possible alteration of the physical characteristics of the plastic, especially upon long-term exposure. Because plastics are composed of crystalline and amorphous materials, differences in degree of sorption, diffusion and other properties are governed by the proportions of these materials.

Permeation refers to the passage of molecules from the solution through the plastic to the outside or to like passage from without into the solution. The amount and/or rate of permeation will depend upon the plastic used. Examples illustrating the variability might be cited.[12] The transmission rate of Saran and polyvinyl chloride plasticized, at 23°C and one atmosphere pressure was: O_2, 16 and 3100 ml, respectively; N_2, 2.5 and 810 ml, respectively; CO_2, 50 and 19,000 ml, respectively, over a 24-hr period per square meter of film. The rate of passage of a gas through a plastic film will depend upon the molecular weight, branching,

degree of crystallinity, and the amount of amorphous zone through which the gas must travel. Highly crystalline materials exhibit low rates of permeation. The stability of a pharmaceutical preparation could be significantly affected by the permeation characteristics of the plastic used.

Leaching for practical purposes refers to the passage of some ingredient or ingredients from the plastic into the drug preparation contained therein. The extent of the leaching depends in part on the type of plastic used, whether it is composed of only a single polymer or copolymer or compounded from several ingredients such as polymer, plasticizer, antioxidant, colorants, and so forth. The single polymer plastics, sometimes called pure plastics, ordinarily are much less apt to release material into the drug. The formulated plastic, containing many ingredients, is much more likely to release some material into the drug and the identification of such a contaminant is much more difficult. The constituent leached may be a plasticizer or stabilizer rather than the polymer. An interesting illustration of leaching came to light when polyvinyl tubings were substituted for glass in a heart perfusion device.[13] Some constituent was introduced which proved toxic to the heart perfusion preparation. Further study led to the conclusion that it was a stabilizer used in the formulation which was causing the untoward reaction. Of further interest is the fact that several different sources of polyvinyl chloride tubings were used in the preparation but not all exhibited the cardiotoxic activity. This emphasizes the fact that all polyvinyl chloride formulations are not the same, a fact readily discernible but too often not recognized.

The nature of the drug or solvent may, of course, have a significant effect upon the migration of some constituent from the plastic into the drug. Closely related to leaching is the problem of sorption.

Sorption is used to include adsorption and absorption of the drug or solute. The phenomena here referred to, as Autian points out, are closely related to the process of dyeing of synthetic yarns. The rate of diffusion of the solute or drug in the matrix of the plastic is the determining factor in the over-all process of sorption. The amount adsorbed is perhaps insignificant compared to the amount absorbed. The chemical structure of the plastic as well as the chemical nature of the drug or solute are all important factors in the problem of drug sorption. Saski has shown that sorbic acid can be bound to cellulose acetate to varying degrees.[14] Studies by Autian, *et al*, have indicated that many weak organic acids may be sorbed by nylon.[15–17] These include phenol, salicylic acid, the parabens, sorbic acid, benzoic acid, and derivatives of benzoic acid. It should be pointed out that other weak acids are not significantly bound, eg, acetic acid, glycine or tyrosine. These observations emphasize the fact that to date one can at best only hazard an educated guess about sorption. The drug–plastic combination must be proven by test because serious consequences could arise if a potent drug, with a low concentration in the solution, was absorbed or adsorbed on the plastic, effectively removing it from the preparation.

pH can significantly alter the amount of sorption of a drug especially with a plastic such as nylon, a polyamide structure with both amino and carboxylic sites.[10] The solvent can also influence the rate of sorption primarily by causing the plastic to swell and soften, increasing the amount of passageways for the solute molecules. Again the prediction of solvent–plastic–

solute interaction is impossible.   It should be remembered that any organic solvent system which will increase the amorphous content of the plastic will increase the sorption of the plastic.

Concentration of solute has also been shown to influence some plastic sorption characteristics.   Phenol below a critical concentration, for instance, is sorbed by nylon, but when the critical concentration is exceeded, a very sharp increase in sorption takes place, due principally to the swelling and softening effects of phenol on nylon.

Temperature affects the sorption in two ways. With increase in temperature there is an increased rate of sorption but the equilibrium level is below that for lower temperatures.   This was found to be true with nylon and salicylic acid.[11]

It is abundantly clear, then, that only by thorough testing of the particular plastic formulation, both by biological and toxicological and other carefully selected drug–plastic tests, can a plastic be properly chosen for a particular device or drug container for pharmaceutical dispensing.

Batch Lot Tests—After a plastic formulation has cleared all of the initial evaluation tests, it is important to remember that each batch of the substance made up represents a separate entity.   The control over the chemical reactions taking place in the usual complex formulation batch is not such as to guarantee that every batch made to a given formula will be the same with respect to inherent toxicity.   For this reason an abbreviated test procedure must be applied to every batch of material.   The term *batch* here refers to a given mixing or preparation lot and not to the several sublots or batches which may result from a single mixing and processing batch.   There are, of course, sterility and pyrogen tests which are required according to the labeling of the finished package.

The present compilation can not expect to cover all aspects of the use and testing of plastics.   However, in the absence of more formal regulatory stipulations the procedures set forth do offer a logical, systematic approach to the evaluation of any plastic regardless of its chemical nature when its use is contemplated in a therapeutic device or container.

In view of the very complex nature of plastics and in view of the foregone conclusion that there will be many more plastics to come, good pharmaceutic and therapeutic practice requires that a formulation be classified as nontoxic and satisfactory for use only after it has been proved so by careful evaluation tests.

References

1. Wesolowski, S. A., *Evaluation of Tissue and Prosthetic Vascular Grafts*, C. C Thomas, Springfield, Ill., 1962.
2. Simonds, H. R., and Church, J. M., *A Concise Guide to Plastics*, 2nd ed, Reinhold, New York, 1963.
3. Meals, R. N., and Lewis, F. M., *Silicones*, Reinhold, New York, 1959.
4. *Plastic Engineering Handbook*, Society of the Plastics Industry, Inc., Reinhold, New York, 1960.
5. Skeist, I., and Somerville, G. R., *Epoxy Resins*, Reinhold, New York, 1958.
6. Brewer, J. H., and Bryant, H. H., *J. APhA, Sci. Ed.*, **49**, 652 (1960).
7. Report of Pharmaceutical Manufacturers Association (PMA) Committee on Plastics, Mar. 1964.
8. Brewer, J. H., and Bryant, H. H., *J. APhA, Sci. Ed.*, **49**, 654, 655 (1960).
9. McLaughlin, J., *Toxicol. Appl. Pharmacol.*, **5**, 760 (1963).
10. Autian, J., *J. Pharm. Sci.*, **52**, 1, (1963).
11. Autian, J., *J. Pharm. Sci.*, **52**, 105 (1963).
12. Brown, W. E., and Sauber, W. J., *Mod. Plastics*, **36**, 107 (Aug. 1959).
13. Thomas, J. J., and Lagrange, G. J., *Pharm. Belg.*, 3–4, 59 (1962).
14. Saski, W., "Adsorption of Sorbic Acid by Plastic Cellulose Acetate." Presented to Scientific Section, APhA, Las Vegas Meeting, 1962.
15. Marcus, E., *et al*, *J. Pharm. Sci.*, **48**, 457 (1959).
16. Kim, H. K., and Autian, J., *J. Pharm. Sci.*, **49**, 227 (1960).
17. Autian, J., and Shaikh, Z. I., *Drug Std.*, **28**, 103 (1960).

92 | Control

Principles, organization, and functions of quality control

This chapter was prepared by

H. D. Piersma, PhD, *Director, Quality Control Section, Lederle Laboratories, Pearl River, N.Y. 10965, and*
R. W. Elkas, PhD, *Manager, Pharmaceutical Quality Control and Services, Lederle Laboratories, Pearl River, N.Y. 10965*

Large-scale pharmaceutical production presents many problems which are not associated with prescription compounding in a pharmacy, where the quantities of medicaments prepared are usually small and all the work is carried out by the pharmacist himself. Prescription compounding in a pharmacy requires skill and integrity, but the control involved in these assignments is relatively simple. In the manufacture of drugs by an industrial pharmaceutical firm, however, the variety and complexity of operations make it necessary to assign to a separate and independent group of scientists within each company the responsibility for controlling the quality of the final product.

Since one of the primary considerations of a responsible drug manufacturer is a deep concern for the reliability and integrity of the finished products distributed to the market under his name, the quality of each lot of each final product is checked for many characteristics. For this purpose each manufacturer employs a group of highly qualified scientists and technicians, referred to collectively as Quality Control, who examine and check each lot of each product during and upon completion of manufacturing operations for identity, purity, uniformity, and drug content. In addition, this group augments its testing function with continuous auditing of the standard operating procedures, referred to in general as the Control System. Further, after a product has been distributed to the market, a responsible manufacturer will perform appropriate tests designed to assure its stability and performance upon exercise of reasonable care in handling.

The general principles governing control of the quality of drugs are identical for all reputable drug manufacturers, regardless of size of organization or types of product made. Hence, among reliable companies, the execution of the quality-control function differs only in detail. In this connection the following excerpt is taken from a statement on the general principles of total control of quality in the drug industry, as adopted on May 3, 1961, and revised on June 22, 1967, by the Board of Directors of the Pharmaceutical Manufacturers Association (PMA).*

"The quality of a product is its degree of possession of those characteristics designed and manufactured into it which contribute to the performance of an intended function when the product is used as directed. The quality of medicinal and related products is the sum of all factors which contribute directly or indirectly to the safety, effectiveness, and acceptability of the product. Quality must be built into the product during research, development, and production.

"Total control of quality as it applies to the drug industry is the organized effort within an entire establishment to design, produce, maintain, and assure the specified quality in each unit of product distributed. The effort should not only establish specifications for product acceptance but should provide procedures and methods for achieving conformance with such specifications.

"The large variety of substances used in this industry, the complexity of its products, and the various types of company organization make it impossible to design in detail a single universally applicable system for the total control of quality.

"The ultimate objective of a program for the total control of quality in a drug company is the attainment of perfection in meeting specifications for a product of high quality. It is a program designed to assure the professional user or ultimate consumer that every lot of a product conforms to specifications and that each dose distributed will fulfill the representations made in the labeling and will meet all legal requirements and such additional standards as the management of a firm may adopt."

The statement made by the PMA also describes the basic working relationship between Quality Control and Production functions in a responsible drug house. Finally, it outlines in detail the systems and procedures under which a quality control organization operates in executing its responsibilities.

On June 20, 1963, the US Food and Drug Administration (FDA) published several new regulations, among which were criteria for current good manufacturing practice in the manufacture, processing, packing, and holding of finished pharmaceuticals. Since they represent a signal official step in interpreting good manufacturing practice and quality control functions, these regulations are presented hereunder. (The FDA is currently proposing to amend these regulations to clarify and strengthen them and to make them more specific. Because of the delays associated with such an immense project, the final revised regulations will not be promulgated in time to be included in our final printing. The revisions, when completed, will be published in the *Federal Register* and will be available from the US Food and Drug Administration, Washington, D.C.)

Finished Pharmaceuticals; Manufacturing Practice

Section 133.2 Current good manufacturing practice.

The criteria in sections 133.3–133.13, inclusive, shall apply in determining whether the methods used in, or the facilities or controls used for, the manufacture, processing, packing, or holding of a drug conform to or are operated or administered in conformity with current good manufacturing practice to assure that a drug meets the requirements of the act as to safety, and has the identity and strength, and meets the quality and purity characteristics, which it purports or is represented to possess, as required by section 501(a)(2)(B) of the act. (*Ed note:* "act" means the Federal Food, Drug, and Cosmetic Act, sections 201–902, 52 Stat. 1052 (21 U.S.C. 321–392), with all amendments thereto.) The regulations in this Part 133 permit the use of precision automatic mechanical or electronic equipment in the production of drugs when adequate inspection and checking procedures are used to assure proper performance.

Section 133.3 Buildings.

Buildings in which drugs are manufactured, processed, packaged, labeled, or held shall be maintained in a clean and orderly manner and shall be of suitable size, construction, and location in relation to surroundings to facilitate maintenance and operation for their intended purpose. The buildings shall:

(a) Provide adequate space for the orderly placement of equipment and materials used in any of the following operations for which it is employed, to minimize any risk of mix-ups between different drugs, their components, packaging, or labeling:

---

* Pharmaceutical Manufacturers Association, Washington, D.C.

(1) The receipt, sampling, and storage of components.

(2) Any manufacturing and processing operations performed on the drug.

(3) Any packaging and labeling operations.

(4) Storage of containers, packaging materials, labeling, and finished products.

(5) Control and production-laboratory operations.

(b) Provide adequate lighting and ventilation, and when necessary for the intended production or control purposes, adequate screening, filtering, dust, humidity, temperature, and bacteriological controls, as for example, to prevent contamination of products by extraneous adulterants; to prevent the dissemination of micro-organisms from one area to another; to facilitate the sterilization of special work areas, such as those used for production of parenteral preparations; to provide suitable housing for any animals; and to avoid other conditions unfavorable to the safety and integrity of the product.

(c) Provide for adequate washing, cleaning, toilet, and locker facilities.

Section 133.4 Equipment.

Equipment used for the manufacture, processing, packaging, labeling, holding, or control of drugs shall be maintained in a clean and orderly manner and shall be of suitable design, size, construction, and location in relation to surroundings to facilitate maintenance and operation for its intended purpose. The equipment shall:

(a) Be so constructed that any surfaces that come into contact with drugs are suitable, in that they are not reactive, additive, or absorptive to an extent that significantly affects the identity, strength, quality, or purity of the drug or its components.

(b) Be so constructed that any substances required for the operation of the equipment, such as lubricants or coolants, may be employed without hazard of becoming additive to drug products.

(c) Be constructed to facilitate adjustment, cleaning, and maintenance as necessary to assure the reliability of control procedures, to assure uniformity of production, and to assure the exclusion from drugs of contaminants, including those from previous and current manufacturing operations.

(d) Be of suitable size and accuracy for use in any intended measuring, mixing, or weighing operations.

Section 133.5 Personnel.

The key personnel involved in the manufacture and control of the drug shall have a background of appropriate education or appropriate experience or combination thereof for assuming responsibility to assure that the drug has the safety, identity, strength, quality, and purity that it purports to possess.

Section 133.6 Components.

Components used in the manufacture and processing of drugs, regardless of whether they appear in the finished product, shall be identified, stored, examined, tested, inventoried, handled, and otherwise controlled in a manner to assure that they conform to appropriate standards of identity, strength, quality, and purity, and are free of contaminants at time of use, and to provide that appropriate records are maintained of their origin, receipt, examination, testing, disposition, and use in drug manufacture or processing.

Section 133.7 Master-formula and batch-production records.

(a) For each drug product, master-formula records shall be prepared, endorsed, and dated by a competent and responsible individual and shall be independently checked, reconciled, endorsed, and dated by a second competent and responsible individual. The record shall include:

(1) The name of the product, a description of its dosage form, and a specimen or copy of the label and each other portion of the labeling contained in a retail package of the drug.

(2) The weight or measure of each ingredient per dosage unit or per unit of weight or measure of the finished drug, and a statement of the total weight or measure of any dosage unit.

(3) A complete batch formula for each batch size to be produced from the master-formula record, including a complete list of ingredients designated by names or codes sufficiently specific to indicate any special quality characteristic; an accurate statement of the weight or measure of each ingredient, regardless of whether it appears in the finished product, except that reasonable variations may be permitted in the amount of components necessary in the preparation in dosage form, provided that the variations are stated in the master formula; an appropriate statement concerning any calculated excess of an ingredient; appropriate statements of theoretical weight or measure at various stages of processing; and a statement of the theoretical yield.

(4) A description of the containers, closures, packaging, and finishing materials.

(5) Manufacturing and control instructions, procedures, specifications, special notations, and precautions to be followed.

(b) A separate batch-production and control record shall be prepared for each batch of drug produced and shall be retained for at least 2 years after distribution has been completed. The batch-production and control record shall include:

(1) An accurate reproduction of the appropriate master-formula record, checked and endorsed by a competent, responsible individual.

(2) Records of each step in the manufacturing, processing, packaging, labeling, and controlling of the batch, including dates, specific identification of each batch of components used, weights or measures of components and products in course of processing, in-process and laboratory-control results, and the endorsements of the individual actively performing or the individual actively supervising or checking each step in the operation.

(3) A batch number that permits determination of all laboratory-control procedures and results on the batch and all lot or control numbers appearing on the labels of drugs from the batch.

Section 133.8 Production and control procedures.

Production and control procedures shall include all reasonable precautions, including the following, to assure that the drugs produced have the identity, strength, quality, and purity they purport to possess.

(a) Each critical step in the process, such as the selection, weighing, and measuring of components; the addition of active ingredients during the process; weighing and measuring during various stages of the processing; and the determination of the finished yield shall be performed by a competent, responsible individual and checked by a second competent, responsible individual, or if such steps in the processing are controlled by precision automatic mechanical or electronic equipment their proper performance is adequately checked by one or more competent, responsible individuals.

(b) All containers and equipment used in producing a batch of drugs shall be clearly labeled at all times to identify fully and accurately their contents, the stage of processing, and the batch, and shall be stored and handled in a manner adequate to prevent mixups with other drugs.

(c) Equipment, utensils, and containers shall be thoroughly cleaned and previous identification removed between batches and in continuous batch operations at suitable intervals, to prevent contamination and mixups.

(d) Appropriate procedures to minimize the hazard of contamination with micro-organisms in the production of parenteral drugs, ophthalmic solutions, and any other drugs purporting to be sterile.

(e) To assure the uniformity and integrity of products, there shall be adequate in-process controls, such as checking the weights and disintegration time of tablets, checking fill of liquids, and checking the adequacy of mixing, the homogeneity of suspensions, and the clarity of solutions.

(f) Competent and responsible personnel shall check actual against theoretical yield of a batch of drug, and in the event of any significant unexplained discrepancies, key personnel shall prevent distribution of the batch in question and other associated batches of drugs that may have been involved in a mixup with it.

Section 133.9 Product containers.

Suitable specifications, test methods, cleaning procedures, and, when indicated, sterilization procedures shall be used to assure that containers, closures, and other component parts of drug packages are suitable for their intended use, in that they are not reactive, additive, or absorptive to an extent that significantly affects the identity, strength, quality, or purity of the drug, and furnish adequate protection against its deterioration or contamination.

Section 133.10 Packaging and labeling.

Packaging and labeling operations shall be adequately controlled to assure that only those drugs that have met the specifications established in the master-formula records shall be distributed; to prevent mixups between drugs during the packaging and labeling operations; to assure that correct labeling is employed for the drug; and to identify finished products with lot or control numbers that permit determination of the history of the manufacture and control of the batch of drug. Packaging and labeling operations shall:

(a) Be performed with adequate physical segregation of such operations from operations on any other drugs to avoid mixups.

(b) Provide that each type of labeling used shall be stored in a manner that avoids mixups between labelings and shall be carefully checked for identity and conformity to the labeling specified in the batch-production records.

(c) Provide adequate control of the quantities of labeling issued for use with the drug. (Competent, responsible personnel shall reconcile any discrepancy between the quantity of drug finished and the quantity of labeling issued. In the event of any significant unexplained discrepancy, key personnel shall prevent distribution of the batch in question and other associated batches of drugs that may have been involved in a mixup.)

(d) Provide for an inspection of the facilities to be used prior to labeling a drug to assure that all the previously used labeling and other drugs have been removed.

(e) Provide for adequate examination or laboratory testing of adequately representative samples of finished products after packaging and labeling to safeguard against any error in the finishing operations, and to prevent distribution of any batch until all specified tests have been met.

Section 133.11   Laboratory controls.

Laboratory controls shall include the establishment of adequate specifications and test procedures to assure that components, drug preparations in the course of processing, and finished products conform to appropriate standards of identity, strength, quality, and purity. Laboratory controls shall include:

(a) The establishment of master records containing appropriate specifications for each component used in drug production and a description of the test procedures used to check them, including provision for testing adequately representative samples. Such records shall also provide for appropriate retesting of materials subject to deterioration.

(b) The establishment of appropriate specifications, when needed, for drug preparations in the course of processing, and a description of the test procedures to check them, including provision for testing adequately representative samples.

(c) The establishment of appropriate finished-product specifications and a description of laboratory test procedures to check them, including provision for testing adequately representative samples.

(d) Adequate provision for checking the identity and strength for all active ingredients of drugs, for assuring the sterility of articles purporting to be sterile, and the freedom from pyrogens of articles that should be tested for freedom from pyrogens.

(e) Adequate provision to check the reliability, accuracy, and precision of any laboratory test procedures used.

(f) A reserve sample of at least twice the quantity of drug required to conduct all the tests performed on the batch of drug shall be retained at least 2 years after distribution has been completed.

(g) Provision for complete records of all data concerning laboratory tests performed, including the dates and endorsements of individuals making the tests, and provision for specifically relating the tests to each batch of drug to which they apply. Such records shall be retained for at least 2 years after distribution has been completed.

Section 133.12   Distribution records.

Complete records shall be maintained of the distribution of each batch of drug in a manner that will facilitate its recall if necessary. Such records shall be retained for at least 2 years after distribution has been completed, and shall include the name and address of the consignee, the date and quantity shipped, and the lot or control numbers identifying the batch of drug.

Section 133.13   Stability.

Adequate provision shall be made for testing the stability of components, drug preparations in the course of processing, when needed, and finished drugs. Such stability tests shall:

(a) Make adequate provision for determining the reliability and specificity of stability test methods employed.

(b) Make adequate provision to determine the stability of products in the containers in which they are marketed to assure, among other things, that the container is suitable, in that it is not reactive, additive, or adsorptive to an extent that significantly affects the identity, strength, quality, or purity of the drug.

(c) Provide for stability studies of any solutions prepared as directed in the drug labeling at time of dispensing.

(d) Provide for suitable expiration dates to appear in the labeling of the drug when needed to assure that the drug meets appropriate standards of identity, strength, quality, and purity at time of use.

Section 133.14   Complaint files.

Records shall be maintained of all written or verbal complaints for each product. Complaints shall be evaluated by competent and responsible personnel and, where indicated, appropriate action taken. The record shall indicate the evaluation and action.

Organization of Quality Control

The individual directly responsible for the quality of drug products in a drug manufacturing company is generally known as the Director of Quality Control. He should report to the President or a Vice-President, and should be on the same organizational level as the Production Manager. His decisions on quality should be subject to review only by the highest level of management.

The Quality Control organization is usually subdivided into several departments, as shown in the chart, Fig. 767. In a large drug company considerably more detail may be required to depict the interaction between various groups within the Quality Control organization and with other functions in the company.

The Specifications and Assay Development Function—Since the quality of a finished medicament may often depend on the quality of the raw materials used in manufacturing operations, the establishment of specifications for raw materials is an important function. Such specifications are developed jointly by scientists involved in research, product development, and quality control. In addition to the usual criteria such as description, solubility, identification, melting point, loss on drying, residue on ignition, specific rotation, refractive index, specific gravity, and assay, special consideration should be given to the advisability of additional critical features such as particle size, crystal shape, surface tension, viscosity, rate of solution, irritation, related foreign substances, allergenic substances, toxicity, and peculiarities such as crystalline vs amorphous forms. In addition it is necessary to develop and improve specifications for the quality characteristics of the final products being manufactured. These specifications originate by joint effort of quality control, research, product development, production, sales, and management. In addition to the usual criteria such as description, identification, moisture content, pH, specific gravity, surface tension, alcohol content, hardness, disintegration, weight variation, sterility, pyrogenicity, safety, and assay, special consideration should be given to the advisability of additional critical features such as dissolution rate, uniformity of individual unit content, related foreign substances, irritation, microbial content, and stability. All specifications should include at least those requirements, whenever applicable, of the federal and state governments and the official compendia.

The assay methods used to test many raw materials and final products are published in the USP and NF. For those raw materials and final products not described in either of these official compendia, it is necessary for the manufacturer to develop his own methods of testing. Since many pharmaceutical products contain more than one active ingredient, and since many of the inactive ingredients in a formulation may be tested qualitatively and quantitatively, it is essential that an active group of qualified scientists constantly engage in the development of new assay methods. The major cost of quality control lies in the testing of products throughout manufacturing operations, and it is not difficult to understand that considerable attention and effort are directed toward the improvement of assay methods. Variations or complete changes in assay methods may produce greater accuracy in testing, or more rapid results, and thus contribute to reduction in the cost of operations. There is also growing use of automation in the testing of drug products since the mechanical performance of certain tests, or portions of a test, may not only yield accurate results but also permits an increase in the number of samples tested without an increase in cost or time.

Chemical Testing Laboratory—Every lot of every shipment of raw material and every lot of finished product which can be controlled by chemical and physical tests, should be tested in the chemical testing laboratory of the Quality Control organization. This requires a well-equipped chemical laboratory, properly staffed for performance of a great number of chemical analyses. It should be located in an accessible area and protected from the noise and vibration common to manufacturing operations. In addition to the usual gravimetric and volumetric analyses, laboratory personnel should be skilled in the special instrumentation of ultraviolet and infrared spectrophotometry, nonaqueous titrimetry, chromatography (column, gas, paper, and thin-layer), polarography, x-ray diffraction, x-ray fluorescence, spectrophotofluorimetry, and radioactive tracer techniques. See the chapters on *Official Requirements and Tests*, page 585, and *Analysis of Medicinals*, page 596.

Biological Testing Laboratory—A number of finished products require biological assays, even though chemical tests may be required for other components of the formulation. Biological tests are not confined to the group of products recognized as biologics in the drug industry, since a number of pharmaceutical products, such as parenterals, for example, require sterility and pyrogen tests before release to the market. An adequate biological testing laboratory must provide facilities for a variety of pharmacological and bacteriological testing procedures. It is essential to have several species of animals available, and the care and maintenance of them should be under the supervision of a veterinarian. The staff in a biological testing laboratory should be well trained and experienced since many of the procedures used are complex and the biological interactions in many tests are incompletely understood. A high degree of skill and judgment are required to perform and evaluate microbiologic and pharmacologic assays, as well as sterility, pyrogenicity, bacteriologic, irritation, and safety or acute toxicity tests. See the chapters on *Sterilization*, page 1501, *Parenteral Preparations*, page 1519, *Fundamentals of Biological Pharmacy*, page 1417, and *Biological Testing*, page 630.

Central Release Office—The records resulting from the exercise of quality control functions throughout all steps of manufacturing and packaging operations are voluminous. It is mandatory that the quality control organization assume responsibility for the meticulous examination of these records and for the determination of their completeness and accuracy, as well as for their maintenance and storage, for they are of great value in many ways. They provide a complete history of each lot of each product manufactured and, therefore, make it possible to reconstruct the pertinent features of any package distributed in the market. This fact gives these records scientific and legal status. Further, there is much interest in the statistical evaluation of results obtained from the various tests, and the availability of records over extended periods of time makes it possible to evaluate the reliability of analytical tests in routine use, as well as the uniformity of products from lot to lot. See the chapter on *Statistics*, page 122.

The handling of records in quality-control operations may be expedited and simplified by means of electronic data-processing facilities. The speed, accuracy, and reduction in space and personnel made possible by this equipment greatly improves the handling of all records.

The easy access of the central release office to records, together with its liaison with all manufacturing and packaging operations, makes it possible for this office to investigate customer complaints or inquiries on product quality. The results of these investigations are made available in the form of technical reports, which are forwarded to the sales organization for use in reply. Inquiries concerning the therapeutic or clinical performance of a product are referred to the medical section for reply by a physician. Whenever the investigation of a complaint reveals an aspect that provides a basis for improvement of a product, it is brought to the attention of the appropriate development group for consideration and action.

Complete and accurate records are maintained of the receipt and distribution of every lot of raw material and finished product. Further, in order to permit additional analyses, if necessary, retention samples of these products are held in locked areas, under conditions of storage comparable to those to which the finished products are subjected in the market. These retention samples are examined at regular intervals to check on the physical appearance of the lots that have been distributed in the market. Additionally, another collection of retention samples is held for periodic chemical or biological testing for stability of the active components of the preparations under study.

Inevitably, some finished packages are returned by community pharmacies and hospitals for one reason or another, and it is important that all such returns be properly recorded and handled. The disposition of returned goods, whether it be salvage or outright discard, should depend on consultation with the Quality-Control group, in order to assure the continued control of quality and distribution of all lots of every product.

Inspection and Checking—The responsibility for inspection and sampling of every shipment of raw materials received and every lot of finished goods turned over for distribution falls within the province of the Quality-Control Inspectors. The selection of samples of raw materials and finished goods is an important aspect of the quality-control function, since the work of many scientists, the expenditure of substantial sums of money, and the evaluation of the quality of manufactured goods may be directly affected by the suitability and adequacy of the sampling. This function should be performed under the supervision of alert individuals who have had experience in pharmacy and who are familiar with the physical characteristics of the materials they sample and well versed in sampling techniques. Such inspectors also examine every shipment of packaging supplies, which involves primarily the checking for conformity to those physi-

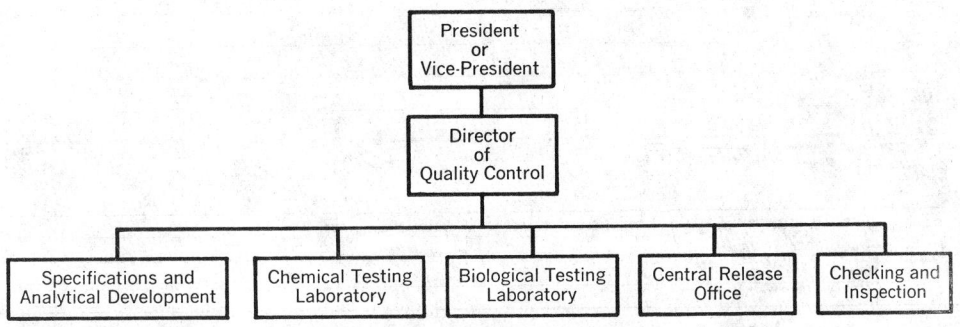

Fig. 767. Quality control organization chart (courtesy, Lederle).

cal characteristics that are important in packaging operations and in maintaining the integrity of the package contents. The inspectors are also responsible for examining and checking all manufacturing, filling, and labeling operations, as well as maintaining periodic examinations on the quality of inventories throughout all phases of storage, shipping, and distribution. These responsibilities of the inspectors are independent of the responsibilities of production and packaging personnel and consist of an independent audit of the work done by operational personnel.

The Control Functions

The fundamental aims of quality control and "good pharmaceutical practice" are identical. Both embrace the idea of building high quality into a product by the use of good raw materials and adherence to a rigid set of manufacturing controls at every step of the production cycle. It is important to recognize that the only way to achieve high quality is to manufacture a product correctly; it cannot be achieved merely by checking, examination, and testing.

Since the formal organization known as Quality Control consists of a relatively small group of individuals, it is impossible for them to check every operational step. Actually, the total control of quality is a plantwide activity. Every employee in a drug manufacturing company must be made aware that his future is directly associated with the quality of his work, and this in turn is reflected in the quality of the finished product. It is a cardinal function of quality control to keep the importance of this idea before every worker in the organization.

Raw Material Control—As each batch of incoming raw material is received, it should be given a Receiving Number by which it will be identified in subsequent operations. This number should have distinguishing characteristics, which will prevent possible confusion with any number previously placed on the container by the supplier.

A Receiving Tally Report should be prepared for every shipment received, indicating the Receiving Number, the date of receipt, the purchase order number, the vendor, the manufacturer's lot number, the receiving drug company's raw material code number, the name of the material, the quantity received (expressed as total weight), and the number of containers and weight of each. A typical Receiving Tally Report is shown in Fig. 768. If a shipment consists of more than one manufacturing lot number, a separate Receiving Number is assigned to each lot. The Receiving Tally Reports should be distributed to all groups within a company directly concerned with the purchase, inventory, use, and control of raw materials.

Each container of each shipment should be identified with the appropriate Receiving Number. All shipments are sampled by inspectors, and all containers sampled should be resealed with a special seal or with a special tape. These samples are then forwarded to the Central Release Office for distribution to the Chemical and/or Biological Testing laboratory to ascertain the conformity of the raw material to specifications.

Manufacturing Control—Upon receiving its copy of the Receiving Tally Report, the production group enters information about the material on a Raw Material Stock Record by code number, receiving number, name of item, total quantity, number and size of containers, date of receipt, vendor, vendor's lot number, and, if applicable, the expiration date. When all testing has been completed, the Central Release Office ascertains that each item in the specifications has been satisfactorily met before it notifies the production group of the acceptability of the raw material. A Quality Control Assay Report is shown

RECEIVING TALLY REPORT

DELIVER TO: Dept. 682-120
LOCATION CODE: Bldg. 120
PURCHASE ORDER NO.: PRT 4269
VENDOR: American Cyanamid-Bound Brook
DATE RECEIVED: 1/8/68 07-100
SHIPPED VIA: Oostdyk Truck Co. PPD 1 COLL X PRO NUMBER: P14152
CAR NUMBER:

ITEM CODE NO.	SUF.	ACCOUNT TO CHARGE	UNIT CODE	VENDOR LOT OR PRECODE NO.	RN NO.	CONTAINER BREAKDOWN	QUANTITY RECEIVED / DEC.	INVOICE AMOUNT	AN NO.
		DESCRIPTION							
		DESCRIPTION							
		DESCRIPTION							
		DESCRIPTION: Sulfadiazine USP							
1846			13	9487	A4802	20 X 50 kg			
		DESCRIPTION							
		DESCRIPTION							
		DESCRIPTION							

CONDITION OF SHIPMENT OR OTHER REMARKS: Containers and Contents Satisfactory — Sampled by Quality Control 1/12/68
CHECKER

QUALITY CONTROL SECTION — MATERIAL RELEASED ☒ Signature DATE 1/18/68 DEPT. 820 — CONDITIONAL RELEASE ☐ — MATERIAL REJECTED ☐ Reason Signature DATE DEPT.
ADDITIONAL INFORMATION

LPR 142-7 PT. REV. 7/67

Fig. 768. Receiving tally report (courtesy, Lederle).

QUALITY CONTROL ASSAY REQUEST

	ANALYTICAL NO.	CODE NO.	BATCH NO.	MATERIAL	POTENCY	MFG. DATE		EXP. DATE		F.O. NO.	
1	7J0726	1846	A4802	SULFADIAZINE USP		682		10000	8078A	01/08/68	G.Virga

	DEPT. CHARGE	COUNTRY	VENDOR	MONOGRAPH	DATE RECEIVED	REVIEWED BY

ACCT. CODE	DAYS TO TEST	DATE DUE	SAMPLE SIZE	RETENTION SIZE	BATCH SIZE/FILL WGT.	PRODUCT TYPE CODE	DISPOSITION	
1061013	5	01/17	1x60cc, 2x100cc	1x60cc	20x50 Kg.	x	1	01/18/68

DISPOSITION: 1,2,3,4-RELEASE 5-REPROCESS 6-REPORT 7-REFER TO FILE 8,9,0-REJECT

TEST DEPT. 822   SPECIAL INSTRUCTIONS

	NO.	ASSAY CODE	TEST FOR	RESULTS	SPECIFICATIONS	LINE CODE	# DET	HOURS	BADGE	W.S.	DATE
2	1	0001-	DESCRIPTION	WHITE, ODORLESS POWDER, FREE FROM FOREIGN MATTER.	WHITE OR SLIGHTLY YELLOW ODORLESS POWDER. FREE FROM FOREIGN MATTER.	10	01				01/16
3	5	3485	LOSS ON DRYING (105°C. 2 HRS.)	0.01%	NMT 0.50%.	10	02				01/16
3	7	9495	HEAVY METALS (NMT 20 PPM)	NMT 20 ppm	NMT 20 PPM.	10	01				01/16
3	8	2398-	SULFADIAZINE % DRY BASIS	100.1%	NLT 99.0% ON DRY BASIS.	10	02				01/16
3	9	9384-	FOREIGN MATTER (COMPRESSION METHOD)	FIVE WAFERS ARE SUBSTANTIALLY FREE FROM DIRT MOTTLING, SPOTS AND DISCOLORATION.	FIVE WAFERS ARE SUBSTANTIALLY FREE FROM DIRT MOTTLING, SPOTS AND DISCOLORATION.	10	01				01/16
3	10	9479	IDENTIFICATION (SULFADIAZINE)	POSITIVE	POSITIVE.	10	01				01/16
3	11	3471-	A.D.M.A. BULK DENSITY	6 cc/Gm.	NMT 6cc/Gm.	10	02				01/16

DEPT. 829

PREPARED BY	APPROVED BY	DATE 01/19/68	COMMENTS		COPY 1

Fig. 769. Quality control assay report (courtesy, Lederle).

WEIGHING ORDER

LABEL PRODUCT WITH THE PREFIX "S" DURING WEIGHING, GRANULATION, DUMPING, SCREENING AND BATCHING. UPON COMPRESSION REMOVE "S" AND LABEL TO AGREE WITH THE NUMBER ON THE PRODUCTION ORDER.

☐ Light   ☒ Heavy   PAGE 3 OF 15

PRODUCT NAME		FORMULA #	PRODUCT #	BATCH #
Sulfadiazine Tablets USP		USF #1	3919	211

BATCH SIZE	DEPT. #	DATE ISSUED	DATE COMPL.
1,200,000 Tablets	650	12/28/67	2-7-68

ITEM CODE	U/M CODE	CK.	INGREDIENT	Step	Part	QUANTITY		UNIT	R.N.	Weighed	Checked
1846	13	2540	Sulfadiazine USP	1	A	200	000	Gm.	A4802	8099	0980
1846	13	2540	Sulfadiazine USP	6	B	200	000	Gm.	A4802	8099	0980
1846	13	2540	Sulfadiazine USP	11	C	200	000	Gm.	A4802	8099	0980
46109	13	2540	Starch USP - Screened	1	A	13	400	Gm.	#305	9644	0980
46109	13	2540	Starch USP - Screened	6	B	13	400	Gm.	#305	9644	0980
46109	13	2540	Starch USP - Screened	11	C	13	400	Gm.	#305	9644	0980
			For Paste								
46109	13	2540	Starch USP - Screened	2	A	20	000	Gm.	#305	9644	0980
46109	13	2540	Starch USP - Screened	7	B	20	000	Gm.	#305	9644	0980
46109	13	2540	Starch USP - Screened	12	C	20	000	Gm.	#305	9644	0980
			For Batching								
46109	13	3783	Starch USP - Screened	19		21	006	Gm.	#305	9644	0980

I have checked the receiving number or lot number of every ingredient used herein and have ascertained that each number is correctly identified with its corresponding code number and title. I have further ascertained that all ingredients have been tested and released by Lederle's Quality Control Section.

Signed E. Shields Date 2/13/68
Quality Control Services Department

Fig. 770. Production order (courtesy, Lederle).

in Fig. 769. If a shipment of raw material is found to be unsatisfactory, the material is rejected and returned promptly to the vendor.

Production Orders, which have been prepared previously by the Production Formula Office, are sent to the proper production department for compounding. A page from a typical Production Order is shown in Fig. 770.

As the various ingredients are measured by weight or volume, the Receiving Number of each one is listed on the Production Order in a space provided opposite the name of the ingredient. The number of the batch of drug being processed and the amount of raw material used are entered on the Raw Material Stock Record. In general, it is well to have two individuals check the weight or volume of each ingredient in order to avoid errors.

The total weight or volume of each batch should be determined at various stages of the production cycles. In tablet production, for example, as the material passes from one processing area to the next, it should be weighed by the supervisor in the area releasing it and the weight verified by the supervisor in the area receiving it. The total weight of the finished tablets should be determined and checked against the weight of the material processed. Any discrepancy in weight at any point should be investigated and explained satisfactorily before processing is continued.

Assays should be made routinely at various steps in the manufacture of all types of products. If a tablet or capsule is being made, it is desirable to assay the blended ingredients prior to tableting or encapsulation to ascertain that the proper amount of all ingredients is present and uniformly distributed. The finished dosage form should be carefully checked for uniformity of weight, disintegration, and general appearance, in addition to the assay for the active ingredients. The first page of a typical Quality Control Assay Report is shown in Fig. 771, and an Assay Summary Sheet is shown in Fig. 772.

Each batch of each product manufactured should be subjected to the most careful scrutiny and testing possible. Nothing should be overlooked or taken for

SEND REPORT TO Pharmaceutical Production Section Technical Office

QUALITY CONTROL ASSAY REPORT

MATERIAL Sulfadiazine Tablets U.S.P.		ANALYTICAL NO.	
SUPPLIER		RECEIVING NO.	BATCH NO. 3919-211
P. R. NO.	CAR NUMBER	LOCATION OF MATERIAL	
POTENCY OR GRADE U.S.P.	NO. AND TYPE OF CONTAINER 51 Containers	TOTAL AMOUNT 1,174,800 Tablets	
CODE NO. OR RESEARCH PROJECT NO.	DATE NEEDED ASAP / DEPT. CHARGE 650	REQUESTED BY L. M. Paterson	DATE 2/7/68

NOTES FOR SPECIAL TESTS:

Quality Control Release of Bulk Lot.

DO NOT WRITE BELOW THIS LINE-RESERVED FOR LABORATORY REPORT

600 Tablets Examined
2 Spotted
2 Chipped
Total Defects less than 1%

INSPECTION FOR APPEARANCE
AND IDENTITY DEPT. 824
Satisfactory TM
2/7/68

SIGNED

DATE

LPR 511-5 PT. REV. 10/66

Fig. 771. Quality control assay report (courtesy, Lederle).

QUALITY CONTROL ASSAY REQUEST POTENCY MFG. DATE EXP. DATE F.O. NO.

1	ANALYTICAL NO. 8B0803	CODE NO. 3919	BATCH NO. 211	MATERIAL SULFADIAZINE TABLETS USP		DEPT. CHARGE 650	COUNTRY	VENDOR	MONOGRAPH 8549	DATE RECEIVED 02/08/68	REVIEWED BY (signature)
	ACCT. CODE 1041064	DAYS TO TEST 3	DATE DUE 02/12	SAMPLE SIZE B 1x60,1x100cc	RETENTION SIZE 1x200cc	BATCH SIZE/FILL WGT. 1,174,800	PRODUCT TYPE CODE b	DISPOSITION 1 (1,2,3,4-RELEASE 5-REPROCESS 6-REPORT)	7-REFER TO FILE 8,9,0-REJECT		DISPOSITION DATE 02/13/68
	TEST DEPT. 822	SPECIAL INSTRUCTIONS									

	NO.	ASSAY CODE	TEST FOR	RESULTS	SPECIFICATIONS	LINE CODE	# DET	HOURS	BADGE	W.S.	DATE
2	1	0001-	DESCRIPTION	ROUND CONVEX SCORED WHITE TABLETS 7/16 in. IN DIAMETER. NO TABLETS ARE CHIPPED, SPOTTED OR OFF COLOR.	ROUND CONVEX SCORED WHITE TABLETS 7/16 in. IN DIAMETER. NMT AN OCCASIONAL TABLET IS CHIPPED, SPOTTED OR OFF COLOR.	10	01				02/12
3	2	9368-	HARDNESS (10 tabs.) AVERAGE, HIGH, LOW	Kg. AVERAGE 7.4 HI 8.8 LO 6.0	AVERAGE NLT 5 kg. and NMT 12 kg. INDIVIDUAL MIN. 4 kg. MAX. 13 kg.	10	01				02/12
3	3	9376	DISINTEGRATION	7 MINUTES	MEETS REQUIREMENTS IN NMT 30 min. IN WATER AT 37°C	10	01				02/12
3	4	3447-	WEIGHT VARIATION (20 tabs.) AVERAGE WT., HIGH DEV., LOW DEV.	AVERAGE Gm. 0.6132 HI 2.0% LO 1.5%	NMT 2 tabs. DEVIATE BY MT 5% of AVERAGE NONE DEVIATE BY MT 10% of AVERAGE	10	01				02/12
3	5	9481	IDENTIFICATION (SULFADIAZINE) TEST A, B, C. MELTING RANGE	POSITIVE 252.5 to 253.1°C	POSITIVE	10	01				02/12
3	6	2398-	ASSAY (VOLUMETRIC)	505.2 mg./tab. 101.0% L.S.	NLT 475 mg. and NMT 525 mg. of SULFADIAZINE/TAB. (95.0-105.0% L.S.)	10	02				02/12

DEPT. 822

PREPARED BY | APPROVED BY (signature) | DATE 2/14/68 | COMMENTS A.M. | COPY 1

Fig. 772. Assay summary sheet (courtesy, Lederle).

granted. Quality Control inspectors should be free to examine all production operations, and it should be their duty to check housekeeping conditions, machinery, and equipment, in addition to checking the over-all appearance of products during all stages of manufacture. In the event of a difference of opinion on issues affecting the quality of a product, the supervisor of the inspectors should be called for consultation with the supervisor of the production department in question.

Packaging Control—All packaging supplies, including bottles, caps, vials, stoppers, and ointment tubes, should be examined carefully on receipt of each shipment. The Packaging Development laboratory within each company is generally responsible for the package specifications of each product. The inspectors in Quality Control are expected to work closely with the Packaging Development laboratory, the vendor of packaging supplies, and the Packaging department in establishing the tolerance limits for packaging supplies. A separate code number should be used to identify each type of packaging component, and many of the controls previously described for receiving of raw materials should be exercised also with packaging supplies.

On completing the production of a drug dosage form, a Finishing Order (Fig. 773) is sent to the Packaging department by the Production Planning department. The Finishing Order specifies by code number the various items of packaging supplies which are to be used in the packaging operations. Each item should be checked by a Quality Control inspector as well as by the Packaging department supervisor. Quality Control inspectors should also ascertain that the product being packaged is the one specified in the order, and that correct labels are being used. They should also make periodic checks throughout the packaging operations to be certain that filled containers have the proper volume, weight, or count, and that they are satisfactory in over-all appearance, including both the contents and the total packages.

Occasionally a final bulk preparation will undergo undesirable changes after release for packaging operations. It is the responsibility of the Quality Control inspectors to be alert for such changes and arrange for corrections prior to further processing.

After packaging operations have been completed the packaged drugs must be held until given a release for distribution by Quality Control. Tests involving identity, which are designed to differentiate the product in question from any other product produced by the manufacturer, constitute the most important of the final tests. Finally, a check is made of all the tests performed on the lot under consideration, and if these are satisfactory, the product is released for commercial distribution.

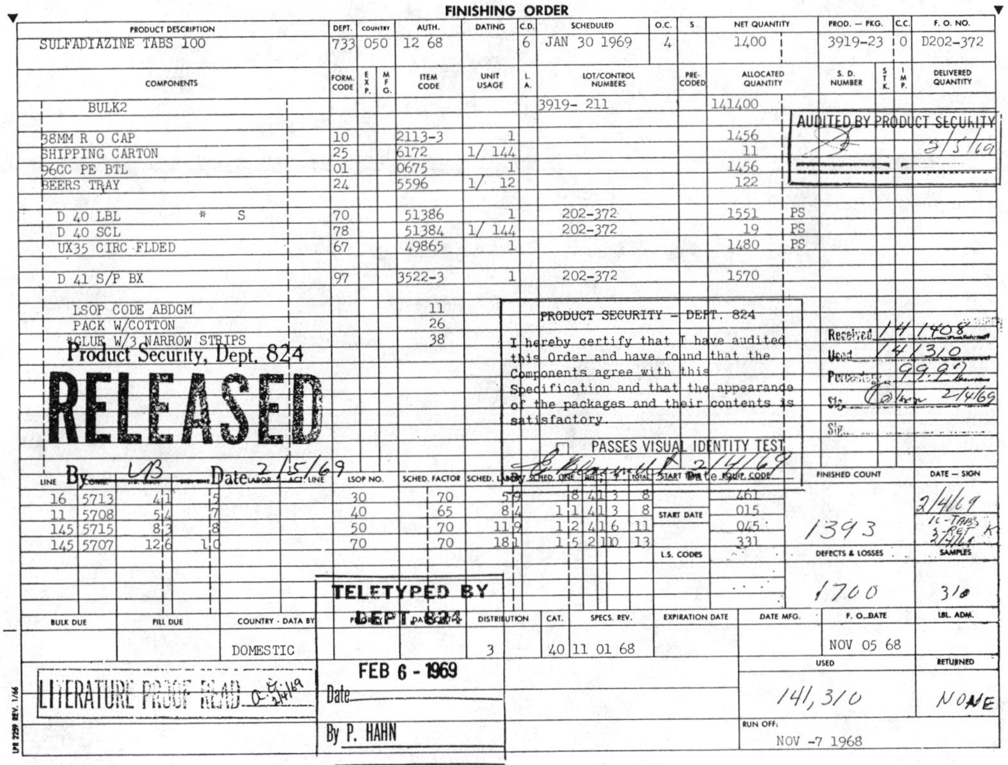
FINISHING ORDER

PRODUCT DESCRIPTION	DEPT.	COUNTRY	AUTH.	DATING	C.D.	SCHEDULED	O.C.	S	NET QUANTITY	PROD. – PKG.	C.C.	F. O. NO.
SULFADIAZINE TABS 100	733	050	12 68		6	JAN 30 1969	4		1400	3919-23	0	D202-372

COMPONENTS	FORM. CODE	ITEM CODE	UNIT USAGE	LOT/CONTROL NUMBERS	ALLOCATED QUANTITY	
BULK2				3919- 211	141400	
38MM R O CAP	10	2113-3	1		1456	
SHIPPING CARTON	25	6172	1/ 144		11	
96CC PE BTL	01	0675	1		1456	
BEERS TRAY	24	5596	1/ 12		122	
D 40 LBL * S	70	51386	1	202-372	1551	PS
D 40 SCL	78	51384	1/ 144	202-372	19	PS
UX35 CIRC FLDED	67	49865	1		1480	PS
D 41 S/P BX	97	3522-3	1	202-372	1570	
LSOP CODE ABDGM		11				
PACK W/COTTON		26				
*GLUE W/3 NARROW STRIPS		38				

AUDITED BY PRODUCT SECURITY 3/5/69

PRODUCT SECURITY – DEPT. 824
I hereby certify that I have audited this Order and have found that the Components agree with this Specification and that the appearance of the packages and their contents is satisfactory.
PASSES VISUAL IDENTITY TEST 2/4/69

Received 141408
Used 141310
Percentage 99.9
2/4/69

Product Security, Dept. 824
RELEASED
By LB Date 2/5/69

FINISHED COUNT 1393
DATE – SIGN 2/4/69
DEFECTS & LOSSES 1700
SAMPLES 31

TELETYPED BY DEPT. 824
FEB 6 - 1969
By P. HAHN

LITERATURE PROOF READ 2/4/69

COUNTRY – DATA BY: DOMESTIC
DISTRIBUTION: 3
CAT.: 40
SPECS. REV.: 11 01 68
F. O. DATE: NOV 05 68
USED: 141,310
RETURNED: NONE
RUN OFF: NOV -7 1968

Fig. 773. Finishing order (courtesy, Lederle).

Distribution Control—After products have been released for commercial distribution the responsibilities of Quality Control are not ended. A sample from each lot of drug distributed to the market is retained for several years, in order to examine or retest the material for any purpose deemed necessary. This retention sample is selected during packaging operations, and the packages are usually identical to those marketed, except when large size packages are involved. Storage conditions for the retention samples are identical to those recommended for the trade packages. The retention samples are inspected periodically for stability, since it is occasionally necessary to recall certain lots of material because of loss of potency or because of physical changes that are not acceptable.

Quality Control should be prepared to assume the responsibility of recommending, if and when necessary, the recall from distribution of any lots of product subsequently found to be unsuitable. The key by which the administrative control of each lot of product is maintained is the control numbering system. This involves the marking of each package of a manufactured lot of product with a control number, by which the manufacturer can establish the entire history of any given lot, including its distribution.

It is also the responsibility of Quality Control to make periodic checks of branch warehouses to oversee the storage and turnover of stock. The objective, of course, is to ascertain that the stock is satisfactory in every respect at the time it is distributed to the customer, and that it is fresh enough to remain satisfactory during the course of time it may reasonably be expected to be dispensed and administered.

Part IX

GENERAL PRACTICE

EDITOR

Richard A. Deno, PhD,[*] *Professor of Pharmacognosy, College of Pharmacy, University of Michigan, Ann Arbor, Mich. 48104*

* Deceased, October 30, 1969.

93 | Hospital Pharmacy

Education and training—the hospital's development and expansion, organization and administration, and financing—the hospital pharmacy's standards of practice and administration

This chapter was prepared by

Clifton J. Latiolais, MSc, *Director of Pharmacy, The Ohio State University Hospitals, Columbus, Ohio 43210*

Hospital Pharmacy may be defined as the practice of pharmacy in a hospital setting. It also may be defined as that department of the hospital wherein the procurement, preservation, storage, compounding, manufacturing, packaging, controlling, assaying, dispensing, and distribution of medications to hospitalized and ambulatory patients are performed by professionally competent and legally qualified pharmacists. Basically, this is also what the pharmacist in community practice does. Essentially, what then makes the practice of pharmacy in a hospital different from private or community practice?

Uniqueness of Hospital Pharmacy—A major factor is the organizational structure of a hospital: a formalized pattern of authority, responsibility, and coordination which affects every department of the over-all health care team. The administrator implements the policies and philosophies of the governing board; he delegates authority and passes on responsibility to department heads to carry out the patient care, teaching, research, and public health objectives of the hospital; department heads are expected to coordinate their services and activities with other department heads; the business and accounting department handles the financial affairs; the building services department provides the essential maintenance, housekeeping, and security functions; the personnel department implements personnel policies; dozens of other departments influence and affect the services of all hospital departments. All of these activities are brought to bear on the hospital pharmacy.

In addition to the traditional physician–pharmacist–patient relationship which exists in the private practice of medicine and pharmacy, there is a physician–pharmacist–nurse–patient relationship in the hospital. Between the physician–pharmacist roles the nurse interjects her professional role in the care of the patient. Thus the hospital pharmacist must work not only with the physician but also with the nurse since she administers practically all medication to patients in a hospital.

In addition to the internal forces operating within the hospital there are some external forces which affect, in various ways, the practice of pharmacy in the hospital setting. For example, accreditation agencies exert their influence on professional standards of practice as they affect patient care; licensing agencies exert legal influences on hospital operations; third party (hospitalization insurance) agencies exert their influence on the methods by which hospitals may be reimbursed for services rendered to patients; social agencies and governmental welfare agencies influence the services provided to medically indigent and totally indigent patients; the governing board and public opinion exert their influences over the policies, objectives, and philosophies of hospital operation and practice.

These are but a few examples of the socio-medico-economic and organizational forces acting on the practice of pharmacy in the hospital setting. These, among many others, are cogent reasons why hospital pharmacy practice differs significantly from community pharmacy practice.

The hospital pharmacy must be considered as one of the many departments of a hospital and as such it has several basic general functions. These functions have been outlined in a document approved by the American Hospital Association, a "Statement on Functions of a Hospital Department."[1] This Statement reads as follows:

"A department carries out its functions according to the philosophy and objectives of the hospital. The philosophy and objectives are established by the governing board. Accordingly, the department head is responsible to the administrator of the hospital. Within the organizational pattern, the functions of the department are:

1. To provide and evaluate service in support of medical care pursuant to the objectives and policies of the hospital.
2. To implement for departmental services the philosophy, objectives, policies, and standards of the hospital.
3. To provide and implement a departmental plan of administrative authority which clearly delineates responsibilities and duties of each category of personnel.
4. To participate in the coordination of the functions of the department with the functions of all other departments and services of the hospital.
5. To estimate the requirements for the department and to recommend and implement policies and procedures to maintain an adequate and competent staff.
6. To provide the means and methods by which personnel can work with other groups in interpreting the objectives of the hospital and the department to the patient and community.
7. To develop and maintain an effective system of clinical and/or administrative records and reports.
8. To estimate needs for facilities, supplies, and equipment and to implement a system for evaluation, control, and maintenance.
9. To participate in and adhere to the financial plan of operation for the hospital.
10. To initiate, utilize and/or participate in studies or research projects designed for the improvement of patient care and the improvement of other administrative and hospital services.
11. To provide and implement a program of continuing education for all personnel.
12. To participate in and/or facilitate all educational programs which include student experiences in the department.
13. To participate in and adhere to the safety program of the hospital."

It is within this framework that the hospital pharmacist practices his profession. The responsibility is his to develop pharmaceutical service comprehensive in scope and high in quality, properly coordinated to meet the needs of the numerous diagnostic and therapeutic departments, the nursing service, the medical staff, and the hospital as a whole in the interest of better patient care.

The remarkable development of the hospital system paralleled by the great achievements in medical science during the 20th century have made it necessary for hospital pharmacy to keep up with the ever-increasing demands being placed upon it. Hospital pharmacy has so developed in recent years that it has personnel with special education and training at the graduate level; it has its own vigorous professional society— The American Society of Hospital Pharmacists; it has been developing a useful body of specialized knowledge through its documented literature; it has developed a strong corps of well-qualified career hospital practitioners who have adopted a sound philosophy of professional service and have developed high standards of practice.

Education and Training—The setting within which the hospital pharmacist practices requires that he have special education and training if he is to function with maximum effectiveness. Unlike his colleague in community practice, the hospital pharmacist must function within an organization which has additional objectives beyond patient care *per se*. These objectives are education, research, and public health. In addition, there is another basic difference between the practice of pharmacy in a hospital and community pharmacy: the hospital in America is a nonprofit institution, while the community pharmacy must realize a net income over expense if it is to survive. This is not meant to imply that the community pharmacist should not realize a profit; on the contrary, the American free enterprise system is based on this philosophy. It does imply, however, that the hospital pharmacist, not necessarily by his own choosing, is in a fortunate position in that he does not need to concern himself with the profit motive; rather, he concerns himself primarily with the public good in the practice of his profession.

The hospital pharmacist must concern himself on a daily basis with professional contacts with other highly specialized and skillfully trained professionals. He meets with physician specialists on equal grounds in formal pharmacy and therapeutics committee meetings in all matters relating to drug therapy; he meets with the nursing profession constantly in his daily practice; he meets with bacteriologists, biochemists, and clinical chemists in regards to diagnostic medicine as it relates to drugs; he meets with physicists and radiologists in relation to radioactive medicaments, diagnostic agents, and contrast media; he meets with clinical pharmacologists and research physicians in matters relating to investigational drugs and drug reactions; he meets with specialists who have graduate degrees in medical sociology, medical record librarianships, medical dietetics, methods engineering, and hospital administration on a routine basis in the operation of a modern hospital pharmacy. Hospital pharmacists long recognized the need for additional education and training and developed internship and residency training programs to accomplish these ends. It was also recognized that additional education on a formal basis was desirable and some colleges of pharmacy developed master of science degree programs in hospital pharmacy. A number of colleges also offer a professional degree of doctor of pharmacy (Pharm D).

The American Association of Colleges of Pharmacy and The American Society of Hospital Pharmacists through a Joint Committee developed a *Statement on the Abilities Required of Hospital Pharmacists*.*[2] This statement outlines the following six abilities: (1) a thorough knowledge of drugs and their actions; (2) ability to develop and conduct a pharmaceutical

manufacturing program; (3) an intimate knowledge of control procedures; (4) ability to conduct and participate in research; (5) ability to conduct teaching and in-service training programs; and (6) ability to administer and manage a hospital pharmacy.

Hospital pharmacists long recognized the need for an additional period of supervised training after graduation from a college of pharmacy. Internship training programs in hospital pharmacy were developed in many hospitals. Since the internships were designed to train the hospital pharmacist beyond the basic requirements for licensure, the designation has been changed to "residency training in hospital pharmacy." Hospital pharmacists charged their national professional organization to develop an accreditation program based on the *Accreditation Standard for Residency in Hospital Pharmacy*.*[3] The standard outlines the qualifications of the training hospital, pharmacy service, preceptor, and applicant, as well as selection of applicant, residency training schedule, certification, and application for accreditation.

The Accreditation program, based on this Standard, is explained in the *Statement on Accreditation of Hospital Pharmacy Residency Programs*.*[4]

Colleges of Pharmacy have recognized the need for providing an educational program for students interested in hospital pharmacy. Most of the colleges offer an undergraduate course in hospital pharmacy, while a number of colleges offer a graduate educational program leading to a Master of Science degree in hospital pharmacy. Most of the graduate programs are coordinated so that the student serves a residency in a hospital pharmacy concurrently with his graduate work at the university. These combined programs started in 1947 at the Philadelphia College of Pharmacy and Science and the Jefferson Medical College Hospital, and at the University of Maryland and the John Hopkins Hospital; the University of Michigan initiated its combined program in 1948. These combined educational and training programs have contributed much to provide career-minded, well-trained hospital pharmacists. Graduates of such programs have gone into hospitals throughout the country and proved their capabilities through the development of a pharmaceutical service of broad scope and high quality.

Hospital pharmacists further recognized the need for continuing education as a result of the demands of professional practice. Such continuing educational programs are referred to as "Institutes." These institutes were initiated in 1946 as a cooperative venture between The American Hospital Association and The American Society of Hospital Pharmacists. Thousands of hospital pharmacists have attended the week-long institutes which are now conducted by the Department of Education and Training of The American Society of Hospital Pharmacists. The nature of this continuing education program for practitioners is embodied in the American Society of Hospital Pharmacists *Statement on Continuing Education*.*[5]

There is a trend toward specialization within hospital pharmacy. Hospital pharmacy residency training programs in years past have trained pharmacists primarily as generalists, with a so-called major in administration. While there is a place for the specialty of administrative hospital pharmacist, there is also the need for other specialists. Certainly, the drug-information specialty is developing into a key position in hospital pharmacy. The specialist in drug-distribution systems and unit-dose dispensing has emerged. The manufacturing and product develop-

* Available from the American Society of Hospital Pharmacists, 4630 Montgomery Ave., Washington, D.C. 20014.

ment specialist is also needed for investigational-drug studies and for product formulations to meet new medical and surgical techniques, such as kidney, heart, and other organ transplants. There is a need also for a radiopharmaceutical specialist to handle, prepare, and formulate new dosage forms, and to conduct research on the large number of diagnostic and therapeutic radioactive pharmaceutical preparations available today. There is a need for a research specialist to participate in the wide variety of challenging research opportunities in hospital pharmacy.

Thus, we see a healthy trend developing toward so-called "group practice" in hospital pharmacy, analogous to group medical practice. A number of these specialists in different areas of hospital pharmacy practice make up the team of pharmacists in today's progressive hospital. It is the advancement of this concept which will strengthen the professional role of the hospital pharmacist and which will give him entry to the group of specialists who make up the health-care team.

The Hospital

The hospital pharmacist must practice within the framework of an organizational structure called a hospital. In order for him to function effectively, it is essential that he understand thoroughly what a hospital is, how it is organized, what its functions are and how the pharmacy service fits into the over-all program.

Definition—Traditionally, a hospital has been defined in terms of its *form;* that is, its physical makeup and the quantitative nature of its services. This definition is best exemplified by the "registration of hospitals program" of the American Hospital Association. In order to be registered under this program an institution must meet certain requirements which constitute the definition of a hospital. Thus, the program differentiates between a hospital and other institutions such as extended-care facilities, convalescent homes, and homes for the aged.

The American Hospital Association's *Requirements for Accepting Hospitals for Registration*[6] serve as a comprehensive definition of a hospital and are as follows:

1. The hospital shall have at least six beds for the care of patients who are nonrelated, who are sick, and who stay on the average in excess of 24 hours per admission.
2. The hospital shall be constructed, equipped, and maintained to insure the safety of the patients, and shall provide uncrowded and sanitary facilities for the treatment of individuals accepted for care.
3. Doctors of medicine, doctors of osteopathy, and doctors of dentistry may admit patients to the hospital. (Patients admitted to the hospital by doctors of dentistry must have an admission history and physical examination done by a doctor of medicine or doctor of osteopathy on the staff of the hospital, and the doctor of medicine or doctor of osteopathy shall be responsible for the patient's medical care throughout his stay.)
4. There shall be an organized medical staff (which may include doctors of osteopathy and of dentistry) governed by bylaws adopted by said staff and approved by the governing board of the hospital.
5. The hospital shall submit evidence of regular care of the patient by a doctor of medicine, doctor of osteopathy, or doctor of dentistry and of general supervision of the clinical work by doctors of medicine.
6. Records of clinical work shall be maintained by the hospital on all patients and shall be available for reference.
7. Registered nurse supervision and such other nursing service as is necessary to provide patient care round the clock shall be available at the hospital.
8. The hospital shall offer services more intensive than those required merely for room, board, personal services, and general nursing care.
9. Minimal surgical or obstetrical facilities (including operating or delivery room), or relatively complete diagnostic facilities and treatment facilities for all patients, shall be available at the hospital.
10. Diagnostic x-ray services shall be regularly and conveniently available.
11. Clinical laboratory services shall be regularly and conveniently available.

On the other hand, a hospital may be defined in terms of its broad *purpose* or *mission* instead of its physical form. The contemporary hospital is a community institution which is an instrument of society. It serves as the citadel or focal point for the coordination and delivery of patient care to its community. A hospital may be viewed as an organized structure which pools together all the health professions, the diagnostic and therapeutic facilities, equipment and supplies, and the physical facilities into a coordinated system for delivering health care to the public.

While the hospital was once considered only as a place where patients were treated, today it is considered as a viable institution which extends its services to the patient wherever he may be located. For example, hospitals provide services to patients: within the institution itself (hospitalized patients), in outpatient clinics and emergency rooms, in physicians' offices at hospitals, in extended-care facilities and nursing homes either affiliated with or owned by the hospital, at home who require home health-care services, at community or neighborhood health clinics.

Certain other definitions are required for proper understanding of the differences between hospitals and patient-care institutions other than hospitals. In its accreditation program the Joint Commission on Accreditation of Hospitals (JCAH) divides *Extended-Care Facilities* into three categories; (1) extended care, (2) nursing care and (3) resident care. These categories are defined as follows:[7]

Extended-Care Facilities—"Establishments with organized medical staff and with continuous professional nursing service that are established to provide comprehensive inpatient care (which is usually postacute hospital care), for the most part of relatively short duration, and to serve convalescent patients who are not in an acute episode of illness or in a stable stage of illness and who have a variety of medical conditions."

Nursing-Care Facilities—"Establishments with medical staffs or a medical staff equivalent and with continuous nursing service under professional nurse direction. They provide, usually, long-term inpatient care (not necessarily posthospital) to patients who have a variety of medical conditions requiring service."

Resident-Care Facilities—"Establishments providing safe, hygienic, sheltered living for residents not capable of or desiring independent living. They furnish regular and frequent but not continuous medical and nursing services and they furnish continuous supportive, restorative, and preventive health services."

A *clinic* is an establishment where ambulatory patients are admitted for special study and treatment by a group of physicians practicing together, and where the patient is not confined as in a hospital. The term *clinic* is also used to indicate the outpatient diagnostic facility operated by a hospital and also facilities operated by other agencies for the care of indigent and medically indigent patients. In the past the term clinic has usually been reserved for facilities of a teaching nature where medical students or intern or resident staff offered treatment to patients unable to afford private practitioners. This concept has changed in recent years with the growing trend of physicians to locate their offices in or adjacent to the hospital, and a so-called private outpatient service has been added to the regular clinic facilities.

Development and expansion—Hospitals had their origin in Indian and Egyptian culture during the sixth century B.C. Evolution of the hospital is related to the sociological development of the individual's expansion of interest beyond himself and his family to the welfare of the community. Although early hospitals were really places to remove people from society to protect society, ie, the insane, the incurables, and the contagious, other hospitals were developed through religious and divine motives. The temples of the gods in early Greek and Roman civilization were used as hospitals where healing was associated with divine powers, while continued illness or death was associated with a lack of purity. Greek temples were forerunners of the modern hospital in the sense that they provided refuge and treatment for the sick and also provided for the teaching of young medical students. Such temples as the Temple of Aesculapius (Greek god of Medicine) existed in 1134 B.C., while the temple at Kos, Greece was where Hippocrates (born about 460 B.C.) practiced.

One of the dominant factors in the development and expansion of hospitals was the religious influence. Prior to the Christian era, hospitals were temples dedicated to the god of medicine in which care of the sick was accompanied by magical, mystical, and religious ceremonies. The doctrines of Jesus Christ intensified the emotions and virtues of love, pity, and charity. These strong motivating forces toward one's fellow man gave impetus to the expansion of hospitals.

Another major factor in the development and expansion of hospitals devolves from a military influence. Much of the impetus toward medical and surgical progress over the centuries has come from the urgent need for care of the wounded on the battlefield. This was true during the Roman empire; it was also true in the United States before, during, and after the Civil War. The Civil War, however, focused attention on the inadequacy of hospital construction and also on the lack of nursing care. Lincoln requested Catholic Sisters to care for wounded army personnel because hospital care was so poor. The work done in the army set a pattern for improvement in patient care and combined the military and religious influence on hospital development.

Other factors which have influenced the development and expansion of hospitals were: (1) the Flexner report on medical education (1910) which caused revolutionary developments in medical education *per se* and in medical internship training which helped the development of minimum standards for patient care in hospital surroundings, (2) the activities of Florence Nightingale during and after the Crimean War which served as the basis for revolutionizing the quality of nursing care in hospitals and for the development of schools of nursing, and (3) the public interest in hospitals through greater dependence and improved confidence in hospital care. With public dependence and confidence came public support and this support provided the finances for further development, expansion, and improvement in hospital facilities. This public interest extended its influence into private hospitalization insurance and into government participation in health care through social security and other health-related agencies. One of the most significant governmental programs which has affected the development and expansion of hospital facilities in the United States was the adoption (in 1946) by the Congress of the Hospital Survey and Construction Act. Commonly known as the Hill–Burton program, this act was passed to provide federal funds for hospital construction on a matching basis with local communities. Since 1946 hundreds of new hospitals have been built while hundreds of other hospitals have undertaken major expansion programs of existing facilities through the availability of government finances through the Hill–Burton Act.

Since that time a number of legislative amendments have been adopted by the Congress which made funds available for construction and improvement of various health-care facilities, including medical and nursing schools, outpatient facilities, extended-care facilities, and specialized diagnostic and therapeutic facilities in hospitals. In addition, the Social Security Amendments of 1965 (Medicare) will have a long-range impact on the development and expansion of hospitals because funds are made available to pay for services of medically indigent patients lacking means to pay hospitals for services rendered.

The first hospital on the American continent was built by the Spaniards (led by Cortez) in 1524—The Hospital of the Immaculate Conception in Mexico City. In 1663 it's name was changed to The Hospital of Jesus of Nazareth and it still exists today. In the American colonies a hospital was built in 1663 on Manhattan Island for sick soldiers. The first incorporated hospital in the United States was the Pennsylvania Hospital, established in 1751 through the efforts of Dr. Thomas Bond to provide physicians in Philadelphia with a place to treat their private patients. In 1769 New York, with a population of 300,000, had no hospital. Since 1873 the population of the United States has more than doubled but the number of hospitals has increased 44 times—from only 149 to approximately 7000.

Beyond the three basic essentials of human existence (food, clothing, and shelter) the hospital has become a necessary instrument for providing a fourth basic element of survival—health. The hospital serves as a major instrument through which the health professions are able to provide health to the people of the community. It is because of the increasing complexity of health care—diagnostic, preventive, and therapeutic—that the necessary trained personnel in the health services and the facilities and equipment being made available through our dynamic technologic industry are consolidated into what is known as the hospital in order to provide the quality of care the public expects, demands, and deserves.

Classification—Hospitals may be classified in different ways, by:

1. type of service
2. length of stay
3. ownership
4. bed capacity

Hospitals are classified by *type of service* as either general or special hospitals. A general hospital provides care to patients with any type of illness: medical, surgical, pediatric, and maternity. On the other hand, special hospitals are those which restrict the care they provide to special conditions, such as tuberculosis, cancer, maternity, or psychiatric.

Hospitals are classified by *length of stay* as either short-term or long-term. A short-term hospital is one in which the average length of stay of the patient is less than 30 days. Patients with acute disease conditions and emergency cases are usually hospitalized for less than 30 days. On the other hand, a long-term hospital is one in which the average length of stay of the patient is 30 days or more. Such patients have long-term illnesses such as tuberculosis, cancer, or psychiatric conditions. Usually general hospitals are also short-term, because acutely ill patients usually recover in a shorter period of time than 30 days, while special hospitals by the very nature of the disease conditions which they treat are usually long-term hospitals. There are exceptions to this, however. For example, a pediatrics hospital is a special hospital but it normally is a short-term rather than a long-term hospital.

Hospitals are classified by *ownership* usually as governmental or nongovernmental. Hospitals falling into these categories of ownership are as follows:

Governmental Hospitals	Nongovernmental Hospitals
Federal (Armed Forces, Veterans Administration & US Public Health Service)	Nonprofit Church related or operated Other nonprofit
State	For profit
County	Individual
City (municipal)	Partnership
City-County	Corporation
Hospital district	

Hospitals are generally classified by *bed capacity* according to the following pattern:

Under 50 beds
50– 99 beds
100–199 beds
200–299 beds
300–399 beds
400–499 beds
500 beds & over

According to these four general classifications, the approximately 7000 hospitals in the United States are 80% nongovernmental, short-term, general or special; roughly half are under 100 beds.

The 7000 hospitals represent approximately 1,700,000 beds, admit about 30 million patients annually, and service approximately 150 million outpatient visits per year.

Federal hospitals are owned and operated by various branches of the Federal Government. The US Army and Navy hospitals are usually general medical and surgical hospitals, provided to care for military personnel, although there are specialized mental institutions within these groups. The Veterans Administration and Public Health Service hospitals provide care for additional specialized groups of our population, and operate general medical and surgical hospitals, and also some mental hospitals. The Public Health Service, in addition to its general hospitals, operates a hospital for the treatment of lepers (Carville, La.) and a hospital for the treatment of narcotic addicts (Lexington, Ky.).

State hospitals are owned by the state and controlled by a board of control or division of the state government, or a similar organization responsible to state government. They are maintained by state appropriations, and consist mainly of mental, nervous, and tuberculosis hospitals. In some instances, state hospitals are general hospitals affiliated with a university.

County hospitals are owned by the county and are financed and controlled similarly to state hospitals, only on a county level. They are usually general hospitals caring for the indigent sick, although they may be mental, tuberculosis, chronic, or communicable disease hospitals.

City hospitals are owned by the city and financed and controlled similarly to state hospitals, only on a city level of responsibility. They are usually general hospitals, caring for the indigent sick, although there may be a chain of city-owned and operated hospitals encompassing, as in New York City, hospitals for mental, neurological, and tubercular patients and also for alcoholics and other addicts.

In the nongovernmental hospital group, the majority of institutions are general medical and surgical hospitals, varying only in their control and their eligibility for receipt of state funds for charity or indigent patient care. The *proprietary* or *private hospital organized for profit* is usually a corporation composed of physicians, although other businessmen may be involved in the corporate profit-making structure. This type hospital is not eligible for state aid and does not usually provide free care. There are approximately 1000 proprietary hospitals in the United States.

In the *nonprofit*, nongovernmental grouping of hospitals, some are *church hospitals*, supported financially by fees from paying patients or by contributions from the several religious orders or churches. These hospitals are owned and controlled either by the religious order, as in the Catholic churches, or by a separate governing board, as in churches of all other denominations.

Community hospitals or private nonprofit hospitals are owned and operated by members of the community, but with no relationship to the local government. They are financed by fees from patients and by subscriptions from residents of the community and surrounding area. The cost of providing medical care for the indigent is a problem for the community hospital that is met through state assistance.

Functions—Traditionally, the hospital's basic purpose for existence has been the treatment and care of the sick and injured. In conjunction with this basic function, hospitals have been concerned with teaching, particularly of medical students, ever since the pre-Christian era of Greek medicine. Research has been another function of the hospital. In modern times a fourth function has been assumed by hospitals, namely, public health. Thus the four fundamental functions of hospitals are patient care, teaching, research, and public health.

Patient Care—The modern hospital is charged with maintaining and restoring health to the community which it serves. The other three functions are really the handmaidens of patient care since they exist only because they contribute either directly or otherwise to the care of the sick and injured. Emergency care of the injured commands prime attention in any hospital—fully as important as the care of the inpatient. Outpatient care, although becoming more important as a function of the hospital's responsibility to the community, is usually subordinate to inpatient and emergency care. Patient care involves the diagnosis and treatment of illness or injury, preventive medicine, rehabilitation, convalescent care, dental care, and personalized services.

In providing patient care, hospitals usually have two basic types of accommodations based on the patient's ability to pay, namely the full-pay or private patient and the partially or totally medical indigent (charity) patient. With the marked increase in prepaid hospitalization insurance (through commercial insurance carriers and Blue Cross) there has been a great increase in the number of private (or semiprivate) patients. The Federal government's involvement with medical care through Medicare and Medicaid expands coverage for a broad population group who previously were partially or totally medical indigents, including nonindigent groups.

Education—Education is an important function of the modern hospital whether it is or is not affiliated with a university. Education as a hospital function is of two major forms:

    1. Education of the medical and paramedical professions. This form includes physicians; nurses; medical social service workers; medical record librarians; dieticians; x-ray and laboratory technicians; medical technologists; inhalation, physical and occupational therapists; hospital administrators; hospital pharmacists; and others. The hospital's educational program for these groups includes formal programs (such as medical and nursing schools), in-service training programs for professional personnel such as internships and residencies, and on the job training programs for non-professional personnel. Such educational programs are essential; it is only in a hospital that facilities are available to provide the necessary practical learning experience for dealing with the saving of human life.

    2. Education of the patient. This form is an important hospital function the scope of which is seldom realized by the public. It includes providing general education for children confined to long-term hospitalization; special education in the area of rehabilitation—psychiatrically, socially, physically, and occupationally; and special education in health care, for example, teaching a diabetic or a cardiac patient to care for his ailment or teaching the colostomy patient who requires a reorientation in caring for his personal needs.

Research—Hospitals carry out research as a vital function for two major purposes: the advancement of medical knowledge against disease and the improvement of hospital services. Both purposes are directed toward the basic aim of better health care for the patient. Examples of research activities in the hospital include devising new diagnostic procedures, conducting laboratory and clinical experiments, developing and perfecting new surgical procedures and techniques, and evaluating investigational drugs. Other examples include research to improve administrative procedures for greater efficiency and for lower cost to the patient, improvement of accounting procedures for more equitable cost distribution of services, and designing, developing, and evaluating new equipment and facilities for providing better patient care. Research in hospitals has been carried on primarily by medical staffs in the past. However, in recent years there has been a significant increase in research activities in the various hospital departments by other than medical personnel. Nursing, for example, is now engaged in significant research activities designed to improve patient care. Although pharmacy has played a limited role in hospital research in the past, there are signs of increasing activity in this area. For example, any drug must be tested in a hospital before it is marketed, and thus the clinical evaluation of investigational drugs presents many opportunities for the hospital pharmacist to participate in research.

Public Health—The prime objective of this fourth and relatively new hospital function is to assist the community in reducing the incidence of sickness and to increase the general health of the population. Examples of public health activities are the close working relationships many hospitals have with public health departments of communicable diseases; the participation in disease detection programs as for tuberculosis, diabetes, and cancer; the participation in mass public innoculation programs such as against influenza and poliomyelitis; and the participation of hospital outpatient departments in teaching better routine hygienic practices, as well as ways in which patients should care for themselves when illness strikes. Hospital pharmacists have an opportunity to contribute to this function by providing health information brochures and services to outpatients and by instructing them on the safe use of drugs and on poison prevention measures.

Standards of Practice—In the United States the public is able to determine whether a hospital provides a minimum quality of patient care through its "accreditation" status. The accreditation program is conducted on a national basis and its purpose is to determine the quality of care rendered to patients. This is achieved through the establishment of minimum standards of quality of patient care and then to invite all hospitals to meet or surpass these standards by improving their services and facilities.

The Accreditation program is carried out by the Joint Commission on the Accreditation of Hospitals (JCAH). This is an independent, voluntary, non-profit corporation made up of representatives (commissioners) from and financed by the following organizations:

American College of Physicians	3 members
American College of Surgeons	3 members
American Medical Association	7 members
American Hospital Association	7 members
American Association of Homes for the Aging	1 member
American Nursing Home Association	1 member
	22 members

The Joint Commission is independent and its actions are not subject to ratification by the organizations represented by its component members. One of its objectives is to make known to the public the names of those hospitals which have invited its scrutiny and have been accredited by it through meeting the minimum standards established for good patient care. The net effect of the program is to enable the public to discriminate between hospitals that are accredited and those that are not.

Accreditation of hospitals began in 1918 when The American College of Surgeons initiated its hospital standardization program. The purpose was to elevate the quality of surgical care provided in hospitals. The program involved setting up minimum standards of practice for the operating rooms, but it also pointed up the need for similar standards in all departments of the hospital. The first list of approved hospitals, published in 1919, contained 89 approved hospitals out of 692 surveyed. Today approximately 5000 of the 7000 hospitals are accredited. The American College of Surgeons standardization program was taken over by the Joint Commission on Accreditation of Hospitals in 1953.

During the years the American College of Surgeons carried out the accreditation program, the pharmacy was not included among the essential divisions of the hospital but, rather, was listed as a complementary division. The Joint Commission on Accreditation of Hospitals continued this classification for several years. However, in 1956 the pharmacy department was included among the essential services of the hospital and thus official recognition was given to the importance of the pharmacy. In 1965 the JCAH amended its standards for medical staff functions by requiring a pharmacy and therapeutics committee. Previously, the JCAH had only considered this committee to be a desirable one rather than an essential committee.

Another major impetus to the development of standards of practice in hospitals came about with the enactment of the Social Security Amendments of 1965 (Medicare). This law sets forth certain conditions which hospitals are required to meet for purposes of participating as providers of services in the Health Insurance for the Aged program. These requirements are published as a manual entitled, *Conditions of Participation—Hospitals.** This manual includes the conditions of participation for the various departments of the hospital, including the pharmacy department. These conditions have played a major role in challenging small hospitals to consider appointing pharmacists to their staffs and to establish pharmacy and therapeutics committees.

Organization and Administration—No matter what the type of organization and control of a hospital there is always a governing body of some sort to which the administrator, director, superintendent, medical director, chief administrative officer, or whatever the individual be titled must report. In the case of the Federal hospitals, this is usually not a group on a local area level. In state, county, and city hospitals the governing body is usually from the political subdivision in which the hospital is located, but need not be so where persons of special ability are concerned or in cases where political pressure is applied. In the nonprofit, nongovernmental hospital, there is usually a governing board, board of trustees, board of governors, or other titled group which assumes over-all responsibility for the proper operation of the hospital so that adequate service can be rendered to the sick and injured at as low a cost as is compatible with efficiency. In some hospitals there is also a second board advisory to the governing board, aimed at providing greater representation of the community in the operation of the hospital. This advisory board is controlled by the governing board, however.

Specifically, the duties of the governing board, performed through the chief administrative officer, are the responsibility for selection of competent personnel including the medical staff, the control of hospital funds, and the supervision of the physical plant. By reason of recent court decisions the responsibility for injury or other act by a member of the hospital staff on the hospital grounds reverts back to the governing board, although the individual hospital personnel is involved.

The governing body, acting on recommendations of the chief administrative officer, must establish the working hours and conditions, salary schedules, and proper checks on personnel. Again, acting on the recommendations of the chief administrative officer, the governing board must establish a schedule of room rates and other charges for hospital inpatient and outpatient care. The board must devise methods for obtaining endowments and other grants that will supplement income from paying patients and help to balance the hospital budget. The board must wisely invest endowment funds and other grants from which the interest is to be used for operating or other expenses. It must make certain that there is established an adequate accounting system and provide for routine audit of the accounts. This board must determine the needs for additional or replacement construction of the physical plant of the hospital and must contract with the most advantageous bidder.

The governing board has its own internal organization, comprised of a president or chairman, vice-chairman, secretary, and treasurer. On many boards the chief administrative officer of the hospital serves as secretary. There are usually certain standing committees appointed, such as the executive committee;

the house or hospital committee dealing with personnel appointments and especially those of the medical staff, and with other activities of departmental nature; the finance committee which is concerned with the hospital budget, room rates, and other financial matters; a nursing committee concerned with the operation of this important service and with nursing education; and a committee on public relations which is concerned with educating the community on the value of the hospital and with maintaining a desirable relationship with the community. There may be other committees appointed as the need arises such as an expansion and development committee where the hospital is concerned with the need for construction of additional hospital beds.

The chief administrative officer of the hospital is directly responsible to the governing board. He is appointed by this board and must produce a two-way channel of communication between the board and the hospital staff and personnel insofar as the needs or desires of both are concerned. He is often the secretary of the governing board, but if not, he is a member of the board and reports to it all essential facts concerning the operation of the hospital and receives from the board all directives it issues. The hospital administrator must have initiative and leadership as well as supervisory ability in order to carry out the details of his responsibility. He must see that all functions of professional care of the patient are carried on within budgetary limitations, and that there is interdepartmental cooperation and harmony.

In order for the administrator to carry out the over-all responsibilities assigned by the governing board he needs assistance. Depending on the site of the hospital he may appoint one or more assistant administrators. He also appoints heads of departments. To the department heads he turns over the responsibility (with commensurate authority) to operate the departments effectively and properly, within the over-all policies and philosophies established by the hospital's governing board.

Among the many departments which make up the modern hospital there are some in which the services involve primarily the *professional care* of the patient while the services of other departments involve mainly the *business management* of the hospital.

Some of the departments which deal with the professional care of the patient (diagnostic or therapeutic) are as follows:

Anesthesia	Medical Records
Blood Bank	Medical Social Service
Central Sterile Supply	Nurseries
Clinical Laboratories	Nursing Service
Delivery Room	Occupational Therapy
Dental Service	Operating Room
Dietary	Out Patient Service
Electrocardiograph Laboratory	Pharmacy Service
Electroencephalograph Laboratory	Physical Medicine
Emergency Room	Post Operative Recovery Room
Inhalation (Oxygen) Therapy	Radioisotopes Laboratory
Medical Library	Radiology & X-Ray Therapy

Departments which deal with the business management or administrative side of the hospital include:

Accounting	Housekeeping
Admitting	Information Service
Business Office	Personnel & Payroll
Cafeteria & Coffee Shop	Post Office
Central Transportation	Purchase & Supply
Credit & Collection	Telephone Switchboard
Data Processing Service	Volunteer Service
Engineering & Maintenance	

---

* Available from the US Dept. of Health, Education, and Welfare, Social Security Admin., Washington, D.C.

The Medical Staff—The medical staff of a hospital falls in a different category organizationally than the departments listed previously. Physicians are independent agents taking care of their patients and they utilize the hospital, its departments, facilities, and services to care for these patients. The governing board of the hospital and the community which it represents exercise effective control over the medical staff. Although the governing board neither originates nor implements medical policy it is responsible for it, and while the board members are not competent to pass judgment on the professional care of the patient they are, as representatives of the ownership of the hospital, liable for dereliction of duties established by law. Thus the board delegates a portion of its duties and responsibilities to its appointed medical staff to originate medical policy honestly and to carry out this policy in good faith. To do this requires that the medical staff be organized to govern itself and appraise its own work, and yet be responsible to the governing board for the details of its work.

In order for a physician to be appointed to the medical staff of a hospital, normally he must make an application for membership. His application along with his credentials are considered by the credentials committee of the medical staff which determines whether he is competent to practice in his claimed specialty. The Credentials Committee, if favorably impressed, makes its recommendation to the medical staff for appointment. Assuming this is approved, the recommendation goes to the governing board for final approval. Upon approval of the board the physician is designated a member of the medical staff of the hospital for a specified period of time, usually 1 year, subject to renewal.

The organized medical staff of a hospital has certain duties: (1) providing professional care of the sick and injured in the hospital, (2) maintaining its own efficiency, (3) self-government, (4) participating in the educational program of the hospital, (5) auditing its own professional work, and (6) advising and assisting the administrator and the governing board regarding medical policies.

There are two main types of hospital staffs, the *open* and the *closed*. An *open* staff is one in which certain physicians other than those on the attending or active medical staff are allowed to utilize the private room facilities, providing they comply with all rules and regulations of the institution. These physicians are termed members of the "courtesy" medical staff; the hospital is termed an *open staff* hospital.

A *closed* staff is one in which all professional services, private and charity, are provided and controlled by the attending or active medical staff. A hospital with this type of staff is termed a *closed staff* hospital. The closed staff, though it has minor drawbacks, is the more desirable for the average hospital and especially for the teaching hospital, because it allows careful selection of a group of specialists with excellent reputation.

The medical staff consists of the following groups: (1) an honorary staff, (2) a consulting staff, (3) an active staff, (4) an associate staff, (5) a courtesy staff, and (6) a resident staff. The *honorary medical staff* is composed of physicians who have been active in the hospital but who are retired, and of those to whom it is desired to do honor because of outstanding contributions. The *consulting medical staff* consists of specialists who are recognized as such by right of passing specialty boards or belonging to the national organization of their specialty, and who serve as consultants to other members of the medical staff when called upon. The *active* or *attending medical staff* is the group primarily concerned with care of the indigent sick. It is the group most actively interested in the hospital. In internal staff government it is the authoritative body. The *associate medical staff* is composed of junior or less experienced members of the staff. Appointment to this group is the first step toward active or attending staff membership. The *courtesy medical staff* consists of those physicians who desire the privilege of attending private patients but who do not desire active staff membership. The *resident medical staff* is composed of residents and interns, who are full-time employees of the hospital. These persons provide specific services in the care of the patient, for which they receive education and experience.

The clinical departments of the hospital are usually three in number: (1) Department of Medicine, (2) Department of Surgery, and (3) Department of Obstetrics and Gynecology.

The Department of Medicine may be subdivided into specialty services as follows:

Allergy	Hematology
Cardiology	Internal Medicine
Communicable Diseases	Pediatric Medicine
Dermatology	Preventive Medicine
Endocrinology	Psychiatry & Neurology
Gastroenterology	Pulmonary Diseases
Geriatrics	Renal Diseases

The Department of Surgery may be subdivided into specialty services as follows:

Anesthesiology	Otolaryngology
General Surgery	Pediatric Surgery
Neurosurgery	Plastic Surgery
Ophthalmology	Proctology
Oral Surgery	Thoracic Surgery
Orthopedic Surgery	Urology

The Department of Obstetrics and Gynecology may be subdivided into specialty services as follows:

Care of the Newborn
Gynecology
Obstetrics

There are other specialties which are classified as clinical departments in some hospitals. These are the Department of General Practice, the Department of Pathology, and the Department of Physical Medicine and Rehabilitation. Radiology may also be designated as a separate clinical department.

Financing Hospital Care—The technological developments of our industrialized society and the rapid advances of the medical sciences annually increase the financial burdens of hospitals. Hospitals, in order to provide the best care available, at the insistence of the public must keep up with these advances by obtaining the newest diagnostic and therapeutic equipment, facilities, and products. In addition, the increasing cost of labor is reflected in the increased cost of the personalized services made available in the modern hospital. The cost of hospital care is a direct reflection of these developments. In 1947 the total cost of operating all US hospitals was $2.4 billion; by 1967 the total cost had reached $16.4 billion.

Perhaps the most widely used statistic to describe hospital costs is the total expense per patient day. In 1952 the average cost per patient day in nonfederal general and special hospitals was $18.35; in 1962 the cost per patient day averaged $36.83, while in 1967 it increased to $54.99. With the trend toward more equitable salaries for hospital personnel, there is every indication that hospital costs will continue to rise dramatically.

For centuries hospitals have struggled with the problem of finances adequate to cover total operating expenses. The fact that, basically, the public does not care to pay for something it does not want has been a major factor in this struggle for financial survival. Individuals resist having to pay hundreds of dollars for an operation or a long hospital stay which they do not want. At one time hospitals were a place where people went to die; the public cared little about their financial struggles. But as the hospital developed into a place where people went to get well the public took a more positive interest in the financial problems. In other words, the public has come to recognize that although it dislikes paying hospital bills it must do so if the hospital is to continue to exist to protect the public health.

Sources of Income—There are several main sources of income for hospitals: patients, government, voluntary contributions, endowment funds and investments.

Since the majority of hospitals in the United States are private, nongovernmentally operated the bulk of income to these institutions is from the patient. Funds may come from the patient directly or they may come through hospitalization insurance (usually referred to as third party payments). A large segment of the population is covered by hospitalization insurance.

Another third-party principle involves the workmen's compensation regulations in the various states. These regulations vary among the states but essentially each regulation involves the employer taking out an accident insurance policy which will pay for emergency treatment or hospitalization of the employee in case of accident or injury on the job.

Medically indigent patients are those who do not have sufficient income to pay for their own personal health needs. Although some private organizations provide assistance to this group of patients, the bulk of the financial assistance comes from tax funds through local, state, and federal governmental agencies. The list of public tax-supported programs for health care assistance is formidable and becomes complex in determining what department, division, or agency of the federal, state, county, or city government is involved. For example, some of the assistance programs are the Kerr-Mills law, Old Age Assistance (OAA), Aid to Dependent Children (ADC), Aid to the Blind (AB), Aid to Permanently and Total Disabled (APTD), Aid for the Aged (AFA), and County and City welfare programs for the poor and needy. In addition, dependents of members of the Armed Forces, members of the Public Health Service and their families, and veterans of foreign wars receive health care through public tax funds. Thus a substantial portion of hospital costs are provided under governmental auspices.

The Social Security Amendments of 1965 extend the benefits for hospitalization, physicians services, and outpatient services from the original Social Security Law. The full implementation of Title 19 of the Social Security Amendment on a state-by-state basis is scheduled to be operational by 1970. It is left up to each state to decide whether it wants to participate in the plan and also to decide which of its citizens should be classed as indigent or medically indigent and thus entitled to benefits. This program, in addition to the benefits of Title 18 of the Act, will provide one of the major sources of income to hospitals for hospitalization as well as ambulatory services.

Another source of income to hospitals comes from the voluntary contributions of individuals, corporations, and foundations and through community fund raising campaigns. Some of these are direct contributions to the hospital; others are made available in the form of grants for research; still others are given for major expansion or remodeling programs. Private health assistance agencies assist individuals who need help by subsidizing the cost of their hospitalization and other health care needs.

Many hospitals are fortunate in receiving substantial sums for the purpose of setting up endowment trust funds and for use by the hospital in other ways. In addition some hospitals receive some income through investments, such as in real estate.

Another category of miscellaneous income to hospitals is the gift shop, small food service facility, or beauty parlor, many of which are operated by a Women's Auxiliary on a voluntary basis.

The Hospital Pharmacy

The separation of pharmacy from medicine took place in charitable institutions operated under governmental or ecclesiastic authority.[8] The fact that business interests played no part in the delivery of care to patients in these institutions led to an eventual division of labor in order to improve the quality of care. This division of labor in the physician–apothecary led to the recognition of pharmacy as a discipline separate from medicine. Since the division occurred in hospitals, the hospital pharmacist was the first recognized practitioner of the profession of pharmacy.

The development of hospital pharmacy in different countries was vitally affected by educational standards and by the caliber of its practitioners. Thus hospital pharmacy as an important professional specialty was virtually neglected in America for almost 168 years, from the time that Jonathan Roberts became the first hospital pharmacist at the Pennsylvania Hospital (Philadelphia) in 1752, to approximately 1920. After naming Charles Rice (1841–1901) of Bellevue Hospital in New York City, and Martin I. Wilbert (1865–1916) of the German Hospital in Philadelphia, it is difficult to recall other equally prominent contemporary hospital pharmacists of the same period.

A National Professional Society—Although the existence of the American hospital covers a span of more than 200 years, only during the past three decades or so have we witnessed the rapid expansion leading to our present vast and complex hospital system. As the movement toward the organization, expansion, and growth of the hospital system in the United States began to take shape, there also developed a movement toward the organization of hospital pharmacists. As Niemeyer, *et al*,[9] point out, the critical years for hospital pharmacy were the two decades from 1920 to 1940. The "awakening in the twenties" came about as a result of a growing realization by hospital pharmacists of the problems, potentialities, and importance of their speciality. The "advances in the thirties" resulted from their determination for organization, recognition, and establishment of higher standards of practice.

The activities of hospital pharmacists during these two critical decades resulted in the formation of The American Society of Hospital Pharmacists in 1942. The development of the Society within the sphere of American pharmacy has been due in large part to the adoption of a philosophy of service by hospital pharmacists which places the patient as the focal point for the existence of pharmacy and which minimizes the professional man's self interests. The unity which binds hospital pharmacists through their national professional society stems from their being a goal-oriented group. The common bond among them is the development of higher standards of professional prac-

formulate the programs which should be carried out by the staff department. The chairmen of the Councils are members of the Board of Directors.

Despite its relative youth, The American Society of Hospital Pharmacists has made significant contributions toward the improvement of hospital pharmacy. The *American Journal of Hospital Pharmacy* is one of the best professional publications in international pharmaceutical circles. The *International Pharmaceutical Abstracts* was introduced by the ASHP because of the need for such a publication. This was done only after international and national pharmaceutical associations had failed to meet the obligation to provide such a service to the profession as a whole. The *American Hospital Formulary Service* is one of the most comprehensive and unbiased sources of current information on drugs available. It serves as a basis for the pharmacist to extend his role as pharmaceutical consultant to the medical profession. *Mirror to Hospital Pharmacy* provides the findings from an exhaus-

American Society of Hospital Pharmacists

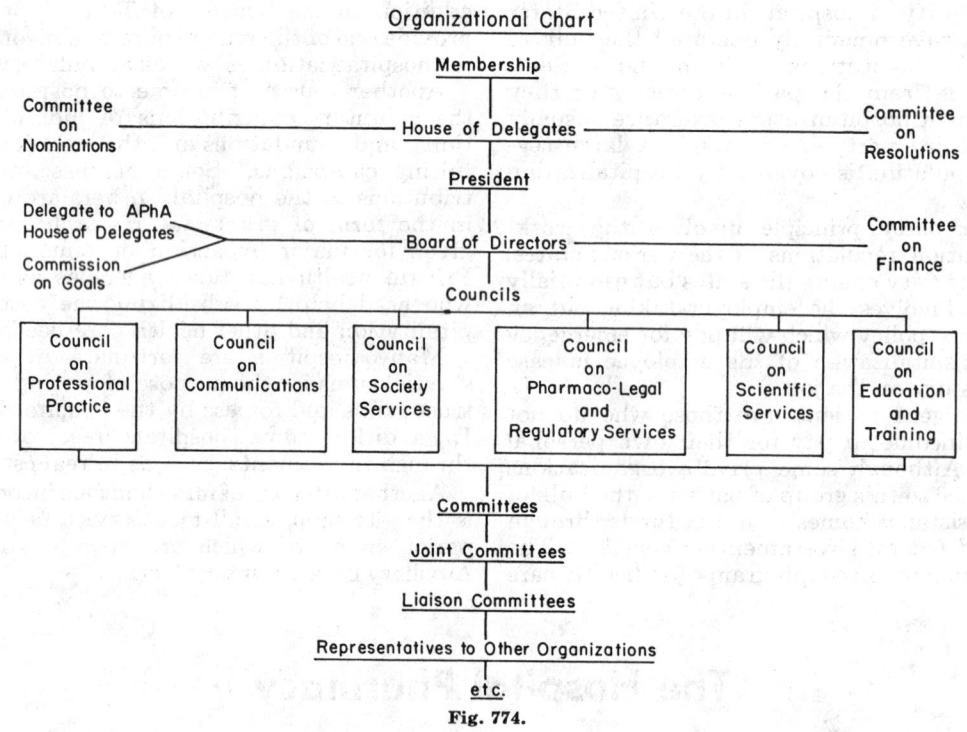

Fig. 774.

tice and service, *because the patient needs it*. Because of this common goal, the American Society of Hospital Pharmacists has made significant progress during the first 25 years of its existence.

Fig. 774 illustrates how the Society is structured to accomplish its objectives. The membership controls the organization; the House of Delegates formulates policies; the six Councils coordinate the vast workings of standing, special and joint committees. Analogous to the six Councils are six Departments of the headquarters staff of the Society. There is an additional Department of Administrative Services. Professionally trained hospital pharmacists serve as full-time directors of these various Departments to carry out staff level responsibilities. They work closely with the chairmen of the corresponding Councils wherein the membership through its various committees

tive study of hospital pharmacy in the United States. The whole basis for this study was to find out existing practices in hospital pharmacy and to determine ways in which to improve the quality and expand the scope of its pharmaceutical service. The *Continuing Education Program*, known as "Institutes," has served to help the hospital pharmacy practitioner keep up with current trends of professional practice. The success of this program has been the envy of other segments of the profession. The *Residency Training Programs* in hospital pharmacy are accredited by the Society and serves as a basis for insuring a high quality of training of future practitioners. The profession as a whole would profit greatly if it were to adopt a similar positive program to insure good internship training. The *Minimum Standard for Pharmacies in Hospitals* with *Guide to Application* provides a helpful set of principles upon which to develop good professional practices within the hospital. Many other contributions dealing with specific phases of hospital pharmacy have been made by the Society and still others are currently under study. Thus the strengths of a goal-oriented Society are readily apparent in the ASHP's contributions to American hospital pharmacy.

Goals for Hospital Pharmacy—If progress is to be made it is essential that the group dedicate itself to achieve idealistic goals. In order to continue its forward thrust, organized hospital pharmacists felt the need to spell out some of these long-range and idealistic goals. Thus, the ASHP has adopted the following Statement on Goals:[10]

Preamble

The membership of the *American Society of Hospital Pharmacists*, recognizing that vigilance and vision are essential elements of any profession, established the Commission on Goals as an advisory body to the Board of Directors for the purpose of analyzing studies, recommending broad goals for hospital pharmacy and outlining plans for achieving such goals.

Serving as a conscience, the Commission on Goals is the *Society's* means of providing some degree of assurance that fundamental principles and basic truths will serve as beacons to hospital pharmacists as they strive for excellence, adhere to a philosophy of service and develop a deep understanding and appreciation of human suffering.

Objectives

The objectives of the *American Society of Hospital Pharmacists* as stated in the Constitution and By-laws are:

1. To provide the benefits and protection of a qualified hospital pharmacist to the patient, to the institution which he serves, to the members of allied health professions with whom he is associated, and to the profession of pharmacy.
2. To assist in providing an adequate supply of such qualified hospital pharmacists.
3. To assure a high quality of professional practice through the establishment and maintenance of standards of professional ethics, education, and attainment.
4. To promote research in hospital pharmacy practices and in the pharmaceutical sciences in general.
5. To disseminate pharmaceutical knowledge by providing for interchange of information among hospital pharmacists and members of allied specialties and professions.

Basic Truths

In striving to fulfill these objectives through the development of long-range goals for hospital pharmacy, any thrust would prove fruitless unless there is first an acceptance of fundamental principles or basic truths. Among these are:

1. A profession is an associative society whose members possess and pass on a special field of knowledge acquired by extensive study and practice.
2. The field of specialized knowledge of pharmacists is pharmacy itself; that is, the science and art of those matters related to the procurement, preparation, control, and distribution of drugs, including the numerous elements that comprise these entities.
3. Possession of this knowledge and skill, and their use for the benefit of humanity are the prime bases for the existence of pharmacists.
4. Pharmacy will receive professional recognition from society only to the extent that its practitioners make use of their specialized scientific and professional knowledge.
5. True professional growth in hospital pharmacy will result only when the hospital pharmacist expands areas of practice which enable him to utilize the specialized professional and scientific knowledge and skills which are uniquely his.
6. The hospital environment provides opportunities in great measure for the pharmacist to utilize his unique knowledge and skills.
7. Education and training form the bedrock upon which hospital pharmacy must build in order to bring knowledge and experience to bear upon practice.
8. Professional advancement is fostered when a professional organization produces and makes widely available information and services which its members cannot provide for themselves.
9. Professional advancement is possible only when practitioners commit themselves to their professional ideals as the vital truths upon which their professional work on earth is made whole.
10. The purpose of a health profession is to serve the health needs of the people.

Goals

With these considerations in mind and consistent with the constitutional objectives of the *Society*, six broad goals can be identified and should be the focus of attention for hospital pharmacists during the next several decades. Coordinated plans must be drawn and implemented to:

1. Teach hospital pharmacists by word and precept the philosophy and ethics of hospital pharmacy as one of the healing arts and their personal, individual accountability to assume responsibility for professional practice.
2. Strengthen and expand the scientific and professional aspects of the practice of hospital pharmacy, including the consulting role of the hospital pharmacist, his teaching role, and his activities in the field of investigation and research.
3. Strengthen and perfect the administrative or management skills and tools essential to the hospital pharmacist in his role as a department head.
4. Attract a greater number of well-trained pharmacists to hospital practice, including those with specialized education and training in hospital pharmacy.
5. Promote payment of realistic salaries to hospital pharmacists in both staff and managerial positions in order to attract and retain the services of career personnel.
6. Utilize the resources of hospital pharmacy to assist in the development and improvement of the profession as a whole.

Goals Into Reality

Transforming these goals into reality will require the concerted efforts of all hospital pharmacists guided by inspired leadership under a carefully drawn plan vigorously executed. From these broad general goals will spring many projects that will provide tangible assistance to pharmacists in hospitals. In the course of time, existing projects will be modified, new projects will be developed, some projects will be discarded, but all projects will provide evidence of the *Society's* intention to drive forward persistently in attaining established goals.

History shows that groups which unite with a purpose, which give a selfless service for the greater good, which make plans and keep driving forward, which set immediate objectives yet maintain a degree of flexibility, which prepare themselves for the future—are those which make tremendous progress.

Standards of Practice

The movement to develop standards of practice in the hospital was initiated by the American College of Surgeons during the early 1900's when surgeons recognized the need to standardize and improve on surgical procedures, operating room techniques, and medical records on surgical operations. The College found that to improve the over-all care of surgical patients standards needed to be developed in other departments of the hospital as well as in the operating room. As a result of their initiative, the first Minimum Standard for Pharmacies in Hospitals was presented to the eighteenth Hospital Standardization Conference of The American College of Surgeons in 1935.[11] In 1942, when The American Society of Hospital Pharmacists was organized, a standing committee on Minimum Standards was appointed for the purpose of maintaining and developing better minimum standards. The original standard of the American College of Surgeons was revised by The American Society of Hospital Pharmacists in 1950. This revised Standard was approved by The American Pharmaceutical Association, American Hospital Association, Catholic Hospital Association, and received editorial endorsement by the American Medical Association. The latest revision of the *Minimum Standard for Pharmacies in Hospitals with Guide to Application** was eventually amended in November, 1962, to delete the words "Division of Hospital Pharmacy of the American Pharmaceutical Association." The Division had been dissolved by mutual APhA-ASHP agreement.

---

* Available from the American Society of Hospital Pharmacists, 4630 Montgomery Ave., Washington, D.C. 20014

The Ohio State University Hospitals
Department of Pharmacy

Functional Organization Chart

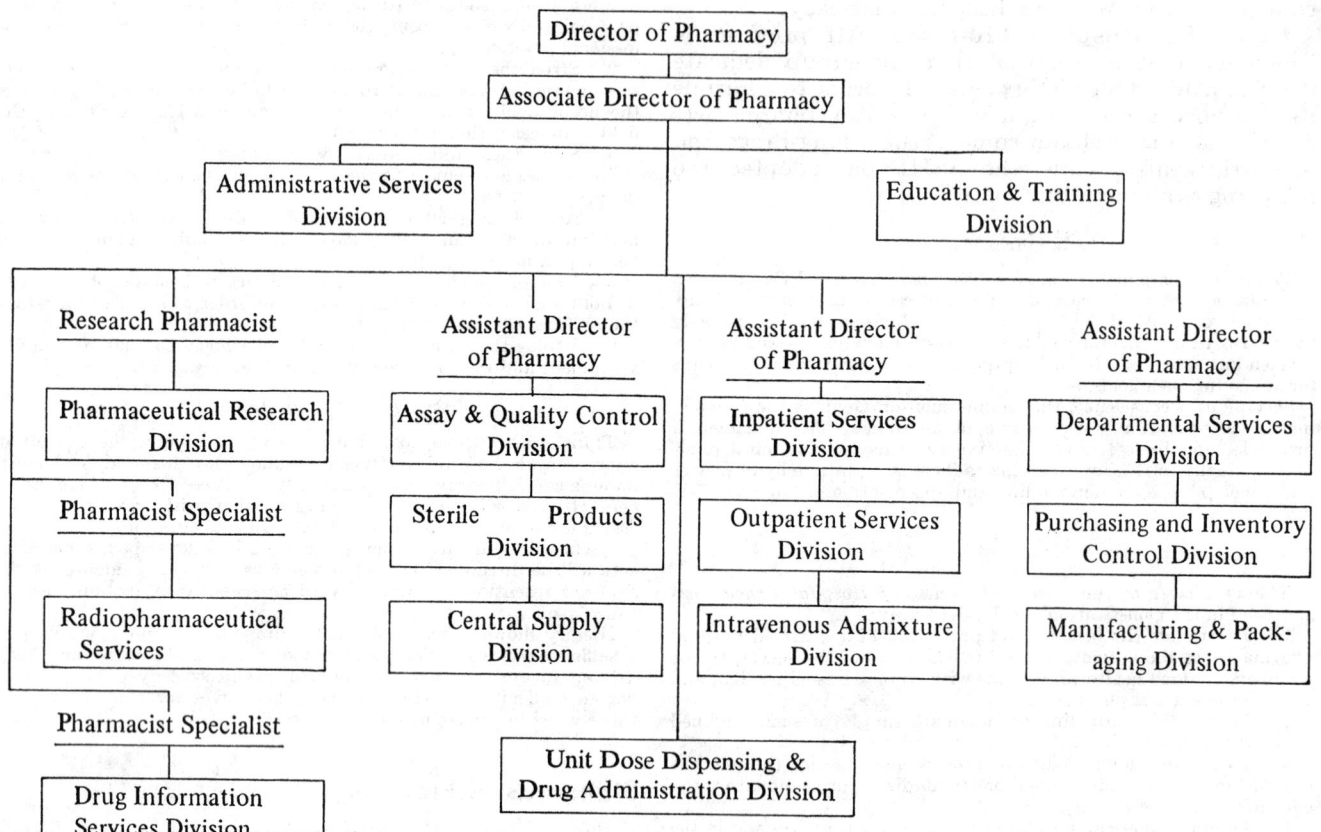

Fig. 775.

Administrative Services Division

1. Plan and coordinate departmental activities, special projects and research studies designed to improve administrative and professional practices and procedures.
2. Develop policies and schedule personnel and provide over-all supervision.
3. Coordinate pharmaceutical services within the hospitals.
4. Revise the policy and procedure manual.
5. Prepare and implement the budget and it's controls.
6. Coordinate the administrative needs of the Pharmacy & Therapeutics Committee and the Pharmacy-Nursing Committee activities.
7. Maintain records and reports and analyze and interpret data for effective management.
8. Supervise the IBM data drug processing activities and plan pharmaceutical aspects of the total Hospital Information System.
9. Supervise secretarial, receptionist and office activities.
10. Revise and update the Formulary of Accepted Drugs.

Education and Training Division

1. Assist in laboratory instruction and supervision of undergraduate pharmacy students enrolled in Hospital Pharmacy 515 each quarter.
2. Instruct graduate pharmacists who are serving a two-year residency in hospital pharmacy.
3. Instruct and supervise pharmacy interns.
4. Participate in formal instruction of student nurses, graduate nurses and medical students.
5. Instruct staff nurses (newly employed) as part of Nursing Service's formal orientation program.
6. Conduct conferences and educational activities for the pharmacy staff.
7. Participate in Nursing Service's Staff Development Program.
8. Coordinate new pharmacy employee orientation and training program.
9. Coordinate instruction in Clinical Pharmacy for students in College of Pharmacy.
10. Train newly employed pharmacists, pharmacy technicians and clerical staff.

Pharmaceutical Research Division

1. Develop research studies in biopharmaceutics, physical pharmacy, pharmaceutical technology, investigational drugs, drug stability and pharmaceutical analysis.

2. Develop new product formulations for special dosage forms of drugs not commercially available and of investigational drugs.
3. Improve the formulation and stability characteristics of products manufactured in the hospital pharmacy.
4. Handle special research projects involving drugs in cooperation with the medical research investigators.

Assay and Quality Control Division

1. Perform qualitative and quantitative analyses on products manufactured and purchased.
2. Coordinate the sterility and pyrogen testing on sterile irrigating, injectable, ophthalmic and other sterile products manufactured.
3. Check in-process controls on the manufacturing and packaging program.
4. Inspect and release finished products.
5. Develop and revise assay procedures.
6. Assist Pharmaceutical Research Division in special formulations, stability problems, etc.
7. Control the quality of all department activities and services.
8. Perform qualitative identification tests on "unknown" drugs to aid in their identification.

Manufacturing and Packaging Division

1. Manufacture different types of pharmaceutical dosage forms of drugs, diagnostic agents, germicidal solutions, laboratory diagnostic stains, and ointments, aerosols, etc.
2. Carry out the manufacturing and packaging in-process controls system.
3. Carry out the overall drug packaging and prepackaging program on manufactured and purchased drugs for the inpatient and outpatient divisions.
4. Maintain the manufacturing and packaging equipment in good operating and clean condition.
5. Perform product development and formula reevaluation activities on non-sterile dosage forms.
6. Develop Manufacturing Work Sheets on non-sterile formulations.
7. Maintain a unit dose drug packaging program for inpatients.

Sterile Products Division

1. Compound and manufacture small volume injectable medications.
2. Prepare sterile irrigation solutions for specific therapeutic applications.
3. Manufacture sterile ophthalmic solutions.

Fig. 775—Continued

4. Compound sterile special preparations for inpatient dispensing and research projects.
5. Perform the aseptic dilution of lyophilized and other "unstable" sterile injections for administration to patients.
6. Package unit doses of specific injectable and ophthalmic therapeutic agents.
7. Perform product development and formula reevaluation activities on sterile dosage forms.
8. Develop and revise Manufacturing Work Sheets on sterile formulations.

Inpatient Services Division

1. Compound and dispense prescriptions for all inpatients in University Hospitals.
2. Prepare extemporaneous prescriptions of dosage forms not commercially available.
3. Handle, control and dispense investigational drugs for single and double blind studies and other research studies.
4. Inspection and control of drugs on all treatment areas.
5. Provide total pharmacy service during evenings, nights, weekends and holidays (24 hours/day, 365 days/year).
6. Prepare the necessary information and material for the Pharmacy-Nursing Committee.
7. Provide a comprehensive drug reconstitution service for inpatients.
8. Check and replenish drugs on the emergency carts and emergency trays.
9. Implement and maintain the hospital formulary system.
10. Coordinate the Pharmacy-Nursing liaison program.

Outpatient Services Division

1. Compound and dispense outpatient prescriptions in the outpatient and clinic pharmacies.
2. Compound and dispense home visit medications for Upham and Dodd Hall patients.
3. Inspect and control outpatient clinic and emergency room medication stations.
4. Provide information and consultation services to medical students, interns and residents in the outpatient clinics.
5. Maintain the patient Prescription Record Service.
6. Maintain records and work with welfare agencies regarding medication for recipients.
7. Keep the health information literature rack current and properly filled.

Drug Information Services Division

1. Provide information and consultation services on drug therapy to the medical staff, medical students, interns, residents, student and staff nurses.
2. Maintain the Drug Information Center current through selection, classification, indexing and filling of pertinent medical, pharmacological and pharmaceutical literature.
3. Prepare material for inclusion in the *Pharmacy Bulletin* for distribution to the medical and nursing staff.
4. Prepare material for inclusion in the *Investigational Drug Bulletin*.
5. Select, classify and replace monographs on new drugs for the American Hospital Formulary Service Reference Books on all patient treatment areas of the hospital.
6. Prepare detailed information on investigational drugs for the professional staff.
7. Maintain the technical information file for use by department staff.
8. Prepare the necessary information and material for Pharmacy and Therapeutics Committee activities.
9. Select and obtain the necessary brochures for the outpatient health information program.
10. Conduct research studies involving the drug literature, including drug information retrieval and drug communication.

Departmental Services Division

1. Dispense and control intravenous solutions and administration set through the automatic replacement system.
2. Handle and control the narcotic and barbiturate drug distribution system in the hospitals.

3. Prepare, compound and dispense drugs for the hospital and other University departments.
4. Coordinate and control the floor stock drug dispensing activities.
5. Coordinate and supervise the drug delivery services to nursing units, outpatient clinics, emergency room and other hospital buildings.
6. Develop special drug requisition forms for other departments and standardize the packaging of drugs for interdepartmental use.
7. Coordinate the housekeeping activities for the department.

Purchasing and Inventory Control Division

1. Maintain the drug inventory control program in each of the pharmacy divisions.
2. Supervise the receiving, checking and proper storage of all drugs, biologicals and chemicals.
3. Inspect the expiration-dated drugs and other unstable drugs for deterioration.
4. Interview medical service representatives.
5. Supervise the removal and return of outdated, deteriorated and other drugs to manufacturers for credit.
6. Supervise the purchasing of pharmaceuticals, supplies and equipment for the department.
7. Supervise the clerical and record keeping activities related to the over-all pharmacy purchasing program.
8. Coordinate the annual drug inventory programs.
9. Supply pharmaceuticals to Means Hall pharmacy.

Central Supply Services Division

1. Plan and coordinate Central Supply services, special projects and research studies designed to improve administrative and professional practices and procedures.
2. Schedule personnel and provide over-all supervision.
3. Develop and coordinate Central Supply services within the hospitals.
4. Develop and revise policy and procedure manuals for Central Supply services.
5. Coordinate the setting up and issuing of special sterile trays to meet the needs of the medical and surgical staffs in special procedures.
6. Supervise the processing and issuing of emergency carts.
7. Clean and maintain sterile and non-sterile mechanical apparatus required in treatment and diagnostic procedures on nursing units.
8. Maintain in-processing controls over the processing of sterile supplies and equipment.
9. Maintain appropriate charging procedures for Central Supply services.
10. Supervise and coordinate the Central Supply services in Means Hall.

Radiopharmaceutical Services Division

1. Centralize the procurement, storage and dispensing of radiopharmaceuticals used in clinical practice in University Hospitals.
2. Perform quantitative analyses and determine the isotopic purity of all radiopharmaceuticals dispensed to assure their quality, potency and purity.
3. Formulate sterile and non-sterile radioactive dosage forms to meet the current needs of the medical staff.
4. Maintain appropriate records as required by the Atomic Energy Commission relative to handling and dispensing of pharmaceuticals.
5. Assist the medical and paramedical staffs in calculating doses of radiopharmaceuticals.
6. Conduct research studies involving various aspects of radiopharmaceutical formulation development, stability, tagging and biological distribution patterns.

Intravenous Admixture Division

1. Centralize the preparation of intravenous solution admixtures for use throughout the hospital.
2. Review each I.V. admixture physician's order for physico-chemical incompatibilities.
3. Schedule the time frequencies for each additional I.V. admixture to be administered to each patient.

To assist hospital administrators and hospital pharmacists to review their pharmacy service in terms of the Minimum Standard, the Committee on Hospital Pharmacy Practice of The Catholic Hospital Association developed a "Point Rating Plan for Hospital Pharmacy Service." Based on the Minimum Standard the Point Rating Plan provides a means for hospital pharmacists to evaluate their pharmacy service through a comprehensive scoring method which points out deficiencies needing correction or improvement. Criteria embodied in the Point Rating Plan include an evaluation of the objectives of the pharmacy department, its organization, committees, policies and regulations, staff, facilities, professional services, administration, educational activities, library, and research activities. This self-evaluation guide has been presented by The

Catholic Hospital Association to The American Society of Hospital Pharmacists.*

The Joint Commission on Accreditation of Hospitals has used the Minimum Standard for Pharmacies in Hospitals as a guide in its hospital accreditation program. Although the Joint Commission has not utilized the Minimum Standard to the fullest extent, the Standard has been influential in promoting better hospital pharmacy practice. For example, the large number of hospitals in the US with a pharmacy and therapeutics committee may be attributed to a great extent to the Joint Commission's view that this committee is essential in every hospital.

Organization—Within the organizational structure of the hospital the chief pharmacist, as a department head, reports to the administrator of the hospital on the proper operation and management of the pharmacy. The chief pharmacist formulates and implements departmental administrative policies of the pharmacy subject to the approval of the administrator. The professional policies relating to hospital pharmacy practice that have a direct relationship to the medical staff are formulated and developed through the pharmacy and therapeutics committee and are subject to administrative approval (see *Pharmacy and Therapeutics Committee*).

The organizational structure of the hospital pharmacy may be illustrated by Fig. 775. This chart lists the functions of a typical hospital pharmacy. A close examination of this functional organizational chart shows the many ramifications of the practice of pharmacy in today's modern hospital.

In a small hospital with only one pharmacist it is a challenge to him to be knowledgeable in all these activities of hospital pharmacy. In a large hospital with a number of pharmacists who specialize in certain areas of practice each may become expert in one or more fields. The staffing pattern in hospital pharmacy varies, depending on the scope and quality of pharmaceutical service being offered. Some hospitals with less than 100 beds employ a pharmacist on a full-time basis while there are few hospitals between 200–300 beds with no pharmacist. The American Society of Hospital Pharmacists has been working diligently to get hospitals with less than 100 beds to appoint a pharmacist to the hospital staff. This is important because approximately half of the hospitals are less than 100 beds and these hospitals urgently need pharmaceutical service. As the size of the hospital increases, so does the personnel in the pharmacy. For example, in a 300-bed progressive hospital the pharmacy may be staffed with a chief pharmacist, an assistant chief pharmacist, from two to four staff pharmacists, one to three nonpharmacists and a full-time department secretary. On the other hand, one may find 300-bed hospitals where the pharmacy is staffed with only one pharmacist and one helper. Thus it is not difficult to visualize the difference in the quality of service rendered between these two hospitals. In the very large hospitals with several hundred beds, one may find the staffing pattern in the hospital pharmacy to consist of a director of pharmacy, an associate director, one or more assistant directors, one or more supervisor pharmacists, as many as 20 or more staff pharmacists, up to 10 or 12 pharmacy residents, and about as many nonpharmacist helpers, technicians, and secretarial personnel.

In order to schedule the workload of the department equitably and to insure that all the functions are carried out various methods are devised, such as the Work Distribution Chart of the Springfield City Hospital, illustrated in Fig. 776. In addition, job descriptions, policy and procedure manuals, functional organizational charts, and other management aids are utilized by the director of pharmacy in a large department to insure that all the services and functions are fulfilled adequately.

Facilities—There are great variations in the amount of floor space devoted to the pharmacy in hospitals of the same size and type. Such variations have a direct bearing on the scope of service which can be developed in the pharmacy.

In the 50-bed hospital, with one pharmacist, only one room is usually required for the pharmacy, a combination of dispensing, manufacturing, administrative, and all other features of a complete pharmaceutical service with the exception of the preparation of sterile products. If sterile products are prepared, and it has on many occasions been proved to be essential, then there should be a separate room for their manufacture. This type of facility is needed for the reconstitution of lyophilized injections, for ophthalmic preparations, and for the preparation of intravenous admixtures, all of which must remain sterile. A small safeguarded portion of the general storeroom should be reserved for excess pharmaceuticals.

In the 100-bed hospital there should be one pharmacist and one or more trained assistants. There will probably be two rooms, one for administration, dispensing, and manufacturing, and an adjacent storeroom. There should again be available a small area in the general storeroom for bulk purchases or excess supplies unless adequate additional space is made available in the pharmacy. If parenteral preparations are manufactured there should be a separate room for this activity.

In the 200-bed hospital there will usually be need for two pharmacists and probably two or more trained assistants. Though many pharmacies in 200-bed hospitals are staffed with but one pharmacist, this person is handicapped in his ability to utilize his specialized training to the utmost. This is especially true where there is a busy outpatient service. In these cases the pharmacist usually depends on nonprofessional personnel to carry out duties that should be assigned to a pharmacist. Such situations should not be tolerated, and the pharmacist should press the administration for an additional full- or part-time pharmacist so that he may properly execute his responsibilities.

Hospitals of 200 beds and larger provide the opportunity for departmentalization of pharmacy activities. There should be a separate area for outpatient service, an office for the chief pharmacist, a manufacturing room, a storeroom, a sterile products room, and a separate area for drug information services.

As the hospital size advances to 500, 1000, or more beds, so, of course, will the ramifications of pharmaceutical service increase. Modern concepts of a total hospital pharmacy include the following: (1) waiting room, (2) office of the chief pharmacist, including a library and drug information center, (3) office for the secretary and bookkeeper, (4) inpatient dispensing laboratory, (5) outpatient dispensing laboratory plus a consultation area to instruct outpatients on the safe and appropriate use of prescription medication, (6) manufacturing laboratory, (7) sterile products laboratory, divided into a "clean-up" room and a "sterile techniques" room, (8) product formulation, control, and research laboratory, (9) prepackaging and labeling laboratory, (10) allergenic products laboratory, (11) pharmacy storeroom (active stock), (12) alcohol and volatile liquids vault or room, (13) narcotic, investigational drugs, and other restricted drug vault or safe, (14) additional bulk storage facilities either separate or as a part of the general storeroom, and (15) a radioactive pharmaceuticals laboratory. In such large-scale operations the chief pharmacist or director of pharmacy service must be an exceptional person to be able to supervise such an elaborate plant and provide in addition the educational and other services that are his responsibility to the patient, to the professional staffs, and to the hospital.

If parenteral solutions or other sterile products are being manufactured, a segregated, restricted-entry area is required, and the rigid controls described in Chap-

WORK DISTRIBUTION CHART—SPRINGFIELD CITY HOSPITAL, SPRINGFIELD, OHIO

Activity	Tot. Hr. Wk.	Chief Pharmacist	Hr. per Wk.	Associate Pharmacist	Hr. per Wk.	Clerk	Hr. per Wk.	Secretary	Hr. per Wk.	Technician	Hr. per Wk.
Prescription Service	65	Prescription dispensing: (a) Inpatient. (b) Outpatient. (c) Personnel.	30	Compound, prepare or dilute, all special prescriptions.	30	Pick-up and delivery service. Assist dispensing pharmacist. Obtain and package items called for.	6	Prepare all charges for drugs to individual patients. File prescriptions and maintain material cost and billing records.	24	Clean and process all bottles and utensils.	3
Ward Stock Service	87½	Supervise clerk. Check filled orders. Check barbiturates. Periodic check of drugs stocked at nursing stations.	½	Perform all bulk compounding and sterilizing procedures. Supervise technician in filling and labeling of stock containers. Train and supervise technician to assist with procedures and preparations.	30	Pick-up and delivery service. Fill orders for nursing stations. Fill and label ward stock containers. Rinse, return empty containers.	25	Tabulate distribution of drugs. Price requisitions for material cost.	4	Bottle and label ward stock products from bulk compounded stock. Wash and process and sterilize returned empty bottles. Clean equipment and utensils. Assist Pharmacist in compounding.	28
Other Miscellaneous Dispensing	10	Dispense narcotics and antibiotics. Maintain narcotic inventory.	2½	Supervise technician in dilution of antibiotics.	2	Delivery service.	½	Billing and tabulation.	2	Unpack and remove seals. Dilute antibiotics.	3
Procurement and Inventory	20	Interview detailmen and salesmen. Compose purchase orders. Check requisitions typed by secretary.	2	Assume responsibility for procurement and inventory when chief pharmacist is not present. Responsible for stocks of basic drugs used in compounding.	6	Obtain and check orders received from purchasing department. Assist pharmacists in stock control and storage of majority of inventory.	4	Type letters and requisitions. Enter receipt of merchandise on card file.	4	Obtain and check orders received from purchasing department. Advise secretary of receipts of shipments according to requisition. Mark material and place in stock.	4
Records and Reports	10½	Compose reports, memoranda to executive director and other departments. Review and check reports and records prepared by secretary.	2	Tabulate production records. Maintain control records of compounded products.	1	Assist secretary with simple tasks, and errands.	2½	Maintain barbiturate inventory. Prepare and type monthly financial reports.	4	Assist with all responsibilities of clerk, when clerk is absent.	1
Administrative and Management	14½	Establish policy and procedure of all transactions of department. Interview, indoctrinate, train, and supervise all employees of the department.	4	Assist in training and supervision of employees. Assist in plans and projects of department. Direct department in absence of chief pharmacist.	2½	Responsible for order and cleanliness of dispensing area. Supplies of soap, towels, and drug containers.	3	Personnel time records. Filing and typing. Answer and channel all telephone calls.	3	Responsible for order and cleanliness of compounding and storage areas.	2
Information Service & Education	3½	Lecture to student nurse pharmacology class. Code literature for filing. Supervise answers to questions of physicians and nurses.	2	Assist chief pharmacist.	½			Typing. File coded literature.	1		
Inter- & Intra-Professional Relations	3	Pharmacy and Therapeutics Committee secretarial duties. Edit Formulary and News Letter. Medical intern discussion. Pharmacy intern program.	1					Typing.	2		
	214		44		44		41		44		41

Fig. 776.

ter 82 on *Parenteral Preparations* (page 1519) should be maintained.

Alcohol and flammable solvents should be specially stored according to the individual specifications of the local fire underwriters and the Alcohol and Tobacco Tax Division of the Internal Revenue Service. There should be a storeroom for drugs, chemicals, and solutions purchased in bulk containers. A properly equipped laboratory should be provided for the maintenance of adequate control of manufactured products and for such research as the pharmacist may undertake.

For the short-term general hospital a *minimum* of 6 square feet per hospital bed is required for effective, efficient pharmacy operation. This may be varied to provide more than 6 square feet per bed in the small hospital of 50 beds or slightly below this minimum in the 1000-bed hospital. A specialized hospital will usually not require as much floor space for the pharmacy as will a general hospital. Estimates for the pharmacy of a 100-bed hospital vary from 500 to 1000 square feet as *minimum* floor space, increasing 6 square feet per bed over 100 beds. Revised floor plans and planning guides for hospital pharmacies are available from the Health Facilities Planning and Construction Service, US Public Health Service, Washington, D.C.

Pharmacy and Therapeutics Committee—The relationship between the community pharmacist and the physicians in the area is a direct person-to-person contact. There is a physician–pharmacist–patient relationship which is uncomplicated by organizational lines. On the other hand, the hospital pharmacist is responsible for maintaining proper relationships with from dozens to a few hundred physicians on the medical staff of one hospital. This is further complicated by the introduction of the nursing profession within the physician–pharmacist–patient relationship. Experience has shown that there is a need for a formal organizational line of communication and liaison between the medical staff and the pharmacy department of a hospital. This was recognized by the American College of Surgeons when they adopted the first Minimum Standard for Pharmacies in Hospitals. It is also recognized by the Joint Commission on Accreditation of Hospitals as an essential committee of the hospital's medical staff.

The American Hospital Association and The American Society of Hospital Pharmacists has formulated and adopted a statement embodying the definition, purpose, organization, functions, and scope of a pharmacy and therapeutics committee in the hospital. This statement (Fig. 777), is an effective guide in organizing such a committee within a given hospital.

It has been thought by many that the sole purpose of a pharmacy and therapeutics committee was to develop a formulary and operate a formulary system. It can be seen from the preceding Statement that there are many important functions of this committee in addition to the formulary system. A hospital's medical staff could have an effective pharmacy and therapeutics committee without having a formulary system. On the other hand, a hospital could not properly operate a formulary system without a pharmacy and therapeutics committee, unless the medical staff served as a "committee of the whole."

Formulary System—The formulary system and formularies have existed in the United States since the days of the American Revolution; they existed in European hospitals for centuries prior to this. The need for hospital formularies becomes increasingly

great because of (1) the increasing number of new drugs being marketed, (2) the increasing influence of biased advertising and unscientific "scientific" drug literature, (3) the increasing complexity of untoward effects of the newer more potent drugs, (4) the highly competitive marketing practices of the pharmaceutical industry and (5) the public's interest in seeing that the health professions are conscientiously providing the best possible care at the lowest possible cost.

The formulary system—because it has attempted to outline the scientific data on a drug, including its toxicities, untoward side effects, and beneficial effects—has been a controversial method of appraising drug therapy. Such a rational and scientific basis of selecting drugs for use in a hospital does not necessarily work to the advantage of a particular pharmaceutical company and it is understandable why the pharmaceutical industry has sometimes opposed the formulary system. While the pharmaceutical industry promotes the virtues of a trade-named drug, the formulary system evaluates the virtues and defects of that drug in comparison to other trade-named brands of the same basic drug. While the pharmaceutical industry has sometimes maintained that the formulary system is detrimental to the free enterprise system, the proponents of the formulary system maintain that it challenges the individual

---

statement on the
PHARMACY & THERAPEUTICS COMMITTEE
Approved by the Board of Trustees of the American Hospital Association and the Executive Committee of the American Society of Hospital Pharmacists February 1959

Preamble

► HOSPITALS ORGANIZE AND MARSHAL the best professional skills and judgment available to provide care and treatment of patients. The treatment of these patients in many cases is dependent upon the effective use of drugs. The multiplicity of drugs available today makes it mandatory that an organized sound program of activity be developed within the hospital to insure that patients receive the best care and protection possible.

One of the most effective ways of providing this kind of care and protection is by organizing a Pharmacy and Therapeutics Committee. This committee is designed to make maximum use of available professional skills and judgment. The establishment of a Pharmacy and Therapeutics Committee is strongly recommended to all hospitals. It is a measure which supports and enhances the principle of self-government in the area of high drug standards and practices for the medical staff connected with a hospital. Ultimate benefits accrue to the patient in improved patient care and treatment as established voluntarily by the medical staff.

The Pharmacy and Therapeutics Committee

The Pharmacy and Therapeutics Committee is an advisory group of the medical staff and serves as the organizational line of communication or liaison between the medical staff and the pharmacy department. This committee is composed primarily of physicians and the pharmacist and is selected under the guidance of the medical staff. It is also a policy-recommending body to the medical staff and to the administration of the hospital on all matters related to the use of drugs. (This committee does not have intrinsic authority or power of action unless specifically granted such authority.)

PURPOSES

The primary purposes of the Pharmacy and Therapeutics Committee are:

A. *Advisory.* The committee recommends the adoption or assists in the formulation of broad professional policies regarding evaluation, selection, procurement, distribution, use, safe practices, and other matters pertinent to drugs in hospitals.

B. *Educational.* The committee recommends or assists in the formulation of programs designed to meet the needs of the professional staff (doctors, nurses and the pharmacist) for complete current knowledge on matters related to drugs and drug practices.

ORGANIZATION

While the composition of the Pharmacy and Therapeutics Committee may vary from hospital to hospital, the following is offered as a guide:

A. The Pharmacy and Therapeutics Committee of the medical staff should be composed of no less than three physicians and the pharmacist, appointed by a governing unit or elected official of the organized medical staff. The hospital administrator and his designated representative should be an ex officio member of the committee.

B. A chairman from the physician representatives should be appointed. The pharmacist is generally designated secretary.

C. The Pharmacy and Therapeutics Committee should meet regularly, no less frequently than twice per year, and should meet on call when necessary.

D. The committee should feel free to invite to its meetings persons within or without the hospital who can contribute from their specialized knowledge or experience.

E. An agenda is desirable and should be prepared and submitted to members of the committee in sufficient time before the meeting.

F. Minutes should be kept by the secretary and should be maintained in the permanent records of the hospital.

G. Recommendations of the Pharmacy and Therapeutics Committee shall be presented to the medical staff or its appropriate committee for adoption or recommendation.

FUNCTIONS AND SCOPE

The basic organization of the hospital and medical staffs will determine the functions and scope of the Pharmacy and Therapeutics Committee. The following list, which is not necessarily comprehensive, is offered as a guide:

A. To serve in an advisory capacity to the medical staff and hospital administration in all matters pertaining to the use of drugs.

B. To serve in an advisory capacity to the medical staff and the pharmacist in the selection or choice of drugs which meet the most effective therapeutic quality standards.

C. To evaluate objectively clinical data regarding new drugs or agents proposed for use in the hospital.

D. To prevent unnecessary duplication of the same basic drug or its combinations.

E. To recommend additions and deletions from

the list of drugs accepted for use in the hospital.

F. To develop a basic drug list or formulary of accepted drugs for use in the hospital and to provide for its constant revision.

G. To make recommendations concerning drugs to be stocked in hospital patient units or services.

H. To establish or plan suitable educational programs for the professional staff on pertinent matters related to drugs and their use.

I. To recommend policies regarding the safe use of drugs in hospitals, including a study of such mat-

ters as investigational drugs, hazardous drugs, and others.

J. To study problems involved in proper distribution and labeling of medications for inpatients and outpatients.

K. To study problems related to the administration of medications.

L. To review reported adverse reactions to drugs administered.

M. To evaluate periodically medical records in terms of drug therapy.

Fig. 777.

pharmaceutical manufacturers to meet the competition which is the basis of the free enterprise system.

In order to outline precisely what the formulary system is and is not, a *Statement of Guiding Principles on the Operation of the Hospital Formulary System* was developed and approved by The American Medical Association, American Hospital Association, American Pharmaceutical Association, and American Society of Hospital Pharmacists. This Statement differentiates between the formulary system and the hospital formulary, and lists a number of guiding principles designed to help physicians, pharmacists, and administrators to operate a hospital formulary system.

Statement of Guiding Principles on the Operation of the Hospital Formulary System[12]

Preamble

The treatment of patients in hospitals in many cases is dependent upon the effective use of drugs. The multiplicity of drugs available makes it mandatory that a sound program of drug usage be developed within the hospital to ensure that patients receive the best care and protection possible.

In the interest of better patient care, there should be a program of objective evaluation, selection and use of medicinal agents in the hospital. This program is the basis of rational drug therapy. The hospital formulary concept is a method for providing such a program in hospitals and has been utilized as such over the years.

The hospital formulary system is based upon its approval by the organized medical staff, the concurrence of individual staff members and the functioning of a properly organized Pharmacy and Therapeutics Committee of the medical staff. The basic policies and procedures governing the hospital formulary system should be incorporated in the medical staff bylaws, or in the medical staff rules and regulations.

The Pharmacy and Therapeutics Committee, composed of physicians and pharmacists, selected under the guidance of the medical staff, represents the official organizational line of communication and liaison between the medical staff and the pharmacy. The Committee is responsible to the medical staff as a whole and its recommendations are subject to approval by the organized medical staff, as well as to the normal process of administrative approval.

This Committee assists in the formulation of broad professional policies relating to drugs in hospitals, including their evaluation or appraisal, selection, procurement, storage, distribution, use and safety procedures.

Definition of Hospital Formulary and Hospital Formulary System

The hospital formulary is a continually revised compilation of pharmaceuticals which reflects the current clinical judgment of the medical staff.

The hospital formulary system is a method whereby the medical staff of a hospital, working through a Pharmacy and Therapeutics Committee, evaluates, appraises and selects from among numerous available medicinal agents and dosage forms those that are considered most useful in patient care.

The hospital formulary system provides for the procuring, prescribing, dispensing and administering of drugs under either their nonproprietary or proprietary names in instances where drugs have both names.

Guiding Principles

The following principles may serve as a guide to physicians, pharmacists and administrators in hospitals utilizing the hospital formulary system:

1. The medical staff shall appoint a Pharmacy and Therapeutics Committee composed of physicians and pharmacists, and outline its purposes, organization, function and scope.

2. The hospital formulary system shall be sponsored by the medical staff based upon the recommendations of the Pharmacy and Therapeutics Committee. The medical staff should adapt the principles of the hospital formulary system to the needs of the particular hospital.

3. The medical staff shall adopt written policies and procedures governing the hospital formulary system as developed by the Pharmacy and Therapeutics Committee. Action of the medical staff is subject to the normal process of administrative approval.

These policies and procedures shall afford guidance in the evaluation or appraisal, selection, procurement, storage, distribution, use, safety procedures, and other matters relating to drugs in the hospital

and shall be published in the hospital's formulary or other media available to all members of the medical staff.

4. To insure the maintenance of the responsibility and prerogatives of the physician in the exercise of his professional judgment, the hospital formulary system shall not contain any policies or procedures which, prior to the time of prescribing, provide for consent by the physician to the dispensing of a nonproprietary drug or to the dispensing of a proprietary brand different from the brand which he prescribed. However, it shall be within his discretion at the time of prescribing to approve or disapprove the dispensing of a nonproprietary drug or the dispensing of a different proprietary brand.

5. The medical staff shall adopt the policy of, and formulate the procedure for, including drugs in the formulary by their nonproprietary names, even though proprietary names are and will continue to be in common use in the hospital. Physicians may be encouraged to prescribe drugs under their nonproprietary names, although the nomenclature used is entirely a matter of the individual medical practitioner's discretion.

6. In the absence of written policies approved by the medical staff relative to the operation of the hospital formulary system, and authorization from the prescribing physician, the pharmacist must dispense the brand prescribed, bearing in mind his professional prerogative to confer with the physician should the prescribed brand be unavailable.

7. A hospital shall make certain that its nursing personnel are informed in writing (through its established means of communication) about the existence of the formulary system in the hospital and the procedures governing its operation.

8. In the formulation of policies and procedures, the terms "substitute" and "substitution" should be avoided, since these terms have been used to imply the unauthorized dispensing of a brand different from that prescribed or the dispensing of an entirely different drug, neither of which takes place under a properly operated hospital formulary system.

9. Provision shall be made to apprise the medical staff of changes in the working of the hospital formulary system or in the content of the hospital formulary.

10. Provision shall be made for the appraisal and use by members of the medical staff:

(a) of drugs not included in the formulary.

(b) of investigational drugs.

11. The pharmacist, with the advice and guidance of the Pharmacy and Therapeutics Committee, shall be responsible for specifications as to quality, quantity, and source of supply of all drugs, chemicals, biologicals and pharmaceutical preparations used in the diagnosis and treatment of patients, and for assuring that quality is not compromised for economic considerations. When applicable, such products shall meet the standards of quality of the *United States Pharmacopeia* or *National Formulary*.

12. The labeling of a medication container with the nonproprietary name of the contents is always proper. The use of a proprietary name other than that describing the actual contents is improper if it is used in a manner that can be taken as descriptive of the contents, even though personnel familiar with the hospital formulary system may understand that it is not descriptive. The following format is recommended for labeling individual patient's containers used within hospitals:

(Nonproprietary Name)
(Name of Manufacturer or Distributor)
Note for information of staff:
Prescription or order for
(Proprietary Name)
dispensed as per formulary policy; contents are
same basic drug as prescribed but may be of another brand.

Recommendation

A hospital formulary system, based upon these guiding principles, is considered to be important in drug therapy in hospitals. In the interest of better patient care, its adoption by hospital medical staffs is recommended.

In addition to these Guiding Principles, most hospital pharmacy and therapeutics committees adopt various regulations governing the admission of drugs to the hospital formulary. The following list is typical of such additional regulations:

The Pharmacy and Therapeutics Committee Regulations

The following rules will govern admission of drugs to the Hospital Formulary:

1. Simple official substances will be admitted unless they have become superfluous. This will include those substances official in the

current revisions of the *United States Pharmacopeia* and the *National Formulary.*

2. No nonofficial drug will be admitted, except for controlled research, before its therapeutic value has been established. Drugs not admitted to the Formulary, however, may be supplied to ward patients and outpatients if paid for by the department concerned.

3. No preparation of secret composition will be admitted.

4. No preparation which is sold under a proprietary name will be admitted under such a name if a preparation of identical composition can be obtained under a nonproprietary name.

5. No mixture of two or more active drugs will be admitted unless evidence is submitted that the mixture presents therapeutic advantages over the simple drug.

6. Any nonofficial drug may be temporarily admitted for controlled research upon recommendation of the Research Committee of the medical staff, providing cost of said drug is paid for by the department concerned.

7. Heads of clinical departments may request inclusion of a drug or preparation in the Formulary by submitting a request to the secretary of this committee and listing the following basic information plus other pertinent facts:

   (a) Official title of drug with proprietary titles, if any.
   (b) Specific pharmacologic action and use of the drug which warrants its admission.
   (c) Reason why this drug is superior to present official formulary drugs.
   (d) Drug or preparation which this new drug will replace.

8. Heads of clinical departments are to be notified whenever any preparation is considered for elimination from the Formulary, in order that they may submit evidence for its retention.

9. A majority of the committee must agree upon the admission of a drug to the formulary, or deletion of a drug from the formulary, following which said recommendations must be presented to a meeting of the medical staff for approval. Following such approval, the drug will be added to or deleted from the Hospital Formulary.

One of the most useful references to help a Pharmacy and Therapeutics Committee develop its own formulary is the *American Hospital Formulary Service.* This service, available from the American Society of Hospital Pharmacists, is a loose-leaf collection of individual drug monographs (Fig. 778). Each monograph contains the nonproprietary and trademark names of the drug, chemical structure, pharmacology and mechanism of action, therapeutic indications, cautions and side effects, dosage, and preparations available. Each monograph is classified according to an extensive pharmacologic–therapeutic classification system. This makes it convenient to compare all the drugs in the same therapeutic classification.

The intent of the Formulary Service is to provide a selective unbiased evaluation of the numerous medicinal agents available, and to encourage the medical staff of the individual hospital to select those drugs its members consider most useful therapeutically, together with the preparations in which they may be administered most effectively. Thus, a compilation of these specific monographs would represent the Formulary of that particular hospital.

Availability of the *American Hospital Formulary Service* offers the medical, pharmacy, and administrative staffs of hospitals an incentive to review the organization and the policies of their Pharmacy and Therapeutics Committee. It would be well to determine, for example, whether clearly written policies and procedures governing the *formulary system* have been approved by the medical staff. Does the Pharmacy and Therapeutics Committee concern itself with broad professional policies regarding the evaluation, selection, procurement, distribution, use, safety procedures, and other matters related to the use of drugs in hospitals? Does the hospital's formulary reflect the clinical judgment of the medical staff and is it, in fact, a critical selection of those drugs considered most useful therapeutically? Have procedures which are fair, simple, reasonable, and expedient been formulated for obtaining nonformulary drugs for evaluation by the medical staff? These and other matters concerned with the use of drugs could be reviewed with profit by the staff of almost every hospital.

One of the principal advantages of the ASHP *Formulary Service* is to give the hospital pharmacist and the Pharmacy and Therapeutics Committee additional time: to work with the medical staff in the selective evaluation of new drugs, to organize and plan for interesting and stimulating meetings of the Pharmacy and Therapeutics Committee, to work with the nursing staff in the elimination of practices and procedures which may lead to medication errors, to encourage the medical staff to undertake an objective audit of the discriminate use of therapeutic agents and to enter other areas for the promotion of rational drug therapy, and to cooperate with the medical and nursing staffs in numerous areas involving broad policies concerning the use of drugs in the hospital.

The ASHP *Formulary Service* complements, it does not replace, the work of the Pharmacy and Therapeutics Committee. It is a tool which can be used by physicians and pharmacists to make the formulary system of each hospital a dynamic ever-changing compilation of modern medicinals selected with discrimination. It is, indeed, a service to the nation's hospitals.

Purchasing—While the pharmacist may be the actual buyer in a small hospital, his principal function in purchasing is to establish standards and specifications for all drugs, chemicals, diagnostic agents, and other preparations used in patients, and pharmaceutical equipment.* He alone is responsible for the quality of drugs dispensed to patients. Especially in the average governmental hospital, the pharmacist does not purchase directly but through a purchasing agent, the hospital's purchase and supply officer. The pharmacist must be prepared to reject purchases not meeting the standards he has prepared. The Pharmacy and Therapeutics Committee serves as a potent

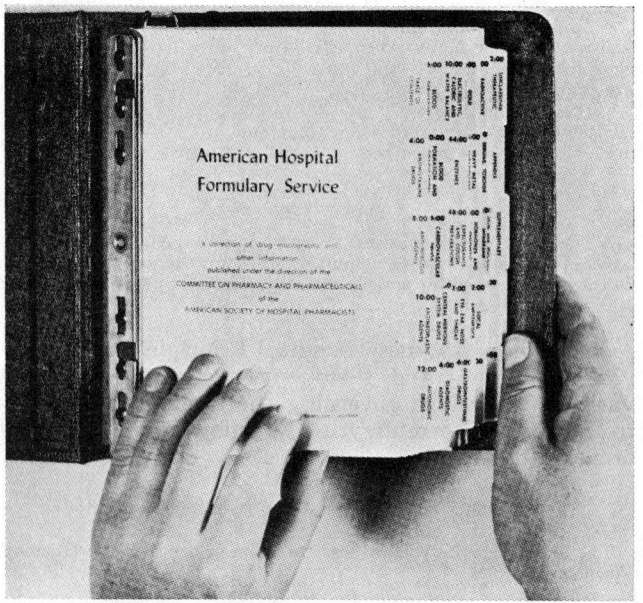

Fig. 778. The American Hospital Formulary Service (courtesy, The American Society of Hospital Pharmacists).

---

* See also *Minimum Standard for Pharmacies in Hospitals,* page 1783.

I. A Hospital Purchasing Policy for Pharmaceuticals

This hospital requires each supplier to certify under oath the following:

A. The company maintains a quality control program equal to or exceeding a standard published by the hospital.

B. The ingredients meet official, national and state standards.

C. The finished product is manufactured, packaged, and handled according to official, national and state standards and that ALL finished products, official and nonofficial, conform to official tests where applicable, i.e., disintegration time for tablets, general requirement for injections, et cetera.

D. That the company in the past two years has (or has not) produced a new product and holds thereon an effective new drug application under Sections 404 and 505 of the Federal Food, Drug, and Cosmetic Act.

E. The company grants permission for a representative from the hospital to visit the company premises at any time during regular business hours for the purpose of determining compliance with provisions of items A, and B above.

F. The hospital requires that, on demand, assay data will be produced by the suppliers.

G. The hospital further requires that successful bidders must post a bond to allow the hospital to assay samples of products of questionable potency or composition at company expense.

II. A Purchasing-Quality Control Program for Hospital Pharmacists

I. Qualifications of Supplier

A. Purchase from manufacturers which are known to participate in research in their own institutions and which are known to support research at nonprofit institutions.

B. If possible, do not purchase from mail-order houses, distributors or agents, or where the company has no representative. Local drug wholesalers, of course, are excluded from this requirement.

C. Where there is some question as to the propriety of purchasing from a company, and where the company is conveniently located, inspect the facilities of the company while production is being carried out. Where the company is out of town, write a hospital pharmacist in that area and ask for the same facts.

II. Organoleptic Properties of the Products

A. Spot check all bulk-purchase products to observe that:
   1. Tablets have not chipped or crumbled.
   2. Injections have not discolored or precipitated.
   3. Injection suspensions have not clumped or are too viscous.
   4. Labeling is specific and correct for your institution.

B. Maintain close liaison with nursing service personnel and record all comments concerning drug dosage forms and difficulty therewith, as:
   1. Difficulty in withdrawing suspensions.
   2. Clogging of needle.
   3. Pain of injection.
   4. All items in II-A, 1, 2, 3, 4.

III. Qualitative and Quantitative Properties

A. Where there is a low-priced product, include the cost of an assay for potency in the purchase price; if this is still a low price, then purchase the product, request copy of company's assay and control data and have your own assay accomplished outside the hospital as a check. Specify this in the original purchase order, and hold invoice for payment until results of your assay corroborate those of the company and indicate a product assaying 100 percent of labeled amount or better.

B. Remember that a single assay done once on a company's product is not sufficient to justify continued purchasing of the same or other products from said company. As a pharmacist you know that in a manufacturing process, there can be variations in every batch of a product; although a reputable manufacturer will not issue a product where the variation is below a standard.

IV. General Principles

A. Where product is not satisfactory, insist on full return for credit, with manufacturer's representative assisting in packaging. Where local representative claims manufacturer will not accept return of spoiled or unusable products, write company direct. If no progress, then make no further purchases from the company.

B. When the chips are down, and the State Board of Pharmacy, or a pharmaceutical manufacturer, or your medical staff, or a complainant's lawyer is opposing you, remember that YOU, the pharmacist, are the person legally responsible for the quality of drugs purchased for your hospital. YOU alone will be held negligent.

Fig. 779. A typical statement of purchasing policy and quality control program for hospital pharmacies.

---

force in helping the pharmacist to set up adequate specifications for the purchase of quality pharmaceuticals.

In setting specifications for drugs, the pharmacist should be guided by one of the recommendations made in the ASHP's *Statement on Hospital Drug Distribution Systems.*[13] This recommendation states:

"Drugs dispensed should be as ready for administration to the patient as the current status of pharmaceutical technology will permit, and must bear adequate identification including (but not limited to): name or names of drug, strength or potency, route(s) of administration, expiration date, control number, and such other special instructions as may be indicated."

This statement places added significance on the need for purchasing drugs in unit-dose and unit-of-use packages where the stability of the drug in those specific packaging materials has been assured.

Increasing numbers of pharmacists are formalizing standards for purchasing. Such standards are especially necessary in governmental institutions where often the purchasing is not accomplished on the premises but by a central purchasing agent for the state or other governmental agency. The statement of purchasing policy and quality control (Fig. 779) is offered as an example of an approach to this problem.

Quantity buying is often advantageous from a price or availability standpoint. Before making large purchases, however, the pharmacist should determine the stability of the items and consider the possibility of a change in policy that might render their use obsolete.

Many persons feel that a turnover of stock of four to eight times annually is desirable. Turnover, reduction in purchase cost, and storage space must be considered in determining the advisability of large purchases of an item.

The Bid—The use of competitive bidding is considered good practice where an item is used in large amounts and where future continued use seems certain. A quotation request is directed to manufacturers dealing in the commodity desired. The company with the lowest price and yet with standard quality usually receives the order for the material, after which the purchase order is prepared. Typical information found in a quotation request follows:

You are hereby invited to quote the lowest net prices for which you are prepared to furnish the merchandise or services described below. Bids will be received until . . . .

Please quote prices as indicated. Quotations will be understood to include all delivery charges to hospital door unless otherwise specified. If merchandise or services cannot be furnished at once kindly specify length of time required for delivery.

Where a bid is asked for a certain article which may be substituted by another "equal thereto" and the bidder intends to furnish an article which he considers equal to the one named, he must specify in his bid the name and grade of said article and submit a sample, if possible, with the bid. This form is only an invitation to bid. IT IS NOT AN ORDER.

Many hospitals have adopted the practice of preparing estimates of drug usage for a given period. Thus, manufacturers are requested to submit their bid quotations on the total quantity of drugs to be used for a 1-year period; or in the case of intravenous solutions, even a 2-year period. The stipulation is that the hospital has the option to determine when and how much will be shipped at any time during the one- or 2-year period.

Upon review of these bids, the hospital pharmacist determines which vendor will receive the contract and a purchase order is sent to the respective manufacturers. Thus, by issuing an annual purchase order to each of the major pharmaceutical manufacturers, the hospital pharmacist eliminates significant amounts of paper work and unnecessary frequent bidding.

Purchase Record—It is desirable that a purchase record be maintained for all items purchased routinely. Each purchase record card should include specifications for the item. With such information at hand, one is at a distinct advantage in obtaining duplicate material on successive purchases.

The purchase record card (Fig. 780) provides a record of the quantity used over a period of time, a control, and simplification of purchasing procedures. This information is of particular value when the pharmacist is faced with a rising market, as it gives him a fairly accurate picture of the immediate future needs and enables him to buy at current prices without overstocking. In addition, such a record furnishes the information necessary so that he may purchase only enough of an item for a predetermined time. The purchase record card provides information on quantities purchased in previous months, quarters, or years, and is required for efficient purchasing, whether by contract or otherwise.

Fig. 781 illustrates the procedures involved in purchasing and receiving.

Annual inventories should be taken as a check on the theoretical inventory record maintained by either pharmacy or accounting. Various procedures are used to take a drug inventory. Many hospitals are using electronic data processing in inventory value determinations.

In many hospitals it has been observed that proprietary duplications abound and clutter the shelves, increasing inventory and decreasing turnover rate and efficiency. The pharmacist should review such inventory periodically and return outmoded and outdated drugs to the manufacturer for credit. In addition, he should bring this matter to the attention of the Pharmacy and Therapeutics Committee since one of its responsibilities is to delete outmoded drugs from the approved inventory.

Drug Distribution Systems—The organizational structure of the hospital has placed certain constraints on the manner in which hospitalized patients receive their drugs. These constraints revolve around professional prerogatives and traditions, as well as legal responsibilities, established for medicine, nursing, pharmacy, and hospital administration.

Physicians prescribe, pharmacists dispense, and nurses administer drugs. However, in order to get this simple tripartite order executed, many things must take place. The over-all drug distribution and utilization process in the hospital involves an infinite number of procedures, personnel, departments, equipment, and storage. As an illustration, trace the history of a drug from procurement to administration to the patient.

Before a drug can be purchased, specifications must be prepared. This is usually done through the medical staff and the pharmacist by means of a Pharmacy and Therapeutics Committee. Requisitions outlining the specifications for the drugs selected are prepared and processed in the pharmacy and

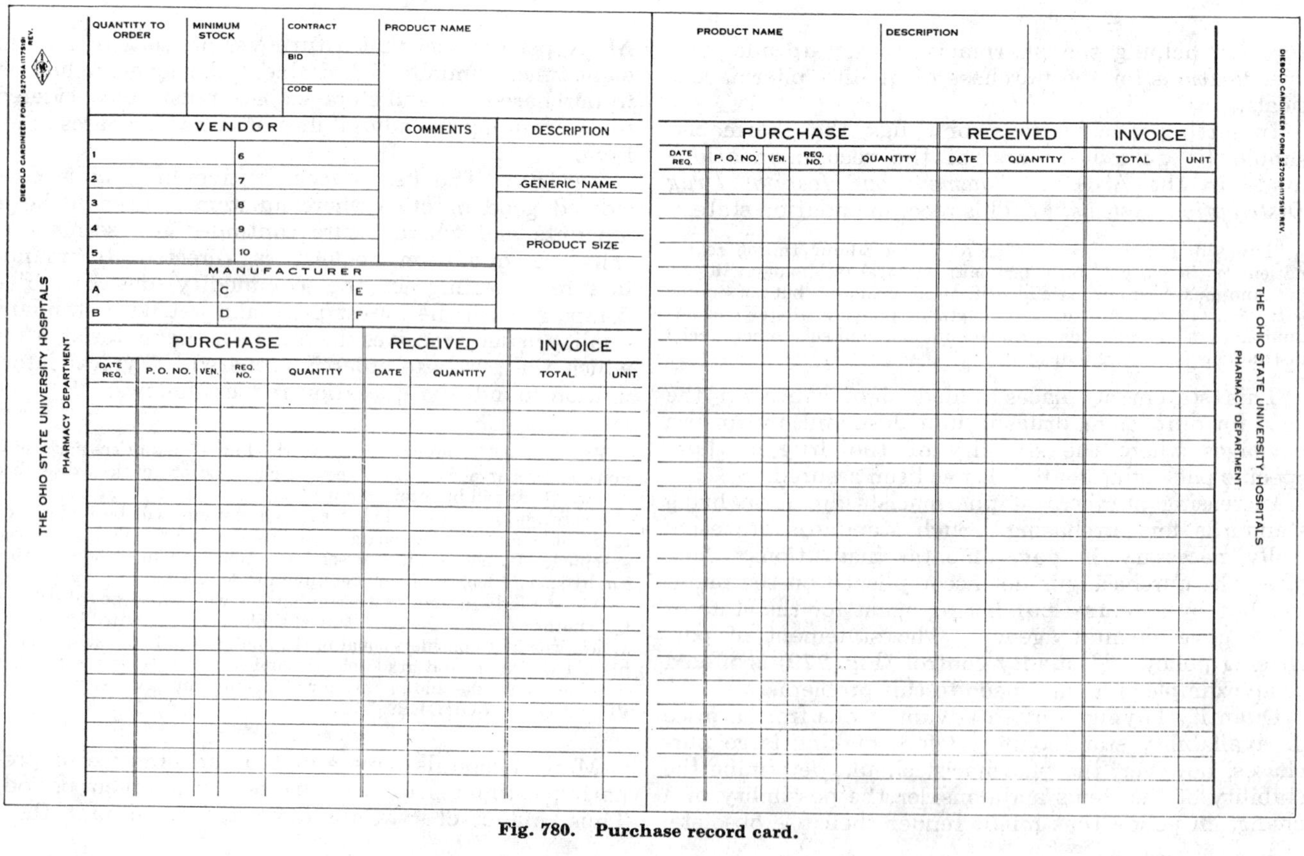

Fig. 780. Purchase record card.

forwarded to the purchasing department for procurement. Drug shipments are received by the receiving department and distributed to the pharmacy. Pharmacy checks these shipments and stores them for future use. Inventory control procedures must be set up. In the meantime, invoicing for payment must be processed through the accounting department through a coordination of efforts among pharmacy, purchasing, receiving, and business offices.

Physicians must prescribe drugs before they can be administered. Nurses must carry out these medication orders and requisition the necessary drugs from the pharmacy. In the pharmacy the drugs are transferred from the storage area to the dispensing area. There they may have to be prepackaged (for future use), may have to be compounded or manufactured and assay and control procedures performed, must be bottled in proper quantities for use by the nurse to administer to the patient, labeled properly, checked for accuracy, and distributed to the nursing unit. At the nursing unit the drugs are stored again for continuous use by the patient according to physicians' orders. The nurse prepares the drug for administration, brings it to the patient, returns to the nursing unit, and records this information on the patient's record.

In the meantime the pharmacy processes the nurses' drug orders for billing purposes and sends these charges to the business office. There, they are posted to the patient's account. Then, through coordination between pharmacy and accounting, data is accumulated on the cost of drugs issued, reduction of drug inventory and income received to offset expenses incurred.

While the mechanics of this operation is taking place, other activities must be completed. Problems must be resolved in the procurement phase regarding overshipments or undershipments or other shipping errors; errors in billing may have to be rectified. Outdated or deteriorated drugs may have to be returned to the manufacturer. Further information may be required from the physician or nurse before the prescription can be filled; that is, information as to dosage, toxicity, and side effects. Perhaps the staff physician may cancel the intern's medication order and the nurse must return the drug to the pharmacy for credit. Thus, the cycle starts all over again!

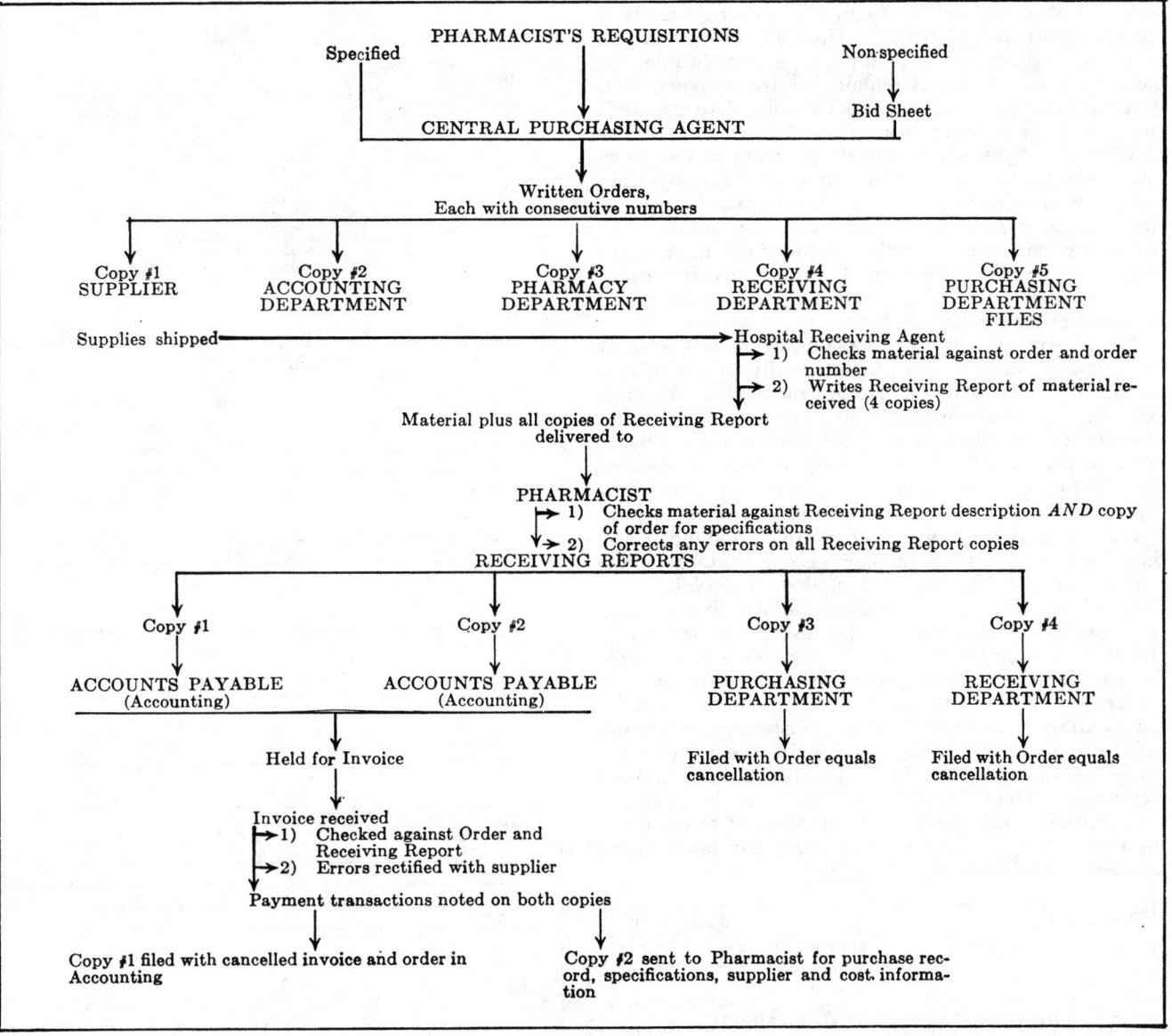

Fig. 781. Purchasing procedure.

How many people are involved in the history of one drug from the time of its specification to the time it reaches the patient? The pharmacist and five or more physicians on the pharmacy and therapeutics committee in preparing drug specification; the pharmacist in selecting the drug to be ordered; the pharmacy secretary in making out the requisition; the purchasing agent in ordering the drug; the receiving clerk in accepting shipment; the delivery clerk from receiving to pharmacy; the pharmacy stock clerk in checking and storing the drug; the physician in prescribing the drug; the nurse in ordering the drug; the pharmacist in preparing and dispensing the drug; the pharmacy delivery clerk in transporting the drug to the nursing unit; the ward clerk in storing the drug; the nurse in preparing and administering the drug and in charting the data; the pharmacy clerk in recording the charge and sending it to the business office; the account clerk in the receiving and processing of the invoices; the business officer in preparing the check for payment; the posting clerk in posting the charge to the patient's bill; the credit manager in collecting the bill. There must be over 20 people involved in some manner or other with one drug order!

Medication is administered to a hospital patient only upon the written order of a physician. Thus, a prescription order originates in the patient's medical record, where the physician writes out all the orders he wants carried out on or for the patient. Since the patient's medical record remains at the nursing unit, it is essential that some means be utilized to transmit the prescription order from the nursing unit to the pharmacy. These orders are transmitted to the pharmacy usually in one of three ways: (1) the physician writes the medication order on a separate blank, (2) the medical record has a duplicate copy so that the pharmacy can obtain a carbon copy of the physician's original medication order, or (3) the physician's order is transcribed by nursing personnel onto an inpatient prescription or requisition form.

The pharmacy department makes drugs available at the nursing unit for patient use usually in one of five ways: (1) individual prescription medication for each patient, (2) a complete floor stock system, (3) a combination of numbers 1 and 2, (4) unit-dose dispensing either centralized in the pharmacy or decentralized at the nursing unit level, and (5) a pharmacy coordinated unit-dose dispensing and drug-administration system.

Individual patient medications are compounded and dispensed in the usual manner except that the name and strength of the drug are included on the label. In hospital practice all medications are kept in a nursing unit medication cabinet and are under the custody of the nurse in charge. She or her assistant is responsible for administering the appropriate medication to each patient on the nursing unit. Thus it is important for her to know what drug she is administering for it is her professional responsibility to observe the patient for untoward reactions and to report this to the patient's physician. Thus the patient never sees the prescription container dispensed by the pharmacist to the nursing unit. A typical inpatient prescription label would contain the following information:

Mr. John Jones		Room 608E
	Tetracycline HCl Capsules, 250 mg	
Doctor's Name	Pharmacists Name	Date
	THE GENERAL HOSPITAL PHARMACY	

In some hospitals the pharmacist will place the *American Hospital Formulary Service* therapeutic classification code number on the label. This is done to help the nurse refer to the monograph of that drug in the AHFS so that she can review the cautions, contraindications, side effects, dosage, or other pertinent information about the particular drug.

Some hospital pharmacists prepare a condensed summary of the pertinent information which the nurse should know about a drug. This information is placed on a small card, usually referred to as a "medication tip," "pharma-tip" or other descriptive title. An example of a medication tip issued with the drug for use by the nurse is shown in Fig. 782.

In order to expedite the dispensing of inpatient prescription medication hospital pharmacists have adopted the practice of prepackaging frequently used drugs in standard dispensing quantities. It is not unusual for a majority of the inpatient prescription medications to be prepackaged. Prepackaging drugs requires accurate procedures, controls, and records in order to

```
                    MEDICATION TIP
                 PENTAZOCINE INJECTION
                       (Talwin)

ACTION:  Non-narcotic analgesic
for acute and chronic disorders.
May be used pre-op and post-op.

DOSE:   30 mg. every 3-4 hours.
Infrequently 60 mg. is given.

ROUTES:  I.M., S.C., & I.V.

DILUENT:  Not required.

STABILITY:  Room temperature.

SIDE EFFECTS:  Nausea, vertigo,
dizziness, vomiting, respiratory
depression, euphoria.
PRECAUTIONS:  Do not mix in syringe
with soluble barbiturate; ppt.
will occur.  Use with caution in
patients with cerebral disease,
pregnancy, asthma, narcotic addic-
tion, renal or hepatic disease.
6/68    OSU HOSPITAL PHARMACY
```

Fig. 782.

THE OHIO STATE UNIVERSITY HOSPITALS
PHARMACY DEPARTMENT

PREPACKAGING DATA RECORD

Control Number _____

Name of Drug _____ Size or Strength _____

Manufactured By _____ Mfgr. Lot No. _____

Expiration Date _____ Checked By _____
(Pharmacist)

PRODUCTION DATA

Number Per Unit	Size & Type Container	No. of Units Prepackaged	Total Time Spent	Prepackaged By	Sample of Control Label

COST DATA

Number Per Unit	Cost per Unit of:			Total Labor Cost Per Unit	TOTAL COST PER UNIT
	Container & Label	Ingredient	Total (Raw Cost)		

Remarks:

Rev. 11/63

Fig. 783. Prepackaging data record.

trace the identity of the drug at all times. Thus a prepackaging control record form, as shown in Fig. 783, is utilized for documentation of manufacturer's control numbers, expiration date, pharmacy control number which appears on each prepackaged container label, and the pharmacist responsible for the prepackaging operation. In the case of a drug recalled by a manufacturer, the pharmacist can easily trace prepackaged quantities of the drug in question.

Drugs dispensed under a floor stock system are of two classes: free and charge. Free floor stock consists of a predetermined list of medications which are available on every nursing unit of the hospital for use at no charge to the patient. Since these drugs are used in large quantities they are prepackaged in standardized containers. In many hospitals these drugs are ordered by means of a preprinted requisition by the nurse, and the pharmacist dispenses the medication which is usually delivered in a drug basket. Orders are usually received from each nursing unit of the hospital each day of the week. In other hospitals the

THE OHIO STATE UNIVERSITY HOSPITALS
PHARMACY DEPARTMENT
PHARMACY FLOOR STOCK DRUG REQUISITION

	1	2	3	4	5	6	Cost	Total
Enema, Fleet's 4½ oz.								
Enema, Fleet's Oil Retention 4½ oz.								
Lubricating Jelly 5 gm Tube #48								
Mouth Wash 1000 cc								
Talcum Powder 240 gm								
Body Lotion 4 oz.								
Hexagerm 1000 cc								
Vinegar Douche Solution 1000 cc								
Acetone 250 cc								
Xylocaine 1% 20 cc								
Xylocaine 2% 20 cc								
Xylocaine-Epinephrine 1% 20 cc								
Xylocaine-Epinephrine 2% 20 cc								
Epinephrine (Topical) 1:1000, 30 cc (8C & 10E)								
Neosporin Ophthalmic Ointment ⅛ oz.								
Initials								
						Total Rec'd		

Month.................................19........ Nursing Unit...............

Fig.784. Pharmacy floor stock drug requisition.

pharmacy assumes the responsibility for maintaining the proper inventory of free floor stock drugs on each nursing unit through an automatic floor stock replacement system. Under such a system the nurse is relieved of having to maintain an inventory control system, fill out a daily requisition order, and return the drug basket items to the shelves. The pharmacy personnel goes to the nursing unit with an adequate supply of each free floor stock drug, takes an on-the-spot inventory, brings the inventory to a predetermined level, and records the quantities on a preprinted requisition which lists the drugs in the order in which they are stocked in the drug cabinets. This requisition (see Fig. 784) is used by the pharmacy to total the usage per nursing unit. Adequate controls thus can be set up on the basis of usage in relation to number of patient days per given interval of time. Some hospitals have adopted electronic data processing procedures to handle the totaling and cost extension of drugs issued and the preparation of monthly drug usage reports for each nursing unit.

Charge floor stock is medication available at each nursing unit of the hospital and for which a charge is made to the patient. Certain medications are required to be used almost immediately after the physician prescribes them, and it is not practical to go to the pharmacy to obtain them in each instance, yet the cost and the volume of usage necessitates a charge to the patient. Such medications are usually injections or other single dose forms. A common method of handling charge floor stock drugs is to attach a small removable label bearing the name of the drug to the charge floor stock drug. When the nurse needs the drug she merely removes the label and affixes it to the usual inpatient prescription or requisition slip. This is then used for charging purposes and for replacement of the drug on the nursing unit.

In hospitals where patients pay for their hospitalization the pharmacy usually employs a combination of the individual inpatient prescription system and the floor stock drug system. Drugs which are free floor stock are charged against the nursing service and, in the final analysis, the patient does pay for the drugs since the cost is included as a part of the nursing service portion of the daily room and board rate.

Because of the large number and variety of drugs stored on nursing units—including individual patient prescriptions, free and charge floor stock, narcotics and other controlled drugs, investigational drugs, and emergency drug tray—it is an important responsibility of the pharmacist to inspect these drugs routinely. Proper storage conditions must be adhered to, dated drugs must be checked, narcotic drugs must be safeguarded, and discontinued drugs must be removed from the nursing unit. To insure proper control of a nursing station drug cabinet, a standardized checklist form is used as a guide by the pharmacist and the head or supervisor nurse making the inspection. This form (see Fig. 785) is used to prepare a written report to

THE OHIO STATE UNIVERSITY HOSPITALS
PHARMACY DEPARTMENT

NURSING STATION MEDICATION REVIEW

The nursing station on ______ was visited by a member of the pharmacy staff on ______ for the purpose of reviewing the contents and condition of the nursing station medication unit as well as procedures for the procurement and storage of drugs. ______ RN, assisted in the review. The results of the review are given below.

		REVIEW SUBJECT	√	COMMENTS Use Reverse Side
Drugs, Containers and Labels	1	Internal separated from external drugs?		
	2	Patient medication separated from floor stock?		
	3	Non-drug items segregated from drug items?		
	4	Clean (labels soiled, marked or defaced?)		
	5	Arrangement and general neatness satisfactory?		
	6	Excessive quantities of drugs? (duplicated special Rx's for patients, unreturned drug credits)		
	7	Charge floor stock inventory level posted?		
	8	Free floor stock inventory level posted?		
	9	Reconstituted drugs properly labeled with expiration date, concentration, diluting material and initials of person making dilution?		
	10	Do charge floor stock items bear voucher card labels?		
	11	Parenteral fluids spot checked for vacuum & clarity?		
	12	Outdated or deteriorated drugs present?		
	13	Investigational drugs present not labeled by pharmacy? If so, name: ______. Is information available?		
Cabinets and Refrig.	14	Clean? (free of dust, spilled liquids, ect.?)		
	15	Locked?		
	16	Drugs requiring refrigeration stored in refrigerator?		
	17	Drugs not requiring refrigeration stored in refrigerator?		
	18	Refrigerator thermometer reading		
Narcotics and Barbiturates	19	Narcotic cabinets locked?		
	20	Narcotics or barbiturates maintained for long periods with no evidence of use?		
	21	Narcotic counters being used properly?		
	22	Certificate of disposition agree with physical inventory? (item checked ______)		
	23	Completed certificates of disposition not returned?		
	24	Automatic stop-orders on narcotics observed?		
Emer. Tray	26	Complete and in good order? Storage noted.		
	27			
	28			
Other Specify	29			
	30			
	31			
	32			
	33			
	34			
	35			
	36			

Rev. 10/60; 4/64 Date ______ Reviewed by: ______ (Pharmacist)

Fig. 785. Nursing station medication review.

the directors of nursing and of pharmacy. The condition of a nursing unit medication station may warrant remedial attention by personnel from both departments. In some hospitals, the pharmacists are assigned to specific nursing units to coordinate all the drug and drug therapy problems at the nursing unit level. Rather than simply checking drug storage conditions, they are developing new roles which brings them closer to the patient care team.[14]

A newer trend for dispensing drugs to hospitalized patients is called "unit-dose dispensing." In this system the pharmacist prepares every dose of medication ready for administration, rather than issuing containers of drugs to nursing units where the nurse must prepare the drug for administration. For example, tablets and capsules are labeled for each patient, liquids are premeasured, lyophilized injections are diluted and accurately measured into sterile syringes, parenteral admixtures are added to intravenous solutions prior to use, and oral powders and other unusual dosage forms are measured and mixed appropriately. Most of these procedures involve pharmaceutical techniques which are properly the pharmacist's responsibility. Hospital pharmacists are studying various methods involving centralized pharmacy versus decentralized pharmacies on the nursing units, using automated systems of communication, information scheduling, and retrieval to provide more accurate and effective over-all drug distribution and utilization in the hospital.

The unit-dose dispensing concept has changed many of the traditional functions of the hospital pharmacist. For example, the traditional prepackaging system of multiple doses of drugs has been changed to include the use of tablet and capsule strip packaging and labeling machines and liquid unit-dose packaging equipment. This is necessary since all drugs are not available from the industry in unit-dose packages. The traditional individual inpatient prescription is also eliminated and thereby eliminates prescription label typing. Thus, the unit-dose-dispensing operation enhances the need for pharmacy technicians to assist in the procedural aspects of this function. Free and charge floor-stock drug activities are essentially eliminated.

Some hospitals have used automated drug-dispensing devices which are located on the nursing unit. These mechanical dispensing machines are usually loaded with prefilled packages of drugs. When activated by means of keys and name plates, a package of the drug is released and thus it becomes the "individual inpatient prescription." However, unit-dose dispensing essentially eliminates the need for this type of automated mechanical dispensing device. Some manufacturers, however, are experimenting with unit-dose dispensing devices.

Unit-dose dispensing lends itself to certain automation procedures, particularly with electronic data processing and computers. On-line computers are used to program patients' total drug-therapy profile, program the times for administering scheduled doses of drugs, maintain records of drugs administered and initiate the drug charges to patients. This eliminates the traditional nurses' drug kardex, medication ticket, and record-of-drug-administered-manual-system of keeping tract of patients drug-therapy profiles. Thus, the hourly reports of the on-line computer on patients drug-therapy profiles can be used both by the pharmacy for unit-dose dispensing and by the nurse for drug administration.

There is a developing trend to consider merging drug dispensing and drug administration into a coordinated system under pharmacy control. This makes sense particularly when one considers the fact that when a physician writes a medication order for a hospitalized patient, it is essentially a pharmaceutical order and pharmaceutical orders should be carried out under the supervision of pharmacists. This system was initiated at the Providence Hospital in Seattle.[15] Registered nurses have been employed by the Pharmacy Department and in conjunction with a unit-dose dispensing system by the pharmacists and technicians, nurses are responsible for administering all the drugs to hospitalized patients. Thus, such a coordinated system effects certain efficiencies and eliminates many steps from the traditional drug distribution and utilization system. A pharmacy-coordinated unit-dose-dispensing and drug-administration system has been initiated at the Ohio State University Hospitals. This system differs from the Providence Hospital program in that pharmacy technicians have been trained to administer the drugs instead of using registered nurses. These pharmacy technicians assist in the unit-dose dispensing phase as well as the drug-administration phase of the coordinated system which is directly controlled and supervised by registered pharmacists. Thus, pharmacists work directly with physicians on the nursing unit to carry out pharmacy's mainstream function of the safe and appropriate use of drugs in patients. This is the interacting role which hospital pharmacists are beginning to develop under the umbrella term, "clinical pharmacy."

One of the significant new developments in hospital pharmacy is the concept embodied in clinical pharmacy. In one sense, clinical pharmacy is merely a new term used to describe good professional hospital pharmacy practice. In another sense, the term clinical pharmacy embodies a broader philosophic approach to the practice of pharmacy than what has been taught traditionally in colleges of pharmacy over the past quarter century and as it has been and is still being practiced today. Pharmacy practice has been almost predominantly product-oriented and the delivery of pharmaceutical services has been primarily a "technician"-oriented task rather than "professionally and patient"-structured.

Clinical pharmacy embodies a patient-oriented approach to the delivery of pharmaceutical services with drug knowledge as the base from which these services emanate. Traditionally, the main purpose of the pharmacist has been "to fill prescriptions." With the dynamic changes taking place, pharmacists are finding that the mechanical aspects of filling prescriptions can be performed easily by technicians.

As the pharmaceutical industry develops the unit-dose-packaging concept and as physicians and the Food and Drug Administration continue their drive to provide patients with drugs labeled with the name of the medication in the original manufacturer's package (to insure stability and identity) this will virtually eliminate the count-and-pour and labeling operations in "filling prescriptions." It substantiates the need to use technicians in the physical handling of drugs. It is obvious that this main purpose of the pharmacist must change if he wants to remain a health professional.

There is, however, a challenging professional role which the pharmacist can assume as a member of the health-care team. This role involves the safe and appropriate use of drugs in patients. Taken in a broad context, this implies a high-level role indeed. This is the mainstream purpose for the existence of pharmacy as a health profession. Thus, the concept behind the clinical pharmacy movement is directed toward the development of this role as the mainstream function of the profession.

Providing pharmacy service at night has been a problem in most hospitals. During recent years a number of hospitals have instituted 24-hour service, with pharmacists on duty seven days a week. However, most hospitals have not felt able financially to justify this essential service and have resorted to other procedures.

Many ingenious methods have been devised for providing night or emergency service. A so-called "night pharmacy on wheels" was invented by one pharmacist. This unit is mobile, contains all emergency drugs and a representative amount of certain other medicines. It is wheeled to the nursing supervisor's office when the pharmacy closes at night and is returned in the morning. The nursing supervisor has the only key to this unit at night. When she dispenses an item she leaves a

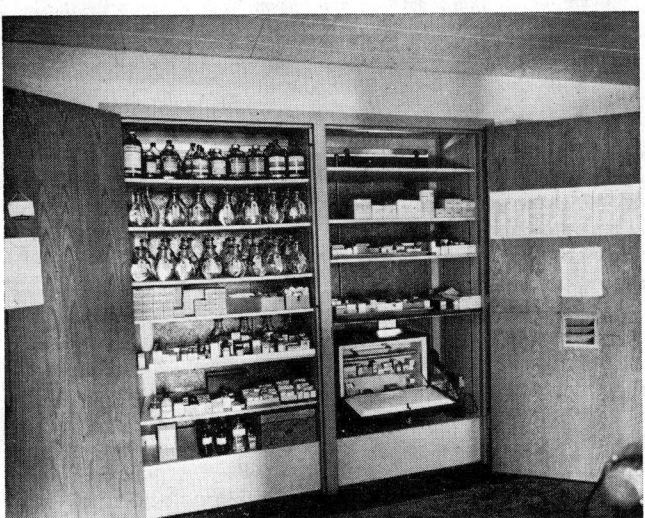

Fig. 786. Method for after-hours pharmacy service, Mary Fletcher Hospital, Burlington, Vt., showing locked area accessible only to night supervisor of nurses, and including refrigerator.

charge for it. In the morning the pharmacist replaces the charges with new stock, the charge is sent to the accounting office, and the "night pharmacy" is ready for another night. The chief pharmacist maintains control of all items in this unit. Another method is to place the night supplies in an after-hours storage area that is accessible only to the nursing supervisor at night (see Fig. 786). Charges are placed therein for all items withdrawn. In both circumstances there is an alphabetical index of items contained in the emergency units.

One might raise the very important philosophic question about the essentiality of having a registered pharmacist on duty during the daytime and then having after-hours services turned over to registered nurses. Thus, hospital administrators, medical staffs, and nurses can logically ask, "why can't the nurse provide pharmacy service during the day just as well as she does at night?" If this were so, then why have a pharmacist during the day? Pharmacists who wish to practice in a hospital and to become a more important member of the health-care team must realize that this team must deliver its services 24 hours/day,

because sick people are sick 24 hours/day, not from 8 am to 5 pm.

Special attention should be given to drugs in the emergency suite or accident ward. Every hospital should have a list of antidotal drugs approved by the professional staff. It should be the duty of the pharmacist to see that drugs on this list are in proper condition and readily available in the emergency suite.

Outpatient Dispensing—Many hospitals provide services to ambulatory patients through their emergency departments and outpatient clinics. Patients receive all the diagnostic and therapeutic services necessary for good patient care. In many of these hospitals the pharmacy department is called upon to provide prescription medication for the outpatients. There are a number of cogent reasons why these hospitals provide outpatient prescription service. Among the major ones are: (1) many of the patients are totally or partially medically indigent, (2) many of the patients are recipients of welfare assistance programs in which the agencies contract with the hospital to provide total medical care, including drugs, (3) some patients are taking investigational drugs and these drugs are not available from community pharmacies. In addition, some hospital pharmacies provide prescription service to hospital employees as part of the over-all hospital benefits. Some patients who are seen in emergency units or outpatient clinics are able to pay for their medication and their prescription orders may be dispensed at the hospital pharmacy.

Some controversy has existed among community and hospital pharmacists regarding the dispensing of outpatient prescription medication. The controversy is not about medication for indigent patients, but rather for those outpatients who are able to pay for their medication. Some years ago one or two state boards of pharmacy indicated an interest in trying to prevent hospital pharmacists from dispensing medication to outpatients. Hospital pharmacists objected on the basis of two fundamental principles: (1) a registered pharmacist is qualified legally to dispense prescriptions regardless of the setting in which he practices, whether community pharmacy or hospital pharmacy, and (2) in a democratic society patients have a right to choose which pharmacist shall provide pharmaceutical services to them. In 1960 The American Society of Hospital Pharmacists adopted the following resolution stating its position on outpatient prescription service:

Whereas ministering to the needs of the sick has always been a matter both for charitable endeavor and for economic gain, and
Whereas members of the public health professions have traditionally ministered to both prince and pauper, and
Whereas people of all economic strata utilize the facilities and services of the modern hospital, of which the pharmacy and its pharmacist are, and must remain, integral and inseparable parts, and
Whereas it is inevitable that, due to the complexities of modern medical care, all members of the health professions serving in hospitals will be called upon to play an increasingly important role in ministering to the health needs of the people, working through the organized hospital wherein each profession must fulfill its destiny, be it therefore
Resolved that The American Society of Hospital Pharmacists, in annual convention assembled, asserts and believes that hospital pharmacists have unquestionable and unchallengeable moral, legal and ethical rights to serve patients, both indigent and nonindigent, by filling prescriptions written by members of the hospital's medical staff for outpatients.[16]

In *Mirror to Hospital Pharmacy*[17] a recommendation was made to establish a Commission on Outpatient Dispensing "...broadly representative of the profession to study the effects the dispensing of prescriptions to indigent and nonindigent outpatients has upon pharmacy as a profession...." Such a commission was established in 1965 and a final report was prepared in 1966 entitled *The Challenge to Pharmacy in Times of Change*. This thought-provoking report outlines the radical changes taking place in the delivery of health care to the American public and the multifaceted relationship of pharmaceutical services to this over-all system. A number of conclusions, guidelines, and recommendations are made in this report. One of the most thought-provoking conclusions is stated this way:[18]

Pharmacy's stewardship: Contemporary social change has brought all professions to a time of self-examination. Pharmacy is called to a higher level of professional stewardship than it has known in the past, one that will require adaptation to a new code of socio-economic responsibility by all health professions. If the service of pharmacy to society continues to be dominated by its distributive function of which it has become a captive, it canot fulfill the needs of a new social order. Only when pharmacy's contribution to society is dominated by the capacity of its practitioners to apply their scientific knowledge to the needs of society and by their concern for public health and safety will the profession be justified in claiming all the privileges of an essential health service.

Investigational Drugs—The hospital pharmacist is in a strategic position to participate in an evaluation program on investigational drugs because such drugs must be tried in a hospital setting where the necessary laboratory and other medical facilities are available. It is thus a prime responsibility of the pharmacy and therapeutics committee to establish policies and procedures relative to the handling and control of investigational drugs in the hospital. To assist pharmacy and therapeutics committees, the American Hospital Association and the American Society of Hospital Pharmacists developed a statement (Fig. 787) embodying basic principles applicable to the safe handling of investigational drugs in the hospital.

There are many problems associated with the use of investigational drugs in the hospital some of which are:

1. Legal problems may result if a hospital does not exercise due care in the proper handling of investigational drugs in the over-all care of the patient.
2. Nurses, as agents of the hospital, are usually responsible for administering investigational drugs to patients. In performing this act it is essential that sufficient information on the proper dosage, route of administration, possible toxic reactions and side effects, precautions, and proper labeling be available to them.
3. Investigational drugs, as they are made available from the manufacturer to the principal investigator, are not labeled sufficiently in many instances to prevent the possibility of error in their administration to patients.
4. Because investigational drugs fall in the area of research in contrast to accepted methods of treatment there are legal implications revolving around the need for written consent by patients.
5. In the case of double blind studies it is essential that the person holding the code be readily available 24 hours a day, seven days a week, in case the patient's condition warrants a breaking of the code.
6. The legal requirements for proper records on the use of investigational drugs have been delineated by the Food and Drug Administration. In case of a recall because of severe permanent toxicity resulting from an investigational drug, it is essential that records of its use on specific patients in a hospital be readily available. In cases where the lot number of the drug is a significant factor such records should also be available.
7. In cases where investigational drugs are used on outpatients it is essential that such drugs be labeled to conform to legal requirements. It should be obvious that information must be readily available to assist physicians in other hospitals who may be required to treat patients suffering from accidental overdosage or toxic symptoms.
8. It is essential that the supply of an investigational drug be available during the night and weekends as well as when the principal investigator is at the hospital if nurses are to maintain uninterrupted dosage schedules in the best interest of the patient.

Thus the problems associated with the proper han-

**Statement of Principles
Involved in the Use of
Investigational Drugs in Hospitals**

Hospitals are the primary centers for clinical investigations on new drugs. By definition these are drugs which have not yet been released by the Federal Food and Drug Administration for general use.

Since investigational drugs have not been certified as being for general use and have not been cleared for sale in interstate commerce by the Federal Food and Drug Administration, hospitals and their medical staffs have an obligation to their patients to see that proper procedures for their use are established.

Procedures for the control of investigational drugs should be based upon the following principles:

1. Investigational drugs should be used only under the direct supervision of the principal investigator who should be a member of the medical staff and who should assume the burden of securing the necessary consent.

2. The hospital should do all in its power to foster research consistent with adequate safeguard for the patient.

3. When nurses are called upon to administer investigational drugs they should have available to them basic information concerning such drugs including dosage forms, strengths available, actions and uses, side effects, and symptoms of toxicity, etc.

4. The hospital should establish, preferably through the pharmacy and therapeutics committee, a central unit where essential information on investigational drugs is maintained and whence it may be made available to authorized personnel.

5. The pharmacy department is the appropriate area for the storage of investigational drugs, as it is for all other drugs. This will also provide for the proper labeling and dispensing in accord with the investigator's written orders.

Fig. 787.

dling of investigational drugs provide ample justification to warrant the establishment of sound policies and procedures governing their use in the hospital. This is a responsibility of the medical staff. The pharmacy and therapeutics committee is a committee of the medical staff and, therefore, it should be the responsibility of this committee to formulate policies and procedures relative to the handling of investigational drugs. The hospital pharmacist as a key member of the Pharmacy and Therapeutics Committee makes a real contribution to better patient care and safety by participating in formulating policies and procedures for handling investigational drugs in the hospital.

It is a common practice for physicians to obtain written consent from the patient prior to use of an investigational drug. A typical form for obtaining patient consent for such special therapy is shown in Fig. 788.

When the hospital pharmacist is called upon to handle an investigational drug he needs to maintain adequate dispensing records. A typical form which provides the controls necessary for the handling of investigational drugs by the pharmacy is shown in Fig. 789.

A single prescription for a single patient does not raise the question of investigational-drug use. The Federal law can be violated by preparing large quantities of drugs which have not been approved for human use by the Food and Drug Administration (FDA). To avoid legal violation, a sponsor of a drug investigation must file with the FDA a "Notice of Claimed Investigational Exemption for a New Drug" (IND). Such a form is usually filed by a pharmaceutical manufacturer; however, others may serve as the sponsor, such as a physician, pharmacist, or an institution such as a hospital, or the hospital pharmacy department.

An abbreviated form of IND is acceptable to the FDA where a physician wants to study a drug which no manufacturer wants to sponsor. The physician may serve both as sponsor and investigator; or the hospital pharmacy may serve as sponsor and the physician as investigator. Some hospital pharmacy departments serve as sponsors on many abbreviated IND's for special drug dosage forms that are not available commercially. The required forms for the sponsor and investigator plus the new-drug regulations are available from the FDA in Washington, D.C. Additional information is given in Chapter 73, *Introduction of New Drugs*.

Bulk Compounding or Manufacturing—A manufacturing laboratory is essential to a well-run hospital pharmacy for economy and to provide facilities for research and for the making of special preparations which cannot be purchased. One of the functions of the pharmacist is to cooperate with the medical staff in preparing the most efficacious preparations for use of the patients. Research by staff pharmacists should be encouraged by the chief pharmacist and by the hospital. In many instances, research will more than repay for the time and labor expended by providing a better and a more economical product for both hospital and patient. A properly equipped and staffed manufacturing laboratory also makes possible better pharmaceutical service. Physicians in hospitals order preparations which are not available commercially and therefore must be prepared in the pharmacy. A pharmacy which has no manufacturing equipment and whose staff has had no experience in manufacturing will not be able to meet these requests. This is especially true when special sterile preparations for injection are requested.

Sterile Products—One of the important duties of a hospital pharmacist is the preparation of parenteral solutions and other sterile products. In the small hospital the chief pharmacist will probably be called upon to do this work personally, while in the larger hospital it may be done by a capable pharmacist and technicians under supervision of the chief pharmacist.

Form 6954

THE OHIO STATE UNIVERSITY
UNIVERSITY HOSPITAL

CONSENT FOR SPECIAL THERAPY OR PROCEDURE

Date

Room No.

Patient's No.
Name
Address
City

I have been informed by Doctor.................................... at University Hospital that my medical condition makes advisable the use of special drugs or procedures and that the expected results of this treatment or these procedures have been explained to me. I hereby give my consent for this treatment or these procedures.

Date..................... Patient's Signature.....................
Witness.....................

(Place in Patient's Chart When Signed)

I have been informed by Doctor.................................... at University

Hospital that the medical condition of.................................... (Patient's Name)

my.................... (relationship), makes advisable the use of special drugs or procedures and that the expected results of this treatment or these procedures have been explained to me. I hereby give my consent for this treatment or these procedures.

Date..................... Signature of parent, guardian or responsible relative.....................

Witness.....................

(Place in Patient's Chart When Signed)

Fig. 788.

THE OHIO STATE UNIVERSITY HOSPITALS
PHARMACY DEPARTMENT

INVESTIGATIONAL DRUG DISPENSING RECORD

Name and Synonyms.....................

Strength and Dosage Form.....................

Manufacturer.....................

Principal Investigator.....................

Date	Patient Name	℞ # or Location	Physician	Lot Number	Amount Dispensed	Amount On Hand

Rev. 12/66

Fig. 789.

This subject is completely discussed in the chapters on *Sterilization* (page 1501) and *Parenteral Preparations* (page 1519). General methods of procedure in preparing, sterilizing, and handling solutions are essentially those outlined in the aforementioned chapters.

The preparation of parenteral solutions is one of the most exacting services the hospital pharmacist undertakes ordinarily. He should not assume this responsibility unless he has been adequately trained, has been provided the special laboratory space and equipment described in the chapter on *Parenteral Preparations* (page 1519) and enforces the rigid controls described therein.

Sterile Intravenous Admixtures—A large number of drugs are added to intravenous (IV) solutions in order to be administered to patients. Some of these drugs must be given in dilute form; others must be given over an extended period; while still others are given in an infusion because it is an effective way to administer them to patients. The majority of IV solutions administered to patients have one or more (as many as 4 or 5) additives. Preparing these IV admixtures requires aseptic technique in order to maintain the sterility of the drug additive as well as of the IV solution. In the majority of hospitals this pharmaceutical compounding procedure has been carried out by physicians and nurses. Recent trends show that a number of hospital pharmacists have developed a pharmacy-based IV admixture service for their entire hospital. A 700-bed teaching hospital may require as many as 350 IV admixtures to be compounded daily by the pharmacy. A complete policy and procedural manual on the operation of a centralized parenteral admixture service is available from the Department of Pharmacy, The Ohio State University Hospitals, Columbus, Ohio 43210.

Control—Rigid controls for all preparations manufactured in the hospital pharmacy are required. Master formulas, working sheets for the manufacturing procedures, samples of the finished product, and the control report all should bear a control number that should follow the finished preparation through the packaging procedures. The appropriate number should appear or be coded on every stock container in the pharmacy and on every prepackaged unit of outpatient or floor stock (including sterile) products. When dispensed, the control number should preferably be transferred to and should appear on the prescription order. Every step in the manufacturing procedure should be checked and initialed by the manufacturer and the checker. The working sheets and control reports should be so filed that they are readily available for future reference.

Master formula manufacturing work sheets should be preprinted so that there is no opportunity for error in the quantities of ingredients specified on a working sheet. Likewise, the specific equipment to be used in the process should be listed. The procedure should be outlined step by step so that no portion of the over-all procedure will be omitted. Packaging and labeling directions should be specified. A sample master formula manufacturing worksheet is illustrated in Fig. 790.

Pharmaceutical manufacturers are responsible for adhering to Part 133—Good Manufacturing Practice, of the Food, Drug, and Cosmetic Act. This part of the Act outlines current good manufacturing practices in the manufacture, processing, packing, or holding of drugs.[19] Although bulk compounding activities in individual hospital pharmacies have not come under the scrutiny of the FDA in the past, it would seem that hospital pharmacists should follow these guidelines in the operation of their manufacturing programs. See also Chapter 92, *Control* (page 1762).

In addition to the inprocess control systems used in manufacturing it is important to outline the quantitative assay control procedures to be performed on the finished product. Fig. 791 shows an example of a quality control worksheet helpful to personnel assigned to the assay and control division of the hospital pharmacy.

Drug-Information Services—*The Minimum Standard for Pharmacies in Hospitals* (page 1783) outlines one of the hospital pharmacists responsibilities as, "furnishing information concerning medications to physicians, interns and nurses." In the section on Facilities, the Minimum Standard states that facilities shall be provided for, "an adequate library and filing equipment to make information concerning drugs readily available to both pharmacists and physicians." The hospital setting provides a unique opportunity (not so readily available in other phases of practice) for the pharmacist to develop a comprehensive drug information service for the medical staff, residents, interns, medical students, nursing staff, student nurses, dentists, and dental residents.

To assume this responsibility the pharmacist will make use of his educational background in the biological and physical sciences which underlie his whole pharmaceutical training. Not only is the hospital pharmacist called upon to provide pharmacological information, but he is called upon also to provide information on the physical and chemical aspects of drugs. Another important responsibility of the hospital pharmacist is to provide biopharmaceutical information. He is in a strategic position to bridge the gap between the biological and the pharmaceutical aspects of dosage forms.

THE OHIO STATE UNIVERSITY HOSPITALS
PHARMACY DEPARTMENT

MANUFACTURING WORK SHEET

Name of Preparation ALCOHOL - MEDICATED 70% ______ Pharmacy Control No. ______

Package Size 1,000 and 4,000 ml. Manufactured by ______ Date ______

No.	Ingredients	Amount	Manufacturer's Name	Manufacturer's Lot No.	Measured By	Checked By
1.	Ethyl Alcohol 95%	265,000 ml.				
2.	Distilled Water q.s.	103,000 ml.				

EQUIPMENT

1. Stainless steel mixing tank with mixer, 100 gallon.
2. Graduate, cylindrical 500 ml.
3. Thermometer
4. Alcoholometer
5. Vacuum filling unit (2 and 3 spout) and transfer pump, Ertel.
6. Polyethylene tank, 30 gallon.
7. Carboy liquid trap.
8. Large (12" x 1") gas dispersion tube (coarse).
9. Approximately 240 empty amber quart containers labeled: Alcohol-Medicated 70%.
10. Approximately 30 empty amber gallon containers labeled: Alcohol-Medicated 70%.

PROCEDURE

____ 1. Check to see if the necessary equipment and an adequate supply of chemicals are available.
____ 2. Obtain a manufacturing control number and place in the appropriate space above.
____ 3. Rinse down the 100 gallon stainless steel mixing tank with distilled water and drain.
____ 4. Place approximately 265,000 ml. (14 five gallon cans - wipe the top of the cans first with a damp cloth) of ethyl alcohol 95% in the 100 gallon mixing tank.
____ 5. Add a sufficient quantity of distilled water to make approximately 350,000 ml. as indicated on the graduated rod placed at the back side of the tank (approximately 1/2 inch below 360,000 ml.).
____ 6. Mix well for 15 minutes with the tank mixer.
____ 7. Collect approximately 500 ml. of the hydroalcoholic solution in a 500 ml. cylindrical graduate as a representative sample.
____ 8. Take the temperature of the sample solution with a thermometer. TEMPERATURE ______.
____ 9. Immerse an alcoholometer in the sample solution and take the proof reading directly from the alcoholometer. PROOF READING ______.
____ 10. Alcoholometer proof readings must correspond within 2 proof degrees of standard (chart on reverse side) in relation to the temperature of the solution. If there is a deviation greater than 2 proof degrees, distilled water or ethyl alcohol 95% must be added to adjust the proof readings to within a 2 proof degree range of the standard (the addition of 5,000 ml. quantities of distilled water or ethyl alcohol 95% will affect the proof reading by approximately 1 proof degree).
____ 11. Mix the hydroalcoholic solution for a minimum of 10 minutes after the addition of any distilled water or alcohol.
____ 12. FINAL PROOF READING ______.

Rev. 9/63

TEMPERATURE Degrees F.	TEMPERATURE Degrees C.	PROOF READING (These proof readings all correspond to 70% at 21 degrees C.)
70	21	143
75	24	145
80	27	146.5
85	29.5	147
90	32	149
95	35	150.5

PACKAGING

____ 1. Rinse out the Ertel vacuum filling unit with distilled water.
____ 2. Rinse down a 30 gallon polyethylene tank with distilled water.
____ 3. Fill the 30 gallon polyethylene tank with the manufactured alcohol solution by gravity feed via the drain hose of the 100 gallon mixing tank. Refill the polyethylene tank as needed.
____ 4. Attach the bottom hose (vacuum) of the Ertel filling unit (2 or 3 spout) to the carboy liquid trap and connect the trap to the Ertel transfer pump.
____ 5. Attach a clean, large (12" x 1") gas dispersion tube (coarse) to the end of the top hose (liquid inlet) of the Ertel filling unit and immerse it in the alcohol solution in the 30 gallon polyethylene tank.
____ 6. Line up the empty "Alcohol-Medicated" bottles (quarts and gallons) side by side.
____ 7. Turn on the Ertel transfer pump and discard the first half gallon delivered by each spout. Fill approximately 240 quarts and 30 gallons (the ratio of quart to gallon usage is 8 to 1. This ratio of bottles filled should be maintained unless the present demands are otherwise).
____ 8. Immediately place white caps on the filled bottles and, if necessary, clean the exterior surface of the bottles with a damp cloth.
____ 9. Place a yellow cellulose sealing band around the caps of the quart bottles and a white cellulose sealing band around the caps of the gallon bottles.

LABELING

____ 1. Replace all soiled or wrinkled labels with new aluminum labels. An example label is shown below.
____ 2. Print a sufficient quantity of Monarch labels with the proper control number.
____ 3. Label the bottles with the Monarch label (attach Monarch label on the shoulder of the bottle opposite the main label).
____ 4. Affix a sample Monarch label in the appropriate space below.

ALCOHOL-MEDICATED
70%
FOR HOSPITAL USE ONLY, RETURN BOTTLE TO PHARMACY
THE OHIO STATE UNIVERSITY
UNIVERSITY HOSPITAL
PHARMACY DEPARTMENT

Lot No.
63090602

No. of Units Packaged ______ Container Check ______ Clarity Check ______
Label Check ______ Assay Results ______
Approval of Quality Control Pharmacist ______ (signature) Date Released ______

Fig. 790.

THE OHIO STATE UNIVERSITY HOSPITALS
PHARMACY DEPARTMENT

QUALITY CONTROL SHEET

Name of
Preparation DILUTED SODIUM HYPOCHLORITE SOLUTION

Pharmacy
Control No. _____

Source of Assay N.F. XI   Assayed By _____ Date _____

EQUIPMENT AND CHEMICALS

1. Acetic acid
2. Burette, 25 ml., clamped on ringstand
3. Erlenmeyer flask, 125 ml.
4. Graduate, 25 ml.
5. Potassium Iodide
6. Sodium thiosulfate solution, 0.1 N.
7. Starch test solution
8. Volumetric pipette, 5 ml.
9. Volumetric pipette, 10 ml.

ASSAY PROCEDURE

_____ 1. Transfer exactly fifteen (15) ml. of the sample to the erlenmeyer flask.
_____ 2. Add twenty-five (25) ml. of distilled water to the sample.
_____ 3. Add two (2) Gm. of potassium iodide to the sample.
_____ 4. Add ten (10) ml. of acetic acid to the sample.
_____ 5. Rinse the burette with a small quantity of the sodium thiosulfate solution.
_____ 6. Run in fifteen (15) ml. of the sodium thiosulfate from the burette to the sample.
_____ 7. Add three (3) drops of fresh starch T.S.
_____ 8. Titrate dropwise, stirring constantly, until the disappearance of the blue color.
_____ 9. Perform the above titration three (3) times.
_____ 10. _____ ml. of _____ N sodium thiosulfate required for titration No. 1.
_____ 11. _____ ml. of _____ N sodium thiosulfate required for titration No. 2.
_____ 12. _____ ml. of _____ N sodium thiosulfate required for titration No. 3.
_____ 13. Average ml. of _____ N sodium thiosulfate required. _____ ml.

CALCULATIONS

Each ml. of 0.1 N sodium thiosulfate is equivalent to 3.722 mg. of NaClO. First determine the equivalent amount of diluted sodium hypochlorite needed to neutralize one (1) ml. of the sodium thiosulfate solution used, then determine the percentage strength of the diluted sodium hypochlorite solution, and then calculate the percent of labeled potency of the diluted sodium hypochlorite solution. Perform all calculations in the indicated space on the back of this sheet.

Example

Sodium thiosulfate standardized at 0.1005 N.
Average ml. sodium thiosulfate used 19.5 ml.

Sodium thiosulfate standardized at _____
Average ml. sodium thiosulfate used _____

$$\frac{0.1 N}{3.722 mg./ml.} = \frac{0.1005 N}{X mg./ml.}$$
X = 3.7406 mg./ml. dil. sod. hypochlorite

$$\frac{0.1 N}{3.722 mg./ml.} = \frac{X mg./ml.}{X mg./ml.}$$
X= _____ mg./ml.

Percent Strength

$$\% = \frac{19.5 ml. Na_2S_2O_3 \times 3.7406 mg./ml. \times 100}{1000 \times 15}$$

$$\% = \frac{ml. Na_2S_2O_3 \times mg./ml. \times 100}{1000 \times 15}$$

% = 0.486   % = _____

11/63

Percent of labeled potency

$$\% = \frac{0.486 \times 100}{0.5}$$

% = 97.2

Tolerance range 90% to 100% of labeled potency, (0.450% to 0.500% NaClO)

Percent of labeled potency

$$\% = \frac{\% \times 100}{0.5\%}$$

% = _____

Assayed Potency

OTHER PHYSICAL AND CHEMICAL TESTS

1. Visual inspection (clarity, container, label).

DISPOSITION

_____ O.K. for use   Date of release _____
_____ Reject and dispose of material
_____ Other (Remarks) _____
_____
_____

Approval of Quality Control Pharmacists _____ Date _____

Attach this form to the Manufacturing Work Sheet and file.

CALCULATIONS

Fig. 791.

Assuming that the pharmacist has the educational background to provide an extensive drug information service, there is a need for developing the necessary resource material, namely, an adequate reference library on drugs. A systematic approach to developing adequate drug reference information involves accumulating current journal literature in addition to standard texts, drug-therapy references, indexes, etc. New knowledge on drugs is uncovered every day and therefore one cannot rely solely on texts as authoritative sources for current information. The hospital pharmacist cannot rely entirely on a medical library in a different building of the health center to provide the drug information called for daily. There is a need for developing source materials in the hospital pharmacy proper if he is to provide an effective service. He can, however, utilize the medical library for support on queries of an involved nature.

A manual entitled *Drug Information Center*, used by the Pharmacy Department of the Ohio State University Hospitals, may be helpful in developing such a center.

As an extension of the Drug Information Center, the pharmacy can make available periodic *Pharmacy Bulletins* or *Newsletters* to the medical and allied staffs on matters pertaining to drugs. Many hospital pharmacists have developed *Pharmacy Bulletins* which have gained the respect of their medical staffs. Some have been reprinted in medical pharmacology journals because of the valuable information contained therein. While some of these bulletins are prepared entirely by the pharmacy staff, others are prepared under the auspices of the pharmacy and therapeutics committee of the hospital. A bulletin is an effective means of promoting the rational use of drugs in the hospital setting, and it provides the hospital pharmacist with a challenging opportunity to utilize his educational background effectively.

The establishment of drug-information centers in a number of hospitals has created the opportunity for pharmacists so inclined to become drug-information specialists, in contrast to those who want to specialize in administration, manufacturing, drug distribution, radiopharmaceuticals, or other specialized areas of hospital pharmacy practice. The developing trend toward clinical pharmacy strengthens the need for and value of a drug-information center in the hospital pharmacy. An essential part of a clinical pharmacist's role is to deliver his knowledge about drugs at the patient's bedside and to the other members of the health-care team. In order for him to do this, he needs the vast resources of drug literature. This places a new significance on the development and expansion of the drug-information-center concept. Practitioners in this area prevailed upon the American Society of Hospital Pharmacists to prepare a statement on *The Hospital Pharmacist and Drug Information Services*. The following statement was adopted by the ASHP House of Delegates.

The Hospital Pharmacist and Drug Information Services[20]

Two of the fundamental characteristics of a profession are (1) mastery of a specific body of basic knowledge and (2) development of a unique expertise by means of which scientific principles are employed in the practical application of such knowledge for the benefit of society.

A vigorous and responsible application of this professional expertise, and a continuing exploration of innovative services for effective response to the changing needs of society are essential to the growth of a profession, its continued franchise as a social institution, and the realization of maximum contributions to society.

As an integral part of the system for drug utilization in health care, the hospital pharmacist is well acquainted with the increasingly complex problems of pharmacotherapy, the biomedical community's difficulties in trying to cope with an overwhelming drug literature, and the limitations of existing drug experience surveillance systems for assessing efficacy and safety of investigational as well as newly marketed drugs. Recognizing the implications for professional responsibility in this situation, many hospital pharmacists are exploring new service roles through which they can contribute more effectively to the resolution of these patient care problems. Prominent among these new services are the growing numbers and increasing effectiveness of drug information services which have been established by hospital pharmacy programs throughout the United States and Canada.

The American Society of Hospital Pharmacists has encouraged and supported this exploration of an innovative pharmacy service which promises to further the exploitation of current scientific knowledge of clinical drug efficacy and toxicity. The SOCIETY does not view rational therapeutics as a unique concern of any single element of the biomedical community, industry, or government. Rather, it takes the position that safe and effective health care with drugs demands the efforts of an increasingly heterogenous complex of health workers. Thus the hospital pharmacist shares with those who create, investigate, test, market, prescribe, administer and regulate the use of therapeutic agents an irreducible obligation to introduce into patient care the maximum extent of our scientifically proven knowledge of drug capabilities and limitations.

There is logical, even compelling, justification for hospital pharmacists to pursue vigorously their responsibilities to rational drug therapy:

1. Traditionally the service orientation of the pharmacist has been related to drugs—their efficacy, safety and control. Therefore, pharmacy encumbers by reason of tradition a special obligation to accept these new challenges.

2. Pharmacy is unique among the health professions in that it possesses an established, but unchallenged, capability to adapt its services for specific contributions to drug therapy. Full utilization of the hospital pharmacist's professional potential represents a more efficient and economical application of health manpower resources.

3. There exists today a nucleus of hospital pharmacy practitioners who are engaged in the functional establishment of a service foundation for drug information activities and responsibilities. Increasing clinical involvement of the heretofore cloistered hospital pharmacist has precipitated a growing demand for this drug information support to those in immediate contact with drug care needs of the patient.

4. Increasingly sophisticated concepts of pharmacodynamic and biochemical complexities of drug actions, a burgeoning drug literature, and the scientific and medicolegal difficulties attending clinical surveillance of drug experiences constitute adequate grounds for advocacy of interprofessional teamwork in the clinical use of drugs. Pharmacy's acceptance of its share of responsibility will lessen the formidable burden placed on other components of the health care community.

Its many continuing educational programs, contributions to the literature, and official statements attest to the *American Society of Hospital Pharmacists'* belief in the inherent obligations of hospital pharmacists to exercise their professional responsibilities in behalf of rational pharmacotherapeutics. To provide appropriate leadership in developing this aspect of pharmaceutical services, the *Society* now attempts to express here the explicit responsibilities which drug information pharmacists are preparing to assume, seeks to identify and characterize the qualitative dimensions of such services, and apprises allied health professions of hospital pharmacy's determination to perform with unprecedented professional distinction in this emerging facet of clinical services.

The hospital pharmacist who proffers his services as a drug information specialist shall be capable of performing responsibly as a professional person in the following respects:

1. He demonstrates professional and technical competence in the evaluation, critical selection, and utilization of the drug literature. He presents to those whom he serves the maximum relevant information with a minimum volume of pertinent supporting documentation so as to permit independent, informed conclusions and decisions.

2. His knowledge of institutional and extramural library facilities, literature utilization, and librarian services will permit his taking full advantage of all such resources available to him.

3. He possesses verbal and written communications skills which enable him to contribute effectively to intra- and inter-institutional dialogue relative to pharmacotherapeutic information.

4. He has the capacity for substantial contributions to the continuing education of all health professions.

5. He is involved directly and indirectly in patient care with drugs as a contributor to its continuing quality and as a monitor of its characteristics.

6. He is familiar with electronic data processing methodology to the extent necessary for him to utilize its services for information storage, processing and retrieval.

7. He is qualified to provide professional services in support of the pharmacy and therapeutics committee.

8. He supports, complements and supplements the efforts of colleagues in pharmacy who are now attempting to marshal the knowledge, skills, scientific acumen and professional judgment necessary to bring appropriately effective pharmaceutical services of all types into the mainstream of patient care with drugs. Thus he contributes to and is an integral part of clinical pharmacy practice and the education of clinical pharmacy practitioners.

9. He contributes to the drug literature through appropriate participation in research activities which include, but are not restricted to, (a) clinical and preclinical drug studies, (b) surveillance of clinical drug experiences in his institution, and (c) experimentation in professional services.

Although recognizing that there are today few hospital pharmacists who fully meet the performance standards which it postulates for drug information specialists, the SOCIETY believes that a lesser expertise can neither provide the requisite services of the clinical community nor meet the aspirations of professional pharmacy. The pursuit of these projected standards represents a commitment on the part of hospital pharmacists to develop a novel service with a quality of performance commensurate with the needs of allied health professionals in their quest for optimum patient care with drugs.

American hospital pharmacy commits itself to the development of practitioners with the aforementioned capabilities as its contribution to a demonstrable and often expressed need of the health professions. The impossibility of a unilateral implementation of this objective is acknowledged.

We solicit the cooperative support of other professional groups whose sympathetic interaction and assistance are essential to the refinement of this new health manpower resource. We appropriate for this purpose a resolution adopted by the American Medical Association's House of Delegates at its 1967 annual meeting: "The [American Society of Hospital Phamacists] should continue to study the effect of new interrelationships and interdependencies between health professionals, as well as the impact of innovative concepts on the organizational structure evolving in the general system of health care delivery."

Pharmaceutical education is petitioned to accept this challenge to which hospital pharmacists unreservedly commit themselves. The educator is urged to join with the clinically experienced drug information specialist who can assist curriculum restructuring to meet the needs of a higher order of professional practice.

With a corporate conviction in the need for newer dimensions of clinical services, and with resolute determination to meet its collective responsibilities in the extraction of maximum benefits of drug therapy in patient care, hospital pharmacy resolves to bring reliable, unbiased drug information services to operate effectively in the interests of rational therapeutics. A reciprocally supportive interaction is solicited from those who utilize their knowledge, skills and judgment in ministering to the specific needs of the patient and those whose mission it is to educate health professionals to meet their responsibilities to society.

Pharmacy Service in Small Hospitals and Nursing Homes—Nearly half of the 7000 hospitals in the United States do not have the services of a pharmacist. This means that personnel other than pharmacists are handling drugs in these institutions. This situation warrants serious attention by the profession of pharmacy. Many of these hospitals are not large enough to appoint a pharmacist on a full-time basis. They need the services, however, of a pharmacist on a part-time basis, and this need can be met only by interested community pharmacists. Guides have been published to help orient community pharmacists to to the pharmaceutical needs of small hospitals and to help hospital administrators become more aware of the services which pharmacists can provide. *Pharmacy Service in Smaller Hospitals*, by Berman and Zugich, and *A Guide for Pharmacists —— Smaller Hospitals*, by C. Lord,† are excellent references for community* pharmacists who wish to provide pharmaceutical service to a small hospital. In 1959 The American Hospital Association and The American Society of Hospital Pharmacists approved a statement entitled *Suggested Principles of Relationship Between Smaller Hospitals and Part-Time Pharmacists who Provide Pharmacy Service*. This statement serves as an excellent guide for a community pharmacist and hospital administrator to develop a good working relationship for providing pharmaceutical service in a small hospital.

---

* Available from the College of Pharmacy, University of Michigan, Ann Arbor, Mich. 48104.
† Available from the Georgia Pharmaceutical Association, 610 Grand Theatre Bldg., Atlanta 3, Ga.

In addition to the small hospitals there are estimated to be 25,000 institutions other than hospitals in the United States in the category of extended-care facilities, nursing homes, and homes for the aged. As the older population increases in the US, so does the number of nursing homes. Since so many of the patients in nursing homes are afflicted with chronic and debilitating illnesses, a tremendous amount of drugs is used in these institutions. The profession of pharmacy has not yet recognized its responsibility for seeing that drugs are properly handled in this large number of institutions. The American Pharmaceutical Association, American Society of Hospital Pharmacists, and American Nursing Home Association prepared a booklet entitled *Pharmaceutical Service in Nursing Homes,** for use as a guide to community pharmacists and nursing home administrators to establish adequate pharmaceutical service.

Suggested Principles of Relationship Between Smaller Hospitals and Part-Time Pharmacists Who Provide Pharmaceutical Services[21]

Approved by the Board of Trustees of the American Hospital Association and the Executive Committee of the American Society of Hospital Pharmacists February 1959.

Preamble

All hospitals should be cognizant of the contribution made by a sound and organized pharmaceutical service for improved patient care and treatment. The introduction annually of numerous potent drugs requires that all hospitals have the full or part-time service of a registered pharmacist. In small hospitals which cannot obtain or afford a full-time hospital pharmacist, the services of a pharmacist on a part-time or consultative basis may be obtained.

If the services of a hospital pharmacist of another hospital are not obtainable, the services of a local registered pharmacist should be utilized whenever possible. When pharmaceutical service from a local pharmacy is considered, the part-time pharmacist and the hospital might consider certain guiding principles of affiliation. The Principles of Relationship Between Smaller Hospitals and Part-time Pharmacists are suggested to achieve the objective of better patient care.

Basic Principle

1. *The pharmaceutical service of the hospital shall be organized and maintained primarily for the benefit of hospital patients.*

In any hospital, the individual elements which are maintained and coordinated are all subordinate to the main objective of providing care to the sick and injured. Any function either newly added or strengthened, as in this instance drug or pharmaceutical services (from any source whatever or by any arrangement), must be in agreement with this basic principle.

Organization

1. *The hospital pharmaceutical service should be under the direction of a professionally competent, legally qualified pharmacist.*

The hospital must exercise due care in its selection of personnel. The hospital safeguards the patient and its public trust by fixing the responsibility for its varied functions by appointing adequately qualified individuals.

2. *A part-time pharmacist, as a professional member of the hospital staff and as the head of a hospital function or department, must assume the responsibilities involved.*

Recognition as a member of the hospital organization will be in direct proportion to the responsibility which the individual is capable of accepting on a part-time basis.

3. *The part-time pharmacist shall be responsible to the proper administrative authority of the hospital for developing, supervising and coordinating the activities of the pharmaceutical services to hospital patients and departments.*

With hospital affiliation, an attendant responsibility is placed on the part-time pharmacist to preserve the unity and coordination of the hospital's component activities as directed by the administrator in policies laid down in behalf of the public which the hospital governing board represents. Thus the part-time pharmacist subscribing to a hospital connection in terms of relationships, is primarily responsible

to the hospital administrator for those services provided to hospital patients and departments.

Rules, regulations and procedures regarding drug services to hospital patients and departments should not be counter to or in opposition to the hospital's policies for patients as interpreted and approved by the hospital administrator in behalf of the medical staff, and of the hospital governing board and the public it represents.

4. *The organization of hospital pharmaceutical services, the relationship to the hospital and its elements, and the specific services to be provided should be outlined and reviewed periodically by the hospital administrator and the part-time pharmacist who provides pharmaceutical services to hospital patients and departments.*

To keep abreast of changing developments of staff demands for high standards of service and to obviate misunderstandings, relationships should be outlined initially and reviewed periodically. This appears to be particularly necessary in those situations where certain elements of services are provided on the hospital premises, and others in varying degrees emanate from sources away from the hospital environment arranged by delegation to others who may be unfamiliar with hospital safeguards and policies.

5. *The organization of pharmaceutical services should include the utilization of an organized Pharmacy and Therapeutics Committee responsible for the development of rules and regulations pertaining to professional policies related to pharmaceutical services for hospital patients.*

Following the usual practice in hospitals, the medical and pharmacy staffs acting in an advisory capacity are the most qualified to recommend to the hospital such policies as relate to selection, evaluation and distribution of drugs used in the hospital. The composition and specific objectives of the Pharmacy and Therapeutics Committee as well as its appointment may be developed to best meet the needs of the hospital and its standards.

Functions

1. *The primary functions of the service provided by a part-time pharmacist should be to furnish drugs with sufficient dispatch so that patient care will not be hindered, to provide adequate safeguards for the patient and hospital personnel, and to provide therapeutic agents of respected quality.*

Responsibilities do not begin or end with filling prescriptions or furnishing drugs remotely from the hospital. The well-rounded and minimum responsibility might include such personal services by the part-time pharmacist as staff education related to safeguards in use of drugs on the premises, contribution to educational or research programs where extant, provision of maximum consultation services to nursing and medical staffs, inspection of drug storage and distribution throughout the hospital, attendance at committee and department meetings, preparation of fiscal and professional reports where necessary, maintenance of an approved stock of emergency drugs, provision for 24-hour drug services, elimination of waste, etc.

2. *Records concerned with hospital patient services should be maintained separately, preserved for the period prescribed by legal or hospital requirements, and be readily available.*

Such records as narcotic, barbiturate, alcohol, prescription, and requisition requests differ between hospitals and retail pharmacy practice. Identification with a hospital transaction or treatment may be of prime importance.

3. *The relationship between the hospital and the part-time pharmacist in the function of drug procurement or purchasing for both patient and general hospital use should be based on fixed responsibilities and meet the following principles on Business Relationships.*

The smaller hospital generally purchases supplies through a modified central channel in the organization. The need for expert evaluation of specifications in the drug field is recognized. Hospitals contributing services to indigent patients enjoy special price privileges, and drugs in this category ethically should not be diverted to other outlets. The complexity in the area of procurement and possibility of abuses by either the hospital or the part-time pharmacist require careful evaluation of the procedure.

a. *That basis of financial arrangement between a hospital and part-time local pharmacist should be followed which would best meet the local situation. It is recognized that no one basis would seem applicable or suitable in all instances.*

The hospital and the part-time pharmacist must have a thorough appreciation of each other's business systems and controls. This may involve detailed exploration.

b. *Arrangements involving services to patients through voluntary insurance, indigent patients, or employees should be established in accordance with accepted hospital relationships and philosophies involving such programs.*

Some insurance plans vary between localities, and in some instances the so-called "no-pay or part-pay" patients comprise a sizable number of persons. Special financial arrangements in accord with hospital policy for other services provided may be required.

c. *Arrangements for a regular schedule for the personal services of*

---

* Available from the American Pharmaceutical Association, 2215 Constitution Ave., N.W., Washington, D.C. 20037.

the part-time pharmacist on the hospital premises should be made on a flexible basis related to time spent and services provided.

The hospital schedule and its 24-hour service to patients demands a varying amount or period spent during regular visits or to meet emergency requirements. In general, an average amount of time may be considered initially. Such an arrangement should be included in a plan, even though many services are provided remotely from the hospital premises.

d. Solicitation of patients or rendering services to the medical staff for their private practice through hospital channels by any person connected with the hospital is unethical.

The privilege of hospital affiliation should not be used to gain unfair advantage over other members of the profession. Patients and physicians are attracted to a particular pharmacy because of its known merit and established reputation for satisfactory service. Implied or open solicitation through hospital connections should not be indulged in by part-time pharmacists.

e. Relationships between a part-time pharmacist and the hospital are considered on the merit of reputable, prompt service to patients at reasonable cost, ability to serve the hospital in all phases of pharmacy service demanded by hospital requirements, and should subscribe to the suggested principles.

In communities where several pharmacies are available, a hospital may hesitate to engage the services of any one pharmacist because of pressures and ill-feeling against the hospital by other pharmacists. Intra-professional rivalry should not place the hospital in a position of not raising its own pharmacy service standards. The hospital as a community institution should be allowed the privilege of judging its future relationships for expanded services on the basis of a part-time pharmacist's ability to provide those services in the spirit in which patient care is provided in that hospital.

Conclusion

These Principles of Relationship Between Smaller Hospitals and Part-time Pharmacists for Hospitals are suggested. These recommended guides for further development and discussion are a beginning for those hospitals and pharmacists who wish to explore possibilities for developing higher standards of pharmaceutical service in institutions without full-time pharmacists.

A combination of such principles and the Minimum Standard for Pharmacies in Hospitals can provide both smaller hospitals and part-time pharmacists a working basis for a higher level of pharmaceutical service.

The Social Security Amendments of 1965 (Medicare) generated much interest within the profession to improve pharmaceutical service in small hospitals and in extended-care facilities. Hospital and nursing home administrators intensified their interest in pharmacy service also primarily because of certain requirements which Medicare imposed on these institutions. These requirements are included in documents called *Conditions of Participation for Hospitals* and *Conditions of Participation for Extended Care Facilities.* Thus, in order for these institutions to receive payment for services rendered to Medicare recipients, they must be certified by the Department of Health Education and Welfare. This means that these institutions must meet these "Conditions of Participation." These conditions are helpful guides to administrators and pharmacists in developing a meaningful pharmaceutical service in hospitals and nursing homes.

Condition of Participation For Hospitals Pharmacy or Drug Room

The hospital has a pharmacy directed by a registered pharmacist or a drug room under competent supervision. The pharmacy or drug room is administered in accordance with accepted professional principles.

Standard A

There is a pharmacy directed by a registered pharmacist or a drug room under competent supervision.

Factor 1. The pharmacist is trained in the specialized functions of hospital pharmacy.
Factor 2. The pharmacist is responsible to the administration of the hospital for developing, supervising, and coordinating all the activities of the pharmacy department.
Factor 3. If there is a drug room with no pharmacist, prescriptions are compounded by a qualified pharmacist elsewhere, and

only storing and distributing are done in the drug room. A consulting pharmacist assists in drawing up the correct procedures, rules, and regulations for the drug room.

Standard B

Facilities are provided for the storage, safeguarding, preparation, and dispensing of drugs.

Factor 1. Drugs are issued to floor units in accordance with approved policies and procedures.
Factor 2. Drug cabinets on the nursing units are routinely checked by the pharmacist. All floor stocks are properly controlled.
Factor 3. There is adequate space for all pharmacy operations and the storage of drugs at a satisfactory location provided with proper lighting, ventilation, and temperature controls.
Factor 4. If there is a pharmacy, equipment is provided for the compounding and dispensing of drugs.
Factor 5. Special locked storage space is provided to meet the legal requirements for storage of narcotics, alcohol, and other prescribed drugs.

Standard C

Personnel competent in their respective duties are provided in keeping with the size and activity of the department.

Factor 1. The pharmacist is assisted by an adequate number of additional registered pharmacists and such other personnel as the activities of the pharmacy may require to insure quality pharmaceutical services.
Factor 2. The pharmacy, depending upon the size and scope of its operations, is staffed by the following categories of personnel:
(I) Chief pharmacist; (II) One or more assistant chief pharmacists; (III) Staff pharmacists; (IV) Pharmacy trainees (where a program has been activated); (V) Nonprofessionally trained pharmacy helpers; (VI) Clerical help.
Factor 3. Provision is made for emergency pharmaceutical services.
Factor 4. If the hospital has only a drug room, a designated individual(s) has responsibility for its operation.

Standard D

Records are kept of the transactions of the pharmacy (or drug room) and correlated with other hospital records where indicated. Such special records are kept as are required by law.

Factor 1. The pharmacy establishes and maintains, in cooperation with the accounting department, a satisfactory system of records and bookkeeping in accordance with the policies of the hospital for:
(I) Maintaining adequate control over the requisitioning and dispensing of all drugs and pharmaceutical supplies;
(II) Charging patients for drugs and pharmaceutical supplies.
Factor 2. A record of the stock on hand and of the dispensing of all narcotic drugs is maintained in such a manner that the disposition of any particular item may be readily traced.

Standard E

Policies are established to control the administration of toxic or dangerous drugs with specific reference to the duration of the order and the dosage.

Factor 1. The medical staff has established a written policy that all toxic or dangerous medications, not specifically prescribed as to time or number of doses, will be automatically stopped after a reasonable time limit set by the staff. The classifications ordinarily thought of as toxic or dangerous drugs are narcotics, sedatives, anticoagulants, and antibiotics.

Standard F

There is a committee of the medical staff to confer with the pharmacist in the formulation of policies.

Factor 1. A pharmacy and therapeutics committee (or equivalent committee), composed of physicians and pharmacists, is established in the hospital and serves as the liaison between the medical staff and the pharmacist.
Factor 2. The committee assists in the formulation of broad professional policies regarding the procurement, distribution, use, safety procedures, and other matters relating to drugs in hospitals.
Factor 3. The committee performs the following specific functions:
(I) Serves as an advisory group to hospital medical staff and the pharmacist on matters pertaining to the choice of drugs; (II) Develops and reviews periodically a formulary or drug list accepted for use in the hospital; (III) Establishes standards concerning the use and control of experi-

mental drugs and research in the use of recognized drugs; (IV) Evaluates clinical data concerning new drugs or preparations requested for use in the hospital; (V) Makes recommendations concerning drugs to be stocked on the nursing unit floors and by other services; and (VI) Prevents unnecessary duplication in stocking the same basic drug and its preparation.

Factor 4. The committee meets at least quarterly and reports to the executive committee and the medical staff.

Standard G

Drugs dispensed are included (or approved for inclusion) in the United States Pharmacopeia, National Formulary, United States Homeopathic Pharmacopeia, New Drugs, or accepted Dental Remedies (except for any drugs unfavorably evaluated therein), or are approved for use by the pharmacy and drug therapeutics committee (or equivalent committee) of the hospital staff.

Factor 1. The pharmacist, with the advice and guidance of the pharmacy and therapeutics committee, is responsible for specifications as to quality, quantity, and source of supply of all drugs.

Factor 2. There is available a formulary or list of drugs accepted for use in the hospital which is developed and amended at regular intervals by the pharmacy and therapeutics committee (or equivalent committee) with the cooperation of the pharmacist (consulting or otherwise) and the administration.

Factor 3. The pharmacy or drug room is adequately supplied with preparations so approved.

Condition of Participation for Extended Care Facilities Pharmaceutical Services

Whether drugs are generally procured from a community pharmacy or stocked by the facilities, the extended care facility has methods and procedures for its pharmaceutical services that are in accord with accepted professional practices.

Standard A

Procedures for Administration of Pharmaceutical Services

The extended care facility provides appropriate methods and procedures for the obtaining, dispensing, and administering of drugs and biologicals, developed with the advice of a staff pharmacist, a consultant pharmacist, or a pharmaceutical advisory committee which includes one or more licensed pharmacists.

Factor 1. If the extended care facility has a pharmacy department, a licensed pharmacist is employed to administer the pharmacy department.

Factor 2. If the facility does not have a pharmacy department, it has provision for promptly and conveniently obtaining required drugs and biologicals from community pharmacies.

Factor 3. If the facility has only a drug room where bulk drugs are stored:

(I) The consultant pharmacist is responsible for the control of all bulk drugs and maintains records of their receipt and disposition.

(II) The consultant pharmacist dispenses drugs from the drug room, properly labels them and makes them available to appropriate licensed nursing personnel. Wherever possible, the pharmacist in dispensing drugs works from the prescriber's original order or a direct copy.

(III) Provision is made for emergency withdrawal of medications from the drug room.

Factor 3. An emergency medication kit approved by the facility's group of professional personnel is kept readily available.

Standard B

Conformance With Physicians' Orders

All medications administered to patients are ordered in writing by the patient's physician. Oral orders are given only to a licensed nurse, immediately reduced to writing, signed by the nurse and countersigned by the physician within 48 hours. Medications not specifically limited as to time or number of drugs, when ordered, are automatically stopped in accordance with written policy approved by the physician or physicians responsible for advising the facility on its medical administrative policies.

Factor 1. The charge nurse and the prescribing physician together review monthly each patient's medications.

Factor 2. The patient's attending physician is notified of stop order policies and contacted promptly for renewal of such orders so that continuity of the patient's therapeutic regimen is not interrupted.

Factor 3. Medications are released to patients on discharge only on the written authorization of the physician.

Standard C

Administration of Medications

All medications are administered by licensed medical or nursing personnel in accordance with the medical and nurse practice acts of each state. Each dose administered is properly recorded in the clinical record.

Factor 1. The nursing station has readily available items necessary for the proper administration of medication.

Factor 2. In administering medications, medication cards or other State approved systems are used and checked against the physician's orders.

Factor 3. Medications prescribed for one patient are not administered to any other patient.

Factor 4. Self-administration of medications by patients is not permitted except for emergency drugs on special order of the patient's physician or in a predischarge program under the supervision of a licensed nurse.

Factor 5. Medication errors and drug reactions are immediately reported to the patient's physician and an entry thereof made in the patient's clinical record as well as on an incident report.

Factor 6. Up-to-date medication reference texts and sources of information are provided, such as ASHP Hospital Formulary and Physicians Desk Reference.

Standard D

Labeling and Storing Medications

Patients' medications are properly labeled and stored in a locked cabinet at the nurses' station.

Factor 1. The label of each patient's individual medication container clearly indicates the patient's full name, physician's name, prescription number, name and strength of drug, date of issue, expiration date of all time-dated drugs, and name, address, and telephone number of pharmacy issuing the drug. It is advisable that the manufacturer's name and the lot or control number of the medication also appear on the label.

Factor 2. Medication containers having soiled, damaged, incomplete, illegible, or makeshift labels are returned to the issuing pharmacist or pharmacy for relabeling or disposal. Containers having no labels are destroyed in accordance with State and Federal laws.

Factor 3. The medications of each patient are kept and stored in their originally received containers and transferring between containers is forbidden.

Factor 4. Separately locked, securely fastened boxes (or drawers) within the medicine cabinet are provided for storage of narcotics, barbiturates, amphetamines, and other dangerous drugs.

Factor 5. Cabinets are well lighted and of sufficient size to permit storage without crowding.

Factor 6. Medications requiring refrigeration are kept in a separate, locked box within a refrigerator at or near the nursing station.

Factor 7. Poisons and medications for "external use only" are kept in a locked cabinet and separate from other medications.

Factor 8. Medications no longer in use are disposed of or destroyed in accordance with Federal and State laws and regulations.

Factor 9. Medications having an expiration date are removed from usage and properly disposed of after such date.

Standard E

Compliance With Laws
Controlling Narcotics, etc.

The extended care facility complies with all Federal and State laws relating to the procurement, storage, dispensing, administration, and disposal of narcotics, hypnotics, amphetamines, certain psychosomatic medications, and other legend drugs.

Factor 1. A narcotic record is maintained which lists on separate sheets for each type and strength of narcotic the following information: date, time administered, name of patient, dose, physician's name, signature of person administering dose, and balance.

References

1. *Hospitals*, **38**, 109 (Jan. 1, 1964).
2. *Am. J. Hosp. Pharm.*, **19**(9), 493 (1962).
3. *Am. J. Hosp. Pharm.*, **20**(8), 378 (1963).
4. *Am. J. Hosp. Pharm.*, **20**(8), 377 (1963).
5. *Am. J. Hosp. Pharm.*, **20**(2), 105 (1963).
6. *Hospitals* (Guide Issue), **42**, 17 (Aug. 1, 1968).
7. *Hospitals*, **41**, 113 (Dec. 16, 1967).
8. Urdang, G., *Bull. Am. Soc. Hosp. Pharm.*, **9**(4), 281 (1952).
9. Niemeyer, G. F., *et al*, *Bull. Am. Soc. Hosp. Pharm.*, **9**(4), 287 (1962).
10. *Am. J. Hosp. Pharm.*, **21**(11), 535 (1964).

11. Spease, E., and Porter, R. M., *J. APhA,* **25,** 65 (1936).
12. *Am. J. Hosp. Pharm.,* **21,** 40 (1964).
13. *Am. J. Hosp. Pharm.,* **21**(11), 535 (1964).
14. Godwin, H., *Drug Intelligence,* **2**(6), 152 (1968).
15. Beste, D., *Am. J. Hosp. Pharm.,* **25**(8), 396 (1968).
16. *Am. J. Hosp. Pharm.,* **17**(12), 813 (1960).
17. Francke, D. E., *et al, Mirror to Hospital Pharmacy,* Mack Printing Co.,

    Easton, Pa., 1964, p. 4.
18. Brodie, D. C., *The Challenge to Pharmacy in Times of Change,* APhA
    Ann. Mtg., Washington, D.C., 1966, pp. 4,5.
19. *Am. J. Hosp. Pharm.,* **21**(9), 399 (1964); also *Fed. Register* (28 F.R.
    6385), 1 (June 20, 1963).
20. *Am. J. Hosp. Pharm.,* **25**(7), 381 (1968).
21. *Am. J. Hosp. Pharm.,* **16**(3), 124 (1959).

94 | The Prescription

Form of the prescription order—handling the prescription—prescription containers—legal considerations—incompatibilities (types, manifestations, correction and prevention, and examples)

This chapter was prepared by

Daniel A. Hussar, PhD, *Associate Professor of Pharmacy, Philadelphia College of Pharmacy and Science, Philadelphia, Pa. 19104*

The term prescription refers either to an order for medication or to the medication dispensed by the pharmacist as a result of the order. A prescription order may be issued by a physician, dentist, veterinarian, or other properly licensed medical practitioner. It is specific in character in that it designates a particular medication for a particular individual at a particular time. The order may be written and signed or it may be dictated to a pharmacist by telephone or other device. When a pharmacist receives an oral prescription order, he is obligated to transcribe it into written form and, if necessary, must obtain the prescriber's signature at a later time.

The following discussion concerning the form and handling of the prescription order pertains primarily to those prescription orders received in a community pharmacy. Medication orders such as those that might be received in a hospital pharmacy for inpatients will not be specifically covered in this chapter, although much of the material considered may be applied to these orders also.

Form of the Prescription Order

It is the responsibility of the pharmacist to interpret the wishes of the prescriber, and thus he should be familiar with the typical form of the written prescription.

For the purpose of examination or study a prescription order may be discussed under eight headings.

1. The name, address, and age of the patient
2. The date prescribed
3. The superscription
4. The inscription
5. The subscription
6. The signa
7. The renewal instructions
8. The name of the prescriber

A model complete prescription order appears below.

John Doe, M.D.		Medical Building Columbus, Ohio	
For:	Mr. Harry Smith 903 Park Place	Date:	April 15, 1970
℞	Codeine Phosphate		0|5
	Ammonium Chloride		6|0
	Cherry Syrup		30|0
	Purified Water sufficient to make		60|

Mix and make solution.
Sig. One teaspoonful every three hours.

Dr. John Doe
Registry No. 1234

In actual practice any or all of these parts, except for the inscription and the name of the prescriber, may sometimes be omitted. The pharmacist then obtains the missing information from the patient or the physician.

The Name, Address, and Age of the Patient—The name and address serve to identify the prescription. Also, placing the full name on the label may serve to prevent a mixup of medication within a household. Federal law requires that both the full name and address be included on narcotic prescriptions. The age generally need only be designated as adult or child, although in the case of a young child the exact age should be included. This information should be placed on the prescription by the prescriber, preferably at the top. When omitted, the pharmacist should always obtain the information and place it on the prescription.

The Date Prescribed—This is important from the standpoint of keeping accurate records of narcotics and other drugs controlled by special laws and regulations. For example, the Drug Abuse Control Amendments specify that no prescription order (for a drug controlled by these amendments) can be dispensed or renewed more than 6 months after the date of issue. The date dispensed often differs from the date prescribed and is a more accurate indication of the age of the dispensed medication.

The Superscription—This consists of the symbol ℞, generally understood to be a contraction of the Latin verb *recipe* (take thou). Some historians believe this symbol originated from the sign of Jupiter, ♃, employed by the ancients in requesting aid in healing. Gradual distortion through the years led to the symbol as currently used. However, regardless of its meaning or origin, this symbol remains today as representative of both the prescription and pharmacy itself.

The Inscription—This, the body or principal part of the prescription order, contains the names and quantities of the prescribed ingredients. It is the portion of the prescription that requires most of the pharmacist's time and attention.

The names of the ingredients are written generally in English, although Latin is occasionally used, particularly in prescriptions requiring compounding. The use of Latin and English abbreviations is common, although this practice is not recommended. It can lead to serious errors unless extreme care is employed by the pharmacist in interpreting the abbreviations.

The quantities of the ingredients are written in either the apothecary or metric system of weights and measures, although the use of the apothecary system is lessening. Both the elimination of the apothecary system from the USP and NF (except for a table of approximate equivalents) and the adoption by drug manufacturers of the metric system for establishing dosage regimens have provided a strong impetus toward ending the use of this system. Medical schools, hospitals, and health agencies in most cases employ only the metric system. However, in spite of this, the use of the apothecary system still lingers on to some extent in prescription writing. As a result, the pharmacist must be familiar with the symbols and abbreviations and with calculations in both systems and be able to dispense prescription orders written in either, or a combination of both, as sometimes occurs. Conversion from one system to the other for the purpose of calculating or compounding is not recommended since this increases the chance of error.

In the use of the metric system the decimal is often replaced by a vertical line that may be imprinted on the prescription blank. The symbols Gm or ml are often eliminated, and it is understood that solids are dispensed by weight and liquids by volume.

In the apothecary system quantities are designated by a symbol followed by a Roman numeral, as Sucrose ℥ iv, indicating 4 drams of sucrose. Chapter 9 on *Metrology*, page 77, lists other apothecary symbols.

The Subscription—This comprises directions to the pharmacist for compounding the prescription. However, the present custom is for the practitioner to omit specific compounding instructions to the pharmacist. This practice results from the reduction in the number of prescriptions requiring compounding as well as a recognition of the skill and knowledge of the pharmacist. In a large majority of prescriptions the subscription serves merely to designate the dosage form and number of doses to be supplied, as M. or misce; D.T.D. capsulae numero xii; F. or fiat solutio; dispense 12 such suppositories.

The Signa—The directions for the patient, sometimes called Signatura, are usually introduced by Sig. or S. (mark thou). It is the responsibility of the pharmacist to place this information on the label of the container in order that the patient have available necessary instructions concerning the quantity, frequency of dose, and manner of administration of the medication. The use of the phrase "as directed" or similar designation is not a satisfactory signa and should be avoided whenever possible. When a physician employs such phrases, he generally supplies the patient with separate written or oral instructions. However, directions delivered orally to the patient or not attached to the prescription container often lead to confusion and misunderstanding, and the pharmacist should assure himself that the patient understands how to employ the medication properly.

In addition to instructions to the patient many practitioners include the name and strength of the prescribed drug in the signa. The practitioner signifies this by either one of the following:

1. Including the name and strength of the drug in the signa; eg, Sig. Cap. i q4h, Achromycin 250 mg.
2. Using the word "label" in the signa or elsewhere on the face of the prescription; eg, Sig. Cap. i q4h, label.

The intended purpose of this procedure is to make the identity of the prescription medication readily available for the physician when

1. Facing an emergency such as an accidental or purposeful overdose.
2. Adjusting dosage levels for a patient.
3. Seeing a patient when unfamiliar with the medication previously prescribed.
4. Meeting situations where a knowledge of the prescription medication is required but it is not possible or practical to contact the pharmacy where it was dispensed.

A principal objection to the use of this procedure is that hazardous self-medication or even "prescribing" by one patient for another may result.

The prescriber may also request that the expiration date of the drug be placed on the label if such information is included on the original package. In at least one state the law requires that this be done. The purpose of this is obvious, especially in view of reports of toxic effects resulting from administration of degraded outdated drugs. However, Deputy Commissioner W. B. Rankin of the Food and Drug Administration points out that the expiration date is predicated on proper storage and it is not reasonable to expect that these conditions always will be maintained by the patient. A more meaningful expiration date might be one based on the probable duration of treatment. Statements such as "do not use after . . ." or "discard after . . . days" serve this purpose.

The decision to place the product name on the label must be made only by the prescriber, based on his judgment of the individual situation. However, the situation of placing the expiration date on the label is not as clear. Some suggest that it is desirable for the pharmacist to include this information on the label whether the prescriber requests it or not, whereas others feel that it should not be routinely included (except for preparations that rapidly lose potency such as oral suspensions of the penicillin derivatives) unless specifically requested by the prescriber or required by law.

The Renewal Instructions—It is recommended that the prescriber indicate on every prescription order whether it may be renewed and, if so, how many times. Many prescription blanks have a small form printed on them where this information may be quickly designated. This matter will be considered in more detail in this chapter under "Legal Considerations."

The Name of the Prescriber—In most instances the name, address, and registry number (the number assigned to the medical practitioner by the Federal Bureau of Narcotics) are imprinted on the prescription blank. The State license number of the prescriber also may be included.

Federal law requires that narcotic prescriptions be validated by the full signature of the prescriber, and many states require a similar validation on all written prescriptions.

Handling the Prescription

The manner in which a pharmacist handles a prescription can enhance his image in the eyes of both the physician and the patient. Proper procedures are given below for receiving, reading, checking, pricing, numbering, dating, labeling, preparing, packaging, rechecking, delivering, recording, and filing prescriptions.

Receiving the Prescription—It is desirable that the patient hand the prescription order directly to a pharmacist since this serves to indicate to the patient its importance and to emphasize the professionalism of the prescription service. However, in situations where this is not possible, the individual receiving the order should be trained to accept it in a professional manner, obtain the correct name, address, and, if necessary, age of the patient, and determine whether the patient wishes to wait, call back, or have the medication delivered. If the pharmacist is unable to receive the prescription order personally, he should be readily available to give an estimate of the length of time required to dispense the prescription and to price it if requested by the patient. Many pharmacists make it a habit to price before dispensing, especially in the case of more expensive medication, to avoid subsequent discussions concerning cost.

In order to identify the finished prescription properly some pharmacies, especially where several pharmacists are on duty, employ a prescription claim check. Such a check might be divided into three parts, each part bearing identical numbers. One part is given to the patient, the second is attached to the prescription order, and the third is attached to the final container. Identification is made more frequently by means of the patient's name and address. This latter procedure tends to give a more personal touch to the service.

Reading and Checking the Prescription—The prescription order first should be completely and carefully read in the privacy of the prescription laboratory. There should be no doubt as to the ingredients or quantities prescribed. The pharmacist has justifiably earned the reputation of being able to read the handwriting of most physicians. It is most essential, however, that he never allows his pride in this reputation to prevent his admitting an inability to decipher a prescription. He should never guess at the meaning of an indistinct word or ambiguous abbreviation. To dispense mercuric chloride for mer. chl., without verification, or Achromycin for Achro when Achrocidin or Achrostatin may be intended, is courting trouble. Other types of abbreviations are also used. For example, the abbreviation "SSKI" represents the use of a "shorthand" for saturated solution and the chemical symbols for potassium iodide.

The use of Latin words, phrases, and abbreviations may also present a problem in understanding parts of the prescription order. Latin is considered the language of the medical world and was used extensively in writing prescription orders until the early part of the 20th century. Its use has gradually been abandoned although it is still employed to some extent, usually in the form of abbreviations in the subscription and signa. Because of their continued occasional use, some Latin terms and abbreviations are listed in Table I. Additional information may be obtained from references on pharmaceutical Latin.[1]

Another problem that confronts the pharmacist in his interpretation of the prescription order is that the names of many drugs look and/or sound like those of other drugs. Examples of such drugs are listed in Table II. More inclusive lists have been published.[2]

In checking the prescription for potential problems, many pharmacists now utilize patient record cards. Such records are a valuable aid to the pharmacist in making sure that the patient is not allergic to the prescribed medication or is not taking other medication with which the newly prescribed medication might interact.

The pharmacist must take great care and use his broad knowledge of drug products to prevent dispensing errors. A call to the physician, made so as not to alarm the patient, will serve to verify the meaning of a prescription that is not clearly written and at the same time serve to bolster the professional reputation of the pharmacist as an alert and valuable member of the medical team.

Omissions, such as failure to specify the potency of a medication or the particular dosage form, should be noted and proper insertions made. In such a case the pharmacist should never elect to dispense the *usual* dose or dosage form, but should consult the prescriber. For example, the decision to dispense 500-mg tablets

when a prescription for Diuril is received and no strength is specified cannot be justified on the basis that this is the usual dose. Likewise, when a prescription for Fiorinal is received and the dosage form is not specified, the pharmacist should inquire as to whether the tablets or capsules are preferred. It should be noted, however, that the pharmacist must be familiar with the available strengths and dosage forms of prefabricated medicinal agents in order to be able to detect such omissions and supply the physician with the necessary information.

Size and frequency of dose must be carefully noted and checked. In determining the safety of the dose of a potentially toxic material, the age or the weight of the patient, the dosage form prescribed, possible synergism, and the frequency of administration must all be considered. Because of the many factors involved in the calculation of an individual dose there are no hard and fast rules on which the pharmacist can rely. However, a number of guides are available to the pharmacist as aids in determining the safety of a prescribed dose. The official compendia list usual doses and dosage ranges. Catalogs, file cards, and package inserts from manufacturers serve as a complete source of dosage information on their products. Reference texts such as *Physicians' Desk Reference, Merck Index,* and *United States Dispensatory* are useful general sources of such information (see Chapter 7 on *Literature,* page 55). In the case of an apparent error in dose, pertinent sources of information should be checked before consulting the physician.

Problems may arise when a reasonable dose is administered too frequently. A prescription calling for "Dexamyl Spansules, Sig. One every three hours" should raise a question in the pharmacist's mind since such a medication is usually only given once daily. Medications might also be administered at a time that is not considered desirable. It is recommended that certain antibiotics should not be given with meals since a significantly decreased absorption of the drug may result.

An estimation of doses for children and infants can be obtained from several empirical rules based on age or weight (see page 108 in Chapter 10 on *Calculation*).

Butler and Richie[3] pointed out that a dose is not always a simple linear function of body weight and that its calculation as so much per kilogram of body weight is often inaccurate. Experience has shown that the doses of many drugs are more nearly proportional to the surface area* of the body. Although there has been some criticism of the surface area method of dosing, its practicality and usefulness have been confirmed and many recommend that it be employed as a basis for determining dosages for children (Table III). A further discussion of pediatric dosage and a table of pediatric doses related to body weight and to body surface area may be found in the Dosage-Posology Handbook published (1965) by the American Pharmaceutical Association.

Unusual doses may be prescribed, and the practitioner may indicate he wishes such a dose by underlining it or by the use of the symbols Q.R. (quantum rectum). However, since there is no uniformly accepted method of indicating unusual doses, the pharmacist must assure himself of the intent of the prescriber. Courts have held pharmacists liable for harm resulting from dis-

---

* Body surface area in square meters (M^2) is approximately equal to body weight in kilograms (Kg) raised to the 0.7 power; ie, Surface area (M^2) = body weight $(Kg)^{0.7}$.

Table I—Latin Abbreviations

Word or phrase	Contraction	Meaning	Word or phrase	Contraction	Meaning
A, aa	...	Of each	Contra	...	Against
Ad	Ad	To, up to	Contusus	...	Bruised
Adde, addantur	...	Add, or let them be added	Cujus, Cujuslibet	Cuj.	Of which, or any
Ad libitum	Ad lib.	At pleasure	Cum	c̄.	With
Admove	Admov.	Apply			
Ad tertiam vicem	...	For three times	Da, detur	D., det.	Give, let be given
			De	...	Of, or from
Adversum	Adv.	Against	Decem, Decimus	...	Ten, the tenth
Agita	Agit.	Shake, stir			
Albus	Alb.	White	De die in diem	De d. in d.	From day to day
Aliquot	...	Some, a few	Dentur tales doses No. iv	D.t.d. No. iv	Let four such doses be given
Alter	...	The other	Detur in duplo	...	Let twice as much be given
Alternis horis	...	Every other hour			
Amplus	...	Large	Dexter, Dextra	...	The right
Ana	A., āā	Of each	Diebus alternis	Dieb. alt.	Every other day
Ante	a	Before	Diebus tertiis	Dieb. tert.	Every third day
Ante cibos	a. c.	Before meals	Dilue, Dilutus	Dil.	Dilute (thou), diluted
Aqua	Aq.	Water			
Aqua aerata	Aq. aerat.	Carbonated water	Dimidius	Dim.	One-half
Aqua astricta	Aq. astr.	Frozen water	Directione propria	D. P. or direc. prop.	With a proper direction
Aqua bulliens	Aq. bull.	Boiling water			
Aqua communis	Aq. comm.	Common water	Dividatur in partes aequales	D. in p. æq.	Let it be divided into equal parts
Aqua fervens	Aq. ferv.	Hot water	Dividendus, -a, -um	...	To be divided
Aqua marina	Aq. mar.	Sea water			
Argentum	arg.	Silver			
Aures utræ	a.u.	Each ear	Eadem (fem.)	...	The same
Aurio dextra	a.d.	Right ear	Ejusdem	Ejusd.	Of the same
Aurio læva	a.l.	Left ear	Emulgens	...	An emulsifying agent
Aut	...	Or			
			Emulsum	Emuls.	Emulsion
Bacillum	...	A bougie	Enema	En.	An enema, a clyster
Bene	...	Well	Et	...	And
Bibe	Bib.	Drink	Etiam	...	Also, besides
Biduum	...	Two days	Ex or E	E.	From one of
Bis	...	Twice	Ex modo prescripto	E. m. p.	After the manner prescribed, as directed
Bis in die	B. i. d.	Twice a day			
Bolus	Bol.	A large pill			
Bonus	...	Good			
Brevis	...	Short			
Bulliat, bulliant	Bull.	Let boil	Fac, Fiat. Fiant	F., Ft.	Make, let it be made, let them be made
Capiat	Cap.	Let him (or her) take			
			Fac pilulas duodecim	F. pil. xii	Make 12 pills
Capsula	Caps.	Capsule	Febris	...	Fever
Cataplasma	Catapl.	Poultice	Fervens	Ferv.	Boiling
Ceratum	Cerat.	Cerate	Fiant pilulæ xii	Ft. pil. xii	Let 12 pills be made
Charta	Chart.	Paper	Fiat pulvis et divide in chartulas xii	Ft. pulv. et. div. in char. xii	Let a powder be made and divide in 12 powders
Charta cerata	Chart. cerat.	Waxed paper			
Chartula	...	Small paper			
Cibus	...	Food	Fiat pulvis in chartulas xii dividenda	...	Let 12 powders be made
Cito dispensetur	Cito disp.	Dispense quickly			
Cochlear or cochleare, Cochleatim	Coch., Cochleat.	A spoonful, by spoonfuls	Fiat secundum artem regulas	F. S. A. R.	Let it be made according to the rules of art
Cochleare amplum	Coch. amp.	A tablespoonful	Flavus	Flav.	Yellow
			Folium	Fol.	A leaf
Cochleare magnum	Coch. mag.	A tablespoonful	Fortis	fort.	Strong
Cochleare medium or modicum	Coch. med.	A dessertspoonful	Gargarisma	Garg.	A gargle
			Granum, Grana	...	Grain, grains
Cochleare parvum	Coch. parv.	A teaspoonful	Grossus	...	Large, coarse
Cola	Col.	Strain	Gutta	Gtt.	A drop
Colatus	Colat.	Strained	Guttæ	Gtt.	Drops
Coletur	Colet.	Let it be strained	Guttatim	Guttat.	By drops
Collunarium	...	A nose wash			
Collutorium	Collut.	A mouth wash	Hic, Hæc, Hoc	...	This
Collyrium	Collyr., Coll.	An eye wash	Hora	H.	An hour
Coloretur	...	Let it be colored	Hora decubitus	hor. dec.	At bedtime
Commisce	...	Mix together	Hora somni	H. S. or Hor. som.	At bedtime
Compositus	Comp.	Compounded			
Congius	Cong.	A gallon	Hydrargyrum	hydrarg.	Mercury
Consperge	Consperg.	To dust or sprinkle			

Table I—Continued

Word or phrase	Contraction	Meaning	Word or phrase	Contraction	Meaning
Idem	...	The same	Pulvis, Pulverizatus	Pulv.	A powder, powdered
Identidem	...	Repeatedly			
In dies	In d.	From day to day, daily	Quaque, quisque	q.	Each, every
Injectio	...	An injection	Quantum rectum	q.r.	The quantity is correct
Inter	...	Between			
			Quantum sufficiat, Quantum satis	Q. S.	As much as is sufficient
Kalium	K	Potassium			
			Quater in die	q.i.d.	Four times a day
Lac	...	Milk			
Lævo	L.	Left	Recens	rec.	Fresh
Lamella	...	Eye disk	Recipe	...	Take
Levis	Lev.	Light	Repetatur, Repetantur	Rept.	Let it be repeated, let them be repeated
Leviter	...	Lightly			
Linimentum	lin.	Liniment			
Liquor	liq.	Solution	Respondere	...	To answer
			Ruber, rubra, rubrum	rub.	Red
Magnus	Mag.	Large			
Mane	man.	Morning			
Masea, Massa pilularis	...	A mass, a pill mass	Saepis	...	Often, frequently
			Secundum artem, Secundum naturam	S. A., S. N.	According to art, according to nature
Minimum	M. or Min.	A minim			
Minutum	...	A minute			
Misce	M.	Mix	Secundum legem	s.l.	According to law
Mistura	mist.	Mixture			
Mitte, Mittatur, Mittantur	...	Send, let it be sent, let them be sent	Semis	ss.	A half
			Siccus	...	Dry, dried
Mitte tales	...	Send of such or this	Signa	Sig. S.	Mark thou
Modo dictu	m. dict.	As directed	Sine	s̄	Without
Modo præscripto	Mod. præsc.	In the manner prescribed	Si opus sit	Si op. sit	If necessary
			Sit	...	Let it be
More dictu.	M. dict.	In the manner directed	Solve, solvere, solutus	...	Dissolve to dissolve, dissolved
Natrium	Na	Sodium	Solutio	sol.	Solution
Nebula	nebul.	A spray	Solutio saturata	sat. sol.	Saturated solution
Niger	nig.	Black	Somnus	...	Sleep
Non	...	Not	Spiritus vini rectificatus	S. V. R.	Rectified spirit of wine (alcohol)
Non repetatur	Non. rep.	Do not repeat			
Nocte maneque	noct. maneq.	Night and morning	Statim	Stat.	Immediately
Nox, noctis	...	Night	Stet, Stent	St.	Let it stand, let them stand
Numerus	No.	Number			
			Suppositorium	supp.	Suppository
Octarius	O	A pint			
Oculo Utro	O.U., O₂	Each eye	Tabella	tab.	Tablet
Oculus dexter	O. D.	Right eye	Talis	t.	of such
Oculus lævus	O. L.	Left eye	Ter in die	T.i.d., or t.d.	Three times a day
Oculus sinister	O. S.	Left eye	Trochiscus	troch.	Troche
Oleum	Ol.	Oil			
Omni hora, Omni bihorio	Omn. hor., Omn. bih.	Every hour, every two hours	Uncia	...	An ounce
			Unguentum	ung.	Ointment
Omni quadrante horæ	Omn. quadr. hor.	Every quarter of an hour	Ut dictum	Ut Dict.	As directed
Omni quarta hora	Omn. 4 hr.	Every 4 hours	Unus	i, I	One
Omni mane	...	Every morning	Duo	ii, II	Two
Omni nocte	...	Every night	Tres	iii, III	Three
Omni secunda hora	Omn. 2 hr.	Every 2 hours	Quattour	iv, IV	Four
			Quinque	v, V	Five
			Sex	vi, VI	Six
			Septem	vii, VII	Seven
Omni tertia hora	Omn. 3 hr.	Every 3 hours	Octo	viii, VIII	Eight
Os, oris	...	Mouth	Novem	ix, IX	Nine
			Decem	x, X	Ten
Pars, partis	...	A part			
Partes æquales	P. æ.	Equal parts	Duodecim	XII	Twelve
Parvus	...	Little	Quindecim	XV	Fifteen
Per os	p.o.	By mouth	Viginti	XX	Twenty
Pilula	...	A pill	Triginta	XXX	Thirty
Placebo	...	To please, satisfy			
Ponderosus	pond.	Heavy	Quinquaginta	L	Fifty
Post cibos	p. c.	After eating	Centum	C	One hundred
Potus	...	Drink	Quingenti	D	Five hundred
Pro re nata	p. r. n.	When necessary	Mille	M	One thousand

Table II—Look-alike and/or Sound-alike Drugs

Achrocidin	Achrostatin
Ananase	Orinase
Apresoline	Priscoline
Compocillin	Ampicillin
Daricon	Darvon
Digitoxin	Digoxin
Doriden	Doxidan
Indocin	Lincocin
Marax	Atarax
Orinase	Ornade
Pabalate	Robalate
Persantine	Trasentine
Prednisone	Prednisolone
Protamide	Protamine
Vigran	Wigraine

pensing overdoses, and the presence of a line under such a dose may not absolve him of his responsibility.

Measurement of the medication may lead to dosage variation. The problems associated with teaspoonful dosage have long been recognized and various suggestions have been made to correct them.

A compounding and dispensing problem arises because of the continuing use of f3i, the symbol for one fluid dram. This represents one-eighth of an apothecary fluid ounce but is frequently interpreted as one teaspoonful when the physician uses this designation in his instructions to the patient.

An American standard teaspoon has been established by the American Standards Association as containing 4.93 ± 0.24 ml. Thus, one fluid ounce (29.57 ml) of a medicated liquid will provide approximately six standard teaspoonful doses. The difficulty occurs in compounding a prescription or formulating a pharmaceutical product. When the following prescription is considered, the problem becomes evident.

R Atropine sulfate	gr 1/250
Flavored vehicle q.s. ad	f 3i
Disp. f 3ii	
Sig. f 3i t.i.d.	

The physician probably intends to give his patient 16 doses of medication. However, if an ordinary household teaspoon is used to measure each dose, only 12 doses will be obtained. It is obvious that if the prescription were compounded to provide 16 doses and the instructions to the patient were to administer one teaspoonful, a significant dosage error would result.

Table III—Determination of Children's Doses[a]

Based on Surface Area of Average Adult

Weight		Surface area,	Fraction of
Kg	lb	M²	adult dose[b]
2	4.4	0.15	0.09
4	8.8	0.25	0.14
6	13.2	0.33	0.19
8	17.6	0.40	0.23
10	22.0	0.46	0.27
15	33.0	0.63	0.36
20	44.0	0.83	0.48
25	55.0	0.95	0.55
30	66.0	1.08	0.62
35	77.0	1.20	0.69
40	88.0	1.30	0.75
45	99.0	1.40	0.81
50	110.0	1.51	0.87
55	121.0	1.58	0.91

[a] Modell, W., ed, *Drugs of Choice*, C. V. Mosby Co., St. Louis, 1968–1969. p. 53
[b] Based on an average adult surface area of 1.73 M².

One method of handling this prescription is to compound on the basis of 12 5-ml doses, each containing 1/250 gr, and instruct the patient to use a household teaspoon or, preferably, a device calibrated to measure 5 ml. Another alternative is to compound on the basis of 16 one-fluid-dram doses, each containing 1/250 gr, and supply the patient with a device to measure accurately one fluid dram (either a teaspoon which is calibrated to contain one fluid dram or a small measuring glass). It is the feeling of this author that the latter method is preferred for in such a procedure the pharmacist follows exactly the compounding and dosage instructions of the physician and by so doing avoids any misinterpretation of the prescription or possible dosage error.

Teaspoonful dosage problems are not confined to prescriptions that must be compounded by the pharmacist. For example, when the following two prescriptions are compared, a discrepancy is evident.

R Achromycin V syrup
Disp. 60 ml
Sig. f 3i q6h

R Chloromycetin palmitate susp.
Disp. 60 ml
Sig. f 3i q6h

Both of these products have been formulated to provide 125 mg of the medication in each teaspoonful. However, Lederle bases its formulation of Achromycin V syrup on a 5-ml teaspoonful whereas Parke-Davis bases its formulation of Chloromycetin suspension on a 4-ml teaspoonful. Without attempting to pass judgment on which method is preferable, the problem can be seen readily. If a physician writes for Chloromycetin suspension intending to have his patient receive 125 mg in each teaspoonful, the patient probably will receive at least 150 mg per teaspoonful if a household teaspoon is used.

Although most pharmaceutical manufacturers base their formulations on 5-ml doses, there are still some who formulate on the basis of 4-ml doses for certain products. Still others formulate some products using apothecary measure.

It is unquestionably the pharmacist's responsibility to insure the patient's receiving the proper amount of medication in each dose. At the present time, the best solution appears to be for the pharmacist to dispense the appropriate measuring device with each liquid prescription.

Several suggestions for long-term improvement of the current situation can be made.

1. All prescriptions should be written and all products formulated using the metric system of measure. It is recognized that presently this is an unrealistic proposal since it is unlikely that the metric system will be used exclusively in the near future.
2. The use of the symbol for one fluid dram in the dosage instructions should be officially recognized as actually indicating one fluid dram or one teaspoonful containing 5 ml. Since the trend is away from the use of the apothecary system, an official 5-ml dose should be recognized. Once such a dose has been established, all pharmaceutical manufacturers should conform by basing all their formulations on this dosage.
3. Physicians should be requested to designate on the prescription the number of milliliters and/or the milligram quantity desired in each dose.
4. Pharmacists should dispense a standard teaspoon that will contain a 5-ml volume with each prescription for an oral liquid where such a dosage is used.

Several pharmaceutical manufacturers are individually taking steps to help reduce the teaspoonful dosage problem. A recently introduced over-the-counter pediatric analgesic product—Dial-a-gesic syrup (Borden)—is packaged in a bottle having a special cap that can be rotated to dispense exactly either $\frac{1}{4}$, $\frac{1}{2}$, $\frac{3}{4}$, or 1 teaspoonful (5 ml).

The use of the medicine dropper may also lead to dosage errors. A recent article[4] reviews the factors that can influence dropper dosage and illustrates the wide variations existing among commercially available droppers.

Pricing the Prescription—The pharmacist, although primarily a professional man, must be proficient in handling the business aspects of his prescription practice. In order for him to be able to provide the high type of pharmaceutical service demanded by the community, he must make a fair and equitable profit. It is, therefore, equally important both to the pharmacist and to the community that a profit be made. Unless the pharmacist's economic future is secure the professional service received by a community may suffer.

The prescription laboratory is becoming increasingly important economically and accounts for a large part of the net profit of most pharmacies. Thus, it is evident that this area must be efficiently operated. It is extremely important that some uniform system of pricing be established within each pharmacy to insure a profitable operation of the prescription laboratory and, also, to avoid complaints from patrons. It is just as wrong to have prices too low as it is to have prices too high and a price fair to both the patient and pharmacist should be developed.

Numerous investigations have clearly pointed out the need for the adoption of scientific business methods in deciding on the price to be charged for prescription medication. The fundamental principles of business demand that in order for one to be successful, the price charged must be sufficient to compensate for the ingredients and containers used, the employment of skilled professional personnel, and the payment of all other costs and expenses, yet still provide for a reasonable profit.

Many systems of pricing have been developed in the past based on (1) arbitrary fees dependent on the type of dosage form and number of doses supplied, (2) percentage markup on the cost of the ingredients, or (3) factors such as overhead, cost of ingredients, time required for compounding, and a professional fee. Most of these methods or combinations of them are currently being employed. However, only methods based on (3) will be considered in detail.

A Prescription Costing and Pricing Method was developed by S. B. Jeffries and H. M. Soba based on the determination of the actual cost of dispensing each prescription. This method takes into account exact cost of ingredients, cost of containers, cost of compounding time, cost of overhead chargeable to the prescription, and profit or professional fee.

A *Calculator* has been developed* to simplify the use of the above system. With this device the pharmacist can quickly determine the price of the prescription once he has determined the cost of *ingredients* and the *container*, plus the *time* required to handle the prescription, including receiving, reading, assembling the ingredients, compounding, packing, labeling, bookkeeping, and delivery to the patient. The cost of compounding time and the overhead chargeable to the prescription are set into the calculator. In the case of

most compounded prescriptions such as powders, capsules, ointments, and suppositories a "time schedule" must be established in order to maintain pricing consistency within a pharmacy.

The Jeffries Method enables the pharmacist to calculate a "break-even cost" that represents all the cost chargeable to the prescription (ingredients, container, overhead, and time). The pharmacist adds to this a fee representing the return for his skill, knowledge, investment, and professional service. This may be determined as a percentage of the break-even cost or applied as a flat fee.

The NARD Suggested Pricing Schedules for Prescriptions were developed, established, and distributed with the help of many local pharmaceutical organizations. These schedules generally took into consideration all of the factors of the Jeffries Method. They also established arbitrary fees necessary for the calculation of the price of compounded prescriptions. However, Federal courts in several states have since ruled that the adoption and the distribution of such schedules by pharmaceutical organizations is a violation of the Sherman Antitrust Act. Thus, while the use of these schedules by *individual* pharmacies was not ruled illegal (they are still in use in many pharmacies throughout the country), their distribution was halted because of these adverse court rulings.

The True Professional Fee Method has received impetus as a result of the above-mentioned court rulings since such a method of pricing may not be subject to antitrust laws. The term "professional fee" is not new. It has been employed in many pricing systems used through the years. However, in spite of the use of this term, prescription pricing was still based on a markup on the cost of ingredients. In contrast the *true* professional fee method of prescription pricing, the addition of a predetermined fee to the wholesale cost of the medication, does not involve such a markup. The three basic tenets of this concept are:[5, 6]

1. A prescription drug is not an ordinary article of commerce, capable of being bought and sold by anyone.
2. The functions performed by a pharmacist in dispensing medication are professional services requiring specialized knowledge and judgment and a degree of responsibility greater than that associated with mere commercial transactions.
3. The cost of providing prescription services is not now, nor has it ever been, a function of the cost of the physical ingredients.

The true professional fee, therefore, is the same for all prescriptions, regardless of the cost of the ingredients used. Of necessity it must be sufficient to cover all costs involved in the preparation and delivery of the prescription, as well as to provide the pharmacist with a livelihood. This fee now represents a charge for service rendered, just as does the fee charged by a physician, dentist, or other practitioner. The pharmacist no longer uses the traditional pricing procedure employed by most merchants, that is, a markup based on the cost of goods. Instead, he now charges for service and the knowledge and skill that permit him to perform this service.

Establishment of the fee should be based on sound principles and requires first an estimate of the pharmacist's anticipated net income. Professional education, qualifications, skill, experience, and the neighborhood or community in which the pharmacy is located are some of the main factors to be considered in establishing this income figure. Once the total net income is established, the expenses of the prescription laboratory are added. This represents the gross income that must come from

---

* Becton, Dickinson & Co., Rutherford, N.J. 07070.

the total number of prescriptions filled over a period of time covering this income and expense.

Professional fee =

$$\frac{\text{Expected net income} + \text{R}\!\!\!/ \text{ laboratory expenses}}{\text{Number of prescriptions dispensed}}$$

Unfortunately, very few pharmacists have adequate financial records pertaining to the operation of the prescription laboratory and thus the use of the above equation and others that have been developed requires considerable guesswork.

The trial and error method for determining a fee is based on the premise that the income derived from the prescriptions should be the same under the fee method as under the markup method. The pharmacist selects a fee that appears satisfactory and uses it to reprice a representative selection of prescriptions previously priced by the markup method. Several hundred should be used, distributed equally over each calendar quarter. The total income obtained under the two methods is compared and any discrepancy is corrected by proper adjustment of the trial fee.

The use of a professional fee decreases the cost to the patient of the more expensive prescription items such as antibiotics and corticosteroids. It concurrently increases the cost of the less expensive prescription items but does not materially alter the average cost of the prescription.

Pharmacists employing a true professional fee method are in the minority but their numbers are increasing. Many governmental units, such as state welfare agencies, have adopted this method of payment for prescriptions handled by local pharmacists. It is currently the opinion of many pharmaceutical leaders that the use of this method of prescription pricing is a necessary requirement if pharmacy is to retain full professional stature. Myers[7] has reviewed the advantages of adopting the professional fee method, the problems involved in implementing it, and the reluctance of some pharmacists to accept it.

After pricing a prescription pharmacists often place a code on the prescription order to indicate to those who later renew it the cost to the patient. Some word or combination of characters is selected and memorized. The word selected has ten letters and no duplicate letters. For example, the following code has been used by some pharmacists

R E P U B L I C A N
1   2   3   4   5   6   7   8   9   0

Such a coding method can also be used to indicate the cost of items in the pharmacy for inventory purposes.

Numbering and Dating—It is universal practice to number the prescription order and to place the same number on the label. This serves to identify the bottle or package and to connect it with the original order should it be necessary to refer to it or to renew the prescription. Consecutive numbers may be assigned by use of a numbering machine. These machines (Fig. 792) can be set to number consecutively, in duplicate or triplicate, so that the same number can be clearly and neatly stamped on the prescription order, label, and record book as desired. Numbers also can be assigned from a consecutive listing written or preprinted in one of the several types of record books available.

Dating of the prescription also helps to establish its identity and should never be omitted. This informa-

tion may prove of importance in the case of subsequent discussion and as an alternate means of locating the prescription order if the number is lost.

Labeling—The prescription label is usually prepared by the pharmacist, although in some large prescription pharmacies a typist may be employed exclusively for this purpose. In either situation the pharmacist is responsible for the correctness of the information on the label. It is necessary that a prescription have an esthetic and professional appearing label. It is important to remember that the patient judges prescription medication by the finished product presented to him. If the label and the container are not neat and professional in appearance, the patient may conclude that the prescription medication was compounded in a careless manner. This may result in loss of confidence in the pharmacy.

Since the label is a significant factor in the appearance of the finished prescription, a quality label should be used. A lithographed or engraved label on high-grade paper is a wise investment (Fig. 793). The size of the label should be commensurate with the size of the prescription container. The name, address, telephone number, and narcotic registry number of the pharmacy are generally imprinted on the label. The prescription number, date of dispensing, patient's name, directions for use, and prescriber's name are typed on the label. The pharmacist should make a particular effort to make the directions for use as clear and complete as possible. For example, "One (1) tablet four (4) times a day" would be preferred to "One 4 times a day." In the case of a narcotic prescription, in addition to the above, the patient's address and prescriber's address and narcotic registry number must be included. When there is insufficient space on a label to include this additional information required by law, an auxiliary label is used on which this can be typed. Several states require that the name or initials of the pharmacist dispensing the medication appear on the label. Renewal information might also be included on the label. Some labels provide a space where the number of renewals authorized by the prescriber may be designated. This information could also be included on an auxiliary label. It has been recommended that the manufacturer's lot number for the medication dispensed be entered on the prescription label. This would aid in the rapid identification of medication that might be recalled.

Where the container is too small to accommodate

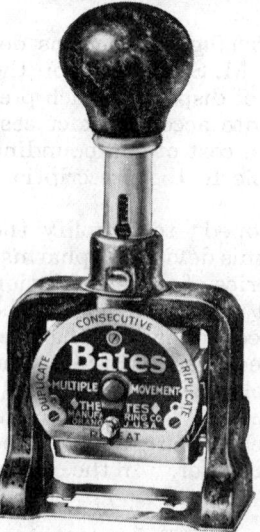

Fig. 792. Multiple-movement numbering machine (courtesy, Bates).

a full-sized label, a strip label, which is longer but narrower than a standard label, may be used. An alternate procedure is to place the prescription number on the immediate container and a complete label on a larger package into which the immediate container is placed. A wide strip of cellophane tape is useful both to protect the label from damage and to secure it in place. All prescription labels should be typewritten to make them neat, attractive, and legible.

Auxiliary labels serve a variety of purposes, including the important one of explaining a property or use of the prescription medication. A "shake-well" label is certainly indicated for a prescription containing material that may separate on standing, such as mixtures, lotions, and emulsions, or where there is the possibility of precipitation or separation occurring at a later date. For example, it is recommended that a "shake-well" label be used for Phenergan Expectorant even though it appears to be a clear solution. The use of labels such as "For the Ear," "For the Eye," and "External Use" is recommended because of the added safety they offer, even when directions indicate proper use. The use of a "poison" label is rarely indicated since it may cause the patient to become unduly alarmed and fearful of using the medication, even according to instructions. Instead, the use of other precautionary labels is indicated to warn that the medication should not be swallowed or used internally or should be kept out of reach of children and others for whom it is not intended.

Auxiliary labels are available in a variety of colors to give them special prominence. Their position on the prescription container is a matter of personal preference, but they should be placed conspicuously. Fig 794. shows examples of some commonly used auxiliary labels.

Preparing the Prescription—After reading and checking the prescription order the pharmacist should decide on the exact procedure to be followed in dispensing or compounding the ingredients. Although the number of prescriptions that now require compounding represents only a very small percentage of the total, the pharmacist must be able to recognize problems that may develop in the preparation of such prescriptions and must maintain the skills necessary to prepare them accurately. When a prescription requiring compounding is received he should take into consideration the order of mixing, the selection of adjuvants, and the need for special techniques. Once he has decided on the procedure he assembles the necessary materials in a single location on the prescription counter. As he uses each ingredient, he moves it to some other established location on the counter (transfer from the left side of the balance to the right side is often suggested). The use of this technique provides the pharmacist with a mechanical check on the introduction of each ingredient. If he is interrupted during the compounding of the medication, there is then no doubt as to which ingredients have already been used. When he has finished with all ingredients, he returns them to their proper location. He has therefore had the opportunity to read the label of each ingredient three times; once when the container is removed from the shelf, again when the contents are weighed or measured, and finally when the container is returned to the shelf.

Any information necessary for renewing should be noted during the course of preparation on the face of the prescription order. Adjuvants used, order of mixing, amount of each ingredient, capsule size, type and size of container, name and product identification number of the manufacturer, auxiliary labels used, the price charged, clarification of illegible words or numbers, and any special notations should all be entered as necessary. Failure to do this may result in a difference in the appearance of a renewed prescription and possibly create doubt and apprehension in the mind of the patient.

Packaging—Selection of a proper container is based on the particular dosage form employed, quantity prescribed, storage requirements, dose, and method of administration. Prescription containers will be discussed in more detail later in this chapter, but the importance of the selection of the proper container should be recognized as an important factor in properly handling a prescription. The dispensing of capsules or tablets in a pasteboard box may result in loss of potency from degradation due to absorbed moisture. A viscous lotion or magma dispensed in a narrow-necked bottle may make withdrawal of the proper dose difficult or impossible. A dusting powder dispensed without a shaker top may result in waste of medication and, in some cases, overdosage. A prescription for drop dosage dispensed in an ordinary prescription bottle will certainly result in inconvenience to the patient and possibly in contamination of the medication. Thus, not only is the patient's impression of a pharmacy influenced by the prescription package, but his safety and the efficacy of the medication as well.

Rechecking—The importance of this step cannot be overemphasized. Every prescription should be

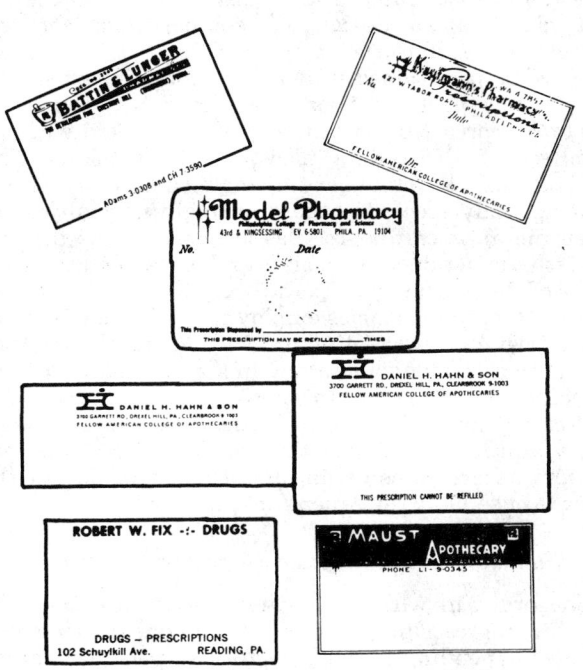

Fig. 793. Typical prescription labels.

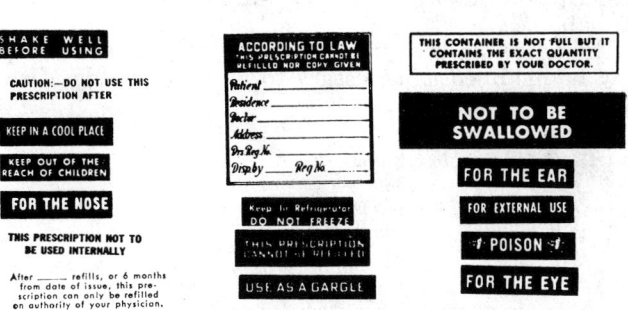

Fig. 794. Typical auxiliary labels.

rechecked. The ingredients and amounts used should be verified by the compounder. All details of the label should be rechecked also against the prescription order to verify directions, patient's name, prescription number, date, and prescriber's name. Ideally, this is accomplished by two pharmacists, one reading the prescription order and the other verifying the information. However, where only one pharmacist is on duty, he can still accomplish this by following the rechecking procedure outlined above.

Delivering the Prescription—Casually dispensed or carelessly wrapped prescription medication can create the impression that the product has been treated throughout in a similar manner. The pharmacist should personally deliver the prescription medication unless it is to be delivered to the home or office of the patient. This gives the pharmacist an opportunity to assure himself that the patient understands how to use the medication properly and emphasizes the importance the pharmacist places on the handling of prescription drugs. At this time the pharmacist should also call attention to any auxiliary instructions such as storage of the medication in a refrigerator and he should alert the patient to any unexpected effects such as the ability of some drugs to color the urine. In situations where personal delivery is not possible the pharmacist should be available to answer any questions the patient may have.

The prescription medication may be wrapped or placed in specially designed and imprinted prescription bags. Many pharmacists prefer to prewrap the completed prescription and place the patient's name, address, prescription number, and price on a label attached to the package or directly on the prescription bag. The patient may find it convenient to retain this label or bag for purposes of tax records.

Recording—Some states require that a record of the prescriptions dispensed be maintained, although the manner in which this is to be done may not be stipulated. Aside from complying with regulations, some method of record keeping is desirable. These records are helpful to the pharmacist, the physician, and the patient. They serve to keep the pharmacist informed as to the number of prescriptions handled, the ratio of renewals to new prescriptions, and related information. They can also serve as a means of locating prescription orders rapidly, making information concerning previously dispensed prescriptions available to the physician, providing a family prescription record of allergies and idiosyncrasies, and permitting compilation of information needed by the patient for tax and insurance purposes.

There are several ways by which prescription orders may be recorded. *The prescription order number method* of indexing is used in many pharmacies. The numbers are preprinted, written, or stamped consecutively in a standard-type prescription record book. Each number is usually followed by the patient's name and address, physician's name, type of prescription medication, price, and initials of the pharmacist dispensing the medication. This method maintains a complete record of the prescriptions dispensed in any single period, but it is not particularly useful in locating a prescription order for renewal if the number or date is not available.

The patient or family record card method is often used as a supplement to the prescription order number method. A file card is generally used for each patient or family. The name is typed on the top of the card and as each prescription is dispensed, the number,

date, name and amount of the medication, and price are placed on the card. The purchase of medications available without a prescription order should also be noted on the card; thus, this card serves as a complete record of medication obtained by each member of the family. Any special information concerning the patient, such as allergies to particular medications or the presence of a particular disease state (eg, diabetes, glaucoma), should also be recorded. Having the above information available, the pharmacist will be able more readily to detect problems related to drug therapy. Such problems may arise when a patient is seeing more than one physician or is taking a medication that is contraindicated in a particular disease state or that might interact with other prescription or over-the-counter medication that is being taken simultaneously. The use of this method also permits rapid location of prescription orders without the need of either number or date, and facilitates the supplying of a listing of all medication dispensed for income tax or insurance purposes. This method, when properly employed, will serve as a complete record of a family's or individual's medication and will permit the pharmacist to perform a valuable service to both the patient and physician.

Filing—A variety of prescription files are available which serve to maintain and preserve original prescription orders. Metal or cardboard units, which conveniently store about 1000 orders, are the most common. In using these files the orders are first punched, slipped onto two metal rods firmly attached to the file, and placed in a designated compartment for safe storage and rapid retrieval.

Suitably partitioned drawers are sometimes used for filing. The partitions may be placed between every 200 or 300 prescription orders, plainly marked with the numbers of the orders filed in that section. This method permits removal of a single sheet without preventing ready access to others, as might normally occur when metal or cardboard files are used. The drawers are esthetic in appearance and can be designed to fit the decor of the pharmacy.

Some large pharmacies employ microfilming for filing and retrieving prescription orders. While this method results in a tremendous saving in storage space, its cost precludes general acceptance.

Prescription orders for narcotics must be filed separately and many pharmacies also maintain a separate file for prescriptions calling for drugs specified in the Drug Abuse Control Amendments.

Summary of Prescription Handling Procedure

The order in which the various steps are taken in handling a prescription will vary from one pharmacy to another depending on such factors as personal habits, methods of record keeping, physical arrangement of the prescription laboratory, and number of employees available.

The following is a suggested order of procedure that may be modified as necessary to meet the needs of an individual situation.

1. Receive the prescription order
2. Read and check the prescription order
3. Price the prescription medication
4. Number and date the prescription order
5. Prepare the label
6. Establish the method and order of preparation
7. Assemble all ingredients
8. Prepare the prescription medication
9. Package and label the completed prescription medication

10. Recheck the completed prescription medication
11. Return the materials to their proper places
12. Deliver the prescription medication to the patient
13. Record the prescription order
14. File the prescription order

Prescription Containers

Selection of containers for prescription medication should receive special care and attention. In making a selection the pharmacist should choose a container that:

1. Protects the efficacy of the medication during the time of its use.
2. Allows convenient and proper use of the medication.
3. Is the most suitable type for the particular dosage form and the quantity dispensed.
4. Represents through its appearance the care employed in preparing the medication.

Prescription Bottles and Jars—Glass containers for dispensing liquid and semisolid dosage forms are available in a variety of sizes, shapes, and colors. Most containers used today are of clear, green, or amber light-resistant glass. The use of amber containers is increasing since there is growing recognition that many drugs are more stable when protected from light. A survey* of the 200 most commonly used drugs in 1967 (representing 65% of all prescription orders written in that year) indicated that 85 of these products, or 42.5%, needed protection from light.

Plastic closures are used on most prescription bottles and jars since they are durable and less reactive than metal closures. The use of suitable closures is also important and the survey mentioned above indicates that 139 products, or 69.5% of the top 200, require tight, protective packaging.

Standard prescription bottles (Figs. 795 and 796) are used for both internal and external solutions, suspensions, and emulsions of low or normal viscosity.

Ointment jars (Fig. 797) are used to dispense ointments, creams, or extremely viscous suspensions or emulsions.

Wide-mouthed powder jars (Fig. 798) are used to package bulk powders, large quantities of tablets or capsules, and viscous liquids that cannot be poured readily from a narrow-necked bottle.

Capsule vials (Fig. 799) are used for capsules, tablets, or small quantities of bulk powders.

Dropper bottles are used for dispensing ophthalmic, oral, nasal, or otic preparations administered by the drop or fraction of a teaspoon. Dropper assemblies are available with glass or plastic pipets which may be calibrated or uncalibrated. Various styles are illustrated in Fig. 800. Ball- or curve-tipped droppers are well suited for eye drops. The blunt-tipped type is commonly used for nasal drops.

Applicator bottles have a small glass or plastic rod attached to the closure. These are useful for applying medication to a wound or skin surface, as in the case of antiseptic solutions.

Plastic Containers—These are of two basic types: flexible polyethylene and rigid polystyrene.

The flexible polyethylene or squeeze bottle is useful for packaging medication to be administered as drops or in the form of a spray. Containers designed for drop dosage and nose and throat sprays are available. Lotions, shampoos, and creams are also conveniently

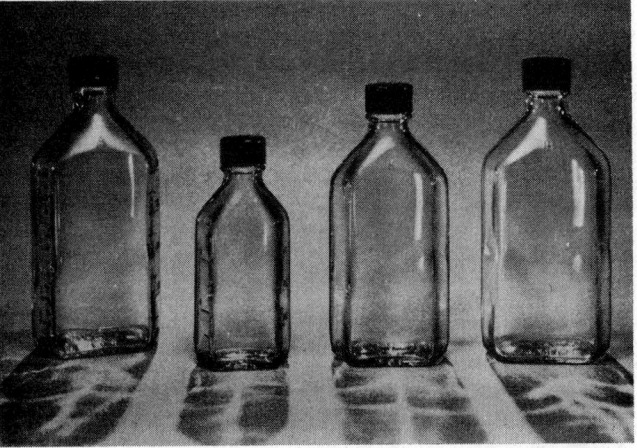

Fig. 795. Prescription liquid containers. Graduated bottles on the left and plain on the right (courtesy, Armstrong Cork).

dispensed in the flexible polyethylene type. Some of these are illustrated in Fig. 801.

Rigid polystyrene vials are used to dispense capsules and tablets (Fig. 802). Ointment jars and containers for dispensing large quantities of capsules and tablets are also available in this type of material.

Advantages of plastic containers are their light weight, durability, and nonreactivity with many medicinal agents. Aqueous solutions of fluorides are more stable when dispensed in plastic containers. Ointments containing compounds that tend to react with the metals of ointment tubes usually can be dispensed in plastic tubes. However, investigations show plastic may absorb or adsorb many drugs and cause a loss of potency. Furthermore, plastics do not offer the protection against moisture and air that is afforded by glass containers. Considerable research is currently being conducted in attempts to eliminate these problems.

Pasteboard Containers—These are available for a variety of dosage forms. Powder boxes for dispensing folded powders and pill boxes for dispensing capsules or tablets are available in several sizes and styles. Suppository boxes may be obtained which will hold either 6, 12, or more suppositories. Sifter-top boxes for dispensing dusting powders are available. The major drawback to pasteboard containers is their inability to protect medication against both air and moisture.

Collapsible Tubes—These are occasionally used by the pharmacist to dispense semisolid dosage forms

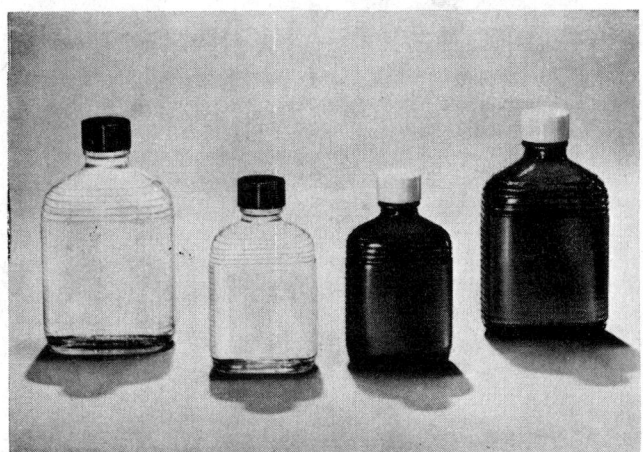

Fig. 796. Phenix bottles, clear glass and amber glass. Front is plain while back is ribbed to provide a good gripping surface (courtesy Armstrong Cork).

---

* "Protective Packaging Indications," compiled by the Armstrong Cork Co. utilizing the Gosselin National Prescription Audit of 1967.

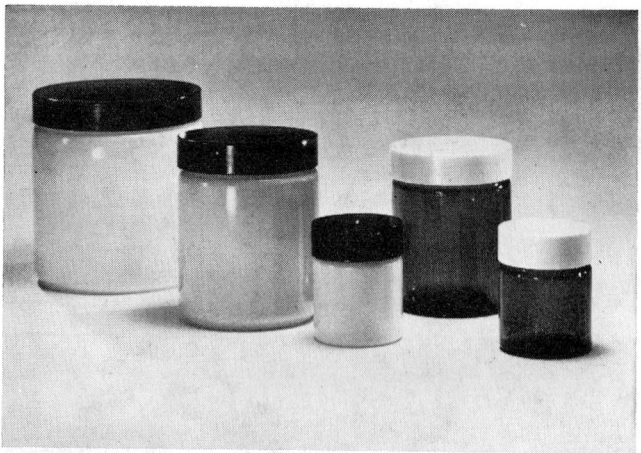

Fig. 797. Ointment jars, white ceramic coated glass on left and amber glass on right (courtesy, Armstrong Cork).

intended for local use. They are made of metal or plastic. Metal tubes are usually composed of tin or aluminum. In the use of metal tubes the pharmacist must always consider the possibility of a chemical reaction between the tube and the contained material, especially if moisture is present. Where this possibility exists, either a metal tube that has been coated with a protective film to prevent such reactions or a plastic tube should be employed.

Child-Proof Containers—Because of the high number of accidental poisonings following the ingestion of large quantities of medication by children, efforts have been directed towards the development of a medication container that a small child cannot open. Several have been developed recently. One, the Palm-N'-Turn (*Med-A-Safe*) may be opened by holding the vial in one hand and pressing the cap into the opposite palm. The vial is then turned counterclockwise. The Armstrong Stay-Tight Cap (*Armstrong*) works on a principle of interlocking ratchets. Downward pressure is applied to the cap to remove it from the bottle. Two other similar products are Screw-Loc (*Owens-Illinois*) plastic vials and Pop-Lok (*Safety Packaging*) containers.

Legal Considerations

Prescription Renewal—The renewing of prescriptions is controlled to a large degree by Federal and state laws. According to Federal regulations, drug products

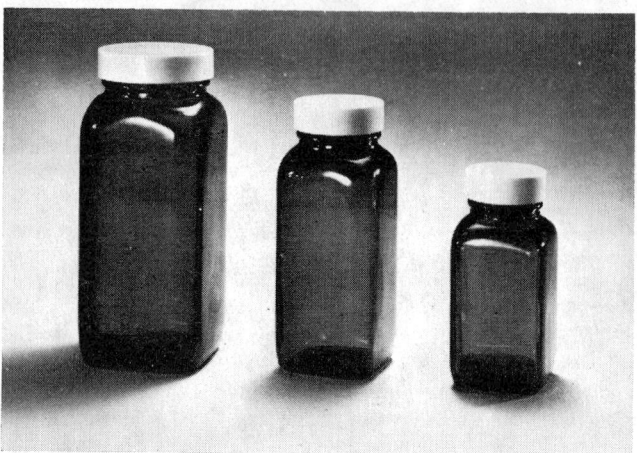

Fig. 798. Wide-mouthed amber glass powder or capsule jars with white plastic caps (courtesy, Armstrong Cork).

are divided into two classes: (1) all drugs which are deemed dangerous or which may be dangerous if used without competent medical supervision and (2) those products which may be used with relative safety by the patient, provided adequate directions for use appear on the label. Drug products in the first group are designated by a label bearing the following statement: *CAUTION—Federal law prohibits dispensing without prescription.* These items require a prescription order before they may be dispensed and also require specific authorization by the prescriber before prescriptions containing them may be renewed.

Prescription orders containing the second group of drugs may be renewed at the discretion of the pharmacist, unless otherwise directed by the physician, since essentially they are items which may be sold over the counter without a prescription. This group includes such preparations as simple vitamin formulas, antacid preparations, laxatives, and other medications which are considered relatively safe.

The American Pharmaceutical Association has proposed a reclassification of drugs into the following four classes:

1. To be dispensed on prescription order and renewable at the prescriber's discretion only.
2. To be initially dispensed on prescription order only, but renewable at the pharmacist's discretion.
3. To be dispensed personally by the pharmacist at the request of the patient.
4. To be directly available to the public without professional direction or control.

However, these recommendations are still being considered and no official action has been taken.

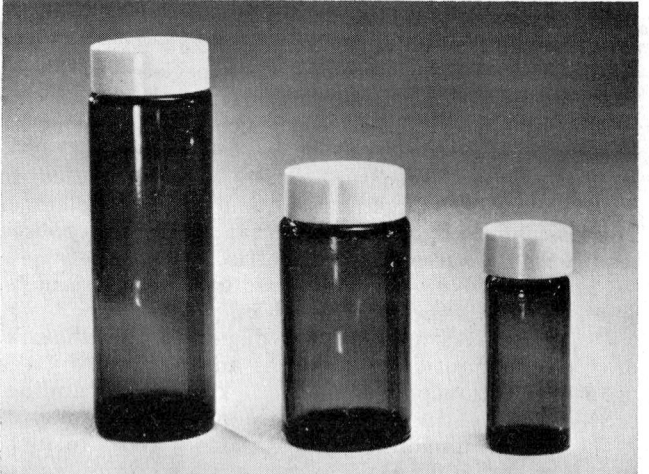

Fig. 799. Amber glass capsule bottles with white plastic caps (courtesy, Armstrong Cork).

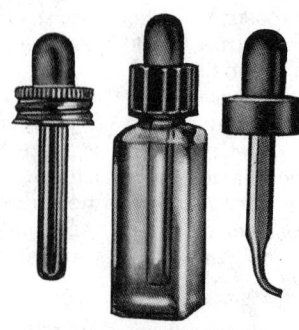

Fig. 800. Dropper bottles and assemblies.

Narcotic drugs are classified under Federal law as Class A, Class B, Class X, and Class M.

Class A narcotic drugs require a prescription order signed by the prescriber and placed in the hands of the pharmacist prior to the delivery of the medication to the patient. Class A narcotic prescriptions cannot be renewed.

Class B narcotic drugs may be prescribed by either a written or an oral order from the prescriber. In the case of an oral (eg, telephone) prescription, the pharmacist is obligated to reduce the order to a written form and add all information that is required by law to be present on a narcotic prescription order. Class B prescription orders also cannot be renewed.

Classes X and M include pharmaceutical preparations which fulfil the Federal requirements for exemption. Although many of these preparations may be dispensed without a prescription order, some bear the Federal legend prohibiting dispensing without either an oral or written order.

Class X (exempt) preparations must contain, in addition to the narcotic, one or more *nonnarcotic active* medicinal agents. Records of sales must be maintained.

Class M preparations contain *active or inactive non-narcotic* ingredients, and there is no limit on the quantity of the narcotic drug included. No records of sales need be maintained.

It should be recognized that in some instances state regulations may be more restrictive than Federal regulations. For example, Paregoric is classified by Federal law as a Class X narcotic but several states have classified it as a Class B narcotic.

In an attempt to eliminate confusion involving renewing of the so-called "legend drugs"—ie, those bearing the *CAUTION—Federal law prohibits dispensing without prescription*—efforts have been made to have the physician indicate renewal instructions on every prescription order. Various professional groups have endorsed this plan and have actively promoted

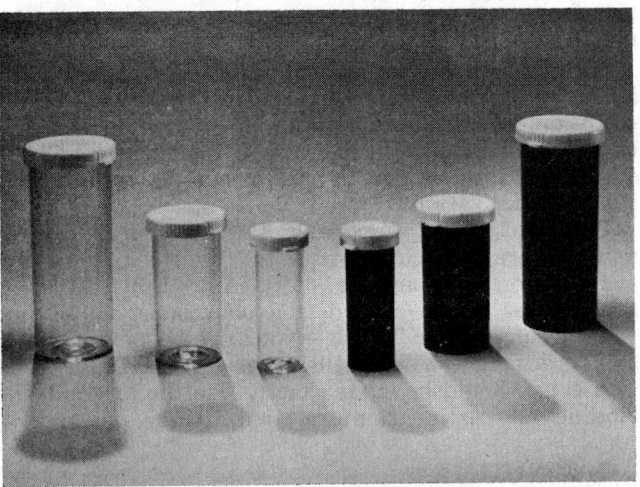

Fig. 802. Rigid polystyrene clear and amber vials with snap-on caps (courtesy, Armstrong Cork).

it. It is suggested that one of the corners of the prescription blank be printed with the following or a similar form whereby the physician need only signify his instructions by checking, underlining, or filling in his desires in the form provided; eg:

NON-REP.	This prescription may be refilled __ times.

However, the use of renewal instructions such as "Renew PRN" or "Renew Ad Lib" to indicate an unrestricted number of renewals is looked on with disfavor. The legality of such designations is in doubt since their use seemingly transfers the decision as to when or how often a prescription may be renewed from the prescriber to the patient. The law gives this authority only to the prescriber and does not permit him to delegate it. Since the law is not specific on the use of these designations, the pharmacist in renewing prescriptions so marked must use care and professional judgment. He should renew such prescriptions only with a frequency consistent with the directions for use and should check with the prescriber after a reasonable time to assure himself that he is complying with the actual intent of the prescriber.

Renewals should be noted on the face or reverse side of the prescription order, the date, the quantity dispensed if different from the original, and the name or initials of the pharmacist dispensing the renewal being designated. If special authorization for renewal has been obtained from the prescriber, this should also be noted.

The maintenance of accurate records of renewals is particularly important since in many cases the physician's record for a patient will have incomplete information as to the number of renewals authorized. The introduction of the Drug Abuse Control Amendments also dictates care in keeping renewal records since the drugs covered under these amendments may be renewed no more than five times (if the prescriber authorizes) during the six-month period after the prescription order was written.

Additional information can be found in Chapter 101 on *Laws Governing Pharmacy*.

Copies of Prescription Orders—These are on occasion requested by a patient or a pharmacist in

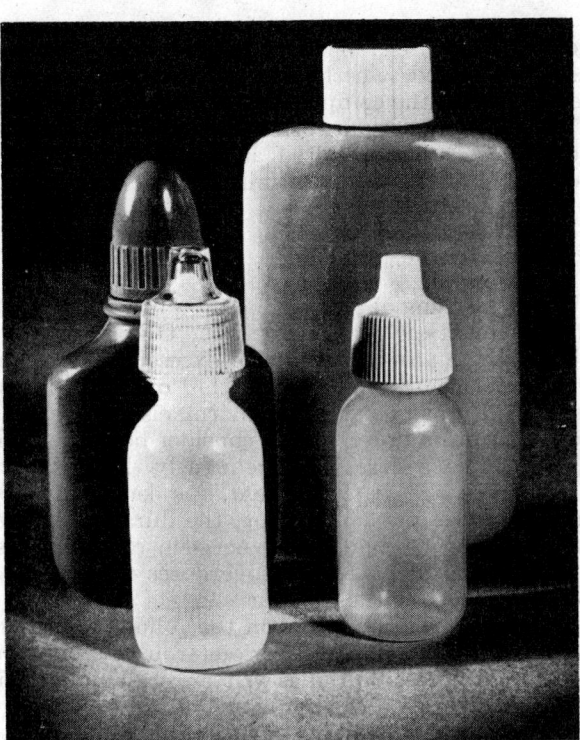

Fig. 801. Flexible polyethylene prescription bottles.

behalf of a patient. Such *bona fide* requests should be honored, unless prohibited by law.

Prescription orders for drugs bearing the Federal legend, which prohibits their dispensing without a prescription order, cannot be renewed without authorization from the prescriber. It follows that copies of such prescription orders cannot be honored without the same authorization.

Copies of prescription orders that are not legally renewable are sometimes requested by the patient for examination by a physician. To insure that the use of such copies is not abused, the pharmacist supplying the copy may write "Copy—Not to be Dispensed" or a similar designation across the top.

A copy should be made exactly like the original, including all pertinent information that a pharmacist might need in dispensing the prescription in exactly the same manner as the original. The copy preferably should be written or typed on a preprinted form identifying the pharmacy. The word "copy" should be clearly placed on the face of the form.

Ownership of the Prescription Order—This has not been completely resolved in the courts. However, it is generally conceded that the ownership of the prescription order passes from the patient to the pharmacist when the medication is dispensed by the pharmacist and accepted by the patient. State laws in most cases require that the pharmacist retain and file the original prescription order for a specified period of time (1 to 5 years). However, the patient still retains the right to obtain a renewal or a copy when not otherwise prohibited by law.

Incompatibility

The term incompatibility may be applied to pharmaceuticals when problems arise during the compounding, dispensing, or administration of these products. Usually, the problems will develop as a result of using two or more drugs but problems involving the use of only one drug, such as dosage errors, may be included under this topic also. The type of incompatibility may be therapeutic, physical, or chemical in nature or, as is often the case, a combination of types. These categories are convenient in studying incompatibilities individually, but it must be recognized that an interrelationship exists among them and in practical situations they cannot always be separated.

The importance of the subject of incompatibility has increased in spite of the reduction in the percentage of compounded prescriptions. The continual marketing of new and complex drugs has made it more important than ever that the pharmacist employ all his fundamental knowledge of chemistry, pharmacology, and pharmacy in dealing with incompatibilities. An understanding of the phenomenon of solubility, chemical reactivity, drug stability, and therapeutic activity from a theoretical as well as a practical viewpoint is essential. Ideally, by properly employing this knowledge the pharmacist should be able to predict the occurrence of incompatibility and to take proper steps to prevent or minimize it, whether he is practicing pharmacy or engaged in pharmaceutical research.

*Therapeutic Incompatibility**

A therapeutic incompatibility exists when the response to one or more drugs in the patient is of a different nature or intensity than that intended by the prescriber. Adverse drug reactions might be considered as therapeutic incompatibilites, and these are considered in detail in Chapter 72.

Therapeutic effectiveness may be reduced or delayed as the result of a physical or chemical reaction. Hydrolysis or oxidation of a drug in a mixture may result in loss of activity. Complexation or combination of a drug with proteins, tannins, surfactants, and other large molecules may result in delay in the release and absorption of a drug. These incompatibilities will be considered in more detail later, but it should be noted here that physical and chemical incompatibilities may lead to therapeutic incompatibilities.

Many therapeutic incompatibilities result from errors in writing or interpreting the prescription order, and the pharmacist is often in a position to detect and help avoid such problems.

The alteration of a prescription order to correct or prevent therapeutic incompatibility generally requires permission of the prescriber. Before contact with him is made, however, the pharmacist should be certain such incompatibility exists and that the effect on the therapeutic activity of the drug is significant. He should then determine how the incompatibility can best be avoided, whether by elimination or replacement of one of the components, change in dose, change in dosage form, or some other way. Only then should the physician be consulted and a suggestion for the prevention of the incompatibility given to him.

Dosage Errors

The dispensing of an overdose of a medication is the most serious type of dosage error. Overdoses can result from the administration of excessive single doses or the too frequent administration of usual doses as mentioned previously. The pharmacist in evaluating the prescription order should consider how much drug is given in each dose, how frequently the medication is given, the age of the patient, the sensitivity of an individual to a particular drug, the duration of activity, and the possibility of synergism or antagonism. It should also be noted that overdoses of medications used externally can also occur.

The problem represented in the following prescription is one that could cause serious trouble if not recognized. As the prescription is written, the amounts indicated are those that are to be included in each capsule. The quantities of phenobarbital and aspirin represent reasonable single doses of these agents. How-

---
* For further information, see Chapter 72, page 1381.

℞ Atropine sulfate   0.006
    Phenobarbital   0.015
    Aspirin   0.300

M. ft.   Cap. #1
Disp.   #12
Sig.   One capsule t.i.d.

ever, the quantity of atropine sulfate is far in excess of the usual and maximum recommended doses. Although in this particular case it appears that the quantity of atropine sulfate specified might be reasonable for the entire 12 capsules, the pharmacist should contact the prescriber to clarify the matter.

Another type of problem might be experienced if this prescription was written slightly differently.

℞ Atropine sulfate   0.006
    Phenobarbital   0.015
    Aspirin   0.300

M. ft.   Div. Cap. #12
Sig.   One capsule t.i.d.

If this prescription were filled as written, the dose of atropine sulfate would be reasonable but the doses of aspirin and phenobarbital would be very small and probably without therapeutic effect. Although the situation might not be as dangerous as that occurring if the former prescription were to be filled as written, nevertheless, the patient would be deprived of the benefits of the therapeutic doses of these ingredients. In addition to analyzing the prescription for dosage problems, the pharmacist should exercise extreme care in performing the calculations necessary to dispense the prescription. The importance of this cannot be too strongly emphasized, since careless calculation errors have resulted in the administration of fatal doses of certain drugs.

Confusion may exist occasionally concerning the dosage strengths of a drug that are commercially available. For example, a pharmacist may receive a prescription order calling for "Diuril tablets, 50 mg." It is unlikely that the prescriber actually wants to give a 50-mg dose of Diuril (*MSD*), and it is the pharmacist's responsibility to consult with the prescriber to determine what is actually desired. In this case the physician probably wanted 500-mg tablets of Diuril to be dispensed, although he may have wanted 50-mg tablets of HydroDiuril (*MSD*).

Wrong Drug or Dosage Form

The fact that many drugs have names that are very similar to those of other drugs has been mentioned earlier in this chapter and examples are cited in Table II. This has led to increasing difficulty in accurately identifying the name of the medication prescribed in many situations and there is a danger that the wrong drug may be dispensed.

In some instances the prescriber may hastily write a prescription for a medication that he does not actually desire. For example, when the prescriber was questioned about the quantity of belladonna tincture requested in the following prescription, he indicated that he had meant to write Donnatal elixir (*Robins*) instead of belladonna tincture.

℞ Belladonna Tinct.   40.0
    Maalox qs ad   120.0

Sig. One tablespoonful every four hours

In cases such as this the pharmacist would have no way of knowing that the wrong drug had been prescribed unless there was a dosage discrepancy or some other clue that might raise a question as to the use of the prescribed drug for the condition being treated.

Many drugs are available in a variety of dosage forms, and when it is not clear which one should be dispensed the prescriber should be consulted. A prescription order requesting a 15-Gm tube of Cordran (*Lilly*) that does not specify whether the ointment or cream should be supplied should not be dispensed until the prescriber is contacted.

The consequences of dispensing the wrong form of a drug can be quite serious. Several deaths have resulted because ipecac fluidextract was dispensed and administered instead of ipecac syrup. Such instances are rare, but the pharmacist should be aware of the potential of their occurrence.

Contraindicated Drugs

The use of a certain drug may be contraindicated in a particular disease state or in situations where an individual has previously shown an allergic response to it. For example, the use of corticosteroids is contraindicated in patients having an active peptic ulcer condition and similar contraindications are listed for many other drugs. An awareness of these potential problems is essential for the pharmacist to serve the patient best.

Formation of Toxic Compounds

While toxic substances are rarely formed because of an incompatibility, prescriptions must be scrutinized for such a possibility. Mercurous salts in combination with other drugs, for example, may possibly be converted to highly poisonous mercuric compounds. Calomel (HgCl) can be oxidized to mercuric chloride by iodine, by excess halide ions in the presence of moisture, by exposure to sunlight, or by heavy trituration.[8]

Synergistic or Antagonistic Effects

Many drugs exhibit synergism and antagonism when administered in combination. Although this could lead to problems, it should be recognized that such combinations may be prescribed deliberately to make use of synergism or antagonism to modify the drug actions. The combination of an amphetamine derivative with a barbiturate to aid in weight control illustrates the use of an apparently antagonistic combination in modern therapy. Other examples of drug antagonism and synergism are cited in the following discussion of drug interactions.

Drug Interactions

During the past several years there has been an increasing awareness of a rather subtle type of interaction, that arising when one drug alters the expected therapeutic response to another drug that has been administered simultaneously. Several reviews[9-16] of these interactions have been published and reports of individual interactions consistently appear in the current literature. There have been a number of mechanisms suggested as possible causes for these interactions and some of these are discussed here.

Mechanisms

Alteration of Gastrointestinal Absorption— Two ways in which gastrointestinal absorption may be altered are alteration of pH and complexation.

Alteration of pH—Since many drugs are weak acids or weak bases, the pH of the gastrointestinal tract will influence the site at which absorption takes place and the extent of absorption. It is recognized that the nonionized form of a drug will be more readily absorbed than the ionized form. Therefore, acidic drugs such as aspirin and phenobarbital will be more readily absorbed from the stomach (having a lower pH) where they primarily exist in a nonionized form. If a drug such as an antacid is given that will raise the pH of the stomach contents, it is possible that the absorption of such acidic drugs can be delayed and/or partially inhibited.

Complexation—The interaction between tetracycline derivatives and certain metal ions is well known. Tetracycline can combine with metal ions such as calcium or aluminum in the gastrointestinal tract to form complexes that are poorly absorbed. Thus, the administration of certain dietary items (milk containing calcium) or drugs (antacids containing aluminum salts) to patients on tetracycline therapy could cause a significant decrease in the amount of tetracycline absorbed. It should be noted that in some instances a physician may suggest that milk be used when taking these drugs to help avoid gastrointestinal side effects that frequently accompany their use. In these situations he may be willing to sacrifice some of the drug's activity in order to have it better tolerated.

Other interactions involving complexation might be anticipated when the drug cholestyramine [Cuemid (*MSD*), Questran (*Mead-Johnson*)] is used. Cholestyramine is a high-molecular-weight resin that is used to complex with bile acids in the gastrointestinal tract, thus preventing their reabsorption. Because cholestyramine could complex with other medications given orally, thus preventing their absorption, it is recommended that it be given at least several hours after the administration of other drugs.

Stimulation of Enzyme Systems—It has been demonstrated by many investigators that phenobarbital can stimulate or increase the activity of liver microsomal enzymes. These enzymes are involved in the metabolism of many drugs. For example, it has been shown that the rate of metabolism of coumarin anticoagulants is increased in patients also being treated with phenobarbital.[17] The result of this interaction would be a decreased response to the anticoagulant since it is being more rapidly metabolized and excreted. Therefore, to compensate for this loss of effect, the dose of the anticoagulant would have to be increased until the desired activity was obtained. A potentially dangerous situation could arise if the patient were to discontinue taking the phenobarbital and the dose of the anticoagulant was not correspondingly reduced.

Many drugs, including other barbiturates, aminopyrine, phenylbutazone, and meprobamate have been shown to stimulate certain liver microsomal enzymes that are involved in drug metabolism.[18,19] The result of this enzyme stimulation may be a more rapid metabolism and excretion of other drugs that are simultaneously administered.

The altering of liver enzyme activity is not only a factor in combination therapy but also may be responsible for the development of tolerance to certain drugs. It has been suggested that tolerance may develop to meprobamate[20] and tolbutamide[21] as a result of the ability of these agents to stimulate liver enzymes and thus actually to stimulate their own metabolism. Therefore, during long-term therapy with these drugs the dose would have to be continually increased to compensate for the loss in pharmacological activity.

Inhibition of Enzyme Systems—There are also drugs that can inhibit the activity of liver enzymes. Such compounds as iproniazid [Marsilid (*Roche*)—withdrawn from the market] and SKF 525A (an agent used in many experimental studies) can potentiate the activity of many drugs by inhibiting the activity of liver enzymes and delaying the metabolism of the drugs.

The monoamine oxidase (MAO) inhibitors [Marplan (*Roche*), Niamid (*Pfizer*), Nardil (*Warner-Chilcott*), Parnate (*SK&F*), and Eutonyl (*Abbott*)] have been shown to inhibit various enzyme systems that may be responsible for metabolizing certain drugs. Many interactions involving the concurrent administration of MAO inhibitors with other drugs and dietary items have been reported, and it is probable that enzyme inhibition plays a role in many of these.

The use of disulfiram [Antabuse (*Ayerst*)] in the treatment of alcoholism also involves enzyme inhibition. Evidence indicates that disulfiram inhibits the activity of aldehyde dehydrogenase, thus inhibiting the oxidation of acetaldehyde (an oxidation product of ethanol) resulting in the accumulation of excessive quantities of this agent.

Displacement of Drugs from Proteins—An interaction of this type may occur when two drugs that are capable of binding to proteins are administered concurrently. Since there are only a limited number of protein binding sites, a competition will exist and the drug that has the greater affinity for the binding sites will displace the other from the plasma or tissue proteins. Both phenylbutazone [Butazolidin (*Geigy*)] and warfarin [Coumadin (*Endo*)] are bound to plasma proteins. However, apparently phenylbutazone has a greater affinity for the binding sites, resulting in a displacement of the warfarin, making increased quantities of the free drug available, both to specific sites of biological action and drug metabolizing enzymes.[22] In these cases the activity of the anticoagulant would be increased, possibly resulting in a hemorrhaging state. To avoid this problem the dose of the anticoagulant would have to be reduced.

Alteration of Urinary Excretion—This may be accomplished by altering the urinary pH and by interfering with tubular excretion.

Alteration of Urinary pH—The alteration of urinary pH, either intentional or unknowing, can influence the activity of certain drugs. For example, acidifying agents are administered with methenamine to enhance its antibacterial activity. The administration of sodium bicarbonate with several of the older sulfonamides has been recommended to provide an alkaline urine in which the drugs are more soluble, thus reducing the incidence of crystalluria.

One manner by which the urinary pH can influence the activity of a drug is by altering the rate of excretion. When a drug is in its nonionized form, it will more readily diffuse from the urine back into the blood. Thus, for an acidic drug such as aspirin, there will be a larger proportion of the drug in the nonionized form in an acid urine than in an alkaline urine where it will exist as an ionized salt. The result is that more aspirin will diffuse back into the blood from an acid urine resulting in prolonged activity.

The opposite will be true for a basic drug such as amphetamine or mecamylamine [Inversine (*MSD*)]. An alkaline urinary pH will favor reabsorption, whereas an acid pH will provide a faster excretion of these agents. It has been noted that the effects of a single dose of amphetamine can last for several days if the urinary pH is sufficiently alkaline.

Interference with Tubular Excretion—It has been known for many years that probenecid [Benemid (*MSD*)] can increase the serum levels and prolong the activity of penicillin derivatives by blocking their tubular excretion. A recent report indicates, however, that other factors may also be involved.[23] These investigators observed a significant decrease in the apparent volume of distribution of certain penicillin derivatives in the presence of probenecid. This decrease in distribution volume would result in higher serum levels.

Alteration of Electrolyte Levels—One of the problems associated with the use of many of the newer diuretics is that they can produce an excessive loss of potassium. This may present a problem in patients being treated with digitalis, many of whom would be candidates for diuretic therapy. If a potassium loss remains uncorrected, the heart may become more sensitive to the effects of digitalis.

Alteration of Receptor Site Interaction—This mechanism has been suggested to explain the potentiated activity of warfarin in patients receiving dextrothyroxine [Choloxin (*Flint*)]. Studies have shown that dextrothyroxine apparently does not affect the absorption, distribution, or rate of metabolism of warfarin; neither does it apparently displace it from protein binding sites or reduce the plasma concentration of Vitamin K-dependent clotting factors.[24] Therefore, it has been suggested that dextrothyroxine can potentiate the effect of warfarin by increasing the affinity of the drug for the receptor site.

Potentiation—It has been shown that alcohol will potentiate the central nervous system depressant effect of the barbiturates and certain tranquilizers in patients taking these medications. Many other examples of potentiation are also known.

Drug Classes

The following discussion reviews some of the interactions that have been observed with several classes of drugs whose members have frequently been implicated in problems of this type.* These particular drugs are considered to give an indication of the frequency with which such interactions can occur unless drug therapy is carefully monitored.

In considering these interactions it should be recognized that just because two drugs interact does not mean that they cannot be administered together. Although there are instances where one drug is specifically contraindicated when another is being given, there are many situations where two drugs that are known to interact can be given concomitantly as long as adequate precautions are taken (such as a change in the dose of one or both of the drugs to compensate for the altered therapeutic response).

Analgesics—Drug interactions are evident not only among drugs having different therapeutic actions but also among drugs that can be used for the same condition. There are several examples of this latter type interaction where instead of obtaining an en-

hanced therapeutic effect by using two drugs, a response is obtained that is less than that obtained from either drug given alone.

The classic example of such an antagonism is seen when probenecid [Benemid (*MSD*)] and aspirin are administered together. Either drug given alone will produce a significant reduction in serum urate levels, but when given together there is a marked inhibition of uricosuric activity regardless of which one is given first or how long the patient is pretreated with the first drug before the second one is introduced.[25]

A recent study indicates that probenecid may interfere with the renal excretion of indomethacin [Indocin (*MSD*)] an agent that may also be used in the treatment of gout.[26] However, in these situations the uricosuric action of probenecid is not antagonized as is seen when aspirin and probenecid are administered together.

One of the effects noted with salicylate therapy is that these agents may cause a lowering of blood prothrombin. Because of this, these drugs must be used carefully, if at all, in patients on anticoagulant therapy. Antlitz *et al*,[27] indicate that another analgesic, acetaminophen, may potentiate the effects of orally administered anticoagulants.

The fact that some of these interactions can occur following the administration of a nonprescription drug (aspirin) with a prescription drug should alert the pharmacist to his particular responsibility in recognizing the possibility of such an interaction, since many times he is more aware than the physician of what nonprescription medications an individual is taking.

Interactions have also been associated with the use of propoxyphene [Darvon (*Lilly*)] when it has been administered concurrently with orphenadrine [Norflex, component of Norgesic (*Riker*)]. Since mental confusion, anxiety, and tremors have been reported in patients on therapy with both of these drugs, their concomitant use is not recommended.[28]

Barbiturates—There have been many reports of an altered therapeutic response to a particular drug when it is administered in combination with one of the barbiturates. Although most of the studies have involved the use of phenobarbital, it should be anticipated that other barbiturates may cause similar problems.

The role of phenobarbital in stimulating liver enzyme systems that metabolize the coumarin anticoagulants has been discussed, and reports indicate that barbital, heptabarbital [Medomin (*Geigy*)], and butabarbital [Butisol (*McNeil*)] act in a similar manner.[29]

Phenobarbital and diphenylhydantoin [Dilantin (*Parke-Davis*)] are often prescribed together for the control of epilepsy, but occasionally there is difficulty in establishing suitable dosages for these agents. It has been shown that phenobarbital can decrease the plasma levels of diphenylhydantoin;[30] however, usually this does not present a significant problem since phenobarbital also has anticonvulsant activity.

Phenobarbital has been reported also to reduce the blood levels of griseofulvin.[31] Thus, the dose of griseofulvin, when administered with phenobarbital, might have to be altered to obtain the desired antifungal activity.

Anticoagulants—The interactions of anticoagulants with other drugs have been reported by many investigators. The consequences of such interactions can be quite serious since it is possible that severe hemorrhaging may result. Most of these interactions have involved the coumarin anticoagulants, primarily

---

* Table IV, page 1835, gives a more complete tabular compilation of drug interactions.

bishydroxycoumarin and warfarin, although several problems have also developed following use of the indandione derivatives; eg, phenindione [Hedulin (*National*)], diphenadione [Dipaxin (*Upjohn*)], and anisindione [Miradon (*Schering*)].

The decreased response to the coumarin anticoagulants in patients on phenobarbital therapy has been discussed and it has been observed that chloral hydrate[32] [Noctec (*Squibb*)] and glutethimide[33] [Doriden (*Ciba*)] show a similar effect. Other agents such as meprobamate and griseofulvin also cause a decreased activity of the coumarin anticoagulants, requiring an increased dose of the latter when both drugs are administered simultaneously.

These drugs apparently decrease the activity of anticoagulants by increasing the rate at which they are metabolized. However, the opposite also may be true. It has been noted that phenyramidol [no longer marketed; formerly marketed as Analexin (*Neisler*)] may inhibit the metabolism of anticoagulants and thereby increase their effect.[34]

Other drugs can also potentiate the effect of anticoagulants. It has been mentioned that phenylbutazone can displace warfarin from protein binding sites making increased quantities of free warfarin available. The same effect should be expected with oxyphenbutazone [Tandearil (*Geigy*)]. It is thought that diphenylhydantoin and clofibrate [Atromid-S (*Ayerst*)] also potentiate the activity of concurrently administered anticoagulants by interfering with protein binding.[34] The manufacturer of clofibrate suggests that it may be necessary to reduce the dose of the anticoagulant by $\frac{1}{3}$ to $\frac{1}{2}$.

Problems may also develop when certain antibiotics such as chloramphenicol and the tetracyclines are administered to patients on anticoagulant therapy.[35] Apparently these antibiotics can increase the anticoagulant effect by interfering with the production of Vitamin K, which would antagonize the activity of the anticoagulants, by certain bacteria in the gastrointestinal tract.

A potentiated anticoagulant effect has been observed when certain anabolic steroids are taken concomitantly. Although the mechanism has not been clarified, it has been noted that norethandrolone[24] [Nilevar (*Searle*)] and methandrostenolone[36] [Dianabol (*Ciba*)] can increase the response to certain coumarin anticoagulants. Quinine and quinidine also may produce this effect.

Dextrothyroxine and the salicylates can also increase the response to anticoagulants, as has been previously mentioned.

The use of certain enzyme products with anticoagulants is not recommended. For example, the use of Papase (*Warner-Chilcott*) is contraindicated in patients on anticoagulant therapy,[37] and it is advised that Ananase (*Rorer*) be given cautiously when prothrombin-depressing drugs are administered concurrently.

The use of anticoagulants warrants careful supervision even when they are given alone. Certainly, when they are administered with other drugs, particular attention should be given to the possibility of an interaction. It would be wise to avoid the concomitant use of an anticoagulant with another drug with which it is known to interact, but frequently such combinations can be administered if adequate precautions are taken.

Antidepressants—The potential danger of concurrent administration of MAO inhibitors—isocarboxazid [Marplan (*Roche*)], nialamide [Niamid (*Pfizer*)], phenelzine [Nardil (*Warner-Chilcott*)], tranylcypromine [Parnate (*SK&F*)], and pargyline [Eutonyl (*Abbott*)]—and sympathomimetic amines is well documented. Although many of these amines (eg, amphetamine) are available only by prescription, others such as ephedrine, phenylephrine, and phenylpropanolamine are found in many popular over-the-counter cold remedies. Certainly it would be wise for patients being treated with MAO inhibitors to avoid using products containing these sympathomimetic agents, and the pharmacist should be alert to his responsibility in helping to prevent such problems.

There have also been reports of serious reactions (hypertensive crises) occurring in people being treated with MAO inhibitors following the ingestion of certain foods having a high tyramine content. These foods include certain cheeses and alcoholic beverages, pickled herring, and chicken livers. Tyramine is metabolized by the monoamine oxidases and normally these enzymes in the intestinal wall and in the liver protect against the pressor actions of amines in foods. However, when these enzymes are inhibited, large quantities of unmetabolized tyramine can accumulate.

MAO inhibitors also should not be administered concurrently with the tricyclic antidepressants—amitriptyline [Elavil (*MSD*)], nortriptyline [Aventyl (*Lilly*)], protriptyline [Vivactil (*MSD*)], imipramine [Tofranil (*Geigy*)], and desipramine [Pertofrane (*Geigy*)]. It is recommended that therapy with one of these agents should not be initiated until at least two weeks after therapy with the other has been discontinued.

It is of interest to note that furazolidone [Furoxone (*Eaton*)], a chemotherapeutic agent, can also inhibit the monoamine oxidases, and it has been suggested that the warnings applying to the use of the other MAO inhibitors should be heeded for this drug also.[38]

Other interactions have been reported with the tricyclic antidepressants. One report has indicated that the antihypertensive effect of guanethidine [Ismelin (*Ciba*)] can be significantly reversed by desipramine and protriptyline.[39] Other studies have suggested that sympathomimetic drugs such as amphetamine and ephedrine, as well as methylphenidate [Ritalin (*Ciba*)] can also reverse the antihypertensive effect of guanethidine.[40]

Antidiabetic Agents—The importance of carefully adjusting the dosage of insulin and oral antidiabetic agents is well recognized. However, it also must be realized that the administration of other drugs with these agents might alter the hypoglycemic response and precipitate a toxic reaction.

It has been reported that sulfaphenazole [Sulfabid (*Purdue*)] can cause hypoglycemic reactions in tolbutamide-treated patients.[41] Since both tolbutamide and sulfaphenazole are bound to serum albumin, it was thought that the additional hypoglycemic activity might be due to a displacement of the tolbutamide from serum-albumin by sulfaphenazole. However, further work indicates that this is probably not the primary mechanism by which this reaction occurs since other sulfa drugs, which are also strongly protein-bound, do not show the same response.

Other drugs that have been shown to enhance the action of tolbutamide include phenylbutazone, oxyphenbutazone, salicylates, phenyramidol, bishydroxycoumarin, and the MAO inhibitors.[42] It has been suggested that probenecid may also enhance the activity of tolbutamide, but a recent study has indicated that this drug does not influence the metabolism of tolbutamide in man.[43]

The potentiation of acetohexamide [Dymelor (*Lilly*)] hypoglycemia by phenylbutazone has been described[44] and it has been suggested that phenylbutazone produces this response by interfering with the renal excretion of hydroxyhexamide, the active metabolite of acetohexamide.

The production of a hypoglycemic reaction following the administration of propranolol [Inderal (*Ayerst*)] to insulin-treated diabetics has been observed.[45] It has been warned that this drug may potentiate the action of insulin and oral hypoglycemic agents. An additional danger in these interactions is that the usual hypoglycemic signs associated with catecholamine liberation, such as sweating and tachycardia, may be abolished.[46]

It has been noted that dextrothyroxine [Choloxin (*Flint*)] may increase blood sugar levels in diabetic patients.[47] Because of this it may be necessary to change the dose of insulin or an oral hypoglycemic agent being administered to these patients.

Other Interactions

There are many other interactions that could be discussed, but the ones mentioned give an indication of the potential dangers of using certain combinations. This should impress on those individuals who prescribe, dispense, or administer drugs the importance of exercising extreme caution in the utilization of any drug. The pharmacist, in particular, by keeping abreast of current literature, can enhance the importance of his role in the care of the patient.

Physical Incompatibility

Physical incompatibility is usually the result of insolubility, liquefaction, or physical complexation. The most frequent cause is insolubility and attention will be directed primarily to this problem.

Insolubility

Insolubility manifests itself because of the *inability of a material to dissolve* in a particular solvent system or because of *precipitation*. While both of these phenomena are related, they will be treated separately as a matter of practical convenience.

The theory of solutions as considered in Chapter 19 on *Solutions and Phase Equilibria* is useful in understanding the importance of solute–solute, solvent–solvent and solute–solvent forces. The reasons for their existence and for their varying strengths must be understood if incompatibilities related to solubility are to be predicted and corrected.

Generally, polar solvents such as water are able to dissolve ionic and polar solutes because of:

1. High dielectric constants (water ≈ 80), which reduce the forces of attraction between unlike charged ions. This reduction results in dissociation of ionic species. Thus, water is capable of disrupting even the strong intermolecular forces of ionic salts such as sodium chloride (its melting point of 800°C is an indication of the strength of these intermolecular forces).
2. Ability to disrupt covalent bonds of compounds such as HCl, through an acid–base reaction, resulting in ionization.
3. Solvation of molecules and ions through dipole interactions, principally hydrogen bonding. In the case of associated solvents such as water the solute must be sufficiently polar to compete for a place in this associated structure. Nonpolar compounds which are incapable of hydrogen bonding and cannot compete for a place in the structure of an associated solvent are insoluble in such a solvent.

Inability of a Material to Dissolve

Inorganic Compounds—These usually possess strong intermolecular forces, ionic or covalent in nature, and therefore are soluble in polar or semipolar solvents such as water, alcohol, and acetone. Strong solvation energies are necessary to disrupt these intermolecular forces (high dielectric solvents reduce this energy requirement). Thus, measurements of any parameter related to hydration energy, such as lyotropic number, ratio of charge to ionic radius, or heats of hydration, reflect solubility within a group of inorganic compounds. Relative solubilities of cations in the same periodic group thus can often be based on these values.

The Alkali Metal Cations—NH_4^+, Li^+, Na^+, and K^+ are listed in order of decreasing solubility. With the exception of the ammonium ion (which is included here although it is not a metal), the solubility of the salts of these cations generally follows heats of hydration and charge-to-ionic-radius-ratio data. Lithium salts have the highest heats of hydration and charge-to-ionic-radius-ratio, and potassium salts the lowest. It follows that the lithium salts are more soluble than the potassium salts. These cations form soluble salts with all univalent and divalent anions. As the charge on the anion increases, the strength of the crystal lattice structure, which is ionic in nature, increases and the energy gained in the hydration process is not sufficient now to disrupt the crystal structure. Thus, salts of the trivalent anions such as PO_4^{-3} show a sharp decrease in solubility. The soluble salts of organic acids are in almost all cases salts of these univalent cations. Other cations generally produce insoluble salts with the organic acids.

The Alkali Earth Cations—Ba^{+2}, Sr^{+2}, Ca^{+2}, and Mg^{+2} generally follow hydration energy data in relationship to solubility, though not as well as the univalent cations previously considered. These cations generally form water-soluble salts with univalent anions, except for the hydroxide and bicarbonate anions. Anions of higher charge increase the strength of the crystal lattice. As a result, for practical purposes, the divalent and trivalent anions form insoluble salts with these cations. Magnesium sulfate is a notable exception to this rule. It exhibits considerable water solubility due to the water molecules associated with it even in the solid state ($MgSO_4 \cdot 6 H_2O$).

The Heavy Metals–Zinc and Mercury form salts in which the binding is partially covalent and the strength of the crystal lattices is dependent also on van der Waal's forces and dipole–dipole interaction.

Zinc tends to form insoluble hydroxides with water that are soluble with an excess of OH^- or H^+ by formation of soluble ions such as $Zn(OH)_4^{-2}$ or Zn^{+2}. It forms soluble salts with univalent and divalent anions. These salts tend to hydrolyze because of the strong attraction of water for this cation, an expected effect based on the high charge-to-ionic-radius-ratio. The oxy-salts which result from hydrolysis are insoluble in water.

Inorganic mercury salts, with the exception of the chloride and oxide, are rarely used in medicine. These salts exist in the oxidation states of +1 (mercurous) and +2 (mercuric). The mercurous salts are insoluble in water. Mercuric salts of univalent anions are slightly soluble but tend to hydrolyze to basic insoluble salts. The chloride is the most stable of the mercuric salts because of its slight ionization in water. The iodide is only sparingly soluble but can be solubilized by the addition of excess iodide ion through the formation of a complex.

Boron and Aluminum—In pharmacy the only boron compounds used to any degree are boric acid, H_3BO_3 (a hydrate of boron anhydride, B_2O_3), and sodium borate (borax), $Na_2B_4O_7 \cdot 10\ H_2O$. Most borates are water soluble; however, an alkaline medium may favor the formation of insoluble basic borates.

Aluminum is frequently used in pharmacy as the chloride, sulfate, phosphate, and hydroxide, and as double sulfate salts with potassium or ammonium (alums). It has a strong ability to bond with water as a result of its very high charge-to-ionic-radius-ratio, an effect manifested by very high heats of hydration. Thus, the tendency for Al^{+3} to form soluble salts is great. Univalent and divalent anions generally form soluble salts. The most commonly used in pharmacy are the chloride and sulfate. Trivalent salts are insoluble. Aluminum acetate is soluble but tends to hydrolyze readily to basic salts and finally to the insoluble hydroxide. This insoluble hydroxide, in the form of a colloidal gel, is used as an antacid. The hydroxide is amphoteric.

Tin and Lead—Tin exists in a valence of +2 and +4, with the +4 state, stannic, the more stable. This metal has found little use in pharmacy, stannous fluoride being the only salt currently used to any extent. This compound has gained wide acceptance in the control of dental caries. It is freely soluble in water, with a strong tendency to hydrolyze to the insoluble basic salt or hydroxide. For this reason it is recommended that solutions of stannous fluoride be freshly prepared.

Lead exists in a valence of +2 and +4, with the +2 state (plumbous) the more stable. Only lead acetate and subacetate are used, and these rarely. Both of these salts are water-soluble, although they tend to hydrolyze rapidly to yield insoluble hydroxides.

Arsenic and Bismuth—The use of arsenic has declined through the years to the point where it is relatively unimportant in modern medicine. It is a constituent of Fowler's Solution (Potassium Arsenite Solution NF XI), a basic solution of arsenic trioxide. It is rarely prescribed in combination with other drugs, so incompatibilities are rarely encountered.

Bismuth salts used in pharmacy are all insoluble oxy-salts, such as the subnitrate, subcarbonate, subgallate, and subsalicylate. These salts tend to hydrolyze in aqueous systems.

Iron—This metal exists in a valence of +2 and +3, with the +3 state the more stable. Because of a very high charge-to-ionic-radius-ratio and subsequently high hydration energies, iron tends to form soluble salts which readily hydrolyze to insoluble hydroxides. The phosphate and carbonate are insoluble. Complex iron salts, because of their limited ionization, are used to avoid hydrolysis and subsequent precipitation. Salts such as iron and ammonium citrate, ferric citrochloride, and iron peptonate may be employed for this purpose, unless the astringent effect of the ionized species is essential for the therapeutic effect.

The Nonmetals—Sulfur and Iodine—The two forms of sulfur generally used in pharmacy, precipitated and sublimed, are insoluble in water and in most common solvents and difficulty is sometimes experienced in compounding aqueous preparations containing this material.

Iodine is essentially insoluble in water, although the commonly used iodide salts are quite soluble. Solutions of iodides, such as potassium iodide, can be used to dissolve larger quantities of iodine because of the formation of the $I_3{}^-$ ion, which is formed by the union of I_2 and an iodide ion.

Acids and Alkalies—Problems involving these compounds are not usually related to their solubility. They are considered in greater detail in the section on *Chemical Incompatibilities*.

Organic Compounds—Except for the hydrocarbons which are nonpolar, organic compounds generally possess both polar and nonpolar parts. As a result, their solubility depends on a balance between these two parts. Organic molecules which are soluble in water to any appreciable extent must possess groups which are capable of hydrogen bonding, being polarized or ionizing. Solubility in water results from hydration of this portion of the molecule through association via hydrogen bonding, induced dipole–dipole interaction, or ion–dipole interaction. The extent of this solubility is the function of the type of water–organic molecule bonding and the ratio of polar to nonpolar portions of the molecule. The ion–dipole bond is the strongest in most cases, and thus greater solubility is demonstrated by compounds which dissolve as a result of this type of bonding.

Hydrocarbons—Because these are completely nonpolar, they are not capable of associating with water. However, they are soluble in nonpolar solvents and possess approximately the same intermolecular forces as benzene, vegetable oils (those without hydroxyl groups), and chloroform. Liquid petrolatum and petrolatum are the only important pharmaceutical compounds that fit into this category. These are unreactive substances and problems associated with their use are generally related to their solubility.

Compounds Solubilized through Hydrogen Bonding and Polarization—Alcohols, phenols, carboxylic acids, amines, aldehydes, ketones, and esters possess water solubility as a result of their ability to form hydrogen bonds and compete successfully for a place in the associated water molecule structure. Compounds in this group are generally assumed to be water-soluble for pharmaceutical purposes if the ratio of functional group to carbon atoms is 1 to 3, slightly soluble if the ratio is 1 to 5, and insoluble if the ratio is 1 to 6 or greater. These compounds show increased solubility in ethanol because of additional nonpolar bonding. They exhibit some ethanol solubility when the ratio is as high as 1 to 16. The usefulness of ethanol as a cosolvent with water to increase the solubility of these compounds is obvious.

Nonpolar atoms other than carbon exert a hydrophobic effect on the solubility approximately proportional to their molecular weights as compared with the molecular weight of carbon. Thus the presence of halogens and metals in organic molecules tends to reduce the solubility in water considerably more than does the addition of a methylene group, except where these atoms introduce significant inductive effects.

Monofunctional Alcohols—Ethyl and isopropyl alcohols are the most important pharmaceutical members of this group. Both alcohols exhibit complete water-miscibility. Alcohols with four or more carbon atoms show a sharp decrease in water solubility, although butyl and amyl alcohols are soluble to some extent. Ethanol is employed in pharmacy as a solvent and cosolvent with water for such compounds as amines (including the alkaloids), phenols (including resinous compounds), carboxylic acids, and barbituric acid derivatives.

Polyfunctional Alcohols—Additional hydroxyl groups serve to increase the water solubility of organic compounds of higher molecular weight by maintaining the 3 or 4 to 1 ratio of carbon atoms to functional groups necessary for this solubility.

Glycols and Carbohydrates—These exhibit water solubility because of their favorable ratio of functional groups to carbon atoms. Glycerin, ethylene glycol, polyethylene glycols, gums such as acacia, agar, and tragacanth, and cellulose derivatives such as methyl and carboxy-methyl cellulose all belong to this group and are water soluble or dispersible.

Phenols—These are weakly acid compounds which owe their water solubility to hydrogen bonding rather than to their limited ionization. Phenol itself, which possesses one hydroxyl group on a benzene ring (equivalent in hydrophobic properties to about four nonconjugated carbons), exhibits only slight water solubility, about 7%. Increase in hydroxyl groups without an increase in the number of carbon atoms results in increased water solubility. Thus resorcinol is considerably more water soluble than phenol. Phenolic compounds that either have more carbon atoms than phenol or maintain the same hydroxyl to carbon ratio show limited solubility. Hexylresorcinol, betanaphthol, thymol, and chlorothymol all are such examples. All of these compounds possess ethanol solubility as would be expected.

Carboxylic Acids—These compounds depend on hydrogen bonding for their water solubility rather than on their limited ionization. Monofunctional acids below a ratio of functional group to carbon atoms of 1 to 3 are infinitely soluble in water; up to a ratio of 1 to 5 they exhibit slight water solubility; beyond that, for practical purposes, none. Thus formic, acetic, and propionic acids are infinitely soluble, while butyric and valeric acids are soluble to the extent of 6 and 4%, respectively. As with the phenols, many of the pharmaceutically important higher acids are alcohol soluble, up to stearic acid (17 carbon atoms). The aromatic carboxylic acids follow a similar pattern.

Benzoic acid, which has the hydrophobic equivalent of five nonconjugated carbons, is soluble to the extent of 0.4%, slightly less than might be predicted from the general rule. The polyfunctional, dicarboxylic, or hydroxy acids are solids rather than liquids, an indication of increased intermolecular hydrogen bonding. Thus while many of the pharmaceutically important acids in this group are water soluble, they are not soluble to the extent that might be expected from the functional group to carbon atom ratios. Oxalic, citric, and tartaric acids are examples. Salicylic acid (*o*-hydroxybenzoic acid) is soluble in water to the same extent as benzoic acid in spite of the presence of the hydroxy group. Intramolecular bonding in this case offsets the effect of this grouping.

Tannic acid, because of the large number of hydroxyl groups present in the molecule, exhibits considerable water solubility.

Amines—These also depend on their ability to hydrogen bond for their water solubility, and as the ratio of carbon atoms to amine groups increases, water solubility drops off sharply. However, because the hydrogen bonding occurs between the unshared electrons on the nitrogen atom of the amine and the hydrogen atom of the water, anything which affects the availability of these electrons will affect the water solubility of the compound. The aliphatic amines show slightly higher solubility limits than the alcohols, while the aromatic amines show about the same limits. However, the effect of substituent groups in the aromatic amines is quite dramatic on solubility.

Aldehydes—Formaldehyde and chloral hydrate are pharmaceutically important members of this group. Both possess considerable water solubility via hydrate formation. Paraldehyde, although it is an acetal, can regenerate acetaldehyde under certain conditions and thus exhibits incompatibilities characteristic of this compound. Paraldehyde is soluble in about eight parts of water and is readily soluble in alcohol.

Ketones—Acetone and camphor are examples of pharmaceutical ketones. Acetone is completely water miscible; camphor, as would be expected, is insoluble in water and soluble in ethanol.

Esters—The lower esters, such as methyl and ethyl acetate, or polyfunctional esters, such as resorcinol monoacetate and glycerylmonoacetate, are very soluble in water. Higher esters such as phenyl salicylate, benzyl benzoate, aspirin, the parabens, and esters of fatty acids, are water insoluble.

Compounds Solubilized through Ionization—Many organic compounds are sufficiently acidic or basic to form salts with bases or acids, respectively. The salts show considerable water solubility as a result of ionization. The organic salts of the alkali metals are in most cases capable of ionizing in water and thus show considerable water solubility, while those of other metals generally do not ionize to any extent and thus do not exhibit water solubility. Organic compounds of very low molecular weights, such as acetates and formates, and organic compounds possessing additional functional groups that increase solubility, such as the citrates, lactates, and tartrates, are exceptions to this rule and will form water-soluble salts with most of the metal cations. Salts formed between organic bases and mineral or relatively strong organic acids are water soluble due to their ionization.

The strength of the ion–dipole bond formed in the solubilization of these compounds is greater generally than the bonding exhibited by the previously considered organic compounds. As a result, many very large organic molecules will exhibit considerable water solubility if they have a functional group capable of ionizing.

Salts of Phenols and Carboxylic Acids—Phenols and carboxylic acids that are normally insoluble in water will dissolve readily in aqueous solutions of bases of the alkali metals through salt formation. These salts demonstrate considerable water solubility through their ability to ionize, whether they are formed as just noted or added to water as previously produced salts. However, as in the case of a mixture of any ionizable species, the tendency is for the compound with the smallest solubility product to form. Thus, in the presence of an ionized acid, these soluble ionized salts will tend to form the least soluble species, the unionized insoluble organic acid. The soluble sodium salts of phenol, resorcinol, benzoic acid, and salicylic acid, for example, exhibit this behavior, and in the presence of acids will precipitate the free acid.

Salts of Sulfonamides—Sulfonamides are sufficiently acid to form salts with strong bases, although only the bases of the alkali metals yield water-soluble salts. As in the case of the phenols and carboxylic acids, the soluble ionized salts react with acids to precipitate the insoluble acidic sulfonamide. The soluble sodium salts of the sulfonamides, such as sodium sulfathiazole and sodium sulfacetamide, react in this manner in an acidic medium.

Salts of Amines—Amines, depending on their basicity, will form water-soluble salts in the presence of mineral and organic acids. Since the ability of the amines to form salts depends on the availability of the unshared electrons on the nitrogen, any substituents which affect the availability of the electrons will affect the salt-forming ability, and thus the water solubility, of these compounds. Alkaloids, many local anesthetics, surface-active agents, phenothiazine derivatives, and other nitrogen containing compounds form soluble salts in the presence of acids. All of these salts tend to precipitate the free base in the presence of alkalies.

Precipitation

Another manifestation of insolubility differs from the first category in that materials previously in solution are forced out of solution, generally as a result of dehydration or salting out, change in solvent system, or temperature change.

Dehydration or salting out of slightly soluble nonelectrolytes from aqueous media occurs on the addition of an electrolyte. The ability of the electrolyte to compete successfully for water results in a reduction in water available for solution of the nonelectrolyte, with subsequent salting out. The stronger the ability of the electrolyte ions to hydrate, as measured by factors such as lyotropic number, hydration energies, and charge-to-ionic-radius-ratios, the greater the effect. Thus cations of the alkali metals Li^+, Na^+, and K^+ show a strong tendency to salt out nonelectrolytes.

The separation of alcohol from a hydroalcoholic vehicle on the addition of large amounts of an electrolyte and the salting out of electrolytes from an aqueous solution by alcohol are examples of this phenomenon. Which will occur depends on which constituent is better able to compete for the water.

Sugars and hydrophilic colloids are precipitated from aqueous solution on the addition of alcohol or electrolytes through this dehydration process. The alcohol or the electrolyte, better able to compete for a place in the associated water structure, actually squeezes out the other compound or dehydrates it. Gums, such as acacia, tragacanth, and agar, sugars, and many hydrocolloids are thus precipitated from aqueous solutions by alcohol and by salts.

Change in Solvent System—The mixing of a preparation having an organic solvent with one in an aqueous medium results in precipitation. Thus the mixing of tinctures or fluidextracts with syrups or other aqueous solutions will generally result in precipitation. This is another reflection of the solubility of the material and often can be predicted from a knowledge and understanding of solubility principles.

Temperature Change—Concentrated or saturated solutions of materials which dissolve endothermically (absorb heat), such as potassium iodide, boric acid, and most common electrolytes and nonelectrolytes, when stored below room temperature will precipitate. Materials which dissolve exothermically (release heat), such as calcium hydroxide, show this effect when stored at temperatures above room temperature.

Liquefaction

Liquefaction of dry material may result from eutexia, release of water of hydration, or absorption of water.

Eutexia—A depression in the melting point of a solid in contact with certain other components, resulting in liquefaction at room temperature is known as eutexia.

Many commonly used drugs containing a phenol, aldehyde, or ketone group exhibit this phenomenon. Many of these compounds themselves possess low melting points, indicative of weak intermolecular forces. Phenol, menthol, thymol, salol, antipyrine, aminopyrine, betanaphthol, and aspirin are common examples of drugs which in combination with one another form eutectic mixtures. Phase diagrams of various combinations of these drugs, when available, are helpful in determining concentrations which result in eutexia.

Water of Hydration—Many chemicals form hydrates, compounds with water of crystallization, that are stable at room temperature and within the range of humidities normally encountered. These compounds will tend to release their water of hydration, however, under the influence of increasing temperature or decreasing humidity. The opposite effect may be expected for some materials from decreasing temperature and increasing humidity. A pasty solid may result in either situation. Under certain conditions heavy trituration also may release water of hydration with a resultant moist product.

Qualitative information that may be useful in predicting incompatibilities of this type may be found in the official compendia. For example, the statements "effloresces in warm, dry air" and "the hydrous form is efflorescent in dry air" appear in the descriptions for magnesium sulfate and citric acid, respectively.

Physical Complexation

Although both inorganic and organic complexes are recognized, generally only the organic complexes present problems with respect to pharmaceutical incompatibilities.

The organic complex, often referred to as a coordinate compound (since the bond formed is a coordinate one and not ionic or covalent) or molecular complex, is a compound in which the constituents are held together by weak donor–acceptor bonds (in some instances this may be a hydrogen bond). They differ from true organic compounds in that they are not held together by primary valence bonds, but rather by an over-all attraction between molecules resulting from polarization forces. The attraction energies are in the range of 5 Kcal/mole and thus may be considered as resulting from physical rather than chemical interaction. Butesin picrate is an example of a molecular complex formed between picric acid and butesin, an aniline derivative.

Marcus[48] has attributed many of the reported problems with nonionic polyether surfactants and phenols, carboxylic acids, and cyclic alcohols to a loose interaction or complex. He noted a loss in elegance and acceptability in preparations containing Carbowax* and phenols, salicylic acid, or tannic acid. He explained this complexation on the basis of hydrogen bonding between the hydroxyl groups of the active ingredient and the ether oxygens of the polyether chain. Other workers have reported not only loss of elegance as a result of this type of interaction but often a delay in drug absorption.[49] Hurwitz, et al,[50] detected similar interactions of cations of chlorpromazine, promethazine, tetracaine, and methylrosaniline, and of anions of naphthalene sulfonate and methyl orange

---

* Carbowax (*Union Carbide*) is a trademark for a series of solid polyethylene glycols.

with polysorbate 80 (a nonionic surfactant). These workers attributed the interactions to mixed micelle formation, with the drugs penetrating into the micellar structure of the surfactant. Modification of drug release and absorption could no doubt be expected from such interactions. Complexes between benzoic acid, salicylic acid, sulfonamides, and barbiturates have been reported with urea.[51]

Often, this type of incompatibility may occur without any physical evidence. Precipitation, which might be expected, may not occur because of solubilization of the complex within the micelles of the surfactant, slow reaction rate, and consequent delay in formation of the complex in any appreciable concentration, or low concentrations of reactants resulting in amounts of the complex which do not exceed solubility. Prediction of such incompatibilities may be difficult. The pharmacist should be aware, nevertheless, that nonionic compounds are capable of interacting with ionic or polarizable species, and that such interaction may result in therapeutic as well as physical incompatibilities.

Treatment of Physical Incompatibility

Physical incompatibilities should be prevented before they occur, whenever possible. When they do not involve a therapeutic incompatibility, they may be corrected simply in any manner that meets the intent of the prescriber.

Insolubility or Immiscibility—These may be treated basically by adjusting the solvent system to permit dissolution, changing the order of mixing, or suspending or emulsifying the material. The remedial procedure may be followed whether the troublesome compound was added initially or formed as the result of a chemical reaction. The selection of a particular procedure depends on whether it will form a product that is not only satisfactory in appearance but will also allow the patient to obtain a proper and uniform dose without difficulty or inconvenience.

Adjusting the Solvent System—An additional solvent or solubilizing agent may be added to dissolve the insoluble material. Unless this adjustment is minor, permission of the prescriber usually must be obtained. The solvents employed in extemporaneous pharmacy are limited and as a result the pharmacist is restricted in his selection. Ethanol, glycerin, and inert oils such as olive oil and mineral oil may be added in moderate amounts as cosolvents. However, when extreme changes are made in the solvent system or it becomes necessary to use less commonly accepted agents such as polyethylene glycol or propylene glycol or solubilizing surfactants such as the Tweens* and Spans,* the permission of the prescriber is necessary.

Before these procedures are employed in an attempt to solubilize insoluble materials, the intent of the prescriber must be considered. Many times insoluble materials are added to a prescription or formed in a chemical reaction deliberately. For reasons of stability or for therapeutic efficacy, the prescriber may intend that insoluble compounds be suspended rather than solubilized. The following prescriptions are examples in which the prescriber intended that suspensions be prepared. A suspension is prepared, in the first case, because a solubilized aspirin shows poor stability,

while the suspended drug is reasonably stable[52] and in the second case, because the active ingredients are the insoluble polysulfides formed by the reaction of the two soluble compounds employed.

℞	Aspirin	gr v
	Cherry Syrup qs ad	℥ i
D.T.D. No. 24		

℞	Zinc Sulfate	4.0
	Sulfurated Potash	4.0
	Rose Water qs ad	60.0

Changing the Order of Mixing—Dissolution of materials separately in the maximum amount of available solvent (selecting the available solvent most effective for each compound) before mixing them together will often minimize or prevent precipitation. If a precipitate does form, it will be in a fine, readily dispersible state. Phenobarbital Elixir USP affords a good example of this technique. The phenobarbital is dissolved in alcohol, and glycerin is added to aid in maintaining the phenobarbital in solution when diluted with water. The water is added last in order to maintain the highest possible alcoholic concentration at all times. A change in this order of mixing might result in precipitation or extremely slow rate of dissolution.

Suspending or Emulsifying the Material—Many times insoluble solids are of sufficiently small particle size (often true when they are precipitated from dilute cold solutions) or the dispersing liquid is of sufficiently high viscosity as to require no suspending agent. The criterion is for shaking the mixture to cause the particles to become suspended and to remain suspended long enough for the patient to obtain a uniform dose. Where suspensions do not meet this criterion, a finer form of the drug may be used or suspending agents may be added. Suspending agents usually function by increasing the viscosity of the vehicle, thus slowing the rate of settling of the solids. Acacia, tragacanth, the methylcellulose derivatives, bentonite and other clays, glycerin, and syrup are examples of compounds that may serve as suspending agents. Generally, any of these may be added in small amounts without the prescriber's permission.

Immiscible liquids, such as mixtures of oils and aqueous liquids, require emulsification. Acacia, tragacanth, or gelatin may be employed without permission of the prescriber. The newer and often more efficient emulsifiers, such as the Tweens and Spans have not been generally accepted in extemporaneous preparations and their use requires prior permission. It is the responsibility of the pharmacist to select an emulsifier that will produce a satisfactory emulsion without affecting therapeutic activity.

Liquefaction of Solids—This can usually be corrected by the addition of inert diluents. Magnesium carbonate, light magnesium oxide, starch, kaolin, or talc may be employed to separate potentially incompatible materials, as in the case of eutectics, or to absorb moisture coming from water of crystallization or from the atmosphere. These techniques are considered in more detail in Chapter 86 on *Powders*.

Physical Complexation—When this results in a significant alteration of therapeutic activity, the preparation should not be dispensed. Permission should be obtained from the prescriber to make the necessary change in the formulation. Precipitates that might result from this incompatibility and apparently do not effect therapeutic efficacy may be treated as previously noted for insoluble material.

---

* Tween and Span are trademarks (*Atlas*) for a series of polyoxyethylene derivatives of sorbitan fatty acid esters and for sorbitan fatty acid esters, respectively.

Chemical Incompatibility

Chemical incompatibility may be the result of oxidation–reduction, acid–base, hydrolysis, or combination reactions. The occurrence of these reactions is sometimes manifested by a change in color, by an evolution of a gas, or by a physical incompatibility such as precipitation; often, the final effect may be a therapeutic incompatibility.

These manifestations, however, are not in themselves an indication of the type of chemical reaction involved. A precipitate may result from any of these reactions. Evolution of a gas may result from either an acid–base reaction (eg, release of carbon dioxide) or a hydrolytic reaction (eg, release of nitrous oxide by hydrolysis of ethyl nitrite in an alkaline medium). A color formation or change in color may result from an acid–base reaction (eg, color changes of indicator dyes), or a redox reaction (eg, oxidation of epinephrine to red adrenochrome). In some instances a chemical incompatibility may result in a therapeutic incompatibility without any physical manifestations (eg, hydrolysis of penicillin and other antibiotics in aqueous media).

Oxidation–Reduction

Oxidation, in a limited way, can be defined as the gain of oxygen or loss of hydrogen, and reduction as the reverse. However, a more general definition in which oxidation is defined as the loss of electrons and reduction as the gain of electrons is less restrictive and will be employed here. Oxidation and reduction must occur together, and thus depend not only on the ability of a compound to donate an electron but also on the ability of a companion compound to accept the electron. This is demonstrated by many compounds normally considered to be readily oxidized, such as the phenothiazine tranquilizers. These drugs are oxidized by Fe^{+3} but not by Cu^{+2}, although both of these cations are capable of accepting electrons. The Fe^{+3} obviously more readily accepts the electrons than does the Cu^{+2}, ie, the iron is more easily reduced. Thus, only certain combinations of oxidizing agents and reducing agents will result in a redox reaction, depending on their relative abilities to take part in these reactions. Certain generalities can be made concerning the redox systems usually found in pharmaceutical mixtures.

Of the inorganic compounds of pharmaceutical importance only relatively few exhibit redox incompatibilities. Almost all of the cations used in pharmacy that exist in more than one valence state will be oxidized from their lower to higher valence states by strong oxidizing agents such as permanganates, chlorates, and peroxides. Only redox reactions involving milder oxidizing agents, therefore, will be covered specifically.

Mercurous salts are easily reduced to free mercury in the presence of moisture, iron, light, or heat. They may be oxidized to the more soluble and more toxic mercuric salts in the presence of moisture and excess anion or oxidizing agents such as Fe^{+3}.

Stannous salts, of which the fluoride is the most important, are readily oxidized by air and most mild oxidizing agents to the stannic form. In the case of the fluoride the stannic form is considered to be a less active anticariogenic agent.

Bismuth compounds are easily reduced to metallic bismuth by organic compounds such as glycerin, natural gums, and other easily oxidized materials.

Iron in the ferric state is an oxidizing agent; in the ferrous state it is a reducing agent. Ferric salts are sufficiently strong oxidizing agents to oxidize organic compounds such as the phenolic compounds and phenothiazine drugs. Complexation of ferric iron with citrates, lactates, phosphates, and EDTA, for example, changes the oxidation potential to the extent that the iron no longer possesses the ability to oxidize most of these compounds.

Silver salts are reduced to metallic silver by light and by compounds such as the reducing sugars.

All organic compounds can be oxidized by strong oxidizing agents such as permanganates, chlorates, and peroxides. These reactions may be extremely violent, especially when the reagents are mixed in dry or concentrated form. Heavy trituration of a permanganate or chlorate with organic material has been known to result in violent explosions.

The oxidation of organic compounds by milder oxidizing agents, such as metallic cations or atmospheric oxygen, depends on the ability of the compound to donate electrons. Compounds with hydroxyl, ketone, amine, and sulfide groups are generally subject to the action of mild oxidants because of the availability of the unshared electrons on these functional groups. These groups in conjugation with aromatic rings yield colored compounds on oxidation due to the formation of quinoid structures. Conditions that make the electrons more readily available will tend to increase the ease of oxidation of these compounds.

Sugars are readily oxidized, especially the so-called reducing sugars containing free ketone groups, by Bi^{+2}, Cu^{+2}, Ag^+, and $Fe(CN)_6^{-3}$ ions in alkaline solutions.

Phenolic compounds, because of the availability of the unshared electrons on the oxygen, are readily oxidized by air and mild oxidants such as Fe^{+3}. The tendency to become oxidized increases in alkaline media where the electrons are less tightly held.

Aldehydes such as formaldehyde and chloral hydrate are subject to the action of oxidizing agents, resulting in the formation of the corresponding acids.

Amines, including many alkaloidal compounds, local anesthetics, and tranquilizers, are readily oxidized. The presence of the unshared electrons on the nitrogen atom makes all of these compounds subject to oxidation. Light, moisture, and metallic ions such as Fe^{+3}, all serve as oxidants. Generally the oxidation is accelerated in alkaline medium, as in the case of the phenols.

Oils and fats develop rancidity as a result of autoxidation, generally catalyzed by light.

Most of the vitamins likely to be used in extemporaneous preparations are subject to oxidative processes. The oxidation of ascorbic acid is catalyzed by traces of copper and iron, to some extent even in the dry state. Its aqueous solutions are subject to air oxidation, especially in the presence of alkali, light, and heat. Thiamine is sensitive to both oxidizing and reducing agents and is converted to inactive forms in the presence of both. Alkaline solutions accelerate this decomposition. Riboflavin is subject to reduction to a leuco form, but it is quite resistant to oxidizing agents.

Incompatibilities resulting from mixing of oxidants and reductants generally can be prevented only by removal of one of the species. This always requires the permission of the prescriber. Light-catalyzed air oxidations can be minimized by storage in light-resistant completely filled containers or by the addition of materials which will be preferentially oxidized, such as sodium bisulfite. However, in most extemporaneous preparations, because of the rapid consumption of the product, no preservatives are generally necessary to prevent air oxidation.

Acid–Base

Most incompatibilities due to acid–base reactions manifest themselves by precipitation, gas formation, or color formation or change.

Precipitation—Soluble inorganic salts, except for the alkali metals, react with basic hydroxides to yield water-insoluble compounds. Soluble salts of the phenols, carboxylic acids, and barbituric acids, whether they were originally dissolved in water or formed there by dissolving the acid form in an alkaline solution, will yield the free acid in the presence of relatively strong acids. Depending on the solubility of these acids in the particular solvent system, they may remain in solution or precipitate. Soluble salts of amine drugs will release the free base in the presence of relatively strong bases. Precipitation will depend on the solubility of this base in the solvent system.

It must be noted that the formation of the free acid or free base depends on the ability to compete for the proton. Thus sodium phenobarbital will form phenobarbital, an acid, only if the phenobarbital ion can compete successfully for the proton. In other words, the base remaining after the formation of phenobarbital must be a weaker base than phenobarbital ion. In the case of an alkaloidal salt, such as quinine hydrochloride, the reverse is true. Quinine base will result only if the acid formed is a weaker acid (holds on to the proton more firmly) than is the quinine hydrochloride. Thus the prediction of acid–base incompatibilities requires a knowledge of relative acid–base strengths as well as of solubilities of the acidic and basic forms of the particular compounds involved.

Evolution of Gas—Carbonates in the presence of acids stronger than carbonic acid will form carbon dioxide, with subsequent evolution of the gas. Weak acids, such as boric acid, will not react with carbonates. In the presence of glycerin, however, glyceroboric acid forms, which is a sufficiently strong acid to react.

Change or Formation of Color—Most dyes or indicators employed in pharmacy are acidic or basic and generally form water-soluble ionized salts with anions (bases) or cations (acids), respectively. The color of these materials is influenced by their ionization and thus a change in the pH of the solution that is sufficient to affect ionization will generally change the color. Phenolphthalein is a colorless acidic compound. On addition of an aqueous solution of a base, such as sodium hydroxide, a red ionized disodium salt with a quinoid structure forms. Gentian violet is a basic purple compound. However, on the addition of sufficient acid to tie up basic groups, the compound changes color through green to yellow, as all the groups become tied up.

Correction or prevention of acid–base reactions may be achieved in several ways. The addition of a buffer or a change of vehicle may be used to prevent the formation of the free acid or base from the salt. The pH-sensitive coloring agents can be treated in a similar manner or by replacement with another coloring agent. In general, these procedures require prior permission.

If the procedures necessary to avoid the incompatibility cannot be resorted to and no therapeutic incompatibility is involved, corrective procedures should be used. Precipitation can be treated as noted previously. A reaction resulting in the release of carbon dioxide can

be carried to completion so that the amount of gas remaining in solution is not sufficient to rupture the container. In some instances the formation of carbon dioxide is desired since it serves to mask the taste of salty and bitter drugs.

Hydrolysis

The reaction of a compound with water may be divided into two broad categories: ionic and molecular hydrolysis.

Ionic hydrolysis involves the reaction of an ionized species with either H^+ or OH^- of water to form an un-ionized insoluble product, and may be considered as a special type of acid–base reaction. This tying up of the H^+ or OH^- results in a change in the pH of the solution. Both inorganic and organic salts may undergo this type of hydrolysis. Salts of a weak acid and a strong base, a strong acid and a weak base, and a weak acid and a weak base tend to hydrolyze. The incompatibilities resulting from this type of hydrolysis generally manifest themselves as precipitates of basic salts or hydroxides.

Zinc salts, salts of a strong acid and a weak base, tend to hydrolyze to form insoluble basic salts.

$$ZnCl_2 + HOH \rightleftharpoons ZnOHCl\downarrow + H^+$$

All zinc salts, with the exception of the sulfate and the nitrate, hydrolyze readily. The addition of H^+ to the solution reverses this reaction, as in the use of boric acid to prevent hydrolysis of zinc borate.

Aluminum salts hydrolyze, yielding insoluble basic salts and the hydroxide. The precipitation of $Al(OH)_2$-CH_3COO from solutions of aluminum acetate and subacetate is a manifestation of the hydrolysis of these soluble salts. Chlorides and sulfates of aluminum also show a slight tendency to hydrolyze. Addition of H^+ or excess anion reverses this hydrolysis.

The insoluble bismuth salts, except for the subcarbonate, hydrolyze to yield an acid when dispersed in water. The subnitrate and subsalicylate yield nitric and salicylic acids, respectively. The formation of these acids results in further incompatibilities due to acid–base reactions.

Soluble salts of barbituric acid derivatives and sulfonamides hydrolyze slowly in water to yield the insoluble free acids.

Molecular hydrolysis is a term applied to the reaction of water with organic compounds such as amides, esters, and lactams. This type of hydrolysis proceeds at a much slower rate than the ionic type, and the rate is often a function of H^+ or OH^- concentration (catalysis). Because of the relatively slow rate of reaction, molecular hydrolysis is generally not of major concern to the community pharmacist. In most cases the prescription will have been consumed before significant hydrolysis occurs. However, since this hydrolysis often reduces the therapeutic efficacy of the drug and is not always detectable by a physical change, the pharmacist should be aware of compounds that may exhibit this type of incompatibility.

Disaccharides hydrolyze in the presence of H^+ to yield monosaccharides. The inversion of sucrose to levulose and dextrose is a typical example of a H^+-catalyzed hydrolysis.

Esters are subject to hydrolysis, yielding the corresponding alcohols and acids. This hydrolysis is usually catalyzed by H^+ or OH^-. Phenyl salicylate hydrolyzes in basic media to phenol and salicylic acid. The rationale behind the former use of this compound as an intestinal antiseptic was based on this hydrolysis. Aspirin is readily hydrolyzed to acetic and salicylic acids in the presence of moisture. This will occur to some extent even in the dry state. Resorcinol monoacetate, the parabens, and glyceryl triacetate are examples of other pharmaceutically important esters which undergo hydrolysis. Nitrite and nitrate esters such as ethyl nitrite, amyl nitrite, glyceryl trinitrate, and pentaerythritol tetranitrate are rapidly hydrolyzed in alkaline media to nitrous or nitric acids and the corresponding alcohol.

Glycosides are subject to hydrolysis which splits them into their sugar and nonsugar (aglycon) portions. Acids and high temperatures accelerate this hydrolysis.

Some antibiotics tend to hydrolyze to inactive forms in aqueous solutions, the rate usually depending on H^+ or OH^- concentration. However, because of the manner in which these drugs are generally prescribed, most products will maintain their strength for the period of time necessary for consumption. In situations where antibiotics are prescribed in combination with other drugs in a mixture, the pharmacist should ascertain that the mixture is stable and that the potency is not affected. The patient should be informed of any special storage requirements that will help retard deterioration.

Vitamins are generally prescribed as prefabricated solid or liquid dosage forms; however, several of the B vitamins are occasionally prescribed in combination with other ingredients.

Thiamine hydrochloride (vitamin B_1) hydrolyzes to inactive or less active forms in solutions of neutral or alkaline pH. Thus, carbonates, bicarbonates, acetates, soluble salts of the barbiturates, and sulfonamides accelerate the hydrolysis of this vitamin. Riboflavin (vitamin B_2) is also subject to hydrolysis in alkaline media. Vitamin B_{12}, although rarely prescribed in extemporaneous combinations, is hydrolyzed by strong acids and bases.

Ionic hydrolysis usually can be prevented or reversed by the addition of any of the species formed as a result of the hydrolysis. Prevention of molecular hydrolysis is more involved and requires a knowledge of conditions that effect stability of the drug involved. Whenever the rate of hydrolysis is sufficiently fast to cause significant degradation of the drug before it would normally be expected to be consumed, correction or prevention of the incompatibility is essential. Permission of the prescriber to make the needed changes is generally required in these situations.

Combination

This may be considered as an ionic reaction in which a pair of ions is removed from the sphere of activity by precipitation or by the formation of a very slightly ionized species.

Precipitation of soluble inorganic salts in the presence of ions which combine to yield insoluble salts is a common cause of incompatibilities. A knowledge of the solubility of the various inorganic salts will enable one to predict this type of incompatibility. Knowing that silver chloride is insoluble is sufficient to forewarn a pharmacist that a solution of silver nitrate cannot be made isotonic with sodium chloride.

Organic salts in the presence of metal cations, other than the alkali metals, will form water-insoluble compounds through combination. Acetates are an exception to this rule. Thus, sodium phenobarbital or sodium benzoate will combine with ions of calcium, zinc, and aluminum to yield water-insoluble organic salts.

Combination reactions of ionized organic species with each other can be predicted by the method suggested by Miller.[53] This method excludes compounds of low molecular weight, which yield soluble compounds even after combination. Organic compounds of high molecular weight that take part in this type of reaction may be divided into anionic and cationic types. Organic salts of metals such as sodium and potassium are anionic, while chlorides, hydrochlorides, sulfates, phosphates, and acetates are cationic. Any mixture containing both an anionic and cationic organic compound of fairly high molecular weight can be considered to be a potentially incompatible mixture. The possibility of precipitation and/or inactivation exists in these mixtures, and similar problems may exist in ointments and lotions where there may be no physical manifestation of their occurrence. Whether or not an incompatibility occurs in a given combination depends on the solubility of the new compound formed, the concentrations of all species involved, and the presence of crystal inhibitors such as sugar.

The precipitation and inactivation of the quaternary antibacterial agents, such as benzalkonium chloride by anionic detergents, is a common example of this type of combination. Amine salts, including most alkaloids, antihistamines, and tranquilizers, may combine with salts of sulfonamides, barbiturates, and anionic detergents to form insoluble and often inactive species.

Prevention of these incompatibilities may be achieved by elimination of or marked reduction in the concentration of one of the ionic species, diluting the solution or adjusting the solvent system to keep the new species in solution. The insoluble compound, if it cannot be redissolved, may be suspended, as in the case of other insoluble compounds. However, if the possibility exists that the new species is inactive or less active, prevention by elimination of one of the species should be employed.

Examples of Incompatibilities

Insolubility

1

℞	Potassium iodide	℥ i
	Phenobarbital	gr xvi
	Thiamine HCl Elixir qs ad	f℥ viii
	M. Ft. Sol.	

The alcoholic concentration of the elixir is not sufficient to dissolve the phenobarbital or to maintain it in solution. A suspension might be prepared but, because of the potency of the phenobarbital and the danger involved if the patient did not uniformly disperse this drug before taking a dose, dissolution is preferable. The concentration of alcohol required to maintain this amount of phenobarbital in solution, as calculated from data obtained by Leuallen,[54] is about 27%. Knowledge of the alcoholic concentration of the elixir would permit calculation of the amount of alcohol that must be added. The phenobarbital is dissolved in this alcohol; the thiamine lost by replacement of the elixir and the potassium iodide are dissolved in the elixir, and the two solutions are mixed. Sodium phenobarbital could not be substituted in this system because the acidity of the elixir will precipitate free phenobarbital and the alkalinity of the sodium phenobarbital may cause some hydrolysis of the thiamine.

Additional solubility data on phenobarbital in mixed solvent systems have been reported by Krause and Cross,[55] Peterson and Hopponen,[56] and Barr and Tice.[57] Similar data on terpin hydrate in alcohol–water vehicles have been reported by Mascardo and Barr.[58]

	2	
℞	Ephedrine Sulfate	0.25
	Menthol	0.02
	Mineral oil, light qs	30.00
	M. Ft. Sol.	

The alkaloidal salt is not oil soluble. Substitution of an anhydrous ephedrine base will permit preparation of a clear solution.

	3	
℞	Phenyl salicylate	5.00
	Olive oil	30.00
	Purif. water qs ad	60.00
	M. Ft. sol.	

The phenyl salicylate is soluble in the oil. However, even without instructions from the physician, it is obvious that the oil solution of phenyl salicylate and the water must be emulsified. The use of acacia or tragacanth would permit satisfactory emulsification.

	4	
℞	Potassium bromide	8.0
	Camphor water qs ad	60.0
	M. Ft. sol.	

Camphor is salted out of the saturated camphor water by the electrolyte, which is better able to compete for the water. Solution of the bromide in a minimum amount of purified water prior to the addition of the camphor water would eliminate the incompatibility.

	5	
℞	Peru Balsam	2.0
	Petrolatum qs	30.0
	M. Ft. oint.	

A granular ointment results because the semipolar (phenolic) components of the balsam are not miscible with the completely nonpolar base. Compounds possessing the proper balance of polar and nonpolar groups, so that they can associate with both the petrolatum and the balsam, will permit the preparation of a smooth product. Castor oil will serve this function. Thus, if the balsam is first mixed with about an equal amount of castor oil and this mixture incorporated into the petrolatum, a smooth ointment results.

	6	
℞	Magnesium carbonate	7.5
	Sodium bicarbonate	15.0
	Citric acid	15.0
	Purif. water qs ad	500.0
	M. Ft. sol.	

The final appearance of this prescription depends on the order of mixing. If the sodium bicarbonate is added to a solution of the citric acid, and the magnesium carbonate is added last, the solution will be incomplete. However, if the magnesium carbonate is added to the solution of citric acid first, soluble magnesium citrate will be formed. The sodium bicarbonate will be soluble in this mixture and a clear solution will be obtained.

	7	
℞	Tr. Benzoin Compound	5.0
	Glycerin	15.0
	Rose Water qs ad	100.0
	M. Ft. lotion	

The resins and other components of the tincture are soluble only in high alcoholic vehicles. The change in solvent system results in an unavoidable precipitate. Addition of the tincture with rapid stirring or in a fine stream under pressure (as with a pipet to the glycerin rose water solution) yields a fine colloidal dispersion. No suspending agent is necessary.

Liquefaction

	8	
℞	Phenyl salicylate	℥ ii
	A.S.A.	℥ i
	Antipyrine	℥ i
	M. Ft. cap. no. 24	

A combination of any two of these ingredients will produce a wet mass or even complete liquefaction. The use of approximately gr ii of magnesium carbonate or light magnesium oxide per capsule to physically separate the ingredients will prevent liquefaction for about two weeks. Gentle trituration and the use of a capsule large enough to permit loose packing is essential.

Physical Complexation

	9	
℞	Phenol	1.0
	Polyethylene glycol-400	10.0
	Zinc oxide	15.0
	Purif. water qs ad	100.0
	M. Ft. lotion	

The complexation of the phenol with the ether oxygens of the polyethylene glycol-400 (PEG) will produce an unsatisfactory suspension, as well as inactivate the phenol. Substitution of bentonite magma for the PEG will permit preparation of a satisfactory product.

Oxidation–Reduction

	10	
℞	Tr. Ferric Chloride	20.0
	Syrup Thorazine qs ad	120.0
	M. Ft. soln.	

The ferric chloride will rapidly oxidize the Thorazine to the inactive sulfoxide. The two preparations must be dispensed separately.

	11	
℞	Sodium salicylate	8.00
	Sodium bicarbonate	16.00
	Peppermint water qs ad	180.00
	M. Ft. Sol.	

This solution darkens on standing. The change is attributed to the alkaline catalyzed oxidation of the salicylate to a quinoid form.[59] A number of substances are useful as antioxidants in retarding the color development and, in this formula, 0.1% sodium bisulfite serves this purpose.

12

℞	Mild mercurous chloride	gr xviii
	Potassium bromide	gr xxx
	Sucrose	gr xxiv
M. Ft. powders 12		

In the presence of moisture the mercurous chloride reacts with the bromide, resulting in both oxidation and reduction of the mercurous salt to mercuric bromide and free mercury. This is potentially a dangerous combination and should not be dispensed.[60]

Acid–Base Reactions

13

℞	Cocaine HCl	gr v
	Boric acid	
	Sodium borate aa	gr xx
	Purified water qs ad	f℥ ii

The alkalinity imparted to the solution by the sodium borate causes precipitation of the water-insoluble cocaine base. Elimination of the sodium borate prevents this incompatibility. This reaction is typical of most amine salts in the presence of bases or basic salts.

14

℞	Sodium bicarbonate	
	Bismuth subnitrate aa	ℨ ii
	Water qs ad	f℥ iii
M. Ft. susp.		

Hydrolysis of the bismuth subnitrate yields nitric acid, which reacts with the bicarbonate to yield carbon dioxide. The gas formed would be sufficient to rupture the container. Completion of the reaction prior to dispensing is not feasible because of the slow rate of acid production from the hydrolysis. A satisfactory remedy is to replace the subnitrate salt with the subcarbonate.

15

℞	Sodium sulfathiazole	gr x
	Boric acid sol. 2% qs ad	f℥ ss
M. Ft. sol.		

The acidity of boric acid will cause the formation of free sulfathiazole. Since this product is intended for use as ear drops, dispensing of a suspension might be considered. However, a more suitable procedure is to eliminate the boric acid and dispense a clear solution.

16

℞	Sodium salicylate	15.0
	Elix. Lactated Pepsin qs ad	120.0
M. Ft. sol.		

The acidic vehicle results in the formation and precipitation of salicylic acid. A change to a neutral or alkaline vehicle or the addition of sufficient alcohol to dissolve the salicylic acid will correct this incompatibility.

Hydrolysis Reactions (Ionic)

17

℞	Zinc sulfate	gr ss
	Sodium borate	gr ii
	Rose water qs ad	f℥ i

The formation of and subsequent hydrolysis of zinc borate results in a precipitate. Zinc sulfate alone will also hydrolyze gradually to precipitate a basic salt. The use of boric acid in place of the sodium borate will prevent the hydrolysis of the zinc salts.

18

℞	Ferric chloride	40.0
	Water qs ad	120.0
M. Ft. sol.		

On standing, a precipitate of ferric hydroxide results from the hydrolysis of the ferric chloride. The addition of a small amount of hydrochloric acid will prevent the hydrolysis.

Hydrolysis Reactions (Molecular)

19

℞	Sodium salicylate	ℨ ii
	Phenobarbital sodium	gr ix
	Vitamin B Complex Elix.	f℥ viii

Vitamin B complex elixir has an acidic pH. The alkalinity of the salts causes deterioration of the B vitamins via hydrolysis as well as eventual precipitation of the acids of these sodium salts. Dispensing of the salts separately is suggested.

20

℞	Penicillin G sodium	1,000,000 u
	Syrup of Cherry qs ad	30.0 ml
M. Ft. sol.		

Hydrolysis of the penicillin salt occurs in the acidic medium as well as precipitation of penicillin as the free acid. A vehicle of aluminum hydroxide gel would serve to slow down the rate of hydrolysis and would also protect the penicillin against degradation in the stomach.

Combination Reactions

21

℞	Butyn sulfate	gr x
	Silver nitrate	gr i
	Distilled water qs ad	f℥ i
M. Ft. sol.		

The silver and sulfate ions will combine to form insoluble silver sulfate. Elimination of one of the compounds is necessary.

22

℞	Benzalkonium chloride	1:5000
	Amaranth solution to color	
M. Ft. sol. 30 ml		

Amaranth (a sodium salt) is an anionic dye and will combine with the cationic antibacterial agent to precipitate as well as inactivate it. Elimination of the amaranth solution is necessary.

References

1. Muldoon, H. C., ed, *Pharmaceutical Latin*, 4th ed, Wiley, New York, 1946.
2. Teplitsky, B., *Am. Profess. Pharmacist*, **34**, 30 (Apr., 1968).
3. Butler, A. M., and Richie, R. H., *New Engl. J. Med.*, **262**, 903 (1960).
4. Hirschorn, J. O., and Silverman, H. I., *Am. J. Pharm.*, **140**, 52 (1968).
5. Fuller, H. J., *Can. Pharm. J.*, **91**, 36 (1958).
6. Abrams, R. E., *Am. J. Pharm.*, **134**, 87 (1962).
7. Myers, M. J., *Am. J. Pharm.*, **139**, 7 (1967).
8. Martin, E. W., ed., *Husa's Pharmaceutical Dispensing*, 6th ed., Mack Publ. Co., Easton, Pa., 1966, p. 555.
9. Ellenhorn, M. J., and Sternad, F. A., *J. APhA*, **NS6**, 62 (1966).
10. Block, L. H., and Lamy, P. P., *J. APhA*, **NS8**, 66 (1968).
11. McIver, A. K., *Pharm. J.*, **199**, 205 (1967).
12. *Patient Care*, **1**, 32 (Nov., 1967).
13. Hartshorn, E. A., *Drug Intelligence*, **2**, 4 (1968).
14. *Ibid*, **2**, 58 (1968).
15. *Ibid*, **2**, 174 (1968). (Other articles are to follow in this series.)
16. Hussar, D. A., *Am. J. Pharm.*, **139**, 215 (1967).
17. Robinson, D. S., and MacDonald, M. G., *J. Pharmacol. Exptl. Therap.*, **153** 250 (1966).
18. Conney, A. H., *et al.*, *J. Pharmacol. Exptl. Therap.*, **130**, 1 (1960).
19. Kato, R., and Chiesara, E., *Brit. J. Pharmacol.*, **18**, 29 (1962).
20. Douglas, J. F., *et al*, *Proc. Soc. Exptl. Biol. Med.*, **112**, 436 (1963).

21. Beaser, S. B., *J. Am. Med. Assoc.*, **187**, 887 (1964).
22. Aggeler, P. M., *et al*, *New Engl. J. Med.*, **276**, 496 (1967).
23. Gibaldi, M., and Schwartz, M. A., *Clin. Pharmacol. Therap.*, **9**, 345 (1968).
24. Schrogie, J. J., and Solomon, H. M., *Clin. Pharmacol. Therap.*, **8**, 70 (1967).
25. Pascal, L. R., *et al*, *J. Lab. Clin. Med.*, **45**, 771 (1955).
26. Skeith, M. D., *et al*, *Clin. Pharmacol. Therap.*, **9**, 89 (1968).
27. Antlitz, A. M., *et al*, *Current Therap. Res.*, **10**, 501 (1968).
28. *Physicians' Desk Reference*, 22nd ed, Medical Economics, Inc., Oradell, N.J., 1967, p. 970.
29. Antlitz, A. M., *et al*, *Current Therap. Res.*, **10**, 70 (1968).
30. Cucinell, S. A., *et al*, *J. Pharmacol. Exptl. Therap.*, **141**, 157 (1963).
31. Busfield, D., *et al*, *Lancet*, **2**, 1042 (1963).
32. Cucinell, S. A., *et al*, *J. Am. Med. Assoc.*, **197**, 366 (1966).
33. Corn, M., *Thromb. Diath. Haemorrhag.*, **16**, 606 (1966).
34. Solomon, H. M., and Schrogie, J. J., *J. Pharmacol. Exptl. Therap.*, **154**, 660 (1966).
35. *The Medical Letter*, **9**, 97 (1967).
36. Dresdale, F. C., and Hayes, J. C., *J. Med. Soc. N.J.*, **64**, 609 (1967).
37. *Physicians' Desk Reference*, 22nd ed, Medical Economics, Inc., Oradell, N.J., 1967, p. 1204.
38. Pettinger, W. A., *et al*, *Clin. Res.*, **14**, 258 (1966).
39. Mitchell, J. R., *et al*, *J. Am. Med. Assoc.*, **202**, 973 (1967).
40. Gulati, O. D., *et al*, *Clin. Pharmacol. Therap.*, **7**, 510 (1966).
41. Christensen, L. K., *et al*, *Lancet*, **2**, 1298 (1963).
42. *Physicians' Desk Reference*, 22nd ed, Medical Economics, Inc., Oradell, N.J., 1967, p. 1180.
43. Brook, R., *et al*, *Clin. Pharmacol. Therap.*, **9**, 314 (1968).
44. Field, J. B., *et al*, *New Engl. J. Med.*, **277**, 889 (1967).
45. Kotler, M. N., *et al*, *Lancet*, **2**, 1389 (1966).
46. *Lancet*, **1**, 939 (1967).
47. *Physicians' Desk Reference*, 22nd ed, Medical Economics Inc., Oradell, N.J., 1967, p. 673.
48. Marcus, A., *Drug Cosmetic Ind.*, **79**, 456 (1956).
49. Ahsan, S. S., and Blaug, S. M., *Drug Std.*, **28**, 95 (1960).
50. Hurwitz, A. R., *et al*, *J. Pharm. Sci.*, **52**, 893 (1963).
51. Bolton, S., *J. Pharm. Sci.*, **52**, 1071 (1963).
52. James, K. C., *J. Pharm. Pharmacol.*, **10**, 363 (1958).
53. Miller, O. H., *J. APhA, Pract. Ed.*, **13**, 657 (1952).
54. Leuallen, E. E., *J. APhA, Pract. Ed.*, **10**, 722 (1949).
55. Krause, G. M., and Cross, J. M., *J. APhA, Sci. Ed.*, **40**, 137 (1951).
56. Peterson, C. F., and Hopponen, R. E., *J. APhA, Sci. Ed.*, **42**, 540 (1953).
57. Barr, M., and Tice, L. F., *Am. J. Pharm.*, **129**, 332 (1957).
58. Mascardo, L. B., and Barr, M., *JAPhA, Pract. Ed.*, **14**, 772 (1953).
59. Grill, F., *J. APhA*, **21**, 765 (1932).
60. Martin, E. W., ed, *Husa's Pharmaceutical Dispensing*, 6th ed, Mack Publ. Co., Easton, Pa., 1966, p. 556.

Appendix

Compilation of Drug Interactions

In using this table it should be recognized that even though two drugs are capable of interacting, they frequently may be given concurrently. Although there are situations where the use of one drug is specifically contraindicated while another is being given, there are many cases where one drug that is known to alter the response of a second agent can be given with it, as long as adequate precautions are taken (such as a change in the dose of one or both of the drugs). In some instances a second drug may be given deliberately to modify the effects of another, such as the administration of an antiparkinson agent to control the extrapyramidal effects caused by a phenothiazine, and several examples of this type are included in this table.

It should also be noted that some of the reports of drug interactions have been based on animal studies and others have resulted from observations of a limited number of humans. Therefore, it should be anticipated that some of these actions may not be clinically significant in many patients. However, an awareness of the potential for difficulty should be maintained.

In considering the interactions of a class of drugs, those that are characteristic of the entire class are listed first. Those additional interactions that are characteristic of an individual member of the drug class are then listed under the appropriate heading.

In compiling a table of this length it is inevitable that certain interactions that should be included will be overlooked. Therefore, it should not be assumed that this represents a complete listing of all interactions that have been reported in the literature.

Table IV—Drug Interactions

Drug	Comment
Analgesics	
Acetaminophen (Tylenol) with	
Oral anticoagulants	An increased response to the anticoagulant has been reported.
Carbamazepine (Tegretol) with	
Monoamine oxidase inhibitors	Since carbamazepine is structurally related to the tricyclic antidepressants, it should not be used with or for at least 1 week after discontinuing therapy with a MAO inhibitor.
Colchicine with	
Central nervous system depressants	Animal studies indicate an increased sensitivity to the depressants.
Sympathomimetics	Animal studies indicate that an enhanced response to sympathomimetic agents may result.
Vitamin B_{12}	Colchicine may interfere with the absorption of Vitamin B_{12} from the GIT; however, there has been no evidence of deficiency as a result of concurrent use.
Dipyrone (Narone, Pyrilgin) with	
Chlorpromazine (Thorazine)	Should not be used together; antipyretic effect is potentiated possibly resulting in severe hypothermia.

Drug	Comment
Indomethacin (Indocin) with	
Oral anticoagulants	Has been suggested that the anticoagulant response is enhanced due to displacement from protein binding sites.
Probenecid (Benemid)	Probenecid interferes with the renal excretion of indomethacin; the uricosuric action of probenecid is not blocked.
Methotrimeprazine (Levoprome) with (see also *Phenothiazines* under *Tranquilizers*)	
Analgesics (salicylates, narcotics)	Effects are additive; dose of one or both agents may have to be reduced.
Hypotensives	Concurrent use with methotrimeprazine is contraindicated.
Monoamine oxidase inhibitors	
Succinylcholine (Anectine)	Fall in blood pressure may occur and CNS effects may be aggravated.
Narcotic analgesics with	
Oral anticoagulants	Prolonged use of narcotics may enhance the anticoagulant effect.
Levallorphan (Lorfan)	
Nalorphine (Nalline)	Will reverse the respiratory depression produced by narcotic analgesics; however, they will not reverse respiratory depression caused by sedatives, hypnotics, anesthetics, etc.

Table IV—Continued

Drug	Comment	Drug	Comment
Monoamine oxidase inhibitors	Effects of the narcotic may be enhanced; dosage should be reduced.	*Chloroform* with Epinephrine Norepinephrine (Levophed)	Chloroform sensitizes the myocardium to the action of these agents; increased likelihood of ventricular tachycardia or fibrillation when used in combination.
Respiratory depressant drugs (anesthetics, barbiturates, phenothiazines, sedatives, hypnotics)	Enhanced respiratory depression may result; dosage of the narcotic should be reduced.		
Oxyphenbutazone (Tandearil) and *phenylbutazone* (Butazolidin) with		Propranolol (Inderal)	Propranolol should not be used to treat arrhythmias associated with the use of anesthetics that produce myocardial depression such as chloroform.
Oral anticoagulants	Anticoagulant response may be increased due to displacement from protein binding sites.	*Cyclopropane* and *halothane* (Fluothane) with Doxapram (Dopram)	Doxapram may cause an increase in epinephrine release to which the heart is more sensitive in the presence of these anesthetics.
Potent chemotherapeutic agents	Increased possibility of toxicity.		
Chloroquine (Aralen) Hydroxychloroquine (Plaquenil)	Phenylbutazone and other agents known to cause drug sensitization and dermatitis should not be given concurrently with chloroquine and hydroxychloroquine.	Epinephrine Norepinephrine (Levophed)	Cyclopropane and halothane sensitize the myocardium to the action of these agents; increased likelihood of ventricular tachycardia or fibrillation when used in combination.
Diphenylhydantoin (Dilantin)	Phenylbutazone has been reported to enhance the effect of diphenylhydantoin by inhibiting its metabolism.	Tubocurarine	Enhanced effect of tubocurarine; dosage should be reduced
Hypoglycemic agents (insulin, sulfonylureas)	Enhanced hypoglycemic effect; phenylbutazone has been reported to interfere with the excretion of the active metabolite of acetohexamide (Dymelor); protein displacement may also be involved.	*Ether* with Propranolol (Inderal)	Propranolol should not be used to treat arrhythmias associated with the use of anesthetics that produce myocardial depression such as ether.
Methandrostenolone (Dianabol)	Methandrostenolone has been shown to cause increased plasma levels of oxyphenbutazone.	Tubocurarine	Enhanced effect of tubocurarine; dosage should be reduced.
Salicylates	In treating arthritic patients combined use may increase danger of GIT ulceration.	*Fluroxene* (Fluoromar) with Tubocurarine	Enhanced effect of tubocurarine; dosage should be reduced.
Sulfonamides	Activity of the sulfonamide may be enhanced.	*Methoxyflurane* (Penthrane) with Tubocurarine	Enhanced effect of tubocurarine; dosage should be reduced.
Tricyclic antidepressants	A study in rats has indicated that imipramine (Tofranil) or desipramine (Pertofrane) may inhibit the intestinal absorption of phenylbutazone.	*Local anesthetics* with Central nervous system depressants Cardiovascular depressants	Effects of these drugs may be enhanced when used simultaneously with local anesthetics.
Phenyramidol (Analexin) with Oral anticoagulants Diphenylhydantoin (Dilantin) Sulfonylureas	Phenyramidol may enhance the effects of these agents due to inhibition of metabolism.	Vasoconstrictors Oxytocics	If hypotension occurs during obstetrical procedures (anesthetics can cause hypotension), the use of an oxytocic with a vasoconstrictor may result in severe persistent hypertension.
Propoxyphene (Darvon) with Analeptics (eg, amphetamine, caffeine and sodium benzoate)	Should not be used to treat propoxyphene overdosage since convulsions may be produced.	*Procaine* with Monoamine oxidase inhibitors Succinylcholine (Anectine)	Effects of procaine may be enhanced. Intravenous injections of procaine may potentiate the effect of succinylcholine.
Orphenadrine (Disipal, Norflex)	Mental confusion, anxiety, and tremors have been reported in patients receiving these agents concurrently.		
Salicylates with Urinary alkalinizers	Decreased effect of salicylate due to increased rate of excretion.	**Antianemics**	
Aminosalicylic Acid (PAS)	Increased danger of causing salicylate toxicity.	*Iron salts* with Allopurinol (Zyloprim)	Concurrent use should be avoided since an increase in hepatic iron concentration has been reported in animals.
Anticoagulants	May enhance anticoagulant effect especially if given in doses exceeding 1 Gm/day.	Ascorbic acid	Large doses of ascorbic acid have been claimed to improve the absorption of orally administered iron.
Corticosteroids	In treating arthritic patients combinations should be used cautiously because of the increased danger of GIT ulceration.	*Dextriferron* (Astrafer) and *iron sorbitex* (Jectofer) with Oral iron therapy	Patient's iron binding capacity may be exceeded resulting in iron toxicity.
Diphenylhydantoin (Dilantin)	Large doses of aspirin have been reported to enhance the effect of diphenylhydantoin.		
Methotrexate	Methotrexate may be displaced from albumin binding sites resulting in increased toxicity.	**Antiarrhythmics**	
Phenobarbital	Decreased effect of salicylates due to enzyme induction.	*Propranolol* (Inderal) with Alpha-adrenergic blocking agents	Should be used together in treating pheochromocytoma to avoid a serious rise in blood pressure.
Phenylbutazone (Butazolidin)	In treating arthritic patients combined use may increase danger of GIT ulceration.	Chloroform Ether	Propranolol should not be used to treat arrhythmias associated with the use of anesthetics, such as chloroform and ether, that produce myocardial depression.
Probenecid (Benemid) Sulfinpyrazone (Anturane)	Salicylates can antagonize the uricosuric activity of these agents.		
Sulfonylureas	Hypoglycemic response may be enhanced due, in part, to displacement of sulfonylurea from protein binding sites.	Hypoglycemics	May cause hypoglycemia; potential danger may be increased because propranolol may prevent the premonitory signs and symptoms of acute hypoglycemia.
Anesthetics		Isosorbide dinitrate (Isordil)	Synergistic effects in treating angina pectoris have been reported; however, the potential benefit of using this combination has been disputed.
General anesthetics with Hypotensive agents and other agents that can lower blood pressure (rauwolfia, alkaloids, phenothiazines, MAO inhibitors, etc)	Hypotensive effect may be enhanced.	Monoamine oxidase inhibitors	Propranolol should not be used concurrently or during the two week withdrawal period from MAO inhibitors.
Kanamycin (Kantrex) Neomycin Streptomycin	These antibiotics could cause neuromuscular paralysis with respiratory depression when given intraperitoneally to patients who have been given anesthetics.	Reserpine (Serpasil, etc)	Added catecholamine blocking action may cause an excessive reduction of the resting sympathetic nervous activity.

Table IV—Continued

Drug	Comment	Drug	Comment
Quinidine with Anticoagulants	Quinidine may depress prothrombin formation in the liver and enhance anticoagulant effect.	Mineral oil	Variable alterations of the anticoagulant effect have occurred on rare occasions.
Muscle relaxants [decamethonium (Syncurine), succinylcholine (Anectine), tubocurarine]	Potentiation of muscle relaxants may occur.	Monoamine oxidase inhibitors	Have been reported to enhance the effects of the indandione anticoagulants.
Rauwolfia alkaloids	Combination should be used cautiously since cardiac arrhythmias may occur.	Narcotics	Prolonged use of narcotics may enhance the anticoagulant effect.
Veratrum alkaloids	Caution should be observed when used together.	Norethandrolone (Nilevar)	May cause an enhanced anticoagulant effect.
		Oral contraceptives	May cause a decreased anticoagulant effect; larger doses of the anticoagulant may be needed.

Anticholinergics

Drug	Comment	Drug	Comment
Anticholinergics with Antihistamines Phenothiazines Tricyclic antidepressants	These agents possess some anticholinergic activity and thus may enhance the anticholinergic effect.	Oxyphenbutazone (Tandearil) Phenylbutazone (Butazolidin)	Anticoagulant response may be increased due to displacement from protein binding sites.
Neostigmine (Prostigmin)	Anticholinergics may slow the intestinal motility and alter the absorption of orally administered neostigmine.	Phenyramidol (Analexin)	Enhances the effect of anticoagulants by inhibiting their metabolism.
		Propylthiouracil	May enhance the anticoagulant effect.
		Proteolytic enzymes extracted from Carica papaya (Papase)	Concurrent use with anticoagulants is contraindicated.

Anticoagulants

Drug	Comment	Drug	Comment
Oral anticoagulants[a] with Barbiturates Chloral hydrate Glutethimide (Doriden) Griseofulvin (Fulvicin, Grifulvin) Meprobamate	These agents can cause enzyme induction resulting in a more rapid metabolism of the anticoagulant; larger doses of the anticoagulant may be required.	Quinidine Quinine	May depress prothrombin formation in liver and enhance anticoagulant effect.
Acetaminophen (Tylenol)	An increased response to the anticoagulant has been reported.	Salicylates	May enhance anticoagulant effect especially if given in doses exceeding 1 Gm/day.
Alcohol	May cause an alteration in the anticoagulant effect but the response is unpredictable.	Sulfonamides	Can enhance the anticoagulant effect; probably due, in part, to interference with the synthesis of Vitamin K by microorganisms in the gastrointestinal tract and protein displacement.
Anesthetics	May enhance anticoagulant effect.		
Antacids	Large doses may decrease the anticoagulant effect by inhibiting absorption.	Tolbutamide (Orinase)	Hypoglycemic effect of tolbutamide can be potentiated due to inhibition of metabolism.
Antibiotics (chloramphenicol, neomycin, tetracyclines)	Enhance the effect of anticoagulants; effect develops in part, due to interference with the synthesis of Vitamin K by microorganisms in the gastrointestinal tract.	Vitamin K	Will antagonize the anticoagulant effect.
Antihistamines	Have been reported to cause a decreased anticoagulant effect.	Xanthines	Large doses may cause an alteration of the anticoagulant effect.
Bromelains (Ananase)	May enhance the anticoagulant effect.		
Chlordiazepoxide (Librium)	Variable alterations in the anticoagulant response have been reported.		

Anticonvulsants

Drug	Comment	Drug	Comment
Chlorpropamide (Diabinese)	Anticoagulants may enhance the effect of chlorpropamide.	*Anticonvulsants* with Diazepam (Valium)	When diazepam is used as an adjunct in treating convulsive disorders, an increase in the dose of standard anticonvulsant medication may be necessary.
Cholestyramine (Cuemid, Questran)	May decrease the effect of anticoagulants by inhibiting or delaying absorption; however, Vitamin K absorption may also be decreased; it is recommended that the anticoagulant be administered at least one hour before cholestyramine.	Haloperidol (Haldol)	The dose of the anticonvulsant should not be altered when haloperidol therapy is initiated; however, subsequent adjustment may be necessary.
Chymotrypsin-trypsin (Chymoral)	Caution should be observed when using concomitantly.	Monoamine oxidase inhibitors	The influence of MAO inhibitors on the convulsive threshold is variable; the dosage of anticonvulsants may have to be altered.
Clofibrate (Atromid-S)	Increased anticoagulant response; a reduction of the anticoagulant dose (by 1/3 to 1/2) may be necessary when clofibrate therapy is initiated.	Phenothiazines Rauwolfia alkaloids Thioxanthenes	These agents can lower the convulsive threshold in susceptible individuals; an increase in the dosage of the anticonvulsant may be necessary.
Corticosteroids Corticotropin (ACTH)	May cause an alteration in the anticoagulant response.	Tricyclic antidepressants	High doses of a tricyclic may precipitate seizures; dosage of the anticonvulsant may have to be changed.
Dextrothyroxine (Choloxin)	Enhances the effect of anticoagulants, possibly by increasing affinity for the receptor site; dose of anticoagulant should be reduced by 1/3 when dextrothyroxine therapy is initiated, and then subsequently adjusted as necessary.	*Barbiturate anticonvulsants* [metharbital (Gemonil), mephobarbital (Mebaral), phenobarbital] with Anticoagulants	Barbiturates may cause enzyme induction resulting in a more rapid metabolism of the anticoagulant.
Diphenylhydantoin (Dilantin)	May enhance the effect of anticoagulants by causing displacement from protein binding sites; anticoagulant can increase serum levels of diphenylhydantoin, possibly leading to toxicity of the latter.	Haloperidol (Haldol) Phenothiazines	Although these agents will potentiate the depressant effect of the barbiturates, the anticonvulsant action is not potentiated.
Disulfiram (Antabuse)	May cause an enhanced anticoagulant effect.	Each other	When two barbiturates are used concurrently the dose should be about 1/2 the amount of each used alone.
Ethchlorvynol (Placidyl)	Has been reported to decrease the anticoagulant response, probably by enzyme induction.	*Diphenylhydantoin* (Dilantin) with Aminosalicylic acid (PAS)	When given concurrently with isoniazid (INH) there has been an inhibition of metabolism of diphenylhydantoin.
Haloperidol (Haldol)	Has been reported to antagonize the anticoagulant effect of phenindione.	Anticoagulants	Bishydroxycoumarin (Dicumarol) has been reported to increase the effects of diphenylhydantoin by inhibiting its metabolism; the anticoagulant effect may also be increased.
Heparin	Increased anticoagulant effect.		
Indomethacin (Indocin)	Has been suggested that the anticoagulant response is enhanced due to displacement from protein binding sites.	Corticosteroids	Diphenylhydantoin has been shown to stimulate the metabolism of hydrocortisone by enzyme induction.
Methandrostenolone (Dianabol)	May cause an enhanced anticoagulant effect.	Disulfiram (Antabuse) Isoniazid (INH) Phenylbutazone (Butazolidin) Phenyramidol (Analexin) Sulfaphenazole (Sulfabid)	May enhance the effect of diphenylhydantoin by inhibiting its metabolism.
Methylphenidate (Ritalin)	An enhanced anticoagulant effect may occur due to inhibition of metabolism.		

Table IV—Continued

Drug	Comment	Drug	Comment
Methylphenidate (Ritalin)	A recent report has indicated that methylphenidate can increase the blood levels of diphenylhydantoin.	Hypoglycemics	An enhanced hypoglycemic effect may result.
Phenobarbital	Can decrease the effect of diphenylhydantoin by increasing its rate of metabolism (enzyme induction); is usually not of clinical significance because phenobarbital also has anticonvulsant activity.	Hypotensives	Enhanced response can occur and may result in hypotension.
		Methotrimeprazine (Levoprome)	Concurrent use is contraindicated.
Salicylates	Large doses of aspirin have been reported to enhance the effect of diphenylhydantoin.	Methyldopa (Aldomet)	Headache, hypertension and related symptoms may develop; combined use should be avoided.
Ethotoin (Peganone) with Phenacemide (Phenurone)	Caution is advised since paranoid symptoms have been reported during therapy with this combination.	Methylphenidate (Ritalin)	Combination should be used cautiously.
		Narcotics	Effects of the narcotic may be potentiated; dosage should be reduced.
Phenacemide (Phenurone) with Ethotoin (Peganone)	Paranoid symptoms have been reported.	Other monoamine oxidase inhibitors	Two MAO inhibitors should not be given simultaneously; it is recommended that two weeks should elapse between the discontinuation of therapy with the one and initiation of therapy with the other.
Other anticonvulsants	Special caution is advised in patients with a history of allergy.		
		Phenothiazines	Additive hypotensive effects may be experienced.
Antidepressants		Procaine	Effects of procaine may be enhanced.
		Propranolol (Inderal)	Propranolol should not be used concurrently or during the 2-week withdrawal period from MAO inhibitors.
Monoamine oxidase inhibitors [isocarboxazid (Marplan), nialamide (Niamid), phenelzine (Nardil), tranylcypromine (Parnate), pargyline[b] (Eutonyl), and furazolidone[c] (Furoxone)] with		Rauwolfia alkaloids	MAO inhibitors inhibit the destruction of serotonin which may be released from tissue stores by Rauwolfia alkaloids; reserpine should not be administered parenterally during, or for 1 week following, treatment with pargyline.
Alcohol	Effects of alcohol may be potentiated; alcoholic beverages should be avoided; disulfiram-like reactions have been reported with furazolidone.	Sympathomimetics (including amphetamine, ephedrine, phenylephrine, phenylpropanolamine)	Concurrent use has resulted in severe hypertensive reactions; should not be used simultaneously.
Amphetamine and derivatives	Combined use could result in hypertensive crisis; simultaneous use should be avoided.	Tricyclic antidepressants	Tricyclics should not be given with or for at least 2 weeks after discontinuing therapy with a MAO inhibitor; combined use may produce severe atropine-like reactions, tremors, convulsions, and delirium.
Anesthetics	MAO inhibitors may enhance the hypotensive effect of anesthetic agents; they should be discontinued prior to surgery.		
Anticonvulsants	The influence of MAO inhibitors on the convulsive threshold is variable; the dosage of anticonvulsants may have to be altered.	*Tricyclic antidepressants* [amitriptyline (Elavil), desipramine (Pertofrane), imipramine (Tofranil), nortriptyline (Aventyl), and protriptyline (Vivactil)] with	
Antihistamines	Response to the antihistamine may be exaggerated.	Alcohol	Effects of alcohol and the tricyclic may be enhanced.
Antiparkinson agents	Caution is advised since severe reactions have been reported following simultaneous use.	Anticholinergics Antiparkinson agents	Since the tricyclics possess weak anticholinergic activity this effect may be enhanced.
Barbiturates	Effects of barbiturates may be enhanced; dosage should be reduced.	Anticonvulsants	High doses of a tricyclic may precipitate seizures; dosage of the anticonvulsant may have to be changed.
Caffeine	Dosage of caffeine-containing medications should be reduced and beverages containing caffeine should be used in moderation; excessive amounts of caffeine can cause hypertensive reactions.	Barbiturates (and other CNS depressants)	Studies in animals indicate that the tricyclics can potentiate the effect of barbiturates.
		Ethchlorvynol (Placidyl)	Transient delirium has been reported with the combination of amitriptyline and ethchlorvynol.
Carbamazepine (Tegretol)	Since this agent is structurally related to the tricyclic antidepressants, its concurrent use with the MAO inhibitors is not recommended.	Guanethidine (Ismelin)	Antihypertensive effect of guanethidine may be antagonized.
Central nervous system depressants [alcohol, barbiturates, chloral hydrate, ethchlorvynol (Placidyl), sedatives, hypnotics, tranquilizers, etc]	An enhanced depressant effect may result; dosage of the depressant should be reduced.	Hypotensive Agents (eg, thiazide diuretics, phenothiazines, vasodilators)	Since the tricyclics may cause orthostatic hypotension caution should be observed when other agents that lower the blood pressure are given concomitantly.
Cocaine	Effects of cocaine may be enhanced.	Methyldopa (Aldomet)	Decreased hypotensive effect.
Diuretics (eg, thiazides)	Hypotension may result; it should be noted that pargyline and methyclothiazide are used in combination (Eutron) for the enhanced antihypertensive effect.	Methylphenidate (Ritalin)	A recent report indicates that methylphenidate may impair the metabolism of imipramine and desipramine.
Doxapram (Dopram)	An enhanced pressor effect may occur.	Monoamine oxidase inhibitors	Tricyclics should not be given with or for at least 2 weeks after discontinuing therapy with a MAO inhibitor; combined use may produce severe atropine-like reactions, tremors, convulsions, delirium.
Ephedrine and derivatives	Simultaneous use should be avoided; hypertension and related symptoms could develop.		
Ethamivan (Emivan)	An additive stimulant effect may result.	Norepinephrine (Levophed)	Tricyclics may increase the pressor effect of norepinephrine.
Foods containing high concentrations of pressor substances such as tyramine (strong or aged cheese, wines, pickled herring, chicken livers, canned figs, yeast extract, pods of broad beans)	Pressor effects may be enhanced and hypertensive crisis could result.	Phenothiazines	Tricyclics and phenothiazines are frequently used in combination (Etrafon, Triavil) in treating agitated forms of depression.
		Phenylbutazone (Butazolidin)	A study in rats has indicated that imipramine or desipramine may inhibit the intestinal absorption of phenylbutazone.
Ganglionic blocking agents	Pargyline should not be used in combination because it will potentiate the effect of these agents.	Reserpine (Serpasil, etc)	Tricyclics may block or reverse the depressive effect of reserpine.
Guanethidine (Ismelin)	Guanethidine should not be given with or for at least one week after discontinuing therapy with a MAO inhibitor.	Sympathomimetics	Enhanced activity of either the tricyclic or sympathomimetic agent may result.
		Thyroid medications	Enhanced activity of either agent may result.

Table IV—Continued

Drug	Comment	Drug	Comment
Antihistamines		Lincomycin (Lincocin)	Antagonism between erythromycin and lincomycin *in vitro* has been reported.
Antihistamines with Oral anticoagulants	Antihistamines may cause a decreased anticoagulant effect.	Probenecid (Benemid)	Probenecid has been shown to inhibit tubular reabsorption of erythromycin in animals.
Anticholinergics	Since many antihistamines possess anticholinergic activity, this effect may be enhanced.	*Griseofulvin* (Fulvicin, Grifulvin, Grisactin) with Oral anticoagulants	Griseofulvin can cause enzyme induction resulting in a more rapid metabolism of the anticoagulant; larger doses of the anticoagulant may be required.
Betahistine (Serc)	Betahistine is a histamine-like agent and concurrent use with antihistamines is not recommended.		
Central nervous system depressants (alcohol, sedatives, hypnotics, narcotics, tranquilizers, etc)	Enhanced sedative effect.	Barbiturates	Phenobarbital has been shown to decrease the effect of griseofulvin due to enzyme induction.
Monoamine oxidase inhibitors	MAO inhibitors may enhance the antihistaminic effect due to inhibition of metabolism.	*Kanamycin* (Kantrex), *neomycin, and streptomycin* with Anesthetics Muscle relaxants	Neuromuscular paralysis with respiratory depression may occur when these antibiotics are administered intraperitoneally concurrently with anesthetics or muscle-relaxing drugs; they should not be administered until the patient has fully recovered from the effects of the anesthetic or muscle relaxant.
Chlorcyclizine (in Fedrazil) and *diphenhydramine* (Benadryl) with Barbiturates	Chlorcyclizine and diphenhydramine and probably other antihistamines can cause enzyme induction which may decrease the activity of the barbiturate; however, sedative effect may be initially enhanced.		
Corticosteroids (and possibly other drugs that are metabolized by liver microsomal enzymes)	Decreased effect of steroids due to enzyme induction.	Urinary Alkalinizers	An alkaline urinary pH enhances urinary antibacterial activity; alkalinization is probably only necessary when streptomycin is used to treat urinary tract infections.
Dimenhydrinate (Dramamine) with Kanamycin (Kantrex) Neomycin Streptomycin	Dimenhydrinate may mask ototoxic symptoms caused by these antibiotics.	Dimenhydrinate (Dramamine)	Dimenhydrinate may mask ototoxic symptoms caused by these antibiotics.
Phenothiazine antihistamines—see *Phenothiazines* under *Tranquilizers*		Each other	Possibility of cumulative ototoxic effects exists when these drugs are given concurrently or in series.
Anti-infectives		*Lincomycin* (Lincocin) with Cyclamate-containing beverages Kaopectate	These agents have been shown to markedly reduce the absorption of lincomycin from the gastrointestinal tract; it is recommended that nothing be given by mouth except water for a period of 1 or 2 hours before and after oral administration of lincomycin.
Anthelmintics			
Piperazine (Antepar) with Phenothiazines	Possible exaggeration of extrapyramidal effects.		
Tetrachloroethylene with Alcohol	Tetrachloroethylene can cause symptoms of inebriation; alcohol may enhance these effects and should not be ingested 24 hours before or after its use.	Erythromycin (Erythrocin, Ilosone)	Antagonism between erythromycin and lincomycin *in vitro* has been reported.
		Penicillins with Bacteriostatic antibacterials (chloramphenicol, sulfonamides, tetracyclines, etc)	Penicillins are bactericidal and only effective against multiplying bacteria; bacteriostatic antibiotics may inhibit their antibacterial effect.
Antibiotics		Dactinomycin (Cosmegen)	*In vitro* studies indicate that the bactericidal action of penicillin G can be antagonized.
Amphotericin B (Fungizone) with Antibiotics Antimetabolites Corticosteroids Mechlorethamine (Mustargen)	Deep fungal infections sometimes emerge in patients being treated with these agents; they should not be given concurrently with amphotericin B unless absolutely necessary to control reactions to amphotericin B or to treat underlying disease.	Probenecid (Benemid)	Probenecid can enhance the effects of penicillin derivatives by interfering with their tubular excretion and decreasing their volume of distribution.
Chloramphenicol (Chloromycetin) with Penicillins	Chloramphenicol is bacteriostatic whereas the penicillins are bactericidal; since the penicillins are only effective against multiplying bacteria, chloramphenicol may inhibit their antibacterial effect.	*Tetracyclines* with Anticoagulants	Enhance the effect of anticoagulants; effect develops, in part, due to interference with the synthesis of Vitamin K by microorganisms in the GIT.
Other drugs that may cause bone marrow depression	Concurrent use should be avoided	Cations (di- and trivalent such as Ca^{+2}, Mg^{+2}, and Al^{+3}) Antacids Milk	These cations can combine with the tetracyclines in the GIT to form complexes that are not readily absorbed; it is claimed that the absorption of doxycycline (Vibramycin) is not markedly influenced by the simultaneous ingestion of milk.
Phenobarbital	Animal studies indicate that pretreatment with phenobarbital can reduce blood levels and chemotherapeutic activity of chloramphenicol.	Hepatotoxic drugs	Tetracyclines have been known to cause hepatotoxicity; if they are given IV, other potentially hepatotoxic drugs should be avoided if possible.
Colistimethate (Coly-Mycin M) and *polymyxin B* (Aerosporin) with Muscle relaxants Kanamycin (Kantrex) Neomycin Streptomycin Dihydrostreptomycin	These agents can interfere with nerve transmission at the neuromuscular junction; since colistimethate and polymyxin B can also cause this effect they should be used only with great caution since increased interference of transmission may occur, resulting in muscle weakness and apnea.	Penicillins	Penicillins are bactericidal and are only effective against multiplying bacteria; the tetracyclines are bacteriostatic and may inhibit the bactericidal effect of the penicillins.
		Antimalarials	
		Chloroquine (Aralen) and *hydroxychloroquine* (Plaquenil) with Hepatotoxic drugs	Chloroquine is known to concentrate in the liver and should be used with caution when hepatotoxic drugs are given.
Erythromycin (Erythrocin, Ilosone) with Urinary alkalinizers	Antibacterial activity is enhanced when the urinary pH is more alkaline.	Phenylbutazone (Butazolidin) Gold	Phenylbutazone, gold and other agents known to cause drug sensitization and dermatitis should not be given concurrently with chloroquine or hydroxychloroquine.

Table IV—Continued

Drug	Comment	Drug	Comment
Primaquine with Quinacrine (Atabrine)	Primaquine should not be given simultaneously with or to patients who have received quinacrine recently since the toxicity may be increased.	Methotrexate	Sulfonamides may displace methotrexate from albumin binding sites; increased toxicity of methotrexate may result.
Quinine with Anticoagulants	Quinine may depress prothrombin formation in the liver and enhance the anticoagulant effect.	Penicillins	Sulfonamides are bacteriostatic whereas the penicillins are bactericidal; the penicillins are only effective against multiplying bacteria and thus the sulfonamides may inhibit rather than enhance their antibacterial effect.

Antituberculars

		Oxyphenbutazone (Tandearil) Phenylbutazone (Butazolidin)	Activity of the sulfonamides may be increased due to displacement from protein binding sites.
Antituberculars with Corticosteroids	Corticosteroids are usually contraindicated in patients with tuberculosis; however, the concurrent administration with antitubercular agents may be lifesaving in certain cases.	Probenecid (Benemid)	Probenecid increases total sulfa plasma levels.
		Sulfinpyrazone (Anturane)	Effect of the sulfonamides may be enhanced.
Each other	It is recommended that several antitubercular agents be used in combination to improve effectiveness of therapy and to reduce the possibility of bacterial resistance developing.	Sulfonylureas	Hypoglycemic response may be enhanced, possibly due to displacement from protein binding sites; the most conclusive studies have involved the use of sulfaphenazole (Sulfabid) and tolbutamide (Orinase).
Aminosalicylic acid (PAS) with Diphenylhydantoin (Dilantin)	Metabolism of diphenylhydantoin has been inhibited when PAS has been given in combination with isoniazid.		

Miscellaneous Anti-infective Agents

		Furazolidone—see *Monoamine oxidase inhibitors* under *Antidepressants*	
Isoniazid (INH)	PAS may increase and prolong the blood levels of isoniazid.	*Methenamine* (Mandelamine, Hiprex) with Urinary alkalinizers	An acidic urine is necessary for methenamine to liberate formaldehyde and be effective; alkalinization of the urine will decrease its effectiveness.
Probenecid (Benemid)	Probenecid decreases urinary excretion of PAS resulting in increased plasma levels.		
Salicylates	Increased danger of causing salicylate toxicity.	Sulfonamides	The sulfonamides are less soluble in an acid urine that is necessary for methenamine to be effective; crystalluria may result with certain of the sulfonamides.
Isoniazid (INH) with Aminosalicylic Acid (PAS)	PAS may increase and prolong the blood levels of isoniazid.		
Diphenylhydantoin (Dilantin)	Effect of diphenylhydantoin may be enhanced due to inhibition of metabolism.	*Metronidazole* (Flagyl) with Alcohol	Disulfiram-like reactions have been reported following the ingestion of alcohol.

Antivirals

		Disulfiram (Antabuse)	Combined use has led to the development of acute psychoses or confusional states.
Amantadine (Symmetrel) with CNS stimulants Psychopharmacologic agents	Since amantadine may exhibit CNS and psychic side effects, these agents should be used cautiously in combination.		

Antiseptics

		Acrisorcin (Akrinol) with Soap	Soap should be completely removed from area of application since it can considerably reduce the activity of acrisorcin.
Idoxuridine (Stoxil) with Boric acid	Boric acid may cause irritation in the presence of idoxuridine and should not be administered during the course of therapy with the latter.		
Corticosteroids	Corticosteroids can accelerate the spread of a viral infection; they should not be used in combination with idoxuridine unless absolutely necessary.	*Boric acid* with Idoxuridine (Stoxil)	Boric acid may cause irritation in the presence of idoxuridine and should not be administered during the course of therapy with the latter.

Sulfonamides

		Quaternary ammonium antiseptics with Anionic agents Soap	Anionic agents and soap are incompatible with the cationic quaternary ammonium compounds.
Sulfonamides with Urinary alkalinizers	With some of the older sulfonamides (sulfadiazine, etc.) it was necessary to alkalinize the urine to prevent crystalluria; since the sulfonamides are weak acids, alkalinization of the urine will increase the rate of excretion and possibly decrease the effectiveness of the drug.		

Antilipemics

		Clofibrate (Atromid-S) with Oral anticoagulants	Increased anticoagulant response; a reduction of the anticoagulant dose (by $\frac{1}{3}$ to $\frac{1}{2}$) may be necessary when clofibrate therapy is initiated.
Aminobenzoic Acid (PABA)	Sulfonamides are effective antibacterials because they compete with PABA and prevent its normal utilization by microorganisms; an increased concentration of PABA will decrease the activity of the sulfonamides. It is possible that certain local anesthetics that have a PABA nucleus will exhibit the same effect.	Sulfonylureas	Caution should be observed in giving clofibrate to diabetic patients since there has been one report of an enhanced hypoglycemic effect in a patient taking tolbutamide (Orinase).
Antacids	Absorption of the sulfonamides from the GIT may be reduced.	*Dextrothyroxine* (Choloxin) with Oral anticoagulants	Enhances the effect of anticoagulants, possibly by increasing affinity for the receptor site; dose of anticoagulant should be reduced by $\frac{1}{3}$ when dextrothyroxine therapy is initiated, and then subsequently adjusted as necessary.
Oral anticoagulants	Anticoagulant effect may be enhanced; probably due, in part, to protein displacement and to interference with the synthesis of Vitamin K by microorganisms in the GIT.		
Diphenylhydantoin (Dilantin)	Sulfaphenazole has been reported to enhance the effect of diphenylhydantoin by inhibiting its metabolism.	Epinephrine	Injections of epinephrine in patients with coronary heart disease may precipitate an episode of coronary insufficiency. The likelihood of this occurring may be increased in patients taking dextrothyroxine.
Methenamine (Mandelamine, Hiprex)	For methenamine to be effective the urine must be acidic; the sulfonamides are less soluble in an acid urine and crystalluria may result.		

Table IV—Continued

Drug	Comment	Drug	Comment
Hypoglycemics	Dextrothyroxine can cause an increase in blood glucose levels; increased doses of the hypoglycemic agents may be necessary.	*Methylphenidate* (Ritalin) with Anticoagulants	An enhanced anticoagulant effect may occur due to inhibition of metabolism.
Thyroid preparations	Dosage of other thyroid preparations may have to be altered.	Diphenylhydantoin (Dilantin)	Methylphenidate may increase the blood levels of diphenylhydantoin.
		Guanethidine (Ismelin)	Hypotensive effect of guanethidine may be decreased.

Antineoplastics

		Monoamine oxidase inhibitors Pressor agents	Combination should be used cautiously. Pressor response may be enhanced.
Antineoplastics with Other drugs that can cause bone marrow depression	Excessive bone marrow depression may result; some antineoplastics are used in combination but with others concurrent use with a second agent is contraindicated.	Tricyclic antidepressants	Methylphenidate has been reported to impair the metabolism of imipramine (Tofranil) and desipramine (Pertofrane).

Digitalis Glycosides

Azathioprine (Imuran) with Allopurinol (Zyloprim)	Allopurinol inhibits the metabolism of azathioprine; dose of the latter should be reduced to ⅓ to ¼ of the usual dose.	*Digitalis glycosides* with Calcium salts (parenterally)	Elevated calcium levels can result in an increased sensitivity of the heart to digitalis.
Cyclophosphamide (Cytoxan) with Chloramphenicol (Chloromycetin)	Animal studies indicate that chloramphenicol pretreatment can reduce the lethality of cyclophosphamide; effect is apparently due to an inhibition of microsomal enzymes which are responsible for the *in vivo* activation of cyclophosphamide.	Diuretics [thiazides, furosemide (Lasix), ethacrynic acid (Edecrin), etc]	Diuretics can cause hypokalemia; if the potassium loss is not corrected the heart becomes more sensitive to the effects of digitalis, possibly resulting in digitalis toxicity.
Corticosteroids	Animal studies suggest that the activation of cyclophosphamide can be inhibited by prednisolone.	Guanethidine (Ismelin) Isoproterenol (Isuprel)	Both drugs decrease the heart rate. Isoproterenol is contraindicated in patients with tachycardia caused by digitalis intoxication.
Dactinomycin (Cosmegen) with Penicillin G	*In vitro* studies indicate that the bactericidal action of penicillin G can be antagonized.	Potassium salts Spironolactone (Aldactone) Triamterene (Dyrenium)	Spironolactone and triamterene are potassium-conserving diuretics; hyperkalemia may result leading to a decreased effectiveness of digitalis.
Mercaptopurine (Purinethol) with Allopurinol (Zyloprim)	Allopurinol inhibits the metabolism of mercaptopurine; dose of the latter should be reduced to ⅓ to ¼ of the usual dose.	Rauwolfia derivatives Veratrum alkaloids	Cardiac arrhythmias are more likely to occur in patients receiving digitalis concurrently.

Diuretics

Methotrexate with Aminobenzoic acid (PABA) Salicylates Sulfonamides (Antibacterial, diuretic, or hypoglycemic)	These agents may displace methotrexate from albumin binding sites; increased toxicity of methotrexate may result.	*Thiazides, chlorthalidone* (Hygroton), *ethacrynic acid* (Edecrin), *furosemide* (Lasix), and *quinethazone* (Hydromox) with Alcohol	Orthostatic hypotension may be potentiated.
Leucovorin	Will antagonize the effects of methotrexate and can be used as an antidote for overdosage.	Ammonium chloride	Ammonium chloride should not be used to correct hypochloremic alkalosis (caused by the diuretic) in patients with hepatic insufficiency.
Thiotepa with Chloramphenicol (Chloromycetin) Sulfonamides	Increased depression of the bone marrow may result.	Barbiturates	Orthostatic hypotension may be potentiated.
		Corticosteroids Corticotropin (ACTH)	Excessive potassium depletion may occur since these agents and the diuretics can cause hypokalemia.

Antitussives

Chlophedianol (Ulo) with Central nervous system depressants or stimulants	Chlophedianol is a centrally acting drug and should be used cautiously with other such agents.	Digitalis	Diuretics can cause hypokalemia; if the potassium loss is not corrected the heart can become more sensitive to the effects of digitalis, possibly resulting in digitalis toxicity.
Pipazethate (Theratuss) with Barbiturates	Pipazethate is chemically related to the phenothiazines; possibility of enhancing barbiturate activity exists.	Hypoglycemics	Diuretics can cause an increase in blood glucose levels; increased doses of the hypoglycemic agents may be necessary.
		Hypotensives	Enhanced hypotensive effect; diuretic will frequently permit a reduction in dosage of the hypotensive agent.

Bronchodilators

Xanthine preparations (Choledyl, Elixophyllin, Quibron, etc) with Oral anticoagulants	Large doses of xanthine derivatives may cause an alteration of the anticoagulant effect.	Monoamine oxidase inhibitors	Hypotension may result; it should be noted that pargyline and methyclothiazide are used in combination (Eutron) for the enhanced hypotensive effect.
Other xanthine preparations Sympathomimetics	Excessive CNS stimulation may occur.	Narcotics	Orthostatic hypotension may be potentiated.
		Norepinephrine (Levophed)	Arterial responsiveness to norepinephrine may be decreased.

Central Nervous System Stimulants

CNS stimulants with Amantadine (Symmetrel)	Amantadine may exhibit CNS side effects and should be used cautiously in combination.	Potassium salts	Potassium salts are frequently given to correct diuretic-induced hypokalemia; the use of enteric-coated dosage forms of potassium salts should be avoided, if possible, since ulceration of the small intestine may occur.
Doxapram (Dopram) with Monoamine oxidase inhibitors Sympathomimetics	These agents should be used cautiously with doxapram since an enhanced pressor effect may occur.	Spironolactone (Aldactone) Triamterene (Dyrenium)	Triamterene and spironolactone are potassium-conserving diuretics and may be combined with other diuretics (eg, thiazides) to reduce potassium loss and to enhance the diuretic effect.
Cyclopropane Halothane (Fluothane)	Doxapram may cause an increase in epinephrine release; since these anesthetics may sensitize the myocardium to catecholamines, the administration of doxapram should be delayed until the anesthetic is discontinued.	Tubocurarine	Diuretics may enhance the effect of tubocurarine.
Ethamivan (Emivan) with Monoamine oxidase inhibitors	An additive stimulant effect may result.	Uricosuric agents	Diuretics decrease the renal excretion of uric acid; higher does of uricosuric agents may be required.

Table IV—Continued

Drug	Comment	Drug	Comment
Mercurial diuretics with Ammonium chloride	Mercurial diuretics may cause hypochloremic alkalosis resulting in a reduced effectiveness of the diuretic; the administration of ammonium chloride may restore responsiveness to the mercurial.	Oral anticoagulants	May cause an enhanced anticoagulant effect.
		Oxyphenbutazone (Tandearil)	Increased plasma levels of oxyphenbutazone have resulted.
		Norethandrolone (Nilevar) with Oral anticoagulants	May cause an enhanced anticoagulant effect.
Spironolactone (Aldactone) and *triamterene* (Dyrenium) with Other diuretics	Spironolactone and triamterene are frequently combined with a thiazide diuretic to reduce potassium loss and to enhance the diuretic effect.	*Testosterone* with Phenobarbital	Effect of testosterone may be decreased due to enzyme induction.
Hypotensive agents Each other	Enhanced hypotensive effect. Hyperkalemia may result.		

Corticosteroids

Drug	Comment
Corticosteroids with Antacids	Corticosteroids may cause hyperacidity or peptic ulcer; antacids should be given as a prophylactic measure during prolonged therapy.
Oral anticoagulants	May cause an alteration in the anticoagulant response.
Antitubercular agents	Corticosteroids are usually contraindicated in patients with tuberculosis; however, the concurrent administration with antitubercular agents may be life saving in certain cases.
Barbiturates	Effect of corticosteroids may be decreased due to enzyme induction.
Diphenylhydantoin (Dilantin)	Diphenylhydantoin has been shown to stimulate the metabolism of hydrocortisone by enzyme induction.
Diuretics	Excessive potassium depletion may occur since both the corticosteroids and diuretics can cause hypokalemia.
Hypoglycemics	Corticosteroids can cause an increase in blood glucose levels; increased dosage of the hypoglycemic agents may be necessary.
Idoxuridine (Stoxil)	Corticosteroids can accelerate the spread of a viral infection; they should not be used in combination with idoxuridine unless absolutely necessary.
Salicylates	In treating arthritic patients combination should be used cautiously because of increased danger of GIT ulceration.

Enzymes

Drug	Comment
Bromelains (Ananase) with Anticoagulants	Anticoagulant effect may be enhanced.
Chymotrypsin-trypsin (Chymoral) with Anticoagulants	Caution should be observed when using concomitantly.
Proteolytic enzymes extracted from Carica papaya (Papase) with Anticoagulants	Combined use is contraindicated.
Streptokinase-streptodornase (Varidase) with Antibiotics	The intramuscular use of streptokinase should be accompanied by the administration of a broad-spectrum antibiotic.

Estrogens

Drug	Comment
Estrogens and estrogen–progestin combinations (oral contraceptives) with Anticoagulants	Oral contraceptives may cause a decreased anticoagulant effect; larger doses of the anticoagulant may be needed.
Hypoglycemics	Blood glucose levels may be increased; higher dosage of the hypoglycemic agent may be necessary.

Gastrointestinal Agents

Drug	Comment
Antacids with Acidic drugs (sulfonamides, etc)	Antacids may decrease the absorption of weak acids from the GIT by increasing pH.
Oral Anticoagulants	Large doses of an antacid may decrease the anticoagulant effect by inhibiting absorption.
Basic drugs [amphetamine, meperidine (Demerol), etc]	Antacids may increase the absorption of weak bases from the GIT by increasing pH.
Corticosteroids	Corticosteroids may cause hyperacidity or peptic ulcer; antacids should be given as a prophylactic measure during prolonged therapy.
Enteric-coated medication [bisacodyl (Dulcolax), etc]	Increased pH may cause disintegration of the enteric coating and release of the drug in the stomach; many enteric coated drugs are irritating and may cause nausea and vomiting.
Tetracyclines	Cations of the antacid combine with the tetracyclines to form complexes that are not readily absorbed.

Thyroid

Drug	Comment
Thyroid preparations with Dextrothyroxine (Choloxin)	Dosage of thyroid preparation may have to be altered.
Tricyclic antidepressants	Enhanced activity of either the tricyclic or thyroid may result.

Antidiarrheals

Drug	Comment
Diphenoxylate–atropine combination (Lomotil) with Barbiturates	Action of barbiturates may be enhanced.

Hypoglycemics

Drug	Comment
Insulin, phenformin (DBI), *sulfonylureas* [*acetohexamide* (Dymelor), *chlorpropamide* (Diabinese), *tolazamide* (Tolinase), and *tolbutamide* (Orinase)] with Corticosteroids Dextrothyroxine (Choloxin) Diuretics [(thiazides, chlorthalidone (Hygroton), ethacrynic acid (Edecrin), furosemide (Lasix)] Estrogens Nicotinic acid (large doses) Oral contraceptives	These agents can cause an increase in blood glucose levels; increased doses of the hypoglycemic agents may be necessary
Alcohol	Response is unpredictable; disulfiram-like reactions have been reported with the sulfonylureas; an increased metabolism of tolbutamide in alcoholic patients has been reported; response probably depends on the amount of alcohol taken, whether the patient is a chronic alcoholic, etc.
Monoamine oxidase inhibitors	Enhanced hypoglycemic effect.
Propranolol (Inderal)	May cause hypoglycemia; potential danger may be increased because

Cathartics

Drug	Comment
Bisacodyl (Dulcolax) with Antacids	Bisacodyl should not be taken within 1 hour after antacids since disintegration of the enteric coating and release of the drug in the stomach may cause irritation and vomiting.
Dioctyl sodium sulfosuccinate (Colace) and *poloxalkol* (Polykol) with Mineral oil	Absorption of mineral oil may be increased; should not be given concurrently for long periods.
Mineral oil with Oral Anticoagulants	Variable alterations of the anticoagulant effect have occurred on rare occasions.
Dioctyl sodium sulfosuccinate (Colace) Poloxalkol (Polykol)	These surface-active agents may increase the absorption of mineral oil and should not be given with it for prolonged periods.
Vitamins	Prolonged administration of mineral oil may reduce the absorption of fat-soluble vitamins (A, D, E, K)

Hormones

Androgens

Drug	Comment
Methandrostenolone (Dianabol) with	

Table IV—Continued

Drug	Comment	Drug	Comment
	propranolol may prevent the premonitory signs and symptoms of acute hypoglycemia.	*Methyldopa* (Aldomet) with Amphetamines	Decreased hypotensive effect.
Sulfonylureas with Oral anticoagulants	The coumarin anticoagulants have been shown to enhance the hypoglycemic effect of the sulfonylureas due to inhibition of metabolism.	Diuretics (eg, thiazides)	Enhanced hypotensive effect; the diuretic also counteracts weight gain and edema which may occur with methyldopa therapy.
Barbiturates (and other sedatives and hypnotics)	Sulfonylureas may prolong the effect of these CNS depressants.	Monoamine oxidase inhibitors	Headache, hypertension and related symptoms may develop; combined use should be avoided
Clofibrate (Atromid-S)	Caution should be observed in giving clofibrate to diabetic patients since there has been one report of an enhanced hypoglycemic effect in a patient taking tolbutamide.	Norepinephrine	Enhanced effect of norepinephrine.
		Tricyclic antidepressants	Decreased hypotensive effect.
Insulin	Enhanced hypoglycemic effect.	*Pargyline*—see *Monoamine oxidase inhibitors* under *Antidepressants.*	
Oxyphenbutazone (Tandearil) Phenylbutazone (Butazolidin)	Enhanced hypoglycemic effect; phenylbutazone has been reported to interfere with the excretion of the active metabolite of acetohexamide; protein displacement may also be involved in these interactions.	*Rauwolfia Alkaloids* [alseroxylon (Rauwiloid), rauwolfia serpentina (Raudixin), reserpine (Serpasil, etc), deserpidine (Harmonyl), rescinnamine (Moderil), and syrosingopine (Singoserp)] with	
Phenformin (DBI)	Enhanced hypoglycemic effect.	Anesthetics	Rauwolfia derivatives should be discontinued 2 weeks prior to surgery to avoid excessive hypotension during anesthesia.
Phenyramidol (Analexin)	May enhance the hypoglycemic response due to inhibition of metabolism.	Anticonvulsants	Convulsive threshold may be lowered in susceptible individuals; an increase in the dosage of the anticonvulsant may be necessary.
Probenecid (Benemid)	Enhanced hypoglycemic response has been reported; however, one study indicates that probenecid has little effect on the metabolism of tolbutamide.	Digitalis	Should be used cautiously in combination since cardiac arrhythmias may occur.
Salicylates	May enhance hypoglycemic response due, in part, to displacement from protein binding sites.	Guanethidine (Ismelin)	Concomitant use may exaggerate orthostatic hypotension, bradycardia, and psychic depression.
Sulfinpyrazone (Anturane)	Hypoglycemic effect may be enhanced.	Monoamine oxidase inhibitors	MAO inhibitors inhibit the destruction of serotonin which may be released from tissue stores by Rauwolfia alkaloids; reserpine should not be administered parenterally during, or for 1 week following treatment with pargyline.
Sulfonamides	May enhance hypoglycemic response, possibly due to displacement from protein binding sites; the most conclusive studies have involved the use of sulfaphenazole (Sulfabid) and tolbutamide.		
		Norepinephrine (Levophed)	May increase arterial responsiveness to norepinephrine.
Hypotensives		Propranolol (Inderal)	Added catecholamine blocking action may cause an excessive reduction of the resting sympathetic nervous activity.
All hypotensive agents with Anesthetics Diuretics (thiazides, etc) Other hypotensives Phenothiazines Monoamine oxidase inhibitors Tricyclic antidepressants Vasodilators	Hypotensive effect may be enhanced. These agents can also cause a lowering of the blood pressure and there may be an enhanced hypotensive effect; reduced dosage of the hypotensive agent is frequently necessary.	Quinidine	Should be used cautiously in combination since cardiac arrhythmias may occur.
		Tricyclic antidepressants	Tricyclics may block or reverse the depressive effect of reserpine.
Guanethidine (Ismelin) with Alcohol	Alcohol may aggravate orthostatic hypotension that is frequently seen with guanethidine therapy.	*Veratrum alkaloids* with Digitalis	Cardiac arrhythmias are more likely to occur in patients receiving digitalis concurrently.
Amphetamines	May decrease the hypotensive effect of guanethidine.	Morphine	Bradycrotic effect of veratrum alkaloids is additive to that produced by morphine and related drugs.
Anesthetics	Guanethidine should not be given during the 2 weeks prior to surgery to avoid the possibility of vascular collapse during anesthesia.	Quinidine	Caution should be observed when used together.
Digitalis	Both drugs decrease the heart rate.		
Ephedrine Methylphenidate (Ritalin)	May decrease the hypotensive effect of guanethidine.	**Muscle Relaxants**	
Monoamine oxidase inhibitors	Guanethidine should not be given with or for at least 1 week after discontinuing therapy with a MAO inhibitor.	*Antiparkinson agents* with Monoamine oxidase inhibitors	Caution is advised since severe reactions have been reported following simultaneous use.
Norepinephrine (Levophed)	Responsiveness to norepinephrine is increased; guanethidine should not be used in patients with pheochromocytoma.	Haloperidol Phenothiazines Rauwolfia derivatives Thioxanthenes	Antiparkinson agents are frequently given concurrently to control extrapyramidal symptoms.
Rauwolfia alkaloids	Concomitant use may exaggerate orthostatic hypotension, bradycardia, and psychic depression.	*Mephenesin* (Tolserol) with Barbiturates	Combination may cause marked sedation and respiratory depression.
Tricyclic antidepressants	Hypotensive effect of guanethidine may be antagonized.	*Orphenadrine* (Disipal, Norflex) with	
Vasopressors	An increased likelihood of occurrence of cardiac arrhythmias may exist.	Propoxyphene (Darvon)	Mental confusion, anxiety, and tremors have been reported in patients receiving these agents concurrently.
Hydralazine (Apresoline) with Epinephrine	Pressor response to epinephrine may be reduced.		
Mebutamate (Capla) with Alcohol Central nervous system depressants	Mebutamate may enhance the effect of these agents.	*Succinylcholine* (Anectine) and *decamethonium* (Syncurine) [depolarizing muscle relaxants] with	
Mecamylamine (Inversine) with Urinary acidifiers	Possible decreased effect of mecamylamine due to an increased rate of excretion.	Anticholinesterases [echothiophate (Phospholine iodide), edrophonium (Tensilon), hexafluorenium (Mylaxen), neostigmine (Prostigmin), phosphorus insecticides, etc]	Effects of succinylcholine and decamethonium can be potentiated.
Urinary alkalinizers	Possible increased effect of mecamylamine since rate of excretion is slowed.		

Table IV—Continued

Drug	Comment	Drug	Comment
Antibiotics [colistimethate (Coly-Mycin M), kanamycin (Kantrex), neomycin, polymyxin B (Aerosporin), streptomycin, dihydrostreptomycin, and possibly bacitracin]	These antibiotics can interfere with nerve transmission at the neuromuscular junction; effects of the muscle relaxant may be potentiated.	Hypnotics	Possible enhancement of sedative effects; however, may speed up the metabolism of the hypnotic by causing enzyme induction.
Dexpanthenol (Ilopan)	Dexpanthenol should not be given within 1 hour after succinylcholine administration.	Chlorinated insecticides	May decrease the effects of barbiturates due to enzyme induction.
		Mephenesin (Tolserol)	Combination may cause marked sedation and respiratory depression.
Methotrimeprazine (Levoprome)	Fall in blood pressure and aggravation of CNS effects may occur when given with succinylcholine.	Monoamine oxidase inhibitors	Effects of barbiturates may be enhanced, necessitating a reduction in dosage.
Procaine	Intravenous injections of procaine may potentiate the effect of succinylcholine.	Steroid hormones	May decrease the effects of the hormone due to enzyme induction.
		Sulfonylureas	Effects of the barbiturates may be prolonged.
Quinidine	Potentiation of muscle relaxants may occur.	Tricyclic antidepressants	Studies in animals indicate that tricyclics can enhance the effect of barbiturates.
Tubocurarine (nondepolarizing muscle relaxant) with		*Chloral hydrate* with	
Anesthetics [ether, cyclopropane, fluoroxene (Fluoromar), halothane (Fluothane), and methoxyflurane (Penthrane)]	Enhanced effect of tubocurarine; dosage should be reduced.	Oral anticoagulants	Decreased anticoagulant effect due to enzyme induction.
Antibiotics [colistimethate (Coly-Mycin M), kanamycin (Kantrex), neomycin, polymyxin B (Aerosporin), streptomycin, dihydrostreptomycin, and possibly bacitracin]	These antibiotics can interfere with nerve transmission at the neuromuscular junction; effects of the muscle relaxant may be potentiated.	Monoamine oxidase inhibitors	Effects of chloral hydrate may be enhanced, necessitating a reduction in dosage.
		Ethchlorvynol (Placidyl) with	
		Amitriptyline (Elavil)	Transient delirium has been reported with this combination.
Anticholinesterases [edrophonium (Tensilon), neostigmine (Prostigmin), etc]	These agents antagonize the effects of tubocurarine.	Oral anticoagulants	Has been reported to decrease the anticoagulant response, probably by enzyme induction.
Diuretics (thiazides, etc)	Diuretics may enhance the effect of tubocurarine.	Monoamine oxidase inhibitors	Enhanced sedative effect; dosage of ethchlorvynol should be reduced.
Quinidine	Effect of tubocurarine may be enhanced.	*Glutethimide* (Doriden) with	
		Oral anticoagulants	Decreased anticoagulant effect due to enzyme induction.
		Methaqualone (Quaalude) with	
		Methscopolamine (Pamine)	Action of methscopolamine may be prolonged.

Parasympathomimetics

Sympathomimetics

Drug	Comment	Drug	Comment
Parasympathomimetic agents with		*Sympathomimetic agents* with	
Dexpanthenol (Ilopan)	Dexpanthenol should not be given for 12 hours after use of a parasympathomimetic because of possibility of hyperperistalsis.	Doxapram (Dopram)	An enhanced pressor effect may occur.
		Monoamine oxidase inhibitors	Concurrent use has resulted in severe hypertensive reactions; should not be used simultaneously.
Anticholinesterases [*ambenonium* (Mytelase), *echothiophate* (Phospholine Iodide), *insecticides, neostigmine* (Prostigmin), *pyridostigmine* (Mestinon), etc] with		Tricyclic antidepressants	Enhanced activity of either the tricyclic or sympathomimetic agent may result.
Succinylcholine (Anectine) and decamethonium (Syncurine)	Effects of succinylcholine and decamethonium can be potentiated.	Xanthine preparations	Excessive CNS stimulation may occur
Tubocurarine	Effects of tubocurarine can be antagonized.	*Amphetamine derivatives* with	
		Urinary alkalinizers	Enhanced activity of amphetamine may result due to a decreased rate of excretion.
Each other and other parasympathomimetic agents	Effects may be enhanced.	Guanethidine (Ismelin)	Hypotensive effect of guanethidine may be decreased.
Echothiophate (Phospholine Iodide) with		Methyldopa (Aldomet)	Decreased hypotensive effect.
Pilocarpine	A preliminary report indicates that prior pilocarpine administration may have a protective effect with respect to the action of echothiophate therapy on the lens.	*Epinephrine* with	
		Chloroform, cyclopropane, and halothane (Fluothane)	These anesthetics seem to sensitize the myocardium to the action of epinephrine; possibility of ventricular tachycardia or fibrillation exists with combined use.
Neostigmine (Prostigmin) with		Dextrothyroxine (Choloxin)	Injections of epinephrine in patients with coronary heart disease may precipitate an episode of coronary insufficiency; the likelihood of this occurring may be increased in patients taking dextrothyroxine.
Anticholinergics	Anticholinergics may slow the intestinal motility and alter the absorption of orally administered neostigmine.		
Kanamycin (Kantrex) Neomycin Streptomycin	Neostigmine can be used to reverse the respiratory depression that may be caused by these antibiotics.	Haloperidol (Haldol) Phenothiazines Thioxanthenes	Epinephrine should not be used to treat hypotension caused by these agents since they may reverse its action, resulting in further lowering of blood pressure.
		Isoproterenol (Isuprel) with	

Sedative–Hypnotics

Drug	Comment	Drug	Comment
All sedative–hypnotics with		Digitalis	Isoproterenol is contraindicated in patients with tachycardia caused by digitalis intoxication.
Central nervous system depressants (alcohol, narcotics, tranquilizers, other sedative–hypnotics, etc)	Enhanced sedative effect.	Epinephrine	These agents should not be used simultaneously since both are direct cardiac stimulants and combined use may produce arrhythmias; however, they may be used alternately.
Barbiturates with			
Alcohol	Enhanced sedative effect.	Other sympathomimetic agents	Dose of other agents should be reduced to avoid excessive response.
Oral anticoagulants	Decreased anticoagulant effect due to enzyme induction; larger doses of the anticoagulant may be required.	*Norepinephrine* (Levophed) with	
Antihistamines	Decreased antihistamine effect due to enzyme induction.	Chloroform Cyclopropane Halothane (Fluothane)	These anesthetics sensitize the myocardium to the action of norepinephrine; possibility of ventricular tachycardia or fibrillation exists with combined use.
Diphenoxylate (in Lomotil)	Action of barbiturates may be enhanced.		
Diphenylhydantoin (Dilantin)	Phenobarbital can decrease the effect of diphenylhydantoin due to enzyme induction; is usually not of clinical significance because phenobarbital also has anticonvulsant activity.	Diuretics (thiazides, etc)	Arterial responsiveness to norepinephrine may be decreased.
Griseofulvin (Fulvicin, Grifulvin, Grisactin)	Decreased effect of griseofulvin due to enzyme induction.	Guanethidine (Ismelin)	Responsiveness to norepinephrine is increased.

Table IV—Continued

Drug	Comment	Drug	Comment
Methyldopa (Aldomet) Rauwolfia alkaloids	Enhanced effect of norepinephrine. Arterial responsiveness to norepinephrine may be increased.		urine; alkalinization decreases the possibility of formation of uric acid stones.
Tricyclic antidepressants	Tricyclics may increase the pressor effect of norepinephrine.	Aminosalicylic acid (PAS)	Probenecid decreases urinary excretion of PAS resulting in increased plasma levels.
		Erythromycin (Erythrocin, Ilosone)	Probenecid has been shown to inhibit tubular reabsorption of erythromycin in animals.

Tranquilizers

Drug	Comment	Drug	Comment
All tranquilizers with Central nervous system depressants (alcohol, barbiturates, narcotics, sedative-hypnotics, other CNS depressants)	Enhanced sedative effect; degree of enhancement depends on the particular tranquilizer used.	Indomethacin (Indocin)	Probenecid interferes with the renal excretion of indomethacin; the uricosuric action of probenecid is not blocked.
Monoamine oxidase inhibitors	MAO inhibitors may enhance the effect of the tranquilizers; an additive hypotensive effect may be seen with the phenothiazines.	Penicillins	Probenecid can enhance the effects of penicillin derivatives by interfering with their tubular excretion and decreasing their volume of distribution.
Chlordiazepoxide (Librium) with Oral anticoagulants	Variable alterations in the anticoagulant response have been reported.	Salicylates	Salicylates antagonize the uricosuric activity of probenecid.
Diazepam (Valium) with Anticonvulsants	When diazepam is used as an adjunct in treating convulsive disorders, an increase in the dosage of standard anticonvulsant medication may be necessary.	Sulfonamides	Probenecid increases total sulfa plasma levels.
		Sulfonylureas	Enhanced hypoglycemic response has been reported; however, one study indicates that probenecid has little effect on the metabolism of tolbutamide (Orinase).
Haloperidol (Haldol) with Anesthetics Oral anticoagulants	Effects of anesthetics are enhanced. Haloperidol has been reported to antagonize the effect of phenindione.	*Sulfinpyrazone* (Anturane) with Citrates Salicylates	Effect of sulfinpyrazone is antagonized.
Anticonvulsants	The dose of the anticonvulsant should not be altered when haloperidol therapy is initiated; however, subsequent adjustment may be necessary.	Insulin Sulfonylureas	Hypoglycemic effect may be enhanced.
Antiparkinson agents	May be used concurrently with haloperidol to control extrapyramidal symptoms.	Sulfonamides	Effect of the sulfonamides may be enhanced.

Uterine drugs

Drug	Comment	Drug	Comment
Epinephrine	Epinephrine should not be used to correct hypotension caused by haloperidol since the latter may block its vasoconstrictor effect.	*Oxytocics* [oxytocin (Pitocin), ergonovine (Ergotrate), methylergonovine (Methergine)] with Vasopressors	Excessively high blood pressure could result.
Meprobamate (Equanil, Miltown) with Oral anticoagulants	Decreased anticoagulant effect due to enzyme induction.	*Oxytocin* (Pitocin) with Sparteine sulfate (Spartocin)	Synergistic action of sparteine sulfate and oxytocin may result in tetanic uterine contractions; several hours should elapse after the last dose of sparteine sulfate before giving oxytocin.

Vasodilators

Coronary Vasodilators

Drug	Comment	Drug	Comment
Phenothiazines and *thioxanthenes*[d] [chlorprothixene (Taractan) and thiothixene (Navane)] with Anesthetics, general	Effects of anesthetic are enhanced.	*Nitrates* with Alcohol	Alcohol may enhance sensitivity to the hypotensive effects of these compounds.
Anticholinergics (atropine, etc)	Effects of anticholinergics may be enhanced.	Acetylcholine	Nitrates can act as physiological antagonists to these substances
Anticonvulsants	Phenothiazines and thioxanthenes can lower the convulsive threshold in susceptible individuals; an increase in the dosage of the anticonvulsant may be necessary.	Histamine Norepinephrine Hypotensive agents	Potent hypotensive agents should be given cautiously since their use with nitrates may produce severe hypotension.
Antiparkinson agents	Are frequently used concurrently with the phenothiazines and thioxanthenes to control extrapyramidal symptoms.	*Isosorbide dinitrate* (Isordil) with Propranolol (Inderal)	Synergistic effects in treating angina pectoris have been reported; however, the potential benefit of using these agents in combination has been disputed.
Dipyrone (Narone, Pyrilgin)	Dipyrone should not be used with chlorpromazine (Thorazine); antipyretic effect is potentiated possibly resulting in severe hypothermia.	*Dipyridamole* (Persantine) with Digitalis	It has been claimed that dipyridamole can enhance the effect of digitalis; however, this finding has been questioned.
Epinephrine	Epinephrine should not be used to treat hypotension caused by a phenothiazine or thioxanthene since these agents have been found to reverse its action, resulting in a further lowering of blood pressure.		

Peripheral Vasodilators

Drug	Comment	Drug	Comment
Hypotensives (including diuretics)	Hypotensive effect may be enhanced.	*Alpha-Adrenergic blocking agents* [phenoxybenzamine (Dibenzyline), tolazoline (Priscoline), etc] with Epinephrine	Epinephrine should not be used to treat overdosage since a further drop in blood pressure may occur (epinephrine reversal).
Insecticides (phosphorus)	Effects of the insecticide may be potentiated.		
Pentylenetetrazol Picrotoxin	Should not be used as stimulating agents in treating overdosage since they may cause convulsions.	Propranolol (Inderal)	These agents should be used with propranolol in treating pheochromocytoma to avoid a serious rise in blood pressure.
Piperazine	Exaggeration of extrapyramidal effects has occurred when piperazine was administered with a phenothiazine.		
Tricyclic antidepressants	Tricyclics and phenothiazines are frequently used in combination (Etrafon, Triavil) in treating agitated forms of depressions.		

Uricosurics

Vitamins

Drug	Comment	Drug	Comment
Uricosuric agents with Diuretics (thiazides, etc)	Diuretics decrease the renal excretion of uric acid; higher doses of uricosuric agents may be required.	*Aminobenzoic acid* (PABA) with Gold therapy	Dermatitis and/or fever associated with gold therapy of arthritis may be aggravated.
Probenecid (Benemid) with Urinary alkalinizers	Urates tend to crystallize out of an acid		

Table IV—Continued

Drug	Comment	Drug	Comment
Sulfonamides	Since sulfonamides are effective antibacterials because they compete with PABA, an increased concentration of the latter will decrease their activity.	*Arginine glutamate* (Modumate) with	
		Other drugs	Many drugs, including barbiturates, narcotics, and diuretics may produce ammonia or interfere with its excretion.
Dexpanthenol (Ilopan) and *salts of pantothenic acid* with		*Betahistine* (Serc) with	
Parasympathomimetics	Dexpanthenol should not be given for 12 hours after use of a parasympathomimetic because of possibility of hyperperistalsis.	Antihistamines	Betahistine is a histamine-like agent and concurrent use with antihistamines is not recommended.
Succinylcholine (Anectine)	Dexpanthenol should not be given within 1 hour after succinylcholine administration.	*Cholestyramine* (Cuemid, Questran) with	
Fat-soluble vitamins (A, D, E, K) with		Other drugs	Cholestyramine can bind with other drugs in the GIT and inhibit their absorption; it has the greatest affinity for acidic drugs and might absorb neutral and basic drugs to a slight extent; the interval between administration of cholestyramine and another drug should be as long as possible.
Cholestyramine (Cuemid, Questran)	Absorption of these vitamins may be impaired.		
Mineral oil	Prolonged administration of mineral oil may impair the absorption of these vitamins.	Fat-soluble vitamins	Absorption of these vitamins may be impaired.
Miscellaneous		*Disulfiram* (Antabuse) with	
Allopurinol (Zyloprim) with		Alcohol	Disulfiram interferes with the degradation of alcohol, resulting in an increased concentration of acetaldehyde and the development of characteristic symptoms.
Azathioprine (Imuran) Mercaptopurine (Purinethol)	Allopurinol can inhibit the metabolism of these agents; dose of these agents should be reduced to $\frac{1}{3}$ to $\frac{1}{4}$ of the usual dose.		
Iron salts	Concurrent use should be avoided since an increase in hepatic iron concentration has been reported in animals.	Oral anticoagulants	May cause an enhanced anticoagulant effect.
Uricosuric agents	Concurrent administration may result in a decreased urinary excretion of oxypurines as compared to their excretion with allopurinol alone; however, combination therapy may provide the best control for many patients.	Diphenylhydantoin (Dilantin)	May enhance the effect of diphenylhydantoin by inhibiting its metabolism.
		Metronidazole (Flagyl)	Combined use has led to the development of acute psychoses or confusional states.
		Paraldehyde	Should not be used concurrently.

[a] Most of the reported interactions involving anticoagulants have been associated with the use of coumarin anticoagulants.

[b] Pargyline is used primarily as a hypotensive agent.

[c] Furazolidone is an antibacterial agent that can cause monoamine oxidase inhibition; however, significant inhibition of these enzymes does not usually occur during the first five days of therapy.

[d] Most of the following interactions have involved the use of phenothiazine derivatives. However, since the thioxanthenes are so closely related to the phenothiazines, it is likely that they will exhibit the same effects.

95 | Dental Services

Dental pharmacy—dental formulas used in general practice—
preparations for surgery and exodontia

This chapter was prepared by

Austin H. Kutscher, DDS, *Head, Section on Therapeutics and Clinical
Pharmacology, School of Dental and Oral Surgery, Columbia University,
New York, N.Y. 10032, and*
Edward V. Zegarelli, MS, DDS, *Director, Division of Stomatology, School of
Dental and Oral Surgery, Columbia University, New York, N.Y. 10032*

Mutual interest in health problems ties pharmacy to medicine, dentistry, nursing, and other branches of the healing arts. The practice of dentistry bears a strong similarity to the practice of medicine. Nevertheless, certain important dissimilarities are encountered which must be appreciated if the pharmacist is to fulfill his obligations to dental practice, to the dental practitioner, and to patients requiring drug therapy for dental and oral diseases.

While pharmacists have always been closely associated with medical practice, only within recent years has a similar cooperation with the dental profession been visualized, although not yet fully realized.

Therapy of Mouth and Jaw Diseases

The practice of dentistry is a specialty within the sphere of medicine. The dentist is responsible for the therapy of a wide variety of oral diseases. By virtue of his training in the basic sciences and his knowledge and skills obtained from the study of specialized sciences such as oral histology, pathology, microbiology, diagnosis, and therapeutics, he is well qualified to detect, diagnose and treat nearly all diseases of the mouth and jaws.

He can note the clinical features of many diseases by direct visual observation. Furthermore, he can usually palpate the lesion. Historical data are also usually easy to obtain and even more significant insofar as interpretation is concerned, since the patient usually becomes aware of the mouth or jaw disease early in the course of its existence. Thus, the dentist can readily fulfill his peculiar responsibilities for the diagnosis and treatment of diseases of the mouth and jaws of his patients.

Since a considerable number of mouth and jaw diseases are associated with or result from systemic disturbances (eg, erosive lichen planus, oral pemphigus and oral herpes simplex infections) dental diagnosis and treatment of mouth and jaw diseases has necessarily had to include systemic–oral manifestations and relationships. The initial manifestations of numerous systemic diseases are often clinically observable in the mouth prior to their appearance elsewhere in the body. The gingival enlargements and infections associated with acute leukemia, the pallor of the gingivae in anemia, the impressive glossitis of vitamin B deficiency, and the pigmentation of oral mucosal tissues in Addison's disease are just a few such instances.

The dentist fulfils his responsibilities to his patients by becoming thoroughly familiar not only with those systemic diseases which may manifest themselves intraorally, but also by becoming knowledgeable concerning drugs which are used for controlling these diseases elsewhere—agents with which dentistry had not previously been concerned. He is familiar with the principles involved in the administration of not only the older drugs (local anesthetics, analgesics, sedatives, antibiotics, certain general anesthetics, and other drugs which have long been important and commonly employed in dental practice), but also the newer drugs (corticosteroids, tranquilizers, hormones and anticoagulants)—and even the placebo. Furthermore, since allergic and toxic reactions of systemically administered drugs may manifest themselves in the mouth, the dentist has had to become familiar with them. He has also had to acquire knowledge concerning groups of drugs such as the chemotherapeutic agents which are employed in the management of malignant neoplasms. For example, aminopterin (a folic acid antagonist) may cause or lead to ulcerations of the oral mucosa.

Thus, the sphere of interest and responsibility of the dentist is intimately associated with (although by no means restricted to) the following disease states and their treatment:

Local Diseases

Dental caries
Periodontitis (pyorrhea)
Acute ulcerative necrotizing gingivitis (Vincent's infection, trench-mouth)
Periapical infection (tooth abscess)
Periodontal infection (pyorrhea abscess)
Allergy
Tumors and neoplasms
Cysts
Local infections: pulpal infection, pericoronitis, osteomyelitis, causes of bacteremia and septicemia, focal infection, actinomycosis, moniliasis
Traumatic ulcers (canker sores)
Chemical burns
Recurrent ulcerative stomatitis
Keratotic diseases including hyperkeratosis and leukoplakia
Osteoradionecrosis
Angular stomatitis
Denture stomatitis
Hypersalivation and hyposalivation
Sialoliths
Halitosis

Systemic Disturbances with Oral Manifestations

Allergy
Hypovitaminosis A, B, C, D, and K
Tumors and neoplasms, metastatic
Hormonal aberrations including Addison's disease, hyperparathyroidism, hypo- and hyperthyroidism, hypo- and hyperpituitarism, diabetes mellitus, hypo- and hypergonadism, pregnancy gingivitis
Dermatologic diseases including erythema multiforme, Stevens-Johnson syndrome, Behcet's syndrome, lichen planus, scleroderma, pemphigus, systemic lupus erythematosus, psoriasis

Malnutritional deficiency diseases including (in addition to vitamin deficiencies) celiac disease, sprue, and cystic fibrosis of the pancreas

Hematologic disorders including anemia, polycythemia, leukemia, leukopenia, purpura, hemophilia

Infectious diseases of a systemic nature including syphilis, tuberculosis, acute primary herpes, herpangina, infectious mononucleosis

Recurrent ulcerative stomatitis (systemic background)

Serum and infectious hepatitis

Keratotic diseases including hyperkeratosis and leukoplakia

Toxic lesions (bismuth, gold, etc)

Osteoradionecrosis

Neurological disturbances including Bell's palsy, Parkinson's disease, trigeminal neuralgia, atypical neuralgia, convulsive disorders

Maxillary sinusitis

Tonsilitis

Laryngitis

Angular stomatitis (systemic background)

Denture stomatitis (systemic background)

Hypo- and hypersalivation

Sialoliths

Glossodynia

Halitosis

Oral Disturbances Directly Related to Drugs

Toxic lesions resulting from therapy with bismuth, gold, etc

Mucosal lesions following therapy with cancer chemotherapeutic agents such as aminopterin

Dilantin fibromatosis

Tetracycline discoloration of the teeth

Fluorine intoxication (endemic or iatrogenically induced fluorosis of teeth)

Systemic Diseases Which May Influence Dental Care

Cardiovascular diseases including those requiring anticoagulant therapy, rheumatic heart disease, subacute bacterial endocarditis

Respiratory tract disease

Urinary tract disease

Central nervous system disease

Hematopoietic disturbances

Gastrointestinal disease

Skin diseases

Neuromuscular disturbances

Malignancies

Serum and infectious hepatitis

Pregnancy

Pharmacist–Dentist Relationship

Restrictions of space prohibit other than the mere mention for illustrative purposes of the various diseases which are of interest and concern to the dentist with regard to therapeutics. Also, it must be assumed that the pharmacist has access to descriptions concerning the nature of these many disease processes[1-5] wherein a knowledge of them appears to be pertinent.

It is of particular importance, insofar as the pharmacist—dentist relationship is concerned, that the pharmacist be thoroughly familiar with the vastly expanded responsibilities of the dentist for the diagnosis and treatment of diseases affecting the tissues of the mouth and jaws.

Numerous cooperative relationships have arisen over the years between the pharmacist and the dentist. For example, dentists have found that pharmacists can best prepare many of the dental products which are commonly used either at the dental chair or in the dental laboratory. It is also of interest to mention that in recent years prescription writing on the part of the dentist has increased markedly, undoubtedly because of the introduction of such useful drugs as the antibiotics, corticosteroids, and tranquilizers.

Pharmacists frequently render invaluable service to the dental profession by cooperating in matters pertaining to the dental education of the public. The dissemination of information concerning the values of fluoridation of public water supplies, the effectiveness of oral hygienic measures, and the dental implications of halitosis are but a few of the benefits to the dental profession obtainable through the aid of the pharmacist.

To play his proper role in advising patrons, the pharmacist must keep in touch with sources of information relating to dental drugs and adjuncts. His best sources of such information are, in general, the *Journal of the American Dental Association* and *Accepted Dental Remedies* (ADR), publications of the American Dental Association. The latter is published annually and is the result of deliberations of the Council on Dental Therapeutics of the Association (available through the Association's office at 222 E. Superior St., Chicago, Ill. 60611). This book provides the pharmacist with information about various kinds of dental products.

It seems to be almost axiomatic that people develop toothache only after the dentist's office is closed. They then obtain from the pharmacist toothache drops and similar preparations. Once relief is obtained, many afflicted people fail to seek the requisite dental treatment. The pharmacist should encourage such persons to consult the dentist promptly, for early treatment is nearly always simpler and less painful, and in the best interests of the patient's general health.

Pharmacology and Therapeutics[6-8]

This section deals with a *few* of the many broad generalizations which are possible concerning the pharmacology of drugs and their applications in the treatment of diseases of the mouth and jaws. Of particular interest in this respect, from the viewpoint of the pharmacist, are considerations pertinent to the following classes of drugs: antibiotics, other antibacterial agents, antihistaminics, corticosteroids, hemostatics, local anesthetics (topical and injectable), protectant-vehicles, sedatives and hypnotics, tranquilizers, and vitamins.

Although the basic course in pharmacology as taught to dental students is similar in most respects to that taught to medical students, the clinical applications of drugs and the art of therapeutics are often markedly different in dentistry in comparison with medicine.

For instance, the therapeutic index of drugs becomes of particular significance when concerned with drugs employed in dentistry since safety *per se* usually must be of paramount importance in dental practice. This aspect assumes even greater significance when it is realized that the clinical training and experience of the dentist in the management of acute allergic or toxic drug reactions are considerably less comprehensive and effectual than that of the physician.

As another example, although the oral route of drug administration is generally the most convenient and economical for both physician and dentist, it is particularly suited to dental practice as the safest from the standpoint of severe allergic and toxic reactions to drugs. Furthermore, the oral route of administration more suitably fits the pattern of dental practice, the parenteral routes being generally avoided for one reason or another, such as lack of training in the necessary techniques, lack of suitable office facilities, or lack of office nursing care.

The distribution, fate, and elimination of drugs are of as much interest to dentists as to members of the medical profession. But again, there are areas in these fields which are of specific interest to dentistry, such as the evaluation of the advantages and hazards of drugs excreted into the saliva. For example, the presence of broad spectrum antibiotics in the saliva undoubtedly exerts a considerable influence on the oral microbial flora. This influence may affect caries incidence or calculus formation, or may predispose to or trigger the onset of oral lesions such as moniliasis.

Drug synergism, addition, and potentiation, as well as chemical, physiological, and specific competitive antagonism are also of interest to dentists, but the areas of application of these concepts are less frequently encountered because of the nature of the usual general dental practice. Nevertheless, certain combinations of drugs are commonly and even routinely utilized, but these combinations more often involve the pairing of a local anesthetic with a vasoconstrictor (eg, lidocaine with epinephrine) or groups of analgesics (eg, aspirin with phenacetin and codeine). Furthermore, the specific competitive antagonists which are more often encountered by the dentist are not those agents he employs but those administered by medical practitioners.

Until recent years little attention has been directed toward the improvement of vehicles which might afford a more effective medium for the application of drugs topically to the surface tissues of the mouth—an approach which might be useful in the treatment of mouth diseases or which might serve as another means of administering systemic therapy. Recently, an adhesive paste, Orabase, and an adhesive powder, Orahesive, have been introduced as vehicles for the oral topical administration of active agents with the result that a wholly new and potentially valuable technique has been made available for the application of drugs to the oral mucous membranes. It is hoped that these as well as other special vehicles (such as long-lasting lozenges, formulations which are now under definitive clinical investigative study) will soon assume their rightful role in the armamentarium of the various healing professions for the treatment of certain mouth diseases.

In summary, although no attempt has been made to present a comprehensive comparative concept of dentistry as it resembles and as it differs from medicine in regard to principles of pharmacology and therapeutics, it is hoped that on the basis of the above discussion the pharmacist will appreciate, understand, and make allowances for the meaningful differences which do exist.

Drugs Used for Oral Lesions and in Routine Practice

Although the topical application of drugs continues to be the favored route of therapy, both in the dental office and in prescriptions written by dentists, in recent years there has been a marked increase in the systemic use of drugs by dental practitioners.[1]

The following discussion of the various classes of drugs is by no means intended to circumvent the need for reading and understanding classical concepts of pharmacology and therapeutics. It is offered, rather, to place proper emphasis and perspective on specific therapeutic agents as they relate to the practice of dentistry.

Analgesics

Dentistry utilizes nearly all of the various techniques available for relieving pain associated with the oral structures. In addition, the dentist concerns himself as often as possible with the removal of the cause of the pain, namely the excavation of dental caries, the extirpation of a diseased pulp, or the extraction of an infected tooth. In other words, the dentist frequently resorts to an instrumental or surgical approach to the relief of pain, in addition to employing drug therapy.

Among the analgesics, particular dependence is placed on aspirin, APC formulations, codeine, Darvon, demerol, methadone, and morphine. Codeine with aspirin and Darvon Compound are frequently prescribed in dental practice. Darvon *per se* has assumed an especially widespread popularity since a narcotics license is not required for its prescription.

Demerol, a drug which has been found highly effective in controlling many and severe types of dental pain, remains a popular prescription item.

Although morphine is occasionally used in dentistry, in recent years methadone has been suggested and utilized as a substitute since it is more reliably effective when administered perorally.

The new and presumably nonaddictive agent, pentazocine [Talwin (Winthrop)], will probably have a substantial impact on dental practice since its use will no longer depend on whether or not the dentist will put aside his aversion to agents which must be administered by parenteral injection. This agent, now available in oral dosage form *and* not requiring a narcotic license, may fill a great void in the dental armamentarium.

A discussion of the following substances is included in ADR 1967:

Aspirin
Phenacetin
Acetaminophen
Ethoheptazine Citrate
Morphine Sulfate
Codeine Phosphate
Codeine Sulfate
Meperidine Hydrochloride
Methadone Hydrochloride
Anileridine

Consult also Chapter 63, page 1120, for a more complete discussion of analgesic agents.

Antibacterial Agents Other than Antibiotics and Sulfonamides

Antibacterial agents are frequently used in dental practice

1. To disinfect penetrating and nonpenetrating instruments,
2. to control superficial infections of the skin or bone either for prophylactic purposes or as a distinct therapeutic procedure, and
3. to disinfect tooth cavities prior to the insertion of a filling material in routine tooth preparations, pulp capping, pulpotomy, or endodontic (root canal) procedures. A brief discussion of the role and efficacy of the more commonly used antibacterial agents as they pertain to dental practice is in order.

Ethyl alcohol as an intraoral antibacterial agent is seldom used. Boric acid and boric acid formulations are far less frequently employed today than heretofore. The dyes, such as gentian violet and methylene blue, are still widely used antiseptic agents for the treatment of mouth infections and lesions in spite of the fact that their clinical efficacy leaves much to be desired.

Formaldehyde finds its most effective role in dental therapeutics as the active component of a desensitizing toothpaste prescribed for the relief of pain and discomfort associated with the sensitive necks of teeth. A 10% solution is also employed in dental offices as a fixative of surgical biopsies and excised specimens.

Weak solutions of sodium hypochlorite are often used as effective antibacterial agents in combatting the organisms adherent to denture appliances and causing denture stomatitis.

Iodine is widely used as a prophylactic agent for preoperative use on intraoral injection sites and as an antiseptic following a dental prophylaxis. Iodoform impregnated gauze drains continue to enjoy widespread usage in oral surgical procedures despite the fact that the clinical effectiveness of the iodoform *per se* is open to question. Povidone-iodine formulations are becoming more popular in dental practice.

Hydrogen peroxide is frequently used. A 1–3% solution is often employed in combatting mouth infections (used as a mouth wash as well as by topical application) although its effectiveness has been found to result more from its cleansing action than from its germicidal potency. Hydrogen peroxide (30%) is employed as a tooth-bleaching agent.

Chromic acid and silver nitrate are used much less frequently today as antibacterial agents since their detrimental caustic actions far outweigh their beneficial values and since safer and more effective antibacterial agents are presently available. Zinc chloride and aluminum acetate, astringents with some antibacterial action, are seldom used as such.

Despite inferior potency as antibacterial agents, irritating action and high systemic toxicity, mercury preparations such as Merbromin, Mercresin, Metaphen, and Merthiolate are still occasionally utilized.

Phenol is infrequently used since it possesses only a weak antiseptic action, is not self-limiting, and possesses a high tissue toxicity potential. However, a number of chemically related compounds are widely employed including thymol, the cresols, guaiacol, creosote, and particularly eugenol. Eugenol, a constituent of essential oils, has been found to be highly effective not only as an antiseptic but also as a topical analgesic and as a substance which possesses desirable counterirritant properties. It is of particular benefit as a component of temporary dressing formulations, eg, zinc oxide and eugenol, which is commonly employed as a temporary filling material for one or more of the above reasons.

Hexachlorophene is also used in dentistry, just as it is in medicine, in the form of hexachlorophene-containing soaps. In addition, it has also been incorporated in toothpastes.

Wide use is made of anionic and cationic surfactants, particularly Zephiran chloride, which is frequently employed as a cold sterilizing solution. Ceepryn, as Cepacol mouthwash and Cepacol lozenges, is another surfactant which is quite commonly used in dental practice. However, it is essential to note that cold sterilization is ineffective for the eradication of the viruses of serum and infectious hepatitis.

A discussion of the following substances is included in ADR 1967:

Arsenic Trioxide
Boric Acid
Dyes
Cresolated Formaldehyde
Paraformaldehyde
Chloramine-t
Chloroazodin
Sodium Hypochlorite Solution
Diluted Sodium Hypochlorite Solution
Iodine
Povidone-Iodine
Iodoform
Thymol Iodide

o-Hydroxyphenylmercuric Chloride
Merbromin
Mercocresols
Nitromersol
Thimerosal
Chromium Trioxide
Hydrogen Peroxide, 30%
Hydrogen Peroxide Solution
Urea Peroxide
Sodium Perborate
sec-Amyltricresol
Parachlorophenol
Camphorated Parachlorophenol
Creosote
Eugenol
Guaiacol
Phenol
Liquefied Phenol
Thymol
Silver Nitrate
Toughened Silver Nitrate
Ammoniacal Silver Nitrate Solution
Ethylene Oxide
Formaldehyde Solution
Mercury Bichloride
Phenylmercuric Borate
Potassium Mercuric Iodide
Cresol
Saponated Cresol Solution
Hexachlorophene
Sodium Pentachlorophenate
Benzalkonium Chloride
Dichlorobenzalkonium Chloride
Benzethonium Chloride
Methylbenzethonium Chloride
Cetyl Dimethyl Ethyl Ammonium Bromide

Consult also Chapter 67, page 1174, for a more complete discussion of antibacterial agents.

Antibiotics

Perhaps even more so than in medicine, the frequency of penicillin reactions, particularly those which are life endangering, has often compelled dentists to resort to the use of broad spectrum antibiotics rather than the penicillins. The frequency of penicillin reactions has been such that many dentists will use penicillin only when this agent is the antibiotic of choice (mandatory) or when it can be employed in hospital environments where resuscitative equipment is instantly available to treat emergency situations. Nevertheless, practically all of the available penicillins find some use in dental practice. Benzathine penicillin, however, is used only rarely. Penicillin in troche form has lost all of its previous extensive popularity because of its frequent role as an antigenic agent when thus employed. Oxacillin, which can be given by mouth, is being used by increasing numbers of dentists to manage resistant staphlococcus infections. Staphcillin, used for similar purposes, has a drawback; it must be administered parenterally.

Because of the above, dentists have turned to the use of the broad spectrum antibiotics, particularly those which can be administered orally with full assurance of effectiveness—namely, chlortetracycline, demethylchlortetracycline, oxytetracycline, and tetracycline.

Chloramphenicol and streptomycin are rarely employed in dental practice in accordance with the officially stated positions of the American Dental Association and the American Medical Association. Mycostatin is widely employed as an antifungal agent and is particularly effective in the management of oral monilial infections. Amphotericin B is probably as effective as mycostatin and in addition lacks its disagreeable taste. If it should be marketed in a suitable formulation, it may well challenge the position of mycostatin for intraoral usage.

Dentists have frequently made use of the erythromycins and at present are encouraged to prescribe erythromycin base rather than Ilosone, in view of the recently appreciated potential hazards of hepatic damage associated on rare occasions with Ilosone therapy. Erythromycin is commonly employed to "back up the line."

Lincomycin has excited some investigational effort and use of marketed forms in dental therapeutics.

Vancomycin and ristocetin are looked upon as agents of last resort, and should be employed only by physicians.

Topical applications of antibiotics intraorally are occasionally employed but are restricted to those antibiotics (bacitracin, neomycin, tyrothricin, and polymyxin B) which lack hazardous local or systemic side-reactions. The development of resistance to these agents by microorganisms is of substantially less consequence since they are not employed for systemic use.

It is to be noted that all topical antibiotic formulations are severely restricted in regard to their efficacy of action in the management of oral lesions. Deep-seated, well-entrenched oral infections which require antibiotic therapy will nearly always require systemically administered agents, with or without supplemental topical antibacterial medication.

It is further to be emphasized that tyrothricin should not be employed in tooth socket formulations since it may be hemolytic.

Dentists are particularly conversant with the necessity for prophylactically administering antibiotics (penicillin, wherever possible) to patients with a history of rheumatic fever, rheumatic heart disease, congenital heart defect, or subacute bacterial endocarditis. However, as stated above, erythromycins or tetracyclines are employed whenever a history of allergy to penicillin is uncovered.

The dentist is called upon occasionally to prescribe for the treatment of an iatrogenic oral allergic or toxic reaction resulting from the use of antibiotics. A variety of therapeutic approaches may be employed. Mouthwashes of antihistamines, such as elixir of Pyribenzamine, may be used. After being distributed throughout the mouth, these may be swallowed for systemic action also. Mycostatin is used for combatting monilial superinfections. Multivitamin formulations are frequently employed to overcome any deficiency aspects of the problem. Topical protectants are also often used. When indicated, a corticosteroid may be employed, preferably in an adhesive vehicle. Thus, plain Orabase or Orahesive may be used as adhesive protectants, and Kenalog in Orabase may be employed, with the latter acting as a vehicle.

A discussion of the following substances is included in ADR 1967:

Benzathine Penicillin G
Potassium Penicillin G
Sodium Penicillin G
Phenoxymethyl Penicillin
Potassium Phenethicillin
Procaine Penicillin G
Chlortetracycline Hydrochloride
Oxytetracycline
Oxytetracycline Hydrochloride
Tetracycline
Tetracycline Hydrochloride
Demethylchlortetracycline Hydrochloride

Erythromycin
Erythromycin Estolate
Bacitracin
Chloramphenicol
Neomycin Sulfate
Nystatin
Polymyxin B Sulfate
Tyrothricin

Consult also Chapter 67, page 1174, for a more complete discussion of antibiotics.

Antihistamines

Antihistamines are commonly employed in dental practice although some of their proposed merits have not been realized. They are most often used in controlling allergic reactions involving the oral tissues and structures. Pyribenzamine elixir and other similar formulations have been found to be beneficial in providing a means of obtaining a mild topical anesthetic action in addition to local and systemic antiallergic effects.

Chlortrimeton and Benadryl are other commonly employed antihistaminic agents. Phenergan is appreciated not only as a highly useful antihistaminic but also as an antiemetic, antisialogogue, sedative, and tranquilizer.

The use of antihistaminics in the management of postoperative sequelae associated with oral surgical procedures (edema, facial swelling, trismus, etc.) has been quite disappointing.

A discussion of the following substances is included in ADR 1967:

Chlorpheniramine Maleate
Dexchlorpheniramine Maleate
Pyrrobutamine Phosphate

Consult also Chapter 64, page 1142, for a more complete discussion of antihistamines.

Corticosteroids

No group of drugs has changed the pattern of drug therapy of noninfectious diseases of the mouth more remarkably than the corticosteroids. These agents have been found to be highly effective in the management of a large number of acute and chronic lesions of the oral mucosae.

Perhaps one of the more efficacious corticosteroids and one which is enjoying widespread intraoral use is Kenalog (triamcinolone acetonide). One of the more important reasons for its popularity is that it is the only corticosteroid marketed in an adhesive vehicle (Orabase), thus assuring more adequate adherence to moistened oral mucosal lesions. Some dentists, unfortunately, are reluctant to prescribe corticosteroids, even as topical agents, for fear of their side effects. It should be borne in mind, however, that the employment of corticosteroids should be restricted to those patients who do not exhibit or give a history of contraindications to their use. It should also be emphasized that the local or systemic side effects from the use of topically applied corticosteroids, administered in proper dosages, are essentially nil, at most minimal.

Systemically administered corticosteroids, however, are seldom prescribed by dentists, the exceptions being in severe allergic reactions or conditions which are more commonly thought of as associated with systemic disease states.

As with the treatment of other diseases, so, too, in corticosteroid therapy of acute and chronic oral mucosal disease states, such agents are primarily ameliorative or suppressant in their actions.

Consult also Chapter 55, page 955, for a more complete discussion of corticosteroids.

Hemostatic Agents

There are many approaches, exclusive of drugs, which are employed by dentists for controlling bleeding episodes within the mouth. For example, various pressure-packing techniques, sutures, and refrigerants are utilized frequently and are commonly found to be effective.

However, on occasion, drugs must be utilized in controlling oral bleeding. Those that are more commonly used are Gelfoam, oxidized cellulose, carboxymethylcellulose, epinephrine, and thrombin. These are employed as topical agents for promoting blood coagulation. They are contraindicated when the bleeding is due to the rupture of a larger blood vessel or when the coagulating agent may lead to the formation of a thrombus.

Epinephrine is a particularly effective agent in controlling the ooze associated with capillary bleeding; for instance, to eliminate oozing of blood during dental operative procedures such as the insertion of a filling material at the gum line.

Systemic approaches for controlling oral bleeding are seldom employed by the dentist. Whole blood transfusions or fresh frozen plasma are not commonly utilized in the dental office. However, they are frequently employed in the hospital as prophylactic or therapeutic measures for controlling oral hemorrhagic incidents such as may occur in hemophiliacs who are to undergo or who have undergone the extraction of teeth, or other oral surgical procedures.

In the management of patients who are on anticoagulant therapy, the dentist seeks the aid of and collaborates closely with the physician, who may wish to administer a vitamin K preparation prior to dental intervention.

A discussion of the following substances is included in ADR 1967:

Epinephrine Solution
Vitamin K
Menadione Sodium Bisulfite
Menadiol Sodium Diphosphate
Thrombin
Absorbable Gelatin Sponge
Oxidized Cellulose
Oxidized Regenerated Cellulose
Aluminum Compounds
Ferric Subsulfate

Consult also Chapter 45, page 815, for a more complete discussion of hemostatic agents.

Local Anesthetics

There are many local anesthetic agents and formulations at the disposal of the dentist (a number of which are used almost exclusively in dentistry, for example, Primacaine, Monocaine, Unacaine, and Ravocaine) which will be found to be suitable for practically every conceivable situation. Almost invariably the therapeutic index of these agents is extremely high.

The desirability of including a vasoconstrictor in all local anesthetic solutions for intraoral use, even for patients with cardiovascular disease, is now well established and has the endorsement of the American Heart Association. There appears to be no specific superiority amongst the various available vasoconstric-

tors, which include epinephrine, norepinephrine, and Nordefrin.

Although procaine long enjoyed a widespread popularity, in more recent years dentists have turned to other local anesthetics such as Xylocaine, Carbocaine, and Primacaine, found to be far more effective as anesthetic agents and, in general, as nontoxic as procaine. Other, but less commonly employed, local anesthetics include Monocaine, Unacaine, Ravocaine, and Oracaine.

Carbocaine, in a 3% solution without epinephrine, has been found to be an effective injectable local anesthetic which satisfactorily avoids the necessity for the use of a vasoconstrictor.

Citanest (prilocaine) enjoys considerable use as an injectable local anesthetic due to its well-documented effectiveness during extensive clinical trials.

Allergic reactions in dentists resulting from the constant handling of local anesthetics are not rare. These generally are local inflammatory reactions of the fingers or face. Allergic reactions are usually avoided when anesthetics of a chemical family other than that causing the reaction are substituted. The dentist therefore, enjoys a high degree of flexibility in the general use of injectable local anesthetics.

A wide variety of topical anesthetic formulations is also available for dental practice. It includes such agents as Pontocaine, Nupercaine, benzocaine, Butyn sulfate, Dyclone, and Pyribenzamine. Adequate and sometimes profound topical anesthesia can be obtained, particularly through the use of tetracaine and dibucaine, but these agents will not produce sufficient depth of anesthesia to permit the painless entry of a hypodermic needle past the superficial epithelial structures. Overdosage of tetracaine and dibucaine may cause hazardous consequences following systemic absorption through the mucosae. Spray formulations of tetracaine have been advocated, but such use intraorally should be discouraged. Benzocaine in high concentrations may produce an oral mucosal slough.

Ethyl chloride is occasionally employed as a spray, particularly for obtaining anesthesia prior to lancing a fluctuant and superficially located abscess. Ethyl chloride is also used in certain temporo-mandibular joint dysfunction states.

Benzocaine Solution

Ethyl Aminobenzoate	3 Gm
Propylene Glycol,	
To make	30 ml

Warm slightly if desired to hasten solution of the ethyl aminobenzoate. The solution may be colored if desired.

A topical anesthetic for application to the mucous membrane before inserting the needle. Apply and wait for 2 minutes.

Butacaine Sulfate Solution

Butacaine Sulfate	1.5 Gm
Purified Water, a sufficient quantity,	
To make	30 ml

Benzocaine Troches

Ethyl Aminobenzoate	0.75 Gm
Vanillin	0.03 Gm
Sucrose	8.00 Gm
Tragacanth	0.25 Gm
Carmine	0.01 Gm
Purified Water,	
To make	12 troches

A troche dissolved on the tongue is very useful in preventing gagging when impressions are being taken and similar operations are being performed.

A discussion of the following substances is included in ADR 1967:

Procaine Hydrochloride
Lidocaine
Lidocaine Hydrochloride
Mepivacaine Hydrochloride
Pyrrocaine Hydrochloride
Butethamine Hydrochloride
Metabutethamine Hydrochloride
Meprylcaine Hydrochloride
Isobucaine Hydrochloride
Tetracaine Hydrochloride
Propoxycaine Hydrochloride
Metabutoxycaine Hydrochloride
Benzocaine
Butacaine Sulfate
Naepaine
Chlorobutanol
Cocaine Hydrochloride
Ethyl Chloride

Consult also Chapter 59, page 1065, for a more complete discussion of anesthetic agents.

Vehicle-Protectants

Attempts to treat acute and chronic lesions of the oral mucous membranes (including chronic marginal gingivitis, the keratoses, desquamative stomatitis, recurrent ulcerative stomatitis, pemphigus, erythema multiforme, and drug eruptions) with topical medications have in the past been severely hampered by the difficulty in maintaining a medication at the site of application.

Orabase, an adhesive-vehicle protectant preparation, was designed especially for the purpose of retaining topically applied drugs on the oral mucous membranes. Studies with this preparation have indicated that it adheres to oral mucosal sites for periods varying from 15 minutes to 2 hours or longer, the duration depending on the degree of mobility of the oral tissues, the "washing action" of saliva, and the amount of vehicle applied.

Orabase, gelatin, pectin, carboxymethylcellulose, a mineral oil–polyethylene base—and the combination of these drugs, have been found to be free of deleterious, toxic, or allergenic properties.

Owing to its physical properties, which favor prolonged adherence, Orabase offers the following potential advantages over previously used vehicles: (1) increased contact–duration time of the tissues with the active component, (2) increased effectiveness of the active component by maintenance of higher concentration at the desired site, (3) decreased amount of an active material which need be applied at any one time, (4) decreased total dosage of active medication—highly desirable in many instances from a systemic-activity point of view, and (5) marked protective action.

Approximately 60 to 250 mg of the adhesive vehicle, with or without a therapeutic agent incorporated therein, is usually applied to the lesion site, in the form of a thin film, after meals and before retiring.

Further study of Orabase, however, has shown that its efficacy as a vehicle or protectant is somewhat limited. For example, erosions or ulcerations which are more than 2 cm in diameter cannot be easily or effectively coated with this vehicle. Still another problem is the inability to apply the paste to lesions in the less accessible areas of the mouth, such as the uvula, soft palate, anterior pillars, and the posterior tongue.

In an effort to overcome these problems, a powder adhesive-vehicle formulation has been prepared, using the same components as in Orabase except for the mineral oil–polyethylene base. This powder, Orahesive, is used and applied by a spray insufflator dispensing device, a No. 119 De Vilbiss spray atomizer.

Adhesion of this powder vehicle to the oral mucosae has also been found to be highly satisfactory. It has proved to be more effective than the paste for reaching less accessible oral lesions, since by properly manipulating the spray dispenser nearly every specific site of the oral cavity can be reached. The powder vehicle has proved to be advantageous in still another respect; ie, it can be applied evenly to as large an area as is indicated. Furthermore, the thinness of the film which is applied is easily controlled, of particular importance when the total dosage of active drug incorporated in the vehicle is best kept at minimal levels.

The therapeutic results obtained through the use of active drugs incorporated in the adhesive powder vehicle (Orahesive) parallel closely the results obtained from the use of the same drugs in equal concentrations prepared in the paste (Orabase).

An intraoral adhesive bandage (Orahesive bandage) is used as a protectant.

Long-lasting lozenges, having dissolution–duration times in the mouth of the order of several hours, are currently under detailed investigation representing a logical extension of the above principles to the topical and transmucosal administration of drugs.

Black currant glycerin pastilles are also used as a surface protectant. Tincture of benzoin compound, when properly applied by the dentist, also provides a soothing although transient coating.

Consult also Chapter 71, page 1316, for a more complete discussion of vehicle-protectants.

Sedatives and Hypnotics

Sedatives and hypnotics are widely employed in dental practice for purposes of decreasing anxiety, improving patient cooperation, lowering the level of reflex excitability, and facilitating postoperative sleep.

Barbiturates are frequently used for these purposes. The most commonly employed members of this family are sodium secobarbital, sodium pentobarbital, sodium amobarbital, and phenobarbital.

These are usually administered by mouth, but on occasion the dentist employs the intramuscular route. Intoxication with barbiturates is seldom a problem in dental practice, since the dosage prescribed and the period of administration are generally restricted.

Chloral hydrate is an excellent sedative–hypnotic but has not achieved widespread popularity in dentistry. Paraldehyde is rarely if ever used.

A discussion of the following substances is included in ADR 1967:

Phenobarbital
Sodium Phenobarbital
Amobarbital
Sodium Amobarbital
Sodium Pentobarbital
Pentobarbital
Calcium Pentobarbital
Secobarbital
Sodium Secobarbital
Hexobarbital
Sodium Thiopental
Sodium Methohexital
Promethazine Hydrochloride

Consult also Chapter 60, page 1077, for a more complete discussion of sedatives and hypnotics.

Stimulants

The dentist usually administers aromatic ammonia spirit by inhalation for the initial treatment of syncope. In severe cases of shock where collapse occurs, a differential diagnosis is obviously the essential initial procedure. Thereafter, management follows accepted medical emergency therapeutic techniques—matters beyond the scope of this section.

A discussion of the following substances is included in ADR 1967:

Oxygen
Aromatic Ammonia Spirit
Ammonium Carbonate
Caffeine
Caffeine and Sodium Benzoate

Consult also Chapter 65, page 1154, for a more complete discussion of stimulants.

Tranquilizers

Although the administration of a tranquilizer is most often under the direction of the physician, occasionally the dentist will prescribe one or another member of this group, particularly Phenergan.

The over-all usefulness of Phenergan, both as an antihistaminic and tranquilizer, has been previously noted. In dentistry, meprobamate is probably the most widely utilized of the minor tranquilizers, and has been described as being effective for dental and oral indications when employed in adequate dosages for suitable periods of time. Both Librium and Valium would seem worthy of equivalent usage in these areas.

Chlorpromazine is rarely administered by dentists. Promazine, prochlorperazine, perphenazine, and triflupromazine are even less frequently employed. The prolonged time required for the onset of action of the rauwolfia alkaloids has made their role in dental therapeutics of minimal importance.

When considering the over-all usefulness and applicability of tranquilizers to oral pharmacotherapeutics, the dentist must consider the following questions: (1) are tranquilizers really effective for office use, (2) when indicated, how reliable are they, (3) from a time standpoint, are they practical, (4) how long does the tranquilizer remain effective, and what are the hazards to the patient after leaving the office, (5) are changes required in the choice or dosage of agents which are concomitantly employed for the management of oral and allied disease states, (6) does a useful response necessitate a large dose?

Over-all, the desirability of using the tranquilizers in routine oral pharmacotherapeutics remains in considerable doubt.

Consult also Chapter 62, page 1104, for a more complete discussion of tranquilizers.

Vitamins

Dentists frequently prescribe vitamins. The mouth may be the initial site of signs of vitamin deficiency. Since the clinical features are nonspecific, the dentist may even prescribe vitamins as a diagnostic procedure.

Although the multivitamin approach to deficiency states is usually favored, there are instances wherein single vitamins or restricted vitamin formulations are utilized in dentistry. For example, high dosages of vitamin A have been employed in the treatment of certain keratotic diseases of oral mucosal surfaces with some therapeutic success. Vi-Dom-A lozenges in dosages of up to 600,000 units per day have been found to be of some value when allowed to dissolve at the site of the oral lesion, followed by swallowing of the resultant "solution." Such therapy is *never* employed where the possibility of a true leukoplakia or malignancy has not been ruled out conclusively by a suitable biopsy procedure except when the patient refuses *all* other forms of therapy (including the biopsy). It is conjectured that the vitamin A in such instances may manifest a pharmacodynamic action other than that attributable to its being a vitamin.

The following substances are listed in ADR 1967:

Vitamin A
Oleovitamin A
Cod Liver Oil
Calciferol
Activated 7-dehydrocholesterol
Synthetic Oleovitamin D
Vitamin B Complex
Thiamine Hydrochloride
Nicotinic Acid
Nicotinamide
Riboflavin
Folic Acid
Cyanocobalamin
Pantothenic Acid
Pyridoxine hydrochloride
Biotin
Choline
Inositol
Vitamin C
Vitamin E
Vitamin K
Vitamin mixtures

Consult also Chapter 56, page 1011, for a more complete discussion of vitamins.

Other Remedies for Local Application

While the consultative function of the pharmacist is important, it is his ability to undertake the formulation of individualized dental preparations that particularly distinguishes him. There are many sources of formulas available. A number of articles on dental formulas have been published in the *Journal of the American Pharmaceutical Association* by various authors. *Accepted Dental Remedies*[5a] is another good source and one which has official backing. *Dental Formulas*[5b] is a rich source of formulas which can be used as such or as points of departure for making improvements. Standard texts in dental pharmacology and operative dentistry and reference books in dental materials also frequently contain formulas. Lastly, professional and research periodicals in dentistry and pharmacy may be consulted.

The more frequently used dental preparations can often be supplied by dental supply houses at less cost than the pharmacist can make them. Nevertheless, the pharmacist can still provide a real service by compounding those preparations which are less readily available. Furthermore, the dentist, upon consultation, often may wish a modified preparation which gives better penetration, is more adhesive, has greater stability, or possesses some other property not available in the original product to the desired degree.

Many of the medicines used in dental practice, especially those dissolved in volatile solvents, should be dispensed in quantities not greater than one ounce, since they are used in very small amounts.

The formulas which follow are not to be considered the ideal, necessarily. Rather they are to be considered prototypes and representative of dental preparations which have been and are used in practice.

Dental Caries Prophylactic Materials

Topical Fluoride Solution

Sodium Fluoride............................	2 Gm
Purified Water,	
To make..................................	100 ml

It is important to use a good quality of sodium fluoride. In general the USP reagent grade is satisfactory. ADR lists acceptable brands. The solution should be stored in Plax (plastic), paraffin-lined, or Pyrex bottles. It may be supplied to dentists in quantities of 100 ml or less in ordinary pharmaceutical glass bottles, since such amounts will be used up within a few months in the ordinary course of dental practice. The sodium fluoride reacts with ordinary glass at a slow but appreciable rate. The reaction may result in the formation of sediment, but does not decrease the sodium fluoride content of the solution significantly. The preparation should be dispensed for office use only, and should bear a "poison" label.

Tablets, each consisting of pure sodium fluoride in quantity sufficient to make 2 ml of topical fluoride solution, are available commercially. Their use permits the extemporaneous preparation of fresh solution.

Stannous fluoride 8% is being used with greatly increased frequency.

Desensitizers for Dentin

The following preparations tend to decrease hypersensitivity of teeth when applied to their outer surface, especially where erosion has occurred near the gum line:

Ammoniacal Silver Nitrate Solution
Formaldehyde Solution
Liquefied Phenol
Zinc Chloride, 80% Solution
Sodium Fluoride Paste

Sodium Fluoride Powder......................	10 Gm
Kaolin.....................................	10 Gm
Glycerin...................................	10 Gm
To make a paste.	

Add more or less glycerin as needed to make a smooth but rather stiff paste.

Thermodent toothpaste is not infrequently prescribed.

Cavity Liners (Varnishes)

Cavity liners or varnishes are used in the dental office to seal the dental tubuli in deep-seated cavities so as to protect the pulp from acid-containing dental cements. Cavity-lining preparations which depend solely upon the development of a film intended to be impervious to aqueous acid are believed to be inadequate because of the difficulty in maintaining the integrity of the film under filling conditions. Cavity liner preparations should be kept in a tightly stoppered bottle to prevent undue evaporation of solvent. The following preparations may be of limited usefulness:

Copal Varnish

Copal.....................................	5 Gm
Chloroform................................	100 ml

Powder the copal mix with 5 Gm of dry washed sand, place in a flask, add the chloroform, and shake occasionally during at least 24 hours, frequently breaking up the gummy mass to facilitate extraction. Filter, and add chloroform to make 100 ml. If necessary, add 5 Gm of purified talc and again filter.

Mastic Varnish

Mastic....................................	30 Gm
Peruvian Balsam............................	30 ml
Chloroform, a sufficient quantity,	
To make...................................	100 ml

Dissolve the mastic and Peruvian balsam in about 50 ml of chloroform and add sufficient chloroform to make 100 ml.

Rosin Varnish

I

Rosin, fragments...........................	7 Gm
Chloroform.................................	100 ml

Make a solution.

II

Rosin.....................................	6.7 Gm
Sodium Carbonate, Monohydrate............	1.7 Gm
Acetone...................................	100 ml

Mix. Do not filter.

Several commercial preparations are available which utilize the chemical effect of calcium hydroxide for neutralizing the acid derived from acid dental cements. These are stated to contain various percentages of calcium hydroxide suspended in aqueous methylcellulose solution. A brand of calcium hydroxide paste produced by Rower Dental Manufacturing Co., Boston 16, Mass., is called *Pulpdent Paste* and is stated to contain 48.6% calcium hydroxide suspended in an aqueous methylcellulose solution. *Pulpdent Liquid* contains 8.7% calcium hydroxide in the same vehicle.

Pulp Cappings or Temporary Cements

Zinc Oxide and Eugenol Cement

Make a thick, putty-like paste of zinc oxide and eugenol. Protect from air and moisture. The zinc oxide and eugenol are supplied separately.

Zinc Oxide and Thymol Cement

Zinc Oxide.................................	67 Gm
Thymol....................................	33 Gm

Melt the thymol in a porcelain evaporating dish on a water bath. Add the zinc oxide and rub the mixture to a smooth paste. Spread in a thin layer over the dish and cool. Break into small pieces and keep in a well-closed container.

Calcium Hydroxide Paste

Disinfectants for Root Canals

Chloroazodin Solution
Creosote
Formocresol
Camphorated Parachlorophenol

Disinfectants for Instruments

Chemical disinfectants which are safe and practical for use on dental instruments will usually not kill all bacterial spores, including those of pathogens. Many of them will not kill *Mycobacterium tuberculosis*. In addition, chemical agents may in one concentration kill bacteria and in another dilution, or under a different set of conditions, merely inhibit or perhaps even stimulate bacterial growth. The Council on Dental Therapeutics of the American Dental Association strongly discourages the use of chemical solutions for the disinfection of dental instruments which might be contaminated with a *hepatitis virus* since there have been reports of many well-documented cases of *viral hepatitis* following the use of nonsterile injection needles or syringes, or other instruments contaminated with blood containing the virus of serum or infectious hepatitis. There is no evidence that chemical solutions will destroy these viruses.

Recognizing these and numerous other limitations of chemical solutions, the following are presented for limited use:

Benzalkonium Chloride Solution 1:1000
Benzethonium Chloride Solution 1:1000
Metaphen Disinfecting Solution
Saponated Cresol Solution

Denture Preparations

Denture Adherent Powder

Tragacanth, fine powder	75	Gm
Sterculia Gum, fine powder	25	Gm
Sassafras Oil	1.5	ml

Mix. To be sprinkled sparingly on the denture before placing it in the mouth. Powdered gum tragacanth alone will serve as well. but its flavor may not be as pleasant.

Adherent powders which are used in connection with denture service are made from finely powdered gums such as karaya, acacia or tragacanth as well as

other newly introduced materials. These materials swell to many times their original volume on the addition of water and assume mucilaginous or gelatinous properties. The powders are prepared by mixing several of the gums or by the use of one alone. They may be flavored with suitable volatile oils and may contain antiseptic agents as well.

Denture Cleanser

Trisodium Phosphate	120	Gm
Cinnamon Oil	0.30	ml
Amaranth Solution	2	ml

Mix. Dissolve ¼ teaspoonful in half a glass of water and use with a brush.

Note—The cellulose acetate type of denture is decomposed by alkaline substances. Phenol-formaldehyde and acrylic types withstand most chemical agents.

Formulas Used in General Practice

Abrasives

These preparations are used by the dentist in cleaning and polishing teeth. They are not suitable for use by the laity, since they may be entirely too harsh for continued or unsupervised use.

Paste Abrasive

I

Pumice, in very fine powder	40	Gm
Methyl Salicylate	1	ml
Amaranth Solution	2	ml
Starch Glycerite	60	Gm
To make about	100	Gm

The amaranth provides a pink color which disguises the color of blood, and the starch glycerite base gives a product which clings well to the brush.

II

Pumice, in very fine powder	61.8	Gm
Sodium Borate	10.8	Gm
Carmine	0.1	Gm
Glycerin	27.2	ml
Spearmint Oil	0.1	ml
To make about	100	Gm

Mix the glycerin and carmine with the sodium borate and add the pumice a little at a time. The final consistency may be adjusted by the addition of further amounts of pumice or glycerin.

Powder Abrasive

Pumice, in very fine powder	80	Gm
Starch	16	Gm
Methyl Salicylate	4	ml
Carmine	0.3	Gm
To make about	100	Gm

For office use only. May be dispensed in capsules, each to contain about 1.5 Gm for convenience in the treatment of the individual patient. Contents of one or more capsules used as an *abrasive*. After removing contents of capsule, add a small quantity of water or glycerin to powder before use.

Dentifrices

A dentifrice is a substance used with a toothbrush for the purpose of cleaning the accessible surfaces of the teeth. Commercial dentifrices are available in the form of pastes and powders.

Many dentifrices contain flavors and soap or synthetic detergents. The powders and pastes contain abrasives such as calcium carbonate, one or more of

the calcium phosphates, calcium sulfate, insoluble sodium metaphosphate, hydrated aluminum oxide, magnesium carbonates and phosphates, sodium bicarbonate and sodium chloride. Tooth pastes contain liquids such as glycerin, propylene glycol, sorbitol solution, water, and alcohol, and thickeners such as starch, tragacanth, algin, and cellulose derivatives. Dentifrices usually contain noncarbohydrate sweetening agents, but a few contain sugar.

It has been shown that individuals vary markedly in their need for an abrasive in dentifrice. Generally speaking, commercial dentifrice powders are more abrasive than pastes. Some individuals who require only a slight degree of abrasion to keep the teeth from staining may find that a mixture of baking soda and finely powdered table salt is satisfactory. Others may require a more abrasive substance, but the Council on Dental Therapeutics of the American Dental Association maintains that there is no valid reason for the use of a dentifrice with a greater abrasiveness than necessary to prevent residual accumulations on the teeth.

The primary purpose of a dentifrice is to assist the toothbrush in cleaning the teeth. This cleansing process of brushing *per se*, with or without a dentifrice, is beneficial to dental health.

There is a continuing effort to obtain additional dental benefits from dentifrices through the inclusion of agents designed to have some specific biological or therapeutic action. For the most part, when such dentifrices are employed as adjuncts to supervised toothbrushing in controlled clinical investigations, their superiority over conventional dentifrices has not been clearly established. Among such dentifrices are those which are claimed to "remineralize" the tooth substance, those which include urea and dibasic ammonium phosphate in their formulas, penicillin dentifrices, foaming agents, and others which have been promoted as "antienzyme" and "antibacterial" agents. In most of these instances, the Council has indicated that more extensive evidence will be required for an accurate evaluation of the claims made by the various manufacturers. *Accepted Dental Remedies*, 1964, discusses this subject in considerable detail and gives references to several source materials.

In 1960 a dentifrice containing stannous fluoride was approved by the Council as a result of controlled studies in which its usefulness as an anticaries agent was demonstrated. This dentifrice is said to contain

0.4% stannous fluoride, 39% calcium pyrophosphate, 30% glycerin, 1.0% stannous pyrophosphate, 4.63% miscellaneous agents, and 24.97% water. It is marketed under the tradename Crest (*Proctor & Gamble*). More recently, Cue (*Colgate*) and Fact (*Bristol-Myers*) have been granted Council acceptance.

Liquid Dentifrice

Hard Soap, powdered	60 Gm
Saccharin	2 Gm
Amaranth Solution	10 ml
Cinnamon Oil	5 ml
Peppermint Oil	5 ml
Clove Oil	10 ml
Alcohol	750 ml
Purified Water, a sufficient quantity,	
To make	1000 ml

Dissolve the soap, the saccharin, and the oils in the alcohol; add the amaranth solution and sufficient water to make 1000 ml. Sprinkle on the moistened toothbrush and use as a dentifrice.

Dentifrice NF XI

[Dentifricum NF; NF Tooth Powder]

Hard Soap, in fine powder	50 Gm
Precipitated Calcium Carbonate	935 Gm
Saccharin Sodium	2 Gm
Peppermint Oil	4 ml
Cinnamon Oil	2 ml
Methyl Salicylate	8 ml
To make about	1000 Gm

Thoroughly triturate the saccharin sodium, the oils, and the methyl salicylate with about one-half of the precipitated calcium carbonate, and mix the soap with the remainder of the precipitated calcium carbonate. Mix the two powders thoroughly, and pass through a fine sieve.

Uses—This is a basic powder used only as a general cleanser. It is not medicated but it forms a splendid vehicle for medication, eg, with sodium perborate or astringent substances.

Oxidizing, astringent, and alkaline qualities may be provided by additions as may be indicated. Only ingredients listed in ADR should be used. In selecting abrasives, eg, calcium carbonate or calcium phosphate, it is safer to use brands and grades listed in ADR since others may be unduly harsh.

Paste Dentifrice

CMC 120 H	0.9 Gm
Glycerin	1.0 Gm
Propylene Glycol	18.0 Gm
Purified Water	13.5 Gm
Methyl Paraben	0.1 Gm
Saccharin Sodium Solution 50%	0.1 Gm
Peppermint Oil	0.3 Gm
Mineral Oil	1.0 Gm
Sodium Lauryl Sulfate	2.5 Gm
Dicalcium Phosphate, in very fine powder	54.0 Gm

Mouth Washes

Dental and medical dictionaries in general define a mouth wash as a medicated liquid used for cleansing the mouth or treating diseased states of the oral mucous membranes. Unfortunately, advertisers attempt to imply wider uses for many such products. *Accepted Dental Remedies* questions the use of the term "antiseptic" in connection with mouth washes and states that the only legitimate use of a mouth wash for the general public is as an adjunct in the toilet of the mouth. Claims that certain mouth washes overcome mouth odors should be viewed with reserve. Most persistent abnormal mouth odors must be recognized as symptoms of diseases or detritus in the mouth, nose, sinuses, chest, or intestinal tract. The elimination of these symptoms

cannot be accomplished by the use of a mouth wash. Neither does it appear that odors arising from certain ingested foods can be eliminated by this means. In dental practice mouth washes may be employed as a part of postoperative treatment, and during the course of certain operative procedures—when such use adds to the comfort or oral hygiene of the patient.

In addition to the preparations which are formulated below, the following solutions are frequently employed as mouth rinses: Sodium Chloride Solution USP (page 843), Mouthwash NF XII, Antiseptic Solution NF XII, Compound Sodium Borate Solution NF XI, and sodium bicarbonate solution (2%).

Peppermint Mouth Rinse

Peppermint Spirit	43.20 ml
Saccharin Sodium	0.07 Gm
Purified Water,	
To make	240 ml

Hypertonic Saline Mouth Rinse

Sodium Chloride	2 Gm
Purified Water,	
To make	100 ml

Alkaline Saline Mouth Rinse

Sodium Chloride	2 Gm
Sodium Bicarbonate	1 Gm
Amaranth Solution	2 ml
Peppermint Water,	
To make	240 ml

Saline Mouth Rinse Powder

Calcium Oxide	2 Gm
Phenolphthalein	0.1 Gm
Saccharin Sodium	0.3 Gm
Cinnamon Oil	0.5 Gm
Sodium Chloride,	
To make	100 Gm

Mix thoroughly. The calcium oxide and the phenolphthalein produce a pink color in the product. Use ¼ teaspoonful to a cup of warm water as a mouth wash.

Irrigation Solutions for Exodontia

The dental surgeon employs Sodium Chloride Solution USP (page 843) as an irrigating solution.

Alveolar Analgesics

Several formulas are given below for liquids and pastes to be employed by the dental surgeon for the symptomatic relief of pain arising from postextraction alveolitis, commonly called "dry socket."

Compound Acetylsalicylic Acid Paste

Ethyl Aminobenzoate Ointment
Benzocaine Paste

Ethyl Aminobenzoate	3 Gm
Clove Oil	3 Gm
Hydrous Wool Fat	12 Gm
Yellow Wax	15 Gm
Petrolatum	15 Gm

Mix the last three ingredients together on a water bath, and then add the benzocaine and clove oil with stirring.

Benzocaine-Guaiacol Solution

Ethyl Aminobenzoate	3 Gm
Guaiacol	3 Gm
Peruvian Balsam	9 Gm

Triturate the benzocaine with the guaiacol to form a smooth paste and then incorporate the Peruvian balsam.

Other formulations include:

Liquids

1. Guaiacol and glycerin, equal parts
2. Chlorobutanol, 25 Gm
   Clove oil to make 100 ml

Pastes

1. Ethylaminobenzoate, 750 mg
   Petrolatum to make 15.00 Gm
2. Ethylaminobenzoate, 1.5 Gm
   Chlorobutanol, 1.5 Gm

Methyl salicylate, 5 drops
Petrolatum or lanolin to make 30.0 Gm

References

1. Kutscher, A. H., *et al*, *Pharmacotherapeutics of Oral Disease*, McGraw Hill, New York, 1964.
2. Burket, L. W., *Oral Medicine*, Lippincott, Philadelphia, 1961.
3. Bernier, J. L., *The Management of Oral Disease*, Mosby, St. Louis, 1959.
4. Shafer, W. G., *et al*, *A Textbook of Oral Pathology*, Saunders, Philadelphia, 1963.
5. (a) *Accepted Dental Therapeutics*, 29th ed, American Dental Association, 1964; (b) Grossman, L. I., *Dental Formulas*.
6. Dobbs, E. C., *Pharmacology and Oral Therapeutics*, Mosby, St. Louis, 1961.
7. Dille, J. M., *Drug Therapy for Dentists*, Year Book, Chicago, 1963.
8. Francis, L. E., and Wood, D. R., *Dental Pharmacology and Therapeutics*, Saunders, Philadelphia, 1961.

This chapter was prepared by

Richard A. Huebner, VMD, *Director, Veterinary Service, Wyeth Laboratories,*
Philadelphia, Pa. 19101

The interprofessional relationship between the pharmacist and the veterinarian should be close to provide the optimum in effectiveness for both. Cognizance of the veterinary medical profession and its responsibilities is helpful to the pharmacist who, not unusually, serves as confidante, adviser, and source of medical reference knowledge for the lay community.

The practicing pharmacist is expected to be completely familiar not only with the general medical circumstances and the local physicians but also with all aspects of public health in order that the best interests of the community may be served. Ever more frequently, aspects of animal medicine are intermingled with other considerations of the public benefit.

Since the end of World War II, the activities and responsibilities assigned to and accepted by the veterinary medical profession have recast the earlier "animal doctor" image. Today's veterinarians, in a multiplicity of operations, function as qualified members of the "health team."

Veterinary Medicine

The domestication of man's animals constitute one of the greatest and farthest-reaching advances in civilization. However, only too infrequently has humankind considered its obligations to the animals lower on the evolutionary scale who are sacrificed to provide food, clothing, and medicinal products; who, during their lives, serve as laborers in our work, participants in our sports, performers in our spectacles, companions in our relaxation, supporters in our friendlessness, protectors in war, guardians in peace, and helpful contributors to our medical knowledge.

The optimum husbandry of animals and their medical care, therefore, is necessary not only for their benefit but also for our own selfish purposes. In many instances in past civilizations, illness in animals received more attention than that given to human beings. Unquestionably, the economics of the circumstances were among the deciding factors, for a good ox often was valued more highly than an ordinary human being.

History—The earliest mention of man's interest in the welfare of his beasts of burden appears in the *Assyrian Code of Hammurabi*, prepared in Babylon about 2100 B.C. The possible relationship to religion is an intriguing speculation, for the Assyrians worshiped gods who were half animal. The code includes a regulatory system for the breeding of animals, the treatment of their diseases, and the fees for the work performed.

The Mosaic doctrines on clean and unclean flesh are considered the first recorded evidence of systematic meat inspection to protect human health. The restrictions established by Moses are understandable when it is considered that the insanitary hog lot may serve as a source of not only tapeworm and trichina infestation but also of tuberculosis, erysipelas, salmonella, and pasteurella infections. Oyster beds contaminated with human excrement are excellent carriers of typhoid fever. The menace of cysticerci and other infestations and infections among pastoral people before the days of the toilet may well be imagined.

The flocks and herds of the Egyptians were completely wiped out by the "Fifth Plague" in 1451 B.C., while those of the Israelites escaped. Divine displeasure against Pharaoh IV, enemy of the favored people, is the Biblical explanation. However, Moses practiced simple rules of livestock sanitation typical of his understanding and knowledge of hygiene, while Pharaoh IV, King of Egypt, maintained a miserable animal industry, characteristic of those dynasties that gradually brought that nation to inevitable extermination.

The maintenance of corps of serviceable animals for military purposes also provided a motivating factor. Xenophon, the Greek historian and soldier (430–355 B.C.), was the first military veterinarian. He commanded the "Ten Thousand" Greek troops in their retreat from the Tigris and Euphrates rivers to the Black Sea after the termination of the Peloponnesian War (400 B.C.). Apsyrtus (*circa* 300–350 A.D.) served as veterinary officer in the cavalry of Constantine the Great in Asia Minor; in addition to veterinary service he instructed the officers and cavalrymen in animal husbandry and sanitation.

Education—Imprisoned with all other sciences during the dark ages, veterinary medicine escaped from its chains during the 18th century. Actually, the military requirements and the demands of army commanders were essential factors in the establishment of recognized veterinary schools in various parts of Europe, beginning in 1761 with the Royal Veterinary School of Lyons, France. Between 1769 and 1842 many veterinary schools were founded in various countries on the continent and in Great Britain.

In colonial America livestock were important in everyday life but there was no veterinary profession—nor was the need for one recognized. Wastes from animal slaughter, dead animals, excrement, and garbage cluttered the towns; swine and dogs roamed unrestricted. Meat from diseased animals and spoiled or fly-blown food products were common in the markets.

Dr. Benjamin Rush—a prominent Philadelphia physician and one of the signers of the Declaration of Independence—urged the establishment of a veterinary department at the University of Pennsylvania in 1806, but only discussion resulted.

America's earliest legally organized veterinary

schools were founded between 1850 and 1860 in Philadelphia, Boston, and New York. The first successful school on the North American continent was the Ontario Veterinary College in Toronto, established in 1862. The New York College of Veterinary Surgery (1864), the Montreal Veterinary College (1866), and Iowa State College (1879) followed in succession.

American Veterinary Medical Association (AVMA)—Veterinarians soon recognized the need for a professional association. Although early attempts at organization failed, the United States Veterinary Medical Association was formed in 1859 and first met in 1863. In 1898 the Association's name was changed to American Veterinary Medical Association.

The AVMA today, as the national representative of the profession, makes its headquarters at 600 S. Michigan Ave., Chicago, Ill. 60605. Of the total of approximately 21,650 veterinarians in the US and its territories, 18,581 are members of the AVMA. The organization's membership in Canada is about 570 and in foreign countries about 230.

As constituents of the AVMA, each of the states and US territories, and the Canadian provinces, has its own Veterinary Medical Association; these associations, in turn, may be supplemented by local associations depending on the size of each smaller area itself.

The AVMA has been active in improving veterinary education and in raising the standard requirements for the schools and for the admission of their students. Through 1967 the AVMA Council on Education accredited 21 schools of veterinary medicine (18 in the US and 3 in Canada). A list of these institutions and additional information on each may be obtained from the AVMA.

Postgraduate Education—Opportunities for graduate work (leading to MS or PhD degrees) are currently available at ten US veterinary medical schools. Several institutions accredited by the American Public Health Association (APHA) to give the degree of Master of Public Health, Doctor of Public Health, and Master of Public Health Education (other than the MPH) accept veterinarians to degree courses.

Continuing Education—From a continuing education standpoint one of the most significant functions of the AVMA is its annual national meeting. Professional intercourse in veterinary medical knowledge has not remained continental, however. The first International Veterinary Congress was held in 1863 in Hamburg, Germany, primarily to discuss the threats of animal disease plagues and their distribution at that time; the most recent Congress (18th) was held in 1967 in Paris. The first Pan American Congress of Veterinary Medicine was held in 1951 in Lima, Peru; the most recent Congress (5th) was held in 1966 in Caracas, Venezuela.

Licensure—Each state and each Canadian province has its own Veterinary Practice Act with which the applicant must comply in order to be granted licensure for the practice of veterinary medicine. In general, submission of appropriate credentials is required and a fee is charged for admission to the examination. Annual registration and citizenship requirements vary with the individual state; reciprocity between the states is the exception.

In 1950 the National Board of Veterinary Medical Examiners was organized, under the sponsorship of the AVMA, to help provide state examining boards with an objective and comprehensive examination for use in place of the usual essay type of examination. Use of the objective examination does not affect the control of licensure by the state boards, who may add such additional oral or practical tests as they deem necessary. Under the advice of the National Board, this examination is prepared and graded by the Professional Examination Service of the American Public Health Association, 1790 Broadway, New York, N.Y. 10019. During 1964, 26 state licensing boards used this examination service for 1170 candidates, and its acceptance continues to widen.

Responsibilities—The primary responsibilities of veterinarians encompass all aspects of the welfare of animals and products harvested or prepared from their bodies, their secretions, or excretions for human food, clothing, or medication. In addition, these obligations continually involve the extrapolation and application of specialized veterinary medical knowledge and information on animal diseases to human diseases.

A measure of the veterinarian's responsibility may be found in US Department of Agriculture reports in the total number of livestock and poultry, on farms and ranches only, as of Jan. 1, 1968: 650,883,000 (valued at $22,766,460,000).

To this number should be added an estimated dog population of approximately 27,500,000 and cats numbering about 29,000,000, of inestimable dollar value because of the sentiment involved. It is readily understandable, then, that the burden of responsibility on veterinary practitioners is enormous.

The Future—To provide the maximum benefit for humankind, the cooperation of and coordination among the many members of the health team must continue to grow and to mature. Although their activities and limits seemed clearly defined and disparate only a generation ago, now the physician, the pharmacist, the nurse, the dentist, the veterinarian, together with all of their supporting personnel, must function as an articulated accumulation of abilities.

The medical knowledge gathered over the past 50 years, with its tantalizing glimpses of potential further progress, has overwhelmed our individual limited mental capacities. The generalist no longer is fully effective and, within each profession, specialization becomes more and more necessary. Because this text is brief, only a few veterinary medical specialties are mentioned under *Activities of Veterinarians*, below; the AVMA Directory lists 33 classifications.

Intense and detailed application to a restricted area of effort improves and burnishes performances but brings the risk of parochialism. It is imperative, therefore, that intra- and interprofessional communications and associations continue to be nurtured and to expand so that each may see with another's eyes.

The obligation of all of medical science is to contribute positively to the general health of mankind. This immense responsibility must be met collectively if it is to be met effectively. Past performance supports the expectation that the veterinary medical profession will respond to fulfill its share of the assignment.

Activities of Veterinarians

The current scope of veterinary medicine includes not only the prevention and treatment of animal diseases as such but also embraces the public health. Within this widely inclusive field each veterinarian must be a specialist within one of such broad groups as:

veterinary medical practitioners, veterinarians in public health and/or service, and veterinarians in industry.

Veterinary Medical Practitioners

The practitioners of veterinary medicine currently number about 14,000 in the US. They may be subdivided into the following categories:

1. The General Practitioner—whose practice includes all species of animals.
2. The Large Animal Practitioner
   a. The General Large Animal Practitioner—who treats all animals other than pet animals and fowl
   b. The Special Practitioner, Bovine
   c. The Special Practitioner, Equine
   d. The Special Practitioner, Porcine
3. The Small Animal Practitioner—whose practice is devoted primarily to the medical and surgical treatment of dogs and cats but usually includes small pet birds (canaries, parakeets)
4. The Special Practitioner, Avian—usually associated with a teaching and/or service facility or devoted to commercial poultry production
5. The Special Practitioner, Zoological Gardens Inhabitants
6. The Special Practitioner, Fur-Bearing Animals (mink, chinchillas, skunks, etc)
7. The Special Practitioner, Laboratory Animal Medicine

Veterinarians in Public Health and/or Service

The roles of veterinarians grouped in this widely inclusive category are exerted in broad fields embracing many disciplines.

There are more than 100 animal diseases transmissible to man; periodically new ones are recognized. For many of them, such as brucellosis and rabies, the eradication or control of the disease in animals is the only known means of eliminating human infection.

Some diseases of animals are contracted from man and in turn are transmitted back to man (eg, milkborne septic sore throat). Many diseases are spread from animal to animal and ultimately to man by arthropod vectors. Others are contracted by human beings either through direct contact or by consumption of meat and food products of animal origin; in the broad sense this includes not only specific transmissible diseases but also changes that may occur during the processing and storage of food products sufficient to cause adverse effects on the consumer.

Federal Government Service—The activities of veterinarians in the many branches of government service vary markedly with each agency's responsibilities but, in general, their work is oriented towards animal diseases transmissible to man, to instances where specialized veterinary medical knowledge and information on animal diseases (naturally occurring or artificially induced) is extrapolative or applicable to human diseases, and to communal economic interests.

It is readily understandable, therefore, that under such broad concepts many types of efforts that may seem individually and separately disparate are found to relate one to the other and to the whole.

Especially during the last 20 years the broadening embrace of government activities, the widening of each department's responsibilities, and the creation of new agencies of vigorous growth and of extending functions have intensified their requirements for veterinarians.

Within the federal government veterinarians are utilized in the following areas (numbers in parentheses):

US Department of Agriculture (925)
  Agricultural Research Service
    Animal Disease and Parasite Research Division
    Animal Health Division
    Veterinary Biologics Division

Consumer and Marketing Service (1416)
    Livestock Slaughter Inspection Division
    Processed Meat Inspection Division
    Poultry Division
    Technical Services Division
  Federal Extension Service (67)
US Department of Health, Education and Welfare
  Food and Drug Administration, Bureau of Veterinary Medicine (47)
    Division of Veterinary Medical Review
    Division of Veterinary New Drugs
    Division of Veterinary Research
  Public Health Service, Veterinary Public Health Branch (115)
US Department of Defense
  Department of the Army, Veterinary Corps (576)
  Department of the Air Force, Veterinary Corps (400)

State, County, and Municipal Government Service—The individual state, county, and municipal governments place varying requirements on their local veterinary public health services but, on the whole, their functions are generally similar to and intermeshed with those of the Federal government. Particularly is this true in the case of meat inspection where these governments control local animal slaughter and examination and in the control of animal diseases transmissible to man.

Each state has its own market milk control laws and its own cooperative agreement with the Federal government for the control of tuberculosis and brucellosis in cattle. Veterinarians are involved in implementing these ordinances.

Veterinarians in Industry

The recent emergence of the specialty of laboratory animal medicine is additional evidence that the veterinarian's role is changing.

Enactment of Public Law 89-544, the *Laboratory Animal Welfare Act* (US Congress, 1966), recognized its importance by requiring that "Programs of disease control and prevention, euthanasia, and adequate veterinary care shall be established and maintained under the supervision and assistance of a doctor of veterinary medicine."

Specifications for the humane handling, care, treatment, and transportation of dogs, cats, guinea pigs, rabbits, hamsters, and nonhuman primates held by dealers or in research facilities have been promulgated by the US Department of Agriculture, whose Animal Health Division (this page) has been charged with enforcement of the law. Additional legislation is pending.

About 500 veterinarians are engaged in laboratory animal medicine on a full- or part-time basis, serving not only commercial laboratory enterprises but also human hospitals and diagnostic laboratories, charitable organizations and foundations, teaching institutions, and government functions (see *Veterinarians in Public Health and/or Service*, this page).

There are about 800 "industrial veterinarians" in the US associated fully with commercial enterprises. The type of industry in which the employing corporation is engaged is the deciding factor, of course, on individual responsibilities which vary, too, between the specific companies within each commercial group.

Animal Diseases

The many species of animals maintained under domestication or confinement complicate the difficulties of disease identification and control. Some infectious diseases affect but a single animal species; others affect two or more—and, of the latter, one may be man. Some are readily transmissible by direct or indirect contact, others are transferable only under direct and unique circumstances (eg, rabies through bite wounds), and still others require an intermediate host in whose body the attacking organism must undergo developmental change to reach its pathogenic potential for the definitive victim (eg, Rickettsia of typhus in fleas and lice).

Transmission

The practitioner of veterinary medicine is deeply involved in maintaining public health, especially in preventing the transfer of diseases from animals to man, either directly or via insects acting as carriers of organisms. However, an important aspect commonly overlooked is that man may transmit some of his diseases to animals, either directly or via insects. Insects may act as hosts and transmit to men or animals the diseases which they carry or they can bite infected men or animals—often withdrawing the infection—and transmit it to other men or animals by means of subsequent bites.

Transmission of pathogenic organisms by all routes is especially important to the veterinarian since it is essential that the source of infection be determined to avoid reinfection of his animal patients and to prevent further spread of the disease.

Examples of diseases transmitted from man to domestic animals are:

1. *Tuberculosis*, with few exceptions, occurs in dogs and cats as a result of their continued exposure to, or association with, cases of open tuberculosis in the human family. Tuberculosis may occur in cattle as a result of continued exposure to an infected human being.
2. *Variola* (pox) may occur in cattle as a result of association with children recently vaccinated. In the US today this may be considered one of the more important origins of outbreaks of pox in cattle.
3. *Ringworm* in the human family is readily transferable to cats, monkeys, dogs, and cattle.
4. *Scabies* (sarcoptic mange) is easily spread from infected humans to pets and other domesticated animals.

Types

Veterinarians, particularly those engaged in public health work, are concerned with animal infections capable of occurring in many different hosts and in man. As previously mentioned, although the list is extensive, many occur very rarely and others are of minor importance. The more important ones which have occurred in the US are presented here.

Diseases Transmitted by Direct Contact with Living Animals

Virus Diseases

Rabies—Occurs from bites of dogs, cats, and wild carnivores. Canine vaccination with modern vaccines is both safe and effective.

Psittacosis and Ornithosis—Psittacosis occurs in birds belonging to the parrot family, principally parrots and parakeets. The disease in nonpsittacine birds is called ornithosis and occurs mainly in pigeons. For man, the virus derived from the psittacine species is generally the more virulent. The syndrome in man is a severe atypical pneumonia with a high death rate.

Cowpox—True cowpox is now rare or nonexistent in the United States and those parts of the world where smallpox is controlled by vaccination. Recently vaccinated persons may infect herds of cattle during the milking process.

Newcastle Disease, a common respiratory disease of poultry, appears in man as an acute conjunctivitis which disappears in a few days leaving no sequelae. In children the disease may be more severe; parotitis may develop.

Infectious Ecthyma, a virus disease of sheep, also known as "sore mouth," is prevalent in many western states. Hot painful swelling frequently appears on the hands and faces of persons handling infected sheep. These lesions eventually ulcerate and heal after several weeks.

Rickettsial Diseases

Q Fever is thus far prevalent only in cattle and sheep in the western states. The rickettsiae of this disease are apparently disseminated in infected droplets from the respiratory tract. Some cases may occur as a result of drinking unpasteurized infected milk. The disease in man is manifested by fever, prostration, and atypical pneumonia; the death rate is not high.

Bacterial Diseases

Anthrax—In the soil-infected regions most cases are seen in animals during the pasture season; winter cases may occur if roughage contains spores. In man, anthrax may occur as a result of wound infection, usually on the hands ("malignant pustule"), in persons who handle carcasses or conduct autopsies; generalization may occur.

Brucellosis, in man, is called "undulant fever" and may occur from contact with discharges of infected animals, from contact with blood or tissues of freshly slaughtered swine, and from raw milk.

Erysipeloid—Man may become infected with the organism, *Erysipelothrix rhusiopathiae* from contact with affected swine, sheep, and turkeys and even from fish, although the organism is not pathogenic for fish. Human infections occur in wounds and are manifested by local swelling, pain, ulceration, and slow healing; occasionally, generalization may occur.

Tularemia is primarily a disease of rabbits also occurring in ground squirrels, beavers, muskrats, and other rodents and occasionally in young lambs. Often called rabbit fever, it is frequently contracted through handling of freshly killed rabbits or through bites of blood-sucking flies, ticks, and other vectors. Mortality in man is high although the use of antibiotics has greatly reduced the death rate.

Glanders is now practically extinct in the United States, but human cases occur from contact with infected members of the horse family. The disease is usually an acute pyemia in man and fatal within two or three weeks, although there have been a few chronic cases.

Leptospirosis—*Leptospira icterohemorrhagiae* may occur in humans and dogs through contact with the urine of wild rats. Dogs infected in this way may transmit the disease to man. *Leptospira canicola* in dogs may spread from dog to dog, and to man, through infected urine. *Leptospira pomona* of cattle affects swine, horses, and humans.

Fungus Diseases and Animal Parasites

Ringworm Infections—*Microsporum canis* (and *felineum*) is identical with *Microsporum lanosum* of man, and clinical evidence suggests that transfer occurs from animals to man and from man to animals. *Trichophyton spp.* of herbivorous animals seems to have greater host specificity, but human infections have been described.

Scabies, Itch, or Sarcoptic Mange are spread by horses, cattle, and others.

Diseases Transmitted through Infected Milk

Bacterial Diseases

Tuberculosis, of the bovine type, is contracted from infected cattle.

Brucellosis is contracted from infected cattle and goats.

Scarlet Fever (Septic Sore Throat) is contracted from cattle suffering with udder infection with hemolytic streptococci of Lancefield, Type A (*Streptococcus pyogenes*). The organism generally thrives on the mucosa of the throat of man, producing severe angina. The toxin produces severe constitutional effects including a skin rash. In some cases the skin eruption is absent; this form of the disease is "septic sore throat."

Staphylococcus Intoxication causes an acute intestinal intoxication—the most common type of food poisoning in man. Most cases are caused by eating contaminated foods. Occasionally milk has been incriminated.

Diseases Transmitted through Raw or Imperfectly Cooked Meat

Bacterial Diseases

Anthrax occurs in human beings usually as a result of handling infected carcasses during skinning and associated dressing procedures.

Tularemia may occur in human beings as a result of handling freshly killed infected wild rabbits.

Brucellosis may occur in human beings as a result of handling freshly slaughtered infected hog carcasses.

Diseases Caused by Animal Parasites

Trichinosis may occur from eating undercooked infested pork.

Tapeworm Disease is caused by *Cysticercus cellulosae* from undercooked infested pork and by *Cysticercus bovis* from undercooked infested beef.

Diseases Transmitted by Invertebrate Vectors

Virus Diseases

Equine Encephalomyelitis—Both the western and eastern types of encephalomyelitis of horses occur in man. Birds of many species appear to be the natural hosts of these viri. Several species of mosquitoes, bird mites and ticks appear to be vectors. Human infections apparently are almost always the result of bites of infected mosquitoes.

St. Louis Encephalitis, a virus disease of man, occasionally in epidemic form, is not known to affect any domestic or wild mammals. In epidemic areas high titers are usually found in birds. Mosquitoes are believed to be the primary transmitting agents.

Rickettsial Diseases

Typhus Fever—A severe and often fatal form not common in the US is transmitted from man to man by the body louse. Another form is called "murine typhus" because rats are the reservoir of infection for man and the rat flea transmits the disease. This form is epidemic in some cities of the East and South, is much milder than the classic form, and apparently is caused by an attenuated virus.

Rocky Mountain Spotted Fever—The carrier is *Dermacentor andersoni*, "the spotted fever tick" in the Northwest and *Dermacentor variabilis*, a dog tick, in the South and East. The disease is severe with a high death rate in the northern Rocky Mountain region.

Bacterial Diseases

Plague of the bubonic and sylvatic varieties is caused by *Pasteurella pestis*. Cases contracted from rat flea bites generally take the bubonic form (Black Death) of European history; parts of modern Asia still have occasional outbreaks. Mortality is high but less than that seen in the pneumonic form which occurs in colder climates and is transmitted from man to man through droplet infection. When rodents other than rats spread the disease, the disease becomes a rural menace and is called "sylvatic plague."

Tularemia may be spread by bloodsucking flies, ticks, and lice from rodents to man.

Treatment

The veterinary medical practitioner uses, in general, drugs employed in the treatment of human diseases, and basic work in veterinary therapeutics refers to the USP or NF. Doses differ with animal species, of course.

Strangely, the general public seems to be of the opinion that animals require different agents for the treatment of their ailments; possibly, the basis for this fallacious thinking is mankind's own high opinion of itself, encouraging the flattering thought that human beings require a special group of medicinal agents to alleviate their diseases.

Obviously, there are special products and formulations specifically for veterinary purposes and for individual species; this is true particularly with biological products (see *Veterinary Biologicals*, this page). However, on the whole, the dissimilarities are exceptions.

Animal species may vary markedly in their response to drugs and to other chemicals. Knowledge of these departures from those which might be anticipated is incomplete, and this problem of species variation is a continual one for the practicing veterinarian. As examples:

1. *Phenol* and *cresol* derivatives, widely used for the disinfection of animal quarters, are satisfactory when properly employed. Cats, however, show a marked sensitivity to these compounds if the drugs are applied topically.
2. *Morphine* and other opium derivatives depress the central nervous system in dogs similarly to the effect in man. However, morphine produces marked excitement in the cat and, to a lesser degree, in most other species of domestic animals.
3. *Strychnine* is relatively well tolerated in birds in comparison with mammals in whom convulsive seizures are produced by small quantities.
4. *Sodium bicarbonate*, in therapeutic amounts—generally considered almost innocuous in man and animals—may be toxic in fowl. Solutions of 1% or less (used as a laxative in birds) cause symptoms resembling those of uremic poisoning and hepatic degeneration.
5. *Belladonna* is toxic to most species of animals and frequently causes fatal poisoning in swine, yet the rabbit tolerates large quantities. This difference is explained by the presence of an enzyme in the

rabbit liver which decomposes atropine. Death has been reported in dogs who consumed the muscles of rabbits fed belladonna leaf experimentally for a long period.

6. *Digitalis* can be administered orally in most species of animals, but ruminants will not respond. It is presumed that the glycoside is destroyed by maceration in the ruminant forestomach.
7. *Red squill* has long been employed as a rodent poison. The rodents cannot vomit after ingesting red squill, but most dogs will vomit and escape fatality.
8. *Penicillin* has increased toxicity for the guinea pig as compared with that reported for other animals and humans. This toxicity is manifested by an acute necrosis involving the adrenal gland, particularly the cortex.
9. The use of *carbon tetrachloride* in ruminants is hazardous because of a peculiar susceptibility to the toxic action of the drug. There is considerable skepticism regarding the indications for its administration to cattle. Sheep show idiosyncrasy to carbon tetrachloride less frequently than cattle, yet losses in this species occur often. The drug is not used in swine because of its toxicity.
10. An additional example of species variation, aside from drug actions, involves *tetanus toxin*. Calculated on equivalent body weight bases the equine species, apparently with the least resistance, is said to be 350,000 times more susceptible to tetanus toxin than are fowl, 600 times more susceptible than are dogs, and 12 times more susceptible than are mice. Some consider sheep and goats to be more susceptible than other ruminants and swine, while the carnivores (dogs and cats) are known to be quite resistant.

Other factors alter drug response in the various species of animals, including:

1. The type and condition of the digestive tract
2. Individual variation

a.	Weight	e.	Drug idiosyncrasy
b.	Age	f.	Temperament
c.	Sex	g.	Tolerance
d.	Time of administration	h.	Pathologic condition

Drug response is affected also by drug variation with respect to:

1.	Route and frequency of administration	3.	Drug synergism
2.	Cumulation	4.	Drug antagonism

Veterinary Biologicals

The uses and doses of many pharmaceutical products used for both man and animals are given in the monographs as they appear in Part VI, *Pharmaceutical and Medicinal Agents*, page 725.

The information in *Fundamentals of Biological Pharmacy*, page 1417, and the basic principles of active and passive immunization in *Immunizing Agents*, page 1426, are equally applicable as background for understanding veterinary biological products.

Biological products for use in animals may be useful in a single species or in more than one, depending on the disease to be controlled; in some instances, differently prepared biologicals may be required in various species to control the same illness.

Descriptions of biological products which follow are intended to provide an over-all general examination of their composition, preparation, and availability. Because the requirements for these products may vary, depending on disease incidence and on scientific and/or technological advances, these listings do not provide a complete survey of the market. More detailed and current information on biological products may be found in the catalogs of suppliers to the veterinary medical profession.

Veterinary Sera*

All veterinary biological products that enter into interstate commerce are produced under license issued by the US Department of

---

* Species dose abbreviations used: H(horses), M(mules), C(cattle), D(dogs), G(goats), Sh(sheep), Sw(swine).

Agriculture, Animal Inspection and Quarantine Branch, and in accordance with the regulations set forth in a virus, serum, toxin act. Details of production and methods of testing to establish identity, safety, and potency are filed with this department by the licensee.

Veterinary antisera are prepared by hyperimmunizing normal healthy animals against specific organisms or agents. Horses, cattle, hogs, and dogs are most commonly used, but other species of animals may be utilized when necessary. All animals are carefully selected on the basis of health and vigor. Complete records are kept on each animal, including temperatures, physical findings, inoculations, hyperimmunizations, bleedings, and treatment.

The use of homologous serum in treatment always is preferable to reduce the danger of anaphylaxis. However, all antisera are pasteurized or undergo processing that may cause significant change in the protein structure. Even homologous serum, therefore, may sensitize certain individuals to subsequent injection of the same serum. When there is reason to suspect that sensitization has occurred, it is advisable to inject a few animals with small doses of serum and to observe them for evidence of anaphylactic reaction.

Some antisera have been found to be only slightly effective. Most of them, however, provide some passive immunity of short duration and thus are useful prophylactic and therapeutic agents.

Antisera may be used in conjunction with, or as supportive therapy to, other types of treatment, especially the antibiotics and sulfonamides; actually, the increased use of these two classes of drugs has reduced the formerly heavy requirements for antisera.

Antibacterial Serum, Canine (Canine Origin) is obtained from healthy distemper-immune dogs hyperimmunized against *Salmonella enteritidis*, *Salmonella schottmuelleri*, *Escherichia coli*, and pyogenic streptococci. *Use:* An aid in the control of infection caused by the microorganisms named. *Dose: Prophylactic*, D, 20–50 ml. *Therapeutic*, D, 20–50 ml, or more, repeated if necessary.

Anti-Canine Distemper Serum (Canine Origin) (Concentrated) is obtained from healthy dogs hyperimmunized against canine distemper (Carre's Disease) virus. *Use:* An aid in the prevention or control of canine distemper and in the simultaneous method of distemper immunization, in which the patient is given a dose of distemper virus and a dose of antiserum at the same time. In clinical cases of distemper it is used in combination with chemotherapeutic or antibiotic agents and supportive treatment when necessary. *Dose: Prophylactic*, D, 1 ml/5–10 lb of body weight. *Therapeutic*, D, 0.5 ml/lb of body weight daily until the crisis has passed.

Anti-Canine Distemper Serum and Anti-Canine Infectious Hepatitis Serum (Bivalent, Canine Origin) (Concentrated) is produced from dogs that have been hyperimmunized against canine distemper virus and canine infectious hepatitis virus. *Use:* Prevention and treatment of canine distemper and infectious canine hepatitis. *Dose: Prophylactic*, D, 1 ml/5–10 lb of body weight. *Therapeutic*, D, 1 ml/lb of body weight, repeated if necessary.

Anti-Feline Distemper Serum is obtained from young cats that have been hyperimmunized against virulent strains of feline distemper virus. Some commercial preparations are produced from cats also hyperimmunized against *Pasteurella feliseptica* (*multocida*), *Salmonella schottmuelleri*, *Staphylococcus aureus* and *albus*, and/or pyogenic streptococci. *Use:* An effective prophylactic agent of therapeutic value when given early in the disease course. *Dose for Cats: Prophylactic*, 2–5 ml. *Therapeutic*, 5-ml minimum.

Anti-Fox Encephalitis Serum is prepared from the blood of dogs that have been hyperimmunized by repeated doses of virulent fox encephalitis virus. *Use:* Production of passive immunity in dogs to encephalitis. *Dose: Prophylactic*. 1 injection of 0.5 ml/lb of body weight, subcutaneously. *Therapeutic*, recommended dose is 0.5 ml/lb of body weight for dogs, which may be repeated in 3 to 4 days.

Anti-Equine Encephalomyelitis Serum: Eastern, Western, and Eastern-Western Combined is prepared from the blood of horses hyperimmunized against eastern, western, or both types, of equine encephalomyelitis virus. *Use:* Prophylaxis and treatment of equine encephalomyelitis. The appropriate preparation is used when the type of infecting virus is known, and the bivalent serum is employed when the type virus is not known or both viruses are known to be present. *Dose: Prophylactic*, H and M, 100–250 ml. *Therapeutic*, H and M, 250–1000 ml.

Anti-Hemorrhagic Septicemia Serum is obtained from horses and cattle hyperimmunized against organisms of the *Pasteurella* group. It is tested for potency by a standard mouse-unit method in addition to the usual sterility and safety tests. *Use:* Prevention or treatment of hemorrhagic septicemia in all species of animals. *Dose: Prophylactic*, H and C, 25–50 ml. *Therapeutic*, Double the prophylactic dose or more.

Anti-Hog Cholera Serum is obtained from the blood of healthy hogs hyperimmunized against hog cholera. Hog cholera antiserum production is conducted under the supervision of inspectors of the USDA and meets the requirements for safety and effectiveness. *Use:* Either alone to confer temporary passive immunity or simultaneously with hog cholera vaccine or modified hog cholera vaccines to induce extended active immunity. *Dose:* The minimum doses recommended by the USDA for use simultaneously with hog cholera vaccine are

Suckling pigs	20 cc
20–40-lb pig	30 cc
40–90-lb pig	35 cc
90–120-lb pig	45 cc
120–150-lb pig	55 cc
150–180-lb pig	65 cc
180-lb pig and over	75 cc

The dose of serum recommended for use with modified hog cholera vaccines varies with the specific product used and with the circumstances under which it is administered. Frequently, it is less than the above recommended dose for use with virulent virus. Increases in the above recommendations may be made by the veterinarian in order more adequately to control the virus reaction and also to provide greater protection against other infections.

This serum is available in concentrated form from several manufacturers; the dose is reduced, of course, and is specified on the label.

Anti-Infectious Hepatitis Serum (Canine Origin) is obtained from the blood of dogs that have been hyperimmunized with virulent infectious canine hepatitis virus. *Use:* Prevention and treatment of infectious canine hepatitis. *Doses: Prophylactic*, D, 5 ml/lb of body weight produces a passive immunity lasting for 3 or 4 weeks. *Therapeutic*, D, 5 ml/lb of body weight. A second dose may be given in 3 or 4 days.

Normal Serum (Bovine Origin) is obtained from normal healthy cattle. *Use:* Nonspecific treatment of animal infections, hemophilialike conditions, debilitating diseases, sweet clover poisoning, and to increase the coagulability of blood. *Dose:* C, 100–500 ml, repeated if necessary. In sweet clover poisoning the dose should range from 200 to 500 ml, intravenously, depending on the weight and age of the animal and the severity of the condition. In severe cases the dose may be repeated in 12 hr. Apparently normal cattle in the same herd should be given 100–200 ml of the serum subcutaneously, pending change of ration.

Normal Serum (Canine Origin) is prepared from sterile blood obtained from healthy dogs. *Use:* Treatment of surgical and traumatic shock, external and internal hemorrhage, dehydration, and hypoproteinemia. It also may be used as an aid in nonspecific treatment of infections, hemophilialike conditions, and to increase the coagulability of the blood. *Dose:* D, 20–100 ml administered intravenously, intraperitoneally, or subcutaneously. The dose may be repeated or increased based upon the size and condition of the dog.

Normal Serum (Equine Origin) is obtained from normal, healthy horses. Horses used in its production are mallein tested and immunized against tetanus. *Use:* An aid in the nonspecific treatment of animal infections, hemophilialike conditions, debilitating disease, and to increase the coagulability of the blood. *Dose:* H, 100–500 ml administered subcutaneously or intravenously.

Anti-Streptococcus Serum is produced by hyperimmunizing various species of animals with repeated injections of streptococcus cultures. Usually additional organisms are included in the antigen for the production of polyvalent antibacterial sera.

Anti-Swine Erysipelas Serum is obtained from horses hyperimmunized by repeated injections of *Erysipelothrix rhusiopathiae*. It is potency tested in mice or pigeons. *Use:* Prevention and treatment of swine erysipelas and for the simultaneous method of vaccination. *Dose: Prophylactic*, Sw, up to 50 lb, 5 ml; 50–75 lb, 10 ml; 75–100 lb, 15 ml; over 100 lb, 20 ml or more. *Therapeutic*, Double the prophylactic dose, repeated if necessary. In the simultaneous method of vaccination erysipelas culture is given in conjunction with a prophylactic dose of antiserum.

Antivenin (North American Antisnakebite Serum)—*Use:* Treatment of ophidism. *Dose:* Dogs may require 1–8 syringefuls according to the size of the animal and the severity of symptoms. The smaller the animal, the more antivenin required. In large animals an initial dose of 1–2 syringefuls may be injected in and around the site of the fang wounds.

Veterinary Antitoxins

Botulinus Antitoxin (Types A, B, and C)—Polyvalent botulinus antitoxin is obtained by hyperimmunizing animals (usually horses) with repeated sublethal doses of Types A, B, and C botulinus toxin. It is standardized by means of biological assay on guinea pigs; each cubic centimeter of the finished product contains not less than 150 combined antitoxic units against Types A, B, and C toxins. *Uses:* Prevention and treatment of botulism in fowl and domestic and fur-bearing animals. *Dose: Prophylactic*, H and C, 40–50 ml (6000–7500 units); Sw and Sn, 5–10 ml (750–1500 units); D and Fox, 5–10 ml (750–1500 units); Mink, 5 ml (750 units); Fowl, 1–2 ml (150–300 units). *Therapeutic*, Double the prophylactic dose, repeated or increased as indicated.

Clostridium Perfringens Antitoxin (Types B, C, and D) (Equine Origin)—Polyvalent antitoxin from horses hyperimmunized with *Clostridium perfringens*, Types B, C, and D. *Uses:* An aid in the prevention and treatment of enterotoxemias of cattle, sheep, and swine due to toxins of this organism. *Doses:* (Subcutaneously) *Prevention:* C, 10–30 ml; Sh and Sw, 5–10 ml; *Treatment:* C, 20–90 ml; Sh and Sw, 10–30 ml.

Tetanus Antitoxin—*Use:* Prevention and treatment of tetanus. *Dose: Prophylactic,* H and C, 1500 units. When the date of injury is in doubt, 3000–5000 units are recommended. Newborn foals should receive 500 units; Lambs, Sh, G, and Pigs, 250–500 units; D, 500–1500 units. Prophylactic doses of tetanus antitoxin are administered intramuscularly or subcutaneously. *Therapeutic,* From 20 to 60 times the propylactic dose is administered and repeated as indicated. This antitoxin may be administered intramuscularly, intravenously, or intraspinally.

Veterinary Vaccines

Because of the risks of unintentional spread of disease inherent in the use of vaccines containing viable organisms or viri, many of these products are under the strict control of federal, state, and/or local governments. It is imperative that the individual handling of these products be completely familiar with the applicable legal restrictions. Also, it is essential that the directions of the manufacturer enclosed with the product be carefully followed and that deviations from these directions be made only by or under the supervision of a licensed veterinarian.

Anthrax Spore Vaccine—There are a number of different anthrax vaccines composed of living attenuated anthrax spores available commercially: anthrax spore vaccine; single, double, and triple injection spore vaccine; intradermal anthrax spore vaccine; and anthrax spore vaccine in saponin solution or alum solution. Occasionally, a highly susceptible animal may contact the disease through vaccination. These vaccines should not be used in anthrax-free areas. Spore vaccine may be used alone or in combination with serum. *Use:* Preventive vaccination against anthrax. *Dose:* Methods of administration and other directions regarding the use of these vaccines vary with the product used. The manufacturer's instructions should be consulted for details.

Bluetongue Vaccine, Modified Live Virus (Chick Embryo Origin) is a live virus modified by adaptation so that it no longer possesses a disease-causing property yet retains high immunogenic activity; it is vacuum dried. *Use:* Immunization of sheep against bluetongue. *Dose:* Sh, 2 ml, subcutaneously.

Brucella Abortus Vaccine is a saline suspension of living Strain 19 *Br. abortus* organisms. *Use:* Stimulation of increased and prolonged resistance against infection with *Br. abortus* (Bang's disease or brucellosis) of cattle. It may be used on calves between 4 and 8 months of age and on noninfected nongravid females and on females not more than 4 months pregnant, provided such use does not conflict with existing state regulations. *Dose:* The dose depends on the product used. Manufacturer's directions and state regulations should be consulted for details.

Canine Distemper–Hepatitis Vaccine (in L. Canicola, L. Icterohemorrhagiae, and BST Bacterins) is prepared from inactivated viri of canine distemper and of canine hepatitis from infected canine tissue in cultures of *L. canicola, L. icterohemorrhagiae,* and *Brucella bronchisepticus* 40%, *streptococcus* (pyogenic) 40%, *Salmonella typhimurium* 20% isolated from dogs. *Use:* Immunization of healthy dogs against distemper, hepatitis, and leptospiral infections and for increasing resistance to the bacterial organisms in the formula. *Dose:* 3 doses of 5 ml, subcutaneously or intramuscularly, 10–14 days apart.

Canine Distemper–Hepatitis Vaccine, Modified Live Virus (Tissue Culture Origin) contains live canine distemper and infectious canine hepatitis viri attenuated by serial passage in tissue culture. *Use:* Immunization of dogs against distemper and hepatitis. It develops rapid immunity (3–4 days) in vaccinated dogs. *Dose:* 2 ml, intramuscularly or subcutaneously.

Canine Distemper–Hepatitis Vaccine, Modified Live Virus (Tissue Culture Origin) with Leptospira Canicola Bacterin contains live canine distemper and infectious canine hepatitis viri modified by serial passage n tissue culture, plus inactivated *Leptospira canicola* bacterin. *Use:* Immunization of dogs against distemper, hepatitis, and leptospirosis caused by *L. canicola. Dose:* 2 ml, intramuscularly or subcutaneously.

Canine Distemper Vaccine (Killed Virus) is a formalinized 20% suspension of virus-bearing tissue obtained from young dogs at the height of the disease. *Use:* Active immunization of dogs against the virus of canine distemper. *Dose:* D, 2 or 3 doses of 5 ml each 9–15 days apart.

Canine Distemper Vaccine in Bronchisepticus–Streptococcus–Typhimurium Bacterin consists of the following, all of canine origin:

Killed canine distemper virus (tissue origin)		20%
in a bacterin consisting of:		
Brucella bronchisepticus	40%	
Streptococcus (pyogenic)	40%	80%
Salmonella typhimurium	20%	
		100%

Use: Production of immunity, in dogs, against canine distemper and secondary invaders usually associated with clinical distemper. *Dose:* 3 doses of 5 ml, administered subcutaneously or intramuscularly at 9–15-day intervals.

Canine Distemper Vaccine and Infectious Canine Hepatitis Vaccine –Bronchisepticus–Streptococcus–Typhimurium Bacterin (See preceding product) is prepared from virulent canine distemper virus, infectious canine hepatitis virus, *B. bronchisepticus, streptococci,* and *S. typhimurium,* formalin-treated for inactivation. *Use:* Vaccination of healthy dogs against canine distemper, infectious canine hepatitis, and their usual bacterial complications. *Dose:* See preceding product.

Canine Distemper Vaccine, Modified Live Virus (Chick Embryo Origin) is a live virus vaccine modified by adaptation so that it no longer possesses the ability to cause distemper, yet retains high immunogenic property. *Use:* Prevention of distemper. *Dose:* 1 injection of 2 ml subcutaneously.

Equine Encephalomyelitis Vaccine (Eastern, Western, and Eastern-Western Combined) is a chemically killed suspension of encephalomyelitis virus which has been propagated on chick embryos. *Use:* Immunization of equines against encephalomyelitis. *Dose:* Eastern or western—usually 1 ml is given intradermally and repeated in 7–14 days. Eastern, western combined—the dose is doubled and given in the same way. Manufacturer's directions should be consulted for details.

Erysipelothrix Rhusiophathiae Vaccine is a living whole culture of *Erysipelothrix rhusiopathiae,* available in liquid or desiccated form. *Use:* Only with anti-swine erysipelas serum for establishment of active immunity against swine erysipelas. *Dose:*

Pigs	Vaccine, ml	Serum, ml
Under 50 lb	¼	5
50–75 lb	½	10
75–100 lb	¾	15
100 lb and over	1	20

Administered subcutaneously.

Feline Distemper Vaccine is a suspension of virus-bearing tissue obtained from cats artificially infected with this disease, inactivated with formalin. *Use:* Active immunization of cats against the virus of feline distemper (infectious enteritis, malignant panleucopenia, infectious feline agranulocytosis). *Dose:* Cats, 2 doses of 2 ml each, 7–10 days apart.

Fowl Laryngotracheitis Vaccine (Chick Embryo Origin) is prepared from laryngotracheitis virus propagated on the chorioallantoic membrane of incubating chicken eggs. *Use:* Active immunization of chickens against infectious laryngotracheitis. *Dose:* Following reconstitution, a small amount of the vaccine is applied to the cloacal mucous membrane by means of a brush.

Infectious Bovine Rhinotracheitis Vaccine (Desiccated) is a modified live virus vaccine attenuated by serial passage in tissue culture. *Use:* Immunization of cattle, particularly feedlot animals, against infectious bovine rhinotracheitis (IBR, Red Nose). *Dose:* 2 ml, given intramuscularly.

Infectious Canine Hepatitis Vaccine is an inactivated suspension of infectious canine hepatitis virus of tissue origin. *Use:* To induce active immunity of the virus of canine hepatitis in healthy dogs. *Dose:* 2 doses of 2 cc each, subcutaneously or intramuscularly, 2–3 weeks apart.

Hog Cholera Vaccine—Four methods of immunization have been developed for the protection of hogs against cholera: Two (Boynton and crystal-violet) employ killed vaccine; one employs culturally modified, live virus vaccine (with or without antiserum) incapable of producing the disease; and the fourth employs fully virulent hog cholera virus administered simultaneously with antihog cholera serum. *Use:* Active immunization of hogs against hog cholera. *Dose:* Considerable variation exists in dose and method of administration. Manufacturer's instructions should be consulted for details.

Newcastle Disease Vaccine is marketed in two types: (1) live virus vaccine—administered into the wing web, dropped into the eye or nasal passage, given in the drinking water, or injected intramuscularly; (2) killed-virus vaccine—formalin-inactivated, aluminum hydroxide-adsorbed virus for intramuscular injection. *Use:* Active immunization of poultry against Newcastle disease. *Dose:* There is considerable variation in dose and immunizing procedure. Manufacturer's directions should be consulted for details.

Ovine Ecthyma Vaccine (Ovine Origin) consists of powdered ecthyma-scab virus, suspended in a diluent just prior to use. *Use:* Vaccination of lambs, sheep, and cattle against ecthyma (sore mouth). *Dose:* Approximately 1 drop of the suspension is rubbed vigorously into a slightly scarified area of the skin.

Pox Vaccine, Avian (Chick Embryo Origin)—Both fowl pox and pigeon pox vaccines are prepared by propagation of virus on the chorioallantoic membranes of incubating chicken eggs. *Use:* Fowl pox vaccine is used for the vaccination of healthy young chickens and turkeys from 8 to 16 weeks of age and susceptible adult birds not in heavy production. Pigeon pox vaccine may be used on fowl of any age, particularly on flocks in egg production and for those showing devitalization or disease. *Dose:* Usually a small amount of vaccine is administered into the wing web by a specially prepared two-tined stabbing instrument. Occasionally, the vaccine is rubbed into 3 or 4 feather follicles by means of a small brush.

Rabies Vaccine (Phenolized 20% Suspension) is a fine emulsion of phenolized brain and spinal cord tissue containing fixed rabies virus, *Prophylactic,* H and C, 50 ml lb; D under 25 lb, 5 ml; over 25 lb, 1 ml for each 5 lb of body weight or fraction thereof; Cats, 3 ml. *After exposure:* H and C, 3 doses of 50 ml 48-hr apart; D, daily injection of prophylactic dose for 7–14 days. Rabies vaccine is administered subcutaneously or intramuscularly.

Rabies Vaccine, Modified Live Virus (Chick Embryo Origin) is a live virus vaccine modified by adaptation so that it no longer possesses the ability to cause rabies yet retains high immunogenic property. *Use:* Prevention of rabies in dogs over 5 months of age. *Dose:* One intramuscular or subcutaneous injection of 3 ml.

Wart Vaccine is prepared from wart tissue obtained from cattle or from virus grown on incubating chicken eggs. *Use:* Control of warts on horses, cattle, and dogs. *Dose:* There is considerable variation in dose and the method of administration. Manufacturer's instructions should be consulted for details.

Veterinary Bacterins

Autogenous bacterins prepared with organisms isolated from individual patients provide the most satisfactory product for this type of treatment. However, their preparation is time-consuming, expensive, and inconvenient, thus stock bacterins are used more commonly.

Although highly popular and extensively used in the health professions a few years ago, bacterins have shown a progressive decline in clinical use. This is true particularly of the stock mixed bacterins prepared from standard laboratory cultures of different pathogens. The development of more effective vaccines and the advancements made in the field of chemotherapy have led to replacement of bacterins for many prophylactic and therapeutic purposes.

Avisepticus–Gallinarum Bacterin (Fowl Cholera–Fowl Typhoid Bacterin) is a mixture of equal parts of killed *Pasteurella avicida* (aviseptica) and *Shigella gallinarum* organisms. *Use:* Aids in the control of fowl cholera and fowl typhoid. *Dose: Prophylactic,* Fowl, 1 ml; young fowl 6–8 weeks of age, 0.5 ml; turkeys over 10 lb, 2 ml. For greater immunity 3 injections 3–7 days apart may be given.

Blackleg Bacterin (Alum Precipitated) is a sterile, whole culture of *Clostridium chauvei.* It contains the organisms and cultural agressin. *Use:* Prevention of blackleg in bovines and other ruminants. *Dose:* Cattle of all ages, 5 ml; Sh and G, 2–3 ml, injected intramuscularly or subcutaneously.

Blackleg–Hemorrhagic Septicemia Bacterin (Alum Precipitated) is a mixture of equal parts of killed cultures of *Clostridium chauvei* and *Pasteurella* strains. *Use:* For the prevention of blackleg and hemorrhagic septicemia in susceptible animals. *Dose:* Cattle of all ages, 5 ml; Sh and G, 3 ml administered subcutaneously or intramuscularly. Calves under 3 months of age at the time of vaccination should be revaccinated within 6 months.

Clostridium Chauvei–Septicum Bacterin (Alum Precipitated) contains equal parts of killed cultures of *Clostridium chauvei* and *Clostridium septicum.* *Use:* Prevention of blackleg and malignant edema in susceptible animals. *Dose:* Calves, 5 ml; lambs, kids, Sh and G, 3 ml. Calves under 6 months of age when vaccinated should be revaccinated within 6 months for greater protection.

Clostridium Chauvei–Septicum–Pasteurella Bacterin (Alum Precipitated) contains killed cultures of *Clostridium chauvei, Clostridium septicum,* and *Pasteurella multocida,* types 1, 2, and 3. *Use:* Immunizing cattle and sheep against blackleg, hemorrhagic septicemia, and malignant edema. *Dose:* Cattle of all ages, 10 ml; Sh and G, 3–5 ml, administered subcutaneously or intramuscularly. Calves under 3 months of age at time of vaccination should be revaccinated within 6 months.

Clostridium Perfringens Type D Bacterin (Alum Precipitated Whole Culture) consists of killed cultures of *Clostridium perfringens,* Type D. *Use:* Production of active immunity in sheep and lambs 2 months of age or older against enterotoxemia. *Dose:* Feeder lambs and adult sheep, 5 ml, injected subcutaneously.

Coli–Staphylococcus–Streptococcus Bacterin is prepared from chemically killed saline suspensions of

Staphylococcus aureus	40%
Streptococcus agalactiae	40%
Escherichia coli	20%

all of bovine origin. *Use:* An aid in the control of mastitis or other infection due to organisms listed in the formula. *Dose:* C, 5 ml,

for animals of average size, subcutaneously or intramuscularly; dose may be repeated or increased as indicated.

Corynebacterium–Pasteurella Bacterin consists of killed, whole cultures of *Pasteurella* and *Corynebacterium pseudodiphthericum* (bovine and porcine). *Uses:* Prevention of hemorrhagic septicemia and the diphtheroid complications in cattle, swine, and sheep. *Dose: Prophylactic,* C and calves, 5 ml; Sh and Sw, 2–5 ml, injected intramuscularly or subcutaneously. In infected herds or flocks, the dose may be increased and repeated as indicated.

Erysipelas Bacterin is a killed, whole culture of *Erysipelothrix rhusiopathiae,* aluminum hydroxide adsorbed. *Use:* Immunization of swine and turkeys against erysipelas. *Dose:* Turkeys, 2 ml, intramuscularly; Sw, 5 ml, subcutaneously.

Hemorrhagic Septicemia Bacterin is usually prepared from cultures of *Pasteurella* obtained from buffaloes, horses, cattle, sheep, and swine (20% each). *Use:* Prevention of hemorrhagic septicemia (shipping fever, shipping pneumonia) in horses, cattle, sheep, goats, and swine. *Dose:* Animals in noninfected herds, 5 ml. The dose may be repeated in 3–7 days, if deemed advisable.

Leptospira Pomona Bacterin is a suspension of chemically killed cultures of antigenic strains of *Leptospira pomona* adsorbed on and suspended in aluminum hydroxide gel. *Use:* To stimulate active immunity against leptospirosis in cattle and swine. *Dose:* C and Sw, 5 ml for animals of average size administered subcutaneously or intramuscularly, preferably the latter. Dose may be repeated as indicated. Booster injections every 6 months are suggested.

Mixed Bacterin, Avian (Chicken Formula) is usually made from cultures of *Pasteurella aviseptica, Staphylococcus* (*albus* and *aureus*), *Streptococcus* (nonhemolytic), and *Pseudomonas aeruginosa,* 25% each. *Use:* Prevention of infection by the organisms named in the formula. *Dose:* Birds of average size, 1 ml; young birds, ¾ ml; geese, 2 ml. For healthy birds in infected flocks the dose is increased.

Mixed Bacterin, Bovine, Formula 1 contains formalin-killed undiluted whole-broth cultures of the following, isolated from cattle:

Pasteurella bovisepticus	50%
Corynebacterium (including 15% *Corynebacter pyogenes*)	30%
Staphylococcus albus and *aureus* (each 5%)	10%
Streptococcus (pyogenic)	10%

Use: To aid in the prevention of conditions attributed to the organisms named in the formula. *Dose:* Mature animals of average size, 5 ml; calves and smaller animals, 2.5 ml, administered subcutaneously or intramuscularly. In infected herds the dose for noninfected animals may be increased and repeated as indicated.

Mixed Bacterin, Bovine, Formula 2 contains formalin-killed undiluted whole-broth cultures of

Streptococcus (pyogenic)	50%
Corynebacterium pyogenes	30%
Staphylococcus aureus	10%
Escherichia coli	10%

all of bovine origin. *Use:* To aid in the treatment of mastitis and other conditions due to infection by organisms named in the formula. *Dose:* Animals in infected herds, 10 ml; in noninfected herds, 5 ml, administered subcutaneously or intramuscularly and repeated as indicated.

Mixed Bacterin, Bovine, Formula 3 is made from formalin-killed undiluted whole-broth cultures of

Escherichia coli	30%
Salmonella enteritidis	30%
Aerobacter aerogenes	20%
Pasteurella boviseptica	20%

all isolated from calves affected with scours (diarrhea). *Use:* Prevention and treatment of calf scours. *Dose: Prophylactic,* 3–5 ml as soon as possible after birth. Dose may be increased and repeated after a 3-day interval. Administered subcutaneously or intramuscularly and repeated as indicated.

Mixed Bacterin, Equine, Formula 1 is prepared from cultures of

Streptococcus (pyogenic)	30%
Pasteurella equiseptica	30%
Staphylococcus albus and *aureus* (each 10%)	20%
Escherichia coli	20%

all of equine origin. *Use:* Prevention of infections caused by the organisms named in the formula. *Dose:* Mature horses of average size, 5 ml; colts, 2.5 ml, administered subcutaneously or intramuscularly. Dose may be increased and repeated as indicated.

Mixed Bacterin, Feline, Formula 1 is prepared from cultures of

Pasteurella felisepticus	60%
Streptococcus (pyogenic)	10%
Salmonella schottmuelleri	20%
Staphylococcus albus and *aureus* (each 5%)	10%

all of feline origin. *Use:* To aid in developing resistance to infection by the organisms named in the formula. *Dose:* ½–1 ml, administered subcutaneously and repeated as indicated.

Mixed Bacterin, Ovine, Formula 1 is prepared from cultures of

Corynebacterium ovis	30%
Pasteurella oviseptica	30%
Salmonella schottmuelleri	20%
Staphylococcus albus and aureus (each 10%)	20%

Use: To aid in the prevention of infections caused by the organisms named in the formula. *Dose:* Mature sheep of normal size, 5 ml; lambs, 2–5 ml, depending on age and weight. In infected flocks the above doses are increased and repeated as indicated.

Mixed Bacterin, Porcine, Formula 1 is prepared from cultures of

Pasteurella suiseptica	30%
Salmonella cholerasuis	30%
Streptococcus (pyogenic)	20%
Corynebacterium pseudodiphthericum	20%

all of porcine origin. *Use:* To aid in the prevention of infections caused by the organisms named in the formula. *Dose:* Sw and shoats, 5 ml; suckling pigs, 2.5 ml. In infected droves the amount of bacterin is increased and repeated as indicated.

Mixed Bacterin, Porcine, Formula 2 is prepared from cultures of

Salmonella schottmuelleri	30%
Salmonella cholerasuis	30%
Pasteurella suiseptica	20%
Escherichia coli	10%
Streptococcus (pyogenic)	10%

all of porcine origin. *Use:* To aid in the control of swine enteritis attributed to the organisms named in the formula. *Dose:* Sw and shoats, 5 ml; small pigs, 2.5 ml. For healthy animals in infected droves the dose is increased and repeated as indicated.

Streptococcus Equi Bacterin (Strangles Bacterin) is a chemically killed suspension of *Streptococcus equi*. *Use:* In healthy individuals of the equine species as an aid in prevention of infection due to *Streptococcus equi* (Strangles). *Dose:* Three 10-ml doses, administered intramuscularly at weekly intervals.

Veterinary Toxoids

Clostridium Perfringens, Type D Toxoid is a purified, concentrated and detoxified culture filtrate of *Clostridium perfringens*, Type D. *Use:* In healthy sheep as an aid in the prevention of enterotoxemia (pulpy kidney disease). *Dose:* 2 ml, preferably subcutaneously, posterior to the elbow, or intramuscularly in the mid-cervical area; a second injection within 10–14 days aids in enhancing and prolonging protection.

Staphylococcus Aureus Toxoid—*Use:* Prevention or treatment of infections due to *Staphylococcus aureus*. It should not be used in severely acute cases. *Dose:* C, 5 ml, injected subcutaneously, repeated at intervals of 5–7 days. D and Cats, 0.5–2 ml, injected subcutaneously, repeated at intervals of 5–7 days.

Tetanus Toxoid (Alum Precipitated)—*Use:* Active immunization of animals against tetanus. *Dose:* H, 10 ml, intramuscularly. A second injection within 3 months is advisable to enhance the immunity and prolong its duration. All animals, 1 ml/100 lb of body weight.

A concentrated toxoid with the advantage of a smaller dose is available. The manufacturer's instructions should be consulted for details.

Veterinary Diagnostic Antigens

Brucella Abortus Stained Antigen (Rapid Plate Method) is prepared from cultures of *Brucella abortus* furnished by the USDA, Animal Inspection and Quarantine Branch, and in accordance with the directions outlined by this department. The test is conducted by mixing 0.03 ml of the antigen with the proper amounts of diluted suspected blood serum on a glass plate. The reaction is indicated by a clumping or grouping of the stained bacteria in the antigen; negative tests and controls remain unchanged.

Leptospira Antigen is a chemically killed, refined, concentrated, standardized suspension of any one of the three serotypes *L. pomona*, *L. canicola*, or *L. icterohemorrhagiae*. Antigen may be used in a rapid plate–screen test to differentiate positive serum from negative or in a capillary tube test to determine positive serum titer. The rapid plate–screen test is accomplished by mixing 1 drop of antigen with a loopful of serum to be tested on a glass plate. Protected against evaporation, it is permitted to stand for 6 min after which the plate is rotated in a circular motion. With positive sera, agglutinated organisms gather at the edge of the serum–antigen drop. Titration of positive serum samples requires dilution of the serum in saline followed by mixture of 0.03 ml of each dilution with 1 drop of antigen; the previously described technique is followed.

Mallein Ophthalmic—*Use:* For the diagnosis of glanders in equines. Mallein is the fluid of the interior part of *Malleomyces mallei*, the offending organism in glanders in equines, extracted following heat treatment and inactivation of *M. mallei* cultures. 0.1 ml is brushed into the conjunctival sac: positive reaction is indicated by an intense reddening of the mucous membrane accompanied by a definite purulent discharge from the eye, usually within 6–8 hr.

Pullorum Disease Stained Antigen, Polyvalent (Rapid Plate Method)—K-Formula is prepared from selected strains of *Salmonella pullorum* obtained from the USDA and in accordance with their specifications. This antigen is used in testing poultry for pullorum disease by the whole blood, rapid plate method. The essentials of the test consist of mixing a wire loopful (0.02 ml) of freshly drawn blood with a drop (0.05 ml) of antigen on a glass or porcelain plate. A positive test is indicated by the agglutination or clumping of the red blood cells; in a negative test, the blood remains unchanged.

Pullorum Tube Antigen (Concentrated), Unstained is a concentrated diagnostic antigen to be diluted as directed for use in the tube method test for pullorum disease in poultry. The proper amount of diluted antigen is mixed in a test tube with serum obtained from suspected birds and the mixture is incubated. A positive reaction is indicated by clumping in the bottom of the tube with clearing of the test mixture.

Tuberculin (Intradermal)—Each 0.1 ml is equivalent to 0.025 Gm Koch's OT. This preparation has superseded other types of tuberculin for the diagnosis of tuberculosis because of ease of administration and sharply defined reaction. In cattle, 0.1 to 0.2 ml is injected intradermally in the skin of the caudal fold and/or in the thin skin of the vulva at its juncture with the mucous membrane. A positive reaction consists of local edematous swelling 72 hr after injection.

This chapter was prepared by

Albert A. Stonehill, PhD, *Manager, Product Research Department, Ethicon, Inc., Somerville, N.J.   08876*

A professional service rendered by many pharmacists consists in supplying surgical instruments, sutures, surgical dressings, and other equipment employed by the surgeon prior to, during, and after a surgical operation. Some pharmacists, who have obtained the necessary background of information, carry a complete line of such supplies, and are even able to provide operating tables and other heavy equipment.

There are comparatively few such completely equipped pharmacies; the major outlet is through surgical supply houses. Every pharmacist, however, should be familiar with two of the products mentioned above, namely, *Surgical Dressings* and *Sutures*, which are discussed in detail below. The selection of the correct type of surgical dressing or suture is a critical factor in safeguarding the welfare of the patient undergoing surgery. Many items belonging in these categories are handled routinely by the pharmacist and all of these items come within the purview of his professional responsibility.

Surgical Dressings

Definition—*Surgical dressing* or *curatio* is a term applied to a wide range of materials used for the dressing of wounds. They are employed as coverings, absorbents, protectives, or supports for injured or diseased parts.

Classification—Dressings may be classified as:

1. Primary wound dressings
2. Adsorbents
3. Bandages
4. Adhesive tapes
5. Protectives

Specifications—Surgical dressings and sutures are required to meet specific requirements of the USP for many characteristics. For these specific requirements and the performance of several of the official tests, eg, *Absorbency test* and *Fiber length* of cotton, the *Diameter* of sutures and the *Tensile strength* of sutures, textile fabrics, and films, the reader is directed to the detailed instructions provided in the USP.

Primary Wound Dressings

This term refers to those dressings that are designed to be placed next to a wound surface and are usually reinforced by materials of various types to absorb the wound secretion and minimize maceration.

Gauze compresses of suitable mesh and thickness have long been widely used as primary wound dressings, but they have the drawback of adherence to other than clean, incised wound surfaces. To minimize this difficulty, various types of dressings have been designed to avoid the pain and trauma caused when a dressing which is stuck to a wound surface is removed.

Petrolatum-impregnated gauze has been widely used for this purpose on the theory that since it possesses hydrophobic characteristics it should not adhere. However, this often does not prove to be the case, and in addition this material very frequently causes maceration and is difficult to sterilize.

In an effort to eradicate these problems, a new type of gauze, specially woven from pure, regenerated cellulose (viscous rayon) and impregnated with a bland, hydrophilic, oil-in-water emulsion in such a way that all pores remain open, has proved to have an extremely low degree of adherence to all types of wounds. It is known as Adaptic Non-Adhering Dressing (*J&J*). Each dressing is packaged sterile in a unique envelope that guarantees sterility and, at the same time, can be opened easily under sterile conditions. Each envelope of the 3 × 8-in. size contains three dressings; the 3 × 16-in. size contains one dressing.

The weave is tight enough so that the growth buds of new skin cannot grow through the dressing and become entangled in the filaments. The dressing has a sidewise stretch which allows conformability to all contours without wrinkling.

The versatility of this dressing makes it excellent for all types of wounds such as burns, skin grafts, plastic surgery, colostomies, ileostomies, open ulcers, and cases where packing is needed.

Another device used to minimize wound adherence is a dry nonadhering dressing consisting of an absorbent pad faced with a soft plastic film having openings. These are large enough to allow fluids to pass through, but too small to allow adhesion of the wound to take place. This dressing is available both in the form of a pad having a perforated film backing and in the form of pads on extra large adhesive bandages. A modification for hospital use consists of the nonadherent flutter valve film covering an absorbent pad which is affixed to a vented adhesive tape. It is designed primarily to cover incisions, small wounds, and abrasions. The excellent nonadhering properties of the flutter valve film permit removal of the dressing from the wound without danger of disturbing the healing area.

It is obviously important to use some type of nonadherent dressing next to any wound surface wherever possible, both as a matter of patient comfort and to minimize interference with wound healing when the dressing is removed. Absorbent cotton, bandages, and similar materials should never be used directly on a wound surface as primary dressings.

Spray-on Wound Dressing—A quick drying aerosol spray that forms a clear, plastic film is available as Scan Spray-On Wound Dressing (*J&J*). The spray forms a smooth, tough transparent protective film which is insoluble in water or body fluids. It is easily removed without pain and is useful in minor surgery, small abrasions, and hard to bandage areas such as fingers, toes, and elbows.

Absorbents

Surgical Cotton—Cotton is the basic surgical absorbent. It is official in the USP under the title *Purified Cotton* (page 1876).

Domestic cotton grown in the southern United States is suitable for surgical purposes. The domestic cotton plant reaches a height of from 2 to 4 ft. Growing from the seeds is a pod or boll which bursts open upon ripening, exposing a mass of white cotton fibers. Each of these fibers is a minute, hair-like tube, the outer wall being pure cellulose, the opening filled with plant juices. When the boll bursts open, the fiber collapses into a flat ribbon-like form, twisted and doubled upon itself more than a hundred times from end to end.

The picking season for cotton begins in the late summer. Most cotton is now picked by machine. The cotton, clinging to its seed, is piled onto the cotton farmer's cart and is hauled to the gin. After the seeds have been removed by the gin, the cotton is compressed and secured with bagging and steel strips into bales weighing about 500 lb.

All cotton grades are standardized by the US Department of Agriculture. Samples of each bale are classified into one of six color groups, then given a "staple length" according to the length of the average fibers, and finally graded as to the amount of foreign matter present and the condition and ripeness of the fibers. From these hundreds of possible grading combinations, each bale is given a "quality rating" which determines its price.

The raw cotton fiber, mechanically cleaned of dirt and carded into layers, but not otherwise treated, has a limited use for paddings and coverings of unbroken surfaces. This form is supplied under the name of *nonadsorbent cotton*. It is also frequently used as cotton plugs in the bacteriological laboratory because of its nonabsorbency.

Absorbent cotton is prepared from the raw cotton fiber by a series of processes which remove the natural waxes and all impurities and foreign substances and render the fibers absorbent. Briefly summarized the processes may be described as follows. Each cotton bale goes through a mechanical cleaning process. Foreign matter, dust, seed hulls, and soil, etc, are removed by means of "openers," "pickers," etc. From the mechanical cleaners, the cotton is blown through large pipes to the boiling kier and the bleaching tub where it is made absorbent and bleached. In these processes it is freed from the waxes, resins, fats, and coloring matter normally present in the raw fiber.

During the chemical treatment, all surgical cotton is thoroughly washed using a fresh supply of water for each washing. A practically pure, white cellulose fiber is the result.

Cotton thus treated is dried by being passed, on a moving screen, through long drying ovens. The dried cotton is then ready for the "lapping" process. This process is similar to the cleaning process. The beaters tear the tufts of cotton to smaller pieces. The grid bars eliminate the short fibers and foreign matter.

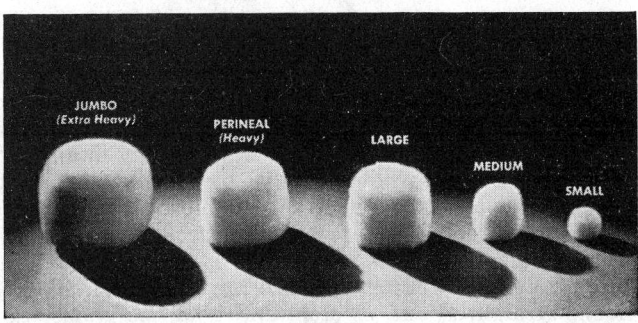

Fig. 803. Sizes of cotton balls.

The rollers press the cotton into a continuous lap in which form it passes through the carding machine. There, thousands of wire needles remove the short fibers and straighten out the longer cotton fibers, forming a thin web. This is the familiar roll cotton. Other cards fold the web which is then cut into uniform strips and automatically rolled into cotton balls.

Besides the familiar roll form, Purified Cotton may be obtained in various prepared forms such as cotton balls (Fig. 803), cotton-tipped applicators, etc.

Cotton balls can be prepared by hand but they are more advantageously made on special machines. Machine-made balls are firm, compact, and uniform in size, shape, and weight. They are produced in several sizes. The larger size balls are made for obstetrical uses, in the delivery room, or when changing perineal pads. The medium cotton ball is particularly useful for applying antiseptics or medication locally, cleansing the skin, and in the nursery where manifold uses are apparent. The small cotton ball is often used for skin cleansing before hypodermic or intravenous injections, and in applying local medications to small areas.

Absorbent balls made of a uniform surgical viscose fiber are also available under the brand name Preptic (*J&J*). These absorbent balls absorb fluids faster and retain their shape better than those made of cotton.

In addition to the long fiber USP grade of cotton, which is primarily used for specialized work and similar uses where high quality is essential, cheaper grades are available for less exacting uses. For example, in gauze-covered dressings and padding for splints, the lower grades are efficient yet more economical.

One such grade consists of a combination of medium and shorter length fibers. Another consists of medium short length fibers and is used particularly by hospitals for drainage pads, padding for splints, and other uses where a long-fibered cotton is not required.

Nonabsorbent bleached cotton, prepared by a modified bleaching process, wherein the water-repellent natural oils and waxes are retained, is also available. This cotton is easily identified by its silky feel. Because it is repellent to water, it does not become matted or inelastic. Consequently it is well adapted to packing, padding, and cushioning of dressings over traumatized areas and as nonabsorbent backing on sanitary napkins, combines, and drainage dressings.

Comber cotton is the uneven fiber pulled out by combing machines in textile mills which make fine yarns or thread. Though not suitable for spinning, comber cotton is clean, of high quality and excellent for many surgical uses. *Linters* are short cotton fibers resulting from the second ginning of the cotton seeds. These and other second-grade cottons are baled, graded, and sold through regular waste cotton markets.

Surgical Gauzes—The function of surgical gauze is to provide an absorbent material of sufficient tensile strength for surgical dressings. It is official in the USP under the title *Absorbent Gauze* (page 1876).

In the process of making surgical gauze, the raw cotton fiber is mechanically cleaned and then spun or twisted into a thread, and the thread, in turn, woven into an open-mesh cloth. This cloth is gray in appearance and nonabsorbent. It is bleached white and rendered absorbent by much the same processes as those used in the preparation of surgical cotton.

The gauze thus treated is dried by passing in a continuous length through a tentering machine. Tenter hooks straighten out, stretch, and hold the gauze taut as it is dried. When it leaves this apparatus, the dried gauze is cut into lengths, folded, rolled, and packed into various sized packages.

Gauze is classified according to its mesh or number of threads per square inch. Some types of surgical dressing require a close-meshed gauze for extra strength and greater protection, while other uses such as primary wound dressings, absorbent secondary dressings, and larger dressings to absorb purulent matter or other drainage require softer, more absorbent gauzes, having a more open mesh. For this reason surgical gauze is woven in some 10 different types or mesh sizes (Fig. 804). The USP recognizes 8 types ranging from 44 × 36 down to 14 × 10. The lengthwise or "warp" threads are mentioned first; the crosswise, or "fill" threads, second (see page 1877). For ascertaining the mesh or threads per inch, a small hand apparatus known as a "thread counter" is used.

Various forms of pads, compresses, and dressings are made from surgical gauze, alone or in conjunction with absorbent cotton.

Filmated Gauze is a folded absorbent gauze with a thin, even film of cotton or rayon distributed over each layer. This filmation fluffs up and gives ample dressing volume, yet costs less than gauze alone of equivalent volume. It possesses quick absorption and unusual softness.

Antiseptic or *Medicated Surgical Gauze* came into vogue in the Listerian era of surgery, and it is still used to some extent but with the advent of antibiotics, other therapeutic agents, and better surgery its popularity is decreasing. The gauze of this type most commonly used is iodoform gauze, which contains 5% iodoform and is largely used as a packing or drainage material. The so-called *Penrose drain*, which is very commonly used for draining surgical cases, is made by drawing a piece of plain or iodoform gauze through a thin-walled tube of latex and cutting to the desired length.

Selvage Edge Gauze Strips in widths of ¼ in. to 2 in. are specially designed and woven for use both as packing strips in surgery of the nose and sinuses, nasal haemostasis, etc, and as drainage wicks in the treatment of boils, abscesses, fistulas, and other draining wounds. The ravel-proof, selvage edges on both sides eliminate all loose threads. These selvage edge gauzes are available unmedicated, or medicated with iodoform 5%. All these gauze strips are obtainable in sterile form packed in sealed glass jars.

Gauze pads or *sponges* are folded squares of surgical gauze. These pads are so folded that no cut gauze edges or loose threads are exposed. This prevents loose fibers from entering the field of operation or the wound. The edges are so folded that each size may be unfolded to larger sizes without exposing cut edges or loose threads. See Fig. 805. Most popular sizes are:

2 × 2-inch—12-ply
3 × 3-inch—12-ply
4 × 4-inch— 8-ply
4 × 4-inch—16-ply
8 × 4-inch—12-ply
8 × 4-inch—24-ply

Patient-Ready sterilized packages of these frequently used all-gauze sponges are available in tamperproof packages of 2's. Such sterile units are particularly well suited to the numerous tray sets prepared in hospitals.

The *Topper Sponge* is a postoperative dressing made of a gauze covering enclosing a web of rayon and a filler of soft absorbent cellulose. Dressings of this type are not used in direct contact with a wound but are used as secondary dressings to absorb drainage, and offer a considerable economy in cost.

Adhesive (Absorbent) Bandage is official in the USP (see page 1875). The compress is composed of layers of absorbent gauze. Dyes or bacteriostatic agents or both, if nontoxic and harmless in the concentration employed, may be added to the compress. The weight of the compress is not less than that of a compress of the same area composed of four layers of Type I absorbent gauze. The absorbent gauze is substantially free from loose threads or ravelings. The adhesive plaster may be perforated over the compress, and the back may be coated with a water-repellent film. The adhesive surface is protected by overlapping strips of

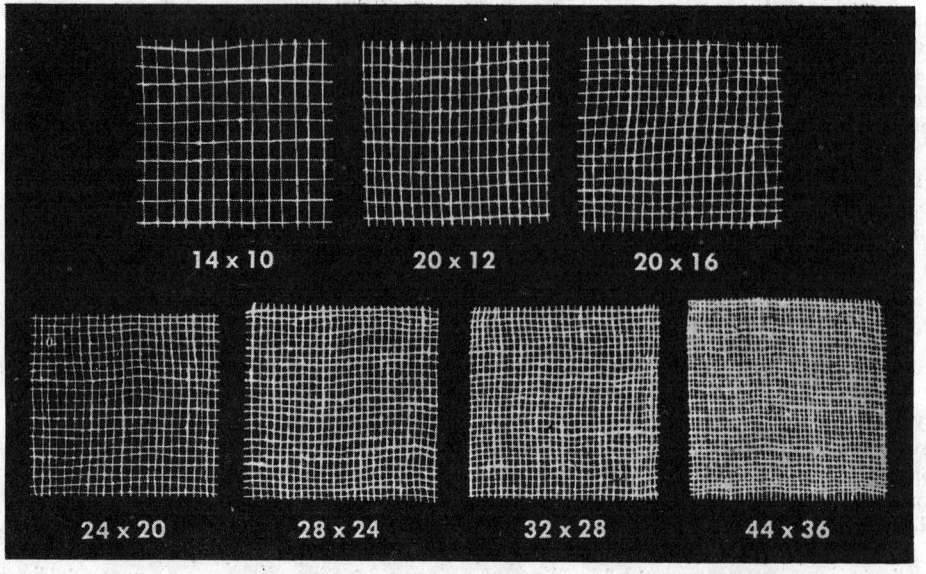

14 x 10   20 x 12   20 x 16

24 x 20   28 x 24   32 x 28   44 x 36

Fig. 804. Actual sizes of standard mesh gauze.

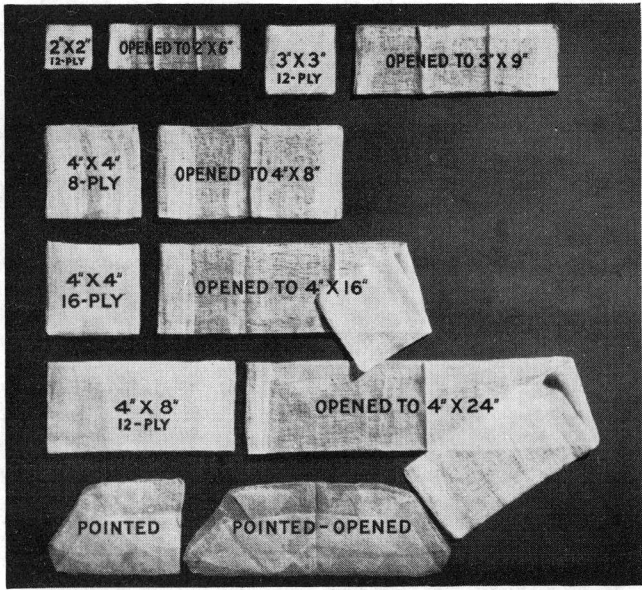

Fig. 805.   Gauze pads.

crinoline or other protective material of a width not less than that of the dressing.

Adhesive absorbent bandages must be sterile and be protected from contamination by suitable packaging.

Adhesive absorbent bandages wherein the gauze compress is medicated with mercurochrome or other antiinfective agents are also available. Dressings of this type are very widely sold under a variety of tradenames as a convenient household dressing for small wounds. Various modifications in larger sizes are also provided for professional and major surgical use.

X-ray Detectable Gauze pads are similar to all-gauze pads but contain inserts treated with barium sulfate. They are nontoxic, soft, and nonabrasive. They remain permanently detectable because they do not deteriorate in the body nor are they affected by either sterilization or time.

Ray-Tec X-Ray Detectable Sponges (*J&J*) contain a nonabrasive vinyl plastic monofilament which remains permanently detectable within the sponge.

Dressing Combines are designed to provide warmth and protection and to absorb large quantities of blood, pus, or other fluids that may drain from an incision or wound. Each combine consists of a layer of absorbent cotton about one inch thick and a layer of nonabsorbent cotton. They are held together and enclosed in a gauze covering. The nonabsorbent side of the pad is used, of course, away from the wound and helps prevent excretions from coming through to soil the linens and bed clothes. Other types of combines are supplied with cellulose filler and without nonabsorbent back, or with all-absorbent cotton filler.

One brand, Surgipad (*J&J*), is constructed of cotton and cellulose. The cellulose is inserted between two thick layers of cotton and serves to diffuse drainage throughout the complete dressing. These packs are available individually wrapped, sterile and Patient-Ready.

Special sterile prepackaged drainage and redressing Patient-Ready packs are also available. Listers J-D Heavy Dressing Pak (*J&J*) is a profuse drainage pack for dressing colostomies, ileostomies, suprapubic cystostomies and other surgical procedures involving profuse drainage. Listers Dressing Pak No. 5 (*J&J*) is a

complete redressing pack for cholecystectomies, thyroidectomies, simple breast operations, as well as other types of surgical procedures involving medium drainage. Both type packs contain Sofnet Cleaner (*J&J*) for cleaning the wound and applying fresh medication, Topper Sponges (*J&J*) and the Surgipad Combine Dressing (*J&J*).

A convenient and disposable instrument pack has been designed for easy removal of sutures. Lister Suture Removal Pak (*J&J*) contains a sterile precision metal scissor which will cut any suture material, and forceps with firm grip, wrapped in the folds of a drape which can be used as a sterile field.

Laparotomy Packs, also known as *Abdominal Packs, Tape Pads* or *Packs, Walling-Off Mops, Stitched Pads, Quilted Pads, Gauze Mops,* etc, are used to form a nonabrasive wall which will prevent abdominal or other organs from escaping into the field of operation and to help maintain body temperature during exposure. They are made of four layers of 28×24-mesh gauze. The edges are folded in and hemmed. The entire pack is cross-stitched and a looped tape ½ in. wide and 20 in. long is attached to one corner of it. A desirable feature of one type is an x-ray detectable insert, so firmly incorporated into the gauze that it cannot become detached. Treated with barium sulfate, the monofilament is nontoxic and, were it to be left inadvertently *in situ*, would cause no more foreign body reaction than an ordinary dressing. If a lap pack is lost in the operative field, the barium-impregnated insert will aid in its detection by means of x-ray.

Sanitary Napkins, intended for special hospital use, otherwise known as *V-Pads, Obstetrical (OB) Pads, Perineal Pads, Maternity Pads,* etc, are used in obstetrical, gynecological, or maternity cases. Boat-type napkin which has repellent tissue on the side and back surfaces of the napkin is usually preferred because of its greater fluid holding capacity. Sanitary napkins generally come with two sizes of filler, 3×9 or 3×11 in. The napkin cover is generally made from a nonwoven fabric or a nonwoven fabric supported with an open mesh scrim. Modess Pad Super (*Personal Products*) are 11-in. pads made with a macerated fluff filler and a soft nonwoven cover 22 in. long.

Sanitary napkins should retain absorbent capacity, color, and volume after the sterilization to which they are subjected when intended for hospital or surgical use.

Sanitary napkins are widely sold under various trade names.

Absorbent Cellulose, a paper product made from wood pulp, is an ideal substitute for cotton when used as a filler for drainage pads, underpads, and sanitary napkins. Rolls are made from many layers of thin absorbent cellulose in widths of 12 and 24 in. and wound in continuous lengths. The cellulose is soft, very absorbent, and bleached white. However, it lacks the elasticity of cotton fiber and when wet becomes sodden.

Cellulose Tissues are small white sheets of soft, strong, absorbent cellulose. Sheets are usually packed in specially slotted boxes from which they are dispensed conveniently, one at a time. In addition to their surgical and personal use, they are sometimes used for cleaning delicate instruments, lenses, and for general purposes in laboratories and clinics.

Disposable Cleaners composed of pure rayon and an inert binding material are manufactured under the brand name Chix Cleaners (*Chicopee*). They have great strength, wet or dry, and have considerable sidewise stretch. Their 300 holes/sq in. impart a cloth-like feel and cleaning action. These cleaners are especially useful in the nursery and maternity departments and are packaged in sizes from 7⅝ × 9 to 13½ × 13½ in.

Face Masks for use in the operating room are made of 4-ply, fine mesh surgical gauze. This construction provides for comfort and adequate absorbency and does not muffle the voice when the surgeon wishes to give instructions. These masks are shaped to fit correctly over the nose and mouth and to extend under the chin to prevent perspiration from dropping onto the operative field. Johnson's O. R. Masks (*J&J*) are made from strong, preshrunk, bleached cloth to withstand repeated laundering. The finely woven, bleached fabric serves as an efficient filter. A new disposable mask is also available under the name Regent Micro Filter Disposable Mask (*J&J*). This mask has been shown to minimize the danger of infection by bacteria from the nasopharynx of the physician, nurse, or patient. The mask is molded to provide a leakproof fit and is set away from the face so that neither the nose nor the mouth touches the filter material which contains an effective bacteriostatic agent.

Bandages

The function of bandages is to hold dressings in place or to provide slight pressure or support. They may be classed as inelastic and elastic. Still another class includes the bandages filled with hardening material, such as plaster of Paris bandages, which are used for purposes of immobilization.

Common Gauze Roller Bandage is official in the USP as a form in which *Absorbent Gauze* may be provided (page 1876). It is prepared from *Type I Absorbent Gauze* in various widths and lengths. Each bandage is in one continuous piece, tightly rolled, and substantially free from loose threads and ravelings.

Muslin Bandage Rolls are made of heavier unbleached material (56 × 60 mesh). They are supplied in the same widths as the regular gauze bandage. Muslin bandages are very strong and are used wherever gauze bandages do not provide sufficient strength or

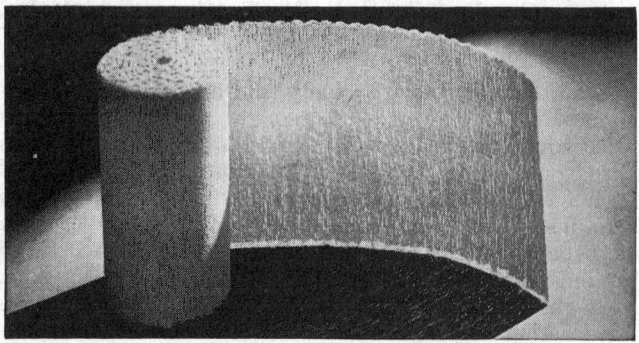

Fig. 806.   Hard-coated plaster of Paris bandage.

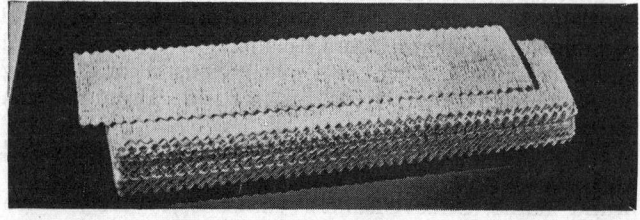

Fig. 807.   Hard-coated plaster of Paris splints.

support. They are frequently used to hold splints or bulky compression dressings in place.

Elastic Bandages are made in 4 types:

1. *Woven Elastic Bandage* is made of heavy elastic webbing containing rubber threads. Good support and pressure are provided by this type of rubber elastic bandage.

2. *Crepe Bandage* is elastic, but contains no rubber. Its elasticity is due to a special weave that allows it to stretch to practically twice its length, even after repeated launderings. This elasticity makes the crepe bandage especially serviceable in bandaging varicose veins, sprains, etc, because it conforms closely to the skin or joint surfaces, lies flat and secure, yet allows limited motion and stretches in case of swelling so that circulation is not impaired.

3. *Conforming Bandage* is a new type of readily conforming bandage made from two plies of specially processed, high quality, 14 × 10 cotton gauze folded to the center. This type of bandage is much easier to use and apply than ordinary roller bandage since it tends to cling to itself during application, thus preventing slipping. It readily conforms to all body contours without the necessity of "reversing" or twisting. A further advantage is the fact that there can be no rough or frayed edge. Kling Elastic Gauze (*J&J*) is a conforming bandage available in a variety of sizes up to 6 in. wide.

4. *Elastic Adhesive Bandage* is a specially woven, all-cotton elastic bandage spread on one surface with a special surgical adhesive mass. Like the crepe bandage its special weave permits it to be stretched to almost twice its original length. The adhesive surface keeps the bandage in place with the desired degree of support and pressure. It is used extensively for conditions requiring a close-fitting bandage support, such as sprains, strains, rib fractures, and certain muscular and ligamentous involvements. When applied to the chest wall to hold dressings in place, its elasticity offers minimal interference with respiration and minimizes the possibility of subsequent hypostasis of the lung.

Triangular Bandages are usually made by cutting a square of bleached muslin diagonally from corner to corner, forming two right triangles of equal size and shape. The length of the base is approximately 54 in. These bandages were brought into prominence by Esmarch and still bear his name. They are used in first aid work for head dressings, binders, arm slings, and as temporary splints for broken bones.

Plaster of Paris Bandages are used to provide immobilization and support in treatment of broken bones and in certain conditions of bones and joints. There are two types of ready-made plaster of Paris dressings.

1. *Hard-coated plaster of Paris bandages* are made from a thick creamy suspension of plaster of Paris spread on cloth and dried to a hard-coated mass. The bandage is cut to various widths and given a serrated, nonraveling edge. This method makes possible a very uniform spread which facilitates the preparation of strong, dependable casts. See Fig. 806.

2. *Hard-coated plaster of Paris splints* are ready-cut lengths of the hard-coated bandage. They are often preferred because they eliminate unrolling and folding from the rolled bandage. Their use greatly simplifies splint- and cast-making technique. They are specially useful as cast reinforcements. They can be cut to any desired size or shape before saturating without loosening the plaster. Usually, from 3 to 7 splints will give the desired thickness for cast reinforcement; 6 to 9 for making an individual splint. These are simply immersed and applied as 1 unit. See Fig. 807.

Individually packaged plaster of Paris bandages and splints are available in a wide variety of sizes. The Specialist (*J&J*) brand is made from specially treated plaster, uniformly spread and firmly bonded to the fabric. This results in a high strength to weight ratio in casts made from such bandages. After saturation, these bandages still possess the firm "body" and good handling qualities desirable in cast preparation.

A plaster of Paris bandage when wet becomes plastic and upon drying or "setting" a cast or splint is formed. The explanation of this reaction is as follows:

Plaster of Paris is manufactured from a solid, crystalline material known as gypsum or calcium sulfate dihydrate. Gypsum is pulverized to break up the crystals and then subjected to intense heat to drive off most of the inherent water of crystallization. The resulting powder is plaster of Paris. When water is added to plaster of Paris the plaster recrystallizes, or "sets," back into solid gypsum. Long, thin crystals form rapidly and interlock closely—and it is this tight interlocking that gives plaster much of its ultimate strength. However, if the plaster is disturbed by excessive molding or bending during the time when plaster is going from a fluid to a solid state, short stubby crystals, only loosely interlocked, are formed and a weak, flabby cast results.

Setting-Time.—Most plaster bandages and splints today fall into one of two categories as far as setting-time is concerned—fast-setting (5–8 min) and extra-fast-setting (2–4 min). The "built-in" setting-time may be modified by outside factors. Warm water will hasten the setting process, while cool water slows it up. Using a bandage "sloppy-wet" will delay setting, while wringing it dry will hasten setting. Various accelerators (potassium sulfate, common salt) or retarders (sodium citrate, borax) may be added to the saturation water to adjust setting, but the addition of these foreign materials may have a deleterious influence on cast strength and it is difficult to fix the setting time.

Thermal Reactions—The chemical reaction which takes place when plaster is combined with water to recrystallize back into gypsum is an exothermic one. The evolution of heat is not very noticeable in thin casts but in over-thick casts the temperature rise may be enough to cause the patient apprehension and, under extreme conditions, actual damage to the skin.

These conditions are within the control of the person applying the cast because, while the quantitative amount of heat produced by a given amount of plaster is a constant figure, the maximum temperature reached will vary with the techniques of application and conditions surrounding the individual cast. The thicker the cast, the higher the maximum temperature reached. Bandages with faster setting time will reach a higher temperature than bandages with a slower setting time. Generally speaking, the higher the room temperature and humidity, the higher the temperature rise.

One of the most important factors in this situation is the amount of ventilation or free circulation of air around the cast. For example, overwrapping the freshly applied cast with an elastic or gauze bandage, placing it on a pillow or mattress, and covering it with a blanket or otherwise insulating the cast from free access to the air, causes a sharp increase in temperature rise. Conversely, the most effective way to reduce the temperature of a cast is to increase circulation of air such as by blowing air over the cast with a circulating fan. This increases the evaporation of excess water, and evaporation consumes heat and, therefore, has a cooling effect. Most casts will reach maximum temperature in 5–15 min after application and then begin to cool off rapidly.

Saturation and Application—Plaster bandages should be saturated in water at room temperature (70–75°F). The excess water picked up in saturation should then be expelled by squeezing. In applying bandages to the patient, a moderate rubbing of the successive turns or layers of each bandage into the layers below will help to form a solid, well-fused cast. In moving a patient with a freshly applied cast, care must be taken to avoid possible distortion of the cast during the "green" period immediately following application.

A type of plaster of Paris bandage which is waterproof, very hard, and easier to keep clean, was introduced to the market in 1952. In this type of product, melamine formaldehyde is incorporated in the dry bandage along with the plaster of Paris. The bandage is dipped in water in the usual manner.

Stockinette Bandages are made of stockinette material knitted or woven in tubular form without seams. Surgical stockinette is unbleached and non-absorbent. Because it is soft and will stretch readily to conform comfortably to the arm, leg, or body it is used to cover the skin prior to the application of a plaster of Paris bandage.

Surgical Wadding is a soft protective padding used under plaster of Paris casts. It consists of bleached, nonabsorbent cotton, glazed on both sides to provide tensile strength and body and to keep moisture from the skin. Surgical wadding is supplied in uncut sheets 36 in. by 6 yd and in rolls 3–8 in. wide by 6 yd long.

Cotton Tipped Applicators are used to apply medications or cleanse an area. Machine-made cotton-tipped applicators are uniform in size, resulting in no waste of cotton or medications. The cotton is firmly attached to the stick and may be readily sterilized without affecting the anchorage of the cotton. These applicators are available in 3- or 6-in. lengths.

Eye Pads are scientifically shaped (2¼ × 2½ in.) to fit comfortably and to completely cover the eye, thus protecting the eyebrow when taped. These pads are made with Masslinn nonwoven fabric (*Chicopee*). Two sides are enclosed to prevent the cotton from escaping and the pad from distorting. Where desired the pad may be folded and used as a pressure dressing. Eye pads are especially useful in the outpatient clinic of the hospital, the industrial medical department, and the doctor's office. They are sealed in individual envelopes, sterilized, and packed in boxes of 50.

Nursing Pads are designed in a contour shape to fit comfortably under the nursing brassiere or breast binder. Johnson's Nursing Pads (*J&J*) are made of soft, absorbent cellulose with a protective backing. Both sides of the pad are enclosed in Masslinn nonwoven fabric (*Chicopee*).

Disposable Underpads, sold under several trade names, are used for incontinent patients, maternity patients, and other cases where there is heavy drainage and linen is soiled. One brand, for instance, known as Tri-Pads (*J&J*), 18 × 24 in., is made with a soft covering of extra-large, fire retardent Masslinn nonwoven fabric (*Chicopee*). This covering adds greatly to the comfort of the patient and the waterproof plastic-film back prevents moisture from striking through the bedding, thus reducing the number of linen changes required each day. Such pads cost less than the average hospital-made pad and provide a neat, clean, easy-to-handle pad that is quickly changed and is easily disposed of.

Disposable Nursery Diapers—One brand, Chux (*J&J*) sterile Nursery Diapers, is designed for hospital infants and will accommodate babies up to 11 lb. A soft, strong, and porous covering allows for rapid absorption and drainage. These sterile diapers have a soft polyethylene backing with exceptional pinning strength. They are packed 12 per bag.

Adhesive Tape

The use of adhesive masses and plasters, which later evolved into modern adhesive tapes, appears to be as old as medicine itself. There is evidence of the use of adhesive, or at least sticky mixtures, in ancient times as a healing preparation applied directly to the local lesion, and the Greeks are known to have used, for this purpose, a paste consisting of olive oil, lead oxide, and water.

Among ancient writings one finds a reference to the popularization of this mixture by Menecrates, a physician to Tiberius. Its applications were many, and it was considered not only nonirritating, but actually soothing for a variety of local ills.

During the middle of the nineteenth century an important improvement was introduced with the addition to the formula of India rubber. This resulted in better adhesive qualities, better support, easier application by virtue of "quicker stick," and cleaner removal.

In 1899 the modern zinc oxide type of adhesive mass was developed. This inaugurated the era of modern adhesive tape masses since it made possible a tape of greatly improved strength and excellent, quick-sticking qualities. Tapes of this type rapidly became an indispensable adjunct to modern surgical and medical practice.

Subsequently, other improvements and modifications have been developed, eg, increased strength of the backing materials used in the various types of tapes with greater lightness and adaptability; waterproofing; uniformity of mass spread and control of flow properties; better anchorage to the backing, minimizing transfer of the mass to the outer surface of adjacent layers or to the skin; and vastly improved aging characteristics.

For a description of *Adhesive Tape* USP, see its monograph on page 1877.

Composition of Adhesive Masses—Modern adhesive tape masses consist of varying mixtures of several basic classes of substances. These are composed essentially of an elastomer (Para or pale crepe rubber in the case of the natural rubber tapes, and substances such as certain polymers of polyisobutylene and similar synthetic elastomers in the case of the so-called synthetic rubber tapes); one of several types of rosin, or modified rosins, which are available in many forms under various trade names; antioxidants; plasticizers; fillers; and coloring agents, to give the tape the desired tint or whiteness.

The elastomers most commonly used in the so-called synthetic tapes, and occasionally in admixture with natural rubber, are polymers of polyisobutylene or the copolymers of butadiene and styrene.

The fillers and whitening agents are usually simple substances such as starch, zinc oxide, talcum, and titanium dioxide.

Use—A primary use of adhesive tape is to pull something into place and then hold it there, as illustrated by traction; a second use is to affix something in place, as a protective covering for dressings.

Every medical specialty finds specific applications for adhesive tape. The orthopedic surgeon has developed countless therapeutic uses for adhesive tape in the treatment of sprains, strains, rupture of a muscle or tendon, fascitis, tendinitis, myositis, separation of certain joints, and other spontaneous or traumatic conditions of the connective and supportive tissues.

In such conditions adhesive strapping may be applied for the purpose of immobilization of a part, to permit more rapid healing, and to alleviate discomfort by the moderate fixation of soft tissues such as fascia, muscles, tendons, and ligaments. These structures can be held in normal or corrective positions, which permit only limited movement, by means of adhesive tape. Similarly, in protecting injured joints the objective is to prevent component structures of the joint from exceeding normal physiologic limits and to provide gentle compression where indicated.

One of the greatest values of adhesive tape lies in its use as a protective covering during short periods of time. The edges of small wounds can be approximated; small blisters, certain skin lesions, and many wounds can be covered and protected from contamination by the proper use of tape.

Adhesive tape enjoys wide use for purposes other than protection and support, particularly as a means of holding in position such items as catheters, endotracheal tubes, intravenous needles, and radium molds. It is used for sealing opened packages, as a label, and for a variety of other purposes.

General Principles—When using adhesive tape for therapeutic purposes, the following simple principles should be kept in mind:

1. The skin, if hairy, should be shaven and should be clean and dry.
2. The skin should be free from oily contamination, but preparation with irritant organic solvents which remove all the natural oils from the skin should be avoided.
3. Skin should not be treated with benzoin or similar preparations. It is unnecessary and may increase irritation.
4. The part must be placed and held in an overcorrected position while applying the strapping.
5. The part should be strapped so as to give firm support but avoid constriction. When strapping is finished, check the circulation.
6. After strapping, if movement of the part causes undue tension with pain, the part should be restrapped.
7. Tape should be left in place sufficiently long to assure healing. If necessary, reinforce from time to time.

Technique of Application—Tape should be applied only to a clean, not a devitalized or chemically dehydrated, skin. Small traces of oil, grease, glycerin, or other substances interfere with adhesion. The same is true of moist surfaces or surfaces covered with a film of dust or powder. The use of counterirritants (iodine tincture, liniments, etc) must be avoided before adhesive tape is applied.

Occasionally, when a strapping does not adhere, examination will reveal that the adhesive surface is covered with a film of desquamated epidermis. In such cases the area should be cleansed with neutral soap and thoroughly dried and the tape reapplied.

When applying adhesive tape to curved surfaces, wrinkles can be avoided by using several narrow strips in place of one wide strip. A similar effect can be obtained by tearing a wide strip at either end to make several narrow tabs, which unite at the middle of of the strip.

In all strappings one should apply the first strips parallel with the fibers of the muscle, fascia, tendon, or ligament for good anchorage. Subsequent strips may run in any logical direction.

Technique of Removal—The proper removal of adhesive tape deserves much consideration and care. The first suggestion toward effecting a relatively painless removal is to be gentle and not to "rip or tear" the tape off, even though the patient requests such heroic measures. Such a procedure often results in considerable irritation and even justifiable anger on the part of the patient.

One should remove adhesive tape along the longitudinal axis of the strapping rather than across it. The edges, which are sometimes difficult to loosen, can be easily peeled back by holding the skin taut and pulling it away from the tape. It is often easier to push the skin away from the adhesive tape than to pull the tape from the skin.

In removing strips of adhesive tape which hold a dressing in place, it is wise to cut across the strips at the gauze edge and then remove the strips by pulling away from the line of cut.   When removing tape near a wound, pull towards the wound, not away from it.

Removal of adhesive tape can be made easy and painless by the use of a suitable solvent.   Carbon tetrachloride and other chlorinated hydrocarbons do not present the dangerous fire hazard of ether, benzine, and similar inflammable solvents.   However, proper ventilation precautions must be taken to avoid toxic concentrations of vapor.   These solvents may remove the natural oils from the skin and may be irritating, so that tape should not be reapplied to areas so treated without thorough washing, drying, and exposure to the air.   Mineral oil works almost as well as an aid to removal as organic solvents, and not only is it completely safe to use, but it also has the advantage of lubricating and soothing the skin beneath the tape.

Large strappings are easily removed with mineral oil or solvents as follows: first, swab along the end and edges of the strip of adhesive tape with cotton saturated with the agent; next, pull up the end so loosened, and continue to swab along the junction of the tape with the skin, peeling the tape back gently as the solvent loosens it.

The part should be cleansed with alcohol or mineral oil, allowed to dry, and dusted with powder, unless adhesive tape is to be reapplied.

Adhesive Tape Reactions—While skin reactions were formerly accepted by the medical profession as a natural accompaniment of the use of adhesive tape, with better understanding of the mechanisms of such reactions and vast progress in research and technology, the objective of hyporeactivity has in large degree been attained.

Because adhesive tape masses consist of such a heterogeneous and complex mixture of organic compounds, it is little wonder that many workers have placed most reactions to the substance on an allergic basis.   More recent work, however, has shown that a true allergic response to the modern adhesive tape mass or its components is present in only a small proportion of the cases, although other forms of dermatitis, infection, and chemical contact irritation do occur.   However, newer tapes containing a smaller number of ingredients produce fewer skin reactions.

More and more attention is being given to the utilization of ingredients having the least possible sensitizing potential.   In any specified case of sensitivity, however, no ingredient should be omitted from suspicion.   It is not uncommon to demonstrate reactivity to the composite mass when no reactivity to individual ingredients can be elicited.   But it is important to emphasize that in the minds of both the profession and the laity considerable confusion in terminology exists, there being more than a tendency to describe all types of reactions as "allergic."   Actually, irritative re-

sponses to adhesive tape may arise from many causes, and in only a very small percentage of the cases is allergy a factor.   Thus the term "hyporeactive" or "hypoirritative" is broader and of greater practical significance than the more restrictive term "hypo-allergenic."

Protectives

Protectives are employed to cover wet dressings and hot or cold compresses, and are also used as a covering for poultices, and for the retention of heat.   They prevent the escape of moisture from the dressing or compress.   In common use as protectives are plastic sheeting, rubber sheeting, and waxed or paraffined paper.

Plastic Sheeting is used to cover wet dressings and hot and cold compresses.   It prolongs retention of heat and prevents escape of moisture from dressing or compress to clothing or bed linens.   It is used extensively to cover hot packs applied in the Kenny treatment of poliomyelitis.

Rubber Sheeting is a rubber-coated cloth, waterproof and flexible.   It is supplied in various lengths and widths for use as a covering for bedding.   One form used as a protection blanket is provided with eyelets for lacing under the bed.   A so-called "nursery sheeting" is supplied, coated only on one side.

Waxed Paper is prepared by passing a parchment-like sheet of paper through melted wax or paraffin.   It is used largely as an economical substitute for more expensive protectives.

Care of Surgical Dressings

The USP provides that all sterile surgical dressings bear a warning statement that the sterility of the contents cannot be guaranteed if the package bears evidence of damage or has been previously opened.   Surgical dressings therefore must be properly cared for in order to preserve the sterility of the contents.   The most suitable storage places are dustproof cases of glass, metal, or wood.   The storage place should be dry and not near steam or furnace heat.   The absorbency and color of cotton, gauze, and cellulose are affected by prolonged contact with heat.

Packages containing sterile surgical dressings should be delivered to the consumer in the original sealed condition.   The packages should not be opened and the contents exposed except at the time of use.   Exposure of surgical dressings to dust, and especially to unnecessary handling, is likely to be a means of conveying infection.   The greatest aseptic care should be used in applying sterile surgical dressings.

Official Surgical Dressings

Adhesive Bandage USP

[Adhesive Absorbent Bandage, USP XVI; Adhesive Absorbent Compress; Adhesive Absorbent Gauze; Band-Aid (*J&J*); Curad (*Bauer & Black*); Quik-Bands (*Rexall*)]

Description—Sterile individual dressing consisting of a plain absorbent compress affixed to a film or fabric coated with a pressure-sensitive, adhesive composition.   One or more colors or bacteriostatic agents or other nontherapeutic materials or combinations thereof, if nontoxic and harmless in the concentration employed, may be added to the compress.   The compress is equivalent in absorbency to a compress of the same area composed of four layers of Type I *Ab-*

sorbent Gauze (page 1876).   The compress is substantially free from loose threads or ravelings.   The adhesive strip may be perforated, and the back may be coated with a water-repellent film.

The adhesive surface is protected by a removable covering of a width not less than that of the bandage.

Gauze Bandage USP

Gauze Bandage is sterile Type I absorbent gauze.   Its length is not less than 98.0% of that declared on the label, and its average width is not more than 1.6

mm less than the declared width. It contains no dye or other additives.

Description—One continuous piece, tightly rolled, in various widths and lengths and substantially free from loose threads and ravelings.

Note—*Before determining the thread count, dimensions and weight, hold the bandage, unrolled, for not less than 4 hours in a standard atmosphere of 65% ± 2% relative humidity at 21° ± 1.1° (70°F ± 2°F).*

Oxidized Cellulose USP

[Absorbable Cellulose; Absorbable Cotton; Cellulosic Acid; Oxycel (*Parke-Davis*)]

Oxidized Cellulose, dried in a vacuum over phosphorus pentoxide for 18 hours, contains 16.0–24.0% of carboxyl groups (COOH). It is sterile.

Description—In the form of gauze or lint. Is slightly off-white in color, is acid to the taste, and has a slight, charred odor.

Solubility—Insoluble in water and in acids; soluble in dilute alkalies.

Uses—Oxidized Cellulose is a gauze or cotton which has been chemically oxidized so as to make it both *hemostatic* and absorbable. The value of oxidized cellulose in various surgical procedures is based upon its properties of absorbability when bured in tissues and its remarkable hemostatic effect. Absorption occurs between the second and seventh day following implantation of the dry material, depending on the adequacy of the blood supplied to the area and the degree of chemical degradation of the implanted material. Complete absorption of large amounts of blood-soaked gauze may take 6 weeks or longer and serious surgical complications have been reported as the result of failure to absorb, and cyst formation. Hemostasis depends upon the marked anity of *cellulosic acid* for hemoglobin. When exposed to blood, either *in vitro* or in surgical conditions, the oxidized gauze or cotton turns very dark brown or black and forms a soft gelatinous mass which readily molds itself to the contours of irregular surfaces and controls surgical hemorrhage by providing an artificially induced clot. Pressure should be exerted on the gauze or cotton for about 2 minutes in order to facilitate the sealing off of the mouths of the bleeding vessels.

Two factors require emphasis: (1) cellulosic acid does not enter the physiological clotting mechanism *per se* but forms what might be termed an "artificial clot," as described and, therefore, is effective in controlling the bleeding hemophiliac, and (2) the hemostatic action of cellulosic acid is not enhanced by the addition of other hemostatic agents, such as thrombin (which in any case would be destroyed by the pH of the gauze unless some means of neutralization were practicable). The hemostatic effect of either one alone is greater than the combination.

Oxidized Cellulose is useful as a temporary packing for the control of capillary, venous, or small arterial *hemorrhage*, but since it inhibits epithelialization, it should be used only for the immediate control of hemorrhage and not as a surface dressing. Recently a purer and more uniform product prepared from oxidized regenerated cellulose has been developed and is available as SURGICEL Absorbable Hemostat. This product offers many advantages over the older, less uniform oxidized cellulose derived from cotton and, because of its chemical uniformity assures dependable performance and overcomes many of the difficulties encountered with the older type of cotton product.

The knitted fabric strips do not fragment, may easily be sutured in place if necessary, and provide prompt and complete absorption with minimum tissue reaction.

Purified Cotton USP

[Gossypium Purificatum; Absorbent Cotton]

Purified Cotton is the hair of the seed of cultivated varieties of *Gossypium hirsutum* Linné, or of other species of *Gossypium* (Fam. *Malvaceae*), freed from adhering impurities, deprived of fatty matter, bleached, and sterilized in its final container.

For a discussion of the preparation and uses of Purified Cotton, see page 1869.

Description—White, soft, fine filament-like hairs appearing under the microscope as hollow, flattened, and twisted bands, striate and slightly thickened at the edges. It is practically odorless and tasteless.

Solubility—Insoluble in ordinary solvents; soluble in ammoniated cupric oxide TS.

Absorbable Dusting Powder USP

[Starch-derivative Dusting Powder; Bio-Sorb (*Ethicon*)]

Absorbable Dusting Powder is an absorbable powder prepared by processing cornstarch and intended for use as a lubricant for surgical gloves. It contains not more than 2.0% of magnesium oxide.

Description—A white, odorless powder. Its pH is between 10.0 and 10.8, in a 1 in 10 suspension.

Uses—This is used as a *surgeon's glove lubricant.*

Absorbent Gauze USP

[Carbasus Absorbens; Gauze]

Absorbent Gauze is cotton in the form of a plain woven cloth conforming to the standards set forth in the USP. Absorbent Gauze that has been rendered sterile is packaged to protect it from contamination. The length of standard-width Absorbent Gauze is not less than 98% of the length declared on the label, and the width is within 1.27 cm (½ inch) of the standard for the type of gauze concerned.

Description—White cotton cloth of various thread counts and weights. May be supplied in various lengths and widths, and in the form of rolls or folds.

Table I designates for each commercial type the thread count and the standard weight in Gm per square meter. The standard width of Type I gauze is 97.8 cm (38.5 inches); that of all other types is 91.4 cm (36 inches).

Note—*Condition all Absorbent Gauze for at least 4 hours in a standard atmosphere of 65 ± 2% relative humidity at 21 ± 1.1° (70 ± 2°F), before determining the weight, thread count, and absorbency. Remove the Absorbent Gauze from its wrappings before placing it in the conditioning atmosphere, and if it is in the form of bolts or rolls, cut the quantity necessary for the various tests from the piece, excluding the last two meters when the total quantity of Gauze available so permits.*

Gauze, Petrolatum—see page 765.

Purified Rayon USP

Purified Rayon is a fibrous form of sterile, bleached, regenerated cellulose. It may contain not more than 1.25% of titanium dioxide.

Description—White, lustrous or dull, fine, soft, filamentous fibers, appearing under the microscope as round, oval, or slightly flattened translucent rods, straight or crimped, striate and with serrate cross-sectional edges. Is practically odorless and practically tasteless.

Table I—Specifications for Gauze

Type	Threads per 2.54 cm		Average count, threads per cm²	Standard weight, Gm per M²
	Warp	Filling		
I	41 to 47[a]	33 to 39	76 to 84[b]	49.8
II	30 to 34	26 to 30	57 to 63	37.4
III	26 to 30	22 to 26	49 to 55	32.3
IV	22 to 26	18 to 22	41 to 47	27.8
V	20 to 24	16 to 20	37 to 43	25.7
VI	18 to 22	14 to 18	33 to 39	22.5
VII	18 to 22	10 to 14	29 to 35	20.6
VIII	12 to 16	8 to 12	21 to 27	13.8

[a] As is stated in the General Notices, the upper limits of a range are inclusive so that the range consists of the two values themselves and all intermediate values.
[b] For Type I rolled gauze, the range is 75 to 85 threads per 6.54 cm².

Solubility—Very soluble in ammoniated cupric oxide TS and dilute sulfuric acid (3 in 5); insoluble in ordinary solvents.

Uses—See *Absorbent Gauze* and *Gauze Bandage*.

Adhesive Tape USP

[Adhesive Plaster USP XVI; Sterile Adhesive Plaster; Sterile Adhesive Tape]

Adhesive Tape consists of fabric and/or film evenly coated on one side with a pressure-sensitive, adhesive mixture. Its length is not less than 98.0% of that declared on the label, and its average width is not more than 1.6 mm less than the declared width. If Adhesive Tape has been rendered sterile, it is protected from contamination by appropriate packaging.

For a comprehensive discussion of the manufacture, usefulness, and utilization of Adhesive Tape, see page 1873.

Sutures and Suture Materials

In a narrow sense, a surgical suture is a strand or fiber used to hold wound edges in apposition, and the process of applying such a strand is called *suturing*. When such material, without a needle, is used to stop bleeding by tying off severed blood vessels, the strand is called a *ligature*, and the process is known as *ligating*. Suture materials, however, have uses beyond those involved in the repair of wounds. They are often used in corrective and repair procedures in tissues.

Surgical sutures were first listed in the second supplement of USP XI in a monograph on catgut sutures, which were then officially designated, "Surgical Gut." USP XII carried also a similar monograph on surgical silk. USP XVI contained, in addition to surgical gut, a generalized monograph designed to cover all sutures except catgut, and this is also true of USP XVIII. These monographs have the force of law, establish the standards by which legal acceptability of sutures is judged, and are the final reference in cases of complaint and dispute concerning properties covered by them.

Since there are many available histories of the development and use of sutures, no attempt will be made here to review the subject. Let it suffice to say that, at one time or another, nearly every form of fibrous material or wire that offered any promise at all has been used as a suture, and indeed many materials which by present standards offer no promise have been thus employed. Cotton and linen were among the earliest suture materials, but the use of animal intestines also claims great antiquity. As in many other fields of science, there have been numerous fads in the use of various materials, so that their use waxed and waned through the centuries. Frequently the acceptance of a given suture material depended on its successful use by an eminent surgeon whose authority carried weight and encouraged emulation. In many cases there appeared to be legitimate scientific justification for such uses. Possibly the most important factor in the acceptance or discard of suture materials has been their characteristics in the presence of infection. As knowledge of bacteriology increased and methods of sterilization improved, the earlier disadvantages of certain sutures in this regard have been overcome, so that currently a wide variety of surgical suture materials may be sterilized in forms suitable for the surgeon's use. It is not inappropriate to point out that boiling is still depended upon in some circles, although it is not clearly effective against spore-forming organisms. Among widely accepted methods for the sterilization of sutures are: autoclave sterilization with free access of water vapor, applicable only for those sutures which are not harmed by this process; dry heat at 310°F; ethylene oxide; and irradiation sterilization by the use of either beta or gamma rays. Irradiation sterilization has many advantages over older methods insofar as commercial production is concerned. The sutures are sterilized in their final sealed packages, eliminating any danger of recontamination. The dose rate is 40% greater than necessary to kill even the most resistant spore-forming organisms.

One great advantage of this method lies in the lack of deteriorating effect upon the suture. Irradiation sterilized surgical gut is stronger, more pliable and easier to handle than ordinary surgical gut sutures.

Suture materials are divided into two principal classes, *absorbable* and *nonabsorbable*. In the first and more important class are found those materials which are capable of being broken down or digested by the enzymes in animal tissues. All useful materials in the absorbable class belong to the proteins, so that it appears that the proteolytic enzymes in tissues are responsible for the digestion of catgut and its disappearance from the wound area.

Absorbable Sutures

Surgical Gut—Catgut is probably still the most widely used suture material and is, therefore, of great importance to surgery generally.

The basic constituent of surgical catgut is collagen. Collagen sutures are produced from connective tissue obtained from healthy animals, usually sheep and cattle.

In the older and still widely used method the collagen is derived from the submucous connective tissue of the small intestine. The intestines from the freshly killed animal are cleaned of their contents and split longitudinally into two ribbons. Mechanical processes remove the innermost mucosa, which was in contact with the food, and the muscularis and serosal layers, which were outside the submucosa, leaving essentially only the submucosa. This appears as a thin, strong network consisting chiefly of collagen, whose orientation and strength are increased markedly by subsequent processing. From one to five or six such ribbons are stretched, spun or twisted under tension, and dried under tension to form a uniform strand. These strands are polished and cut into appropriate lengths for packaging and sterilization.

In the newer method collagen sutures are produced from collagen derived from beef tendon. The tendons are suitably treated and dispersed. The dispersed collagen is extruded, precipitated, and reconstituted as fine strands which are then twisted, stretched, tanned, and otherwise treated to give absorbable sutures with the desired characteristics.

In the United States practically no unsterilized surgical gut is sold, although in other countries this is a common item and requires chemical or heat sterilization by the surgeon.

Diameter and strength requirements for absorbable surgical suture (surgical gut), as specified in the USP, are shown in Table II.

In the USP will be found descriptions of the apparatus and methods for measuring diameters and tensile strengths and for carrying out other tests on sutures.

Plain and Chromicized Surgical Gut—The description given above applies for the following two varieties as distinguished by their resistance to absorptive action by tissue enzymes, *Type A*, plain or untreated, and *Type C*, medium treatment. This reflects the surgeon's requirements for catgut that will retain its tensile strength for varying periods of time, or that will show an increased resistance to the proteolytic substances found in certain organisms or body tissues. Surgical gut may be treated by the deposition in it of chromium oxide or by other chemicals so as to prolong its survival in tissues. Such products were formerly designated as 10-, 20-, or 40-day catgut, it being assumed that these sutures would remain for such periods in normal tissues. The variations in catgut as a natural product, variations in patients as regards the rate of attack of their tissues on catgut and the variation in sites of implantations

Table II—Diameter and Tensile Strength of Absorbable Surgical Sutures

Size	Limits on diameter, mm		Limits on knot-pull tensile strength, Kg
	Min	Max	
9–0	0.018	0.038	0.023
8–0	0.038	0.064	0.045
7–0	0.064	0.089	0.07
6–0	0.089	0.127	0.18
5–0	0.127	0.179	0.38
4–0	0.179	0.241	0.77
3–0	0.241	0.318	1.25
2–0	0.318	0.406	2.00
1–0	0.406	0.495	2.77
1	0.495	0.584	3.80
2	0.584	0.673	4.51
3	0.673	0.762	5.90
4	0.762	0.864	7.00
5	0.864	0.978	9.00

make such a designation merely qualitative, so that it was replaced by the more general statement now in use. While many tests for the expected duration of resistance have been proposed, none is fully accepted as being comparable to digestion in animal tissues, and none has been included in the USP.

Approximately half the surgical gut used in the United States has been chromicized or otherwise treated. Raw catgut is similar chemically to rawhide, while chromicized catgut is comparable to chrome-tanned leather. This tanning process is applied either to the submucosa ribbons before they have been twisted into the strand form or to the finished dried strand. Treatment in the ribbon form is reported to result in a more uniform deposition of chromium oxide throughout the entire cross section of the suture, while string chromicization sometimes causes the deposition of relatively heavier concentrations of the tanning agent near the periphery of the strand, with less penetration to its center. Deficient tanning of catgut may result in its premature absorption with possible wound disruption, although such incidents are now often recognized as effects of nutritional inadequacies with resultant weakness of the tissues themselves. Excessive chrome concentrations in surgical gut may produce sutures that are extremely slow to digest, since they survive in normal tissues for a long time and may indeed appear as knot extrusions some months after an operation. The mechanism of such knot extrusions by highly tanned catgut or by nonabsorbable sutures is not yet clear, but surgeons encounter such extrusions from time to time.

Tissue Reaction to Catgut—Following any surgical incision, there is an outpouring of blood and lymph into and through the wound. These fluids clot, and fibrils form a network upon which new cells may build. The capillaries in the area dilate, and the blood supply in the vicinity of the wound is increased.

The leukocytes in the area increase in number. Tissue fluids increase and bring in fibroblasts and other cells, generally about the fourth day after an operation. As the small blood vessels regenerate and build new blood channels, the fibroblasts produce new tissue and the wound is gradually sealed and closed off.

The absorption of surgical gut takes place along with the tissue repair processes. The leukocytes, which appear early in any wound, produce proteolytic enzymes which, among other functions, carry out the digestion of absorbable catgut sutures. After this process is well along, fibroblasts appear and begin to lay down the collagen fibers essential for the growing strength and healing of the wound. In the first phase the number and character of the debriding cells, together with such secondary effects as swelling, pain and redness constitute "tissue reaction." The surgeon strives to minimize tissue reaction which tends to retard the healing process and may lead to the formation of excessive scar tissue with reduced strength and other objectionable characteristics. It is thus seen that while the wound healing proceeds in two stages, the digestion of catgut is continuous after its implantation. Chromic catgut elicits less tissue reaction of a leukocytic or exudative type than does the plain variety.

Plain gut is digested by enzymes at a faster rate than is chromic gut. The surgeon chooses either plain or chromic gut, depending on the type of tissue involved, the condition of the patient and the estimated healing period of the wound. Small sizes of surgical gut cause less tissue reaction and irritation than large sizes. There is less digestive work for the enzymes to do. For this reason surgeons make it a rule never to use a suture that is stronger than the tissue in which it is to be used. The larger sutures merely add to tissue irritation without supplying any needed strength to the wound.

The wound, is usually about one-third healed on the sixth postoperative day and two-thirds healed on the eighth postoperative day. Ten days is the minimum repair period for healing an ordinary clean wound. Up to 14 and 16 days are required for the wound to obtain maximum strength. The condition of the individual patient and particular tissues in the patient's body can cause wide variances in these figures for wound healing.

Selection of Absorbable Sutures—The sizes of surgical gut sutures used vary with the technique of the surgeon, but, in general, plain gut should be used in tissues that heal quickly; chromic gut should be employed where slower healing and longer support of the suture line are indicated, but there appears to be a growing preference for the use of chromic gut in suitable sizes under most circumstances. Some surgeons prefer a double line of fine sutures rather than a single strand of heavier gut.

There is now a definite trend toward the use of surgical gut of finer gages for all surgical purposes. One reason for this is that finer sutures may be tied into smaller knots. Another point in favor of the use of smaller sizes is the fact that the surgeon is less likely to tie too tightly and less apt to interfere with circulation. There is also less danger of necrosis from strangulation of tissues.

There is abundant evidence that chromic catgut, properly chromicized and free from soluble chromium compounds, is less irritating and causes less foreign body reaction than does plain catgut. Many surgeons are now routinely using medium chromic catgut in the finer gages, and their reports indicate that healing is more rapid and the frequency of wet wounds is minimized. This is of particular importance in thyroidectomy. Table III, for chromic gut, has been compiled in consultation with eminent surgeons.

Sterilization and Packaging of Surgical Gut—Disappointing experiences with many attempts to sterilize gut by means of chemicals has created widespread distrust of the effectiveness of any chemical, so that catgut sutures after dehydration are sterilized by exposure to high temperatures or by irradiation. An important property of catgut, which determines many of its treatments and methods of preparation and use, is its ability to react with water. This reaction is called *proteolysis* and is a special form of the general hydrolysis reactions. It consists of the addition of water at reactive bonds in the protein chain with swelling, loss of tensile strength and solubilization of the catgut. This reaction is accelerated by high temperature, acids, alkalies, or suitable proteolytic enzymes and makes necessary a complete drying of the catgut before its exposure to the high-temperature sterilization. It also determines the methods and fluids employed in packaging.

At one time most surgical gut was produced and labeled as *boilable*. It was packaged in glass tubes with the strands immersed in a water-free high-boiling tubing fluid—usually xylol. Exteriors of the tubes could be sterilized at the hospital by autoclaving—hence, the term *boilable*.

The disadvantage of boilable catgut is that the drying necessary to permit high-temperature sterilization produces a stiff strand, which is still stiff as removed from the tube, and which requires soaking for several minutes in sterile water before surgeons find it pliable enough to use. This is no longer used (with isolated exceptions).

Table III—Chromic Surgical Gut[a]

Use	Size of surgical gut	No. of pieces into which 54-in. strand is cut
Ligatures		
Small deeper vessels	00, 0, 1	4
Small main vessels	1, 2	4
Small subcutaneous vessels	3-0, 00	4
Sutures		
Bones	3, 4	2
Cervix Uteri	1	2
Fascia	00, 0, 1	2
Intestines, tubes	4-0, 000,	2
ovaries	00	
peripheral nerves	5-0, 6-0	
Kidneys	0, 1	2
Muscles, tendons, ligaments	0, 1, 2	2
Peritoneum	00, 0, 1	2
Rectum	1	2
Skin (through-and-through)	0, 1	2
Skin	00	2
(subcutaneous)	0	2
Stomach	00, 0	2
Vagina	1	2

[a] Plastic surgeons uniformly use smaller gages than those described in this table.

The present method of packaging catgut produces sutures ready for use as removed from the packet and is designated as *nonboilable*. The catgut, contained in either a foil or plastic packet, is immersed in a pliabilizing fluid which generally consists of an alcohol or mixtures of an alcohol with a small percentage of water. The water has a pliabilizing effect on the catgut, but would ruin the gut if the latter is subjected to high-temperatures—therefore, the designation *nonboilable*.

For even greater convenience, all foil or plastic packets are now overwrapped in a secondary package. Both the contents of the inner packet and the outside of the packet are rendered sterile. By peeling open the overwrap package, the inner packet can be delivered ready for use in a sterile condition in the operating room.

Surgical Needles—Catgut is sold in standard tubes containing lengths in excess of 54 in. without needles, and, on being opened, these strands are cut in two or three pieces for ligating or are cut in three or four pieces to be threaded on eyed needles for suturing. While formerly only eyed needles were available, there is an increased trend to the use of eyeless needles, one or two being attached to each individual strand. One such needle is provided with an open channel into which the suture can be placed, and the channel is then swaged around the strand. Another type, known as "seamless," has a very delicate threaded hole drilled in the shank into which the suture is actually screwed. To prevent pull-out the shank is then pressed firmly about the suture. These sutures offer great advantage in minimizing trauma. With an eyed needle an opening in tissue must be made large enough to accommodate the needle and two thicknesses of suture, but with the eyeless needle, the opening need only accommodate the needle, slightly larger than the single suture which follows. This is greatly esteemed in fine surgery such as plastic and eye work. Suitable eyeless needles on catgut and other materials are now available to meet most of the demands of the modern surgeon.

Sterility Testing—Freedom from contamination is the most important property of any suture. Every lot of sutures furnished by reputable manufacturers is subjected to a series of physical and chemical tests, as well as to complete bacteriological examination for aerobic, anaerobic and mold organisms. No lot of sutures is released until all of these tests have been successfully passed; hence, the surgeon has come to have justified confidence in the adequacy and sterility of these products.

Operating Room Procedures with Sutures—Before a scheduled operation, the assigned nurse usually selects the necessary types of sutures as designated by the operating surgeon. The required amount of overwrapped packages are opened by peeling apart the outer package and flipping or otherwise removing in an aseptic manner the inner sterile packets and placing them on the Mayo stand. The packets are opened by tearing if foil and by cutting with sterile scissors if plastic. Straightening out of the nonboilable suture is accomplished by a gentle pull, but jerking may produce irreparable damage and pulling catgut sutures through rubber-gloved fingers will also harm the suture. Nonboilable sutures are commonly used as removed from the packet, but with boilable catgut the coil is placed directly from the packet, without straightening, into water or other softening solution. After softening is complete, straightening is safely done without breaking the bond between the plies, which might happen if the anhydrous sutures were first straightened. Abuse of catgut sutures may lead to their failure in tissues, with serious consequences to the patient. Although surgical gut is one of the strongest natural materials and equals the strength of soft steel, it still may be ruined by improper handling or application.

Catgut ribbons are offered by some manufacturers. They are prepared from the submucosa of sheep intestines and are sold in ribbons ⅝ inch wide and 18 inches long, plain or chromic, in a boilable tubing. Ribbon gut distributes pressure over a broader surface, permitting the application of tension to certain parenchymatous tissues without cutting through and with minimum circulatory constriction. The ribbons have been applied successfully in the closure of kidney wounds, the repair of hernias, operations designed for the correction of incontinence, operations in vascular surgery, and elsewhere.

Kangaroo Tendons—These are obtained from the tail of wallabies. The bundle of tendons is split into various sizes, usually larger than catgut. The tendons may be used plain or chromicized, and are available in boilable or nonboilable tubing. The tendons consist of compact fibrous bundles of connective tissue, characterized by a relatively low affinity for water so that the presoaking of such tendons before use is a matter of some importance. Kangaroo tendons vary in length from about 10 to 17 in. or over. They are generally fairly resistant to tissue enzymes and are commonly used to suture the broken ends of bones, support fracture lines and effect the radical cure of hernia, the latter being the principal use of the finer gauge tendons. There are also available kangaroo bands in which the central portion of the tendons have been flattened into a bandlike area ¾ in. in width. These are designed to hold in apposition the broken ends of certain types of bones and to provide proper support to the fracture line.

Cargile Membrane—This is a thin sheet of pliable tissue obtained from the appendix ("blind gut") of the steer or ox. It is designed primarily to cover surfaces from which the peritoneum has been removed, especially where a sterile membrane would lessen the formation of adhesions. The membrane is available in sterile sheets of approximately 4 × 6 in. and is sometimes used as a packing or protective sheath. At the present time the use of such material is limited.

Fascia Lata—This is obtained from ox fascia and is designed for use as a heavy suture or repair in hernia and similar cases. It is usually attached firmly to some strong fascial structure by means of a nonabsorbable suture. Fascia lata is supplied in the form of sterile strips approximately ½ in. wide and 8 in. long and also in sheets about 3 × 5 in.

Insultoic Membrane—This is prepared from the allantoic membrane of bovine embryos. It serves as cargile membrane does, as an interposed insulating material for the temporary protection of denuded surfaces, which are normally nonadherent. It has found applications in the surgery of nerves, tendons, joints, dura, and fallopian tubes.

It should be emphasized, in connection with the above, that catgut strands and ribbons are the only ones which are completely and readily absorbable. The other materials may be absorbed very slowly or may be incorporated in the tissues by invasion of fibroblasts and a kind of replacement process. The same is probably true of live fascial grafts taken from the patient himself to repair abdominal hernia.

Nonabsorbable Sutures

The second principal class of sutures consists of those nonabsorbable suture materials which are not appreciably attacked, or are not broken down and digested by normal tissue fluids. Such sutures will survive apparently unchanged for many years in animal tissues, and may either be encapsulated as tissues react to most foreign bodies, or, if the fibrous structure permits, may be intergrown with fibroblasts and collagenous connective tissue. When such sutures are used in the skin, they are removed after the incision or wound is healed.

Silk is an important nonabsorbable surgical suture. Selected grades of degummed commercial silk fibers are utilized, and consist chiefly of the protein fibroin as extruded by the silkworm. Many such fibers are twisted into a single strand and sold in the natural color or after dyeing. Of increased popularity is braided silk in which several twisted yarns are braided into a compact structure favored for its firmness and disinclination to broom out at the cut ends and thus interfere with needle threading. Most braided silk is dyed and also given a treatment to render it noncapillary. In use as a skin suture this minimizes the rise of tissue fluids to the surface and thus the counterpassage inward of organisms from the surface. Further objects of such treatments are to impart a degree of stiffness to improve the handling and tying properties, to minimize attachment of tissue cells that would cause pain on removal of the suture and to lubricate the implantation and removal of the silk. When silk or any other suture is dyed, the USP requires that such dyeing be done with an iron dye, a harmless vegetable dye or a certified coal-tar color.

Specifications—The USP prescribes in the monograph for Nonabsorbable Surgical Suture (which now includes cotton, linen, metallic wire, nylon, rayon, dacron, and silk) that the respective sizes have the diameter and tensile strength shown in Table IV.

Table IV—Diameter and Tensile Strength of Nonabsorbable Surgical Sutures

	Limits on diameter, mm		Limits on knot-pull tensile strength,[a] Kg		
Size	Min	Max	Class I	Class II	Class III[b]
10–0	0.013	0.025	0.020	..	0.05
9–0	0.025	0.038	0.045	0.03	0.06
8–0	0.038	0.051	0.08	0.05	0.11
7–0	0.051	0.076	0.14	0.08	0.16
6–0	0.076	0.102	0.25	0.14	0.27
5–0	0.102	0.152	0.50	0.29	0.54
4–0	0.152	0.203	0.75	0.57	0.82
3–0	0.203	0.254	1.120	0.82	1.36
2–0	0.254	0.330	1.80	1.27	1.80
1–0	0.330	0.406	2.70	1.81	3.40
1	0.406	0.483	3.40	2.26	4.76
2	0.483	0.559	4.00	3.17	5.90
3	0.559	0.635	5.00	3.85	7.26
4	0.635	0.711	6.10	..	9.11
5	0.711	0.813	7.70	..	11.4
6	0.813	0.914	9.1	..	13.6
7	0.914	1.016	11.3	..	15.9

[a] The limits on tensile strength apply to nonsterilized Nonabsorbable Surgical Suture that has not been sterilized; for sterilized Sutures of Class I and Class II, the limits are 20% lower.
[b] The tensile strength of sizes larger than 2–0 of monofilament *Class III* (metallic) Nonabsorbable Surgical Suture is measured by straight pull.

Nonabsorbable sutures are generally packaged much as catgut in sealed glass tubes, foil or plastic packets, while unsterilized silk is sold on spools containing 25 to 100 yd. To attempt to sterilize any suture on the wooden spools on which the suture is supplied will often cause contamination by waxes and resins which leach out of the wood, and the possibility of sterilizing wooden objects by autoclaving has been questioned. It is common practice to wind silk on special paddles in such a way that a single cut across the coil will provide many sutures of the lengths demanded by the surgeon. Sterilization in the hospital is commonly and most efficiently done by autoclaving.

Uses of Silk—Silk sutures are easily handled, resistant to repeated sterilizations (it is not desirable to sterilize silk sutures more than three times) and well tolerated by body tissue. In the presence of infection, however, the interstices of silk strands protect organisms from antiseptics and from the body's defense mechanisms, so that chronic sinuses may form which do not heal until the silk is removed or is sloughed out by the tissues. Silk, as well as any other nonabsorbable suture, often migrates from the site of implantation and comes to the surface for extrusion months after the operation. In certain sites, the suture knots or ends may serve as centers for the formation of concretions or for other irritating action. The best silk technique may require as much as 50% more operating time than the same operation performed with catgut. Silk usually becomes encapsulated and remains permanently in the tissues. Silk sutures are used in a wide variety of surgical procedures, as in the brain, eye, gastrointestinal tract, nerves, blood vessels, or in general in any wound which is not infected. Many surgeons, using catgut or other materials in tissues, employ silk for skin closure, either braided or as the artificial silkworm gut or dermal sutures described below.

Silkworm Gut—This interesting material comes from a province in Spain where it originated, and where most of the less than 1000 population derive their subsistence from its manufacture. The caterpillars, which would normally proceed to the formation of a cocoon from which the familiar silk is obtained, are killed by being plunged into a vinegar bath, and the proteinaceous substance which would have formed the fine fibers of a cocoon is drawn out from the two tubular sacs as a single short thread. These threads are bleached, polished, sorted into sizes, and bundled for shipment to America. This provides a strong, smooth inert suture of the same composition as ordinary silk, but as a single monofilament instead of the usual multifilament forms. The 12- to 16-in. strands are sterilized by autoclaving and may require additional boiling in water to soften them sufficiently for use. They are used chiefly as a stay or tension suture, placed somewhat back from the incision and often through more than one layer of tissue so as to take up most of the stress that might otherwise disrupt the incision. Silkworm gut is marketed as fine, medium or coarse and in sterile or unsterilized forms.

Artificial Silkworm Gut or Dermal Sutures—These sutures consist of natural twisted silk encased in a nonabsorbable coating of tanned gelatin or other protein. This coating must withstand autoclaving without stripping, and its purpose is to prevent the ingrowth of tissue cells which would interfere with its removal after use as a skin or dermal suture. This product is marketed sterile in tubes or unsterilized in boxes, and its chief uses are as stay sutures and skin sutures.

Nylon—Nylon came into use as a suture partly as a result of World War II shortages of high-grade silk and partly because of its own merits. It is a synthetic protein-like plastic (obtained from the condensation of adipic acid and hexamethylene diamine) of low tissue reactivity, and appears to be quite unaffected by tissue fluids. It is available in the form of monofilaments in the useful range of sizes, as well as in the form of multifilament fibers braided into strands of comparable diameter. It is strong and water-resistant, and has come into some use for all suturing or ligating but has the disadvantages for some purposes of considerable elasticity and knot slippage. While most surgeons tie a flat or reef knot in other sutures, this is inadequate with monofilament nylon, which requires three or even four single throws instead of the two throws sufficient for catgut and silk. Multifilament braided nylon, however, appears not very different from braided silk in knot-holding power. Monofilament nylon is used as a skin or stay suture or for plastic surgery. Braided nylon is more often buried in tissues and is subject to the same limitations as braided silk in the presence of infection.

Linen—This suture material is one of the oldest known, but is currently used to only a limited extent. The advantage of linen resides in its high tensile strength and its stability during sterilization. Its diameter uniformity, however, leaves something to be desired, and it tends to cause sinuses in the presence of infection. An important modification of linen is produced by coating it with collodion. Such linen is known as *Pagenstecher's linen*, and is used principally for the purse string suture at the base of the appendix following an appendectomy. A few surgeons use both forms of linen in general surgery in preference to silk.

Cotton—This material has recently regained a large degree of popularity and its military use has been extensive, although it, too, is among the oldest sutures used. It is readily available and of good resistance to heat sterilization. As provided by suture manufacturers it has good uniform tensile strength. Some surgeons still depend upon household sewing cotton which is cheap but lacks the tensile strength, uniform diameter and smoothness of surface to be found in the cotton sutures prepared especially for surgery. Like silk, the use of cotton tends to slow the operation.

Horsehair Sutures—These come from the tail and, to a limited extent, from the mane of the horse. They are characterized by fine gauge, a flexibility which makes them easy to handle, noncapillarity, and a minimal tissue reaction. They are, however, of varying diameter along the strand and possess relatively low tensile strength. They require thorough sterilization, and are used primarily for skin closure and plastic surgery because of the inconspicuous residual scar.

Polyester Fiber

Of the numerous multifilament synthetic fibers that were introduced after the advent of Nylon, only polyester fiber has been accepted as a suitable braided nonabsorbable suture. Polyester fiber is a polymer of ethylene glycol and terephthalic acid. Its potential use as a suture material came to light when Oppenheimer[1] and his co-workers implanted various plastic films, including polyester fiber, in rats and were unable to produce sarcomas when polyester fiber was embedded. Following these studies many investigators established the merits of polyester fibers as a suture material. Polyester fiber is available in fine filaments which make it advantageous for braiding in a multiple number of suture sizes. In general, the tensile strength of polyester braided sutures is superior to braided silk, braided nylon and twisted cotton. In contrast with braided silk and braided nylon, polyester fiber braided sutures are not weakened by wetting in water. Also in contrast with braided silk it is not treated with waxes or other stiffening and water repellent agents. Its advantage over Nylon sutures is particularly exemplified by its reduced knot slippage, which has always been a problem with Nylon sutures. Mersilene (*Ethicon*) polyester fiber braided sutures are dyed with D & C Green No. 6 for maximum visibility in the operating area.

Recent developments have seen the commercialization of braided polyester fiber sutures coated or impregnated with nontoxic lubricants such as polytetrafluoroethylene or silicone resin. These sutures present the advantage of a smoother surface which gives the suture improved handling properties and permits an easier and more gentle passage through tissue.

Polyolefin Fibers

Of recent interest in the nonabsorbable suture field are the use of the polyolefin fibers—polyethylene and polypropylene. Polyethylene is produced by polymerization of ethylene under heat and pressure to build up predominantly linear chains of CH_2 groups with molecular weights ranging between 1000 and 40,000. Polypropylene is produced by polymerization of propylene to form linear chains of $\left(-CH-CH-CH_2-CH-CH_3 \atop \quad\; CH_3 \qquad\quad CH_3 \right)$

Both fibers as sutures are used in the form of monofilaments. Polyethylene fibers have a lower melting point than polypropylene fibers, and melt when subjected to sterilization by autoclaving. Polypropylene fibers successfully withstand autoclaving temperatures. Their chief advantages over Nylon monofilament sutures are greater pliability, reduced tissue reaction, and better knot-holding properties.

Metallic Sutures and Appliances

In recent years increased attention has been paid to the use of various metal wire sutures and of other metallic devices to assist surgical repair. Notable in connection with this type of suture is the extensive development with *vitallium*, and more recently *tantalum* for many purposes.

Silver—Among the older materials which are still used to some extent are silver wire, foil, hemostatic clips, and other forms. Relatively little work has been reported recently on these items. Silver is readily available and is alleged to have some antiseptic action, but in some tissues is definitely irritating. Irritation has been shown by a great many metals and alloys, and is now regarded as a controlling consideration in the choice of substances for implantation in tissues.

Stainless Steel—This ferrous alloy, which has so long been usefully employed in industrial and other applications where resistance to chemical attack is essential, has been used widely in the form of wire sutures, fixation plates, screws, and other items. Stainless steel is a rather general term covering a wide variety of materials, and many of the early alloys were attacked by body fluids. Corrosion of the alloy liberated metallic ions which caused pain, and where the metal was in the form of a screw or nail in bone, the bone around such stainless steel was broken down, so that the screw would be removed easily. This destruction of tissue sometimes necessitated removal of the implant. The proper selection of stainless steel compositions seems to provide a material essentially inert in tissues and free from the earlier disadvantages. It still remains true that metallic parts that are not homogeneous may give rise to local cells or galvanic couples so that certain areas of the piece corrode (are cathodic) and produce harmful metallic ions in tissues. Physical properties of modern stainless steels are generally quite satisfactory for surgical purposes.

Vitallium—This metal, which is an alloy of cobalt, chromium and molybdenum, has been applied to many surgical problems in various forms since 1937, although not in the form of sutures or ligatures. The alloy has shown some variability in strength and stiffness and is incapable of much modification at the time of operation, but generally shows negligible tissue reactions. In addition to some use for dentures, surgical forms of vitallium include: fracture plates, screws, bolts, nails and appliances, orbital implants, nasal skeletal supports, tendon rods, tubes for blood vessel anastomosis and for bile duct repair, and skull plates.

Tantalum—Although tantalum (page 418) was discovered in 1802, its use in surgery did not begin until 1936. Thereafter it gained tremendous impetus from its adoption by the Army and Navy for many purposes. Tantalum is a steel-gray, malleable metallic element, and owes its industrial acceptance to its inertness to strong nitric acid, sulfuric acid and many other chemicals. Thousands of implantations have also demonstrated its inertness in animal and human tissue.

Tantalum wire for sutures is available in diameter from 0.003 to 0.040 in. and is used in many types of surgery ranging from the repair of peripheral nerves to the fixation of large bone fractures. Foil is offered in thicknesses 0.0005 to 0.00075 in. and is used as a cuff around peripheral nerve anastomoses, in repair of some membranes, and for similar purposes. Tantalum sheet in thicknesses from 0.002 to 0.020 in. is finding applications in orthopedic, plastic and other surgical procedures, but its chief use has been in the form of plates 0.0125 or 0.015 in. thick for the repair of defects of the skull. Such plates are shaped to duplicate the original skull contours and are laid in a chiselled-out ledge of the bone, being secured by triangular glazier points, screws or tantalum wire. Tantalum ribbon is formed into hemostasis clips, which in brain operations have been shown to produce no tissue reaction as compared with the extensive reaction shown by the silver clips formerly used.

Tantalum gauze is prepared from 0.003-in. wire woven 50 × 50 to the inch. It is pliable, and has come into wide use for the repair of extensive hernias not readily amenable to other procedures. After removal of attenuated tissues the surgeon prepares an appropriate piece of the gauze by bending its edge under all around and attaching this doubled edge to surrounding strong tissues. Artificial eyes are constructed with this gauze as backing, so that the muscles can be attached and impart motion to the prosthesis. The gauze is being used also to fill voids, cover defects and in general where it is desired to produce a smooth tough tissue replacement.

Numerous papers on the applications of tantalum have appeared, and many special forms are finding unique applications. An outstanding feature of tantalum seems to be that fibroblasts adhere to it tenaciously when it is implanted in tissue and a layer of connective tissue forms about the metal. This reaction seems to be self-limiting so that, even when used as a repair for the dura, scar tissue and adhesions do not form. This reaction is observed also when tantalum is used in contact with bone where the repair tissue is soon penetrated by osteoblasts which form new bone structure which adheres firmly to the tantalum implant. Around other metallic forms there is often sufficient corrosion to break down the bone structure and permit easy removal of an object such as a screw. This has not been reported, however, for tantalum, which usually tends to be covered by a firm overgrowth of bone which must be chiselled away for removal.

Bone Wax—Bone wax, while not a suture, is generally classed among suture materials. It is composed of a mixture of various waxes, mainly beeswax, and used to stop bleeding and oozing on the surface of severed bones. It requires a certain amount of moulding in the hand to warm it and make it spread easily over the moist bone wound.

Absorbable Dusting Powder USP

It has been repeatedly demonstrated that talcum powder when introduced into tissues is capable of causing extensive fibrosis, resulting in strictures of vessels, abdominal adhesions, and general granulomas. Many materials have been suggested to replace talc, and the most satisfactory appears to be a mixture of amylose and amylopectin derived from corn starch and treated chemically to assure good lubricating properties after sterilization. This is marketed under the name *Biosorb*. It may be sterilized by autoclaving and has been shown to have no deleterious effect on rubber gloves. A growing literature points out the hazards of talc in the operating room and the advantages of using *Absorbable Dusting Powder USP* (see page 1876) as its replacement.

To overcome the dustiness of absorbable dusting powder, a cream suspension of the powder has been placed on the market under the name Bio-Sorb Cream which dries quickly and leaves a lubricating film.

Official Sutures

Absorbable Surgical Suture USP

[Surgical Catgut; Catgut Suture; Surgical Gut; Chorda Chirurgicalis Absorbenda; Sterilized Surgical Catgut BP; Sterilized Surgical Ligature]

Absorbable Surgical Suture is a sterile strand prepared from collagen derived from healthy mammals. Its length is not less than 95.0% of that stated on the label. Its diameter and tensile strength correspond to the size designation indicated on the label, within the limits prescribed herein (see page 1878). It is capable of being absorbed by living mammalian tissue, but may be treated to modify its resistance to absorption. It may be impregnated with a suitable antimicrobial agent. It may be colored by a color additive approved by the federal Food and Drug Administration.

Caution—Do not subject Absorbable Surgical Suture marked "Nonboilable" to heat.

Description—Flexible strand varying in treatment, color, size, packaging, and resistance to absorption, according to the intended purpose. It is either *Type A* Suture or *Type C* Suture. Both Types consist of processed strands of collagen, but *Type C* Suture is processed by physical or chemical means so as to provide greater resistance to absorption in living mammalian tissue.

Note—If the Suture is packaged in a fluid, make the required measurements for the appropriate USP tests within 2 min after removing it from the fluid.

Nonabsorbable Surgical Suture USP

[Surgical Sutures; Surgical Silk; Sterile Surgical Silk; Chorda Chirurgicalis Non-absorbenda]

Nonabsorbable Surgical Suture is a strand of material that is suitably resistant to the action of living mammalian tissue. Its length is not less than 95.0% of that stated on the label. Its diameter and tensile strength correspond to the size designation indicated on the label, within the limits prescribed herein (see page 1881). It may be nonsterilized or sterile. It may be impregnated or coated with a suitable antimicrobial agent.

Nonabsorbable surgical suture may be modified

with respect to body or texture, or to reduce capillarity, and may be suitably bleached. It may be colored by a color additive approved by the federal Food and Drug Administration.

Description—Flexible, monofilament, or multifilament, continuous strand, placed in an envelope, tube or other suitable container or wound on a reel or spool. If it is a multifilament strand, the individual filaments may be combined by spinning, twisting, braiding, or any combination thereof. Nonabsorbable Surgical Suture is classed and typed as follows: *Class I* Suture is composed of monofilament or twisted or braided silk or synthetic fibers. *Class II* Suture is composed of cotton or linen fibers or coated natural or synthetic fibers where the coating forms a casing of significant thickness but does not contribute appreciably to strength. *Class III* Suture is composed of monofilament or multifilament metal wire.

Note—If the Suture is packaged in a fluid, make the required measurements for the appropriate USP tests within 2 min after removing it from the fluid.

Reference

1. Oppenheimer, B. S., *et al, Proc. Soc. Exptl. Biol. Med.,* **67,** 366 (1952).

98 | **Medical Emergencies**

Principles of first aid—stoppage of breathing—bleeding—shock—
fainting—fractures—wounds—foreign bodies—injuries caused by heat
and cold—bandaging

This chapter was prepared by

Albert A. Stonehill, PhD, *Manager, Product Research Department, Ethicon,
Inc., Somerville, N.J. 08876*

First aid is the immediate, temporary emergency aid given by a layman to a sufferer in case of a medical emergency (accident or sudden illness) before regular medical or surgical attention can be rendered. Proper first aid may save the life of the patient, and should reduce his suffering, and place him in the hands of the physician in a better condition to receive professional treatment. The sole duty of the first-aider is to render more or less skilled assistance until the arrival of a physician; thereupon his responsibility ceases and the medical practitioner is in complete charge.

For a thorough discussion of the emergency treatment of poisonings, see Chapter 100, *Poison Control*, page 1947.

Need for Training—Every year the need for first aid in the United States is greatly increasing. In spite of national safety programs, the trend of accidents is ever upward. During the year 1966, according to the National Safety Council, 53,000 persons were killed and 1,800,000 injured in auto accidents. This means that the automobile casualties alone, for a single year, numbered many times the total US casualties for World War I and even outnumbered the total US casualties for World War II. During the year 1966 fires were responsible for the death of 8000 persons, 28,000 were killed in home accidents, 6800 by drowning, and 2200 by firearms. When these figures are added to those for the accidents in the home, in industry, and on the farm, one readily appreciates the great need for extensive first-aid training programs as well as the desirability of national safety campaigns.

Purpose of Training—Every first-aid training program strives to accomplish three main objectives:

1. To prevent accidents. This is accomplished by means of safety campaigns and instruction in the fundamentals of first aid wherever possible.
2. To teach the first-aider how to determine the type and extent of an injury, not with the thoroughness of a medically trained diagnostician, but with sufficient accuracy to prevent harm resulting to the patient when assistance is rendered.
3. To teach the first-aider how to act quickly and efficiently in case of an emergency. This includes training in what not to do as well as instruction in the recognized methods of treatment.

Cardinal Principles—The four most important rules of first aid, in order of importance, are:

1. Supply oxygen to the lungs
2. Stop bleeding
3. Prevent and treat shock
4. Prevent further injury.

Every victim of an accident should be regarded with these principles uppermost in the mind. Always keep the patient lying down quietly and comfortably, allay his fears with a reassuring manner, and keep him warm. Look for *stoppage of breathing, hemorrhage, evidence of poisoning, wounds, burns, fractures,* and *dislocations,* in this order. If a patient is semiconscious or unconscious

following an accident, an injury to the head is often the cause. Remove and loosen the clothing; cut it rather than aggravate an injury.

The following outline of general principles explains the more important fundamental considerations.

General Principles

Whether or not the injured person is conscious:

1. Make sure whether or not he is breathing; if not, begin artificial respiration immediately.
2. When an injured person is breathing satisfactorily, look carefully for any visible bleeding, and if you find it, take measures to control it either by pressure and bandaging or by a tourniquet.
3. When breathing is satisfactory and there is no evidence of bleeding, look for signs of shock and fractured bones.

1. Always treat the most dangerous and urgent condition first. It is helpful to remember the four "B's," eg, *breathing, bleeding, broken bones,* and *burns.*
2. Obtain medical aid quickly—get someone to call the doctor, or get the injured to doctor or hospital.
3. Keep cool and work fast, but carefully.
4. Loosen tight clothing—collar, waistband, or belt.
5. If the injured person vomits, lower head and turn it to one side, so that the vomited material cannot go into the lungs.
6. Don't fail to remove any loose objects from the mouth of an unconscious patient (gum, tobacco, teeth).
7. Don't attempt to give an unconscious person anything to drink.
8. Do not aggravate injury by unnecessary movements.
9. Don't allow the injured with a fracture or suspected fracture to be moved until splints have been applied.
10. Don't overlook shock.
11. Don't burn the injured with an unwrapped hot water bottle or other heated object.
12. Keep the injured quiet, warm, and as comfortable as possible; do not move him except to avoid further injury until you are sure of the nature of the injury and have adequate help to move him properly.

Stoppage of Breathing

Causes

In cases of stoppage of breathing, there is immediate need for artificial respiration. It may occur in:

Suffocation or strangulation
Electric shock
Drowning

Gas poisoning (illuminating gas, coal gas, exhaust gas)
Foreign body in throat

Delay in starting artificial respiration may result in death.

Suffocation by Strangulation—Suffocation is commonly produced by a foreign body such as a bolus of food or a small toy that is sucked into the windpipe and, therefore, blocks it. This is particularly common in children. The object must be removed very quickly, but do not try to remove it with your fingers unless you are *positive* you can reach it and hook it out without pushing it farther into the air passages. Hold the child upside down by his legs or ankles and give him one or more smart blows with the flat of the hand on his back between his shoulder blades. This will often jar the object loose. As soon as the object comes out, see if the breathing has stopped or is very irregular. If this is the case, give artificial respiration at once.

If the victim is an adult or too heavy to hold, hang him head down over the edge of a table and hit hard with the fist between his shoulder blades.

If you are unable to remove the obstruction very quickly, the only recourse is to rush the victim to the hospital where facilities are available to make an emergency opening in the windpipe and permit the patient to breathe while the object is being extracted.

Electric Shock—Shut off the current at once, if possible, and pull the victim away. If current is still on release the victim from source of current, exerting care not to come in contact yourself. In releasing the victim, do not touch wire, source of current, or victim's body. Do not touch with bare hands anything made of metal.

Stand on a dry board or other dry, nonconducting material (such as dry rubber soles or rubbers) and drag the patient from the contact with one hand that has been thickly insulated in some nonconducting material such as rubber, dry cloth, or several layers of heavy paper or newspaper; or make a loop of dry rope on a dry stick and, by looping this over the victim's hand or foot, drag him away from contact. Sometimes the wire can be pulled from the patient by similar means, or even cut, if a suitable, thoroughly insulated tool is available.

As soon as contact is broken, start artificial respiration immediately. This should be continued until the patient is breathing normally, or it is certain, beyond question, that he is dead—*you cannot be sure for at least four hours.*

After respiration has been resumed, keep the patient warm and quiet in a semirecumbent position, and watch for signs of secondary shock—depressed body state. Such patients, upon recovery, are prone to hysterical outbursts, and may attempt to run about completely disoriented. The patient must be guarded against himself if he becomes violent.

Drowning—Do *not* waste time trying to roll the patient over a barrel or anything else in an attempt to get the water out of him; you are wasting precious seconds which could better be devoted to starting artificial respiration. It has been stated that *no more than 10 seconds* should be spent in preparing the patient for artificial respiration, and this is an excellent goal to try to attain.

As soon as the patient has been put into the proper position, with the head slightly lower than the rest of the body, and artificial respiration has been started, a helper should do the following things as quickly as possible, in sequence:

1. Free the patient's mouth and upper respiratory tract of all foreign bodies such as chewing gum and false teeth. Specifically delegate some one to call a doctor and a first-aid squad.
2. Loosen all tight clothing; if the patient is wet, remove as much clothing as possible without interfering with the procedure of artificial respiration.
3. Cover the patient with blankets, or some substitute, to conserve body warmth. Get a blanket under the patient if possible; newspapers are better than nothing.
4. Obtain and apply some suitable means of supplying external heat such as hot-water bottles, warm stones or bricks, or heating pads. Be sure that precautions are taken not to burn the patient.

5. Keep the tongue pulled forward and the air passages as free and clear as possible. Carefully watch the mouth and nose for discharges of water, stomach contents, or mucus.
6. Stand by to aid in any way requested in administering oxygen from an inhalator or resuscitator as soon as this equipment arrives.

Artificial respiration should be continued—*without interruption for any reason whatever—until the victim is again breathing normally or until he has been pronounced dead by a physician.*

Gas Poisoning—This occurs from the escape of ordinary coal gas, illuminating gas, the fumes from a charcoal fire, the choke-damp of mines, gases from sewers and wells, exhaust from automobiles or other internal combustion engines operated without adequate ventilation, or the fumes from a burning building. Most smoke poisoning is in reality carbon monoxide poisoning. Carbon monoxide is the commonest cause of gas poisoning.

Symptoms

In mild cases: headache, yawning, nausea, loss of muscular activity. In severe instances: the victim may become unconscious. The skin may become cherry red.

Treatment

Open doors and windows. Do not use lighted match or candle; use flashlight. Get the victim to fresh air quickly. Perform artificial respiration. Send for the doctor. In cases of illuminating gas, phone the gas company in your district. Loosen tight clothing.

Resuscitation Methods

Back-Pressure–Arm-Lift Method of Artificial Respiration—The Holger-Nielsen or Back-Pressure–Arm-Lift method of artificial respiration is generally recognized as an effective technique for artificial respiration (Figs. 808–810). The injured person is placed facedown, elbows bent, arms overhead with one

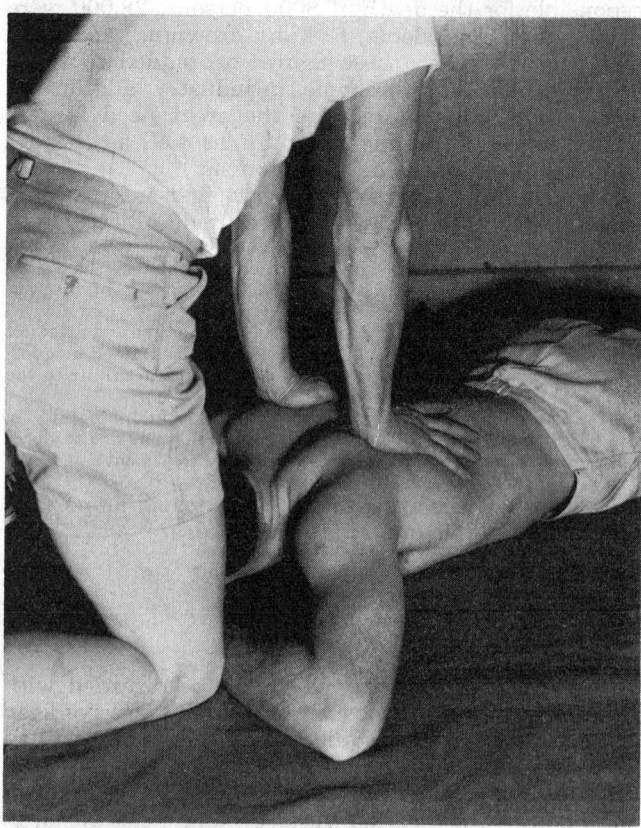

Fig. 808. Proper position, back-pressure–arm-lift method, beginning of exhalation phase (courtesy, J & J).

hand upon the other. The cheek is placed on the hand with the face turned slightly to one side. Kneel on one knee at the head of the victim and put the foot of the opposite leg near the elbow. Put your hands on the victim's back in such a way that the thumbs just touch, the heels of the hands being just below a line running between the armpits. Rock slowly forward, elbows straight, until your arms are approximately vertical, exerting steady pressure upon the back of the chest. Rock back slowly sliding your hands to the victim's arms just above the elbows. Raise the arms until definite resistance is felt from the victim's shoulders. Release the arms. This completes a full cycle and should be repeated at a rate of at least 12 times per min.

Mouth-to-Mouth Breathing Method—Another method, which is rapidly achieving much popularity because of its simplicity and high efficiency, is the so-called *mouth-to-mouth*, or expired air, breathing method. It is an easily learned life-saving procedure and is being widely adopted by the Armed Forces, utility companies, and other bodies, since studies indicate it to be definitely superior to manual resuscitation methods.

Aesthetic objections to oral contact with a victim or patient now can be overcome by the use of a simple device consisting of a mouth-to-mouth airway,* which provides both an artificial oropharyngeal airway and a mouthpiece for the operator.

The increased tidal volumes obtained by this method rapidly overcome initial oxygen deficiency and carbon dioxide accumulation and prevent their recurrence. Obstruction of the air passageway above the larynx—the most common cause of failure in artificial respiration—is prevented because the hands are free to keep

the head extended (sniffing position) and the lower jaw is displaced forward.

Mouth-to-mouth breathing is the only technique which allows the rescuer to be stationed at the patient's head for constant monitoring of the air passageway and its patency. Partial or complete obstruction can be detected on a breath-to-breath basis and corrected immediately by extending the neck, supporting the jaw properly, clearing the air passages, or readjusting the breathing tube.

From his position at the victim's head, the rescuer can (1) observe the movements of the victim's chest and thereby detect and correct inadequate inflation, (2) keep the head extended and support the jaw with both hands, and (3) clean the oropharynx when necessary with little loss of time. In addition, the rescuer can (4) sense resistance if the air passages become obstructed, (5) overcome reduced lung–chest distensibility or partial air passageway obstruction by blowing more forcefully in the case of adults, (6) feel and hear the gurgling of accumulated secretions, and (7) feel the return of spontaneous breathing.

Four to five inflations (5–20 sec) restore the victim's pulmonary oxygen concentration to normal. Reoxygenation of arterial blood depends on the circulatory state and may take from 15 sec to about 3 min. Alveolar carbon dioxide concentration is lowered to control values in from 3 sec to 2 min.

By taking an inspiration just before each insufflation, the rescuer converts his exhaled air to a suitable resuscitating gas. The rescuer's mild hyperventilation provides for normal oxygenation of the victim and adequate carbon dioxide removal.

The energy expenditure in mouth-to-mouth resuscitation is less than that of any manual method. Small or young individuals can satisfactorily perform

---

* Resusitube Airway (J & J).

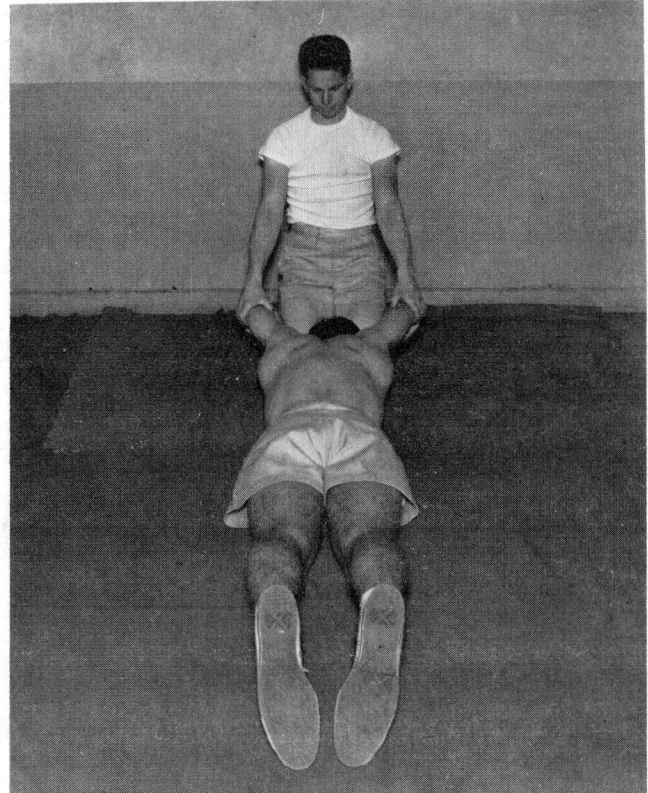

Fig. 809. Lifting of arms at about the halfway point through the inhalation phase (courtesy, J & J).

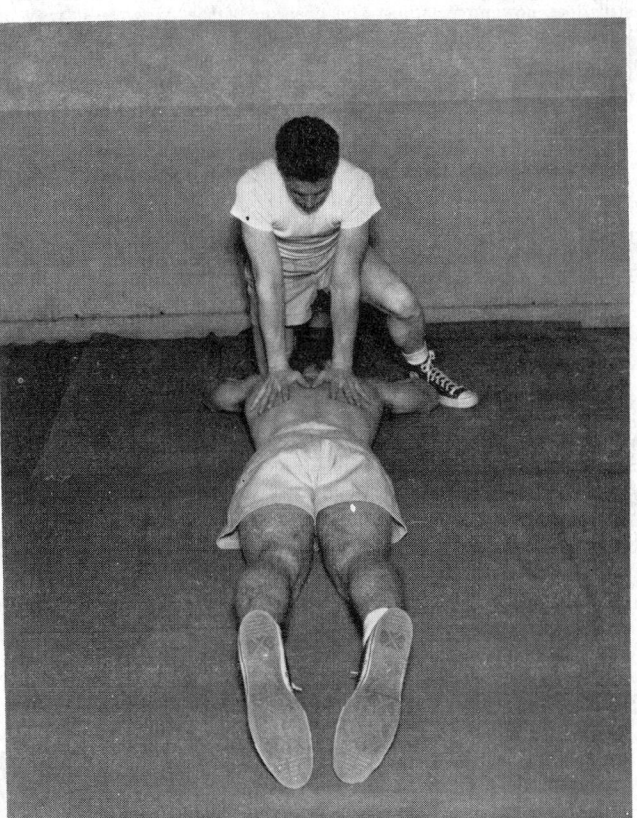

Fig. 810. Inhalation phase completed and beginning of new exhalation phase (courtesy, J & J).

mouth-to-mouth breathing for an hour without undue fatigue on subjects much larger than themselves. This technique permits rescuers to breathe for a victim while he is being transported.

The operator can assist each spontaneous respiration as the victim resumes breathing. Full inflations can be interposed between the patient's own breaths if the rate is slow.

Directions for Mouth-to-Airway Resuscitation of Nonbreathing Victims

Step 1. Insert the breathing tube.

Place the victim on his back (face up). Take up your position at the top of his head (vertex). If foreign matter is visible at his mouth, turn his head to the side, force his mouth open, and wipe his throat clean with your fingers or a piece of cloth. Insert the Airway over his tongue until the flange of the tube rests upon his lips.

Do not push the tongue back into the throat; hold it forward with your finger. If the victim is an adult, insert the long end. If the victim is a child over 3 years of age, insert the short end. With children, the flange positioning is unnecessary as the hands will prevent air leakage. In children under 3 years, do not use this tube, but use direct mouth-to-mouth breathing.

Step 2. Hold lower jaw forward. Keep head extended (front of neck stretched). Prevent air leakage.

Pull victim's jaw upward and toward yourself. *Never let his chin sag.* Keep front of neck stretched so his head is in "sniffing position." Prevent air leakage by pinching his nostrils with your thumbs, and by pressing the flange firmly over his lips with your index fingers.

Step 3. Blow into tube.

Take a deep breath, and blow into the mouthpiece of the tube. Blow quite forcefully into an adult and gently into a child. Watch the victim's chest. When his chest moves, take your mouth off the Airway and let the victim exhale passively. When his exhalation is finished, blow in the next deep breath. The first few breaths you blow must be deep and at a rapid rate. Thereafter, about one breath every 4 seconds is adequate.

If the chest does not move, increase the "chin-up" position, improve the position of your fingers and blow more forcefully. If the chest still does not move, adjust the position of the Airway—it may be inserted too deeply or not deeply enough. The flange must rest firmly on the lips. When you assist shallow natural breathing, blow at the moment when the victim inhales and take your mouth off quickly when he exhales.

Points to Remember

1. Always keep jaw forward and head extended.

In any unconscious victim, breathing or not breathing, the air passageway becomes blocked when the neck is flexed (chin down). Therefore, keep pulling the chin up, even when the Airway is in place. Leave the Airway in until the victim tries to expel it or reacts by retching or coughing.

2. Air in stomach.

If the air passageway is blocked by improper support of head and lower jaw or if the blowing is too forceful, inflation of the stomach may occur. If the stomach is seen to bulge, the rescuer should interrupt blowing momentarily and press with his hand between the victim's navel and breastbone. This causes the air to be "burped." If this makes the victim vomit, his mouth and throat should be cleaned at once.

3. Snoring.

Noisy breathing indicates partial blockage of the air passageway.

4. Apparent "breathing."

Movements of the victim's chest and abdomen may occur while there is actually no air moving into his lungs. This is due to complete blockage of the air passageway caused by improper positioning of the head and jaw. Determine whether or not there is movement of air in and out of the mouth and nose by listening closely or feeling with the fingers.

5. Transportation of victim.

The rescuer must remain at the victim's head during transportation in order to keep his air passageway open and to start mouth-to-airway breathing at once if the victim ceases to breathe.

6. Drowning.

It is most important to get air into the lungs of the victim without delay. Water cannot be removed from the lungs satisfactorily by any means. Valuable seconds should not be wasted in turning the victim to clear the lungs or empty the stomach. The rescuer should empty the stomach—by pressing with his hand between the navel and breastbone—only when it is obviously bulging or when the throat continues to fill up with regurgitated material.

7. Recovery.

The onset of breathing is often prefaced by slight twitching movements of the fingers, followed by a sigh-like catching of the breath. This is a good sign, but the operator must continue until regular breathing has been re-established. It is important to stand by and be ready to start again on a second's notice, as sometimes the patient will cease breathing, and he must again receive artificial respiration.

When breathing is well established and it is certain that the patient is fully conscious, he should be given some stimulant by mouth. A teaspoonful of aromatic spirits of ammonia in a glass of cool water is good. The patient may appreciate some hot coffee or tea. At this point he should not be allowed to stand or sit up, but his head may be raised a little to help in taking liquids. As he may not yet be able to swallow well, he should be fed with a teaspoon until he is able to drink by himself without choking.

Until recovery is complete the case should be handled as a potential case of shock, and the patient should be removed with proper precautions to a hospital where adequate facilities for observation and further treatment are available.

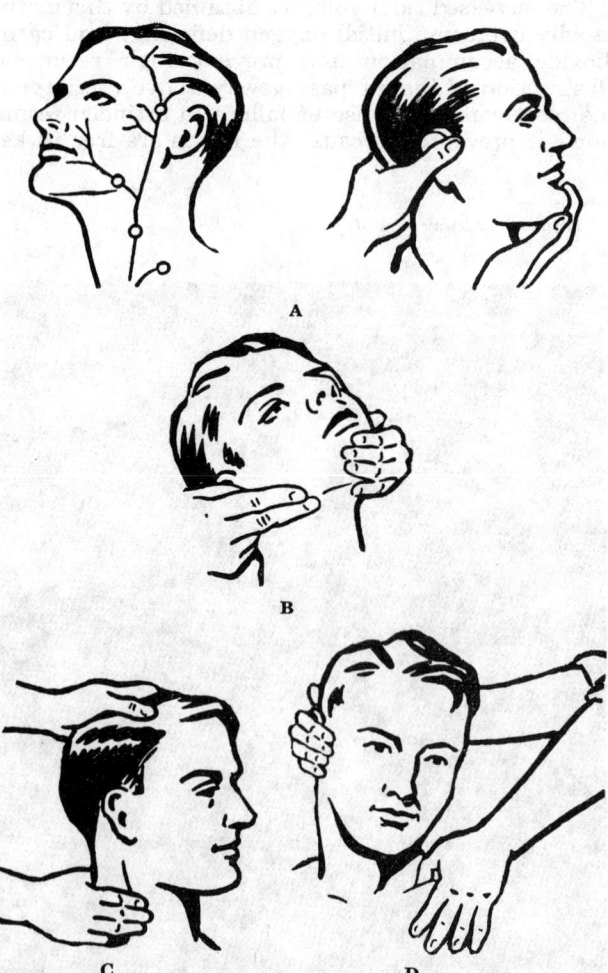

Fig. 811. Pressure points; control bleeding by finger compression on these points. *A:* Bleeding from scalp or forehead; press thumb in front of opening of ear on side of bleeding. *B:* Bleeding from face; press side of lower jaw in front of angle of jaw bone. *C:* Bleeding from neck or cut throat; place fingers on neck beside windpipe and press toward backbone. *D:* Bleeding from shoulder or armpit; tip head toward injured side and press down with thumb at side of neck (courtesy, J & J).

Bleeding

Second only to correcting cessation of breathing, the control of bleeding is the most urgent first-aid requirement.

Serious bleeding must be treated as soon as possible. The body holds about five quarts of blood. About 1 pint can be lost without serious effect; loss of 2 pints, plus the effects of injury, may be serious. When a man has many cuts or a deep cut severing a vein or an artery, enough bleeding may occur to endanger his life. When an injured man is bleeding heavily, he will soon become unconscious and go into shock; if the bleeding is not checked promptly, he will die.

Loss of half the total blood volume is almost always fatal; loss of 3 pints may prove fatal, particularly if the loss has been very rapid. Loss of 2 pints, coupled with the effects of injury, is serious and will quite probably lead to shock.

There are four main categories of bleeding: arterial, venous, capillary, and internal; the latter may consist of any of the three preceding types. For practical purposes, the same general control measures are used for the first three types, although capillary bleeding is rarely serious.

The best way to control bleeding is to elevate the bleeding part and apply pressure with a clean cloth or handkerchief directly to the cut or laceration from which the blood is coming. The pressure must be strong enough to stop the flow of blood. Then the cloth (a sterile gauze pad is best if available) can be firmly bandaged or otherwise pressed down on the wound making it tight enough to stop the bleeding.

Another method which may be used quite satisfactorily at times is to apply pressure on the main vessel supplying the injured part as it passes over a bony structure, providing a so-called "pressure point." This method, of course, requires an anatomical knowledge of the main arteries and veins (Figs. 811–813). Sufficient pressure must be applied to stop the flow in the vessel completely; otherwise, the bleeding from the wound site will be made worse.

Get medical attention as soon as possible. Give water, tea, or coffee if the injured can drink, but do not give whisky or other alcoholic drinks.

If the bleeding is severe and the wound is such that this procedure fails to stop the flow, apply a tourniquet close to the wound but between it and the heart, and tighten it until the bleeding stops (Fig. 814). Contrary to older teaching, after a tourniquet has been applied it should never be released except by a phy-

sician, and when necessary it may be kept in place for as long as 3–4 hr. It has been shown that frequent release of a tourniquet predisposes to severe shock and the modern theory therefore is that it is "better to lose a limb than a life." *A tourniquet should only be used for severe hemorrhage* which cannot be controlled by such means as are outlined above.

Internal Bleeding—This may come from the stomach, bowels, or lungs. In the first two instances the victim should be placed on his back and kept quiet. He should not be moved. The head may be turned to one side for vomiting or coughing. Apply warmth, but do not give stimulants. Call a physician immediately. In lung injuries, where breathing is difficult, the head and shoulders may be elevated and supported.

Do not have the injured sit up, except in lung injuries and nosebleed. Do not give a stimulant in severe bleeding until the bleeding has been checked.

Nosebleed—Nosebleed is common and usually occurs as the result of a blow on the nose, or high blood pressure in older people; it is frequent during childhood—particularly in adolescent girls who are beginning menstruation. Contributory causes may be excessive nose picking, certain blood conditions, and various contagious diseases.

Most cases, however, simply occur because the network of veins very near the surface of the mucous

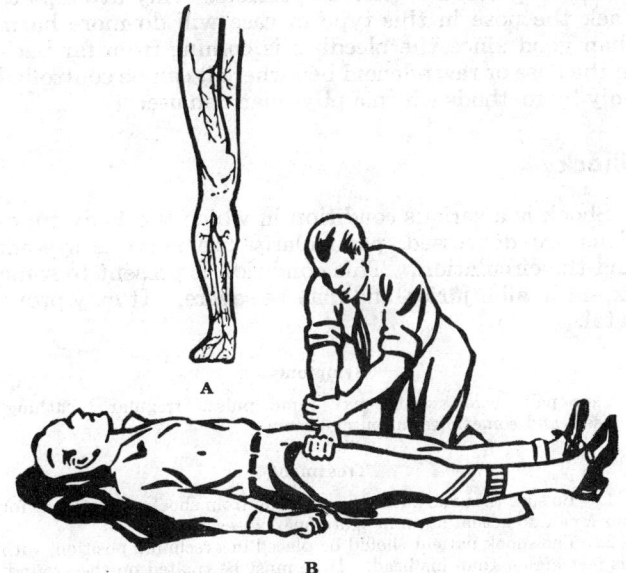

Fig. 813. *A:* **Course of main arteries of leg.** *B:* **Bleeding from leg; place patient on back and press down the heel of the hand into middle of groin (courtesy, J & J).**

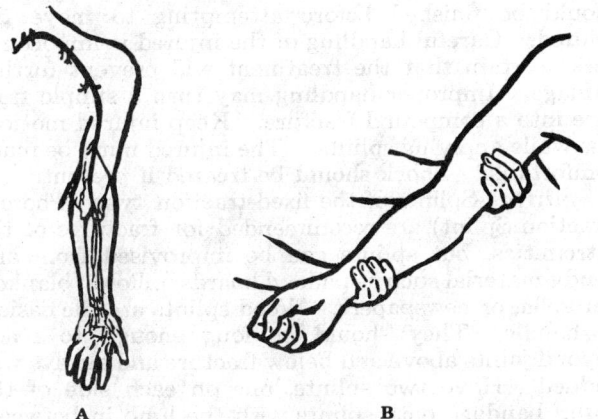

Fig. 812. *A:* **Course of main arteries of the arm and shoulder.** *B:* **Bleeding from arm; press with fingers on inner side of arm below armpit (courtesy, J & J).**

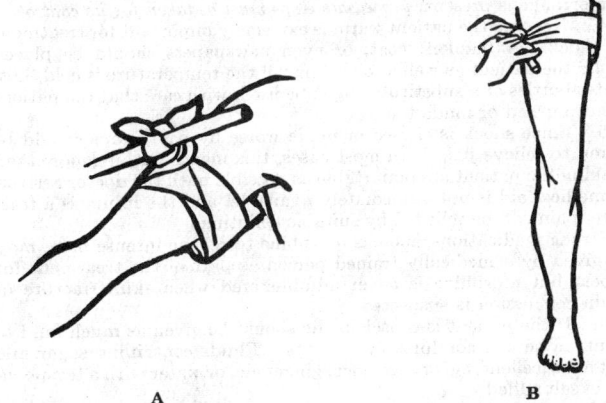

Fig. 814. *A:* **Tourniquet for upper arm.** *B:* **Tourniquet for the thigh (courtesy, J & J).**

membrane just inside the nose is rather delicate and may easily rupture.

The simplest method of treatment is to gently insert a small wad of sterile absorbent cotton or gauze into each nostril so that a small amount still protrudes, and gently but firmly compress the nostrils between the thumb and fingers steadily for at least six minutes *by the clock.* Keep the patient in a sitting position—*not lying down.* After six minutes, gradually relax the pressure and watch for further bleeding. Do not remove the cotton for several hours because the bleeding may start up again; work the cotton out very gently.

Sometimes the bleeding can be stopped by simply exerting very firm pressure with the thumbs against the tissues just below the nose.

In certain severe types of cases in older people, the bleeding cannot be controlled by simple first-aid measures; in cases of this type a physician should be called or the patient taken to a hospital immediately, since in rare cases nasal bleeding may become serious.

It should be emphasized that the severe nosebleed which may occur a few days after a tonsillectomy or an adenoidectomy cannot be controlled by simple first aid and, therefore, requires the prompt attention of the nose and throat surgeon. In the meantime, keep the child quiet in a sitting position, and apply an ice bag to the back of the neck—prevent the child from swallowing blood insofar as possible. Any attempt to pack the nose in this type of case will do more harm than good since the bleeding is coming from far back in the nose or raw adenoid bed where it can be controlled only by methods which a physician can use.

Shock

Shock is a serious condition in which the body functions are depressed, particularly the nervous system and the circulation. This condition is present to some extent in all injuries, and may be severe. It may prove fatal.

Symptoms

Face pale, cold sweat, weak rapid pulse, irregular breathing, nausea, and sometimes unconsciousness.

Treatment

1. Be sure that the patient is suffering from shock—treatment for shock can do actual harm in acute heart disease.
2. The shock patient should be placed in a reclining position, with his feet higher than his head. If he must be treated on the ground, feet and legs may be elevated with blankets, boxes, or any available substitute. If a bed is used, some sort of "blocks" placed under the legs of the bed at the foot will suffice.
3. Be sure to note any significant external bleeding. If such a hemorrhage is present, *immediate steps must be taken for its control.*
4. Keeping the patient warm is extremely important for treatment of shock. A blanket, coat, or even newspapers should be placed *under* the patient as well as over him; if the temperature is cold, hot-water bottles or a substitute might be used, with care that the patient is not burned or made too warm.
5. Since shock is caused or made worse by pain, steps should be taken to relieve pain. In most cases, this means nothing more than making the patient as comfortable as possible until the doctor arrives. If medical aid is not immediately available, and the injury is a fracture, pain can be relieved by suitable splinting.

Strong medications, such as morphine to relieve intense pain, may be given by a medically trained person as part of the treatment for shock, but morphine is never administered when skull fracture or brain concussion is suspected.

6. If the patient is conscious, he should be given as much fluid to drink as he can comfortably tolerate. Fluids containing sugar and salt are excellent, eg, orange juice, ginger ale, or water with a teaspoonful of salt added.

If medical aid is not immediately available, and if the patient is unable to take fluids by mouth, a sugar or salt solution may be administered by rectum in the form of a retention enema. The solution should be a concentration of about one teaspoonful to a glass of room temperature water run very slowly into the rectum through a tube inserted about 6 inches.

First-aid squads could use this sort of equipment in their vehicles to begin administration of fluids in this manner for accident cases, on the way to the hospital.

Fainting

Treatment

Loosen all tight clothing. Place body flat on back with head slightly lowered. Apply cold water to face, and warmth to the extremities. Insure a plentiful supply of fresh air, rest, and quiet. Ammonia inhalants or smelling salts held to the nose are useful. When consciousness returns, give stimulants. When a seated person is about to faint, do not move him unless there is room to lay him down. Bend his head down between his knees until the pallor is replaced by flushing of the face and he obviously feels better. However, if patient can be stretched full-length on the floor as in shock, this is preferable. See Fig. 815.

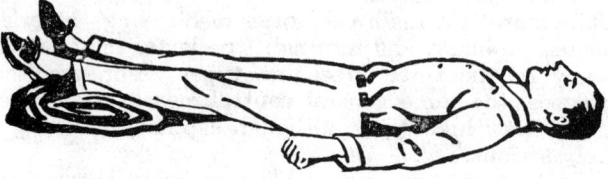

Fig. 815. Lay patient at full length on back with head low and feet raised for the treatment both of shock and common syncope (fainting) (courtesy, J & J).

Fractures (Broken Bones)

Types

Simple Fracture—This is a fracture in which the bone is broken but the skin is not pierced.

Compound Fracture—These fractures are more serious because the bone is broken and, in addition, there is a wound from the fracture to the skin surface. Sometimes the bone may protrude through the skin wound. In fractures there is pain, loss of use of the limb or part, deformity, and swelling.

Treatment

"Splint Them Where They Lie."—In simple fractures, apply splints. Never move a patient with a broken bone until the break has been adequately splinted by whatever means available. Rolled blankets or newspapers firmly bound in place are far better than nothing. For compound fractures, first stop the bleeding and bind the wound by applying sterile gauze held in place by bandage or adhesive plaster; apply splints. Never try to set or reduce the fracture. Splinting should be finished before attempting to move the injured. Careful handling of the injured is important; make certain that the treatment will prevent further damage. Improper handling may turn a simple fracture into a compound fracture. Keep injured motionless while applying splints. The injured must be made comfortable. Shock should be treated if present.

Splints—Splints of the fixed-traction type (Thomas Traction Splint) are recommended for fractures of the extremities, but splints can be improvised from any handy material such as padded boards, pillows, blanket, umbrella, or newspapers. Wood splints are the easiest to handle. They should be long enough to reach beyond joints above and below fracture and always well padded. Have two splints, one on each side of the limb; bandage both splints with the limb in between. For padding, absorbent cotton is the best material. To improvise padding, use soft cloth or soft garment. For binding, use the triangular or roller bandage or handkerchiefs, towels, garters, tape, suspenders, straps, or adhesive plaster.

If necessary to bring a fracture victim to the doctor's office, do not transport him until he has been properly and completely splinted.

Use a stretcher where necessary.

In a suspected fracture, use the same treatment as in fracture.

Location

Skull—Place the patient in a reclining position with his head slightly raised and supported. Do not administer stimulants. If scalp wounds are present, apply sterile gauze dressing and cover it with a bandage. In severe head injury and suspected fracture, the treatment is the same. Do not attempt to move the patient until adequate help is available.

Nasal Bones—Cover the injury with a gauze dressing held in place with a bandage or adhesive tape. Do not attempt to splint. Bring the patient to a physician.

Lower Jaw—Bring lower jaw to upper and while thus supported, apply either triangular or roller bandage around the chin to the top of the head (Figs. 822–824).

Spine—First-aid treatment of a fracture of the spine centers largely around properly moving the patient to a hospital and preventing others from improperly moving him. Transportation is a very grave problem and should not be undertaken until you are sure just how you are going to do it. There also should be at least three strong persons available to help you.

If the patient has a *broken neck*, he must be transported on a rigid support, flat on his back, *face up*. If he is not already lying on his back, he must be turned into that position. This must be done as a coordinated effort of at least three persons so that his head and neck are kept at all times in line with the rest of his body, without twisting. It is better to wait to turn the patient until the rigid support on which you are going to transport him is ready; then he can be turned and placed on the support in one operation.

An ordinary stretcher is not suitable for transporting a patient with a broken neck, as even the firmest ones are too flexible.

1. Procure a board or boards, at least 7 ft long and wide enough to amply accommodate the patient. If two boards are used, leave a space of at least 2 in. down the center.

2. Unless the boards are very heavy they must be reinforced with cross pieces nailed or tied crosswise at points corresponding approximately to where the patient's shoulders, hips, and heels will be.

3. Pad the support with blankets, and arrange the ties in such a way that they may be tied over the patient at frequent intervals so as to hold him absolutely firm and immobile during transportation.

4. Place the improvised stretcher as close as possible to the patient.

5. Assign one person to do nothing but hold the victim's head and keep it in line with the rest of the body at all times, or do this job yourself.

6. Assign one person to the shoulders, one to the hips, and another, if available, to the legs and feet; if not, the hip man will have to be responsible for the legs as well.

7. At a prearranged signal, gently lift the patient just enough so that the stretcher can be slid under him, or, if insufficient help is available, he can be lifted onto it.

8. Be sure the entire body moves as a unit without any twisting of, or pushing or pulling on, the vertebral column.

9. When the patient is on the stretcher, secure him firmly with the prearranged ties and cover him with blankets.

10. Do *not* use a pillow of any kind under the head, but *do* use sandbags, rolled newspapers, sweaters, or coats on each side of the head to keep it from moving during transit.

11. Someone should guard the head during the trip to the hospital, and until released by a doctor to be sure that it does not move.

A similar procedure is followed for a *broken back*, with this important exception: the patient is transported in the *face-down* position. The injury which produces a broken back often occurs when the victim is bent forward so that he is often found lying on his abdomen. In that case:

1. Gently straighten the victim in accordance with the principles outlined above, and place him face down on a rigid stretcher.

2. If he should be found lying wholly or partially on his back, attempt to apply the splint *before* turning him.

3. After the splint is firmly secured to the victim along the *front of his body*, he may then be safely and easily turned.

4. If it is not possible to do this, turn and place him on the stretcher as described for a broken neck, except that he is placed in the facedown position.

5. Finally, if insufficient help or materials are available to move the patient, cover him with a blanket and wait for adequate help. *It is better to do nothing than to do harm.*

Elbow—If the arm is straight, apply a well-padded splint on the front side, and hold it in place with a bandage or adhesive plaster strips. If the elbow is bent, apply a sling to the elbow and bandage the arm to the body as in Fig. 816*A*.

Upper Arm—Bend the arm at the elbow and hold it close to the body. Tie a well-padded splint alongside the upper arm, reaching from the shoulder to the elbow or below. Place the forearm in a sling. Tie the arm to the side of the body with a wide bandage (Fig. 816*B*).

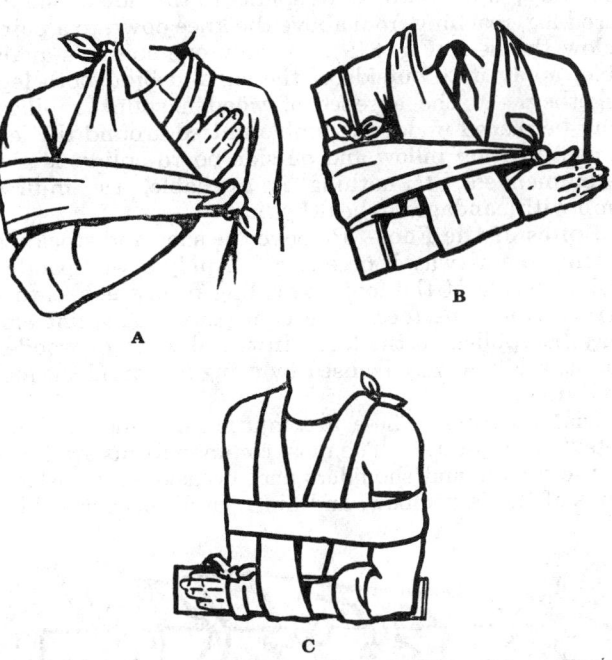

Fig. 816. *A*: **Triangular bandage and sling for fractured arm or collar bone.** *B*: **Splint for fractured upper arm.** *C*: **Splint for fractured hand or fingers (courtesy, J & J).**

Forearm and Wrist—Apply two well-padded splints, one from the elbow to the finger tips on the front, and another on the back of the forearm and hand. Hold the splints in place with a bandage or adhesive plaster. In the absence of wood splints, use newspaper, magazine, telephone book, or any material that will encircle the forearm and wrist and provide support. Suspend in a sling. The bandage may be tied around the arm to the side of the body.

Hand or Fingers—Apply a well-padded splint to the front of the hand extending from the middle of forearm to beyond the finger tips. Hold the splint with a bandage and support it with a sling (Fig. 816*C*).

Collar Bone—Place a pad in the armpit. Push the arm upward. Support the arm in a sling. Tie the arm to the side of the body with a strong bandage (Fig. 816*A*).

Ribs—Lay the victim on his uninjured side, with his head and chest elevated. Wrap with wide bandages around the chest, covering painful or tender areas.

Pelvis (Hip)—Place the victim in a comfortable position and support him with a cushion under and around his hips. Apply a wide bandage, bed sheet, or blanket around his hips to give support. Tie both ankles and knees together with bandages. Do not move him unless necessary and then in the same manner as if he had a fractured back.

Thigh—Grasp the injured limb at the heel and pull gently so that it is brought in line with the body. Apply two well-padded splints, a longer one outside extending from the armpit to the foot, the inner one from the crotch to the foot. Fasten splints with bandages around waist, hips, crotch, above and below knee, and at the ankle. Where only one splint is available, apply it to the outside. Place cushion or pillow between the thighs and legs, and tie the two limbs together (Fig. 817).

Knee-Cap—Straighten the injured limb. Apply a splint on the back of the leg, reaching from high up on the thigh to the heel (Fig. 818).

Leg—Gently grasp the foot and pull it in line with the body; apply two board splints to the side of the injured leg, reaching from above the knee down to a point below the heel (Fig. 819). If only one splint is available, apply it to outside of the leg and bind both legs together. In the absence of wooden splint a pillow may be placed under the limb and tied around the leg. A combination pillow and outside board splint, is also recommended. If nothing is available, tie injured limb with bandages to healthy limb.

Bones of the Foot—Remove the shoe and stocking, cutting them away if necessary. Apply a well-padded splint to sole of the foot, extending from the heel to a little beyond the toes. Tie it in place. A splint also may be applied to the leg. In the absence of wooden splint, a pillow may be used by tying it around the foot and ankle.

Dislocations—These are injuries in which a bone gets "out of joint." The most common forms are those of the fingers and shoulders and, occasionally, dislocations of the jaw, elbow, and hip. In dislocations there is pain and deformity of the joint and swelling. A dislocation can be treated like a fracture with splints or sling. Do not attempt to correct the dislocation. Send for a physician.

Concussions—A concussion of the head is due to head injury and to all intents and purposes it is treated like a skull fracture. Keep the patient quiet until examined by a physician. If there is bleeding from the scalp, apply sterile gauze and a bandage. Do not give stimulants. Avoid unnecessary handling. Keep the patient warm.

Wounds

There are several kinds of wounds: abrasions (made by rubbing or scraping of the skin surface); incised (caused by sharp cutting instruments); lacerated or torn (caused by blunt instruments); punctured wounds and stabs (caused by penetrating device such as wire or a bullet). Those wounds in which bleeding is slight can be simply cleaned with soap and water, covered with sterile gauze, using a nonadherent dressing next to the wound, and bandaged. In bleeding wounds, if not severe, the pressure of the dressing will stop hemorrhage. Where hemorrhage is severe, check bleeding and then dress the wound.

In large wounds such as those caused by machinery, and in railroad and automobile accidents, cover the wound with sterile gauze and a bandage. In the case of crushed hands, feet, fingers, or toes, cover with sterile gauze, bandage, and rest the limb on a folded blanket or cushion. In case of crushed arms, legs, or other parts, lay the patient down, cut away clothing, wrap him in plenty of sterile gauze, and thoroughly splint and support the part before moving him. Call medical aid immediately.

Remove foreign substances only when it can be done easily. Avoid contaminating the wound. It is safer, as a rule, to bind up the wound temporarily than to handle it with unclean hands or instruments. Grease, soot, and dirt from machinery may be wiped away from around the wound with benzine or turpentine applied on sterile gauze. If fractures are present, cover wound with sterile dressings before applying splints.

Bruises—If the bruise is severe, with swelling, apply cold moist dressings.

Splinters—If the splinter is near the surface and can be removed easily, take tweezers or ordinary sewing needle, boil in water, or pass several times through a flame, and remove foreign body without digging into the wound. If a splinter or other foreign body is buried deeply and cannot be removed easily, do not attempt removal. Apply antiseptic, sterile gauze pad, bandage, and send for a physician.

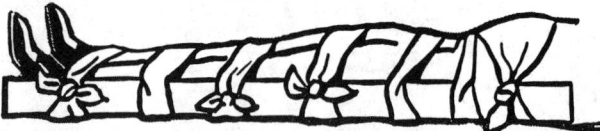

Fig. 817.   Splints for fractured thigh (courtesy, J & J).

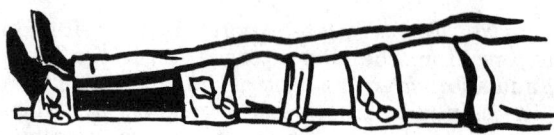

Fig. 818.   Splint for fractured knee cap (courtesy, J & J).

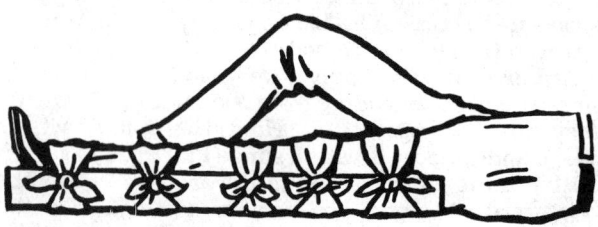

Fig. 819. Improvised wooden splint for fractured leg (courtesy, J & J).

Wound Dressing Hints

Do not handle the wound with fingers.

Do not touch the wound with the hand, mouth, clothing, or any unclean material. Sterile gauze should be used where possible.

Do not wash into the wound; wash *away* from it; use clean soap and water, being very gentle, but thorough.

Do not disturb blood clots.

Do not attempt to stitch a wound—leave that for the doctor.

Do not use absorbent cotton directly over a wound or burn.

Do not use collodion or similar preparation directly on a wound.

Do not use iodine near the eyes or body cavities.

Do not use iodine on a burn.

Do not cover a tourniquet with a bandage or splint; it may be forgotten.

Do not apply a wet bandage.

Do not bandage too loosely (except in burns) or too tightly.

Do not tear a dressing from a wound; if it sticks, it can usually be painlessly removed by soaking with hydrogen peroxide.

Poisoned Wounds

Snake Bite—Bandage the limb or apply a tourniquet tightly enough above the wound to check venous return circulation but *not* to shut off circulation *to* the limb. If necessary, keep moving tourniquet upward as swelling extends. Open the holes made by the snake's fangs with a sharp knife or razor blade which first has been sterilized by passing it through a flame if possible. Cut across and lengthwise. Let the blood run from the knife-cut. Sucking the wound and expectorating the poison answers the same purpose, but less effectively. Treat for shock, but do not give whisky or other forms of alcohol. Move the patient to a doctor as soon as possible. Keep pressure applied. Never travel in snake-infested country without having an emergency snakebite kit with you.

Bites of Dogs, Cats, and Other Animals—Wash the wound thoroughly. Apply iodine and sterile gauze, and bandage. Move the patient to a doctor rapidly. Have someone check on the animal that bit the victim so that it may be watched for signs of rabies by the health authorities for the legally required period.

Insect Bites and Stings—Apply compress soaked in weak ammonia water (1%) or baking soda paste. The stinger of a bee is usually seen in the wound and should be removed by scraping. Plucking out with the thumb and forefinger empties the contents of the poison sac into the wound.

Foreign Bodies

Eye—Do not rub the eye. Keep it closed and let tears gather to wash the foreign substance to corner. Attempt to remove it with the corner of a piece of sterile gauze. If a foreign body is imbedded, see a physician.

If a foreign body is under the lid, pull the lid up and, with a wisp of clean gauze or absorbent cotton twisted on the end of match, attempt removal.

Nose—Blow the nose gently while pressing on opposite nostril to close it. Sneezing sometimes expels a foreign body. If the body cannot be expelled, a few drops of olive oil may be dropped in the nose to relieve irritation until injured is brought to a physician.

Ear—Put a few drops of warm oil into the ear. Do not probe with wire, needles, or pins. Send for a doctor.

Injuries Caused by Heat and Cold

Burns and Scalds—Burns are classified according to the nature of damage to the tissues, not according to size, eg, first-degree: reddening of the skin; second-degree: blistering of the skin; and third-degree: destruction of the skin or underlying parts.

The danger to the body does not correspond necessarily to the degree, but rather to the extensiveness. A mild burn over a large area is more dangerous than a second-degree burn of small size. Shock is usually severe in burns over a large area. As a general rule the first aid treatment of burns involves relief of pain and the treatment of shock. Call the doctor immediately.

All burns are painful. Mild burns of the first degree

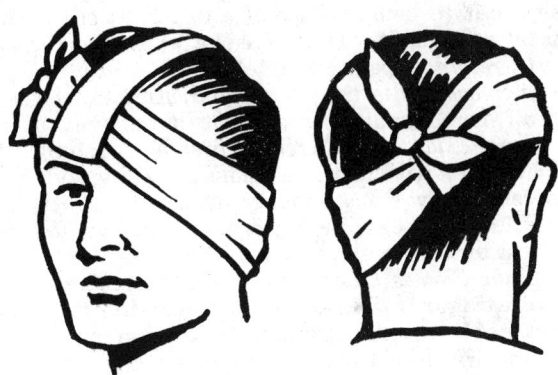

Fig. 821. Bandage for the eye (courtesy, J & J).

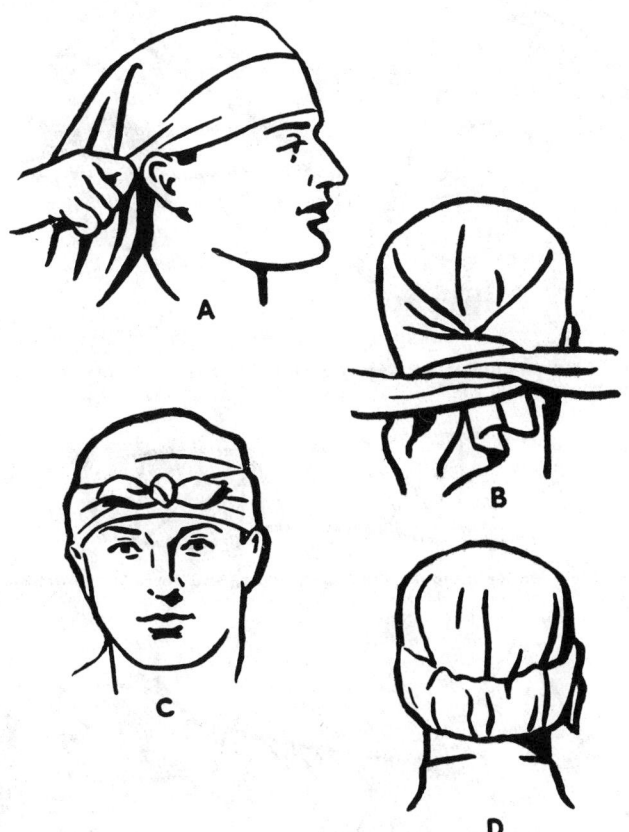

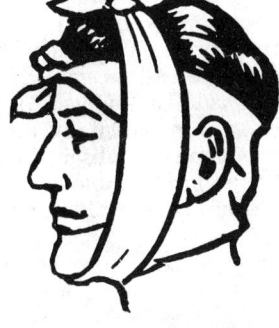

Fig. 822. Roller bandage for head or jaw (courtesy, J & J).

Fig. 823. Bandage for chin (courtesy, J & J).

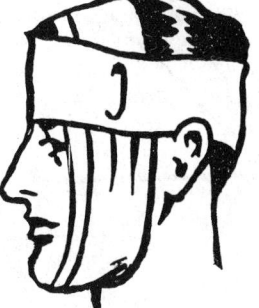

Fig. 820. Head bandage made with triangular bandage (courtesy, J & J).

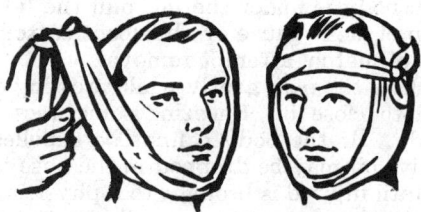

Fig. 824. Cravat bandage for chin or side of face (courtesy, J & J).

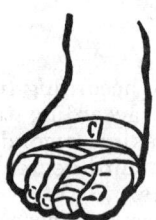

Fig. 825. Roller bandage for toe (courtesy, J & J).

are sometimes relieved by the application of a good burn ointment or a solution of baking soda. Second- and third-degree burns are best treated by applying sterile gauze saturated with a slightly warm baking soda solution. To make a solution, add 2 or 3 heaping tablespoonsful of baking soda to 1 quart of water, previously boiled. The gauze dressing, a primary nonadherent dressing, can be held in place by a lightly applied bandage or by covering it with a large cloth (see also *Primary Wound Dressings*, page 1868).

In *chemical burns* use large quantities of water to wash off the chemical and treat as above. Burns from *strong acids* can be treated first by washing with water and then with warm solutions of baking soda. In burns caused by *strong alkalies* wash with water and apply diluted vinegar or boric acid solution, followed by a burn ointment.

When the Clothes Catch Fire—Roll the person on the floor to extinguish the flames or envelop him in a coat, blanket, table cover, or similar article conveniently at hand, and roll him from side to side. Cut away any loose clothing and treat as above.

Sunburns—Apply calamine lotion, bland oil, or a suitable first-aid ointment. In case of blistering do not open the blister. Apply a dressing of sterile gauze.

Do not apply iodine to a burn.

Frostbite—This is caused by exposure to unusually cold temperatures, resulting in freezing of parts of the body, usually fingers, toes, nose, and other exposed areas. Pain is usually present in freezing of hands or feet, but may be absent in freezing of the ears and nose. Get the victim immediately into a warm place and undress him, preferably putting him in a warm bed. The

best and perhaps the easiest treatment is to cover the affected part with soft sterile toweling, cloth, or gauze dressing. Be extremely gentle. In the case of a hand it might be held against some warm part of the body such as the thigh or the armpit until medical aid can be obtained. This can be done until the circulation is re-established and the pain is lessened. Cover the area with toweling or cloth. Rubbing with snow or applying hot water or exposure to extreme heat is dangerous and produces further injury.

Heat Cramps—This condition occurs in those who are subject to high temperatures and who drink large amounts of water, sweat excessively, and lose a great deal of body salt. Heat cramps can be prevented by maintaining an adequate intake of salt.

The *symptoms* are severe muscle cramps in the calf and abdominal muscles, slight dizziness, and exhaustion.

Treatment consists simply of the administration of adequate amounts of salt. In mild cases 5 or 10 grains, taken in coated tablets, allays the symptoms.

Heat Exhaustion—This condition occurs in those persons who have a tendency to perspire very freely.

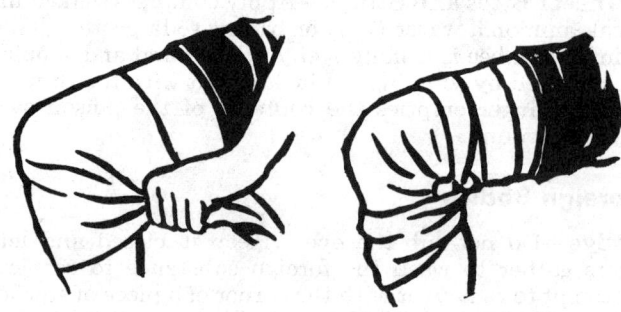

Fig. 827. Cravat bandage for knee (courtesy, J & J).

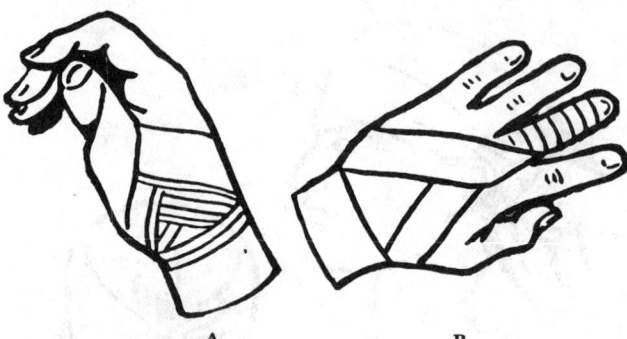

A   B

Fig. 828. *A:* Roller bandage for thumb. *B:* Roller bandage for finger (courtesy, J & J).

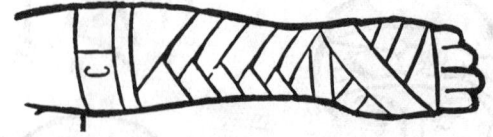

Fig. 829. Roller bandage for hand, wrist, and forearm (courtesy, J & J).

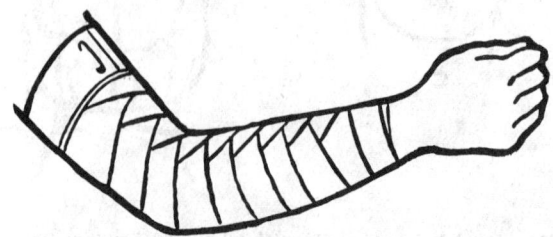

Fig. 830. Roller bandage for elbow joint (courtesy, J & J).

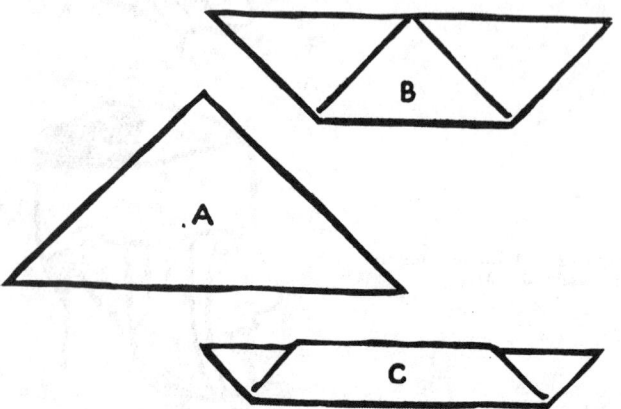

Fig. 826. Triangular bandage folded as a cravat (courtesy, J & J).

Symptoms

Heat exhaustion is characterized by fatigue, lassitude, and a general feeling of faintness. The patient breaks out in a profuse cold perspiration, turns white, and faints. The skin feels cold and clammy, the pulse is weak and thready, and breathing is shallow. Although the skin may feel cold, the body temperature is often slightly above normal.

Treatment

1. Move the patient to a cool place. Loosen his clothing or take it off, and put him in shock position (legs higher than head). Apply cool moist cloths to the patient's forehead and wrists.
2. Hold aromatic spirits of ammonia near his nose to act as a stimulant.
3. If these measures are not effective, further elevate the legs and bandage each leg tightly from the ankles towards the body to force the blood back into circulation.
4. Give salt solution or salt tablets by mouth if the patient is conscious; if not, give it by retention enema.
5. The patient should rest in a cool place until completely recovered. Give cool, sweetened drinks, especially coffee containing sugar, because it acts as a stimulant. *Do not give alcohol.*

Heatstroke—Heatstroke, sometimes referred to as sunstroke, is far more serious than heat exhaustion. At the same temperatures an attack is much more likely under conditions of physical exertion and high humidity than under low humidity.

Symptoms

The skin is flushed, very dry, and very hot. If circulatory collapse follows, the face turns gray. The body temperature may reach 106°F or higher, which is the clue to the diagnosis. Any body temperature over 105°F occurring during hot weather in a collapsed person with a red, hot dry skin is more than likely to be heat stroke.

Treatment

This is a grave emergency! The danger lies in the actual cooking of the tissues caused by the high temperature.
1. Place the patient in a tub of very cold (ice) water.
2. When the body temperature has come down to about 100°F, put him in bed and wrap him in sheets wet with cold water. Fanning increases the rate of evaporation and, hence, the cooling effect. If the temperature tends to rise again, return the patient to the cold-water tub.
3. If cold-water tubs are not available, wrap the patient in wet sheets and fan him in any manner possible. Electric fans are best. Give retention enemas of ice water. Anything that can be done to lower the excessively high body temperature may be life-saving.
4. Heat stroke is a complicated medical problem, and the patient should receive medical help as soon as possible.

Bandaging

Types of Bandages

Two kinds of bandages are generally used in first-aid work. These are the roller bandage and the triangular (Esmarch) bandage.

Roller Bandages may be prepared from muslin or gauze. These are available packed in special containers and sterilized. The new conforming-type bandages are a special type of roller bandage which more readily conforms to any part and are much easier to apply. Roller bandages can be used for bandaging of wounds, for support and for improvised slings. They are prepared in several widths.

Fingers and toes—1 in. wide (Figs. 825 and 828).
Head, hands and limbs of children—2 in. wide (Figs. 829 and 830).
Head, hands, and limbs of adults—2 and 3 in. wide (Figs. 822 and 823).
Thigh, groin, and trunk—3 in. wide.

The Triangular (Esmarch) Bandage is extremely useful. It may be applied as a covering, as a wide-folded bandage (wide cravat), or as a narrow-folded bandage (narrow cravat). It may be used for tying splints to limbs, for holding a splinted limb to the body, as a hand bandage, as a wide sling for arm, as a head and scalp covering, and as a head and face bandage. It similarly can be applied over other parts of the body—the forehead, chest, knee, and foot. It can be used as a narrow sling or wide sling. In other words it can be improvised for use as a bandage, support, or covering for nearly every part of the body (see Figs. 816, 820, 821, 824, and 827).

Bandaging Sprains and Strains

Twist or Wrench at the Joint—This is usually accompanied by pain and swelling.

Wrap in folded gauze or towel and apply cold water or ice. Keep the part elevated and at rest. If a fracture is suspected, treat as previously described.

Muscle Wrench or Tear—Apply heat and massage. Supporting the injured part with a bandage or adhesive plaster will relieve the pain. Medicated plasters, whole or cut in strips, are useful in affording support and warmth.

99 | Health Accessories

Dressings and first-aid supplies—supplies for the infant and older baby—thermometers—inhalers, atomizers, and insufflators—hypodermic equipment—sickroom appliances—invalid and geriatric services—trusses and orthopedic aids—supplies for diabetic patients—invalid and other special foods—analytical and chemical departments—proprietary and over-the-counter preparations—veterinary medicines and supplies—insecticides, fungicides, and rodenticides—toilet articles and preparations—hypoallergenic cosmetics and dermatological pharmaceuticals—hearing aids—the pharmacist and venereal disease control

This chapter was prepared by

John N. McDonnell, DSc, *Consultant to the Pharmaceutical Industry,* *Meadowbrook, Pa. 19046*

In addition to filling prescriptions a well-trained pharmacist is qualified to give technical and professional advice and assistance in many matters dealing with sickness and health. There must be a sharp line drawn between the kind of information and help rendered by the physician and that offered by the pharmacist. For instance, the pharmacist does not determine by symptoms or clinical tests that a patient is suffering from diabetes, and advise the administration of insulin. That is strictly the physician's responsibility. However, it is the pharmacist's province, when he is asked by the physician, to supply information and guidance to the latter as to the respective properties and advantages of parenteral unmodified insulin, protamine zinc insulin, NPH insulin, the Lente insulins, and globin zinc insulin, and the relationship they hold to oral antidiabetic preparations. Then, as to the patient, when the physician has ordered insulin in specific unit doses, it would be within the province of the pharmacist to assist in the selection of the syringe and needles, perhaps to demonstrate special devices like the Busher automatic syringe, to offer a proper type of alcohol for sterilizing needles and the skin, to explain and sell a dietary scale, and to supply the insulin.

The more important departments where such helpful services may be rendered are described below.

Dressings and First-aid Supplies

Wound Dressings—The pharmacist is the proper distributor of sterile materials for treating wounds. His training enables him to appreciate the care necessary in their handling and storage, and he is often called upon for advice, or instruction as to their use. The following items fall in this class: absorbent cotton; cotton balls and buds; sterile pads of gauze; bandages—muslin, elastic (web and rubber), gauze; disposable fabric tissues and underpads; eye pads, sponges, tissues, and towels; gauze diapers for adults; plaster of Paris; adhesive plaster; adhesive elastic bandages; aerosol adherent; spray dressings; first-aid kits; scissors; tweezers; and applicators.

Sanitary Aids—This department might well be organized under the supervision of one of the women pharmacists or female clerks who could be specially trained to offer the necessary assistance and advice to women customers. This department would stock sanitary belts, napkins, pads, tampons, aprons, deodorants, etc.

The Family Medicine Closet—There is a place in every home for some simple medicines; these should be kept in one place, preferably in a locked closet.

The medicine closet should always be kept *out of reach of children.* Prescriptions in current use may be kept in the closet, but should be destroyed after the patient is well. *Every bottle or box should be clearly labeled.* Some pharmacists provide folders containing information on first aid, poison antidotes, and simple home medication for use by their patrons so that the pharmacy's name is always in view in the medicine cabinet. This is also accomplished by providing a gummed "family prescription record" for the inside of the cabinet door, or an "emergency label" bearing space for entry of telephone numbers for doctor, pharmacy, hospital, fire and police service, to be attached to the telephone set or telephone book.

The neighborhood pharmacist may properly recommend the installation in every home of a first-aid cabinet. The following items for a family medicine chest were suggested in the American Medical Association magazine, *Today's Health.* These should be in every home.

Drugs	Supplies
Glycerin, Seidlitz Powders, Boric Acid Solution, Quinine Sulfate, Acetylsalicylic Acid (Aspirin), Castor Oil, Iodine Tincture (2%), Mercurial or Nitrofuran Antiseptic Solution, Cascara Extract Tablets, Bismuth Subgallate or Subcarbonate, Sodium Bicarbonate, Compound Benzoin Tincture, Boric Acid Ointment, Mineral Oil and Petrolatum, Milk of Magnesia.	Suitable books on First Aid, Nursing and Diets for the Layman, Clinical Thermometer, Drinking Tubes, Medicine Glass, Medicine Dropper, Bedpan, Enema Syringe, Sterile Gauze "Sponges," Sterile Absorbent Cotton, Disposable Tissues and Towels, Vaporizers, Cotton Wadding, Hot Water Bottle, Ice Bag, Adhesive Plaster, Sterile Gauze.

These items may be replaced by any others intended for the same purpose as may be selected by the pharmacist. In addition, in this automobile age, the pharmacist should urge that every family car in his community be equipped with a small but adequate first-aid kit, in addition to a flash light, flares, and a hand fire extinguisher.

Every hospital pharmacist should have a chart of disaster unit equipment required for a hospital and all pharmacists should be familiar with the requirements and needs of disaster units.

Scales or Balances—The pharmacist provides a suitable distribution center for special types of scales, such as those for bathroom use, or those for weighing

1896

babies, and also those used for weighing food for diabetics (see Figs. 831–833). Modern bathroom scales are available with capacities up to 250 to 300 pounds, are made of plastic or metal, are adjustable, colorful, with an adjustable exact zero scale, carrying a free factory-repair warranty, and are quite accurate. Principal suppliers are Brearley and Borg-Erickson.

Supplies for the Infant and Older Baby

The pharmacist is especially qualified to furnish many of the supplies required for the health and well-being of babies and children. He is also in position to impart information to the mother supplemental to that given by the physician.

There are approximately 4 million babies born annually in the US. In the decade and a half following World War II, America's birth rate increased rapidly, from a 1946 figure of 3,426,000 births.

In 1957, the peak year, the birth rate reached a crest of 25.3 per thousand, the fertility rate (number of births per 1000 women aged 15 to 44) climbed to 122.7, and the year brought a bumper crop of 4.3 million babies. However, the trend changed downward, and in 1968, according to US Bureau of the Census estimates, the total number of births was 3.4 million, or about 82 births per 1000 women. This is at a rate of about 17.6 live births for every 1000 Americans of both sexes and all ages.

A discernible tendency of young people to postpone marriage, and to form smaller families may be reflected in the lowering trend in birth rate.

In 1965 there were 20.4 millions of infants and babies 4 years of age or younger in this country. Reliable estimates[1] set this figure at 21.3 millions for 1970; 27.2 millions for 1975 and 31.04 millions in 1980. These numbers are equally divided between males and females.

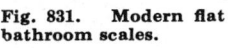

Fig. 831. Modern flat bathroom scales.

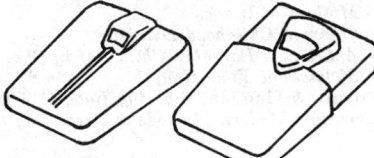

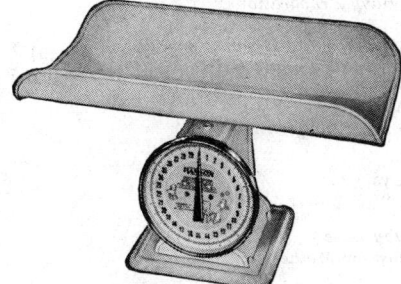

Fig. 832. Baby scales.

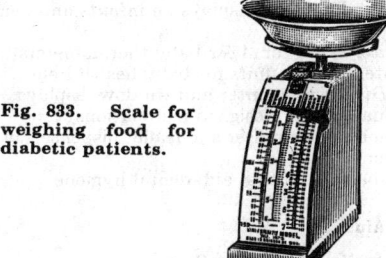

Fig. 833. Scale for weighing food for diabetic patients.

It is important, however, to distinguish between the birth rate and the actual number of babies born. The number of women of childbearing age has been rising.

Between 1965 and 1975 the number of people from 18 to 24 years of age will increase by more than 35%,[2] or more than twice as fast as the increase in the total population. This will be at the expense of the middle-aged group (35 to 54 years) as those 55 years and over will approximate the average for all ages. And more people should mean more babies even though the birth rate itself is dropping off.

Current predictions of US population for 1970 and thereafter vary.[3] The 1970 estimate is approximately 206 millions, while that for the end of the century is about 300 million.

The pharmacy, by nature of its unique professional-retailing position and close working relationship with the medical profession, has an excellent advantage over other types of retail businesses in capturing and holding the baby market. If the community pharmacist is to retain his present competitive position in this area, greater knowledge must be his weapon. The American public spends a great deal each year on baby needs. *Drug Topics* estimates that in 1967 the American public spent $161 million in community pharmacies for baby needs. This amounts to about $3,580 for every pharmacy in the country, but actually only 52% of the total spent for baby needs is received by pharmacists. Department stores, supermarkets, variety stores, and even mail order houses garner over half of all the average family spends each year on baby supplies, prescription accessories, first-aid supplies, and equipment, which in 1967 amounted for the whole country to more than $780 million, according to *Drug Topics*.

If alert to this opportunity a pharmacist will logically make the Baby Department most attractive, he will stock and display every item which an expectant mother will need immediately upon the arrival of the new baby, and will emphasize these items by seeing that she receives one of the many available booklets written by experts on the care of the baby. Such booklets are made available for distribution by many firms.

Specialized Departments—Organizing a retail pharmacy into departments has become an accepted procedure and is utilized wherever possible, reaching its greatest height of efficiency in the Baby Department.

In opening space for a sales-producing Baby Department, many pharmacists become interested in a complete store revision for more efficient self-selection selling. Anyone contemplating reorganization or modernization of a pharmacy should recognize the fact that each store should be analyzed individually. Certain aspects of self-service may be practical in one and not in another retail store. Physical facilities, type of location, nature of clientele are all to be considered.

The five essentials of a good Baby Department are as follows:

1. It should be complete.
2. It should be prominent.
3. It should be a self-selection department.
4. It should reflect a "baby atmosphere."
5. It should be visibly priced.

A long list of supplies is indicated, some of which are mentioned below. It is also desirable to have available and on display a complete "layette" ready for emergency, including the surgical and other emergency supplies needed by the mother and baby at the time of birth.

Women Attendants—A trained woman attendant is especially valuable in this department. The opportunity for a woman pharmacist to develop service in this field is obvious and many pharmacist–owners have discovered that a woman pharmacist retained not only for dispensing activity but also for supervising the operation of departments set aside for baby's and mother's needs, for sanitary supplies, etc, will soon develop a large measure of community recognition.

Booklets and Displays—A vast amount of merchandising material is now available to retail druggists from interested manufacturers. It involves not only the Baby Department, but almost every other section in the retail drugstore.

An excellent example of wholesaler cooperation is the store-modernizing program of McKesson and Robbins, which has sought to devise a method for simplifying the selling process while at the same time contributing to the atmosphere of the pharmacy.

The scheme is designed to provide two kinds of display of drug merchandise:

1. Narrow step-shelves permitting a vertical display of a small number of items to produce a mass effect.
2. Sections at hand level for displaying of small items such as hand lotions, toothpaste, shaving creams, etc.

The departments into which the scheme is divided are the major drug and toiletry departments representing over 40% of the sales volume in the nation's drug stores. They are: Hair Care, Cough and Cold, First Aid, Baby Needs, Cosmetics, Oral Hygiene, and Vitamins. By providing for display of these high volume departments at about 30 inches from the floor and below eye level at the wrapping counter, McKesson has found that sales increases of up to 50% and more of the store's volume are possible, and an average increase of 25% has been recorded. These increases have been realized with a very slight increase in overhead, at the same time freeing the pharmacist from the tedious and unrewarding work of seeking and carrying merchandise and permitting a greater amount of his time to be expended in actually dealing with the customer and in compounding prescriptions.

Agencies of the Federal government provide valuable assistance to pharmacists for nursing and expectant mothers in the form of informative pamphlets available from the Superintendent of Documents, Government Printing Office, Washington, D.C. 20042. Some of them are:

Prenatal Care, 1962, 96 p. il, Catalog No. FS 14.111:4, 20¢.
When Your Baby Is on the Way, 1961, 32 p. il, Catalog No. FS 14.111:391, 15¢.
Your Premature Baby, 1954, 13 p. il, Catalog No. FS 14.118:40, 10¢.
Infant Care, 1963, 108 p. il, Catalog No. FS 14.111:8, 20¢.
Your Baby's First Year, 1962, 32 p. il, Catalog No. FS 14.111:400, 15¢.
Your Child from 1 to 3, 1965, 24 p. il, Catalog No. FS 14.111:413, 20¢.
Your Child from One to Six, 1962, 98 p. il, Catalog No. FS 14.111:30, 20¢.
When You Adopt a Child, 1965, 27 p. il, Catalog No. FS 14.118:13/2, 15¢.
Your Child from 3 to 4, 1966, 26 p. il, Catalog No. FS 14.111:446, 25¢.
Home Play and Play Equipment for Young Children, Rev. 1959, 23 p. il, Catalog No. FS 14.111:238/2, 15¢.
Foods Your Children Need, Rev. 1958, 16 p. il, Catalog No. FS 14.118:14, 10¢.
Nutrition and Healthy Growth, 1955, 35 p, Catalog No. FS 14.111:352, 20¢.
Day Care Services, 1965, 44 p. il, Catalog No. FS 14.111:420, 25¢.
The Care of Your Children's Teeth, 1966, 12 p. il, Catalog No. FS 14.111:439, 15¢.
The Child with a Speech Problem, 1964, 24 p. il, Catalog No. FS 14.118:52, 15¢.
Accidents and Children, Reprinted 1965, 20 p. il, Catalog No. FS 14.118:48/2, 15¢.

Every pharmacist interested in a Baby Department should also get a copy of "Infant Care."[4] Display this invaluable aid to every mother coming into your pharmacy and offer them for sale, or, better still, give one to every regular customer for baby supplies. Obtain a copy of "Advice to the Mother-to-be"[5] and have copies made for distribution. It may be well for the pharmacist to obtain a selection of popular books on child health and care, and to establish a library for the use of expectant and nursing mothers.

Some of the booklets which are freely available to pharmacists as single copies or in quantity from commercial and other sources and which may be distributed *gratis* are listed below.

Baby Department Material

Booklets

Davol—
    Baby Feeding Made Easier
    Pssst! Need a New One?
    Baby Loves Baby Foods
Gerber—
    Infant Nutrition Manual
    Nutritive Values of Gerber Baby Foods
    Current Practices in Infant Feeding folder (written especially for the physician, pharmacist, nurse, and dietitian)
    Foods for Baby and Mealtime Psychology (designed for distribution by physicians to their patients) (1967)
Hankscraft—*The Simple Sanitary Way to Bottle Feed Your Baby*
Mead-Johnson—
    Pregnancy . . . A Time for Healthful Habits
    A Formula Center for Better Baby Care
    Preparing Formula and Feeding Baby
    What You Should Know about Breast Feeding
    Helpful Hints for Traveling with Baby
    Timely Tips for the Father-to-be
    Helpful Hints for Naming Your Baby
Metropolitan Life—
    Your Child
    Understanding Your Young Child
    To Parents about Immunization
    Memo to Parents . . . About Immunization
    Memo to Parents about Your Child's Eyesight
    Memo to Parents about Your Child's Sleep
    Mothers at Work
    Common Childhood Diseases
    A Letter to Parents—Child Safety Check List
    Sickness at Your House?
Proctor & Gamble—*Bathing Baby* (1959)
Evenflo—*Modern Methods of Preparing Baby's Formula*

Folders

Breck—*Breck Baby Prepdrations*
Davol—
    Terminal Sterilization of Baby's Formula
    Every Mother Needs a Little Help
Holland-Rantos—
    for *Rantex Masks*
    H-R Diaper Rash Baby Cream

Counter Displays

Breck—
    for *Breck Baby Lave*
    for *Breck Soap for Mothers and Babies*
Chicopee—
    Common Sense in Dressing Baby
    Trip Tip—Take One
    Helpful Hints for Home Nursing
Davol—counter and window displays on infants and health essential products
Faichney—counter stand for *Apex* baby thermometers
Faultless—counter display units for baby health items
Homemakers—*Diaperene* counter and window displays—by arrangement, individual custom-designed installations
J & J—baby lotion merchandiser and leaflet dispenser, baby products merchandiser
    Literature on baby care, first aid, dental hygiene

Merchandising Aids

Davol—*How to Increase Drugstore Profits*

Baby Department Supplies

Medicines

Alcohol (70%), for washing and sterilizing
Boric Acid, crystal and solution
Boric Acid Ointment
Burn Emollient
Calcium Lactate
Camphorated Oil
Castile Soap
Castor Oil, plain and aromatic
Cod Liver Oil Concentrates
Compound Benzoin Tincture
Cough Medicines
Glycerin Suppositories
Green Soap, Tincture
Iodine Tincture, 2%
Lactic Acid, to make acid milk
Lanolin or Wool Fat
Liquid Petrolatum
Lime Water
Mercurial or Nitrofuran Antiseptic Solution
Milk of Magnesia or other laxatives
Olive Oil
Peppermint Spirit
Petroleum Jelly, plain and medicated
Rubbing Alcohol
Sodium Bicarbonate
Teething Lotions
Zinc Oxide Ointment
Zinc Stearate

Baby Foods

Baby Soups, Vegetables, and Meats
Prepared Foods, in disposable containers
Whole, Modified, and Malted Milk Preparations

Antiseptic Dressings and Surgical Supplies

Bandage, plain and medicated
Absorbent Cotton
Gauze, plain and medicated
First Aid Outfit
Adhesive Tape
Dental Floss
Nursing Pads
Tongue Depressors
Wooden Applicators
Umbilical Tape
Oil Silk
Layettes and Maternity Kits
Applicators, cotton-tipped

Infant and Maternal Supplies

Nursing Bottles (narrow neck, wide neck, disposable, screw top)
Electric Bottle Warmers
Bottle Caps
Bottle Racks
Bottle Brushes and Cleaners
Graduates
Funnels
Measuring Glasses and Spoons
Covered Jars
Bibs, washable and disposable
Droppers, medicine
Strainers
Humidifiers
Straws, drinking
Pacifiers
Lights, night
Toys
Milk Pasteurizers
Milk-bottle Sterilizers
Nursery Tongs
Atomizers
Thermometers (clinical, bath, house, and dairy)

Canned Heat (Sterno)
Alcohol Stoves
Vacuum Bottle
Safety Pins, assorted sizes
Baby Scales
Hot Plates
Toilet Paper
Starch-Free Foods
Protein Foods
Carbohydrate Foods
Sugar Substitutes
Malted Milk Powder
Malt Syrup
Milk Substitutes
Milk Sugar
Evaporated Milk
Vitamin Foods, Concentrates, and Compounds

Baby Toiletries

Baby Cream, jars and tubes
Baby Oil
Baby Soaps
Baby Talc, plain or borated
Dusting Powder
Medicated Powder
Nose Drops
Toilet Gift Sets
Tooth Brushes
Hair Brushes
Nail Brushes
Combs
Sponges
Covered Jars, plain and decorated
Powder Puffs
Soft Wash Cloths
Manicuring Scissors
Thumb Guards or other thumb sucking preventive appliances
Safety Strap with leader
High Chair Pads (rubberized)
Baby Toilet Seats or Commodes
Diapers (disposable)
Croup Kettles and Vaporizers
Heating Pads
Disposable Towels
Disposable Wash Cloths

Rubber Sundries

Nipples
Teething Rings
Rattles
Bottle Caps
Nipple Covers for terminal sterilization
Nipple Shields
Breast Pumps
Rubber Pants
Diaper Bags
Sheeting and Crib Sheets, rubber or plastic
Infant Nasal Aspirators
Infant Syringes
Ear and Ulcer Syringes
Baby Hot Water Bottles
Eye and Medicine Droppers
Rectal Syringes
Rubber Gloves

Medicines and Supplies for the Baby—Care is essential not only in the preparation and labeling of medicines for administration to infants but also in making certain that the mother understands their use. There are many strictly professional services rendered by pharmacists for babies. None is more important than dispensing prescriptions or in filling an order for prevention or cure of disease. Inasmuch as babies are highly responsive to medication, mark every prescription plainly *For Baby.* Be sure that the parents understand what they are using and that these materials are exactly as prescribed by the physician.

Baby's Needs—Upon his arrival into the home the new baby will need food, with bottles, nipples, sterilizer, clothing and items for the bath. Often these articles, other than food, have been obtained well in advance of the blessed event. The physician will prescribe the type and quantity of infant food he deems best for the specific needs of the new arrival. Meanwhile, mother should be provided with at least a minimum supply of the essentials.

The *Baby Department* centers around six basic products. Talc neutralizes irritants due to diaper moisture, guards against excess moisture, and protects against prickly heat rash. An antiseptic emulsion lotion is a protective cleanser. Castile soap and a bland, soothing cream are essentials, the latter for chapped cheeks, crawlers' knee, and rubbed elbows. A nontoxic shampoo for baby's hair, that will not irritate sensitive eyes, and a baby oil to lubricate, protect, and cleanse the skin are the others. Some manufacturers provide these items already packaged as gift items. Preparations for prevention and treatment of diaper rash, packed as aerosols for more effective administration, have been introduced.

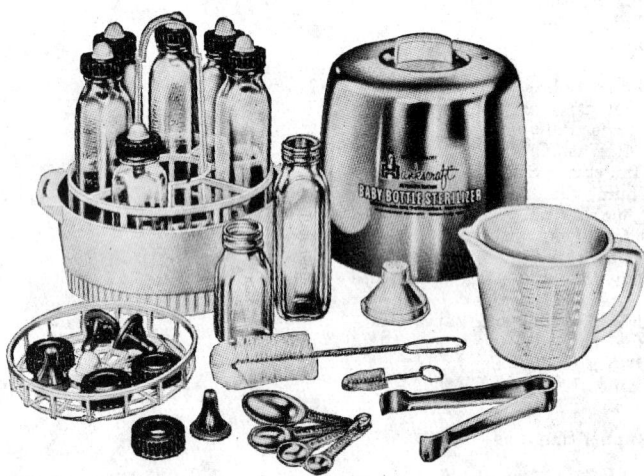

Fig. 834. Complete unit for preparation of baby food formula (Hankscraft) with interim or terminal sterilizer, bottle rack, milk formula bottles, tray for parts, funnel, measuring cup, measuring spoons, bottle and nipple brushes, clamp.

A "list" of medicines and supplies which will permit the mother to check her needs without forgetting any essential item is useful. The listing above and the following suggestions may be helpful and can be copied and distributed by the pharmacist.

Aids for Feeding the Baby—There are many types of apparatus needed by a mother for preparing the baby's food. More than 37% of the baby population today have feeding problems. Large *measuring jars* of about one quart or one liter capacity are available in glass or enamel, with printed, molded, or blown markings in various volume scales. Although measuring jars are frequently supplied, graduates are more exact in measuring and should be recommended. Standardized *spoons* for measuring milk sugar are available. A small *graduate* is an essential for measuring cream or top milk. However, this is no longer common practice, as Foman[11] in 1965 estimated that only 3% of babies 1-month old were fed on whole cow's milk.

Nursing Bottles—Two types of nursing bottles are used principally: the narrow neck, used with pull-on nipples and preferred by hospitals, and the more popular reversible screw-top nurser bottle for complete assembly of nipple, plastic collar, and protective seal.

Manufacturers of bottles today have accounted for principles of easy cleaning, heat resistance, and compact storage in both narrow-neck and screw-top styles. Wide-neck or wide-mouth nursers have an added advantage of a larger neck opening which facilitates filling and cleaning. See Figs. 834–836.

Most sterilizers have been designed to take all popular nursers and bottles.

The pharmacist should always suggest the use of nylon or bristle nipple brushes and bottle brushes when nursing bottles are purchased (Fig. 834 and 837).

Nipples—Fitting the "small-mouth" or "narrow-neck" bottles are the Davol *Anti-Colic* nipples with convenient, sanitary tab for easy assembly. Standard nipples are made with three feeding holes. These nipples keep the baby's mouth shapely. *Sani-Tab* nipples are manufactured with a special vent which prevents nipple collapse and assures continuous flow of formula. Inasmuch as the wrong kind of soft, long flexible nipple will deform the baby's mouth and jaw, it is essential that the short, firm type be employed to simulate the areola of the breast (see Figs. 841 – 843).

Modern tastes have taken to the "screw-top" or wide-neck nurser, which is designed for complete assembly of bottle, nipple, screw-on plastic collar, and protective cap or seal. The *Nurser* unit can be made up with nipple inverted in the bottle, or upright if assembled with the new rubber nipple covers for sterile protection.

If stored with nipple inverted, the mother must remove the plastic collar, and upright the nipple for feeding. Rubber nipple covers, on the other hand, allow for sterile protection of both nipple and formula right up to feeding time with no need for touching the nipple

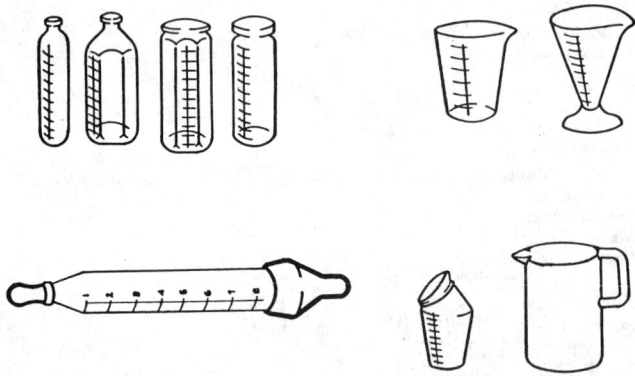

Fig. 835. Nursing bottles (upper left); measuring glasses (upper right); measuring glass and jar (lower right); Brecht feeder (lower left).

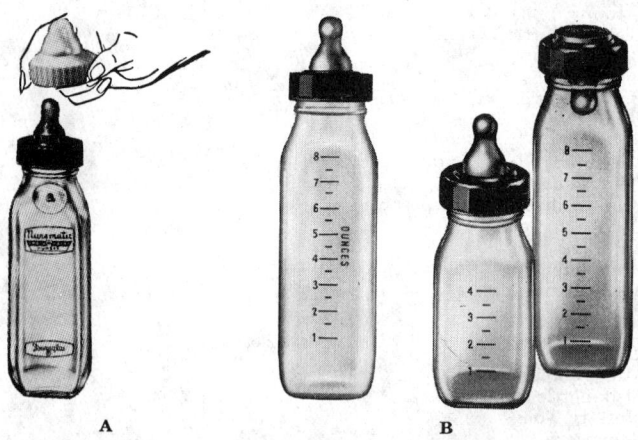

Fig. 836. Nursing bottles. *A:* Improved nursing bottle with nipple, flow control, cover for refrigeration-sterility. *B:* Screw-top nursing bottles. Nursing bottle with nipple and cap cover.

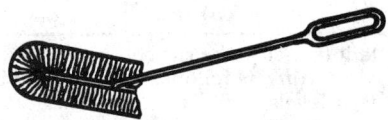

Fig. 837.   Bottle brush.

after sterilization (Fig. 844).   The Hankscraft *Nurs-matic* widemouthed bottle features a stainless steel control valve (*Insta-Valve*) which prevents excessive air swallowing which causes colic, and a leakproof nipple which regulates flow of the formula (*Les-Air Nipple*).

Screw-top nursers are available with both eight- and four-ounce bottles.   The assembly parts such as collars, seals, nipple covers, and nipples, should be made standard stock in the Baby Department.

Nipple Shields and Breast Pumps—The mother may frequently find it necessary to protect the breast areola with a nipple shield.   This is a glass vessel which fits around the nipple, and has attached an ordinary rubber nipple for baby feeding.   This prevents irritation.   Plain breast shields of soft rubber, plastic, metal, or fabric may be supplied without the nipple, to prevent breast injury.   When the baby is unable to suckle, a breast pump may be employed.   This may also be used in developing the mammary glands before the baby's arrival (Figs. 840, 846, and 847).

Preparing the Baby's Milk—As milk is an excellent culture medium many so-called summer complaints and similar digestive disturbances may be traced to infected milk.   But as sterilization requires a temperature of at least 100°C and as high temperatures destroy most of the vitamin content of milk and lessen its digestibility, sterilized milk is not a complete food and should not be fed regularly.   However pasteurization, heating at 70°C for 30 minutes, destroys most of the offending organisms likely to be present in milk, and without injuring its food value.

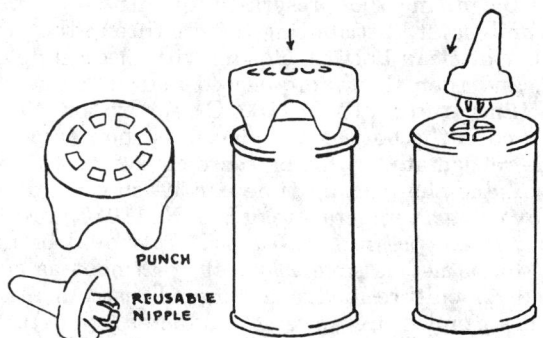

Fig. 838.   "Instant Nurser" kit for canned ready-to-use infant formula (Mead Johnson's "Enfamil") where mixing, pouring, and breakage are avoided—a center-hole punch opens the can, the nipple with nipple cover is inserted, and the can is ready for baby.

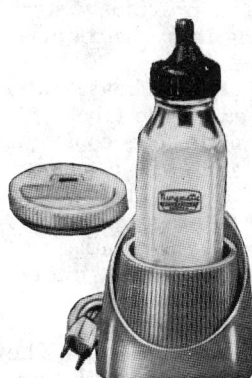

Fig. 839.   Lightweight, break-resistant plastic, automatic, thermostatically controlled bottle warmer with vaporizer attachment for steam for cold relief (Hankscraft).

Pasteurization of milk can be done with ordinary kitchen equipment or with *pasteurizers*.   *Nonabsorbent cotton* was formerly used to plug the baby bottle necks.   Rubber or glass *caps* should be placed over the top of the milk bottles after pasteurization to keep the contents free from icebox odors (Fig. 845).

No food is so suited for healthy babies as mother's milk.   A most informative article is "Helping Mothers to Nurse Their Babies."[6]   However, it is frequently necessary to supplement or replace mother's milk with artificial preparations.

According to a survey of mothers of children under two years of age conducted by *Parents Magazine* (1966) 61% of all new mothers feed their babies via the bottle only.   Breast feeding is done by 4.2% of the mothers, with the remainder (34.8%) using both feeding methods.

Fewer and fewer mothers in Western countries are breast-feeding their babies.   Studies in the Chicago area, plus the findings of investigators here and abroad,

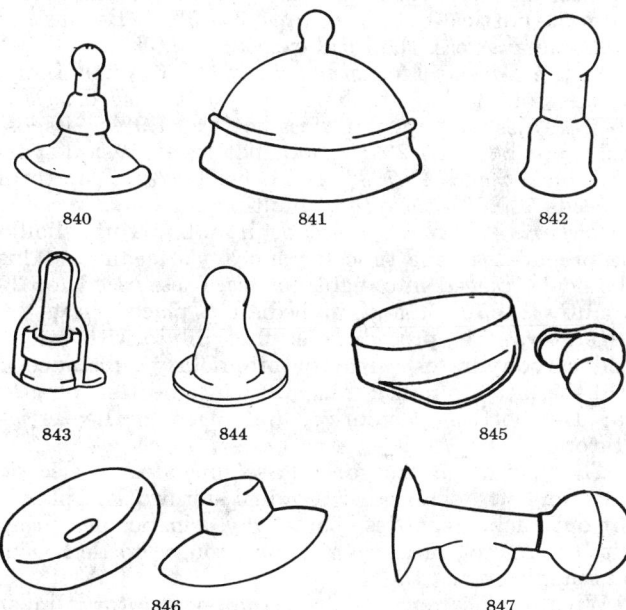

Fig. 840.   Wide-neck glass nipple shield with nipple attached.   Fig. 841.   Nipple (wide mouthed).   Fig. 842.   Nipple (narrow neck).   Fig. 843.   Anticolic nipple showing top and internal construction.   Fig. 844.   Rubber nipple cover.   Fig. 845.   Milk bottle caps.   Fig. 846.   Nipple shields.   Fig. 847.   Breast pump.

report Drs. Michael Newton, clinical professor of obstetrics and gynecology, University of Chicago Medical School, and his wife, Niles Newton, assistant professor of psychology, Northwestern University Medical School, show that the percentage of American mothers who nurse their children was cut in half in a 10-year period.[7, 8]   In Bristol, England, the percentage dropped more than half in 20 years.   And a survey in France showed that the percentage of infants that received breast milk fell about a quarter during a 5-year period.   They maintain that the reasons for the phenomenon are largely psychological and social and not due to any change in the physical capacity of mothers.

Milk Mixtures—The essential differences between cow's milk and human milk is the former's larger (2½:1) percentage of protein and smaller percentage of lactose.   Also, while human milk flocculates, cow's milk is likely to form a clot when coagulated with rennin.   Human milk and cow's milk are usually slightly alkaline when raw, but cow's milk has changed to a slightly acid state by the time it has reached the consumer.

Constituents of Human and Cow's Milk

%	Protein	Fat	Lactose	Salt	Water
Human	1.4	3.7	7.2	0.2	87.5
Cow	3.4	3.9	4.9	0.7	87.1

If cow's milk is diluted to simulate human milk, the remaining percentages of fat and sugar are too low for the baby's needs. The cow's milk is diluted, therefore, with water, and the deficiency in fat brought up by adding a proportion of cream or "top milk." The deficiency in milk sugar can be overcome by adding *lactose* (milk sugar) or other carbohydrates such as dextrose or maltose.

Mothers using bottle feeding reported (1966) that they used the following products: fresh milk 18.1%; evaporated milk 24.6%; ready prepared formula mix, powder 13.4%, liquid 59.1%; pre-filled disposable formula bottles 3.1%; and other 4.5%. Because of multiple answers, the total exceeds 100.0%.

In the *Parents Magazine* survey (1966) of mothers, it was found that mothers using bottle feeding for their babies used regular glass bottles 81.9%; disposable glass bottles 1.2%; plastic bottles 42.3%; disposable plastic sacs 15.7%; and other 0.3%. The total exceeds 100.0% because of multiple answers.

Preparing the Mixture—Enough milk mixture should be prepared at one time for one day's feeding. This should be placed into eight bottles, pasteurized for 30 minutes at 70°C, and immediately placed in a refrigerator. The procedure is: first, dilute with water; add carbohydrates (sugar or proprietary substances); add the fat (top milk); distribute into bottles, plug or cap the bottles, pasteurize, and place in the refrigerator.

The typical nursing formula set includes an electric unit for both regular and terminal sterilization, plastic lift-out rack, 8 bottles, parts tray, plastic measuring pitcher, funnel, measuring spoons, tongs, bottle brush, and nipple brush.

When milk is removed from the refrigerator it must be warmed to body temperature by placing it in hot water or in an *electric bottle warmer*. For traveling parents there is available an insulated heating-pad-type carrying case which keeps bottle cold until feeding time, then heats it quickly when plugged into any automobile 6-volt or 12-volt lighter.

Feeding dishes heated either by electricity or by hot water for keeping bulk foods warm are also available.

Formula Preparation—Regardless of the infant food prescribed for the baby the formula is generally prepared in the home by one of two methods, either the *aseptic technique* or the *terminal heating method*. The purpose of either is to help assure a formula of low bacterial content, free of pathogens. In child-caring institutions, terminal heating and other safeguards are usually required to prevent possible spread of disease.

In using the aseptic technique, the clean bottles, nipples, utensils (such as measuring pitcher, spoon, funnel, tongs, etc) are sterilized by boiling in water. The water for the formula also is boiled. The prescribed amounts of infant food and of cooled sterilized water are mixed in the measure and distributed in the prescribed number of sterilized bottles, the bottle nipples (generally with covers) applied, and the closed bottles put in the refrigerator as soon as possible.

Table I

Infant formula intended to be the sole source of nutrition for infants should contain the following *minimum* vitamin, mineral, and protein levels/100 Kcal of intake. (Values given in mg except where otherwise noted.)

	Minimum amount/ 100 Kcal
Vitamins	
Vitamin A (IU)	250
Vitamin D (IU)	40
Vitamin E (IU)	0.3
Ascorbic Acid (Vitamin C)	8
Thiamine (Vitamin B_1)	0.025
Riboflavin (Vitamin B_2)	0.06
Niacin	0.8[a]
Vitamin B_6	0.035
Folic acid (mcg)	4
Pantothenic acid	0.3
Vitamin B_{12} (mcg)	0.15
Minerals	
Calcium	50
Phosphorus	25
Magnesium	6
Iron	1
Iodine (mcg)	5
Copper	0.06

Protein (per 100 Kcal)

Not less than 1.8 Gm of protein of quality equivalent to that of casein (Protein Efficiency Ratio); or an amount and quality of protein such that the quality of the protein expressed as a fraction of that of casein, multiplied by the Gm weight of the protein/100 Kcal, is not less than 1.8; and the protein is of a quality not less than 70% of that of casein.

[a] The niacin value is comprised of 0.25 mg niacin and 0.55 mg niacin equivalent, the latter from tryptophan supplied by the 1.8 Gm protein.

In using the terminal heating method the formula is made by mixing the prescribed quantities of infant food and water, distributing the mixture in the proper number of clean bottles, closing with clean nipples or caps, and then the whole heated at the temperature of boiling water 212°F (100°C) for 25 or 30 min. When cool, the bottles are placed as soon as possible in the refrigerator. If a pressure cooker or autoclave is available the heating time can be shortened to 10 min by using a temperature of 230°F (110°C) resulting from a steam pressure of 6.1 psi. It should be noted that this is not as severe a heat treatment as is employed for culture media or surgical instruments etc. Infant formulas are adversely affected by excessive, unnecessary heating resulting in partial degradation of the protein by combination with carbohydrate, and in partial destruction of some of the vitamins.

In the home a single bottle of formula may be prepared extemporaneously by using a previously sterilized bottle and nipple and placing in it the required amounts of sterile water and infant food.

A few specialized foods are not to be heated and where this is the case it is indicated on the label.

When the formula has been made and cooled it should be refrigerated as soon as possible passing through the temperature range of rapid bacterial growth 140°F to 40°F as quickly as practicable.

When feeding the infant, the bottle is usually first gently warmed to body temperature but many infants will take formula at room temperature.

Infant Food Product Forms—Infant foods are marketed primarily as canned liquid or as a powder. The liquid may be in concentrated form requiring dilution,

Table II[a]

| | Age, years | | Weight | | Height | | | | Fat-soluble vitamins | | |
	from	up to	Kg	(lb)	cm	(in.)	Kcal	Protein, Gm[b]	Vitamin A activity, IU	Vitamin D, IU	Vitamin E activity, IU
Infants	0	–	⅙	4	9	55	22	Kg × 120	Kg × 2.2	1500	400	5
	⅙	–	½	7	15	63	25	Kg × 110	Kg × 2.0	1500	400	5
	½	–	1	9	20	72	28	Kg × 100	Kg × 1.8	1500	400	5

| Water-soluble vitamins | | | | | | | Minerals | | | | |
Ascorbic acid, mg	Folacin, mg.[c]	Niacin mg equiv.[d]	Ribo-flavin, mg	Thia-mine, mg	Vitamin B_6, mg	Vitamin B_{12}, mcg	Cal-cium, Gm	Phos-phorus, Gm	Iodine, mcg	Iron, mg	Mag-nesium, mg
35	0.05	5	0.4	0.2	0.2	1.0	0.4	0.2	25	6	40
35	0.05	7	0.5	0.4	0.3	1.5	0.5	0.4	40	10	60
35	0.1	8	0.6	0.5	0.4	2.0	0.6	0.5	45	15	70

[a] Food and Nutrition Board, National Academy of Sciences-National Research Council recommended daily dietary allowances, revised 1968; designed for the maintenance of good nutrition of practically all healthy people in the USA.

[b] Assumes protein equivalent to human milk. For proteins not 100% utilized factors should be increased proportionately.

[c] The folacin allowances refer to dietary sources as determined by *Lactobacillus casei* assay. Pure forms of folacin may be effective in doses less than ¼ of the RDA.

[d] Niacin equivalents include dietary sources of the vitamin itself plus 1 mg equivalent for each 60 mg of dietary tryptophan.

usually with an equal volume of water, or it may be ready for use, with the water supplied in the formula by the producer. The latter product possesses a convenience in use but at the cost of freight transportation of half its volume of water, frequently over distances of thousands of miles. In preparing formula from concentrated liquid the mother adds the water at point of use. Either the ready-to-use or concentrated liquids may be commercially manufactured by the traditional canning and retorting process or by aseptic canning, both methods producing a sterile commercial product in the can or bottle.

Powdered infant foods are manufactured in the US today by spray-drying. Contrary to general belief, powders are not sterile but are of high quality bacteriologically and may be relied upon as a safe food for baby.

Considering both economy and convenience, the concentrated liquid is widely accepted as representing the optimum compromise.

In recent years, ready-to-feed formulas have been introduced primarily in hospitals where their use results in some savings in labor costs and elimination of formula rooms. However, the container cost added to each feeding of the infant, together with freight costs on water, place some economic limitation on widespread consumer acceptance.

Other systems have been introduced for use exclusively in hospitals and innovations have been marketed in feeding containers for use in the home.

Infant Nutrition—Optimum nutrition is vital to the individual. From the moment of conception, during the 9 months of his life before birth, and during the months after he is born, proper nutrition is essential to his welfare and lack of it may produce irreversible damage.

Malnutrition in the mother during the gestational period can interfere with the eventual physical and intellectual ability of the child.

Experimental studies with animals have shown that growth proceeds by increase of cell number at first, followed by a period of increasing cell size together with increasing numbers of cells, and then a period of increasing cell size only. Deficient nutrition of the young in the nursing period results in a lesser number of cells in the brain and other organs. Some effects of malnutrition can be reversed by subsequent good nutrition but the damage to mental development is irreversible and permanent.

With this brief discussion in mind, one can appreciate the importance of nutrition to the infant at all stages of his early development.

The prescribing of nutrition for the infant is in the province of the physician. Nevertheless it is most desirable for the pharmacist to possess at least an elementary knowledge of infant feeding in order that he may intelligently supply the modern foods available.

Because the infant is changing greatly each day in weight, length, development, and maturity, he requires close attention to his changing nutritional intake. This requirement includes a supply of energy for resting metabolism, synthesis of body tissues, physical activity, heat balance, etc; protein to provide amino acids for building body protein and for other nitrogen containing substances; fat and carbohydrate to give energy; minerals, such as calcium and phosphorus for bones and teeth, and iron for hemoglobin; and the vitamins with their various functions; all in adequate but not excessive amounts. Sufficient water for the baby's needs also must be supplied, in his formula and additionally, especially in hot weather.

Human milk is quite logically considered ideal for the human infant, and infant formulas have traditionally been patterned generally upon it. Cow's milk contains almost 3 times the protein of human milk and if used for feeding the infant the milk is diluted and carbohydrates such as *milk sugar*, *Dextri-Maltose*, *Karo*, or *table sugar* added. This must be supplemented with *vitamins* and *iron*. In this manner, whole milk or evaporated milk have formerly enjoyed a popularity in such formula preparation. However, the simplicity, convenience, and economy of the modern, concentrated, complete infant formula which needs only dilution with, usually, an equal volume of water has enabled it to displace home prepared milk modification in most of the US.

Normal infants up to about 2 months of age are often fed an energy intake of 55 Kcal/lb/day (120 Kcal/Kg) and from 2 to 6 mos. of age, 50 Kcal/lb day (110 Kcal/Kg).

The Food and Nutrition Board of the National Research Council has established *Recommended Dietary*

Allowances deemed to be adequate for good nutrition.[9] Those for infants are set forth in Table II. Allowances for males and females of all other ages, and the special requirements for pregnancy and lactation are given in the NRC publication.

The various nutrient levels mentioned here, together with the general principles of nutrition[10-13] are utilized in the design of the modern complete infant food.

It will be noted that many variables are changing as the infant increases in age: weight, height, fluid requirement, energy requirement (Kcal), and requirement for protein, some of the vitamins, and minerals. Further, the ratios of calories to body weight decrease. Other factors which change are the infant's capacity for each feeding and the number of feedings per day.

Formulas for the normal infant are generally fed at a concentration of 20 Kcal/fl oz. The total number of calories supplied/day is usually based upon the body weight. This volume of formula is distributed into bottles according to the number of feedings/day (commonly 6/day for the first 1 or 2 months, then 5/day) which are roughly correlated with the volume of intake by the infant (approximately 220 ml/Kg shortly after birth, decreasing to approximately 170 ml/Kg at 3 months). The modern infant formula is designed to meet the daily requirements on this basis.

The reader will rightfully conclude that assigning a feeding program for the infant is best left to the expert, and the feeding must be tailored to the individual infant.

Milk-Based Formulas—The greatest volume of infant formulas is that based on cow's milk as the source of protein. In addition, the fat component (which may be vegetable oil), carbohydrate, vitamins, and minerals make up the product which when ready for the infant supplies 20 Kcal of energy/fl oz. Examples are *Bremil*, *Baker's*, *Enfamil*, and *Similac*.

SMA 26 has a lactalbumin-casein ratio of 60:40, by using whey which has been demineralized by electrodialysis as one of its sources of protein.

Milk-intolerant Infants—Not all infants tolerate formulas based upon cow's milk. A substantial number are intolerant of or allergic to the protein of cow's milk. For these infants, milk-free formulas are available, such as *Mull-Soy* and *Sobee*, which are based upon the vegetable protein of the soybean. Another product, *Soyalac*, is made from a soybean extract as the protein source. In recent years, soybean protein isolate fortified with methionine has gained wide usage as the protein source because the resulting product has a white, milk-like color. *Neo-Mull-Soy* and *Pro-Sobee* are products of this class.

Proteins other than that of soybean have been used to avoid milk protein; for example, *Meat Base Formula* from beef hearts and *Lambase* from lamb. *Nutramigen* depends upon an enzymatic hydrolysate of casein for the protein ingredient. Finally, *goat's milk* should be mentioned as having enjoyed popularity as a substitute for cow's milk.

Other Nutritional Disorders of the Infant—Occasionally the physician may call upon the pharmacist to supply a food for one of the less frequently occurring conditions. Some examples follow.

In disaccharide intolerance the infant cannot utilize disaccharides such as lactose. The product *CHO-Free* enables the physician to add various carbohydrates to aid in diagnosing and managing the problem.

For the infant with galactosemia, in which galactose, resulting from the splitting of lactose, is not metabolized, soy-based formulas or *Nutramigen* are used.

In phenylketonuria, phenylalanine must be restricted. The product *Lofenalac* in which casein is enzymatically digested and its phenylalanine removed meets the nutritional needs, but a metabolic disorder of this type requires continuing professional supervision.

Other products for the infant include *Dryco*, *Maltsupex*, *Probana*, and many others.

For more detailed information on nutrition in infancy consult the references.

Vitamin Products—If the physician is feeding the infant a formula based upon modified whole or evaporated milk, or an incomplete commercial formula he will necessarily prescribe vitamin drops and iron.

The use of fluoride in some vitamin products precludes the use of such products in localities where the drinking water contains more than 0.7 ppm of fluoride.

Other Apparatus for Baby Care—Newborn babies have no teeth, but a *soft toothbrush* is essential, to remove clots of milk from the inner surface of the baby's cheek. Such oral hygiene aids in preventing sore mouths, bacterial infections, and digestive disturbances. A *thermometer*, in a wooden case to prevent breakage, is necessary to test the temperature of the baby's bath.

Pediatricians say that weight is an important indication of adequate nutrition. Therefore, a *baby scale* for regular daily use is an essential.

Talc and zinc stearate are used as *dusting powders*. In every case an automatic, self-closing device should be employed on the powder can to prevent inflammation of the baby's lungs or asphyxiation from the light dusting powder should it be accidentally released.

Rectal syringes and *ice throat collars* are essential, as are *crib sheets* (made of pure gum rubber or heavy plastic) for the bassinet or crib.

Premature and feeble infants are frequently fed by means of a *Brecht feeder*. *Diet scales* are likewise necessary adjuncts in the home of the new baby.

Sterilizers—Apparatus for sterilization of milk and prepared foods for the baby are marketed by Hankscraft, Formulette, Pyramid, Jones Metal, and Electric Steam.

Thermometers

Hippocrates in 460 B.C. recognized that abnormal human temperature was a disease symptom. In 1610 A.D. Sanctorius developed the first clumsy oral thermometer. The thermometer was unreliable until 1714, when Fahrenheit developed the first dependable scale and instrument. It had standard graduations and mercury was used as the heat-measuring liquid. In 1835, two Frenchmen, Becquerel and Breschet, established the mean, or average, temperature of a healthy man as 98.6° on the scale devised by Fahrenheit. A Hollander, Antoon Van Haen, in 1754 had developed the first practical clinical thermometer. Thermometers were seldom depended on in medical practice until about 100 years ago, when, in 1865, a Scottish physician named Aitken invented a self-registering thermometer.

Thermometers for Home Use—The various types of thermometers usually employed in the home are: (1) the *household thermometer* (Fig. 848) or common type for reading interior or outside air temperature, (2) *bath thermometers* for recording the temperature of bath water, and (3) *clinical* or *fever thermometers* (Fig. 849). The temperature of the atmosphere at the surface of the earth varies more than 200°F, but man's body temperature rarely varies beyond 97° to 104°F, with danger at either extreme.

The change in temperature of the patient is one of the important symptoms upon which the physician bases his diagnosis and treatment. The instrument employed for body temperature determination is the *clinical* or more popularly called *fever thermometer*.

An abnormal temperature is nature's warning that something is wrong. Rapid rise or fall and substantial deviations from normal are danger signals. Every home should have a fever thermometer available at all times.

The essential difference between an ordinary thermometer and one designed for determining body temperature is the self-registering feature of the fever thermometer. When the mercury column has risen to the maximum temperature, it remains until shaken back into the reservoir at the bottom of the instrument. This is due to a constriction which acts as a tiny check valve in the thermometer bore, just above the bulb, and permits passage of the mercury on expansion but does not permit return on contraction.

Clinical or Fever Thermometers—Three bulb types of fever thermometers are available: (1) the *oral type*, characterized by the slender mercury reservoir, most senstive for mouth use; (2) the *rectal*, with a blunt, strong, pear-shaped bulb for safety and to insure

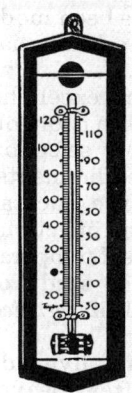

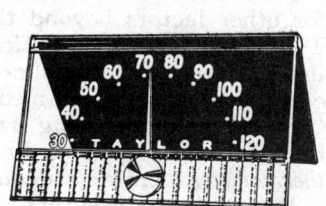

Fig. 848. **Household thermometers** (courtesy, Taylor).

retention in the rectum; and (3) a small, sturdy "universal," "security," "snub," or "stubby" type with a short stubby bulb, for oral or rectal use, and safer for babies or irrational patients. See Fig. 849.

All fever thermometers have a magnifying lens front which renders the mercury column visible against an opaque background. Some have a colored line which by reflection helps detect the mercury column, or guide lines which center the eye on the image of the column. Others are flat in shape so that the markings are on the same plane as the mercury when the thermometer is held in normal reading position.

Taking Body Temperature—Fever thermometers should always be sterilized and shaken down below 97° before taking a reading. For *oral* temperatures, the thermometer should be placed in the mouth with the bulb under the rear edge of the tongue and rotated once or twice to assure complete contact. Transfer of body heat to the thermometer is speeded by then shifting the bulb to the opposite rear edge of the tongue. The lips should be kept closed and the thermometer left in the mouth for at least three minutes. Regardless of length of initial oral exposure, it is always well after the initial reading to return the thermometer to the patient's mouth for another minute, to provide a check or verification of the original temperature reading. Oral temperatures should not be taken for thirty minutes

after exercising, smoking, eating, or taking hot or cold drinks.

Rectal temperature should be taken only with a rectal or stubby bulb thermometer. The bulb should be lubricated and gently inserted deeply enough to pass the constricting muscle, leaving about half the thermometer exposed. Babies should be held firmly face down, their buttocks separated with one hand and the thermometer held in place with the other. The thermometer should be left in place at least four minutes.

A longer time may be necessary for temperature readings if the thermometer is cold or if the patient is anemic or aged, with poor blood circulation. Axillary (under-arm) temperature is not recommended except when all other methods are impossible.

Normal Temperatures—The average normal mouth temperature is 98.6°F but some variations are natural. Healthy persons may have temperatures as much as 1°F above or below the average normal temperature. One's temperature may range from about 97.3°F at 2 to 5 a.m. to about 98°F in the morning and to about 99°F in the late afternoon. One should determine his normal temperature by a series of readings while in good health for comparison as a personal standard when one is ill.

Fig. 849. **Diagram of thermometer construction.**

Normal rectal temperatures are usually 1°F higher, or 99.6°, though the "normal" mark on all types of fever thermometers, including the rectal type, is at 98.6°, because this marking is apparently preferred by the medical profession.

The normal body temperatures of other animals, frequently of importance in veterinary medicine, average as follows: fowl, 107.6°F; monkey, 99.2°F; horse, 100.4°F; rabbit, 100.8° to 102.0°F; guinea pig, 101.3° to 103.1°F; and dog, 103.1°F. Special heavier and longer thermometers, some with ring tops, are available for veterinary use. Regular fever thermometers with rectal or stubby bulbs may be used and are quite suitable for small animals.

Basal Temperature Graph—A woman who wishes to become pregnant may increase her chances of conception greatly by having intercourse at the time of ovulation, or she may decrease the chance of conception by avoiding intercourse then. And one may use her knowledge of the fertile interval for avoidance of conception for some time by natural means, then use it for a planned pregnancy (*natural child spacing*).

Basal temperature graphs are helpful in determining whether and when ovulation occurs. Ovulation, the release of an egg (ovum) from the ovary, ordinarily happens only once in each menstrual cycle. Conception can take place only if intercourse takes place at or near this time, during the interval of transition between low and high temperature levels.

The basal temperature graph* reflects slight body changes taking place during the menstrual cycle. The "basal" *resting* temperature in the first part of the cycle is usually well below normal; in the last 2 weeks or so of the cycle the basal temperature is closer to 98.6. Most important, *the shift from the lower to the higher temperature level occurs about the time of ovulation.* See Fig. 850.

The variations in the temperature before and after ovulation are slight, often only a few tenths to a half degree, so it is important that the temperature be taken carefully and recorded accurately. Special thermometers are available for this purpose; they are manufactured by Becton-Dickinson and by Zeal, Ltd. They record temperatures within the usual range of cyclic variation (from 96° to 100° only) and are graduated in tenths of a degree and are easier to read than the ordinary fever thermometers, although the latter may be used.

References to the medical literature on this subject are available.[13-16]

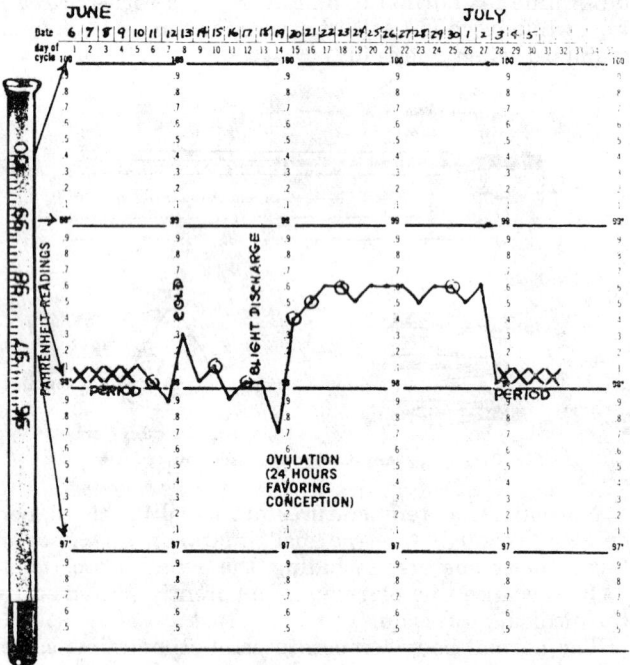

Fig. 850. Basal temperature graph for determination of ovulation period in the female.

Temperature Comparisons—In the United States, Canada, and most of the United Kingdom, the Fahrenheit scale is employed. However, many hospitals and physicians as well as foreign-born laymen prefer the Centigrade scale and Centigrade thermometers are available from US manufacturers. The normal mark on a Centigrade thermometer is at 37°C. A comparison of temperatures on the two scales appears in the table below.

Throughout Latin America and the rest of the non-English-speaking world, the Centigrade scale clinical thermometer is used.

Accuracy—The critical factors in obtaining maximum accuracy are: the thermometer must be properly designed, it must be sufficiently accurate to meet each specific requirement, and it must be properly used.

* Charts for plotting the daily temperatures are available from Schering, Becton-Dickinson, and elsewhere.

Temperature Comparison

Fahrenheit	Centigrade
96.0°	35.55°
97.0	36.11
97.5	36.38
98.0	36.65
98.6	37.0
99.0	37.22
99.5	37.50
100.0	37.77
101.0	38.33
102.0	38.88
103.0	39.44
104.0	40.0

In general, the accuracy of fever thermometers is established by either federal standards, issued by the US Department of Commerce and developed by the trade under the procedure of the Commodity Standards Division, or by states, local authorities, and sometimes private institutions, usually operating for hospital groups. The national standard is known as CS1-52 (Commercial Standard No. 1, 1952 revision).[17] Special "state seal" standard requirements for thermometers are required in Connecticut, Massachusetts, and Michigan for thermometers sold in these states. Since issuance of CS1-52, state requirements have been modified to be in close conformity with the commercial standard.

Thermometers are offered for sale which excel the standards, and usually bear specific information on the certificate indicating special accuracy or selection for other factors beyond the minimum requirements. They are valuable for critical temperature use, such as in diagnosis of certain pulmonary diseases and infectious cases, both surgical and medical, also for basal temperature studies, now being used widely in the study of human fertility. For ordinary use the CS1-52 *certified thermometer* is entirely adequate.

It must be realized that even the most carefully made thermometer is subject to normal hazards after it leaves the factory. It may be overheated or dropped, and while not externally damaged the contraction inside may have been shattered. A minute break in the constricted area may block the capillary tube or the contraction to develop a "hard shaker" or produce a "retreater."

Few actual hard-shaking or retreating thermometers escape from the rigid inspection guards of reputable manufacturers. The retreaters are more serious because they may endanger human life. Such dangerous thermometers are destroyed by reliable manufacturers when detected and should be disposed of immediately if the condition develops in use.

All well-made fever thermometers are "aged" before certification to remove most of the strains in the glass which would cause later shrinkage and errors in readings. This is done by laying the unfinished thermometers away for several months or by an accelerated heat-treating method which removes stress in the whole instrument, and anneals the contraction as well as the bulb.

Reading the Thermometer—Next to accuracy, the most important feature of a fever thermometer is its ease of reading. This is especially true for the inexperienced home user, who will appreciate being shown thermometers with easy-reading features, as offered by many manufacturers. Always demonstrate how to hold the thermometer for reading, which should be done with the back to good light and the instrument held horizontally in the right hand, about 12 inches from the eyes. The bulb should never be held while reading, but the thermometer may be steadied by the left hand index finger placed behind it. With the markings to the front, the thermometer should be rotated slowly until the mercury is visible.

To enable the user to read a clinical thermometer more easily the Bard *Magna Therma* oral or rectal thermometer is supplied with a special case which lights up and magnifies the numerals when the thermometer is inserted in the case (Fig. 851).[18]

Care of the Thermometer—After the thermometer has been read and the temperature recorded, it should always be shaken down so that it is ready for use the next time it is needed. In shaking down the mercury column, the thermometer should be grasped firmly between the thumb and the forefinger at the scale end and shaken vigorously by several snaps of the wrist until the reading is below 97°. This is effective and a good way to describe this method is to liken it to shaking water off the bulb, which the customer can visualize. The thermometer should *never* be held in the fingers while the hand is struck upon a solid surface to jar down the mercury column. Such rough handling is almost certain to cause breakage or a rupture of the constriction, even though it may appear unbroken. If dropped, even though apparently unbroken, the thermometer should be tested before using. Fever thermometers should never be exposed to heat, to the sun's rays, or to a heat unit, or be displayed in a shop window.

Disinfection of Thermometers—After using, and before re-use, thermometers should be carefully cleansed to avoid the possibility of carrying infection from one patient to another. They must never be washed in hot water. Sommermeyer and Carroll,[19] who studied the disinfection of oral thermometers, recommend the following procedure:

1. Wipe the contaminated oral thermometer with a cotton ball moistened with a solution of equal parts of 95% ethyl alcohol and tincture of green soap.
2. Rinse the soap from the thermometer with cold running water.
3. Place the thermometer in a solution containing 0.5 to 1% iodine in either 70% ethyl alcohol or 70% isopropyl alcohol. (Other authorities suggest that phenol, 1:1000 mercury oxycyanide or 1:1000 mercuric chloride solutions can also be employed. Strong alkaline

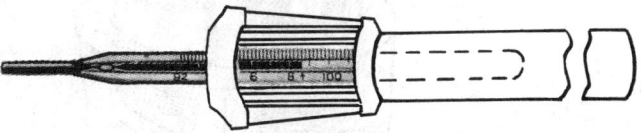

Fig. 851. Bard *Magna Therma* clinical thermometer with special magnifying lens and battery-powered illumination for easier reading.

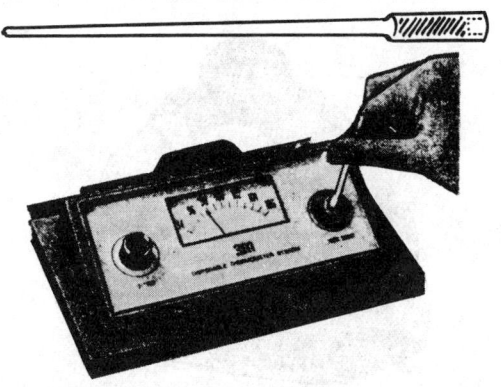

Fig. 852. 3-M brand clinical thermometer system with economical, disposable wax probes and battery-powered portable sensing unit.

disinfecting solutions should be avoided.) Before re-use, rinse in cold water.

Thermometers should never be placed on a hard surface but are preferably stored at the bedside, placed upright and resting on a pad of absorbent cotton in a sterilizer jar or in a tumbler. It is highly desirable to clean them immediately after use and, if possible, restore them to their cases. A thermometer which has not been thoroughly cleansed should never be used.*

Special Types of Thermometers—A number of special types of fever thermometers are available, including one intended for dermatologic use and having a special, flat-bladed, thin-glass, mercury reservoir for contact with the skin surface.† Veterinary and basal-temperature thermometers are mentioned above. Other types have been developed for special uses, including remote-reading dial and recording instruments for continuous records. Thermocouples are employed extensively in some biological testing (see Fig. 421, page 645).

A disposable, economical thermometer system has been developed for taking and reading human temperatures, replacing routine use of conventional glass thermometers. The *3M brand Disposable Thermometer* consists of a supply of presterilized, single-use probes and a portable sensing unit (Fig. 852).

The large end of the probe corresponds to the bulb end of a glass thermometer. It contains an inert, tasteless wax which assumes and holds the patient's temperature until the reading is taken by insertion in the probe socket on the unit.

First depress and turn the test knob to 105°F to assure calibration accuracy. Then insert the probe in the socket, where the sensor pierces the probe, "measures" the temperature and records the temperature on the meter.

Because these probes are made of plastic and can be used only once, they are free from accidental breakage and offer maximum protection from possible cross-infection.

The most common case for fever thermometers is of plastic, similar to a fountain pen, with or without clip. An inner spring is usually provided so that the thermometer will not fall out easily. Special cases holding a pair of thermometers, one oral and one rectal, are available; also cases which permit the storage of an antiseptic solution in which the thermometer is immersed. Some cases are designed to help shake down the thermometers easily, an aid to the aged or inexperienced user. Hospitals usually employ centrifugal devices which hold a quantity of thermometers and whirl the mercury down.

A thermometer, designed to make quantitative temperature measurements directly from the surface of the skin, has been developed at the University of Colorado, Craig Rehabilitation Hospital.

The instrument is accurate to within one-tenth of a degree when measuring the difference in heat generated by an arthritic joint and that generated by a healthy tissue.

Its probe is about 6 in. long and about ⅝ in. in diameter. Its hollow aluminum barrel holds a spring mechanism—like a ballpoint pen—that permits the

---

* Literature for distribution to the public on clinical thermometers is available as follows: *Facts on Fever* (Kessling); *Facts about Fever, There's a Big Difference in Clinical Thermometers, What is Your Normal Temperature, When You Are Ill, Fever Thermometers*, and *Some Helpful Questions and Answers* (Becton-Dickinson); *Fever, What It Means, What To Do About It* (Taylor).

† Becton-Dickinson, Faichney, Kessling, and Taylor are some of the major manufacturers of thermometers in the US.

user to exert uniform pressure when measuring skin temperature.

Inhalers, Atomizers, and Insufflators

Atomizers are instruments used to reduce liquid medication to fine particles in the form of a spray or aerosol. They are most frequently employed in the treatment of diseases of the respiratory tract.

The modern atomizer is an outgrowth of an apparatus developed in Berlin, Germany, in the year 1860 by a Dr. Bergson. In that instrument a current of vapor, produced by the action of heat from a flame on water in an enclosed vessel, drew up medicament from a reservoir by suction. The jet carried the vaporized medicament to the funnel-shaped apparatus and then to the nostril or mouth. This apparatus embodied the basic principles of an inhaler and an atomizer.

Inhalers—Few remedial agents have as soothing an effect in acute inflammations of the nasal and bronchial tract as do warmth and moisture. To obtain the therapeutic value of moist heat in the treatment of acute diseases of larynx, trachea, or bronchi, steam inhalers are used.

In Bergson's original atomizer, the method of force and suction was steam pressure. The patient received the medication plus heat and water vapor. Steam atomizers are still used for laryngitis in some cases, but they are cumbersome and have been largely superseded by more efficient forms.

The original inhaler, employed long before Bergson's time, was merely a tin can with a stovepipe arrangement. The can is half filled with water, and heated. Steam eventually is emitted from the spout. A medicament is then added through a small hole in the cover or lid and the latter closed and portions of the drug are carried over with the steam, with or without vaporization. An adaptation of this is the *Myrick inhaler* (Fig. 853).

Naturally enough, the spout must be sufficiently long to allow the vapor to cool somewhat before coming into contact with the nasal membranes. The pharmacist must always be sure to caution the patient regarding this, to avoid scalding.

The common *benzoin inhaler* is one well-known type. This apparatus has the disadvantage that it has no heating unit and is not readily portable. Its advantage lies in its inexpensive construction. Nearly equally valuable results can be obtained from a folded towel and a basin of steaming water.

Croup Kettles—A modification of the inhaler is the croup kettle. "Croup" is any laryngitis severe enough to cause difficulty in breathing, and is especially common in children.

In the croup kettle the water in the kettle is caused to boil and kept boiling by an alcohol lamp underneath. After adding medication through a funnel, the patient inhales the vapor from a long spout. The advantages of this apparatus lie in its own heat-unit enabling its use for longer periods of time, and its greater capacity.

Steam Vaporizers—The modern steam inhaler is essentially the same as the croup kettle except that it uses electricity to generate heat and steam. The advantage of this more modern adaptation lies in the attainment of a constant temperature. Also most forms of this apparatus are equipped with a regulator so that when they run dry, the heating unit shuts off simultaneously. These are also easier to handle in the home, especially at night.

Many mothers are confused about the differences between the vaporizer and the humidifier.

The familiar vaporizer provides the conventional, hot-steam therapy for the relief of upper respiratory illnesses. Physicians recommend it for colds, sinusitis, and similar ailments.

The portable room humidifier, on the other hand, provides a cool mist to compensate for the lack of sufficient moisture in the air in dry, steam-heated rooms.

Some vaporizers are used solely for their warm, moist spray while others are provided with a chamber or cup in which a volatile medication can be placed in liquid form or on cotton. The steam passes over this material, as in Bergson's original vaporizer, causing the medication to volatilize and pass out of the spray.

Steam inhalers do not deliver a spray and can carry medication in their vapors only when such medication is volatile at the temperature of boiling water. In Bergson's original atomizer the medication was carried

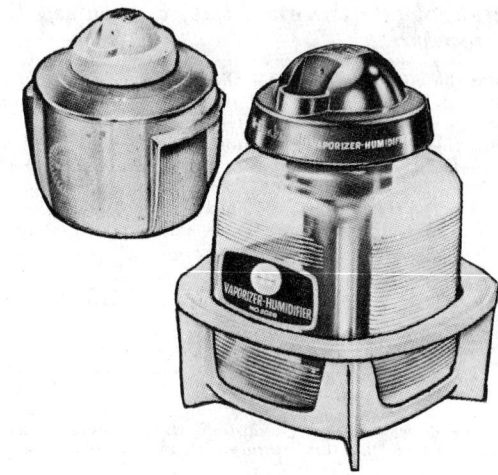

Fig. 854. Combination Hankscraft vaporizer–humidifier units.

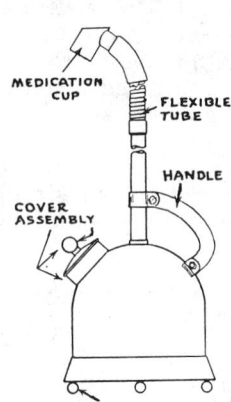

Fig. 853. "Myrick" inhaler (Rochester Products).

MEDICATION CUP

FLEXIBLE TUBE

HANDLE

COVER ASSEMBLY

FEET

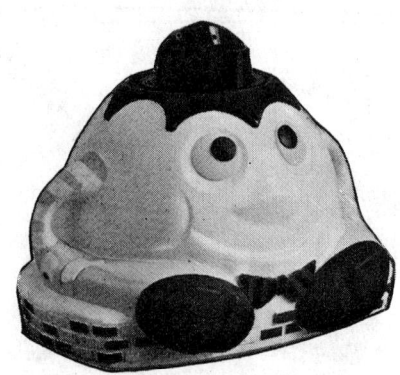

Fig. 855. *Steemy*, a vaporizer designed especially for children (courtesy, Prak-T-Kal).

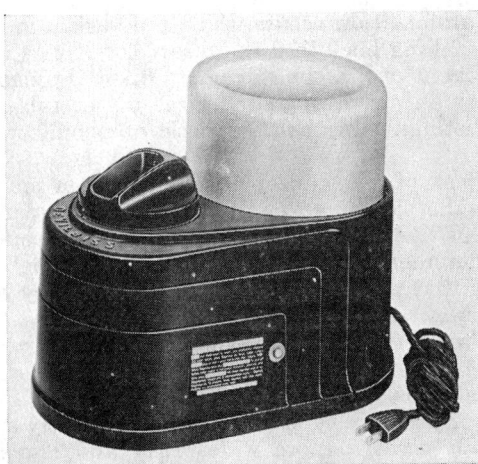

Fig. 856. DeVilbiss vaporizer.

into the spray by the atomizing principle and a large variety of drugs could be applied. However, steam vaporizers are valuable for ordinary home treatment of colds, coughs, and other respiratory diseases (Fig. 856).

In the electrode-type vaporizer, two electrodes are separated from contact by an insulating nonconductor. When mineral-containing water is added to the reservoir, an electric current passes between the electrodes and heats the water to boiling. The mineral content is necessary to permit the passage of electricity. The content of minerals should be kept to a

minimum, however, as an excess of dissolved material will cause foaming, frothing, and spilling over. Distilled water, to which a small quantity of salt has been added, is preferable. Hard water is usually not satisfactory. Electrode-type vaporizers should be cleaned periodically.

In heater-type vaporizers, an ordinary heating element connected to 115 volt, 50 cycle, ac electric current is immersed in a reservoir of water. Most heater type vaporizers now have thermostatic controls. A cup or chamber is provided for volatile medication. Any kind of water is satisfactory and the reservoir can be replenished at will. The value of this type of vaporizer rests almost entirely with its warmth and moist spray. See Fig. 858.

Vaporizers are used extensively in the home today to humidify bedrooms or chambers where patients suffering from various bronchial conditions may rest. Cool-vapor humidifiers provide effective high-humidity inhalation therapy for respiratory patients, and can be used as well to restore proper humidity to rooms dried out by winter heating. They are of breakproof metal or plastic, in modern colorful designs. Prominent among such humidifiers is the versatile heat, moisture and medication vaporizer, *Croupaire* (produced by Air-Shields), and those supplied by Hankscraft.

Types of electrode and heater vaporizers are shown in Figs. 856–859.

Atomizers—The basic principle of Bergson's first atomizer was that a current of air or vapor passing over an open tube creates suction in that tube toward the orifice. If the other end of the tube is immersed in a liquid, it is drawn up and when in contact with the air current is turned into a spray.

The larger the air orifice, the larger will be the volume of finely dispersed droplets. The larger the fluid opening, the larger the volume of fluid delivered and the coarser the spray. Likewise a narrower and shorter tube for the fluid means a faster flow.

In 1865 Dr. Clark of London improved upon the original cumbersome model by substituting a compressible rubber bladder or "bulb" for the elaborate steam jet engine. This was the precursor of the atomizer of today. The compressed bulb satisfactorily produced a

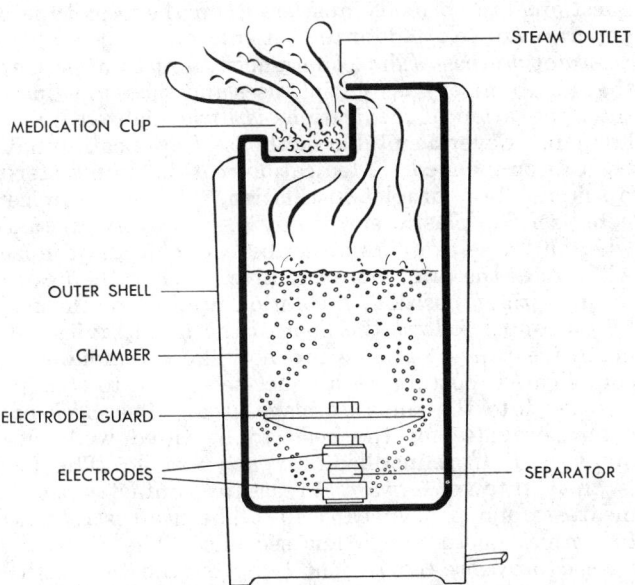

Fig. 857. Electrode-type vaporizer.[20]

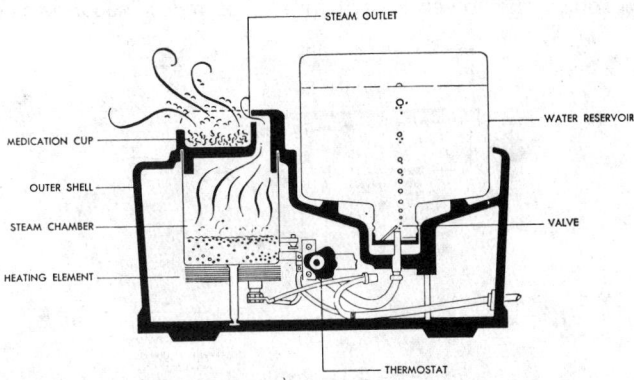

Fig. 858. Heater-type vaporizer.[20]

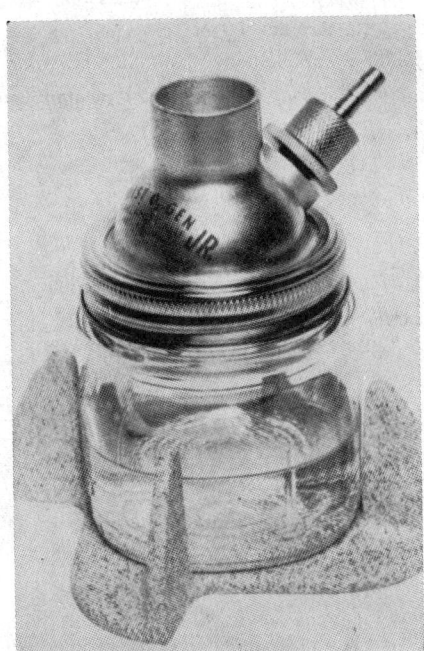

Fig. 859. "Mistogen" Junior nebulizer (Mist-O₂-Gen).

current of air but it lost the soothing value of the warmth.

Types of Atomizers—There are two basic types of atomizers as follows:

The *vacuum type* operates on the basic principles of atomization, depending upon suction at the tip of the atomizer to cause the formation of a fine spray. These apparati are intermittent in action. They employ either oils or aqueous solutions and are characterized by their larger opening and emission of more fluid.

The *pressure type* of atomizer is one which employs a greater volume of air and smaller fluid resulting in a more finely divided spray. It backs up the suction phase of the atomization by allowing some of the air to be pumped into the container of fluid, providing additional pressure on the surface of the liquid. These forms of apparatus are usually employed for oleaginous fluids and are continuous in flow.

The vacuum and pressure type atomizers employ the principle of Bernoulli's theorem. This postulates that, in an area of increased air velocity, there will also exist an area of decreased pressure. The diminished pressure allows the liquid to be forced into a smaller diameter tube due to the greater pressure on its surface. This liquid is then forced into contact with the air stream which, in turn, causes dispersion of the liquid into minute suspended drops. The efficiency of an atomizer depends on the smallness of the size of particles. The more uniform the diameter of drops the more effective is the medication. The features of the two types of atomizers are shown schematically in Fig. 860.

Nebulizer—The *nebulizer* acts on a slightly more complex principle than the atomizer. Within the container of the apparatus is built a small atomizing unit,

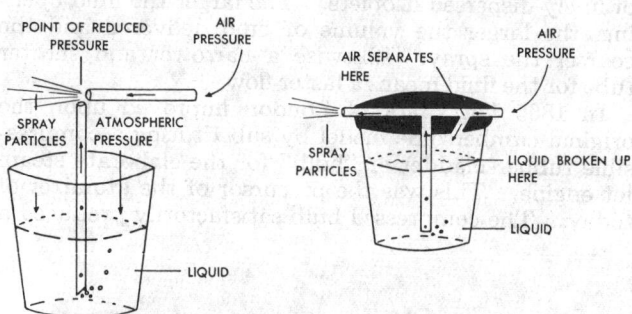

Fig. 860. Vacuum- and pressure-type atomizers.[20]

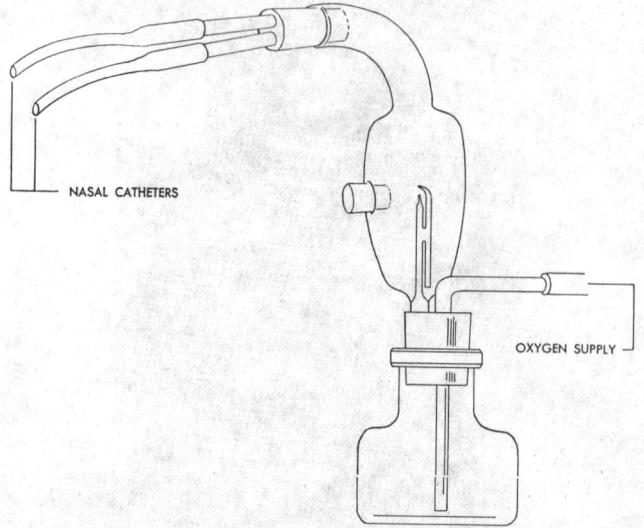

Fig. 861. Nebulizer with twin top outlet.[20]

so that atomization occurs inside the flask, the heavier droplets falling back into the reservoir. Since there is some current of air, the extremely finely divided cloud floats out on air through the large outlet tube. This is the distinguishing characteristic of nebulizers. See Fig. 861.

The flask of a nebulizer always carries a mark part way up the side. Never fill the container with fluid above this line, for atomization will fail to occur if the unit is submerged. Many persons return nebulizers, claiming that they do not work properly, solely because of this error.

Use and Application—The terms atomizers and nebulizers are not interchangeable, and the therapeutic purposes of the two designs are not the same. The continuous or pressure type of atomizer is slightly superior because it gives a more widespread and less intense medication, and a finer subdivision which carries it easily into the deeper cavities of the nose and throat.

The nebulizer is not as useful as the atomizer for applying medication to nose and pharynx. Yet, because it is very finely subdivided, the medication can be inspired and carried into the deeper parts of the respiratory tract, even as far as the bronchi. The nebulizer is especially valuable for diseases of the larynx and trachea.

Purchasing Atomizers—The pharmacist's first question of a prospective purchaser of an atomizer is "What is to be its use?" Is an *oil* or *water* solution to be employed? What portion of mucous membrane and respiratory tract is to be reached? Only when these questions are correctly answered can the best type of apparatus be selected for the patient.

Effectiveness—The pharmacist must appreciate that an atomizer has multiple uses and that its value in the application of medications is little realized by the layman. Several suitable methods of application have been recommended. Medication may be administered by liquid flow, droplet instillation, tampon, atomizer, nebulizer, or plastic spray bottle. In every instance where a "nose drop" is prescribed or sold, an atomizer will render the drug more effective. When the head is in an upright position, a solution applied to the nose by a dropper follows the floor of the nasal cavity. In home treatment patients are not likely to follow the complicated posture technique necessary to get the solution into the sinus drainage area. The *Beck procedure* provides for the head to be tilted well back, and several drops instilled into each nostril. The head is then thrown forward to assure contact with the meatuses and pharyngeal wall. The head is returned to normal posture in a few seconds. The *Parkinson method* provides the patient lying on the side with a pillow under the lower shoulder so that the head is bent downward and sidewise. The drops are instilled through the lower nostril and after a few seconds the

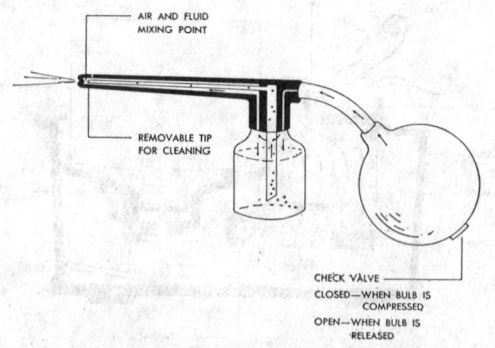

Fig. 862. Simple outlet atomizer.[20]

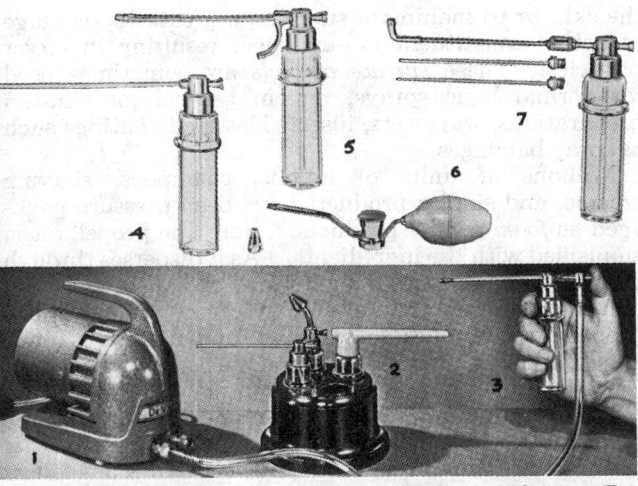

Fig. 863. Physician's set for nasal–oral–respiratory therapy (De-Vilbiss); useful for clinics. (1) Portable 115 volt AC 60 cycle air compressor; (2) bottle rack; (3) cut off with tubing; (4) aqueous atomizer; (5) adjustable tip atomizer; (6) atomizer head with bulb; (7) aqueous or oil atomizer with nose guard, three interchangeable tubes. A number of other units, powder blowers, syringes, and irrigators are also available.

position is reversed. The flow of dropped solutions also tends to carry an infection from comparatively superficial regions to deeper areas. A solution sprayed into the nose reaches all the walls of the nasal passages including the sinus drainage area. In home treatment, the patient may hold his head in a natural upright position.

When a solution is gargled, it reaches only a small area of the throat because the soft palate necessarily closes tightly against the tongue, preventing the solution from reaching deep-seated areas affected. A sprayed solution in the throat passes the soft palate since it is quite possible to inhale while spraying, and allows the sprayed solution to reach all affected throat regions.

Pharmacists who dispense considerable quantities of "nose drops" will find that an inexpensive, convenient, and compact atomizer or plastic spray bottle may be provided free or sold at each occasion.

Instructions—Nasal guards, either smooth or vented, are placed over the tip of the atomizer to protect delicate membranes and to limit back flow. Grooved surfaces prevent any undesirable excess of air pressure in the cavities. To clean, place a finger over the spray tip tightly and compress the bulb to force out any sediment lodged in the tubes. Cleaning wires are employed if the foregoing does not remove the foreign material. To sterilize, pass the spray tube through a flame or boil the metal parts.

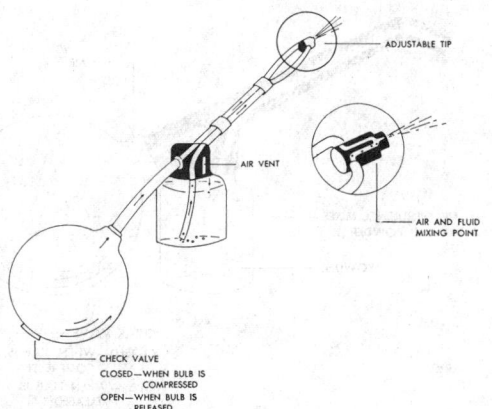

ADJUSTABLE TIP

AIR VENT

AIR AND FLUID MIXING POINT

CHECK VALVE
CLOSED—WHEN BULB IS COMPRESSED
OPEN—WHEN BULB IS RELEASED

Fig. 864. Vacuum-type atomizer.[20]

Variations in Atomizers—Many types of atomizers are supplied. Some use single outlet tubes, particularly for solutions which tend to crystallize. Others have twin tubes and a spray atomizing tip. Hard rubber atomizers are available for use where solutions employed will attack metal or deteriorate in its presence as is true of many modern antiseptics or sulfonamide solutions. Some atomizers have an unusually small reservoir, where the total volume of the medication is small. These are especially adaptable to such items as hormone solutions where concentration or cost and potency may be factors. Leakproof attachments are also available for travelers.

Physicians' and surgeons' atomizers represent refinements desired for specific purposes. Some employ ordinary compression bulbs while others use a motor-driven air pump under controlled pressure (Fig. 863).

Cautions—Pharmacists should caution the patient to refrain from using any caustic medication in nasal or throat passages. Any solution which is intended for atomization, should first be warmed to body temperature, to facilitate action and to avoid chills.

Wax Sprayers—For liquefying and spraying paraffin and wax-like preparations, a wax sprayer or *theromer* is employed. It is only occasionally used today in the treatment of burns, giving relief by application of a coating. To operate the spray the wax must be melted.

Ether Dispensers—Sprays for minor operations, as ether dispensers, or for removal of adhesive tape, are also supplied.

Perfume Atomizers—The principle of atomization for medicinals is employed as well for perfumes, and elaborate and fancifully designed apparatus are available. Many purse-sized containers of perfume are now provided with atomizer stoppers of relatively inexpensive construction.

Plastic Bottle Atomizers—Several firms are now offering solutions, intended for the treatment of the nasal passages, in plastic containers or accompanied with plastic atomizers. These bottle-like containers are flexible and when pressed produce an atomized spray or, when inverted and pressed, force out the solution in drops. Where a very potent drug is to be employed infrequently, with a single inhalation generally affording control of an acute attack, as in bronchial asthma, emphysema, or bronchitis, a modified form of aerosol device may be employed. Typical of these are the *Mistometer* (Winthrop) or *Medihalor* (Riker). The *Mistometer* and *Medihalor* are similar in construction and the former is shown as assembled for use (Fig. 865).

Aerosol Therapy—Although atomizers, nebulizers, vaporizers, and inhalers have been employed for many years, the most recent development in dispersed medication, aerosol mists, or sprays from pressure packed containers, has been rapidly accepted as a most effective means of administering medication as well as dispersing many common products such as insecticides, lotions, and deodorants.

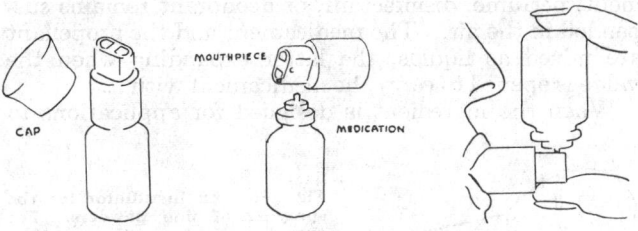

CAP

MOUTHPIECE

MEDICATION

Fig. 865. "Mistometer" type of inhaler, used by Isuprel (courtesy, Winthrop).

The use of aerosol therapy and a nebulizer in the treatment of asthma and with asthma preparations has become increasingly important of late. A special form of all-glass atomizer is available for nebulizing certain drug solutions, whereby the liquid is reduced to submicroscopic particles, 0.5 to 2 microns in diameter, which are inhaled through the mouth or nostrils and drawn deeply into all of the nasal cavities and pharynx.

This type of apparatus is supplied by several pharmaceutical laboratories. A pocket nebulizer is available for use in aerosol therapy. It is a small pocket-size version of the standard nebulizer with equal performance. It meets the need for an easily portable unit when it is necessary to have a nebulizer available at all times.

The term *aerosol* has come into use to indicate a nebulized solution made up of very fine particles carried by means of a propellant gas or liquid under pressure. The objective originally, in vaporizers, was to obtain sprays which would penetrate into the alveoli of the lungs. To accomplish this to the optimum extent the liquid had to be dispersed as droplets with a diameter of 5 microns or less. Aerosols may contain a surface-active agent to aid in the subdivision of the liquid.

Aerosols in the form of pressure packaging are also not new. Certain gases and volatile solvents have been used as propellants for other materials in the past. The recent popularity of pressure packaging, however, is due to the ease or convenience of application, uniformity and speed of application, elimination of manual contact, avoidance of contamination, elimination of air in the preparation, and formation of a light mist where desired for inhalation.

Pressure packaging requires a product or medicament in liquid, semiliquid, or powder form, a compressed liquefied or dissolved gas as a propellant, a pressure resistant container, and an appropriate dispensing valve. The propellant and the medicament are contained in the package. When the valve is opened the gas expands and escapes, carrying the medicament with it in the form of fine particles.

Widely used as propellants are the fluorinated hydrocarbons. These are harmless, stable, nonirritating to the skin, odorless, and stainless. Du Pont markets several propellants of this type under the trade name "Freon." They vary slightly in chemical formulation. There are others available from other sources such as Allied, Pennwalt, Stauffer, Union Carbide, and Thiokol.

Carbon dioxide, nitrogen, and nitrous oxide have been used. Certain gases which are flammable are used in industrial aerosols but not with medicaments. Typical of these are dimethyl ether and butane. Because of their contained pressure, unexpended aerosol packages should not be heated, incinerated, or punctured.

Aerosols by type are classified as "space," "surface," "foam," and "powder."

Space aerosols release a mist in which the medicament, perfume, disinfectant, or deodorant remains suspended in the air. The medicament and the propellant are mixed as liquids, the latter expanding when the valve is opened to carry the medicament with it.

When the ingredient is designed for applications to the skin or to inanimate surfaces, a greater percentage of active constituent is employed, resulting in larger particles. These *surface aerosols* are sometimes used for dermatologic sprays, but in general for sun-tan preparations, wave-sets, insecticides, and coatings such as spray bandages.

Millions of units of lotions, shampoos, shaving creams, and similar products have been pressure packaged as *foam aerosol* products. Here, the propellant is emulsified with the ingredients. As it disperses through the valve it produces a light foam or ball of suds-like material which can be employed as desired. The propellant continues to vaporize, and maintains pressure until exhausted. Here, as little as 10% propellent is employed.

Where powders are pressure packaged, they are suspended in liquefied propellant. Release of the material in a *powder aerosol* through the valve must follow shaking to insure adequate dispersion and suspension of granules.

Aerosol pressure packaging has been successfully adapted to burn treatment, to topical antiseptics and to dermatologic preparations. Antibiotic products, vasodilators, steroids, and bronchodilators are also widely prescribed and accepted in this form by physician and patient. It is likely that the surface application or inhalation of many different medications in the future will be facilitated by the use of aerosol packaging. See also Chapter 90, *Aerosols*.

Insufflators—Apparatus for the production of a finely divided cloud of a dry powder are called insufflators. The older type, in limited use today, operate with a bulb and a nozzle, the powder being placed in the bulb or on a trough in the nozzle and when the bulb is compressed the current of air divides the powder into a fine cloud (see Fig. 866).

Finely powdered drugs are also occasionally administered by the oral or nasal route, by inhalation. Special insufflators are provided into which a cartridge of the sterile drug is inserted and then opened or, in some cases, each dose is aseptically sealed in an insufflator-like container which is discarded after use. The seal is broken, the apparatus applied to the mouth or nose and deep breaths taken. The incoming air causes a loose inside section to sharply tap the drug cartridge, releasing a small amount of the powder which is then immediately drawn into the respiratory tract with the incoming air. The Abbott insufflator of this type is known as an *Aerohalor*. For a period of time, insufflators were widely used for penicillin therapy. Although the *Aerohalor* was used for this purpose it is now generally employed for administration of *Norisodrine*, an antiasthmatic preparation.

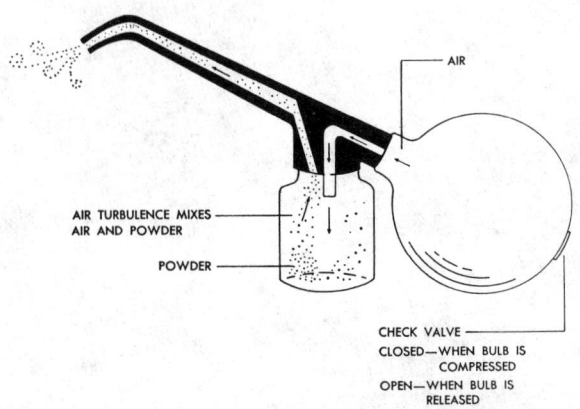

Fig. 867.   **Principle of the powder insufflator.**

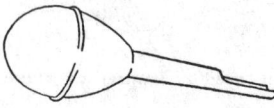

Fig. 866.   **An insufflator for the spraying of fine powders.   For throat, vaginal, or other medication.**

A streamlined insufflator is also available with a bottle for the powder being used. This new design makes the powder insufflator a versatile instrument because powder can now be easily applied to ear, nose, throat, body surfaces, and tooth sockets.

Hypodermic Equipment

Syringes are instruments intended for the injection of water or other liquids into the body or its cavities. They are classified according to differences in principle of action into three categories: (1) *plunger syringes*, such as the hypodermic syringes; (2) *bulb syringes*, of which the ear and ulcer syringes are a type; and (3) *gravity syringes*, characterized by the fountain syringes.

On the basis of capacity, syringes may also be classified into three groups: (1) *small*, those of 10 ml or less capacity, such as the hypodermic type; (2) *medium*, those from 10 ml to 100 ml in volume, of which the ear and ulcer syringes are examples (although some special hypodermic syringes are available in sizes up to 500-ml capacity); and (3) *large*, such as enema or vaginal syringes.

Hypodermic Syringes—These syringes are used to administer medication *subcutaneously* (under the skin) or *intradermally, intravenously* (into a vein or artery), or *intramuscularly* (into the muscle).

Hypodermic syringes are seldom used by the average patient, with the exception of diabetics. Because of their illicit application in the administration of narcotics, in some states it is illegal for hypodermic syringes to be found in the possession of laymen.

Parenteral therapy or injection of medication under the skin and through tissues dates from the beginning of the 19th century. The first crude instrument of this type was a needletrocar, developed to deposit morphine in paste form. The principle of introducing medication under the skin, however, became popular in the first half of the 20th century.

The basic principle of the *hypodermic syringe* uses a combination of a glass barrel through which a carefully fitted glass plunger passes and a needle attachment which pierces the skin. Two developments led to the basic principle of hypodermic medication. At first, glass syringes were merely drawn to a glass needle point, a dangerous device due to breakage. The application by Pravaz in 1853 of a separate needle and a separate syringe led to the later development of the all-glass syringe and metal needle. Screw-joint connections of needle and syringe did not prove satisfactory. These required washers to prevent leakage and their attachment was time-consuming. The familiar friction connection of metal on ground glass was later developed and proved safer, more practical, and provided a secure fastening.

Luer Syringes—The inventor of this type of apparatus, Dr. Luer, patented his syringe; now the letters patent have long since expired but today most of the hypodermic syringes of this style bear his name. The outstanding feature of the Luer syringe was its ground-glass surfaces. In many instances, the inside of the glass barrel and the outside of the glass plunger were ground individually. Later, they have been ground together so that they will provide a perfect fit but prevent back leakage. The plunger must accurately fit and securely close the barrel or cylinder. The latest type of Luer syringe has an unground glass barrel with a fitted ground glass plunger. The clear glass barrel is tougher, stronger, more resistant to breakage, and eliminates the loss from friction or erosion that occurs with the ground-glass barrel. Although Luer syringes are comparatively expensive and easily broken, they have many superior qualities. They are accurate in measuring medication for administration, they can be sterilized readily by boiling the pieces separately, and they may be adapted to many purposes and needs.

Luer syringes are customarily prepared of *resistance* or *Pyrex glass*. The latter is more fragile. Shock-resistant glass can withstand rapid temperature changes from freezing to boiling. Manufacturers customarily place identical matching numbers on each paired plunger and cylinder to insure that the user will properly match or "pair" the parts. It is not always necessary to "pair" the plunger and barrel. Several manufacturers are now making syringes with interchangeable barrels and plungers. The *Multi-Fit* syringes made by Becton-Dickinson and by some other manufacturers under differing brand names, are all ground uniformly and the plungers and barrels of each brand are interchangeable. Most syringes are reinforced at the barrel's shoulders, to withstand shock of the moving plunger, and have flared barrel mouths to facilitate rapid and easy entry of the plunger (Fig. 868).

Plungers may be supplied in blue glass to facilitate scale reading. Some plungers have a black or colored line at their tip to make their passage through the barrel more evident and thus permit easier dosage reading.

Hypodermic syringes are always of the plunger type, characterized by the type of piston and difference of size or capacity. The *tuberculin syringe* is a small syringe not exceeding 1 ml in capacity, and graduated in 0.1- or 0.01-ml divisions. The *hypodermic syringe* is usually of 2-ml to 50-ml capacity. There are larger piston syringes, ranging up to 200 ml, for various purposes such as transfusions and veterinary medicine. Graduations may be in fractions of a ml or in *minims*. Syringes may also be prepared with special graduations, such as *units* of insulin (Fig. 869).

To test the efficiency of a hypodermic syringe, close the tip with a finger and attempt to withdraw the

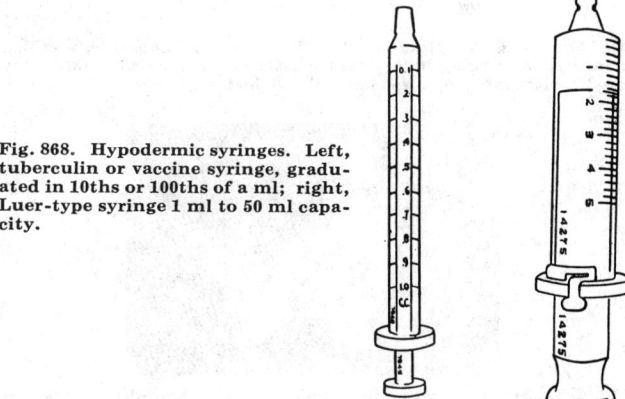

Fig. 868. Hypodermic syringes. Left, tuberculin or vaccine syringe, graduated in 10ths or 100ths of a ml; right, Luer-type syringe 1 ml to 50 ml capacity.

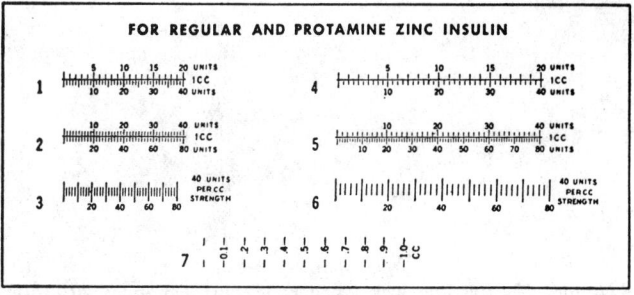

Fig. 869. Relative scale sizes of insulin syringes.

plunger. If the plunger and barrel fit perfectly the vacuum created in the cylinder will prevent withdrawal of the plunger. Do not allow the plunger to return rapidly, due to the vacuum created, or the barrel may be broken.

Nylon Syringes—Hypodermic syringes made of processed nylon are available and said to be unbreakable, leak-proof, autoclavable, and interchangeable.

Disposable Hypodermic Syringes—Various types of disposable hypodermic syringes, each carrying a single dose of sterile medication, are now supplied as a standard dosage container by many pharmaceutical manufacturers. They have become popular for the administration of penicillin, and other antibiotics, antihistamines, tranquilizers, heparin, narcotics, biologicals, and the vitamins.

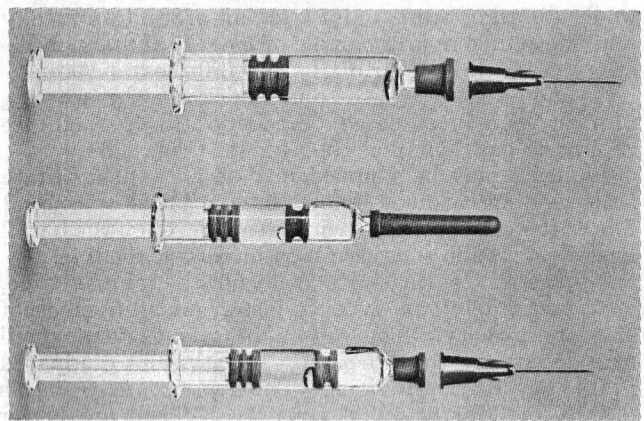

Fig. 870. Commercially available sterile, disposable, ready-to-use hypodermic syringes, in bulk empty (Becton-Dickinson *Hypak* units) or prefilled with medication (Becton-Dickinson *Parentopak* service).

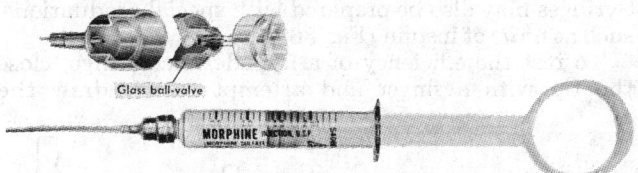

Fig. 871. *Dosette* syringes. Unit dose, sterile, disposable, prefilled, glass hypodermic syringe; with plastic and rubber plunger; steel needle with patented glass ball-valve (courtesy, Intra).

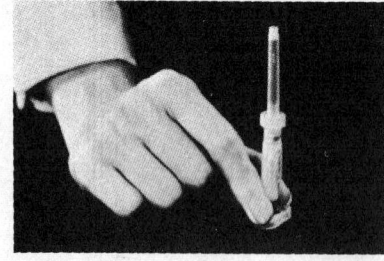

Fig. 872. Sterile, plastic, disposable *Unimatic* (Squibb) syringe with sealed cartridge of medication, and needle.

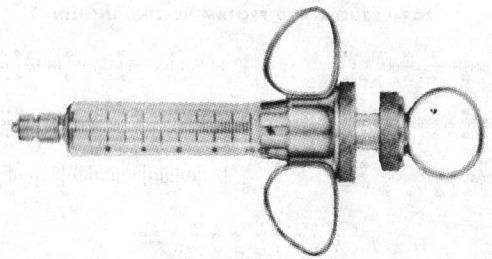

Fig. 873. Multifit luer-lock hypodermic control syringes with interchangeable metal parts, and replaceable glass barrel and plunger.

Syrettes and Ampins—During World War I, a form of disposable injector was developed, called the *Syrette*. These were pure tin collapsible tubes containing medication (usually morphine) with a fixed, covered, sterile hypodermic needle. When in an emergency they were inserted subcutaneously, intramuscularly, or even intravenously, and squeezed, the medication was injected. They were revived in field packs in World War II.

A Spanish development of the early 1940's was the *Ampin*. This was a sterile, glass ampul partially filled with a measured amount of medication in solution (usually narcotic or anesthetic), with an inert gas under pressure filling the remaining space, and a flexible impervious plastic or rubber tube leading to a sterile, covered hypodermic needle. The secret was the fiber plug in the tube. When pointed downward, the needle inserted into the tissue, and the tubing squeezed around the plug, the compressed gas forced the fluid past the plug through the needle into the tissue.

Carpules and Tubex—For a number of years, a form of disposable unit for injection was available to the dental surgeon. Known as *Carpules* these were cylindrical tubes of glass, stoppered at each end with rubber inside closures. A stainless steel case was employed, with a barrel into which the Carpules were fitted. A plunger is forced in at one end of one of the rubber closure, and so forces the other rubber closure on to a double ended hypodermic needle, and the medicament (usually a narcotic or anesthetic solution) passes out through the needle.

A later modification of and improvement on this device is the *Tubex* system of Wyeth. Here the stainless steel barrel is hinged. The disposable sterile glass tube of medicine carrying its own sterile disposable needle with cover is slid into it, and the plunger portion folded back, ready to plunge. See Fig. 874.

Disposable hypodermic syringes empty, without medication, are available from several sources, including Becton-Dickinson Co.; some are plastic, others are glass. Separate disposable needles, packed sterile in envelopes, are also available. See Figs. 875–877.

Disposable products used by physicians in addition to hypodermic syringes and needles, include gauze, gauze dressing and tape, disposable paper towels, drapes, gowns, covers and cups, polyvinyl and pliofilm surgical and examination gloves, and various laboratory

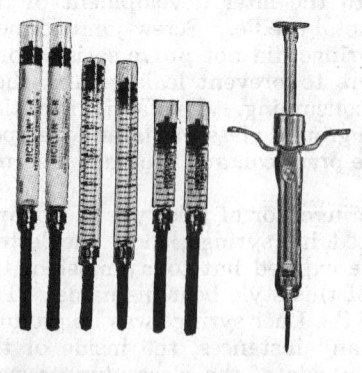

Fig. 874. Tubex (Wyeth) syringe and disposable tube-and-needle units.

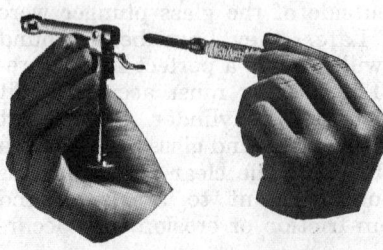

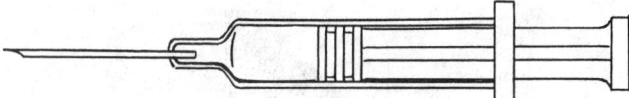

Fig. 875. Disposable glass syringe, Hypak Discardit type (Becton-Dickinson).

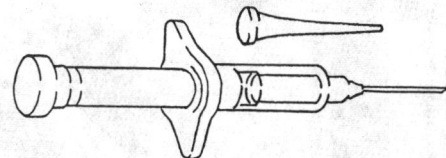

Fig. 876. Single-dosage disposable syringe.

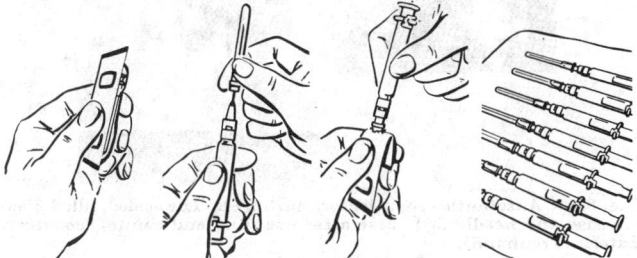

Fig. 877. Sterile disposable needles.

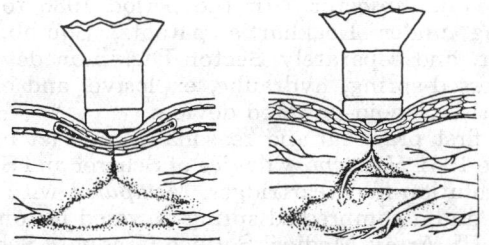

Fig. 878. The pressure of the jet injector on the skin compresses superficial veins so that the medication passes through, leaving no detectable amount in the lumen. By the time the jet has penetrated to the deep veins, it lacks sufficient force to enter them (courtesy, Hypospray).

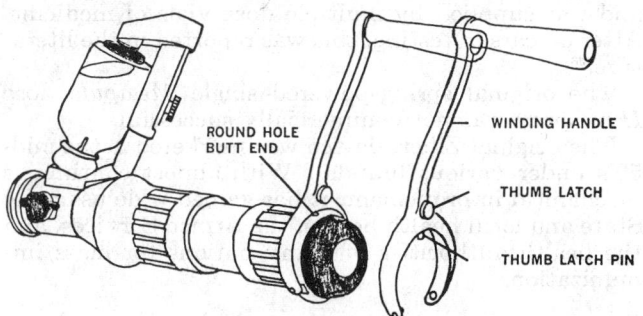

ROUND HOLE
BUTT END

WINDING HANDLE

THUMB LATCH

THUMB LATCH PIN

Fig. 879. *Hypospray* multidose jet injector, adapted from original single-dose unit.

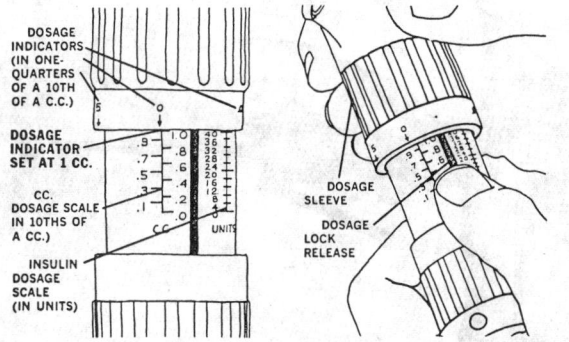

DOSAGE INDICATORS (IN ONE-QUARTERS OF A 10TH OF A C.C.)

DOSAGE INDICATOR SET AT 1 CC.

CC. DOSAGE SCALE IN 10THS OF A CC.)

INSULIN DOSAGE SCALE (IN UNITS)

DOSAGE SLEEVE

DOSAGE LOCK RELEASE

Fig. 880. Dosage indicators and regulators, *Hypospray* multidose jet injector.

devices such as pregnancy and urine tests, blood sample tubes, and lancets. The volume of sales of these items is rapidly increasing. A decade ago, disposables represented only 3% of the market.[21-26] But in 1968 their volume reached 80% of the total purchases of these materials. This represents about $200 million for the year.

The sale of disposable and other surgical supplies can be a major contribution to the success of a community pharmacy if the latter devotes sufficient capital, space and attention to it. In 1968, one supplier estimated that its physician's supply pharmacy distributors had averaged purchases of $15,000 or approximately $23,000 in sales volume.

A physician's supply pharmacy should have at least 30 and preferably as many as 50 practicing physicians in its immediate neighborhood upon whom it can depend for sales, prescription, and reference volume. It is not advisable to institute a physician's and surgical supply business if the needs of the area are already being adequately served by other establishments.

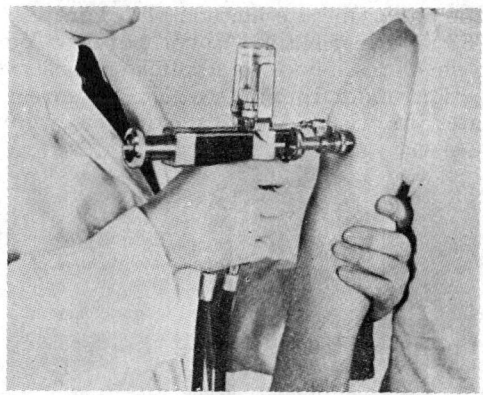

Fig. 881. *Scientific* multidose jet injection apparatus in use with commercial vial as reservoir (courtesy, Sci. Equip.).

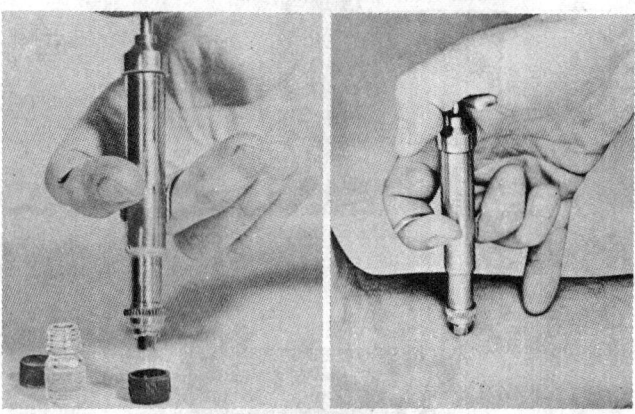

Fig. 882. *Sterineedle* tuberculin test instrument, with disposable multineedle cartridge at tip, is dipped into a cap containing concentrated Tuberculin PPD solution, placed on the forearm, and the handle is pressed. The device also can be employed for smallpox vaccination.

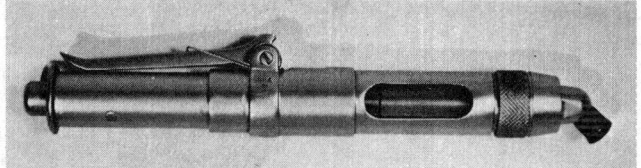

Fig. 883. Type of jet injector adapted to dental use; it also may be employed in podiatry and in dermatologic conditions. It is capable of administering 0.1 ml of solution to a depth of 2 to 6 mm in the surface membranes. Several similar models are available (courtesy, Ormont).

The economic projection of such a department is based on the capital which will have to be invested in inventory and space rental, the pharmacist's or trained clerk's expenses for an initial 2-year period, the sales volume which the department is expected to reach within 2 years, and the anticipated net profits in dollars and percentages for the same period.

Disposable syringes and needles present a serious problem of multiplication of inventory, turnover and storage space requirement, however, all disposable items are increasing in volume and importance. One leading Mid-Western pharmacy which a few years ago operated satisfactorily with about $1000 inventory contained in 6 linear feet of shelf space now finds that 30 times as much space and 4 times the investment are required. Another leading pharmacist warns of economic difficulties in this area for the average establishment.

Jet Injection—The first jet injection was described by F. Beclard and M. Galante in 1866,[27] and M. J. Servajan based his thesis in medicine at the University of Paris in 1872 on the "douche filiforme" principle.[28] Bartholow[29] in 1879 first drew attention in the US to the aquapuncture method of Guerart.

In 1933 Sutermeister and Roberts of New York first tried to develop a device to administer anesthetics by jet injection under compressed air pressure. Three years later, M. L. Lockhart, a New Jersey inventor,

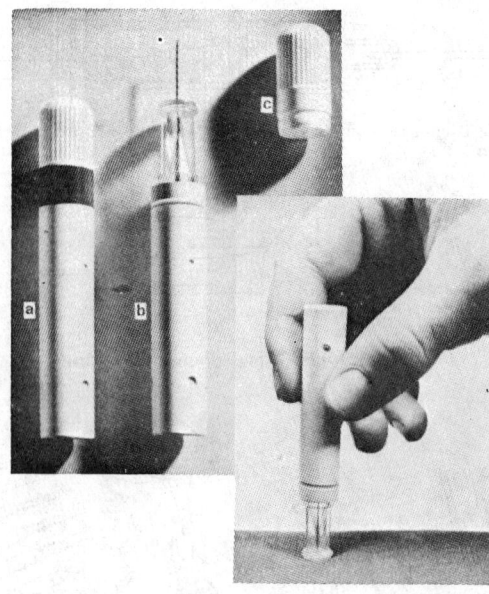

Fig. 885. Automatic self-injector, *Autinject*. The sealed, filled plastic case and needle (a); case after use (b); and cap (c) (courtesy, Intern. Treuhand).

developed the first working explosive-powered piston operated jet injector. In the period 1936 to 1941, working under Lockhart's patents, Squibb, with Scherer, and separately Becton-Dickinson developed compressed-spring, hydraulic, explosive, and electromagnetic solenoid-powered devices.

The first practical and reasonably safe jet injector was the 1951 *Hypospray* device of Scherer and Squibb, using solution-filled cartridges, *Metapules*, with a tiny orifice, and a compressed spring-powered piston.

The US Army Medical Service Graduate School in 1951 at the request of the Commission on Immunization of the Armed Forces Epidemiological Board studied the problem of mass immunization, and developed a powered, practical device that was self-cocking and was supplied by multiple dose vials of medicine. After 3 years of testing, this was reported in the literature.[30]

The original spring-powered single *Metapule* dose *Hypospray* was not commercially successful.

The original Ziherl device was marketed in the mid-50's under various brands. With almost continuous mechanical improvement, it has gained wide usage by State and local health bodies, the Armed Services, and the health authorities of many nations for mass immunization.

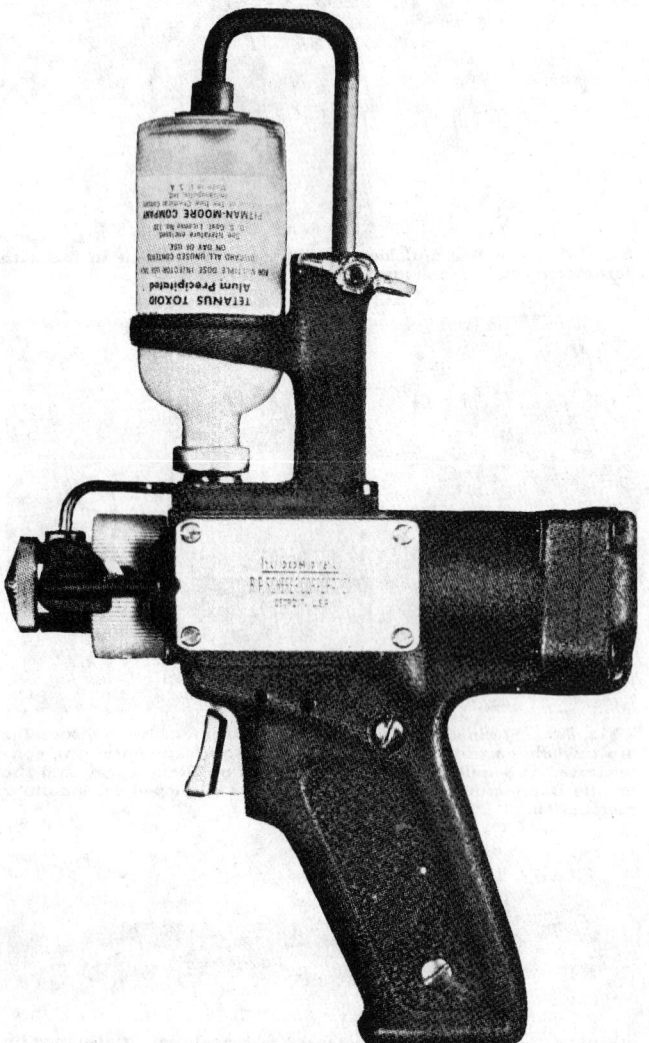

Fig. 884. Multitype, automatic, electrically powered Hypospray hypodermic injector of the "K Series" which handle vials of 50 ml of medicament and a standardized dose, or are as shown allow for graduated dosages and a range of reservoir vial sizes.

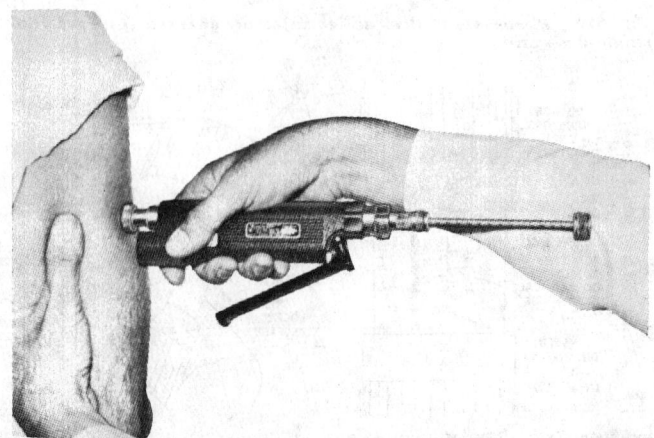

Fig. 886. *Press-O-Jet* multidose jet inoculator (courtesy, Z &W).

The advantages of jet injection to the patient are removal of danger of cross-infection, no needle penetration, sharply reduced pain sensation, and accelerated injection procedure. The physician appreciates the elimination of danger of serum hepatitis, elimination of patient emotional trauma, reduction in patient physical trauma, markedly lower cost, and greatly speeded administration.

Principle and Physiology of Jet Injection—The principle of jet injection is based upon the development of a high velocity jet of fluid projected through a micro-orifice. The fluid is ejected in the form of a fine spray which pierces the skin and penetrates the tissue to a depth determined in advance by the amount of pressure. About 2,200 psi pressure is required to penetrate the skin (Fig. 878).

High pressures have been obtained by means of springs, electromagnetic solenoids, compressed air, nitrogen or carbon dioxide, and explosive powder or nitroglycerin cartridges.

Pump-automated, multidose jet injectors develop a maximum pressure of about 2,400 psi and an injector spring load of 280 psi. This gives at full recoil position 3,734 psi and a jet velocity at the nozzle of 700 fps with normal saline and an orifice of 0.005 in.

Technique of Jet Injection—Jet injectors are precision medical instruments and should be handled accordingly. If the jet injector is improperly used, the injector, the patient and even the person using the device can be damaged or injured.

A jet injector should never be discharged without ejection of liquid. The injector should never be pointed at oneself or at another person unless an injection is being given, as the force of the jet may cause harm. Jet injectors are not toys, and should be kept out of the hands of older as well as young children.

Safety of Jet Injection—Although initially there was some fear expressed concerning the possibility of serious injury occurring to physician or patient, such did not occur. Patient apprehension of jet injection has been a problem. Skin laceration was at one time an occasional occurrence. It still can be if the jet is handled by a careless or unskilled operator and the nozzle of the jet is tangential to the skin surface or if it moves during the inoculation cycle. In a small percentage of cases, a droplet of blood will appear, and in an additional small percentage a fine trickle of blood will result if the injection site is not compressed, covered with cotton or dressed with a small tape.

Commercial Jet Injectors—The jet injectors available for use today fall into three major classes:

1. Hydraulic pump-operated, automatic-recocking, compressed-spring action, multidose, pistol-type jet injectors, with either electric motor or foot-treadle power;
2. Hand-cranked or lever-powered, single-shot, compressed-spring action, multidose jet injectors; and
3. Hand-lever-powered, limited-dosage, single-shot, compressed-spring action, multidose or single cartridge jet injectors.

A hand-cranked, multidose but single-shot, compressed-spring action jet injector is marketed as the *Hypospray* injector by Scherer. To it is attached a multiple dose pharmaceutical vial of medication. A hand crank is used to build up the necessary spring power, which when released drives a piston that forces a measured dose of liquid out through an orifice into the skin (Figs. 879 and 880).

The *Press-O-Jet Varidose* multidose jet injector is a rectangular shaped instrument with a stainless steel reservoir syringe projecting from the rear. The latter is filled (15 ml) from standard vials of solutions, micro-

nized suspensions, or vaccines. Dosage delivered is 1 ml. It is activated by a spring-driven hollow piston which is cocked by a handle. It is marketed by Z & W.

There are two high-capacity, motor-driven, hydraulic-pump, multidose jet injectors available. The *Scientific* multidose injection apparatus operates from a motor-driven hydraulic oil pump. It accommodates standard pharmaceutical sterile product vials, and can be adjusted to provide dosages of from 0.1 to 1.0 ml. A foot-powered hydraulic pump is also available for this device. It is marketed by Sci. Equip. (Fig. 881).

The other, the Scherer *Model K3 Hypospray* multidose jet injector, is somewhat similar in design. It also accommodates pharmaceutical vial packages and can be adjusted to administer from 0.1 to 1.0 ml. dosages (Fig. 884).

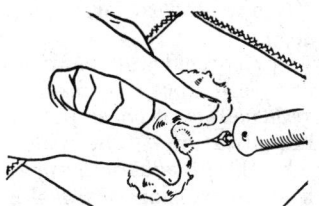

1. The area is anesthetized with a local anesthetic.

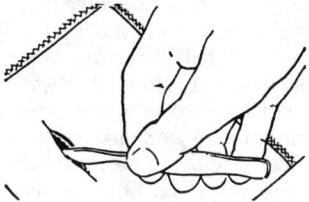

2. A small incision is made into the skin to allow free passage of the large injector needle.

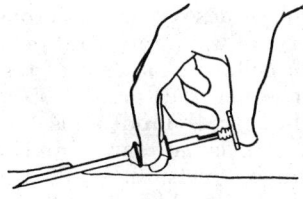

3. The injector needle, with sharp plunger in place, is inserted into the subcutaneous tissue. Sharp plunger is then withdrawn.

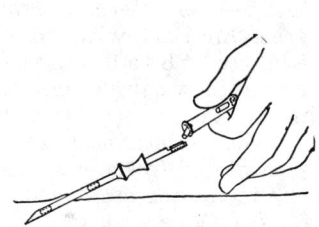

4. Pellets are inserted into the injector.

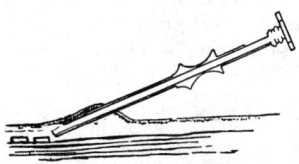

5. The pellets are gently forced with the blunt plunger into the prepared pocket.

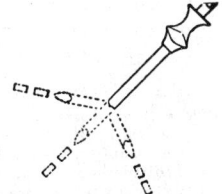

6. Injector is withdrawn and incision closed with suture, clip or adhesive bridge.

Fig. 887. Pellet implantation.

Other Jet Injectors—The value of jet injection in other fields, such as dentistry, is evident in the use of these devices in intramucosal injection. Three similar injectors are available, consisting of a sterilized glass cylinder reservoir, containing from 1 to 4 ml. of medicament, which is fed into it by syringe from a vial of solution (see Fig. 883). A hand crank serves to tighten the spring which provides the driving force to the jet. The jet must always be used with the jet bulb downward and the crank handle pointed upward. The device can be sterilized by autoclaving, boiling, or chemical fluid. It can be used in dentistry, podiatry, or dermatology. This style of jet was developed by Wright Dental. It is marketed as *Panjet* (Acrodent); as *Dermo-Jet* (Robbins Instr.); and as *SyriJet* (Mizzy).

Capacity—The capacity for administration of doses for the various jet injectors varies, the 5-ml reservoir *Dermo-Jets* can inject 300 doses/hour; the hand-powered 15-ml reservoir *Press-O-Jets*, 600 doses/hour; and the electric-powered motor hydraulic pump jets as the *Scientific* or *Model K3 Hypospray*, 1,200 doses/hour.

Other Injectors—Low-cost screening of large groups of adults or children for the Mantoux test for "hidden" tuberculosis can be accomplished with the *Sterineedle* intradermal multiple puncture device. As many as 450 individuals can be tested per hour. The device (by Panray) is employed with a highly purified concentrated (Connaught) PPD, giving a painless, more uniform, and reliable test. Disposable cartridges eliminate danger of cross infection, using six sharp points to pierce the skin to uniform depth of 1 mm. This device can also be readily adapted to large-scale smallpox vaccination (Fig. 882).

Pellet Injector—Wherever prolonged and continuous absorption of testosterone, estradiol, or desoxycorticosterone acetate is desired, pellets of these potent hormones are employed by implantation. The pellets are implanted subcutaneously by the physician using an injector (Fig. 887) or by making an incision in the skin of the thigh. They provide active hormone effects which last for many months and thus the patient does not need repeated parenteral or oral therapy. Over a long period of time, this type of therapy is the most economical for the patient. The pellets of pure crystalline free testosterone, estradiol, or desoxycorticosterone are cylindrical, with a diameter of 3.2 mm ($\frac{1}{8}$ in.) and a length of 8 to 9 mm. Each pellet in the case of testosterone weighs 75 mg and has a surface area of 95 sq mm. They are packed sterile in individual vials.*

Pellets of steroid hormones are also implanted in the posterior infrascapular region by incision.[31] This is the technique employed with sterile, disc-shaped desoxycortisone acetate 125 mg (Ciba).

Hypodermic Needles—Hypodermic needles used with Luer syringes are of metal, and consist of a hub, which locks to the ground-glass tip by friction, and a needle point which varies in diameter and length. Needles are also called *cannulas*. Hypodermic needles may be made of stainless steel, hyperchrome steel,

carbon steel, chromium, nickeloid, platinum, platinum—iridium, silver, or gold.

Hypodermic needles are characterized by their different points, which have a long, tapering reinforced point and beveled cutting edges of varying degree. A *long bevel* or long *taper* needle is used for local anesthesia, aspirating, hypodermoclysis, and subcutaneous administration. A *short bevel* needle is used for intravenous administration, infusions, and transfusions. A *special short bevel* needle is employed for intradermal and spinal administration (Fig. 888).

Size of Hypodermic Needles—Selection of a size is governed by four factors—safety, rate of flow, comfort of patient, and depth of penetration. There are three standard dimensions—length, outside diameter of the cannula and wall thickness. Regular needles are measured for length from where the cannula joins the hub to the tip of the point (hub not included). Special needles that have a "bead" or stop on the cannula (such as the B-D "Security") are measured from the "bead" to the tip of the point; always the working part of the cannula.

The gauge of a needle is measured by the outside diameter of the cannula or needle shaft. The measuring device universally employed is the standard Stubb's English wire gage. Gauge numbers are often stamped on the flat of the hub for ready reference. The usual range of diameter for needles is from 13-gauge (largest diameter) to 27-gauge. Needles seldom are less than $\frac{1}{4}$ in. in length or longer than $3\frac{1}{2}$ in.

There are many special needles, designed for a variety of purposes. Various *biopsy* and *bone marrow transfusion* needles range from 16-gauge to 19-gauge and $\frac{1}{2}$ in. to $3\frac{1}{2}$ in. in size. They are characterized by their heavy shaped hubs.

Needles for *local anesthesia* range from 26-gauge $\frac{1}{2}$ in. to 20-gauge 6 in. *Intravenous, blood transfusion* needles, some with fitted cannulae, range from 19-gauge $1\frac{1}{4}$ in. to 15-gauge $2\frac{1}{2}$ in.

There are also special needles and cannulae for *abscess, eye, hemorrhoidal, tonsil, laryngeal,* and *pneumothorax* use.

These many types of special purpose hypodermic needles, are of varying sizes in diameter, and varying

---

* Pellets of hormones are supplied by Schering and by Ciba and were originally inserted with the Kearns Pellet Injector, developed by Dr. Walter Kearns of Milwaukee, Wis., a three-part device consisting of a hollow needle with inside diameter of 3.2 mm and a sharp and a blunt plunger. The Kearns Pellet Injector can be obtained from Marco. A modification of this injector, designed by Dr. William H. Perloff of Philadelphia, is available from Pilling.

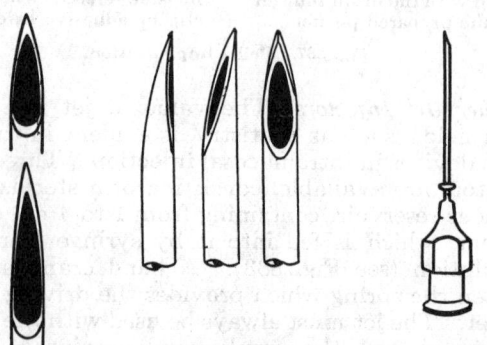

Fig. 888. Hypodermic needles. Left, short bevel and long bevel needle points; left center, the Huber point with closed bevel and side opening to avoid producing tissue plugs; right center, regular point showing features which insure less cutting, more distention of tissue, reduced trauma, seepage, and after-pain; right, needle with security button which prevents a broken cannula from becoming lost in the issues.

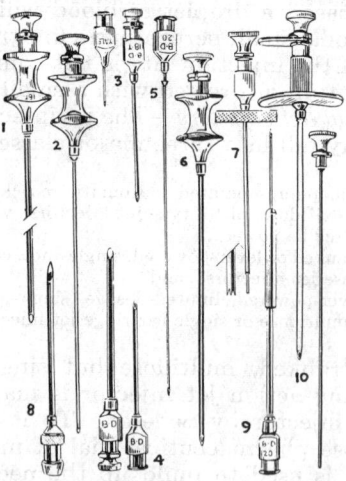

Fig. 889. Special hypodermic needles—1: caudal needle; 2: epidural needle for single-shot anesthesia; 3: intravenous anesthesia short-bevel and long needles (with vinyl tubing); 4: blood transfusion needles (with vinyl tubing); 5: short-bevel beaded local anesthesia needle; 6: spinal needle with large spool hub; 7: biopsy needle for bone marrow aspirations; 8: infusion needle, with female luer slip; 9: hemorrhoidal needle with threaded adjustable gauge to adjust depth of puncture; 10: cerebral angiography needle with thin-walled outer cannula, corrugated shield, and inner cannula (courtesy, Becton-Dickinson).

lengths. Some of these are shown in the accompanying illustration. These are intended for single-shot anesthesia, epidural; long-needle and short-bevel needles for *intravenous anesthesia; caudal* needles; *blood transfusion* needles; short-bevel beaded needles for *local anesthesia; biopsy* needle for bone marrow aspirations; *infusion* needle, with female luer slip; *hemorrhoidal injection* needle, with threaded adjustable gauge to adjust depth of puncture; *cerebral angiography* needle with thin-walled outer cannula, corrugated shield, and inner cannula. There are many others, such as specially shaped needles for pneumothorax, electroencephalography, aortography, arteriography, cholangiography, discography, lymphangiography, myelography, ventriculography, and tracheotomy.

For continuous pipetting, an ordinary luer-lock glass syringe is fitted into a *metal pipetting holder*, and a *metal filling assembly* slipped into the luer-lock. The latter comprises an automatic valve, metal sinker, and 2 feet of rubber tubing. Two regular metal *cannulae* complete the outfit, and fit on the end of the filling assembly.

Needle Locks—In order to prevent hypodermic needles from slipping off or jumping off the tip of the syringe, patented locking devices have been developed. These are valuable where pressure or manipulation of the needle is required while in the tissue. A metal tip with a slip and a metal collar with a circular internal groove engage the needle hub, and in a half turn locks the needle in place (Fig. 890).

The tip of a hypodermic syringe may be eccentric, that is, "off center," to facilitate placement of the needle and barrel against skin or tissue.

Ampuls and Vials—Injectable sterile solutions are customarily supplied in *glass ampuls*. These ampuls contain slightly more (approximately 10%) than the desired dosage or stated contents. This additional quantity of medication insures that the total proper

dosage can be removed. It allows for the loss of medication caused by "wetting" of the inside of the glass.

To open an ampul, make a small nick on the neck of the ampul with a file By gentle pressure from the side the ampul may be broken. There are also available automatic ampul cutters which grasp the ampul and when rotated cut the neck.

There are also available glass ampuls which have a special mark or ring around their neck, which provides a "weak point" to facilitate breakage, permitting the physician or nurse to open the ampul by gentle pressure of the finger only, and insuring a clean, even break.

It is always desirable to withdraw into a syringe slightly more of a medication than is necessary for dosage. Then hold the syringe with the needle uppermost, and press on the plunger until the first of the medication issues from the needle tip. This avoids an air pocket in the needle which might be forced into a vein. For more detailed information see the chapter on *Parenteral Preparations* (page 1519).

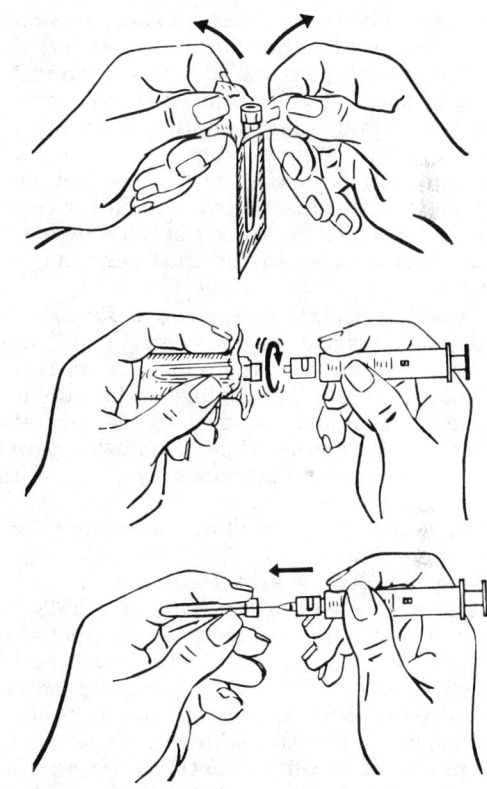

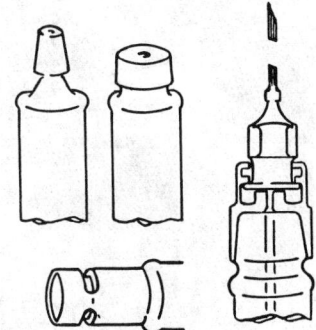

Fig. 890. **Syringe tips. Upper left, ordinary glass tip and a large tip designed for Luer-Lok tip; right, cross section of a Luer-Lok syringe tip with needle in place.**

Fig. 892. **Sterile disposable hypodermic needles, packed in foil envelopes, are exposed at hub end, the hub twisted on to syringe hub to fasten, then the needle guard is removed. One brand (Becton-Dickinson) shows needle gauge by color of hub: tan, 26 g; blue, 25 g; light green, 23 g; black, 22 g; green, 21 g; yellow, 20 g; dark brown, 19 g; and pink, 18 g.**

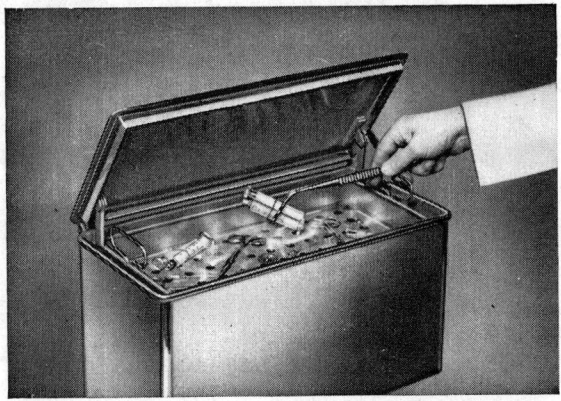

Fig. 891. **Sterilizing syringes by boiling.**

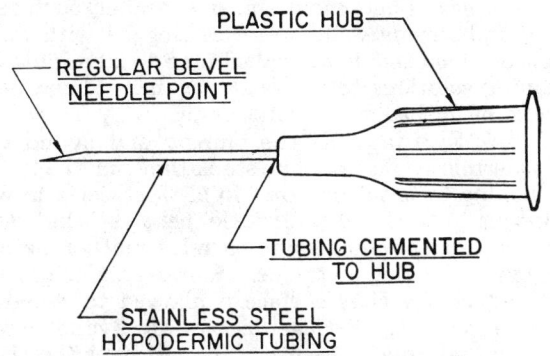

PLASTIC HUB

REGULAR BEVEL
NEEDLE POINT

TUBING CEMENTED
TO HUB

STAINLESS STEEL
HYPODERMIC TUBING

Fig. 893. **Construction of disposable plastic hub hypodermic needle (courtesy, Autian and Brewer[32]).**

Care of Hypodermic Equipment

Immediately after use, syringes and needles should be flushed two or three times, or until all traces of medication have disappeared, with a commercially accepted neutral (pH 7) cleaning solution. Needle and syringe parts then should be separated and soaked in the cleaning solution from 5 to 20 minutes. Abrasive cleaners must be avoided.

If used for blood work, syringes and needles should be flushed first with cold tap water to minimize the introduction of blood into the cleaning solution. When used for oily solutions, they should be allowed to soak from 1 to 1½ hours. Any soiling that is not removed should be brushed or wiped away.

After soaking, the syringe should be assembled and flushed with cleaning solution, rinsed thoroughly under running tap water, and flushed with distilled water or alcohol. The syringe is then ready for sterilization.

Needles may be removed from the cleaning solution, rinsed with alcohol or ether, and dried in air prior to sterilization. They should be kept sharp by honing.

Rustless needles require no lubrication but the ordinary carbon steel type must be coated with mineral oil when not in use. It is customary to pass and keep a cleaning wire through any cannula, to insure removal and elimination of foreign bodies. (Always insert wire through hub, not from the point.) Carbon steels are not as flexible as rustless steels. The latter require less care and are not affected by iodine salts or most acids. Stainless steels, while highly rust-resisting, are not fully rustless.

Most hospital central supply rooms furnish the floor or ward with a small stainless steel pan containing cleaning solution for immediate flushing of hypodermic equipment after use. The syringe and needle often are left in the solution and returned to the central supply for preparation for sterilization. Enameled pans should be avoided since small particles may chip off and clog the needle and syringe.

Improper care and handling of syringes leads to several types of failure.

Removal of Stains and Deposits—A 10% nitric acid solution is used for removal of alkali deposits. Arsenic and iron stains are removed by the use of 10% solution of hydrochloric acid, and gentian violet by 10% solution of nitric acid. For blood stains 10% solution of nitric acid, sodium citrate, or concentrated ammonia is used, or with soaking in the newer biologic enzyme preparations offered to the consumer for fabric cleaning. In the above cases, swabbing carefully with a cotton applicator dipped in the solution and rinsing thoroughly with distilled water after each swabbing is satisfactory.

Needle stains can be removed by the use of fine powdered or caked household abrasive cleaner, such as Bon Ami, and rinsing well. Needles clogged with medications or blood should be soaked for 5 to 20 minutes with cleaning solutions before final washing. Then needles should be flushed with alcohol or air.

Stuck Syringes—If the plunger and cylinder of a hypodermic syringe become stuck they may be loosened by boiling for a few minutes in 25% glycerin in water. Allowing nitric acid to trickle between the ground-glass surfaces of plunger and barrel is another method of removing clogging materials. However, this procedure may affect the glass surface if allowed to remain too long in contact. *Syringe openers* are available which employ hydraulic pressure. They fit over the tip of a clogged syringe and by firm steady pressure warm

water is forced against the tip of the plunger and is made to infiltrate between plunger and barrel. The plunger of the stuck syringe is thus driven backward (Fig. 894).

Stuck Needles—To remove stuck needles the syringe and needle are soaked for 5 to 20 minutes in a commercially accepted neutral (pH 7) cleaning solution such as the B-D Yale Cleaner. The square part of the needle hub is grasped firmly in a pair of pliers or with forceps. (Never grasp the round part of hub.) The syringe (*not the forceps*) is rotated counter-clockwise. Force must not be used.

Sterilization of Equipment—Medications intended to be administered parenterally must be sterile, also the hypodermic syringes and needles by which the medication is administered. Syringes should be sterilized by first separating the plunger from the cylinder, washing the pieces in warm water, and then by boiling. Do not boil syringes in alkaline type water, bicarbon-

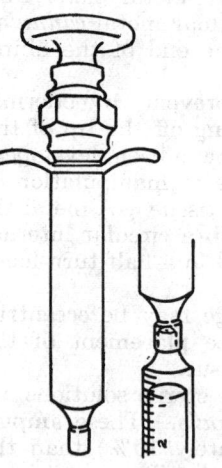

Fig. 894. Metal syringe opener. Right, showing how a stuck syringe is opened by employing the metal syringe opener which applies uniform hydraulic pressure with warm water to open the syringe.

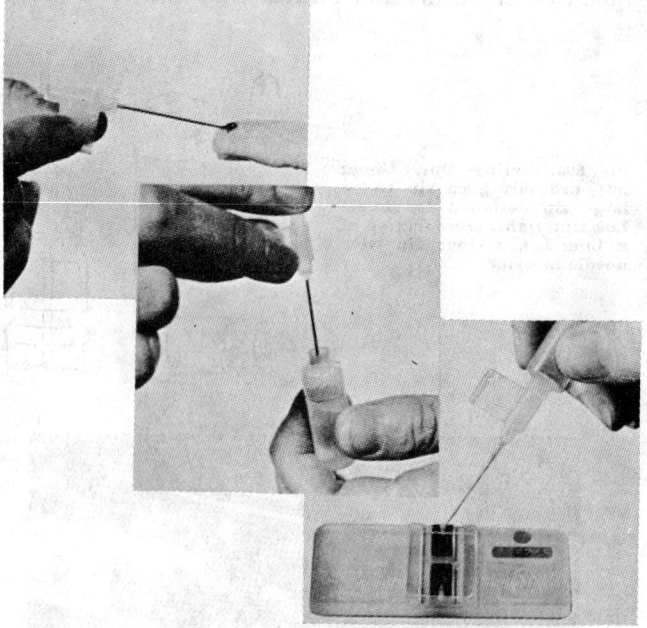

Fig. 895. *Unopette* disposable blood-diluting pipette (courtesy, Becton-Dickinson).

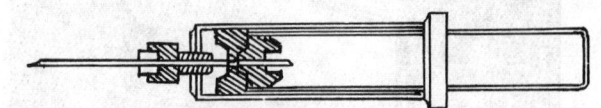

Fig. 896. *Vacutainer* blood-collecting system functions as an aspirating syringe (courtesy, Becton-Dickinson).

ate solution, or solutions containing sterilizing tablets. After use, wash in warm water, rinse in alcohol or ether, and dry the pieces separately. Physicians frequently allow sterile syringes to remain in the sterilizer until needed (Fig. 891). Only distilled water should be used in the sterilizer and the sterilizer frequently cleansed, so as to avoid the presence of foreign particles which might get into the syringe and needle and thus into the solution to be injected.

Other sterilization methods employ dry heat or hot air. The temperature usually used is 320°F, and the time 1 hour. The instructions of the particular hot-air sterilizer should be followed. Chemical sterilizing is sometimes used if it is believed that there are no resistant spores present. The agents used should be kept at recommended strengths and immersion prolonged.

Sterilization by autoclaving is accomplished as follows: After cleaning, the syringe with the barrel and plunger separated is wrapped between layers of gauze, then wrapped in a double layer of muslin and pinned or tied. The size of the syringe is marked on the muslin for easy identification. The wrapped syringe is then sterilized for 30 minutes under 15 to 17 pounds pressure at 250°–254°F unless specific instructions are given for a particular autoclave.

Needles may be sterilized in the usual physical or chemical fashion. Many hospitals prefer hot-air sterilization because the needles are always dry. Sterilize for 1 hour at 320°F unless otherwise specified by the manufacturer. Platinum–iridium needles may be sterilized by flaming. Users should test the temper of needles frequently.

In the use of a hypodermic syringe and needle the surface of the skin through which the needle will pass must also be sterilized by 70% alcohol or some other antiseptic.

Blood Sampling Devices—For expediting blood cell counts, a disposable blood collecting unit is available consisting of a glass capillary tube of uniform bore and length, fitted with a plastic adapter, and an attachable plastic reservoir containing a premeasured diluent. It is *Unopette* (Becton-Dickinson).

Widely used as an efficient and rapid means of taking blood samples in fair amounts is the B-D *Vacutainer* which has a sterile glass vacuum plunger, with a rubber diaphragm stopper. This fits into a sterile barrel in the end of which is a metal cap through which passes a steel screw cannula. When the plunger is pushed forward the inner needle point is embedded in the rubber stopper. When the outside sterile needle is unsheathed, and inserted in the vein, the diaphragm puncture is completed and the blood rushes into the vacuum.

Plunger Syringes

At one time *piston* or *plunger syringes* were cumbersome and of little value. They consisted principally of glass or metal barrels through which passed metal or glass rods bearing leather, rubber, or string washers. Pressure on the plunger forced liquids out of the barrel through the opening or aperture at the end. These syringes were employed for crude irrigation of body cavities.

It was impossible for the syringe to operate without a tightly fitting washer. Syringes of this type are still manufactured, because they are satisfactory for some purposes and are inexpensive. They are not to be recommended for general use, however, because they

cannot be sterilized and the washers soon deteriorate and fail to operate, thus allowing leakage. *All-metal syringes*, Fig. 897, with the plunger approximating the inside diameter of the barrel, are used in veterinary medicine. *Hard rubber syringes* of the plunger type are today only employed occasionally for rectal irrigation (Fig. 898). These syringes may be satisfactory if the washer is accurately ground or constructed to prevent leakage. However, they have the disadvantage of opacity and the volume injected cannot be measured accurately. They have the advantages, however, of being unbreakable and easily sterilized.

Urethral Syringes—These customarily have glass barrels, because they must be sterilized before and after use. Piston-type syringes for this purpose may use asbestos, rubber, leather, or thread-wrapped washers. Rubber is not recommended for washers, however, because it deteriorates rapidly. These syringes may be used as well for irrigation of body cavities, for moistening dressings, and for similar purposes.

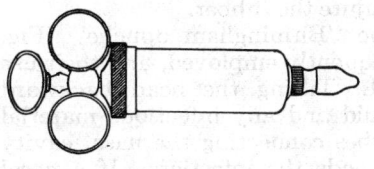

Fig. 897. Metal plunger syringe. Used for irrigating body cavities but not recommended for home use.

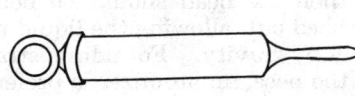

Fig. 898. Hard rubber or vulcanite syringe operating on the plunger principle. The piston consists of a leather washer which must be kept greased to prevent leakage around it.

Bulb Syringes

Bulb syringes are frequently preferred for use where sterility is not necessary or where plunger-type syringes, because of their force, would be dangerous to use. Bulb syringes are of particular value in the nose and ear.

The Asepto Syringe—This type, modifications of which are produced by several firms, consists of a glass barrel with a tip shaped to meet a particular need, with a small rubber bulb whose compression provides the necessary force. The rubber bulb is fitted inside one end of the barrel, instead of outside as is usually the case in bulb syringes. The rubber does not stretch and the syringe is less likely to get out of order. The size of the bulb is gauged to the capacity of the barrel, so that the fluid is not drawn into the rubber bulb. The bulb is readily movable and the barrel can be easily cleansed and sterilized. Various modifications of this type of syringe are available for bladder, urethra, cervix, ear, nose, and larynx treatment (Fig. 899).

A sterile, disposable syringe with finger grips and printed calibrations on the shatterproof polypropylene barrel is the *Medaseptic D* unit with catheter tip and tip protector, packed in peel-pack envelope (Baxter—Canada).

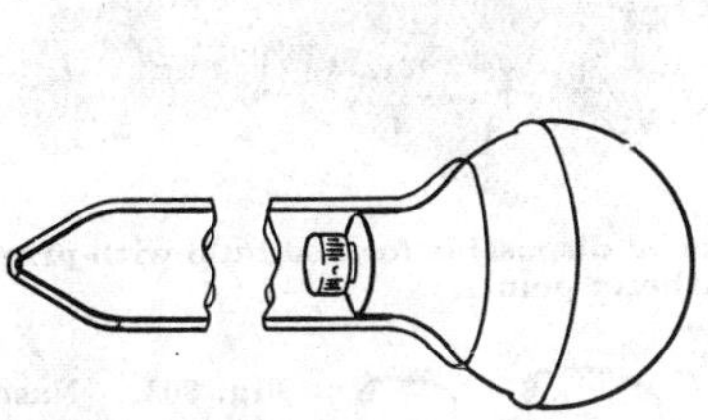

Fig. 899. The Asepto syringe with improved bulb and plastic plug for easy cleaning.

Other Bulb Syringes—These syringes are customarily known by the name of the part of the body for which they are intended.

Nasal syringes or *nasal aspirators* are soft rubber bulbs of about 1 ounce capacity, with an acorn-shaped nasal tip to fit the nostril. The tip may be either glass or hard rubber. Glass is more popular as the transparency allows visual examination of the mucous removed from the nostril. (Fig. 903.)

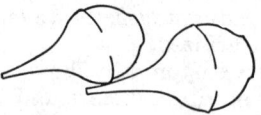

Fig. 900. Infant's and adult's soft rubber ear and ulcer syringes.

Ear syringes and *ulcer syringes* are one-piece molded bulbs of soft, flexible rubber, with long, narrow nozzles and are employed in treating the eye, ear, and nose, and for irrigation of any open cavity or ulcer.

If necessary, bulb syringes should be sterilized with germicidal solutions, such as saponated cresol solution. Prolonged boiling will injure the rubber.

Nasal douches as the "Birmingham douche" (Fig. 904) are now only infrequently employed, and their use should be discouraged. Tilting the head backward forces the irrigating fluid and any infectious material into the Eustachian tubes connecting the nasal cavity and the ear. This spreads the infection. If a nasal syringe must be used, then the head should be bent forward and the nose washed out, allowing the liquid to flow out of the nose freely by gravity. For administration of medication into the nose, an atomizer is preferably employed.

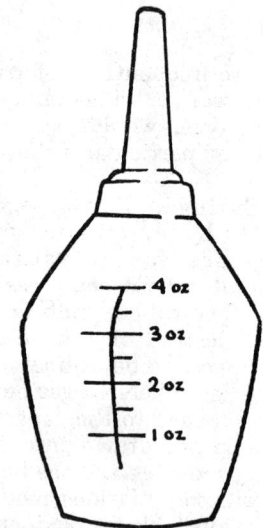

Fig. 901. Bulb-type graduated transparent infant enema syringe.

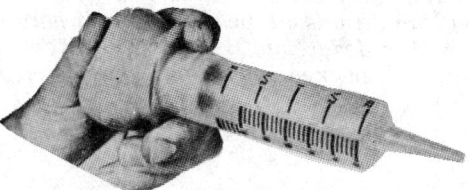

Fig. 902. Special disposable formed bulb with printed polyethylene barrel and catheter point.

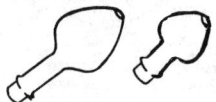

Fig. 903. Nasal aspirator tips (either glass or hard rubber).

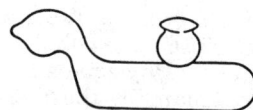

Fig. 904. Birmingham style nasal douche.

Rectal syringes are customarily of the bulb type, with a long narrow nozzle. They are frequently employed in the administration of enemas to infants. These are the safest and least expensive of syringes with little to get out of order. Infants' syringes customarily are of 1- to 2-ounce capacity; babies' syringes of 4-ounce capacity. Although many syringes provide hard rubber or vulcanite tips, the use of hard tips should be discouraged because of occasional injury to the soft tissues from their use (Fig. 905).

Vaginal syringes, used for irrigation of the vagina, are half-pint to 10-ounce capacity bulb syringes with a large vulcanite or rubber spray tube. Pressure on the bulb forces the medicated or irrigating liquid through the tip of the syringe either in a direct stream or with a "whirling" motion. These syringes in white or various colors are provided with rubber sleeve-shaped round or oval shields to prevent leakage when in use. Caps sealing the nozzles are provided to avoid leakage or loss of the contents before use (Fig. 906). One model has a convenient plastic stopper at the bottom of the bulb opening with a removable strainer, which permits mixing of medicaments.

Enema Syringes—*Enema syringes* are of two types, the more popular and preferable *fountain syringe*, and the other, the *valve syringe*. The latter has a rubber bulb with two openings to which are connected flexible rubber tubes, one leading to the reservoir and the other to the spray tip. Alternate constriction of the bulb creates vacuum to draw up the irrigant from the reservoir into the bulb and then forces the liquid through the tube to the nozzle and the process is repeated. The intermittent flow of the latter may provide too great a force. This type is inferior to the fountain syringe although it is convenient for traveler's use (Fig. 907).

Fountain syringes consist of a reservoir with a capacity of 1 to 3 quarts, a 5-foot rubber tube, and a vaginal or rectal nozzle. These are used for irrigation with water, salt solution, soap suds, or special medications.

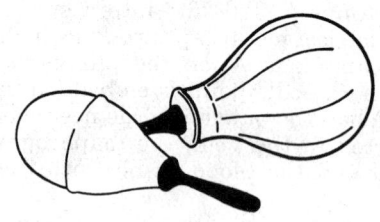

Fig. 905. Infant's and adult's rectal syringes; soft rubber bulb and hard tip.

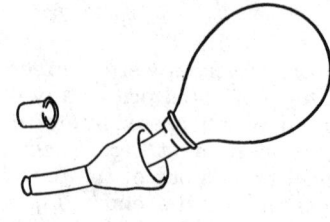

Fig. 906. Vaginal syringe.

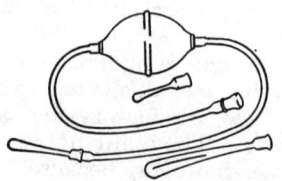

Fig. 907. Valve syringe for giving enemas or for vaginal irrigation; convenient for travelers.

The reservoir may be of rubber, which requires little storage space, and some grades are guaranteed to last a long time. Glass or enamelware reservoirs are also employed and are more readily cleaned and more sanitary.

Precautions to be observed by pharmacists in cautioning users of enema syringes are: the "drop" must not exceed 4 feet, to prevent excessive gravity pressure; the fluid should be maintained at body temperature to avoid chills or burns; and the tube is customarily closed with a mechanical metal pinchcock. Before using the syringe, the cut-off should be released for a moment until some liquid issues from the nozzle. The user must be certain that no air remains which might be forced from the tube into the body cavity. Hard rubber nozzles are frequently supplied with enema syringes but as they may cause damage to the rectum they are preferably replaced by catheters or tubes of soft rubber, about $\frac{3}{16}$ inch in diameter by 15 in. in length.

There are also available disposable enema administration units, non-spill plastic bags, tubing, tube clip, containers of castile soap and of lubricating jelly. A rectal tip is provided. In the case of disposable barium enema administration units, a special barium tip of molded plastic is supplied (Davol).

Enemas—In simple constipation, whenever evacuation of the lower bowel is indicated, and when proctologic examination or surgery is indicated, an enema is customarily given because of its local, comfortable, and safe action in minutes time. Castile soapsuds and other similar evacuants have long been employed but are now partially replaced by preparations whose hypertonic and surfactant properties insure rectal peristalsis and softening of impacted feces. Some aqueous solutions, 4 to 6 ounces in quantity, contain sodium phosphate and biphosphate or sodium citrate and laurylsulfoacetate, sorbitol and sorbic acid, and glycerin. Liquid petrolatum is also employed. Either an unbreakable vinyl plastic squeeze bottle, or a plastic container and 30 to 60 inches of tubing, each with a smooth 2-inch rectal tip, is provided. Enemas should not be used when nausea, vomiting, or abdominal pain is present, nor, more often than necessary, to avoid dependence. Available as well are transparent, plastic, graduated (in half-ounces), 4-ounce transparent or opaque infant enema syringes which allow accurate filling, mixing and use of the physician's prescribed formulas. Prepared enemas are available f r use in simple constipation or whenever evacuation of the lower bowel is indicated, such as in proctologic or sigmoidoscopic examinations; small, disposable units comprising flexible plastic bottles of 6 to 50 ml aqueous or oil solutions, with self-fitted comfortable plastic or rubber tip (Fleet; J&J).

Snake-Bite Kits—Anyone in snake, bee, or wasp country should carry a snake-bite kit (Fig. 908). Usually available in a compact plastic or metal case is a tourniquet, rubber or other lymph constrictor, antiseptic, razor blade or knife, and one or several suction cups or syringes. These are available from Cutter or

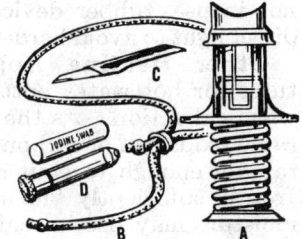

Fig. 908. Pocket snake bite kit contains (A) suction device, (B) tourniquet, (C) incision blade, and (D) antiseptic swab.

Becton-Dickinson. Many lives are saved each year by prompt action at the spot where the snake attacks, and relief from the pain and swelling of severe insect stings is also important.

Snake bites are medical emergencies that require immediate treatment. Most common of poisonous snakes are the rattlesnakes, found in almost every area. Copperheads are common in the Great Lakes region and from the Plains States eastward. Water moccasins or cottonmouths are common to the swamps and lakes of the South. About 2000 to 2500 people are bitten annually and of these about 15 die (*Dept. of Publ. Health, Indiana Univ. School of Med.*). Snake bites are most common in summer months. Most frequently involved are children, or adults engaged in camping, hunting or fishing. The majority of snakebites (57%) occur on the legs, and 40% of these occur on the foot.

surgical supplies

Absorbable hemostat
Adhesive dressings
Bandages, elastic and cotton
Bandage scissors, blades and blade handles
Cold sterilization solutions
Crutches and canes
Diagnostic examination lights— such as otoscopes, etc.
Disposable examination gloves
Disposable tissues
Dressings, absorbent and non- adhering
Elastic supports
Face masks
Finger cots
Hypodermic needles and syringes
Pharmaceuticals and injectibles
Porous elastic tape
Presurgical antiseptic
Professional leather goods
Rubber doughnuts and sponge sheeting
Rubber and plastic sheeting
Scales
Sterile lubricants
Surgical tape
Sutures—professional put-ups
Underpads

Fig. 909. List of items commonly available in community pharmacies serving physicians' needs.

Sickroom Appliances

The value of counterirritation as a remedial measure in deep-seated inflammations of the chest and abdomen has been recognized for centuries. The local application of heat and cold has been termed the best domestic therapeusis. It is particularly valuable for relief of neuralgic and rheumatic pains, cramps, etc. It also exerts curative effects in inflammation of thoracic and abdominal regions. Counterirritation also has the general advantage of producing no harmful effects.

Moist heat is applied by hot water compresses and poultices, and is employed for superficial relief from inflammation of the skin and subcutaneous areas.

Dry heat is used for the reflex effects it produces in deep-seated organs.

Hot Water Bottles—The best instruments for applying dry heat are the hot water bottle and the electric heating pad. Made of rubber, hot water bottles may be of the usual 2-quart size, or of pint capacity in the form of a "face bottle" for neuralgia of the head and for infant conditions. Each hot water bottle has an opening through which warm water is added and a stopper securely sealed with a washer. It is more convenient to permanently attach the stopper to the bottle

Table III

Surgical supplies

1—Hospital beds, sick room furniture.	8—Oxygen and respiratory equipment.	18—Laboratory supplies.
2—Wheelchairs, invalid walkers.	9—Traction equipment.	19—Syringes, thermometers.
3—Commodes.	10—Stainless steel ware.	20—Aerosols.
4—Walkers.	11—Enamel ware.	21—Whirlpool equipment, bathtub equipment.
5—Crutches, canes.	12—Plastic ware.	22—Bed boards, bed tables and trays.
6—Surgical garments and appliances.	13—Surgical instruments.	23—Therapeutic and other lamps.
7—Colostomy, urinary and like appliances.	14—Elastic bandages.	24—Rubber and plastic sheeting.
	15—Catheters.	25—Armslings.
	16—Disposable syringes, needles.	26—Patient lift.
	17—Blood pressure and like equipment.	

Surgical suppliers[a,b]

20	Aeroceuticals	2, 3, 4	Erie	5, 9, 13	Ortho. Equip.
14	Arbeka	2, 4, 5	Everest & Jennings	18	Pfeiffer
6, 9	Atco	23	Frohock-Stewart	12	Plasta-Medic
1	Atlas Hosp.	2, 3	Gendron	26	Plymouth
6	Baka	8	Gen. Dynamics	5, 9, 14, 16, 18, 26	Popper
15, 16	Bard	6	Glove	26	Porto-Lift
14, 16	Bauer & Black	7	Gricks	6	Posey
17	Baum	1	Hard	18	Profex
14, 16, 19	Becton-Dickinson	4, 5	Hosp. & Ortho. Aides	13, 15, 17	Propper
12	Bel-Art	19	Hypo	24	Replogle
24	Better Sleep	23	Ille	15	Rusch
6	Bittner	1	Inland Bed	6	Salk
12	Buck	2, 3, 4, 26	Inst. Ind.	9	Sani-Pac
5	Calley & Currier	11	Jones Metal	21	Schuco
13	Cardiosonic	25	Kadan	1	Shampaine
1	Carrom	3, 4, 5	Levy	1	Superior
13	Christy	6	Little	6	Surg. Hosiery
8, 2	Colson	25	Luxo	6	Surg. Prod.
14	Conco	3, 4, 5	Mah-Zell	24	Tuco
8, 26	Continental Hosp.	6	Melrose	10	Vollrath
5	Cove-Craft	21	Menda	7	Wagner
7, 15, 16	Davol	13	Miltenberg	10, 11	Weiss
16	Dennison	8	Monaghan	16	Whitestone
19	DeVilbiss	8	Nageldinger	4	Winfield
4	Edco	6	Noveltex		

^a Figures at left of supplier correspond to the number at left on the list of supplies. They indicate the kind of supplies provided by the firm.
^b For complete names and addresses of these firms, see page 2023.

to prevent loss. Some have screw stopper attachments, which permit conversion of the bottle into a fountain syringe (Fig. 910).

Leakage must be guarded against. If the patrons are not familiar with the use of hot water bottles they should be directed to fill the bottle with water to not more than one-half of its capacity. After the hot water is poured into the bottle, the latter should be compressed to remove the remaining air, and then the bottle securely closed. This removal of excess air provides a more flexible bottle, one which shapes well to the body.

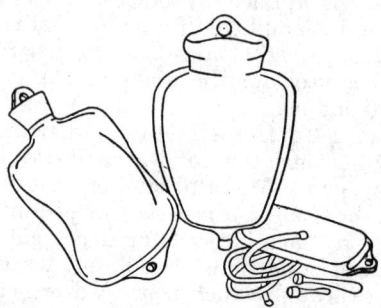

Fig. 910. Hot water bottle (left); standard-type fountain syringe (center); travel style syringe (right).

When filling a water bottle, hold it against the back of hand or forearm to insure that the temperature is not too high. Never allow bare rubber to come in contact with the skin, or burns may result. Rubber pads, flannelette bags, or even a towel wrapped around the hot water bottle will give adequate passage of heat with comfort and convenience.

A type of hot water bottle is now available with one side made of special corrugated construction which allows direct contact with the skin surface without burning. This feature offers the possibility of both dry and moist heat application with the same bottle.

After using, empty the hot water bottle and hang it by the tab at its bottom to thoroughly drain. Do not permit water of boiling temperature, oil, grease, alcohol, or turpentine to come in contact with rubber. When not in use, rubber devices should be protected from direct light to avoid hardening of the rubber.

Other Heating Appliances—Ingenious substitutes for hot water bottles depend upon the heat of chemical action. As the temperature of fire is due to rapid oxidation of carbon particles, so iron may oxidize rapidly enough to emit appreciable amounts of heat. Iron in sufficiently fine subdivision in the presence of moisture may rise in temperature within 3 to 10 minutes to over 190°F. Formulas[33] for this purpose are as follows:

Powdered iron	92.0
Ferrous sulfate	3.0
Copper sulfate	5.0

or

Powdered iron	10.0
Potassium chlorate	10.0

The maximum temperature will last for 10 minutes and the material will be hot enough for therapeutic action for several hours.

Sodium acetate is also used. It is placed in a metal container and heated until anhydrous and liquid. The cap is then replaced and the container set aside until required. When the cap is removed, crystallization takes place rapidly with the development of much heat.

Electric Heating Pads—Electric heating pads are now commonly employed. Their advantage lies in the fact that there is no possibility of leakage or spilling, and the temperature is constant and controlled. Most are wet-proof for wet or dry application, have cushion-soft thick foam padding and washable flannel covers. Some have adjustable heating elements which permit the temperature to be set at the desired level and illuminated temperature control panel. Quantity production now permits these devices to overcome the disadvantage of expensive construction and they are available at low cost. All such electrical devices customarily are inspected by the Insurance Underwriters Bureau to insure safe operation. However, short circuits and breakage of the heating element may result from constant use.

Automatic heat bonnets for scalp treatments; heat bandage for sprains, bursitis, arthritis; neck and throat heating pads for stiff neck or whiplash cases; sinus masks for heat therapy of sinus areas; and even thermal massages are available now from sources such as Casco.

Cold Application—In deep inflammation the effects of external application of either heat or cold are essentially similar, due to reflexes arising from the stimulation of the nerves conducting temperature sensation. Experience has shown that there are some conditions (such as appendicitis) where the application of cold is the more desirable.

Appliances for local application of cold are: the cumbersome rubber coil and freezing unit chiefly used in hospitals and the familiar *ice bag* or *ice cap*. The latter is usually a circular rubber or rubberized mackintosh cloth bag, circular in shape, with a large opening to admit cracked ice. Occasionally thick rubber is employed similar to that used in hot water bottles. Icecaps usually require a cover of some type to protect the skin.

The contents of an icecap are less flaccid than the liquid in hot water bottles. Therefore, thin rubber or cloth construction is preferable in order to insure better conformation with the body. The pleated shape common to many icecaps avoids bulginess and allows introduction of large amounts of ice (Fig. 911).

An adaptation of the icecap is used for throat inflammation. It is the collar-shaped rubber bag known as a *tonsillectomy bag*. It fits snugly around the neck, holding the ice upon the parts. There are two styles, one with a spring clip and the other tying into place with strings or laces. Ice bags are also made in a long narrow shape for use around the throat and along the spine. Throat or spine bags are of thicker material because firmness and retention of shape under stress are desired.

Instead of ice, some hospitals keep their ice bags filled with glycerin or an isopropyl alcohol–ice mixture. These *redi-freeze ice packs* are stored in refrigerators until needed and are exchanged in the wards for bags which have become warm in use. Thus cold bags are immediately available at all times, and the liquid contents conform more readily to the body contours.

Ice packs of soft rubber or plastic, filled with a nontoxic solution of 10% propylene glycol and water are available in the usual designs. When stored in the freezing compartment or in deep-freeze compartment of the refrigerator, the contents freeze to a semisolid or slush which provides greater comfort in use and longer retention of cold temperature than ice cubes. Fitted with tabs and tie-tapes, they are available in throat and body shapes.

Comfort Aids—Discomfort in a patient causes unhappiness and delays recovery. Any aids relieving pain are of real therapeutic value both because of the psychological factor and from the actual physical effect.

Air cushions distribute the pressure of a sitting or recumbent body. All operate on the principle of a "pillow of air." There is considerable variation in the size and shape of air cushions. Patients lacking adipose covering suffer discomfort and local injury from long recumbency. The knees, hips, and buttocks of bedridden patients should be protected. Various types of air cushions are supplied for use in bed or in chairs. The circular type is superior in some cases, giving better distribution of pressure and preventing slipping. Circular air cushions vary in outside diameter from 12 to 17 in. The smallest type is for use between the knees; ther 12-in. size is best for hips and buttocks. If the opening is too large the air cushion will not properly support the weight (Fig. 912).

Patients sitting for long periods of time in chairs should use *circular*, *oval*, or *horseshoe-shaped cushions*. The sitting person has his greatest weight on one spot, that part of the pelvic bone known as the *tuberosity of the ischium*. In the adult these bones are customarily 4 to 6 in. apart. The inside diameter of a cushion should parallel these bones, or be not more than 2 in. wider. The hole in the center of circular air cushions is generally slightly more than one-third the outside diameter—the 12-in. cushion having a 4½-in. diameter hole, the 16-in. cushion having a 6½-in. opening. Therefore, a 12- to 14-in. diameter air cushion is usually too small. Small air cushions force the bones apart and cause rectal and anal discomfort. If the recommended cushion is too large, the bones are forced together, closing the rectum and anus and causing pain, particularly when hemorrhoids are present. Circular

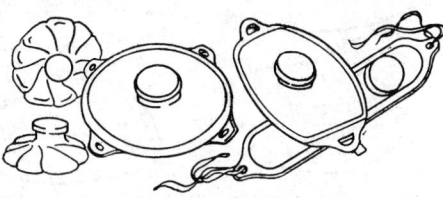

Fig. 911. Icecaps and bags. Left, mackintosh cloth and rubber collapsible icecap; center, icebags; right, spinal and throat icebags.

Fig. 912. Air cushions, circular type, pillow type, and horsehoe style.

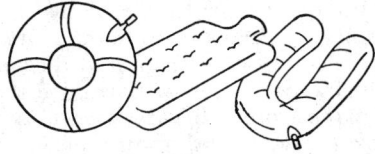

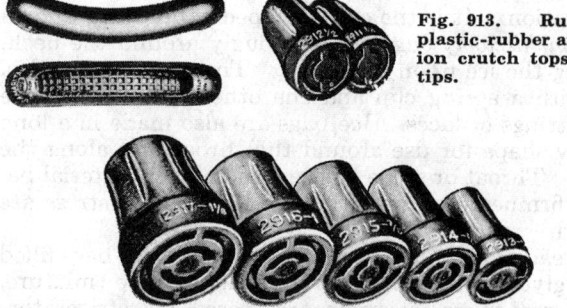

Fig. 913. Rubber or plastic-rubber air cushion crutch tops; cane tips.

Fig. 914. Rubber or plastic crutch tips.

cushions frequently become very warm due to the radiation of heat from the patient's body and the consequent raising of the temperature of the air in the opening.

The horseshoe type of air cushion is preferable because it is flexible and adjustable, conforms better to the body, and provides adequate ventilation. Do not blow air cushions too tight. They will then become quite hard. Inflatable ring or horseshoe-style cushions may be of airtight soft rubber or durable vinyl. Featherweight latex-foam cushions are also available in medium and large sizes, with polyethylene or fabric cover bags. They are available from Davol, Faultless, or others.

Air pillows are used to support the hollow of the back. Sponge rubber cushions are also available for this purpose.

Sponge rubber "dumb-bell" shaped pillows are useful in relieving the weight of the patient's head. Also, large pillows with armrests are used for patients who need support while sitting up in bed.

Crutch pads, *crutch tips*, and *cane tips* of rubber or plastic are frequently-called-for "stock items" in many pharmacies. Pads, molded to fit the crutch head, usually have inside grill design to provide an air cushion. Crutch tips usually are supplied ⅝ to 1⅛ in. inside diameter, cane tips are ⅜ in. and ½ in. diameter. Finger "cots" or pads of rubber are supplied in various sizes.

Suppliers of all types of rubber and plastic sundries include Davol, Goodrich, and Faultless.

Feeding Cups—Of the various types of feeding instruments the glass or porcelain feeding cups are the most commonly employed. Those with a long spout are superior and avoid spilling or leakage. Feeding instruments are a necessity for bedridden patients. Either bent or straight glass tubes are frequently prescribed. Cellulose acetate or plastic straws also serve today to meet this problem (Fig. 915).

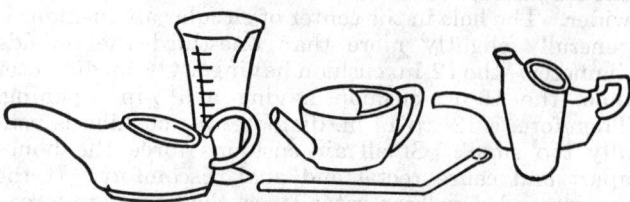

Fig. 915. Feeding cups, graduate, and glass or plastic "straw."

Collection of Excreta—The collection and sanitary removal of excreta and body discharges are an important health problem in the sickroom and hospital. Pharmacies should stock receptacles for the collection of excreta and discharges. There are three principal types of normal discharges from the body: *urine* from the kidneys, *sputum* from the mouth, and *feces* from the intestines. An abnormal discharge

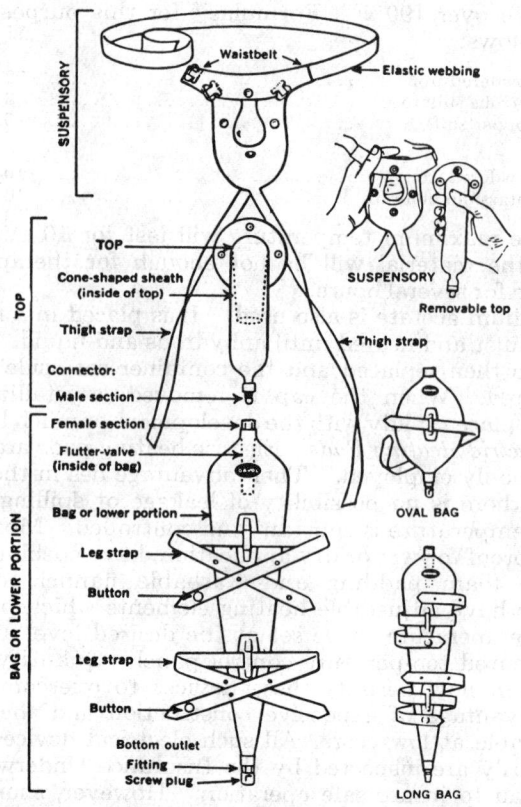

Fig. 916. Nomenclature of urinal components (Davol).

which may appear at any location on the body is *pus* which consists of broken tissue elements and microorganisms.

A very valuable publication has been prepared by Bergstrom and Grendahl.[34]

Urinals—These containers are employed to collect urine. They differ in shape according to male or female use. They are ordinarily made of glass, agateware, or white enamelware (Fig. 917). The latter are light and durable. Hospitals frequently employ glass urinals which facilitate close examination. Occasionally, glass urinals may be calibrated to facilitate measurement of the volume of urine. Urinals are readily cleaned by washing, and sterilized with the usual sterilizing solutions. Rubber urinals, to be worn by the patient, strapped to the leg, are also available (Figs. 918, 919, and 920). This type of urinal is becoming more widely used and is available in a number of different styles. The selection of any one style is usually a matter of personal preference or physician's recommendation.

The complete urinal consists of two parts, the top fitting portion, and the lower bag. Special drip urinals for patients suffering from partial incontinence comprise only the top with an outlet drain plug.

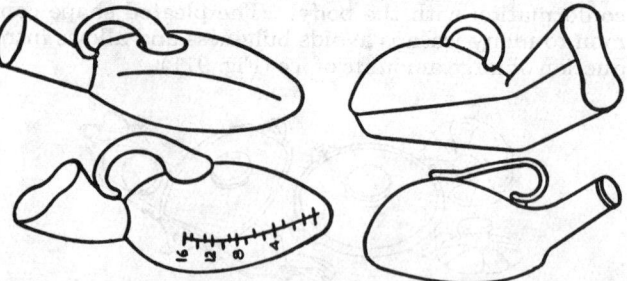

Fig. 917. Urinals, upper left, glass male type; lower left, glass female type with graduated scale; upper right, enamelware female type; lower right, galvanized iron male type.

Urinals for males are for wear during the day or night, while erect or reclining, asleep or awake. Female urinals are for use when the body is in an upright position, standing or walking (Fig. 920).

Male urinals for night use have a sheath in the top to prevent back flow of urine. All urinals have another valve at the inlet of the lower bag to prevent back flow.

Urinal bags come in different capacities, and two styles, long and oval-short. A bag may be emptied easily by a half turn of its outlet cap. Adjustable, elastic leg straps hold the bag against the leg, where it is not conspicuous. Urinals are supplied by Dean,

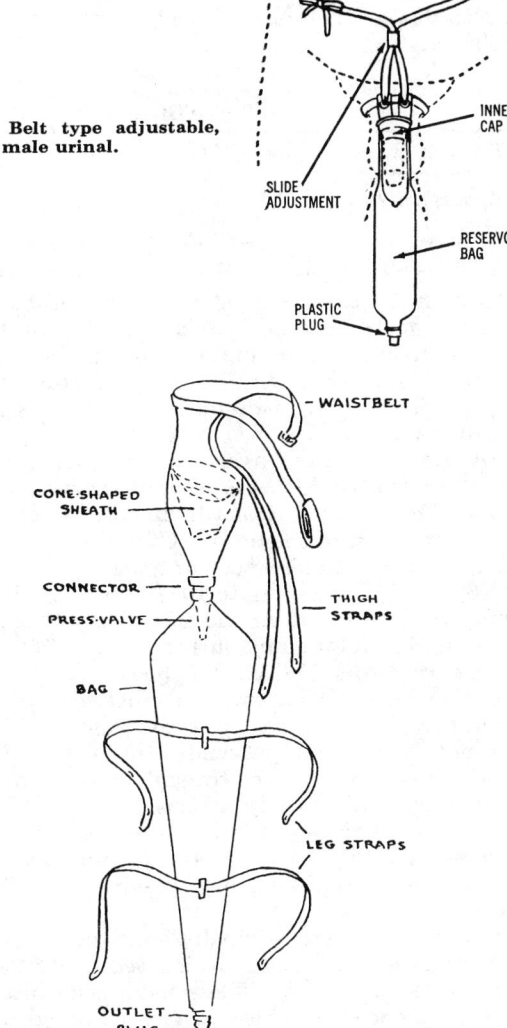

Fig. 918. Belt type adjustable, leakproof, male urinal.

Fig. 919. Male suspensory urinary, Davol type.

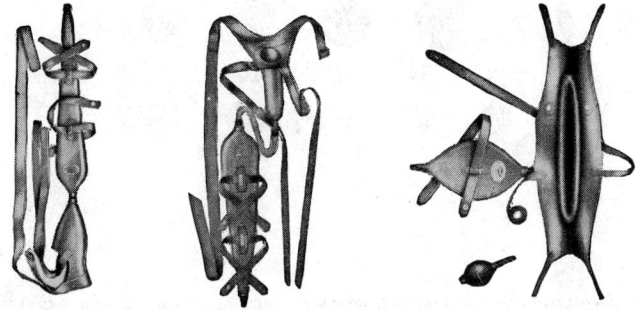

Fig. 920. Types of urinals for ambulatory patients. Male urinals (left and center) and female urinal (right).

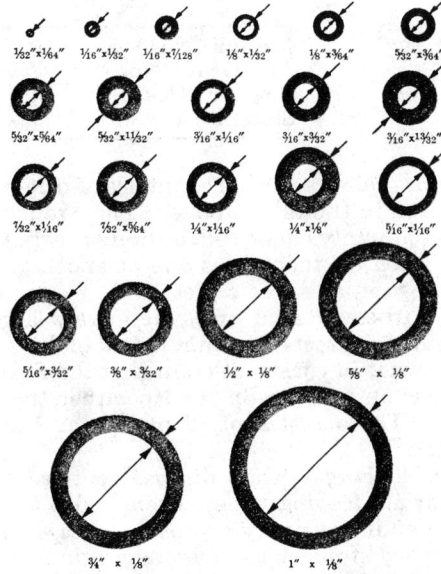

Fig. 921. Actual diameter and thickness of standard medical tubing.

United Surgical, and Davol. The *Weimer Urinal* of the United Surgical Supplies Co., is leakproof, comfortable, and easy to apply. The Dean device is noted for its convenience.

Davol also offers a special *Raiche Drain* for female incontinence, for intermittent drainage, or with urine reservoir for constant drainage. It is for use while upright or reclining. The top is an indwelling inflated balloon type to insure seal of the urethra.

Incontinence—Available are body-contoured incontinence pants for men, women, and children of all ages and sizes. Most are of outer soft fabric with plastic or rubber inner surfaces, which remain soft, pliable, and sanitary after repeated washings or even boiling. Bacteria-resistant flannel controls odor, mold, mildew, and bacterial growth. These garments are provided with snap-in flannel or other absorbent fillers. Elasticized waist and legs prevent leakage.

Catheters—To collect urine from the bladder of the patient unable to void naturally, catheters are employed. Nonflexible catheters of glass, or of metals such as silver, are used for females but are rarely employed in males except for special diseases or where constriction of the urethra has occurred. They are narrowly limited in use. The flexible soft rubber type is commonly preferred for male patients.

The insertion of catheters is a dangerous procedure customarily handled by physicians. Serious infections of the bladder and damage to the urethral and bladder tissues may result from improper insertion.

Flexible soft rubber catheters consist of small rubber tubes with a closed solid tip. At one end is a flaring funnel-shaped opening to facilitate attachment of the catheter to a glass junction or another tube. The central channel opens for entry of urine through a wide opening near the other end. Catheters of rubber with tiny balloon attachments near the tip enable the prolonged insertion of a catheter in the urethra and bladder where the patient is bed-ridden. These are termed *balloon catheters* (Fig. 924). Newer modifications of the balloon catheter are more desirable, such as the *Bardex Foley Catheter*, which provides consistent, dependable performance as it expands in an area just short of the tip. It is supplied by Bard. Varying in size, the diameter of catheters has not been formally standardized. The three chief scales used for catheters have been

Catheter Scales

French (Nos.)	10	12	14	16	18	20	22
American (Nos.)	7	8	10	11	12	14	15
English (Nos.)	4	5	6	7	9	11	12
Size (in.)	$13/100$	$15/100$	$18/100$	$20/100$	$23/100$	$26/100$	$29/100$

named from their respective countries of origin. They are compared in the table above. The French scale is the most commonly employed, although catheters may bear imprinted on their sides one or another, or even scale readings in all three styles.

Rectal Tubes—Rectal tubes are merely larger catheters intended for rectal use in removal of feces. They differ somewhat in construction in that the flexible rubber tube has an opening on the tip rather than on the side only. Three scales of diameters are employed. See Fig. 923.

Hospital Tubing—Other disposable plastic tubing includes sterile feeding tubes, French size 5 to 8 and from 15 to 42 in.; urinary drainage tubes with $3/16$- or $9/32$-in. lumen; stomach tubes for aspiration of stomach content and for feeding, French scale 12 to 18 and 50 in. in length; rectal or enema tubes for gas expulsion (French 24, 20 in.) or colonic evacuation (French 24, 60 in.); and sterile suction tubes (French 10 to 18, 22 in.) with nylon adapters. In addition there are oxygen, sterile extension, and connecting tubes.

The medical grade vinyl tubing is used for intubation, spinal and epidural anesthesia, intravenous infusion, perfusion, and general fluid transfers. A medical grade polyethylene tubing is used for intubation, arterial and aortic catheterization, intravenous and intra-arterial infusion, and arteriography. It is white and opaque. Polypropylene tubing, stiffer but workable, is used for cardiac intubation. Medical grade Teflon translucent tubing is noncompliant, and used for pressure recording and injection. A medical grade silicone tubing is translucent and elastic for IV use, and blood handling, where ultimate nonreactivity and nontoxicity are desired.

Blood Collecting Equipment—Sterile disposable blood donor sets comprising intravenous needles, stopper-puncturing needle, holder clamp, and tubing are available as units. For this and other purposes, disposable plastic tubing is provided, medical grade polyethylene or vinyl tubing, and vinyl laboratory tubing. These medical grade tubings preclude basic incompatibility between materials used and human tissue. They are tested for toxicity, skin reactivity, tissue sensitivity, and pyrogenicity.

The polyethylene tubing is generally available in 12- to 36-in. length and 0.25- to 2.67-mm diameter. The medical vinyl is available from 0.51- to 7.93-mm diameter and up to 48 in. in length.

Rectal Tube Scales

French (Nos.)	22	24	26	28	30	32
American (Nos.)	15	16	17	19	20	21
English (Nos.)	12	14	15	17	18	20
Size (in.)	$9/32$	$10/32$	$10.5/32$	$11/32$	$12/32$	$13/32$

Colon Tubes—These are large rectal tubes, employed for the removal of feces from the lower colon. See Fig. 923. Their size varies according to the scales as follows:

Colon Tube Scales

French (Nos.)	30	32	34
American (Nos.)	20	21	22
English (Nos.)	18	20	21
Size (in.)	$12/32$	$13/32$	$14/32$

Duodenal Tubes—Duodenal tubes, rubber or plastic tubes of 48-in. length over-all, are supplied with glass connector. Opaque to x-ray, the tubes are marked 4 in. apart beginning $17\frac{1}{2}$ in. from distal tip. They are measured in diameter on the French scale from 10 to 20.

Pus Basins—Pus basins, *emesis basins*, *discharge basins*, or *kidney basins* are small curved elongated basins of a kidney shape which permits them to fit close to any part of the body. Of white enamel, monel metal, plastic, stainless steel, or glass, they vary in size from $6\frac{1}{2} \times 5\frac{1}{2} \times 1\frac{1}{2}$ in. to $10\frac{3}{4} \times 5 \times 2\frac{1}{4}$ in. These basins are very useful in the sickroom or hospital and can be employed for many purposes (Fig. 927).

Sputum Cups—While the chief duty of the physician is to cure his patient, he must also protect the community from his patient's contagion. The public does not generally appreciate the fact that many diseases may be spread through mouth discharges. Sputum cups are usually associated with tuberculosis by the laity. However, other diseases which may be conveyed in this manner are pneumonia, measles, scarlet fever, diphtheria, and possibly infantile paralysis.

Sputum cups were originally constructed of enamelware, porcelain, or metal, which required sterilization by chemical solutions. These have been discarded in favor of paper cups which can be disposed of readily

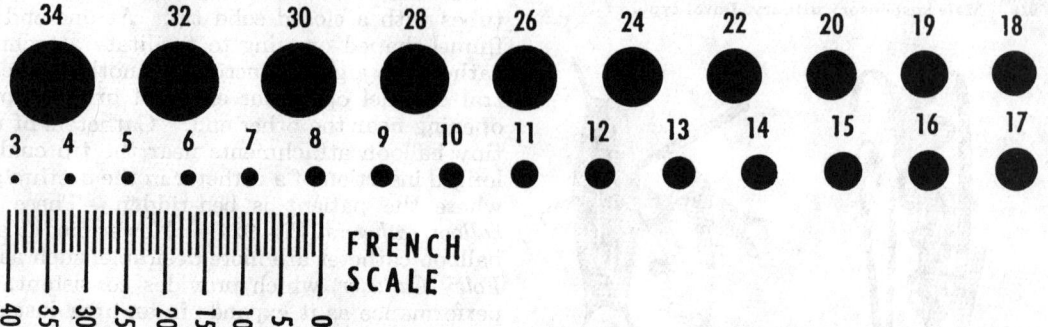

Fig. 922.   Standard French Scale for hospital tubing, catheters, rectal and colon, stomach feeding, suction, urinary drainage and oxygen tubes (courtesy, Becton-Dickinson). To determine French size if instruments are oval or other shape, use strip of paper to measure the periphery—then lay on the scale at the left.

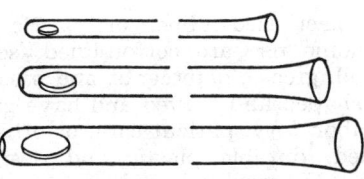

Fig. 923. Rubber catheter (above); rubber rectal tube (center); rubber colon tube (bottom).

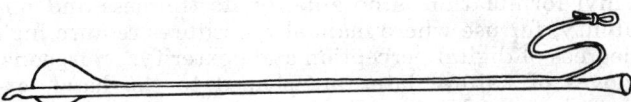

Fig. 924. Balloon catheter, for prolonged insertion through the urethra into the bladder.

by burning. Such waterproof paper sputum cups customarily have paper or metal lids for esthetic reasons.

Bedpans and Douche Pans—For the collection of feces, bedpans are employed. They may be round, oval, or of the special "individual shaped" type. The round type has been succeeded by the oval which is more comfortable, and by the "individual" which is more efficient. Bedpans are constructed of enamelware, plastic, porcelain, or rubber. A soft, red-rubber, inflatable bedpan like an invalid cushion, is also available (Davol), reinforced rubber bottom, drainage tube and bulb and tube for inflation, over-all opening 4½ in. × 8 in. and outside 14 in. × 16 inches. The inflatable, rubber bedpan is far more comfortable than those made from metal or porcelain and is recommended especially for the use of bed-ridden patients. There is also available a smaller, sloping, flatter fracture bedpan for use with immobilized or overweight patients. Glass bedpans are uncommon, because they are breakable and unesthetic. Bedpans frequently have covers for preserving the feces for later examination by the physician or pathologist.

Douche pans of enamelware, plastic, or porcelain are employed for the collection of washes or solutions following administration of a medicated douche (see Fig. 927).

Other frequently requested items for the sick room for patient care are wash basins, oval foot basins, buckets and covers, sponge bowls, solution bowls, beakers, iodine cups, funnels, applicator and thermometer jars, pitchers, dressing jars with lids, and instrument trays in metal, plastic or glass. (Vollrath is a supplier of such medical ware.)

Ostomy Products—Pharmacists frequently find it necessary to service the needs of patients who have undergone surgical treatment and removal of certain of their internal organs with resultant surgical formation of an ostomy.

The word "ostomy," as it applies to intestinal or bladder surgery, has been in use for a few years. As it relates to this type of surgery, it is a contraction of several words, ie, *dry colostomy, ileostomy, cutaneous ureterostomy, wet colostomy* with ureteral transplants, and *ileal-bladder* where both ureters are brought to an inside sack created from tissue of the small intestine (ileum). "Ostomy," as used today, can be, or have to do with any of these operations. An ostomy patient, therefore, is one who has undergone any one of the operations mentioned. An "ostomy product" is one

that is made for the specific use of a patient who has had the type of surgery that creates an artificial opening in the body for drainage from the kidney, the small intestines, or the colon.

An "ostomy product" consists mainly of a specially shaped and fitted ring surrounding the artificially created body opening. A cup covers the ring and attached to it is provision for drainage into a portable, attached receptacle or for removal and dispersion on suitable occasions. The ring is generally of soft rubber or plastic material, the cup of metal or plastic and the container of rubber or polyethylene plastic. A number of different models of ostomy products are available, suited to the patient's surgical reconstruction. See Figs. 928–930.

Pharmacists should be familiar with these devices and be in a position to advise patients, where necessary, and to provide complete products or parts and give the necessary information concerning irrigation, cleaning, and proper fitting.

A most informative technical discussion of the subject is the article, "Self Care for Patients—Learning Colostomy Control."[35]

Very informative and encouraging booklets for the patient are *The Management of a Colostomy* (Davol) and *A Message to All New Ileostomy, Colostomy and Ileal-Bladder Patients* by Wayne Brubaker (United Surgical). Pharmacists should have quantities on hand for distribution to the public; and, for the pharmacist, the following publications are available from United Surgical: *Instruction Manual for all of the Colostomies, United Ostomy Educational Folder, Miniature Visual Ostomy Demonstrator*, and *Instructions for the Deddish Colostomy Irrigator*.

Ostomy products and devices, stoma pads, disposable bags, lubricants, lotions, deodorants, and other articles, and full information as to their use may be obtained from United Surgical, Davol, and others.

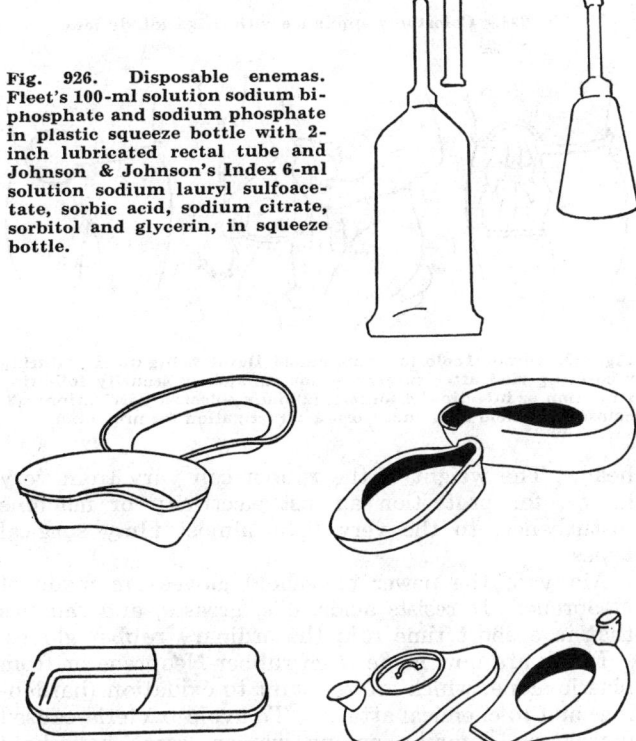

Fig. 926. Disposable enemas. Fleet's 100-ml solution sodium biphosphate and sodium phosphate in plastic squeeze bottle with 2-inch lubricated rectal tube and Johnson & Johnson's Index 6-ml solution sodium lauryl sulfoacetate, sorbic acid, sodium citrate, sorbitol and glycerin, in squeeze bottle.

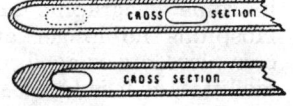

Fig. 925. Cross-section views of colon tubes (above) with dual-spaced openings, and rectal tubes (below).

Fig. 927. Pus or emesis basins (upper left); bed pans (upper and lower right); douche pan (lower left).

With the usual colostomy and ileostomy appliance, in addition to the rubber or plastic frame, belts, and rings, rubber or disposable plastic bags are supplied and surgical adhesive, and antiseptic, deodorant soap.

Rubber Gloves—Rubber or household gloves have become standard basic items in baby care and in the sickroom.

Household rubber and rubber–plastic gloves are essential. Modern styles have naturally shaped fingers to lessen fatigue and extra fullness at the knuckles for comfort. Fitted wrists prevent bunch-up and reversible cuffs protect from dripping when working over-

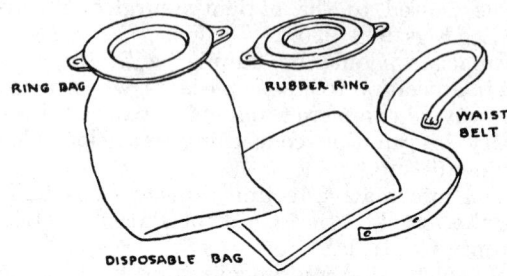

Fig. 928. Colostomy appliance, Davol type.

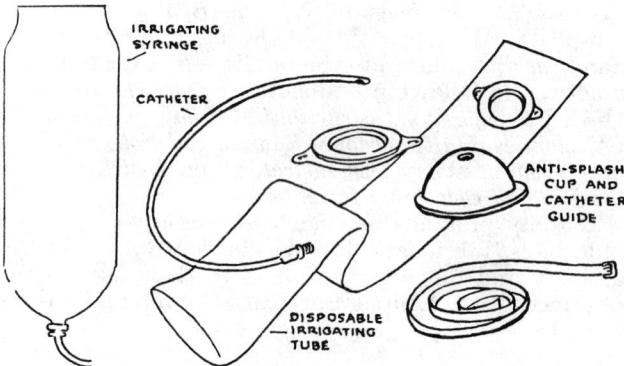

Fig. 929. Colostomy appliance with irrigation devices.

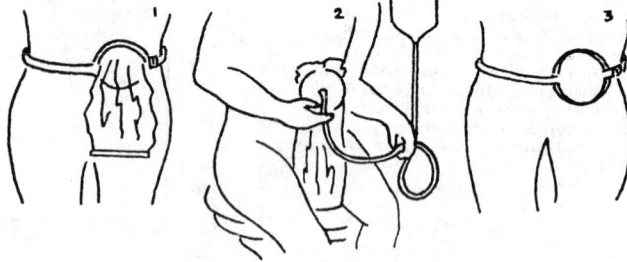

Fig. 930. Disposal colostomy appliance (Davol) being worn (1) during recovery period after surgery or for emergency security following irrigation or intestinal disorder; (2) daily colostomy irrigation; (3) colostomy shield appliance worn after irrigation for protection.

head. The weight of the rubber can vary from very heavy, for protection against electricity or machine disturbance, to the very light almost filmy surgical types.

Many of the newer household gloves are made of Neoprene. It resists acids, oils, greases, and caustics that in a short time ruin the ordinary rubber gloves.

Many are now made from rubber-Neoprene or from plastic alone, which are resistant to oxidation (hardening) and to chemical attack. To avoid bacteria-caused dermatitis, common among women, some household gloves are impregnated with hexachlorophene or other antiseptics.

Ordinary plasticized-rubber or plastic (Neoprene) gloves for home use are cotton-lined, soft and impervious to oil, grease, detergents, and most chemicals. Fingers are shaped and curved and have grid surfaces. Gloves for laboratory, patient care, or other use are of tough seamed, durable plastic and designed to fit either hand. Disposable vinyl examination gloves, designed to fit either hand, are molded to provide a tight skin fit, maximum comfort, and sensitivity. The vinyl formulation is notable for its thinness and pliability, for use where manual procedures require high degrees of digital perception and dexterity. Surgeons' gloves of natural latex are shaped to the hand, extremely rugged but medium weight, usually with rolled wrist. The latter are usually available in glove sizes 6 to 10, while other gloves are offered in small (7 and 7½), medium (8 and 8½), and large (9).

Another glove development is a rough surface on the palms and fingers that reduces substantially the chances of dropping soapy or wet items. For the housewife who objects to the feel of rubber gloves, there are three new types of treatment to the inside of household gloves. Some are now permanently satinized inside, others have a flock lining which gives them a dress glove feeling, and some of the finer gloves actually have a knit cloth lining inside that gives the greatest possible comfort to the hands. But the basic reason for all of these treatments is to make the gloves easy to put on and remove without talcum.

Since rubber or Neoprene gloves can be boiled with the other items that the housewife is sterilizing, she can be sure that the baby or sick person is not exposed to organisms that may be carried on her hands. During sickroom care the attendant eliminates chances of picking up communicable bacteria that might be transferred to friends or members of the family.

Allergy Masks—Allergy masks made of soft urethane foam shaped to conform to facial contour and with head straps afford protection against dust, pollen, and sprays for sensitive allergic patients. Washable filters are re-usable.

Invalid and Geriatric Services

Increased life expectancy has produced an increase in the number of aged persons and a corresponding increase in the number of ill and infirm persons in this segment of our population. The number of people of 65 years of age and over is increasing (July 1967) at the rate of 1000/day, and will have risen from 18.8 millions in 1967 in the United States to more than 25 millions in 1980. The growing number of aged persons, the trend toward their greater subsidization, and the rapid increase in nursing homes portends an ever increasing number of potential candidates for sickroom supplies and convalescent aids in the future. However, the ills which afflict the aged are not all of the nature to cause hospitalization, or even nursing home care. Many aged persons live at home and are quite capable of attending to their own needs or require only a minimum of assistance from members of the family or the Visiting Nurse services. This is also true of many people who are not aged but are ill or infirm.

Nursing homes do care for a substantial number of such patients, and their capacity is rapidly increasing, in some geographic areas in excess of actual need. Hospitals no longer attempt to provide services to convalescents or aged patients not in need of acute care facilities, as it is too costly for the patient and hospital, especially in efficient utilization of the latter's extremely limited and expensive personnel. As a result, the trend is to transfer the patient to home care as soon as possible. This is creating a growing demand upon some community pharmacies for surgical appliances and sick-room needs.

Professional Approach—Not every pharmacist should hastily conclude that he will be successful in this field, regardless of his estimate of the local market, his inventory, and his display facilities. Unless the pharmacist is willing to devote time and intelligent effort to the venture, he may fail. He must be interested in helping the aged, infirm, sick patients. His attitude must be professional and his approach to the prospective referring physicians and the public must be made on that basis, not on mere availability or price. If he is willing to accept the responsibilities, put in the investment, and promote his service, success will come to him.

The surgical supply department is recognized by physician and layman alike as a most professional extension of the pharmacist's professional service. The physician quickly learns to depend on it, and the much talked of and sought after relationship of "consultant to the physician" comes to the pharmacist in due course.

Volume of Service—The volume of sale of such supplies, devices, and appliances is large and growing rapidly. More than $270 million was expended in pharmacies in 1967 for such items, and an almost equal amount in non-pharmaceutical supply houses and hospitals. Important is the fact that the average purchase of such items is $25, with sales of $100 to $150 not unusual. Through such lines, the margin of gross profit is 50 to 60%. Of course, the service of selection and fitting is either a part of that profit margin, or in some instances pharmacists charge a fitting fee in addition.

In the average pharmacy, 30.2% of the volume of sale of such items comes from physicians' prescriptions or referrals. In the specializing surgical supply pharmacy, the physician is responsible for 40.5%.

Other Opportunities—Aside from patients coming to the pharmacy for supplies and appliances, there are three other major market areas which should be developed, no matter how difficult and competitive. These are the community physicians, small industrial plants, and clinics and nursing homes. The average physician sees 27 patients a day (geriatric specialists see 29 daily), and purchases over $230 worth of surgical supplies annually. Most industrial plants of from 4 to 499 employees are large users of supplies, and most prefer to buy their needs locally. There were in 1966 1.6 million such industries in the country (*Statistical Abstract of the US*, 1968), and another 1.94 million firms with 3 or less employees. Clinics and nursing homes rank in between in volume in a community, and are stable, prompt-paying customers. In 1963 more than a half million older citizens lived in 13,514 nursing homes, figures which are estimated to have almost doubled by 1969. Extended-care facilities in 1967 numbered an additional 3,669 units, with 262 thousand beds (*Statistical Abstract of the US, 1968*).

Sources of Supply—Pharmacists can obtain fine quality and complete lines of various types of surgical supplies from numerous sources, although some surgical trade companies refuse or are reluctant to supply pharmacists at first. This is because of the inclination of many retail druggists to "cut" prices on these items as they do, unfortunately, on ordinary merchandise.

Most leading pharmacist suppliers have found that this is not necessary or desirable, nor is it necessary to sell supplies to physicians at or near cost.

As a check list of such items Table III may help the interested pharmacist.

Sixty-six to 90% of all such supplies and appliances are prescribed or ordered by the physician. Yet department stores, mail order houses and even supermarkets are now getting some sales volume.

A 1962 survey of several hundred prescription pharmacies showed that the larger the prescription volume the better the chances for surgical business. Among those doing 40% or more of their volume in prescriptions, two out of three were selling over $1000 per year in surgical supplies, and 40% of those were gaining over $2500 per year. Presented another way, of the 40% prescription volume pharmacies, half were doing better than 4% of their volume in surgical supplies and 16% were enjoying better than 10% of their volume from this source.

The larger the pharmacy's total volume, the better its chances to succeed in surgical supplies. Pharmacies grossing annually $150,000 or more showed half doing better than $2500 in surgical supplies, and another 33% gaining from $1000 to $2500 per year. For smaller volume pharmacies, the number enjoying these volumes of sales were 33% and 29%, respectively.

Pharmacists should obtain and carefully study the available literature which deals with the market before making any decision as to entrance into it. Some of these publications are: "Expanding Surgical Appliances in Your Pharmacy,"[36] Expanding Pharmacy's Health Services,"[37] Selling Surgical Accessories and Sickroom Needs,"[38] "Sales and Rentals of Invalid Equipment in a Professional Pharmacy,"[39] "The Orthotic Support and Appliance Market,"[40] "The Development and Operation of the Medical Appliance Aspect of the Retail Pharmacy."[41]

Trusses and Orthopedic Aids

The handling of sales of trusses, suspensories, foot, ankle, and wrist supporters, rubber and other elastic stockings, belts and supporters, crutches, canes, and invalid chairs properly belongs to the list of specialized services offered by the pharmacist.

Hernias and Trusses—Hernias are as old as mankind. The first trusses were nothing more than a rope or strap and a rock. Celsus developed the use of a plate and in medieval times a form of plaster and plate were used. The spring and belt type truss, practically as it is today in principle, was developed by the Netherlands physician Camper in 1785.

Abdominal hernias are exceedingly common. Infants in the first year of life show an incidence of 19.6/1000. Between ages 20 and 24, the incidence is lowest, rising to 24.2/1000 in the 70 to 74 age group.

Of all males afflicted with hernias, 96% suffer from the inguinal type, the corresponding incidence among females being 44.3%. A hernia may undergo a spontaneous cure, but on the other hand, strangulation is a frequent occurrence and one which requires quick and forceful surgical action.

The pharmacist should visit an established "surgical pharmacy" and discuss with his colleague there the latter's problems, procedures, and experiences with the sale of such items. He should study carefully the available literature on the fitting, use, and characteristics of appliances and aids.

The pharmacist who will be in charge of the service

and department may well benefit from attending a fitting school conducted by one of the appliance manufacturers. This requires time and travel but it firmly grounds the pharmacist in the anatomy involved. Such courses for pharmacists are given by Horn & Bro. and by OTC.

These courses are given at intervals throughout the year and train the pharmacist or his assistant on the definition, location, varieties, frequency, symptoms, predisposing and direct causes, complications, prognosis, treatment, and anticipated results in:

Hernia —inguinal, scrotal, femoral, umbilical, ventral, labical and irreducible	Sacro-lumbar support
	Dorso-lumbar support
	Varicocele, hydrocele support
Postoperative support	Varicose veins
Ptosis, uterine support	Sprains, swellings
Obesity support	Dislocations
Postnatal support	Fractures
Sacro-iliac support	Conditions requiring traction

Reference should be made by every interested pharmacist to the literature available from the appliance manufacturers, such as: *Physical Requirements for a Professional Surgical Appliance Department in Todays Pharmacy* (OTC), *Surgical Appliances in Your Pharmacy* (OTC), *The Faultless Way* (Faultless), and *Make Customers Stop-by Promotions.*[42] There are also several texts which should be in the Pharmacy's library.[43, 44]

Inguinal and Umbilical Trusses for infants, of gum rubber, are occasionally called for. Inguinal devices, with button fasteners for adjustment, are available in single right or left, or double, in three sizes, 10 to 12 inches, 14 to 16 inches, and 18 to 22 inches. Umbilical trusses also are available in 3 sizes.

Supports and Suspensories—In the male, arduous physical work and exercise require supportive assistance for the scrotum and penis and the back and abdomen. Of elastic webbing, made of yarn-covered rubber thread or nylon, athletic supports provide an upward and inward lift. Available in three sizes (waist measurements 26–32, 32–38, and 38–44) some have light-weight straps and narrow waistband, others heavier tailored stretch bands with removable stays.

Suspensories are frequently prescribed, in four sizes, with adjustable nonelastic waistband, adjusting elastic strip in yoke or drawstring, and cotton-mesh pouch held by diagonal pull from the sides. These items are available from a number of suppliers such as Bauer & Black, J & J, Horn & Bro., OTC, Jung, Ritter, Camp, and others.

Wristlets—For sprained wrists, tenosynovitis, or wrist injuries of any kind, the physician frequently prescribes a wristlet. These may be of leather, with straps and buckles, or leather or cotton laces to insure adequate rigidity, or more popularly rubber, rubberized fabric or specially woven cotton. They are used in place of elastic bandages. Wristlets have side openings as thumb openings for use on the hand itself; with a second wristlet an excellent pressure bandage is supplied. A temporary splint for the wrist can be provided by slipping a tongue depressor under the hand and another over the hand. A wristlet on the foot with the opening at the heel and a second one over the arch or ankle provides good arch support. Athletes are frequent customers for wristlets. Knee braces and knee supports are also in frequent demand when the tendons and ligaments which usually stabilize the knee become deficient because of injury or disease. These items are available from many sources, such as Baka.

Elastic and Support Stockings—Six of every ten women and four of every ten men suffer from varicose

veins at some time in their lives. It is not a condition affecting only older people. One fifth of sufferers begin to have trouble in their early 20's and many women under 30 years of age begin to develop varicose veins.

When the human body is subjected to strains over prolonged periods of time, such as a clerk in a store who is on her feet all day—or a pharmacist, the leg veins enlarge as it becomes increasingly difficult for the heart to pump the blood from the extremities. The veins, most often directly under the skin, show as bluish cords, knots or sacs, due to stagnating waste-laden blood. As the veins swell, pain increases with fatigue, the vein walls stretch and the valves leak. If untreated or unsupported, the veins protrude, rupture, ulcerate, and may cause an embolism.

Varicose veins are also frequently observed in expectant mothers. Overweight individuals also tend to the condition, naturally or when they affect tight girdles. Tight leg garters may also cause problems.

For many years patients employed ordinary bandages to provide support for varicose veins. With the advent of wide knitted or elastic bandages, these replaced the older forms. Then, because of the esthetic problem, women demanded some other form of support, and special hose were supplied.* At first these were bulky, of woven rubberized fabric and unsatisfactory. Now various styles of hosiery are generally employed which are more acceptable. Depending on the condition of the patient, the physician will determine the degree of support from the elastic stockings that is indicated. Mild cases where prophylactic support is desired to assist fluid dynamics or post phlebitis syndrome usually only require support. Simple varicose veins and chronic venous insufficiency are more serious matters and demand special treatment. It is a matter of holding power or uniformity and amount of pressure to be exerted on the protruding veins.

Today a range of stockings is available which provide styles ideal for street or social wear, being fully fashioned, seamless, and of sheer nylon, or nylon and cotton, comfortable, easy to launder, and will not discolor. White stockings of these types are available for nurses. Knee-length, seamless elastic hosiery for men has recently been introduced and has also become popular with women for wear with bermuda shorts or slacks. There are also available less expensive stockings for home wear, alone or under other stockings, and heavier forms for wear where the condition requires extreme pressure.

Elastic stockings are fitted by measuring the circumference of the thigh, knee, calf and ankle, and the length of the leg, from base of heel to 5 inches above the knee. Sizes are designated as small (S), medium (M), large (L), medium extra length (MXL), and large extra length (LXL). The foot style may be above or below knee or thigh length, open toe or full foot.

Space here does not permit a more detailed discussion of elastic support hose. However, for additional information† on the historical aspect, anatomical considerations, and etiologic factors of compression therapy in varicose veins, and other data of value in the fitting and marketing of elastic hose for men and women, the pharmacist is referred to the helpful literature available from manufacturers.

---

* Literature on elastic stockings for the layman is available from Horn & Bro., Bauer & Black, and Ritter.

† *Orthopedic Therapeutic Corrective Professional Appliances* (OTC) and *Elastic Stocking Compression in the Therapy of Varicose Veins* (Kendall), with bibliography.

Developing a Full Professional Service

Surgical supports and orthopedic appliances, commodes, walkers, wheelchairs, oxygen apparatus, hospital beds, and traction and other corrective devices are also prescribed by physicians. Although the physician's prescription or order may specify the brand or model number of the appliance, it is almost always necessary for the pharmacist to personally demonstrate or fit the device to insure its appropriateness and patient acceptability.

It was estimated that in 1962 more than $219 million was expended by the public for all individual health supports, including surgical and orthopedic supports and accessory items. Of $66 million spent for surgical elastic goods in that year only 32% was received by pharmacists. A study (S. H. Camp and Co., Jackson, Mich.) indicated that the market for back and abdominal supports, maternity supports and girdles, orthopedic and corrective supports, braces and collars, traction apparatus and breast prostheses amounted to over $80 million annually.

Abdominal and postoperative supports are used chiefly (60 to 65%) by females. They are distributed to them 28.2% through department stores, 21.0% by surgical dealers, and only 7.2% by pharmacies. Corset shops (14.1%), mail order houses (18.2%), and physicians (5.2%) and other outlets account for the rest.

Orthopedic and corrective supports are about equally divided between men and women, and surgical dealers supply about one-third of each. Mail order houses supply 16.2%, corset shops supply 13.5%, and pharmacies and department stores each supply 10.8%.

Five-sixths of all elastic stockings are purchased by women. Department stores gain 31%, pharmacies and surgical dealers equally divide 45%, while supermarkets sell 10% of the remaining 24%.

Two-thirds of all braces and collars are bought by men, all on physicians' prescriptions. Surgical dealers account for 35%. Thirty per cent are supplied by brace shops and 23% by physicians. Pharmacies supply only 12%.

Pharmacies do better with trusses, 91% of which are used by men. Pharmacies supply 30% but mail order houses sell 41%. Surgical dealers supply only 17%. The rest are supplied by various other dealers.

When considering the establishment of a full-line invalid, surgical, and sickroom supply department, the community pharmacist must be careful to evaluate the needs of his neighborhood or area, and determine if at present they are being cared for adequately. His interest should be in response in part to a demand for such aids and services. He should study his location, as to proximity to other suppliers, to a medical building, and to a hospital. Will patients travel to the pharmacy or must the fitter go to the home? How well does the pharmacist know the physicians? What about deliveries and returns?

When the pharmacist is ready to provide service, he will have to promote it to the physicians, usually in person, and to the public. It will take time, as both physician and patient must have built up their confidence in the pharmacist's ability, knowledge, and extent of service and stock. The latter is important, for in usually needed sizes and types of simple sickroom and surgical appliances, the initial inventory may well represent an investment of several thousand dollars. In patient aids, walkers, crutches, and other items, a minimal inventory may well exceed that figure. The pharmacist can usually obtain out-sizes or unusual items readily from wholesale suppliers or direct from their sources. However, he must remember that the patient is ill and wants immediate relief. Delays are detrimental to patient and physician confidence.

Keep a service record by patient, with data on physician's instructions, appliances fitted, reorders or repairs, for reference but as well for follow-up at intervals. Also keep a record by physician as a key to increase or decrease in volume of orders.

The Fitting Room—For such a department, an adequate *private* fitting room and stock space nearby are absolutely necessary. The fitting room or rooms may be no more than 8 feet x 8 feet, soundproof, clean, and free of any stock or display, with an inward swinging door to shield the fitting table from view. As most fittings are done with the patient in a horizontal position, a table 72 × 26 × 30 in. high, padded with moistureproof covering and a pillow is needed. A hinged, center drop leaf is useful. Also needed are a chair, clothes tree, small dressing table and mirror, and a four-legged stool. Professional simplicity and cleanliness are most important. The use of rolled paper on table and floor is practical and economical. A Trendelenberg stand, an angular wedge for under the patient's buttocks, is very useful as well. The device elevates the hips and returns abdominal contents to normal position.

Conveniently near to the fitting room should be the stock. The inventory depends on volume of sales, types and number of physicians prescribing appliances, extent of the pharmacist's promotion, and whether the service is for men only or for both sexes. An estimate of stock space required for each fitting room is about 20 square feet if for men's service, 30 to 40 square feet if for both sexes.

Fitting appliances is a professional service. The pharmacist must treat it and the patient as such. While it is well to have trained women deal with female patients, most fitting of both sexes is by men. Pharmacists fitting appliances today in proper environment almost never experience a complaint or unpleasant occurrence with female patients.

The fitter must impress upon the patient, by manner more than by words, that he is confident and seriously interested in the patient's problem. The latter resents the need for an appliance and wants the whole matter treated most confidentially.

Patient Aids and Comforts—For patient comfort aids, display space must be set aside. In the average prescription pharmacy this is difficult because of the existing excessive demand for space. However, if these items are to be supplied, they must be shown, and either provision made for them by elimination of other nonprofessional stock, or additional adjoining space obtained. Patients and others acting for them will not select these relatively expensive items from catalogs. The features and functions of the items must be demonstrated.

One pharmacist successful in this field has recommended the following as a basic inventory of items of major importance for this department.

    1 wheelchair with adjustable foot and leg rests, brakes
    1 wheelchair with adjustable foot rests, brakes
    1 invalid walker with arm crutches
    1 walkerette
    1 commode
    3 pair adult metal forearm crutches
    6 assorted wooden canes
    1 metal hospital bed with catch spring
    1 orthopedic mattress with plastic cover
    1 pair bedsides
    1 overbed table

In addition to the usual familiar items, air pillows, pads, urinals, ostomy appliances described earlier, together with back and abdominal supports, maternity supports, girdles, corrective supports, braces and collars, hernia trusses, traction appliances, the supplementary supplies may include retention catheters, bed blocks, abdominal and drainage pads, whirlpool baths, bed trays, infusion stands, and oxygen equipment, depending on the ultimate growth of the department's volume.

Standardization of equipment from one or a few sources is important, to allow for ready interchangeable replacement, repair and optional feature parts, especially if a rental service is provided and periodic refurbishing of items becomes necessary.

Many pharmacies rent equipment, with charges depending on the item's initial cost, frequency of use, transportation cost, and the competition. Wheelchairs rented by the month cost from $10 to $50; an invalid walker from $10 to $25 per month, with or without inclusion of delivery and pick-up charges. Other items are in proportion. Commodes and mattresses are not rented. Companion and sequential sales or rentals are customary, as the patient progresses from hospital bed to wheelchair, walker, walkerette, and crutches.

As people usually want the best quality in such items, showing these first rather than the cheaper ones is desirable. Best quality in rental merchandise in the long run is usually more economical as well. A checklist of suggested appliances and materials for home health care rental or sale is provided in Table IV.[45]

Sales and Rentals of Invalid Equipment—Not every pharmacy should have an invalid rental and sales department. The retail sources for invalid equipment are few. In order of their importance, surgical supply houses are probably the largest suppliers; second come rental agencies; and third are such organizations as Sears-Roebuck, Montgomery-Ward, etc. Retail and professional pharmacies are natural outlets, but today they probably rank last as a supplier to the public for these products.

With a small amount of training, any conscientious pharmacist can intelligently inform a prospective buyer about the type of wheel chair an invalid requires, the reason for the selection, and limitations and advantages for the invalid. There are wheelchairs for amputees, chairs for partially paralyzed patients, chairs for patients with fractured extremities, chairs which recline, chairs for the obese patient, electric-powered chairs, youth chairs, chairs for patients from 6 to 16 years, and chairs for patients 3 to 6 years. In addition to this, there are from 10 to 15 features which can be added to any of the forementioned chairs, such as special arm rests, special tires, special foot rests, head rests, restraining and safety straps, special hand rims, and number of accessories which enables an invalid with certain infirmities to operate his or her wheel chair in a more satisfactory manner.

One Oklahoma pharmacy, for instance, has available in stock for rental, wheel chairs, glide-about chairs, invalid walkers, hospital beds with mattresses, bed rails, commode chairs, belt vibrators, trapeze bars, Hoyer lifters, walking aids, buck's extensions, over-door traction, hospital bed table, and Croupaire. This pharmacy established its rental department more than 15 years ago with a relatively small inventory. Recently the inventory comprised 121 pieces on rental and 69 not on rental.

The gross profit margin on equipment for sale is usually 40% or better. If a piece of equipment costs $60.00, the retail price is $100.00. The annual gross profit is figured by multiplying the monthly gross profit figure by 12. This department brings into the pharmacy approximately 50 to 100 people a month who would ordinarily not patronize it.

The department covers 4 to 8 square feet of display area plus one display window showing only wheel chairs and invalid walkers. The promotion of the invalid equipment department is accomplished by newspaper advertising, radio "spot" announcements, a telephone directory "Yellow Page" listing, a sign on the face of the building, and descriptive pamphlets made available by manufacturers.

There are a half dozen major manufacturers of wheel chairs, patient lifters, and invalid walkers, such as Hoyer, whose distributors operate on a nonfranchise basis, such as Everest & Jennings, who then operate through approved dealerships. Others are Cary, Am. Wheel Chair, Colson, DeLucien, Erie, and Gendron (whose products are distributed by Howmet). A most valuable reference booklet by Fahland and Grendahl[46] is available on this subject.

Insurance Protection—As these additional services and responsibilities expand, the pharmacist must be certain that his professional and public liability insurance coverage is increased proportionately. Here the services of an impartial insurance advisor and agent are essential.

Supplies for Diabetic Patients

There is no other disease that over a period of years requires more frequent visits to the pharmacy than *diabetes mellitus*. It is reported that there are over 1½ million diabetics in the United States, who use insulin regularly, and this number is increasing annually. There are also estimated to be nearly 10 million persons suffering from diabetes who are being treated with oral antidiabetic agents or being maintained on diet control. This large and well-defined group requires constant treatment and many medical supplies.

It has been estimated that the average diabetic will make from 24 to 48 trips per year to the pharmacist for insulin alone. This does not take into consideration many other items which the diabetic uses constantly nor does it include his purchases of the many other drugstore commodities he may require.

The family of a diabetic spends 78% more than the nondiabetic family in the drugstore every year, according to a booklet published as a service to pharmacists by Ames called *The Why, Where and How of a Separate Diabetic Department for Your Pharmacy;* the booklet cites the opportunities to be gained with a special department to service the "million or more" known American diabetics.

The pharmacist has a special service opportunity in this specialized field and should be prepared to render intelligent and efficient aid to such patients.

Establishing a Diabetic Department—The items frequently purchased by the diabetic patient should be displayed in a special section of the pharmacy, and all pharmacists meeting physicians and patients interested in diabetic service should be especially and fully instructed so that they have a knowledge of the following:

1. The disease of diabetes.
2. Dietetics and food content.
3. All types of insulin and the synthetic antidiabetic agents.
4. Foods, drugs, and accessories used by the diabetic.

5. Hypodermic equipment, such as the proper sizes of needles and syringes.

6. Testing of urine for sugar.

7. The care and sterilization of syringes and needles.

8. Hypodermic technique.

9. Scales and other diabetic equipment.

10. The common faults that a lay user usually exhibits with diabetic equipment.

Some of the items usually found in a diabetic department are:

Insulin (all strengths and varieties)—kept in a refrigerator
Synthetic Antidiabetic Agents—kept in dispensing stock
Insulin Syringes of assorted types
Insulin Needles (assorted sizes and rustproof)
Insulin Carrying Case
Busher Injector
Isopropyl Alcohol for sterilizing the skin
Absorbent Cotton
Test Sets for sugar and acetone in urine
Saccharin (tablets and the granular form)
Sucaryl, Sweeta or other synthetic sweetening agents
Diet Scale
Diet Charts and books on diabetes
Dusting Powder (for dusting feet of diabetics)
Lanolin Cocoa Butter (for the feet)

Testing for Sugar in Urine—Since an excess of sugar in either the urine or the blood is a danger signal for the diabetic patient, the physician frequently directs the patient to regularly test the urine for sugar. A blood test for sugar is much more complicated, as a sample of blood must be drawn and the sugar content determined by the physician or a trained technician employing special analytical procedures.

However, sugar (glucose) can be detected in urine by a simple test which the pharmacist can teach the patient to conduct at home. A standard test tube is filled to about one-quarter capacity (5 ml) with *Benedict's Qualitative Reagent*. This should be warmed over an alcohol lamp, and not more than 8 to 10 drops of the patient's urine added. Boil for 1 to 2 minutes or keep in boiling water for 5 minutes.

If glucose is present an opaque red, yellow, or green precipitate appears. If no glucose is present, the solution will remain clear or on cooling show a gray flocculent precipitate due to urates.

Test Solutions and Kits—The pharmacist should supply the patient with home test kits, consisting of Benedict's qualitative solution, several tubes, a test tube holder, a test tube brush, and medicine dropper. Pharmacists should have at hand for physician's use *Benedict's Quantitative Reagent*, together with the essential glassware and apparatus.

For home use, Benedict's Reagent has been largely replaced by simple test sets. Some of these indicate only the presence or absence of sugar in the urine while others are useful in determining the percentage, the color developed in the test being matched against a color chart.

For simply determining the presence of abnormal amounts of sugar in the urine, Ames supplies a test set

---

Table IV—Checklist of Appliances and Materials for Home Health Care Rental or Sale[a]

Beds and bed accessories	Wheel chairs, walking aids	Toilet seat extensions
Standard 2 crank hospital beds	Standard wheel chair w/footrests	Shower stools
Hilo 3 crank hospital beds	Standard wheel chair w/legrests	Sitz baths
Electric hospital beds	Junior wheel chair w/footrests	Whirlpool baths
Innerspring mattresses	Junior wheel chair w/legrests	Steam baths
Foam rubber mattresses	Child wheel chair w/footrests	
Safety side rails	Child wheel chair w/legrests	**Automobile items**
Trapeze (clamp on type)	Removable arm wheel chairs	Auto patient lifts
Trapeze (free standing)	Reclining back wheel chairs	Auto back rests
Traction for bed use	Lightweight wheel chairs	Handicapped driver apparatus
Traction for chair, door, etc.	Arthritic wheel chairs (get-abouts)	Stretcher for station wagon
Overbed tables	Geriatric chairs	
Bedside tables	Rolling walkers	**Exercise, massage equipment**
Bed trays	Jump walkers (variety)	Electric cycles
Bed boards	Child's walkers	Manual cycles
Foot stools	Standard crutches (wood, aluminum)	Walking machines
Back rests	Forearm crutches (Canadian)	Rowing machines
Draw sheets	Canes (2, 3, and 4 toed)	Belt vibrators
Bed pans	Canes (large selection)	Massage rollers
Urinals (male and female)	Cane and crutch accessories	Hand massagers
Bedside commodes	Chair cushions	
Rolling commodes	Ring cushions	**Miscellaneous items**
Blanket supports		Paraffin baths
Foot boards	**Inhalation, respiratory items**	Blood pressure machines
Alternating pressure pads	Oxygen	Thermometers
Patient lifts	Oxygen masks and catheters	Hypothermy machines
Perineal lamps	Oxygen tests and canopies	Incontinent garments
Heat lamps	Oxygen emergency kits	Colostomy supplies
Sun lamps	Croup tents	Disinfectants
Hair rinsers	Nebulizers (humidifiers)	Autoclaves
Hair dryers	Dehumidifiers	Stair ramps
Bed wetting device	Pulmonary ventilators (I.P.P.E. for tank)	Waste can liners
Room dividers (screens)	Intermittent pressure breathing equipment	Nurses garments
Intravenous stands	Suction equipment (aspirator)	
Emesis basins	Defibrillators	**Allied items**
Wash basins		Rollaway beds
Sputum cups	**Bathroom items**	Baby beds
Air cleaners	Bath tub patient lift	Baby scales
Air deodorizers	Bath tub safety rails	High chairs
Fans	Grab bars (good selection)	Strollers
	Toilet safety frames	Bed boards

a Courtesy, Institutional Industries, Inc.[45]

called *Clinistix*. For determining both the presence and the percentage of sugar in the urine other test sets consisting of droppers, test tubes, and reagent tablets, are available for the use of the physician or for the home use of patients. Among these are Ames' *Clinitest* and *Uristix* and Lilly's *Tes-tape*.

Of particular interest is the inexpensive kit available under the name of *Selftester*, a modification of the *Clinitest*, designed for home testing for diabetes and developed as a part of a nationwide campaign to discover latent diabetes, by the American Diabetes Association.

Testing for Acetone in Urine—The diabetic patient is also required to make frequent tests at home for the presence of acetone in the urine. For this purpose Ames offers a paper reagent strip, *Ketostix*.

Special Diabetic Foods—The selection of products and items for the diabetic department should have careful consideration, particularly those preparations which are outside the list of actual necessities. In this selection, it is advisable to be guided by the opinions of physicians in your community.

Special diabetic food products are many and varied. Although many physicians now put their diabetic patients on special diets from the table, diabetic foods still have considerable demand. There are different kinds and brands of flour for baking purposes, canned fruits and fruit juices, canned vegetables, specially prepared cookies, crackers, candies, and chewing gum. The extent to which such special diabetic items should be stocked will depend, of course, upon the number of customers as well as upon the preferences of the local physicians.

It must be borne in mind that most special foods contain definite amounts of carbohydrate, protein, and fat, and consequently their food values must be considered in calculating menus. The mere fact that a special bread has a low carbohydrate content is not enough to justify its indiscriminate use by the diabetic patient. Many such breads contain a correspondingly greater protein content, over half of which may be utilized as sugar in the body.

The diabetic's diet is just as important a part of his treatment as his dose of insulin—one must be balanced against the other, and alterations must not be made without consulting the physician in charge.

Too often diabetic patients think of the grocery store as the main source of these special foods while, as a matter of fact, they should be buying them from the pharmacist. Once a diabetic learns that he can purchase special diabetic foods from his local pharmacist, he usually can be depended upon to continue as a customer.

Promotion of the Diabetic Department—In addition to establishing a special Diabetic Department, many pharmacists have increased the sales of diabetic merchandise by personally contacting physicians and informing them of their facilities for serving the needs of diabetics. Special mention of the Diabetic Department can also be made in the store advertising. This affords a means of reaching many diabetic customers who otherwise might not know about these services. A card-index file of all known diabetics may be kept and a letter emphasizing some feature in the department sent periodically. A well coordinated, consistent publicity program directed to both the physicians and the public is certain to bring gratifying results.

Reference Works—In a Diabetic Department the pharmacist should have available and advise the patient to read such publications as the following:

Diabetic Literature

American Diabetes Association, *Diabetes Guide Book*, New York, N. Y. 10017.

Atwater and Bryant, *The Chemical Composition of American Food Materials*, Bulletin No. 28, US Dept. of Agriculture, Washington, D. C.

Bowes, *Food Values of Portions Commonly Used*, College Offset Press, Philadelphia, Pa.

Bradley, *Tables of Food Values*, Manual Arts Press, Peoria, Ill.

Chatfield and McLaughlin, *Proximate Composition of Fresh Fruits*, Circular No. 50, US Dept. of Agriculture, Washington, D.C.

Chatfield and Adams, *Proximate Composition of Fresh Vegetables*, Circular No. 146, US Dept. of Agriculture, Washington, D.C.

Duncan, *Diabetics Mellitus and Obesity*, Lea & Febiger, Philadelphia, Pa.

Duncan, *Modern Pilgrim's Progress for Diabetics*, Saunders, Philadelphia, Pa.

Joslin, *A Diabetic Manual*, Lea & Febiger, Philadelphia, Pa.

Joslin, Root, White and Marble, *The Treatment of Diabetes Mellitus*, Lea & Febiger, Philadelphia, Pa.

Podolsky and Weil, *The Diabetes Specialist*, Allied Medical Publications, New York.

Rudy, *Practical Handbook for Diabetic Patients*, M. Barrows and Co., Boston, Mass.

Sansum, *Diabetes Mellitus*, Harper, New York, N.Y.

Sevringhaus, *Guide for Diabetic Patients*, Pharmacy of the University of Wisconsin Medical Center Hospital, Madison, Wis.

Sindoni, *The Diabetes Handbook*, Ronald Press, New York, N. Y.

Watt and Merrill, *Composition of Foods*, US Dept. of Agriculture, *Agricultural Handbook No. 8*, Washington, D.C.

Williams, *Diabetes*, Paul B. Hoeber, Inc., New York, N.Y.

Other professional educational material on diabetes that is available are the following:

Diabetes, The Journal of the American Diabetes Association, a monthly scientific publication of at least 80 pages, of which more than one half is devoted to major scientific papers and review articles. About 6 pages are set aside for abstracts of papers dealing with diabetes published throughout the world. It also contains case reports, book reviews, editorials, and Association news, including committee reports. *The Journal* was published bimonthly from January-February 1952 to November-December 1964.

ADA Forecast, A bimonthly magazine without advertising, 32 pages, printed in color, devoted entirely to the interests of people with diabetes and their families. Each issue contains authoritative, up to date medical and scientific articles, personal experiences of people with diabetes, and a recipe and menu department. Other popular features are "Not 'Good for Diabetes,'" "Dave's Diary," "Young Folks Corner," "Letter Box," and "The Funny Side."

Diabetes Mellitus: Diagnosis and Treatment, a new series of books developed under the aegis of the Committees on Scientific Publications and Professional Education and edited by T. S. Danowski, M.D. Forty-one physicians and life scientists contributed to Volume I and 47 to Volume II. The former contains 224 pages and the latter, 266.

Meal Planning with Exchange Lists, Booklet, 20 pages, illustrated; "Diabetic Diet Card for Physicians"; Meal Plans 1-9; Bland, Low-Fiber Diet; Sodium Restricted Diet; prepared for distribution to the diabetic patient by the physician.

A Cookbook for Diabetics, A 172-page cookbook with more than 200 recipes which appeared in the *ADA Forecast* over a period of 12 years. Contains more than 28 pages of dessert recipes alone. Indexed and spirally bound for easy use.

Facts About Diabetes, (1966 edition; 28 pages in color). A booklet of basic information about diabetes, answering the questions most frequently asked. Easy to read and to understand; illustrated.

ADA Forecast Reprint Series comprises 55 reprints of published articles available at 10¢ each under the following titles:

1 *Why Single-scale Insulin Syringes*
2 *Diabetes and Abdominal Operations*
3 *Beware of Fake Diabetes Cures*
4 *Urine Testing: Its Methods and Its Importance*
5 *Renal Diabetes*
6 *Fractures in the Diabetic*
7 *Lente: The New Insulin*
8 *Payoff in Numbers*
9 *When Diabetics Have Ulcers*
10 *Meals on Wheels*
11 *The Diabetic Foot*
12 *Food Values for Passover Dishes*
13 *Hypoglycemic Reactions from Insulin or Oral Compounds*
14 *The Care and Handling of Insulin Syringes*
15 *The Food We Eat*
16 *The Six Exchange Lists*
17 *The Child with Diabetes*
18 *Overcoming a Common Ailment*

These publications are available from the American Diabetes Association.

Available from Lilly is a 66-page handbook (January 1967) entitled *A Guide for the Diabetic.*

Varieties of Insulin—The forms of insulin most frequently prescribed are described on pages 976 to 980.

The pharmacist should be familiar with all of the various brands of insulin on the market and he should carry more than one brand as they differ in some respects. One may be prepared only from beef pancreas while others are prepared from the pancreas of both beef and hogs. Sometimes idiosyncrasies to one of these proteins appear.

Storing Insulin—Insulin is a stable product *if kept in a cool place*, preferably in a refrigerator. Before the expiration of the patents controlling insulin, it was made under a license of the University of Toronto and conformed to the standards established and maintained by the University's Insulin Committee. Now, these standards have been provided by the USP and are used by the US Food and Drug Administration. Each lot, before distribution, must be tested and standardized by the latter by authority granted to it under an amendment to the Food, Drug and Cosmetic Act. The pharmacist should check the expiration date, as stated on the label, so that outdated insulin will not be sold or used.

Administering Insulin—Insulin is injected subcutaneously into the arm or thigh, or into the adipose tissue of the upper abdomen, after sterilization of the surface area. Because of its "depot effect," insulin should not be administered on two successive occasions in the same area.

Sterilization of syringes in boiling distilled water and of needles in alcohol should be carried out by the usual methods. Needles and syringes may be kept sterile, when not in use, by immersing them in ethyl alcohol containing 1% of glycerin and then boiling them at least once a week. Needles and syringes should be dry inside before use. Insulin can be administered by the patient or by a member of the family and is usually given in prescribed dosage one-half hour before meals. Insulin can be given by inunction but requires much greater dosage. In order to facilitate administration a *Busher Automatic Injector* has many advantages over the regular insulin syringe. The injection is painless, the area of injection is not bruised, and a patient can make the injection much more easily than when using an ordinary syringe (Fig. 931). See page 976 for further information about insulin.

Another special insulin syringe, known as *TruSet*, is marketed by MacGregor. This device attaches to the standard syringe and ensures the exact dose of insulin when the adjustable bar has been set to deliver the desired volume.

Synthetic Antidiabetic Agents—The discovery of the synthetic antidiabetic agents or oral hypoglycemics revolutionized the treatment of diabetes. It is estimated that nearly 750,000 patients in the US are being treated with the synthetic antidiabetic drugs *Orinase Tablets* (tolbutamide—Upjohn), *Diabinese Tablets* (chlorpropamide—Pfizer), *DBI Tablets* and *DBI-TD Capsules* (timed release) (phenformin—USV), *Dymelor Tablets* (acetohexamide—Lilly) and *Tolinase Tablets* (tolazamide—Upjohn) in uncomplicated *diabetes mellitus*. Yet the usage of the various forms of insulin has held constant since 1963 (to 1968) at $23 million at manufacturers' level. The synthetics rose in volume in the same period from $50 million to $70 million. See page 980 for further information about synthetic antidiabetic agents.

Invalid and Other Special Foods

The pharmacist is frequently called upon for special-purpose foods, prepared in advance and designed to meet the needs of invalids and others whose conditions indicate that they must omit certain portions of the normal diet. The pharmacist is especially qualified to handle such foods.

Special purpose foods are often of importance to the diabetic who is deprived of sugar- and dextrose-forming substances. Other foods are frequently prescribed for the mother and child. Loeb Dietetic and Chicago Dietetic are among the principal suppliers of *diabetic foods, gluten flour, starch-free, flour, starch-free bran,* and *sugarless candy, sweets, taffy,* and *sweeteners*. Most of these employ a substitute for sugar such as *saccharin*, saccharin and sodium cyclamate, as *Sweeta*

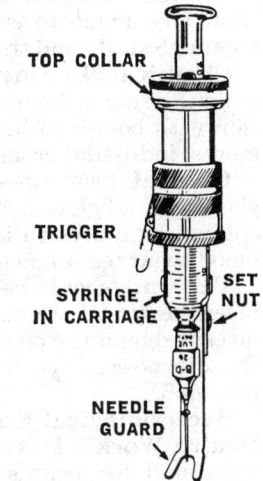

Fig. 931. Structure of the Busher Automatic Hypodermic Needle Injector (Becton-Dickinson).

TOP COLLAR

TRIGGER

SYRINGE IN CARRIAGE

SET NUT

NEEDLE GUARD

(Squibb), *Sucaryl* (Abbott), or other synthetic sweeteners and pharmacists must bear in mind that in many states, laws require that any foodstuff containing these sweeteners must bear a statement to that effect in large letters on the label of each package. The use of *dulcin*, another sugar-like substance, was forbidden by the Food and Drug Administration (1949).

Where other normal diet components are objectionable and fat-free or protein-free foods are required, or when seasoning and condiments are restricted, or the use of table salt forbidden, the pharmacist has an opportunity for special assistance. For instance, where salt must be avoided, patients may use substitutes such as *Neocurtasal* (Winthrop), *Co-Salt* (USV), *Diasal* (Fougera), and *Adolph's Salt Substitute* (Adolph). *Lonalac* (Mead-Johnson) is a low sodium high-protein dietary milk used by patients who need a low-sodium diet, but can still have a diet which is protein adequate.

Where actual nutritional deficiencies occur, special-purpose foods are not to be recommended. Vitamin deficiency or general health conditions should be diagnosed and treated by a physician who should prescribe the desired replacement therapy.

In many instances when the patient cannot obtain adequate nourishment by mouth, tube feeding offers the logical solution to supplying his nutritional needs during this critical period. A product suited to tube feeding is *Sustagen*, a complete, well-tolerated nutrient administered with a specially designed plastic tube feeding set. Sustagen is a powder containing vitamins A and D, B_6, cyanocobalamin, ascorbic acid, thiamine hydrochloride, riboflavin, niacinamide, calcium pantothenate, choline bitartrate, iron, calcium, sodium, potassium, phosphorus, fat, protein, and carbohydrate and flavoring (Mead-Johnson).

The geriatric use of *Maltsupex* (nondiastatic malt extract neutralized with potassium carbonate) for constipation in elderly patients, is advocated by Borcherdt. Borden and Gerber have found their specially prepared foods of special interest to healthy but aging patients, chronic special-diet patients, and short-term special diet patients, in addition to the extensive use given these products in pediatrics.

Analytical and Chemical Departments

Elsewhere in this book will be found chapters dealing specifically with most of the items mentioned below. These will frequently bring reputation and profit to the pharmacy and its special laboratories, but it must be emphasized that special training is required to develop the technical skills required and no attempt should be made to engage in these activities without thorough study and training.

Chemical Testing—Equipment and facilities for making general chemical tests are essential for cooperation with boards of health, food officials, police departments, industrial groups, and individuals.

Clinical Testing—Sufficient chemical reagents and glassware, a balance, a microscope, and other necessary equipment are essential for conducting urine analyses, blood sugar tests, and other clinical tests.

This work should be undertaken only by one who has received special training to insure reliable results. In no case should the pharmacist make or attempt to make the diagnosis. See the chapter on *Clinical Analysis*, page 646.

Bacteriological Examinations and Other Public Health Work—This offers a valuable service to physicians and for boards of health in evaluating water,

milk, sewage, and items of the diet. Also facilities for preparing autogenous vaccines and other extemporaneous biological products may be developed.

Chemicals for Use in the Arts and Sciences—In some places there are many calls for these chemicals and the pharmacist possesses the necessary knowledge to handle such supplies properly.

Proprietary and "Over-the-counter" Preparations

The pharmacist who is endeavoring to assist the physicians of his community in their treatment of the sick or in the maintenance of general health must adopt a policy for the handling of proprietary medicines which will be in the best interest of the public and fully cooperative with the physician. The advertising and active promotion of the use of proprietary medicines for the treatment of diseases would naturally be resented by members of the medical profession. *Such practices are contrary to the principles of a professional pharmacy.* There are, however, certain simple home medicines, as already suggested, for which there is a legitimate use, but some products in this class may be specialties and even assume the character of proprietary medicines. Well-known mouth washes, some germicides, and simple cathartics fall within this class. Such medicines are usually bought by the public to treat self-diagnosed ailments. The pharmacist must not under any circumstances attempt to diagnose an illness or prescribe medical treatment unless as first aid in emergencies, and then a physician must be summoned as soon as possible.

The rapid growth of the "over-the-counter" pharmaceuticals in recent years has not only proved to be economically important to the prescription pharmacist, but as well has represented a new and important challenge to his professional integrity. Sales of prescription pharmaceuticals at manufacturer's levels in 1967 exceeded $2.1 billion. The public spent $3.9 billion for these products almost all of it in pharmacies,[47] excepting of course the volume dispensed in hospital pharmacies. These are preparations bearing the "Prescription Legend" (Caution: Federal law prohibits dispensing without prescription) and are restricted to dispensing. However, the Durham-Humphrey Amendment to the Federal Food, Drug and Cosmetic Act saw the creation of the new "over-the-counter" category of non-consumer-advertised products, most of which were formerly prescription items. Total sales of non-prescription packaged medication sold in 1967 reached an annual volume of sale of $2.27 billion (two thirds in pharmacies), at manufacturer's level more than $1 billion. The pharmaceutical products which are not advertised directly to the public but which are sold in many instances on the recommendation of physicians and without a prescription and in some instances by the pharmacist himself now exceed the continuing volume of sale at manufacturer's level of proprietary drugs. The latter represents a volume of about $950 million per year.

However, for the protection of the public, it is preferable that packaged medicines be distributed by registered pharmacists. *Remember that pharmacists are not qualified to, and should not, assist in the specification of treatment of self-diagnosed ailments,* but registered pharmacists, by their specialized knowledge of therapeutics can and do assist in the promotion of public health when the distribution of packaged medicines is placed in their hands.

Veterinary Medicines and Supplies

The pharmacist is frequently called upon to suggest simple medicines for animals of various kinds. It may be a simple cathartic or a worm medicine, or perhaps something to destroy fleas. Veterinary pharmaceuticals are customarily classified into those which are used, dispensed, or prescribed by licensed veterinarians and those which are advertised to the public, farmer, poultryman, cattle raiser, etc. The total volume of sale of veterinary products in consumer dollars in 1967 was $280 million, of which only $82 million or 29% was through pharmacies. The companies directing their marketing efforts principally to veterinarians are Pitman-Moore (now transferred to J & J), Cutter, Schering, and Jensen-Salsbery. These products may be handled by some pharmacists who serve the needs of their local veterinarians. Much of this type of medication, however, is sold direct to the veterinarian or through veterinary supply houses. The veterinarian administers the drugs, and charges the animal's owner accordingly.

Proprietary veterinary manufacturers, such as Glover, Salsbury, Polk-Miller (Sergeant's Remedies), and others, advertise their products directly to the public and distribute through retail pharmacists, pet shops, hardware stores, and other local distributors.

Some manufacturers, such as Squibb, Lederle, and Pfizer (Globe), manufacture both veterinary specialties and proprietaries, selling the former through professional channels to the veterinarians and advertising their consumer products directly to the public. See the chapter on *Veterinary Services*, page 1859.

In farming districts there are many helps which the pharmacist who is properly informed can offer in the care of animals. Here again, however, the pharmacist must not assume responsibility for the treatment of a serious sickness in an animal for he does not have the necessary training or the legal right, and he may find himself accountable for a financial loss, especially when larger animals, such as cows and horses, are involved.

Insecticides, Fungicides, and Rodenticides

An entire chapter on *Pesticides*, (page 1274), has been devoted to this subject. The pharmacist, by being well informed will become an important distributor of information on the extermination of pests, which will prove of value and great service to his customers, and assist in establishing him as an important health factor in the community.

Toilet Articles and Preparations

Most of these products are merely distributed by the pharmacist. Very often a woman assistant may be employed who is well informed in the uses of cosmetics and can develop a particularly valuable department. The sale of many of these products to men should not be overlooked. Dental and shaving outfits, depilatories, treatments for the hair, face, and hands, perfumes, etc., fall within this department.

The total volume of consumer dollars paid for these products is tremendous, amounting to over $5.54 billion in 1967[47] of which pharmacies accounted for only 26%.

Hypoallergenic Cosmetics and Dermatological Pharmaceuticals

Hypoallergenic cosmetics are cosmetics especially designed to reduce the possibilities of creating allergic reactions and irritations caused by cosmetic allergens in sensitive users. Allergens are substances causing abnormal sensitivities in individuals, both male and female. These are over 60 known ingredients once commonly used in cosmetics which are allergenic and several hundred other substances which are known to be allergenic and which are occasionally found in cosmetic formulations even today (Table V[48-50]).

Some of the chief offenders among the cosmetic ingredient allergens were orris root, lanolin, starches, oils, gums and dyes. Naturally, there are some offenders among the newer synthetic ingredients now employed, but their identity in formulations is usually a trade secret of the maker. There is little distinction today among established lines of cosmetics as to their sensitization potential.

A cosmetic has varied interpretations—a one-dimensional use categorization by industry, with subdivisions by product form; and a two-dimensional definition for the physician, based on its reactivity on skin tissue, or lack of it. Under the latter pathologic categorization is another subgrouping, based upon the methodology of reactivity (Table VI[51]).

Among physicians, there is considerable difference of opinion as to the incidence of sensitivity to cosmetics, dermatologists and allergists finding continuing instances which require study. However, the American Medical Association in *Today's Health* (Apr. 1963) declared the term "hypoallergenic" obsolete but it is still in general use.

A much-publicized list[50] of 10 criteria for the formulation of hypoallergenic cosmetics is as follows:

1. Use of only the purest, most highly refined ingredients.
2. Preclusion of any substances reported in the medical and technical literature to be an irritant or a frequent sensitizer.
3. Clinical pretesting of each cosmetic product on a panel of persons known to be allergic to that type of cosmetic, with at least a 95% degree of probability of safety.
4. Availability of the qualitative formula to the medical and pharmaceutical professions.
5. Use of substances shown to have an occasional or minor sensitizing index *only* when no satisfactory substitute is available.
6. Absence of any medication.
7. Absence of any scenting agent.
8. Absence of any perfume, either natural or synthetic.
9. Absence of any ingredients possessing a physiologic action.
10. Elimination from product of the word "nonallergic," as nothing can be truthfully and scientifically considered as such.

It has been estimated that one out of every ten women is sensitive to cosmetics. The major groups of women who use hypoallergenic cosmetics are those who experience allergic reactions to the specific cosmetic ingredients themselves, those women who experience allergic reactions to ragweed, house dust, or certain foods, where standard cosmetics will usually add to the severity of the reaction, and those women who have husbands and children who are allergic to certain standard cosmetics. Children and adult males often suffer many of the same symptoms as allergic women, merely by coming in close contact with the cosmetics containing certain allergens.

When your customer complains about itching, irritation, or a breaking out of the surface of the skin, frequently this can be traced to the allergenic components of the cosmetics she is using. She probably has not heretofore given any thought to this possibility. In some instances, the skin condition can become so serious that it assumes systemic characteristics, even to the point where the strongly sensitive person may require hospitalization. Dermatologists and allergists, and the more perceptive practitioners, have learned to suspect skin irritations on the face, hands, feet, and underarm

Table V—Sensitizing Ingredients of Cosmetics[a]

Acacia	Linseed oil
Acetone	Lycopodium
Alizarin	
Alkyd resins	Methacrylate resins
Almond oil	Methenamine
Alum	Methylheptene carbonate
Aluminum acetate	Methylheptene ketone
Aluminum chloride	Methylnonylacetaldehyde
Aluminum sulfate	Morpholine
p-Aminophenol	
Amidol (dye)	Oil of bergamot
Ammonium carbonate	Oil of cananga
Ammoniated mercury	Oil of cassia
Amylmetacresol	Oil of citronella
Angelica root	Oil of coriander
Antimony compounds	Oil of heliotrope
Arnica flowers	Oil of hydroxycitronellal
Arrow root	Oil of lavender
Arsenic compounds	Oil of lemon
	Oil of lemongrass
Balm of Gilead	Oil of lime
Balsam of Peru	Oil of limonene
Barium sulfide	Oil of linalool
Bay oil	Oil of mandarin orange
Bayberry oil	Oil of neroli
Bay laurel	Oil of orange
Beeswax	Oil of orange peel
Benzaldehyde	Oil of origanum
Benzoic acid	Oil of orris
Benzoyl peroxide	Oil of peppermint
Benzyl benzoate	Oil of spearmint
Betanaphthol	Oil of tuberose
Bismuth compounds	Oil of wintergreen
Boric acid	Oil of ylang-ylang
Bromfluorescein	Orris root
Bromo acid	Orris root powder
	Orthophenol phenol
Calcium sulfide	Oxalic acid
Canada balsam	
Cantharides	Phenol
Carvacrol	Phenol-formaldehyde resins
Castor oil	p-Phenylenediamine
Cedarwood oil	Potassium carbonate
Chlorothymol	Potassium sulfide
Cinnamic aldehyde	Potassium sulfite
Citral	Pyrogallol
Clove oil	Pyrogallic acid
Coconut oil	
Corn starch	Quinine salts
Cresol	
	Rice powder
Dibromfluorescein	Rice starch
Diethylphthalate	Resin
	Resorcinol
Eosin dyes	Rosin
Ethanolamines	
Eucalyptus oil	Salicylic acid
Eugenol	Sodium carbonate
	Sodium persulfate
Formaldehyde	Sodium zirconium lactate
	Strontium sulfide
Geranium rose oil	Sulfonamide resins
Gum arabic	
Gum benzoin	Terpenes
Gum karaya	Terpineol
Gum olibanum	Tetrabromfluorescein
Gum tragacanth	Thioglycollic acid salts
	Thymol
Heliotropin	m-Toluenediamine
Henna	p-Toluenediamine
Hyacinth oil	
	Vanilla beans
Jasmine oil	
Jonquil oil	Wheat starch
Lanolin	Zinc chloride
Lavender oil	Zinc formate
Lead compounds	Zinc salicylate
	Zinc sulfate

[a] After Theodore,[48] Feinberg,[49] and Kahn.[50]

areas as cosmetic allergies.   These allergies evidence themselves in various ways.

Irritations of the skin are commonly caused by cosmetics, causing it to become red, cracked, or chafed, or there may be skin eruptions or hives.   Disturbances of the respiratory tract appear, causing the nasal passages to become irritated, and often creating a condition similar to a common cold.   Upset of the digestive tract also may be seen, causing diarrhea or headaches.

Many pharmacists have found the establishment of a hypoallergenic cosmetic department particularly advantageous to both the cosmetic department and the prescription department.   The close relationship between dermatological pharmaceuticals, some of which are prepared in the prescription department, and prefabricated hypoallergenic cosmetics, enables the pharmacist to render special services, and increases his professional stature.

Since almost all hypoallergenic cosmetics are sold through pharmacies, the pharmacist is expected to have a working knowledge of their need by the sensitive or allergic woman.   Men are also susceptible to the allergens found in many cosmetics and sensitive to the ingredients found in shaving lotions, shaving creams, as well as to the cosmetics used by their wives, children, mothers, friends, etc.   The pharmacist may do well to recommend hypoallergenic cosmetics to the wife of an allergy-ridden husband.

Dermatologists have long been aware of the role of cosmetics in dermatological sensitivity.   Allergists have revealed cosmetics as causative factors in many acute and chronic cases of obscure etiology.   Otolaryngologists are tracing an increasing incidence of respiratory disturbances to cosmetics.   Ophthalmologists, too, are finding many minor eye inflammations and other minor ocular irritations due to minute traces of nail polish

Table VI—Industry and Dermatologic Definitions of Cosmetic Groups[51]

Industry	Dermatology	
	Nonreactive	Active
Skin		
Creams	X	
Soaps	X	
Lotions	X	
Powders	X	
Colors	X	
Hair		
Shampoos	X	
Lotions	X	
Oils	X	
Pomades	X	
Waving agents		X
Fixatives		X
Bleaches		X
Dyes		X
Dye remover		X
Nails		
Lotions		X
Polishes	X	
Colors	X	
Accessories		X
Hygiene and Psyche		
Deodorants		X
Antiperspirants		X
Depilatories		X
Oral preparations	X	
Suntan products		X
Perfumes	X	
Other aromatics	X	
Lipsticks		X

scratched into the area surrounding the eye or due to particular eye make-up used. Gastroenterologists have observed gastritis and colitis from the small amount of lipstick licked from the lips.

As hypo-allergenic cosmetics are especially formulated with the express purpose of minimizing allergic reaction, ingredients are used that have a low index of sensitivity. The physician, therefore, will recommend or prescribe hypo-allergenic cosmetics in conjunction with dermatological preparations or alone for the allergic or sensitive patient. In most instances, the allergist and dermatologist will immediately place the patient on the use of hypoallergenic cosmetics or have the patient's wife, etc, with whom the patient is in daily contact use hypoallergenic cosmetics.

A study by both the physician and the pharmacist of the formulas of hypoallergenic cosmetics will indicate the ingredients used and those omitted are an important adjunct to the successful treatment of allergic patients. In the formulation of hypoallergenic cosmetics, inorganic rather than organic ingredients are used whenever possible. This, again, is specifically done to minimize the possibility of allergic reaction. In the use of organic ingredients, especially those obtained from animals such as sheep and cattle, allergens normally causing irritation or sensitization are formulated into the cosmetic product. Avoiding the use of such organic ingredients, and substituting inorganic ingredients, the possibility of incorporating known allergens into the formulation is reduced and the hypoallergenic cosmetic is therefore virtually free of known sensitizers.

Hypoallergenic cosmetics are marketed by Texas Pharmacal, Ar-Ex, Marcelle, Almay, and others.

Hearing Aids[52]

According to the Office of Health, Education, and Welfare, one out of every 12 persons has some loss of hearing. Of these, two out of five, or more than 6 million people, require some help. Only 2 million persons wear hearing aids; the Hearing Aid Industry Conference believes that the average hard of hearing person waits 5 years before seeking help. The expanding use of hearing aids offers an excellent opportunity to the pharmacist for additional sales volume.

Supplying and servicing the hearing aids for the deaf is a proper paramedical service for the community pharmacist. The pharmacist must be prepared, however, to devote sufficient time and attention to the selection and adjustment of these devices. The problems of the hard of hearing and today's highly sensitive transistorized

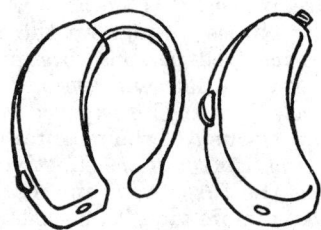

Fig. 932. Behind-the-ear battery-powered transitor hearing aids, with and without sound earphone.

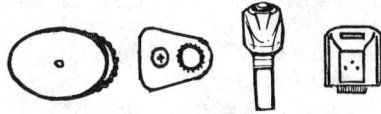

Fig. 933. Several types of self-contained in-the-ear hearing aids.

instruments require careful handling. It includes the initial selection and fitting of the equipment and the subsequent furnishing of batteries and replacement of worn parts. A small, quiet room, furnished with tables and chairs, must be available for satisfactory testing and fitting.

Needed are an audiometer, air and bone conduction hearing aids, batteries, cords and replacement parts, including impression material for custom-made earmolds. Hearing aids are worn in the ear, behind the ear (weighing but a fraction of an ounce), and in the form of inconspicuous eyeglass temple installations. They may be monaural or binaural.

The *eyeglass hearing aid* or bone conduction listener is more suitable for severe loss threshold levels, is self-contained with battery, transistors, switch and automatic telephone pickup, and set in the temple bow of one's eyeglasses.

A *behind-the-ear* or *at-the-ear hearing aid* is available that by electronic circuitry and multitransistor low-voltage battery power, gives greater clarity and realism, and has a magnet that switches off and on when needed for the telephone. These have built-in earphone, and battery with volume control and weigh only half an ounce.

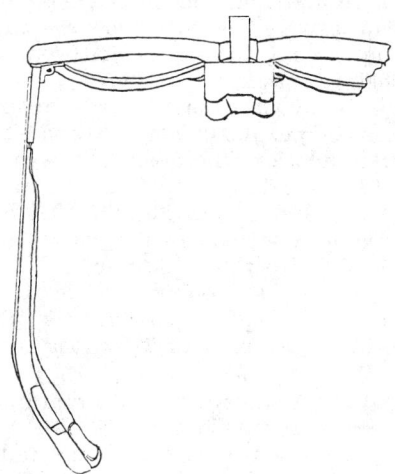

Fig. 934. Battery-powered adjustable transistor hearing aid in eyeglass temple, with plastic wedge across nose to bring unit in touch with conducting bone.

In-the-ear hearing aids also have no cords or tubing, but slip in or out without difficulty and are inconspicuous, especially suited for persons who suffer with a small but exasperating hearing loss.

Valuable information on hearing aids is available in the following pamphlets: *Caring for a Child's Hearing Aid* (Zenith), *An Informative Guide for the Hard-of-Hearing* (Zenith), *The Joy of Better Hearing* (Zenith), *Reference and Data Folder, Sonotone Hearing Aids* (Sonotone), *Otarion Electronics Bulletins* (Otarion). An interesting article on the subject is "Lifting the Curtain of Silence."[53]

Manufacturers of hearing aids provide training courses for the pharmacist by correspondence and special courses at factory centers.

Major suppliers of hearing aid instruments are Zenith, Sonotone, Otarion, and Dahlberg.

The Pharmacist and Venereal Disease Control

Venereal disease is the nation's number one communicable disease problem in the United States today. In the immediate post-World War II period, an enlightened government public health program made growing provision for venereal disease (VD) control.

This marked the end of evasion by the general public of recognition of venereal disease as one of the nation's greatest health problems, and focused public attention on the prevalence and devastating effects of syphilis. In 1938 Congress had enacted the VD Control Act establishing a national policy of aid to the states for "the prevention, treatment, and control of the venereal diseases." By January of 1950 nearly all states had enacted adequate legislation for the control of prostitution, one of the major factors in the spread of VD.

Statistics—Before the Federal VD Control Act was passed in 1938 few states and cities had VD Control services of any kind. During the decade 1936–1945, through the improved laboratory tests available everywhere, the nation learned how many people have syphilis. Every selectee and recruit for the US Army was given a blood test. Blood tests of candidates for marriage licenses were required in most states and blood testing became a routine practice in most hospitals. Prenatal blood tests for syphilis were required by 45 states by 1960.

VD rates, held low during wartime, however, rose sharply in 1946 and 1947, declined again to the beginning of 1954, but recently have showed a rapid rate of rise especially among teen-agers and young men and women in their twenties.

The number of *syphilis* cases reported among civilians declined from 357 per 100,000 in 1940 and a peak of 440 per 100,000 population when penicillin was introduced in 1943 to 51.9 per 100,000 population in 1967 (*VD Statistical Letter*, Feb., 1968, No. 96, USPHS).

The number of reported cases of *gonorrhea* decreased from a peak of 275 per 100,000 population in 1947 to about 130 per 100,000 population in 1957. More recent figures (*VD Statistical Letter*) for 1967 show a sharp continuing rise to over 228.3 per 100,000 however.

Experts of the Veneral Disease Program, National Communicable Disease Center, USPHS, Atlanta, say the statistics, as bad as they are, do not tell the whole story. The volume of reported cases of both syphilis and gonorrhea are startling enough.

In 1968 venereal disease (specifically syphilis and gonorrhea combined) was the leading communicable disease in the country, with about 3000 new cases per day. In fact, the incidence of gonorrhea is so great that it is a close contender to the common cold as the most prevalent disease condition affecting man.[54–56]

A 1968 survey[57] on venereal disease indicated that the spread of gonorrhea is reaching epidemic proportions in the US while the battle to eradicate infectious syphilis is showing early signs of success.

At a conference[58] held in October, 1968, by the American Social Health Association it was agreed that syphilis would eventually be "eradicated" from the US and that this goal would be achieved by the 1972 "target date" set by the US Surgeon General of Public Health's task force in 1961.

The 1968 project, entitled "National Survey of VD Incidence," was supported with funds provided by the US Public Health Service and was conducted by the American Social Health Association, a national voluntary health agency, in cooperation with the American Medical Association, the National Medical Association, and the American Osteopathic Association.

All 206,283 medical and osteopathic physicians in private practice in the US and Puerto Rico received questionnaires late in 1967 asking them to report how many VD cases they treated during the 3-month period from April to June that year. A high percentage, 65.3% of the doctors, responded.

Statisticians then estimated the number of people treated for both diseases during the year from July, 1967, to June, 1968. The tally included projections for the doctors who did not return the questionnaires as well as the known number of cases handled by public health clinics.

Gonorrhea was found to be rampant, with 1,499,584 cases for the year. The estimate for syphilis was put at 75,207 cases treated.

Compared with a nearly identical study carried out in 1962 by the American Social Health Association, the current incidence of gonorrhea was up 35.3%, while the rate for syphilis was down by 29.3%.

Most doctors simply do not report to health officials the number of cases of venereal disease they treat each year, the study found. It was estimated that eight out of nine cases of gonorrhea cured or treated by private doctors went unreported, while seven out of eight cases of syphilis were similarly hushed up. Doctors do not want to embarrass their patients, the report said.

The estimates given above are confirmed by actual figures on reported[56, 59] cases of gonorrhea in the US, which are shown to have increased each year since 1957 with the exception of 1962, and to have reached a new high of 431,380 cases in fiscal year 1968, according to data supplied by the National Communicable Disease Center's venereal disease program. The total for 1957 was 216,476 cases.

The 100% increase in cases between 1957 and 1968 was reflected in cases reported by private medical facilities as well as in those reported by tax-supported hospitals and venereal disease clinics.

Cases reported from private medical facilities during that period increased by 232%, from 37,295 to 123,756, while cases reported by public medical facilities increased by 71%, from 179,181 to 307,624.

The 431,380 cases in 1968 represented an increase of 55,774 cases, or 14.8% over the number reported in 1967. In 1968, cases reported from private medical facilities and public medical facilities increased 14.7 and 14.9%, respectively.

The reason why gonorrhea is on the upsurge and the incidence of syphilis is going down is because the emphasis in recent years has been on syphilis, the more dangerous disease, and the problem has been one of where to allocate available funds.

The effort to eliminate syphilis is an expensive procedure because of the manpower needed to conduct the "contact tracing process." Contact tracing, practiced by public health clinics throughout the country, is the attempt to get infected persons to supply the names and addresses of all others with whom they have had recent sexual relations. The exposed individuals are then traced and warned of their contamination.

Contact tracing is often more effective in combating syphilis because the three-week incubation period for the disease allows more time to seek out the infected men and women than for gonorrhea, which has an incubation period of 3 to 9 days.

There is now available as well a reasonably reliable and inexpensive diagnostic culture medium which can be used both as a test of cure to evaluate the efficacy of gonorrhea therapy schedules and for detecting gonorrhea in the female.[57]

The resurgence of gonorrhea, according to some health authorities may be due to increased sexual promiscuity among teen-agers.   Experts at the Atlanta center give these reasons for the upsurge in venereal disease:

Actual increase was cited by many states as the reason; more intensive laboratory follow-up and investigation were given as other reasons.

Steadily increasing urbanization of the population—that is, the move to the big cities, where venereal disease rates have always run highest.

Increased mobility of the population, such as in migrant labor groups, and also the increased use of the airplane and automobile.

False feelings of security against the threat of contracting venereal disease. These notions result from the well-known fact that penicillin and other antibiotics have been successful in syphilis or gonorrhea. The trouble is that too many people forget to make use of the cure after they have had exposure, especially in the case of syphilis, where early symptoms may pass unnoticed.

The agency's venereal disease experts say the upsurge "is not confined to any race, sex, socioeconomic group, or geographic area" but has occurred generally throughout the nation.

Incidence of venereal diseases among females is highest at age 18.   The peak reported among males is at age 23.   Although the teen-agers and young adults (15–24 age group) comprise only 13% of the total population they account for more than 15% of reported cases of gonorrhea and syphilis (1957).

Accomplishment—In 1936 the standard treatment of syphilis required at least 18 months. Treatment of gonorrhea required at least three months and was often ineffectual.   Only 25 to 30% of the VD patients completed treatment of either infection. The great majority became discouraged, lapsed treatment, continued to spread disease, and suffered the grave effects of neglect.

In contrast to this dismal picture, during a period of 1936 to 1945 many important advances were made:

The "5-day intravenous drip" and other extensive arsenical treatments of syphilis were developed and widely applied.

The penicillin treatment of syphilis was developed and made generally available.

The sulfonamide treatment of gonorrhea was discovered, tested, and applied throughout the nation.

The penicillin treatment of gonorrhea was discovered and made universally available.

The treatment time of early syphilis has been reduced from *1½ years*, with few completing treatment, to *1 week*, with nearly all completing treatment.   The treatment time of gonorrhea has been reduced from *3 months* with few completing treatment to *1 day*, with cures in better than 8 out of 10 cases, and all completing treatment.

Penicillin is still the drug of choice in the treatment of venereal diseases.   It is effective in over 95% of patients with early syphilis.   It is also most effective in neurosyphilis.

However, recently (1969) there have been indications[60] that penicillin therapy for gonorrhea will have to be re-evaluated because of the importation from Southeast Asia of gonococci resistant to the drug, most cases being also complicated by other organisms.

Among Servicemen who developed gonorrheal urethritis, a single intramuscular dose of 2.4 million units of aqueous penicillin G was ineffective in 46%.   This was reduced to a failure rate of only 11% by following

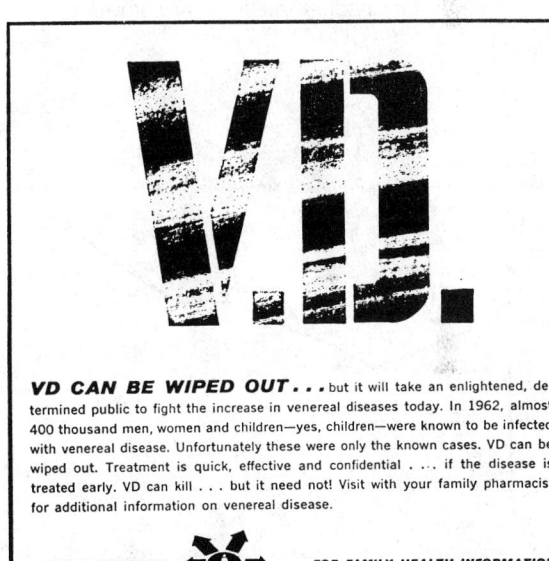

Fig. 936.

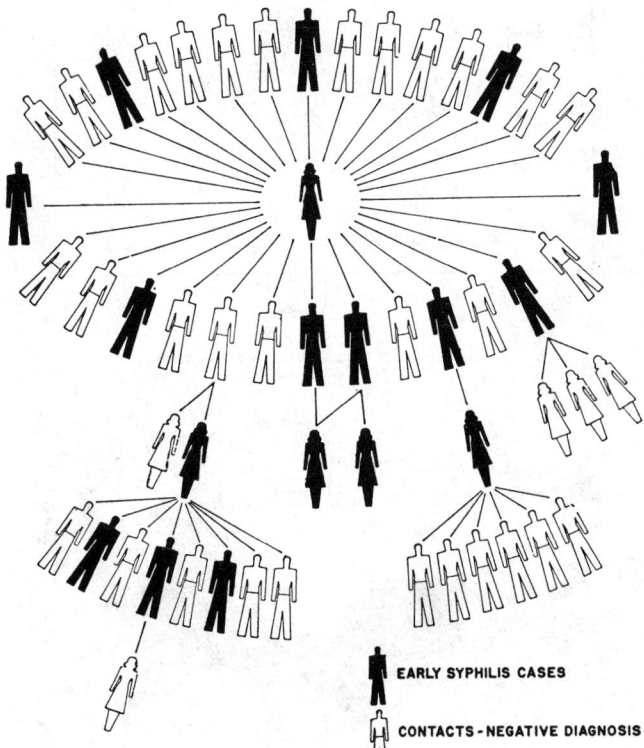

■ EARLY SYPHILIS CASES

☐ CONTACTS - NEGATIVE DIAGNOSIS

Fig. 935.   Chart showing an epidemiological study of early syphilis among white teenagers made January through May in one year (reproduced from "Today's VD Control Problem" through the courtesy of The American Social Hygiene Association, Inc., New York City).

VD information where to get it

The following brochures on venereal disease are available for distribution to your pharmacy patrons—

▶**Some Questions And Answers About VD** (8-page, color leaflet; single copies free; $4 per 100 copies; available from American Social Health Association, 1799 Broadway, New York, N.Y.)

▶**Today's VD Control Problem** (79-page, illustrated booklet; 50¢ a copy; $35 per 100 copies; available from American Social Health Association)

▶**Teenagers and Venereal Disease** (4-page, color leaflet; single copies free; $2.00 per 100 copies; available from American Social Health Association)

Fig. 937.

the penicillin with tetracycline hydrochloride 250 mg orally qid for 5 days. Other effective regimens were tetracycline orally 500 mg qid for 5 days; procaine penicillin 1.2 million units intramuscularly plus tetracycline orally; and procaine penicillin 2.4 million units intramuscularly twice, 48 hours apart.

The great advantages of rapid treatment with penicillin and other antibiotics which are effective against the gonococci and spirochetes are—nearly all cases complete treatment, and they are all under control while undergoing treatment. Rapid treatment, which renders syphilis noninfectious, will go far toward wiping out syphilis if new cases can be found and brought under treatment fast enough.

The Pharmacist's Role—Pharmacists must constantly keep in mind the fact that venereal disease is an epidemiological rather than merely therapeutic problem. Antibiotic therapy cannot eradicate syphilis, nor can it be controlled alone by treatment of patients. In fact, there is a rapidly increasing reservoir of resistant strains of infectious organisms observed in VD treatment. Every attempt must be made to find the source of patient infection. Intensive contact, case studies, and investigations are necessary to uncover hidden infectors.

Probably the most significant reason for the prevalence of VD is the lack of education about the seriousness of the disease. Increased sexual promiscuity among various groups is another. Overconfidence about the ease of treatment and lack of fear of infections are other factors.

Fortunately, both syphilis and gonorrhea can be completely cured quickly and effectively with penicillin. But VD has always carried a stigma with it and those infected often are reluctant to seek treatment.

If we could find and treat every infected person early, we could control syphilis and gonorrhea effectively. The problem is acute, and unless we as a nation join in the fight against VD, the problem will become worse.

The Joint Committee of the American Pharmaceutical Association and the American Social Hygiene Association has played an important part in arousing the interests of pharmacists throughout the country and enlisting their participation in efforts to combat the venereal diseases. Large and successful educational programs have been carried out by the American Social Hygiene Association with the advice and under the sponsorship of this Joint Committee. Only persistent effort by physicians and official agencies, aided by the

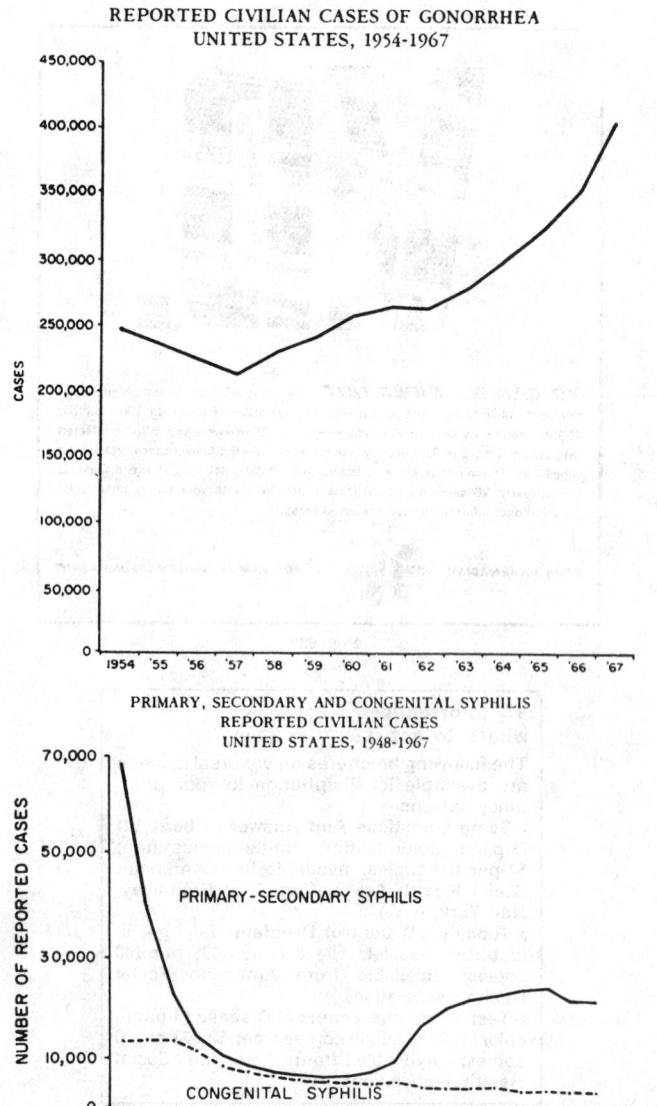

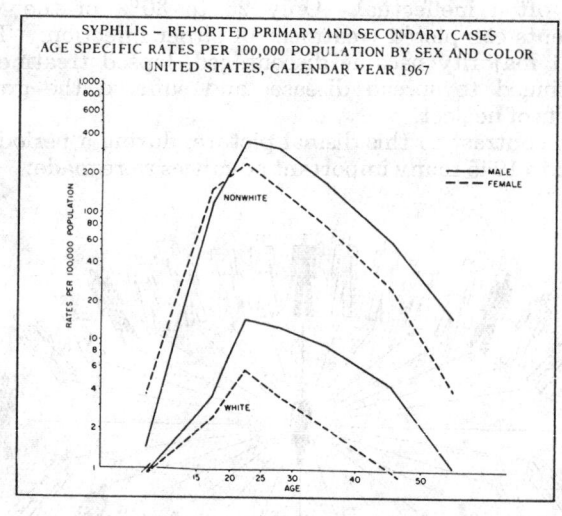

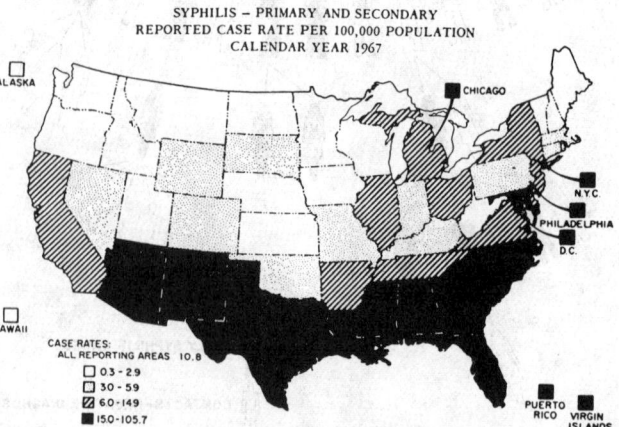

Figs. 938–941. US venereal disease trends. The shape of the venereal disease uptrends since 1957 and the age and geographic distribution of syphilis in 1967 are shown in charts from the 1967 *Annual Supplement to Morbidity and Mortality Weekly Report* of the USPHS's National Communicable Disease Center.

pharmacist and other socially minded citizens, can stamp out VD. Only thus can the gains already made be held.

1. Pharmacists should become fully acquainted with the pertinent laws and ordinances of the state, county, and city in which they practice, insofar as these relate to the dispensing of medicines and appliances, without a physician's prescription, for the treatment of venereal diseases, and also with reference to the sale of proprietary medicines and appliances for the same purpose. The observance of these laws by the pharmacist becomes a first consideration.

2. Pharmacists should prevail on persons applying to them for treatment to go to skilled physicians for the necessary advice and treatment and under no circumstances should they treat patients themselves.

3. The sale of appliances for the prevention of disease only, if construed to authorize the sale of disinfectants for the prevention of disease only, is a matter of particular concern for the reason that unless there are full instructions for the use of the disinfectants and unless the disinfectants have been thoroughly approved as efficient in the way in which the instructions indicate they should be used, it is likely that they would have very little if any value in preventing disease.

4. Pharmacists can best aid in the prevention of disease by referring all persons seeking advice or treatment to physicians, or to the City Board of Health if they are indigents. It should be kept in mind that these diseases may affect any part of the body, that blindness may result from acute infection of an adult's eye, that syphilis is transmissible congenitally, and that inadequate and delayed treatment is the reason why so many lesions of the nervous system, the cardiovascular system, etc, develop and cause such great loss of earning capacity and so many disabilities.

5. Since enactment of the national Venereal Disease Control Act of 1938, local, state, and Federal health agencies have developed a nation-wide system of venereal disease clinics and hospitals, and the interest of private physicians in venereal disease control has greatly increased. It has been found, however, that venereal diseases cannot be controlled effectively unless other important elements of the community cooperate wholeheartedly. Wherever local and state control programs have been most successful, it is usually found that the pharmacists are participating actively.

6. With the discovery that the sulfonamide drugs were effective to some extent in the treatment of gonorrhea and that penicillin was effective for both gonorrhea and syphilis, there has been an increasing tendency for the general public to become exceedingly careless and fearless of the consequences of venereal infection, and when infected to attempt self-medication. Because of this trend, the cooperation of the pharmacists with the medical profession and public health authorities as outlined above becomes even more necessary for the protection of both individual and public health.

Health Information Service—Public Health officials and medical authorities have long recognized the importance and potential of the community pharmacist in educating the public on health matters, and the need for early diagnosis and early medical treatment.

The community pharmacist's great number of contacts with the general public gives him a potential, as a source of health information through personal contact, far greater than any combined force of the other health professions.

The community pharmacist has been looked upon by the public as a reliable source for health information. Because of the undesirable and unhealthy effect of increased nonprofessional information from many printed sources, medical quackery, and by word of mouth from many nonprofessionals in nonprofessional outlets, the public is often misled and sorely in need of proper guidance.

It is important, therefore, for the pharmacist to have not only the knowledge and be equipped to advise the public on such matters, but as well to be in a position to provide literature and other informational material as a community health information center. Through such a service pharmacists find that they develop greatly increased patron confidence and loyalty.

In support of this local pharmaceutical effort, the American Pharmaceutical Association through its Health Education Center Service,[61] provides at nom-

inal cost a large assortment of informative pamphlets on a variety of health subjects, from a number of authoritative sources, for distribution to a pharmacy's patrons.

Several states have also initiated similar services for pharmacists in the interest of better community health. The Pennsylvania Pharmaceutical Association,[62] with the cooperation of the Commonwealth of Pennsylvania Health Department, provides free supplies of such pamphlets prepared by the Department, for distribution to the public.

References

1. *Stat. Abstr. US*, 89th ed., US Dept. of Commerce, Stat. Inform. Div., Washington, D.C., 1968 (includes current and projected population, by age and sex: 1960–1980).
2. *NY Times* (Jan. 6, 1969).
3. *US News & World Rept.* (June 24, 1968).
4. *Infant Care* (Publ. No. 8), Children's Bur., Soc. Sec. Admin., US Dept. of HEW, Washington, D.C., 106 pp; available from USGPO, Washington, D.C. 20402.
5. Apgar, V., *Am. Baby*, **53,** 23 (Jan., 1963).
6. Grossman, E., *Am. Family Physician*, 8(5), 32 (May, 1965).
7. Newton, M., and Newton, N., *New Engl. J. Med.*, **277**(22), 1179 (Dec., 1967).
8. *Med. World News*, **8,** 5 (Dec. 29, 1967).
9. *Recommended Dietary Allowances* (Publ. 1694: Natl. Acad. Sci.), 7th rev. ed., Food & Nutr. Board, Natl. Res. Council, Washington, D.C., 1968.
10. *Present Knowledge in Nutrition*, 3rd ed., The Nutr. Found., Inc., 99 Park Ave., New York, N.Y. 10016, 1967.
11. Fomon, S. J., *Infant Nutrition*, Saunders, Philadelphia, 1967, p. 196.
12. Burton, B. T., *Heinz Handbook of Nutrition*, McGraw-Hill, New York, 1959, Chap. 17.
12a. Various publications of the American Academy of Pediatrics, 1801 Hinman Ave., Evanston, Ill. 60204.
13. *J. Am. Med. Assoc.*, **124,** 698 (1944).
14. *J. Obstet. Gynaecol. Brit. Empire*, **52,** 241 (June, 1945).
15. *Med. Clin. N. Am.*, **29,** 1425 (Nov., 1945).
16. *How To Use the Basal Temperature Thermometer*, Becton-Dickinson, Rutherford, N.J., 1952; rev. 1966.
17. *Clinical Thermometers, A Recorded Voluntary Standard of the Trade* (Commercial Std. 1-52), Commodity Std. Div., Office of Tech. Serv., US Dept. of Commerce, in cooperation with the Natl. Bur. Std., 1952; available from USGPO, Washington, D.C. 20402.
18. "Bard Magna-Therma-Thermometer," *Drug. Merch.* (Can.) (Jan., 1968).
19. Sommermeyer, L., and Carroll, D., Natl. Res. Lab., USPHS, Atlanta, Ga.; see *Nursing Res.*, **1,** 32 (1952).
20. Neuroth, M. L., *Am. Profess. Pharmacist*, **26,** 238 (1960).
21. Shaw, R. N., *Looking Ahead: The Physicians' Supply Field—An Opportunity for Expanding Professional Service*, Symp. Am. Coll. of Apoth., Chicago, Ill., Apr. 28, 1961.
22. Shaw, R. N., *Disposable Equipment—Present and Future*, Symp. Am. Coll. of Apoth., White Sulphur Springs, W. Va., Oct. 28, 1963.
23. Loeher, J. F., *Am. Surg. Trades Assoc. J.*, **51,** 40 (June, 1964).
24. Kenna, F. R., *Ill. Pharmacist*, **28,** 410 (May–June, 1964).
25. *Mod. Med. Topics*, **26**(5), 1 (May, 1965).
26. Ritter, F. T., Jr., *Drug Cosmetic Ind.*, **97**(5), 671 (Nov., 1965).
27. Beclard, F., *Bull. Imp. Acad. Med.* (*Paris*), **32,** 327 (1866) and Galante, H., *Notice sur quelques Nouveaux instruments et Appareils de Chururgie*, Paris, 1866, p. 43.
28. Servajan, M. J., *Bull. Gen. Therap.*, **83,** 234 (1872).
29. Bartholow, R., *Manual of Hypodermic Injection*, 2nd ed., Lippincott, Philadelphia, 1879, pp. 22 *ff*.
30. Warran, J., *et al*, *J. Am. Med. Assoc.*, **157,** 633 (Feb. 19, 1955).
31. Thorn, G., *Clin. Endocrinol.*, **1,** 76 (1941).
32. Autain, J., and Brewer, J. H., *Am. J. Hosp. Pharm.*, **15,** 313 (Apr. 1958).
33. *Pharm. J.*, **144,** 3980 (4th ser., vol. 90), 96 (Feb. 10, 1940).
34. Bergstrom, D. A., and Grendahl, B., *Care of Patients with Bowel and Bladder Problems*, Am. Rehabil. Found., Inc., Kenny Inst., and Univ. of Minn. School of Med., under a grant from the Div. of Chronic Dis., USPHS.
35. Katona, E. A., *Mod. Med.*, **36**(4), 164 (Feb. 12, 1968).
36. Dease, J. C., *J. APhA*, NS4, 72 (1964).
37. McAuliffe, P. J., *J. APhA*, NS4, 67 (1964).
38. *Mid-Atlantic Apoth.*, **13,** 27 (Oct., 1963).
39. Scheffe, W. P., Symp. Am. Coll. of Apoth., White Sulphur Springs, W. Va., Oct., 1963.
40. Yesalis, C. E., *The Orthotic Support and Appliance Market*, Symp. Am. Coll. of Apoth., White Sulphur Springs, W. Va., Oct., 1963 (statistical information compiled on market for surgical supports and appliances, S. H. Camp & Co., Jackson, Mich.).
41. Allen, J. G., Can. Pharm. Assoc. Ann. Mtg., Toronto, Ont., Aug. 15, 1967.
42. Kazin, L. E., and Loughlin, L., *Make Customers Stop-by Promotions*, J & J, New Brunswick, N.J., 1959.
43. Boyland, H. W., *Surgical Appliance Technician's Handbook*, Surg. Appl. Ind., Inc., Cincinnati, 1963.
44. Bloomberg, M. H., *Orthopedic Braces*, Lippincott, Philadelphia, 1964.
45. *NARD J.*, **90**(3), 32 (Feb. 5, 1968).
46. Fahland, B., and Grendahl, B. C., *Wheelchair Selection: More Than Choosing a Chair with Wheels*, Am. Rehabil. Found., Inc., Minneapolis, prepared under a grant from the Div. of Chronic Dis., USPHS.
47. *Drug Trade News* (Aug. 12, 1968).

48. Theodore F. H., *NY State J. Med.*, **58**, 2233 (July 1, 1967).
49. Feinberg, J. G., *Cosmetic Sci.*, **293**, 310 (1959).
50. Kahn, J. B., *NARD J.*, **89**(9), 45 (May 1, 1967).
51. Sppor, H. J., *NY State J. Med.*, **60**(12), 1940 (June 15, 1960).
52. Stuart, R. C., *J. APhA*, **NS4**, 83 (1964).
53. Ratcliff, J. D., *Today's Health*, **45**, 66 (Nov., 1967).
54. *AMA News*, **11**, 5 (Nov. 4, 1968).
55. *Med. Tribune*, **10**(8), 12 (Jan. 27, 1969).
56. *AMA News*, **12**, 7 (Jan. 13, 1969).

57. *Med. Tribune*, **10**(91), 1 (Nov. 11, 1968).
58. *Med. World News*, **9**, 58 (Nov. 8, 1968).
59. *VD Stat. Letter*, No. 80 (Nov., 1963), No. 95 (Nov., 1967), and No. 96 (Feb., 1968), Venereal Dis. Program, Nal. Communicable Dis. Ctr., Bur. of Dis. Prevent. & Environ. Control, USPHS, Atlanta, Ga. 30333.
60. *Med. Tribune*, **9**(57), 3 (July 15, 1968).
61. *J. APhA*, **NS6**, 423 (1966).
62. *Pa. Pharmacist*, **49**(7), 10 (Feb., 1968).

This chapter was prepared by

Alan K. Done, * **MD,** *Director, Poison Information and Therapy Center, University of Utah Medical Center, Salt Lake City, Utah   84112*

At all ages of childhood and during early adulthood (up to about 36 years of age), accidents are the leading cause of death and disability in the US. Among children beyond the first year of life, accidents cause more deaths than do the five leading fatal diseases combined. Between ages 15 and 24 years, accidents claim more lives than do all other causes combined. Also among the most common causes of death of pre-adolescents, adolescents, and adults is suicide. Both accidents and suicides frequently involve poisons. Even though the reporting, especially of suicides, undoubtedly is incomplete, there are known to be nearly 10,000 deaths in the US each year attributable to accidental or suicidal poisoning.

In addition to the fatalities due to poisoning, there are staggering numbers of nonfatal cases requiring treatment. The toll in terms of manpower, expense, and occupation of medical facilities cannot be estimated, but must be tremendous. It is estimated that approximately one million individuals are victims of poisoning in this country each year.

While notable progress has been made in reducing morbidity and mortality from disease, the incidence of accidental and suicidal poisoning has increased so that its relative importance has become magnified in recent years. The increased incidence of both fatal and nonfatal poisonings is related in part to increased availability of potentially toxic materials and to an increase in susceptible population.

At least the accidental poisonings should be preventable in most instances. Especially is this true of accidental poisonings of young children by drugs and chemicals in the home. This is a problem of great public-health significance the solution of which will require efforts of individuals in many disciplines. Among these are pharmacists, who can play a key role in preventing or mitigating the consequences of accidental poisonings, especially those due to drugs.

Epidemiology

Effective preventive measures require a knowledge of what and who are involved, and under what circumstances. Consideration must be given to predisposing and contributory factors; otherwise, little progress can be expected. These factors often have been ignored in the past, with the result that efforts aimed only at superficially obvious solutions have proved to be ineffectual. For example, the important admonition to parents to keep potentially toxic materials under lock and key is thwarted by the fact that parents do not consider many of the most frequently involved materials to be toxic. In addition, they underestimate the ability of a young child to acquire the material and, as noted below, potential toxins ingested by children are most often not in their usual place of storage at the time of the accident.

Table I presents an approximation of the annual number of deaths known to be due to poisoning in the US. Interpretation of these data should take into account the fact that many poisonings are not recognized as such and many suicides are termed accidents. For example, a sizable but unknown number of the "accidental" cases in persons over 5 years of age undoubtedly are actually suicides. The figures shown also have the limitation that data from different years had to be used in various categories because they were all that was available; consequently, the totals shown can be considered only as approximations of the usual yearly rates. They do, however, give an idea of the order of magnitude of the poisoning problem as it involves various substances.

Of considerable epidemiologic interest is the relationship between accidental poisoning fatalities in young children (Table I) and the frequency of acci-

Table 1—Annual Number of Deaths Due to Poisoning in the US

Substance	"Accidental"[a] Under 5 years	"Accidental"[a] Over 5 years	Suicidal[b]	Totals
Barbiturates & derivatives	8	378	2,052	2,438
Salicylates	115	53	83	251
Morphine & derivatives	3	72	18	93
Other analgesic & soporific drugs	13	228	277	518
Other or unspecified drugs	45	311	236	592
Total drugs	184	1,042	2,666	3,892
Alcohol	3	276		
Lead & its compounds	57	17		
Petroleum products	48	7		
Corrosives	18	31		
Industrial solvents	12	32		
Arsenic, antimony, & compounds	17	19		
Mercury & compounds	2	6		
Noxious foodstuffs	1	5		
Fluorides	2	3		
Other & unspecified solid & liquid substances	70	167		
Total nondrug solids & liquids	230	563	733	1,526
Total: solids & liquids	414	1,605	3,399	5,418
Gases and vapors	30[c]	1,618[c]	2,386	4,034
Totals	444	3,223	5,785	9,452

[a] Yearly average for the decade, 1957–1966: data from the National Clearinghouse for Poison Control Centers.
[b] 1963: data from Berger, F. M.[1]
[c] 1966 only: data from National Center for Health Statistics, US Public Health Service.

* The author acknowledges gratefully the influence of the preceding author of this chapter, the late Dr. Harold Jacobziner, whose pioneering efforts and leadership did much to promote poison control.

Table II—Substances Most Frequently Involved in 72,661 Accidental Ingestions Among Children Under 5 Years of Age in 1967[a]

	% of cases
Medicines	52.8
Internal	46.9
Aspirin	23.2
Vitamin & iron preparations	4.1
Other analgesics	2.3
Tranquilizers	2.3
Hormones	1.9
Amphetamines	1.4
Antihistamines	1.3
Laxatives	1.3
Cough medicines	1.2
Cardiac preparations	1.0
External	5.9
Liniments & rubbing alcohol	1.2
Antiseptics	1.2
Cleaning & polishing agents	14.3
Soaps, detergents, and cleaners	4.3
Bleach	3.0
Disinfectants & deodorizers	2.5
Furniture polish	2.0
Lye & caustics	1.3
Cosmetics	6.4
Perfumes and toilet water	2.4
Pesticides	5.6
Insecticides	2.9
Rodenticides	1.3
Paint Products	5.0
Petroleum Products	4.6
Plants	4.0
Gases and vapors	0.1

[a] Reported by National Clearinghouse for Poison Control Centers: data from 395 centers in 43 states.

dental ingestion (Table II). The latter data are presented as percentages of the total number of accidental ingestions because the absolute numbers are not known (not all poison centers report their data and not all accidentally poisoned patients are seen at poison centers).

The number of accidental ingestions involving children under the age of 5 years is estimated at 500,000 annually in this country. It is especially noteworthy that the bulk of ingestions and of fatalities do not involve substances which are considered classically to be poisons by the layman. Such a commonplace material as aspirin is responsible for the largest number of accidental ingestions and fatalities. No other substance even comes close to aspirin as a cause of accidental poisoning. Common household materials, such as cleaning and polishing agents and cosmetics, are frequently ingested accidentally by children but rarely cause fatalities; exceptions are furniture polish and lye and other caustic materials, which have a high rate of morbidity and mortality.

With the exception of gases and vapors (most commonly, carbon monoxide), barbiturates and related compounds are the most commonly involved substances in fatal suicidal poisoning. In recent years the frequency of involvement of other sedative or tranquilizing agents has been increasing rapidly. Pesticides are a highly significant cause both of fatal and nonfatal poisoning; however, differences in nomenclature used in the tabulation of data for ingestions and for fatalities make comparisons difficult. Many of the heavy metals and other inorganic nonmedicinal materials listed in Table I are undoubtedly from pesticides. A major exception is lead poisoning, especially in young children, where the most common source is paint, chewed because of the perversion of appetite known as pica.

Among accidental poisonings, comparisons of ingestion and fatality rates provide some indication of the degree of toxicity of various agents (Tables I and II). The commonest offender, aspirin, is involved in 23% of the ingestions by young children, and it and other salicylates are responsible for 26% of the accidental poisoning deaths in individuals under the age of 5 years. With some other materials the mortality rate is far out of proportion to the ingestion rate, suggesting higher degrees of toxicity. Examples are the petroleum products, involved in 4.6% of ingestions in this age group but responsible for 11% of the deaths.

Even more striking is the fact, not demonstrated by the data shown here, that a child who ingests kerosene or other volatile petroleum distillates has more than one chance in three of requiring hospitalization (for aspirin the hospitalization rate is 12% and for cosmetics it is 3%). Another example is the corrosives such as lye, involved in 1.3% of ingestions by young children but responsible for about 4% of the fatalities (and leading to hospitalization in nearly half the cases of ingestion).

The importance of the fact that most of the difficulty is caused by drugs or common household products and not by classical poisons lies in the misdirection of preventive efforts and in a lack of recognition of the real hazards. Anyone not bent on self-destruction is likely to be most cautious about the handling or storage of cyanide, arsenic, or similar poisons, but many fail to appreciate the toxic potential of such materials as aspirin, kerosene, and caustics. Most reasonable people know enough to keep a pesticide stored in a relatively safe place but may not realize that electric dishwasher detergent, furniture polish, or drain cleaner may be equally hazardous to a child.

Many people fail to recognize aspirin not only as a potential poison but even as a drug. This is evidenced by the fact that in the taking of medical histories it is usual for patients (or parents, in the case of a child) to say no when asked whether drugs are being taken, until they are specifically asked about aspirin and other common nonprescription medications. It is small wonder, therefore, that these materials are frequently not treated with sufficient respect and are so frequently placed where they are available to children.

Also of importance is therapeutic overdosage with such common household medications as aspirin; this factor has important preventive implications for the pharmacist, as is discussed below. It is not at all uncommon for a parent who has never been told of the toxic potential of such a commonplace item to administer several times the safe dose of aspirin to a small infant over a period of several days. In fact, such unintentional overdoses are responsible for many of the most serious cases of aspirin poisoning.

Particularly tragic are accidental poisonings due to materials which are either outmoded, excessively toxic for their intended use, or for which there is only questionable rationale. Oil of wintergreen (methyl salicylate) is one of the most dangerous causes of salicylate poisoning, a teaspoonful being a potentially lethal dose for a 2-year-old child; yet its elimination from household medicinal use would not create a significant therapeutic void. Camphorated oil is another outmoded form of treatment which is excessively toxic. The inclusion of iron in many hematinic and tonic preparations is of questionable rationale and represents an unnecessary hazard; needed iron therapy is better prescribed separately.

Carbon tetrachloride, although recently removed from most cleaning and anthelmintic preparations, is still available and is excessively dangerous. Some pesticides, while valuable to the professional exterminator, are excessively toxic for routine household use. For example, there is little reason for employing highly dangerous inorganic materials such as arsenic, phosphorus, and thallium as rodenticides when warfarin, practically devoid of acute human toxicity, will do the job unless the animals have become resistant.

Influential Factors

Emphasis here will be upon accidental poisoning in children because these are the cases which are most readily preventable if enough is known about the reasons for their occurrence. A number of factors that should be considered in any preventive endeavors are enumerated in Table III, which presents composite data from the experience of the author over a period of several years.

Age—Approximately 70% of poisonings occur in children and are accidental; a majority of the 30% which occur in adults represent suicide attempts. Much has been said about poisoning accidents among adults resulting from such events as the inadvertent taking of some material instead of a medication or accidental overdosage of a proper medication. Actually, such accidents are rather rare. This is not to suggest that people should not be cautioned to read labels carefully before taking medications, not to take medications in the dark, not to transfer materials from their original containers, to protect medication labels against destruction, and to follow recommended dosage schedules assiduously. It is important, however, to recognize that factors which are not so often discussed are actually more important, numerically speaking.

Accidental poisoning is relatively rare under the age of 1 year or beyond 5 or 6 years of age. The critical age period is between 1 and 3 years, where approximately 46% of the accidental poisonings occur. Indeed, at that age poisoning accounts in this institution for more than 40% of the accidents of sufficient severity to require treatment in an emergency ward.

Between 1 and 3 years of age, poisoning is more likely to bring a child to the hospital for emergency treatment than any other single cause. The reasons for the high incidence at that age relate to certain characteristics of child development. During these early years the youngster is inquisitive and accustomed to mouthing everything within reach. By 1 year of age he is also usually able either to creep or to walk, yet he is too young to recognize danger. It is to be expected that he will attempt to ingest any substance left within reach.

It is the universal experience of those who treat children that nothing, no matter how distasteful, is exempt. While flavoring may be responsible for a child's ingesting a larger dose, it has little bearing on the likelihood that he will attempt to ingest the material. During the first 2 or 3 years of life, texture is at least as important as flavor in determining acceptability of something to be eaten. Materials that would gag an older individual may be accepted readily by the young child. Indeed, even highly caustic substances such as lye are not uncommonly ingested without hesitation by children at this age.

Table III—Epidemiologic Factors in Accidental Childhood Poisoning[a]

	% of total poisonings	Poisoning as % of home accidents[b]
Age		
Less than 1 year	2	13
(given by older sibling in 47%)		
1–3 years	46	41
3–6 years	18	19
6–12 years	1	2
12–16 years	3	5
Over-all figure for children	70	22
Previous history of ingestion accident	9%	
Place of occurrence		
At home, inside	83%	
Kitchen	32%	
Bedroom	30%	
Bathroom	11%	
Other rooms	10%	
At home, outside (or in garage)	11%	
Away from home	6%	
Accessibility		
In usual storage space	40%	
Left out	60%	
Before use	24%	
After use	36%	
Container		
Original	91%	
Changed	6%	
Supervision		
By parent(s)	95%	
By others	5%	

[a] Poison Information and Therapy Center, University of Utah College of Medicine, and the emergency service of the University Hospital.
[b] Accidents sufficiently severe to merit Emergency Room treatment.

Among children less than 1 year old, it is of interest to note that in our experience the infant was given the material by an older sibling in nearly half the cases. Thus, it is important to keep potentially toxic materials inaccessible not only to very young children but to their older brothers and sisters as well. In addition, children must be educated not to give things to the baby without a parent's permission.

It is of interest also that among children older than 3 years of age ingestions occur as group activities in nearly half the cases. A group of children will share the material in some form of play, where they perhaps would be unlikely to ingest it by themselves. At this age, children are becoming more educable than earlier, so that instruction plays a fairly important preventive role.

A certain number of supposedly accidental poisonings in teenage and younger children are actually suicide attempts or gestures. It is important in this connection to realize that serious suicide attempts occur at much younger ages than is generally appreciated; serious attempts at 9 or 10 years of age have been known to occur. Suicidal attempts or gestures are, of course, quite common among adolescents and in the few years immediately before and after this important transitional stage of life.

"Accident Proneness"—This is a somewhat overrated concept. As can be seen in Table III, less than 10% of our patients who were treated for poisoning had a previous history of having been involved in similar accidents. Much has been said and written about the poisoning repeater, but he actually accounts for only a small percentage of the cases seen. On the other hand, a child who has ingested something surreptitiously, especially if some effort was required in the act, does represent a greater future risk and should be treated accordingly. The idea that there are accident-prone children is probably less valid than that there are accident-prone situations and surroundings.

Location—The majority (over 80%) of accidental childhood poisonings occur in the home. Many people have the mistaken idea, however, that most of them occur in the bathroom because that is the location of the medicine cabinet in most homes. As is pointed out below, materials which become involved in accidental childhood poisoning usually have been left out while in use, rather than being in their usual place of storage at the time they were taken. This, plus the fact that common household products are involved so frequently, dictates that other rooms are even more dangerous. Most preventive efforts and educational campaigns have emphasized the bathroom medicine cabinet.

As noted in Table III, the kitchen and the bedroom are the rooms in which the majority (62%) of childhood poisonings occur. The bathroom runs a poor third. Among various locations there are differences both in the types of materials that are likely to be involved and in the time of peak occurrence during the day.

The highest incidence of accidental poisoning is in the late morning hours, just before lunch; the majority of these occur in the kitchen and the substances most frequently involved are common household products such as cleaning agents, polishes, and other materials commonly kept in the kitchen. Another peak in incidence occurs in the early afternoon (at naptime); the majority of these occur in the bedroom and involve cosmetics and, to a lesser extent, medications. Another peak in the early evening (at bedtime) has similar relationships. Bathroom incidents are scattered throughout the day and tend usually to involve either medications or cosmetics.

Among the cases which occur outside of the home, the family automobile and the garage are common sites of accidental poisoning in young children. Involved most frequently in the automobile are medications which have been left either in the glove compartment or in mother's purse. In the garage, pesticides, petroleum products, cleaning agents, and paint products are most often involved. A small but significant percentage of cases occuring outside the home involve plants which are growing either in the yard or wild in the fields. Children sometimes are poisoned when they visit the homes of others (especially grandparents) who leave things within reach because they are not accustomed to having children about.

Accessibility—Many poisoning prevention campaigns have focused upon the provision of a locked medicine cabinet. While the availability of such a place for the safe storage of medicines is desirable, it should be recognized that this would prevent less than half the cases of accidental childhood poisoning (unless the presence of a locked cabinet increases the likelihood that materials will be replaced there, a factor which has not been studied fully).

In approximately 60% of cases, the materials involved in accidental childhood poisoning have been left out within reach of a child. It is most common for material to be left out after being used, but in nearly ¼ of the total cases, materials which have been taken out but not yet used are involved. In many of the latter instances, ingestion occurs when the individual responsible for the care of a child is interrupted in his use of the material in question.

From the foregoing, it is apparent that people must be instructed not only to provide a storage place for potentially toxic materials, but also to return these materials immediately thereto and not to let them out of their sight even for a moment until so secured. In an alarming number of instances, ingestion takes place so quickly that the individual responsible for the care of the child is within a few feet of him at the time of the accident. It is also important that the products themselves or their containers be made as safe as possible, since people undoubtedly will continue to leave materials within reach of children.

The Container—Removal of potentially toxic materials from their original containers is a significant factor in increasing the risk of accidental poisoning, especially with certain compounds. The common practice, for example, of storing a small quantity of kerosene in a soft-drink bottle is especially hazardous, for obvious reasons. Other hazardous materials with which this is frequently done are cleaning solutions, paint products, turpentine, and pesticides. Sometimes the container to which they are transferred is a drinking glass or dish. In all such instances, a material is made to seem more attractive to the child because of the resemblance to something which has given pleasure in the past.

In addition to the foregoing, transfer of materials from their original containers creates problems of accurate identification if and when poisoning does occur. A similar problem exists when materials, particularly medications, are not properly identified in their original containers. Medically speaking, there is rarely a defensible reason for failing to identify even prescription medications on the label.

Most people are sufficiently sophisticated medically that they can and should be informed about the medications that they receive (at the instigation of the physician, not the pharmacist). This would greatly ease the burden upon the individual who might later be called upon to treat a case of poisoning due to the product. In addition, the labeling of prescription products makes for more meaningful medical histories and more rational use of the products by lay persons. (They will use them anyway; why not at least help them to avoid mistakes?)

There are occasional problems that result from the placing of containers of similar size, shape, and/or color in proximity, either in medicine cabinets, pharmacies, or nursing stations. This invites errors and should be discouraged. Such accidents have been particularly common in hospitals, and one of the responsibilities of the pharmacist and the Drug or Formulary Committee should be to eliminate such hazards. Bottles of distilled water which are to be used in the mixing of solutions should not, for example, be kept near bottles containing other materials. It sometimes helps either to place such materials in colored bottles or else to add coloring to such solutions as rubbing alcohol.

Supervision—The vast majority of children are nominally under the supervision of one or of both their parents at the time accidental poisoning occurs. Thus, adult supervision as it is usually practiced is not adequate to prevent poisoning accidents in young children. As was noted before, this is due in part to the fact that parents underestimate the ability of the child to obtain and to ingest a potentially toxic material with lightning rapidity. As also noted above, children frequently ingest materials that are in the open and are being used. Often this is because of an interruption; for example, a mother may leave a cleaning solution or furniture polish unattended for a moment while answering the telephone or the door bell.

Parents should be cautioned that when such interruptions occur, they should either replace the material in safe storage or take it or the child with them. With amazing frequency, children get into things in the presence of their parents, even without such interruptions. It is essential that when potentially toxic materials are being used in the presence of small children either the child or the material or both be in sight at all times.

All too often, children are invited to become poisoned by being given a potentially dangerous material to play with by an adult who underestimates the child's ability to gain access to the contents of almost any container. An unwary mother may, for example, give a fussing child an aspirin bottle thinking that he will be unable to remove the cap. Another common error is to leave medications on a bedside stand after administering them to a young child; the child for whom it was intended or a sibling may ingest the entire contents.

A significant number of childhood poisonings occur when there is a disruption in the normal household routine. Times of moving or painting, holidays, visits by friends or relatives, or death or illness in the family are occasions when increased caution should be exercised. Another matter that invites unsupervised access of children to potentially toxic materials is when they are sent through the mail or discarded into a refuse container.

The practice of sending drug samples through the mail either should be discouraged or the packages should be made tamperproof. They are frequently delivered when parents are not available or else are left within reach in the home after delivery. When deteriorated or unwanted materials are discarded, the safest procedure for potentially toxic liquids or powders is either to pour them down a drain or flush them down a toilet. With some highly concentrated and highly toxic materials, such as pesticide concentrates, even the amount left remaining in an "empty" bottle may be sufficient to cause serious poisoning. Such containers should be rinsed before being discarded.

Optimal supervision of self or others involves also attention to detail in the legitimate use of potentially hazardous materials. As previously noted, drug labels always should be examined carefully to ensure accurate identification before a medication is administered. Care must be taken that deteriorated or outdated drugs are not used, since some may have significantly altered effects. Self-medication or prescription of a child's treatment by the parents should be discouraged.

There is a tendency for many to believe that if a material were significantly hazardous it would not be available for over-the-counter sales, but nothing could be further from the truth. All too frequently, parents overmedicate a child, either because they underestimate the potential hazard or are given inadequate instructions. It is incumbent upon physicians who order medications, and indeed upon pharmacists who dispense them, to provide and emphasize specific instructions concerning proper use.

Though seemingly unlikely, it is not at all uncommon for a patient who has been advised to take or administer "some aspirin every once in a while" to use two or three times the safe dose every few hours for several days until serious intoxication occurs. Instructions on the label are meaningful to the cautious and the inquisitive, but these are rarely the people who become poisoned. Person-to-person conversation is far more effective and can well take place at the time a material is prescribed or dispensed.

Treatment

The management of poisoning is so steeped in erroneous tradition and influenced by anachronism that either maltreatment or no treatment at all is frequent outside of hospitals. On the one hand, there is the widespread but erroneous belief that there is an effective antidote for all or most poisons, and that without it other measures are to no avail. On the other hand, there is the mistaken notion that a great deal can be accomplished with simple household remedies.

Actually, there are very few poisons for which there are effective antidotes; for most cases of poisoning, good supportive care is all that can be offered. Even in those instances where antidotes are available, supportive care is at least as important; indeed, the best antidote in the world is of little value without good supportive care. Most of the home remedies which have been recommended from time to time actually are of little value, and most tend to waste valuable time that could better be devoted to proper treatment under adequate medical supervision.

Unfortunately, many of the lay publications, including first-aid texts, are outmoded in this respect and continue to recommend all sorts of elaborate but ineffective procedures to be carried out in the home. Even where recommendations can be made for truly effective procedures, the necessary material usually cannot be found readily in the home. The same criticism can be leveled at many of the instructions provided on the many rather complicated antidote lists and first-aid treatment charts that are disseminated for use of the public, often by pharmacists or pharmaceutical organizations.

The cardinal rule for the first-aid treatment of poisoning is to remove the poison from contact with the patient (unless such removal is contraindicated) *and to obtain definitive medical care at the earliest possible moment.*

The more simplified one can make any instructions for home treatment, the more likely they are to be followed and the less likely they are to either delay or be substituted for proper care by a physician. Thus, general procedures that can be carried out simply and are applicable almost irrespective of the nature of the poison are to be recommended until medical help can be obtained.

Pharmacists do not and should not perform or recommend treatment for poisoning except for simple first-aid measures. It is nonetheless important to outline some of the recommended procedures. Pharmacists are frequently called upon to provide instructions when poisoning occurs, and sometimes they provide such instructions to their clients as a prophylactic measure.

Pharmacists also play a key role in the development and the management of many poison control and treatment centers and in establishing the availability of proper treatment materials for use by physicians and in hospitals. In addition, the pharmacist is often the resource person to whom the physician turns for information, especially about poisoning due to drugs or about the availability of drugs for the treatment of poisoning. Thus, while the pharmacist should not be involved in prescribing a specific antidote, he can be of great help in informing the physician as to whether one is available. Details about how to use the material then can be obtained readily from conventional reference sources.

Recommended procedures for lay use in the first-aid treatment of poisoning are those suggested by the Subcommittee on Accidental Poisoning of the American Academy of Pediatrics (Table IV). The principal elements are (1) obtaining medical advice immediately to determine whether unusual procedures are indicated or usual procedures are contraindicated, and (2) terminating exposure of the victim by removal of the poison, usually through induction of vomiting. In regard to the latter point, it should be noted that induction of vomiting has been shown to be superior to gastric lavage in the removal of ingested poisons. Many of the measures recommended in the past for the induction of vomiting, such as mechanical stimulation

Table IV—First-Aid Treatment for Poisoning
(*American Academy of Pediatrics, Subcommittee on Accidental Poisoning*)

1. Swallowed poisons
   A. Call physician, hospital, poison control center, or rescue unit promptly.
   B. Dilute poison by giving water, one or two glassfuls.
   C. Make patient vomit if so directed, *but not if:*
      1. Patient is unconscious or having fits.
      2. Swallowed poison was a strong corrosive (lye, strong acid, drain cleaner, etc).
      3. Swallowed poison contained kerosene, gasoline, or other petroleum distillates (unless containing a dangerous pesticide as well, which must be removed).
   D. *Directions for making a patient vomit:*
      1. Give one tablespoonful (½ ounce) of syrup of ipecac for a child 1 year of age or older, plus at least 1 cup of water. If no vomiting occurs in 20 min, this dose may be repeated *once only.*
      2. If no ipecac syrup is available, try to induce vomiting by tickling back of throat with a spoon handle or other blunt object, after giving water.
      3. Do not waste time waiting for vomiting, but transport patient promptly to a medical facility. Bring package or container with intact label.
2. Fumes or gases (fuel gases, auto exhaust, dense smoke from fires, or fumes from poisonous chemicals, for example)
   A. Get victim into fresh clean air.
   B. Loosen clothing.
   C. If victim is not breathing, start artificial respiration promptly. Do not stop until patient is breathing well, or help arrives.
   D. Have *someone else* call a physician, hospital, poison control center, or rescue unit.
   E. Transport victim to a medical facility promptly.
3. Eye
   A. Gently wash eye out immediately, using plenty of water (or milk in an emergency), for 5 min with eyelid held open.
   B. Remove contact lenses if worn; never permit the eye to be rubbed.
   C. Call physician, poison control center, or rescue unit, and transport victim to a medical facility promptly.
4. Skin (acids, lye, other caustics, pesticides, etc)
   A. Wash off skin immediately with a large amount of water; use soap if available.
   B. Remove any contaminated clothing.
   C. Call physician, hospital, poison control center, or rescue unit, and transport victim to a medical facility if necessary.

of the posterior pharynx or the giving of mustard water or salt water, are usually not effective although they may be worthwhile if other more effective materials are not available. Probably the most serviceable emetic for first-aid use is syrup of ipecac, which is highly effective if used in the doses recommended here. Patients who will not cooperate by taking syrup of ipecac can be induced to vomit by the parenteral use of apomorphine.

In recent years there has been a movement, in some instances instigated or promoted by pharmaceutical organizations, to encourage the keeping of a first-aid treatment kit containing syrup of ipecac and activated charcoal in homes where there are children of poisoning-prone age. The kit promoted by the University of Utah Poison Information and Therapy Center in cooperation with the Utah Pharmaceutical Association is shown in Fig. 942.[2] It should be noted that a prominent part of the kit is the instruction on the lid to call a doctor or the local poison control center.

Activated charcoal is a highly effective adsorbent of a large number of poisons. (A notable exception is cyanide, which poisons charcoal.) Most organic and inorganic materials are adsorbed to a greater or lesser extent by this material and so its use more-or-less routinely in cases of poisoning by ingestion is worthwhile. It should be noted, however, that if activated charcoal is given before syrup of ipecac, it will inactivate the latter; consequently, it is advisable to induce vomiting first before administering the charcoal. Activated charcoal is worthwhile as a nonspecific antidote not only for home use but also for use in hospitals and in poison treatment centers.

Antidotes—Before discussing specific antidotes, it should be emphasized that while activated charcoal is an effective, nonspecific adsorbent of a large number of materials, there is no true "universal antidote." The classical universal antidote which has been in use for a long period of time consists of activated charcoal, tannic acid, and magnesium oxide (or, in the home: burnt toast, strong tea, and milk of magnesia). It now has been well established that the last two constituents have no significant efficacy and may actually impede the one active ingredient, activated charcoal. The long-advocated preparation of activated charcoal in the home by burning toast has no merit; the material does not have significant adsorptive properties.

It is important for information to be available readily concerning antidotes; not only so that they can

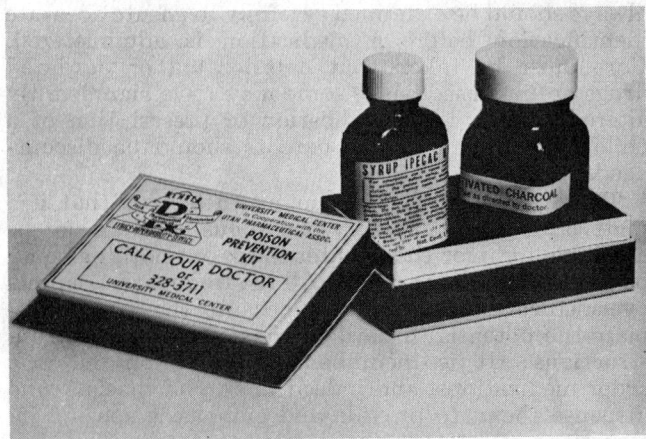

Fig. 942. A poison prevention kit containing syrup of ipecac (one ounce) and activated charcoal, developed by the Utah Pharmaceutical Association with the assistance of the University of Utah Poison Information and Therapy Center. (Courtesy, *JAPhA*[2]).

be used properly at the earliest possible moment, but also so that time is not wasted in searching for a nonexistent antidote. For a number of poisons, there are chemical antidotes that react with the poison in the stomach either to inactivate it or to retard its absorption. These are listed in Table V. Most such materials are sufficiently innocuous that they safely can be included in first-aid efforts by persons other than physicians.

Table VI lists those antidotes that are available for systemic administration to counteract the effects of poisons which have already been absorbed. Information is not given here concerning doses or other details of administration. These matters must be decided by a physician and are readily obtainable once the nature of the antidote is known.

Other measures—Aside from removal or inactivation of the poison and the use of antidotes when available, the treatment of poisoning is mainly supportive. The symptomatic or supportive approach to treatment does not differ significantly from that encountered in other medical problems, and its details are beyond the scope of this text. Common problems requiring supportive care include coma, respiratory insufficiency, convulsions, shock, vomiting, diarrhea, fluid and electrolyte disturbances, cerebral edema, kidney failure, and damage to other organs.

A number of procedures may be utilized to hasten elimination of a poison. In some instances this can be accomplished through diuresis induced either by increased fluid intake, alkalinization of the urine, or the use of pharmacologic or osmotic diuretics. With poisons that are dialyzable, either peritoneal dialysis or extracorporeal hemodialysis (use of the artificial kidney) may be employed. These procedures are especially worthwhile when normal excretory processes fail or prove to be inadequate, or when the degree of poisoning portends a fatal outcome unless the level of poison in the body is reduced rapidly.

Peritoneal dialysis can be performed in nearly any hospital setting and offers the advantages of simplicity, lack of requirement for elaborate equipment or extensive experience, and rapidity with which it can be instituted. Extracorporeal dialysis is far more efficient, but requires some hours to prepare and exceptional equipment and experience. Centers which are likely to be called upon to treat cases of poisoning should have the necessary supplies and equipment for performance of peritoneal dialysis and, if a hemodialysis setup is not available, should have information concerning the nearest location of such equipment.

Needed Materials—Because pharmacists are frequently the professionals responsible for the establishment or operation of poison centers and for the provision of facilities for the treatment of poisoning in hospitals, Table VII was constructed. It includes the antidotes and other pharmaceutical agents, equipment, supplies, and references that should be included in any poison treatment center (poison treatment centers are described further in the subsequent section). Whether or not a poison treatment center is established, most of the listed materials should be available in any medical facility that is likely to be called upon to treat cases of poisoning. (It should be noted, however, that some of the substances in the list of antidotes and other pharmaceutical agents are recommended only if so dictated by the presence of particular local hazards.) It is suggested further that such materials be kept either in a kit or in a specified location so that dangerous delays in the institution of proper treatment can be avoided.

Prevention

A number of preventive measures have been suggested or alluded to previously. It is important that preventive efforts take into account the "anatomy" of childhood poisoning. As is depicted in Fig. 943, the

Table V—Locally Acting Antidotes against Unabsorbed Poisons

| Poison | Antidote | |
	Substance and dose or concentration	Mechanism of action
Acids, corrosive	Weak alkali (magnesium oxide or hydroxide)	Neutralization
Alkali, caustic (eg, lye)	Weak acid (1:4 vinegar, 1% acetic acid, or lemon juice)	Neutralization
Alkaloids	Potassium permanganate, 1:10,000 (lavage)	Oxidation
Coniine		
Quinine		
Physostigmine[a]		
Strychnine		
Arsenic[a]	Protein (milk, egg white, etc)	Adsorption
Barium salts	Sodium sulfate, 2%	Precipitation
Chlorine gas	Sodium bicarbonate aerosol	Neutralizes HCl
Detergents, cationic	Soap	Inactivation
Fluoride[a]	Calcium (milk, lime water, calcium lactate or gluconate)	Precipitation
Formaldehyde	Ammonia water, 0.2%, or ammonium acetate or carbonate, 1% (lavage)	Form methenamine
Iodine	Starch, 1–10%	Inactivation
Iron[a]	Sodium bicarbonate, 5%; deferoxamine, 5–10 Gm	Form ferrous carbonate; chelates
Kerosene	Mineral oil	Increase viscosity (less aspiration hazard)
Mercury[a]	Sodium formaldehyde sulfoxylate, 5% (lavage), or protein (eg, milk)	Precipitation
Oxalic acid[a]	Calcium (see fluoride)	Precipitation
Petroleum hydrocarbons	Mineral oil	Increase viscosity (less aspiration hazard)
Phenol	A vegetable oil (olive, etc)	Retards absorption
Phosphorus	Copper sulfate, 0.2% (lavage)	Precipitation
Silver nitrate	Normal saline	Precipitation
Unknown and miscellaneous	Activated charcoal (as slurry in water)	Adsorbs many poisons

[a] Systemic antidotes also available (see Table VI).

Table VI—Systemic Antidotes

Poison	Antidote	Mechanism of Action
Acetanilid	(see *Nitrites*)	
Alphaprodine	(see *Narcotics*)	
Amanita muscaria	(see *Muscarine*)	
Amphetamines	Chlorpromazine	Blocks excitation
Aniline dyes	(see *Nitrites*)	
Arecoline	(see *Muscarine*)	
Arsenic	Dimercaprol (BAL)	Chelation
Benzedrine	(see *Amphetamines*)	
Bishydroxycoumarin	Vitamin K	Reverses hypoprothrombinemia
Black widow spider	Latrodectus antivenom	Inactivates venom
Botulinus	Botulinus antitoxin	Inactivates toxin
Bromide	Na or NH$_4$ chloride	Hastens excretion
Cadmium	Edathamil (?)	Chelation
Carbachol	(see *Muscarine*)	
Chlorates	Methylene blue	Reduces Methemoglobin
Chlorpromazine	(see *Phenothiazines*)	
Codeine	(see *Narcotics*)	
Copperhead (snake)	(see *Crotalidae*)	
Coral snake	Microcrurus antivenom	Inactivates venom
Coumadin	(see *Bishydroxycoumarin*)	
Crotalidae (snakes)	Crotalid antivenom	Inactivates venom
Cyanide	Amyl &/or Na nitrite	Methemoglobin iron (3+) competes with cytochromes for cyanide
	Na thiosulfate	Form thiocyanate
Demerol (meperidine)	(see *Narcotics*)	
Demeton	(see *Organophosphates*)	
Dexedrine	(see *Amphetamines*)	
Dextropropoxyphene	(see *Narcotics*)	
DFP	(see *Organophosphates*)	
Digitalis	Potassium Chloride	Physiologic antagonist
	Versene	Chelates calcium
Dilaudid	(see *Narcotics*)	
Dipterex	(see *Organophosphates*)	
ENP	(see *Organophosphates*)	
Ethyl biscoumacetate	(see *Bishydroxycoumarin*)	
Ethylene glycol	Ethanol	Retards metabolism to oxalate
Ferrous sulfate	(see *Iron*)	
Fluoride	Calcium	Precipitates; also corrects hypocalcemia
Fluoroacetate	Glycerol monoacetate	Bypasses metabolic block
Formaldehyde	Ammonium salts	Form methenamine
Heroin	(see *Narcotics*)	
HETP	(see *Organophosphates*)	
Hydrocyanic acid	(see *Cyanide*)	
Iron	Deferoxamine	Chelation
Latrodectus (spider)	(see *Black widow spider*)	
Lead	Dimercaprol plus edathamil	Chelation
Levopropoxyphene	*Do not* use levallorphan or nalorphine	
Malathion	(see *Organophosphates*)	
Mecholyl	(see *Muscarine*)	
Meperidine	(see *Narcotics*)	
Mercury	Dimercaprol	Chelation
Methacholine	(see *Mecholyl*)	
Methadone	(see *Narcotics*)	
Methamphetamine	(see *Amphetamines*)	
Methanol	Sodium bicarbonate	Reverses acidosis
	Ethanol	Retards formation of toxic metabolites
Moccasin snakes	(see *Crotalidae*)	
Morphine	(see *Narcotics*)	
Muscarine	Atropine	Parasympatholytic
Mushrooms (toxic)	(see *Amanita muscaria*)	
Narcotics	Levallorphan or Nalorphine	Specific antagonism
Neostigmine	(see *Prostigmin*)	
Nickel	Dimercaprol	Chelation
Nitrites	Methylene blue	Reduces methemoglobin
Nitrobenzene	(see *Nitrites*)	
OMPA	(see *Organophosphates*)	
Opiates	(see *Narcotics*)	
Organophosphates	Atropine	Parasympatholytic
	Pralidoxime chloride	Regenerates cholinesterase
Oxalate	Fluoride	Precipitates; also corrects hypocalcemia
Parathion	(see *Organophosphates*)	
Phenacetin	(see *Nitrites*)	
Phenindione	(see *Bishydroxycoumarin*)	

Table VI—Continued

Poison	Antidote	Mechanism of Action
Phenothiazines	Diphenhydramine	Blocks neuromuscular reaction (only)
Physostigmine	(see *Prostigmin*)	
Pilocarpine	(see *Muscarine*)	
Polymyxin	Antihistaminics	Block histamine effects
Potassium chlorate	(see *Chlorates*)	
Prochlorperazine	(see *Phenothiazines*)	
Propoxyphene	(see *Dextropropoxyphene* or *Levopropoxyphene*)	
Prostigmin	Atropine	Parasympatholytic
	Pralidoxime chloride	Regenerates cholinesterase
Prussic acid	(see *Cyanide*)	
Racemorphan	(see *Narcotics*)	
Rattlesnakes	(see *Crotalidae*)	
Sarin	(see *Organophosphates*)	
Scorpions	Antivenom	Inactivates venom
Snakes	(see *Crotalidae* or *Coral snake*)	
Sodium chlorate	(see *Chlorates*)	
Sodium fluoride	(see *Fluorides*)	
Sodium fluoroacetate	(see *Fluoroacetate*)	
Sodium nitrite	(see *Nitrites*)	
Soman	(see *Organophosphates*)	
Strychnine	Barbiturates	Sedation
Systox	(see *Organophosphates*)	
TEPP	(see *Organophosphates*)	
Thallium	Potassium chloride Activated charcoal	Hasten excretion
	Dithiocarb or dithizone	Chelation
Trifluoperazine	(see *Phenothiazines*)	
Trifluopromazine	(see *Phenothiazines*)	
Urecholine	(see *Muscarine*)	
Warfarin	(see *Bishydroxycoumarin*)	

majority of accidental poisonings in children involve common household articles or ubiquitous drugs. Materials that would be recognized universally as being poisons are not frequently involved, and it is a mistake to think that provision of an inaccessible storage place will solve the problem. This is not to say that classical poisons are not a serious problem or that locked medicine cabinets should not be provided. We must, however, view the problem realistically; much previous effort has been concentrated on the superficially obvious, and insufficient attention has been given to more influential epidemiologic factors.

Total prevention through education is an ideal worth striving for. When done in the usual way, however, it can be expected to affect only part of the problem. One difficulty is that educational efforts have been too general; the public has not really known precisely what it should do. Instruction is most effec-

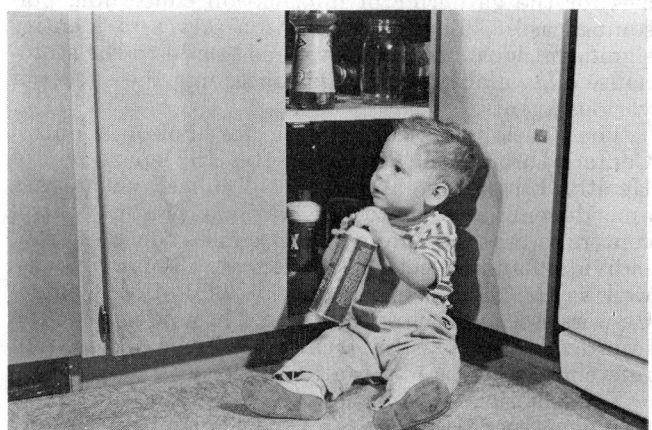

Fig. 943. The anatomy of accidental childhood poisoning. The majority are due to common household articles or drugs which are left within the reach of toddlers.

tive when it includes specific directions that can and should be followed. For instance, announcing to parents that they should "keep things out of the reach of small children" helps little until they are told what to keep out of reach, and of whom, and how.

The commonest histories obtained in cases of childhood poisoning are that the parents were not aware that the material was potentially poisonous, or that they took no special precautions because their child had been no problem previously, or that they thought the material was inaccessible to the child. Aiming educational efforts specifically at the various epidemiologic factors mentioned previously has far more effectiveness. General admonitions about preventing poisoning are likely to be as ineffective as have been such slogans as "safety first" in preventing other types of accidents.

Consonant with the theory of specific instruction is the issuing of directions with individual products. This can come from a number of sources (including the pharmacist, as discussed later) and in several ways. Precautionary labeling is of limited value because, unless it is so vivid as to be inescapable, it is likely to be read and heeded only by those individuals who represent the least risk. Precautionary labeling is already so ubiquitous that there is a tendency for it to be ignored; further steps in this direction are not likely to be very effective. They are effective in directing individuals to proper treatment, but their preventive value leaves something to be desired. Person-to-person instruction by the physician or dispensing pharmacists is preferred.

Limiting availability of highly toxic materials or directing the consumer to the least toxic material that will serve the intended purpose are of considerable value. Outmoded materials which have high degrees of toxicity should be eliminated, if necessary by fiat, as safer substitutes become available. Those who serve

Table VII—Recommended Antidotes, Equipment, and References for Poison Treatment Centers

Antidotes and other pharmaceutical agents

Acetic acid, 5% (or vinegar)	Mannitol, 25% (intravenous)
Activated Charcoal USP (Powder)	Metaraminol bitartrate (parenteral)
Ammonia water, 0.2%	Methylene blue, 1% aqueous (parenteral)
Amyl nitrite pearls[a]	Mineral oil
Amytal sodium (parenteral)	Nalorphine or levallorphan
Antivenins[b]	Norepinephrine (parenteral)
Apomorphine (parenteral)	Olive oil
Atropine sulfate (parenteral)	Paraldehyde
Botulinus antitoxin, polyvalent	Phenobarbital sodium (parenteral)
Calcium chloride, 5% (or lime water)	Phenylephrine hydrochloride (parenteral)
Calcium gluconate, 10% (parenteral)	Picrotoxin and/or bemegride (parenteral)
Copper sulfate, 0.2%	Potassium chloride (tablets and parenteral)
Deferoxamine	Potassium permanganate, 1:10,000
Dexamethasone (parenteral)	Pralidoxime chloride
Dimercaprol (BAL)	Procainamide (parenteral)
Diphenhydramine (parenteral)	Sodium bicarbonate, 5%
Dithizone[c] and/or dithiocarb[c]	Sodium formaldehyde sulfoxylate, 5%
Edathamil calcium disodium (Ca EDTA)	Sodium nitrite, 3% (parenteral)[a]
Ephedrine sulfate (parenteral)	Sodium sulfate
Ethanol (parenteral)	Sodium thiosulfate, 25% (parenteral)[a]
Glyceryl monoacetate (monacetin)[d]	Starch
Ipecac syrup	Tromethamine (parenteral)
Magnesium hydroxide (milk of magnesia)	Vitamin K_1 or K_1 oxide

Equipment and supplies

Catheters & stomach tubes	Containers for storage of aspirated gastric contents
Syringes 2, 5, 10, 20, 50 ml, & needles	Poison report forms
Mouth gags	Resuscitation, endotracheal intubation, tracheotomy,
Restraint sheets, blankets	suction, and dialysis equipment, as prescribed
Emesis basins	

References (minimal)[e]

Clinical Toxicology of Commercial Products
Supplemental Card Index on Toxicity of Trade Name Products
Poisonous Plants of the United States and Canada
Modern Drug Encyclopedia and Therapeutic Index
Physicians' Desk Reference
Merck Index
Standard pharmacology text(s)
Recommended Antidotes, Supplies and References for Poison Control Centers

[a] Materials for the antidotal treatment of cyanide poisoning (amyl nitrite, sodium nitrite, and sodium thiosulfate) can be obtained ready for use in a kit specifically designed for this purpose from the Eli Lilly Co. The kit includes instructions concerning its use.
[b] Polyvalent crotalin (rattlesnakes and moccasins), elapid (coral snakes), *Latrodectus* (black widow spider), scorpion, depending upon endemic hazards.
[c] Preliminary observations suggest usefulness in severe thallium poisoning; availability suggested if thallium is a significant local hazard.
[d] Experimental evidence of usefulness in fluoroacetate poisoning; availability suggested if fluoroacetate is a significant local hazard.
[e] See *Bibliography*.

the purchasing public should be in a position to advise about comparative safety as well as efficacy of the materials that they purvey.

Safety packaging offers preventive possibilities that have not been exploited fully. For instance, various means of packaging solid dosage forms of medications are proving to be significant obstacles for children. While innumerable innovations of this type have proved to be impractical by reason of expense or inconvenience, some have been developed which are both inexpensive and effective in preventing or retarding ingestions by children. Some of these are shown in Fig. 944. This method of prevention is deserving of additional exploration.

Poison Control Centers*—Such centers, of which there are now more than 500 in this country, have played an important role both in preventing and mitigating poisoning problems. There are two major types of centers: those which give information only (Poison Information Centers) and those which provide both information and treatment (Poison Treatment Centers).

---

* The latest directory of poison control centers is available to interested persons.[3]

Most of the treatment centers are based in hospitals; the information centers may be operated by hospitals, health departments, universities, civic organizations, or pharmacies. Both types of centers accumulate reference materials from which prognostic and treatment information can be obtained and serve as agencies for the gathering of information concerning poisoning cases. The latter function serves to identify significant local hazards as well as to add to the storehouse of available knowledge concerning the effects of various agents.

The National Clearinghouse for Poison Control Centers, through the auspices of the US Department of Health, Education, and Welfare, collects such data and disseminates it to the various poison control centers so that maximum benefit can be achieved from individual and collective experiences. This agency as well as the American Association of Poison Control Centers assists in the establishment of new centers, the improvement of existing facilities and the provision of reference material on a continuing basis.

The American Association of Poison Control Centers has developed standards for poison control centers which include, in addition to the functions mentioned above, the provision of 24-hour-a-day service, neces-

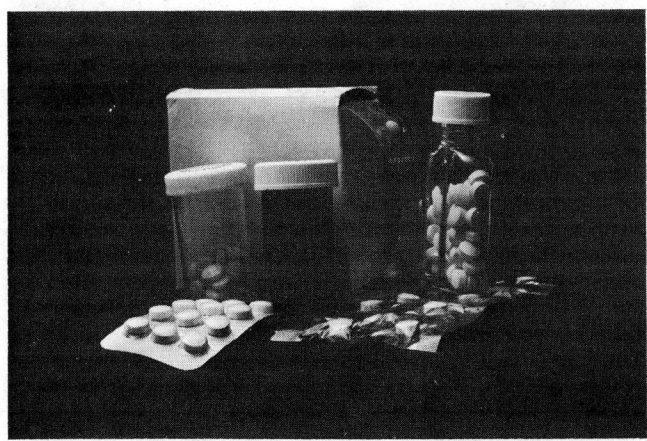

Fig. 944. Economical and effective forms of safety packaging. Each of the vial or bottle caps is of the pressure-release type requiring considerable downward pressure while turning in order to be removed (courtesy, specimens, Sterling, Wyeth, Plough, Walgreen, and Owens-Illinois).

sary treatment (or information as to where it can be obtained, in the case of information centers), the keeping of records concerning poisoning cases, and participation in educational programs both for the community and for those responsible for the care of poisoned patients.

National Poison Prevention Week—Since 1962 the third week of March has been designated National Poison Prevention Week. In addition to giving annual emphasis to the problem of poison control, this week provides an opportunity for concentrated educational efforts directed to the public. Pharmacists can and should play an active role in the activities of this period. Special displays in pharmacies have been one type of effective weapon. Other worthwhile activities have included television or radio messages, special meetings, and newspaper articles, all of which can be made more effective by interested pharmacists.

Role of the Pharmacist—There is much that the pharmacist can do to help prevent poisoning and to improve the treatment thereof. He should not become involved in the therapy of poisoning except for necessary first aid, but he plays a key role in ensuring that adequate equipment and information are available. Indeed, it is often the pharmacist of a hospital or medical group who initiates the development of adequate facilities and materials for the treatment of cases. Some states (Utah, for example) require that pharmacies maintain a certain amount of poisoning treatment information, and it need hardly be said that this information should be accurate.

Undoubtedly, the most important role can be played by the pharmacist in the area of prevention. His role should relate to all types of material within his province; however, it is particularly critical with regard to nonprescription items. With prescription medications, there is involvement of a physician who should provide instructions and precautionary advice. However, with over-the-counter materials, the pharmacist is usually the only person who is in a position to serve these functions.

The pharmacist can and should provide, explain and amplify directions for the proper use of potentially toxic materials. He should bear in mind that the concern is not only for the safety of the patient but also for other individuals in the household. Thus, the dispensing of a toxic medication provides an opportunity to warn the buyer about the hazards of leaving the material within reach of children.

In some instances it is desirable to affix warning labels on the products that a pharmacist dispenses. The dispensing of a drug provides an opportunity also to inquire and to give advice about facilities for safe storage. Because of his intimate knowledge of his patrons the pharmacist has a personalized role to play in cautioning about many prescription drugs and a host of commercial products. He can and should advise his patrons not to indulge in potentially dangerous self-medication. If unable to discourage the latter, the pharmacist can at least do much to improve self-treatment.

He can do much to remove the aforementioned limitations of labeling. While the public often may not read or appreciate precautions on labels, the effectiveness of the latter are increased significantly if they are explained by a pharmacist or similar individual.

When the pharmacist is consulted about a poisoning, he can best advise the individual to contact a physician immediately. In the meantime, he can help to ensure proper first-aid treatment and, more importantly, help to prevent injurious maltreatment by disseminating such advice as that contained in Table IV. He can be most effective in his advisory capacity if he has acquainted himself thoroughly with the existing poison information and treatment facilities of his area. He can assist greatly if he avoids diverting the services of functioning poison control centers to local pharmacies.

There has been a tendency for the development of too many small and ineffectual poison centers the activities of which could be carried out more effectively and efficiently if they were amalgamated with others in the same area. A trend toward centralization of poison information and treatment facilities should be encouraged.

The pharmacist has a unique role to play in detecting improper and defective labeling on hazardous products. He has an obligation to call the attention of legal enforcement agencies to any labeling defects.

Pharmacists can assist greatly in the educational efforts of a community by distributing literature provided by himself or by the local medical or pharmaceutical societies, and by providing space for displays related to poisoning prevention.

Finally, the pharmacist must do everything possible to eliminate unsafe practices in the dispensing of drugs. Some of these have been mentioned previously.

References

1. Berger, F. M., *Clin. Pharmacol. Therap.*, **8**, 219 (1967).
2. Done, A. K. *J. APhA*, **NS7**, 472 (1967).
3. *Directory: Poison Control Centers*, (PHS Publ. #1278) US Dept. of Health, Education, and Welfare, Washington, D.C. (for sale by the Superintendent of Documents, US Government Printing Office, Washington, D.C. 20402).

Bibliography

Arena, J. M., *Poisoning*, Thomas, Springfield, Ill., 1963.
Done, A. K., in Shirkey, H. C., ed., *Pediatric Therapy*, 3rd ed., Mosby, St. Louis, 1968.
Dreisbach, R. H., *Handbook of Poisoning: Prognosis and Treatment*, 6th ed., Lange Med. Publ., Los Altos, Calif., 1961.
Gleason, M., *et al*, *Clinical Toxicology of Commercial Products*, 3rd ed., Williams & Wilkins, Baltimore, 1969.
Goodman, L., and Gilman, A., *The Pharmacological Basis of Therapeutics*, 3rd ed., Macmillan, New York, 1965.
Kingsbury, J. M., *Poisonous Plants of the United States and Canada*, Prentice-Hall, Englewood Cliffs, N.J., 1964.
Merck Index, 8th ed., Merck & Co., Rahway, N.J., 1968.
Modern Drug Encyclopedia and Therapeutic Index, 10th ed., Donnelley, New York, 1965.
Physicians Desk Reference, 23rd ed., Medical Economics, Oradell, N.J., 1969.
Recommended Antidotes, Supplies, and References for Poison Control Centers, Am. Assoc. of Poison Control Centers, c/o Acad. of Med. of Cleveland, 1965.
Supplemental Card Index on Toxicity of Trade Name Products, National Clearinghouse for Poison Control Centers, Food & Drug Admin., Washington, D.C. 20201.
von Oettingen, W. F., *Poisoning. A Guide to Clinical Diagnosis and Treatment*, 2nd ed., Saunders, Philadelphia, 1963.

101 | Laws Governing Pharmacy

Commercial law—composite pharmacy law—labeling of drugs

This chapter was prepared by

Sidney H. Willig, JD, *Professor of Law and Director of Drug Law Unit,*
Temple University, Philadelphia, Pa.   19122

The pharmacist—whether he be a community practitioner in a retail establishment, a hospital pharmacist employed to prepare and dispense drugs to inpatients and outpatients, or occupied with the pharmaceutical industry in the manufacture or sale of drugs, devices, or cosmetics—must be aware of statutory law and legal relationships that affect his sphere of activity.

Essentially, this subdivides into three areas for consideration.

1. The pharmacist and his achievement and maintenance of licensure, with the requirements, responsibilities, and prerogatives that pertain. (The Pharmacy Practice Act, Regulations, and Rules of the State Board of Pharmacy).

2. The statutory outlines of fulfilment of his particular function as a pharmacist as set out in the Federal Food, Drug, and Cosmetic Act; the State Drug, Device, and Cosmetic Act and the regulations thereunder, plus any local laws that similarly pertain; and the Federal and State Narcotic laws and their regulations. This includes special laws and regulations that apply to groups of drugs deemed abusable and/or habituating on the federal, state, and local level.

3. The pharmacist practices a dynamic role in society. As a professional member of the health sciences and as an employer or employee engaged in supplying products and services to the public, he must be aware of certain legal considerations that have developed out of historic common law traditions and courtroom decisions, and which overlay his daily activities.

Commercial Law

Business Laws—The pharmacist should understand the general principles of the law of contracts, so that he will realize his responsibility when he undertakes a business obligation. The law of agency concerns him in the management of his employees. In deciding on the proper methods of conducting his business, raising capital, etc, he should know the applicable principles of partnership and corporation law. As he is engaged in a profession which demands a high degree of care, competency, and skill, he should be familiar with the law of negligence as it applies to the practice of pharmacy and the operation of a community pharmacy.

It is impossible in a general treatise of this kind to lay down in detail the legal subjects upon which the pharmacist should keep posted. All that can be attempted is a general outline.

Diversity of Laws—The American Union is composed of fifty distinct and separate sovereignties, each supreme within its own territory, excepting only so far as the people by their Constitution have granted certain powers to the Federal Government. Pharmacists are, of necessity, subject to a multiplicity of state and federal laws. While these laws, when seen in the aggregate, are aimed at bettering public health and surrounding the distribution of drugs and medicines with every necessary safeguard, they differ greatly in detail. There are, however, fundamental principles upon which the laws of nearly all the states agree. These are the principles of the "common law" of England, brought to this country by our forefathers, and either consciously or unconsciously followed since by the lawmakers of the several states as they sought to enact legislation to meet the changing needs of their communities. Therefore it is possible for the business man, by a study of the "common law" as it affects his business, to acquire, with a little help from a lawyer of his own state, an adequate grasp of the rules of law which must govern him in the management of his business and professional affairs.

The Contract—In looking into the operation of the "common law" on this subject, it is found that:

A Promise Is Not a Contract—It is difficult for the layman to grasp the idea that the law will not necessarily enforce a promise. Originally, only those promises which were written "under seal"—attested by the solemnity of a waxen or written seal—could be enforced. Later, the principle was accepted that if the person to whom the promise was made lost something because of that promise, then it was not fair that the other party should break his word: so it became the law that if "consideration" passed—if value passed from the promisee because of the promise made to him—then the contract should be as binding as though it had been in writing and under seal.

Size of Consideration Is Not a Factor—The law is not interested in the value of the consideration. If there is consideration, the contract stands. One who has made a bad bargain may not ordinarily invoke the law to escape from the consequences of that bargain. Contracts are supposed to be made by men "standing at arm's length" so that each one is required to use his wits to see that he makes the best terms possible for himself.

When there is "a meeting of the minds" with respect to the aims and purposes of the contract, as they bear upon the contracting parties, then a contract may be said to have ensued.

Where the parties to a contract do not stand on an equal footing with one another, the utmost good faith is required from the person standing in the superior position. Thus a father's contract with a son, a lawyer's contract with a client, a physician's contract with a patient—all require that the utmost good faith be shown, so that no advantage will be taken of the person who has a right to expect such good faith.

Fraud, However, May Make a Contract Void—Fraud may render any contract void. If a man induces another by fraud to enter into a contract, the courts will interfere and in appropriate cases declare the contract null and void. It is therefore important to know what constitutes fraud. As a general proposition fraud consists of misrepresentation of a material fact. If a man should say, "I am engaged to marry So-and-So," and thereby gain an extension of credit—this statement if false would amount to fraud. If, on the other hand, he should say, "I hope to marry So-and-So," this would not be fraud, as a statement of a hope or wish is not a statement of fact.

The tendency of the law today, however, is to broaden the definition of fraud by making it embrace every statement made with intent to deceive—for, as was recently said by an eminent English judge, "The state of a man's mind is as much a question of fact as the state of his digestion."

It is therefore important before deciding whether a contract is invalid because of fraud, to consult the law of the state where the contract was made and the decisions of the court bearing on the subject.

Contracts entered into for the purpose of doing some unlawful act are void, and no court will entertain a suit for damages resulting from nonperformance.

Contracts calling for the performance of contract terms which are unconscionable, unduly harsh, or impossible to be done are void or voidable upon appeal to the appropriate judicial body.

Parties—The parties to a contract should be of full age and of sound mind; and the contract itself, to be enforceable, must be for the doing of a thing which is lawful. It is well to remember, however, that a minor can *make* a contract (with an adult); but such a contract is not enforceable against a minor, except for the furnishing of necessaries.

Written Contracts—It is not necessary that contracts—save in a few excepted cases—be in writing. They may be expressed or implied, depending upon the facts in the case. If, however, the parties elect to put their agreement in writing, the writing must disclose the entire contract. Should there be a dispute later about its terms, they would each be limited to whatever rights they held under the written instrument. Oral testimony of an understanding or enlarging or changing the terms of the written contract, is not ordinarily admissible at a trial to enforce rights under the contract. Ignorance of this principle has often resulted in serious loss.

Sale transactions in the pharmacy are contractual in nature even though they are informal and hopefully frequent. Therefore, certain rights may remain to both buyer and seller. The latter has the right to expect that the payment given him or promised to him will not be defaulted. If the pharmacist is paid by check, he rightfully expects that the payer has the authority to write it and the funds to back it.

The purchaser has the right to expect that the articles purchased are as represented, that they are fit for the purpose intended and are of satisfactory quality, and that the seller had a right to sell them. While some of these rights arise from actual conversation or advertisement and are express warranties, others have been implied from general morality and conduct and common law.

What Contracts Must Be in Writing—There are certain contracts, however, which the law requires to be in writing. These are, generally speaking, contracts to guarantee or stand surety for another, contracts dealing with rights in real estate, and contracts for the sale of goods over a certain figure. The local state laws need to be consulted on this point.

Remedies for Breach of Contract—If a contract is broken, the party wronged may in nearly all cases sue the other in a court of law, asking money damages as compensation for loss sustained. In some cases, however, where money damages would not compensate, he has the right to go into a court of equity and ask that the other party be compelled to carry out his agreement.

A lease, which in all cases should be in written form, is merely a contract between the owner (called the lessor) of the property and the person (known as the lessee) who wishes to lease the property, setting forth the essential details governing the duration of the lease, the amount of the rent, when payable, renewability, and other facts and conditions bearing upon the use and occupancy of the leased building or quarters.

The amount of rent is determined in a number of ways. It may be for a definite amount annually, payable in monthly installments. It may also be for a flat sum per year, plus a share of the sales volume of the store, as agreed to by the parties involved. In some cases the lessee agrees to pay to the lessor a stated percentage of sales, the percentage to be increased as the volume grows.

The pharmacist should study all phases of the lease very carefully so that he may take every precaution necessary for the protection of his interests. He should give serious consideration to the time element.

It is well not to enter into a term longer than is prudent and safe. In all cases, however, the lease should be renewable for a definite term on conditions agreed upon when the lease is originally written.

It should be borne in mind, too, that as a general rule, where controversy arises over the meaning of any term in the lease, or where the conditions governing the use and occupancy of the leased quarters are not clearly stated, the law favors the lessor on the theory that his is the greater and more dominant interest.

Agency—Contracts involving agency are very important, as it is necessary for every businessman to transact a great part of his work through agents. These may be general agents, with full power to act for their principals, or special agents, whose authority is limited by the contract of employment.

Duty toward Agent—The principal owes to the agent the duty of payment for services rendered and remuneration for expenses properly incurred. If the agent is an employee, he has other obligations toward him, looking to his safety and health. These obligations are generally defined in the various workmen's compensation laws which are in force in practically every state. Under these laws, the employee is paid compensation for injuries resulting from accidents suffered while engaged in the employer's business, such payment being made according to a schedule set forth in the law. The amounts of payment depend upon the severity of the injury and the earning power of the employee. The principal is further required to be insured against the risk of liability for such payment.

Duty toward Employer—The agent owes to the principal the duty of loyalty and service. He may not make a secret profit out of his employment; he may not "serve two masters."

Duty toward Third Parties—The principal is bound by contracts made by his agent within the scope of the agent's actual authority. The principal is also bound by contracts made by the agent within the scope of his *apparent* authority—even though such contracts be in direct violation of the agent's instructions—unless, of course, such violation be known or should be known by the person with whom the agent is dealing. That "the act of the agent is the act of the principal," is well established in the law.

Agency by Estoppel—If a person without any authority whatever claims to be an agent of a certain principal, it is the duty of that principal to speak out and deny the agency so as to put all other persons on their guard. If the so-called principal remains silent and third parties are by his silence deceived into thinking that the person claiming to be such agent is telling the truth—then there is danger that the principal will become liable "by estoppel" for any loss suffered by such third party. The innocent party, in cases such as this, is entitled to the protection of the law.

Liability for Torts and Crimes—The principal is further liable to third parties for torts (wrongs) committed by the agent while seeking to further the employer's business, and this is also true whether or not such wrongs were committed in violation of instructions. A principal, however, is not criminally responsible for crimes committed by the agent, unless he instructed the agent to commit the crimes and thereby was a party to them.

In some urban areas pharmacists have organized themselves into labor unions, or joined labor unions which represent various categories of health-care personnel. Federal and much state labor law mirrors the view held by the legislatures that the business of a nonprofit hospital is so affected with the public interest as to require continuous and uninterrupted service to the public and has been historically loath to give such employees and such unions the right to organize, collectively bargain, and strike. Today, the prohibition in the main goes only to the latter. In states such as New York, which have been more responsive to labor's needs, the statute and its amendments are designed to avoid labor disputes in voluntary hospitals by prohibiting hospital employees from striking or picketing, but providing substitutes of mediation, fact-finding, and binding arbitration.

The Partnership—The simplest form of doing business is that of personal ownership, which has few complications. If, however, a partnership is formed, the law deems each partner both a principal and an agent—each partner is agent for all the others, within the scope of partnership business. It follows, therefore, that each partner can bind the partnership by contract; further, that each partner is responsible for all contracts made by the partnership and all debts incurred by it. This is true irrespective of the size of the interest of the partner in the business—*he is responsible for every cent of the firm's debts*, no matter what that interest is, so long as he is a partner.

Partnership contracts, because of the highly personalized relationships which they involve, should be carefully drawn and entered into only after a full understanding of the legal burdens imposed.

Dissolution of Partnership—Upon dissolution of a partnership, it is more important that the retiring partner or partners cause public notice to be made of the fact of such dissolution; in addition specific notice should be given to all firms or individuals with whom the partnership has been accustomed to do business. If such notice is not given, there is the possibility of a "liability by estoppel" as previously discussed.

The Limited Partnership—If individual liability is sought to be avoided, the device of a limited partnership may be employed. This is brought about by making application to the proper authority of the state, naming the contribution of each partner toward the business capital. There must always be at least one general partner in a limited partnership, whose liability is unlimited.

The Corporation—The corporation is formed by authority of the state, which, upon application, grants a charter to the incorporators. This charter states the powers of the corporation. In its activities, the corporation is held to the powers expressly stated in the charter, and the obvious implications inherent therein.

Capital Stock—The capital stock of the corporation is divided into shares, and the number of shares held by each stockholder is evidenced by the certificate of stock issued to him. The stockholders elect a board of directors who, with the officers, conduct the affairs of the corporation.

Stock is either common or preferred. Common stock is the ordinary voting stock of the company. Its holders share in the profits of the company, whenever dividends are declared by the directors. Preferred stockholders are entitled to receive stated dividends before any payments or declarations whatever are made to the holders of common stock. The rights of all stockholders, so far as receipt of dividends is concerned, are printed on the certificates of stock issued to them.

Liability of Stockholders—In case a corporation becomes insolvent, stockholders are liable for only the amount of stock subscribed for by them, with certain exceptions with regard to banking corporations, etc., where the state law must be consulted. Some state laws provide that when a corporation becomes insolvent, the stockholders are held individually liable for payment of wages to employees.

Bonds—Bonds of corporations are evidences of debt, that money has been borrowed. The terms of payment, the nature of the security, all questions of priority, etc., are stated on the bond. Bondholders, of course, must be paid in accordance with these terms, before any money is paid to stockholders.

Commercial Paper—Practically every state has enacted the "Uniform Negotiable Instruments Law." It provides that "negotiable paper," ie, bills of exchange, checks, promissory notes, etc, shall be negotiable by endorsement or delivery, so that a person who has given value for such negotiable paper, before the maturity date named thereon, has a right to proceed for nonpayment, not only against the maker but also against all prior endorsers. Such nonpayment is termed *dishonor* and the *Negotiable Instruments Law* is very specific in detailing how, when, and to whom such notice of dishonor must be given. Unless notice is given in strict accordance with this law, there can be no recovery against prior endorsers—though there can still be recovery against the original maker.

Notice of Dishonor—Formal "notice of dishonor" must be given to all prior parties on the note in order to hold them responsible. This notice must be given by a Notary Public, in a form called a "protest," and such protest must be made at or immediately after the actual dishonor of the note. Consult local statutes for manner and time for such notice. Unless such notice is given in strict accordance with the statute, there can be no recovery under the law.

If one desires to endorse commercial paper without incurring any liability thereunder, he should place over his signature the words "without recourse."

Negligence—A pharmacist is responsible if anyone is injured by the negligent act of himself or his agent, provided such act is done within the scope of the agent's real or apparent authority. Negligence is the absence of proper care. What is proper care is a question depending on the facts in each case.

In general, where the preparation, storage, or dispensing of a drug can be shown to be the proximate cause of harm to the patient, liability may be imposed. Any instrumentality of putting such an unsafe or ineffective drug into a patient's hands for use is liable to be named as defendant by an irate plaintiff. This includes along with the manufacturer, the pharmacist and/or the physician. This is aside from the issue of prescribing.

Courts generally characterize the duty of care reasonably anticipated from health science professionals such as pharmacists as being, minimally, that degree of care that a reasonably prudent person would have exercised under the same or similar circumstances. However, while this seems an average standard of care, it is higher than the care required in most other activities by which the public's health is neither directly benefited nor jeopardized. There is no question that the law holds those engaging in activities requiring unique knowledge and ability (such as labeling, dispensing, manufacturing, and compounding potent drugs) to perform in a manner commensurate with their undertaking.

The professional, however, also will be liable where his conduct is unreasonable and imprudent as compared to how any ordinary reasonable person might act, without considering the professional implications.

In the latter event, the testimony of experts is certainly not essential to resolve the great bulk of the factual questions. Even where professional duties and standards are involved—while expert testimony of pharmacists and physicians generally may be indicated—there are occasions when the acts or omissions of pharmacists might on their face be found to fall below the layman's standard of reasonably prudent care.

Liability for Error in Filling Prescriptions—If a pharmacist fills a prescription according to its terms, ordinarily he is not responsible if the medicine fails to cure or even does harm to the person taking it. Cases, however, may arise where a pharmacist is under a special duty to guard the patient from harm. Where unusual circumstances show that the physician who wrote the prescription could not have been aware of the dangerous nature of the ingredients prescribed, a duty rests upon the pharmacist to refuse to fill the prescription. The pharmacist should be especially careful to see that the dosage is safe under the conditions prescribed, as failure to observe this caution would, in all probability, constitute negligence on his part.

The rule is universal that prescriptions may be filled only by a registered pharmacist or by some other person acting under his direct and immediate personal supervision.

Preservation of Prescriptions—All prescriptions should be preserved by the pharmacist for at least five years as they are subject to inspection by federal or state officials, should there be some public need for such inspection. Special care must be observed in the numbering, filling, and preservation of prescriptions for *narcotics*. The state and federal regulations on this point must be followed most carefully.

Ownership of Prescriptions—The question arises from time to time respecting the ownership of the prescription. There is some authority vesting the ownership in the physician who wrote it or in the pharmacist who, as a matter of law, must keep it on file.

The better view, however, is that the patient has that kind and degree of qualified ownership which gives him the right to have the prescription renewed, whenever such renewal is legal, or to receive a copy, except in those cases where the giving of copies is forbidden by statute.

Poisons—It is held that a violation of a statute governing the care or use of the thing which does the damage is in itself negligence. It therefore is proper at this place to consider the special statutes concerning the sale of poisons. *A poison has been defined as any drug known to the pharmaceutical or medical profession, which is liable to be destructive to adult human life if taken in quantities of 60 grains or less.* This general definition is helpful in indicating the substances customarily regarded as poisonous, but it is not followed in many of the state poison laws. It is difficult, if indeed not impossible, to formulate a definition of the term "poison" which will be found satisfactory under any and all conditions.

In some state poison laws, the substances covered are arbitrarily selected, thus avoiding the futility of definitive phraseology. As there is a vast lack of agreement among the state poison laws, the law of each state should be consulted whenever transactions in any given state are involved.

Forbidden to Send by Mail—Under federal law the pharmacist is prohibited from transmitting poisons through the mails without special authority from the Postmaster-General.

Labels—The laws of practically all states provide that whenever a poison is sold or delivered by a pharmacist the bottle, package, or other container of the substance must bear a label giving the name of the article, the word "poison" and the name and place of business of the seller. A pharmacist is further forbidden to sell any poison to a person without satisfying himself that the person understands the nature of the poison and intends to put it to proper use.

Record of Sale Required—Pharmacists are required, under specific state laws, to register all retail sales of poisons in a book especially kept for that purpose known as "The Poison Register." The record of sale must include the name and address of the purchaser, the name of the seller, the date of sale, the name and quantity of the poison, and the purpose for which it is intended.

In Maryland and Wisconsin, the purchaser must affix his signature to the record of purchase, the effect of which not only is to give the seller a receipt for the poisons sold but also to emphasize the dangerous nature of the item being purchased.

It is interesting to note that courts have held that "The Poison Register" must be used exclusively for that purpose. It must be preserved for the number of years stipulated in the state act, and is subject to inspection by the proper state authorities.

Abortifacients—By virtue of a United States law, it is forbidden to send through the mails any drug or device tending to produce abortion. The current view is that abortifacients are "dangerous drugs," as this term is defined in the Food, Drug and Cosmetic Act, and are required to bear the legend "Caution—federal law prohibits dispensing without prescription." The sale of such drugs is prohibited by law in several states, except when prescribed by physicians in the course of their professional practice.

Advertising—The advertising and promotion of drugs on an interstate commerce basis is a shared commitment of numerous federal agencies, including the Post Office, Federal Communications Commission, Federal Trade Commission, and Food and Drug Administration. The latter two bear the brunt of the responsibility. The FDA oversees prescription drug advertising and the FTC does the same for OTC products. However, there is considerable overlap because of statutory definitions of labeling and by mutual agreement among the agencies.

In intrastate commerce, frequently analogous controls exist both in terms of substantive law and enforcement apparatus. However, limitations imposed mainly by budget make this less than a proportional effect in comparison to federal activities.

Pharmacists, however, are bound by federal legal restrictions that may exist. Therefore, promotional displays and mailings, especially as regards prescription drugs, should be cleared in terms of federal and state regulations. While federal law does not inhibit price advertising *per se* of prescription drugs, in some jurisdictions prescription price advertisements are legal while in many they are not.

In 1968 a joint meeting of APhA and NARD officials addressing itself to the question summarily noted the opinion that consumer advertising of prescription drug prices is a danger to public health and safety. It was emphasized that this served to place prescription products within the general description of commercial goods. Among important differences, aside from the legal controls applicable, are that historically and traditionally no professional practitioner is expected to solicit professional practice.

The selection of a personal pharmacist should be based on factors other than an advertised price for a specific product. These factors are confidence in and professional reputation of the pharmacist, services available, and conveniences offered, depending on the location and type of pharmacy involved. That is how other professional services are selected.

The now famous *Fred Meyer* decision rendered by the US Supreme Court, March 18, 1968, made clear that a distributor who gives promotional allowances to a direct-buying retailer has an obligation to do likewise for retailers who buy indirectly through wholesalers, and are in competition with the direct-account retailers.

Resulting from this has come an omnibus proposal by the Federal Trade Commission to establish guidelines as a "useful and comprehensive tool for assessing the impact of legal requirements and applying them to affected business practices." Its affect on pharmacy and toilet good promotions is obvious since the bulk of distribution is accomplished by "nondirects."

This has been finalized, effective June, 1969, and was published in the *Federal Register*, June 2, 1969. To obviate difficulties some manufacturers have abandoned direct selling in favor of uniform distribution through wholesalers.

Under the terms of the Wheeler-Lea Amendment to the Federal Trade Commission Act, false or deceptive advertising of food, drugs, devices, and cosmetics is made a federal offense. For the purpose of the amendment "false advertising" is defined as follows:

The term "false advertisement" means an advertisement, other than labeling, which is misleading in a material respect; and in determining whether any advertisement is misleading, there shall be taken into account (among other things) not only representations made or suggested by statement, word, design, device, sound, or any combination thereof, but also the extent to which the advertisement fails to reveal facts material in the light of such representations or material with respect to consequences which may result from the use of the commodity to which the advertisement relates under the conditions prescribed in said advertisement, or under such conditions as are customary or usual.

In many states, truthful advertising laws are in effect, and these should be consulted by every pharmacist who engages in promotion or advertising in the usual manner.

Insurance Programs—Many prescription prepayment plans have been elaborated in recent years which would tend to give subscribers the same type of insurance advantages available in the case of other medical services.

A typical plan (Maryland Blue Cross) sets forth the understanding that for dispensing prescriptions the pharmacy will receive the cost of the merchandise, based on charges by independent service wholesalers, plus a professional fee of $1.85. The plans contain certain quantitative limitations on prescription size and do not cover proprietary drugs (OTC's) or devices. These plans overcome the objection of limiting a patient's selection of a pharmacy by inviting all registered pharmacists in the state to participate.

Defamation—Another group of torts which may on occasion involve the pharmacist is of the intentional variety and generally termed the "defamatory" torts. These include slander, libel, and product libel; we may treat them generally without detailed legal differentiation.

Defamatory statements, whether oral, written, or otherwise communicated, are described as those which tend to expose a person to hatred, contempt, or aversion, or lower the community opinion of him. It affects reputation and the law is concerned since this in turn may hinder the earning of a livelihood, the enjoyment of normal social life, and the possibilities of profit and promotion. Therefore, it must be "published," that is, communicated to a third party.

An employer pharmacist may call his employee lazy, unchaste, or careless. A physician may call the pharmacist and say he is overcharging patients or does not have a modern inventory of drugs. It only becomes legally defamatory if these statements are made to others or in the presence of others than to whom the critical or insulting comment is directed.

Every subsequent publication creates a new cause of action and liability. Everyone who repeats a slander or libel is responsible for the damage caused by the repetition, even though he indicates he is merely opining or that it was told him by someone else, and even though he has every reason to believe it to be true. Malice may be imputed from the nature of the libelous statement where it clearly tends to injure.

While "truth" is the perfect defense to a charge of defamation, partial truth or honest error are to no avail. There are certain qualified privileges which permit communication of defamatory statement; however, these are few and, if malicious, are often disqualified.

It should be obvious that pharmacists have a special stake in refraining from slanderous opining about co-professionals, customers, and products. They should respect the confidential and fiduciary nature of their calling.

The pharmacist also must bear in mind that every member of the health-care team is expected to serve the patient with decency and respect, and to prevent invasion of his privacy to the greatest degree possible. The patient has the right to have information relating to his condition and treatment kept secret insofar as any other persons are concerned unless he authorizes its release.

Other Special Legislation—Stringent laws govern the possession and sale of narcotics. These laws are discussed on page 1970. The Federal Food, Drug and

Cosmetic Act, which prohibits adulteration or misbranding, is discussed on page 1976. The *Federal*

Hazardous Substances Labeling Act is discussed on page 1986.

Laws Governing the Practice of Pharmacy

The regulation of the practice of pharmacy is a function of the states, and not of the Federal Government. It rests upon the power vested in the state to protect the health, safety, and welfare of its citizens.

Like every profession, the practice of pharmacy is a privilege bestowed by the state under the constitutional reservation of "Police Powers." However, this is a privilege available to a class of persons who satisfy stated minimal parameters within the concept of practice subject to mandatory licensure requirement. No one may practice pharmacy without a license, except for those exempted by specification within the Act. However, anyone may achieve such licensure by carrying through successfully the statutory pattern of qualification which the state has set forth and administers by an agency generally termed a Board of Pharmacy. In some instances the board of pharmacy is a subagency in that it exists as part of a larger state agency, such as a Department of Health.

Once licensure is gained it may not be taken lightly by either the state or the licentiate. The former may suspend, revoke, or terminate it after due process and for just cause as set out in the Act. At the same time, the state undertakes to protect the public and the licensed members of the pharmacy profession from practice by unlicensed (hence, unqualified) parties in its jurisdiction.

As to the licensed pharmacist, he has gained a profession the practice of which is safeguarded by the federal and state constitutions as a property right. While he must abide by the Act to preserve it, must pay fees required to accomplish initial and continuing registration, must satisfy the legal, moral, and ethical standards of his peers as set out in law and regulations, he does have the right to legal redress against any who would seek to deprive him of the profits and prerogatives of licensure.

While pharmacy laws of the different states may vary among themselves, they are in agreement with respect to the fundamental principles, purposes, aims, and objectives of pharmaceutical practice.

The Basic Laws Regulating Pharmacy

Pharmacy laws generally provide for:

1. The educational and experience qualifications which pharmacists must meet at the time of examination or registration.
2. The agency, usually known as the State Board of Pharmacy, charged with the enforcement and administration of the law.
3. The granting of permits for the conduct of a community pharmacy or drug store. In most states permits are issued for one year and application must be made for their renewal.
4. The minimum of professional and technical equipment and apparatus which the pharmacy must, at all times, possess. The USP and the NF are generally included in this requirement.
5. Periodic re-registration of pharmacists. In most states, certificates of registration are granted for the period of one year.
6. The conditions under which certificates of registration or store permits may be canceled or revoked.
7. The prominent display of the certificate of registration in the store or pharmacy in which the holder is employed.
8. Penalties for violations. Infractions of pharmacy laws are punishable by fines in most instances.
9. Reciprocal registration. A pharmacist licensed by examination in one state may, by conforming to more or less nominal rules, become registered in another state, the latter registration being without examination.
10. The discretion vested in boards of pharmacy. While the Board is authorized to make rules and regulations for the enforcement and administration of the pharmacy law, such rules and regulations must be strictly in accord with the expressed or implied purposes of the law. The Board is an administrative, not legislative, agency. It may not exercise any power or authority not clearly delegated to it, or which by reasonable implication is necessary to the proper functioning of the pharmacy law.
11. The sale of proprietary and patent medicines, and commonly used household and domestic remedies by dealers other than pharmacists. As a rule, such dealers are unrestricted in the sale of preparations falling in these classifications, although in some states permits by the Board of Pharmacy are required.

Reciprocity—Reciprocal registration, referred to in item 9 above, is in effect in 47 states, the District of Columbia, and Puerto Rico.

In the year 1970 there were only three states, namely, California, Florida, and Hawaii, which did not grant reciprocal registration. Pharmacists considering reciprocal registration should obtain in advance full information regarding the specific requirements for reciprocity in the state in which registration is sought. For such information, write to Secretary of the National Association of Boards of Pharmacy, 77 W. Washington St., Chicago, Ill. 60602.

Composite Pharmacy Law

As the pharmacy laws in the several states vary in minor details, a composite pharmacy law is here given. This will afford the student an opportunity to grasp their over-all objectives and purposes. Pharmacists must, of course, be versed in the statutory requirements of their state. This is essential if violation of the pharmacy laws is to be avoided.

The quoted paragraphs are taken verbatim either from state pharmacy acts or the so-called *Uniform State Pharmacy Act* sponsored by the Committee on the Modernization of Pharmacy Laws of the American Pharmaceutical Association. The source of the quoted

paragraphs is given in each instance, and in order to distinguish the quoted material from the explanatory portions of the text, the former is placed in smaller type.

Title

An Act to repeal Article . . . . . . of the Code of Public General Laws of . . . ., and to enact in lieu thereof a new Article entitled, the "Uniform State Pharmacy Act."

The title is an important part of all bills submitted to the legislature and to all laws passed by it. The title must, in a very precise sense, give the purpose of the measure and some indication of the means by which the purpose is to be accomplished.

Finding and Declaration of Policy and Purpose

"The Legislature (or whatever other designation is used in referring to the lawmaking body) of the State (or Commonwealth) of . . . . , hereby finds that it is essential to the public health and safety to regulate and control the manufacture, sale and distribution of drugs, cosmetics and medical supplies as defined in this Act:

"It is, therefore, hereby declared to be the policy and purpose of this Act to vest in an administrative agency composed of specially trained, competent and skilled persons the power and authority to administer and enforce the provisions of this Act, to the end that the manufacture and distribution of drugs, medical supplies and cosmetics and the compounding and dispensing of prescriptions may be properly regulated and supervised in the interest of public health and safety." (*Uniform State Pharmacy Act*)

While it is not necessary that a legislative act, such as the State Pharmacy Law, include a declaration of policy and purpose, such declaration often proves advantageous. It is of aid to the court when the constitutionality of the measure is involved, and also throws much light upon the meaning of the various provisions of the law. Also, it serves to inform the members of the legislature having the measure under consideration the objectives sought by the passage of the law.

Enacting Clause

Section 1

Be it enacted by the general assembly of . . . .(or whatever the proper designation of the lawmaking body may be), That Article . . . . . .of the Code of Public General Laws of . . . . (or whatever the proper designation may be) title . . . . , be and the same is hereby repealed.

Section 2

And be it further enacted, That a new Article be added to the Code of Public General Laws of . . . .(or whatever the proper designation may be), to be known as Article . . . . .of said Code, entitled "Uniform State Pharmacy Act" with appropriate subtitles. Said new Article to read as follows:

As a general rule, the state constitutions do not require an enacting clause but courts have very generally held that an accurate enacting clause is essential to valid legislation.

In presenting bills to the legislature of any state, the enacting clause should be so drawn as to meet the requirements of that particular state. For instance, a bill introduced in the Pennsylvania legislature should conform with Pennsylvania custom and usage with respect thereto.

Short Title

This Act shall be known as the "Uniform Pharmacy Act of the State of . . . ."

The "Short Title," as the term itself suggests, is a convenient device by means of which legislation may be referred to in a brief, concise manner.

Definitions

"For the purpose of this Act:

"(a) The term '*pharmacy*' shall be held to mean and include every store or shop or other place where (1) drugs are dispensed, or sold at retail, or displayed for sale at retail; or (2) where physicians' prescriptions are compounded; or (3) which has upon it or displayed within it, or affixed to or used in connection with it, a sign bearing the word or words 'Pharmacist,' 'Pharmacy,' 'Apothecary,' 'Drug Store,' 'Druggist,' 'Drugs,' 'Medicines,' 'Medicine Store,' 'Drug Sundries,'

'Remedies,' or any word or words of similar or like import; or (4) where the characteristic show bottles or globes filled with colored liquids or otherwise colored, are exhibited; or (5) any store or shop or other place, with respect to which any of the above words are used in any advertisement." (*Uniform State Pharmacy Act*)

Basic definitions are essential to the clarity, administration, and enforcement of any law. Thus, the term "pharmacy," as here given, is meant to be broadly inclusive of all places, functions, and public representations having any bearing upon the compounding, dispensing, or distribution of drugs and medicines.

In the foregoing definition, it is interesting to note that a pharmacy may conform to all of the numbered qualifications or it may be a pharmacy if it conforms to any one of them. For instance, a store or shop or other place where drugs are dispensed or sold at retail, or displayed for sale at retail, because a pharmacy quite aside from whether it does any of the other things provided for in the definition. The point is that each of the numbered requirements is exclusive of the other, and is sufficient in itself to constitute a pharmacy under this definition.

In contrast with the definition given above, the Pennsylvania Pharmacy Act defines "pharmacy" as follows:

"The term 'pharmacy' when not otherwise limited, shall, for all the purposes of this Act, be taken to mean a retail drug store or any place where drugs, medicines, or poisons are compounded, dispensed, prepared, or sold at retail."

"The term '*drug*' means (1) articles recognized in the official United States Pharmacopeia, official Homeopathic Pharmacopoeia of the United States, or official National Formulary, or any supplement to any of them, intended for use in the diagnosis, cure, mitigation, treatment, or prevention of disease in men or other animals; and (2) all other articles intended for use in the diagnosis, cure, mitigation, treatment, or prevention of disease in man or other animals; and (3) articles (other than food) intended to affect the structure or any function of the body of man or other animals; and (4) articles intended for use as a component or any articles specified in clause (1) (2), or (3); but does not include devices or their components, parts or accessories." (*Uniform State Pharmacy Act*)

The definition of the term "drug" as here used, is identical with that in the Federal Food, Drug and Cosmetic Act, with one exception. Under the federal law, the term "drug" means "articles recognized in the official United States Pharmacopeia, official Homeopathic Pharmacopœia of the United States, or official National Formulary, or any supplement to any of them."

This definition is essential to the purposes of the Food, Drug and Cosmetic Act which, among other things, is established to prevent interstate commerce in adulterated or misbranded drugs. For this reason the high courts frequently have upheld the government's determination that a surgical ligature is a drug, that a phonograph record is a drug so that the stricter requirements of the Act may apply. Once a product is declared a drug, if it is "new" and the FDA believes it is not yet proven safe and effective, it can be thus forced to gain approval through the Act's New Drug Approval Section (Sec. 505).

The Pharmacy Act, however, is concerned more with matters of distribution and seeks to include within the term "drugs" only those articles recognized in the official compendia that are "intended for use in the diagnosis, cure, mitigation, treatment, or prevention of disease in man or other animals."

Hence, under the Food, Drug and Cosmetic Act, such substances as sugar, salt, lard, distilled water, and other similar products, are drugs; but they would not be so considered under this definition, as to include them would be inconsistent with the theory and purposes of the Pharmacy Law.

"The term '*cosmetic*,' which shall be held to include 'dentifrice' and 'toilet article,' means (1) articles intended to be rubbed, poured, sprinkled, or sprayed on, introduced into, or otherwise applied to the human body, or any part thereof for cleansing, beautifying, promoting attractiveness, or altering the appearance; and (2) articles intended for use as a component of any such articles; except that such term shall not include soap." (*Uniform State Pharmacy Act*)

This definition of "cosmetic" is identical with that in the Food, Drug and Cosmetic Act.

"*Medical supplies* means, in addition to drugs, biological products and all other parenteral medication, absorbent cotton, bandages, gauze, sutures, compacts, compresses, surgical dressings of all kinds and descriptions, and all other products, preparations, other than foods, used in the diagnosis, cure, mitigation, or prevention of disease in man or other animals, or intended to affect the structure of any function of the body of man or other animals, but shall not include instruments, appliances, or devices used by physicians, dentists, nurses, or veterinarians in the pursuit of their professional practice." (*Pennsylvania Pharmacy Act*)

This definition closely follows that set forth in the Uniform State Pharmacy Act, and is another expression of the belief that the production and distribution of medical supplies, together with drugs and medicines generally, need to be brought under permit control.

"The term '*prescription*' as used herein means an order for drugs or medicines or combinations or mixtures thereof, written or signed by a duly licensed physician, dentist, veterinarian, or other medical practitioner licensed to write prescriptions intended for the treatment or prevention of disease in man or animals, and includes orders for drugs or medicines or combinations or mixtures thereof transmitted to pharmacists through word of mouth, telephone, telegraph, or other means of communication by a duly licensed physician, dentist, veterinarian, or other medical practitioner licensed to write prescriptions intended for the treatment or prevention of disease in man or animals, and such prescriptions received by word of mouth, telephone, telegraph, or other means of communication shall be recorded in writing by the pharmacist and the record so made by the pharmacist shall constitute the original prescription to be filed by the pharmacist." (*New Jersey Pharmacy Act*)

This definition is designed to reach and include every situation likely to arise with respect to the prescribing of drugs and medicines upon the part of duly licensed physicians, dentists, veterinarians, or other qualified medical practitioners.

Without exception, the pharmacy laws limit the compounding and dispensing of prescriptions to the registered pharmacist or to persons acting under his immediate and personal supervision.

"The term '*person*' shall be held to mean and include 'person,' 'copartnership,' 'association,' or 'corporation.'" (*Uniform State Pharmacy Act*)

This definition is customary as it provides broad coverage without undue repetition.

Administration

"There shall exist and be maintained within this State, a Board of Pharmacy to be known as the '.....................Board of Pharmacy' with duties and powers as hereinafter defined and provided. The said Board of Pharmacy shall consist of five (5) members, and the now existing State Board of Pharmacy, heretofore appointed, shall continue in the office and shall act as the......... .... Board of Pharmacy, with all the duties and powers as herein provided, until the terms of its present members respectively expire, the vacancies as they occur to be filled in keeping with the requirements of this Act." (*Uniform State Pharmacy Act*)

The numerical strength of the Boards varies greatly. For instance, the majority of states have a Board consisting of 5 members, while Louisiana has 19, New York 9, California 7, and South Carolina and Texas each have 6. On the other hand, eight states have Boards consisting of 3 members only.

"Hereafter, only registered pharmacists who have been licensed in this State for at least five (5) years and are actively engaged in retail pharmacy shall be eligible for appointment to the said Board of Pharmacy." (*Uniform State Pharmacy Act*)

As one of the duties of the Board is to pass upon the fitness of applicants to engage in the practice of pharmacy, it is generally required that its members shall have been actively engaged in pharmaceutical practice for a designated period of years.

The State Pharmacy Acts customarily provide for the submittal of a list of nominees by the state pharmaceutical association to the Governor from which he may select the persons to constitute the Board. In some states the Governor is limited to the list so submitted, but in most states the list is advisory only. As a practical matter, however, the Governor usually shows proper courtesy by confining his appointees to the association list.

As the Board is a functioning agency, it must be organized so as to conform to parliamentary usage. While the secretary of the Board should be a registered pharmacist, he need not necessarily be a member of the Board. In fact, in many states he is not a member, but is chosen by the Board because of his peculiar fitness for the duties to be performed.

The Board must have the technical and clerical aid and assistance necessary for the proper conduct of the office.

As the secretary is the executive officer of the Board, it is necessary that his duties be defined and his specific responsibilities fixed in so far as these can be done by legislative act.

"The secretary of the said Board shall furnish a bond, the amount of such bond to be fixed by the Board, conditional upon the faithful performance and discharge of the duties of his office according to law.

"The secretary shall receive a salary to be fixed by the Board, and all necessary expenses incurred in the performance of his official duties.

"The president and the secretary of the Board shall be empowered to administer oaths in connection with the duties of the Board." (*Uniform State Pharmacy Act*)

These are mere routine matters, and are customary in legislation of this kind.

Courts generally give much weight to the records, activities, and findings of the Board of Pharmacy and hence the books, registers, and records which the Board is required to keep constitute *prima facie* evidence in any court proceedings in which they are involved.

"The said Board of Pharmacy shall hold meetings for the examination of applicants for registration and for the transaction of such other business as may legally come before it, at least three (3) times a year and such additional meetings as may be deemed necessary. Three members shall constitute a quorum for the transaction of any and all business. Due public notice of all meetings shall be given at least thirty (30) days in advance of said meetings." (*Uniform State Pharmacy Act*)

It is interesting to note that a Board may not conduct any private or special examination. Therefore, it is required that due public notice be given of all meetings at which examinations are conducted.

"The Board shall make a written report annually to the Governor of the state and to the State Pharmaceutical Association, of its proceedings and of its receipts and disbursements under this Act, including also the names of all registrants duly licensed to practice under this Act and record of permits and renewals." (*Uniform State Pharmacy Act*)

The purpose here is again twofold: One, to account to the Governor, as the head of the state, with respect to the Board's proceedings, activities, and financial matters; and two, to keep the State Pharmaceutical Association informed with respect to the conduct of those pharmaceutical affairs entrusted to the Board.

"The Board may refuse an application for examination or may suspend or revoke the certificate of a registered pharmacist or a registered assistant pharmacist for any of the following causes: When the application or registration is shown to have been obtained by misrepresentation or fraudulent means or when the applicant or registrant is guilty of chronic or persistent inebriety, or addiction to the use of narcotic drugs, or has been convicted of violating any law of this or any other state or of the United States relating to narcotic drugs, or has been convicted of violating the provisions of any law relating to the sale of liquors, or has been twice convicted of violating any law relating to the practice of pharmacy, or has been convicted of a crime involving moral turpitude, or has impersonated an applicant for registration before the Board. Before a certificate shall be refused, suspended, or revoked, the accused person shall be furnished with a copy of the complaint and given a hearing before the Board. Any person to whom a certificate shall be denied by the Board or whose certificate shall be suspended or revoked by the Board shall have the right to appeal by certiorari to the supreme court for a review of such action." (*New Jersey Pharmacy Act*)

As the pharmacist, of necessity, is engaged in matters of vital concern to the public welfare, it is assumed that his professional conduct is consistent with his professional and civic obligations.

However, the law takes cognizance of the frailties of human nature and provides for the suspension or revocation of the pharmacist's registration in cases of gross dereliction of his professional duties.

The Pennsylvania Pharmacy Act deals with this matter in the following language:

"The registration of any pharmacist or assistant pharmacist, under this act of Assembly, may be revoked by the Pennsylvania Board of Pharmacy, when the registration is proved to have been obtained by fraudulent means, or suspended or revoked upon being convicted for a second violation, in connection with the practice of pharmacy, or any law of this Commonwealth or of the United States.

"Before any registration is suspended or revoked, the holder of such registration certificate shall be given a hearing before the Board of Pharmacy, after notice of the time and place of such hearing and of the charges made against him. At such hearing the accused may be represented by counsel, and shall be entitled to compulsory attendance of witnesses." (*Pennsylvania Pharmacy Act*)

Boards of Pharmacy are customarily empowered to make such rules and regulations as are necessary to the enforcement and administration of the Pharmacy Law. However, the power to make rules and regulations may not be used to accomplish, in the name of the Pharmacy Act, that which the legislature has not specifically sanctioned. The power to revoke for cause any permit granted by the Board is essential to the enforcement of the Act, and for the protection of the public in all matters to which Board permits are applicable.

Qualifications for Registration

"Every applicant for examination and registration as a pharmacist shall be not less than twenty-one (21) years of age, of good moral character and temperate habits, a graduate of a school or college of pharmacy or department of a university recognized and approved by the...................... Board of Pharmacy, and shall file proof satisfactory to the Board, substantiated by proper affidavits, of a minimum of one year of experience in a retail pharmacy, under the supervision of a registered or licensed pharmacist and shall pass an examination by the........................... Board of Pharmacy: PROVIDED, that all applications for examinations shall be made on a form to be supplied by the....................... Board of Pharmacy and shall be filed with the said Board at least .... days before any stated meeting of the Board at which examinations are to be held. Each application must be accompanied by an examination fee of $............" (*Uniform State Pharmacy Act*)

With the exception of one or two states, college of

pharmacy graduation is required for registration as a pharmacist. In determining whether a school or college of pharmacy is worthy of recognition and approval, a board of pharmacy may not base its conclusions upon its own arbitrary or capricious standard.

In the case of Mauldin v. Matthews (41 S.C. 414) the Court declared "the statute does not confer upon the board of pharmaceutical examiners the power to exact of a college compliance with its own standards. On that point, the general assembly has directed that licenses be issued to graduates of reputable colleges— that is, colleges of whose character those of the public having general acquaintance with the subject, entertain a good opinion.

"The . . . College of Pharmacy, being a college of which such good opinion is entertained, is a reputable college; the board of examiners had, therefore, no discretion to refuse to issue the license to the petitioner who is one of its graduates."

Practical drug-store experience is looked upon as an essential ingredient in the training of a pharmacist, and is required under the laws of every state.

In some states, experience, to be acceptable to the Board, may not be obtained prior to one's sixteenth birthday. In Maryland, it is specifically provided that vacation periods may be counted towards meeting the experience requirement, while in New Jersey, practical drug-store experience is on an accreditation basis and may be obtained only after completion of the college course.

The experience requirement is sometimes referred to as *pharmacy internship*, and to be worthy of credit must be obtained only in those drug stores recognized for that purpose by the Board of Pharmacy.

In Wisconsin, the obtaining of practical experience by the Trainee is accomplished during periods of "externship" and "internship" under the preceptorship of pharmacists who have been certified as Preceptors in Pharmacy by the Board. Furthermore, no training may be acquired by the future pharmacist prior to the completion of the first professional year at an accredited college of pharmacy, and six months of the training (the internship period) must be obtained subsequent to graduation.

Under the practical experience requirement, as set forth in the agreements between the states holding membership in the National Association of Boards of Pharmacy, experience in a hospital pharmacy will be accepted as the equivalent of the same period in a retail pharmacy.

Records purporting to set forth practical drug-store experience must be validated under oath so as to enable the Board to satisfy itself with respect to the practical experience claimed by the applicant for examination.

Renewal of Certificates

In the majority of the states, certificates of registration expire annually, but may be renewed upon the payment of a specific fee. Annual re-registration aids law enforcement by providing a current list of all eligible to practice pharmacy within any calendar year.

Reciprocal Registration

"It shall be within the power of the...................Board of Pharmacy to enter into reciprocal relations with the boards of pharmacy or similar agencies of such other States as do likewise, and to register as a pharmacist any person registered by examination in another State without further examination, provided such applicant's qualifications are such that he would have been eligible for registration by examination by the .... Board of Pharmacy at the time he became registered in such other State. Applicants for registration under this clause to produce satisfactory documents bearing upon his previous examination from the secretary of that Board, and paying the secretary of the .... Board of Pharmacy the accustomed fee. Applicants, in addition, will be required to furnish satisfactory record as to his morality, sobriety, and close observance of the more important laws touching the life of a pharmacist." (*Maryland Pharmacy Act*)

Reciprocal registration is based upon equality of treatment, that is, a person registered in Pennsylvania in any given year would be eligible for registration in Nebraska, provided the requirements were equal to those in effect in Nebraska during the year in question. At present reciprocity is available from all Boards except California, Florida, and Hawaii, according to the National Association of Boards of Pharmacy.

While it is rather common for the state acts to require every pharmacist to be in possession of the United States Pharmacopeia and the National Formulary, only a few states empower the Boards of Pharmacy to determine the professional and technical equipment and apparatus essential to maintaining adequate standards of pharmaceutical practice. In those states, however, in which the Boards are vested with this power by law, they have the authority to see to it that pharmacies and retail drug stores are adequately equipped for the compounding and dispensing of prescriptions, and for the manufacturing of pharmaceutical preparations.

There can be no doubt that the minimum equipment provision can be most helpful in maintaining pharmaceutical work at the proper professional level.

Permits

"From and after this .... day of ....19.., it shall be unlawful

"For any person to operate, maintain, open or establish any pharmacy within this State, without first having obtained a permit so to do, from the .... Board of Pharmacy.

"On evidence satisfactory to the said.................... Board of Pharmacy: (*a*) that the pharmacy for which the permit is sought will be conducted in full compliance with the law and the rules and regulations of the said .... Board of Pharmacy; (*b*) that the location and appointments of said pharmacy are such that it can be operated and maintained without endangering the public health or safety; and (*c*) that said pharmacy will be constantly under the personal and immediate supervision of a registered pharmacist, a permit shall be issued to such persons as the said .... Board of Pharmacy shall deem qualified to conduct such pharmacy." (*Maryland State Pharmacy Act*)

In most states retail pharmacies or drug stores may be operated only under permits issued by the Board of Pharmacy. While many of the permit sections are not very explicit with respect to the degree of discretion vested in the Board, it would seem reasonable to assume that the discretion was intended to play an active part in the enforcement and administrative duties and activities of the Board.

In addition to requiring all retail pharmacies to operate under permits issued by the State Board of Pharmacy, the Uniform State Pharmacy Act includes sections applying the permit principle to the following: dispensing physicians; clinics; dispensaries; auctioneers—when dealing in drugs, medicines, or similar products; house-to-house canvassers of drugs, medicines, and related items; itinerant vendors of health care preparations and supplies; persons engaged in the business of distributing samples of drugs or medicinal products.

The permit principle is, of course, applicable to any phase of the manufacture or distribution of drug products on the theory that it gives the agency issuing the permit closer contact with the field, and therefore a better law enforcement position.

In considering this whole subject of permits, the opinion is growing among pharmacy law enforcement officials that the power to grant the permit includes the power to deny. It also embraces the power to revoke or suspend as occasion may warrant or demand. This power, not necessarily expressed in the Pharmacy Act, is based upon the conviction that the conditions precedent to the issuance of the permit remain in effect as long as the privileges inherent in the permit are exercised. In other words, a permit holder may not, after the permit has been issued, conduct himself in such a manner which would have justified the Board in refusing the permit in the first instance.

If one of the qualifications for a drugstore permit, for instance, was that the applicant must not be addicted to narcotic drugs or alcohol, the permit would seem automatically to become inoperative once the permit-holder did become so addicted. The same principles would also apply to the Certificates of Registration issued by the Board as evidence that the holder had complied with all the conditions set forth in the Pharmacy Act. Failure to observe these conditions would afford legal grounds for the revocation or suspension of such certificates.

Some states have included in their statutes specific provisions pertaining to the right of their Board of Pharmacy to cancel a pharmacy permit. The Wisconsin Statutes, for example, provide that:

"Issuance or continuation of the permit for the conduct of a drug store, pharmacy or any similar place of business may be refused when the applicant for the registration thereof has been found to be in violation of ch. 151 or 161." (*ch. 151-Pharmacy Law; ch. 161-Narcotic Law*).

Pharmacists to be in Charge

"Except as otherwise provided in this article, every pharmacy shall be at all times, when open for business, under the personal supervision and management of a duly licensed and registered pharmacist." (*New York Pharmacy Act*)

The New Jersey Pharmacy Law requires that every drug store or pharmacy shall be operated or managed at all times by a registered pharmacist.

Under the Pharmacy Act of Ohio, and this applies to pharmacy acts in general, it is provided that a pharmacy must be "in full and actual charge of a registered pharmacist."

The Pharmacy Act of Maryland specifically demands that "no pharmacy shall be at any time left in charge of any person who is not a registered pharmacist."

The question is frequently asked, "What is meant by *being in charge?*"

In a case directly involving this point (Haas v. People, 27 Ill. App. 416), the Supreme Court of Illinois has had this to say:

"The law makes it the duty of the owner to have in charge of his store a registered pharmacist. It is the corresponding duty of the latter to take charge, if he accepts the employment. Taking charge of the store in this instance means something more than nominal representation of the owner. He is the person who must decide and control as to the sale of drugs, medicines, and poisons. The owner cannot pretend to put him in charge, and at the same time employ an unskilled person in the same store who is independent of him as to such sales. The registered pharmacist who enters upon the charge of such a store, upon such conditions, does so at his peril."

Prescription Files Required

"There shall be kept in every pharmacy a suitable book or file, in which shall be preserved for a period of not less than five (5) years.

every prescription compounded or dispensed at said pharmacy and said book or file of prescriptions shall at all times be open to inspection of the members of the .... Board of Pharmacy, or its duly authorized agents or employees." (*Uniform State Pharmacy Act*)

This is a routine provision in State Pharmacy laws. By preserving all prescriptions dispensed, the pharmacist has in his possession the best evidence should he be called upon to defend a damage suit based upon the allegation that a prescription has been imperfectly or incompetently dispensed.

It is also necessary that enforcement officials have access to the pharmacist's prescription files when and if the occasion occurs.

Qualifications of Manufacturing Personnel

There is a growing disposition to limit the manufacture and/or repackaging of drugs and medicines to persons having the necessary professional and technical qualifications.

Often the responsibility of ensuring such protection to the public in this area is given to the State Board of Pharmacy, as in Wisconsin where the law provides:

"No person shall manufacture, package or prepare within this state any drugs or medicines except under the personal and immediate supervision of a registered pharmacist or such other person as is approved by the board after an investigation and a determination that such other person is qualified by scientific training and education to perform such supervision in a manner adequate to protect the public health and safety. No person shall manufacture, package or prepare any drugs or medicines within this state without first obtaining a permit from the board. For the issuance of such permit there shall be paid an inspection fee of $15 together with a registration fee of $30. Upon annual renewal of registration all permit holders shall pay a fee of $30, payable on May 31 of each year. The issuance of such permit shall be subject to such rules as the board may from time to time adopt for the protection of the public health and safety."

Distributors Licensed

Laws have been passed to place the distributors of dangerous drugs under licensure by the State Board of Pharmacy, as in Wisconsin where the law provides that anyone engaging in the sale or distribution at wholesale of dangerous drugs (those bearing the statement: "Caution–federal law prohibits dispensing without prescription") must first obtain a license to do so from the State Board of Pharmacy. A minimal license fee of $10 is charged and the Board is given great latitude in implementing this requirement of the law by the statutory provision which states "Such license or renewals thereof shall be issued in the discretion of the board to responsible applicants of good reputation."

Exemptions Favoring Physicians, Patent, and Proprietary Medicines

"Nothing in this Act shall apply to, nor in any manner interfere with the business of a regularly licensed physician in compounding for and supplying his patients with such medicines as may seem to him proper in his professional capacity as a physician;

"And...nothing in this Act shall apply to, nor in any manner interfere with the business of a general merchant in selling any of the following articles, to wit: Medicines of secret composition, and which are advertised to the general public, and popularly known as patent or proprietary medicines, providing said medicines are not poisonous." (*Indiana Pharmacy Act*)

The Pharmacy Acts of all states recognize the right of the physician to dispense drugs and medicines to his patients in the course of his professional practice. Also, these acts are so written as not to interfere with the sale of patent or proprietary medicines. Generally, the

Pharmacy Acts permit the indiscriminate sale of commonly used household or domestic remedies.

However, when physicians are in the regular practice of dispensing drugs, they are required to undertake the same responsibilities in labeling and record-keeping as is the pharmacist's obligation in accordance with pertinent state and federal laws. The extent to which the physician may delegate this prerogative is not delineated for the most part. However, in cases of alleged injury, and in negligence and malpractice actions, the court will define it according to the facts and circumstances underlying the complaint.

Non-Pharmacy Permit Control

"Any store, not licensed as a pharmacy, may sell, in original packages put up by a licensed pharmacist whose name and business address shall be displayed upon the package, any drugs, chemicals, or medicinal compounds or preparations, when a permit to do so shall have been obtained from said commission." (*Connecticut Pharmacy Act*)

"Any person of good moral character over twenty-one years of age, who conducts a retail business at a place more than five miles from a drug store employing a registered pharmacist, may procure from the Board, upon application and payment to said Board of a fee of three dollars annually, a license which shall permit such retailer to keep for sale, and sell in original packages, the simple household remedies and such other emergency medicines and poisons as may from time to time be approved for sale by the Board." (*North Dakota Pharmacy Act*)

While the comparable provisions of the Uniform State Pharmacy Act have not been adopted in any state, the Connecticut and North Dakota Pharmacy Acts, as indicated above, do require that all nonpharmacy outlets handling drugs and medicines operate under permit regulation and control. Under the provisions of state and federal food, drug, and cosmetic acts, all drug products sold without prescription, must bear adequate directions for use. This requirement is being written into state pharmacy laws. The Pharmacy Acts of Arizona and Kansas, not to mention others, are examples of this modern trend.

Forms, Fees, Renewals, and Revocation

"Application for permits required under the preceding section shall be made on a form to be provided and furnished by the said .... Board of Pharmacy and shall be accompanied by the required fee hereinafter required in this section, which amount shall be paid as a fee for each annual renewal of such permit.

"Separate application shall be made and separate permits issued for each separate place at which is carried on any of the operations for which a permit is required in the preceding section.

"The fees required for the issuing of the permits required in the preceding section are as follows:

(a)—$............	(d)—$............	(g)—$............
(b)—$............	(e)—$............	(h)—$............
(c)—$............	(f)—$............	(i)—$............

"Permits issued under the provisions of the preceding section shall be conspicuously exposed in the place for which the permit was granted. Such permits shall not be transferable; shall expire on the last day of December following the date of issuance, and shall be renewed annually." (*Uniform State Pharmacy Act*)

As previously stated, registration and permit fees vary in the several states. The Uniform State Pharmacy Act, however, groups all fees in one section merely as a means of convenience and ready reference.

While ordinarily the actions or rulings of a Board of Pharmacy dealing with mere matters of discretion are not subject to judicial review, it is thought desirable for the plaintiff to have access to the court in all cases involving refusal to grant a drugstore permit or a revocation thereof.

Valuable property may be jeopardized and the Board should not, as a matter of sound administration, have exclusive authority over the matter.

Penalties

"Any person violating any of the provisions of this Act, shall upon conviction before any court of competent jurisdiction in this State, be fined a sum not to exceed............Dollars($......), for each violation, and each and every day such violation continues shall constitute a separate and distinct offense. Upon conviction of a permittee hereunder, his permit shall also forthwith be revoked and become null and void.

"*Note: This Section should be drawn to conform with the law of each State and should also provide to whom the fines should be paid.*" (*Uniform State Pharmacy Act*)

Penalties are customarily prescribed for violations of the State Pharmacy Act. There is, however, no uniformity in this respect. As a very general rule, however, a pharmacist's drugstore permit is not revocable merely because of a single or even occasional violation of the Pharmacy Act.

The provision of the Uniform State Pharmacy Act is quoted here merely to indicate that severe penalties may be prescribed if deemed necessary to effectuate the general purposes of the law.

Relief by Injunction

"The State Board of Pharmacy, created under the provisions of this Act, may, in its discretion, in addition to the remedy set forth in the preceding section, apply to a court having competent jurisdiction over the parties and subject matter, for a writ of injunction to restrain repetitious violations of the provisions of this Act." (*Uniform State Pharmacy Act*)

In addition to penalties for specific violations of the Pharmacy Law, courts of equity are sometimes empowered to grant an injunction restraining a pharmacist from repetitious violations of the Act.

While such courts are not inclined to grant an injunction so as to prevent prospective violations of law, they should be resorted to in those cases where a drugstore or pharmacy is continuously operated contrary to the terms of the Pharmacy Act, and where it can be shown that the public interest is jeopardized thereby.

Severability Clause

"*And be it further enacted*, That if any clause, sentence, paragraph, or section of this article shall, for any reason, be adjudged by any court of competent jurisdiction, to be unconstitutional and invalid, such judgment shall not affect, repeal, or invalidate the remainder thereof, but shall be confined in its operation to the clause, sentence, paragraph, or section thereof so found unconstitutional and invalid." (*Uniform State Pharmacy Act*)

This is known as the severability clause, and is designed to prevent a law being declared unconstitutional in its entirety merely because some portions may be found invalid. The value of the severance clause may be doubted other than being indicative of the legislature's intent that as much of the Act be given effect as is consistent with Constitutional principles.

However, aside from the severance clause, courts are burdened with the obligation to so interpret a legislative act as to give it validity whenever the results reached would appear to be consistent with the legislative purpose.

Inconsistencies Repealed

"*And be it further enacted*, That all laws or part of laws, general or local, of the State of ...., inconsistent with the provisions of this Act, be and the same are hereby repealed to the extent of such inconsistency." (*Uniform State Pharmacy Act*)

While, as a general rule, a later enactment is tantamount to the repeal of all previous enactments inconsistent therewith, it is considered good draftsmanship to repeal specifically such inconsistent legislation.

While there are rare questions attached to pharmacy acts and to drug, cosmetic, and device acts other than those addressed to their constitutionality, not infrequently Board rules, procedures, or regulations are attacked as excessive or unauthorized.

So long as the underlying statute adequately indicates the nature and scope of regulations to effectuate the legislative intent, the courts are apt to uphold them. Similarly, the statute's provision for standards and guidelines under which the administering agency (the pharmacy board) can promulgate and adopt rules should withstand controversy where violators of the rules, after a hearing before the board, make such a challenge. The purpose of having boards so constituted, is to have knowledgeable and experienced people act effectively on behalf of the public and to safeguard its interests.

In statutes, therefore, that deal with public health, professional practice, and the like, it is neither practical nor realistic to expect the legislature to spell out in minute detail the parameters of qualification, testing, disqualification, grant, maintenance, and revocation of licenses and permits. It is often said that the power to grant a license implies the right to suspend or revoke it.

Therefore, so long as a board acts for good cause and public purpose after due notice and a fair hearing in accordance with constitutional due process, and acts without arbitrariness or caprice out of some substantial evidentiary findings, the courts will find them with the inherent power to develop rules and regulations and deal with violations thereunder as an expression of the police power of the state for the protection of the public weal.

Standards of Professional Practice

Most pharmacy boards by rule or regulation declare it improper for a pharmacist to advertise that his professional services are superior to those of other pharmacists in the community, and disallow distribution of trading stamps or other rebates offered or given with dispensing of prescriptions. They also oppose use of the terms "cut-rate," "discount," "bargain," or terms of similar connotation in conjunction with the offering of pharmaceutical service. There have been instances where courts have upheld the right of a board to suspend a license where, through catalogue advertising or signs, the licensee offered a discount on such services.

Other violations which may have like effect are providing medical practitioners with prescription blanks bearing a pharmacist's or pharmacy's name and address thereon, or entering agreements to solicit or channel business to a particular pharmacy in denial of the patient's right of free choice of pharmacist.

Most state boards see pharmacists as responsible for providing complete pharmaceutical service by compounding or dispensing all prescription medications which the public may reasonably expect, and to this end require pharmacists to meet certain minimums of stock, equipment, space, and advisory materials. Courts have shown unwillingness to allow boards to refuse the right to register pharmacies in areas where the board has felt pharmaceutical services are already overly abundant. The hornbook rule for professional practitioners is that they can extend their service at will and can refuse to serve if they choose. However, this is being modified by state laws and regulations which do not allow the choice to be a discriminatory one which is an affront to civil rights.

The Pennsylvania regulation for pharmacists in this regard does not prohibit patient choice, but rather states that the pharmacist has a responsibility to make his professional service available:

1. In a nondiscriminatory manner, so that he gives the same quality and quantity of professional service to all individuals or groups of individuals based on the amount of service and facilities he has available. This involves his inventory, equipment and personnel, within their limitations. Hospital and institutional pharmacists need give pharmaceutical service only to inpatients. This, however, does not preclude serving outpatients.

2. The pharmacist is responsible to make his professional services available without requiring the potential recipient to be a member of any organization or to pay or contribute any enrollment, membership, or participation fee as a condition for obtaining professional services. This does not mean he cannot serve professionally unions or organizations that do use such procedures on their own.

3. The pharmacist has the responsibility to offer complete pharmaceutical service by having sufficient equipment and inventory to cover reasonable prescription dispensing volume. (I know of no attempt at disciplinary enforcement of this type of rule, although many discount operations rely on inventory savings and short inventories to keep down operating costs. On the other hand, wholesaler service and proximity might be a factor. Reasonable expectation has never been defined in this regard.)

4. Pharmacists have the responsibility to safeguard the storage and distribution of all drugs, keep proper records and recommend or advise as required concerning contents, therapeutic values, and uses of such articles. This restricts statutory obligations to receive, hold, and dispense unadulterated, nonmisbranded products.

As other professionals, pharmacists may not use agents or solicitors to collect and forward to them prescriptions gathered at nonlicensed pharmacy locales (union medical services or industrial installations that have no dispensing service).

The pharmacist or pharmacy may not participate in any plan to solicit business in the doctor's office or enter into any agreement that eliminates or hurts the pharmacist–patient–prescriber relationship. How this would be variously affected by the pharmacist's relationship with numerous state, welfare board, and other arrangements is speculative and possibly rendered unenforceable, unless the state board has made prior arrangements or is highly courageous.

Pharmacists and pharmacies must exclude taboo words and phrases in conjunction with pharmaceutical service (undefined); eg, "cut-rate," "discount," "bargain," "buy for less." Some of the guiding principles of business morality laws on the federal and state level discourage the use of "bait" advertisements and promotions: advertising or offering merchandise at "loss leader" prices for the purpose of obtaining leads or prospects, or "switchover" to more profitable goods.

One may not represent directly or by implication, orally or in writing, that any of the merchandise offered for sale is guaranteed, unless able to provide a guarantee in fact which identifies its nature and extent, the name of the guarantor, and the manner in which he will perform in accordance with the extent and representations set forth.

One may not misrepresent to those sold to or bought from that the establishment is controlling or part of a chain of stores unless, of course, it is true. While the federal and state drug laws spell it out statutorily in certain instances, in general the use of advertising material or other documents which simulate official or governmental forms or documents or misrepresent in any manner the originator, source or authority of advertising materials is prohibited.

Put briefly, these laws forbid the use of any advertising which unfairly takes advantage of business competitors and those the pharmacist does business with by adopting promotional methods, sales plans, or procedures involving the use of false, deceptive, or misleading statements or representations.

The Durham–Humphrey Amendment clearly defined drugs which may be distributed only with the prescription legend on the manufacturer's label: "Caution: Federal law prohibits dispensing without prescription."

Should a drug of such definition go into interstate commerce and be subsequently held or transferred locally and not bear the legend on the label, it is a misbranded drug. Only when, as a dispensed product authorized by a qualified prescriber under state law, the pharmacist puts the prescription labeling thereon may it go to another's hand minus the full labeling otherwise set out in Section 502 of the Federal Act. Two recent additions to this category of drugs are nitroglycorin tablets and amyl nitrite.

If, therefore, there is no physician's authority for the original dispensing of prescription medication containing such a drug or for its refill, the product is misbranded and the pharmacist issuing it is a misdemeanant in federal law.

At the same time, both he and the product are at least similarly violative of state law, although under the latter additional infractions may attach. Therefore, among the punitive possibilities involved may be seizure of the product, an injunction against such further action by the pharmacist, criminal prosecution with fine up to $1000 and sentence up to one year, and suspension or revocation of store registration and/or of personal pharmacist licensure.

In one recent case where the highest state court upheld the right of a state board of pharmacy to punish a pharmacist for violating any drug laws, federal or state, that were applicable to his unauthorized refilling of a prescription presented to him by an agent of the pharmacy board, the court indicated that a 1-year suspension is a reasonable penalty. This court held, as have many others before it, that when a board agent gives a suspect an opportunity to break the law without coercing him or enticing him to do so, the state's case is not disqualified by a charge of entrapment. (Arkansas State Board of Pharmacy vs Patrick, 423 S.W. 2nd 263, 1968.)

The Harrison or Federal Narcotic Law and Regulations*

The Act of December 17, 1914 (known as the Harrison Narcotic Law), as amended by Sections 1006 and 1007 of the Revenue Act of 1918 (these sections re-

---

* Enforcement of all Federal Narcotic Laws and the Drug Abuse Control Amendments of 1965 which relate to nonnarcotic drugs of abuse (eg, amphetamines, barbiturates, and hallucinogens) are now carried out by the Bureau of Narcotics and Dangerous Drugs of the Department of Justice.

enacted in the Revenue Acts of 1921 and 1924, section 432 of the Revenue Act of 1928, the Act of January 22, 1927, Section 806 of the Revenue Act of 1936 (approved June 22, 1936) and the Act of April 22, 1960 (known as the Narcotics Manufacturing Act of 1960), which amended the Internal Revenue Code of 1954, controls the importation, manufacture, production, compounding, selling, dealing in, dispensing, and giving away of opium and coca leaves and all compounds, manufactures, salts, derivatives, and preparations thereof. Every person, prior to engaging in any of the foregoing activities, is required to register with the Director of Internal Revenue for his district and pay tax as provided in the Act. In order to register in any class it is necessary for the applicant to be lawfully entitled to engage in the activity involving the use of narcotic drugs, in connection with which registration is desired. Classes of registrants with the special taxes imposed are as follows:

Class I. The tax is at the rate of $24 per annum. It covers importers, manufacturers, producers, and compounders.

Class II. The tax is at the rate of $12 per annum. It covers persons buying and selling stamped packages of narcotic drugs or preparations produced by others.

Class III. The tax is at the rate of $3 per annum. It includes persons selling narcotic drugs from the original stamped package, in pursuance of bona fide prescriptions issued by registered practitioners.

Class IV. The tax is at the rate of $1 per annum or fraction thereof. It applies to physicians, dentists, veterinary surgeons, and other practitioners lawfully entitled to distribute, dispense, give away, or administer narcotic drugs to patients upon whom they, in the course of their professional practice, are in attendance.

Class V. The tax is $1 per annum or any fractional part of a year. It covers manufacturers of and dealers in narcotic preparations and remedies not subject to stamp tax.

Class VI. The tax is $1 per annum. It includes persons not registered in Class 1, but lawfully entitled to obtain and use in a laboratory narcotics for purposes of research, instruction, or analysis.

Under the Federal Narcotic Act (the Harrison Act) as amended, narcotic drugs which have narcotic properties similar to morphine, or the other narcotics expressly mentioned in the act, automatically became subject to its provisions as they come upon the market. The effect of this is to make the Harrison Act flexible enough to keep step with developments in this field as they come along, without the need for additional legislation.

Registration—Persons seeking to engage in any narcotic business must first file application for registry and special tax stamp on Form 678 with an inventory for each class in which registration is desired except Classes I and II. Blank forms are procurable from the Director for the district. Application on Form 678 must be made within the month within which business is commenced. Persons already registered must *on or before July 1* of each year file application in the same manner for the renewal of their registration. Directors will annually mail blank forms without request to all registered persons as soon as practicable prior to July 1. Failure of any person to receive these blank forms will be no excuse, however, for failure to make application for reregistry and special tax stamp within the required time. Address the Director of Internal Revenue for the district if blank forms are not received.

Inventories—An inventory on the reverse of Form 678 is required for each class except Classes I and II. No inventory whatever is required of nontaxable (exempt) narcotic preparations and remedies. Form 678 may be used for Classes II and V, listing the taxable narcotic drugs and preparations on hand with the notation "No taxable narcotic drugs on hand in Class V" written at the bottom of the list.

Requisitions for Narcotic Drugs—Every registered person, except dealers in nontaxable or exempt narcotic preparations and remedies only, is qualified to obtain blank official order forms from the Director of Internal Revenue at a price of ten cents per book of ten, requisition therefor to be made on blank Form 679, obtainable from the Director for the district without charge. Only one book will be furnished at a time except to persons registered in Class I or II. Official order forms for the purchase of narcotic drugs may be filled only by persons qualified as manufacturers or wholesale dealers, except an order form calling exclusively for a one-ounce quantity of an aqueous or oleaginous narcotic solution which may be filled by a pharmacist qualified in Class III provided the narcotic content does not exceed a greater proportion than 20% of the complete solution, to be used in legitimate office practice. Order forms must be made out according to the instructions printed on the cover of the book. They must be returned by the manufacturer or wholesale dealer if not properly prepared in every detail. The duplicate copy of every order form issued must be kept on file for a period of two years. The original of all order forms for one-ounce quantities of aqueous or oleaginous solutions must be kept on file by retail dealers likewise for two years.

Disposition of Narcotics—Pharmacists qualified only in Class III may dispose of narcotic drugs only upon properly prepared prescriptions with the exception of one-ounce quantities of aqueous or oleaginous narcotic solutions as above stated. Prescriptions for taxable narcotic drugs or preparations may be issued by registered physicians, dentists, veterinarians, or other practitioners, and each prescription must be dated as of the date on which signed, shall be signed by the issuing physician, dentist, veterinary surgeon, or other practitioner, and shall bear the full name and address of the patient, and the name, address, and registry number of the issuing practitioner. A physician may sign prescriptions for narcotics in the same manner as he would sign a check or legal document, as, for instance, J. H. Smith, John H. Smith, or John Henry Smith. Merely signing it as "Smith" or "J. H. S." would not suffice. Prescriptions for narcotics must be written with ink or indelible pencil or on a typewriter and they all must be signed by the practitioner with ink or indelible pencil. The pharmacist upon dispensing the prescription must preserve it in a separate file for a period of two years from the date indicated thereon. A prescription for taxable narcotic drugs or preparations is not renewable, and as a general rule such prescription must not be dispensed in part. If, however, a pharmacist is unable to supply the full quantity called for in a prescription, he may, if an emergency exists and he later advises the issuing practitioner, supply a portion of the drugs called for by the prescription, provided he makes a suitable notation on the face of the prescription of the quantity furnished and a suitable explanation of the reason for not supplying the full quantity on the back of the prescription. No further quantity will be supplied except upon a new prescription.

Prescriptions by Telephone—Where written prescriptions signed by the practitioner are required, the furnishing of narcotics pursuant to telephone advice of practitioners is prohibited, whether signed prescriptions covering such orders are subsequently received or not, but in an emergency a pharmacist may deliver or have delivered through his responsible employee or agent narcotics pursuant to a telephone order, provided a properly prepared signed prescription is supplied before delivery is made, which shall be filed by the pharmacist as required by law. Those narcotic preparations for which a written prescription signed by the practitioner is required are known as "Class A Narcotics."

"Class B Narcotics" are those for which a pharmacist may accept an oral prescription communicated to him by a duly registered practitioner. In issuing an oral prescription, the prescriber shall furnish the dealer with the same information as is required in the case of a written prescription except for the written signature of the prescriber. The oral prescription, including the information required to be furnished by the prescriber, shall promptly be reduced to writing by the pharmacist, who shall file and preserve the writing in his narcotic prescription file.

The Federal narcotic law and regulations convey no authority to fill an oral prescription in violation of a state or territorial narcotic law. Although many states have amended the state narcotic law to allow the acceptance of oral narcotic prescriptions in conformity with the Federal law and regulations, it is necessary that the pharmacist refer to the narcotic law of the state in which he is practicing to determine the status of the compounds for which he will be accepting oral prescriptions.

Classification of Narcotic Drugs

As a result of the passage of the "Narcotics Manufacturing Act of 1960" narcotic drugs are now divided into four control groups—A, B, X, and M.

Class A and Class B include taxable drugs or compounds which must bear tax stamps and for which order forms are required for their transfer and a practitioner's prescription for their dispensing. For those preparations in Class B, a pharmacist may accept a practitioner's oral or telephoned prescription; all other taxable narcotic drugs are Class A products for which a pharmacist must obtain a written, signed prescription from a practitioner before he may dispense the drug or preparation.

Classes X and M contain preparations for which no tax stamp is needed—exempted preparations. Preparations of either class may be sold without a narcotic prescription, but only for *bona fide* medical use. Persons buying these preparations for resale must be registered in Class V-D and must supply their registry number when purchasing these preparations for resale.

Class A is the basic narcotic drug class used to control products that possess great addiction liability. Class B contains those narcotic preparations for which an oral prescription may be given. Class X is the exempt narcotic category in which preparations with only a slight addiction liability is placed and Class M contains preparations with an addiction liability less than that of the preparations in Class X. Both Class X and Class M preparations may be sold over-the-counter, but appropriate sales records must be maintained by persons selling Class X preparations while no such sales records are required for the sale of Class M preparations.

Class X preparations are those which contain not more than 2 gr of opium, ¼ gr of morphine, 1 gr of codeine, ½ gr of dihydrocodeine or ½ gr of ethylmorphine or any of their salts per ounce of the product, combined with active nonnarcotic medicinal ingredients in sufficient proportion to confer on the preparation medicinal qualities other than those possessed by the narcotic alone. Also included are preparations in solid form containing not more than 2.5 mg of diphenoxylate

and not less than 25 micrograms of atropine sulfate per dosage unit.

Class M preparations are those which contain noscapine (narcotine), papaverine, narceine, cotarnine or nalorphine or any of their salts, without limit as to quantity, combined with active or inactive nonnarcotic ingredients of the type used in medicinal preparations.

Neither Class X nor Class M include any straight or pure narcotic drug or any of its salts. Only pharmaceutical preparations in which the narcotic is combined with other ingredients are included in these categories. Hence, pure opium, morphine, codeine, dihydrocodeine, and ethylmorphine and their salts are Class A, and pure noscapine, papaverine, narceine, cotarnine, and nalorphine and their salts are Class B preparations.

Labeling—Each package of narcotic drugs or preparations dispensed on prescriptions must bear a label showing the name and registry number of the pharmacist, the serial number of the prescription, the name and address of the patient, and the name, address, and registry number of the practitioner.

A narcotic prescription may be dispensed only if issued for legitimate medical purposes. If the pharmacist to whom a prescription is presented for dispensing has any knowledge or entertains any suspicion which would cause him to believe that the narcotics will not be used for such purposes, he should not dispense it. The mere presentation of a prescription issued by a registered physician or other practitioner does not compel the pharmacist to whom it is presented to supply the drugs requested. A prescription issued to a person for a narcotic drug for the purpose of satisfying his craving for the drug and not for any legitimate medical purpose does not come within exception (b) of Section 2 of the law and must not be dispensed. Any pharmacist who dispenses such a prescription may be held correspondingly liable with the physician who issued it.

Public officials, such as officials of the United States, District of Columbia, the various states and cities, who, in the exercise of their official duties, dispense or handle narcotic drugs, are not thereby required to register and pay special tax. Prescriptions issued by such officials for narcotics for official patients must be prepared on blanks provided by the Government or Department of which the issuing practitioner is an official, or, if no special blanks are provided, such prescriptions must be prepared on official stationery. Each prescription must show the name, title, and official address of the officer by whom executed.

Nontaxable (Exempt) Narcotic Preparations—Exempt narcotic preparations and remedies may be sold without a prescription but a record of sale must be kept as follows:

Date of Sale	Name of Purchaser	Address	Name of Preparation	Quantity

The term *"exempt preparation"* is really a misnomer, as preparations lawfully coming within this category are more accurately designated as *"conditionally exempt."* That is, they may be sold or otherwise disposed of only on the condition that they are to be used as medicines and not for the purpose of evading the intentions and provisions of the law.

To emphasize and reinforce this understanding, a new federal regulation was placed into effect November 1, 1969, which tightens the criteria of permissibility surrounding such retail sales somewhat along the lines required in many states at the present time. We have given some typical state law examples at a further point in this chapter.

No exempt narcotic may be sold to one under 18 years of age and the pharmacist is urged to use his professional discretion in challenging a purchaser for proof of age. Further, the licensed pharmacist has the sole prerogative to make such a retail sale. He must also restrict the quantity sold, in the absence of more stringent local requirements, to no more than 4 ounces of Class "X" preparations for one person in a 48-hour span. During the same period of time however no more than 2 ounces of paregoric or no more than 8 ounces of other Class "X" products containing exempt quantities of opium (eg, antidiarrheal preparations) could be sold according to the federal regulations.

The foregoing applies to sales of Class "X" products at retail, so that none of these limitations apply to prescriptions which call for dispensing exempt narcotic preparations in whole or in part.

A person registered in class III must also be registered in class V in order to dispose of exempt preparations although the payment of the $1 tax is not required. Exempt preparations may be dispensed on prescriptions and such prescriptions may be renewed.

There is no specified limit as to the quantity of exempt preparations which may be sold by a pharmacist at retail. However, as heretofore stated, such preparations may be sold as medicines only. A pharmacist would be liable to the penalties imposed by the Act if he sold any quantity of an exempt preparation knowing that it would be consumed for other than legitimate medical purposes, that is for addiction purposes.

A pharmacist must be registered as a wholesaler in Class II if he desires to fill order forms of other registered persons for stamped packages of narcotic drugs. The stock of stamped packages maintained for the purpose of sale on order forms must be kept separate from the Class III stock. A wholesale monthly return, together with a statement of stock and totals of receipts and dispositions must be sworn to and transmitted to the Director of Internal Revenue for the district on or before the 15th of the month subsequent to that for which rendered in the manner provided in the instructions and regulations printed on Form 811.

Community pharmacists desiring to dispense order forms of other registered persons with packages of their own manufacture, production, or packing must be registered in Class I as manufacturers. Each package manufactured, produced, or packed must be separately stamped. The tax is at the rate of one cent per ounce or fraction thereof on the gross contents of the package. The stamps are procurable only by Class I registrants. Requisitions therefor on Form 786 should be made to the district Director of Internal Revenue. Stocks of narcotic drugs used for Class I purposes must be kept separate from all other stocks. Manufacturers must keep daily records on Form 810a of all receipts for the Class I stock, and on Form 810b of all dispositions from the Class I stock. They must also keep a daily record on Form 810c of drugs used for production and of drugs or preparations produced. They must likewise keep a daily record on Form 810d of drugs or preparations used for packaging or repackaging and of the packages resulting from such processes. Monthly returns on these forms with a summary on Form 810 must be made to the Director of Internal Revenue similarly as monthly returns are required from whole-

sale dealers but in accordance with the instructions and regulations printed on Form 810. Manufacturers who import raw opium must render a special return to the Commissioner of Narcotics, using Forms 163, 163a, and 163b, in accordance with the instructions on these forms, accounting for all such importations and for all manufacture from such raw or crude opium.

Both manufacturers and wholesale dealers must render annual inventories of the narcotic drugs on hand as of December 31 of each year, such inventories to be made a part of the December return.

Manufacturers must place serial numbers on all packages produced by them which contain one ounce or more of morphine or cocaine. Both manufacturers and wholesale dealers must record the serial numbers of such packages and the names and addresses of the purchasers thereof, keeping such as a part of their permanent records.

The Safe Storage of Narcotic Drugs—Pharmacists must accept the obligation to store narcotic drugs in their possession in the most secure manner possible. They must take extra precautions to prevent such drugs from falling in the hands of illicit dealers, dope peddlers, and others who engage in the illegal distribution of narcotic drugs.

Proper storage facilities include a safe, protected by a lock which can be opened only by those who have the combination.

Other pharmacists prefer to disperse narcotic drugs so widely throughout their prescription stock as to make it impossible for these drugs to be obtained through theft or burglary. It is believed that any procedure which assures safe storage of narcotics would meet the requirements of federal and state narcotic laws, and be approved by the appropriate officials charged with the enforcement of these laws.

Inquiries Concerning Narcotics—Inquiries relative to registration or re-registration under the law and the payment of taxes thereunder should be addressed to the Director of Internal Revenue for the district in which the taxpayer is located. Inquiries dealing with the dispensing of individual prescriptions should be addressed to the Narcotic District Supervisor of the district in which the pharmacist is located. All other questions pertaining to the Harrison Narcotic Law, as amended, or the regulations thereunder, should be addressed to the Commissioner of Narcotics, Washington, D.C. All questions pertaining exclusively to the importation into, the exportation from, or the trans-shipment of narcotic drugs through the United States from one country to another should be addressed to the Commissioner of Narcotics, Bureau of Narcotics, Washington, D.C.

Narcotic Drugs Import and Export Act—The Narcotic Drugs Import and Export Act, approved May 26, 1922, as amended, limits importations of narcotic drugs to crude opium and coca leaves in sufficient quantities to meet medical and legitimate requirements only. No opium may be imported for manufacturing heroin. Permits to import are issued only to manufacturers having apparatus or equipment for producing drugs or medicines from opium or coca leaves, and who have been approved for this purpose by the Commissioner of Narcotics. Permits to export are issued only to duly qualified manufacturers and wholesale dealers. All the permissive features of the Act are administered by the Commissioner of Narcotics.

State Narcotic Acts—The procurement, manufacture, use, and distribution of narcotics are also regulated and controlled by state laws. In general, however, the state acts harmonize with federal laws. The state requirement that records of all transactions in narcotics be kept is usually complied with by the keeping of the records demanded by the federal law. Official state order forms are generally not required, although in some states a special official order form is provided pharmacists, physicians, and others, for the lawful purchase of exempt narcotics.

Many of the states, primarily those in which the Uniform State Narcotic Act is in effect, provide for the licensing of persons engaged in the manufacturing and wholesaling of narcotic drugs. This requirement together with those providing for the licensing of physicians, dentists, veterinarians, and pharmacists, gives the state much stricter control over the persons lawfully authorized, in any manner, to deal in narcotics. As with drug laws generally, where the local requirements are stricter than the federal, the pharmacist is bound to observe them.

The state laws provide for the suspension or revocation of any of the foregoing licenses for designated infractions or violations of federal or state narcotic acts.

As a person's eligibility to register under the federal narcotic law is predicated upon his right to engage in his calling or practice his profession in the state in which he lives, it follows that revocation of the state license automatically cancels whatever rights or privileges had been accorded him under the federal narcotic laws.

Descriptive List of Drugs Subject to Federal Narcotic Laws

Class "A" (Fully Controlled) Narcotic Drugs

(Require a written, signed prescription)

I. OPIUM and its derivatives and compounds, including but not limited to the following:

a. Raw, granulated, powdered, deodorized OPIUM, tincture of OPIUM, powdered or solid extracts of OPIUM and OPIUM preparations.†

b. Mixed alkaloids of OPIUM and their salts. (Pantopon, Spasmalgin)

II. Phenanthrene opium alkaloids, their salts, derivatives and compounds, including but not limited to the following:

a. ACETYLCODONE (acetyldihydrocodeine), its salts, compounds, and preparations.‡

b. BENZYLMORPHINE, its salts, compounds and preparations.‡

c. CODEINE (methylmorphine) and its salts.*†

d. CODEINE-N-OXIDE, its salts, compounds and preparations.‡

e. DESOMORPHINE (dihydrodesoxymorphine-d), its salts, compounds and preparations.‡

f. DESOXYMORPHINE, its salts, compounds and preparations.‡

g. DIACETYLMORPHINE or HEROIN, its salts, compounds and preparations.† (Manufacture, sale, distribution or possession is prohibited in the United States.)‡

h. DIHYDROCODEINE (drocode, Parzone, Rapacodin), its salts, compounds and preparations.*†

i. DIHYDROMORPHINE (Paramofan), its salts, compounds and preparations.

j. ETHYLMORPHINE (Dionin) and its salts.*†

k. HYDROCODONE (dihydrocodeinone), its salts, compounds and preparations.*

l. HYDROMORPHINOL (14-hydroxydihydromorphine), its salts, compounds and preparations.‡

m. HYDROMORPHONE (dihydromorphinone, Dilaudid), its salts, compounds and preparations.

n. METHYLDESORPHINE (6-methyl-Δ⁶-desoxymorphine), its salts, compounds and preparations.‡

o. METHYLDIHYDROMORPHINE (6-methyldihydromorphine), its salts, compounds and preparations.‡

p. METOPON (methyldihydromorphinone), its salts, compounds and preparations.

q. MORPHINE alkaloid, MORPHINE salts, MORPHINE compounds and preparations.†

r. MORPHINE METHYLBROMIDE, its salts, compounds and preparations.‡

s. MORPHINE METHYLSULFONATE, its salts, compounds and preparations.‡

t. MORPHINE-N-OXIDE (genomorphine), its salts, compounds and preparations.‡

u. MYROPHINE (myristyl benzyl morphine), its salts, compounds and preparations.‡

v. NICOCODINE (6-nicotinylcodeine), its salts, compounds and preparations.‡

w. NICOMORPHINE (nicophine, Vilan), its salts, compounds and preparations.‡

x. NORMORPHINE, its salts, compounds and preparations.‡

y. OXYCODONE (dihydrohydroxycodeinone, Eucodal), its salts, compounds and preparations.*

z. OXYMORPHINE (dihydrohydroxymorphine), its salts, compounds and preparations.‡

aa. OXYMORPHONE (dihydrohydroxymorphinone, Numorphan), its salts, compounds and preparations.

bb. PHOLCODINE (betamorpholinylethylmorphine, homocodeine), its salts, compounds and preparations.

cc. THEBACON (acedicone, acetyldihydrocodeinone), its salts, compounds and preparations.‡

dd. THEBAINE, its salts, compounds and preparations.

III. COCA LEAVES, their alkaloids, derivatives, extracts or compounds, including but not limited to the following:

a. COCAINE, its salts, compounds and preparations.

b. ECGONINE, its salts, compounds and preparations.

c. TROPOCOCAINE, its salts, derivatives, compounds and preparations.‡

IV. MARIHUANA (Cannabis sativa), its derivatives or compounds. (Marihuana is not presently used for medicinal purposes in the United States.)‡

V. PETHIDINE (isonipecaine, meperidine, Demerol, Dolantin), its salts, compounds and preparations.

VI. Opiates, their salts, derivatives and compounds.

1. *Pethidine Group:*

a. ALLYLPRODINE (Alperidine, NIH-7440, RO-2-7113), 3-allyl-1-methyl-4-phenyl-4-propionoxypiperidine, its salts, compounds and preparations.‡

b. ALPHAMEPRODINE or NU-1932, a-1-methyl-3-ethyl-4-phenyl-4-propionoxypiperidine, its salts, compounds and preparations.‡

c. ALPHAPRODINE or NU-1196 (Nisentil, Nisintil, Prisiliden), a-1,3-dimethyl-4-phenyl-4-propionoxypiperidine, its salts, compounds and preparations.

d. ANILERIDINE (Leritine, Lerinol), ethyl 1-[2-(p-aminophenyl)ethyl]-4-phenylpiperidine-4-carboxylate, its salts, compounds and preparations.

e. BENZETHIDINE, ethyl 1-(2-benzyloxyethyl)-4-phenyl-4-piperidinecarboxylate, its salts, compounds and preparations.‡

f. BETAMEPRODINE or NU-1932, B-1-methyl-3-ethyl-4-phenyl-4-propionoxypiperidine, its salts, compounds and preparations.‡

g. BETAPRODINE or NU-1779, B-1,3-dimethyl-4-phenyl-4-propionoxypiperidine, its salts, compounds and preparations.‡

h. DIPHENOXYLATE, ethyl 1-(3-cyano-3,3-diphenylpropyl)-4-phenyl-4-piperidinecarboxylate, its salts, compounds and preparations.‡

i. ETOXERIDINE (Atenorax, Atenos, Cargetidine), 1-[2-(2-hydroxyethoxy)-ethyl]-4-phenylpiperidine-4-carboxylic acid ethyl ester, its salts, compounds and preparations.‡

j. FURETHIDINE, ethyl 1-(2-tetrahydrofurfuryloxyethyl)-4-phenyl-4-piperidinecarboxylate, its salts, compounds and preparations.‡

k. HYDROXYPETHIDINE (bemidone, oxypetidin), 1-methyl-4-(3-hydroxyphenyl)-piperidine-4-carboxylic acid ethyl ester or 1-methyl-4-metahydroxyphenylpiperidine-4-carboxylic acid ethyl ester, its salts, compounds and preparations.‡

l. KETOBEMIDONE (Ketogan, Cliradon). 4-(3-hydroxyphenyl)-1-methyl-4-piperidyl ethyl ketone or 1-methyl-4-metahydroxyphenyl-4-propionylpiperidine, its salts, compounds and preparations. (Production not authorized in United States.)‡

m. MORPHERIDINE (morpholinoethylnorpethidine), 1-(2-morpholinoethyl)-4-phenylpiperidine-4-carboxylic acid ethyl ester

---

* See Class B for compounds permissible on oral prescription.
† See Class X for compounds permissible as exempt preparations.
‡ Manufacture not authorized; no basic Classes for these drugs.

or 1-(2-morpholinoethyl)-4-carbethoxy-4-phenylpiperidine, its salts, compounds and preparations.‡

n. NORPETHIDINE (Normeperidine, Pethidine Intermediate-B), ethyl-4-phenylpiperidine-4-carboxylate or 4-phenylpiperidine-4-carboxylic acid ethyl esters, its salts, compounds and preparations.‡

o. PETHIDINE-INTERMEDIATE-A, 4-cyano-1-methyl-4-phenylpiperidine, its salts, compounds and preparations.‡

p. PHENOPERIDINE, 1-(3-hydroxy-3-phenylpropyl)-4-phenylpiperidine-4-carboxylic acid ethyl ester, its salts, compounds and preparations.‡

q. PIMINODINE (Alvodine, Anopridine, Cimadon, NIH-7590, WIN-14098), ethyl 4-phenyl-1-[3-(phenylamino)-propyl]-4-piperidinecarboxylate, its salts, compounds and preparations.‡

r. PROPERIDINE (Gevelina, Ipropethidine, Isopedine, Spasmodolosina), isopropyl 1-methyl-4-phenylpiperidine-4-carboxylate, its salts, compounds and preparations.‡

s. TRIMEPERIDINE (Promedol), 1,2,5-trimethyl-4-phenyl-4-propionoxypiperidine, its salts, compounds and preparations.‡

2. *Methadone Group:*

a. ACETYLMETHADOL (methadyl acetate), 4,4-diphenyl-6-dimethylamino-3-acetoxyheptane or 6-dimethylamino-4,4-diphenyl-3-acetoxyheptane, its salts, compounds and preparations.‡

b. ALPHACETYLMETHADOL, a-6-dimethylamino-4,4-diphenyl-3-acetoxyheptane, its salts, compounds and preparations.‡

c. ALPHAMETHADOL, a-6-dimethylamino-4,4-diphenyl-3-heptanol, its salts, compounds and preparations.‡

d. BETACETYLMETHADOL, B-6-dimethylamino-4,4-diphenyl-3-acetoxyheptane, its salts, compounds and preparations.‡

e. BETAMETHADOL (Betametadol), B-4,4-diphenyl-6-dimethylamino-3-heptanol or B-6-dimethylamino-4,4-diphenyl-3-heptanol, its salts, compounds and preparations.‡

f. DEXTROMORAMIDE (Palfium, Jetrium, Pyrrolamidol, R-875, SKF-d-5137), d-3-methyl-2,2-diphenyl-4-morpholino-butyrylpyrrolidine or d-2,2-diphenyl-3-methyl-4-morpholino-butyrylpyrrolidine, its salts, compounds and preparations.‡

g. DIMENOXADOL (NIH-7577, Lokarin), dimethylaminoethyl 1-ethoxy-1,1-diphenylacetate or dimethylaminoethyl diphenyl-a-ethoxyacetate, its salts, compounds and preparations.‡

h. DIMEPHEPTANOL (Methadol, Pangerin, Amidol, NIH-2933), 4,4-diphenyl-6-dimethylaminoheptanol-3 or 6-dimethyl-amino-4,4-diphenyl-3-heptanol, its salts, compounds and preparations.‡

i. DIOXAPHETYL BUTYRATE (Amidalgon, Spasmoxale), ethyl 2,2-diphenyl-4-morpholinobutyrate, its salts, compounds and preparations.‡

j. DIPIPANONE (Pipadone, Phenylpiperone, Fenpidon, Pamedon, piperidylamidone, piperidylmethadone), 4,4-diphenyl-6-piperidino-3-heptanone, its salts, compounds and preparations.‡

k. ISOMETHADONE (Isoadanon, Isoamidon), 4,4-diphenyl-5-methyl-6-dimethylaminohexanone-3 or 6-dimethylamino-5-methyl-4,4-diphenyl-3-hexanone, its salts, compounds and preparations.

l. LEVOMORAMIDE, l-3-methyl-2,2-diphenyl-4-morpholino-butyrylpyrrolidine, its salts, compounds and preparations.‡

m. METHADONE (Adanon, Amidone, Dolophine, Methadon), 4,4-diphenyl-6-dimethylaminoheptanone-3 or 6-dimethyl-amino-4,diphenyl-3-heptanone, its salts, compounds and preparations.

n. METHADONE-INTERMEDIATE, 4-cyano-2-dimethyl-amino-4,4-diphenylbutane, its salts, compounds and preparations.‡

o. MORAMIDE-INTERMEDIATE, 2-methyl-3-morpholino-1,1-diphenylpropanecarboxylic acid, its salts, compounds and preparations.‡

p. NORACYMETHADOL, a-d-3-acetoxy-6-methyl-amino-4,4-diphenyl heptane, its salts, compounds and preparations.‡

q. NORMETHADONE (Deatussan, Mepidon, Normedon, Phenyl-dimazone, Ticarda, Veryl), 4,4-diphenyl-6-dimethylamino-3-hexanone, its salts, compounds and preparations.‡

r. PHENADOXONE or CB-11 (Hepagin, Heptalgin, Heptalin, Heptan, Heptazone, Heptone), 4,4-diphenyl-6-morpholinoheptanone-3 or 6-morpholino-4,4-diphenyl-3-heptanone, its salts, compounds and preparations.‡

s. RACEMORAMIDE (R-610), d-3-methyl-2,2-diphenyl-4-morpholinobutyrylpyrrolidine, its salts, compounds and preparations.‡

3. *Morphinan Group:*

a. DEXTRORPHAN, d-3-hydroxy-N-methylmorphinan, its salts, compounds and preparations.‡

b. LEVOMETHORPHAN, l-3-methoxy-N-methylmorphinan or (−)-3-methoxy-N-methylmorphinan, its salts, compounds and preparations.

c. LEVOPHENACYLMORPHAN (NIH-7525, RO-4-0288), l-3-hydroxy-N-phenacylmorphinan or (−)-3-hydroxy-N-phenacyl-morphinan, its salts, compounds and preparations.‡

d. LEVORPHANOL (Dromoran, Levo-Dromoran, Levorphan, Aromarine), l-3-hydroxy-N-methylmorphinan or (−)-3-hydroxy-N-methylmorphinan, its salts, compounds and preparations.

e. METAZOCINE (methobenzorphan, NIH-7539), 2′-hydroxy-2,5,9-trimethyl-6,7-benzomorphan, its salts, compounds and preparations.

f. NORLEVORPHANOL (NIH-7539), l-3-hydroxynormor-phinan or (−)-3-hydroxynormorphinan, its salts, compounds and preparations.

g. PHENAZOCINE (phenobenzorphan, Prinadol, NIH-7519, SKF-6574), 2′-hydroxy-5,9-dimethyl-2-(2-phenylethyl)-6,7-benz-orphan, its salts, compounds and preparations.

h. PHENOMORPHAN (NIH-7274), 3-hydroxy-N-phenethyl-morphinan, its racemic and levorotatory forms (but excepting its dextrorotatory form), their salts, compounds and preparations.‡

i. RACEMETHORPHAN, dl-3-methoxy-N-methylmorphinan, its salts, compounds and preparations.

j. RACEMORPHAN (Citarin, Methorphinan), dl-3-hydroxy-N-methylmorphinan, its salts, compounds and preparations.

4. *Thiambutene Group:*

a. DIETHYLTHIAMBUTENE (diethibutin, Themalon, diethylambutene), 3-diethylamino-1,1-di-(2-thienyl)-1-butene, its salts, compounds and preparations.‡

b. DIMETHYLTHIAMBUTENE (aminobutene, dimethibutin, Kobaton, Ohton, Skikiton, Takaton), 3-dimethylamino-1,1-di-(2-thienyl)-1-butene, its salts, compounds and preparations.‡

c. ETHYLMETHYLTHIAMBUTENE (Emethibutin,ethyl-methiambutene), 3-ethylmethylamino-1,1-di-(2-thienyl)-1-butene, its salts, compounds and preparations.‡

5. *Others:*

a. CLONITAZENE, 2-(p-chlorobenzyl)-1-diethylaminoethyl-5-nitrobenzimidazole, its salts, compounds and preparations.‡

b. DIAMPROMIDE, N-[2-(methylphenethylamino)-propyl]-propionanilide, its salts, compounds and preparations.‡

c. ETONITAZENE, 2-(p-ethoxybenzyl)-1-diethylaminoethyl-5-nitrobenzimidazole, its salts, compounds and preparations.‡

d. PHENAMPROMIDE, N-(1-methyl-2-piperidinoethyl)-propionanilide, its salts, compounds and preparations.‡

e. PROHEPTAZINE (Proheptazone), 1,3-dimethyl-4-phenyl-4-propionoxyhexamethyleneimine, its salts, compounds and preparations.‡

Class "B" (Oral Prescription) Narcotic Drugs

(Authorized for "oral prescription")

1. Isoquinoline alkaloids of opium, or any of their salts.
   a. NARCOTINE (Noscarpine) §
   b. PAPAVERINE §
   c. COTARNINE §
   d. NARCEINE §
   e. MECONIN‡

2. APOMORPHINE or any of its salts, alone or in combination with other active non-narcotic medicinal ingredients.

3. NALORPHINE (N-allyl-normorphine) or any of its salts.§

4.
   a. Compounds of CODEINE (methylmorphine), or any of its salts, with equal or greater quantity of isoquinoline alkaloid where codeine content does not exceed eight (8) grains per fluid ounce or one grain per dosage unit. (Copavin, etc.)
   b. Compounds of CODEINE (methylmorphine), or any of its salts, with one or more active non-narcotic ingredients in therapeutic amounts where codeine content does not exceed eight (8) grains per fluid ounce or one grain per dosage unit. (Codesal, Codempiral, Edrisal with Codeine, etc.)

5.
   a. Compounds of HYDROCODONE (dihydrocodeinone) or any of its salts, with a four-fold quantity of any isoquinoline alkaloid where hydrocodone content does not exceed one and one-third grains per fluid ounce or one-sixth grain per dosage unit.
   b. Compounds of HYDROCODONE (dihydrocodeinone) or any of its salts, with one or more active non-narcotic ingredients in therapeutic amounts where hydrocodone content does not exceed one and one-third grains per fluid ounce or one-sixth grain per dosage unit (Tussionex, etc.)

6. Compounds of DIHYDROCODEINE, or any of its salts, with one or more active non-narcotic medicinal ingredients in therapeutic amounts where the dihydrocodeine does not exceed eight (8) grains per fluid ounce or one grain per dosage unit.

7. Compounds of OXYCODONE (dihydrohydroxycodeinone, Eucodal, etc.), or any of its salts, with one or more active non-narcotic ingredients in therapeutic amounts where the oxycodone does not exceed two-thirds grain per fluid ounce or one-twelfth grain per dosage unit.

8. Compounds of ETHYLMORPHINE, or any of its salts, with one or more active non-narcotic ingredients in therapeutic amounts where the ethylmorphine content does not exceed one and one-third grains per fluid ounce or one-sixth grain per dosage unit.

---

§ See Class M for preparations classified as exempt.

Class "X" Narcotic Drugs (Exempt Preparations)

(Exempted preparations may be sold without prescription.)

1. OPIUM Preparations: containing not more than two grains of opium per fluid or avoirdupois ounce along with therapeutically active non-narcotic ingredients.
2. MORPHINE Preparations: containing not more than one-fourth grain morphine, or any of its salts, per fluid or avoirdupois ounce.
3. CODEINE Preparations: containing not more than one grain codeine, or any of its salts, per fluid or avoirdupois ounce.
4. DIHYDROCODEINE Preparations: containing not more than one-half grain dihydrocodeine, or any of its salts, per fluid or avoirdupois ounce.
5. ETHYLMORPHINE Preparations: containing not more than one-fourth grain ethylmorphine, or any of its salts, per fluid or avoirdupois ounce.
6. DIPHENOXYLATE Preparations: pharmaceutical preparations in liquid or solid forms containing not more than 2.5 mg diphenoxylate and not less than 25 micrograms of atropine sulfate per dosage unit.

Class "M" Narcotic Drugs (Especially Exempted Preparations)

1. NARCOTINE (Noscapine) Preparations: any pharmaceutical preparation containing narcotine, without limit in quantity, along with either active or inactive non-narcotic ingredients of the type used in medicinal preparations.
2. PAPAVERINE Preparations: any pharmaceutical preparation containing papaverine, without limit in quantity, along with either active or inactive non-narcotic ingredients of the type used in medicinal preparations.
3. NARCEINE Preparations: any pharmaceutical preparation containing narceine, without limit in quantity, along with either active or inactive non-narcotic ingredients of the type used in medicinal preparations.
4. COTARNINE Preparations: any pharmaceutical preparation containing cotarnine, without limit in quantity, along with either active or inactive non-narcotic ingredients of the type used in medicinal preparations.
5. NALORPHINE Preparations: any pharmaceutical preparation containing nalorphine, without limit in quantity, along with either active or inactive non-narcotic ingredients of the type used in medicinal preparations. (Nalline, etc.)

(from General Circular No. 262, Federal Bureau of Narcotics—July 25, 1962)

Federal Food, Drug and Cosmetic Act

The First Federal Food and Drugs Act went into effect on June 30, 1906, and, after several amendments, was completely rewritten and re-enacted by Congress in 1938. The present Food, Drug and Cosmetic Act dates from June 23, 1938, and amendments have followed placing insulin, penicillin, streptomycin, bacitracin, chlortetracycline, and chloramphenicol under the control of the Food and Drug Administration, the agency established by the Congress to enforce the Act. The major requirements of the Act, so far as they regulate the quality and movement of drugs and devices in interstate commerce, are quoted in the following pages. An attempt has been made to supply interpretations, but the law presents a very complex picture and rulings and regulations often depend upon special conditions surrounding each individual problem and upon the application of new court decisions.

Manufacturers and others who must operate under federal or state drug and cosmetic laws usually delegate the problems arising from the necessity of compliance, to specially trained individuals in their organization or to legal experts specializing in such laws.

Two major revisions of the Act have occurred in the past 6 years:

1. New Drug Amendments of 1962
2. Drug Abuse Control Amendments of 1965.

For this reason we would recommend that an up-to-date copy of the Act and its effectuating regulations—21 CFR, Part 1 to end—should be examined. We have set forth immediately following, however, their main effect on the pharmacy practitioners, along with state and narcotic laws, as they bear on the stocking and dispensing of drugs.

The Pharmacist's Stock in Trade

We have noted elsewhere that boards of pharmacy have in many instances determined within reasonable parameters the quantity of inventory minimally required to support registration as a pharmacy. Obviously, this stock must be legitimately acquired and maintained and dispensed in accordance with pertinent laws.

The usual inventory of drugs is divided between over-the-counter (OTC) drugs and prescription drugs. The former is subdivided in many ways, such as proprietary drugs, heavily advertised for sale or demand, and household remedies which may be non-proprietaries, packaged from bulk by the pharmacist himself or put up by a supplier. He may have an "own goods" line or an "unknown brand" line of drugs to use on special promotions or to sell against branded proprietaries where price and profit are at issue. He may have OTC's from well-known manufacturers which are only sold through ethical promotion. All of these categories of goods have legal implications which vary slightly.

So far as prescription drugs are concerned, there is also a similar differential chart possible. There are prescription drugs of usual variety, either new or old, classed as stimulants or depressants, dangerous drugs, narcotics, orals, parenterals, enzymes, animal or plant extractives, antibiotics, etc. As this material comes into the pharmacy or is stored there it must have complete and correct labeling according to the Act. It may not be misbranded or adulterated. It may be seized if it in any way violates the Sec. 301 series of prohibitions set forth.

In general, if it is an article intended for human use with any antibiotic or antibiotic salt or derivative, or insulin, it has to come from a batch tested and certified by the FDA (Sec. 506,507). There are some exemptions available to this in terms of both human and veterinary drugs set out in exemptive regulations.

A "new" drug as defined in the Act is one which is not yet generally recognized by medical experts as being both safe and effective for the intended use. This might be by virtue of its having new drug substances as ingredients, or having an older chemical ingredient for which a new use, new dosage level, or new period of usage has been essayed. Sometimes, a combination of old drugs placed together in a new dosage form with claims for use that go beyond each ingredient individually is considered a new drug. Some articles are recognized as safe, but have not yet been proven effective (Sec. 505).

We have noted previously that Sec. 503(b) established the legal differences between prescription drugs and nonprescription drugs. Prescription drugs must be labeled with the restrictive legend until dispensed on prescription. Nonprescription drugs, no matter what their source or nature, do not bear the legend on the basis that they may be safely employed in self-treatment if properly labeled with adequate descriptions of usage and limitations, directions for uses represented or which may be reasonably anticipated, and any cautions required for their safe and effective utilization.

The label in any case must have the name and address (zip code) of the manufacturer, packer, or distributor and reflect his true status. It must have an accurate statement of the net amount of the drug in the package, expressed in usual and understandable units that will make for a fair and nonmisleading representation of true content. It must show the active ingredients, using in conjunction the established name for each, if there is one. If a proprietary product, it describes the category of use. If the label bears the names of certain listed drugs that require the specialized "Warning—May be habit forming," that must be in immediate juxtaposition. Quantities of ingredients contained which are potent alkaloids, coal tar derivatives, alcohol, etc, must be stated.

In the case of prescription drugs, besides the legend, the label must bear the quantity and proportion of each active ingredient, and if for other than oral use, the names of all other ingredients. If it is for parenteral use, the label must bear the names and quantities of all ingredients. Further, when it is a prescription drug, it should bear a statement of recommended or usual dosage and the package insert must include all the information needed to enable the physician to use or prescribe its use safely and effectively.

If it is a drug subject to Sec. 201(v) because of its stimulant or depressant character, and has not been exempted from the requirements of Sec. 511, the label must further bear the special control symbol of an R within a large C.

Everything on the label is generally required on the immediate outer container or carton wrapper, unless it is windowed. In the case of proprietary drugs, the label and outer carton or a leaflet associated with the package must bear adequate directions for use, including adequate warning, quantity, and frequency of dosage. No aspect of the label or accompanying labeling may be false or misleading in any respect, including qualitative and quantitative representations.

The pharmacist's stock is in a great sense controlled by the authorities who interpret and enforce good manufacturing practices insofar as suppliers are concerned, and require registration of all who distribute drugs. Pharmacies need not be so registered unless they do repackaging to supply other outlets.

The pharmacist must store and handle his stock according to his knowledge, compendial requirements, and package statements. If the drugs deteriorate in any manner, contain any filthy, putrid, or decomposed substances, or show evidence of inadequate or decomposed containers that may render the contents injurious to health, they will be considered adulterated in federal and state law and be subject to seizure and condemnation. The pharmacist involved is also subject to prosecution and penalty.

The law recognizes the USP, NF, and HP as official compendia. All drugs named therein are required by law to meet the standards of strength, quality, and purity described in the compendia, and should be packaged and labeled as prescribed therein as they await usage. If the drug differs in strength, quality, or purity from the compendial standard, that exact difference must be evident on the label. Otherwise, variant drugs that do not meet compendial standards, or do not reflect the strength, quality, or purity they purport to have, are adulterated. Obviously, in such an instance they are misbranded as well.

Devices also stocked by the pharmacist are subject to much of the same requirements. They too divide into "prescription devices" and nonprescription devices (which bear no cautionary Federal legend). They are also subject to misbranding violations.

Cosmetics, too, are subject to appropriate safeguards against misbranding and adulteration in their manufacture, stocking, and distribution. Their labels also must state the name and address of those who place them into commerce and an accurate statement of the net contents and general category of use.

The Pharmacist and Prescription Drugs

While such drugs are in his possession prior to the act of dispensing, they must be kept in a manner that will not allow adulteration. Products that become deteriorated or lose labeled strength and potency are in violation of both federal and state laws. They are subject to seizure. Either the holding or the dispensing of adulterated products is in violation of the law: sale, manufacture, delivery, offer for sale or possession of adulterated or misbranded drugs, devices, cosmetics. Of course, those who manufacture adulterated products, or cause them to be introduced or introduce them into interstate or intrastate commerce, violate federal and/or state law.

Also, the drug prior to dispensing must be in a properly labeled container. In most cases this means either the manufacturer's original labeled container or one that has what amounts to a facsimile of such labeling, including control and other identifying numbers.

The Order to Dispense

Federally (Sec. 503(b)), the order to dispense a legend drug must be received either orally or in writing by the pharmacist before the drug is dispensed. It should represent an order by one licensed to prescribe such drugs in the state where the dispensing act is to take place. Reasonable exceptions are the occasional prescriptions of physicians immediately adjacent to that state or prescriptions by physicians attending patients in governmental institutions. The orders should result from a *bona fide* patient relationship that would not be suspect to an ordinary prudent pharmacist. They may be communicated to the pharmacist by the physician's agent under the physician's supervision and authority, unless the state requires only direct communication from the doctor. The pharmacist should be satisfied in such instances that the prescriptive communication is actually an act of agency. Such satisfaction may require more substance where dangerous drugs and narcotics are involved; here, the physician has sole authority and cannot delegate this prescribing function to anyone else. His agents may only transmit his order.

The Sec. 503(b) exemption is not available where the prescription is not dispensed according to 503(b)(1) or where it arises out of the conduct of a business of dispensing drugs pursuant to diagnosis by mail. It is also invalidated by unauthorized "substitution" of ingredients ordered by the doctor.

There are three classes of legend drugs (Sec. 503(b)) intended for use by man:

> 1. Habit-forming drugs to which Sec. 502(d) applies and those declared subject to abuse according to the DACA amendments of 1965.
> 2. Drugs which require physicians to supervise their use or administer them because they are potentially toxic, potent, harmful, or must be used by means that require a physician's assistance.
> 3. Drugs established as legend drugs by the NDA approval.

These are to be dispensed only on a written or oral prescription order (reduced promptly to writing) and filed by the pharmacist (federal).

The label must bear (federal) the name and address of the dispenser, the serial number and date of the prescription order or its dispensing, and the name of the prescriber. If stated in the prescription order, the label must also bear the name of the patient, directions for use, and any cautionary statements.

In the case of narcotic prescriptions these requirements are subordinate to the more stringent requirements of the Harrison Narcotic Act. Where state laws are more stringent, practitioners in such jurisdiction must comply with their extra requirements.

Renewal may be written, as indicated on the original prescription order, or by an oral order reduced immediately to writing and filed (federal).

In the case of DACA* drugs, a prescription order has a life of 6 months and may not be refilled more than 5 times, if so ordered, within that period. After 6 months, the pharmacist needs a new prescription order or a new oral prescription which he must reduce immediately to writing and file. Since all prescription orders for drug-abuse drugs must be accountable and reconcilable with inventory and purchases, the files for such prescription orders are available for inspection, whether kept separately or as part of regular prescription files (federal).

In some states (eg, Pennsylvania), dangerous drugs are all drugs other than narcotics which are legend drugs in federal law or which the state describes as legend drugs, as well as drugs for investigational use.

Only a pharmacist or a physician can dispense a legend drug, although certain classes of their agents (pharmacy interns, medical interns, nurses) may do so under supervision and pursuant to direction of the licensed pharmacist or physician.

The oral prescription with the date of its communication, the name and address of the prescriber, and other information required by law or pharmacy regulations for written prescriptions must be reduced promptly to writing and filed for 2 years, so it will be accessible to inspection by state authorities. (Federal law requires prescription orders for legend drugs to be kept 5 years).

Generally, in state laws the prescriber should confirm an oral prescription in writing within 72 hours of issuing it. If he does not do so, the pharmacist should remind him of the requirement and make note of this on the back of the prescription order. If circumstances are suspicious to an average prudent pharmacist, he may want to be even more diligent and take additional steps. Some pharmacists feel it is not being careful or prudent to accept an oral refill order for an unconfirmed original oral prescription,

unless they are very sure of the prescriber's authenticity and reliability.

Whether on oral or written order, the pharmacist must affix a label to the prescription container which bears the (1) pharmacist's name and address, (2) patient's name and address, (3) date compounded and consecutive number under which the prescription is recorded, and (4) prescribing practitioner's name.

As to narcotic prescription orders, they must be dated as of the day on which signed and must be signed by the issuing prescriber. Orders for Class A or Class B narcotics should be issued following a physical examination of the person or animal for whom the drugs are intended. Prescription orders are to be kept on file for 2 years.

A pharmacist federally and in most states may accept an oral order for a narcotic if it is Class B (or of lesser risk) from an authorized practitioner. The oral order plus its date of communication, the name and address of the prescriber, and such other information as may be required by law or regulation in the case of written prescriptions shall be reduced promptly to writing by the pharmacist. The written order must be filed and preserved and held accessible for inspection for 2 years. In most states using the triplicate system (eg, California) one copy of the narcotic prescription order goes to the state board promptly.

No narcotic prescription order can be refilled. However, for Class B narcotics a new oral order can be given where state law allows. The dispensing label for oral or written narcotic prescriptions must have thereon the (1) date plus the pharmacist's name, address, and registry number; (2) employing pharmacist's name, address, and registry number; (3) patient's (or animal owner's) name and address; (4) prescriber's name, address, and registry number; and (5) directions for use.

A pharmacist must keep a record of all purchases and sales of narcotics. Prescription files serve for sales. Paid bills and narcotic order form copies serve for purchases.

Dispensing Physicians

A physician dispensing a dangerous drug must label the container in which he dispenses it to the patient. (This does not apply where he merely gives a correctly labeled physician's sample.) In brief, if he regularly undertakes the pharmacist's function, he undertakes also some of his labeling and record-keeping responsibilities such as the (1) physician's name and address, (2) date dispensed, (3) patient's name and address, and (4) directions for use.

If a physician dispenses a narcotic (Class A or B), it must be issued following a physical examination of the person or animal for whom intended. He must label the container with the (1) date plus his name, address, and registry number and (2) patient's (or animal owner's) name and address.

A doctor, dentist, or veterinarian in most states must keep a record for 2 years of Class A and B narcotics dispensed or distributed by him, showing the (1) amount administered, dispensed, or distributed and (2) date plus the patient's (or animal owner's) name and address. No records are needed for any such drugs administered in emergencies. This is like Class 4 prerogative in hospital circumstances.

In some state laws, there is an additional class of drugs termed nonproprietary drugs which may be sold by a registered pharmacist in a retail pharmacy.

---

* Drugs classified under the Drug Abuse Control Amendments of 1965.

These also can be sold by a hospital pharmacist in a hospital pharmacy, by a dispensing doctor in his office, and by a manufacturer, wholesaler, or other agent to pharmacists and other authorized recipients. A nonproprietary drug is one containing any quantity of any narcotic drug, a drug containing biologicals or substances of glandular origin (except intestinal enzymes and all liver products), drugs administered by LT, IM, or IV, but not any such drugs which are prepackaged with complete dosage instructions in the labeling limiting their use to the care or treatment of poultry and livestock. In common parlance, proprietary drugs are those which are sold with instructions for lay use OTC. Nonproprietary drugs are prescription drugs.

Class X and M narcotics may be sold, dispensed, distributed, or given away by a registered pharmacist in a licensed pharmacy without a prescription. However, every licensed pharmacy should maintain an appropriate registry to list such sales of Class X narcotic drugs and it should have the (1) purchaser's name and address and the date of purchase; (2) name of medication and quantity; and (3) dispensing pharmacist's name.

Class X preparations dispensed without prescription orders cannot be sold in amounts to exceed 4 fluid or avoidupois ounces in any 72-hour period. While this includes mixtures containing paregoric as an ingredient, paregoric by itself, although federally Class X, is treated as Class B in Pennsylvania; therefore, it requires an oral or written prescription order.

Certain classes of persons may acquire more than 4 ounces of Class X narcotics in 72 hours (eg, manufacturers, wholesalers, importers or exporters of drugs, registered pharmacists in licensed pharmacies, *bona fide* owners of pharmacies or drug stores, doctors, dentists, other accredited prescribers, government officials, warehouse-men for handling, nurses under physician's supervision; laboratory supervisors where such drugs are going to be used for scientific purposes such as teaching or analysis, captains or other proper officers of ships, and persons in employ of the foregoing. All these and patients by virtue of prescription orders validly executed and dispensed may have possession of dangerous drugs, narcotics, and exempt narcotics in excess of 4 ounces per 72 hours.

In addition to violations characterized as misbranding or adulteration under federal and state law, under the latter there most often is spelled out the offense of substitution. While the definitions vary somewhat depending upon who is trying to prevent or to justify the act of substitution, quite simply it means what it stands for literally. It represents the replacement of the written or orally specified needs of a patient with any other commodity, without notice, authority, or consent.

This has important legal implications beyond the punishment set out in the state acts which view it either as a palpable misdemeanor or as an abrogation of professional conduct requirements. In either event therefore, it is punishable by fine or by suspension or revocation of licensure.

Aside, however, from the fact that it is unethical to fail, without physician consent in the case of prescription drugs (and without buyer consent in the case of nonprescription drugs), to carry out the express order of the prescriber or orderer, these are elements of fraud and misrepresentation present in such cases of nondisclosure. This is not only immoral, but poses further problems, especially in the event the substi-

tuted product fails the user as to safety and/or effectiveness. While numerous cases have been decided in instances where substitution has been accidental rather than intentional, the prudent and ethical practitioner will have the danger of substitution on his mental checklist for himself and his employees, and will never substitute except in those instances where the substitution is authorized by one with a right to exert such authority.

For more detail as to product liability and decisional views on substitution, see "Ethical and Legal Implications of Drug Substitution," in the *Food, Drug, and Cosmetic Law Journal*, CCH (June, 1968).

The officials of the Federal Food and Drug Administration, at Washington, are also very cooperative when consulted on general or specific questions of interpretation or compliance and it is a wise precaution to take advantage of their willingness to assist and advise when in doubt about the proper course to follow.

The Federal Food, Drug and Cosmetic Act, as suggested by its title, is "an act to prohibit the movement in interstate commerce of adulterated and misbranded food, drugs, devices, and cosmetics and for other purposes."

The Act must be regarded as an act to protect the consumer, and must be read and studied in this light.

Courts have universally held that the Act is a "consumer act" and that it will be interpreted and construed so as to serve this purpose.

In construing statements made on the labels of products subject to the provisions of the Act, courts have said repeatedly that they should be read with due regard to "the man on the street" as it was for his protection that the Act was passed by Congress in the first instance.

Definitions—The following definitions set forth in the Act are basic to an understanding of the theory and purpose of the law:

"The term *food* means (1) articles used for food or drink for man or other animals, (2) chewing gum, and (3) articles used for components of any such article.

"The term *drug* means (A) articles recognized in the official United States Pharmacopeia, official Homeopathic Pharmacopœia of the United States, or official National Formulary, or any supplement to any of them; and (B) articles intended for use in the diagnosis, cure, mitigation, treatment, or prevention of disease in man or other animals; and (C) articles (other than food) intended to affect the structure or any function of the body of man or other animals; and (D) articles intended for use as a component of any article specified in clause (1), (2), or (3); but does not include devices or their components, parts, or accessories.

"The term *counterfeit drug* means a drug which, or the container or labeling of which, without authorization, bears the trademark, tradename, or other identifying mark, imprint, or device, or any likeness thereof, of a drug manufacturer, processor, packer, or distributor other than the person or persons who in fact manufactured, processed, packed, or distributed such drug and which thereby falsely purports or is represented to be the product of, or to have been packed or distributed by, such other drug manufacturer, processor, packer, or distributor."

"The term *device* (except when used in paragraph (*n*) of this section and in sections 301 (*i*), 403 (*f*), 502 (*c*), and 602 (*c*)) means instruments, apparatus, and contrivances, including their components, parts, and accessories, intended (1) for use in the diagnosis, cure, mitigation, treatment, or prevention of disease in man or other animals; or (2) to affect the structure of any function of the body of man or other animals.

"The term *cosmetic* means (1) articles intended to be rubbed, poured, sprinkled, or sprayed on, introduced into, or otherwise applied to the human body or any part thereof for cleansing, beautifying, promoting attractiveness, or altering the appearance, and (2) articles intended for use as a component of any such articles; except that such term shall not include soap.

"The term *label* means a display of written, printed, or graphic matter upon the immediate container of any article; and a requirement made by or under authority of this Act that any word, statement, or other information appearing on the label shall not be considered to be complied with unless such word, statement, or other information also appears on the outside container or wrapper, if any there be, of the retail package of such article, or is easily legible through the outside container or wrapper.

"The term *immediate container* does not include package liners.

"The term *labeling* means all labels and other written, printed, or graphic matter (1) upon any article or any of its containers or wrappers, or (2) accompanying such article.

"If an article is alleged to be misbranded because the labeling is misleading, then in determining whether the labeling is misleading there shall be taken into account (among other things) not only representations made or suggested by statement, word, design, device, or any combination thereof, but also the extent to which the labeling fails to reveal facts material in the light of such representations or material with respect to consequences which may result from the use of the article to which the labeling relates under the conditions of use prescribed in the labeling thereof or under such conditions of use as are customary or usual.

"The representation of a drug, in its labeling, as an antiseptic shall be considered to be a representation that it is a germicide, except in the case of a drug purporting to be, or represented as, an antiseptic for inhibitory use as a wet dressing, ointment, dusting powder, or such other use as involves prolonged contact with the body.

"The term *new drug* means—(1) Any drug (except a new animal drug or an animal feed bearing or containing a new animal drug) the composition of which is such that such drug is not generally recognized, among experts qualified by scientific training and experience to evaluate the safety and effectiveness of drugs, as safe and effective for use under the conditions prescribed, recommended, or suggested in the labeling thereof, except that such drug not so recognized shall not be deemed to be a *new drug* if at any time prior to the enactment of this Act it was subject to the Food and Drugs Act of June 30, 1906, as amended and if at such time its labeling contained the same representations concerning the conditions of its use; or (2) Any drug (except a new animal drug or an animal feed bearing or containing a new animal drug) the composition of which is such that such drug, as a result of investigations to determine its safety and effectiveness for use under such conditions, has become so recognized, but which has not, otherwise than in such investigations, been used to a material extent or for a material time under such conditions."

Adulterated Drugs and Devices—"A drug or device shall be deemed to be adulterated—

a. "(1) If it consists in whole or in part of any filthy, putrid, or decomposed substance; or (2)(A) if it has been prepared, packed, or held under insanitary conditions whereby it may have been contaminated with filth, or whereby it may have been rendered injurious to health; or (B) if it is a drug and the methods used in, or the facilities or controls used for, its manufacture, processing, packing, or holding do not conform to or are not operated or administered in conformity with current good manufacturing practice to assure that such drug meets the requirements of this Act as to safety and has the identity and strength, and meets the quality and purity characteristics, which it purports or is represented to possess; or (3) if it is a drug and its container is composed, in whole or in part, of any poisonous or deleterious substance which may render the contents injurious to health; or (4) if (A) it is a drug which bears or contains, for purposes of coloring only, a color additive which is unsafe within the meaning of section 706(a), or (B) it is a color additive the intended use of which in or on drugs is for purposes of coloring only and is unsafe within the meaning of section 706(a); or (5) if it is a new animal drug which is unsafe within the meaning of section 512; or (6) if it is an animal feed bearing or containing a new animal drug, and such animal feed is unsafe within the meaning of section 512.

b. "If it purports to be or is represented as a drug the name of which is recognized in an official compendium, and its strength differs from, or its quality or purity falls below, the standard set forth in such compendium. Such determination as to strength, quality, or purity shall be made in accordance with the tests or methods of assay set forth in such compendium, except that whenever tests or methods of assay have not been prescribed in such compendium, or such tests or methods of assay as are prescribed are, in the judgment of the Secretary, insufficient for the making of such determination, the Secretary shall bring such fact to the attention of the appropriate body charged with the revision of such compendium, and if such body fails within a reasonable time to prescribe tests or methods of assay which, in the judgment of the Secretary are sufficient for purposes of this paragraph, then the Secretary shall promulgate regulations prescribing appropriate tests or methods of assay in accordance with which such determination as to strength, quality, or purity shall be made. No drug defined in an official compendium shall be deemed to be adulterated under this paragraph because it differs from the standard of strength, quality, or purity therefor set forth in such compendium, if its difference in strength, quality, or purity from such standard is plainly stated on its label. Whenever a drug is recognized in both the

United States Pharmacopeia and the Homeopathic Pharmacopœia of the United States it shall be subject to the requirements of the United States Pharmacopeia unless it is labeled and offered for sale as a homeopathic drug, in which case it shall be subject to the provisions of the Homeopathic Pharmacopœia of the United States and not to those of the United States Pharmacopeia.

c. "If it is not subject to the provisions of paragraph (b) of this section and its strength differs from, or its purity or quality falls below, that which it purports or is represented to possess.

d. "If it is a drug and any substance has been (1) mixed or packed therewith so as to reduce its quality or strength or (2) substituted wholly or in part therefor."

Misbranded Drugs and Devices—"A drug or device shall be deemed to be misbranded—

a. "If its labeling is false or misleading in any particular.

b. "If in package form unless it bears a label containing (1) the name and place of business of the manufacturer, packer, or distributor; and (2) an accurate statement of the quantity of the contents in terms of weight, measure, or numerical count: *Provided*, That under clause (2) of this paragraph reasonable variations shall be permitted, and exemptions as to small packages shall be established, by regulations prescribed by the Secretary.

c. "If any word, statement, or other information required by or under authority of this Act to appear on the label or labeling is not prominently placed thereon with such conspicuousness (as compared with other words, statements, designs, or devices, in the labeling) and in such terms as to render it likely to be read and understood by the ordinary individual under customary conditions of purchase and use.

d. "If it is for use by man and contains any quantity of the narcotic or hypnotic substance alpha-eucaine, barbituric acid, beta-eucaine, bromal, cannabis, carbromal, chloral, coca, cocaine, codeine, heroin, marihuana, morphine, opium, paraldehyde, peyote, or sulphonmethane; or any chemical derivative of such substance, which derivative has been by the Secretary, after investigation, found to be, and by regulations designated as, habit forming; unless its label bears the name, and quantity or proportion of such substance or derivative and in juxtaposition therewith the statement 'Warning—May be habit forming.'

e. "(1) If it is a drug, unless (A) its label bears, to the exclusion of any other nonproprietary name (except the applicable systematic chemical name or the chemical formula), (i) the established name (as defined in subparagraph (2)) of the drug, if such there be, and (ii), in case it is fabricated from two or more ingredients, the established name and quantity of each active ingredient, including the quantity, kind, and proportion of any alcohol, and also including whether active or not, the established name and quantity or proportion of any bromides, ether, chloroform, acetanilide, acetophenetidin, amidopyrine, antipyrine, atropine, hyoscine, hyoscyamine, arsenic, digitalis, digitalis glucosides, mercury, ouabain, strophanthin, strychnine, thyroid, or any derivative or preparation of any such substance, contained therein: *Provided*, That the requirement for stating the quantity of the active ingredients, other than the quantity of those specifically named in this paragraph, shall apply only to prescription drugs; and (B) for any prescription drug the established name of such drug or ingredient, as the case may be, on such label (and on any labeling on which a name for such drug or ingredient is used) is printed prominently and in type at least half as large as that used thereon for any proprietary name or designation for such drug or ingredient: and *Provided*, That to the extent that compliance with the requirements of clause (A)(ii) or clause (B) of this subparagraph is impracticable, exemptions shall be established by regulations promulgated by the Secretary.   (2) As used in this paragraph (e), the term "established name", with respect to a drug or ingredient thereof, means (A) the applicable official name designated pursuant to section 508, or (B), if there is no such name and such drug, or such ingredient, is an article recognized in an official compendium, then the official title thereof in such compendium, or (C) if neither clause (A) nor clause (B) of this subparagraph applies, then the common or usual name, if any, of such drug or of such ingredient: *Provided further*, That where clause (B) of this subparagraph applies to an article recognized in the United States Pharmacopeia and in the Homeopathic Pharmacopeia under different official titles, the official title used in the United States Pharmacopeia shall apply unless it is labeled and offered for sale as a homeopathic drug, in which case the official title used in the Homeopathic Pharmacopeia shall apply.

f. "Unless its labeling bears (1) adequate directions for use; and (2) such adequate warnings against use in those pathological conditions or by children where its use may be dangerous to health, or against unsafe dosage or methods or duration of administration or application, in such manner and form, as are necessary for the protection of users: *Provided*, That where any requirement of clause (1) of this paragraph, as applied to any drug or device, is not necessary for the protection of the public health, the Secretary shall promulgate regulations exempting such drug or device from such requirement.

g. "If it purports to be a drug the name of which is recognized in an official compendium, unless it is packaged and labeled as prescribed therein: *Provided*, That the method of packing may be modified with the consent of the Secretary. Whenever a drug is recognized in both the United States Pharmacopeia and the Homoeopathic Pharmacopœia of the United States, it shall be subject to the requirements of the United States Pharmacopeia with respect to packaging and labeling unless it is labeled and offered for sale as a homoeopathic drug, in which case it shall be subject to the provisions of the Homoeopathic Pharmacopœia of the United States, and not to those of the United States Pharmacopeia.

h. "If it has been found by the Secretary to be a drug liable to deterioration, unless it is packaged in such form and manner, and its label bears a statement of such precautions, as the Secretary shall by regulations require as necessary for the protection of the public health. No such regulation shall be established for any drug recognized in an official compendium until the Secretary shall have informed the appropriate body charged with the revision of such compendium of the need for such packaging or labeling requirements and such body shall have failed within a reasonable time to prescribe such requirements.

i. "(1) If it is a drug and its container is so made, formed, or filled as to be misleading; or (2) if it is an imitation of another drug; or (3) if it is offered for sale under the name of another drug.

j. "If it is dangerous to health when used in the dosage, or with the frequency or duration prescribed, recommended, or suggested in the labeling thereof.

k. "If it is, or purports to be, or is represented as a drug composed wholly or partly of insulin, unless (1) it is from a batch with respect to which a certificate or release has been issued pursuant to section 506, and (2) such certificate or release is in effect with respect to such drug.

l. "If it is, or purports to be, or is represented as a drug composed wholly or partly of any kind of penicillin, bacitracin, streptomycin, chlortetracycline, and chloramphenicol or any derivatives thereof, unless (1) it is from a batch with respect to which a certificate or release has been issued pursuant to section 507, and (2) such certificate or release is in effect with respect to such drug: *Provided*, That this paragraph shall not apply to any drug or class of drugs exempted by regulations promulgated under section 507 (c) or (d).

m. "If it is a color additive the intended use of which in or on drugs is for the purpose of coloring only, unless its packaging and labeling are in conformity with such packaging and labeling requirements applicable to such color additive, as may be contained in regulations issued under section 706.

n. "In the case of any prescription drug distributed or offered for sale in any State, unless the manufacturer, packer, or distributor thereof includes in all advertisements and other descriptive printed matter issued or caused to be issued by the manufacturer, packer, or distributor with respect to that drug a true statement of (1) the established name as defined in section 502(e), printed prominently and in type at least half as large as that used for any trade or brand name thereof, (2) the formula showing quantitatively each ingredient of such drug to the extent required for labels under section 502(e), and (3) such other information in brief summary relating to side effects, contraindications, and effectiveness as shall be required in regulations which shall be issued by the Secretary in accordance with the procedure specified in section 701(e) of this Act: *Provided*, That (A) except in extraordinary circumstances, no regulation issued under this paragraph shall require prior approval by the Secretary of the content of any advertisement, and (B) no advertisement of a prescription drug, published after the effective date of regulations issued under this paragraph applicable to advertisements of prescription drugs, shall, with respect to the matters specified in this paragraph or covered by such regulations, be subject to the provisions of sections 12 through 17 of the Federal Trade Commission Act, as amended (15 U.S.C. 52-57). This paragraph (n) shall not be applicable to any printed matter which the Secretary determines to be labeling as defined in section 201(m) of this Act.

o. "If it is a drug and was manufactured, prepared, propagated, compounded, or processed in an establishment in any State not duly registered under section 510."

Certification of Coal-Tar Colors for Drugs—

"The Secretary shall promulgate regulations providing for the listing of coal-tar colors which are harmless and suitable for use in drugs for purposes of coloring only and for the certification of batches of such colors, with or without harmless diluents."

New Drugs—

a. "No person shall introduce or deliver for introduction into interstate commerce any new drug, unless an approval of an application filed pursuant to subsection (b) is effective with respect to such drug.

b. "Any person may file with the Secretary an application with respect to any drug subject to the provisions of subsection (a). Such persons shall submit to the Secretary as a part of the application (1) full reports of investigations which have been made to show whether or not such drug is safe for use and whether such drug is effective in use; (2) a full list of the articles used as components of such drug; (3) a full statement of the composition of such drug; (4) a full description of the methods used in, and the facilities and controls used for, the manufacture, processing, and packing of such drug; (5) such samples of such drug and of the articles used as components thereof as the Secretary may require; and (6) specimens of the labeling proposed to be used for such drug.

c. "Within one hundred and eighty days after the filing of an application under this subsection, or such additional period as may be agreed upon by the Secretary and the applicant, the Secretary shall either—(1) approve the application if he then finds that none of the grounds for denying approval specified in subsection (d) applies, or (2) give the applicant notice of an opportunity for a hearing before the Secretary under subsection (d) on the question whether such application is approvable. If the applicant elects to accept the opportunity for hearing by written request within thirty days after such notice, such hearing shall commence not more than ninety days after the expiration of such thirty days unless the Secretary and the applicant otherwise agree. Any such hearing shall thereafter be conducted on an expedited basis and the Secretary's order thereon shall be issued within ninety days after the date fixed by the Secretary for filing final briefs.

d. "If the Secretary finds, after due notice to the applicant in accordance with subsection (c) and giving him an opportunity for a hearing, in accordance with said subsection, that (1) the investigations, reports of which are required to be submitted to the Secretary pursuant to subsection (b), do not include adequate tests by all methods reasonably applicable to show whether or not such drug is safe for use under the conditions prescribed, recommended, or suggested in the proposed labeling thereof; (2) the results of such tests show that such drug is unsafe for use under such conditions or do not show that such drug is safe for use under such conditions; (3) the methods used in, and the facilities and controls used for, the manufacture, processing, and packing of such drug are inadequate to preserve its identity, strength, quality, and purity; (4) upon the basis of the information submitted to him as part of the application, or upon the basis of any other information before him with respect to such drug, he has insufficient information to determine whether such drug is safe for use under such conditions; or (5) evaluated on the basis of the information submitted to him as part of the application and any other information before him with respect to such drug, there is a lack of substantial evidence that the drug will have the effect in purports or is represented to have under the conditions of use prescribed, recommended, or suggested in the proposed labeling thereof; or (6) based on a fair evaluation of all material facts, such labeling is false or misleading in any particular; he shall issue an order refusing to approve the application. If, after such notice and opportunity for hearing, the Secretary finds that clauses (1) through (6) do not apply, he shall issue an order approving the application. As used in this subsection and subsection (e), the term "substantial evidence" means evidence consisting of adequate and well-controlled investigations, including clinical investigations, by experts qualified by scientific training and experience to evaluate the effectiveness of the drug involved, on the basis of which it could fairly and responsibly be concluded by such experts that the drug will have the effect it purports or is represented to have under the conditions of use prescribed, recommended, or suggested in the labeling or proposed labeling thereof.

e. "The Secretary shall, after due notice and opportunity for hearing to the applicant, withdraw approval of an application with respect to any drug under this section if the Secretary finds (1) that clinical or other experience, tests, or other scientific data show that such drug is unsafe for use under the conditions of use upon the basis of which the application was approved; (2) that new evidence of clinical experience, not contained in such application or not available to the Secretary until after such application was approved, or tests by new methods, or tests by methods not deemed reasonably applicable when such application was approved, evaluated together with the evidence available to the Secretary when the application was approved, shows that such drug is not shown to be safe for use under the conditions of use upon the basis of which the application was approved or (3) on the basis of new information before him with respect to such drug, evaluated together with the evidence available to him when the application was approved, that there is a lack of substantial evidence that the drug will have the effect it purports or is represented to have under the conditions of use prescribed, recommended, or suggested in the labeling thereof; or (4) that the application contains any untrue statement of a material fact: *Provided*, That if the Secretary (or in his absence the officer acting as Secretary) finds that there is an imminent hazard to the public health, he may suspend the approval of such application immediately, and give the applicant prompt notice of his action and afford the applicant the opportunity for an expedited hearing under this subsection; but the authority conferred by this priviso to suspend the approval of an application shall not be delegated. The Secretary may also, after due notice and opportunity for hearing to the applicant, withdraw the approval of an application with respect to any drug under this section if the Secretary finds (1) that the applicant has failed to establish a system for maintaining required records, or has repeatedly or deliberately failed to maintain such records or to make required reports, in accordance with a regulation or order under subsection (j), or the applicant has refused to permit access to, or copying or verification of, such records as required by paragraph (2) of such subsection; or (2) that on the basis of new information before him, evaluated together with the evidence before him when the application was approved, the methods used in, or the facilities and controls used for, the manufacture, processing, and packing of such drug are inadequate to assure and preserve its identity, strength, quality, and purity and were not made adequate within a reasonable time after receipt of written notice from the Secretary specifying the matter complained of; or (3) that on the basis of new information before him, evaluated together with the evidence before him when the application was approved, the labeling of such drug, based on a fair evaluation of all material facts, is false or misleading in any particular and was not corrected within a reasonable time after receipt of written notice from the Secretary specifying the matter complained of. Any order under this subsection shall state the findings upon which it is based.

f. "Whenever the Secretary finds that the facts so require, he shall revoke any previous order under subsection (d) or (e) refusing, withdrawing, or suspending approval of an application and shall approve such application or reinstate such approval, as may be appropriate.

g. "Orders of the Secretary issued under this section shall be served (1) in person by any officer or employee of the Department designated by the Secretary or (2) by mailing the order by registered mail or by certified mail addressed to the applicant or respondent at his last-known address in the records of the Secretary.

h. "An appeal may be taken by the applicant from an order of the Secretary refusing or withdrawing approval of an application under this section. Such appeal shall be taken by filing in the United States court of appeals for the circuit wherein such applicant resides or has his principal place of business, or in the United States Court of Appeals for the District of Columbia Circuit, within sixty days after the entry of such order, a written petition praying that the order of the Secretary be set aside. A copy of such petition shall be forthwith transmitted by the clerk of the court to the Secretary, or any officer designated by him for that purpose, and thereupon the Secretary shall certify and file in the court the record upon which the order complained of was entered, as provided in section 2112 of title 28, United States Code. Upon the filing of such petition such court shall have exclusive jurisdiction to affirm or set aside such order, except that until the filing of the record the Secretary may modify or set aside his order. No objection to the order of the Secretary shall be considered by the court unless such objection shall have been urged before the Secretary or unless there were reasonable grounds for failure so to do. The finding of the Secretary as to the facts, if supported by substantial evidence, shall be conclusive. If any person shall apply to the court for leave to adduce additional evidence, and shall show to the satisfaction of the court that such additional evidence is material and that there were reasonable grounds for failure to adduce such evidence in the proceeding before the Secretary, the court may order such additional evidence to be taken before the Secretary and to be adduced upon the hearing in such manner and upon such terms and conditions as to the court may seem proper. The Secretary may modify his findings as to the facts by reason of the additional evidence so taken, and he shall file with the court such modified findings which, if supported by substantial evidence, shall be conclusive, and his recommendation, if any, for the setting aside of the original order. The judgment of the court affirming or setting aside any such order of the Secretary shall be final, subject to review by the Supreme Court of the United States upon certiorari or certification as provided in section 1254 of title 28 of the United States Code. The commencement of proceedings under this subsection shall not, unless specifically ordered by the court to the contrary, operate as a stay of the Secretary's order.

i. "The Secretary shall promulgate regulations for exempting from the operation of the foregoing subsections of this section drugs intended solely for investigational use by experts qualified by scientific training and experience to investigate the safety and effectiveness of drugs. Such regulations may, within the discretion of the Secretary, among other conditions relating to the protection of the public health, provide for conditioning such exemption upon—(1) the submission to the Secretary, before any clinical testing of a new drug is undertaken, of reports, by the manufacturer or the sponsor of the investigation of such drug, of preclinical tests (including tests on animals) of such drug adequate to justify the proposed clinical testing; (2) the manufacturer or the sponsor of the investigation of a new drug proposed to be distributed to investigators for clinical testing obtaining a signed agreement from each of such investigators that patients to whom the drug is administered will be under his personal supervision, or under the supervision of investigators responsible to him, and that he will not supply such drug to any other investigator, or to clinics, for administration to human beings; and (3) the establishment and maintenance of such records, and the making of such

reports to the Secretary, by the manufacturer or the sponsor of the investigation of such drug, of data (including but not limited to analytical reports by investigators) obtained as the result of such investigational use of such drug, as the Secretary finds will enable him to evaluate the safety and effectiveness of such drug in the event of the filing of an application pursuant to subsection (b). Such regulations shall provide that such exemption shall be conditioned upon the manufacturer, or the sponsor of the investigation, requiring that experts using such drugs for investigational purposes certify to such manufacturer or sponsor that they will inform any human beings to whom such drugs, or any controls used in connection therewith, are being administered, or their representatives, that such drugs are being used for investigational purposes and will obtain the consent of such human beings or their representatives, except where they deem it not feasible or, in their professional judgment, contrary to the best interests of such human beings. Nothing in this subsection shall be construed to require any clinical investigator to submit directly to the Secretary reports on the investigational use of drugs.

j. "(1) In the case of any drug for which an approval of an application filed pursuant to this section is in effect, the applicant shall establish and maintain such records, and make such reports to the Secretary, of data relating to clinical experience and other data or information, received or otherwise obtained by such applicant with respect to such drug, as the Secretary may by general regulation, or by order with respect to such application, prescribe on the basis of a finding that such records and reports are necessary in order to enable the Secretary to determine, or facilitate a determination, whether there is or may be ground for invoking subsection (e) of this section: *Provided, however,* That regulations and orders issued under this subsection and under subsection (i) shall have due regard for the professional ethics of the medical profession and the interests of patients and shall provide, where the Secretary deems it to be appropriate, for the examination, upon request, by the persons to whom such regulations or orders are applicable, of similar information received or otherwise obtained by the Secretary. (2) Every person required under this section to maintain records, and every person in charge or custody thereof, shall, upon request of an officer or employee designated by the Secretary, permit such officer or employee at all reasonable times to have access to and copy and verify such records.

The Durham-Humphrey Act—Of special interest to pharmacists are the changes in the Federal Food, Drug, and Cosmetic Act popularly known as the Durham-Humphrey Amendment.

Under this amendment drugs fall into two classes—(1) those which may be dispensed only on prescription, and (2) those which fall into the category of over-the-counter drug products.

Drugs in group (1) are known as "prescription legend drugs" and may be supplied only on prescription. Every such drug must bear this statement on its label: "Caution: Federal law prohibits dispensing without prescription."

If the label of a drug or drug product is not required by the law to bear the prescription legend, it may be sold at will without prescription.

Under the provisions of the Durham-Humphrey Act, the prescription legend, as a matter of legislative compulsion, must appear upon all drugs to which it properly and appropriately applies. Conversely, it is a violation of the act to place the prescription legend caution upon drugs which, by their very nature, may be used with relative safety without medical supervision or advice.

The Durham-Humphrey Act permits the physician to give and the pharmacist to receive prescriptions for legend drugs over the telephone thus contributing to the convenience of the physician, pharmacist, and patient.

The pharmacist, in all such cases, must record and file the prescription giving the drug prescribed, the directions, name of the patient, and all other facts and data telephoned to him by the physician.

Prescriptions for legend drugs may not be refilled except in those cases where the refilling is authorized and directed by the physician involved. Here, too, the authorization to refill may be telephoned. The pharmacist must make a record of the whole transaction, just as he is required to do when taking a telephoned prescription for a legend drug in the first instance.

Several devices are being resorted to by both physician and pharmacist in order to facilitate the refilling of prescriptions under the Durham-Humphrey Act.

Among these is to have the physician indicate that the prescription, either oral or written, may be refilled for a designated number of times. Or that it may be refilled at will during a specified time, usually a relatively short period.

But, whatever the devices, the pharmacist should not allow these to lead him into practices which he knows are in conflict with good professional procedure.

The point to bear in mind is that the refilling of prescriptions calling for legend drugs must be authorized by the physician, and this means an affirmative authorization. The pharmacist who relies upon some general authority or formula assumes the risk of violating the law if enforcement officials should hold that such generalization or formula does not meet the statutory requirements.

Imports and Exports—"The Secretary of the Treasury shall deliver to the Secretary of Health, Education and Welfare, upon his request, samples of food, drugs, devices, and cosmetics which are being imported or offered for import into the United States, giving notice thereof to the owner or consignee, who may appear before the Secretary of Health, Education and Welfare and have the right to introduce testimony. If it appears from the examination of such samples or otherwise that (1) such article has been manufactured, processed, or packed under unsanitary conditions, or (2) such article is forbidden or restricted in sale in the country in which it was produced or from which it was exported, or (3) such article is adulterated, misbranded, or in violation of section 505, then such article shall be refused admission. This paragraph shall not be construed to prohibit the admission of narcotic drugs the importation of which is permitted under section 2 of the Act of May 26, 1922, as amended (U. S. C., 1946 ed., title 21, sec. 173).

"A food, drug, device, or cosmetic intended for export shall not be deemed to be adulterated or misbranded under this Act if it (1) accords to the specifications of the foreign purchaser, (2) is not in conflict with the laws of the country to which it is intended for export, and (3) is labeled on the outside of the shipping package to show that it is intended for export. But if such article is sold or offered for sale in domestic commerce, this subsection shall not exempt it from any of the provisions of this Act."

The Labeling of Repackaged Drugs—Under the Sullivan Case, the Food and Drug Administration has direct jurisdiction over the sale to consumers of drugs which have moved in interstate commerce.

For instance, a drug taken from a container which has been shipped in interstate commerce must be labeled in strict accord with the label on the original container.

The pharmacist can make certain that he is complying with the law if he repackages an over-the-counter drug and offers it in good faith under the same labeling that was used on the interstate package in which it was received.

The repackaging of drugs now, however, subjects the repackager to more extensive controls by the Food and Drug Administration than heretofore existed as a result of legislation passed in 1962.

Drug Amendments of 1962—The passage of the Kefauver–Harris bill, officially known as the "Drug Amendments of 1962," made some major changes in the Federal Food, Drug and Cosmetic Act.

The law now requires that persons and firms engaged in the manufacture, repacking, or relabeling of drug products "register" annually with the Food and Drug Administration, a requirement which applies equally to those engaged solely in intrastate business as well as those engaged in interstate business. Pharmacies engaged in the customary activity of dispensing prescriptions and selling drugs at retail are exempt from the registration requirement.

The law now requires that the Food and Drug Administration inspect every registered establishment at least once every two years. It also provides that all such establishments make available for inspection by the FDA all their files, records, and process and control information. Pharmacists engaged in their customary activity of dispensing prescription drugs need not make their files and records available for inspection, however.

The Kefauver–Harris amendent to the Federal Food, Drug and Cosmetic Act specifically requires that the facilities, methods and control procedures used by a manufacturer conform with "current good manufacturing practice" as established by the Food and Drug Administration to insure the integrity of drug products being manufactured and distributed. Drugs manufactured under conditions which fail to meet established minimum requirements are considered to be "adulterated."

Labeling of drugs is also further controlled by the provisions of the 1962 Act which require that the label of each drug bear the nonproprietary or generic name of the drug as well as the trade name. The new law also requires that all prescription drug advertising contain the generic name of the drug as well as its trade name wherever the trade name appears, and that the type for the generic name be at least half as large as the type used for printing the trade name.

The new law requires that a "new drug" not only be safe for use but that it be effective for its intended purpose and also authorizes the Food and Drug Administration to require manufacturers and distributors of new drugs to submit reports of adverse effects of the drugs, even after the drug has been cleared. The new law further provides for more extensive control by the Food and Drug Administration over drugs intended for clinical investigation.

Antibiotic drug certification provisions were altered by the 1962 amendment in that previously only products containing penicillin, streptomycin, bacitracin, chlortetracycline and chloramphenicol or their derivatives were subject to certification. Full certification required that a sample from each batch of the antibiotic had to be tested and a certificate for the particular batch issued by the Food and Drug Administration, if the drug had the proper potency, purity, etc. Now, all antibiotics intended for human use are subject to certification procedures. The new law, however, authorizes the Food and Drug Administration to establish exemptions so that a particular antibiotic could be exempted from batch certification if the manufacturer could comply with the FDA's exempting provisions.

The only veterinary antibiotic drug preparations subject to certification are those containing penicillin, streptomycin, bacitracin, chlortetracycline, chloramphenicol or derivatives thereof.

Stilbestrol or ingredients known to be capable of inducing cancer may be approved for use in medicated feeds if the available evidence shows that the medicated feed does not adversely affect the health of the animal and no residue of the drug remains in the edible portions of the animal or in any food produced by the animal, (eg, milk or eggs).

Enforcement of the Act—The Act is enforced and administered by the Food and Drug Administration of the Department of Health, Education and Welfare. This body is staffed with physicians, chemists, pharmacologists, bacteriologists, pharmacists, lawyers, and other technical and professional personnel essential to its regulatory duties. The Food and Drug Administration is, in conformity with the limitations set forth in the Act, empowered to make rules and regulations for that kind and degree of enforcement contemplated by the embrasive language and broad purposes of the legislation.

The Food and Drug Administration, while vested with wide powers of regulation, discipline, and control, has no authority to inflict punishment or impose penalties. By this is meant that all issues of fact are triable in court, the final disposition of the case being determined according to the rules of evidence and customary judicial procedure.

Violations of the Act are misdemeanors and are punishable by "imprisonment for not more than one year, or a fine of not more than $1000, or both such imprisonment and fine." For second or subsequent convictions, the penalty is increased "to imprisonment for not more than three years, or a fine of not more than $10,000, or both such imprisonment and fine."

Many states have enacted food, drug, and cosmetic acts closely conforming to the federal law. In these instances uniformity has been sought, and, looking to this end, the states have adopted for the purpose of intrastate enforcement, the regulations of the Food and Drug Administration in so far as they are applicable to local problems.

The foregoing discussion is by no means meant to encompass the broad sweep of the Food, Drug and Cosmetic Act. Rather, it is intended only to suggest the public policy which the Act is intended to serve, and to outline some of the provisions, prohibitions, and cautions by means of which its purposes may be achieved.*

Both federal and state agencies that implement the drug laws carry out active registration and inspection programs. These have been traditionally without warrant despite the fact that criminal prosecution and penalties are therein provided. This has caused some extensive litigation and review in recent years.

While there is little doubt that the public's interest is served by cooperation between those who regulate and those who are regulated, it is also in the public interest to assure fair play and to provide remedies for intrusion as well as obstruction when its justification is questionable.

In See vs Seattle, the US Supreme Court tackled the question of Fourth Amendment protection against warrantless inspection of business premises. Their conclusions have given a fair blueprint of the degree of immunity businessman may enjoy.

"The businessman, like the occupant of a residence, has a constitutional right to go about his business free from unreasonable official entries upon his private commercial property. The businessman, too, has that right placed in jeopardy if the decision to enter can be made and enforced by the inspector in the field without official authority evidenced by a warrant."

---

* A copy of the *Federal Food, Drug and Cosmetic Act*, with the general regulations for its enforcement and any new amendments, may be obtained by writing to the US Department of Health, Education and Welfare, Food and Drug Administration, Washington 25, D.C.

The court indicated that procurement of a warrant for "probable cause" in the case of a residential inspection will utilize the traditional depth of understanding of that basis, while "probable cause" in the case of a commercial premise might be subject to a more simplistic evaluation. So that while all administrative inspections are seen subject to the Fourth Amendment, the dwelling is differentiated from the business establishment.

"Probable cause" has certain key ingredients to be compounded by a warrant-seeker. There should be some basis to believe that the public's health or safety is jeopardized by noncompliance with some substantive or procedural element of public law. Further, the observation or confirmation of such a circumstance has been or will be denied to enforcement personnel; or surprise will be of the essence, with some show of probable cause for such a likelihood. To this the court has emphasized and added that the request for a warrant has to be organizational rather than that of the enforcement agent or inspector in the field. The language of the court has, however, modified the weight of probable cause for administrative inspections of commercial property.

First, where an establishment seeks licensure and the prerequisite is an inspection spelled out in the regulations, then the businessman has indicated his willingness to accede. While the case is not quite so clear on permitting inspections for maintenance of licensure, it has been expanded in some quarters to have such an interpretation. Whether this means prior agreement to warrantless inspection or routine grant of warrants for inspection on the simplest "probable cause" (namely, license status requirements) probably will see further high-court clarification.

Second, where an establishment is one such as is covered by a law and the law authorizes or indicates a need for inspection, agency supervisors may anticipate that their application for the "Fourth Amendment" warrant will be granted. Again, the matter of a warrant issued subsequent to an initial refusal, a pattern of refusal or because of the likelihood of need of surprise may all require different material submissions. On the other hand, a show of a specific routine of inspection as an effectuation of the statute and a procedure of the agency might be entirely sufficient.

In food and drug inspections, there are many instances where the inspector under orders or on his own enters areas of discovery that are not clearly accessible to him under the statute. It has been suggested that if the agency must go to the procedure of applying for a warrant, they should specify therein access to particular documents, files, or other records. However, there is reason to suppose that search prerogatives set forth in the warrant would not be granted to exceed statutory authority sought to be vested.

There is also reason to believe that the inspected not only has a right to qualify or withdraw consent given in the absence of a warrant, but also that he can limit inspection to the exact specifications of a warrant. The courts take a dim view of the rare attempts by enforcement officials to expand or distort the license given by the warrant.

As for specifications in a particular warrant, Alvin A. Gotlieb, Deputy Assistant General Counsel, FDA, expressed them summarily—in an address at the 1968 Meeting of the Central Atlantic States Association of Food and Drug Officials, Philadelphia, May 27, 1968 —to encompass answers to five questions:

1. Who is to inspect? That is, the identity of the Inspectors and their official authorization.
2. What to inspect? The identity of the firm to be inspected, and a description of its operations as coming within the purview of the statute.
3. Why to inspect? The statute or agency declarations of authority and necessity; that is, the inspection is routinely scheduled, as required by statute, or to determine if violative conditions exist.

4. When to inspect? The data and time of day.
5. Where to inspect? The specific address or addresses.

Obviously these specifics set the parameters for opposition to the warrant, whether expressed in disobedience and after-trial for same or moving to quash it.

Patents and Proprietary Medicines

Patents—A patent is a license issued by the United States Government, giving to the holder thereof the exclusive right to make, use, and sell the thing or process patented for a period of 17 years. This license is issued by the Patent Office in Washington. In order to secure it, an applicant must file with the office an affidavit, with appropriate charts, drawings, models, etc, showing the exact composition of the thing or process which he has invented or discovered. "Letters patent" should be issued only when the Patent Office is of the opinion that the invention or discovery is both novel and useful.

The right conferred by the letters patent is an exclusive right, and all others besides the patentee and his assignees are prohibited from infringing on that right during the life of the patent. At the expiration of the seventeen-year period, the right passes to the public generally. Thereafter any person is at liberty to make, use, and deal with the thing or process patented, without any restraint whatever imposed by the patentee.

Proprietary Medicines—The manufacturer of a proprietary medicine takes the risk of its being made and sold by anybody who can duplicate it. Unless he is protected by a patent he cannot prevent anyone from dealing at will with the article.

Trade-Marks—The protection given to the owner of a trade-mark exists by virtue of common law, ie, irrespective of any right conferred by statute. If the maker of any article chooses to mark it with a distinctive device or brand to designate the source or origin of the article, such device is a trade-mark, and it cannot be copied or used by anyone else without permission of the owner. The right to the exclusive use of the trade-mark, however, lasts only as long as the owner or his assignees actually make general use of it in trade. The following material was obtained from the US Patent office.

Definition of Trade-marks—A "trade-mark," as defined in Section 45 of the Trade-Mark Act of July 5, 1946, "include any word, name, symbol, or device, or any combination thereof adopted and used by a manufacturer or merchant to identify his goods and distinguish them from those manufactured or sold by others."

Functions of Trade-marks—The primary function of a trade-mark is to indicate origin. However, trade-marks also serve to guarantee the quality of the goods bearing the mark, and through advertising, to create and maintain a demand for the product. Rights in a trade-mark are acquired only by use, and the use must ordinarily continue if the rights so acquired are to be preserved. Registration of a trade-mark in the Patent Office does not in itself create or establish any exclusive rights but is recognition by the Government of the right of the owner to use the mark in commerce to distinguish his goods from those of others.

Selecting a Mark—The selection of a trade-mark is very important since many marks are not subject to registration. Among these are marks which consist of or comprise immoral, deceptive, or scandalous matter; or matter which may disparage or falsely suggest a connection with persons, living or dead, institutions, beliefs, or national symbols, or bring them into contempt, or disrepute; the flag or coat of arms or other insignia of the United States, or of any State or municipality, or any foreign nation, or any simulation thereof. Registration of a name, portrait, or signature identifying a particular living individual except by his written consent, or the name, signature or portrait of a deceased President of the United States during the life of his widow, if any, except by the written consent of the widow is prohibited. A mark is not registrable which so resembles a mark registered in the Patent Office or a mark or trade name previously used in the United States by another and *not* abandoned as to cause confusion or mistake or to deceive purchasers.

Marks which are descriptive or deceptively misdescriptive of the applicant's goods; marks which, when applied to the goods of the applicant are primarily geographically descriptive or deceptively misdescriptive of them, except as indications of regional origin; or marks which are primarily merely surnames, are registrable on the Principal Register only when they have become distinctive of the applicant's goods through use in commerce.

How to Obtain Registration—A trade-mark may be registered only by the owner of the mark, and the mark must be in use in commerce. A trade-mark is deemed to be used in commerce when it is placed in any manner on the goods or their containers or the displays associated therewith or on the tags or labels affixed thereto and the goods are sold or transported in commerce. The word "commerce" means all commerce which may lawfully be regulated by Congress, such as commerce between the states or commerce between the United States and its territories or the Indian Tribes. Use in commerce within the District of Columbia will also qualify a mark for registration.

Prerequisites for Registration—A complete application for registration consists of a written application, a drawing of the mark, the required fee, and specimens or facsimiles showing the mark as actually used on or in connection with the goods.

Term and Renewal—Registrations granted under the 1946 Act remain in force for twenty years from the date of registration and may be renewed for periods of twenty years from the date of expiration. Existing registrations which were granted under the Trade-Mark Acts of 1881 and 1905 continue in full force and effect for their unexpired terms and may be renewed under the provisions of the New Act. Registrations which were granted under the Act of 1920 either expired on January 5, 1948, or will expire twenty years from the date of registration, whichever date is later. Registrations granted under the 1920 Act which must be maintained in order to support a foreign registration may be renewed on the supplemental register of the new Act.

The applicant for renewal must be the owner of the mark and the mark must be in use in commerce which may be regulated by Congress. The application must be in affidavit form and must be accompanied by the required fee. The renewal affidavit may not be executed earlier than six months prior to the date of expiration, but must be filed within said six-month period. A late renewal application may be filed during the three-month period following the date of expiration upon the payment of an additional fee.

Assignments—A registered mark or a mark for which application to register has been filed is assignable with the good will of the business with which the mark is used, or with that part of the good will of the business connected with the use of and symbolized by the mark. It is not necessary to include the good will of the business connected with any other mark.

Trade Names—Undoubtedly words or devices may be adopted as trademarks which are not original inventions of him who adopts them, and courts of equity will protect him against any fraudulent appropriation or imitation of them by others. Property in a trade-mark, or rather in the use of a trademark or name, has very little analogy to that which exists in copyrights, or in patents for inventions. Words in common use, with some exceptions, may be adopted, if at the time of their adoption, they were not employed to designate the same, or like articles of production. The office of a trademark is to point out distinctively the *origin, or ownership of the article to which it is affixed;* or, in other words, to give notice who was the producer. This may, in many cases, be done by a name, a mark, or a device well known, but not previously applied to the same article.

"But though it is not necessary that the word adopted as a trade name should be a new creation, never before known or used, there are some limits to the right of selection. This will be manifest when it is considered that in all cases where rights to the exclusive use of a trademark are invaded, it is invariably held that the essence of the wrong consists in the sale of the goods of one manufacturer or vendor as those of another; and that it is only when this false representation is directly or indirectly made that the party who appeals to a court of equity can have relief. This is the doctrine of all the authorities" (Per Mr. Justice Strong, US Supreme Court, in *Canal Company v. Clark*, 13 Wall. 311).

The Federal Hazardous Substances Labeling Act—In 1960 the act passed to replace the Federal Caustic Poison Act to enable better regulation of the interstate distribution and sale of packages of hazardous substances intended or suitable for household use was published as Public Law 86-613 and officially known as the "Federal Hazardous Substances Labeling Act."

The Act provides control over "hazardous substances" which includes any substance or mixture of substances which is toxic, corrosive, an irritant, a strong sensitizer, is flammable, or generates pressure through decomposition, heat or other means, if such substance or mixture of substances may cause substantial personal injury or substantial illness during or as a proximate result of any customary or reasonably foreseeable ingestion by children. The act exempts economic poisons subject to the Federal Insecticide, Fungicide, and Rodenticide Act; foods, drugs, and cosmetics subject to the Federal Food, Drug and Cosmetic Act; and substances intended for use as fuels when stored in containers and used in the heating, cooking or refrigeration system of a house.

The label of a hazardous substance should contain:

1. The name and place of business of the manufacturer, packer, distributor, or seller.
2. The common or usual name or the chemical name (if there be no common or usual name) of the hazardous substance or of each component which contributes substantially to its hazard, unless by regulation the use of a recognized generic name is permitted.
3. The word DANGER on substances which are extremely flammable, corrosive, or highly toxic.
4. The word WARNING or CAUTION on all other hazardous substances.
5. An affirmative statement of the principal hazard or hazards such as "Flammable," "Vapor Harmful," "Causes Burns," "Absorbed Through Skin," or similar wording descriptive of the hazard.
6. Precautionary measures describing action to be followed or avoided.
7. Instruction, when necessary or appropriate, for first-aid treatment.
8. The word "poison" for any highly toxic hazardous substance.
9. Instructions for the handling and storage of packages which require special care in handling or storage.
10. The statement "keep out of the reach of children" or its practical equivalent.

The enforcement of this Act is the responsibility of the Food and Drug Administration and it is that agency which will issue regulations to implement and explain the provisions of the Act.

For further information about the "Federal Hazardous Substances Labeling Act," the reader is advised to obtain a copy of the Act and regulations under the Act by request directed to the Food and Drug Administration, US Department of Health, Education and Welfare, Washington, D.C.

Labeling of Drugs

Much of the material presented in this chapter has been copied, with permission, from a pamphlet issued to registered pharmacists in the State of New Jersey. This information was issued as a joint project of the New Jersey Department of Health, the New Jersey State Board of Pharmacy, and the New Jersey Pharmaceutical Association. Some of the original material has been modified at the suggestion of officials of the Food and Drug Administration, Washington, D.C. The pharmacist desiring specific information on special applications of the Food, Drug, and Cosmetic Act should write for information to the Commissioner, Food and Drug Administration, Washington, D.C.

Below are stated in nonlegal terms some of the principal requirements of the Federal Food, Drug, and Cosmetic Act as they relate to the labeling of drugs. These statements* are not meant to be exhaustive, nor do they indicate the various exceptions and special cases in which they may not be applicable. For complete information, reference is made to the act itself and to the regulations. The sections of the law and the applicable regulations are mentioned in connection with the various subjects discussed.

General Provisions

1. Information required by the law to appear on the label must appear also on the wrapper or carton of the retail package, or be easily legible through it. (Sec. 201(k))

---

* The labeling of drugs under the provisions of the Federal Food, Drug, and Cosmetic Act" issued by the Department of Health, Education, and Welfare, Food and Drug Administration.

2. All data required to appear on the label or labeling must be prominently and conspicuously placed thereon so as to be readily available under customary conditions of purchase and use. Prominence and conspicuousness of required information should not be sacrificed for any other phraseology, pictures, etc. (Sec. 502(c))
3. All information required on the label or labeling must appear in English; if any statement is made in a foreign language, all required information should appear in that language also as well as in English. (Regulation (c) under Sec. 502(c))
4. New drugs must not be marketed before an application has been filed with the Secretary and has become effective. (Secs. 201(p), 301(d), 505)
5. Drugs containing insulin, penicillin, streptomycin, bacitracin, aureomycin (chlortetracycline), or chloramphenicol must not be marketed until they have been certified as prescribed by the Secretary. (Secs. 506 and 507)
6. A person who ships a drug in interstate commerce is responsible for compliance of that drug with the law unless he holds a guaranty in proper form. (Secs. 301(a), 303(c))
7. Any person who causes a drug to be adultered or misbranded while it is in interstate commerce violates the law. (Sec. 301(b))
8. Any person who receives a drug in interstate commerce and thereafter sells it or offers to sell it or give it away is responsible for compliance with the act, unless he is protected by a guaranty in proper form. (Secs. 301(c), 303(c))
9. Any act with respect to a drug or to its labeling while it is held for sale after shipment in interstate commerce, if this results in causing the article to be adulterated or misbranded, constitutes a violation of the law. (Sec. 301(k))
10. A drug sold under an official name (Sec. 201(g)) or under circumstances creating the impression that it is an official drug must comply with the official requirements except that it may differ from the official requirements in strength, quality, or purity only. If it does so differ, the label must indicate the nature and extent of each such difference. Difference from official specifications in the identity of ingredients is not permitted. (Sec. 501(b))
11. Official drugs must be packaged and labeled as prescribed in the official texts. Unofficial drugs should be packaged so as to prevent deterioration. (Sec. 502(g) and (h))
12. Drugs must not be packaged in unnecessarily large or otherwise deceptive containers. (Sec. 502(i))

13. Drugs required to bear the legend "Caution: Federal law prohibits dispensing without prescription" must not be sold without prescription and prescriptions for these drugs must not be refilled except as authorized by the physician. (Sec. 503(b))

13a. Some drugs intended for use in pets, livestock, etc., are classed as veterinary prescription drugs which must be labeled with the legend "Caution! Federal law restricts this drug to sale by or on the order of a licensed veterinarian." Such drugs may not be sold without a prescription from a licensed vetrinarian. (Regulation 1.106(c))

Label and Labeling

14. The "label" is the principal display portion or portions of the container and the outside carton or wrapper. (Sec. 201(k))

15. "Labeling" includes all printed or written matter accompanying the article at any time. (Sec. 201(m))

The Label Must Contain—

16. The name and address of the manufacturer, packer, or distributor. (Sec. 502(b))

17. A statement of the quantity of the drug in the package. (Sec. 502(b))

18. A statement of the quantity and percentage of certain habit-forming drugs, together with the statement "Warning—May be habit forming." (Sec. 502(d))

19. The common or usual name of the drug. (Sec. 502(e))

20. If it is composed of two or more ingredients, the common name of each active ingredient and the proportions of certain specified ingredients. (Sec. 502(e)) Abbreviations should be avoided in listing ingredients. If all ingredients are mentioned the statement should clearly show which are active and which are merely solvents, diluents, flavorings, etc.

21. The legend "Caution: Federal law prohibits dispensing without prescription" if the drug is unsuitable for use in self-medication. (Sec. 503(b))

The Label or Other Labeling Must Contain—

22. Adequate directions for use. (Sec. 502(f))

23. Adequate warnings against unsafe use by children and against use in conditions where warnings are required to insure against harm. (Sec. 502(f))

24. Warning against use in an amount or for a length of time or by method of administration which may make it dangerous to health. (Sec. 502(f))

25. A clear indication of therapeutic limitations. The labeling should not mention the useful effects of a drug only but should disclose any harmful or deleterious effects also. (Sec. 201(n))

The Label or Other Labeling Must Not Contain—

26. Any false or misleading statement regarding the composition of the article or the effects it will produce. (Sec. 502(a))

27. Any false or misleading statement regarding any other drug or device. (Regulation (b) under Sec. 502(a))

28. The legend "Caution: Federal law prohibits dispensing without prescription" on drugs safe and suitable for use in self-medication. (Sec. 503(b))

Approval of Labeling or Formulas—

29. The act does not authorize the Food and Drug Administration to approve labels or formulas. It places upon manufacturers and distributors full responsibility for distributing their products in harmony with its provisions. Before undertaking the preparation or revision of labeling, the proprietor should inform himself of the provisions of the law and regulations. If he does not have expert knowledge concerning the treatment of the diseases for which a drug is recommended and concerning the physiological effects and therapeutic limitations of the ingredients of which it is composed, he should obtain advice from those who have such expert knowledge. The facilities available to the Administration will not permit review of any considerable number of labels or extensive labeling for a single manufacturer, but comment will be offered on details concerning which a proprietor may have doubt after he has made a careful study of the terms of the law as they apply to his preparations. When labeling is submitted for comment, the complete labeling and the formula, showing the amount of each active ingredient contained in a stated dose or other unit of the medicine, together with other pertinent factual information, should be submitted, preferably in triplicate.

Advertising, Use of Mails, and State Laws

30. The Food and Drug Administration cannot supply information concerning the requirements of Federal laws pertaining to the advertising, other than labeling, of food, drugs, and cosmetics, or to the requirements of postal laws. These statutes are enforced by the Federal Trade Commission and by the Post Office Department, respectively.

31. A list of State officials from whom information concerning State laws may be obtained will be furnished, upon request, by the Food and Drug Administration.

Labeling Regulations

Proposed by the Department of Health, Education, and Welfare, Food and Drug Administration*

Department of Health, Education and Welfare

Food and Drug Administration

[21 CFR Part 131]

Interpretative Statements Re Warnings on Drugs and Devices for Over-the-Counter Sale

Notice of Proposed Rule Making

The Commissioner of Food and Drugs, under authority vested in the Secretary of Health, Education, and Welfare by the Federal Food, Drug, and Cosmetic Act (secs. 503(b) (1) A), (C) and (3), 506, 507, 701; 52 Stat. 1052 as amended; 61 Stat. 11; 63 Stat. 409; 67 Stat. 489; 21 U.S.C. 353(b) (1) (A), (C) and (3), 356, 357, 371) and delegated to him by the Secretary (21 CFR 130.101(b); 22 F.R. 1045; 23 F.R. 9500),

proposes to amend Title 21, Chapter I, by adding thereto the following new part:

Subpart A—Definitions and Interpretations

Sec.
131.1 Purpose of issuance.
131.2 Definitions.
131.3 Warnings required on drugs exempted from prescription-dispensing requirements of section 503 (b) (1) (C).
131.4 Warnings required on drugs by formal or informal statements of policy.
131.5 Warnings required on insulin intended for over-the-counter sale.
131.6 Warnings required on certifiable antibiotics exempted from prescription-dispensing requirements.
131.7 Warnings required by official compendia.
131.8 Warning statements in relation to conditions for use.
131.9 General warnings re accidental ingestion by children.
131.10 Conspicuousness of warning statements.
131.11 Warnings on veterinary drugs intended for administration to diseased animals.

Subpart B—Drugs for Human Use

131.15 Drugs for human use; recommended warning and caution statements.

---

* *Federal Register*, Vol. **24,** No. 59, Washington, March 26, 1959, p. 2361.

131.16 Drugs for human use; warning and caution statements required by regulations.
131.17 Drugs for human use; warning and caution statements specifically required by law.

Subpart C—Drugs for Veterinary Use

131.20 Drugs for veterinary use; recommended warning and caution statements.
131.21 Drugs for veterinary use; warning and caution statements required by regulations.

Subpart D—Devices

131.25 Devices; recommended warning and caution statements.

AUTHORITY: §§ 131.1 to 131.25 issued under secs. 503, 506, 507, 701, 52 Stat. 1052, as amended; 55 Stat. 851; 59 Stat. 463, as amended; 52 Stat. 1055, as amended; 21 U.S.C. 353, 356, 357, 371. Interprets or applies sec. 502, 52 Stat. 1050, as amended; 53 Stat. 854; 21 U.S.C. 352.

CROSS REFERENCES: For interrelated regulations issued under the Federal Food, Drug, and Cosmetic Act, see Parts 1 (Drugs), 3, 130, 146, 146c, 146d, 146e, 164, 165.

Subpart A—Definitions and Interpretations

§ 131.1   Purpose of issuance.

The warning and caution statements suggested in Subparts B, C, and D of this part, for inclusion in the label or labeling of drugs and devices subject to section 502(d) and (f) (2) and other relevant provisions of the Federal Food, Drug, and Cosmetic Act are issued for the purpose of assisting industry in preparing proper labeling for these articles for over-the-counter sale and in meeting the legal requirements of the act that the label or labeling of drugs and devices bear adequate warnings, in such manner and form as are necessary for the protection of users. Only section 502(d) of the act requires use of the specific language included in these suggested warning and caution statements. These suggested warning or caution statements are illustrative of those that may be necessary or desirable: It is the responsibility of the manufacturer, packer, shipper, or distributor in interstate commerce to see that such statements are adequate for compliance with the provisions of the law. Omission of any article from this suggested list does not relieve drugs and devices subject to provisions of the act from bearing adequate warning or caution statements where such statements are necessary or desirable for the protection of the user.

§ 131.2   Definitions.

(a) As used in this part, the term "act" means the Federal Food Drug, and Cosmetic Act.
(b) The terms "drugs" and "devices" are defined in section 201 (g) and (k) of the act.
(c) Official compendia are defined in section 201 (j) of the act.

§ 131.3   Warnings required on drugs exempted from prescription-dispensing requirements of section 503(b) (1) (C).

Drugs exempted from prescription-dispensing requirements under section 503(b) (1) (C) of the act are subject to the labeling requirements prescribed in § 130.102(a) of this chapter. Although, for convenience, warning and caution statements for a number of the drugs named in § 130.102 of this chapter (cross-referenced in the text of this part) are included in Subpart B of this part, the inclusion of such drugs in §§131.15, 131.16, 131.17 in no way affects the requirements for compliance with § 130.102 (a) of this chapter, or the provisions of an effective application pursuant to section 505(b) of the act.

§ 131.4   Warnings required on drugs by formal or informal statements of policy.

The warning and caution statements included in Subpart B in no way affect any warning statement suggested for such drugs or devices by any statement of policy or interpretation in Part 3 of this chapter.

§ 131.5   Warnings required on insulin intended for over-the-counter sale.

Warning and caution statements for insulin products sold over the counter must comply with the specific labeling provisions of the act and § 164.6 of this chapter.

§ 131.6   Warnings required on certifiable antibiotics exempted from prescription-dispensing requirements.

Certain certifiable antibiotic drugs are exempted from prescription-dispensing requirements under section 507 of the act, but are subject to the specific labeling requirements, including warning or caution statements, of the applicable section of the antibiotic regulations.

§ 131.7   Warnings required by official compendia.

Any drug included in the official compendia defined by the act shall bear such warning or caution statement as may be required by such compendia, and no statement in Subpart B or Subpart C of this part is intended to alter, modify, or permit the omission of any such statement required by such compendia.

§ 131.8   Warning statements in relation to conditions for use.

The mention in any warning or caution statement included in Subparts A, B, and C of this part, of a disease condition does not imply a finding on the part of the Food and Drug Administration that any drug or device is efficacious in such condition; nor is any drug or device bearing labeling referring to such disease condition precluded from regulatory action under the applicable provisions of the act if such claim is considered to be misbranding.

§ 131.9   General warnings re accidental ingestion by children.

Section 131.15 includes at the present time under certain items but not all medicines, the statement "Keep this and all medications out of the reach of children" or "Keep out of the reach of children." However, in view of the possibility of accidental ingestion of drugs, it is not only suggested but is recommended that one of these statements be used in the labeling of all drug products.

§ 131.10   Conspicuousness of warning statements.

Necessary warning statements should appear in the labeling prominently and conspicuously as compared to other words, statements, designs, and devices in order to comply with the provisions of section 502 (c) and (f) (2) of the act. The warning statements should be placed in the labeling in juxtaposition with the directions for use, and in any case should appear on the label when there is sufficient label space in addition to other mandatory label information.

§ 131.11   Warnings on veterinary drugs intended for administration to diseased animals.

None of the warning or caution statements recommended for use in the labeling of drugs intended for administration to diseased animals shall be construed to suggest or imply that any product of a diseased animal is suitable for food use. (See section 402(a) (5) of the act.)

Subpart B—Drugs for Human Use

Since changes occur in this category with great frequency, any specific problem should be checked against the latest copy of 21 CFR, Part 131.15.

§ 131.15   Drugs for human use; recommended warning and caution statements.

ACETANILID.
Warning—Do not exceed recommended dosage. Overdosage or continued use may result in serious blood disturbances.

ANESTHETICS FOR EXTERNAL USE (LOCAL ANESTHETICS). (See also § 130.102(a) (19) of this chapter.)
Caution—Do not use in the eyes. Not for prolonged use. If the condition for which this preparation is used persists or if a rash or irritation develops, discontinue use and consult physician.

ANTIBIOTICS FOR EXTERNAL USE FOR PREVENTION OF INFECTION. (See also §§ 130.102(a) (5), 146c.202, 146e.402, 146e.407, 146e.409, 146e.411, 146e.422 of this chapter.)
Caution—In case of deep or puncture wounds or serious burns consult physician. If redness, irritation, swelling, or pain persists or increases or if infection occurs, discontinue use and consult physician. Do not use in the eyes.

ANTIHISTAMINICS FOR EXTERNAL USE (EXCEPT PREPARATIONS FOR OPHTHALMIC USE).
Caution—Do not use in the eyes. If the condition for which this preparation is used persists or if a rash or irritation develops, discontinue use and consult physician.

ANTIHISTAMINICS, ORAL. (See also § 130.102(a) (4), (6), and (13) of this chapter.)
Caution—This preparation may cause drowsiness. Do not drive or operate machinery while taking this medication. Do not give to children under 6 years of age or exceed the recommended dosage unless directed by physician.
The reference to drowsiness is not required on preparations for the promotion of sleep or on preparations that are shown not to produce drowsiness.

ANTIPERSPIRANTS.
Do not apply to broken skin. If a rash develops, discontinue use.

ANTIPYRINE.
Warning—Do not exceed recommended dosage. If skin rash appears, discontinue use and consult physician.

ANTISEPTICS FOR EXTERNAL USE. (See also §130.102(a) (18) of this chapter.)
Caution—In case of deep or puncture wounds or serious burns, consult physician. If redness, irritation, swelling, or pain persists or increases or if infection occurs discontinue use and consult physician.
The reference to wounds and burns is not required on preparations intended solely for diaper rash.

ARSENIC PREPARATIONS.
Warning—Frequent or prolonged use may cause serious injury. Do not exceed recommended dosage.

BELLADONNA PREPARATIONS AND PREPARATIONS OF ITS ALKALOIDS (ATROPINE, HYOSCYAMINE, AND SCOPOLAMINE (HYOSCINE)); HYOSCYAMUS, STRAMONIUM, AND RELATED DRUG PREPARATIONS.
Warning—Not to be used by elderly persons or by children under 6 years of age unless directed by physician.
Caution—Do not exceed recommended dosage. Not for frequent or prolonged use. If dryness of the mouth occurs, decrease dosage. Discontinue use if rapid pulse, dizziness, or blurring of vision occurs.
See also Rectal Preparations for additional warnings.
Scopolamine or scopolamine aminoxide preparations for insomnia should include one of the following:
Warning—Not to be used by elderly persons or by children under 12 years of age unless directed by physician; or
Warning—Not to be used by persons having glaucoma or excessive pressure within the eye (conditions that occur most often in the elderly), or by children under 12 years of age, unless directed by physician.
In addition to either of the above statements, the following should be included:
Caution—Do not exceed recommended dosage. Not for frequent or prolonged use. If dryness of the mouth occurs, decrease dosage. Discontinue use if rapid pulse, dizziness, or blurring of vision occurs.
Scopolamine or scopolamine aminoxide preparations for motion sickness should include the following:
Warning—Not to be used by children under 6 years of age unless directed by physician.
Caution—Do not exceed recommended dosage. Discontinue use if rapid pulse, dizziness, or blurring of vision occurs.

BORIC ACID (POWDERED, CRYSTALLINE, OR GRANULAR).
Warning—Do not use as a dusting powder, especially on infants, or take internally. Use only as a solution. Do not apply to badly broken or raw skin, or to large areas of the body.

BROMIDES.
Caution—Use only as directed. Do not give to children or use in the presence of kidney disease. If skin rash appears or if nervous symptoms persist, recur frequently, or are unusual, discontinue use and consult physician.

CARBOLIC ACID (PHENOL) PREPARATIONS (MORE THAN 0.5 PER-CENT) FOR EXTERNAL USE.
Warning—Use according to directions. Do not apply to large areas of the body. If applied to fingers or toes, do not bandage.

CATHARTICS AND LAXATIVES—IRRITANTS AND OTHER PERISTALTIC STIMULANTS.
Warning—Do not use when abdominal pain, nausea, vomiting, or other symptoms of appendicitis are present. Frequent or prolonged use of this preparation may result in dependence on laxatives.
Mercury preparations should have added to the "frequent use" statement, the words "and serious mercury poisoning."
Phenolphthalein preparations should bear, in addition to the general warning, the following statement:
Caution—If skin rash appears, do not use this or any other preparation containing phenolphthalein.
See also Mineral Oil Laxatives.

CHLORATES: MOUTH WASH OR GARGLE.
Avoid swallowing.

COBALT PREPARATIONS. (See also § 3.48 of this chapter.)
Warning—Do not exceed the recommended dosage. Do not administer to children under 12 years of age unless directed by physician. Do not use for more than 2 months unless directed by physician.
This warning is not required on articles containing not more than 0.5 milligram of cobalt as a cobalt salt per dosage unit and which

recommended administration of not more than 0.5 milligram per dose and not more than 2 milligrams per 24-hour period.

"COUGH-DUE-TO-COLD" PREPARATIONS. (See also § 130.102(a) (14) and (20) of this chapter.)
Warning—Persons with a high fever or persistent cough should not use this preparation unless directed by physician.

COUNTERIRRITANTS AND RUBEFACIENTS.
Caution—Do not apply to irritated skin or if excessive irritation develops. Avoid getting into the eyes or on mucous membranes.
If offered for use in arthritis or rheumatism, in juxtaposition therewith, the statement:
Caution—If pain persists for more than 10 days, or redness is present, or in conditions affecting children under 12 years of age consult a physician immediately.
See also "Salicylates" in this section for additional warnings for preparations containing methyl salicylate.

CREOSOTE, CRESOLS, GUAIACOL, AND SIMILAR SUBSTANCES IN PREPARATIONS FOR EXTERNAL USE.
Caution—Do not apply to large areas of the body.

CREOSOTE, CRESOLS, GUAIACOL, AND SIMILAR SUBSTANCES IN DOUCHE PREPARATIONS.
Warning—The use of solutions stronger than those recommended may result in severe local irritation, burns, or serious poisoning. Mix as directed before pouring into douche bag. Do not use more often that twice weekly unless directed by physician.

DIARRHEA PREPARATIONS.
Warning—Do not use for more than 2 days or in the presence of high fever or in infants or children under 3 years of age unless directed by a physician.

DISPENSERS PRESSURIZED BY GASEOUS PROPELLANTS FOR DRUGS FOR EXTERNAL USE. (See also § 130.102(a) (11) and (18) of this chapter.)
Warning—Keep away from eyes or other mucous membranes. Avoid inhaling.
This warning is not necessary for preparations specifically designed for use on mucous membranes.
Where indicated, in order to prevent chilling the tissues, a caution should be included against holding the dispenser too close to the body.
Warning—Contents under pressure. Do not puncture or throw into fire or incinerator. Exposure to high temperature may cause bursting.
If the preparation is flammable, the following additional statement should be included: "WARNING: FLAMMABLE. Keep away from open flame."

DOUCHE PREPARATIONS.
Warning—Do not use more often than twice weekly unless directed by physician.
See also Creosote * * * Douche for additional warning.

DRESSINGS, PROTECTIVE SPRAY-ON TYPE. (See also § 130.102(a) (11) and (18) of this chapter.)
Warning—In case of deep or puncture wounds or serious burns consult physician. If redness, irritation, swelling, or pain persists or increases or if infection occurs consult physician. Keep away from eyes or other mucous membranes. Avoid inhaling.
See also Dispensers Pressurized by Gaseous Propellants * * * for additional warnings to be included for products under pressure.

EPHEDRINE PREPARATIONS (ORAL)
Warning—Do not exceed the recommended dosage. Reduce dosage if nervousness, restlessness, or sleeplessness occurs. Do not use if high blood pressure, heart disease, diabetes, or thyroid disease is present unless directed by physician.

EPINEPHRINE INHALATION 1:100 (NOT FOR INJECTION).
Warning—For inhalation only. Reduce dosage if bronchial irritation, nervousness, restlessness, or sleeplessness occurs. Do not use if high blood pressure, heart disease, diabetes, or thyroid disease is present unless directed by physician. If prompt relief is not obtained consult physician. Do not use epinephrine inhalation if it is brown in color or contains a precipitate.

GENTIAN VIOLET (METHYLROSANILINE CHLORIDE) TABLETS.
Caution—Do not bite or chew tablets before swallowing. If nausea develops, discontinue for 1 or 2 days; then resume treatment with reduced dosage. This preparation should not be used by persons with heart, kidney, or liver disease or intestinal disorders. Abstinence from alcohol during treatment is advisable.

HEXYLRESORCINOL ANTHELMINTICS.
Warning—Do not chew or break in the mouth.

IODINE AND IODIDES (ORAL).
Caution—If a skin rash appears, discontinue use and consult physician.

MERCURY PREPARATIONS FOR EXTERNAL USE.
Warning—Discontinue use if irritation develops. Frequent or prolonged use, or application to large areas may cause serious mercury poisoning.
Ammoniated mercury bleach cream:
Warning—Discontinue use if skin irritation develops. Do not apply to irritated or damaged skin (cuts, bruises, sunburn) or after shaving or using a depilatory. Do not apply to children under 12 years of age.

MINERAL OIL LAXATIVES.   (See also § 3.4 of this chapter.)
Caution—Take only at bedtime. Avoid prolonged use. Do not administer to infants or young children, or in pregnancy unless directed by physician. Administer with caution to bed-ridden or aged persons.

NASAL PREPARATIONS: OIL BASE.
Warning—Do not exceed recommended dosage nor use for prolonged period. Do not administer to infants or children unless directed by physician. Do not use as a spray.

NASAL PREPARATIONS IN PLASTIC SPRAY CONTAINERS.
Avoid overdosage. Follow directions for use carefully.

NASAL PREPARATIONS: VASOCONSTRICTORS (AMPHETAMINE, EPHEDRINE, EPINEPHRINE, METHAMPHETAMINE AND OTHERS OF SIMILAR ACTIVITY). (See also § 130.102(a) (16) of this chapter.)
Caution—Do not exceed recommended dosage. Overdosage may cause nervousness, restlessness, or sleeplessness. Do not use for more than 3 or 4 consecutive days unless directed by physician.

NASAL PREPARATIONS: VASOCONSTRICTORS (PHENYLEPHRINE HYDROCHLORIDE, HYDROXYAMPHETAMINE, PHENYLPROPANOLAMINE, AND OTHERS OF SIMILAR ACTIVITY).
Caution—Do not exceed recommended dosage.

NUX VOMICA AND STRYCHNINE PREPARATIONS.
Warning—Do not exceed the recommended dosage. Keep out of the reach of children.

OPHTHALMIC PREPARATIONS.   (See also § 3.28 of this chapter.)
Warning—If irritation persists or increases, discontinue use and consult physician. Keep container tightly closed.
Solutions should include statement: Do not touch dropper tip to any surface since this may contaminate solution.

PHENYLEPHRINE HYDROCHLORIDE PREPARATIONS, ORAL.
Caution—Individuals with high blood pressure, heart disease, diabetes, or thyroid disease should use only as directed by physician.

PHENYLPROPANOLAMINE HYDROCHLORIDE PREPARATIONS, ORAL.
Caution—Individuals with high blood pressure, heart disease, diabetes, or thyroid disease should use only as directed by physician.

QUININE AND OTHER CINCHONA DERIVATIVES (EXCEPT FOR USE IN MALARIA).
Caution—Discontinue use if ringing in the ears, deafness, skin rash, or visual disturbances occur.

RECTAL PREPARATIONS FOR EXTERNAL USE.   (See also § 130.102(a) (3) of this chapter.)
Warning—In case of rectal bleeding, consult physician promptly. See also Belladona Preparations * * * for additional warnings.

RESINS, OLEORESINS, AND VOLATILE OILS.
Caution—If nausea, vomiting, abdominal discomfort, diarrhea, or skin rash occurs, discontinue use and consult physician.

RESORCINOL (NOT THE MONOACETATE) HAIR PREPARATIONS.
Caution—Excessive use of this preparation may temporarily discolor blond, white, or red hair.

SALICYLATES, INCLUDING ASPIRIN AND SALICYLAMIDE (EXCEPT METHYL SALICYLATE, EFFERVESCENT SALICYLATE PREPARATIONS, AND PREPARATIONS OF PARAAMINOSALICYLIC ACID AND ITS SALTS). (See also §§ 3.43 and 3.509 of this chapter.)
Warning—Keep out of the reach of children; or
Warning—Keep this and all medications out of the reach of children.
The above information should appear on the label.

Caution—For children under 3 years of age consult physician ; or
Caution—For younger children consult your physician.
One of the two statements immediately preceding is required on the label of all aspirin tablets, but such a statement is not required on the labels of other salicylates clearly offered for administration to adults only.
If offered for use in arthritis or rheumatism, in juxtaposition therewith, the statement:
Caution—If pain persists for more than 10 days, or redness is present, or in conditions affecting children under 12 years of age consult a physician immediately.

SALICYLATES: METHYL SALICYLATE (WINTERGREEN OIL).   See also §§ 3.35 and 3.509 of this chapter.
Warning—Do not use otherwise than as directed. Keep out of the reach of children to avoid accidental poisoning.
If the preparation is a counterirritant or rubefacient the statement:
Caution—Discontinue use if excessive irritation of the skin develops. Avoid getting into the eyes or on mucous membranes.
If offered for use in arthritis or rheumatism, in juxtaposition therewith, the statement:
Caution—If pain persists for more than 10 days, or redness is present, or in conditions affecting children under 12 years of age consult a physician immediately.

SILVER.
Caution—Frequent or prolonged use of this preparation may result in permanent discoloration of skin and mucous membranes.

SODIUM PERBORATE MOUTH WASH AND GARGLE AND TOOTHPASTE.
Caution—Discontinue use if irritation or inflammation develops, or increases. Avoid swallowing.

SULFONAMIDE NOSE DROPS.
Caution—Do not use if a known allergy to sulfonamide drugs exists.

SULFUR PREPARATION FOR EXTERNAL USE.
Caution—If undue skin irritation develops or increases, discontinue use and consult physician.

THROAT PREPARATIONS FOR TEMPORARY RELIEF OF MINOR SORE THROAT: LOZENGES, TROCHES, WASHES, GARGLES, ETC.   (See also § 3.510 of this chapter.)
Warning—Severe or persistent sore throat or sore throat accompanied by high fever, headache, nausea, and vomiting may be serious. Consult physician promptly. Do not administer to children under 3 years of age unless directed by physician.

TOOTHACHE PREPARATIONS.
For temporary use only until a dentist can be consulted.

ZINC STEARATE DUSTING POWDERS.
Warning—Keep out of the reach of infants and children; avoid inhaling.

§ 131.16   Drugs for human use; warning and caution statements required by regulations.

ACETAMINOPHEN (*N*-ACETYL-*p*-AMINOPHENOL).   (See § 130.12(a) (1) of this chapter.)
Warning—Do not give to children under 3 years of age or use for more than 10 days unless directed by a physician.
If offered for use in arthritis, or rheumatism, in juxtaposition therewith, the statement:
Caution—If pain persists for more than 10 days, or redness is present, or in condition affecting children under 12 years of age consult a physician immediately.

ALCOHOL RUBBING COMPOUND.   (See 26 CFR 182.855(a) (5); The National Formulary, Eleventh Edition 1960; and section 502(g) of the act.)
Warning—For external use only. If taken internally serious gastric disturbances will result.

ANTIBIOTIC-CONTAINING DRUGS FOR EXTERNAL USE FOR PREVENTION OF INFECTION.
Caution—If redness, irritation, swelling, or pain persists or increases or if infection occurs, discontinue use and consult physician. Do not use in the eyes.

ANTIHISTAMINICS, ORAL (PHENYLTOLOXAMINE DIHYDROGEN CITRATE, MECLIZINE HYDROCHLORIDE, AND DOXYLAMINE SUCCINATE PREPARATIONS).   (See § 130.102(a) (4), (6), and (13) of this chapter.)
Caution—This preparation may cause drowsiness. Do not drive or operate machinery while taking this medication. Do not give to children under 6 years of age or exceed the recommended dosage unless directed by physician.

If offered for symptoms of colds, the statement:
Caution—If relief does not occur within 3 days, discontinue use and consult physician.

BACITRACIN-CONTAINING OINTMENTS. (See §§ 146e.402, 146e.407, 146e.411 of this chapter.)
For use only in the prevention of infection in minor cuts and abrasions.
Use of the drug should be discontinued and a physician consulted if signs of infection or irritation appear.

BACITRACIN (ZINC BACITRACIN)-POLYMYXIN OINTMENT; BACITRACIN-POLYMYXIN-NEOMYCIN OINTMENT. (See §§ 146e.409 and 146e.422 of this chapter.)
For use only in the prevention of infection in minor cuts and abrasions. Use of the drug should be discontinued and a physician consulted if signs of infection or irritation appear.
If it is in liquid form, also the statement "Not for injection."

CARBETAPENTANE CITRATE PREPARATIONS. (See Cough-Due-to-Cold Preparations.)

"COUGH-DUE-TO-COLD" PREPARATIONS (DEXTROMETHORPHAN HYDROBROMIDE AND CARBETAPENTANE CITRATE). (See § 130.102(a) (14) and (20) of this chapter.)
Warning—Keep out of the reach of children. Do not administer to children under 2 years of age unless directed by physician. Persistent cough may indicate the presence of a serious condition. Persons with a high fever or persistent cough should not use this preparation unless directed by physician.

DEXTROMETHORPHAN HYDROBROMIDE PREPARATIONS. (See Cough-Due-to-Cold Preparations.)

DIAMTHAZOLE DIHYDROCHLORIDE FOR EXTERNAL USE. (See § 130.102(a) (7) of this chapter.)
Warning—Do not apply to children under 6 years of age because serious reactions may occur. Do not apply to children 6 to 12 years of age unless directed by physician. Do not use on mucous membranes. Discontinue use and consult physician if irritation develops or relief is not obtained. Keep out of the reach of children.

DICYCLOMINE HYDROCHLORIDE WITH AN ANTACID (See § 130.102(a) (8) of this chapter.)
Warning—Do not exceed the recommended dosage. Do not administer to children under 12 years of age or use for a prolonged period unless directed by physician, since persistent or recurring symptoms may indicate a serious disease requiring medical attention.

DIPHEMANIL METHYLSULFATE FOR EXTERNAL USE. (See § 130.102(a) (22) of this chapter.)
Caution—If redness, irritation, swelling, or pain persists or increases, discontinue use and consult physician.

DYCLONINE HYDROCHLORIDE. (See § 130.102(a) (23) of this chapter.)
Caution—Do not use in the eyes. Not for prolonged use. Do not apply to large areas of the body. If redness, irritation, swelling, or pain persists or increases, discontinue use unless directed by physician. Do not use, but consult physician for deep or puncture wounds or serious burns. Do not use in case of rectal bleeding, as this may indicate serious disease.

HEXADENOL. (See § 130.102(a) (11) of this chapter.)
Caution—Do not use for treatment of serious burns or skin conditions or for conditions which persist for prolonged periods. In such cases, consult your physician. Do not spray in vicinity of eyes, mouth, nose, or ears. Do not store above 120° F.

INSULIN. (See § 164.4(c) of this chapter.)
Insulin (40, 80, or 100 U.S.P. units per milliter):
Caution—Do not remove stopper. Not for intravenous nor intramuscular use. Do not use after expiration date shown on outside wrapper or container. Do not use if drug has become viscous or if its color has become other than water clear.
In addition to the above warnings, the following statements should be included in the labeling: "Keep in a cold place, avoid freezing. Failure to follow directions for use may lead to infection." Protamine zinc insulin, isophane insulin, lente insulin, semilente insulin, or ultralente insulin:
Caution—Do not remove stopper. Not for intravenous nor intramuscular use. Do not use after expiration date shown on outside wrapper or container. Do not substitute for any other insulin-containing drug unless directed by physician. Do not use when precipitate has become lumped or granular in appearance or has formed a deposit of solid particles on the wall of the container.
In addition to the above warnings for protamine zinc insulin * * *, the following statements should be included in the labeling of these

preparations: "Keep in a cold place, avoid freezing"; "Shake carefully" or "Shake well before using" or "Shake well" or "Shake carefully to suspended all particles"; "Failure to follow directions for use may lead to infection."
Globin zinc insulin:
Caution—Do not remove stopper. Not for intravenous nor intramuscular use. Do not use after expiration date shown on outside wrapper or container. Do not use if any turbidity or precipitate has developed in the solution. Do not substitute for any other insulin-containing drug unless directed by physician.
In addition to the above warnings for globin zinc insulin, the following statements should be included in the labeling: "Keep in a cold place, avoid freezing. Failure to follow directions for use may lead to infection."

ISOAMYLHYDROCUPREINE AND ZOLAMINE HYDROCHLORIDE RECTAL PREPARATIONS FOR EXTERNAL USE. (See § 130.102(a) (3) of this chapter.)
Warning—Do not use this preparation in case of rectal bleeding, as this may indicate serious disease.

NEOMYCIN SULFATE WITH A VASOCONSTRICTOR, IN NASAL PREPARATIONS (SPRAY OR DROPS). (See § 130.102 (a) (9) of this chapter.)
Caution—Do not exceed recommended dosage. Do not administer to children under 3 years of age unless directed by physician.

OXYTETRACYCLINE AND POLYMYXIN B SULFATE. (See Antibiotic-Containing Drugs for External Use * * *.)

PRAMOXINE HYDROCHLORIDE FOR EXTERNAL USE. (See § 130.102(a) (19) of this chapter.)
Caution—Do not use in the eyes or nose. Not for prolonged use. Do not apply to large areas of the body. If redness, irritation, swelling, or pain persists or increases, discontinue use unless directed by a physician.

SODIUM FLUORIDE DENTIFRICE POWDER. (See § 130.102(a) (10) of this chapter.)
Caution—Children under 6 years of age should not use this drug.

SODIUM GENTISATE. (See §§ 3.43, 3.509, 130.102(a) (2) of this chapter.)
Warning—Do not give to children under 6 years of age or use for prolonged period unless directed by physician.
Warning—Keep this and all medications out of the reach of children, or
Warning—Keep out of the reach of children.
If offered for use in arthritis or rheumatism, in juxtaposition therewith, the statement:
Caution—If pain persists for more than 10 days, or redness is present, or in conditions affecting children under 12 years of age, consult a physician immediately.

SODIUM MONOFLUOROPHOSPHATE DENTIFRICE SOLUTION. (See § 130.102(a) (15) of this chapter.)
Caution—Children under 6 years of age should not use this drug.

TUAMINOHEPTANE SULFATE NASAL PREPARATIONS. (See § 130.102(a) (16) of this chapter.)
Caution—Do not exceed recommended dosage. Overdosage may cause nervousness, restlessness, or sleeplessness. Individuals with high blood pressure, heart disease, diabetes, or thyroid disease should use only as directed by physician. Do not use for more than 3 or 4 consecutive days unless directed by physician.

VIBESATE PREPARATIONS. (See § 130.102(a) (18) of this chapter.)
Caution—Do not use but consult physician for deep or puncture wounds or serious burns. If redness, irritation, swelling, or pain persists or increases, discontinue use and consult physician.
Warning—Contents under pressure. Do not puncture or throw into fire or incinerator. Exposure to high temperatures may cause bursting.

WARNING—FLAMMABLE. Keep away from open flame.

§ 131.17 **Drugs for human use; warning and caution statements specifically required by law.**

PREPARATIONS CONTAINING HABIT-FORMING DERIVATIVES OF SUBSTANCES NAMED IN SECTION 502(d) OF THE ACT. (See §§ 1.104, 1.108, and 165.1 of this chapter and 26 U.S.C. 3220 and 3238(b), and regulations thereunder.)
The statement "*Warning*—May be habit forming" is required to appear on the label of all drugs containing derivatives designated in § 165.1 of this chapter as habit forming, including exempt narcotic preparations described in § 151.2 of Title 26 of the Code of Federal Regulations (26 CFR 151.2) and preparations containing one or

more derivatives of barbituric acid, unless such drug is not suitable for internal use and is distributed and sold exclusively for such external use as involves no possibility of habit formation.

Subpart C—Drugs for Veterinary Use

§ 131.20 Drugs for veterinary use; recommended warning and caution statements.

ACETYLAMINONITROTHIAZOLE FOR POULTRY.
Warning—Discontinue use at least 1 week before slaughtering birds for human consumption to permit elimination of the drug from edible tissues.

AMINONITROTHIAZOLE   (2-AMINO-5-NITROTHIAZOLE) FOR POULTRY.
Warning—Discontinue use at least 1 week before slaughtering birds for human consumption to permit elimination of the drug from edible tissues.

ANESTHETICS FOR EXTERNAL USE (LOCAL ANESTHETICS).
Caution—Not for prolonged use. If the condition for which this preparation is used persists or if a rash or irritation develops, discontinue use and consult veterinarian.

ANTHELMINTICS.
Caution—Consult veterinarian before using in severely debilitated animals.

ANTHELMINTICS CONTAINING CADMIUM OXIDE AND CADMIUM ANTHRANILATE.
Caution—Consult veterinarian before using in severely debilitated animals.
Warning—Treated hogs must not be slaughtered for human consumption for at least 30 days following treatment to permit elimination of cadmium residues from edible tissues.

ANTHELMINTICS: NICOTINE.
Caution—Consult veterinarian before using in severely debilitated animals.

ANTHELMINTICS: PHENOTHIAZINE.
Warning—Do not treat lactating dairy animals.
Caution—Consult veterinarian before using in severely debilitated animals. Individual animals are occasionally sensitive to phenothiazine.

ANTIBIOTICS FOR EXTERNAL USE. (See also §§ 3.25 and 146.1(k) of this chapter.)
Warning—Avoid adulteration of milk with this drug applied to udders or teats of dairy animals.
Caution—If redness, irritation, or swelling persists or increases, discontinue use and consult veterinarian.

ANTIBIOTICS (INTRAMAMMARY). (See also § 146.1(k) of this chapter.)
Warning—Milk taken from dairy animals within — hours after the latest treatment for mastitis must not be used for human consumption.
The blank is filled in with the number 72, unless the person has submitted to the Commissioner information adequate to prove that milk from dairy animals treated with the drug as prepared by him contains no antibiotics after a time period that is shorter than 72 hours after the latest treatment. In such cases, the blank shall be filled in with the number 60, 48, 36, or 24, as authorized by the Commissioner.
This statement should appear on the label of the immediate container, if it is intended for use in the prevention or treatment of mastitis in dairy animals by intramammary infusion.

ANTIHISTAMINICS FOR EXTERNAL USE.
Caution—If the condition for which this preparation is used persists or if a rash or irritation develops, discontinue use and consult veterinarian.

ANTISEPTICS FOR EXTERNAL USE.
Caution—In case of deep or puncture wounds or serious burns consult veterinarian. If redness, irritation or swelling persists or increases, discontinue use and consult veterinarian.

ARSENICALS (ORGANIC, FOR POULTRY AND SWINE). (See also § 146.26(b) of this chapter.)
Warning—Do not administer to laying hens. Discontinue use at least 5 days before slaughtering animals for human consumption to permit elimination of the drug from edible tissues.
The above warning concerning laying hens is not required on arsenic preparations that have been shown to leave no residue in eggs.

CARBOLIC ACID (PHENOL) PREPARATIONS (MORE THAN 0.5 PER-CENT) FOR EXTERNAL USE.
Caution—Use only as directed. Avoid contact with the eyes and mucous membranes. Do not apply to large areas of the body. Do not use on cats.

CORTISONE, HYDROCORTISONE, PREDNISOLONE, AND PREDNISONE PREPARATIONS FOR EXTERNAL USE.
Caution—Do not use where infection (pus) is present, since the drug may allow infection to spread. If redness, irritation, or swelling persists or increases, discontinue use and consult veterinarian.

COUNTERIRRITANTS AND RUBEFACIENTS.
Caution—Do not apply to irritated skin or if excessive irritation develops. Avoid getting into eyes or on mucous membranes.

CREOSOTE, CRESOLS, GUAIACOL, AND SIMILAR SUBSTANCES IN PREPARATIONS FOR EXTERNAL USE.
Caution—Use only as directed. Avoid contact with eyes and mucous membranes. Do not apply to large areas of the body. Not recommended for use on cats.

DIARRHEA PREPARATIONS.
Caution—If symptoms persist after using this preparation for 2 or 3 days, consult veterinarian.

DIENESTROL DIACETATE FOR POULTRY.
Warning—Discontinue use at least 24 hours before slaughtering birds for human consumption to permit elimination of the drug from edible tissues.

DIETHYLSTILBESTROL IN ANIMAL FEEDS.
Warning—Discontinue use at least 48 hours before slaughtering animals for human consumption to permit elimination of the drug from edible tissues.

DISPENSERS PRESSURIZED BY GASEOUS PROPELLANT FOR DRUGS FOR EXTERNAL USE.
Caution—Keep away from eyes or other mucous membranes. Avoid inhaling.
This warning is not necessary for preparations especially designed for use on mucous membranes.
Warning—Contents under pressure. Do not puncture or throw into fire or incinerator. Exposure to high temperature may cause bursting.
If the preparation is flammable, the following additional statement should be included:
WARNING—FLAMMABLE. Keep away from open flame.

DRESSINGS, PROTECTIVE SPRAY-ON TYPE.
Caution—In case of deep or puncture wounds or serious burns or if redness, irritation, or swelling persists or increases, consult veterinarian.
Keep away from eyes or other mucous membranes. Avoid inhaling.
See also Dispensers Pressurized by Gaseous Propellant * * * for additional warnings to be included for products under pressure.

ESTROGEN PELLETS IN CATTLE AND SHEEP.
Warning—Implant pellets in the _____ (name of the anatomical area) only. Any other location may result in violation of Federal law. Do not attempt salvage of implanted site for human or animal food.

ESTROGEN PELLETS IN POULTRY.
Warning—Implant pellets within ½ inch of the skull. Any other location may result in violation of Federal law. Do not attempt salvage of implanted site for human or animal food.

GLYCARBILAMIDE FOR POULTRY.
Warning—Do not feed to laying hens in production. Discontinue use at least 4 days before slaughtering birds for human consumption to permit elimination of the drug from edible tissues.

NICARBAZIN FOR POULTRY.
Warning—Do not feed to laying hens in production. Discontinue use at least 4 days before slaughtering birds for human consumption to permit elimination of the drug from edible tissues.

NITHIAZIDE FOR POULTRY.
Warning—Do not feed to laying hens in production. Discontinue use at least 24 hours before slaughtering birds for human consumption to permit elimination of the drug from edible tissues.

OPHTHALMIC PREPARATIONS.
Caution—If condition persists or increases discontinue use and consult veterinarian. Keep container tightly closed.
Solutions should also include the following statement: "Do not touch applicator tip to any surface, since this may contaminate solution."

SALMONELLOSIS TREATMENTS FOR POULTRY.

Important—Poultry that have survived salmonella outbreaks should not be kept for laying-house replacements or breeders, unless tests show that they are not carriers.

STREPTOMYCIN AND DIHYDROSTREPTOMYCIN (INTRAMUSCULAR) IN POULTRY.

Caution— Do not exceed recommended dosage.

SULFONAMIDE PREPARATIONS (SYSTEMIC).

Caution—If symptoms persist after using this preparation for 2 or 3 days consult veterinarian.

SULFONAMIDES FOR EXTERNAL USE.

Caution—If redness, irritation, or swelling persists or increases, discontinue use and consult veterinarian.

If the preparation has not been sterilized, the following statement should also be used:

Caution—This preparation has not been sterilized. Do not use in body cavities or deep wounds.

§ 131.21   Drugs for veterinary use; warning and caution statements required by regulations.

ANIMAL FEED CONTAINING PENICILLIN, STREPTO- MYCIN, DIHYDROSTREPTOMYCIN, CHLORTETRACY- CLINE, TETRACYCLINE, CHLORAMPHENICOL, OR BACITRACIN, WITH OTHER DRUGS. (See § 146.26 of this chapter.)

The following warnings are required when animal feeds containing any of the above-named antibiotics also contain the following drugs:

Arsanilic acid, sodium arsanilate, or 3-nitro-4-hydroxyphenol arsonic acid (3-nitro-4-hydroxyphenylarsonic acid) for poultry and swine. (See § 146.26(a) and (b) of this chapter.)

Warning—Do not administer to laying hens. Discontinue use 5 days before the treated animals are slaughtered for human consumption.

Chlortetracycline for leptospirosis of swine. (See § 146.26(b) (41) of this chapter.)

The following warning is required on preparations containing, per ton of feed, 400 grams of chlortetracycline:

Warning—Discontinue use 10 days before the treated animals are slaughtered for human consumption.

Dienestrol diacetate for poultry. (See § 146.26(b) of this chapter.)

Warning—Do not use in laying hens. Discontinue use 24 hours before the treated birds are slaughtered for human consumption.

Diethylstilbestrol for sheep. (See § 146.26(b) of this chapter.)

Warning—Discontinue use 48 hours before the treated animals are slaughtered for human consumption.

3,5-Dinitrobenzamide for poultry. (See § 146.26(b) of this chapter.)

Warning—Do not feed to laying hens. Discontinue use 48 hours before the treated animals are slaughtered for human consumption.

Glycarbylamide (4,5-imidazole-dicarboxamide) for chickens. (See § 146.26(b) of this chapter.)

Warning—Do not feed to laying hens. Discontinue use 4 days before the treated chickens are slaughtered for human consumption.

Hygromycin B for swine. (See § 146.26(b) of this chapter.)

Warning—Discontinue use 48 hours before the treated swine are slaughtered for human consumption.

Nithiazide (1-ethyl-3-(5-nitro-2-thiazolyl) urea) for poultry. (See § 146.26(b) of this chapter.)

Warning—Do not feed to laying hens. Discontinue use 24 hours before treated birds are slaughtered for human consumption.

Nystatin for turkeys. (See § 146.26(b) of this chapter.)

Warning—If used in laying hens, eggs are to be used for hatching purposes only.

ANTIBIOTIC-CONTAINING PREPARATIONS FOR VET- ERINARY USE. (See parts 146a, 146b, 146c, 146d, and 146e of this chapter.)

All drugs containing penicillin, streptomycin, dihydrostrepto- mycin, chlortetracycline, tetracycline, chloramphenicol, or baci- tracin or any of their derivatives, labeled solely for veterinary use and bearing directions for use by the laity, are required to bear the label statement "For veterinary use only."

ANTIBIOTICS (INTRAMAMMARY). (See § 146.1(k) of this chapter.)

"*Warning*—Milk taken from dairy animals within _____ hours after the latest treatment for mastitis must not be used for human consumption," the blank being filled in with the number 72 unless the person who requests certification has submitted to the Com- missioner information adequate to prove that milk from dairy animals treated with the drug as prepared by him contains no anti- biotics after a time period that is shorter than 72 hours after the latest treatment. In such cases, the blank shall be filled in with the number 60, 48, 36, or 24, as authorized by the Commissioner. This statement shall appear on the label of the immediate container.

BACITRACIN-CONTAINING PREPARATIONS FOR VET- ERINARY USE ONLY. (See Part 146c of this chapter.)

All bacitracin-containing drugs labeled solely for veterinary use by the laity are required to bear the label statement "For veterinary use only."

BACITRACIN-CONTAINING OINTMENTS. (See Part 146e of this chapter.)

All bacitracin-containing ointments are required to bear the label statements:

For use only in the prevention of infection in minor cuts and abrasions. Use of the drug should be discontinued and a veterinarian consulted if signs of infection or irritation appear.

BACITRACIN-CONTAINING PREPARATIONS WITH VASOCONSTRICTOR; BACITRACIN OPHTHALMIC. (See §§ 146e.405, 146e.408, 146e.414, 146e.424 of this chapter.)

Warning—Not for injection.

BACITRACIN- (OR ZINC BACITRACIN-) NEOMYCIN- POLYMYXIN POWDER TOPICAL. (See § 146e.430 of this chapter.)

This drug is required to bear the label statement: "Not sterile."

BACITRACIN- (OR ZINC BACITRACIN-) POLYMYXIN OINTMENT; BACITRACIN-POLYMYXIN-NEOMYCIN OINTMENT. (See §§ 146e.409 and 146e.422 of this chapter.)

These drugs are required to bear the label statements: "For use only in the prevention of infection in minor cuts and abrasions. Use of the drug should be discontinued and a veterinarian consulted if signs of infection or irritation appear."

If they are in liquid form they also bear the statement: "Not for injection."

BACITRACIN OR FEED GRADE BACITRACIN POWDER ORAL VETERINARY; BACITRACIN METHYLENE DI- SALICYLATE AND STREPTOMYCIN SULFATE CAP- SULES, POWDER, OR TABLETS ORAL VETERINARY. (See §§ 146e.417, 146e.425, 146e.426, 146e.427, 146e.428 of this chapter.)

These drugs are required to bear the label statement: "For oral veterinary use only."

CHLORAMPHENICOL-CONTAINING PREPARATIONS FOR VETERINARY USE ONLY. (See Part 146d of this chapter.)

All chloramphenicol-containing drugs labeled solely for veterinary use and bearing directions for use by the laity are required to bear the label statement "For veterinary use only."

CHLORAMPHENICOL OPHTHALMIC. (See § 146d.304 of this chapter.)

Warning—Not for injection.

CHLORAMPHENICOL OTIC; CHLORAMPHENICOL TOPICAL. (See § 146d.308 of this chapter.)

Warning—For external use only.

CHLORAMPHENICOL SOLUTION; CHLORAMPHENI- COL FOR AQUEOUS INJECTION. (See § 146d.307 of this chapter.)

The label of this drug is required to bear the statement "For intra- muscular use only."

CHLORTETRACYCLINE OR TETRACYCLINE-CON- TAINING PREPARATIONS FOR VETERINARY USE ONLY. (See Part 146c of this chapter.)

All drugs containing chlortetracycline or tetracycline or their derivatives, labeled solely for veterinary use and bearing direc- tions for use by the laity, are required to bear the label statement "For veterinary use only."

CHLORTETRACYCLINE- OR TETRACYCLINE-CON- TAINING PREPARATIONS FOR OPHTHALMIC, OTIC, OR ORAL USE; CHLORTETRACYCLINE- OR TETRA- CYCLINE-CONTAINING PREPARATIONS WITH VASO- CONSTRICTOR. (See §§ 146c.206, 146c.208, 146c.215, 146c.-217, 146c.226, and 146c.240 of this chapter.)

Warning—Not for injection.

CHLORTETRACYCLINE GAUZE PACKING; CHLOR- TETRACYCLINE DRESSING. (See §§ 146c.213 and 146c.214 of this chapter.)

These drugs are required to bear the label statement "Sterility cannot be guaranteed if package shows evidence of damage or has been previously opened."

CHLORTETRACYCLINE ORAL VETERINARY (CRUDE); CHLORTETRACYCLINE SEED. (See §§ 146c.219 and 146c.241 of this chapter.)

These drugs are required to bear the label statement "For oral veterinary use only."

TETRACYCLINE HYDROCHLORIDE FOR INTRAMUSCULAR USE. (See § 146c.221 of this chapter.)

This drug is required to bear the label statement "For intramuscular use only."

PENICILLIN-CONTAINING PREPARATIONS FOR VETERINARY USE ONLY. (See Part 146a of this chapter.)

All penicillin-containing drugs labeled solely for veterinary use and bearing directions for use by the laity are required to bear the label statement "For veterinary use only."

BUFFERED CRYSTALLINE PENICILLIN. (See § 146a.37 of this chapter.)

If represented for use as a treatment for mastitis, the statement: "Important—Milk from treated segments of udders should be discarded or used for purposes other than human consumption for at least 72 hours after the last treatment."

BUFFERED PENICILLIN POWDER, PENICILLIN POWDER WITH BUFFERED AQUEOUS DILUENT; DIBENZYLAMINE PENICILLIN AND POTASSIUM PENICILLIN POWDER, BUFFERED; PENICILLIN POWDER, BUFFERED; PENICILLIN WITH VASOCONSTRICTOR. (See §§ 146a.32, 146a.51, and 146a.95 of this chapter.)

Warning—Not for injection.

CAPSULES PENICILLIN-TETRACYCLINE PHOSPHATE COMPLEX-NOVOBIOCIN–NYSTATIN VETERINARY. (See § 146a.21 of this chapter.)

This drug is required to bear the label statement, "For oral veterinary use only in the treatment of susceptible bacterial infections in dogs and cats."

CRYSTALLINE PENICILLIN-STREPTOMYCIN- (OR DIHYDROSTREPTOMYCIN-) POLYMYXIN-OXYTETRACYCLINE-CARBOMYCIN POWDER VETERINARY. (See § 146a.112 of this chapter.)

These drugs are required to bear the label statement "For udder instillations of cattle only."

EPHEDRINE PENICILLIN TABLETS. (See § 146a.49 of this chapter.)

Warning—Not for injection or oral use.

PENICILLIN-CONTAINING PREPARATIONS FOR INTRAMUSCULAR USE ONLY. (See §§ 146a.25, 146a.41, 146a.43, 146a.47, 146a.50, 146a.58, 146a.65, 146a.66, 146a.67, 146a.75, 146a.77, 146a.78, 146a.80, 146a.84, 146a.85, 146a.86, 146a.90, 146a.91, 146a.110 of this chapter.)

All these preparations are required to bear the label statement "For intramuscular use only."

PENICILLIN-CONTAINING OINTMENTS. (See Part 146a of this chapter.)

If these preparations are labeled solely for udder instillations of cattle and are packaged in glass containers, they are required to bear the label statements: "Not for injection. For udder instillations of cattle only."

PENICILLIN FOR SURFACE APPLICATION. (See § 146a.33 of this chapter.)

If the drug is not sterile, the statements: "Not sterile—Not for injection—Not to be used in deep wounds or body cavities."

PENICILLIN-NEOMYCIN OINTMENT. (See § 146a.62 of this chapter.)

This drug is required to bear the label statement "For udder instillation of cattle only."

PROCAINE PENICILLIN AND STREPTOMYCIN (OR DIHYDROSTREPTOMYCIN) IN OIL; DIBENZYLAMINE PENICILLIN AND STREPTOMYCIN (OR DIHYDROSTREPTOMYCIN) IN OIL; PROCAINE PENICILLIN-STREPTOMYCIN- (OR DIHYDROSTREPTOMYCIN-) POLYMYXIN IN OIL (OR OINTMENT). (See § 146a.57, 146a.97, and 146a.108 of this chapter.)

These drugs are required to bear the label statements: "For udder instillations of cattle only" or "For subcutaneous injection in fowl only. Inject in the neck immediately behind the head."

PROCAINE PENICILLIN IN OIL; PROCAINE PENICILLIN AND STREPTOMYCIN (OR DIHYDROSTREPTOMYCIN) IN OIL; PENICILLIN-STREPTOMYCIN- (OR DIHYDRO-STREPTOMYCIN-) NEOMYCIN IN OIL; BENZATHINE PENICILLIN G IN OIL; BENZATHINE PENICILLIN G-PROCAINE PENICILLIN G-STREPTOMYCIN (OR DIHYDRO-STREPTOMYCIN) IN OIL. (See §§ 146a.45, 146a.52, 146a.57, 146a.100, 146a.101, 146a.102 of this chapter.)

These drugs are required to bear the label statements:
"For udder instillations of cattle only" (if intended for such use); or "For subcutaneous injection in fowl only. Inject in the neck immediately behind the head" (if packaged and labeled solely for subcutaneous injection in fowl).

STREPTOMYCIN- AND DIHYDROSTREPTOMYCIN-CONTAINING PREPARATIONS FOR VETERINARY USE ONLY. (See Part 146b of this chapter.)

All streptomycin- or dihydrostreptomycin-containing drugs or their derivatives labeled solely for veterinary use and bearing directions for use by the laity are required to bear the label statement "For veterinary use only."

STREPTOMYCIN- AND DIHYDROSTREPTOMYCIN-CONTAINING PREPARATIONS FOR ORAL, VETERINARY USE ONLY. (See §§ 146b.115, 146b.119, and 146b.129 of this chapter.)

These drugs are required to bear the label statement "For oral veterinary use only."

STREPTOMYCIN (OR DIHYDROSTREPTOMYCIN) FOR INHALATION THERAPY; STREPTOMYCIN-DIHYDRO-STREPTOMYCIN FOR INHALATION THERAPY. (See §§ 146b.112 and 146b.125 of this chapter.)

Warning—Not for injection. For use only in the prevention or treatment of chronic respiratory disease (air-sac infection) in chickens.

STREPTOMYCIN FOR TOPICAL USE. (See § 146b.105 of this chapter.)

Caution—Not for intravenous or systemic medication.

STREPTOMYCIN- (OR DIHYDROSTREPTOMYCIN) PENICILLIN-SULFONAMIDE WITH KAOLIN AND PECTIN. (See § 146b.118 of this chapter.)

Warning—Not for injection.

STREPTOMYCIN (OR DIHYDROSTREPTOMYCIN) AND PARA-AMINOBENZOIC ACID POWDER FOR INHALATION THERAPY. (See § 146b.130 of this chapter.)

Warning—Not for injection.
Caution—Discontinue use 24 hours before birds are slaughtered for human consumption.

Subpart D-Devices

§ 131.25 Devices; recommended warning and caution statements.

INFRARED GENERATORS (INCLUDING HEATING PADS).

Warning—Use carefully. May cause serious burns. Do not use over insensitive skin areas or in the presence of poor circulation. The unattended use of infrared heat by children or incapacitated persons may be dangerous.

MECHANICAL MASSAGERS AND VIBRATORS.

Warning—This device should not be used over swollen or inflamed areas or skin eruptions. Do not use in unexplained calf pain. Consult physician.

STEAM OR TURKISH BATH.

Warning—Elderly persons or those suffering from heart disease or high blood pressure should not use this device unless directed by physician.

ULTRAVIOLET GENERATORS.

Warning—Wear protective goggles during use to avoid eye injury. Serious burns may be caused by exposure in excess of recommended dosage. Do not use over skin eruptions unless directed by physician.

DISPENSERS PRESSURIZED BY GASEOUS PROPELLANTS FOR DRUGS FOR EXTERNAL USE.

Warning—Contents under pressure. Do not puncture or throw into fire or incinerator. Exposure to high temperature may cause bursting.

If the preparation is flammable, the following additional statement should be included:
WARNING—FLAMMABLE. Keep away from open flame.

Where indicated, in order to prevent chilling the tissues, a caution should be included against holding the dispenser too close to the body.

Economics of health care—pharmaceutical economics—the community pharmacy—pharmacy management: planning, administration, and operation—trends

This chapter was prepared by

James W. Richards, MBA, *Associate Professor of Pharmacy Administration, College of Pharmacy, University of Michigan, Ann Arbor, Mich. 48104*

The economic impact of the health care industry on our society is difficult to evaluate. It is accepted that advances made by the industry during the past few decades have reduced morbidity and mortality rates which, in turn, have increased productivity and added to the gross national product. At the same time, the cost of health care is rising at a faster rate than is the consumer price index, and this cost continues to represent an increasing share of the gross national product.

Economics of Health Care

Total US expenditures for health services, facilities, products, administration, and research reached $45.4 billion in 1966.[1] The total expenditures represented about 6% of the gross national product, at a per capita cost of $231. A breakdown of national health expenditures for a recent 5-year period is given in Table I.

Health expenditures rose 173% between 1950 and 1966, from a per capita expenditure of $84 to the $231 figure. Total expenditures are influenced by a variety of factors, including the following:

Population increases
Rising cost of services
Increased utilization of facilities and services
Increased governmental involvement in health care
Increased quality of care from new techniques, equipment, and drugs

However, even when adjusted for increased population and higher price levels, the 1966 expenditures represent an increase of 57% over 1950 in terms of 1966 constant dollars. Since 1963, expenditures have shown an average annual increase of 6% in constant dollars.

Further analysis of national health expenditures reveals that in 1966 a noticeable upward shift occurred in the portion of total health expenditures paid for with public funds. Medicare accounted for most of the increased governmental spending. However, state Medicaid and Office of Economic Opportunities health programs also contributed to the $12.9 billion public expenditure for health care.

The magnitude of health care expenditures in the US and the growing governmental involvement as a third-party payer of health care costs are evidence of our society's commitment to providing the best care possible for all citizens. Those involved in the delivery of health care share society's commitment and, therefore, must be concerned with the economics of the delivery system.

The pharmaceutical segment of the health care industry entails the third largest type of expenditure. In 1966 $5.2 billion were spent for drugs and drug sundries in the US. The 1966 expenditure for drugs and pharmaceutical services represented 11.5% of the nation's health bill. The health expenditures of private consumers for drugs represented almost 17% of out-of-pocket health payments in 1966.

Through 1966 a relatively small share of total drug costs was paid by third-party payers, such as health insurance carriers and governmental programs. How-

Table I—National Health Expenditures by Type of Expenditure: 1962–1966 (In Millions)[a]

	1966	1965	1964	1963	1962
Hospital care	$15,429	$13,807	$12,621	$11,642	$10,598
Physicians' services	9,392	8,745	8,065	6,891	6,498
Dentists' services	3,015	2,808	2,648	2,277	2,234
Other professional services	986	960	940	921	902
Drugs and drug sundries	5,235	4,813	4,446	4,235	4,095
Eyeglasses and appliances	1,594	1,223	1,072	952	908
Nursing home care	1,502	1,324	1,214	891	695
Expenses for prepayment and administration	1,629	1,298	1,176	1,097	1,088
Government public health activities	810	696	608	538	503
Other health services	2,242	1,837	1,673	1,545	1,445
Research and medical facilities construction	3,587	3,382	3,086	2,640	2,438
Total	$45,421	$40,893	$37,544	$33,629	$31,404

ever, the expansion of Title XIX Medicaid programs in a majority of the states and the prepayment program for drugs which was negotiated for the nation's automobile workers strongly suggest that third-party payment for drugs will increase substantially.

In view of the level of expenditures for drugs and pharmaceutical services and of the trend of health care costs, it is apparent that those involved in the delivery of pharmaceutical services must be aware of their responsibility to provide high-quality services in the most economical way. Although some experts look on third-party payment as a mechanism for solving the high cost of health care, including the drug-cost segment, it should be understood that third-party payment does not reduce the cost. It simply spreads it over a larger population.

Actually, third-party payment increases the total cost of health care; additional administrative costs and increased utilization of services are inherent in third-party payment programs. It follows that third-party payers, whether governmental or private, have an obligation to their constituents to ensure the delivery of quality services at reasonable prices. In this regard health professionals will find their services under scrutiny by a sophisticated group of agencies representing a large portion of the general public.

In the past the economics of health care was given little attention by the providers of health services. It was assumed that the primary obligation of the provider was to ensure the physical well being of the patient, without regard to cost. It is now apparent that it does little good to develop a level of health care which is unsurpassed in the world if a sizable segment of the population cannot afford to pay for it.

The obligation of health professionals to consider the economic dimensions of health care is now recognized. In recent years the American Medical Association has sponsored a series of conferences on the socioeconomics of health care. The American Pharmaceutical Association, through its Committee on Social and Economic Relations, has called upon the profession of pharmacy to concern itself not only with the level of pharmaceutical services but with cost as well.

The concern of health professionals with the cost of health care now reinforces the efforts of consumer groups, government, and others involved in financing health care, to the end of providing the best care for all, regardless of economic status.

According to the Health Insurance Council, comprehensive health service planning and delivery should be based upon the following guidelines.[2]

Health services cost money, and good health service costs a good deal of money. Agencies which spend money on behalf of others have a responsibility to get their money's worth for their beneficiaries.

Financing methods for health service should encourage efficient organization and management of the professional personnel and institutions.

Financing methods should distribute the burden of medical care costs in the way which best assures proper care of the entire population.

Health personnel and institutions must be reimbursed in amounts and by methods which permit them to maintain standards and achieve efficiency.

Although the guidelines of the Health Insurance Council are intended for the total health care system, they may be applied to any segment of the system. The guidelines include concepts which well may be applicable to pharmacy practice. The guidelines suggest that health insurers promote the efficient organization and management of personnel and facilities. It follows that pharmacists should promote efficient organization and management. With the utilization of carefully developed organizational plans and modern management techniques, pharmacists in community practice can contribute to the solution of the problems of the cost of health care.

The Community Pharmacy

The majority of consumer expenditures for prescription drugs, proprietary medicines, and health appliances are channeled through the approximately 52,000 community pharmacies in the US. Although heterogeneous in some respects, as in type of ownership and type of goods and services offered, community pharmacies are generally recognized by the public as the most accessible source of drugs and of information about drugs.

Community pharmacy, as used here, is defined broadly to include all of those establishments that are privately owned and whose function, in varying degrees, is to serve society's need for drug products and for pharmaceutical services. It is difficult to characterize or describe the typical pharmacy because of the great variance among pharmacies. They range from the corporately-owned chain pharmacy, resembling a small department store, to the independently owned pharmaceutical center, providing prescription service along with a relatively few lines of health-related products.

In 1967 sales in community pharmacies totaled about $11 billion. Of this total, approximately $3.5 billion came from charges for the nearly 1.1 billion prescription medications dispensed by community pharmacists. The remaining $7.5 billion was derived from sales of proprietary medicines, health appliances, cosmetics, and sundry items. Nonpharmacy outlets continue to increase their sales of nonprescription drugs and other pharmaceutical products, and sales to the institutional market are also increasing.

The community pharmacy, however, continues to be the major outlet for the distribution of drugs and related health products. According to a report issued by the US Department of Health, Education, and Welfare in 1967, at least two-thirds of consumer expenditures for nonprescription medication occurred in community pharmacies. During the same year approximately 75% of domestic sales of prescription drugs by US manufacturers was to drug wholesalers and community pharmacists.

According to the operating data submitted to the *Lilly Digest* by over 2,000 community pharmacy owners, the average independent community pharmacy generated sales of $188,429 in 1967.[3] The data reported represent a summary of individual pharmacy operating figures which were supplied voluntarily by pharmacy managers and owners.

It should be noted that the editors of the *Lilly Digest* make no attempt to structure the sample that comprises the data input and, therefore, citations therefrom are subject to the statistical limitations

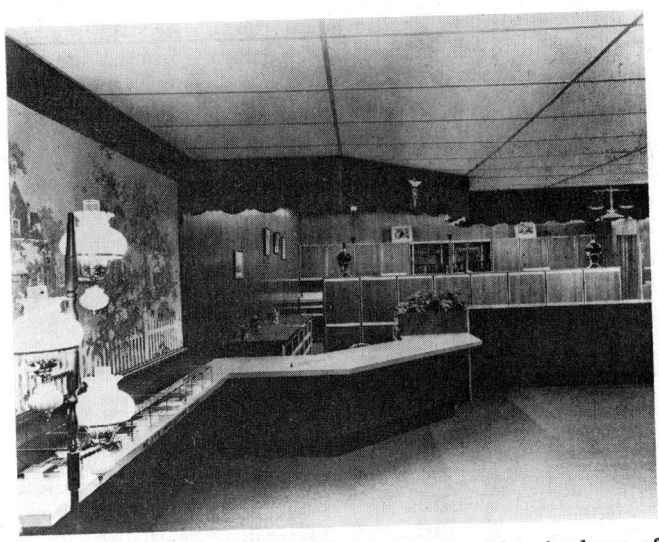

Fig. 945. A pharmaceutical center (courtesy, APhA Academy of General Practice).

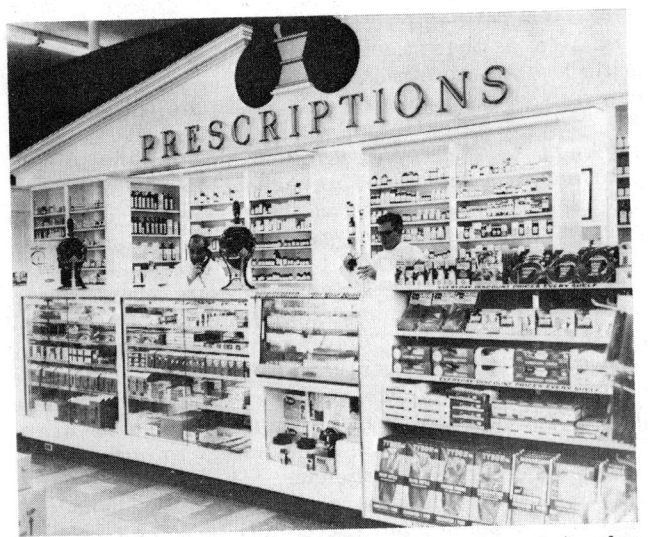

Fig. 946. The prescription laboratory in a modern chain pharmacy (courtesy, Walgreen).

inherent in the collection of unstructured voluntary data. It appears, however, that the figures reported serve to describe fairly accurately the economics of the independent community pharmacy.

Other studies, such as those done by *American Druggist* and *Drug Topics*, show slightly higher average annual sales than the *Lilly Digest*. These sources, however, include more of the large, corporately owned chain pharmacies which typically have much larger annual sales volumes.

The data from the *Lilly Digest* and from other sources indicate that approximately 40% of the revenues of the independent pharmacy are derived from prescription medication. Over a recent 20-year period the average annual number of prescription medications dispensed from the independent community pharmacy has more than doubled. During the same period the average prescription charge has risen from $1.51 in 1948 to $3.66 in 1967.[4]

It should be noted that the average prescription charge is not an accurate measure of the price changes for prescription drugs. Over a period of years the mix of drugs dispensed changes as do the prescribing habits of physicians for quantities of drugs ordered. Therefore, the average prescription charge in 1967 was for a different kind of medication and for a different quantity than was the average charge in 1948.

Trends in the data related to prescription activity in *Lilly Digest* pharmacies are given in Table II. Increased per capita utilization of prescription drugs and availability of more efficacious drugs with higher costs have contributed to the growing importance of prescription medication revenues in the economics of community pharmacy practice.

Chain Pharmacies

The foregoing discussion has dealt mainly with the independent community pharmacies which represent about 88% of the total number of pharmacies in the US. Chain pharmacies, which number near 6,000, are also an important factor in the delivery of pharmaceutical services and products to the public.

Table II—Prescription Trends in *Lilly Digest* Pharmacies: 1948–1967 (Averages per Pharmacy)[3]

Year	Sales			% of prescription sales to total sales	Number of prescriptions	% Renewals	Prescription charge
	Prescription	Other	Total				
1948	$14,745	$ 63,881	$ 78,626	18.8	9,742	42.9	$1.51
1949	14,806	63,007	77,813	19.0	9,258	41.5	1.60
1950	15,987	62,203	78,190	20.4	9,020	42.2	1.77
1951	18,617	66,852	85,469	21.8	9,875	42.5	1.90
1952	21,735	69,799	91,534	23.7	10,436	40.6	2.08
1953	22,546	70,511	93,057	24.2	10,295	40.1	2.19
1954	25,054	75,732	100,786	24.9	11,037	42.3	2.27
1955	27,688	73,905	101,593	27.3	11,273	43.2	2.46
1956	31,430	75,268	106,698	29.5	11,985	44.5	2.62
1957	38,477	86,107	124,584	30.9	13,502	45.7	2.85
1958	40,454	84,403	124,857	32.4	13,693	47.0	2.96
1959	45,319	87,930	133,249	34.0	14,656	48.0	3.09
1960	47,825	90,517	138,342	34.6	14,972	49.3	3.19
1961	49,144	90,032	139,176	35.3	15,135	51.1	3.25
1962	52,578	93,607	146,185	36.0	15,817	52.1	3.32
1963	58,688	94,574	153,262	38.3	17,320	52.0	3.39
1964	63,157	98,616	161,773	39.0	18,532	53.7	3.41
1965	68,587	99,060	167,647	40.9	19,708	53.7	3.48
1966	71,586	103,060	174,646	41.0	19,962	53.6	3.59
1967	78,789	109,640	188,429	41.8	21,544	54.5	3.66

A universal definition for a chain pharmacy is not available, as there appears to be question as to what criteria are appropriate for classifying a group of centrally owned pharmacies as chain pharmacies. To some, the matter of central ownership is itself sufficient to classify the individual units as chain pharmacies. Another approach is to classify individual units which are centrally owned as chain pharmacies only when there is also centralized organization and management.

The number of centrally owned units has also been used as a method of defining chain pharmacies. However, this criterion does not provide a satisfactory answer to the question; many multiple units are centrally owned and yet each unit functions independently from the central ownership. In mode of operation these pharmacies are more similar to individually owned community pharmacies. On the other hand, as the number of units under a central ownership increases, at some point there must be some coordination of policies and activities which results in more central management.

Although it is not possible to establish an exact number of units as the point where all units assume the characteristics of a true chain pharmacy operation, it appears that there is some relationship between the number of units owned and the definition of a pharmacy chain. The US Department of Commerce defines a pharmacy chain as those units with prescription departments which are centrally owned by individuals or organizations who own four or more units.

Although chain pharmacies represent only 12% of the community pharmacies in the US, they generated approximately one-third of the total sales volume reported for all community pharmacies in 1967.[5] Over the past decade, the chain pharmacies have demonstrated a much larger growth rate in sales volume than the independently owned community pharmacies. Among the factors that have contributed to the better than average growth of chain pharmacies are the following:

Preferred Locations—The drug chains are able to compete effectively for good locations in the larger shopping centers. For the most part, independent pharmacists have not been able to qualify for leases in regional and community shopping centers.

Low Price Image—Through the use of quantity buying, mass merchandising techniques, and effective advertising the drug chains are able to establish an atmosphere of low prices to the public.

Effective Management—The larger drug chains are able to employ and utilize management specialists to promote efficient large-scale operations.

In addition, the chain pharmacy operates from a broader base in the variety of goods offered for sale than does the independent pharmacy. The kinds of goods offered for sale in chain pharmacies are almost limitless, and include innumerable durable consumer goods in addition to health-related products.

In this regard it may be somewhat misleading to compare sales in the chain pharmacy with sales in the independent community pharmacy. However, when trends over the past few years are studied, it is apparent that the chain pharmacies are also improving their relative position in such areas as income from prescription medications and from nonprescription drugs. The evidence suggests that the chain pharmacies may be leading the way towards more efficient distribution of health products.

Efficiency in the distribution of health products and in the providing of pharmaceutical services is an obligation of all those engaged in community pharmacy practice. At the same time the quality of products and services cannot be compromised for the sake of efficiency and economy. Yet, it is increasingly apparent, as the level of health expenditures grows, that each segment of the health care industry needs to re-examine its delivery system with the objective of improving efficiency and economy. In this regard the owners and managers of community pharmacies should be knowledgable about modern management and administrative techniques that can contribute to the development of an economically sound delivery system for quality pharmaceutical products and services.

Establishment of a Community Pharmacy

During the 5-year period, 1963–1967, approximately 12,300 new community pharmacies were established in the US.[6] During the same period a few more pharmacies discontinued operation, resulting in a small drop in the total number. This decrease along with the fact that the population increased significantly, suggests that there is not a shortage of pharmacies to serve the needs of society.

There are shortages of pharmacy practitioners and facilities in certain geographic areas, such as rural communities and the inner areas of our larger cities. However, most experts agree that the existing number of pharmacies is adequate if the distribution problem could be solved.

It is increasingly difficult for the marginal pharmacy to continue in the face of rising operating costs. Further, the magnitude of health costs dictates that society can no longer afford to support the "pharmacy on every corner" concept. In some communities pharmacists have recognized the economic waste involved in maintaining two facilities when one would serve the needs of the population and have consolidated two or more pharmacies into one unit on a group-practice basis.

The foregoing factors suggest that a pharmacist considering the establishment of a new pharmacy should subject the basic decision to an objective analysis. The analysis should include a consideration of community needs—does the community really need another facility for pharmaceutical services?

The question may have both a quantitative and a qualitative dimension. Perhaps a given community has a sufficient number of pharmacies and yet none of them is providing the full scope of modern services. If a community need is identified, the analysis should continue in terms of evaluating the various alternatives that are available for satisfying the need. Perhaps an existing pharmacy could be purchased and made to provide more extensive pharmaceutical services. There may be an opportunity to join with another pharmacist in the ownership of an existing pharmacy and to establish a group practice.

Such alternatives provide the opportunity for improving services to the community while promoting the most efficient use of professional manpower and facilities.

If the analysis indicates that a new pharmacy should be established, the pharmacist must then consider a number of questions, some of them simultaneously; eg, What is the appropriate legal organization for the enterprise? What specific location should be chosen? How may the necessary capital be obtained? Although each of the foregoing questions is related to the others and cannot be isolated in a practical situation, for purposes of this discussion each will be treated by itself.

Organization

The pharmacist may choose from three widely recognized forms of legal organization for the community pharmacy enterprise. Traditionally, the majority of pharmacies have been organized as individual or sole proprietorships, with relatively little governmental control applied to the organizational structure.

In recent years, because of the increase in the joint ownership of pharmacies by two or more individuals, the partnership and corporate forms of organization have become more significant. The partnership as a form of business organization enjoys relative independence from governmental control. The corporation, as a creation of the state government, is subject to rather strict governmental regulation. Each form of organization presents advantages that must be weighed against the advantages, disadvantages, and limitations that become apparent when comparison is made with the alternative forms of organization.

The business enterprise owned and managed by an unincorporated sole proprietor is not considered in law to be a separate legal entity; rather, the owner and the enterprise are considered as one. It follows, then, that the risk inherent in establishing a business enterprise in this way has implications for the non-business assets of the proprietor.

The unincorporated sole proprietor has unlimited personal liability. His personal assets are available to satisfy business obligations and his business assets may be used to satisfy personal debts. In return for assuming unlimited liability, the sole proprietor enjoys the freedom to conduct his enterprise in any lawful manner he deems appropriate.

Further, except for required licenses, the sole proprietor may begin or quit operations without legal formality or governmental permission. Some states do require that a statement of ownership be filed with a designated office when the owner's name is not indicated in the name of the enterprise. The sole proprietor receives all profits from his enterprise and as a general rule income taxes are at a minimum level for this form of business organization.

Size or scope of operation is not necessarily a determining factor in the decision to organize as a sole proprietorship as opposed to one of the other forms of organization. However, due to the risks involved and to the fact that few men possess all of the abilities and capacities necessary for carrying on a large complex enterprise, the sole proprietorship is most often associated with smaller, less complex, operations.

Historically, the majority of community pharmacists are independent by nature, and have chosen this rather informal form of organization. Further, the typical community pharmacy being geographically local and only moderately complex in scope of operation generally succeeds under the unincorporated sole-ownership system.

When the resources of one individual are not sufficient to provide a proper base for establishing a pharmacy or when the individual does not wish to assume the entire risk associated with the entrepreneurial function, joint ownership may be considered. Partnership arrangements and incorporation are mechanisms that may be utilized to broaden the financial or talent base for an enterprise and may also serve to spread the risk involved. The partnership may be described as an association of two or more individuals based on an expressed or implied contract. They combine their resources as co-owners of an enterprise for their mutual profit. This provides a way for the individuals to do jointly what they could not do separately.

As to liability, a partnership may be described as an association of sole proprietors, because at law the partnership is not considered separate from those who compose it. As with the sole proprietorship, each partner is liable for all debts of the partnership, even to the extent of his personal assets. Within the scope of partnership activities, each general partner is considered an agent of the other general partner and as such each has the right to bind or commit the partnership in business affairs. Because of the mutual agency concept and the unlimited liability inherent in partnership associations, it is especially important that the full implications of such an arrangement be understood before adopting this form of organization.

Although it is a contractual arrangement, there are relatively few legal restrictions or regulations applied to the partnership association. No expressed governmental consent is required to establish or to dissolve a partnership, and the contract may be written or simply based on a handshake, as long as the elements of a valid contract are present. This is not to imply that the partnership should be consummated on the basis of an informal verbal agreement. The contractual relationship between partners should be attested by a written document, drafted with the assistance of a lawyer.

The close personal relationship among partners tends to foster a disregard for formalized written documents relating to the operation of the partnership. In the interest of producing a smoothly functioning organization and to help prevent disagreements among the partners, it is most important that a written partnership agreement be prepared at the outset.

Such matters as the investment of each partner, duties, responsibilities, and division of profits and losses should be considered and incorporated into the partnership agreement. The agreement not only provides a reference for solving future misunderstanding but also serves to compel the partners, at the inception of the agreement, to consider matters that might otherwise remain hidden until a specific problem arises.

The partnership as a form of business organization provides a mechanism for joint ownership of an enterprise which is relatively free of governmental regulation and which embodies the same flexibility of operation enjoyed by the sole proprietorship. As the partnership is not considered a legal entity, it is not required to pay income taxes on profits; rather, the individual partners are assigned their share of profits and pay income taxes on them as individuals.

When compared to the corporate form of joint ownership, the partnership usually presents an advantage to the co-owners with regard to income tax liability. The partnership has been a popular form of organization for the co-ownership of community pharmacies.

Co-ownership may also be effected through a more formal type of organization known as the corporation. The corporation is a separate legal entity, created by the expressed authority of the state. A properly constituted corporation offers the stockholders the advantage of limited liability.

In contrast to the sole proprietorship and the partnership, the incorporated business enterprise is considered as separate from the persons who own it. Consequently, in the absence of a statute to the contrary, corporate stockholders are liable only to the extent of their contributions to the capital of the enterprise. As a general rule, creditors of the corporation cannot proceed against the individual stockholders for debts of the corporation.

As a legal entity created by the state, the corporation enjoys continuity of life subject only to limitation included in its charter. The death or incapacity of a stockholder or the transfer of ownership in no way effects the corporate existence.

The corporation provides a way for individuals to invest in a business venture without placing their personal assets in jeopardy. It also provides a convenient, highly organized mechanism for accumulating a large amount of capital from several individuals in order to establish a business enterprise.

In terms of initial organization, the formation of a corporation is more complex and formal than other types of ownership. Each state has a required procedure to be followed in the creation of a corporation, and once franchised, the corporation is subject to regulation and control by the state.

By definition, the corporation has only those powers and can do only those things that are authorized by the state, in contrast to the partnership, which may do any lawful thing agreed to by the partners. The corporation may be dissolved only by or with the expressed consent of the state.

Further, the status of the corporate enterprise as a legal person makes it subject to local, state, and federal income taxes upon its earnings. When the earnings after corporate income taxes are distributed to the stockholders as dividends, the individual stockholders are required to pay personal income taxes upon them. As a result, the owners of corporations are said to be subject to double taxation, a factor which in many cases has deterred sole proprietorships and partnerships from adopting the corporate form of organization.

In the field of community pharmacy, the majority of chain pharmacy organizations are corporations. The corporate form provides the protection of limited liability which is especially important for larger multiunit operations. In addition, a fair number of the larger nonchain pharmacies are also incorporated, although it should be noted that neither size nor scope of operation is necessarily the only determinant in the decision to incorporate.

In establishing a new pharmacy, the prospective owner or owners must decide at the outset which form of organization to follow. The factors of liability, flexibility of operations, governmental regulation, continuity of life, and income taxes should be considered in relationship to the scope of the operation and the personal circumstances of the organizers. It is especially important to seek legal counsel in arriving at a decision.

Site Selection

Much has been written on the criteria that should be employed in choosing a specific community as the site for a new pharmacy. Such factors as population in the trading area, distribution of income among the population, type of industry, and the competitive climate have been cited as being important in site selection. In fact, many chain pharmacies are established and located according to these factors.

Often, an independent pharmacy is established in a community because the pharmacist-owner is determined to own his own pharmacy and wants a specific community because of personal factors such as family ties, climate, or other appeals of the community. In both cases, the decisions are often made without regard to the key issue of whether or not the community needs another facility for pharmaceutical services. As stated previously, the selection of a community as a site for a new pharmacy should turn on an objective analysis of community need.

If a need is identified in a given town or city, the selection of a specific site within the community will require careful consideration. The degree of success of a community pharmacy may depend upon the choice of the location most suitable among those available. In some cases, the choice of a specific site is extremely limited; the pharmacist must choose from what is available rather than that which is most desirable.

The majority of consumers choose the pharmacy they will patronize on the basis of convenience and accessibility, as long as the pharmacy offers adequate service and fair prices. Therefore, the primary emphasis in site selection should be on obtaining a location that is central to the population to be served. Further, the modern pharmacy must provide easy access and adequate parking for a motorized society. The growth of shopping centers may be cited as evidence of the importance of these factors.

As a general rule, shopping centers are located centrally in relation to the neighborhood, community, or region they serve and they provide easy access and adequate free parking. Pharmacies located in shopping centers represent slightly less than 15% of all US pharmacies, yet they enjoy approximately 40% of total pharmacy sales.[7] Interestingly, the growth in prescription volume is greater among neighborhood and community shopping centers than in the larger regional centers. This tends to substantiate the impression that consumers wish to obtain professional pharmacy services near home.

Although a site in a neighborhood or community shopping center may be considered to be a choice location for a new pharmacy, as a practical matter few independent community pharmacists are able to obtain such locations. Because of the nature of the system used to finance new shopping centers, preference is given by the developers of the centers to large well-established chain pharmacies.

However, it appears that there are other suitable locations for a traditional pharmacy that emphasizes professional services rather than the sale of non-health-related merchandise.

The island type of location, where the pharmacy sits by itself on a main traffic artery into a suburb and surrounded by adequate parking facilities, has proven to be attractive to consumers. A location within a large medical clinic may also prove to be valuable, although, because of the tendency of patients to obtain prescription service near home, the clinic location may not be so significant as some believe it to be. The selection of a site solely because it is readily or inexpensively available should be avoided. Usually a bargain location in terms of rent proves in the long run to be a liability rather than an asset.

The selection of the proper site for a new pharmacy is especially important because it is a decision that the pharmacist may have to live with for 5, 10, or more years, depending on the terms of the lease. Whenever possible, advice should be obtained from others regarding site selection. Some wholesale drug firms provide counsel in this regard, or a business consulting firm may be engaged to assist in making an objective evaluation of alternatives.

Capital Requirements

Planning and assembling the capital requirements for a new pharmacy are predicated upon a careful evaluation of projected sales volume, breadth and depth of inventory requirements, and estimated operating expenses. The amount of capital required for the operation of a successful pharmacy is a function of the productivity of the pharmacy.

Although certain of the assets required represent a fixed core necessary for any pharmacy, regardless of sales volume, beyond these the amount of assets required depends, in large measure, upon the scope of operation and the volume anticipated. As illustrated in Table III, as sales volume increases, investment in inventory, fixtures and other assets also increases.

Other factors also have an impact on capital requirements. For example, the policy of the pharmacy owner toward offering credit may require more or less working capital. The mix of sales volume may also affect capital requirements. As a general rule, prescription revenues can be generated with proportionately less capital than can revenues from other sources.

The problem of determining capital requirements for a new pharmacy is difficult. Most of the underlying factors are based on conjecture and forecasts regarding the future, for which there is no reliable basis at the outset. However, some judgement must be made as to what assets are required for a specific venture so that the pharmacist may explore the feasibility of assembling a definite amount of capital.

When making the forecasts and estimates needed to establish the basis from which to estimate capital requirements, a sense of conservatism should prevail. The projected sales volume should be estimated in terms of minimum level, while operating expenses should be projected at maximum level. It is usually easier to add new capital if sales exceed expectation than it is to recall committed capital if sales are less than anticipated. When operating expenses are estimated on the high side and planned for accordingly with adequate capital, a margin of safety is provided. If expenses are estimated at a level lower than is actually realized, financial difficulty may be encountered.

The method of estimating the capital requirements for a new pharmacy can be described by example. Assume that a conservative estimate indicates that a new pharmacy can produce $200,000 in sales volume during the first year of operation. The question becomes: What kinds of capital will be necessary to support the estimated volume and in what amounts? The kinds of capital are as follows: cash, inventory, fixtures, and equipment. The assumption made here is that the pharmacy owner will not own the building or land used for the pharmacy. The amount of capital required in each category is in varying degrees related to the anticipated sales volume, and may be estimated as follows.

Cash—Sufficient cash is required to pay preopening expenses, operating expenses for a stated period of time, and some excess for emergency use. Preopening expenses include license fees, legal fees, utility deposits, and advertising. These expenses, with the possible exception of advertising, are relatively fixed for any new pharmacy and are not related to sales volume. They are easily determined and usually total $1,000 to $2,000. Let us here assume the higher figure.

Table III—Balance Sheets for *Lilly Digest* Pharmacies under 5 Years Old (Averages per Pharmacy)[3]

	Sales under $100,000 (107 stores)	Sales $100,000 to $200,000 (243 stores)	Sales over $200,000 (135 stores)
Assets			
Current assets			
Cash.........................	$ 3,164— 10.3%	$ 6,702— 12.4%	$ 11,238— 12.7%
Accounts receivable.............	3,969— 12.9%	6,020— 11.2%	10,819— 12.3%
Inventory.....................	16,689— 54.0%	29,484— 54.6%	47,567— 53.9%
Total current assets............	$23,822— 77.2%	$ 42,206— 78.2%	$ 69,624— 78.9%
Fixed assets			
Fixtures and equipment and leasehold improvements (net after reserve for depreciation).................	6,045— 19.6%	10,090— 18.7%	15,635— 17.7%
Other assets			
Prepaid expenses, deposits, etc......................	972— 3.2%	1,681— 3.1%	3,016— 3.4%
Total assets[a].....................	$30,839—100.0%	$ 53,977—100.0%	$ 88,275—100.0%
Liabilities			
Current and accrued liabilities			
Accounts payable...............	$ 4,748— 15.4%	$ 8,280— 15.3%	$ 14,907— 16.9%
Notes payable (within one year).....................	2,733— 8.9%	2,978— 5.5%	4,578— 5.2%
Accrued expenses and other liabilities...............	770— 2.5%	2,187— 4.1%	4,640— 5.3%
Total current and accrued liabilities..............	$ 8,251— 26.8%	$ 13,445— 24.9%	$ 24,125— 27.4%
Long-term liabilities			
Notes payable (due more than one year later)........	8,614— 27.9%	12,637— 23.4%	17,211— 19.5%
Total liabilities.................	$16,865— 54.7%	$ 26,082— 48.3%	$ 41,336— 46.9%
Net Worth........................	13,974— 45.3%	27,895— 51.7%	46,939— 53.1%
Total liabilities and net worth[a]........	$30,839—100.0%	$ 53,977—100.0%	$ 88,275—100.0%
Net working capital..............	$15,571	$ 28,761	$ 45,499
Sales...........................	$75,861	$145,435	$278,396
Purchases.......................	$47,650	$ 94,968	$188,356
Net profit (before taxes).........	$ 3,095	$ 7,739	$ 13,393

[a] Excludes land, buildings, investments, and goodwill and corresponding liabilities.

It is considered good practice to start a new business venture with sufficient cash to pay the first 2- to 3-months operating expenses, on the theory that the first months of operation may be extremely slow. For a new pharmacy, the amount required may be determined by relating estimated monthly sales volume to operating expense statistics, available from such sources as the *Lilly Digest*. Only cash expense items are used in the calculation. Such noncash expenses as depreciation and bad debt losses are not considered.

For a pharmacy in the volume category of our example, the *Lilly Digest* indicates that approximately 30% of sales go to cover cash operating expenses, including a salary for the pharmacy owner. Applying this percentage to 3-months sales of a pharmacy with annual sales of $200,000 gives a figure of $15,000 needed to pay operating expenses for a 3-month period. There are no guidelines in regard to emergency requirements. However, we will arbitrarily set aside $1,000 for this purpose. The total amount of cash required equals $18,000. In addition, cash will be needed to provide the other kinds of capital described below.

Inventory—The amount of inventory necessary to support a $200,000 sales volume may be determined by referring to data that give averages for cost of goods sold and annual stock-turnover rates. Again referring to the *Lilly Digest*, the cost of goods sold for a pharmacy with sales of $200,000 is about 64%, or $128,000. The average annual stock-turnover rate is given as 3.5, and is determined by dividing cost of goods sold by average inventory at cost. Knowing the cost of goods sold and the stock-turnover rate, it is possible to estimate the average inventory; in this case, $36,600.

Fixtures and Equipment—The fixtures and equipment necessary for a new pharmacy are also related to estimated volume. Larger volume means more inventory, which in turn requires more fixtures and equipment to facilitate storage and display. The size of the building to be furnished and the quality of fixtures chosen will also effect the total expended. On occasion, savings may be realized by purchasing good used fixtures and equipment, usually available at a fraction of the cost of new fixtures and equipment. A reasonable expenditure for these items for a pharmacy properly equipped to generate annual sales of $200,000 would be about $12,000.

Total Investment and Sources of Capital

The total investment required for a new pharmacy with estimated sales per year of $200,000 would be approximately $66,600, broken down as follows:

Cash (for preopening and operating expenses)	$18,000
Inventory	36,600
Fixtures and equipment	12,000
Total investment	$66,600

The total represents the cash value of the assets required to establish the new pharmacy in this example. However, the amount of actual cash needed will be somewhat less than the total amount stated. In most cases, the pharmacy owner will be able to assemble the required assets by utilizing a combination of equity capital, borrowed capital, and credit.

Equity capital consists of the investment of the owner or owners, and comes from personal savings or from other sources that require no security and no commitment as to date of repayment. Relatives may be a source of equity capital, either on a co-ownership basis or simply by providing unsecured undated loans. It is thought that at least one-half to two-thirds of the total requirement should be equity capital, although many successful pharmacies have been established with much lower equity investments. The amount of equity capital provided will influence the availability of borrowed capital and the level of credit that may be obtained by the pharmacy owner.

Commercial lending institutions, such as banks and savings and loan associations, usually require a substantial equity interest in a new business venture before they will consider lending the funds necessary to supplement the owner's contribution. As a general rule, commercial lending institutions should not be depended upon for a significant portion of initial capital needs. Such institutions are limited in the amount of risk they are willing to assume, especially for new ventures.

Trade sources, such as suppliers of fixtures and wholesale drug firms, present the best opportunity for obtaining nonequity capital for the new pharmacy. It is common for wholesalers to supply the opening inventory requirements for a new pharmacy on the basis of approximately 50% of the total cost as a down-payment, with the balance to be paid over an extended period of time. The period of time allowed varies with the individual circumstances. Usually, if the time exceeds 90 to 180 days, the supplier will attach an interest charge to the unpaid balance.

The amount of cash required for inventory may be further reduced by cutting back the level of inventory at the outset and then building it up to the required level as operations continue and sales volume increases. Two cautions should be considered in obtaining any significant amount of capital through the use of trade credit: (1) the interest factor should be studied; depending upon the rate and the method of calculation, interest charges can be surprisingly high; (2) the use of credit simply postpones the underlying obligation to some future date or dates. Repayment of credit obligations should be considered in terms of the practical feasibility of meeting the obligations when they are due.

Fixtures and equipment may be obtained by relatively long-term financing through suppliers, or in some cases through finance companies by a mechanism similar to the one used to finance a personal automobile. Underlying this form of financing is a chattel mortgage which places title to the fixtures and equipment in the hands of the lender as security.

The interest charges from this type of financing may be especially significant, sometimes reaching an effective rate of 10% or more annually. Usually a down-payment of one-quarter to one-third of the value of the fixtures is required, with the balance to be paid in instalments over as many as 5 years. The scheduled instalment payments should be included in long-range financial budgeting and planning.

After the potential sources of capital have been carefully evaluated, it may be necessary to make compromises or adjustments regarding the amounts estimated originally. In some cases the pharmacist-owner will reduce his withdrawals or salary during early operations to reduce the amount of cash needed for operating expenses. Inventories may also be reduced at the outset. In fact, it is considered good practice to hold about 20% of the amount budgeted for inventory in abeyance until the needs of the particular community are identified.

The amount required for fixtures and equipment may be reduced by purchasing some used fixtures and equipment. By these means, and through the judicious use of borrowed funds and credit, a new pharmacy may be established with less cash than is indicated by the figure for the total investment.

Pharmacy Management

In an era of increasing specialization, the owner of the typical community pharmacy continues to function as a generalist, in both his professional and business activities. More often than not, he is owner, manager, staff pharmacist, and salesman. As a result, the management function, by practical necessity, is relegated to a part-time activity. Under such circumstances, it becomes especially important for the pharmacist to make the best use of the time and energy that he is able to devote to the management function.

In general terms the management function may be described as all those activities involved in the organization and direction of the elements of an economically productive enterprise. Money, material, equipment, and people must be brought together in the proper relationships to one another to achieve the objectives and goals that management has identified. Management practices predicated upon predetermined goals and objectives provide for more efficient operation and provide a basis for measuring the effectiveness of management activities.

The management activities of the pharmacist too often consist of handling day-to-day problems and crises. Much of the activity labeled management in the typical community pharmacy is actually routine administrative work that can and should be delegated to nonmanagement personnel. Perhaps this point is best illustrated by the axiom "management's job is not to do, but to get others to do."

The traditional casual approach to community pharmacy management consisting of the *ad hoc* handling of problems as they arise is not consistent with the nature or responsibilities of modern practice. The sum total of all activities in a pharmacy are becoming increasingly complex, due to increased volume of operations and to outside pressures for more effective delivery of pharmaceutical services and products.

All health workers are being called upon to develop a social conscience, and to assume more responsibility for the economic impact of their activities. Although technological changes may relieve some of the pressure on health care costs, better management and administrative techniques can also contribute significantly to solving the problem.

The impact of more effective management may also be reflected in improved professional services to the public. For example, a management decision to assign certain record-keeping functions in the prescription department to nonprofessional personnel allows a more economical use of professional staff. At the same time, it provides the pharmacist with more time for consultation with the patient.

The Role of Management

The first role of management for any business enterprise should be to establish the objectives and goals for the organization. Concurrently, management must provide the policies which will serve as the framework for accomplishing the stated objectives.

For example, an atmosphere of patient orientation might be stated as one of the objectives for a given community pharmacy. The elements of patient orientation would need to be identified: proper record-keeping procedures, facilities for consultation with patients, and patient-oriented personnel would be prerequisite for carrying out the stated objective.

Working with predetermined objectives provides the manager with a basis for establishing policy and assists in decision making. As in the example cited, the objective of patient orientation has implications in the area of personnel policies and practices. Recruitment and selection techniques geared toward obtaining professional and supporting staff who can function effectively in a patient-oriented environment would have to be developed by the manager.

The kinds of objectives to be established by management might be divided into two categories: (1) a set of rather basic, almost philosophical objectives need to be developed; for example, will the pharmacy stress low prices rather than full service? (2) objectives concerned with more specific operational matters are needed, as meeting a projected sales volume level during a given year. In either case, it is management's responsibility to provide a sense of direction by setting forth both basic and specific objectives as guidelines for current and future activities.

Objectives lie in the future and, therefore, are subject to adjustments dictated by forces outside the control of management. Management personnel should keep abreast of those technological, economic, and social changes that relate to stated organizational objectives. In this regard the role of management in establishing objectives and goals must include a mechanism for continuing re-evaluation and updating of objectives.

Organization of the material and human resources necessary to pursue the objectives of the enterprise represents the second management function. The kinds and amounts of resources required are dictated in large measure by the nature of the organizational objectives. The ability to obtain capital, generally considered to be an entrepreneurial rather than a managerial function, may also influence this management responsibility.

For the typical community pharmacy, it is neither possible nor practical to divorce the acquisition of capital from its application and management. In most cases, the same person is charged with both functions. Assuming that the required inventories, equipment, and people can be assembled, it remains for management to provide the organizational structure and the coordination necessary to mold these resources into an efficiently functioning community pharmacy.

The third management function is that of planning. Although a major share of the manager's time must be devoted to the fourth function (controlling day-to-day operations), he must maintain a balance between the present and the future. The control of current operations far too often becomes the sole management function of many pharmacy managers, who devote little or no time to planning for future operations.

Lack of planning often compounds the problems associated with day-to-day operations, resulting in a situation where the controlling function requires all of the management effort. For example, many pharmacy managers spend a disproportionate amount of time ordering merchandise and maintaining the inventory when, through a properly planned inventory-control program, this routine activity could be delegated to others.

The brief and simplistic description of management functions given here tends to understate the complexity and significance of these functions. Management may be considered an art rather than a science. There are no established laws or formulas for solving the problems inherent in conducting an economically productive enterprise. It is especially difficult to make the numerous and varied decisions required in exercising the management functions. Although there have been attempts to quantify management decisions through the use of mathematics and mathematical models, in the last analysis, the human element still dominates the management decision-making process.

As management decisions are made and implemented by human beings to affect human beings, it is apparent that those who manage need to consider and study the behavioral and social sciences in order to function effectively. For the community pharmacist who performs the dual role of health professional and manager, such a background is especially appropriate.

Essentially, management is an excercise in group dynamics. The manager must be able to organize, direct, and control a group of individuals toward the stated objectives of the organization. The manager who is unable to get the cooperation of his subordinates or who fails to delegate the responsibility for routine operational matters to others is not functioning effectively.

In the community pharmacy setting the human dimension of management practice is especially crucial. The nature of the typical community pharmacy is such that the manager is constantly in close personal contact with his employees, suppliers, and patrons.

In such an environment it is difficult to make consistently objective management decisions. Further, the dual role of the pharmacist–manager tends to create situations involving conflicts between sound management decisions and professional responsibilities. For example, in the management role the pharmacist establishes policies regarding the extension of credit to patrons. Yet when a patron with a poor credit rating has an immediate need for prescription medication, the established policies may be waived or adjusted to satisfy the professional obligation of the pharmacist to the patron.

These rather unique characteristics, and the need for the pharmacist–manager to be more flexible than those performing the management function in other types of organizations should not be construed to minimize the importance of effective management in community pharmacy practice. In the current socio-economic climate, with increasing costs of operation and pressures to reduce the costs of health care, the management function takes on greater rather than lesser significance.

The functions of management provide a somewhat theoretical basis for understanding the over-all role of management in the continuing operation of an economically viable enterprise. For practical purposes, however, it may be more valuable to examine the role of management as it relates to the various resources and activities which go to comprise the business entity.

In the community pharmacy the following items require effective management: money, inventory, facilities, personnel, credit, and risk. The management functions of establishing objectives, organization, planning, and control apply to each of these items as well as to the pharmacy as a unit. At this level the objectives will be more specific, and the organization, planning, and control more definitive.

Consideration of the management of the specific elements that in total represent the community pharmacy does not imply that each element is managed in isolation from the others. There are many interrelationships among the various elements, and a management decision regarding one element often has an impact on one or more of the others. For example, the decision to expand the inventory of the pharmacy may have implications to the management of money, facilities, personnel, and risk.

Money

To a large extent, the success of the community pharmacy depends upon the ability to obtain money from a variety of sources in sufficient quantity to acquire and to support the resources necessary for operation. Once the money is obtained it becomes management's function to employ it in the most appropriate way to achieve the objectives of the pharmacy.

In its simplest and most pragmatic form the objective of money management is to maximize the rate of return on investment. Such an objective may appear inconsistent with the responsibilities of professionals engaged in providing health services, yet in the long run the economical use of money is beneficial to society.

In theory, money is in limited supply and demand exceeds supply. In the competition for the limited supply, only the most efficient users of money will be able to obtain it. Applying this concept to community pharmacy practice would suggest that only those pharmacy owners who can effectively manage money in all its forms will succeed. In a sense the foregoing concept is simply a statement of the basis of our economic system, where efficiency is rewarded and inefficiency is not.

In the broad sense money management applies not only to cash but to all those materials and services which are utilized in the operation of a pharmacy and are purchased with money. Given a limited amount of money, the pharmacy manager must make judgments and decisions about the use of the money in terms of the stated objectives.

In this regard conflicts may develop between basic objectives. For example, the objective of maximizing return on investment may conflict with the objective of offering full services, as in the case where a decision must be made regarding the purchase of a delivery vehicle. The money invested in a delivery vehicle represents an inefficient use of money for many pharmacies and thus is contrary to the objective of maximizing return on investment. Yet, in order to meet the goal of providing full services to the patrons of the pharmacy such an investment may be necessary.

The effectiveness of money management may be

measured to some extent by the progress made toward meeting noneconomic objectives. For the most part, however, the most meaningful measure of effectiveness is in economic terms, specifically, by the return on investment. The return on investment for a pharmacy may be expressed in two ways:

1. *Return on Total Assets*—The rate of return on total assets is determined by dividing the sum total of all assets employed in the pharmacy into the net profit. No distinction is made between owner's equity and borrowed capital in this calculation. This ratio describes the productivity of the total asset investment.

2. *Return on Owner's Equity*—The rate of return realized on the owner's investment in the pharmacy is determined by dividing the difference between total assets and total liabilities (owner's equity) into the net profit. This ratio describes how well the funds provided by the owners are being utilized.

The pharmacy manager may calculate these rates for his pharmacy and compare them with national data to obtain some idea of the effectiveness of his money management policies. Rates below the national averages, such as those reported in the *Lilly Digest*, may indicate too much investment for the level of operation or inefficient management of other operational features of the pharmacy.

In either event, by utilizing the return on investment concept and analyzing the operation of the pharmacy, the pharmacy manager is able to identify a problem requiring attention and can take appropriate steps to correct the problem.

The management of money in terms of the total commitment of capital and in terms of the application of the owner's equity represents only one dimension of the management function in this area. In a narrower sense, money management is also concerned with the day-do-day inflow and outflow of cash from operations. The maintenance of a balanced cash flow requires application of the management function of planning and control.

Advance planning through the budgeting mechanism is necessary in order to assure that sufficient cash will be available to meet such obligations as accounts payable, wages, and taxes. To a large extent, cash needs can be anticipated in advance by an analysis of past experiences combined with projections regarding the level of operations in the future.

The inflow of cash may be estimated in the same way. Matching of cash revenues with cash expenditures is of more than academic significance: both excessive and deficient cash balances may prove to be uneconomical. In the case where more cash is maintained than is necessary for normal operations, the excess amount represents earning power which is not being utilized.

For the pharmacy that consistently maintains a balance of several thousand dollars in the firm's checking account, it may be possible to transfer some of the cash to a savings account or to convert the cash into high-quality marketable securities. In this way, the excess cash will be earning interest or otherwise appreciating and yet still will be easily available for emergency use. A deficient cash position presents some obvious problems, including a possible impairment of the firm's credit rating which may have long-term implications.

One specific problem associated with an unfavorable cash position is the inability to pay bills on time. In many cases this results in a loss of cash discounts. It is common practice for suppliers to allow a 1 or 2% discount for payment of invoices within a given time. The usual terms allow the discount to be taken

if the amount is paid within 10 days of a specified date; otherwise the full amount is due in 30 days. The buyer is offered what appears to be a small discount for paying the bill 20 days early. In terms of interest rates, however, the 2% cash discount for paying 20 days early represents an annual interest rate of 36%.

For the typical pharmacy, cash discounts can amount to $1,000 or more each year. Too often, pharmacy managers do not recognize the significance of taking advantage of all cash discounts, and consequently they do not devote sufficient thought to alternative courses of action when faced with an unfavorable cash position. It may be possible to borrow money on a short-term basis at 6 to 7% annual interest in order to take advantage of a 2% cash discount representing an effective annual interest rate of 36%.

To some extent, the manager is able to control the cash flow in the pharmacy. Although certain obligations such as payrolls and taxes are relatively fixed as to time of payment, the manager may be able to influence other aspects of cash flow. Good management of credit and collection procedures, for example, can increase the cash inflow. Proper scheduling of purchases of inventory can effect a degree of control over the timing of the outflow of cash for such purposes.

The manager makes the decisions regarding acquisition of new fixtures and equipment that requires outflows of cash either in a lump sum or in instalments. Depending upon future prospects for cash inflow, the manager can decide whether or not to proceed with such acquisitions. He can then decide upon the best way to budget the expenditures.

In actual practice, cash inflow for a given period should be estimated and known fixed obligations for the same period should be deducted. If a balance remains, this represents discretionary cash available for expenditure. If a negative figure results, it is management's responsibility to attempt to increase the inflow or decrease the outflow of cash in order to achieve a balance. During periods of temporary cash deficiencies, management may be required to obtain additional funds through borrowing. Knowledge of the sources of funds and the cost of such funds is a prerequisite for the effective management of money.

Inventory

The merchandise inventory represents the largest single asset on the balance sheet for the typical community pharmacy. About 52% of all assets excluding real estate holdings were reported as merchandise inventory for *Lilly Digest* pharmacies in 1967. The extent of this investment plus the fact that the inventory requirements for a given pharmacy are in a constant state of flux forces a need for continuing management attention to this area of operation.

It has been stated that the community pharmacist is the buying agent in his community for health-related products. He must provide the right products in the right quantities at the right time at the right prices to serve the needs of his patrons.

Due to varying consumer preferences and geographical differences in the prescribing habits of physicians, the management of inventory becomes a highly individualized management function in each community pharmacy. Given a limited amount of capital and the responsibility to utilize the capital economically, the pharmacy manager must develop systems and policies that will ensure a continuous flow of needed goods while avoiding the problems of excessive inventory levels.

Although the objective of effective inventory management is simply stated here, in practice it represents one of the most challenging responsibilities of management.

In the community pharmacy the management of inventory is complicated by the fact that a major portion of the inventory consists of prescription legend drugs. This factor makes the problem of inventory control in the pharmacy unique in comparison with control in other enterprises that distribute products at the retail level.

The demand for prescription drugs is generated by physicians and other health practitioners rather than by the ultimate consumer. When dealing directly with the consumer, it is easier to manage inventory. Excessive inventory levels can be reduced by special sales and markdowns. These techniques cannot be utilized to effect reduction in overstock of prescription drugs.

On the other hand, the successful pharmacy depends on maintaining a breadth and depth of prescription drug inventory which is adequate to handle all prescription orders received. Usually the need for a prescription drug is immediate. The patient cannot wait until the drug is ordered, to be delivered in a few days. The dilemma of the manager in this situation is apparent: that of providing a continuous supply of products that are characterized by an unpredictable and uncontrollable demand.

The management of other segments of the merchandise inventory such as proprietary drugs, cosmetics, and sundry items, while not subject to the limitations inherent in the prescription drug segment, present no less a problem to the manager. Changing consumer preferences and pressures by suppliers to buy greater quantities and greater assortments of nonprescription drugs and nondrug items increase the need for careful attention to this area of management.

Three basic decisions are required for the effective management of inventory: the specific items to be included in the inventory, the quantity of each item required, and the best source of supply.

The specific items included in the inventory should be chosen according to the needs of the community served by the pharmacy. Although there is a core of items common to every pharmacy, a significant portion of the inventory will be dictated by local demand. In this regard the pharmacy manager must be objective in his selection of goods. He must ignore those personal preferences that might influence his decisions. For the newly established pharmacy it is important that a portion of the capital budgeted for the initial inventory be held in reserve until the preferences of the local community are identified. As operations continue, the manager will constantly be faced with decisions on additions to the original selection.

Some managers adopt the policy of stocking all new items immediately, as long as the items are related to current merchandise assortments. Other managers adopt the wait-and-see policy, stocking new items only when a local demand is definitely established. Both approaches have advantages and drawbacks.

The wait-and-see manager runs the risk of losing considerable sales volume and perhaps, more importantly, the pharmacy develops a reputation for not having in stock what the patrons desire. On the other hand, the manager who indiscriminately adds all new items to his inventory runs the risk of an over commitment of capital to inventory, with its serious economic implications. Striking a balance between these two extremes presents a challenge to the manager.

Perhaps as important as the specific items to be included in the inventory is the quantity of each item carried in stock. Assuming that a given item should be stocked, the manager must decide what quantity is necessary. At this point, a number of decisions must be made, based on a consideration of sources of supply, extent of demand for the products, and such financial factors as quantity discounts and buying terms.

In most instances the pharmacy manager may choose from alternative sources of supply. Most manufacturers of prescription drugs and many producers of the other goods distributed through pharmacies will sell directly to the pharmacy. The pharmacist may also obtain a majority of his inventory needs from indirect sources, such as drug wholesale companies.

Direct sources offer the advantage of lower prices while indirect sources offer the advantage of faster delivery. As a general rule, direct purchasing requires a larger commitment to inventory investment because of minimum order requirements established by the manufacturer and increased delivery time.

Indirect sellers, such as wholesale drug firms, do not usually establish a minimum order level and emphasize rapid and frequent delivery service. The quantity of a given item carried in the pharmacy's stock, therefore, will be influenced to some degree by the source of supply.

Quantity-purchase discounts play an important role in decisions regarding inventory levels. As a general rule, the purchase of larger numbers or larger sizes of the items stocked in the pharmacy will effect lower cost per item or unit. Such cost savings can be beneficial to both the owner of the pharmacy and to the public being served. It should be noted, however, that cost savings on the purchase of goods in larger quantities can be offset by additional expenses that accrue from excessive inventory levels.

The costs associated with maintaining a merchandise inventory include implicit and explicit interest, obsolescence, deterioration, storage, property taxes, and insurance. Generally these costs increase in direct proportion to the level of inventory.

The capital invested in inventory represents money that could be utilized in other ways to earn a return. To the extent that such an investment is necessary to generate sales and to earn a profit, it may be said that the investment is economically sound. However, when the investment in inventory exceeds what is actually required for the level of operation realized, the excess represents an uneconomical use of capital.

For example, assume that a pharmacy has $40,000 invested in inventory. The safest alternative use of this capital might be to buy time savings certificates at an effective annual rate of 5%. At this rate, the $40,000 would earn $2,000/year and it can be said that this inventory investment has an implicit interest cost of $2,000. To the extent that the inventory produces net profit in excess of $2,000, the capital represented is being used economically.

Assume further that it can be shown that the $40,000 inventory could be reduced to $35,000 without adversely affecting sales or net profit. In terms of the safest alternative use of funds, the excess inventory of

$5,000 is costing $250/year in interest that could be earned and added to net profit.

An explicit interest cost may also result from excess inventory levels if the capital tied up in inventory is needed to pay other operational expenses. The pharmacy owner may be forced to borrow money at current interest rates in order to support current activities. To the extent that the need to borrow is caused by excessive inventory investment, the cost of borrowing should be considered as a cost of the excess inventory.

The possibility of obsolescence and deterioration are risks associated with the maintenance of an inventory, and although such risks may result in some unavoidable losses, these losses are minimized at optimum inventory levels. When the costs of storage, insurance, and taxes are added to the interest factors and to the risk of obsolescence and deterioration, the cost of each dollar invested in inventory can be significant. An awareness of the costs associated with inventory investment will prove useful to the pharmacy manager as he makes decisions regarding the types and quantities of goods to be included in the merchandise inventory.

The effectiveness of inventory management has traditionally been measured by the stock-turnover rate (the annual rate of turnover for the inventory). The rate is calculated using the following formula:

$$\frac{\text{cost of goods sold for the year}}{\text{average inventory at cost}} = \text{stock-turnover rate}$$

The stock-turnover rate denotes the number of times, on the average, that the inventory has been sold and replaced during a given year. It represents the turnover of dollars invested in inventory, but tells nothing of the turnover of specific items or units that go to make up the inventory. As presented here, the stock-turnover rate relates to the entire inventory of the pharmacy. However, the same concept may be applied to departments if appropriate data are available.

The stock-turnover rate may be calculated for a specific pharmacy and then compared with national averages such as those reported in the *Lilly Digest*. The average stock-turnover rate reported by the *Lilly Digest* pharmacies for the past several years has been about 3.7 times/year. It is generally assumed that a stock-turnover rate of approximately 4 times/year is indicative of adequate management of inventory. Rates considerably below this level may indicate an overinvestment in inventory.

It should be noted that pharmacies with rather low sales volumes typically have stock-turnover rates much lower than the average. For these pharmacies, increased sales represent the only real opportunity for improving their position in this area.

The typical community pharmacy with a sales volume near the national average of about $200,000/year should show an annual stock-turnover rate of about 4 times/year. If the rate falls significantly below the average, the management of inventory should be re-examined.

The rate may be improved in two ways. Attempts can be made to increase sales while the inventory level is held constant. Generating more sales with the same inventory increases the rate. In the event it is not possible to increase sales, the alternative is to reduce the inventory level. With constant sales, this will produce a faster rate of turnover.

A combination of the two alternatives, increasing sales while reducing inventory levels, can have a profound effect on the stock-turnover rate. As a practical matter, the manager may be best able to work toward a reduction of the inventory level as an immediate means of improving the rate. Certain items in the inventory may be returned to suppliers for refunds or credit. Items that cannot be returned may be sold at reduced prices. Most importantly, buying practices should be reviewed with the objective of reducing purchases until a more favorable rate is achieved.

If a stock-turnover rate of 4 is adequate, a rate of 7 or 8 might appear to be excellent. In some cases this is a valid assumption. However, unless the merchandise inventory is managed carefully, high rates may cause problems that are as serious as those resulting from low rates. An extremely high rate may be achieved by ultraconservative buying policies. Conservative buying will better the rate for capital invested in inventory, but the improvement may prove to be uneconomical in the long run.

When undue emphasis is placed upon maintaining a high stock-turnover rate, quantity discounts may be lost, resulting in an increase in cost of goods sold. As a general rule, a pharmacy can afford to do at least some quantity buying, thus realizing the benefits accruing from quantity discounts. Frequently, buying in small quantities increases the time and effort involved in the buying process. More orders must be submitted and checked in, and more accounting time is required to process several small orders as compared with a few large ones.

Finally, and perhaps most importantly, the pharmacy manager who attempts to control the inventory level too closely runs the risk of frequently being out of items called for by patrons. The disadvantages of being out of goods requested by patrons include a reduced sales volume and accompanying gross margin. Further, a reputation for being out of stock may result in the loss of patrons to other pharmacies where their needs will be met more consistently.

Through good management, however, it is possible to realize an annual stock-turnover rate higher than the accepted norm without creating the problems described here, and many successful pharmacies do this. However, unusually high rates reduce the likelihood of meeting the objective of having on hand the right goods at the right time in the right quantity at the right price.

In the final analysis the key to effective management of merchandise is stock control on a day-to-day basis. The manager is responsible for designing policies, procedures, and systems for controlling and maintaining the proper selection and level of goods carried in stock. Proper training of employees in the importance of stock control and proper use of established control systems in the pharmacy is the responsibility of management.

The pharmacy manager must take the time to impress upon the employee the need to maintain a continuous supply of goods. Otherwise, the employee may be careless or apathetic about following the established inventory control systems. Most pharmacies use the want-list or want-book system for recording those items that need to be reordered. Unless each employee is made aware of the importance of recording items on the list or in the book, the system will fail to serve its purpose.

There are a number of fairly sophisticated formal systems that may be employed to assist in inventory control. Many large chain pharmacies, for example, maintain and control stock by using computer-based reorder systems. Other firms utilize the perpetual inventory method of stock control. At the present time, however, most of these formal systems are not practical for the average community pharmacy. This is not to imply that a system of inventory control cannot or should not be utilized in the community pharmacy.

The pharmacy manager can effect a reasonable control over inventory by implementing a well-organized visual stock-control system. By predetermining the number of units of each item to be carried in stock, based on estimated sales and adequate turnover, the manager can establish minimum and maximum stock levels for each item. The indicated levels for each item are recorded in an inventory control book or on the shelf where the item is stored. It becomes a simple task for an employee to check the stock on a regularly scheduled basis and to note those items that should be reordered.

There is nothing profound about such a system, but it does formalize an important function and provides a mechanism for maintenance of inventory levels. Such a system also forces the manager to think in terms of minimum and maximum stock levels for each item. This in itself effects a degree of control over the total inventory.

Very often, the overcommitment of capital to inventory is not apparent until the end of an accounting period, when a physical inventory is made. In many cases the inventory level creeps upward without a corresponding increase in sales. When little attention is given to a comparison of the inflow of goods against the outflow, it is easy to accumulate excessive inventory.

One mechanism that may be used to combat this problem is the buying budget. In its simplest form the buying budget provides a means of dollar control of inventory based upon matching purchases with sales. In a pharmacy, each dollar of sales generally represents about 65 cents in inventory at cost prices. Assuming a balanced inventory level at the outset, about $650 would be required to restore the inventory level after $1,000 worth of goods had been sold at retail.

The buying budget concept is most effective when used to plan purchases in the near future. A budget is determined by estimating sales for a future period, as for the next month, then calculating the amount of new inventory that will be necessary to support the anticipated sales. The resulting figure becomes the merchandise or buying budget for the period involved.

As purchases of inventory items are made during the period, they are subtracted from the budgeted amount. The balance is termed the open-to-buy allowance for the remainder of the period. Although the budgeted figure represents neither an absolute minimum nor maximum, it does provide a guide for management control of the dollars invested in inventory. The real advantage of the buying budget lies in the fact that continuing management attention is directed toward an important operating problem. One form of a monthly buying budget is given in Fig. 947.

Facilities

On the average approximately 20% of the capital required for a typical community pharmacy is invested in fixtures, equipment, and leasehold improvements.

Charges for housing the pharmacy are second only to wages among the costs of operation. Expressed as a percentage of annual net sales, rent represents about 2.5%.

Over-all, the cost of the facilities necessary to operate a pharmacy represents a significant portion of total costs. Management of these costs is especially difficult, because they are based on long-term commitments from which there is little opportunity for retreat. Rent, for example, is most often agreed upon in advance for a 5- to 10-year period. The lease which establishes the level of rent to be paid is a legal contract which, once agreed to, is enforceable for its term. Fixtures and equipment, once purchased, represent costs that can only be recovered by long-time use.

FORM OF MONTHLY BUYING BUDGET

Month of———

	Total Store	Departments		
		I	II	III
Estimated sales this month	$	$	$	$
Amount of purchases to be made this month	$	$	$	$
Subtract amount of overbuying from preceding month, or add amount of underbuying	$	$	$	$
Subtotal	$	$	$	$
Subtract amount of advance orders for merchandise to be sold this month	$	$	$	$
NET amount of purchases to be made this month	$	$	$	$
Bought 1st				
Balance				
Bought 2d				
Balance				
Bought 3d				
Balance				
Bought 4th				
Balance				
Bought 29th				
Balance				
Bought 30th				
Balance				
Bought 31st				
Balance				
Actual amount of sales this month	$	$	$	$
Actual amount of merchandise purchases this month	$	$	$	$
DESIRED amount of purchases for this month	$	$	$	$
Amount of overbuying or underbuying this month	$	$	$	$
Overbuying or underbuying preceding months	$	$	$	$
Total overbuying or underbuying	$	$	$	$

Fig. 947.

Management's main role in the effective and economical utilization of facilities lies in a careful consideration of the original commitment to these assets. In a sense, facilities must be managed in advance.

Rental Agreements

As is the case in most areas of management, decisions regarding the types and amounts of facilities depend in large measure upon projections and forecasts of future operations. Basic decisions on size of building and quantities of fixtures and equipment are intimately related to anticipated sales volume. The nature of the pharmacy also plays a role in these decisions. An exclusive prescription pharmacy usually requires less space than does a pharmacy that emphasizes general merchandise. Table IV shows some of the relationships among size of the pharmacy, annual sales volume, and rent.

In negotiating the rental agreement the manager must have some notion of anticipated sales and the relationship of rent to sales. Although such information may be useful as a guideline for negotiating with potential landlords, as a general rule landlords refuse to be bound by statistics. When used as a guide, information such as that given in Table IV does provide the pharmacy manager with a rough idea of the amount to be allocated for rent in projected operating budgets.

As with any typical or average data, care must be taken to revise the data to fit the specific case. In many cases rental figures for two or more pharmacies are difficult to compare because the services provided by the landlords may vary. A pharmacy located in a medical clinic may pay rent considerably in excess of the average figure for a pharmacy doing a similar volume in another location. However, it may be that the rent includes janitorial services, centralized heating, air conditioning, or other services not normally provided.

When negotiating a rental agreement or renewing a lease, the manager may be able to get a stabilization of the rental charge as a percentage of sales by obtaining a percentage lease arrangement. The percentage lease provides that the landlord will receive rent based on a percentage of net sales. Such an arrangement is especially attractive for a new pharmacy where there is doubt about the level of sales volume that may be realized.

Landlords are increasingly receptive to percentage lease arrangements. In most cases, however, they will insist on a guaranteed minimum rent, with a percentage to be added after a specified sales volume has been realized. If the guaranteed minimum rent is set at a modest figure, this arrangement may prove to be advantageous for the community pharmacy.

It would be inaccurate to infer that the pharmacy manager has significant command of the alternatives and terms of the rental agreement. More often than not, the landlord dictates the terms of the lease. Management's main role is to avoid gross errors in judgement, resulting in long-term overcommitments for space and rent.

Fixtures and Equipment

To a greater extent than with the rental agreement, the manager is able to "manage" concerning fixtures and equipment. The original commitment for these items should be made only after careful analysis of requirements, and after searching the market for the most economical and suitable fixtures and equipment. The pharmacy manager has options regarding quantity, quality, and sources of supply for these facilities. It is good practice to secure bids from several sources before making the final decision on purchase of fixtures and equipment. Further, many suppliers will provide counsel and advice.

Once acquired, the problem of proper arrangement of the fixtures and equipment requires additional management decisions. For example, should the prescription laboratory be located in the front or the rear of the pharmacy? When located in the front, it is visible from the street and tends to emphasize prescription service to passers-by. When located in the rear of the pharmacy, the prescription laboratory provides a private atmosphere, free from congestion and activity.

Numerous other decisions regarding layout must be made, and the pharmacy manager is well advised to utilize the services of experts in store design before making these decisions. Studies have demonstrated that the arrangement of fixtures and the proper departmentalization of goods can help increase sales

Table IV—Rent Correlated with Various Factors for *Lilly Digest* Pharmacies:[3]

Annual sales	Average sales	Size of store (sq ft)	Sales/ sq ft	Average rent	Rent/ sq ft	Rental percentage
Under $40,000	$ 29,407	1,011	$ 35.06	$ 1,285	$1.27	4.4%
$ 40,000 to $ 50,000	45,038	1,390	32.51	1,994	1.43	4.4%
$ 50,000 to $ 60,000	55,059	1,148	47.99	1,608	1.40	2.9%
$ 60,000 to $ 70,000	65,297	1,168	55.97	2,562	2.19	3.9%
$ 70,000 to $ 80,000	75,691	1,291	58.72	2,265	1.75	3.0%
$ 80,000 to $ 90,000	85,114	1,506	56.49	2,518	1.67	3.0%
$ 90,000 to $100,000	94,751	1,523	62.16	2,724	1.79	2.9%
$100,000 to $120,000	109,964	1,518	72.57	2,925	1.92	2.7%
$120,000 to $140,000	129,701	1,692	76.68	3,213	1.90	2.5%
$140,000 to $160,000	150,027	1,923	78.01	3,668	1.91	2.4%
$160,000 to $180,000	170,114	2,092	81.29	3,969	1.89	2.3%
$180,000 to $200,000	189,114	2,268	83.37	4,649	2.04	2.5%
$200,000 to $225,000	212,489	2,492	85.24	5,060	2.03	2.4%
$225,000 to $250,000	237,030	2,416	98.25	5,538	2.29	2.3%
$250,000 to $300,000	273,019	2,766	98.71	6,546	2.36	2.4%
$300,000 to $400,000	340,154	3,291	102.63	7,789	2.37	2.3%
Over $400,000	529,268	4,445	117.85	13,210	2.97	2.5%
Lily Digest average	188,429	2,147	86.16	4,662	2.17	2.5%

volume, promote employee efficiency, and make the pharmacy more pleasant and convenient for the patrons. With modern fixtures designed for flexibility, the manager is able to experiment with various arrangements and layouts until the most efficient combination is achieved. Proper management of facilities can play a significant role in the efficient and profitable operation of a community pharmacy.

Personnel

One of the most important aspects of developing an efficiently operating community pharmacy is a well-conceived program of personnel administration. The uniquely personal nature of the atmosphere in the typical community pharmacy dictates that the proper selection, training, and maintenance of employees be given top priority as management functions. Each employee represents the pharmacy in daily interaction with patrons, physicians, and suppliers. The ability of employees to reflect and to carry out the objectives of the pharmacy may mean the difference between financial success and failure.

In view of the obvious benefits of sound personnel management, it is surprising to observe that many pharmacy managers look upon good personnel administration as an area for which they have neither inclination nor time. Deficiencies in this area arise in part from the numerous and diverse responsibilities assumed by most pharmacy managers. Yet, time and attention devoted to personnel administration would, in the long run, free more time for other management functions. The properly selected and well-trained employee can assume many duties that may otherwise be the responsibility of the manager.

The nature of retail employment also contributes to the complexity of personnel management in the pharmacy. In general, retail concerns experience significant variations in the demand for employees. Seasonal variations in sales during certain periods of the year require adjustments in staff needs. Further, retail activity is often concentrated during certain days of the week and certain hours of the day. Under such conditions, it is difficult to manage payroll costs without extensive use of part-time help.

While part-time employees may be used to meet the problem of irregular demand, such employees are rarely committed to their jobs and are often less than satisfactory. Extensive use of part-time employees also presents problems in employee turnover and adds a general instability to the staff.

Due to the extensive use of part-time employees, many of the people employed by retail firms are young people without previous work experience. Quite often they are immature and have little understanding of the economic value of the services they are expected to render. Personnel of this type presents special problems in training and orientation, not only to a specific job but also to the general obligation of an employee to an employer.

Attracting competent employees is further made difficult by the need for the owners of retail stores to cater to the desires of the public regarding store hours. Modern consumers expect to shop 7 days a week and into the late evening hours. The retail employee, therefore, is expected to work during hours and on days when others in society are free to shop and play. Although a relatively recent trend in retailing as a whole, 7-day/week operations have been traditional in the community pharmacy.

Other problems associated with obtaining good employees are inherent in the nature of retailing. Retail employees are continually meeting the public, so these employees must be of at least average intelligence, present a good appearance, and have an acceptable personality. Add to these factors the fact that wages paid to retail employees are ordinarily well below those paid in other industries and it becomes apparent that the effective management of retail personnel requires devotion and imagination.

Selection

Although the nature of retail employment is unique in many respects, the basic principles of personnel administration may be applied in the development of a program for selecting, training, and maintaining employees for the retail field and specifically for the community pharmacy. Proper selection techniques must be developed in order to ensure that employees will be compatible with the job to be done and with the objectives of the pharmacy.

A high rate of turnover in a pharmacy often makes the attitude of management towards selection of employees rather casual. Managers rationalize that the employee will not be staying very long; therefore, why worry about selectivity. Further, the manager is frequently faced with the problem of replacing employees on relatively short notice. In such emergencies selectivity is often ignored.

Improper selection of employees has the effect of perpetuating and intensifying the turnover problem, and the employee who is not suited to his job can be detrimental to the operation of the pharmacy. Two general rules should be incorporated into the personnel policies regarding selection.

First, minimum standards for qualifications of employees should not be allowed to fall below the minimum standards for service established for the pharmacy. To "underhire" for a given position can only serve to undermine the reputation of the pharmacy. Second, "overhiring" should be avoided: obviously superior people should not be hired for inferior jobs. Such personnel rapidly become discontented and may have an adverse effect on staff morale and efficiency.

Proper selection of personnel for a specific job is predicated on an understanding of the duties and responsibilities involved and on knowledge of the individual characteristics required for efficient performance. The manager should develop a job description and a job specification for each position in the pharmacy.

The job description is a brief summary of the scope of the job, its relationship to other jobs, and such details as working hours and pay scales. The job description also serves to prevent misunderstandings about the nature or duties of a particular job. The job specification sets forth the characteristics and competencies required in the individual who fills the position.

With these materials the manager is in a position objectively to evaluate the candidates who apply for the position. Selection also requires a knowledge of the sources of potential employees. For some jobs, promotion from within the pharmacy staff may be appropriate. In most cases external sources must be used, such as employment agencies, placement offices of schools and universities, or classified newspaper advertising.

A growing source of part-time employees are the co-op work–study programs being instituted in many high schools. An availability file should be established in the pharmacy—a record of qualified people who applied for jobs when no openings existed.

The pharmacy manager should develop an application blank to assist in the selection process. Although the application blank serves basically to provide information about the applicant, it can serve other purposes as well. For example, it provides a means for observing the applicant's ability to follow simple written instructions.

The application blank also serves as a guide in the employment interview. If no openings are currently available, it can go into the availability file. Finally, the application blank serves a practical purpose as a part of the employee's permanent record, and as a source of information for social security and withholding tax reports.

A properly designed application form can serve as an effective screening device for prospective employees. The information supplied on the application form will often indicate that the applicant does not meet the job specifications and thus should not be considered further. If the information supplied suggests that the applicant is a good prospect, the selection procedure should continue with an interview.

Often the employment interview is the sole selection procedure used by pharmacy managers, and this is not advisable. At the very least, the references provided by the applicant should be checked thoroughly to substantiate the impressions generated by the interview. The interview, however, is a key step in most selections. It should be conducted in an unhurried manner, in privacy, and in a relatively informal atmosphere. Much can be learned about the prospective employee through a properly conducted interview.

The pharmacy manager might also consider developing some simple tests to be utilized in the selection process. Testing is used as a selection technique by many larger firms and it can be most useful. In the pharmacy, simple arithmetic tests can be utilized in selecting personnel for sales or clerking positions. These positions require that the person be able to handle the simple problems involved in making change and computing sales taxes.

Orientation and Training

Proper selection needs to be followed by adequate orientation and training of the employee. Proper orientation and training can serve to increase productivity and reduce employee turnover. The orientation process should include a give-and-take discussion with the employee on the following questions:

What are the basic philosophies of the pharmacy (toward patrons, toward other health professionals, toward employees)?
What hours will the employee be expected to work (evenings, weekends, holidays)?
How long is the lunch hour?
How is overtime handled?
What is the policy regarding coffee breaks?
What are the regulations about smoking?
What are the rules regarding punctuality?
Are uniforms required? If so, who buys them and who pays for laundering?
What are the safety and security regulations?
May this employee answer the telephone? If so what information is he authorized to give?
Can the telephone be used for personal calls?
What is the vacation policy?
What is the policy regarding leave (sick, personal business)?

What are the opportunities and procedures for advancement?
What are the policies on employee purchases and discounts?

The preceding questions are by no means all-inclusive on those matters that might be of concern to both the employer and the employee, but the use of such a list will provide a basis for posing additional specific questions. Although some of the questions may appear to be trivial, studies show that these are the kinds of matters that often cause problems between employers and employees.

In an extreme case disagreements over such matters may lead to termination of employment. In other cases employee resentment may be reflected in attitudes toward and dealings with patrons of the pharmacy. This could be the most serious consequence of such disagreement. If these matters are discussed in advance, misunderstandings may be minimized, to the mutual benefit of both parties.

After a general orientation to the pharmacy the employee needs specific training in the duties and responsibilities of his job. Too often the new pharmacy employee is trained by the sink-or-swim method. He is simply put to work and is expected to pick up knowledge about his job as best he can. Obviously, such a method of training is inefficient and in the long run costly, although it does offer the advantage of requiring little or no management time or effort.

Even though the typical community pharmacy has neither staff nor facilities for sophisticated training programs, there are effective simple training methods that can be used. For example, the sponsor system of training is most appropriate for a pharmacy. A new employee is assigned to a capable experienced employee who explains and demonstrates the job in question.

The conference method also may be used, by itself or to supplement the sponser system. Here the new employee meets privately with the pharmacy manager or a designated employee to discuss the techniques of his job. In either case the management responsibility lies in organizing and structuring the training so that all aspects of the employee's duties are considered.

Compensation

Retaining good employees is one of the most difficult problems faced by the community pharmacy manager. There are many elements in the employment environment that may help in keeping employees, but most important among them is the compensation program. Adequate compensation is necessary not only to retain employees but also to encourage them to work toward the over-all goals and objectives of the pharmacy. The basic elements of a sound compensation plan are as follows:

Adequacy—The amount of compensation should be commensurate with the responsibility of the job and sufficient to provide the employee with a reasonable standard of living. Adequacy also may be viewed in a legal sense in terms of state and federal minimum wage laws. The applicability of such laws varies with individual circumstances. Recent amendments to the Federal Labor Standards Act bring certain retail and service firms under its coverage. The pharmacy manager should investigate the applicability of minimum wage laws to his situation.
Simplicity—Compensation plans that are uncomplicated are easily understood by the employee and have the further advantage of being easy to administer.
Progressiveness—A compensation plan should recognize and reward initiative, productivity, and increasing value of the employee to the pharmacy. The plan should provide incentive for doing a better job. Periodic review of performance and salary should be provided for in the compensation program.

Patron Protection—The plan should not encourage acts that are detrimental to the best interests of the patrons of the pharmacy. For example, it is inappropriate to offer extra commission for promoting the sale of nonprescription drugs. If commissions are paid on these drugs, the employee may be tempted to place personal economic gain ahead of the real needs of the patron.

Traditionally, the compensation program for pharmacy employees has consisted of an hourly or weekly salary plus the employers legally required social security contribution for each employee. Modern personnel management calls for a broader compensation program in order to compete effectively for the limited number of good employees.

Increasingly, even small pharmacies are offering compensation programs that include not only salary but such fringe benefits as health insurance, life insurance, paid vacation and sick days, and supplemental retirement benefits. When such benefits are provided, the employer should calculate the value of the benefits in terms of pre-income tax dollars in order to demonstrate to the employee the real economic value of the benefits.

Although pharmacists have been slow in general to recognize the benefits of effective personnel management, recent evidence indicates improvement in this area. Social pressures resulting in labor legislation and increased union activities have drawn attention to this aspect of management. In recent years the presence of a sellers' market for qualified employees has also had an impact on attitudes toward personnel practices. Given the importance of the human element in community pharmacy practice, it is apparent that continued attention to the management of personnel will be required.

Credit

According to a survey conducted by *American Druggist* in 1968, 90.4% of all community pharmacies offered direct charge accounts to patrons.[8] The same survey indicated that, on the average, 17% of the patrons of a typical pharmacy maintain charge accounts, and that these account for more than 30% of the total sales. These data are representative of what has been termed a trend toward a "cashless" society, where it is predicted that the majority of goods and services eventually will be provided on a credit basis. It is apparent that consumers like credit; in many cases they need credit.

The need for credit is especially apparent when health products and services are involved. The need for drugs and pharmaceutical services is often immediate and independent of the cash position of the patient. Further, a charge account statement provides the patient with a mechanism for keeping track of expenditures for drugs for insurance and income tax purposes.

These factors suggest that the community pharmacy will be increasingly involved in the delivery of goods and services on a credit basis. Further evidence of this trend is shown by the fact that chain pharmacies, traditionally operated on a cash-and-carry basis, are now investigating methods of providing credit to their patrons.

Credit management in the community pharmacy, on occasion, presents a conflict between sound business practice and professional responsibility. Sound business practice may indicate that credit should not be given to a particular patron, while professional responsibility may dictate that credit must be given. It is not possible to develop inflexible credit policies that will solve such problems. However, it is possible to develop policies and procedures that will be effective in a majority of situations. There are two general areas that require attention in credit management.

The first general area of concern is that policies and procedures must be established for granting credit. Included here are the matters of eligibility, limits on credit, credit terms, maintaining accurate records, and identification of credit patrons. Deciding which patrons are eligible for credit is the most troublesome problem for the pharmacy manager.

It is difficult to make a decision without knowing the credit history of the patron. Data on past credit experiences must be obtained and should be checked. The patron can be asked to supply the necessary information and usually will do so. However, verification presents a serious practical problem. Some managers attempt to verify the information personally by contacting each credit reference. Such a procedure is time-consuming and the information received is often incomplete.

A better approach appears to lie in the use of professional credit bureaus. Most localities are now served by such bureaus; agencies which, for a fee, will investigate prospective credit customers and supply a report on their ratings. With this information the manager is able to make better decisions and minimize the problems associated with the granting of credit.

The second general area is that of collection. The best policies can be thwarted by careless collection procedures. The terms of credit granted should be made clear to the grantee at the outset. If the terms are not compiled with, appropriate and prompt action should be taken. The manager is responsible for establishing the guidelines and procedures necessary to ensure prompt payment of credit accounts. Collection policies that result in prompt payment offer a number of advantages.

Prompt payment means rapid turnover of capital invested in accounts receivable; this permits a given level of operations to be supported with less capital. Operating expenses are lower when accounts are paid on time; delinquent accounts cost money in terms of employee time and supplies required for followups.

Finally, there is a definite relationship between the length of time accounts are outstanding and bad debt losses; as a general rule the longer an account is outstanding, the less likely it is to be collected.

Although guidelines and procedures should be established for collecting past-due accounts, rarely is the same procedure appropriate for all such accounts. New accounts, for example, should be handled firmly in order to impress the patron with the importance of prompt payment. Casual handling or lack of followup of delinquent new accounts sets a precedent that may be hard to overcome.

For established accounts, more individualized treatment is indicated. Some patrons fail to pay promptly simply out of negligence. Usually a simple reminder will stimulate payment. Other patrons may be willing to pay their debts but for reasons beyond their control are unable to do so. The pharmacy manager may be able to work out a budget plan for those in this category to help solve their problems.

A small group of patrons may fall into the category of those who simply do not wish to pay. Outside collection agencies or legal action may be the only alternative for this group. In any event, policies and procedures for collection should be included as part of the credit management function.

A recent innovation in the credit field is the bank charge-card system. Although dating back to the early 1950's, this system only recently has grown significantly. The system involves the establishment of a line of credit for an individual with a participating bank or group of banks. The individual is issued a charge card which will be honored by participating businesses for goods or services. The participating business then forwards the receipts for sales of goods or services to the bank and receives immediate payment, less a service charge of between 2 and 7% of the sales amount.

The advantages of this system lie in the fact that bad-debt losses are reduced almost to zero; the cost of billing is assumed by the bank. Even though the amount realized from the sales transaction is reduced by the amount of the service charge, some pharmacy owners view the bank charge-card system as the answer to problems associated with credit transactions. In fact many pharmacies attempt to use such systems as their only credit program.

As a practical matter, however, many people who require drugs and pharmaceutical services cannot qualify, and some people refuse to participate in this type of charge-account system. As a result, most pharmacies use such systems simply as a supplement to their own charge-account system. In addition, increasing numbers of pharmacies are accepting nationally recognized credit cards such as Carte Blanche, American Express, and Diners' Club.

In order to measure the effectiveness of management control over credit sales, it is useful to calculate the average collection period of customers' accounts receivable. Average daily credit sales are divided into the total of accounts receivable at the end of a period, giving the average collection period for accounts receivable. In theory this figure should be about 40 days if all accounts are paid on time. Figures in excess of 60 days indicate deficiencies in credit policies and credit management, and call for prompt action.

Risk

As a commercial enterprise, a community pharmacy presents numerous risks in terms of economic gain or loss. Certain of the risks inherent in the operation are speculative in nature. For example, will operations produce a profit or a loss? With this type of risk there is an uncertainty that may work to the detriment or to the benefit of the pharmacy owner. Such risks can only be managed indirectly by careful attention to the management of all of the elements comprising the pharmacy. Even then there is no guarantee of success.

Other risks associated with the operation of a pharmacy may be termed pure risks.[9] Pure risk involves uncertainty and chance of loss but does not directly provide a gain if the loss is not realized. Tangible destructible property is subject to pure risk; its destruction is always possible but not certain. For example, there is a risk that the merchandize inventory owned by the pharmacy may be destroyed by fire. If a fire occurs a loss will surely be suffered, but if a fire does not occur no direct increase in value or profit is realized. Pure risk may be controlled or protected against by appropriate direct management action.

Types

The first function of management related to controlling pure risk is to identify and analyze the several perils to which business assets are subject. Some perils are common to all pharmacies while others are unique to specific situations. It is important, therefore, that the analysis of risk be individualized. There are four common categories of perils to be considered.

Actual Loss of Property—All tangible property is subject to being lost. For the pharmacy most such losses are due to dishonesty such as shoplifting, burglary, robbery, or embezzlement.

Damage or Destruction of Property—Most tangible property is exposed to possible destruction or damage by fire, the elements, civil commotion, and a variety of other causes.

Civil Liability—Every pharmacy is subject to a variety of risks associated with dealing with the public and with employing people. Negligence or breach of responsibility, alleged or proven, can cause financial losses to the pharmacy. Injuries to individuals in the pharmacy, malpractice by pharmacists, and product liability are examples of these perils.

Contractual Liability—Legal liability beyond that imposed by the law may be assumed in a contractual relationship between a pharmacist and other persons. The lease signed by the pharmacist to obtain the building for the pharmacy is an example of contractual liability.

Methods of Handling Risks

Each peril identified by the pharmacy manager must be further analyzed to determine the probability of occurrence of an actual loss as follows: the loss must be quantified in terms of its impact on the total assets of the pharmacy and the ability to handle the loss; the manager must decide which of the alternative methods or combination of methods should be utilized to protect against each peril or loss. The three commonly recognized ways to handle risks are as follows:

Self-Insurance—Self-insurance may be utilized to protect against relatively small losses with a low probability of occurrence. A reserve is established and in the event such losses occur they are paid for out of the reserve. The reserve is created by systematically setting aside money for this purpose. A major danger is that a large loss may occur before a sufficient reserve has been established. Except for large multiunit pharmacies, self-insurance is not practical for community pharmacies.

Assumption of Risk. When the probability of loss is low and the loss is of small magnitude, it may be economically advantageous for the owner to assume the risk. For example, when the cost of insuring plate glass against perils other than fire and the elements is compared with the probability of loss from these perils, most pharmacy owners decide to assume the risk involved. Assumption of risk differs from self-insurance in that no reserve is established. Obviously, this method of risk management must be used carefully.

Insurance through Others. The majority of pure risks associated with community pharmacy practice are of sufficient magnitude to dictate the placement of risks with other parties such as insurance companies. Insurance companies offer service to the insured and provide indemnity in the event a loss is suffered. Such firms provide the technical knowledge and the legal experience required to settle losses quickly and efficiently. Often the services of insurance companies are as important as the indemnification they provide, as is the case in liability suits.

Too often the management of risk is considered to be adequate when proper provision has been made to insure indemnification in the event of a loss. A complete-risk management program should include a consideration of loss prevention as well as protection. An attempt to prevent losses can be beneficial in many ways.

Insurance companies are beginning to recognize clients with good records and to reward them by reductions in premiums. A direct cash savings is thus effected by reducing or preventing losses. More importantly, most tangible losses result in other losses that cannot be handled by insurance. For example, when an error is made in dispensing prescription medication and a malpractice suit is brought, the tangible dollar cost of such a suit may be paid by the insurance company.

The intangible loss due to damage to the reputation of the pharmacy can not be alleviated by cash payment. Prevention of such occurrences is the best way to avoid all of the losses involved. Loss prevention, both philosophically and practically, should be an integral part of risk management programs.

The services of an insurance counselor may prove valuable to the manager of a pharmacy in developing a risk management program. The complexities involved in evaluating risks and in understanding the various types of insurance policies and terminology call for expert advice. The insurance counselor is generally the best source of unbiased information.

The insurance counselor does not usually order policies. His function is to evaluate the risks of a specific individual or firm and to make recommendations regarding the best way to deal with them. The insurance counselor receives his fee from the insured rather than the insurer. Expenditures of money for this service may prove to be extremely economical in the long run.

Insurance

Among the types of insurance coverage required for the community pharmacy are:

    Fire insurance
    Malpractice insurance
    General public liability insurance
    Products liability insurance
    Employer's liability or workmen's compensation
    Crime insurance
    Business interruption insurance

The specific coverages described above may be acquired separately, or a number of them may be included in a package policy, similar to the well-known homeowner's policy. Package policies have the advantage of offering broader coverage at the same or even at lower cost than do the individual policies purchased separately. Such policies should be evaluated carefully; the multiple coverage involved may leave gaps in protection that are not readily apparent until a loss occurs. It is often difficult to know exactly what is covered, and to what extent, under package "all risks" policies.

Perhaps the most important coverage for the tangible assets of the pharmacy is fire insurance. Although most pharmacies are protected to some degree, often the amount of the fire insurance falls below the actual value of the property.

This is particularly important because most fire insurance policies contain a co-insurance clause. This clause requires that insurance equal to a specified percentage of the value of the property be carried at all times. A common requirement is 80% of the value.

Under co-insurance, if at the time of a loss the amount of insurance carried is below the required amount, the insured will have to bear part of the loss. For example, if the insurable value of the property owned by a pharmacist is $50,000 and the fire insurance policy has an 80% co-insurance clause, the pharmacist must carry $40,000 worth of insurance on the property. If only $30,000 is carried and a $10,000 loss is suffered, the insurer is required to pay only $7,500. The pharmacist must assume the balance of the loss because he maintained only 75% of the required amount of insurance.

The standard fire insurance policy should be supplemented by an extended coverage endorsement. For a small additional fee this endorsement has the effect of extending protection to cover damage by windstorm, hail, explosion, riot, smoke, and from land vehicles and aircraft. It should be noted that usually neither the standard fire insurance policy nor the extended coverage endorsement covers losses of documents, accounts receivable, prescription files, or currency.

Several types of liability insurance are becoming increasingly important in modern practice. The pharmacy owner may be required to answer a suit arising out of the negligence or alleged negligence of himself or of his employees. In addition, the pharmacy is a public facility where there are innumerable opportunities for injury to patrons.

Product liability may arise out of claims of patrons that they have suffered injuries from products purchased in the pharmacy. Although the pharmacist may be able to fall back upon the manufacturer under the concept of implied warranty, such claims must be answered by the pharmacist. Insurance can provide the financial and legal resources necessary to answer suits of this type.

The pharmacy owner must obtain coverage of sufficient scope and of dollar amounts adequate to protect against liability claims. It is not unusual for such claims to result in awards of $50,000 or more. Without insurance coverage, an unfavorable judgment from one such claim may be sufficient to bankrupt the owner.

Insurance coverage against dishonesty and criminal acts also should be obtained. In addition, the pharmacy manager is in an excellent position to utilize loss prevention as a means of minimizing these risks. Minimizing the amount of cash carried on the premises, installation of burglar alarm systems, and carefully observed security measures can greatly reduce losses in this area.

The dishonesty of employees can be controlled best by adequate systems and policies regarding the handling of cash and other assets of the pharmacy. Shoplifting losses can be reduced by proper surveillance and proper training of employees; as a rule, insurance is not available to cover these losses.

When a pharmacy suffers losses because of fire or other causes that interrupt operations, the actual loss goes beyond the property that is damaged or destroyed. Profits will be lost during the period when the pharmacy is closed. Certain business expenses continue, even during interrupted operations. Key employees may be forced to seek other employment. Such losses may be covered by business interruption insurance. This insurance is designed to indemnify the pharmacy owner for lost profits, continuing expenses, and salaries of key employees during a reasonable period of interrupted operations.

Life insurance may also have a role in a comprehensive risk-management program for a community pharmacy. If a pharmacist is the sole owner of a pharmacy, insurance on his life can provide funds to take care of the debts of the pharmacy in the event of his death. If the pharmacist is the co-owner of the pharmacy as a partner, arrangements should be made for life insurance on each partner with the other partner or partners named as beneficiaries. The amount of such insurance should be sufficient to pay for each partner's equity in the enterprise.

In the event of the death of a partner, the surviving partner or partners can use the proceeds from the insurance to buy a deceased partner's interest in the pharmacy from his heirs. Such an arrangement reduces the possibility that the enterprise would be dissolved in order to settle the estate of a deceased partner. The premium payments made for partnership life insurance policies are regarded as a business expense.

There are a variety of other risks that may be covered effectively by insurance. Some of these are peculiar to individual circumstances and must be analyzed and managed in terms of the specific pharmacy. Effective management of all the insurable risks associated with modern community pharmacy practice must be combined with effective management of the uninsurable speculative risks inherent in entrepreneurial activity.

Records

For a variety of reasons—some legal, some financial and some professional—the maintenance of records in the pharmacy is becoming increasingly important. The types of records required may be classified as follows:

Records required by law regarding the acquisition and disposition of drugs
Records regarding patient utilization of drugs
Records regarding the past and present financial status of the pharmacy

Management's role in the record-keeping function is to identify the specific records required, to develop systems for keeping them, and to delegate the responsibility for day-to-day record keeping to capable personnel.

Legal Records

According to federal and state law, the pharmacy owner or manager is charged with maintaining accurate up-to-date records on specific classes of drugs and poisons. For many years narcotic drug records have been required. Under the 1965 Drug Abuse Control Ammendments to the Federal Food, Drug, and Cosmetic Act, the pharmacist is charged with maintaining accurate records related to the acquisition and disposition of psychotoxic drugs and chemicals. Several states have enacted legislation that requires accurate records on the distribution of poisons and other hazardous substances.

The legal implications of record keeping as it relates to these drugs are serious. Improperly maintained or incomplete records can bring legal action and penalties. For further details regarding the legal record-keeping requirements see Chapter 101 on *Laws Governing Pharmacy.*

Patient Records

In recent years many pharmacists have broadened their record-keeping activities to include patient drug histories. Although the form of patient record varies, the basic idea is to establish a record, usually on a family-unit basis, that will allow the pharmacist to monitor the drug usage of each member of the family. It is increasingly apparent that, because of the kinds and amounts of drugs being taken by the average patient, there is need for a drug history for each individual.

In order to reduce the problems associated with drug interactions and individual idiosyncrasies to drugs, the pharmacist has a professional obligation to maintain records of this type. In addition, patient records may also serve economic purposes, as sources of information for insurance claims and for income tax deductions of the patient.

There are a number of patient record systems available, some of which are copyrighted. A prototype is shown in Fig. 948. The basic information required for a family-type patient record system is as follows:

Name of each member of the family
Birthdate for each child
All known drug sensitivities for each member of the family
All known chronic medical problems for each member of the family
Prescription order file numbers
Prescription charges
Physician's name
Address and telephone number of the family
Prescription medication dispensed, with dates

All of the foregoing information may be useful in a specific situation and should be obtained when the record is established. An all-inclusive record also should include all nonprescription medication purchased for use by members of the family. Properly developed and maintained, the patient record system can prove to be beneficial to both patient and family pharmacist.

It should be noted that when a pharmacist assumes the responsibility for maintaining patient records and drug histories he may increase his liability. At present there is no legal requirement that the pharmacist know the patient's drug history regarding idiosyncrasies or drug allergies. In the absence of such knowledge it would be difficult to hold a pharmacist liable in the event a patient suffered a serious drug reaction. However, when the pharmacist inquires into such matters and establishes a record of drug sensitivities, it appears that he may assume more civil liability for the proper use of such information in his possession.

For example, a patient may be sensitive to penicillin. If his family pharmacist did not know of this sensitivity, he probably would not be held liable if he dispensed prescription medication containing penicillin to this patient and a reaction occurred. If, however, the pharmacist inquires into the matter of sensitivities and records them on the patient record, he assumes a

Husband's Name	Children	Birthdate
Wife's Name		
Street		
City Phone		
Sensitivities and other information		

Date	℞ No.	Patron	Physician	Medication – ℞ and o-t-c	Remarks	Ph	Fee

Fig. 948. One prototype for a family medication record (courtesy. APhA Academy of General Practice).

greater responsibility. In the example cited a pharmacist with the sensitivity information on file might be held liable if he dispensed penicillin for the use of the patient. Any increased liability occurring from the maintenance of patient records, however, should not deter a pharmacist from offering his patients the benefits inherent in the system.

Financial Records

Financial records derived from properly collected and organized accounting data serve a variety of important uses in the community pharmacy. Such records are of value to the pharmacy owner in measuring return on investment. Management personnel require financial records to evaluate past operations and to plan for the future. Potential granters of credit and loans to the pharmacy base their decisions upon the financial records of the pharmacy. Federal, state and local governmental agencies may be interested in certain financial records as they relate to income and personal property tax levies.

Accountability through adequate financial records is an increasingly important management responsibility in current pharmacy practice. Accounting data and the statements that summarize such data provide basic tools for efficient management. Sound decisions regarding future cash needs, inventory requirements, personnel matters, and expansion of facilities can be made only if adequate financial records are available.

Future planning and forecasting by management is based upon accounting data. Effective control of current operations also may be expedited by proper financial records. Such records provide a basis for analyzing revenues and expenses to the end of maintaining a balance that will ensure a profitable operation. Finally, adequate financial records provide the main criteria for measuring the effectiveness of community pharmacy management.

As a general rule, the manager no longer acts as bookkeeper in the community pharmacy. Although some pharmacists themselves continue to maintain an outmoded single-entry accounting system, modern managers for the most part delegate the responsibility for accounting either to a qualified employee or to an outside public accounting firm.

Considering the complexities of contemporary business practice and the importance of good financial records, the pharmacist is well advised to employ experts to assist in the development and maintenance of his accounting system. The experts can help to develop an individualized system that meets the accepted criteria for good financial records: objectivity, conservatism, consistency, and comparability.

Financial records should reflect insofar as is possible an objective evaluation of the transactions and data upon which they are based. Personal opinion and judgment should not be allowed to prevail over an objective analysis of financial data. For example, the cost of fixtures in the pharmacy should be reported in the financial statement on the basis of acquisition cost as evidenced by a bill of sale or an invoice.

The value of these fixtures should not be increased on the statements simply because management feels they are worth more than the original cost because of increasing price levels. Convincing objective evidence of the dollar amounts reported on the financial statement is a prerequisite to maintaining the integrity of such statements.

The generally optimistic attitude of many owners and managers of business enterprises may be in conflict with the principle of conservatism as it relates to financial records. A moderately conservative approach should be employed in reporting financial data; otherwise, the data may tend to overstate earnings and assets and to understate liabilities. The consequences of overstated earnings include the possibility of excess income tax liability in a given year.

If a choice must be made between understatement or overstatement of income or assets, the principle of conservatism would dictate understatement. This does not imply that earnings or assets should be deliberately understated. However, when estimates or opinions must be utilized in making decisions regarding financial records, a conservative attitude should prevail. For example, many pharmacy managers are reluctant to admit that a certain percentage of accounts receivable will prove to be uncollectable.

They are inclined to report accounts receivable in the financial records without a realistic reduction for bad debts. To report accounts receivable without adjustment based on recognition of the likelihood of some not being collected is to violate the principle of conservatism.

Although there is no hard and fast rule for accounting for financial transactions, it is important that a given enterprise be consistent in its accounting system. Consistency is also closely linked to the final criterion for good financial records: comparability.

There are various methods of recording and reporting financial transactions, and decisions must be made regarding the best method for a given enterprise. Once a method is chosen, it should be applied consistently throughout the life of the enterprise so that financial records will be comparable from period to period. For example, there are several ways to allocate depreciation charges to expense. If the policy on depreciation is changed from one period to the next, the net income may be altered significantly. Such a change would have an impact on the comparability of the financial statements for the two periods.

Attention to consistency and comparability should not necessarily rule out all changes in accounting methods. When valid reasons dictate a change in method, such change should be made. However, the nature of the change should be clearly indicated on future financial statements.

Comparability of financial records is also important in the broader sense of ability to compare records between firms in the same field. It is advantageous for a pharmacy manager to be able to compare the financial statements for his pharmacy with similar statements as reported in the *Lilly Digest* and other references. Such comparisons are facilitated if relatively standard accounting systems are used. The pharmacy manager could instruct his accountant to classify expenses according to the system used in the *Lilly Digest*. He then would be able to analyze the expenses of his pharmacy in relation to national trends and averages.

The day-by-day financial transactions are summarized in the statements prepared at the end of the accounting period. Among the statements most important to those concerned with the financial progress of the pharmacy are the balance sheet and the income statement. Assuming that the underlying data have been treated objectively and conservatively, the balance sheet should represent fairly accurately the financial position of the pharmacy at the end of a given period. The balance sheet reflects the basic accounting equation: assets = liabilities + owner's equity.

Assets are the items of value owned by the enterprise, listed at cost prices less any allowances for depreciation or doubtful accounts. The liabilities and owner's equity represent the claims against the assets.

The balance sheet is of interest to the owners of the pharmacy in terms of the total value of their investment and the value of specific assets that make up the total investment. Managers are especially interested in such items as total merchandise inventory and accounts receivable.

Future management decisions regarding inventory control and credit policies may be influenced by the information included on the balance sheet. Those who are asked to grant credit to the pharmacy will be interested in the current liabilities and the owner's equity, as reported on the balance sheet. A formal detailed balance sheet should be prepared at least once a year.

The income statement describes in detail the effects of revenue and expense transactions during a given accounting period. Unlike the balance sheet, which describes the financial position of an enterprise on a given date, the income statement summarizes only those transactions directly related to income production for a specific period of time, usually a year. For most purposes the income statement is used in concert with the balance sheet, each supplementing the other.

The owners of the pharmacy are interested not only in total investment but also in the net profit which represents return on investment. The manager cannot judge accurately the appropriatness of the level of merchandise inventory reported in the balance sheet without knowing the sales revenue generated by the inventory as reported in the income statement.

The information included in the income statement can be utilized by the manager to plan for future operations and as a means for controlling current operations. When the information is compared against past years and national averages, trends will be observed and problem areas may be identified. The manager then can make decisions and take actions intended to improve the profit-making potential of the pharmacy.

Record keeping in the pharmacy is certain to assume greater importance in the years ahead. The traditional casual approach to record keeping is not consistent with the increasing internal and external demands upon the pharmacist for information. As has been indicated previously, effective internal management of the pharmacy is based upon adequate financial records. These same records are required by governmental agencies for tax purposes.

In the future certain financial records will probably be required from those pharmacies participating in governmental third-party drug payment programs. Evolving systems of health care also may place more record-keeping responsibility upon the pharmacist. Already, some experimental health-care programs being developed under governmental sponsorship require detailed record keeping by participating pharmacists. Complete patient records and renewal calendars for prescription orders are among the requirements of these programs.

The progressive pharmacy manager will anticipate these developments by planning a system and training personnel to maintain adequate records.

Trends

During the past several years the economic dimension of community pharmacy practice has improved greatly. Steady, uninterrupted growth in total sales volume and increasing revenues from larger numbers of prescription orders have resulted in greater dollar income for most owners. Even though operational and other expenses have risen, it appears that increased sales have compensated for most of these higher costs. Net profit as a percentage of net sales has been declining slightly in recent years, but return on owner's investment, a truer indicator of successful operations, has remained at about 20%.

A generally healthy national economy during the past decade has contributed to the success of community practice. During this period the number of community pharmacies in the US has remained relatively fixed while population has increased. The per capita prescription rate has increased in recent years, rising from 4.2 in 1962 to about 5 in 1967. When these factors are considered, along with the trend toward larger pharmacies with more diverse merchandise offerings, the growth in community pharmacy sales and profits is easily explained.

Growth of Chain Pharmacies

Further analysis of the economics of community pharmacy operation indicates that a definite trend is developing in favor of chain pharmacies. Independent pharmacies accounted for 75% of total pharmacy sales in the US in 1962. In 1967 the independents' share had dropped to about 67%.

The R. A. Gosselin & Co. National Prescription Audit for 1967 indicated that all pharmacies in the US showed a growth of 1.3% in the number of prescription orders dispensed, while *Chain Store Age* estimated an increase of 14.2% for chain pharmacies during the same year. Buying advantages held by such large buyers as the drug chains plus efficient management have allowed the chains to sharpen their low-price image to the public. Coupled with location advantages derived from the preference given to drug chains for shopping center locations, these factors account for the better than average growth of chain pharmacies.

There are some who view the growth of chain pharmacies with alarm and who feel that they will eventually control the market for drugs and pharmaceutical services. The evidence indicates, however, that the well-managed independent community pharmacy will continue to be a significant factor in the distribution of drugs and pharmaceutical services.

The independent pharmacist offers the flexibility inherent in local ownership and management, and he generally enjoys prestige as one of the leading businessmen in the local community. Further, it appears that a sizable segment of the American public continues to demonstrate a preference for the convenient service-oriented community pharmacy.

Outpatient Services by Institutions

A trend toward the increasing involvement of institutions in the distribution of drugs and pharmaceutical services is also apparent. Although more than 90% of outpatient prescription medication was dispensed by community pharmacists in 1966, a significant increase in the amount of medication dispensed from outpatient hospital pharmacies has been noted in recent years. Over half of the nation's more than 7,000 hospitals now provide outpatient pharmacy services.

In addition, a growing number of government-sponsored health care institutions are providing "in house" pharmaceutical services. Mental health clinics, Regional Heart, Cancer, and Stroke Centers and a variety of facilities related to the "War on Poverty" provide pharmaceutical services to their clients in varying degrees.

The economic implications to the community pharmacy of the increasing involvement of institutions in pharmacy practice are not yet clear. Considerable opposition to this trend has been voiced by pharmacists and their professional organizations. In the long run, however, only society can decide whether present institutions or others yet to be developed can best meet the health needs of the public.

Pharmacy Manpower

Related to the trends toward greater involvement of chains and institutions in pharmacy practice is the availability and utilization of pharmacy manpower. The present supply of licensed pharmacists does not meet the demand for such personnel. It can be argued that better utilization of professional manpower would alleviate this situation. Nevertheless, increasing demands for pharmaceutical services, both quantitative and qualitative, indicate that new approaches are needed in order to solve the manpower problem.

More and more pharmacists are entering institutional practice, because of greater emphasis on pharmaceutical services in hospitals, extended-care facilities and group-practice clinics. With a higher percentage of pharmacists entering institutional practice and a seemingly inadequate number graduating from the colleges of pharmacy, there will be great competition for community practitioners. The implications of this situation will be manifested in higher salaries for professional staff in the community pharmacy. This will be passed on to consumers of drugs and pharmaceutical services.

The shortage of professional manpower also may serve to reduce the rate of growth of the drug chains. According to many experts, the drug chains would be even more dominant if they could obtain sufficient pharmacists to staff additional units. The manpower shortage also will have an impact on independent community pharmacy practice. There will be fewer pharmacists available to purchase established pharmacies when present owners retire.

In addition, the newly licensed pharmacist is now able to choose from a variety of professionally and financially rewarding positions which, when weighed against the risks and problems associated with the ownership of a pharmacy, may deter him from assuming the entrepreneurial function.

The quantitative aspect of the pharmacy manpower problem represents only one dimension of the situation. A trend toward improved quality of pharmaceutical services is also apparent. The traditional function of the pharmacist as a drug-distribution specialist is only a part of modern, comprehensive high-quality service. Increasingly, the pharmacist is being expected to serve as a drug-utilization counsellor for patients and as a source of drug information for other health professionals.

Services of this type require more of the pharmacist's time and effort and compound the manpower shortage. Such services also have implications for the economics of pharmacy management. Additional costs are incurred when better services are provided. Meeting the increased costs of better pharmaceutical services is a major challenge to the owners and managers of community pharmacies.

One approach to the manpower problem and its economic implications is through increased utilization of subprofessional personnel in the community pharmacy. Although a complex subject with many ramifications legally and ethically, the use of pharmacy aids or technicians in the community pharmacy presents some interesting possibilities for a partial solution to both the quantitative and qualitative aspects of the pharmacy manpower problem.

Subprofessionals may be able to assume the increasing paperwork and record-keeping function now a part of the pharmacist's responsibility. A properly trained pharmaceutical secretary to handle third-party drug payment records may prove to be economically and professionally advantageous. Adequately supervised aides might be utilized to prepackage drugs into commonly ordered quantities to be dispensed by the pharmacist. In specific cases there may be other routine functions that can be assumed by nonpharmacists.

Admittedly, care must be exercised in the utilization of nonprofessional personnel, lest the quantitative aspect of the manpower problem be solved at the expense of the quality of pharmaceutical services. It appears, however, that the judicious use of such personnel can contribute toward alleviating the manpower problem and improving the over-all quality of pharmaceutical services offered by the community pharmacy.

Third-Party Payment

The application of third-party payment to drugs and pharmaceutical services represents one of the most economically significant trends in community practice. Third-party payment emerging from governmental programs and contracts negotiated by labor unions will have an impact on the practice of community pharmacy yet to be completely defined. If such programs prove to be feasible and economically sound, many of the trends discussed previously probably will be affected.

The growth of chain pharmacies may be slowed; under third-party plans, the patient may be more inclined to seek service and convenience because price is no longer of direct concern to him. Further, third-party programs mean more record keeping, with claim forms to be completed and patient eligibility determinations to be required. As the volume of third-party claims increases, the community pharmacist will need to investigate more thoroughly the use of nonprofessional personnel to assist with the record-keeping function.

Although the concept of third-party payment for drugs and pharmaceutical services is not new, the projected scope of third-party involvement in pharmacy practice is almost unlimited. In the past the community pharmacist has participated to a limited extent in local welfare programs and for a number of years in the VA hometown drug program.

For the most part these programs were rather limited and accounted for only a small portion of the total revenues of the typical pharmacy. Current developments in this area suggest the possibility that in the future a sizable portion if not the majority of revenues for professional services will come from third-party payers. Some experts predict that by 1980 as much as 75% of the community pharmacy's prescription revenues will come from third-party programs.

When the growing involvement of governmental agencies, through such programs as Medicare, Medicaid, and a variety of antipoverty programs is considered, plus the efforts of trade unions to obtain comprehensive prepaid health services for their members, such estimates are probably well founded.

Although third-party programs take the direct burden of the cost of drugs off the consumer, it should be noted that such programs do not reduce the responsibility of the pharmacist to provide quality services in an efficient and economical manner.

As representatives of that segment of the public which they serve, whether public or private agencies, third-party payers have an obligation to obtain the best quality health services at the most economical cost. In this regard, third-party payers will be in a position to dictate standards of service and levels and methods of reimbursement for pharmaceutical services. The concentration of economic power inherent in a system dominated by third-party payers is of legitimate concern to all those engaged in community pharmacy practice.

As third-party programs are developed, it is important that pharmacists, individually and collectively, assist the architects of such programs to ensure an equitable result for society and for the profession. Further, as such programs are implemented, the tendency to become inefficient when a large impersonal agency is paying the bill must be avoided.

In the event that third-party programs—which utilize the independent and chain pharmacies as providers of pharmaceutical services—prove to be too costly, the alternative of in-house institutional pharmacies is available. Governmental drug programs could consist of a number of government-operated clinics, where drugs and pharmaceutical services could be made available. The benefits to the community pharmacy inherent in increased utilization of third-party prepaid drug programs can only be realized if efforts are made to ensure efficient and economical pharmacy practice.

Determination of Prescription Charges

The trend toward third-party payment for pharmaceutical services has resulted in a re-examination by pharmacists of the methods employed to determine prescription charges.

Traditionally, prescription charges have been determined by what may be termed a commodity approach to pricing. Prescription medication has been viewed as a commodity or product, subject to the pricing techniques that are used for toothpaste and mouthwash. Under this approach a pre-determined percentage markup is applied to the cost of the prescription drug, resulting in a final charge that is related directly to the wholesale cost of the drug being dispensed.

The approach ignores two important differences between prescription drugs and other products: (1) prescription drugs are not ordinary commodities, in the sense that toothpaste and mouthwash are; (2) the skill, training, and responsibility associated with dispensing prescription medication is not directly proportional to the wholesale cost of the medication.

Although these differences have been apparent for years and many pharmaceutical economists have called attention to the inconsistencies of using commodity pricing techniques for professional services, it has taken the recent involvement of third-party payers to bring pharmacists to a reappraisal of their traditional approach to prescription charges.

For the most part third-party payers do not reimburse pharmacists on the commodity pricing basis. Rather, most third-party programs provide for reimbursement based upon acquisition cost of the medication plus a dispensing or professional fee. The fee, in theory, is sufficient to reimburse the pharmacist for the overhead cost of operating the prescription laboratory and to provide adequate compensation for his services.

The advantages of the fee approach to determining prescription charges include the more equitable allocation of the cost of providing pharmaceutical services to all patients. Under the commodity approach, patients receiving prescription medication with a high wholesale cost tend to subsidize patients receiving low-cost medication. The fee approach tends to eliminate wholesale drug cost as the major factor in drug selection by the pharmacist.

For generic prescription orders the pharmacist using the percentage markup approach may be tempted to dispense drugs with higher wholesale costs in order to realize a higher gross profit. With the fee approach the drug cost becomes irrelevant except as it reflects quality. Utilizing the fee approach, the pharmacist can satisfy his obligation to provide quality drugs at the lowest possible cost to the patient.

Although the commodity approach to determining prescription charges still dominates in the field of community pharmacy, there appears to be a trend toward the increased use of the professional fee method.

The interrelationship of the trends and changes occurring in community pharmacy practice make it difficult to chart the future of the community pharmacy in health care. When the intraprofessional trends are combined with the extraprofessional changing social attitudes toward health care, the future is even less predictable. The community pharmacist can only attempt to keep up-to-date with changing patterns in health care and to make every effort to meet the needs of society as they relate to his services.

To some degree, the future of community practice lies with those who own and manage the nation's pharmacies. To the extent that community practitioners can anticipate and adjust in an efficient and economical way to the growing needs of society for pharmaceutical services, the next decade promises continued professional and economic growth for community pharmacy.

References

1. *National Health Expenditures 1950–66*, Social Security Bull., Social Security Admin., Washington, D.C., Apr., 1968, p. 3.
2. *Health Insurance Viewpoints*, Health Insurance Council, New York, Dec., 1967.
3. *The Lilly Digest for 1967*, Lilly, Indianapolis, Ind., p. 5.
4. *The Lilly Digest for 1967*, Lilly, Indianapolis, Ind., pp 52, 53.
5. *Am. Druggist*, **158**, 23 (Apr. 8, 1968).
6. *Drug Topics*, **112**, 38 (Apr. 1, 1968).
7. *Am. Druggist*, **158**, 69 (Oct. 7, 1968).
8. *Am. Druggist*, **158**, 13 (Mar. 25, 1968).
9. Mowbray, A. H., and Blanchard, R. H., *Insurance*, 4th ed., McGraw-Hill, New York, 1955, p. 7.

Part
X

APPENDIX

Manufacturers Index

An alphabetical list of pharmaceutical and other manufacturers who have graciously supplied illustrations, processes, descriptions of specialties, and other valuable help and information for RPS XIV

Names and addresses	Abbreviations[a]

A

Abbe, Paul O., Inc., Abbe & Center Aves., Little Falls, N.J. 07424 . . . . Abbe
*Abbott Laboratories, Abbott Park, North Chicago, Ill. 60064 . . . . Abbott
Aceto Chemical Co., Inc., 126–02 Northern Blvd., Flushing, N.Y. 11368 . . . . Aceto
Acrodent Div., Ormont Drug & Chemical Co., Inc., 223 S. Dean St., Englewood, N.J. 07631 . . . . Acrodent
Adolph's Food Products Mfg. Co., Magnolia St., Burbank, Calif. 91503 . . . . Adolph
Advance Div., Carlisle Chemical Works, Inc., 500 Jersey Ave., New Brunswick, N.J. 08901 . . . . Advance
Advance Solvents & Chemical Div.—see *Advance* . . . . Advance Solvents
Aeroceuticals, Inc., 104 Sillman Ave., Bridgeport, Conn. 06605 . . . . Aeroceuticals
Agricultural Biologicals, 35 Wilburn St., Lynbrook, N.Y. 11563 . . . . Agr. Biol.
Air Control, Inc., 125 Noble St., Norristown, Pa. 19401 . . . . Air Control
Air-Shields, Inc., 4 County Line Rd., Hatboro, Pa. 19040 . . . . Air-Shields
*Alcon Laboratories, Inc., P.O. Box 1959, Fort Worth, Tex. 76101 . . . . Alcon
Alkalol Co., 141 Washington St., Taunton, Mass. 02780 . . . . Alkalol
Allen-Bradley Co., 1201 S. 2nd St., Milwaukee, Wis. 53204 . . . . Allen-Bradley
*Allergan Pharmaceuticals, Inc., 1000 S. Grand Ave., Santa Ana, Calif. 92705 . . . . Allergan
Allied Chemical Corp., 61 Broadway, New York, N.Y. 10006 . . . . Allied
Allis-Chalmers Mfg. Co., 864 S. 70th St., Milwaukee, Wis. 53214 . . . . Allis-Chalmers
Almay Hypo-Allergenic Cosmetic Div., Schieffelin & Co., 41 E. 42nd St., New York, N.Y. 10017 . . . . Almay
Almor Corp., 23343 Sherwood St., Warren, Mich. 48091 . . . . Almor
Alphaden Co., Inc., 6413 W. Irving Park Rd., Chicago, Ill. 60634 . . . . Alphaden
Alsop Engineering Corp., 1969 Norton St., Milldale, Conn. 06467 . . . . Alsop
Aluminum Co. of America, 1200 Alcoa Bldg., Pittsburgh, Pa. 15219 . . . . Alcoa
Amaco, Inc., 2601 W. Patterson Ave., Chicago, Ill. 60645 . . . . Amaco
Amchem Products, Inc., Box 33, Ambler, Pa. 19002 . . . . Amchem
American Air Filter Co., Inc., 200 Central Ave., Louisville, Ky. 40208 . . . . Am. Air
American Can Co., Drugs & Cosmetics Marketing, US Hwy. 22, Union, N.J. 07083 . . . . . Am. Can
American Chicle Co., 201 Tabor Rd., Morris Plains, N.J. 07950 . . . . Am. Chicle
American Cyanamid Co., Wayne, N.J. 07470 . . . . Am. Cyanamid
American Diabetes Association, 18 E. 48th St., New York, N.Y. 10017 . . . . Am. Diabetes
American Felsol Co., 200½ 9th St., Lorain, Ohio 44052 . . . . Am. Felsol
American Ferment Co., Inc., 90 Park Ave., New York, N.Y. 10016 . . . . Am. Ferment
American Instrument Co., Inc., 8130 Georgia Ave., Silver Spring, Md. 20910 . . . . Am. Instrument
American Machine & Foundry Co., 261 Madison Ave., New York, N.Y. 10016 . . . . Am. Machine
American Optical Corp., 14 Mechanic St., Southbridge, Mass. 01550 . . . . Am. Optical
American Pharmaceutical Co., 120 Bruckner Blvd., Bronx, N.Y. 10454 . . . . APC
American Sterilizer Co., 2400 W. 23rd St., Erie, Pa. 16506 . . . . Am. Sterilizer
American Viscose Div., FMC Corp., 1617 John F. Kennedy Blvd., Philadelphia, Pa. 19103 . . . . Am. Viscose
American Wheel Chair, 5500 Muddy Creek Rd., Cincinnati, Ohio 45238 . . . . Am. Wheel Chair
*Ames Co., 1127 Myrtle St., Elkhart, Ind. 46514 . . . . Ames
Amfre-Grant, Inc., 924 Rogers Ave., Brooklyn, N.Y. 11226 . . . . Amfre
Anderson-Stolz Corp., Inc., 1731 Walnut St., Kansas City, Mo. 64108 . . . . Anderson-Stolz
Anderson, V. D., Co., 1935 W. 96th St., Cleveland, Ohio 44102 . . . . Anderson
Antara Chemicals—see *GAF* . . . . Antara
Applied Physics Corp., 2724 S. Peck Rd., Monrovia, Calif. 91016 . . . . Applied Physics
Approved Pharmaceutical Corp., 114 Gifford St., Syracuse, N.Y. 13202 . . . . Approved
Aqua-Chem, Inc., Box 421, Milwaukee, Wis. 53201 . . . . Aqua-Chem
Arbeka Webbing Co., 1151 Roosevelt Ave., Pawtucket, R.I. 02865 . . . . Arbeka
Ar-Ex Products Co., 1036 W. Van Buren St., Chicago, Ill. 60607 . . . . Ar-Ex
*Armour Pharmaceutical Co., P.O. Box 1022, Chicago, Ill. 60690 . . . . Armour
Armstrong Cork Co., W. Liberty St., Lancaster, Pa. 17603 . . . . Armstrong
*Arnar-Stone Laboratories, Inc., 601 E. Kensington Rd., Mt. Prospect, Ill. 60056 . . . . Arnar-Stone
*Ascher, B. F., & Co., Inc., P.O Box 827, Kansas City, Mo. 64141 . . . . Ascher
Associated Concentrates Div., American Lecithin Co., Inc., 32-30 61st St., Woodside, N.Y. 11377 . . . . Assoc. Concentrates
*Astra Pharmaceutical Products, Inc., 7 Neponset St., Worcester, Mass. 01606 . . . . Astra
Atco Surgical Supports, Inc., 450 Portage Tr., Cuyahoga Falls, Ohio 44221 . . . . Atco
Atlantic Richfield Co., 260 S. Broad St., Philadelphia, Pa. 19102 . . . . Atlantic
Atlas Chemical Industries, Du Pont Bldg., Wilmington, Del. 19899 . . . . Atlas
Atlas Hospital Equipment Co., Inc., Windber, Pa. 15963 . . . . Atlas Hosp.
Atomic Accessories, Inc., 104 S. Central Ave., Valley Stream, N.Y. 11580 . . . . Atomic Accessories
Atomic Energy of Canada, Ltd., P.O. Box 93, Ottawa, Canada . . . . Atomic-Canada
Avondale Div., Hewlitt-Packard, Route 41, Avondale, Pa. 19311 . . . . Avondale
*Ayerst Laboratories, 685 3rd Ave., New York, N.Y. 10017 . . . . Ayerst

---

* Member, Pharmaceutical Manufacturers Association.
[a] This abbreviation is used in the text, immediately after the names of specialties, to indicate the name of the manufacturer.

Names and addresses	Abbreviations[a]

B

Baird-Atomic, Inc., 33 University Rd., Cambridge, Mass. 02138	Baird-Atomic
Baka Mfg. Co., Inc., 7-11 Cross St., Plainville, Mass. 02762	Baka
Baker, Co., Inc., Biddeford, Me. 04005	Baker
*Baker, J. T., Chemical Co., 600 N. Broad St., Phillipsburg, N.J. 08865	J. T. Baker
Baltimore Biological Laboratory, P.O. Box 175, Cockeysville, Md. 21030	BBL
Bard, C. R., Inc., 731 Central Ave., Murray Hill, N.J. 07974	Bard
*Barnes-Hind Pharmaceuticals, Inc., 895 Kifer Rd., Sunnyvale, Calif. 94086	Barnes-Hind
Barnstead Still & Sterilizer Co., 38 Rivermoor St., West Roxbury, Mass. 02132	Barnstead
Baroid Div., National Lead Co., Box 1675, Houston, Tex. 77001	Baroid
*Barry Laboratories, Inc., 461 N. E. 27th St., Pompano Beach, Fla. 33064	Barry
Bartlett-Snow, Inc., 6250 Harvard Ave., Cleveland, Ohio 44105	B & S
Bates Mfg. Co., 18 Central Ave., West Orange, N.J. 07051	Bates
Battle & Co., 3910 Lindell Blvd., St. Louis, Mo. 63108	Battle
Bauer & Black, 309 W. Jackson Blvd., Chicago, Ill. 60606	B & B
Baum, W. A., Co., Inc., Copiague, N.Y. 11726	Baum
Bausch & Lomb, Inc., 626–69 Lomb Park, Rochester, N.Y. 14602	B & L
*Baxter Laboratories, Inc., 6301 Lincoln Ave., Morton Grove, Ill. 60053	Baxter
Baxter Laboratories of Canada, Ltd., Malton, Ontario, Canada	Baxter-Canada
Baybank Drug Co., Inc., 1000 Stewart Ave., Garden City, N.Y. 11530	Baybank
Beckman Instruments, Inc., 2500 Harbor Blvd., Fullerton, Calif. 92634	Beckman
*Becton, Dickinson & Co., Stanley St., Rutherford, N.J. 07070	BD & Co.
Bel-Art Products, 6 Industrial Rd., Pequannock, N.J. 07440	Bel-Art
Bell-Craig, Inc., 41–14 27th St., Long Island City, N.Y. 11101	Bell-Craig
Belmont Laboratories Co., 4730 Market St., Philadelphia, Pa. 19139	Belmont
Benet Drug Corp., DARA Products, 1817 Mentor Ave., Cincinnati, Ohio 45212	Benet
Bentex Oil Corp., Benedum-Trees Bldg., Pittsburgh, Pa. 15222	Bentex
Best Foods, 10 E. 56th St., New York, N.Y. 10022	Best Foods
Better Built Machinery Corp., 441 Market St., Saddle Brook, N.J. 07662	Better Built
Better Sleep Mfg. Co., Berkeley Heights, N.J. 07922	Better Sleep
Bilhuber, E., Inc.—see *Knoll*	Bilhuber
Biochemical Research Laboratories, Inc., 1 E. Walton Pl., Chicago, Ill. 60611	Biochemical Research
*BioQuest, P.O. Box 175, Cockeysville, Md. 21030	BioQuest
Bio-Rad Laboratories, Richmond, Calif. 94002	Bio-Rad
Bird Machine Co., Racaduc Rd., South Walpole, Mass. 02071	Bird Machine
Bischoff, Ernst, Co., Inc.—see *Miles*	Bischoff
Bishop Laboratories, Inc., 374 50th St., Brooklyn, N.Y. 11220	Bishop
Bittner Industries, Inc., 639 Diaz St., Prichard, Ala. 36610	Bittner
*Blue Line Chemical Co., 302 S. Broadway, St. Louis, Mo. 63102	Bluline
Borcherdt Co., 217 N. Wolcott Ave., Chicago, Ill. 60612	Borcherdt
Borden Co., Pharmaceutical Div., 350 Madison Ave., New York, N.Y. 10017	Borden
Borg-Erickson Corp., 1133 N. Kilbourn Ave., Chicago, Ill. 60651	Borg-Erickson
Bowen Engineering, Inc., 3 Station Rd., North Branch, N.J. 08876	Bowen Eng.
*Bowman, Inc., 965 Cleveland Ave., N.W., Canton, Ohio 44702	Bowman
Boyle & Co., 6330 Chalet Dr., Los Angeles, Calif. 90203	Boyle
Bradley-Sun Div.—see *Am. Can*	Bradley-Sun
*Brayten Pharmaceutical Co., 1715 W. 38th St., Chattanooga, Tenn. 37409	Brayten
Brearley Co., 2107 Kishwaukee St., Rockford, Ill. 61105	Brearley
Breck, John H., Inc., Berdan Ave., Wayne, N.J. 07470	Breck
*Breon Laboratories, Inc., 90 Park Ave., New York, N.Y. 10016	Breon
Brewer & Co., Box 190, Mystic, Conn. 06355	Brewer
Brinkmann Instruments, Inc., Cantiague Rd., Westbury, N.Y. 11590	Brinkmann
*Bristol Laboratories, Inc., P.O. Box 657, Syracuse, N.Y. 13201	Bristol
British Drug Houses, Ltd., Graham St. L, London N 1, England	British Drug
Brookfield Engineering Laboratories, Inc., 240 Cushing St., Stoughton, Mass. 02072	Brookfield
Brown Co., 150 Causeway St., Boston, Mass. 02114	Brown
Buck, E. R., Chain Co., Clinton, Mass. 01510	Buck
Buffington's, Inc., 328 Shrewsbury St., Worcester, Mass. 01604	Buffington
Builders Sheet Metal Works, Inc., 108 Wooster St., New York, N.Y. 10012	Builders
Bundy, C. M., Co., 329 Perry St., Cincinnati, Ohio 45202	Bundy
Burnham Soluble Iodine Div., Morgan Products Corp., 160 E. 127th St., New York, N.Y. 10035	Burnham
Burrough Bros. Pharmaceuticals, Inc., 714 E. Pratt St., Baltimore, Md. 21202	Burrough Bros.
*Burroughs Wellcome & Co. (USA) Inc., 1 Scarsdale Rd., Tuckahoe, N.Y. 10707	Burroughs-Wellcome
Burton, Parsons & Co., Inc., 7351 86th Ave., Washington, D.C. 20027	Burton, Parsons

C

C. S. C. Pharmaceuticals, 245 Madison Ave., New York, N.Y. 10016	CSC
Cabot Corp., 125 High St., Boston, Mass. 02110	Cabot
Calley & Currier Co., Bristol, N.H. 03222	Calley & Currier
Ca-Ma-Sil Co., 52 "O" St., N.W., Washington, D.C. 20001	Ca-Ma-Sil
Cambridge Filter Corp., 7647 7th North Rd., Syracuse, N.Y. 13201	Cambridge
Camp, S. H., & Co., P.O. Box 89, Jackson, Mich. 49201	Camp
Campbell, G. M., Products Co., 125 W. 40th St., New York, N.Y. 10018	G. M. Campbell
Campbell Pharmaceuticals, Inc.—see *Ayerst*	Campbell
Cannon Instrument Co., Box 812, University Park, Pa. 16802	Cannon
Carbide & Carbon Chemicals Co.—see *Union Carbide*	Carbide
*Carbisulphoil Co., 2917 Swiss Ave., Dallas, Tex. 75204	Carbisulphoil
Cardiosonic Instruments, Medical Products Div., 3M Co., 23 Bay State Rd., Cambridge, Mass. 02138	Cardiosonic
Carlisle Chemical Works Inc., West St., Cincinnati, Ohio 45215	Carlisle
Carnes, A. H., Co., 75 E. Wacker Dr., Chicago, Ill. 60601	Carnes
*Carnrick Laboratories, 65 Horse Hill Rd., Cedar Knolls, N.J. 07927	Carnrick

Names and addresses	Abbreviations[a]
Carrom Div., Affiliated Hospital Products, Inc., Box 310, Ludington, Mich. 49431	Carrom
Carron Products Co., 331 N. Lawrence St., Philadelphia, Pa. 19106	Carron
Carter Products, Inc., 2 Park Ave., New York, N.Y. 10016	Carter
Cary Line, The—see *Inst. Ind.*	Cary
Casco Products Corp., 512 Hancock Ave., Bridgeport, Conn. 06602	Casco
Castle Co., 1777 E. Henrietta St., Rochester, N.Y. 14623	Castle
Cavendish Pharmaceutical Corp., 1460 Chestnut Ave., Hillside, N.J. 07205	Cavendish
Celanese Chemical Co., 245 Park Ave., New York, N.Y. 10017	Celanese
*Central Pharmacal Co., 116–128 E. 3rd St., Seymour, Ind. 47274	Central
Central Scientific Co., 2600 S. Kostner Ave., Chicago, Ill. 60623	Central Scientific
Century Laboratories, Inc., 4936 Veterans Memorial Hwy., Metairie, La. 70004	Century
Chase-Logeman Corp., 633 Bergen St., Brooklyn, N.Y. 11238	Chase-Logeman
Chatham Pharmaceuticals, Inc., 901 Broad St., Newark, N.J. 07102	Chatham
Chemagro Corp., P.O. Box 4913, Kansas City, Mo. 64120	Chemagro
Chemical & Pharmaceutical Industry Co., Inc., 260 W. Broadway, New York, N.Y. 10013	ChemiPharm
Chemicolloid Laboratories, Inc., 55 Herrick Rd., Garden City Park, N.Y. 11040	Chemicolloid
Cherry-Burrell Corp., 105 W. Adams St., Chicago, Ill. 60603	Cherry-Burrell
Chesebrough-Pond's, Inc., 485 Lexington Ave., New York, N.Y. 10017	Chesebrough-Pond's
Chester-Kent, Inc., P.O. Box 3383, St. Paul, Minn. 55101	Chester-Kent
Chevron Chemical.—see *Ortho-Chevron*	Chevron
Chicago Dietetic Supply House, Inc., 405 E. Shawmut Ave., La Grange, Ill. 60525	Chicago Dietetic
Chicopee Mills, Inc., Baby Products Div., 1450 Broadway, New York, N.Y. 10018	Chicopee
Chipman Chemicals, Ltd., 519 Parkdale Ave., N., P.O. Box 100, Postal Station C, Hamilton, Ontario, Canada	Chipman
Christina, Vincent, & Co., Inc., 401 Troy Ave., Brooklyn, N.Y. 11213	Christina
Christy Machine Co., 108 Brichard Ave., Fremont, Ohio 43420	Christy
*Ciba Pharmaceutical Co., 556 Morris Ave., Summit, N.J. 07901	Ciba
Cleary, W. A., Corp., P.O. Box 749, New Brunswick, N.J. 08903	Cleary
Coastal Pharmaceutical Co., Inc., 1022 W. 27th St., Norfolk, Va. 23517	Coastal
Cochrane Div., Crane Co., P.O. Box 191, King of Prussia, Pa. 19406	Cochrane
*Cole Pharmacal Co., Inc., 3721 Laclede Ave., St. Louis, Mo. 63108	Cole
Colgate-Palmolive Co., 300 Park Ave., New York, N.Y. 10022	Colgate
Colson Corp., 39 S. La Salle St., Chicago, Ill. 60603	Colson
Colton, Arthur, Co.—see *Colton-Kiefer*	Colton
Colton-Kiefer Div., Cherry-Burrell Corp., 656 Busse Hwy., Park Ridge, Ill. 60068	Colton-Kiefer
*Commercial Solvents Corp., 245 Park Ave., New York, N.Y. 10017	Commercial Solvents
*Conal Pharmaceuticals, Inc., Chicago Pharmacal Div., 5547 N. Ravenswood Ave., Chicago, Ill. 60640	Conal
Conco, Inc., Conco Rd., Mendota, Ill. 61342	Conco
Consolidated Electrodynamics, N. Sierra Madre Villa & Foothill Blvd., Pasadena, Calif. 91109	Consol. Electrodynamics
Consolidated Midland Corp., CMC Research Div., 15 Parkway, Katonah, N.Y. 10536	Consolidated
Consolidated Packaging Machinery Corp., 1900 West Ave., Buffalo, N.Y. 14213	Consolidated Packaging
Consolidated Products Co., Inc., 156 Observer Hwy., Hoboken, N.J. 07030	Consolidated Prod.
Contamination Control, Inc., 100 Forty Fort Rd., Kulpsville, Pa. 19443	Contamination Control
Continental Can Co., 633 3rd Ave., New York, N.Y. 10017	Continental Can
Continental Hospital Industries, Inc., 18636 Detroit St., Cleveland, Ohio 44107	Continental Hosp.
Controlled Environment Equipment Corp., 344 South Ave., Whitman, Mass. 02382	Controlled Environment
Cooper Laboratories, Inc., P.O. Box 190, Mystic, Conn. 06355	Cooper
Corning Glass Works, 80 Houghton Park, Corning, N.Y. 14830	Corning
Coulter Electronics, Inc., 2601 Mannheim St., Franklin Park, Ill. 60131	Coulter
Cove-Craft, Inc., P.O. Box 307, Laconia, N.H. 03246	Cove-Craft
Cozzoli Machine Co., 403 E. 3rd St., Plainfield, N.J. 07060	Cozzoli
Crane Co., 4100 S. Kedzie Ave., Chicago, Ill. 60632	Crane
Crookes-Barnes Laboratories, Inc., 328 Shewsbury St., Worcester, Mass. 01604	Crookes-Barnes
Crown Cork & Seal Co., Inc., 9300 Ashton Rd., Philadelphia, Pa. 19114	Crown
*Cutter Laboratories, 4th & Parker Sts., Berkeley, Calif. 94710	Cutter

D

DCA Food Industries, Inc., 45 W. 36th St., New York, N.Y. 10018	DCA
*DPI Div., Eastman Chemical Products, Inc., Kingsport, Tenn. 37662	DPI
Dade Reagents, Inc., 1851 Delaware Pkwy., Miami, Fla. 33125	Dade Reagents
Dahlberg Electronics, Inc., Miracle Ear Dept., 7735 6th Ave., N., Minneapolis, Minn. 55427	Dahlberg
Dartell Laboratories, Inc., 1226 S. Flower St., Los Angeles, Calif. 90015	Dartell
*Davies, Rose Hoyt Pharmaceutical Div., Kendall Co., 633 Highland Ave., Needham, Mass. 02194	Davies-Rose
*Davis & Geck, Inc., Pearl River, N.Y. 10965	Davis & Geck
Davol, Inc., 69 Point St., Providence, R. I. 02901	Davol
Day, J. H., Co., 4932 Beech St., Cincinnati, Ohio 45212	Day
Dean Rubber Mfg. Co., 1601 Iron St., North Kansas City, Mo. 64116	Dean
De Lucien, Inc., 417 E. Madison St., South Bend, Ind. 46622	De Lucien
Dennison Mfg. Co., 67 Ford Ave., Framingham, Mass. 01701	Dennison
Denver Chemical Mfg. Co., Inc., 35 Commerce Rd., Stamford, Conn. 06902	Denver
De Pree Co., 130 Central Ave., Holland, Mich. 49423	De Pree
Desitin Chemical Co.—see *Leeming/Pacquin*	Desitin
DeVilbiss Co., P.O. Box 552, Somerset, Pa. 15501	DeVilbiss
Dewey & Almy Chemical Div., W. R. Grace & Co., 62 Whittemore Ave., Cambridge, Mass. 02140	Dewey & Almy
Dietene Co.—see *D. M. Doyle*	Dietene
*Difco Laboratories, 920 Henry St., Detroit, Mich. 48201	Difco
Dios Chemical Co., 4200 Laclede Ave., St. Louis, Mo. 63108	Dios

Names and addresses	Abbreviations[a]

Doak Pharmacal Co., Inc., 2000 Shames Dr., Westbury, N.Y. 11590.................Doak
Doho Chemical Corp.—see *Ayerst*..Doho
*Dome Laboratories, 400 Morgan Ln., West Haven, Conn. 06516................Dome
Donley-Evans & Co., 5239 Brown Ave., St. Louis, Mo. 63115..................Donley-Evans
Dorr-Oliver, Inc., 77 Havemeyer Ln., Stamford, Conn. 06904.................Dorr-Oliver
*Dorsey Laboratories, N.E. US 6 & I-80, Lincoln, Neb. 68501.................Dorsey
Dow Chemical Co., Midland, Mich. 48640...................................Dow
Dow Chemical Co., P.O. Box 1656, Indianapolis, Ind. 46206.................Dow-PM
Dow Corning Corp., Midland, Mich. 48640..................................Dow-Corning
Doyle, D. M., Pharmaceutical Co., 2330 Hwy. 100 S., Minneapolis, Minn. 55416..D. M. Doyle
Drug Products Co., Inc., 230 Broad St., Bloomfield, N.J. 07003.............Drug Products
Drugmaster, Inc., 2700 Wagner Pl., Maryland Heights, Mo. 63042............Drugmaster
Dubin, H. E., Laboratories, 800 2nd Ave., New York, N.Y. 10017............Dubin
Duke Laboratories, Inc., Duke Pl., South Norwalk, Conn. 06854.............Duke
Dumas-Wilson & Co.—see *Mallinckrodt*...................................Dumas
*Du Pont Pharmaceuticals Div., E. I. du Pont de Nemours & Co., Inc., 1007
    Market St., Wilmington, Del. 19898...............................Du Pont
Durex Products, Inc., 684 Broadway, New York, N.Y. 10012.................Durex
*Durst, S. F., & Co., Inc., 5317 N. 3rd St., Philadelphia, Pa. 19120......Durst
Dynac Corp., Thompson's Point, Portland, Me. 04102.......................Dynac

E

Eaton Laboratories, 17 Eaton Ave., Norwich, N.Y. 13815...................Eaton
Edco International Corp., 19302 W. Grand River St., Detroit, Mich. 48223..Edco
Edcraft Industries, Inc., 618 Commerce Rd., Linden, N.J. 07036...........Edcraft
Elder, Paul B., Co., P.O. Box 31, Bryan, Ohio 43506......................Elder
Electro-Air Div., Emerson Electric Co., Olivia & Sproul Sts., McKees Rocks, Pa. 15136..Electro-Air
Elkins-Sinn, Inc., 22 Cherry Hill Industrial Ctr., Cherry Hill, N.J. 08034..Elkins-Sinn
Emkay Chemical Co., 321 2nd St., Elizabeth, N.J. 07206...................Emkay
Emko Co., 7912 Manchester Ave., St. Louis, Mo. 63143....................Emko
Emulsol Equipment, Inc., 300 W. Washington St., Chicago, Ill. 60606.....Emulsol
*Endo Laboratories, Inc., 1000 Stewart Ave., Garden City, N.Y. 11530.....Endo
Entoleter, Inc., P.O. Box 1919, New Haven, Conn. 06509..................Entoleter
Envirco, P.O. Box 6098, Albuquerque, N.M. 87107.........................Envirco
Erie City Mfg. Co., 1030 W. 12th St., Erie, Pa. 16501...................Erie
Ertel Engineering Co., 20 Front St., Kingston, N.Y. 12401...............Ertel
Esta Medical Laboratories, Inc., 902 Broadway, New York, N.Y. 10010.....Esta
*Ethicon, Inc., US Hwy. 22, Somerville, N.J. 08876......................Ethicon
Evenflo Products, 771 N. Freedom St., Ravenna, Ohio 44266...............Evenflo
Everest & Jennings, Inc., 1803 Pontius Ave., Los Angeles, Calif. 90025..Everest & Jennings
Evron Pharmaceutical Co., Inc., 7475 N. Rogers Ave., Chicago, Ill. 60626..Evron

F

F & M Scientific Corp.—see *Avondale*...................................F & M
Faichney Instrument Corp., Gray-Landon Bldg., Watertown, N.Y. 13601.....Faichney
Farastan Co., Inc., 2126 E. Somerset St., Philadelphia, Pa. 19134.......Farastan
Faultless Rubber Co., 268 E. 4th St., Ashland, Ohio 44805...............Faultless
Fecker, J. W., Div., American Optical Co., 4709 Baum Blvd., Pittsburgh, Pa. 15213..Fecker
Fellows Medical Mfg. Co., Inc., 1354 W. Lafayette Blvd., Detroit, Mich. 48226..Fellows
Fellows-Testagar—see *Fellows*...Fellows-Testagar
*Ferndale Laboratories & Surgical, Inc., 780 W. 8 Mile Rd., Ferndale, Mich. 48220..Ferndale
*Fine Chemicals Dept., American Cyanamid Co., Pearl River, N.Y. 10965...Fine Chemicals
First Machinery Corp., 209 10th St., Brooklyn, N.Y. 11215...............FMC
*First Texas Pharmaceuticals, Inc., P.O. Box 5026, Dallas, Tex. 75222...First Texas
Fisher Scientific Co., 203 Fisher Bldg., Pittsburgh, Pa. 15219.........Fisher
Fitzpatrick Co., 812 Industrial Dr., Elmhurst, Ill. 60126..............Fitzpatrick
*Fleet, C. B., Co., Inc., P.O. Box 1100, Lynchburg, Va. 24505..........Fleet
Fleming & Co., 9730 Reavis Pk. Dr., St. Louis, Mo. 63123...............Fleming
*Flint Laboratories, Inc., 6301 Lincoln Ave., Morton Grove, Ill. 60053..Flint
Fluid Chemical Co., Inc., 878 Mt. Prospect Ave., Newark, N.J. 07104....Fluid Chemical
Fluid Energy Processing & Equipment Co., 153 Penn Ave., Hatfield, Pa. 19440..Fluid Energy
Foremost Dairies, Inc., 111 Pine St., San Francisco, Calif. 94111......Foremost
Formulette Co., 47-25 27th St., Long Island City, N.Y. 11101...........Formulette
Foster-Milburn Co., 468 Dewitt St., Buffalo, N.Y. 14213................Foster-Milburn
*Fougera, E., & Co., Inc., P.O. Box 73, Hicksville, N.Y. 11802.........Fougera
Freeda Pharmaceuticals, 110 E. 41st St., New York, N.Y. 10017..........Freeda
Fritzsche Brothers, Inc., 76 9th Ave., New York, N.Y. 10011............Fritzsche
Frohock-Stewart Co., Box 648, Worcester, Mass. 01601...................Frohock-Stewart
Frosst, Charles E., & Co., 350 Selby St., Montreal 6, Quebec, Canada...Frosst

G

GAF Corp., 140 W. 51st St., New York, N.Y. 10020.......................GAF
Galen Co.—see *Nopco*..Galen
Gane's Chemical Works, Inc., 535 5th Ave., New York, N.Y. 10017........Gane's
Gardner, R. W., Firm of, Inc., 372 Henry St., Orange, N.J. 07050.......Gardner
Garret Laboratories, Inc., 448 Equitable Bldg., Baltimore, Md. 21202...Garret
Gebauer Chemical Co., 9410 St. Catherine Ave., Cleveland, Ohio 44104...Gebauer
*Geigy Pharmaceuticals, Saw Mill River Rd., Ardsley, N.Y. 10502........Geigy
Gelatin Products Co., 9425 Grinnell Ave., Detroit, Mich. 48213.........Gelatin Prod.
Gelman Instrument Co., 600 S. Wagner Rd., Ann Arbor, Mich. 48106.......Gelman
Gendron Wheel Co.—see *Howmet*...Gendron
General Aniline & Film Corp.—see *GAF*.................................Gen. Aniline

Names and addresses	Abbreviations[a]

General Dynamics Corp., 1 Rockefeller Plaza, New York, N.Y. 10020.................Gen. Dynamics
George Glove Co., Inc., 27 Haynes Ave., Newark, N.J. 07114.....................George Glove
Geoscience Instruments Corp., 435 E. 3rd St., Mt. Vernon, N.Y. 10553.............Geoscience
Gerber Products Co., 445 State St., Fremont, Mich. 49412.......................Gerber
Glenbrook Laboratories, 90 Park Ave., New York, N.Y. 10016....................Glenbrook
Glenwood Labs, Inc., 83 Summit St., Tenafly, N.J. 07670........................Glenwood
Glidden-Durkee Div., SCM Corp., 900 Union Commerce Bldg., Cleveland, Ohio 44115. Glidden
Glyco Chemicals, Inc., P.O. Box 330, Williamsport, Pa. 17701....................Glyco
Gold Leaf Pharmacal Co., Inc., 223 S. Dean St., Englewood, N.J. 07631...........Gold Leaf
Goldschmidt Chemical Div., Wilson Pharmaceutical & Chemical Corp., 153
  Waverly Pl., New York, N.Y. 10014...Goldschmidt
Gotham Pharmaceutical Co., Inc., 1840 McDonald Ave., Brooklyn, N.Y. 11223........Gotham
Grace, W. R., & Co., Agricultural Products Div., 3 Hanover Sq., New York, N.Y.
  10004..Grace
Graham Mfg. Co., 56 Canal St., Holyoke, Mass. 01040...........................Graham
Grand Rapids Sectional Equipment Co., 200 Fuller Bldg., Grand Rapids, Mich. 49503. Grand Rapids
Grant Chemical Co., Inc., 924 Rogers Ave., Brooklyn, N.Y. 11226.................Grant
Gray Pharmaceutical Co., Inc., 50 Axminster St., Yonkers, N.Y. 10701.............Gray
Gricks, Inc., 202-11 Jamaica Ave., Hollis, N.Y. 11423...........................Gricks
Guard Chemical Co., Inc., N. Water St., Ossining, N.Y. 10562....................Guard
Guardian Chemical Corp., 41-45 Crescent St., Long Island City, N.Y. 11101.........Guardian

H

Haag, Inc., 1503 E. Main St., Richmond, Va. 23219.............................Haag
Hall, C. P., Co., 414 Broadway, Akron, Ohio 44308.............................C. P. Hall
Hankscraft Co., P.O. Box 120, Reedsburg, Wis., 53959..........................Hankscraft
Hard Mfg. Co., 50 Watts St., Buffalo, N.Y. 14207..............................Hard
Harshaw Chemical Co., 1933 E. 97th St., Cleveland, Ohio 44106..................Harshaw
Hart, E. J., & Co., Ltd., 508 Chartres St., New Orleans, La. 70130................E. J. Hart
Harvey, G. F., Co., Inc., 99-101 Sawmill River Rd., Yonkers, N.Y. 10701...........Harvey
Haskell, Charles C., & Co., Inc.,—see *Arnar-Stone*.............................Haskell
*Haver-Lockhart Laboratories, 12707 W. 63rd St., Shawnee Mission, Kan. 66201........Haver-Lockhart
Heun, E. W., Co., 2303 Schuetz Rd., St. Louis, Mo. 63141........................Heun
Heyden Div., Tenneco Chemicals, Inc., 280 Park Ave., New York, N.Y. 10017.........Heyden
Hobart Laboratories, Inc., 900 N. Franklin St., Chicago, Ill. 60610...............Hobart
*Hoechst Pharmaceutical Co., 1385 Tennessee Ave., Cincinnati, Ohio 45229.............Hoechst
*Hoffman-La Roche, Inc., 340 Kingsland St., Nutley, N.J. 07110...................Hoffman-La Roche
Holland-Rantos Co., Inc., 393 7th Ave., New York, N.Y. 10001...................Holland-Rantos
*Hollister-Stier Laboratories, 3525 N. Regal St., Spokane, Wash. 99207..............Hollister-Stier
Homemakers Products Div.—see *Breon*.......................................Homemakers
Hormann, F. R., Co., Inc., Milldale, Conn. 06467..............................Hormann
Horn, Wm. H., & Brother, 451 N. 3rd St., Philadelphia, Pa. 19123................Horn & Bro.
Horton & Converse, 621 W. Pico Blvd., Los Angeles, Calif. 90015.................Horton & Converse
Hospital Liquids, Inc.—see *McGaw*...Hospital Liquids
Hospital & Orthopedic Aides Co., 3640 N.W. 41st St., Miami, Fla. 33142...........Hosp. & Ortho. Aides
Howmet Corp. of Ohio, Hospital Div., Lugbill Rd., Archbold, Ohio 43502...........Howmet
Hull Corp., Davisville Rd., Hatboro, Pa. 19040...............................Hull
Humble Oil & Refining Co., Box 2180, Houston, Tex. 77001.......................Humble
*Hyland Div., Travenol Laboratories, Inc., 4501 Colorado Blvd., Los Angeles, Calif.
  90039..Hyland
*Hynson, Westcott & Dunning, Inc., Charles & Chase Sts., Baltimore, Md. 21201.....Hynson
Hypo Surgical Supply Corp., 11 Mercer St., New York, N.Y. 10013.................Hypo
Hy-Tape, Surgical Hosiery Corp., 4090 Broadway, New York, N.Y. 10032............Hy-Tape

I

Ille Electric Corp., Reach & Quality Sts., Williamsport, Pa. 17701................Ille
Industrial Dynamics Div., American Sterilizer Co., 2400 W. 23rd St., Erie, Pa. 16512..Industrial Dynamics
Ingram Pharmaceutical Co., 202 Green St., San Francisco, Calif. 94111............Ingram
Inland Bed Co., 2900 W. 36th St., Chicago, Ill. 60632..........................Inland Bed
Institutional Industries, 5500 Muddy Creek Rd., Cincinnati, Ohio 45238............Inst. Ind.
Interchemical Corp., 1133 Ave. of the Americas, New York, N.Y. 10036............Interchemical
International Flavors & Fragrances, Ltd., Enfield, Middlesex, England............Intern. Flavors
Internationale Treuhand AG, Basel, Switzerland.............................Intern. Treuhand
*Ives Laboratories, Inc., 685 3rd Ave., New York, N.Y. 10017.....................Ives

J

Jackson-Mitchell Pharmaceuticals, Inc., P.O. Box 30055, Santa Barbara, Calif. 93105..Jackson
Jamieson Pharmacal Co., Inc., 310 Madison Ave., New York, N.Y. 10017...........Jamieson
Jewell Pharmaceuticals, Inc., 508 Franklin Ave., Mt. Vernon, N.Y. 10553..........Jewell
*Johnson & Johnson, 501 George St., New Brunswick, N.J. 08901..................J & J
Jones Metal Products Co., 59 Donovan St., West Lafayette, Ohio 43845............Jones Metal
Jung Products, Inc., 312 E. Court St., Cincinnati, Ohio 45202....................Jung

K

Kadan, D. A., Co., Inc., 29 Clinton St., Yonkers, N.Y. 10701.....................Kadan
Kahlenberg Laboratories, P.O. Box 3318, Sarasota, Fla. 33578....................Kahlenberg
Kartridg Pak Co., 807 W. Kimberly Rd., Davenport, Iowa 52808..................Kartridg-Pak
Kelco Co., Clark, N.J. 07066...Kelco
Keleket/CGR Corp., 1603 Trapelo Rd., Waltham, Mass. 02154..................Keleket

	Names and addresses	Abbreviations[a]

Kent Machine Works, Inc., 37 Gold St., Brooklyn, N.Y. 11201.................**Kent**
Kenwood Laboratories, Inc., 39 Lawton St., New Rochelle, N.Y. 10801..........**Kenwood**
Kessler Chemical Co., State Rd. & Cottman Ave., Philadelphia, Pa. 19111.......**Kessler**
Kessling, E., Thermometer Co., Inc., 682 Jamaica Ave., Brooklyn, N.Y. 11208......**Kessling**
Ketchum Laboratories, Inc., 26 Edison St., Amityville, N.Y. 11701.............**Ketchum**
Key Pharmaceuticals, 50 N.W. 176th St., Miami, Fla. 33169..................**Key**
Kiefer, Karl, Machine Co.—see *Colton-Kiefer* ....**Kiefer**
Kimble Glass Co.—see *Owens-Illinois*..................................**Kimble**
*Kinney & Co., Inc., P.O. Box 307, Columbus, Ind. 47201....................**Kinney**
Knapp Mills, Inc., 23-15 Borden Ave., Long Island City, N.Y. 11101............**Knapp**
Knight, Maurice A., 171 Kelly Ave., Akron, Ohio 44306......................**Knight**
*Knoll Pharmaceutical Co., 377 Crane St., Orange, N.J. 07050................**Knoll**
Kontes Glass Co., 9000 Spruce St., Vineland, N.J. 08360....................**Kontes**
*Kremers-Urban Co., P.O. Box 2038, Milwaukee, Wis. 53201...................**Kremers-Urban**

L

*Lafayette Pharmacal, Inc., 526 N. Earl Ave., Lafayette, Ind. 47904...............**Lafayette**
*Lakeside Laboratories, Inc., 1707 E. North Ave., Milwaukee, Wis. 53201..........**Lakeside**
Laminaire Corp., 1575 Irving St., Rahway, N.J. 07065.......................**Laminaire**
LaMotte Chemical Products Co., Chestertown, Md. 21620....................**LaMotte**
Lanteen Medical Laboratories, Inc.—see *Esta*...........................**Lanteen**
LaWall & Harrisson Research Laboratories, 1921 Walnut St., Philadelphia, Pa. 19103..**LaWall**
*Lederle Laboratories, Pearl River, N.Y. 10965............................**Lederle**
Leeds & Northrup Co., 4901 Stenton Ave., Philadelphia, Pa. 19144.............**Leeds, Northrup**
Leeming, Thos., & Co., Inc.—see *Leeming/Pacquin*.......................**Leeming**
Leeming/Pacquin Divs., Chas. Pfizer & Co., Inc., 235 E. 42nd St., New York,
   N.Y. 10017...**Leeming/Pacquin**
Lehn & Fink Consumer Products, 225 Summit Ave., Montvale, N.J. 07645.........**Lehn & Fink**
*Lemmon Pharmacal Co., P.O. Box 30, Sellersville, Pa. 18960.................**Lemmon**
Levy, Harry, Co., 118 E. 129th St., New York, N.Y. 10035....................**Levy**
Lewal Pharmaceutical Co., 4149 N. Milwaukee St., Chicago, Ill. 60641...........**Lewal**
Liberty Vitamin Corp., 924 Rogers Ave., Brooklyn, N.Y. 11226................**Liberty**
*Lilly, Eli, & Co., Box 618, Indianapolis, Ind. 46206.........................**Lilly**
Lincoln Laboratories, Inc., P.O. Box 1139, Decatur, Ill. 62525.................**Lincoln**
Little Mfg. Co., Box 202, Wadesboro, N.C. 28170...........................**Little**
Lloyd Brothers, Inc.—see *Hoechst*...................................**Lloyd**
Lloyd, Dabney & Westerfield, Inc., 3941 Brotherton Rd., Cincinnati, Ohio 45209.....**Lloyd, D & W**
Lobica-Debruille, Inc.—see *Consolidated*..............................**Lobica-Debruille**
Loeb Dietetic Food Co., Inc., 4378 Broadway, New York, N.Y. 10033............**Loeb Dietetic**
Loeb Equipment Supply Co., 4131 S. State St., Chicago, Ill. 60609..............**Loeb**
Luxo Lamp Corp., 100 Dock St., Port Chester, N.Y. 10573...................**Luxo**

M

M & D Store Fixtures Div., Walter Kidde & Co., Inc., 650 W. Duarte St., Arcadia,
   Calif. 91006..**M & D**
MacGregor Instrument Co., 1000 Highland Ave., Needham Heights, Mass. 02194......**MacGregor**
Magnus, Mabee & Reynard Div., BFM Corp., 16 Desbrosses St., New York, N.Y.
   10013..**Magnus**
Mah-Zell Precision Products Co., 115 Lexington Ave., Brooklyn, N.Y. 11238........**Mah-Zell**
*Mallard, Inc., 3021 Wabash Ave., Detroit, Mich. 48216......................**Mallard**
*Mallinckrodt Pharmaceuticals, 3600 N. 2nd St., St. Louis, Mo. 63147...........**Mallinckrodt**
Manton Gaulin Mfg. Co., Inc., 67 Garden St., Everett, Mass. 02149.............**Manton Gaulin**
Marcelle Hypo-Allergenic Cosmetics, 350 Madison Ave., New York, N.Y. 10007.....**Marcelle**
Marco & Son, Inc., P.O. Box 102, Oakhurst, N.J. 07755......................**Marco**
*Marion Laboratories, Inc., P.O. Box 963, Kansas City, Mo. 64141..............**Marion**
Marschall Div., Miles Laboratories, Inc., P.O. Box 188, Clifton, N.J. 07015.........**Marschall**
Marvell Pharmacal Co., 55 W. 16th St., New York, N.Y. 10011................**Marvell**
*Massengill, S. E., Co., 527 5th St., Bristol, Tenn. 37620....................**Massengill**
Mathe Chemical Co., 171 Millbank St., Lodi, N.J. 07644.....................**Mathe**
Matthews Research, Inc., S. Gordon & Wheeler Sts., Alexandria, Va. 22304........**Matthews Res.**
Maywood Div., Stepan Chemical Co., 100 W. Hunter Ave., Maywood, N.J. 07607....**Maywood**
McCourt Label Cabinet Co., 42-54 Bennett St., Bradford, Pa. 16701.............**McCourt**
McGaw Laboratories, Milledgeville, Ga. 31061............................**McGaw**
*McKesson Laboratories, P.O. Box 548, Bridgeport, Conn. 06602...............**McKesson**
*McNeil Laboratories, Inc., Camp Hill Rd., Fort Washington, Pa. 19034..........**McNeil**
*Mead Johnson Laboratories, 2404 Pennsylvania St., Evansville, Ind. 47721........**Mead-Johnson**
Mears-Kane-Ofeldt, Inc., Church St., Bridgeport, Pa. 19405..................**Mears**
Med-A-Safe Div., Hayes-Albion Corp., Route 2, Whitmore Lake, Mich. 48189.......**Med-A-Safe**
Medical Arts Supply Co., Inc., 706 4th Ave., Huntington, W. Va. 25701...........**Medical Arts**
Medical Chemicals, Inc., 406 E. Water St., Baltimore, Md. 21202...............**Medical Chemicals**
Medical Times Overseas, Inc., Professional Service Div., Manhasset, N.Y. 11030....**Medical Times**
Medico Chemical Corp. of America, 274 Madison Ave., New York, N.Y. 10016......**Medico**
Medicone Co., 225 Varick St., New York, N.Y. 10014.......................**Medicone**
Medics Instrument Corp., 4221 Ft. Hamilton Pkwy., Brooklyn, N.Y. 11219.........**Medics**
Melrose Mfg. Co., 95 Commercial St., Brooklyn, N.Y. 11222..................**Melrose**
Menda Co., 53 W. Union St., Pasadena, Calif. 91101........................**Menda**
Menley & James Laboratories, 1500 Spring Garden St., Philadelphia, Pa. 19101......**Menley & James**
*Merck & Co., Inc., 126 E. Lincoln Ave., Rahway, N.J. 07065.................**Merck**
*Merck Chemical Div., Merck & Co., Inc., 126 E. Lincoln Ave., Rahway, N.J. 07065..**Merck Chemical**
*Merck Sharp & Dohme, West Point, Pa. 19486............................**MSD**
*Merrell, Wm. S., Co., Lockland Station, Cincinnati, Ohio 45215...............**Merrell**
Metropolitan Life Insurance Co., 1 Madison Ave., New York, N.Y. 10010.........**Metropolitan Life**

Names and addresses	Abbreviations[a]

Meyer Laboratories, Inc., 22601 Mack Ave., St. Clair Shores, Mich. 48080...........Meyer
Miles Laboratories, Inc., 1127 Myrtle St., Elkhart, Ind. 46518.....................Miles
Millipore Corp., 200 Walsh Rd., Bedford, Mass. 01730...........................Millipore
Miltenberg, E., Inc.—see *Miltex*...Miltenberg
Miltex Instrument Co., 300 Park Ave., S., New York, N.Y. 10010..................Miltex
Miranol Chemical Co., Inc., 279 Coit St., Irvington, N.J. 07111..................Miranol
Mist-O₂-Gen Equipment Co., 2711 Adeline St., Oakland, Calif. 94607.............Mist-O₂-Gen
Monaghan, J. J., Co., 2500 W. 5th Ave., Denver, Colo. 80204....................Monaghan
Monsanto Co., 800 N. Lindbergh Blvd., St. Louis, Mo. 63166....................Monsanto
Morton Chemical Co., 110 N. Wacker Dr., Chicago, Ill. 60606...................Morton
Mulford Colloid Laboratories, Inc., P.O. Box 30, Sellersville, Pa. 18960.........Mulford Colloid

N

NRC Equipment Div.—see *Norton*..NRC
Nageldinger, John, & Son, Inc., 366 E. 153rd St., Bronx, N.Y. 10455.............Nageldinger
Nalco Chemical Co., 180 N. Michigan Ave., Chicago, Ill. 60601..................Nalco
National Aniline—see *Allied*...National Aniline
National Bureau of Standards, Washington, D.C. 20234.......................NBS
National Cash Register Co., Main at K Sts., Dayton, Ohio 45409................NCR
*National Drug Co., 4663 Stenton Ave., Philadelphia, Pa. 19144................National Drug
Neisler Laboratories, Inc., P.O. Box 1110, Decatur, Ill. 62525.................Neisler
Neoco Corp., 1000 N. Highland Ave., Los Angeles, Calif. 90038.................Neoco
New England Nuclear Corp., 575 Albany St., Boston, Mass. 02118..............New England Nuclear
New York Pharmaceutical Co., P.O. Box 322, Mystic, Conn. 06355..............N.Y. Pharmaceutical
Niagara Chemical Div., FMC Corp., 10 Niagara St., Middleport, N.Y. 14105......Niagara
*Nion Corp., 1000 N. Highland Ave., Los Angeles, Calif. 90038.................Nion
Nopco Chemical Div., Diamond Shamrock Corp., 60 Park Pl., Newark, N.J. 07102....Nopco
Norden Laboratories, Inc., 601 W. Cornhusker Hwy., Lincoln, Neb. 68501.........Norden
Norgine Laboratories, Inc., 207 E. 37th St., New York, N.Y. 10016.............Norgine
North American Pharmacal, Inc., 6851 Chase Rd., Dearborn, Mich. 48126.........N. Am. Pharmacal
Norton Co., Vacuum Equipment Div., 160 Charlemont St., Newton, Mass. 02161....Norton
*Norwich Pharmacal Co., 17 Eaton Ave., Norwich, N.Y. 13815...................Norwich
Noveltex Paper Products Co., 2346 Amsterdam Ave., New York, N.Y. 10033........Noveltex
Novocol Chemical Mfg. Co., Inc., 2911 Atlantic Ave., Brooklyn, N.Y. 11207.......Novocol
*Noyes, P. J., Co., Inc., 101 Main St., Lancaster, N.H. 03584..................Noyes
Nuclear Associates, Inc., 35 Urban Ave., Westbury, N.Y. 11590.................Nuclear Associates
Nuclear Measurements Corp., 2470 N. Arlington Ave., Indianapolis, Ind. 46218......Nuclear Measurements
Nulomalene Div., Sucrest Corp., 120 Wall St., New York, N.Y. 10005............Nulomalene
Numotizine, Inc.—see *Hobart*...Numotizine

O

OTC Div., Surgical Appliances Industries, Inc., Erie Ave., Cincinnati, Ohio 45209......OTC
Od Peacock Sultan Co., 1 Fairchild Ct., Hicksville, N.Y. 11803.................Od Peacock
Ohio Chemical & Surgical Equipment Co., 1400 E. Washington Ave., Madison, Wis. 53703..Ohio Chemical
Olin Mathieson Chemical Corp., Chemicals Div., 745 5th Ave., New York, N.Y. 10022.Olin Mathieson
Onyx Chemical Corp., 190-T Warren St., Jersey City, N.J. 07302...............Onyx
*Organon, Inc., 375 Mt. Pleasant Ave., West Orange, N.J. 07052...............Organon
Ortega Pharmaceutical Co., Inc., P.O. Box 6212, Jacksonville, Fla. 32205........Ortega
Ortho Div., Chevron Chemical Co., Lucas Ave. & Ortho Way, Richmond, Calif. 94804.Ortho-Chevron
*Ortho Pharmaceutical Corp., Hwy. 202, Raritan, N.J. 08869.................Ortho
Orthopedic Equipment Co., Inc., Bourbon, Ind. 46504.......................Ortho. Equip.
Otarion Electronics, Inc., Scarborough Park, Ossining, N.Y. 10562.............Otarion
Owens-Illinois Glass Co., 405 Madison Ave., Toledo, Ohio 43604................Owens-Illinois

P

PPG Industries, Inc., 1 Gateway Ctr., Pittsburgh, Pa. 15222..................PPG
Packard Instrument Co., Inc., 2200 Warrenville Rd., Downers Grove, Ill. 60515......Packard Instrument
Pacquin Div.—see *Leeming/Pacquin*.......................................Pacquin
Pangborn Corp., 10 Pangborn Blvd., Hagerstown, Md. 21740..................Pangborn
Panray Div., Ormont Drug & Chemical Co., Inc., 223 S. Dean St., Englewood, N.J. 07631..Panray
*Parke, Davis & Co., P.O. Box 118, Detroit, Mich. 48232....................Parke-Davis
Parr Instrument Co., 209 53rd St., Moline, Ill. 61262.......................Parr Instrument
Patterson-Kelley Co., Inc., 105 Warren St., East Stroudsburg, Pa. 18301.........Patterson-Kelley
Patterson-Ludlow Div., Banner Industries, Inc., P.O. Box 1069, East Liverpool, Ohio 43920...PFM
Paxton, F. H., & Sons, Inc., P.O. Box 729, Evanston, Ill. 60204................Paxton
*Penick, S. B., & Co., 100 Church St., New York, N.Y. 10007.................Penick
Pennsylvania Engineering Corp., Dept. T, New Castle, Pa. 16103...............Pa. Eng.
Pennwalt Corp., 3 Penn Ctr., Philadelphia, Pa. 19102.......................Pennwalt
Perry Industries, Inc., New South Rd. & Commerce Pl., Hicksville, N.Y. 11802......Perry
Personal Products Co., Milltown, N.J. 08850...............................Personal Products
Pfanstiehl Labs., Inc., 1219 Glen Rock Ave., Waukegan, Ill. 60089.............Pfanstiehl
Pfaudler Co., West Ave. & Clark St., Rochester, N.Y. 14611..................Pfaudler
Pfeiffer Glass, Inc., 140 Bennington Dr., Rochester, N.Y. 14616...............Pfeiffer Glass
*Pfizer, Chas., & Co., Inc., 235 E. 42nd St., New York, N.Y. 10017............Pfizer
Pharmacia Laboratories, Inc., 800 Centennial Ave., Piscataway, N.J. 08854.......Pharmacia
Pharmaseal Laboratories, 1015 Grandview Ave., Glendale, Calif. 91201.........Pharmaseal
Phenix Box & Label Co., 4118 Penn St., Kansas City, Mo. 64111..............Phenix
Philadelphia Quartz Co., 1123 Public Ledger Bldg., Philadelphia, Pa. 19106......Phila. Quartz

Names and addresses	Abbreviations[a]
Philips Electronics & Pharmaceutical Industries Corp., Instruments Div., 750 S. Fulton Ave., Mt. Vernon, N.Y. 10550	Philips
*Philips Roxane Laboratories, 330 Oak St., Columbus, Ohio 43216	Philips-Roxane
Phillips Petroleum Co., Phillips Bldg., Bartlesville, Okla. 74003	Phillips
Picker X-Ray Corp., Nuclear Div., 1275 Mamaroneck Ave., White Plains, N.Y. 10605	Picker
Pictorial Paper Package Corp., 232 S. Lake St., Aurora, Ill. 60506	Pictorial
Pitman-Moore Co.—see *Dow-PM*	Pitman-Moore
Pittsburgh Plate Glass Co.—see *PPG*	Pittsburgh
Pilling Co., Delaware Dr., Fort Washington, Pa. 19034	Pilling
Pinoleum Co.—see *Baybank*	Pinoleum
Plasta-Medic, Inc., 154 W. 131st St., Los Angeles, Calif. 90061	Plasta-Medic
Plessner, Paul, Co., P.O. Box 7087, St. Petersburg, Fla. 33734	Plessner
Plough Laboratories, Inc., 3022 Jackson Ave., Memphis, Tenn. 38101	Plough
Plymouth Rubber Co., Inc., 59 Revere St., Canton, Mass. 02021	Plymouth
Pneumatic Scale Corp., 68 Newport Ave., Quincy, Mass. 02171	Pneumatic Scale
Pope Scientific Co., 13602 W. Reichert Ave., Menomonee Falls, Wis. 53051	Pope
Popper & Sons, Inc., 300 Park Ave., S., New York, N.Y. 10010	Popper
Porter, H. K., Co., Inc., Porter Bldg., Pittsburgh, Pa. 15219	Porter
Porto-Lift Mfg. Co., Higgins Lake, Mich. 48627	Porto-Lift
Posey, J. T., Co., 39 S. Santa Anita Ave., Pasadena, Calif. 91107	Posey
*Poythress, Wm. P., & Co., Inc., P.O. Box 2158, Richmond, Va. 23217	Poythress
Prak-T-Kal Div., Purepac Corp., 200 Elmora Ave., Elizabeth, N.J. 07202	Prak-T-Kal
Precision Scientific Co., 3737 W. Cortland St., Chicago, Ill. 60647	Precision
Precision Valve Corp., 702 Nepperhan Ave., Yonkers, N.Y. 10703	Precision Valve
Premier Mill Corp., 224-A 5th Ave., New York, N.Y. 10001	Premier
Premo Pharmaceutical Laboratories, Inc., 111 Leuning St., South Hackensack, N.J. 07606	Premo
Price, R. N., 59 Mill Spring Rd., Manhasset, N.Y. 11030	Price
Proctor & Gamble Distributing Co., Toilet Goods Div., P.O. Box 599, Cincinnati, Ohio 45201	Proctor & Gamble
Proctor & Schwartz, Inc., 7th St. & Tabor Rd., Philadelphia, Pa. 19120	Proctor & Schwartz
Professional Drugs, Inc.—see *Lemmon*	Prof. Drugs
Profex Div., Shampaine Industries, Inc., 1920 S. Jefferson Ave., St. Louis, Mo. 63104	Profex
Propper Mfg. Co., 10-34 44th Dr., Long Island City, N.Y. 11101	Propper
Pulverizing Machinery Div., Slick Industrial Co., 26 Chatham Rd., Summit, N.J. 07901	Pulverizing
*Purdue Frederick Co., 99-101 Saw Mill River Rd., Yonkers, N.Y. 10701	Purdue
Puritan Compressed Gas Corp., 2014 Grand Ave., Kansas City, Mo. 64106	Puritan
Pyramid Rubber Co., 771 N. Freedom St., Ravenna, Ohio 44266	Pyramid

R

*Rx Pharmaceuticals, P.O. Box 1656, Indianapolis, Ind. 46206	Rx
Rachelle Laboratories, Inc., 700 Henry Ford Ave., Long Beach, Calif. 90810	Rachelle
Rawl Chemical Co., Inc., 303 Park Ave., S., New York, N.Y. 10010	Rawl
Raymond, Charles, & Co., Inc., 381 Park Ave., S., New York, N.Y. 10016	Raymond
Raymond Pulverizer Div., Combustion Engineering, Inc., 427 W. Randolph St., Chicago, Ill. 60601	Raymond Pulverizer
Read Corp., 901 S. Richland Ave., York, Pa. 17403	Read
Recordak Corp., 770 Broadway, New York, N.Y. 10003	Recordak
Recsei Laboratories, 633 Tabor Ln., Santa Barbara, Calif. 93103	Recsei
*Reed & Carnrick, 30 Boright Ave., Kenilworth, N.J. 07033	Reed & Carnrick
Reed Machinery Co., Inc.—see *Read*	Reed
Reitz Mfg. Co., Box 690, West Chester, Pa. 19380	Reitz
Replogle Globes, Inc., 1901 N. Naragansett Ave., Chicago, Ill. 60639	Replogle
Repp Industries, Inc., Route 209, Gardiner, N.Y. 12525	Repp
Republic Seitz Filter Corp., Milldale, Conn. 06467	Republic
Research Products Corp., 1017 E. Washington Ave., Madison, Wis. 53703	Research
Research Supplies Pharmaceutical Corp., P.O. Box 8025, Pine Station, Albany, N.Y. 12203	Res. Supplies
Rexall Drug & Chemical Co., 8480 Beverly Blvd., Los Angeles, Calif. 90048	Rexall
Rhodes Pharmacal Co., Inc., 41 E. Oak St., Chicago, Ill. 60611	Rhodes
Riches-Nelson, Inc., Greenwich, Conn. 06830	Riches-Nelson
Richlyn Laboratories, 3725 Castor Ave., Philadelphia, Pa. 19124	Richlyn
*Riker Laboratories, Inc., 19901 Nordhoff St., Northridge, Calif. 91324	Riker
Risdon Mfg. Co., 250 Risdon St., Naugatuck, Conn. 06770	Risdon
Ritter, F. A., Co., 4624 Woodward Ave., Detroit, Mich. 48201	Ritter
Robbins Instruments Co., Inc., 236 Main St., Chatham, N.J. 07928	Robbins Instr.
*Robins, A. H., Co. Inc., 1407 Cummings Dr., Richmond, Va. 23220	Robins
Robinson Div., Painter St., Muncy, Pa. 17756	Robinson
Robinson Wagner Co., Inc., 626 Waverly Ave., Mamaroneck, N.Y. 10543	Robinson Wagner
Roche Laboratories Div., Hoffman La Roche, Inc., Roche Park, Nutley, N.J. 07110	Roche
Rochester Medical Equipment Co., Inc., 300 1st St., N.E., Rochester, Minn. 55901	Rochester
Rochester Products Co.—see *Rochester*	Rochester Products
Roerig, J. B., & Co., 235 E. 42nd St., New York, N.Y. 10017	Roerig
Rohm & Haas Co., Washington Sq., Philadelphia, Pa. 19105	Rohm & Haas
*Rorer, Wm. H., Inc., 500 Virginia Dr., Fort Washington, Pa. 19034	Rorer
*Ross Laboratories, 625 Cleveland Ave., Columbus, Ohio 43216	Ross
Roussel Corp., 155 E. 44th St., New York, N.Y. 10017	Roussel
*Rowell Laboratories, Inc., Baudette, Minn. 56623	Rowell
Royco Instruments, Inc., 141 Jefferson Dr., Menlo Park, Calif. 94025	Royco
Rusch, Inc., 17 W. 17th St., New York, N.Y. 10011	Rusch
Ruson Laboratories, Inc., 506 S.W. 6th St., Portland, Ore. 97204	Ruson
Rystan Co., 47 Center Ave., Little Falls, N.J. 07424	Rystan

Names and addresses	Abbreviations[a]

S

Safety Packaging Corp., Morristown, N.J. 07960	Safety Packaging
Salk, Murray, Inc., 119 Braintree St., Boston, Mass. 02134	Salk
Sandia Corp., P.O. Box 5800, Albuquerque, N.M. 87115	Sandia
*Sandoz Pharmaceuticals, Route 10, Hanover, N.J. 07936	Sandoz
Sani-Pac Corp., 45 W. 25th St., New York, N.Y. 10010	Sani-Pac
*Savage Laboratories, Inc., P.O. Box 700, Bellaire, Tex. 77401	Savage
*Scherer, R. P., Corp., 9425 Grinnell Ave., Detroit, Mich. 48213	Scherer
*Schering Corp., 1011 Morris Ave., Union, N.J. 07083	Schering
*Schieffelin & Co., Pharmaceutical Laboratories Div., Apex, N.C. 27502	Schieffelin
Schleicher & Schuell, Inc., 541 Washington St., Keene, N.H. 03431	Schleicher
Schmid, Julius, Inc., 423 W. 55th St., New York, N.Y. 10019	Schmid
Schuco Industries, Inc., 250 W. 18th St., New York, N.Y. 10011	Schuco
Schuemann-Jones Co., 3030 W. 117th St., Cleveland, Ohio 44111	Schuemann-Jones
Schuylkill Chemical Co., 2346 Sedgley Ave., Philadelphia, Pa. 19132	Schuylkill
Scientific Equipment Mfg. Corp., 20 North Ave., Larchmont, N.Y. 10538	Sci. Equip.
*Searle, G. D., & Co., P.O. Box 5110, Chicago, Ill. 60680	Searle
Sears, Roebuck & Co., 925 S. Homan Ave., Chicago, Ill. 60624	Sears
Selas Corp. of America, Dresher, Pa. 19025	Selas
Shampaine Industries, Inc., 1920 S. Jefferson Ave., St. Louis, Mo. 63104	Shampaine
Sharples Div., Pennwalt Corp., 955 Mearns Rd., Warminster, Pa. 18974	Sharples
Sheffield Chemical Co., 2400 Morris Ave., Union, N.J. 07083	Sheffield
*Sherman Laboratories, Inc., 5031 Grandy Ave., Detroit, Mich. 48211	Sherman
Shield Laboratories, 99-101 Saw Mill River Rd., Yonkers, N.Y. 10701	Shield
Shriver, T., & Co., 854 Hamilton St., Harrison, N.J. 07029	Shriver
*Smith Kline & French Laboratories, 1500 Spring Garden St., Philadelphia, Pa. 19101	SK&F
Smith, Martin H., Co., P.O. Box 322, Mystic, Conn. 06355	M. H. Smith
*Smith, Miller & Patch, Inc., 902 Broadway, New York, N.Y. 10010	Smith, Miller & Patch
Smith, Upsher, Co.—see Upsher Smith	Smith, Upsher
Sonoral Laboratories, 1910 Webster Ave., Bronx, N.Y. 10457	Sonoral
Sonotone Corp., Saw Mill River Rd., Elmsford, N.Y. 10523	Sonotone
Southern Drug & Mfg. Co., P.O. Box 2506, Knoxville, Tenn. 37902	Southern
Spanner, G. O., Inc., 20 Church St., Montclair, N.J. 07042	Spanner
Spinco Div., Beckman Instruments, Inc., Palo Alto, Calif. 94304	Spinco
Sprout, Waldron & Co., Inc., 60 Logan St., Muncy, Pa. 17756	Sprout
*Squibb Beech-Nut, Inc., 745 5th Ave., New York, N.Y. 10022	Squibb
Staley, A. E., Mfg. Co., Box 151, Decatur, Ill. 62525	Staley
Standard Collapsible Tube Co., P.O. Box 271, Rochester, Pa. 15074	Standard Tube
Standard Laboratories, 201 Tabor Rd., Morris Plains, N.J. 07950	Standard Labs.
*Standard Pharmacal Co., 1300 Abbott Dr., Elgin, Ill. 60120	Standard
Standard Products, US—see US Standard Products	Standard Products
Standard Specialty & Tube Co.—see Standard Tube	SST
Stauffer Chemical Co., 299 Park Ave., New York, N.Y. 10017	Stauffer
Stecker Chemicals, Inc., P.O. Box 326, Ridgefield, N.J. 07657	Stecker
Stepan Chemical Co., Northfield, Ill. 60093	Stepan
Sterling Products, 416 W. Washington St., Monticello, Ill. 61856	Sterling
Stiefel Laboratories, Inc., Oak Hill, N.Y. 12460	Stiefel
Stoddard, G. S., & Co., Inc., 295 Lafayette St., New York, N.Y. 10012	Stoddard
Stokes Div., Pennwalt Corp., 5500 Tabor Rd., Philadelphia, Pa. 19120	Stokes
Storck Pharmaceuticals, Inc.—see Arnar-Stone	Storck
*Strasenburgh Laboratories, P.O. Box 1710, Rochester, N.Y. 14603	Strasenburgh
Stratford-Cookson Co., 550 Commercial Dr., Yeadon, Pa. 19051	Stratford
*Strong Cobb Arner, Inc., 11700 Shaker Blvd., Cleveland, Ohio 44120	Strong Cobb
Strong, F. H., & Co., 112 W. 42nd St., New York, N.Y. 10036	Strong
*Stuart Div., Atlas Chemical Industries, Inc., 3360 E. Foothill Blvd., Pasadena, Calif. 91109	Stuart
Sturtevant Div., Westinghouse Electric Corp., Damon St., Boston, Mass. 02136	Sturtevant
Success Chemical Co.—see Ketchum	Success
Summers Laboratories, Inc., Morris Rd. & Wissahickon Creek, Fort Washington, Pa. 19034	Summers
Superior Sleeprite Corp., 750 W. Washtenaw Ave., Chicago, Ill. 60612	Superior
Supermatic Packaging Machines, Inc., 979 Lehigh Ave., Union, N.J. 07083	Supermatic
Supreme Pharmaceutical Co., Inc., 354 Mercer St., Jersey City, N.J. 07302	Supreme
Surface Combustion Div., Midland-Ross Corp., 2389 Dorr St., Toledo, Ohio 43601	Surface Combustion
Surgical Hosiery Corp.—see Hy-Tape	Surg. Hosiery
Surgical Products, Inc., 95 Bridge St., Lowell, Mass. 01852	Surg. Prod.
*Sutliff & Case Co., Inc., P.O. Box 838, Peoria, Ill. 61601	Sutliff & Case
*Syntex Laboratories, Inc., 3401 Hillview Dr., Palo Alto, Calif. 94304	Syntex

T

Tablax Div., Day-Baldwin, Inc., 1460 Chestnut Ave., Hillside, N.J. 07205	Tablax
Tailby-Nason Co., Inc., 50 N. Dupont Blvd., Dover, Del. 19901	Tailby-Nason
Takamine Laboratory, Inc.—see Marschall	Takamine
Tarbonis Co.—see Reed & Carnrick	Tarbonis
Tavolek Laboratories, Inc., Camp Hill Rd., Fort Washington, Pa. 19034	Tavolek
Taylor Instrument Cos., Olson & Ames Sts., Rochester, N.Y. 14601	Taylor
Technicon Co., Inc., Saw Mill River Rd., Chauncey, N.Y. 10502	Technicon
*Tenneco Chemicals, Inc., 300 E. 42nd St., New York, N.Y. 10017	Tenneco
Testagar & Co., Inc.—see Fellows	Testagar
Texas Pharmacal Co., P.O. Box 1659, San Antonio, Tex. 78206	Texas Pharmacal
Thayer Laboratories, Inc., 666 5th Ave., New York, N.Y. 10019	Thayer
Thermovac Industries Corp., 41 Decker St., Copiague, N.Y. 11726	Thermovac
Thiokol Chemical Corp., Bristol, Pa. 19007	Thiokol

Names and addresses	Abbreviations[a]
Thomas, Arthur H., Co., P.O. Box 779, Philadelphia, Pa. 19105	Thomas
Thomas Engineering, Inc., P.O. Box 198, Hoffman Estates, Ill. 60172	Thomas Eng.
Thompson, M. R., Inc., 711 5th Ave., New York, N.Y. 10022	MRT
*Tilden-Yates Laboratories, Inc., Box 1548, Worcester, Mass. 01601	Tilden-Yates
Torigian Laboratories, Inc., 218 98th Ave., Queens Village, N.Y. 11429	Torigian
Torsion Balance Co., 35 Monhegan St., Clifton, N.J. 07013	Torsion
Tosse, E., & Co., Inc., 924 Rogers Ave., Brooklyn, N.Y. 11226	Tosse
Tracerlab Div., Lab for Electronics, Inc., 547 Commerce Dr., Yeadon, Pa. 19051	Tracerlab
Travenol Labs, Inc., 6301 Lincoln Ave., Morton Grove, Ill. 60053	Travenol
Trent, Inc., 201 Leverington Ave., Philadelphia, Pa. 19127	Trent
Tri-Homo Corp., 6 Colby St., Salem, Mass. 09170	Tri-Homo
Troemner, Henry, Inc., 6825 Greenway Ave., Philadelphia, Pa. 19142	Troemner
Tuco Work Shops, Inc., 43 Upson Pt., Lockport, N.Y. 14094	Tuco
Tutag, S. J., & Co., 19180 Mt. Elliott Ave., Detroit, Mich. 48234	Tutag
Tyler Laboratories, 917 W. 5th Ave., Gary, Ind. 46402	Tyler
Tyree, J. S., Chemist, Inc., 7351 86th Ave., Washington, D.C. 20027	Tyree

U

*USV Pharmaceutical Corp., 800 2nd Ave., New York, N.Y. 10017	USV
Ulmer Pharmacal Co., 1400 Harmon Pl., Minneapolis, Minn. 55403	Ulmer
Ultra Chemical Works, Inc.—see *Witco*	Ultra
Union Carbide Corp., 270 Park Ave., New York, N.Y. 10017	Union Carbide
United Laboratories, 333 S. Fair Oaks Ave., Pasadena, Calif. 91101	United Laboratories
United Products Co., 451-T S. Jefferson St., Orange, N.J. 07050	United Products
United Shoe Machine Corp., 140 Federal St., Boston, Mass. 02107	United Shoe
US Bottlers Machinery Co., 4023 N. Rockwell St., Chicago, Ill. 60618	US Bottlers
US Government Printing Office, Washington, D.C. 20402	USGPO
US Industrial Chemicals Co., 99 Park Ave., New York, N.Y. 10016	US Ind. Chem.
US Standard Products Co.—see *Arnar-Stone*	US Standard Products
United Surgical Co., 11775 Starkey Rd., Largo, Fla. 33540	United Surgical
*Upjohn Co., 7171 Portage Rd., Kalamazoo, Mich. 49002	Upjohn
Upsher Smith Co., 529 S. 7th St., Minneapolis, Minn. 55415	Upsher Smith

V

*Vale Chemical Co., Inc., 1201 Liberty St., Allentown, Pa. 18102	Vale
Valentine Co., Inc., P.O. Box 7360, Richmond, Va. 23221	Valentine
Vanderbilt, R. T., Co., Inc., 230 Park Ave., New York, N.Y. 10017	Vanderbilt
Van Dyk & Co., Inc., 11 William St., Belleville, N.J. 07109	Van Dyk
Van Patten Pharmaceutical Co., 4450 Ravenswood Ave., Chicago, Ill. 60640	Van Patten
Van Pelt & Brown, Inc.—see *Mallinckrodt*	Van Pelt & Brown
Varian Associates, 611 Hansen Way, Palo Alto, Calif. 94303	Varian
Vestal Laboratories Div., W. R. Grace & Co., 4963 Manchester Ave., St. Louis, Mo. 63110	Vestal
Victor Chemical Works, 155 N. Wacker Dr., Chicago, Ill. 60607	Victor
Vineland Chemical Co., W. Wheat Rd., Vineland, N.J. 08360	Vineland
Virtis Co., Inc., Route 200, Gardiner, N.Y. 12525	Virtis
Visking Corp.—see *Union Carbide*	Visking
Vitabex Products Co., 64 E. 34th St., New York, N.Y. 10016	Vitabex
Vitamix Pharmaceuticals, 5051 Lancaster Ave., Philadelphia, Pa. 19141	Vitamix
Vitarine Co., Inc., 227-15 N. Conduit Ave., Springfield Gardens, N.Y. 11413	Vitarine
Vogel Laboratories, 47 Bluebird Dr., Congers, N.Y. 10920	Vogel
Vollrath Co., 1236 N. 18th St., Sheboygan, Wis. 53061	Vollrath

W

WTS-Pharmacraft, Box 1212, Rochester, N.Y. 14603	WTS
Wagner Industries, Inc., 272 Spencer St., Rochester, N.Y. 14608	Wagner
Walgreen Co., 4300 W. Peterson Ave., Chicago, Ill. 60646	Walgreen
*Walker, Corp. & Co., Inc., P.O. Drawer 1320, Syracuse, N.Y. 13201	Walker, Corp.
Walker Laboratories, Inc.—see *National Drug*	Walker
*Wallace Pharmaceuticals Div., Carter-Wallace, Inc., Half Acre Rd., Cranbury, N.J. 08512	Wallace
*Wallerstein Co., 6301 Lincoln Ave., Morton Grove, Ill. 60053	Wallerstein
*Wampole Laboratories, 35 Commerce Rd., Stamford, Conn. 06902	Wampole
*Warner-Chilcott Laboratories, 201 Tabor Rd., Morris Plains, N.J. 07950	Warner-Chilcott
*Warren-Teed Pharmaceuticals, Inc., 582 W. Goodale St., Columbus, Ohio 43215	Warren-Teed
Webster, William A., Co., P.O. Box 18358, Memphis, Tenn. 38118	Webster
Weiss, Max, & Sons, Inc., 45 Cedar St., Stamford, Conn. 06904	Weiss
Welch Scientific Co., 7300 N. Linden Ave., Skokie, Ill. 60076	Welch
Wendt-Bristol Co., 1159 Dublin Rd., Columbus, Ohio 43212	Wendt-Bristol
West Co., Inc., Phoenixville, Pa. 19460	West
*Westerfield Laboratories, Inc., 3941 Brotherton Rd., Cincinnati, Ohio 45209	Westerfield
West-ward, Inc., 745 Eagle Ave., Bronx, N.Y. 10456	West-ward
*Westwood Pharmaceuticals, 468 Dewitt St., Buffalo, N.Y. 14213	Westwood
Wheaton Glass Co., Wheaton Ave., Millville, N.J. 08332	Wheaton
White Laboratories, Inc., Galloping Hill Rd., Kenilworth, N.J. 07033	White
Whitehall Laboratories, 685 3rd Ave., New York, N.Y. 10017	Whitehall
Whitestone Products Corp., 595 Broad Hollow Rd., Farmingdale, N.Y. 11735	Whitestone
Whittaker Laboratories, Inc., P.O. Box 551, Peekskill, N.Y. 10566	Whittaker
Will Scientific, Inc., P.O. Box 1050, Rochester, N.Y. 14603	Will Scientific, Inc.
Wilmot Castle Co.—see *Castle*	Wilmot

Names and addresses	Abbreviations[a]
*Wilson Pharmaceutical & Chemical Corp., 4221 S. Western Blvd., Chicago, Ill. 60609	Wilson
Winfield Co., Inc., 3062 46th Ave., N., St. Petersburg, Fla. 33714	Winfield
*Winthrop Laboratories, 90 Park Ave., New York, N.Y. 10016	Winthrop
Witco Chemical Co., Inc., 2 Wood St., Paterson, N.J. 07524	Witco
Wood Ridge Chemical Corp., Park Pl., E., Woodridge, N.J. 07075	Wood Ridge
Wright Dental Co., Ltd., Dundee, Scotland	Wright Dental
Wyandotte Chemicals Corp., Alkali Sq., Wyandotte, Mich. 48192	Wyandotte
*Wyeth Laboratories, P.O. Box 8299, Philadelphia, Pa. 19101	Wyeth
Wynn Pharmacal Corp., 2900 N. 17th St., Philadelphia, Pa. 19132	Wynn
Wynn Pharmaceuticals, Box 190, Mystic, Conn. 06355	Wynn Pharmaceuticals

Y

Young, F. E., & Co., 8057 Stony Island Ave., Chicago, Ill. 60617	Young

Z

Zeal, G. H., Ltd., Lombard Rd., Merton, London S.W. 1, England	Zeal
*Zemmer Co., Inc., 231 Hulton Rd., Oakmont, Pa. 15139	Zemmer
Zenith Hearing Aid Sales Corp., 6501 W. Grand Ave., Chicago, Ill. 60635	Zenith

Alphabetic Index

M